■ CARDIAC NURSING

■ ■ ■ A Companion to Braunwald's Heart Disease

Debra K. Moser, DNSc, RN, FAHA, FAAN

Professor and Gill Chair of Nursing

Co-Director, RICH Heart Program

University of Kentucky College of Nursing

Lexington, Kentucky

Editor, *Journal of Cardiovascular Nursing*

Barbara Riegel, DNSc, RN, CS, FAHA, FAAN

Associate Professor

School of Nursing

University of Pennsylvania

Philadelphia, Pennsylvania

Editor, *Journal of Cardiovascular Nursing*

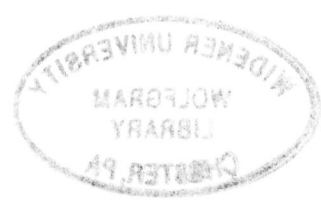

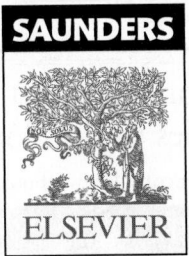

SAUNDERS

ELSEVIER

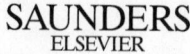

SAUNDERS
ELSEVIER

11830 Westline Industrial Drive
St. Louis, Missouri 63146

CARDIAC NURSING: A COMPANION TO BRAUNWALD'S HEART DISEASE   978-1-4160-2934-2

Notice

Knowledge and best practice in this field are constantly changing. As new research and experience broaden our knowledge, changes in practice, treatment and drug therapy may become necessary or appropriate. Readers are advised to check the most current information provided (i) on procedures featured or (ii) by the manufacturer of each product to be administered, to verify the recommended dose or formula, the method and duration of administration, and contraindications. It is the responsibility of the practitioner, relying on their own experience and knowledge of the patient, to make diagnoses, to determine dosages and the best treatment for each individual patient, and to take all appropriate safety precautions. To the fullest extent of the law, neither the Publisher nor the Editors assume any liability for any injury and/or damage to persons or property arising out or related to any use of the material contained in this book.

The Publisher

ISBN-13: 978-1-4160-2934-2

Executive Publisher: Barbara Nelson Cullen
Managing Editor: Maureen R. Iannuzzi
Senior Developmental Editor: Jennifer Ehlers
Publishing Services Manager: John Rogers
Senior Project Manager: Kathleen L. Teal
Senior Designer: Teresa McBryan
Cover images copyright Dennis Kunkel Microscopy, Inc.

Printed in Canada

Last digit is the print number: 9   8   7   6   5   4   3   2   1

This book is dedicated to all the cardiovascular nurses
working daily in their myriad settings who make this field
the most exciting, dynamic, and rewarding of all.

Mohannad Eid Abu-Ruz, PhD, RN
Assistant Professor, College of Medicine
Sultan Qaboos University
Muscat, Oman
Inflammation

Nancy Albert, PhD(c), CCNS, CCRN, CAN, FAHA
Director, Nursing Research-Division of Nursing and
 Clinical Nurse Specialist
George M. and Linda H. Kaufman Center for Heart
 Failure
Cleveland Clinic
Cleveland, Ohio
Dysrhythmia Monitoring and Recognition

Bradley E. Aouizerat, PhD
Assistant Professor, School of Nursing
University of California, San Francisco
San Francisco, California
Genetic and Environmental Basis of Cardiac
 Disease

Nancy T. Artinian, PhD, RN, BC, FAHA
Professor and Director of Doctoral and Postdoctoral
 Programs
College of Nursing
Wayne State University
Troy, Michigan
Hypertension as A Risk Factor
Management of Hypertension

Susan J. Appel, PhD, CCRN, APRN, BC
(ACNP and FNP)
Associate Professor, School of Nursing
University of Alabama–Birmingham
Birmingham, Alabama
Care of Patients with Complications of Acute
 Myocardial Infarction

Karen Badellino, PhD, RN
Assistant Professor, School of Nursing
University of Pennsylvania
Philadelphia, Pennsylvania
Pathogenesis of Atherosclerosis

Kathy Berra, RN, MSN, FAHA, FAAN
Clinic Coordinator, Stanford Prevention Research Center
Stanford University School of Medicine
Stanford, California
Interdisciplinary Team in Cardiac Rehabilitation
Cardiac Rehabilitation

Martha Biddle, PhD(c), RN, ARNP, CCNS
Director of Operations
RICH Heart Program
University of Kentucky
Lexington, Kentucky
Interdisciplinary Team in Cardiac Rehabilitation

Kristi Borowski, MD
University of Iowa Hospitals and Clinics
Department of Obstetrics and Gynecology
Iowa City, Iowa
The Cardiovascular System and Pregnancy

Lynne T. Braun, PhD, RN
Nurse Practitioner
Preventive Cardiology Center
Chicago, Illinois
Sedentary Lifestyle
Management of Dyslipidemia

Beth Broering, MSN, RN, CEN, CCRN
Trauma Coordinator
Vanderbilt University Medical Center
Nashville, Tennessee
Care of Patients with Cardiac Trauma

Rosemary S. Bubien, PhD, RN, CNS, CCRC, FAHA I
Nurse Research Manager, Arrhythmia Section
Department of Medicine, Division of Cardiovascular
 Disease
University of Alabama–Birmingham
Birmingham, Alabama
Care of Patients with Sudden Cardiac Death,
 Cardiac Arrest, and Life-Threatening
 Dysrhythmias
Care of Patients with Implanted Cardiac Rhythm
 Management Devices

Lora E. Burke, PhD, RN
Professor, School of Nursing
University of Pittsburgh
Pittsburgh, Pennsylvania
Obesity

Mary A. Caldwell, PhD, RN
Healdsburg, California
Patient Delay in Seeking Treatment for Cardiac
 Symptoms

Mary M. Canobbio, RN, MN, FAAN
Ahmanson UCLA Adult Congenital Heart Disease Center
Lecturer, UCLA School of Nursing
Los Angeles, California
Care of Adults with Congenital Heart Disease

Diane L. Carroll, PhD, RN
Clinical Nurse Specialist
Massachusetts General Hospital
Boston, Massachusetts
The Impact of Cardiac Disease on Psychological State

Taletha Carter, RN, MS, CRN
Clinical Nurse Specialist
Cleveland Clinic Foundation
Cleveland, Ohio
Care of Patients with Pericardial Diseases

Dennis J. Cheek, PhD, RN, FAHA
Abell-Hanger Professor
Texas Christian University
Harris School of Nursing & School of Nurse Anesthesia
Fort Worth, Texas
Regulation of Cardiac Output and Blood Pressure

Jina Choo, PhD, RN
School of Nursing and Graduate School of Public Health
University of Pittsburgh
Pittsburgh, Pennsylvania
Obesity

Sharon K. Christman, PhD, RN
Assistant Professor
Cedarville University
Cedarville, Ohio
Care of Patients with Peripheral Vascular Disease

Deborah A. Chyun, PhD, RN
Associate Professor, Yale School of Nursing
New Haven, Connecticut
Diabetes and the Cardiovascular System

Tracey J. F. Colella, BSN
Associate Professor, School of Nursing
Laurentian University
Toronto, Ontario, Canada
Relationship Between Social Support and Cardiac Disease

Rebecca Cross, RN, MSN, FNP
Doctoral Student
School of Nursing
University of California, Los Angeles
Los Angeles, California
Impact of Depression on Cardiac Disease

Patricia Davidson, PhD, RN
Associate Professor of Nursing, Nursing Research Unit
School of Nursing, Family, & Community Health,
College of Social and Health Sciences
University of Western Sydney and Western Sydney Area
   Health Service
Area Nurse Education Centre
Cumberland Hospital, Paramatta, New South Wales
Australia
Palliative Care

Leslie L. Davis, MS, RN
Nurse Practitioner
Division of Cardiology
University of North Carolina at Chapel Hill
Chapel Hill, North Carolina
Care of Patients with Acute Coronary Syndrome

Marla J. DeJong, PhD, RN
Lt. Colonel
United States Air Force
Wilford Hall Medical Center
San Antonio, Texas
Impact of Anxiety on Cardiac Disease

Shelly Devillier, BSN, RN
North Richland Hills, Texas
Care of Children with Heart Disease

Holli A. DeVon, PhD, RN
Assistant Professor
Marquette University College of Nursing
Milwaukee, Wisconsin
Chest Pain

Victoria V. Dickson, CRNP, MSN
Lecturer, School of Nursing
University of Pennsylvania
Philadelphia, Pennsylvania
Optimal Outpatient Education and Counseling

Lynne Doering, RN, DNSc
Associate Professor and Chair, Acute Care Section
School of Nursing
University of California, Los Angeles
Los Angeles, California
Impact of Depression on Cardiac Disease

Kathleen Dracup, PhD, RN, FAHA, FAAN
Professor and Dean
University of California San Francisco, School of Nursing
San Francisco, California
Patient Delay in Seeking Treatment for Cardiac Symptoms

Barbara J. Drew, PhD, RN, FAAN
Professor of Nursing and Clinical Professor of Medicine
University of California San Francisco
San Francisco, California
ST Segment Monitoring

Jennifer Dungan, PhD(c), RN, MS
Doctoral Student, Office for Research Support
University of Florida, College of Nursing
Gainesville, Florida
*Hypertension as a Risk Factor
Management of Hypertension*

Joann Eastwood, PhD, RN
Assistant Professor, School of Nursing
University of California, Los Angeles
Los Angeles, California
*Nurse's Role in the Cardiac Catheterization
Laboratory*

Lorraine S. Evangelista, PhD, RN
Assistant Professor
University of California, Los Angeles School of Nursing
Los Angeles, California
Promoting Adherence to Treatment

Barbara Fletcher MN, RN
Jacksonville, Florida
Sedentary Lifestyle

Lorraine Frazier, PhD, RN
University of Texas Health Science Center at Houston
Houston, Texas
*Novel and Emerging Risk Factors for Coronary
Heart Disease*

Susan K. Frazier, PhD, RN
Assistant Professor, College of Nursing
University of Kentucky
Lexington, Kentucky
*Pulmonary Circulation
Hemodynamic Monitoring*

Maureen M. Friedman, PhD, RN
Professor of Nursing
Nazareth College of Rochester, Department of Nursing
Rochester, New York
Fatigue

Marjorie Funk, PhD, RN, FAAN, FAHA
Professor and Director, Yale-Howard Partnership Center
Yale University School of Nursing
New Haven, Connecticut
Epidemiology of Heart Failure

Laurie G. Futterman, ARNP-c, MSN, CCRN
Cardiac Transplant
Highland Professional Building
Miami, Florida
Electrocardiography: Abnormal Electrocardiogram

Jana Glotzer, MSN, RN
Heart Failure Nurse Practitioner
University of North Carolina-Chapel Hill
Chapel Hill, North Carolina
Nursing Assessment in the Inpatient Setting

Kathleen L. Grady, PhD, RN, FAHA, FAAN
Director, Center for Heart Failure
Northwestern Cardiovascular Institute
Division of Cardiac Surgery
Chicago, Illinois
*Care of Patients with Circulatory Assist Devices
Care of Patients Undergoing Cardiac
Transplantation*

Meg Gulanick, PhD, APRN, FAAN, FAHA
Professor, Neihoff School of Nursing
Loyola University-Chicago
Maywood, Illinois
*Interdisciplinary Team in Cardiac Rehabilitation
Cardiac Rehabilitation*

Cynthia Hambach, MSN, RN, CCRN
Adjunct Clinical Faculty
Drexel University College of Nursing and Health
Professions
Philadelphia, Pennsylvania
Care of Patients with Acquired Valvular Disease

Diane A. Hawley, PhD, RN, CCNS
Harris School of Nursing
Fort Worth, Texas
Regulation of Cardiac Output and Blood Pressure

Laura L. Hayman, PhD, RN, FAHA, FAAN
Professor
New York University Division of Nursing
The Steinhardt School of Education
New York, New York
Primary Prevention in Childhood

Patricia Kunz Howard, PhD, RN, CEN
(2004-2005, President of the Emergency Nurses
Association)
Staff Development Specialist, Emergency Department
University of Kentucky Hospital
Research Protocol Clinical Manager, Cardiovascular
Nursing
University of Kentucky College of Nursing
Lexington, Kentucky
*Emergency Department Nursing Care
of the Cardiac Patient*

Jill Howie, PhD, RN, NP
Associate Clinical Professor, School of Nursing
University of California-San Francisco
San Francisco, California
*Cardiomyopathy and Myocarditis
Care of Patients with Endocarditis*

Suzanne Hughes, MSN, RN
AGMC Health & Wellness
Women's Heart Advantage
Akron, Ohio
*Dyslipidemia
Novel and Emerging Risk Factors for Coronary
Heart Disease
Management of Dyslipidemia*

Tiny Jaarsma, PhD, RN
Department of Cardiology
Thoraxcenter
University Hospital Groningen
Groningen, The Netherlands
Impact of Cardiovascular Disease on Sexuality

Sharon Josephson-Keeven, RN, MS, CRNP
Cardiology Nurse Practitioner
Kaiser Permanente Mid-Atlantic States
Silver Spring, Maryland
Nursing Assessment in the Outpatient Setting

Corrine Y. Jurgens, PhD, RN
Stony Brook University, School of Nursing
Stony Brook, New York
Dyspnea

Stacen Keating, PhD, RN
School of Nursing
University of Pennsylvania
Philadelphia, Pennsylvania
Collaborative Care

Kathryn M. King, PhD, RN
Associate Professor and Heritage Population Health
   Investigator
Faculty of Nursing and Department of Community
   Health Sciences
University of Calgary
Calgary AB, Canada
*Relationship Between Social Support and Cardiac
   Disease*

Deborah G. Klein, MSN, RN, CCRN, CS
Clinical Nurse Specialist, Cardiac ICU and Heart Failure
   Specialty Unit
Division of Nursing
Cleveland Clinic Foundation
Cleveland, Ohio
Nurses in Intensive Care

Mary Jo Kocan, RN, MSN
Clinical Nurse Specialist
University of Michigan Health System
Ann Arbor, Michigan
*Neurological Disorders and the Cardiovascular
   System*

Varda Konstam, PhD
Professor, Department of Counseling and School
   Psychology
Graduate College of Education
University of Massachusetts, Boston
Boston, Massachusetts
*Role of the Cardiac Health Psychologist: Expanding
   Opportunities*

Cindy Lamendola, RN, MSN/ANP
Clinical Research Coordinator
Stanford University School of Medicine
Stanford, California
*Insulin Resistance, Diabetes, and Cardiovascular
   Disease*

Mary C. Langford, MS, RN, ACNP, CDE
Bethesda, Maryland
Cardiorenal Syndromes

William R. Law, PhD
Chair, Department of Biological Sciences
University of the Sciences in Philadelphia
Philadelphia, Pennsylvania
Cardiovascular Physiology: The Myocardium

Dorothy Lee, MSN, APRN, BC
Doctoral Student, Wayne State University
Research Coordinator
Wayne State University–Pulmonary Hypertension
   Research
Detroit, Michigan
*Pulmonary Hypertension and the Cardiovascular
   System*

Leanne L. Lefler, MSN, APN, CCRN
Clinical Assistant Professor
University of Arkansas for Medical Sciences
Little Rock, Arkansas
Women and Cardiovascular Disease

Terry A. Lennie, PhD, RN, FAHA
Associate Professor, College of Nursing
University of Kentucky
Lexington, Kentucky
Inflammation
*Fundamentals of Nutrition for Cardiovascular
   Health*

Anne Leonard, RN, MPh, FAHA
Coordinator, UTHSCA Stroke Program
University of Texas Health Sciences Center
   at San Antonio
San Antonio, Texas
Care of Patients with Stroke

Mary Elizabeth Mancini, PhD, RN, CAN, FAAN
Professor
Associate Dean for Undergraduate Nursing Programs
University of Texas at Arlington, School of Nursing
Arlington, Texas
*Care of Patients with Sudden Cardiac Death,
   Cardiac Arrest, and Life-Threatening
   Dysrhythmias*

Kathleen McCauley, PhD, RN
Associate Professor and Associate Dean for Academic
   Programs
University of Pennsylvania School of Nursing
Philadelphia, Pennsylvania
Dysrhythmia Monitoring and Recognition

Janet P. McMahon, MSN, MS, APRN, BC
Heart Failure Intervention Nurse
College of Nursing
University of Pennsylvania
Philadelphia, Pennsylvania
Optimal Patient Education and Counseling

Jean C. McSweeney, PhD, RN, FAHA, FAAN
Professor
University of Arkansas for Medical Sciences
College of Nursing
Little Rock, Arkansas
Women and Cardiovascular Disease

Wendy Mercier, PhD, RN
Chair, Department of Biokinetics
Eastern University
St. Davids, Pennsylvania
Cardiovascular Adaptations to Exercise

Nancy Houston Miller, BSN, RN
Associate Director
Stanford Cardiac Rehabilitation Program
Department of Medicine–Cardiovascular Medicine
Stanford University
Stanford, California
Smoking

Philip Moons, PhD, RN, NFESC
Assistant Professor
Advanced Practice Nurse, Congenital Cardiology
Center for Health Services and Nursing Research
Katholieke Universiteit Leuven
Leuven, Belgium
Care of Adults with Congenital Heart Disease

Debra K. Moser, DNSc, RN, FAHA, FAAN
Professor and Gill Chair of Nursing
Co-Director, RICH Heart Program
University of Kentucky College of Nursing
Lexington, Kentucky

Editor; *Journal of Cardiovascular Nursing*

Regulation of Cardiac Output and Blood Pressure
Care of Patients with Acute Coronary Syndrome
Care of Patients with Acute Coronary Syndrome:
ST-Segment Elevation Myocardial Infarction
Care of Patients with Chronic Heart Failure

Michelle J. Nickolaus, CRNP
Program for Adults with Congenital Heart Disease
Lipid and Cardiovascular Wellness Program
Penn State Milton S. Hershey Medical Center
Division of Cardiology
Hershey, Pennsylvania
Care of Adults with Congenital Heart Disease

Jessica Novak, BSN, RN
Staff Nurse
University of Pittsburgh
Pittsburgh, Pennsylvania
Obesity

Sara Paul, RN, MSN, FNP
Nurse Practitioner
Western Piedmont Heart Centers
Hickory, North Carolina
Nurses in Outpatient Clinics
Care of Patients with Acute Heart Failure

Michele M. Pelter, PhD, RN
Director of Nursing Research and Outcomes
Washoe Health System
Reno, Nevada
Electrocardiography: Normal Electrocardiogram

Mariann R. Piano, PhD, RN, FAHA
Associate Professor
University of Illinois–Chicago
Nursing College
Chicago, Illinois
Cardiovascular Physiology: The Myocardium
Pathophysiology of Heart Failure

Nancy A. Pike, RN, MN, FNP
Nurse Practitioner
Marina Del Ray, California
Promoting Adherence of Treatment

Terry Preuss
Hamilton, New Jersey
Care of Patients with Acquired Valvular Disease

Marie Raia, RN
Nurses and Home Care

Sally H. Rankin, PhD, RN, FAAN
Associate Professor and Director
Family NP Program
University of California–San Francisco
Family Health Care Nursing
San Francisco, California
The Impact of Cardiac Disease on the Family

Nancy S. Redeker, PhD, RN, CS
Professor and Associate Dean for Resarch
UMDNJ School of Nursing
Newark, New Jersey
Sleep, Sleep Disorders, and Cardiac Disease

Michael W. Rich, MD
Associate Professor of Medicine
Washington University School of Medicine
St. Louis, Missouri
The Impact of Aging on Cardiac Function

Barbara Riegel, DNSc, RN, FAHA, FAAN
Associate Professor, School of Nursing
University of Pennsylvania
Philadelphia, Pennsylvania

Editor, *Journal of Cardiovascular Nursing*

Evidence-Based Practice: Practicing What is Known,
Not What is Believed
The Impact of Cardiac Disease on Psychological
State
Care of Patients with Acute Coronary Syndrome
Care of Patients with Chronic Heart Failure
Care of Patients with Pericardial Diseases

Marianne Roncoli, PhD, RN
Quality Management
Visiting Nurse Regional Health Care System
Empire State Home Care Service
New York, New York
Nurses and Home Care
Home Care and Heart Disease

Joseph A. Rubertone, PT, PhD
Associate Professor
Health Sciences Program
College of Nursing and Health Professions
Drexel University
Philadelphia, Pennsylvania
Anatomy of the Cardiovascular System

Connie B. Scanga, PhD
Practice Assistant Professor
School of Nursing
University of Pennsylvania
Philadalphia, Pennsylvania
Stress

Rose Schaffer, RN, MSN, ACNP-CS, CCRN
Cardiology Nurse Practitioner
Thomas Jefferson University Hospital
Philadelphia, Pennsylvania
Care of Patients Undergoing Fibrinolytic Therapy
and Percutaneous Coronary Intervention

Dorie W. Schwertz, PhD, RN, FAHA, FAAN
Associate Professor
College of Nursing
University of Illinois
Chicago, Ilinois

Kristine Anne Scordo, PhD, RN, CS, ACNP
Professor and Director
Acute Care Nurse Practitioner Program
Wright State University
Dayton, Ohio
Nurse's Role in Exercise Testing and Noninvasive
Imaging

Patricia C. Seifert, RN, MSN, CRNFA, FAAN
Education Coordinator
CV Operating Room
Inova Heart and Vascular Institute
Falls Church, Virginia
Nurses in Peri-Operative Settings
Care of Patients Undergoing Cardiac Surgery

Kristen Sethares, PhD, RN
Associate Professor
College of Nursing
University of Massachusetts–Dartmouth
North Dartmouth, Massachusetts
Care of Patients Undergoing Cardiac Surgery

Suzette Sewell, RN, MS
Nurse Practitioner
Kentuckiana Center for Better Bone and Joint Health
Louisville, Kentucky
Rheumatic Diseases and the Cardiovascular System

Julie A. Shinn, RN, MA
Cardiovascular Critical Care
Stanford University Medical Center
Palo Alto, California
Care of Patients with Circulatory Assist Devices

Heather Smith, RN
Operations Director
Penn E-lert
Philadelphia, Pennsylvania
Care of Patients Undergoing Cardiac Surgery

Patricia S. A. Sparacino, RN, MS, FAAN
Vice Chair, Administration and Academic Coordinator
Family Health Care Nursing
University of California–San Francisco
San Francisco, California
Nurses and Home Care
Home Care and Heart Disease

Elaine E. Steinke, PhD, RN
Professor
School of Nursing
Wichita State University
Wichita, Kansas
Impact of Cardiac Disease on Sexuality

Sharon A. Stephens, PhD, GNP, RN
Post-Doctoral Fellow
School of Nursing
Oregon Health & Science Center
Portland, Oregon
Fatigue

Simon Stewart, PhD, RN
NHF Chair of Cardiovascular Nursing
University of South Australia

Professor of Health Research
University of Queensland
Queensland, Australia
Epidemiology of Coronary Artery Disease

Wendy Gattis Stough, PharmD
Duke Clinical Research Institute
Durham, North Carolina
Contributions of Clinical Pharmacists

Anna Strömberg, PhD, RN, NFESC
Senior Lecturer, Heart Failure
Nurse Specialist
Department of Medicine and Care
Nursing Science
Linköping University
Linköping, Sweden
Heart Failure Disease Management

Tanna Thomason, MSN, RN
Clinical Nurse Specialist
Sharp Memorial Hospital
San Diego, California
Nurses in Progressive Care Units

Robin J. Trupp, MSN, RN
Doctoral Student
Ohio State University
Columbus, Ohio
*Evidence-Based Practice:What is Known, Not What
is Believed*
*Care of Patients with Implanted Cardiac Rhythm
Management Devices*
Cardiorenal Syndromes

Amy Verstappen, MA
President
Adult Congenital Heart Association
Raleigh, North Carolina
Care of Adults with Congenital Heart Disease

Lisa Vollano, MS, PA-C
Western Piedmont Heart Centers
Hickory, North Carolina
Care of Patients with Acute Heart Failure

Melanie T. Warziski, BSN
Health and Community Systems Department
School of Nursing
University of Pittsburgh
Pittsburgh, Pennsylvania
Obesity

Megan White, RN, MSN, ACNP
Northwestern Memorial Hospital
San Francisco, California
Care of Patients with Endocarditis

Connie White-Williams, PhD, RN, FAAN
University of Alabama–Birmingham
Birmingham, Alabama
*Care of Patients Undergoing Cardiac
Transplantation*

**Debra Lynn-McHale Wiegand, PhD, RN, CCRN,
FAAN(B)**
Assistant Professor
Department of Organizational Systems and Adult Health
School of Nursing
University of Maryland–Baltimore
Baltimore, Maryland
Care of Patients with Acquired Valvular Disease

Sue Wingate, RN, DNSc, CRNP, CS
Cardiology Nurse Practitioner
Kaiser-Permanente Mid-Atlantic States
Silver Spring, Maryland
Nursing Assessment in the Outpatient Setting

Catherine G. Winkler, RN, BSN, PhD (cand.)
College of Nursing
Yale University
New Haven, Connecticut
Epidemiology of Heart Failure

Mary A. Woo, DNSc, RN
Professor, School of Nursing
University of California, Los Angeles
Los Angeles, California
Central Nervous System and the Heart

Shu-Fen Wung, PhD, RN
Associate Professor, College of Nursing
University of Arizona
Tucson, Arizona
*Genetic and Environmental Basis of Cardiac
Disease*

Jerome Yankowitz, MD
Director
Division of Maternal-Fetal Medicine and Fetal
and Diagnosis Treatment Unit
Department OB/GYN
University of Iowa Hospitals and Clinics
Iowa City, Iowa
The Cardiovascular System and Pregnancy

Lawrence H. Young, MD
Professor of Internal Medicine
Director of Cardiac Metabolism Research Program
Yale University School of Medicine
New Haven, Connecticut
Diabetes and the Cardiovascular System

Carolyn B. Yucha, RN, PhD, FAAN
Professor and Dean
School of Nursing
University of Nevada
Las Vegas, Nevada

Editor, *Biological Research for Nursing*
Hypertension as a Risk Factor
Management of Hypertension

Cheryl Hoyt Zambroski, PhD, RN
Assistant Professor
School of Nursing
University of Louisville
Louisville, Kentucky
Palliative Care
Hospice and Palliative Care

Vicki L. Zeigler, MSN, RN
Doctoral Student
Azle, Texas
Care of Children with Heart Disease

Cynthia D. Adams, RN, MSN, APRN-BC
The Indiana Heart Hospital
Indianapolis, Indiana

Nancy M. Albert, PhD, CCNS, CCRN, CAN
The Cleveland Clinic Foundation
Cleveland, Ohio

Nancy F. Altice, RN, MSN, CCRN, CCNS
Carilion Roanoke Memorial Hospital
Roanoke, Virginia

Diane M. Anderson, RN, MSN
Cardiovascular Associates of Northern Wisconsin
Wausau, Wisconsin

Rebecca L. Angerstein, RN, BSN, MA, MSN, BC, CCRN, CNS
The Heart Group, Inc.
Akron General Medical Center
Akron, Ohio

James M. Badger, PhD, APRN, BC
Rhode Island Hospital
Providence, Rhode Island

Susan Bell, RN, MS, CNP, CNRN
The Ohio State University Medical Center
Columbus, Ohio

Linda Benson, RN, MS, APRN-BC, CCRN
Bronson Methodist Hospital
Kalamazoo, Michigan

Martha Biddle, ARNP, CCNS
Georgetown Community Hospital
Georgetown, Kentucky

Roger S. Blumenthal, MD
Johns Hopkins University School of Medicine
Baltimore, Maryland

Theresa M. Boley, RN, MSN, APN/FNP
Southern Illinois University School of Medicine
Springfield, Illinois

Jill E. Bormann, PhD, RN, CS
VA San Diego Healthcare System
San Diego, California

Elizabeth Burlew, RN, MSN, APN, CCNS, APN-Cardiology
Methodist University Hospital
Memphis, Tennessee

Diane C. Byrum, RN, MSN, CCRN, CCNS, FCCM
Carolinas Medical System
Charlotte, North Carolina

Catherine Y. Campbell, MD
Johns Hopkins University School of Medicine
Baltimore, Maryland

Diane L. Carroll, RN, PhD, FAHA
Massachusetts General Hospital
Boston, Massachusetts

Jessie Casida, MS, RN, CCRN, APN-C
Department of Adult Health Nursing
Seton Hall University
South Orange, New Jersey

Judith A. Cavanaugh, RN, MSN
Advocate Christ Medical Center
Oak Lawn, Illinois

Amy Chorzempa, RN, MS, ANP-BC
St. Luke's Roosevelt Hospital Center
New York, New York

Patricia Chriss, MSN, CRNP
Philadelphia Veterans Affairs Medical Center
Philadelphia, Pennsylvania

Suzanne H. Clark, MSN, MA, RNP
Kaiser Permanente
Woodland Hills, California

Bernice Coleman, PhD
Cedars-Sinai Medical Center
Los Angeles, California

Pat Comoss, RN, BS, FAACVPR
Nursing Enrichment Consultants
Harrisburg, Pennsylvania

Vicki J. Coombs, RN, PhD
Midatlantic Cardiovascular Associates
Baltimore, Maryland

Peggy A. Davis, MSN, RN, CNS
Department of Nursing
The University of Tennessee at Martin
Martin, Tennessee

Fabienne Dobbels, MPsy, PhD
Katholieke Universiteit Leuven
Leuven, Belgium

Diane K. Dressler, RN, MSN, CCRN
Marquette University College of Nursing
Milwaukee, Wisconsin

Arabella Droullard, RN, MS, CCRA
Genetech, Inc.
San Francisco, California

Sandra B. Dunbar, RN, DSN, FAAN
Nell Hodgson Woodruff School of Nursing
Emory University
Atlanta, Georgia

Margaret Eckert-Norton, MS, APRN.BC
State University of New York Downstate/New York
    University
New York, New York

Joseph M. Filakovsky, MSN, APRN, BC, CCNS, FAHA
Greenwich Hospital
Greenwich, Connecticut

Mary Kay Flynn, DNSc, RN, CCRN
Grand Canyon University
Phoenix, Arizona

Susan K. Frazier, PhD, RN
The Ohio State University College of Nursing
Columbus, Ohio

Robyn Gallagher, BA, MN, PhD
Faculty of Nursing, Midwifery, and Health
University of Technology
Sydney, New South Wales, Australia

Cecilia D. Garrison, RN, BSN, MS, CCRN
Baptist Memorial Healthcare Corporation
Memphis, Tennessee

Scott E. Glosner, PharmD, BCPS
Pfizer, Inc.
Midwestern University-Chicago College of Pharmacy
    and Purdue University School of Pharmacy
Elmurst, Illinois

Susan F. Goran, RN, MSN
Southern Maine Medical Center
Biddeford, Maine

Kathleen L. Grady, PhD, RN, APN, FAAN
Northwestern Memorial Hospital
Feinberg School of Medicine
Northwestern University
Chicago, Illinois

Marshall Hammond, MSN
Ocean Springs Hospital
Singing River Hospital System
Ocean Springs, Mississippi

David J. Hartman, MSN, CRNP
Hospital of the University of Pennsylvania
Philadelphia, Pennsylvania

Frank D. Hicks, PhD, RN
Rush University College of Nursing
Chicago, Illinois

Leslie Holmberg, RN, MS
St. Joseph's Hospital Health Center
Syracuse, New York

Patricia Kunz Howard, PhD, RN, CEN
University of Kentucky Hospital
University of Kentucky College of Nursing
Lexington, Kentucky

Louise S. Jenkins, PhD, RN, FAHA
School of Nursing
University of Maryland
Baltimore, Maryland

Ann N. Jessup, RN, MSN, APRN-BC
School of Nursing
University of North Carolina–Chapel Hill
Chapel Hill, North Carolina

Colleen Keller, PhD, RN, FNP, RN-C, FAHA
Boerne, Texas

Jeanette Kernicki, RN, PhD, ANP
Texas Women's University
Houston, Texas

Laura P. Kimble, PhD, RN
Georgia State University
Atlanta, Georgia

Karen A. Larimer, MSN, APRN, BC
Northwestern University
Chicago, Illinois

Barbara Leeper, RN, MN, CCRN, FAHA
Baylor University Medical Center
Dallas, Texas

Terry A. Lennie, PhD, RN
College of Nursing
University of Kentucky
Lexington, Kentucky

Ruth A. Lindquist, PhD, RN, FAAN, APRN, BC
School of Nursing
University of Minnesota
Minneapolis, Minnesota

Janet B. Long, MSN, APRN, BC, ACNP
Rhode Island Cardiology Center
Providence, Rhode Island

Gina Maiocco, PhD, RN, CCRN, CCNS
West Virginia University
Morgantown, West Virginia

Kathleen McCauley, PhD, RN, BC, FAAN, FAHA
University of Pennsylvania School of Nursing
Philadelphia, Pennsylvania

Susan D. McConnell, MSN, ANP
Emory University School of Medicine
Atlanta, Georgia

Kathleen M. McCormick, PhD, FACSM
Department of Exercise and Nutrition Sciences
University at Buffalo, SUNY
Buffalo, New York

Catherine J. Morse, MSN, CRNP, CCRN
The Chester County Hospital
West Chester, Pennsylvania

Caitlin Nassn, MSN
Waterbury Hospital
Waterbury, Connecticut

Andrea I. Neumark, MN, RN
Cedars-Sinai Medical Center
Los Angeles, California

Jennifer Niederstadt, MS, APRN, BC
St. Francis Hospital
Milwaukee, Wisconsin

Patricia Anne O'Malley, PhD, RN, CCRN, CNS
Indiana University East
Wright State University
Dayton, Ohio

Robert Lee Page, II, PharmD, FASCP, BCPS
Departments of Clinical Pharmacy and Physical
   Medicine
University of Colorado at Denver
Health Sciences Schools of Pharmacy and Medicine
Denver, Colorado

Lori A. Pennell, MS, APNC
Department of Cardiovascular and Thoracic Surgery
St. Michael's Medical Center
Newark, New Jersey

Kristine Jo Peterson, RN, MS, CCRN, CCNS
Methodist Hospital
Park Nicollet Health Services
St. Louis Park, Minnesota

Ann Petlin, RN, MSN, CCRN, CCNS, CSC
Barnes-Jewish Hospital at Washington University
   Medical Center
St. Louis, Missouri

Nancy A. Pike, RN, PhD, FNP
University of California–Los Angeles School of Nursing
Children's Hospital Los Angeles
Marina Del Rey, California

Marie S. Pilz, MSN, RN, CCNS
St. Joseph's/Candler
Savannah, Georgia

Sita S. Price, ARNP-BC, BS, BSN, MSN
Orlando Regional Medical Center
Orlando, Florida

Kathleen Rawlins, RN, MSN, CNS
Kaiser Foundation Hospital
San Francisco, California

Mary Beth Reid, PhD, RN, CNS-AD, CCRN, CEN
Presbyterian Hospital of Plano
Plano, Texas

Regina M. Renaud, MSN, RN, CCRN, CEN
St. Vincent Hospital at Worcester Medical Center
Worcester, Massachusetts

Joyce A. Ross, RN, BSN, MSN, CRNP, CS
University of Pennsylvania Health System
Cardiovascular Risk Intervention Program
Philadelphia, Pennsylvania

Catherine Ryan, PhD, RN, APN, CCRN
College of Nursing
University of Illinois at Chicago
Chicago, Illinois

Kristen E. Sandau, RN, PhD
Allina Health System
Minneapolis, Minnesota

Linda H. Schakenbach, MSN, RN, CNS, CCRN, CWCN, CS
Inova Alexandria Hospital
Alexandria, Virginia

Roberta W. Scherer, PhD
University of Maryland School of Medicine
Baltimore, Maryland

Audra Summers, RN, MSN, ARNP
University of Kentucky
Lexington, Kentucky

Linda M. Tamburri, RN, MS, APNC, CCRN
Robert Wood Johnson University Hospital
New Brunswick, New Jersey

Ruth E. Taylor-Piliae, RN, PHN, CNS, BSN, MN, PhD
Stanford Prevention Research Center
Stanford University
Stanford, California

Linda Teplitz, RN, PhD
Independent Cardiovascular Nursing Consultant
Palos Park, Illinois

Lorie Thomas, RN, MS
Sharp HealthCare
San Diego, California

Nancy C. Tkacs, RN, PhD
University of Pennsylvania School of Nursing
Philadelphia, Pennsylvania

Julie A. van Wyke, RN, MSN, APRN-BC, CCRN
Great Plains Regional Medical Center
North Platte, Nebraska

Rosemary Volosin, MSN, RN, APN
University of Pennsylvania
Philadelphia, Pennsylvania

Eileen M. Walsh, PhD, APRN, CVN
Jobst Vascular Center
Toledo, Ohio

Julie M. Waters, RN, MS, CCRN
Stanford Hospital and Clinics
Stanford, California

Deborah A. Whalen, APRN, BC, MBA
Boston Medical Center
Boston, Massachusetts

Connie White-Williams, RN, MSN
University of Alabama Hospital–Birmingham
Birmingham, Alabama

Sue Wingate, RN, DNSc, CRNP, CS
Kaiser Permanente Mid-Atlantic States
Silver Springs, Maryland

Susan L. Woods, PhD, RN, FAAN, FAHA
University of Washington
Seattle, Washington

Jane Nelson Worel, RN, MS, FAACVPR
University of Wisconsin Hospital and Clinics
Preventive Cardiology Program
Madison, Wisconsin

As we approach the second decade of the century, several important predictions in cardiovascular disease made more than 50 years ago have come to pass. First, the cardiovascular pandemic, which was so feared in the 1950s and 1960s, is now squarely upon us. Despite advances in the quality of cardiovascular care, the very high overall prevalence of cardiovascular disorders in North America, Western Europe, and other industrialized nations has remained stubbornly unchanged, although cardiac patients are now older and have more co-morbidities than heretofore. At the same time, cardiovascular disease in developing nations is climbing at an alarming rate. Indeed, it is now certain that during the next 15 years cardiovascular disease will, for the first time in human history, become the most frequent cause of death worldwide. Second, the prevalence of obesity and diabetes is also rising rapidly, especially among young people, leading to the concern that if these twin risk factors are left unchecked, the cardiovascular pandemic may not recede for many decades.

On a more positive side, very substantial basic and clinical research has provided knowledge to combat cardiovascular disease. Virtually all disorders can now be diagnosed quite accurately, usually by noninvasive techniques. Most can be treated effectively, albeit not cured. Furthermore, we are beginning to understand the underlying causes of atherosclerosis, hypertension, heart failure, and cardiac arrhythmias. Most importantly, we now know how to prevent or at least to defer many of these conditions. However, the results of numerous observational studies and registries have shown that we are not using this recently acquired information sufficiently to prevent or treat cardiovascular disease. In other words, there is a growing gap between our knowledge and its application.

At a time when there is a growing shortage of cardiologists, and when the opportunity to improve care to an increasing number of patients with cardiovascular disease, or who are at risk for developing it, is increasing, the role of nurses who understand and can apply new information to the diagnosis, treatment, and prevention of cardiovascular disease has never been more important. Braunwald's *Heart Disease: A Textbook of Cardiovascular Medicine* has provided such information to physicians for 30 years. Fifteen years ago, it became apparent that with the enormous growth of the field, all-important information could not be contained within a single book—even a very large one. Hence the decision was made to develop a Companion series to the "mother text." Given the ever-expanding role of nurses in the diagnosis, treatment, and prevention of cardiovascular disease, the editors recommended the development of *Cardiac Nursing* as a Companion to *Braunwald's Heart Disease*.

Drs. Debra K. Moser and Barbara Riegel, who are recognized internationally as leaders in cardiac nursing, have edited this splendid new text. They and their talented authors—almost all of whom are also experienced cardiac nurses with specialized skills—should be congratulated on the clarity, depth, and breadth of this book. Every area of cardiovascular medicine, nursing, and relevant basic science is described lucidly. We hope and anticipate that this Companion, *Cardiac Nursing*, will be useful not only to practicing nurses, but also to nursing educators and their trainees. By enhancing their knowledge and skills, we anticipate that this book will improve the care of the patient with, or at risk for, cardiovascular disease.

Eugene Braunwald, MD
Peter Libby, MD
Robert O. Bonow, MD
Douglas L. Mann, MD
Douglas P. Zipes, MD

The dominance of cardiovascular disease as a major cause of death and disability is now a worldwide phenomenon.[1] There is good news, however, with the recent findings that death rates from heart disease have dropped.[2] But this news is tempered by the fact that the incidence and prevalence of a number of important cardiovascular risk factors are escalating at alarming rates not only in the United States and in other industrialized countries, but also in developing countries.[2] For example, rising rates of obesity in developed countries and increasing tobacco use in developing countries threaten any progress made in decreasing the hold that cardiovascular disease has on the world population.

Given the global impact of cardiovascular disease and its preventable nature, it is essential that all health care providers be prepared to provide state-of-the-art, evidence-based care to individuals with, and at risk for, this chronic condition. Nurses, in particular, are at the forefront in providing preventive and restorative care at all stages in the continuum of cardiovascular disease development, progression, and rehabilitation. To provide this care requires a nursing workforce highly knowledgeable about the physiologic, psychosocial, and behavioral aspects of cardiovascular disease management.

Cardiac nursing is the largest specialty within nursing. Among critical care nurses alone, up to 70% of the more than 250,000 critical care nurses in the United States identify their specialty as cardiac. This book was developed and written to give nurses the knowledge and skills needed to deliver the highest quality, most up-to-date, and most comprehensive cardiac care possible. The text was developed for all the nurses who care for, or direct the care of, cardiac patients, including bedside, community-based, and advanced practice nurses. The book is intended to serve as a resource for nurses who work in a variety of settings, from in-hospital intensive care units to outpatient clinics to schools to hospice. The book is also intended to serve as a textbook for graduate students in critical care nursing, cardiac nursing, and Cardiac Nurse Practitioner or Clinical Nurse Specialist programs.

This book is intended to be a resource that allows nurses with varied expertise to augment their knowledge in specific areas of content. It was not that long ago when a "good" nurse could master all the information that she or he needed to care capably for a particular type of patient. Recent years have seen a knowledge explosion, however. The Internet has increased our access to information. More nurses are educated at the doctoral level with in-depth knowledge in specific, relevant areas of content such as genetics, pharmacology, and psychology. This expertise has permeated all levels of nursing, raising the bar of expectations and anticipation. Expert, advanced practice nurses are now common in nursing. These expert clinicians routinely use the knowledge produced by scientists in nursing and other related fields for the benefit of patients. In most settings, staff nurses are caring for increasingly complex patients, and the knowledge produced by nurse scientists and access to clinical experts supports them in the provision of excellent care.

The book is divided into six sections. The first section, *Foundations of Cardiac Care*, gives the reader an overview of the epidemiology, physiology, and pathophysiology of cardiac disease, as well as an understanding of the broader impact of cardiac disease on quality of life and the family. The second section is titled *Core Competencies of Clinicians Practicing Across the Continuum of Care*. In this section, the roles and skills of the various practitioners who work together with a common goal of improving patient outcomes are described. From bedside nurses to advanced practice nurses and other disciplines on the team, these chapters emphasize working as a team. Varied and unique subspecialty and disciplinary perspectives and contributions to improving outcomes are detailed.

In the third section, *Risk Factor Modification in Primary, Secondary and Tertiary Prevention*, the various risk factors are discussed. This section emphasizes the gender, ethnic/racial, and age-related differences associated with each risk factor. Emphasis in these chapters is on nurse-led interventions. Behavioral change is addressed in each chapter in this section, with an underlying theme of motivating behavioral change.

The fourth section, on *Cardiac Conditions*, is the largest section in the book. This section discusses the assessment and management of symptoms, conditions, and complications of cardiac disease. In the fifth section, *Using Evidence-Based Practice to Improve Outcomes in Outpatient Settings*, evidence and the use of published clinical guidelines are discussed. This section also addresses treatment adherence and patient education as key approaches underlying outpatient care. Finally, the last section, titled *Interactions Between the Heart and Other Systems*, discusses the relationship between heart disease and other system disorders.

Key Features of this book are authority, organization, presentation, and practical application. In terms of authority, the book is edited by two of the leading names in cardiac nursing along with the "father of modern cardiology." Leaders in cardiovascular nursing from across the world have contributed chapters. The organization is unique, with comprehensive coverage of cardiac nursing and with an emphasis on nursing care rather than medicine. The presentation includes a full-color design, which allows the highlighting of key content and specific features. There are full-color illustrations, photographs, and images that better mirror the conditions seen in practice and will enhance a nurse's understanding of the underlying pathology and related assessment findings. Liberal use of easy-to-read tables and figures illustrates important points and makes reading this comprehensive text easier and appealing to a wide range of readers. A key feature is the emphasis on the practical application of research to clinical practice. The text is supplemented by boxes addressing Technology, Clinical Conundrums, and Evidence-Based Practices that can be applied immediately.

Given the massive volume of information one would need to find and organize to stay current, most individuals feel overwhelmed by the task of keeping up to date. This text represents the state of our current knowledge in cardiovascular nursing, thus substantially easing that task. If the next few years are anything like the past decade, we expect that knowledge to increase exponentially. This text (and future revisions) will be here to provide cardiovascular nurses with the tools they need to stay abreast of the body of knowledge they need to optimize patient outcomes.

Debra K. Moser
Barbara Riegel

References

1. Gaziano TA: Reducing the growing burden of cardiovascular disease in the developing world. *Health Aff (Millwood)* 26:13-24, 2007.
2. Weisfeldt ML, Zieman SJ: Advances in the prevention and treatment of cardiovascular disease. *Health Aff (Millwood)* 26:25-37, 2007.

ACKNOWLEDGMENTS

The contributions and support of many people make such a book possible. We would like to thank Dr. Eugene Braunwald, the editor of *Braunwald's Heart Disease,* and his co-editors, Drs. Robert O. Bonow, Peter Libby, Douglas L. Mann, and Douglas P. Zipes, for having the vision to suggest a cardiovascular nursing companion to the Braunwald book series. The spirit of collaboration epitomized by this vision is fundamental to ensuring optimal patient outcomes. Each of the contributors of chapters to this book committed much in terms of time, intellectual contribution, and devotion to the support of the profession of cardiovascular nursing. This book would have been impossible without their contributions. We are indebted to the many reviewers who gave freely of their time and expertise in reviewing each chapter of this book and making it better for their comments. Barbara Cullen, our publisher at Elsevier, was endlessly supportive and a great champion of this project, and we greatly appreciate her support and dedication to the book. We could never have completed the monumental task of organizing this effort, revising, and editing without the help of our project manager, Kathy Teal, and our editors, Catherine Harold and Jennifer Ehlers. Finally, we would be remiss if we omitted thanking our families and loved ones for their unwavering support and patience during this Herculean effort.

Debra K. Moser
Barbara Riegel

CONTENTS

■ **SECTION V**
Using Evidence-Based Practice to Improve Outcomes in Outpatient Settings

Barbara Riegel and Debra K. Moser

■ **SECTION VI**
Interactions Between the Heart and Other Systems

Debra K. Moser and Barbara Riegel

Foundations of Cardiac Care

DEBRA K. MOSER and BARBARA RIEGEL

One of the greatest compliments a nurse can hear is that she or he is "the best nurse I know." Nurses strive to be the best and to be considered excellent by those who work with them. But what is the best? How does one reach this pinnacle of success? Exactly how does one deliver the best nursing care?

Exceptional nurses are distinguished not only by good technical and organizational skills but also by seemingly magical problem-solving abilities and talent for knowing which patients will develop complications and which patients will do well. They have all of the same information as the rest of us, but they always seem to be able to do more with it.

Exceptional nurses are the ones who put together apparently disparate bits of information to figure out exactly why a previously stable patient now mysteriously is deteriorating. They are the ones who know when and when not to call the family to soothe a suddenly disoriented patient. They figure out why the same patient is readmitted repeatedly to the intensive care unit with a digoxin overdose. They are the ones who point out the laboratory work that everyone else ignored as inconsequential but that now might explain that persistent dysrhythmia. They seem instinctively to know how to do the patient teaching that finally works with the chronically nonadherent heart failure patient. Some have called this special ability intuition. Is this truly just intuition? Or is something more complex at play?

We would argue that what passes, in many cases, as intuition actually is clinical experience shaped and informed by a comprehensive and well-integrated knowledge of relevant physiology, pathophysiology, psychology, sociology, epidemiology, and behavioral science. More than two decades ago, Patricia Benner[1] described the road from novice to expert for nurses and explicated the development of experiential wisdom on the foundation of scientific knowledge. She described expert nurses as those who successfully combine intuition with science. Although some have critiqued Benner's work as promoting intuition over science, in fact her work beautifully illustrated the importance of recognizing how intuition interacts with, develops from, and builds upon a strong scientific base.[1,2]

Truly outstanding nurses know that nursing is both an art and a science and that one is not sufficient to make an exceptional nurse without the other. To become one of the best, nurses must have a strong scientific foundation in physiology, pathophysiology, psychology, sociology, epidemiology, and behavioral science upon which to develop the art of nursing. The chapters in this section provide the scientific knowledge and context essential to the promotion of cardiovascular nursing excellence.

---

1. Benner P: *From novice to expert: excellence and power in clinical nursing practice*, Reading, Mass, 1984, Addison-Wesley.
2. Benner P: A response by P. Benner to K. Cash, "Benner and expertise in nursing: a critique," *Int J Nurs Stud* 33:669-674, 1996.

chapter 1

Evidence-Based Practice: Practicing What is Known, Not What is Believed

Robin J. Trupp
Barbara Riegel

CHAPTER ABBREVIATIONS

AACN   American Association of Critical-Care Nurses
ACE   angiotensin-converting enzyme
ADHERE   Acute Decompensated Heart Failure Registry
ANOVA   analysis of variance (statistics)
RCT   randomized clinical trials

"There are two classes of people in this world—those who take the best and enjoy it and those who wish for something better and try to create it. The world needs the appreciation of the first and the discontent of the second."

Florence Nightingale

Clinical practice must be based on current and sound scientific evidence. Yet in nursing, many patient care practices and decisions are founded on ritualistic patterns of behavior and unfounded beliefs. Although clinically relevant and scientifically reliable information may be available, in many instances there is a knowledge gap within the practice of nursing such that new evidence does not produce considerations for a change in behavior. In many situations, there is an absence of information altogether, resulting in nursing practice that is based on folklore or scientific knowledge being "borrowed" from other disciplines, leading to devaluation of the profession of nursing by others.

Even with the best intentions, keeping current with the latest research is challenging. Rapid advances in biomedicine, the tendency to overlook information not used routinely, and the necessity of learning new information while relearning forgotten information contribute to the difficulty of remaining current. Reforming opinions on efficacy of therapies and filtering out outdated information are monumental undertakings.

The concept of evidence-based practice has become increasingly prominent in the literature. Evidence-based practice begins with critical appraisal of findings from clinically relevant and scientifically sound studies before the adoption or rejection of any new evidence. Clinical practice guidelines are developed from this approach and are intended to assist clinicians by providing explicit recommendations for clinical practice along with the rationales for those recommendations.

Evidence-based practice is particularly challenging in nursing. Not only is there an absence of sufficient rigorous research to guide practice, but also there are significant barriers to using the evidence that is available. The purpose of this chapter is to describe the barriers that exist and to suggest ways that nurses can overcome them so that the growing body of evidence is used to improve patient outcomes.

The ultimate goal of nursing is to provide "evidence-based care that promotes quality outcomes for patients, families, health care providers, and the health care system."[1] Although nurse researchers must generate knowledge that directly or indirectly influences nursing practice, nurses also must embrace evidence-based approaches to patient care in order to promote optimal outcomes.

WHAT IS EVIDENCE-BASED PRACTICE? WHY IS IT IMPORTANT?

Evidence-based practice is the process of integrating evidence obtained from systematic research into clinical practice. Sackett and colleagues[2] defined evidence-based practice as "the conscientious and judicious use of current best evidence in making decisions about the care of individual patients." Two approaches to evidence-based practice are (1) individual efforts to evaluate and use new research in practice (i.e., research utilization) and (2) changing practice to reflect published clinical guidelines.

Evidence-based practice should be a goal and an outcome for the nursing profession and for the practicing nurse. Early nursing research focused on nursing issues (e.g., asking, "Is staffing sufficient?"). However, since the mid-1980s, nursing research has emphasized clinical issues or research on the outcomes associated with nursing care. Increasing emphasis is being placed on the importance of research. New journals highlight nursing research, scholarships are offered to support the conduct of research and dissemination of research findings, and resources are available for teaching and implementing evidence-based practice.[3] Additionally, several models have been published that illustrate how to incorporate research into clinical practice to improve the quality of care.[4-6] Even with the increasing awareness of and apparent agreement on the importance of research, nurses still are not practicing as the evidence directs them.

Unfortunately, much of nursing practice is founded on folklore rather than on scientific evidence, and large gaps still exist between research and clinical practice. Examples of failure to change practice or to follow the most current scientific evidence abound in nursing. For example, in surveys on nursing practice, the American Association of Critical-Care Nurses **(AACN)** found that nurses failed to practice according to the most current science available. Despite supporting evidence to the contrary, critical care nurses reported in 2003 that they still used a standard lead for monitoring patients, regardless of diagnosis; failed to prepare the skin properly before attaching electrodes; and improperly placed electrodes when monitoring patients. Other examples cited in "practice alerts" by the AACN include the following: suctioning secretions from intubated patients without elevating the head of the bed to at least 30 degrees, thus increasing the risk of ventilator-acquired pneumonia; the addition of food dye to enteral feedings as a method for detecting aspiration; and the confirmation of gastric tube placement using auscultation rather than radiography. Hence, the AACN now includes practice alerts on their website and in e-mail to members with the goals of closing the gap between research and practice, standardizing practice, and providing updates of new advances or trends in patient care.[7]

Failure to use evidence in practice is not limited to nursing. Other disciplines, including medicine, struggle with this issue as well. As an example, over the past decade many pharmacological and nonpharmacological treatment strategies for heart failure have been evaluated in large, multisite, randomized clinical trials that enrolled thousands of patients. The good news is that many of these strategies are effective, giving those with heart failure an improved prognosis with reduced morbidity and mortality and better quality of life.[8] Based on this overwhelming evidence, the American College of Cardiology and American Heart Association published "Guidelines for the Evaluation and Management of Chronic Heart Failure in the Adult" in 2001 and updated it in 2005.[9] These guidelines can be used as "quality markers" for the evaluation of patient care. The guidelines firmly promote angiotensin-converting enzyme **(ACE)** inhibitors—or alternatively, angiotensin receptor blockers—and beta blockers as the cornerstones of therapy in heart failure. Yet even with explicit recommendations for practice, gaps continue to exist between best evidence and clinical practice in implementation of the guidelines.

Data from the **ADHERE Registry,** the Acute Decompensated Heart Failure Registry, which currently has information on more than 150,000 patients, demonstrates continued underutilization of ACE inhibitors and beta blockers. ACE inhibitors are prescribed in approximately 72 percent of patients at the time of hospital discharge and beta blockers in approximately 68 percent.[10] Studies suggest that 30 to 40 percent of patients with chronic heart failure are not receiving care based on current scientific evidence and that as much as 25 percent of the care provided to these patients is unnecessary or potentially harmful.[11]

Other illustrations of the challenge of evidence-based practice include the following:

- A study by Switzer and colleagues[12] showed that adherence to the guidelines for treatment of community-acquired pneumonia was only 56 percent in low-risk persons. (Ironically, physicians with more clinical experience in treating pneumonia were less likely to follow the recommendations.)
- According to *Healthy People 2010,* which promotes a goal of decreasing smoking rates from 25 percent of adults to 12 percent by 2010, cigarette smoking is the single most preventable cause of disease and death.[13] Although the importance of smoking cessation counseling is well recognized, two studies have demonstrated that fewer than half of providers routinely counsel patients to quit smoking.[14,15]
- From the National Registry of Myocardial Infarction, despite repeated evidence supporting the use of beta blockers in acute myocardial infarction, between 1997 and 1999 only 60 percent of patients were receiving beta blockers at the time of hospital discharge.[16] In addition, the treatment gap between hospital arrival and definitive treatment time fell only marginally between 1990 and 1999.[17] The major factor explaining a delay in treatment was the "data-to-decision time"—the time spent with emergency department personnel and other physicians, such as a primary care physician or cardiologist, discussing which treatment should be given.[18]

DECISION MAKING IN HEALTH CARE

Making decisions is a routine part of everyday life and encompasses the spectrum from the mundane (What shall I wear today?) to the life-altering (Should I get married?). Advantages and disadvantages of options are weighed before a choice is made. Positive, negative, or neutral consequences occur as a result of these choices. However, in health care decision making, the consequences can be far greater and have lasting repercussions, not just for the individual making the decision but, more importantly, for the recipient of that decision—the patient. Decisions about treatment are most effective when the providers and the patient work together. The experience, knowledge, and evidence of the clinician, when combined with the patient's knowledge, experiences, wishes, and values, should lead to the best and most appropriate choices.

Nurses make clinical decisions routinely. Some examples of these decisions include intervention selection (Should I use acetaminophen or morphine to treat the pain?), interpretation of clinical issues (Is that ventricular tachycardia?), and communication (Do I page the physician now or wait until rounds?). Advanced practice nurses engage in more sophisticated and complex decisions, analogous to medical judgments about diagnosis, treatment, testing, and interpretation. Nurses also make administrative and organizational decisions relating to processes of care and staffing ratios. These important decisions influence the quality of care delivered and should involve nurses as key stakeholders and patient advocates.

Clinical practice guidelines, developed after a critical appraisal of clinically relevant and scientifically sound research by experts in the area, are intended to increase adherence or compliance with the evidence and to assist with evidence-based practice. Attention now is focused on the importance of provider adherence to guidelines. In fact, the National Institutes of Health, through the National Heart, Lung, and Blood Institute, issued a call for assessment of innovative strategies to improve evidence-based clinical practice.[19]

BARRIERS TO EVIDENCE-BASED PRACTICE

Clinical practice is well known to deviate from published guidelines.[20] Why are clinicians slow or reluctant to follow guidelines? Knowledge and attitudes affect clinicians' practices in relation to clinical guidelines. A report by Cabana and Kim[21] identifies multiple barriers to use of guidelines, including "inertia of previous practice due to habit or custom" (p. 146) and low outcome expectancy with "low likelihood that patient outcomes will improve" (p. 144). Individual perception of adherence to the evidence is also subject to bias. In one study, physicians overestimated their adherence to guidelines 87 percent of the time.[22]

Barriers to evidence-based clinical decision making include habits or routines that have been established, lack of understanding about the evidence presented, judgments about the efficacy of new therapies, and poor motivation for change. Changing behavior is difficult even with awareness of the need to do so. External barriers include time constraints associated with implementing and subsequently evaluating change, organizational structures, and lack of staff support to assist with amending clinical practice.

In nursing, the body of evidence is not yet extensive enough to generate comprehensive clinical practice guidelines. Thus evidence-based practice typically involves the evaluation of groups of studies in specific areas (i.e., research utilization). Nurses face numerous barriers to evidence-based practice that seem to revolve around three main issues: access to new evidence; support for utilization of new information; and interpretation of new clinical findings.

Access to New Evidence

Access to new evidence includes the availability of evidence supporting practice, the ability and time to retrieve the evidence, and availability of forums for sharing best clinical practices. In many cases there is simply a lack of evidence to support a particular nursing practice. When no evidence in nursing exists, nurses borrow information from other disciplines or maintain a "that's the way we've always done it" approach to patient care. When tradition and rituals guide practice, no compelling reason to change is encountered. Embedded in rituals is the belief that patient care is "routine," so why is change necessary in the first place?[23]

Although academicians value and are stimulated by new information, bedside caregivers, with heavy patient assignments, place more value on the "real world" of direct patient care. Bedside nurses may have limited access to current journals and articles, a shortage of computers with Internet resources, limited access to information sites within the work environment, or lack of skill in navigating the Internet. When these barriers are combined with patient assignments that leave nurses exhausted or under stress, it is no surprise that evidence-based practice is not routine.

Support for Use of New Information

Health care institutions have multiple financial constraints that, when combined with a nursing shortage and the need to spend funds on registry nurses just to staff the units, make evidence-based practice a low priority when allocating resources. This is especially true if the research plan or change to clinical practice creates additional strain on or confiscates the already limited resources for direct patient care. Consequently, few resources are spent on evidence-based practice or helping staff to become familiar with the latest science to update their knowledge base and practice.

Nursing leadership plays a critical role in evidence-based practice. In particular, nurse managers can influence the staff greatly by role modeling evidence-based practice. Evaluating variations in outcomes or quality data provides a perfect starting point for investigating clinical practice and exploring alternatives. Fostering a milieu that encourages nurses to question nursing rituals, seek new knowledge, critically appraise the evidence, and then use it to make decisions demonstrates commitment to quality care. Sharing responsibilities in a team-based environment allows for equal participation in decision making and validates the importance of evidence-based practice.[23] Effectively involving staff in the process of change will increase the likelihood of success.

Interpretation of New Clinical Findings

The adoption of research into clinical practice is a lengthy process; implementation of new evidence into practice takes 17 years, on average.[24] This fact is not surprising to cardiovascular nurses who see that medications with demonstrated abilities to influence outcomes positively for patients with heart failure, hypertension, and dyslipidemias still are not routinely prescribed for appropriate patients.[25]

Evidence-based practice is based on the "best available evidence."[2] Before a change in practice is made from the latest reported findings, however, new evidence first must be appraised critically. Not all evidence is created equal. Developing skills for critical assessment of the literature enables the practicing nurse to examine the credibility and integrity of the research and its applicability to nursing practice. Although reading published articles or attending programs can increase awareness of recent studies, those activities alone are typically insufficient. A thorough critique of research is needed before nurses can judge clinical relevance. Important considerations for evaluating research are listed in Table 1-1. A range of evidence, from the gold standard of randomized clinical trials to meta-analyses to expert opinion, is used in evidence-based practice (Table 1-2). The evidence has a hierarchy, however, and randomized clinical trials are given the most weight, followed by meta-analyses.

■ ■ ■

TABLE 1-1   CRITIQUING RESEARCH: QUESTIONS TO ASK YOURSELF

AREA OF CRITIQUE	QUESTIONS TO ASK
Overall	What is the problem being studied?
	What is the purpose of the study?
	Do you feel that you now know what is known and not known about this topic?
	Is the theoretical framework clear?
	Are the hypotheses clear, correct, and testable?
	Are the major terms labeled and defined?
Methods	How was the sample obtained?
	What is the sample size? What is the power analysis? Is the sample sufficient to avoid a type II error?
	If more than one group was studied, do the groups appear equivalent?
	What was the research design? Was it appropriate? Was it powerful?
	How well did the researchers follow the protocol? How did they make decisions?
Measurement and analysis	How were the variables measured? How were validity and reliability described?
	How were the data collected? Were the data flawed?
	Did sources of bias limit internal validity?
	What statistical tests were used? Were they appropriate? What was the match between functional words and analyses:
	• Effect or difference—ANOVA, t-test, chi-square
	• Relationship—correlation coefficient
	• Prediction—regression analysis
Results	What were the results? Does the researcher limit discussion to findings or go beyond the data?
	Are the hypotheses supported?
	Are the results related to the theoretical framework?
	Restate the question(s). Does the analysis match the question? The design?
	Were there unexpected (serendipitous) findings?
	Are the findings consistent with prior research?
Limitations	What study limitations were identified?
	Are there limitations that were not mentioned?
	What is the external validity of the study?
	Are there expressed and unexpressed assumptions? Do you agree with them?
	Are there uncontrolled extraneous variables that may have influenced findings?
	Were there errors in reporting or methods?
Final questions	How much confidence can be placed in these results?
	What other questions emerge from the findings? What remains to be discovered?
	Is this a study that you would use to support a change in practice?

ANOVA, Analysis of variance (statistics).

■ ■ ■

TABLE 1-2   LEVELS OF EVIDENCE AND EFFECTIVENESS

LEVEL	SOURCE OF EVIDENCE
I	Evidence from a systematic review or meta-analysis of all relevant randomized controlled trials (RCTs) or evidence-based clinical practice guidelines based on systematic reviews of RCTs *or three or more RCTs of good quality that have similar results*
II	Evidence obtained from at least one well-designed RCT
III	Evidence obtained from well-designed controlled trials without randomization
IV	Evidence from well-designed case-control or cohort studies
V	Evidence from systematic reviews of descriptive and qualitative studies
VI	Evidence from a single descriptive or qualitative study
VII	Evidence from the opinion of authorities and/or reports of expert committees

LEVEL	EFFECTIVENESS OF NURSING ACTIVITY
Effective	Research validates the effectiveness of the nursing activity, preferably with level I evidence or with a combination of level II or lower evidence and expert opinion.
Possibly effective	Some research studies validate the effectiveness of the nursing activity but not enough to recommend that nurses institute the activity at this time. Generally, more research is needed.
Not effective	Research has shown that the nursing activity is not effective and generally should not be used.
Possibly harmful	Some studies show harm to patients when using the nursing activity, and the nurse should evaluate carefully whether the activity is appropriate.

Adapted from Melnyk BM: *Worldviews on Evidence-Based Nursing* 1:194-197, 2004.

Nurses enter the profession from a variety of educational perspectives with varying levels of knowledge and understanding of research. Course work on research, theory, and statistics is, by and large, included at the baccalaureate level and higher, leaving a large proportion of bedside clinicians without the ability to interpret and apply research findings.

Critical appraisal of scientific evidence is a learned skill that requires a basic level of understanding of research types, study designs and methods, statistics, and clinical issues related to the study in question. If beginning this process, good forums for learning how to critique research are journal clubs and research symposia. Published studies cannot be assumed to reflect truth, regardless of the journal that published the article; published research is only as good as the scientists who provided peer review.

Guidelines, however, include research already appraised by content experts. As such, they allow nurses to bypass the step of critiquing individual studies. Guidelines promote evidence-based practice by providing explicit information on which to base practice and how to manage patients.

STRATEGIES FOR IMPROVING EVIDENCE-BASED PRACTICE

Interventions aimed at improving evidence-based practice include provider-directed, health care system-directed, and patient-directed strategies. Provider-directed approaches include increasing awareness about guidelines and their usefulness in clinical practice. Brush and colleagues[26] argued that busy clinicians use heuristics or mental shortcuts in decision making, but guidelines are typically lengthy documents that require time to study. They recommend the use of memory aids such as standard order sets, acronyms, and discharge checklists to make evidence-based practice part of the routine in clinical practice.

Health care system–directed strategies for promoting evidence-based practice include the use of standard orders, checklists, and the electronic medical record to increase the use of guidelines in clinical practice. External benchmarking is used in pay-for-performance efforts that evaluate the performance of hospitals and their providers, as a group, and use this performance to contract with high-quality providers. Provider and hospital performance have been publicized for several years.[29,30]

Other system-level strategies include the current efforts of the American College of Cardiology/American Heart Association Task Force on Clinical Guidelines to develop methods for updating clinical guidelines in a rapid and ongoing fashion. A system for doing so is currently in pilot testing.

Patient-directed systems for improving evidence-based practice are reflected in current efforts to share clinical guidelines with patients so that they can evaluate the care they receive. Pay-for-performance efforts also publicize provider and hospital performance measures to help consumers select high-quality providers.

Evidence-based practice has evolved quickly over the past decade. What began as a movement inappropriately labeled "cookbook medicine"[31,32] has evolved into a worldwide and shared focus on using research to make decisions about patient care and to improve outcomes. At this point, nurses are optimistic that the future will find them practicing what is known. Evidence-based practice is what patients expect and deserve.

Pay-for-performance efforts use financial and nonfinancial incentives to motivate providers to improve patient care.[27] Nonfinancial incentives for quality—any stimulus for improving quality that is not linked directly to a monetary payment[28]—are used alone and in combination with financial incentives to stimulate evidence-based practice. In performance measurement, one form of nonfinancial incentive—feedback—is given to providers on the quality of care they provide. The 2001 Institute of Medicine Report, *Crossing the Quality Chasm*, suggested the following six dimensions of health care in which improvement is needed to better meet patient needs and that could be used as performance measures: safety, effectiveness, patient-centeredness, timeliness, efficiency, and equitability.[28] In theory, performance measurement and feedback provides an incentive for providers to compare their performance with that of others and to improve quality accordingly. Efforts to use performance measurement to improve the quality of cardiovascular care have met with varying degrees of success.

REFERENCES

1. Craig JV, Smyth RL: *The evidence-based practice manual for nurses,* Edinburgh, 2002, Churchill Livingstone
2. Sackett DL, Rosenberg WMC, Gray JAM et al: Evidence-based medicine: what it is and what it isn't, *Br Med J* 312(7023):71-72, 1996.
3. University of Iowa Hospitals and Clinics. The Iowa Model of Evidence-Based Practice. Retrieved November 24, 2006 from http://www.uihealthcare.com/depts/nursing/rqom/evidencebasedpractice/iowamodel.html
4. Horsley JA, Crane J, Bingle JD: Research utilization as an organizational process, *J Nurs Adm* 8(7):4-6, 1978.
5. Stetler CB: Updating the Stetler model of research utilization to facilitate evidence-based practice, *Nurs Outlook* 49:272-279, 2001.
6. Titler MG, Kleiber C, Steelman V et al: Infusing research into practice to promote quality care, *Nurs Res* 43:307-313, 1994.
7. American Association of Critical-Care Nurses: Practice alert. Retrieved November 24, 2006, from http://www.aacn.org/AACN/practiceAlert.nsf/vwdoc/pa2
8. Scow DT, Smith EG, Shaughnessy AF: Combination therapy with ACE inhibitors and angiotensin-receptor blockers in heart failure, *Am Fam Physician* 68:1795-1798, 2003.
9. Hunt SA, Abraham WT, Chin MH et al. ACC/AHA 2005 guideline update for the diagnosis and management of chronic heart failure in the adult: summary article, *Circulation* 112:1825-1852, 2005.
10. Fonarow GC, on behalf of the Steering Committee: The Acute Decompensated Heart Failure Registry (ADHERE): opportunities to improve care of patients hospitalized with acute decompensated heart failure, *Rev Cardiovasc Med* 4(suppl 7):S21-S30, 2003.
11. Grol J, Grimshaw J: From best evidence to best practice: effective implementation of change in patients' care, *Lancet* 362:1225-1230, 2003.
12. Switzer GE, Halm EA, Chang CC et al: Physician awareness and self-reported use of local and national guidelines for community-acquired pneumonia, *J Gen Intern Med* 18:816-823, 2003.

13. Healthy People 2010. Healthy People. Retrieved November 24, 2006, from www.healthypeople.gov/

14. Kawachi I, Colditz GA, Stampfer MJ et al: Smoking cessation and time course of decreased risks of coronary heart disease in middle-aged women, *Arch Intern Med* 154:169-175, 1994.

15. Thorndike AN, Rigotti NA, Stafford RS et al: National patterns in treatment of smokers by physicians, *JAMA* 279:604-608, 1998.

16. Bradley EH, Herrin J, Mattera JA et al: Quality improvement efforts and hospital performance: rates of beta-blocker prescription after acute myocardial infarction, *Med Care* 43:282-292, 2005.

17. Rogers WJ, Canto JG, Lambrew CT et al: Temporal trends in the treatment of over 1.5 million patients with myocardial infarction in the US from 1990 through 1999: the National Registry of Myocardial Infarction 1, 2 and 3, *J Am Coll Cardiol* 36:2056-2063, 2000.

18. National Registry of Myocardial Infarction: *Data trends.* Retrieved January 24, 2006, from www.nrmi.org/nrmi_data.html

19. National Heart, Lung, and Blood Institute: *Trials assessing innovative strategies to improve clinical practice through guidelines in heart, lung, and blood diseases,* 2001. Retrieved February 5, 2005, from http://grants.nih.gov/grants/guide/rfa-files/RFA-HL-01-011.html

20. Grimshaw JM, Shirran L, Thomas R et al: Changing provider behavior: an overview of systematic reviews of interventions, *Med Care* 39:II2-II45, 2001.

21. Cabana MD, Kim C: Physician adherence to preventive cardiology guidelines for women, *Womens Health Issues* 13:142-149, 2003.

22. Adam AS, Soumerai SB, Lomas J et al: Evidence of self-report bias in assessing adherence to guidelines, *Int J Qual Health Care* 56:187-192, 1999.

23. Udod SA, Care WD: Setting the climate for evidence-based nursing practice: what is the leader's role? *Nurs Leadersh* 17:64-75, 2004.

24. Frist WH: Overcoming disparities in US health care, *Health Aff* 24:445-451, 2005.

25. Pearson TA, Blair SN, Daniels SR et al: AHA guidelines for primary prevention of cardiovascular disease and stroke: 2002 update—consensus panel guide to comprehensive risk reduction for adult patients without coronary or other atherosclerotic vascular disease, *Circulation* 106:388-391, 2002.

26. Brush JE, Radford MJ, Krumholz HM: Integrating clinical practice guidelines into the routine of everyday practice, *Critical Pathways in Cardiology* 4:161-167, 2005.

27. Salaway T, Burris C: Service line assessment and performance management through information integration: the case for cardiovascular services, *Top Health Inf Manage* 22:79-91, 2001.

28. Institute of Medicine: *Crossing the quality chasm: a new health system for the 21st century,* Washington, DC, 2001, National Academies Press.

29. Bufalino V, Peterson ED, Burke GL et al: Payment for quality: guiding principles and recommendations—principles and recommendations from the American Heart Association's Reimbursement, Coverage, and Access Policy Development Workgroup, *Circulation* 113:1151-1154, 2006.

30. Keckley PH: Evidence-based medicine in managed care: a survey of current and emerging strategies, *MedGenMed* 6:56, 2004.

31. Jones GW: Credibility, cookbook medicine, and common sense, *Ann Intern Med* 121:898-899, 1994.

32. Parmley WW: Practice guidelines and cookbook medicine: who are the cooks? *J Am Coll Cardiol* 24:567-568, 1994.

■ ■ ■ chapter **2**
Epidemiology of Coronary Artery Disease

Simon Stewart

CHAPTER ABBREVIATIONS

CAD coronary artery disease

CI confidence interval

DALY disability-adjusted life-year

ECG electrocardiogram

IDACC Identifying Depression as a Comorbid Condition

MONICA Monitoring Trends and Determinants in Cardiovascular Disease

NHANES National Health and Nutrition Examination Survey

OR odds ratio

WHO World Health Organization

As the overall wealth of the world's population steadily increases, there is an inevitable trade-off with a parallel increase in the total burden and impact of the diseases of affluence.[1] These diseases mark a transition in human history from the traditional killers of malnourishment, infectious disease, and violence that severely limited life expectancy to conditions that emerge in the latter years of an expanded life span. An increasing burden imposed by diseases of affluence has been exacerbated by advancing treatment options that prolong the inevitable in an aging body rather than provide an immortality elixir that defies the natural aging process.

In the past few decades, cardiovascular disease has spread from its traditional home in middle-aged men in affluent societies to children and adults of both sexes in affluent and poorer societies around the globe. The temptation is to regard cardiovascular disease as the exclusive domain of an aging cardiovascular system and, therefore, an inevitable killer of human beings at the end of their allotted life. However, data from the World Health Organization (**WHO**) indicate that cardiovascular disease is responsible for 10 percent of healthy life-years lost (expressed as disability-adjusted life-years [**DALYs**]) in low- to middle-income countries and almost double that figure (18 percent) in the most affluent countries. Cardiovascular disease is now the single largest cause of death in the world today.[2]

The biggest contributor to cardiovascular-related morbidity and mortality is coronary artery disease (**CAD**). CAD is a complex condition characterized predominantly by internal narrowing of the coronary arteries caused by atherosclerotic lesions, complicated by endothelial and platelet dysfunction that lead to a prothrombotic state (see Chapter 10). CAD is responsible for a spectrum of conditions correlated to the level of underlying myocardial ischemia and damage to the structural and functional integrity of the heart.[2] During the natural history of CAD, affected persons typically experience multiple manifestations of the underlying disease process that range from mildly debilitating to immediately life-threatening.[3] These manifestations include the following:

- Chronic exertional angina pectoris
- Chronic refractory angina pectoris
- Unstable angina pectoris
- Acute myocardial infarction
- Chronic heart failure
- Acute heart failure/cardiogenic shock
- Sudden cardiac death (as from sustained ventricular fibrillation)

In terms of disability, the number of DALYs currently attributable to CAD on a global basis (about 47 million/annum) is projected almost to double by the year 2020. Figure 2-1 shows the singular importance of CAD in contributing to the percentage of DALYs lost in men and women age 15 and older around the globe.

Within that context this chapter outlines the major features of the epidemiology of CAD. Because the field of epidemiology often is limited by the lack of systematic data collection on a whole-population basis, it relies on scientific rigor in data collection and interpretation. Given the enormous and intensive focus on CAD and the inherent risk of providing misleading information from highly selective studies, the information presented in this chapter is derived largely from large-scale population studies. The chapter focuses on key features of the epidemiology of CAD rather than providing exhaustive comparisons from the enormous and expanding array of conflicting data now available in the literature.

Table 2-1 summarizes the key terms used to describe the epidemiological profile of any disease state. Strict use of these key terms ensures that standardized and adjusted comparisons (e.g., per head of population on an age and sex-specific basis) can be made. The major uncertainty, therefore, lies in defining the index condition and ensuring that an accurate diagnosis is made based on its agreed definition. Fortunately, the term *coronary artery disease* and its various clinical manifestations are far less susceptible to misclassification than, for example, heart failure (see Chapter 3).

The broad objectives of this chapter are as follows:
1. To summarize major and evolving features of CAD from the whole-population perspective
2. To highlight significant studies that contribute to our current understanding of the epidemiology of CAD

To achieve these objectives, the following are presented:

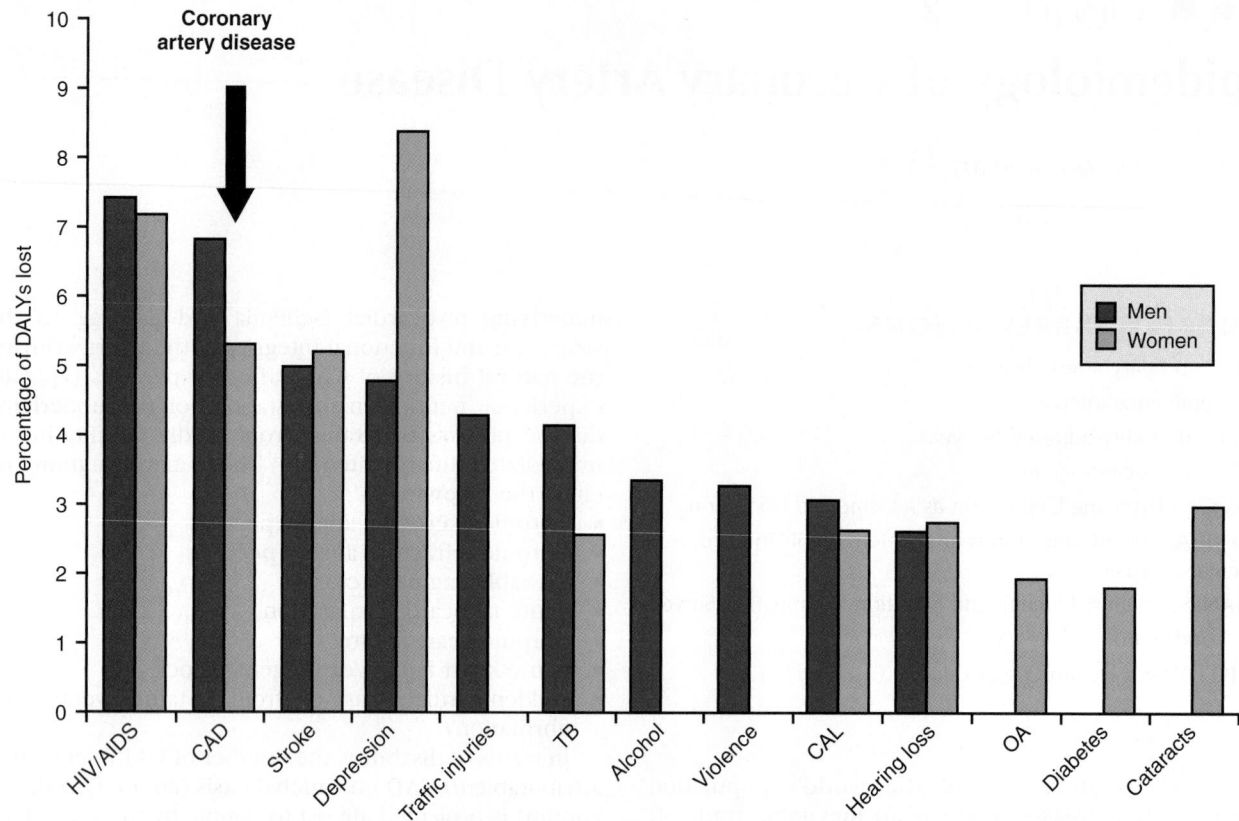

FIGURE 2-1 ■ Global impact of coronary artery disease on disability-adjusted life-years lost relative to the top 10 morbidities in men and women age 15 and older worldwide. *CAD,* Coronary artery disease; *CAL,* chronic airflow limitation; *HIV-AIDS,* human immunodeficiency syndrome; *OA,* osteoarthritis; *TB,* tuberculosis. (Data from World Health Organization: *Atlas of heart disease and stroke.* Retrieved November 2006 from www.who.int/cardiovascular_diseases/resources/atlas/en/index.html)

■ ■ ■

TABLE 2-1   KEY TERMS AND DEFINITIONS IN CLINICAL EPIDEMIOLOGY

TERM	DEFINITION
Incidence	The number of new cases occurring over a specific period relative to the number of persons at risk of being affected during that time (e.g., 200 new cases of coronary artery disease [CAD] per 100,000 persons per year)
Case-fatality	A death arising from a particular disease. It can be expressed as a percentage (e.g., 21% case-fatality at 12 months after acute myocardial infarction) or a population rate (e.g., 50 CAD-related deaths per 100,000 persons per year).
Prevalence	A product of incidence (rate of new cases) and survival (how long they survive), prevalence is the number of affected cases at any one time (point prevalence) relative to the total population (e.g., 100 cases of CAD per 1000 persons in 2004).
Risk factor	A factor demonstrated to be strongly associated (in epidemiological and pathophysiological terms) with an increased risk of developing a particular disease
Absolute (attributable) risk	The actual (or calculated) difference in the risk of an event (e.g., 10% versus 5%) occurring in the presence of a particular factor compared with its absence. Another valid definition often used is the proportion of cases that can be ascribed to the specific risk factor.
Relative risk	The proportional difference in the risk of an event occurring in the presence or absence of a risk factor (e.g., 10% versus 5% equates to a 50% difference in relative risk)
Population-attributable risk	The product of the absolute risk of developing a disease for any given risk factor by the proportion of persons affected, it provides a measure of what proportion of a disease may be avoided by avoiding or minimizing the given risk factor (e.g., a risk factor that imparts a very low attributable risk for CAD will have a very large population-attributable risk if it is present in more than 50% of the population).
Borderline risk factor	In nondichotomous risk factors that are expressed via a range of continuous values (e.g., systolic blood pressure or serum lipid levels), there may be a definitive threshold at which a high risk for developing a particular disease is established and attributable and relative risks calculated. However, an artificial cutoff in risk often fails to take into account the continuous nature of risk. Studies now also focus on borderline values that have a low attributable risk but, because of their high prevalence, have a high population-attributable risk.

- The major features of the incidence and prognostic impact of CAD in a range of populations
- The overall prevalence and morbidity profile (e.g., health care utilization rates and related expenditures) of CAD
- Common risk factors associated with CAD, with a particular focus on their population impact and influence on the overall epidemiological profile of CAD in the world today
- Key issues relating to potential differences in the epidemiology of CAD based on gender and diverse ethnic and cultural groups

INCIDENCE OF CORONARY ARTERY DISEASE

Determining the true incidence of CAD within whole populations is problematic given that the gold standard for determining its presence involves an invasive coronary angiogram[3] or postmortem examination.[4] In unusual circumstances, it is sometimes possible to obtain information that highlights the inadequacy of existing data to describe the natural history and epidemiological profile of a complex disease state. For example, a study of the coronary arteries of young male U.S. soldiers killed in action in Korea found evidence of CAD in 232 of 300 postmortem examinations (CAD prevalence of 77 percent). A severe form of the disease was found in 5 to 6 percent of cases overall.[5] Most investigators focus on older individuals in whom CAD has resulted in nonfatal symptoms (e.g., angina pectoris), an acute nonfatal event (e.g., an acute myocardial infarction) or sudden cardiac death. Thus, they miss individuals who remain asymptomatic or die without a postmortem examination. As a result, the true incidence and prevalence of CAD is commonly underreported. Only studies in which the health of coronary arteries and markers of CAD are tracked throughout a person's life span reveal the true natural history and incidence of CAD in whole populations.

Population Studies

Despite the aforementioned limitations, a number of key population studies have revealed important aspects of the epidemiological profile of predominantly symptomatic and fatal CAD-related events.

Framingham Heart Study

The Framingham Heart Study is an ongoing prospective population cohort study in which the incidence of CAD over a prolonged period has been described. The study began in 1948 when 5209 residents of Framingham, Massachusetts, ages 28 to 62, were enrolled in the study.[6,7] Participants were assessed every 2 years via medical histories, physical examinations, and selected laboratory tests. In 1971, the study was extended to include 5124 of the original participants' offspring and their spouses, who were followed every 4 years.[8] In 1991, the Framingham investigators reported the 12-year incidence of CAD in middle-aged men ($n = 1663$) and women ($n = 1714$) as part of the offspring cohort. These participants were ages 30 to 59 and were determined to be free from the disease at baseline examination (1972 to 1974).[9] In that study, CAD was defined as the occurrence of angina pectoris, acute myocardial infarction, coronary insufficiency, or coronary death.

During study follow-up, 156 men (10.4 percent) and 55 women (3.3 percent) were found to have developed CAD. The average age of those men and women was 44.6 and 47.2 years, respectively. In comparison, their male and female counterparts who remained free from detectable CAD were ages 40.8 and 40.5 years, respectively. These data reconfirmed a higher incidence of CAD among men compared with women in middle age. On average, women who developed incident CAD were about 4 years older than their male counterparts. Overall, 10-year age-adjusted incident rates in the cohorts ranged from 2 to 16 percent in men and 1 to 8 percent in women, depending on each person's baseline risk factor profile.[9]

In a later report the Framingham investigators analyzed the lifetime risk of CAD using data from all 7733 study participants who had attended at least one examination between 1971 and 1975 and who had no signs of the disease at initial assessment. The original criteria for determining incident CAD until the study census date of July 1996 were applied. During 109,948 person-years of follow-up, 684 men and 473 women between ages 40 and 94 manifested incident CAD (Figure 2-2). From these data, age- and gender-specific risks for developing incident CAD were generated. They showed that in adults younger than age 40, the risk of developing CAD was extremely low (1.2 percent in men and 0.2 percent

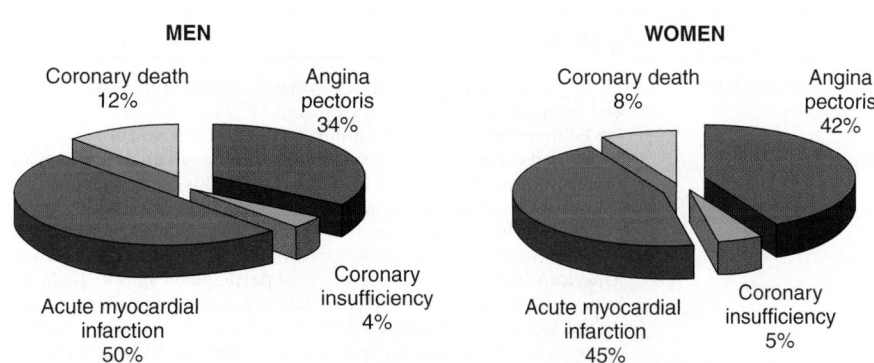

FIGURE 2-2 ■ Composition of incident coronary artery disease–related events in the Framingham cohort. (Data from Lloyd-Jones DM, Larson MG, Beiser A et al: *Lancet* 353[9147]:89-92, 1999.)

in women). Figure 2-3, however, shows study data indicating that beyond age 40, men and women are at high risk of developing CAD. Beyond age 70, the risk of subsequently developing CAD falls dramatically in those men and women who have survived without manifesting any forms of the disease.[10]

Although these data underestimated the significance of sudden cardiac death as a marker of CAD, they did highlight the importance of acute myocardial infarction as a marker of the disease in the late 20th century. As will be discussed later, evolving definitions of acute myocardial infarction and ischemia[11] make direct comparisons with data derived from 21st–century epidemiological studies problematic.

Because Framingham Heart Study data were derived from a semi-rural, white population, generalizing them to today's more diverse populations is problematic, particularly given the potential race-based differences. Furthermore, treatment advances and better risk-management programs call into question their relevance to the present day.

To fully explore and compare the detailed findings of the increasing number of prospective population studies that have examined the incidence of CAD is beyond the scope of this chapter, particularly given the differ-

ent methods used to detect the disease. Nevertheless, studies outlined in Table 2-2, in addition to those specifically described later in this chapter, are indicative of the range of studies that have examined the incidence of CAD.

Recent advances in detection (e.g., troponin testing[11]), treatment (e.g., thrombolysis and primary angioplasty[16]), and more sensitive delineation of the extent of myocardial ischemia and necrosis (e.g., nuclear imaging[17]) probably will require a more detailed examination of the range of acute coronary syndromes that reflect underlying CAD in future epidemiological studies. Recently published data from Scotland are indicative of the difficulty in comparing past and current data when the evolving epidemiology of CAD and the definitions used to identify its presence are considered.

Scottish Morbidity Surveillance Data

Whole-population data from the Scottish population, using unique data from the Scottish Morbidity Record scheme, highlight the evolving nature of the incidence of nonfatal CAD events when the full range of events included in acute coronary syndrome are examined. This linked data set provides information on all National Health Service hospital discharges in Scotland (total population approximately 5.1 million). Data are collected and collated by the Information and Statistics Division of the National Health Service and are linked to the Registrar General's death certificate data to provide individualized tracking of morbid and fatal events.[18]

Using these data, Murphy and colleagues[19] examined 225,512 incident hospitalizations for acute myocardial infarction, unstable angina pectoris, and for suspected cases of acute coronary syndrome (i.e., chest pain presentation) from 1990 to 2000. These hospitalizations included 96,026 cases of acute myocardial infarction (43 percent of total cases); 37,403 cases of unstable angina (17 percent); and 92,083 cases of chest pain (41 percent). Overall, observed changes in the annual incidence of each diagnosis between 1990 and 2000 were as follows:

- Acute myocardial infarction: 260 cases versus 173 cases per 100,000 population (an adjusted decline of 33 percent)

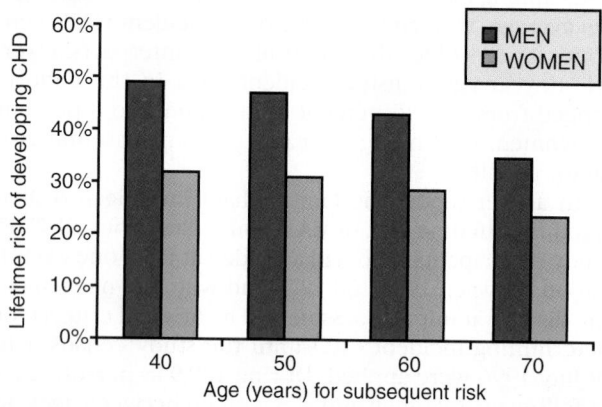

FIGURE 2-3 ■ Age- and gender-specific lifetime risk of developing coronary heart disease (CHD) according to the Framingham cohort. (Data from Lloyd-Jones DM, Larson MG, Beiser A et al: *Lancet* 353[9147]:89-92, 1999.)

TABLE 2-2   KEY STUDIES OF EXAMINING INCIDENCE OF CAD

STUDY	KEY FEATURES
Prospective Cardiovascular Munster Study[12]	Study of a working population in Germany: 20,060 employees recruited from 52 companies and local government authorities from 1979 to 1985. The cohort was periodically followed up every 2 years (minimum 10 years of follow-up).
The San Antonio Heart Study[13]	Diabetes and cardiovascular disease studied in Mexican-Americans and non-Hispanic whites from low-, middle-, and high-income households in Texas from 1984 to 1988. Follow-up examinations were performed from 1991 to 1996 (median 7.5 years). Coronary artery disease incidence was examined in 2569 persons who were free of diabetes at baseline.
The Strong Heart Study[14]	This study commenced in 1988 to examine cardiovascular disease and its risk factors in American Indians. The cohort of 4549 participants ages 45 to 74 initially was screened between 1989 and 1992 with periodic screening and follow-up thereafter.
The Adventist Health Study[15]	Included 34,198 non-Hispanic white Seventh-Day Adventists in California from 1974 to 1976. Subjects were followed for more than 12 years to determine coronary artery disease-related morbidity and mortality.

CAD, Coronary artery disease.

- Unstable angina: 59 cases versus 105 cases per 100,000 population (an adjusted rise of 78 percent)
- Chest pain: 114 cases versus 296 cases per 100,000 population (an adjusted rise of 110 percent)[19]

Figure 2-4 represents the trends in incidence rates for acute myocardial infarction and unstable angina over the study period on a gender-specific basis. The overall decline in confirmed acute coronary syndromes was a relatively small 12 percent (319 versus 278 cases per 100,000 population) over the study period. Significantly, this decline may be counterbalanced by the rising number of true cases of CAD "hidden" within those diagnosed with chest pain alone.[19]

Minnesota Heart Survey

These data were consistent with data reported from the Minnesota Heart Survey of the population living in the Twin Cities (Minneapolis and St. Paul) in the United States. In the Minnesota Heart Survey, a 20 percent decline was reported in incident admissions for acute myocardial infarction from 1985 to 1995. This decline was offset by a 56 percent and 30 percent increase in admissions for angina pectoris in men and women, respectively.[20] Table 2-3 represents the comparison of incident rates of hospitalization for acute myocardial infarction in the Minnesota and Scottish populations in 1990 and 1995. Although incidence rates in men were similar in these two studies, there was a large absolute difference in women. Overall, there were similar adjusted declines in incidence rates in men and women during the 5-year study period.

It is also important to examine the "hidden" component of incident CAD—sudden cardiac death. The most comprehensive study of sudden cardiac death in a whole population was derived from the Scottish Morbidity Record scheme. Figure 2-5 represents observed age- and sex-specific changes for fatal cardiac events from 1986 to 1995. The incidence of sudden cardiac death increases dramatically with age. Overall, there were significant declines (between 20 percent and 50 percent) in sudden fatal events in men and women and all adult age groups.[21]

Data from the Framingham Heart Study for the period 1950 to 1999 also showed that the risk of sudden cardiac death had declined by 39 percent from 1990 to 1999 relative to the original reference period in subjects without a history of CAD. In subjects with known CAD, the decline was 57 percent. Of the 811 deaths attributed to CAD (571 men and 240 women), 358 (44 percent) were sudden cardiac deaths. About half of these fatal events (173 out of 358) occurred in those without known CAD.[22]

In summary, it appears that the incidence of CAD, as reflected by decreased rates of acute myocardial infarction and sudden cardiac death, is rapidly declining in developed countries. Alternatively, the incidence of "milder" and more chronic forms of CAD is potentially rising. The rise in chronic forms of CAD may be due to an evolving natural history that is modulated by the introduction of more effective modern treatments and

TABLE 2-3 COMPARISON OF INCIDENT ADMISSIONS (PER 100,000 POPULATION) FOR ACUTE MYOCARDIAL INFARCTION: MINNESOTA, UNITED STATES, VERSUS SCOTLAND, UNITED KINGDOM

POPULATION COHORT	MEN		WOMEN	
	1990	1995	1990	1995
Scotland	320	274	205	180
Minnesota	289	272	111	106

Data from Murphy NF, MacIntyre K, Capewell S et al: *BMJ* 328:1413-1414, 2004; and McGovern PG, Jacobs DR, Shahar E et al: *Circulation* 104:19-24, 2001.

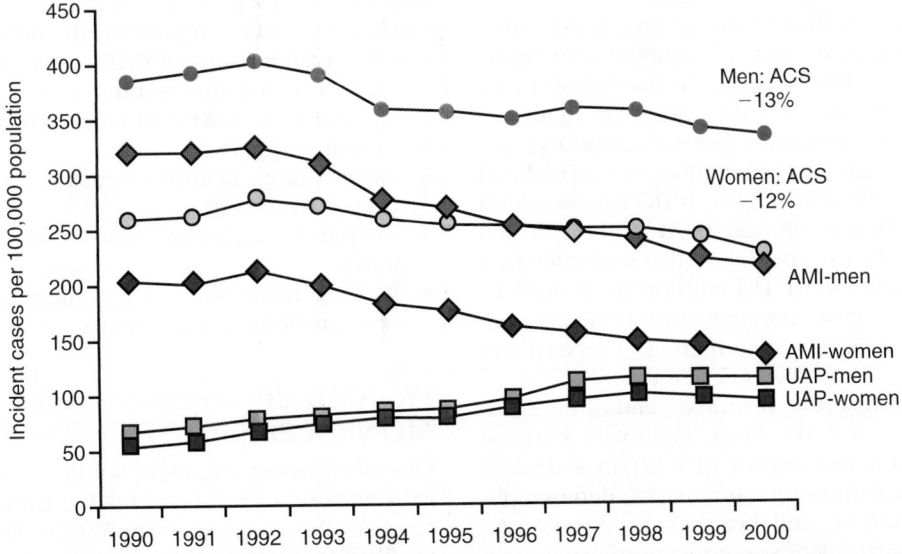

FIGURE 2-4 ■ Ten-year trends in the incidence of unstable angina pectoris (UAP), acute myocardial infarction (AMI), and the two combined (acute coronary syndrome, ACS) in the Scottish population. (Data from Capewell S, MacIntyre K, Stewart S et al: *BMJ* 328:1413-1414, 2004.)

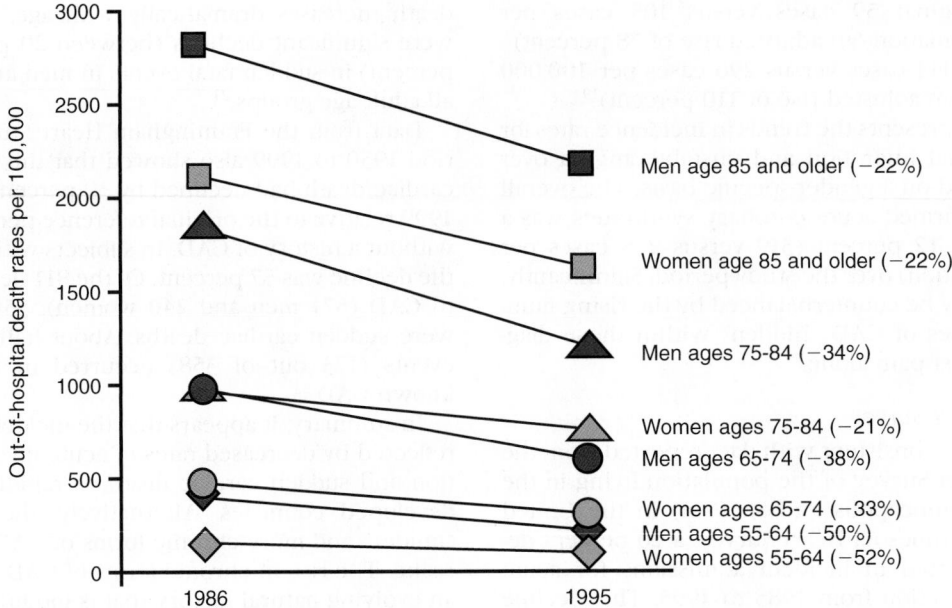

FIGURE 2-5 ■ Population rates for out-of-hospital sudden cardiac deaths in Scotland from 1986 to 1997. (Data from Capewell S, MacIntyre K, Stewart S, et al: Lancet 358:1213-1217, 2001.)

substantial lifestyle changes. The net effect is most likely a modest decline in the overall incidence of CAD in Western developed countries. Thus, the reported lifetime risk of a middle-aged man (1 in 2) or woman (1 in 3) developing CAD in his or her remaining lifetime is likely to remain constant in the foreseeable future.

CORONARY ARTERY DISEASE–RELATED CASE-FATALITY

As described, some data suggest a declining incidence of CAD, at least in the United States and Western Europe. However, observed declines in acute myocardial infarction and sudden cardiac death appear to be offset by an increase in milder and more chronic forms of the disease. The American Heart Association has estimated that CAD still accounts for nearly 700,000 deaths yearly in the United States alone.[23] Similarly, the British Heart Foundation has estimated that the equivalent figure for the United Kingdom remains close to 120,000 yearly, with an absolute decline in the number of CAD-related deaths of around 3000 yearly.[24] The WHO has estimated that CAD currently contributes to 7.1 million deaths yearly on a global basis. The WHO also estimates that this figure will increase to 11.1 million by 2020.[25] In Europe, CAD is the most common cause of death, contributing to one in six deaths in men (17 percent) and one in seven deaths in women (15 percent).[23]

Case-fatality is a discrete, definitive, and often inevitable consequence of CAD. Thus, fatality is a useful outcome to monitor the impact of CAD in a diverse range of countries with unique population demographics, risk factor profiles, and health care systems. As such, direct comparisons of sex- and age-adjusted case-fatality rates on a country-by-country basis for the same period provide the most compelling data concerning the global impact of CAD. Analysis of major trends over time (positive or negative) provides important information in terms of the likely strategies required to combat CAD burden in whole populations. Figure 2-6 (adapted from original WHO surveillance data[25]) represents observed declines in age-adjusted case-fatality rates in men in four developed countries since the 1970s.

One of the key questions arising from the declining case-fatality rates is whether these observations are a true reflection of the fatal impact of the disease. If so, what are the reasons for the decline? If we knew the reasons for the decline, they could be reinforced or reproduced. Are the reasons for decline universal (i.e., applicable to countries around the globe and for men and women?) Figure 2-7 (adapted from original WHO surveillance data[25]) represents the most recent between-country comparisons of CAD-related case-fatality rates. Overall, it demonstrates a number of marked gradients (from higher to lower) in case-fatality rates in the following directions:

- Eastern (e.g., Belarus) versus Western Europe (e.g., United Kingdom)
- Northern (e.g., Ireland) versus Southern Europe (e.g., Italy)
- Western hemisphere (e.g., United States) versus Eastern hemisphere (e.g., Japan)

World Health Organization's MONICA Project

One of the most extensive studies of the epidemiological transition of CAD and related trends in case-fatality rates around the globe is the WHO's **MONICA** (Monitoring Trends and Determinants in Cardiovascular Disease) Project.[26] The MONICA Project emanated from the Bethesda Conference on the Decline in Coronary Heart

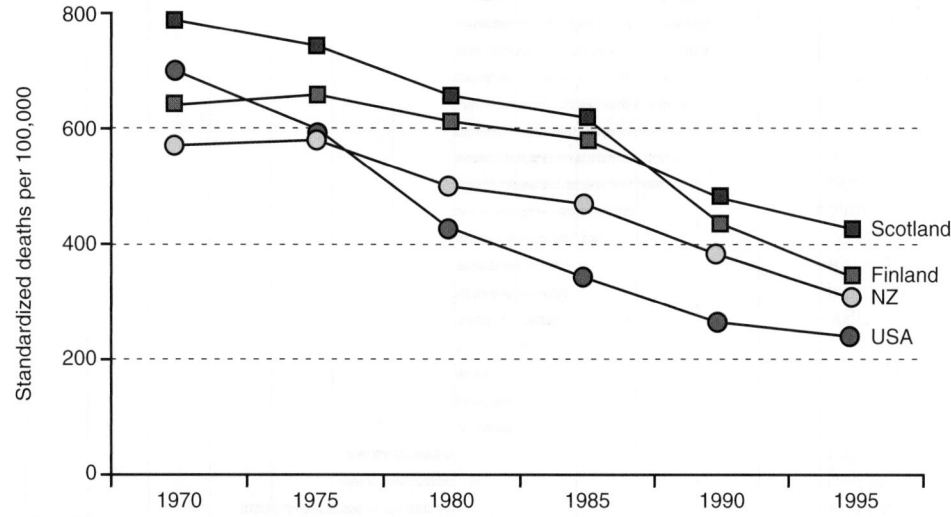

FIGURE 2-6 ■ The decline in age-adjusted case-fatality rates for coronary artery disease in men of Scotland, Finland, New Zealand (NZ), and the United States (USA). (Data from Salomaa V, Keonen M, Koukkunen H et al: *Circulation* 10:691-696, 2003.)

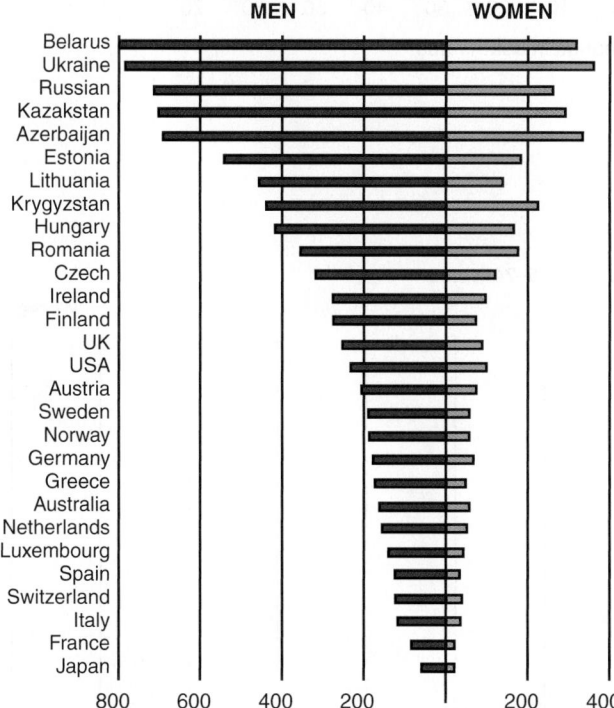

FIGURE 2-7 ■ Comparison of global coronary artery disease-related case-fatality rates in men and women ages 35 to 74 in 1999. (From World Health Organization: *Atlas of heart disease and stroke*, 2002. Retrieved November 2006 from http://www.who.int/cardiovascular_diseases/en/cvd_atlas_13_coronaryHD.pdf)

Disease Mortality in 1978. The MONICA project has provided ongoing surveillance of well-defined population cohorts of men and women ages 35 to 64 in a large range of countries around the globe. The study has provided key data used to generate comparative tables relating to current population rates of CAD-related case-fatality (Figure 2-7). Significantly, the study also has provided a comparison of long-term trends in this re-

gard, as shown in Figure 2-8 (adapted from WHO data[25]).

Analysis of 166,000 coronary events that occurred during 8 to 14 years of follow-up of the MONICA population cohorts (core data from 1985 to 1991 in all countries) showed that North Karelia, Finland, had the highest 10-year CAD event rates in men, whereas Bejing, China, had the lowest. In women, the highest rates occurred in Glasgow, Scotland, and the lowest in Catalonia, Spain. In most countries, CAD event rates declined.

A comparison of MONICA event rates that relied on strict qualifying criteria for the presence of CAD showed that routinely reported case-fatality rates from official death registries consistently overestimate declines in CAD-related deaths. Unfortunately, despite the detailed nature of the MONICA Study, the broad range of populations studied produced heterogeneous and complex data. As a consequence, the investigators were unable to provide definitive insight into factors that have contributed to apparent changes in CAD-related case-fatality rates around the globe.[26]

Close examinations of the trends observed in individual population cohorts can provide insights about the causes and consequences of changes in CAD-related case-fatality. Apart from Australia, Norway, and Luxemburg, the most impressive improvements in case-fatality have occurred in the male and female population of Finland located in northeastern Europe. The study, an extension of the MONICA Project, involved an analysis of trends in out-of-hospital deaths in four geographic areas in that country in order to explain observed declines in CAD-related case-fatality.[27] Consistent with Scottish data,[21] the rate and absolute proportion of sudden cardiac deaths increased with age, particularly in women. Analysis of 3494 fatal events recorded during 1983 to 1997 showed that age-standardized case-fatality from sudden cardiac death fell by 6.1 percent and 7.0 percent in men and women, respectively. These declines contributed to a 70 percent and 58 percent im-

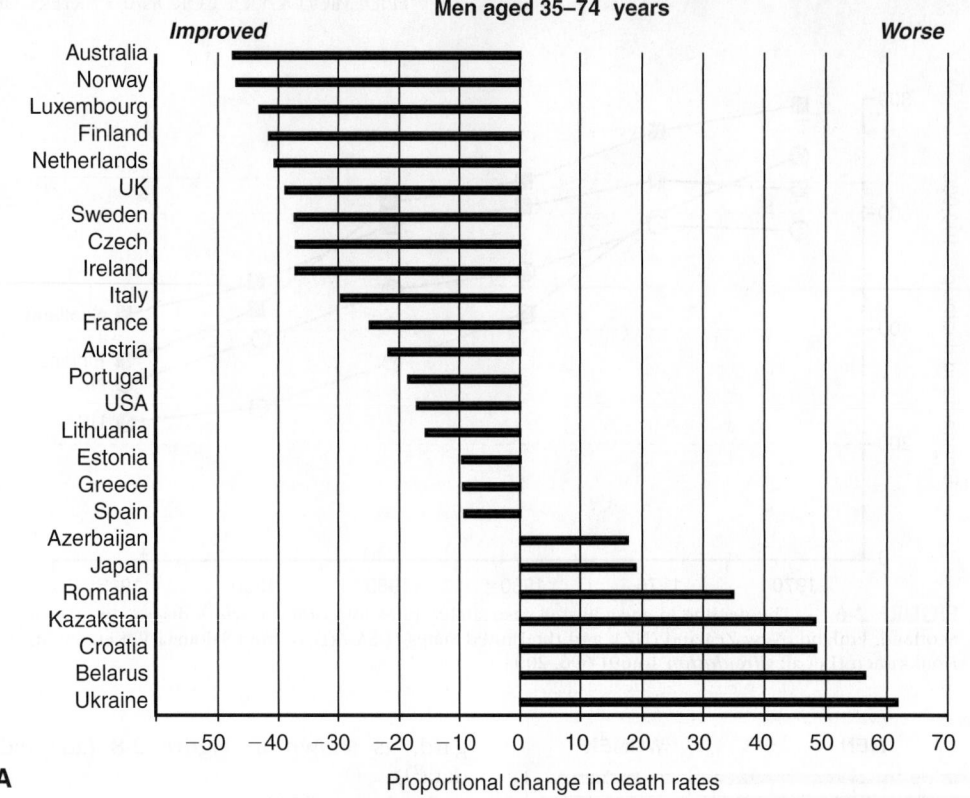

Men aged 35–74 years

Improved   *Worse*

Proportional change in death rates

A

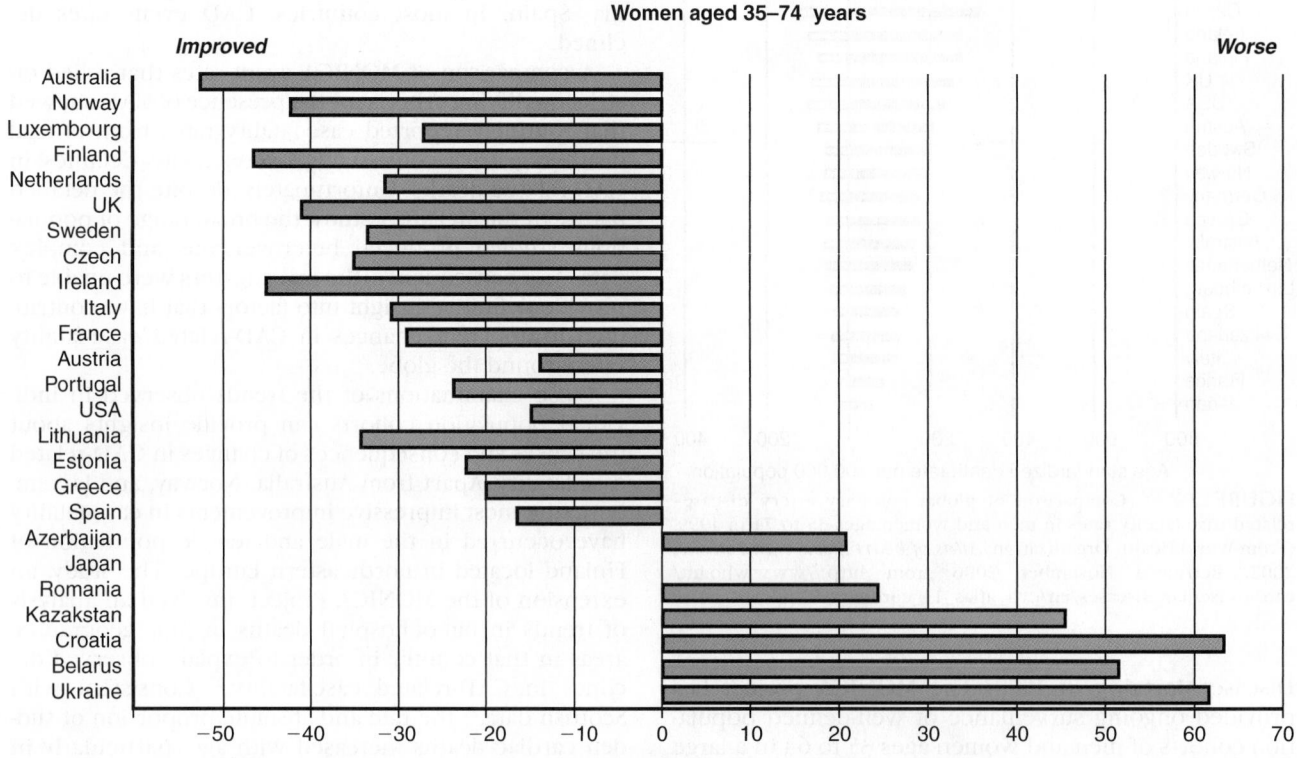

Women aged 35–74 years

Improved   *Worse*

Proportional change in death rates

B

FIGURE 2-8 ▇ Trends in age-standardized coronary artery disease–related case-fatality rates per 100,000 population (1968 to 2001). 8a, Men ages 35 to 74. 8b, Women ages 35 to 74. (From World Health Organization: *The Global Burden of Coronary Heart Disease* 2002. Retrieved November 2006 from www.who.int/cardiovascular_diseases/resources/atlas/en/print.html)

provement in male and female CAD mortality rates in those ages 35 to 64 overall.[27] Despite these positive findings, almost half of the documented cases of out-of-hospital death were the *first* clinical manifestation of CAD.

Minnesota Heart Survey

Case-fatality related to acute coronary syndrome was examined in the Minnesota Heart Survey, in a hospitalized cohort of patients ages 30 to 74 between 1985 and 1997.[20] Comparable with overall U.S. data at the time, a 3 to 4 percent annual decline was observed in CAD-related case-fatality rates during the mid-1980s. This decline accelerated to almost 6 percent yearly between 1985 and 1997. Overall, these trends contributed to a 50 percent decline in case-fatality rates between 1985 and 1997. During the periods of 1985 to 1991 and 1991 to 1997, in-hospital case-fatality rates declined by 43 percent and 39 percent in men (absolute decline from 100 to 35 fatal events per 100,000 males during 1985 to 1997) and by 39 percent and 49 percent in women (absolute decline from 40 to 15 fatal events per 100,000 females during 1985 to 1997). In addition to a decline in the rate of presenting cases of acute coronary syndromes, there was a parallel decline in subsequent case-fatality rates (in-hospital and sudden cardiac death combined). Specifically, the following were found:

- In men, 3-year age-adjusted case-fatality following an index hospitalization for an acute coronary syndrome declined from 28 to 19 percent during the period 1985 to 1995.
- In women, the equivalent figures were 35 percent and 21 percent, respectively.[20]

Worcester Heart Attack Study

Investigators from the Worcester Heart Attack Study examined trends in hospital and long-term case-fatality rates from incident acute myocardial infarction in a Massachusetts community (*n* = 5270) in the United States from 1975 to 1995.[28] Initially, age-adjusted incidence rates for acute myocardial infarction increased (from 244 to 272 per 100,000 in 1975 to 1981) and then declined thereafter (from 272 to 184 per 100,000 in 1981 to 1995). Significantly, crude in-hospital case-fatality declined from 17.8 percent in 1975/1978 to 11.7 percent in 1993/1995. Overall, the age-adjusted risk of dying in the later versus earliest period of follow-up was 0.44 (95 percent confidence interval [**CI**], 0.35 to 0.57). This figure was only slightly less (relative risk, 0.43; 95 percent CI, 0.32 to 0.58) when adjusted for all other clinical and demographic variables. Unlike the Minnesota Heart Survey,[20] the Worcester Heart Attack Study did not show absolute improvements in long-term case-fatality.[28]

Scottish Population Data

Investigators using data from the Scottish Morbidity Record scheme compared case-fatality rates in Scottish men and women hospitalized for acute myocardial infarction (*n* = 96,023) or unstable angina pectoris

(*n* = 37,401) from 1990 to 2000.[29] Crude 30-day case-fatality was reported to be considerably higher for acute myocardial infarction than unstable angina pectoris in men (16 percent versus 2 percent) and women (26 percent versus 2 percent). However, Table 2-4, which represents short- to long-term unadjusted case-fatality in those who survived to 30 days, shows that the fatal and progressive nature of CAD led to equivalent poor outcomes in the longer term irrespective of the initial form of acute presentation.

To explain the observed decline in CAD-related case-fatality rates further, it is necessary to consider a number of factors that may influence the natural history of CAD. In this context, Unal and colleagues[16] applied an advanced population model of CAD in the United Kingdom to help explain the type of changes observed in the MONICA Project. The model integrated data on the number of cases of CAD, treatment advances, risk factor profile changes, and median survival in those affected in England and Wales during the period 1981 to 2000. Based on this model, the investigators reported 68,230 fewer coronary deaths in 2000 compared with 1981. They also reported a population gain of about 925,415 life-years in people ages 25 to 84 in these two countries. Figure 2-9 represents the contributions of better treatments and risk factor management to the reported declines in CAD-related case-fatality during the study period. Alternatively, it also displays the counter-effects of increasing obesity, diabetes, and physical inactivity rates within this population that have contributed to more CAD-related deaths. A more detailed examination of the impact of risk factor modification regarding the overall prevalence of CAD is included later in this chapter.

Data from the MONICA Project suggest that age- and sex-adjusted CAD-related case-fatality rates have declined dramatically in many countries. Evidence also suggests that declines in sudden cardiac deaths have made a strong contribution to these trends, as have declines in short- to medium-term case-fatality rates following admission for acute coronary syndrome. However, CAD remains a major cause of death in most

■ ■ ■

TABLE 2-4 SHORT- AND LONG-TERM CASE-FATALITY RATES FOR MEN AND WOMEN IN SCOTLAND WHO INITIALLY SURVIVED AN ADMISSION FOR ACUTE MYOCARDIAL INFARCTION OR UNSTABLE ANGINA PECTORIS

CASE-FATALITY	MEN		WOMEN	
	AMI	UAP	AMI	UAP
1 year	6.4%	6.5%	8.9%	6.4%
5 years	21.6%	23.9%	26.0%	23.5%
10 years	36.0%	39.8%	40.6%	41.5%

AMI, Acute myocardial infarction; *UAP,* unstable angina pectoris.
From MacIntyre K, Murphy N, Capewell S et al: *Population survival after emergency admission with chest pain compared to angina and myocardial infarction: "chest pain" is not a benign condition.* Data presented at the British Cardiac Society, 2003.

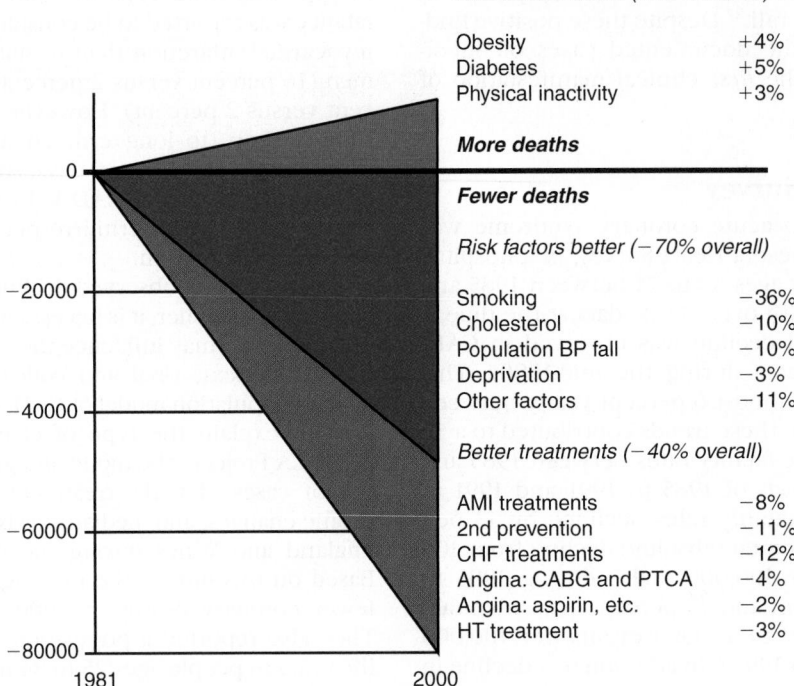

FIGURE 2-9 ■ Factors contributing to a decline in coronary artery disease–related case-fatality rates (68,230 fewer deaths) in England and Wales from 1981 to 2000. *AMI,* Acute myocardial infarction; *BP,* blood pressure; *CABG,* coronary artery bypass graft; *CHF,* congestive heart failure; *HT,* hypertension; *PTCA,* percutaneous coronary angioplasty. (Data from Unal B, Critchley JA, Fidan D et al: *Am J Public Health* 95[1]:103-108, 2005.)

developed countries. Moreover, some evidence suggests that even milder forms of CAD are associated with high long-term case-fatality. Modern treatments and strategies likely are delaying rather than avoiding the inevitable morbidity and mortality of CAD. Few investigators have examined trends in men and women over age 75. Absolute prevention of CAD is important in reducing its impact at the whole-population level.

Prevalence of Coronary Artery Disease

The increase in the impact of diseases of affluence seen as the wealth of the world's population steadily increases is often referred to as *epidemiological transition.* In urban areas of India, Latin America, and the former socialist countries, where increased CAD incidence and case-fatality rates already have been documented, the prevalence of CAD is undoubtedly increasing.[1]

Given the declines in age-adjusted incidence and case-fatality rates previously outlined, it would be natural to assume that the absolute number of persons affected by CAD in parts of Western Europe, North America, Australia, and New Zealand also is declining dramatically. This is certainly not the case. Firm predictions are that the overall number of deaths caused by CAD will increase dramatically between 1990 and 2020 in developing countries in women (by 120 percent) and men (by 137 percent). That is, CAD-related case-fatality rates are predicted to continue to rise in those countries where the trends suggest that CAD is in decline (by 29 percent in women and 48 percent in men).[23] The British Heart Foundation currently estimates that 2.7 million of the 60 million persons living in the United Kingdom (4.5 percent) yearly are living with CAD, with the numbers expected to rise each year.[24] Using population studies, the American Heart Association estimates that 13 million Americans (6.9 percent) yearly, making up 7.1 million men (8.4 percent of male population) and 5.9 million women (5.6 percent), are affected by CAD. Of these prevalent cases, 4.1 million men and 3 million women are reported to have experienced an incident acute myocardial infarction.[23]

What are the potential reasons behind what can be described only as a "sustained epidemic" of CAD? The future prevalence of CAD in whole populations that initially have thwarted its fatal effects is now widely acknowledged to be influenced largely by a combination of the following:

1. An aging population in whom incidence rates for CAD are highest[30]
2. An evolving natural history of CAD from acute and fatal events to milder, more chronic forms of the disease[1]
3. A steady improvement in case-fatality rates[2,21,26]

Consistent with these factors, it has been estimated that by the year 2020 in the United States, the average life expectancy for men will have risen to 82 years for women and 74.2 years for men. By 2040, these averages are expected to have risen to 83.1 years for women and 75 years for men.[30] An extended life span inherently places a larger number of persons at risk of developing symptomatic forms of CAD; even at age 70, the lifetime risk of incident CAD is still 25 percent to 35 percent.[11] In Western countries, the aging of the large postwar baby boomer cohort (born between 1946 and 1964) now has reached the stage where evidence of CAD is most likely to emerge and affect overall CAD population prevalence. The American Heart Association estimates that 3 percent of men and 1.6 percent of women ages 45 to 54 in the United States already are affected by CAD.[23]

NHANES III

The prevalence of nonfatal CAD in the United States was estimated with data gathered during the third National Health and Nutrition Examination Survey, called **NHANES III**. This survey involved a representative sample of 17,705 participants older than age 17 studied during the period 1988 to 1994. The presence of CAD was determined from self-report of anginal symptoms or past myocardial infarction and electrocardiogram (**ECG**) data. Table 2-5 represents key findings from the 1125 persons with angina or a history of acute myocardial infarction (6.4 percent of the total cohort, 53 percent of which were men), the 746 persons with a combined history of acute myocardial infarction or ECG-detected myocardial infarction (4.2 percent and 63 percent), and 1072 persons with a combination of angina, a history of myocardial infarction, or ECG evidence of myocardial infarction (6.1 percent and 43 percent).[31] These data summarize the most conservative estimates and suggest that CAD affected at least 3 percent to 4 percent of adult Americans in the early 1990s.

MONICA Project Data

During a similar period (1986 to 1994), the underlying prevalence of angina pectoris in the 2459 middle-aged cohort of men and women living in Northern Sweden and participating in the MONICA Project was examined.[32] In this study the presence of angina was determined formally using a specific instrument (Rose Angina Questionnaire) that was presumed to be more sensitive to the true presence of angina pectoris. During the study period, the proportion of participants with a history of myocardial infarction declined from 4.6 to 2.0 percent. Similarly, the underlying prevalence of angina pectoris in men declined from 3.4 to 3.1 percent and significantly declined in women from 5.9 to 2.8 percent.[33] These observed declines in the prevalence of angina pectoris were consistent with data derived from the MONICA cohort in Iceland (the Reykjavik Study).[34]

■ ■ ■

TABLE 2-5   PREVALENCE OF CORONARY ARTERY DISEASE IN THE ADULT AMERICAN POPULATION ACCORDING TO RACE

	ANGINA PECTORIS	SELF-REPORTED MI	ECG-AMI
Black	4.0%*	7.0%	4.5%
Mexican-American	5.0%	7.0%	3.0%
White	5.5%	9.5%	4.0%

MI, Myocardial infarction; *ECG-AMI,* acute myocardial infarction confirmed by electrocardiogram.
*Figures rounded to nearest 0.5%.
Data from Ford ES, Giles WH, Croft JB: *Am Heart J* 139:371-377, 2000.

The observed declines in the prevalence of angina in middle-aged cohorts is predictable given that CAD (and, therefore, absolute number of affected individuals) is more likely to occur in older age groups. This age differential is best illustrated by studies that include persons of all ages. For example, a more contemporary study from four registries of CAD patients in the primary care setting in London examined the prevalence of CAD within the local population of 378,021 men and women during a 6-month period in 2000 to 2001. The presence of CAD was confirmed by an initial diagnosis made by the person's primary care physician and the presence of supporting documentation and investigations (e.g., coronary angiography or exercise testing). This study, therefore, not only examined clinically manifest cases of CAD, but those who had been diagnosed and treated for CAD. A proportion of those studied were asymptomatic as a result of optimal treatment. Figure 2-10 represents the age- and gender-specific prevalence of CAD in this large United Kingdom population cohort. The overall age-adjusted prevalence of CAD was 7.8 percent in men (95 percent CI, 7.6 to 8.3 percent) and 4.2 percent in women (95 percent CI, 4.0 to 4.3 percent).[35]

Australian Longitudinal Study of Aging

An increasing prevalence of CAD in very old persons also has been observed in the Australian Longitudinal Study of Aging.[36] Significantly, it is in the Australian population that the greatest advances in reducing CAD-related case-fatality have been documented. These advances are seen in the substantial public health gains in reducing the CAD risk profile of the population (Figure 2-8).[26] Investigators examined a representative community sample of 3263 men and women older than age 70. Angina pectoris occurred in 5.1 percent of males and 2.9 percent of females, whereas 21.6 percent of males and 13.8 percent of females had a history of myocardial infarction. The prevalence of CAD who had survived to old age was 23.8 percent in men and 15.0 percent in

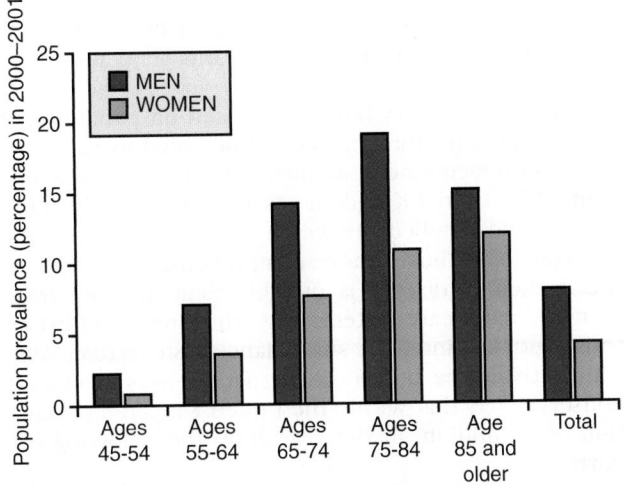

FIGURE 2-10 ■ Prevalence of coronary artery disease in a large United Kingdom population cohort (2000-2001). (Data from Carroll K, Majeed A, Firth C et al: *J Public Health* 25:29-35, 2003.)

women (combined prevalence of 18.7 percent). Prevalence of CAD was highest in men and women older than age 80, at an approximate prevalence of 25 percent and 20 percent, respectively.[3] See the accompanying Conundrum feature.

CORONARY ARTERY DISEASE–RELATED MORBIDITY

Given the multiple manifestations and consequences of CAD, calculating the overall burden of the sustained epidemic of CAD is problematic. The following parameters provide a comprehensive, but not always reliable, indication of the burden imposed by CAD within a whole population:

- Hospital stay
- Diagnostic investigations
- Surgical procedures
- Pharmacotherapy
- Hospital outpatient management
- Specialist cardiac rehabilitation
- Primary care management
- Residential aged care
- Loss of employment and income
- Quality of life
- Premature life-years lost (calculated by subtracting age of death from normal age- and gender-specific life expectancy)

The contemporary burden imposed on patients suffering angina pectoris has been calculated using many of the aforementioned parameters for the United Kingdom.[37] The United Kingdom has a universal health care system, and detailed utilization and expenditure data are available. Thus a more comprehensive analysis of the burden of disease is possible than in more fragmented health care systems (e.g., the United States) or those with less intensive surveillance systems (e.g., Australia). Using the best available data, it was estimated conservatively that within the United Kingdom population of 60 million, in the year 2000 the following occurred:

- 634,000 patients (1.1 percent of the total population) were managed for angina pectoris by their local primary care physician.

- These patients required 2.4 million primary care visits for angina pectoris.
- There were 250,000 referrals to hospital outpatient clinics for specialist investigation and management.
- There were 16 million prescriptions to treat angina pectoris (mainly nitrate therapy).
- The total cost of community management of angina pectoris was £172 million ($310 million or the equivalent of almost £3 per person).
- There were almost 150,000 admissions for angina and unstable angina (not including acute myocardial infarction).
- There were almost 120,000 coronary angiograms, coronary artery bypass grafts, and percutaneous coronary angioplasty procedures, with or without a coronary stent.
- Hospitalized patients required more that 500,000 outpatient visits (not including cardiac rehabilitation).
- The total cost of hospital-based management of angina pectoris was almost £500 million ($900 million, or the equivalent of more than £8 per person).[37]

Angina pectoris consumed more that 1 percent of the health service budget in the United Kingdom in the year 2000. The major cost components were bed occupancy and revascularization procedures (more than 70 percent of expenditure).[37] Figure 2-11 compares this expenditure to two closely related cardiac conditions: atrial fibrillation[38] and chronic heart failure.[39] Both conditions commonly are caused by underlying CAD. Given that revascularization procedure rates are far below those commonly seen in the United States and Europe,[40] sensitivity analyses were performed to determine the extra cost of equivalent procedure rates in the United Kingdom. These analyses showed that revascularization procedures would increase the cost of man-

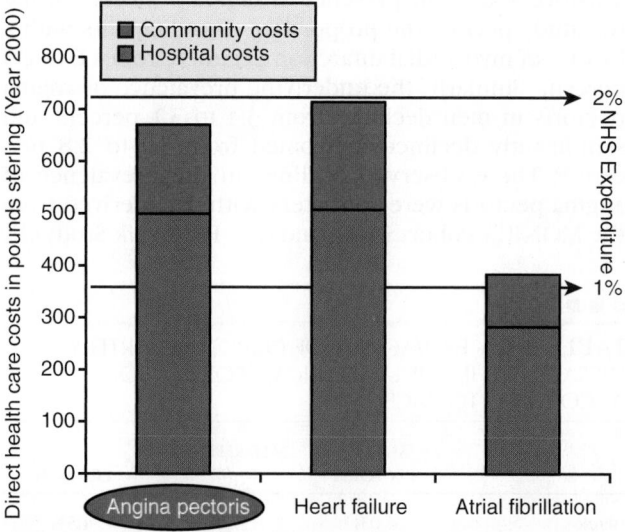

FIGURE 2-11 ■ Comparison of the cost of angina pectoris, chronic heart failure, and atrial fibrillation to the National Health Service (NHS) in the United Kingdom (year 2000). (Data from Stewart S, Murphy N, McGuire A et al: *Heart* 89:848-853, 2003; Stewart S, Murphy N, McGuire A et al: *Heart* 90:286-292, 2004; and Stewart S, Jenkins A, Buchan S et al: *Eur J Heart Fail* 4:361-371, 2002.)

aging patients with angina pectoris by more than 15 percent if applied at the same rate and that cardiac rehabilitation most probably would cost an additional 11 percent in health care expenditure if more widely applied.[37]

The British Heart Foundation estimates that the total number of persons with a history of angina in 2000-2001 was 2 million (3.3 percent of the total population). Also that year there were 275,000 myocardial infarctions that would have cost an additional £1.5 billion ($2.7 million), representing 4 percent of National Health Service expenditure. Therefore in the United Kingdom, CAD was associated with £7.5 billion ($13.5 million, or $255,000 per million persons) in direct and indirect expenditures in the year 2000.[24] In comparison, CAD currently is estimated to cost the United States $142.1 billion yearly ($980,000 per million persons). In 1999 alone, Medicare beneficiaries were paid $11 billion for CAD-related costs. Moreover, the number of coronary angiograms rose exponentially, along with other invasive procedures, in the past 2 decades (from 300,000 in 1979 to 1.4 million in 2002).[23]

Coronary Artery Disease and Quality of Life

As shown in Figure 2-1, CAD is a major contributor to the global burden of disease. The WHO estimates that CAD results in about 6 percent of healthy years of life lost (DALYs) in low- to middle-income countries and more than 10 percent in high-income countries.[2] As the natural history of CAD evolves from a fatal disease in middle-aged men and women to a more chronic form that undoubtedly will influence the affected person's quality of life, there is increasing focus on measuring the individual impact of the disease. Patients who require active treatment for CAD, particularly those who need coronary revascularization,[41] have poorer health-related quality of life scores, as measured by generic instruments, relative to age-matched men and women without the disease.[42] General measures of quality of life in persons with acute and chronic forms of the disease highlight typical problems associated with CAD:

- Sleep disturbance
- Low energy levels
- Exercise intolerance
- Emotional disturbance
- Social isolation[41-43]

IDACC STUDY

In recent years, there has been increasing awareness of the role of depression and anxiety in CAD-related morbidity and mortality. The Identifying Depression as a Comorbid Condition (**IDACC**) study monitored depression over a 12-month period in 1541 patients hospitalized for an acute coronary syndrome at four major general hospitals in Australia. On initial examination, 46.3 percent of 1455 study participants had some evidence of depression (Epidemiological Studies-Depression Scale score of 16 or greater, or Hospital Anxiety and Depression Scale score of 8 or greater), and one-fifth of patients had moderate to severe depression. During a 12-month

follow-up, depression documented at baseline persisted in 35 percent of cases subject to routine medical treatment compared with 25 percent in those exposed to a tailored psychiatric intervention.[44]

With an increasingly older group of persons suffering from symptomatic CAD and its common consequences (e.g., chronic heart failure), there is a strong possibility that average CAD-related quality of life will worsen. For example, those who develop chronic heart failure experience a lower quality of life than seen in any other form of chronic disease.[45] The true impact of CAD on quality of life will be better understood with the publication of prospective longitudinal studies that systematically track this important health outcome using a CAD-specific instrument.[46]

In summary, the true burden imposed by CAD on whole populations is impossible to calculate. Its overall impact on health care utilization rates and social disruption is complex, largely as a result of premature mortality and, conversely, chronic disease in older adults who survive an acute cardiac event. Contemporary data suggest that CAD directly consumes at least 5 to 10 percent of health care expenditures in developed countries. Based on increasing prevalence rates and the application of more expensive therapeutics, it is forecast that CAD-related expenditure will grow exponentially in the next decade.

RISK FACTORS FOR CORONARY ARTERY DISEASE

Given the enormous impact of CAD at an individual and a population level, it is clearly preferable to prevent the progression of coronary atherosclerosis and the resulting clinical cascade of debilitating symptoms, significant morbidity, and premature mortality. Longitudinal population studies such as the Framingham Heart Study[6-8] and those outlined in Table 2-2 provide clear therapeutic targets for risk minimization and, therefore, prevention of CAD in progressively aging populations. Worth noting is that the various associations established between CAD and the major risk factors vary not only in their intensity but also in the length of exposure needed to stimulate the development of CAD. As such, there are more proximate risk factors (e.g., smoking, with its immediate and potentially reversible effects on platelet aggregation and endothelial function) that clearly differ from long-term risk factors (e.g., systolic hypertension) that often mediate more permanent pathophysiological changes over a prolonged period.

Nonmodifiable Risk Factors

Three major, nonmodifiable risk factors for the development of CAD are advancing age, male gender, and family history. Any analysis of the true impact of the modifiable risk factors described next would be meaningless without adjustment for age and gender. Although there is some evidence that underlying CAD, in the form of coronary atherosclerosis, develops much earlier in the human life cycle than initially thought,[5] the cumulative exposure to underlying risk factors with advancing age leaves the heart more susceptible to advanced forms of CAD. Overall, men have about a 1.5 times higher risk of developing CAD in their lifetimes compared with women.[10] Men typically develop external manifestations of the disease about 5 to 10 years earlier than women, who start to catch up to men only after reaching menopause (see the following discussion).[46-51]

INTERHEART Study

A family history of CAD conveys a strong risk for developing the disease. The INTERHEART Study was a large, international, standardized case control study of similar cohorts in 52 countries designed to examine the importance of risk factors for CAD on a worldwide basis. During the study, 262 centers recruited men and women with a first-ever acute myocardial infarction who were taken to their local coronary care unit. At least one age- and sex-matched control was recruited for each case of acute myocardial infarction. Overall, 12,461 cases and 14,637 controls were analyzed.[52] Individuals with a positive family history had a 50 percent greater risk of having an acute myocardial infarction.[53] However, this observation was explained largely by the influence of modifiable risk factors. Probably, therefore, family history is linked to CAD through shared genetic pathways *and* lifestyle choices. This leaves the strong possibility of enhanced CAD prevention via a dual approach to proactive risk modification and genetic-based therapeutics in persons with a strong family history of CAD.

Modifiable Risk Factors

Many potentially modifiable risk factors are linked directly to the development and progression of CAD. These risk factors commonly are referred to as causal risk factors based on strong evidence of their involvement in the pathological processes underlying CAD. These factors represent important targets for primary and secondary prevention strategies. Many associated factors also are linked to an increased risk of developing CAD by contributing to its underlying pathophysiology and by worsening the effects of causal risk factors. Table 2-6 summarizes the most important modifiable risk factors in the prevention of CAD.

In addition to the major risk factors summarized in Table 2-6 (all of which are prominent in studies, such as the INTERHEART Study,[52] that attempt to explain the population risk profiles and their consequences), a number of other key risk factors have been identified as important in any attempts to monitor or prevent CAD. Individual targets for risk prevention include exercise, homocysteine level, stress, psychological status, and socioeconomic deprivation.

Exercise

The benefits of exercise in improving general cardiovascular fitness (e.g., a lower resting heart rate and blood pressure), reducing weight, lowering blood glucose and cholesterol levels, and improving endothelial and platelet function, are well documented.[61,62] However, in afflu-

ent countries, only one-third of the population exercises moderately for the recommended 30 minutes, 5 times each week.[23] See Chapter 38 for a complete discussion of sedentary lifestyle as a CAD risk factor.

Homocysteine Level

Homocysteine is a metabolite of an essential amino acid that can enter the body only via ingested food (mainly animal protein). In population studies, elevated homocysteine levels have been associated independently with cardiovascular outcomes. For example, in elderly participants in the Framingham Study, a serum homocysteine level in the upper quartile range of recorded values was associated with a 1.54 (95 percent CI, 1.31 to 1.82) increased risk of cardiovascular mortality relative to the remaining cohort.[63] Hyperhomocysteinemia is linked closely to platelet activation, endothelial function, and atherogenesis.[64] Folate, which is required for metabolism of homocysteine, is derived mainly from vegetables. Therefore, risk minimization involves promoting a vegetable-rich diet with less meat and possibly supplements of folic acid and B vitamins.

Stress and Psychological Status

The importance of stress and other psychosocial factors in the development of CAD has been increasingly recognized. Expert groups have concluded from systematic reviews of the literature that there is strong and consistent evidence of a risk relationship of depression, social isolation, and lack of quality social support with development and progression of CAD. Less convincing has been the role of chronic life events, work-related stressors, and certain behavioral and personality types.[65] In support of this, the INTERHEART Study found that psychosocial factors (as measured by four simple questions about stress at work and home, financial stress, and major life events in the past year) independently predicted the risk of acute myocardial infarction.[66]

Socioeconomic Deprivation

The recognition that equitable access to health foods, healthful messages, more healthful lifestyle choices (e.g., safe areas to exercise), and optimal health care will reduce the risk and consequences of CAD is increasing.[23] Population studies consistently demonstrate that those from lower socioeconomic circumstances have a worse risk factor profile that their more affluent counterparts. Figure 2-12 shows key results of a population-based analysis of sudden cardiac deaths and 30-day case-fatality following an acute myocardial infarction in the Scottish population. A social gradient in the population rate of fatal and nonfatal events was clear, almost double in the poorest (score of 5) relative to the most affluent persons (score of 1).[67]

Clearly, there are major interactions between causal and associated risk factors for CAD that vary according to a person's age and gender. To quantify the individual risk of a fatal or nonfatal CAD event, a number of scoring algorithms have been developed based on age, sex, and major risk factor profile. These prediction models calculate the "absolute risk" of experiencing a CAD event within 10 years. The most commonly applied of

■ ■ ■

TABLE 2-6 MAJOR MODIFIABLE RISK FACTORS FOR CORONARY ARTERY DISEASE

MAJOR RISK FACTORS	KEY FEATURES
Smoking tobacco	Smoking (inhaled and passive) is the single most important target for CAD prevention. The contaminated smoke from cigarettes contains ammonia, benzene, carbon monoxide, and nicotine, which have multiple effects directly related to the development of CAD, including tachycardia, vasoconstriction, hypoxia, and atherogenesis.[54] Case-fatality rates for cardiovascular disease are more than double in smokers, with a disproportionate number of premature life-years lost.
Abnormal lipid profile	The link between dietary cholesterol and CAD has long been known and confirmed by studies such as the PROCAM,[12] Framingham,[7] and Helsinki Heart studies.[27] Initial fatty streaks and lipid recruitment into atherosclerotic lesions in the coronary arteries are key to CAD development. On this basis, statins are used to normalize the lipid profiles of persons with[55] and without[56] established CAD.
	Rather than concentrate on overall cholesterol or triglyceride levels, there are clear differential targets to optimize the lipid profile of at-risk persons. For example, in the Prospective Cardiovascular Munster Study, triglyceride levels were not an independent predictor of incident CAD. However, there was a very-high-risk group that had an LDL/HDL cholesterol ratio of greater than 5. In this group, those with triglyceride levels greater than 200 mg/dl had more than double the number of CAD events over 6 years compared with participants with triglyceride levels less than 200 mg/dl.[12]
	Similar results were found in the Helsinki Heart Study, where subjects with a high LDL/HDL cholesterol ratio and a triglyceride level greater than 200 mg/dl had a threefold increased risk of cardiac events.[27] LDL cholesterol is a particularly atherogenic lipoprotein, whereas HDL cholesterol is antiatherogenic.
	Recent years have seen increasing interest in apolipoproteins and their role in atherosclerosis and CAD events.[57] Apolipoprotein B (APO B) is found in all atherogenic lipoproteins (including LDL), whereas APO A-I is one of the major constituents of HDL. In the recent Apolipoprotein-Related Mortality Risk Study (AMORIS), 175,553 men and women were followed for about 5½ years. During follow-up the risk of an acute myocardial infarction was highest in those with the worst versus most optimal APO B/APO A-I ratio. The risk of acute myocardial infarction was 4.8 times higher in men and fourfold higher in women. On multivariate analysis the APO B/APO A-I ratio was a better predictor of acute myocardial infarction (fatal and nonfatal) than total cholesterol or triglyceride levels.[58]
Hypertension	Hypertension, an abnormal lipid profile, and smoking form the traditional triad of CAD risk factors. A highly prevalent condition (50 million Americans and 1 billion persons worldwide are affected), hypertension greatly increases the risk of cardiovascular disease. For individuals age 40 to 70, each increment of 20 mm Hg in systolic and 10 mm Hg in diastolic blood pressure doubles the risk of disease across the entire blood pressure range.[59]
Diabetes	More than 2% of the world's population has diabetes, a number estimated to double by the year 2025. The prevalence of diabetes (including type 2 diabetes, the more common form) is particularly high in Europe and North America: about 4% and rising. The number of adults with high fasting glucose levels or impaired glucose tolerance is rising in parallel to the increasing consumption of high-fat and high-carbohydrate diets, obesity, and sedentary lifestyles. A triad of hypertriglyceridemia, low HDL cholesterol levels, and elevated LDL cholesterol levels is common in a prediabetic state (called metabolic syndrome) and established adult-onset type 2 diabetes.[60] Insulin resistance also is associated closely with endothelial and platelet dysfunction. In the United States, 17% of men and 15% of women age 60 and older are diagnosed with this condition.[23]
Obesity	The World Health Organization defines overweight as a body mass index that exceeds 25 kg/m² and obesity as a body mass index that exceeds 30 kg/m². In most affluent countries the prevalence of overweight is increasing dramatically, with about 40% of the adult population affected. The British Heart Foundation recently estimated that the number of obese adults in the United Kingdom doubled in the last decade, from 14% to 22%.[24] Among adults ages 40 to 59 in the United States, a startling 75% of men and 65% of women are overweight.[23] Those with a waist circumference greater than 35 inches and 40 inches, respectively, are at high risk for developing CAD. Obesity is linked closely to an abnormal lipid profile, insulin resistance, diabetes, and hypertension.[62] The proportion of overweight American children was estimated at 25% and rising.[23]

CAD, Coronary artery disease; *LDL*, low-density lipoprotein; *HDL*, high-density lipoprotein.

these risk scores is the 10-year Framingham Coronary Heart Disease Risk Score, which was derived mainly from the Framingham Heart Study. A contemporary analysis of the Framingham cohort based on this score showed that, at age 40, those with risk scores in tertiles 1, 2, and 3 had a 38.4 percent, 41.7 percent, and 50.7 percent (men) and a 12.2 percent, 25.4 percent, and 33.2 percent (women) *lifetime* risk of developing CAD. This scoring algorithm was most sensitive in older persons and women.[68] A European equivalent of the Framingham risk score also has been developed with data from 12 cohort studies in that region.[69]

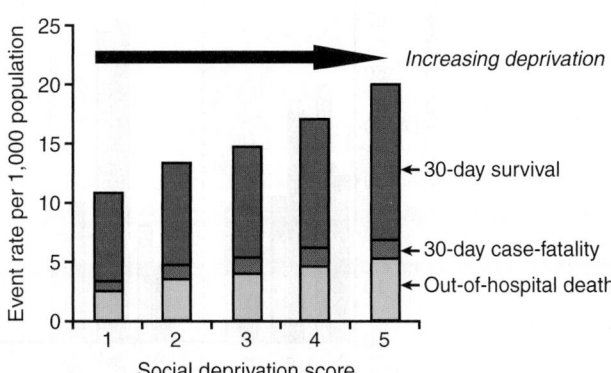

FIGURE 2-12 ■ The link between social deprivation, sudden cardiac death, and acute myocardial infarction case-fatality in the Scottish population. (Data from MacIntyre K, Stewart S, Capewell S et al: *BMJ* 322:1152-1153, 2001.)

POPULATION IMPACT OF RISK FACTORS FOR CORONARY ARTERY DISEASE

Apart from calculating individual risk, it is highly desirable to calculate the overall risk of CAD at the whole-population level to inform public health policies. Recognition is increasing that studying risk factors from the perspective of a series of absolute cutoff values (i.e., systolic blood pressure of 140 mm Hg or more equals systolic hypertension and an increased risk of CAD) is of limited value. For example, it has been suggested that the 10 percent of the population most at risk of cardiovascular disease only accounts for 20 percent of related events.[70] When considering the high population-attributable risk associated with borderline risk factors (see Table 2-1 for a working definition), where the risk is relatively small but the population prevalence is high, it has been proposed that treating the entire population age 55 and older with a preventive polypill (composed of a statin, aspirin, an antihypertensive, and folic acid) would reduce cardiovascular disease rates by more than 80 percent.[71] This compares with the approximately 10 percent reduction in cardiovascular events resulting from aggressive pharmacological management of the 6 percent of the population with a 10-year Framingham event risk of more than 30 percent.[72]

Investigators have combined data from the Framingham Heart Study and NHANES III to estimate the absolute contributions of borderline and elevated risk factors to the population burden of CAD in that country.[73] This study was based on the knowledge that known risk factors account for more than three quarters of cases of CAD in the United States. Figure 2-13 shows the risk profile of the men ($n = 681$) and women ($n = 807$) who participated in NHANES III according to whether they had an "optimal" profile, a borderline risk, or established risk for CAD in relation to their blood pressure,

lipid profile, glucose tolerance, and smoking history. The key findings of this study were as follows:

- Overall, 26 percent of men and 41 percent of women had at least one borderline risk factor.
- Isolated borderline risk factors (i.e., those in the absence of high risk factors) accounted for only 10 percent of age-adjusted, 10-year CAD events.
- Borderline risk factors in the presence of other established risk factors increased the risk of CAD events incrementally. For example, the presence of one "high" risk factor in men conveyed a 2.73 percent increased risk of a CAD event within 10 years (all ages). The presence of two, three, or four borderline risk factors increased this risk to 5.31 percent, 8.05 percent, and 14.46 percent, respectively.[73]

Based on these data, it appears clear that borderline risk factors also should be targeted for preventive measures in those individuals with other more established risk factors.

The enormous potential for population-based risk management and prevention of CAD is emphasized further by the results of the INTERHEART Study.[52] After multivariate analysis the following five modifiable risk factors were found to be associated most strongly with incident myocardial infarction relative to case-controls:

1. Current smoking (odds ratio [**OR**] 2.87; 99 percent CI, 2.58 to 3.19)
2. Increased apolipoprotein B/apolipoprotein A-I ratio* (OR 3.25; CI, 2.81 to 3.76)
3. Diabetes (OR 2.37; CI, 2.07 to 2.71)
4. Hypertension (OR 1.91; CI, 1.74 to 2.1)
5. Psychosocial stress (OR 2.67; CI, 2.21 to 3.22)

---

*Top versus lowest quintile. Combined index comparing exposure versus nonexposure to depression, high perceived stress, poor locus of control, and major life events.

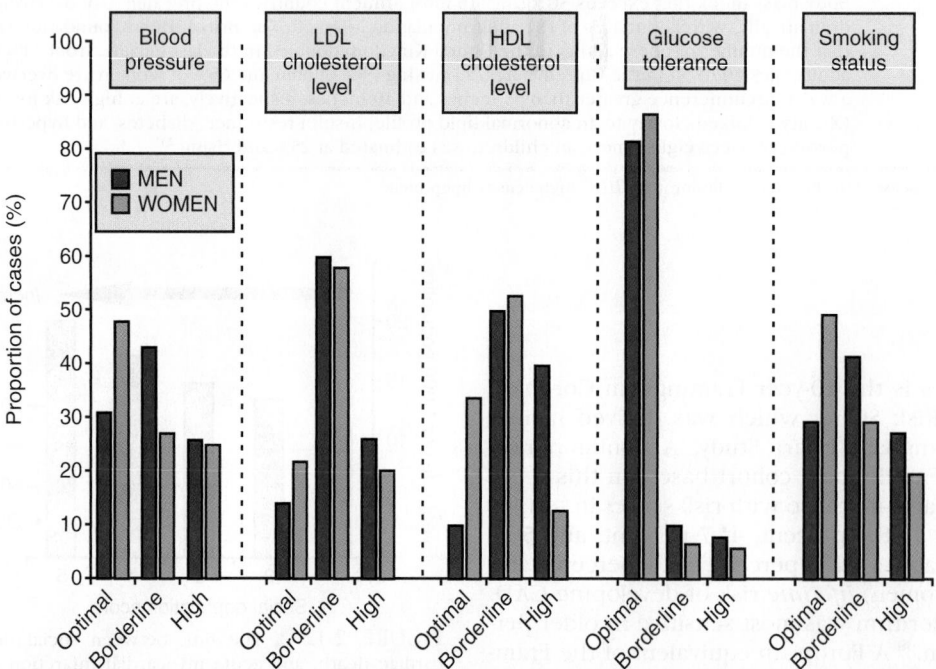

FIGURE 2-13 ■ Coronary artery disease risk factor profile of the NHANES III cohort. *HDL,* High density lipoprotein; *LDL,* low density lipoprotein. (Data from Vasan RS, Sullivan LM, Wilson PF et al: *Ann Intern Med* 142:393-402, 2005.)

When combined, current smoking, hypertension, and diabetes increased the OR of an acute myocardial infarction to 13.01 (10.69 to 15.83) compared with persons without these risk factors. Adding an abnormal apolipoprotein B/apolipoprotein A-I ratio (highest versus lowest quintile) increased this risk to 42.3 (33.2 to 54.0). When abdominal obesity was added to these four risk factors, the population-attributable risk increased to 80.2 percent. Figure 2-14 shows population-attributable risks for the nine major risk factors examined in the study on a gender-specific basis. Collectively, these risk factors accounted for 90 percent (men) and 94 percent (women) of the population-attributable risk for acute myocardial infarction.[53]

POTENTIAL RISK FACTORS

As suggested by reports from the INTERHEART Study, there is a logical argument to suggest targeting the nine key risk factors summarized in Figure 2-14 will yield the greatest results in reducing the population impact of CAD. However, a number of other potentially modifiable factors may contribute significantly to an increased risk of developing the disease via independent or associated pathological pathways. These factors include the following:

- Low-grade infections
- Endothelial inflammation/insulin resistance
- Carotid intima-media thickness
- Serotonin and other prothrombotic factors
- Coronary artery calcification
- Environmental pollution

As described in much greater detail in Chapter 9, there is increasing evidence that inflammation plays a key pathogenetic role in atherogenesis. For example, in a recent analysis of 3037 men and women in the Framingham Offspring Study, metabolic syndrome and elevated C-reactive protein were associated with a greater risk of a cardiovascular event during 7-year follow-up. The adjusted hazard risk for men and women with levels in the highest versus lowest C-reactive protein quartiles were 1.9 (95 percent CI, 1.2 to 2.9) and 1.8 (95 percent CI, 1.4 to 2.5) in the presence of metabolic syndrome.[74] An expert review of the literature concluded that inflammatory markers such as high-sensitivity C-reactive protein (see Chapter 43) should be used routinely to increase the accuracy of risk assessment in those with known risk factors rather than for population screening.[75] The role of other novel markers and risk factors for CAD remains undetermined at this time.

The major risk factors for CAD are well documented. Data from prospective population studies suggest that risk minimization strategies have the potential to reduce CAD events dramatically over and beyond targeting only high-risk individuals. The costs, benefits, and feasibility of applying a population approach currently are being examined.

GENDER DIFFERENCES IN CORONARY ARTERY DISEASE

Any analysis of the epidemiological profile of CAD has to account for significant age and gender differences in its development and progression. Women are more likely to develop symptomatic or fatal CAD at a later stage in life (a major reason for their more prolonged life expectancy); however, it is difficult to account for all the key differences in the epidemiology of CAD based on age alone.[47] Overall, women lag about 5 to 10 years behind men in their risk of developing symptomatic CAD after age 40. Probably, the protective effects of endogenous estrogen are lost when a women reaches menopause.[48] However, the potential cardioprotective effects of exogenous replacement of the hormone remain controversial.[49,50]

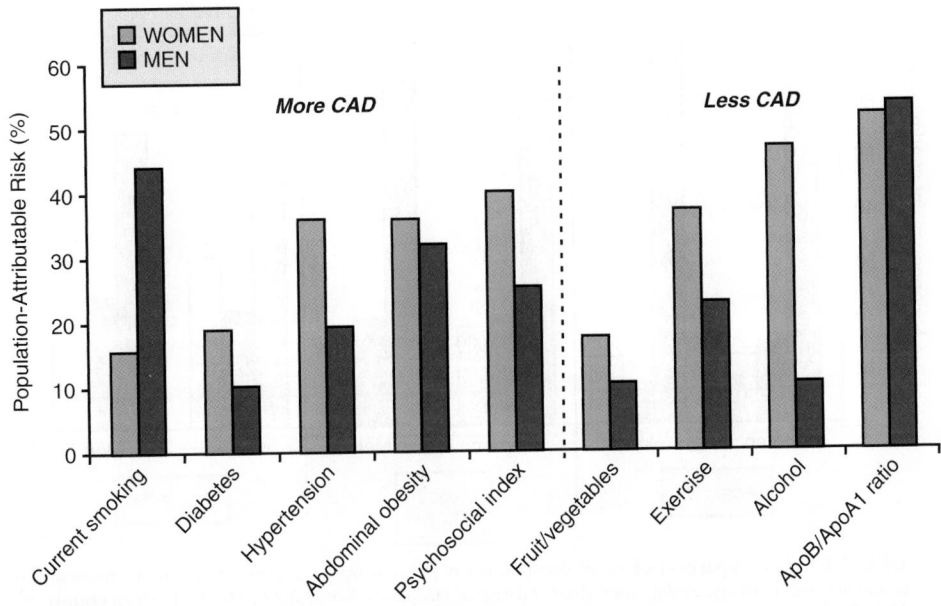

FIGURE 2-14 ■ Population-attributable risk of the nine major modifiable risk factors identified in the INTERHEART Study. *CAD,* Coronary artery disease. (Data from Yusuf S, Hawken S, Ôunpuu S et al: *Lancet* 364:937-952, 2004.)

Important gender differences influence the pattern of modifiable risk factors for CAD. Although the negative impact of hypertension, family history, obesity, and physical inactivity appears to be similar for men and women, some data suggest that smoking does not appear to be as strong a risk factor for women, possibly because of lower nicotine consumption. Conversely, lower high-density lipoprotein cholesterol levels and higher glucose levels or the presence of diabetes confer a greater risk of developing cardiovascular disease in women compared with men.[47] In postmenopausal women, newer risk factor markers (including C-reactive protein, homocysteine, and lipoprotein apolipoprotein A-I) have been found to play a greater role in predicting risk compared with age-matched men.[51]

Once a woman develops symptomatic CAD, evidence suggests that she is less likely to experience and express symptoms of the classic type seen in men. Observed differences in the extent of myocardial ischemia in women compared with men may reflect important differences in plaque type, clotting mechanisms, and coagulability. A recent analysis of data from 881 women (43 percent) and 1192 men and women arriving at a hospital with a confirmed acute myocardial infarction in 1997 and 1999, as part of the Worcester Heart Attack Study, examined potential gender differences in this regard. Figure 2-15 shows the major features of presentation for men and women separately. Overall, women were less likely to have a chief complaint of chest pain, the difference in men and women being more accentuated with advancing age.[76] The risk of misdiagnosis from a lack of definitive symptoms during episodes of acute myocardial ischemia, therefore, appears to be higher in women than

men. A recent study of 515 women who were hospitalized with an acute myocardial infarction found that a large proportion experienced unusual fatigue (71 percent), sleep disturbance (48 percent), dyspnea (42 percent), indigestion (39 percent) and anxiety (35 percent) in the month leading to the acute event.[77] See chapter 52 for further discussion of symptoms in women.

A series of reports from the Worcester Heart Attack Study showed an important interaction between age and gender that affected in-hospital case-fatality, with younger, but not older, women having higher case-fatality rates than men of a similar age. Women also had a higher case-fatality within 2 years of discharge. The increased risk of case-fatality was 15.4 percent per 10-year decrease in age for women relative to men.[78]

Data from the MONICA Project (involving patients ages 35 to 74)[79] and the Scottish Morbidity Record scheme (all ages)[80] confirmed some important trends in this regard. In the latter study, 201,114 incident cases of acute myocardial infarction (out-of-hospital fatal events and survivors who reached the hospital) occurring in Scotland from 1986 to 1995 were analyzed. Consistent with the Worcester Heart Attack Study, clinically important gender-based differences in survival according to age were found in men and women who survived to reach the hospital. Younger women had a higher 30-day case-fatality rate than men (6.5 percent versus 4.8 percent case-fatality in those younger than age 55). However, when out-of-hospital deaths from an incident acute myocardial infarction were considered, 30-day case-fatality rates associated with *all* forms of immediately fatal and nonfatal acute myocardial infarction were lower in women compared with men (adjusted risk 0.9;

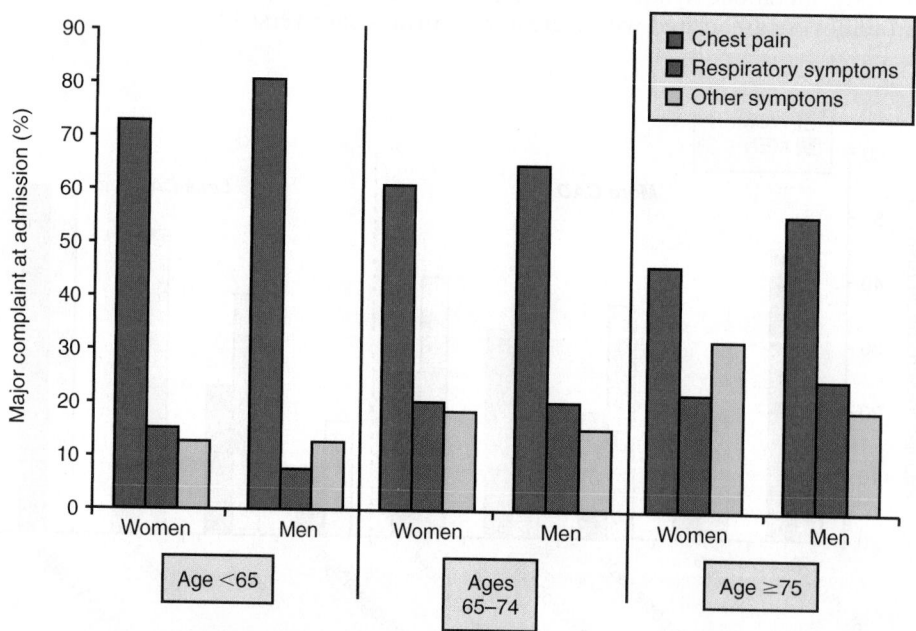

FIGURE 2-15 ■ Comparison of chief complaint on presenting to hospital with acute myocardial infarction according to age and gender. *Aust,* Australia; *HK,* Hong Kong; *MEC,* Middle Eastern countries; *NZ,* New Zealand; *SE,* South East. (Data from Vaccarino V, Krumholz HM, Yarzebski J et al: *Ann Intern Med* 134[3]:173-181, 2001.)

95 percent CI, 0.89 to 0.93). Figure 2-16 shows the important features of these data. The figure illustrates the fact that although female gender increases the probability of surviving to the hospital with an incident acute myocardial infarction, it also confers an increased risk of in-hospital death. Overall, however, younger men fare worse than younger women in terms of combined out-of-hospital and 30-day post acute hospitalization case-fatality. These important differences suggest the potential benefits of applying gender-specific strategies to improve case-fatality rates in acute myocardial infarction.[81]

Important gender differences are found in the epidemiology of CAD. Gender differences may largely reflect the cardioprotective effects of endogenous estrogen delaying onset of symptomatic CAD for an average of 5 to 10 years compared with men. Yet, there are significant age-adjusted differences in the pattern of antecedent risk factors, clinical presentation, and case-fatality.

ETHNIC AND RACIAL DIFFERENCES IN CORONARY ARTERY DISEASE

As suggested by Table 2-4 and the data presented in Figure 2-7, there are potentially important racial and ethnic differences in the prevalence and prognostic impact of CAD in different communities and populations. As demonstrated by studies in North America[14] and Australia,[82] indigenous populations fare worse in developed countries where primary prevention and health care services are usually widely available and applied. These data raise an important question. Are there significant genetic differences between the major racial groups of the world, or do cultural and ethnic differences in respect to lifestyle and CAD risk behaviors explain observed differences in CAD-related incidence and case-fatality?

Certainly, the recognition of an epidemiological transition of CAD in many developing countries shows that affluence and the adoption of Western lifestyles often is accompanied by the emergence of an epidemic of CAD.[1] The most obvious example of this is the former socialist states in Eastern Europe, which have emerged from extremely austere conditions to develop greater levels of affluence. There appear to be important racial differences in the development and progression of CAD, although the apparent importance of race and ethnicity often is weakened considerably once confounding variables are considered. For example, there is evidence that the link between an abnormal lipid profile and CAD is less important in South Asians.[83] Alternatively, the consequences of hypertension in relation to CAD appear to be more important in black Americans[23] and the Chinese.[84]

The INTERHEART Study suggested that nine risk factors amenable to modification accounted for about 90 percent of the risk of an incident myocardial infarction. Moreover, it demonstrated that the effect of these risk factors was consistent across a wide range of ethnic, cultural, and geographic regions across the globe. Figure 2-17 shows regional differences in the population-attributable risk (reflective of the relative prevalence and risk associated with each risk factor) associated with smoking (range 25 to 45 percent), abnormal lipid profile (55 to 75 percent), and hypertension (5 to 40 percent).[53]

Racial and ethnic differences in the epidemiological pattern of CAD have been reported. The true role of inherent genetic risk compared with confounding cultural and environmental factors that increase the underlying prevalence and impact of major risk factors remains uncertain. Data from the INTERHEART Study suggest that the same risk factors drive an epidemic of CAD in different populations.

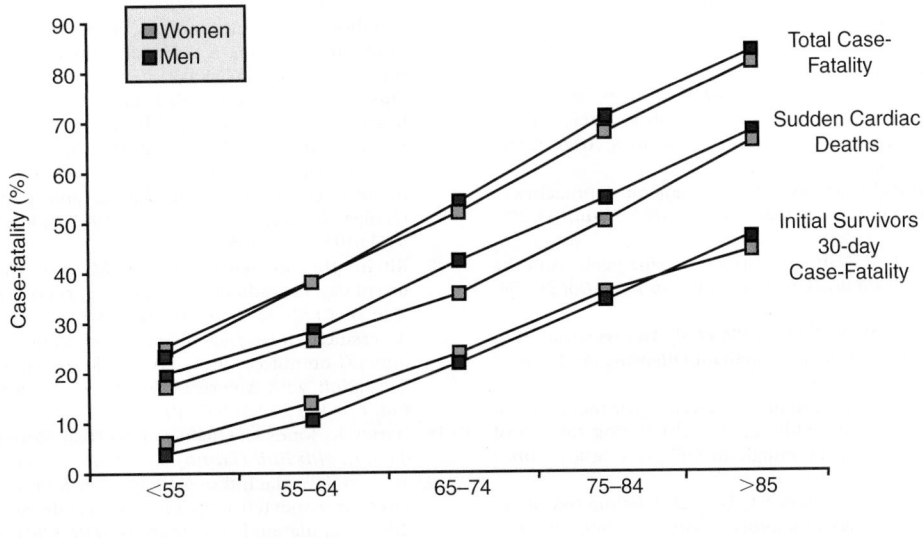

FIGURE 2-16 ▪ Sex-based differences in acute myocardial infarction case-fatality in the Scottish population. (Data from MacIntyre K, Stewart S, McMurray JJV et al: *J Am Coll Cardiol* 38:729-735, 2001.)

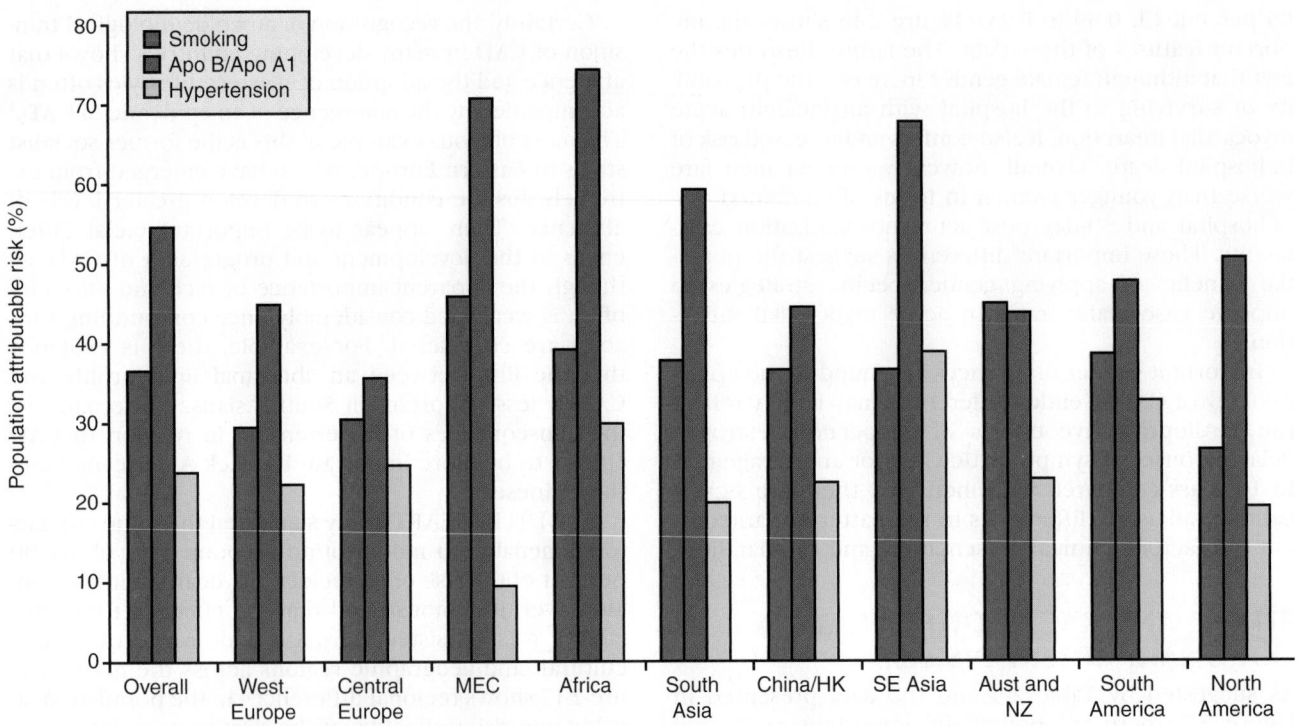

FIGURE 2-17 ■ Global comparison of the population-attributable risk of coronary artery disease for smoking, dyslipidemia, and hypertension. (Data from Yusuf S, Hawken S, Ôunpuu S et al: *Lancet* 364:937-952, 2004.)

REFERENCES

1. Yusuf S, Reddy S, Ôunpuu S, Anand S: Global burden of cardiovascular diseases. I. general considerations, the epidemiologic transition, risk factors and impact of urbanization, *Circulation* 104:2746-2753, 2001.
2. World Health Organization: *Atlas of heart disease and stroke.* Geneva, 2005, World Health Organization. Retrieved November 2006, from www.who.int/cardiovascular_diseases/resources/atlas/en/print.html
3. Scanlon PJ, Faxon DP, Audet AM et al: ACC/AHA guidelines for coronary angiography: a report for the American College of Cardiology/American Heart Association Task Force on Practice Guidelines (Committee on Coronary Angiography), *J Am Coll Cardiol* 33:1756-1824, 1999.
4. Fox CS, Evans JC, Larson MG et al: A comparison of death certificate out-of-hospital coronary heart disease death with physician adjudicated sudden cardiac death, *Am J Cardiol* 95:856-859, 2005.
5. Virmani R, Robinowitz M, Geer JC et al: Coronary artery atherosclerosis revisited in Korean war combat casualties, *Arch Pathol Lab Med* 111:972-976, 1987.
6. Dawber TR, Meadors GF, Moore FE: Epidemiologic approaches to heart disease: the Framingham study, *Am J Public Health* 41:279-286, 1951.
7. Kannel WB, Feinleib M: Natural history of angina pectoris in the Framingham study: prognosis and survival, *Am J Cardiol* 29:154-163, 1972.
8. Kannel WB, Feinleib M, McNamara PM et al: An investigation of heart disease in families: the Framingham Offspring Study, *Am J Epidemiol* 110:281-290, 1979.
9. Wilson PF, Anderson KM, Castelli WP: Twelve-year incidence of coronary heart disease in middle-aged adults during the era of hypertensive therapy: the Framingham Offspring Study, *Am J Med* 90:11-16, 1991.
10. Lloyd-Jones DM, Larson MG, Beiser A, Levy D: Lifetime risk of developing coronary heart disease, *Lancet* 353(9147):89-92, 1999.
11. Antman EM, Anbe DT, Armstrong PW et al, for the American College of Cardiology; American Heart Association Task Force on Practice Guidelines: ACC/AHA guidelines for the management of patients with ST-elevation myocardial infarction: executive summary—a report of the American College of Cardiology/American Heart Association Task Force on Practice Guidelines (Writing Committee to Revise the 1999 Guidelines for the Management of Patients with Acute Myocardial Infarction), *Circulation* 110:588-636, 2004.
12. Voss R, Cullen P, Schulte H, Assmann G: Prediction of risk of coronary events in middle-aged men in the Prospective Cardiovascular Munster Study (PROCAM) using neural networks, *Int J Epidemiol* 31:1253-1262, 2002.
13. Hanley AJG, Williams K, Stern MP, Haffner SM: Homeostasis model assessment of insulin resistance in relation to the incidence of cardiovascular disease: the San Antonio Heart Study, *Diabetes Care* 25:1177-1184, 2002.
14. Resnick HE, Jones K, Ruotolo G et al: Insulin resistance, the metabolic syndrome, and risk of incident cardiovascular disease in nondiabetic American Indians: the Strong Heart Study, *Diabetes Care* 26:861-867, 2003.
15. Fraser GE, Shavlik DJ: Risk factors for all-cause and coronary heart disease mortality in the oldest old: the Adventist Health Study, *Arch Intern Med* 157:2249-2258, 1997.
16. Unal B, Critchley JA, Fidan D, Capewell S: Life-years gained from modern cardiological treatments and population risk factor changes in England and Wales, 1981-2000, *Am J Public Health* 95(1):103-108, 2005.
17. Ritchie JL, Batemen TM, Bonow RO et al: Guidelines for clinical use of cardiac radionuclide imaging: report of the American College of Cardiology/American Heart Association Task Force on Assessment of Diagnostic and Therapeutic Cardiovascular Procedures (Committee on Radionuclide Imaging), developed in collaboration with American Society of Nuclear Cardiology, *J Am Coll Cardiol* 25:521-547, 1995.
18. Harley K, Jones C: Quality of Scottish Morbidity Records (SMR) data, *Health Bull (Edinb)* 54:410-417, 1996.
19. Murphy NF, MacIntyre K, Capewell S et al: Hospital discharge rates for suspected acute coronary syndromes between 1990 and 2000: population based analysis, *BMJ* 328:1413-1414, 2004.
20. McGovern PG, Jacobs DR, Shahar E et al: Trends in acute coronary heart disease mortality, morbidity and medical care from 1985 through 1997: the Minnesota Heart Survey, *Circulation* 104:19-24, 2001.

21. Capewell S, MacIntyre K, Stewart S et al: Age, sex and social trends in out-of-hospital cardiac deaths in Scotland 1986-1995: a retrospective cohort study, *Lancet* 358:1213-1217, 2001.

22. Fox CS, Evans JC, Larson MG et al: Temporal trends in coronary heart disease mortality and sudden cardiac death from 1950 to 1999: the Framingham Heart Study, *Circulation* 110(5):522-527, 2004.

23. American Stroke Association, American Heart Association: *Heart disease and stroke statistics: 2005 update*. Retrieved January 2006, from www.americanheart.org/ downloadable/heart/ 1105390918119HDSStats2005Update.pdf

24. British Heart Foundation: *British Heart Foundation coronary heart disease statistics 2006*. Retrieved January 2006, from www.bhf.org.uk/

25. World Health Organization:*The Global Burden of Coronary Heart Disease*. Retrieved November 2006, from http://www.who.int/ cardiovascular_diseases/en/cvd_atlas_13_coronaryHD.pdf

26. Tunstall-Pedoe H, Kuulasmaa K, Tolonen H et al: Contribution of trends in survival and coronary event rates to changes in coronary heart disease mortality: 10-year results from 37 WHO MONICA Project populations, *Lancet* 353:1547-1557, 1999.

27. Salomaa V, Keonen M, Koukkunen H et al: Decline in out-of-hospital coronary heart disease deaths has contributed the main part to the overall decline in coronary heart disease mortality rates among persons 35 to 64 years of age in Finland, *Circulation* 10:691-696, 2003.

28. Goldberg RJ, Yarzebski J, Lessard D, Gore JM: A two-decades (1975 to 1995) long experience in the incidence, in-hospital and long-term case-fatality rates of acute myocardial infarction: a community-wide perspective, *J Am Coll Cardiol* 33:1533-1539, 1999.

29. Capewell S, Murphy NF, MacIntyre K, et al: Short and long-term outcomes in 133,429 emergency patients admitted with angina or myocardial infarction in Scotland 1990-2000, *Heart* 2006: In press.

30. Schneider EL, Gurainik JM: The aging of America, *JAMA* 263:2335-2340, 1990.

31. Ford ES, Giles WH, Croft JB: Prevalence of nonfatal coronary artery disease among American adults, *Am Heart J* 139:371-377, 2000.

32. Glader EL, Stegmayr B: Declining prevalence of angina pectoris in middle-aged men and women: a population-based study within the Northern Sweden MONICA Project, *J Intern Med* 246:285-291, 1999.

33. Rose GA: *Cardiovascular survey methods*, ed 2, Monograph Series No 56, Geneva, 1982, World Health Organization.

34. Sigurdsson E, Thorgeirsson G, Sigvaldson H, Sigfusson N: Prevalence of coronary heart disease in Icelandic men 1968-86: the Reykjavik Study, *Eur Heart J* 14:584-591, 1993.

35. Carroll K, Majeed A, Firth C, Gray J: Prevalence and management of coronary heart disease in primary care: population-based cross-sectional study using a disease register, *J Public Health Med* 25:29-35, 2003.

36. Harris J, Giles L, Finucane P, Andrews G: Prevalence of coronary heart disease and cardiovascular risk factors in a sample of older Australians: Australian Longitudinal Study of Aging, *Aust J Aging* 23:25-32, 2004.

37. Stewart S, Murphy N, McGuire A, McMurray JJV: The current cost of angina pectoris to the National Health Service in the United Kingdom, *Heart* 89:848-853, 2003.

38. Stewart S, Murphy N, McGuire A, McMurray JJV: The cost of an emerging epidemic: an economic analysis of atrial fibrillation in the UK, *Heart* 90:286-292, 2004.

39. Stewart S, Jenkins A, Buchan S et al: The current cost of heart failure in the UK: an economic analysis, *Eur J Heart Fail* 4:361-371, 2002.

40. Maier W, Windecker S, Boersma E et al: Evolution of percutaneous transluminal coronary angioplasty in Europe (1992-1996), *Eur Heart J* 22:1733-1740, 2001.

41. Lukkarinen H, Hentinen M: Assessment of quality of life with the Nottingham Health Profile among women with coronary artery disease, *Heart Lung* 27:189-199, 1998.

42. Pfisterer M, Buser P, Osswald S et al, for the Trial of Invasive versus Medical Therapy in Elderly Patients (TIME) Investigators: Outcome of elderly patients with chronic symptomatic coronary artery disease with an invasive vs optimized medical treatment strategy: one-year results of the randomized TIME trial, *JAMA* 289:1117-1123, 2003.

43. Kaul P, Armstrong PW, Fu Y et al, for GUSTO-IIb Investigators: Impact of different patterns of invasive care on quality of life outcomes in patients with non-ST elevation acute coronary syndrome: results from the GUSTO-IIb Canada-United States substudy, *Can J Cardiol* 20:760-766, 2004.

44. Schrader G, Cheok F, Hordacre AL et al: Effect of psychiatry liaison with general practitioners on depression severity in recently hospitalised cardiac patients: a randomized controlled trial, *Med J Aust* 182:272-276, 2005.

45. Harrison MB, Browne GB, Roberts J et al: Quality of life of individuals with heart failure, *Med Care* 40:271-282, 2002.

46. Oldridge N, Saner O, McGee H, for the HeartQoL Study Investigators: The Euro Cardio-QoL Project: an international study to develop a core heart disease health-related quality of life questionnaire, the HeartQoL, *Eur J Cardiovasc Prev Rehabil* 12:87-94, 2005.

47. Knopp RH: Risk factors for CAD in women, *Am J Cardiol* 89:28E-35E, 2002.

48. Kannel WB, Wilson PW: Risk factors that attenuate the female coronary disease advantage, *Arch Intern Med* 155:57-61, 1995.

49. Shakir YA, Samsioe G, Nyberg P et al: Cardiovascular risk factors in middle-aged women and the association with use of hormone therapy: results from a population-based study of Swedish women—the Women's Health in the Lund Area (WHILA) Study, *Climacteric* 7:274-283, 2004.

50. Kuh D, Langenberg C, Hardy R et al: Cardiovascular risk at age 53 years in relation to the menopause transition and use of hormone replacement therapy: a prospective British birth cohort study, *BJOG* 112:476-485, 2005.

51. Ridker PM, Hennekens CH, Buring JE, Rifai N: C-reactive protein and other markers of inflammation in the prediction of cardiovascular disease in women, *N Engl J Med* 342:836-843, 2000.

52. Ôunpuu S, Negassa A, Yusuf S, for the INTERHEART Investigators: INTERHEART: a global study of risk factors for acute myocardial infarction, *Am Heart J* 141:711-721, 2001.

53. Yusuf S, Hawken S, Ôunpuu S et al: Effect of potentially modifiable risk factors associated with myocardial infarction in 52 countries (the INTERHEART Study): case-control study, *Lancet* 364:937-952, 2004.

54. Wells AJ: Passive smoking as a cause of heart disease, *J Am Coll Cardiol* 24:546-554, 1994.

55. The Long-Term Intervention with Pravastatin in Ischaemic Disease (LIPID) Study Group: Prevention of cardiovascular events and death with pravastatin in patients with coronary heart disease and a broad range of initial cholesterol levels, *N Engl J Med* 339:1349-1357, 1998.

56. Downs JR, Clearfield M, Weis S et al: Primary prevention of acute coronary events with lovastatin in men and women with average cholesterol levels: results of AFCAPS/TexCAPS, *JAMA* 279:1615-1622, 1998.

57. Hamsten A, Silveira A, Boquist S et al: The apolipoprotein CI content of triglyceride-rich lipoproteins independently predicts early atherosclerosis in health middle-aged men, *J Am Coll Cardiol* 45:1013-1017, 2005.

58. Walldius G, Junger I, Holme I et al: High apolipoprotein B, low apolipoprotien A-I, and improvement in the prediction of fatal myocardial infarction (AMORIS) study: a prospective study, *Lancet* 358:2026-2033, 2001.

59. Chobanian AV, Bakris GL, Black HR et al, and the National High Blood Pressure Education Program Coordinating Committee: The Seventh Report of the Joint National Committee on Prevention, Detection, Evaluation and Treatment of High Blood Pressure: the JNC 7 Report, *JAMA* 289:2560-2572, 2003.

60. American Heart Association: *Diabetes mellitus*. Retrieved January 2006, from www.americanheart.org/presenter.jhtml? identifier=4546

61. Anfossi G, Russo I, Massucco P et al: Impaired synthesis and action of anti-aggregating cyclic nucleotides in platelets from obese subjects: possible role in platelet hyperactivation in obesity, *Eur J Clin Invest* 34:482-489, 2004.

62. Liese AD, Schulz M, Moore CG, Mayer-Davis EJ: Dietary patterns, insulin sensitivity and adiposity in the multi-ethnic Insulin Resistance Atherosclerosis Study population, *Br J Nutr* 92:973-984, 2004.

63. Spencer CG, Martin SC, Felmeden DC et al: Relationship of homocysteine to markers of platelet and endothelial activation in "high risk" hypertensives: a substudy of the Anglo-Scandinavian Cardiac Outcomes Trial, *Int J Cardiol* 94:293-300, 2004.

64. Bostom AG, Silbershatz H, Rosenberg IH et al: Nonfasting plasma total homocysteine levels and all-cause and cardiovascular disease mortality in elderly Framingham men and women, *Arch Intern Med* 24(159):1077-1080, 1999.

65. Bunker SJ, Colquhoun DM, Esler MD et al: "Stress" and coronary heart disease: psychosocial risk factors, *Med J Aust* 178:272-276, 2003.

66. Rosengren A, Hawken S, Ôunpuu S et al, for the INTERHEART Investigators: Association of psychosocial risk factors with risk of acute myocardial infarction in 11,119 cases and 13,648 controls from 52 countries (the INTERHEART Study): case control study, *Lancet* 364:953-962, 2004.

67. MacIntyre K, Stewart S, Capewell S et al: Heart of inequality: the relationship between socio-economic deprivation and death from a first acute myocardial infarction—a population-based analysis, *BMJ* 322:1152-1153, 2001.

68. Lloyd-Jones DM, Wilson PW, Larson MG et al: Framingham risk score and prediction of lifetime risk for coronary heart disease, *Am J Cardiol* 94:20-24, 2004.

69. Conroy RM, Pyorala K, Fitzgerald AP et al, for the SCORE project group: Estimation of ten-year risk of fatal cardiovascular disease in Europe: the SCORE project, *Eur Heart J* 24(11):987-1003, 2003.

70. Law MR, Wald NJ: Risk factor thresholds: their existence under scrutiny, *BMJ* 324:1570-1576, 2002.

71. Wald NH, Law MR: A strategy to reduce cardiovascular disease by more than 80%, *BMJ* 326:1419, 2003.

72. Emberson J, Whincup P, Morris R et al: Evaluating the impact of population and high-risk strategies for the primary prevention of cardiovascular disease, *Eur Heart J* 25:484-491, 2004.

73. Vasan RS, Sullivan LM, Wilson PF et al: Relative importance of borderline and elevated levels of coronary heart disease risk factors, *Ann Intern Med* 142:393-402, 2005.

74. Rutter MK, Meigs JB, Sullivan LM et al: C-reactive protein, the metabolic syndrome, and prediction of cardiovascular events in the Framingham Offspring Study, *Circulation* 110:380-385, 2004.

75. Pearson TA, Mensah GA, Alexander RW et al: Markers of inflammation and cardiovascular disease, *Circulation* 107:499-511, 2003.

76. Milner KA, Vaccarino V, Arnold AL et al: Gender and age differences in chief complaints of acute myocardial infarction (Worcester Heart Attack Study), *Am J Cardiol* 93:606-608, 2004.

77. McSweeney JC, Cody M, O'Sullivan P et al: Women's early warning symptoms of acute myocardial infarction, *Circulation* 108(21):2619-2623, 2003.

78. Vaccarino V, Krumholz HM, Yarzebski J et al: Sex differences in 2-year mortality after hospital discharge for myocardial infarction, *Ann Intern Med* 134(3):173-181, 2001.

79. Tunstall-Pedoe H, Morrison C, Woodward M: Sex differences in myocardial infarction and coronary deaths in the Scottish MONICA population of Glasgow 1985 to 1991, *Circulation* 93:1981-1992, 1996.

80. MacIntyre K, Stewart S, McMurray JJV et al: Gender and survival: a population-based study of 208,527 men and women following a first acute myocardial infarction, *J Am Coll Cardiol* 38:729-735, 2001.

81. Hochman JS, McCabe CH, Stone PH et al: Outcome and profile of women and men presenting with acute coronary syndromes: a report from the TIMI IIIB TIMI investigators. *J Am Coll Cardiol* 30:141-148, 1997.

82. Australian Institute of Health and Welfare: *The health and welfare of Australia's Aboriginal and Torres Strait Island peoples,* Canberra 2003, Australian Bureau of Statistics.

83. Pais P, Pogue J, Gerstein H et al: Risk factors for acute myocardial infarction in Indians: a case control study, *Lancet* 348:358-363, 1996.

84. Yusuf S, Reddy S, Ôunpuu S, Anand S: Global burden of cardiovascular diseases. II. Variations in cardiovascular disease by specific ethnic groups and geographic regions and prevention strategies, *Circulation* 104:2855-2864, 2001.

chapter 3

Epidemiology of Heart Failure

Marjorie Funk
Catherine G. Winkler

CHAPTER ABBREVIATIONS

A-HeFT African-American Heart Failure Trial

BEST Beta-Blocker Evaluation of Survival Trial

BMI body mass index

CAD coronary artery disease

COMET Carvedilol or Metoprolol European Trial

CONSENSUS Cooperative North Scandinavian Enalapril Survival Study

NHANES National Health and Nutrition Examination Survey

SAVE Survival and Ventricular Enlargement Study

SHEP Systolic Hypertension in the Elderly Program

SOLVD Study of Left Ventricular Dysfunction

Despite recent improvements in its management, heart failure remains a major clinical and public health problem responsible for significant disability and health care expenditures. As mortality from coronary disease—the most common precursor of heart failure—declines, the prevalence of heart failure appears to be increasing. This increase is occurring in part because prolonged survival with coronary disease is likely to result in a higher incidence of heart failure.

Accurate description of the epidemiology of heart failure is made difficult by the variety of ways heart failure has been defined in different studies. Traditionally, the term *heart failure* refers to the common clinical syndrome that results from circulatory failure of any cause. Heart failure is characterized by the signs and symptoms of inadequate "forward" cardiac output (e.g., fatigue, cardiac cachexia, and hypotension) and those of "backward" circulatory congestion (e.g., dyspnea, ascites, and dependent edema). Left ventricular dysfunction underlies the clinical syndrome of heart failure in most cases, although heart failure with preserved ejection fraction and diastolic dysfunction may account for as many as 30 to 50 percent of cases. With recent advances in diagnostic technology, the presence of asymptomatic left ventricular dysfunction has increased. Asymptomatic left ventricular dysfunction is defined as decreased ventricular function with few or no overt clinical signs or symptoms.[1]

In response to this evolution in the concept of heart failure, the American College of Cardiology/American Heart Association guidelines for the evaluation and management of heart failure proposed a staging system that includes presymptomatic stages.[2] Figure 3-1 illustrates the four stages of heart failure. This staging system turns attention to the prevention of symptomatic heart failure. Persons in stage A have risk factors for heart failure but no structural heart disease or symptoms. Those in stage B have structural heart disease but no history of symptoms of heart failure. Only those in stages C (structural heart disease with prior or current symptoms) and D (refractory heart failure requiring specialized interventions) qualify for the traditional clinical diagnosis of heart failure. Patients at risk of developing heart failure—particularly those with structural abnormalities but no overt symptoms (stage B)—perhaps should be included in any epidemiological study, but often are not.[3] (See the accompanying Conundrum box, *Detection of Preclinical Heart Failure.*)

Heart failure also can be conceptualized as systolic versus diastolic dysfunction. Systolic heart failure is characterized by impaired pump function and reduced left ventricular ejection fraction. Diastolic failure is characterized by increased resistance to filling of the left ventricle. With diastolic heart failure, patients experience symptoms of heart failure but have normal ejection fractions. Increasingly, epidemiological studies are addressing diastolic and systolic heart failure.

■■■ CONUNDRUM

DETECTION OF PRECLINICAL HEART FAILURE

The four stages of heart failure illustrated in Figure 3-1 raise important questions about screening for heart failure in persons who have no symptoms.

- For *stage A* (risk factors, but no structural heart disease or symptoms), screening is primarily by health history, followed by management of risk factors.
- For *stage B* (structural heart disease, but no symptoms), screening is challenging. Echocardiogram is prohibitively costly and impractical on a large scale. B-type natriuretic peptide (BNP) is not accurate in this population, which does not have overt heart failure. BNP has a poor positive predictive value but good negative predictive value: if the BNP value is less than 18 pg/ml, it is unlikely that ventricular dysfunction is present, but if it is greater than 18 pg/ml, ventricular dysfunction is not necessarily present. The availability of effective treatment for asymptomatic systolic ventricular dysfunction with angiotensin-converting enzyme inhibitors has pointed to the need for cost-effective and accurate methods of screening so that early pharmacological intervention can be initiated and progression of disease retarded.

Questions

- How do you cost-effectively screen in stage B heart failure?
- How do you balance the risk-to-benefit ratio of treatment in asymptomatic heart failure patients?
- How do you promote adherence to treatment in patients who feel good?

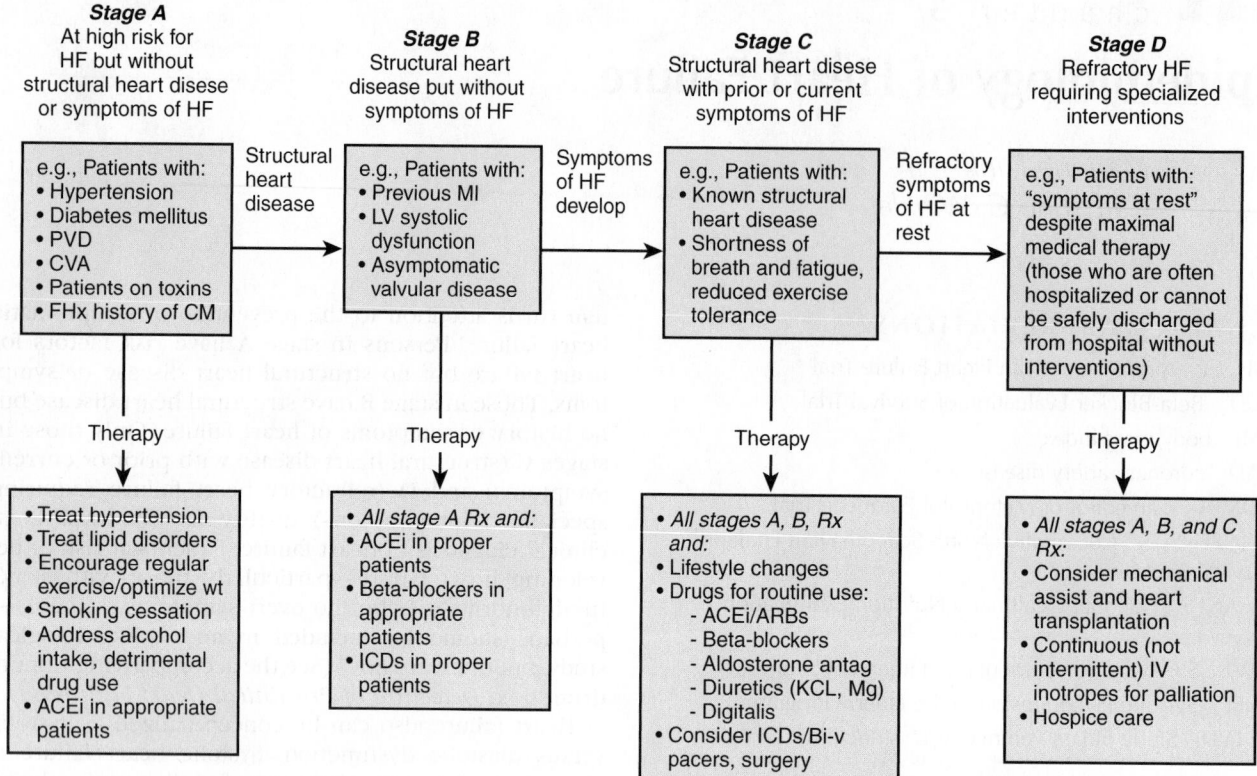

FIGURE 3-1 ▪ Staging of heart failure. *ACEi,* Angiotensin-converting enzyme inhibitors; *ARB,* Angiotensin receptor blockers; *BiV,* Biventricular; *CM,* Cardiomegaly; *CVA,* Cerebrovascular accident; *FHx,* Family history; *HF,* Heart failure; *ICDs,* Implantable cardioverter-defibrillators; *IV,* Intravenous; *KCL,* Potassium chloride; *LV,* Left ventricular; *Mg,* Magnesium; *MI,* Myocardial infarction; *PVD,* Peripheral vascular disease; *Rx,* Therapy; *wt,* weight. (Modified from American College of Cardiology/ American Heart Association *Guidelines for Heart Failure Diagnosis and Management.* Data from Young JB: *Med Clin North Am* 88:1135-1143, 2004.)

INCIDENCE

Incidence refers to the number of new cases detected in a given period. Incidence can be determined by two approaches:

- Reexamination of persons within a cohort at intervals to identify those who have developed heart failure (e.g., the Framingham Heart Study)
- Identification of subjects who develop heart failure for the first time using a population-based surveillance system (e.g., the Rochester, Minnesota Study)[4]

The number of studies that have assessed a population-based cohort repeatedly for the appearance of heart failure is small, and all incidence calculations have been based on the presence of clinical signs and symptoms of heart failure. No population-based studies examining the incidence of heart failure have used echocardiographic measurements of ventricular structure or function at each examination as a criterion.[5]

The Framingham Heart Study provided the first estimates of the incidence of heart failure. The Framingham Study began in 1948 and initially consisted of a community-based cohort but has evolved subsequently to include offspring of the original cohort and spouses of these offspring. Extrapolation of data from the Framingham Study reveals that about 550,000 new cases of heart failure occur each year in the United States.[6]

The incidence of heart failure in the Framingham study increased dramatically with age and was higher in men than women (Figure 3-2). From ages 35 to 64 and ages 65 to 94, the annual incidence rate in men increased from 3 per 1000 to 12 per 1000. In women the corresponding rates were 2 and 9 per 1000, respectively. The higher incidence of heart failure with advancing age and in men is primarily attributable to the elevated rates of coronary artery disease (**CAD**) in older persons and in

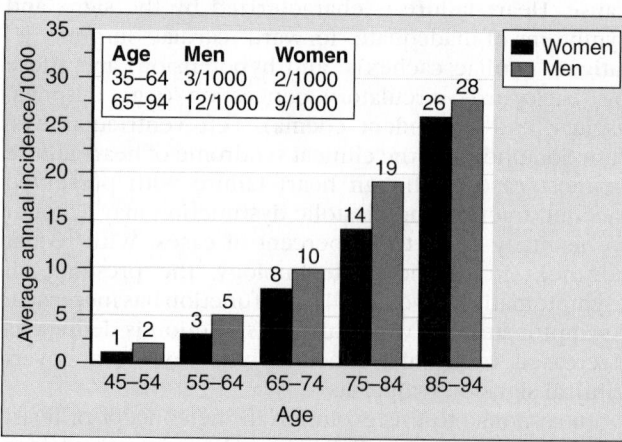

FIGURE 3-2 ▪ Annual incidence of congestive heart failure in women *(dark bars)* and men *(light bars)* in the Framingham study. (From Kannel WB, Vasan RS: Epidemiology of heart failure. In Mann DL, editor: *Heart failure: a companion to Braunwald's heart disease,* Philadelphia, 2004, WB Saunders.)

men.[5] These findings have been confirmed in population-based studies in Rochester[7,8] and eastern Finland.[9]

The concept of lifetime risk allows consideration of the absolute cumulative risk of a person developing a given disease during his or her remaining lifetime. Framingham data reveal that at age 40, the lifetime risk of developing heart failure is about 1 in 5 for men and women. At age 40 and in the absence of myocardial infarction, the lifetime risk of heart failure is 1 in 9 for men and 1 in 6 for women. Lifetime risk of heart failure doubles for persons with hypertension.[10]

In an examination of temporal trends in the incidence of heart failure among subjects in the Framingham Study during a 50-year interval from the 1950s through the 1990s, Levy and colleagues[6] found no significant change over time in the age-adjusted incidence of heart failure among men. Among women, however, the age-adjusted incidence of heart failure declined by 31 to 40 percent in the decades following the first time period (Table 3-1). In the Rochester cohort the incidence of heart failure remained stable for men and women during the 20-year interval between 1979 and 2000 (Table 3-2).[8]

Although it is commonly thought that improved survival after acute myocardial infarction results in a higher incidence of heart failure, an analysis of data from the Rochester study indicates that the occurrence of heart failure after myocardial infarction has declined by 28 percent over a period (1979 to 1994) coinciding with the increased use of reperfusion therapy.[11] Although more persons are surviving acute myocardial infarction and are at risk of developing heart failure, the diminishing severity of myocardial infarction attributable to early reperfusion seems to have attenuated this risk.

PREVALENCE

Prevalence is the number of existing cases of a disease at a particular point in time. Prevalence is determined by factors that affect the occurrence of disease (incidence) and those that affect the severity or duration of disease (mortality). Prevalence rates can vary widely across investigations depending on the source of data, geographic region, population demographics, and diagnostic criteria for heart failure.[4]

Table 3-3 presents an overview of the prevalence of heart failure by age and sex in studies published since 1992. In general, prevalence increased with advancing age and was similar in men and women or higher in men. Because it is a broad-based community survey, the National Health and Nutrition Examination Survey (**NHANES**) may provide the best estimate of the prevalence of heart failure in the United States. Extrapolation of the NHANES heart failure prevalence rates to include institutionalized and older persons (and accounting for current demographic characteristics of the population) provides the basis for the recent estimate of 5 million Americans or 2.3 percent of the U.S. population currently living with heart failure.[21]

With the exception of the Glasgow study,[16] Strong Heart Study,[18] and Rochester study,[20] estimates of the prevalence of heart failure from all the studies outlined in Table 3-3 were based on the presence of overt clinical

■ ■ ■

TABLE 3-1   TEMPORAL TRENDS IN THE AGE-ADJUSTED INCIDENCE OF HEART FAILURE: FRAMINGHAM COHORT

	MEN		WOMEN	
PERIOD	INCIDENCE OF HEART FAILURE (PER 100,000 PERSON-YEARS)	RATE RATIO	INCIDENCE OF HEART FAILURE (PER 100,000 PERSON-YEARS)	RATE RATIO
1950-1969	627 (475-779)	1.00	420 (336-504)	1.00
1970-1979	563 (437-689)	0.87 (0.67-1.14)	311 (249-373)	0.63 (0.47-0.84)
1980-1989	536 (448-623)	0.87 (0.67-1.13)	298 (247-350)	0.60 (0.45-0.79)
1990-1999	564 (463-665)	0.93 (0.71-1.23)	327 (266-388)	0.69 (0.51-0.93)

Note: All values are adjusted for age (less than 55, 55 to 64, 65 to 74, 75 to 84, 85 years or older). Values in parentheses are 95 percent confidence intervals. The 1950-1969 period served as the reference period.
Data from Levy D, Kenchaiah S, Larson MG et al: *N Engl J Med* 347:1397-1402, 2002.

■ ■ ■

TABLE 3-2   TEMPORAL TRENDS IN THE AGE-ADJUSTED INCIDENCE OF HEART FAILURE: ROCHESTER COHORT

	PERIOD			
GROUP BY GENDER	1979-1984	1985-1990	1991-1995	1996-2000
Men				
Incidence per 100,000 (95% CI)	360 (323-396)	390 (354-425)	375 (340-409)	383 (351-415)
RR (95% CI)	1.00	1.07 (0.94-1.22)	1.01 (0.88-1.15)	1.04 (0.92-1.18)
Women				
Incidence per 100,000 (95% CI)	284 (260-307)	292 (270-315)	260 (238-282)	315 (292-338)
RR (95% CI)	1.00	1.04 (0.93-1.16)	0.93 (0.83-1.05)	1.11 (1.00-1.24)

CI, Confidence interval; *RR,* relative risk.
Data from Roger VL, Weston SA, Redfield MM et al: *JAMA* 292:344-350, 2004.

■■■

TABLE 3-3   PREVALENCE OF HEART FAILURE

STUDY (PUBLICATION DATE) AGE GROUPS	CASE ASCERTAINMENT	MEN (%) Sx	Asx	WOMEN (%) Sx	Asx	TOTAL (%) Sx	Asx
NHANES I (1992)[12]	Questionnaire						
25-54		0.4		0.3		0.4	
55-64		2.2		2.0		2.1	
65-74		3.7		3.2		3.4	
NHANES I (1992)[12]	Physical examination						
25-54		0.8		1.3		1.1	
55-64		4.5		3.0		3.7	
65-74		4.8		4.3		4.5	
Framingham study (1993)[13]	Physical examination						
50-59		0.8		0.8		0.8	
60-69		2.2		2.2		2.2	
70-79		5.1		4.3		4.7	
80-89		6.6		7.9		7.3	
Cardiovascular Health Study (1993)[14]	Interview; physical examination; medical record review						
65-69		2.2		1.2		1.6	
70-74		1.9		1.5		1.7	
75-79		3.2		2.4		2.7	
80-84		3.2		2.5		2.8	
85+		2.9		2.2		2.6	
Helsinki Ageing Study (1997)[15]	Physical examination						
75-86		5.2		9.3		8.2	
Glasgow, U.K. (1997)[16]	Survey; echocardiogram (LVEF less than or equal to 30%)	Sx	Asx	Sx	Asx	Sx	Asx
25-34		0	0	0	0	0	0
35-44		0	0.7	0	0	0.3	0
45-54		1.4	4.4	1.2	1.2	1.3	2.7
55-64		2.5	3.2	2.0	0	2.3	1.6
65-74		3.2	3.2	3.6	1.3	3.4	2.2
Göteborg, Sweden (2001)[17]	Physical examination						
55-64		0.6		—		—	
65-74		2.8					
75-79		6.2					
Strong Heart Study (2001)[18]	Echocardiogram						
	LVEF 40%-54%	—		—		11.1%	
	LVEF less than 40%					2.9%	
National Health Interview Survey (2003)[19]	Survey						
18-39		<0.1		0.1		0.1	
40-64		1.2		1.1		1.1	
65-74		4.5		2.9		3.6	
75+		5.7		5.5		5.5	
Rochester, Minn. (2003)[20]	Echocardiogram (LVEF less than or equal to 50%)						
45-54		5.1		1.0		3.0	
55-64		7.4		2.2		4.8	
65-74		10.6		3.8		7.1	
75+		22.8		6.6		12.9	

LVEF, Left ventricular ejection fraction; *NHANES,* National Health and Nutrition Examination Survey; *Sx,* symptomatic; *Asx,* asymptomatic.

signs and symptoms of left ventricular dysfunction. They did not include objective assessment of ventricular structure and function. This is important in light of clinical trials[22] that have demonstrated the benefit of medical therapy, not only in symptomatic patients with left ventricular ejection fractions less than 35 percent but also in asymptomatic patients with low ejection fractions. The finding that asymptomatic patients with systolic dysfunction may benefit from medical therapy has changed heart failure epidemiology and placed greater emphasis on the prevention of left ventricular dysfunction.[1] Therefore, it is important to determine the prevalence of heart failure based on an objective assessment of ventricular structure and function (e.g.,

echocardiography). This strategy would increase the prevalence because it would include not only those persons in stages C and D but also those in stage B with asymptomatic left ventricular dysfunction (Figure 3-1).

Prevalence figures are clearly higher when asymptomatic persons are included, as they were in the Glasgow,[16] Strong Heart Study,[18] and Rochester[20] Cohorts. Although Table 3-3 shows the prevalence of definite left ventricular dysfunction (ejection fraction of 30 percent or less) in the Glasgow study, McDonagh and colleagues[16] report that 7.7 percent of their total sample had ejection fractions of 35 percent or less, and 77 percent of these subjects had no symptoms. Rodeheffer[1] proposes that this high prevalence rate may reflect the high prevalence of CAD in this area of Scotland. It also should be noted that these figures represent prevalence in a relatively young cohort; those age 75 and older were excluded. In the older Rochester cohort[20] (age 45 and older), the overall prevalence of left ventricular dysfunction (defined as an ejection fraction of 50 percent or less) was 6.0 percent. Data from the Strong Heart Study of American Indians[18] showed a higher prevalence of left ventricular dysfunction, with 11.1 percent having an ejection fraction of 40 to 54 percent and 2.9 percent having an ejection fraction less than 40 percent. In addition to variances by population studied, these investigations varied in echocardiogram measurement methods, definition of left ventricular dysfunction (the cutoff value for abnormal ejection fraction), and the age range of the cohort.[1]

Just as it is important to include asymptomatic persons with low ejection fractions in estimates of the prevalence of heart failure, it is also essential to consider symptomatic persons with normal ejection fractions. This latter syndrome commonly is referred to as *diastolic heart failure.* Until recently, the prevalence of diastolic heart failure in the community has been uncertain. Case finding to ascertain the prevalence of diastolic heart failure has relied on the occurrence of clinically overt heart failure in persons with a normal ejection fraction. Using this method of case ascertainment, it has been estimated that about 30 to 50 percent of patients with heart failure symptoms have a normal or nearly normal ejection fraction, thus meeting the definition of diastolic heart failure.[5] According to this definition, diastolic dysfunction more often is detected in women. This definition is inadequate, however, because it is not based on any specific measurement of diastolic function.[1]

The Rochester group[20] was the first to use semiquantitative Doppler imaging techniques to measure diastolic dysfunction in a community-based cohort. They found that 20.8 percent of their cohort of randomly selected subjects age 45 and older had mild diastolic dysfunction, 6.6 percent had moderate diastolic dysfunction, and 0.7 percent had severe diastolic dysfunction. The prevalence of diastolic dysfunction increased with age and, contrary to past observations, was equally common in men and women.

The expansion of the definition of heart failure so that now persons with asymptomatic, or preclinical, ventricular dysfunction (stage B) also are considered to have heart failure has resulted in higher estimates of prevalence. To appreciate the full scope of heart failure better, it is also important to consider those with risk factors for heart failure but without evidence of structural or functional heart disease (stage A).

CAUSES AND RISK FACTORS

Although these terms often are used interchangeably in discussions about heart failure, the distinction between a *cause* and a *risk factor* is important. To be considered a cause, the characteristic must meet certain criteria—such as a strong association, biological credibility, consistency across investigations, appropriate temporal sequence,

and a dose-response relationship. In contrast, a risk factor is a characteristic that is suspected to have a relationship to the occurrence of a specific disease but is neither a necessary nor sufficient cause of the disease (Box 3-1).[4]

Also important is to recognize the subtle difference between a *risk factor* and a *marker.* The term *marker* is used to describe biological characteristics, such as a low serum sodium level, and clinical factors, such as cachexia. A marker does not appear to be a characteristic that influences disease development but rather is an indicator of a decline in clinical condition.

Causes of Heart Failure

The causes of heart failure can be categorized into myocardial, volume, pressure loading, and restrictive. Myocardial causes of heart failure include ischemia resulting from CAD and chamber dilatation that can be idiopathic or caused by toxins, inflammation, or pregnancy. Disorders causing volume changes, such as aortic and mitral regurgitation and anemia, also can cause heart failure. Conditions resulting in pressure loading of the left ventricle, such as hypertension and aortic stenosis, often lead to heart failure. Lastly, restrictive conditions, which include constrictive pericarditis, amyloidosis, and sarcoidosis, although rarely seen in the Western world, are more common causes of heart failure in less developed areas of the world.

BOX 3-1 ▪ ▪ ▪
HEART FAILURE CAUSES AND RISK FACTORS

Causes
- Myocardial
  - Chamber dilatation (idiopathic, toxins, inflammatory, peripartum)
  - Ischemic (coronary artery disease)
- Volume
  - Anemia
  - Aortic and mitral regurgitation
- Pressure loading
  - Aortic stenosis
  - Hypertension
- Restrictive
  - Amyloidosis
  - Constrictive pericarditis
  - Sarcoidosis

Risk Factors
- Modifiable
  - Diabetes
  - Left ventricular hypertrophy
  - Less than high school education
  - Obesity
  - Physical inactivity
  - Smoking
  - Valve disease
- Nonmodifiable
  - Age
  - Gender
  - Race
- Novel or potential
  - Alcohol
  - Depression
  - Metabolic syndrome
  - Sleep disordered breathing
  - Toxins

Of all of these possible causes, hypertension and CAD are currently the most common causes of heart failure. They also can be considered modifiable risk factors. In the general population, there is an attributable risk of 13 percent for developing heart failure from CAD or hypertension.[23] These diseases, although not preventable, may be modified to slow the progression of the heart failure trajectory through reducing cardiovascular risk by pharmacological means, coronary artery revascularization, and lifestyle adjustments. Levy and colleagues[6] note that the incidence of heart failure is reduced by about 50 percent when hypertension is treated.

With CAD and hypertension as the main causes of heart failure in the general population, it is difficult to determine which condition prevails because they coexist in about 40 percent of patients with heart failure.[5] Findings from NHANES point to CAD as the chief cause of heart failure,[24] whereas data from the Framingham Study suggest that hypertension is the key contributor.[25] By conceptualizing both diseases as part of the heart failure trajectory, Kannel and Vasan[5] propose that CAD is a step along the causal pathway beginning with hypertension and ending with heart failure.

The cause of heart failure varies according to geographic location. Although hypertension and CAD account for most cases of heart failure in developed countries, rheumatic valve disease and nutritional cardiac disease are much more common as precursors to heart failure in the developing world.[4]

Hypertension

Hypertension, based on its severity and the length of time it is experienced, will increase the incidence of heart failure in the general population. Data from the Framingham Study showed a twofold increase in heart failure risk for men and a threefold increase for women with hypertension.[25] More specifically, the Framingham data indicate a greater influence of systolic than diastolic pressure at all ages and in both sexes.[26] Furthermore, persons with hypertension who also have had a myocardial infarction have an almost sixfold increased independent risk of heart failure. Some 34 to 52 percent of patients with hypertension and heart failure also have sustained a myocardial infarction.[5] Moreover, hypertensive persons who also have diabetes and left ventricular hypertrophy have a twofold to threefold increase in the risk of heart failure.

Coronary Artery Disease

In some studies, CAD represents the leading cause of heart failure. Alone, CAD occurs in 19 percent of men and 7 percent of women.[5] In NHANES,[24] the population-attributable risk for CAD accounted for 61.6 percent of the heart failure incident cases, with 67.9 percent in men and 55.9 percent in women. Of note, hypertension remains the leading cause of heart failure in women, whereas myocardial infarction is the predominate cause in men.[25] Although consensus is lacking regarding the predominate cause of heart failure, clearly both diseases alone and together are significant contributors to heart failure risk and provide the greatest opportunity for the practitioner to intervene.

Modifiable Risk Factors

Other risk factors are also modifiable. Therefore, it is important that practitioners focus on these factors to prevent heart failure, if possible, and if not, to slow the progression of the disease and improve the patient's prognosis.

Diabetes

Diabetes is associated with an acceleration of CAD, hypertension, and obesity, thereby predisposing patients to heart failure. Diabetes is also an independent predictor of heart failure even without hypertension and imposes a twofold greater hazard of heart failure in women than in men.[5] Diabetes affects the heart functionally, structurally, and through metabolic changes that suggest the existence of a diabetic cardiomyopathy. It may be that microangiopathy affects the myocardium in the same way that it affects the retina, skin, and kidneys.[4] In NHANES, diabetes was identified as a significant risk factor for the development of heart failure.[24] In addition, the risk of heart failure in the context of diabetes increases when glycemic control is poor or when there is evidence of microalbuminuria.[5]

Valvular Disease

In general, valvular disease increases the risk of heart failure 2 to 2.5 times but only explains 7 to 8 percent of the population burden.[5] Therefore, the impact of valvular disease is minimal compared with hypertension and CAD. However, in the elderly, valvular disease has become increasingly common. NHANES revealed that a history of valvular disease was positively and significantly associated with an increased risk of heart failure, with a population-attributable risk of 2.3 percent.[24] Rheumatic heart disease, with later valvular dysfunction, is a more common precursor of heart failure in developing countries than in the developed world, although it still occurs.[4]

Obesity

Framingham data showed that the risk of heart failure increased with a higher body mass index (**BMI**), even when controlling for other variables. A 5 percent increase of heart failure in men and a 7 percent increase in women were found with each unit increase in the BMI. In addition, 66 percent of obese patients had left ventricular dysfunction, as indicated by ejection fractions of less than 50 percent.[27]

The exact way in which obesity influences heart failure risk is unknown, although it may be by several different paths. Heart failure is associated directly with CAD, and increased BMI—with its associated risks of hypertension, diabetes mellitus, and dyslipidemia—is a risk factor for CAD. Moreover, excessive weight is associated with hemodynamic overload, which is characterized by increased blood supply and cardiac output. Obesity also adversely affects cardiac diastolic function. These processes—along with activation of the neuroendocrine system, deficiencies in natriuretic pathways, and the generation of proinflammatory cytokines by adipose tissue—contribute to an increased risk of heart failure. These changes may be associated with myocardial depression and sodium retention disorders.[27]

The relationship of obesity and heart failure is yet more complex. Obesity is a definitive risk for the *development* of heart failure, whereas it may have a positive influence on survival *after the onset* of heart failure. (See Reverse Epidemiology later in the chapter.)

Hypercholesterolemia

Hypercholesterolemia is a well-defined risk factor for CAD, which a lower cholesterol level may prevent. Surprisingly, a high total serum cholesterol level is only weakly associated with heart failure, whereas dyslipidemia characterized by a high ratio of total cholesterol to high-density lipoprotein cholesterol has a strong relationship with heart failure for men and women.[5]

However, two groups[28,29] found that in patients with already established heart failure, a lower cholesterol level independently was associated with a worse prognosis. (See Reverse Epidemiology.) As a result of these findings, lowering cholesterol should be a goal in preventing heart failure; however, after the onset of heart failure, cholesterol reduction needs to be considered carefully by weighing the potential benefits and harm in the context of the overall cardiovascular disease process.

Left Ventricular Hypertrophy

Left ventricular hypertrophy is associated with heart failure risk regardless of its cause (e.g., hypertension, obesity, CAD, diabetes, or valvular disease). Furthermore, the risk of heart failure increases in relationship to the severity of the hypertrophy. Therefore, it is imperative that left ventricular hypertrophy be identified and treated early in the disease trajectory. About 20 percent of heart failure events in the general population are preceded by electrocardiograhic evidence of left ventricular hypertrophy, but left ventricular hypertrophy appears on the echocardiograms of 60 to 70 percent of heart failure cases.[5]

Additional Risk Factors

Other factors are associated significantly with heart failure but more weakly than hypertension, CAD, and diabetes. They include cigarette smoking, physical inactivity, and lower socioeconomic status.

An analysis of data from NHANES[24] indicated that cigarette smoking—an independent risk factor for heart failure—is associated with a 45 percent higher risk of heart failure in men and 88 percent in women after adjusting for CAD and other known heart failure risks. This same study also reported that 17 percent of incident heart failure cases in the U.S. general population may be attributable to cigarette smoking. Ex-smokers accrued benefits within 2 years of quitting and had a 30 percent reduction in mortality compared with current smokers in the Study of Left Ventricular Dysfunction (**SOLVD**) trials.[30]

Physical inactivity was identified as another risk factor in NHANES and accounted for about 9.2 percent of heart failure cases after adjusting for other risk factors in the U.S. population. Strength training and endurance exercise have been shown to decrease fatigue and dyspnea and increase functional activity and quality of life in patients with established heart failure.[31]

Having less than a high school education (an index of lower socioeconomic status) increases the risk of heart failure. This may relate to limited access to health care and poor compliance with treatment of diabetes, hypertension, and other modifiable risk factors that lead to the development of heart failure.[24]

Nonmodifiable Risk Factors

Gender, race, and age are nonmodifiable risk factors for heart failure. Gender differences have been studied inadequately until recently; still, the impact on both genders is significant, with a lifetime risk of heart failure of 21 percent for men and 20 percent for women based on Framingham data.[5] Additionally, the impact of race on heart failure is important to note because of the particular risk that may exist for groups that otherwise may go unnoticed if not studied independently. Recognition that race is self-designated and may be viewed as a sociopolitical factor rather than a physiological indicator is important.[32] Age has long been identified as a risk factor for the development of heart failure.[1] Older patients experience age-related changes in the cardiovascular system and are more likely to experience comorbid conditions that heighten their risk for heart failure. Not only do these factors influence the risk of heart failure, but also they affect how patients experience heart failure (morbidity).

Gender

Hypertension is the primary precursor for heart failure in women, whereas CAD—specifically myocardial infarction—is the primary cause of heart failure in men.[6] Until recently, little was known about the extent of the differences between men and women in relation to heart failure because of the historical underrepresentation of women in clinical trials.

The Beta-Blocker Evaluation of Survival Trial (**BEST**)[33] emphasized recruitment of women, and randomization was stratified by cause, left ventricular ejection fraction, ethnicity, and gender. The design makes this study particularly useful for examining gender differences in heart failure. Significant gender differences were found in several baseline characteristics, such as a better prognosis associated with women's increased prevalence of nonischemic disease, higher ejection fractions, lower incidence of atrial fibrillation, and lower plasma norepinephrine level. Women had a survival advantage when heart failure was nonischemic. Female sex was also a significant independent predictor of survival for those with heart failure, regardless of clinical profile or beta blocker treatment, in the Cardiac Insufficiency Bisoprolol Study.[34]

In the National Heart Failure Project, women were less likely than men to have CAD, chronic obstructive pulmonary disease, and prior coronary revascularization. Additionally, women had lower mortality rates than men up to 1 year after hospitalization.[35]

The Framingham study has shown an improvement in survival rates after the onset of heart failure for both sexes over the past 50 years. Despite the overall improvement in survival rates; however, the incidence of heart failure in men has not declined as it has in women.[6] A decline in the incidence of heart failure in women may be from earlier and more effective treatment for hypertension. In contrast, men have a greater vulnerability to CAD and the resulting myocardial damage that places them at greater risk of heart failure.

Race and Ethnicity

Although race may represent a social construct rather than describe a demographic variable for epidemiological study, research indicates that race is an important risk factor for heart failure. The prevalence of heart failure in blacks is reported to be higher than for other groups. The age-adjusted prevalence rate for non-Hispanic black men is 3.5 percent, whereas the rate for non-Hispanic white men is 2.3 percent. The trend follows in women, with non-Hispanic blacks having a prevalence rate of 3.1 percent in contrast to a rate of 1.5 percent in non-Hispanic whites.[5]

Blacks also have a different heart failure profile. They are younger, have more hospital admissions and readmissions, and have a higher incidence of hypertension and left ventricular hypertrophy than whites.[3] Although some studies have found that blacks with heart failure have a higher mortality rate than whites,[36] others report no racial difference in mortality.[37]

In addition to racial differences in the prevalence and cause of heart failure, and in morbidity and possibly mortality, there also is evidence of racially based biological variations that may influence the response to various heart failure medications. Blacks may have a less active renin-angiotensin system and a lower bioavailability of nitric oxide than whites. Based on these suggested biological differences, the African-American Heart Failure Trial (**A-HeFT**) was undertaken. This trial revealed that the addition of a fixed dose of isosorbide dinitrate plus hydralazine to standard therapy for heart failure, including neurohormonal blockers, is effective and increases survival among black patients with advanced heart failure.[38] Whether race is a surrogate marker for biological differences and whether the differences observed in the causes and outcomes of heart failure are linked to race alone remain unclear.

Age

Heart failure disproportionately affects older persons. In this group, age is associated with poorer outcomes, especially when patients have concurrent diseases, and results in a fivefold increase in sudden cardiac arrest.[39] The increased prevalence of age-related cardiovascular diseases and the changes that occur in the cardiovascular system as a person ages contribute to the exponential rise in heart failure prevalence with advancing age. Changes in the cardiovascular system include the following[4]:

- Reduced responsiveness to beta-adrenergic stimulation
- Increased vascular stiffness
- Increased stiffness of the heart itself
- Altered myocardial energy metabolism

In the Framingham and Rochester studies, the incidence of heart failure increased exponentially with advancing age.[1] The mean age for the initial diagnosis of

heart failure also has increased over the last 50 years. In the Framingham study the mean age at diagnosis was 62.7 in the 1950s, compared with a mean age of 80.0 in the 1990s.[6] Fifty percent of persons with heart failure are older than age 65, with the prevalence of the condition increasing from 3 per 1000 in men ages 50 to 59 to 27 per 1000 for men ages 80 to 89.[3] In a British population-based study, mortality was associated independently with age and increased by 26 percent for every decade after the onset of heart failure.[40] Hospitalized elderly Medicare patients with heart failure also suffer from additional illnesses, with 40 percent having diabetes and 33 percent having chronic obstructive lung disease.[41]

Novel and Potential Risk Factors

New and evolving risk factors may be indicators for heart failure risk. These potential risk factors include toxin exposure, metabolic syndrome, sleep-disordered breathing, depression, and alcohol intake.

Toxins

Certain toxins, such as chemotherapeutic drugs, have long been known to predispose persons to heart failure because of their adverse effect on the pumping mechanism of the heart.[3] Clinical monitoring and ongoing cardiac assessment must take place when patients are treated with these drugs. Serial echocardiograms with measurement of left ventricular ejection fraction are useful to track the effect of these toxic drugs on cardiac function.

Recently, nonsteroidal antiinflammatory drugs have been considered cardiotoxic. Concomitant use of nonsteroidal antiinflammatory drugs and diuretics is a risk factor for the onset of heart failure because of the inhibition of prostaglandin synthesis and consequent sodium and water retention.[42]

Metabolic Syndrome

Metabolic syndrome has not been established firmly as a direct risk factor for heart failure. However, it is important to note that characteristics of metabolic syndrome are associated independently with CAD, which is an important antecedent of heart failure. These characteristics include elevated BMI with insulin resistance, glucose intolerance, low high-density lipoprotein cholesterol level, and hypertriglyceridemia.[27]

Sleep-Disordered Breathing

No prospective studies have linked sleep-disordered breathing to the development of heart failure; however, a large cross-sectional survey showed a doubling of the odds of self-reported heart failure in the presence of sleep-disordered breathing.[43] Further, in patients with obstructive sleep apnea, an increase in pulmonary artery hypertension causing right ventricular failure, combined with an increase in sympathetic activity and blood pressure, can cause heart failure to progress.[27]

Depression

In the Systolic Hypertension in the Elderly Program (**SHEP**),[44] depression was associated independently with a substantial increase in the risk of heart failure among older persons with isolated systolic hypertension. This association does not appear to be mediated by myocardial infarction. In another longitudinal, community-based study of elderly persons, depression was identified as an independent risk factor for heart failure in women, but not in men.[45] The association of depression with heart failure is still inconclusive. The link between depression and cardiac dysfunction may be mediated by behavioral mechanisms, such as poor adherence with medical therapies.

Alcohol Intake

The relationship of alcohol intake to the development of heart failure remains controversial. Although alcohol abuse has been associated with the development of dilated cardiomyopathy,[46] when consumed in moderation, alcohol appears to protect against heart failure.[47,48] When compared with no alcohol consumption, low to moderate levels were associated with lower heart failure risk when controlling for other factors, such as CAD.[48] Other evidence indicates that light drinking is safe and may be beneficial for patients with ischemic left ventricular dysfunction, but not for those with nonischemic dysfunction.[49] Because research findings are inconsistent, drinking of alcohol should not be encouraged. If patients do drink, limiting intake to low or moderate amounts is preferable.

Reverse Epidemiology

The classic cardiac risk factors of obesity, hypercholesterolemia, and hypertension are associated independently with the development of heart failure.[27] Recently, however, paradoxical observations have been reported. These factors—traditionally associated with the development of heart failure in the general population—have been found to be strongly associated with decreased mortality and morbidity in patients with *existing* heart failure. (See the accompanying Conundrum box, *Obesity, Hypercholesterolemia, and Hypertension May Be*

Protective in Heart Failure.) These findings, in contrast to the usual associations, are referred to as *reverse epidemiology* (Table 3-4).[50] Although the basis for this reverse relationship in patients with heart failure is unknown, it also has been observed in patients with end-stage renal disease, elderly patients in nursing homes, and patients with malignancies.

Obesity

Recent studies have reported that in patients with existing heart failure, those who are overweight or obese have better outcomes than patients whose weight is in the normal or low range. Clearly, involuntary weight loss in the setting of severe heart failure (cachexia) is a poor prognostic sign; however, being overweight or mildly to moderately obese does not seem to be associated with higher mortality.[27] In the SHEP study,[51] being overweight

---

■■■ CONUNDRUM

OBESITY, HYPERCHOLESTEROLEMIA, AND HYPERTENSION MAY BE PROTECTIVE IN HEART FAILURE

Recent research has indicated that obesity, hypercholesterolemia, and hypertension—conditions known to be risk factors for the *development* of heart failure—actually may be protective for persons with *existing* heart failure. Possibly, patients with these risk factors eventually may suffer from consequences of these conditions if they live long enough.

Questions
- Is deliberate weight loss and treatment for hypercholesterolemia and hypertension advisable for patients with heart failure?
- At what point in the trajectory of heart failure should these conditions not be treated?
- Is there a point in the trajectory of heart failure that efforts should be directed to increasing weight, cholesterol, and blood pressure?
- What parameters should be used to decide whether it is appropriate to shift the approach for the management of weight, cholesterol, and blood pressure?

■■■

TABLE 3-4   REVERSE EPIDEMIOLOGY OF CARDIOVASCULAR RISK FACTORS IN HEART FAILURE

RISK FACTORS FOR CARDIOVASCULAR DISEASE	DIRECTION OF THE ASSOCIATIONS BETWEEN RISK FACTORS AND OUTCOMES		COMMENTS
	GENERAL POPULATION	PATIENT WITH HEART FAILURE	
Body mass index (BMI)	High BMI and obesity are deleterious.	High BMI and obesity are protective.	Increased BMI is a risk factor for heart failure. Elderly persons, smokers, patients on maintenance dialysis, and hospitalized patients have an adverse association similar to patients with heart failure.
Serum cholesterol level	Hypercholesterolemia, high LDL cholesterol level, and low HDL cholesterol level are deleterious.	Hypercholesterolemia (and maybe high LDL cholesterol level) is protective.	Associations between low cholesterol and mortality may be similar in elderly persons, smokers, and patients with AIDS or who are undergoing dialysis.
Blood pressure	Hypertension is deleterious.	A low systolic blood pressure often indicates a poor outcome.	Similar reverse associations between blood pressure and outcome have been described in dialysis patients.

LDL, Low-density lipoprotein; *HDL,* high-density lipoprotein; *AIDS,* acquired immunodeficiency syndrome.
Data from Kalantar-Zadeh K, Block G, Horwich T et al: *J Am Coll Cardiol* 43:1439-1444, 2004.

was linked to a decreased rate of stroke and reduced total mortality in patients with heart failure. Cardiac death and all-cause mortality were lower in obese patients with heart failure in the Rotterdam Study cohort.[39] Curtis and colleagues[52] confirmed the presence of an "obesity paradox" in the Digitalis Investigation Group trial, in which those who were overweight or obese had a lower risk of mortality compared with patients at a healthy weight. It may be possible that increased cardiac output and myocardial demands, in combination with a higher prevalence of endothelial dysfunction, lead overweight patients to be diagnosed earlier in their disease process, resulting in lower mortality rates. Other hypotheses are being investigated, however, for all studies to date that suggest a link between obesity and lower mortality in heart failure have been observational.

Hypercholesterolemia

Hypercholesterolemia is another well-established risk factor for heart failure, but in patients with existing heart failure, hypercholesterolemia may be cardioprotective. Vredevoe and colleagues[53] found that a low total cholesterol level was predictive of mortality in patients with heart failure. In patients with severe heart failure, lower total cholesterol levels are associated with lower albumin levels, left ventricular ejection fractions, and cardiac output values.[54]

Hypertension

Hypertension is another recognized risk factor for cardiovascular and cerebrovascular events in the general population. In contrast, in several studies,[39,55] hypertension was not an independent risk factor for mortality in patients with previously diagnosed heart failure. In the Carvedilol or Metoprolol European Trial (**COMET**), a randomized trial of patients with heart failure, Poole-Wilson and colleagues[56] found that a higher systolic blood pressure at baseline was associated with lower mortality. Similarly, Cowie and colleagues[40] reported that higher systemic arterial pressure was associated with better survival in patients with heart failure. It may be that the hypertension reflects the ability of the circulatory system to compensate for low cardiac output with an adequate perfusion pressure.

Possible Explanations

Kalantar-Zadeh and colleagues[50] propose several possible explanations for the reverse epidemiology phenomenon. These explanations include time discrepancies among competitive risk factors, malnutrition-inflammation complex syndrome, the endotoxin-lipoprotein hypothesis, survival bias, and reverse causation.

Time Discrepancies Among Competitive Risk Factors

Patients with heart failure have a shortened life expectancy. Therefore, they may experience improved short-term survival with any risk factor that exerts a positive effect on longevity. Factors that typically are associated with long-term survival may not apply. This time discrepancy favors the patient with heart failure in the short term, outweighing the harmful effects of these same cardiovascular risk factors in the long term. In the

United States and most industrialized countries, manifestations of overnutrition, such as obesity and hypercholesterolemia, are major risk factors for cardiovascular mortality. In these countries, people have a longer life expectancy compared with people in other parts of the world. People in developing countries, where malnutrition is a powerful determinant of morbidity and mortality, have a shortened life expectancy—much like people with heart failure.[50]

Malnutrition-Inflammation Complex Syndrome

Cardiac cachexia is an independent risk factor for mortality in patients with heart failure.[57] An important feature of cardiac cachexia is related to the inflammatory syndrome.[58] In the setting of severe heart failure, a chronic inflammatory state may result from bacterial or endotoxin translocation from bowel wall edema.[50] This inflammatory response may be responsible for the cachexia that can develop in patients with heart failure.

Patients who are underweight or who have low cholesterol may be suffering from malnutrition-inflammation complex syndrome and be prone to its poor outcome. Being underweight or having a low serum cholesterol level may indicate a state of malnutrition, which may predispose the person with heart failure to infection or inflammatory diseases. Therefore, any condition that attenuates the magnitude of the inflammatory response, such as obesity, hypercholesterolemia, and hypertension, should be favorable to patients with heart failure.[50]

Endotoxin-Lipoprotein Hypothesis

Lower serum cholesterol and lipoprotein levels are associated with impaired survival in patients with heart failure. A higher serum cholesterol level may be a marker for a richer pool of lipoproteins that can bind actively to and remove circulating endotoxins, which can cause inflammation and subsequent atherosclerosis. This phenomenon may explain the paradoxical effect of high cholesterol. In patients with heart failure, there is an optimal lipoprotein level below which intervention to reduce lipids would be detrimental.[50]

Survival Bias

Patients with heart failure also may have characteristics that differ from the general population because of the "survival of the fittest" phenomenon. More than 50 million persons with cardiac disease are at risk for developing heart failure, but only 5 million persons actually have been diagnosed with clinically evident heart failure.[50] Many persons with heart disease and its associated risk factors do not survive to develop heart failure. Patients who survive to the point of developing heart failure, despite having some traditional risk factors, may have other protective traits that negate the adverse effects.

Reverse Causation

Lastly, perhaps the causal pathway in patients with heart failure may be reversed. Low BMI, low total cholesterol level, and low blood pressure may be associated with a chronic disease that has advanced to heart failure. Hence, it may not be hypotension per se that is detrimental, but rather the underlying cause of hypotension (i.e., progressive cardiac pump failure). Conceivably, the risk factors are not etiologically linked to a higher mortality in heart failure patients; rather they serve as markers for a more severe illness and an impending poor outcome. Nevertheless, even if the direction of the associations are unclear, interventions aimed at avoiding weight loss, low cholesterol level, and hypotension may be beneficial to the survival of patients with heart failure.[50]

Summary

The presence of multiple risk factors dramatically and disproportionately increases the risk of heart failure. An exponential, rather than merely additive, effect occurs when a person has multiple risk factors. In persons with hypertension, cardiac conditions, or diabetes, the risk of heart failure varies with the associated burden of modifiable risk factors and indicators of left ventricular dysfunction.[59] Therefore, a multipronged approach to identify and modify risk factors early in the illness trajectory, as well as throughout treatment of heart failure, is important.

MORBIDITY

Heart failure is associated with substantial morbidity and is a major reason for hospital admissions and readmissions. Hospitalizations for heart failure have risen considerably over time, from 377,000 in 1979 to 970,000 in 2002, an increase of 157 percent.[21] Although hospitalization for heart failure is increasing, the total number of hospital days for this diagnosis has leveled off, probably because of a substantial decline in length of stay. One possible consequence of decreasing length of stay is an increase in hospital readmission.[4] Several investigators have reported that patients who survive hospitalization for heart failure are particularly vulnerable to readmission.[60-62] In one large study of Medicare beneficiaries in Connecticut,[61] 44 percent were readmitted within 6 months after hospitalization for heart failure. In a study from Scotland,[60] 85 percent of patients in a national database were readmitted for heart failure or died within 3 years after a first admission for heart failure. Cardiovascular events (e.g., myocardial infarction and atrial fibrillation) and noncardiovascular events (e.g., renal failure and acute respiratory infection) precipitated these readmissions. The high hospital readmission rates emphasize the vulnerability of persons with heart failure to recurrent illness.

Although hospitalization for heart failure traditionally is considered the best marker of morbidity, these data relate only to persons who require treatment in a hospital and do not completely reflect what it is like to live with heart failure. Heart failure often significantly impairs the performance of activities of daily living. The diagnosis of heart failure brings with it a constellation of activity-limiting symptoms, such as dyspnea, fatigue, and fluid retention.[63] These symptoms can affect the quality of one's life. In addition to quality of life, other psychosocial factors, such as social support, anxiety, and depression, have emerged as important independent predictors of morbidity in persons with heart failure.[63,64]

MORTALITY

Heart failure has a high mortality rate. In fact, heart failure has a shorter life expectancy than many types of cancer.[13,65] Until recently, data indicated that the death rate from heart failure was increasing over time. Now it appears that, depending on the source of the data, this trend may be reversing.

Data regarding mortality are derived from various types of sources, such as population-based studies (e.g., Framingham or Rochester), national mortality statistics (e.g., National Center for Health Statistics), hospital-based studies, and drug trials (e.g., Cooperative North Scandinavian Enalapril Survival Study [**CONSENSUS**], Survival and Ventricular Enlargement [**SAVE**], and **SOLVD**). Each of these sources has advantages and disadvantages and can produce different mortality figures. Population-based studies reflect deaths from heart failure in the particular community under study and may not be generalizable to areas with different demographic characteristics. National mortality statistics are based on information from death certificates. The fact that heart failure is often a contributing cause of death, rather than an underlying cause of death, must be considered when interpreting national mortality statistics. Hospital-based studies are biased by limiting inclusion to sicker patients requiring hospitalization. In many cases, heart failure is diagnosed outside the hospital. Hospital-based studies evaluate survival after hospitalization for heart failure, not after the first occurrence of heart failure, so the mortality rate may seem higher. Drug trials are composed of a highly select group of patients, so even examining mortality just in the placebo group may not be generalizable to the entire population with heart failure.

The latest Framingham data revealed that age-adjusted 30-day mortality rates for men and women were 11 percent and 10 percent, respectively; 1-year mortality rates were 28 percent and 24 percent, respectively; and 5-year mortality rates were 59 percent and 45 percent, respectively (Table 3-5).[6] Table 3-5 also reveals that after a slight increase in the 1970s, mortality in persons with heart failure has declined in men and women over the last five decades. The reason for the decline in mortality is uncertain. Contributing factors could be time-dependent shifts in heart failure causes (CAD versus valvular disease or hypertension) or improved medical management.[1] Similar trends in mortality rates were reported in the Rochester study.[8]

From clinical trials[22,66-68] it is clear that the use of angiotensin-converting enzyme inhibitors improves survival in persons with heart failure. Population-based studies suggest that the efficacy of angiotensin-converting enzyme inhibitors found in clinical trials may be having a benefit at the community level.[1]

In general, mortality rates are higher in men than women and higher in blacks than whites. The National Center for Health Statistics has reported that among persons age 65 and older, age-adjusted mortality rates for 1995 were 126.1 per 100,000 for black men, 117.0 for white men, 107.6 for black women, and 101.2 for white women.[69]

■ ■ ■

TABLE 3-5   TEMPORAL TRENDS IN AGE-ADJUSTED MORTALITY AFTER THE ONSET OF HEART FAILURE AMONG MEN AND WOMEN AGES 65 TO 74*

	30-DAY MORTALITY PERCENT (95 PERCENT CONFIDENCE INTERVAL)		1-YEAR MORTALITY PERCENT (95 PERCENT CONFIDENCE INTERVAL)		5-YEAR MORTALITY PERCENT (95 PERCENT CONFIDENCE INTERVAL)	
PERIOD	MEN	WOMEN	MEN	WOMEN	MEN	WOMEN
1950-1969	12 (4-19)	18 (7-27)	30 (18-40)	28 (16-39)	70 (57-79)	57 (43-67)
1970-1979	15 (7-23)	16 (6-24)	41 (29-51)	28 (17-38)	75 (65-83)	59 (45-69)
1980-1989	12 (5-18)	10 (4-16)	33 (23-42)	27 (17-35)	65 (54-73)	51 (39-60)
1990-1999	11 (4-17)	10 (3-15)	28 (18-36)	24 (14-33)	59 (47-68)	45 (33-55)

*All values adjusted for age (less than 55, 55 to 64, 65 to 74, 75 to 84, 85 years or older).
Data from Levy D, Kenchaiah S, Larson MG et al: *N Engl J Med* 347:1397-1402, 2002.

Data about the relative effect of diastolic versus systolic dysfunction on mortality are conflicting. In the Framingham study, diastolic heart failure was associated with better long-term survival,[70] whereas in the Rochester study it was a more powerful predictor of mortality than was systolic dysfunction.[71] This difference could result from differences in the way diastolic heart failure was defined and measured in the particular studies.

The mechanism of death in heart failure varies. Most persons with heart failure experience sudden death or die of progressive pump or circulatory failure. Sudden death usually is defined as death within 1 hour of the onset of symptoms. Sudden death is at least as common in the setting of heart failure as it is in CAD and is responsible for up to half of all deaths in persons with heart failure. This represents 6 to 9 times the rate of sudden death in the general population.[21] Although progressive pump failure accounts for most of the remainder of deaths, noncardiac illnesses also contribute. Patients with heart failure often tolerate conditions such as pneumonia, systemic and pulmonary embolism, and stroke poorly and may die of one of these conditions, with heart failure as a contributing rather than underlying, cause of death.[3,5]

SUMMARY

About 550,000 new cases of heart failure are diagnosed each year in the United States. The incidence of heart failure increases with age and is higher in men than in women. About 5 million Americans—2.3 percent of the population—currently are living with heart failure. Prevalence increases with age and may be slightly higher in men.

A number of potential risk factors have emerged recently. In addition to the factors long known to cause or increase the occurrence of heart failure (e.g., hypertension, CAD, diabetes, valve disease, hypercholesterolemia, left ventricular hypertrophy, black race, and older age), toxins, metabolic syndrome, sleep-disordered breathing, depression, and alcohol intake may play an increasingly important role in the development of heart failure in the future.

Recently, the phenomenon of reverse epidemiology has been noted. Traditional risk factors for the development of cardiovascular disease in general, and heart failure in particular (obesity, hypercholesterolemia, and hypertension) have been found to increase survival in patients with existing heart failure.

Hospital admission and readmission for heart failure are commonly cited indicators of morbidity. Both have been increasing over the last 20 years. Mortality is declining, although heart failure is still a highly lethal condition.

The epidemiology of heart failure has evolved considerably in the last decade. The scope of heart failure has expanded to include not only persons with symptomatic heart failure but also those with asymptomatic, or preclinical, ventricular dysfunction. Including these asymptomatic individuals has exposed the submerged portion of the heart failure iceberg. The prevention of clinical heart failure with accurate and cost-effective screening techniques for preclinical ventricular dysfunction and the early initiation of therapeutic intervention is now the highest priority.[1] The early identification of patients at risk for heart failure (stage A) and asymptomatic patients with structural heart disease (stage B) is critical to begin to reverse the epidemic of heart failure and decrease the population burden of heart failure morbidity and mortality.

REFERENCES

1. Rodeheffer RJ: The new epidemiology of heart failure, *Curr Cardiol Rep* 5:181-186, 2003.
2. Hunt SA, Baker DW, Chin MH et al: ACC/AHA guidelines for the evaluation and management of chronic heart failure in the adult: executive summary—a report of the American College of Cardiology/American Heart Association Task Force on Practice Guidelines (Committee to Revise the 1995 Guidelines for the Evaluation and Management of Heart Failure), *Circulation* 104: 2996-3007, 2001.
3. Young JP: The global epidemiology of heart failure, *Med Clin North Am* 88:1135-1143, 2004.
4. Funk M, Milner KA, Krumholz HM: Epidemiology of heart failure. In Moser DK, Riegel B, editors: *Improving outcomes in heart failure: an interdisciplinary approach*, Gaithersburg, Md, 2001, Aspen.
5. Kannel WB, Vasan RS: Epidemiology of heart failure. In Mann DL, editor: *Heart failure: a companion to Braunwald's heart disease*, Philadelphia, 2004, WB Saunders.
6. Levy D, Kenchaiah S, Larson MG et al: Long-term trends in the incidence of and survival with heart failure, *N Engl J Med* 347:1397-1402, 2002.

7. Senni M, Tribouilloy CM, Rodeheffer RJ et al: Congestive heart failure in the community: trends in incidence and survival in a 10-year period, *Arch Intern Med* 159:29-34, 1999.

8. Roger VL, Weston SA, Redfield MM et al: Trends in heart failure incidence and survival in a community-based population, *JAMA* 292:344-350, 2004.

9. Remes J, Reunanen A, Aromaa A et al: Incidence of heart failure in eastern Finland: a population-based surveillance study, *Eur Heart J* 13:588-593, 1992.

10. Lloyd-Jones DM, Larson MG, Leip EP et al: Lifetime risk for developing congestive heart failure: the Framingham Heart Study, *Circulation* 106:3068-3072, 2002.

11. Hellermann JP, Goraya TY, Jacobsen SJ et al: Incidence of heart failure after myocardial infarction: is it changing over time? *Am J Epidemiol* 157:1101-1107, 2003.

12. Schocken DD, Arrieta MI, Leaverton PE et al: Prevalence and mortality rate of congestive heart failure in the United States, *J Am Coll Cardiol* 20:301-306, 1992.

13. Ho KKL, Pinsky JL, Kannel WB et al: The epidemiology of heart failure: the Framingham study, *J Am Coll Cardiol* 22(suppl A): 6A-13A, 1993.

14. Mittelmark MB, Psaty BM, Rautaharju PM et al: Prevalence of cardiovascular diseases among older adults: the Cardiovascular Health Study, *Am J Epidemiol* 137:311-317, 1993.

15. Kupari M, Lindroos M, Iivanainen AM et al: Congestive heart failure in old age: prevalence, mechanisms and 4-year prognosis in the Helsinki Ageing Study, *J Intern Med* 241:387-394, 1997.

16. McDonagh TA, Morrison CE, Lawrence A et al: Symptomatic and asymptomatic left ventricular systolic dysfunction in an urban population, *Lancet* 350:829-833, 1997.

17. Wilhelmsen L, Rosengren A, Eriksson H et al: Heart failure in the general population of men: mortality, risk factors and prognosis, *J Intern Med* 249:253-261, 2001.

18. Devereux RB, Roman MJ, Paranicas M et al: A population-based assessment of left ventricular systolic dysfunction in middle-aged and older adults: the Strong Heart Study, *Am Heart J* 141:439-446, 2001.

19. Hanyu N: Prevalence of self-reported heart failure among US adults: results from the 1999 National Health Interview Survey, *Am Heart J* 146:121-128, 2003.

20. Redfield MM, Jacobsen SJ, Burnett JC et al: Burden of systolic and diastolic ventricular dysfunction in the community, *JAMA* 289:194-202, 2003.

21. Thom T, Haass N, Rosamond W et al: Heart disease and stroke statistics: 2006 update, *Circulation* 113:85-151, 2006.

22. The SOLVD Investigators: Effect of enalapril on mortality and the development of heart failure in asymptomatic patients with reduced left ventricular ejection fractions, *N Engl J Med* 327:685-691, 1992.

23. Gottdiener JS, Arnold AM, Aurigemma GP et al: Predictors of congestive heart failure in the elderly: the Cardiovascular Health Study, *J Am Coll Cardiol* 35:1628-1637, 1996.

24. He J, Ogden LG, Bazzano LA et al: Risk factors for congestive heart failure in US men and women: NHANES I Epidemiologic Follow-Up Study, *Arch Intern Med* 161:996-1002, 2001.

25. Levy D, Larson MG, Vasen RS et al: The progression from hypertension to congestive heart failure, *JAMA* 275:1557-1562, 1996.

26. Kannel WB: Needs and prospects for prevention of cardiac failure, *Eur J Clin Pharmacol* 49:3-9, 1996.

27. Kenchaiah S, Gaziano JM, Vasen RS: Impact of obesity on the risk of heart failure and survival after the onset of heart failure, *Med Clin North Am* 88:1273-1294, 2004.

28. Rauchhaus M, Clark AL, Doehner W et al: The relationship between cholesterol and survival in patients with chronic heart failure, *J Am Coll Cardiol* 42:1933-1940, 2003.

29. von Haehling S, Anker SD: Statins for heart failure: at the crossroads between cholesterol reduction and pleiotropism, *Heart* 91:1-2, 2005.

30. Suskin N, Sheth T, Negressa A et al: Relationship of current and past smoking to mortality and morbidity in patients with left ventricular dysfunction, *J Am Coll Cardiol* 37:1677-1682, 2001.

31. Mondoa CT: The implications of physical activity in patients with chronic heart failure, *Nurs Crit Care* 9:13-20, 2004.

32. Yancy CW: Does race matter in heart failure? *Am Heart J* 146:203-206, 2003.

33. Ghali JK, Krause-Steinrauf HJ, Adams KF et al: Gender differences in advanced heart failure: insights from the BEST Study, *J Am Coll Cardiol* 42:2128-2134, 2003.

34. Simon T, Mary-Krause M, Funck-Brentano C et al: Sex differences in the prognosis of congestive heart failure, *Circulation* 103:375-380, 2000.

35. Rathore SS, Foody JM, Wang Y et al: Sex, quality of care, and outcomes of elderly patients hospitalized with heart failure: findings from the National Heart Failure Project, *Am Heart J* 149:121-128, 2005.

36. Dries DL, Exner DV, Gersh BJ et al: Racial differences in the outcome of left ventricular dysfunction, *N Engl J Med* 340:609-616, 1999.

37. Dunlap SH, Mallemala S, Sueta CA et al: Survival rates are similar between African American and white patients with heart failure, *Am Heart J* 146:265-272, 2003.

38. Taylor AL, Ziesche S, Yancy C et al: Combination of isosorbide dinitrate and hydralazine in blacks with heart failure, *N Engl J Med* 351:2049-2057, 2004.

39. Mostard A, Cost B, Hoes AW et al: The prognosis of heart failure in the general population: the Rotterdam Study, *Eur Heart J* 22:1318-1327, 2001.

40. Cowie MR, Wood DA, Coats AJ et al: Survival of patients with a new diagnosis of heart failure: a population based study, *Heart* 83:505-510, 2000.

41. Havranek EP, Masoudi FA, Westfall KA et al: Spectrum of heart failure in older patients: results from the National Heart Failure Project, *Am Heart J* 143:412-417, 2002.

42. Kenchaiah S, Narula J, Vasen RS: Risk factors for heart failure, *Med Clin North Am* 88:1145-1172, 2004.

43. Shahar E, Whitney CW, Redline S et al: Sleep-disordered breathing and cardiovascular disease: cross-sectional results of the Sleep Heart Health Study, *Am J Respir Crit Care Med* 163:19-25, 2001.

44. Abramson J, Berger A, Krumholz HM et al: Depression and risk of heart failure among older persons with isolated systolic hypertension, *Arch Intern Med* 161:1725-1730, 2001.

45. Williams SA, Kasil SV, Heiat A et al: Depression and risk of heart failure among the elderly: a prospective community-based study, *Psychosom Med* 64:6-12, 2002.

46. Gavazzi A, DeMaria A, Parolini M et al: Alcohol abuse and cardiomyopathy in men, *Am J Cardiol* 85:1114-1118, 2000.

47. Walsh CR, Larson MJ, Evans JC et al: Alcohol consumption and risk for congestive heart failure in the Framingham Heart Study, *Ann Intern Med* 136:181-191, 2002.

48. Abramson JL, Williams SA, Krumholz HM et al: Moderate alcohol consumption and risk of heart failure among older persons, *JAMA* 285:1971-1977, 2001.

49. Piano MR: Alcohol and heart failure, *J Card Fail* 8:239-246, 2002.

50. Kalantar-Zadeh K, Block G, Horwich T et al: Reverse epidemiology of conventional cardiovascular risk factors with chronic heart failure, *J Am Coll Cardiol* 43:1439-1444, 2004.

51. Wassertheiel-Smoller S, Fann C, Allman RM et al: Relation of low body mass to death and stroke in the Systolic Hypertension in the Elderly Program: the SHEP Cooperative Research Group, *Arch Intern Med* 160:494-500, 2000.

52. Curtis JP, Selter JG, Wang Y et al: The obesity paradox: body mass index and outcomes in patients with heart failure, *Arch Intern Med* 165:55-61, 2005.

53. Vredevoe DL, Woo MA, Doering LV et al: Skin test anergy in advanced heart failure secondary to either ischemic or idiopathic dilated cardiomyopathy, *Am J Cardiol* 82:323-328, 1998.

54. Horwich TB, Fonarow GC: The impact of obesity on survival in patients with heart failure, *Heart Fail Monit* 3:8-14, 2002.

55. Ghali JK: Contemporary issues in heart failure, *Am Heart J* 138:5-8, 1999.

56. Poole-Wilson PA, Swedberg K, Cleland JG et al: Comparison of carvedilol and metoprolol on clinical outcomes in patients with chronic heart failure in the Carvedilol or Metoprolol European Trial (COMET): randomised controlled trial, *Lancet* 362:7-13, 2003.

57. Ajayi AA, Adigun AQ, Ojofeitimi EO et al: Anthropometric evaluation of cachexia in congestive heart failure: the role of tricuspid regurgitation, *Int J Cardiol* 71:79-84, 1999.

58. Conraads VM, Bosmans JM, Vrints CJ: Chronic heart failure: an example of a systemic chronic inflammatory disease resulting in cachexia, *Int J Cardiol* 85:33-49, 2002.

59. Kannel WB: Lessons from curbing the coronary artery disease epidemic for confronting the impending epidemic of heart failure, *Med Clin North Am* 88:1129-1133, 2004.

60. Khand AU, Gemmell I, Rankin AC et al: Clinical events leading to the progression of heart failure: insights from a national database of hospital discharges, *Eur Heart J* 22:153-164, 2001.

61. Krumholz HM, Parent EM, Tu N et al: Readmission after hospitalization for congestive heart failure among Medicare beneficiaries, *Arch Intern Med* 157:99-104, 1997.

62. Philbin EF, Rocco TA Jr, Lindenmuth NW et al: Clinical outcomes in heart failure: report from a community hospital-based registry, *Am J Med* 107:549-555, 1999.

63. Moser DK, Worster PL: Effect of psychosocial factors on physiologic outcomes in patients with heart failure, *J Cardiovasc Nurs* 14:106-115, 2000.

64. Moser DK: Psychosocial factors and their association with clinical outcomes in patients with heart failure: why clinicians do not seem to care, *Eur J Cardiovasc Nurs* 1:183-188, 2002.

65. Stewart S, MacIntyre K, Hole DJ et al: More 'malignant' than cancer? Five-year survival following a first admission for heart failure, *Eur J Heart Fail* 3:315-322, 2001.

66. The CONSENSUS Trial Study Group: Effects of enalapril on mortality in severe congestive heart failure: results of the Cooperative North Scandinavian Enalapril Survival Study (CONSENSUS), *N Engl J Med* 316:1429-1435, 1987.

67. Pfeffer MA, Braunwald E, Moye LA et al: Effect of captopril on mortality and morbidity in patients with left ventricular dysfunction after myocardial infarction: results of the Survival and Ventricular Enlargement trial—the SAVE investigators, *N Engl J Med* 327:669-677, 1992.

68. The SOLVD Investigators: Effect of enalapril on survival in patients with reduced ejection fractions and congestive heart failure, *N Engl J Med* 325:293-302, 1991.

69. Centers for Disease Control and Prevention: Changes in mortality from heart failure: United States, 1980-1995, *MMWR Morb Mortal Wkly Rep* 47:633-637, 1998.

70. Vasan RS, Larson MG, Benjamin EJ et al: Congestive heart failure in subjects with normal versus reduced left ventricular ejection fraction: prevalence and mortality in a population-based cohort, *J Am Coll Cardiol* 33:1948-1955, 1999.

71. Pritchett AM, Mahoney DW, Jacobsen SJ et al: Diastolic dysfunction and left atrial volume: a population-based study, *J Am Coll Cardiol* 45:87-92, 2005.

Anatomy of the Cardiovascular System

Joseph A. Rubertone

CHAPTER ABBREVIATIONS

AV   atrioventricular

SA   sinoatrial

The cardiovascular system consists of the heart and its associated vessels. The unique structure of the cardiovascular system allows for the distribution of blood throughout the body, a process that supplies all cells with oxygen and nutrients and removes metabolic wastes and carbon dioxide from the tissues. The cardiovascular system also provides a conduit for hormones and cells of the immune defense system and participates in the regulation of body temperature.

The heart consists of two dual-chambered muscular pumps that contract synchronously and continuously at about 70 times a minute throughout life. The right and left pumps consist of an intake chamber (atrium) and an outflow chamber (ventricle) each. The atria receive blood from the great veins, and the ventricles pump blood through the arterial trunks. Each set of chambers is separated by valves, which greatly enhance the pumping action of the chambers. The right atrium receives oxygen-depleted blood from the body (Figure 4-1). The blood then passes through the right atrioventricular **(AV)** valve to the right ventricle, which pumps it to the lungs. Oxygenated blood returns to the heart via the left atrium, passes through the left atrioventricular valve, and is pumped into the aorta by the left ventricle.

The vascular system consists of miles of channels uniquely adapted for transporting fluids, gases, nutrients, metabolic waste, cells, and hormones. The channels vary by histological structure and luminal diameter according to function. The lymphatic system is a parallel circulatory system that functions to return excess interstitial fluid to the heart.

The purpose of this chapter is to describe the structure of the heart and vascular system with an emphasis on clinically relevant functional anatomy and histology. See Chapter 5 for a discussion of cardiovascular physiology.

GROSS ANATOMY OF THE HEART
Location and Position

The heart resides within the mediastinum. This central area of the thoracic cavity contains all the viscera of the chest except the lungs and visceral pleura. The heart, pericardium, and origins of the great vessels form the *middle mediastinum* (Figure 4-2).

The position of the heart can be delineated further by descriptions of its base, apex, anatomical surfaces, and margins. The *base* of the heart is formed by the left atrium, pulmonary veins, and origins of the great vessels (Figure 4-3). The base of the heart faces posteriorly and to the right and lies anterior to thoracic vertebrae 5 to 8 in supine or 7 to 9 in erect posture. The *apex* of the heart, formed mainly by the tip of the left ventricle, faces anteriorly to the left (Figure 4-4). The apex of the heart resides deep to the 5th intercostal space at about the midclavicular line (Figure 4-5).

The anterior or *sternocostal surface* of the heart faces forward and upward and is formed mainly by the right atrium and right ventricle. Sulci or grooves visible in this surface include the anterior portion of the atrioventricular or *coronary sulcus* and the *anterior interventricular sulcus* (Figure 4-6, *A*). The inferior or *diaphragmatic surface* rests on the diaphragm (Figure 4-6B). The diaphragmatic surface is formed mainly by the left ventricle. The *posterior interventricular sulcus* separates the left ventricle from the right ventricle. The posterior portion of the coronary sulcus separates the diaphragmatic surface from the base or posterior aspect of the heart. The left surface consists of the *obtuse margin* of the left ventricle and is bounded laterally by the left phrenic nerve and pleura of the left lung. The right surface consists of the right atrium above and the right ventricle below. The right surface is bordered laterally by the right phrenic nerve and the pleura of the right lung. The *acute margin* courses horizontally toward the apex where the right ventricle meets the diaphragm (Figure 4-7).

Surface Projection

Surface projections, as all areas of anatomical science, are subject to variations. The surface projection of the heart (Figure 4-5) can vary according to gender, age, stature, posture, and ventilation.[1] To draw the surface projection on a colleague's chest, you would place dots 1 cm lateral to the sternum on each of the following landmarks: (a) the second left costal cartilage, (b) the third right costal cartilage, and (c) the sixth right costal cartilage. Place a fourth dot in the 5th intercostal space at the midclavicular line at the point of the apex of the heart (d). Connecting the dots reveals the borders of the heart. The *superior border* is a sloping line connecting dots *a* and *b*. The *right border* is a laterally curved line from *b* to *c*. The *inferior border* forming the acute margin of the heart runs from *c* to *d*. The *left border,* corresponding to the obtuse margin, is a line that curves laterally as it runs from *d* to *a*. *Text continued on p. 50*

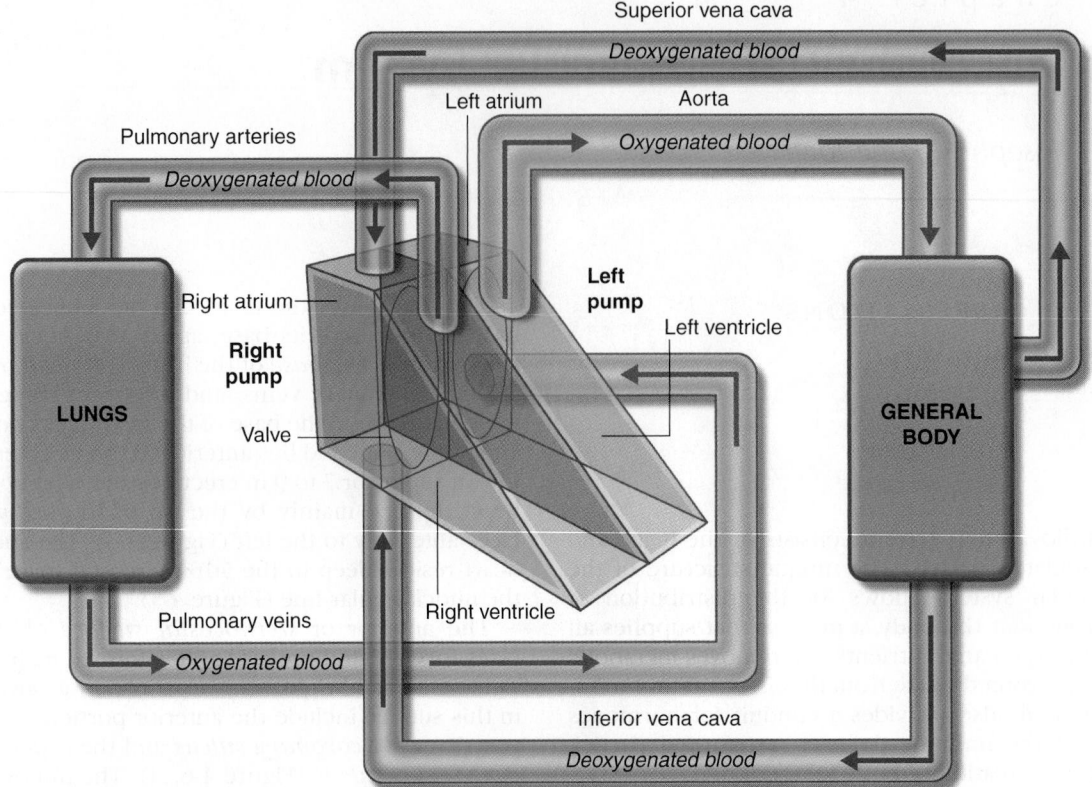

FIGURE 4-1 ■ Cardiovascular system. (From Drake R, Vogl W, Mitchel AWM: *Gray's anatomy for students,* Edinburgh, 2005, Elsevier Churchill Livingstone.)

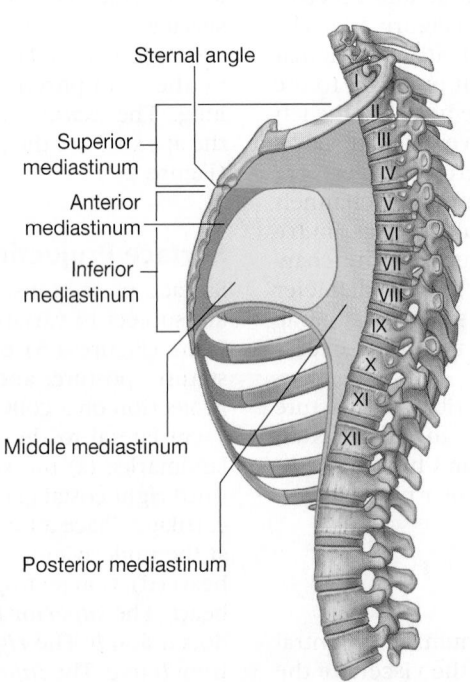

FIGURE 4-2 ■ Subdivisions of the mediastinum. (From Drake R, Vogl W, Mitchel AWM: *Gray's anatomy for students,* Edinburgh, 2005, Elsevier Churchill Livingstone.)

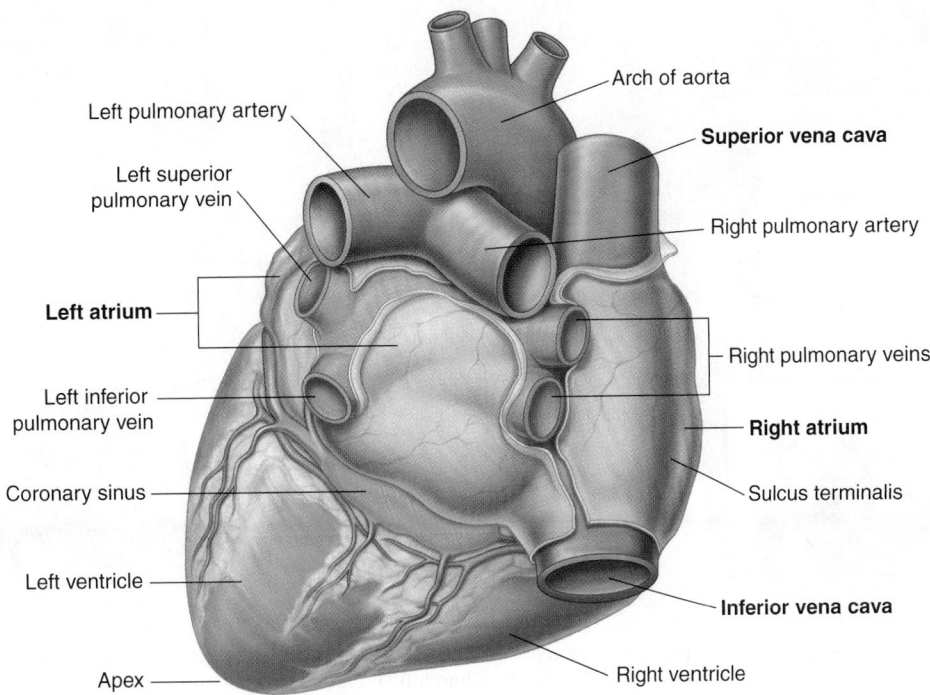

FIGURE 4-3 ▪ Base of the heart. (From Drake R, Vogl W, Mitchel AWM: *Gray's anatomy for students,* Edinburgh, 2005, Elsevier Churchill Livingstone.)

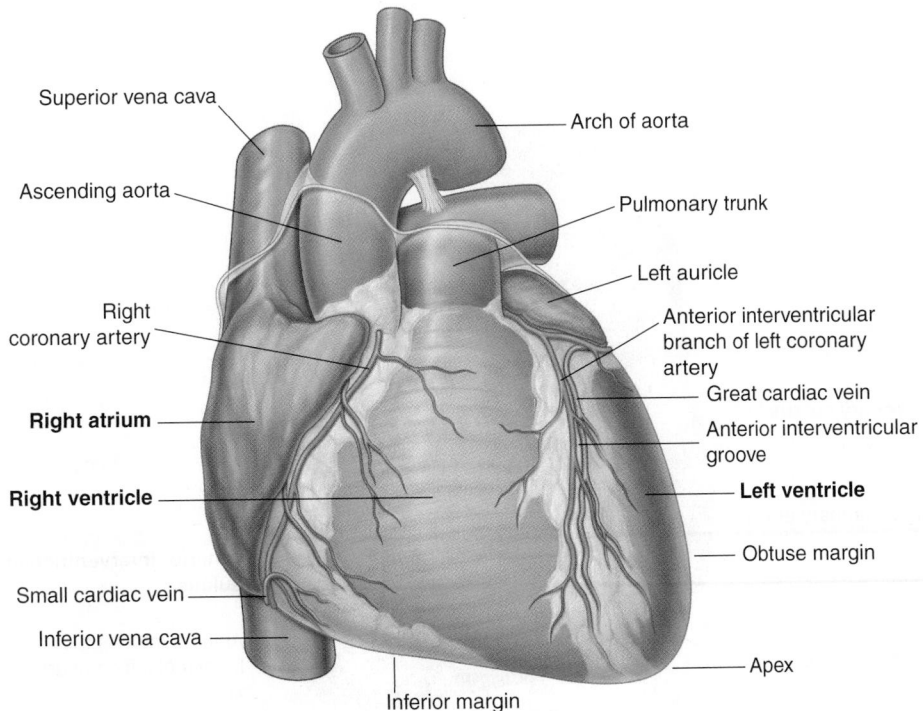

FIGURE 4-4 ▪ Apex of the heart. (From Drake R, Vogl W, Mitchel AWM: *Gray's anatomy for students,* Edinburgh, 2005, Elsevier Churchill Livingstone.)

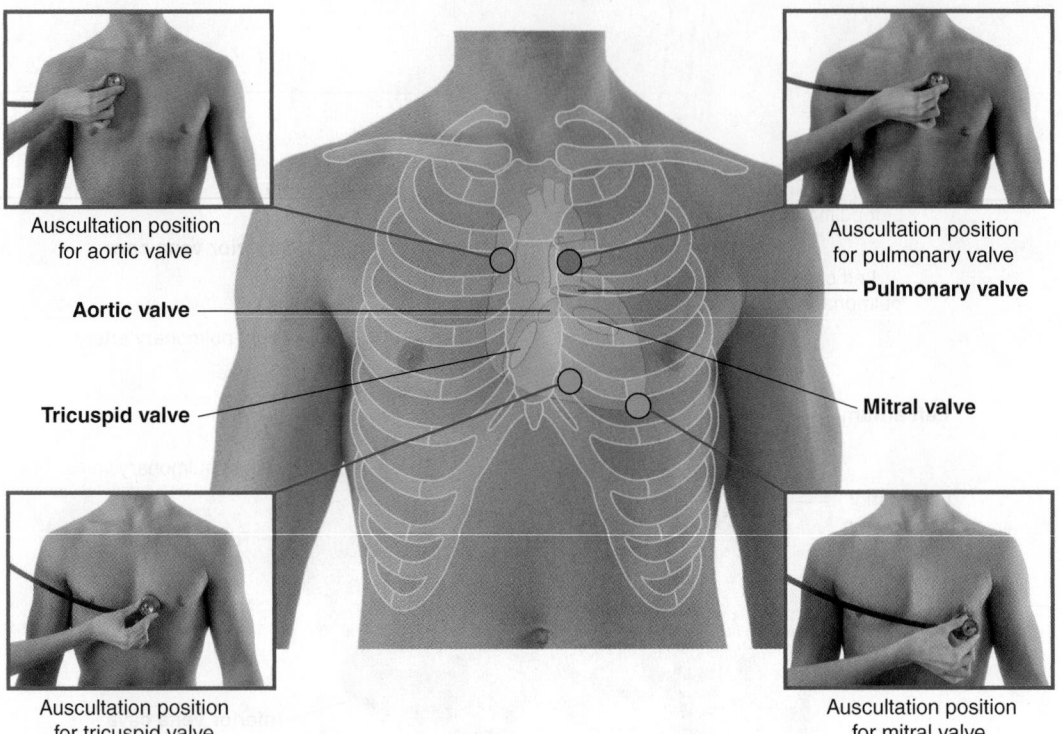

Auscultation position for aortic valve

Aortic valve

Tricuspid valve

Auscultation position for pulmonary valve

Pulmonary valve

Mitral valve

Auscultation position for tricuspid valve

Auscultation position for mitral valve

FIGURE 4-5 ■ Surface projection of the heart. (From Drake R, Vogl W, Mitchel AWM: *Gray's anatomy for students,* Edinburgh, 2005, Elsevier Churchill Livingstone.)

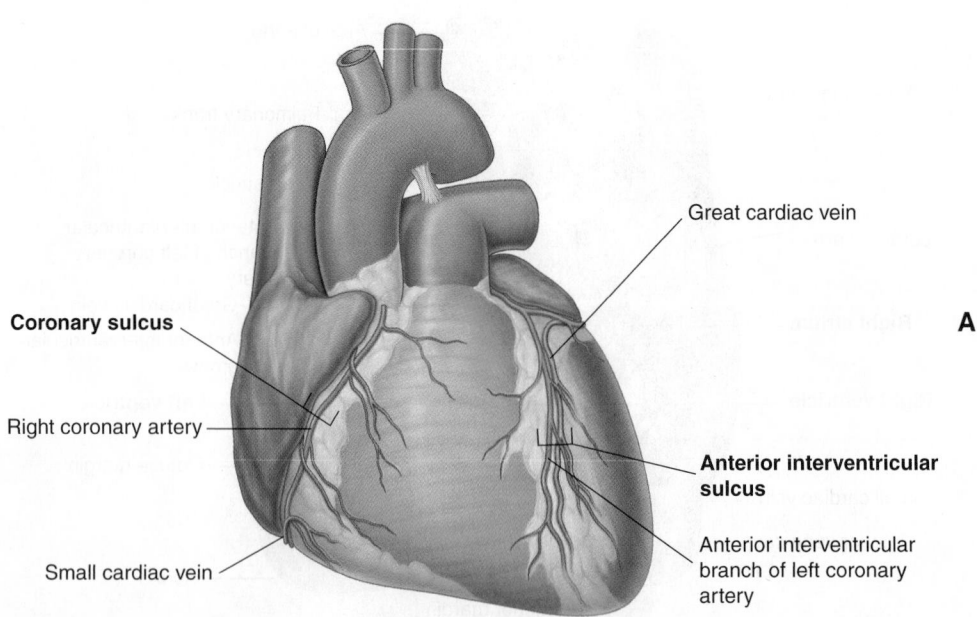

Great cardiac vein

Coronary sulcus

Right coronary artery

Small cardiac vein

Anterior interventricular sulcus

Anterior interventricular branch of left coronary artery

A

FIGURE 4-6 ■ Surfaces of the heart. **A,** Sternocostal surface. (From Drake R, Vogl W, Mitchel AWM: *Gray's anatomy for students,* Edinburgh, 2005, Elsevier Churchill Livingstone.)

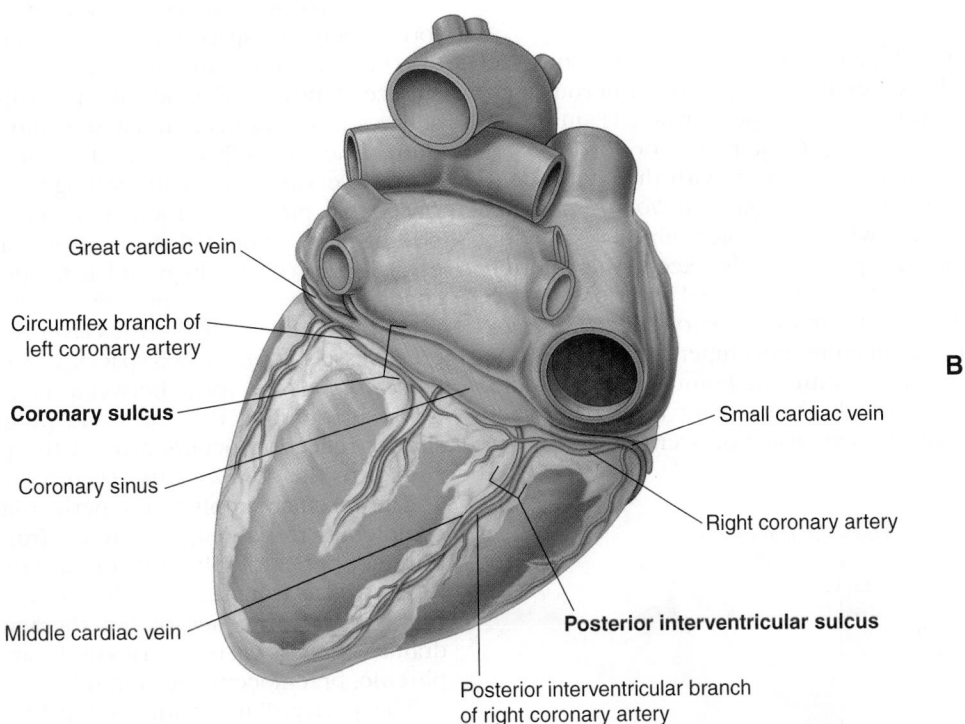

Great cardiac vein

Circumflex branch of
left coronary artery

Coronary sulcus

Coronary sinus

Middle cardiac vein

Small cardiac vein

Right coronary artery

Posterior interventricular sulcus

Posterior interventricular branch
of right coronary artery

B

FIGURE 4-6, cont'd ■ **B,** Diaphragmatic surface. (From Drake R, Vogl W, Mitchel AWM: *Gray's anatomy for students,* Edinburgh, 2005, Elsevier Churchill Livingstone.)

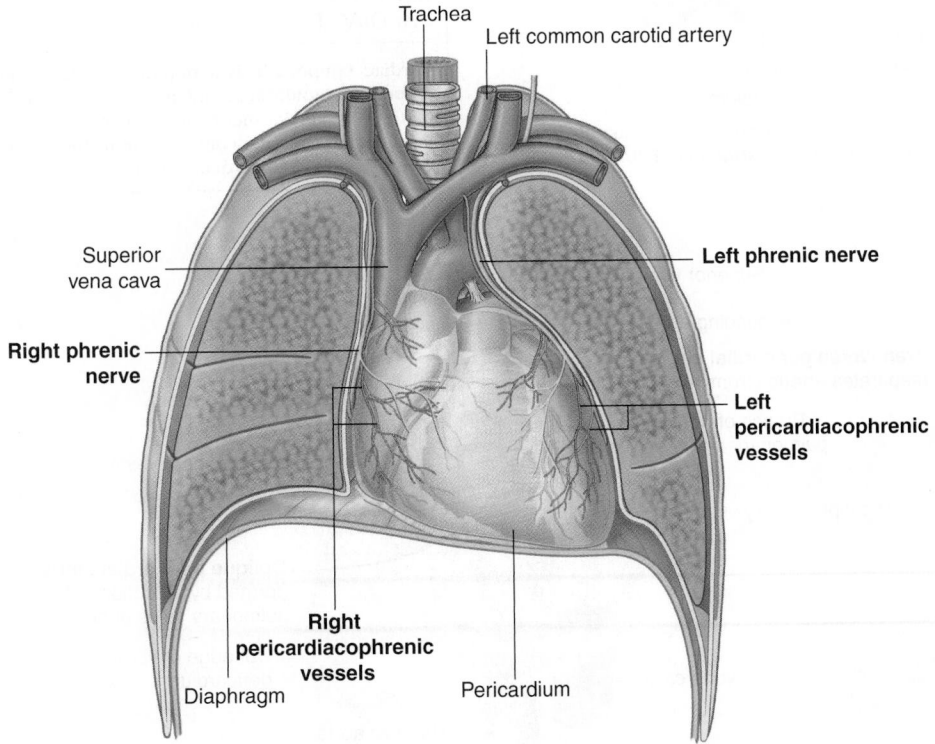

Trachea

Left common carotid artery

Superior
vena cava

**Right phrenic
nerve**

Left phrenic nerve

**Left
pericardiacophrenic
vessels**

**Right
pericardiacophrenic
vessels**

Diaphragm

Pericardium

FIGURE 4-7 ■ Margins of the heart. (From Drake R, Vogl W, Mitchel AWM: *Gray's anatomy for students,* Edinburgh, 2005, Elsevier Churchill Livingstone.)

Pericardium

The heart is enveloped by a double-walled serous sac that is strengthened externally by a tough fibrous connective tissue layer. This sac or pericardium (Figure 4-8) consists of three layers. The outer layer, or *fibrous pericardium,* is continuous inferiorly with the central tendon of the diaphragm via the *pericardiophrenic ligament* and blends with the outer fibrous layer or adventitia of all the great vessels except the inferior vena cava. The outer layer is attached anteriorly to the sternum by the highly variable *sternopericardial ligaments.* These ligamentous attachments keep this incredibly active organ within the bounds of the middle mediastinum. The tough fibrous outer layer also is believed to limit cardiac expansion or overfilling.[2]

The double-walled serous layer reflects upon itself to form a potential space known as the *pericardial cavity.* The outer layer, or *parietal pericardium,* lines the inner surface of the fibrous pericardium. The inner visceral layer adheres to the myocardium and is known as the *epicardium.* The serous fluid secreted by these specialized epithelial layers forms a thin lubricating film in the pericardial cavity that provides a friction-free environment for the beating heart. Abnormal accumulation of fluid in the pericardial space can produce cardiac tamponade (Box 4-1), a condition covered in Chapters 59, 68, and 75.[3]

As the double-walled serous layer reflects around the great vessels, it forms two spaces, or sinuses. The *transverse sinus* is the space between the pericardial reflections surrounding the aorta and pulmonary trunk. A similar reflection occurs around the pulmonary veins and forms the *oblique sinus* (Figure 4-9).

The vascular supply to the pericardium is varied and complex. Arterial supply stems from the musculophrenic, pericardiophrenic, and inferior phrenic arteries, as well as from the bronchial, esophageal, and superior phrenic branches of the thoracic aorta. Venous drainage occurs via tributaries of the azygos, pericardiophrenic, brachiocephalic, and internal thoracic veins.

The pericardium is innervated by branches of the sympathetic trunk, vagus, and phrenic nerves. Although the sympathetic innervation is known to be vasomotor, function of the vagal fibers is uncertain. Pericardial pain is carried by afferent fibers in the phrenic nerve (Box 4-2). Assessment of cardiac pain is described in depth in Chapter 53.

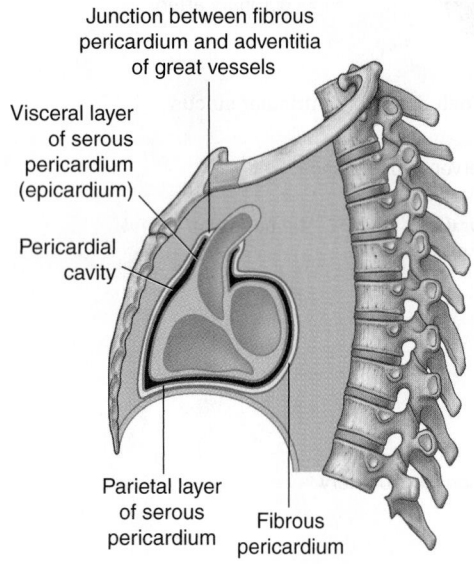

FIGURE 4-8 ■ Pericardium of the heart. (From Drake R, Vogl W, Mitchel AWM: *Gray's anatomy for students,* Edinburgh, 2005, Elsevier Churchill Livingstone.)

BOX 4-1 ■■■
CARDIAC TAMPONADE

Cardiac tamponade is a potentially fatal condition that occurs when fluid rapidly accumulates in the pericardial cavity as a result of trauma, aortic aneurysm, or cardiac surgery. The increased fluid causes external compression of the heart, which decreases venous return and cardiac output.

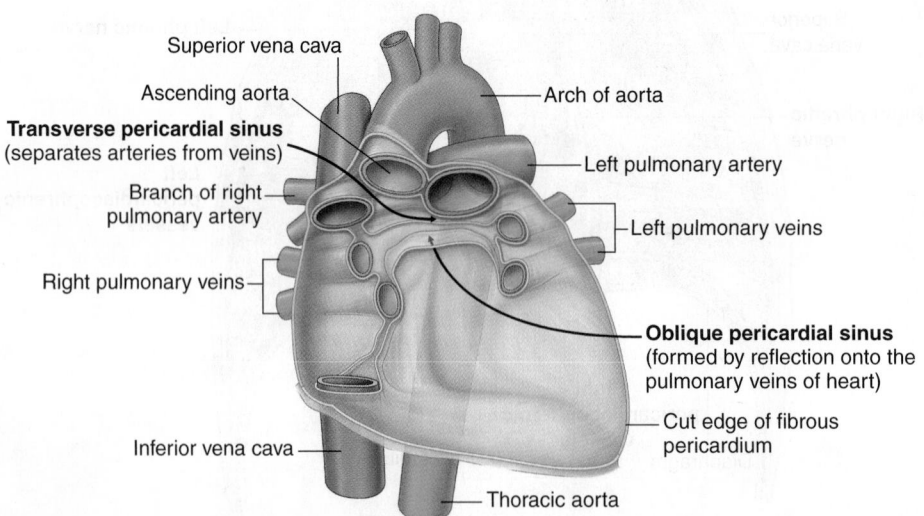

FIGURE 4-9 ■ Pericardial sinuses. (From Drake R, Vogl W, Mitchel AWM: *Gray's anatomy for students,* Edinburgh, 2005, Elsevier Churchill Livingstone.)

Heart Chambers
Right Atrium

The right atrium (Figure 4-10) receives deoxygenated blood from the systemic and coronary circulatory systems. Blood from the superior and inferior venae cavae enter the smooth-walled area of the atrium known as the *sinus venarum*. During the fetal period, the crescent-shaped *valve of the inferior vena cava* (eustachian valve) shunts oxygenated blood from the umbilical veins through the foramen ovale to the left atrium. This opening usually is closed at birth by the septum primum to form a shallow depression known as the *fossa ovalis*. This thumb print–sized depression on the interatrial septum is bounded superiorly by a ridge known as the *limbus of the fossa ovalis.* The opening of the coronary sinus shunts the greater part of the coronary venous return back into the right atrium. The *valve of the coronary sinus* (thebesian valve) is contiguous with the valve of the inferior vena cava.[4]

The *crista terminalis* or terminal crest is a vertical muscular ridge that separates the sinus venarum from the anterior portion of the chamber, which is derived from the primordial embryonic atrium. Fine muscular ridges (musculi pectinati, or *pectinate muscles*) leave the crest at right angles to course anteriorly to infuse the wall of the *right auricle.* This area is subject to a number of atrial septal defects (Box 4-3).[5] Congenital cardiac defects are described fully in Chapters 70 and 71.

Right Ventricle

The right ventricle (Figure 4-11) also can be divided into muscular and smooth-walled areas. The muscular portion of the ventricle consists of ridge-like and bridge-like configurations of muscle known as *trabeculae carneae.* The right ventricle receives deoxygenated blood from the right atrium via the open right atrioventricular or tricuspid valve.

The *tricuspid valve* consists of anterior, septal, and posterior cusps. Each cusp is attached to its correspond-

---

BOX 4-2 ■ ■ ■
PERICARDIAL PAIN

Pericardial pain may be described as substernal and sharp. Because pain from the pericardium is carried by the phrenic nerve (C3 to C5), it may be referred to the ipsilateral shoulder. The pain may be relieved by leaning forward and worsened by lying back or to the left side. The relief or exacerbation of pain by these maneuvers allows pericardial pain to be distinguished from other types of cardiac pain.

BOX 4-3 ■ ■ ■
ATRIAL SEPTAL DEFECTS

Atrial septal defects are associated with heart murmurs and are the most common congenital cardiac anomalies in adults. Untreated, they may cause pulmonary hypertension and a significant shortening of life.

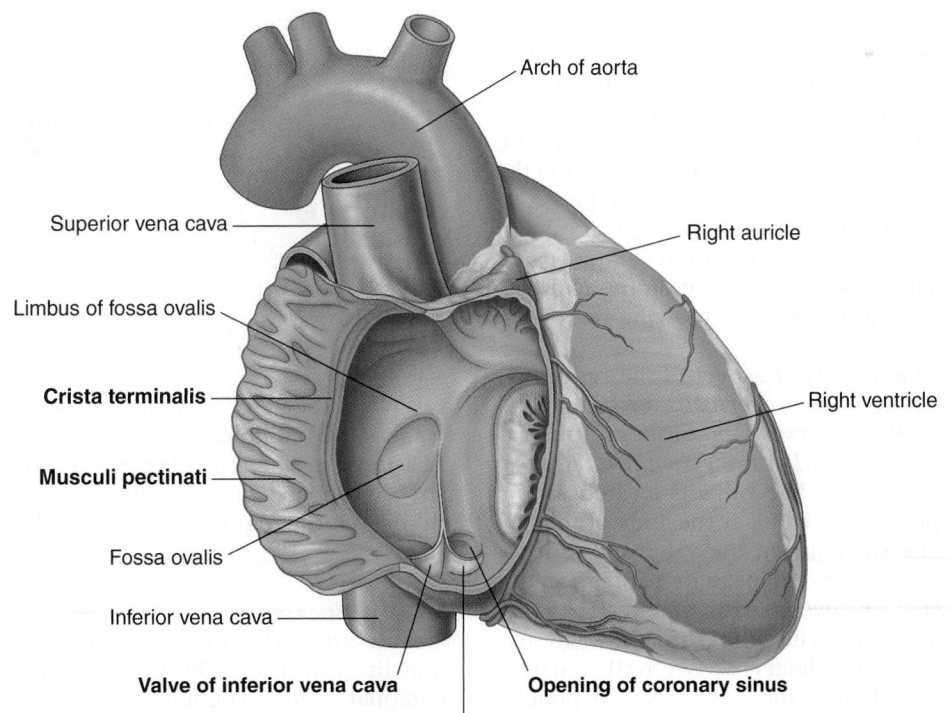

FIGURE 4-10 ■ Right atrium, internal view. (From Drake R, Vogl W, Mitchel AWM: *Gray's anatomy for students,* Edinburgh, 2005, Elsevier Churchill Livingstone.)

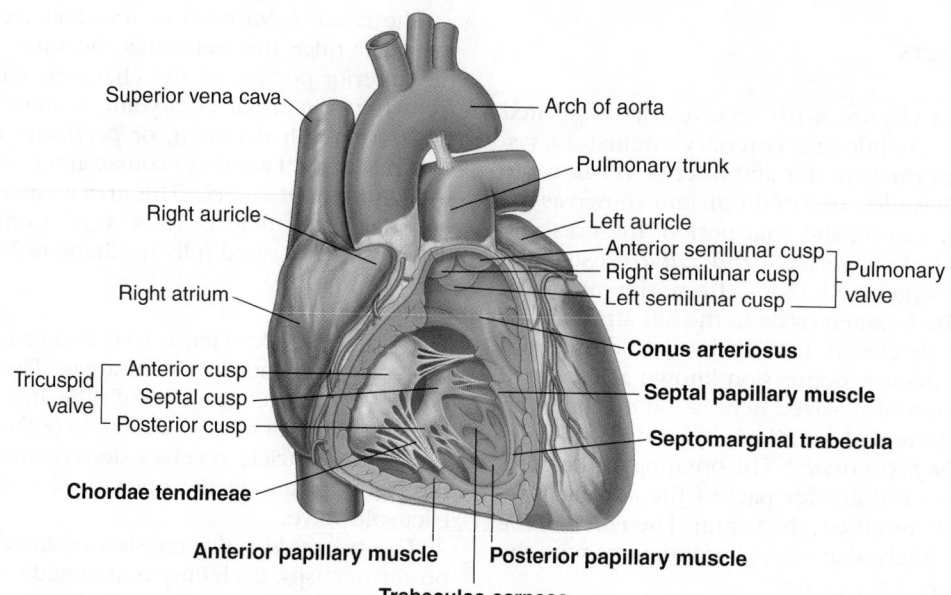

FIGURE 4-11 ■ Right ventricle, internal view. (From Drake R, Vogl W, Mitchel AWM: *Gray's anatomy for students,* Edinburgh, 2005, Elsevier Churchill Livingstone.)

ingly named papillary muscle by fibrous cords known as *chordae tendineae.* The papillary muscles are conical extensions of the muscular wall into the ventricular lumen. The *anterior papillary muscle* is the largest of the three and originates from the anterior ventricular wall. The anterior papillary muscle is continuous with the *septomarginal trabecula* (moderator band), which extends into the interventricular septum. The *posterior papillary muscle* may be bifurcated or trifurcated and arises from the diaphragmatic surface of the ventricle. The *septal papillary muscle* is typically small, variable in number, and occasionally absent. Chordae tendineae typically arise from the apical one-third of the papillary muscles and fan out to insert on adjacent valve cusps. In some instances, chordae tendineae may arise directly from the muscular walls or septum. The valve prevents reflux of blood into the right atrium during ventricular systole. Papillary muscles begin to contract at the beginning of systole. The tension they place on the chordae tendineae prevents the cusps from blowing back into the atrium.

The smooth-walled superior aspect of the right ventricle is known as the *conus arteriosus,* or infundibulum. The infundibulum funnels blood into the pulmonary trunk via the open *pulmonary semilunar valve* during ventricular systole. The valve is located at the entrance of the pulmonary trunk at the apex of the conus arteriosus. The structure of the valve allows it to function without chordae tendineae or papillary muscles (Figure 4-12). The valve consists of anterior, right, and left semilunar cusps. The *pulmonary sinuses* are the spaces between the dilated vessel wall and the cusps. Each cusp and sinus forms a pocket or pouch. The free margins of each pouch are reinforced by a centrally placed *nodule* and laterally associated *lunula.* These thickened areas of connective tissue help form a tight seal when the valve is closed and prevent the valve cusps from being totally compressed against the vessel

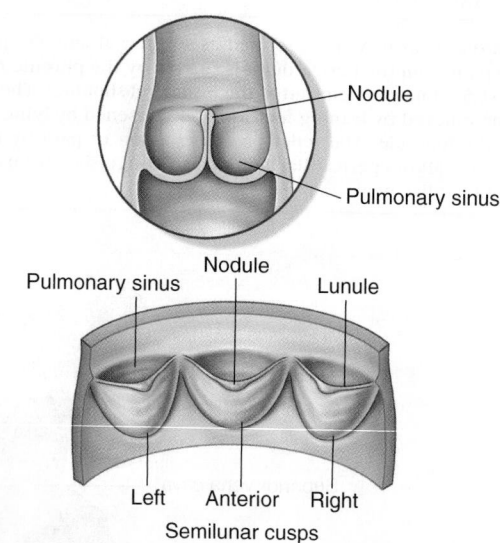

FIGURE 4-12 ■ Pulmonary semilunar valve. (From Drake R, Vogl W, Mitchel AWM: *Gray's anatomy for students,* Edinburgh, 2005, Elsevier Churchill Livingstone.)

wall when the valve is open. During diastole the elastic recoil of the pulmonary trunk forces blood back toward the ventricle. The returning blood fills and expands the partially opened pockets, effectively closing the valve and preventing regurgitation of blood back into the ventricle.

Left Atrium

The left atrium (Figure 4-13) receives oxygenated blood from the valveless right and left superior and inferior pulmonary veins. The left atrium is similar to the right atrium in having smooth and trabeculated areas. The smooth region is formed embryologically by the proximal portions of the pulmonary veins. Unlike the right atrium, trabeculae only occur in the *left auricle,* and there is no structure similar to the crista terminalis.

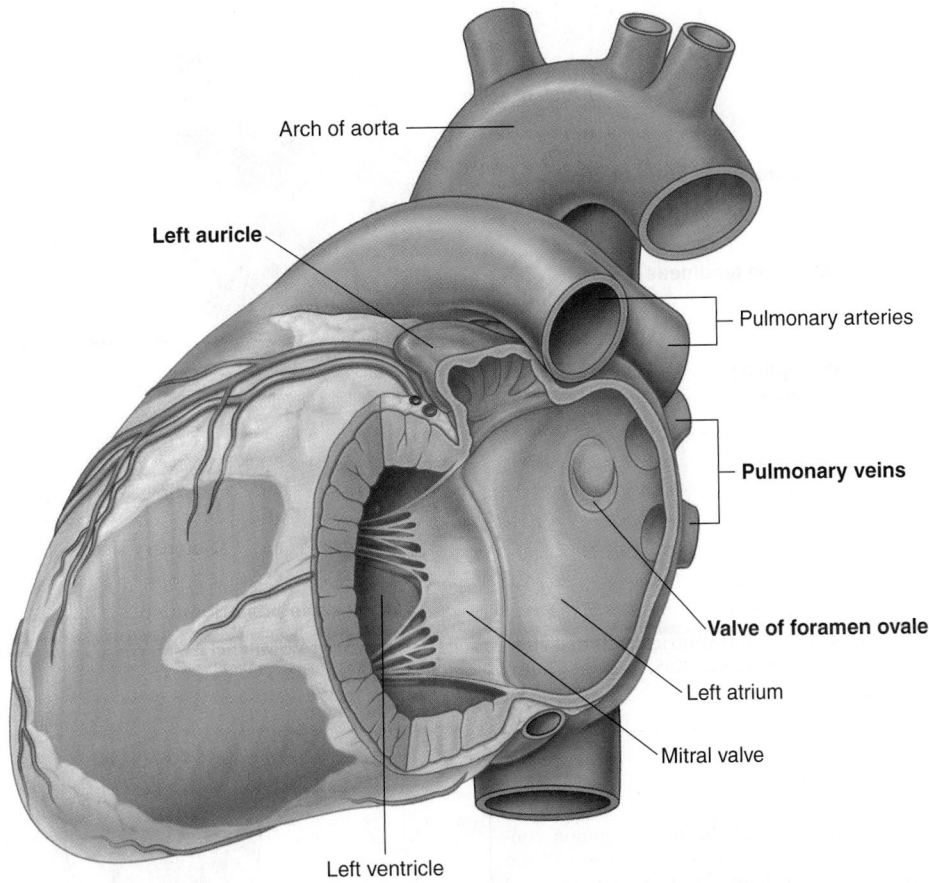

FIGURE 4-13 ■ Left atrium, internal view. (From Drake R, Vogl W, Mitchel AWM: *Gray's anatomy for students,* Edinburgh, 2005, Elsevier Churchill Livingstone.)

BOX 4-4 ■ ■ ■
PATENT FORAMEN OVALE

Probe-patent foramen ovale occurs in about 15 to 25 percent of persons. The condition appears as a small, flap-like opening associated with the valve of the foramen ovale and is often of little hemodynamic significance.

BOX 4-5 ■ ■ ■
MITRAL VALVE STENOSIS

Mitral valve stenosis is associated with rheumatic heart disease, systemic lupus erythematosus, and rheumatoid arthritis. Valve cusps are thicker and have shortened and thickened chordae tendineae. Resultant regurgitation causes left atrium dilatation and consequent formation of mural thrombi.

A thin area of depression in the interatrial septum represents the fossa ovale. The fossa ovale is bounded superiorly by a ridge or brim and inferiorly by the crescent-shaped *valve of the foramen ovale* (Box 4-4).

Left Ventricle

The walls of the left ventricle (Figure 4-14) are about 2 to 3 times thicker than those of the right ventricle. This is a direct reflection of the difference in the amount of work needed to overcome the peripheral resistance of the systemic versus pulmonary circulatory systems. The trabeculae carneae are more numerous and more delicate. These characteristics result in a more intricate mesh-like pattern in the walls of the left ventricle.

Oxygenated blood enters the left ventricle through the left atrioventricular (*bicuspid* or *mitral*) valve. The term *mitral* is derived from the resemblance of the valve to a bishop's hat or miter. The valve consists of an *anterior* and *posterior cusps* with several accessory cusps usually interposed between them. The associated papillary muscles vary in size and are often bifurcated. The anterior and posterior papillary muscles take origin respectively from the sternocostal and diaphragmatic walls of the left ventricle. Chordae tendineae arising from each muscle insert on adjacent cusps. Systole begins with contraction of the papillary muscles, and the consequent increased tension on the chordae tendineae prevents valvular eversion into the left atrium. Box 4-5 introduces one of the abnormalities possible in the mitral valve.

The *interventricular septum* separates the left and right ventricles and consists of muscular and membranous components. The *muscular septum* bulges into the cavity of the right ventricle. The muscular septum extends from the apex of the heart to the level of the origin of the septal cusp of the tricuspid valve. The *membranous component* is superior to the septal cusp and separates the right atrium from the portion of the left ventricle that funnels into the aortic orifice known

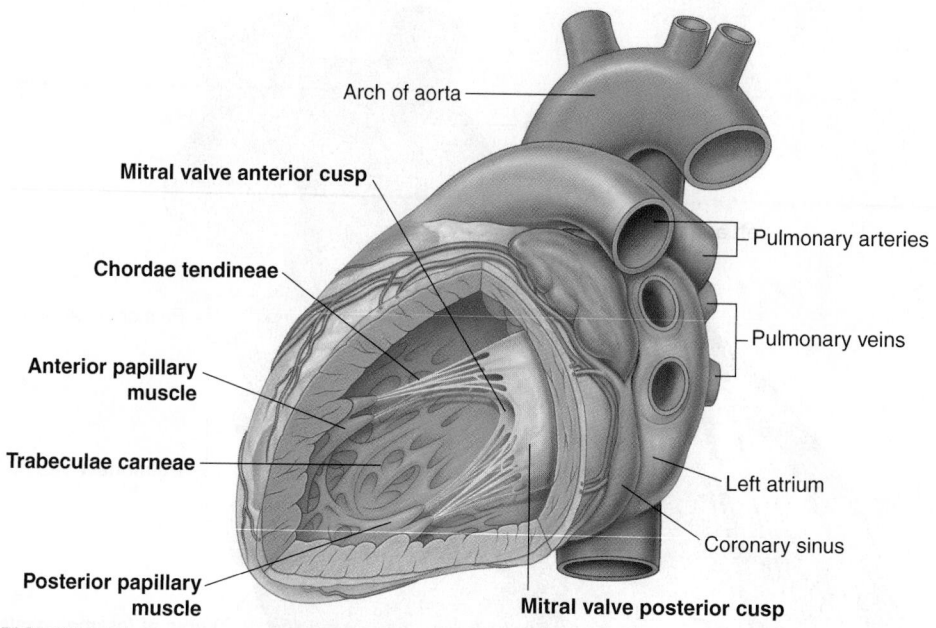

FIGURE 4-14 ■ Left ventricle, internal view. (From Drake R, Vogl W, Mitchel AWM: *Gray's anatomy for students*, Edinburgh, 2005, Elsevier Churchill Livingstone.)

BOX 4-6   ■ ■ ■
VENTRICULAR SEPTAL DEFECTS

Ventricular septal defects are some of the most common congenital anomalies in children. The membranous portion of the septum most often is involved. The left-to-right shunting of blood results in right ventricular hypertrophy and pulmonary hypertension.

---

as the *aortic vestibule*. Like the atria, the ventricles are subject to a number of congenital defects described in detail in Chapters 70 and 71 (Box 4-6).

The *aortic semilunar valve* consists of a right, left, and posterior cusps and associated sinuses (Figure 4-15). The cusps have nodules and lunulae to reinforce their free margins. The *right and left aortic sinuses* contain the openings, or ostia, for the right and left coronary arteries. For this reason the right, left, and posterior cusps often are referred to as the right coronary, left coronary, and noncoronary cusps, respectively. The valve not only functions to prevent the backflow of blood into the left ventricle during diastole but also indirectly regulates the pressure of blood flowing into the coronary arteries. The open valve cusps direct the full force of ventricular systole away from the ostia of the coronary arteries. During diastole, the elastic recoil of the ascending aorta fills the pockets of the valves and simultaneously supplies blood to the right and left coronary arteries through their respective ostia.

Coronary Circulation

The heart is supplied by the left and right coronary arteries (Figures 4-16 and 4-17). These vessels are the first branches of the ascending aorta. Venous blood enters the right atrium through the coronary sinus. This struc-

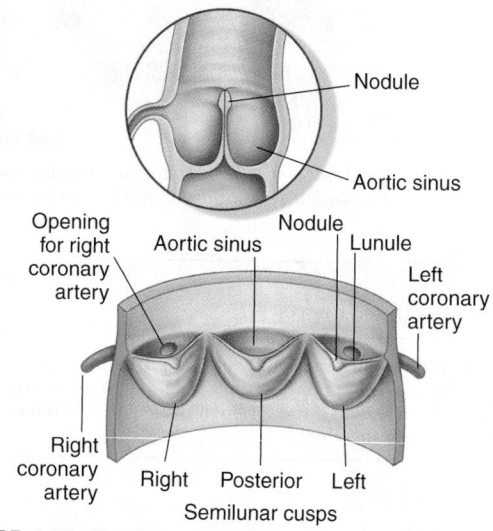

FIGURE 4-15 ■ Aortic semilunar valve. (From Drake R, Vogl W, Mitchel AWM: *Gray's anatomy for students*, Edinburgh, 2005, Elsevier Churchill Livingstone.)

ture receives most of the venous return from the larger cardiac veins and their tributaries.

Arterial Supply

The *right coronary artery* typically supplies the right atrium and ventricle, the sinoatrial and atrioventricular nodes, and the interventricular septum. The vessel arises from the right aortic sinus, courses through the coronary sulcus, and gives rise to the following branches. The *conal artery* supplies the conus arteriosus. This vessel may arise as a separate entity from the right aortic sinus. When this occurs, the conal artery is known as the third coronary artery. The *sinoatrial* (**SA**) *nodal artery* courses posteriorly in the space between the right auricle and ascending aorta to loop behind the

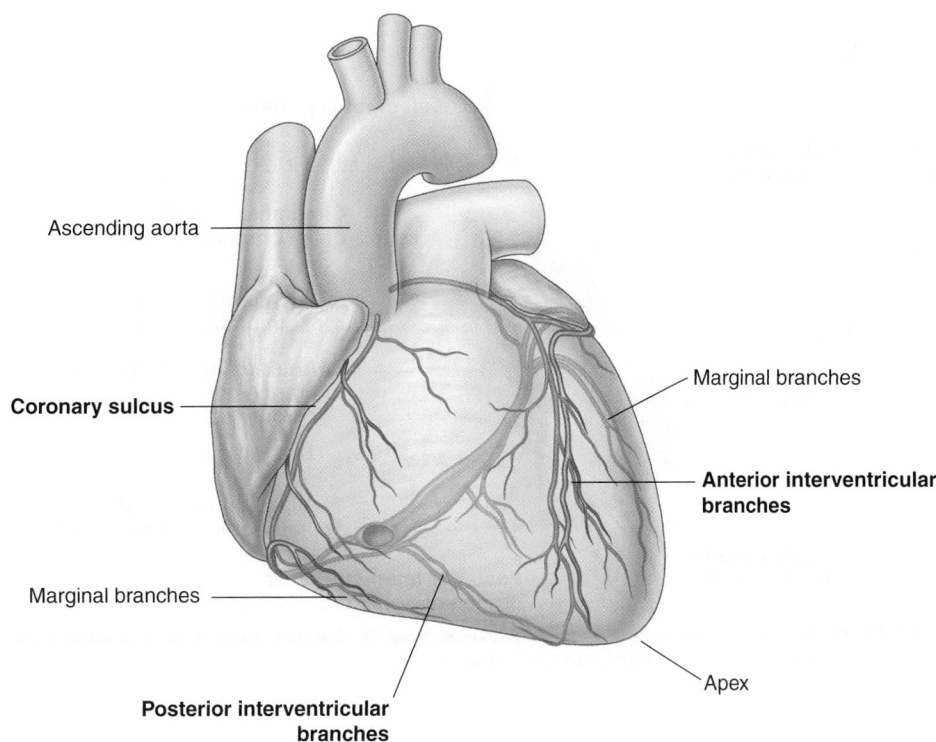

Ascending aorta

Coronary sulcus

Marginal branches

Posterior interventricular branches

Marginal branches

Anterior interventricular branches

Apex

FIGURE 4-16 ▪ Cardiac vasculature, anterior view. (From Drake R, Vogl W, Mitchel AWM: *Gray's anatomy for students,* Edinburgh, 2005, Elsevier Churchill Livingstone.)

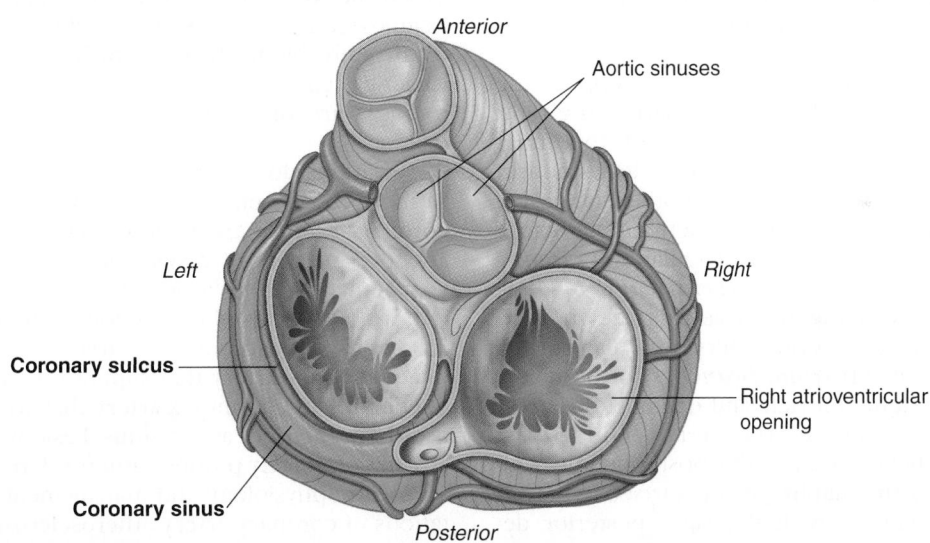

Anterior

Aortic sinuses

Left

Right

Coronary sulcus

Right atrioventricular opening

Coronary sinus

Posterior

FIGURE 4-17 ▪ Cardiac vasculature, cross-section at coronary sulcus. (From Drake R, Vogl W, Mitchel AWM: *Gray's anatomy for students,* Edinburgh, 2005, Elsevier Churchill Livingstone.)

superior vena cava to supply the sinoatrial node. This artery typically arises from the right coronary artery but also may be a branch of the left coronary artery. A variable number of anterior atrial and ventricular branches are given off before the origin of the *right marginal artery.* This vessel follows the acute margin of the heart to reach the apex. The right coronary artery continues in the coronary sulcus to the diaphragmatic surface, where it gives rise to the atrioventricular nodal and posterior interventricular arteries. The *atrioventricular nodal branch* enters the myocardium at the crux of the

heart. This is the cross formed by the interatrial and interventricular grooves as they intersect with the coronary sulcus on the diaphragmatic surface of the heart. The atrioventricular nodal artery also may arise from the left coronary artery. The *posterior interventricular branch* descends in the posterior interventricular sulcus and clinically is referred to as the right posterior descending artery. This artery supplies both ventricles and gives rise to *short septal branches,* which supply the posterior one third of the interventricular septum. The right posterior descending artery commonly anas-

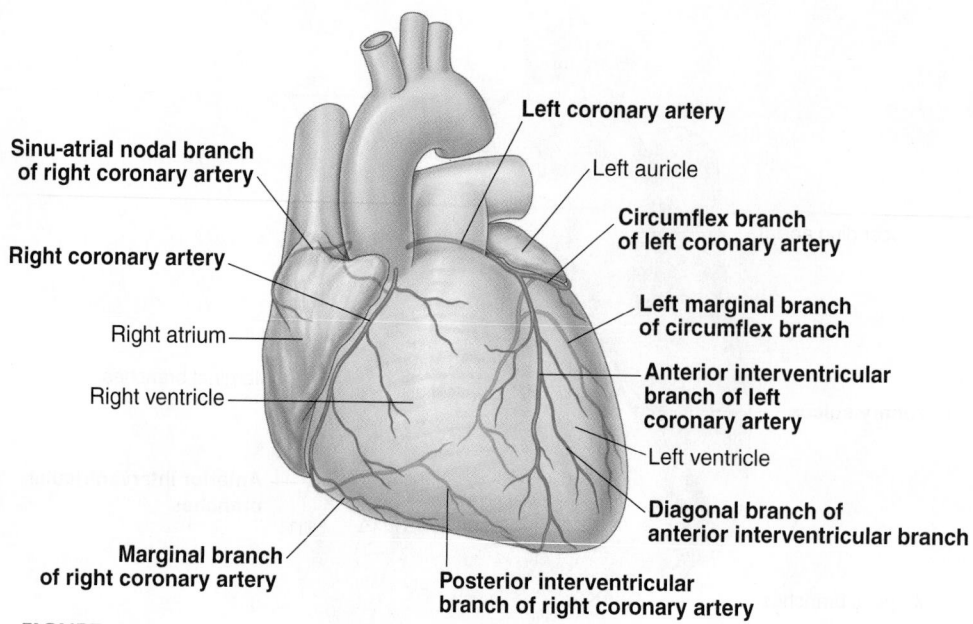

FIGURE 4-18 ▪ Coronary arteries. (From Drake R, Vogl W, Mitchel AWM: *Gray's anatomy for students,* Edinburgh, 2005, Elsevier Churchill Livingstone.)

tomoses with the left anterior descending branch of the left coronary artery. After giving off the posterior descending branch, the right coronary artery continues for a short distance in the coronary sulcus and typically anastomoses with the circumflex branch of the left coronary artery.

The *left coronary artery* (Figure 4-18) supplies the left atrium, most of the left ventricle, part of the right ventricle, and the anterior two-thirds of the interventricular septum. The artery begins at its ostium in the left aortic sinus and courses a short distance between the pulmonary trunk and the left auricle before dividing into the anterior interventricular and circumflex branches. The *anterior interventricular branch,* or left anterior descending artery as it is known clinically, descends in the anterior interventricular sulcus, where it often gives off *conal branches* to the conus arteriosus of the right ventricle and diagonal or lateral branches to the left ventricle. The artery continues past the apex of the heart to enter the posterior interventricular groove on the diaphragmatic surface, where it commonly anastomoses with the right posterior descending artery. The *circumflex branch* circumnavigates the heart in the coronary or atrioventricular groove. This branch provides small branches to the left atrium and a large marginal branch. This *left marginal branch* follows the obtuse margin of the heart to supply the left ventricle. The circumflex artery continues in the coronary sulcus to the diaphragmatic surface of the heart, where it commonly anastomoses with branches of the right coronary artery.

The right and left coronary arteries often are categorized as end arteries. End arteries do not benefit from collateral circulation formed through anastomoses with other arteries. Anastomoses do occur between the branches of the right and left coronary arteries. These anastomoses typically are formed by small-caliber ves-

sels that are not large enough to provide adequate collateral circulation in the event of a sudden occlusion. However, with the slowly progressive pathological condition that often accompanies coronary artery disease, hemodynamic changes in the diseased vessels often shunt more blood through small anastomosed vessels, causing them gradually to enlarge. These enlarged anastomoses are of greater functional value in occlusive disease.

Variations do occur in the coronary arterial supply. In most cases, branching patterns of the right and left coronary arteries are as described before. However, in about 15 percent of cases studied, the posterior interventricular artery is a branch of the circumflex artery (Figure 4-19). This phenomenon is known as *left dominance.* Two less common variations include a single large coronary artery that supplies the entire heart and a separate left circumflex artery that arises from its own ostium in the right aortic sinus. Lesions of the coronary arteries ultimately produce atherosclerotic plaques (Box 4-7). Pathophysiology and management of the manifestations of coronary artery atherosclerosis are described in chapters throughout this book.

Venous Return

The vast majority of venous return (Figure 4-20) enters the right atrium through the valve of the *coronary sinus.* Tributaries of the coronary sinus include the great,

---

BOX 4-7   ▪ ▪ ▪
CORONARY ARTERY ATHEROSCLEROSIS

Coronary artery atherosclerosis and resulting plaque formation is the principle cause of myocardial infarction. Myocardial infarction can result from occlusive or ruptured plaques. Ruptured plaques that are often less than 50 percent occlusive may play a significant role in acute myocardial infarction.

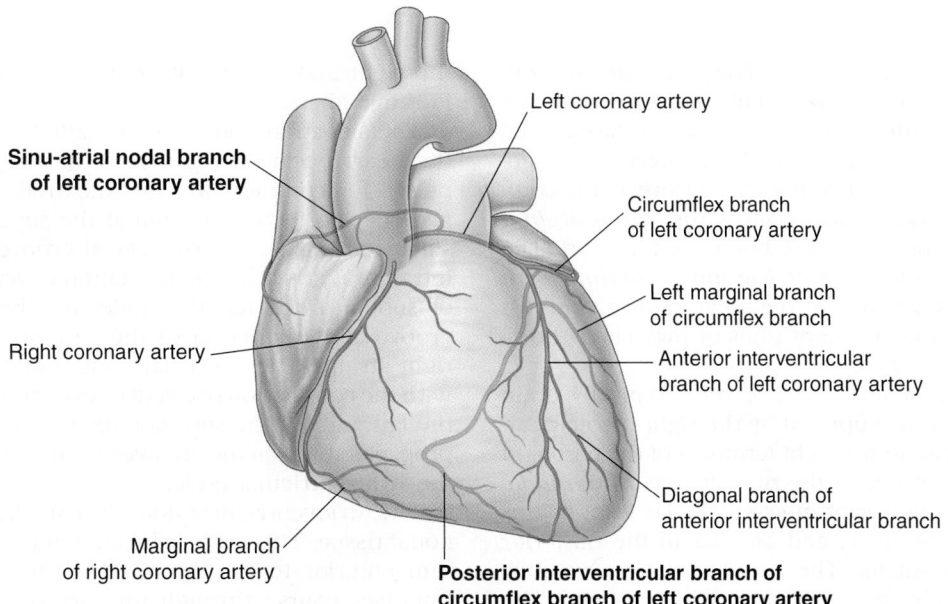

FIGURE 4-19 ▒ Left coronary artery dominance. (From Drake R, Vogl W, Mitchel AWM: *Gray's anatomy for students,* Edinburgh, 2005, Elsevier Churchill Livingstone.)

Labels in Figure 4-19:
- Left coronary artery
- Sinu-atrial nodal branch of left coronary artery
- Circumflex branch of left coronary artery
- Left marginal branch of circumflex branch
- Anterior interventricular branch of left coronary artery
- Right coronary artery
- Diagonal branch of anterior interventricular branch
- Marginal branch of right coronary artery
- Posterior interventricular branch of circumflex branch of left coronary artery

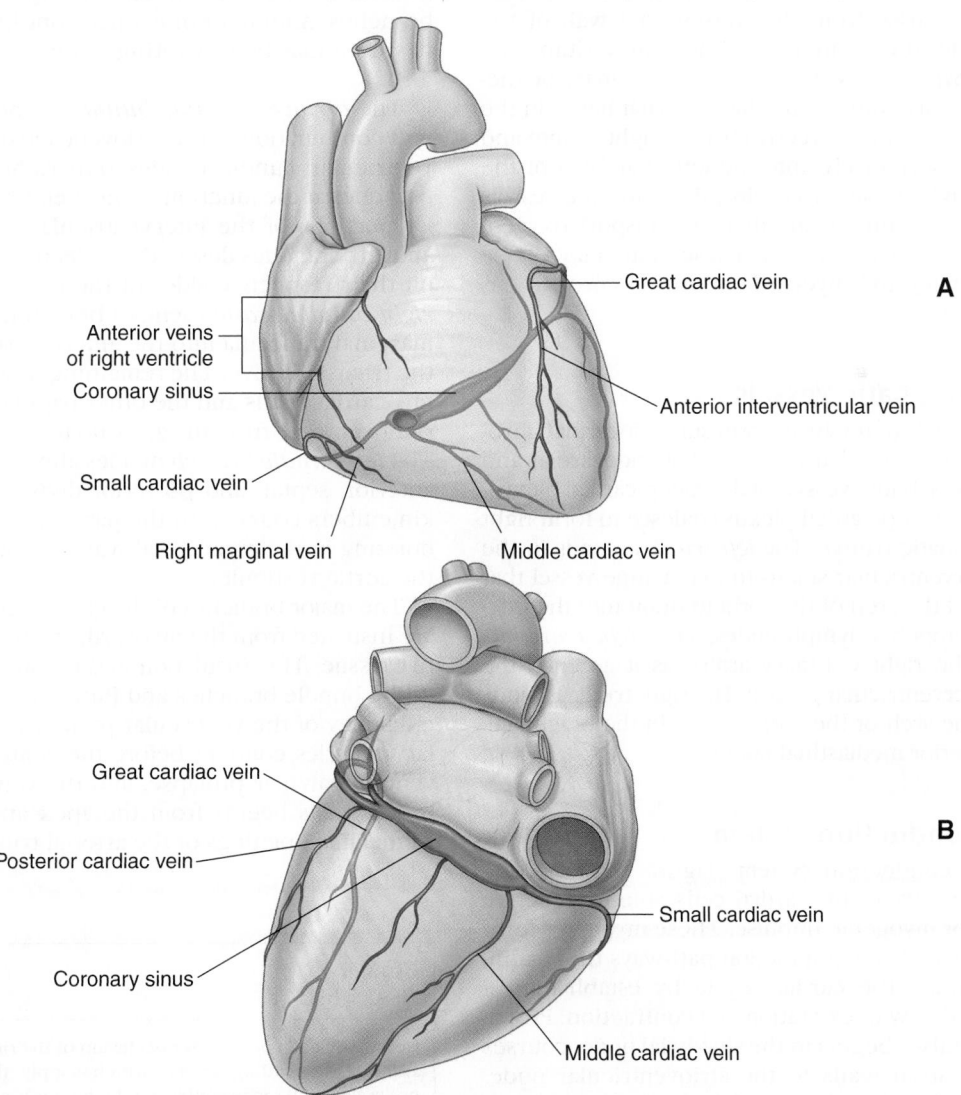

A

Labels (A, Anterior view):
- Great cardiac vein
- Anterior veins of right ventricle
- Coronary sinus
- Anterior interventricular vein
- Small cardiac vein
- Right marginal vein
- Middle cardiac vein

B

Labels (B, Posterior view):
- Great cardiac vein
- Posterior cardiac vein
- Small cardiac vein
- Coronary sinus
- Middle cardiac vein

FIGURE 4-20 ▒ Venous return. **A,** Anterior view. **B,** Posterior view. (From Drake R, Vogl W, Mitchel AWM: *Gray's anatomy for students,* Edinburgh, 2005, Elsevier Churchill Livingstone.)

middle, and small cardiac veins. The *great cardiac vein* ascends the anterior interventricular sulcus. In this position the great cardiac vein receives venous blood from both ventricles and often is called the anterior interventricular vein. As the vein courses posteriorly in the coronary sulcus, it commonly receives the *left marginal vein,* which drains the obtuse border of the heart. The *posterior vein of the left ventricle* and the *oblique vein of the left atrium* may join the great cardiac vein just before it enters the coronary sinus or may enter the sinus as separate entities.

The middle and small cardiac veins typically drain the area of the heart supplied by the right coronary artery and terminate in the right terminus of the coronary sinus just before it enters the right atrium. The *middle cardiac vein,* or posterior interventricular vein, begins at the apex of the heart and ascends in the posterior interventricular sulcus. The *small cardiac vein* may begin as the right marginal vein, which ascends the acute margin of the heart. The right marginal vein may enter the coronary sinus or the right atrium directly.

The anterior and smallest cardiac veins drain directly into the chambers of the heart. Three or four *anterior cardiac veins* arise from the sternocostal wall of the right ventricle to end directly in the right atrium. The *smallest cardiac veins* (venae cordis minimae, or thebesian veins) form numerous channels that begin in the myocardium and enter directly into the right atrium and ventricle or, more rarely, into the left chambers of the heart. Although classified as veins, these minute vessels form valveless communications that transport oxygenated and deoxygenated blood. These veins may play a role in supplying the myocardium during coronary artery occlusion.

Cardiac Lymphatic Vessels

Lymphatic vessels of the heart form subendocardial, myocardial, and subepicardial plexuses. Subendocardial and myocardial vessels join vessels of the subepicardial plexus. Vessels of the subepicardial plexus coalesce to form right and left lymphatic trunks. The *left trunk* ascends in the anterior interventricular sulcus to join a large vessel that passes behind the arch of the aorta to drain into the inferior tracheobronchial lymph nodes. The *right trunk* accompanies the right coronary artery as it ascends the posterior interventricular groove. The right trunk ascends anterior to the arch of the aorta to end in the brachiocephalic or anterior mediastinal nodes.

Cardiac Conduction System

The cardiac conduction system (Figure 4-21) is composed of specialized myocardial cells able to generate an intrinsic or myogenic impulse. These myocytes form nodes and specialized conduction pathways that exquisitely coordinate the cardiac cycle by establishing a unidirectional flow of excitation and contraction. Propagation of impulses begins in the sinoatrial node, courses through the atrial walls to the atrioventricular node, and then is relayed to the ventricles through a succession of pathways formed by the atrioventricular bundle,

the right and left bundle branches, and the terminal Purkinje fibers.

The sinoatrial node often is called the pacemaker of the heart because it generates and regulates the impulses for contraction. The sinoatrial node is located just deep to the epicardium at the superior end of the sulcus terminalis, the superficial groove formed by the intramural crista terminalis. Often covered by a plaque of subepicardial fat, the node may be visible in the groove at the junction of the superior vena cava and right atrium. The sinoatrial node initiates atrial systole with the contraction of circular myocardial fibers around the entrance of the superior vena cava. The impulse is propagated myogenically over both atria until it enters the atrioventricular node.

The atrioventricular node is a smaller collection of nodal tissue. This node is located in the interatrial septum anterior to the opening of the coronary sinus. Impulses course through internodal pathways in the atria and converge on the atrioventricular node to trigger a response. Impulses propagated in the atrioventricular node are relayed to the ventricles through the atrioventricular bundle and its right and left bundle branches. A number of cardiac conditions can produce dysrhythmias by disrupting impulse propagation (Box 4-8).

The *atrioventricular bundle* (bundle of His) is a direct continuation of the atrioventricular node. The atrioventricular bundle divides into right and left bundle branches at the junction of the membranous and muscular portions of the interventricular septum. The right and left branches descend just deep to the endocardium on their respective sides of the muscular septum. The *right bundle branch* sends a branch through the septomarginal trabecula into the anterior papillary muscle of the tricuspid valve. The remaining fibers arborize in the myocardial walls and the other papillary muscles of the right ventricle from the apex up to the conus arteriosus. The *left bundle branch* divides almost immediately into anterior, septal, and posterior divisions. Terminal Purkinje fibers course into the papillary muscles before arborizing in the myocardial walls as they ascend toward the aortic vestibule.

The major branches of the cardiac conduction system are insulated from the myocardium by a layer of connective tissue. This insulation and the arborization pattern of the bundle branches and Purkinje fibers enhance the efficiency of the ventricular pumping action. The papillary muscles contract before the ventricular walls, preventing valvular prolapse, and the wave of contraction in the walls begins from the apex and ascends to the funnel-like openings of the arterial trunks.

BOX 4-8 ■ ■ ■
HEART BLOCK

Heart block can occur after occlusion of the right coronary or left anterior descending artery, which supply the atrioventricular node. Ventricles may contract independently at a slower rate after being disconnected from the sinoatrial node.

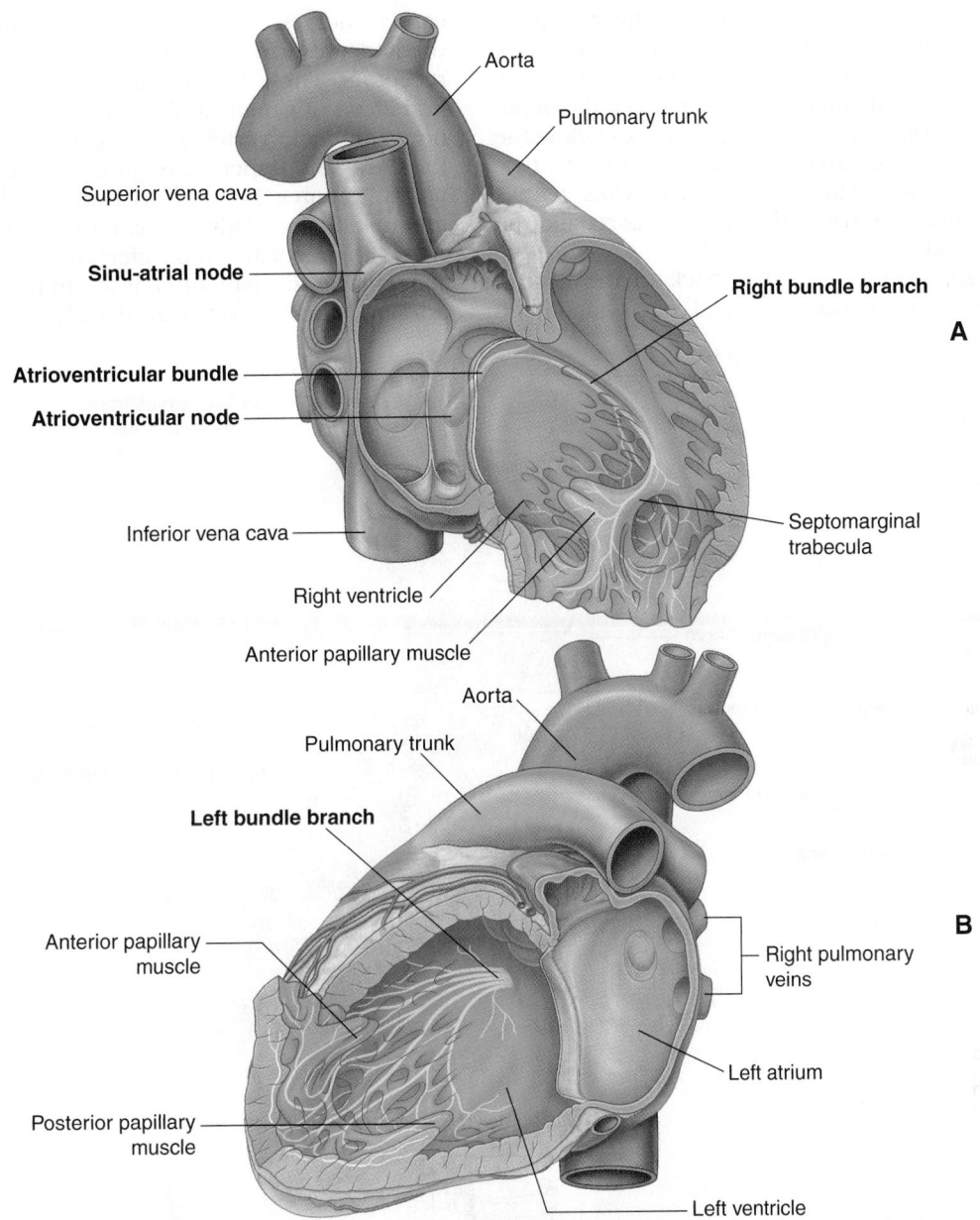

FIGURE 4-21 ■ Cardiac conduction system. **A,** Right side. **B,** Left side. (From Drake R, Vogl W, Mitchel AWM: *Gray's anatomy for students,* Edinburgh, 2005, Elsevier Churchill Livingstone.)

Cardiac Innervation

The heart propagates its own beat, but heart rate, force of contraction, cardiac output, and coronary artery luminal diameter are controlled by the autonomic nervous system (Figure 4-22). The sympathetic and parasympathetic divisions of this system work in concert to allow the heart to meet changes in physiological demands. Visceral afferents course back to the central nervous system via autonomic nerves to provide the sensory limb of cardiac innervation.

The *sympathetic supply* takes origin from preganglionic cell bodies in the intermediolateral cell column (lateral horn) of the spinal gray in thoracic spinal cord segments T1 to T4 or T5. Fibers from these cells pass through white rami communicantes to synapse on postganglionic neurons in upper thoracic and cervical para-

vertebral ganglia. Postganglionic fibers form the cardiac nerves that enter the cardiac plexuses. The net effect of sympathetic innervation is accelerated heart rate, increased force of contraction, increased cardiac output, and dilatation of the coronary arteries.

Fibers arising from preganglionic *parasympathetic neurons* located in the dorsal motor nuclei of cranial nerve X give rise to the cardiac branches of the right and left vagus nerves. These fibers synapse on postganglionic neurons located in the cardiac plexuses or in the walls of the atria. The net effect of parasympathetic innervation is coronary artery vasoconstriction and decreased cardiac output by slowing the heart rate and decreasing the force of contraction.

The *cardiac plexus* is mixed in that it contains postganglionic sympathetic fibers, postganglionic parasympathetic neurons, and visceral afferent fibers. Fibers from both autonomic divisions distribute to the sino-atrial and atrioventricular nodes. The plexus can be divided into superficial and deep interconnected components. The *superficial cardiac plexus* resides below the concavity of the aortic arch just to the right of the ligamentum arteriosum. The larger *deep cardiac plexus* lies in the connective tissue between the aorta and the tracheal bifurcation.

Visceral afferent fibers travel back to the central nervous system in sympathetic and parasympathetic cardiac nerves. Afferent fibers traveling with sympathetic nerves carry impulses generated by visceral pain receptors. These fibers course through the paravertebral chain of ganglia and enter the spinal nerves of the upper thoracic vertebrae. Somatic sensory fibers from the chest and upper extremities course through spinal nerves to enter the same areas of spinal gray as the autonomic fibers. This overlap of sensory distribution serves the mechanism of referred pain. This is the reason why cardiac pain often is felt in the chest and ulnar border of the left arm (Figure 4-23).

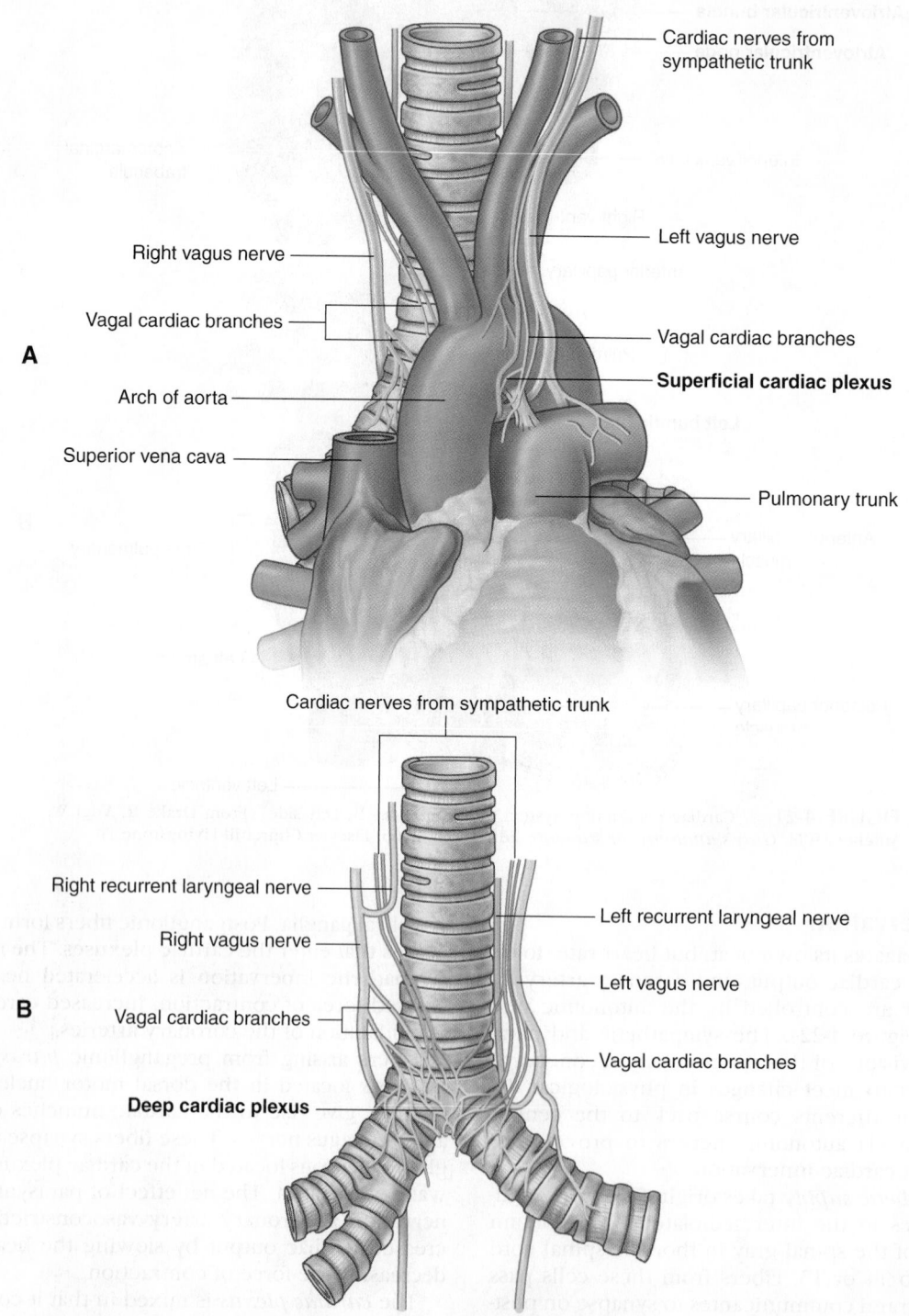

FIGURE 4-22 ■ Cardiac innervation. **A,** Superficial plexus. **B,** Deep plexus. (From Drake R, Vogl W, Mitchel AWM: *Gray's anatomy for students,* Edinburgh, 2005, Elsevier Churchill Livingstone.)

MICROANATOMY OF THE HEART
Connective Tissue and Skeleton

Connective tissue is found throughout the myocardium. This relationship is similar to that found in skeletal muscle in that the connective tissue components are related intimately to a skeletal structure, allowing for a directed force of muscle contraction. An *endomysium* ensheathes individual muscle cells, a *perimysium* surrounds larger fascicles of myocardium, and an outermost layer, or *epimysium,* envelopes the whole muscle. These components meld with the dense fibrous connective tissue skeleton of the heart.

The *cardiac skeleton* (Figure 4-24) consists of the annuli fibrosi, trigones, and the connective tissue cores of the membranous portions of the interatrial and interventricular septa. The *annuli fibrosi* are four relatively complete rings that surround the orifices of the atrioventricular and semilunar valves. The thickened areas of dense connective tissue that interconnect the annuli fibrosi are the trigones. The *left trigone* connects the ring surrounding the aortic semilunar valve with the left atrioventricular ring. The *right trigone* joins the aortic annulus with the right atrioventricular ring. The central fibrous body of the cardiac skeleton is formed by the right trigone and the connective tissue core of the intramembranous septum. The septum is pierced by the atrioventricular bundle.

The connective tissue skeleton serves structural and electrophysiological functions.[1] Structurally, the connective tissue allows for attachment of atrial and ventricular muscle from its superior and inferior surfaces. This relationship enhances the wringing action of the spirally oriented ventricular musculature, forcing blood up from the apex through the ostia of the arterial trunks. The annuli fibrosi maintain the patency of the orifices of their respective valves and provide a quasi-rigid point of attachment for the valve cusps. Electrophysiologically, the cardiac skeleton plays an important role as an insulator in the cardiac conduction system. The cardiac skeleton separates atrial from ventricular musculature, effectively blocking continuous impulse conduction from the atria to the ventricles. As the atrioventricular bundle pierces the central fibrous body, it and its bundle branches become ensheathed in an insulating coat of connective tissue, allowing the impulse to reach the apex and papillary muscles before general ventricular contraction.

Cardiac Muscle

Cardiac muscle differs histologically from skeletal muscle in a number of ways that underscore its continuous function (Figure 4-25). Cardiac myoblasts do not fuse to form a single continuous fiber as do their skeletal counterparts. Consequently, each myocardial fiber consists of a single cell connected to other cells by specialized junctional complexes known as *intercalated discs.* Each cell has a *centrally placed nucleus* unlike the multiple peripheral pattern associated with skeletal fibers. Cardiac cells *branch* and these arborizations are connected to those of other cells to form a mesh-like weave that aids in the expulsion of blood.

Myocardial cells contain abundant, large mitochondria interspersed between contractile proteins (Figure 4-26). This configuration is needed to maintain a high level of oxidative metabolism.

Cardiac muscle is sandwiched between two layers of specialized tissue. The *epicardium,* or visceral pericardium, is the superficial layer. The *endocardium* lines the inner surface of all four chambers and is continuous with the endothelial lining of the cardiovascular system. Infection of this endothelial lining can produce endocarditis (Box 4-9).[6] See Chapter 73 for a full discussion of care of the patient with endocarditis.

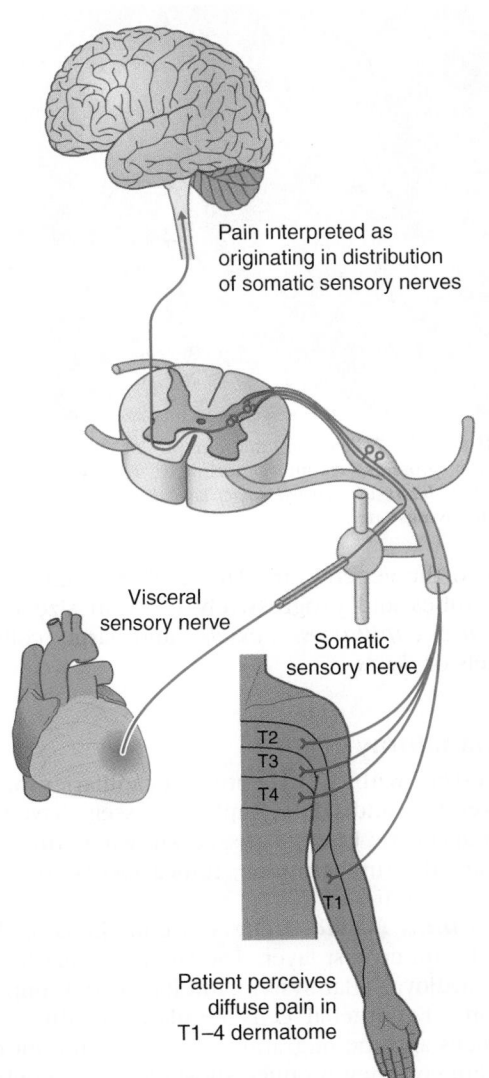

Pain interpreted as originating in distribution of somatic sensory nerves

Visceral sensory nerve

Somatic sensory nerve

T2
T3
T4

T1

Patient perceives diffuse pain in T1–4 dermatome

FIGURE 4-23 ■ Pathway for referred pain. (From Drake R, Vogl W, Mitchel AWM: *Gray's anatomy for students,* Edinburgh, 2005, Elsevier Churchill Livingstone.)

BOX 4-9   ■ ■ ■
INFECTIVE ENDOCARDITIS

Infective endocarditis is an infection of the endocardial lining of the heart that can lead to myocardial abscess, valvular insufficiency, and congestive heart failure. Infective endocarditis is typically a *Staphylococcus aureus* infection that gains entrance by invasive vascular procedures or intravenous drug abuse.

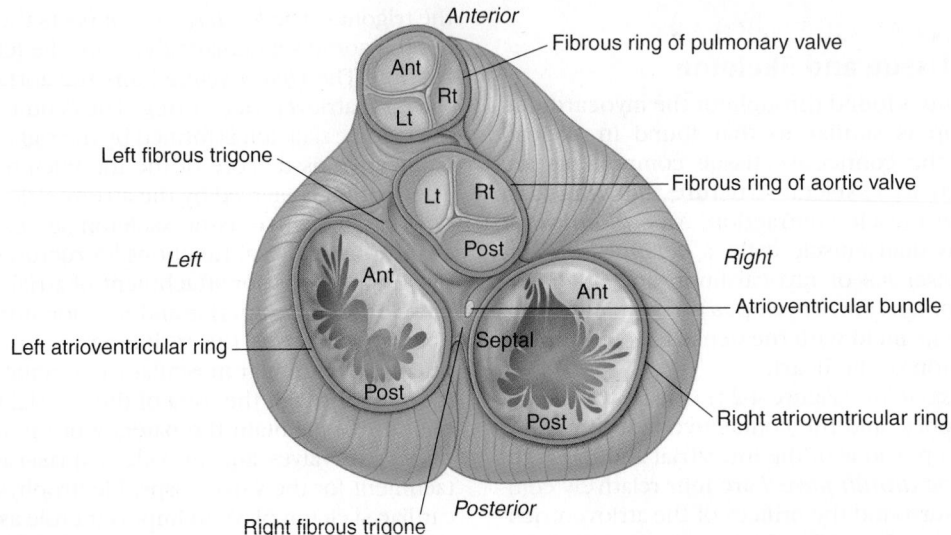

FIGURE 4-24 ■ Cardiac skeleton. *Ant,* Anterior; *Lt,* left; *Post,* posterior; *Rt,* right. (From Drake R, Vogl W, Mitchel AWM: *Gray's anatomy for students,* Edinburgh, 2005, Elsevier Churchill Livingstone.)

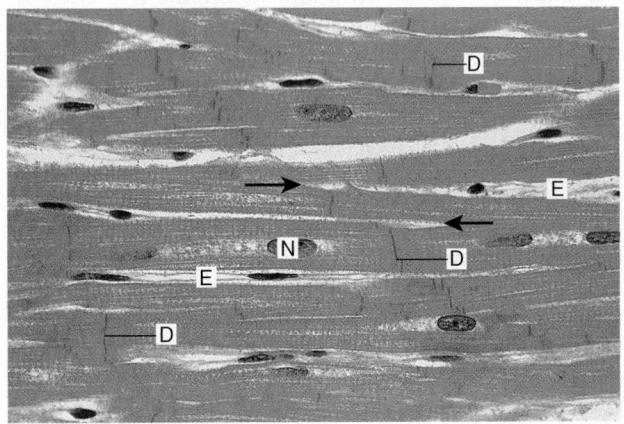

FIGURE 4-25 ■ Myocardium. (From Standring S: *Gray's anatomy: the anatomical basis of clinical practice,* Edinburgh, 2005, Elsevier Churchill Livingstone.)

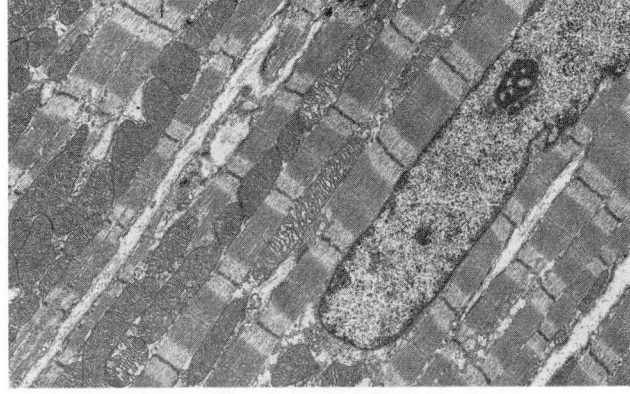

FIGURE 4-26 ■ Electron micrograph of mitochondria and contractile proteins. (From Standring S: *Gray's anatomy: the anatomical basis of clinical practice,* Edinburgh, 2005, Elsevier Churchill Livingstone.)

ANATOMY OF THE VASCULAR SYSTEM
Gross Anatomy

The vascular system consists of arteries, veins, and lymphatic vessels. Arteries distribute oxygen, nutrients, and hormones to the tissues. To serve these functions, arteries increase in number and become progressively smaller as they move distally. The increase in number occurs through repeated divisions. The reduction in size occurs through decreases in luminal dimension and wall thickness. This pattern of arborization begins with the *large elastic arteries* such as the aorta, pulmonary trunk, and brachiocephalic arteries. These vessels undergo subsequent divisions to form *muscular arteries, arterioles,* and *capillaries.*

Veins return carbon dioxide to the lungs and absorbed nutrients to the liver. They increase in size and diminish in number as they course back to the heart. Beginning as *postcapillary venules,* these vessels increase in size to become *muscular venules* and *veins.*

Lymphatic vessels return excess interstitial fluid or lymph to the general circulation. They begin as endothelial tubes and progressively grow in size to form *lymphatic capillaries, vessels,* and large collecting channels or *ducts.*

Microanatomy

Most vessels, with the exception of capillaries, postcapillary venules, and small lymphatic vessels, have two or three concentric layers of tissue known as tunics. The layers are the tunica intima, tunica media, and tunica adventitia (Figure 4-27).

The *tunica intima* consists of endothelial cells and forms the innermost layer. The tunica intima lines the entire cardiovascular system and has several important functions. Endothelial cells regulate the diffusion of substances and the migration of cells in and out of the vessel lumen. They produce substances that control luminal diameter and clot formation and secrete autocrine growth factors that stimulate angiogenesis for growth and repair.

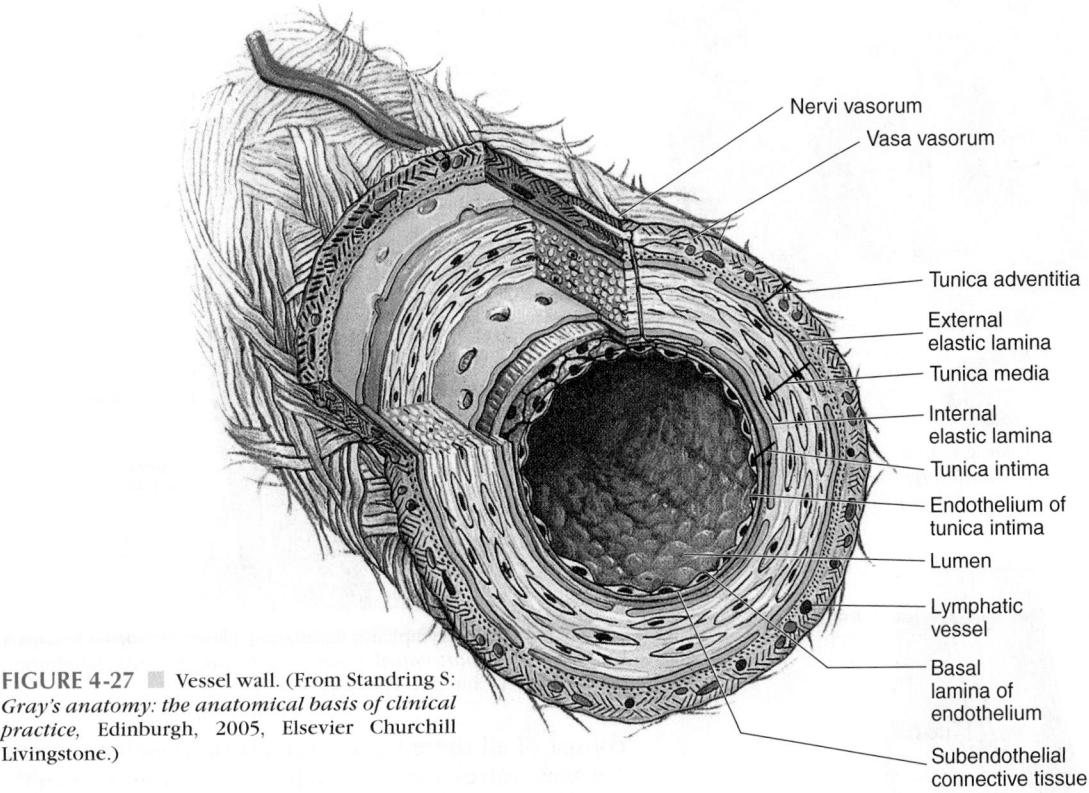

Nervi vasorum
Vasa vasorum
Tunica adventitia
External elastic lamina
Tunica media
Internal elastic lamina
Tunica intima
Endothelium of tunica intima
Lumen
Lymphatic vessel
Basal lamina of endothelium
Subendothelial connective tissue

FIGURE 4-27 ■ Vessel wall. (From Standring S: *Gray's anatomy: the anatomical basis of clinical practice,* Edinburgh, 2005, Elsevier Churchill Livingstone.)

The *tunica media* or intermediate layer is made up of smooth muscle cells, elastic fibers, and collagen. The layer is not found in capillaries and is relatively reduced in size in veins. Smooth muscle cells function to control luminal diameter and have the capacity to secrete elastin and collagen that lend elasticity and strength to the vessel wall.

The outermost coat is the *tunica adventitia.* This layer is composed mainly of connective tissue. The tunica adventitia functions to link the vessels to surrounding tissue and provide a platform for the blood supply or vaso vasorum and innervation to the walls of the larger vessels. The composition of the vessel wall allows for histological classification of the various types of vessels in the arterial, venous, and lymphatic systems.

The aorta, brachiocephalic, common carotid, subclavian, and common iliac arteries are examples of *large elastic arteries* because of the large concentration of elastin in their walls. Elastin forms a subendothelial layer associated with the intima and an internal elastic lamina between the intima and media. The media is infused completely with elastin, with elastic lamellae alternating with layers of smooth muscle and collagen. Elastic fibers also are found in the adventitia, which also contains fibroblasts, macrophages, and mast cells. This pervasive elastin component serves the important function of elastic recoil. The expansion of the vessels during systole and recoil during diastole allows for a sustained flow of blood. Weaknesses in the layers of arterial vessel walls can produce aneurysms (Box 4-10).[7]

The tunica media of *muscular arteries* contains abundant smooth muscle. In larger vessels, an external elastic lamella may be found between the media and adventitia. Muscular arteries serve the important function of shunting blood to areas of higher physiological need, such as from the abdomen to the muscles of the

extremities and brain during increased stress or physical activity.

The media of *arterioles* consists of only one or two layers of smooth muscle. The surrounding adventitia is very thin. Arterioles function as precapillary sphincters in that they regulate the flow of blood to the capillary bed.

The entire wall of *capillaries* consists of endothelium and its associated basal lamina sparsely surrounded by mesenchymal contractile cells known as pericytes. The endothelium may or may not contain openings known as fenestrations. The luminal diameter of capillaries is just large enough to permit passage of a single blood cell (Figure 4-28). The thinness of the capillary wall enhances the diffusion of blood gases, nutrients, and metabolic wastes.

Postcapillary venules are formed when two or more capillaries merge to form a larger vessel. They are similar to capillaries in structure and function. They consist of endothelial cells surrounded by a basal lamina and pericytes and are just as permeable to substances as capillaries. During the inflammatory response, they are the site for leukocyte migration and locus for increased

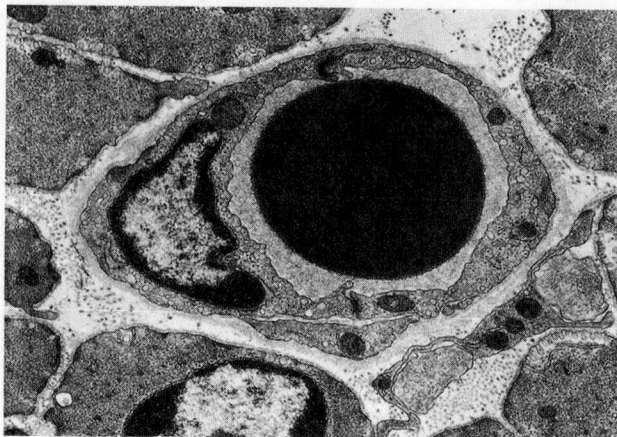

FIGURE 4-28 ■ Electron micrograph of capillary with red blood cell. (From Standring S: *Gray's anatomy: the anatomical basis of clinical practice,* Edinburgh, 2005, Elsevier Churchill Livingstone.)

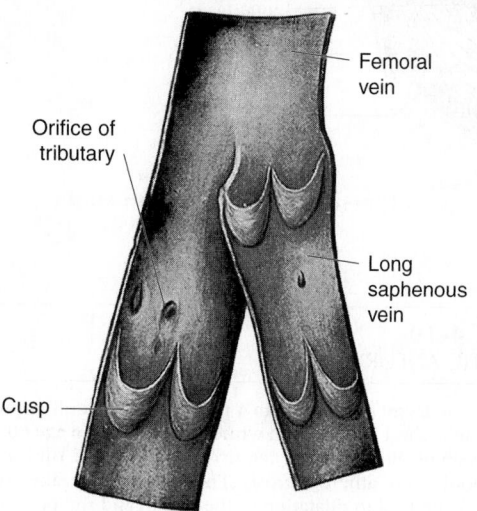

FIGURE 4-29 ■ Valves in veins. (From Standring S: *Gray's anatomy: the anatomical basis of clinical practice,* Edinburgh, 2005, Elsevier Churchill Livingstone.)

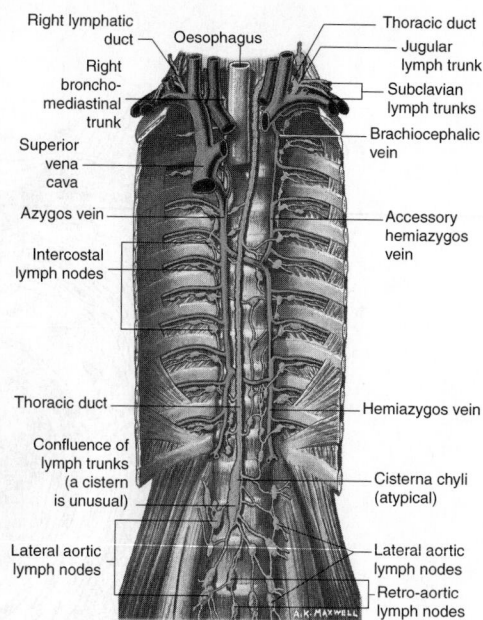

FIGURE 4-30 ■ Lymphatic circulation. (From Standring S: *Gray's anatomy: the anatomical basis of clinical practice,* Edinburgh, 2005, Elsevier Churchill Livingstone.)

permeability of fluids. Postcapillary venules converge and form progressively larger-diameter vessels known as *venules.* Smooth muscle begins to appear in the tunica media of larger venules. These *muscular venules* converge to form larger vessels called veins.

The walls of veins are composed of all three tunics, but the tunica media of veins contains considerably less smooth muscle and elastin than arteries of the same diameter. The adventitia connects the outer vessel wall with surrounding tissue. This connection keeps the walls of veins from collapsing during times of low blood pressure. Veins have a series of valves consisting of two or three cusps. They are inward projections of the walls and lined superficially by endothelium. Venous blood is moved toward the heart by the intermittent contraction of adjacent musculature. The one-way valves function to maintain this unidirectional flow (Figure 4-29).

Lymphatic capillaries arise from plexuses and merge to form larger vessels. These endothelial channels are covered by a connective tissue layer as they increase in size. Like veins, the walls of larger lymphatic vessels

consist of all three tunics. Lymphatic vessels also have one-way valves for the unidirectional flow of lymph. Lymph is returned to the venous circulation through the right lymphatic and thoracic ducts. The *right lymphatic duct* carries lymph from the head and neck and upper extremity on the right, and the *thoracic duct* typically receives trunks from the left side of the rest of the body. Both ducts enter the subclavian vein at its junction with the internal jugular vein on their respective sides (Figure 4-30).

A thorough knowledge of cardiovascular anatomy is essential for conceptualizing the various pathophysiological processes that affect the heart and vessels. This information also provides a foundation for understanding data obtained from diagnostic tools commonly used in cardiac angiography, echocardiography, electrocardiography, and nuclear cardiology. The cardiovascular anatomy and microanatomy detailed in this chapter should serve as a basis for further study and provide for a better understanding of current and future research.

REFERENCES

1. Standring S: *Gray's anatomy: the anatomical basis of clinical practice,* Edinburgh, 2005, Elsevier Churchill Livingstone.
2. Broderick LS, Brooks GN, Kuhlman JE: Anatomic pitfalls of the heart and pericardium, *Radiographics* 25:441-453, 2005.
3. Fitzgerald M, Spencer J, Johnson F et al: Definitive management of acute cardiac tamponade secondary to blunt trauma, *Emerg Med Australas* 17:494-499, 2005.
4. Jirasek JE: *An atlas of human prenatal developmental mechanics: anatomy and staging,* London, 2004, Taylor & Francis.
5. Raja SG: Atrial septal defect in infancy: to close or not to close? *J Thorac Cardiovasc Surg* 130:1483, 2005; author reply, p 1483.
6. Cowie MR: Infective endocarditis: new guidance recommends a more aggressive approach, *Clin Med* 4:489-490, 2004.
7. Fleming C, Whitlock EP, Beil TL et al: Screening for abdominal aortic aneurysm: a best-evidence systematic review for the US Preventive Services Task Force, *Ann Intern Med* 142:203-211, 2005.

Cardiovascular Physiology: The Myocardium

Mariann R. Piano
William R. Law

CHAPTER ABBREVIATIONS

ATP adenosine triphosphate

AV atrioventricular

Ca^{++} calcium

FAT/CD 36 fatty acid translocase

g$_{Ca}$ calcium conductance

g$_{Na}$ sodium conductance

I$_{Ca}$ inward calcium current

I$_{Ca-L}$ long-lasting component of inward calcium current

I$_{Ca-T}$ transient component of inward calcium current

I$_f$ inward pacemaker current

I$_K$ outward potassium current

I$_{KR}$ rapid delayed rectifier potassium current

I$_{KS}$ slow delayed rectifier potassium current

I$_{Na}$ sodium current

I$_{to}$ transient outward potassium current

K$^+$ potassium

K$_{ir}$ or K$_1$ inward rectifier potassium channel

K$_V$ voltage-gated (delayed rectifier) potassium channel

Na$^+$ sodium

RMP resting membrane potential

SA sinoatrial

SERCA2a sarco[endo]plasmic reticulum Ca^{++}-ATPase

Cardiovascular physiology is a broad topic that typically encompasses aspects of anatomy, hemodynamics, the cardiac cycle, the microcirculation and lymphatic vessels, and the arterial and venous systems. The primary aim of this chapter, however, is to detail the molecular events that underlie force generation (contraction), relaxation, and the development and spread of electrical current through the myocardium. Many therapeutic modalities are aimed at altering or improving the molecular mechanisms that underlie such physiological processes.

The myocardium is made up of several cell types. They include cardiomyocytes (contractile cells that generate force), P cells (cells responsible for the generation of action potentials), fibroblasts (cells residing in the extracellular matrix), and endothelial and smooth muscle cells (cells found in blood vessels). The focus of this chapter is the function of cardiomyocytes and P cells. The chapter is divided into four parts. The first part details the membrane and cellular components important in contraction and relaxation. The second part reviews the actual process of contraction, cross-bridge cycling, and relaxation. The third part details myocar-

dial electrophysiology. And the final section presents aspects of myocardial substrate utilization and the different metabolic fuels that the myocardium uses under different conditions.

CELLULAR BASIS OF MYOCARDIAL CONTRACTION AND RELAXATION

The myocardium is composed mainly of striated muscle cells called cardiomyocytes. The main function of the cardiomyocyte is to develop force and shorten, which allows the ventricles to develop pressure, contract, and eject blood. Cardiomyocytes represent one-third of the total myocardial cell population; however, they occupy at least 75 percent of the total myocardial structural space,[1] because relative to the other cell types—such as the fibroblast—the cardiomyocyte is a very large cell.

During the first several weeks of life, the number of cardiomyocytes doubles by means of mitotic division. After this, any growth that occurs is primarily a result of individual myocyte hypertrophy.[2] The inability of the myocardium to regenerate was once attributed to the fact that the adult myocyte is a terminally differentiated cell type. More recent evidence, however, suggests that there may be some degree of mitosis and new myocyte formation and that, within the myocardium, there are some resident stem cells (cells capable of extensive proliferation).[3,4] Even though the myocardium may have the capacity for regeneration, this capacity is not enough to sustain new myocyte regeneration after an event such as myocardial infarction.[4]

Unique aspects of the cardiomyocyte plasma membrane and intracellular organelles are reviewed separately. Table 5-1 also provides a summary.

Sarcolemma

Similar to all cell types, each cardiomyocyte is enclosed by a plasma membrane, termed the sarcolemma. The sarcolemma of the cardiomyocyte is characterized by the presence of T tubules, which are extensive invaginations of the sarcolemma (Figure 5-1).[1] T tubules serve to increase the surface area and facilitate the propagation of the action potential. The T tubules are in contact with the sarcomeres at the region of the Z disc (t-sarcoplasmic reticulum junction). Along the T tubules are many L-type **Ca^{++}** voltage-dependent channels (also referred to as dihydropyridine receptors) located at the junction of the sarcolemma and sarcoplasmic reticulum. L-type Ca^{++} channels are classified as voltage-dependent channels because a change in sarcolemma electrical potential (voltage) modulates the opening and

TABLE 5-1   INTRACELLULAR ORGANELLES AND CELLULAR AND MEMBRANE COMPONENTS IMPORTANT TO CARDIOMYOCYTE FUNCTION

INTRACELLULAR ORGANELLE	STRUCTURE AND FUNCTION
Mitochondria	Mitochondria have a spherical shape and are found in the cytoplasm.
	Compared with other cell types, such as skeletal myocytes, cardiomyocytes contain many mitochondria, and mitochondria occupy at least 33% of the cell volume of the cardiomyocyte. These features are typical of cells requiring a continuous supply of ATP.
	Their major function is oxidative phosphorylation (i.e., major site for generation of ATP).
	At excessive levels of intracellular calcium, the mitochondria accumulate calcium, thus preventing the intracellular calcium level from becoming too high.
Sarcoplasmic reticulum (SR)	This specialized form of the endoplasmic reticulum is the major site for calcium storage and release.
	Calcium entry during the action potential stimulates calcium release from the SR.
SERCA2a	This integral SR-membrane–spanning protein pump is a Ca^{++}-ATPase–activated magnesium protein pump that couples ATP hydrolysis to the active transport of calcium from the cytosol back into the SR.
	Reuptake of calcium back into the SR is critical for relaxation.
Phospholamban	This protein is an integral part of the SERCA2a pump and regulates SERCA2a activity.
Calcium-release channel (ryanodine receptor)	The calcium release channel is part of the SR and is in proximity to the T tubules.
	Calcium entry during the plateau phase of the action potential stimulates calcium released from the SR.
	Calcium released from the calcium-release channel binds troponin C.
Nucleus	Cardiomyocytes contain a single nucleus (unlike skeletal muscle cells, which have multiple nuclei).
	The nucleus is a spherical, membrane-bound organelle usually located in the middle of the cell.
	Its main function is the storage and transmission of genetic information (i.e., DNA transcription).
Lysosome	This spherical organelle is enclosed by a single membrane.
	It contains many enzymes responsible for proteolysis.
Cardiomyocyte Proteins	
Myofibril	Myofibrils are composed of the contractile proteins actin and myosin.
Actin (thin filament)	Globular actin proteins coil around a tropomyosin protein.
Troponin complex	The troponin complex consists of three troponin proteins: troponin T, troponin I, and troponin C.
	Troponin T attaches the whole troponin complex to tropomyosin.
	Troponin I binds to actin.
	Troponin C binds Ca^{++}.
Myosin (thick filament)	Myosin is composed of myosin II molecules.
	Each myosin head contains the actin-binding site and the enzymatic site (myosin ATPase) that hydrolyzes ATP to adenosine diphosphate and inorganic phosphate during cross-bridge cycling.

ATP, Adenosine triphosphate.

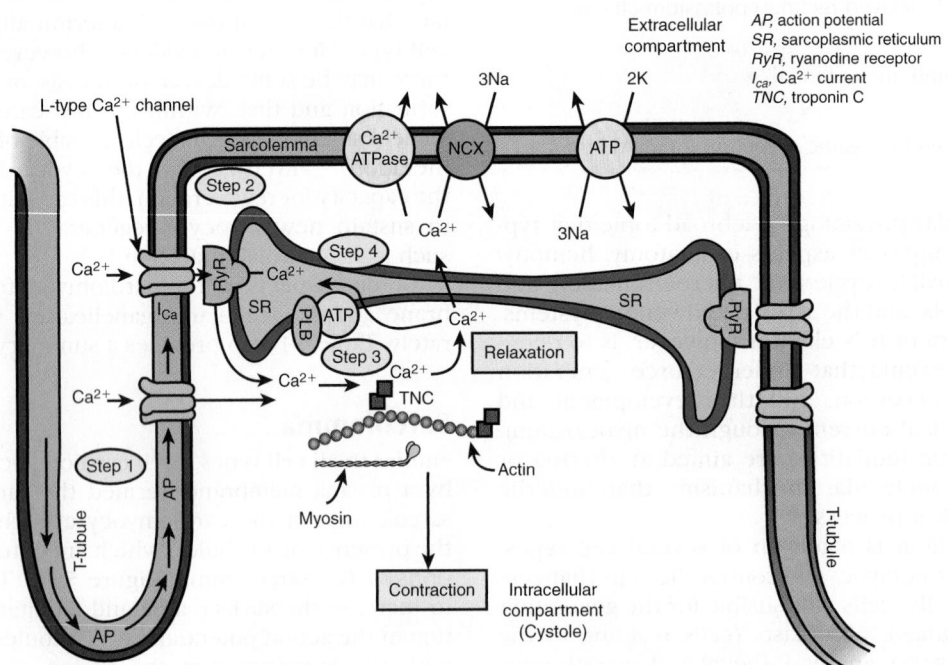

FIGURE 5-1 ▪ A summary of key events during the excitation-contraction coupling cycle of a myocyte. Depolarization of the membrane stimulates the opening of voltage-dependent Ca^{++} channels and an increase in Ca^{++} current (I_{Ca}; step 1). Ca^{++} entry through the L-type Ca^{++} channels stimulates the release of Ca^{++} from the sarcoplasmic reticulum (SR) ryanodine receptor (RyR; step 2). Ca^{++} released from the SR binds troponin C (TNC), which elicits a conformational change in the actin filament that exposes the myosin binding sites (step 3). This allows the strong cross-bridge formation between actin and myosin and force generation. Relaxation is an active process and is brought about by the release of Ca^{++} and reuptake back into the SR via the SERCA2a pump. Depending on the levels of intracellular Ca^{++}, some Ca^{++} is also removed via the sarcolemmal Ca^{++} ATPase pump and sodium-calcium exchanger (NCX).

closing of these channels. T tubules are in approximation to the sarcoplasmic reticulum calcium-release channel (also known as the ryanodine-sensitive channel and labeled RyR in Figure 5-1).[5,6]

Sarcomere

The sarcomere is the contractile unit of the cardiomyocyte and is composed of two groups of protein filaments: the thin filaments and thick filaments (Figure 5-2). Thick filaments are composed mainly of myosin molecules, whereas thin filaments are composed of actin molecules, troponin proteins, and a tropomyosin protein. The thick and thin filaments are also known as myofibrils.[7]

Myosin filaments are located in the middle of the sarcomere and are attached to the Z line of the sarcomere by the protein titin.[7] In addition, myosin-binding protein C (or C-protein) is attached to myosin filaments.[7,8] Myosin-binding protein C also is attached to titin, and the interaction among these proteins may be important in cross-bridge function and in the generation of passive tension. For example, when the sarcomere is stretched, titin elongates and exerts a passive force. When the sarcomere relaxes (shortens), titin is important in restoring the force during early diastole.[9] Actin filaments, which are attached to the Z lines, overlap the myosin filaments from opposite ends of the sarcomere.

As noted before, the thin filament is composed mainly of helical chains of globular actin proteins that are coiled around a tropomyosin protein (Figure 5-3A).[7,10] At regularly spaced intervals (43 nm), the troponin heterotrimer (troponin complex) is attached to actin proteins.[7,10,11] The troponin heterotrimer consists of three troponin proteins: troponin T, troponin I, and troponin C.[10,11] Collectively, these proteins are referred to as regulatory proteins because they control the interaction between actin and myosin and therefore cross-bridge cycling.[10] Troponin T attaches the whole troponin complex to tropomyosin, the long filamentous protein that in the resting state covers the myosin-binding sites on actin. Troponin I binds to actin, and troponin C binds Ca^{++}.[7] As detailed later, the binding of Ca^{++} to troponin C regulates the actin/myosin interaction and cross-bridge cycling.

The thick filament is composed of myosin II molecules. The myosin heavy chain has three distinct regions: the tail, hinge, and head (Figure 5-3B).[7,10,11] The tail and hinge regions are composed of two intertwined myosin heavy chains, which branch into two head regions. Each head region (also referred to as the S_1 fragment) contains one alkali (blue) and one regulatory (red) light chain. The regulatory and alkali light chains serve two important functions: regulation of myosin adenosinetriphosphatase (ATPase) activity and stabilization of the myosin head region, respectively. The myosin head region also contains the actin binding site and

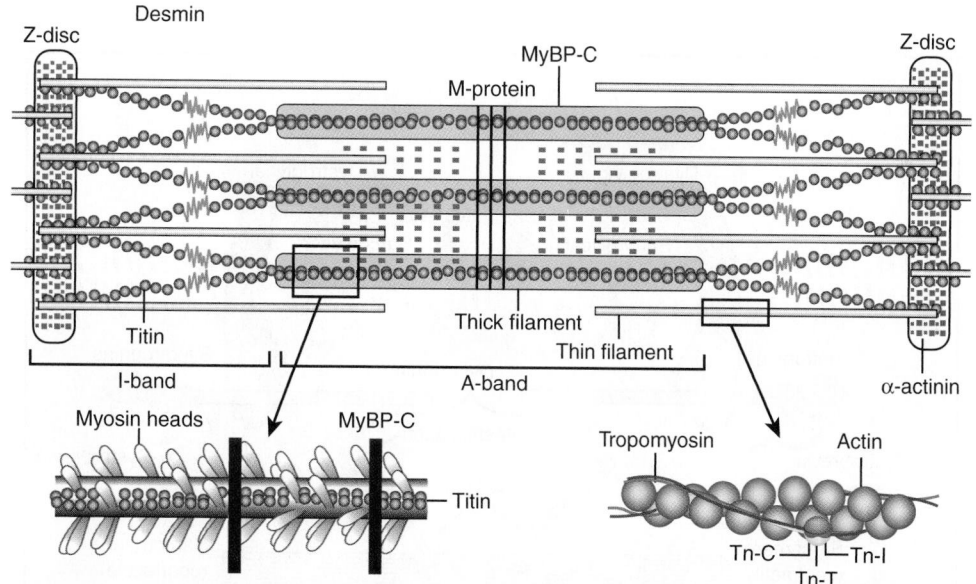

FIGURE 5-2 ▥ Arrangement of thick and thin filaments within a single sarcomeric unit. In the cardiomyocyte the thick (myosin) and thin (actin) filaments are arranged in repeating sarcomeric units. Myosin is located in the middle of the sarcomere. Actin filaments are bound to the Z disc (line). The Z disc is a composite of interconnecting proteins such as desmin and alpha-actinin. These proteins link the actin filaments to the Z disc. Titin is another protein attached to the Z disc. Titin serves to anchor myosin to the Z disc, while myosin binding protein (MyBP-C) attaches to myosin toward the middle of the sarcomere. All of these intracellular proteins are critical in stabilizing the myofilaments during and after cross-bridge formation and in the transduction of force. When viewed through a light electron microscope, the sarcomere has an alternating light and dark appearance that is due to the composition and arrangement of the myofibrils. The dark band also designated as the A band is composed only of myosin filaments. The light band or I band lies between the A bands of two neighboring sarcomeres and is composed of portions of two actin filaments that do not overlap myosin filaments. (From Anand IS, Florea VG: Alterations in ventricular structure: role of left ventricular remodeling. In Mann DL, editor: *Heart failure: a companion to Braunwald's heart disease*, Philadelphia, 2004, Saunders.)

A THIN FILAMENT

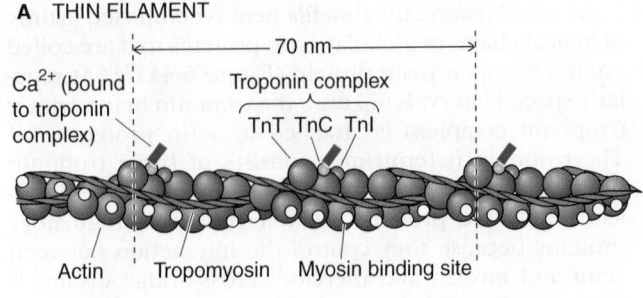

B MYOSIN MOLECULE

C INTERACTION OF THIN AND THICK FILAMENTS

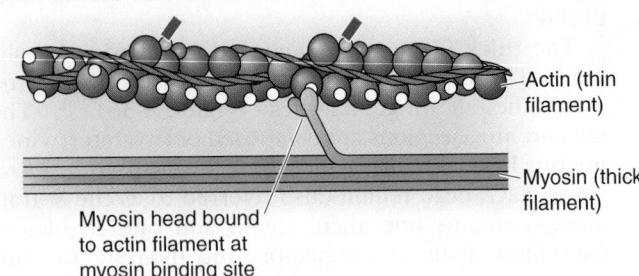

FIGURE 5-3 ■ **A,** The thin filament is composed of many globular actin molecules, a long filamentous tropomyosin protein, and three troponin proteins: TNC—troponin C, TNI—troponin I, TNT—troponin T. In a weak cross-bridge state the tropomyosin protein covers the myosin binding sites on the actin filament. **B,** The myosin filament consists of three regions: the head, which is composed of the regulatory and alkali light chains; the hinge region; and the tail region. The head region is where actin binds and ATP is hydrolyzed to adenosine diphosphate and inorganic phosphate. **C,** Calcium binding to troponin C elicits a conformational change in the actin filament, such that the myosin binding sites on actin are exposed, which allows the myosin head to bind to the actin filament at the myosin binding site. (From Apkon M: Cellular physiology of the skeletal, cardiac, and smooth muscle. In Boron WF, Boulpaep EL, editors: *Medical physiology,* Philadelphia, 2005, Elsevier Saunders.)

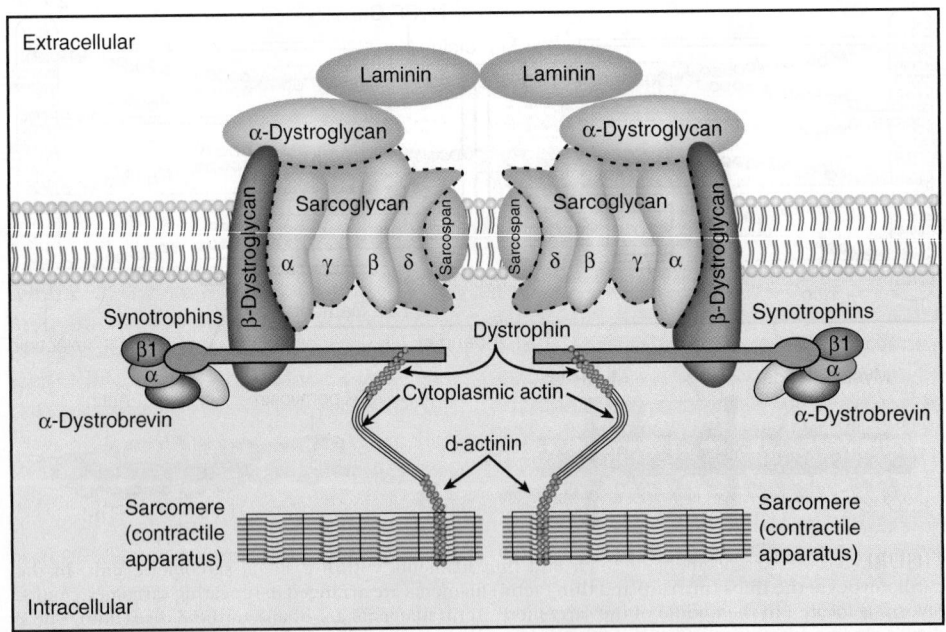

FIGURE 5-4 ■ Membrane and cytoskeletal proteins. The cytoskeleton is a group of intracellular proteins that form an intracellular architectural scaffold that serves to connect sarcomeric proteins to each other, as well as to other proteins in the extracellular matrix. Extracellular matrix proteins include laminin and alpha-dystroglycan. These are bound to integral sarcolemma proteins (proteins spanning the sarcolemma, also referred to as integrins) such as beta-dystroglycan and sarcoglycan. The integral sarcolemma protein beta-dystroglycan is linked to cytoskeletal proteins such as dystrophin, which in turn is linked via alpha-actinin and actin to the sarcomeric contractile apparatus. (Adapted from Towbin JA, Bowles NE: Heart failure as a consequence of genetic cardiomyopathy. In Mann DL, editor: *Heart failure: a companion to Braunwald's heart disease,* Philadelphia, 2004, Saunders.)

the enzymatic site (myosin ATPase) that hydrolyzes **ATP** to adenosine diphosphate and inorganic phosphate.[7]

Cytoskeleton

The cytoskeleton is a group of intracellular proteins that form an intracellular architectural scaffold that connects sarcomeric proteins to each other and to sarcolemmal proteins and other proteins in the extracellular matrix.[11,12] The spectrum of cytoskeletal proteins includes, but is not limited to, desmin, integrins, and dystrophin. Classified as an intermediate filament, desmin surrounds the Z discs and connects sarcomeres to each other and the sarcolemma. Integrins form a group of transmembrane proteins that bind extracellular matrix proteins. Dystrophin binds to cytosolic actin and to dystroglycans in the sarcolemma (Figure 5-4).[12,13] The cytoskeleton is critical in providing a structural framework for the lateral transmission of force, not only among sarcomeres but also from the sarcomeres to the sarcolemma and into the extracellular matrix.[12]

As shown in Figure 5-4, extracellular matrix proteins such as laminin and alpha-dystroglycan are bound to integral sarcolemma proteins (proteins spanning the sarcolemma, also referred to as integrins) such as beta-dystroglycan and sarcoglycan. The integral sarcolemma protein beta-dystroglycan is linked to cytoskeletal proteins such as dystrophin.[12,13] Dystrophin is linked via other cytoskeletal proteins (e.g., alpha-actinin and actin) to the sarcomeric contractile apparatus. These connections among the extracellular matrix proteins, sarcolemma, and sarcomeric proteins are critical for the coordination of force generation and the unified contraction of the myocardium.

Sarcoplasmic Reticulum

The sarcoplasmic reticulum is the major site for Ca^{++} storage, release, and reuptake (sequestration); consequently, the sarcoplasmic reticulum plays a central role in cardiac contraction and relaxation.[11] The sarcoplasmic reticulum is a large intracellular structure that is surrounded by actin and myosin filaments and is coupled to the sarcolemma via the T tubules. The sarcoplasmic reticulum has two components: the junctional sarcoplasmic reticulum (terminal cisternae) and the longitudinal tubules. The junctional sarcoplasmic reticulum is close to the sarcolemma and contains the calcium-release channel or ryanodine-sensitive channel (Figure 5-1).[14,15]

Mitochondria

In cardiomyocytes, mitochondria occupy a large proportion of the cytosolic compartment and are located between myofibrils. Mitochondria are the major sites for oxidative phosphorylation (adenosine triphosphate [ATP] generation), as well as oxidative metabolism of fatty acids, pyruvate, and amino acids. A continuous supply of ATP is required to sustain contraction and relaxation, support sarcolemmal ion pumps, and fuel many enzymatic reactions. Another mitochondrial function is to buffer high concentrations of cytosolic Ca^{++}. In conditions of Ca^{++} overload that occur during prolonged periods of ischemia, the mitochondria will accumulate Ca^{++}. However, too much Ca^{++} accumulation in the mitochondria eventually impairs the proton gradient across mitochondrial membranes, reducing ATP synthesis and overall mitochondrial function and viability.[11]

MOLECULAR MECHANISMS OF CONTRACTION, CROSS-BRIDGE CYCLING, AND RELAXATION

Contraction

The process of contraction begins with depolarization of the sarcolemma and the entry of Ca^{++} during phase 2 of the action potential. As shown in Figure 5-1, step 1, a propagated action potential leads to depolarization of the sarcolemma and opening of voltage-dependent L-type Ca^{++} channels. Under physiological conditions the intracellular concentration of Ca^{++} is in the nanomolar range (10^{-9} M), whereas the extracellular Ca^{++} concentration is in the millimolar range (10^{-3} M); therefore, Ca^{++} enters the cell down a steep electrochemical gradient.[11] The extracellular Ca^{++} that enters the cell during phase 2 of the cardiac action potential is the trigger for Ca^{++} release from the sarcoplasmic reticulum, referred to as calcium-induced calcium release (Figure 5-1, step 2). Ca^{++} is released from the sarcoplasmic reticulum through the ryanodine receptor. An important note is that the amount of Ca^{++} that enters the cell during phase 2 of the action potential is not sufficient for myofilament activation. However, this Ca^{++} is sufficient to activate the release of Ca^{++} from the ryanodine receptor. In fact, the amount of Ca^{++} entering through the L-type channel is an important determinant of how much Ca^{++} is released from the ryanodine receptor. For example, with a greater Ca^{++} current, the ryanodine receptor is more activated, resulting in a greater rise in the total intracellular Ca^{++} concentration.[5,6] An increase in cardiomyocyte action potential duration is associated with an increase in phase 2 Ca^{++} influx and therefore an increase in total intracellular Ca^{++}, enhancing myocardial contractility.

Ca^{++} binds to the regulatory protein troponin-C and induces a conformational change in another regulatory protein, troponin I (Figure 5-1, step 3). The conformational change in troponin I allows actin to interact with myosin, inducing a strong cross-bridge formation and force generation. Once actin and myosin interact, ATP is hydrolyzed to form adenosine diphosphate and inorganic phosphate, supplying the energy required for movement of myosin along the actin molecule and thereby contraction.[7,16] This phenomenon is repeated during contraction and is referred to as cross-bridge cycling.

Cross-Bridge Cycling

Myocardial contraction and subsequent force development occur as a result of cross-bridge cycling or the re-

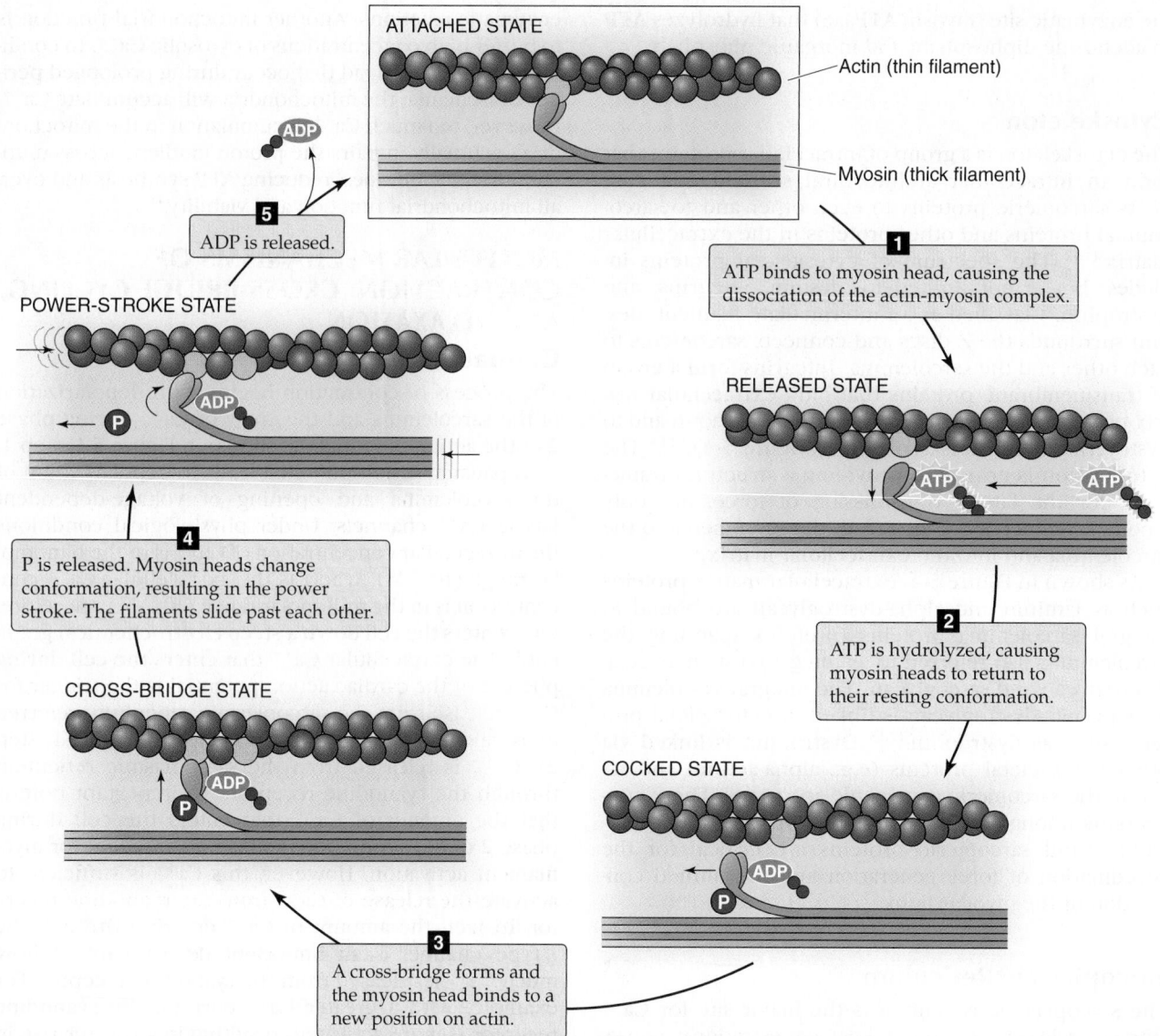

FIGURE 5-5 ■ Cross-bridge cycling. See text for details. (From Apkon M: Cellular physiology of the skeletal, cardiac, and smooth muscle. In Boron WF, Boulpaep EL, editors: *Medical physiology,* Philadelphia, 2005, Elsevier Saunders.)

petitive binding and interaction between actin and myosin and the sliding of these filaments past each other (previously referred to as the sliding filament theory). Cross-bridge cycling involves interactions among the contractile proteins (actin and myosin) and regulatory proteins (troponin and tropomyosin). In the relaxed state (diastole), troponin I inhibits the interaction between actin and the myosin heads because it keeps the tropomyosin protein aligned over the myosin-binding sites of actin.[7,16] When intracellular Ca^{++} increases as a result of Ca^{++} entry, Ca^{++} binds to troponin C. The interaction between Ca^{++} and troponin C causes troponin I to bind to troponin C, eliciting a conformational change in troponin T that pushes the tropomyosin away from the myosin-binding sites on actin.[6] This process allows for cross-bridge formation between actin and myosin.

As shown in Figure 5-5 *(step 1),* in the released or resting state, ATP is bound to the head of myosin. ATP is hydrolyzed by myosin ATPase to adenosine diphosphate and phosphate. The free energy of ATP hydrolysis is used for the mechanical work (Figure 5-5, *step 2*). As a result of the hydrolysis, the myosin head is in a more favorable or strong binding conformation, which allows it to align with a binding site further down on the actin filament (Figure 5-5, *step 3*). Myosin binds with actin, and a cross bridge forms. This cross-bridge formation in itself may promote more actin-myosin cross-bridge reactions by a cooperative feedback mechanism. The release of phosphate corresponds to flexion of the myosin head and bending of the myosin hinge, such that the actin filament slides toward the tail of myosin (Figure 5-5, *step 4*). The conformational change that causes the actin filament to be moved along the myosin filament (cross-bridge formation) produces force and motion. Adenosine diphosphate is released, and a regenerated ATP binds to the same site on myosin, stimulating the dissociation of actin and myosin (*steps 5 and 1,* Figure 5-5). ATP binding to myosin returns myosin to its original resting 90-degree position or weak-binding conformation. Lack of ATP, such as occurs after lack of oxygen, causes rigor mortis. Rigor mortis, or muscle rigidity, is caused by the permanent attachment of the actin and myosin filaments.[7]

Relaxation

Relaxation, or diastole, comes about by the intracellular Ca^{++} concentration being lowered back to basal levels $(10^{-9}$ M).[5] In human hearts the predominant relaxation mechanism is Ca^{++} reuptake (sequestration) by the sarcoplasmic reticulum (Figure 5-1). That relaxation is an energy-dependent (ATP-dependent) process is important to note. Ca^{++} uptake occurs via a Ca^{++}- and magnesium-dependent ATPase pump located in the longitudinal section of the sarcoplasmic reticulum. This pump is referred to as the sarco[endo]plasmic reticulum Ca^{++}-ATPase (**SERCA2a**).[5,6] SERCA2a transports Ca^{++} against a high concentration gradient from the cytosol back into the lumen of the sarcoplasmic reticulum (step 4, Figure 5-1). The Ca^{++} is stored within the lumen of the junctional sarcoplasmic reticulum, whereby it is in approximation to the ryanodine receptor and is bound to a number of calcium-binding proteins, including calsequestrin, calreticulin, and glycoproteins.[11]

Regulation of Ca^{++} uptake by the sarcoplasmic reticulum occurs through the phosphorylation state of the protein phospholamban (PLB in Figure 5-1), which is a large protein colocalized with SERCA2a.[11] Under basal conditions, phospholamban is not phosphorylated (i.e., does not have the addition of a phosphate) and exerts an inhibitory effect on (slows down) SERCA2a activity. Many beta-adrenergic agents (e.g., isoproterenol and epinephrine) stimulate phosphorylation of phospholamban by cyclic adenosine monophosphate–dependent protein kinase A, which relieves the inhibition and allows for a faster uptake of Ca^{++} and faster decline in the intracellular level of Ca^{++}.[5,6] This translates into a faster rate of relaxation or lusitropic effect. An increase in sarcoplasmic reticulum Ca^{++} uptake also leads to greater filling of the sarcoplasmic reticulum with Ca^{++}. The physiological effect is such that, during the subsequent cycle, more Ca^{++} is released, which leads to an increase in contractile force and therefore cardiac output.

The sarcolemmal Na/Ca exchanger (NCX in Figure 5-1) and Ca^{++}-ATPase also removes Ca^{++} from the cytosol. During relaxation, SERCA2a removes about 70 percent of activator Ca^{++}, the Na/Ca exchanger removes about 28 percent, and about 1 percent is removed by the sarcolemmal Ca^{++}-ATPase.[5]

Factors that Modulate Contraction and Relaxation

The mechanisms that alter contraction (force generation) and relaxation can be organized into three catego-ries: (1) increased activation of cross bridges by Ca^{++} ions, which results in stronger cross-bridge forming and cycling; (2) phosphorylation or dephosphorylation of contractile proteins (altering the cross-bridge response to Ca^{++} affecting force and relaxation); and (3) the length/alignment of the sarcomere (Frank-Starling relationship).[11]

Because Ca^{++} is the most important regulator of contraction, modulating intracellular Ca^{++} levels is an important mechanism by which to increase force. Under basal physiological Ca^{++} conditions (that is, on a beat-to-beat moment), sarcomeres generate about 25 percent of their possible peak force.[11] Stated another way, the heart has a large contractile reserve such that, with each contraction, not every actin and myosin participate in cross-bridge cycling. Increasing the intracellular (cytosolic) free Ca^{++} concentration during systole increases the amount of Ca^{++} that interacts with troponin C, thereby increasing the amount and rate of cross-bridge cycling and force generation. An increase in intracellular Ca^{++} also can be accomplished by increasing sarcoplasmic reticulum release of Ca^{++}, which can occur following an increase in Ca^{++} current through the L-type Ca^{++} channel.

Another way to modulate force and relaxation is through phosphorylation and dephosphorylation reactions.[6,10] Sarcomeric proteins (e.g., troponin I), proteins associated with intracellular structures (e.g., phospholamban), and membrane channels (e.g., L-type Ca^{++} channels) can be phosphorylated (adding a phosphate group) or dephosphorylated (deleting a phosphate group). These phosphorylation/dephosphorylation reactions alter the function of the protein. For example, as noted before, phosphorylation of phospholamban relieves SERCA2a inhibition, promoting faster Ca^{++} uptake. This translates into a faster decline in the intracellular level of Ca^{++} and a faster rate of relaxation, allowing diastole to happen more quickly (lusitropic effect). A longer diastole allows for adequate and complete perfusion of the myocardium. In particular, the left ventricle receives most of its coronary artery blood flow during diastole. In addition to phospholamban, troponin I and the regulatory myosin light chain (in the myosin heavy chain head) are targets for phosphorylation. Troponin I phosphorylation causes an adjacent decrease in the Ca^{++} affinity of troponin C and increased dissociation of Ca^{++} from the troponin C protein. This also enhances the rate of relaxation because the release of Ca^{++} causes a conformational change in actin and its dissociation from myosin, hence relaxation.[10] How are phosphorylation/dephosphorylation reactions initiated in cardiomyocytes? Many conditions and drugs can stimulate phosphorylation/dephosphorylation reactions; however, most relevant to the myocardium are beta-adrenergic agents. In brief, beta-adrenergic agents lead to an increase in cyclic adenosine monophosphate–dependent protein kinase A, an enzyme that adds a phosphate moiety to cellular proteins.[11]

Finally, altering the length/alignment of the sarcomere (Frank-Starling relationship) also modulates sarcomere force development. As the ventricle contracts and relaxes, the sarcomeres are stretched to various lengths. Increased sarcomere stretch (up to a point) is associated

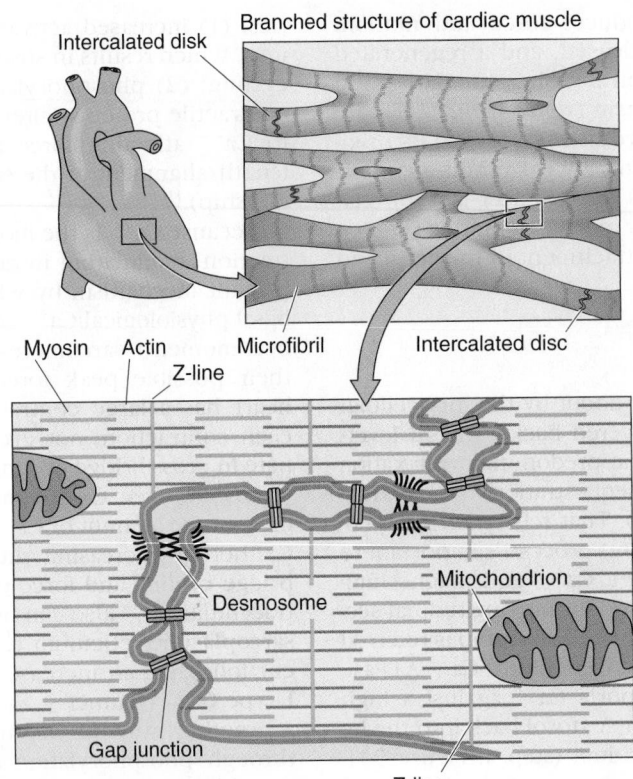

FIGURE 5-6 ▪ Intercalated disc and gap junction. (From Apkon M: Cellular physiology of the skeletal, cardiac, and smooth muscle. In Boron WF, Boulpaep EL, editors: *Medical physiology,* Philadelphia, 2005, Elsevier Saunders.)

with corresponding increases in force/tension.[17] The mechanism that underlies this relationship is not understood completely but may involve improved geometrical overlap between the myofilaments or increased myofilament sensitivity to Ca^{++}. Under physiological conditions, extreme stretching of the sarcomere usually does not occur. Proteins such as titin serve to oppose excessive stretch and restore force as the sarcomere shortens.[18]

MYOCARDIAL ELECTROPHYSIOLOGY

In 1883, Ringer demonstrated that, once removed from the body and perfused with a physiological solution containing electrolytes and other substrates, the isolated heart could beat and contract spontaneously. Unlike other muscle types such as skeletal muscle, the heart does not require neural innervation for excitation. The molecular basis for how electrical current is propagated, develops (automaticity), and results in the excitation of all cardiomyocytes is discussed next.

Cellular Basis for Propagation of Electrical Current

Depolarization of P cells in the sinoatrial node leads to the eventual depolarization of all other cardiomyocytes. Cardiomyocytes are tightly apposed to each other via intercalated discs where the sarcolemmas of adjacent cells are in proximity. Three kinds of junctional complexes connect adjacent cardiomyocytes at the intercalated disc: fascia adherens, desmosomes, and gap junc-

tions.[19] The fascia adherens serves as an anchor for cytoplasmic actin, whereas desmosomes attach to intermediate filaments (such as desmin) and the Z line of the sarcomere (Figure 5-6). Fascia adherens and desmosomes are, therefore, attachment points for the cytoskeleton that connects the myofilaments and sarcolemma.

Gap Junctions and Desmosomes

Gap junctions are pores that mediate the cell-to-cell propagation of ions and current flow (Figure 5-6). Gap junctions are composed of connexin proteins. The major connexin expressed in the heart is connexin 43, which is found in abundance in ventricular and atrial cardiomyocytes.[19] The connexins form pores that connect adjacent cardiomyocytes at the intercalated disc and allow for the movement of ions and small molecules between cardiomyocytes. The low electrical resistance of gap junctions allows rapid and orderly propagation of current from cardiomyocyte to cardiomyocyte, facilitating synchronous contraction of the myocardium. Gap junction permeability depends on several factors, including pH, intracellular Ca^{++} concentration, and transjunctional and transmembrane voltage. Interestingly, during ischemia, when there is a rise in intracellular Ca^{++}, the connexin proteins close, which is thought to seal off injured cells from uninjured cells, preventing lethal increases in intracellular Ca^{++} in neighboring uninjured cardiomyocytes. Alterations in gap junctions and connexin protein expression can occur in a number of cardiac pathological states, and these changes may be important in the genesis of cardiac arrhyth-

A CONDUCTION PATHWAYS THROUGH HEART

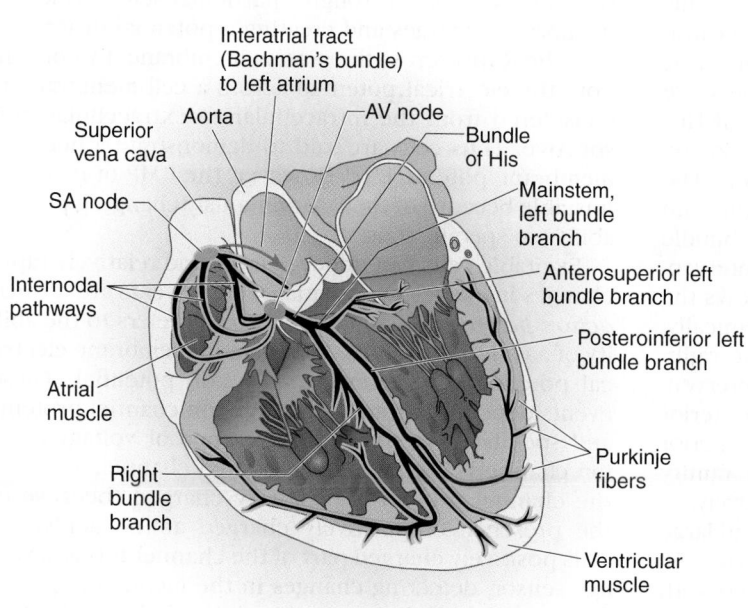

B CARDIAC ACTION POTENTIALS

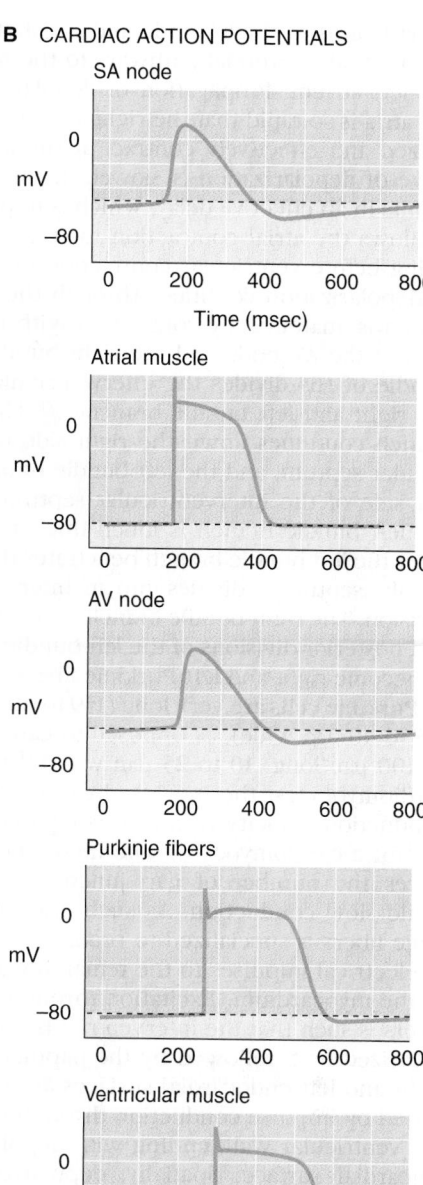

FIGURE 5-7 ■ **A,** Conduction pathways through the heart and in relationship to the different anatomical sections of the heart. Impulses that originate in the sinoatrial (SA) node via intranodal pathways are conducted to the atrioventricular (AV) node and then are conducted along both bundle branches. **B,** Cardiac cellular action potentials originating from different anatomical locations. (From Lederer WJ: Cardiac electrophysiology and the electrocardiogram. In Boron WF, Boulpaep EL, editors: *Medical physiology,* Philadelphia, 2005, Elsevier Saunders.)

mias.[20] Disturbances in gap junction organization could impair and slow cell impulse propagation, giving rise to areas of inhomogeneous and slowed conduction, contributing to dysrhythmogenesis.[19,20]

P Cells and the Conduction System

Electrical activity in the myocardium begins with a group of specialized cells that spontaneously depolarize and therefore are referred to as automatic cell types or P cells (pacemaker cells). Unlike the cardiomyocytes (con-

tractile cells), P cells are void of organized sarcomeres. P cells are found in the sinoatrial (**SA**) node and atrioventricular (**AV**) node of the myocardium and are named for their generalized anatomical location.[21] The SA node is a small area located in the right atrium, just posterior to the junction of the right atrium, the coronary sinus, and the superior vena cava. The AV node is situated on the right side of the partition that divides the atria, at the base junction of the atria and ventricles.

Electrical activity precedes mechanical activity. As shown in Figure 5-7, the organized depolarization of the heart begins in the SA node and simultaneously travels down atrial internodal pathways to the AV node and to the left atrium. Propagation of depolarization through the atria is so rapid that the right and left atria are depolarized and effectively contract at the same time. The wave of depolarization is slowed in the AV node. This results in an effective delay, which is important because it allows the atrial contraction to complete ventricular filling before ventricular contraction begins. The wave of depolarization continues through the bundle of His, which is anatomically continuous with the anterior region of the AV node and the right bundle branch. The bundle of His divides the interventricular septum into the right and left bundle branches.[21] The right bundle branch continues down the right side of the interventricular septum, and the left bundle branch follows the left side of the interventricular septum. Anatomically, the left bundle branch is much thicker than the right. After the left bundle branch penetrates the left interventricular septum, it divides into an anterior and posterior division. The right bundle branch, as well as the anterior and posterior divisions of the left bundle branch, ramify to become right and left Purkinje fibers, respectively.

Purkinje cells are very long (159 to 200 μm) and large (35 to 40 μm wide), as opposed to cardiomyocytes (50 to 100 μm long, 10 to 25 μm wide).[11] Compared with cardiomyocytes, the increased cell diameter increases conduction velocity (2 m/sec compared with 0.60 m/sec for a cardiomyocyte), and increased cell length reduces the number of gap junctions that potentially could slow conduction. As such, the structure of Purkinje fibers is specialized to promote rapid conduction of electrical impulses to the remaining areas and layers of the myocardium. Excitation through the myocardial layers is such that the interventricular septal area is depolarized first, followed by the papillary muscles. The right and left endocardial surfaces are depolarized, followed by impulse conduction through the thickness of the ventricular wall, ending with depolarization of the epicardial surface. Spatially, depolarization proceeds through the myocardium, such that contraction of the ventricles begins at the apex of the ventricle. Because the right ventricle is thinner than the left, the right ventricular epicardial surface depolarizes slightly before the left. The organized propagation of electrical activity through the conduction system is necessary for the sequential and coordinated contraction of the atria and ventricles. This produces a strong, efficient contraction that moves blood up and out of the ventricle toward the outflow tracts.[11,21]

Resting Membrane Potential, Excitability, Automaticity, and Rhythmicity

All cells demonstrate an electrical potential difference across the plasma membrane, termed the resting membrane potential (**RMP**). This potential difference arises because of differences in the intracellular and extracellular concentration of ions such as **Na⁺** and **K⁺** and to differences in permeability of the resting plasma membrane to those ions. At rest, the concentration of K⁺ inside the cell is more than 30 times greater than the

concentration of K⁺ outside the cell. In addition, the resting membrane possesses far greater permeability to K⁺ than to any other ion. This combination of properties sets the stage for small amounts of K⁺ to diffuse out of the cell, leaving behind excess negative, impermeant (i.e., unable to pass through a particular semipermeable membrane) charges and creating a potential difference (i.e., the RMP) across the plasma membrane. By convention, the electrical potential across a cell membrane is considered from the intracellular to extracellular perspective. Thus cells are said to demonstrate a negative membrane potential.[11,21] However, the RMP of P cells is unstable because of their continuously changing permeability to specific ions.

Excitable cells can undergo large and relatively rapid changes in electrical potential. These events are termed *action potentials.* Excitability broadly refers to the ability of a cell to respond to a change in membrane electrical potential and generate an action potential. These events depend on transmembrane ion channel proteins and specifically require the presence of voltage-gated ion channels. Within a voltage-gated channel, a part of the channel protein is positively charged (because of the presence of positively charged amino acids).[21,22] This positively charged part of the channel acts as a voltage sensor, detecting changes in the membrane potential that in turn elicit a conformational change leading to opening of the channel.

P cells and cardiomyocytes are excitable cell types. P cells are responsible for initiating and propagating electrical activity, whereas cardiomyocytes are responsible for propagating electrical activity and for contraction. The RMP of a quiescent contractile cell is around −80 to −90 mV, whereas the RMP of a P cell is between −50 and −60 mV.[11,21] For an action potential to occur, the RMP must decrease (become more positive) and reach an activation (depolarizing) threshold value of approximately −65 mV in a contractile cell and −40 mV in a P cell.[11,21] When each cell type reaches its activation threshold potential, voltage-gated channels are activated, triggering a propagated action potential.

The action potential of the P cells and contractile cells is associated with changes in the transmembrane ionic conductance of Na⁺, K⁺, and Ca⁺⁺ ions through their respective channel types. Because these ions are electrically charged, their movement across the membrane generates a current: a current is the flow of charge in some direction. The response of a membrane to ion movement across the membrane is described in terms of conductance and depends on the permeability of the membrane to the ion and the ion concentration difference across the membrane. As noted in the following sections, the magnitude, change, and duration of Na⁺, K⁺, and Ca⁺⁺ conductance and current through their respective channels are different between P and contractile cells.[21]

Ion Movements During the Action Potential of P Cells

P cells have two unique electrical features: automaticity and rhythmicity.[11,21] The unique rhythmic and automatic (spontaneous depolarization) properties of P cells allow the myocardium to continue beating independently of the nervous system. The terms *automaticity* and *rhythmicity* frequently are used interchangeably. Automaticity refers to the ability of the cell to depolarize spontaneously, whereas rhythmicity refers to the regularity of this spontaneous depolarization.[11] As shown in Figure 5-8, the spontaneous depolarization of P cells and subsequent action potential development arises from changes in the Ca^{++}, Na^+, and K^+ currents through specific voltage-gated sarcolemmal channels.[11,21]

The pacemaker activity of the SA and AV nodal P cells is attributed to changes in the inward Ca^{++} current (I_{Ca}), outward K^+ current (I_K), and inward pacemaker current (I_f; this current is due to Na^+ and K^+ conductance).[11] The RMP is around -60 mV, and the activation threshold is about -40 mV. Two components to the I_{Ca} are activated at different threshold potentials. The first is a transient component (I_{Ca-T}) activated at a threshold potential between -60 and -50 mV and a more prominent and long-lasting component (I_{Ca-L}) with a threshold of about -40 mV (Figure 5-8). The I_K (delayed rectifier) is chiefly due to an outward K^+ current. The I_f (also referred to as the hyperpolarization-activated cyclic nucleotide-gated current) is due to an increase in inward Na^+ current and to a lesser extent by changes in an inward K^+ current.[11,21] I_K is referred to as the hyperpolarization-activated cyclic nucleotide-gated channel/current because the current is not fully operative until the SA node is hyperpolarized. Increases in I_{Ca-T} and I_f give rise to the slow diastolic depolarization or phase 4 (gentle upstroke) of the action potential.[11] When the threshold is reached, the cell fully depolarizes, giving rise to the rapid upstroke or phase 0 of the action potential. During phase 3, the repolarization phase, the outward K^+ (I_K) current is activated and predominates. The ion fluxes and corresponding changes in the action potential are summarized in Figure 5-8.[21]

The reason that the SA node is designated as the pacemaker of the heart is because P cells in the SA node undergo diastolic depolarization (phase 4) at a faster rate than other P cells located in the AV node.[11] However, if P cells in the SA node are dysfunctional because of disease or ischemia, cells in the AV node become the primary pacemakers of the heart. AV node cells have a spontaneous frequency of depolarization of 40 to 60 times a minute, resulting in a heart rate of 40 to 60 beats per minute when the pacemaker shifts to the AV node. If the P cells in the AV node are destroyed, Purkinje cells would be the next to depolarize spontaneously; however, their frequency of depolarization is equal to or less than 40 times per minute.[11,21] At this heart rate, blood pressure falls and cardiac output becomes insufficient to meet the oxygen and metabolic demands of the brain, resulting in syncope.

Control of the Rate of Spontaneous Depolarization

The electrical activity of P cells can be influenced by changes in electrolyte concentrations, hormones such as neurotransmitters and paracrine/endocrine substances, as well as drugs. Under physiological condi-

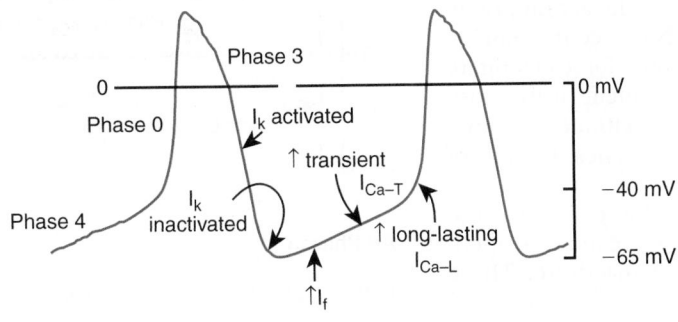

AP Phases

RMP	• -50 to -60 mV
Activation threshold (or depolarizing threshold)	• -35 to -40 mV
Phase 4	• Also referred to as phase 4 diastolic depolarization • Arises from ↑ inward I_{Ca} (transient I_{Ca-T}) and inward I_f and a slowing (decay) of the ↑ outward I_K currents
Phase 0	• Primarily attributed to ↑ inward I_{Ca} (long-lasting inward I_{Ca-L})
Phase 3	• ↑ Outward I_K current predominates

FIGURE 5-8 ■ Summary of the ionic fluxes during the action potential of a P cell. An important note is that the term *inward* indicates the flow of ions into the cell and the term *outward* indicates the flow of ions out of the cell. I_f, Inward pacemaker current; I_{Ca-T}, transient calcium current; I_{Ca-L}, long-lasting calcium current; I_K, potassium current; RMP, resting membrane potential.

tions, however, the SA node is under the tonic influence of both divisions of the autonomic nervous system. Parasympathetic stimulation dominates and exerts an inhibitory effect, and the sympathetic nervous system enhances automaticity. Acetylcholine, the neurotransmitter of the parasympathetic nervous system, decreases the amplitude, rate of increase, and duration of the SA action potential (Figure 5-9). The latter effects of acetylcholine are primarily attributable to activation of K^+ channels, outward flow of K^+, and more negative membrane potential (hyperpolarization). The net effect is that it takes the cell longer to reach its activation threshold, and this slows the rate of diastolic depolarization and hence the heart rate.[11] The net effect of sympathetic stimulation via an increase in the neurotransmitter norepinephrine is an increase in the heart rate. The slope of diastolic depolarization increases, and a slight increase occurs in the maximal diastolic potential. The way in which norepinephrine stimulates an increase in heart rate may involve numerous mechanisms, some of which include activation of latent pacemaker cells in the SA node (more cells begin to depolarize) and an increase in amplitude of the Ca^{++} current.[11,23] The K^+ current also increases, which leads to a faster rate of repolarization.[24] All of these effects increase heart rate.

Ion Movements During the Action Potential of the Cardiomyocyte

In cardiomyocytes a decrease in the RMP to the threshold voltage of -65 mV opens voltage-dependent fast Na^+ channels, giving rise to an increase in Na^+ conductance (g_{Na}) and current (I_{Na}). An increase in I_{Na} corresponds to the upstroke, or phase 0, of the action potential (Figure 5-10). The influx of Na^+ occurs quickly because concentration and electrostatic forces facilitate its movement into the cell. The movement of the positively charged Na^+ ions into the cell continues to depolarize the cell, such that the RMP reaches a value of about $+20$ mV.[21]

The fast Na^+ channels of contractile cells have the property of rapid opening; however, once they are open, the channels also rapidly close and inactivate. These channels cannot reopen until they are reset by repolarization of the membrane back to a negative membrane potential. Therefore, when the transmembrane potential reaches a positive potential of about $+20$ to $+30$ mv, Na^+ channel inactivation abruptly decreases I_{Na}. The initial rapid phase of depolarization is followed by a brief period of repolarization (phase 1). During phase 1, I_{Na} has subsided, and there is a decrease in the I_K (specifically a decrease in the transient outward K^+ current [I_{to}]). The membrane potential becomes less positive ($+20$ mV to $+10$ mV). At this positive membrane potential, voltage-dependent L-type Ca^{++} channels open, increasing Ca^+ conductance (g_{Ca}) and I_{Ca}. The Ca^{++} current through L-type channels gives rise to the most distinguishing feature of the cardiomyocyte action potential, which is phase 2, or the plateau phase. The entry of Ca^{++} through L-type channels can be blocked by drugs such as verapamil and diltiazem, which results in a decrease in heart rate and conduction velocity.[23] As noted before, Ca^{++} entering the cell during the plateau phase stimulates Ca^{++} release from the sarcoplasmic reticulum and ultimately initiates contraction.

The plateau phase is followed by repolarization (phase 3), which is due to a decrease in inward Ca^+ and Na^+ currents and an increase in I_K. Myocardial cells have several types of K^+ channels, including voltage-gated (delayed rectifier; K_V) or inward rectifier channels (K_{ir} or K_1).[21] Some K^+ channels appear to be hybrids between the inward rectifier and an ATP-binding type of channel, such as the ATP-sensitive K^+ channel. How-

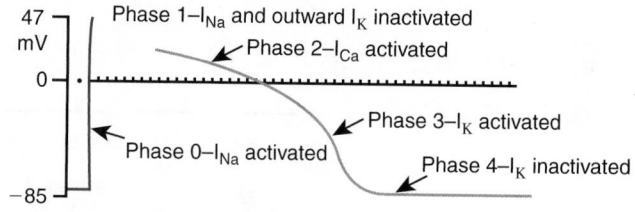

AP Phases

RMP	• -75 to -90 mV
Activation threshold (or depolarizing threshold)	• -55 to -65 mV
Phase 0	• Rapid ↑ in inward I_{Na}
Phase 1	• ↓ in inward I_{Na} and outward I_K
Phase 2	• ↑ inward I_{Ca}
Phase 3	• Beginning of repolarization, primarily attributable to an ↑ in the outward I_K current and ↓ in inward I_{Na} and I_{Ca}
Phase 4	• Repolarization and return to RMP

FIGURE 5-10 ■ Summary of the ionic fluxes during the action potential of a cardiomyocyte (ventricular) cell. An important note is that the term *inward* indicates the flow of ions into the cell and the term *outward* indicates the flow of ions out of the cell. I_{Na}, sodium current; I_{Ca}, calcium current; I_K, potassium current; RMP, resting membrane potential.

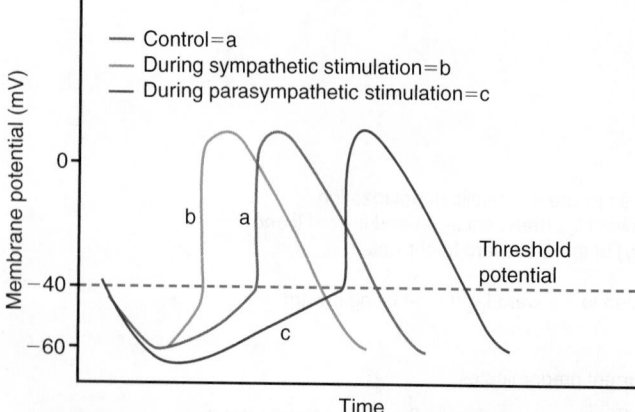

FIGURE 5-9 ■ Effects of control basal conditions, *(line a)*, sympathetic stimulation *(line b)*, and parasympathetic stimulation *(line c)* and on the action potential of a P cell.

ever, the ATP-sensitive K^+ channel is only active under pathophysiological conditions, such as ischemia. Under physiological conditions, at least three different outward K^+ currents flow through the different K^+ channels, and all collectively participate in repolarization. The K^+ currents include the rapid (I_{KR}) and slow (I_{KS}) delayed rectifier current or, the early transient outward current (I_{to}), and the inward rectifier (I_{K1} or I_{Kir}).[22,23] These currents are activated at different membrane potentials and are critical for cell repolarization and maintenance of the RMP. In the final phase of repolarization (phase 4), the membrane potential returns to a resting value of -80 to -90 mV (Figure 5-10).

Refractoriness

Refractoriness is a property of contractile cells and P cells. Refractoriness, or the refractory period, refers to the period during the action potential in which the cell does not respond to a further excitatory stimulus with a normal action potential. The refractory period is divided into two phases: the absolute refractory period and relative refractory phase. In a contractile cell, the beginning of the absolute refractory period corresponds to phase 1 of the action potential and inactivation of the fast Na^+ channels (Figure 5-11). During the absolute refractory period, regardless of the stimulus intensity, the contractile cell cannot accept another action potential, and therefore the cell cannot be excited.[23] There follows a relative refractory period during which the cell is not fully repolarized but could be depolarized by a strong, supraphysiological excitatory stimulus. The period encompassed by the absolute refractory period and the relative refractory period is referred to as the effective refractory period because a normal physiological stimulus cannot result in an action potential. In the heart the effective refractory period lasts longer than a contractile event. This results in an inability to achieve tetany in the heart, thus preventing interference with effective pumping of blood.

MYOCARDIAL SUBSTRATE UTILIZATION
Substrate Availability and Use

Myocardial oxygen extraction is among the highest per gram of tissue in the body. As a result, increases in oxygen demand require increased oxygen delivery, so adequacy of coronary perfusion is associated intimately with the metabolic requirements of the heart.

Human hearts can metabolize a variety of substrates, including fatty acids, carbohydrates, lactate, pyruvate, and ketone bodies. The relative utilization of each individual substrate is readily altered, depending on conditions such as food intake, exercise, and disease conditions.[24] On average, however, fatty acids account for 60 to 70 percent of myocardial oxygen consumption for energy production, with carbohydrates and lactate providing the balance. The glucose-fatty acid balance strongly influences the preference of substrate utilization. When adipose lipolysis is increased, as in fasting, increased fatty acid availability inhibits glucose metabolism. Conversely, when circulating glucose and insulin increase, lipolysis is inhibited, thereby reducing fatty acid inhibition of myocardial glycolysis. Thus glucose can become the dominant substrate used by the myocardium, for example, after a high-carbohydrate meal.

Fatty Acid Availability

The uptake of fatty acids by the myocardium from the blood is a highly regulated transport process that is just beginning to be understood. Some of the mechanisms and pathways in myocardial fatty acid metabolism are outlined in Figure 5-12. The extracellular source of fatty acids can be (1) circulating fatty acids associated with plasma albumin and (2) triacylglycerol cores of lipoproteins, including chylomicrons and very low-density lipoproteins (VLDLs). Fatty acids are transferred from blood to cardiac myocytes by transport proteins, including lipoprotein lipase, fatty acid binding protein, fatty acid translocase (**FAT/CD 36**), and fatty acid transport pro-

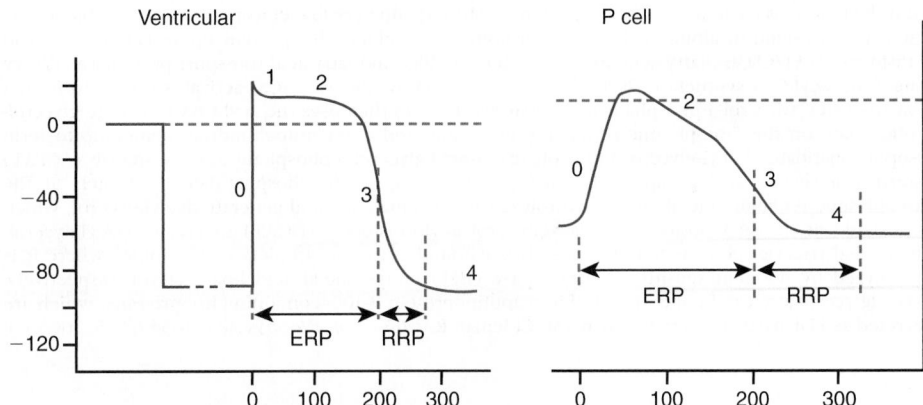

FIGURE 5-11 ▪ Effective refractory period (ERP) and relative refractory period (RRP) during the action potentials of a cardiomyocyte and P cell. (Adapted from Berne RM, Levy MN, editors: *Principles of physiology*, St Louis, 1990, Mosby.)

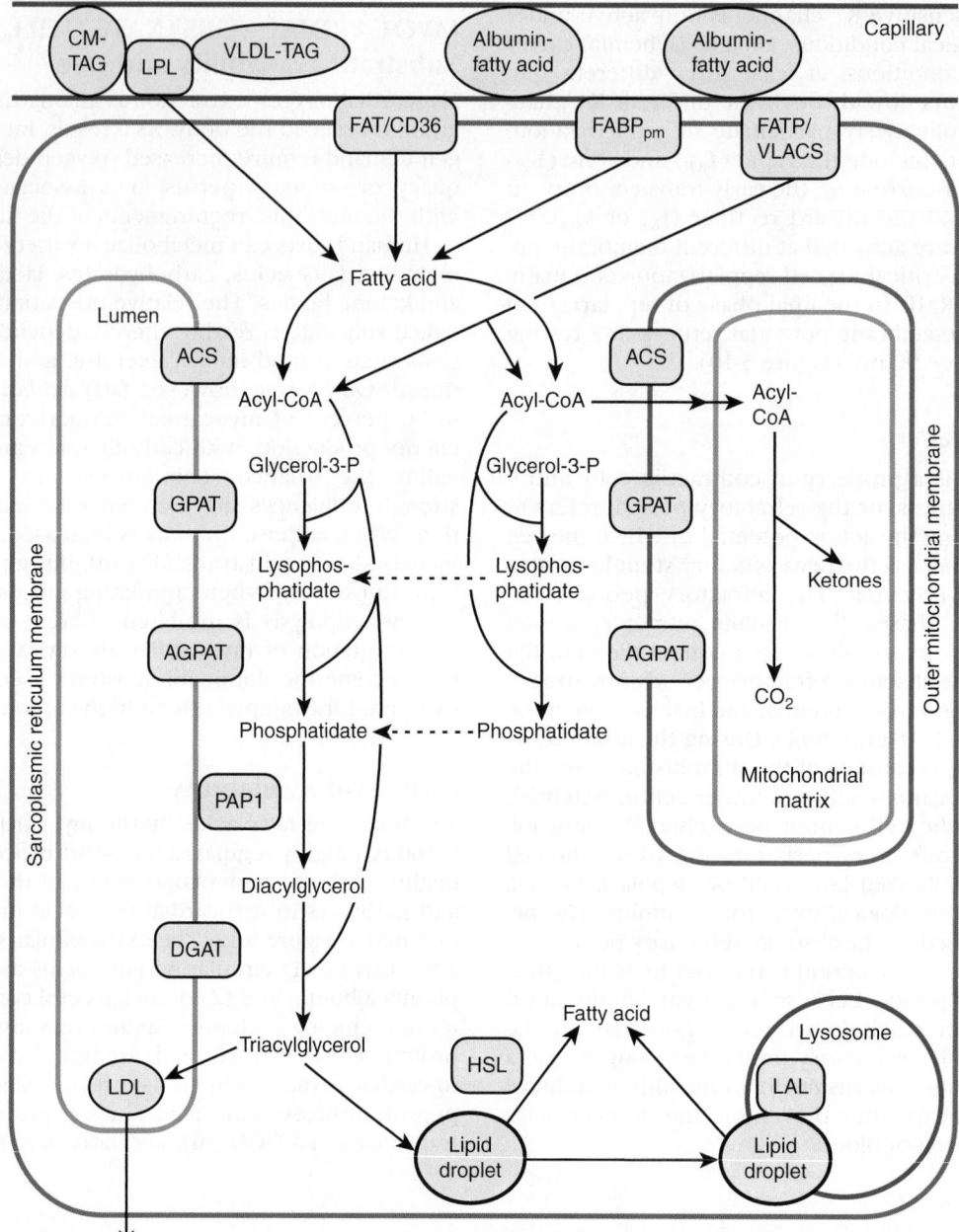

FIGURE 5-12 ▪ Proteins required for myocardial free fatty acid uptake, triacylglycerol (TG) synthesis, lipolysis and lipoprotein secretion. The proteins involved in the transfer of fatty acids (FAs) from the blood (as chylomicron-triacylglycerol [CM-TAG] and very low-density lipoprotein TAG [VLDL-TAG], or FA bound to albumin) into the cardiomyocyte include lipoprotein lipase (LPL), fatty acid translocase (FAT/CD36), fatty acid binding protein (FABP), and fatty acid transport protein/FATP/very long-chain acyl-CoA synthetase (FATP/VLACS). Acyl-CoA synthetase (ACS) activates the FA to form a CoA thioester. Glycerol-3-phosphate acyltransferase (GPAT) then uses the acyl-CoA to acylate glycerol-3-phosphate on the sarcoplasmic reticulum membrane and outer mitochondrial membrane to form lysophosphatidate (1-acyl-glycerol-3-phosphate). 1-Acyl-glycerol-3-phosphate acyltransferase (AGPAT) esterifies a second acyl group at the sn-2 position to generate phosphatidate. PAP1 acts at the sarcoplasmic reticulum membrane to hydrolyze the phosphatidate and generate diacylglycerol, which is acylated at the sn-3 position by diacylglycerol acyltransferase (DGAT) to create triacylglycerol. Myocardial triacylglycerol is found in membrane-bound cytosolic droplets or lysosomes where it is hydrolyzed by hormone-sensitive neutral lipase (HSL) or lysosomal acid lipase (LAL), respectively. Triacylglycerol also can be incorporated into apolipoprotein B-100–containing lipoproteins, which are secreted as LDL particles. (From Lewin TM, Coleman RA: *Biochem Biophys Acta* 1634:63-75, 2003.)

tein. As much as 70 percent of long-chain fatty acids in the blood can be taken up by myocytes in a single pass through a capillary bed.[25]

In isolated perfused hearts, it has been reported that fatty acids are taken up preferentially over triacylglycerols; however, the evidence in vivo indicates a preference for blood-borne triacylglycerols. The transport of the fatty acids contained in triacylglycerols from chylomicrons and VLDLs to the heart is mediated by lipoprotein lipase. Lipoprotein lipase is synthesized by cardiac myocytes and can translocate to capillary endothelial surfaces to mobilize fatty acids from lipoproteins into the myocardial interstitial space. Evidence for the importance of lipoprotein lipase can be found in physiological and pathophysiological conditions. Lipoprotein lipase is elevated with fasting and diabetes, contributing to higher cardiac triacylglycerol stores in those conditions. When lipoprotein lipase is inhibited or removed from the heart, glucose oxidation increases to meet the energy demands; uptake of long-chain fatty acids associated with albumin does not appear to increase substantially.[26,27] Thus although fatty acids associated with albumin are available for use by the heart, this appears to be a secondary source of fatty acid supply for the myocardium.

The transport of fatty acids into the cardiomyocytes involves fatty acid binding protein, FAT/CD 36, and fatty acid transport protein to varying degrees. A role for FAT/CD 36 in this regard is clear, and recent work suggests that this membrane protein is required for long-chain fatty acid use.[26,27] The specific roles of fatty acid binding protein and fatty acid transport protein are less clear. These proteins also are thought to be involved in the uptake of fatty acids by cardiomyocytes but may be more important as means of maintaining fatty acid availability in the aqueous cytoplasmic environment.

Stores of triacylglycerols within cardiac myocytes are used and replenished constantly such that intracellular triacylglycerols provide 10 to 50 percent of the energy requirements of the heart for oxidative metabolism. Drawing from stored triacylglycerols continues even when provision of triacylglycerols or fatty acids is high,[28] suggesting constant turnover of myocardial triacylglycerols.

Glycolysis

Glycolysis is the metabolic pathway by which glucose is converted to pyruvate. Glucose moves across the sarcolemma by facilitated diffusion via glucose transporter-1 (GLUT1) and GLUT4.[29,30] Once in the cell, glucose is phosphorylated readily by hexokinase to form glucose-6-phosphate, keeping cytosolic glucose very low and maintaining the gradient for glucose influx. The glucose-6-phosphate is directed to glycogen synthesis or glycolysis. Of the various enzymes in the glycolytic pathway, phosphofructokinase has a major influence on the fate of glucose-6-phosphate metabolism. When phosphofructokinase activity is increased, as in the ab-

sence of fatty acids or during hypoxia and ischemic conditions, glucose-6-phosphate is converted at a higher rate to fructose 1,6-bisphosphate, which is metabolized further to pyruvate. Another product of glycolysis, fructose 2,6-bisphosphate plays an important role in the heart by stimulating phosphofructokinase activity. Fructose 2,6-bisphosphate is not a glycolytic intermediate but a specific product of the enzyme phosphofructokinase-2. The cellular concentration of fructose 2,6-bisphosphate contributes to the regulation of the glycolytic rate in response to the presence of fatty acids, ketone bodies, insulin, and changes in workload to the myocardium.[30]

When plasma glucose is elevated, the relative contribution of glycolysis to total cardiac energy requirements increases. The myocardium is one of the most sensitive of insulin-sensitive organs,[31] which contributes to increased glycolysis during periods of higher plasma glucose concentration. In addition to increasing glycolysis, insulin also increases the number of GLUT1 and GLUT4 in the sarcolemma to accommodate increased glucose utilization.

In the presence of adequate oxygen, pyruvate produced from glycolysis enters the citrate cycle. The heart also can use lactate as a fuel, so pyruvate also can be formed by lactate dehydrogenase from lactate extracted from the blood by the heart. The contribution of lactate to the total energy requirements of the heart can be up to 60 percent during or immediately after anaerobic exercise and can rise to 90 percent during infusion of lactate-containing solutions. Like glucose, the movement of lactate across the sarcolemma is transporter-mediated, in a process that involves monocarboxylate transporter-1 and other transport proteins.[32] When oxygen delivery is inadequate to meet the total energy demands of the heart, pyruvate in excess of that which can be oxidized is converted to lactate, which leaves the heart. Indeed, lactate efflux from the heart in vivo has been used as an indicator of myocardial ischemia.

Glycolysis also appears to be important in the adaptation of the heart to a variety of cardiac-centered pathological conditions, including myocardial atherosclerotic processes and associated reductions in oxygen delivery, overt ischemia, and hypertrophic heart failure.[33] In heart failure, increased expression of glucose transporters and other metabolic enzymes that favor glycolysis has been associated with hypertrophic compensation, whereas progression into decompensated heart failure is associated with decreased expression of these critical proteins.[34] The importance of cardiac glucose metabolism during hypoxic or anoxic conditions has long been a focus of investigators. GLUTs translocate to the sarcolemma, and glycolysis is stimulated. Evidence indicates that glycolysis becomes compartmentalized in the cell and that glycolysis can be vital to supporting membrane pump function during anaerobic conditions and may be important in supporting contractile function during periods of modest to severe flow restrictions.[3;36]

SUMMARY

The myocardium is composed of cardiomyocytes and P cells, which work in synchrony to produce coordinated depolarization and contraction of the myocardium. Intracellular events, such as increases in Ca^{++} and cross-bridge cycling, are the molecular underpinnings of force generation and contraction. Relaxation is an equally important event, requiring the rapid reduction of intracellular Ca^{++}, which is predominately an energy-dependent process. The myocardium also can modulate its substrate utilization of fatty acids, carbohydrates, lactate, pyruvate, and ketone bodies, depending on conditions such as food intake, exercise, and pathological states. In many ways, various pathophysiological states of the myocardium result in the breakdown or malfunction of many of the molecular mechanisms described. To understand the pathophysiology and the rationale that underlie different treatment modalities, the practitioner must understand the physiology.

REFERENCES

1. Sommer JR, Jennings RB: Ultrastructure of cardiac muscle. In Fozzard HA, Haber E, Jennings RB, et al editors: *The heart and cardiovascular system,* ed 2, New York, 1991, Raven Press.
2. Nadal-Ginard B, Kajstura J, Leri A et al: Myocyte death, growth, and regeneration in cardiac hypertrophy and failure, *Circ Res* 92:139-150, 2003.
3. Anversa P, Kajstura J: Ventricular myocytes are not terminally differentiated in the adult mammalian heart, *Circ Res* 83:1-14, 1998.
4. Orlic D, Hill JM, Arai AE: Stem cells for myocardial regeneration, *Circ Res* 91:1092-1102, 2002.
5. Bers DM: Cardiac excitation-contraction coupling, *Nature* 425:198-205, 2002.
6. Trafford AW, Eisner DA: Excitation-contraction coupling in cardiac muscle. In Solaro RJ, Moss RL, editors: *Molecular control mechanisms in striated muscle contraction,* Boston, 2002, Kluwer Academic Publishers.
7. Apkon M: Cellular physiology of the skeletal, cardiac, and smooth muscle. In Boron WF, Boulpaep EL, editors: *Medical physiology,* Philadelphia, 2005, WB Saunders.
8. Anand IS, Florea VG: Alterations in ventricular structure: role of left ventricular remodeling. In Mann DL, editor: *Heart failure: a companion to Braunwald's heart disease,* Philadelphia, 2004, WB Saunders.
9. Granzier H, Labeit S: The giant protein titin: a major player in myocardial mechanics, signaling, and disease, *Circ Res* 94:284-295, 2004.
10. Solaro RJ: Modulation of cardiac myofilaments activity by protein phosphorylation. In Page E, Fozzard H, Solaro RJ, editors: *Handbook of physiology,* vol 1, *The heart,* New York, 2002, Oxford Press.
11. Opie LH: *Heart physiology from the cell to circulation,* ed 4, New York, 2004, Lippincott Williams & Wilkins.
12. Clark KA, Mittal B, Sanger JM, Sanger JW: Striated muscle cytoarchitecture: an intricate web form and function, *Annu Rev Cell Dev Biol* 18:637-706, 2002.
13. Towbin JA, Bowles NE: Heart failure as a consequence of genetic cardiomyopathy. In Mann DL, editor: *Heart failure: A companion to Braunwald's heart disease,* Philadelphia, 2004, WB Saunders.
14. Mikami A, Imoto K, Tanabe T et al: Primary structure and functional expression of the cardiac dihydropyridine-sensitive calcium channel, *Nature* 340:230-234, 1989.
15. Movsesian MA, Leveille C, Krall J et al: Identification and characterization of proteins in human cardiac sarcoplasmic reticulum, *J Mol Cell Cardiol* 22:1477-1485, 1990.
16. Rayment I, Holden EM, Whittaker M: Structure of the actin-myosin complex and its implications for muscle contraction, *Science* 261:58-65, 1993.
17. Konhilas JP, Irving TC, De Tombe PP: Frank-Starling law of the heart and cellular mechanisms of length-dependent activation, *Pflugers Arch* 445:305-310, 2002.
18. Walker JS, De Tombe PP: Titin and the developing heart, *Circ Res* 94:505-513, 2004.
19. Severs NJ, Coppen SR, Dupont E et al: Gap junction alterations in human cardiac disease, *Cardiovasc Res* 62:368-377, 2004.
20. Spray DC, Suadicani SO, Srinivas M et al: Gap junction in the cardiovascular system. In Page E, Fozzard H, Solaro RJ, editors: *Handbook of physiology,* vol 1, *The heart,* New York, 2002, Oxford Press.
21. Lederer WJ: Cardiac electrophysiology and the electrocardiogram. In Boron WF, Boulpaep EL, editors: *Medical physiology,* Philadelphia, 2005, WB Saunders.
22. Sah R, Ramirez RJ, Oudit GY et al: Regulation of cardiac excitation-contraction coupling by action potential repolarization: role of the transient outward potassium current, *J Physiol* 546:5-18, 2003.
23. Berne RM, Levy MN: *Cardiovascular physiology,* ed 8, St Louis, 2001, Mosby.
24. Deal KK, England SK, Tamkun MM: Molecular physiology of the cardiac potassium channels, *Physiol Rev* 76:49-79, 1996.
25. Grynberg A, Demaison L: Fatty acid oxidation in the heart, *J Cardiovasc Pharmacol* 28(suppl 1):S11-S17, 1996.
26. Brinkmann JF, Abumrad NA, Ibrahimi A et al: New insights into long-chain fatty acid uptake by heart muscle: a crucial role for fatty acid translocase/CD36, *Biochem J* 367:561-570, 2002.
27. Augustus A, Yagyu H, Haemmerle G et al: Cardiac-specific knockout of lipoprotein lipase alters plasma lipoprotein triglyceride metabolism and cardiac gene expression, *J Biol Chem* 279:25050-25057, 2004.
28. Augustus AS, Kako Y, Yagyu H et al: Routes of FA delivery to cardiac muscle: modulation of lipoprotein lipolysis alters uptake of TG-derived FA, *Am J Physiol Endocrinol Metab* 284:E331-E339, 2003.
29. Saddik M, Lopaschuk GD: Myocardial triglyceride turnover and contribution to energy substrate utilization in isolated working rat hearts, *J Biol Chem* 266:8162-8170, 1991.
30. Young LH, Renfu Y, Russell R et al: Low-flow ischemia leads to translocation of canine heart GLUT-4 and GLUT-1 glucose transporters to the sarcolemma in vivo, *Circulation* 95:415-422, 1997.
31. Depre C, Rider MH, Hue L: Mechanisms of control of heart glycolysis, *Eur J Biochem* 258:277-290, 1998.
32. Law WR, McLane MP, Raymond RM: Adenosine is required for myocardial insulin responsiveness in vivo, *Diabetes* 37:842-845, 1988.
33. Evans RK, Schwartz DD, Gladden LB: Effect of myocardial volume overload and heart failure on lactate transport into isolated cardiac myocytes, *J Appl Physiol* 94:1169-1176, 2003.
34. Taegtmeyer H: Energy metabolism of the heart: from basic concepts to clinical applications, *Curr Probl Cardiol* 19:59-113, 1994.
35. Razeghi P, Young ME, Ying J et al: Downregulation of metabolic gene expression in failing human heart before and after mechanical unloading, *Cardiology* 97:203-209, 2002.
36. Fang HK, Sturgeon C, Segil LJ et al: Cardiac contractile function during coronary stenosis in dogs: association of adenosine in glycolytic dependence, *Am J Physiol* 272:H2195-H2203, 1997.

chapter 6

Cardiovascular Adaptations to Exercise

Wendy Mercier

CHAPTER ABBREVIATIONS

AACVPR American Association of Cardiovascular and Pulmonary Rehabilitation

ACSM American College of Sports Medicine

CAD coronary artery disease

CDC Centers for Disease Control and Prevention

CO cardiac output

HR heart rate

IOM Institute of Medicine

SV stroke volume

TPR total peripheral resistance

VO$_2$ volume of oxygen consumption

VO$_2$ max maximal oxygen consumption

VO$_2$ R volume of oxygen consumption reserve

A continuous hemodynamic competition goes on in the body, a rivalry for a finite circulating blood volume. The moment exercise begins, the competition intensifies. The heart beats faster and with more force to meet increasing metabolic demands, but not all tissues receive this increased flow. Organs less vital to exercise (e.g., kidneys and visceral organs) receive less blood flow, whereas working muscles (cardiac and skeletal) receive more. If body temperature rises, as it usually does with exercise, then the skin needs an increasing share of the limited blood flow to dissipate the heat. The brain requires a constant delivery of blood, or the whole competition is off.

The heart and vessels are regulated predominantly by the autonomic nervous system, but in certain tissues and at certain times the vessels may be *autoregulated* by local factors. The cardiovascular system responds to exercise by increasing cardiac output (flow) and redistributing that flow. However, in order to understand fully the complexities of these cardiovascular responses, one must consider these responses within the context of hemodynamic changes associated with exercise. Blood pressure (which drives blood flow) and vessel resistance (which opposes that driving force) are altered during exercise. The rate and force of cardiac contraction increases to augment cardiac output. All of these factors—flow, pressure, resistance, heart rate, and contractility—are regulated during exercise by a coordinated interplay between neural mechanisms (central and peripheral) and local factors in the exercising tissue. With chronic exercise the blood, heart, and vessels adapt over time to respond more efficiently and effectively to the stress of exercise.

The goal of this chapter is to explore the acute responses of the cardiovascular system to exercise and the regulatory mechanisms that coordinate them. Included is a discussion of the adaptations of the cardiovascular system to chronic exercise that enhance the function of cardiac, vascular, and regulatory mechanisms and allow for an improvement in exercise capacity.

REGULATORY MECHANISMS OF CARDIOVASCULAR RESPONSES TO EXERCISE

The appropriate responses to exercise are regulated primarily by the activity of the autonomic nervous system. Responses to acute exercise are mediated centrally, in specific brain and brain stem command centers, and peripherally through receptor reflexes. The former mechanism, termed the *central command theory,* refers to cortical influence in cardiovascular centers in the medulla. In the latter mechanism the peripheral baroreceptor and chemoreceptor responses are reflex arcs that respond to peripheral chemical, mechanical, and pressure changes to mediate effectors through the same cardiovascular medullary centers.[1] Together, central command and peripheral receptor mechanisms regulate cardiovascular responses to increased activity through sympathetic and parasympathetic modulation. Additionally, autonomic influence may be dominated by local vasodilatory metabolites in exercising muscle.[2] Figure 6-1 depicts the relationship between higher central command mechanisms, peripheral receptors, and exercise-induced changes in arterial pressure.[1]

Central Command Theory

The central command theory suggests that the cerebral cortex is involved in signaling cardiovascular responses from the onset of exercise. Specifically, the motor cortex, which signals voluntary skeletal muscle contraction, sends efferent signals to the cardiovascular neuronal circuits in the medulla. These efferent signals generate an almost immediate increase in heart rate (and respiratory rate) via the autonomic nervous system as soon as muscle contraction begins. Accompanying these responses is an augmented blood flow *to* working skeletal muscle and *away from* less active tissue.[1,3]

The pathways of the central command mechanism remain ill defined, though some details have been clarified. An increase in heart rate and blood pressure are initiated at the same time skeletal muscle activity is attempted.[4,5] Muscle tension development, however, does not appear necessary in order for these centrally mediated cardiovascular responses to occur; studies in which

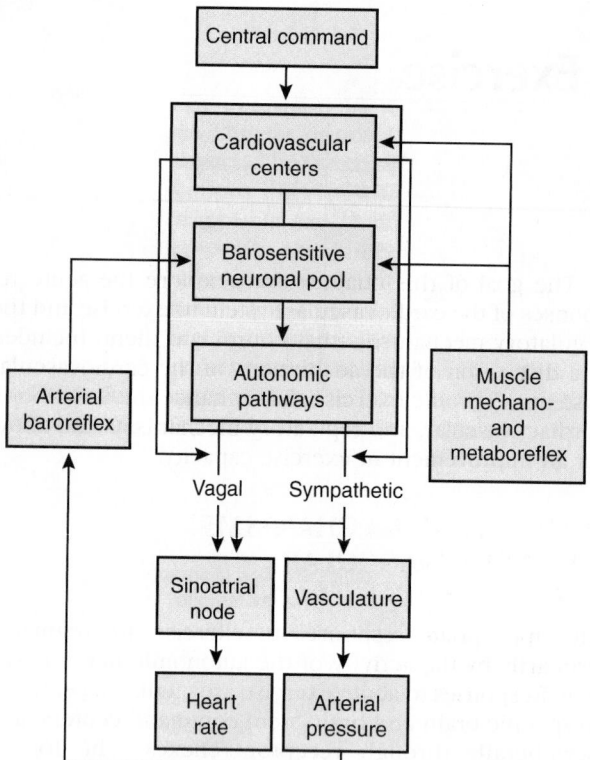

FIGURE 6-1 ◾ Schematic diagram illustrating the main neural mechanisms of cardiovascular regulation during exercise. Also depicted is a feedback mechanism to arterial baroreceptors by exercise-induced changes in arterial pressure and the influence of muscle mechanoreflexes and metaboreflexes. (From Iellamo F: *Ital Heart J* 2[3]:200-212, 2001.)

muscles have been paralyzed by neuromuscular block and then signaled to contract have confirmed this.[5-7] These studies demonstrate that even when the muscle could not develop tension, there was a diminished but significant increase in heart rate and blood pressure. In other words, the central command activation occurs independently of muscle contraction and for this reason, the mechanism sometimes is referred to as "feed-forward" regulation.[2]

Evidence indicates, however, that some "feedback" afferent nerves from the contracting muscles signal cortical areas to *modify* the cardiovascular responses to exercise. Central command responses are abolished in cases of T_8 to T_{12} cord transection,[8] so an intact spinal pathway appears essential to the central command responses.

It is likely that the hypothalamus is involved in mediating central command activity in response to acute stress such as exercise. The patterned response to threatening stimuli seen in human beings is similar to those responses described before: increased heart rate, blood pressure, and ventilation. These responses are regulated by hypothalamic nuclei (dorsomedial) via the autonomic nervous system. Forebrain areas such as the amygdala appear to play an important role in the central mediation of these responses.[9] Whether the central command mechanism is involved in the hypothalamic

responses to stress or whether the hypothalamus generates the stress responses itself is unknown, but there is speculation that a common set of "command neurons" within the dorsomedial hypothalamus triggers cardiovascular responses to the motor cortex (with exercise) and the amygdala (with stressful stimuli).[2]

The central command signal affects the heart and vessels via the autonomic nervous system. With the onset of exercise, parasympathetic signals to the heart are inhibited and sympathetic signals are activated, leading to an increase rate and force of contraction. The effects on heart rate reflect a concomitant withdrawal of parasympathetic stimulation and activation of sympathetic fibers. The sympathetic fibers release the neurotransmitter norepinephrine, which has its effect primarily on the sinoatrial node. Specifically, norepinephrine increases the slope of the pacemaker potential that leads to increased frequency of depolarization and thereby increased heart rate. Sympathetic fibers are also invested in the myocardium, usually along the coronary fibers. Norepinephrine binds to beta-adrenergic receptors on myocardial cells and operates through the cyclic adenosine monophosphate second messenger system to raise cytosolic levels of calcium. Contractility is determined by the amount of free intracellular calcium, so when levels rise, the heart contracts with more force. Additionally, sympathetic stimulation shortens systole and increases the rate of ventricular relaxation (lusitropic effect), which enhances ventricular filling.[10]

Sympathetic innervation extends to blood vessels, but the vascular changes that occur with exercise are not entirely due to this autonomic control. Sympathetic activity predominates in nonexercising tissues, such as those in the renal, splanchnic, and hepatic (visceral) regions.[2,11] In these regions the tonic secretion of norepinephrine is increased with the onset of exercise. Norepinephrine binds to alpha-adrenergic receptors on vascular smooth muscle cells to cause contraction, vasoconstriction, and an increase in resistance. This effect shunts blood flow away from these tissues to the highly metabolic muscles.[10] Other humoral vasoactive substances may influence vascular resistance in nonexercising tissues (e.g., hormonal norepinephrine), and local factors that are less subservient to central control are at play in tissues that autoregulate their blood flow during exercise (discussed in the section on redistribution of blood flow).[1]

Receptor Reflexes

Receptor reflexes are *feedback* (versus feed-forward) neuroregulatory processes. Two major feedback mechanisms play a role in cardiovascular responses to exercise; they are the *arterial baroreceptor reflex* and the *muscle mechanoreceptor/metaboreceptor reflexes.* Both reflex mechanisms involve peripheral receptors that respond in a reflex arc to specific internal homeostatic disturbances brought about by exercising muscles. These mechanisms in turn activate cardiovascular centers in the brain stem. In addition, these mechanisms influence, and are influenced by, the central command signals.[2]

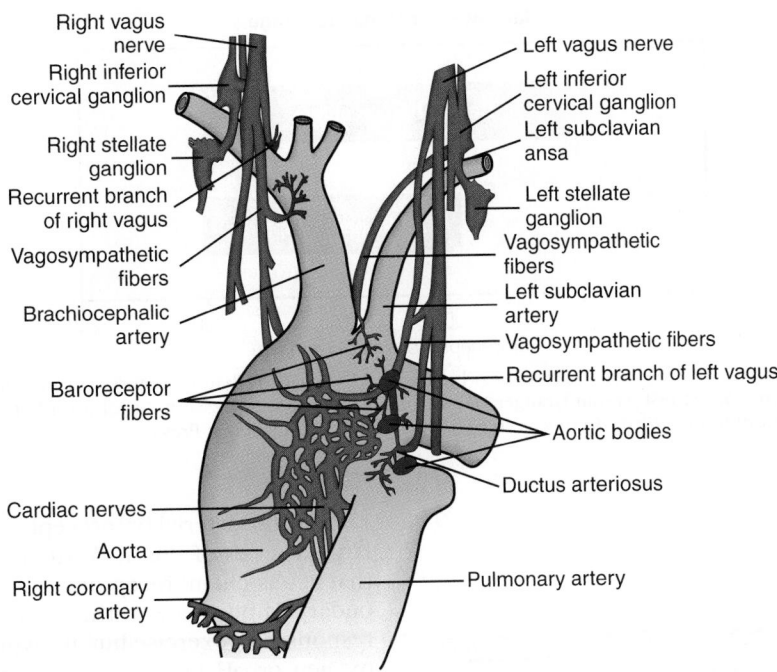

FIGURE 6-2 ■ Anterior view of the aortic arch showing the aortic bodies and innervation that make up the aortic baroreceptor reflex. (From Berne R, Levy M: *Cardiovascular physiology,* ed 8, St Louis, 2001, Mosby.)

Arterial Baroreceptors

Arterial baroreceptors are stretch receptors located in the aortic arch and near the carotid artery sinuses (Figures 6-2 and 6-3). At rest, and during exercise, these receptors are involved in the modulation of vascular resistance and heart rate in order to maintain appropriate blood pressure. When arterial pressure (or pulse pressure) increases at rest, the walls of the aorta and carotid sinuses stretch and activate the baroreceptors. Signals are sent via the vagus nerve (aortic arch) and via the glossopharyngeal nerve (carotid sinus) to medullary nuclei (tractus solitarius) in the vasomotor center. This activation of baroreceptors inhibits sympathetic nerve impulses to the peripheral blood vessels. Vasodilatation occurs, blood pressure drops, and the negative feedback loop is completed. Afferent fibers from the arterial baroreceptors extend to the medullary cardiac center as well, where in the face of increasing pressure, they cause a parasympathetic-mediated decrease in heart rate. The arterial baroreceptors are primarily responsible for short-term adjustment of blood pressure. They respond beat-by-beat to relatively abrupt fluctuations in pressure such as those that occur with postural changes.[10] They are less effective at regulating long-term pressure because they appear to reset or become insensitive when subjected to prolonged elevated blood pressure (Figure 6-4).[2]

During exercise the arterial baroreceptor reflex is altered as evidenced by an increase (rather than decrease) in heart rate when mean arterial pressure rises (Figure 6-5).[1] Most studies indicate that the reflex resets such that it operates in a higher pressure range. In addition, this resetting occurs in a direct relationship to the intensity of exercise, from rest to maximum effort. The

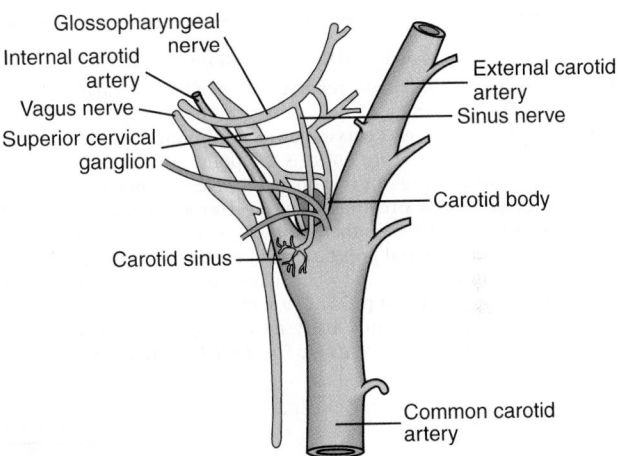

FIGURE 6-3 ■ Anterior view of the carotid bifurcation showing the carotid body and innervation that form the carotid baroreceptor reflex. (From Berne R, Levy M: *Cardiovascular physiology,* ed 8, St Louis, 2001, Mosby.)

slope of the curve of baroreceptor pressure to mean arterial pressure (heart rate) is unchanged, so there appears to be no change in the gain of the reflex. In other words, the minimum-maximum pressure response range shifts to the right, and the minimum-maximum operating range shifts upward.[12,13] This allows the baroreceptors to affect vessels and the heart at an appropriately higher pressure during exercise. Whether exercise has the same effect on baroreceptor vasoactivity as it does on heart rate response or whether aortic baroreceptors reset similarly to carotid baroreceptors is still unclear.[1,12] Higher brain centers, such as central command, may have a role in the resetting of the carotid baroreflex during exercise (Figures 6-6 and 6-7).[12,14,15]

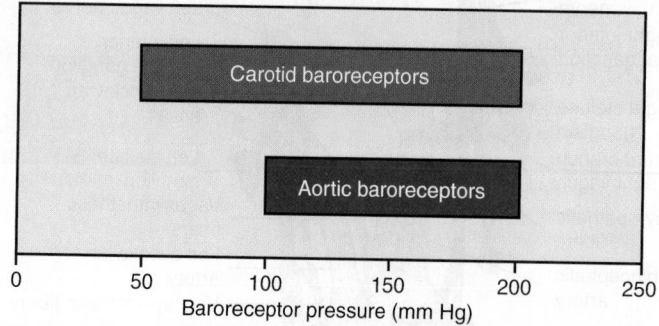

FIGURE 6-4 ■ Pressure ranges over which carotid and aortic baroreceptors can monitor mean arterial pressure at rest. (From Granger DN: Regulation of arterial pressure. In Johnson L, Gerwin T, editors: *Essential medical physiology,* ed 3, New York, 2004, Academic Press.)

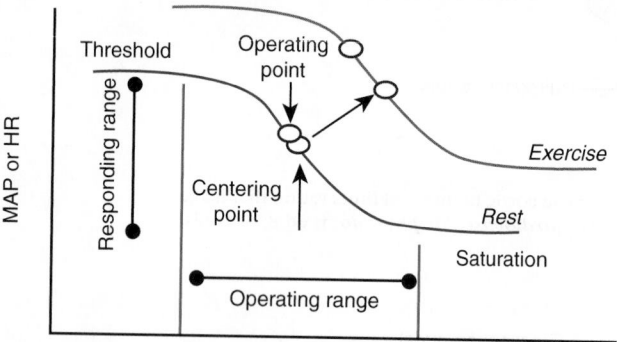

FIGURE 6-5 ■ A schematic representation of the carotid baroreflex function curve at rest and its subsequent reset during exercise. *Responding range* is the maximum to minimum change in mean arterial pressure. *Centering point* is the point at which there is an equal depressor and pressor response to a given change in pressure. *Operating point* is the prestimulus mean arterial pressure or carotid sinus pressure. *Threshold* is the point where no further increases in heart rate or mean arterial pressure are elicited by further reductions in pressure. *Saturation* is the point where no further decreases in heart rate or mean arterial pressure are elicited by further increases in pressure. *HR,* Heart rate; *MAP,* mean arterial pressure. (From Raven PB, Fadel PJ, Smith SA: *Exerc Sport Sci Rev* 30:40, 2002.)

Near the arterial baroreceptors in the aortic arch and large arteries of the neck are aortic and carotid bodies that act as chemoreceptors. These receptors are of secondary importance in the regulation of cardiovascular responses to exercise but are worthy of mention. When oxygen or pH levels drop or carbon dioxide levels increase, they transmit signals to the cardioacceleratory center and the vasomotor center in the medulla. The cardioacceleratory center sends signals via the sympathetic efferent nerves to the sinoatrial node to increase heart rate. The vasomotor center transmits signals, also sympathetic, to blood vessels to cause vasoconstriction. The net result is an increase in arterial pressure. These chemoreceptors serve a primary role in the regulation of respiratory rate (Figure 6-8).[1,2]

Muscle Mechanoreceptor/Metaboreceptor Reflexes

Skeletal muscles contain receptors within their interstitium that are sensitive to mechanical and chemical stimuli. Myelinated afferent nerves are more sensitive to mechanical changes (i.e., muscle tension), and unmyelinated afferent nerves tend to be activated by local chemical stimuli (i.e., metabolic byproducts), though

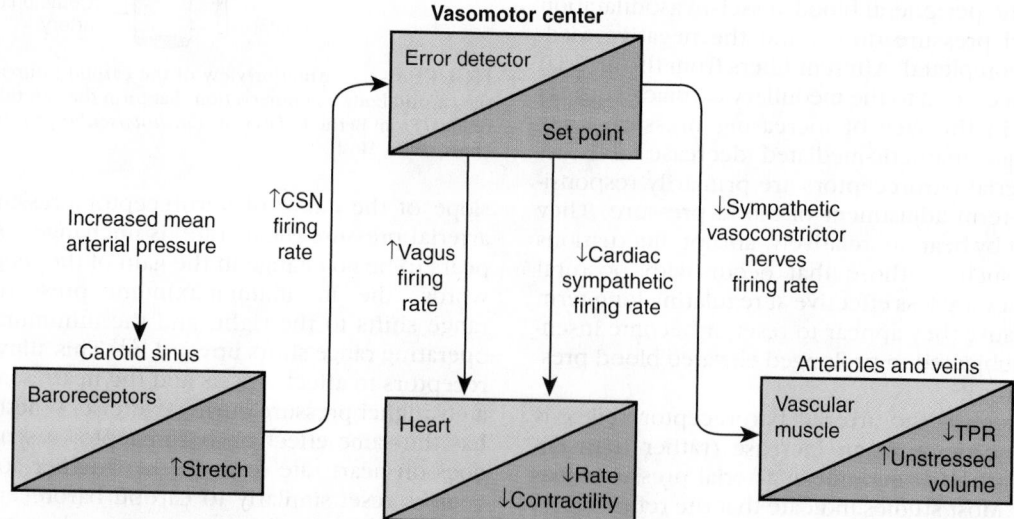

FIGURE 6-6 ■ Functional organization of the carotid sinus reflex. CSN = carotid sinus nerve; TPR = total peripheral resistance. (From Granger DN: Regulation of arterial pressure. In Johnson L, Gerwin T, editors: *Essential medical physiology,* ed 3, New York, 2004, Academic Press.)

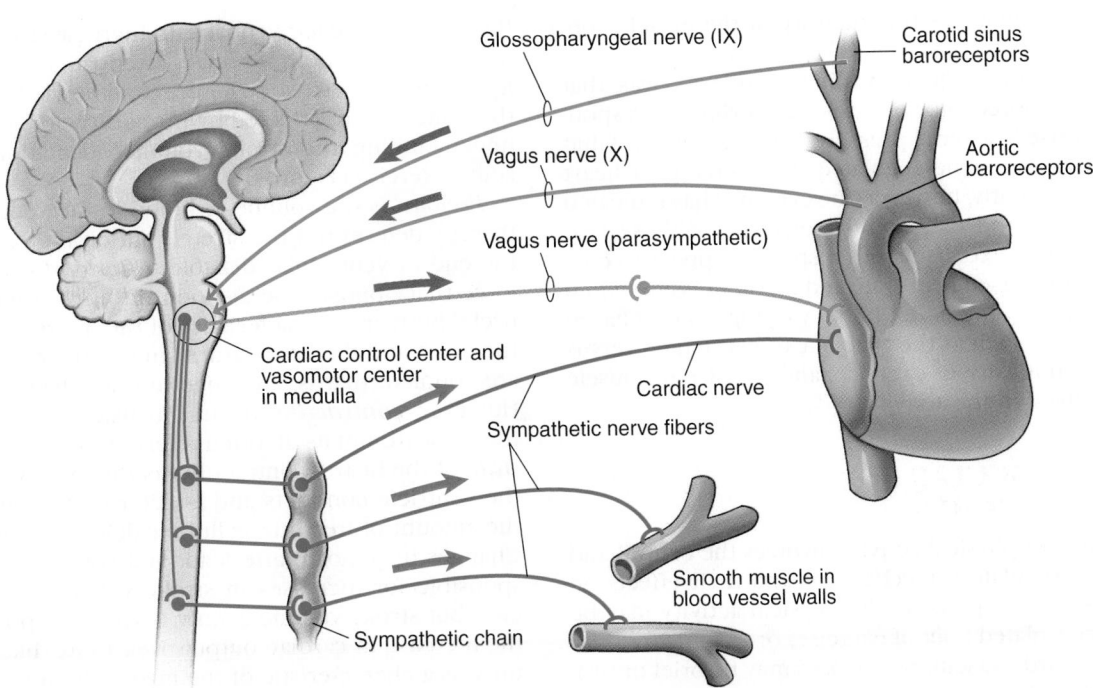

FIGURE 6-7 ■ Vasomotor baroreflexes. Carotid sinus and aortic baroreceptors detect changes in mean arterial pressure and feed the information back to the cardiac control center and the vasomotor center in the medulla. In response, these control centers alter the ratio between sympathetic and parasympathetic output.

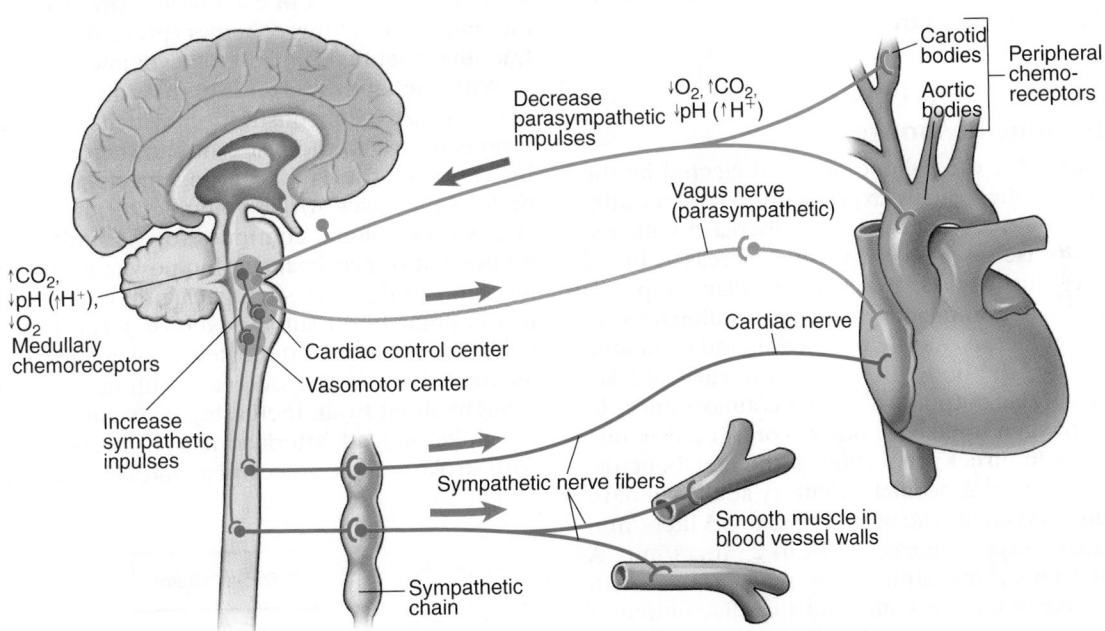

FIGURE 6-8 ■ Chemoreceptor reflexes. Chemoreceptors in the carotid and aortic bodies, as well as chemoreceptive neurons in the vasomotor center of the medulla itself, detect increases in carbon dioxide (CO_2), decreases in oxygen (O_2), and decreases in pH. This information feeds back to the cardiac control center and the vasomotor control center of the medulla, which in turn alter the ratio of parasympathetic and sympathetic output.

both respond to either stimulus. The mechanism of the mechanoreceptor response is unknown. Evidence indicates that muscle contractions during dynamic exercise activate the receptors to contribute to the rise in heart rate and arterial pressure that is observed.[1,16]

Much more is known about the muscle metaboreceptor reflex during exercise. As muscle activity begins, blood flow and oxygen delivery to muscle tissue becomes insufficient, and chemical byproducts of metabolism accumulate (e.g., lactic acid). The chemicals activate the myelinated and unmyelinated afferent nerves, which trigger a sympathetically mediated increase in blood pressure. Mechanoreceptors and metaboreceptors provoke an increase in heart rate and mean arterial pressure that matches the intensity of the muscle contractions.[1,14]

For some time the prevailing consensus was that muscle metaboreceptor reflexes were primarily responsible for a rise in arterial pressure with exercise and that the central command regulated the increase in heart rate. More recently, however, the evidence has indicated an integrated and overlapping response of these two mechanisms to exercise. Both responses appear to contribute to increased heart rate and blood pressure when physical activity increases, but to varying degrees based on conditions such as the type of exercise (static versus dynamic), intensity of exercise, and the size of muscle mass involved in the activity.[1,14,16]

CARDIOVASCULAR RESPONSE TO ACUTE EXERCISE

Any change in physical activity involves the central and peripheral regulatory mechanisms and their effects on cardiovascular responses. The physical activity may be acute (one isolated bout of exercise) or chronic (regular exercise); cardiovascular responses may be brief or prolonged. Whether acute or chronic exercise or brief or prolonged cardiovascular responses, the cardiovascular system responds to the activity through alterations in cardiac output, vascular resistance, blood pressure, and local factors. The following section explains these responses in relation to exercise.

Cardiac Output and Other Hemodynamic Responses

Cardiac output is the volume of blood ejected by the ventricle over time, usually expressed in liters per minute. Cardiac output must, and does, increase with the onset of exercise in order to provide increased blood flow to working tissues. A resting cardiac output is about 4.5 to 6 liters/min and variable depending on size, age, and other factors. As exercise begins and metabolic needs increase, the body increases its oxygen uptake. The rise in cardiac output that occurs is almost linear to the rise in oxygen uptake. In other words, cardiac output increases in direct proportion to the metabolic demand of the body.[17] A normal sedentary adult will have a maximum oxygen uptake of about 3.0 to 3.5 liters/min and a cardiac output increase to 18 to 23 liters/min. A well-trained endurance athlete may reach a maximum oxygen uptake of 6.2 liters/min and a cardiac output of 42 liters/min.[11] A patient with left ventricular failure may be unable to increase cardiac output to meet any exercise demand and actually may experience a decrease in cardiac output with the onset of physical work.[18]

Cardiac output (**CO**) is the product of *stroke volume* (**SV**) and *heart rate* (**HR**):

$$\text{CO (liters/min)} = \text{SV (ml/beat)} \times \text{HR (beats/min)}$$

Stroke volume is the amount of blood ejected from the ventricle per beat, and heart rate is the number of times the heart beats per minute. The ability of the heart to increase cardiac output with exercise is really the ability of the left ventricle to increase stroke volume or heart rate or both. Preload, afterload, and contractility determine stroke volume, so knowledge of how these factors are affected by physical work is critical to understanding the stroke volume adaptations during acute exercise (Figure 6-9).[10,11,18]

Preload is the volume of blood in the ventricle (and thereby determines the stretch put on the ventricle) at the end of ventricular diastole. *Afterload* is a counterforce that opposes the ejection of blood from the ventricle. Both are characteristics of the interplay between the heart and the vasculature, and so their adjustments are coupled; that is, a change in one affects the other. However, *contractility* is an intrinsic characteristic of the myocardium itself, often referred to as the *inotropic state* of the heart. Contractility is the force with which the ventricle contracts and is determined primarily by the amount of free intracellular calcium during systole. Changes in preload, afterload, and contractility are responsible for increases in stroke volume during exercise, but stroke volume is only partially responsible for the increase in cardiac output. Heart rate, like contractility, is a characteristic of the myocardium itself. Heart rate is modulated during exercise by neural and humoral factors that affect sinoatrial node excitation of the heart.[10,18] Stroke volume and heart rate increase with exercise to cause increased cardiac output, though they are not independent of each other. Any change in heart rate modifies the three factors (preload, afterload, contractility) that determine stroke volume.[10]

With the onset of exercise, the sympathetic nervous system causes venoconstriction, which leads to a greater venous return to the heart and an increase in preload. By virtue of the Frank-Starling mechanism, a greater preload increases stroke volume. During upright exercise, stroke volume continues to rise until about 40 to 60 percent of maximal aerobic power, at which time it levels off or declines slightly (Figure 6-10). (This effect is less dramatic in supine exercise.) The physiological explanation for the attenuated stroke volume at a submaximal level is the decreased filling time (diastole) brought about by an increasing heart rate.[17,19]

Unlike preload, afterload has an inverse relationship with stroke volume and cardiac output. Systolic pressure

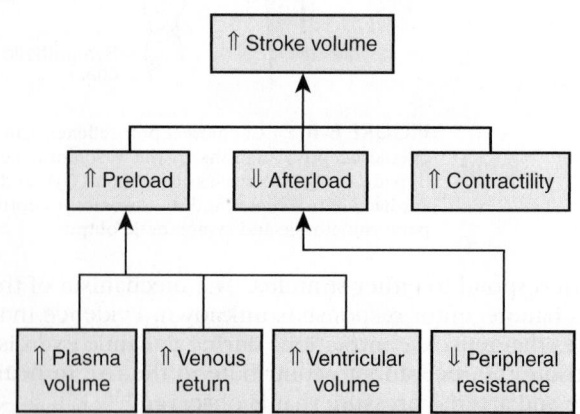

FIGURE 6-9 ■ Summary of mechanisms that affect stroke volume during exercise.

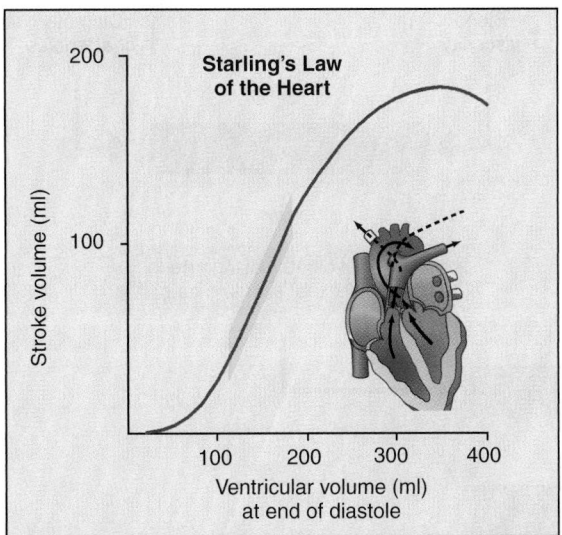

FIGURE 6-10 ■ Frank-Starling law of the heart. The curve represents the relationship between stroke volume and end-diastolic volume (preload). Typically, the heart operates in the shaded range on the graph. (From Thibodeau G, Patton K: *Anatomy & physiology*, ed 5, St Louis, 2003, Mosby.)

is the primary determinant of afterload; as systolic pressure rises with exercise, so does afterload, although the increase in afterload is normally minimal compared with other hemodynamic changes. This rise in afterload would diminish stroke volume if not for the compensation provided by increased preload and contractility.[17,19]

Contractility of the heart is enhanced in response to acute exercise and causes a more forceful contraction of the ventricle independent of preload. This lowers end-systolic volume and consequently increases stroke volume. The maintenance of preload and contractility that occurs during exercise is enough to offset the small increase in afterload. The net result is an increase in cardiac output in response to acute exercise.[17,19]

Because the increase in cardiac output parallels oxygen consumption and oxygen consumption continues to rise throughout exercise, clearly, stroke volume, with its plateau at 40 to 60 percent of maximum, does not entirely explain cardiac output. Once maximal stroke volume is reached during exercise, heart rate *alone* causes further increases in cardiac output. During exercise, heart rate increases linearly with oxygen consumption, reaching a maximum of about 200 beats/min. This is true for exercise-trained and untrained adults. This linear correlation between the two makes the measurement of heart rate a simple, convenient, and reliable index for cardiovascular strain during exercise. A clinician, therefore, can use heart rate responses to determine the intensity of the exercise and to assess the effects of an exercise training regimen, recognizing the distinct variability of heart rate from one person to another. For this reason, heart rate responses should be evaluated on an individual basis only.[19,20] The autonomic nervous system and humoral factors that regulate heart rate during exercise are discussed later in this chapter.

Blood flow is determined by two hemodynamic factors: blood pressure (the force that propels the blood)

and vascular resistance (the opposition to this driving force presented by the vasculature). The basic flow equation demonstrates the relationship between the hemodynamic factors of blood flow, blood pressure, and vascular resistance:

$$\text{Blood flow} = \text{Blood pressure/Vascular resistance}$$

Blood flow through the entire body is cardiac output. Blood pressure changes that occur with acute exercise are due to alterations in cardiac output and vascular resistance. Often, *mean arterial pressure* is used as an index of blood pressure because it is a weighted average of the systolic blood pressure and diastolic blood pressure and therefore best reflects perfusion pressures to the tissues. Vascular resistance through the entire systemic circuit is called *total peripheral resistance* and is the friction placed on blood flow by the vessel walls. To understand blood pressure changes with acute exercise, the basic flow equation (just given) can be manipulated algebraically to produce the Ohm equation:

$$\text{Blood pressure} = \text{Blood flow} \times \text{Vascular resistance}$$

Substituting the whole body indices of cardiac output and total peripheral resistance (**TPR**), the equation looks like this[11,19]:

$$\text{Mean arterial pressure} = \text{CO} \times \text{TPR}$$

Systolic pressure increases dramatically during exercise and may exceed 200 mm Hg before it plateaus. This increase is due to an increasing cardiac output and a rise in vascular resistance in tissues that are less metabolically active. Diastolic blood pressure, however, rises minimally, does not rise at all, or may fall slightly; subsequently, mean arterial pressure increases only modestly with exercise. The minimal change in diastolic blood pressure and mean arterial pressure is due to the *decrease* in vascular resistance that occurs in the vasodilated (more precisely, less constricted) arterioles of exercising muscle, so there is a *net* decrease in total peripheral resistance. A well-trained endurance athlete, for instance, actually may drop the diastolic blood pressure to 50 mm Hg. Conversely, someone with an abnormal exercise diastolic blood pressure response experiences an elevation in diastolic blood pressure greater than 10 mm Hg from rest.[19,20] So the Ohm equation, with arrows inserted to indicate relative changes during exercise, could be represented this way:

$$\uparrow \text{Mean arterial pressure} = \uparrow\uparrow\uparrow \text{CO} \times \downarrow\downarrow \text{TPR}$$

Mean arterial pressure is directly proportional to arterial blood volume. Cardiac output affects arterial blood volume by changing the amount of blood *entering* the arterial vessels. So when heart rate or stroke volume increases, cardiac output increases, and that in turn increases arterial blood volume and pressure. Total peripheral resistance affects blood volume by altering the amount of blood *leaving* the arterial vessels (arteriole runoff). When total peripheral resistance increases because of an increase in blood viscosity or narrowing of arteriolar diameter, less blood leaves the arterial system, and arterial blood volume and pressure increase (Figure 6-11).[20,21]

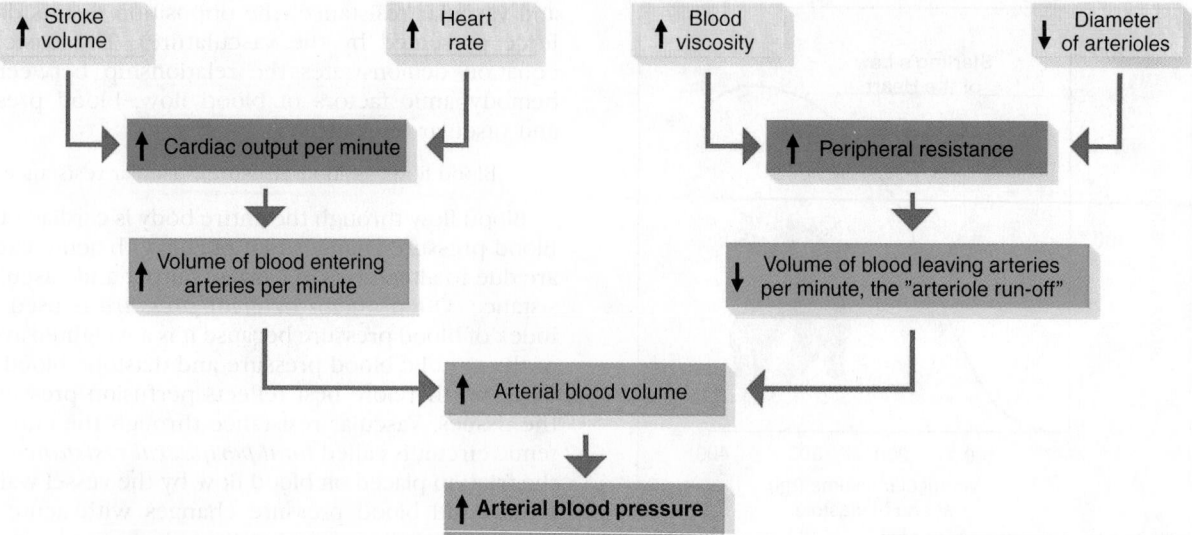

FIGURE 6-11 ■ Relationship between arterial blood volume and blood pressure. Mean arterial pressure is directly proportional to arterial blood volume. Cardiac output (CO) and total peripheral resistance (TPR) are directly proportional to arterial blood volume, but for opposite reasons: CO affects blood entering the arteries, and TPR affects blood leaving the arteries. If CO increases, the amount of blood entering the arteries increases and tends to increase the volume of blood in the arteries. If TPR increases, it decreases the amount of blood leaving the arteries, which tends to increase the amount of blood left in them. Thus an increase in CO or TPR results in an increase in arterial blood volume, which increases mean arterial pressure. (Thibodeau G, Patton K: *Anatomy & physiology*, ed 5, St Louis, 2003, Mosby.)

Redistribution of Blood Flow

As stated previously, exercise intensifies the dynamic competition of the body for blood flow. Although an increase in cardiac output is essential to meet the demands of an exercising body, a redistribution of that flow is just as critical to sustaining the work. Blood flow to any region in the body depends on the vascular resistance exerted by the vessels in that region and the mean arterial pressure. Vascular resistance is mediated by neural factors, local factors, or a balance of the two depending on the tissue involved. The final result is that local blood flow is matched to the metabolic demands of the tissue.

At rest, skeletal muscle receives approximately 20 percent (1200 ml/min) of cardiac output, whereas the efficient heart receives 4 percent (250 ml/min). The brain must maintain its 750 ml/minute, which is about 15 percent of resting cardiac output, and the skin gets approximately 7 percent (500 ml/min). The remainder of the resting blood flow is delivered to the visceral organs (kidneys, gastrointestinal tract, liver, pancreas, and spleen). With the onset of exercise, blood flow is redistributed away from the visceral organs to the more metabolically active organs. Skeletal muscle receives the largest proportion of blood flow, ranging from 47 percent (4500 ml/min) during light exercise to as high as 88 percent (22,000 ml/min) at maximal work capacity. Absolute blood flow to the cardiac muscle increases, but it remains at about 4 to 5 percent of cardiac output even with increasing exercise intensity. Blood flow to visceral organs is attenuated with increasing reduc-

tions as the intensity of work rises until maximal exercise when the blood flow is less than 5 percent (Figure 6-12).[10,20]

Shunting of blood away from nonexercising tissue to active tissues during exercise is accomplished through a careful balance of autonomic nervous system regulation and local autoregulatory factors.[11,20] As exercise begins and heart rate rises to greater than 100 beats/min, sympathetic stimulation increases to vascular smooth muscle of passive tissue. Also, plasma norepinephrine levels rise, and the net effect is vasoconstriction of arterioles serving visceral organs. At rest, these organs receive blood flow in excess of their metabolic needs, so when that flow is diverted away, it greatly augments flow to active tissue.[10,11,20]

In the more metabolically active tissues, primarily skeletal muscle, the onset of exercise activates local signals that cause arteriolar smooth muscle relaxation and vasodilatation. Local autoregulation during physical activity is termed *exercise hyperemia*. Several factors are at play. First, working muscles produce metabolites such as carbon dioxide, potassium ions, hydrogen ions, lactic acid, and adenosine. In addition, tissue oxygen levels fall. Most likely, some combination of these factors acts to relax arterioles and cause exercise hyperemia in the muscle tissue.[20,22] Second, the endothelial cells of muscle vessels produce nitric oxide and other *endothelial-derived relaxing factors* during exercise. Local chemical factors (e.g., low oxygen levels and norepinephrine) or mechanical factors (e.g., sheer stress) stimulate the release of nitric oxide, which seems to cause local arterial and arteriolar dilatation.[20,23,24] Lastly,

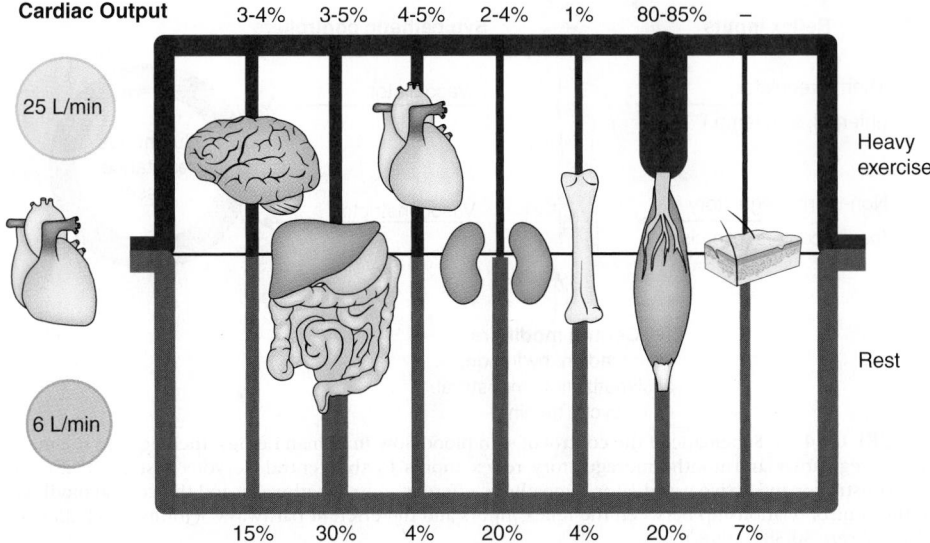

FIGURE 6-12 ■ Distribution of cardiac output during rest and maximal exercise, when cardiac output increases from 5 to 25 liters/min. (From Powers SK, Howley ET: *Exercise physiology,* ed 6, New York, 2006, McGraw-Hill.)

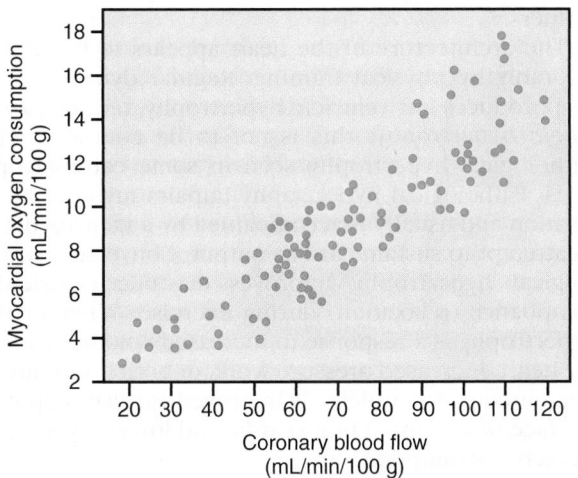

FIGURE 6-13 ■ Relationship between myocardial oxygen consumption and coronary blood flow during a variety of interventions that increased or decreased myocardial metabolic rate. (From Berne R, Levy M: *Cardiovascular physiology,* ed 8, St Louis, 2001, Mosby.)

sympathetic vasoconstrictor activity is supervened by local vasodilatory factors. Although sympathetic activity rises with increasing levels of exercise, the local vasodilatory metabolites have a more potent effect on local blood vessels. Ultimately, blood flow to skeletal muscle matches exercise intensity and the metabolic needs of the tissue are met.[10,20]

The most remarkable aspect of coronary blood flow is how closely it matches metabolic requirements of the myocardium. This relationship is linear, as depicted in Figure 6-13. At rest, the sympathetic nervous system exerts a basal vasoconstriction of coronary arterioles. During exercise (and other conditions that alter myocardium metabolism), the coronary circulation is primarily under local control. The most potent signal for coronary vasodilatation is oxygen need. Whether the signal is a decrease in blood flow or an increase in oxygen demand, the signal causes the release of local vasodilatory factors (e.g., adenosine) and coronary blood flow increases. As exercise intensity increases, absolute blood flow to the myocardium rises, though it usually remains about 4 percent of total cardiac output.[10,23]

Skeletal muscle and cardiac muscle need enhanced blood flow during exercise to nourish working tissue. Skin, however, requires relatively little metabolic nourishment, even during exercise, but is still likely to experience high flows. This occurs because the primary function of skin blood flow during exercise is to maintain body temperature. Because heat is released by contracting muscles, body temperature usually rises during exercise. In addition, if the external environment is warm, skin temperature will rise. Also, nonthermoregulatory signals are sent to the central nervous system from peripheral receptors involved with exercise. The hypothalamus integrates these core and surface temperature afferent nerve signals, with afferent nerve signals from central and peripheral modifiers, and sends signals that inhibit sympathetic influence to cutaneous arterioles. This results in cutaneous vasodilatation. In addition, parasympathetic efferent signals cause nearby sweat glands to secrete sweat, and the sweat contains bradykinins that cause local vasodilatation. As exercise intensity increases, body temperature is likely to rise, and a dynamic battle for blood flow ensues. Working muscles need augmented blood flow that delivers oxygen, and skin needs enhanced blood flow that delivers heat to the body surface (Figure 6-14).[10,24,25]

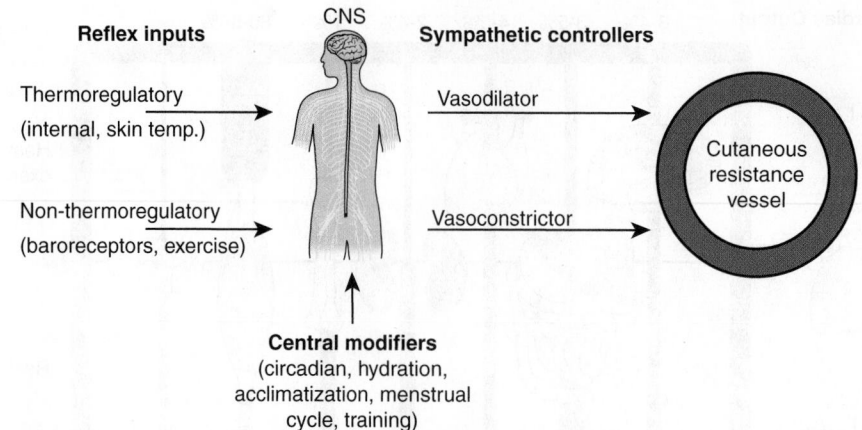

FIGURE 6-14 ▌ Schematic of the control of skin blood flow in human beings. Included are the major thermoregulatory and nonthermoregulatory reflex inputs to the central nervous system (CNS), the vasoconstrictor and active vasodilator sympathetic efferent control pathways, and the central modifiers of the control relationship between the reflex inputs and the efferent pathways. (Johnson JM: *Med Sci Sports Exerc* 30:383, 1998.)

CARDIOVASCULAR RESPONSE TO CHRONIC EXERCISE

Chronic dynamic exercise (physical training) provokes favorable alterations in the heart, the vasculature, the blood, and the mechanisms involved in cardiovascular regulation. A general and accepted definition of chronic exercise is regular physical activity that is of moderate intensity at least 2 to 3 times weekly for 20 to 30 minutes per session.[19] The favorable alterations are manifested in hemodynamic changes that make exercise more efficient. Cardiac function improves because of a larger stroke volume and a notable bradycardia, vascular function improves because of enhanced vasodilatory capacity, and plasma volume is significantly expanded. Most noticeable to the exercising individual is the increasing ease of doing the same physical work. Together these adaptations and changes in central and local regulatory mechanisms improve the ability of the cardiovascular system to deliver oxygen to working muscles as manifested by an increase in maximal oxygen uptake.

Cardiac Function

Exercise training increases stroke volume and maximal cardiac output, which improves systemic oxygen transport. This effect is due to alterations in the factors that affect stroke volume: preload and afterload. Exercise training improves diastolic filling and therefore increases end-diastolic volume (preload). This is accomplished through an expansion of circulating plasma volume, prolongation of diastolic filling time, and increase in ventricular volume. All of these adaptations enlarge preload and, through the Frank-Starling mechanism, increase stroke volume.[26,27] Afterload is reduced with physical training and is attributed to an exercise-induced lowering of total peripheral resistance. The combination of enhanced preload and reduced afterload allows the heart to maintain stroke volume at a lower myocardial oxygen consumption, making the heart more efficient. Most studies indicate no change in intrinsic contractility because of training,[28] though there is evidence of enhanced contractile performance in runners.[29]

The architecture of the heart appears to be altered favorably by physical training. Regular dynamic exercise produces left ventricle hypertrophy, termed *physiologic hypertrophy;* this is not to be confused with pathological hypertrophy seen in some cardiomyopathies. Pathological hypertrophy impairs myocardial relaxation and usually is accompanied by a tachycardia in an attempt to sustain cardiac output. Conversely, physiological hypertrophy improves diastolic ventricular compliance (relaxation) during exercise. Whether the hypertrophy is a response to increased volume work of the heart, increased pressure work, or both is unknown. The outcome for athletes is improved cardiac output in the face of a training bradycardia and lower myocardial oxygen consumption.[18,30]

Improved coronary circulation resulting from vascular remodeling is yet another favorable consequence of chronic exercise. The effect of training on the coronary vasculature has been studied in large and small coronary arteries, arterioles, and capillaries and reveals a varied type and time course of changes in each segment. There appears to be growth of more capillaries and small arterioles that leads to longitudinal extension of the coronary network with training, and circumferential expansion of resistance and large conduit arteries. Figure 6-15 depicts the coronary vascular segments and the effects of training on each segment. The net result in the trained heart is a larger and more profuse arterial supply.[31,32]

Several stimuli have been identified that directly or indirectly trigger coronary vascular remodeling. Mechanical stress, as imparted by the stretching myocardium (increased diastolic filling) and myocardial compression of vessels (during more forceful contractions), stimulate changes in the endothelial and smooth muscle of the vessel wall. Increased blood flow leads to elevated

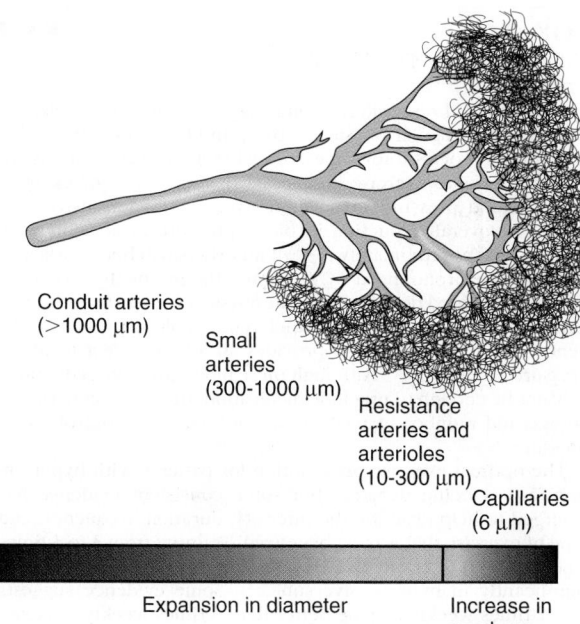

Conduit arteries
(>1000 μm)

Small
arteries
(300–1000 μm)

Resistance
arteries and
arterioles
(10–300 μm)

Capillaries
(6 μm)

Expansion in diameter   Increase in numbers

FIGURE 6-15 ■ Schematic diagram of the coronary arterial vascular tree and capillaries showing which segments are remodeled in response to exercise by proliferation in numbers of vessels and increase in size of vessels. (From Brown MD: *Exp Physiol* 88[5]:649, 2003.)

shear stress and wall tension on the coronary vessels affecting the endothelium and smooth muscle to increase vessel diameter and thickness. Growth factors have been implicated as direct or indirect mediators in the remodeling process. Growth factors may be stimulatory, such as endothelial growth (e.g., vascular endothelial growth factor), and/or fibroblast growth factors (e.g., fibroblast growth factors 1 and 2). Ultimately, coronary circulation remodeling is believed to assist arterial flow capacity to the heart and thereby improve oxygen transport.[32]

The importance of endothelial-released vasodilators, especially nitric oxide, has received particular attention in exercise studies. Shear stress during episodic increases of blood flow, as occurs during exercise, is thought to signal the release of nitric oxide. Nitric oxide is considered the most important mediator of flow-induced vasodilatation. Nitric oxide also may be directly or indirectly responsible for endothelial growth with chronic exercise.[31,32]

Autonomic Nervous System

Whether chronic exercise alters sympathetic activation and mean arterial pressure at rest is unclear. The consensus, however, is that exercise training leads to diminished sympathetic outflow to the heart and vasculature during submaximal exercise. Because sympathetic outflow, vascular resistance, and mean arterial pressure are coupled, vascular resistance and mean arterial pressure also are diminished during submaximal exercise.[24] The reduced sympathetic activation at a given workload is at least partially due to an increased stroke volume that occurs with chronic exercise.[26,33,34]

Diminished sympathetic activation with training has its most dramatic effect on vascular resistance. Evidence indicates that visceral organ sympathetic activity and regional vascular resistance (as mediated by baroreceptors) are decreased by chronic exercise. Also, the sympathetically mediated rise in mean arterial pressure is attenuated. A training-induced increased plasma volume may explain this. The volume expansion is enough to stimulate the baroreceptors such that they inhibit sympathetic efferent nerves arising from the vasomotor center in the medulla. The subsequent vasodilatation and reduced vascular resistance leads to the attenuation of mean arterial pressure.[1,26]

Sympathetic activity induced by muscle metaboreceptor and muscle chemoreceptor reflexes is diminished as well. This reduction is most likely due to improved muscle metabolism, oxidative capacity, and perfusion. Whether chronic exercise alters peripheral reflexes, central command efferent nerves, or both remains unclear. What is clear is that improved cardiac pumping and muscle metabolism contribute to alterations in central and peripheral mechanisms that regulate cardiac function and vascular resistance. In turn, sympathetic outflow is diminished with training during submaximal exercise.[1,26]

The most obvious cardiovascular adaptation observed with chronic exercise is a reduction in resting and submaximal heart rate, called *training bradycardia*. The primary contributor to resting bradycardia is an enhanced parasympathetic signaling to the heart (*vagal* tone). This increased vagal tone is especially prominent early in exercise training. A higher stroke volume (augmented by enhanced preload and diminished afterload) allows for a lower heart rate to maintain the same cardiac output.[35] Enhanced parasympathetic signaling to the heart does not entirely explain the profound bradycardia, especially in highly trained athletes. Training bradycardia also may be due to decreased sympathetic outflow to the heart or a lowering of the intrinsic automaticity of the sinus atrial node with intense training, but these mechanisms remain unclear.[33-35]

Systemic Vascular Function

Exercise training improves vascular function and blood flow dynamics in part because of autonomic regulatory changes. The attenuated sympathetic activation of certain arterioles increases their diameter during exercise and results in a reduction in vascular resistance. With training, blood flow is higher to exercising muscles than to nonexercising muscles and visceral organs.[34,36]

Local vasoregulatory adaptations to chronic exercise occur as well. In muscle, structural and functional adaptations have been documented with endurance training that preferentially direct blood to exercising muscles. Training increases resting and exercising arterial diameters and contraction-induced vasodilatation, which causes increased maximal perfusion and oxygen delivery where it is needed most—exercising muscle. In addition, vasodilatation of terminal arterioles occurs more rapidly in the transition from resting to exercising, leading to a more rapid increase in muscle blood flow.[37]

Exercise training challenges temperature regulation by way of cutaneous circulation. Regular dynamic exercise causes increased skin blood flow at a given body temperature at rest and during exercise. This change is likely due to an increase in the sensitivity of the skin blood flow–internal temperature relationship and/or a shift in the threshold at which skin blood flow increases. In any case, the adaptations enhance the capacity of the body to transport and dissipate heat.[24,25]

In all vessels of the vascular tree, the endothelium plays an important role in the vasoactivity of underlying smooth muscle. Long thought of as a passive lining, endothelium now is known to actively produce many vasoactive substances; perhaps the most studied is nitric oxide. Nitric oxide is a vasodilator with known antiatherogenic properties. Regular dynamic exercise has been shown to improve endothelium-dependent vasodilator function locally (in exercising muscle) and systemically because of the upregulation of endothelial nitric oxide bioactivity. How this benefits the vasculature is unclear, but this may be another factor in the cardioprotective actions of regular exercise.[38]

Chronic exercise also improves arterial compliance generally. Because arterial stiffness has an impact on resistance and afterload, the training effect offsets the elevated arterial pulse amplitude caused by enhanced stroke volume. As a result, exercise blood pressure in the trained person does not increase higher than the untrained person, despite a higher stroke volume.[39]

Perhaps the most clinically relevant vascular response to chronic exercise is the lowering of blood pressure (Box 6-1). Regular physical activity leads to modest decreases in blood pressure (about 2 to 3 mm Hg) in normotensive subjects and more dramatic decreases (about 7 to 8 mm Hg) in hypertensive subjects. Even the modest 2 to 3 mm Hg reduction is enough to confer protection against cardiovascular morbidity and mortality. These adaptations can be accomplished when training is at least 3 to 5 times weekly for 30 to 60 minutes per session at a moderate intensity. Table 6-1 outlines an exercise prescription guideline for hypertensive individuals. Further evidence indicates that 7 times per week may confer an even greater reduction in blood pressure; it has not been demonstrated that greater intensity increases blood pressure reductions.[40] As mentioned previously, vascular resistance, blood pressure, and sympathetic outflow are closely linked. The reduction in sympathetic activation with chronic exercise is thought to enhance vasodilatation and reduce vascular resistance and blood pressure. In addition, training reduces plasma norepinephrine and the activity of plasma vasopressin and renin during exercise, all of which can lead to a vasoconstriction.[34,43]

EXERCISE AND CARDIOVASCULAR DISEASE

Exercise training bestows cardioprotective effects that reduce cardiovascular morbidity and mortality (Box 6-2).[19,44,45] Many structural and functional changes in the heart, coronary vasculature, systemic vessels, and regulatory mechanisms are responsible for improved performance and cardiovascular health. Training enhances

---

BOX 6-1 ■ ■ ■
EXERCISE AND HYPERTENSION

Epidemiological research has long suggested an inverse relationship between regular physical activity and blood pressure.[40,41] A recent review of 68 studies measuring blood pressure response to dynamic aerobic exercise concluded that this type of exercise lowers blood pressure in normotensive and hypertensive subjects. The overall reduction in blood pressure in normotensive subjects was approximately −3/−2 mm Hg (small but significant) and a more pronounced −7/−6 mm Hg in the hypertensive group.[40] An added benefit of regular physical activity to the hypertensive patient is weight loss, which reduces blood pressure independent of exercise and so provides an add-on effect to blood pressure reduction.[40-42] Although these blood pressure reductions may not be enough to preclude medication, they can decrease the dosage and number of medications necessary to control blood pressure.

The optimal exercise prescription for patients with hypertension still is being debated, but some consistent evidence has emerged to help describe the intensity, duration, frequency, and type of exercise that is most beneficial. Training from 3 to 5 times weekly for 30 to 60 minutes per session reduces blood pressure significantly in hypertensive subjects. Some evidence suggests that 7 times weekly may be better than 3 times weekly. An exercise intensity of about 40 to 50 percent heart rate maximum (moderate) appears to be as effective in reducing blood pressure as 70 percent (high) intensity. Insufficient data are available on exercise of light (less than 40 percent) or very high (more than 70 percent) intensities. Therefore, the suggestion is that intensity be prescribed at a moderate level because patients are more comfortable exercising at a moderate versus high intensity and thus are more likely to prolong their exercise session and adhere to the prescription.[40-42] Special attention must be given to the interaction of antihypertensive medications and exercise.

The most beneficial type of exercise is one that is dynamic aerobic (uses large muscle groups in a rhythmic, continuous fashion) such as walking, jogging, bicycling, or swimming. In the past, resistance exercise was thought to be harmful for patients with hypertension because heavy resistance exercises combined with breath-holding (Valsalva maneuver) can lead to acute spikes in systolic and diastolic blood pressure.[19] However, appropriate resistance training enhances muscle strength and endurance, which helps the hypertensive patient perform endurance and strength activities (including occupational) more effectively. A beneficial resistance training regimen, therefore, is one that includes low weights, a high number of repetitions, and proper breathing technique (exhaling on exertion) and that is performed *at least* twice weekly.[19,42]

Exercise (along with other lifestyle modifications) continues to be the foundation of nonpharmacological therapy for high blood pressure.[40,41] Substantial evidence is available on appropriate *dose* and type of exercise. The challenge remains to motivate hypertensive patients to adopt a lifestyle that includes regular physical activity.

---

stroke volume, reduces heart rate and mean arterial pressure, increases coronary blood flow, improves arterial endothelial function, and diminishes myocardial oxygen consumption. In essence, with regular exercise training the cardiovascular system performs the same work more efficiently and effectively. Additionally, regular physical activity has been shown to reduce risk factors for heart disease, such as hyperlipidemia,[44] type 2 diabetes,[44,49] and obesity.[44,50] For these reasons, moderate to vigorous exercise has become a major component of treatment for patients with cardiovascular disease.[19,44,45]

The clinical implication is that regular exercise should be prescribed as therapy for persons with cardio-

■■■

TABLE 6-1 EXERCISE PRESCRIPTION FOR PATIENTS WITH HYPERTENSION

PARAMETER	PRESCRIPTION
Intensity	40%-50%
Duration	30-60 minutes
Frequency	3-5 times per week (or most days)
Type	Dynamic aerobic; modified resistance training

BOX 6-2 ■■■
EXERCISE AND CORONARY ARTERY DISEASE

Patients with coronary artery disease (**CAD**) experience improvements in functional capacity and reductions in clinical symptoms with exercise training. Decreases in submaximal heart rate at any given workload and a reduction, or even disappearance, of anginal pain with regular exercise have been demonstrated consistently. However, patients with CAD are at greater risk for cardiovascular complications during exercise, so an appropriate exercise prescription must be carefully modified and individualized to ensure safety.[46]

Before starting exercise, patients with CAD should have a complete physical examination, medical history, and graded exercise stress test. Of particular importance is a careful medical evaluation of clinically relevant pathophysiological conditions: left ventricular dysfunction, myocardial ischemia, or cardiac dysrhythmias. These problems should be controlled before the patient is cleared to begin exercise. The exercise prescription then is developed, with supervision and monitoring, based on initial medical evaluation and data collected from the exercise stress test.[19,46]

Aerobic exercise using large muscle groups in continuous motion (e.g., walking, jogging, bicycling, and swimming) provides the best cardiovascular improvements. Aerobic exercise increases functional capacity and the threshold for negative signs and symptoms. The intensity should begin at about 40 percent of maximal functional capacity (or maximal oxygen consumption—VO_2 max) below the level that provokes angina, myocardial ischemia, or exercise intolerance. Patients should be taught to self-rate their intensity (rating of perceived exertion) and cease exercise if angina or other negative signs and symptoms occur. The duration should be 20 to 40 minutes and the frequency at least 3 nonconsecutive days per week. Resistance training is not contraindicated for patients with CAD. Increases in functional strength and endurance can be obtained working 10 to 12 muscle groups using lower weights at higher repetitions at least twice a week.[19,46-48]

Along with functional improvements, exercise provides other health benefits to patients with CAD. Exercise training can contribute to blood pressure control, especially in patients with hypertension; promote weight loss; and decrease cardiovascular mortality. Moreover, exercise training has been shown to reduce depression in clinically depressed patients following acute myocardial infarction. Finally, patients who engage in exercise rehabilitation after revascularization surgery or myocardial infarction experience a significant reduction in medical care costs compared with nonparticipants. So there may be a cost advantage to rehabilitative exercise.[46]

■ **EVIDENCE-BASED PRACTICE**

EXERCISE PRESCRIPTION RESOURCES FOR NURSES

Exercise has become a primary therapeutic intervention for cardiovascular disease, cardiovascular risk factors (e.g., diabetes, obesity, and hyperlipidemia), and disease prevention. The science and art of prescribing exercise to patients with cardiac disease has progressed to include increasingly sophisticated and diversified programs that enable patients to engage in safe and effective physical activity. However, only an estimated 11 to 38 percent of patients needing cardiac rehabilitation services actually receive them.[48] In reality, many health care professionals, including nurses, are called upon to provide advice, education, and even management of patient exercise.

Fortunately, there are resources that can help health care professionals keep abreast of the up-to-date, evidence-based information in the field of exercise science. The American College of Sports Medicine (ACSM), founded in 1954, has become the interface between exercise science and medical practice. According to its mission statement, "the ACSM advances and integrates scientific research to provide educational and practical applications of exercise science and sports medicine." The most widely read and referenced text of the ACSM, *ACSM's Guidelines for Exercise Testing and Prescription,* in its seventh edition,[19] provides a "virtual pharmacopoeia of exercise guidelines for a broad spectrum of patients"; of particular interest is the section on exercise prescription for cardiac patients. This text is considered the gold standard of its kind in the exercise science field. *Guidelines* is complemented by a companion publication, *ACSM's Resource Manual for Guidelines for Exercise Testing and Prescription* (third edition),[51] which offers a more detailed treatment of topics in *Guidelines.* Both textbooks offer frameworks by which health care professionals can develop, implement, and maintain individualized exercise programs with their cardiac patients.

The ACSM also provides resources through its *Pronouncements,* which delivers position stands, joint position statements, and opinion statements.[46] A position statement has the support of extensive scientific research, whereas an opinion statement has less scientific data available; both carry significant weight with rule-making committees for policies and standards regarding exercise and health. All ACSM pronouncements appear first in the official ACSM journal *Medicine & Science in Sports & Exercise,* another useful source of current exercise science research. The ACSM website presents other professional and community resources and education opportunities (*www.acsm.org*).

Another important agency linking exercise and cardiovascular medicine is the American Association of Cardiovascular and Pulmonary Rehabilitation (**AACVPR**). Founded in 1985, the stated mission of AACVPR is "To reduce morbidity, mortality, and disability from cardiovascular and pulmonary diseases through education, prevention, rehabilitation, research, and aggressive disease management."[48] The AACVPR offers members networking and educational opportunities and other health professionals access to practical information for daily practice. In addition the *Journal of Cardiopulmonary Rehabilitation* is the bimonthly publication of the association that provides timely clinical and practical information from the current scientific research in the field.

vascular disease, much as medication is prescribed. (See the evidence-based practice feature.) Prescribed exercise forms the foundation of *cardiac rehabilitation,* defined by the U.S. Public Health Service as "comprehensive, long term programs involving medical evaluation, prescribed exercise, cardiac risk factor modification, education, and counseling."[45] Chapter 80 details the topic of cardiac rehabilitation; the basic principles of prescribed exercise are introduced in this last section.

The question is, "What amount of exercise is safe yet effective in improving cardiovascular functioning in persons with cardiovascular disease?" Determining the appropriate "dosage" or amount of exercise is a highly individualized process that depends on a patient's medical history, clinical status, symptoms, and medication regimen (Box 6-3). (See the pharmacology feature, p. 95) The exercise prescription will include recommendations for *intensity* (how hard), *frequency* (how often), *duration* (how long), and *type* (what kind) of

BOX 6-3 ■ ■ ■
HOW MUCH EXERCISE IS ENOUGH?

Most persons know that exercise is beneficial, but it is not clear how much exercise is necessary to realize these benefits. Early publicized guidelines by the American College of Sports Medicine (ACSM) recommended vigorous exercise for at least 20 minutes per day and 3 times per week. More recently (1995), the ACSM and Centers for Disease Control and Prevention (**CDC**) modified their guidelines to recommend at least 30 minutes of moderate-intensity physical activity on most, preferably all, days of the week. The U.S. surgeon general endorsed this standard the following year. In 2002 the Institute of Medicine (**IOM**) increased the recommended duration to 1 hour per day, citing that 30 minutes was not sufficient to maintain a healthy body weight (body mass index of 18.5 to 25 kg/m^2) or to maximize the health benefits of the exercise. Considering that only 27 percent of American women and 34 percent of American men engage in regular exercise,[52] it is hard to imagine an effective strategy for motivating persons to exercise 1 hour every day!

The well-intentioned recommendations of the IOM appear to contradict those of the ACSM, CDC, and surgeon general, but the IOM simply presents a different perspective on physical activity. The goal of the IOM was to offer guidelines that maximize the health benefits of exercise and help with appropriate weight loss. The ACSM recognizes that a longer duration of exercise at lower intensity is a preferable strategy for weight loss for persons who are overweight or obese. The ACSM also recognizes that longer duration of exercise reaps even greater cardiovascular fitness and health benefits.[19] However, what the ACSM recommendations are more likely to accomplish, and the IOM recommendations fail to do, is strike a balance between optimal efficacy and feasibility.

The public health message from the ACSM/CDC guidelines is that even modest increases in physical activity can convey significant and measurable improvements in cardiovascular health, independent of weight loss.[19,52,53] Still, weight loss also may occur as demonstrated in two studies in which walking regularly[54] and walking with modest caloric restriction,[55] lead to significant weight reduction. Walking is the most common leisure activity among U.S. adults. Additionally, moderate exercise reduces blood pressure, raises glucose tolerance and insulin sensitivity, and improves blood lipid levels.[52,53]

The take-home message is that any physical activity is better than none. Moderate aerobic exercise of 30 minutes per day, at least 3 days per week, provides measurable cardioprotective effects, decreases morbidity and mortality, and helps with appropriate weight maintenance. More activity (longer duration, greater frequency) is better as long as it is accomplished safely.

exercise. The optimal amount of exercise, like the optimal amount of medication, enhances cardiovascular health with little or no untoward side effects.[19,44]

Intensity describes the physical stress put on the cardiovascular system by exercise, and *duration* describes the length of time of an exercise session. Together these terms express the total work accomplished in an exercise session. Intensity is assessed as a percentage of the maximal ability of the body to do work, called the maximal aerobic capacity or maximal oxygen consumption (**VO$_2$ max).** Oxygen consumption increases as intensity increases, so **VO$_2$** is a reliable and reproducible measure of the capacity of the cardiovascular system to deliver blood to working muscles.[17,19,45] Intensity, therefore, is prescribed as a percentage of VO$_2$ max (%VO$_2$ max). Recently, the American College of Sports Medicine (**ACSM**) revised its guidelines to recommend the usage of percentage of VO$_2$ *reserve* (%VO$_2$ R instead of %VO$_2$ max) for cardiac patients.[19] **VO$_2$ R** is

the difference between resting VO$_2$ and VO$_2$ max, so it accounts for the oxygen consumption used at rest. Using %VO$_2$ R to prescribe intensity for persons with cardiac disease, especially those who have low fitness levels, improves accuracy of calculating an appropriate intensity level or *target* VO$_2$.[19,45]

Heart rate is used as a standard guide to setting exercise intensity because the relationship between VO$_2$ and heart rate is relatively linear and heart rate is an easily obtained measurement. Heart rate maximum (which corresponds with VO$_2$ max) can be obtained by exercise stress test (recommended for all cardiac patients) or can be calculated using the following equation[19]:

$$\text{Heart rate max} = 220 - \text{age (years)}$$

Heart rate reserve is maximal heart rate minus the resting heart rate and corresponds with the VO$_2$ R.[45] Thus the heart rate reserve can be calculated and used to prescribe exercise intensity.

The ACSM recommends a minimal exercise intensity of 45 percent VO$_2$ R for persons with cardiovascular disease[19] (Table 6-2). Higher-intensity training offers additional benefits (e.g., greater improvements in VO$_2$ max), provided it does not lead to adverse signs or symptoms (e.g., angina, ischemia, or ventricular dysrhythmias).[45,53,56] In fact, epidemiological research has demonstrated a lower all-cause mortality for those exercising at vigorous versus moderate versus lower intensities.[57,58] However, higher-intensity exercise may lead to discouragement, especially for low-fit patients, because of discomfort, injury, or lack of success.[44] Therefore the realistic goal is to initiate exercise intensity at approximately 40 to 45 percent VO$_2$ R and progressively increase it as tolerated.

The *duration* of the exercise session necessary to achieve a training effect varies inversely with the intensity; that is, if exercise is being performed at a high intensity, then the duration can be shorter. If exercise is performed at a relatively low intensity, then a longer duration is necessary to achieve improvements in cardiorespiratory fitness.[19,53] At the recommended 45 percent VO$_2$ R intensity, approximately 30 minutes of exercise is recommended for persons with cardiovascular disease. Some cardiac patients, especially those who are sedentary, may not be able to achieve 30 minutes of exercises at the start of an exercise program. In this case, cardiorespiratory benefits still can be gained by breaking up the exercise sessions into two to three sessions daily, accumulating at least 30 minutes per day.[44,53]

The minimum recommended *frequency* of aerobic-type exercise is three sessions per week.[44,53] Ideally, however, the goal should be to exercise every day. Improvements in cardiorespiratory fitness occur as a function of frequency of training (though VO$_2$ max tends to plateau when training exceeds 3 days weekly).[19] Additionally, other health benefits can be gained with daily physical activity, particularly for persons with cardiovascular disease.[19,44,45]

An exercise prescription should include aerobic and resistance exercise; this is the recommendation for cardiac patients[44,45] and for the general population.[53] Aero-

■■■ PHARMACOLOGY

DRUG THERAPY AND EXERCISE

Patients with cardiovascular disease are likely to be on a regimen of cardiac drugs that potentially interact with their exercise. Knowing and accommodating for the actions of these medications is an important part of developing an exercise prescription. For example, beta-adrenergic antagonists, or beta blockers, commonly are prescribed for patients with hypertension and/or coronary artery disease. These drugs reduce resting and exercise heart rate and blood pressure. (Certain calcium channel blockers also may reduce heart rate.) The benefit for patients with angina is the ability to achieve a higher *functional* capacity with fewer adverse signs and symptoms (e.g., ST segment changes and angina) during exercise.[47] Patients with hypertension who are taking beta blockers can reduce exercise-related increases in blood pressure.[42] The trade-off is a blunting of the normal heart rate response and exercise capacity; this makes heart rate a less reliable index of exercise intensity for these patients. Therefore, heart rate maximum and target heart rate should be determined by exercise stress test (not by a calculated method), and exercise intensity should be prescribed from these data. Also, these patients should be taught a subjective rating of effort (rating of perceived exertion) as an additional intensity guide.[19,47]

There are special considerations for other cardiac drugs. The following table outlines some common cardiac medications and their effects on heart rate, blood pressure, and exercise capacity, with comments.

MEDICATION	HEART RATE	BLOOD PRESSURE	EXERCISE CAPACITY	COMMENTS
ACE inhibitors	$\leftrightarrow$ R $\leftrightarrow$ E	$\downarrow$ R $\downarrow$ E	$\leftrightarrow$, except $\uparrow$ or $\downarrow$ in patients with CHF	Recommended for endurance athletes
Alpha-adrenergic blockers	$\leftrightarrow$ R $\leftrightarrow$ E	$\downarrow$ R $\downarrow$ E	$\leftrightarrow$	Negligible interactions with exercise
Beta blockers	$\downarrow$ R $\downarrow$ E	$\downarrow$ R $\downarrow$ E	$\uparrow$ in patients with angina $\downarrow$ or $\leftrightarrow$ in patients without angina	Fatigue; use target HR from exercise stress test plus perceived exertion rating
Calcium channel blockers Amlodipine, felodipine, isradipine, nicardipine, nifedipine, nimodipine, nisoldipine	$\uparrow$ or $\leftrightarrow$ R and E	$\downarrow$ R $\downarrow$ E	$\uparrow$ in patients with angina $\leftrightarrow$ in patients without angina	Slow onset; watch for hypotension
Diltiazem, verapamil	$\downarrow$ R and E	$\downarrow$ R $\downarrow$ E	$\uparrow$ in patients with angina $\leftrightarrow$ in patients without angina	Fatigue; use target HR from exercise stress test plus perceived exertion
Digitalis	$\downarrow$ with aFib and possibly with CHF	$\leftrightarrow$ R $\leftrightarrow$ E	$\uparrow$ in patients with angina $\uparrow$ in patients with CHF	Bradycardia; patients with aFib may experience a low resting HR
Diuretics	$\leftrightarrow$ R $\leftrightarrow$ E	$\leftrightarrow$ or $\downarrow$ R and E	$\leftrightarrow$, except possibly in CHF	Decreased plasma volume and stroke volume; susceptible to impaired thermoregulation and dehydration
Nitrates	$\uparrow$ R $\uparrow$ or $\leftrightarrow$ E	$\downarrow$ R $\downarrow$ or $\leftrightarrow$ E	$\uparrow\uparrow$ in patients with angina $\leftrightarrow$ in patients without angina $\uparrow$ or $\leftrightarrow$ in patients with CHF	Orthostatic hypotension, particularly when dehydrated
Vasodilators	$\uparrow$ or $\leftrightarrow$ R and E	$\downarrow$ R $\downarrow$ E	$\leftrightarrow$, except $\uparrow$ or $\leftrightarrow$ in patients with CHF	Orthostatic hypotension, particularly when dehydrated

ACE, angiotensin-converting enzyme; *R,* rest; *E,* exercise; *CHF,* congestive heart failure; *HR,* heart rate; *aFib,* atrial fibrillation.
Data from American College of Sports Medicine: *ACSM's guidelines for exercise testing and prescription,* ed 6, Baltimore, 2000, Lippincott Williams & Wilkins.

bic work is exercise involving large muscle groups involved in dynamic, usually continuous and rhythmic, motion.[17] Fast walking often is recommended for aerobic activity because it is a familiar and easy-to-perform activity for most persons, requires little additional cost in equipment or facility, is easy to quantify in amount (dosage), and may be done alone, with a partner, or in a group. Walking also can be incorporated into a busy day.

Resistance exercise (or strength training) is work that overloads specific muscle groups (through lifting weights or pulling against resistance) in order to enhance or maintain muscular strength and endurance.[17] Resistance training can be performed safely by persons with cardiovascular disease as long as certain guidelines are followed. The ACSM recommends that cardiac patients start at a low weight (less than 50 percent of their maximal ability in one repetition/lift) and perform the lift/pull 10 to 15 times (repetitions) in sets of 2 or 3

times. The recommended set is 8 to 10 different exercises/lifts involving approximately four to five upper extremity exercises and four to five lower extremity exercises. The suggested frequency for strength training is twice weekly.[19,44]

The benefits of enhanced muscular fitness include improved cardiovascular function, enhanced psychosocial and physical well-being, and favorably modified

■■■

TABLE 6-2   EXERCISE PRESCRIPTION FOR PATIENTS WITH CORONARY ARTERY DISEASE

PARAMETER	PRESCRIPTION
Intensity	40% (limited by angina and other symptoms)
Duration	20-40 minutes
Frequency	3 nonconsecutive times per week (or daily)
Type	Dynamic aerobic; modified resistance training

coronary risk factors. In addition, daily weight lifting activities (e.g., carrying groceries and occupational tasks) can be performed with greater safety and effectiveness.[44,45] Cardiac patients should be advised to exhale with exertion and to raise the weights slowly, in a controlled movement to full extension. Also, they should avoid straining, bearing down (the Valsalva maneuver), and tight gripping of handles/bars to prevent a sudden rise in blood pressure.[19]

A person with cardiovascular disease should not start an exercise program without medical clearance from a physician. Ideally, a new cardiac patient is enrolled in a cardiac rehabilitation program before independently pursuing exercise. The supervision and education provided in such a program help patients safely and confidently progress in their physical activity (see Chapter 80). Not all cardiac patients should engage in exercise. Contraindications include abnormal blood pressure (too high or too low), unstable angina, critical aortic stenosis, acute systemic illness, uncontrolled dysrhythmias, third-degree heart block (without a pacemaker), recent vascular event (embolism or thrombophlebitis), uncontrolled diabetes, severe orthopedic conditions that prohibit exercise, and other acute metabolic conditions.[19]

Finally, Lee and Paffenbarger[59] give this advice for the prevention of coronary artery disease: "at least 30 minutes of moderate intensity physical activity on most days of the week would be a good starting point for those who are sedentary. When previously sedentary individuals can adopt this regimen comfortably, they should strive for the goal of more vigorous exercise, provided there are no contraindications."

SUMMARY

Acute exercise signals a shift in priorities for the cardiovascular system. Hemodynamic changes in stroke volume, heart rate, cardiac output, and total peripheral resistance are vital to sustain mean arterial pressure and adequate blood flow. Just as critical is the redistribution of that blood flow away from nonexercising tissues to active muscles. Central, peripheral, and local mechanisms accomplish this through cooperative regulation. The autonomic nervous system, through changes in sympathetic and parasympathetic activation, is a key player in this shift. The short- and long-term benefits of regular exercise extend to patients with cardiovascular disease. In this population, exercise is not only possible but also strongly recommended. An appropriately designed exercise prescription (as part of a complete cardiac rehabilitation program) can lead to enhanced cardiorespiratory fitness, muscular strength, psychosocial well-being, and improved morbidity and mortality. Daily exercise should be a goal toward the prevention of cardiovascular disease.

REFERENCES

1. Iellamo F: Neural control of the cardiovascular system during exercise, *Ital Heart J* 2:200-212, 2001.
2. Dampney R, Coleman MJ, Fontes MP et al: Central mechanisms underlying short- and long-term regulation of the cardiovascular system, *Clin Exp Pharmacol Physiol* 29:261-268, 2002.
3. Porta A, Baselli G, Rimoldi O et al: Assessing baroreflex gain from spontaneous variability in conscious dogs: role of causality and respiration, *Am J Physiol* 279:H2558-H2567, 2000.
4. Goodwin GM, McCloskey DI, Mitchell JH: Cardiovascular and respiratory responses to changes in central command during isometric exercise at constant muscle tension, *J Appl Physiol* 226:173-190, 1972.
5. Gandevia SC, Killian K, McKenzie DK: Respiratory sensations, cardiovascular control, kinesthesia and transcranial stimulation during paralysis in humans, *J Appl Physiol* 470:85-107, 1993.
6. Leonard B, Mitchell JH, Mizuno M et al: Partial neuromuscular blockade and cardiovascular responses to static exercise in man, *J Appl Physiol* 359:365-379, 1985.
7. Victor RG, Pryor SL, Scher NH et al: Effects of partial neuromuscular blockade on sympathetic nerve responses to static exercise in humans, *Circ Res* 65:468-476, 1989.
8. Hobbs SIF, Gandevia SC: Cardiovascular responses and the sense of effort during attempts to contract paralyzed muscles: role of the spinal cord, *Neurosci Lett* 57:85-90, 1985.
9. DiMicco JA, Stolz-Potter EH, Monroe AJ et al: Role of the dorsomedial hypothalamus in the cardiovascular response to stress, *Clin Exp Pharmacol Physiol* 23:171-176, 1996.
10. Berne R, Levy M: *Cardiovascular physiology,* ed 8, Philadelphia, 2001, Mosby.
11. Secher N, Kagaya A, Saltin B et al: *Exercise and circulation in health and disease,* Champaign, Ill, 2000, Human Kinetics.
12. Raven PB, Fadel JP, Smith SA: The influence of central command on baroreflex resetting during exercise, *Exerc Sport Sci Rev* 30:39-44, 2002.
13. Fadel PIJ, Ogoh S, Keller DM et al: Recent insights into carotid baroreflex function in humans using the variable pressure neck chamber, *Exp Physiol* 88:671-680, 2003.
14. Sullivan SE, Bell C: The effects of exercise and training on human cardiovascular reflex control, *J Auton Nerv Syst* 81:16-24, 2000.
15. Timmers H, Wieling W, Karemaker J et al: Cardiovascular responses to stress after carotid baroreceptor denervation in humans, *Ann N Y Acad Sci* 1018:515-519, 2004.
16. O'Leary DS: Heart rate control during exercise by baroreceptors and skeletal muscle afferents, *Med Sci Sports Exerc* 28:210-217, 1996.
17. Powers S, Howley E: *Exercise physiology,* ed 4, New York, 2001, McGraw-Hill.
18. Opie LH: *The heart: physiology from cell to circulation,* ed 3, Baltimore, 1998, Lippincott Williams & Wilkins.
19. American College of Sports Medicine: *ACSM's guidelines for exercise testing and prescription,* ed 6, Baltimore, 2000, Lippincott Williams & Wilkins.
20. Foss ML, Keteyian SJ: *Fox's physiological basis for exercise and sport,* ed 6, New York, 1998, McGraw-Hill.
21. Thibodeau G, Patton KT: *Anatomy & physiology,* ed 5, St Louis, 2003, Mosby.
22. Johnson PD, Wagner PD, Wilson DF: Regulation of oxidative metabolism and blood flow in skeletal muscle, *Med Sci Sports Exerc* 28:305-314, 1996.
23. McAllistor RM, Hirai T, Musch TI: Contribution of endothelium-derived nitric oxide to the skeletal muscle blood flow response to exercise, *Med Sci Sports Exerc* 27:1145-1151, 1995.
24. Johnson JM: Physical training and the control of skin blood flow, *Med Sci Sports Exerc* 30:382-386, 1998.
25. Vissing S: Neural control of skin circulation. In Saltin B, Boushel R, Secher N, Mitchell J, editors: *Exercise and circulation in health and disease,* Champaign, Ill, 2000, Human Kinetics.
26. Saltin B, Boushel R, Secher N, Mitchell J, editors: *Exercise and circulation in health and disease,* Champaign, Ill, 2000, Human Kinetics.
27. Keul J, Konig D, Huonker M et al: Adaptation to training and performance in elite athletes, *Res Q Exerc Sport* 67:S29-S36, 1996.
28. Huoker M, Schmid A, Sorichter S et al: Cardiovascular differences between sedentary and wheelchair-trained subjects with paraplegia, *Med Sci Sports Exerc* 30:609-613, 1998.
29. Jensen-Urstad M, Bouvier F, Nejat M et al: Left ventricular function in endurance runners during exercise, *Acta Physiol Scand* 162:167-172, 1998.
30. DiBello V, Santoro G, Talarico L et al: Left ventricular function during exercise in athletes and in sedentary men, *Med Sci Sports Exerc* 28:190-196, 1996.

31. Laughlin MH, Oltman CL, Bowles DK: Exercise training-induced adaptations in the coronary circulation, *Med Sci Sports Exerc* 30:352-360, 1998.

32. Brown MD: Exercise and coronary vascular remodeling in the healthy heart, *Exp Physiol* 88(5):645-658, 2003.

33. Bonaduce D, Petretta M, Cavallaro V et al: Intensive training and cardiac autonomic control in high level athletes, *Med Sci Sports Exerc* 30:691-696, 1998.

34. Ray CA: Sympathetic adaptations to one-legged training, *J Appl Physiol* 86:1583-1587, 1999.

35. O'Sullivan S, Bell C: The effects of exercise and training on human cardiovascular reflex control, *J Auton Nerv Syst* 81:16-24, 2000.

36. McAllistor RM: Endothelial-mediated control of coronary and skeletal muscle blood flow during exercise, *Med Sci Sports Exerc* 27:1122-1124, 1995.

37. Lash JM: Training-induced alterations in contractile function and excitation-contraction coupling in vascular smooth muscle, *Med Sci Sports Exerc* 30:60-66, 1998.

38. Maiorana A, O'Driscoll G, Taylor R et al: Exercise and the nitric oxide vasodilator system, *Sports Med* 33:1013-1035, 2003.

39. Stewart JM, Zu Z, Ochoa M et al: Exercise decrease epicardial coronary artery wall stiffness: roles of cGMP and cAMP, *Med Sci Sports Exerc* 30:220-228, 1998.

40. Fagard RH: Exercise characteristics and the blood pressure response to dynamic physical training, *Med Sci Sports Exerc* 33:S484-S492, 2001.

41. *Seventh Report of the Joint National Committee on the Detection, Evaluation, and Treatment of High Blood Pressure (JNC 7)*, Washington, DC, 2004, National Institutes of Health; National Heart, Lung, and Blood Institute.

42. Snowise M, Dexter WW: Hypertension and exercise: a review, *Am J Med Sports* 4:291-297, 2002.

43. Shoemaker JK, Green HJ, Ball-Burnett et al: Relationships between fluid and electrolyte hormones and plasma volume during exercise with training and detraining, *Exerc Sport Sci Rev* 30:497-505, 1998.

44. Shephard RJ, Balady GJ: Exercise as cardiovascular therapy, *Circulation* 99:963-972, 1999.

45. Franklin VA, Swain DP, Shephard RJ: New insights in the prescription of exercise for coronary patients, *J Cardiovasc Nurs* 18(2):116-123, 2003.

46. American College of Sports Medicine: *Pronouncements: the official position stands, joint position statements, and opinion statements of the ACSM,* ed 13, Indianapolis, 2000, The College.

47. Fardy RS, Franklin BA, Porcari JP et al: *Training techniques in cardiac rehabilitation,* Champaign, Ill, 1998, Human Kinetics.

48. American Association of Cardiovascular and Pulmonary Rehabilitation: *Guidelines for cardiac rehabilitation and secondary prevention programs,* ed 4, Champaign, Ill, 2004, Human Kinetics.

49. Kriska A: Can a physically active lifestyle prevent type 2 diabetes? *Exerc Sport Sci Rev* 31(3):132-137, 2003.

50. Ross R, Freeman JA, Janssen I: Exercise alone is an effective strategy for reducing obesity and related comorbidities, *Exerc Sport Sci Rev* 28(4):165-170, 2000.

51. Roitman JL, editor: *ACSM's resource manual for guidelines for exercise testing and prescription,* Baltimore, 1998, Williams & Wilkins.

52. Bassuk SS, Manson JE: Physical activity and cardiovascular disease prevention in women: how much is good enough? *Exerc Sport Sci Rev* 31(4):176-181, 2003.

53. American College of Sports Medicine: Position stand on the recommended quantity and quality of exercise for developing and maintaining cardiorespiratory and muscular fitness and flexibility in healthy adults, *Med Sci Sports Exerc* 30:975-991, 1998.

54. Irwin ML, Yasui Y, Ulrich CM et al: Effect of exercise on total and intra-abdominal body fat in postmenopausal women: a randomized trial, *JAMA* 289:323-330, 2003.

55. Hill JO, Wyatt HR, Reed GW et al: Obesity and the environment: where do we go from here? *Science* 299:853-855, 2003.

56. Swain DP, Franklin BA: Is there a threshold intensity for aerobic training in cardiac patients? *Med Sci Sports Exerc* 34:1071-1075, 2002.

57. Lee IM, Hsieh CC, Paffenbarger RS: Exercise intensity and longevity in men: the Harvard Alumni Health Study, *JAMA* 215:1179-1184, 1995.

58. Lee IM, Paffenbarger RS: Associations of light, moderate, and vigorous intensity physical activity with longevity: the Harvard Alumni Health Study, *Am J Epidemiol* 151:293-299, 2000.

59. Lee IM, Paffenbarger RS: The role of physical activity in the prevention of coronary artery disease. In Thompson PD, editor: *Exercise and sports cardiology,* New York, 2001, McGraw-Hill.

chapter 7

Regulation of Cardiac Output and Blood Pressure

Dennis J. Cheek
Diane A. Hawley
Debra K. Moser

CHAPTER ABBREVIATIONS

BSA   body surface area
CI   cardiac index
LVEDP   left ventricular end-diastolic pressure
MVO_2 myocardial oxygen consumption
PVR   pulmonary vascular resistance
SVR   systemic vascular resistance

Hemodynamics is a term used to describe the complex interplay of physical principles controlling pressure, flow, and resistance of blood specifically as they relate to the circulatory system. The propulsion of blood through the circulatory system is complex and relies on the heart, a unique cyclical pump that propels blood into a convoluted branching highway of blood vessels with various dimensions and distensibilities. The ultimate purpose of the circulatory system is to transport sufficient oxygen and nutrients to tissues to maintain viability and ongoing metabolism. This chapter addresses the many variables that affect hemodynamics of the circulatory system.

CARDIAC CYCLE

In 1 day the heart moves more than 7000 liters of blood through the body. This is done by means of the rhythmic pumping action of the heart. The cardiac cycle refers to the time from the beginning of one beat of the heart to the next, and includes systole, a period of cardiac muscle contraction, and diastole, a time of muscle relaxation. The heart cycles as two separate pumps that deliver blood to the pulmonary and systemic vascular systems in a synchronous manner.

The primary mechanism responsible for the forward movement of blood through the heart is the trans area pressure gradient; blood flows throughout the body from areas of higher pressure to areas of lower pressure.[1] The greater the pressure gradient between areas, the greater the blood flow (Figure 7-1).

Most of the blood volume is in the venous system, and it is that deoxygenated blood that spills into the thin-walled right atrium from the superior vena cava, inferior vena cava, and coronary sinus. Because there are no valves between the junctions of the central veins and the atria, atrial filling occurs during systole and diastole. Atrial pressure is controlled by the ability of the corresponding ventricle to empty itself adequately and

intrathoracic pressures that move blood from the pulmonary or venous circulation (venous return) into the atria.

The right myocardial pump is a low-pressure, low-resistance circuit that usually consumes small amounts of myocardial oxygen. The left myocardial pump, however, is a high-pressure, high-resistance circuit. The left ventricle must supply adequate quantities of oxygenated blood to the pulmonary and systemic circulations. In the performance of this task, most of the available myocardial oxygen is consumed.

The atria are reservoir chambers that serve to deliver blood to the receiving ventricles passively and through contractile movement. During a complete cycle, the ventricles are in systole (ventricular ejection) approximately one-third of each cycle and in diastole (filling) two-thirds of the same cycle.[1] The diastolic phase is crucial because it is during this time of rest that the epicardium, myocardium, and endocardium are perfused via the coronary arteries and microcirculation. The cyclical process of ventricular filling and ejection apply to both sides of the heart.

Diastole

Until recently, diastolic function was thought of as of secondary importance compared with systolic function. In fact, diastolic function has an equally important role in the cardiac cycle, and it substantially influences preload and afterload.[2] A major influence on diastolic function is heart rate, which determines how much time is available for filling during diastole. Tachycardia shortens diastolic filling time and reduces coronary artery blood flow to the myocardium.

Physiological diastole begins with the reduced ejection of blood from the ventricle. For a very brief moment there is a reversal of blood flow back within the root of the pulmonary artery and aorta as the pressure in the aorta and pulmonary artery exceeds the falling pressures in the ventricles. This retrograde blood flow closes the pulmonary artery and aortic valves. The closures of these two valves create the second heart sound. At this point, ventricular pressures are higher than atrial pressures, so the atrioventricular valves remain closed. Because all valves are closed during this moment in time, the ventricular volumes do not change. This time frame within the cardiac cycle is referred to as the isovolumetric relaxation phase because although there is no change in volume in the ventricles, the pressures decrease and the ventricles continue to relax (Figure

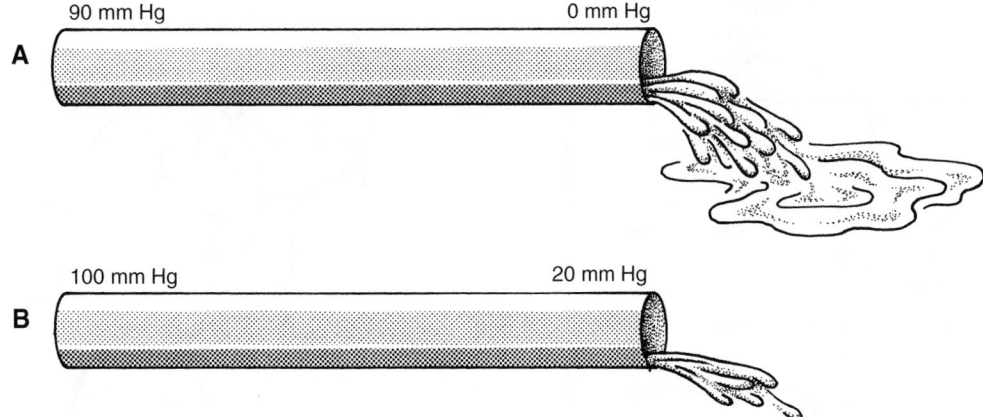

FIGURE 7-1 ■ Blood flow throughout the body is a function of pressure gradients. **A,** A pressure gradient of 90 mm Hg drives fluid through the tube. **B,** Despite a 10-mm Hg increase in pressure at the beginning of the tube, fluid flow rates are decreased because pressure at the end of the tube is increased to 20 mm Hg. This decreases the pressure gradient, or fluid-driving force, to 80 mm Hg. (From Darovic GO: *Hemodynamic monitoring: invasive and noninvasive clinical application,* ed 3, Philadelphia, 2002, WB Saunders.)

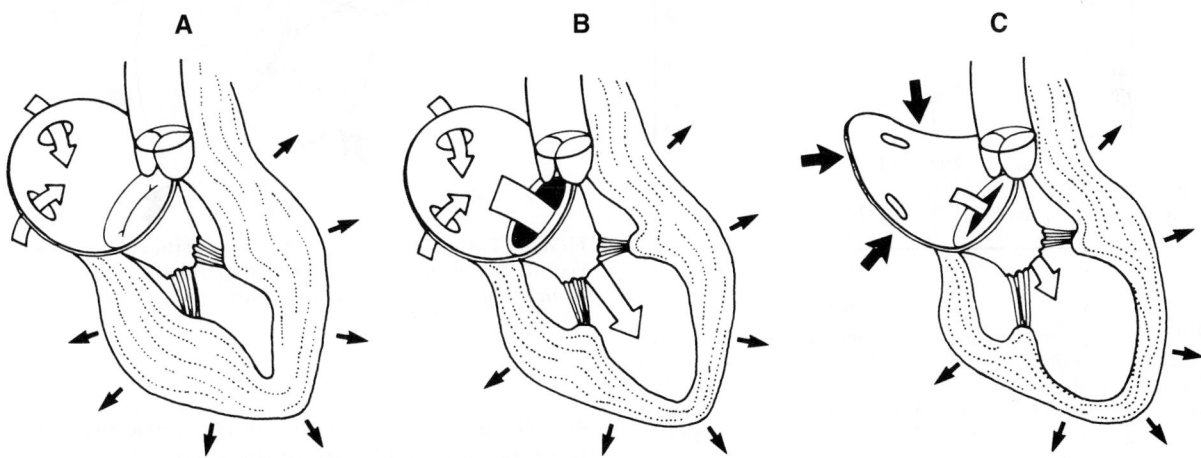

FIGURE 7-2 ■ **A** to **C,** Diastolic phases of the cardiac cycle. (From Darovic GO: *Hemodynamic monitoring: invasive and noninvasive clinical application,* ed 3, Philadelphia, 2002, WB Saunders.)

7-2A). During this phase, blood continues to flow from the veins and pulmonary venous system into the atria (Figure 7-3).

When ventricular pressures fall below atrial pressures, the atrioventricular valves passively open and blood flows into the ventricle. This is called the passive filling phase, and 70 to 90 percent of ventricular filling occurs during this time (Figure 7-2B). As atrial and ventricular pressures equalize, ventricular filling ceases. Well-supported data suggest that the ventricles create suction or recoil during the early filling phase to pull volume actively from the atria.[2] The ventricles appear to spring outward to cause a drop in diastolic filling pressure that augments filling.

Continued filling of the ventricle requires a pressure gradient from the atrium to the ventricle that is achieved with atrial systole. With atrial systole, blood flow into the ventricle is the result of atrial contraction (Figure 7-2C). Blood flow from atrial contraction follows the path of least resistance, forward into the ventricle as is usually the case, or retrograde into the great veins if pressures are too high in the ventricle (as occurs in heart failure). The blood volume ejected during contraction adds 10 to 30 percent to the ventricular end-diastolic volume, enhancing cardiac output by increasing stroke volume.[1,3,4] Individuals with atrial fibrillation may suffer a decrease in cardiac output by as much as 25 percent (particularly in the setting of a damaged myocardium) because their heart's cannot augment ventricular end-diastolic volume with each atrial contraction. Atrial contraction becomes important during periods of increased activity when diastolic filling time is decreased because of an increase in heart rate or when the ventricle fails to relax normally as in left ventricular hypertrophy.

Systole

Physiological systole begins with the isovolumetric contraction phase. At this moment in the cardiac cycle, ventricular myocardium is creating tension without

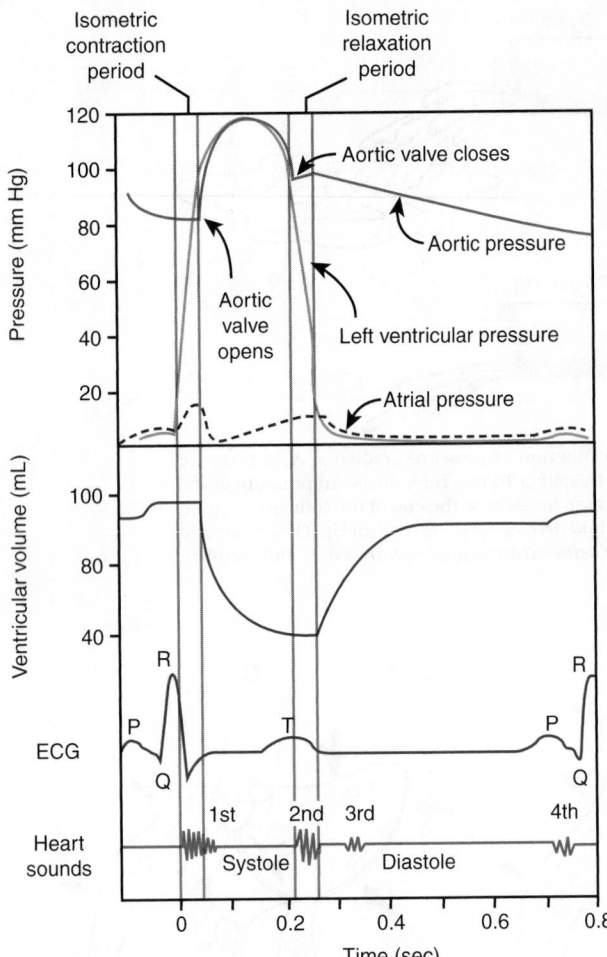

FIGURE 7-3 ■ Volume and pressure changes in the cardiac cycle. At the beginning of the isometric contraction and relaxation period, all valves are closed, so there is no change in volume yet tremendous changes in pressure. *ECG,* Electrocardiogram. (From Porth CM: *Essentials of pathophysiology,* Philadelphia, 2004, Lippincott Williams & Wilkins.)

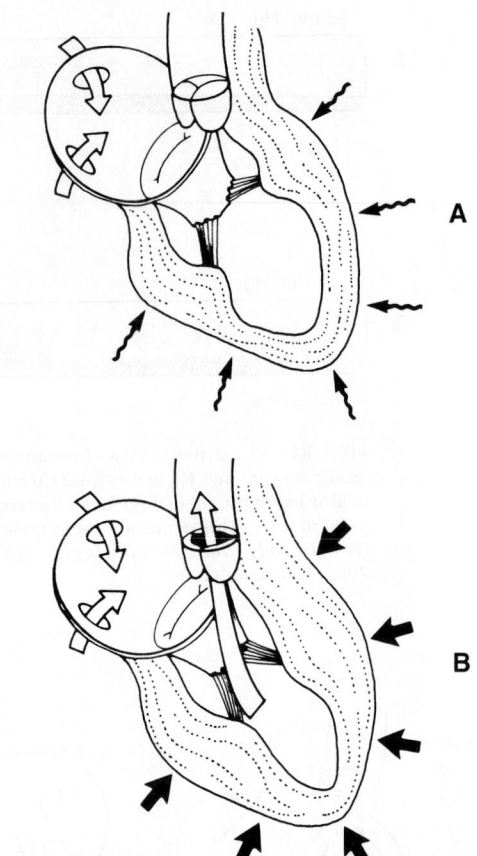

FIGURE 7-4 ■ **A** and **B,** Systolic phases of the cardiac cycle. (From Darovic GO: *Hemodynamic monitoring: invasive and noninvasive clinical application,* ed 3, Philadelphia, 2002, WB Saunders.)

changing the muscle fiber length or volume amount, thus the term *isovolumetric* (Figure 7-3). The ventricles quickly create enough pressure to exceed atrial pressure, and shortly thereafter the atrioventricular valves close (Figure 7-4A). The closure of the atrioventricular valves creates the first heart sound. In relation to mitral valve closure, it is commonly thought that valve closure coincides with the crossover point at which left ventricular pressure exceeds left atrial pressure. In fact, closure of the mitral valve is delayed slightly because of the sheer inertia of blood flow out of the left ventricle, creating a potential split S1 heart sound.

The next phase of systole is maximal ejection that results in opening of the semilunar valves. The ventricles have created the required systolic pressure and thus contract to thrust blood out into the aorta and pulmonary artery (Figure 7-4B).[1,3,4] The strength of ejection depends on not only the pressure gradient between the ventricles and the semilunar valves but also the elastic properties of the aorta, pulmonary artery, and systemic/pulmonary vasculature that expand during systole. The aortic pressure begins to fall during the last quarter of

systole, and there is a notch in the aortic pressure tracing representing closure of the aortic valve. At the end of systole, the ventricles begin to relax, and as this occurs, blood flows from the large arteries back toward the ventricles. As a consequence, the ventricles never completely empty. At the end of systole, there is approximately 50 ml remaining in the ventricles.[1]

Right ventricular ejection occurs primarily as a bellow-like action rather than a muscle shortening movement. This accomplishes adequate systolic ejection because of the high-volume, low-resistance environment. Efficient right ventricle wall movement becomes a problem when there are pressure loads on the ventricle as in pulmonary emboli or pulmonary hypertension.[1]

The left ventricle functions by reducing its chamber circumference significantly. The law of Laplace states that the muscle tension necessary to maintain a level of pressure is reduced as the radius decreases. A chronically dilated yet hypertrophied ventricle requires greater muscle tension and energy to reduce its circumference. When a ventricle is subject to excess volume loads, the enlarged and hypertrophied ventricle compromises left ventricular efficiency.[1,3,4]

Ejection fraction is a term used to represent the percentage of diastolic volume that is ejected from the heart during systole. The formula is as follows:

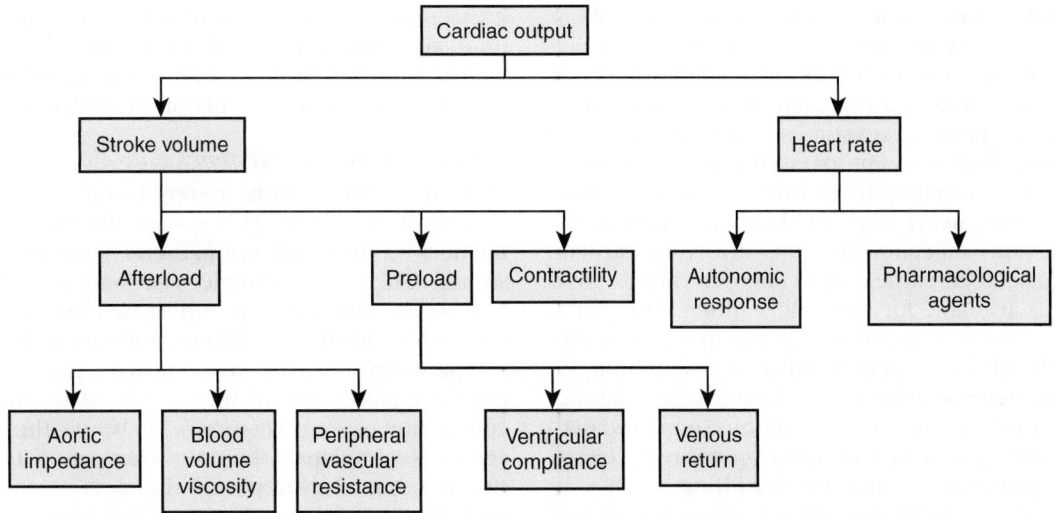

FIGURE 7-5 ▪ Determinants of cardiac output. (Adapted from Michaelson CR: *Congestive heart failure,* St Louis, 1983, Mosby.)

$$\text{Ejection fraction} = \frac{\text{End-diastolic volume} - \text{End systolic volume}}{\text{End-diastolic volume} \times 100\%}$$

Normal values for left ventricular ejection fraction are 0.55 to 0.75 when measured angiographically or by echocardiography. The normal values are lower (0.50 to 0.65) when measured via radionuclide angiography. Ejection fraction normally declines with age and does not differ based on gender.[2]

DETERMINANTS OF CARDIAC PERFORMANCE

The work of the heart as an efficient pump is measured in terms of cardiac output, or the amount of blood the heart pumps each minute. The hemodynamic determinants of cardiac output are heart rate and stroke volume, which are expressed as the the following equation: cardiac output = heart rate × stroke volume (Figure 7-5). The heart is two separate pumping systems with different volume loads. The usual volume is approximately 1.5 liters in the right ventricle and 3.5 liters in the left ventricle.[5]

Cardiac output can vary substantially within minutes based on the metabolic need of the tissues and the physical activity of the person. The average cardiac output in healthy adults ranges from 3.5 to 8.0 liters/min.[5] Because cardiac output varies considerably in accordance with body size, the cardiac index (**CI**) is used to achieve an accurate estimate of blood flow in proportion to body surface area (**BSA**). The formula is CI = cardiac output/BSA. The average CI is 2.4 to 4 liters/min/m².

A normal cardiac output for a highly trained athlete can increase threefold to fivefold during maximum exercise, with the percentages of blood flow being redistributed according to need during exercise (Table 7-1). Cardiac reserve is a concept that refers to the maximum percentage of increase in cardiac output that can be achieved above normal resting level. Healthy young adults have a cardiac reserve of 300 to 400 percent

▪ ▪ ▪

TABLE 7-1 COMPARISON OF ORGAN PERFUSION PERCENTAGES OF CARDIAC OUTPUT AT REST AND WITH EXERCISE

AT REST CARDIAC OUTPUT: 5 liters/min	ORGAN PERFUSED	EXERCISE CARDIAC OUTPUT: 25 liters/min
13%	Brain	4%
5%	Heart	5%
22%	Liver and gastrointestinal tract	5%
25%	Kidneys	4%
25%	Muscles and skin	80%
10%	Bone and bone marrow	2%

Adapted from Folkow D, Neil E: *Circulation,* New York, 1971, Oxford University Press.

above baseline. The ability of the heart to adjust and increase cardiac output almost on a beat-to-beat basis depends primarily on heart rate and the parameters that determine stroke volume: preload, afterload, and contractility.

Heart Rate

Heart rate is determined by the number of times the ventricles contract in 1 minute. Heart rate is controlled by the spontaneous electrical pacemaker activity (automaticity) of cells in the sinoatrial node. Automaticity depends on the passage of ions through ionic channels located throughout the sinoatrial node and the entire myocardium. The sodium, potassium, calcium, and chloride ions are the major charge carriers, and their movement across the cell membranes creates the flow of current that generates an excitation signal and subsequent mechanical contraction.[2,6,7] A heart rate of 60 to 100 beats per minute usually can maintain an adequate resting cardiac output.

The intrinsic heart rate at rest, without neurohormonal influences is 100 to 120 beats/min. A healthy person's heart rate at rest of 60 to 100 beats/min reflects a balance between sympathetic (stimulating) and parasympathetic (inhibiting) responses, with the parasympathetic predominating. The parasympathetic nervous system creates a usual resting heart rate that is lower than the intrinsic heart rate. The heart rate can be altered by several mechanisms, thus affecting cardiac output. As discussed earlier, heart rate determines how much time is available for ventricular filling. At normal heart rates, diastole composes a greater portion of the cardiac cycle (about 65 percent) than systole (about 35 percent). An increase in heart rate shortens the diastolic filling time. Under tachycardic conditions, impaired diastolic functioning can be improved by reducing heart rate, which provides a longer time for filling.[2]

With increasing heart rate there is an influx of calcium into the sarcoplasmic reticulum, resulting in increased force of contraction (the treppe phenomenon). The treppe phenomenon counteracts the reduction in diastolic filling time at faster heart rates. When heart rates exceed 180 beats/min, the diastolic filling time is so short that cardiac output usually falls. Also at very high heart rates, overuse of cellular substrates begins to cause a decrease in the strength of contraction.[2]

The oxygen demands of a critically ill person in a physiologically stressful, hypermetabolic situation stimulate a heart rate of 100 to 130 beats/min to maintain an adequate cardiac output.[3] Because heart rate is such a pivotal determinant of cardiac output, one would think that changes to heart rate would affect cardiac output considerably. To the contrary, surprisingly few changes to cardiac output occur when the heart rate is within physiological limits (Figure 7-6). Maintenance of cardiac output is a result of changes in venous return, which significantly affects cardiac output in the normal heart. When heart rate increases slightly, venous return decreases as a consequence of a reduction in stroke volume, and cardiac output is maintained. The reciprocal is also true. When heart rate is decreased slightly, venous return increases to maintain cardiac output.[4]

Autonomic Nervous System Control

The autonomic nervous system is a major factor in the control of heart rate. This system has two opposing influences on the heart, sympathetic and parasympathetic stimuli. These two influences act on the heart so that a balance is achieved. A group of neurons—the vasomotor center—in the cerebral medulla form the origin for sympathetic fibers that travel down a tract in the spinal cord and pass outward into the heart to innervate the conduction system (Figure 7-7). When the vasomotor center is stimulated, the neurotransmitter norepinephrine is released. Norepinephrine acts on the sinoatrial node to increase heart rate, on the myocardium to increase contractility, and in the vasculature to produce vasoconstriction. Also located in the vasomotor center is another group of neurons that are cardioinhibitory; these neurons function in opposition to cardiac acceleration and vasoconstriction. Parasympathetic fibers originate in this inhibitory center and reach the cardiac conduction system by means of the vagus nerve. Nerve impulses traveling along the parasympathetic fibers cause release of the neurotransmitter acetylcholine, which decreases heart rate (Figure 7-7).[6,7]

The sympathetic nervous system exerts its effects by acting on adrenergic receptor sites. These receptors are classified as alpha, beta$_1$, and beta$_2$. The response to sympathetic nervous system activation depends on the activation of one or more of these types of receptors, and the distribution of these sites within an organ or tissue. Alpha-adrenergic receptor sites respond to the release of norepinephrine and epinephrine causing vascular effects but little direct cardiac effect.[7] Beta-adrenergic receptors are classified into three categories: beta$_1$, beta$_2$, and beta$_3$. Beta$_1$ receptors are located predominantly in the heart. Their stimulation causes an increase in conduction velocity, thus increasing heart rate and increasing myocardial contractility. Beta$_2$ receptors are located primarily in the lungs, and their stimulation results in peripheral vasodilatation and bronchodilatation with little direct cardiac effect.[6,7] A new beta receptor, beta$_3$, has been proposed to reside in the myocardium and is postulated to mediate cardioinhibitory responses via a nitric oxide pathway in a counterbalance to excessive adrenergic stimulation.[2]

Nerve cells that are responsive to changes in blood pressure or chemical changes in blood are called baroreceptors (also known as baroreflexes) and chemoreceptors, respectively. Their primary locations are in the carotid sinus and the aortic root, although there are other locations. Chemoreceptors react to cellular oxygen deficiencies or an increase in carbon dioxide levels in blood, and the result is sympathetic stimulation to increase heart rate. When blood pressure increases and stretches a location, the baroreceptors are activated and send an impulse to stimulate the cardioinhibitory center and suppress cardiac acceleration. Consequently, more parasympathetic impulses travel by way of the vagus

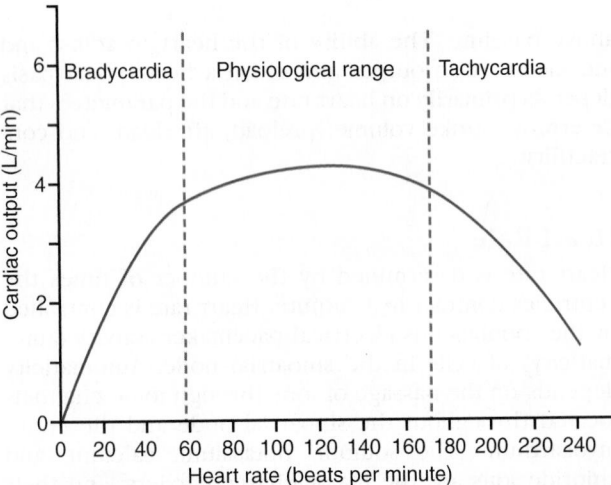

FIGURE 7-6 ■ The impact of different heart rates on cardiac output. Cardiac output is relatively insensitive to changes in heart rate within the physiological range. Cardiac output decreases substantially at both high and low ranges of heart rate. (From Johnson LR: *Essential medical physiology,* Boston, 2003, Elsevier Academic Press.)

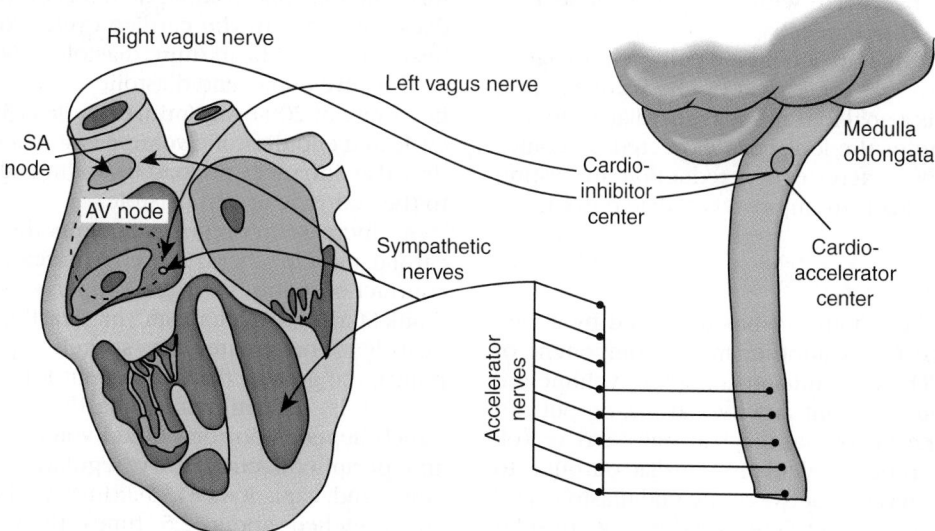

FIGURE 7-7 ■ Sympathetic and parasympathetic activity on the heart. *AV,* Atrioventricular; *SA,* sinoatrial. (From Michaelson CR: *Congestive heart failure,* St Louis, 1983, Mosby.)

nerve to the heart than sympathetic stimuli.[6,7] The result is a decrease in heart rate and force of contraction, which leads to a drop in blood pressure. This response is a normal compensatory mechanism to keep blood pressure from rising too high or too precipitously. Conversely, if blood pressure drops below normal, the compensation is a reflex acceleration of the heart and strengthened cardiac contraction. The baroreceptor response is observed when reduced circulating volume results in an increase in heart rate and blood pressure.

An autonomic disorder known as chronotropic incompetence is an overexaggeration of parasympathetic effect without sufficient sympathetic response.[2] Chronotropic incompetence is manifested by decreased heart rate sensitivity to the normal increase in sympathetic tone during exercise. Chronotropic incompetence is defined as the inability to increase heart rate to at least 85 percent of age-predicted maximum heart rate.

Strong emotions such as fear, anxiety, and anger stimulate the vasomotor center located in the medulla of the brain stem. As a result, sympathetic impulses can increase heart rate and produce peripheral vasoconstriction, causing an increase in blood pressure. The opposite effect can be triggered with a Valsalva maneuver, in which a person forcibly expires against a closed glottis in a straining manner. With this maneuver, intrathoracic pressure rises, causing venous return, stroke volume, and blood pressure to decrease, leading to sympathetic stimulation. On release of the strain, there is a sudden rise in cardiac output as the blood pooled in the venous system returns to the heart. An overshoot of parasympathetic stimulation occurs to counteract the initial sympathetic response to the maneuver, which leads to a profound, although usually transient, bradycardia.[4,6,7] Vasovagal stimuli such as retching, severe coughing, pain, carotid massage, bearing down for a bowel movement or any significant rectal stimuli such

as with endoscopic examination can produce a Valsalva response in some individuals.

Alterations in Heart Rate

Heart rate is the most important determinant of myocardial oxygen consumption (**MVO$_2$**). When heart rate doubles, myocardial oxygen uptake approximately doubles. The resulting supply-demand balance becomes a problem for two reasons. First, increased heart rate increases MVO$_2$. Second, an increased heart rate also reduces coronary blood flow because of decreased diastolic filling time. When heart rates increase, systolic time of ejection stays relatively constant, while diastolic filling time and coronary blood flow are reduced (Figure 7-8). The end result is an ischemia prone myocardium.[5] Tachycardia in any form can reduce cardiac output. For these reasons much of the pharmacological management of myocardial ischemia prone individuals is geared

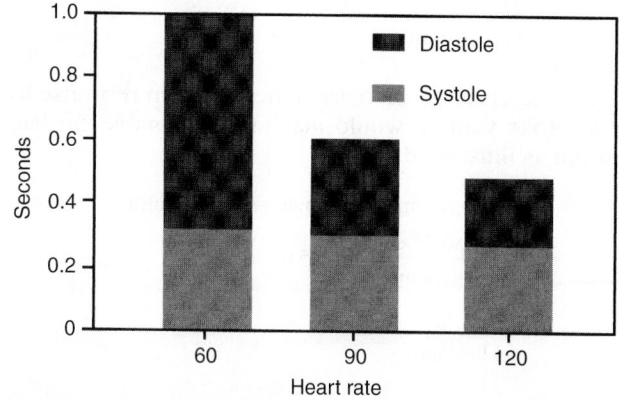

FIGURE 7-8 ■ Response of heart rate on the cardiac cycle. Diastole in normal heart rate ranges is two-thirds of every beat. As heart rate increases, the diastolic time is shortened substantially. (From Darovic GO: *Hemodynamic monitoring: invasive and noninvasive clinical application,* ed 3, Philadelphia, 2002, WB Saunders.)

toward reducing heart rate with drugs such as beta-adrenergic blockers.

Bradycardia, down to an individual's physiological limit, will improve cardiac output by the Frank-Starling mechanism and is a goal for improving cardiac function. For example, one of the long-term expected outcomes of routine aerobic exercise is a reduction in resting heart rate, which leads to improved cardiac output.

Stroke Volume

Stroke volume, the amount of blood ejected by a ventricle during systole, is another major component of cardiac output. The determinants of stroke volume are preload, afterload, and contractility. Cardiac output can be divided by the heart rate to yield one's stroke volume. Another method of calculating cardiac output is to determine the difference between the end-diastolic and end-systolic volumes. This calculation does not consider the normal beat-to-beat variation in chamber size resulting from respiration, nor does it reflect the impact of atrial dysrhythmias. A normal stroke volume ranges from 60 to 130 ml.[1,5] Consider the following formula:

Stroke volume × Heart rate = Cardiac output

$$\frac{70 \text{ ml} \times 75 \text{ beats}}{\text{beat} \times \text{minute}} = 5250 \text{ ml/min}$$

or

Normal cardiac output of 5.3 liter/min

Stroke volume is decreased when cardiac muscle is damaged, as can be the case in acute coronary syndrome or cardiomyopathy. Extracardiac causes of reduced stroke volume such as hypovolemia or pericardial dysfunction also inhibit cardiac performance. Under these circumstances, cardiac output is reduced as represented in the following formula:

Stroke volume × Heart rate = Cardiac output

$$\frac{45 \text{ ml} \times 75 \text{ beats}}{\text{beat} \times \text{minute}} = 3375 \text{ ml/min}$$

or

3.4 liter/min

A compensatory increase in heart rate in response to low stroke volume would maintain acceptable cardiac output as illustrated:

Stroke volume × Heart rate = Cardiac output

$$\frac{45 \text{ ml} \times 95 \text{ beats}}{\text{beat} \times \text{minute}} = 4275 \text{ ml/min}$$

or

4.3 liter/min

Preload

Preload refers to the stretch on a relaxed muscle before contraction. In the heart, preload is a function of the pressure and volume in the left ventricle at the end of diastole. Because ventricular filling occurs during dias-

tole, end-diastolic volume depends on the length of the diastolic phase of the cardiac cycle. For example, at a heart rate of 72 beats/min, diastole is 60 percent of the cardiac cycle and end-diastolic volume is greater. At a heart rate of 200 beats/min, diastole is 35 percent of the cycle and end-diastolic volume is smaller. Atrial contraction also enhances preload by adding additional volume to the ventricle at end diastole.

An increase in preload augments the stretch on myocardial muscle fibers, thereby increasing the force of contraction. This physical property is known as the Frank-Starling mechanism or Starling's law of the heart.[1,6,7] The greater the stretch (up to an optimal point), the greater the subsequent force of contraction. Preload is determined primarily by venous return, which depends on total blood volume, cardiac output, and peripheral circulatory regulation (vascular resistance and capacitance). Maximally, the muscle fibers are stretched about 2.5 times their normal resting length. The Frank-Starling mechanism is the mechanism whereby the heart makes beat-by-beat adjustments in cardiac output to manage changing volume loads from venous return (Figure 7-9).

There is no way to measure myocardial fiber length or directly to measure left ventricular end-diastolic volume; however, normally a close correlation exists between ventricular end-diastolic volume and ventricular end-diastolic pressure.[1,2,4,5] Left ventricular end-diastolic pressure (**LVEDP**) can be estimated at the bedside using a pulmonary artery catheter. Assuming no mitral valve disease, pulmonary artery occlusion pressure (measured using the distal pulmonary artery port with the

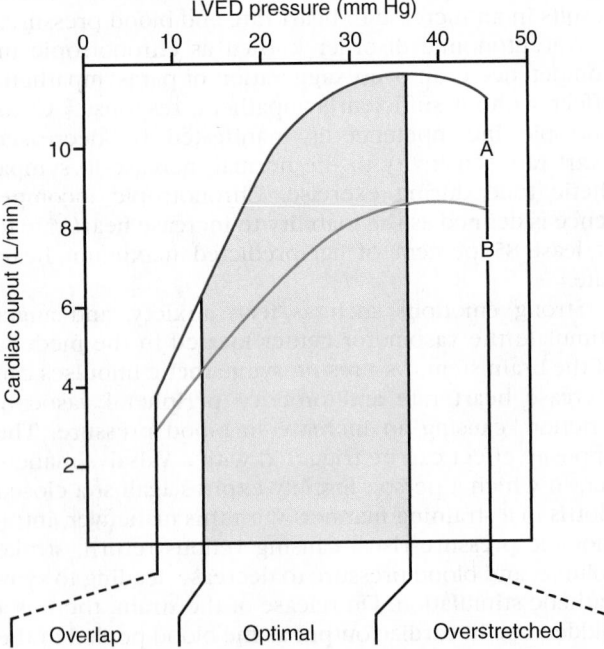

FIGURE 7-9 ■ Optimal preload for the heart. The maximum force of contraction and increased stroke volume are achieved when diastolic filling causes the muscle fibers to be stretched about 2.5 times their resting length. Overlap and overstretched refer to stretching of the actin and myosin filaments at different left ventricular end-diastolic (LVED) filling pressures. (From Porth CM: *Essentials of pathophysiology*, Philadelphia, 2004, Lippincott Williams & Wilkins.)

balloon inflated, and commonly called pulmonary artery wedge pressure) correlates with LVEDP. This measurement is a glimpse at the ventricular end-diastolic volume. Clinicians should be wary of applying this correlation every time; there are instances when ventricular compliance is altered and there is an inverse relationship between ventricular volume and pressure, as can be noted in Figure 7-10.

The Frank-Starling mechanism also explains why ventricular function improves with increased preload, up to a point. During heart failure, compensatory mechanisms that promote sodium and fluid retention capitalize on the relationship between increased preload and increased cardiac output. Sodium and fluid retention increase preload to better stretch the myocardial filaments, causing a stronger contraction, up to an individual's physiological limit. The usual upper limit for improving left ventricular function is an LVEDP of 15 to 18 mm Hg (although this pressure is subject to considerable variation depending on ventricular compliance and other factors).[4,5] Ultimately, continually increasing preload is ineffective in augmenting myocardial contraction, and pulmonary and systemic congestion result (see Chapter 62).

Factors Influencing Preload

Blood volume and venous tone are two components that determine pressure in the venous system. Although the venous system is a low-pressure system, two-thirds of the circulating blood volume is found in this system, and thus venous return is a major determinant of preload. For this reason, hemorrhage or dehydration can exert a major negative effect on preload and cardiac output.

The pumping action of skeletal leg muscles on deep veins causes the propulsion of blood toward the heart, and as a result, venous pooling normally does not interfere with venous return and adversely affect preload. An exception can occur when a person stands still without moving the legs for long periods. Under these circumstances, the blood pools in the extremities, and an individual suddenly can faint because of a lack of blood flow to the cerebrum as cardiac output falls from a decrease in preload. This example demonstrates the importance of the skeletal pump mechanism in maintaining venous return and preload to preserve adequate cardiac output and blood pressure.

Another component of preload is ventricular compliance. Compliance refers to the distensibility or stiffness of the ventricles. Conditions that contribute to reduced compliance (such as myocardial infarction) result in elevated ventricular filling pressure without a proportionate increase in ventricular filling volume. The stiff ventricle cannot respond to accommodate the increase in blood volume. Conditions in which ventricular compliance increases result in ventricular filling pressure becoming disproportionately decreased relative to significant volume loads. Box 7-1 describes conditions that increase and decrease compliance of the ventricle.

MVO_2 correlates with the diameter of the heart. A twofold increase in the size of the heart results in a twofold increase in MVO_2, thus ventricular hypertrophy or dilatation could have detrimental effects on the ischemia-prone heart.[5] A dilated heart with a large end-diastolic volume must develop more wall tension than a normal-sized heart. To adapt to this demand, the ventricles increase in muscle mass. This process is known as ventricular hypertrophy. Decreasing heart size by reducing the ventricular volume through the use of diuretics or venodilator agents (such as nitroglycerine) decreases MVO_2.

Afterload

Afterload is the tension or force facing ventricular muscle after contraction begins or during the shortening phase of contraction.[1,2,4,5] Afterload reflects the sum of the forces against which the ventricle must act to eject blood. Afterload can be represented as the pressure work of the heart just as preload reflects the volume

Interventricular septum

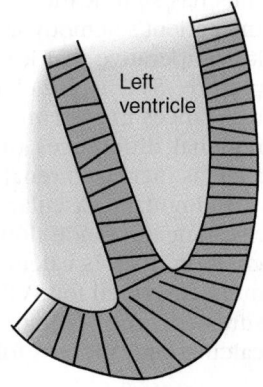

A Normal compliance
End-diastolic volume 120 ml

B Reduced compliance
End-diastolic volume 120 ml

FIGURE 7-10 ■ **A** and **B,** Volume and pressure differences related to compliance. Volume and pressure do not have a definitive relationship. There are times in picture A where volume is increased and pressure is normal. Picture B shows an instance in which volume is increased and pressure also is increased. (From Darovic GO: *Hemodynamic monitoring: invasive and noninvasive clinical application,* ed 3, Philadelphia, 2002, WB Saunders.)

BOX 7-1   ■ ■ ■
FACTORS THAT ALTER VENTRICULAR COMPLIANCE

Decreased Compliance
- Ventricular hypertrophy
- Myocardial fibrosis
- Pericardial tamponade
- Pericardial disease
- Advanced age
- Hypoxia
- Ventricular ischemia
- Acidosis

Increased Compliance
- Ventricular dilatation

Altered Compliance
- Any drug that significantly decreases ventricular diastolic pressure alters ventricular compliance, i.e., nitroglycerin and calcium channel blockers.

Adapted from Darovic GO: *Hemodynamic monitoring: invasive and noninvasive clinical application,* ed 3, Philadelphia, 2002, WB Saunders.

work of the heart. The term *afterload* refers to the work required of the heart after the volume has stabilized in the ventricles. Left ventricular afterload is a function of the ventricle primarily responding to systemic arterial blood pressure through the aortic valve.

Factors Influencing Afterload

Factors that can affect afterload include semilunar valve stenosis, blood viscosity, systemic vascular resistance (**SVR**), and hypertensive conditions. A stenotic valve that has a narrowed opening causes resistance to the ejection of blood from the ventricle. The work effort on the part of the ventricle is substantial in stenosis.

Blood viscosity increases afterload and thus physically can affect stroke volume. Conditions that increase viscosity, such as polycythemia or dehydration, cause an increase in afterload because of the sluggish nature of blood being resistant to ejection movement.

SVR is the resistance to blood flow by means of the force of friction between blood and the walls of the blood vessels. SVR can be determined by looking at the diameter of the blood vessels and applying Poiseuille's law, which determines resistance to blood flow. This law states that the resistance to blood flow increases substantially with reduced blood vessel radius.[3-5] For example, if vasoconstriction decreases the radius of the arterial circulation by one-fourth, the resistance to flow increases by 8 times.

A concept related to SVR is that of the impact of hypertension. When arterial pressures, specifically diastolic pressures are high, the ventricle has to work considerably harder to overcome the diastolic pressures that are on the opposing side of the aortic valve. As afterload increases, the ventricular muscle still needs to respond to eject blood effectively. In a normal resting state of the heart, 90 percent of myocardial oxygen is consumed to create the necessary force or tension in the left ventricle.[6,7] Little myocardial oxygen reserve is left to respond to stress such as that of increased afterload. Interventions to reduce blood pressure decrease afterload and improve ventricular functioning. (See Special Feature Box.)

■ ■ ■ TECHNOLOGY

BLOOD PRESSURE MEASUREMENT

The standard method of measuring a person's blood pressure involves a mercury sphygmomanometer and stethoscope or aneroid and electronic blood pressure cuff. This measurement involves a one-time snapshot of a person's blood pressure in a 24-hour period. This methodology has some intrinsic problems related to the high potential for measurement error from the operator or instrument.

New technological advances in 24-hour ambulatory blood pressure devices are providing important insights into the true nature of blood pressure in the natural environment. A 24-hour ambulatory blood pressure device is worn by an individual with a cuff attached to a monitoring unit that collects blood pressure data over a 24-hour period. The ambulatory blood pressure device can be coupled with another new technological device, the ambulatory impedance monitor. The combination provides valuable hemodynamic data such as heart rate, blood pressure, calculated cardiac output and systemic vascular resistance for a 24-hour period, noninvasively.[8-11]

The aortic blood pressure is essentially equal to left ventricle pressure during the ejection phase of systole, thus afterload generally can be represented by this index. Another clinically significant index for cardiac afterload is SVR. Vascular resistance cannot be measured directly but can be calculated with the following formula that may be applied to systemic or pulmonary circulation:

$$\frac{\dfrac{\text{Mean outflow}}{\text{pressure}} - \dfrac{\text{Mean inflow}}{\text{pressure}}}{\substack{\text{Volume of blood flow in 1 minute} \\ \text{(cardiac output)}}} = \text{Vascular resistance}$$

SVR is the average resistance to blood flow throughout the entire systemic circulation. Clinically, SVR is calculated by subtracting central venous pressure (CVP) as a mean inflow pressure from mean arterial pressure (MAP), which is an outflow pressure measurement. This number is the pressure gradient across the systemic vascular bed and a summation of all pressures in the vasculature. This quantity then is divided by the cardiac output, which represents the rate of flow through the vascular bed. The result then is multiplied by a constant of 80, which is a conversion factor for dyne-sec·cm^{-5}.[4-6] Thus the formula for calculating SVR is as follows:

$$\frac{\text{MAP} - \text{CVP (or right atrial pressure [RAP])}}{\text{Cardiac output}} \times 80 = \text{SVR dyne-sec} \cdot \text{cm}^{-5}$$

Example

$$\frac{95 \text{ mm Hg} - 6 \text{ mm Hg}}{5 \text{ liters/min}} \times 80 = 1424 \text{ dyne-sec} \cdot \text{cm}^{-5}$$

Normal SVR values range from 770 to 1500 dyne-sec·cm^{-5}.[5] When SVR is increasing, it represents generalized vasoconstriction; and reciprocally, when SVR is decreasing, vasodilatation is occurring. The SVR value thus has significance in vasoactive therapy to optimize the patient's hemodynamic status. When analyzing SVR, it is imperative that it is taken in context of the clinical picture. SVR is a global representation of the various resistances in systemic circulation. SVR may not reflect regional differences that can be clinically significant, such as increased renal vascular resistance.

Pulmonary vascular resistance (**PVR**) is the average resistance to blood flow throughout the pulmonary circulation. PVR is calculated by essentially the same formula described for SVR but is translated to reflect pressures in the pulmonary circuit. The formula for calculating PVR is as follows:

$$\frac{\text{Mean pulmonary artery pressure} - \text{PAOP}}{\text{Cardiac output}} \times 80 = \text{SVR dyne-sec} \cdot \text{cm}^{-5}$$

Where

PAOP is pulmonary artery occlusion pressure

The pulmonary arterial circulation is a low-resistance circulation that produces right ventricular afterload. Normal values for PVR range from 20 to 120 dyne-sec·cm^{-5}.[5]

In clinical conditions such as emphysema or pulmonary artery hypertension that increase PVR, the right ventricle must overcome this increased resistance to eject the necessary volume of blood into the pulmonary system and then forward to the left side of the heart.

When the myocardium is damaged, the ventricles do not respond well to changes in afterload. The more significant the ventricular dysfunction, the greater the impact that increased afterload has on the myocardial ability to control stroke volume. In overt heart failure, for example, cardiac output is very afterload dependent such that increases in afterload substantially reduce cardiac output. This is one reason vasopressor therapy to increase blood pressure in cardiogenic shock can have negative consequences on cardiac function. As SVR increases, so does MVO_2. The ability of the heart to adapt to higher afterload is limited with left ventricular dysfunction, and heart failure may worsen with vasoconstriction. Conversely, vasodilatation decreases afterload by decreasing SVR, which often helps optimize ventricular performance.

Contractility

Contractility refers to the ability of the heart to develop maximum muscle shortening velocity regardless of the components of the Frank-Starling mechanism. Contractility is often referred to as the intrinsic ability of the heart to cause a greater magnitude and velocity of shortening and thereby augment stroke volume.

The contractile state of the myocardial muscle is controlled by biochemical and biophysical properties that govern the activation, formation, and cycling of cross bridges between actin and myosin filaments. Contractility reflects the availability of calcium to the myofilaments and the sensitivity of the myofilaments to calcium. Calcium binding to troponin C induces a conformational change in troponin C that causes it to elongate during systole compared with diastole. Troponin I and troponin T migrate closer to troponin C, and the normal inhibitory effect of troponin I and troponin T on actin-tropomyosin is reduced. This repositioning of tropomyosin relative to actin, and the exposure of the actin site to which a myosin head can attach, allows the cross-bridging cycle to begin.[2,6,7]

Factors Influencing Contractility

Myocardial contractility can be affected by various biochemical processes that can change the inotropic state of the heart, increasing cardiac output and tissue perfusion. A positive inotropic stimulus produces a ventricular function curve that improves ventricular performance significantly for any given preload volume. Examples of a positive inotropic effect include epinephrine and norepinephrine released from cardiac sympathetic nerves into the circulation, increased heart rate (i.e., the treppe effect), or pharmacological effects as with digoxin. Negative inotropic stimuli reduce contractility even with increases in preload (Figure 7-11). Negative inotropic stimuli include reduction of high-energy phosphate availability, reduced sensitivity of contractile proteins to calcium as in acidotic states, or generation of lactate because of reduction of oxygen availabil-

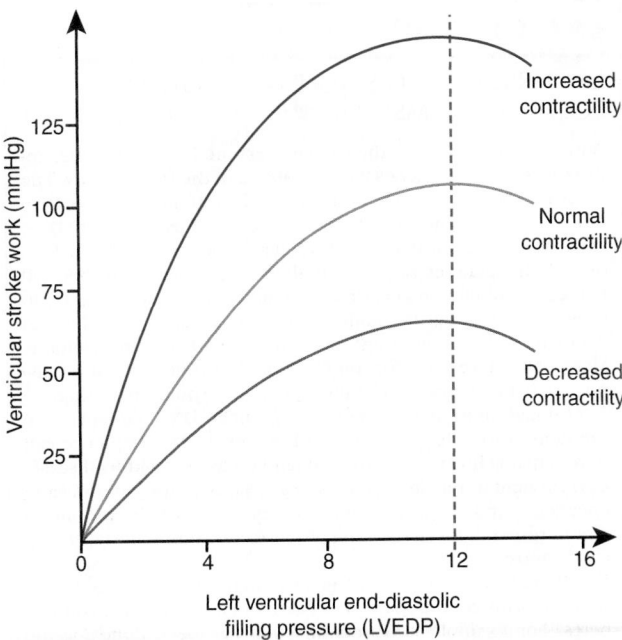

FIGURE 7-11 ■ Effects of contractility on ventricular function curve. (From Michaelson CR: *Congestive heart failure,* St Louis, 1983, Mosby.)

BOX 7-2   ■ ■ ■
CONTRACTILITY CONDITIONS AFFECTING THE HEART

Decreased Contractility
- Parasympathetic stimulation
- Negative inotropic drug therapy
  - Beta blockers
- Metabolic states
  - Hyperkalemia
  - Myocardial ischemia/infarct
  - Acidosis

Increased Contractility
- Sympathetic stimulation
- Positive inotropic drug therapy:
  - Epinephrine
  - Dopamine (moderate/high doses)
  - Digoxin
  - Calcium
- Metabolic state:
  - Hypercalcemia

---

ity.[2,4,6,7] Box 7-2 describes the various factors leading to negative and positive inotropic conditions.

EXTRINSIC REGULATION OF THE HEART
Autonomic Control of Contractility

Although the heart is regulated intrinsically via hemodynamic and mechanical mechanisms, it also is regulated extrinsically via autonomic innervation, with subsequent autonomic control of contractility and blood pressure regulation. The autonomic nervous system is composed of two branches, the sympathetic branch and parasympathetic branch. Sympathetic stimulation increases the activity of the heart by increasing the heart rate and the force of contraction. This sympathetic response is mediated by the release of the neurotransmitter norepinephrine and its subsequent binding to the beta-adrenergic receptor, more specifically the beta[1]

UNDERSTANDING SINGLE NUCLEOTIDE POLYMORPHISMS

With the completion of the Human Genome Project in 2002, approximately 39,000 genes were identified in the human body. The focus of researchers now has turned to identifying single nucleotide polymorphisms, or SNPs, pronounced "snips." SNPs are DNA sequence variations that occur when a single nucleotide (A, T, C, or G) in the genome sequence is altered. SNPs make up about 90 percent of all human genetic variation, and they occur every 100 to 300 bases along the 3-billion-base human genome. SNPs can occur in coding (gene) and noncoding regions of the genome. Many SNPs have no effect on function, but others could predispose persons to disease or influence their response to a drug.

Although more than 99 percent of human DNA sequences are the same across the population, variations in DNA sequence can have a major impact on how human beings respond to disease; environmental insults such as bacteria, viruses, toxins, and chemicals; and drugs and other therapies. Thus SNPs are important in research for developing pharmaceutical products or medical diagnostics.

SNP maps may help in the identification of multiple genes associated with conditions such as cardiovascular disease and diabetes. For example, SNP identification has been done for the beta-adrenergic receptor. Some the more prevalent and common SNPs of the beta$_2$ receptor located in the vasculature include the polymorphism located at codon of the 16th and 27th amino acid. This polymorphism results in beta-adrenergic receptor desensitization that can produce hypertension.[12,13]

receptors. The beta$_1$ receptors are responsible for the increase in rate and force of contraction. Stimulation of the parasympathetic nervous system results in a slowing of the heart rate and a decrease in the force of contraction. The parasympathetic response is mediated by the release of acetylcholine and its binding with M$_2$ muscarinic receptors.

Sympathetic Control

The sympathetic vasomotor nerves leave the spinal cord through the thoracic vertebrae and the first two lumbar spinal nerves. They pass immediately into a sympathetic chair, one of which lies on each side of the vertebral column[7] (see Figure 7-7 and Figure 7-12). They then pass by two routes to the circulation—one through sympathetic nerves that innervate mainly the vasculature of the heart and internal viscera, and into peripheral portions of the spinal nerves and are distributed to the vasculature of the peripheral area such as blood vessels.[7]

Strong sympathetic stimulation can increase the heart rate in young adults from a resting rate of 70 beats/min up to 180 beats/min and even as high as 250 beats/min. Sympathetic stimulation increases the force of contraction, thereby increasing cardiac output, which results in an increase in blood pressure[6] (see Figure 7-6).

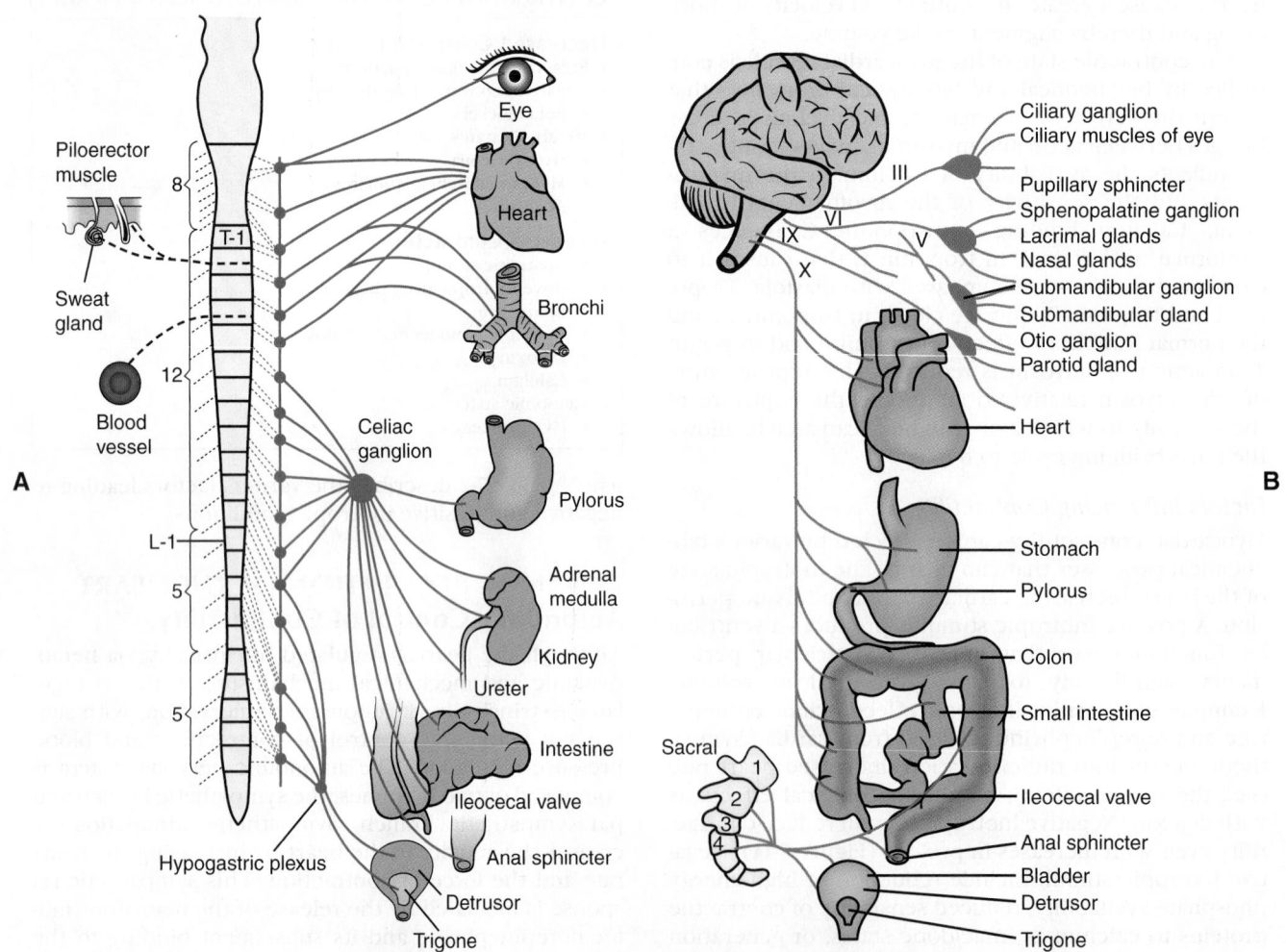

FIGURE 7-12 ■ Sympathetic (**A**) and parasympathetic (**B**) nervous system. (From Guyton A, Hall J: *Textbook of medical physiology*, ed 11, Philadelphia, 2006, WB Saunders.)

Activation of Beta₁ Receptors

Signal transduction in the sympathetic nervous system is initiated when the naturally occurring catecholamine norepinephrine agonist binds to the cardiac beta receptors, specifically the beta₁ receptor subtype. Activation of the beta₁ receptor then activates the intracellular G protein and the adenylate cyclase system.[2]

Adenylate cyclase is a transmembrane enzyme system also referred to as adenylyl or adenyl cylase that responds to input from G proteins. Gs is the stimulatory protein complex that passes the signal from the beta receptor to adenylate cyclase (Figure 7-13). Adenylate cyclase, stimulated by Gs, produces the second messenger cyclic AMP, which then acts through an additional series of signals via another messenger, protein kinase A, to increase cytosolic calcium.[2] The hypothesized sequence of events describing the positive inotropic effects of catecholamines is as follows. Catecholamine binds to beta₁ receptors and the receptor is activated. G protein stimulates adenylate cyclase with formation of cyclic AMP with activation of cyclic AMP–dependent protein kinase and phosphorylation of sarcolemmani protein 27. The consequence is increased entry of calcium through voltage-dependent L-type calcium channels, greater calcium-induced calcium release via ryano-dine receptors with increased calcium-troponin C interaction and deinhibition of tropomyosin effect on actin-myosin interaction. The end result is an increased rate and number of cross bridges resulting in increased rate and peak of force development.[2]

Endothelial Control of Circulation

Endothelial cells, or endothelium, line the blood vessels of the body. These cells together weigh about 1 kg of a 70-kg person. Endothelial cells are arranged in a single layer (monolayer) with the edges of one cell touching the edges of the cells surrounding it without overlap. This monolayer of endothelium begins in the heart, surrounds the endocardium, travels down through the aorta, the arteries, and into the capillaries where the vasculature itself is only composed of this single endothelial layer, then back through the venous system and into the right atrium. Researchers now are learning that this single layer of cells is important to the functioning of the body, especially regarding the regulation of blood pressure.[14-16]

Endothelium is not inert; it is metabolically active, as described in chapter 9. The endothelium produces, releases, and generates vasoactive substances. The endothelium is analogous to an input/output device that

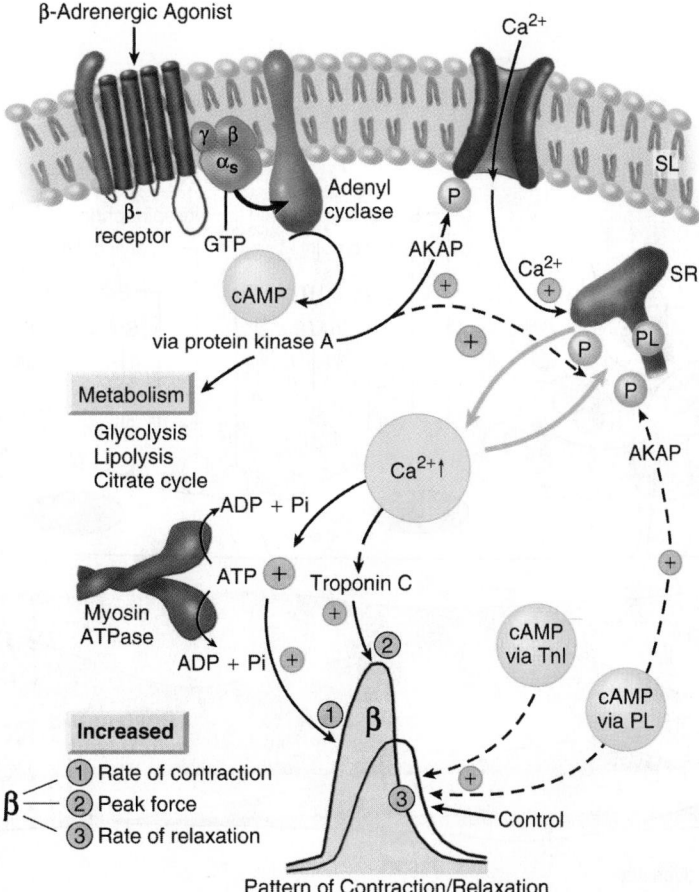

FIGURE 7-13 ■ Signal systems involved in positive inotropic and lusitropic (enhanced relaxation) effects of beta-adrenergic stimulation. *ADP,* Adenosine diphosphate; *AKAP,* A-kinase anchoring protein; *cAMP,* cyclic adenosine monophosphate; *GTP,* guanosine triphosphate; *P,* phosphorylation; *Pi,* inorganic phosphate; *PL,* phospholamban; *SR,* sarcoplasmic reticulum; *TnI,* treponin I. (From Zipes DP, Libby P, Bonow RO, Braunwald E, editors: *Heart disease: a textbook of cardiovascular medicine,* ed 7, Philadelphia, 2005, WB Saunders.)

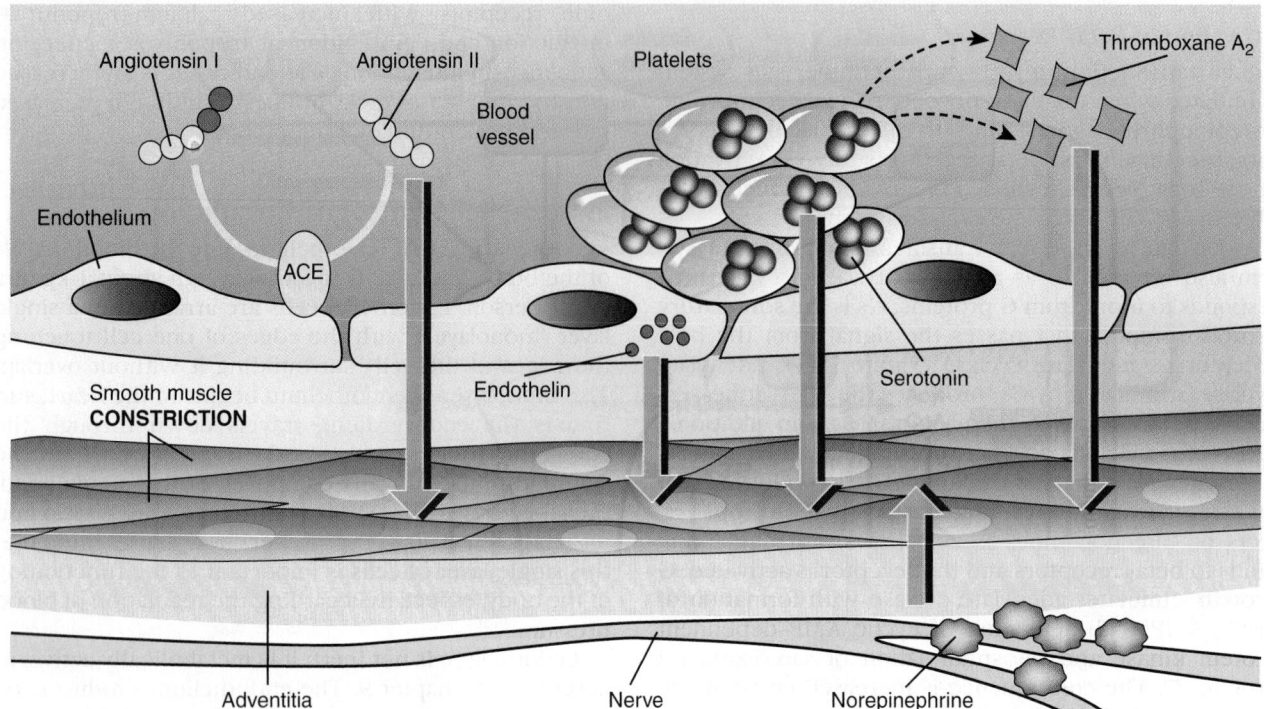

FIGURE 7-14 ■ The endothelium regulates vasomotion (constriction and dilatation) and platelet aggregation by releasing a variety of constricting and dilating substances. *ACE,* Angiotensin-converting enzyme. (From Huether S, McCance K: *Understanding pathophysiology,* ed 3, St Louis, 2004, Mosby.)

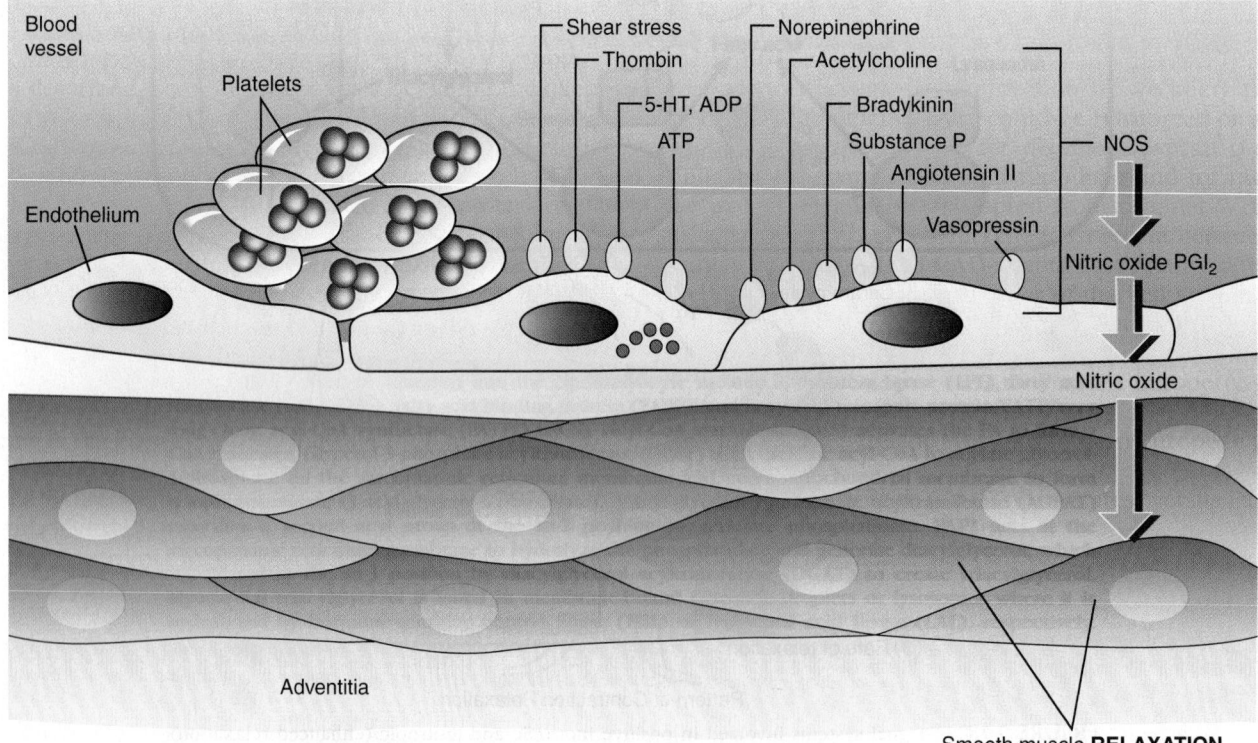

FIGURE 7-15 ■ Factors causing endothelium-dependent vasodilatation. *ADP,* Adenosine diphosphate; *ATP,* adenosine triphosphate; *NOS,* nitric oxide synthetase. (From Huether S, McCance K: *Understanding pathophysiology,* ed 3, St Louis, 2004, Mosby.)

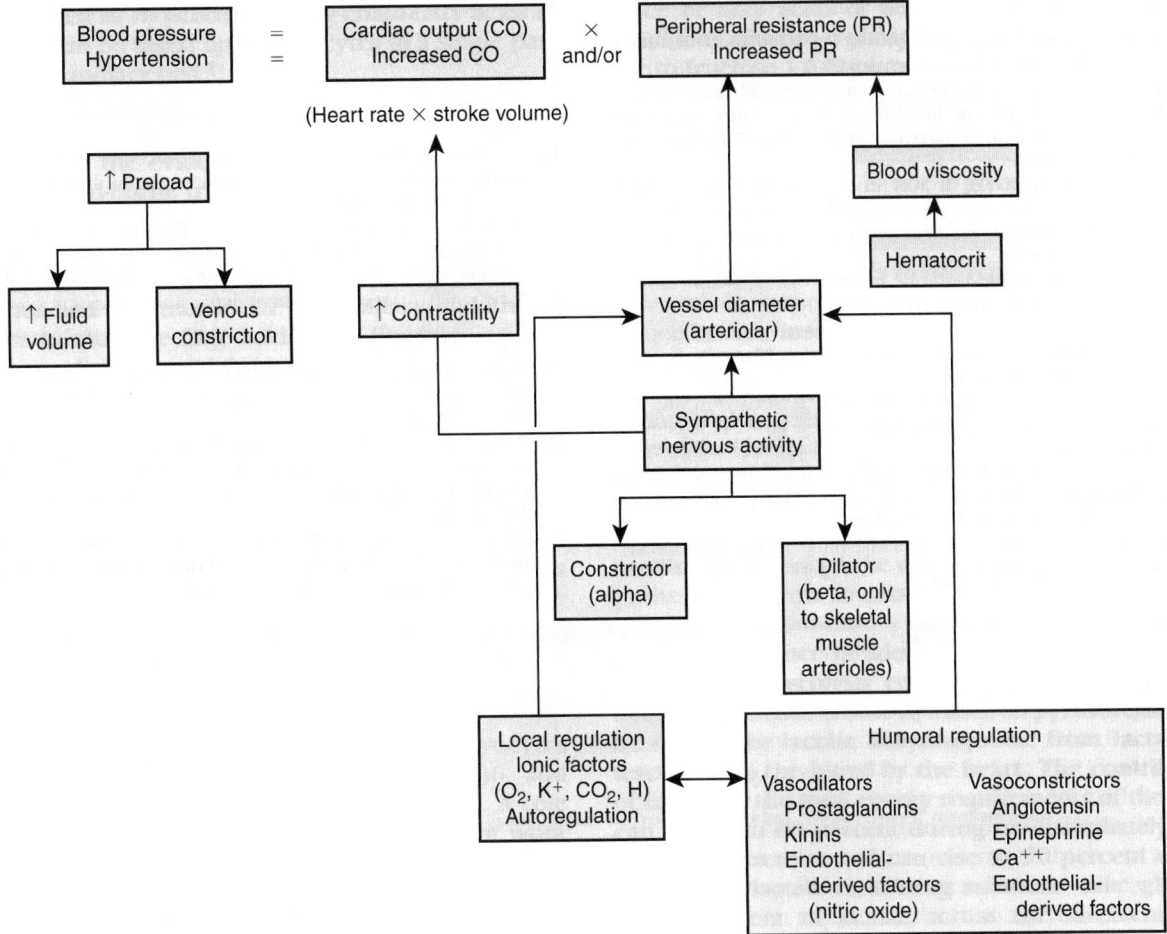

FIGURE 7-16 ■ Factors regulating blood pressure. (From Huether S, McCance K: *Understanding pathophysiology*, ed 3, St Louis, 2004, Mosby.)

senses changes in the vessel lumen and in the vascular smooth muscle and responds accordingly. Endothelial cells interact with a host of factors such as platelets, leukocytes, cytokines, coagulation factors, macrophages, and other circulating mediators. Smooth muscles beneath the endothelium also induce the release of biological mediators from the endothelium. Endothelial cells release not only nitric oxide but also a host of other agents in response to their environment (Figures 7-14 and 7-15).

Normally, vessels are in a homeostatic, anticoagulant, profibrinolytic, platelet inhibitory, and vasodilatory state produced by the generation and release of nitric oxide, the anticoagulant thrombomodulin, and profibrinolytic tissue plasminogen activator. Norepinephrine, acetylcholine, bradykinins, substance P, and serotonin have receptors on endothelium that induce relaxation[14-17] (see Figures 7-14 and 7-15).

The functional vasculature endothelium can shift or be activated to a dysfunctional endothelium. Dysfunctional endothelium switches the vascular milieu to a procoagulant, antifibrinolytic, platelet-activating, and vasoconstrictive state by the generation and release of endothelin, thromboxane A$_2$, and increased conversion of angiotensin I by angiotensin-converting enzyme lo-

cated on the surface of the endothelial cells to angiotensin II, a potent vasoconstrictor. The dysfunctional endothelium also produces the procoagulant, tissue factor. The dyfunctional endothelium and fibrin have binding sites for various circulating coagulation factors and adhesion molecules. The dysfunctional endothelium also begins to generate additional antifibrinolytic mediators such as plasminogen activator inhibitor, as well as platelet activators such as von Willenbrand factor and platelet activating factor.[14-17] (See Figures 7-14 and 7-15 and Chapters 9 and 10.)

SUMMARY

Blood pressure and caloric output are determined by the interplay of the heart rate and volume (Figure 7-16).[17] Blood pressure also is affected by alterations in the autonomic nervous system and beta receptor sensitivity. Blood pressure may be affected by changes in peripheral resistance in the microcirculation, specifically via the endothelial-generated release of a host of vasoactive mediators. The cooperative interplay of all these systems is necessary to maintain tissue perfusion through the microcirculation and ultimately tissue physiological homeostasis.

REFERENCES

1. Porth CM: *Essentials of pathophysiology,* Philadelphia, 2004, Lippincott Williams & Wilkins.
2. Opie LH: Mechanism of cardiac contraction and relaxation. In Zipes DP, Libby P, Bonow RO, Braunwald E, editors: *Heart disease: a textbook of cardiovascular medicine,* ed 7, Philadelphia, 2005, WB Saunders.
3. Kinney MR, Dunbar SB, Brooks-Brunn JA et al: *AACN clinical reference for critical care nursing,* ed 4, St Louis, 1998, Mosby.
4. Johnson LR: *Essential medical physiology,* Boston, 2003, Elsevier Academic Press.
5. Darovic GO: *Hemodynamic monitoring: invasive and noninvasive clinical application,* ed 3, Philadelphia, 2002, WB Saunders.
6. Davies A, Blakeley A, Kidd C: *Human physiology,* New York, 2001, Churchill Livingstone.
7. Guyton AC, Hall JE: Cardiovascular system. In Guyton AC, Hall JE, editors: *Textbook of medical physiology,* ed 11, Philadelphia, 2006, WB Saunders.
8. Sherwood A, Hughes JW, McFetridge J: Ethnic differences in the hemodynamic mechanisms of ambulatory blood pressure regulation, *Am J Hypertens* 16:270-273, 2003.
9. McFetridge JA, Sherwood A: Hemodynamic and sympathetic nervous system responses to stress during the menstrual cycle, *AACN Clin Issues* 11:158-167, 2000.
10. McFetridge JA, Sherwood A: Impedance cardiology for noninvasive measurement of cardiovascular hemodynamics, *Nurs Res* 48:109-113, 1999.
11. Sherwood A, McFetridge J, Hutcheson JS: Ambulatory impedance cardiography: a feasibility study, *J Appl Physiol* 85:2365-2369, 1998.
12. Johnson JA, Terra SG: β-adrenergic receptor polymorphisms: cardiovascular disease associations and pharmacogenetics, *Pharm Res* 19:1779-1787, 2002.
13. Dishy V, Sofowora GG, Xie HG et al: The effect of common polymorphisms of the beta2-adrenergic receptor on agonist-mediated vascular desensitization, *N Engl J Med* 345:1030-1035, 2001.
14. McHugh JC, Cheek DJ: Nitric oxide and regulation of vascular tone: pharmacological and physiologic considerations, *Am J Crit Care* 7:131-140, 1998.
15. Oxhorn B, Cheek DJ, Buxton ILO: Role of nucleotides and nucleosides in the regulation of cardiac blood flow, *AACN Clin Issues* 11:241-251, 2000.
16. Buxton ILO, Kaiser RA, Oxhorn BC et al: Evidence supporting the nucleotide axis hypothesis: ATP release and metabolism by coronary endothelium, *Am J Physiol Heart Circ Physiol* 281:1657-1666, 2001.
17. Huether SE, McCance KL: Alteration in cardiovascular function. In Huether SE, McCance KL, editors: *Understanding pathophysiology,* ed 2, St Louis, 2000, Mosby.

Pulmonary Circulation

Susan K. Frazier

The respiratory system functions to provide a regular supply of oxygen for cellular metabolism and cyclical removal of carbon dioxide. Normal respiratory system function requires ventilation or the movement of gas in and out of the lungs, regulation of ventilation, diffusion of gases at the alveolar capillary membrane (external respiration) and the cellular level (internal respiration), and perfusion for transport of gases to and from the alveolar capillary membrane. This chapter focuses on bronchial and pulmonary circulation and pulmonary perfusion.

PULMONARY AND BRONCHIAL CIRCULATION

The pulmonary system is different from most other body systems because it has a dual circulation. The lungs receive blood flow through the bronchial and pulmonary circulations. Both vascular circuits are required for normal pulmonary function, but they differ in structure and function.

Bronchial Circulation

The function of the bronchial circulation is to deliver oxygen and nutrients to the airways (down to the terminal bronchioles), the visceral pleura, the outer adventitial layer of larger pulmonary blood vessels, pulmonary sympathetic ganglia, and hilar lymph nodes (Figure 8-1). Bronchial blood flow totals only about 1 to 2 percent of total cardiac output, as little as 50 to 100 ml of blood per minute. Bronchial arterial vessels arise from the thoracic aorta and are similar in structure to other systemic arteries. Compared with pulmonary vessels, bronchial vessels have more smooth muscle and thicker walls. The bronchial circulation is a low-compliance, high-resistance system with pressures similar to aortic pressure.

Once oxygenated blood is delivered to lung structures, deoxygenated or venous blood drains into the bronchial veins. Deoxygenated blood from the bronchial veins flows into the pulmonary veins and the azygous veins. The azygous veins are one component of the systemic venous system and empty into the right atrium, whereas blood from the pulmonary veins flows into the left atrium. This small volume of deoxygenated bronchial venous blood and another small volume from the coronary veins is termed a venous admixture. The addition of this small volume of blood accounts for the slightly greater output of the left ventricle compared with the right ventricle.

The presence of chronic infection and inflammatory lung diseases produces significant hypertrophy of the bronchial circulation. In addition, pulmonary neoplasms and granulomas receive blood flow from this circuit. With chronic pulmonary pathological conditions, connections or anastamoses form between the bronchial and pulmonary circulations, and up to 30 percent of cardiac output may be shunted through the bronchial circulation.[1] Hypoxemia results because this blood bypasses the alveolar capillary membrane and the volume of venous admixture significantly increases. Hemoptysis and serious hemorrhage may be produced with bronchial vessel disruption because the pressure in this system is similar to systemic pressure.

Pulmonary Circulation

The function of the pulmonary circuit is to deliver deoxygenated blood to the alveolar capillary membrane for gas diffusion. This high-compliance, low-pressure circuit of vessels receives the entire output of the right ventricle (Figure 8-2). The main pulmonary artery extends only 5 cm from the right ventricle before dividing into the right and left pulmonary arteries. Normally, the walls of these large arteries are structurally different from systemic arteries of the same caliber with primarily elastic fibers and little smooth muscle. The walls of large pulmonary vessels are composed of eight elastic layers and are ideal for accommodation of larger blood volumes without significant increases in pressure. The vessel media of the larger arteries contains only a thin layer of smooth muscle, but the amount of smooth muscle increases in the smaller pulmonary arterioles, particularly those between 100 and 200 μm in diameter. The pulmonary vessels continue to branch into smaller and smaller vessels until they form approximately 100 billion pulmonary capillaries. These capillaries are approximately 12 μm in length and 7 to 8 μm in diameter and surround alveoli in sheets.

The smooth muscle in the thin-walled pulmonary arteries inserts into short elastic fibers, which allows the vessel to distend easily and accommodate changes in right ventricular cardiac output. The compliance of the main pulmonary vessels is only 1 mm Hg increase for each 2-ml increase in blood volume.[1,2] The global pulmonary compliance is approximately 30 ml/1 mm

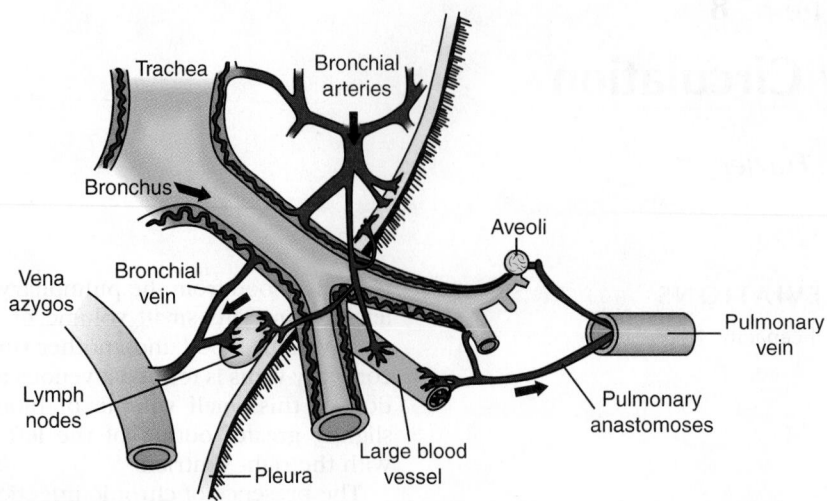

FIGURE 8-1 ■ Bronchial circulation provides oxygen and nutrients to airways (down to terminal bronchioles), the visceral pleura, hilar lymph nodes, and outer adventitial layer of large blood vessels.

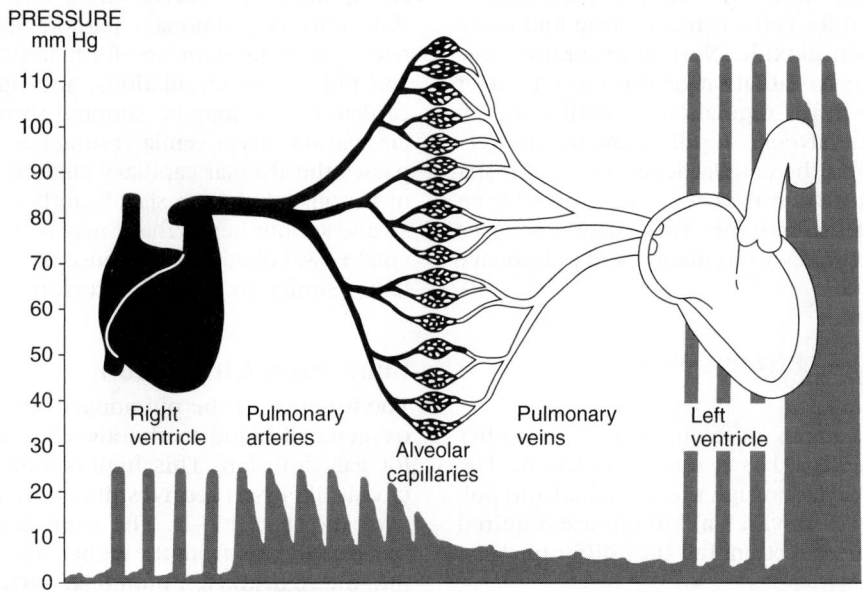

FIGURE 8-2 ■ Pulmonary circulation. (From Darovic G: *Hemodynamic monitoring: invasive and noninvasive clinical application,* ed 3, St Louis, 2002, Saunders.)

Hg pressure, so large changes in volume are not accompanied by large changes in pressure. Pulmonary vessel compliance varies during the ventilatory cycle.[3]

The greatest degree of pulmonary vessel compliance is found at end-inspiration; the least compliance is found at end-expiration. This compliance is due to shifts of blood volume between alveolar and extraalveolar blood vessels with the ventilatory cycle. Alveolar vessels are those that are located around the alveoli and are exposed directly to varying alveolar distention and pressure. Extraalveolar vessels are located in lung parenchyma outside of the alveolar wall, and they are surrounded by elastic connective tissue. As the thoracic cavity expands or reduces in size with ventilation, the elastic tissue stretches or recoils and exerts an influence on these extraalveolar vessels. At end-inspiration, alveolar vessels are compressed by inflated alveoli, radial traction increases extraalveolar vessel diameter, and

blood is shifted to extraalveolar vessels. Thus, pulmonary arterial compliance is increased. At end-expiration, elastic recoil has reduced the diameter of extraalveolar vessels, alveoli have deflated, and blood is propelled into alveolar vessels for gas exchange. Pulmonary arterial compliance then is reduced.

PULMONARY BLOOD VOLUME, PRESSURE, AND VASCULAR RESISTANCE

The pulmonary circulation contains approximately 10 percent of total blood volume or about 500 ml.[1] This volume is distributed about equally between the arteries, veins, and microcirculation. The pulmonary circulation is designed to receive deoxygenated blood from the right ventricle and to distribute this volume continuously to the microcirculation for gas exchange purposes. Right ventricular work and oxygen consumption are significantly lower than left because of the high compliance, low pressure, and low resistance in this circuit. This is ideal for the small-muscled right ventricle that must only generate enough pressure to deliver blood to the apices of the lungs. Significant increases in volume normally are not accompanied by increases in pressure because the vessels are able to distend and accommodate more volume (compliance). Additionally, under normal conditions, a number of pulmonary microvessels are closed or open, but without blood flow, and a small increase in vascular pressure recruits these vessels.

Mean blood pressure in the pulmonary circulation is only about 15 mm Hg. Pulmonary systolic pressure is approximately 25 mm Hg and the diastolic, 10 mm Hg. Low pulmonary pressures are primarily due to low pulmonary vascular resistance (20 to 120 dynes-sec·cm^{-5} or 0.25 to 1.7 R units).[1,4] The vascular resistance of the pulmonary circuit is only about one-tenth to one-twelfth of the systemic circulation or approximately 1.5 mm Hg/liter/min in a normal adult. Active and passive mechanisms alter pulmonary vascular resistance and influence pulmonary blood flow (Box 8-1). Under normal conditions, pulmonary blood flow is dominated primarily by passive mechanisms.

Passive mechanisms produce changes in pulmonary vascular tone because of a mechanical influence on vessel caliber. These mechanisms include changes in pulmonary artery pressure, blood volume, left atrial pressure, lung volume, and blood viscosity. As pulmonary blood volume and pulmonary vessel pressures increase, vascular resistance decreases. Because of the degree of pulmonary vessel compliance, right ventricular cardiac output must increase by 2.5 times before any change in pressure is detected.[2] Ordinarily, an increase in right ventricular output results in the recruitment of underperfused vessels and distention of perfused vessels, so resistance to blood flow decreases.

An increase in left atrial pressure also decreases vascular resistance. The pressure in the pulmonary circuit must remain higher than that in the left atrium to establish a pressure gradient for forward flow of blood. An increase in left atrial pressure without a concomitant increase in pulmonary pressure produces distention of pulmonary vessels, which reduces vascular resistance. However, vessel distention may increase capillary hydrostatic pressure sufficiently to produce movement of fluid into the interstitium.

Blood viscosity is the internal friction produced by fluid molecules in response to a change in form or relative position. Blood viscosity is associated directly with hematocrit. With a hematocrit of 40 to 45 percent, blood viscosity is nearly 4 times greater than that of water. According to Poiseuille's law (i.e., flow rate, Q, is dependent on fluid viscosity, η = viscosity, pipe length, L, and the pressure difference between the ends, ΔP, thus $Q = \pi R^4 \Delta P/8\eta L$), as hematocrit and blood viscosity increase, resistance to blood flow increases, and for every 1 percent increase in hematocrit, pulmonary vascular resistance increases by 4 percent.[5]

Lung volume passively influences vascular resistance. Ordinarily, the relationship between resistance and volume is U-shaped, with vascular resistance lowest at functional residual capacity (Figure 8-3).[5] As lung volume increases, radial traction on the extraalveolar vessels increases vessel caliber, and alveolar vessels are compressed and resistance increases. Because the alveolar and extraalveolar vessels are located in series, the total resistance is the sum of these two resistances, and total vascular resistance increases. At lung volumes less than functional residual capacity, radial traction on extraalveolar vessels is significantly reduced, as is vessel diameter, whereas alveolar vessels have a greater diameter. Again the total resistance increases. In areas with atelectasis and loss of lung volume, vascular resistance is increased passively due to tissue recoil and collapse. In this situation, there are also active mechanisms that influence vascular resistance.

Active mechanisms that influence pulmonary vascular resistance acutely alter the diameter of pulmonary vessels and include autonomic tone, hypoxia, acidosis, and release of several vasoactive molecules from the endothelial layer or from platelets.[1] Normally, the effect of the autonomic nervous system on pulmonary vascular tone is minimal. Sympathetic stimulation slightly in-

---

BOX 8-1
FACTORS THAT INFLUENCE PULMONARY
VASCULAR RESISTANCE

- Acidosis
- Autonomic tone
- Endothelial and platelet-derived vasoactive substances
- Hematocrit/viscosity of blood
- Hypoxemia
- Left atrial pressure
- Lung volume
- Vascular pressure

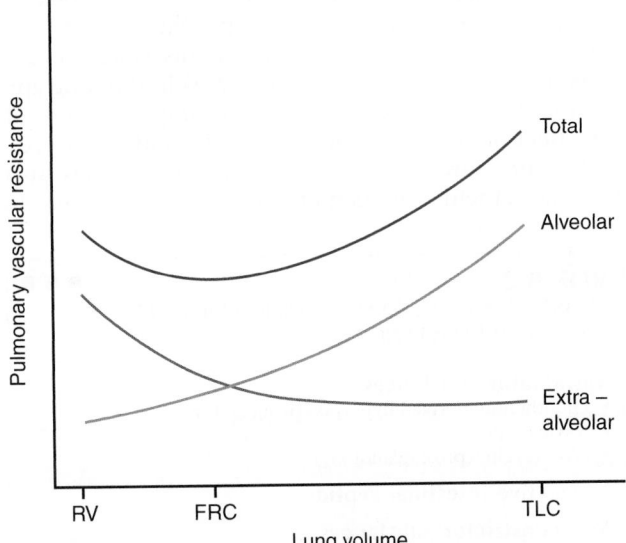

FIGURE 8-3 ■ Effect of changes in lung volume on pulmonary vascular resistance. *FRC,* Functional residual capacity; *RV,* residual volume; *TLC,* total lung capacity. (From Taylor AE, Rehder K, Hyatt R, Parker JC: *Clinical respiratory physiology,* Philadelphia, 1989, Saunders.)

creases vasoconstriction and resistance, whereas parasympathetic stimulation produces slight vasodilatation and decreased resistance. Other active mechanisms have a much greater influence on vascular resistance.

Hypoxia is the most important influence on vascular tone in pulmonary vessels. Hypoxia in adjacent alveoli inhibits one or more voltage-gated potassium channels located in the small pulmonary arteries.[6-9] The result is membrane depolarization and opening of voltage-dependent calcium channels. Intracellular calcium rises and produces smooth muscle contraction and vasoconstriction called hypoxic pulmonary vasoconstriction. The intent of this mechanism is appropriate matching of perfusion with ventilation. Hypercapnia and subsequent acidosis often occur concurrently with hypoxia. Hypercapnia produces acidosis, and pulmonary vascular resistance increases by 50 percent for each 0.1 pH decrease below 7.35.[2,4] A significant synergistic effect occurs when hypoxia and hypercapnia/acidosis are present. The hypoxic pulmonary vasoconstriction response is 3 times more potent in the presence of alveolar hypoxia and a pH reduction by 0.1 to 0.2 units.[2] A number of substances also are produced by pulmonary endothelial cells that influence the degree of smooth muscle contraction and thus pulmonary vascular resistance (Box 8-2). These substances are produced primarily by the pulmonary endothelium; however, some are produced and released by platelets.

DISTRIBUTION OF PULMONARY BLOOD FLOW

The distribution of pulmonary blood flow is influenced by gravity, the pressure surrounding the vessels, and the degree of pulmonary vascular resistance. In an upright individual, blood flow decreases in a linear fashion from lung base to lung apex. The primary reason is the effect of gravity on hydrostatic pressure. The difference between the vascular pressure measured at the apex of the lung to that at the lung base is approximately 23 mm Hg.[5] Because the mean pressure of this system is approximately 15 mm Hg, there are areas in the lung apices that will not receive blood flow simply because of the effect of gravity on the blood hydrostatic pressure.

The pressure surrounding pulmonary vessels also influences the distribution of pulmonary blood flow. As alveolar pressure increases, vessels may be compressed and blood volume moved to other areas of the pulmonary vasculature. West[5] and West and others[10] described the factors that influence pulmonary blood flow distribution and determined that these factors produce differential distribution of blood flow in the lung because of changes in the gradient for blood flow. These are described as zones (Figure 8-4).

Zone 1: No-Flow Zone

The no-flow zone may be found in the uppermost portion of the lung. In this area, alveolar pressure is higher than pulmonary arterial and venous pressure. For example, the mean arterial pressure may be 5 mm Hg because of hydrostatic effects, and the average venous pressure is 5 mm Hg. Alveolar pressure may be 7 mm Hg in certain situations. The high alveolar pressure compresses vessels, and blood flow is obliterated. Because gas exchange cannot occur in this situation, this is alveolar dead space. This type of zone is not common in the normal lung. However, this situation may occur with significant hyperinflation or with high alveolar pressures developed because of the application of positive pressure ventilation, particularly with the application of positive end-expiratory pressure or with a reduction in pulmonary vascular pressure seen with any type of shock state.

Zone 2: Intermittent-Flow Zone

In the intermittent-flow zone, arterial pressure is greater than alveolar pressure. However, alveolar pressure is still greater than venous pressure. Flow only occurs in these vessels during systole because alveolar pressure collapses these vessels during diastole. Blood flow in this zone is determined by the arterial alveolar pressure gradient, and the venous pressure has no effect. This area may be considered underperfused. This zone has been likened to a waterfall where the height of a waterfall has no effect on the flow of water, and the top of the waterfall is not influenced at all by the situation at the

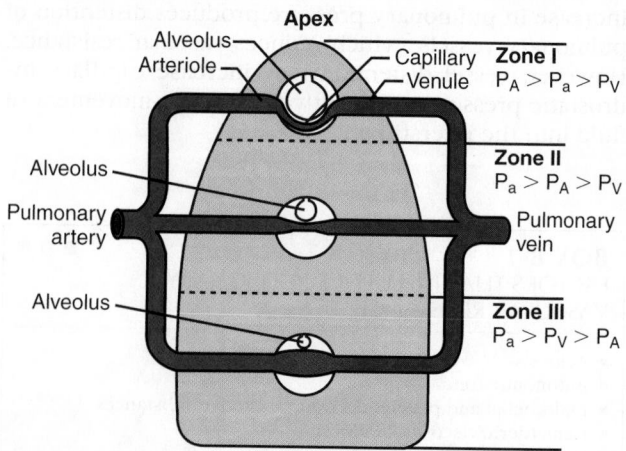

FIGURE 8-4 ■ West's lung zones demonstrating the relationship between alveolar (P$_A$), arterial (P$_a$), and venous pressure (P$_V$). (From McCance K, Huether S: *Pathophysiology: the biologic basis for disease in adults and children*, ed 4, St Louis, 2002, Mosby.)

bottom. This type of perfusion zone can be produced by any situation that increases alveolar pressure (positive pressure ventilation, hyperventilation). Hypovolemia also may increase this type of perfusion, and volume loading, or volume resuscitation in this instance, reduces this type of flow zone.

Zone 3: Continuous Blood Flow

In the dependent portions of the lung, arterial and venous pressures are greater than alveolar pressure. Thus, the typical arterial venous pressure gradient is responsible for blood flow. Vessels in this zone remain open continuously. Normally, two-thirds of the lung exhibits zone 3 blood flow. Vascular resistance is low because of distention of vessels in this zone, and this is the area with greatest blood flow.

METABOLIC FUNCTION OF PULMONARY CIRCULATION

The pulmonary vasculature is uniquely suited for metabolic activity because only the lungs and heart receive the entire blood volume.[5] A number of substances are converted, metabolized, inactivated, and removed as blood passes through pulmonary vessels. Angiotensin I is cleaved by angiotensin-converting enzyme produced by pulmonary endothelium. Angiotensin II is one product of this enzymatic action. Concurrently, bradykinin is almost totally inactivated by angiotensin-converting enzyme. Serotonin also is inactivated in pulmonary vessels, but rather than enzymatic breakdown, serotonin is taken up by the endothelium and stored. Some serotonin possibly is transferred to platelets, and some of the stored serotonin is released during anaphylaxis. Prostaglandin E_2 and $F_{2\alpha}$ are substances that are removed completely as blood passes through the pulmonary vessels. Histamine, dopamine, angiotensin II, prostaglandin A_2 and vasopressin pass through the pulmonary circulation unchanged.

SUMMARY

The pulmonary vascular system has a dual circulation that provides oxygen to the conducting airways and pulmonary parenchyma (bronchial circulation), as well as to the alveolar capillary membrane for gas exchange (pulmonary circulation). The pulmonary circulation is a low-pressure, low-resistance circuit that contains about 10 percent of total blood volume at any point in time. Pulmonary blood volume, vessel pressure, and vascular resistance are influenced by passive and active mechanisms.

Pulmonary blood volume is distributed differentially in pulmonary vessels. The primary influences of this distribution are gravity, the pressure surrounding the vessels, and the degree of pulmonary vascular resistance. The differential distribution of pulmonary blood flow is described as zones (zone 1, no flow; zone 2, intermittent flow; zone 3, continuous flow) and is determined by the relationship between these factors and their influence on the pressure gradient for forward flow. The pulmonary circulation also has an important metabolic function. A number of vasoactive substances are converted, metabolized, inactivated, and/or removed as they pass through the pulmonary circuit. The pulmonary circulation is uniquely suited for this role because it receives and transports the entire blood volume.

REFERENCES

1. Ali J, Summer W, Levitzky M: *Pulmonary pathophysiology,* New York, 2005, Lange.
2. MacNee W: Pathophysiology of cor pulmonale in chronic obstructive pulmonary disease, *Am J Respir Crit Care Med* 150: 1158-1168, 1994.
3. Grant B, Lieber B: Compliance of the main pulmonary artery during the ventilatory cycle, *J Appl Physiol* 72:535-542, 1992.
4. Darovic GO: *Hemodynamic monitoring: invasive and noninvasive clinical application,* ed 3, Philadelphia, 2002, Saunders.
5. West JB: *Pulmonary physiology and pathophysiology: an integrated, case-based approach,* Philadelphia, 2001, Lippincott Williams & Wilkins.
6. Humbert M, Morrell NW, Archer SL et al: Cellular and molecular pathobiology of pulmonary arterial hypertension, *J Am Coll Cardiol* 43:13S-24S, 2004.
7. Sweeney M, Yuan JX: Hypoxic pulmonary vasoconstriction: role of voltage-gated potassium channels, *Respir Res* 1:40-48, 2000.
8. Platoshyn O, Remillard CV, Fantozzi I et al: Diversity of voltage-dependent K+ channels in human pulmonary artery smooth muscle cells, *Am J Physiol Lung Cell Mol Physiol* 287:L226-L238, 2004.
9. Lopez-Barneo J, del Toro R, Konstantin L et al: Regulation of oxygen sensing by ion channels, *J Appl Physiol* 96:1187-1195, 2004.
10. West JB, Dollery CT, Naimark A: Distribution of blood flow in isolated lung: relations to vascular and alveolar pressures, *J Appl Physiol* 19:713, 1964.

chapter 9

Inflammation

Mohannad Eid Abu Ruz

Terry A. Lennie

CHAPTER ABBREVIATIONS

ACE   angiotensin-converting enzyme

CRP   C-reactive protein

hs-CRP   high-sensitivity C-reactive protein

ICAM   intracellular adhesion molecule

IL   interleukin

IL-1ra   interleukin-1 receptor antagonist

LDL   low-density lipoprotein

LPS   lipopolysaccharide

MCP   monocyte chemoattractant protein

MMP   matrix metalloproteinase

NF   nuclear factor

NO   nitric oxide

TNF   tumor necrosis factor

VCAM   vascular cell adhesion molecule

Inflammation is defined as a nonspecific immunological defense against injury or infection that is marked by the classic signs of rubor (redness), tumor (swelling), calor (heat), dolor (pain), and functiolaesa (loss of function). From this perspective, inflammation is considered to serve a protective role. Since this definition originally was derived, the medical community has developed a greater understanding of biological and molecular mechanisms involved in the inflammatory process.

Inflammation now is recognized as playing a pathological role in many conditions, including the development and progression of cardiovascular diseases. In these cases, inflammation begins as a protective response to injurious stimuli such as oxidized lipids, cigarette smoking, or hypertension. Continued exposure to these stimuli, however, results in a chronic inflammatory response that produces pathological changes. These changes result in cardiovascular diseases such as atherosclerosis, as well as clinical syndromes such as heart failure. The broadened understanding of inflammation also has led to the identification of inflammatory markers associated with development of cardiovascular disease. In this chapter the role of inflammation in the development and progression of atherosclerosis, acute coronary syndrome, and heart failure are reviewed as they represent three key stages in cardiovascular disease. In addition, the clinical implications of new inflammatory markers are addressed..

The structure of a normal artery wall is depicted in Figure 9-1. The wall is composed of three layers: the intima, media, and adventitia. Several features are important to highlight for the following discussion. First, endothelial cells form the inner surface of the vessel. These endothelial cells can express surface receptors and produce biologically active chemicals such as nitric oxide that control smooth muscle activity. Although the endothelial cells along the vessel surface are fitted tightly together, junctions between cells provide openings for smaller molecules and cells, including small proteins and monocytes, to enter the intima. Larger proteins and lipoproteins enter through endocytic vesicles. Smooth muscle cells and elastic connective tissue compose the majority of the remainder of the wall. These cells normally align linearly along the lines of tension, which is essential for controlling vessel lumen size. In the absence of inflammation, macrophages are resident in the adventitia but migrate to inner layers in response to inflammatory stimuli.

ROLE OF INFLAMMATION IN ATHEROSCLEROSIS

Once thought to be a simple consequence of lipid accumulation in the intimal space, atherosclerosis now is considered a chronic inflammatory condition. Inflammation plays an essential role in all steps of atherogenesis, from foam-cell development, to plaque formation, plaque rupture, and finally thrombosis formation (Figure 9-2).[1]

Vascular endothelial cells serve as primary sources of inflammatory mediators and, when injured, initiate the inflammatory cascade. The inflammatory response is adaptive in the case of acute vascular injury, but it becomes pathological in the presence of chronic inflammatory stimuli such as low-density lipoproteins (**LDLs**). The initiation of atherosclerosis begins in plaque-prone regions with vascular endothelial dysfunction from sheer stress or other causes. This dysfunction results in endothelial cells releasing inflammatory mediators that stimulate plaque formation (Table 9-1). Contributing to, or co-initiating, the process of atherosclerosis is the diffusion of LDLs from the blood through gaps in vascular endothelial cells into the intimal layer. The mechanisms responsible for sheer stress and lipoprotein movement into the intimal layer are described in more detail in Chapter 10.

Once in the intimal layer, LDLs attach to proteoglycans, which are large molecules composed of proteins and carbohydrates that serve multiple functions within the cell. Proteoglycan binding traps LDL in the intima and promotes oxidation. The oxidation of LDLs stimulates the release of proinflammatory cytokines such as interleukin-1β (**IL-1β**) and tumor necrosis factor-alpha (**TNF**-α) from endothelial cells and macrophages (Table 9-1). IL-1β and TNF-α are responsible for multiple com-

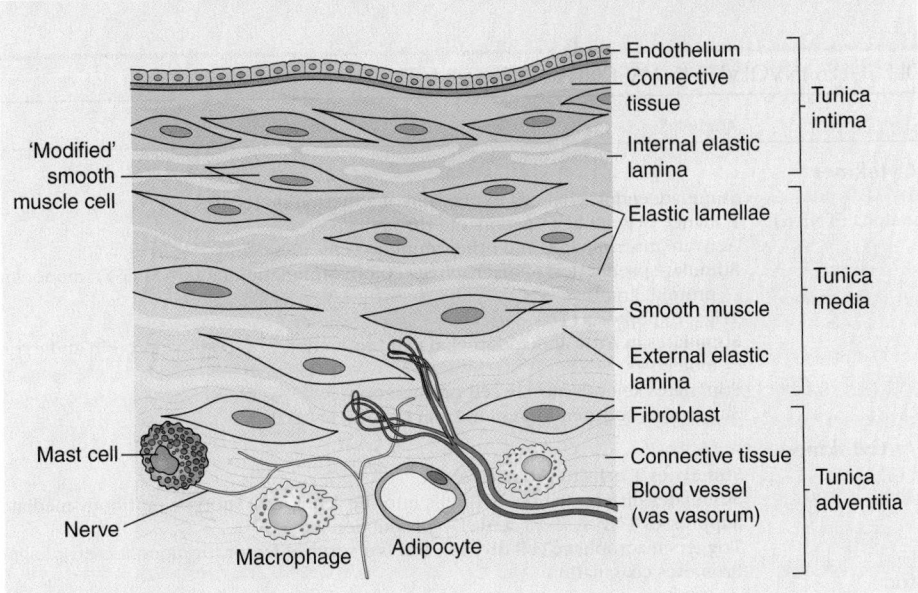

FIGURE 9-1 ■ Cross-section of the wall of a normal artery. (From Hansson K, Nilsson J: Pathogenesis of atherosclerosis. In Crawford MH, DiMarco JP, editors: *Cardiology,* London, 2001, Mosby.)

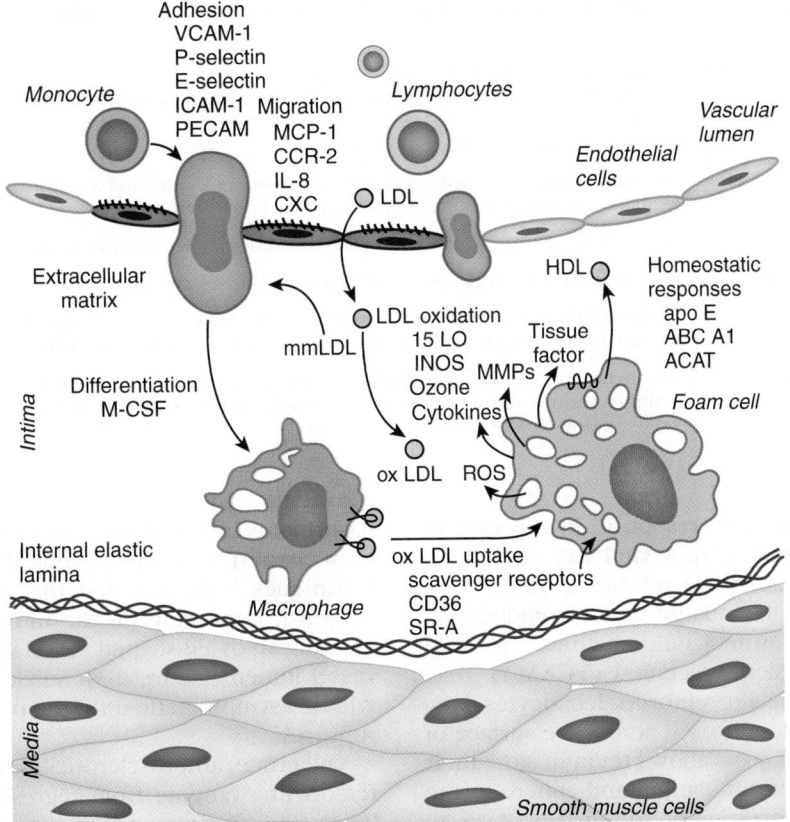

FIGURE 9-2 ■ *Top panel:* The initial stage of inflammation in the intima. Monocytes attach to vascular epithelial adhesion molecules, migrate into the intima, and differentiate into macrophages. These macrophages take up oxidized low-density lipoprotein molecules. Over time, macrophages change into foam cells that release additional proinflammatory molecules. *Middle panel:* Ongoing inflammation with development of a stable atherosclerotic lesion. The lesion is characterized by a collection of foam cells capped by a layer of smooth muscles that are covered by a fibrous cap. *Bottom panel:* A mature, unstable plaque that has ruptured. Platelets aggregate at the site of rupture, releasing growth and clotting factors. Two outcomes are possible: development of an occlusive clot that causes a myocardial infarction or an enhanced inflammatory response that produces a larger lesion that restabilizes over time. *apoE,* Apolipoprotein E; *ABC,* Al ATP binding cassette transporter; *ACAT,* acyl-CoA: cholesterol O-acyltransferase; *CxC,* alpha chemokines; *CCR-2,* chemokine (c-c) receptor 2; *CD 36,* cell differentiation receptor 36; *HDL,* high-density lipoprotein; *ICAM-1,* intracellular adhesion molecule-1; *IL-8,* interleukin-8; *INOS,* inducible nitric oxide synthase; *LDL,* low-density lipoprotein; *MCP,* monocytic chemoattractant protein; *MCSF,* macrophage colony-stimulating factor; *mmLDL,* minimally modifid LDL; *PECAM,* platelet/ endothelial cell adhesion molecule; *ROS,* reactive oxygen species; *SR-A,* class A scavenger receptor; *VCAM-1,* vascular cell adhesion molecule-1. (From Scott J: *Curr Opin Genet Dev* 124:271-279, 2004.)

■ ■ ■

TABLE 9-1   MOLECULES INVOLVED IN VASCULAR INFLAMMATION

MOLECULE	ACTIONS
Proinflammatory Cytokines	
Interleukin-1β (IL-1β)	Stimulate endothelial cell expression of adhesion molecules
Tumor necrosis factor-alpha (TNF-α)	Enhance platelet aggregation and thrombosis
	Activate macrophages and other immune cells
	Stimulate production of macrophage colony-stimulating factor (M-CSF), monocyte chemoattractant protein, and IL-8
	Trigger apoptosis (TNF-α)
Interleukin-6	Stimulates hepatic and endothelial cell production of C-reactive protein and expression of adhesion molecules
	Stimulates smooth muscle cell proliferation
Interferon-γ	Suppresses collagen formation from endothelial cells
Immune-Regulatory Cytokines	
Interleukin-2	Stimulates T cells to proliferate
Interleukin-4	Stimulates differentiation of T cells into the T helper 2 subtype (antibody-mediated immunity)
Interleukin-10	Suppresses TNF-α, IL-1β, and IL-6 production
M-CSF	Triggers macrophage cell division and is a survival factor for mononuclear phagocytes
Protein Tissue Factor	Promotes coagulation
Adhesion Molecules	
E-selectin	Involved in leukocyte rolling, in which rapidly passing leukocytes attach to receptors and slowly roll
Vascular adhesion molecule-1	along the endothelium, promoting ability to attach to adhesion molecules
Intracellular adhesion molecule	Bind leukocytes to vascular endothelial cells, allowing them to migrate into the intima
Chemoattractant Proteins	
Monocyte chemoattractant protein-1	Chemokines that provide chemical signals
Interleukin-8	Stimulate adherent leukocytes to move into the intimal layer through gaps in vascular endothelial cells
	Attract neutrophils to site of inflammation
C-Reactive Proteins	Stimulate endothelial cells to express adhesion molecules and macrophages to secrete cytokines
	Enhance macrophage uptake of low-density lipoproteins
CD40 Ligand	Promotes endothelial cell expression of adhesion molecules and secretion of TNF-α and IL-1β
Matrix Metalloproteinases	Cause enzymatic breakdown of collagen, weakening tissue or plaque structure
Nuclear Factor κB	A transcription factor that activates gene transcription of proinflammatory cytokines, cellular adhesion molecules, chemoattractant proteins, and thrombogenic factors
Nitric Oxide	Gas synthesized in vascular epithelium that promotes vasodilatation at low concentrations
	Inhibits contractility and promotes myocardial apoptosis at higher concentrations

ponents of the inflammatory response. In the case of atherosclerosis, they may play a vital role in linking LDLs to plaque formation. The release of these cytokines in response to LDL oxidation induces endothelial cells to express adhesion molecules such as E-selectin and vascular cell adhesion molecule-1 (**VCAM**-1). E-selectin molecules provide a receptor for leukocytes passing by rapidly in the blood to roll across the surface of the vascular epithelium. This allows them to slow their movement, come out of circulation, and adhere to the epithelium. VCAM-1 expression on the surface of vascular endothelial cells provides receptors for adherence of monocytes to the vascular endothelial membrane. Chemotactic molecules such as monocyte chemoattractant protein-1 (**MCP**-1), which also is released during inflammation, then promote the migration of monocytes into the intima. These monocytes differentiate into intimal macrophages with specialized receptors that take up oxidized LDLs. Intimal macrophages subsequently are transformed into foam cells as LDLs accumulate.

The development of an atherosclerotic lesion occurs over many years and is not a continuous process. Origi-

nally it was believed that plaque initially grew into the vessel lumen, restricting blood flow. Improved imaging techniques have revealed that plaque initially grows outward, impinging on the intima media and thereby creating an ovoid-shaped vessel with a relatively normal vessel lumen (Figure 9-3). Subsequently, most persons will be asymptomatic until the plaque becomes large or ruptures.

Over time, atherosclerotic lesions undergo periods of remodeling ranging from regression to growth during bursts of inflammatory activity. The repeated remodeling produces plaques that are stable at times but that become unstable during periods of inflammation. Stable plaques are dominated by smooth muscle cells embedded in a dense collagen matrix. Unstable plaques contain a large number of inflammatory cells. In these plaques, inflammatory cells release enzymes such as matrix metalloproteinases (**MMPs**) that digest the collagen matrix. Other mediators such as interferon-gamma inhibit new collagen secretion from smooth muscle cells. This results in degradation of the fibrinous cap. Apoptotic signals from macrophages trigger death of

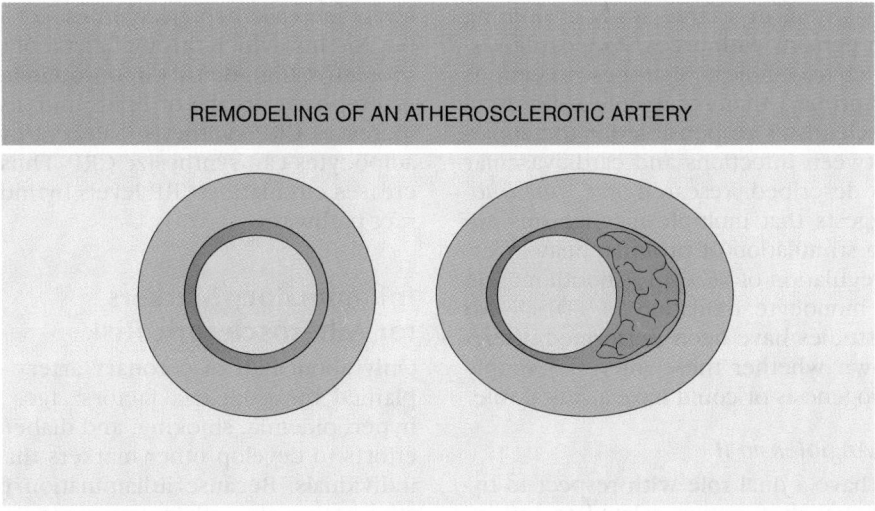

REMODELING OF AN ATHEROSCLEROTIC ARTERY

FIGURE 9-3 ■ During the early stages of plaque development, the artery may maintain the lumen opening and compensate for increased intimal thickness by remodeling of the extracellular matrix in the median and adventitia. The result is an oval-shaped vessel. (From Hansson K, Nilsson J: Pathogenesis of atherosclerosis. In Crawford MH, DiMarco JP, editors: *Cardiology,* London, 2001, Mosby.)

smooth muscle cells, further weakening the plaque and increasing the risk of rupture.

Plaque rupture exposes blood components to protein tissue factor and other procoagulation factors. The result is platelet aggregation and thrombus formation. Plaque rupture with thrombus formation can produce two clinical outcomes. One is the development of an acute coronary event. The other outcome is a silent event with no clinical symptoms. During silent events, the thrombus is absorbed into the existing plaque. This process produces several growth factors that stimulate migration and proliferation of smooth muscle cells, production of collagen matrix, and reformation of a fibrinous cap. This process results in a larger, restabilized lesion. As this process is repeated, plaques increase in size.

Many cardiac events occur in individuals with normal LDL levels.[2] This suggests that other factors work in concert or independently of LDLs to stimulate the inflammatory process associated with atherosclerosis. Several factors have been identified as playing at least contributory roles.

Additional Triggers of Inflammation in Atherosclerosis
C-Reactive Protein

C-reactive protein (**CRP**) is a hepatic acute-phase protein that may play an active role in the inflammatory process associated with atherosclerosis. In addition to hepatic synthesis, arterial endothelial cells have been shown to produce CRP.[3] Local concentrations of CRP in atherosclerotic lesions are much higher than circulating concentrations. CRP serves as an opsonin for LDL, thereby enhancing uptake of LDL by macrophages. CRP also triggers macrophages to release IL-6, IL-1β, and TNF-α. IL-6 stimulates the release of CRP from hepatic and endothelial cells. Higher levels of IL-6 in the lesion

result in a local positive feedback loop in which additional CRP is produced by endothelial cells. At high concentrations, CRP stimulates VCAM-1 and MCP-1 expression by endothelial cells, which as noted before, is an initial step in the inflammatory process leading to plaque formation.

Infectious Agents

Chronic nonvascular infections could provide additional inflammatory triggers that promote plaque formation. Periodontal disease (e.g., gingivitis), prostatitis, and bronchitis are three such chronic infections. Of the three, periodontal disease has the most evidence to establish a relationship with atherosclerosis. Periodontal disease, which itself is inflammatory, could provide a secondary inflammatory stimulus that increases circulating proinflammatory cytokines.[4] Higher cytokine levels may enhance vascular inflammation and accelerate generation of atherosclerotic plaques. Alternatively, episodes of bacteremia from periodontal microbes such as *Porphyromonas gingivalis, Actinobacillus actinomycetemcomitans, Treponema denticola, Bacteroides forsythus,* and a number of other organisms associated with periodontal disease may seed atherosclerotic plaques.[5] Growth of these bacteria in the plaque would produce additional inflammation. This may be one cause of inflammatory bursts that lead to plaque instability and potential rupture.

Vascular infections with microbes such as *Chlamydia pneumoniae* and *Helicobacter pylori* or with viruses such as *Cytomegalovirus* and herpes simplex have been hypothesized to cause endothelial dysfunction and subsequent development of vascular inflammation. These microbes have been found frequently in atherosclerotic plaques.[6] Investigators also have shown an association between *C. pneumonia* and *Cytomegalovirus* infections and risk of myocardial infarction, cardiac-related death, and stroke.[7-9] This association was not found to be as strong in a large study examining recurrent events in persons with preexisting cardiovascular disease,[10] which may indicate that these infections are more related to primary than recurrent cardiovascular events. The mechanisms responsible for the apparent association between infections and cardiovascular events are not fully described. Research on *C. pneumonia* infections suggests that multiple mechanisms are involved, including stimulation of proinflammatory cytokine release, upregulation of VCAM-1, smooth muscle proliferation, and monocyte oxidation of LDLs.[11] No large prospective studies have been performed; therefore, it is not known whether these microbes simply contribute to atherogenesis or could have a causal role.

Hypertension and Angiotensin II

Inflammation may have a dual role with respect to hypertension. Endothelial dysfunction related to inflammation causes vessel wall thickening and decreased production of nitric oxide (**NO**), an important local vasodilator. These result in vessel stiffness and a predominantly vasoconstrictive state, both of which contribute to hypertension.[12,13] However, hypertension may accelerate atherosclerosis by enhancing inflammation.[14] Elevated intravascular pressures associated with hypertension contribute to endothelial dysfunction resulting in release of adhesion molecules, attachment of monocytes to vascular endothelium, movement of monocytes into the intima, and initiation of the inflammatory cascade described before.

In addition to a well-recognized role in hypertension, angiotensin II is proinflammatory.[15] Angiotensin II stimulates nuclear factor κB (**NF-κB**), an important proinflammatory transcription factor. NF-κB regulates gene expression of key mediators involved in inflammation, including TNF-α, IL-6, intracellular adhesion molecule-1 (**ICAM**-1), and VCAM. Thus, the ability of angiotensin II to stimulate NF-κB conveys broad proinflammatory properties on this molecule. Angiotensin II also promotes inflammation by a secondary pathway. Angiotensin II stimulates the production of superoxide dismutase, which rapidly converts vascular NO to peroxynitrite, a potent oxidant.[13,16] NO has vasodilator and antiinflammatory activities. Loss of NO activity results in vasoconstriction, enhanced LDL oxidation, endothelial cell release of VCAM-1 and NF-κB, and smooth muscle migration and proliferation.

Obesity

Adipose tissue, once considered a passive energy storage depot, now is recognized to have endocrine-like activities with important metabolic effects. Among these activities is the secretion of CRP and proinflammatory cytokines, particularly TNF-α and IL-6.[17,18] Levels of both cytokines are elevated in obese individuals in direct relationship to amount of body fat in general and abdominal fat in particular.[19] Several consequences arise from these elevated levels. The higher circulating cytokine levels create a proinflammatory state that could promote atherogenesis. TNF-α increases lipolysis and inhibits lipoprotein lipase synthesis, resulting in increased free fatty acid levels.[20] Higher free fatty acid levels increase hepatic synthesis of very low-density lipoproteins, which through metabolic interaction, lower protective high-density lipoprotein levels. IL-6 increases macrophage uptake of lipids and, as previously noted, increases CRP synthesis.[21] Recent evidence shows that adipocytes can synthesize CRP. Thus, adipose tissue increases circulating CRP levels by indirect (IL-6) and direct pathways.

Inflammatory Markers for Atherosclerotic Risk

Only about half of coronary artery disease can be explained by usual risk factors: age, sex, hypertension, hyperlipidemia, smoking, and diabetes.[2] This has led to efforts to develop other markers that identify high-risk individuals. Because inflammation plays a key role in atherosclerosis, inflammatory mediators have been examined as potential markers (Table 9-2).[22] The most prominent of these are discussed next.

C-Reactive Protein

CRP has received considerable attention as a systemic marker of vascular inflammation and as a prognostic indicator for coronary events. CRP has several properties that make it particularly attractive as a biomarker. CRP has a long half-life, remains stable in the plasma, has minimal circadian variation, and is measured easily. Multiple investigators have shown that persons with elevated circulating CRP levels have up to double the risk of a coronary event compared with those with normal levels.[23] Elevated CRP levels are predictive of future coronary events in persons with no history of coronary artery disease, with normal LDL levels, and with a history of acute myocardial infarction.

The Centers for Disease Control and Prevention/American Heart Association workshop guidelines recommend CRP as the inflammatory marker of choice because it has the strongest supporting evidence as a prognostic indicator.[22] The high-sensitivity CRP (**hs-CRP**) assay is the recommended laboratory test because it is standardized, accurate, widely available, and less expensive than other risk assessment methods such as vascular imaging. The association between hs-CRP level and risk for coronary events remains significant even after adjustment for traditional risk factors including age, sex, total cholesterol, smoking, body mass index, diabetes, hypertension, and family history of coronary artery disease.[24,25] The averaged value of two measurements (fasting or nonfasting) taken 2 weeks apart should be used. Current recommended cutoff points for determining risk are the following[22]:

- Low risk: less than 1.0 mg/liter
- Average risk: 1.0 to 3.0 mg/liter
- High risk: greater than 3.0 mg/liter

Hs-CRP levels greater than 10.0 mg/liter indicate the need for repeat testing or further evaluation to rule out ongoing infection or other inflammatory conditions. If other causes are ruled out, these high levels are associated with very high cardiovascular risk.

Several factors should be considered when using CRP as a risk marker. First, CRP is a nonspecific marker

■ ■ ■

TABLE 9-2 INFLAMMATORY MARKERS AS PROGNOSTIC INDICATORS IN ATHEROSCLEROSIS

MARKER	FUNCTION
Acute-Phase Reactants C-reactive protein Fibrinogen Serum amyloid A	Synthesized in the liver in response to inflammatory mediators, such as interleukin-6. Levels increase in proportion to degree of inflammation but are nonspecific.
Soluble Adhesion Molecules E-selectin Intracellular adhesion molecule-1 Vascular cell adhesion molecule	Molecules are shed into blood from cell membranes. Higher levels may indicate greater inflammatory activity in vascular endothelial and smooth muscle cells.
Proinflammatory Cytokines Tumor necrosis factor-alpha Interleukin-1β Interleukin-6	Higher levels indicate greater inflammation.
Immune Elements Leukocyte count	Greater numbers may indicate inflammatory process. Nonspecific.
Inflammatory Mediators CD40 ligand	Higher levels indicate increased monocyte migration into intima and greater proinflammatory cytokine activity.
Matrix myeloperoxidase	Higher levels indicate increased enzyme activity leading to greater risk of plaque instability and rupture.

of inflammation. Any stimulus, including cigarette smoking, infection, injury, cancer, and possibly psychological stress, can stimulate production of CRP. Therefore, a 2-week history of any factors that can cause inflammation must be ruled out before a CRP level is drawn. Second, combining CRP with LDL cholesterol, total cholesterol, or Framingham score provides additive predictive value.[26] This emphasizes that multiple factors are involved in the development of atherosclerosis, and reliance on a single marker to determine a person's risk should be avoided. Third, CRP does not provide a gauge of the extent of atherosclerosis. Studies have shown a poor correlation between hs-CRP and plaque quantification by Doppler ultrasound and computerized tomography scanning.[27,28] Fourth, treatment with statins, which have antiinflammatory and lipid-lowering effects, can decrease CRP levels. The relationship between CRP levels and risk for future coronary events in patients treated with statins has not been clearly established. However, a drop in CRP levels following the start of statin therapy may be an indicator of the antiinflammatory effects of therapy.

Proinflammatory Cytokines

Given the difficulty of measuring cytokines and the high degree of variability in circulating levels among patients, there is little practical value in using them as clinical markers. Regardless, they frequently are reported in research studies that guide clinical practice and thus merit discussion. TNF-α and IL-1β have short half-lives (less than 30 minutes) and operate mainly locally in paracrine or autocrine manners. Therefore, high levels of these cytokines are not detected consistently in the blood, and they are not reliable systemic markers of inflammation, atherosclerosis, or cardiovascular risk. The two membrane receptors for TNF-α (TNF-R1 and TNF-R2) are shed from the cell surface

into the blood after TNF-α binding and become soluble receptors (sTNF-R1 and sTNF-R2). Both soluble receptors have longer half-lives, are detected more easily in the blood, and have been used as surrogate markers for TNF-α activity in research studies.

The gene for IL-1 receptor antagonist (**IL-1ra**), a counterregulatory molecule that binds to cell receptors and blocks IL-1 binding, is activated by the same transcription factors as IL-1β and is thus co-produced with IL-1β. IL-1ra is detected more readily in the blood with levels that are proportionate to the magnitude of IL-1β. Therefore, IL-1ra has been deemed a surrogate serum marker of IL-1β activity.[29] Soluble TNF receptors and IL-1ra have been shown to be elevated in persons with atherosclerosis and in those with unstable angina.[30] Their clinical utility as markers of inflammation in atherosclerotic lesions, however, is still under investigation.

IL-6 is considered a circulating mediator of local inflammation. Elevated levels of IL-6 are predictive of future coronary events in persons with and without coronary heart disease,[31] but levels have not been shown to be consistent independent markers of risk.[32] IL-6 is a primary stimulator of CRP production in the liver and vascular tissue, and levels of IL-6 and CRP are likely to co-vary. Moreover, IL-6 is a nonspecific marker of inflammation. Higher circulating levels are found in nearly all conditions associated with inflammation.

Cellular Adhesion Molecules

Cellular adhesion molecules include E-selectin, ICAM-1, and VCAM-1. Levels of these molecules can increase up to tenfold in endothelial cells activated by inflammatory mediators such as CRP or IL-1. The extracellular portion subsequently is released into the blood, making circulating levels of these molecules an indicator of the extent of inflammatory activity in endothelial cells. In the

Physician's Health Study,[33] healthy men with the highest levels of ICAM-1 had 1.6 times higher risk for future myocardial infarction than those with the lowest levels. The Atherosclerosis Risk in Communities investigators[34] showed that baseline levels of ICAM-1 were independent predictors of risk for future atherosclerosis in healthy persons. VCAM-1 and ICAM-1 have been shown to be predictive of future cardiovascular death in patients with coronary artery disease.[35]

Use of Inflammatory Markers in Practice

The evidence to support routine use of inflammatory markers in clinical practice is limited, and therefore only general recommendations can be made. Further, only one marker, hs-CRP, has published cutoff values for risk assessment. Based on current evidence, the maximum potential benefit from measuring hs-CRP appears to be for primary prevention[22]; that is, to identify patients who are at risk but currently not on a protective treatment for coronary artery disease (e.g., lipid-lowering or antiplatelet drugs, lifestyle changes, and other cardioprotective therapies). This marker may be most useful for patients who are at moderate or intermediate risk in which an additional marker would support a decision to implement interventions.

Measuring hs-CRP or other markers for secondary prevention in patients receiving treatment is not advocated. CRP levels are not correlated with extent of atherosclerotic plaque, so serial testing of hs-CRP to measure disease progression is not helpful. Similarly, CRP levels have limited usefulness for selecting patients who would benefit from invasive coronary or peripheral arterial procedures.

Two potential additional uses for hs-CRP measurement have been suggested. First, hs-CRP may be useful for monitoring statin therapy. If hs-CRP levels do not decrease after therapy begins, treatment may need to be adjusted. Second, sharing hs-CRP levels with patients may motivate high-risk patients to adhere to drug therapy or modify risk factors such as smoking, diet, excess body weight, and sedentary lifestyle. The utility of these approaches requires future testing in randomized controlled trials to demonstrate effectiveness.

Therapeutic Interventions for Inflammation in Atherosclerosis

The beneficial effects of several therapeutic interventions are thought to be due to antiinflammatory actions in addition to their primary indication. Several of the key agents are discussed next (Box 9-1)

Statins

Drug trials have shown that the decreased morbidity and mortality associated with statin therapy is due to the lipid-lowering and antiinflammatory effects of these drugs.[1,2,36-38] Statins decrease CRP levels, number of cellular adhesion molecules, level of chemoattractant molecules, and amount of proteases and other inflammatory mediators in the vascular endothelium and smooth muscle cells. These drugs appear to have the greatest benefit in patients with the highest CRP levels, who

---

BOX 9-1 ■ ■ ■
ANTIINFLAMMATORY THERAPIES AND INTERVENTIONS
Drug Therapies
Angiotensin-converting enzyme inhibitors
Antibiotics
Aspirin
Statins
Thiazolidinediones
Thienopyridines
Lifestyle Interventions
Exercise
Moderation of alcohol intake
Smoking cessation
Weight loss

---

presumably have the greatest degree of inflammation. Statins also have vasodilating effects that may be related to increased local production of NO.

Aspirin

In addition to inhibiting platelet aggregation, aspirin has well-known antiinflammatory effects. The antiplatelet and antiinflammatory effects of aspirin likely are linked because platelet aggregation is triggered by inflammatory mediators. As with statins, the beneficial effects of aspirin therapy in prevention are greatest in those with higher CRP levels.[39]

Angiotensin-Converting Enzyme Inhibitors

Given the proinflammatory actions of angiotensin II described earlier, it is not surprising that angiotensin-converting enzyme (**ACE**) inhibitors have antiinflammatory effects. ACE inhibitors decrease the incidence of atherosclerotic plaques, indicating a primary prevention role. The use of ACE inhibitors has benefit in secondary prevention as well. ACE inhibitors given after acute myocardial infarction decrease the incidence of heart failure, recurrent ischemia, reinfarction, and new onset of angina, all of which have an inflammatory component.[40]

Antibiotics

The antiinflammatory effects of antibiotics follow from their treatment of potential infective agents such as *Chlamydia pneumonia, P. gingivalis,* or other bacteria discussed previously. In a 1-year follow-up randomized control trial, 325 patients admitted with acute myocardial infarction or unstable angina received amoxicillin or placebo. Patients treated with amoxicillin had significantly lower CRP levels. Death or readmissions for acute coronary syndrome in this group were 36 percent lower at 3 months and at 1 year than in patients receiving placebo.[41]

ROLE OF INFLAMMATION IN ACUTE CORONARY SYNDROME

Inflammation plays a role in the onset of and recovery from acute coronary syndrome. The role of inflammation in the onset of acute coronary syndrome, including plaque instability, plaque rupture, and thrombus formation, is described in the first section of this chapter. In this section the role of inflammation in acute coronary syndrome is described.

As with any cellular injury, ischemic myocardial cell damage triggers an inflammatory response.[42] The outcome of this inflammatory response can be positive, leading to healing and restoration of function. Alternatively, inflammation can cause additional cell death and cardiac remodeling, leading to heart failure. The amount of myocardial tissue involved appears to be the primary factor influencing which outcome occurs. Smaller areas of tissue damage typically result in an inflammatory response that resolves as damaged tissue is removed and the myocardium is repaired. Larger areas of tissue damage can trigger exaggerated inflammatory mediator release. Higher levels of inflammatory mediators in combination with the large volume of damaged tissue promote the development of a chronic inflammatory state. Chronic inflammation can lead to additional cell death and myocardial remodeling that can extend into healthy tissue, thereby enlarging the area of damage.

The onset of inflammation is marked by the release of TNF-α, IL-1β, and IL-6 in the ischemic and surrounding tissue. Multiple stimuli are thought to trigger cytokine release by myocardial and immune cells:

- Mechanical stress from stretching of myocardial fibers in the ischemic and adjacent tissue triggers a series of intracellular signals that ultimately activate NF-κB and other gene transcription factors responsible for cytokine production.
- Ischemia causes oxidative stress through the production of reactive oxygen species that act as secondary messengers and trigger gene transcription factors for cytokine synthesis.
- Changes in cell membranes caused by impaired perfusion—including hypoxia, altered osmotic balance, and production of free radicals—activate other intracellular signaling pathways that lead to cytokine production.

The greater the tissue damage, the greater the inflammatory stimulus. In cases of extensive tissue damage, the inflammatory response can become exaggerated and self-perpetuating. Chemoattractant factors (e.g., MCP-1 and IL-8) draw monocytes to the site in proportion to the severity of tissue injury. These monocytes migrate into damaged tissue and transform into macrophages. During the acute stage of injury, neutrophils are drawn to the site in large numbers. Mast cells accumulate in surrounding ischemic tissues that regain perfusion or in tissue that is reperfused following intervention. Together, macrophages, neutrophils, and mast cells produce significant amounts of cytokines, growth factors, and other mediators that enhance the inflammatory response. TNF-α can be released from damaged myocardial cells in sufficient quantities to stimulate adjacent healthy myocytes to release additional TNF-α.

TNF-α has positive and negative effects on myocytes. These variable effects are in part dependent on which of the two membrane-bound receptors (TNF-R1 or TNF-R2) binds TNF-α. TNF-α binding to either receptor can trigger signaling pathways that lead to activation of NF-κB, resulting in induction of growth factors and cell survival. In this case, TNF-α and other cytokines play important roles in several components of wound healing, including phagocyte removal of necrotic tissue, stimulation of tissue growth factors, synthesis of collagen, myoblast proliferation, and angiogenesis. Other beneficial effects of TNF-α include upregulation of myocardial free radical scavengers and enhanced production of protective heat shock proteins. At higher levels these cytokines also promote myocyte hypertrophy.

The binding of TNF-α to TNF-R1 can trigger alternate pathways that lead to apoptosis (cell death) of myocytes. For this ability—first discovered in tumor cells—TNF was named. Although not fully understood, the apoptosis pathway appears to be triggered in cells that are altered or damaged or in which the NF-κB pathway is blocked.[43] Although triggering of the apoptotic pathway leads to death of a single cell, other negative consequences of TNF-α, IL-1β, and IL-6 have more global effects on the myocardium.

TNF-α and IL-6, but particularly TNF-α, can decrease myocardial contractility. These cytokines alter the function of the sarcoplasmic reticulum, resulting in decreased calcium. Compounding the effects of decreased calcium availability, TNF-α also can decrease the sensitivity of myofilaments to calcium. Prolonged TNF-α exposure further alters contractility by decreasing calcium pumps (i.e., sarcoplasmic/endoplasmic reticulum calcium adenosinetriphosphatase) in the sarcoplasmic reticulum, which limits calcium reuptake and delays myofilament relaxation following contraction. This last effect has been proposed as one cause of heart failure.[44] TNF-α, IL-1, and interferon-gamma contribute to oxidative stress by promoting the production of free radicals and inhibiting antioxidants. Results of oxidative stress include impaired contractility, DNA damage, myocyte fibrosis, and hypertrophy.

Over time, TNF-α, IL-1β, and IL-6 can affect myocytes distant from the site of infarction, resulting in inflammation-induced changes in regions not initially affected by ischemic injury.[45] Clinically significant consequences of cytokine activity in these areas include collagen formation and hypertrophy. This results in not only scar formation and remodeling of necrotic tissue but also remodeling of otherwise healthy myocardial tissue.

In summary, ischemia triggers inflammation in the myocardium that is proportionate to the extent of tissue damage. TNF-α, IL-1β, IL-6, interferon-gamma, and other cytokines mediate multiple components of the inflammatory response. This response is essential for recovery and is responsible for clearing necrotic cells, promoting angiogenesis in damaged tissue, stimulating proliferation of new myocytes, and ensuring structural integrity through formation of scar tissue in necrotic areas. In cases of extensive tissue damage, a chronic inflammatory response can be elicited. Negative consequences of chronic inflammation include cell death, impaired cardiac contractility, hypertrophy, fibrosis, and collagen formation in healthy myocardial tissue. When the inflammatory response is sufficiently severe or prolonged, structural and functional changes within the myocardium can cause, or at least significantly contribute to, heart failure.

ROLE OF INFLAMMATION IN HEART FAILURE

The conceptualization of heart failure pathophysiology has evolved significantly over the past 50 years. In the 1950s, it was considered a problem related to the cardiorenal axis in which focus was placed on controlling symptoms by reducing sodium and water retention. Over the next few decades, the focus shifted to improving cardiac function and hemodynamics to reverse forward and backward failure. Recently, appreciation of the neurohormonal components of heart failure resulted in emphasis on the control of sympathetic nervous system activation, the renin-angiotensin-aldosterone system, and other vasoactive and counterregulatory hormones. Most recently, evidence that proinflammatory cytokines such as TNF-α and IL-6 are elevated in patients with heart failure has changed the definition of heart failure to that of a multisystem disorder in which the overriding pathological process is inflammation.[46] The discussion of inflammation in heart failure can be divided into myocardial and systemic effects.

Myocardial Effects

The same chronic inflammatory processes described above in the section on acute coronary syndrome persist after the development of heart failure. Chronic inflammation results in continued impaired cardiac function and further remodeling. One effect of long-term inflammation is increased activity of MMP.[47] Increased MMP activity is not due to increased amounts of MMP but to decreased amounts of tissue-derived inhibitors of these enzymes. The net result is enzymatic loss of the collagen fibril matrix surrounding myocytes. This leads to rearrangement and slippage of myofilaments with subsequent ventricular dilatation. A second deleterious consequence of long-term inflammation is progressive loss of functional tissue. Ongoing activation of intracellular apoptotic pathways by TNF-α results in progressive loss of myocytes that are replaced with fibrous tissue. IL-6 may contribute to remodeling by inducing myocyte hypertrophy in functional areas of the ventricles.

Systemic Effects

Levine and colleagues[48] were the first to report that patients with heart failure had elevated levels of circulating TNF-α. Since then, TNF-α has been shown to be a major mediator, directly and indirectly, of many components of heart failure pathology.[49] Although IL-1β has received less attention as an inflammatory mediator in heart failure, it also may play a role. TNF-α can stimulate the release of IL-1β,[50] and both can stimulate the release of IL-6.[51] Moreover, IL-1β and TNF-α act synergistically in autocrine and paracrine manners to induce many of the metabolic alterations that occur during the systemic inflammatory response.[50] In contrast, IL-6 is a systemic mediator of local inflammation. Interestingly, IL-6 ap-

pears also to serve a counterregulatory role of capping the magnitude of TNF-α and IL-1β activity.

The origin of TNF-α and other proinflammatory cytokines in the blood of patients with heart failure is not known for certain, but several sources have been proposed. One source may be proinflammatory cytokines synthesized in the myocardium that leak out into circulation. Given the amount of circulating cytokines measured in some patients, myocardial-derived cytokines may contribute, but are not the sole source of systemic cytokines. A second source is thought to be cytokines produced by immune and other cells in ischemic tissues. Ischemia leads to hypoxic tissue injury, which initiates a cascade of events that stimulate immune, epithelial, and other cells in the ischemic tissue to produce proinflammatory cytokines. A third source may be stimulation of immune cells by lipopolysaccharide (**LPS**) from the cell wall of gram-negative bacteria. Gram-negative bacteria are suspected of translocating across the ischemic gut into the blood, where LPS binds to immune cells. LPS is a potent stimulator of TNF-α production in immune cells.[52] Patients with heart failure, particularly those with edema, have been reported to have elevated blood levels of LPS that are associated with higher circulating TNF-α levels. With treatment to reverse edema in these patients, LPS levels decreased.[53]

The most prominent consequence of systemic inflammation associated with heart failure is the development of cardiac cachexia. Researchers have established a positive relationship between proinflammatory cytokines levels and severity of cardiac cachexia, indicating that cytokines play an important role.[54,55] Proinflammatory cytokines operate by direct and indirect actions on peripheral tissues and in the brain. Because proinflammatory cytokines are too large to pass through the blood-brain barrier, multiple ways for peripherally produced cytokines to enter the brain have been proposed. Cytokines can enter the brain via saturable transports along the vasculature. They can enter directly through areas without a blood-brain barrier such as the circumventricular organs in the hypothalamus and brain stem.[56] Circulating lymphocytes that are activated in ischemic tissue can migrate to the brain and secrete cytokines.[35] Brain cells located in key hypothalamic areas can synthesize cytokines in response to peripheral neural signals.[25] The combined effects of cytokine activity in the periphery and brain include decreased food intake, catabolism of muscle and adipose tissue, stimulation of catabolic hormones such as epinephrine and cortisol, increased metabolism, and fatigue.

Decreased Food Intake

Although it has not been definitively demonstrated, proinflammatory cytokines are believed to play a role in decreased food intake observed in many patients with heart failure. Evidence indicates that cytokines can have a direct effect on nuclei in the hypothalamus that are involved in controlling food intake. In the lateral hypothalamus, IL-1β suppresses the activity of glucose-sensitive neurons, whereas in the ventromedial hypothalamus, it excites glucose-sensitive neurons. Suppression of neurons in the lateral hypothalamus prolongs the interval between meals, whereas excitation of the ventromedial hypothalamic neurons decreases the amount of food eaten per meal.[57]

The paraventricular nucleus also plays an important role in controlling food intake. TNF-α and IL-1β activate pathways responsible for corticotropin-releasing hormone synthesis. Corticotropin-releasing hormone inhibits the synthesis of neuropeptide Y, a potent stimulator of food intake. Leptin, an important energy regulatory hormone, is released in greater amounts from adipose tissue in response to proinflammatory cytokines. This hormone travels to the hypothalamus and causes further suppression of neuropeptide Y. Suppression of neuropeptide Y limits the development of hunger in response to food deprivation. Chronically decreased neuropeptide Y levels, which would occur with chronic inflammation, impair one of the primary hypothalamic mechanisms responsible for promoting food intake in response to negative energy states. Peripheral effects of inflammation include delayed gastric emptying and stimulation of the gut hormone cholecystokinin.[58] Delayed emptying prolongs sensations of fullness, which prolongs the time between meals by inhibiting hunger sensations. Cholecystokinin acts on central feeding centers to produce sensations of satiety that can result in the person feeling satisfied or full after eating only a small amount of food.

Tissue Catabolism

The stimulation of corticotropin-releasing hormone by cytokines activates the hypothalamic pituitary axis, resulting in release of glucocorticoids and activation of the sympathetic nervous system. In combination, proinflammatory cytokines, catecholamines, leptin, and glucagon inhibit lipase enzymes and activate lipolytic enzymes in adipose tissue. This produces a state of decreased fat storage with enhanced release of stored fatty acids, resulting in accelerated loss of body fat. Proinflammatory cytokines also work in concert with glucocorticoids, oxidative stress, and proteolysis-inducing factor to activate the ubiquitin-proteasome pathways in skeletal muscle. These are the major pathways responsible for breakdown of proteins in cells. Cellular proteins are marked by attachment of ubiquitin molecules. The marked protein then is transported to the 26S proteasome, where it is degraded into small peptides. Glucocorticoids further enhance catabolism of muscle tissue by inhibiting muscle protein synthesis and promoting conversion of amino acids to glucose in the liver.[59] Another major cause of muscle loss in heart failure is TNF-α–triggered apoptotic pathways in skeletal myocytes that cause cell death.[60]

Increased Metabolism

Proinflammatory cytokines increase sympathetic nervous system activity and release of catecholamines. Important consequences of sympathetic activity include increased metabolic rate and promotion of tissue catabolism. Blood catecholamine levels are associated with severity of cachexia in patients with heart failure, and patients with the most severe symptoms have been show to have the highest metabolic rate.[61]

Fatigue

Fatigue is among the most common symptoms of heart failure. Multiple factors are responsible for this symptom. Inflammation plays a role in several of these factors. The loss of skeletal muscle mass as described before is a major contributor. Proinflammatory cytokines are associated with impaired vasodilatation of skeletal muscle, which limits exercise capacity. Proinflammatory cytokines also act in the brain to produce symptoms of malaise, decreased motivation, and increased slow wave sleep.[62] Collectively, these symptoms produce sensations of fatigue. In cases of chronic inflammation, the neuronal changes induced by proinflammatory cytokines that cause these symptoms are suspected of producing depression.

Counterregulation of Proinflammatory Cytokines

As a part of homeostasis, the systemic actions of proinflammatory cytokines are opposed by antiinflammatory cytokines, including IL-4, IL-10, and IL-12. IL-10, in particular, has potent antiinflammatory properties including down-regulation of TNF-α, IL-1β, and IL-6 production.[63] Unfortunately, patients with heart failure may not produce enough IL-10 to counter proinflammatory cytokine activity. One study showed that although IL-10 levels were higher in patients with heart failure than similarly aged controls, patients had a lower ratio of IL-10 to TNF-α.[64] Thus, despite having higher IL-10 levels, proinflammatory cytokine activity was apparently greater in patients with heart failure. This conclusion is supported by additional studies that show the lowest ratio of IL-10 to TNF-α is found in the most symptomatic patients.[65,66]

Activation of the hypothalamic-pituitary-adrenal axis is the second major counterregulatory mechanism to control proinflammatory cytokine activity. As noted before, proinflammatory cytokines, especially IL-1β, stimulate the hypothalamic-pituitary-adrenal axis resulting in release of glucocorticoids, primarily cortisol. The antiinflammatory properties of cortisol are well known and include suppression of proinflammatory cytokine and stimulation of IL-10 production from immune cells. Thus, proinflammatory cytokines trigger one of the primary negative feedback loops for their production.

Inflammatory Markers in Heart Failure
Proinflammatory Cytokines

Currently, assessing proinflammatory cytokine levels has limited clinical utility because of the difficulty with measurement and lack of standardized criteria to guide clinical management. As was the case with atherosclerosis, measurement of these molecules is confined to research studies. The results of these studies, however, have clinical implications, and therefore these molecules merit discussion.

Similar to atherosclerosis, TNF-α and IL-1β levels are not elevated consistently in patients with heart failure. IL-6 is found more consistently in the serum of patients with heart failure than TNF-α.[67] The soluble TNF receptors sTNF-R1 and sTNF-R2 can similarly serve as surrogate markers for TNF-α activity in heart failure. Elevated levels may reflect the combined consequence of cytokines produced in peripheral tissues indicating greater ischemia and from the myocardium indicating worsening ventricular function. Analysis of cytokine and receptor levels of patients from the Vesnarinone (VEST) trial showed that sTNF-R1 and sTNF-R2 levels were higher in patients at New York Heart Association Classes III and IV.[68] Levels in men and women differed. Men showed a linear relationship with increasing age, whereas levels in women remained flat (comparable to levels of 20- to 30-year-old men) until the age of 50, after which there was a sharp increase to levels comparable to 70-year-old men. Race and smoking status were not related to circulating levels. Both receptors and IL-6 levels were independent predictors of survival when individually combined with key clinical variables in a predictive model. However, when all cytokines, receptors, and clinical variables were entered together into a predictive model, only sTNF-R2 emerged as an independent predictor of mortality. A smaller study reported sTNF-R1 was the stronger predictor of mortality.[69] These discrepancies emphasize the need for additional research before proinflammatory cytokine markers can be used clinically to manage patients with heart failure.

Uric Acid

Elevated levels of uric acid have been reported in patients with heart failure independent of factors such as diuretics and renal impairment that can affect blood levels. Cell death and tissue hypoxia activate xanthine oxidase. This enzyme converts purine to uric acid and stimulates the production of oxygen free radicals. Increased free radicals stimulate the production of proinflammatory cytokines. Thus, high uric acid levels reflect tissue hypoxia and the associated inflammatory process. A graded relationship between serum uric acid levels and survival has been demonstrated.[70] Survival rate decreased progressively as serum uric acid levels exceeded normal levels of 400 μmol/liter. For every 100-μmol increase in uric acid over 400 μmol/liter, the risk of death is estimated to increase by 53 percent. Because uric acid level is obtained easily, it has been suggested as a useful clinical marker to monitor therapies that improve metabolic and hemodynamic status.

C-Reactive Protein

In one prospective study of 76 patients admitted for heart failure treatment, there was a trend for CRP levels measured on admission to be higher with poorer New York Heart Association function classification. Patients with CPR levels greater than 0.9 mg/dl were readmitted up to 5 months sooner that patients with levels less than 0.9 mg/dl. The relative risk for readmission within 18 months in patients with CRP levels of 0.9 mg/dl or greater was 1.4. CRP levels exceeding 3.0 mg/dl carried a relative risk for readmission of 1.96. Additional larger studies controlling for multiple clinical factors are needed to determine the utility of CRP as a clinical marker in heart failure.

Therapeutic Interventions for Inflammation in Heart Failure

Given the important role TNF-α plays in mediating the inflammation associated with heart failure, blocking the activity of this cytokine is an attractive treatment option. Two large randomized controlled studies were conducted to test the effectiveness of using the drug etanercept as a treatment for heart failure.[71] Etanercept is a molecule that functionally resembles sTNF-R2 by binding TNF-α in the blood and tissues. Both trials were ended early because of lack of evidence of benefit. One reason for lack of benefit of etanercept in treatment of heart failure may be related to the functions of soluble receptors. At high concentrations, soluble TNF receptors bind TNF-α and function primarily to limit its activity. However, by binding to TNF-α, these receptors also stabilize its trimeric structure, preventing degradation. This effectively prolongs the half-life of TNF-α. By binding to TNF-α, etanercept actually may prolong rather than inhibit TNF-α activity. In another trial, infliximab, a monoclonal antibody that binds TNF-α in the circulation and TNF-α bound to membranes, was tested as an antiinflammatory therapy.[72] This trial also was ended early because of lack of demonstrated benefit. One reason suggested for failure to show benefit is that plasma levels of infliximab were much higher than expected for the dose provided. Another reason for lack of benefit for all drug trials is that TNF-α is only one component of the inflammatory cascade associated with heart failure. For antiinflammatory therapy to be effective it may require blocking multiple cytokines or other inflammatory mediators.

Statins

As noted in the section on atherosclerosis, statins possess antiinflammatory actions in addition to their anticholesterol activity. Statin therapy has been shown to decrease mortality in patients with preserved and nonpreserved systolic function.[73,74] Interestingly, doses of statins that produce antiinflammatory effects but do not lower cholesterol levels may be the most effective in heart failure.[52] Recall that patients with heart failure have elevated circulating levels of LPS, which is suspected of originating from gram-negative bacteria that translocate into the blood across the ischemic gut. Research has shown that circulating lipoproteins can bind LPS in the blood, preventing it from attaching to immune cells to stimulate TNF-α release. In this respect, higher lipoprotein levels may be beneficial for patients with heart failure because they limit LPS-stimulated TNF-α release.[75] Several studies have shown a positive relationship between high cholesterol levels and survival of patients with heart failure. The largest study of more than 1100 patients showed the highest survival in patients with cholesterol levels greater than 250 mg/dl.[74]

Angiotensin-Converting Enzyme (ACE) Inhibitors and Beta Blockers

ACE inhibitors and beta blockers have antiinflammatory actions in heart failure. They have indirect antiinflammatory effects by virtue of improving metabolic and hemodynamic function, which limits the systemic inflammation associated with poor tissue perfusion. As noted previously, ACE inhibitors also block angiotensin II stimulation of NF-κB, which subsequently limits gene transcription of TNF-α, IL-1β, IL-6, and other inflammatory mediators. The addition of beta blockers has been shown to decrease proinflammatory cytokine levels further in patients already optimized on ACE inhibitor, diuretic, and digoxin therapy. Evidence suggests that for ACE inhibitors and beta blockers, the antiinflammatory effects are due in part to blocking sympathetic nervous system effects on the immune system.[76]

SUMMARY

Inflammation is involved in the development of atherosclerosis, onset of acute coronary syndrome, recovery and remodeling of the myocardium following ischemic damage, and the development and progression of heart failure. In addition to local effects in the vascular epithelium and myocardium, inflammation has important systemic effects in heart failure that lead to development of cardiac cachexia. Given the pathological roles inflammation plays in a full spectrum of cardiac conditions, a considerable amount of research has been devoted to identifying markers of inflammation that indicate cardiovascular risk and treatments that target the inflammatory cascade. Several inflammatory markers have been identified as important indicators of cardiovascular risk. New inflammatory markers that allow earlier identification of patients at risk for cardiovascular diseases likely will be determined in the future. To date, no successful treatments that specifically target the inflammatory cascade have been developed for any cardiovascular condition. Because inflammation also plays important protective roles in the body, successful antiinflammatory treatments will need to bridge a fine line between allowing acute inflammatory responses that are protective while blocking chronic inflammatory responses associated with pathological cardiovascular conditions.

REFERENCES

1. Shishehbor MH, Bhatt DL: Inflammation and atherosclerosis, *Curr Atheroscler Rep* 6:131-139, 2004.
2. Spence JD, Norris J: Infection, inflammation, and atherosclerosis, *Stroke* 34:333-334, 2003.
3. Venugopal SK, Devaraj S, Jialal I: Macrophage conditioned medium induces the expression of C-reactive protein in human aortic endothelial cells: potential for paracrine/autocrine effects, *Am J Pathol* 166:1265-1271, 2005.
4. Haynes WG, Stanford C: Periodontal disease and atherosclerosis: from dental to arterial plaque, *Arterioscler Thromb Vasc Biol* 23:1309-1311, 2003.
5. Beck JD, Eke P, Heiss G et al: Periodontal disease and coronary heart disease: a reappraisal of the exposure, *Circulation* 112:19-24, 2005.
6. Danesh J, Collins R, Peto R: Chronic infections and coronary heart disease: is there a link? *Lancet* 350:430-436, 1997.
7. Arcari CM, Gaydos CA, Nieto FJ et al: Association between *Chlamydia pneumoniae* and acute myocardial infarction in young men in the United States military: the importance of timing of exposure measurement, *Clin Infect Dis* 40:1123-1130, 2005.
8. Eryol NK, Kilic H, Gul A et al: Are the high levels of cytomegalovirus antibodies a determinant in the development of coronary artery disease? *Int Heart J* 46:205-209, 2005.
9. Masoud SA, Arami MA, Kucheki E: Association between infection with *Helicobacter pylori* and cerebral noncardioembolic ischemic stroke, *Neurol India* 53:303-306, 2005; discussion, pp 306-307.
10. Smieja M, Gnarpe J, Lonn E et al: Multiple infections and subsequent cardiovascular events in the Heart Outcomes Prevention Evaluation (HOPE) Study, *Circulation* 107:251-257, 2003.
11. Langheinrich AC, Bohle RM: Atherosclerosis: humoral and cellular factors of inflammation, *Virchows Arch* 446:101-111, 2005.
12. Pelat M, Balligand JL: Statins and hypertension, *Semin Vasc Med* 4:367-375, 2004.
13. Larose E, Ganz P: Statins and endothelial dysfunction, *Semin Vasc Med* 4:333-346, 2004.
14. Li JJ, Chen JL: Inflammation may be a bridge connecting hypertension and atherosclerosis, *Med Hypotheses* 64:925-929, 2005.
15. Libby P, Ridker PM, Maseri A: Inflammation and atherosclerosis, *Circulation* 105:1135-1143, 2002.
16. Reckelhoff JF, Romero JC: Role of oxidative stress in angiotensin-induced hypertension, *Am J Physiol Regul Integr Comp Physiol* 284:R893-R912, 2003.
17. Hotamisligil GS, Arner P, Caro JF et al: Increased adipose tissue expression of tumor necrosis factor-alpha in human obesity and insulin resistance, *J Clin Invest* 95:2409-2415, 1995.
18. Purohit A, Ghilchik MW, Duncan L et al: Aromatase activity and interleukin-6 production by normal and malignant breast tissues, *J Clin Endocrinol Metab* 80:3052-3058, 1995.
19. Yudkin JS, Stehouwer CD, Emeis JJ, Coppack SW: C-reactive protein in healthy subjects: associations with obesity, insulin resistance, and endothelial dysfunction: a potential role for cytokines originating from adipose tissue? *Arterioscler Thromb Vasc Biol* 19:972-978, 1999.
20. Beutler B, Cerami A: The biology of cachectin/TNF—a primary mediator of the host response, *Annu Rev Immunol* 7:625-655, 1989.
21. Yudkin JS, Kumari M, Humphries SE, Mohamed-Ali V: Inflammation, obesity, stress and coronary heart disease: is interleukin-6 the link? *Atherosclerosis* 148:209-214, 2000.
22. Pearson TA, Mensah GA, Alexander RW et al: Markers of inflammation and cardiovascular disease: application to clinical and public health practice—a statement for healthcare professionals from the Centers for Disease Control and Prevention and the American Heart Association, *Circulation* 107:499-511, 2003.
23. Danesh J, Whincup P, Walker M et al: Low grade inflammation and coronary heart disease: prospective study and updated meta-analyses, *BMJ* 321:199-204, 2000.
24. Koenig W, Sund M, Frohlich M et al: C-Reactive protein, a sensitive marker of inflammation, predicts future risk of coronary heart disease in initially healthy middle-aged men: results from the MONICA (Monitoring Trends and Determinants in Cardiovascular Disease) Augsburg Cohort Study, 1984 to 1992, *Circulation* 99:237-242, 1999.
25. Ridker PM: High-sensitivity C-reactive protein: potential adjunct for global risk assessment in the primary prevention of cardiovascular disease, *Circulation* 103:1813-1818, 2001.
26. Ridker PM, Rifai N, Rose L et al: Comparison of C-reactive protein and low-density lipoprotein cholesterol levels in the prediction of first cardiovascular events, *N Engl J Med* 347:1557-1565, 2002.
27. Redberg RF, Rifai N, Gee L, Ridker PM: Lack of association of C-reactive protein and coronary calcium by electron beam computed tomography in postmenopausal women: implications for coronary artery disease screening, *J Am Coll Cardiol* 36:39-43, 2000.
28. Hunt ME, O'Malley PG, Vernalis MN et al: C-reactive protein is not associated with the presence or extent of calcified subclinical atherosclerosis, *Am Heart J* 141:206-210, 2001.
29. Dinarello CA: Biologic basis for interleukin-1 in disease, *Blood* 87:2095-2147, 1996.
30. Patti G, D'Ambrosio A, Dobrina A et al: Interleukin-1 receptor antagonist: a sensitive marker of instability in patients with coronary artery disease, *J Thromb Thrombolysis* 14:139-143, 2002.
31. Lind L: Circulating markers of inflammation and atherosclerosis, *Atherosclerosis* 169:203-214, 2003.
32. Pai JK, Pischon T, Ma J et al: Inflammatory markers and the risk of coronary heart disease in men and women, *N Engl J Med* 351:2599-2610, 2004.

33. Ridker PM, Hennekens CH, Roitman-Johnson B et al: Plasma concentration of soluble intercellular adhesion molecule 1 and risks of future myocardial infarction in apparently healthy men, *Lancet* 351:88-92, 1998.

34. Hwang SJ, Ballantyne CM, Sharrett AR et al: Circulating adhesion molecules VCAM-1, ICAM-1, and E-selectin in carotid atherosclerosis and incident coronary heart disease cases: the Atherosclerosis Risk In Communities (ARIC) study, *Circulation* 96:4219-4225, 1997.

35. Blankenberg S, Rupprecht HJ, Bickel C et al: Circulating cell adhesion molecules and death in patients with coronary artery disease, *Circulation* 104:1336-1342, 2001.

36. Ridker PM, Rifai N, Pfeffer MA et al: Inflammation, pravastatin, and the risk of coronary events after myocardial infarction in patients with average cholesterol levels—Cholesterol and Recurrent Events (CARE) Investigators, *Circulation* 98:839-844, 1998.

37. Schwartz GG, Olsson AG, Ezekowitz MD et al: Effects of atorvastatin on early recurrent ischemic events in acute coronary syndromes: the MIRACL study—a randomized controlled trial, *JAMA* 285:1711-1718, 2001.

38. Downs JR, Clearfield M, Weis S et al: Primary prevention of acute coronary events with lovastatin in men and women with average cholesterol levels: results of AFCAPS/TexCAPS—Air Force/Texas Coronary Atherosclerosis Prevention Study, *JAMA* 279:1615-1622, 1998.

39. Ridker PM, Cushman M, Stampfer MJ et al: Inflammation, aspirin, and the risk of cardiovascular disease in apparently healthy men, *N Engl J Med* 336:973-979, 1997.

40. Yusuf S, Sleight P, Pogue J et al: Effects of an angiotensin-converting-enzyme inhibitor, ramipril, on cardiovascular events in high-risk patients: the Heart Outcomes Prevention Evaluation Study Investigators, *N Engl J Med* 342:145-153, 2000.

41. Stone AF, Mendall MA, Kaski JC et al: Effect of treatment for *Chlamydia pneumoniae* and *Helicobacter pylori* on markers of inflammation and cardiac events in patients with acute coronary syndromes: South Thames Trial of Antibiotics in Myocardial Infarction and Unstable Angina (STAMINA), *Circulation* 106:1219-1223, 2002.

42. Nian M, Lee P, Khaper N, Liu P: Inflammatory cytokines and postmyocardial infarction remodeling, *Circ Res* 94:1543-1553, 2004.

43. Pimentel-Muinos FX, Seed B: Regulated commitment of TNF receptor signaling: a molecular switch for death or activation, *Immunity* 11:783-793, 1999.

44. Mayosi B, Kardos A, Davies C et al: Heterozygous disruption of SERCA2a is not associated with impairment of cardiac performance in man: implications for SERCA2a as a therapeutic target in heart failure, *Heart* 92:105-109, 2005.

45. Nakamura H, Umemoto S, Naik G et al: Induction of left ventricular remodeling and dysfunction in the recipient heart after donor heart myocardial infarction: new insights into the pathologic role of tumor necrosis factor-alpha from a novel heterotopic transplant-coronary ligation rat model, *J Am Coll Cardiol* 42:173-181, 2003.

46. Conraads VM, Bosmans JM, Vrints CJ: Chronic heart failure: an example of a systemic chronic inflammatory disease resulting in cachexia, *Int J Cardiol* 85:33-49, 2002.

47. Mann DL: Stress-activated cytokines and the heart: from adaptation to maladaptation, *Annu Rev Physiol* 65:81-101, 2003.

48. Levine B, Kalman J, Mayer L et al: Elevated circulating levels of tumor necrosis factor in severe chronic heart failure, *N Engl J Med* 323:236-241, 1990.

49. Mann DL: Activation of inflammatory mediators in heart failure. In Mann DL, editor: *Heart failure,* Philadelphia, 2004, WB Saunders.

50. Dinarello CA, Cannon JG, Wolff SM et al: Tumor necrosis factor (cachectin) is an endogenous pyrogen and induces production of interleukin 1, *J Exp Med* 163:1433-1450, 1986.

51. Le JM, Vilcek J: Interleukin 6: a multifunctional cytokine regulating immune reactions and the acute phase protein response, *Lab Invest* 61:588-602, 1989.

52. Michie HR, Manogue KR, Spriggs DR et al: Detection of circulating tumor necrosis factor after endotoxin administration, *N Engl J Med* 318:1481-1486, 1988.

53. Niebauer J, Volk HD, Kemp M et al: Endotoxin and immune activation in chronic heart failure: a prospective cohort study, *Lancet* 353:1838-1842, 1999.

54. Anker SD, Clark AL, Teixeira MM et al: Loss of bone mineral in patients with cachexia due to chronic heart failure, *Am J Cardiol* 83:612-615, 1999.

55. Steele IC, Nugent AM, Maguire S et al: Cytokine profile in chronic cardiac failure, *Eur J Clin Invest* 26:1018-1022, 1996.

56. Banks WA, Kastin AJ, Durham DA: Bidirectional transport of interleukin-1 alpha across the blood-brain barrier, *Brain Res Bull* 23:433-437, 1989.

57. Plata-Salaman CR: Cytokines and feeding, *Int J Obes Relat Metab Disord* 25(suppl 5):S48-S52, 2001.

58. Lennie TA: Anorexia in response to acute illness, *Heart Lung* 28:386-401, 1999.

59. Mitch WE, Goldberg AL: Mechanisms of muscle wasting: the role of the ubiquitin-proteasome pathway, *N Engl J Med* 335:1897-1905, 1996.

60. Sharma R, Anker SD: Cytokines, apoptosis and cachexia: the potential for TNF antagonism, *Int J Cardiol* 85:161-171, 2002.

61. Anker SD, Chua TP, Ponikowski P et al: Hormonal changes and catabolic/anabolic imbalance in chronic heart failure and their importance for cardiac cachexia, *Circulation* 96:526-534, 1997.

62. Dantzer R: Somatization: a psychoneuroimmune perspective, *Psychoneuroendocrinology* 30:947-952, 2005.

63. Asadullah K, Sterry W, Volk HD: Interleukin-10 therapy: review of a new approach, *Pharmacol Rev* 55:241-269, 2003.

64. Yamaoka M, Yamaguchi S, Okuyama M, Tomoike H: Anti-inflammatory cytokine profile in human heart failure: behavior of interleukin-10 in association with tumor necrosis factor-alpha, *Jpn Circ J* 63:951-956, 1999.

65. Aukrust P, Ueland T, Lien E et al: Cytokine network in congestive heart failure secondary to ischemic or idiopathic dilated cardiomyopathy, *Am J Cardiol* 83:376-382, 1999.

66. Stumpf C, Lehner C, Yilmaz A et al: Decrease of serum levels of the anti-inflammatory cytokine interleukin-10 in patients with advanced chronic heart failure, *Clin Sci (Lond)* 105:45-50, 2003.

67. MacGowan GA, Mann DL, Kormos RL et al: Circulating interleukin-6 in severe heart failure, *Am J Cardiol* 79:1128-1131, 1997.

68. Deswal A, Petersen NJ, Feldman AM et al: Cytokines and cytokine receptors in advanced heart failure: an analysis of the cytokine database from the Vesnarinone trial (VEST), *Circulation* 103:2055-2059, 2001.

69. Rauchhaus M, Doehner W, Francis DP et al: Plasma cytokine parameters and mortality in patients with chronic heart failure, *Circulation* 102:3060-3067, 2000.

70. Anker SD, Doehner W, Rauchhaus M et al: Uric acid and survival in chronic heart failure: validation and application in metabolic, functional, and hemodynamic staging, *Circulation* 107:1991-1997, 2003.

71. Anker SD, Coats AJ: How to RECOVER from RENAISSANCE? The significance of the results of RECOVER, RENAISSANCE, RENEWAL and ATTACH, *Int J Cardiol* 86:123-130, 2002.

72. Chung ES, Packer M, Lo KH et al: Randomized, double-blind, placebo-controlled, pilot trial of infliximab, a chimeric monoclonal antibody to tumor necrosis factor-alpha, in patients with moderate-to-severe heart failure: results of the anti-TNF Therapy Against Congestive Heart Failure (ATTACH) trial, *Circulation* 107:3133-3140, 2003.

73. Fukuta H, Sane DC, Brucks S, Little WC: Statin therapy may be associated with lower mortality in patients with diastolic heart failure: a preliminary report, *Circulation* 112:357-363, 2005.

74. Horwich TB, MacLellan WR, Fonarow GC: Statin therapy is associated with improved survival in ischemic and non-ischemic heart failure, *J Am Coll Cardiol* 43:642-648, 2004.

75. Rauchhaus M, Coats AJS, Anker SD: The endotoxin-lipoprotein hypothesis, *Lancet* 356:930-933, 2000.

76. Gage JR, Fonarow G, Hamilton M et al: Beta blocker and angiotensin-converting enzyme inhibitor therapy is associated with decreased Th1/Th2 cytokine ratios and inflammatory cytokine production in patients with chronic heart failure, *Neuroimmunomodulation* 11:173-180, 2004.

chapter 10

Pathogenesis of Atherosclerosis

Karen Badellino

CHAPTER ABBREVIATIONS

aa amino acid

ABCA1 ATP-binding cassette protein A1

ACAT acyl CoA:cholesterol acyltransferase

APO apolipoprotein

ATP adenosine triphosphate

DGAT diacylglycerol acyltransferase

HDL high-density lipoprotein

HMG-CoA hydroxymethylglutaryl-coenzyme A

IDL intermediate-density lipoprotein

LDL low-density lipoprotein

LRP LDL receptor-related protein

MCP-1 monocyte chemoattractant protein-1

M-CSF macrophage colony-stimulating factor

MMP matrix metalloproteinase

NPC1L1 Niemann-Pick C1 Like 1 protein

PAF-AH platelet-activating factor acetylhydrolase

PDGF platelet-derived growth factor

PG proteoglycan

PPAR peroxisome proliferator-activated receptor

RNA ribonucleic acid

ROS reactive oxygen species

SREBP sterol-responsive element binding proteins

VLDL very low-density lipoprotein

Occlusive vascular disease is one of the most common causes of morbidity and mortality in developed countries. Atherosclerosis is the term applied to the pathophysiological process underlying the development of occlusive disease of the cerebral, coronary, and peripheral vasculature. Atherosclerosis increasingly is recognized as a chronic inflammatory process, a response to injury of the arterial intima initiated by deposition of cholesterol and lipids. Diets high in saturated fat, sedentary lifestyles, genetics, and environmental influences combine to promote lipid deposition in the walls of elastic arteries (aorta, iliac, and carotid), and medium-sized muscular arteries (coronary and popliteal). The process begins in the 1st decade of life, generally becoming symptomatic in the 5th decade and later. The risk of clinically symptomatic atherosclerosis is likely to be the result of genetic predisposition responding to environmental factors.

Nurses interact daily with patients who have risk factors for atherosclerosis but no overt disease. A thorough understanding of the pathological process can provide the foundation for counseling patients to modify their risk. With ever greater frequency, nurses provide care for those being treated with pharmaceutical agents and dietary supplements for hypertriglyceridemia and hypercholesterolemia. Many of these agents target specific parts of cholesterol and lipid synthesis and degradation pathways. Other strategies for prevention and treatment address the inflammatory and procoagulant processes that lead to arterial occlusion.

This chapter addresses the elements of the pathogenesis of atherosclerosis: increased plasma cholesterol leading to intimal lipid deposition and inflammation. To understand the alterations responsible for elevations in plasma cholesterol, it is necessary to review what currently is known about lipid metabolism and lipid transport between the intestine, the liver, and the periphery. This includes a discussion of the process by which elevated plasma cholesterol results in the initiation and progression of atherosclerotic lesions in the vessel wall. Throughout this chapter, the influence of the more established genetic abnormalities on lipid metabolism and the development of atherosclerosis are addressed.

INCREASED PLASMA CHOLESTEROL: PRIMARY CAUSE OF ATHEROSCLEROSIS

Histological examination of an atherosclerotic plaque reveals a complex lesion containing a lipid core surrounded by macrophages, T lymphocytes, and smooth muscle cells. Early lesions are primarily lipid-filled macrophages, also known as foam cells. Advanced lesions may show layers of fibrotic tissue and calcification, perhaps with an associated thrombosis. The composition of these lesions suggests that cholesterol may be central to their development.

Numerous investigators have demonstrated a strong positive correlation between low-density lipoprotein (**LDL**) cholesterol levels and atherosclerosis. The Framingham study reported a strong inverse relationship between high-density lipoprotein (**HDL**) levels and development of the disease. The reason for the different effects of the two types of lipoprotein has been the focus of intense investigation over the last 25 years.

Cholesterol circulates in plasma in association with triglycerides, phospholipids, apolipoproteins (lipid-binding proteins), and other proteins, organized into particles called lipoproteins. Lipoproteins can be classified according to size, density, and associated apolipoproteins. As shown in Figure 10-1, the major classifications are chylomicrons, very low-density lipoproteins (**VLDLs**), intermediate-density lipoproteins (**IDLs**), LDLs, and HDLs. Lipoproteins also are characterized based on their major associated apolipoproteins and lipid content (Table 10-1).[1-4]

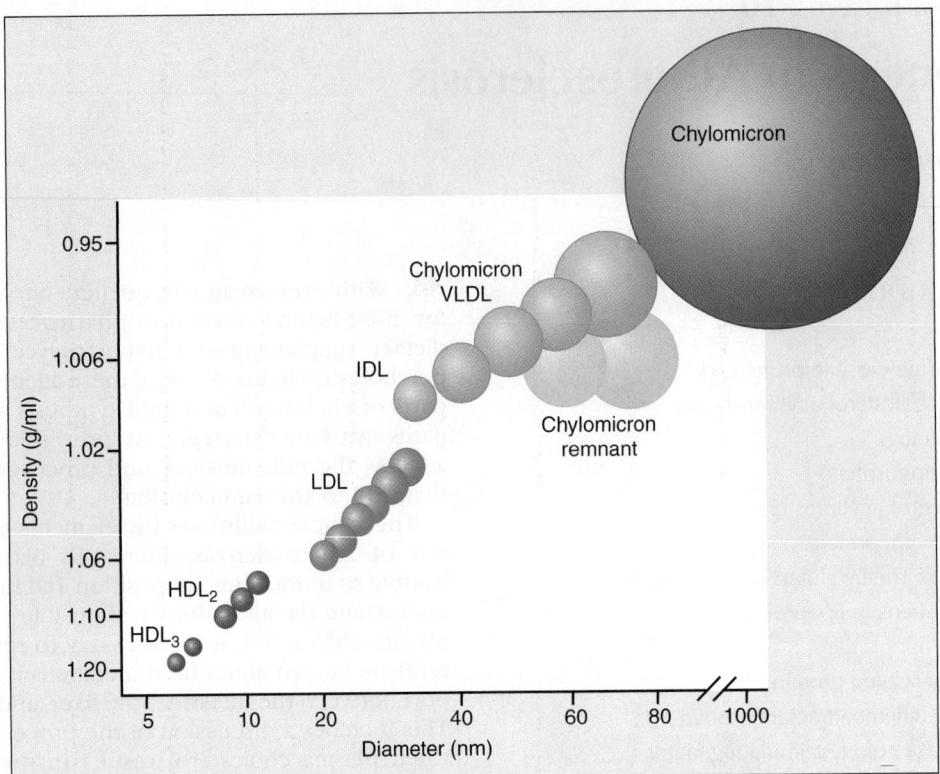

FIGURE 10-1 ■ Lipoproteins can be classified according to size, density, lipid content, and associated apolipoproteins. As density increases, size decreases and the percentage of protein content increases. Low-density lipoprotein (LDL) is the primary carrier of cholesterol in the plasma compartment. High-density lipoprotein (HDL) has an inverse relationship with the incidence of atherosclerosis. *IDL,* Intermediate-density lipoprotein; *VLDL,* very low-density lipoprotein. (From Zipes DP, Libby P, Bonow RO, Braunwald E: *Braunwald's heart disease,* ed 7, Philadelphia, 2005, Elsevier Saunders.)

■ ■ ■

TABLE 10-1   PROTEIN AND LIPID CONTENT OF LIPOPROTEINS

APOLIPOPROTEIN/ LIPID	PLASMA CONCENTRATION (mg/dl)	HDL (%)	LDL (%)	IDL (%)	VLDL (%)	TISSUE SOURCE
APO A-1*	130	6				Liver, intestine
		4				Liver
APO A-II	40	2				Liver
		0				
APO A-IV	—					Liver
APO B-48	—					Intestine
APO B-100*	80		95	63	36	Liver
APO C-I	6	6		1	3	Liver
APO C-II	3	1		4	7	Liver
APO C-III	12	4		15	40	Liver
APO D	10	3		—	—	Liver
APO E	5	2	Less than 5	14	13	Liver, plasma, vascular cells
Cholesteryl ester	250					Liver, plasma, vascular cells
Phospholipid	230					Liver, intestine
Triglyceride	140					Liver, diet

*Although APO A-I is found exclusively on high-density lipoprotein particles, APO B-100 is solely a low-density lipoprotein.
APO, Apolipoprotein; *HDL,* high-density lipoprotein; *IDL,* intermediate-density lipoprotein; *LDL,* low-density lipoprotein; *VLDL,* very low-density lipoprotein.
Data from Plasma lipoproteins: structure, nomenclature and occurrence. In Gotto A, Pownall H: Manual of lipid disorders, 2003, Philadelphia, Lippincott Williams and Wilkins.

The structures of triglyceride, phospholipids, and cholesterol are shown in Figure 10-2. Triglyceride and phospholipid differ in the replacement of a fatty acid with a phosphatidyl acylamine. A phosphatidyl acylamine introduces a charge on the phospholipid, making it partially water soluble. Apolipoproteins have hydrophobic, lipid-binding regions and hydrophilic regions capable of interacting with the surrounding plasma. With these properties, apolipoproteins stabilize the lipoprotein particle and mediate cell-surface binding, lipid transfer, and lipid hydrolysis.[5]

Lipoproteins containing apolipoprotein B-100 and apolipoprotein B-48, VLDL, IDL (remnant particles), and LDL are considered atherogenic. Lipoproteins con-

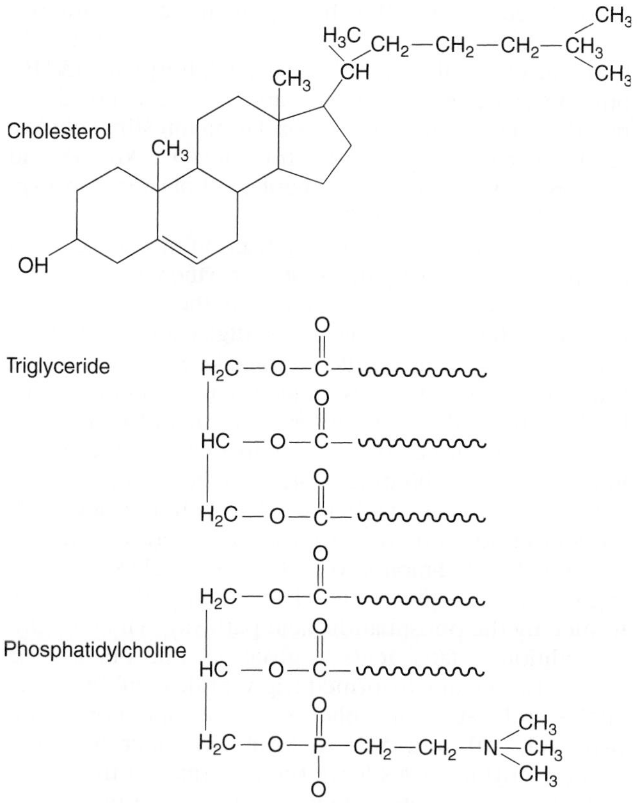

FIGURE 10-2 ■ Lipoproteins contain a central core of cholesteryl ester and triglyceride surrounded by phospholipids and smaller amounts of free cholesterol. The structures of cholesterol, triglyceride, and phospholipids are shown.

taining apolipoprotein A-I, HDL usually are considered protective. As is discussed in some detail later, these different effects are related to the cell-surface receptors with which the two classes of lipoproteins interact and to the proteins associated with them. The relative amounts of each type of lipoprotein in plasma are a result of the balance between production and clearance from the circulation through receptor- and non–receptor-related processes.

Production of the lipids and apolipoproteins in lipoproteins is a complex process involving control over the transcription of genes encoding the apolipoproteins, lipolytic enzymes, transfer proteins, and cell-surface receptors, as well as the activity of these various proteins toward the different lipid molecules. A brief review of these processes follows.

SOURCES OF CHOLESTEROL AND SYNTHESIS OF LIPIDS

The two sources of plasma fat and cholesterol are intestinal absorption of ingested lipids and hepatic synthesis. The levels of cholesterol and triglyceride are controlled in the body, such that a decrease in dietary fat intake results in an increase in de novo synthesis of triglyceride and cholesterol by the liver. Specific pathways also exist for clearance of excess cholesterol through bile synthesis and receptor- and non–receptor-mediated lipoprotein clearance in the liver.

Intestinal cholesterol absorption is a relatively slow process that occurs mainly in the jejunum. The probable receptor, Niemann-Pick C1 Like 1 protein (**NPC1L1**), mediates the majority of cholesterol absorption and is located mainly in the proximal jejunum.[6] A new pharmaceutical agent, ezetimibe, significantly decreases dietary cholesterol absorption, although the nature of its interaction with NPC1L1 has not been characterized. Pharmaceutical agents that modify absorption and production of cholesterol and triglycerides are summarized in the accompanying Pharmacology feature, *Agents Used to Treat Dyslipidemia.*

■ ■ ■ PHARMACOLOGY

AGENTS USED TO TREAT DYSLIPIDEMIA

CLASSIFICATION	AGENT	MECHANISM OF ACTION
Bile acid sequestrant	Colesevelam	Decreases bile acid reabsorption Increases cholesterol 7α hydroxylase expression and bile synthesis Increases HMG-CoA reductase and LDL receptor expression
Cholesterol absorption inhibitor	Ezetimibe	Decreases cholesterol absorption, in conjunction with statins
Fibric acid derivative	Fenofibrate, gemfibrozil	Activates peroxisome proliferator-activated receptor-alpha, resulting in increased lipoprotein lipase and APO A-I expression Decreases APO C-III expression Produces decreased LDL Increases high-density lipoprotein
HMG-CoA reductase inhibitor	Atorvastatin, fluvastatin, lovastatin, pravastatin, rosuvastatin, simvastatin	Blocks hepatic cholesterol synthesis
Niacin	Niaspan (brand)	Increases expression of hepatic LDL receptor Reduces hepatic triglyceride synthesis Increases APO B degradation Decreases LDL Decreases clearance of APO A-I
Thiazolidinedione	Pioglitazone, rosiglitazone	Adipogenesis Improves insulin sensitivity because of increased glucose transporter 4 expression

APO, Apolipoprotein; *HMG-CoA,* hydroxymethylglutaryl coenzyme A; *LDL,* low-density lipoprotein.

In a typical Western diet, about 1800 mg of cholesterol enters the small intestine daily, 300 to 500 mg of which is derived from the diet, the rest from bile acids and sloughed mucosal cells. About 50 percent of the total cholesterol is absorbed,[7] where it subsequently is esterified to cholesterol ester through the addition of a fatty acid, coenzyme A (CoA) by acyl CoA:cholesterol acyltransferase (**ACAT**). Subsequently, this cholesterol

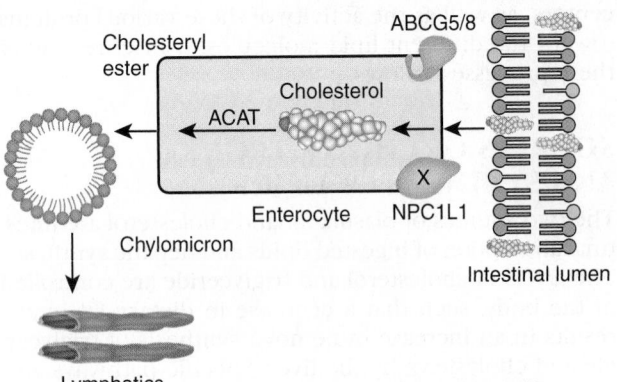

FIGURE 10-3 ▪ Intestinal cholesterol absorption most likely occurs through the Niemann-Pick C1 Like 1 protein (NPC1L1) located in the proximal jejunum. The pharmaceutical agent ezetimibe blocks cholesterol absorption by interacting with this receptor. *ABCG,* ATP-binding cassette protein G5/8; *ACAT,* acyl CoA: cholesterol acyltransferase; *NPC1L1,* Niemann-Pick Like1 protein.

ester is combined with other lipids into a chylomicron (Figure 10-3). Recently, two new members of a lipid transporter family, the adenosine triphosphate (**ATP**)-binding cassette transporter family, have been identified that may be involved in regulating intestinal cholesterol absorption. These two transporters, ABCG5 and ABCG8, may cooperatively regulate cholesterol absorption and bile excretion.[8,9]

Dietary triglyceride is catabolized to monoglycerides and free fatty acids by the action of pancreatic lipase in the small intestine. Bile salts emulsify the phospholipids, free cholesterol, monoglycerides, diglycerides, and fatty acids into a structure called a micelle. Because of their low water solubility, these micelles are absorbed easily by the intestinal brush border. Long-chain free fatty acids are transported to the smooth endoplasmic reticulum by fatty acid binding proteins, where they are acylated by acyl CoA synthetase. Through the action of monoglyceride and diglyceride acyltransferases, they are combined with 2-monoglycerol to form diglycerides and triglycerides, respectively. Triglyceride also can be formed by the phosphatidic acid pathway, which begins by addition of fatty acids to glycerol-3-phosphate[5] (Figure 10-4). The newly formed triglyceride combines with cholesterol ester, phospholipids, and apolipoproteins B-48, A-I, A-II, and A-IV to form chylomicrons. Once formed, chylomicrons leave the intestine via the lymph and enter the venous system through the thoracic duct.

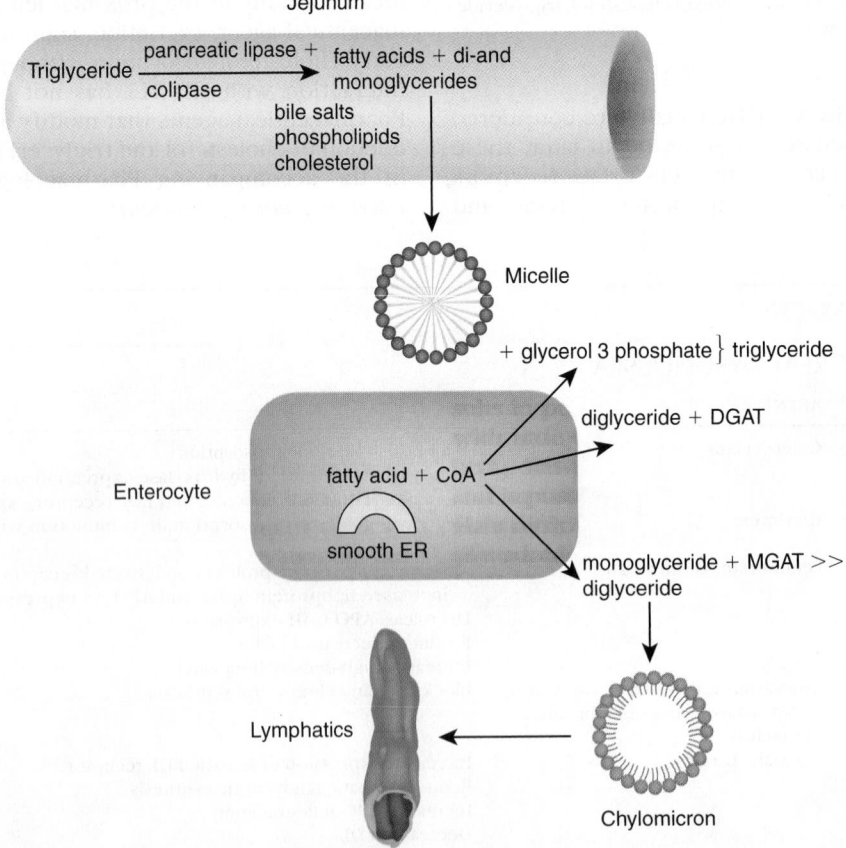

FIGURE 10-4 ▪ Digestion of triglyceride in the small intestine by pancreatic lipase results in production of free fatty acids, monoglycerides, and diglycerides. Because of their lipid solubililty, they are absorbed easily into the enterocyte. Triglyceride is resynthesized and then combines with phospholipids and apolipoproteins to form chylomicrons. *CoA,* Coenzyme A; *DGAT,* diacylglycerol acyltransferase; *ER,* endoplasmic reticulum; *MGAT,* monoacylglycerol acyltransferase.

When intestinal sources of triglyceride are absent, the liver can synthesize fatty acid from glucose. Glucose is converted to acetyl CoA by the citrate lyase reaction and from amino acids, which also are converted to acetyl CoA. Acetyl CoA is the substrate used by fatty acid synthase ultimately to produce palmitate, a 16-carbon saturated fatty acid. Palmitate can be elongated and desaturated to produce a variety of fatty acids that subsequently are incorporated into triglycerides and phospholipids

Triglyceride is formed in the liver by the glycerol phosphate pathway (Figure 10-5). Two fatty acyl CoA molecules combine with glycerol-3-phosphate to form phosphatidic acid. The phosphate group is hydrolyzed, forming diacylglycerol. A third fatty acid is added by the action of acyl CoA: diacylglycerol acyltransferase (**DGAT**). The enzymatic activity of DGAT is found in two proteins from different families: DGAT1 and DGAT2.[10] DGAT also is found at high levels in adipocytes and all cell types using triglyceride for cellular needs. Genetic studies investigating the relevance of DGAT1 and DGAT2 to plasma lipid levels are relatively few. DGAT is, along with other lipid-hydrolyzing and transfer proteins, a potential target for pharmacological modification (Table 10-2).

Like cholesterol, phospholipids are essential components of the membranes of all cells. They are also surface elements of all lipoproteins because of the hydrophobic (not water soluble) fatty acids and the charged phosphate group on their side chain, which interacts with the surrounding plasma. When fatty acid concentrations are low, phospholipids are produced through the transfer of cytidine 5′ diphosphate-choline or 5′ diphosphate-ethanolamine to the diacylglycerol formed from phosphatidic acid.

Cholesterol also is formed in the liver from acetyl CoA derived from glucose and amino acids. Two molecules of acetyl CoA combine to form acetoacetyl CoA, which condenses with another acetyl CoA to form hydroxymethylglutaryl CoA (**HMG-CoA**). This molecule is reduced to mevalonic acid by HMG-CoA reductase. Mevalonic acid is phosphorylated and decarboxylated to form a five-carbon structure called isopentenyl phosphate. Three C-5 units eventually condense to form a structure called lanosterol, which becomes cholesterol after a series of enzymatic steps (Figure 10-6). The statin drugs specifically inhibit cholesterol synthesis by inhibiting HMG-CoA reductase. (See the Pharmacology feature, *Agents Used to Treat Dyslipidemia*.)

Newly formed cholesterol can be incorporated into a lipoprotein for secretion. Cholesterol added to apolipoprotein B–containing lipoproteins in the liver is esterified by addition of a fatty acid to the hydroxyl group through the action of ACAT. Similar to DGAT, there are two ACAT enzymes encoded by separate genes. ACAT2 is present in the lumen of the endoplasmic reticulum, where it contributes cholesterol to newly formed VLDL. ACAT1 is present on the cytoplasmic side of the endoplasmic reticulum in macrophages, where it promotes cholesterol storage.[11,12] ACATs and DGAT are potential targets for pharmacological inhibition as well.[10,13]

Lipid synthesis is controlled on the genetic and the protein level (Figure 10-7). Sterol-responsive element binding proteins (**SREBPs**) regulate a number of enzymes involved in fatty acid and cholesterol synthesis, as well as the LDL receptor. SREBP-2 regulates cholesterol synthesis. In the absence of cholesterol, a protein called SREBP cleavage-activating protein (SCAP) mediates the action of an enzyme, PCSK9, which cleaves SREBP-2.[14] The cleavage product migrates to the cell nucleus and increases the transcription of genes involved in cholesterol homeostasis.[15] Two other SREBPs, SREBP-1a and SREBP-1c, regulate enzymes involved in fatty acid metabolism.[16] They are responsive to insulin and to saturated fatty acids. Oleic acid (olive oil) downregulates SREBP-1 and SREBP-2, whereas fish oil down-

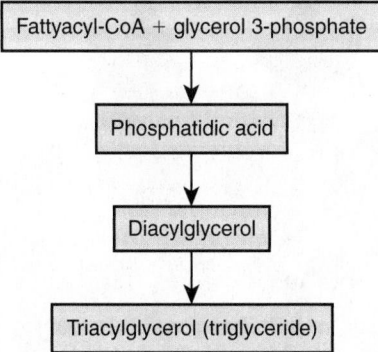

FIGURE 10-5 ■ Triglyceride is synthesized in the liver from two fatty acids that combine with glycerol-3-phosphate. The product, phosphatidic acid, undergoes hydrolysis of its phosphate group, resulting in formation of diacylglycerol. A third fatty acid is added to form triglyceride.

TABLE 10-2   PHARMACOLOGICAL TARGETS UNDER INVESTIGATION*

PHYSIOLOGICAL TARGET	ACTION	EFFECT OF INHIBITION (I) OR UPREGULATION (U)
Acyl CoA acyltransferase	Esterification of cholesterol	I—increased bile secretion, decreased plasma cholesterol
Diacylglycerol acyl transferase	Triglyceride synthesis	I—decreased plasma triglycerides, decreased APO B and APO B–containing lipoproteins
Microsomal transfer protein	Triglyceride synthesis	I—decreased plasma triglycerides, decreased APO B and APO B–containing lipoproteins
ABCA1	Excretion of cholesterol from macrophages in the vessel wall	U—increased HDL levels, promotion of reverse cholesterol transport and lesion regression
Recombinant APO A-I Milano	Increase HDL synthesis	U—increased HDL levels, increased reverse cholesterol transport and antiinflammatory properties of HDL
APO A-I mimetic peptides	Increase synthesis of lipid-poor APO A-I discs	U—increased reverse cholesterol transport

*Agents that modulate many enzymes involved in the synthesis and modification of lipids are being tested in animal models or human clinical trials. The agents listed are under consideration or are being studied actively in human beings.
APO, Apolipoprotein; *ABCA1*, ATP-binding cassette transporter A1; *HDL*, high-density lipoprotein.

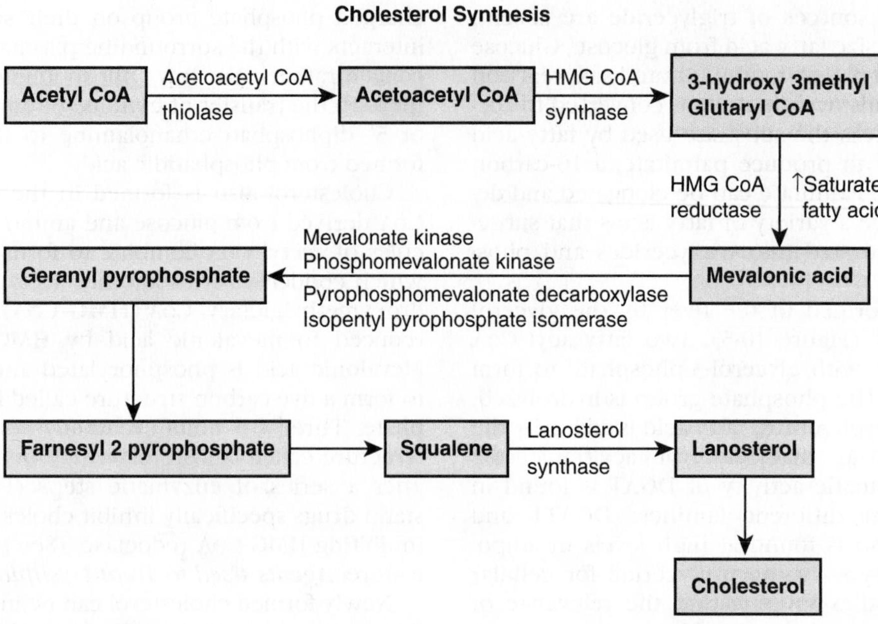

Cholesterol Synthesis

Acetyl CoA →[Acetoacetyl CoA thiolase]→ Acetoacetyl CoA →[HMG CoA synthase]→ 3-hydroxy 3methyl Glutaryl CoA

3-hydroxy 3methyl Glutaryl CoA →[HMG CoA reductase] [↑Saturated fatty acids]→ Mevalonic acid

Mevalonic acid →[Mevalonate kinase / Phosphomevalonate kinase / Pyrophosphomevalonate decarboxylase / Isopentyl pyrophosphate isomerase]→ Geranyl pyrophosphate

Geranyl pyrophosphate → Farnesyl 2 pyrophosphate → Squalene →[Lanosterol synthase]→ Lanosterol → Cholesterol

FIGURE 10-6 ■ Cholesterol is formed in the liver from the combination of molecules of acetyl coenzyme A. The rate-limiting step in this reaction is hydroxymethylglutaryl (HMG) CoA reductase, an enzyme that is inhibited by the statin drugs.

regulates SREBP-1. This is one mechanism by which dietary lipid intake can modulate cholesterol and triglyceride levels.

In the presence of excess cholesterol, the cell can downregulate cholesterol synthesis and increase cholesterol esterification. Similarly, the cell can increase the removal of cholesterol by increasing the synthesis of a protein called ATP-binding cassette protein A1 (**ABCA1**). ABCA1 synthesis is increased by 22-OH cholesterol stimulation of a nuclear receptor called LXR.[17] Pharmaceutical agents capable of stimulating increased ABCA1 synthesis are currently under investigation.

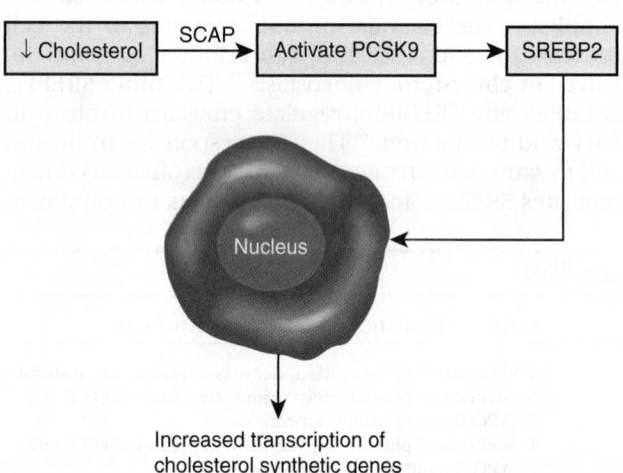

↓ Cholesterol →[SCAP]→ Activate PCSK9 → SREBP2 → Nucleus → Increased transcription of cholesterol synthetic genes

FIGURE 10-7 ■ Cholesterol synthesis is under the control of proteins called sterol responsive element binding proteins (SREBPs). With low cholesterol concentrations, a protein called SREBP cleavage-activating protein (SCAP) activates an enzyme, proprotein convertase subtilsin/kexin type 9 (PCSK9), that subsequently cleaves and activates SREBP-2. SREBP-2 migrates to the nucleus and increases transcription of genes involved in cholesterol synthesis.

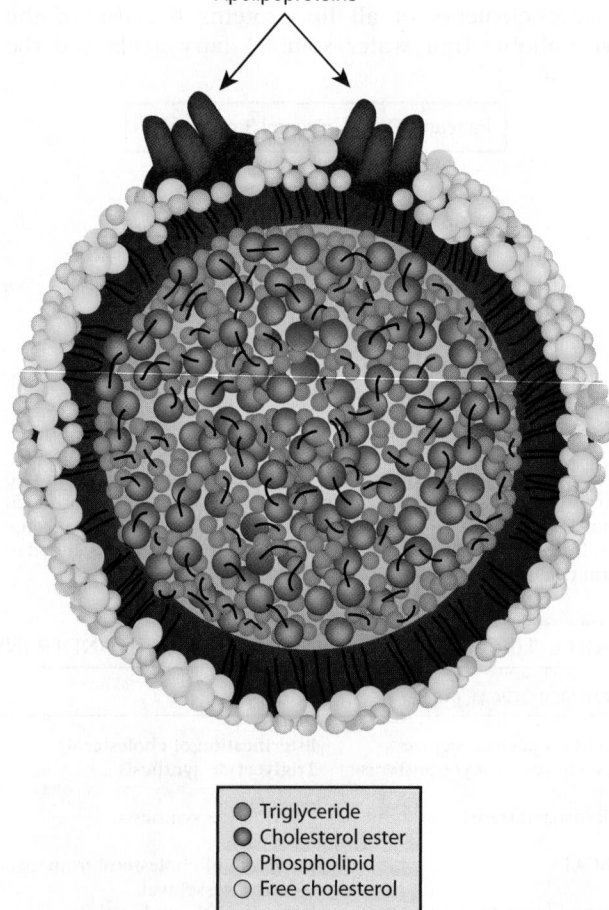

Apolipoproteins

- ● Triglyceride
- ● Cholesterol ester
- ○ Phospholipid
- ○ Free cholesterol

FIGURE 10-8 ■ Lipoprotein particles contain a core of the neutral lipids: triglyceride and cholesteryl ester. Surrounding the core are phospholipids, free cholesterol, apolipoproteins, and other associated proteins. (Modified from a figure courtesy Daniel Rader, MD.)

LIPOPROTEIN FORMATION

The formation of a nascent lipoprotein requires the presence of apolipoproteins to which the lipids bind, resulting in a complex spherical particle. The core of a lipoprotein contains neutral lipids, i.e., triglyceride and cholesterol ester (Figure 10-8). The core is surrounded by phospholipids and proteins. The triglyceride-rich particle formed in the liver is VLDL. VLDL is formed by the fusion of two particles. One particle is formed by addition of triglyceride as its primary apolipoprotein, apolipoprotein B-100 (**APO** B-100), is being synthesized on the rough endoplasmic reticulum, and the other is formed from cholesterol and triglyceride in the smooth endoplasmic reticulum. The newly formed VLDL is released into the space of Disse and migrates through the sinusoids into the bloodstream.[18-20]

The creation of the lipid droplets included in VLDL requires microsomal transfer protein, the absence of which causes a disease known as abetalipoproteinemia. Addition of triglyceride to the developing APO B molecule is essential to the proper folding of the protein. In the absence of microsomal transfer protein, the APO B molecule is degraded and the VLDL particle is not secreted.[21] For homozygous persons, this results in failure to thrive because of deficiencies in fat-soluble vitamins. Heterozygous persons have low levels of LDL cholesterol and are free from atherosclerosis. Inhibition of microsomal transfer protein is under investigation as a means of treating the most severe cases of hypercholesterolemia.[22]

APO B is essential to the formation of VLDL particles and remains the structurally important apolipoprotein on LDL. APO B is a protein, with 4536 amino acids known as APO B-100, when expressed in the liver. In the intestine a unique messenger **RNA** (ribonucleic acid) editing machinery, APO B mRNA editing enzyme catalytic complex 1 (apobec-1), introduces a stop codon, thus truncating the protein to 48 percent of the total length.[19] Apo B-48 lacks the receptor-binding domain located on the carboxyterminus of APO B-100.

The formation of HDL particles is not as well characterized. Through the process of reverse cholesterol transport (Figure 10-9), HDL particles represent the primary means by which the cells of the body rid themselves of excess cholesterol. The majority of APO A-I is produced by the liver with small amounts also produced by the intestine. Nascent HDL particles, APO A-I with small amounts of associated triglyceride, are released from the liver.[23] These lipid-poor small HDL particles bind to a receptor called ATP-binding cassette transporter A1 (ABCA1), which mediates cholesterol transfer to HDL.[24] Through the action of lecithin:cholesterol acyltransferase,[25] cholesterol ester transfer protein,[26] and phospholipid transfer protein,[27] HDL enlarges and matures. Lecithin:cholesterol acyltransferase is an enzyme that hydrolyzes the fatty acid from phosphatidylcholine and transfers that fatty acid to cholesterol

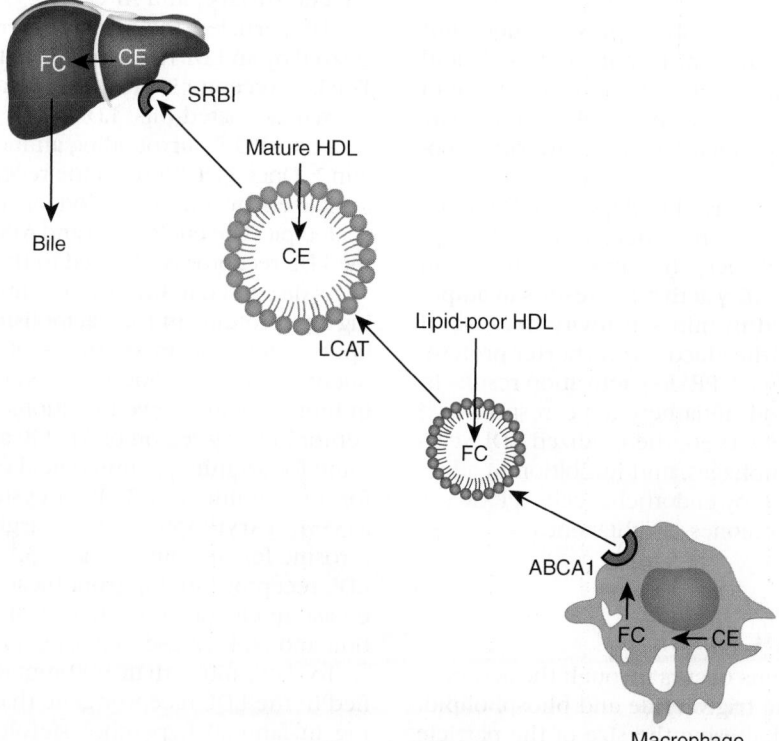

FIGURE 10-9 ■ Lipid-poor apolipoprotein A-I particles bind to ATP-binding cassette protein A1 (ABCA1) in the macrophage. ABCA1 transports free cholesterol (FC) out of the cell to the apolipoprotein A-I particle. Through the action of lecithin:cholesterol acyltransferase, the cholesterol is esterified. The high-density lipoprotein (HDL) particle matures, obtaining triglyceride from low-density lipoprotein (LDL) and very low-density lipoprotein (VLDL), mediated by cholesterol ester (CE) transfer protein and phospholipids, mediated by phospholipid transfer protein. The HDL particle can bind to the SR-B1 receptor on the liver, thus returning cholesterol for excretion. *LCAT,* Lecithin cholesterol acyltransferase.

where it is esterified.[24] Cholesterol ester transfer protein carries the cholesterol ester to LDL and VLDL in exchange for triglyceride.[25] Phospholipid transfer protein mediates the transfer of phospholipids from chylomicron and VLDL remnants to HDL.[26] Deficiencies of either ABCA1[28,29] or phospholipid transfer protein are associated with HDL deficiencies.

ROLE OF PEROXISOME PROLIFERATOR-ACTIVATED RECEPTORS IN LIPID METABOLISM

Peroxisome proliferator-activated receptors (**PPAR**s) are transcription factors belonging to the superfamily of nuclear receptors.[30] As transcription factors, they regulate expression of a number of proteins involved in lipid and glucose metabolism. They can be activated by fatty acids and their derivatives and by the pharmacological agents, fibrates, and glitazones. Three distinct subtypes have been identified: alpha, beta/delta, and gamma.[31] PPAR-α is expressed in liver, kidney, skeletal muscle, heart, and all the cell types active in the atherosclerotic lesion: endothelial cells, smooth muscle cells, macrophages, and lymphocytes. PPAR-α regulates beta-oxidation of fatty acids, increases expression of lipoprotein lipase, decreases expression of its inhibitor, APO C-II, and increases expression of APO A-I and ABCA1. The effects of PPAR-α activation include decreased plasma triglycerides, increased reverse cholesterol transport, and antiinflammatory effects in the arterial wall. PPAR-α is activated by fibrates.

PPAR-β, although ubiquitously expressed, does not have a clearly defined function. In animal models and cell culture systems, it has been shown to have a role in lipid metabolism, inflammation, and fertility, and it may be involved in the development of gastrointestinal neoplasia.

PPAR-γ has two isoforms: PPAR-γ2 and PPAR-γ3. PPAR-γ2 is expressed solely in adipose tissue. PPAR-γ3 is expressed in macrophages, the large intestine, and white adipose tissue. PPAR-γ activation results in adipogenesis and in improved insulin sensitivity because of increased expression of the glucose transporter protein, GLUT4. In the vascular wall, PPAR-γ activation results in both proatherogenic and antiatherogenic responses.[32] There is upregulation of CD 36, the oxidized LDL scavenger receptor in macrophages, and inhibition of adhesive molecule expression by endothelial cells. PPAR-γ is activated by thiazolidinediones, or glitazones.

LIPOPROTEIN CATABOLISM AND CHOLESTEROL CLEARANCE

Catabolism of lipoproteins occurs through the action of enzymes that cleave the triglyceride and phospholipid, releasing fatty acid and altering the size of the particle and promoting changes in its composition. These lipases are members of the triglyceride lipase enzyme family, which includes pancreatic lipase. Lipoprotein lipase, hepatic lipase, and endothelial lipase are found on the vascular endothelium, bound to proteoglycans. Lipoprotein lipase is produced by skeletal and cardiac muscle, adipocytes, and macrophages. Its hydrolysis of triglycerides releases fatty acids that are used for energy or storage in adipocytes.[33,34] In contrast to lipoprotein lipase, hepatic lipase is found mainly in the liver,[35] and endothelial lipase is found in liver, lung, steroidogenic tissues such as the adrenal gland, and in endothelial cells, including vessels in the heart.[36] Each enzyme also has differences in activity. Lipoprotein lipase hydrolyzes triglycerides. Hepatic lipase hydrolyzes triglycerides but has some activity in hydrolyzing phospholipids. Endothelial lipase, with some triglyceride hydrolase activity, is primarily a phospholipase. This suggests that each enzyme has a distinct physiological role in the metabolism of lipoproteins.

After a meal, chylomicrons enter the bloodstream through the thoracic duct. On entering the circulation, the triglycerides in these particles are hydrolyzed by lipoprotein lipase. Chylomicron remnant particles bind through an APO E–mediated process to a chylomicron remnant receptor in the liver and are thus cleared from circulation.[5]

VLDL particles are cleared through a similar process via a VLDL receptor. VLDL also is hydrolyzed by lipoprotein lipase to a VLDL remnant, IDL. IDL loses its C apolipoproteins and acquires APO E. IDL can be cleaved further by hepatic lipase in the liver, to form an LDL particle, or can be cleared via two different receptors, a remnant receptor or the LDL receptor-related protein (**LRP**). Binding to LRP is mediated through proteoglycans, such as heparan sulfate proteoglycans, present on the cell surface, and APO E.

LDL particles, the primary carriers of cholesterol, are cleared by an LDL receptor present on the surface of cells. The LDL receptor is present in areas of the cell membrane known as coated pits. LDL binds to the receptor via an area on APO B surrounding amino acid 3500 on the protein.[37] Once LDL binds to the receptor, the complex is internalized by the formation of an endosome from the coated pit. The cholesterol and APO B are hydrolyzed, and the LDL receptor is recycled to the cell membrane.

As discussed in Chapter 13, mutations in genes encoding key proteins in the catabolism of APO B–containing lipoproteins and in synthesis of HDL particles are frequent causes (1 in 500 persons) of lipid disorders found in human beings. Five mutations are common in the receptor-binding region of APO B: a substitution of a glutamine for arginine at amino acid (**aa**) 3500, a tryptophan for an arginine at aa3500, a cysteine for an arginine at aa3531, a tryptophan for an arginine at aa3480, and a tyrosine for histidine at aa3543.[3] The resultant defect in LDL receptor binding from these mutations causes a decrease in clearance of these LDL particles from circulation and an increase in plasma LDL concentration.[38]

To date, more than 900 mutations have been identified in the LDL receptor gene that are functional, resulting in familial hypercholesterolemia.[39] The worldwide frequency of this disorder is 1:500 for heterozygotes and 1:1,000,000 for homozygotes. Some of these mutations produce a defective receptor; others result in a receptor completely incapable of binding and uptake of LDL. Still others affect the gene promoter so that affected individuals have no detectable LDL receptors on cell surfaces. Those with familial hypercholesterolemia have extremely high plasma total cholesterol, with the highest levels seen in homozygotes. They have early onset of symptomatic coronary artery disease, with myocardial infarctions occurring as early as their teens.

Defects in the APO A-I gene can result in severe HDL deficiencies. Because there is a well-documented inverse relationship between HDL levels and atherosclerosis, defects and deficiencies in APO A-I result in premature arteriosclerosis. The number of carriers of the 40 known defects in APO A-I is limited. Consequently, data on the incidence of premature cardiovascular disease are also limited.

One process by which HDL is atheroprotective is known as reverse cholesterol transport (see Figure 10-9). HDL is the acceptor of the free cholesterol released from the cell via the ABCA1 transporter. ABCA1 is a unidirectional transporter of cholesterol, carrying cholesterol out of the cell to a nascent HDL particle. ABCA1 is abundant in macrophages, liver, and placenta, with lesser amounts in small intestine, lung, stomach, trachea, and kidney and at low levels in brain, heart, and pancreas.[40] As described before, the free cholesterol transported from the cell is esterified by lecithin:cholesterol acyltransferase. The HDL particle then acquires phospholipids and triglyceride by the action of the two transfer proteins. HDL travels through the bloodstream to the steroidogenic tissues such as the adrenal glands and to the liver, where it binds to a receptor called scavenger receptor B1 (SR-B1) via regions in APO A-I. This receptor, through selective uptake, removes the cholesterol from the HDL particle. Lipid-poor HDL, including APO A-I, is cleared through the kidney. Other as yet unrecognized clearance processes for HDL are also possible.

In the absence of ABCA1, cholesterol accumulates in peripheral tissues. A genetic disease, called Tangier disease, is caused by a defective or absent ABCA1 transporter.[28,29] Persons with Tangier disease have low levels of an abnormal HDL particle and accumulate cholesterol ester in tonsils and spleen, with ocular abnormalities and neuropathies. They also experience early onset of atherosclerosis.

HDL also has been shown to have antiinflammatory properties because of two proteins that are carried on the particle: paraoxonase and platelet-activating factor acetylhydrolase (**PAF-AH**). Paraoxonase is a calcium-dependent ester hydrolase that cleaves oxidized long-chain fatty acids from phospholipids. In test tube assays, it has been shown to decrease the inflammatory properties of oxidized lipids and, in epidemiological studies, to have an inverse relationship with atherosclerosis.[41] PAF-AH is an enzyme that cleaves shorter acyl chains, including PAF, and longer aldehydes. PAF-AH inhibits the proatherogenic and proapoptotic effects of LDL phospholipid oxidation.[42]

PATHOLOGICAL PROCESS OF ATHEROSCLEROSIS

How does the presence of cholesterol in the intimal space result in pathological lesions that occlude blood flow? Cholesterol normally is found in the intima of blood vessels. Studies done on vessels of newborns have shown cholesterol depositions in their vessel walls. It has been proposed that the amount of cholesterol found in the walls of infants correlates with the plasma cholesterol levels of their mothers.[43] This suggests that cholesterol deposition may vary with plasma concentrations in children and adults also. The plasma cholesterol levels deemed normal in industrialized societies may indeed be higher than is physiologically necessary. Because the incidence of atherosclerosis is lower in agrarian societies where grain is the major food source, it is possible that we do not have the appropriate metabolic pathways to handle a high-fat diet.

The factors responsible for initiating the process of atherosclerosis continue to be the focus of intense investigation. In laboratory animals, initiation of a high-cholesterol "Western" diet quickly produces an accumulation of cholesterol in the vessel wall. An examination of different atherosclerotic plaques in deceased persons of varying ages suggests that there is a developmental process that, upon reaching a specific morphology, becomes an additive, positive feedback loop. The American Heart Association Committee on Vascular Lesions of the Council on Arteriosclerosis[44-46] developed a numerical classification system to standardize the manner in which different lesion types are described. These classes are introduced with the description of the process of atherosclerosis.

An infectious agent also has been considered as a possible initiating factor. *Chlamydia pneumoniae,* cytomegalovirus, herpes simplex virus, and *Helicobacter pylori* have been considered, based on their ability to infect endothelial cells, macrophages, and smooth muscle cells, causing alterations in the uptake and metabolism of cholesterol. Recent evidence suggests that neither herpes simplex virus[47] nor *H. pylori*[48] seropositivity is associated with an increased risk of coronary artery disease. Several investigators have found an association between cytomegalovirus seropositivity[47,49] or *C. pneumoniae*[50] infection and atherosclerotic disease.

LOCATION OF ATHEROSCLEROTIC LESIONS

Atherosclerosis tends to develop more quickly and result in symptomatic lesions in certain areas of the body. To comprehend the process, it will be helpful to understand the histological structure of elastic and muscular arteries (Figure 10-10). Arteries contain three discrete layers: the intima, media, and adventitia. The intima is composed of a layer of endothelial cells resting on a basement membrane primarily of type IV collagen, laminin, and fibronectin. Beneath the basement membrane is a layer of proteoglycans, proteins with highly sulfated sugar chains containing negative charge. In elastic arteries the media contains layers of smooth muscle cells embedded in lamina of elastic tissue composed primarily of elastin. In muscular arteries the smooth muscle cells are surrounded by a collagen-rich extracellular matrix. The adventitia is a thinner layer of fibroblasts and mast cells in a connective tissue matrix, which also contains nerve endings and vasa vasorum, the network

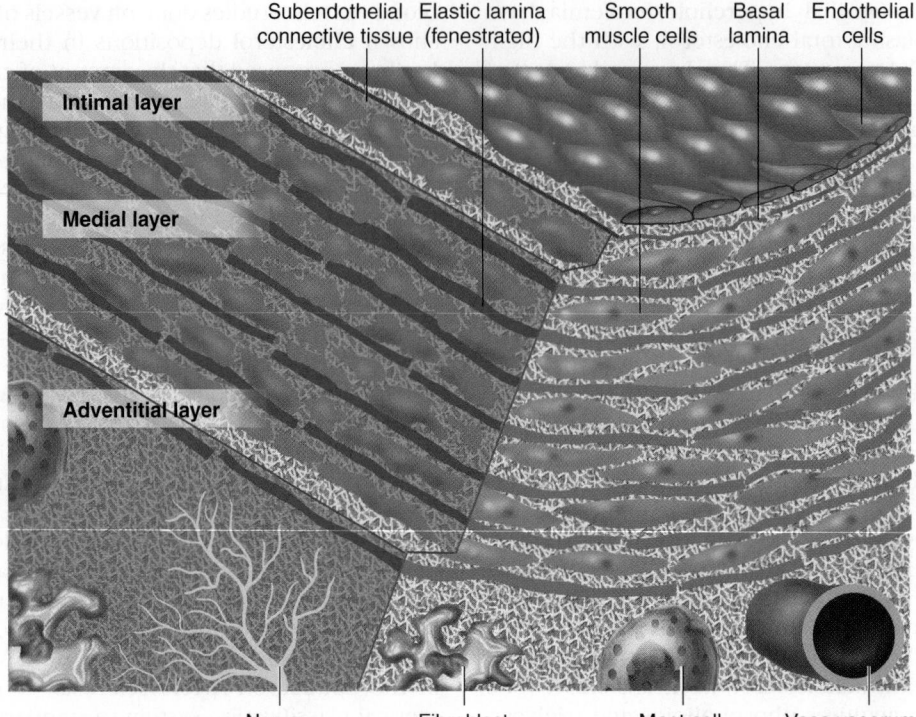

FIGURE 10-10 ■ Elastic arteries contain an intima composed of endothelial cells, few smooth muscle cells, and a proteoglycan layer. A thick medial layer is composed of smooth muscle cells separated by layers of elastin, laminin, and fibronectin. The artery has a relatively thin adventitial layer of connective tissue, nerves, and vasa vasorum. (From Zipes DP, Libby P, Bonow RO, Braunwald E: *Braunwald's heart disease,* ed 7, Philadelphia, 2005, Elsevier Saunders.)

of tiny vessels found in the walls of medium and large arteries and veins.

Early in life, the intimal composition begins to change at arterial bifurcations and other areas where blood flow changes direction. In these areas, endothelial and smooth muscle cell turnover increases and a protective cushion develops, causing intimal thickening. LDL concentrations are increased in these areas. With increasing age, there are changes in these and other areas that include an increase in the number of smooth muscle cells and a change to the more fibrillar collagens type I and II, resulting in what is known as *diffuse intimal thickening.* Certain areas of the blood vessel are more prone to the development of diffuse intimal thickening. These areas include bifurcations, the aortic arch, the left coronary artery, and other areas where blood flow changes directions. These same areas are more likely to develop atherosclerosis.

Why does atherosclerosis develop in some areas of a given artery and not others? With higher plasma cholesterol concentrations the gradient between the plasma cholesterol level and the vessel wall would favor cholesterol movement across the endothelium. Because the endothelial layer is considered to be a significant barrier, differences must exist between one part of the artery and another. Blood flow through parts of some arteries can be variable because of bending and other changes in body position, as well as their location. This results in differences in transmural pressure and pulsatile stretch. Flow characteristics differ at arterial bifur-

cations versus more linear portions of the vessel. Flow is laminar with high sheer stress across the linear parts of the blood vessel, but becomes turbulent, with decreased sheer stress at branch points. Endothelial cells now are known to respond to sheer stress by increasing production of antithrombotic and antiatherogenic genes and their subsequent proteins. Superoxide dismutase is an enzyme that catabolizes O_2^-. Nitric oxide synthase produces nitric oxide, a potent vasodilator and inhibitor of platelet adhesion.[51] Nitric oxide also inhibits inflammatory molecules the expression of which is regulated by the nuclear factor κB and by adhesion molecules that mediate monocyte and T lymphocyte binding to the endothelium.[52]

For atherosclerosis to develop, there must be a change from the antithrombotic, antiinflammatory surface to one that is inflammatory. This occurs when the lipid content in the intima becomes oxidized. LDL particles bind to proteoglycans on the endothelial surface and in the subendothelial area of the intima (Figure 10-11, *1*). Particles bound to the cell surface are subject to enzymatic modification by lipoprotein, hepatic and endothelial lipase, becoming smaller. Small, dense LDL particles are considered more atherogenic,[53] perhaps because they are more capable of traversing the endothelial cell barrier and becoming deposited in the subintimal space. Innate and adaptive immune responses attempt to control the amount of cholesterol and neutralize the damaging effects of oxidized lipid in the vessel wall.

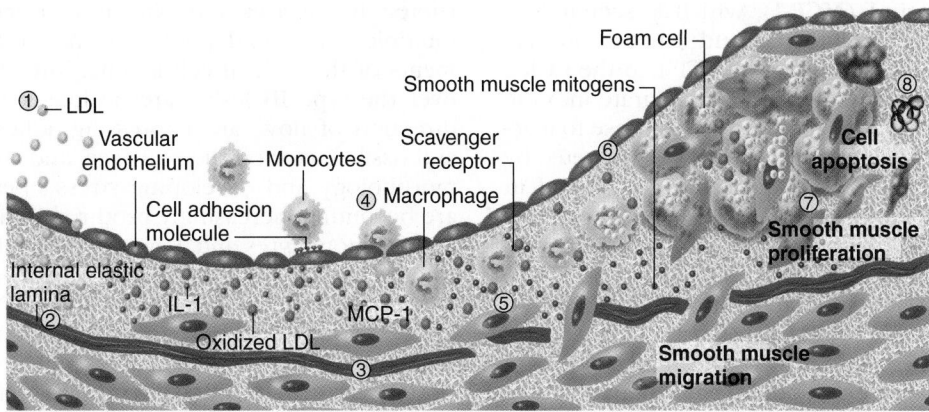

FIGURE 10-11 ■ The pathogenesis of atherosclerosis begins with oxidation of phospholipids in low-density lipoprotein (LDL) that has traversed the endothelial layer. A dysfunctional endothelium expresses adhesion molecules that allow monocytes and lymphocytes to bind and move into the intimal space by diapedesis. The monocyte differentiates into a macrophage, which expresses scavenger receptors and CD36, the oxidized LDL receptor. Uptake of lipids causes the formation of foam cells. The lesion progresses through further accumulation of lipid, inflammatory, and adaptive immune responses. See text for further explanation. *MCAP-1,* Monocyte chemoattractant protein-1. (From Zipes DP, Libby P, Bonow RO, Braunwald E: *Braunwald's heart disease,* ed 7, Philadelphia, 2005, Elsevier Saunders.)

OXIDATIVE STRESS AS THE INITIATING FACTOR

How does cholesterol deposition cause atherosclerotic plaque formation? To answer this, it is necessary to consider the second key component of atherosclerosis: inflammation. A large body of evidence supports the theory that oxidation of phospholipid in LDL is the initial process that triggers inflammation in the vascular wall[54-60] (Figure 10-11, *2*). During normal metabolic processes, enzymatic byproducts are released that are capable of oxidizing phospholipids and proteins present in the subintimal space. Oxidation of LDL also may result from interaction with reactive oxygen species (**ROS**) produced through the action of enzymes upregulated by fatty acid components of the diet, smoking, infectious agents, and other, as yet ill-defined environmental influences. Arachidonic acid, released from phospholipids by macrophage phospholipase A_2 enzymes,[61] can stimulate production of nicotinamide adenine dinucleotide/nicotinamide adenine dinucleotide phosphate (NADH/NADPH) oxidase activity. NADH/NADPH oxidase is a membrane-bound enzyme that produces superoxide anions. NADH/NADPH oxidase is produced by macrophages and by other cells in the vascular wall. Its production is increased in endothelial cells, smooth muscle cells, and adventitial fibroblasts by angiotensin II, thrombin, platelet-derived growth factor (**PDGF**), and tumor necrosis factor-alpha.[55] Lysophosphatidylcholine, the product of lipase hydrolysis of one fatty acid, also can activate the NADH/NADPH oxidase system to produce ROS. In areas of variable or nonlaminar flow, NADH/NADPH oxidase undergoes a sustained increase in expression.[62] The endothelium in these areas becomes dysfunctional, with decreased nitric oxide production and subsequent increased vascular tone. Nitric oxide reacts with the superoxide anion, O_2^-, to produce peroxynitrite, a reactive nitrogen species with strong oxidizing and nitrating properties.[63] The leukotrienes 12(S)-hydroxyeicosatetraenoic acid (12[s]-HETE) and 15(s)-HETE, which stimulate inflammatory gene expression and smooth muscle cell growth, also can be produced from arachidonic acid by 12/15 lipoxygenase.[64] Importantly, ROS also can mildly oxidize the phospholipid and APO B in the LDL particles present in the intima.[65]

These ROS have been implicated in the initiation of endothelial injury and dysfunction that leads to increased uptake of oxidized LDL and monocyte recruitment to the vessel wall. Endothelial cell exposure to oxidized LDL has been shown to upregulate endothelial lipase expression,[36] which may be one contributing factor to the low HDL levels correlated with increased risk of atherosclerosis.

The following discussion uses the numerical classification system developed by the American Heart Association Committee on Vascular Lesions of the Council on Arteriosclerosis[44-46] in describing the development of vascular lesions.

DEVELOPMENT OF A TYPE I LESION

Although the specific process is not known completely, clearly the result of oxidative stress is endothelial dysfunction. One possible mechanism was described by Napoli and colleagues,[58] who found that oxidized and glycated LDL downregulated nitric oxide synthase in coronary endothelial cells. Endothelial cell exposure to oxidized phospholipids results in the expression of P-selectin, which promotes leukocyte rolling, and the adhesion molecules, vascular cell adhesion molecule-1 and intercellular adhesion molecule, which bind to the very late antigen-4 integrin on monocytes and T lymphocytes. Once bound to the endothelial cell, the monocyte responds to a protein called monocyte chemoattractant protein-1 (**MCP-1**), which is secreted by cytokine-stimulated endothelial and smooth muscle cells in the intima. The binding of MCP-1 to the CCR-2 receptor on the monocyte causes it to migrate into the subendothelium[62] (Figure 10-11, *3*). In response to macrophage colony-stimulating factor (**M-CSF**), secreted by endothelial cells, fibroblasts, and other cells found in the arterial wall, the monocyte differentiates into a macrophage. In the macrophage, expression of the scavenger receptor SR-A and the oxidized LDL receptor, CD36, are increased. CD36 binds and internalizes oxidized lipids resulting in the formation of foam cells (Figure 10-11, *4*). Small, microscopically visible, lipid-laden foam cells constitute a type I lesion. They commonly are found in infants and young children but also can be found in vascular areas in adults that are more resistant to the development of atherosclerosis.[45]

PROGRESSION TO TYPE II LESION

The macrophage response to M-CSF includes cell division and proliferation, as well as scavenger receptor upregulation (Figure 10-11, *5*). The macrophage also produces a variety of substances capable of further oxidizing lipids in the intimal space. The resulting cycle of foam cell formation, lipid oxidation, further monocyte recruitment, macrophage differentiation, and proliferation produces an accumulation of cell-contained lipid that is visible on gross inspection of the involved artery. Accumulation of lipid-free macrophages, mast cells, and T lymphocytes begins in the lesion as well. T cells are attracted to the area by endothelial cells, macrophages, and dendritic cells, which function as antigen-presenting cells.

In the proinflammatory environment created by macrophage-secreted cytokines and chemokines, the smooth muscle cells divide and alter their phenotype to one with fewer contractile fibers and increased amounts of rough endoplasmic reticulum, where protein is synthesized. In type II lesions, a few lipid-laden smooth muscle cells begin to develop.

The principal lipids found in type II lesions are cholesteryl ester, cholesterol, and phospholipid. The lipid is contained within the macrophage and smooth muscle cell. These lesions are found primarily in children but, again, can be found in regions of the adult artery where advanced lesions are uncommon. These lesions are more likely to regress in response to decreased plasma LDL cholesterol levels. The type II lesion located in areas of diffuse intimal thickening is more likely to progress to a more advanced lesion.[45] The more turbulent blood flow in these areas promotes LDL binding to the vessel wall, increasing the local concentration of cholesterol and promoting lesion formation.

TYPE III LESION OR PREATHEROMA

As lipid continues to accumulate in the vessel wall, extracellular lipid droplets begin to appear, attached to the walls of macrophages and smooth muscle cells and in pools that displace the proteoglycans and extracellular matrix. The layers of smooth muscle cells are disrupted. In one area of the involved artery, there may be multiple small lipid pools causing localized derangements of the intimal cell lamina. The endothelial cells over the type III lesion are no longer oriented in the direction of flow, are expressing adhesion molecules and tissue factor on their surface, and are altering their morphology and developing stress fibers. These cells are becoming increasingly prothrombotic and adhesive toward monocytes and T lymphocytes. Proliferation of smooth muscle cells continues and can be found deeper within the intimal layer (Figure 10-11, *6*). Smooth muscle cell uptake of lipid is mediated by the LRP-1.[66] In response to the increased intracellular lipid content, smooth muscle cells have hyperplasia of the rough endoplasmic reticulum, smooth endoplasmic reticulum, and Golgi apparatus with increased synthesis of type I collagen, the chondroitin sulfate proteoglycan (**PG**) versican, the dermatan sulfate PG biglycan, the heparan sulfate PG perlecan,[64] and other intercellular matrix components. Numerous macrophage foam cells form, partly from proliferation and partly from continued chemotaxis. The principal lipid in the foam cells of the type III lesion is cholesteryl ester, because of increased expression of lipoprotein lipase,[65] which promotes holoparticle LDL uptake, and ACAT1. The foam cells produce significant quantities of tumor necrosis factor-alpha, interleukin-1, MCP-1, PDGF, M-CSF, CD antigens that promote differentiation of the TH1 type of T cell, tissue factor, and matrix metalloproteinases (**MMPs**). The MMPs are secreted as proenzymes that can be activated by tryptase and chymase released from tissue mast cells.[67] Once activated, the MMPs can degrade the proteoglycans and collagen in the intercellular matrix.[68] Evidence suggests that breakdown of the matrix surrounding smooth muscle cells promotes their proliferation. TH1 lymphocytes secrete copious amounts of interferon-gamma and CD-40, which activate macrophages, with resulting scavenger receptor expression and oxidized lipid uptake.

The type III lesion is considered a preatheroma because it does not occlude the vessel lumen and because the lesion cap is intact. This kind of lesion is considered a precursor to a type IV lesion, the initial atheroma that may produce clinical symptoms.

TYPE IV ATHEROMA

The type IV atheroma is the first lesion type considered to be advanced, based on the extent of intimal thickening, lipid accumulation, the derangement of the intimal lamina, alterations in matrix composition, and mineralization and vessel wall deformity.[46] The individual lipid pools of the type III lesion have coalesced into a large extracellular lipid core. Lipid continues to accumulate in the core from LDL in the plasma. Any narrowing of the vessel lumen is a result of the size of the lipid core. If the lipid accumulates slowly, the media adapts such that there is an outward widening of the vessel wall. If, however, lipid accumulates quickly because of a high plasma LDL concentration, the lumen can be narrowed.

The intimal cap underlying the endothelial layer, but overlying the lipid core, contains macrophages with and without lipid accumulation, mast cells, T lymphocytes, and few smooth muscle cells. The lack of smooth muscle cells and collagen makes the intimal cap susceptible to development of fissures in response to turbulent blood flow in these lesion-prone areas. In response to vascular endothelial growth factor and other angiogenic molecules, capillaries begin to form, mainly on the edges of the lesions. A hematoma or thrombus may develop if the intima is disrupted in these areas. With the development of a surface defect and thrombus formation, a type IV lesion can progress to a type VI lesion.[69]

TYPE V LESION

The type V lesion is characterized by a fibrous cap containing increased amounts of collagen type I produced from a larger number of smooth muscle cells enriched in rough endoplasmic reticulum (Figure 10-11, 7). The lesion has more capillaries, in the fibrous cap and along the margins of the lesion. As the involved area of the vessel wall thickens, tissue hypoxia stimulates the growth of an increased number of vasa vasorum.[70] Capillaries sprout from these vessels to perfuse the thickened intima. The repeated disruption of the intimal cap, with subsequent hematoma or thrombus formation, results in layers of lipid cores separated by fibrous tissue. This lesion, because of the multiple fibrous layers, opposes outward expansion and narrows the vessel lumen.

TYPE VI OR COMPLICATED LESION

A type IV or V lesion with a surface disruption, hematoma, or thrombosis is considered a type VI lesion. A type VI lesion may also develop from an earlier lesion type. Surface disruption can occur from apoptosis of smooth muscle cells and macrophages,[71,72] releasing proteolytic enzymes that destabilize the cap, causing small to large fissures and ulcerations. Exposure of tissue factor or von Willebrand factor can result in thrombus formation. Hemorrhage from newly formed capillaries can produce a hematoma.

Fibrinogen is cleaved by thrombin, cross-links, and forms fibrin and a platelet plug. Fibrinogen is an acute-phase reaction protein.[73] Fibrinogen increases with age[74] and in response to IL-6.[75] In the chronic inflammatory milieu of atherosclerosis, fibrinogen levels increase. The elevated fibrinogen level results in progression of the atherosclerotic plaque, most likely by promotion of thrombus formation with subsequent deposition of fibrous tissue. Prolonged thrombus formation also may contribute to the loss of vessel patency. There is increased expression of plasminogen activator inhibitor-1 and levels of lipoprotein (a), an APO B with an attached protein similar to plasminogen but without its fibrinolytic activity. The binding of these two proteins may compete for plasminogen binding to fibrin and may interfere with resolution of the clot.

Repeated episodes of thrombosis or hematoma with successive dissolution can produce type V lesions with decreasing lumen patency as the fibromuscular layers continue to increase. Lesions are dynamic, responding to changes in lipid levels and inflammatory processes.

LESION TYPES VII AND VIII

Over time, cells in the atheroma necrose or undergo apoptosis. The release of cell contents, including calcium, can result in a calcified plaque. The phosphatidylserine present in the ruptured cell membranes also can bind calcium. Evidence also is increasing that, in the plaque, calcifying vascular cells, which may be differentiated smooth muscle cells, are capable of depositing bone-like structures and calcium[76] (Figure 10-11, 8). Elastin also binds calcium with high affinity, and the affinity increases with age.[77] This type of lesion, with or without a lipid core, is considered a type VII lesion. Type VII and type VIII lesions, in which fibromuscular changes predominate, have been seen in lesions with lipid regression.

THE VULNERABLE PLAQUE

The thrombosis that occurs over an atherosclerotic plaque and leads to vessel occlusion and myocardial infarction is produced by a superficial erosion of the intima or plaque disruption. Both scenarios expose platelets to collagen, resulting in their activation and the initiation of a thrombus. Exposure of tissue factor with binding of factor VIIa initiates the coagulation cascade, thrombin formation, and more platelet activation.[78]

Activated macrophages overexpress matrix metalloproteases and cathepsins,[79] causing proteolytic digestion of the proteoglycans, collagen, fibronectin, and laminin in the intracellular matrix. Interferon-gamma, released from TH1 lymphocytes,[80] inhibits collagen synthesis by smooth muscle cells. A few smooth muscle cells are present because of apoptosis mediated by T lymphocytes.

A plaque prone to rupture is one that cannot withstand the force applied by flowing blood. The vulnerable plaque is one with a large lipid core, less collagen, and more activated macrophages releasing matrix-degrading enzymes. The narrowing of the vessel lumen causes turbulence and altered pressure in the vessel wall. As cells in the plaque die, there is less deposition of extracellular matrix and more degradation by proteases. This occurs more acutely at the edge of the plaque, which is exposed to the greater force from the turbulent blood flow. Therefore, it is the edge of the plaque that most commonly ruptures.

The development of an atherosclerotic plaque in the arterial wall stimulates angiogenesis, the production of a network of new vasa vasorum that function to sustain the growth of the intima beyond the critical limits of diffusion from the artery lumen.[81] These new blood vessels also may function to deliver leukocytes and other inflammatory mediators that foster the development of more lesion. Plaque rupture also can result in intraplaque hemorrhage from disruption of this vulnerable network of small arteries.

SUMMARY

The pathophysiological process of atherosclerosis involves the complex interaction of vascular biology, lipid metabolism, and innate and adaptive immunity. Symptomatic disease is advanced disease. Therefore, the emphasis must be placed on prevention to decrease disability and death on an individual basis.

Atherosclerosis continues to be the leading cause of disability and death in industrialized societies. Our understanding of the physiology of cholesterol and lipid metabolism has expanded tremendously over the last 20 years, allowing the development of pharmacological treatments with great potential to alter disease progression. Similarly, our understanding of the pathophysiology of the atherosclerotic process and of genetic alterations that disrupt normal lipid metabolism is opening new areas for drug discovery and for the development of meaningful lifestyle modifications.

Nurses are in the ideal position of being able to counsel patients about lifestyle changes and pharmacological management. The exciting and rapid expansion of our understanding of the causative nature of elevated triglycerides and cholesterol in developing atherosclerosis allows us realistically to hope that prevention can become a reality.

REFERENCES

1. Hussain MM: A proposed model for the assembly of chylomicrons, *Atherosclerosis* 148:1-15, 2000.
2. Cohn JS, Marcoux C, Davignon J: Detection, quantification, and characterization of potentially atherogenic triglyceride-rich remnant lipoproteins, *Arterioscler Thromb Vasc Biol* 19:2474-2486, 1999.
3. Dormans TP, Swinkels DW, de Graaf J et al: Single-spin density-gradient ultracentrifugation vs gradient gel electrophoresis: two methods for detecting low-density lipoprotein heterogeneity compared, *Clin Chem* 37:853-858, 1991.
4. O'Connell BJ, Genest J: High-density lipoproteins and endothelial function, *Circulation* 104:1978-1983, 2001.
5. Gotto A, Pownall H: *Manual of lipid disorders,* Philadelphia, 2003, Lippincott Williams & Wilkins.
6. Altmann SW, Davis HR, Zhu LJ et al: Niemann-Pick C1 Like 1 protein is critical for intestinal cholesterol absorption, *Science* 303:1201-1204, 2004.
7. Turley SD, Dietschy JM: Sterol absorption by the small intestine, *Curr Opin Lipidol* 14:233-240, 2003.
8. Hubacek JA, Berge KE, Cohen JC et al: Mutations in ATP-cassette binding proteins G5 (ABCG5) and G8 (ABCG8) causing sitosterolemia, *Hum Mutat* 18:359-360, 2001.
9. Lee MH, Lu K, Hazard S et al: Identification of a gene, ABCG5, important in the regulation of dietary cholesterol absorption, *Nat Genet* 27:79-83, 2001.
10. Yu YH, Ginsberg HN: The role of acyl-CoA:diacylglycerol acyltransferase (DGAT) in energy metabolism, *Ann Med* 36:252-261, 2004.
11. Temel RE, Gebre AK, Parks JS et al: Compared with acyl-CoA: cholesterol O-acyltransferase (ACAT) 1 and lecithin:cholesterol acyltransferase, ACAT2 displays the greatest capacity to differentiate cholesterol from sitosterol, *J Biol Chem* 278:47594-47601, 2003.
12. Smith JL, Rangaraj K, Simpson R et al: Quantitative analysis of the expression of ACAT genes in human tissues by real-time PCR, *J Lipid Res* 45:686-696, 2004.
13. Raal FJ, Marais AD, Klepack E et al: Avasimibe, an ACAT inhibitor, enhances the lipid lowering effect of atorvastatin in subjects with homozygous familial hypercholesterolemia, *Atherosclerosis* 171:273-279, 2003.
14. Abifadel M, Varret M, Rabes JP et al: Mutations in PCSK9 cause autosomal dominant hypercholesterolemia, *Nat Genet* 34:154-159, 2003.
15. McPherson R, Gauthier A: Molecular regulation of SREBP function: the Insig-SCAP connection and isoform-specific modulation of lipid synthesis, *Biochem Cell Biol* 82:201-211, 2004.
16. Lin J, Yang R, Tarr PT et al: Hyperlipidemic effects of dietary saturated fats mediated through PGC-1beta coactivation of SREBP, *Cell* 120:261-273, 2005.
17. Francis GA, Annicotte JS, Auwerx J: Liver X receptors: Xcreting Xol to combat atherosclerosis, *Trends Mol Med* 8:455-458, 2002.
18. Olofsson SO, Asp L, Boren J: The assembly and secretion of apolipoproteins B-containing lipoproteins, *Curr Opin Lipidol* 10:341-346, 1999.
19. Davis RA: Cell and molecular biology of the assembly and secretion of apolipoprotein B-containing lipoproteins by the liver, *Biochim Biophys Acta* 1440:1-31, 1999.
20. Fisher EA, Ginsberg HN: Complexity in the secretory pathway: the assembly and secretion of apolipoprotein B-containing lipoproteins, *J Biol Chem* 277:17377-17380, 2002.
21. Berriot-Varoqueaux N, Aggerbeck LP, Samson-Bouma M et al: The role of the microsomal triglyceride transfer protein in abetalipoproteinemia, *Annu Rev Nutr* 20:663-697, 2002.
22. Ueshima K, Akihisa-Umeno H, Nagayoshi A et al: Implitapide, a microsomal triglyceride transfer protein inhibitor, reduces progression of atherosclerosis in apolipoprotein E knockout mice fed a Western-type diet: involvement of the inhibition of postprandial triglyceride elevation, *Biol Pharm Bull* 28:247-252, 2005.
23. Colvin P, Moriguchi E, Barrett H et al: Production rate determines plasma concentration of large high density lipoprotein in non-human primates, *J Lipid Res* 39:2076-2085, 1998.
24. Oram JF, Lawn RM, Garvin MR et al: ABCA1 is the cAMP-inducible apolipoprotein receptor that mediates cholesterol secretion from macrophages, *J Biol Chem* 275:34508-34511, 2000.
25. Ayyobi AF, McGladdery SH, Chan S et al: Lecithin:cholesterol acyltransferase (LCAT) deficiency and risk of vascular disease: 25 year follow-up, *Atherosclerosis* 177:361-366, 2004.
26. Barter PJ, Brewer HB, Chapman MJ et al: Cholesteryl ester transfer protein: a novel target for raising HDL and inhibiting atherosclerosis, *Arterioscler Thromb Vasc Biol* 23:160-167, 2003.
27. Huuskonen J, Olkkonen VM, Jauhiainen M et al: The impact of phospholipid transfer protein (PLTP) on HDL metabolism, *Atherosclerosis* 155:269-281, 2001.
28. Bodzioch M, Orso E, Klucken J et al: The gene encoding ATP-binding cassette transporter 1 is mutated in Tangier disease, *Nat Genet* 22:347-351, 1999.
29. Brooks-Wilson A, Marcil M, Clee SM et al: Mutations in ABC1 in Tangier disease and familial high-density lipoprotein deficiency, *Nat Genet* 22:336-345, 1999.
30. Duval C, Chinetti G, Trottein F et al: The role of PPARs in atherosclerosis, *Trends Mol Med* 8:422-430, 2002.
31. Kota BP, Huang TH, Roufogalis BD: An overview on biological mechanisms of PPARs, *Pharmacol Res* 51:85-94, 2005.
32. Castrillo A, Tontonoz P: PPARs in atherosclerosis: the clot thickens, *J Clin Invest* 114:1538-1540, 2004.
33. Stein Y, Stein O: Lipoprotein lipase and atherosclerosis, *Atherosclerosis* 170:1-9, 2003.
34. Mead JR, Ramji DP: The pivotal role of lipoprotein lipase in atherosclerosis, *Cardiovasc Res* 55:261-269, 2002.
35. Deeb SS, Zambon A, Carr MC et al: Hepatic lipase and dyslipidemia: interactions among genetic variants, obesity, gender, and diet, *J Lipid Res* 44:1279-1286, 2003.
36. Jaye M, Lynch KJ, Krawiec J et al: A novel endothelial-derived lipase that modulates HDL metabolism, *Nat Genet* 21:424-428, 1999.
37. Vrablik M, Ceska R, Horinek A: Major apolipoprotein b-100 mutations in lipoprotein metabolism and atherosclerosis, *Physiol Res* 50:337-343, 2001.
38. Whitfield AJ, Barrett PH, van Bockxmeer FM, Burnett JR: Lipid disorders and mutations in the apoB gene, *Clin Chem* 50:1725-1732, 2004.
39. Dedoussis GV, Schmidt H, Genschel J: LDL-receptor mutations in Europe, *Hum Mutat* 24:443-459, 2004.
40. Kielar D, Dietmaier W, Langmann T et al: Rapid quantification of human ABCA1 MRNA in various cell types and tissues by real-time reverse transcription-PCR, *Clin Chem* 47:2089-2097, 2001.

41. Watson AD, Berliner JA, Hama SY et al: Protective effect of high density lipoprotein associated paraoxonase: inhibition of the biological activity of minimally oxidized low density lipoprotein, *J Clin Invest* 96:2882-2891, 1995.

42. Caslake MJ, Packard CJ: Lipoprotein-associated phospholipase A2 (platelet-activating factor acetylhydrolase) and cardiovascular disease, *Curr Opin Lipidol* 14:347-352, 2003.

43. Palinski W, Napoli C: The fetal origins of atherosclerosis: maternal hypercholesterolemia, and cholesterol-lowering or antioxidant treatment during pregnancy influence in utero programming and postnatal susceptibility to atherogenesis, *FASEB J* 16:1348-1360, 2002.

44. Stary HC, Blankenhorn DH, Chandler AB et al: A definition of the intima of human arteries and of its atherosclerosis-prone regions: a report from the Committee on Vascular Lesions of the Council on Arteriosclerosis, American Heart Association, *Circulation* 85:391-405, 1992.

45. Stary HC, Chandler AB, Dinsmore RE et al: A definition of advanced types of atherosclerotic lesions and a histological classification of atherosclerosis: a report from the Committee on Vascular Lesions of the Council on Arteriosclerosis, American Heart Association, *Circulation* 92:1355-1374, 1995.

46. Stary HC, Chandler AB, Glagov S et al: A definition of initial, fatty streak, and intermediate lesions of atherosclerosis: a report from the Committee on Vascular Lesions of the Council on Arteriosclerosis, American Heart Association, *Arterioscler Thromb* 14:840-856, 1994.

47. Sorlie PD, Nieto FJ, Adam E et al: A prospective study of cytomegalovirus, herpes simplex 1, and coronary heart disease, *Arch Intern Med* 160:2027-2032, 2000.

48. Folsom AR, Nieto FJ, Sorlie PD et al: *Helicobacter pylori* seropositivity and coronary heart disease incidence, *Circulation* 98:845-850, 1998.

49. Muhlestein JB, Horne BD, Carlquist JF et al: Cytomegalovirus seropositivity and C-reactive protein have independent and combined predictive value for mortality in patients with angiographically demonstrated coronary artery disease, *Circulation* 102:1917-1923, 2000.

50. Liu C, Water DD: *Chlamydia pneumoniae* and atherosclerosis: from Koch's postulates to clinical trials, *Prog Cardiovasc Dis* 47:230-239, 2005.

51. Cines DB, Pollak ES, Buck CA et al: Endothelial cells in physiology and in the pathophysiology of vascular disorders, *Blood* 91:3527-3561, 1998.

52. Tsao PS, Buitrago R, Chan JR et al: Fluid flow inhibits endothelial adhesiveness: nitric oxide and transcriptional regulation of VCAM-1, *Circulation* 94:1682-1689, 1996.

53. Coresh J, Kwiterovich PO, Smith HH et al: Association of plasma triglyceride concentration and LDL particle diameter, density, and chemical composition with premature coronary artery disease in men and women, *J Lipid Res* 34:1687-1697, 1993.

54. Witztum JL, Steinberg D: Role of oxidized low density lipoprotein in atherogenesis, *J Clin Invest* 88:1785-1792, 1991.

55. Ross R: Atherosclerosis: an inflammatory disease, *N Engl J Med* 340:115-126, 1999.

56. Subbanagounder G, Leitinger N, Shih PT et al: Evidence that phospholipid oxidation products and/or platelet-activating factor play an important role in early atherogenesis: in vitro and in vivo inhibition by WEB 2086, *Circ Res* 85:311-318, 1999.

57. Napoli C, de Nigris F, Palinski W: Multiple role of reactive oxygen species in the arterial wall, *J Cell Biochem* 82:674-682, 2001.

58. Napoli C, Lerman LO, de Nigris F et al: Glycoxidized low-density lipoprotein downregulates endothelial nitricoxide synthase in human coronary cells, *J Am Coll Cardiol* 40:1515-1522, 2002.

59. Madamanchi NR, Vendrov A, Runge MS: Oxidative stress and vascular disease, *Arterioscler Thromb Vasc Biol* 25:29-38, 2005.

60. Morrow JD: Quantification of isoprostanes as indices of oxidant stress and the risk of atherosclerosis in humans, *Arterioscler Thromb Vasc Biol* 25:279-286, 2005.

61. Ghesquiere SA, Gijbels MJ, Anthonsen M et al: Macrophage-specific overexpression of group IIa sPLA2 increases atherosclerosis and enhances collagen deposition, *J Lipid Res* 46:201-210, 2005.

62. Takahara N, Kashiwagi A, Maegawa H et al: Lysophosphatidylcholine stimulates the expression and production of MCP-1 by human vascular endothelial cells, *Metabolism* 45:559-564, 1996.

63. Rubbo H, O'Donnell V: Nitric oxide, peroxynitrite and lipoxygenase in atherogenesis: mechanistic insights, *Toxicology* 208:305-317, 2005.

64. Wight TN, Merrilees MJ: Proteoglycans in atherosclerosis and restenosis: key roles for versican, *Circ Res* 94:1158-1167, 2004.

65. Ichikawa T, Liang J, Kitajima S et al: Macrophage-derived lipoprotein lipase increases aortic atherosclerosis in cholesterol-fed Tg rabbits, *Atherosclerosis* 179:87-95, 2005.

66. Llorente-Cortes V, Badimon L: LDL receptor-related protein and the vascular wall: implications for atherothrombosis, *Arterioscler Thromb Vasc Biol* 25:497-504, 2005.

67. Johnson JL, Jackson CL, Angelini GD et al: Activation of matrix-degrading metalloproteinases by mast cell proteases in atherosclerotic plaques, *Arterioscler Thromb Vasc Biol* 18:1707-1715, 1998.

68. Newby AC: Dual role of matrix metalloproteinases (matrixins) in intimal thickening and atherosclerotic plaque rupture, *Physiol Rev* 85:1-31, 2005.

69. Stary HC: Natural history and histological classification of atherosclerotic lesions: an update, *Arterioscler Thromb Vasc Biol* 20:1177-1178, 2000.

70. Moulton KS, Olsen BR, Sonn S et al: Loss of collagen XVIII enhances neovascularization and vascular permeability in atherosclerosis, *Circulation* 110:1330-1336, 2004.

71. Napoli C: Oxidation of LDL, atherogenesis, and apoptosis, *Ann N Y Acad Sci* 1010:698-709, 2003.

72. Stoneman VE, Bennett MR: Role of apoptosis in atherosclerosis and its therapeutic implications, *Clin Sci (Lond)* 107:343-354, 2004.

73. de Maat MP, Kastelein JJ, Jukema JW et al: -455G/A polymorphism of the beta-fibrinogen gene is associated with the progression of coronary atherosclerosis in symptomatic men: proposed role for an acute-phase reaction pattern of fibrinogen: REGRESS group, *Arterioscler Thromb Vasc Biol* 18:265-271, 1998.

74. Folsom AR, Wu KK, Rasmussen M et al: Determinants of population changes in fibrinogen and factor VII over 6 years: the Atherosclerosis Risk In Communities (ARIC) study, *Arterioscler Thromb Vasc Biol* 20:601-606, 2000.

75. Gervois P, Vu-Dac N, Kleemann R et al: Negative regulation of human fibrinogen gene expression by peroxisome proliferator-activated receptor alpha agonists via inhibition of CCAAT box/enhancer-binding protein beta, *J Biol Chem* 276:33471-33477, 2001.

76. Doherty TM, Asotra K, Fitzpatrick LA et al: Calcification in atherosclerosis: bone biology and chronic inflammation at the arterial crossroads, *Proc Natl Acad Sci U S A* 100:11201-11206, 2003.

77. Bailey M, Pillarisetti S, Jones P et al: Involvement of matrix metalloproteinases and tenascin-C in elastin calcification, *Cardiovasc Pathol* 13:146-155, 2004.

78. Lee RT, Libby P: The unstable atheroma, *Arterioscler Thromb Vasc Biol* 17:1859-1867, 1997.

79. Yasuda Y, Li Z, Greenbaum D et al: Cathepsin V, a novel and potent elastolytic activity expressed in activated macrophages, *J Biol Chem* 279:36761-36770, 2004.

80. Gupta S, Pablo AM, Jiang X et al: IFN-gamma potentiates atherosclerosis in ApoE knock-out mice, *J Clin Invest* 99:2752-2761, 1997.

81. Moulton KS, Vakili K, Zurakowski D et al: Inhibition of plaque neovascularization reduces macrophage accumulation and progression of advanced atherosclerosis, *Proc Nat Acad Sci U S A* 100:4736-4741, 2003.

Central Nervous System and the Heart

Mary A. Woo

Cardiovascular disease is a major cause of morbidity and mortality throughout the world, and considerable efforts have been made to examine and evaluate its most prominent component, the heart. However, this emphasis on the heart and, to a lesser extent, other organs in the thoracic cavity, ignores the profound influence of the central nervous system (**CNS**) on cardiovascular symptoms and disease. The influence of the CNS on all aspects of heart disease is unmistakable, and testimony to its impact is present in many of the chapters in this book, including Chapters 6, 7, 8, 17, 39, 40, 41, and 42. In addition, multiple reports exist of brain abnormalities in cardiovascular disease. For example, scattered cerebral infarcts, decreased brain volumes, changes in hypothalamic function, and abnormalities in the forebrain renin-angiotensin system have been described in heart failure patients.[1-3] In addition to these physiological brain abnormalities, there have been reports of alterations in emotion and motivation in many persons with cardiovascular disease.

The CNS can dramatically affect all parts of the cardiovascular system (heart, blood vessels, blood components) and influence expression of symptoms of cardiovascular disease (blood pressure, heart rate, cardiac contractility, perception of chest pain, dyspnea, depression, sleep, thirst). Also, the heart and other cardiovascular components have important influences on CNS activity and function (embolic events, supplies of nutrients/oxygen to the brain). Thus, there is extensive communication and interface between the functions of the CNS and heart.

To better evaluate and care for patients with cardiovascular disease, health care providers need to understand the influences and interactions between the CNS and the heart. The CNS and the heart communicate in four ways: direct nerve connections (Figure 11-1), chemicals/hormones, pressures, and behaviors.

DIRECT NERVE CONNECTIONS

The heart is the only part of the cardiovascular system that is innervated by the sympathetic and parasympathetic divisions of the autonomic nervous system (**ANS**). In contrast, direct links between the CNS and the blood vessels are via the sympathetic nervous system (Table 11-1).

Autonomic Nervous System

The portion of the nervous system that regulates the visceral functions of the body is the ANS. This system helps to control blood pressure, heart rate (and rhythm), pupillary responses to light, temperature, smooth muscle and glandular tissue, and many other bodily functions. The ANS often is viewed as an involuntary system. In other words, the actions and functions of the ANS are not under constant, conscious control. The ANS can be divided into central (brain) and peripheral (spinal cord and parts outside of the head/neck areas) components, as well as sympathetic and parasympathetic sections. The ANS is activated mainly by sites located in the spinal cord, brain stem, hypothalamus, cerebral cortex, and insula.[4] Impulses from these regions are transmitted to the rest of the body via the two subdivisions of the ANS, the sympathetic and parasympathetic nervous systems.

A great deal of interplay occurs among all parts of the ANS and between the voluntary (somatic) and ANS systems. The primary aim of the ANS, and all of these system interactions, is to maintain homeostasis. For example, running up the stairs requires instantaneous responses from the body, such as an increase in cardiac output, redistribution of blood flow, and enhancement of blood glucose release. All of these rapid responses of the body to increased or decreased activity (whether physical or mental/emotional) are coordinated by the ANS. Thus, without the efficient activities of an intact ANS, an individual attempting to sit up or stand could have a syncopal episode, because of the inability of the body to provide adequate nutrients and oxygen to respond to changes in bodily demands.

Traditionally, the two parts of the ANS, the sympathetic and parasympathetic nervous systems, are considered to have antagonistic actions on cardiac function. The sympathetic nervous system is associated with the need of the body to respond to internal and external stimuli and increases in catabolic (energy-using) activity. The parasympathetic nervous system often is concerned with a reduction in energy expenditure (return or maintenance of a baseline or resting state) and anabolic (energy-storing) activity. However, not all ANS responses are momentary operations or are restricted to isolated reflex adjustments to stimuli. Instead, both branches of the ANS must maintain a minimal level of operating tone. The presence of this tonic ANS activity provides continuous control of heart rate, cardiac output, and other cardiovascular functions.

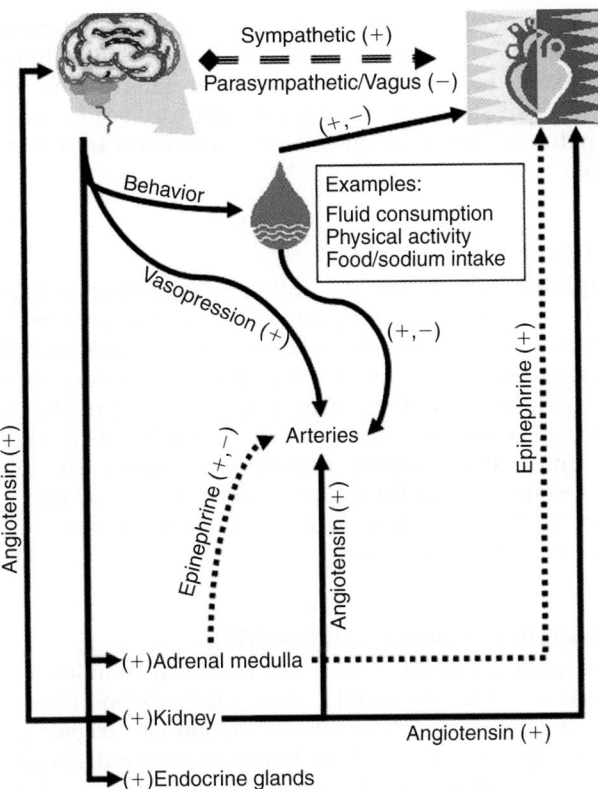

FIGURE 11-1 ■ Figure illustrating the communication and interaction between the central nervous system and the heart.

Sympathetic Nervous System

The sympathetic nervous system is associated with "flight or fight" responses. Stimulation of the sympathetic nervous system increases heart rate and cardiac contractility (thus increasing cardiac output), and lowers the threshold (thereby increasing the risk) for some types of cardiac tachydysrhythmias. Basal sympathetic innervation to the heart originates primarily from the rostral ventrolateral medulla in the brain. However, the right insular lobe in the brain plays an important role in "dampening" sympathetic activity. Human and animal studies have demonstrated that infarctions in the right insular cortex greatly diminish heart rate variability (an indirect indication of higher sympathetic tone). The primary sympathetic nervous system efferent receptors in the heart, which mediate between the brain and heart activity, are beta$_1$ receptors.

In contrast to the heart, which has sympathetic and parasympathetic connections, blood vessels are innervated only by the sympathetic nervous system, particu-

larly at the precapillary arterioles. In general, sympathetic nervous system activation causes arterioles to constrict (via alpha-adrenergic receptors), whereas reductions in sympathetic traffic (or stimulation of beta-adrenergic receptors) induce vascular relaxation. Sympathetic nervous system control of the vasculature is complex; the sympathetic nervous system is not activated as one unit, rather discrete sections of the vasculature receive differing levels of sympathetic input. Therefore, different parts of the vascular system can have varying levels of sympathetic stimulation and thus can have different amounts of vasoconstriction. For example, sympathetic stimulation of blood vessels in the gastrointestinal area can cause vasoconstriction, but simultaneous activation of sympathetic receptors (beta-adrenergic receptors) in skeletal muscle vasculature would cause vasodilatation. The primary neurotransmitter for postganglionic sympathetic nervous system neurons is norepinephrine.

Parasympathetic Nervous System

The parasympathetic nervous system promotes return to baseline states. Activation of the parasympathetic nervous system (via the M2 muscarinic receptors located in the heart) decreases heart rate (by reducing conduction velocity of the sinoatrial and atrioventricular nodes) and cardiac contractility (in the atria) and increases cardiac conduction times (thus decreasing the risk for tachydysrhythmias). Traditionally, parasympathetic nerve control is believed to be located primarily in the brain stem. However, the CNS also exerts significant influence over the ANS. The left insular cortex in the brain controls much of the parasympathetic nerve activity. Human and animal studies have demonstrated that damage in the left insular cortex decreases parasympathetic tone.

The vagus is the principle nerve that mediates CNS parasympathetic activity to the heart. The principal neurotransmitter associated with parasympathetic activity is acetylcholine. Under baseline/nonstimulation conditions, parasympathetic tone predominates in the heart, which causes the resting heart rate to be lower than that of the intrinsic rate of the cells of the sinoatrial node. Heart rate can be decreased by escalating parasympathetic activity (or decreasing sympathetic activity), and it can be increased by removal of parasympathetic tone (or increasing sympathetic stimulation).

The CNS can influence the heart and cardiovascular system independent of the direct nerve connections of the ANS. Indirectly, the CNS influences the cardiovascular system using chemicals/hormones, pressures, and behaviors.

■ ■ ■

TABLE 11-1   SYMPATHETIC AND PARASYMPATHETIC INFLUENCES ON THE HEART AND VASCULAR SYSTEMS

| | SYMPATHETIC NERVOUS SYSTEM | | PARASYMPATHETIC NERVOUS SYSTEM | |
	ACTION	RECEPTOR	ACTION	RECEPTOR
Heart rate	Increase	Beta$_1$	Decrease	M$_2$
Contractility	Increase	Beta$_1$	Decrease	M$_2$
Atrial or ventricular tachydysrhythmias	Increase	Beta$_1$	Decrease	M$_2$
Vasculature diameter	Decrease	Alpha	Increase	—

CHEMICALS AND HORMONES

Many chemicals and hormones are associated with communication between the CNS and the heart. These substances are described in detail below.

Catecholamines

The sympathetic nervous system can influence the heart and blood vessels through stimulation of chromaffin cells in the adrenal medulla. These cells release catecholamines into the general circulation. When catecholamines are released into the bloodstream, they can elicit sympathetic-like responses in other parts of the body. Chromaffin cells release more epinephrine than norepinephrine, and beta-adrenergic receptors are more sensitive than alpha-adrenergic receptors to epinephrine stimulation. Sympathetic stimulation of the adrenal medulla increases heart rate and produces vasodilatation in the blood vessels supplying skeletal muscle tissue.

Renin

Renin is a key component in the renin-angiotensin-aldosterone system (**RAAS**), which is an important factor in the control of blood pressure and of volume homeostasis. When the RAAS is activated in the periphery (i.e., areas outside of the brain), sympathetic outflow acts on beta-adrenergic receptors in the kidney, causing the release of renin into the bloodstream. Renin induces the production of angiotensin, which is a potent vasoconstrictor. Although many clinicians are aware of the activities and impact of the peripheral RAAS, few realize that the brain has its own RAAS, which often acts and reacts independent of the peripheral RAAS.

In the brain RAAS, angiotensin II is the primary effector that induces increased sympathetic outflow. Angiotensin II receptor binding sites have been identified in specific areas in the forebrain and brain stem. Angiotensin II acts through at least two receptors (i.e., AT_1 and AT_2). Most of the classic actions (blood pressure control, drinking behavior/thirst, natriuresis, and release of vasopressin into the circulation) of angiotensin II in the brain are mediated by the AT_1 receptors.[5] Thus, inhibition of AT_1 receptors in the brain contributes to the blood pressure–lowering effects of peripheral AT_1 receptor blockers and may reduce brain ischemic injury in stroke. The AT_2 receptors are involved primarily in brain development and in neuronal regeneration and protection. Although not directly associated with action in the cardiovascular system, the AT_2 receptors modulate the effects of the AT_1 receptors on the cardiovascular and renal systems.

Thyroid

Thyroid hormone is produced from the thyroid gland in response to stimulation, especially from the pituitary gland. Thyroid gland influences the metabolic activity of every cell in the body. In relation to the heart and the cardiovascular system, increased thyroid activity/hormone release increases heart rate and blood pressure. Hyperthyroid states are associated with increased incidence of cardiac tachydysrhythmias, higher blood pressure, and elevated myocardial oxygen demand. Hypothyroid states are associated with cardiac bradydysrhythmias, lower blood pressure, and decreased metabolic rates.

Arginine Vasopressin

Arginine vasopressin (or antidiuretic hormone) is released by the posterior pituitary gland and actively increases blood pressure by acting on the arteriolar V_1 vasopressin receptors in the arterioles to induce vasoconstriction. Another way arginine vasopressin increases blood pressure is to act on the V_2 vasopressin receptors in the kidney to suppress diuresis. The hormone also acts on the CNS to potentiate the baroreceptor reflex, thus exaggerating heart rate responses to changes in blood pressure.

Hypoxemia and Hypercapnia

Although not often viewed as a chemical stimulus, low oxygen levels (hypoxemia) and/or high carbon dioxide levels (hypercapnia) in the circulation can trigger potent responses in the brain. Hypoxemia stimulates arterial chemoreceptors, located primarily in the carotid bodies, which then communicate with the nucleus of the solitary tract in the CNS to trigger vasoconstriction in a large area of the body, thus increasing blood flow to the brain. The carotid bodies also respond to changes in hydrogen ion concentration (which is linked to the level of carbon dioxide in the blood). Central chemoreceptors are located primarily in the pons and medulla.

PRESSURES

An important negative feedback reflex for cardiovascular homeostasis is the baroreceptor reflex. This reflex is activated by changes in blood pressure. Pressure sensors (baroreceptors) for this reflex are located in the aortic arch and carotid sinuses. As blood pressure increases, the pressure sensors (which are made up of stretch receptors) are activated (i.e., generate a greater number of action potentials) as the walls of the blood vessels in these areas expand. The increase in baroreceptor activity is transmitted to the nucleus of the solitary tract, which in turn communicates to the caudal ventrolateral medulla and eventually stimulates parasympathetic (vagal) tone in the sinoatrial node. Vagal activation decreases heart rate and cardiac output, which contributes to a decrease in blood pressure and lessens stimulation of the stretch receptors in the aortic arch and carotid sinuses.

BEHAVIORS

The brain can be viewed as the "organ of behavior." Behavior can be defined as the actions or reactions of a person in response to external or internal stimuli. A person's behavior (adherence to health care instructions, dietary choices, drinking in response to thirst, activity, and health promotion activities) can have a profound impact on cardiovascular status and well-being. Yet the question is, does the brain influence behavior or vice versa? In other words, "nature vs. nurture". Some controversy exists on whether biology (such as genotype or brain stucture) ultimately controls behavior ("nature") or if it is behavior and other environmental influences ("nurture") that ultimately influence and modify biology and the brain. Considerable evidence indicates that genes and external influences (such as traumatic brain injury; light, seasons) can alter brain function. Also, little doubt exists that serious brain damage and changes in brain chemistry (by factors such as medications) can alter behavior. Yet there are also multiple reports of how behavior can alter brain chemistry. For example, psychological or physical stress causes changes in brain chemistry activity. Reports also indicate that psychosocial interventions, such as cognitive behavioral therapy, can alter brain function (and possibly structure). Thus, it would appear likely that there are multiple interactions among behavior, the brain, and the environment. However, at this time there is little research in persons with cardiovascular disease to allow us fully to understand the interactions between behavior, environment, and the brain in these high-risk groups.

EVIDENCE OF CENTRAL NERVOUS SYSTEM CHANGES IN HEART DISEASE

There are reports that link cardiovascular risk factors to brain structure changes. According to Cook and colleagues,[6] greater control of factors associated with increased cardiovascular disease such as diabetes, hypertension, high cholesterol, and smoking, is associated with decreased incidence of adverse brain structure changes, such as atrophy and white matter lesions.

Direct evidence of alterations in brain structure in persons with heart disease has been reported by a variety of investigators. Using structural magnetic resonance imaging (**MRI**) techniques, Schmidt and colleagues[7] found greater cortical and ventricular atrophy in a heterogeneous group of heart failure patients relative to healthy individuals. They also reported multiple scattered areas of cerebral infarcts in the patients with heart failure but did not identify specific sites of regional brain cell injury nor associated clinical symptoms or ANS abnormalities to their CNS findings.

Studies by our investigative team have identified specific sites of structural gray matter loss and functional abnormalities in persons with heart failure.[8,9] Heart failure patients in our samples showed significant, and largely lateralized, gray matter injury in ANS and respiratory-related areas, including the insula (Figure 11-2). These areas of gray matter injury may contribute to the inappropriate ANS regulation often observed in heart failure patients. Other brain sites in which heart failure patients exhibited less gray matter volumes compared with healthy individuals included the deep cerebellar nuclei, right cingulate, thalamus, and right frontal cortex.

These areas of structural loss also reflected functional abnormalities.[9] Application of ANS challenges

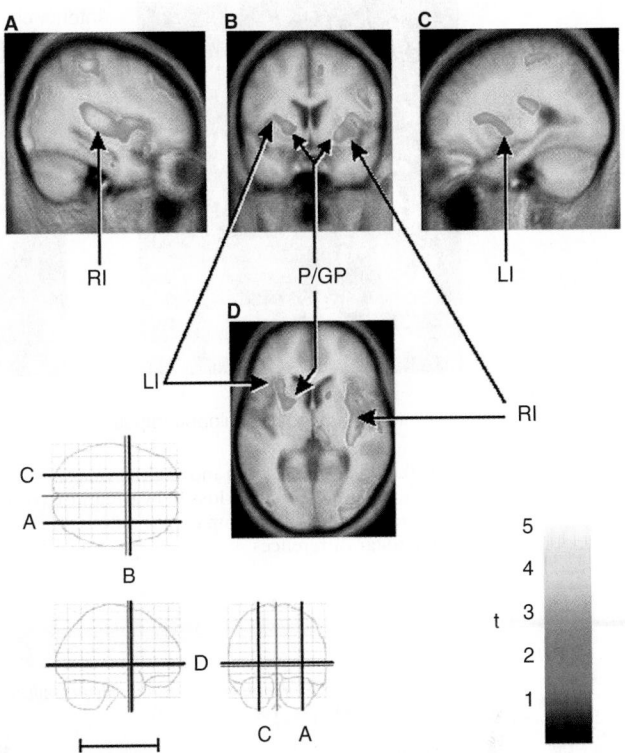

FIGURE 11-2 ■ Regions of gray matter injury for insular areas are shown in heart failure versus healthy controls and are overlaid on an averaged anatomic image of all subjects. **A, B,** and **D,** Gray matter injury in the right insula (RI). **B,** Extension of the loss to the ventral putamen and globus pallidus (P/GP) for the RI. **B, C,** and **D,** Loss in the left anterior insula (LI). **B** and **D,** Extension of these injuries to the basal ganglia (P/GP). The scale represents t-statistic values, with all indicated regions exceeding the significance threshold of $p < 0.005$ and minimum cluster size of 200 voxels. The locations of sagittal, coronal, and axial planes of slices **A** to **D** are indicated in the outline drawing, where the brain outline is in Talairach space.

(cold pressor test and Valsalva maneuver) elicited aberrant responses in the anterior and posterior hypothalamus, bilateral amygdala, hippocampus, cerebellar cortex, insular cortex, and mid/posterior cingulate cortex, right ventral frontal cortex, and temporal and frontal cortices. Many of these areas neighbored or overlaid regions of previously demonstrated gray matter damage (Figure 11-3). In these functional MRI studies, activity in the right insula, in response to potent sympathetic stimuli, was reduced dramatically in heart failure compared with controls. This damage likely contributes to the wildly variable heart rates in the heart failure patients during ANS challenges, such as during the cold pressor test (Figure 11-4, left panel). These differences in heart rate response may result from the changes observed in the right insula, which usually dampens sympathetic response, and when damaged, sympathetic nervous system activation is less controlled. As seen in Figure 11-4, the averaged heart rate values show increased beat-to-beat variation, as well as increased heart rate related to the high sympathetic tone.

Yet are these changes in the brain restricted to persons with heart failure? The answer is probably not.

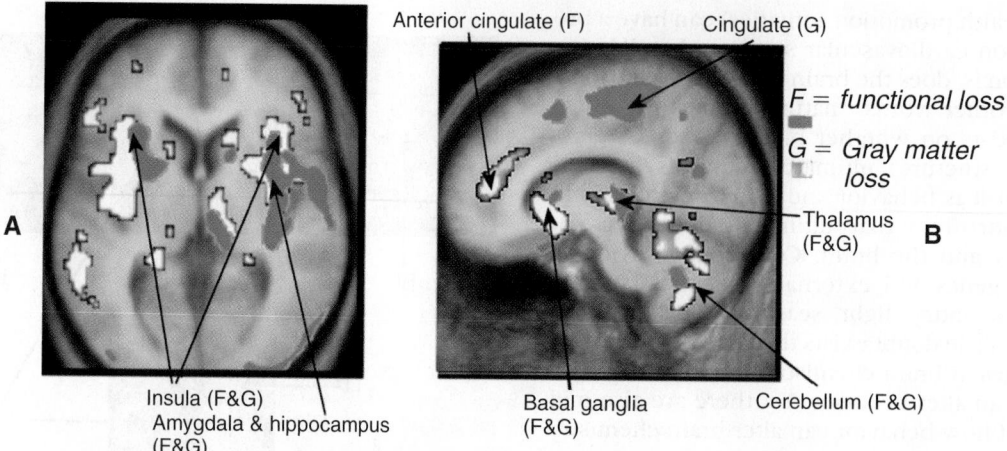

FIGURE 11-3 ■ Axial and sagittal images showing functional abnormalities in response to Valsalva maneuver and structural loss in heart failure patients in comparison to controls. **A,** Axial view of insula, amygdala, and hippocampal differences. **B,** Sagittal view of basal ganglia, cingulate, thalamus, and cerebellar differences.

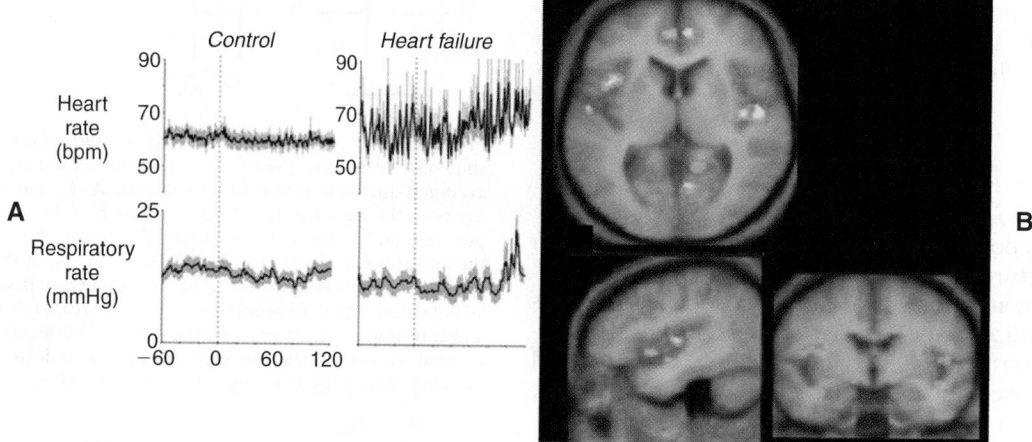

FIGURE 11-4 ■ **A,** Mean heart and respiratory rate changes (S.E.) to cold pressor application to the forehead (application at time 0). Heart and respiratory rates increase late in the challenge in heart failure patients. The heart rates and respiratory rates illustrated are the mean rates for the groups. The heart rates for the heart failure subjects varied widely from moment to moment, unlike the control subjects, in response to the cold pressor stimulus. Thus, the variability seen in the heart rate plot is not due to artifact or signal noise but to actual heart rate responses. **B,** Axial, sagittal, and coronal images showing left and right insular damage in the heart failure patients to the cold pressor challenge. *BPM,* Beats per minute.

Persons with obstructive sleep apnea, who are at high risk for developing cardiovascular disease, share many of the functional MRI abnormalities observed in heart failure patients.[10]

Although there are multiple reports of changes in brain structure and function among individuals with cardiovascular conditions, it is uncertain whether these CNS alterations are linked to clinical symptoms or prognosis. Also, it is unclear whether these structural and functional changes in the CNS are due to changes or abnormalities in the cardiovascular system or if the alterations in the CNS precede and contribute to cardiovascular dysfunction. Whatever the underlying cause for the CNS changes seen in persons with cardiovascu-

lar disease, there is extensive evidence for the existence of strong interactions between the brain and the heart.

EVIDENCE OF BRAIN-HEART INTERACTIONS

The impact of brain-heart interactions often is ignored by clinicians. Yet these two systems can have a profound impact on each other. The brain plays a key role in ANS regulation of cardiovascular activity (through the release of catecholamines and other hormones and by direct nerve connections), which can be reflected in the areas of cardiac dysrhythmias, alterations in cardiovascular risk, and changes in heart rate variability.

Cardiac Dysrhythmias and Sudden Death

Most cardiovascular clinicians are familiar with the risk of cardiac sudden death, especially in the setting of structural heart disease. However, often there is less awareness of the fact that there are cerebrogenic causes of cardiac dysrhythmias and sudden death that can occur without the presence of structural heart disease. Electrocardiographic changes, without association with acute cardiac events, have been noted in persons with subarachnoid hemorrhage (40 to 70 percent), intracranial hemorrhage (60 to 70 percent), and ischemic stroke (15 to 40 percent).[11] Similar electrocardiographic patterns have been reported in other brain conditions, such as head trauma, brain tumors, meningitis, and hydrocephalus. These electrocardiographic changes include prolonged QT intervals, ST segment depression, inverted T waves, ST segment elevation, Q waves, U waves, and increased QRS complex amplitude. These electrocardiographic changes may evolve over several days, during the acute phase of the brain abnormality, whereas some electrocardiographic changes, such as QT interval prolongation or U waves, may be permanent.

Persons with cerebrogenic electrocardiographic changes (i.e., in the absence of any acute cardiac events) often have creatine kinase myocardial isoenzyme elevations. These cardiac-specific isoenzymes are linked closely to the magnitude of the electrocardiographic changes and cardiac dysrhythmias, especially in persons with acute stroke. Of interest is the fact that the cardiac-specific isoenzymes gradually increase during the first 4 days of the stroke, which is in distinct contrast to their behavior after an acute myocardial infarction, in which they gradually decrease.

Cardiac dysrhythmias commonly are reported in all types of stroke. The dysrhythmias that have been reported after stroke include bradycardia, supraventricular tachycardia, atrial fibrillation/flutter, premature ventricular beats, multifocal ventricular tachyardia, torsade de pointes, and ventricular fibrillation/tachyardia.[11,12]

Another, also often ignored, factor that can contribute to cerebrogenic sudden death is behavior. Behavioral factors are associated with the development of malignant dysrhythmias and sudden cardiac death. Emotional stressors, particularly anger, have been linked to increased incidence of sudden cardiac death.[13,14]

Thus structural, ANS, and behavioral components of the CNS can affect survival directly, particularly related to the risk for sudden cardiac death. Although sudden cardiac death is one of the more severe adverse effects of the CNS on the cardiovascular system, the brain also can influence cardiovascular risk factors negatively, which could increase the incidence of cardiovascular disease.

Increased Cardiovascular Risk Related to the Brain

Traditionally, cardiovascular risk factors are viewed as being directed by external (e.g., diet) and genotype issues. However, the brain may influence cardiovascular risk factors dramatically. This influence can be via behavior, as discussed earlier. Additionally, there now are indications that alterations in the ability of the brain to control hormone secretion could increase the risk for developing cardiovascular problems, such as atherosclerotic heart disease and stroke. For example, in a study by Heikens and colleagues,[15] adult survivors of childhood brain cancer had higher blood pressures and cholesterol levels, and were more likely to accumulate fat at the waistline. The investigators believed that these body changes were due to radiation treatment for childhood brain cancer that interfered with brain control of several hormones because of altered function of the pituitary gland. Levels of human growth hormone, produced by the pituitary gland, were abnormally low in 58 percent of these brain cancer survivors. The group with growth hormone deficiency showed the highest low-density lipoprotein cholesterol levels and waist-to-hip ratios.

In addition to increasing cardiovascular risk factors, changes in the brain (especially of the insular lobes) are related to increased risk for cardiac disease states. For example, there are now reports that myocardial injury can occur after stroke in the absence of primary cardiac causes.[16]

Heart Rate Variability and the Central Nervous System

Heart rate variability, a measure of R-R interval behavior (time interval between heart beats), reflects ANS tone. Multiple investigators have reported that reduced heart rate variability is associated with disease progression and outcome in many cardiovascular diagnoses, such as myocardial infarction, heart failure, and hypertension.[17,18] Although peripheral ANS activity influences heart rate variability, there are indications that CNS components also exert strong control over heart rate variability. In animal models and in humans with stroke, heart rate variability is altered in association with structural changes in the insular lobes.[19-22]

SUMMARY

Prevailing evidence suggests that changes in CNS structure and function play an important role in the pathogenesis and progression of cardiovascular disease. Clinicians should be aware of this brain-heart interaction and should carefully assess CNS status in their patients. However, further investigations are needed to increase our understanding of the structural and functional characteristics of the CNS in persons with cardiovascular disease. An increased understanding in this area will help health care providers to elucidate the relationships between the peripheral and CNS abnormalities commonly seen in these patients and holds the potential for correction of the adverse accompaniments of cardiovascular disease states. Such correction may alter disease progression and mortality in this ever-growing patient population.

REFERENCES

1. Shanoudy H, Soliman A, Moe S et al: Early manifestations of "sick euthyroid" syndrome in patients with compensated chronic heart failure, *J Card Fail* 7:146-152, 2001.
2. Weiss ML, Kenney MJ, Musch TI et al: Modifications to central neural circuitry during heart failure, *Acta Physiol Scand* 177: 57-67, 2003.
3. Wei SG, Felder RB: Forebrain renin-angiotensin system has a tonic excitatory influence on renal sympathetic nerve activity, *Am J Physiol Heart Circ Physiol* 282:H890-H895, 2002.
4. Ferguson DW, Mark AL: Clinical neurocardiology: role of the autonomic nervous system in clinical heart failure. In Armour JA, Ardell JL, editors: *Neurocardiology,* Oxford, Great Britain, 1994, Oxford University Press.
5. Culman J, Blume A, Gohlke P et al: The renin-angiotensin system in the brain: possible therapeutic implications for AT$_1$-receptor blockers, *J Hum Hypertens* 16(suppl 3):S64-S70, 2002.
6. Cook IA, Leuchter AF, Morgan ML et al: Longitudinal progression of subclinical structural brain disease in normal aging, *Am J Geriatr Psychiatry* 12:190-200, 2004.
7. Schmidt R, Fazekas F, Offenbacher H et al: Brain magnetic resonance imaging and neuropsychologic evaluation of patients with idiopathic dilated cardiomyopathy, *Stroke* 22:195-199, 1991.
8. Woo MA, Macey PM, Fonarow GC et al: Regional brain gray matter loss in advanced heart failure, *J Appl Physiol* 95:677-684, 2003.
9. Woo MA, Macey PM, Keens PT et al: Functional abnormalities in brain areas which mediate autonomic nervous system control in advanced heart failure, *J Card Fail* 11:437-446, 2005.
10. Henderson LA, Woo MA, Macey PM et al: Neural responses during Valsalva maneuvers in obstructive sleep apnea syndrome, *J Appl Physiol* 94:1063-1074, 2003.
11. Cheung RTF, Hachinski V: The insula and cerebrogenic sudden death, *Arch Neurol* 57:1685-1688, 2000.
12. Oppenheimer SM, Cechetto DF, Hachinski VC: Cerebrogenic cardiac arrhythmias: cerebral electrocardiographic influences and their role in sudden death, *Arch Neurol* 47:513-519, 1990.
13. Mittelman MA, Maclure M, Sherwood JB et al: Triggering of acute myocardial infarction onset by episodes of anger, *Circulation* 92:1720-1725, 1995.
14. Kovach JA, Nearing BD, Verrier RL: Angerlike behavioral state potentiates myocardial ischemia-induced T-wave alternans in canines, *J Am Coll Cardiol* 37:1719-1725, 2001.
15. Heikens J, Ubbink MC, van der Pal et al: Long term survivors of childhood brain cancer have an increased risk for cardiovascular disease, *Cancer* 88:2116-2121, 2000.
16. Ay H, Koroshetz WJ, Benner T et al: Neuroanatomic correlates of stroke-related myocardial injury, *Neurology* 66:1-5, 2006.
17. Kleiger RE, Stein PK, Bigger JT: Heart rate variability: measurement and clinical utility, *Ann Noninvasive Electrocardiol* 10: 88-101, 2005.
18. Frenneaux MP: Autonomic changes in patients with heart failure and in post-myocardial infarction patients, *Heart* 90:1248-1255, 2004.
19. Cechetto DF, Chen SJ: Subcortical sites mediating sympathetic responses from insular cortex in rats, *Am J Physiol* 258:R245-R255, 1990.
20. Oppenheimer SM, Wilson JX, Guiraudon C et al: Insular cortex stimulation produces lethal cardiac arrhythmias: a mechanism of sudden death? *Brain Res* 550:115-121, 1991.
21. Oppenheimer SM, Gelb A, Girvin JP et al: Cardiovascular effects of human insular cortex stimulation, *Neurol* 42:1727-1732, 1992.
22. Oppenheimer SM, Kedem G, Martin WM: Left-insular cortex lesions perturb cardiac autonomic tone in humans, *Clin Auton Res* 6:131-140, 1996.

▪▪▪▪ chapter 12

Fundamentals of Nutrition for Cardiovascular Health

Terry A. Lennie

CHAPTER ABBREVIATIONS

AHA   American Heart Association

BMI   body mass index

DASH   Dietary Approaches to Stop Hypertension

DHA   docosahexaenoic acid

EPA   eicosapentaenoic acid

HDL   high-density lipoprotein

HOPE   Heart Outcomes Prevention Evaluation

IBW   ideal body weight

INTERSALT   International Study of Sodium, Potassium, and Blood Pressure

LDL   low-density lipoprotein

LPS   lipopolysaccharide

MAC   midarm circumference

MAMC   midarm muscle circumference

MUFA   monounsaturated fatty acids

PUFA   polyunsaturated fatty acids

TSF   triceps skin fold

USDA   U.S. Department of Agriculture

On the most basic level, eating is a simple act to meet the primal goal of relieving hunger pangs. This is coupled with an innate appetite for varying the types of foods eaten to promote a diet that includes all necessary nutrients. Research, technology, commercialization, and in some instances, politicization of food have transformed eating into a complex act aimed at obtaining the correct combination of various nutrients in the correct amount to optimize health. When addressing nutrition, foods are no longer viewed with respect to color, texture, taste, or other qualities that make eating enjoyable. Rather, foods are viewed from the perspective of their composition of various macronutrients and micronutrients.

The challenge for clinicians working with patients to improve their nutrition is that recommendations for the optimal combination of macronutrients and micronutrients in the diet are in continuous flux. Some foods that previously were vilified now are considered acceptable, whereas others that once were recommended now are deemed undesirable. The list to which a particular food is delegated can depend more on the interpretation of available evidence than the evidence itself. This emphasis on individual nutrients has initiated a popular trend to focus on dietary supplements rather than on whole foods as the best means to achieve health. Dietary supplement companies have capitalized on this trend, turning supplements into a multibillion-dollar industry.

This chapter describes individual nutrients thought to affect cardiovascular health and reviews the evidence to support their role in promoting cardiovascular health. The recommendations and guidelines presented, however, advocate whole-food/dietary pattern approaches to promoting nutrition for cardiovascular health. These recommendations are intended to apply to all patients at risk for or with cardiovascular disease. Detailed guidelines for specific cardiovascular diseases that have a nutrition-related component, such as hypertension and dyslipidemia, are presented in their respective chapters. Because heart failure is a consequence of cardiovascular diseases, not a cardiovascular disease itself, an overview of nutrition-related factors for heart failure is presented at the end of this chapter.

MACRONUTRIENTS

The three categories of macronutrients are fats, carbohydrates, and proteins (Table 12-1). Each of these categories can be subdivided further according to chemical structure, food source, and metabolic need or effect. Of the three, fats have received the most attention with respect to cardiovascular disease. Carbohydrates have received attention for their potential effects on plasma lipoproteins and triglycerides. Proteins have received the most attention for prevention of cardiovascular disease and as a potential replacement for dietary carbohydrates.

Fats

Dietary fats exist mainly as triglycerides that are made up primarily of fatty acids. Fatty acids, of which there are 24, provide energy and serve as important structural components of cell membranes. Fatty acids are found in fat-soluble vitamins and steroid hormones. Fats are the most energy-dense of the macronutrients, providing 9 kcal/g, which is more than double the calories in carbohydrates and proteins. Fats can be subdivided into the following categories based on chemical structure: saturated, *trans*, polyunsaturated, and monounsaturated (Box 12-1). The distinction between different categories of fats is made based on the number of bonds between carbon atoms and the number and location of hydrogen atoms bound to carbon in the fatty acid chains.

Earlier research, such as the Framingham studies, showed an association between lipids and cardiovascular disease. This led to the development of the dietary fat-blood lipid-coronary artery disease hypothesis.[1] A broad recommendation to limit all dietary fats was advocated to prevent cardiovascular disease.[2] More recent research has shown that although some fats (i.e., satu-

■ ■ ■

TABLE 12-1   MACRONUTRIENTS

	SOURCES	COMMENTS
Saturated fats	Animal: fatty meats, butter Plant: coconut and palm oil Commercial: margarine, processed foods	Increase LDL High intake associated with cardiovascular disease
Trans fats	Margarine Processed foods with partially hydrogenated oils	Increase LDL Decrease HDL Alter structure of cell walls Proinflammatory
Polyunsaturated fats	Plants and fatty fish, canola, soybean, corn, sunflower, and safflower oils	Omega-3 antiinflammatory Omega-6 proinflammatory Lower cholesterol and LDL but also HDL
Monounsaturated fats	Plants, olive oil, peanut oil, canola oil, almonds, peanuts, pecans, avocados	Decrease LDL without affecting HDL
Carbohydrates	Pasta, potatoes, rice, fruits, vegetables, whole grains	May decrease HDL Effects vary by carbohydrate source (e.g., glycemic index)
Animal protein	Fish, meats, dairy products, eggs	Fatty meats high in cholesterol High-protein diets may decrease cholesterol, LDL, and VLDL
Vegetable protein	Nuts, seeds, legumes, grains, cereals, soy products	Most are incomplete proteins that lack one or more essential amino acids Soy decreases total cholesterol, LDL, and triglycerides

HDL, High-density lipoprotein; *LDL,* low-density lipoprotein; *VLDL,* very low-density lipoprotein.

BOX 12-1   ■ ■ ■
UNDERSTANDING THE NOMENCLATURE OF *TRANS,* MONOUNSATURATED, AND POLYUNSATURATED FATTY ACIDS

Principles
- The first number is the number of carbon atoms in the fatty acid.
- The second number is the number of carbons with double bonds.
- The third and any subsequent numbers indicate the carbons where the double bonds occur.
- *Cis* means the hydrogen atoms are on the same side at the site of the double bond.
- *Trans* means the hydrogen bonds are on opposite sites.

Examples

18:1(9)	Oleic acid There are 18 carbons in the fatty acid. One location (at carbon 9) has a double bond (monounsaturated fat).
18:3(3 *cis*)	Alpha-linolenic acid There are 18 carbons in the fatty acid. Three locations have carbon pairs with double bonds (polyunsaturated fat). The first double bond occurs at carbon 3 (omega-3 fatty acid). The hydrogen atoms are on the same (*cis*) side. Shorthand is n-3 or ω-3.
20:2(3 *trans*)	There are 20 carbons in the fatty acid. Two locations have double bonds. The first double bond is at carbon 3. The hydrogens are on opposite (*trans*) sides.

*cis**

*trans**

rated and *trans* fats) increase health risks such as cardiovascular disease, other fats (i.e., monounsaturated and polyunsaturated fats) have beneficial effects. Current dietary recommendations provide a more balanced approach to dietary fat intake. Concerns about limiting some dietary fats now are related more to their high calorie content than to negative cardiovascular effects.

Saturated Fats

Saturated fats have a single bond between all carbons in the chain. Each carbon has a hydrogen atom bound at all available binding sites, hence the designation *saturated.* This formation makes the carbons along the fatty acid chain align in a straight line, resulting in the fats fitting closely together. As a result, saturated fats (with the exception of coconut oil) are stable and solid at room temperature. Saturated fats can be divided further into animal and plants sources. Saturated fats from animals are in the form of solid fats in meats. Plant sources are limited to palm kernel and coconut oils used mostly in manufactured foods and snacks. Saturated fats have long been the fats to avoid. These fats raise blood cholesterol, including low-density lipoprotein (**LDL**), which is linked to atherosclerosis. Saturated fat, however, also can increase beneficial high-density lipoprotein (**HDL**).

Trans *Fats*

Some *trans* fats are made naturally in the stomachs of ruminants and are found in beef, lamb, and whole milk. These account for only a small amount of total *trans* fats in the diet, however. The most common sources of *trans* fats are margarines, manufactured or premade foods, fried fast foods, and snacks.[3] The *trans* fats in these foods are created by hydrogenation of unsaturated fats to make them more stable. The hydrogenation process changes the location of the hydrogen atoms along the fatty acid chain (Box 12-1). This process changes their curved structure to a straight line resembling saturated fats. Subsequently, they function like saturated fats and carry similar cardiovascular risks. In fact, *trans* fats are considered to have more deleterious effects than saturated fat because they increase triglycerides and LDL while also decreasing HDL. When incorporated into cell membranes, *trans* fats may promote inflammation, including that associated with atherosclerosis.[4] Epidemiological studies have shown a strong association between *trans* fat intake and increased risk of sudden cardiac death. Evidence from other research suggests that additional, as yet unknown, effects of *trans* fats contribute to the high risk of cardiac death associated with these fats.[5]

Trans fats compose about 4 to 7 percent of the fats in a typical Western diet. Data are insufficient to establish a specific level of *trans* fat intake,[6] but a general rule is to limit *trans* fats to 2 percent or less of fat intake.[7] Avoiding fried fast foods, processed and premade foods, and commercially prepared snacks is the best way to avoid *trans* fats. In some foods, however, the beneficial effects of other ingredients outweigh the effects of the *trans* fats. For example, most commercial peanut butters contain a small amount of *trans* fats that are produced during the hydrogenation process to prevent oil separation. The positive effects of the high amount of beneficial fats and protein in peanut butter far exceed any negative effects of the *trans* fats.

Monounsaturated Fats

Monounsaturated fatty acids (**MUFAs**) have a single pair of carbons with a double bond between them, hence the name *monounsaturated*. The carbons in the double bond have an open site where a hydrogen atom could bind (Box 12-1, *cis* structure). This configuration causes the fatty acid chain to curve at the site of the double bond. The curved structure of these fats in the cell membrane increases membrane fluidity and provides pathways between the cytosol and extracellular fluid. The configuration also results in the fatty acids having an electrical charge, making them useful for electron transport. Neither of these functions is present in saturated or *trans* fats because of their straight structure. The curved structure also makes MUFAs align loosely, resulting in their being liquid at room temperature. Oleic acid is the dominant monounsaturated fat.

MUFAs are considered "heart friendly." Replacement of saturated fats with MUFAs in the diet decreases cholesterol and LDL levels in the blood. In addition to lowering LDL levels, MUFAs appear to increase the size of remaining LDL and decrease their susceptibility to oxidation, both of which suppress atherogenesis.[8] MUFAs also are being investigated as a caloric substitute for carbohydrates in diabetic diets because they appear to improve glycemic control.

Polyunsaturated Fats

Polyunsaturated fatty acids (**PUFAs**) have two or more carbon pairs with double bonds. Because there are multiple pairs of double bonded carbons with open sites that potentially could bind a hydrogen atom, these fatty acids are referred to as polyunsaturated. PUFAs have multiple curves (at each double bond) along their structure and are liquid at room temperature.

Replacing dietary carbohydrates or saturated fats with PUFAs produces a decrease in LDL levels. The effect is greater for saturated fat replacement than for carbohydrates. The two main classes of PUFAs are omega-6 and omega-3. The distinction between these two fatty acids is the location of the first pair of carbons with a double bond. For omega-6, it is the 6th and 7th carbons; for omega-3, it is the 3rd and 4th carbons. Both are considered essential fatty acids because the body cannot synthesize them and because pathological changes are associated with dietary deficiency. These fatty acids have received considerable attention because of their actions in the cardiovascular system.

Linolenic acid is the primary omega-6 fatty acid. This fatty acid can be metabolized into gamma-linolenic acid and arachidonic acid. Arachidonic acid is the major precursor for the inflammatory prostaglandins.

Alpha-linolenic acid is the primary omega-3 fatty acid. This fatty acid can be metabolized into docosahexaenoic acid (**DHA**) and eicosapentaenoic acid (**EPA**). DHA and EPA serve important biological functions throughout the body, including many related to cardiovascular health.

Omega-6 and omega-3 fatty acids are incorporated into cell walls. During tissue injury or stress, metabolic pathways are triggered that convert these fatty acids into biologically active metabolites. Linolenic acid (omega-6) forms arachidonic acid metabolites such as prostaglandins of the E_2 series (PGE_2), thromboxanes of the A_2 series (TXA_2), and leukotrienes of the B_4 and C_4 series (LTB4 and LTC4). These metabolites are potent mediators of inflammation and promote vasoconstriction and platelet aggregation.[9] The alpha-linolenic (omega-3) metabolites EPA and DHA produce the less inflammatory three series prostaglandins, PGE_3 and PGI_3, TXA_3, and LTB_5 and LTC_5. These metabolites also suppress platelet aggregation and promote vasoconstriction.

Omega-6 and omega-3 fatty acids compete for the same enzymes during the process of forming their respective metabolites. When the proportion of omega-3 fatty acids in the diet increases to about one-third the amount of omega-6 fatty acids, they replace a proportionate amount of omega-6 fatty acids in cell membranes. In response to inflammatory stimuli, omega-3 fatty acids, by right of greater number, successfully compete with omega-6 fatty acids for the enzyme pathways. Subsequently, tissues with higher amounts of omega-3 fatty acids produce less inflammation than tissues with a greater proportion of omega-6 fatty acids. Benefits of increased omega-3 fatty acids in the vascular epithelium include slowed progression of atherosclerosis and decreased platelet aggregation. Additional positive effects attributed to omega-3 fatty acids include antivasopressor, antihypertension, and antiarrhythmic activities.[10]

Individuals who eat a lot of processed foods obtain less of these essential fatty acids because the hydrogenation of the polyunsaturated fats (i.e., conversion to *trans* fats) alters the location of hydrogen atoms, making them unusable as essential fatty acids by the body. Western diets typically contain a much greater proportion of omega-6 fatty acids than is thought to be beneficial. This is because omega-6 fatty acids compose a large component of the oils (corn, safflower, cottonseed, peanut, and soybean) used for cooking and in prepared foods. In contrast, the primary source of omega-3 fatty acids is oily fish such as sardines, mackerel, trout, and salmon.[9] Alpha-linolenic acid is found in flaxseed oil. Humans convert only about 15 percent of alpha-linolenic acid to the more active DHA or EPA. In contrast, fish are efficient at converting alpha-linolenic acid to DHA and EPA, which is why they are a good source of these fatty acids. The American Heart Association (**AHA**) recommends eating at least two servings of fatty fish per week. Fish with high amounts of omega-3 fatty acids include mackerel, lake trout, herring, sardines, albacore tuna, and salmon. An important note is that canned tuna is not a good source of omega-3 fatty acids. This is true even for tuna packed in oil because manufacturers typically replace the tuna oil with a vegetable oil that is not as high in omega-3 fatty acids. Plus, vegetable oil leaches omega-3 fatty acids from the tuna and then is drained off. Consequently, tuna packed in water may be higher in omega-3 fatty acids.

Given these positive effects, it is tempting to recommend a diet high in PUFAs. As with most nutrients, however, excessive amounts can produce negative effects that counter the positive effects observed at lower levels of dietary intake.[1] Omega-3 and omega-6 fatty acids can promote insulin secretion. Insulin activates the pathway leading to arachidonic acid release from the cell membrane with the resultant production of inflammatory mediators. These fatty acids are prone to oxidation, which can increase oxidative stress. Moreover, incorporation of high amounts of PUFAs in LDL particles promotes LDL oxidation and the subsequent inflammation associated with atherosclerosis. Thus, the universal axiom of "everything in moderation" holds for PUFA intake as well.

Fish Oil

The AHA recommends a dietary approach to obtaining adequate amounts (about 1000 mg/d) of EPA and DHA for everyone.[11] For patients with coronary artery disease in which this amount cannot be achieved readily through diet alone, the use of fish oil supplements may be considered, in consultation with a physician, to reduce cardiovascular disease risk. Supplements also may be considered for medical management of hypertriglyceridemia, but larger doses (2 to 4 g/d) are required. A 1000-mg fish oil capsule contains about 350 mg of EPA and DHA combined. Three capsules provide a total of about 1000 mg of EPA and DHA. High-potency capsules contain higher amounts. A test by *Consumer Reports* showed that the inexpensive fish capsules available at drug stores and supermarkets provide the same amounts of EPA and DHA as many of the more expensive products.[12] None of the capsules contained significant amounts of mercury. For vegetarians, flaxseed oil is an alternative source. Flaxseed oil contains omega-3, omega-6, and omega-9 fatty acids. The omega-3 fatty acid in flaxseed is alpha-linolenic acid, which must be converted to the beneficial EPA and DHA. As noted previously, human beings are not efficient at this conver-

sion. Although flaxseed capsules are touted to contain twice as much omega-3 fatty acid as fish oil capsules, they probably provide lower amounts of EPA and DHA.

Carbohydrates

Carbohydrates provide energy for muscle and other metabolically active tissues and are the main source of energy for brain cells and erythrocytes. Carbohydrates also are combined with proteins to form important structural and functional molecules in cells such as glycoproteins in cell membranes. The inclusion of carbohydrates into cell membrane proteins makes them more hydrophilic, which enhances interaction with the extracellular environment and promotes folding into their tertiary (functional) structure. Carbohydrates are less energy dense than fats, providing only 4 kcal/g. Energy from carbohydrates is stored as glycogen in liver and muscle, and as triglycerides (fat) in adipose tissue. Human beings store only 25 g of carbohydrates in the form of glycerol, meaning that the majority of carbohydrates consumed in excess of energy need are stored as fat.

Carbohydrates vary from simple three- to seven-carbon sugars (monosaccharides) to large complex molecules (polysaccharides) containing up to 10,000 or more monosaccharides. This structure provides a convenient way to classify carbohydrates as simple versus complex. However, this classification has little relevance to the effects of carbohydrates on the cardiovascular system. Developing an alternative classification has been challenging because carbohydrates are found in many foods.

Many of the foods high in carbohydrates—such as fruits, vegetables, cereals, and legumes—have been shown to have beneficial effects on the cardiovascular system. However, diets excessively high in carbohydrates may lower HDL levels and increase the amount of small LDL.[13] Additional negative effects of carbohydrates are related to their role in promoting excess weight and obesity. The debate regarding low-carbohydrate versus high-carbohydrate diets is discussed in a later section. The related, hotly debated issue of whether protein should replace carbohydrates in the diet also is reviewed in more detail in a later section.

Glycemic Index

The glycemic index has been advocated as a way to classify carbohydrates that has relevance for diabetes and cardiovascular disease. Given the degree of interest and number of diet books published based on the glycemic index, a discussion is merited. The glycemic index rates carbohydrates based on their effect on blood glucose levels over the 2 hours following ingestion. Common glycemic indices rate foods against glucose or white bread as the standard food. Foods that receive a 100 on the scale have the same effect on blood glucose as white bread or glucose. Foods with a rating less than 55 are considered to have a low glycemic index. Those that rate 55 to 70 have a moderate glycemic index. Those with an index higher than 70 are considered to have a high glycemic index. The most recent comprehensive glycemic index table of foods was published in 2002.[14]

To account for differences in the amount of carbohydrates available in different foods, the concept of glycemic load was developed. The glycemic load takes the glycemic index for a particular food and adjusts it for the amount of carbohydrates available in a serving. Foods that have a low glycemic index are absorbed more slowly and therefore produce a lower, more sustained rise in blood glucose level. Slower absorption is thought to lengthen the time before a person feels hungry again, prolong the suppression of free fatty acid release into the blood, and avoid a large peak in blood glucose and insulin. This metabolic state should be consistent with decreased daily calorie intake, better blood lipid profiles, and improved glucose tolerance. Yet a systematic review of the available evidence showed that low-glycemic-index diets did not affect triglyceride, LDL, or HDL levels or decrease the risk for cardiovascular disease.[15]

An important note is that most of the trials in which low-glycemic-index diets were tested were short-term with small sample sizes. Larger, better-controlled trials may show a benefit. To date, however, there is insufficient evidence to support recommending low-glycemic-index diets as a way to decrease cardiovascular risk factors. Also important to note is that meals usually contain a mixture of proteins and fats that can alter the absorption of carbohydrates, effectively changing their glycemic index. Further, glycemic index is not to be used as the sole means of choosing carbohydrates. One must balance the nutrient quality of the food against its glycemic index. For example, ice cream has a lower glycemic index than carrots.

Fiber

One classification of carbohydrates for which there is no debate regarding the effects on cardiovascular disease risk factors is fiber. The fiber found naturally in foods such as fruits, vegetables, whole-grain cereals, and legumes is termed *dietary fiber*. The fiber added as a food supplement is labeled *added fiber*. Fiber is divided into soluble and insoluble forms. Closely related are resistant starches. Resistant starches are slow to be digested, and significant amounts pass into the large intestine. Now, considerable evidence exists supporting the beneficial effects of fiber on cardiovascular risk factors. In fact, the Food and Drug Administration allows the health claim that soluble fiber from oats and psyllium can decrease the risk of developing cardiovascular disease when included as part of a diet low in saturated fat and cholesterol. The positive effects of various fibers are outlined in Table 12-2.[16]

It should be noted that some of the beneficial effects of high-fiber intake result from other changes in the diet needed to obtain adequate fiber. Foods high in fiber tend to have a low glycemic load. Further, foods high in fiber usually replace foods high in saturated fat and refined carbohydrates in the diet. As noted before, diets low in saturated fat and refined carbohydrates, independent of fiber intake, can decrease cardiovascular disease risk. However, when combined with high fiber, these diets should have added benefit.

■ ■ ■

TABLE 12-2 BENEFICIAL EFFECTS OF FIBER

TYPE	EFFECT
Fiber in general	Slow intestinal glucose absorption, minimizing postprandial spikes in blood glucose
	Improve insulin sensitivity
	Promote gastric formation of propionate, which inhibits a key enzyme (HMG-CoA reductase) in hepatic cholesterol synthesis
Soluble fiber	Decrease total cholesterol
	Decrease low-density lipoproteins
Cereals, fruits, vegetables	Decrease incidence of coronary events
	Decrease total cholesterol
Oats	Decrease small, dense, low-density lipoproteins
	Promote cholesterol removal through bile acid synthesis
Legumes	Slow intestinal lipoprotein absorption

HMG-CoA, 3-hydroxy-3-methylglutaryl coenzyme A.

Proteins

Proteins are composed of various combinations of 20 different amino acids. In addition to carbon, hydrogen, and oxygen also found in fats and carbohydrates, amino acids contain nitrogen and sulfur. The presence of nitrogen in proteins allows them to assume several hundred different forms. The form a protein takes dictates its function. Protein is considered the totipotent nutrient because the constituent amino acids are the only molecules that can be transformed into all three macronutrients: proteins, carbohydrates, and fats.[17] Proteins serve many essential functions in the body. They are a major component of all body tissues and the main component of lean body mass. Proteins provide the structure for hormones and enzymes. They serve as major blood transporters of molecules that are not water soluble, such as drugs and vitamins, as well as fat in the form of lipoproteins. Protein depletion leads to impaired metabolism, altered immune function, muscle wasting, and in severe cases, death.[18]

Debate is ongoing regarding the optimal level of protein in the diet. Although diets high in protein may reduce cardiovascular disease risk factors, high-protein diets (i.e., more than 30 percent of total energy) increase urinary calcium loss and the risk of osteoporosis and raise the urea load on the kidneys, increasing the risk of renal damage.[19,20] The two major sources of protein, animal and plant, are discussed separately.

Animal Protein

Early epidemiological studies showed that animal protein intake increased the risk of death from cardiovascular disease.[21] At the time these studies were conducted (1950s), high-fat or marbled meats were considered most desirable. As such, animal protein in these studies was strongly associated with higher saturated fat and cholesterol intake. Subsequent studies using lean (low-fat) sources of animal proteins showed that high-protein diets were associated with reductions in triglycerides, total cholesterol, LDL, and very low-density lipoprotein and a modest increase in HDL. This finding is seen in persons with elevated lipids and in those with normal lipid levels.[22,23] In sum, animal protein from sources that are low in saturated fat and cholesterol appear to be cardioprotective. An important note is that the recommendation to use low-fat animal protein sources does not apply to fish, which contain polyunsaturated fats that are beneficial.

Plant-Based Protein

The amount of protein in fruits and vegetables is lower than in meat. However, it is possible to obtain all essential amino acids required for protein formation by eating a variety of fruits and vegetables. Vegan (entirely plant-based) diets are naturally low in saturated fat, *trans* fats, and cholesterol and are high in fiber, all of which are heart healthy. Vegetarian diets, which may include milk and eggs, are also lower in fats and higher in fiber. A complete discussion of these diets or making specific dietary recommendations regarding the ideal plant-based diet is beyond the scope of this chapter. Soy protein, however, is one vegetable protein that merits further discussion. The addition of soy protein to the diet has implications for all individuals regardless of whether their diet is completely plant based or includes animal protein.

Soy Protein

Soy-based products such as soy milk, tofu, and protein drinks are now readily available. The increased popularity of soy protein is due in large part to research showing that diets high in soy protein are associated with a lower incidence of cardiovascular disease. Research showing the beneficial effects of soy protein was sufficient for the Food and Drug Administration to approve the following health claim in 1999: *25 grams of soy protein a day, as part of a diet low in saturated fat and cholesterol, may reduce the risk of heart disease.*[24] Routine dietary intake of soy protein (e.g., tofu) has been shown to decrease triglyceride, total cholesterol, and LDL levels. However, supplementation also appears beneficial. A study comparing 15- or 25-g soy protein supplementation with placebo in hypercholesterolemic patients showed that 8 weeks of supplementation decreased total cholesterol, LDL, and apolipoprotein B levels.[25] The 25-g dose of soy protein was almost twice as effective as the 15-g dose. Soy protein appears to be most effective in persons with elevated LDL or cholesterol levels. In persons with normal LDL levels, soy protein will not cause a further reduction. Thus, soy protein supplementation in persons with normal LDL levels is of limited benefit, although supplementation could help keep their levels in the normal range. The decision to replace protein sources that contain saturated fats and cholesterol with soy would be beneficial for everyone.

The mechanisms by which soy protein decreases cardiovascular disease risk are not fully known. The isoflavones contained in soy are thought to play a role. Isoflavones are naturally occurring molecules that modulate estrogen receptors. A meta-analysis of 23 studies was conducted to determine the effects of soy protein supplementation with different levels of isoflavones on plasma lipids.[26] Overall, soy protein with isoflavones was more effective in lowering triglyceride, total cholesterol, and LDL levels. A small increase in HDL level also was found. The effects were greatest among men and postmenopausal women. Soy supplements that provided 80 mg/d of isoflavones were more effective than those that provided less than 40 mg/d of isoflavones. The authors noted a high degree of variability in outcomes among the studies because of considerable heterogeneity in study design, which indicates that the effects of soy protein were influenced by multiple, as yet unidentified, environmental and behavioral factors. Factors that were identified as affecting the response to soy supplementation included sex (more effective in men), initial lipid levels, duration of supplementation, and dietary patterns of individuals. These factors emphasize that recommendations focused on manipulating a single nutrient without consideration of personal and lifestyle factors are not effective strategies for reducing cardiovascular disease risk.

MICRONUTRIENTS

Two major categories of micronutrients are vitamins and minerals. They are called micronutrients because they are present in food at amounts that are 100 to more than 10,000 times lower than proteins, fats, and carbohydrates. Several of these micronutrients have been promoted as important to cardiovascular health (Table 12-3).

Vitamins

Vitamin A and Beta-Carotene

Vitamin A is a fat-soluble vitamin that has antioxidant actions. Beta-carotene is a vitamin A precursor. Vitamin A is incorporated into LDL molecules and may play a role in preventing LDL oxidation. LDL oxidation stimulates inflammation in the vascular epithelium, leading to atherosclerosis (see Chapter 9). The AHA does not recommend vitamin A supplementation because of lack of evidence that it helps prevent cardiovascular disease or stroke.[35] In fact, there is evidence that vitamin A intake may be associated with an increased risk of cardiovascular disease, especially in persons with other risk factors.[36] The reason for the increased risk is unknown. Studies of beta-carotene show similar outcomes. The Alpa-Tocopherol, Beta-Carotene Cancer Prevention Study and the Beta-Carotene and Retinol Efficacy trials showed an increased risk of lung cancer and ischemic cardiovascular disease with beta-carotene supplementation.[37,38]

Vitamin C

Vitamin C is an important antioxidant and also helps maintain tissue levels of vitamins A and E.[39] Like vitamin A, vitamin C is thought to limit LDL oxidation. Vitamin C may improve vascular endothelial function by minimizing oxidative stress and preserving nitric oxide. The latter is accomplished when vitamin C scavenges reactive oxygen species that otherwise would be scavenged by nitric oxide. Observational studies and clinical trials, however, show no evidence that vitamin C decreases cardiovascular disease risk.[40-42] Current AHA guidelines

■ ■ ■

TABLE 12-3   MICRONUTRIENTS IMPORTANT TO CARDIOVASCULAR HEALTH

	SOURCES		RECOMMENDED INTAKE[27-32]
Vitamin A	Dark orange, yellow, and red fruits and vegetables	Females older than age 14	700 µg
	Dark green leafy vegetables	Males older than age 14	900 µg
		UL	
		Ages 14-18	2800 µg
		Ages 19-70	3000 µg
		Older than age 70	2000 µg
Vitamin C	Fruits and vegetables, especially papaya, strawberry, orange,	Females ages 14-18	65 mg*
	kiwi, cantaloupe, mango, red bell pepper, and brussels	Females older than age 18	75 mg
	sprouts	Males ages 14-18	75 mg
	Juices, especially orange, grapefruit, and tomato	Males older than age 18	90 mg
		UL	
		Ages 14-18	1800 mg
		Older than age 19	2000 mg
Vitamin E	Whole grains, nuts, peanut butter	Adults	15 mg
	Salad dressings, vegetable oil	UL	1000 mg
Calcium	Milk, cheese, yogurt	Females ages 18-50	1000 mg
	Broccoli, spinach, oranges	Females older than age 50	1200 mg
	Almonds	Males	
	Foods fortified with calcium	UL	1000 mg
			2500 mg
Folate or folic acid	Green leafy vegetables, legumes, nuts	Adults	400 µg
	Liver	UL	
	Fortified grain products	Ages 14-18	800 µg
		Older than age 19	1000 µg
Thiamine	Foods made with fortified whole grains	Females	1.1 mg
	Meat, poultry, fish	Males	1.2 mg
	Fruits, vegetables	UL	ND
Magnesium	Nuts, especially almonds, soy, cashews, and peanuts	Females	
	Soybeans, tofu, legumes, wheat germ	Ages 14-18	360 mg
	Chocolate	Ages 19-30	310 mg
	Dark green vegetables	Older than age 30	320 mg
	Yogurt and dairy products	Males	400 mg
		Ages 19-30	420 mg
		Older than age 30	
		UL	
		Older than age 9	350 mg*
Potassium	Apricots, bananas, orange juice, cantaloupe	Older than age 14	4700 mg
	Almonds	UL	NS
	Chicken, turkey		
	Yogurt, milk		
Selenium	Plants (amount varies depending on soil content of selenium in	Adults	55 µg
	growing region)	UL	
	Organ meats, seafood	Ages 9-13	280 µg
		Older than age 13	400 µg
Sodium	Commercially prepared food or added during cooking	Older than age 6	500 mg
		UL	Less than 2400 mg[33,34]

*Applies to supplementation beyond that obtained from food sources.
ND, Not determined; *NS,* no upper limit set, but supplementation should be taken only under medical supervision; *UL,* safe upper limit of intake.

do not recommend vitamin C supplementation as a means of preventing cardiovascular disease.[43]

Vitamins B₆, B₁₂, Folate, and Homocysteine

Homocysteine is an intermediate metabolite of the essential amino acid methionine. Homocysteine can follow two intracellular pathways.[44] One pathway, which requires folate and vitamin B₁₂, converts homocysteine back to methionine. The other pathway, which requires vitamin B₆, degrades homocysteine to the nonessential amino acids cysteine and taurine. Deficiencies in vitamins B₆, B₁₂, and folate impair homocysteine metabolism and lead to an accumulation of intracellular homocysteine. Elevated levels of homocysteine are associated with increased risk of coronary artery disease, stroke, and thromboembolism.[45]

At least three effects of homocysteine may be responsible for the association between elevated levels and cardiovascular disease. Homocysteine can alter vascular endothelial function by decreasing the bioavailability of endothelium-derived nitric oxide, alter the clotting cascade by increasing expression of platelet adhesion molecules, and stimulate inflammation by promoting oxidation of LDL and release of cytokines.[46] Surprisingly, lowering homocysteine levels does not appear to affect inflammation markers that are associated with its suspected roles in atherosclerosis. In a randomized, controlled trial of men and postmenopausal women, folic acid supplementation (800 µg/d) for 1 year decreased homocysteine levels by 28 percent but did not affect levels of C-reactive protein, oxidized LDL, or intracellular adhesion molecule-1,[47] which play roles in atherosclerosis (see Chapter 9).

The minimum daily dose of folic acid that lowers homocysteine levels is 400 μg, which can lower homocysteine levels by about 25 percent.[48] Vitamin B$_6$ and B$_{12}$ supplements have much less effect on homocysteine levels. Although some data suggest that supplementation is more effective than dietary folate, the AHA does not recommend widespread use of folic acid or vitamin B supplements to reduce the risk of cardiovascular disease or stroke.[35] Instead, the AHA recommends a balanced diet that includes at least five daily servings of grain products, citrus fruits, tomatoes, and other vegetables. Products made with wheat are good sources because wheat flour is fortified with folic acid. Wheat sources in the typical American diet provide about 25 percent of the recommended amount of daily folic acid.

The recommendation to focus on food sources is supported by data from large population studies. These studies showed that a diet of whole-grain bread, fresh fruit, olive oil, mushrooms, cruciferous vegetables (e.g., broccoli, cauliflower, cabbage, and greens), wine, and nuts was associated with higher plasma vitamin B$_6$ and folate levels and lower homocysteine levels.[49] This dietary pattern is similar to the Mediterranean diet discussed in a later section. Folic acid supplementation of 400 μg/d is reserved for persons unable to obtain at least 400 μg of dietary folate. The Food and Nutrition Board recommends no more than 1 mg per day of folic acid supplementation.[27] Higher levels can mask vitamin B$_6$ deficiency.

Vitamin E

Vitamin E contains eight active forms, each with varying activity. The most active form of vitamin E is alpha-tocopherol. Vitamin E in supplements frequently is supplied in the synthetic form, alpha-tocopheryl acetate, although natural forms are available. The activity of the synthetic form is about half that of the natural form.[50] Vitamin E has potent antioxidant properties. With respect to cardiovascular disease, vitamin E limits the oxidation of LDL. Lower amounts of oxidized LDL in turn should decrease the inflammation in vascular epithelium responsible for the development of atherosclerosis (see Chapter 9). Early observational studies showed that persons with higher dietary intake of vitamin E or who electively took vitamin E supplements had a lower incidence of cardiovascular disease. Therefore, vitamin E supplementation was popularized as a means to prevent atherosclerosis.[51]

Most clinical trials of vitamin E, however, have shown no benefit of vitamin E supplementation in preventing cardiovascular events. Several recent studies have raised questions regarding the safety and effectiveness of vitamin E supplements in preventing cardiovascular disease. The Women's Health Study included a large randomized controlled trial to determine the effectiveness of natural-source vitamin E supplementation (600 units every other day) for prevention of cardiovascular disease or cancer. More than 39,000 healthy women age 45 and older were divided equally between vitamin E or placebo treatment and followed for an average of 10 years. Overall, vitamin E supplementation showed no benefit in reducing cardiovascular death,

myocardial infarction, or stroke. Age may make a difference in the effectiveness of vitamin E. A subgroup analysis of women age 65 and older showed a 26 percent reduction in cardiovascular events among the group taking vitamin E, a finding that was related largely to a reduction in myocardial infarctions in the vitamin E group. The **HOPE** (Heart Outcomes Prevention Evaluation) and the extension HOPE-TOO trials enrolled patients with preexisting cardiovascular disease or diabetes.[52] Participants received 400 units/d of natural-source vitamin E or placebo and were followed for an average of 7 years. No benefit was demonstrated for vitamin E supplementation in preventing myocardial infarction, angina, stroke, or cardiovascular death. Moreover, the vitamin E group had a higher incidence of patients who developed heart failure and were hospitalized for heart failure. The reasons for this observation are not known.

A meta-analysis of 19 clinical trials raised further concerns about the safety of vitamin E supplementation. The results of the analyses showed that daily vitamin E in doses of 400 units/d or higher were associated with increased risk of all-cause mortality.[53] The 400-unit dose associated with increased mortality is considerably lower than the maximal safe dose of 1600 units set by the Institute of Medicine Food and Nutrition Board, which was established before the publication of recent studies.[27] The methodology used for the meta-analysis received considerable critique, including bias in the selection of studies included and excluded. Further, many of the studies included had methodological weaknesses, including small, heterogeneous samples; short follow-up time; and failure to verify adherence to daily vitamin E intake. Additional studies are needed to establish the safety of high-dose vitamin E.

Based on the available evidence, vitamin E supplementation cannot be recommended for primary or secondary prevention of cardiovascular disease. The AHA does not endorse use of vitamin E or any other antioxidant for the prevention of cardiovascular disease because of insufficient evidence showing benefit. Further, there is some evidence that vitamin E doses of 400 units or higher may increase the risk of death and heart failure.

Several mechanisms have been suggested as possible reasons for increased mortality associated with vitamin E supplementation.[52,53] First, the alpha-tocopherol form of vitamin E has the potential to act as a prooxidant in environments with high oxidative activity, which would promote vascular endothelial inflammation. Second, high doses of a single form of vitamin E could displace other forms of vitamin E that have important antioxidant and antilipid activities. Third, vitamin E can promote hemorrhagic stroke and other forms of bleeding by interfering with vitamin K-dependent coagulation pathways. Fourth, vitamin E can interfere with cellular enzymes involved in detoxifying drugs and endogenously formed toxins.

Thiamin

Thiamin is a coenzyme in many metabolic functions, including carbohydrate metabolism and the maintenance of myelin needed for proper nerve and muscle function. The most prominent effect of thiamin deficiency on the cardiovascular system is development of high-output heart failure. Other effects of deficiency include muscle weakness, neuropathy, and edema.[54] The body has a limited ability to store thiamin, making regular dietary intake necessary. Patients taking loop diuretics are at risk for thiamin deficiency because of increased thiamin excretion in the urine and may need more than the current recommended daily intake.

Minerals

Calcium

Calcium is a major component of bone metabolism. In addition, calcium plays pivotal roles in the coupling of electrical and contractile activity in the myocardium. Electrical stimulation of the cell membrane promotes movement of calcium into the cell by opening calcium channels. The influx of calcium stimulates the release of additional calcium from the sarcoplasmic reticulum, resulting in myofilament shortening and contraction. Calcium deficiencies can produce asynchrony between electrical and contractile activity and are associated with life-threatening cardiac dysrhythmias.

Calcium also promotes nitric oxide synthase activity, resulting in increased formation of nitric oxide, which is an important vasodilator. Subsequently, calcium supplementation has been investigated as a means to lower blood pressure. Meta-analyses of intervention trials showed only a modest effect of 1000 mg of calcium on blood pressure. Some data suggested that populations with drinking water high in calcium had lower incidences of myocardial infarction. However, a well-designed population-based study showed that high amounts of calcium in the water did not protect against myocardial infarction.[55]

The current recommendations for daily calcium intake are based on the prevention of deficiency and osteoporosis. Loop diuretics can increase calcium loss, which may increase the daily requirement. No evidence exists that calcium supplementation is beneficial in treatment or prevention of cardiovascular disease. Recommendations for supplementation, therefore, should be limited to prevention of deficiencies rather than prevention of cardiovascular disease.

Magnesium

Magnesium plays an important role in activating cellular sodium-potassium pumps. Magnesium also inactivates calcium channels and affects cellular calcium currents, thereby serving as an endogenous calcium channel blocker. Magnesium deficiencies contribute to the development of hypokalemia and cardiac dysrhythmias. Concerns about magnesium deficiency are greatest in patients with heart failure and patients who take loop and thiazide diuretics because these drugs increase magnesium loss.[54] In addition, dietary deficiencies may be common in patients with heart failure. Use of serum levels of magnesium are not a good reflection of level of depletion. Whole-body deficiencies must be severe before hypomagnesmia occurs.[56] Magnesium, like calcium, was thought to be protective against myocardial infarc-

tion when present in higher amounts in drinking water. However, high amounts of magnesium have been found not to be protective against myocardial infarction.[55] A number of intervention studies have examined the potential of magnesium supplementation to lower blood pressure. The weight of evidence shows that magnesium is not effective in lowering blood pressure in patients who are not depleted by diuretic therapy or dietary deficiency.

Potassium

Potassium is needed to maintain the normal function of nerve and muscle cells. Potassium plays an important role in maintaining the electrical voltage difference across cell membranes. The voltage difference is needed to generate the electrical impulse to produce a contraction. Data from the Nurses Health Study II showed that potassium supplementation produced a modest reduction in blood pressure.[57] However, the evidence is not sufficient to recommend potassium supplements as an intervention for hypertension. The regulation of potassium is tied closely to sodium. Our bodies are designed to prioritize the retention of sodium at the expense of potassium. Fortunately, there is sufficient potassium in foods to compensate. Potassium supplements are reserved for patients at risk for potassium deficiency, a consequence mainly of drug therapy, such as potassium-wasting diuretics. Potassium levels are also a concern in hospitalized patients, for whom physiological stress can lead to sodium retention and potassium depletion. The dysrhythmogenic consequences of potassium depletion and potassium excess are among the first pearls of wisdom learned and among the few rarely forgotten by practitioners. This emphasizes that supplementation should be provided only under medical supervision.

Selenium

Selenium is a trace mineral found in plants and animals. The amount and quality of selenium in the diet depends on the amount of selenium in the soil. Therefore, there are regional differences in selenium in local diets. Selenium is incorporated into a number of selenoproteins that are antioxidants involved in preventing cellular free radical damage. In the vascular endothelium, glutathione peroxidase (which is dependent on selenium) limits the damage associated with the byproducts of LDL oxidation. Studies of regions with low selenium content have shown a relationship between selenium deficiency and development of carotid and cardiovascular disease.[58] Selenium supplementation in regions with adequate selenium levels does not appear to convey cardioprotective effects. This implies that when an adequate amount of selenium is obtained in the diet, additional selenium is not beneficial.

Sodium

Sodium was once a scarce commodity. Our physiology accordingly was designed to conserve sodium at the expense of potassium, which is more naturally abundant. Our appetite for sodium is high, presumably to encourage the ingestion of foods that contain sufficient sodium to meet physiological needs. These adaptations do not serve us well in the current environment, in which sodium is abundant. Sodium plays important roles in maintaining fluid balance and cell function, including muscle contraction and impulse conduction. Thus, it is not surprising that diets high in sodium intake affect the cardiovascular system.

The **INTERSALT** (International Study of Sodium, Potassium, and Blood Pressure) was a large international study that examined the relationship between urine sodium, as a measure of dietary sodium intake, and blood pressure. Results of the study firmly established a strong connection between dietary sodium and blood pressure. Sodium intake greater than 2300 mg was associated with increased blood pressure.[59] A follow-up meta-analysis of observational studies determined that the effect of sodium on blood pressure was greatest in older adults and persons with higher baseline blood pressures.[60]

Salt sensitivity is an arbitrary distinction based on a person's response to sodium restriction. A reduction in mean arterial pressure of at least 10 mm Hg in response to a 10 percent reduction in dietary sodium defines a person as salt sensitive. About 50 percent of persons with hypertension and 25 percent of persons with normal blood pressure are salt sensitive. It has been suggested that the ancestors of these persons had an adaptive advantage when sodium was less available, but this adaptation increases the risk of hypertension now that sodium is abundant.[61] No clinical markers are readily available to identify persons who are salt sensitive. The most rationale approach is to recommend a reduction in dietary sodium to everyone.

The new U.S. Department of Agriculture (**USDA**) dietary guidelines recommend sodium intake of less than 2300 mg per day.[62] The AHA recommends dietary sodium intake of 2400 mg or less per day.[34] This is equivalent to 1 tsp or 6 g of salt per day (Box 12-2). These guidelines effectively eliminate the concept of the low-sodium diet. Practitioners and their patients with hypertension and heart failure should have diets with comparable amounts of sodium. One of the most common suggestions to decrease dietary sodium is to remove the salt shaker from the table. The estimated sources of sodium in American diets listed in Box 12-3 show that this strategy has limited impact.[63] The only effective strategy is to focus on identifying and substituting high-sodium processed foods, fast foods, and most restaurant foods with low-sodium foods or preferably with fresh foods. Fresh, unprocessed foods—including all meats, fruits, nuts, and vegetables—are naturally low in sodium. For example, a hamburger has about 70 mg of sodium. Lean ham has only 60 mg of sodium per serving. In contrast, bacon has 600 to 1000 mg, cured or canned ham has 850 to 1100 mg, and Canadian bacon has 1200 to 2500 mg per serving.

DIETS
Low-Carbohydrate, High-Fat, and High-Protein Diets

The AHA recommended that fat compose 30 percent or less of total calories. Much of the problem with this diet was not related to the recommendation per se but with its implementation by the public and health professionals. The focus became solely on replacing high-fat foods with low-fat alternatives rather than a more comprehensive approach to managing all dietary macronutrients. The food industry responded by making low-fat and fat-free products that typically were high in carbohydrates and equally high in calories. The limited fat in these products usually was saturated or *trans* fats. Subsequently, implementation of these recommendations has had little effect on the growing incidence of obesity and related cardiovascular disease risks.

Alternatively, low-carbohydrate, high-protein diets such as the Atkins diet were found to induce significant weight loss without adversely affecting lipid profiles.[2,64] The surprising success of these diets raised questions regarding whether low-fat diets were the best approach to decreasing obesity and cardiovascular disease risk factors. The low-carbohydrate, high-protein diet has been criticized because it allows free latitude with foods high in protein and fat but severely restricts carbohydrates. As a result, the diet may be incomplete in some vitamins and minerals present in high-carbohydrate foods. The available research evidence has been used to support both positions.[2,19,20] A comparison of the pros and cons of the low-fat, high-carbohydrate with the low-carbohydrate, high-protein diet is provided in Table 12-4. In summary, there is no long-term evidence of the safety and efficacy of low-carbohydrate, high-fat diets. Alternatively, there is limited evidence that following the lower-fat diet recommendations of the AHA is effective in decreasing cardiovascular mortality. Clearly, additional research is needed before this controversy can be settled definitively.

Mediterranean Diet

Interest in the Mediterranean diet was generated when epidemiological studies showed that people in the Mediterranean region had a lower incidence of cardiovascular disease than people in Western countries.[65] The Mediterranean diet has the following components:[66]

- High consumption of olive oil, legumes, cereals, fruits, and vegetables

---

BOX 12-2 ▪▪▪
CONVERTING SALT TO SODIUM

Conversion formula: salt (g) × 400 = sodium (mg)
- 1 g salt = 400 mg of sodium
- 6 g of salt = 2400 mg of sodium
- 1 tsp = 6 g = 2400 mg sodium

BOX 12-3 ▪▪▪
SOURCES OF SODIUM IN THE AMERICAN DIET

Added during cooking	5%
Added at the table	6%
Naturally occurring in foods	12%
Processed foods	77%

■ ■ ■

TABLE 12-4 COMPARISON OF DIETS

	HIGH-PROTEIN, LOW-CARBOHYDRATE	LOW-FAT, HIGH-CARBOHYDRATE
Pros	Causes weight loss Lowers cholesterol, low-density lipoprotein, and very low-density lipoprotein levels	Nutritionally complete Sufficient food variety to promote life-long adherence
Cons	Risk of micronutrient deficiency High in saturated fat and cholesterol Low in fiber May cause liver and renal damage Long-term safety not established High attrition rate	No evidence that diet decreases cardiovascular disease risk May lower high-density lipoprotein level May increase triglyceride level

- Moderate to high consumption of fish
- Moderate consumption of wine, dairy (cheese and yogurt), beans, nuts, and seeds
- Low consumption of eggs, meat, and meat products

A number of large randomized controlled trials of diets that follow the Mediterranean pattern have been conducted.[67] These trials have shown significant reductions in cardiac mortality compared with Western and other diets. Multiple components of the diet are likely responsible for decreased cardiovascular mortality. The diet is low in saturated fat and cholesterol and high in monounsaturated fats, fiber, and carbohydrates that have a low glycemic index. The diet provides a good balance between omega-3 and omega-6 fatty intake, and it contains adequate amounts of the cardioprotective beta-carotene, vitamin C, vitamin E, and selenium. In addition, the phenol compounds found in olive oil, the primary oil in the diet, decrease oxidative stress and inflammation and increase nitric oxide.[68] The AHA position statement on the Mediterranean diet notes that lifestyle differences in the region also may account for decreased cardiovascular mortality.[69] The differential effects of lifestyle from diet have not been fully determined. This distinction may not be crucial. No dietary intervention alone is sufficient; diet must be coupled with lifestyle modifications that promote cardiovascular health.

DASH Diet

The **DASH** (Dietary Approaches to Stop Hypertension) diet was developed as a comprehensive approach to lowering dietary sodium by focusing on promoting a food pattern rather than limiting dietary sodium. The DASH diet emphasizes intake of whole grains, vegetables, fruits, low-fat dairy products, poultry, fish, and nuts. Foods to limit include red meats, sweets, and beverages with sugar. The diet is low in saturated fat and cholesterol; high in fiber, potassium, calcium, and magnesium; and moderately high in protein. A more detailed description of the diet can be found in Chapter 78. The diet with a complete eating plan can be downloaded free from the National Heart, Lung, and Blood Institute from the following website: *www.nhlbi.nih. gov/health/public/heart/hbp/dash/new_dash.pdf*. Clinical trials have shown that the diet is effective in lowering blood pressure in normotensive and hypertensive persons.[70,71] The effects were more pronounced in hypertensive persons. Other studies have shown that the DASH diet can lower total cholesterol and LDL levels.[72,73] However, the diet also may lower the HDL level. Overall, the diet is considered safe, nutritious, and consistent with goals of USDA and AHA dietary guidelines. To date, no studies have been done to demonstrate long-term adherence, and only limited evidence is available showing sustained effects of the diet.[74]

NUTRITION GUIDELINES
Estimating Caloric Need

Food labels and many dietary recommendations are based on percentages of total energy intake, making it necessary to estimate caloric need before developing individual nutrition guidelines. The AHA provides a simple method to estimate the number of calories needed per day that can be used clinically.

Multiply weight in pounds by 13 calories if a person is not active and by 15 calories if a person is moderately active.

Persons with high activity levels will need additional calories depending on their level of activity. These individuals, however, typically are involved in planned programs of activity or have an established exercise routine in which they already account for caloric intake and thus are less likely to require guidance with estimating caloric intake. An important note is that this method will provide an excessively high estimate of caloric need in persons who are obese. In these cases, estimate caloric need based on an adjusted body weight using the following formula:

$$\text{Adjusted body weight} = \text{Ideal body weight} + \\ [(\text{Actual body weight} - \text{Ideal body weight}) \times 0.25]$$

This formula accounts for the fact that adipose tissue, which is the major component of weight difference between actual and ideal body weight, is less metabolically active.

Assessment of Body Fat for Cardiovascular Risk

An association has been established between body fat, particularly visceral fat, and the risk of cardiovascular disease. Methods to quantify the amount of lean and fat tissue require sophisticated equipment and trained technicians, which makes these methods clinically impractical. Fortunately, there are two simple methods of estimating body fat that have been shown to be predictive of cardiovascular risk: body mass index (**BMI**) and waist circumference. BMI provides a good index of total body fat mass in persons who are not active body builders. Waist circumference provides a good index of how much of the excess body fat is located in the abdominal area. This is an important distinction because excess abdominal body fat is associated with the greatest increase in cardiovascular disease risk. This holds even for persons whose BMI is in the normal range but who carry a disproportionate amount of abdominal body fat.

The methods for determining BMI and waist circumference are outlined in Box 12-4. Their relationship to cardiovascular risk is listed in Table 12-5. The waist-to-hip ratio has been used as another index of body fat distribution, but BMI and waist circumference are better predictors of cardiovascular risk, and this method is no longer recommended.[35] Treatment guidelines recommend initiating weight-loss strategies for persons with a BMI of 30 kg/m² or higher and a waist circumference greater than 40 inches (men) or 35 inches (women) and who have two or more additional risk factors (cigarette smoker, hypertension, dyslipidemia, impaired fasting glucose, family history of cardiovascular disease, age

older than 45 [men] or 55 [women], and postmenopausal women).[75]

U.S. Department of Agriculture Guidelines

The new USDA guidelines represent an extension of the philosophical approach to nutrition established by the USDA in the 1980s.[33] It was then that the food-pattern approach to nutrition was implemented. The new guidelines incorporate the food-pattern approach but encourage other lifestyle modifications, especially increased activity. Although activity is promoted, general caloric requirements are based on a sedentary lifestyle to limit the risk of overestimating caloric need. Important changes from the original pyramid include the following[62]:

- Separating fats into groups of solid fats and oils, with most (60 percent) discretionary fats derived from oils (monounsaturated and polyunsaturated)
- Increasing the amounts of legumes and vegetables, particularly dark green vegetables
- Increasing the amount of whole grain foods to at least half of all grains

The best approach to using these guidelines is to take advantage of the interactive website: *www.mypyramid.gov*. This site allows practitioners or patients themselves to determine the daily amount of foods in each category based on age, sex, and activity level. Specific foods in each category are listed, as well as tips for following the guidelines. The guidelines produce a low-fat, high-carbohydrate diet in which low-fat or fat-free choices are advocated. It is important to emphasize to patients that high-quality, nutrient-dense foods should be used as low-fat substitutes. The previous public focus on selecting alternatives simply because they were low fat without regard for caloric or nutrient content is suspected of contributing to the increase in obesity.[2]

American Heart Association Guidelines

The AHA Dietary Guidelines for Healthy Americans follow a similar philosophy to the USDA guidelines in that lifestyle modifications are recommended along with the dietary guidelines.[34] The number of daily servings of fruit, vegetables, and grains is similar to the USDA guidelines as well. The AHA guidelines make a specific recommendation for at least two servings of fish per week, which the USDA guidelines do not include. The AHA guidelines also offer recommendations for specific populations, including children, older adults, and patients with cardiovascular disease, elevated lipids, diabetes, renal disease, and heart failure. Of note is the distinction made between avoiding saturated and *trans* fats and ensuring adequate intake of monounsaturated and polyunsaturated fats. This distinction is important because it emphasizes the need for practitioners to reorient the public away from the previous axiom that all fats should be avoided. The reorientation also needs to include wise selection of foods that are high in proteins and carbohydrates rather than focusing only on dietary fat, as was previously done. As noted before, it was this selective interpretation of the guidelines that has led to poor food

---

BOX 12-4
MEASUREMENT OF BODY MASS INDEX AND ANTHROPOMETRICS   ■ ■ ■

Body Mass Index (BMI)

Weight in kilograms/(height in meters)²

or

704.5 × (weight in pounds/[height in inches]²)

A program to calculate BMI for varying heights and weights is available from the following website address: *www.nhlbi.nih.gov/health/public/heart/obesity/lose_wt/index.htm* (National Heart, Lung, and Blood Institute, 1999).

Anthropometric Measures
Waist circumference: Locate the upper hip bone and the top of the iliac crest. Place a tape measure horizontally, level with the iliac crest. Pull the tape so it is snug but not compressing the skin. Take the measurement at the end of expiration.
Triceps skin fold (**TSF**): Take the measurement while the arm is hanging freely. Use your thumb and forefinger to grasp a fold of skin and subcutaneous fat slightly above the midpoint. Apply a caliper to the area and, after 2 to 3 seconds, measure to the nearest 1.0 mm. Repeat the procedure 2 more times, and average the measurements.
Midarm circumference (**MAC**): Take the measurement on the nondominant arm at the midpoint between the olecranon process and acromion process (where the scapula joins the shoulder). Using a nonstretchable tape, measure the circumference to the nearest millimeter while the forearm is flexed 90 degrees.
Midarm muscle circumference (**MAMC**) *formula:* Use the following formula to remove the contribution of subcutaneous fat and bone from the circumference of the arm. This provides an indication of the muscle mass of the arm.

$$MAMC (cm^2) = \frac{[MAC\ cm - (3.13 \times TSF\ cm)]^2}{12.52}\ or$$

− 10 (males) *or* − 6.5 (females)

■ ■ ■

TABLE 12-5   NATIONAL HEART, LUNG, AND BLOOD INSTITUTE DISEASE RISK CLASSIFICATION OF OVERWEIGHT AND OBESITY BY BODY MASS INDEX AND WAIST CIRCUMFERENCE

			WAIST CIRCUMFERENCE	
DESCRIPTION	CLASS	BODY MASS INDEX (kg/m²)	MEN: ≥102 cm WOMEN: ≥88 cm	LESS THAN 102 cm (40 inches)* LESS THAN 88 cm (35 inches)*
Underweight		Less than 18.5		
Normal		18.5-24.9		
Overweight		25.0-29.9	Increased†	High†
Obesity	I	30.0-34.9	High†	Very high†
	II	35.0-39.9	Very high†	Very high†
Extreme obesity	III	Less than 40	Extremely high†	Extremely high†

*Increased waist circumference also can be a marker for increased risk even in persons of normal weight.
†Disease risk for type 2 diabetes, hypertension, and cardiovascular disease.
Data from National Heart, Lung, and Blood Institute Obesity Education Initiative Expert Panel on the Identification Evaluation and Treatment of Overweight and Obesity: *Obes Res* 6(suppl 2):51S-209S, 1998.

choices. Table 12-6 compares the components of diets considered to be heart healthy.

HEART FAILURE, OBESITY, AND CARDIAC CACHEXIA
Obesity in Heart Failure

Weight loss has been recommended for obese patients with heart failure, but a series of studies has raised questions about the value of body weight reduction for these patients. The population-based Rotterdam study showed that patients with high body mass indices (BMI of 25 kg/m² or higher) had the same risk for death from heart failure as persons with normal BMIs.[76] In the same year a retrospective review of a large sample of heart failure patients awaiting cardiac transplantation showed that patients with above-normal BMI had longer survival than normal-weight patients.[77] A prospective study of 580 patients treated at a heart failure clinic showed that survival rates were highest in those who were overweight (BMI of 28 to 31 kg/m²) followed closely by those who were obese (BMI higher than 31 kg/m²).[78] In another prospective study, 3-year survival rates of 2707 patients following their first hospitalization for heart failure were determined. The survival rates were best in patients with a BMI higher than 34 kg/m² and poorest in patients with a BMI of 24.3 kg/m² or lower.[79] In sum, as least six studies with a combined total of more than 10,500 patients have shown better outcomes among overweight and obese patients compared with normal

or underweight patients.[76-81] These studies provide evidence that higher body fat is associated with longer survival in patients with heart failure.

Although obesity may increase the risk of developing heart failure, it may be beneficial once heart failure develops. Why this is the case is not clear. One reason may be that greater amounts of body fat provide a metabolic reserve that allows these patients to tolerate the metabolic-catabolic stress of heart failure for a longer time.[78] Another reason may be related to high blood cholesterol levels in overweight and obese patients, which also have been shown to be associated with improved survival.[82] Endotoxin in the form of lipopolysaccharide (**LPS**) is derived from the cell wall of gram-negative bacteria. LPS is a potent stimulator of inflammatory mediator tumor necrosis factor-alpha (TNF-α) release from immune cells. Higher levels of TNF-α are associated with decreased survival.[83] Patients with heart failure have elevated circulating levels of LPS, which is suspected of originating from gram-negative bacteria that translocate into the blood across the ischemic gut.[84] Circulating lipoproteins can bind LPS in the blood, preventing it from attaching to immune cells and stimulating TNF-α release. The higher lipoprotein levels associated with increased adipose tissue in obese patients[85] may provide a protective mechanism by limiting TNF-α release.[86] Additional research is needed to establish firmly that higher body fat is beneficial to patients with heart failure and to determine the mechanisms. The current evidence, however, questions the wisdom of

■ ■ ■

TABLE 12-6   COMPARISON OF MACRONUTRIENT COMPOSITION AMONG HEART-HEALTHY DIETS

	AHA	USDA	DASH	MEDITERRANEAN
Total fats	Less than 30%	20%-35%	22%-33%	30%-40%
Saturated fat	7%-10%	Less than 10%	Less than 11%	Less than 9%
Monounsaturated		11%	10%	18%
Polyunsaturated		9%	6%	
Cholesterol	Less than 300 mg	Less than 300 mg	Less than 200 mg	
Carbohydrates	55%	55%	57%	
Proteins	15%	18%	21%	

AHA, American Heart Association; *DASH*, Dietary Approaches to Stop Hypertension; *USDA*, U.S. Department of Agriculture.

universally recommending weight loss for overweight and obese patients with heart failure.

Cardiac Cachexia

At the opposite end of the scale, the data overwhelmingly show that patients with cachexia have poor outcomes and shorter survival times.[87] These patients are most likely to be malnourished. Unintentional weight loss is associated with malnutrition and produces the syndrome called cardiac cachexia.

A number of mechanisms have been proposed to contribute to development of cachexia and muscle loss in heart failure (Table 12-7).[88,89] Poor dietary intake is common in patients with advanced heart failure and is related to decreased appetite (anorexia) caused by intestinal edema, inflammation, drug toxicities, and factors related to aging. In addition to causing anorexia, gut edema, hypoperfusion, and intestinal hypomotility cause malabsorption of ingested nutrients. Inactivity promotes muscle atrophy and decreased skeletal muscle protein synthesis. Elevated circulating catecholamines further enhance muscle protein breakdown.

Cachexia in heart failure is related closely to the cytokine-mediated inflammation that underlies pathological heart failure. Proinflammatory cytokines, TNF-α, interleukin-1, and interleukin-6 are elevated in patients with heart failure.[90] These inflammatory cytokines play a role in suppressing food intake, accelerating catabolism of skeletal muscle, and impairing the ability to store energy as fat (see Chapter 9).

Changes that occur with aging can contribute to decreased spontaneous food intake and loss of muscle. Decreases in the sense of taste and smell result in a diminished desire to eat.[91] Older adults release higher amounts of cholecystokinin, an intestinal hormone released as food enters the gut. Cholecystokinin diminishes the desire to continue eating, resulting in smaller meals being ingested.[92] Delayed gastric emptying that occurs as a normal part of growing older can lengthen the time after a meal before hunger sensations return. Other changes can contribute to decreased food intake in older adults as well. These include social isolation, depression, poverty, and a limited ability to shop for and prepare foods. Sarcopenia is defined as an age-related loss of muscle mass.[93] Sarcopenia is due to changes in physical activity and lower circulating anabolic hormones and can compound the loss of protein-based tissues from heart failure.

Nutrition Assessment

Early detection and treatment of patients at risk for malnutrition may reduce the incidence of cardiac cachexia. No consensus exists regarding the definition of cardiac cachexia, and multiple definitions have been offered (Table 12-8). If the patient has severe weight loss and tissue wasting, visual assessment is all that is required. In the remaining patients the following clinically useful definition has been suggested: unintentional weight loss of more than 6 percent of previous normal (premorbid) dry body weight over a period of 6 or more months.[89] Further distinctions can by made. Involuntary weight loss of more than 5 percent in 30 days is defined as a clinically significant health risk requiring aggressive intervention.[18] Regardless of the time period, a 10 percent involuntary weight loss typically indicates a mild level of malnutrition, a 15 to 25 percent weight loss is considered a sign of moderate malnutrition, and weight loss exceeding 25 percent indicates severe malnutrition.

An important note is that, based on these definitions, persons who are overweight or obese but have a history of significant involuntary weight loss are defined as having cachexia. These patients have a similar risk of poorer outcomes as the underweight patients nurses most commonly associate with cachexia.

■ ■ ■

TABLE 12-7 POTENTIAL MECHANISMS CONTRIBUTING TO THE DEVELOPMENT OF CARDIAC CACHEXIA

MECHANISM	POSSIBLE CAUSE
Poor dietary intake	Anorexia from hepatic and gut edema
	Anorexia from drug toxicities
	Anorexia from proinflammatory cytokines: tumor necrosis factor-alpha and interleukin-1
	Micronutrient deficiencies altering metabolism and cardiac function
Increased energy and protein requirements	
Accelerated muscle protein breakdown because of catecholamines and proinflammatory cytokines: tumor necrosis factor-alpha and interleukin-1	
Malabsorption	Delayed emptying
	Intestinal hypomotility
	Intestinal edema
	Intestinal tissue hypoperfusion
Protein-losing enteropathy	
Sympathetic nervous system activation	
Decreased skeletal muscle protein synthesis	Decreased sense of taste and smell
	Early satiety from increased cholecystokinin release from the gut
Effects of aging on appetite and muscle	Altered nutrient digestion from decreased hydrochloric acid in the stomach
	Psychosocial factors, such as social isolation, depression, limited transportation, and poverty
	Sarcopenia (muscle loss resulting from aging)

■ ■ ■

TABLE 12-8 DEFINITIONS OF CARDIAC CACHEXIA

PARAMETER	DEFINING VALUE
Blood chemistry	Albumin less than 3.0 mg/dl[94,95]
Lean tissue	Documented loss of 10% skeletal muscle size[96]
Ideal body weight (IBW)	Less than 90% IBW[94,95]
	Less than 85% IBW[97]
	Less than 80% IBW[98]
Weight loss (dry)	Weight loss of 10% over past year[99]
	Weight loss of 7.5% of normal over 6 months[87]
	Moderate: greater than 7.5% but ≤15% weight loss and greater than 85% IBW[100]
	Severe: greater than 15% weight loss or greater than 7.5% weight loss and less than 85% IBW[87]

Another easily obtained clinical indicator of malnutrition is BMI. A BMI of less than 23.5 kg/m^2 in men and less than 22 kg/m^2 in women carries an increased risk of mortality. A BMI of less than 21 kg/m^2 for either sex indicates the need for immediate nutritional intervention.

Anthropometric measures are another indicator of malnutrition but are not as easily obtained (Box 12-4). Table 12-9 provides guidelines for interpreting these measures. Biological markers, such as the serum proteins albumin, transferrin, and prealbumin, as well as total lymphocyte count, provide additional data about nutritional status. The clinical significance of altered levels of these markers is outlined in Table 12-10. Low serum prealbumin levels have been divided further into subcategories to guide clinical practice. Patients with a level less than 15 mg/dl should be referred for a dietary consult. Those with a level less than 11 mg/dl are at significant nutritional risk and require aggressive nutritional intervention. Those with a prealbumin level less than 5 mg/dl are at high risk and require immediate nutrition intervention.[101]

Interventions to Promote Nutrition

Research-based treatment strategies to promote nutritional intake in patients with heart failure are limited. Table 12-11 outlines a number of interventions with available evidence to support them. The goal of these interventions is to ensure sufficient intake of calories, protein, and micronutrients to maintain body weight and optimize nutritional status. The nutrients most likely to be deficient in patients with heart failure are outlined in Table 12-12. Many of these potential nutrient deficiencies can be addressed by providing a multivitamin with minerals. The best approach, however, is to promote intake of whole foods. This is particularly true for promoting adequate protein and caloric intake. One important principle to keep in mind when planning treatments to improve nutrition and reverse cachexia is that it takes about 3 times as long to replace tissue lost during illness as it took to lose it.[18] The rate at which protein and fat are used during illness is estimated to be 5 to 10 times faster than the rate at which these tissues are restored during recovery. Patients who develop another illness or subsequent exacerbation of their disease before fully recovering will lose additional body tissue and require a more prolonged period of recovery. Patients who are unstable will develop a progressive downward spiral of weight loss because they are unable to recover adequately before the next exacerbation. A second important principle to remember is that patients with heart failure appear to need 20 percent more calories and protein than the current recommended daily intakes.[99]

Providing small, frequent meals addresses the early satiety that occurs with illness and aging. Calorie-dense foods are best because the amount of food eaten has a greater effect on feelings of satiety in older adults than the calorie content. If necessary, nutritional supplements can provide a good source of additional calories, protein, and other important nutrients. These may be particularly effective in older adults because supple-

■ ■ ■

TABLE 12-9   MIDARM MUSCLE AREA IN ADULTS AGES 55 TO 74

ASSESSMENT OF MUSCLE MASS	MEN (cm^2)	WOMEN (cm^2)
Adequate	43 to 64 cm^2	27 to 44 cm^2
Marginal	$\leq$40 cm^2	$\leq$25 cm^2
Depleted	Less than 35 cm^2	Less than 21 cm^2
Wasted	Less than 30 cm^2	Less than 18 cm^2

Data from Beers MH, Berkow R, editors: Nutrition: general considerations and nutrition in clinical medicine. In *The Merck manual of diagnosis and therapy,* ed 17, Hoboken, NJ, 1999, John Wiley & Sons.

■ ■ ■

TABLE 12-10   BIOLOGICAL INDICATORS OF MALNUTRITION

	MILD	MODERATE	SEVERE
Albumin (g/dl)	2.8-3.5	2.1-2.7	Less than 2.1
Transferrin (mg/dl)	151-200	100-150	Less than 100
Prealbumin (mg/dl)	15-30	10-15	0-10
Total lymphocyte count (mm^3)	1200-1500	800-1199	Less than 800

Data from Demling RH, DeSanti L: *Involuntary weight loss and protein-energy malnutrition: diagnosis and treatment.* Retrieved from www.medscape.com/viewprogram/713_pnt

■ ■ ■

TABLE 12-11   INTERVENTIONS TO IMPROVE INTAKE IN PATIENTS WITH HEART FAILURE

INTERVENTION	RATIONALE	EVIDENCE
Minimize additional stressors.	Decrease release of catabolic counterregulatory hormones.	CD
Eat small, frequent meals.	Inflammatory mediators produce early satiety.	CD, SC
Increase calorie and nutrient density of food.	Volume of food has greater effect on satiety than caloric density.	CD, SC, SH
Provide foods that vary in color, texture, and taste.	Appeal to appetitive factors prevents sensory-specific satiety.	SH
Eat meals when hunger sensations are present.	Hunger sensations are cyclical and may diminish if meal is delayed.	CD
Promote socialization during meals.	Persons eat less when alone.	CD
Add flavor enhancers.	If taste sense is diminished, flavor enhancers may increase enjoyment of food.	SC
Provide diet counseling and goal setting.	Increase incentives to eat even if not hungry.	SC
Eat diets high in omega-3 fatty acids.	Decrease inflammatory response and other components of heart failure.	CT
Identify and treat drug toxicities.	Detection and treatment of drug toxicities reduces associated anorexia.	CD

Data from Lennie TA: *Heart Lung* 28:386-401, 1999.
CD, Clinical deduction based on causes of anorexia; *CT,* clinical trials; *SC,* small clinical studies or case reports; *SH,* studies using healthy subjects.

■ ■ ■

TABLE 12-12 NUTRIENTS MOST LIKELY TO BE DEFICIENT IN PATIENTS WITH HEART FAILURE

NUTRIENT	RECOMMENDED DAILY INTAKE
Calories	Underweight: 32 kcal/kg[99] Normal weight: 28 kcal/kg[99]
Protein	1/g kg[99]
Vitamin D	Less than age 70: 10 μg[28] Older than age 70: 15 μg[28]
Thiamin	Males: 1.2 mg[29] Females: 1.1 mg[29] Patients taking loop diuretics may need more than recommendation.
Calcium	1200 mg[28] Patients taking loop diuretics may need more than recommendation.
Magnesium	Males: 420 mg[28] Females: 320 mg[28] Patients taking loop or thiazide diuretics may need more than recommendation.
Potassium	4700 mg[31] Patients taking loop and thiazide diuretics may need more than recommendation, whereas patients taking angiotensin-converting enzyme inhibitors, angiotensin receptor blockers, and aldosterone inhibitors may need less. Provide supplementation only under medical supervision.

ments do not decrease appetite or lower the amount of food eaten at the meal following supplementation.[102] Even if nutritional supplementation does not fully reverse cachexia, it may break the cycle of progressive weight loss and minimize additional tissue catabolism.

A final potential treatment to improve cachexia may be to decrease systemic inflammation. Two strategies may help. First is to ensure that patients are optimized on their medications. Improvement in hemodynamic status will decrease systemic inflammation (Chapter 9). Second, increasing the amount of omega-3 fatty acids in the diet also may help because of their antiinflammatory effects. Lower levels of inflammatory mediators should lead to improved appetite and decreased protein tissue catabolism.

In summary, patients with heart failure are at risk for altered nutritional intake from the consequences of heart failure and aging, as well as side effects of treatment. Although these patients have a higher risk of specific micronutrient deficiencies than other patient populations, the general dietary guidelines for promoting cardiovascular health apply to this population as well.

CONCLUSION

The current nutritional guidelines outlined by the AHA and USDA are out of step with the popular trend to focus on individual nutrients and take nutritional supplements as the ideal path to optimal health. It will take concerted effort on the part of health care practitioners to overcome this trend and change the focus to eating patterns. The DASH diet, Mediterranean diet, and the nutrition guidelines of the AHA and USDA focus on adoption of food patterns rather than individual nutrients. Following any of these diets provides macronutri-

ents in proportions that the overwhelming majority of evidence shows are beneficial to cardiovascular health. Moreover, they provide adequate micronutrients such that supplementation is not needed. To date, no research has shown convincingly that any of these diets is superior to the others.

Soy protein and fish oil are the only dietary supplements for which there is sufficient evidence to support judicious use. Neither, however, is intended as a substitute for whole foods with comparable nutrients.

Finally, it must be reemphasized that nutritional modification cannot function in isolation but must be combined with other lifestyle changes, including adequate sleep, stress reduction, smoking cessation, regular exercise, and weight loss in those who are overweight. Only with this comprehensive approach are the full benefits of good nutrition achieved.

REFERENCES

1. Dubnov G, Berry EM: Omega-6 fatty acids and coronary artery disease: the pros and cons, *Curr Atheroscler Rep* 6:441-446, 2004.
2. Weinberg SL: The diet-heart hypothesis: a critique, *J Am Coll Cardiol* 43:731-733, 2004.
3. ASCN/AIN Task Force on Trans Fatty Acids: American Society for Clinical Nutrition and American Institute of Nutrition: position paper on trans fatty acids, *Am J Clin Nutr* 63:663-670, 1996.
4. Mozaffarian D, Pischon T, Hankinson SE et al: Dietary intake of trans fatty acids and systemic inflammation in women, *Am J Clin Nutr* 79:606-612, 2004.
5. Dyerberg J, Eskesen DC, Andersen PW et al: Effects of trans- and n-3 unsaturated fatty acids on cardiovascular risk markers in healthy males: an 8 weeks dietary intervention study, *Eur J Clin Nutr* 58:1062-1070, 2004.
6. Institute of Medicine: *Dietary reference intakes for energy, carbohydrate, fiber, fat, protein, amino acids (macronutrients),* Washington, DC, 2002, Academic Press.
7. Oomen CM, Ocke MC, Feskens EJ et al: Association between trans fatty acid intake and 10-year risk of coronary heart disease in the Zutphen Elderly Study: a prospective population-based study, *Lancet* 357:746-751, 2001.
8. Ros E: Dietary *cis*-monounsaturated fatty acids and metabolic control in type 2 diabetes, *Am J Clin Nutr* 78:617S-625S, 2003.
9. Heller AR, Theilen HJ, Koch T: Fish or chips? *News Physiol Sci* 18:50-54, 2003.
10. McCarty MF: Fish oil and other nutritional adjuvants for treatment of congestive heart failure, *Med Hypotheses* 46:400-406, 1996.
11. Kris-Etherton PM, Harris WS, Appel IJ: Fish consumption, fish oil, omega-3 fatty acids, and cardiovascular disease, *Circulation* 106:2747-2757, 2002.
12. Omega-3 oil: fish or pills? *Consumer Reports* pp 30-32, July 2003.
13. Reddy KS, Katan MB: Diet, nutrition and prevention of hypertension and cardiovascular disease, *Public Health Nutr* 71(1A):167-186, 2004.
14. Foster-Powell K, Holt SH, Brand-Miller JC: International table of glycemic index and glycemic load values: 2002, *Am J Clin Nutr* 76:5-56, 2002.
15. Kelly S, Frost G, Whittaker V, Summerbell C: Low glycaemic index diets for coronary heart disease, *Cochrane Database Syst Rev* CD004467, 2004.
16. Erkkilä AT, Lichtenstein AH: Fiber and cardiovascular disease risk: how strong is the evidence? *J Cardiovasc Nurs* 21(1):3-8, 2006.
17. Pasini E, Aquilani R, Gheorghiade M, Dioguardi FS: Malnutrition, muscle wasting and cachexia in chronic heart failure: the nutritional approach, *Ital Heart J* 4:232-235, 2003.
18. Witte KK, Clark AL: Nutritional abnormalities contributing to cachexia in chronic illness, *Int J Cardiol* 85:23-31, 2002.

19. Kappagoda CT, Hyson DA, Amsterdam EA: Low-carbohydrate-high-protein diets: is there a place for them in clinical cardiology? *J Am Coll Cardiol* 43:725-730, 2004.

20. St Jeor ST, Howard BV, Prewitt TE et al: Dietary protein and weight reduction: a statement for healthcare professionals from the Nutrition Committee of the Council on Nutrition, Physical Activity, and Metabolism of the American Heart Association, *Circulation* 104:1869-1874, 2001.

21. Terpstra AH, Hermus RJ, West CE: The role of dietary protein in cholesterol metabolism, *World Rev Nutr Diet* 42:1-55, 1983.

22. Wolfe BM: Potential role of raising dietary protein intake for reducing risk of atherosclerosis, *Can J Cardiol* 11(suppl G):127G-131G, 1995.

23. Wolfe BM, Piche LA: Replacement of carbohydrate by protein in a conventional-fat diet reduces cholesterol and triglyceride concentrations in healthy normolipidemic subjects, *Clin Invest Med* 22:140-148, 1999.

24. Food and Drug Administration: *FDA approves new health claim for soy protein and coronary heart disease.* Retrieved November 24, 2006, from www.fda.gov/bbs/topics/ANSWERS/ANS00980.html

25. Hoie LH, Graubaum HJ, Harde A et al: Lipid-lowering effect of 2 dosages of a soy protein supplement in hypercholesterolemia, *Adv Ther* 22:175-186, 2005.

26. Zhan S, Ho SC: Meta-analysis of the effects of soy protein containing isoflavones on the lipid profile, *Am J Clin Nutr* 81:397-408, 2005.

27. Institute of Medicine: *Dietary reference intakes: applications in dietary assessment,* Washington DC, 2000, National Academic Press.

28. Institute of Medicine: *Dietary reference intakes for calcium, phosphorus, magnesium, vitamin D, and fluoride,* Washington, DC, 1997, National Academic Press.

29. Institute of Medicine: *Dietary reference intakes for thiamin, riboflavin, niacin, vitamin B6, folate, vitamin B12, pantothenic acid, biotin, and choline,* Washington, DC, 1998, National Academic Press.

30. Institute of Medicine: *Dietary reference intakes for vitamin C, vitamin E, selenium, and carotenoids,* Washington, DC, 2000, National Academic Press.

31. Institute of Medicine: *Dietary reference intakes for water, potassium, sodium, chloride, and sulfate,* Washington, DC, 2000, National Academic Press.

32. Institute of Medicine: *Dietary reference intakes for vitamin A, vitamin K, arsenic, boron, chromium, copper, iodine, iron, manganese, molybdenum, nickel, silicon, vanadium, and zinc,* Washington, DC, 2001, National Academic Press.

33. U.S. Department of Agriculture: *Dietary guidelines for Americans 2005.* Retrieved November 24, 2006, from www.healthierus.gov/dietaryguidelines

34. Krauss RM, Eckel RH, Howard B et al: AHA Dietary Guidelines: revision 2000—a statement for healthcare professionals from the Nutrition Committee of the American Heart Association, *Circulation* 102:2284-2299, 2000.

35. American Heart Association. *Vitamin and mineral supplements: A scientific position statement.* Retrieved November 24, 2006, from www.americanheart.org

36. Alissa EM, Bahjri SM, Al-Ama N et al: Dietary vitamin A may be a cardiovascular risk factor in a Saudi population, *Asia Pac J Clin Nutr* 14:137-144, 2005.

37. The effect of vitamin E and beta carotene on the incidence of lung cancer and other cancers in male smokers: the Alpha-Tocopherol, Beta Carotene Cancer Prevention Study Group, *N Engl J Med* 330:1029-1035, 1994.

38. Omenn GS, Goodman GE, Thornquist MD et al: Effects of a combination of beta carotene and vitamin A on lung cancer and cardiovascular disease, *N Engl J Med* 334:1150-1155, 1996.

39. Roberts AJ, O'Brien ME, Subak-Sharpe G: *Nutraceuticals: the complete encyclopedia of supplements, herbs, and healing foods,* New York, 2001, Berkley Publishing Group.

40. Todd S, Woodward M, Tunstall-Pedoe H, Bolton-Smith C: Dietary antioxidant vitamins and fiber in the etiology of cardiovascular disease and all-causes mortality: results from the Scottish Heart Health Study, *Am J Epidemiol* 150:1073-1080, 1999.

41. Klipstein-Grobusch K, Geleijnse JM, den Breeijen JH et al: Dietary antioxidants and risk of myocardial infarction in the elderly: the Rotterdam Study, *Am J Clin Nutr* 69:261-266, 1999.

42. Blot WJ, Li JY, Taylor PR et al: Nutrition intervention trials in Linxian, China: supplementation with specific vitamin/mineral combinations, cancer incidence, and disease-specific mortality in the general population, *J Natl Cancer Inst* 85:1483-1492, 1993.

43. Kris-Etherton PM, Lichtenstein AH, Howard BV et al: Antioxidant vitamin supplements and cardiovascular disease, *Circulation* 110:637-641, 2004.

44. Fowler B: Homocysteine: overview of biochemistry, molecular biology, and role in disease processes, *Semin Vasc Med* 5:77-86, 2005.

45. Wald DS, Law M, Morris JK: Homocysteine and cardiovascular disease: evidence on causality from a meta-analysis, *BMJ* 325:1202, 2002.

46. Bolander-Gouaille C: *Focus on homocysteine and the vitamins involved in its metabolism,* Paris, 2002, Springer.

47. Durga J, van Tits LJ, Schouten EG et al: Effect of lowering of homocysteine levels on inflammatory markers: a randomized controlled trial, *Arch Intern Med* 165:1388-1394, 2005.

48. Verhoef P, de Groot LC: Dietary determinants of plasma homocysteine concentrations, *Semin Vasc Med* 5:110-123, 2005.

49. Weikert C, Hoffmann K, Dierkes J et al: A homocysteine metabolism-related dietary pattern and the risk of coronary heart disease in two independent German study populations, *J Nutr* 135:1981-1988, 2005.

50. USDA Nutrient Laboratory: *Welcome to the Nutrient Data Laboratory home page.* Retrieved November 24, 2006, from www.ars.usda.gov/main/site_main.htm?modecode=12354500.

51. Jialal I, Fuller CJ: Effect of vitamin E, vitamin C and beta-carotene on LDL oxidation and atherosclerosis, *Can J Cardiol* 11(suppl G):97G-103G, 1995.

52. Lonn E, Bosch J, Yusuf S et al: Effects of long-term vitamin E supplementation on cardiovascular events and cancer: a randomized controlled trial, *JAMA* 293:1338-1347, 2005.

53. Miller ER 3rd, Pastor-Barriuso R, Dalal D et al: Meta-analysis: high-dosage vitamin E supplementation may increase all-cause mortality, *Ann Intern Med* 142:37-46, 2005.

54. Witte KK, Clark AL, Cleland JG: Chronic heart failure and micronutrients, *J Am Coll Cardiol* 37:1765-1774, 2001.

55. Rosenlund M, Berglind N, Hallqvist J et al: Daily intake of magnesium and calcium from drinking water in relation to myocardial infarction, *Epidemiology* 16:570-576, 2005.

56. Costello RB, Moser-Veillon PB, DiBianco R: Magnesium supplementation in patients with congestive heart failure, *J Am Coll Nutr* 16:22-31, 1997.

57. Sacks FM, Willett WC, Smith A et al: Effect on blood pressure of potassium, calcium, and magnesium in women with low habitual intake, *Hypertension* 31:131-138, 1998.

58. Alissa EM, Bahjri SM, Ferns GA: The controversy surrounding selenium and cardiovascular disease: a review of the evidence, *Med Sci Monit* 9:RA9-RA18, 2003.

59. Elliott P, Stamler J, Nichols R et al: INTERSALT revisited: further analyses of 24 hour sodium excretion and blood pressure within and across populations: INTERSALT Cooperative Research Group, *BMJ* 312:1249-1253, 1996.

60. Law MR, Frost CD, Wald NJ: By how much does dietary salt reduction lower blood pressure? III. Analysis of data from trials of salt reduction, *BMJ* 302:819-824, 1991.

61. Lev-Ran A, Porta M: Salt and hypertension: a phylogenetic perspective, *Diabetes Metab Res Rev* 21:118-131, 2005.

62. US Department of Health and Human Services, US Department of Agriculture: *Dietary guidelines for Americans, 2005,* ed 6, Washington, DC, 2005, Government Printing Office.

63. Mattes RD, Donnelly D: Relative contributions of dietary sodium sources, *J Am Coll Nutr* 10:383-393, 1991.

64. Brehm BJ, Seeley RJ, Daniels SR, D'Alessio DA: A randomized trial comparing a very low carbohydrate diet and a calorie-restricted low fat diet on body weight and cardiovascular risk factors in healthy women, *J Clin Endocrinol Metab* 88:1617-1623, 2003.

65. Keys A, Menotti A, Karvonen MJ et al: The diet and 15-year death rate in the seven countries study, *Am J Epidemiol* 124:903-915, 1986.

66. Kokkinos P, Panagiotakos DB, Polychronopoulos E: Dietary influences on blood pressure: the effect of the Mediterranean diet on the prevalence of hypertension, *J Clin Hypertens (Greenwich)* 7:165-170, 2005.

67. Parikh P, McDaniel MC, Ashen MD et al: Diets and cardiovascular disease: an evidence-based assessment, *J Am Coll Cardiol* 45:1379-1387, 2005.

68. Ruano J, Lopez-Miranda J, Fuentes F et al: Phenolic content of virgin olive oil improves ischemic reactive hyperemia in hypercholesterolemic patients, *J Am Coll Cardiol* 46:1864-1868, 2005.

69. Kris-Etherton P, Eckel RH, Howard BV et al: AHA Science Advisory: Lyon Diet Heart Study—benefits of a Mediterranean-style, National Cholesterol Education Program/American Heart Association Step I Dietary Pattern on cardiovascular disease, *Circulation* 103:1823-1825, 2001.

70. Appel LJ, Moore TJ, Obarzanek E et al: A clinical trial of the effects of dietary patterns on blood pressure: DASH Collaborative Research Group, *N Engl J Med* 336:1117-1124, 1997.

71. Bray GA, Vollmer WM, Sacks FM et al: A further subgroup analysis of the effects of the DASH diet and three dietary sodium levels on blood pressure: results of the DASH-Sodium Trial, *Am J Cardiol* 94:222-227, 2004.

72. Obarzanek E, Sacks FM, Vollmer WM et al: Effects on blood lipids of a blood pressure-lowering diet: the Dietary Approaches to Stop Hypertension (DASH) Trial, *Am J Clin Nutr* 74:80-89, 2001.

73. Harsha DW, Sacks FM, Obarzanek E et al: Effect of dietary sodium intake on blood lipids: results from the DASH-sodium trial, *Hypertension* 43:393-398, 2004.

74. Ard JD, Coffman CJ, Lin PH, Svetkey LP: One-year follow-up study of blood pressure and dietary patterns in dietary approaches to stop hypertension (DASH)-sodium participants, *Am J Hypertens* 17:1156-1162, 2004.

75. National Heart, Lung, and Blood Institute: *The NHLBI practical guide: identification, evaluation, and treatment of overweight and obesity in adults*, NIH Pub No 00-4084, Bethesda, Md, 2000, National Institutes of Health.

76. Mosterd A, Cost B, Hoes AW et al: The prognosis of heart failure in the general population: the Rotterdam Study, *Eur Heart J* 22:1318-1327, 2001.

77. Horwich TB, Fonarow GC, Hamilton MA et al: The relationship between obesity and mortality in patients with heart failure, *J Am Coll Cardiol* 38:789-795, 2001.

78. Davos CH, Doehner W, Rauchhaus M et al: Body mass and survival in patients with chronic heart failure without cachexia: the importance of obesity, *J Card Fail* 9:29-35, 2003.

79. Hall JA, French TK, Rimmasch HL et al: Obesity paradox validation: elevated body mass index portends better prognosis in heart failure—analysis of 2,707 patients in an integrated healthcare delivery system, *Circulation* 10:S104, 2004.

80. Cicoira M, Iwanowska E, Doehner W et al: Fat tissue mass and prognosis in 486 patients with chronic heart failure, *Circulation* 108(suppl 4):IV-486, 2003.

81. Lavie CJ, Osman AF, Milani RV, Mehra MR: Body composition and prognosis in chronic systolic heart failure: the obesity paradox, *Am J Cardiol* 91:891-894, 2003.

82. Horwich TB, Hamilton MA, Maclellan WR, Fonarow GC: Low serum total cholesterol is associated with marked increase in mortality in advanced heart failure, *J Card Fail* 8:216-224, 2002.

83. Michie HR, Manogue KR, Spriggs DR et al: Detection of circulating tumor necrosis factor after endotoxin administration, *N Engl J Med* 318:1481-1486, 1988.

84. Niebauer J, Volk HD, Kemp M et al: Endotoxin and immune activation in chronic heart failure: a prospective cohort study, *Lancet* 353:1838-1842, 1999.

85. Misra A, Vikram NK: Clinical and pathophysiological consequences of abdominal adiposity and abdominal adipose tissue depots, *Nutrition* 19:457-466, 2003.

86. Rauchhaus M, Coats AJS, Anker SD: The endotoxin-lipoprotein hypothesis, *Lancet* 356:930-933, 2000.

87. Anker SD, Ponikowski P, Varney S et al: Wasting as independent risk factor for mortality in chronic heart failure, *Lancet* 349:1050-1053, 1997.

88. Anker SD, Sharma R: The syndrome of cardiac cachexia, *Int J Cardiol* 85:51-66, 2002.

89. Anker SD, Steinborn W, Strassburg S: Cardiac cachexia, *Ann Med* 36:518-529, 2004.

90. Sharma R, Anker SD: Cytokines, apoptosis and cachexia: the potential for TNF antagonism, *Int J Cardiol* 85:161-171, 2002.

91. Marcus EL, Berry EM: Refusal to eat in the elderly, *Nutr Rev* 56:163-171, 1998.

92. Ballinger A, McLoughlin L, Medbak S, Clark M: Cholecystokinin is a satiety hormone in humans at physiological post-prandial plasma concentrations, *Clin Sci (Lond)* 89:375-381, 1995.

93. Doherty TJ: Invited review: aging and sarcopenia, *J Appl Physiol* 95:1717-1727, 2003.

94. Carr JG, Stevenson LW, Walden JA, Heber D: Prevalence and hemodynamic correlates of malnutrition in severe congestive heart failure secondary to ischemic or idiopathic dilated cardiomyopathy, *Am J Cardiol* 63:709-713, 1989.

95. Milani RV, Mehra MR, Endres S et al: The clinical relevance of circulating tumor necrosis factor-alpha in acute decompensated chronic heart failure without cachexia, *Chest* 110:992-995, 1996.

96. Freeman LM, Roubenoff R: The nutrition implications of cardiac cachexia, *Nutr Rev* 52:340-347, 1994.

97. Levine B, Kalman J, Mayer L et al: Elevated circulating levels of tumor necrosis factor in severe chronic heart failure, *N Engl J Med* 323:236-241, 1990.

98. Otaki M: Surgical treatment of patients with cardiac cachexia: an analysis of factors affecting operative mortality, *Chest* 105:1347-1351, 1994.

99. Aquilani R, Opasich C, Verri M et al: Is nutritional intake adequate in chronic heart failure patients? *J Am Coll Cardiol* 42:1218-1223, 2003.

100. Anker SD, Coats AJ: Cardiac cachexia: a syndrome with impaired survival and immune and neuroendocrine activation, *Chest* 115:836-847, 1999.

101. Prealbumin in Nutritional Care Consensus Group: Measurement of visceral protein status in assessing protein and energy malnutrition: standard of care, *Nutrition* 11:169-171, 1995.

102. Beckoff K, MacIntosh CG, Chapman IM et al: Effects of glucose supplementation on gastric emptying, blood glucose homeostasis, and appetite in the elderly, *Am J Physiol Regul Integr Comp Physiol* 280:R570-R576, 2001.

chapter 13

Genetic and Environmental Basis of Cardiac Disease

Dorie W. Schwertz
Bradley E. Aouizerat
Shu-Fen Wung

CHAPTER ABBREVIATIONS

DNA   deoxyribonucleic acid

HCM   hypertrophic cardiomyopathy

HERG   human ether-a-go-go-related gene

LQT   long-QT

mtDNA   mitochondrial DNA

mRNA   messenger RNA

RNA   ribonucleic acid

SNP   single nucleotide polymorphism

With few exceptions, all cells in the body have the same genetic material *(genotype)* in the form of deoxyribonucleic acid (**DNA**). DNA contains functional subunits called *genes* that provide the template for making all proteins. However, different cell types—such as cardiac muscle cells (myocytes), fibroblasts, and monocytes—express (or synthesize) only a small subset of the total possible proteins encoded by DNA. These differences in protein expression contribute in large part to the tremendous variation found in cell structure and function. In other words, differential protein expression largely influences different cell *phenotypes.* Alterations in the DNA code (variations or *mutations*) can modify proteins, thereby changing cell structure and function. These phenotypic changes can result in cardiac abnormalities, disease, increased susceptibility to disease, or rarely, resistance to disease.

This chapter focuses on the relationship between genetics, environmental factors, and cardiovascular disease. Understanding the contribution of genetics to disease has been greatly facilitated by the Human Genome Project, particularly the sequencing of human DNA and the ongoing identification of specific protein-coding genes. We review DNA structure and regulation of protein expression. Principles of genetic inheritance and types of genetic mutations and polymorphisms are described. The impact of environment-gene and lifestyle-gene interaction on risk, severity, and prognosis of disease are addressed. All of these principles are put into context using the long-QT dysrhythmogenic syndrome and hypertrophic cardiomyopathy as cardiac disease models. We focus particularly on environment-gene interactions because intervention aimed at altering environment and behavior to optimize health and minimize disease is a centerpiece of nursing practice.

GENES AND CHROMOSOMES

Genes are the functional and physical unit of heredity passed from parent to offspring. A gene is a linear segment of DNA that carries instructions for synthesizing proteins. The amino acid sequence of a protein is encoded by four repeating nucleotide bases (adenine, cytosine, guanine, and thymine). The bases are ordered precisely by covalent linkage to a phosphate-sugar (deoxyribose) backbone (Figure 13-1).

The DNA molecule has two strands of nucleotides with the nucleic acids facing inward (like rungs of a ladder), whereas the sugar-phosphate moieties form a backbone (like the sides of a ladder). The ladder structure twists into a double helix for stability. Nucleotide bases on each side of the ladder are linked by hydrogen bonds in a specific way. Adenine (A) always pairs with thymine (T), and guanine (G) always pairs with cytosine (C). For example, if one strand of the DNA molecule has the sequence ACTTGC, the associated strand would have the *complementary* sequence TGAACG.

Each DNA molecule contains hundreds to thousands of genes. DNA molecules are wound around proteins called *histones* that provide structural support and regulatory functions and are packaged into chromosomes. Most cells in the body have 23 pairs of morphologically distinct chromosomes for a total of 46 chromosomes (Figure 13-2). One member of the pair is inherited from the mother, and the other is inherited from the father. Twenty-two of the pairs are *autosomal chromosomes* or *autosomes* that contain gene coding for structural and functional proteins of the somatic cells of the body. The two chromosomes making up each pair are called *homologs.* Each of the *homologous chromosomes* has a gene coding for the same protein (one inherited from the mother and the other from the father). The two copies of the gene are called *alleles.* If the two alleles are exactly the same, they are called *homozygous.* If the alleles are different, they are called *heterozygous.*

The 23rd chromosomal pair (the sex chromosomes) has either an X chromosome from the mother and father (XX chromosomes, coding for proteins associated with the female phenotype) or an X chromosome from the mother and a Y chromosome from the father (XY chromosome, producing a male phenotype). The germ cells (i.e., the egg and the sperm) have only one chromosome from each homologous pair (i.e., 23 unpaired chromosomes) and thereby only one allele. When the egg is fertilized, the resulting zygote (or first embryonic cell)

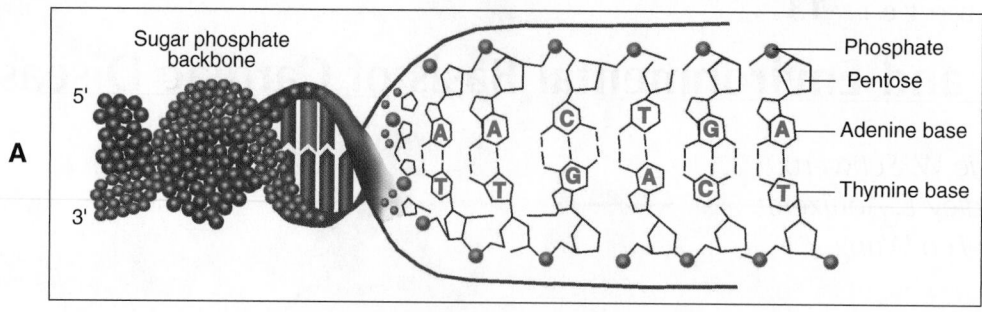

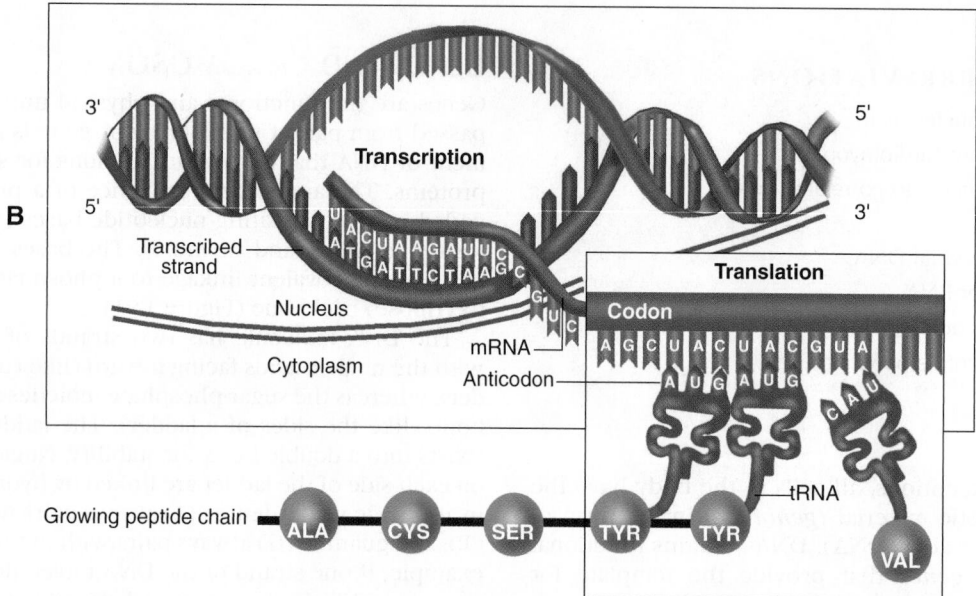

FIGURE 13-1 ■ The structure of deoxyribonucleic acid (DNA) contains information that is *transcribed* into ribonucleic acid (RNA) and subsequently *translated* into proteins. **A,** The DNA molecule consists of two long strands of nucleotides that are complementary and that coil into a double helix for stability. The two strands are held together by hydrogen bonds between complementary nucleic acid bases: adenine (A) is bound to thymine (T), and guanine (G) is bound to cytosine (C). **B,** The double helix opens, and one side is transcribed into a single complementary strand of messenger RNA (mRNA). The resulting mRNA sequence then is translated into amino acids (read in units of three adjacent nucleotides, or *codons*) and a peptide chain is formed at a cell structure called the ribosome. The amino acid chain may be processed further to form a mature protein. *tRNA,* Transfer RNA. (From Zipes DP, Libby P, Bonow RO, Braunwald E: *Braunwald's heart disease,* ed 7, Philadelphia, 2005, Elsevier Saunders.)

again has 23 pairs of chromosomes, half of each pair inherited from each parent. Therefore, every cell in the body arising from the original cell will have a copy of a given gene from the mother and from the father.

Chromosomes can be isolated from the nucleus of cells, stained, and observed under a microscope. This display of all chromosomes is the person's *karyotype* (Figure 13-2). Each of the chromosomes is morphologically distinct, meaning that it can be recognized by its size, shape, staining pattern, and the position of a structure called the *centromere* (Figures 13-2A and B and 13-3). The centromere is a constricted area along the chromosome that is asymmetrically located relative to the long arm of the chromosome. Because of the asymmetrical location, the chromosome appears to have a short arm (labeled *p* for petite) and a long arm (labeled *q*). Chromosome staining results in lighter and darker areas on the arms, corresponding to areas of higher and lower GC nucleotide content, respectively, which is

preferentially bound by the Giemsa dye used in the procedure. This is important because areas with greater GC content harbor the majority of genes in each chromosome. The densely stained areas are labeled consecutively from 1, located closest to the centromere, to increasingly higher numbers as the discretely, densely stained area occurs progressively farther out on the arm. This labeling system is used to identify the location (or *locus*) of a gene of interest.

For example, the chromosomal location of a gene called human ether-a-go-go related gene **(HERG)** (or KCNH2) coding for a potassium channel involved in the long-QT syndrome is 7q3,5 (Figure 13-3). Thus, the gene for this protein would be located at the fifth band in the third region of the long arm of chromosome 7. This annotation would be stated as follows: "chromosome seven 'q' three, five," or "the long arm of chromosome seven band three, five." The use of sub-banding is common and becoming more so; for example, "chromo-

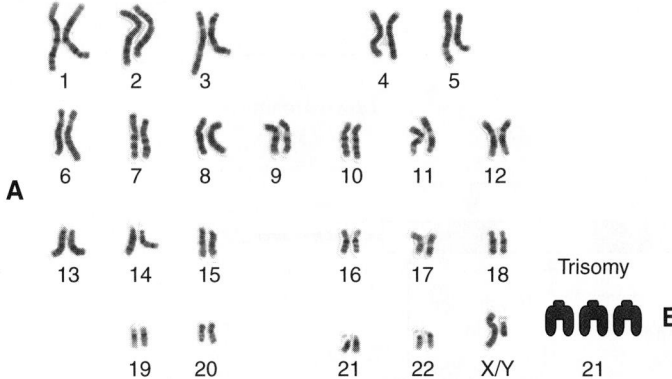

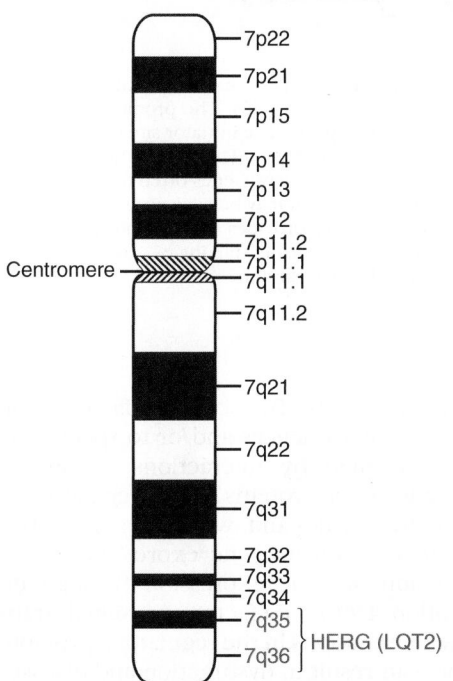

FIGURE 13-2 ■ **A,** The human karyotype. The autosomal chromosomes are numbered from 1 to 22. Each of the chromosomes can be recognized by its size, shape, staining pattern, and the position of the centromere (the constriction area where two identical copies of the chromosomes join together). The largest autosome is number 1 and the smallest is number 21. Historically, the second smallest chromosome has been designated number 22. The Y chromosome is about the same size as chromosome 22, and the X chromosome is larger than the Y chromosome. **B,** An example of a autosomal abnormality that results in cardiac disease. This karyotype is from a male patient with Down syndrome, or trisomy 21, showing three copies of chromosome 21. Congenital heart disease is present in at least one-third of all live-born Down syndrome infants.

FIGURE 13-3 ■ Each chromosome has a landmark constriction called a centromere that is asymmetrically located and demarcates a long (q) arm and a short (p) arm of the chromosome. Darkly stained regions (bands) along the length of the chromosome are numbered and are used to identify the locus of a gene. The long QT2 syndrome (LQT2) disease gene, human ether-a-go-go-related gene (HERG, also called KCNH2), is located on the long arm of chromosome 7, as shown.

some seven q three, five point two" would be written as 7q35.2. Sub-banding is a modification of the standard chromosomal banding procedure that involves staining the chromosomes that have been arrested at a slightly different point during mitosis. Gross chromosomal abnormalities such as extra, missing, or broken chromo-

somes can be identified by examining the karyotype (Figure 13-2).

DNA also is contained in the mitochondria of cells (**mtDNA**). The mitochondria are organelles located outside of the nucleus in the cellular cytoplasm. Each mitochondrion contains several copies of its own unique DNA. Because each cell usually has many mitochondria, the number of mtDNA molecules for each cell can be large. Human mtDNA molecules are circular and contain 37 genes, including two encoding ribosomal **RNAs** and 22 encoding transfer RNAs. Some human diseases are caused by mutations in the mtDNA, including rare forms of dilated or hypertrophic cardiomyopathy caused by deletions and point mutations of mtDNA. As the only gamete that contains cytoplasm and organelles, the egg is the source of mitochondrial transfer, and thus exhibits its *maternal inheritance.* All offspring of a female harboring a disease-causing mitochondrial gene are at risk of inheriting the abnormality, whereas no offspring of an affected male are at risk.

REGULATION OF GENE EXPRESSION

In the process of making proteins, genes are *transcribed* into complementary single-stranded messenger ribonucleic acid (**mRNA**; Figure 13-1). In mRNA the nucleotide base uracil is substituted for thymidine. mRNA then is *translated* into the amino acid sequence of a protein at a cellular structure called the ribosome. However, the entire RNA is not always translated. Genes have nucleotide sequences called *exons* that are transcribed and primarily are translated into proteins. A small portion of the exons located at either end of the mRNA often are left untranslated into protein and are termed the 5'- and 3'-untranslated regions (stated as "five-prime UTR" or "three-prime UTR"), respectively. Genes also have nucleotide sequences called *introns* that although transcribed into message then can be cut out and not translated into the final protein product (Figure 13-4). This allows one gene to form several different proteins by cutting out not only various introns but a subset of exons. The process results in the formation of different species of mRNA and thereby different proteins. This process is called *alternative splicing.* During translation, specific amino acids are encoded for by units of three consecutive nucleotides (nucleic acid sequences) and are termed *codons.* The four nucleic acids can be organized into 64 possible codons (4^3). Because there are only 20 amino acids, some codons are redundant for the same amino acid; i.e., there may be more than one codon for an amino acid (Table 13-1). For example, the codons UUU and UUC code for the same amino acid—phenylalanine.

The transcriptional unit of a gene (Figure 13-5; also see Figure 13-4) not only contains the nucleotide triplicates (codons) that are transcribed into message and translated into amino acids but also contains other nucleotide sequences that provide information about where transcription should begin (i.e., at the transcription initiation site), where it should end (at a transcription stop site), or where it should be spliced (splicing signals). The transcriptional unit of a gene also contains nucleotide

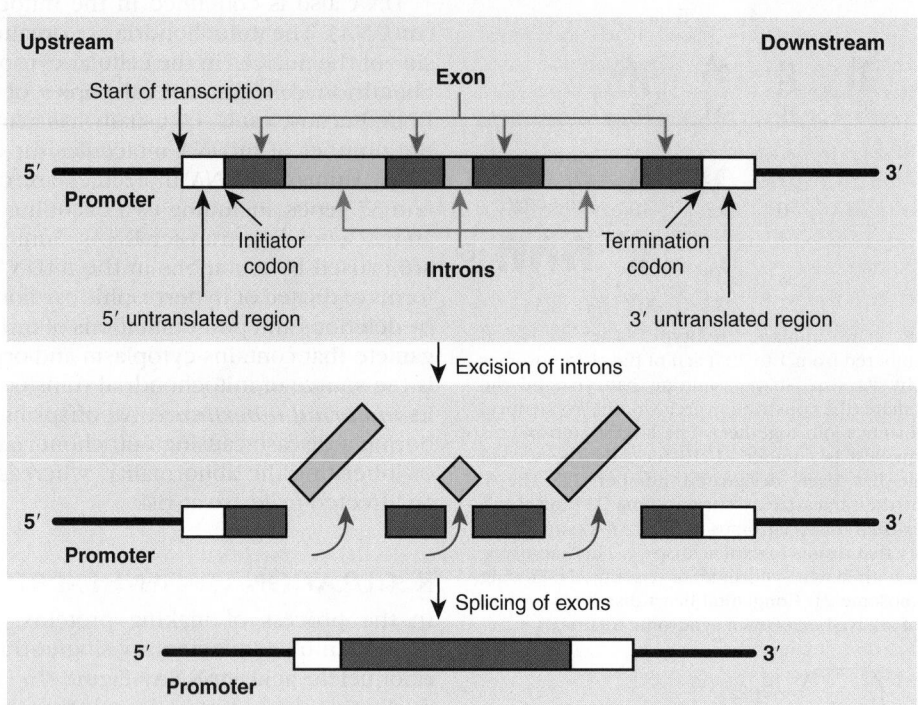

Transcription Unit

FIGURE 13-4 ▪ Transcription unit of a gene. The transcription unit of a gene has nucleotides providing information other than the nucleotide triplicates that code for amino acids. The promoter area is involved with regulation of the rate and tissue distribution of transcription. The initiator site and the initiator codon indicate where transcription and translation begins, respectively. The termination site and stop codon indicates where transcription and translation stops, respectively. Genes often have areas that are not transcribed called introns. Different combinations of exons that may be excised along with the introns and the remaining regions (exons) are spliced together. This provides the possibility for one gene to code for more than one protein (or variations of a protein) by variable splicing of exons. Alternative proteins made from the same gene in this manner are called splice variants.

sequences that regulate tissue specificity, response to environmental stimulus, and rate of transcription of that gene. This area is called the *promoter region.*

Gene expression (the conversion of the nucleotide code into protein) is highly regulated. In a given cell type, some genes are never expressed, others are always expressed at a basal level, and still others may be turned on and off or their rate of transcription modulated. For example, hemoglobin will never be expressed in a cardiomyocyte, whereas the muscle fiber protein, myosin is continually (or constitutively) expressed in cardiomyocytes. Extracellular signals (for example, estrogen) may increase transiently the expression of a protein such as endothelial nitric oxide synthase in vascular endothelial cells.

As mentioned previously, differentiation of cell structure and function results from and is influenced by regulation of gene expression. Regulation occurs at the transcriptional, translational and posttranslational level, and many cellular proteins are involved in the process. *Transcription factors* are one such class of regulatory proteins. Endocrine, paracrine, and autocrine signal molecules (such as steroid hormones, neurotransmitters, and growth factors, respectively) can activate or inactivate

transcription factors. Transcription factors bind to specific nucleotide sequences and/or to specific secondary structures formed by interactions of nucleotide sequences and other proteins in the regulatory/promoter region of target genes and, with the help of other *co-factor proteins,* modulate gene expression (Figure 13-5). Dysregulation of gene expression through defects in transcription factor, co-factor, or signal transduction proteins, or mutations in the regulatory/promoter region of a gene, can result in dysfunction and disease.

CONTRIBUTION OF PARENTAL DNA TO OFFSPRING

Each cell in the body (except germ cells) normally contains 22 homologous pairs of autosomal chromosomes and two sex chromosomes (a total of 46 chromosomes). Human beings inherit one chromosome of each homologous pair from the mother and the other from the father. Cells having these two, paired, homologous chromosomes are referred to as *diploid* (2n). In contrast, the germ cells (egg and sperm) have 23 unpaired chromosomes and are referred to as *haploid* (1n). An in-depth review of the molecular mechanisms by which germ

TABLE 13-1   A. MESSENGER RNA CODONS*

First (5') Letter		SECOND LETTER								Third (3') Letter
		U		C		A		G		
U		UUU	Phe	UCU	Ser	UAU	Tyr	UGU	Cys	U
		UUC		UCC		UAC		UGC		C
		UUA	Leu	UCA		UAA	Ochre†	UGA	Opal†	A
		UUG		UCG		UAG	Amber†	UGG	Trp	G
C		CUU	Leu	CCU	Pro	CAU	His	CGU	Arg	U
		CUC		CCC		CAC		CGC		C
		CUA		CCA		CAA	Gln	CGA		A
		CUG		CCG		CAG		CGG		G
A		AUU	Ileu	ACU	Thr	AAU	Asn	AGU	Ser	U
		AUC		ACC		AAC		AGC		C
		AUA		ACA		AAA	Lys	AGA	Arg	A
		AUG	Met‡	ACG		AAG		AGG		G
G		GUU	Val	GCU	Ala	GAU	Asp	GGU	Gly	U
		GUC		GCC		GAC		GGC		C
		GUA		GCA		GAA	Glu	GGA		A
		GUG		GCG		GAG		GGG		G

*Each codon in messenger RNA specifies the initiation signal, amino acid, or termination signal called for in a given polypeptide chain, or protein.
†Termination codon.
‡Initiation codon.

B. ABBREVIATIONS FOR AMINO ACIDS

AMINO ACID	THREE-LETTER ABBREVIATION	ONE-LETTER SYMBOL
Alanine	Ala	A
Arginine	Arg	R
Asparagine	Asn	N
Aspartic acid	Asp	D
Asparagine or aspartic acid	Asx	B
Cysteine	Cys	C
Glutamine	Gln	Q
Glutamic acid	Glu	E
Glutamine or glutamic acid	Glx	Z
Glycine	Gly	G
Histidine	His	H
Isoleucine	Ile	I
Leucine	Leu	L
Lysine	Lys	K
Methionine	Met	M
Phenylalanine	Phe	F
Proline	Pro	P
Serine	Ser	S
Threonine	Thr	T
Tryptophan	Trp	W
Tyrosine	Tyr	Y
Valine	Val	V

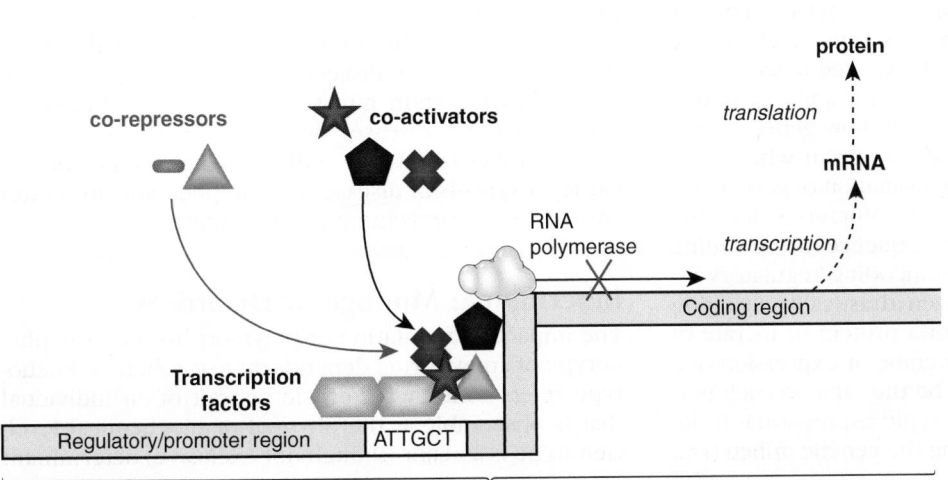

FIGURE 13-5 ▓ Regulation of gene expression. The transcription unit of a gene includes the coding region (containing instructions for the amino acid sequence of a protein) and regulatory/promoter regions that are involved in controlling the rate of gene transcription by RNA polymerase. Cellular proteins called transcription factors and co-activator and co-repressor proteins also are involved in this regulatory process. Transcription factors and other co-factor proteins can be activated or inhibited by extracellular signals. These proteins bind to specific nucleotide sequences, to secondary DNA structure, and/or to other transcription factors in the regulatory/promoter region of the gene, thereby influencing gene expression. *DNA,* Deoxyribonucleic acid; *mRNA,* messenger RNA; *RNA,* ribonucleic acid.

cells become haploid (the process is called meiosis) is beyond the scope of this chapter. However, a few basic principles are described.

During one step of meiosis, each of the 46 chromosomes in progenitor cells replicates. The number of chromosomes is then 92 or 4n. The duplicated chromosomes are called *sister chromatids*. Sister chromatids can exchange chromosomal segments in a process called *meiotic recombination*. This results in each chromosome having gene segments from both parents. The probability that neighboring genes on a single chromosome will become separated by meiotic recombination generally increases with the distance between two gene loci. As a corollary, genes that are close together usually are inherited together and are said to be *linked*. Exchanging genetic material between chromosomes of maternal and paternal origin during meiotic recombination contributes considerably to genetic variation. As a result, each person has a unique genotype.

Following recombination, the 4n progenitor cells undergo two divisions, and the resulting germ cell has an equal probability of receiving one chromosome (1n) that originated from the paternal or the maternal side. This is referred to as the principle of *independent assortment*. When the egg and the sperm unite, they form the first embryonic cell, which is again diploid (2n) with one chromosome of a homologous pair inherited from the mother and the other from the father. However, because of recombination (or sister chromatid exchange) neither parent's chromosome in the embryonic cells is absolutely identical to the parent's chromosome.

MUTATIONS: CHROMOSOMAL AND GENETIC DEFECTS

Cardiac structural abnormalities, dysfunction, and disease can result from chromosomal anomalies or single- or multiple-gene mutations and can be influenced to a greater or lesser degree by environmental factors. Chromosomal abnormalities, such as gain or loss of chromosomes *(aneuploidy)*, often result in congenital heart defects that are discussed in Chapter 71. In some cases a small group of neighboring genes on the same chromosome (undetectable by karyotype analysis) are deleted. The outcome of this type of chromosomal abnormality is referred to as a *contiguous gene syndrome*. An example is Williams syndrome. This disorder results from a microdeletion of chromosomal region 7q11.23 that includes the elastin gene and has cardiovascular consequences.[1]

The following discussion focuses on single-gene mutations, how genes are inherited, and how genetic variation influences phenotype. Errors can occur when chromosomal DNA replicates during formation of germ cells. These errors are called *mutations*. Mutations have the potential to alter the nucleotide sequence of the coding region of a gene or to change noncoding/regulatory regions, thereby minimally or even drastically changing the structure and/or function of a protein or its rate of expression. The phenotypic outcome or expression of a given mutation will not always be the same in each person. As is discussed later, phenotypic expression is influenced by many factors, including the genetic milieu (i.e.,

gene-gene interactions), lifestyle factors, and environmental exposure. Although our main concern in this chapter is the association of gene mutations with cardiac disease and inheritance of cardiac disease, one has to remember that a mutation may have no effect or, rarely, it may improve the structure or function of a protein, thereby conferring a biological advantage.

There are many types of mutations. One type of error that can occur during DNA replication is nucleotide base *substitution* (i.e., one nucleotide base is substituted for another). A nucleotide substitution can alter a codon and cause the substitution of one amino acid for another, thereby influencing protein structure and function. Nucleotide substitution also can alter information inherent in stop codons, initiation sites, or regulatory sequences. If a DNA substitution results in altered protein structure; it is referred to as a *missense mutation*. However, because there are redundant codons for certain amino acids, it is possible that a nucleotide substitution would not alter the amino acid code; as such, it would be called a *neutral mutation*. Base pair substitutions that occur in at least 1 percent of a population are referred to as *single nucleotide polymorphisms* or **SNP**s. More than 11 million SNPs have been identified in the human genome.

Another type of replication error can result in the deletion or insertion of one or more nucleotide bases. Because the genetic code is translated in units of three adjacent nucleotides, deletions and insertions can cause reading *frame shifts* such that the codons that follow the error are read incorrectly. Mutations at sites involved in splicing are called *splice-site mutations* and can have serious consequences for the resulting protein. If a mutation is present in the parent's DNA or if it occurs during meiotic DNA replication (i.e., in the formation of a germ cell), the mutation may be passed on to the offspring.

The Human Genome Project has revealed important information about genetic variability. One of the goals of the project was to sequence all of the 3 billion nucleotide base pairs in human beings. Results of the project have shown about one SNP in every 100 to 300 bases.[2] A long-term goal of the Human Genome Project is to clone and identify specific genes to determine which proteins are coded for by each gene. As previously mentioned, genetic sequence variations, including SNPs, may or may not affect the structure or function of a protein. However, some do alter protein structure or expression. With the information made available from the Human Genome Project, researchers are investigating whether certain mutations or polymorphisms are associated with diseases or susceptibility to diseases. These studies eventually will allow more efficient and earlier diagnosis of disease, with implications for better approaches to prevention and treatment.[3]

Inheritance: Monogenic Disorders

The impact of a mutation or polymorphism on the phenotype of an offspring depends on many factors. Phenotype refers to a characteristic or trait of an individual that is observable at the physical or biochemical level. Genotype is a major (though not exclusive) determinant of phenotype. One factor influencing phenotype is whether a person is homozygous or heterozygous for a given gene. If both alleles (or copies) of a gene are identical, the person is homozygous; if the alleles are different (for example, if one allele has a mutation and the other does not), the person is heterozygous.

Another factor influencing phenotype is whether a trait resulting from a gene exerts a *dominant* or *recessive* influence. In the case of autosomal dominant inheritance, it takes only one mutated allele to express a trait. In other words, if the mutant allele is passed on, the offspring will have the trait. In the case of autosomal recessive inheritance, a recessive trait may not be observable unless the person is homozygous for the recessive gene. In the context of a disease-causing gene, if only a single mutated allele is enough to result in the disease, then the trait is dominant. If both alleles must be mutated for the person to be affected by the disease, then the trait is recessive. To some degree, whether a trait (or disease) is dominant or recessive in its inheritance depends on whether the error in formation of the protein can be compensated for by other factors.

The probability that a *monogenic disease* (disease caused by a mutation in one gene) will be inherited often is assessed by using a Punnent square (Figure 13-6).

Both parents are heterozygous

Father is heterozygous and mother is homozygous dominant

Father is heterozygous and mother is homozygous recessive

FIGURE 13-6 ■ Autosomal recessive inheritance shown with Punnent squares. The letter "h" represents a recessive allele for a heart disease trait on an autosomal chromosome, and "H" represents an autosomal dominant nondisease (normal) allele. **A,** Both parents are heterozygous (Hh), and each offspring has a 1 in 4 chance of having the disease phenotype. **B,** The mother is homozygous for the nondisease "H" allele, and the father is heterozygous. None of the offspring will have the heart disease trait, but offspring have a 50 percent chance of being a carrier. **C,** The mother is homozygous recessive for the trait and has the disease, whereas the father is heterozygous. Each offspring will have a 50 percent chance of having heart disease.

These squares are constructed based on Mendelian principles of inheritance. One principle, termed the *principle of segregation,* is that germ cells will receive only one allele for each autosomal pair from each parent. A second principle, termed the *principle of independent assortment,* is that either allele has an equal chance of being passed on to each offspring. Figure 13-6, *A* shows a Punnent square that predicts the probability that an offspring will inherit an autosomal recessive characteristic (e.g., a disease) if both parents are heterozygous for the disease. In this figure, "H" represents the dominant normal or nondisease allele, and "h" represents the recessive disease allele. Because the disease shows a recessive inheritance pattern, the disease trait is not observable in either parent. In addition, even though both parents carry the "h" allele, there is only a 25 percent (1 in 4) chance that the offspring will receive both recessive alleles (hh) and have the disease phenotype.

In Figure 13-6, *B,* one parent (the mother) is homozygous for the H allele, whereas the father is heterozygous. In this case, none of the offspring will have the disease even though 50 percent will carry the recessive gene. Finally, the Punnent square in Figure 13-6, *C* shows the probability of a child having the disease trait if the mother is homozygous recessive and the father is again heterozygous. Under these conditions, the mother will have the disease phenotype and every offspring will carry the disease gene. The probability that an offspring will express the disease is 50 percent.

An exception to the foregoing examples occurs in males when the trait is *X-linked* (i.e., when the gene for the trait is located on the X chromosome). In this situation, the gene will be expressed in males regardless of whether the trait is dominant or recessive because no homologous allele is found on the Y chromosome. In a female, the trait produced by the same gene can be recognized as dominant or recessive because, with two X chromosomes, the female may be homozygous or heterozygous.

A pedigree chart is used visually to represent the genetic history of a family for a given disease or trait (Figure 13-7, *A*). Pedigree charts are useful for determining patterns of inheritance and the risk that a person will develop a disease. An example of autosomal recessive inheritance from two parents who are heterozygous for a disease allele is illustrated in Figure 13-7, *B.* The square and circle symbols at the top of the chart represent a man and a woman (respectively). A person with the disease phenotype is represented by a solid (filled) symbol, and carrier status (i.e., carrying the disease allele) is represented by a symbol that contains a red dot. The second row of square and circle symbols represents the second generation, and the third row represents the third generation. As shown in Figure 13-6, *A,* when both parents are heterozygous, each of the children (the second generation) has a 25 percent chance of inheriting the recessive allele from both parents and thereby a 25 percent chance of having the disease. In Figure 13-7, *B,* two of the four second-generation children have an observable disease phenotype, and because it is a recessive phenotype, it can be assumed that these two children received a disease allele from each parent. None of the children in the third generation display the disease phenotype because the mates of children from the second generation did not carry the gene.

Figure 13-7, *C* shows a pedigree chart of an autosomal dominant pattern of inheritance through three generations. In this example, the father is heterozygous for the gene responsible for this dominant trait, and the mother does not carry the disease allele. Each child in the second generation has a 50 percent chance of inheriting the gene and, because the trait is dominant, a 50 percent probability of having the disease. Children without the disease who marry persons without the disease have no risk of having offspring with the disease. However, children with the disease who marry persons

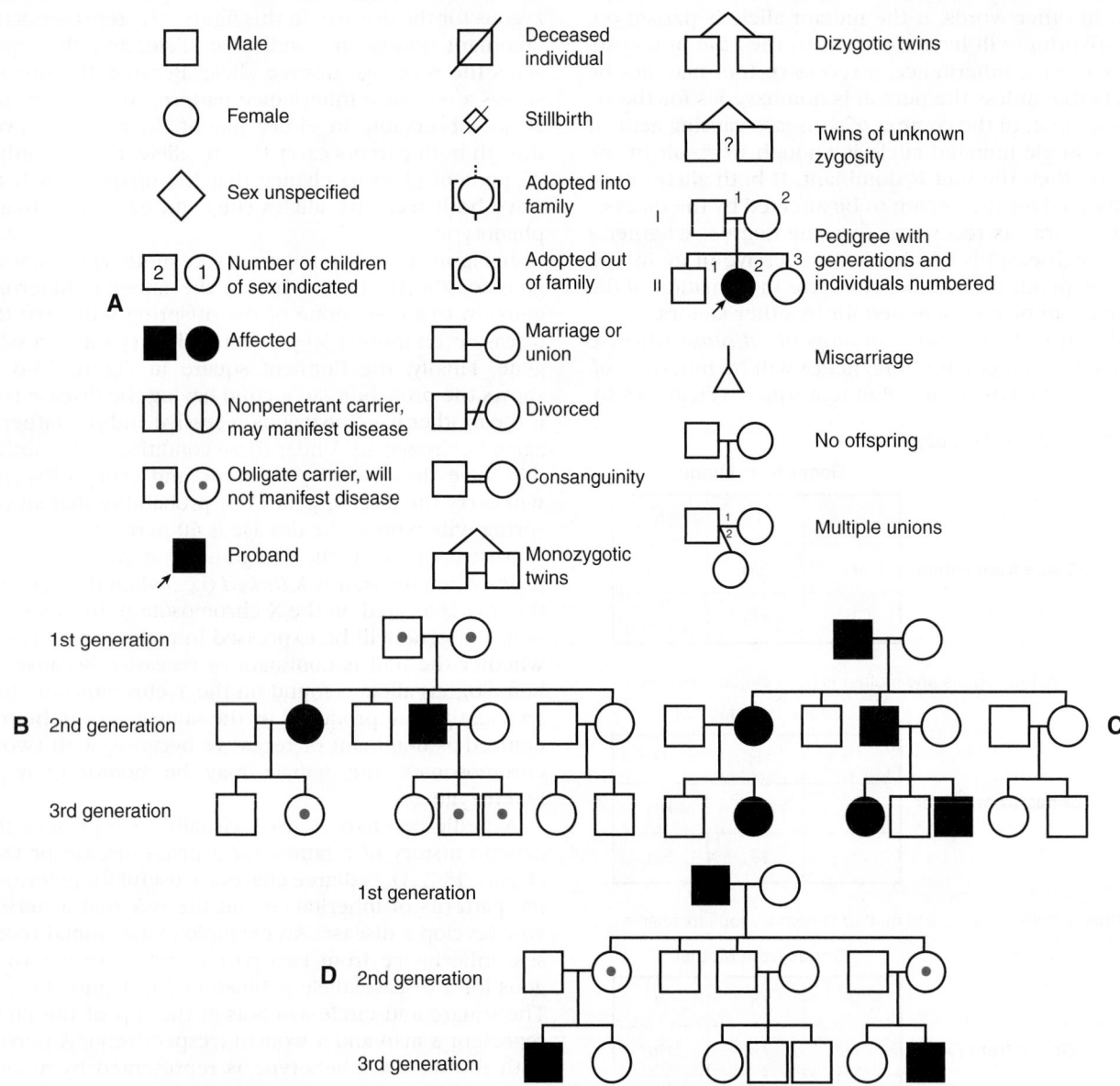

FIGURE 13-7 ▪ **A,** Symbols commonly used in a pedigree. **B,** A pedigree of autosomal recessive inheritance. Autosomal recessive disease occurs only in individuals with two mutant alleles (homozygotes) and no normal allele. In this pedigree, two siblings in the second generation are affected. Both parents of the affected person are carriers (heterozygotes). Each offspring's risk of receiving a recessive allele is one-half from each parent. Therefore, each offspring of two carriers has a 25 percent chance of being affected, a 50 percent chance of being a carrier, and a 25 percent chance of inheriting neither mutant allele. Both genders are equally likely to be affected. **C,** A pedigree of autosomal dominant inheritance. In a typical autosomal dominant inheritance, every affected individual in a pedigree has an affected parent, who also has an affected parent. It also affects several generations. Both sexes are equally likely to be affected, and male-to-male transmission exists. Each offspring of an affected parent has a 50 percent chance of being affected. **D,** A pedigree of X-linked recessive inheritance. There is no male-to-male transmission. All daughters of an affected male are carriers. Sons of a carrier mother have a 50 percent chance of being affected. Daughters of a carrier mother have a 50 percent chance of being carriers.

without the disease, like their parents, will have a 50 percent chance of having children affected by the disease. Figure 13-7, *D* is a pedigree chart of a family with an X-linked mutation. The pedigree chart shows typical characteristics of X-linked inheritance. All daughters of affected males are carriers.

Another pattern of single-gene disorder inheritance is *mitochondrial inheritance.* Several important mitochondrial proteins are encoded on genes from a chromosome found in the mitochondria. Because mitochondrial chromosomes are contributed to the offspring exclusively by the mother, transmission is maternal (i.e., shows maternal inheritance) and affected men do not pass on the trait.

A fraction of those with a genotype that would be predicted to show a trait or disease phenotype (e.g., homozygous for a recessive trait or homozygous or heterozygous for a dominant trait), will not display the trait or disease. Under these circumstances, the mutant allele has what is called *incomplete penetrance.* If the phenotype is always expressed in those carrying the mutant allele, the trait is said to display *complete penetrance.* Finally, if a person carries a mutant allele but shows no observable phenotypic expression, the trait is called *nonpenetrant.* In actuality, nonpenetrance may reflect insufficient sensitivity to measure a small degree of phenotypic expression. Variation in penetrance and phenotypic expression of a mutant gene many be related to gene-gene interactions (one gene exacerbates or attenuates the expression of another) or environment-gene interactions (to be discussed in a later section).

Multifactorial Disorders

Single-gene disorders follow the patterns of inheritance discussed before, but many diseases are complex, *multifactorial disorders.* Not only do these disorders depend on multiple gene mutations and/or polymorphisms, but also their expression is influenced by environment and lifestyle factors. Each allelic mutation or polymorphism that contributes to a complex disease is likely to have low penetrance, and thus the contribution of each polymorphism may be subtle. As a result, the risk for and severity of a complex disease depends on the number of contributing gene variants.

Gene polymorphisms associated with an altered risk for a disease are called *susceptibility genes.* Completion of human DNA sequencing, discovery of the high frequency of single-nucleotide polymorphisms, and ongoing identification of genes by the Human Genome Project have been a huge impetus toward identifying susceptibility genes for complex diseases. Complex disorders cluster in families but do not appear to follow Mendelian principles of inheritance. Of note, multifactorial traits (complex disorders) are composed of a series of genes that each displays a Mendelian pattern of inheritance, but the fact that these susceptibility alleles are co-inherited confounds the observation of Mendelian inheritance patterns when using classical genetics tools (i.e., pedigree analysis). The disorder is expressed when genetic and environmental influences combine to reach a critical threshold. Examples of complex

cardiovascular disorders are coronary artery disease and heart failure.

EFFECT OF LIFESTYLE AND ENVIRONMENT ON EXPRESSION OF COMPLEX DISORDERS

Many genetic mutations have been linked directly to heart disease. Also well known is that environmental influences such as hypoxia, drugs, microorganisms, and radiation can injure the heart directly. However, in most if not all cases of heart disease, genetic, environmental, and/or lifestyle factors interact to alter incidence and severity. Clear evidence of environment-gene interaction can be found in studies documenting increased incidence of cardiovascular disease in those from Asia who move to the West and adopt a Western lifestyle.[4,5] Several models, illustrated in Figure 13-8, have been proposed to explain how genes and environment interact to influence the expression of disease phenotype.[6]

In model 8A (see Figure 13-8), neither the genotype nor the environmental factors alone cause a disease, but the environmental and genetic components are required for the disease phenotype to occur. An example is phenylketonuria. In this disorder, a single mutation of the gene encoding for the enzyme phenylalanine hydroxylase leads to the accumulation of phenylalanine, with resulting neurological damage and mental retardation. Neither phenylalanine ingestion in the absence of the susceptibility gene, nor the presence of the susceptibility gene in the absence of phenylalanine, results in a disease phenotype.

Model 8B (see Figure 13-8), illustrates the situation whereby a known gene variant exacerbates the effect of an existing environmental or lifestyle factor. For example, genes that code for dysfunctional DNA-repair enzymes would increase the risk of skin cancer caused by ultraviolet radiation–induced DNA damage. Model 8C shows how an environment or lifestyle factor can exacerbate a genetic risk factor. For example, dyslipidemia resulting from a gene variant of the low-density lipoprotein receptor would be exacerbated by a high-lipid diet. A final model, illustrated by Figure 13-8, *D,* is when either an environmental factor or a genetic mutation could cause a disease, but the presence of both factors has a synergistic effect on the expression of the disease phenotype. This situation is a combination of models B and C.

The impact of environmental and lifestyle factors on disease phenotype is complicated and often unpredictable. Complexity arises from the fact that multiple environmental factors interact with each individual's susceptibility genes in different ways (Figure 13-9). Each interaction potentially can exacerbate or mitigate the contribution of each susceptibility gene. To add to the complexity, persons are exposed to environmental factors for different periods, which further contributes a dose factor to the environment-gene interaction.

Environmental factors may include temperature, radiation, humidity, barometric pressure, chemicals in the air and water, and microorganisms. Lifestyle factors are associated more closely with behavioral choices such as how much a person exercises, what they choose to eat, whether they smoke or drink alcohol, and the manner

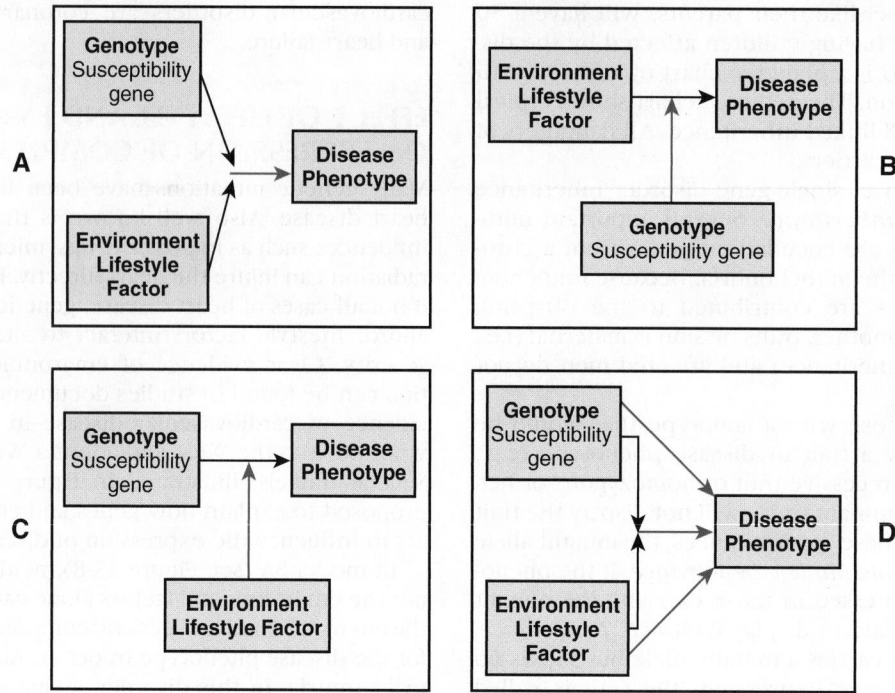

FIGURE 13-8 ■ Models of gene-environment interaction. **A,** Neither the genotype nor environmental factors alone can cause a disease, but together the disease phenotype is observed. **B,** An environment or lifestyle factor alone can cause a disease. Certain genotypes can exacerbate or even mitigate an environmentally initiated disease phenotype. **C,** A gene variant alone can result in a disease phenotype, and environmental factors can exacerbate or mitigate the genetic effect. **D,** Either susceptibility genes or environmental factors can cause a disease, or together they produce a disease phenotype.

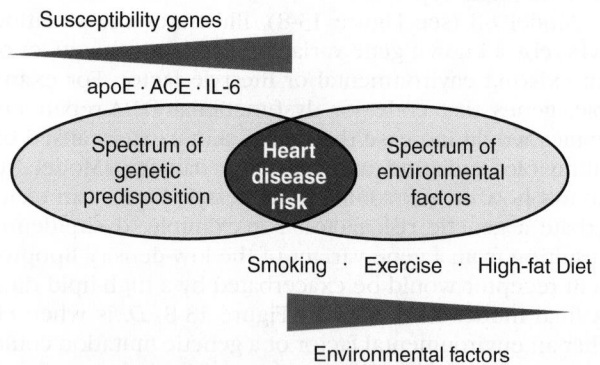

FIGURE 13-9 ■ Genes and environmental factors interact to alter disease risk. Each individual may have a different number of susceptibility genes and a different number of environmental or lifestyle factors that interact to determine disease risk. Eventually the genetic and environmental factors combine to reach a threshold after which the disease phenotype is observed. *apoE,* Apolipoprotein E; *ACE,* angiotensin-converting enzyme; *IL-6,* interleukin-6. (Modified from Talmud JP, Stephens JW: *Diabetes Obes Metab* 6:1-7, 2004.)

in which they respond to stress. The mechanisms by which environmental and lifestyle factors interact with genes are likely to be similar. However, lifestyle factors may be modified more easily; e.g., it may be easier to increase exercise level than to change the barometric pressure. The fact that these factors can be modified provides an opportunity to intervene to reduce disease risk and disease severity.

Regular physical activity produces cardiovascular adaptations that increase exercise capacity, endurance, and skeletal muscle strength. Prospective epidemiological studies of occupational and leisure-time physical activity consistently have documented a reduced incidence of coronary artery disease events in physically active and fit subjects. Physical activity prevents and counteracts many established atherosclerotic risk factors, including elevated blood pressure, insulin resistance, and glucose intolerance. Evidence also indicates that exercise reduces the risk of other chronic diseases, including type 2 diabetes mellitus, osteoporosis, obesity, and depression. The American Heart Association, the Centers for Disease Control and Prevention, and the American College of Sports Medicine advocate engaging in 30 minutes or more of moderate-intensity physical activity on most (preferably all) days of the week.[7]

Environment-gene interactions can occur by multiple mechanisms. In this regard, an environmental or lifestyle factor can be thought of as a *signal.* One mechanism by which this signal can interact with a gene is by modifying the function of a gene product or by exerting a stress on a protein encoded for by a gene. This concept is illustrated by Figure 13-10, which shows a hypothetical cell where a nutrient is metabolized by enzyme A to metabolite A and then by enzyme B to metabolite B. Enzyme B is the rate-limiting enzyme in the pathway. Enzyme B has a slow and a rapid metabolizing isoform encoded for by gene B, allele S, and allele R, respectively. If a person has the gene encoding for the slow-metabolizing isoform of enzyme B *and* ingests an excessive amount of the nutrient, metabolite A will accumulate. Accumulation of metabolite A increases the risk of heart disease. If the person has the slow-metabolizing form of

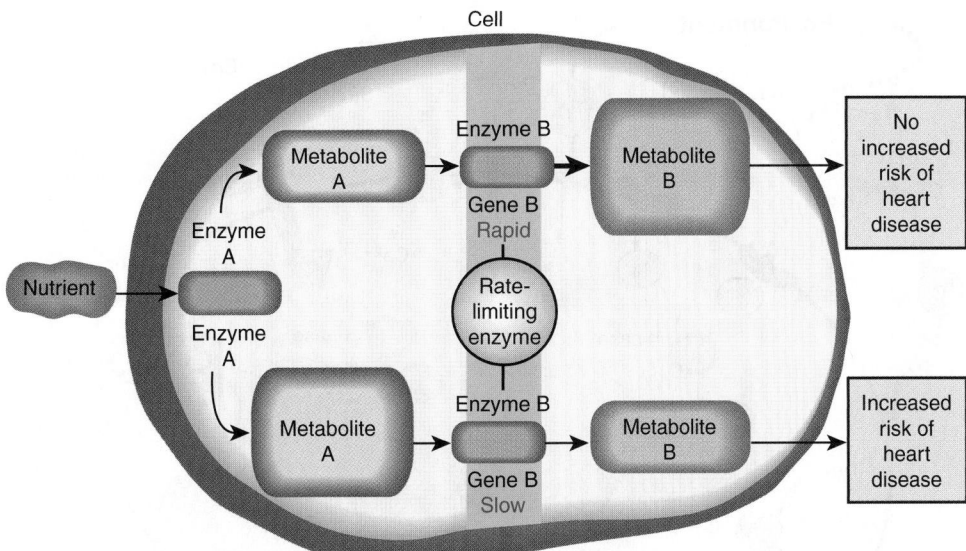

FIGURE 13-10 ■ Environmental or lifestyle factors can surpass the ability of a protein to contribute optimally to the health of the cell, tissue, or even the individual. A nutrient is metabolized by enzyme A to metabolite A and then by enzyme B to metabolite B. Enzyme B is the rate-limiting enzyme in this pathway. Two alleles of the gene code for enzyme B; one encodes a rapid-metabolizing enzyme, and the other encodes a slow-metabolizing enzyme. If the nutrient is metabolized to metabolite B, there is no risk of heart disease. However, if metabolite A accumulates, because the rate-limiting enzyme B is coded for by allele S (enzyme B will have a slow rate of activity), the risk of heart disease will increase. If a person has both the slow-metabolizing allele of enzyme B and ingests a large amount of the nutrient, more metabolite A will accumulate. Under these circumstances, the gene/lifestyle interaction may reach a critical threshold resulting in the expression of a heart disease phenotype. (Modified from Humphries SE, Donati MB: *Ital Heart J* 3:3-5, 2002.)

enzyme B but eats normal amounts of the nutrient, the heart disease phenotype will not be expressed. In the presence of the fast-metabolizing isoform of enzyme B, excessive ingestion of the nutrient will not increase the risk of heart disease. Thus in this example, an environmental/lifestyle factor (level of ingestion of the nutrient) and a genetic factor (presence of a gene encoding the fast or slow isoform of enzyme B) interact to alter the risk of heart disease.

Varying susceptibility to a cardiac dysrhythmia called torsades de pointes provides an example of the concept illustrated in Figure 13-10. Drug-induced torsades de pointes is a significant iatrogenic cause of morbidity and mortality. Torsades de pointes is associated with alterations in potassium channels that mediate cardiac cell repolarization and alterations in the metabolism of drugs that interact with these potassium channels. Like the vast majority of genes in the human genome, genes encoding for potassium channels and metabolizing enzymes harbor mutations and genetic polymorphisms. A growing body of literature provides evidence that a subset of these naturally occurring variations may underlie many cases of drug-induced torsades de pointes, resulting in high plasma drug concentrations or diminished cardiac repolarization reserve, respectively. (See the later discussion of long-QT syndrome and Shah[8] for an in-depth review.)

Another mechanism by which environmental signals influence the risk or severity of disease is by altering gene expression and protein synthesis. This is illustrated schematically in Figures 13-11 and 13-12. Information

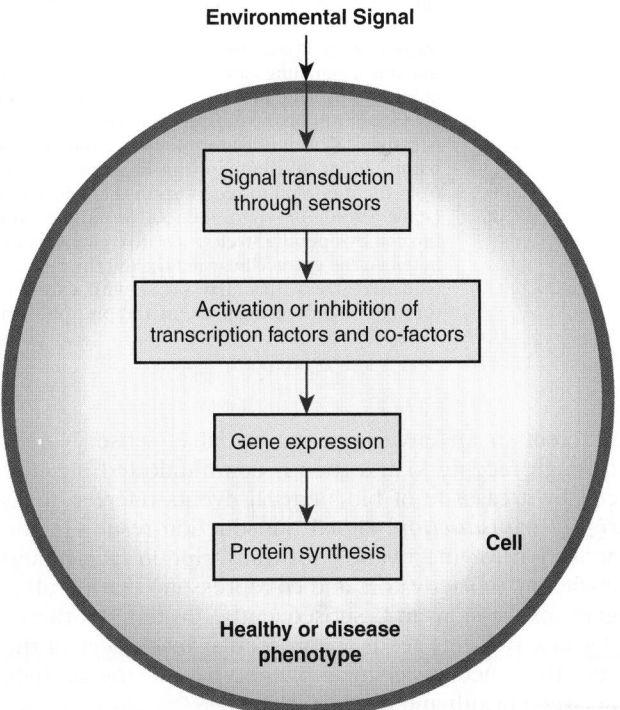

FIGURE 13-11 ■ Environmental signals sensed by the cell alter gene expression. Environmental signals are sensed by the cell through receptors. The signal initiates a cascade of biochemical events that results in activation of transcription factor and co-factor proteins. These proteins have key roles in regulating the rate of gene expression and protein synthesis. Changes in protein synthesis can alter cell phenotype, thereby mediating the expression of a healthy or disease phenotype.

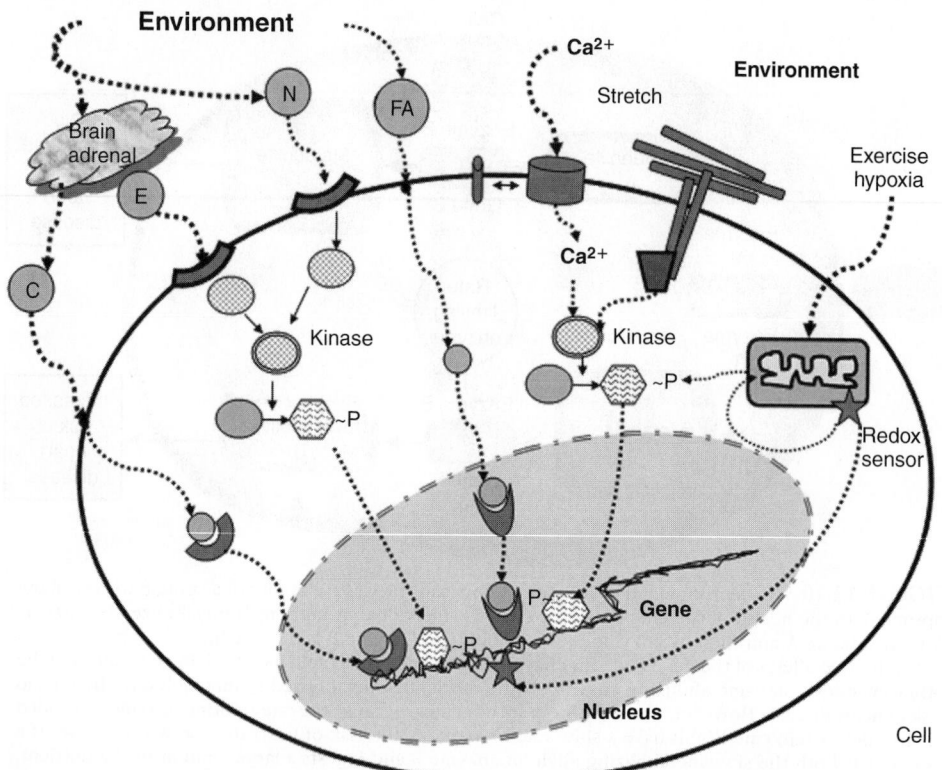

FIGURE 13-12 ■ Schematic examples of environmental factor activation of signal transduction pathways. Stress results in the release of cortisol (C) and epinephrine (E) from the adrenal gland. Cortisol passes into the cell, where it binds to the glucocorticoid receptor. The cortisol/receptor complex acts as a transcription factor that binds to the regulatory region of target genes (i.e., genes with specific nucleotide sequences/secondary structures in the regulatory region [see Figure 13-4]). With additional binding of cell-specific co-factors, the complex increases or decreases the rate of gene transcription. Water-soluble epinephrine binds to cell-surface adrenergic receptors. Receptor binding initiates a signaling cascade that activates an intracellular kinase enzyme. The kinase phosphorylates (adds a phosphate moiety to) a transcription factor protein or co-factor protein. Phosphorylation may activate or inhibit the transcription factor (or co-factor), which then alters the rate of gene transcription. Nicotine (N) from cigarette smoke binds to nicotinic receptors and activates a signal transduction pathway that, like epinephrine-induced signaling, activates kinase enzymes. Specific fatty acids (FA) from the diet bind to receptors in the cell. The fatty acid/receptor complex can act as a transcription factor. Stretch or strain, induced by muscle exercise or fluid overload can transduce information into the cell by opening stretch-sensitive channels or by communicating the stretch/strain via connections between the extracellular matrix and the cytoskeleton. Even changes in cellular redox potential and/or oxidative stress (that may occur with exercise, smoking, or hypoxia) can alter gene transcription through redox-sensing proteins and phosphorylation cascades.[48] Ca^{2+}, Calcium.

inherent in an environmental signal is sensed (often through receptors) and then is communicated into the cell by a cascade of biochemical events referred to as *signal transduction*. Signal transduction results in the activation (or inactivation) of transcription factors and co-factors (co-activators and co-repressors) that regulate gene expression and, subsequently, protein synthesis. Because proteins act as the molecular machinery of the cell, they mediate cellular phenotype and the balance between health and disease.

The next section discusses gene defects and environment-gene interactions using a dysrhythmogenic disorder (long-QT syndrome) and a disorder of cardiac pump function (hypertrophic cardiomyopathy) as examples. The section is not intended to be an exhaustive list of the genes associated with these or other cardiac diseases. For a detailed review of genes

associated with cardiovascular diseases, see *Braunwald's Heart Disease*, Chapter 70.

GENE DEFECTS ASSOCIATED WITH LONG-QT SYNDROME AND HYPERTROPHIC CARDIOMYOPATHY
Long-QT Syndrome

The long-QT (also known as **LQT**) syndrome is a potentially lethal form of cardiac rhythm disturbance that causes 3000 to 4000 sudden deaths in children and young adults each year in the United States. Sudden cardiac death is a frequent outcome of the most dangerous forms of dysrhythmias, including torsades de pointes, ventricular tachycardia, and ventricular fibrillation.[9,10] Torsades de pointes is a French term meaning "twisting of the points" and is characterized by undulations of continually varying QRS complex amplitudes that appear alternately above and below the baseline. Genetic studies have led to the discovery of multiple molecular defects that contribute to dysrhythmogenesis. These defects include mutations in transmembrane cardiac ion channels, intracellular channels, and non-ion conducting proteins.[11]

The LQT syndrome often is recognized by prolonged ventricular repolarization (i.e., prolonged QT interval) on the electrocardiogram and a propensity for syncope, seizures, and sudden death resulting from episodes of malignant ventricular tachycardia or torsades de pointes. The familial LQT syndrome was described first in 1957, when investigators reported an autosomal recessive disease that had clinical features of deafness, QT prolongation, and sudden death in childhood. In the early 1960s, the more common Romano-Ward variant characterized by autosomal dominant inheritance and syncope and/or sudden cardiac death was reported.

LQT syndrome can be congenital or acquired. Congenital LQT syndrome is an inherited disease in children and adolescents who have a structurally normal heart but, with prolongation of the QT interval, have recurrent syncope and/or sudden death. Seven LQT-syndrome genes have been discovered, and more than 300 mutations have been identified.[12] Acquired LQT syndrome, often referred as drug-induced QT syndrome, describes QT prolongation with exposure to an environmental stressor and reversion back to normal following withdrawal of the stressor.[13] For acquired LQT syndrome, it is believed that the main issue is the blockade (often by drugs) of the slow component of the delayed rectifier potassium current (I_{KR}), a major repolarization current in the heart. These I_{KR} blockers have a high propensity to induce torsades de pointes in the presence of other risk factors, such as female gender, bradycardia, and hypokalemia.[12]

Genetic heterogeneity is a distinguishing feature of LQT syndrome. Disease-causing mutations have been identified in genes on six chromosomes, accounting for more than 60 percent of affected patients.[12] Early studies used linkage analysis to map major genetic loci involved in the pathogenesis of LQT syndrome.[14] Linkage analysis (previously described) involves the exploitation of DNA sequence polymorphisms that occur near or within a gene of interest by examining the degree of cotransmission of such variants with a disease or trait within families. Such *linked* variations act as surrogate markers for a nearby disease-causing mutation in that gene.

Another method used to determine the location of polymorphisms associated with LQT syndrome is *positional cloning* (also termed *reverse genetics*). Positional cloning involves the cloning or identification of a gene for a particular disease based on its location in the genome, as determined by a collection of techniques including linkage analysis, physical mapping, and bioinformatics, in situations whereby no information about the biochemical basis of the disease is known.

A third method is the *candidate gene approach,* which involves examining genetic variations and/or mutations in genes that encode for proteins selected because of their biochemical properties or because of their participation in biological processes that are found to be altered in subjects with LQT syndrome.

These methods have aided in the identification of mutations in three genes that code for ion channels (KCNQ1, KCNH2, and SCN5A). Mutations in four additional genes (ankyrin B, KCNE1, KCNE2, and KCNJ2) were identified using the candidate gene approach (Table 13-2). Currently, more than 300 different mutations have been reported, and most are missense mutations.[12] Based on the type of mutation, the congenital form of LQT syndrome can be divided into seven subgroups (LQT1 to LQT7). Most LQT-syndrome genes encode cardiac potassium channels, with the exception of LQT3 and LQT4, which have mutations, respectively, in the gene that encodes the cardiac sodium channel and the gene encoding for an adaptor protein involved in anchoring important proteins in the cell membrane.[15]

LQT1 is the most prevalent genetic form of congenital LQT syndrome, accounting for 50 percent of genotyped patients.[16] LQT1 is caused by mutations in the KCNQ1 gene, resulting in a loss of function of potassium channels and thereby prolonged phase 3 of the action potential. LQT2 is the second most common form of congenital LQT syndrome, being responsible for 35 percent to 45 percent of mutations in LQT syndrome genotyped patients. LQT2 is caused by mutations in a potassium channel gene, called the human ether-a-go-go-related gene (HERG, also known as KCNH2). HERG mutations lead to a reduced potassium current and a delayed repolarization of the action potential. LQT3 is estimated to represent 3 percent to 15 percent of LQT

■ ■ ■

TABLE 13-2   GENETIC DEFECTS LINKED TO CONGENITAL LONG-QT SYNDROME

PHENOTYPE	PROPORTION OF CASES	GENE	PROTEIN FAMILY	GENE MAP	CURRENT	DYSRHYTHMIA ONSET
LQT1	50%	KCNQ1 (KVLQT1)	Ion channels	11p15.5	↓ I_{KS}	Physical exercise
LQT2	35%-45%	KCNH2 (HERG)	Ion channels	7q35-q36	↓ I_{KR}	Auditory stimuli, medications
LQT3	3%-15%	SCN5A	Ion channels	3p21-23	↑ I_{Na}	Rest, sleep
LQT4	Less than 1%	ANK2 (ankyrin B)		4q25-27	↑ late I_{Na^+}	
LQT5	Less than 1%	KCNE1 (*minK*)	Ion channels	21q22.1-22.2	↓ I_{KS}	Exercise
LQT6	Less than 1%	KCNE2 (*MiRP1*)	Ion channels	21q22.1-22.2	↓ I_{KR}	
LQT7	Less than 1%	KCNJ2	Ion channels	17q23	↓ $I_{Kir2.1}$	

I_{KS}, Slowly activating component of delayed rectifier potassium current; *HERG*, human "ether-a-go-go" related gene and a pore-forming protein; I_{KR}, rapidly activating component of delayed rectifier potassium current; *SCN5A*, cardiac voltage–dependent sodium channel gene; $I_{Kir2.1}$, inward rectifier potassium current; I_{Na}, sodium current; *MiRP1*, minK-related peptide 1, a small integral membrane subunit that assembles with HERG.

syndrome genotyped patients. LQT3 syndrome is caused by mutations in the SCN5A gene, which increases inward sodium current and also prolongs action potential duration. LQT4, LQT5, LQT6, and LQT7 each represent less than 1 percent of LQT syndrome. A missense mutation in the ANK2 gene on chromosome 4 was identified in one family with LQT4.[15] LQT5 and LQT6 are caused by mutations in the KCNE1 gene (minK)[16] and KCNE2 gene (MiRP1)[17] located on chromosome 21. KCNJ2, located on chromosome 17, is the gene associated with LQT7.[18]

Available data suggest remarkable phenotypic variability in the clinical presentation of LQT syndrome. Gene variant–specific differences in ST-T wave morphology,[19] specific triggers for potentially lethal dysrhythmia,[20-22] and risk of cardiac events[23] are reported as gene-specific differences. For example, patients with LQT2 have a lower cumulative event-free survival than those with LQT1, and a similar trend was shown between LQT3 versus LQT1 patients.[20] The percentage of genetically affected patients with normal QT interval (called *silent mutation carriers*) is much higher with LQT1 (36 percent) than LQT2 (19 percent) and LQT3 (10 percent). These findings are valuable for genotype-based risk stratification.

Congenital LQT syndrome (Romano-Ward variant) is inherited as an autosomal dominant trait. However, a common feature of LQT syndrome is incomplete penetrance of the disease phenotype. Incomplete penetrance is when a trait (such as long QT on the surface electrocardiogram or syncope, seizures, and sudden death resulting from malignant polymorphic ventricular tachycardia) is not expressed even though the person has the disease-causing genotype. Thus, the person is a carrier but does not have the trait. This incomplete penetrance can severely complicate accurate risk assessment. Variable expressivity refers to a phenomenon whereby a disease trait is not manifested uniformly among individuals carrying the same genetic mutation or variation and often is documented in a family known to carry the same mutations in a single gene.[24] In the same family, one person carrying the mutation may experience sudden cardiac death, whereas another carrying the same genetic mutation may have normal QT intervals and never develop any dysrhythmias.[25] The hypothesis is that the determinants of clinical variability in this scenario likely are mediated by "modifier" factors, either genetic or environmental.[26] Modifier genes do not cause the disease but affect the severity of phenotypic expression. Therefore, in patients with LQT syndrome a genetic mutation may cause a susceptibility to cardiac dysrhythmias, but genetic modifiers or environmental risk factors then are needed actually to trigger the disease phenotype. The recent appreciation of modifiers that also may play a protective role likely will further complicate dissection of these multifactorial traits.

Environmental factors may play an important role in triggering stress-mediated, life-threatening ventricular dysrhythmias. Congenital LQT syndrome-related polymorphic ventricular dysrhythmias most often occur in association with physical activity and emotion (Table 13-1). LQT1 and LQT5 are prone to dysrhythmias in response to exercise. For example, Moss and colleagues[22] studied 19 subjects with LQT syndrome. The available genotype analysis showed that cardiac events related to swimming activity occurred exclusively in all patients with the KVLQT1 mutation (LQT1), suggesting a broader association of LQT1 with exercise-related cardiac events. Individuals with LQT1 are most responsive to standard beta-blocker therapy. The LQT2 patients had an equally distributed pattern of precipitators, including exercise, fright and emotion, and sleep. Wilde and colleagues[27] reported that in HERG-related LQT2 families, sudden cardiac death, ventricular tachyarrhythmias, and unexplained syncope were precipitated by an unexpected auditory stimulus, such as the telephone ringing or an alarm clock sounding, and were less heart-rate dependent. Similar results also were reported by Moss and colleagues,[22] who showed auditory-related cardiac events are associated with the LQT2 genotype. The sudden onset of dysrhythmia, within seconds of a stimulus, suggests that the sudden release of catecholamine plays a role in triggering the event.[27] In contrast, patients with the LQT3 genotype tend to experience events associated with bradycardia, such as during sleep.[28]

Acquired LQT syndrome is a common disorder and has many clinical features similar to those of inherited LQT syndrome. However, acquired syndrome more typically affects older persons and females and often is associated with specific drugs or metabolic abnormalities. Drugs that produce acquired LQT syndrome are structurally heterogeneous, including antidysrhythmics (i.e., quinidine), nonsedating antihistamines (i.e., terfenadine), and psychiatric drugs (i.e., haloperidol).[29] Data support the existence of a pathogenic link between low-penetrant genetic defects of cardiac ion channels and the predisposition to acquired LQT syndrome.[30] Several cases of mediator-triggered "torsade de pointes" and cardiac arrest in individuals with mutations in ion channels have been reported.[17,31-33] Genetic defects are likely to create a substrate that favors the onset of malignant dysrhythmia when an appropriate trigger is also present, such as QT interval–prolonging drugs or low plasma potassium levels. Dysfunction of the HERG channel (LQT2) is a common cause of acquired forms of LQT syndrome.[34] The coexistence of mutations in KCNH2 (LQT2) and KCNE2 (LQT6) appears to modulate the drug sensitivity of the potassium channel.[12] Some phenotypically subclinical KCNQ1 (LQT1) mutations are found in the general population in those who are predisposed to drug-induced ventricular dysrhythmia. For example, a point mutation in the KCNQ1 gene (Val315Cys: substitution of cysteine for valine at the 315th amino acid) was found in a 77-year-old woman who experienced cardiac arrest when receiving cisapride, a drug used to treat gastroesophageal reflux disease that has an apparent interaction with the LQT1 syndrome gene.[33] Three KCNE2 mutations (LQT6) and a SNP mutation in this gene have been associated with antibiotic-induced cardiac dysrhythmia.[17,32]

Common experience with drugs associated with QT-interval prolongation suggests that only a minority of subjects treated with these drugs actually will develop abnormal responses. In addition, only a few with clinically overt LQT syndrome will develop drug-induced "torsade de pointes" each time they accidentally receive potentially harmful drugs. Therefore, the interplay of several of the different critical precipitating factors likely is needed to induce the dysrhythmic event.[30] Patients with LQT1 should avoid strenuous or competitive exercise, particularly swimming and diving. Patients with LQT2 should be advised to remove unexpected sources of loud noise in their environment, such as telephones and alarm clocks.

A diagnosis of congenital LQT syndrome is a life-changing event for patients and their families. They have a possible need for lifelong therapy and medical restriction from competitive sports. A diagnosis of acquired LQT syndrome is usually of limited duration, with prompt resolution following identification and correction of the inciting factor. In-depth and current information for patients, their families, and health care providers can be found at the websites for LQT-syndrome (*www.long-qt-syndrome.com/lqts_links.html*), and the American Medical Association (*www.ama-assn.org/*), and the American Heart Association (*www.americanheart.org*).

Hypertrophic Cardiomyopathy

Hypertrophic cardiomyopathy (**HCM**) is the most common cause of sudden cardiac death in individuals younger than age 35, particularly in competitive athletes.[35] Although previously considered to be a rare disorder, recent population-based studies suggest the prevalence of HCM to be as high as 0.2 percent (or 1 in 500) in the general population of young adults.[36] HCM is a disease of contractile (sarcomeric) proteins with primary defects in thick and thin filaments. The principal histological hallmark is a triad of myocyte hypertrophy without secondary causes, myocyte disarray, and interstitial fibrosis. Clinical diagnosis is based on an unexplained cardiac hypertrophy on an echocardiogram, which can range from subtle to massive. Hypertrophy is classically asymmetrical with particular involvement of the interventricular septum. Asymmetrical septal hypertrophy causes a resting or provocative left ventricular outflow tract obstruction in about 25 percent of affected persons.

The first genetic linkage study of HCM was reported in a large French-Canadian family in 1989.[37] HCM is a heritable disorder that is transmitted as an autosomal dominant trait. Offspring of an affected person have a 50 percent risk of inheriting the mutation. HCM is genetically heterogeneous, with well more than 120 possible mutations in 11 causative genes encoding sarcomeric proteins (Table 13-3).[38] Mutations in nonsarcomeric genes[39] and mtDNA[40] also have been associated with HCM.

Mutations in the genes encoding beta-myosin heavy chain (MYH7), myosin-binding protein C (MYBPC3), and cardiac troponin T (TNNT2) are the three most common primary (causal) genes,[41] collectively responsible for 60 to 70 percent of all HCM cases (Table 13-2). No particular gene predominates in terms of its contribution to HCM, and the frequency of each mutation in the HCM population is relatively low (less than 5 percent).[38] The MYH7 gene on chromosome 14 is one of the most frequently implicated genes, being responsible for about 35 to 50 percent of all HCM cases. More than 80 mutations have been reported, with most located in the globular head or head-rod junction of the beta-myosin heavy chain. These mutations disrupt contractile function.

The MYBPC3 gene on chromosome 11 is the second most common causal gene for human HCM and accounts for about 15 to 30 percent of all cases. More than 40 different mutations in the MYBPC3 gene have been identified, and most are deletion, insertion, or splice mutations.[38] These mutations result in a frame shift or truncation of myosin-binding protein C and lead to severe structural or functional defects in the protein or immediate degradation of expressed proteins. Another relatively common causal gene for human HCM is the TNNT2 gene on chromosome 1, accounting for about 10 to 20 percent of all HCM cases.[38,41] Most mutations in the TNNT2 gene are missense.[42]

A characteristic feature of HCM, like all other autosomal dominant diseases, is the presence of a wide clinical spectrum in its phenotypic expression, ranging from a benign, asymptomatic course, to symptoms of heart failure, to the most serious complication: sudden cardiac death. Specific mutations are associated with different disease severity and prognosis. For example,

■ ■ ■

TABLE 13-3   GENES INVOLVED IN HYPERTROPHIC CARDIOMYOPATHIES

HYPERTROPHIC CARDIOMYOPATHY GENE	SYMBOL	CHROMOSOME LOCUS	PROPORTION OF CASES
Beta-myosin heavy chain	MYH7	14q12	35%-50%
Myosin binding protein-C	MYBPC3	11p11.2	20%-30%
Cardiac troponin T	TNNT2	1q32	10%-15%
Alpha-tropomyosin	TPM1	15q22.1	Less than 5%
Cardiac troponin I	TNNI3	19q13.4	Less than 5%
Essential myosin light chains	MYL3	3p	Less than 5%
Regulatory myosin light chains	MYL2	12q23-24.3	Less than 5%
Cardiac alpha-actin	ACTC	15q14	Less than 5%
Titin	TTN	2q24.3	Less than 5%
Alpha-myosin heavy chain	MYH6	14q12	Rare
Cardiac troponin C	TNNC	3p21.3-3p14.3	Rare

mutations in the MYH7 gene generally cause a severe form of HCM with early onset (about age 20), significant myocardial hypertrophy, complete penetrance, and a higher incidence of sudden cardiac death.[43,44] Variable expressivity also occurs in persons with HCM because different mutations on the same gene also can affect clinical presentation. For instance, affected family members with a phe513cys mutation (that results in replacement of cysteine for phenylalanine on the 513th amino acid) on the MYH7 gene have near-normal life expectancy; whereas affected persons with an arg719trp mutation (substitution of tryptophan for arginine at the 719th amino acid) have a high incidence of premature death and an average life expectancy of 38 years.[45] Mutations in the MYBPC3 gene generally are associated with onset in middle age or late adult life (around the 40s to 50s), a relatively mild hypertrophy, low penetrance, and a low incidence of sudden cardiac death.[43] In contrast, mutations in the TNNT2 gene generally cause only mild or subclinical hypertrophy but are associated with a poor prognosis and a high risk of sudden death.[46]

Similar to LQT syndrome, HCM exhibits intrafamilial phenotypic variation, or variable expressivity, whereby affected individuals from the same family or among families with an identical genetic mutation display distinct clinical and morphological manifestations. This suggests the involvement of factors other than the causal mutations, such as lifestyle factors or modifier genes.[41] Further studies are needed to shed light on the role of these factors in HCM.

HCM is the most common cause of death in young athletes. Sudden death often is precipitated by physical activity,[47] occurring during or immediately after severe exertion on the athletic field. Environmental factors, such as exercise, are thought to contribute to variation in phenotype and prognosis. In addition, acceleration of the evolution of the cardiac phenotype is observed during adolescence and puberty, implicating the involvement of growth factors and perhaps sex hormones in modulating expression of hypertrophy in HCM.[43] Patients with HCM should avoid strenuous or competitive exercise. In-depth and current information for patients, their families, and physicians can be found at the websites for the Cardiomyopathy Association *(www.cardiomyopathy.org/homepage.htm)*, the Hypertrophic Cardiomyopathy Association *(www.4hcm.org/flash/index.html)*, the American Medical Association *(www.ama-assn.org/)*, and the American Heart Association *(www.americanheart.org)*.

CONCLUSION

The integration of genetics into clinical practice is moving rapidly. Completion of the first draft of the human genome sequence and continued analysis has moved the use of genetics in the clinical setting from a rare event to a commonplace diagnostic and prognostic tool. Currently, this shift has occurred mainly at the clinical-research interface. However, it is vital that health care professionals educate themselves in view of the certainty of this evolution in patient care and clinical

practice. Nowhere is this more clear than in the area of cardiovascular disease.

Molecular genetics provides us with a better understanding of many cardiac disorders previously classified as idiopathic. Identification of human mutations associated with cardiovascular disorders, and environmental factors that interact with these mutations, will allow earlier and more accurate diagnosis, enabling a modification of specific lifestyle factors (i.e., avoidance of competitive athletics) and early therapeutics (e.g., implantation of cardioverter-defibrillators) to reduce the serious morbidity and mortality associated with cardiac genetic disorders.[48] The promise of the Human Genome Project, initiated in 1990 but appreciated long before, promises to greatly benefit the lives of health care providers and those they serve.

REFERENCES

1. Morris CA, Mervis CB: Williams syndrome and related disorders, *Annu Rev Genomics Hum Genet* 1:461-484, 2000.
2. Casey D: *Human Genome Project information.* Retrieved March 9, 2005 from www.ornl.gov/sci/techresources/Human_Genome/home.shtml
3. Singh R, Pislaru S, Simari R: ABCs of molecular cardiology and the impact of the Human Genome Project on clinical cardiology, *Cardiol Rev* 10:24-33, 2002.
4. Kagan A, Harris BR, Winkelstein W Jr et al: Epidemiologic studies of coronary heart disease and stroke in Japanese men living in Japan, Hawaii and California: demographic, physical, dietary and biochemical characteristics, *J Chronic Dis* 27:345-364, 1974.
5. Nichaman MZ, Hamilton HB, Kagan A et al: Epidemiologic studies of coronary heart disease and stroke in Japanese men living in Japan, Hawaii and California: distribution of biochemical risk factors, *Am J Epidemiol* 102:491-501, 1975.
6. Ottman R: Gene-environment interaction: definitions and study designs, *Prev Med* 25:764-770, 1996.
7. Thompson PD, Buchner D, Pina IL et al: Exercise and physical activity in the prevention and treatment of atherosclerotic cardiovascular disease: a statement from the Council on Clinical Cardiology (Subcommittee on Exercise, Rehabilitation, and Prevention) and the Council on Nutrition, Physical Activity, and Metabolism (Subcommittee on Physical Activity), *Circulation* 107:3109-3116, 2003.
8. Shah RR: Pharmacogenetic aspects of drug-induced torsade de pointes: potential tool for improving clinical drug development and prescribing, *Drug Saf* 27:145-172, 2004.
9. Priori SG, Barhanin J, Hauer RN et al: Genetic and molecular basis of cardiac arrhythmias; impact on clinical management: study group on molecular basis of arrhythmias of the working group on arrhythmias of the European Society of Cardiology, *Eur Heart J* 20:174-195, 1999.
10. Spooner PM, Albert C, Benjamin EJ et al: Sudden cardiac death, genes, and arrhythmogenesis: consideration of new population and mechanistic approaches from a National Heart, Lung, and Blood Institute workshop, part I, *Circulation* 103:2361-2364, 2001.
11. Cheng CF, Kuo HC, Chien KR: Genetic modifiers of cardiac arrhythmias, *Trends Mol Med* 9:59-66, 2003.
12. Chiang CE: Congenital and acquired long QT syndrome: current concepts and management, *Cardiol Rev* 12:222-234, 2004.
13. Roden DM, Viswanathan PC: Genetics of acquired long QT syndrome, *J Clin Invest* 115:2025-2032, 2005.
14. Keating M, Atkinson D, Dunn C et al: Linkage of a cardiac arrhythmia, the long QT syndrome, and the Harvey ras-1 gene, *Science* 252:704-706, 1991.
15. Mohler PJ, Schott JJ, Gramolini AO et al: Ankyrin-B mutation causes type 4 long-QT cardiac arrhythmia and sudden cardiac death, *Nature* 421:634-639, 2003.
16. Priori SG, Napolitano C: Genetics of cardiac arrhythmias and sudden cardiac death, *Ann N Y Acad Sci* 1015:96-110, 2004.

17. Abbott GW, Sesti F, Splawski I et al: MiRP1 forms IKr potassium channels with HERG and is associated with cardiac arrhythmia, *Cell* 97:175-187, 1999.

18. Tristani-Firouzi M, Jensen JL, Donaldson MR et al: Functional and clinical characterization of KCNJ2 mutations associated with LQT7 (Andersen syndrome), *J Clin Invest* 110:381-388, 2002.

19. Moss AJ: T-wave patterns associated with the hereditary long QT syndrome, *Card Electrophysiol Rev* 6:311-315, 2002.

20. Schwartz PJ, Priori SG, Spazzolini C et al: Genotype-phenotype correlation in the long-QT syndrome: gene-specific triggers for life-threatening arrhythmias, *Circulation* 103:89-95, 2001.

21. Ackerman MJ, Tester DJ, Porter CJ: Swimming, a gene-specific arrhythmogenic trigger for inherited long QT syndrome, *Mayo Clin Proc* 74:1088-1094, 1999.

22. Moss AJ, Robinson JL, Gessman L et al: Comparison of clinical and genetic variables of cardiac events associated with loud noise versus swimming among subjects with the long QT syndrome, *Am J Cardiol* 84:876-879, 1999.

23. Priori SG, Schwartz PJ, Napolitano C et al: Risk stratification in the long-QT syndrome, *N Engl J Med* 348:1866-1874, 2003.

24. Priori SG, Napolitano C, Schwartz PJ: Low penetrance in the long-QT syndrome: clinical impact, *Circulation* 99:529-533, 1999.

25. Neyroud N, Denjoy I, Donger C et al: Heterozygous mutation in the pore of potassium channel gene KvLQT1 causes an apparently normal phenotype in long QT syndrome, *Eur J Hum Genet* 6:129-133, 1998.

26. Keating MT, Sanguinetti MC: Molecular and cellular mechanisms of cardiac arrhythmias, *Cell* 104:569-580, 2001.

27. Wilde AA, Jongbloed RJ, Doevendans PA et al: Auditory stimuli as a trigger for arrhythmic events differentiate HERG-related (LQTS2) patients from KVLQT1-related patients (LQTS1), *J Am Coll Cardiol* 33:327-332, 1999.

28. Schwartz PJ, Priori SG, Locati EH et al: Long QT syndrome patients with mutations of the SCN5A and HERG genes have differential responses to Na+ channel blockade and to increases in heart rate: implications for gene-specific therapy, *Circulation* 92:3381-3386, 1995.

29. Witchel HJ, Hancox JC: Familial and acquired long qt syndrome and the cardiac rapid delayed rectifier potassium current, *Clin Exp Pharmacol Physiol* 27:753-766, 2000.

30. Priori SG, Napolitano C: Genetic defects of cardiac ion channels: the hidden substrate for torsades de pointes, *Cardiovasc Drugs Ther* 16:89-92, 2002.

31. Kubota T, Shimizu W, Kamakura S et al: Hypokalemia-induced long QT syndrome with an underlying novel missense mutation in S4-S5 linker of KCNQ1, *J Cardiovasc Electrophysiol* 11:1048-1054, 2000.

32. Sesti F, Abbott GW, Wei J et al: A common polymorphism associated with antibiotic-induced cardiac arrhythmia, *Proc Natl Acad Sci U S A* 97:10613-10618, 2000.

33. Napolitano C, Schwartz PJ, Brown AM et al: Evidence for a cardiac ion channel mutation underlying drug-induced QT prolongation and life-threatening arrhythmias, *J Cardiovasc Electrophysiol* 11:691-696, 2000.

34. Sanguinetti MC, Jiang C, Curran ME et al: A mechanistic link between an inherited and an acquired cardiac arrhythmia: HERG encodes the IKr potassium channel, *Cell* 81:299-307, 1995.

35. Maron BJ, Shirani J, Poliac LC et al: Sudden death in young competitive athletes: clinical, demographic, and pathological profiles, *JAMA* 276:199-204, 1996.

36. Maron BJ, Gardin JM, Flack JM et al: Prevalence of hypertrophic cardiomyopathy in a general population of young adults: echocardiographic analysis of 4111 subjects in the CARDIA Study—Coronary Artery Risk Development in (Young) Adults, *Circulation* 92:785-789, 1995.

37. Jarcho JA, McKenna W, Pare JA et al: Mapping a gene for familial hypertrophic cardiomyopathy to chromosome 14q1, *N Engl J Med* 321:1372-1378, 1989.

38. Marian AJ: On genetic and phenotypic variability of hypertrophic cardiomyopathy: nature versus nurture, *J Am Coll Cardiol* 38:331-334, 2001.

39. Blair E, Redwood C, Ashrafian H et al: Mutations in the gamma(2) subunit of AMP-activated protein kinase cause familial hypertrophic cardiomyopathy: evidence for the central role of energy compromise in disease pathogenesis, *Hum Mol Genet* 10:1215-1220, 2001.

40. Simon DK, Johns DR: Mitochondrial disorders: clinical and genetic features, *Annu Rev Med* 50:111-127, 1999.

41. Marian AJ: Modifier genes for hypertrophic cardiomyopathy, *Curr Opin Cardiol* 17:242-252, 2002.

42. Forissier JF, Carrier L, Farza H et al: Codon 102 of the cardiac troponin T gene is a putative hot spot for mutations in familial hypertrophic cardiomyopathy, *Circulation* 94:3069-3073, 1996.

43. Niimura H, Bachinski LL, Sangwatanaroj S et al: Mutations in the gene for cardiac myosin-binding protein C and late-onset familial hypertrophic cardiomyopathy, *N Engl J Med* 338(18):1248-1257, 1998.

44. Charron P, Dubourg O, Desnos M et al: Genotype-phenotype correlations in familial hypertrophic cardiomyopathy: a comparison between mutations in the cardiac protein-C and the beta-myosin heavy chain genes, *Eur Heart J* 19:139-145, 1998.

45. Anan R, Greve G, Thierfelder L et al: Prognostic implications of novel beta cardiac myosin heavy chain gene mutations that cause familial hypertrophic cardiomyopathy, *J Clin Invest* 93:280-285, 1994.

46. Watkins H, McKenna WJ, Thierfelder L et al: Mutations in the genes for cardiac troponin T and alpha-tropomyosin in hypertrophic cardiomyopathy, *N Engl J Med* 332:1058-1064, 1995.

47. Maron BJ, Roberts WC, McAllister HA et al: Sudden death in young athletes, *Circulation* 62:218-229, 1980.

48. Chung MW, Tsoutsman T, Semsarian C: Hypertrophic cardiomyopathy: from gene defect to clinical disease, *Cell Res* 13:9-20, 2003.

The Impact of Aging on Cardiac Function

Michael W. Rich

In the 20th century, reductions in infant and maternal mortality, improvements in sanitation, and the introduction of antibiotics led to dramatic improvements in life expectancy in the United States and other developed countries (Table 14-1). These changes have resulted in a significant shift in population demographics, with an increasing proportion of persons surviving to advanced age (Figure 14-1).[1] An important public health consequence of this shift has been the progressive rise in the incidence and prevalence of chronic diseases, including cardiovascular disease, cancer, arthritis, and other chronic conditions, which now account for about 70 percent of all health care expenditures in the United States. In addition, these chronic illnesses are affecting an increasingly aging population, and therapeutic advances have led to improved survival among patients with prevalent chronic diseases.

Cardiovascular disease remains the leading cause of death and major disability in the United States, and the prevalence of cardiovascular disorders increases progressively with age in men and women (Figure 14-2).[2] At the present time, Americans over age 65 compose about 13 percent of the population but account for more than 50 percent of all hospital admissions for cardiovascular causes and more than 50 percent of all major cardiovascular procedures (Tables 14-2 and 14-3).[2,3] Moreover, persons over age 65 account for 85 percent of all cardiovascular deaths in the United States, and more than 50 percent of all deaths occur in the 6 percent of the population over age 75.

From 2010 to 2030, there will be a considerable increase in the number of Americans over age 65, reflecting the aging of the baby boomer generation (those born between 1945 and 1965). As a result, the number of older Americans will swell from 35.1 million in 2000 to about 71.5 million in 2030, by which time nearly 1 in 5 Americans will be age 65 or older. Similarly, the number of persons age 85 or older will increase strikingly from 2030 to 2050, and it is anticipated that the proportion of the population over age 85 will increase from 1.5 percent in 2000 to 5.0 percent in 2050.[4] In addition, with continued advances in the health sciences, it may be anticipated that older persons will live longer, healthier, and more active lives.

As the population ages, it is inevitable that the societal burden of cardiovascular disease will continue to rise. Therefore, it is critically important that health professionals have an appreciation of the intersection between aging and cardiovascular disease. This chapter reviews the major effects of normal aging on cardiovascular structure and function, describes how these changes predispose to the development of cardiovascular disease, and discusses some of the clinical implications of age-related changes for the diagnosis and treatment of cardiovascular disorders in older adults.

EFFECTS OF AGING ON THE CARDIOVASCULAR SYSTEM

Normal aging refers to processes that occur as a function of biological aging alone and are independent of age-related diseases and adverse environmental or behavioral influences (e.g., pollution and smoking). Distinguishing physiological changes inherent to aging from changes arising from external factors often is difficult. Nonetheless, studies in laboratory animals and healthy human beings carefully screened for occult cardiovascular risk factors or preclinical cardiovascular disease have identified a host of biochemical, cellular, and tissue changes that appear to occur as a consequence of normal aging.[5-7] Box 14-1 lists key changes in cardiovascular structure and function that have direct clinical implications for older adults.

Vascular Stiffness

With increasing age comes increased collagen deposition and collagen cross-linking in the media and adventitia of large- and medium-sized arteries. In addition, elastin fibers degenerate. In combination, these changes render older arteries stiffer—less distensible—than healthy younger arteries. As a result, impedance to left ventricular ejection (afterload) is increased. The loss of elasticity of the aorta and other great vessels also results in an increase in pulse wave velocity as blood is ejected from the heart.[8]

TABLE 14-1 LIFE EXPECTANCY IN THE UNITED STATES: 1900-2002

| | LIFE EXPECTANCY FROM BIRTH (YEARS) | | | | | | |
| | ALL RACES | | | WHITE | | BLACK* | |
	TOTAL	MEN	WOMEN	MEN	WOMEN	MEN	WOMEN
1900	47.3	46.3	48.3	46.6	48.7	32.5	33.5
1950	68.2	65.6	71.1	66.5	72.2	59.1	62.9
2002	77.3	74.5	79.9	75.1	80.3	68.8	75.6

*Data for 1900 and 1950 are for the nonwhite population.
Data from Arias E: United States life tables, 2002. *Natl Vital Stat Rep* vol 53, no 6, 2004.

TABLE 14-2 HOSPITAL ADMISSIONS FOR CARDIOVASCULAR DISEASE

| | NUMBER OF ADMISSIONS (IN THOUSANDS) | | |
	TOTAL	AGE ≥65 YEARS	AGE ≥75 YEARS
Acute myocardial infarction	783	500 (63.9%)	284 (36.3%)
Coronary artery disease	1412	790 (55.9%)	378 (26.8%)
Dysrhythmias	670	464 (69.3%)	288 (43.0%)
Heart failure	978	773 (79.0%)	529 (54.1%)
Cerebrovascular disease	1010	746 (73.9%)	493 (48.8%)

Popovic J, Kozak LJ: National hospital discharge survey: annual summary, 1998. National Center for Vital Statistics, *Vital Health Stat* vol 13, no 148, 2000.

TABLE 14-3 MAJOR CARDIOVASCULAR PROCEDURES IN THE UNITED STATES, 2002

| | AGE | | | | | |
| | LESS THAN 45 YEARS | | 45-64 YEARS | | ≥65 YEARS | |
	NO.*	%	NO.*	%	NO.*	%
Cardiac catheterization	133	(9.1)	597	(40.8)	732	(50.1)
Percutaneous coronary revascularization	76	(6.3)	517	(43.0)	608	(50.6)
Coronary bypass surgery	19	(3.7)	217	(42.1)	279	(54.2)
Permanent pacemaker	—	(NA)	21	(10.9)	172	(89.1)
Implanted cardioverter-defibrillator	—	(NA)	21	(36.8)	36	(63.2)
Carotid endarterectomy	—	(NA)	33	(24.6)	101	(75.4)

*In thousands.
NA, not available.
Data from American Heart Association: *Heart disease and stroke statistics: 2005 update*, Dallas, 2004, The Association.

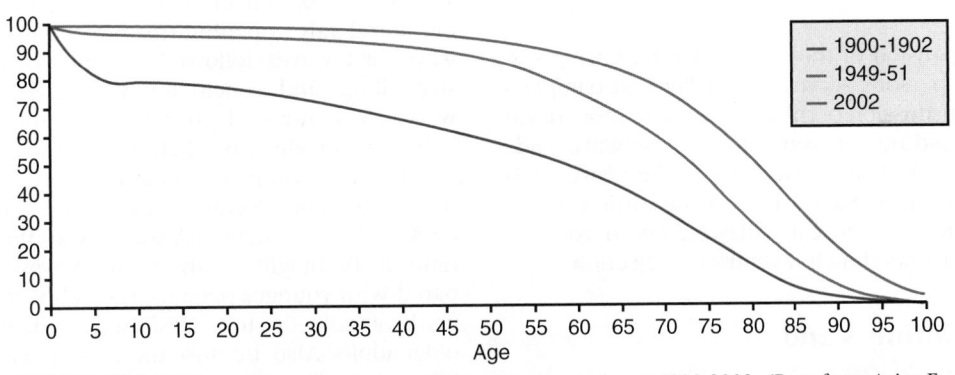

FIGURE 14-1 ■ Proportion of persons surviving to advanced age: 1900-2002. (Data from Arias E: United States life tables, 2002. *Natl Vital Stat Rep* vol. 53, no 6, 2004.)

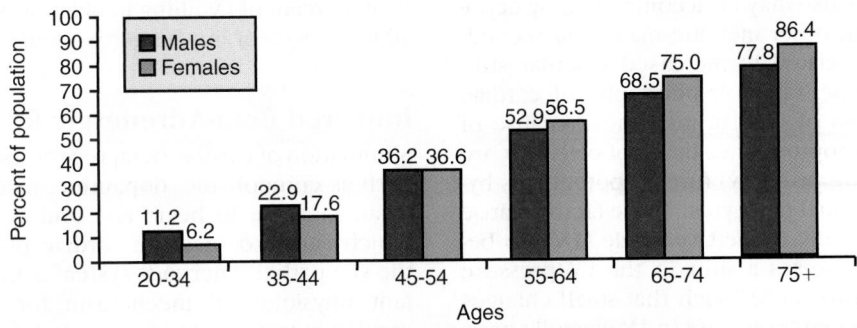

FIGURE 14-2 ■ Prevalence of cardiovascular disease in men and women in the United States. (Data from American Heart Association: *Heart disease and stroke statistics—2005*, Dallas, 2004, The Association.)

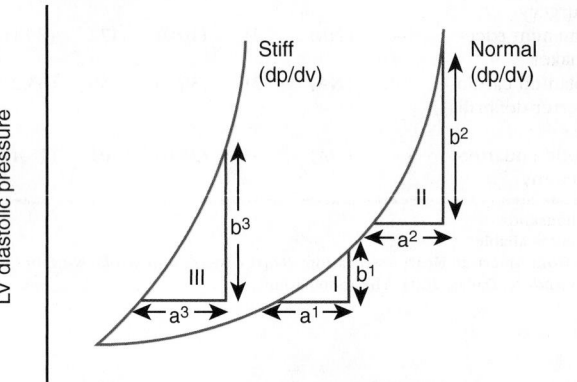

FIGURE 14-3 ■ Left ventricular pressure-volume curves in normal and stiff hearts. Note that in stiff hearts the pressure-volume relation is shifted upward and to the left so that small increases in diastolic volume (a^3) result in greater increases in diastolic pressure (b^3) relative to normal hearts. *dp/dv,* Diastolic pressure/diastolic volume; *lv,* left ventricular. (Adapted from Gaasch WH, Levine HJ, Quinones MA et al: *Am J Cardiol* 38:645-653, 1976.)

By contrast, expansion of the proximal aorta during systole in younger persons serves as a buffer that dampens the speed of transmission of the pulse wave to more distal vessels. More rapid transmission of the pulse wave leads to earlier reflection of the wave back to the heart, such that the reflected pulse wave arrives at the aortic valve in late systole rather than in early diastole (as in younger persons), further impeding left ventricular ejection.

Myocardial Stiffness and Impaired Relaxation

Several factors contribute to increased myocardial stiffness at older age. First, as with the great vessels, there is increased interstitial collagen deposition and collagen cross-linking, which also may be accompanied by deposition of amyloid and other inelastic materials. Second, increased afterload related to increased vascular stiffness results in compensatory hypertrophy of cardiac myocytes. Third, loss of cardiac myocytes because of normal age-related apoptosis (i.e., death of cells that are no longer functioning properly) further potentiates hypertrophy of the residual myocytes. These factors cause the heart, and especially the left ventricle (**LV**), to become stiffer, which causes a shift in the LV pressure volume relation (Figure 14-3),[9] such that small changes in LV volume cause greater changes in LV diastolic pressure in older compared with younger persons.

In addition to being stiffer, older hearts are less able to relax following systolic contraction. Myocardial relaxation at the end of systole is an active, energy-requiring process involving the release of calcium from the contractile proteins and resequestration in the sarcoplasmic reticulum and storage pool. For reasons that have not yet been fully elucidated, this process occurs more slowly in older hearts, which therefore may be viewed as being in a state of residual (mild) contraction at the onset of diastole.

The combination of increased myocardial stiffness and impaired relaxation has a profound effect on the dynamics of LV diastolic filling in older adults. The time to mitral valve opening following aortic valve closure is delayed slightly because LV relaxation progresses more slowly during the isovolumetric relaxation period. More significantly, the rate of ventricular filling during early diastole (the rapid filling phase) is attenuated because of impaired relaxation and increased myocardial stiffness. The rate of ventricular filling during middiastole (the passive filling phase) also is impaired as a result of increased myocardial stiffness. In response to higher LV diastolic pressure, the left atrium undergoes hypertrophy and contracts more forcefully at the end of diastole, which serves to maintain LV end-diastolic volume (preload), an important determinant of LV contractility (via the Frank-Starling mechanism) and stroke volume.

These changes in LV diastolic filling are readily apparent on Doppler echocardiographic interrogation of diastolic inflow velocities from the left atrium across the mitral valve into the LV (Figure 14-4). Figure 14-4, *A* depicts a young person, illustrating rapid filling of the LV following mitral valve opening (manifested by the early filling wave, or E wave), followed promptly by a period of passive filling, and concluding with atrial contraction (A wave). In contrast, Figure 14-4, *B* represents a healthy older person, showing slight prolongation of the isovolumetric relaxation phase, an attenuated early filling wave, prolongation of the downslope of the E wave from LV stiffness, and an augmented A wave. Note the reversal of the ratio of the heights of the E and A waves in older compared with younger persons, the echocardiographic hallmark of mild diastolic dysfunction manifested in most older adults. Also, because the area under the LV diastolic filling curves is proportional to blood volume, it is evident that a greater proportion of the LV end-diastolic volume is attributable to atrial contraction in older compared with younger persons. Thus, the atrial kick may account for 30 to 40 percent of LV filling in older persons compared with 10 to 15 percent in younger persons.

Impaired Beta-Adrenergic Responsiveness

Stimulation of cardiac beta$_1$ receptors by catecholamines such as epinephrine, dopamine, or dobutamine results in an increase in heart rate and contractility, both of which serve to increase cardiac output. Activation of the sympathetic nervous system is thus the most important physiological mechanism for acutely increasing cardiac output in response to increased demands (e.g., physical exertion) or pathological stress (e.g., ischemia).

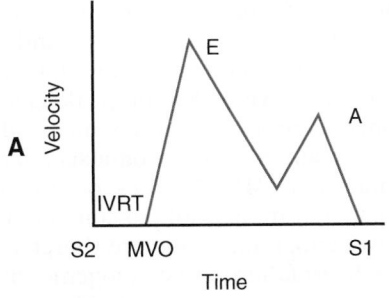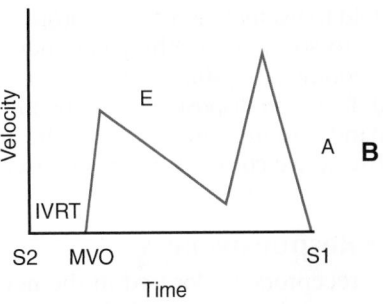

FIGURE 14-4 ■ Schematic diagram of mitral valve inflow patterns in healthy young and older adults. Left ventricular inflow velocities derived from Doppler echocardiograms in younger (**A**) and older (**B**) adults. Note prolongation of isovolumetric relaxation time (IVRT), decreased peak velocity of early filling (E wave), impaired passive filling during middiastole (represented by the downslope after the E wave), and increased magnitude of atrial contraction (A wave) in older compared with younger adults. *MVO,* Mitral valve opening.

Aging is associated with diminished responsiveness to beta-adrenergic stimulation, resulting in declines in the peak heart rate and peak contractile state under conditions of increased demand, thus limiting maximum cardiac output. Under physiological conditions, maximum attainable heart rate (**HR**) may be approximated by the following formula:

$$HR_{max} = 220 - age$$

This equation is used widely to calculate the target HR during exercise testing. Thus, HR_{max} is about 200 beats/min in a 20-year-old but only 140 beats/min in an 80-year-old. Because cardiac output (**CO**) is proportional to HR and LV stroke volume (CO = HR × SV), where *SV* is stroke volume, it is evident that the age-related decline in maximum HR greatly limits peak CO in response to stress. In addition, the decline in beta-adrenergic responsiveness with age also reduces maximum contractility, further impairing peak CO.

The mechanisms underlying the age-related reduction in beta-adrenergic responsiveness have not been elucidated fully, but circulating catecholamine levels, beta-receptor function, and calcium-mediated contractility appear to be well preserved in old age, suggesting a defect in intracellular protein metabolism or function.

Another effect of impaired beta-adrenergic responsiveness is that beta$_2$-mediated peripheral arterial vasodilatation also declines with age. This contributes to the age-related increase in afterload and, more importantly, attenuates peak blood flow to exercising muscles and skin, thereby contributing to diminished exercise capacity and impaired ability to release body heat generated during exercise or febrile illnesses.

Adenosine Triphosphate Production

The mitochondria produce adenosine triphosphate (**ATP**) to meet the energy requirements of the myocardium at rest and during exercise. With increasing age, the maximum ATP-generating capacity of the mitochondria declines. At rest, ATP production is sufficient to meet the metabolic needs of the myocardium in healthy persons of all ages. As a result, myocardial contractility is well preserved at rest, even in the very elderly, and LV ejection fraction is unaffected by age in healthy persons. With exercise, aged mitochondria are less able to increase ATP production commensurate with increased myocardial oxygen demands. This factor, with reduced beta-adrenergic responsiveness, further reduces peak contractility in elderly persons, as manifested by a failure to increase ejection fraction in response to stress to the same degree as observed in healthy younger persons. Decreased peak ATP production thus contributes to reduced exercise capacity in old age.

Sinus Node Dysfunction

At birth the sinoatrial node contains about 5000 cells capable of spontaneous depolarization leading to initiation of a heartbeat. Aging is associated with fibrosis and degenerative changes of the sinus node, leading to a progressive decline in the number of functioning sinus node pacemaker cells. By age 75, only about 10 percent of the original cells retain capacity to initiate a sinus impulse. In addition, degenerative changes involving the transition cells surrounding the sinus node may impair conduction of the impulse to the atrial conduction system (sinus node exit block). Associated changes in the atria and atrioventricular (**AV**) node predispose older persons to develop supraventricular dysrhythmias and AV-nodal conduction disorders, respectively.

Endothelial Dysfunction

Endothelium-independent vasodilatation is not affected by age in healthy persons, and the vasodilatory response to nitroglycerin and nitroprusside are thus well preserved in old age. In contrast, endothelium-dependent vasodilatory capacity declines by about 2 percent per decade after age 40 in men and 5 percent per decade after age 50 in women, apparently from impaired production of nitric oxide.[10] Because endothelial dysfunction plays an important role in the pathogenesis and progression of atherosclerosis, age-related endothelial dysfunction contributes to the development of coronary artery disease and peripheral arterial disease in older adults. Moreover, coronary endothelial cells regulate coronary blood flow, and endothelium-mediated vasodilatation permits a threefold to fivefold increase in coronary blood flow in response to stress in healthy young persons. In older persons, endothelial dysfunction limits maximum coronary blood flow, predisposing to ischemia when myocardial demands are increased, even in the absence of significant obstructive coronary artery disease.

Baroreceptor Responsiveness

The carotid baroreceptors are located in the neck contiguous with the carotid arteries just below the angle of the jaw. These receptors are exquisitely sensitive to changes in blood pressure, and they can initiate a rapid feedback loop to adjust HR and blood pressure to maintain cerebral perfusion within a narrow range. With age, baroreceptor sensitivity declines, permitting wider and more sustained fluctuations in cerebral perfusion pressure and blood flow. This decline in baroreceptor responsiveness is an important factor contributing to the increased risk of orthostatic hypotension, falls, and syncope in older adults.

Net Effect

As discussed later in this chapter, age-related changes in cardiovascular structure and function have important implications for the development, clinical features, and management of cardiovascular disease in older adults. Taken together, the dominant effect of these changes is a marked and progressive reduction in cardiovascular reserve. This effect, which constitutes the hallmark of cardiovascular aging, is illustrated in Figure 14-5.[11] These data, derived from participants in the Baltimore Longitudinal Study on Aging, who were screened carefully to exclude occult cardiovascular disease or risk factors, show that in healthy men and women there is an accelerating decline in maximum oxygen consumption (an objective index of peak cardiovascular and pulmonary aerobic capacity) in men and women. These graphs explain why the prognosis after acute myocardial infarction (**MI**) declines progressively with age. Older patients are less able to compensate in the face of new myocardial injury and are therefore more likely to develop heart failure and cardiogenic shock. The graphs also explain the propensity of older persons to develop heart failure, because the margin between compensation and decompensation becomes narrower with increasing age (a phenomenon often referred to as homeostenosis). In this regard, note that in healthy persons older than age 80, maximum oxygen consumption is often less than 20 ml/min/kg, a level corresponding to New York Heart Association Class II heart failure in younger persons.

EFFECTS OF AGING ON OTHER ORGAN SYSTEMS

Box 14-2 summarizes age-related changes in other organ systems that parallel the cardiovascular aging changes described before.[12] Many of these changes have important effects on the clinical features and treatment of cardiovascular disorders in the elderly.

Kidneys

Glomerular filtration rate (**GFR**) declines at about 8 ml/min per decade after age 30. Because muscle mass also declines with age (see the following), the serum

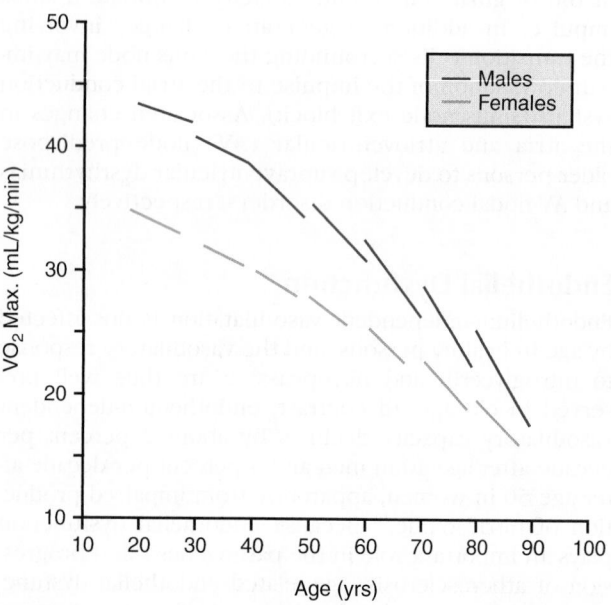

FIGURE 14-5 ■ Age and maximum oxygen consumption (VO₂max) in healthy subjects: the Baltimore Longitudinal Study on Aging. Note the accelerating decline in VO₂max with increasing age in men and women. (Data from Fleg JL, Bos AG, Brant LH et al: *Circulation* 102[suppl 2]:II-602, 2000.)

BOX 14-2   ■ ■ ■
EFFECTS OF AGING ON OTHER ORGAN SYSTEMS

Kidneys
- Decline in glomerular filtration rate (about 8 ml/min per decade)
- Impaired water and electrolyte homeostasis
- Reduced plasma renin and aldosterone activity
- Impaired elimination of renally excreted drugs

Lungs
- Loss of elastic recoil
- Decreased strength of respiratory muscles
- Increased ventilation-perfusion (V/Q) mismatching
- Reduced vital capacity and minute ventilation

Nervous System
- Diminished reflex responsiveness, especially baroreceptors
- Reduced central nervous system autoregulatory capacity
- Impaired thirst mechanism

Musculoskeletal System
- Loss of muscle mass and strength (sarcopenia)
- Loss of bone mass, especially in women (osteopenia)

Hemostatic System
- Increased coagulation factors and platelet activity
- Decreased endogenous fibrinolytic activity
- Increased inflammatory cytokines and C-reactive protein
- Decreased angiogenesis

Altered Pharmacokinetics and Pharmacodynamics of Most Drugs

creatinine level is a relatively poor index of renal function in older adults. Estimating creatinine clearance using the Cockcroft-Gault equation is preferable[13]:

$$\text{Creatinine clearance*} = \frac{(140 - \text{age}) \times (\text{weight in kg})}{72 \times (\text{serum creatinine in mg/dl})}$$

Using this formula, a 40-year-old man weighing 176 lb (80 kg) with a serum creatinine level of 1.0 mg/dl would have an estimated creatinine clearance of 111 ml/min. In contrast, an 85-year-old woman weighing 110 pounds (50 kg) with a serum creatinine level of 1.0 mg/dl would have an estimated creatinine clearance of 32 ml/min. An important corollary of reduced GFR is that aging is associated with impaired elimination of all renally excreted drugs.

In addition to reduced GFR, aging is associated with diminished capacity to preserve fluid and electrolyte homeostasis. As a result, the kidneys are less able to excrete a fluid load (e.g., from a large volume of oral fluid intake or intravenous fluid administration) and less able to conserve fluids (i.e., by concentrating the urine) in a state of volume contraction. Similarly, the kidneys are less able to excrete or conserve electrolytes, including sodium, potassium, and magnesium, predisposing older persons to electrolyte disorders such as hyponatremia or hypokalemia in response to therapy with thiazide or loop diuretics, or hyperkalemia from angiotensin-converting enzyme (ACE) inhibitors or aldosterone antagonists. These alterations in fluid and electrolyte balance are mediated in part by age-related reductions in plasma renin and aldosterone activity.

Lungs

As in blood vessels, aging is associated with increased collagen deposition and degeneration of elastin fibers in the lungs. As a result, the lungs are stiffer (less able to fill with air), and there is a loss of spontaneous elastic recoil. In addition, the strength of the respiratory muscles declines with age, and the chest wall itself tends to become stiffer and less resilient. Taken together, these changes lead to reduced vital capacity, minute ventilation, and maximum ventilatory volume in older adults. Aging also is associated with increased ventilation-perfusion mismatching and impaired gas exchange, predisposing to hypoxia and hypercapnea. Age-related changes in the lungs thus may contribute to or worsen hypoxemia or ischemia in elderly patients with cardiovascular disease, leading to more severe symptoms (e.g., dyspnea and exercise intolerance) and a worse prognosis (e.g., in the setting of acute pulmonary edema or MI).

Nervous System

Aging is associated with diffuse changes in the central and peripheral nervous systems. Changes of particular relevance in older adults with cardiovascular disease include a generalized reduction in reflex responsiveness (i.e., most reflexes become slower with age) so that the "fine tuning" of HR and blood pressure in response to internal and external stimuli is impaired (e.g., diminished baroreceptor responsiveness, as previously discussed). These changes predispose older adults to orthostatic and postural hypotension, which in turn are important causes of dizziness, falls, and syncope.

Aging also is associated with reduced capacity of the central nervous system to maintain cerebral perfusion in the setting of rapid changes in systemic arterial blood pressure. Therefore, older adults are more susceptible to confusion or impaired mental status when blood pressure falls as a result of an acute cardiovascular event (e.g., MI or dysrhythmia), noncardiovascular condition (e.g., sepsis or blood loss), or iatrogenic disturbance (e.g., medications or volume contraction). The thirst mechanism, regulated by the hypothalamus, also is impaired in older adults so that intravascular volume depletion is less likely to stimulate increased fluid intake, thereby contributing to the propensity of elderly persons to become dehydrated.[14]

Musculoskeletal System

A hallmark of aging is the progressive loss of skeletal muscle mass and strength, referred to as sarcopenia. Sarcopenia contributes to age-related weakness and impaired physical capacity, thus aggravating symptom severity and disability in elderly patients with cardiovascular disease, especially heart failure. Sarcopenia also predisposes older adults to falls and related injuries, such as hip fractures.

Bone mass declines with age, especially in women, leading to osteopenia and osteoporosis. As with sarcopenia, loss of bone mass contributes to weakness, exercise intolerance, and frailty. In addition, compression fractures of the thoracic vertebrae further diminish respiratory reserve.

Hemostatic System

Aging is associated with an increase in circulating coagulation factors V, VIII, IX, and XIIIa; von Willebrand factor; and fibrinogen, as well as an increase in platelet activity and platelet aggregability. At the same time, there is an increase in plasminogen activator inhibitor-1. These changes alter the balance between thrombosis and fibrinolysis in favor of thrombosis; as a result, older adults are at increased risk for developing arterial (e.g., coronary artery and left atrial) and venous thrombi and are less capable of spontaneously lysing such thrombi.

Aging also is associated with an increase in inflammatory cytokines, including interleukin-6 and tumor necrosis factor-alpha, as well as C-reactive protein. Inflammation now is recognized as an important factor in the pathogenesis of atherosclerosis and a key mediator in acute coronary syndromes; increased inflammatory activity predisposes older adults to acute and chronic cardiovascular disorders.

Angiogenesis, the formation of new blood vessels, is an important mechanism for restoring perfusion to tissues with inadequate blood supply, including the heart. However, aging is associated with increased production

---

*In women, multiply by 0.85.

of endogenous inhibitors of angiogenesis, including plasminogen activator inhibitor-1, platelet factor 4, and alpha$_2$-antiplasmin. These changes may contribute to the impaired ability of older adults to develop collateral blood vessels in response to repeated episodes of ischemia, an effect referred to as ischemic preconditioning.[15,16] When present, ischemic preconditioning reduces the extent of ischemia and improves the prognosis in patients with acute MI.

Drug Metabolism

Age-related changes in the gastrointestinal system, hepatobiliary system, and kidneys result in altered absorption, distribution, metabolism, and elimination of almost all drugs. As a result, drug dosages suitable for use in middle-aged persons may cause increased toxicity in the elderly. Although the optimal dose of a specific drug in an elderly person is difficult to determine empirically, as a general principal, initial dosages should be reduced (a 50 percent reduction is a common rule of thumb), and the drug titration interval should be increased. However, in the absence of contraindications or side effects, the "target" maintenance dosage of most cardiovascular drugs in elderly patients should be based on those proven to be effective in prospective randomized clinical trials. In other words, age alone should not be used as the sole rationale for giving lower, possibly less effective, drug dosages.

IMPACT OF COMORBIDITIES

Apart from age-related changes in the heart, blood vessels, and other organ systems, another factor that distinguishes elderly from middle-aged patients is the increasing prevalence of comorbid illnesses, many of which affect the clinical presentation, response to therapy, and prognosis of older adults with cardiovascular disease. As shown in Figure 14-6, more than 85 percent of Medicare beneficiaries hospitalized with heart failure have two or more noncardiac comorbidities. Moreover, there is a strong correlation between the number of noncardiac comorbidities and the likelihood of being rehospitalized for any reason (Figure 14-7).[17] Note that patients with six or more comorbidities have more than a 75 percent probability of being rehospitalized within 1 year. In addition, up to 50 percent of hospitalizations are potentially preventable, often through more aggressive intervention in managing noncardiac conditions. Table 14-4 lists common noncardiac comorbidities and their potential implications for management of older adults with cardiovascular disease.

Reduced Renal Function

As previously discussed, renal function declines progressively with age. Moreover, numerous recent studies have documented that renal insufficiency is a powerful predictor of adverse prognosis, including increased mortality, among patients with acute coronary syndromes, stable coronary artery disease, heart failure, and other cardiovascular conditions.[18-23] In addition, renal insufficiency may limit the use of certain cardiovascular drugs or increase the risk of adverse drug effects (e.g., low-molecular-weight heparins, glycoprotein IIb/IIIa inhibitors, ACE inhibitors, angiotensin receptor blockers, and aldosterone antagonists). Conversely, diuretics, ACE inhibitors, angiotensin receptor blockers, and intravenous contrast agents may contribute to worsening renal function.

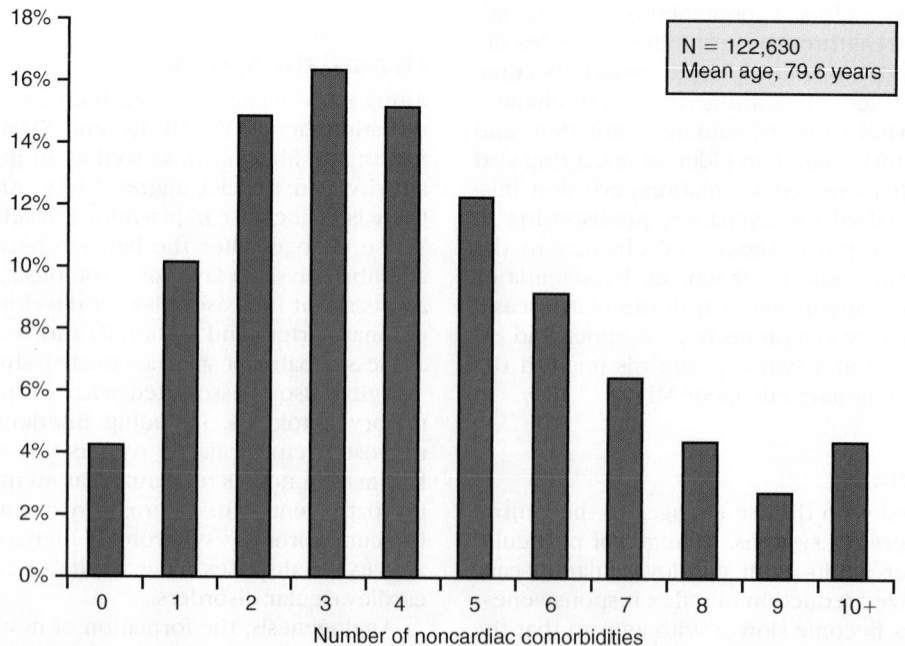

FIGURE 14-6 ■ Prevalence of noncardiac comorbidities in Medicare beneficiaries with heart failure. (Data from Braunstein JB, Anderson GF, Gerstenblith G et al: *J Am Coll Cardiol* 42:1226-1233, 2003.)

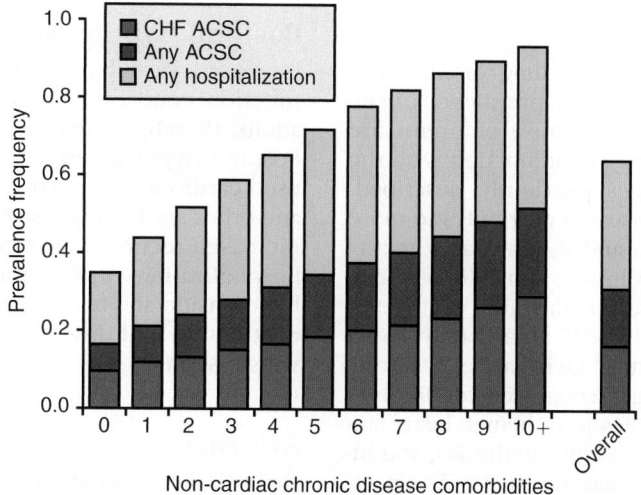

FIGURE 14-7 ■ Impact of noncardiac comorbidities on the annual probability of hospital admission in Medicare beneficiaries with chronic heart failure. *ACSC,* Ambulatory care sensitive conditions; *CHF,* chronic heart failure. (Data from Braunstein JB, Anderson GF, Gerstenblith G et al: *J Am Coll Cardiol* 42:1226-1233, 2003.)

■ ■ ■

TABLE 14-4 COMMON NONCARDIAC COMORBID CONDITIONS IN OLDER PATIENTS

CONDITION	IMPLICATIONS
Renal dysfunction	Potent predictor of adverse prognosis
	Potentially worsened by diuretics, ACE inhibitors, ARBs, intravenous contrast
	May limit use or increase risk of medications, e.g., low-molecular-weight heparin, glycoprotein IIb/IIIa inhibitors, aldosterone antagonists, ACE inhibitors, ARBs
Anemia	Worsens symptoms and prognosis
	Potentially aggravated by antithrombotic and fibrinolytic therapies
Chronic lung disease	Worsens symptoms and prognosis
	Increases risk of dysrhythmias
	Contributes to diagnostic uncertainty
Cognitive dysfunction	Interferes with compliance with diet, medications, activity recommendations
	Often exacerbated by hospitalization (especially in intensive care unit)
	May pose ethical challenges
Depression, social isolation	Worsens quality of life and prognosis
	Interferes with compliance
Postural hypotension, falls	Often exacerbated by cardiovascular medications
	Increased risk during hospitalization
Arthritis	Contributes to activity limitation and impaired quality of life
	May limit diagnostic testing (e.g., exercise test)
	Nonsteroidal antiinflammatory drugs antagonize cardiac medications, may increase cardiovascular risk
Nervous system disorders (e.g., stroke, parkinsonism, and neuropathies)	Limit exercise capacity and quality of life
	May limit diagnostic testing
	Medications may cause cardiac side effects (e.g., levodopa)
Urinary incontinence	Aggravated by diuretics, ACE inhibitors
	Increased risk for infections, decubitus ulcers
Sarcopenia, osteopenia	Contribute to impaired exercise tolerance
	Increase risk of falls and fractures
Sensory deprivation	Interferes with compliance, quality of life
	May increase risk of falls
Nutritional disorders	Exacerbated by dietary restrictions
	Contribute to weakness, impaired activity tolerance, fall risk
Frailty	Exacerbated by hospitalization
	Increased risk of iatrogenic complications, falls
Polypharmacy	Interferes with compliance
	Increased risk for drug interactions

ACE, Angiotensin-converting enzyme; *ARB,* angiotensin receptor blocker.

Anemia

Recent studies also have shown that anemia is associated with adverse prognosis in cardiac patients, independent of renal function.[24-28] Anemia reduces the oxygen-carrying capacity of the blood, thereby worsening symptoms of ischemia and heart failure while reducing exercise tolerance. In addition, patients with lower baseline hemoglobin or hematocrit levels are less able to maintain tissue oxygen delivery if bleeding results from antithrombotic or fibrinolytic drug therapy, and they are therefore at greater risk for developing coronary ischemia or incident heart failure.

Lung Disease

Chronic obstructive and restrictive lung diseases are common in older adults, although the prevalence of emphysema declines after age 75 because of premature death in lifelong tobacco users. In conjunction with the age-related pulmonary changes previously described, superimposed chronic lung disease contributes to more severe symptoms of ischemia and dyspnea and greatly reduces exercise tolerance. Chronic lung disease also increases the risk of supraventricular and ventricular dysrhythmias, including multifocal atrial tachycardia, atrial fibrillation, and ventricular tachycardia. Obstructive sleep apnea, an increasingly recognized condition in cardiac patients, also contributes to ischemia, heart failure, tachydysrhythmias, and bradydysrhythmias, and increases the risk of sudden cardiac death.[29-33] The presence of chronic lung disease also may lead to diagnostic uncertainty because it may be difficult to determine whether symptoms are primarily cardiac or pulmonary.

Cognition Dysfunction

Cognitive dysfunction becomes increasingly common with advancing age, especially after age 80 or 85. Elderly patients with cognitive dysfunction are at increased risk for developing acute delirium during hospitalization for cardiac problems (known as sundowning or intensive care unit psychosis).[34] In addition, significant cognitive dysfunction or delirium increases the hospital stay, increases the risk of iatrogenic complications (e.g., falls), increases the likelihood that the patient will require discharge to an extended care or chronic care facility, and greatly increases hospital mortality.[35] Cognitive impairment also interferes with the patient's capacity to comply with medical advice regarding diet, medications, and activities. In addition, difficult ethical issues often arise in caring for patients with significant cognitive dysfunction, including questions about how aggressive to be in pursuing diagnostic and therapeutic interventions and how best to address end-of-life care.

Depression

Depression affects about 15 to 20 percent of patients with cardiovascular disease. Although the prevalence of depression is lower in older compared to younger cardiac patients, most depressed cardiac patients are over age 65 because of the much higher prevalence of cardiovascular disease in this age group. Social isolation is also highly prevalent in older adults, especially elderly women who have outlived their spouses. Depression and social isolation contribute to impaired quality of life and interfere with compliance in elderly cardiac patients (e.g., as a result of disinclination to take medications, inability to acquire medications because of transportation difficulties, or lack of spousal reminders or assistance).[36,37] In addition, depression has been associated with increased mortality in patients with coronary artery disease or heart failure,[38-40] possibly because of an increased risk of dysrhythmias or recurrent ischemic events.[41]

Postural Hypotension

Increased vascular stiffness and impaired autonomic function contribute to postural hypotension in older adults, thereby increasing the risk of falls and fractures. Postural hypotension often is worsened by commonly used cardiovascular drugs, including diuretics, nitrates, and other antihypertensive and antiischemic drugs. The increased recumbency that often accompanies cardiac hospitalization further increases the risk of postural hypotension and falls as a result of intravascular volume contraction and downregulation of the autonomic nervous system.

Arthritis

Arthritis is the single most common chronic condition affecting the elderly (not cardiovascular disease, as sometimes is stated). Chronic arthritis impairs quality of life and often imposes activity limitations that, in some cases, may interfere with cardiac diagnostic testing. Perhaps more important, the widespread use of prescription and over-the-counter nonsteroidal antiinflammatory drugs (**NSAIDs**) interferes with the actions of many cardiovascular drugs, including diuretics, ACE inhibitors, and beta blockers. NSAIDs also may cause fluid and sodium retention, and the risk of heart failure is increased strikingly in elderly patients using these drugs.[42] NSAIDs also may worsen renal function, and some NSAIDs have been associated with an increased risk of MI and stroke.[43,44]

Central Nervous System Disorders

Central nervous system disorders, such as stroke and parkinsonism, as well as peripheral neuropathies (e.g., diabetic neuropathy), increase in prevalence with advancing age. These conditions limit exercise capacity and quality of life, and they may interfere with cardiac diagnostic testing. In addition, drugs used in treating these disorders may cause cardiovascular side effects (e.g., angina or palpitations caused by levodopa).

Incontinence

Urinary incontinence is common in older adults, especially women, and the condition commonly is overlooked unless the patient is asked specifically. Incontinence often is worsened by diuretics and occasionally by ACE inhibitors (e.g., in patients with ACE inhibitor cough). Fear of incontinence is a common cause of nonadherence to diuretic therapy; to avoid embarrassment, patients will skip their morning diuretic dose when they are going to be away from home. Urinary incontinence also poses an increased risk of urinary tract infections and decubitus ulcers, especially in bedridden patients in a hospital or chronic care facility.

Sarcopenia and Osteopenia

As previously discussed, sarcopenia and osteopenia contribute to impaired exercise tolerance and increase the risk of falls and fractures. Both of these conditions are aggravated by bed rest, even for short periods. Chronic heparin administration worsens osteopenia, and warfarin may contribute to osteopenia in some patients by interfering with the function of vitamin K.

Sensory Decline

Auditory and visual acuity decline with age, as do the sensations of taste, smell, and touch. Significant impairments in hearing or sight may interfere with compliance because patients may not hear directions properly or may not be able to read instructions or labels on pill bottles. Diminished visual and tactile sensations also increase the risk of falls and fractures.

Nutritional Deficiency

Nutritional deficiencies are common in the elderly and may contribute to weakness, impaired activity tolerance, neurological dysfunction (e.g., from vitamin B_{12} deficiency), and an increased risk of falls. Dietary restrictions imposed for treatment of hypertension, dyslipidemia, diabetes, coronary heart disease, heart failure, or advanced renal disease often contribute to nutritional deficiencies and may lead to frank malnutrition (i.e., inadequate caloric and nutritional intake to meet the metabolic needs of the body). Malnutrition, in turn, increases the risk of falls, iatrogenic complications, functional decline, and frailty.

Frailty

Frailty is a syndrome that becomes increasingly common in old age, especially after age 80.[45] The elements of frailty include generalized weakness, slow movement, reduced physical activity, unintentional weight loss, and a sense of exhaustion or low energy.[46] Frailty substantially limits physical function and the ability to perform routine activities of daily living. Frailty is also a potent risk factor for iatrogenic complications during hospitalization. Frailty almost invariably worsens during hospitalization, especially when associated with bed rest or lengthy periods of recumbency, and frail patients rarely return to their previous level of function after a lengthy hospital admission.

Polypharmacy

Polypharmacy may be defined as the regular use of five or more drugs, including prescription and nonprescription drugs. Because coronary artery disease, heart failure, hypertension, and diabetes often are treated with two or more drugs and because these conditions often coexist, the drug regimens of patients with cardiovascular disease, particularly the elderly, often meet the criteria for polypharmacy.

Polypharmacy contributes to inadvertent noncompliance from confusion about which medicines to take and when, a problem that is aggravated when patients are receiving drugs from multiple prescribers. Medication errors are particularly common after hospital discharge, especially if multiple changes have been made to the regimen.

Polypharmacy is also a key risk factor for adverse drug interactions, with the risk of such interactions increasing exponentially with the number of drugs prescribed and exceeding 90 percent in patients receiving 10 or more drugs.[47] As previously noted, NSAIDs are a common source of adverse drug interactions in elderly patients. Other common situations include coadministration of an ACE inhibitor with spironolactone (increased risk of hyperkalemia),[48,49] and the use of warfarin, which interacts with numerous medications.

In summary, older patients with cardiovascular disease almost invariably have other cardiac and noncardiac conditions that influence the diagnosis, clinical features, management, and prognosis of the primary cardiovascular disorder. The number, nature, and severity of these comorbidities, coupled with the somewhat variable rate of aging of the cardiovascular system and other organ systems, leads to considerable heterogeneity in the elderly population with or without cardiac disease.

As a result, optimal management of the elderly patient must be undertaken in the context of these multiple competing comorbidities and risks and must be individualized in accordance with each patient's unique circumstances and personal preferences. It follows that the results of cardiovascular clinical trials conducted in predominantly middle-aged patients are not necessarily applicable to the very elderly,[50,51] and that a "one-size-fits-all" approach to managing elderly cardiac patients is unlikely to yield favorable outcomes on a population-wide basis.

AGING AND CARDIOVASCULAR DISEASE

As shown in Figure 14-2, the prevalence of cardiovascular disease rises progressively with age, such that among men age 75 or older, more than 75 percent have clinically manifest hypertension, coronary heart disease, heart failure, or stroke. Among women age 75 or older, the prevalence of cardiovascular disease is even higher—more than 85 percent—in large part because of the extremely high prevalence of hypertension in elderly women.[2] The two most important factors contributing to the high prevalence of cardiovascular disease at elderly age are the age-related changes in the cardiovascular system described before and the cumulative effects of long-term exposure to traditional cardiovascular risk factors, unhealthy behaviors (e.g., atherogenic diet and physical inactivity), and environmental influences (e.g., pollution and second-hand tobacco smoke).

A secondary factor, but one that is becoming increasingly important, is the increased survival of middle-aged persons with manifest cardiovascular disease or risk factors as a result of advances in diagnosis and therapy. Thus, persons who 50 years ago were dying from coronary heart disease in middle age now are surviving to old age because of treatments such as aspirin, beta blockers, ACE inhibitors, fibrinolytic agents, coronary angioplasty, and bypass surgery. Similarly, persons with severe hypertension who 50 years ago were dying prematurely from stroke now are surviving to older age, where they remain at high risk for coronary heart disease, heart failure, and peripheral arterial disease.

Although a comprehensive review of the interactions between aging and cardiovascular disease is beyond the scope of this chapter, a brief discussion of several common conditions in which aging changes play a pivotal role in the pathogenesis, clinical features, and management is warranted.

Hypertension

Age-related arterial stiffness and loss of elasticity produce a gradual but progressive rise in systolic blood pressure with increasing age (Figure 14-8).[52] Conversely, the diastolic blood pressure tends to plateau in late middle age, declining slightly thereafter, as a result of diminished elastic recoil during diastole. Pulse pressure, the difference between systolic and diastolic pressures, also increases with age, and the magnitude of the pulse pressure may be used as a rough index of the severity of vascular aging.

The prevalence of hypertension increases with age (Figure 14-9),[2] in part from the effects of cardiovascular

aging but with substantial contributions from age-related diseases, including atherosclerosis, renal dysfunction, diabetes, and obesity. Dietary factors, such as high sodium intake, and other behavioral factors, such as physical inactivity, also play a pivotal role. Importantly, isolated systolic hypertension (i.e., elevated systolic blood pressure with normal diastolic blood pressure) becomes the dominant form of hypertension in old age, especially in women.[53]

The rise in systolic blood pressure with increasing age once was viewed as a normal and even desirable phenomenon, giving rise to the aphorism that the systolic blood pressure should be about 100 plus age. However, elevated systolic blood pressure now is recognized as a powerful risk factor for coronary heart disease, stroke, heart failure, and atrial fibrillation in older men and women. Moreover, numerous randomized trials have shown conclusively that antihypertensive therapy greatly reduces cardiovascular risk in elderly persons with systolic or diastolic hypertension (Table 14-5).[54-63] Because several of these trials included patients more

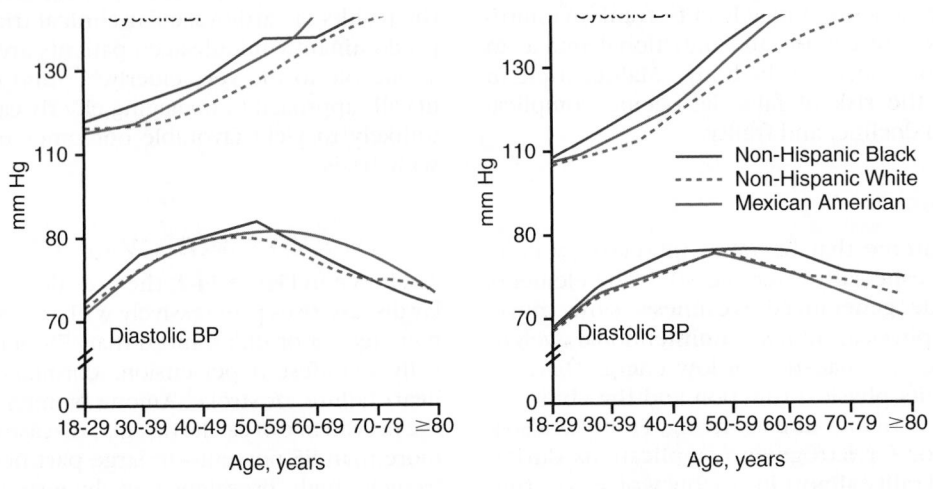

FIGURE 14-8 ■ Mean systolic and diastolic blood pressure in the United States by age, gender, and race. *BP,* Blood pressure. (Data from National Health and Nutrition Examination Survey [NHANES].)

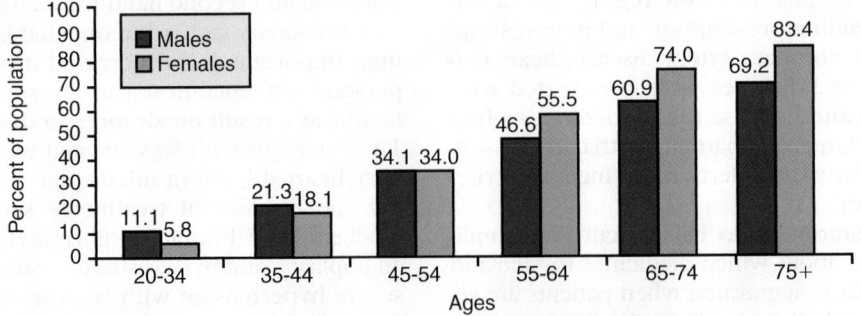

FIGURE 14-9 ■ Prevalence of hypertension in men and women in the United States. (Data from American Heart Association: *Heart disease and stroke statistics—2005,* Dallas, 2004, The Association.)

■ ■ ■

TABLE 14-5   TRIALS OF ANTIHYPERTENSIVE TREATMENT IN THE ELDERLY

			RISK REDUCTION (%)			
TRIAL	n	AGE	STROKE	CAD	CHF	ALL CVD
Australian	582	60-69	33	18	NR	31
EWPHE	840	Less than 60	36	20	22	29
Coope	884	60-79	42	−3	32	24
STOP-HTN	1627	79-84	47	13	51	40
MRC	4396	65-74	25	19	NR	17
HDFP	2374	60-69	44	15	NR	16
SHEP	4736	≥60	33	27	55	32
Syst-Eur	4695	≥60	42	26	36	31
STONE	1632	60-79	57	6	68	60
Syst-China	2394	≥60	38	33	38	37

CAD, Coronary artery disease; *CHF,* congestive heart failure; *CVD,* cardiovascular disease; *EWPHE,* European Working Party on High Blood Pressure in the Elderly; *STOP-HTN,* Swedish Trial in Old Patients with Hypertension; MRC, Medical Research Council; *HDFP,* Hypertension Detection and Followup Program; *SHEP,* Systolic Hypertension in the Elderly Program; *Syst-Eur,* Systolic Hypertension in Europe; *STONE,* Shanghai Trial of Nifedipine in the Elderly; *Syst-China,* Systolic Hypertension in China; *NR,* not reported.

than 80 years of age, we know that treatment of hypertension is warranted for almost all older persons.[64]

Coronary Artery Disease

Vascular aging, endothelial dysfunction, and increased inflammatory activity set the stage for the development and progression of coronary artery disease and generalized atherosclerosis in older adults. The increasing prevalence of major cardiovascular risk factors with age, particularly hypertension, dyslipidemia, and diabetes, serves to perpetuate and accelerate the atherosclerotic process. In addition, age-related changes in the hemostatic system predispose older adults to the development of intravascular thrombosis, increasing the risk of acute coronary syndromes.

The convergence of these factors leads to a striking increase in the prevalence of coronary artery disease at elderly age. In addition, diminished cardiovascular reserve ensures that the prognosis for older patients with acute or chronic coronary heart disease is substantially worse than in younger patients. Thus, as shown in Tables 14-2 and 14-3,[2,3] the 13 percent of the U.S. population over age 65 now accounts for more than 60 percent of all acute MIs, more than half of all revascularization procedures, and more than 80 percent of all deaths attributable to coronary artery disease or its complications. Furthermore, more than half of all such deaths occur in the 6 percent of the population over age 75.

Aging changes also may reduce the efficacy or increase the risk associated with standard therapies for coronary artery disease. For example, age-related vascular, endothelial, and hemostatic changes may reduce the efficacy of fibrinolytic and antithrombotic therapy in elderly patients with acute coronary syndromes. Conversely, the risk of major bleeding, including intracranial hemorrhage, increases with age. Similarly, the risk of major complications and death following percutaneous or surgical coronary revascularization procedures increases greatly after age 80.[65,66] Nonetheless, the elderly compose a large high-risk subgroup of the coronary heart disease population, a group that has potentially much to gain from aggressive treatment. Unfortunately, the very elderly, and especially those with multiple comorbidities, have been greatly underrepresented in clinical trials, so that the optimal approach to managing elderly patients with acute or chronic coronary heart disease remains uncertain.

Valvular Heart Disease

Aging is associated with fibrosis and calcification of the cardiac skeleton and valves, especially the aortic valve and the mitral valve annulus. However, the extent to which these changes may be attributable to inflammation and atherosclerotic processes rather than aging remains a subject of ongoing investigation. In clinical practice, aging is associated with a progressive increase in the prevalence of aortic valve stenosis and mitral valve disorders, especially mitral regurgitation but also nonrheumatic mitral stenosis.

Aortic stenosis in the very elderly typically occurs in the setting of a normal trileaflet aortic valve and usually is associated with considerable calcification and fibrosis of the leaflets without commissural fusion. As in younger patients, elderly patients with severe aortic stenosis may report shortness of breath, chest discomfort (angina), light-headedness, or syncope. Atypical or nonspecific symptoms such as generalized fatigue, weakness, or impaired exercise tolerance occur more often in older than in younger patients. Physical findings include a loud crescendo-decrescendo systolic murmur and an S_4 gallop; the carotid upstrokes often are preserved because of rapid pulse wave transmission resulting from arterial stiffness. Echocardiography is diagnostic in almost all cases. Aortic valve replacement, usually with a bioprosthesis, is the only effective therapy, and long-term results following surgery are excellent, even in octogenarians.[67,68]

Mitral valve annular calcification (**MVAC**) tends to be more common and more severe in elderly women compared with men, particularly those with longstanding hypertension. MVAC commonly is associated with mitral regurgitation, and it is a risk factor for atrial fibrillation, stroke, and heart failure.[69] In severe cases, marked MVAC can encroach on the mitral valve orifice, resulting in nonrheumatic mitral stenosis. Although mitral regurgitation or mitral stenosis caused by MVAC may contribute to exertional dyspnea and impaired exercise tolerance, surgical repair or replacement of the mitral valve rarely is warranted.

Heart Failure

Heart failure (**HF**) is the quintessential disorder of cardiovascular aging, representing the final common pathway arising from age-related cardiovascular diseases (especially hypertension and coronary artery disease) superimposed on the progressive age-related decline in cardiovascular reserve.

As shown in Table 14-6, HF in older adults differs from HF in middle age in many important respects.[12] Not only is the prevalence considerably higher, but there is a predominance of women, most of whom have hypertension rather than coronary artery disease as the primary cause. The clinical features of HF, including symptoms, signs, and laboratory findings, are less sensitive and less specific in the elderly, whereas atypical symptoms, such as confusion and anorexia, are more common in the very elderly. The chest x-ray film is more often nondiagnostic in the elderly because of chronic pulmonary disease and age-related changes in the chest cavity and lungs. B-type natriuretic peptide levels increase with age, especially in women, so that the diagnostic accuracy of B-type natriuretic peptide declines with age.[70]

Perhaps the most important difference between older and younger persons with HF is the considerable increase in prevalence of HF with preserved LV systolic function in the elderly.[71,72] Age-related impairments in LV diastolic relaxation and compliance, coupled with the rise in systolic blood pressure caused by increased vascular stiffness, predispose older persons to clinical HF despite preserved systolic function at rest. As a result, about 40 percent of men and up to two-thirds of women over age 65 with HF have a normal LV ejection fraction.[72] Moreover, although the prognosis for patients with HF in the setting of preserved systolic function

tends to be more favorable than in patients with systolic HF, symptom severity, exercise capacity, and hospitalization rates are similar in patients with either form of HF.[72-74]

Despite the high prevalence of HF with preserved systolic function in the elderly, few clinical trials have addressed this condition, and to date, no pharmacological or nonpharmacological interventions have been shown to improve survival for patients with this disorder. Similarly, although many trials have evaluated a panoply of therapies for systolic HF, the elderly have been greatly underrepresented in these trials, and virtually none of these studies have enrolled elderly subjects with multiple comorbid conditions.[50,51] As a result, treatment of elderly HF patients remains largely empirical rather than evidence-based, and elderly patients are also more likely to be under the care of a generalist physician rather than a cardiologist.

A notable exception to the underrepresentation of elderly subjects in HF clinical trials is in the area of multidisciplinary HF disease management, in which many studies have targeted older adults, including those with complex medical and social problems.[75] Recent meta-analyses of HF disease management trials indicate that these programs reduce hospitalizations, have a favorable effect on quality of life, and have a neutral or favorable effect on overall cost of care.[76-78] Some studies also have documented a reduction in mortality among patients receiving multidisciplinary care.[79]

Dysrhythmias and Conduction Disorders

Age-related changes in the sinoatrial and AV nodes, as well as in the specialized conduction system of the heart, result in age-related increases in bradydysrhythmias and tachydysrhythmias.

As noted before, degenerative changes in and around the sinus node result in a marked decline in the number and effectiveness of sinus node pacemaker cells in older adults. These changes give rise to sick sinus syndrome, manifested by inappropriate resting bradycardia, chronotropic incompetence (inability to increase HR in response to increased demands imposed by normal activities), sinus pauses, and sinus arrest. AV nodal conduction disorders, such as first-degree AV block and Mobitz I second-degree AV block, are also common in patients with sick sinus syndrome and may worsen bradycardia. In addition, many patients also have supraventricular tachydysrhythmias, especially atrial fibrillation, resulting in tachy-brady syndrome, a common variant of sick sinus syndrome.

Sick sinus syndrome is the most frequent indication for permanent pacemaker implantation in the United States. More than 75 percent of all permanent pacemakers are placed in patients age 65 or older,[2] including 50 percent in persons over age 75. Most are for treatment of sick sinus syndrome.

The frequency and complexity of supraventricular and ventricular ectopic activity increase with age. However, in the absence of significant structural heart disease (e.g., coronary artery disease or cardiomyopathy),

■ ■ ■

TABLE 14-6 HEART FAILURE IN THE MIDDLE-AGED VERSUS THE ELDERLY

	MIDDLE-AGED	ELDERLY
Prevalence	Less than 1%	~10%
Gender	M more than F	F more than M
Cause	CAD	HTN
Clinical features	Typical	Atypical
LVEF	Reduced	Normal
Comorbidities	Few	Multiple
RCTs	Many	Few
Therapy	Evidence-based	Empiric
Physician	Cardiologist	Primary care

CAD, Coronary artery disease; *HTN*, hypertension; *LVEF*, left ventricular ejection fraction; *RCTs*, randomized clinical trials.
Data from Rich MW, Kitzman DW: *Am J Geriatr Cardiol* 9(suppl):97-104, 2000.

frequent isolated supraventricular and/or ventricular premature complexes are usually benign phenomena requiring no specific treatment.

Age-related changes in LV diastolic filling and accompanying changes in left atrial size and function predispose older adults to the development of atrial fibrillation. As illustrated in Figure 14-10,[80] the prevalence of atrial fibrillation increases progressively with age, and more than half of all cases of atrial fibrillation occur in the 6 percent of the population older than age 75. In addition, the proportion of strokes attributable to atrial fibrillation increases with age, from less than 2 percent in persons ages 50 to 59 to more than 20 percent in those over age 80.[81] Because older patients with diastolic dysfunction rely on atrial contraction to optimize LV filling, the onset of atrial fibrillation and the associated rapid HR often results in acute HF because of the sudden fall in CO and concomitant rise in LV diastolic pressure.

Although recent studies indicate that asymptomatic or minimally symptomatic atrial fibrillation can be managed effectively with rate-controlling agents (such as beta blockers, diltiazem, verapamil, and digoxin) in conjunction with warfarin,[82,83] management of atrial fibrillation in the elderly often is complicated by the presence of significant symptoms (especially exertional shortness of breath, fatigue, effort intolerance) or by contraindications to warfarin (such as fall risk and bleeding disorders). Therefore, optimal management of atrial fibrillation in the elderly remains the subject of numerous ongoing investigations.

Ventricular dysrhythmias, including ventricular tachycardia, also increase in frequency with age. At present, evaluation and management of ventricular dysrhythmias is similar in younger and older adults. It follows, therefore, that older adults often are considered candidates for implantable cardioverter-defibrillators (**ICDs**). Available evidence indicates that the benefits of ICDs are comparable in appropriately selected patients of all ages; thus age alone should not be considered a contraindication to ICD insertion.

CLINICAL DECISION MAKING IN ELDERLY PATIENTS WITH CARDIOVASCULAR DISEASE

Clinical decision making in elderly patients often is complicated by diagnostic uncertainty, arising from atypical or nonspecific symptoms, signs, and laboratory findings; by a lack of relevant high-quality data on which to base decisions, especially in the very elderly and in nursing home residents; by competing comorbidities that alter the benefit-risk equation, as in the use of antihypertensive drugs in patients with symptomatic orthostatic hypotension; by the inability to obtain informed input from the patient, as in acute delirium; by individual patient preferences regarding, for example, quality versus quantity of life; and by ageism—the tendency to withhold aggressive interventions solely based on advanced age.

In light of these factors, it is not surprising that elderly patients, especially those age 80 to 85 or older, are substantially less likely to receive evidenced-based cardiovascular procedures and therapies than younger patients with similar conditions, even when there is no apparent contraindication to their use.[84-86] At the present time, it is unclear to what extent the disparity in health care provided to the very elderly can be attributed to the various factors listed, and additional research is needed to address these issues. It is evident, however, that failure to undertake a specific intervention (such as thrombolytic therapy for acute MI or im-

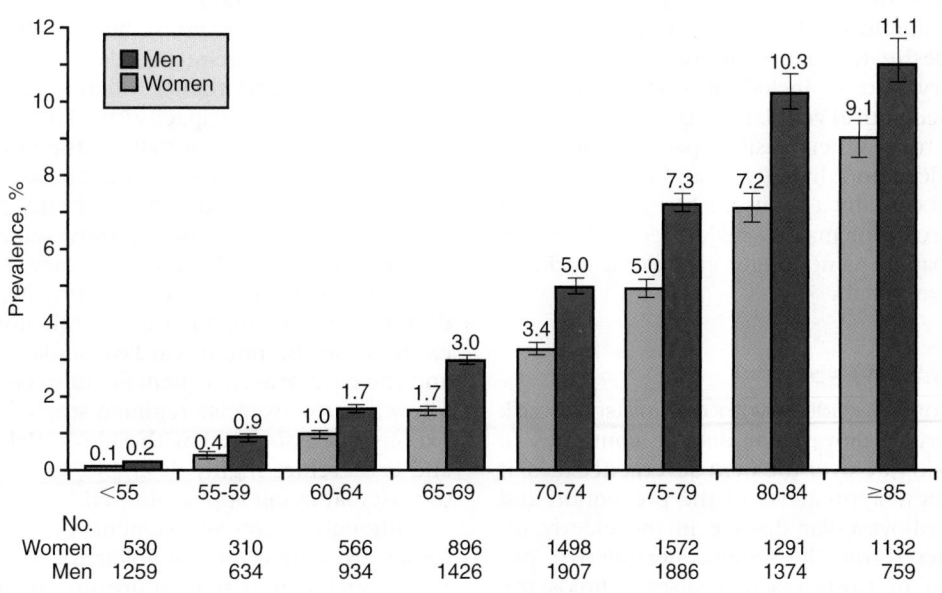

FIGURE 14-10 ■ Prevalence of atrial fibrillation in men and women in the United States. (Data from Go AS, Hylek EM, Phillips KA et al: *JAMA* 285:2370-2375, 2001.)

■■■

TABLE 14-7   EXPECTED REMAINING YEARS OF LIFE AT SELECTED AGES

AGE (YEARS)	REMAINING YEARS	
	MEN	WOMEN
25	51.0	55.8
50	28.3	32.2
65	16.6	19.5
70	13.2	15.8
75	10.3	12.4
80	7.8	9.4
85	5.7	6.9
90	4.2	5.0
95	3.2	3.7
100	2.5	2.8

From Arias E: United States life tables, 2002. *Natl Vital Stat Rep* vol 53, no 6, 2004.

plantation of an ICD) when based on a rational assessment of potential benefits and risks, or on the patient's stated preferences, does not equate with substandard care. Conversely, withholding treatment on the basis of age alone, without discussing the various options with the patient and family, should be avoided. In this regard, it must be recognized that the benefits of almost all proven cardiovascular interventions are realized within (at most) 2 to 3 years of implementation, a time frame that is well within the average remaining life expectancy of even the most elderly patients (Table 14-7).[1]

Considering the complexity of clinical decision making in the elderly, virtually all major nonemergent decisions should be made only after a frank discussion with the patient (and family, when appropriate) that includes a realistic appraisal of the short- and long-term risks and benefits of the various therapeutic options, giving due consideration to the patient's overall health and functional status, prevalent comorbid conditions, and individual preferences regarding treatment options and remaining life goals. In addition, patient preferences for end-of-life care should be discussed and documented, including the desire to receive or forgo specific life-sustaining interventions, including cardiopulmonary resuscitation, mechanical ventilation, renal dialysis, and use of a feeding tube. When feasible, patients should be encouraged to develop a living will and to designate a single individual (usually a spouse, sibling, or child) to serve as their proxy for making major decisions in the event that the patient is no longer capable of deciding on his or her own behalf.

FUTURE DIRECTIONS

As the number of older adults with cardiovascular risk factors and overt cardiovascular disease continues to increase at a rapid rate over the next several decades, it is evident that new approaches to the prevention and treatment of cardiovascular disease in the elderly urgently are needed. From the societal perspective, primary prevention of cardiovascular disease holds the greatest potential for reducing the morbidity, disability, costs, and mortality associated with heart and vascular

disease in older adults. Accordingly, current strategies are focused primarily in two arenas: early diagnosis and treatment of known cardiovascular risk factors in young and middle-aged persons, and the development of novel therapies that have a favorable impact on the aging process itself.

Recent data indicate that in the next half century, the increasing prevalence of obesity and diabetes in the United States may neutralize or even reverse longstanding trends toward increasing life expectancy.[87] Thus, stemming the tide of the obesity epidemic offers perhaps the greatest opportunity for reducing the future epidemic of cardiovascular disease in the elderly. Although extensive basic and clinical research clearly is needed, it is also apparent that there is a compelling need to alter dramatically the dietary and physical activity patterns on a population-wide basis, beginning in early childhood and continuing throughout adult life into old age. Likewise, more effective strategies for the diagnosis and early treatment of other major cardiovascular risk factors, including hypertension, dyslipidemia, and tobacco use, need to be developed and aggressively pursued. Ongoing basic science and translational research designed to elucidate the genetic basis for coronary risk factors also may play a crucial role in lessening the long-term impact of these highly prevalent and potent contributors to the cardiovascular disease burden.

Because cardiovascular aging plays a pivotal role in the development and progression of cardiovascular disease in older adults (including hypertension), a complementary approach to reducing cardiovascular risk factors is to develop strategies that slow the rate of aging in general and cardiovascular aging in particular. To date, research in this area has been directed at evaluating three general types of interventions: exercise, dietary modifications, and pharmaceutical agents. In the future, genetic manipulations (gene therapy) and stem cell therapies also may be used in an effort to alter the aging process favorably.

Regular aerobic exercise helps preserve vascular resilience, reduces age-related diastolic filling abnormalities, improves endothelial function, and increases cardiovascular reserve capacity.[88-92] Thus, lifelong exercise attenuates some (but not all) of the effects of aging on the cardiovascular system, and those who are trained tend to live longer and to have a better prognosis in the face of acute or chronic cardiovascular disease compared with those who are sedentary. Exercise also reduces the risk of obesity, diabetes, hypertension, and dyslipidemia. However, the overall impact of regular exercise on the rate of cardiovascular aging is modest, and the cardiovascular benefits of exercise decline rapidly when the exercise regimen stops.[93] In sum, regular exercise is associated with substantial health benefits and is therefore highly desirable, but its effects on cardiovascular aging appear limited.

Although dietary supplements promoted as antiaging tonics are a multimillion-dollar industry in the United States, such claims remain unsubstantiated and, for the most part, lack a scientific basis. However, a very low-fat vegetarian diet, when combined with other lifestyle changes, has been shown to slow or even reverse the rate of progression of atherosclerosis in some persons with established coronary artery disease,[94,95] implying that dietary factors may have the potential to alter cardiovascular aging favorably. Additional support for this concept comes from multiple studies involving laboratory animals and nonhuman primates, demonstrating that chronic caloric restriction slows the aging process across multiple organ systems and increases longevity by up to 50 percent.[96,97] In addition, recent data indicate that calorie restriction has a favorable effect on blood pressure, LV diastolic function, and inflammatory markers in middle-aged adults.[98] Thus, although the long-term effects of caloric restriction in human beings remain uncertain, the potential for reduced caloric intake to slow the rate of aging is the subject of active investigation.

Pharmacological agents with the potential for modulating the aging process by targeting specific age-related changes are also the subject of ongoing study. One agent, ALT-711, a nonenzymatic advanced-glycation end product (AGE) collagen cross-link breaker, has been shown to enhance vascular compliance in laboratory animals, nonhuman primates, and human beings.[99-102] In human studies, treatment with ALT-711 for 8 weeks was associated with a significant reduction in the aortic pulse pressure and pulse wave velocity, suggesting a favorable effect on vascular aging.[102] Although promising, the long-term effects of this agent are unknown. Other drugs with similar attributes are in development, and there also is ongoing work to develop a pharmaceutical agent that simulates the effects of caloric restriction without requiring major dietary modifications.

SUMMARY AND CONCLUSIONS

The population of the United States and other developed countries is aging rapidly, and the societal burden of cardiovascular disease in the elderly will increase dramatically over the next several decades. The high prevalence of cardiovascular disease in the elderly arises mainly as a result of age-related changes in cardiovascular structure and function, in conjunction with the cumulative effects of highly prevalent major cardiovascular risk factors. Age-related cardiovascular changes alter the clinical features and management of cardiovascular disease in older adults, and the high prevalence of noncardiovascular comorbid conditions also contributes importantly to disease presentation, response to therapy, and prognosis. Optimal diagnosis and treatment of cardiovascular disease in the elderly require consideration of the impact of normal aging changes and associated comorbid illnesses on an individualized basis, often using a multidisciplinary approach involving nurses, dietitians, pharmacists, physicians, social workers, and therapists. Future research focusing on preventing cardiovascular disease through risk factor reduction and by attenuating the effects of aging on the cardiovascular system holds the greatest promise for reducing the burden of cardiovascular disease in our progressively aging society.

REFERENCES

1. Arias E: United States life tables, 2002, *Natl Vital Stat Rep* vol 53, no 6, 2004. Retrieved November 30, 2006 from www.cdc.gov/nchs/data/nvsr/nvsr53/nvsr53_06.pdf
2. Thom T, Haase N, Rosamond W, et al. *Heart disease and stroke statistics—2006 update, Circulation* 113:e85-e151, 2006.
3. Popovic JR, Kozak LJ: National hospital discharge survey: annual summary, 1998. National Center for Health Statistics, *Vital Health Stat* vol 13, no 148, 2000. Retrieved November 30, 2006 from www.cdc.gov/nchs
4. US Census Bureau: *US interim projections by age, sex, race, and Hispanic origin.* Retrieved November 30, 2006 from www.census.gov/ipc/www/usinterimproj/natprojtab02a.pdf
5. Lakatta EG, Levy D: Arterial and cardiac aging: major shareholder in cardiovascular disease enterprises. I. Aging arteries: a "set up" for vascular disease, *Circulation* 107:139-146, 2003.
6. Lakatta EG, Levy D: Arterial and cardiac aging: major shareholders in cardiovascular disease enterprises. II. The aging heart in health: links to heart disease, *Circulation* 107:346-354, 2003.
7. Lakatta EG: Arterial and cardiac aging: major shareholders in cardiovascular disease enterprises. III. Cellular and molecular clues to heart and arterial aging, *Circulation* 107:490-497, 2003.
8. Rogers WJ, Hu YL, Coast D et al: Age-associated changes in regional aortic pulse wave velocity, *J Am Coll Cardiol* 38:1123-1129, 2001.
9. Gaasch WH, Levine HJ, Quinones MA et al: Left ventricular compliance: mechanisms and clinical implications, *Am J Cardiol* 38:645-653, 1976.
10. Celermajer DS, Sorensen KE, Spiegelhalter DJ et al: Aging is associated with endothelial dysfunction in healthy men years before the age-related decline in women, *J Am Coll Cardiol* 24:471-476, 1994.
11. Fleg JL, Bos AG, Brant LH et al: Longitudinal decline of aerobic capacity accelerates with age, *Circulation* 102(suppl 2):II-602, 2000.
12. Rich MW, Kitzman DW: Heart failure in octogenarians: a fundamentally different disease, *Am J Geriatr Cardiol* 9(suppl):97-104, 2000.
13. Cockcroft DW, Gault MH: Prediction of creatinine clearance from serum creatinine, *Nephron* 16:31-41, 1976.
14. Phillips PA, Rolls BJ, Ledingham JG et al: Reduced thirst after water deprivation in healthy elderly men, *N Engl J Med* 311:753-759, 1984.
15. Abete P, Ferrara N, Cacciatore F et al: Angina-induced protection against myocardial infarction in adult and elderly patients: a loss of preconditioning mechanism in the aging heart? *J Am Coll Cardiol* 30:947-954, 1997.
16. Edelberg JM, Reed MJ: Aging and angiogenesis, *Front Biosci* 8: s1199-s1209, 2003.
17. Braunstein JB, Anderson GF, Gerstenblith G et al: Noncardiac comorbidity increases preventable hospitalizations and mortality among Medicare beneficiaries with chronic heart failure, *J Am Coll Cardiol* 42:1226-1233, 2003.
18. Bibbins-Domingo K, Lin F, Vittinghoff E et al: Renal insufficiency as an independent predictor of mortality among women with heart failure, *J Am Coll Cardiol* 44:1593-1600, 2004.
19. Ezekowitz J, McAlister FA, Humphries KH et al: The association among renal insufficiency, pharmacotherapy, and outcomes in 6,427 patients with heart failure and coronary artery disease, *J Am Coll Cardiol* 44:1587-1592, 2004.
20. McAlister FA, Ezekowitz J, Tonelli M et al: Renal insufficiency and heart failure: prognostic and therapeutic implications from a prospective cohort study, *Circulation* 109:1004-1009, 2004.
21. Masoudi FA, Plomondon ME, Magid DJ et al: Renal insufficiency and mortality from acute coronary syndromes, *Am Heart J* 147:623-629, 2004.
22. Sadeghi HM, Stone GW, Grines CL et al: Impact of renal insufficiency in patients undergoing primary angioplasty for acute myocardial infarction, *Circulation* 108:2769-2775, 2003.
23. Lok CE, Austin PC, Wang H et al: Impact of renal insufficiency on short- and long-term outcomes after cardiac surgery, *Am Heart J* 148:430-438, 2004.
24. Nikolsky E, Aymong ED, Halkin A et al: Impact of anemia in patients with acute myocardial infarction undergoing primary percutaneous coronary intervention: analysis from the Controlled

Abciximab and Device Investigation to Lower Late Angioplasty Complications (CADILLAC) Trial, *J Am Coll Cardiol* 44:547-553, 2004.

25. Langston RD, Presley R, Flanders WD et al: Renal insufficiency and anemia are independent risk factors for death among patients with acute myocardial infarction, *Kidney Int* 64:1398-1405, 2003.

26. Anand I, McMurray JJ, Whitmore J et al: Anemia and its relationship to clinical outcome in heart failure, *Circulation* 110:149-154, 2004.

27. Kosiborod M, Smith GL, Radford MJ et al: The prognostic importance of anemia in patients with heart failure, *Am J Med* 114:112-119, 2003.

28. Ezekowitz JA, McAlister FA, Armstrong PW: Anemia is common in heart failure and is associated with poor outcomes: insights from a cohort of 12,065 patients with new-onset heart failure, *Circulation* 107:223-225, 2003.

29. Gami AS, Howard DE, Olson EJ et al: Day-night pattern of sudden death in obstructive sleep apnea, *N Engl J Med* 352:1206-1214, 2005.

30. Alonso-Fernandez A, Garcia-Rio F, Racionero MA et al: Cardiac rhythm disturbances and ST-segment depression episodes in patients with obstructive sleep apnea-hypopnea syndrome and its mechanisms, *Chest* 127:15-22, 2005.

31. Gami AS, Pressman G, Caples SM et al: Association of atrial fibrillation and obstructive sleep apnea, *Circulation* 110:364-367, 2004.

32. Bradley TD, Floras JS: Sleep apnea and heart failure. I. Obstructive sleep apnea, *Circulation* 107:1671-1678, 2003.

33. Leung RS, Bradley TD: Sleep apnea and cardiovascular disease, *Am J Respir Crit Care Med* 164:2147-2165, 2001.

34. McGann PE: Comorbidity in heart failure in the elderly, *Clin Geriatr Med* 16:631-648, 2000.

35. Zuccalà G, Pedone C, Cesari M et al: The effects of cognitive impairment on mortality among hospitalized patients with heart failure, *Am J Med* 115:97-103, 2003.

36. Rumsfeld JS, Havranek E, Masoudi FA et al: Depressive symptoms are the strongest predictors of short-term declines in health status in patients with heart failure, *J Am Coll Cardiol* 42:1811-1817, 2003.

37. Krumholz HM, Butler J, Miller J et al: Prognostic importance of emotional support for elderly patients hospitalized with heart failure, *Circulation* 97:958-964, 1998.

38. Vaccarino V, Kasl SV, Abramson J et al: Depressive symptoms and risk of functional decline and death in patients with heart failure, *J Am Coll Cardiol* 38:199-205, 2001.

39. Welin C, Lappas G, Wilhelmsen L: Independent importance of psychosocial factors for prognosis after myocardial infarction, *J Intern Med* 247:629-639, 2000.

40. Carney RM, Blumenthal JA, Catellier D et al: Depression as a risk factor for mortality after acute myocardial infarction, *Am J Cardiol* 92:1277-1281, 2003.

41. Carney RM, Freedland KE, Rich MW et al: Depression as a risk factor for cardiac events in established coronary heart disease: a review of possible mechanisms, *Ann Behav Med* 17:142-149, 1995.

42. Page J, Henry D: Consumption of NSAIDs and the development of congestive heart failure in elderly patients: an underrecognized public health problem, *Arch Intern Med* 160:777-784, 2000.

43. Solomon DH, Schneeweiss S, Glynn RJ et al: Relationship between selective cyclooxygenase-2 inhibitors and acute myocardial infarction in older adults, *Circulation* 109:2068-2073, 2004.

44. Topol EJ: Failing the public health: rofecoxib, Merck, and the FDA, *N Engl J Med* 351:1707-1709, 2004.

45. Hamerman D: Toward an understanding of frailty, *Ann Intern Med* 130:945-950, 1999.

46. Fried LP, Tangen CM, Walston J et al: Cardiovascular Health Study Collaborative Research Group: frailty in older adults—evidence for a phenotype, *J Gerontol A Biol Sci Med Sci* 56:M146-M156, 2001.

47. Nolan L, O'Malley K: Prescribing for the elderly. I. Sensitivity of the elderly to adverse drug reactions, *J Am Geriatr Soc* 36:142-149, 1988.

48. Schepkens H, Vanholder R, Billiouw JM et al: Life-threatening hyperkalemia during combined therapy with angiotensin-converting enzyme inhibitors and spironolactone: an analysis of 25 cases, *Am J Med* 110:438-441, 2001.

49. Juurlink DN, Mamdani MM, Lee DS et al: Rates of hyperkalemia after publication of the Randomized Aldactone Evaluation Study, *N Engl J Med* 351:543-551, 2004.

50. Masoudi FA, Havranek EP, Wolfe P et al: Most hospitalized older persons do not meet the enrollment criteria for clinical trials in heart failure, *Am Heart J* 146:250-257, 2003.

51. Heiat A, Gross CP, Krumholz HM: Representation of the elderly, women, and minorities in heart failure clinical trials, *Arch Intern Med* 162:1682-1688, 2002.

52. Burt VL, Cutler JA, Higgins M et al: Trends in the prevalence, awareness, treatment, and control of hypertension in the adult US population: data from the Health Examination Surveys, 1960 to 1991, *Hypertension* 26:60-69, 1995.

53. Kannel WB: Prevalence and implications of uncontrolled systolic hypertension, *Drugs Aging* 20:277-286, 2003.

54. Management Committee: Treatment of mild hypertension in the elderly, *Med J Aust* 2:398-402, 1981.

55. Amery A, Birkenhager W, Brixko P et al: Mortality and morbidity results from the European Working Party on High Blood Pressure in the Elderly Trial, *Lancet* 1:1349-1354, 1985.

56. Coope J, Warrender TS: Randomised trial of treatment of hypertension in elderly patients in primary care, *BMJ* 293:1145-1151, 1986.

57. Dahlof B, Lindholm LH, Hannson L et al: Morbidity and mortality in the Swedish Trial in Old Patients with Hypertension (STOP-Hypertension), *Lancet* 338:1281-1285, 1991.

58. MRC Working Party: Medical Research Council Trial of Treatment of Hypertension in Older Adults: principal results, *BMJ* 304:405-412, 1992.

59. Hypertension Detection and Follow-up Program Cooperative Group: Five-year findings of the Hypertension Detection and Follow-up Program. I. Reduction in mortality of persons with high blood pressure, including mild hypertension, *JAMA* 242:2562-2571, 1979.

60. Systolic Hypertension in the Elderly Program (SHEP) Cooperative Research Group: Prevention of stroke by antihypertensive drug treatment in older persons with isolated systolic hypertension: final results of SHEP, *JAMA* 265:3255-3264, 1991.

61. Staessen JA, Fagard R, Thijs L et al: Randomised double-blind comparison of placebo and active treatment for older patients with isolated systolic hypertension: the Systolic Hypertension in Europe (Syst-Eur) Trial Investigators, *Lancet* 350:757-764, 1997.

62. Gong L, Zhang W, Zhu Y et al: Shanghai Trial of Nifedipine in the Elderly (STONE), *J Hypertens* 14:1237-1245, 1996.

63. Liu L, Wang JG, Gong L et al: Comparison of active treatment and placebo in older Chinese patients with isolated systolic hypertension: Systolic Hypertension in China (Syst-China) Collaborative Group, *J Hypertens* 16:1823-1829, 1998.

64. Chobanian AV, Bakris GL, Black HR et al: The Seventh Report of the Joint National Committee on Prevention, Detection, Evaluation, and Treatment of High Blood Pressure: the JNC 7 report, *JAMA* 289:2560-2572, 2003.

65. Batchelor WB, Anstrom KJ, Muhlbaier LH et al: Contemporary outcome trends in the elderly undergoing percutaneous coronary interventions: results in 7,472 octogenarians—National Cardiovascular Network Collaboration, *J Am Coll Cardiol* 36:723-730, 2000.

66. Alexander KP, Anstrom KJ, Muhlbaier LH et al: Outcomes of cardiac surgery in patients > 80 years: results from the National Cardiovascular Network, *J Am Coll Cardiol* 35:731-738, 2000.

67. Gehlot A, Mullany CJ, Ilstrup D et al: Aortic valve replacement in patients aged eighty years and older: early and long-term results, *J Thorac Cardiovasc Surg* 111:1026-1036, 1996.

68. Sundt TM, Bailey MS, Moon MR et al: Quality of life after aortic valve replacement at the age of > 80 years, *Circulation* 102(suppl 3):III70-III74, 2000.

69. Aronow WS, Ahn C, Kronzon I et al: Association of mitral annular calcium with new thromboembolic stroke at 44-month follow-up of 2,148 persons, mean age 81 years, *Am J Cardiol* 81:105-106, 1998.

70. Redfield MM, Rodeheffer RJ, Jacobsen SJ et al: Plasma brain natriuretic peptide concentration: impact of age and gender, *J Am Coll Cardiol* 40:976-982, 2002.

71. Vasan RS, Larson MG, Benjamin EJ et al: Congestive heart failure in subjects with normal versus reduced left ventricular ejection fraction: prevalence and mortality in a population-based cohort, *J Am Coll Cardiol* 33:1948-1955, 1999.

72. Kitzman DW, Gardin JM, Gottdiener JS et al: Importance of heart failure with preserved systolic function in patients − 65 years of age: CHS Research Group, Cardiovascular Health Study, *Am J Cardiol* 87:413-419, 2001.

73. Senni M, Redfield MM: Heart failure with preserved systolic function: a different natural history? *J Am Coll Cardiol* 38:1277-1282, 2001.

74. Kitzman DW, Little WC, Brubaker PH et al: Pathophysiological characterization of isolated diastolic heart failure in comparison to systolic heart failure, *JAMA* 288:2144-2150, 2002.

75. Rich MW, Beckham V, Wittenberg C et al: A multidisciplinary intervention to prevent the readmission of elderly patients with congestive heart failure, *N Engl J Med* 333:1190-1195, 1995.

76. Gonseth J, Guallar-Castillon P, Banegas JR et al: The effectiveness of disease management programmes in reducing hospital readmission in older patients with heart failure: a systematic review and meta-analysis of published reports, *Eur Heart J* 25:1570-1595, 2004.

77. McAlister FA, Stewart S, Ferrua S et al: Multidisciplinary strategies for the management of heart failure patients at high risk for admission: a systematic review of randomized trials, *J Am Coll Cardiol* 44:810-819, 2004.

78. Phillips CO, Wright SM, Kern DE et al: Comprehensive discharge planning with postdischarge support for older patients with congestive heart failure: a meta-analysis, *JAMA* 291:1358-1367, 2004.

79. Stewart S, Horowitz JD: Home-based intervention in congestive heart failure: long-term implications on readmission and survival, *Circulation* 105:2861-2866, 2002.

80. Go AS, Hylek EM, Phillips KA et al: Prevalence of diagnosed atrial fibrillation in adults: national implications for rhythm management and stroke prevention—the AnTicoagulation and Risk Factors in Atrial Fibrillation (ATRIA) Study, *JAMA* 285:2370-2375, 2001.

81. Wolf PA, Abbott RD, Kannel WB: Atrial fibrillation as an independent risk factor for stroke: the Framingham Study, *Stroke* 22:983-988, 1991.

82. Wyse DG, Waldo AL, DiMarco JP et al: A comparison of rate control and rhythm control in patients with atrial fibrillation, *N Engl J Med* 347:1825-1833, 2002.

83. Van Gelder IC, Hagens VE, Bosker HA et al: A comparison of rate control and rhythm control in patients with recurrent persistent atrial fibrillation, *N Engl J Med* 347:1834-1840, 2002.

84. Rathore SS, Mehta RH, Wang Y et al: Effects of age on the quality of care provided to older patients with acute myocardial infarction, *Am J Med* 114:307-315, 2003.

85. Shahi CN, Rathore SS, Wang Y et al: Quality of care among elderly patients hospitalized with unstable angina, *Am Heart J* 142:263-270, 2001.

86. Masoudi FA, Rathore SS, Wang Y et al: National patterns of use and effectiveness of angiotensin-converting enzyme inhibitors in older patients with heart failure and left ventricular systolic dysfunction, *Circulation* 110:724-731, 2004.

87. Olshansky SJ, Passaro DJ, Hershow RC et al: A potential decline in life expectancy in the United States in the 21st century, *N Engl J Med* 352:1138-1145, 2005.

88. Seals DR: Habitual exercise and the age-associated decline in large artery compliance, *Exerc Sport Sci Rev* 31:68-72, 2003.

89. DeSouza CA, Shapiro LF, Clevenger CM et al: Regular aerobic exercise prevents and restores age-related declines in endothelium-dependent vasodilatation in healthy men, *Circulation* 102:1351-1357, 2000.

90. Beere PA, Russell SD, Morey MC et al: Aerobic exercise training can reverse age-related peripheral circulatory changes in healthy older men, *Circulation* 100:1085-1094, 1999.

91. Palka P, Lange A, Nihoyannopoulos P: The effect of long-term training on age-related left ventricular changes by Doppler myocardial velocity gradient, *Am J Cardiol* 84:1061-1067, 1999.

92. Petrella RJ, Cunningham DA, Paterson DH: Effects of 5-day exercise training in elderly subjects on resting left ventricular diastolic function and VO2max, *Can J Appl Physiol* 22:37-47, 1997.

93. Fatouros IG, Jamurtas AZ, Villiotou V et al: Oxidative stress responses in older men during endurance training and detraining, *Med Sci Sports Exerc* 36:2065-2072, 2004.

94. Koertge J, Weidner G, Elliott-Eller M et al: Improvement in medical risk factors and quality of life in women and men with coronary artery disease in the Multicenter Lifestyle Demonstration Project, *Am J Cardiol* 91:1316-1322, 2003.

95. Ornish D, Scherwitz LW, Billings JH et al: Intensive lifestyle changes for reversal of coronary artery disease, *JAMA* 280:2001-2007, 1998.

96. Heilbronn LK, Ravussin E: Calorie restriction and aging: review of the literature and implications for studies in humans, *Am J Clin Nutr* 78:361-369, 2003.

97. Lane MA, Mattison J, Ingram DK et al: Caloric restriction and aging in primates: relevance to humans and possible CR mimetics, *Microsc Res Tech* 59:335-338, 2002.

98. Susic D, Varagic J, Ahn J et al: Crosslink breakers: a new approach to cardiovascular therapy, *Curr Opin Cardiol* 19:336-340, 2004.

99. Asif M, Egan J, Vasan S et al: An advanced glycation endproduct cross-link breaker can reverse age-related increases in myocardial stiffness, *Proc Natl Acad Sci U S A* 97:2809-2813, 2000.

100. Vaitkevicius PV, Lane M, Spurgeon H et al: A cross-link breaker has sustained effects on arterial and ventricular properties in older rhesus monkeys, *Proc Natl Acad Sci U S A* 98:1171-1175, 2001.

101. Kass DA, Shapiro EP, Kawaguchi M et al: Improved arterial compliance by a novel advanced glycation end-product crosslink breaker, *Circulation* 104:1464-1470, 2001.

102. Lane MA, Ingram DK, Roth GS: The serious search for an anti-aging pill, *Sci Am* 287(2):36-41, 2002.

chapter 15

The Impact of Cardiac Disease on Psychological State

Diane L. Carroll
Barbara Riegel

CHAPTER ABBREVIATIONS

AMI   acute myocardial infarction
BDI   Beck Depression Inventory
CABG   coronary artery bypass grafting
CHD   coronary heart disease
HRQL   health-related quality of life
ICD   implantable cardioverter-defibrillator
KCCQ   Kansas City Cardiomyopathy Questionnaire
LHFQ   Minnesota Living with Heart Failure Questionnaire
NYHA   New York Heart Association
SAQ   Seattle Angina Questionnaire
SF-36   Short Form 36 (generic measure of HRQL)
STAI   State Trait Anxiety Inventory

The development of cardiac disease has a profound effect on a person's psychological state and quality of life. Decades of research have illustrated that a cardiac diagnosis can cause anxiety, depression, and poor quality of life. In this chapter, we describe the impact of acute cardiac events on these psychological states and emotions.

Emotions, in general, exist on a continuum from normal to pathological. As a response to a changing environment, emotions allow flexibility in human behavioral responses. When emotions become uncontrollable, accentuated, and persistent, they are destructive. The importance of subjective psychological states is evident in subsequent chapters that discuss how these states negatively affect prognosis. Our purpose is to illustrate the influence of cardiac disease on psychological state.

ANXIETY

Anxiety is a negative affective state resulting from a perceived threat. This extremely distressing emotion is characterized by a perceived inability to predict, control, or mitigate a given situation.[1] Anxiety has cognitive, neurobiological, and behavioral components that arise out of a person's interaction with the environment (Table 15-1).[2]

Anxiety is considered an adaptive process until its magnitude or persistence renders it a dysfunctional response that can have negative consequences. Examples of persistent and dysfunctional anxiety disorders include panic disorder, phobic anxiety, generalized anxiety, anxiety reactions, and chronic anxiety.

With Coronary Heart Disease

Anxiety is common in those who have chronic coronary heart disease (**CHD**) and among those recovering from acute cardiac events.[3] In fact, anxiety is more common than depression. The prevalence of anxiety is about 70 to 80 percent among patients suffering an acute cardiac event and persists chronically in about 20 to 25 percent of those with CHD. Even in persons with chronic CHD who have never had an acute event, the prevalence of anxiety is 20 to 25 percent.[4] Although anxiety is an expected and even normal reaction to an acute cardiac event or the threat of living with a chronic illness, anxiety is not benign if it persists or is extreme.

After Myocardial Infarction

Following acute myocardial infarction (**AMI**), 10 to 26 percent of patients have elevated anxiety, with rates as high as 50 percent during hospitalization and higher-than-normal anxiety levels during the first 2 weeks at home.[5] For example, one sample of 486 patients (mean age 62, 67 percent male, 33 percent female) admitted to a hospital with an AMI completed the Spielberger State Trait Anxiety Inventory (**STAI**) within 72 hours of admission.[6] Their overall mean state anxiety score was significantly higher (39 ± 13) than that seen in normal adults of this age-group (34.5 ± 10.3 men; 32.2 ± 8.7 women). When the data were divided into groups based on time of completion of the STAI, anxiety was highest in the first 12 hours after admission ($p < 0.05$), and women rated their anxiety higher than men ($p < 0.001$). Others have found that patients with AMI had anxiety levels higher than that of patients with a psychiatric disorder.[7,8]

The prevalence and severity of anxiety after AMI have not been studied extensively in international populations, although anxiety is known to be a universal emotion[9] found in every country studied.[10] Additionally, somatization of anxiety—psychological issues expressed as physical symptoms—appears to be a common reaction across cultures.[11] This topic is significant because the population of the United States and of countries around the world is becoming increasingly diverse and multicultural.

In a prospective, comparative, cross-cultural investigation, Moser and colleagues[12] compared anxiety within the first 72 hours of hospital admission for AMI in 912 patients from five different countries: Australia, England, Japan, South Korea, and the United States. Women had higher anxiety levels than men (0.76 ± 0.90 versus 0.57 ± 0.70,

TABLE 15-1 PHYSIOLOGICAL, BEHAVIORAL, COGNITIVE, AND AFFECTIVE RESPONSES TO ANXIETY

RESPONSE	BODY SYSTEM AFFECTED	EFFECT	RESPONSE	BODY SYSTEM AFFECTED	EFFECT
Physiological	Cardiovascular	Decreased blood pressure*	Behavioral	Accident proneness	Hypervigilance
		Decreased pulse rate*		Avoidance	Inhibition
		Fainting*		Flight	Interpersonal withdrawal
		Faintness*		Hyperventilation	Lack of coordination
		Increased blood pressure			Physical tension
		Palpitations			Rapid speech
		Racing heart			Restlessness
	Respiratory	Choking sensation			Startle reaction
		Gasping			Tremors
		Lump in throat		Cognitive	Blocking of thoughts
		Pressure on chest			Confusion
		Rapid breathing			Decreased perceptual field
		Shallow breathing			Diminished productivity
		Shortness of breath			Errors in judgment
	Gastrointestinal	Abdominal discomfort			Fear of injury or death
		Abdominal pain*			Fear of losing control
		Diarrhea*			Flashbacks
		Heartburn*			Forgetfulness
		Loss of appetite			Frightening visual images
		Nausea*			Impaired attention
		Revulsion toward food			Loss of objectivity
	Neuromuscular	Clumsy movement			Nightmares
		Eyelid twitching			Poor concentration
		Fidgeting			Preoccupation
		Generalized weakness			Reduced creativity
		Increased reflexes			Self-consciousness
		Insomnia		Affective	Alarm
		Pacing			Edginess
		Rigidity			Fear
		Startle reaction			Fright
		Strained face			Frustration
		Tremors			Guilt
		Wobbly legs			Helplessness
	Urinary tract	Frequent urination*			Impatience
		Pressure to urinate*			Jitteriness
	Skin	Flushed face			Jumpiness
		Generalized sweating			Nervousness
		Hot and cold spells			Numbing
		Itching			Shame
		Localized sweating (e.g., palms)			Tension
		Pale face			Terror
					Uneasiness

*Parasympathetic response.
From Stuart GW, Laraia MT: *Principles and practice of psychiatric nursing*, ed 7, St Louis, 2001, Elsevier Mosby.

$p = 0.005$ main effect for gender), and this pattern of higher anxiety in women was seen in every country studied. Neither sociodemographic nor clinical variables could explain the differences in anxiety between the sexes.

The mean level of anxiety in the full sample, assessed using the Brief Symptom Inventory, was 0.62 ± 0.76 (range 0 to 3.83), which is 44 percent higher than the normal mean level reported in a sample of healthy adults. The published norms are 0.35 ± 0.45 for nonpatient subjects, 1.5 ± 1.1 for psychiatric inpatients, and 1.7 ± 1.0 for psychiatric outpatients.[13] Levels of anxiety for each country are shown in Figure 15-1. Anxiety following AMI was 54 percent higher than normal in Australia, 34 percent higher than normal in England, 89

percent higher than normal in Japan, 83 percent higher than normal in South Korea, and 97 percent higher than normal in the United States. A total of 46, 35, 43, 52, and 50 percent of patients in Australia, England, Japan, South Korea, and the United States, respectively, reported anxiety levels higher than the normal reference mean.

To evaluate whether there are unique cultural factors that influence the expression of anxiety, De Jong and colleagues[14] reanalyzed these data to test for an interaction between country and sociodemographic and clinical variables. Age, gender, marital status, education level, medical history, Killip classification on admission, use of various therapies in the emergency department, and pain level were examined. None of these variables

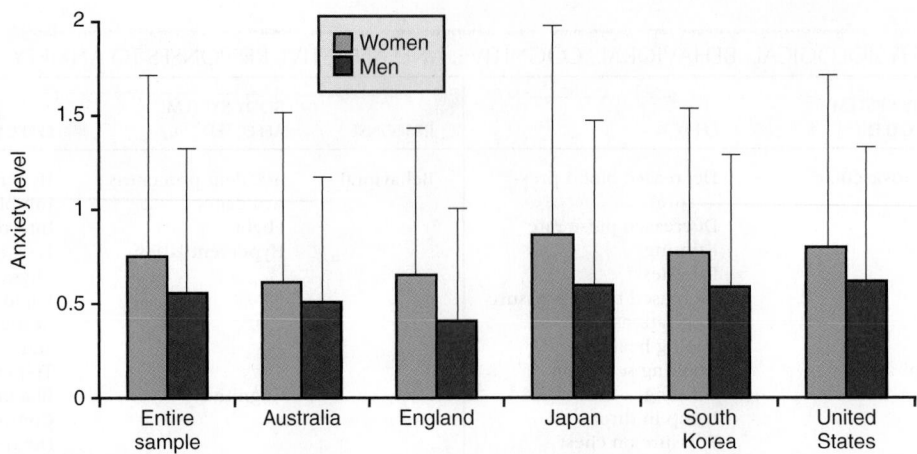

FIGURE 15-1 ■ Gender differences in anxiety overall and in each country. (Data from Moser DK, Dracup K, McKinley S et al: An international perspective on gender differences in anxiety early after acute myocardial infarction, *Psychosom Med* 65:514, 2003.)

interacted with country to affect anxiety. Clearly, AMI causes anxiety, and it is a universal phenomenon unexplained by sociodemographic and cultural differences.

Although anxiety is a universal emotion found in all societies, the expression and communication of anxiety are believed to be culturally different.[11] Others argue, however, that apparent differences are really a reflection of culturally unique schemas or patterns, appraisal propensities, behavior repertoires, or regulation processes.[15,16] That is, emotions are social constructs, but with a specific threat-anticipation of physical danger, a universal response may be generated. Thus, the expectation that there are cultural differences in the experience of anxiety may be unfounded.

In summary, anxiety is elevated following AMI and the diagnosis of chronic CHD, and this is not a uniquely North American response. Cultural responses may influence the manner in which anxiety is expressed, which influences our ability to assess the response. However, patients with CHD or AMI can be anticipated to experience anxiety.

After Coronary Artery Bypass Graft Surgery

Most persons undergoing coronary artery bypass graft (**CABG**) surgery experience it as a life-threatening procedure.[17] Uncertainty about the outcome can make the period before the operation anxiety-producing, especially in patients who are symptomatic.[18,19] Thus, it is not surprising that the recovery process after CABG surgery is neither simple nor consistent. In one study the incidence of anxiety increased from 27 percent preoperatively to 45 percent ($p < 0.001$) postoperatively.[20] In general, patients with elevated levels of anxiety before surgery maintain these levels during recovery.[21] For example, in another study, 55 percent of patients were highly anxious preoperatively, 34 percent were anxious shortly after surgery, and 23 percent still had clinically relevant levels of anxiety 3 months after surgery.[22] By 6 months,[23,24] anxiety can be expected to return to the preoperative level for most, although some patients may require a year to recover fully.[25] Gender differences in

anxiety after CABG surgery have been found by some investigators but not by others.[26]

In one large study of 330 persons undergoing CABG surgery, almost 30 percent of patients failed to experience a favorable resolution of their initial anxiety after 1 year.[24] Researchers have focused on identifying factors associated with anxiety and its resolution after CABG. Cognitive functioning is associated with anxiety in this population.[27] Recent studies suggest that a significant number of persons undergoing CABG may have subtle problems with memory, attention, and executive function (i.e., higher-order cognitive abilities) going into surgery. Postoperatively, elevated anxiety appears to accentuate the subjective perception of these deficits.[28]

Coping style is another factor that influences anxiety related to CABG surgery. In one study the coping style associated with resolution of anxiety in the months after CABG was a sensitizing style, defined as an awareness of internal impulses and feelings.[24] Preoperative state anxiety measured using the trait scale of the STAI resolved best over the year of follow-up in patients using sensitizing, rather than repressive coping.

With Heart Failure

Anxiety in persons with heart failure has been studied only recently. One investigative team found mean anxiety scores in heart failure patients to be only slightly higher than the general population.[29] However, patients who were more functionally compromised (i.e., New York Heart Association [**NYHA**] Class III) had higher anxiety than those with less compromise (NYHA Class I or II). A recent comparison of heart failure patients to other cardiac patient groups and to healthy older adults found that anxiety was similar in the patient groups but higher than that experienced by healthy older adults.[30]

In a recent study of 100 outpatients with systolic heart failure drawn from a community heart failure program in the United Kingdom, the prevalence of anxiety was 18.4 percent by clinical diagnostic interview.[31] Predictors of anxiety included a history of mental illness, comorbid physical illness (diabetes and angina), and

NYHA class. Interestingly, anxiety was not higher in patients with relatively poorer systolic function.

Anxiety levels can vary as a function of the timing of measurement. In a study of 119 persons with heart failure, anxiety was the first emotion experienced immediately after diagnosis. Anxiety levels were high at this time, but they increased even further over the first year after diagnosis.[32] These data illustrate that anxiety is not a temporary response in this patient group. Further research is needed to understand the factors associated with anxiety in those with heart failure. This information is essential for the design of interventions for patients experiencing anxiety as a chronic emotional response.[33]

After Device Implantation

Anxiety has been identified as a prominent emotional response in recipients of implantable cardioverter-defibrillators (**ICDs**). ICD recipients have a 24 to 87 percent incidence of elevated levels of anxiety, with an estimated 13 to 38 percent incidence of clinically significant anxiety disorders.[34] Dunbar and colleagues[35] reported that ICD recipients who had dysrhythmic events had higher psychological distress (specifically anxiety, fatigue, and confusion) compared with those who did not experience such events after implantation.

Psychological response is influenced by the actual activation of the ICD that causes the recipient to receive a shock; anxiety is clearly the most common response to ICD shock.[36] Eckert and Jones[37] performed a thematic analysis of recipients' responses to receiving a shock and identified that the lack of control over ICD shock occurrence precipitated feelings of anxiety and powerlessness.

Comparison of Anxiety in Cardiac and General Populations

Comparisons of anxiety in cardiac patient populations to general population groups are uncommon, but we do know that anxiety is higher in persons experiencing AMI than in patients with a psychiatric disorder[7,8] and in healthy adults.[13] Anxiety in persons with heart failure is similar to that experienced by other cardiac patient groups, at least initially, but higher than that experienced by healthy older adults.[30] Anxiety in persons with heart failure may last longer than that experienced by other cardiac patient groups. More research is needed to compare anxiety in the cardiac population with that experienced by other patient populations and by well elders. This type of research will facilitate clinical assessment and intervention.

Clinical Assessment

Accurate assessment of anxiety in cardiac patients is key to treatment. De Jong and colleagues[14] determined that physiological parameters, such as elevated heart rate and blood pressure, were not correlated with levels of anxiety in AMI patients. These results call into question the longstanding belief that elevated blood pressure and heart rate is evidence of anxiety. An unexpected finding in that study was that higher anxiety was associated with a lower blood pressure. The mechanism explaining this response requires further study.

The study by De Jong and colleagues[14] illustrates the need to assess anxiety using a standardized approach that can be replicated over time. Several short, concise screening instruments are available for assessing anxiety. Table 15-2 gives a list of instruments and the range of scores considered to indicate a level of anxiety requiring further assessment with clinical interview.

A clinical interview is a patient-led interaction in which the health care provider uses communication skills and active listening.[38] The goals of a clinical interview are to identify and explore anxiety, discuss healthful ways of reducing the anxiety response, build a satisfying interpersonal relationship between the clinician and the patient, and provide an opportunity for the patient to feel understood and comfortable. The clinical interview allows for the communication of emotional

■ ■ ■

TABLE 15-2   ANXIETY BEHAVIOR RATING SCALES

SCALE	MEASURES	WHERE TO OBTAIN
Beck Anxiety Scale	21-item questionnaire used to differentiate between anxiety and depression symptoms that minimally overlap with those of anxiety Established reliability	Purchase from *http://harcourtassessment.com/HAIWEB/Cultures/en-us/Productdetail.htm?Pid=015-8018-400&Mode5summary* 1-800-211-8378
Hamilton Rating Scale for Anxiety	13-items that measure global anxiety including cognitive and somatic symptoms	In Hamilton M: The assessment of anxiety state by rating, *Br J Med Psychol* 32: 50-59, 1959
Spielberger State-Trait Anxiety Inventory	Two 20-item questionnaires, one measuring trait (long-standing) and one measuring state (situational) anxiety Easy to use Established reliability	Purchase from *www.mindgarden.com*
Zung Anxiety Scales	20-item self-rating scale	In Zung WWK: A rating instrument for anxiety disorders, *Psychosomatics* 12:371-379, 1971
Hospital Anxiety-Depression Scale	14-item scale that quantifies both anxiety and depression in hospitalized patients Has had limited use in the United States	Purchase from *www.nfer-nelson.co.uk*

concerns in a caring environment, which facilitates the measurement of anxiety.

DEPRESSION

Depression is a highly prevalent and disabling mental illness that is associated with as much disability, dysfunction, and impairment in daily functioning as other chronic illnesses. In one study comparing the costs of various chronic conditions, depression and psychosis had the highest annual costs in a Medicaid population.[39] Yet depression is greatly underdiagnosed and undertreated in the United States, especially in the cardiac patient population.[40,41]

Major depression is defined as the daily presence of at least five of the nine symptoms shown in Box 15-1 for at least a 2-week period.[42] Minor depression is diagnosed when the person has some of the symptoms in Box 15-1 and doing regular activities takes extra effort. These symptoms can be indicated by the subjective account of the patient or by observations of significant others.

With Coronary Heart Disease

About 20 percent of all cardiac disease patients meet the diagnostic criteria for major depression, with higher rates in those with unstable angina and those awaiting CABG surgery.[9] A distinct gender difference is found in the prevalence of depression in cardiac patients, with females reporting about twice as much depression as males.[43]

After Myocardial Infarction

A recent review of 86 original research studies illustrated that about 20 percent of persons hospitalized for AMI have major depression and an additional 10 to 47 percent have significant depressive symptoms.[44] The symptoms of depression are surprisingly stable after AMI. Most patients who experience a major depressive episode after AMI continue to have symptoms 3 or 4 months later, suggesting that these symptoms represent something more serious than a transient reaction.[45] Although depression and anxiety are often highly correlated (e.g., $r = 0.56$ in one study of patients following AMI),[46] both should be screened for.

BOX 15-1   ■ ■ ■
SYMPTOMS OF MAJOR DEPRESSION

- Depressed mood most of the day, particularly in the morning
- Greatly diminished interest or pleasure in almost all activities (anhedonia) nearly every day
- Significant weight loss or gain
- Insomnia or hypersomnia
- Psychomotor agitation or retardation
- Fatigue or loss of energy
- Feelings of worthlessness or guilt
- Impaired concentration, indecisiveness
- Recurring thoughts of death or suicide

Data from American Psychiatric Association: *Diagnostic and statistical manual of mental disorders*, Primary Care Version (DSM-IV-PC), ed 4, Washington, DC, 2000, American Psychiatric Association Press.

After Coronary Artery Bypass Graft Surgery

Depression is common after CABG, as illustrated in a recent study of 137 patients undergoing elective isolated first CABG surgery.[47] Prevalence of major depressive disorder detected by structured diagnostic interview or the Beck Depression Inventory (**BDI**) during the month before surgery was 28.2 percent, but 6 to 12 weeks after surgery, that prevalence decreased to 16.4 percent ($p = 0.04$). When depression was compared in the 72 men and 65 women, women had significantly more depressive symptoms than men before CABG: mean BDI 12.5 (95 percent confidence interval [CI], 10.6 to 14.4) for women versus 8.0 (95 percent CI, 6.3 to 9.8) for men ($p = 0.0001$). After the surgery, depressive symptoms improved almost sixfold more in women than in men. Depression is a particularly important emotional outcome in persons undergoing CABG because it independently predicts cardiac rehospitalizations, continued surgical pain, and failure to return to prior activity at 6 months. The fact that presurgical depression predicts postsurgical depression[48] illustrates the importance of screening for this emotion.

With Heart Failure

The prevalence of depression has been estimated to range from 13 to 77 percent in patients with heart failure, depending on the timing and manner in which depression was measured.[49,50] Higher rates are found in hospitalized patients (point prevalence 37 percent) than those assessed in an outpatient setting (point prevalence 26 percent).[51] Another 16 percent of hospitalized patients meet criteria for minor depression.[52] Together, up to 50 percent of heart failure patients can be expected to have depressive symptoms or minor or major depression.

Depression is higher in persons with heart failure who have a relatively worse severity of illness, poorer functional capacity, more comorbid conditions, and more symptoms.[53] Depression is believed to be approximately equal in men and women with heart failure, although evidence is accumulating to suggest that the women may have higher levels of depression.[54-56]

Differing rates of depression across the various studies may be related to the methods of assessment used. Those who used the Diagnostic Interview Schedule, a tool used by trained interviewers to identify major depression, found lower rates of depression; whereas those using scales designed to measure depressive symptoms (e.g., the BDI) reported higher rates of depression.[33]

After Device Implantation

Early studies of patient response to implantation of a device demonstrated mainly anxiety and impaired quality of life, but depression was reported in a significant number of ICD recipients. Depression is particularly problematic in ICD recipients who experience a defibrillatory shock. In one study of 15 survivors of sudden cardiac arrest who were treated with an ICD, depression—as well as anxiety, anger, and stress—was higher in patients who had received a shock (and in members of those patients' families).[57] In another study, patients who were depressed expressed many fears and concerns; reductions in physical activities were associated consistently with depression in ICD recipients.[35]

■ ■ ■

TABLE 15-3 DIFFERENCES BETWEEN ANXIETY AND DEPRESSION

ANXIETY	DEPRESSION
Predominantly fear or apprehension	Predominantly sad or hopeless with feelings of despair
Difficulty falling asleep (initial insomnia)	Early morning awakening (late insomnia) or hypersomnia
	Diurnal variation (feels worse in the morning)
Phobic avoidance behavior	Slowed speech and thought processes
Rapid pulse and psychomotor hyperactivity	Psychomotor retardation (agitation also may occur)
Breathing disturbances	Delayed response time
Tremors and palpitations	
Sweating and hot or cold spells	
Faintness, light-headedness, dizziness	
Depersonalization (feeling detached from one's body)	Inability to experience pleasure
Derealization (feeling that one's environment is strange, unreal, or unfamiliar)	Loss of interest in usual activities
Selective and specific negative appraisals that do not include all areas of life	Negative appraisals are pervasive, global, and exclusive
Sees some prospects for the future	Thoughts of death or suicide
	Sees the future as blank and has given up all hope
Does not regard defects or mistakes as irrevocable	Regards mistakes as beyond redemption
Uncertain in negative evaluations	Absolute in negative evaluations
Predicts that only certain events may go badly	Global view that nothing will turn out right

From Stuart GW, Laraia MT: *Principles and practice of psychiatric nursing,* ed 7, St Louis, 2001, Elsevier Mosby.

Comparison of Cardiac and General Populations

Major depression is found in about 9.5 percent of the general population,[58] 16 to 47 percent in patients with CHD,[59] and 13 to 75 percent in those with heart failure. Higher rates of depression have been found in women than in men in some studies,[60,61] but not all.[62] In a national sample of adults, blacks and Hispanics have higher rates of major depression relative to whites. When controlling for confounders, white and Hispanic adults had similar rates, and blacks had significantly lower rates of depression than whites.[63] Similar results were found in a sample with heart failure.[56] Further research on the effect of racial and ethnic minority status on rates of depression in cardiac disease is an area greatly needing further study.

Clinical Assessment

It can be difficult to distinguish between anxiety and depression because they often coexist; therefore, their discrete differences are shown in Table 15-3. The clinical interview, described before, is most effective in identifying and diagnosing clinical anxiety and depression. However, simply asking about the two core symptoms of depression (depressed, sad mood and decreased interest or pleasure in almost all activities) can be used for screening.

If more time is available, a number of valid and reliable surveys can be used to screen for depression. Five questionnaires that can be used in the clinical setting to assess for depression are shown in Table 15-4. These

■ ■ ■

TABLE 15-4 DEPRESSION BEHAVIOR RATING SCALES

SCALE	MEASURES	WHERE TO OBTAIN
Geriatric Depression Scale	30-item tool to assess depression in geriatric populations on a scale of 0 to 100 Can be completed in 5 to 10 minutes Scores of 0 to 9 are considered normal, 10 to 19 indicate mild depression, and 20+ indicate severe depression	In Yasavage JA, Brink TL: Development and validation of a geriatric depression screening scale: a preliminary report, *J Psychiatr Res* 17:37-49, 1983
Beck Depression Scale	21-item tool to assess behavioral manifestations of depression on a scale of 0 to 3 Scores of 10 to 18 indicate mild depression, 19 to 29 moderate depression, and 30+ severe depression	Purchase from *http://harcourtassessment.com/HAIWEB/Cultures/en-us/Productdetail.htm?Pid=015-8018-370&Mode=summary* 1-800-211-8378
Hamilton Depression Scale	17-item tool to measure severity of depression Higher score indicate more severe depression Must be administered by a health care professional with clinical experience in depression	In Hamilton M: Rating depressive patients, *J Clin Psychiatry* 41(12):21-24, 1980
Center for Epidemiologic Studies Depression Scales (CESD)	20-item tool to measure depression in community populations	In Radloff LS: The CES-D scale: a self-report depression scale for research in the general population, *Appl Psychol Meas* 1:385-401, 1977
Zung Depression Scale	20-item scale that taps affective, cognitive, behavioral, and physical aspects of depression Lower scores indicate mild depression	In Zung WWK: A self-rating depression scale, *Arch Gen Psychiatry* 12:63-70, 1965

questions and surveys are useful for assessing the degree and duration of depressive symptoms. A recent National Heart Lung and Blood Institute Working Panel recommends the Beck Depression Inventory.[64]

Screening cardiac populations with symptoms that are similar to those of depressed persons (e.g., fatigue and difficulty sleeping) is particularly challenging. An *inclusive* approach allows detection of clinically significant depressive symptoms, regardless of cause. In an inclusive strategy, which captures symptoms in a sensitive fashion, depressive symptoms are rated, regardless of suspected cause. In an *exclusive* approach, symptoms with another possible cause are excluded. The inclusive approach yields a higher rate of major depression (20.7 percent versus 10.4 percent with exclusive approach), although patients vary little in illness severity, treatment, and impairment caused by depression.[65] Therefore, mental health professionals prefer the inclusive approach. Screening questions do not replace a diagnostic interview by a trained professional, but use of screening approaches in clinical practice could improve greatly the rates of referral for this important response to cardiac illness.

QUALITY OF LIFE

In one of the early definitions, the World Health Organization defined quality of life as "a state of complete physical, mental, and social well-being and not merely the absence of disease or infirmity."[66] Since that time, numerous investigators have proposed conceptual models illustrating the physical, psychological, and sociological domains of this multidimensional construct. Health-Related Quality of Life (**HRQL**) refers to those aspects of quality of life that are most influenced by health. A popular model by Wilson and Cleary[67] identified components of HRQL that shift the focus from the biological cell to the organism as a whole, including symptoms, functioning, perceived health, and overall quality of life. This HRQL model was refined recently by Ferrans and colleagues[68] to capture better the influence of individual and environmental characteristics on biological function. This section focuses on research that has assessed the components of HRQL, symptom burden, functioning, general health, and overall HRQL in those with cardiac disease.

In Coronary Heart Disease

Persons with CHD have been found to have impairments in each of the major domains of HRQL: physical, psychological, and sociological. Specific dimensions with difficulties include physical functioning, exercise capacity, vitality, social roles, emotions, perceived health, symptom burden, and bodily pain.[69-71] In a 2-year follow-up of 4484 veterans enrolled from outpatient settings, perceived health status, and specifically physical limitation, was a significant predictor of mortality along with age and presence of heart failure. Subjects with severe physical limitation had 6 times the chance of dying (odd ratio [OR] 6.2; 95 percent CI, 3.8 to 10.5) versus those with minimal limitation. In addition, those reporting

severe angina were 3 times as likely (OR 3.1; 95 percent CI, 1.7 to 5.3) to be admitted to the hospital for acute coronary syndrome than those reporting minimal angina. In women with coronary artery disease, chest pain is associated with lower HRQL scores.[72] These symptoms limited activities of daily living, social activities, and performance of household activities.

After Myocardial Infarction

All the domains of HRQL are affected after AMI. Specific aspects of HRQL that have been found to be compromised after AMI include physical and mental health.[73] After the acute event, though, HRQL improves. For example, in one study using the Medical Outcomes Study Short Form 36 (**SF-36**), a commonly used generic measure of HRQL, the physical composite summary score was 39.3 ± 8.9 during hospitalization but improved to 43.9 ± 10.3 6 months later ($p < 0.001$). The mental health composite summary score was 44.4 ± 10.9 at hospitalization and improved to 48.9 ± 9.5 at 6 months ($p < 0.04$).

Several studies have identified characteristics of AMI patients predictive of HRQL outcomes: age, sex, symptoms, ejection fraction, and comorbid conditions. Increasing age predicts poorer outcomes in some dimensions of HRQL, but psychological well-being is worse in younger patients, who report more depression, anxiety, and worry.[73,74] Men have better HRQL outcomes with the exception of perceived health status.[74]

Patients with continuing symptoms[75] or a low ejection fraction also have continuing impairments in HRQL. In a study of 1848 patients enrolled in the GUSTO-I Angiographic Study, ejection fraction was related significantly to physical ($p = 0.02$) and social ($p = 0.01$) function, psychological well-being ($p = 0.04$), and perceived health status ($p = 0.02$).[74] The presence of comorbidities increased the likelihood of worse outcomes in all dimensions of HRQL.

After Coronary Artery Bypass Graft Surgery

In general, after CABG, patients experience improvements in physical, social, and role functioning and have less bodily pain. However, about 25 percent of patients have recurrent angina after CABG, and 17 percent of post-CABG patients continue to have moderate to severe chest discomfort. Those who have continuing pain or poor sleep quality report poor HRQL.[76] Women undergoing CABG report significantly worse HRQL in the dimensions of physical functioning, symptom burden, and perceived health status compared with men.[77]

With Heart Failure

Symptom burden and functional limitations appear to be the major illness characteristics affecting HRQL in persons with heart failure. In one study, an average of 7.2 symptoms was identified on admission and 4.2 symptoms 6 weeks after a heart failure hospitalization.[78] Initially, shortness of breath was the primary symptom, but by 6 weeks, fatigue was most common and troubling. Low vigor scores were similar to those with cancer.

Persons with heart failure are able to perform basic activities of daily living, but intermediate activities of daily living are limited, which greatly impairs HRQL. Some investigators have found gender differences in HRQL,[79] but others have not.[80] When women with heart failure were compared with the general population, those with heart failure had lower perceived vigor (14.3 ± 6) than a general population (19.5 ± 6), with scores in women with heart failure similar to those of persons with cancer.[79]

Age of onset may be an important contributor to HRQL in persons with heart failure. In one study, women younger than age 65 had poorer HRQL compared with men in the same age-group.[55] This relationship may be related to baseline psychological state or the burden of other illnesses. For example, diabetes and hypertension are common causes of heart failure in younger women. When heart failure is added to the burden associated with these chronic conditions, a measurable influence on HRQL may become evident. In patients older than age 60, the factors associated with low HRQL were poor functional status, depression, low socioeconomic status, and two or more comorbid conditions.[81]

After Device Implantation

Studies that address HRQL after ICD implantation report that most recipients accept their device and consider it essential to their well-being despite fears and concerns about receiving a shock. In one study of 71 ICD recipients followed over the first year after ICD implantation, no significant changes in the mental and physical health composite summary scores of the SF-36 were seen, although significant improvement occurred in the health transition score ($p < 0.001$).[82] Similar to the findings of others,[36] there were significant improvements in ability to assume usual roles, physical functioning, vitality, and social functioning over time.

After an ICD delivers a shock, the recipient is commonly psychologically and physically immobilized.[83] Physical functioning is reduced in hopes of avoiding activities that may trigger another device shock. Whenever an ICD recipient is unable to adjust to the device shock, the person may develop exaggerated perceptions of physical limitations, social isolation, and psychological distress.[34]

Comparison of Cardiac and General Populations

Quality of life appears to be lower in cardiac patients than in healthy comparison samples. Several studies measured HRQL using the SF-36, which provides normative data for comparison. In those normative scores, the mean score for men and women is 71.9 ± 20. Data from a variety of sources found that heart failure patients had a mean score of 47.1 ± 24, post-AMI patients had a mean score of 59.2 ± 19, and hypertensive patients had a mean score of 63.3 ± 20. These scores in cardiac patients are significantly lower than normative data from general populations ($p < 0.05$) and are similar to those with chronic obstructive lung disease and Parkinson disease.

Clinical Assessment

Several valid and reliable measures of HRQL are available. Some measures are broad, assessing each of the broad domains of quality of life. Others are focused on specific dimensions. Guyatt[84] recommends using generic and disease-specific measures of HRQL.

One commonly used generic measure is the SF-36, which has established validity and reliability.[85] The SF-36 represents two of the most important health concepts included on the Medical Outcomes Survey: physical and mental health. The physical health composite summary measures physical functioning, physical role functioning, bodily pain, and general health. The mental health composite summary reflects vitality, social functioning, mental role functioning, and mental health. Scores are standardized on a scale from 0 to 100, with higher scores indicating better physical and mental health.

Disease-specific measures of overall HRQL or health status include the Kansas City Cardiomyopathy Questionnaire (**KCCQ**)[86] and the Minnesota Living with Heart Failure Questionnaire (**LHFQ**).[87] Both are heart failure–specific instruments. The LHFQ contains 21 items and two subscales: physical and emotional. Higher scores indicate poorer quality of life. The 23-item KCCQ quantifies disease-specific physical limitations, symptom frequency, severity and change over time, overall quality of life, social interference, and self-efficacy and knowledge. Recent studies comparing these measures suggest that the KCCQ is 3 times more sensitive to clinical changes in HRQL than LHFQ or the SF-36.[88]

Other measures focus on specific dimensions of HRQL. Emotional and physical symptoms, or perceptions or feelings about an abnormal state, tend to be related. Few symptom questionnaires are standardized, and the relationship between emotional and physical symptoms is not clear in cardiac disease. The Seattle Angina Questionnaire (**SAQ**) assesses the effect of CHD symptoms on quality of life. The 19-item SAQ taps the five domains of treatment satisfaction, angina frequency, angina stability, physical limitation, and quality of life. Higher scores indicate greater treatment satisfaction, fewer symptoms, better physical functioning, and better quality of life.[89]

CONCLUSIONS

The major emotions experienced in response to cardiac illness events are anxiety, depression, and impaired HRQL. These psychological states are affected negatively by all cardiac diagnoses. Women appear to experience more emotional distress than men, regardless of the diagnosis. That is, in general, women have higher anxiety, more depression, and worse HRQL than men when first diagnosed with cardiac disease and women do not adjust as well as men after CABG. Women may have worse HRQL after developing heart failure, but the literature is controversial on this topic.

Looking at this body of literature as a whole, several themes can be identified that predict poor psychological outcomes. Persons who are extremely distressed, with poor coping skills, at the time of diagnosis can be expected to have relatively more and continuing anxiety, depression, and impaired HRQL over time. Patients without social support may not have the resources needed to cope. In addition, persons with other comorbid illnesses and compromised physical functioning may have more distress than others who are not burdened with these extra physiological challenges.

The literature on age-related differences is interesting. From some studies it appears that as persons age, they develop the resources to handle illness, although this is not a consistent finding. It may be that older adults cope better than younger ones only if they have certain resources, such as cognitive skills and social support. The finding that younger adults with cardiac illness have relatively more psychological distress, one component of HRQL, may be explained by a feeling that "it is not time yet." More research on the effect of age on the psychological response to cardiac illness is greatly needed.

Although decades of investigation clearly document the psychological distress experienced by cardiac patients, intervention research is distinctly lagging. Others have noted that anxiety is not assessed systematically by health care providers. Clearly, the vast majority of anxious patients go underdiagnosed and undertreated.[90,91] One may logically assume that depression and impaired HRQL also are not assessed during acute care episodes. For humanistic and clinical reasons, it is time to address the emotional distress experienced by cardiac patients.

REFERENCES

1. Barlow J, Wright C, Sheasby J et al: Self-management approaches for people with chronic conditions: a review, *Patient Educ Couns* 48:177-187, 2002.
2. Kubzansky LD, Kawachi I, Weiss ST et al: Anxiety and coronary heart disease: a synthesis of epidemiological, psychological, and experimental evidence, *Ann Behav Med* 20:47-58, 1998.
3. Sirois BC, Burg MM: Negative emotion and coronary heart disease: a review, *Behav Modif* 27:83-102, 2003.
4. Januzzi JL Jr, Stern TA, Pasternak RC et al: The influence of anxiety and depression on outcomes of patients with coronary artery disease, *Arch Intern Med* 160:1913-1921, 2000.
5. Frasure-Smith N, Lesperance F: Depression and other psychological risks following myocardial infarction, *Arch Gen Psychiatry* 60:627-636, 2003.
6. An K, De Jong MJ, Riegel BJ et al: A cross-sectional examination of changes in anxiety early after acute myocardial infarction, *Heart Lung* 33:75-82, 2004.
7. Crowe JM, Runions J, Ebbesen LS et al: Anxiety and depression after acute myocardial infarction, *Heart Lung* 25:98-107, 1996.
8. Moser DK, Dracup K: Is anxiety early after myocardial infarction associated with subsequent ischemic and arrhythmic events? *Psychosom Med* 58:395-401, 1996.
9. Ballenger JC, Davidson JR, Lecrubier Y et al: Consensus statement on depression, anxiety, and cardiovascular disease, *J Clin Psychiatry* 62(suppl 8):24-27, 2001.
10. Lepine JP: Epidemiology, burden, and disability in depression and anxiety, *J Clin Psychiatry* 62(suppl 13):4-10, 2001; discussion, pp 11-12.
11. Kirmayer LJ: Cultural variations in the clinical presentation of depression and anxiety: implications for diagnosis and treatment, *J Clin Psychiatry* 62(suppl 13):22-28, 2001; discussion, pp 29-30.
12. Moser DK, Dracup K, McKinley S et al: An international perspective on gender differences in anxiety early after acute myocardial infarction, *Psychosom Med* 65:511-516, 2003.
13. Derogatis LR, Wise TN: *Anxiety and depressive disorders in the medical patient,* Washington, DC, 1989, American Psychiatric Press.
14. De Jong MJ, Moser DK, An K et al: Anxiety is not manifested by elevated heart rate and blood pressure in acutely ill cardiac patients, *Eur J Cardiovasc Nurs* 3:247-253, 2004.
15. Mesquita B, Frijda NH: Cultural variations in emotions: a review, *Psychol Bull* 112:179-204, 1992.
16. Mesquita B, Walker R: Cultural differences in emotions: a context for interpreting emotional experiences, *Behav Res Ther* 41:777-793, 2003.
17. Bresser PJ, Sexton DL, Foell DW: Patients' responses to postponement of coronary artery bypass graft surgery, *Image J Nurs Sch* 25:5-10, 1993.
18. McCormick KM, McClement S, Naimark BJ: A qualitative analysis of the experience of uncertainty while awaiting coronary artery bypass surgery, *Can J Cardiovasc Nurs* 15:10-22, 2005.
19. McCormick KM, Naimark BJ, Tate RB: Uncertainty, symptom distress, anxiety, and functional status in patients awaiting coronary artery bypass surgery, *Heart Lung* 35:34-45, 2006.
20. Andrew MJ, Baker RA, Kneebone AC et al: Mood state as a predictor of neuropsychological deficits following cardiac surgery, *J Psychosom Res* 48:537-546, 2000.
21. McCrone S, Lenz E, Tarzian A et al: Anxiety and depression: incidence and patterns in patients after coronary artery bypass graft surgery, *Appl Nurs Res* 14:155-164, 2001.
22. Rymaszewska J, Kiejna A, Hadrys T: Depression and anxiety in coronary artery bypass grafting patients, *Eur Psychiatry* 18:155-160, 2003.
23. Jenkins CD, Stanton BA, Savageau JA et al: Coronary artery bypass surgery: physical, psychological, social, and economic outcomes six months later, *JAMA* 250:782-788, 1983.
24. Boudrez H, De Backer G: Psychological status and the role of coping style after coronary artery bypass graft surgery: results of a prospective study, *Qual Life Res* 10:37-47, 2001.
25. Rothenhausler HB, Grieser B, Nollert G et al: Psychiatric and psychosocial outcome of cardiac surgery with cardiopulmonary bypass: a prospective 12-month follow-up study, *Gen Hosp Psychiatry* 27:18-28, 2005.
26. King KB: Emotional and functional outcomes in women with coronary heart disease, *J Cardiovasc Nurs* 15:54-70, 2001.
27. Gallo LC, Malek MJ, Gilbertson AD, Moore JL: Perceived cognitive function and emotional distress following coronary artery bypass surgery, *J Behav Med* 28(5):433-442, 2005.
28. Raja PV, Blumenthal JA, Doraiswamy PM: Cognitive deficits following coronary artery bypass grafting: prevalence, prognosis, and therapeutic strategies, *CNS Spectr* 9:763-772, 2004.
29. Majani G, Pierobon A, Giardini A et al: Relationship between psychological profile and cardiological variables in chronic heart failure: the role of patient subjectivity, *Eur Heart J* 20:1579-1586, 1999.
30. Moser DK, Zambroski CH, Lennie TA et al: Aging with a broken heart: the effect of heart disease on psychological distress in the elderly, *Circulation* 110(suppl):416, 2004 (abstract).
31. Haworth JE, Moniz-Cook E, Clark AL et al: Prevalence and predictors of anxiety and depression in a sample of chronic heart failure patients with left ventricular systolic dysfunction, *Eur J Heart Fail* 7:803-808, 2005.
32. van Jaarsveld CH, Sanderman R, Miedema I et al: Changes in health-related quality of life in older patients with acute myocardial infarction or congestive heart failure: a prospective study, *J Am Geriatr Soc* 49:1052-1058, 2001.
33. Konstam V, Moser DK, De Jong MJ: Depression and anxiety in heart failure, *J Card Fail* 11:455-463, 2005.
34. Sears SF Jr, Todaro JF, Lewis TS et al: Examining the psychosocial impact of implantable cardioverter defibrillators: a literature review, *Clin Cardiol* 22:481-489, 1999.

35. Dunbar SB, Kimble LP, Jenkins LS et al: Association of mood disturbance and arrhythmia events in patients after cardioverter defibrillator implantation, *Depress Anxiety* 9:163-168, 1999.

36. Schron EB, Exner DV, Yao Q et al: Quality of life in the antiarrhythmics versus implantable defibrillators trial: impact of therapy and influence of adverse symptoms and defibrillator shocks, *Circulation* 105:589-594, 2002.

37. Eckert M, Jones T: How does an implantable cardioverter defibrillator (ICD) affect the lives of patients and their families? *Int J Nurs Pract* 8:152-157, 2002.

38. Varcarolis EM: The clinical interview and communication skills. In Varcarolis EM, editor: *Foundations of psychiatric mental health nursing,* ed 4, Philadelphia, 2002, Saunders.

39. Garis RI, Farmer KC: Examining costs of chronic conditions in a Medicaid population, *Manag Care* 11:43-50, 2002.

40. Nemeroff CB, Musselman DL, Evans DL: Depression and cardiac disease, *Depress Anxiety* 8(suppl 1):71-79, 1998.

41. Guck TP, Kavan MG, Elsasser GN, Barone EJ: Assessment and treatment of depression following myocardial infarction, *Am Fam Physician* 64:641-648, 2001.

42. American Psychiatric Association: *Diagnostic and statistical manual of mental disorders, primary care version* (DSM-IV-PC), ed 4, Washington, DC, 2000, American Psychiatric Association Press.

43. Naqvi TZ, Naqvi SS, Merz CN: Gender differences in the link between depression and cardiovascular disease, *Psychosom Med* 67(suppl 1):S15-S18, 2005.

44. Bush DE, Ziegelstein RC, Patel UV et al: Post-myocardial infarction depression, *Evid Rep Technol Assess (Summ)* pp 1-8, May 2005.

45. Schleifer SJ, Macari-Hinson MM, Coyle DA et al: The nature and course of depression following myocardial infarction, *Arch Intern Med* 149:1785-1789, 1989.

46. Slimmer LM, Lyness JM, Caine ED: Stress, medical illness, and depression, *Semin Clin Neuropsychiatry* 6:12-26, 2001.

47. Mitchell RH, Robertson E, Harvey PJ et al: Sex differences in depression after coronary artery bypass graft surgery, *Am Heart J* 150:1017-1025, 2005.

48. Doering LV, Magsarili MC, Howitt LY et al: Clinical depression in women after cardiac surgery, *J Cardiovasc Nurs* 21:132-139, 2006.

49. Vaccarino V, Kasl SV, Abramson J et al: Depressive symptoms and risk of functional decline and death in patients with heart failure, *J Am Coll Cardiol* 38:199-205, 2001.

50. Thomas SA, Friedmann E, Khatta M et al: Depression in patients with heart failure: physiologic effects, incidence, and relation to mortality, *AACN Clin Issues* 14:3-12, 2003.

51. Koenig H: Depression in hospitalized older patients with congestive heart failure, *Gen Hosp Psychiatry* 20:29-43, 1998.

52. Freedland KE, Rich MW, Skala JA et al: Prevalence of depression in hospitalized patients with congestive heart failure, *Psychosom Med* 65:119-128, 2003.

53. Koenig HG: Depression outcome in inpatients with congestive heart failure, *Arch Intern Med* 166:991-996, 2006.

54. Murberg T, Aarsland T, Svebak S: Functional status and depression among men and women with congestive heart failure, *Int J Psychiatry Med* 28:273-291, 1998.

55. Hou N, Chui MA, Eckert GJ et al: Relationship of age and sex to health-related quality of life in patients with heart failure, *Am J Crit Care* 13:153-161, 2004.

56. Gottlieb SS, Khatta M, Friedmann E et al: The influence of age, gender, and race on the prevalence of depression in heart failure patients, *J Am Coll Cardiol* 43:1542-1549, 2004.

57. Dougherty CM: Psychological reactions and family adjustment in shock versus no shock groups after implantation of internal cardioverter defibrillator, *Heart Lung* 24:281-291, 1995.

58. Katz DA, McHorney CA: Clinical correlates of insomnia in patients with chronic illness, *Arch Intern Med* 158:1099-1107, 1998.

59. Horsten M, Mittleman MA, Wamala SP et al: Depressive symptoms and lack of social integration in relation to prognosis of CHD in middle-aged women: the Stockholm Female Coronary Risk Study, *Eur Heart J* 21:1072-1080, 2000.

60. Blazer DG, Moody-Ayers S, Craft-Morgan J et al: Depression in diabetes and obesity: racial/ethnic/gender issues in older adults, *J Psychosom Res* 53:913-916, 2002.

61. Angst J, Gamma A, Gastpar M et al: Gender differences in depression: epidemiological findings from the European DEPRES I and II studies, *Eur Arch Psychiatry Clin Neurosci* 252:201-209, 2002.

62. Stordal E, Bjartveit Kruger M, Dahl NH, et al: Depression in relation to age and gender in the general population: the Nord-Trondelag Health Study (HUNT), *Acta Psychiatr Scand* 104:210-216, 2001.

63. Dunlop DD, Song J, Lyons JS et al: Racial/ethnic differences in rates of depression among preretirement adults, *Am J Public Health* 93:1945-1952, 2003.

64. Davidson KW, Kupfer DJ, Bigger JT et al: Assessment and treatment of depression in patients with cardiovascular disease: National Heart, Lung, and Blood Institute Working Group Report, *Psychosom Med* 68:645-50, 2006.

65. Koenig HG, George LK, Peterson BL et al: Depression in medically ill hospitalized older adults: prevalence, characteristics, and course of symptoms according to six diagnostic schemes, *Am J Psychiatry* 154:1376-1383, 1997.

66. World Health Organization: *Constitution of the World Health Organization: chronicle of the World Health Organization,* Geneva, 1947, The Organization.

67. Wilson IB, Cleary PD: Linking clinical variables with health-related quality of life: a conceptual model of patient outcomes, *JAMA* 273:59-65, 1995.

68. Ferrans CE, Zerwic JJ, Wilbur JE et al: Conceptual model of health-related quality of life, *J Nurs Scholarsh* 37:336-342, 2005.

69. Kiebzak GM, Pierson LM, Campbell M et al: Use of the SF36 general health status survey to document health-related quality of life in patients with coronary artery disease: effect of disease and response to coronary artery bypass graft surgery, *Heart Lung* 31:207-213, 2002.

70. Ruo B, Rumsfeld JS, Hlatky MA et al: Depressive symptoms and health-related quality of life: the Heart and Soul Study, *JAMA* 290:215-221, 2003.

71. Spertus JA, Jones P, McDonell M et al: Health status predicts long-term outcome in outpatients with coronary disease, *Circulation* 106:43-49, 2002.

72. Olson MB, Kelsey SF, Matthews K et al: Symptoms, myocardial ischaemia and quality of life in women: results from the NHLBI-sponsored WISE Study, *Eur Heart J* 24:1506-1514, 2003.

73. Bengtsson I, Hagman M, Wedel H: Age and angina as predictors of quality of life after myocardial infarction: a prospective comparative study, *Scand Cardiovasc J* 35:252-258, 2001.

74. Coyne KS, Lundergan CF, Boyle D et al: Relationship of infarct artery patency and left ventricular ejection fraction to health-related quality of life after myocardial infarction: the GUSTO-I Angiographic Study experience, *Circulation* 102:1245-1251, 2000.

75. Roebuck A, Furze G, Thompson DR: Health-related quality of life after myocardial infarction: an interview study, *J Adv Nurs* 34:787-794, 2001.

76. Hunt JO, Hendrata MV, Myles PS: Quality of life 12 months after coronary artery bypass graft surgery, *Heart Lung* 29:401-411, 2000.

77. Phillips Bute B, Mathew J, Blumenthal JA et al: Female gender is associated with impaired quality of life 1 year after coronary artery bypass surgery, *Psychosom Med* 65:944-951, 2003.

78. Friedman M: Older adults' symptoms and their duration before hospitalization for heart failure, *Heart Lung* 26:169-176, 1997.

79. Riedinger MS, Dracup KA, Brecht ML: Quality of life in women with heart failure, normative groups, and patients with other chronic conditions, *Am J Crit Care* 11:211-219, 2002.

80. Riegel B, Moser DK, Carlson B et al: Gender differences in quality of life are minimal in patients with heart failure, *J Card Fail* 9:42-48, 2003.

81. Gott M, Barnes S, Parker C et al: Predictors of the quality of life of older people with heart failure recruited from primary care, *Age Ageing* 35:172-177, 2006.

82. Carroll DL, Hamilton GA, Kenney BJ: Changes in health status, psychological distress, and quality of life in implantable cardioverter defibrillator recipients between 6 months and 1 year after implantation, *Eur J Cardiovasc Nurs* 1:213-219, 2002.

83. Carroll DL, Hamilton GA: Quality of life in implanted cardioverter defibrillator recipients: the impact of a device shock, *Heart Lung* 34:169-178, 2005.

84. Guyatt GH: Measurement of health-related quality of life in heart failure, *J Am Coll Cardiol* 22(4 suppl A):185A-191A, 1993.

85. Ware JE Jr, Gandek B: Overview of the SF-36 Health Survey and the International Quality of Life Assessment (IQOLA) Project, *J Clin Epidemiol* 51:903-912, 1998.

86. Green CP, Porter CB, Bresnahan DR et al: Development and evaluation of the Kansas City Cardiomyopathy Questionnaire: a new health status measure for heart failure, *J Am Coll Card* 35:1245-1255, 2000.

87. Rector T, Kubo S, Cohn J: Validity of the Minnesota Living with Heart Failure questionnaire as a measure of therapeutic response to enalapril or placebo, *Am J Cardiol* 71:1106-1107, 1993.

88. Spertus J, Peterson E, Conard MW et al: Monitoring clinical changes in patients with heart failure: a comparison of methods, *Am Heart J* 150:707-715, 2005.

89. Spertus JA, Winder JA, Dewhurst TA et al: Development and evaluation of the Seattle Angina Questionnaire: a new functional status measure for coronary artery disease, *J Am Coll Cardiol* 25:333-341, 1995.

90. Frazier SK, Moser DK, Daley LK et al: Critical care nurses' beliefs about and reported management of anxiety, *Am J Crit Care* 12:19-27, 2003.

91. De Jong MJ, Chung ML, Roser LP et al: A five-country comparison of anxiety early after acute myocardial infarction, *Eur J Cardiovasc Nurs* 3:129-134, 2004.

chapter 16

The Impact of Cardiac Disease on the Family

Sally H. Rankin

CHAPTER ABBREVIATIONS

CABG coronary artery bypass grafting
ICD implantable cardioverter-defibrillator
MI myocardial infarction

Ginger Smith is a 41-year-old, married, childless woman who awoke on a Sunday morning with epigastric pain, nausea, and mild shortness of breath. After showering and dressing, she became more nauseated and vomited twice. Her epigastric pain continued, and worsened, as did her shortness of breath. By one o'clock in the afternoon, her husband was sufficiently worried that he called emergency medical services. The paramedics were unimpressed by Mrs. Miller's symptoms and suggested to her husband that she had gastroenteritis. However, her husband and other family members convinced the paramedics to transport her to a medical center emergency room.

While in the emergency department, Mrs. Smith was worked up for an ectopic pregnancy and cocaine abuse; a complete blood count and differential were ordered, as was an abdominal x-ray series. Mrs. Smith's husband watched the staff and was very concerned about his wife's pain but was unable to advocate for additional testing or a hastened response. Mrs. Smith's pain continued and finally at 9 PM she was premedicated for an exploratory laparotomy, at which time an electrocardiogram was done. Mrs. Smith's electrocardiogram revealed that she had sustained a massive myocardial infarction (**MI**). Mr. Smith blamed himself for lack of a more expedient treatment plan and diagnosis. When Mrs. Smith was discharged from the hospital, she was able to perform her own activities of daily living but was unable to return to heavy household cleaning, caring for an infant niece, or participating in a bowling league with her husband. Mrs. Smith's husband was encouraged by Mrs. Smith's sister to bring suit against the hospital, but he declined to do so, saying that it would not improve her condition and would cause her to be reminded of her problems.

FAMILY-CENTERED CARE

As the preceding case study illustrates, heart disease affects all members of the family system and, likewise, the family affects the patient with heart disease. Family-centered care—which was first developed by pediatric nurses who became aware of the importance of caring for the parents and the child—is an important concept in helping patients and families affected by heart disease. The goal of family-centered care is to maximize the patient's physiological and psychosocial outcomes through family participation in care; collaboration and mutual decision making with the health care team; and care by nurses of the family and the patient. Family-centered care also empowers families through patient education to advocate for themselves and for the family member with heart disease. Indeed, family-centered care provides the "heart and soul" to families and patients dealing with cardiac disease, whether the patient is hospitalized or at home.

This chapter establishes the evidence base for family-centered care with a primary focus on acute MI, cardiac surgery, and heart failure. The first section addresses the concept of family function; family systems and the management of chronic illness in families; the interaction of family members, the patient, and cardiac disease; and how caregiver burden may influence family members. The case study is used to illustrate various concepts. Family roles as a hindrance or enhancement of patient recovery from cardiac events is considered with particular attention being paid to a growing segment of the population affected by cardiac disease, that is, unpartnered (widowed, divorced, and never married) elders. The impact of various cardiac conditions on the family is reviewed, and finally, family-centered interventions to improve family and patient outcomes are examined.

FAMILY FUNCTIONS AND FAMILY FUNCTIONING

When nurses consider families from a functional perspective, there are five functions that families provide:

- Affection and caring
- Economic resources
- Sexuality and reproduction
- Socialization of children and adults
- Health care functions (Table 16-1)

Patterns of Western family life changed during the 20th century so that functions of sexuality, reproduction, and provision of housing and economic support have retreated somewhat in importance and functions of affection and health care have remained significant. The health care system increasingly looks to family members to provide nursing care, appointment scheduling, transportation, medication and symptom monitoring, reinforcement of hospital discharge guidelines, and meal preparation in their homes for members with heart disease. The extension of the health care system into the home has placed a tremendous burden on families, especially on women, who consistently are the

■ ■ ■

TABLE 16-1   FIVE FUNCTIONS OF THE FAMILY

FAMILY FUNCTION	ENHANCING FAMILY FUNCTION
Affection and caring Meeting socioemotional needs	If the needs of the patient or family member are not being met, the family may be referred to counseling.
	Other resources include caregiver support groups and American Heart Association supports, such as Mended Hearts for surgical patients.
Economic resources	If the family lacks economic resources, a referral should be made to medical social work so that Medicaid and Medicare systems are in place.
Sexuality and reproduction	Concerns related to sexuality are common with cardiac patients; nurses should be straightforward with information.
Socialization of children and adults	Families often need help orienting younger members to the hospital environment and to the needs of acutely ill patients.
	Once home, children of cardiac patients may have to assume duties previously assigned to the ill parent.
Health care functions	Because families assume home care responsibilities in most situations, nurses need to provide teaching related to monitoring of symptoms, medications, diet, and exercise.

providers of health care to family members.[1] If a family is assessed as unable to provide the two essential family functions related to affection/caring and health care assistance, the nurse has important data indicating that the family will need additional support.

In addition to assessing a family's ability to provide the five classic functions, the family system itself should be assessed. Family systems theory is a useful approach that includes assessment of family structure and function. The addition of family life cycle stage makes such an assessment approach useful (Figure 16-1). Family structure includes components such as hierarchy, which means who has power and authority in the family; boundaries or subsystems/subgroups in the family, such as a husband/wife subsystem; and family roles, for example, who is responsible for providing health care.

Mrs. Smith's was a large, extended family in which she and her husband lived with her parents and a sister who had an 8-month-old baby. Although the family applied pressure to the paramedics to transport Mrs. Smith, the responsibility for advocacy fell to Mr. Smith. His family role had been an instrumental one, as wage earner, but he was unprepared to function in the health care decision maker role. Family processes involve the family's ability to problem solve, adapt to change, maintain stability, and communicate effectively inside and outside the family system. The Smith family was unable to decide how to respond to Ginger's disability, and the stability of the family was threatened by her inability to care for her sister's child so that her sister could work. Ginger's older parents also depended on her to care for

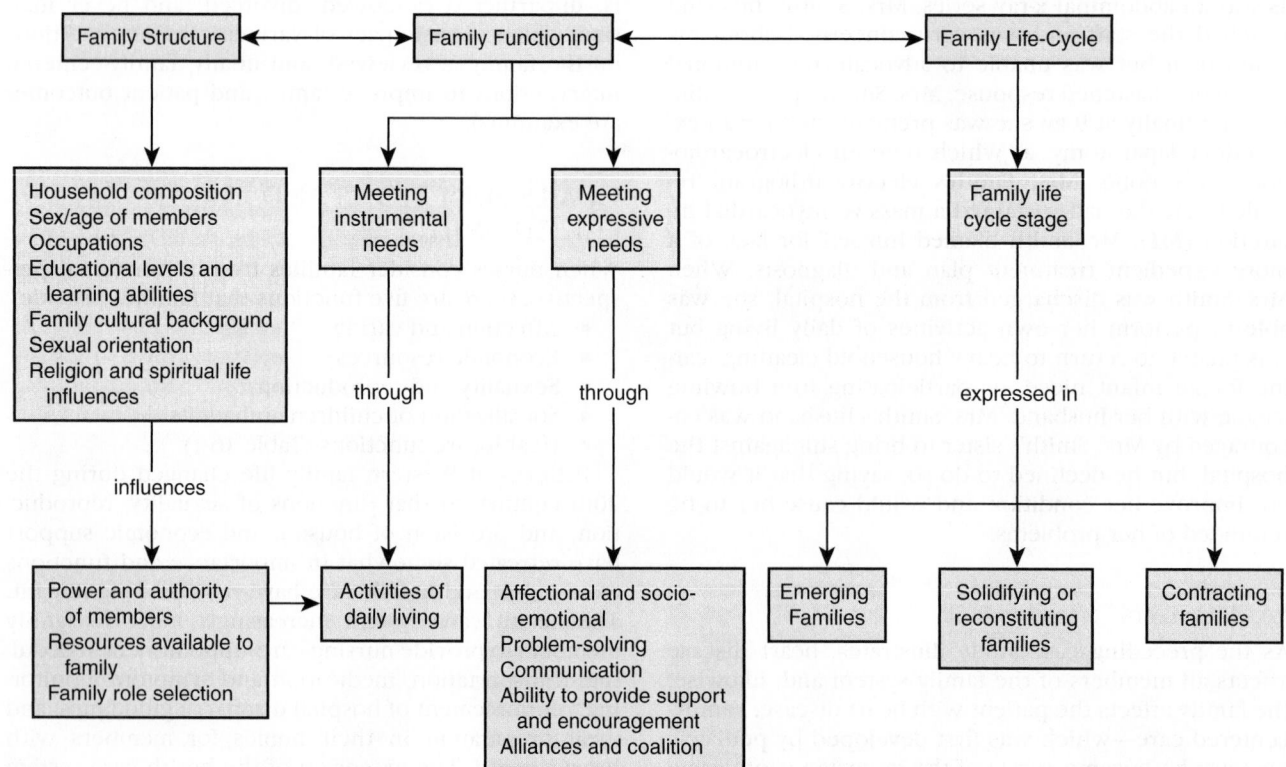

FIGURE 16-1 ■ Assessment of family structure, function, and life cycle.

them and to maintain the household. Because Ginger was unable to do heavy housework, her husband assumed the household chores and continued to be the primary wage earner for the extended family. When Ginger went for an appointment at the cardiology department 6 months after her MI, the family was experiencing severe stress and needed assistance. Table 16-2, *A, B,* and *C* reviews the components of family structure, function, and life cycle that commonly influence a patient's recovery and provide questions useful in assessing these aspects of family.

FAMILY SYSTEM EFFECTS ON THE PATIENT

Heart disease arises from the family of origin, that is, the family into which one is born, and it in turn affects the family of generativity, that is, the family that one creates. A positive family history for heart disease has long been recognized as an independent predictor of coronary artery disease.[2] However, an understanding of this predictor only recently has been elucidated through genetic studies that suggest a "susceptibility" gene for MI.[2] Women appear to be at even higher risk than men for developing coronary artery disease, even when both have a positive family

■ ■ ■

TABLE 16-2   A. QUESTIONS TO ASK WHEN ASSESSING FAMILY STRUCTURE

AREA OF ASSESSMENT	QUESTIONS TO ASK
Household composition	Who is living in the household?
	What other family members are available to help?
Sex/age of members	What is the sex and age of persons living in the household?
	What is the sex and age of other family members who are available to help?
	What is the sexual orientation of family members?
Occupation of members	Do family members work?
	What type of work do they do?
	Does employment provide for insurance?
	Is there flexibility with work so that family members are available to provide home care?
	Is the income from work sufficient to provide for family and household needs?
	Are there additional family members who provide financial help if needed?
Educational levels of members	How much education does each family member have?
	Do all family members have literacy skills?
Health status of members	What is the health status of each family member?
	Who takes care of family members when they are ill?
Family ethnicity and cultural background	What is the family's ethnic background?
	How many generations has the family lived in the United States?
	What is the primary language spoken in the family?
	In which cultural practices does the family engage?
Religion and spiritual life	Do family members participate in a synagogue, church, or mosque?
	Are there religious practices within the home?
Resources available to members	Are there resources available to the family from the extended family? Community? Other?
Family role selection	What roles do family members play?
	How do these roles relate to one another?
	Is there one member in the family who is most likely to be ill?

B. QUESTIONS TO ASK WHEN ASSESSING FAMILY FUNCTIONING

AREA OF ASSESSMENT	QUESTIONS TO ASK
Instrumental Needs	
Activities of daily living	Are any members of the family unable to bathe, toilet, feed, or prepare medications?
	If so, who will do these tasks for them?
Expressive Needs	
Affectional and socioemotional	Is there open expression of affection in the family that is culturally appropriate?
	Do children seek support from adult family members?
	Who spends time with whom in the family?
	Are children socialized to the family expectations?
	Who provides support and encouragement when children or the elderly need it?
Problem solving	How has the family solved problems in the past?
	Who identifies problems, i.e., do persons from inside or outside identify problems?
	Are the problems related to instrumental needs or emotional needs?
Communication	Is communication direct, i.e., is it sent to the intended recipient?
	Is communication clear or distorted, i.e., do all members of the family understand the messages being sent?
	What is the nature of verbal and nonverbal communication between family members?
Power and authority of members	Who makes the rules in the family?
	Who is in control of the family?
Alliances and coalitions	What are the important alliances in the family?
	Are there coalitions in which family members side against others?

Continued

■ ■ ■

TABLE 16-2   C. QUESTIONS TO ASK WHEN ASSESSING FAMILY LIFE CYCLE

AREA OF ASSESSMENT	QUESTIONS TO ASK
Emerging family	Is this a new relationship or marriage? Is a member pregnant? Are there newborn or very young children? What is the role of the extended family? Are there problems for the family in terms of recognition legally or socially (e.g., some gay or lesbian families may "closet" their status because of lack of acceptance of gay/lesbian family life)?
Solidifying or reconstituting family	Is the family in the midst of dissolution? With whom will the children live? Where will financial support come from? Have plans been made for the care of all family members who were once part of the family before dissolution? *If the family is a reconstituting, or blended family:* Who will be living together? Who will meet the affective and instrumental needs of children and adults? How do the adults and children and the reconstituting family relate to one another?
Contracting family	Has a family member recently left because of entering adulthood and leaving home? Death? Other reasons? Does the contracted family have the necessary resources to meet its needs?

history.[3] Moreover, a maternal history of heart disease appears to be more ominous than a paternal history.[4] Therefore, the importance of knowing one's family history is vital so that modifiable risk factors can be amended.

Many inherited cardiovascular risk factors, especially those related to lipids, diabetes mellitus, and hypertension, can be modified;[5] however, few U.S. providers follow national recommendations for the screening of family members.[6] Despite clear family risk factors, members of the family of origin and the family of generativity do not sufficiently reduce their behavioral risk factors or adhere to treatment plans.

The family of generativity is equally important in terms of patient adjustment to the diagnosis and prognosis related to heart disease. The family's reaction to diagnosis and prognosis frequently sets the course for patient adherence to a prescribed treatment plan. For example, family members who respond to the need for lifestyle changes by modifying the entire family's diet, encouraging appropriate exercise, and assisting with medications when necessary are frequently able to normalize the life not only of the patient but also of the entire family. However, families that respond with fear, denial, or efforts to control all aspects of the patient's behavior make poor family adjustments to the required changes in lifestyle. Likewise, patients may be deprived of needed social support or may be subjected to so much surveillance that they resent family assistance.

EFFECTS OF THE PATIENT'S CARDIAC DISEASE ON THE FAMILY SYSTEM

Like many other chronic diseases, heart disease affects the family system in many ways. Changes in roles and patterns of family living require the greatest amount of adjustment. In younger families, wives and children may be forced to take on chores or learn new skills with which they are unfamiliar. In some cases, the primary wage earner may be unable to work or may be delayed in

returning to work, causing a change in family income or requiring that the unaffected spouse, usually a woman in younger families, obtain employment. In older families, men may take on the unfamiliar role of family caregiver to wives recovering from acute MI or cardiac valve replacement. Sexual activity patterns are likely to change after a cardiac event, with most patients reporting less frequent and less satisfaction with sexual activity. Changes in sexual activity patterns affect partners, and this change in intimacy may disrupt the relationship. Chapter 18 addresses issues related to cardiac disease and sexuality.

THE ROLE OF FAMILIES IN ENHANCING OR HINDERING RECOVERY

For many reasons, families may enhance or hinder a patient's recovery from a cardiac event. Some of these reasons are related to caregiving burden, but others are related to the context of family lives. This context is examined most clearly in light of life span development theory, an approach that includes the various cohort and historical influences on persons' lives.

Effects of Life Span Development

The life span development framework has been used by social scientists since the 1970s, and nursing is overdue in recognizing and using this theoretical and methodological framework. The unique focus of the framework on biological (normative age-graded), sociohistorical (normative history-graded), and nonnormative influences (events occurring out of synchrony) provides a constructive approach with individuals and families (Figure 16-2). Important developmental influences that may affect the self-care abilities of patients recovering from MI in the community include the following:

- Normative age-graded factors, that is, person-related biological and environmental variables that exhibit a high correlation with chronological age

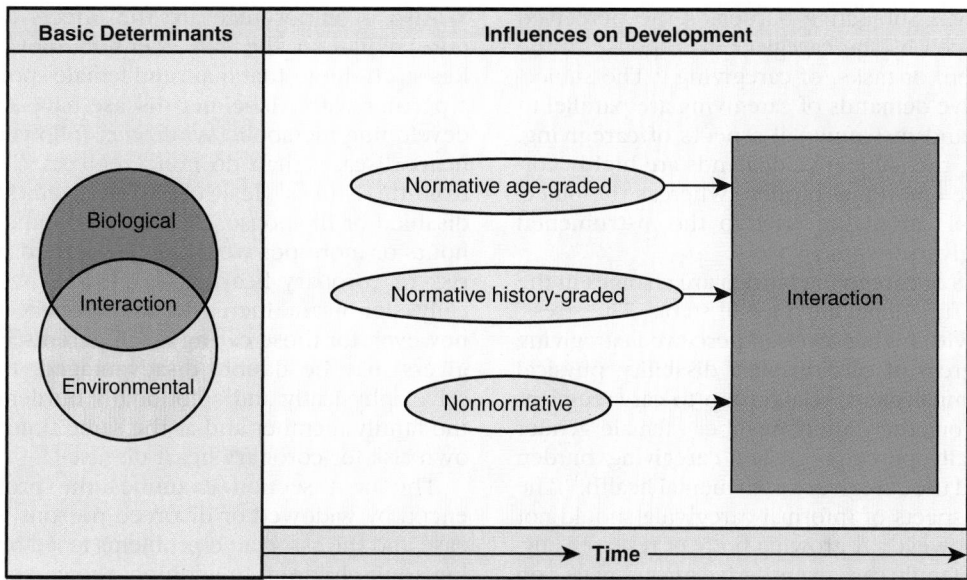

FIGURE 16-2 ■ Determinants of and influences on life span development. (From Baltes PB, Reese HW, Lipsitt LP: Life-span developmental psychology. *Ann Rev Psychol* 31: 65-110, 1980.)

- Normative history-graded factors, for example, the historical events that influence particular birth cohorts
- Nonnormative factors, that is, life events that occur asynchronously with the life course or are not experienced by the population at large. Nonnormative events are the most difficult for families to incorporate. For example, since Ginger Smith's MI occurred asynchronously—not in the usual sequence of health events—one could expect her family to have greater difficulty incorporating it than if the event had occurred later in her life. Thus, the clinician should consider the timing of cardiac events when assessing the family.

Understanding the historical context that today's cardiac patients experienced during their formative years is important to understanding why they may or may not participate in health-promoting activities. Likewise, understanding the historical context of caregiving family members is also essential, for belief systems influenced by historical context may not be congruent across birth cohorts.

Life span development theory suggests that because of normative history-graded influences, or cohort influences, the generation of women currently experiencing heart disease and MI have participated in fewer physical activities before MI and are less likely to be amenable to cardiac rehabilitation programs after MI.[7] Men, however, are more likely to participate in cardiac rehabilitation.[8] Life span theory also suggests that adult children who serve as family caregivers to their parents have had different cohort experiences during their lives than their parents. Therefore, factors such as greater participation in the workforce for caregiving women may mean that they are less accessible as caregivers to their parents than had been true in previous generations.

FAMILIES AND CHRONIC ILLNESS MANAGEMENT

Chronic illness produces long-term stressors for the patient (care-recipient) and the primary family caregiver, as well as for other members of the family system.[9] The first source of chronic stress is the magnitude of the stressors, which is worsened by the number of changes demanded by the patient's illness management. A second source of chronic stress is the ability of the patient and caregiver to make the changes demanded by the illness regimen. A third source of chronic stress is the availability of extrafamilial support resources such as the community and medical system to provide support to the patient and caregiver. The last part of this chapter examines psychoeducational interventions that affect these sources of stress for families managing cardiac disease.

Certain family characteristics—such as hostility within the family, criticism and blame, extrafamilial stress, and lack of extrafamilial support—increase the risk of poor disease management and intrafamilial stress.[10] Negative, critical, or hostile family comments and relationships have a greater negative effect on the patient than supportive relationships.[11,12] Therefore, interventions for caregivers and patients should be targeted at decreasing hostility and critical comments and increasing extrafamilial family support.

CAREGIVER BURDEN

Caregiver burden in families has been examined from a stress and coping perspective in various chronic illness situations, including Alzheimer disease, stroke, cancer, and heart disease. Caregiver burden is a reaction to the subjective and objective onus of providing care and may increase as new care demands arise or as existing demands intensify.[13] Subjective burden is the perceived stress experienced by the caregiver in response to the objective burden, or tasks, of caregiving.[14] The subjective and objective demands of caregiving are parallel to the emotional and instrumental aspects of caregiving. In other words, the subjective demands are highly correlated with the emotional burden, whereas the objective demands of caregiving refer to the instrumental tasks that caregivers assume.

Other aspects of caregiving burden are changes in the care-recipient's functional and mental status. The stressors associated with higher levels of perceived caregiving burden are degrees of care-recipient disability, physical and cognitive impairment, relationship to care-recipient (spouse, child, or other family member), female gender (females generally perceive greater caregiving burden than males), and the caregiver's own mental health.[15] The more positive aspects of informal caregiving should not be neglected, however. A growing body of research suggests that many family caregivers derive great satisfaction and rewards from caring for family members and develop their own particular approaches to caregiving that are rewarding for care-recipient and caregiver.[16,17]

The tasks associated with caregiving for a family member with heart disease generally are not perceived to be as onerous as those associated with caring for a family member with Alzheimer disease, stroke, or cancer. Most patients can care for themselves within a short time after a cardiac event, decreasing the number of objective tasks associated with caregiving. However, if the event was unexpected, such as an acute MI or emergent surgery for coronary artery bypass grafting (**CABG**), then the family must adapt to a new medical regimen that may include changes in the patient's diet, exercise, and medications; such a regimen can be perceived as burdensome. Greater burden may be associated with fears related to the patient's mental and physical health. For example, patients who are depressed after CABG, a not uncommon occurrence, are more likely to increase the caregiver's burden.[15]

Pohl and colleagues[18] examined elder caregiver relationships in shared households and found that the amount and scope of help that caregivers provided had a negative effect on their relationship with the older person. The more assistance that was required by the older person, the more negative the impact of the elder's presence on the household. This relationship may be explained by Skaff and Pearlin's findings[19] that the caregiver may experience psychological strain, such as feeling engulfed by the caregiving role. Being a caregiver affects all areas of a person's life. The greatest effect is on the caregiver's personal life, such as privacy and leisure time, although other areas, such as family relationships and employment, are affected as well.[20] Although caregivers of patients with heart disease may not be as burdened as those caring for patients with Alzheimer disease, stroke, or other disease conditions, the requirements of caregiving for spouses, children, and other relatives must be considered when preparing the patient and family for discharge to the home. If family caregivers can be helped to "reframe" stressors and focus on some of the rewards of caregiving, then the burden may be lessened.

Also of importance are the effects that caregiving burden has on the caregiver's cardiovascular health. Research shows that male and female spouses caring for a partner with Alzheimer disease have a higher risk of developing metabolic syndrome, followed by coronary heart disease, than do noncaregivers.[21] Likewise, data from the Nurses' Health Study showed that caring for a disabled or ill spouse, children, or grandchildren for 9 hours or more per week was associated with increased risk of coronary heart disease; there were no statistically significant increases in coronary heart disease, however, for those caring for ill parents.[22,23] Thus, caregivers may be doubly disadvantaged: they are themselves physically and emotionally burdened by care for the family member and at the same time increase their own risk for coronary heart disease.

The next section examines the problems experienced by widowed or divorced persons with heart disease and the associated problems faced by their caregiving adult children. In addition, the caregiving demands of unpartnered adults who may have been widowed or divorced but never had children are considered. As the divorce rate in Western nations increases and more persons are choosing not to have children, the needs of persons without spouses or children available to them as family caregivers must be considered.

EFFECTS OF CARDIAC DISEASE ON UNPARTNERED PERSONS

Although age and gender often are considered the main markers of vulnerability to cardiac disease, there are other factors pertaining to the family, or lack of significant others that influence cardiac outcomes. Other markers of vulnerability include unpartnered or unmarried status. Social isolation and lack of social support from a spouse have been noted as powerful predictors of recurrent MI for men.[24,25] Fewer investigators have examined psychosocial factors in women's recovery from cardiac events; however, poor psychosocial recovery appears to be related to lack of a social network, such as may be faced by unmarried women without children who may receive caregiving from siblings or nieces or nephews.[26,27] In addition, progress of coronary artery disease is worsened in women when they are socially isolated and lack emotional support. Lack of a marital partner has been associated with limited self-care abilities in heart failure patients[28] and limited knowledge and adherence.[29] Research examining coping resources of disabled elderly persons at home indicates that social networks for married persons are much larger than those for unmarried persons, suggesting the vulnerability of the unmarried during recovery from major cardiac events.[30,31]

Caregiver Burden in Adult Children of Unpartnered Elders

Relationship satisfaction in the caregiver/care-recipient relationship is fundamental to recovery from a cardiac event and important to the satisfaction the caregiver experiences in relationship with the parent care-recipient.

Parents tend to view their relationships more favorably than do offspring across adulthood. Contact frequency and geographic proximity positively affect support,[32] and neither generation in the family prefers a situation in which various generations live together.

When elders need assistance, one person, usually a family member assumes the role of primary caregiver. Others are likely to become secondary or tertiary caregivers, providing less frequent help. In the absence of a spouse, daughters are likely to become the primary caregiver; sons typically assume the role of primary caregiver only when there is no daughter. Aging mothers are more likely to choose daughters as confidantes than they are to choose sons, and daughters are more likely to report strained relationships with their parents than are sons.[33] Additionally, the caregiving role is different between sons and daughters. Daughters are more likely to assist with activities of daily living, whereas sons help more with instrumental activities of daily living.[34] Sons also may be more likely to be a caregiver when the parent's needs are not demanding or are only intermittent.[35] Cross-generational caregiving is more difficult than intergenerational caregiving, making the children of unpartnered elders themselves at risk for depression. Because heart disease usually does not strike earlier than the fifth decade for men and the seventh for women, family caregivers frequently are caring for an elderly person. That the elderly person also may be widowed or divorced increases the caregiving burden. In summary, health care providers should note that caregiving burden is generally the greatest when the patient is not a spouse and when cross-generational caregiving, such as from a child, is required.

SOCIAL SUPPORT IN THE FAMILY SYSTEM

Social support is a multidimensional and instrumental construct that includes various dimensions including sources of support, type of support, and perceived or received support.

Sources of support include the network that is available to the recovering cardiac patient and the social network available to the family caregivers. Impoverished networks for the patient or the family caregiver are associated with greater caregiver burden than social networks that furnish support from many different sources.

One type of support that is fundamental to patients and caregivers is appraisal support.[36] Appraisal support is information one is given related to the circumstances of their situation and how they are doing with the management of situation. Appraisal and informational support together form two significant types of support that are important to persons with heart disease.

Perceived support is the belief that support is available, whereas received support is the actual acquisition of support.[37-40] Reciprocal support is the belief that one can give and take in a relationship.[41-43] Within the family system, emotional concern and warmth is the most important type of support provided by families.[11] Therefore, families that provide higher levels of appraisal and informational support, that are able to reciprocate in

support relationships, and that offer warmth and support are more likely to be able to help the family member recover from a cardiac event and at the same time be less likely to suffer as a family from the caregiving demands. See Chapter 42 for an in-depth discussion of social support.

Social support for caregivers can moderate caregiver depression following spousal cardiac surgery[44] and stroke.[45] In most instances, this support arises from other nuclear or extended family members or from sources in the community, such as religious groups. Most work examining adult caregiving children and social support has used dementia as the disease model; however, findings pertaining to social support also may be pertinent to heart disease populations.

Social support to patients is an important predictor of recovery from cardiac events and is more significant for reducing mortality from heart disease than for reducing the initial incidence of clinical disease.[46] Social support is also important for reducing symptoms[47] and for improving the health-related quality of life in cardiac patients.[48] In one study, socially isolated adults with heart disease had a significantly higher risk for cardiac mortality even when age, disease severity, income, hostility, and smoking status were controlled.[49] Social support is an important variable in adapting to cardiovascular disease.[50,51] This suggests that social support—through warmth and caring provided within the family system by spousal or adult child caregivers—may be essential to cardiac recovery, whereas hostility and annoyance impairs cardiac recovery. Indeed, network and perceived social support reported by women with heart disease was associated significantly with improved health-related outcomes up to 18 months after cardiac events. Married women reported higher levels of physical and psychological health than unmarried women, an indication that social support from a spouse can enhance physical and psychological health outcomes.[52]

IMPACT OF CARDIAC CONDITIONS ON THE FAMILY
Acute Cardiac Events

Although MI and CABG are different types of cardiac events, they are acute and tend to be compared in the literature that examines family responses. Therefore, this section compares and contrasts family responses to MI and CABG.

Acute cardiac events are likely to be frightening experiences for families. Before the patient is hospitalized, family members may participate in decisions to access medical care and thus may participate in delaying treatment for symptoms of MI. Indeed, studies demonstrate that when symptoms of MI occur in the presence of family members, delay time is longer than when in the presence of strangers.[53,54] Later, family members may blame themselves for not recognizing the seriousness of the symptoms and experience guilt that the patient did not access care earlier. Once at the hospital, family members may have to confront emergency rooms, intensive care units, and other hospital locations with which they are unfamiliar. Family education related to symptoms and response to symptoms is an essential intervention for families. The importance of educating female patients and their family members is urgent because women often misinterpret their symptoms even though most studies demonstrate that they do not delay significantly longer than men.[55] Because MI often is followed by CABG surgery, angioplasty, or thrombolysis, it is imperative that family members recognize symptoms so that the most effective treatment can be sought in a timely manner.

During the acute period and hospitalization, family members need reassurance, education, and assistance with discharge planning. Family members of MI and CABG patients should be prepared for possible depression, mood changes, sleeplessness, and role changes for the patient and family members. Studies show that anxiety and depression for spousal pairs are highly correlated and that one often predicts the other.[56,57] Thus, if assessment of the hospitalized couple suggests that the patient or spouse is anxious or depressed, it is likely that the other partner also is anxious or depressed. Because high levels of anxiety before surgery decrease the ability to process information pertaining to the surgical event, it is incumbent on health care providers to try to decrease patient and spousal anxiety so that preoperative teaching can occur.[58]

Following hospitalization, families are most vulnerable to disruption in the areas of role changes and continuing depression. For example, previously employed women may take leave from their paid employment to care for recovering husbands. This may mean decreased income to the family and loss of social support that resides in the wife's work environment. Because women typically are older than men when their first MI or CABG occurs, their husbands commonly are retired and can provide caregiving without a loss of family income. In fact, older caregiving men may embrace a "work model" of caregiving, organizing around it as if it were paid employment.[57] This ability to organize around the instrumental aspects of caregiving—the tasks of caregiving—may protect older caregiving men from some of the emotional burdens of caregiving. Women, however, tend to become involved in the emotional and instrumental aspects of caregiving and may be made more vulnerable to caregiving burden because of this involvement.[22,23]

Research comparing patients recovering in the community from various cardiac conditions shows that marriage can be a protective mechanism. For example, MI patients who are married and living as a couple reported fewer physical problems than unmarried patients, although heart failure and chronic ischemic heart disease patients did not appear to experience this protective effect.[59] Marriage may be more protective for men than women, with one study finding that never-married men had poorer physical and mental health outcomes compared with never-married women after MI.[25]

The acute nature of MI and CAGB surgery, in a strange way, may be a benefit to family systems because the family then is mobilized to confront a recovery trajectory. If health care providers can plot the primary markers of recovery for patients and family members, families are more likely to be prepared for the problems encountered during recovery. Indeed, recovery for families of CABG patients may be less burdensome because surgery commonly is associated in patients' and family members' minds with a complete recovery. Although the process of heart disease continues inexorably, patients and family members commonly believe the patient has been "cured" and move on with their lives. However, acute MI, unless followed by CABG or angioplasty, may not be perceived in the same manner. Thus, families may perceive the MI patient as chronically ill, and the patient himself or herself may be more distressed than the CABG patient during recovery. Family patterns of constant monitoring, surveillance, and overprotection may develop after MI and lead to family dysfunction as a result. Family interventions are presented later in the chapter.

Heart Failure

The term *heart failure* conjures frightening thoughts for families, and the growing recognition that the prognosis is poor over the long term makes this cardiac condition difficult for families. No wonder that when heart failure patients are compared with patients with other cardiac conditions, they report more severe problems than those with other diagnoses.[59] Chapters 3, 62, 63, and 64 discuss heart failure in depth.

Like MI and CABG, heart failure requires role changes on the part of the patient and family. Responding to the demands of illness—including diet, medications, and exercise—requires careful attention from family members. The fragility of heart failure patients means that family members must participate in the medical regimen if optimal outcomes and survival are to be achieved. Because persons with heart failure are usually older than those with MI or CABG, demands on the extended family are often extensive. Although men typically develop heart failure before women, women are also at risk for heart failure and often have different underlying disease etiologies and treatment regimens. Gender influences patient response to heart failure; women tend to find the restrictions on their ability to provide care and support to friends as the most difficult aspect of heart failure, whereas men report the physical and social restrictions are most difficult for them.[60] These findings are not unlike those for men and women with MI and CABG. Thus, families should be prepared for maximizing the male patient's ability to participate in physical and social activities and for providing opportunities for women to respond to their friends and family in ways that are personally meaningful.

Spousal support and belief in the heart failure patient's ability to participate in health-promoting behaviors have been found to predict patient survival, particularly when marital functioning is of high quality.[61] Spousal confidence in the patient's ability to participate in health promotion and marital functioning and satisfaction were stronger predictors of survival than the patient's own self-efficacy expectations. Because management of heart failure is a constant, ongoing process that can be assisted by family involvement, it behooves nurses to help spouses realize that their own confidence in their family member's ability to participate in health-promoting activities may improve the family member's outcome. Because heart failure has an inconsistent trajectory with many ups and downs and an unclear prognosis, caregiving family members need assistance voicing their frustrations, adapting to frequent changes in the patient's condition, and responding flexibly to constant schedule, diet, and medication adjustments. Such demands are stressful for families. Lack of a concrete trajectory strains the family's adaptation skills.[62]

Unpartnered heart failure patients are at even greater risk for poor outcomes because they do not have spousal support, and extended family support may be fragmented. Peer support programs have been attempted with recovering MI and CABG patients, and such programs may be useful also to heart failure patients.[63-65] The provision of peer support from another elder who has experienced the same disease can improve outcomes for vulnerable cardiac patients, although some reports suggest that the nature of heart failure may be less amenable to peer support than other cardiac conditions.[66]

Other Cardiac Conditions

Other cardiac conditions that can be expected to affect the family are cardiac valve replacement or repairs and receipt of an implantable cardioverter-defibrillator (**ICD**). Although the underlying cause of valvular heart disease is different from that underlying the need for CABG, the recovery is not unlike that of CABG patients, and thus the demands on family are similar. Valve replacement patients are often older and more chronically ill when they have surgery compared with CABG patients, but because they have been living with a chronic cardiac condition for a long time, they often respond enthusiastically to the improvement in activity levels that the new valve allows them. Thus, compared with patients who have had CABG surgery in an emergent setting, their distress following surgery may be less, which in turn may diminish caregiver burden.

Implantation of an ICD may follow a sudden cardiac arrest. The arrest itself is a frightening experience for spouses or intimate partners. The needs of family caregivers of ICD patients change over time, with the most acute needs for support and information occurring during the first month after implantation.[67] Once the ICD is implanted, spouses and partners face an uncertain future. The spouses of ICD patients have reported that they worried most about caring for the ICD patient, caring for themselves in the midst of the multiple illness demands of the survivor, and the impact on their relationship in terms of sexuality, role changes, communication, and driving restrictions.[68] The needs of families is an area that deserves greater research as the implantation of ICDs becomes more common.

IMPROVING HEALTH OUTCOMES FOR FAMILY MEMBERS AND CAREGIVERS
Family Psychoeducational Interventions

Psychoeducational interventions are defined for purposes of this chapter as patient education and emotional coping strategies that address disease management and how it affects the caregiver/patient relationship. Psychoeducational programs provide information about how disease management affects family relationships, decision making, and family problem solving during the initial and later stages of disease management. Psychoeducation may be delivered in various formats, including multifamily groups, patients and family members separately, or patients and family members together. Such interventions increase understanding about the disease so that personal and relationship coping is improved.[10]

Family-centered care interventions use psychoeducation as a strategy to improve family relationships. Families of cardiac patients have many needs for information and support. Studies suggest that family caregivers need information, comfort (attention to caregivers' needs for their own health and support), and communication[69,70] at a time when recovering patients may be experiencing anxiety and depression as they adjust to management of their chronic condition. The interactive aspects of caregiving and care-receiving have been recognized in the literature,[69,71,72] but scant attention has been paid to methods of improving the relationship between the two so that outcomes are improved for all.

Strategies for a Family-Centered Intervention

As noted before in the chapter, health care providers often neglect to assess the risk of family members for cardiac disease. A unique approach to working with family caregivers and patients recovering from an acute event, such as CABG or MI, includes incorporating the caregiver and patient into an intervention that seeks to enhance primary and secondary prevention strategies for the caregiver while at the same time enhancing tertiary prevention strategies for the patient. An important aspect of the intervention is the dual focus on reducing caregiver burden and augmenting caregiver and patient psychosocial health. Table 16-3 illustrates the various components of a psychoeducational intervention that focuses on family caregiver and patient fears and concerns following an event such as MI or CABG. Such an intervention can begin in the hospital and then, because hospitalizations typically are short, can continue in an outpatient setting with an advanced practice nurse. Because patients and family members often are disturbed by the lack of recovery milestones following an acute event, this table suggests milestones for both groups during the first 6 weeks after discharge from the hospital. By allowing caregivers an opportunity to voice their needs and concerns, as well as the benefits they receive from caregiving, a shift can occur from the relatively egocentric focus on the patient to the dual needs of caregiver and care recipient.

■ ■ ■

TABLE 16-3   TOPICS FOR ADVANCED PRACTICE NURSE INTERVENTIONS FOLLOWING DISCHARGE AFTER MYOCARDIAL INFARCTION OR CORONARY ARTERY BYPASS GRAFTING

WEEK	PATIENT TOPIC	CAREGIVER TOPIC
1	What to expect early in recovery	Fears related to patient's recovery
	Symptoms	Patient's symptoms
	Medications	Managing patient's medications
2	Fears related to recovery	What to expect during recovery process
	Sleep patterns	Patient's diet
	Physical activity	Patient's physical activity
	Common complications of recovery	Patient's mood
3	Caregiver/patient role changes	Caregiver diet
	Depression	Need for caregiver role changes
4	Diet and nutrition	Helping patient obtain services
	Performance of activities of daily living and independent activities of daily living	Caregiver exercise
		Caregiver monitoring of patient
5	Return to work or household activities	Review of caregiver coronary heart disease risk factors
	Managing stress	Patient's return to work, driving, and other activities
6	Managing risk factors	Managing stress
		Caregiver wellness activities

SUMMARY

The purpose of this chapter, to address the impact of cardiac disease on the family, was accomplished in a number of ways. The interactive effects of patient and family characteristics were discussed, and the importance of considering family roles, chronic illness management in the family system, caregiving burden and rewards, and the unique needs of unpartnered persons were addressed. The influence of life span development on patients and caregivers was offered as an important consideration when working with birth cohorts of different generations. Acute MI, CABG surgery, heart failure, and ICD implantation were reviewed from the perspective of their effects on the family system. Lastly, psychoeducational interventions to improve caregiver and patient outcomes were presented. The rewards to nurses who work with families and cardiac patients can be immense if the needs of the family are considered. Indeed, nurses are privileged to work with families, the "heart and soul" of any patient.

REFERENCES

1. Williams A: Changing geographies of care: employing the concept of therapeutic landscapes as a framework in examining home space, *Soc Sci Med* 55:141-154, 2002.
2. Mayer B, Erdmann J, Schunkert H: Genetics and heritability of coronary artery disease and myocardial infarction, *Clin Res Cardiol* 2006; epub ahead of print.
3. Mansur A, Gomes E, Avakian S et al: Clustering of traditional risk factors and precocity of coronary disease in women, *Int J Cardiol* 81:205-209, 2001.
4. Sesso H, Lee I, Gaziano J, Rexrode K et al: Maternal and paternal history of myocardial infarction and risk of cardiovascular disease in men and women, *Circulation* 104:393-398, 2001.
5. Shammas NW, Lemke JH, Deckert J, et al: Gender differences in adhering to national guidelines in a community lipid clinic, *Prev Cardiol* 9:215-8, 2006.
6. Swanson J, Pearson T: Screening family members of high risk coronary disease: why isn't it done? *Am J Prev Med* 20:50-55, 2001.
7. Rankin S: Going it alone: women managing recovery from acute myocardial infarction, *Fam Community Health* 17:50-62, 1995.
8. Witt B, Jacobsen S, Weston S et al: Cardiac rehabilitation after myocardial infarction in the community, *J Am Coll Cardiol* 44:988-996, 2004.
9. Weihs K, Fisher L, Baird M: Families, health and behavior, *Fam Syst Health* 20:7-46, 2002.
10. Franks MM, Stephens MA, Rook KS, et al: Spouses, J Fam Psychol 20:311-8, 2006.
11. Campbell T: The effectiveness of family interventions for physical disorders, *J Marital Fam Ther* 29:263-281, 2003.
12. Berkhuysen M, Nieuwland W, Buunk B et al: Change in self-efficacy during cardiac rehabilitation and the role of perceived overprotectiveness, *Patient Educ Couns* 38:21-32, 1999.
13. Given C, Stommel M, Given B et al: The influence of cancer patients' symptoms and functional states on patients' depression and family caregivers' reaction and depression, *Health Psychol* 12:277-285, 1993.
14. Biegel D, Sales E, Schulz R: *Family caregiving in chronic illness: Alzheimer's disease, cancer, heart disease, mental illness,* Newberry Park, Calif, 1991, Sage Publications.
15. Sherwood P, Given C, Given B, Von Eye A: Caregiver burden and depressive symptoms: analysis of common outcomes in caregivers of elderly patients, *J Aging Health* 17:125-147, 2005.
16. Schumacher K: Reconceptualizing family caregiving: family-based illness care during chemotherapy, *Res Nurs Health* 19:261-271, 1996.
17. Eldredge DH, Nail LM, Maziarz RT et al: Explaining family caregiver role strain following autologous blood and marrow transplantation, *J Psychosoc Oncology* 24:53-74, 2006.
18. Pohl J, Given C, Collins C, Given B: Social vulnerability and reactions to caregiving in daughters and daughters-in-law caring for disabled aging parents, *Health Care Women Int* 15:385-395, 1994.
19. Skaff M, Pearlin L: Caregiving: role engulfment and the loss of self, *Gerontologist* 32:656-664, 1992.
20. McKinlay J, Crawford S, Tennstedt S: The everyday impacts of providing informal care to dependent elders and their consequences for the care recipients, *J Aging Health* 7:497-528, 1995.
21. Vitaliano P, Scanlan J, Zhang J et al: A path model of chronic stress, the metabolic syndrome, and coronary heart disease, *Psychosom Med* 64:418-435, 2002.
22. Lee S, Colditz G, Berkman L, Kawachi I: Caregiving to children and grandchildren and risk of coronary heart disease in women, *Am J Public Health* 93:1939-1944, 2003.
23. Lee S, Colditz G, Berkman L, Kawachi I: Caregiving and risk of coronary heart disease in US women: a prospective study, *Am J Public Health* 24:113-119, 2003.
24. Kawachi I, Colditz G, Ascherio A et al: A prospective study of social networks in relation to total mortality and cardiovascular disease in men in the USA, *J Epidemiol Community Health* 50:245-251, 1996.

25. Rankin S: Life-span development: refreshing a theoretical and practice perspective, *Sch Inq Nurs Pract* 14:379-387, 2000.

26. Burker E, Blumenthal J, Feldman M et al: Depression in male and female patients undergoing cardiac surgery, *Br J Clin Psychol* 34:119-128, 1995.

27. Rankin S, Fukuoka Y: Predictors of quality of life in women 1 year after myocardial infarction, *Prog Cardiovasc Nurs* 18:6-12, 2003.

28. Carlson B, Riegel B, Moser D: Self-care abilities of patients with heart failure, *Heart Lung* 30:351-359, 2001.

29. Ni H, Nauman D, Burgess D et al: Factors influencing knowledge of and adherence to self-care among patients with heart failure, *Arch Intern Med* 159:1613-1619, 1999.

30. Boaz R, Hu J: Determining the amount of help used by disabled elderly persona at home: the role of coping resources, *J Gerontol B Psychol Sci Soc Sci* 52:S317-S324, 1997.

31. Rankin SH, Butzlaff A, Carroll DL, Reedy I: FAMISHED for support: recovering elders after cardiac events, *Clin Nurs Spec* 19:142-9, 2005.

32. Rossi A, Rossi P: *Of human bonding: parent-child relations across the life course,* Hawthorne, NY, 1990, Aldine de Gruyter.

33. Umberson D: Relationships between adult children and their parents: psychological consequences for both generations, *J Marriage Fam* 54:664-674, 1992.

34. Connidis I, Rosenthal C, McMullin J: The impact of family composition on providing help to older parents: a study of employed adults, *Res Aging* 18:402-429, 1996.

35. Horowitz A: Sons and daughters as caregivers to older parents: differences in role performance and consequences, *Gerontologist* 25:612-617, 1985.

36. House J: *Work stress and social support,* Reading, Mass, 1981, Addison-Wesley.

37. Cobb S: Social support as a moderator of life stress, *Psychosom Med* 38:300-314, 1976.

38. Hobfoil S, Vaux A: Social support: social resources and social context. In Goldberger L, Breznitz S, editors: *Handbook of stress: theoretical and clinical aspects,* ed 2, New York, 1993, Free Press.

39. House J, Kahn R: Measures and concepts of social support. In Cohen S, Syme S, editors: *Social support and health,* New York, 1985, Academic Press.

40. Thiots P: Life stress, social support, and psychological vulnerability: epidemiological considerations, *J Community Psychol* 10:341-362, 1982.

41. Dwyer J, Miller M: Differences in characteristics of the caregiving network by area of residence: implications for primary caregiver stress and burden, *J Appl Fam Child Stud* 39:27-37, 1990.

42. Tilden V, Hirsch A, Nelson C: The interpersonal relationship inventory: continued psychometric evaluation, *J Nurs Meas* 2:63-78, 1994.

43. Tyler KA. The impact of support received and support provision on changes in perceived social support among older adults, *Int J Aging Hum Dev* 62:21-38, 2006.

44. Rankin S, Monahan P: Great expectations: perceived social support in couples experiencing cardiac surgery, *Fam Relat* 40:297-302, 1991.

45. Grant JS, Elliott TR, Weaver M et al: Social support, social problem-solving abilities, and adjustment of family caregivers of stroke survivors, *Arch Phys Med Rehabil* 87:343-50, 2006.

46. Greenwood D, Muir K, Packham C, Madeley R: Coronary heart disease: a review of the role of psychosocial stress and social suport, *J Public Health Med* 18:221-231, 1996.

47. Lindsay G, Smith L, Hanlon P, Wheatley D: Coronary artery disease patients' perception of their health and expectations of benefit following coronary artery bypass grafting, *J Adv Nurs* 32:1412-1421, 2001.

48. Bosworth H, Siegler I, Olsen M et al: Social support and quality of life in patients with coronary artery disease, *Qual Life Res* 9:829-839, 2000.

49. Brummett B, Barefoot J, Siegler I et al: Characteristics of socially isolated patients with coronary artery disease who are at elevated risk for mortality, *Psychosom Med* 63:267-272, 2001.

50. Brummett B, Barefoot J, Siegler I, Steffens D: Relation of subjective and received social support to clinical and self-report assessments of depressive symptoms in an elderly population, *J Affect Disord* 61:41-50, 2000.

51. Welin C, Rosengren A, Welhelmsen L: Social relationships and myocardial infarction: a cast-control study, *J Cardiovasc Risk* 3:183-190, 1996.

52. Janevic M, Janz N, Dodge J et al: Longitudinal effects of social support on the health and functioning of older women with heart disease, *Int J Aging Hum Dev* 59:153-175, 2004.

53. Reilly A, Dracup K, Dattolo J: Factors influencing prehospital delay in patients experiencing chest pain, *Am J Crit Care* 3:300-306, 1994.

54. Rosenfeld A: Women's risk of decision delay in acute myocardial infarction: implications for research and practice, *AACN Clin Issues* 12:29-39, 2001.

55. Moser D, McKinley S, Dracup K, Chung M: Gender differences in reasons patients delay in seeking treatment for acute myocardial infarction symptoms, *Patient Educ Couns* 56:45-54, 2005.

56. Moser D, Dracup K: Role of spousal anxiety and depression in patients psychosocial recovery after a cardiac event, *Psychosom Med* 66:527-532, 2004.

57. Rankin S: Psychosocial adjustments of the CAD patient and spouse: nursing implications, *Nurs Clin North Am* 27:271-284, 1992.

58. Rankin S, Stallings K, London F: *Patient education in health and illness,* ed 5, Philadelphia, 2005, Lippincott Williams & Wilkins.

59. Dixon T, Lim L-Y, Powell H, Fisher J: Psychosocial experiences of cardiac patients in early recovery: a community-based study, *J Adv Nurs* 31:1368-1375, 2000.

60. Stromberg A, Martensson J: Gender differences in patients with heart failure, *Eur J Cardiovasc Nurs* 2:7-18, 2003.

61. Rohrbaugh M, Shoham V, Coyne J et al: Beyond the "self" in self-efficacy: spouse confidence predicts patient survival following heart failure, *J Fam Psychol* 18:184-193, 2004.

62. Dunbar S, Clark P, Deaton C et al: Family education and support interventions in heart failure, *Nurs Res* 54:158-166, 2005.

63. Whittemore R, Rankin S, Callahan C et al: The peer advisor experience providing social support, *Qual Health Res* 10:200-276, 2000.

64. Carroll D, Robinson E, Buselli E et al: Activities of the APN to enhance unpartnered elders self-efficacy after myocardial infarction, *Clin Nurse Spec* 15:60-66, 2001.

65. Winder P, Hiltunen E, Sethares K, Butzlaff A: Partnerships in mending hearts: nurse and peer intervention for recovering cardiac elders, *J Cardiovasc Nurs* 19:184-191, 2004.

66. Riegel B, Carlson B: Is individual peer support a promising intervention for persons with heart failure? *J Cardiovasc Nurs* 19:174-183, 2004.

67. Dougherty C: Family-focused interventions for survivors of sudden cardiac arrest, *J Cardiovasc Nurs* 12:45-58, 1997.

68. Dougherty C, Pyper G, Benoliel J: Domains of concern of intimate partners of sudden cardiac arrest survivors after ICD implantation, *J Cardiovasc Nurs* 19:21-31, 2004.

69. Fleury J, Moore S: Family-centered care after acute myocardial infarction, *J Cardiovasc Nurs* 13:73-82, 1999.

70. Naylor M: Nursing intervention research and quality of care: influencing the future of healthcare, *Nurs Res* 52:380-385, 2003.

71. Riegel B, Dracup K: Does overprotection cause cardiac invalidism after acute myocardial infarction? *Heart Lung* 21:529-535, 1992.

72. Van Horn E, Fleury J, Moore S: Family interventions during the trajectory of recovery from cardiac event: an integrative literature review, *Heart Lung* 31:186-198, 2002.

■■■ chapter **17**

Sleep, Sleep Disorders, and Cardiac Disease

Nancy S. Redeker

CHAPTER ABBREVIATIONS

AHI   apnea/hypopnea index

CBT   cognitive-behavioral therapy

CPAP   continuous positive airway pressure

CSB-CSA   Cheyne-Stokes breathing–central sleep apnea

EEG   electroencephalography

MI   myocardial infarction

NPSG   nocturnal polysomnography

NREM   non–rapid eye movement

OSAHS   obstructive sleep apnea/hypopnea syndrome

REM   rapid eye movement

SHHS   Sleep Heart Health Study

Recent basic and clinical research findings have resulted in exponential growth in knowledge about sleep. With this knowledge has come increased awareness that sleep and sleep disorders are tied integrally to primary, secondary, and tertiary prevention of cardiovascular disease. Sleep disorders contribute to the development of cardiovascular pathophysiological conditions such as hypertension and heart failure and to increased morbidity and mortality. Conversely, poor sleep and sleep-disordered breathing associated with chronic heart failure may worsen pathophysiological processes and have a negative impact on quality of life and daytime functioning.

Disturbed sleep associated with hospitalization and recovery after treatment of cardiovascular conditions also has a significant impact on recovery, functional outcomes, and quality of life. Promoting adequate sleep, and preventing and treating sleep disorders are increasingly important components of nursing and collaborative cardiovascular care. The purpose of this chapter is to explore the scientific evidence supporting the linkages between sleep, sleep disorders, and cardiovascular disease and to examine the cardiovascular nurse's role in sleep promotion and management of sleep disorders across the continuum of primary, secondary, and tertiary prevention.

NORMAL SLEEP
Behavioral and Physiological Characteristics of Sleep

Sleep is a multidimensional phenomenon that has physiological and behavioral attributes. Sleep has been defined in various ways. An often-cited behavioral definition describes sleep as a "recurring state of existence characterized by (a) reductions in awareness of and interactions with the environment, (b) lowered motility and muscular activity, and (c) partial or complete abeyance of voluntary behavior and consciousness"[1] (p. 2).

The two main physiological states of sleep are non–rapid eye movement sleep (**NREM**) and rapid eye movement sleep (**REM**). In adults, REM and NREM sleep (stages 1, 2, 3, and 4) alternate throughout the night in approximately 90-minute cycles (Figure 17-1). As the sleep stages progress from NREM stage 1 through stage 4, the person is more difficult to awaken. During NREM sleep the brain is relatively inactive but actively regulated, and the body is movable.[2] Each stage of NREM sleep is associated with characteristic patterns of brain wave (electroencephalography [**EEG**]) activity. During REM sleep the brain is highly activated, and there is atonia of all skeletal muscles except those of the eyes, middle ear ossicles, and diaphragm.[3] Rapid eye movements and vivid dreams are prevalent during REM sleep.

The circadian pacemaker, or biological clock, controls the daily timing of sleep. This structure is the suprachiasmatic nucleus located in the hypothalamus. Physiological activities, including sleep and wake states, have circadian patterns that occur without external stimuli. However, exogenous factors such as light/dark, the timing of meals, and social cues also influence the pattern of sleep and other circadian physiological events. These factors, called zeitgebers, result in the occurrence of sleep and wake during predictable times during the day or night. For example, in most situations, adults are awake during the day and asleep at night. Loss of zeitgebers at regular times of day may alter circadian rhythms of activity and rest along with many physiological processes.

The need for sleep increases as wake time increases. Prolonged periods of wakefulness cause decreased alertness and increased sleepiness. Once sleep occurs, the accumulated "sleep debt" is replenished. This results in the feeling of being rested. To date, the scientific basis for the restorative nature of sleep has not been explained completely.

Neuroendocrine processes are under circadian control and are active during sleep. Growth hormone peaks in the early part of the night and appears to be linked with slow wave sleep. Prolactin levels are highest during sleep and lowest during wakefulness. Cortisol secretion is inhibited during sleep but has a circadian pattern. Cortisol secretion is lowest in the early stages of sleep and highest in the early morning hours. Thyroid-stimulating hormone has a circadian rhythm, with lowest levels during the day and highest before sleep onset. Thyroid-stimulating hormone is inhibited by sleep.[3] Glucose levels remain fairly stable over the course of the

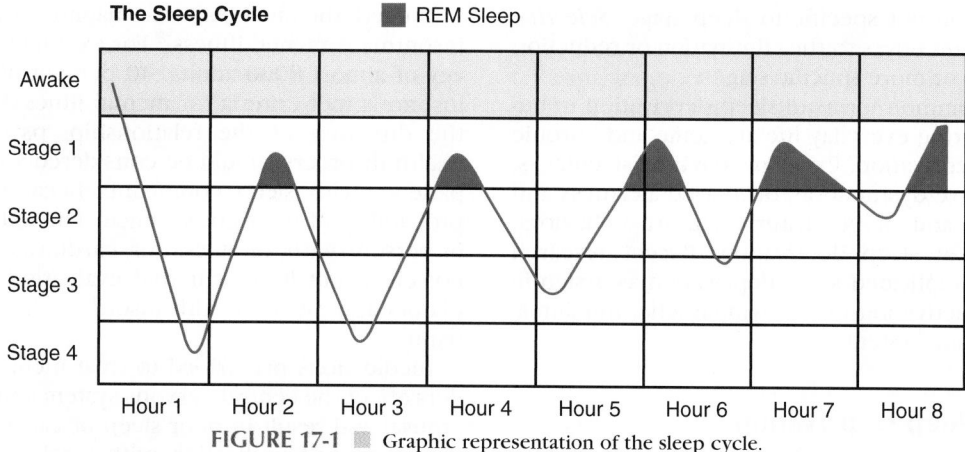

FIGURE 17-1 ■ Graphic representation of the sleep cycle.

nocturnal sleep period, despite the fasting state. Sleep deprivation is associated with impaired glucose tolerance, reduced thyrotropin levels, decreased growth hormone secretion, elevated evening cortisol levels, and sympathetic nervous system activation.[4]

The cardiovascular system undergoes profound changes during sleep. Parasympathetic nervous system activity increases, and sympathetic activity decreases during NREM sleep compared with the waking state. Parasympathetic and sympathetic activity decrease during REM sleep. During REM sleep, parasympathetic activity is dominant; however, there are intermittent surges in sympathetic activity during phasic REM sleep. NREM sleep is associated with autonomic stability and decreases in heart rate, blood pressure, cardiac output, and systemic vascular resistance.[5] During REM sleep the heart rate is highly variable, and there may be episodes of tachycardia and bradycardia. Surges in autonomic activity during REM sleep may explain observations of more frequent ventricular dysrhythmias occurring during this phase of sleep. Cardiac output falls during sleep over the course of the night and reaches its lowest point during the last REM cycle in the early hours of the morning.[3] Decreased cardiac output and increased sympathetic activity during REM sleep, particularly in the early morning hours, may explain the higher occurrence of sudden cardiac death and ischemic cardiac events at this time.

Respiratory changes also characterize progression from waking through NREM and REM sleep. Ventilation decreases during sleep. During wakefulness, breathing is controlled by voluntary and autonomic mechanisms. However, during sleep, voluntary control over ventilation is lost. During NREM sleep, respiratory rate and minute ventilation decrease, PcO_2 rises, and PO_2 and oxyhemoglobin saturation fall. Decreased activity of the pharyngeal dilator muscles causes increased airway resistance that may predispose to snoring, hypopnea, and apnea. Hypoventilation occurs because of the absence of stimuli associated with waking and reduced chemosensitivity to carbon dioxide. Increased blood flow to the brain further decreases chemosensitivity during REM sleep. Skeletal muscle atonia of all but the diaphragmatic muscles during REM sleep further contributes to decreased ventilatory response. Apneas are particularly likely to occur at sleep onset and during REM sleep.[3]

Developmental Changes in Sleep

Normal sleep patterns change over the course of life. Newborns sleep throughout much of the 24-hour day and have brief periods of awakening. As children progress into the toddler and preschool years, their sleep becomes more consolidated during the night, and napping decreases. During middle childhood the nocturnal sleep period decreases. Daily sleep time gradually declines from 10 to about 7 to 8 hours by the end of adolescence.

Young adults typically report sleeping about 7½ hours at night on weekdays and 8½ hours or longer on weekends. However, the amount of sleep is highly variable and is influenced by many factors, including genetics, preference, lifestyle, and environment. Usually there is one long sleep period and little or no daytime napping. REM sleep occupies about 20 to 25 percent of the sleep period and NREM occupies 75 to 80 percent. Slow wave sleep (stages 3 and 4) occurs mostly in the first third of the night, and REM sleep occurs mainly near the end of the night.[2]

As adults age, there is little change in the total amount of sleep, but there is less slow wave sleep. Some research and clinical observations have suggested that older adults may report more insomnia and have more frequent nocturnal awakenings and poorer sleep efficiency than younger adults. However, the sleep disturbance observed among older adults often is associated with medical or mental health illnesses or primary sleep disorders.[6] Therefore, the commonly held belief that sleep disturbance is a normal part of aging is not supported, and reports of disturbed sleep should not be attributed to aging alone.

SLEEP DEPRIVATION

Sleep deprivation is a reduced quantity and quality of sleep. Complete sleep deprivation refers to the absence of sleep. Sleep deprivation also may refer to the loss of the restorative power of sleep through frequent brief arousals. *Partial sleep deprivation* refers to reductions in sleep duration not specific to sleep stage. *Selective sleep deprivation* refers to the elimination or reduction of sleep in one or more specific stages.

The most common forms of sleep deprivation in human beings during everyday life are acute and chronic partial sleep deprivation. Excessive daytime sleepiness, fatigue, cognitive dysfunction, decreased alertness and reaction time, and mood disturbance are behavioral consequences of sleep deprivation. Recent research findings have implicated sleep deprivation as a significant cause of activation of the sympathetic, inflammatory, and immune systems.

Causes of Sleep Deprivation

The sleep-wake system is influenced by a host of environmental, personal, social, occupational, psychological, disease-related, and treatment-related factors. Primary sleep disorders such as insomnia, sleep-disordered breathing, and parasomnias are also significant contributors to sleep deprivation.

Environmental Factors

Environmental factors that may contribute to sleep deprivation include noise, lighting, and ambient temperature extremes. The presence of other persons, such as a bed partner who snores or is restless, or children or pets that may be awake or restless during the night, is a common cause of sleep disruption. Sleeping in an unfamiliar environment (e.g., hospital or hotel room) also may cause sleep deprivation. Hospitalized patients often report excessive levels of lighting and noise, as well as frequent sleep interruptions for patient care activities.

Personal Factors

Personal factors that influence sleep-wake cycles include the person's predisposition to be an "owl" (late bedtime, late rising time) or a "lark" (early bedtime, early rise time) or the tendency to prefer longer or shorter sleep periods. Some of these preferences appear to be genetically determined. Living in a fast-paced "24/7" society also plays a major role in sleep deprivation as work, social, and leisure activities increasingly occupy hours that were once spent sleeping.

Occupational and Social Factors

Occupational and social factors also contribute to sleep deprivation. Shift workers who work night or rotating shifts experience difficulty getting to sleep, decreased total sleep time, and somnolence during working hours.[7] Shift workers appear to be at excess risk for cardiovascular morbidity. Although the mechanism is not known, sleep deprivation and altered circadian timing may be contributing factors.

Mental Health Disorders and Stress

Most mental health disorders are associated with insomnia, a disorder of initiating and maintaining sleep. Likewise, sleep disturbances appear to contribute to the development of many mental health problems, such as depression, anxiety, and substance abuse.

Indeed, the most common diagnosis of patients with insomnia is mental illness.[8] For example, in a large survey of almost 8000 adults, 40 percent of persons with insomnia met criteria for mental illness.[9] Regardless of the direction of the relationship, psychiatric-mental health disorders should be considered when evaluating patients with sleep complaints because of the high probability of their coexistence. The extent of overlap in persons with, or at risk for, cardiovascular disease is not clear, but it is clear that evaluation of sleep complaints and mental health disorders should go hand in hand.

Medications prescribed to treat mental health disorders affect the central nervous system and may heighten arousal and result in poor sleep or cause sedation. Furthermore, self-medication with alcohol is common in persons with insomnia. However, although alcohol initially causes sleepiness, even small quantities have a negative effect on sleep architecture.

Stress—with its associated elevation in sympathetic tone, manifested as hyperarousal, anxiety, elevated heart and respiratory rate—is another important contributor to acute and chronic insomnia.

Medical Disorders

Almost all medical disorders are associated in some way with disturbed sleep. Some examples include asthma, chronic obstructive pulmonary disease, diabetes mellitus, renal failure, and Parkinson disease. Cardiovascular disorders also are associated with sleep disturbance, and the relationships between sleep and cardiovascular disorders are examined in depth later in the chapter. Sleep disturbance may result from an underlying pathophysiological process, but it also may result from the person's disease-related symptoms, emotional reactions to illness (e.g., pain, shortness of breath, and anxiety), characteristics of the health care environment, or medical or surgical treatments.[10] Many prescribed and over-the-counter medications contribute to sleep deprivation. Excess use of caffeine, alcohol, and nicotine contribute substantially to disturbed sleep patterns as well.

Primary Sleep Disorders

Primary sleep disorders are another significant cause of sleep deprivation. The most common sleep disorder in adults is insomnia. Sleep-disordered breathing, periodic limb movement disorders, and parasomnias (e.g., bruxism, sleepwalking, and talking during sleep) also may cause significant sleep disruption.

CONTRIBUTIONS OF SLEEP DISORDERS TO CARDIOVASCULAR MORBIDITY AND MORTALITY

Scientific evidence is increasing that suggests sleep disorders, such as obstructive sleep apnea/hypopnea syndrome (**OSAHS**), insomnia, and sleep deprivation have a significant impact on cardiovascular morbidity and mortality. Although the causal relationships have not been identified completely, sleep disorders have been linked with hypertension, coronary heart disease, heart failure, dysrhythmias, pulmonary hypertension, and stroke.

Obstructive Sleep Apnea/ Hypopnea Syndrome

OSAHS is a respiratory disturbance that results from repetitive intermittent partial or complete obstruction of the pharyngeal airway during sleep. The obstruction occurs on a continuum from snoring and hypopnea (reduced ventilation) to apnea (complete cessation of breathing). The increased effort required to breathe against an obstructed airway results in frequent arousals from sleep. Nocturnal oxygen desaturation often accompanies the respiratory events. The severity of OSAHS is determined by the apnea/hypopnea index (**AHI**), which is the number of apneas and hypopneas per hour of sleep. The AHI corresponds to the following levels of OSAHS severity:

- Less than 5 = normal
- 5 to 15 = mild
- More than 15 to 30 = moderate
- More than 30 or more = severe

Excessive daytime sleepiness is a necessary component of the diagnosis.[11] Bed partners of persons with OSAHS may observe gasping, snorting, and loud snoring, as well as apneas. Persons with OSAHS may report a dry mouth, a sore throat, a headache, or a combination of these problems upon awakening. Daytime consequences include excessive daytime sleepiness, mood alterations, impaired memory, impaired reaction time, and other cognitive deficits. Excessive daytime sleepiness may result in motor vehicle accidents, interfere with performance in work and social activities, and impair quality of life. However, persons with OSAHS may not be aware that their functioning is compromised.

Male gender, postmenopausal status in women, obesity (especially central obesity), smoking, craniofacial abnormalities, and pharyngeal anatomical features (e.g., large uvula and tongue) are risk factors for OSAHS. Smoking also may contribute. A large neck circumference (more than 17 inches in men or 16 inches in women) suggests increased risk. Symptoms are usually more severe after the consumption of alcohol or medications with sedative effects.

Epidemiology of OSAHS and Cardiovascular Disease

OSAHS, defined as more than five apneas or hypopneas per hour of sleep and daytime hypersomnolence, occurs in 4 percent of American middle-aged men and 2 percent of middle-aged women.[12] Using the AHI alone, the prevalence is even higher: 24 percent of men and 9 percent of women. OSAHS is about 3 times more prevalent in men than women, although its prevalence increases in women after menopause. OSAHS also appears to be more prevalent in blacks than whites. Although prevalence estimates vary with measurement methods, scores used for diagnosis, and study populations, sleep specialists believe that OSAHS is underdiagnosed.

Data accumulated since the identification of OSAHS in the 1970s increasingly support its association with cardiovascular morbidity and mortality. Controversy is ongoing among sleep experts regarding the degree of sleep-disordered breathing that may have negative cardiovascular consequences. However, current evidence suggests that snoring and even relatively few apneas and hypopneas may contribute to the development of hypertension, coronary heart disease, stroke, heart failure, dysrhythmias, and cardiovascular disease–related death.

Hypertension

Two population-based studies provide the most powerful epidemiological evidence to date for the linkage between OSAHS and hypertension. Investigators for the Wisconsin Sleep Cohort Study[13] found a linear increase in blood pressure as the AHI increased in a sample of 1060 employed men and women between ages 30 and 60. Longitudinal follow-up of 760 of these participants revealed a dose-response relationship between sleep-disordered breathing at baseline and the development of hypertension 4 years later, thus suggesting a causal relationship.[14]

The Sleep Heart Health Study (**SHHS**)[15] is a federally funded, community-based, prospective study designed to evaluate the linkages between OSAHS and cardiovascular morbidity and mortality. More than 6000 middle-aged participants were recruited from 23,000 participants enrolled in large population-based studies throughout the United States. Data obtained from 6132 middle-aged men and women revealed that mean systolic and diastolic blood pressure and prevalence of hypertension increased significantly at higher AHIs. The odds ratio for hypertension, comparing the highest AHI level (greater than 30/hr) to the lowest (less than 1.5/hr) was 1.37 (confidence interval [CI] = 1.03 to 1.83, $p < 0.005$). Furthermore, the findings revealed a statistically significant relationship between hemoglobin oxygen saturation of less than 90 percent and hypertension, and smaller associations between arousal index (by EEG), self-reported snoring, and hypertension. These relationships were similar for middle-aged and older persons, men and women, and those from varied ethnic backgrounds.[16] The associations were statistically significant even after controlling for co-occurring risk factors for hypertension and sleep-disordered breathing, such as alcohol consumption and body mass index.

Many human and animal studies have focused on the relationship between OSAHS and cardiovascular disease. Apneas and hypopneas cause hypoxemia and nocturnal and daytime sympathetic activation. Nocturnal sympathetic activation, in turn, results in elevated heart rate, increased cardiac output, decreased heart rate variability, peripheral vascular resistance, and tubular sodium reabsorption[17]—all of which may contribute to the development of hypertension. Notable is that the Joint National Committee on Prevention, Detection, Evaluation, and Treatment of High Blood Pressure VII included sleep apnea as a contributor to hypertension.[18]

Coronary Heart Disease

Several studies have implicated OSAHS as a risk factor for ischemic heart disease, and severe OSAHS has been documented in patients who have nocturnal angina.[19] Cross-sectional data obtained from 6424 SHHS participants revealed small to moderate associations between sleep-disordered breathing and manifestations of cardiovascular disease, including heart failure, stroke, and coronary heart disease. There were small to moderate effects of the AHI on the likelihood of having cardiovascular disease, even at AHI ranges often considered normal or mildly elevated.[20]

Many studies have sought to ascertain the processes whereby OSAHS may contribute to the development of vascular pathophysiology and coronary artery disease. Several pathways have been proposed and are supported by human and animal data. The most plausible hypotheses suggest that hypoxia and sleep fragmentation lead to the following:

- Increases in sympathetic activity, manifested by elevations in cortisol level, increased resting heart rate, and decreased heart rate variability
- Endothelial dysfunction associated with endothelin-1, a vasoconstrictive substance
- Increases in inflammatory mediators, including C-reactive protein, interleukin-6, and oxidative stress
- Increases in prothrombotic factors, such as fibrinogen, platelet activation and aggregation, and inhibition of plasminogen activator inhibitor.[17-21] (See Chapters 9 and 10 in this text for a discussion of the pathophysiology of coronary disease.)

One of the difficulties encountered in studying the relationships between OSAHS and cardiovascular disease is the presence of overlapping risk factors (such as obesity, diabetes, and hypertension). Many studies of the links between OSAHS and cardiovascular disease have not controlled for these variables. Therefore, the independent relationship between OSAHS and cardiovascular disease has been difficult to evaluate. Cross-sectional data from the SHHS supported the overlap between sleep-disordered breathing and traditional cardiovascular risk factors. The respiratory disturbance index was related to age, body mass index, waist-to-hip ratio, hypertension, diabetes, and lipid levels.[20]

OSAHS also may lead to coronary heart disease through its influence on the development of diabetes and obesity. Hypoxia and sleep fragmentation associated with sleep-disordered breathing have been linked with impaired glucose tolerance, insulin resistance, and elevated leptin levels. Sleep apnea appears to increase insulin resistance through its effect on cortisol, interleukin-6, and tumor necrosis factor-alpha.[22] Evidence that nocturnal use of continuous positive airway pressure (**CPAP**) improves insulin sensitivity in persons with sleep-disordered breathing provides further support for this hypothesis.[23] These findings also emphasize the idea that sleep-disordered breathing is a systemic disorder.

Heart Failure

OSAHS appears to be common among patients with systolic and diastolic heart failure. The mechanisms are likely multifactorial. OSAHS appears to lead to left ventricular hypertrophy independently of its effect on hypertension.[24] The development of heart failure also is likely to follow from the effect of OSAHS on hypertension and ischemic heart disease.

Stroke

A history of snoring and OSAHS are linked with a higher-than-expected incidence of stroke and transient ischemic attacks. Pathophysiological evidence suggests that the association between OSAHS and stroke is related to hypoxia, alterations in cerebral hemodynamics, and increased coagulability. Obstructive respiratory events cause elevations in intracranial pressure and decreased cerebral perfusion. Changes in cerebral blood velocity may strain blood vessels and may contribute to atherosclerosis. Platelet aggregation increases during the early morning hours in men with severe OSAHS and may contribute further to the likelihood of stroke. This process may explain the frequent onset of stroke symptoms in early morning hours.[25]

Dysrhythmias

Various dysrhythmias appear to be associated with OSAHS. Bradycardia and atrioventricular block may be associated with vagal responses resulting from apneic events. Ventricular and supraventricular tachycardia also may occur. Atrial fibrillation is more common in heart failure and coronary artery surgery patients who have OSAHS than it is in similar patients who do not have OSAHS. Atrial fibrillation also has a higher rate of recurrence after cardioversion in patients with poorly controlled OSAHS.[17]

Treatment of Obstructive Sleep Apnea/ Hypopnea Syndrome

The primary preventive strategy for OSAHS is weight loss.[26] Elimination of alcohol consumption in the evening and avoidance of sedative medications appears to reduce the frequency of respiratory events as well. When OSAHS is more severe in the supine position, sleeping in a lateral position may be effective in reducing respiratory events.

Nasal CPAP, applied during all sleep periods, including naps, is the most effective strategy for reducing apneas and hypopneas during sleep (Figure 17-2). CPAP serves as a splint that prevents the collapse and narrow-

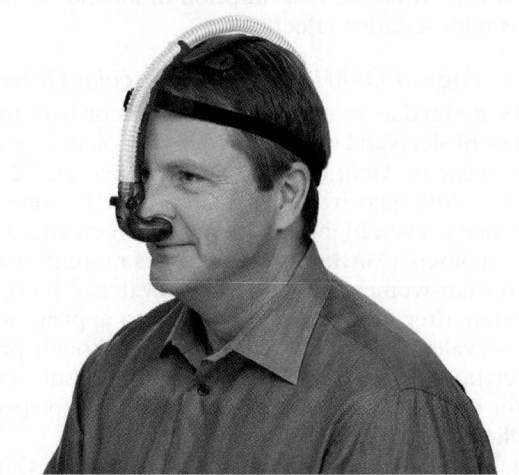

FIGURE 17-2 ■ Continuous positive airway pressure device in use. (Image courtesy Nellcor Puritan Bennett Inc, Pleasanton, Calif.)

ing of the airway during sleep. Dental appliances that cause mandibular advancement and tongue protrusion are successful about 50 percent of the time. Surgical treatments, such as laser-assisted uvulopalatoplasty and reduction of tongue volume, are generally effective in reducing snoring but are not as effective in reducing apneas and hypopneas, particularly in patients with severe OSAHS.

Although CPAP is effective in reducing apneas, hypopneas, and cortical arousals and in reducing nocturnal blood pressure in hypertensive OSAHS patients,[27] its long-term effects on daytime hypertension are less clear.[28] Faccenda and colleagues[29] reported decreases in 24-hour diastolic blood pressure that were greater in persons with more severe oxygen saturation, whereas Narkiewicz and colleagues[30] reported decreases in serum and urine norepinephrine levels. Taken together, these studies suggest that CPAP may reduce hypertension through its effects on oxyhemoglobin saturation and sympathetic traffic. However, researchers also have found small effects of CPAP on blood pressure that may not change the diagnosis of hypertension. For example, Hermida and colleagues[31] found very small, not statistically significant, effects on ambulatory blood pressure in a sample of 122 OSAHS patients, of whom 64 had hypertension. Others found that therapeutic CPAP levels reduced mean arterial ambulatory blood pressure, but reductions in blood pressure were higher in persons with more severe OSAHS.[32] Few studies have been conducted to consider the relative or combined effects of weight loss and CPAP, and no prospective clinical trials have examined the extent to which CPAP reduces cardiovascular morbidity and mortality. No clinical trial could be found that evaluated the extent to which surgical treatment or dental devices used to treat OSAHS affect cardiovascular disease.

INSOMNIA AND SLEEP DEPRIVATION

Insomnia, a form of chronic partial sleep deprivation, is associated with difficulty falling asleep, staying asleep, or the perception of nonrestorative sleep. Insomnia can range in duration from a few days to many months or years. Insomnia may be primary (no identifiable cause) or the result of other problems. According to the National Sleep Foundation, 54 percent of adults surveyed report having had one or more symptoms of insomnia at least a few nights a week in the past year; 33 percent say they have had insomnia every night or almost every night. Insomnia is more common in women, shift workers, those with lower incomes, and those with children. Hypertension, nighttime heartburn/gastroesophageal reflux disease, anxiety, depression, heart disease, arthritis, heart disease, and lung disease were reported to be associated with insomnia.[33]

Insomnia appears to be associated with death from coronary heart disease, independent of sleep-disordered breathing.[34] The Framingham study demonstrated that trouble falling asleep was associated with a threefold risk of developing a nonfatal myocardial infarction (**MI**) or death from coronary heart disease.[35] Longitudinal data from the Piedmont study indicated that restless

sleep and trouble falling asleep predicted incident MI after controlling for age, gender, and race. However, these relationships were diminished after controlling for education, use of prescription medications, self-rated health, and depression.[36] The investigators concluded that insomnia may be a manifestation of underlying mood disturbance or distress. More recently, however, Leineweber and colleagues[37] found that women who had poor sleep quality had 2.5 times the risk of acute MI or unstable angina. This relationship did not appear to be associated with depression. However, women with sleep disturbance and depression had an elevated risk of recurrent cardiac events.

Although the underlying mechanism of the relationship between insomnia and cardiovascular morbidity and death is not understood clearly, insomnia may be a marker for underlying stress and autonomic dysfunction.[34] An alternative explanation for these findings may be that the study participants had undetected sleep-disordered breathing. However, this seems unlikely because they did not report snoring, and one of the insomnia symptoms was prolonged sleep latency, a complaint not usually associated with sleep-disordered breathing.

Evaluation of a complaint of insomnia should include a review for medical disorders and medication use, mental health concerns (e.g., stress, anxiety, depression, and substance abuse), environmental influences, social and occupational concerns, and the presence of other primary sleep disorders (such as sleep-disordered breathing, periodic limb movement disorder, and restless legs syndrome) that may cause frequent nocturnal arousals and nonrestorative sleep. Primary insomnia is less common but may be associated with heightened arousal.

Treatment of Insomnia

Treatment of insomnia includes a variety of behavioral and medicinal approaches and may be most effective when medications are combined with behavioral approaches. Behavioral approaches include sleep hygiene, stimulus control, cognitive-behavioral therapy (**CBT**), and strategies to reduce arousal, such as massage and biofeedback. Sleep hygiene includes strategies to manipulate environmental conditions and personal behaviors to support effective sleep (Box 17-1). CBT combines behavioral interventions for insomnia with cognitive therapy directed at changing perspective and beliefs about sleep and insomnia.[38] CBT is a multicomponent therapy that may include a combination of sleep hygiene, sleep restriction, relaxation training, stimulus control, paradoxical intention, and cognitive restructuring. Various combinations of these strategies have been used.[39]

Hypnotic drugs are most appropriate for treating transient or intermittent insomnia but may be used in chronic insomnia if the effects are monitored closely. Benzodiazepines are the most commonly prescribed. However, the use of nonbenzodiazepine or benzodiazepine receptor agonists, such as zolpidem and zaleplon, is increasing, and these drugs may be less likely to produce tolerance or hangover effects than the benzodiazepines. Many persons use over-the-counter medications containing the antihistamine diphenhydramine, which

---

BOX 17-1 ▪ ▪ ▪
SLEEP HYGIENE INSTRUCTIONS

Do
- Maintain consistent weekday and weekend bedtime and wake-up time.
- Engage in relaxing and enjoyable activity before bedtime.
- Maintain a comfortable bedroom temperature.
- Make the bedroom as quiet and dark as possible.
- Use the bed only for sleeping and sexual activity.
- Exercise in the late afternoon.
- Eat a light snack before bed if hungry.

Don't
- Consume alcohol or caffeine within 6 hours of bedtime.
- Take stimulant medications.
- Take naps during the day and early evening.
- Engage in intellectually stimulating or stressful activity before bedtime.
- Go to bed on a full stomach or hungry.
- Watch the clock.
- Allow pets in the bedroom.
- Keep the television on at night.
- Turn on bright lights if you get out of bed at night.
- Think about the troubles of the past day.

---

causes sedation, drowsiness, and tolerance. Daytime sleepiness is common. Antihistamines may have adverse effects when used with anticholinergic drugs and central nervous system depressants; there is little data supporting their use as hypnotics. Tricyclic antidepressants that have sedating effects also may be used to promote sleep and may be particularly useful in patients with insomnia and depression. However, these drugs should be used with caution in patients with cardiovascular disease. The extent to which treating insomnia with any of these modalities improves cardiovascular morbidity and mortality is unknown.

SLEEP DISORDERS CAUSED BY CARDIOVASCULAR DISORDERS

Cheyne-Stokes Breathing–Central Sleep Apnea

Cheyne-Stokes breathing–central sleep apnea (**CSB-CSA**) refers to the pattern of waxing and waning respiration during sleep, with periods of central apnea. The term *periodic breathing* describes waxing and waning patterns of tidal volume with hypopneas rather than apneas. CSB-CSA may occur in 40 to 63 percent of persons with systolic heart failure,[40] although rates as low as 9 percent have been reported in heart failure patients managed in specialized heart failure disease management programs.[41] However, estimates of prevalence are based on studies that had small samples, of which some have consisted of only men; further, the results of individual studies are difficult to compare because of differences in the clinical characteristics of the patients studied (e.g., ejection fraction and medications). CSB-CSA is associated with a risk for ventricular tachycardia[40] and mortality, although the association may reflect the poorer cardiac status of patients with CSB-CSA.[42] A recent study found that heart failure patients managed in a specialized heart failure center who have CSB-CSA or

OSAHS had increased mortality at 500 days, but there was no difference in mortality at 52 weeks.[43]

Increased ventricular filling pressure, pulmonary congestion, and hyperventilation from vagal stimulation of pulmonary irritant receptors contribute to the development of CSB-CSA. Hyperventilation leads to reductions in $Paco_2$. Central apneas result from hypocarbia and loss of the respiratory stimulus of carbon dioxide. Low cardiac output and prolonged circulation time contribute to the waxing-waning ventilation. Intermittent hypoxia, frequent arousals, sympathetic nervous system activation, and surges in blood pressure and heart rate are consequences. These pathological events exacerbate the pathophysiological processes of heart failure. (See Chapter 62.)

Frequent brief EEG arousals during lighter states of sleep in persons with CSB-CSA prevent its progress into deeper stages. The resulting partial sleep deprivation has daytime functional consequences, such as the perception of nonrestorative sleep and excessive daytime sleepiness.[44] Other consequences are cognitive deficits, disturbed mood, and decreased exercise tolerance.

Like OSAHS, CSB-CSA is associated with nocturnal hypoxia and frequent arousals that may result in reports of nonrestorative sleep. Unlike OSAHS, snoring is not present. Evidence indicates that CSB-CSA and OSAHS coexist in patients with heart failure. Tkacova and colleagues[45] found that obstructive apneic events decreased and central apneic events increased among heart failure patients who had both forms of sleep-disordered breathing. These changes corresponded to increased circulation time and decreased PCO_2 as the night progressed. The risk factors for CSB-CSA appear to be male gender, hypocapnea, and atrial fibrillation,[46] but low ejection fraction also has been implicated.[47]

Treatment

CSB-CSA should be treated when sleep is fragmented and nonrestorative, there are frequent nocturnal oxyhemoglobin desaturations, or the patient has excessive daytime sleepiness. No specific AHI or arousal levels have been identified as goals for treatment. Optimizing medications improves cardiac output and appears to improve CSB-CSA. Small studies have suggested that nocturnal oxygen reduces nocturnal periodic breathing. However, there have been few longitudinal clinical trials. Nocturnal CPAP reduces apneas, periodic breathing, and oxygen desaturation during sleep. Although CPAP is thought to benefit heart failure patients by increasing intrathoracic pressure and decreasing afterload, preload, and venous return to the right atrium, a randomized study of heart failure patients with and without periodic breathing showed improvements in ejection fraction and mortality only in those patients who had periodic breathing.[48] Data on the long-term effects of CPAP are lacking. In a recent small study of heart failure patients with CSB-CSA and left bundle branch block, cardiac resynchronization therapy reduced CSB-CSA and improved oxygen saturation and sleep quality. Although the study findings seem promising, further research is needed to determine the long-term impact of this treatment.[49]

Insomnia

As many as 70 percent of patients with systolic and diastolic heart failure report disturbed sleep.[50, 51] Although some may be attributable to sleep-disordered breathing, the characteristics of self-reported sleep disturbance (prolonged sleep latency, lying awake at night for long periods of time, and early morning awakenings) suggest that insomnia also may be prevalent. Among a group of 223 elderly Swedish patients with New York Heart Association Class II to IV heart failure, 36 percent reported that they did not get enough sleep, and 35 percent perceived that they slept too much. Twenty-three percent reported difficulty falling asleep, and 25 percent reported lying awake for 1 to 3 hours at night. Nocturia occurred in 90 percent of participants, and 9 percent reported nocturnal dyspnea. Females with heart failure had significantly lower sleep sufficiency and more difficulty maintaining sleep than a normative sample who did not have heart failure, and male heart failure patients had more frequent awakenings, more trouble initiating and maintaining sleep, and more frequent early morning awakenings compared with the normative group.[52] Erickson and colleagues[53] reported that 56 percent of a sample of 84 heart failure patients with ejection fractions of 40 percent or less recruited from an outpatient heart failure clinic reported difficulty sleeping, and 32 percent used sleep medications. The most frequent sleep problems were inability to sleep flat (51 percent), restless sleep (44 percent), trouble falling asleep (40 percent), awakening before necessary (39 percent), leg restlessness (38 percent), and trouble returning to sleep (32 percent). Findings from a more recent study[51] indicated that heart failure patients had more prolonged wake periods after sleep onset, but no shorter duration, than a comparison group of people who did not have heart failure. Forty four percent of the heart failure patients reported excessive daytime sleepiness, compared with 18.6 percent of the comparison group.

SLEEP DURING HOSPITALIZATION AND RECOVERY FROM CARDIOVASCULAR DISORDERS

Sleep deprivation is common among adults who are hospitalized for, are being treated for, or are recovering from cardiovascular disorders. The experience of patients undergoing cardiac surgery, especially during the early postoperative period, has been the focus of considerable attention.[54] Many of these patients experience sleep disturbance, manifested as frequent awakenings, short sleep duration, perceptions of poor sleep quality, and daytime napping that may account for as much as 50 percent of the total 24-hour sleep period.[55-57] They have little REM or slow wave sleep[55,58] and frequent awakenings with no apparent cause.

Improvements in sleep appear to correspond with recovery after cardiac surgery and begin during the first postoperative week. In one study of women after coronary artery bypass grafting, sleep was highly fragmented during the early postoperative period but became less fragmented and more consolidated at night (less daytime napping and nocturnal awakening) toward the end of the first postoperative week. Improvements in sleep consolidation and reductions in daytime sleep continued through the sixth month after hospital discharge and appeared to correspond with improvements in postoperative functional status.[57] Similar improvements were seen in men and women followed until the eighth postoperative week. Individual sleep characteristics returned to preoperative levels at 8 weeks. However, overall sleep efficiency and activity occurring during sleep (an indicator of restless sleep) remained worse at 8 weeks than during the preoperative period,[59] which suggests that recovery of sleep may continue beyond this time period. Findings of improvement of sleep at 6 months[60] and 1 year,[61] compared with preoperative sleep, emphasize the potential influence of improved cardiovascular function associated with revascularization on sleep patterns once patients have completed the process of postoperative recovery.

Surprisingly little is known about the factors that contribute to sleep disturbance over the course of recovery during hospitalization or after discharge. However, characteristics of the hospital environment are likely to play a significant role during the early postoperative period. Simpson and colleagues[62] reported positive relationships between the frequency and severity of self-reported sleep-disturbing factors and self-reported sleep disturbance. In another study,[63] 48 percent of 29 postoperative cardiac surgery patients reported that the main reasons for their sleep disturbance were interventions by health care providers and environmental noise.

Although understudied, the nature of the surgical procedures, anesthesia and pain management practices, use of cardiopulmonary bypass, and postoperative pain and medication management are likely to influence differences in postoperative sleep. For example, coronary artery bypass patients who had off-pump procedures had greater sleep efficiency during the first postoperative week than patients who underwent traditional on-pump bypass.[64] Improvements in cerebral perfusion associated with off-pump surgery may reduce the negative impact on sleep. As surgical and medical interventions for coronary revascularization evolve, trends in postoperative sleep and sleep disturbance should be evaluated.

Symptoms of pain and fatigue, as well as emotional distress, are common among hospitalized cardiac patients. However, there is surprisingly little empirical data on the impact of pain management on sleep during the early postoperative period. Data on the relationships among sleep and emotional distress in patients undergoing cardiac surgery are conflicting. Sleep disturbance appears to be associated with disturbed mood during the preoperative period,[58,65] and sleep was related to anxiety[58] but unrelated to postoperative total mood disturbance.[66]

Age, gender, and comorbidity are other factors that may influence sleep. Consideration of these influences should account for the interrelationships among aging, gender, and comorbidity, given that women tend to be older and have more severe cardiac disease at the time of the surgical procedure.[54]

Given the high prevalence of insomnia and sleep-disordered breathing among cardiac patients, primary preoperative sleep disorders may influence sleep during acute care hospitalization[57] but have been the focus of little research. Redeker and colleagues[59] found that preoperative sleep status explained a modest but statistically significant proportion of the variance in sleep in cardiac surgical patients followed up to the eighth postoperative week. This suggests that it may be possible to identify before surgery those patients who are at risk for sleep disturbance after surgery and target them for postoperative sleep-promoting interventions. Suggestions for evaluation and treatment of the sleep disturbances in persons hospitalized for treatment of cardiovascular disorders, including postoperative cardiac surgery patients, are shown in Box 17-2.

BOX 17-2   ■ ■ ■
STRATEGIES TO ASSESS AND PROMOTE SLEEP DURING HOSPITALIZATION

Assessment Topics
- Prehospital influences on sleep
  - Habitual sleep complaints or sleep disorder
  - Treatment patterns (e.g., continuous positive airway pressure and hypnotics)
  - Comorbid medical conditions
  - Mental health disorders
  - Medication history, including complementary therapies
  - Anticipatory stress related to hospitalization and illness
  - Substance use (caffeine, nicotine, alcohol, recreational drugs)
  - Aging, gender
- Influences on sleep during hospitalization
  - Environmental factors
- Lighting, especially at night
- Noise levels in patient care areas
- Frequency and nature of patient care interactions
- Roommate and other patients
- Presence of family or visitors
  - Illness- and treatment-related factors
- Pain, dyspnea, other discomforts
- Anxiety
- Medications
- Medical procedures
- Pathophysiological processes

Interventions
- Target patients who may be at high risk because of prehospitalization risk.
- Reduce light levels, especially at night.
- Minimize unnecessary patient care interactions.
- Cluster patient care to allow uninterrupted periods of sleep.
- Provide massage.
- Play music.
- Provide a warm bath or shower, as appropriate.
- Provide a light bedtime snack.
- Provide comfort measures, such as clean linens, pillows, and repositioning.
- Monitor presence of visitors.
- Use hypnotic drugs judiciously.
- Ensure effective pain and anxiety management.
- For the patient with sleep-disordered breathing, provide continuous positive airway pressure and avoid use of sedating medications.

Evaluation Topics
- Observed and self-reported sleep
- Satisfaction with sleep intervention
- Daytime function, including cognition and mood
- Pain, discomfort, anxiety

Sleep quality and associated circadian rhythmicity of activity-rest were associated with better physical function and shorter length of hospital stay among a sample of 25 female coronary bypass patients.[67] Better sleep was associated with physical function and emotional well-being at 4 and 8 weeks after surgery in a sample of cardiac surgical patients, of whom the majority underwent coronary artery bypass.[68] Persons with self-reported poor sleep at 1 year after surgery were 4.8 times more likely to report poor to very poor quality of life (95 percent CI, 1.66 to 14.0, $p = 0.002$)[69] at 1 year after cardiac surgery. However, improvements in sleep between the preoperative period and 1 year after surgery did not predict 5-year mortality.[56]

QUALITY OF LIFE CONSEQUENCES OF SLEEP DISORDERS

Sleep disorders have a profound impact on many dimensions of quality of life, as demonstrated by community-based studies, clinical observation, and a growing body of literature on the sleep of patients with cardiovascular disorders. A meta-analysis of 19 studies showed that sleep deprivation impairs functioning.[70] Better self-reported sleep quality was associated with fewer psychological and physical complaints, more positive effect, better life satisfaction, increased vigor, and decreased fatigue and confusion in adults ages 40 to 70. Finn and colleagues[71] reported relationships between the severity of sleep-disordered breathing and decrements in mental health, vitality, physical function, social function, role (physical), and general health perception. Severe sleep-disordered breathing was associated with poorer physical role, general health vitality, and social functioning scores (odds ratio [OR]: 1.47 to 1.54, $p < 0.01$), but not poorer physical function, body pain, general health, or mental health scores when these participants in the SHHS were compared with those who had milder or no sleep-disordered breathing.[72] In the same study, persons with disorders of initiating and maintaining sleep were significantly more likely to fall within the lowest quartile of all Medical Outcomes Study Short Form 36 (SF-36) dimensions (physical function, role [physical], body pain, general health, vitality, social functioning, and mental health; OR: 1.36 to 2.11, $p < 0.001$) than persons without disorders of initiating and maintaining sleep. These findings strongly suggest that sleep-disordered breathing and self-reported alterations in the pattern of sleep were important independent contributors to decrements in performance and quality of life.

Recent studies also have underscored the importance of sleep to quality of life among persons with cardiovascular illness. For example, Redeker and colleagues[73] documented relationships between sleep and physical function and emotional well-being among male and female cardiac surgery patients; persons with self-reported poor sleep, measured with a single item at 1 year after surgery, were 4.8 times more likely to report poor to very poor quality of life (95 percent CI, 1.66 to 14.0, $p = 0.002$) 1 year after cardiac surgery.[69] Others have shown that sleep makes a significant contribution to quality of life among persons with heart failure.[52,73]

PRINCIPLES OF SLEEP ASSESSMENT

Nurses provide care to patients across the spectrum of cardiovascular disease. Therefore, specific strategies for evaluation and management vary according to the stage of illness and environmental context in which the care takes place. Given the high prevalence of sleep disorders among patients with cardiovascular conditions and their significant pathophysiological and functional consequences, sleep assessment and intervention should be an integral component of nursing care of the cardiovascular patient, regardless of setting.

Sleep evaluation includes sleep history, physical assessment, and an in-depth review of specific sleep complaints. Characteristics of specific sleep complaints should be reviewed in detail (Box 17-3). Sleep assessment also should include factors that may influence sleep, including the presence of medical disorders, mental health disorders, environmental factors, and primary sleep disorders, the most common of which in adults are insomnia, sleep-disordered breathing, and periodic limb movements during sleep. A detailed review of medications (including over-the-counter medications), alternative therapies, and substances that the patient consumes (such as alcohol and caffeine), as well as an evaluation of activities of daily living and occupational and social activities, is also helpful in evaluating factors that influence sleep. Physical assessment is helpful in detecting abnormalities that may contribute to upper airway obstruction, such as craniofacial abnormalities, recessed chin, and a large tongue or uvula.

The gold standard for evaluation of sleep disorders is nocturnal polysomnography (**NPSG**) conducted in a sleep laboratory (Figure 17-3). NPSG is indicated for the diagnosis of sleep-disordered breathing.[74] Although not routinely indicated for the evaluation of complaints of insomnia,[75] it may be useful in ruling out other causes of sleep disturbance (such as sleep-disordered breathing, nocturnal seizures, and periodic limb movements) in patients whose insomnia is refractory to insomnia treatments. Attended polysomnography is conducted in a specialized sleep laboratory.

Polysomnography consists of EEG, chin electromyelography, and electrooculography to evaluate sleep duration, sleep latency, and sleep architecture (sleep stages). Brief arousals also may be detected through EEG patterns. Central or obstructive apneas and hypopneas are diagnosed with measurement of effort (chest and abdominal expansion), airflow or pressure (thermistor or nasal cannula), and oxygen saturation (pulse oximetry). A continuous electrocardiogram enables evaluation of heart rate changes associated with cardiorespiratory events, dysrhythmias, and their concordance with other sleep-related physiology. Other physiological parameters can be measured as well, such as periodic limb movements or gastric pH, depending on the purposes of the sleep study.

A clinical NPSG report includes information on the duration of sleep, sleep stages, sleep latency (time from lights out until sleep onset), and sometimes an evaluation of the frequency of brief nocturnal arousals. Essential to the diagnosis of sleep-disordered breathing is the AHI or respiratory index (apneas and hypopneas per hour of sleep) and oxygen saturation. Apneas and hypopneas also are described as central or obstructive depending on their association with respiratory effort. (Central apneas and hypopneas are not associated with effort; obstructive apneas are associated with effort.) Other phenomena that may be reported include periodic limb movements, nocturnal seizures, and dysrhythmias that occur during sleep. If a titration of nasal CPAP therapy was conducted, the results and a prescription for the appropriate pressure also is reported.

Evaluation of patients for sleep-disordered breathing may be conducted over one or two nights in a sleep laboratory. The first night may consist of a diagnostic study. If the patient has significant sleep-disordered breathing, titration of CPAP is conducted on the second night. A therapeutic level of CPAP is obtained when apneas and hypopneas are abolished and oxygen saturation is maximized. For patients with severe sleep apnea, the NPSG study and CPAP titration may occur on the same night: the first half of the night is used for diagnosis; the second half for CPAP titration.

Adherence to CPAP is a significant concern because patients may have trouble tolerating the nightly treatment and because nightly use for the duration of the sleep period is necessary for a positive outcome. Some patient education usually is provided in the sleep labora-

---

BOX 17-3
SLEEP ASSESSMENT

Typical Sleep Pattern
- Bedtime (weekdays and weekends)
- Wake-up time (weekdays and weekends)
- Duration of sleep
- Frequency of nighttime awakenings
- Sleep latency (lights out to sleep onset)
- Daytime napping
- Perceived causes of nighttime awakenings
- Events that occur during sleep, such as pain, parasomnias, and snoring
- Limb movements or limb discomfort before or during sleep
- Recent changes in sleep pattern and perception of cause
- Bed partner's reports of snoring, apnea, parasomnias, restlessness, and confusion on awakening

Factors That May Influence Sleep
- Environmental characteristics (presence of bed partner, lighting, ambient noise, pets)
- Social relationships
- Perceived stressors
- Occupation (shift work)
- Medical disorders
- Mental health disorders
- Medications
- Use of caffeine, nicotine, alcohol, and recreational drugs
- Use of alternative or complementary therapies

Consequences of Sleep
- Satisfaction with sleep
- Daytime sleepiness
- Cognitive function
- Memory
- Work performance
- Social relationships
- History of accidents or injury
- Mood
- Quality of life

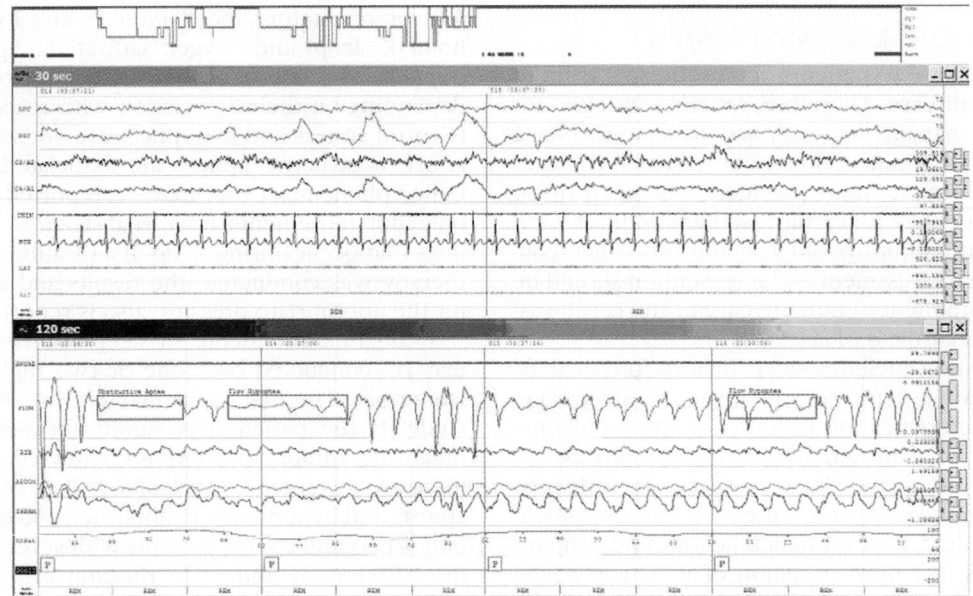

FIGURE 17-3 ▨ Example of polysomnographic recording in a patient with heart failure. The top panel in pink is the hypnogram (graphic display of sleep stages throughout the night). The panel labeled "30 sec" indicates one 30-second epoch of sleep recording with eye movements (two channels), electroencephalogram (two channels), chin electromyogram, electrocardiogram, and right and left leg movements. The bottom panel labeled "120 sec" shows nasal airflow (pressure transducer), respiratory (rib and abdomen) effort, thermistor (nasal airflow), oxygen saturation, and position. Note the obstructive apneas and hypopneas occurring in rapid eye movement sleep. The patient was in the prone position when these events were recorded.

tory at the time of the mask fitting and CPAP titration. However, ongoing patient education and coaching often are needed to promote long-term adherence. This may be especially true for persons with cardiovascular disorders who may need to incorporate OSAHS treatment into an already complex self-management regimen.

Ongoing evaluation of the effects of CPAP treatment should be integrated into long-term patient care. Recurrence of excessive daytime sleepiness after initially successful treatment may indicate nonadherence with treatment or may signal the need for increased CPAP pressure because of failure to treat respiratory events. This is particularly likely for persons who have gained excessive weight.

Because of the high cost and intrusive nature of NPSG, there is growing interest in the use of ambulatory sleep studies for the assessment of sleep-disordered breathing, particularly in settings were NPSG is not readily available. Available monitors are of three general types:

- Devices capable of full portable polysomnography
- Devices that permit modified portable sleep apnea testing (at least two channels of respiratory movement or respiratory movement and airflow, heart rate or electrocardiogram, and oxygen saturation)
- Devices that obtain continuous recordings of oxygen saturation or airflow

These devices may be used in an attended (laboratory) or unattended (home) setting.[76] Validity of the devices depends on whether they are used in attended or unattended settings, the rate of sleep-disordered breathing in the population studied, and the presence of co-

morbid illness. Unattended sleep studies often are associated with technical failures, and the use of these devices currently is not recommended by professional organizations.[77]

Excessive daytime sleepiness can be evaluated by self-report with the Epworth Sleepiness Scale, a measure of sleepiness in everyday life, the Multiple Sleep Latency Test, or the Maintenance of Wakefulness test. The latter two diagnostic tests normally are conducted after NPSG.

Once treatment of sleep disorders begins, long-term patient education and support are critical to ensure positive outcomes. These strategies are most effective if integrated into ongoing health promotion and patient and family self-management programs. Prevention and treatment of sleep disorders holds high promise as a pathway to reduced morbidity and mortality from cardiovascular disease and improved quality of life for persons across the spectrum of cardiovascular disease.

REFERENCES

1. Anch M, Browman CP, Mitler MM, Walsh JK: *Sleep: a scientific perspective*, Englewood Cliffs, NJ, 1988, Prentice Hall.
2. Carskadon MA, Dement WC: Normal human sleep: an overview. In Kryger MH, Roth TC, Dement WC, editors: *Principles and practice of sleep medicine*, ed 3, Philadelphia, 2000, Saunders.
3. Chokroverty S: Physiologic changes in sleep. In Chokroverty S, editor: *Sleep disorders medicine: basic science, technical considerations, and clinical aspects*, ed 2, Boston, 1999, Butterworth.
4. Spiegel K, Leproult R, Van Cauter E: Impact of sleep debt on metabolic and endocrine function, *Lancet* 354:1435-1439, 1999.

5. Verrier RL, Harper RM, Hobson JA: Cardiovascular physiology: central and autonomic regulation. In Kryger MH, Roth TC, Dement WC, editors: *Principles and practice of sleep medicine,* ed 3, Philadelphia, 2000, Saunders.

6. Vitiello MV, Moe KE, Prinz PN: Sleep complaints cosegregate with illness in older adults: clinical research informed by and informing epidemiological studies of sleep, *J Psychosom Res* 53:555-559, 2002.

7. Akerstedt T: Shift work and disturbed sleep/wakefulness, *Occup Med* 53:89-94, 2003.

8. Benca RM: Mood disorders. In Kryger MH, Roth TC, Dement WC, editors: *Principles and practice of sleep medicine,* ed 3, Philadelphia, 2000, Saunders.

9. Ford DE, Kamerow DB: Epidemiologic study of sleep disturbances and psychiatric disorders: an opportunity for prevention? *JAMA* 262:1479-1484, 1989.

10. Redeker NS: Sleep in acute care settings: an integrative review, *J Nurs Scholarsh* 32:31-38, 2000.

11. American Academy of Sleep Medicine Task Force: Sleep-related breathing disorders in adults: recommendations for syndrome definition and measurement techniques in clinical research, *Sleep* 22:667-689, 1999.

12. Young T, Palta M, Dempsey J et al: The occurrence of sleep-disordered breathing among middle-aged adults, *N Engl J Med* 328:1230-1235, 1993.

13. Hla KM, Young TB, Bidwell T et al: Sleep apnea and hypertension: a population-based study, *Ann Intern Med* 120:382-388, 1994.

14. Young T, Peppard P, Palta M et al: Population-based study of sleep-disordered breathing as a risk factor for hypertension, *Arch Intern Med* 157:1746-1752, 1997.

15. Quan SF, Howard BV, Iber C et al: Sleep Heart Health Study: design, rationale, and methods, *Sleep* 20:1077-1085, 1997.

16. Nieto FJ, Young TB, Lind BK et al: Association of sleep-disordered breathing, sleep apnea, and hypertension in a large community-based study: Sleep Heart Health Study, *JAMA* 283:1829-1836, 2000.

17. Parish JM, Somers VK: Obstructive sleep apnea and cardiovascular disease, *Mayo Clinic Proc* 79:1036-1046, 2004.

18. Chobanian AV, Bakris GL, Black HR et al: The Seventh Report of the Joint National Committee on Prevention, Detection, Evaluation, and Treatment of High Blood Pressure, *JAMA* 289:2560-2572, 2003.

19. Shafer H, Koehler U, Ploch T et al: Sleep-related myocardial ischemia and sleep structure in patients with obstructive sleep apnea and coronary heart disease, *Chest* 111:387-393, 1997.

20. Shahar E, Whitney CW, Redline S et al: Sleep-disordered breathing and cardiovascular disease, *Am J Respir Crit Care Med* 163:19-25, 2001.

21. Quan SF, Gersh BJ: Cardiovascular consequences of sleep-disordered breathing: past, present and future, *Circulation* 109:951-957, 2004.

22. Vgontzas AN, Chrousos GP: Sleep-disordered breathing, sleepiness, and insulin resistance: is the latter a consequence, pathogenic factor, or both? *Sleep Med* 3:389-391, 2002.

23. Harsch IA, Schahin SP, Radespiel-Troger M et al: Continuous positive airway pressure treatment rapidly improves insulin sensitivity in patients with obstructive sleep apnea syndrome, *Am J Respir Crit Care Med* 169:156-162, 2004.

24. Hedner J, Ejnell H, Caidahl K: Left ventricular hypertrophy independent of hypertension in patients with obstructive sleep apnoea, *J Hypertens* 8:941-946, 1990.

25. Mohsenin V: Sleep-related breathing disorders and risk of stroke, *Stroke* 32:1271-1278, 2001.

26. Peppard PE, Young T, Palta M et al: Longitudinal study of moderate weight change and sleep-disordered breathing, *JAMA* 284:3015-3021, 2000.

27. Dimsdale JE, Loredo JS, Profant J: Effect of continuous positive airway pressure on blood pressure: a placebo trial, *Hypertension* 35:144-147, 2000.

28. Krieger A, Redeker NS: Obstructive sleep apnea: a risk factor for hypertension, *J Cardiovas Nurs* 17:1-11, 2002.

29. Faccenda JF, Mackay TW, Boon NA et al: Randomized placebo-controlled trial of continuous positive airway pressure on blood pressure in the sleep apnea-hypopnea syndrome, *Am J Respir Crit Care Med* 163:344-348, 2001.

30. Narkiewicz K, Kato M, Phillips BG et al: Nocturnal continuous positive airway pressure decreases daytime sympathetic traffic in obstructive sleep apnea, *Circulation* 100:2332-2335, 1999.

31. Hermida R, Zamarron C, Ayala DE et al: Effect of continuous positive airway pressure on ambulatory blood pressure in patients with obstructive sleep apnea, *Blood Press Monit* 9:193-202, 2004.

32. Pepperell J, Ramdassingh-Dow S, Crosthwaite N et al: Ambulatory blood pressure after therapeutic and subtherapeutic nasal continuous positive airway pressure for obstructive sleep apnea: a randomized trial, *Lancet* 359:204-210, 2001.

33. National Sleep Foundation: 2005 *Sleep in American Poll.* Retrieved November 21, 2006 from www.sleepfoundation.org/hottopics/index.php?secid=16&id=245.

34. Schwartz S, Anderson WM, Cole SR et al: Insomnia and heart disease: a review of epidemiologic studies, *J Psychosom Res* 47:313-333, 1999.

35. Eaker ED, Pinsky J, Castelli WP: Myocardial infarction and coronary death among women: psychosocial predictors from a 20-year follow-up of women in the Framingham Study, *Am J Epidemiol* 135:854-864, 1992.

36. Schwartz SW, Cornoni-Huntley J, Cole SR et al: Are sleep complaints an independent risk factor for myocardial infarction? *Ann Epidemiol* 8:384-392, 1998.

37. Leineweber C, Kecklund G, Janszky I et al: Poor sleep increases the prospective risk for recurrent events in middle-aged women with coronary disease: the Stockholm Female Coronary Risk Study, *J Psychosom Res* 54:121-127, 2003.

38. Stepanski EJ: Behavioral therapy for insomnia. In Kryger MH, Roth TC, Dement WC, editors: *Principles and practice of sleep medicine,* ed 3, Philadelphia, 2000, Saunders.

39. Harvey AG, Tang KY: Cognitive behaviour therapy for insomnia: can we rest yet? *Sleep Med Rev* 7:237-262, 2003.

40. Lanfranchi PA, Somers VK: Sleep-disordered breathing in heart failure: characteristics and implications, *Respir Physiol Neurobiol* 136:153-165, 2003.

41. Redeker NS, Walsleben J, Freudenberger, R et al. Demographic, clinical, and sleep-related correlates of central sleep apnea in stable HF patients. (Abstract). *Sleep, 29,* A176, 2006.

42. Hanly PJ, Zuberi-Khokhar NS: Increased mortality associated with Cheyne-Stokes respiration in patients with congestive heart failure, *Am J Respir Crit Care Med* 153:272-276, 1996.

43. Roebuck T, Solin P, Kaye DM et al: Increased long-term mortality in heart failure due to sleep apnea is not yet proven, *Eur Respir J* 23:735-740, 2004.

44. Hanly P, Zuberi-Khokhar N: Daytime sleepiness in patients with congestive heart failure and Cheyne-Stokes respiration, *Chest* 107:952-958, 1995.

45. Tkacova R, Niroumand M, Lorenzi-Filho G et al: Overnight shift from obstructive to central apneas in patients with heart failure, *Circulation* 103:238-243, 2001.

46. Sin DD, Fitzgerald F, Parker JD et al: Risk factors for central and obstructive sleep apnea in 450 men and women with congestive heart failure, *Am J Respir Crit Care Med* 160:1101-1106, 1999.

47. Javaheri S, Parker TJ, Wexler L et al: Occult sleep-disordered breathing in stable congestive heart failure, *Ann Intern Med* 122:487-492, 1995.

48. Sin DD, Logan AG, Fitzgerald FS et al: Effects of continuous positive airway pressure on cardiovascular outcomes in heart failure patients with and without Cheyne-Stokes respiration, *Circulation* 102:61-66, 2000.

49. Sinha AM, Skobel EC, Ole-Alexander B et al: Cardiac resynchronization therapy improves central sleep apnea and Cheyne-Stokes respiration in patients with chronic heart failure, *J Am Coll Cardiol* 44:68-71, 2004.

50. Jaarsma T, Halfens R, Abu-Saad HH et al: Quality of life in older patients with systolic and diastolic heart failure, *Eur J Heart Fail* 1:151-160,1999.

51. Redeker NS, Stein S; Characteristics of sleep in patients with stable heart failure versus a comparison group, *Heart Lung* 35: 252-261, 2006.

52. Brostrom A, Stromberg A, Dalstrom U et al: Sleep difficulties, daytime sleepiness, and health-related quality of life in patients with chronic heart failure, *J Cardiovasc Nurs* 19:234-242, 2004.

53. Erickson VS, Westlake CA, Dracup KA et al: Sleep disturbance symptoms in patients with heart failure, *AACN Clin Issues* 14:477-487, 2003.

54. Redeker NS, Hedges C: Sleep during hospitalization and recovery after cardiac surgery, *J Cardiovasc Nurs* 17:5-68, 2002.

55. Edell-Gustafson UM, Hetta JE, Aren CB: Sleep and quality of life assessment in patients undergoing coronary artery bypass grafting, *J Adv Nurs* 29:1213-1220, 1999.

56. Hedner J, Caidahl K, Sjoland H et al: Sleep habits and their association with mortality during 5-year follow-up after coronary artery bypass surgery, *Acta Cardiol* 57:341-348, 2002.

57. Redeker NS, Mason DJ, Wykpisz E et al: Sleep patterns in women after coronary artery bypass surgery, *Appl Nurs Res* 9:115-122, 1996.

58. Edell-Gustafson UM, Hetta JE: Anxiety, depression, and sleep in male patients undergoing coronary artery bypass surgery, *Scand J Caring Sci* 13:137-143, 1999.

59. Redeker NS, Ruggiero J, Hedges C: Patterns and predictors of sleep disturbance after cardiac surgery, *Res Nurs Health* 27(4):217-224, 2004.

60. Lukkarinen H: Quality of life in coronary artery disease, *Nurs Res* 47:337-343, 1998.

61. Chocron S, Tatou E, Schjoth B et al: Perceived health status in patients over 70 before and after open-heart operations, *Age Ageing* 29:329-334, 2000.

62. Simpson T, Lee E, Cameron C: Patients' perceptions of environmental factors that disturb sleep after cardiac surgery, *Am J Crit Care* 5:173-181, 1996.

63. Redeker NS, Ruggiero J, Dankanics L et al: *Self-reported sleep of post-operative cardiac surgery patients: preliminary data, 2000.* Retrieved November 21, 2006 from http://rutgersscholar.rutgers.edu/volume02/redesork/redesork.htm

64. Hedges C, Redeker NS: Sleep and mood in post-operative off-pump vs on-pump coronary artery bypass patients. Paper presented at Eastern Nursing Research Society 17th Annual Scientific Session, 2005, New York.

65. Redeker NS, Ruggiero J, Hedges C: Sleep disturbance, mood, and symptom distress of pre-operative cardiac surgery patients. Paper presented at Eastern Nursing Research Society Scientific Sessions, 2001, Atlantic City, NJ.

66. Ruggiero J, Redeker N, Cochrane C: Symptom and mood correlates of activity-rest in cardiac surgery patients, *Sleep* 23(suppl 2):A352, 2000.

67. Redeker NS, Mason DJ, Wykpisz E et al: First postoperative week activity patterns and recovery in women after coronary artery bypass surgery, *Nurs Res* 49:168-173, 1994.

68. Redeker NS, Ruggiero J, Hedges C: Sleep is related to physical function and emotional wellbeing after cardiac surgery, *Nurs Res* 53:154-162, 2004.

69. Hunt JO, Hendrata MV, Myles PS: Quality of life 12 months after coronary artery bypass graft surgery, *Heart Lung* 29:401-411, 2000.

70. Pilcher JJ, Huffcutt AI: Effects of sleep deprivation on performance: a meta-analysis, *Sleep* 19:318-326, 1996.

71. Finn L, Young T, Palta M, Fryback DG: Sleep-disordered breathing and self-reported general health status in the Wisconsin Sleep Cohort Study, *Sleep* 21:701-706, 1998.

72. Baldwin C, Griffith KA, Nieto J et al: The association of sleep-disordered breathing and sleep symptoms with quality of life in the Sleep Heart Health Study, *Sleep* 24:96-105, 2001.

73. Redeker NS, Hilkert R: Sleep and quality of life in patients with stable heart failure, *J Cardiac Fail* 11:700-704, 2005.

74. American Sleep Disorders Association and Sleep Research Society: Practice parameters for the indications for polysomnography and related procedures, *Sleep* 20:406-422, 1997.

75. Reite M, Buysse DJ, Reynolds C et al: The use of polysomnography in the evaluation of insomnia, *Sleep* 18:58-70, 1995.

76. Flemons WW, Littner MR, Rowley JA et al: Home diagnosis of sleep apnea: a systematic review of the literature, *Chest* 124:1543-1579, 2003.

77. Li CK, Flemons WW: State of home sleep studies, *Clin Chest Med* 24:283-295, 2003.

■■■ chapter 18

Impact of Cardiovascular Disease on Sexuality

Elaine E. Steinke
Tiny Jaarsma

Many persons with cardiac disease have concerns about resuming sexual activity after an acute episode or an exacerbation of their illness. Likewise, partners often have considerable anxiety and may be overprotective. Nurses can play a key role in ensuring that questions and concerns are addressed through patient education. Sexual counseling means providing education and specific strategies to address sexual concerns and to facilitate a return to sexual activity. Assessment and evaluation of patient and partner concerns provides direction for the information discussed during sexual counseling.

Sexuality should be viewed within the larger context of intimacy. Intimacy is a warm, meaningful feeling of joy that occurs on a number of levels. Intimacy can be experienced on a social level with family and friends; an intellectual level when discovering that others share common interests; an emotional level that includes friendship and romantic love; and a physical level. Physical intimacy includes (1) nonsexual hugging and touching that is common with close family members and friends and (2) sexual intimacy that involves sexual behaviors such as masturbation or intercourse (Figure 18-1).[1]

When one's need for intimacy is not met, other needs may become more important. For example, if the physical need for closeness is not met, then the nonsexual aspects of intimacy may assume greater importance. Sexuality reflects who we are as a male or female, or in other words, our sexual identity. Duffy states that "like thirst, hunger, and pain avoidance, sex is a life-long instinctive drive. Sex can be fun, intimate, passionate, and a restorative force, bringing healing and renewed energy for life"[2] (p. 66). Therefore, sexuality involves physical and psychosocial components and may contribute to improved quality of life. Patients and their partners may find that frequency and intensity of sexual activity may diminish with a cardiac condition. This may lead to altered sexual satisfaction and performance anxiety. Careful assessment of patient and partner concerns will help clarify these issues and assist the nurse in developing a plan for sexual counseling.

ASSESSMENT OF SEXUAL FUNCTION

Nurses must take a proactive role in addressing sexual concerns. Patients often feel embarrassed to ask questions about this personal topic. When nurses bring up the topic, patients' sexual concerns are acknowledged as normal and common with a cardiac illness. Being aware of one's own biases and approaching the patient in a nonjudgmental manner is crucial. Successful sexual counseling also includes selecting the most appropriate setting and approach for sexual counseling. A private environment, such as a conference room or quiet area, is more conducive to discussion of sensitive topics. Care should be taken to arrange for as much privacy as possible. The patient should be assured that the discussion is confidential, unless sexual issues arise that need further intervention and documentation.

The topic of sexual concerns and cardiac illness can be broached easily within the context of exercise or in a general discussion on consequences of the disease for daily life. After discussing the recommendations for exercise, the topic of return to sexual activity as a component of exercise can be approached. Open-ended questions tend to facilitate discussion and enable the nurse to assess sexual concerns.[3] For example, the nurse might say, "Many people have concerns about resuming sexual activity after a heart attack. What concerns do you have?" This statement implies that it is normal to have these concerns and then allows the patient to bring them up. If the patient is not sexually active or does not have concerns, this usually becomes apparent with the response to this question. The response also allows the nurse to determine the order in which sexual counseling topics might be discussed. Specific questions also are used to clarify sexual concerns and problems (Box 18-1).

All cardiac patients should receive information on returning to sexual activity. Some patients, although not currently sexually active, may want to resume sexual activity at a later time when cardiac symptoms have resolved. Therefore, providing information tailored to the patient's concerns and using the guidelines in this chapter will facilitate a return to sexual activity at a time when the patient feels ready and it is medically safe.

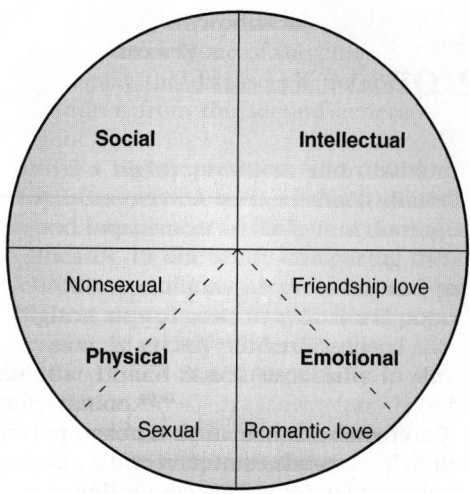

FIGURE 18-1 ■ The circle of intimacy. (From Modigh A: Intimacy and sexuality. In Stone JK, Wyman JF, Salisbury SA, editors: *Clinical gerontological nursing: a guide to advanced practice,* ed 2, Philadelphia, 1999, Saunders.)

BOX 18-1 ■ ■ ■
QUESTIONNAIRE TO ASSESS INTIMACY AND SEXUALITY

1. How would you describe your relationship with your spouse or partner?
2. Are you currently sexually active?
3. Is there any difference in your sexual enjoyment from earlier times? Do you think there is a difference for your partner?
4. If yes, how is your sexual enjoyment different?
5. Do you have any idea why it is different?
6. Do you and your partner discuss sex and intimacy?
7. How important is intimacy in your relationship? Are activities such as hugging, kissing, and just being close an important part of your relationship?
8. Are you satisfied with the kind and amount of intimacy you receive?
9. Do you understand the normal age-related changes that might affect sexual activity?
10. Have you noticed any changes in your sexual performance, such as problems with erections or orgasm, vaginal dryness, or decreased desire for sex?
11. What medications or supplements are you currently taking?
12. Would your partner or spouse be willing to come in with you to discuss these issues?

Adapted from Modigh A: Intimacy and sexuality. In Stone JK, Wyman JF, Salisbury SA, editors: *Clinical gerontological nursing: a guide to advanced practice,* ed 2, Philadelphia, 1999, Saunders.

CARDIOVASCULAR EFFECTS OF SEXUAL ACTIVITY

Patients often are concerned about resuming sexual activity following a cardiac event or revascularization. Some may fear another heart attack, whereas others are not sure when they should resume sexual activity. Nurses can reassure patients by providing information on the energy requirements for sexual activity.

Muller and colleagues[4] found that of 858 patients, 9 percent reported sexual activity in the 24 hours before a myocardial infarction (**MI**) and 3 percent had sexual activity in the 2 hours preceding the MI. Sexual activity was a likely contributor in only 0.9 percent of cases. Regular physical activity has been shown to include a protective effect and may eliminate any increased risk of

---

BOX 18-2 ■ ■ ■
CARDIOVASCULAR RISK AND SEXUAL ACTIVITY

Low Risk
Sexual activity does not present a significant risk.
- Asymptomatic, with less than three risk factors for coronary artery disease (excluding gender)
- Controlled hypertension
- Mild, stable angina that is being treated
- Successful coronary revascularization
- History of myocardial infarction, uncomplicated
- Mild valvular disease
- Left ventricular dysfunction or New York Heart Association (NYHA) Class I status
- Other cardiovascular conditions

Intermediate or Indeterminate Risk
Cardiac evaluation is needed before sexual activity can be recommended or sexual dysfunction can be treated.
- Asymptomatic, three or more risk factors for coronary artery disease (excluding gender)
- Moderate, stable angina
- Recent myocardial infarction (more than 2 and less than 6 weeks)
- Left ventricular dysfunction and/or heart failure, NYHA Class II
- Noncardiac problems, such as stroke or peripheral vascular disease

High Risk
The cardiac condition must be fully evaluated and treated, and the patient must be stabilized before sexual activity can be recommended or sexual dysfunction treated.
- Unstable or refractory angina
- Uncontrolled hypertension
- Heart failure of NYHA Class III to IV
- Recent myocardial infarction (less than 2 weeks)
- High-risk dysrhythmias
- Obstructive hypertrophic cardiomyopathy
- Moderate to severe valvular disease

Data from Kostis JB, Jackson G, Rosen R, Barrett-Connor E, Billups K, Burnett AL, Carson C III, Cheitlin M, Debusk R, Fonseca V, Ganz P, Goldstein I, Guay A, Hatzichristou D, Hollander JE, Hutter A, Katz S, Kloner RA, Mittleman M, Montorsi F, Montorsi P, Nehra A, Sadovsky R, Shabsigh R: Sexual dysfunction and cardiac risk (the Second Princeton Consensus Conference). *Am J Cardiol* 96(12B):85M-93M, 2005.

---

coronary events with sexual activity.[5] However, Hellerstein[6] notes that a return to sexual activity after MI depends on several important factors. These include libido, age, previous functional and cardiac status, myocardial loss, response to medical or surgical treatment, and psychological factors. Muller studied several of these factors as triggers 2 hours before MI. Results from a sample of 1712 patients reinforced the low frequency of sexual intercourse as a trigger for MI (1.5 percent) compared with that of anger (2.4 percent), heavy exertion (4.9 percent), psychological stress (11.6 percent), or after awakening (19.0 percent).[7] A report from the Princeton Consensus Panel[8] also provides guidelines for the risk of sexual activity for cardiac patients and can be used in patient management (Box 18-2).

Changes in vital signs occur in healthy adults with sexual activity. This fact is helpful to remind patients who may be overly concerned about changes in heart rate with sexual activity. Drory and colleagues[9] found that peak heart rate during intercourse (117 ± 21) in patients without ischemia was less than during exercise (150 ± 13). In addition, patients who did not have ischemia with exercise did not have ischemia with intercourse. One-third of patients in the study ($n = 88$) did have ischemia during intercourse (mostly silent ischemia), although in some cases exercise heart rates were higher than with intercourse. Therefore, exercise testing may be warranted in some patients before resuming sexual activity.[10]

The energy cost to the cardiovascular system often is measured in metabolic equivalents (**METs**). METs are determined by exercise testing and are the amount of metabolic energy the person can expend safely at rest or for a given activity. Sexual activity during the preorgasmic phase of sexual responses is equivalent to 2 to 3 METs, similar to walking 2 to 3 miles per hour on a level surface.[8] The energy expended during the orgasmic phase of sexual activity is 3 to 4 METs. This energy expenditure is considerably less than activities such as cycling at 10 miles per hour (6 to 7 METs). Clinically, recommendations for sexual activity based on METs should include "real world" advice to avoid stress, a heavy meal, or excess alcohol consumption before sexual intercourse. Always important is to individualize advice rather than relying only on statistical evidence.[10]

CARDIOVASCULAR MEDICATIONS AND SEXUAL FUNCTION

Medications used in the treatment of cardiovascular disease can have a significant impact on sexual function. Medications exert adverse effects on sexuality through mechanisms such as hormonal effects and actions on the autonomic and central nervous systems. More specifically, the mechanisms that promote dysfunction are adrenergic inhibition, adrenergic receptor blockade, and endocrine, sedative, and anticholinergic effects.[11] For men, adverse effects include decreased or absent libido, difficulty in attaining or maintaining an erection, priapism, retarded ejaculation, retrograde ejaculation, premature ejaculation, and gynecomastia. Women may experience decreased vaginal lubrication, menstrual irregularity, decreased or absent libido, or inability to achieve orgasm.[12,13] Specific medications with sexual side effects are shown in Table 18-1.

Antihypertensives and diuretics are common causes of drug-induced sexual dysfunction. Persons with hypertension can be affected adversely by the disease process itself or by antihypertensives. Persons with uncontrolled blood pressure who also smoke cigarettes and are overweight are at risk because of the additive effect of these factors on their lifestyle in general and with sexual activity, in which blood pressure normally increases. Control of blood pressure is particularly important in a patient with ischemic heart disease.

Medications for treating hypertension are well known for their adverse effects on sexual function. In the Treatment of Mild Hypertension study of 902 hypertensive persons, the incidence of erectile dysfunction (**ED**) was 9.5 percent at 24 months and 14.7 percent at 48 months and was related to the type of antihypertensive prescribed.[14] Decreased libido, impotence, and ejaculatory difficulty also have been noted in men. Thiazide diuretics can cause decreased libido, impotence, and ejaculatory difficulty in men and decreased vaginal lubrication in women.[11,12]

Other cardiovascular drugs, such as calcium channel blockers, beta-adrenergic blockers, vasodilators, and lipid-lowering agents can affect sexual function.[15,16] Some effects are dose-related, which was suggested by one study showing that patients who received propranolol doses exceeding 120 mg developed ED at a higher rate than those who received lower doses.[17] More side effects (such as gynecomastia and menstrual problems) were noted with spironolactone dosages that exceeded 200 mg per day.[11] Many central nervous system drugs, hypoglycemics (including insulin), and antidepressants (particularly tricyclic drugs) may affect libido, potency, and ejaculation adversely.[12]

Health professionals should take a sexual health history before a patient starts any drug that might affect sexual function. This allows for more accurate assessment at follow-up visits, and evidence of sexual dysfunction related to medications will be easier to determine. Little evidence indicates that changing cardiovascular therapy will reverse ED because the underlying disease process might be more important. However, if there is a strong temporal relationship between the start of treatment and the onset of ED (2 to 4 weeks), it is logical to change therapy if it is safe to do so.[10] Sexual dysfunction as a side effect of medications can affect patient adherence to treatment; therefore, a careful patient history and discussion of patient questions and concerns are important considerations.

Sometimes helpful is for patients to know that sexual difficulties can be related to drug therapy rather than personal inadequacy. Suggest that patients have sex at a time when the blood levels of medications, such as antihypertensives, are lowest. Also, instruct patients not to stop any drug that may be affecting sexual function without talking to their physician or other health care professional.

Also, consider the possibility that patient knowledge that cardiac medications may have sexual side effects can lead to a self-fulfilling prophecy; that is, assuming the side effect will occur affects patient anxiety and sexual function. In a study of 96 males with newly diagnosed cardiovascular disease and no previous ED, knowledge of the side effects of beta blockers was related to the incidence of ED. ED was as high as 31 percent in patients who knew the side effects of the drug; for those unaware of the side effects, the incidence of ED was 10 times lower. In most cases, ED was reversed completely with a placebo.[18] These findings do not suggest that patients should remain uninformed about side effects; however, health care providers should be aware of the effect of education on this matter.[19]

Some studies describe beneficial effects of angiotensin II inhibitors in hypertensive patients. In one study of postmenopausal women ages 51 to 55 who had mild to moderate scores for three items related to libido, taking valsartan was related to significant improvements in sexual desire, changes in behavior, and sexual fantasies.[20] Improved sexual function also was found in hypertensive males taking valsartan.[21] These findings also are described for other angiotensin II inhibitors, such as losartan and candesartan.

■ ■ ■

TABLE 18-1 CARDIAC DRUGS THAT CAN CAUSE SEXUAL DYSFUNCTION

DRUG	DECREASED LIBIDO	SEXUAL DYSFUNCTION	ERECTILE PROBLEMS	IMPOTENCE	IMPAIRED EJACULATION
Angiotensin-Converting Enzyme Inhibitors					
Benazepril (Lotensin)	Yes			Yes	
Captopril (Capoten)				Yes (rare)	
Enalapril (Vasotec)			Yes	Yes (rare)	
Fosinopril (Monopril)	Yes			Yes (rare)	
Lisinopril (Zestril)		Yes		Yes (rare)	
Moexipril (Univasc)				Yes	
Quinapril (Accupril)	Yes			Yes	
Ramipril (Altace)	Yes			Yes (rare)	
Alpha-Adrenergic Blockers					
Doxazosin (Cardura)			Yes		
Prazosin (Minipress)[1]			Yes	Yes	
Terazosin (Hytrin)[1]			Yes	Yes	
Dysrhythmics					
Disopyramide (Rhythmodan)				Yes (rare)	
Mexiletine (Mexitil)	Yes			Yes (rare)	
Flecainide (Tambocor)	Yes			Yes (rare)	
Propafenone (Rythmol)				Yes (rare)	
Amiodarone (Cordarone)				Yes (rare)	
Beta-Adrenergic Blockers					
Acebutolol (Sectral)	Yes		Yes	Yes	
Atenolol (Tenormin)				Yes	
Carteolol (Cartrol)				Yes	Yes
Labetalol (Normodyne)[1,2]				Yes	Yes[2]
Metoprolol (Lopressor)[3]				Yes	
Nadolol (Corgard)				Yes	
Pindolol (Visken)				Yes	
Propranolol (Inderal)[3,4]	Yes			Yes	
Sotalol (Betapace)				Yes (rare)	Yes
Timolol (Blocadren)	Yes			Yes	
Calcium Channel Blockers					
Amlodipine (Norvasc)		Yes	Yes		
Felodipine (Plendil)		Yes			
Nicardipine (Cardene)		Yes			
Nifedipine (Adalat)		Yes			
Nisoldipine (Sular)		Yes			
Cardiac Glycoside					
Digoxin (Lanoxin)[5]	Yes			Yes	
Centrally Acting Antihypertensives					
Clonidine (Catapres)[5]			Yes	Yes	Yes
Methyldopa (Aldomet)[5]				Yes	Yes
Guanfacine (Tenex)				Yes	
Diuretics					
Thiazide diuretics	Yes		Yes		Yes
Spironolactone[5,6]	Yes	Yes			
Lipid-Lowering Agents					
Clofibrate				Yes	
Gemfibrozil (Lopid)				Yes	

[1]Priapism (prolonged painful erection lasting several hours or more).
[2]Delayed tumescence.
[3]Peyronie's disease (painful erections and deformity of penis from plaques in dense fibrous tissue surrounding corpus cavernosum of penis).
[4]Effects seen at high doses.
[5]Gynecomastia.
[6]Menstrual irregularities.
Data from Grimm R, Grandits G, Prineas R et al: Long-term effects of sexual function of five antihypertentive drugs and nutritional hygienic treatment of hypertensive men and women, *Hypertension* 29:8-14, 1997; Gutierrez K, Queener S: *Pharmacology for nursing practice,* St Louis, 2003, Mosby.

IMPACT OF CARDIAC CONDITIONS ON SEXUAL FUNCTION

Studies of the relationship between sexual function and cardiac disease are limited, although some clinical articles briefly address sexual counseling in patient education. The recommendations presented for sexual counseling in selected cardiac conditions are based on current evidence and information from clinical practice. Additional patient education resources are listed in Box 18-3.

Coronary Artery Disease
Psychosocial Concerns

Bedell and colleagues[22] studied the need for information about sexual concerns among cardiac patients. Patients (48 women, 188 men) with known coronary artery disease responded to a mailed questionnaire. Most (64 percent women, 81 percent men) believed that the cardiologist should initiate discussion of sexual functioning, although respondents indicated some discomfort in discussing this personal topic. Only 18 percent of women and 3 percent of men believed that they had been informed adequately about sexual functioning by the cardiologist. Similarly, a review of medical records showed that discussion of sexual functioning was documented for only 43 percent of men and 13 percent of women.

Sexual dysfunction, particularly ED, is common in coronary disease. An increased incidence of ED has been noted with diabetes, heart disease, and hypertension.[23] Men with stable angina may be sexually active but limited by ED. Little is known about the impact of coronary disease on the sexual functioning of women.

BOX 18-3 ■ ■ ■
CARDIAC PATIENT EDUCATION RESOURCES

Print Resources
- American Heart Association: *Sex and heart disease,* Dallas, 2001, American Heart Association. Contact your local affiliate for a pamphlet or call 1-800-AHA-USA1.
- Jones K: *Heart smart sex: a guide for heart patients and their partners,* Charlotte, NC, 1995, Mecklenburg Rehabilitation Center. Available from Kathy Jones, Mecklenburg Cardiac Rehabilitation Center, 1718 East 4th St., Suite 401, Charlotte, NC 28204; 704-384-5031.
- Pritchett & Hull Associates: *The sensuous heart: guidelines for sex after a heart attack or heart surgery,* Atlanta, 2004, Pritchett & Hull Associates. Call 1-800-241-4925.
- Krames Communications: *Sex, intimacy and heart disease,* San Bruno, Calif, 2004, Krames Communications. Available from Krames Communications, 1100 Grundy Lane, San Bruno, CA 94066-3030; 1-800-333-3032.

Other Media
- Steinke EE: *Sex after a heart attack: guidelines for you and your partner,* Wichita, Kan, 2000, Wichita State University. Available in VHS or DVD format. Contact Elaine Steinke, School of Nursing, Wichita State University, 1845 Fairmount, Wichita, KS 67260-0041; 316-978-5740.
- American Heart Association: *Sexual activity and heart disease or stroke.* www.americanheart.org/presenter. jhtml?identifier=4714

Guidelines for Resuming Sexual Activity

Guidelines for stable cardiac patients are based on data from normal volunteers, patients who have angina or who are taking antianginal medications, and on post-MI guidelines. Symptomatic patients with exercise restriction may not be able to engage in sexual activity. Those with stable angina should be reassured that sexual activity is unlikely to trigger an MI. Other areas of discussion include sexual functioning, sexual satisfaction, and ED, including the effects of medications on sexual function.[22,23] An assessment of depression may be needed because cardiac disease and sexual dysfunction have been linked to depression.[24]

Myocardial Infarction

Much of the available research and clinical literature describing sexuality and cardiac patients is focused on those with MI. These studies answer questions related to informational needs of patients, psychosocial concerns, and rehabilitation approaches in general. Although only a few studies specifically address the wide range of teaching topics for resuming sexual activity, a number of articles provide teaching guides for health professionals.[11,25-30] Despite these resources, sexual counseling as a part of cardiac rehabilitation may be neglected.

Psychosocial Concerns

Fear, anxiety, and overprotectiveness by the partner are common experiences after MI.[31] Often there is a fear of chest pain or another MI during sexual activity.[32-35] Dhabuwala and colleagues[36] found that 80 percent of male MI patients were afraid to resume sexual activity in the first 6 months post-MI. Likewise, most partners experience anxiety post-MI, and 53 percent had at least some anxiety, and 26 percent had moderate or high anxiety.[37] Fear of death[32,36] is a concern for patients, although the risk of MI during sexual activity is low, occurring in less than 1 percent of patients with acute MI.[4] Patients often have misconceptions about the amount of energy expended for sexual activity, giving rise to these fears. Concealing one's worries can have a negative impact on patients and partners; therefore, open communication with nurses and between patients and partners is needed.[8]

Psychosocial recovery after MI has been linked to patients' feelings of control,[38] and overall emotional distress, anxiety, and depression significantly decreases over time.[39] Anxiety, fear, and depression can be overwhelming for patients and their partners. Patient education and sexual counseling for MI patients can help provide the support and perhaps control desired by these patients.

Guidelines for Resuming Sexual Activity

It is imperative that nurses assess the need for information and provide information on return to sexual activity for MI patients and their partners. Reiley and colleagues[40] found that half of MI patients reported not knowing when to resume normal activities, whereas the nurse believed the patient knew about resuming normal activities in all but one instance.

Beginning counseling with more general aspects is recommended, for example, the effects of an MI on the heart or how to relate to one's partner after an MI. These more general topics are usually less threatening to patients and allow the nurse to progress to more sensitive topics. Partners commonly are concerned about returning to sexual activity, often becoming overprotec-tive, anxious, and fearful. Patient education that includes the partner is recommended to help alleviate any concerns. Encourage the MI patient to discuss with the partner any anxieties about resuming sexual activity.

Specific guidelines for sexual counseling are included in Table 18-2. Explanatory comments for selected guidelines are included in this section. Guide-

■ ■ ■

TABLE 18-2   GUIDELINES FOR SEXUAL COUNSELING AFTER MYOCARDIAL INFARCTION

OBJECTIVE	GUIDELINES	RATIONALE
Assess concerns about the sexual relationship.[3, 25-29]	Do a brief sexual assessment that includes patient and partner concerns about resuming sex, current sexual activity, importance of sex in the relationship, medications taken, and health problems. (See Box 18-1.)	This allows specific concerns to be discussed as part of sexual counseling. Areas of concern are addressed in addition to each guideline listed.
	Encourage open and honest communication between patient and partner about sexuality.	This minimizes stress and anxiety, and promotes intimacy.
	Suggest that the couple take daily walks together.	Exercise improves functional capacity and promotes intimacy.
	Remind the couple that the demand of sexual activity on the heart is similar to other daily activities.	
	Discuss heart rate changes that occur normally with sex.	
	Remember that sexual activity is individually defined, i.e., hugging, kissing, fondling, masturbation, or sexual intercourse.	This recognizes that the type, pattern, and interest in sexual activity vary.
Discuss activity guidelines.	Remind the couple that activities such a kissing, hugging, fondling, and masturbation can be resumed more quickly after MI.[11,30]	Energy requirements for these activities are less than that of sexual intercourse.
	Sexual intercourse can be resumed in about 1 to 2 weeks after an uncomplicated MI,[41] and some recommend 3 to 4 weeks.[8]	
	For a complicated MI, the patient should consult the physician. Sexual activity will need to be resumed gradually.	A complicated MI may involve the following: cardiopulmonary resuscitation, hypotension, serious arrhythmias, and heart failure.[41]
	Encourage the couple to engage in foreplay before sexual activity.	Foreplay focuses on intimacy and not just performance.
Address environmental issues for sexual activity.	Encourage a comfortable, familiar setting for sexual activity.	Familiar settings and being well-rested minimizes stress in resuming sexual activity.[3]
	Avoid unfamiliar surroundings or partners.	
	Remind the patient to be well-rested at the time of sexual activity, such as after a nap.[11]	
	Encourage the patient to use a comfortable position for sexual activity, one that permits unrestricted breathing.[11]	Blood pressure and heart rate may increase in an unfamiliar position.[42]
	Discourage eating or drinking for 1 hour before sexual activity.	Heavy meals and alcohol may contribute to chest pain with sexual activity when blood flow is diverted toward digestion.
	Tell the patient to wait 2 to 3 hours after a heavy meal or alcohol.[11]	
Discuss warning signs of cardiac stress.	Encourage the patient to report any warning signs that occur with sexual activity, such as chest pain, shortness of breath, rapid or irregular heart rate, dizziness, insomnia, or extreme fatigue the day after sexual activity.[11,30,33]	Unrelieved chest pain should be reported to the health care provider, and 911 should be called if necessary.
	Advise the patient to stop, rest, and/or use nitroglycerin (if prescribed) for chest pain with sexual activity and to notify the physician if pain is unrelieved.[11,26,30]	
Discuss medication effects on sexual function based on the patient's medication plan.	Discuss the patient's medications and side effects.	Medications can affect sexual performance.
	Take a sexual history before starting any new medication that might affect sexual function.	
	Advise the patient to report any side effects or sexual problems to the physician.[30]	Discussing side effects and explaining when to call the health care provider can improve adherence to drug therapy.
	Encourage the patient not to stop taking a medication if a side effect is experienced but to consult the health care provider. Substitution or a dosage change of the medication may be possible.	
	See Table 18-1 for side effects and/or refer to a current drug therapy or pharmacology textbook for each medication.	
Review guidelines for anal sex and illicit drugs.	Encourage the patient to avoid anal sex.	Decreased performance and chest pain may result from vagal stimulation.[32,43]
	Avoid illicit drugs such as stimulants, cocaine, and marijuana.[30]	These may lead to sexual dysfunction. Marijuana increases heart rate and myocardial oxygen consumption and decreases libido and testosterone level.
		Cocaine can cause chest pain, produce fatal MI, decrease sex drive, and cause difficulty with erection, orgasm, and ejaculation.

MI, Myocardial infarction.

lines from the American College of Cardiology and the American Heart Association[41] suggest that patients with an uncomplicated MI can resume sexual activity in a week to 10 days. A longer time may be needed before resuming sexual activity if the patient required cardiopulmonary resuscitation or suffered hypotension, serious dysrrhythmias, or heart failure. Recommendations from the Second Princeton Consensus Conference on Sexual Dysfunction recommend resuming sexual activity in 3 to 4 weeks.[8] A return to sexual activity typically occurs within the first month post-MI, although some persons may take more than 6 months to return to prior levels of activity.[35,44,45] Assessing the comfort level of the MI patient and partner in resuming sexual activity is an important component. The patient's response to treatment, the medical history, and current concerns must be considered when making recommendations about resuming sexual activity.

Sexual foreplay can be an ideal way to ease into sexual activity. Simple sensual affection can be relaxing and reassuring to the couple. Anxiety can lead to secondary impotence, so relaxed foreplay can provide an alternative to coitus and can help reassure the man of the quality and duration of his erections. Couples should try to focus more on intimacy and pleasuring behaviors than on sexual performance. This in itself can relieve some of the anxiety about returning to sexual activity.

Sexual positions after MI have been a topic of some debate. In the past, it was thought that certain sexual positions lessened the cardiac workload, for example, lying on the side, lying on the back with the partner on top, or for men, sitting in a wide chair with feet touching the floor.[11] The MI patient was expected to assume a passive position for sexual activity. However, it has been found that heart rate and blood pressure do not change when different positions are used during intercourse,[42] but that blood pressure and heart rate do increase when the patient uses an unfamiliar position.[46] Therefore, patients can be advised to assume their usual position or one that is most comfortable to them.[3]

One topic that most health professionals are reluctant to discuss is anal sex. However, anal penetration stimulates the vagus nerve, which decreases heart rate, rhythm, impulse conduction, and coronary blood flow. Diminished cardiac performance and chest pain can result.[32,43] McCann[43] offers this suggestion for broaching this topic: "Some people enjoy anal stimulation or anal intercourse; if you do, you need to know that those activities may increase your heart's workload" (p. 1138). Patients interested in resuming anal sex should discuss this topic with their cardiologist. The ability to resume anal sex depends on the extent of the MI, the amount of cardiac compromise, and successful management of cardiac symptoms. If anal intercourse is not possible, alternate forms of sexual pleasure should be discussed.

Sexual Counseling after Myocardial Infarction

The informational needs of patients after MI are great and, although sexual function may not be an early concern after MI, questions often arise during the recovery period. The importance of sexual counseling after MI was explored in a study of 91 patients post-MI, with all 14 items specific to sexual activity rated as important over the 6-month period.[35] In general, patient education on sexual activity should begin during hospitalization and continue throughout the recovery period after discharge.

Approaches for sexual counseling have included written materials, verbal information, videotape information, and telephone counseling. Varvaro[47] found that patients who received a nursing instructional program had fewer concerns about sexual activity, better adaptation to family role and work, and increased self-confidence in resuming sexual activity over time. Likewise, Dhabuwala and colleagues[36] found that MI patients who received sexual counseling had less fear about resuming sexual activity. Froelicher and colleagues[44] used a teaching-counseling program on exercise to assess return to usual activities; participants completed eight sessions on risk factor modification and post-MI adjustment. The rate of return to physical activities did not differ significantly between groups, and most patients returned to sexual activity, driving, and outdoor activities by 3 weeks post-MI. A videotape used for sexual counseling after MI showed improved experimental group knowledge at 1 month post-MI.[45] These studies show that a variety of approaches for sexual counseling can be used successfully by nurses and other health professionals. Nurses can develop printed teaching guides or use those in the literature to help in discussing this sensitive topic. It is imperative that health professionals implement assessment and interventions that can facilitate the MI patient's return to usual activities.

Coronary Artery Bypass Surgery
Psychosocial Concerns

Providing sexual counseling after coronary artery bypass grafting (**CABG**) is particularly important. Although some couples may experience no change in sexual satisfaction, others report sexual problems. Stanley and Frantz[48] interviewed 26 spouses after their partner's CABG procedure. Participants reported a low level of satisfaction with their sexual relationship (58 percent), although only 8 percent said this was a change from before surgery, and 54 percent of spouses reported a low level of satisfaction with the frequency of sexual activity after their partner's surgery. Interest in work, hobbies, and sexual activities was mostly stable in more than half of post-CABG patients ($n = 587$), and interest was significantly better for those who had not experienced a cardiac event before CABG.[49] Similarly, sexual satisfaction after CABG ($n = 318$) compared with 1 year before surgery was unchanged for 50 percent and equally divided for the remainder, who reported better or worse satisfaction.[50] For those who had less satisfaction, decreased desire and energy were reported. Speziale and colleagues[51] found no difference in sexual satisfaction between those treated with medical therapy versus CABG at baseline and at 6 months.

Sexual satisfaction is just one component in evaluating the sexual experience. Sexual problems following CABG were noted in 15 percent of 43 young male patients, who had a mean age of 35.[52] Sexual problems may persist over a longer time. Sjoland and colleagues,[53] in a prospective study of quality of life in 2121 CABG patients, reported that although physical capacity was improved, sexual problems were still frequent at 2 years post-CABG. Predictors for sexual problems included postoperative problems, male gender, and diabetes mellitus. These findings highlight the importance of sexual counseling for CABG patients and their partners, although in some studies, sample sizes were small.

Guidelines for Resuming Sexual Activity

Instructions for resuming sexual activity after CABG are similar to those for the MI patient. Instruct the patient to choose familiar surroundings, a comfortable room temperature, to be well rested before sexual activity, and to wait 2 to 3 hours after drinking alcohol or eating a heavy meal before having sex. Encourage the CABG patient and partner to allow plenty of time for sexual activity. The patient also should report if any of the previously described warning signs occur.

Additional time should be spent counseling the CABG patient about incisional pain and how this might affect resumption of sexual activity. Incisional pain usually is described as a dull ache in the midsternal area without radiation to the jaw or left arm. Reassure patients and partners that they are not likely to harm the sternum. Sexual activity usually can be resumed 3 to 6 weeks after surgery.[54]

King and Gortner,[55] in a study of 31 women post-CABG, reported that most women (70 percent) had problems with their chest incision. They included infection, incisional pain with radiating shooting sharp pain to the breasts, difficulty healing, and chest numbness. Similarly, Moore[56] studied a group of 20 post-CABG women who described breast sensations as sharp, burning, heavy, numb, and tingling. Women may be reluctant to discuss breast issues with health care providers. These findings should be considered when discussing post-CABG sex with the female patient and her partner. The patient should choose a position that is most comfortable to her, use pillows or other methods to support the breasts, and take a pain reliever such as acetaminophen or ibuprofen before sex if needed.

Sexual Counseling after Coronary Artery Bypass Grafting

Patients and their partners likely have unanswered questions about returning to sexual activity, similar to couples after MI. Like the findings for MI patients, health professionals have not addressed sexual counseling for CABG patients adequately. One study compared the information needs of patients before, 6 months after, and 1 year after CABG ($n = 432$) or coronary angioplasty (percutaneous transluminal coronary angioplasty; $n = 183$).[57] Psychosocial functioning was the most powerful predictor of informational needs at 6 months and 1 year. CABG patients rated informational support as mostly adequate, although after 1 year, males had a significantly greater need for information about sexual life than did women. Similarly, men needed more information about sexual life at 6 months after percutaneous transluminal coronary angioplasty. Further research on quality of life, psychosocial variables, and sexual concerns of male and female CABG patients is warranted.

Heart Failure
Psychosocial Concerns

Patients with advanced heart failure face several challenges in trying to maintain sexual function. Decreased exercise capacity, fatigue, shortness of breath, fear of death, anxiety, medications, and changes in self-esteem and mood can contribute to changes in sexual function.[58] In European and American samples with advanced heart failure (New York Heart Association [NYHA] Class III or IV), changes in sexual activity have been reported as a result of the disease process.[58-60]

Two specific studies examining sexual function in patients with heart failure have been undertaken in the United States. In a cohort of 62 patients (mean age 53), 75 percent reported a marked decrease in sexual interest and the frequency of sexual problems caused by their typical symptoms of heart failure.[58] In another study of 63 heart failure patients (mean age 56), 62 percent reported slight or marked decrease in their frequency of sexual activity, and 59 percent reported slight or marked loss of interest in sexual activities.[60]

In a European sample of heart failure patients ($n = 73$), fewer sexual problems were reported, although many patients in the study did not answer these questions because they did not want to discuss the subject or thought the questions did not apply to them. In the month preceding their hospital admission, a large number of patients described a marked decrease in sexual interest (47 percent), a decline in frequency of sex (48 percent), severe negative changes in sexual performance (45 percent), and a loss of pleasure or satisfaction related to sexual function (40 percent) as a result of their heart failure. This did not change significantly during the recovery phase after discharge. Most did not report an increase in number of arguments about sex with their partner, nor did the relationship with the partner change because of the illness.[59] A relationship between higher level of daily functioning and fewer sexual problems was established, as was a relationship between the number of comorbidities and sexual problems. Symptoms of dyspnea and fatigue may hinder sexual activity. Patients might fear deterioration and death as a result of sexual activity.

Guidelines for Resuming Sexual Activity

Few guidelines for heart failure patients and sexual activity are available in the literature. Patients can be advised that a semireclining or bottom position may decrease the amount of physical effort needed for sexual activity.[61] The suggestions for MI patients related to the timing of sexual activity also apply to the heart failure patient, such as being well-rested before sex, avoiding sex after a heavy meal or alcohol, and use of familiar surroundings. In addition, patients should be encouraged to stop and rest if shortness of breath occurs with sexual activity.

Sexual foreplay can be beneficial in allowing the patient and the partner to determine tolerance for sexual activity. Encourage patients to express their affection through hugging, kissing, and foreplay. Activities such as mutual masturbation, oral sex, or intercourse may not be possible if exercise capacity is diminished. If needed, advise the patient to adapt the timing of diuretic use to sexual activity, obtaining the benefits of symptom relief from the diuretic while minimizing the disturbance of frequent urination.

Sexual Counseling in Heart Failure

As with all cardiac patients, it is important to discuss sexual activity and the consequences of the disease process on sexual function. Individuals might differ in the importance they attach to resuming sexual activity and on the kind of activities they still want to pursue, considering symptoms and functional status. In patients with heart failure, the 6-minute walk test can be administered easily in the clinical setting as part of patient assessment. The 6-minute walk test measures the distance that a person can walk in 6 minutes and provides an assessment of the patient's effort at submaximal exertion. The test can serve as a guide for overall physical function and for sexual activity. Patients who cannot manage the 6-minute walk or expend about 3 to 5 METs may not be able to handle the exertion required with sexual activity. This should be discussed with the patient and partner.

Patients and nurses may differ in the perceptions of the importance and realism of heart failure education content, including addressing the issue of sexual activity. A significant patient and nurse difference was found in the ratings of information on general activity and sexual activity.[62,63] The authors state that this difference may be due to the wide age range of patients, the large number of patients without traditional sex partners, or that patients may be uncomfortable asking about sexual concerns. Many heart failure patients are older, and the importance of sexual activity for some older adults may not be as great as in their younger years. Frattini and colleagues[64] studied learning needs of heart failure patients and showed that sexual activity was rated higher by nurses than patients. The researchers note that patients likely had been affected by medications and the illness itself, thus negatively influencing sexual function. This study emphasizes the importance of assessing what patients want to learn. In preliminary descriptive research, 18 percent of heart failure patients indicated that they required more information on the side effects of medications, sexual dysfunction as a result of heart failure, and asked for more openness on the subject.[65]

Westlake and colleagues[60] reported that partners and patients differed in their assessment of the amount and kind of sexual problems. The most important sexual relationship issue of patients and partners was related to decreased frequency in sexual relations. They reported the need to receive specific information about sexual activity, rated as moderate to very high, and this was unrelated to the level of need for education and counseling. In other words, even if patients and partners do not experience problems directly in the area of sexual activity, they still require relevant information. Further research and clinical literature describing the sexual concerns and patient education strategies for sexual counseling of the heart failure patient is needed.

Implantable Cardioverter-Defibrillators
Psychosocial Concerns

Patients with an implantable cardioverter-defibrillator (**ICD**) often have concerns about whether the device will function properly. Concerns include anxiety about exercising for fear that the increased heart rate may trigger the device to fire, not knowing when the device may fire, and fear of shocking others if the device fires.[66-68] Vitale and Funk[66] noted that sexual activity was least likely to be affected when considering quality of life issues, with 25 percent of subjects reporting the ICD affected sexual function. Dougherty[69] found that dyadic adjustment was not affected by psychological distress from the ICD and a reduced sexual frequency. Other ICD patients report reduced sexual activity as a concern,[67] including 54 percent of subjects at 1 and 3 months after ICD placement.[70] Additional concerns by patients and partners include overprotectiveness by the partner, erectile difficulties, and lack of interest in sexual activity after ICD placement.[67] Research on partners is limited, although concerns about the ICD, the couple's relationship, and care of the ICD partner are some of the areas being explored.[71]

Fear of ICD firing with sexual activity may be an exaggerated concern. Dunbar and colleagues[72] found that only 1 of 22 subjects had the ICD fire during sexual activity. In another study,[67] ICD discharge with sexual activity occurred for 18 percent ($n = 11$) of 61 subjects. Firing of the ICD during sexual activity is related to the increased heart rate required during sex, which may stimulate firing of the device. Some patients fear that if the device fires, their partner may be shocked by the ICD. In reality, if someone is touching the patient when the ICD fires, the person will feel only a tingling sensation.[73] These findings highlight the importance of discussing sexual concerns with patients and partners.

Guidelines for Resuming Sexual Activity

Few guidelines are available in the literature for sexual counseling for the ICD patient. James[74] advises telling patients that they are not likely to receive a shock during sexual activity. In contrast, Knight and colleagues[73] note that it is possible for the device to fire with increased heart rates and advise telling patients that the device may fire with sexual activity because of the increased heart rate, that they or their partner may or may not feel the device fire, and that it will not injure the partner.[68,75] A change in rate settings for the device may be needed. In general, patients should not restrict their activities after ICD implantation unless there are other cardiac reasons for limitations. White[76] notes that sexual activity can be resumed as long as it does not cause dyspnea, chest discomfort, or dizziness. Additional suggestions for sexual counseling are provided in Table 18-3.

Sexual Counseling after Implantable Cardioverter-Defibrillator Placement

Limited research is available that assesses the extent to which sexual counseling is provided for ICD patients in clinical settings. One study explored the sexual con-

■ ■ ■

TABLE 18-3 GUIDELINES FOR SEXUAL COUNSELING AFTER IMPLANTABLE CARDIOVERTER-DEFIBRILLATOR PLACEMENT

OBJECTIVE	GUIDELINES	RATIONALE
Assess concerns about the sexual relationship.	Follow guidelines and areas of assessment listed in Table 18-2. Discuss feelings of overprotectiveness by the partner and concerns about implantable cardioverter-defibrillator (ICD) discharge during sex.[67] Reinforce positive, protective aspects of living with an ICD.	Open discussion of feelings and concerns can help allay fears and promote adaptation to the ICD.
Discuss activity guidelines.	Sexual activity usually can be resumed after hospital discharge, after incisions are healed and strain on the incisional site is avoided.[77] Discuss the potential of ICD discharge during sexual activity. Tell the patient to report it to the health care provider. Stress that the partner will not be injured if the ICD fires.[75]	There are few limitations for resuming sexual activity as long as other conditions do not prohibit it. Patients and partners should be aware that the ICD could fire with sexual activity. Frequent ICD discharge may require changing the device settings.[73] Frequent ICD discharge may require changing the device settings.[73]
Discuss cardiac warning signs.	Instruct the patient to report problems such as dyspnea, chest discomfort, or dizziness with sexual activity.[76] Also see Table 18-2.	Unrelieved chest pain should be reported to the health care provider, and 911 should be called if needed. Other symptoms also should be reported.
Discuss medication effects on sexual function based on the patient's medication plan.	Follow guidelines in Table 18-2.	
Provide resources to the patient and partner.	Make resources available to the patient and partner, such as an ICD support group, written materials, or a person who has an ICD and is sexually active and is willing to discuss sexual concerns with the patient and partner.	Resources will help with adaptation to the ICD and improve quality of life. A person who has an ICD is the ideal person to discuss living with an ICD, including sexual issues.

ICD, Implantable cardioverter-defibrillator.

cerns and educational needs of ICD patients ($n = 82$) and their partners ($n = 47$).[67] Most patients (60 percent) and partners (62 percent) reported not receiving information on resuming sexual activity after ICD placement. Few patients received information on fears and concerns (20 percent), potential for ICD shock with sexual activity (19 percent), the rate at which the ICD might be triggered (16 percent), or the effects of medications on sexual activity (10 percent). Most patients and partners did not receive specific instructions on resuming sexual activity, and some expressed the need for more information. Further study is needed to examine sexual concerns, educational needs, and effective strategies for sexual counseling.

Heart Transplantation

Disturbances in sexual function for heart transplant patients before and after transplantation are noted in the literature. Difficulty in sexual performance related to end-stage heart disease was rated as one of the most distressing symptoms.[65] After heart transplant, sexual function might improve;[78,79] however, some patients may experience impotency, ejaculatory problems, decreased libido, and low satisfaction with sex life.[80,81] Assessing for iatrogenic, physical, and psychological causes of sexual dysfunction is recommended as part of the health professional's sexual assessment. In addition, perceived health, patient and partner libido, impaired erectile ability, and number of medications taken were found to be related to the amount of sexual disability in heart transplant patients.[82] Factors contributing to sexual dysfunction were fear of overtaxing the heart, concerns about donors' sexuality, feelings of unattractiveness caused by body changes from immunosuppressants, and changing role functions as the patient regains energy after transplantation.

The problem of sexual dysfunction increasingly is documented in the literature for heart transplant, although few suggestions are provided to guide patient education. Nurses must inform themselves of the potential sexual difficulties of heart transplant patients. Assessing sexual concerns, body image changes, and medications are particularly important in guiding patient education.

MANAGEMENT OF SEXUAL DYSFUNCTION

Cardiovascular patients often seek treatment for ED. Proper assessment and appropriate counseling of the patient or couple are of major importance. Beyond sexual activity, the caring, nonsexual aspects of the relationship should be stressed and detailed advice and support provided. Treatment of ED has been transformed by the introduction of phosphodiesterase-5 (**PDE-5**) inhibitors, the first of which was sildenafil (Viagra). Vardenafil (Levitra) and tadalafil (Cialis), with similar mechanisms of action, since have been added to this family of drugs. Success in restoring erectile function is possible in up to 80 percent of patients (depending on cause) with minimal adverse effects.[10] These drugs work by inhibiting production of the liver enzyme phosphodiesterase and its effect on cyclic guanosine monophosphate as a mediator of nitric oxide-induced vasodilatation.[83-86] With sexual stimulation, nitric oxide is generated, promoting penile blood flow and restoring erectile function.

A synergistic hypotensive effect with nitrates, particularly nicorandil, is the only major contraindication.[10] The combination of organic nitrates and the PDE-5 inhibitors can cause severe hypotension, tachycardia, MI, and death. Patients with known coronary artery disease, heart failure, vascular disease, or hepatic or renal disease may be able to take these medications if they are monitored closely.[85] Adverse effects for PDE-5 inhibitors include headaches, flushing, dyspepsia, and rhinitis. Tadalafil is associated with more back pain, and sildenafil with vision changes.[10,83] The nurse must remember several key points for patient education regarding PDE-5 inhibitors (Box 18-4). Although patients may be anxious to try these drugs to relieve sexual problems, health professionals must assess the risks and benefits of using them.

In addition to these medications, patients may use nutraceuticals to enhance sexual desire and function. The common nutraceuticals and potential interactions are shown in Table 18-4. Consult a reputable book on alternative therapy for specific information on amounts taken and potential side effects. Although patients may be anxious to try medications and nutraceuticals to relieve sexual problems, health care professionals must assess carefully the associated risks and benefits. Patient education directed at the action, dose, and adverse effects of medications and alternative therapies for sexual dysfunction is vital. An open and honest discussion of potential side effects related to sexual function, as well as other interventions to enhance sexual function, is of prime importance. Patients also may try other alternative therapies, such as hypnosis, biofeedback, and acupuncture.

Other means of treating sexual dysfunction include intracavernosal penile injections, transurethral alprostadil (Muse), transurethral vacuum constriction devices, and penile implants. Patients must be evaluated carefully, including a full discussion of the benefits and risks of therapies for sexual dysfunction.

SUMMARY

Sexual concerns are evident for many persons experiencing a cardiovascular event. Patients and their partners often have fears and concerns about resuming sexual activity. Providing information in a timely manner in the acute care setting and continuing throughout the recovery period is particularly important to meeting the quality of life needs of the patient and partner. Therefore, health professionals must be actively involved in assessment and education regarding sexual concerns. Further research is needed to better understand patient needs and concerns and to refine educational methods for sexual counseling.

BOX 18-4   ■ ■ ■
CLINICAL CONSIDERATIONS FOR PHOSPHODIESTERASE-5 INHIBITORS

All Drugs in Class
- Overall, these drugs can be used successfully by patients with cardiovascular disease.
- Sexual stimulation is essential for drug effect to occur.
- Administration with nitrates and other nitric oxide substrates is contraindicated.
- Safety and efficacy are similar to sildenafil.
- Drugs should not be taken more than once daily.

Sildenafil (Viagra)
- Recommended dose: 50 mg taken 1 hour before sex; 25 mg is advised for patients older than 80; 100 mg usually is needed by patients with diabetes
- Time to peak effect: 1 hour
- Duration: up to 6 hours
- No excess risk of myocardial infarction, stroke, or mortality
- Avoid within 4 hours of taking doxazosin.
- Also effective for patient with heart failure suitable for erectile dysfunction therapy
- First dose may not be effective; may take seven or eight attempts before sexual intercourse is possible.
- Effects are facilitated by an empty stomach and by avoiding alcohol and cigarettes.
- Short half-life makes this the drug of choice for patients with more severe cardiovascular disease, allowing early support therapy if an adverse clinical event occurs.
- Disadvantage is that sexual activity must be planned because of the quick onset and short duration of the drug.

Tadalafil (Cialis)
- Recommended dose: 10 mg taken before sex
- Time to peak effect: 1 to 2 hours
- Duration: has been recorded beyond 36 hours
- Urge caution with use of doxazosin. (Advise spreading the intake of doxazosin and tadalafil to evening and morning.)
- Be careful with beta blockers.
- Consumption of more than 5 units of alcohol can have additive effects, with signs of orthostatic hypotension, tachycardia, dizziness, and headache.
- Specific recommendations for sildenafil also apply except that food does not effect onset of activity.
- Sublingual nitrates cannot be use for 48 hours after tadalafil.
- Drug may not be the first choice in more complex cardiac patients because nitrates cannot be used for a relatively long time after taking tadalafil.
- Longer duration of action allows greater spontaneity.

Vardenafil (Levitra)
- Recommended dose: 10 mg taken 1 hour before sex; 5 mg to start if patient is older than age 65.
- Time to peak effect: 1 hour, although it may work in as little as 15 minutes
- Duration: 3 to 5 hours, up to 6 hours
- Less data are available on effectiveness and safety.
- Drug should be avoided by patients with congenital QT-interval prolongation and those who take class IA or class III antidysrhythmic drugs.
- Beta blockers are contraindicated.
- Half-life may be increased by a high-fat meal.

Data from Jackson G: Treatment of erectile dysfunction in patients with cardiovascular disease, *Drugs* 64:1533-1545, 2004; Russel S, Khandheria K, Nehra A: Erectile dysfunction and cardiovascular disease, *Mayo Clinic Proc* 79:782-794, 2004; Brock G, MacMahon G, Chen K et al: Efficiency and safety of tadalafil for the treatment of erectile dysfunction: results of integrated analysis, *J Urol* 168:1332-1336, 2002; Porst H, Rosen R, Padma-Nathan H et al: Efficacy and tolerability of vardenafil, a new oral selective phosphodiesterase type 5 inhibitor, in patients with erectile dysfunction: the first at home clinical trial, *Int J Impot Res* 13(4):192-199, 2001; Wooten J: Erectile dysfunction: there are now three effective oral drugs for treating ED, paving the way for nurses to put patients with this condition on the road to good sexual health, *RN* 67:40-4, 2004.

■ ■ ■

TABLE 18-4 NUTRACEUTICALS FOR SEXUAL PROBLEMS*

PROBLEM	NUTRACEUTICAL	CONSIDERATIONS
Depressed libido	Nutmeg	Used as aphrodisiac
		May be potentiated when taken with antidiarrheals, MAO inhibitors, psychotropic drugs, or phenobarbital
	Pau d'arco	Used as aphrodisiac and for sexually transmitted diseases
		Causes increased risk of bleeding with anticoagulants such as heparin, salicylates, and warfarin
	Yohimbe	Used as aphrodisiac and hallucinogenic and for erectile dysfunction and sexual dysfunction
		Interacts with ACE inhibitors, alpha-adrenergic blockers, CNS stimulants, MAO inhibitors, phenothiazines, and SSRIs
Impotence	Bee pollen	Advise caution in those with pollen allergy or diabetes
	Chaste tree	Discourage use with oral contraceptives
		Discourage use during lactation
		May interfere with action of antipsychotics, dopamine agonists, and estrogens
	Damiana	Used as aphrodisiac to increase sexual potency
		May irritate the urethra and increase sensitivity of the penis
		Has diuretic and antidepressant effects
		Discourage use during lactation and pregnancy
		May interfere with diabetes therapy
	Saw palmetto	Used to treat benign prostatic hypertrophy, as a mild diuretic, and to increase breast size, sperm count, and sexual potency
		Discourage use in pregnancy, lactation, and by those hypersensitive to saw palmetto
		May interact with anticoagulants, antiplatelet drugs, estrogens, and oral contraceptives

Data from Skidmore-Roth L: *Mosby's handbook of herbs & natural supplements,* ed 2, St Louis, 2004, Mosby; and Therapeutic Research Faculty: Pharmacist's letter/prescriber's letter natural medicines comprehensive database, ed 6, Stockton, Calif, 2004, Therapeutic Research Faculty.
*Most of the nutraceuticals listed are taken orally and come in a variety of forms and dosages depending on the indication. Consult an alternative therapy handbook for complete dosing and side effect information.
MAO, Monoamine oxidase inhibitor; *ACE,* angiotensin-converting enzyme; *CNS,* central nervous system; *SSRI,* selective serotonin reuptake inhibitor.

REFERENCES

1. Modigh A: Intimacy and sexuality. In Stone J, Wyman J, Salisbury S, editors: *Clinical gerontological nursing: a guide to advanced practice,* ed 2, Philadelphia, 1999, Saunders.
2. Duffy L: Lovers, loners, and lifers: sexuality and the older adult, *Geriatrics* 53:S66-S69, 1998.
3. Steinke E: Sexual counseling after myocardial infarction, *Am J Nurs* 100:38-43, 2000.
4. Muller J, Mittleman M, Maclure M et al: Triggering myocardial infarction by sexual activity, *JAMA* 275:1405-1409, 1996.
5. Muller J: Triggering of cardiac events by sexual activity: findings from a case-crossover analysis, *Am J Cardiol* 86:14F-18F, 2000.
6. Hellerstein D: Sexual activity and the risk of myocardial infarction, *JAMA* 10:782, 1996.
7. Muller J: Sexual activity as a trigger for cardiovascular events: what is the risk? *Am J Cardiol* 84:2N-5N, 1999.
8. Kostis JB, Jackson G, Rosen R, Barrett-Connor E, Billups K, Burnett AL, Carson C 3rd, Cheitlin M, Debusk R, Fonseca V, Ganz P, Goldstein I, Guay A, Hatzichristou D, Hollander JE, Hutter A, Katz S, Kloner RA, Mittleman M, Montorsi F, Montorsi P, Nehra A, Sadovsky R, Shabsigh R: Sexual dysfunction and cardiac risk (the Second Princeton Consensus Conference). Am J Cardiol 96(12B):85M-93M, 2005.
9. Drory Y, Kravetz S, Weingarten M: Comparison of sexual activity of women and men after a first myocardial infarction, *Am J Cardiol* 85:1283-1287, 2000.
10. Jackson G: Treatment of erectile dysfunction in patients with cardiovascular disease, *Drugs* 64:1533-1545, 2004.
11. Seidl A, Bullough B, Haughey B et al: Understanding the effects of a myocardial infarction on sexual functioning: a basis for sexual counseling, *Rehabil Nurs* 16:255-264, 1991.
12. Rerkpattanapipat P, Stanek M, Kotler M: Sex and the heart: what is the role of the cardiologist? *Eur Heart J* 22:201-208, 2001.
13. Russel S, Khandheria K, Nehra A: Erectile dysfunction and cardiovascular disease, *Mayo Clinic Proc* 79:782-794, 2004.
14. Grimm R, Grandits G, Prineas R et al: Long-term effects of sexual function of five antihypertentive drugs and nutritional hygienic treatment of hypertensive men and women, *Hypertension* 29:8-14, 1997.
15. Kotler D: Sexual dysfunction in patients with cardiovascular disease, *J Am Acad Physician Assist* 5:423-431, 1992.

16. Tardif G: Sexual activity after a myocardial infarction, *Arch Phys Med Rehabil* 70:763-766, 1989.
17. Warren S, Warren S: Propranolol and sexual impotence, *Ann Intern Med* 86:112, 1977.
18. Silvestri A, Galetta P, Cerquetani E et al: Report of erectile dysfunction after therapy with beta-blockers is related to patient knowledge of side effects and is reversed by placebo, *Eur Heart J* 24:1928-1932, 2003.
19. Jaarsma T, Moser D: Beta-blockers and sexual problems, *Eur Heart J* 25:617, 2004.
20. Fogari R, Preti P, Zoppi A et al: Effect of valsartan and atenolol on sexual behavior in hypertensive postmenopausal women, *Am J Hypertens* 17:77-81, 2004.
21. Dusing R: Effect of angiotensin II antagonist valsartan on sexual function in hypertensive men, *Blood Press Suppl* 2:29-34, 2003.
22. Bedell S, Superval M, Goldberg R: Cardiologists' discussion about sexuality with patients with chronic coronary artery disease, *Am Heart J* 144:239-242, 2002.
23. Jackson G: Sexual intercourse and stable angina pectoris, *Am J Cardiol* 86:35F-37F, 2000.
24. Roose SP, Seidman SS: Sexual activity and cardiac risk: is depression a contributing factor? *Am J Cardiol* 86:38F-40F, 2000.
25. Baggs J, Karch A: Sexual counseling of women with coronary heart disease, *Heart Lung* 16:154-159, 1987.
26. Boone T, Kelley R: Sexual issues and research in counseling the postmyocardial infarction patient, *J Cardiovasc Nurs* 4:65-75, 1990.
27. Boycoff S: Strategies for sexual counseling of patients following a myocardial infarction, *Dimens Crit Care Nurs* 8:368-373, 1989.
28. Cohen J: Sexual counseling of the patient following myocardial infarction, *Crit Care Nurse* 6:18-26, 1986.
29. Gondek M: Talking about sex: a post-MI script, *RN* 62:52-54, 1999.
30. Steinke E: Talk about sex with MI patients, *AACN News* 18(12):4-5, 2001.
31. Friedman S: Cardiac disease, anxiety, and sexual functioning, *Am J Cardiol* 86:46F-50F, 2000.
32. Briggs L: Sexual healing: caring for patients recovering from myocardial infarction, *Br J Nurs* 3:837-842, 1994.
33. Franklin B, Munnings F: Sex after a heart attack: making a full recovery, *Physicians Sportsmed* 22:84-89, 1994.

34. Hamilton G, Seidman R: A comparison of the recovery period for women and men after an acute myocardial infarction, *Heart Lung* 22:308-315, 1993.

35. Steinke E, Patterson-Midgley P: Importance and timing of sexual counseling after myocardial infarction, *J Cardiopulm Rehabil* 18:401-407, 1998.

36. Dhabuwala C, Kumar A, Pierce J: Myocardial infarction and its influence on male sexual function, *Arch Sex Behav* 15:499-504, 1986.

37. Kettunen S, Solovieva S, Laamanen R et al: Myocardial infarction, spouses' reactions and their need of support, *J Adv Nurs* 30:479-488, 1999.

38. Moser D, Dracup K: Psychosocial recovery from a cardiac event: the influence of perceived control, *Heart Lung* 24:273-280, 1995.

39. Riegel B, Gocka I: Gender differences in adjustment to acute myocardial infarction, *Heart Lung* 24:457-466, 1995.

40. Reiley P, Iezzoni LI, Phillips R et al: Discharge planning: comparisons of patients' and nurses' perceptions of patients following hospital discharge, *Image J Nurs Sch* 28:143-147, 1996.

41. American College of Cardiology, American Heart Association: *ACC/AHA guidelines for the management of patients with ST-elevation myocardial infarction*, 2004. Retrieved November 20, 2006 from http://circ.ahajournals.org/cgi/reprint/110/9/e82

42. Nemac E, Mansfield L, Kennedy J: Heart rate and blood pressure responses during sexual activity in normal males, *Am Heart J* 92:274-277, 1976.

43. McCann M: Sexual healing after a heart attack, *Am J Nurs* 89:1133-1140, 1989.

44. Froelicher E, Kee L, Newton K et al: Return to work, sexual activity, and other activities after acute myocardial infarction, *Heart Lung* 23:423-435, 1994.

45. Steinke E, Swan J: Effectiveness of a videotape for sexual counseling after myocardial infarction, *Res Nurs Health* 27:269-280, 2004.

46. Walbroehl G: Sexual activity and the post coronary patient, *Am Fam Physician* 29:175-177, 1984.

47. Varvaro F: Family role and work adaptation in MI women, *Clin Nurs Res* 9:339-351, 2000.

48. Stanley M, Frantz R: Adjustment problems of spouses of patients undergoing coronary artery bypass graft surgery during early convalescence, *Heart Lung* 17:677-682, 1988.

49. Pintor P, Torta R, Bartolozzi S et al: Clinical outcome and emotional-behavioural status after isolated coronary surgery, *Qual Life Res* 1:177-185, 1992.

50. Jenkins C, Stanton B, Savageau J et al: Coronary artery bypass surgery, *JAMA* 250:782-788, 1983.

51. Speziale G, Bilotta F, Ruvolo G et al: Return to work and quality of life measurement in coronary artery bypass grafting, *Eur J Cardiothor Surg* 10:852-858, 1996.

52. Samuels L, Sharma S, Kaufman M et al: Coronary artery bypass grafting in patients in their third decade, *J Card Surg* 11:402-407, 1996.

53. Sjoland H, Caidahl K, Wiklund I et al: Impact of coronary artery bypass grafting on various aspects of quality of life, *Eur J Cardiothor Surg* 12:612-619, 1997.

54. Relf M: Sexuality and the older bypass patient, *Geriatr Nurs* 12:294-296, 1991.

55. King K, Gortner S: Women's short-term recovery from cardiac surgery, *Prog Cardiovasc Nurs* 11:5-15, 1996.

56. Moore S: CABG discharge information: addressing women's recovery, *Clin Nurs Res* 5:97-104, 1996.

57. Kattainen E, Merilainen P, Jokela V: CABG and PTCA patients' expectations of informational support in health-related quality of life themes and adequacy of information in 1-year follow-up, *Eur J Cardiovasc Nurs* 3:149-163, 2004.

58. Jaarsma T, Dracup K, Walden J et al: Sexual function in patients with advanced heart failure, *Heart Lung* 25:262-270, 1996.

59. Jaarsma T: Sexual problems in heart failure patients, *Eur J Cardiovasc Nurs* 1:61-67, 2002.

60. Westlake C, Dracup K, Walden J et al: Sexuality of patients with advanced heart failure and their spouses or partners, *J Heart Lung Transplant* 18:1133-1138, 1999.

61. Burke L: Cardiovascular disturbances and sexuality. In Fogel C, Lauver D, editors: *Sexual health promotion*, Philadelphia, 1990, Saunders.

62. Hagenhoff B, Feutz C, Conn V et al: Patient education needs as reported by congestive heart failure patients and their nurses, *J Adv Nurs* 19:685-690, 1994.

63. Gerard P, Peterson L: Learning needs of cardiac patients, *J Cardiovasc Nurs* 20:7-11, 1984.

64. Frattini E, Lindsay P, Kerr E et al: Learning needs of congestive heart failure patients, *Prog Cardiovasc Nurs* 13:11-16, 1998.

65. Koops A, Jaarsma T, van Veldhuisen D: Need for information concerning sexual changes in chronic heart failure patients, *Eur J Cardiovasc Nurs* 4(1):77 (abstract); 2005.

66. Vitale M, Funk M: Quality of life in younger persons with an implantable cardioverter defibrillator, *Dimens Crit Care Nurs* 14:100-111, 1995.

67. Steinke E: Sexual concerns of patients and partners after an implantable cardioverter defibrillator, *Dimens Crit Care Nurs* 22:89-96, 2003.

68. Walker R, Campbell K, Sears S et al: Women and the implantable cardioverter defibrillator: a lifespan perspective on key psychosocial issues, *Clin Cardiol* 27:543-546, 2004.

69. Dougherty C: Psychological reactions and family adjustment in shock versus no shock groups after implantation of internal cardioverter defibrillator, *Heart Lung* 24:281-291, 1995.

70. Dunbar S, Jenkins L, Hawthorne M et al: Factors associated with outcomes 3 months after implantable cardioverter defibrillator insertion, *Heart Lung* 28:303-315, 1999.

71. Dougherty C, Pyper G, Benoliel J: Domains of concern of intimate partners of sudden cardiac arrest survivors after ICD implantation, *J Cardiovasc Nurs* 19:21-31, 2004.

72. Dunbar S, Warner C, Purcell J: Internal cardioverter defibrillator device discharge: experiences of patients and family members, *Heart Lung* 22:494-501, 1993.

73. Knight L, Livingston N, Gawlinkski A et al: Caring for patients with a third-generation implantable cardioverter defibrillator: from decision to implant to patient's return home, *Crit Care Nurs* 17:46-63, 1997.

74. James J: Living with a cardioverter defibrillator in the community, *Nurs Times* 95:50-51, 1999.

75. Moser S, Crawford D, Thomas A: Updated guidelines for patients with automatic implantable cardioverter defibrillators, *Crit Care Nurs* 13:62-71, 1993.

76. White E: Patients with implantable cardioverter defibrillators: transition to home, *J Cardiovasc Nurs* 14:42-52, 2000.

77. Wolbrette DL, Naccarelli GV: Management of implantable cardioverter defibrillator patients: role of predischarge electrophysiologic testing and proper patient instruction before hospital discharge, *Curr Opin Cardiol* 16(1):72-75, 2001.

78. Grady K, Jalowiec A, White-Williams C: Improvement in quality of life in patients with heart failure who undergo transplantation, *J Heart Lung Transplant* 15:749-757, 1996.

79. Jalowiec A, Grady K, White-Williams C et al: Symptom distress three months after heart transplantation, *J Heart Lung Transplant* 16:604-614, 1997.

80. Grady K, Jalowiec A, White-Williams C: Predictors of quality of life in patients at one year after heart transplantation, *J Heart Lung Transplant* 18:202-210, 1999.

81. Berman D, Ben-Gal T, Sahar G et al: Functional status and quality of life of heart transplant recipients surviving beyond 5 years, *Transplant Proc* 32:731-732, 2000.

82. Mulligan T, Sheehan H, Hanrahan J: Sexual function after heart transplantation, *J Heart Lung Transplant* 10:125-128, 1991.

83. Brock G, MacMahon G, Chen K et al: Efficiency and safety of tadalafil for the treatment of erectile dysfunction: results of integrated analysis, *J Urol* 168:1332-1336, 2002.

84. Porst H, Rosen R, Padma-Nathan H et al: Efficacy and tolerability of vardenafil, a new oral selective phosphodiesterase type 5 inhibitor, in patients with erectile dysfunction: the first at home clinical trial, *Int J Impot Res* 13(4):192-199, 2001.

85. Wooten J: Erectile dysfunction: there are now three effective oral drugs for treating ED, paving the way for nurses to put patients with this condition on the road to good sexual health, *RN* 67:40, 2004.

86. Gutierrez K, Queener S: *Pharmacology for nursing practice*, St Louis, 2003, Mosby.

SECTION 11

Core Competencies of Clinicians Practicing Across the Continuum of Care

BARBARA RIEGEL and DEBRA K. MOSER

The chapters in the next section of the book describe what clinicians directly caring for patients do every day in their various settings. As such, these chapters are a glimpse into the lives of the practitioners who work in hospice with dying cardiac patients, those who assist cardiovascular surgeons in the operating room, those who are responsible for critically ill patients, and more. We asked the authors to describe their practice setting for others who have never worked there and to define the essential knowledge, skills, and abilities that they need to be successful in their clinical practice. It sounded like an easy task, but the authors struggled with these chapters. Why? Most found it difficult to discern the unique components of the roles they have mastered and the factors that made them successful.

"Competencies" refers to "a cluster of knowledge, attitudes, and skills that affects a major part of one's job, correlates with performance on the job, and can be measured against well-accepted standards."[1] This elusive attribute, competency, is illustrated in the application of knowledge, judgment, interpersonal decision making, personal attributes, and psychomotor skills. In nursing, competencies are used to promote the health, ethical welfare, and safety of the public.[2,3] Competencies differ across practice settings, disciplines, and practice levels. With relatively more education, the advanced practice nurse is expected to demonstrate "a greater depth and breadth of knowledge, a greater degree of synthesis of data, and complexity of skills and interventions" than the entry-level registered nurse.[4] When applicable, we have asked the authors to address how the competencies of clinicians in their settings differ in terms not only of their disciplinary knowledge but also in educational level. As such, our goal was to make these chapters useful to a wide variety of cardiac clinicians.

The chapters in this section reflect the true nature of today's clinical practice: the team. Thus the section begins with a chapter on collaborative care that discusses communication, coordination, and collaboration as essential ingredients of health care delivery. Not so long ago, nurses routinely used the term *multidisciplinary* to describe their practice settings. However, nurses now recognize that simply collaborating with other professionals without evolving into an interdisciplinary or transdisciplinary group is less than ideal for patient care. As described in Chapter 19, in multidisciplinary teams, each health care professional continues to work within the constructs of his or her own disciplinary values and methods (e.g., nursing, social work, or physical therapy).[5] Interdisciplinary collaboration occurs when the disciplines working together on a team stretch beyond their own disciplinary paradigm, integrating information, concepts, and theories to improve patient care.[6] Zerhouni,[7] in the National Institutes of Health Roadmap, calls upon members of the health sciences to move a step further to transdisciplinary collaboration, with a fusion, a melding of disciplinary knowledge into a new hybrid form. That new knowledge will benefit patients and clinicians.

At the time of this writing, the many organizations representing cardiovascular nurses have united to revise and update the American Nurses Association Scope and Standards of Cardiovascular Nursing Practice. We hope that the chapters in this section of the book will be useful in informing us all about the rich and diverse ways that our colleagues practice and that the new standards will reflect this diversity.

1. Parry S: The quest for competencies, *Training* 33:48-56, 1996.
2. National Council of State Boards of Nursing: *Nursing regulation.* Retrieved March 18, 2005, from www.ncsbn.org

3. Canadian Nurses Association: *Advanced nursing practice: a national framework—Canadian Nurses Association.* Retrieved March 17, 2005, from www.cna-nurses.ca/cna/
4. American Nurses Association: *Scope and standards of advanced practice registered nursing,* Washington, DC, 1996, American Nurses Publishing.
5. Bruce A, Lyall C, Tait J et al: Interdisciplinary integration in Europe: the case of the Fifth Framework Programme, *Futures* 36:457-470, 2004.

6. National Academy of Sciences, National Academy of Engineering, Institute of Medicine: *Facilitating interdisciplinary research,* Washington, DC, 2004, National Academies Press.
7. Zerhouni E: The NIH roadmap, *Science* 302:63-72, 2004.

Collaborative Care

Stacen Keating

CHAPTER ABBREVIATION

JNC-VI   Sixth Report of the Joint National Committee on Prevention, Detention, Evaluation, and Treatment of High Blood Pressure

Nurses have a long history of collaborating with professionals from many disciplines to deliver the best possible care for patients. Collaboration has been described as "a complex process that requires intentional knowledge sharing and joint responsibility for patient care."[1] The importance of collaboration was illustrated in 1986 when Knaus and colleagues[2] first published the results of their study regarding the effectiveness of collaboration and communication among the physicians and nurses in intensive care units. They found that the patient death rate was lower in intensive care units with exemplary collaboration and communication among nurses and physicians. Those who were dedicated, well-prepared, and able to achieve high levels of effective communication were the best equipped to work together in a way that could benefit patients profoundly.

As a result of this early work and later studies, nurses now recognize the importance of the *process of care* on patient outcomes.[2] Health care professionals must pay more attention to the ways in which they interact with one another. Communication, coordination, and collaboration are essential in every aspect of health care delivery. Most would agree that nurse-physician collaboration, in particular, is an important factor in the delivery of effective health care. However, nurses also need to build strong collaborative relationships with other professionals (dietitians, physical therapists, and others) who work with complex patients. The need to collaborate successfully on health care teams with multiple disciplines has been noted repeatedly.[3,4]

Cardiovascular care, in particular, is an area with numerous opportunities for nurses to collaborate with colleagues from many disciplines to foster positive outcomes for their patients. To date, many hospitals and clinics have established formal collaborative teams of health care professionals dedicated to working together as a group to treat and care for patients. It is important for nurses and others to understand the full impact of interdisciplinary collaboration in making substantial improvements in cardiac care.

The purpose of this chapter, then, is to discuss interdisciplinary collaboration among health care professionals dedicated to improving health outcomes for cardiac patients. Readers will benefit from learning how existing collaborative practice models work. This knowledge will help clinicians incorporate evidence-based practices into the current working environment and help clinicians and researchers formulate ways in which future models of care can best be constructed. A discussion of how to promote effective collaboration is included to help outline many of the significant challenges that exist. This chapter offers an overview of many of the skills needed to be a collaborator on an interdisciplinary health care team. Finally, this chapter challenges the nurse to give serious thought to the role that the interdisciplinary team has in achieving improved outcomes for cardiac patients and the pivotal role that nurses have in shaping and contributing to the collaborative team.

UNDERSTANDING THE TERMS OF COLLABORATION

Collaboration refers to the sharing of knowledge and the partnering of health care professionals who jointly accept responsibility for improving patient care and outcomes.[1] At the outset, it is probably helpful to acknowledge the most frequently used terms in describing the process of working on collaborative health care teams. Major terms used to describe working with professionals across disciplinary lines include *multidisciplinary, interdisciplinary,* and *transdisciplinary collaboration.* Often these terms are used interchangeably; however, they actually describe different ways of working with colleagues. These differences may appear subtle, but they can be important. A helpful note is that these terms are not mutually exclusive but are instead complementary to one another.[5]

Multidisciplinary collaboration involves professionals working within the construct of their own disciplinary values and methods.[6] For example, nurses working on the team would use concepts from nursing theories and nursing frameworks while caring for patients or taking part in research projects. Social workers who are part of the same team would work in their own disciplinary paradigm, and so on.

Interdisciplinary collaboration is a different form of teamwork. In this model, disciplines come together on a team and stretch beyond their own disciplinary paradigm. Interdisciplinary collaboration occurs when information, concepts, and theories are *integrated* on the team.[7] The team as a collective whole would work together to decide what overarching concepts or theories should inform patient care or frame the research project (Figure 19-1).

Lawrence[5] describes *transdisciplinary* collaboration as a "fusion of disciplinary knowledge with the know-how of lay-people that creates a new hybrid that is different from any specific constituent part" (p. 489). In ef-

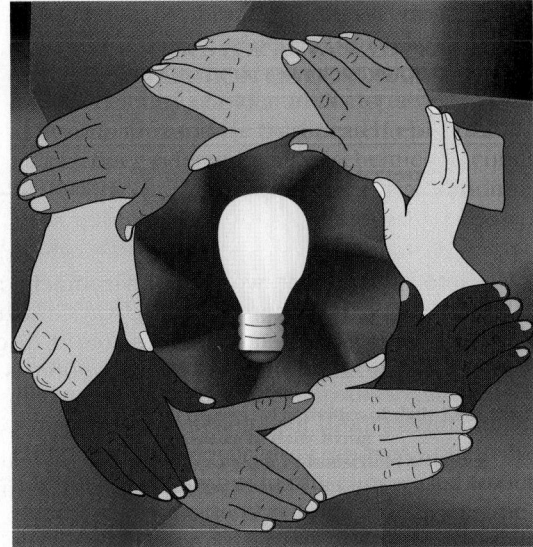

FIGURE 19-1 ■ Joining disciplines to form an interdisciplinary team.

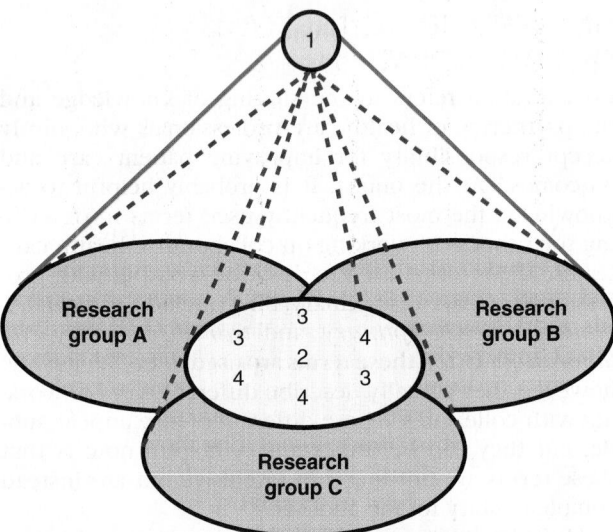

FIGURE 19-2 ■ How disciplinary knowledge is fused to create a new hybrid-transdisciplinary-model that differs from any specific constituent. Collaboration involves transgressing across disciplinary lines and results in an approach that is focused on the problem rather than the disciplines. Different disciplinary concepts and knowledge are melded to form an entirely new entity. (Data from Papst J: *Transdisciplinarity: the unifying paradigm of humanities, natural and social sciences.* Retrieved 12/8/06 from www.inst.at/trans/15Nr/01_6/papst_b_15.htm)

fect, collaboration within this model entails *transgressing* across disciplinary lines and results in an approach that is "problem-oriented, theory-guided and methodologically driven."[8] In other words, transdisciplinary collaboration may be thought of in terms of a melding of different disciplinary concepts and knowledge, resulting in an entirely new entity (Figure 19-2). This concept of collaboration is newer and more difficult to practice than the others and occurs far less often than multidisciplinary or interdisciplinary collaboration.

This chapter refers most often to the terms *multidisciplinary* and *interdisciplinary collaboration.* In fact, interdisciplinary is the term most used when individuals discuss the collaboration of professionals across disciplinary lines. When nurses work on a team with other professionals, it is important to have a basic understanding of how the team collaborates in order to help foster effective communication among group members.

HEALTH CARE PROFESSIONALS IN INTERDISCIPLINARY COLLABORATION

Even without a thorough understanding of the underlying mechanisms that make collaboration successful, multidisciplinary disease management has become accepted in many aspects of health care, including cardiac care. A collaborative team approach is especially necessary for complex illnesses, such as heart failure, as discussed later.[4]

Nurses collaborate with physicians and a number of other disciplines, including pharmacists, dietitians, physical therapists, psychologists, primary care providers, and social workers. This list is not meant to be exhaustive but does suggest the range of professional expertise that may be needed to treat complex patients effectively. In a recent survey of heart failure disease management teams in the Netherlands, 60 percent (85 out of 142 hospitals, 83 of which took part in the study) had established multidisciplinary models of disease management with professionals from various disciplines (Figure 19-3). Cardiologists were present on all teams (100 percent), followed closely by heart failure nurses (81 percent), dietitians (59 percent), and physical therapists (47 percent).[4] Depending on the patient's personal needs, input from certain disciplines can be critical in helping follow the treatment regimen, thereby achieving a better quality of life and health.

Understanding exactly who needs to be on the collaborative team sometimes can be difficult. According to Jaarsma,[4] creating the right mix of health care professionals poses an important challenge because there is no one-size-fits-all model of interdisciplinary care. Individual patient situations and needs vary, demanding a unique approach to treatment and care; building a team requires an assessment of the specific patient population. In other words, deciding who will be on the team is not necessarily a straightforward task. Experienced health care professionals know that, along with the desire to provide optimal care and achieve successful patient outcomes, there remains the need to allocate costly resources wisely, so not everyone can be included.

DEVELOPING COLLABORATIVE PRACTICE MODELS IN CARDIAC CARE

A number of models of collaborative care substantially improve outcomes for cardiac patients and others. Other models have the potential to work but for various reasons fall short of desired goals. Patients with cardiac disease present complex challenges because many are elderly and have multiple risk factors and numerous comorbid conditions.

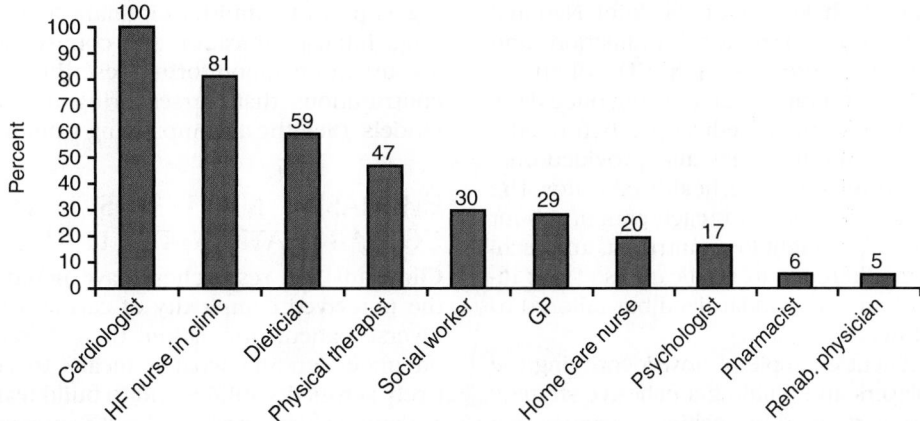

FIGURE 19-3 ▨ Health care professionals involved in heart failure clinics in the Netherlands in 2003 (*n* = 83 hospitals). *GP*, General practitioner. (Data from Jaarsma T: *Eur J Heart Fail* 7:343-349, 2005.)

Nurses have been working in collaboration with other health care professionals on interdisciplinary teams to help patients reduce cardiovascular risk, alter lifestyle behaviors, and engage in secondary prevention.[1-3] Some examples of the contributions of these teams are reviewed next.

Reducing Cardiovascular Risk

Strong scientific evidence indicates that interventions aimed at reducing cardiovascular risk for individual patients may be highly effective and yield positive patient outcomes. Unfortunately, in general, only about 50 percent of persons who could benefit from a risk assessment are assessed by a health care provider.[9] According to Allen and Scott,[10] the reason for this gap in ideal care is largely due to the ineffectiveness of traditional methods of addressing risk reduction, which emphasize the need for physicians to discuss risk reduction during routine office visits. Most physicians face severe time constraints when seeing patients and are not able to spend the time needed to address risk reduction effectively. As discussed later, nurses and other health care professionals now work collaboratively to counsel patients, which has helped patients achieve greater levels of risk reduction than prior models of care.

Altering Lifestyle Behaviors

Motivated persons can achieve lifestyle behavior changes that will decrease their risk factors for cardiovascular disease.[11] To encourage lifestyle behavior change, patients require education on how to make dietary changes (such as eating a low-fat diet), increase physical activity, and reduce or eliminate smoking. Physicians who have tried to get this message across to patients during office visits have had varied success. Conversely, prevention teams made up of multiple disciplines have achieved better levels of success at helping patients alter health behaviors than physicians acting alone. Simpson and colleagues[11] found that multidisciplinary group counseling or a combination of group and individual counseling was effective in helping patients

achieve lifestyle behavior changes. Nurses' expertise in patient education and counseling are integral to interdisciplinary teams searching for innovative ways to improve behavior modification and increase positive lifestyle changes in their patients.

Improving Secondary Prevention

As discussed in other chapters, lipid lowering is an effective method of secondary prevention for cardiac patients. Unfortunately, few patients achieve optimal cholesterol control.[12] Allen and Scott[10] reviewed the effectiveness of collaborative models of care organized to manage dyslipidemia and summarized the evidence of randomized controlled trials supporting the use of nurse-directed multidisciplinary teams in terms of helping patients meet lipid goals and receive effective treatment. They found that, when nurse case managers are part of the interdisciplinary team, there is an increased likelihood that drug management algorithms will be followed strictly. In addition, patients received individualized counseling and regular follow-up more often, which contributed to the success of the multidisciplinary team effort.

Controlling Hypertension

Uncontrolled hypertension is a significant public health problem that increases morbidity, mortality, and health care costs.[13] Tao and colleagues[14] established a multidisciplinary hypertension clinic to address these issues. The team was composed of three general internists, a nurse health educator, a pharmacist, and a dietitian. In 6 months, this team was able to get 58 percent of patients in the practice to reach a blood pressure of less than 140/90 mm Hg. They reported that their overall success might have been even better, but the disadvantaged minority population they served required intense personal and socioeconomic attention, which affected their ability to perform follow-up with others.

In this trial,[14] physicians met with patients to determine the most likely reason for the uncontrolled hypertension. Medication decisions were based on recommendations by the Sixth Report of the Joint National Committee on Prevention, Detention, Evaluation, and Treatment of High Blood Pressure (**JNC-VI**). All efforts were made to simplify therapy, such as using once-daily dosing and maximizing initial medications before adding additional ones to the list. They also provided one-on-one education from the nurse health educator, the pharmacist, and the nutritionist to teach patients about hypertension, exercise, weight loss, nutrition, and techniques to improve adherence to medications. Their intervention curriculum was standardized but tailored to individual patient needs.

This is one excellent example of how identifying the necessary team players and building a cohesive strategy to treat hypertension resulted in positive outcomes in a disadvantaged population with numerous challenges. Nurses added substantively to the collaborative team model. The nurse educator helped patients achieve better medication adherence, monitored patient understanding of the treatment regimen, and explained or clarified potential side effects when speaking with patients.

Managing Atrial Fibrillation

Another collaborative team of providers effectively managed patients with atrial fibrillation after hospital discharge.[15] They designed a nurse-led, home-based intervention with a structured home visit 7 to 14 days after discharge. These visits were done originally by a nurse and a pharmacist and later by a qualified cardiac nurse. The home-based intervention focused on several issues, but of particular interest was the focus on optimizing patient access to effective multidisciplinary management with clear treatment and outcome goals. This access was to the primary care physician, the specialist physician, the community pharmacist, the community nurse, and other allied health professionals where appropriate. The home-based intervention resulted in better outcomes for patients; patients in the intervention groups experienced fewer hospital readmissions and fewer fatal events than those who received the routine postdischarge care.

Managing Heart Failure

Heart failure has been a major focus of study by investigators looking to improve outcomes for this extremely complex, costly, and difficult-to-treat population. As a result, a number of investigators from various fields have conducted randomized controlled trials in multidisciplinary disease management aimed at improving the poor outcomes often associated with heart failure. These results, summarized in recent reviews and meta-analyses,[16-20] and discussed in Chapter 79 of this book, illustrate convincingly that this type of collaborative approach is effective in improving outcomes in this patient group.

In 2005, Jaarsma[4] discussed the importance of a collaborative model of treatment and care for heart failure patients and the challenge that exists in deciding on the optimal mix of health care professionals. The major factors needed to establish successful HF teams, as outlined by Jaarsma, are listed in Box 19-1. Nurses have expertise in a number of these components. Collaborat-

ing as part of a multidisciplinary team, discharge planning, intense education and counseling, providing follow-up and telemonitoring describe some of the major contributions that nurses bring to collaborative care models. (See the accompanying Conundrum box.)

EMPHASIS ON INTERDISCIPLINARY COLLABORATION: THE LARGER PICTURE

Clinicians and researchers have noted that because of the perceived complexity of caring for an increasingly diverse patient population, there is renewed emphasis on understanding what it means to collaborate effectively across disciplines and to build teams that can help patients achieve positive health outcomes. Health care professionals and others generally acknowledge that interdisciplinary collaboration will play a large role in the future of health care. At the national level a number of initiatives have been put forth to encourage health care professionals, especially in areas of research, to forge interdisciplinary relationships with one another to meet the challenges of an ever-changing, complex society.

National Institutes of Health

The National Institutes of Health drew a substantial amount of attention to the call for interdisciplinary collaboration with the recently published *Roadmap Initia-*

BOX 19-1 ■ ■ ■
RECOMMENDED COMPONENTS OF A MULTIDISCIPLINARY PROGRAM FOR PERSONS WITH HEART FAILURE

- Optimal diagnostics
- Optimized medical therapy with guidelines
- Team approach
- Vigilant follow-up starting within 10 days of discharge
- Discharge planning
- Increased access to health care
- Intense education and counseling
- Inpatient and outpatient (home-based)
- Attention to behavioral strategies
- Address barriers to compliance
- Early attention to signs and symptoms (e.g., telemonitoring)
- Flexible diuretic regimen
- Exercise program

Data from Jaarsma T: *Eur J Heart Fail* 7:343-349, 2005.

■ ■ ■ **CONUNDRUM**

WHAT IS THE APPROPRIATE MIX FOR AN OPTIMAL INTERDISCIPLINARY TEAM?

Teams composed of professionals from multiple disciplines can improve outcomes for patients with complex cardiovascular disease. In theory and practice, interdisciplinary collaboration recognizes the expertise and added value of nurses and other health care disciplines to evidence-based practice. Nurses remain unclear, however, about the appropriate mix of professionals needed on the team and factors that facilitate true collaboration. Once these questions are answered, new models of care may arise that will be even more effective in improving health outcomes for cardiac patients.

tive.[21] Concerned with significant roadblocks that may be impeding scientific progress in health care, the roadmap explicitly stated the need to assemble teams that include all key players from across disciplinary boundaries. A major theme of the initiative called for teams of the future that look different from teams of the past. The National Institutes of Health acknowledged that biomedical research problems confronting society today are extremely complex and in need of a more holistic understanding of the problem. As a result, there is a belief that no single discipline will be able to tackle important issues without input from other disciplines. The roadmap initiative has set the tone for a commitment to fostering interdisciplinary research at the national level.

National Academy of Sciences

Similarly, backed by the W.M. Keck Foundation, the National Academy of Sciences began taking significant steps to advance the understanding of interdisciplinary collaboration. In 2003 the Committee on Facilitating Interdisciplinary Research was formed to begin an investigation aimed at improving understanding of a number of key issues related to interdisciplinary collaboration. That initiative focuses on the identification of structural models of interdisciplinary settings, government policies that promote or hinder interdisciplinary research, and how best to evaluate the effect that interdisciplinary collaboration has on research, to name just a few. The committee's report, published in 2004,[7] revealed a number of challenges to successful collaboration. Among the conclusions was the notion that a much better understanding of the social and intellectual processes that promote successful interdisciplinary collaboration is needed.

PROMOTING INTERDISCIPLINARY COLLABORATION IN PRACTICE AND RESEARCH

Developing models of interdisciplinary collaboration to improve cardiovascular care holds great promise. If there is truly a belief and interest in working effectively across disciplines to achieve better outcomes for patients, then it is important that nurses understand how best to facilitate interdisciplinary collaboration. To promote effective interaction among health care professionals, it is helpful to understand better the factors that are important to successful collaboration. A review of some of the nursing, medical, and social work literature on this topic reveals some of the important factors identified by those with experience working across disciplinary boundaries.

Leadership

Anecdotal accounts of interdisciplinary efforts in the nursing, medical, and social work literature have noted the importance of leadership in relation to the success or failure of the team.[21-29] As one would imagine, opinions differ on the best way to construct group leadership in order to achieve the team's purpose. Leadership that is fluid appears to be most desirable,[26,29] even to the point that leadership might be rotated among group

members. Feelings that power should be shared among group members also have been expressed.[22]

Issues surrounding leadership can be highly emotive. Much of the health care literature on this topic of leadership in interdisciplinary teams focuses on issues of respect for one another individually and for disciplinary perspectives as a whole.[29,30] Individuals want to feel empowered and have their voices heard.[31] Fears by some disciplines that there are different levels of "status" on the team seem to lead to conflict.[29,32]

As a result, barriers to interdisciplinary collaboration may arise when one discipline dominates the group and becomes too influential. As one group dominates, others feel that their voices go unheard, and they may become disillusioned with working as part of the team and ultimately leave the group or hold back on communicating valuable insights into practice- and research-related issues for fear of being disrespected or overlooked by the group. Notions of the interdisciplinary team as being a "true partnership" have been expressed because this connotes a group where all members have a voice, feel valued based on their unique expertise, and take joint responsibility for the conduct of a project.[23]

The idea that leadership can be shared or rotated among group members is not expressed by all. Interestingly, McGuire[26] notes the importance of having a clearly designated leader on the team to take the responsibility of making difficult, unanticipated decisions that may confront the team. Even with a designated leader, however, McGuire notes the importance of maintaining democratic leadership and fostering consensual decision making. As a result, the leader would need to set the tone that input from all team members is desirable and essential to overall group functioning.

Professional Autonomy

Similarly, to promote interdisciplinary practice and research, there needs to be an understanding and belief in the professional autonomy of individual disciplines that want to establish their unique identity and contributions to the team.* Members on the interdisciplinary team need to complement one another's knowledge and have their unique contributions valued for their importance to the overall functioning of the group.[23,25,34] In other words, team members want to work collaboratively to achieve group and patient goals, but they also want to maintain their unique professional identity.

Differing Worldviews

Individuals with experience working on an interdisciplinary team have noted a number of factors that seem to impede the overall functioning of the group. A review of some of the health care literature on this topic revealed that certain factors were expressed by multiple disciplines as being barriers to interdisciplinary collaboration. For example, professionals from the disciplines of nursing, medicine, and social work have acknowledged the complex nature of working across interdisci-

---

*References 22, 23, 25, 28, 29, 32, 33.

plinary lines because of the inherent differences in the culture and value systems of these unique disciplines.

Professional disciplines often are socialized differently and learn to see the world through their own unique paradigm or lens.[23,25,27-29,34-37] When collaborating across disciplines, it may become evident that differences in professional values and theoretical bases are large, and wide differences in opinions can result. One must understand that although professional theories and values may be different from one another, these differences do not have to be insurmountable. Acknowledging and respecting another professional's cultural differences are key aspects of interdisciplinary collaboration. In fact, sharing of culture and values across disciplinary lines can foster greater creativity in conceptualizing problems and developing interventions to be tested in the research arena.[37]

Disciplinary Jargon

With the knowledge that professional disciplines learn to view the world through different paradigms, it is no surprise that individual disciplines often have a unique language. This discipline specific jargon helps members of a professional culture communicate with one another quickly and easily but also has the potential to create barriers when collaborating with others across disciplinary lines.* It should be noted that sometimes even when different disciplines use similar terms, communication problems can arise because similar terms often carry different meanings for different professions. On a positive note, disagreement about the use of a term may be inevitable but also can be desirable while one is working on the interdisciplinary team.[22] Differences of opinion can open the lines of communication and act as a catalyst for growth and improvement of communication efforts.

Understanding how to construct effective team leadership, value the professional autonomy of others, respect the differing professional paradigms to which colleagues subscribe, and minimize the use of professional jargon are important aspects of interdisciplinary collaboration. Successful collaboration is more likely to be promoted when these issues and others are acknowledged and addressed (Box 19-2).

---

*References 22, 23, 26-29, 31, 34, 37, 38.

BOX 19-2 ■ ■ ■
FACTORS THAT HELP PROMOTE INTERDISCIPLINARY COLLABORATION

- Effective leadership
- Respect for others on the team
- Allowing all team members to have a voice
- Acknowledgment of the professional autonomy of others
- Working to understand the worldview of another discipline
- Minimizing disciplinary jargon
- Promotion of clear, effective communication
- Identification of the optimal mix of professionals for the team
- Striving for lifelong learning
- Including professionals who are dedicated and well prepared

SUMMARY

Increasingly, health care professionals are acknowledging the complex nature of health care problems and the need for multiple disciplines to work together across professional boundaries to provide the best evidenced-based care for complex patients. Successful interdisciplinary collaboration has the potential to improve health care quality and outcomes for many patients suffering from complex cardiovascular disease. To date, little research has been done to understand the process of interdisciplinary collaboration and how best to formulate teams that will work well together and improve overall patient care. Research in this area is greatly needed.

Health care professionals interested in building successful teams need numerous skills. Building teams where effective leadership and excellent communication pathways exist are important aspects of interdisciplinary collaboration. Those who believe in the need to strive for lifelong learning help promote collaboration. These individuals look constantly to improve their knowledge and skills and to help develop environments where evidence-based best-practice models are used. Development of intellectual skills that allow team members to respect and understand the perspectives and paradigms of other professional disciplines is needed on an interdisciplinary team. Building teams that employ dedicated and knowledgeable professionals will help foster trust among group members.

Lastly, it is important to understand that team building does not happen overnight. Building a successful collaborative team can take a great deal of time and effort, but the ability of interdisciplinary teams to achieve positive outcomes in cardiac care and elsewhere has great potential. Nurses are challenged to gain a thorough understanding of how to collaborate effectively across disciplines in order to become an essential part of the interdisciplinary team. This ability will establish nurses firmly as leaders and innovators in health care.

REFERENCES

1. Lindeke LL, Sieckert AM: Nurse-physician workplace collaboration, *Online J Issues Nurs* 10(1):5, 2005.
2. Knaus WA, Draper EA, Wagner DP, Zimmerman JE: An evaluation of outcome from intensive care in major medical centers, *Ann Intern Med* 4:410-418, 1986.
3. Fairman J: Not all nurses are good, not all doctors are bad, *Bull Hist Med* 78:451-460, 2004.
4. Jaarsma T: Health care professionals in a heart failure team, *Eur J Heart Fail* 7:343-349, 2005.
5. Lawrence RJ: Housing and health: from interdisciplinary principles to transdisciplinary research and practice, *Futures* 36:487-502, 2004.
6. Bruce A, Lyall C, Tait J, Williams R: Interdisciplinary integration in Europe: the case of the Fifth Framework Programme, *Futures* 36:457-470, 2004.
7. National Academy of Sciences, National Academy of Engineering, Institute of Medicine: *Facilitating interdisciplinary research*, Washington, DC, 2004, National Academies Press.
8. Balsiger PW: Supradisciplinary research practices: history, objectives and rationale, *Futures* 36:407-421, 2004.
9. Cooper R, Cutler J, Desvigne-Nickens P et al: Trend and disparities in coronary heart disease, stroke, and other cardiovascular diseases in the United States: findings of the National Conference on Cardiovascular Disease Prevention, *Circulation* 102(25):3137-3147, 2000.

10. Allen J, Scott LB: Alternative models in the delivery of primary and secondary prevention programs, *J Cardiovasc Nurs* 18(2):150-156, 2003.

11. Simpson DR, Dixon BG, Bolli P: Effectiveness of multidisciplinary patient counseling in reducing cardiovascular disease risk factors through nonpharmacological intervention: results from the Heart Healthy Program, *Can J Cardiol* 20(2):177-186, 2004.

12. Yates S, Annis L, Pippins J, Walden S: Does a lipid clinic increase compliance with national cholesterol education treatment program guidelines? report of a case-matched controlled study, *South Med J* 94:907-909, 2001.

13. Whelton PK, He J, Appel LJ et al, the National High Blood Pressure Education Program Coordinating Committee: Primary prevention of hypertension: clinical and public health advisory from the National High Blood Pressure Education Program, *JAMA* 288:1882-1888, 2002.

14. Tao LS, Hart P, Edwards E et al: Treatment of difficult-to-control blood pressure in a multidisciplinary clinic at a public hospital, *J Natl Med Assoc* 95(4):263-269, 2003.

15. Inglis S, McLennan S, Dawson A et al: A new solution for an old problem? effects of a nurse-led, multidisciplinary, home-based intervention on readmission and mortality in patients with chronic atrial fibrillation, *J Cardiovasc Nurs* 19(2):118-127, 2004.

16. Gwadry-Sridhar FH, Flintoft V, Lee DS et al: A systematic review and meta-analysis of studies comparing readmission rates and mortality rates in patients with heart failure, *Arch Intern Med* 164(21):2315-2320, 2004.

17. Phillips CO, Wright SM, Kern DE et al: Comprehensive discharge planning with postdischarge support for older patients with congestive heart failure: a meta-analysis, *JAMA* 291(11):1358-1367, 2004.

18. McAlister FA, Stewart S, Ferrua S, McMurray JV: Multidisciplinary strategies for the management of heart failure patients at high risk for admission: a systematic review of randomized trials, *J Am Coll Cardiol* 44(4):810-819, 2004.

19. Ledwidge M, Barry M, Cahill J et al: Is multidisciplinary care of heart failure cost-beneficial when combined with optimal medical care? *Eur J Heart Fail* 5(3):381-389, 2003.

20. McDonald K, Ledwidge M, Cahill J et al: Heart failure management: multidisciplinary care has intrinsic benefit above the optimization of medical care, *J Card Fail* 8(3):142-148, 2002.

21. Zerhouni E: The NIH roadmap, *Science* 302(5642):63-72, 2004.

22. Bronstein LR: A model for interdisciplinary collaboration, *Soc Work* 48(3):297-306, 2003.

23. Gueldner SH, Stroud SD: Sharing the quest for knowledge through interdisciplinary research, *Holist Nurs Pract* 10(3):54-62, 1996.

24. Martin KM: Coordinating multidisciplinary, collaborative research: a formula for success, *Clin Nurse Spec* 8(1):18-22, 1994.

25. Mock B, Hill MN, Dienemann JA et al: Challenges to behavioral research in oncology, *Cancer Pract* 4(5):267-273, 1996.

26. McGuire DB: Building and maintaining an interdisciplinary research team, *Alzheimer Dis Assoc Disord* 13(suppl 1):S17-S21, 1999.

27. Milligan RA, Gilroy J, Katz KS et al: Developing a shared language: interdisciplinary communication among diverse health care professionals, *Holist Nurs Pract* 13(2):47-53, 1999.

28. Neill KM: A holistic interdisciplinary health care research model, *Holist Nurs Pract* 13(2):54-60, 1999.

29. Reese DJ, Sontag M: Successful interprofessional collaboration on the hospice team, *Health Soc Work* 26(3):167-174, 2001.

30. Bruhn JG: Interdisciplinary research: a philosophy, art form, artifact or antidote? *Integr Physiol Behav Sci* 35(1):58-66, 2000.

31. McCloskey JC, Maas M: Interdisciplinary team: the nursing perspective is essential, *Nurs Outlook* 46:157-163, 1998.

32. Abramson JS, Mizrahi T: Understanding collaboration between social workers and physicians: application of a typology, *Soc Work Health Care* 37(2):71-100, 2003.

33. Klein JT: *Crossing boundaries: knowledge, disciplinarities and interdisciplinarities,* Charlottesville, Va, 1996, University of Virginia Press.

34. Merwin E: Building interdisciplinary mental health services research teams: a case example, *Issues Ment Health Nurs* 16:547-554, 1995.

35. Lattuca LR: Learning interdisciplinarity: sociocultural perspectives on academic work, *Journal of Higher Education* 73(6):711-740, 2002.

36. Mazure CM, Espeland M, Douglas P et al: Multidisciplinary women's health research: the national centers of excellence in women's health, *J Womens Health Gend Based Med* 9(7):717-724, 2000.

37. Stokols D, Fuqua J, Gress J et al: Evaluating transdisciplinary science, *Nicotine Tob Res* 5(suppl 1):S21-S39, 2003.

38. Pellmar TC, Eisenberg L (eds): *Bridging disciplines in the brain, behavioral, and clinical sciences,* Washington, DC, 2000, National Academies Press.

Emergency Department Nursing Care of the Cardiac Patient

Patricia Kunz Howard

CHAPTER ABBREVIATIONS

ACLS advanced cardiac life support

AED automatic external defibrillator

AHA American Heart Association

ECG electrocardiogram

ED emergency department

ENA Emergency Nurses Association

NTG nitroglycerin

The position of Emergency Nurses Association (**ENA**) is that the specialty of emergency nursing is an autonomous profession with an independent scope of practice.[1] Emergency nurses should be responsible and accountable for their own actions and should be supervised and evaluated for the quality and effectiveness of that practice by other professional nurses. Although autonomous, emergency nursing is collaborative and interdependent. Thus, emergency nurses are expected to facilitate open and timely communication with other health care providers. Mutual respect for professional autonomy should guide jointly coordinated emergency care provided by nurses, physicians, and other providers.

Emergency nurses, as all specialty practice groups, are accountable for maximizing their professional practice through identification of self-learning needs and ongoing education. The profession is advanced through research and evidence-based practice. Professional boundaries, outlined by state nurse practice acts, require that emergency nurses maintain legal and ethical responsibility for the delivery of quality patient care.

Quality patient care by nurses in an emergency department (**ED**) is particularly challenging because of the diverse patient populations seen. Emergency nurses must be knowledgeable of many cardiac conditions because cardiac complaints—especially chest pain—are a frequent reason for patients to present to the ED. The ability to prioritize the care these patients receive is even more important today than in years past because EDs are busier than ever before. Indeed, ED visits in the United States reached a record high of nearly 114 million in 2003, whereas the number of EDs decreased by 14 percent from 1993 to 2003.[2]

When a patient with chest pain or another symptom of an acute coronary syndrome presents to the ED, some facilities activate a specific team. Others depend on staff to handle all types of cases. Regardless of the system used, essential competencies for nurses providing care to cardiac patients in the ED include triage, cardiac dysrhythmia interpretation and management, electrocardiogram (**ECG**) interpretation, hemodynamic monitoring, and resuscitation. This chapter provides an overview of the skills and knowledge required of nurses in the ED. The care of patients with specific conditions is detailed in other chapters.

TRIAGE

Rapid assessment and prioritization based on the patient's clinical presentation are skills that are essential for the ED nurse to provide effective triage. The ability to differentiate chest pain–related complaints within the context of the medical history, current appearance, and vital signs requires excellent, refined assessment skills. Patients suspected of having cardiac-mediated chest pain must receive a high triage priority. The actual triage score assigned will vary based on the triage acuity system used. Triage of the patient with chest pain is accomplished best by moving the patient directly to the treatment area.

For patients with acute myocardial infarction, the goal is 1 hour from symptom onset to definitive treatment. This goal is based on data demonstrating increased morbidity and mortality associated with longer times from symptom onset to treatment.[3,4] Delay time is an important predictor of morbidity and mortality.[4] Survival rates are improved by up to 50 percent if reperfusion is achieved within 1 hour of symptom onset, and by 23 percent if reperfusion is achieved within 3 hours of symptom onset.[5] In one trial, delaying treatment by 30 minutes reduced average life expectancy by 1 year.[6] In another study of 565 patients undergoing angioplasty for acute myocardial infarction, those who received the first balloon inflation within 60 minutes of arrival at the hospital had a 30-day mortality rate of 1.0 percent, but for every 15 minutes longer than 1 hour, the odds of death increased 1.6 times.[4]

Treatment-seeking delay phases have been broken down into the time from (1) symptom onset to patient/bystander decision to seek medical attention; (2) transportation time; and (3) in-hospital delays to receiving treatment. The first phase consumes the major proportion of delay time, and delay in arriving at the hospital continues to be the major reason patients do not receive timely treatment. Patient delay in seeking treatment is discussed thoroughly in Chapter 51. Transportation to the hospital consumes only a small proportion of prehospital delay time.[7] Once the patient arrives for care, the in-hospital phase of delay to treatment is relatively small, although hospital transfers still can introduce considerable delay.

Facilities able to triage a patient with chest pain directly to a treatment area minimize the delay in starting definitive diagnostics and interventions to preserve function. Early recognition of the need for diagnostic procedures such as serial ECG and serial measurement of cardiac markers (e.g., troponin) is integral to making decisions about patient disposition. Reliance on nonspecific factors such as age, a single ECG, and medical history should be avoided when making triage decisions. The triage nurse must anticipate recognized (e.g., substernal chest pain) and less recognized (e.g., nausea and vomiting without chest pain) complaints as potentially suspicious for a cardiac condition requiring a high triage priority.

SUPPORTIVE CARE AND DIAGNOSTIC TOOLS

Chest pain or other cardiac chief complaints should elicit a standard management approach. All patients should receive appropriate diagnostic evaluation regardless of age. Evidence has shown that acute coronary syndromes can and do occur in early adulthood. All cardiovascular conditions require a complete assessment (Table 20-1), initiation of monitoring, baseline and repeated vital sign measurements, establishment of intravenous access, and consideration of the need for supplemental oxygen.

The initial approach to a patient with chest pain and a possible cardiac condition includes administration of aspirin, assuming no allergy or contraindications to salicylates exists. Pain level should be assessed with sensitivity to differences in cultural manifestations of pain.[8] Management of pain is dictated by current clinical status and facility protocol or orders from a primary care provider. Patients experiencing chest pain may be anxious; adequate pain control helps reduce anxiety. Ongoing assessment for changes in clinical status, response to interventions, and pain level is essential to provide optimal management. Changes in cardiac status may be reflected in physiological parameters such as changes in vital signs or cardiac rhythm. Nurses must closely monitor the cardiac rhythm, being prepared to intervene and communicate with the health care team to manage the patient appropriately.

RHYTHM RECOGNITION

Cardiac patients often have hemodynamic compromise from rhythm disturbances. Accurate interpretation of cardiac rhythms is an essential competency for the emergency nurse. The ability to integrate the clinical presentation, cardiac rhythm, and necessary management can affect the patient's outcome. Rhythm disturbances that result in clinical compromise are caused by inadequate cardiac output resulting from bradycardia, tachycardia, or pulseless rhythms. Rapid recognition and intervention by the emergency nurse are essential to ensure adequate oxygenation and perfusion to vital organs. Table 20-2 depicts the rhythms that ED nurses encounter commonly and need to be able to interpret accurately and manage. Management of these dysrhythmias should be guided by presenting clinical condition using current American Heart Association (AHA) Advanced Cardiac Life Support (ACLS) Guidelines.[9] The emergency nurse needs to be prepared to implement interventions that will ensure physiological stability.

■ ■ ■

TABLE 20-1 INITIAL ASSESSMENT OF PERSONS PRESENTING TO THE EMERGENCY DEPARTMENT WITH CARDIAC COMPLAINTS

ASSESSMENT TYPE	ELEMENTS
Subjective	Chief complaint • Onset, duration • Precipitating factors Medical history Current medications • Prescription • Over-the-counter Herbal or homeopathic remedies
Objective	General appearance • Level of consciousness • Color Respiratory status • Rate and effort • Breath sounds Circulation • Apical heart rate, heart tones • Peripheral pulses Secondary assessment

■ ■ ■

TABLE 20-2 ESSENTIAL CARDIAC RHYTHMS THAT EMERGENCY NURSES MUST KNOW

TYPE	RHYTHM
Sinus	Normal sinus rhythm Sinus bradycardia Sinus tachycardia Sinus arrhythmia Sinus arrest
Atrial	Atrial fibrillation Atrial flutter Atrial tachycardia Multifocal atrial tachycardia Wandering atrial pacemaker Premature atrial contraction
Junctional	Junctional rhythm Accelerated junctional rhythm Junctional tachycardia Premature junctional contraction
Atrioventricular blocks	First-degree atrioventricular block Second-degree atrioventricular block type I (Mobitz I, Wenckebach) Second-degree atrioventricular block type II Third-degree heart block
Ventricular	Monomorphic ventricular tachycardia Polymorphic ventricular tachycardia Ventricular fibrillation Premature ventricular contraction Idioventricular rhythm
Other	Ventricular paced Atrioventricular sequential paced Asystole Pulseless electrical activity Intraventricular conduction defect

DYSRHYTHMIA MANAGEMENT STRATEGIES

Determination of the cardiac rhythm may guide initial diagnostic and management decisions. Patients with inadequate perfusion related to a dysrhythmia need to receive rapidly the general supportive care measures already described. After the initial assessment and interventions are completed, the appropriate AHA algorithm or facility protocol should be implemented. External defibrillation with an automatic external defibrillator (**AED**) is the standard of care in the management of out-of-hospital pulseless arrests. Prehospital providers may transport a patient to the ED with an AED in use. Upon arrival to the ED, use of the AED may be continued or a standard monitor/defibrillator may be used. Evidence-based guidelines are available for monophasic and biphasic defibrillators. The recommendation for monophasic waveform defibrillation is 360 J for ventricular fibrillation/pulseless ventricular tachycardia. Current recommendations for biphasic defibrillation are 150 to 200 J for truncated exponential biphasic waveform and 120 J for a rectilinear biphasic waveform.[9]

Electrical therapy is often the management of choice for hemodynamically unstable patients (e.g., presence of chest pain, shortness of breath, light-headedness, hypotension) with fast or absent cardiac rhythms. Stable patients with heart rates in excess of 150 beats/min usually require pharmacological intervention to prevent clinical deterioration. Table 20-3 depicts pharmacological strategies commonly used in the ED for stable tachycardias.

Bradycardic patients also may have physiological instability manifested by chest pain, syncope, dizziness, hypotension. Rhythms with rates less than 60 beats/min may be managed emergently with a temporary pacemaker. In the ED, transcutaneous pacing is used more often than transvenous pacing. Box 20-1 illustrates the procedure for transcutaneous pacing.

Pharmacological adjuncts may be used to manage symptomatic bradycardia if a pacemaker is not immediately available. Box 20-2 depicts pharmacological agents commonly used to treat clinically unstable bradycardia. Later sections of the chapter deal with specific cardiac conditions commonly encountered in the ED.

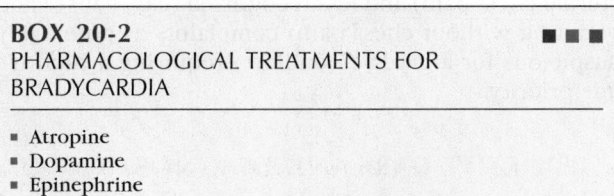

BOX 20-1   ▪ ▪ ▪
USE OF A TRANSCUTANEOUS PACEMAKER

Rate less than 60 beats/min with signs/symptoms
- Apply pacer pads to chest according to manufacturer directions.
- Connect cable to pacing unit.
- Set rate to 70 to 80 beats/min.
- Increase milliamperes until capture is achieved (consistent QRS complex after pacer spike); then add 2 mA.

BOX 20-2   ▪ ▪ ▪
PHARMACOLOGICAL TREATMENTS FOR BRADYCARDIA

- Atropine
- Dopamine
- Epinephrine

ELECTROCARDIOGRAM INTERPRETATION

ECG interpretation is another essential competency of emergency nurses. The ability to recognize acute ischemia, injury, and infarction patterns allows the ED nurse to predict and plan for likely physiological sequelae. (See Chapters 46 to 48.) Knowledge of coronary blood flow and the area of the heart supplied by each vessel also is helpful to anticipation of potential complications with acute myocardial injury.[10] The skill of the ED nurse in recognizing abnormal ECG findings, such as ST segment elevation greater than 1 mm in two or more contiguous leads, may contribute to reducing delays to definitive reperfusion therapy. Although ST segment elevation commonly has been correlated to acute injury patterns, non–ST segment elevation and non–Q-wave injury patterns also may be present. It is essential that the emergency nurse examine contiguous leads for changes and, if available, compare the current ECG to a previous ECG.

Patients with an ECG that is inconclusive or suspicious for right ventricular injury or ischemia need to have additional leads obtained from the right side. This may be limited to obtaining a fourth precordial lead ($_RV_4$) from the right side or, depending on facility protocol, obtaining a 15- or 18-lead ECG to assess for right ventricular injury patterns. It is incumbent on the ED nurse to be able to recognize accurately any abnormal ECG findings to facilitate the patient's progress in the acute care trajectory. (See Chapter 49.)

HEMODYNAMIC MONITORING

Hemodynamic monitoring may need to be considered for a patient with refractory heart failure. Placement of a pulmonary artery catheter may be necessary to manage the patient's volume status optimally. Noninvasive hemodynamic monitoring may be an alternative to placement of a pulmonary artery catheter in some facilities. Ensuring adequate oxygen delivery may be difficult because of pulmonary congestion. Bilevel or continuous positive airway pressure (BiPAP or CPAP) may be used before intubation and mechanical ventilation for patients with severe heart failure.

▪ ▪ ▪

TABLE 20-3   PHARMACOLOGICAL STRATEGIES FOR STABLE TACHYCARDIAS

NARROW COMPLEX	WIDE COMPLEX	ATRIAL RHYTHM
Adenosine	Amiodarone	Diltiazem or other
Diltiazem	Lidocaine	calcium channel
Beta blockers		blocker
Digoxin		Metoprolol or other
		beta blocker
Nonpreserved Cardiac Function		
Amiodarone	Amiodarone	Digoxin
		Diltiazem
		Amiodarone

Data from American Heart Association: *Circulation* 112(suppl):24, 2005.

RESUSCITATION

Management of a patient in cardiac arrest should follow current AHA guidelines. Factors complicating resuscitation of the patient in cardiac arrest can include trauma, chronic renal failure, and presence of assistive devices such as a ventricular assist device. Resuscitation procedures may need to be modified in these situations. For example, modifications to the standard advanced cardiac life support algorithms for chronic renal failure are aimed at correcting underlying acid-base disturbances and potassium abnormalities. The emergency nurse needs to know how to perform basic life support when a ventricular device is in place. These devices have a manual mode that can be selected if the device battery fails or resuscitation begins.

PATIENTS WITH SPECIFIC CONDITIONS
Acute Coronary Syndromes

Chest pain was the second leading reason that patients presented to the ED in 2004.[11] The emergency nurse must to be able to recognize that patients presenting to the ED with chest pain may be experiencing an acute coronary syndrome event. Patients experiencing chest pain upon arrival to the ED need general supportive care measures as described earlier in this chapter and then should receive nitroglycerin (**NTG**) if systolic blood pressure is greater than 90 mm Hg. If pain is unrelieved by NTG and there are no contraindications, administration of morphine may be considered. Recent observational data from a registry has suggested a relationship between morphine administration and poor outcomes in patients with non-ST segment elevation myocardial infarction.[12] This evidence increases the need to be judicious when considering morphine for pain relief with acute coronary events, although further, prospective research is needed and morphine should not be withheld if chest pain is present after treatment with NTG.

Caution should be used when administering NTG or morphine to the patient with ECG changes compatible with acute ischemia or injury in leads II, III, or aVF. Right ventricular injury may compromise cardiac output, and the addition of vasodilating drugs may cause significant hypotension.

The AHA[9] has established guidelines related to the diagnostic management of the patient assumed to be experiencing or at risk for an acute coronary syndrome. Serial ECG, cardiac markers, and patient history are the criteria that should be considered when deciding patient disposition. Patients should be managed as if acute coronary syndrome is present to prevent delays in reperfusion therapies. Those who have acute pain, ECG changes consistent with acute ischemia, injury or infarction need reperfusion therapy. Percutaneous coronary intervention is the gold standard in reperfusion therapy.[13] Glycoprotein IIb/IIIA inhibitors should be given to help maintain adequate coronary flow before and immediately after coronary intervention.

Many facilities do not have the ability to perform interventional angiography. If a cardiac catheterization laboratory is not available within 90 minutes, fibrinolytic therapies (e.g., alteplase, reteplase, anistreplase, or tenecteplase) should be administered. The emergency nurse needs to be familiar with the absolute and relative contraindications to fibrinolytic therapy and the need to avoid unnecessary venipuncture.

Heart Failure

The incidence of heart failure–related visits to the ED is expected to continue to rise as the overall incidence of heart failure in the general population continues to increase. The first point of care for 77 percent of heart failure patients was the ED.[14] Many heart failure patients present to ED triage with a complaint that is not linked immediately to the underlying diagnosis of heart failure. Early recognition of an exacerbation of heart failure is paramount.

Once supportive care has begun, laboratory studies need to include a serum B-natriuretic peptide level. At a cutoff point of 100 pg/ml, B-natriuretic peptide had a sensitivity of 93.1 percent, a specificity of 77.3 percent, a positive predictive value of 51.9 percent, a negative predictive value of 97.7 percent, an accuracy of 80.6 percent, a positive likelihood ratio 4.10, and a negative likelihood ratio 0.09 for the presence of heart failure.[15] Management strategies need to be directed toward optimizing cardiac performance. Diuretic therapy is essential and needs to be started as early as possible in the ED visit. Vasoactive infusions may need to be added for those who do not achieve optimal results with diuretic therapy. Management strategies for the patient with heart failure should be consistent with chronic heart failure guidelines such as those published by the AHA/American College of Cardiology.[16]

Stroke

Immediate treatment also is the goal for patients presenting to the ED with symptoms suggestive of stroke. Relatively shorter time to fibrinolysis substantially improves clinical outcome patients with acute ischemic stroke. Treatment within 3 hours of symptom onset is beneficial,[17] but even within that 3-hour window, benefit from fibrinolysis decreases as time from symptom onset increases.[18] An analysis of six large, randomized, controlled trials of intravenous fibrinolysis revealed that the optimal time for administration of fibrinolytics is within 90 minutes of stroke symptom onset.[19] See Chapter 76 for a discussion of the patient with stroke.

Cardiac Trauma

In the setting of cardiothoracic trauma (discussed in detail in Chapter 68), there may be a need to perform internal defibrillation. Although this is not typically a nursing role, the emergency nurse must be familiar with the location, use, and energy setting requirements for internal defibrillation. Table 20-4 illustrates common electrical therapy management for unstable tachycardic rhythms and pulseless arrest situations.

■■■

TABLE 20-4 ELECTRICAL THERAPY FOR RESUSCITATION

HEART RHYTHM	THERAPY
Pulse present Rate greater than 150 beats/min Hemodynamic compromise	Airway managed/supported Patent intravenous access Consider sedation Synchronized cardioversion (appropriate monophasic or biphasic energy selection for rhythm based on AHA guidelines)
Pulse absent Ventricular fibrillation Ventricular tachycardia	Basic life support measures until a monitor/defibrillator or automatic external defibrillator is present Single defibrillation (appropriate monophasic or biphasic energy selection for rhythm based on AHA guidelines) followed by 2 minutes of effective cardiopulmonary resuscitation

Data from American Heart Association: *Circulation* 112(suppl):24, 2005.

PEDIATRIC CONSIDERATIONS

Congenital cardiac conditions such as anatomical heart defects, conduction disturbances or acquired heart conditions may result in presentation of pediatric patients to the ED with cardiac-related complaints.[20] Knowledge of normal growth and development, normal pediatric vital signs, and perfusion parameters are essential to manage this population effectively. Perfusion in the pediatric patient depends more on heart rate than stroke volume. Early assessment of heart rate with appropriate interventions affects the pediatric patient's outcome. Presenting complaints may be nonspecific, such as poor feeding or an infant who "does not act right." Abnormal behavior or appetite may be the only clue the parent or child can identify. Careful attention to initial assessment, palpation of central versus distal pulses and assessment of capillary refill are essential to identify any underlying cardiac conditions.

GERIATRIC CONSIDERATIONS

Increasingly, older patients are presenting to the ED with cardiac complaints. A study conducted by the ENA demonstrated that 60 percent of the ED managers reported an increase in the number of elderly and nursing home patient visits in 2000.[21]

With the rapidly increasing number of older patients seeking care in the ED, emergency nurses must incorporate knowledge of normal geriatric changes in their assessments. (See Chapter 14.) They must be able to recognize how these changes influence usual illness patterns. Compared with younger patients, elders are more likely to present to the ED with higher acuity levels, to arrive by ambulance, to be admitted to the hospital and specifically to an intensive care unit, to have longer lengths of stay, and to require more staff time and resources.[22-24]

Older adults are more likely to present to the ED with depression, dementia, comorbid illnesses, and polypharmacy—all of which complicate the care required.[23,24] Falls or hip fractures may have resulted from acute cardiac decompensation that resulted in syncope or other physiological instability. The ED nurse needs to be vigilant in assessing the older patient for underlying cardiac conditions. Geriatric assessment may be complicated by chronic medical conditions, multiple medications, and a complicated medical history.[25]

The position of ENA[26] is that the physiological, psychological, sociological, and economic changes that occur in the geriatric population are core areas of knowledge for ED nurses. Emergency nurses should know how these changes influence assessment, interventions, teaching, discharge decisions, and community referrals.

Depression, dementia, comorbidity, polypharmacy, and inadequate assistance with activities of daily living often are unrecognized or are not assessed during the older patient's stay in the ED. Knowledge of how to recognize these changes during assessment and incorporate them into a comprehensive plan of care is necessary to provide quality care to older adults. In addition, the ED is often a point of entry into the health care system for the elderly patient, and the emergency nurse must be able to recognize those in need of assistance from the ED, the institution, the community, and their home.

REFERENCES

1. Emergency Nurses Association: *Emergency Nurses Association position statement: autonomous emergency nursing practice*, Des Plaines, Ill, 2005, The Association. Retrieved November 17, 2006,from http://www.ena.org/about/position/PDFs/3E4FD02D236147FEA22155920C859764.PDF.
2. Centers for Disease Control and Prevention: *Visits to U.S. emergency departments at all-time high; number of departments shrinking,* May 26, 2005. Retrieved November 17, 2006, from www.cdc.gov/od/oc/media/pressrel/r050526.htm
3. Berger AK, Schulman KA, Gersh BJ et al: Primary coronary angioplasty vs thrombolysis for the management of acute myocardial infarction in elderly patients, *JAMA* 282:341-348, 1999.
4. Berger PB, Ellis SG, Holmes DR Jr et al: Relationship between delay in performing direct coronary angioplasty and early clinical outcome in patients with acute myocardial infarction: results from the global use of strategies to open occluded arteries in Acute Coronary Syndromes (GUSTO-IIb) trial, *Circulation* 100:14-20, 1999.
5. Simoons ML, Serruys PW, van den Brand M et al: Early thrombolysis in acute myocardial infarction: limitation of infarct size and improved survival, *J Am Coll Cardiol* 7:717-728, 1986.
6. Rawles JM, Metcalfe MJ, Shirreffs C et al: Association of patient delay with symptoms, cardiac enzymes, and outcome in acute myocardial infarction, *Eur Heart J* 11:643-648, 1990.
7. Dracup K, Alonzo AA, Atkins JM et al: The physician's role in minimizing prehospital delay in patients at high risk for acute myocardial infarction: recommendations from the National Heart Attack Alert Program: Working Group on Educational Strategies to Prevent Prehospital Delay in Patients at High Risk for Acute Myocardial Infarction, *Ann Intern Med* 126:645-651, 1997.
8. Free MM: Cross-cultural conceptions of pain and pain control, *Proceedings of the Baylor University Medical Center* 15:143-145, 2002.
9. American Heart Association: American Heart Association guidelines for cardiopulmonary resuscitation and emergency cardiovascular care, *Circulation* 112(suppl):24, 2005.

10. Barnason S: Cardiovascular emergencies. In Newberry L, editor: *Sheehy's emergency nursing: principles and practice*, ed 5, St Louis, 2003, Mosby.

11. McCraig LF, Burt CW: *National ambulatory medical care survey: 2004 emergency department summary, advance data, 2006.* Retrieved November 17, 2006, from http://www.cdc.gov/nchs/data/ad/ad372.pdf

12. Meine TJ, Roe MT, Chen AY et al: Association of intravenous morphine use and outcomes in acute coronary syndromes: results from the CRUSADE Quality Improvement Initiative, *Am Heart J* 149:1043-1049, 2005.

13. Goldstein P, Wiel E: Management of prehospital thrombolytic therapy in ST-segment elevation acute coronary syndrome >12 hours), *Minerva Anestesiol* 71:297-302, 2005.

14. Peacock WF, Emerman CL: Emergency department management of patients with acute decompensated heart failure. *Heart Fail Rev* 9:187-193, 2004.

15. McCullough PA, Hollander JE, Nowak RM et al: Uncovering heart failure in patients with a history of pulmonary disease: rationale for the early use of B-type natriuretic peptide in the emergency department, *Acad Emerg Med* 10:198-204, 2003.

16. Hunt SA, Abraham WT, Chin MH et al: *2005 guideline for the update and diagnosis of chronic heart failure in the adult: a report of the American College of Cardiology/American Heart Association Task Force on practice guidelines.* Retrieved 11/17/06 from http://content.onlinejacc.org/cgi/reprint/46/6/e1

17. National Institute of Neurological Disorders and Stroke rt-PA Stroke Study Group: Tissue plasminogen activator for acute ischemic stroke, *N Engl J Med* 333:1581-1587, 1995.

18. Marler JR, Tilley BC, Lu M et al: Early stroke treatment associated with better outcome: the NINDS rt-PA stroke study, *Neurology* 55:1649-1655, 2000.

19. Hacke W, Donnan G, Fieschi C et al: Association of outcome with early stroke treatment: pooled analysis of ATLANTIS, ECASS, and NINDS rt-PA stroke trials, *Lancet* 363:768-774, 2004.

20. Martin SA, Morfin MR: Cardiovascular emergencies. In Thomas DO, Bernardo LM, Herman B, editors: *Core curriculum for pediatric emergency nursing,* Sudbury, Mass, 2003, Jones and Bartlett.

21. MacLean SL: *2001 ENA benchmark guide: emergency departments,* Des Plaines, Ill, 2001, Emergency Nurses Association.

22. Ross MA, Compton S, Richardson D et al: The use and effectiveness of an emergency department observation unit for elderly patients, *Ann Emerg Med* 41:668-677, 2003.

23. Richardson B: Overview of geriatric emergencies, *Mt Sinai J Med* 70:75-84, 2003.

24. Aminzadeh F, Dalziel WB: Older adults in the emergency department: a systematic review of patterns of use, adverse outcomes, and effectiveness of interventions, *Ann Emerg Med* 39:238-247, 2002.

25. Doherty KA: Cardiovascular emergencies. In Jordan KS, (editor: *Emergency nursing core curriculum*, Philadelphia, 2000, Saunders.

26. Emergency Nurses Association: *Emergency Nurses Association position statement on care of older adults in the emergency setting,* Des Plaines, Ill, 2003, The Association. Retrieved November 17, 2006, from www.ena.org/about/position/PDFs/Care-of-OlderAdults.pdf

Nurses in Intensive Care

Deborah G. Klein

CHAPTER ABBREVIATIONS

ACLS advanced cardiac life support
CPR cardiopulmonary resuscitation
ECG electrocardiogram
ICU intensive care unit

Intensive care units (**ICUs**) were established to monitor closely the sickest patients within a hospital. Since the first critical care unit opened in the 1960s, significant technological advances have occurred. Care of the critically ill patient incorporates this technology with the psychosocial state, spiritual needs, ethical issues, and the needs of family members. The American Association of Critical-Care Nurses supports the role of the critical care nurse as a patient advocate and has defined nursing competencies for critical care nursing practice (Box 21-1). Incorporated throughout these competencies are the assessment skills and knowledge required to care for the critically ill patient. This chapter focuses on some of these assessment skills used to identify, manage, and prevent complications in the critically ill cardiac patient. Detailed discussion of specific disease states and monitoring devices are discussed in other chapters.

Critical thinking skills and evidence-based practice have become increasingly important in the rapidly changing critical care environment. Critical thinking skills enable the nurse to analyze patient data, evaluate problems, and determine appropriate interventions to solve clinical issues and improve patient outcomes. Critical care nurses are encouraged to participate in clinical decision making and practice improvement activities. Unit protocols should mirror national clinical practice guidelines and standards or should be derived from new evidence obtained from randomized controlled trials. An evidence-based approach to patient care allows the nurse to confirm or challenge the way that care is provided.

INTENSIVE CARE UNIT ENVIRONMENT

The ICU is a stressful environment for the patient because of lack of privacy, artificial lighting 24 hours a day, constant noise from equipment, absence of family members, lack of sleep, difficulty communicating, and physical pain or discomfort from medical and nursing procedures. Factors that influence the response to the ICU environment include age, medications, medical history, culture, prior experiences with illness and hospitalization, family relationships, and personal beliefs about life, death, and spirituality. Assessment of each is important so that effective strategies can be implemented to

mitigate stress. Some strategies to reduce anxiety include frequent reorientation and explanation, effective pain management, provision of alternate methods of communication, dimming the lights and reducing noise levels to promote sleep, and family presence and involvement in care.

PATIENT ASSESSMENT

A thorough history includes subjective data, prior hospitalizations, allergies, and family medical history. In a critically ill cardiac patient, a history of rheumatic fever, diabetes mellitus, hypertension, asthma, renal disease, or cerebrovascular accident is significant. The presence of implantable devices such as an implantable cardioverter-defibrillator or pacemaker and previous surgeries or procedures influence the nursing care provided. Current medications (prescription and over the counter, including alternative or herbal remedies) should be identified, and the patient's understanding of these medications should be assessed if possible.

A psychosocial history, including major stress events and daily stresses, is obtained. Prior or current depression, anxiety, other psychological conditions, and coping skills may help predict the response to medical and nursing interventions. Usual exercise routine (type, amount, and frequency), daily food patterns, sleep patterns, and use of alcohol, tobacco, recreational drugs, coffee, tea, and caffeinated soda intake are important in the nursing assessment.

Physical Assessment

Before the physical assessment, determine recent and recurrent symptoms related to the current problems, including the presence or absence of fatigue, fluid reten-

---

BOX 21-1 ■ ■ ■
DESIRED COMPETENCIES OF NURSES CARING
FOR THE CRITICALLY ILL

- Clinical judgment and clinical reasoning skills
- Advocacy and moral agency in identifying and resolving ethical issues
- Caring practices that are tailored to the uniqueness of the patient and family
- Collaboration with health care team members, including family members
- Systems thinking that promotes holistic nursing care
- Response to diversity
- Clinical inquiry and innovation to promote the best clinical outcomes
- Role as patient/family educator

American Association of Critical-Care Nurses: *AACN Certification Corporation: The AACN synergy model of patient care,* Aliso Viejo, Calif, 2003, The Association.

tion, dyspnea, palpitations, and chest pain. The physical assessment encompasses all body systems, not just the cardiovascular system (Table 21-1). However, a patient whose primary problems are cardiovascular commonly exhibits alterations in circulation and oxygenation. Knowledge of normal cardiac anatomy and physiology, how it manifests in physical signs and symptoms, and how it relates the medical condition is essential. Critical care nurses need skill in assessing heart sounds (see Chapter 45), monitoring hemodynamics (Chapter 50), monitoring rhythm (Chapters 46 to 49), and managing codes. In addition, knowledge of common complications (infection, hypoxemia, bleeding, and dysrhythmias) associated with the patient's medical condition and therapies is imperative. Knowing what to report and when to report changes in the patient's condition to the physician or advanced practice nurse allows early intervention and improves outcomes (Table 21-2).

Auscultation of Heart Sounds

Auscultation of the heart is performed by placing the stethoscope over the valve, chamber, or great vessel being examined. The dominant heart sounds are made by the four heart valves as they close. The first sound, S_1, is made by closure of the mitral and tricuspid valves. S_1 is best heard at the apex (5th intercostal space, left midclavicular line) of the heart and represents the beginning of ventricular systole. The second sound, S_2, is made by the closure of the aortic and pulmonic valves. S_2 is best heard at the 2nd intercostal space at the right or left sternal border and represents the beginning of ventricular diastole. The first and second heart sounds are best heard with the diaphragm of the stethoscope with the patient lying in the supine position.

A third heart sound, S_3, can be normal in a child but usually is abnormal in an adult. The sound may be produced when the heart is overfilled or poorly compliant as with fluid overload or heart failure. The S_3 is low pitched and is best heard with the bell of the stethoscope at the 5th intercostal space at the left midclavicular line. S_3 occurs immediately after S_2.

A fourth heart sound, S_4, is produced from atrial contraction that is more forceful than normal. S_4 can be normal in elders; however, it often is heard after a myocardial infarction when the atria contract more forcefully against ventricles distended with increased blood volume. In the severely failing heart, all four heart sounds may be heard producing a "gallop" rhythm, named because it sounds like the hoof beats of a galloping horse. A gallop is best heard with the bell of the stethoscope at the 5th intercostal space at the midclavicular line.

A heart murmur, caused by turbulence of blood flow through the heart valves, usually is heard as a rumbling, blowing, harsh, or musical sound. It is important to distinguish the sound, anatomical location, loudness, and intensity of a murmur and whether extra heart sounds are heard. In adults, murmurs can be heard when a valve, usually aortic or mitral, is narrow, inflamed, stenosed, or incompetent or when the valve leaflets fail to approximate (insufficiency).

The presence of a new murmur in a patient with an acute myocardial infarction warrants special attention. A papillary muscle may have ruptured, causing the valve to approximate incorrectly. This new murmur can be indicative of severe damage and impending complications such as heart failure and pulmonary edema (see Chapters 59 and 63). Heart murmurs are graded on a scale of grade I (lowest in intensity/loudness) to VI (loudest in intensity). Table 21-3 summarizes abnormal heart sounds.

Cardiac Monitoring

The goals of cardiac monitoring have expanded from simple tracking of heart rate and basic rhythm analysis to the diagnosis of complex dysrhythmias, the detection of myocardial ischemia, and the identification of prolonged QT interval. Over the past 40 years, major improvements have occurred in cardiac monitoring systems, including computerized dysrhythmia detection

■ ■ ■

TABLE 21-1 A SYSTEMS ASSESSMENT OF THE CRITICALLY ILL CARDIAC PATIENT

SYSTEM	ASSESSMENT
Neurological	Level of consciousness, orientation, behavior (restlessness, irritability, cooperativeness), eye movements, response to tactile stimuli, type and location of pain, how pain is relieved, patient complaints
Skin	Color, temperature, dryness, turgor, presence of rashes, pressure areas, areas of skin breakdown, wounds, incision, urticaria
Cardiovascular	Blood pressure; heart rate; rhythm; presence and quality of pulses (carotid, radial, femoral, posterior tibial, dorsalis pedis); capillary refill; monitor leads in correct placement; PR interval, QRS complex, and QT interval; heart sounds (presence of rubs, gallops, or murmurs); neck vein distention; edema (sacral or dependent); hemodynamic measurements and calculations; temporary pacemaker settings; presence of implantable cardioverter-defibrillator; medications to maintain blood pressure or rhythm; laboratory results
Respiratory	Rate, quality, depth of respirations; oxygen; cough; sputum (type, color, suctioning frequency); breath sounds (crackles, rhonchi); arterial blood gases; chest tube (amount and color of drainage, amount of suction); presence of endotracheal tube or tracheostomy; ventilator settings, ventilator rate versus patient's own rate, patient's spontaneous tidal volume
Gastrointestinal	Abdominal size and softness, bowel sounds, nausea and vomiting, bowel movement, dressing and/or drainage, nasogastric tube (type and amount of drainage), feeding tube (type and amount of feedings), drains
Genitourinary	Foley or voiding; urine color, amount, and quality; vaginal or urethral drainage
Intravenous	Fluid volume, type of solution, rate/dosage of medication(s), intravenous site condition, type of intravenous devices and location
Wounds	Dry or with drainage (type, color, amount, odor), hematoma, inflamed, tender, drains, dressing changes, cultures

TABLE 21-2 POTENTIAL COMPLICATIONS OF CRITICALLY ILL CARDIAC PATIENTS

COMPLICATION	POTENTIAL CAUSE	REPORTABLE CONDITIONS
Infection	Invasive devices (tubes, drains, intravascular devices) Immunocompromise Debilitated patient condition Aspiration Prolonged immobility Wounds (traumatic, surgical, pressure ulcer) Redness, swelling, foul odor, and/or exudates from catheter insertion site or wound Decreased tissue perfusion Diabetes mellitus	Fever Redness, swelling, foul odor, and/or exudates from catheter insertion site or wound Increased or decreased white blood cell count Results of cultures (blood, urine, sputum, wound)
Hypoxemia	Low cardiac output state (hypovolemia, cardiogenic shock, cardiac tamponade) Hypoventilation (central nervous system depression, thoracic surgery, pneumothorax) Intrapulmonary shunting (pneumonia, pulmonary edema, atrial or ventricular septal defects) Ventilation/perfusion mismatch (pulmonary embolus, increased secretions, bronchospasm) Diffusion defects (thickened alveolar capillary membrane, increased fluid in interstitial space)	Dyspnea Tachypnea Tachycardia Dysrhythmias Chest pain Hypertension with increased heart rate Hypotension with decreased heart rate Anxiety, restlessness Coma Pallor Cool, dry skin Cyanosis Diaphoresis (late)
Bleeding	External and internal fluid losses (hemorrhage, third spacing sequestration) Expanding hematoma	Hypotension Tachycardia Tachypnea Oliguria Cool, pale skin Decreased hemoglobin/hematocrit Frank bleeding Anxiety, decreased level of consciousness
Dysrhythmias	Electrolyte imbalances Hypoxia Hypothermia Hyperparathyroidism Digitalis toxicity Myocardial ischemia, injury, infarction Acid-base imbalances Medications	Change in heart rate or rhythm Palpitations Syncope Hypotension Abnormal electrolyte values ST segment changes Abnormal cardiac enzymes Chest pain

TABLE 21-3 ABNORMAL HEART SOUNDS

SOUND	CAUSE	TYPICAL UNDERLYING ABNORMALITY
Accentuated S_1	Forceful closure of mitral valve	Mitral valve stenosis Tachycardia from exercise, anemia, or hyperthyroidism
Diminished S_1	Early closure of mitral valve before systole	Prolonged diastole resulting from slowed impulse conduction to or within atrioventricular node
Accentuated S_2	Forceful closure of the aortic or pulmonic valve (closes late and forceful) Stiffness of aortic or pulmonic valve, increasing the impact of closure	Elevated systemic and pulmonary pressure prolongs systole as blood pushed out of ventricles against a higher pressure Aortic valve syphilis
Diminished S_2	Gentle closure of aortic valve Gentle closure of aortic valve caused by incomplete opening	Low blood pressure in the systemic arteries reduces the pressure that pushes the valve leaflets shut Aortic stenosis
S_3 Gallop	"Thud" of blood hitting noncompliant ventricular walls at the start of ventricular filling	Myocardial damage that stiffens heart muscle and prevents relaxation during systole
S_4 Gallop	Ejection of blood into an overfilled ventricle during atrial systole	Incomplete emptying of ventricle during previous systole because of myocardial damage, aortic stenosis, hypertension and/or fluid overload
Murmurs	Turbulent blood flow at high blood pressure	Constriction or dilatation of any structure through which blood flows (valvular stenosis or incompetence, atrial or ventricular septal defect)
Rub	Friction within the pericardium from loss of pericardial fluid	Surgery, infection, inflammation, or adhesion that damages the parietal or visceral pericardium
Click	Sudden, abnormal movement of an aortic or pulmonic valve leflet	Valve prolapse (valve leaflets open backward and forward) from an increase in valve opening
Snap	Opening of a stenotic mitral or tricuspid valve	Mitral or tricuspid stenosis

Adapted from McCance KL: Structure and function of the cardiovascular and lymphatic systems. In McCance KL, Huether SE, editors: *Pathophysiology: the biological basis for disease in adults & children*, Philadelphia, 2002, Mosby.

algorithms, ST segment/ischemia monitoring software, reduced noise, multilead monitoring, and the ability to monitor 12-lead electrocardiograms (**ECGs**) with a minimal number of electrodes.[1]

Patients at significant risk of an immediate, life-threatening dysrhythmia benefit from cardiac dysrhythmia monitoring. These patients should continue on cardiac monitoring with a portable, battery-operated monitor, or monitor defibrillator if they must leave the ICU for diagnostic or therapeutic procedures (see Chapters 48 and 49).[2]

Cardiac monitoring is performed in many different patient care units in the hospital. The medical and nursing leadership in the ICU determine the competencies required to monitor patients safely based on the types of patients typically admitted. Regardless of these policies, critical care nurses should understand specific ECG abnormalities (Box 21-2) and be proficient in monitoring skills (Box 21-3).[2]

Nurses who are responsible for ECG monitoring should be trained on the monitoring system used and

---

BOX 21-2
ELECTROCARDIOGRAM ABNORMALITIES THAT CRITICAL CARE NURSES SHOULD RECOGNIZE

Sinus rhythm
Sinus bradycardia
Sinus dysrhythmia
Sinus tachycardia
Right and left bundle branch block
Aberrant ventricular conduction
Bradydysrhythmias
   Inappropriate sinus bradycardia
   Sinus node pause or arrest
   Nonconducted atrial premature beats
   Junctional dysrhythmia
   Atrioventricular blocks (first degree, second degree [Mobitz I, Mobitz II, advanced], third degree [complete heart block])
   Asystole, pulseless electrical activity
   Sinoventricular rhythm (in severe hyperkalemia)
Tachydysrhythmias (supraventricular)
   Paroxysmal supraventricular tachycardia
   Atrial fibrillation
   Atrial flutter
   Multifocal atrial tachycardia
   Atrial tachycardia with 2:1 block
   Junctional ectopic tachycardia
Ventricular dysrhythmia
   Accelerated ventricular rhythm
   Nonsustained/sustained monomorphic ventricular tachycardia
   Nonsustained/sustained polymorphic ventricular tachycardia
   Prolonged QT interval associated ventricular ectopy (torsades de pointes)
   Ventricular fibrillation
Premature complexes
   Supraventricular (atrial, junctional)
   Ventricular
Pacemaker electrocardiography
   Failure to capture
   Failure to pace (no pacer output)
   Failure to sense
   Failure to capture both ventricles in biventricular pacing
Electrocardiogram abnormalities of acute myocardial ischemia
   ST segment elevation and depression
   T wave inversion
Muscle or other artifacts simulating dysrhythmias

From Drew BJ, Califf RM, Funk M et al: *Circulation* 110:2721-2746, 2004.

BOX 21-3
ESSENTIAL ELECTROCARDIOGRAM MONITORING COMPETENCIES OF A NURSE IN CRITICAL CARE

Operation of monitoring system used in the intensive care unit (dysrhythmia, ST segment monitoring)
Recognition of limitations of computer algorithms
Proper skin preparation for applying electrodes
Accurate electrode placement for system used (e.g., reduced lead set)
Setting heart rate and ST alarm parameters appropriately
Measurement of heart rate
Measurement of intervals (use of electrocardiogram [ECG] calipers)
Recognition of atrial activity
Evaluating pauses
Diagnosis of specific rhythms
Recording of standard 12-lead ECG, landmarks for, and importance of accurate lead placement
Recording from postoperative epicardial wires (including electrical safety)
Ability to intervene (unit protocols for responding to, reporting, and documenting)
Defibrillation/cardioversion
Patient with bradycardia
Patient with tachycardia
Patient with syncope
Patient with cardiorespiratory arrest
Patient with implanted device (new or chronic)
Patient with temporary transvenous pacemaker
Patient with transcutaneous pacemaker

From Drew BJ, Califf RM, Funk M et al: *Circulation* 110:2721-2746, 2004.

---

educated about the monitoring goals specified in unit policies. Training includes didactic content and practice with return demonstrations. Demonstration of accurate electrode placement is especially important because inaccurate lead placement is common and can result in misdiagnosis. Periodic competency evaluation is required to ensure continued proficiency in the critical elements of cardiac monitoring, including electrode placement and rhythm strip interpretation.

Some ICUs use monitor watchers or technicians to observe the monitors, obtain rhythm strips, and give appropriate information to the nurse about each patient's ECG. Those observing the monitors must know the acceptable dysrhythmia patterns for each patient and should be notified of any interruptions in monitoring including changing electrodes or placing a patient on a portable monitor.

Regardless of the process used for monitor observation, certain practices are essential. If the monitor alarm sounds, the nurse evaluates the clinical status of the patient before doing anything else to determine whether the problem is an actual dysrhythmia or a malfunction of the monitoring system. An unattached ECG wire can be mistaken for asystole, and tapping of an electrode can be misinterpreted as ventricular tachycardia. Only when direct care is being provided to the patient can the alarm system safely be put on "standby" mode. This ensures that a life-threatening dysrhythmia does not go unnoticed.

Rhythm strips are documented at least every 8 hours and, if available in the monitoring system, at the onset and offset of tachydysrhythmias and bradydysrhythmias to discover clues as to the mechanism of the dysrhythmia. Documentation can be ensured by setting alarm parameters. Additional documentation may include trend reports or statements about the frequency of the dysrhythmia. Notation on the trend report of medications given is helpful. Folding or winding rolls of ECG strips into the chart is not recommended because data are lost when the chart is copied or scanned.[2]

ST segment monitoring is used to monitor cardiac ischemia (Chapter 49). Immediately after thrombolytic therapy for ST elevation acute myocardial infarction, ST segment monitoring can be used to document recovery of the ST segment elevation. Rapid ST segment recovery indicates that an infarct-related artery is patent. The goal of ST segment monitoring in a patient 48 hours after an acute myocardial infarction is to detect recurrent ischemia that may warrant further intervention. ST segment analysis software was added to cardiac monitoring systems in the mid-1980s; however, many ICUs still do not have this capability.

Unlike dysrhythmia monitoring that is activated automatically, ST segment monitoring must be activated manually. A recent study revealed that ST segment monitoring for myocardial ischemia was underused in patients with acute coronary syndromes.[3] The main reason for nonuse was "lack of physician support," followed by a high number of false ST alarms, and lack of education on how to use the technology and what to do in response to ST alarms. Strategies have been developed to improve the diagnostic accuracy of ST segment monitoring (Box 21-4).

The QT interval is an indirect measurement of ventricular repolarization (see Chapter 46). Acute increases in the QT interval are associated with an increased risk of syncope and sudden cardiac death from torsades de pointes. Clinical conditions that may cause QT interval prolongation include overdosage of QT interval-prolonging drugs, cardiac ischemia/infarction, electrolyte imbalances (severe hypokalemia or hypomagnesemia), sudden decreases in heart rate, and acute neurological events (subarachnoid hemorrhage).[2]

Nurses need to know which medications prolong ventricular repolarization (as evidenced by a prolonged QT interval) and cause torsades de pointes. Antidysrhythmic agents considered prodysrhythmic include quinidine, procainamide, disopyramide, sotalol, dofetilide, and ibutilide. Amiodarone can prolong the QT interval; however, it rarely causes torsades de pointes.[4] No guidelines exist as to how often QT intervals should be measured and what is considered a prolonged QT interval. QT interval measurement should be performed in the same lead each time.

Hemodynamic Monitoring

Hemodynamic monitoring is used in critical care to diagnose various cardiovascular disorders, to guide therapy, and to evaluate response to therapy (Chapter 50). Hemodynamic monitoring includes monitoring of intra-arterial pressures, right atrial pressures (through a triple-lumen catheter), left atrial pressures (through a left atrial catheter), and pulmonary artery pressures (through a pulmonary artery catheter). The nurse caring for a patient with hemodynamic monitoring must understand cardiopulmonary anatomy and physiology, the monitoring system components, and the concepts of preload, afterload, and contractility. Additional knowledge includes normal hemodynamic values, the rationale for therapies used to enhance cardiac output, principles of oxygen delivery and consumption, potential complications, and the ability to distinguish between physiological changes and monitoring system problems. Box 21-5 outlines the skills needed by the nurse to care competently for patients with hemodynamic monitoring.

Pulmonary artery catheters provide information on right and left ventricular function. In addition, cardiac output and pulmonary artery occlusion pressure measurements can be performed, and cardiac index, stroke volume, systemic vascular resistance, and pulmonary vascular resistance can be calculated. Box 21-6 outlines skills needed by the nurse to competently care for a patient with a pulmonary artery catheter. Knowledge of the complications associated with pulmonary artery catheters is essential.

Technology

Technology that assists in patient care in the ICU is improving rapidly. Invasive and noninvasive monitoring systems are used to facilitate patient assessment and to

---

BOX 21-4 ■ ■ ■
STRATEGIES TO IMPROVE THE QUALITY OF ST SEGMENT ISCHEMIA MONITORING

- Identification of ST segment fluctuations resulting from body position changes
- Careful skin preparation (shave hair from electrode sites, remove skin oils with alcohol and rough washcloth)
- Consistent lead placement
- ST alarm parameters individualized to patient's baseline ST level
- Understanding the goals of ST segment monitoring in the individual patient
- Analysis of electrocardiogram printout rather than graphic trends

From Drew BJ, Califf RM, Funk M et al: *Circulation* 110:2721-2746, 2004.

BOX 21-5 ■ ■ ■
ESSENTIAL HEMODYNAMIC MONITORING COMPETENCIES OF A NURSE IN CRITICAL CARE

- Knowledge of equipment (transducer, monitor, flush system)
- Correct "leveling" of the transducer at the phlebostatic axis
- Performance of zero referencing
- Performance of square wave test (dynamic response testing)
- Recognition of appropriate and inappropriate waveforms for pressures monitored (arterial, central venous, left atrial, pulmonary artery, pulmonary artery occlusion)
- Troubleshooting of equipment
- Knowledge of complications
- Assistance with insertion of hemodynamic monitoring catheters
- Articulation and performance of appropriate nursing care for patients with hemodynamic monitoring catheters
- Knowledge of factors that alter hemodynamic monitoring pressures
- Setting alarm parameters appropriately

BOX 21-6
ESSENTIAL SKILLS NEEDED TO CARE FOR A PATIENT WITH A PULMONARY ARTERY CATHETER

- Knowledge of the type of pulmonary artery (PA) catheter present (four lumen, five lumen with venous infusion port, seven lumen with one lumen for continuous cardiac output measurement and one lumen for continuous mixed venous oxygen saturation monitoring)
- Interpretation of right atrial, right ventricular, pulmonary artery, and pulmonary artery occlusive pressure (PAOP) waveforms
- Recognition of abnormal waveforms
- Correct performance of PAOP measurement
- Correct performance of cardiac output measurements and interpretation of cardiac output curves
- Correct calculation of cardiac values
- Knowledge of complications associated with PA catheter (pneumothorax, infection, ventricular dysrhythmias, PA rupture or perforation)
- Knowledge of complications associated with PAOP and cardiac output measurement
- Recognition of problems and implementation of troubleshooting strategies associated with PA catheter pressure monitoring
- Setting alarm parameters appropriately
- Interpretation of hemodynamic monitoring data in relation to patient clinical presentation

evaluate responses to treatment. Laboratory testing performed at the bedside provides immediate values to expedite treatment. Hospitals are implementing computerized records that include physician orders, medication administration records, laboratory results, and ICU flow sheets. As ICUs expand their services, nurses must maintain their cutting edge knowledge of medical conditions and become knowledgeable about new treatments. They must be competent in therapies requiring new equipment, such as intraaortic balloon pump therapy, continuous renal replacement therapy, ventricular assist devices, and extracorporeal membrane oxygenation (Figure 21-1). Comfort in applying technology, troubleshooting devices, and evaluating the accuracy of values is essential; however, critical care nursing is not a lone endeavor, and resources must be in place 24 hours a day for nurses to ensure patient safety.

Code Management

Prompt recognition of cardiac or respiratory arrest and rapid initiation of cardiopulmonary resuscitation (**CPR**) and advanced cardiac life support (**ACLS**) measures are essential to achieve the best patient outcome. All nurses working in an ICU need basic cardiac life support training, including expertise in operating an automatic external defibrillator. Competence is needed in setting up and operating a defibrillator with or without transcutaneous pacing capability. ACLS provider training is available through the American Heart Association and is strongly recommended for the nurse working in an ICU.[5]

The first person to recognize a cardiac or respiratory arrest or code calls for help and begins life support measures. Another team member immediately brings the crash or code cart to the bedside. Crash carts vary in organizational layout; however, they should contain the same basic emergency equipment and medications as outlined by the American Heart Association *ACLS Provider Manual.* Many hospitals have standardized crash carts (Figure 21-2), so any one responding to a code is familiar with the location of the items on the cart. In other hospitals the content and organization of the crash cart are unique to each unit. Whether the carts are standardized or unique to an individual unit, nurses responding to codes must be familiar with the content and how to use each piece of equipment, including the defibrillator and transcutaneous cardiac pacemaker. The ICU nurse must know the ACLS algorithms for the assessment and management of ventricular fibrillation, pulseless ven-

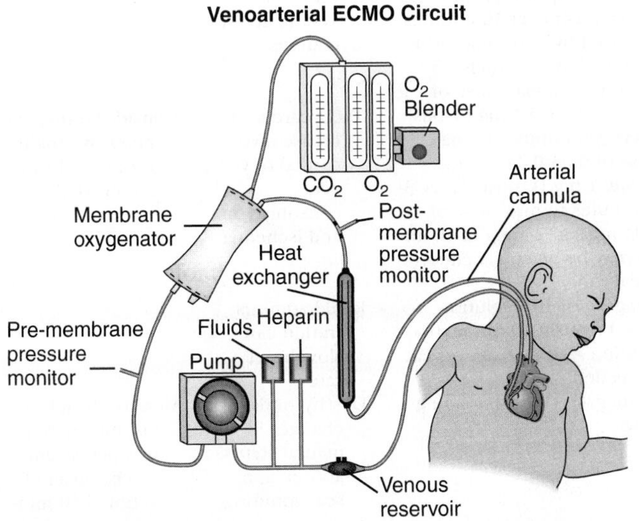

Venoarterial ECMO Circuit
O2 Blender
CO2 O2
Arterial cannula
Membrane oxygenator
Post-membrane pressure monitor
Heat exchanger
Heparin
Pre-membrane pressure monitor
Fluids
Pump
Venous reservoir

FIGURE 21-1 Schematic of extracorporeal membrane oxygenation (ECMO).

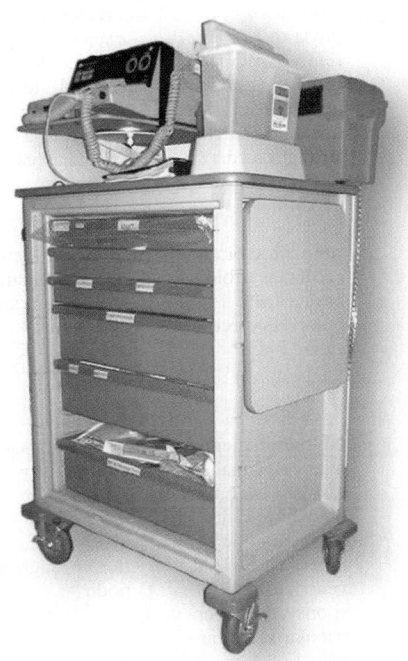

FIGURE 21-2 A crash cart.

tricular tachycardia, pulseless electrical activity, asystole, bradycardias, tachycardias (including electrical cardioversion), acute pulmonary edema, hypotension and shock, acute myocardial infarction, and acute stroke.[6] Medications used in a cardiac arrest and medications frequently used in the ICU are outlined in Table 21-4. Adequacy of resuscitation attempts in hospital settings has been evaluated and found to need improvement.[7,8] (See the Evidence-Based Practice feature.)

Each patient's code status must be known by the nurses caring for the patient. The Patient Self-Determination Act of 1991 recognizes the right of an individual to make decisions about his or her medical care, including the end of life. The patient may have a living will that documents wishes and provides instructions to family members, physicians, and other health care providers. An advanced directive may be prepared based on the patient's living will. Physicians and families should talk with the patient about preferences regarding CPR and life support issues. Frequently, critically ill patients are too ill to participate in decision making. The health care team should determine from the family if the patient has an advanced directive

■ EVIDENCE-BASED PRACTICE

QUALITY OF CARDIOPULMONARY RESUSCITATION

In two studies aimed at evaluating the quality of in-hospital cardiopulmonary resuscitation (CPR), Abella and colleagues[1,2] measured in-hospital chest compression rates and compliance with published international guidelines. Data from 97 cardiac arrests were analyzed with an innovative handheld recording device developed by the investigators to measure chest compression rate as a surrogate for CPR quality. Results revealed that in more than one-third of the segments evaluated, compression rates were inadequate (fewer than 80 compressions per minute), and 21.7 percent had rates of fewer than 70 compressions per minute. Compression depth was too shallow (defined as less than 38 mm) for more than one-third of compressions. Poor quality of CPR was related to poor outcomes.

References
1. Abella BS, Alvarado JP, Myklebust H et al: Quality of cardiopulmonary resuscitation during in-hospital cardiac arrest, *JAMA* 293:305-310, 2005.
2. Abella BS, Sandbo N, Vassilatos P et al: Chest compression rates during cardiopulmonary resuscitation are suboptimal: a prospective study during in-hospital cardiac arrest, *Circulation* 111:428-434, 2005.

■ ■ ■

TABLE 21-4　MEDICATIONS USED OFTEN IN THE INTENSIVE CARE UNIT

MEDICATION	INDICATION	MECHANISM OF ACTION	DOSAGE/ROUTE	SIDE EFFECTS	NURSING IMPLICATIONS
Adenosine (Adenocard)	Initial drug of choice for supraventricular dysrhythmias	Slows conduction in atrioventricular (AV) node and interrupts AV nodal reentry circuits	6 mg IV bolus over 1-3 seconds followed by 20 ml rapid flush; if no response in 1-2 minutes, give 12 mg repeat dose and flush; may repeat 12 mg dose if necessary	Headache, transient flushing, dyspnea, and chest pain; may cause asystole up to 15 seconds	Half-life 10 seconds; higher dose needed with theophylline, lower dose needed with dipyridamole or after cardiac transplantation
Amiodarone (Cordarone)	Treatment and prophylaxis of recurrent ventricular fibrillation and hemodynamically unstable ventricular tachycardia; rapid atrial dysrhythmias	Decreases membrane excitability, prolongs action potential to terminate ventricular tachycardia or ventricular fibrillation	*Cardiac arrest:* 300 mg diluted in 20-30 ml NS or D_5W IV push followed by 150 mg in 3-5 minutes (max dose 2.2 g/24 hr) *Nonarrest, rapid infusion:* 150 mg IV push over 10 minutes followed by 1 mg/min infusion for 6 hours, then 0.5 mg/min to a max dose of 2 g	Bradycardia, hypotension; use with caution with preexisting conduction system abnormalities	Monitor for symptomatic sinus bradycardia, PR interval prolongation
Atropine	Symptomatic bradycardia, asystole, bradycardic pulseless electrical activity	Increases sinoatrial node automaticity and AV conduction activity	*Bradycardia:* 0.5-1 mg IV push every 3-5 minutes to max dose of 0.03-0.04 mg/kg *Asystole:* 1 mg IV push every 3-5 minutes to max dose of 0.04 mg/kg; 2-3 mg in 10 ml NS may be given via endotracheal tube	Tachycardia, increase myocardial oxygen consumption and ischemia	Consider transcutaneous pacing if repeated doses are needed
Calcium chloride	Acute hyperkalemia, hypocalcemia, calcium channel blocker toxicity	Increases myocardial contractility	8-16 mg/kg of 10% solution slow IV push; 10 ml of 10% solution = 10 mg/ml; repeat as needed	Rapid administration can slow heart rate	
Digitalis (digoxin)	Atrial fibrillation or flutter with rapid ventricular response, supraventricular tachycardia	Decreases conduction through AV node	10-15 mcg/kg IV push loading dose	Dysrhythmias, changes in mental status, anorexia, nausea, vomiting	Monitor drug levels; ensure normal potassium levels; onset of action 5-30 minutes, peak 1½-3 hours

MEDICATION	INDICATION	MECHANISM OF ACTION	DOSAGE/ROUTE	SIDE EFFECTS	NURSING IMPLICATIONS
Diltiazem (Cardizem)	Reentrant supraventricular tachycardias, atrial fibrillation and flutter with rapid ventricular response	Calcium channel blocker that slows conduction and prolongs refractoriness in the AV node	0.25 mg/kg over 2 minutes for rapid atrial fibrillation/flutter; repeat in 15 minutes at 0.35 mg/kg if needed; maintenance infusion of 5-15 mg/hr titrated to heart rate	Myocardial depression	Use with caution with left ventricular failure
Dobutamine (Dobutrex)	Depressed cardiac contractility	Inotropic agent with beta-stimulating activity; increases cardiac output by improving stroke volume with minimum increases in heart rate, blood pressure (BP), and dysrhythmias	Continuous IV infusion 0.5-1 mcg/kg/min initially and titrated to 2.5-15 mcg/kg/min for desired response	Myocardial ischemia, chest pain, hypertension, tachycardia	Use extreme caution in myocardial infarction; correct hypovolemia and acidosis before initiating; dilution 250-1000 mg/250 ml D_5W
Dopamine (Intropin)	Hypotension not related to hypovolemia	*Moderate doses* (5-10 mcg/kg/min): increases contractility and cardiac output *High doses* (10-20 mcg/kg/min): causes vasoconstriction and increases systemic vascular resistance	Continuous IV infusion 2-5 mcg/kg/min initially and titrated as needed	Tachycardia, dysrhythmias	Extravasation may cause necrosis and sloughing; dilution 400-800 mg/250 ml D_5W = 1600-3200 mcg/ml
Epinephrine (Adrenalin)	Ventricular fibrillation, pulseless ventricular tachycardia, pulseless electrical activity, asystole	Increases contractility, automaticity, systemic vascular resistance, and arterial BP; vasoconstriction improves coronary and cerebral perfusion	1 mg IV push or 2-5 mg in 10 ml via endotracheal tube; may repeat every 3-5 minutes		In cardiac arrest, may be used as a continuous infusion for hypotension; dilution 1 mg/250 ml NS; infuse at 1-5 mcg/min and titrate as needed
Esmolol (Brevibloc)	Supraventricular tachycardia	Beta₁-selective adrenergic blocker with antidysrhythmic effects; decreases heart rate and BP	500 mcg/kg/min IV loading dose over 1 minute, then 50 mcg/kg/min infusion for 4 minutes; repeat loading dose every 5 minutes and increase infusion by 50 mcg/kg/min until desired therapeutic effect or max dose of 200 mcg/kg/min	Hypotension, heart block	Use with extreme caution in patients with asthma, diabetes, or impaired renal function; dilution 2.5 g/250 ml D_5W = 10 mg/ml
Isoproterenol (Isuprel)	Symptomatic bradycardia in cardiac transplantation patients or if external pacing not available	Beta-agonist increases contractility and heart rate Greatly increases myocardial oxygen demand	Continuous IV infusion at 2 mcg/min, titrated to maintain heart rate of 60 beats/min; dilution 1 mg in 250 ml D_5W = 4 mcg/ml (range 2-10 mcg/min)	Myocardial ischemia, ventricular dysrhythmias	Monitor for myocardial ischemia
Lidocaine (Xylocaine)	Ventricular fibrillation, ventricular tachycardia, premature ventricular complexes	Suppresses ventricular dysrhythmias Raises fibrillation threshold	*Ventricular fibrillation:* 1-1.5 mg/kg IV push followed by 0.5-0.75 mg/kg every 5-10 minutes to max dose of 3 mg/kg; may be given by endotracheal tube at a dose of 2-4 mg/kg; followed by continuous infusion at 2-4 mg/min	Neurological toxicity if drug level excessive	Lower dose if impaired hepatic blood flow; dilution 1 g/250 ml or 2 g/500 ml = 4 mg/ml
Magnesium	Torsades de pointes, hypomagnesemia Decreases post-infarction dysrhythmias	Essential for enzyme reactions and sodium-potassium pump	*Cardiac arrest:* 1-2 g/100 ml D_5W over 1-2 minutes *Nonarrest:* 1-2 g/100 mL D_5W over 5-60 minutes followed by infusion of 0.5-1 g/hr and titrate to control torsades de pointes	Flushing, bradycardia, hypotension, cardiac and central nervous system depression leading to respiratory collapse	Monitor serum levels and respiratory status

Continued

■ ■ ■

TABLE 21-4   MEDICATIONS USED OFTEN IN THE INTENSIVE CARE UNIT—cont'd

MEDICATION	INDICATION	MECHANISM OF ACTION	DOSAGE/ROUTE	SIDE EFFECTS	NURSING IMPLICATIONS
Milrinone (Primacor)	Cardiogenic shock or heart failure	Phosphodiesterase inhibitor with inotropic and vasodilatory effects	Loading dose 50 mcg/kg IV over 10 minutes followed by infusion of 0.375-0.75 mcg/kg/min; dilution: 20-40 mg/100 ml D_5W	Hypotension, dysrhythmias, myocardial ischemia	Reduced dose required in renal impairment
Nitroglycerin	Hypertension, unstable angina	Arterial and venous vasodilator. Decreases myocardial oxygen consumption, preload, and afterload	*Hypertension:* 5 mcg/min IV initially and increase by 5 mcg/min every 3-5 minutes until BP response. *Unstable angina:* 10-20 mcg/min IV initially and increase by 5-10 mcg/min every 5-10 minutes or until desired hemodynamic response	Headache, hypotension	Mix in glass bottles and use non-polyvinyl chloride tubing to reduce drug loss by adsorption into plastics; dilution: 50 mg/250 ml D_5W = 0.4 mg/ml
Nitroprusside, sodium (Nipride)	Hypertensive emergencies, cardiogenic shock, heart failure, acute pulmonary edema	Peripheral vasodilatation of smooth muscle of blood vessels	0.1 mcg/kg/min IV initially and titrate to desired effect (0.5-10 mcg/kg/min)	Hypotension, cyanide toxicity, headache, methemoglobinemia	Dilution: 50-100 mg/250 ml D_5W
Norepinephrine (Levophed)	Hypotension uncorrected by other medications	Alpha and beta agonist. Causes arterial and venous vasoconstriction. Some increases in myocardial contractility	Continuous IV infusion at 0.5-1 mcg/min, titrated upward as needed to max dose of 30 mcg/min. Dilution: 4 mg/250 ml D_5W	Myocardial ischemia	Administer through central line, if possible; extravasation may cause necrosis and sloughing
Procainamide (Pronestyl)	Premature ventricular complexes, ventricular tachycardia uncontrolled by lidocaine, supraventricular tachycardia	Decreases automaticity of ectopic pacemakers. Slows intraventricular conduction	Administer 20 mg/min until dysrhythmia is suppressed, hypotension occurs, the QRS complex widens by greater than 50% of original width or 17 mg/kg has been administered, followed by a continuous infusion of 1-4 mg/min	Hypotension, heart block	Do not exceed recommended infusion dose; dilution 1 g
Sodium bicarbonate	Metabolic acidosis in cardiopulmonary arrest uncorrected by defibrillation, correct cardiopulmonary resuscitation technique, oxygenation, and other medications	Counteracts metabolic acidosis by binding with hydrogen ions to produce water and carbon dioxide	1 mEq/kg IV push initially, may repeat 0.5 mEq/kg every 10 minutes as needed; administration dictated by arterial blood gas results		Ensure adequate cardiopulmonary resuscitation, oxygenation, and ventilation
Vasopressin (Pitressin)	Alternative pressor to epinephrine in ventricular fibrillation, diabetes insipidus, hemodynamic support in vasodilatory shock (septic shock)	Nonadrenergic. Peripheral vasoconstriction. Diuretic	*Cardiac arrest:* 40 units IV push (one dose only). *Septic shock:* 0.01-0.1 units/min (not titrated); dilution 60 units/250 ml D_5W	Hypertension, cardiac ischemia, dysrhythmias, angina, bradycardia, hyponatremia	May also be useful in asystole and pulseless electrical activity, but not yet validated
Verapamil (Calan, Isoptin)	Supraventricular tachycardia unresponsive to adenosine that does require cardioversion	Calcium channel blocker. Decreases myocardial contractility. Slows AN nodal conduction. Vasodilates smooth muscle	Initially 2.5-5 mg IV push over 1-2 minutes; repeat dose at 5-10 mg if needed in 15-30 minutes or 5 mg every 15 minutes to a max dose of 30 mg	Hypotension, myocardial depression, bradycardia	Contraindicated in left ventricular failure; beta blockers have synergistic effect; use with caution in Wolff-Parkinson-White syndrome, atrial fibrillation, and atrial flutter

and, if he or she does not, whether the patient would want to be resuscitated in the event of a cardiac arrest.

Many states have implemented "no CPR" options. The patient, who usually has a terminal illness, signs a document requesting "no CPR" if there is a loss of pulse or if breathing stops. In some states, this document directs the patient to wear a "no CPR" identification bracelet. In the event of a code, the bracelet alerts the responders that CPR efforts are prohibited. The health care team must respect the patient's wishes.

In the past, family members were not allowed to be present at the bedside during a code or resuscitation. However, research now supports the benefits of family presence during a code. Families who have been present during a code describe the benefits as knowing that everything possible was being done for their loved one, feeling supportive and helpful to the patient and staff, sustaining patient-family relationships, providing a sense of closure on a life shared together, and facilitating the grief process.[9-11]

Decisions regarding family presence are made on an individual basis, considering individual preferences and assessment of coping mechanisms.[11,12] If family members are not in the patient's room during the code, a staff member, chaplain, volunteer, or friend should remain with them and keep them informed of the patient's progress. If the family is not in the hospital during the code, the next of kin should be called as soon as possible and informed of the patient's critical status.

If the patient is resuscitated successfully, the family is allowed to see the patient as soon as is feasible. Communication of events and the status of the patient are important. If the patient does not survive, the family should be encouraged to see the patient if they were not present during the code because this may facilitate the grief process.

CONCLUSION

ICUs were established to monitor closely the sickest patients within the hospital. Nurses are specifically educated and trained in critical care nursing care for these extremely vulnerable patients. Knowledge of basic sciences, disease processes, technological advances, and pharmacology is essential to ensure safety and the best patient outcomes.

REFERENCES

1. Drew BJ, Pelter MM, Brodnick DE et al: Comparison of a new reduced lead set ECG with the standard ECG for diagnosing cardiac arrhythmias and myocardial ischemia, *J Electrocardiol* 35: S13-S21, 2002.
2. Drew BJ, Califf RM, Funk M et al: Practice standards for electrocardiographic monitoring in hospital settings: an American Heart Association scientific statement from the Councils on Cardiovascular Nursing, Clinical Cardiology, and Cardiovascular Disease in the Young—endorsed by the International Society of Computerized Electrocardiology and the American Association of Critical-Care Nurses, *Circulation* 110:2721-2746, 2004.
3. Patton JA, Funk M: Survey on the use of ST-segment monitoring in patients with acute coronary syndromes, *Am J Crit Care* 10:23-34, 2001.
4. Malik M, Camm AJ: Evaluation of drug-induced QT interval prolongation: implications for drug approval and labeling, *Drug Saf* 24:323-351, 2001.
5. Klein D: Code management. In Sole ML, Klein D, Moseley M, editors: *Introduction to critical care nursing,* ed 4, Philadelphia, 2005, Elsevier Saunders.
6. American Heart Association: *ACLS provider manual,* Dallas, 2001, The Association.
7. Abella BS, Alvarado JP, Myklebust H et al: Quality of cardiopulmonary resuscitation during in-hospital cardiac arrest, *JAMA* 293:305-310, 2005.
8. Abella BS, Sandbo N, Vassilatos P et al: Chest compression rates during cardiopulmonary resuscitation are suboptimal: a prospective study during in-hospital cardiac arrest, *Circulation* 111: 428-434, 2005.
9. Meyers TA, Eichhorn DJ, Guzzetta CE et al: Family presence during invasive procedures and resuscitation: the experience of family members, nurses, and physicians, *Am J Nurs* 100:32-42, 2000.
10. MacLean SL, Guzzetta CE, White C et al: Family presence during cardiopulmonary resuscitation and invasive procedures: practice of critical care and emergency nurses, *Am J Crit Care* 12:246-257, 2003.
11. Emergency Nurses Association: *Family presence at the bedside during invasive procedures and/or resuscitation,* Des Plaines, Ill, 2001, The Association.
12. Tucker TL: Family presence during resuscitation, *Crit Care Nurs Clin North Am* 14:177-185, 2002.

chapter 22

Nurses in Progressive Care Units

Tanna Thomason

CHAPTER ABBREVIATIONS

AMI acute myocardial infarction

CABG coronary artery bypass grafting

HF heart failure

GWTG Get with the Guidelines

PCCN progressive care certified nurse

PCI percutaneous coronary intervention

PCU progressive care unit

Adult cardiac progressive care units (**PCU**) cover a wide range of patient populations and care demands. Patients in these units require close monitoring for potential physiological instability and rapid status changes. The PCU patient typically requires continuous cardiac monitoring and has a complex treatment plan. Many require technical support with specialized therapy and equipment, invasive monitoring, and possibly mechanical ventilation.

PCUs typically range in size from a few beds to 80 or more beds. Over the past decade, many hospitals have seen growth in the number of beds allocated to the PCU. Select patients are spending less time in the intensive care unit and more time in PCU.[1-3] These units have many different names, including telemetry units, stepdown units, direct observation units, and intermediate care units. Throughout this chapter, PCU is used to refer to all types of cardiac telemetry nursing care units.

The scope of telemetry nursing knowledge, skill, and expertise ranges from specialized to broad. For example, some PCUs provide care for a specific patient population (e.g., heart failure unit), whereas other units have a larger variety of patients including those with multiple diagnoses and multisystem diseases. Most PCU nurses care for three to five patients each shift. Common cardiac diagnoses including coronary artery bypass grafting (**CABG**) surgery, valve replacement surgery, newly diagnosed acute myocardial infarction (**AMI**), pacemaker and implantable cardiac defibrillator insertions, all stages of heart failure including those requiring support from mechanical ventricular assist devices, and patients who undergo percutaneous coronary interventions (**PCIs**) such as coronary angioplasty and intracoronary stent insertion. These complex cardiac patients have the potential for major complications and readmission to the intensive care unit. The PCU nurse uses refined assessment and critical thinking skills for prevention and early identification of complications.

The American Association of Critical-Care Nurses has developed a certification examination for the progressive care certified nurse (**PCCN**) defined as a nurse who delivers care to patients who "are moderately stable with less complexity, require moderate resources and intermittent nursing vigilance or are stable with a high potential for becoming unstable and require increased intensity of care and vigilance."[4] Progressive care nurses who meet the eligibility criteria and pass the written examination can become PCCNs. According to the American Association of Critical-Care Nurses, the PCCN certification denotes to the public those practitioners who possess a distinct and clearly defined body of knowledge called progressive care nursing.

This chapter focuses on two major nurse competencies that are essential to providing evidenced-based nursing care to hospitalized PCU patients. The primary competency is the identification and prevention of complications. The second but equally important competency is the preparation of patients for their transition to the next level of care or home.

IDENTIFYING AND PREVENTING COMPLICATIONS

Few PCU patients have invasive hemodynamic central line monitors, making assessments of preload, afterload, and cardiac contractility challenging. An accurate assessment of blood pressure, heart sounds, volume status using jugular venous distention, and the electrocardiogram are paramount in the skill set of the PCU nurse.

Blood Pressure

On initial examination, blood pressure should be recorded in both arms. Subsequently, the arm with the higher blood pressure should be used and documented. Avoid using the arm with an arteriovenous shunt or fistula and the arm on the affected side after mastectomy. Ensure that the cuff size is appropriate; the lower margin of the cuff should be 2.5 cm above the antecubital space. (See Chapter 45 for the proper procedure for taking blood pressure.)

Assessing Hypotension

Postural (orthostatic) hypotension, an abnormal drop in blood pressure that occurs as the patient changes from a supine to a standing position, is relatively common in PCU patients who have been on bed rest. Signs and symptoms include a 20-mm Hg decrease in systolic blood pressure or a 10-mm Hg decrease in diastolic pressure within 3 minutes of standing.[5] Additional symptoms include weakness, dizziness, and syncope. Postural changes in blood pressure should be measured in patients older than age 65, diabetic patients, those receiving antihypertensive therapy, and anyone complaining of dizziness or syncopy.[6]

A structured history and measurement of blood pressure and heart rate in supine and upright position are necessary for diagnosis of orthostatus hypotension. When assessing for potential postural hypotension, begin by measuring blood pressure and heart rate in the supine position. The normal postural response is a transiently increased heart rate of 5 to 20 beats/min, a drop in systolic pressure of less than 10 mm Hg, and an increase in diastolic pressure of approximately 5 mm Hg.[5] Besides bedrest, a common cause of postural hypotension is intravascular volume depletion, common with aggressive diuretic therapy, inadequate intake, or intravascular to extravascular fluid shifts.[6] Pharmacological agents commonly also cause hypotension. If orthostatic hypotension is found to be chronic and related to a secondary autonomic disorder,[7] the management consists initially of education, with advice and training on various factors that influence blood pressure such as leg crossing, squatting, elastic abdominal binders and stockings, and exercise.[7] If acute, management involves addressing the cause (prolonged bedrest or volume depletion).

The PCU nurse frequently administers antihypertensive agents, calcium channel blockers, angiotensin-converting enzyme inhibitors (ACE), angiotensin II receptor blockers (ARB), and nitrates. Many PCU patients with polypharmacy and underlying left ventricular dysfunction have a baseline systolic blood pressure reading in the 80- to 90-mm Hg range. Routinely, the PCU nurse faces challenges regarding which medications to administer, which to hold, and when to call the primary provider for further discussion. The PCU nurse must be knowledgeable about the pharmacological properties (onset, peak effects, and untoward effects) of each medication type, along with synergistic effects of potential drug-drug interactions. Obtaining drug administration "parameters" from the physician is helpful, but not a substitute for a solid pharmacological knowledge base.

Physical Assessment

Physical assessment skills and knowledge of normal and abnormal heart sounds are essential for nurses working in PCU. See Chapter 45 for a review of heart sound assessment. The PCU nurse may be the first to detect a new S_3 or S_4 heart sound. This new assessment finding would alert the nurse to hemodynamic changes reflecting a decline in ventricular compliance or an increase in ventricular volume. In AMI the auscultation of a new systolic murmur over the 5th intercostal space and mid-clavicular line (mitral valve area) could reflect a newly ruptured papillary muscle; late clinical complications may be associated with the development of new abnormal heart sounds. When study results (e.g., echocardiogram) are available, correlate the diagnostic findings to the heart sound assessment findings. Discuss any new findings with the primary provider, and collaborate to identify the optimal treatment plan.

The normal jugular venous pressure should not exceed 9 cm. H_2O.[8] A higher jugular venous pressure may help to explain other assessment findings such as shortness of breath or auscultation of rales. If an elevated jugular venous pressure appears acutely, collaborate

with the provider to reduce the volume/pressure to prevent worsening of myocardial hemodynamic function.

Electrocardiogram Monitoring

Telemetry monitoring is used widely in hospitals; the importance of being able to monitor, interpret, and treat dysrhythmias has been universally accepted. The PCU nurse must be competent in the recognition and collaborative treatment of advanced dysrhythmias commonly seen in the PCU setting (see Chapters 46-48). Computer algorithms assist early detection; however, the critical thinking of accurate skin electrode preparation, appropriate lead placement, and customized lead selection remain essential PCU nurse skills. See Chapter 49 for a thorough discussion of ST segment monitoring.

Patients with heart failure and AMI are at risk of developing complex ectopy, bundle branch block, and wide complex tachycardias. Although lead II has been a longtime favorite for assessing atrial ectopy and heart blocks, leads V_1 and V_6 are most helpful in diagnosing bundle branch blocks or wide complex tachycardias.[9]

Figure 22-1 shows the correct electrode placement for a standard five-lead cable commonly used in PCU. This type of telemetry system allows for the recording of all limb leads (I, II, III, aV_R, aV_L and aV_F) along with additional monitoring of one precordial or "V" lead. To monitor in a V_1 lead, the "C" electrode must be at the 4th intercostal space, along the right sternal border. Patients commonly are found to have incorrect electrode placement. Correct electrode location should be verified on each shift with the initial head-to-toe assessment of the patient.

Continuous 12-lead electrocardiogram ST segment monitoring has been shown to detect transient myocardial ischemia effectively in PCU patients with AMI, un-

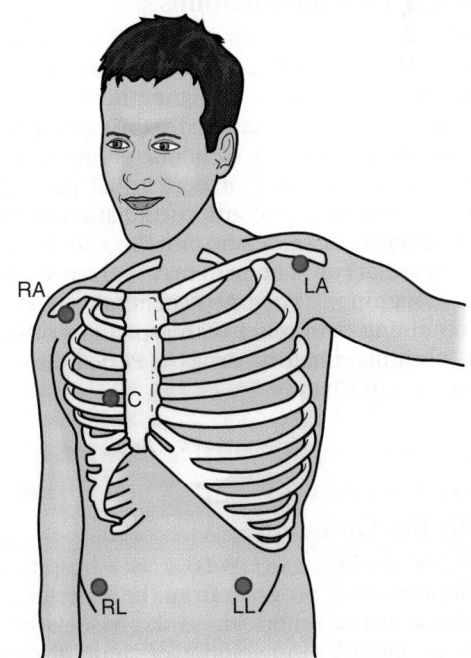

FIGURE 22-1 ■ Standard electrode placement for five-lead electrocardiogram monitoring. *C,* Chest; *LA,* left arm; *LL,* left leg; *RA,* right arm; *RL,* right leg.

stable angina, and coronary artery disease. These patients are more likely to receive an intervention (e.g., PCI) and experience fewer adverse in-hospital events.[10]

Activity Progression

The PCU nurse facilitates activity progression while critically evaluating the balance between myocardial oxygen consumption and demand. The benefits of exercise begin in the hospital recovery phase and continue for years to follow. Studies demonstrate that an early and consistent progression of activity decreases hospital length of stay in the cardiac surgical patient population and continues to show benefits up to 5 years following CABG.[11]

With technological advances in femoral artery closure devices, time spent in bed has been reduced safely in post-PCI patients from the traditional 6 hours to 1 or 2 hours. Early ambulation in these patients also has reduced back pain.[12] The PCU nurse must stay alert to hemodynamic tolerance, femoral vessel hemostasis, and signs and symptoms of potential coronary artery vessel closure during early mobilization.

For AMI patients who are hemodynamically stable, prolonged bed rest is unnecessary and is contraindicated. The physiological consequences of bed rest and inactivity include reductions in plasma volume, which reduces cardiac filling, stroke volume, and cardiac output. Skeletal muscle fiber size, diameter, and capillarity are reduced, as is bone density. These changes reduce physical work capacity.[13] To prevent deconditioning from prolonged bed rest, low-level activities such as toileting, assisted bathing, and light ambulation are encouraged.

Detecting Late Complications

Pericarditis may appear days to several weeks after an AMI. Patients with pericarditis have larger infarcts, lower ejection fractions, and a higher incidence of heart failure.[14] Differentiation between pain caused by pericarditis and that caused by ischemia is important. Distinguishing characteristics of pericardial pain include pleuritic or positional discomfort; radiation to the left shoulder, scapula, or trapezius muscle; and association with a pericardial rub. The pain may worsen with inspiration or coughing.[15] Treatment generally is centered around obtaining pain relief with aspirin or other non-steroidal antiinflammatory drugs.[14] Pericarditis is discussed further in Chapter 75.

FACILITATING PATIENT DISCHARGE FROM THE HOSPITAL
Get with the Guidelines

Get with the Guidelines (**GWTG**)[16] is a hospital-based quality improvement program from the American Heart Association and the American Stroke Association. The program is intended to empower multidisciplinary health care provider teams to treat patients in a manner consistent with the most updated treatment guidelines.

> ### ■ EVIDENCE-BASED PRACTICE
> #### GET WITH THE GUIDELINES
>
> Early results of the Get with the Guidelines program are now available in abstract form. At the 2004 Scientific Sessions, LaBresh and colleagues[21] presented evidence that improvements in quality of care can be sustained over time. Data from 92 hospitals and 59,788 patients (30 consecutive records per participating hospital) were analyzed. Data on 12 quality measures collected quarterly over a 2-year period showed significant progressive improvements in five measures and sustained improvements in another four measures over each of the eight quarters studied.
>
> The largest improvements were seen in early aspirin use, beta blocker use early in hospitalization and upon discharge, and counseling for smoking cessation, weight management, and exercise or cardiac rehabilitation referral. Nurses can take much of the credit for these improvements in counseling because they are the providers who routinely counsel patients about these topics. Aspirin use at discharge did not change. These early results suggest that hospitals participating in the Get with the Guidelines program can improve the quality of care provided to coronary artery disease patients, and they can sustain those improvements over at least a 2-year period.

GWTG is expected to save up to 80,000 lives annually by closing potential treatment gaps in cardiovascular disease and stroke patients.

GWTG-Coronary Artery Disease, an acute care program, focuses on care team protocols to ensure that patients with coronary artery disease are treated and discharged on appropriate medications and with risk modification counseling. Collaborative learning sessions, conference calls, e-mail, and staff support are used to assist hospital teams to improve secondary prevention efforts in hospitals. (See the Evidence-Based Practice feature box.) Twelve performance criteria are tracked, with the following five necessary before discharge for eligible patients with coronary artery disease and without contraindications:

- Smoking cessation counseling for current smokers (or persons who have smoked within the last 12 months)
- Aspirin on discharge
- Beta blocker on discharge
- Angiotensin-converting enzyme inhibitor and/or angiotensin II receptor blocker on discharge
- Lipid-lowering therapy on discharge

Heart Failure Patients

A large proportion of PCU patients have heart failure (**HF**), so the PCU nurse must have the knowledge and educational foundation to teach HF patients. In addition to the five criteria listed in GWTG, the patient and family must understand additional information in the following areas:

- Weight monitoring: Patients are asked to weigh themselves at the same time each morning after urinating, while wearing similar clothing, and using the same scale. The purpose of weighing is to detect fluid accumulation, not adipose tissue. Patients are instructed to advise their primary physician of any

2-day weight gain of 3 lb or a 3- to 5-lb weight gain over 1 week.

■ Sodium-restricted (and possibly fluid-restricted) diet

Strategies for Successful Discharge Teaching

Many clinicians feel that an optimal time to intervene with a smoking cessation program is at the time of major cardiovascular event, such as following AMI, after CABG surgery, or after PCI. Studies have shown that patient adherence to recommended therapies is better when the therapies are started during hospitalization rather than as an outpatient.[16,17]

The PCU nurse provides an ongoing assessment of the patient's and family's interest level regarding educational content while continuously searching for the optimal "teachable moments." The nurse assesses the patient's and family's *willingness* and *ability* to learn new information. Despite having the attention of the patient and evidence of the importance of making lifestyle changes, the hospital setting may not be an optimal environment for patients and families to learn new information. The acutely ill, hospitalized patient is likely to be under considerable stress, and patients/family members may not be able to absorb information concerning the medical condition and required discharge medications and therapies. The decreasing length of hospital stay further challenges the PCU nurse to provide streamlined yet comprehensive patient education.

Despite potential barriers to learning, essential information must be packaged to fit the learning needs of the patient and family. Educational materials should be written in simple terms and should be easy to read. Health literacy, defined as a patient's ability to read, comprehend, and act on medical instructions, is a potent factor influencing retention of material taught.[18] Higher levels of education are associated with better health literacy, but still, approximately 30 percent of taught information is not well comprehended.[19] Poor comprehension challenges the PCU nurse to develop different or additional communication skills that can address problems of low health literacy, especially in patients over age 65, and those with chronic conditions.[20]

Most patients prefer practical information about what to do if symptoms occur at home, how to reach their provider, and information about their medications. Innovative teaching styles (e.g., computerized learning tutorials, Internet management log records, telephonic support, health education television programs, and peer support groups) can increase learning and retention of materials for some patients. Not all patients are ready to learn during hospitalization, and methods of accommodating them until they are ready are greatly needed. Responsibility for some education can be delegated to health care professionals who see the patient after discharge (e.g., cardiac rehabilitation, home health nurse, or office nurse). Inclusion of the spouses or family member in the teaching process increases learning and retention. For example, Karner and colleagues[21] found that spouses lacked understanding concerning important parts of cardiac rehabilitation activities and postulated that these misconceptions could have an important influence on their partner's behavior.

Patients receive numerous written educational materials from multiple disciplines (dietician, physical therapy, cardiac rehabilitation). The use of a single notebook or binder for all educational materials may provide consistency and easy storage of important reference material. To facilitate interdisciplinary communication, each person providing education should document his or her patient education on a single form. When used correctly, this tool can be used to identify educational goals that have been met and those that require follow-up education.

Discharge Medication Teaching

One of the most time consuming but important aspects of discharge teaching centers on discharge medications. Because most patients are receiving multiple medications (often as many as 8 to 15 medications daily), close attention to detailed medication teaching is required. Numerous barriers to education may result in the patients' discharge home with an incomplete or confusing medication list, predisposing the patient to complications and hospital readmission. A recent study by Field and colleagues[22] illustrated that although all of the HF patients they interviewed thought that medication adherence was important, the vast majority of them knew little about the medication purpose and side-effects. Table 22-1 lists a few of the most common schedule barriers along with potential solutions.

Minimizing the dosing frequency of required discharge medications improves treatment compliance. Numerous investigators have studied this phenomenon in a wide variety of drugs and disease states.[23,24] Although medication compliance cannot be assured with once-a-day dosing, forgetting to take medications is one reason why patients fail to adhere to therapy. Collaborate with the provider and pharmacist to simplify the discharge medication regimen. For example, if equivalent in dosing and efficacy, the nurse might recommend a sustained-release (once-a-day medication) to replace one given 2 to 3 times daily. Anecdotal evidence suggests that it is not uncommon for patients to save expired and replaced medications. So, patients need to be reminded to discontinue all medications previously taken and to bring his or her medication list to each outpatient appointment. Patients are strongly advised to avoid taking any nonprescription over-the-counter agents without prior consultation with their primary provider. Even commonly used foods, such as grapefruit, and drinks like coffee and cola can interact with medicines. For example, the polycyclic aromatic hydrocarbon-inducible cytochrome P450 (CYP) 1A2 participates in the metabolism of caffeine as well as certain drugs. Selective serotonin reuptake inhibitors (particularly fluvoxamine), antidysrhythmics (mexiletine), and quinolones (enoxacin)—among others—have been reported to be potent inhibitors of this isoenzyme.[25]

■ ■ ■

TABLE 22-1   MEDICATION SCHEDULE BARRIERS AND SOLUTIONS

POTENTIAL MEDICATION TEACHING AND COMPLIANCE BARRIERS	POSSIBLE SOLUTIONS
Incomplete Medication List Prescription written for newly prescribed medications, but no mention is made of medications that were taken previously at home (e.g., levothyroxine [Synthroid] or hormone replacement therapy). Fragmented medication list: Consulting (specialist) physician writes prescriptions for medicines within scope of practice but makes no evaluation of the full list of discharge medications. Primary provider does not evaluate and refine the comprehensive medication list. Patient is sent home with an incomplete medication list.	**Improved Interdisciplinary Collaboration on Discharge Medications** With an electronic documentation system, consider designing a "discharge medication screen" to incorporate admission medications (those taken at home) and current hospital medications. Establish an electronic method for providers to validate the comprehensive medication list before discharge. This screen could be printed for the patient to take home. With paper documentation systems, establish a "discharge medication" communication tool on which physicians can write in "anticipated" discharge medications followed by a "final" comprehensive medication list. Through interdisciplinary cardiac committees, seek collaborative agreement on the importance of discharging patients with an accurate medication list. Generate innovative ideas to continue to improve of this quality measure.
Confusing or Difficult-to-Read Medication Schedule Discharge medication schedules may have space limitations resulting in medications being typed or handwritten in a small font size. This predisposes to mistakes with home medications. Time frequencies written in medical language (Q.D. or "daily") instead of once a day may be confusing. Lack of clarity on when the medication was last taken on the day of discharge may lead to improper dosing schedule. Duplicate listing of medications may result in potential confusion between generic and trade names (e.g., atenolol and Tenormin). Patient may unknowingly "double dose" on the same medication.	**Reformat Forms and Standardize Medication Schedule Language** Via interdisciplinary committees/councils, strive to improve formatting of medication schedule template allowing for adequate font size (14 pt font or larger is preferred). Standardize the language for medication frequencies. Use lay language for dosage frequency. Provide a column on a medication form that includes "last taken in hospital." Provide generic and trade names.

BRIDGING HOSPITAL EDUCATION TO OUTPATIENT PROGRAMS

Heart Failure Disease Management Program Referrals

Numerous studies have shown a direct relationship between inadequate patient education and frequent hospital readmission in patients with HF. Those factors that contribute most often to otherwise avoidable rehospitalizations generally relate to dietary indiscretions, medication nonadherence, failure to monitor weight daily, lack of detection of worsening symptoms, and failure to see a provider for timely postdischarge follow-up. Recent meta-analyses have demonstrated that comprehensive discharge planning and referral to an outpatient management program improves outcomes from HF.[26,27] In HF patients who are readmitted, the PCU nurse is instrumental in collaborating with the provider to identify community resources that might be available for the patient, if no in-hospital disease management program exists.

Cardiac Rehabilitation Referrals

Patients who have had an AMI or coronary revascularization and those with chronic stable angina benefit from cardiac rehabilitation. This includes elderly patients who are less likely to be referred for these programs. In one study, elderly patients who participated in cardiac rehabilitation had a 13 percent increase in overall quality of life scores.[28]

Approximately 60 percent of adults in the United States do not achieve the recommended amount of physical activity (30 to 60 minutes of moderate to intense activity 3 to 4 times weekly), and an estimated 33 percent are overweight.[29] Weight reduction and exercise are important adjuncts to therapy (e.g., lipid lowering) for cardiac patients. This information is reinforced by the PCU nurse during the transition from hospital to home.

Enrolling in an outpatient cardiac rehabilitation program may improve long-term survival and quality of life following AMI. However, less than half of eligible patients participate, and women are less likely to participate than men.[30] All cardiac patients should be encouraged to consider cardiac rehabilitation and to discuss the benefits of it with their primary provider. The PCU nurse is often the one to recommend referral to the provider.

In summary, the PCU nurse's role is multifaceted but core clinical competencies involve the identification and prevention of complications and preparing patients for transition to the next level of care. Because of the vast range of cardiac patients in the PCU setting, PCU nurses are challenged to maintain a broad knowledge base and read widely if they are to provide evidence-based care to these diverse patients.

REFERENCES

1. Sakallaris BR, Halpin LS, Knapp M et al: Same day transfer of patients to the cardiac telemetry unit after surgery: the rapid after bypass back into telemetry program, *Crit Care Nurse* 20(2):59-68, 2000.
2. Durairaj L, Reilly B, Das K et al: Emergency department admissions to inpatient cardiac telemetry beds: a prospective cohort study of risk stratification and outcomes, *Am J Med* 110(1):7-11, 2001.
3. Estrada CA, Rosman HS, Prasad NK et al: Evaluation of guidelines for the use of telemetry in the non-intensive care setting, *J Gen Intern Med* 15(1):51-55, 2000.
4. American Association of Critical Care Nurses: *Progressive care certified nurse.* Retrieved 11/30/2006 from www.certcorp.org
5. Calkins H, Zipes DP: Hypotension and syncopy. In Zipes DP, Libby P, Bonow RO, Braunwald E, editors: *Heart disease: a textbook of cardiovascular medicine,* ed 7, Philadelphia, 2005, Elsevier Saunders.
6. Levine BS: History taking and physical examination. In Woods S, Froelicher ES, Motzer SU et al, editors: *Cardiac nursing,* ed 5, Philadelphia, 2005, Lippincott Williams & Wilkins.
7. Lahrmann H, Cortelli P, Hilz M, Mathias CJ, Struhal W, Tassinari M: EFNS guidelines on the diagnosis and management of orthostatic hypotension, *Eur J Neurol* 13:930-936, 2006.
8. Bickley LS, Szilagyi PG: *Bates' guide to physical examination and history taking,* ed 8, Philadelphia, 2003, Lippincott Williams & Wilkins.
9. Jacobson C: Electrocardiography. In Woods SL, Froelicher ES, Motzer SU et al, editors: *Cardiac nursing,* ed 5, Philadelphia, 2005, Lippincott Williams & Wilkins.
10. Pelter NM, Adams MG, Drew BJ: Transient myocardial ischemia is an independent predictor of adverse in-hospital outcomes in patients with acute coronary syndromes treated in the telemetry unit, *Heart Lung* 32:71-78, 2003.
11. Trent-Jabocson D, Lindquest RA: Functional recovery and exercise behavior in men and women 5 to 6 years following coronary artery bypass graft surgery, *West J Nurs Res* 26:479-498, 2004.
12. Vlasic W: An evidence-based approach to reducing bed rest in the invasive cardiology patient population, *Evid Based Nurs* 7:100-101, 2004.
13. Krasnoff J, Painter P: The physiological consequences of bed rest and inactivity, *Adv Ren Replace Ther* 6:124-132, 1999.
14. Spodick DH: Acute pericarditis: current concepts and practice, *JAMA* 289:1150-1153, 2003.
15. Barkauskas VH, Baumann LC, Darling-Fisher CS: *Health and physical assessment,* ed 3, St Louis, 2002, Mosby.
16. La Bresh K, Tyler P: A collaborative model for hospital-based cardiovascular secondary prevention, *Qual Manag Health Care* 12:20-27, 2003.
17. Jackevicius CA, Mandani M, Tu JV: Adherence with statin therapy in elderly patients with and without acute coronary syndromes, *JAMA* 288:462-467, 2002.
18. Schillinger D, Grumbach K: Association of health literacy with diabetes outcomes, *JAMA* 288:475-482, 2002.
19. Gausman Benson J, Forman WB: Comprehension of written health care information in an affluent geriatric retirement community: use of the Test of Functional Health Literacy, *Gerontology* 48:93-97, 2002.
20. Schwartzberg J, VanGeest J, Wang CC, editors: *Understanding health literacy: implications for medicine and public health,* Chicago, 2005, American Medical Association Press.
21. LaBresh KA, Waltham MA, Fonarow GE et al: Are improvements in cardiovascular care associated with the American Heart Association's Get with the Guidelines program sustained over time? *Circulation* 110:III-784, 2004 (abstract 3618).
22. Karner A, Dahlgren MA, Bergdahl B: Coronary heart disease: causes and drug treatment—spouses' conceptions, *J Clin Nurs* 13:167-176, 2004.
23. Granger AL, Fehnel SE, Hogue SL, Bennett L, Edin HM: An assessment of patient preference and adherence to treatment with Wellbutrin SR: a web-based survey, *J Affect Disord* 90:217-221, 2006.
24. Recker RR, Gallagher R, MacCosbe PE. Effect of dosing frequency on bisphosphonate medication adherence in a large longitudinal cohort of women. *Mayo Clin Proc.*;80:856-861, 2005
25. Carrillo JA, Benitez J: Clinically significant pharmacokinetic interactions between dietary caffeine and medications, *Clin Pharmacokinet* 39:127-153, 2000.
26. Phillips CO, Wright SM, Kern DE et al: Comprehensive discharge planning with postdischarge support for older patients with congestive heart failure: a meta-analysis, *JAMA* 291:1358-1367, 2004.
27. McAlister FA, Stewart S, Ferrua S, McMurray JJV: Multidisciplinary strategies for the management of heart failure patients at high risk for admission: a systematic review of randomized trials, *J Am Coll Cardiol* 44:810-819, 2004.
28. Lavie C, Milani R: Benefits of cardiac rehabilitation and exercise training programs in elderly coronary patients, *Am J Geriatr Cardiol* 10:323-327, 2001.
29. American Heart Association: *Heart and stroke facts statistical update, 2006,* Dallas, 2006, The Association.
30. Ades P, Green NM, Coello C: Effects of exercise and cardiac rehabilitation on cardiovascular outcomes, *Cardiol Clin* 21:435-448, 2003.

■ ■ ■ chapter **23**

Nurses in Perioperative Settings

Patricia C. Seifert

CHAPTER ABBREVIATIONS

AORN Association of periOperative Registered Nurses

CABG coronary artery bypass grafting

CAD coronary artery disease

CPB cardiopulmonary bypass

GEA gastroepiploic artery

GSV greater saphenous vein

IV intravenous

LIMA left internal mammary artery

OR operating room

SaO$_2$ oxyhemoglobin saturation

Perioperative nursing competencies, outlined by the Association of periOperative Registered Nurses (**AORN**),[1] reflect the basic knowledge, skills, and abilities required by nurses to provide a professional standard of care for patients undergoing operative and other invasive cardiac procedures. The 18 competency statements are divided among the following areas: assessment, nursing diagnosis, outcome identification, planning, implementation, and evaluation. Specific cardiac perioperative nursing competencies, explicated by Seifert,[2] reflect the special needs of cardiac patients. The competency statements are supported by AORN's Perioperative Nursing Data Set,[2] which identifies nursing interventions to achieve patient outcomes.[4]

ASSESSMENT
Physical Health Status and Response

Competency to assess the physical health status and physiological response of the patient. Patients classified as elective cardiac surgical candidates—in contrast to those scheduled for urgent or emergent surgery—usually are tested a few days before admission to the perioperative suite. Table 23-1 lists common preoperative laboratory and diagnostic imaging examinations.[3] Patients requiring urgent/emergent surgery undergo many of the diagnostic tests, albeit urgently. An abbreviated nursing assessment is performed with special consideration of allergies, hemodynamic status, and electrocardiographic changes.

When the patient arrives in the preoperative area, the patient's record is reviewed. Documented allergies are of special concern. In addition to known drug allergies, patients may be sensitive to protamine sulfate, commonly used to reverse the systemic heparinization used during cardiopulmonary bypass. In patients with

known or suspected protamine sensitivity, heparin reversal may be accomplished by allowing the heparin to metabolize naturally without the infusion of exogenous protamine. This process only slightly delays heparin reversal. Patients may be sensitive to latex; supplies such as latex-free intravenous (**IV**) tubing, sterile gloves, and endotracheal tubes should be used. Cold antibodies that can cause red blood cell agglutination at low temperatures may be identified by the blood bank during initial typing and crossmatching of blood products. The presence of these antibodies should be communicated to the surgical team; bypass techniques (such as using crystalloid, rather than blood carrying, solutions, and minimizing the reduction of body temperature) can be adjusted to avoid red cell agglutination in capillary beds. In severe cases of cold sensitivity, surgery may be performed without cardiopulmonary bypass, under normothermic temperatures.

The results of cardiac catheterization and other diagnostic test results are reviewed to plan for the selected procedure. Cardiac catheterization data are used to delineate coronary atherosclerotic lesions; identify the number, source, and proposed anastomotic sites for coronary artery bypass grafting (**CABG**); calculate ejection fraction; illustrate ventricular wall motion; and demonstrate shunts and regurgitant flow. Echocardiography can provide information about the severity of stenotic, regurgitant, or mixed valvular pathological conditions.

Current and past medical diagnoses, previous surgeries, and medication history, particularly drugs that may affect coagulation—such as aspirin, warfarin, clopidogrel, or certain herbal medicines[4] (Table 23-2)—are assessed. A review of cardiac, respiratory, renal, neurological, and other systems includes noting sensory impairments, prosthetic implants—pacemaker, heart valves, joint replacements—and mobility of body parts. Risk factors for infection, such as previous cardiac surgery, hyperglycemia, obesity, and length of preoperative hospitalization, are noted. Obesity is a risk factor for mediastinitis after CABG because of poor distribution of antibiotics in adipose tissue, difficulty in maintaining sterility among multiple skinfolds, and adipose tissue acting as an ideal substrate for bacterial growth. Intraoperative infection-related risk factors, such as duration of surgery, length of cardiopulmonary bypass, and blood transfusion,[5] can be minimized by having necessary supplies and equipment readily available to reduce delays, using blood salvaging procedures (autotransfusion), and maintaining strict aseptic techniques.

The medication records are reviewed to plan for care. Patients with a history of aspirin use, for example, may require platelet transfusion. Patients scheduled for

TABLE 23-1 PREOPERATIVE LABORATORY EVALUATION OF PATIENTS UNDERGOING CARDIAC SURGERY

PREOPERATIVE LABORATORY TEST	ABNORMAL FINDING	COMMENT
Complete blood count	1. Anemia, especially Hct <35%	1. Anticipate that hemodilution will occur on cardiopulmonary bypass, and blood loss will occur intraoperatively. In stable patients, preoperative iron supplementation (weeks) or erythropoietin therapy (days) should be considered. Patients with unstable angina, congestive heart failure, aortic stenosis, and left main coronary artery disease should be advised against autologous donation of blood in the preoperative period.
	2. WBC >10,000	2. Search for possible infection.
Coagulation screen	1. Prolonged bleeding time 2. Elevated PT and/or PTT 3. Thrombocytopenia	Any of these laboratory abnormalities suggest that the patient is at risk for bleeding postoperatively and may have excessive chest tube drainage. Corrective measures (e.g., vitamin K, fresh frozen plasma, platelet transfusions) should be considered preoperatively, and surgery may need to be postponed. Hematological consultation may be required if there is reason to suspect an inherited defect coagulation (e.g., von Willebrand factor deficiency) or heparin-induced thrombocytopenia.
Chemistry profile	1. Elevated BUN/ creatine	1. Abnormal renal function that may worsen in the perioperative period (caused by nonpulsatile flow on cardiopulmonary bypass and potential low flow postoperatively); may necessitate temporary or even permanent hemodialysis.
	2. Potassium <4.0 mEq/liter and/or magnesium <2.0 mEq/liter	2. Electrolyte deficits may place the patient at risk of arrhythmias perioperatively and should be corrected before induction of anesthesia.
	3. Abnormal liver function tests	3. Patient may clear anesthetic agents as well as other cardioactive drugs more slowly. Low albumin level may indicate a state of relative malnutrition that may need to be corrected with nutritional support perioperatively.
Stool Hema test	Positive for occult blood	Because heparinization will take place while on the cardiopulmonary bypass apparatus, the patient may be at risk for GI bleeding perioperatively. The source of GI heme loss should be investigated perioperatively if clinical circumstances permit. The potential for bleeding in the future may influence the choice of prosthetic valve inserted.
Pulmonary function	Reduced VC or prolonged FEV$_1$	Anticipate longer than usual process of weaning from ventilator postoperatively if FEV$_1$ <65% of VC or FEV$_1$ <1.5-2.0 liters. Obtain baseline arterial blood gas analysis on room air to help guide respiratory management postoperatively.
Thyroid function	These tests are not ordered routinely but should be performed in cases of suspected hypothyroidism or hyperthyroidism, known thyroid dysfunction during replacement therapy, and atrial fibrillation.	Hypothyroid patients require prolonged period of ventilatory support postoperatively because of slower clearance of anesthetic agents. Hyperthyroid patients have a hypermetabolic state that places them at increased risk of myocardial ischemia, vasomotor instability, and poorly controlled ventricular rate in atrial fibrillation.
Echocardiography	1. Decreased LV ejection fraction	1. Patients with decreased LV function are at higher perioperative risk for surgery. Selected patients should undergo viability assessment.
	2. Decreased RV function	2. RV function increases perioperative risk, and identification may lead to preoperative assessment of reversibility of pulmonary hypertension.
	3. Aortic stenosis	3. Mild to moderate aortic stenosis (gradient <25 mm Hg) may be treated by prophylactic valve replacement in selected low-risk patients.
	4. Aortic insufficiency	4. Ventricular dimension helps guide decisions to perform valve replacement in addition to revascularization in patients with combined aortic regurgitation and coronary disease.
	5. Mitral insufficiency	5. Moderate or severe mitral regurgitation may warrant valve exploration in patients undergoing coronary revascularization.
	6. LV aneurysm	6. This may alert surgeons to the need of aneurysmectomy in selected patients.
	7. Ventricular septal defect	7. Identification suggests the need for early surgical intervention.
Cardiac catheterization	1. Elevated LV end-diastolic pressure and pulmonary capillary wedge pressure	1. May remain elevated in the early postoperative period and indicate a need for careful attention to maintenance of adequate preload postoperatively.
	2. Elevated right atrial pressure	2. May reflect tricuspid regurgitation or RV dysfunction from prior infarction. Such patients require vigorous volume expansion postoperatively to maintain adequate cardiac output.
	3. Elevated pulmonary artery pressure (and pulmonary vascular resistance)	3. Fixed pulmonary vascular resistance should be suspected when the pulmonary artery diastolic pressure exceeds the mean pulmonary capillary wedge pressure. Vigorous oxygenation and pharmacological support with a pulmonary vasodilator (isoproterenol, prostaglandin E) are important in such cases. Patients with a pulmonary artery diastolic pressure equal to the pulmonary capillary wedge pressure usually have more rapid resolution of pulmonary hypertension postoperatively.
	4. LV mural thrombus	4. Increased risk of stroke perioperatively.
	5. Status of internal mammary arteries	5. Highly desirable arterial conduits for planned revascularization surgery. Particular care is required during reoperation if patent internal mammary artery bypass is in place from previous surgery.
	6. Status of saphenous vein grafts	6. "Pseudoextravasation" of dye outside the lumen in a patent graft with slow flow probably represents thrombus-filled atherosclerotic aneurysm of the graft.

BUN, Blood, urea, nitrogen; *FEV$_1$*; forced expiratory volume in 1 second; *GI*, gastrointestinal; *HCT*, hematocrit; *LV*, left ventricular; *PT*, prothrombin time, *PTT*, partial thromboplastin time; *RV*, right ventricular; *VC*, ventilatory capacity; *WBC*, white blood count. *Continued*

■ ■ ■

TABLE 23-1 PREOPERATIVE LABORATORY EVALUATION OF PATIENTS UNDERGOING CARDIAC SURGERY—cont'd

PREOPERATIVE LABORATORY TEST	ABNORMAL FINDING	COMMENT
Vascular Doppler	1. Carotid stenosis	1. Suggests an increased risk of perioperative stroke. If symptomatic or if stenosis >80%, consideration for combined or staged carotid surgery.
	2. Aortic iliac disease	2. May contraindicate insertion of an intraaortic balloon pump and suggest increased risk of peripheral vascular complications.
	3. Absent or varicosed veins	3. In patients with severe varicosities or who have undergone venous stripping, alternative conduits such as bilateral internal mammary arteries or radial grafts must be considered.

From Adams DH, Filsoufi F, Antman EM: Medical management of the patient undergoing cardiac surgery. In Zipes DP, Libby P, Bonow RO, Braunwald E, editors: *Braunwald's heart disease,* ed 7, Philadelphia, 2005, Saunders.

■ ■ ■

TABLE 23-2 PERIOPERATIVE EFFECTS OF HERBAL MEDICINES

AGENT	PHARMACOLOGIC ACTION	CONCERNS AND CONSIDERATIONS
Echinacea (purple cone-flower root)	Activates cell-mediated immunity	Decreases effectiveness of immunosuppressants; should not be taken by organ transplant patients
Ephedra	Increases heart rate and blood pressure through sympathomimetic effects	Increases risk of stroke and myocardial ischemia; may cause intraoperative hemodynamic instability
Garlic	Inhibits platelet aggregation; increases fibrinolysis	Increases risk of bleeding, especially in combination with other platelet inhibitors
Ginkgo	Inhibits platelet activation	Increases risk of bleeding, especially in combination with other platelet inhibitors
Ginseng	Inhibits platelet activation; lowers blood glucose; has many diverse effects	Increases risk of bleeding; has potential to decrease anticoagulation effect of warfarin; may cause hypoglycemia
St John's Wort	Inhibits neurotransmitter reuptake	Induces enzymes that affect warfarin and many other drugs; may affect calcium channel blockers and decrease serum digoxin levels

From Seifert PC: *Cardiac surgery: perioperative patient care,* St Louis, 2002, Mosby. Modified from Ang-Lee MK, Moss J, Yuan CS: *JAMA* 286:208, 2001; Liu EH, Turner LM, Lin SX et al: *J Thorac Cardiovasc Surg* 120:335-341, 2000; Brumley C: *AORN J* 72:785, 2000; and Association of periOperative Registered Nurses: *Safe medication administration tool kit,* Denver, 2005, AORN. Retrieved November 19, 2006 from www.aorn.org/toolkit/safemed/

valve replacement surgery are reviewed for a history of anticoagulation. In patients with previous anticoagulation therapy for a prior transient ischemic attack or chronic atrial fibrillation, anticipate continuation of anticoagulation therapy postoperatively. Success in prior anticoagulation therapy is one indication for the use of a mechanical prosthetic heart valve. Although mechanical prostheses require postoperative chronic anticoagulation, they have the advantage of long-term durability. Biological prostheses, the second category of prosthetic replacement valves, have the intrinsic advantage of not requiring chronic anticoagulation, but their long-term durability is shorter than that of mechanical valves. Among other considerations for the selection of valvular prostheses are anatomy, age, lifestyle, availability of laboratory facilities for testing, and patient preference.

After reviewing the record, interview the patient to confirm the patient's identity, surgical site, and procedure. Physical signs such as shivering from anxiety or from chilling are significant because anxiety can trigger endogenous catecholamine release, and shivering caused by cooling increases myocardial oxygen consumption. Provide warm blankets and demonstrate concern with soft words and a soft touch to reduce patient (and family) concerns.

Psychosocial Health Status

Competency to assess the psychosocial health status and psychophysiological response of the patient. Psychosocial risk factors are reviewed for their potential negative impact on the patient. The operating room (**OR**) can be a frightening place, in part because of its secluded location and its array of "hi-tech" machines and devices (Figure 23-1). Patients who are fearful or anxious or who recently have undergone stressful life events have an elevated myocardial oxygen consumption from an adrenergic response that increases catecholamine release and subsequently increases heart rate and contractility. Patients with coronary artery disease (**CAD**) may be especially at risk for a cardiac event because their atherosclerotic lesions impair the supply of blood to the myocardium. Interventions to reduce anxiety or fear (talking with patient, answering questions, describing the OR environment, holding the patient's hand, and allowing family members and spiritual advisors into the preoperative area) can promote a balance between myocardial oxygen demand and supply.

Patients demonstrate an array of coping mechanisms[6] and needs. Some want to know as much about the surgery as possible. Questions should be answered succinctly and

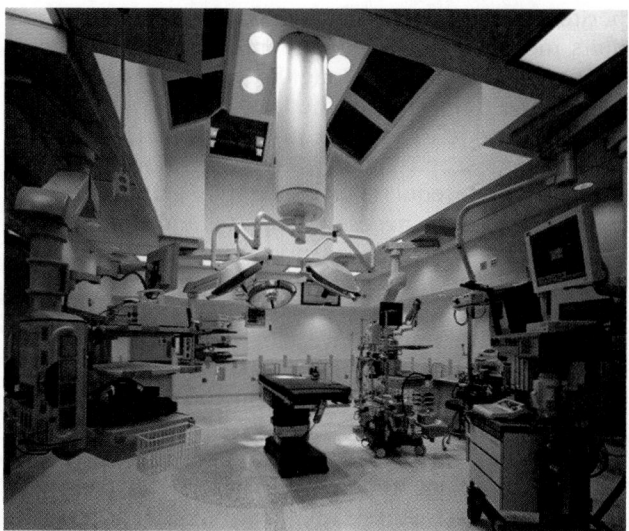

FIGURE 23-1 ■ Operating room offers open and minimally invasive surgery. (From Inova Heart and Vascular Institute, Inova Health System.)

honestly; if the answer is not known, other professionals who can address the question properly should be contacted to respond to the patient. Other patients display anger, denial, or withdrawal. Ascertain the cause of the anger, if possible, and address it. Anger may be part of a grieving process, or it may be related to perceived or actual poor service. If poor service has occurred, the nurse or supervisor should attempt to rectify the situation.

Denial is another coping mechanism that should be respected as long as it does not impede necessary interventions by caregivers. For example, make the patient aware of actions that will occur during the period that he or she is awake and alert: starting an IV infusion or intraarterial pressure monitoring line, and changing into a hospital gown. Some patients want answers to questions about personal concerns (e.g., allergies, previous surgeries, or presence of prosthetic implants). Others may exhibit signs of withdrawal and not desire detailed information. Support these patients by describing what can be expected, minimizing all but essential details, allowing them to retain as much control over their situation as possible. See Chapter 83 for further discussion of "blunters and monitors." Attending family members can provide emotional support to the patient and their participation should be welcomed.

When emergency surgery is imminent, elicit critical information (e.g., allergies) and provide emotional comfort. Family members can accompany the patient to the preoperative area and should be allowed to stay with the patient to provide support up to the moment when the patient is transported to the OR. In these situations, family members who have been present should be updated with news about their loved one as soon as it is feasible.

NURSING DIAGNOSIS
Data Analysis and Interpretation

Competency to analyze and interpret health status data in determining nursing diagnoses. After reviewing the physiological and psychosocial status of the patient, integrate patient-specific information with expected outcomes associated with the operative procedure (e.g., a patient undergoing CABG may have knowledge deficits related to the source of bypass grafts or conduits available, or concerns about the effect of a traditional incision (versus a smaller, minimally invasive incision) on self-image. Patient desires for a specific graft source or a type of incision should be considered jointly among the patient, nurse, and surgeon.

The surgical environment has its own intrinsic risks. Surgery interrupts the skin barrier and increases the potential for infection. This reality is especially important to consider in patients with diabetes mellitus because of impaired healing. Endogenous flora pose a risk for infection, so instruments and supplies used to excise the saphenous leg vein from the groin area are kept separate from items used in the chest. This minimizes cross-contamination.

The potential for injury caused by foreign objects retained in a patient is a special concern of nurses. Multiple small devices and supplies are used during an operation, and these must be accounted for before the incision is closed. Retained endogenous particulate matter (fat globules, calcium particles) can be a source of embolus; efforts to remove particles from instruments and the surgical site are important safety actions.

Among the nursing diagnoses commonly used in the cardiac surgical population are those related to knowledge deficits, anxiety, infection, cardiac output, injury (related to positioning, retained foreign objects, and chemical/physical/electrical hazards), impaired skin/tissue integrity, fluid/electrolyte imbalances, and self-image. Other diagnoses are used as indicated by patients' needs and expectations.

Medical diagnoses, such as *ventricular fibrillation, cardiac arrest,* and *hemorrhage* impede cardiac output. These are collaborative problems considered by all providers because of the close interdisciplinary environment of the OR and the ever-present risk of these conditions to patients. These problems necessitate joint consideration and planning.

OUTCOME IDENTIFICATION
Patient Goals

Competency to establish patient goals based on nursing diagnoses. Perioperative patient outcomes are observable, measurable physiological and psychosocial responses to nursing interventions.[7] Generic surgical patient outcomes include freedom from signs and symptoms of injury (e.g., laser, radiation, electrical, and retained foreign bodies), freedom from signs and symptoms of infection, and adequate pain control. Patients should participate in identifying expected goals. In some cases the patient's goals may be different from the clinician's goals, and these differences should be explored and discussed, particularly if the goals conflict with accepted therapy. For example, a patient with mitral valve regurgitation may want a reparative procedure rather than a prosthetic replacement; however, if the leaflets or chordae tendineae are torn and irreparable, the valve may require replacement. The nurse must provide sufficient information to assist patients in understanding the rationale for decisions. Not only does the explanation promote true informed consent and increase patient satisfaction, but also enables the patient to participate actively in the therapy.

PLANNING
Development of Plan of Care

Competency to develop a plan of care that prescribes nursing actions to achieve patient goals. Developing a plan of care requires that the nurse understand the sequence of events to be expected. Each patient is unique, and the procedure planned is specific to the patient.

In patients undergoing CABG, the nurse communicates with the patient, the surgeon, and other colleagues to provide the most appropriate bypass grafts for bypass grafting. (See the Evidence-Based Practice feature: Patency of Arterial Coronary Bypass Grafts Over 15 Years.) Arterial and venous grafts commonly are required because patients often have multivessel CAD, and there may be insufficient arterial conduits available to achieve complete revascularization. Available arterial conduits include the left and/or right internal mammary artery, the right or left radial artery, and occasionally the gastroepiploic artery (GEA) (which requires entering the

peritoneum with its attendant risk). Veins used as conduits include the greater saphenous and the lesser saphenous veins, located along the medial aspect and the lower posterior aspect of the legs, respectively. The patient may desire to have the greater saphenous leg vein excised endoscopically (versus via traditional open leg incision). Such requests usually can be granted, and the nurse prepares the necessary supplies and equipment to achieve that goal. CABG surgery may be performed with or without the use of cardiopulmonary bypass. If the plan is to perform "off-pump" surgery, the nurse prepares for that procedure. The nurse and the rest of the surgical team also plan for the possibility of instituting bypass promptly if the patient's hemodynamic status suddenly worsens.

In patients who need surgery on a cardiac valve, the nurse ensures that the appropriate type of prosthesis and the sizers, prosthesis holders, and other accessories specific to the type of prosthesis to be used are available. Special requirements (such as basins and normal saline irrigating fluid to rinse the glutaraldehyde storage solution from a biological valve) also are incorporated into the plan.

After entry to the OR, the patient is transferred to the OR bed and is prepared for endotracheal intubation and insertion of central venous pressure and pulmonary artery pressure lines. In some institutions, central venous pressure and pulmonary artery lines are inserted before

---

■ EVIDENCE-BASED PRACTICE

PATENCY OF ARTERIAL CORONARY BYPASS GRAFTS OVER 15 YEARS

Given the excellent long-term patency of the left internal mammary artery (LIMA), there is an expectation that other arterial grafts—the right internal mammary artery (RIMA) and the radial artery (RA)—can provide similar patency rates that are superior to saphenous vein grafts. Two observers[1] reviewed the consecutive postoperative angiograms of 2127 patients with arterial and venous coronary bypass grafts. Angiograms were indicated for cardiac symptoms. Overall, the following patency rates were identified:

- LIMA, 96.4 percent (1296 of 1345)
- RIMA, 88.3 percent (534 of 605)
- RA (aortocoronary bypass), 89.3 percent (158 of 177)

Patency of the LIMA to the left anterior descending coronary artery was 97.1 percent (1131 of 1165), and patency to the obtuse marginal branch of the circumflex coronary artery was 91.7 percent (165 of 180, $p = 0.01$). Patency of the RIMA *pedicle* graft (i.e., remaining attached to the right subclavian artery) was 86 percent (275 of 381); the *free* RIMA (i.e., disconnected from the subclavian artery) had a patency of 91 percent (259 of 284, $p = $ NS). The degree of native coronary stenosis influenced patency rates was as follows: stenoses greater than 60 percent were associated with higher patency rates. LIMA patency at 5 years was 98 percent; at 10 years, 81 percent; and at 15 years, 65 percent. RIMA patency was 96 percent, 81 percent, and 65 percent at 5 years, 10 years, and 15 years, respectively. RA patency was 96 percent at 1 year and 89 percent at 4 years. Of the 3714 vein grafts studied, 61 percent were open (2266 of 3214) overall. Vein graft patencies at 5 years, 10 years, and 15 years, respectively, were 95 percent, 71 percent, and 32 percent. In summary, superior long-term patency of arterial grafts was found when compared with vein grafts.

Reference

1. Tatoulis J, Buxton BF, Fuller JA: Patencies of 2,217 arterial to coronary conduits over 15 years, *Ann Thorac Surg* 77:93-101, 2004.

■ EVIDENCE-BASED PRACTICE

SKIN PIGMENTATION AND THE ACCURACY OF PULSE OXIMETRY

Although pulse oximetry is designed to compute accurately the arterial hemoglobin oxygen saturation independent of skin pigmentation, there have been cases of unacceptable errors in pulse oximetry at low saturation levels in pigmented subjects. The authors[1] of one study tested three finger types of pulse oximeters to determine whether errors at low arterial oxyhemoglobin saturation (SaO_2) correlate with skin color. Twenty-one healthy, nonsmoking subjects were studied; 11 subjects were very darkly pigmented individuals of African-American descent; 10 subjects were light-skinned individuals of northern European descent. Pulse oximeter probes were placed on the fingers, and an indwelling 22-gauge radial artery line was inserted to sample SaO_2. Study results showed that at all SaO_2 levels and with all three types of oximeters, SpO_2 (oxygen saturation measured by pulse oximetry) readings were approximately 1 percent higher in dark- than in light-skinned individuals ($p < 0.0001$). At lower oxyhemoglobin saturation levels (hypoxia), there were differences of up to 8 percent between light- and dark-skinned persons.

The authors suggest that because most pulse oximeters have been designed and calibrated by manufacturers using light-skinned individuals at room air saturation levels, it has been assumed that skin pigment is unimportant. Accurate SaO_2 readings during surgery for acquired or congenital heart disease are necessary to anticipate, monitor, and treat hypoxic episodes. The authors recommend that there be a warning notice on devices to alert clinicians to the possibility of overestimation of arterial oxygen saturation in dark-skinned individuals, especially at low saturation levels.

Reference

1. Bickler PE, Feiner JR, Severinghaus JW: Effects of skin pigmentation on pulse oximeter accuracy at low saturation, *Anesthesiology* 102:715-719, 2005.

intubation occurs. A finger pulse oximeter is used to measure arterial oxygen saturation; stay alert to potential inaccuracies in pulse oximetry readings. (See the Evidence-Based Practice feature Pulse Oximetry.) During induction of general anesthesia, stay alert to hemodynamic changes, particularly in patients with left main CAD or other lesions that may impair left ventricular function. Table 23-3 lists the hemodynamic effects of certain anesthetic drugs, and Table 23-4 lists the desired hemodynamic objectives during anesthesia induction and maintenance.[8] The surgical team is prepared to institute resuscitation measures promptly if cardiac arrest occurs.

A direct blood pressure monitoring line usually is inserted before the patient enters the OR. The radial artery on the nondominant side of the lower arm is a common insertion site. The radial artery selected depends on whether the artery is to be excised for use as a bypass graft. The radial artery of the nondominant arm typically is harvested for use as a conduit; the radial pressure line would be inserted into the dominant/contralateral arm. When use of the radial artery is planned, the surgical assistant ensures adequate collateral (ulnar artery) blood flow.

After anesthesia induction, a urinary drainage catheter is inserted to decompress the bladder and to measure urine output, which serves as an indirect measure of cardiac function. A rectal temperature probe may be inserted. The connections of these probes, catheters, drug infusion, and monitoring lines should be secured. Electrosurgical dispersive pads ("grounding pads") are applied bilaterally to the buttocks to disperse the elec-

■ ■ ■

TABLE 23-3 HEMODYNAMIC EFFECTS OF ANESTHETIC DRUGS

DRUG	HEMODYNAMIC EFFECT					
	CI	BP	SVR	PLVED	HR	CONTRACTILITY
d-Tubocurarine	↓	↓	↓	↓	↑	↔
Diazepam	↓	↓	↓	↓	↔	↔
Dimethyl tubocurarine	↑	↔↑	↔↓	↔↓	↑	↔
Droperidol	↔↑	↓	↓	↓	↑	↔
Enflurane	↓	↓	↓	↔↓	↔↓	↓
Fentanyl	↔	↓	↓	↔	↔	↔
Halothane	↓	↓	↔↓	↔↑	↔↑↓	↓
Innovar	↔↑	↓	↓	↓	↔	↔
Isoflurane	↔	↓	↓	↔	↑	↓
Ketamine	↑	↑	↑	↑	↑	↑
Methoxyflurane	↓	↓	↓	↔	↔	↓
Midazolam	↔	↔	↔↓	↓	↑	↔↓
Morphine	↔↑	↔↓	↓	↔↑	↓	↔
Nitrous oxide	↓	↔↓	↔↑	↑	↔↓	↓
Pancuronium	↑	↑	↔	↓	↑	?
Succinylcholine	↓	↔↓	↓	↓	↑↓	?
Thiopental	↔↓	↔	↑	↔	↑	↓
Vecuronium	↔	↔	↔	↔	↔	↔

From Kouchoukos N, Blackstone EH, Doty DB et al: *Kirklin/Barratt-Boyes cardiac surgery*, vol 1, ed 3, Philadelphia, 2003, Churchill Livingstone.
Key: ↓, Decrease; ↑, increase; ↔, no change; ?, insufficient data; *CI*, cardiac index; *BP*, blood pressure; *SVR*, systemic vascular resistance; *PLVED*, left ventricular end-diastolic pressure; *HR*, heart rate.

■ ■ ■

TABLE 23-4 CARDIAC GRID: DESIRED OBJECTIVES DURING INDUCTION AND MAINTENANCE OF ANESTHESIA

CARDIAC LESION	OBJECTIVE				
	HEART RATE	RHYTHM	CONTRACTILITY	PRELOAD	AFTERLOAD
Coronary artery disease	−	Sinus	+	+	+
Tamponade	++	Sinus	++	++	++
Aortic stenosis	+	Sinus	++	++	++
Aortic regurgitation	++	Sinus	+	+	−−
Mitral stenosis	−	Sinus	+	+	+
Mitral regurgitation	++	Sinus	+	−	−−
Hypertrophic obstructive cardiomyopathy	−	Sinus	−	++	++
Coarctation of the aorta	0	Sinus	+	+	PAO−, PPA+
Aortopulmonary shunt	0	Sinus	0	+	−
Fontan physiology	−	Sinus	+	+	−
Tetralogy of Fallot	+	Sinus	0	+	−

From Kouchoukos N, Blackstone EH, Doty DB et al: *Kirklin/Barratt-Boyes cardiac surgery*, vol 1, ed 3, Philadelphia, 2003, Churchill Livingstone.
Key: +, Increase; −, decrease; *PAO*, systemic (aorta) pressure; *PPA*, pulmonary artery pressure.

trical energy from the cautery machine. Frequently, two cautery units are used for CABG, one for the chest and one for the leg(s).

Patients are placed commonly in the supine position. Cardiac procedures usually last 4 to 5 hours or longer, so measures are taken to minimize the risk of pressure injuries. OR beds are covered with a soft pad. The fingers are placed around a small roll, and the hands and elbows are padded with foam or other soft material. Patients with arthritic joints are positioned as anatomically correctly as possible without injury to the joints. Patients who are obese may require widening of the OR bed with accessory table parts. If the radial artery is to be excised, the affected arm and hand are placed in the supine position (with an upward-facing palm) and placed on a wide arm board to expose the artery. After excision of the conduit, the arm tissue is closed, dressed, padded, and placed along the patient's side.

A small pillow is placed under the head and under the heels (if the feet remain under the drapes, as they would usually during valve surgery). A metal screen often is placed over the head to keep the drapes off the face and to make the airway accessible to the anesthesia provider. A screen may be placed over the feet when they are covered by drapes. During coronary procedures, the feet are wrapped in a towel or other material and are placed on top of the drapes in order to manipulate the feet and legs during conduit excision.

The skin is disinfected and prepared ("prepped") for surgery with an antiseptic solution designed to remove dirt and transient microbes. Care is taken to avoid allowing the cleansing solution to pool under the skin or drip between the skin and the electrical dispersive pads on the buttocks. The patient then is draped to expose the intended incision sites and to cover the rest of the body. A median sternotomy, the most common incision,[9] is made with a powered saw. Although surgery increasingly is performed through smaller incisions, the median sternotomy remains the standard incision because it provides the best exposure of the heart and great vessels and facilitates the institution of cardiopulmonary bypass. In patients undergoing CABG, the bypass grafts are harvested before the institution of cardiopulmonary bypass (**CPB**). At the end of the procedure, the sternal edges are reapproximated with stainless steel wire. An increasing number of sternal closure systems are available; these systems may use single strands of stainless steel, twisted cable wires, plates and screws, or some other design.

The conduits used most frequently during CABG are the left internal mammary artery (**LIMA**) and the greater saphenous vein (**GSV**). Arterial grafts have excellent long-term patency.[10] Thus additional conduits, such as the radial artery, may be used. Although the mammary, radial, and gastroepiploic arteries are used whenever possible, the use of these vessels may not be feasible in a particular patient. In diabetic patients, for example, use of the bilateral mammary arteries as grafts causes discontinuation of blood flow to the sternal wall and increases the risk of poor wound healing.[5] Other patients may have insufficient collateral blood flow in one or both arms, which would cancel plans to use the ra-

dial arteries. Thus, the GSV often is used to provide additional bypass grafts when multiple grafts are needed.

Commonly, the LIMA is grafted to the left anterior descending coronary artery, and GSV grafts are connected to marginal branches of the circumflex coronary artery and/or to the right coronary artery, as indicated. The LIMA is dissected by exposing the retrosternum with a retractor that elevates the left sternal wall. The GSV is excised, increasingly, with video-assisted endoscopic techniques. The radial artery is excised while the LIMA is being dissected. If the gastroepiploic artery (**GEA**) is to be used, special supplies and instruments are used to open the peritoneum to expose the stomach and the right GEA; the proximal portion of the GEA remains attached to its connection to the gastroduodenal artery, and the distal end is brought through a small opening made in the diaphragm. The GEA often is attached to the right main coronary artery or to distal right or circumflex artery branches (such as the posterior descending coronary artery, which may branch from the right or circumflex coronary arteries).

When arterial conduits are dissected, heparin is given systemically before the arteries are clamped and cut in order to avoid thrombus formation. Arterial conduits tend to spasm, so antispasmodic drugs (such as papaverine) frequently are injected into the cut end of the artery. After the conduits are available, the surgeon prepares to institute CPB.

Preparing for CPB includes communication with the perfusionist and the surgeon to confirm how bypass is to be established and with which catheters, tubing, and lines. The goal of CPB is to perfuse the organs so that the heart can be arrested to provide a quiet field in which to work by bypassing the heart (pump) and the lungs (oxygenator). The process of extracorporeal circulation involves temperature manipulation, myocardial preservation, cerebral protection, blood conservation, and organ perfusion. With the application of an ascending aortic cross-clamp, the heart is isolated from the CPB circuit and is not perfused.

Myocardial protection strategies include induced hypothermia (to reduce the metabolic rate and concomitant oxygen demand) and immediate diastolic arrest (achieved with an infusion of hyperkalemic solution to conserve myocardial energy resources). In patients with extensive calcification or atherosclerosis of the ascending aorta, placement of a cross-clamp increases the risk of disruption and subsequent embolization of atheromatous material from the aorta. To avoid manipulating the aorta with a clamp, the surgeon may elect to perform CABG without the use of CPB ("off pump"), which does not require an aortic clamp. Off-pump techniques are suitable for CABG because the chambers of the heart are not entered. In procedures where one or more chambers of the heart is opened—such as valve surgery—an open, beating heart would produce massive air embolus and blood loss.

During CPB, one or two cannulas are used to drain venous return, and another cannula is inserted into a large artery (usually the ascending aorta) to infuse arterialized blood into the systemic circulation. The selec-

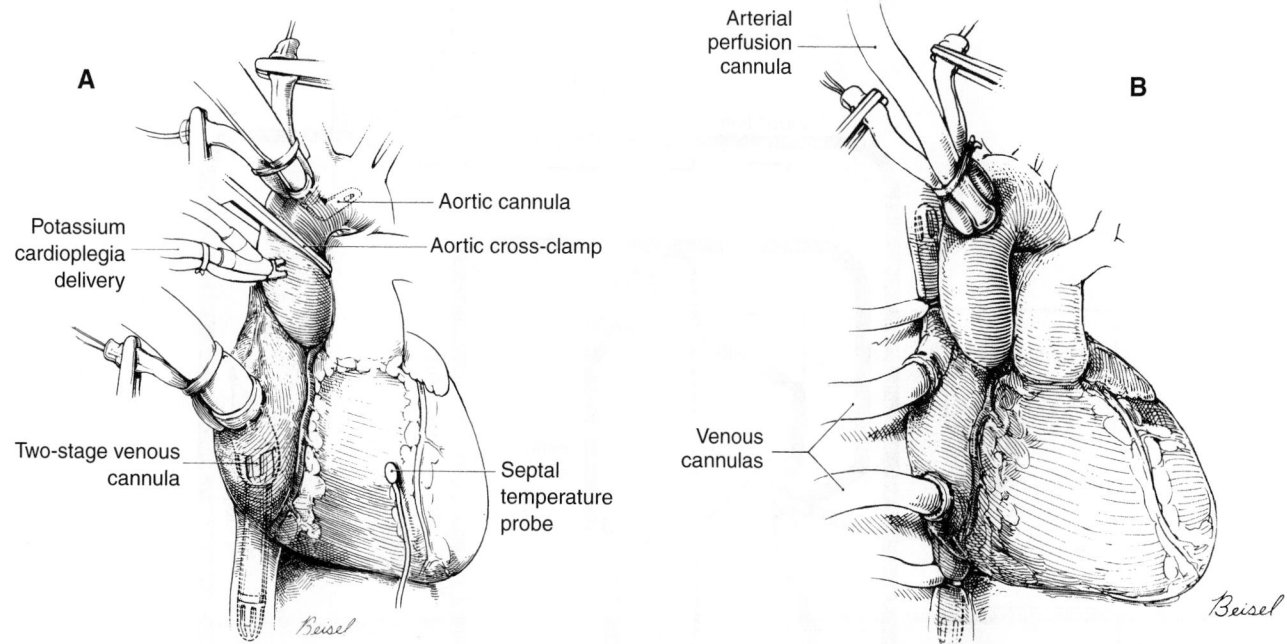

FIGURE 23-2 ■ A, Two-stage venous cannula. The distal openings drain the inferior vena cava, and the proximal openings in the right atrium drain venous return from the superior vena cava and the heart via the coronary sinus in the right atrium. The antegrade cardioplegia delivery catheter and the aortic cross-clamp are in place. A temperature probe is shown in the interventricular septum. **B,** Double venous (bicaval) cannulation of the inferior and superior venae cavae. In procedures performed in the right side of the heart, bicaval cannulation prevents returning venous blood from flooding the surgical field. (**A** from Waldhausen JA, Pierce WS: *Johnson's surgery of the chest,* ed 5, St Louis, 1985, Mosby. **B** from Waldhausen JA, Pierce WS, Campbell DB: *Surgery of the chest,* ed 6, St Louis, 1996, Mosby.)

tion of bypass cannulas is determined by the severity and location of the lesion, the amount of cardiac decompression (ventricular unloading) required, and the anticipated amount of time required for the surgical repair. With most CABG and aortic valve procedures, a two-stage venous drainage cannula is used (Figure 23-2A).[9] This technique allows some venous blood to enter the right side of the heart. When lesions of the right side (e.g., tricuspid valve insufficiency) are repaired, venous return entering the right atrium needs to be drained by individual cannulation of the superior and inferior venae cavae to avoid flooding the right atrium (and the surgical site) with returning blood (Figure 23-2B). The bypass circuit (Figure 23-3)[11] drains venous blood that is oxygenated, cooled or warmed, and filtered; arterialized blood is pumped into the systemic circulation.

To arrest the heart, hyperkalemic antegrade cardioplegia solution is infused into the coronary circulation via a needle in the aortic root (Figure 23-2A); retrograde cardioplegia solution is infused through a catheter inserted through the right atrium and positioned in the coronary sinus. Antegrade and retrograde cardioplegia delivery techniques enable the arresting solution to flow transmurally, even in the presence of coronary atherosclerotic lesions or ventricular hypertrophy.

When CABG surgery is performed on a beating heart, CPB is not used, although a bypass machine and

a perfusionist are commonly immediately available. Off-pump procedures require special planning. Nurses need to be prepared to place the patient on bypass immediately if there is severe hemodynamic deterioration. The location of the attachment of the bypass graft on the heart must be stabilized in order to create a relatively quiescent area on which to perform the anastomosis of the graft to the artery.

IMPLEMENTATION
Patient Transfer

Competency to implement nursing actions in transferring the patient according to the prescribed plan. Whether bringing the patient to the OR from the preoperative area or transporting the patient to the postoperative recovery (surgical intensive care) unit, the nurse ensures that patient transfer is performed safely and smoothly. The selection of transporting personnel is based on the patient's acuity; often postoperative (or unstable preoperative) patients are accompanied by an anesthesia provider, a nurse, and a monitoring technologist. In teaching institutions, a resident physician also may accompany the patient. Sublingual nitroglycerin tablets may be placed on the chart for immediate use if the patient has angina.

Patients with indwelling intraaortic balloon pumps are likely to be transferred in the bed rather than a gurney,

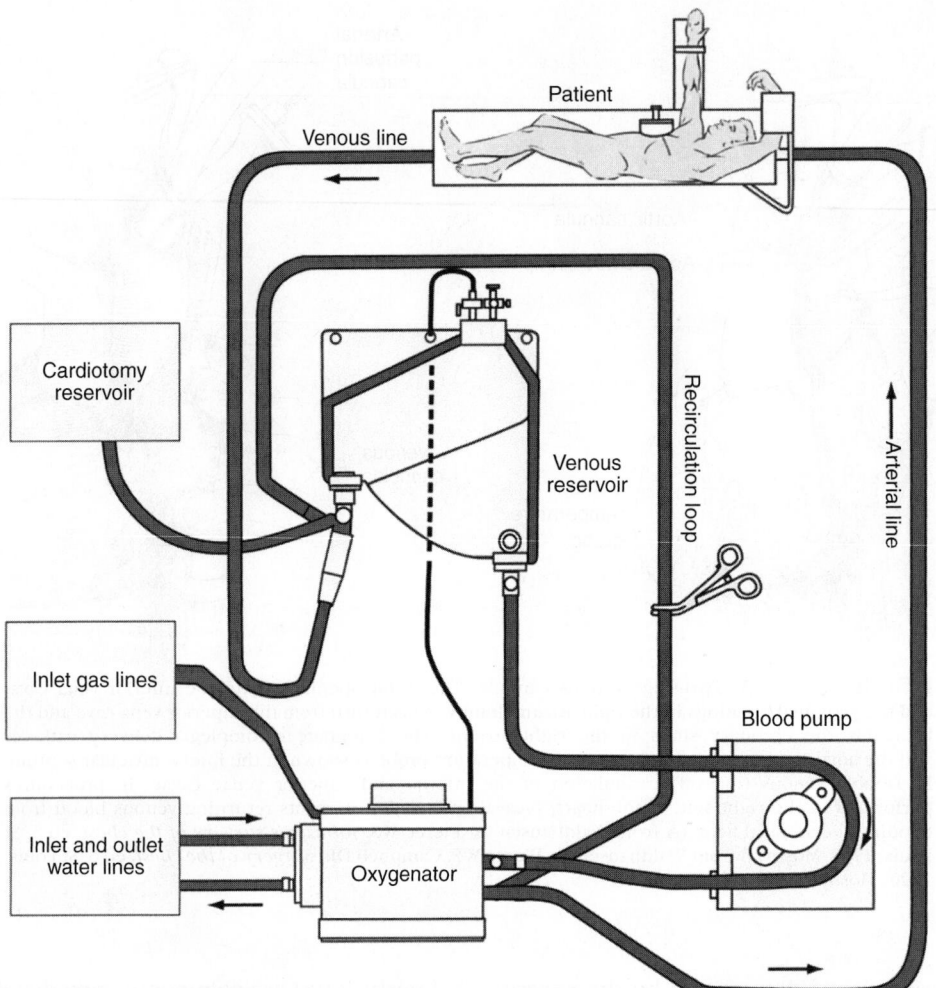

FIGURE 23-3 ▪ Cardiopulmonary bypass circuit. Venous blood drains from the patient through tubing that flows to the venous reservoir and the oxygenator, where gas exchange and cooling/warming occurs. Oxygenated blood is pumped through the arterial line into the patient's systemic circulation. Throughout the bypass circuit, filters and in-line sensors monitor air or particulate matter that may embolize to the brain and other organs. (From Buxton B, Frazier OH, Westaby S [eds]: *Ischemic heart disease: surgical management,* London, 1999, Mosby.)

with the balloon pump being pushed in tandem with the bed. Additional transport devices may include a portable hemodynamic monitor and defibrillator. Consideration of the patient's comfort and dignity mandate that the patient be fully covered during transport; touching and verbally communicating with patients can enhance comfort (even when patients are unconscious). Transferring the patient to and from the OR bed should be accomplished with a minimum of four persons: one at the head, one at the feet, and one person on each side of the patient.

Patient and Family Teaching

Competency to participate in patient/family teaching. Patients and family members awaiting surgery often have many questions about the surgery itself and other aspects of the perioperative experience. Table 23-5 outlines patient teaching content related to preoperative and postoperative CABG and valve surgery issues.[4] Patients are interested especially in information about anesthesia, the surgical procedure, and the OR environment.[12] Nurses can be proactive in asking if there are questions about these subjects. Describing the OR environment (sights, sounds, masked individuals, temperature) can help patients prepare for their entry into this foreign environment.

Questions about anesthesia ("Will I be awake?") and surgery ("How long will the surgery last?") should be answered in an honest and empathetic manner. For example, when asking about the length of surgery, patients may fixate on the time mentioned to them by the surgeon. They should be made aware that this time frame may be shorter than the actual time they are in the OR. Central lines are inserted preoperatively, and dressings are applied at the end of surgery: this may add an additional hour or more to the anticipated time frame. Waiting families may focus on the clock and worry unnecessarily if the time told to them by the surgeon passes. When there are delays (because of the prolonged surgery of a previous patient, for example, or difficulty weaning a patient from CPB), family members should be informed and periodically updated.

■ ■ ■

TABLE 23-5 PATIENT TEACHING CONTENT FOR CORONARY ARTERY BYPASS GRAFT SURGERY AND VALVE SURGERY

TOPIC	CABG SURGERY	VALVE SURGERY
Preoperative Pointers		
Medical diagnosis	Coronary artery occlusive disease	Valve regurgitation, stenosis or mixed
Diagnostic tests	ECG, chest radiograph, nuclear imaging, cardiac catheterization	Same, plus echocardiogram
Routine preoperative tests	CMP, ECG, T&C, pulmonary function, PT, PTT, INR	Same
Incision site	Midsternal or anterior thoracotomy; multiple leg incisions for vein harvest, arm incision for radial artery harvest	Mini- or full sternotomy
Resume eating	2-3 days after removal of ET and NG tubes	Same
Pain control	IM, PO, PCA	Same
Estimated length of procedure	4-6 hours	Same
Estimated length of hospital stay	5-7 days	6-8 days
Long-term effects of surgery	Loss of saphenous vein, possible intermittent lower leg ischemia	Possible chronic anticoagulation; differences between biologic and mechanical prostheses, valve repair
Drains or tubes	2 days: mediastinal chest tube, pleural tube; 2-3 days: leg drains, urinary drainage catheter	2 days: mediastinal and pleural tubes, urinary catheter
Postoperative Pointers/Home Instructions		
Food	Cardiac diet	Same
Wound care	Wounds covered if draining; redress after shower or bath; contact clinician if signs of infection	Same
Bathing	Daily	Same
Driving	4-6 weeks (automatic shift only)	Same
Sex	Restricted by limits of ability to bear weight on upper arms and chest	Same
Return to work	8-12 weeks	Same
Medications	Aspirin anticoagulant, cardiac drugs	Warfarin (Coumadin), cardiac drugs
Follow-up	7-14 days	Same, plus lab tests for determination of bleeding times
Special restrictions	Upper body movement restricted for 6 weeks for sternal healing	Same
Lifestyle changes	Reduction of coronary risk factors; rehabilitation	Risk factor reduction; rehabilitation
Worrisome but normal	Fatigue, swelling in leg; leg discomfort 4-6 weeks; weakness, emotional let down	Fatigue; sound of mechanical valve; weakness; emotional let down

CMP, Comprehensive metabolic panel (includes glucose, blood urea nitrogen, sodium, potassium, chloride, creatinine, albumin, bilirubin, calcium, alkaline phosphatase, total protein); *ECG,* electrocardiogram; *ET,* endotracheal; *IM,* intramuscular; *INR,* international normal ratio; *NG,* nasogastric; *PCA,* patient-controlled analgesia; *PO,* by mouth (per os); *PT,* prothrombin time; *PTT,* partial thromboplastin time; *T&C,* type and cross-match.
Modified from Fox VJ: Patient education and discharge planning. In Meeker MH, Rothrock JC, editors: *Alexander's care of the patient in surgery,* ed 11, St Louis, 1999, Mosby.
From Seifert PC: *Cardiac surgery: perioperative patient care,* St Louis, 2002, Mosby. Modified from Fox VJ: Patient education and discharge planning. In Meeker MH, Rothrock JC, editors: *Alexander's care of the patient in surgery,* ed 12, St Louis, 2003, Mosby.

Patients and family members have become generally well informed about many aspects of the OR and the surgery itself. Access to the Internet has enabled many to learn about their surgery and to communicate with others who share similar experiences. An important educational role for the nurse is to clarify or correct misconceptions or erroneous information that may be found on some Internet websites.

A Sterile Field

Competency to create and maintain a sterile field. The "sterile field" refers to the incised areas of the body and the surrounding tissue. For most cardiac surgery procedures, the field includes a midline sternal incision, the underlying heart and pericardium, and the surrounding anterior chest; right or left lateral chest wall incisions may be used for some procedures (Figure 23-4). Commonly, the operative field also includes the right and left

inguinal folds and surrounding tissue in anticipation of the need to insert a femoral arterial pressure line or an intraaortic balloon. When patients arrive in the OR with a balloon in place, the catheter exit site in the leg will be covered with a sterile impervious drape. The contralateral groin area will be made available should a central line be required. In patients undergoing CABG surgery using the saphenous vein, the legs become part of the field along with the anterior chest and groin areas. In these patients, inadvertent hypothermia is a concern because a large portion of the body is exposed. Therefore, active warming interventions (increasing room temperature, applying warm blankets and/or forced warm air devices, using IV fluid/blood warmers) should be used.

The field/incision sites are cleansed with an antiseptic solution. Often a sterile adhesive plastic drape, impregnated with an iodophor-based antiseptic, is applied to the anterior chest and legs. In iodophor-sensitive patients, nonimpregnated drapes are used. Sterile drapes

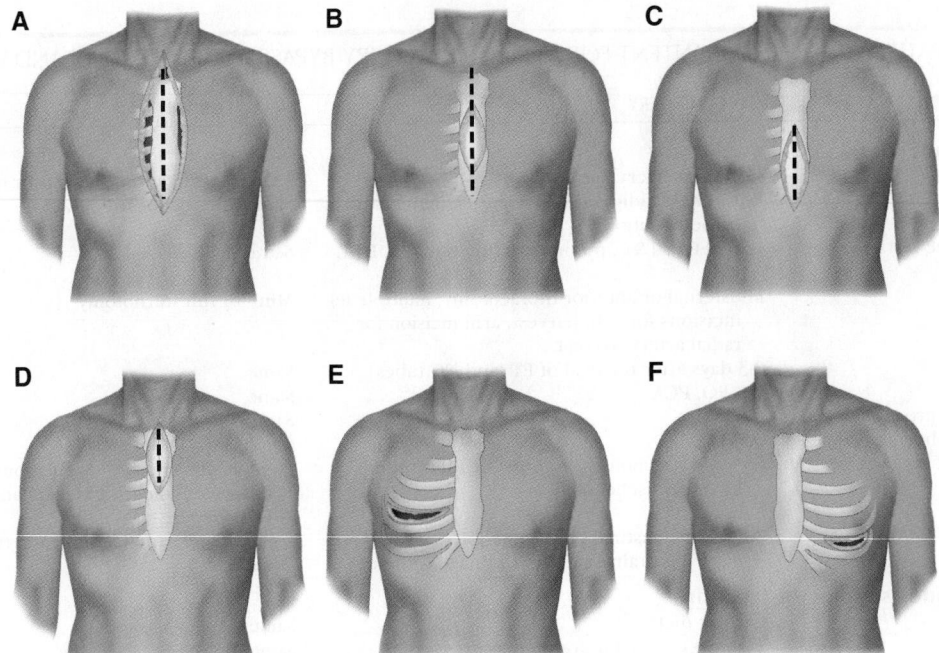

FIGURE 23-4 ■ Schematic representation of traditional incision and sternotomy (**A**) compared with a variety of less invasive incisions (*dotted lines* represent chest wall incisions). Limited skin incisions/full sternotomy (**B**) can offer a more cosmetically appealing appearance. Partial lower or upper sternotomy (**C** and **D**) may be used for pacemaker lead insertion or certain valve procedures. Limited right anterior thoracotomy (**E**) may be used in mitral valve reoperations. Anterior small thoracotomy (**F**) may be used in robotically assisted coronary artery bypass surgery. (From Adams DH, Filsoufi F, Antman EM: Medical management of the patient undergoing cardiac surgery. In Zipes DP, Libby P, Bonow RO, Braunwald E, editors: *Braunwald's heart disease,* ed 7, Philadelphia, 2005, Elsevier Saunders.)

then are placed around the planned incision sites and the potential incision sites (i.e., the groin area). When the patient is fully draped, the only exposed skin areas are the anterior chest, the inguinal areas, and the legs (in non-CABG patients, the legs generally are cleansed to the knee).

Anything coming into contact with the field and the patient's tissue must be sterile. Surgical instruments, supplies, drapes, catheters, internal defibrillator paddles, myocardial septal temperature probes, and other items must be sterilized before coming into contact with the area in which the operation is performed. The tables and other pieces of furniture on which sterile items are placed are covered with sterile drapes so that sterile items contact a sterile surface. Surgical personnel directly involved in the surgery must wear gloves and body-covering gowns that are sterile; hats and masks must be worn, but these are not required to be sterilized because the clinician's head would not make contact with the patient.

Sterilization methods used in health care settings include steam, ethylene oxide gas, peracetic acid, and gas plasma. Manufactured supplies may be sterilized with irradiation techniques.[13,14]

Equipment and Supplies

Competency to provide equipment and supplies based on patient needs. The cardiac OR contains a myriad of equipment used for making incisions, hemostasis, fibrillation, defibrillation, extracorporeal circulation, blood conservation, and irrigating fluids used for warming and cooling (Box 23-1). Much of this equipment is complex and potentially dangerous to patients and staff. Competency in using surgical equipment typically is achieved through a partnership among nurses, surgeons, educa-

---

BOX 23-1 ■ ■ ■
CARDIOVASCULAR OPERATING ROOM EQUIPMENT

- Defibrillator, cords, and paddles (internal and external)
- Fibrillator (to create a period of brief, controlled, fine fibrillation during which suture repairs may be made to anastomoses)
- Sternal saw and power source
- Cardiopulmonary bypass pump
- Headlight and light source
- Endoscopic light source
- Insufflation device for endoscopy
- Autotransfusion system (for autologous blood conservation)
- Discard suction system (for waste fluid disposal)
- Electrosurgical cutting/coagulation unit(s): monopolar and bipolar
- Ultrasonic cutting/coagulating devices
- External pacemaker generator
- Hypothermia/hyperthermia units (for topical solutions)
- Hypothermia/hyperthermia blankets
- Forced warm air units
- Positioning equipment (e.g., arm boards and leg holders)
- Radiofrequency generator, probes/catheters (for dysrhythmia surgery)
- Cryoablation units, probes/catheters (for dysrhythmia surgery)
- Laser (for transmyocardial revascularization)
- Robot (computerized, voice-activated, remotely controlled robotic device that can be used for retraction and digitized surgical manipulation in minimally invasive, endoscopic, video-assisted procedures)

tors, biomedical engineers, and manufacturers' representatives. Including the manufacturer is especially important because frequent change in technology mandates close communication with staff to enable them to retain their skill in the use of the technology. Some highly technical devices, such as the voice-activated, remotely manipulated, computer enhanced robot can be used to perform minimally invasive procedures that, in one study, resulted in significantly reduced length of stay.[15] The success of these newer, innovative techniques is especially dependent on the nurse's ability to communicate with surgical colleagues, to understand the use (and potential misuse) of these devices, and to be able to troubleshoot problems that may arise.

Complex devices and other machines are only one part of the cardiac inventory. An array of disposable and reusable supplies is available that may be no less complex than many of the machines in use. Surgical instruments, the most common reusable items, must be functioning properly to avoid injuring tissue. Vascular clamps, in particular, can tear or otherwise damage blood vessels if the jaws of the instrument are not aligned or have burrs. The care and storage of instruments has implications for the safety of patients. Sterile disposable supplies include the patient draping material, knife blades, syringes, hypodermic needles, gloves, gowns, suture, laparotomy pads and other "sponges," and other small items that are used for hemostasis, retraction, irrigation, suction, and sewing.

Another category of supplies is the prostheses. This inventory includes prosthetic replacement heart valves (mechanical and biological) and annuloplasty rings. Replacement valves and rings require manufacturer-specific sizers and implantation accessories. The perioperative nurse will ensure that the sizers/obturators used to measure the valve annulus correspond to the prosthesis planned for insertion. Using a sizer designed to measure one type of prosthetic valve for another kind of prosthesis can lead to implanting a prosthesis that does not fit properly and will require removal and insertion of a different prosthesis.

Graft material used to repair or replace sections of diseased blood vessels comes in the form of tubes or patches. Tube grafts (commonly Dacron) are available in graduated sizes; sizing accessories are used to determine the appropriate-size graft.

Sponge, Sharps, and Instrument Counts

Competency to perform sponge, sharps, and instrument counts. Accountability for ensuring that all foreign bodies are removed from the patient is an important nursing responsibility. Items, large and small, that may be retained inadvertently are counted before the incision is made (to determine a baseline) and are recounted before closing a body cavity (i.e., the pericardium) and again before the skin incision is closed.

Drug and Solution Administration

Competency to administer drugs and solutions as prescribed. Aside from the multiple drugs managed by anesthesia personnel, there is a wide array of medications and solutions within the surgical field (Table 23-6).[4] Antispasmodic drugs (papaverine) are used to reduce vascular spasm in the internal mammary artery and the radial artery. Topical irrigating solutions (saline, antibiotic drugs) and intracoronary infusions (containing potassium to achieve cardiac arrest) are among the drugs handled by perioperative nurses. All medica-

■ ■ ■

TABLE 23-6   MEDICATIONS USED IN ADULTS DURING CARDIAC SURGERY

MEDICATION	PURPOSE/DESCRIPTION/DELIVERY
Analgesics and Anesthetics	
Thiopental	Induction, ultra-short-acting barbiturate, intravenous bolus
Fentanyl (Sublimaze)	Synthetic narcotic, intravenous bolus and/or infusion
Sufentanil (Sufenta)	Synthetic narcotic, intravenous bolus and/or infusion
Alfentanil (Alfenta)	Synthetic narcotic, intravenous bolus and/or infusion
Morphine	Narcotic, intravenous bolus
Halothane (Fluothane)	Inhalation anesthetic, maintenance
Enflurane (Ethrane)	Inhalation anesthetic, maintenance
Isoflurane (Forane)	Inhalation anesthetic, maintenance
Methohexital (Brevital)	Three times more potent and faster clearance than thiopental
Remifentanil (Ultiva)	Synthetic narcotic, intravenous bolus and/or infusion
Propofol (Diprivan)	Intravenous anesthetic; bolus and/or infusion; very fast acting
Sevoflurane (Ultane)	Inhalation anesthetic, maintenance
Desflurane (Suprane)	Inhalation anesthetic, maintenance
Muscle Relaxants	
Vecuronium (Norcuron)	Intubation, maintenance of muscle relaxation
Pancuronium (Pavulon)	Maintenance of muscle relaxation
Pipecuronium	Maintenance of muscle relaxation; relatively free of circulatory effects
Rocuronium (Zemuron)	Fast-acting muscle relaxant; allows homodynamic stability

From Seifert PC: *Cardiac surgery: perioperative patient care,* St Louis, 2002, Mosby. Modified from Larach DR: Cardiovascular drugs. In Hensley FA, Martin DE, editors: *The practice of anesthesia,* Boston, 1990, Little, Brown; Morrill P: *AORN J* 71:173, 2000; Kervin MW, Wren KR, Haas RE, Farrer D: *CRNA* 9(3):93-98, 1998; and Grogan K, Nyhan D, Berkowitz DE: Pharmacology of anesthetic drugs. In Kaplan JA, editor: *Kaplan's cardiac anesthesia,* ed 5, Philadelphia, 2006, Elsevier Saunders.

Continued

TABLE 23-6   MEDICATIONS USED IN ADULTS DURING CARDIAC SURGERY—cont'd

MEDICATION	PURPOSE/DESCRIPTION/DELIVERY
Amnesiacs	
Midazolam (Versed)	Hypnotic; anxiety-reducing sedative
Scopolamine	Sedative; amnesic
Lorazepam (Avitan)	Hypnotic sedative; premedication
Cardiovascular Agents	
Anticholinergics	
Atropine	Decreases vagal tone; treats sinus bradycardia
Glycopyrrolate (Robinul)	Similar to atropine but has less incidence of dysrhythmias than atropine with slower onset
Vasopressors	
Norepinephrine (Levophed)	Increases force and velocity of contraction; increases systemic and pulmonary vascular resistance
Phenylephrine (Neo-Synephrine)	Arteriolar and venous vasoconstriction; increases blood pressure and systemic vascular resistance
Vasodilators	
Nitroglycerin (Tridil)	Dilates coronary arteries, reduces preload
Phentolamine (Regitine)	Decreases systemic and pulmonary vascular resistance
Prostaglandin E 1 (Prostin VR)	Vascular smooth muscle dilator, potent pulmonary vascular dilator; used to maintain patency of ductus arteriosus in cyanotic neonates, patients with severe pulmonary hypertension
Nitroprusside (Nipride)	Arteriolar and venous vasodilatation; reduces preload and afterload
Inotropic Agents	
Amrinone (Inocor)	Increases cardiac output, force and velocity of contraction
Calcium chloride	In ionized form, increases cardiac output, BP, and contractility
Dopamine (Intropin)	In low doses, increases renal and mesenteric perfusion; with moderate doses increases heart rate, contractility, and cardiac output; in higher doses increases systemic and pulmonary vascular resistance
Dobutamine (Dobutrex)	Increases contractility with less increase in heart rate than occurs with dopamine; has vasodilatation effect on vascular bed
Ephedrine	Increases contractility, cardiac output, and BP
Epinephrine (Adrenalin)	Increases rate and strength of contraction, BP (effective bronchodilator)
Isoproterenol (Isuprel)	Increases heart rate, contractility, cardiac output; decreases systemic vascular resistance
Milrinone	Increases cardiac output, force and velocity of contraction
Antidysrhythmics	
Lidocaine (Xylocaine)	Acts on ventricles; decreases automaticity of ischemic ventricular tissue
Bretylium (Bretylol)	Prolongs duration of action potential and refractory period; useful for ventricular dysrhythmias refractory to therapy
Digoxin (Lanoxin)	Decreases ventricular rate in atrial fibrillation or flutter and other supraventricular dysrhythmias; avoid in patients with Wolff-Parkinson-White syndrome and other accessory atrioventricular pathways
Nifedipine (Procardia)	Calcium channel blocker; reduces coronary artery spasm; produces coronary vasodilatation; extremely light sensitive; must be given PO or via nasal or oral mucosa; antihypertensive
Procainamide (Pronestyl)	Decreases automaticity and conduction in all cardiac tissue (normal and ischemic); stabilizes cellular membranes
Quinidine	Similar to procainamide; atrial and ventricular dysrhythmias
Verapamil (Calan, Isoptin)	Calcium channel blocker; used to treat atrial dysrhythmias; slows ventricular rate in atrial fibrillation or flutter; can be given IV
Adenosine	Supraventricular dysrhythmias
Diuretics	
Furosemide (Lasix)	Decreases renal absorption of sodium and chloride; increases excretion of water and electrolytes, especially potassium, sodium, chloride, magnesium, and calcium
Mannitol	Osmotic diuretic, pulls free water out of organs (reducing cerebral edema); protects kidneys
Anticoagulants/Coagulants	
Heparin	Systemic anticoagulation during CPB; blocks activation of thrombin (and intrinsic clotting cascade)
Protamine sulfate	Heparin antagonist; NPH insulin-dependent diabetic patients may be at increased risk for protamine reaction
Antibiotics	
Cephalosporins (Mandol, Ancef, Keflex, Keflin, Cefadyl)	Broad-spectrum prophylaxis
Tobramycin (Nebcin)	Aerobic gram-negative and gram-positive bacteria
Vancomycin	Severe endocarditis
Bacitracin	Topical irrigation
Miscellaneous	
Diazepam (Valium)	Sedative, induction of anesthesia
Nitric oxide (NO)	Vascular (especially pulmonary) relaxation; inhaled; reduces pulmonary hypertension
Lidocaine 1% (plain)	Local anesthesia
Papaverine	Reduces arterial spasm (e.g., mammary artery)
Potassium	Replaces electrolyte loss
Sodium bicarbonate	Corrects acidosis
Insulin (NPH, etc.)	Corrects hyperglycemia in diabetic patients
Topical hemostatic agents	Intraoperative control of bleeding
Desmopressin (DDAVP)	Pharmacologic hemostatic agent

BP, Blood pressure; *CPB,* cardiopulmonary bypass; *IV,* intravenous; *PO,* by mouth.

tion containers on and off the sterile field should be labeled.

Physiological Monitoring

Competency to physiologically monitor the patient during surgery. Monitoring of the cardiovascular, respiratory, central nervous system, and renal system is needed (Table 23-7).[4] Although monitoring is a primary responsibility of the anesthesia providers, it is a multidisciplinary responsibility with nurses, physicians, and technologists sharing in this essential function. Nurses functioning as the room manager (i.e., the circulating nurse), the scrub nurse, or the surgical assistant remain alert to electrocardiographic and hemodynamic changes as seen on the monitors and compare these with the heart itself. So too does the surgeon correlate waveforms and numbers from monitoring devices to visual functioning of the heart. Cardiovascular technologists may be available to manage the monitoring equipment and troubleshoot equipment problems. For example, perfusionists who run the CPB machine monitor various parameters during the period when the patient is supported by the bypass pump. The surgeon may be focused on a small area of extracardiac anatomy when a patient fibrillates, and the surgical assistant or anesthesia provider may alert the surgeon to the fibrillating heart. All this occurs during a period of 2 to 3 seconds, but it attests to everyone's responsibility to observe and communicate promptly.

■ ■ ■

TABLE 23-7   PHYSIOLOGICAL MONITORING

MONITORING DEVICE	LOCATION	ASSESSES/MEASURES
Cardiovascular System		
Electrocardiogram (ECG)	Electrodes placed on shoulders, hips, and left axillary line	Electrical activity of heart: lead II useful to monitor cardiac rhythm (good visualization of P wave and QRS) and myocardial ischemia (inferior surface); lead V5 useful to detect myocardial ischemia (anterior surface)
Intraarterial catheter	Radial artery (also femoral artery) aorta, bypass circuit, in children, may use superficial temporal or dorsalis pedis arteries; in neonates, may use umbilical artery	Direct arterial blood pressure (BP); blood gases; blood chemistries
Blood pressure cuff	Right or left arm	Indirect BP
Central venous pressure (CVP) line	Right atrium (RA)	RA pressure (CVP); right ventricular (RV) filling pressure; RV preload
Pulmonary artery (PA) catheter (addition of fiberoptics provides additional information about mixed venous oxygen saturation [SVO_2])	PA (proximal and distal)	PA pressures: systolic, diastolic, mean, wedge; pulmonary vascular resistance; left ventricular (LV) filling pressure; LV preload; cardiac output (CO); assessment of stroke volume, stroke work, systemic vascular resistance; mixed venous saturation (continuous indirect assessment of CO and reflection of tissue oxygenation); RV function
Left atrial (LA) catheter (when used)	LA	LA pressure (direct); LV filling pressure; LV preload
Transesophageal echocardiography (TEE)	Esophagus	Valve function before and after repair; LV wall motion, failure; intracardiac air bubbles
Urinary drainage catheter	Urinary bladder	Urinary output, renal perfusion; indirect measure of CO
Respiratory System		
Mass spectrometry	Anesthesia circuit	Inspired/expired O_2, CO_2, and anesthetic gases; used to avoid hypoxia, hypercarbia, anesthetic overdose
Pulse oximeter	Finger or toe cot; earlobe, nose	Oxygen saturation of arterial hemoglobin; tissue oxygenation
Capnography	Anesthesia circuit	End-tidal CO_2; used to detect integrity of anesthesia circuit; avoid disconnections of monitor, endotracheal tube; detect spontaneous ventilation, rebreathing, obstructive pulmonary disease
Central Nervous System		
Temperature	Esophagus, nasopharynx, urinary bladder, rectum, ventricular septum, bypass circuit, PA catheter	Core and peripheral temperature of heart, brain, and other organs
Electroencephalogram	Scalp electrodes	Detect cerebral ischemia, embolus; indication of depth of anesthesia
Renal System		
Urinary drainage catheter	Bladder	Urinary output; indirect measure of cardiac output

BP, Blood pressure.

From Seifert PC: *Cardiac surgery: perioperative patient care,* St Louis, 2002, Mosby. Modified from Charney JR: Cardiothoracic anesthesia. In Baumgartner FJ, editor: *Cardiothoracic surgery,* ed 4, Philadelphia, 1999, Saunders; and Reich DL, Mittnacht AJ, London MJ, Kaplan JA: Monitoring of the heart and vascular system. In Kaplan JA, editor: *Kaplan's cardiac anesthesia,* ed 5, Philadelphia, 2006, Elsevier Saunders.

Environmental Monitoring and Control

Competency to monitor and control the environment. Internal and external (ambient room) temperature control is another safety factor. When a patient enters the OR, warm blankets are applied and the thermostat is set at approximately 70°F to prevent shivering. When CPB is to be used, the heat exchanger within the bypass circuit regulates the temperature of the circulating blood by cooling or warming the blood as indicated. External devices such as forced warm air blankets may be used, but their application may be restricted to placement along the patient's side because most of the anterior body is made accessible for chest and leg incisions. When the legs do not need to be exposed (or when the GSV has been excised and the leg incision is closed), sterile drapes may be placed over the legs to conserve heat. These drapes need to be removable because a femoral artery pressure line or intraaortic balloon may be inserted during the procedure.

Other environmental considerations include controlling traffic in and out of the OR and adhering to safety policies and procedure (such as sanitation, hazardous material, and fire evacuation). Proper waste disposal and cleaning procedures are also part of the perioperative nurse's environmental responsibilities.

Patient Rights

Competency to respect patients' rights. Respect for patients' rights can be demonstrated by actions such as those that ensure confidentiality of information, the competence of caregivers, the safe use of supplies and equipment, adequate information that facilitates true informed consent to surgery, and respect for ethnic, religious, and cultural differences. These rights are articulated in documents such as the American Hospital Association Patient's Bill of Rights, the American Nurses Association *Code of Ethics for Nurses with Interpretive Statements,*[16] and AORN *Explications for Perioperative Nursing,*[17] which interprets and applies the American Nurses Association Code of Ethics provisions to the perioperative setting. For some cardiac patients there may be ethical or religious concerns about receiving blood or blood products or about having a porcine heart valve implanted. Ideally, these patients are identified before surgery so that, whenever possible, care can be tailored to fit the patient's beliefs.

EVALUATION
Accountability

Competency to perform nursing actions that demonstrate accountability. Nurses have a duty to remain current with the newest technologies, scientific evidence, and patient care practices occurring in the OR, and this requires life-long learning in addition to a basic orientation and mandatory continuing education. Flexibility and adaptability are prerequisites for good decision making in situations in which the patient's status suddenly changes or an unanticipated event occurs (such as an electrical power outage or a malfunctioning sternal saw). Contingency planning—such as having a back-up saw immediately available—in anticipation of changes demonstrates professional accountability.

Accountability also is demonstrated by communicating perioperative patient information to the receiving surgical intensive care unit. This communication promotes a smooth transition for the patient and provides information that will assist critical care colleagues to perform their care efficiently and effectively (Box 23-2).[4]

Patient Outcomes

Competency to evaluate patient outcomes. Determining whether patient outcomes have been achieved is predicated on measuring the degree of goal achievement with objective criteria (such a laboratory tests, accounting for all extraneous objects used within the surgical field, morbidity and mortality data), nurses' observations, and subjective assessments such as patients' responses. Box 23-3 lists perioperative patient outcomes in the three domains of safety, physiological responses, and patient and family behavioral responses.[2,7] Safety-related outcomes refer to freedom from injury from environmental, physical, medication,

---

BOX 23-2 ■ ■ ■
PATIENT TRANSFER REPORT

Procedure (include source of autogenous grafts and use of endoscopic vein harvest):

Monitoring Devices

CVP _____	Arterial line _____
Swan _____	Peripheral lines _____
CPB _____	off-pump _____

Intraoperative Occurrences

Blood loss _____	BP _____
Dysrhythmias _____	Bypass problems _____
Defib 3 _____	Lo temp _____
Setting _____	Hi temp _____
Cross-clamp time _____	Pump time _____
CO _____ CI _____	Urine _____

Blood: Given _____   Available _____
Autotransfusion totals: ml   Units
Components: FFP   Platelets   Cryo
Additional ordered (type) _____

Medications

Neo _____	Dopamine _____	Dobutamine _____
Lidocaine _____	Nitro _____	Levophed _____
Epinephrine _____	Nitroprusside _____	Inocor _____
DDAVP _____	Aprotinin _____	other _____

Tubes/drains: Mediastinal   Pleural

Epicardial leads: Atrial _____   Ventricular _____
Pacing: Yes/No   Rate _____

Labs: K$^+$ _____   Na1 _____   Glu _____   Mg^{++} _____
   Hgb _____   Hct _____   Other _____

Patient concerns _____
Additional information _____
ICU bed No.   ETA   Reported by
   To _____   Time _____

From Seifert PC: *Cardiac surgery: perioperative patient care,* St Louis, 2002, Mosby.

BOX 23-3
PERIOPERATIVE PATIENT OUTCOMES   ■ ■ ■

Domain: Patient Safety
- Freedom from signs and symptoms of injury related to the following:
  - Chemical, electrical, laser, and radiation hazards
  - Retained extraneous/foreign bodies
  - Positioning
  - Transfer/transport
  - Medication administration

Domain: Physiological Responses
- Freedom from signs and symptoms of infection
- Wound/tissue perfusion consistent with or improved from preoperative baseline levels
- At or returning to normothermia immediately postoperatively
- Cardiovascular, respiratory, and neurological functions consistent with or improved from preoperative baseline levels
- Fluid, electrolyte, and acid-base balances consistent with or improved from preoperative baseline levels
- Adequate pain control reported or demonstrated throughout the perioperative period

Domain: Behavioral Responses—Patient and Family
- Demonstrates knowledge of the following:
  - Wound healing
  - Expected responses to the operative or invasive procedure
  - Nutritional requirements related to the operative or invasive procedure
  - Medication management
  - Pain management
- Participates in decisions affecting his or her perioperative plan of care
- Care is consistent with perioperative plan of care
- Participates in rehabilitation process
- Right to privacy is maintained
- Receives competent and ethical care within legal standards of practice
- Receives consistent and comparable care regardless of setting
- Value system, lifestyle, ethnicity, and culture are considered, respected, and incorporated into the plan of care

Adapted from Association of periOperative Registered Nurses: Perioperative patient outcomes. In *2005 standards, recommended practices, and guidelines,* Denver, Colo, 2005-2006, The Association.

and other hazards that nurses control to protect patients. Outcome achievement is reflected in the absence of injury. The domain of physiological responses includes nursing interventions to prevent infection or impaired tissue perfusion, to promote adequate pain control, and to maintain adequate cardiovascular, renal, neurological, and other organ function. Outcome achievement can be measured by laboratory reports, hemodynamic records, and patient responses. Patient and family behavioral responses demonstrate whether they have the knowledge needed to participate actively in the perioperative, recovery, recuperation, and rehabilitation periods. This domain also addresses privacy rights, ethical and legal standards, and respect for diversity of values, cultures, and beliefs. Outcome achievement can be demonstrated by patient/family responses to questions eliciting understanding of the planned surgery, patient satisfaction surveys and verbal feedback, and participation in rehabilitation programs.

In addition to specific perioperative nursing outcome statements, there are other ways to measure the prediction and achievement of patient outcomes. The institutional quality indicator reports can provide information

to evaluate patients' outcomes and suggest improvements in the planning and delivery of care. Cardiac programs also may participate in the Society of Thoracic Surgeons *(www.sts.org)* database,[18] which compares the clinical outcomes of the participating institutions' cardiac patients to regional and national standards. A similar database maintained by the American College of Cardiology at *www.acc.org* tracks interventional cardiology. The National Quality Forum publishes 21 National Voluntary Consensus Standards for Cardiac Surgery[19] that reflect hospital-level structure, process, and risk-adjusted outcome consensus standards along with related research and implementation recommendations. The European System for Cardiac Operative Risk Evaluation (EuroSCORE) is a large patient database that was developed for the prediction of in-hospital mortality after adult cardiac surgery,[20] and it has been shown to be valuable in predicting early mortality after heart valve surgery.[21] From the results of these and other databases, clinicians can identify areas of strength and areas for improvement in achieving desired outcomes.

Effectiveness of Nursing Care

Competency to measure effectiveness of nursing care. The ability to measure nursing care is facilitated with quality improvement data, nursing-specific outcome criteria, peer review, patient interviews and surveys, and physical assessment. These resources and processes enable the nurse to scrutinize the effectiveness of actions. If a wound infection develops, for example, review the perioperative care to identify practices that may require improvement. Perhaps antibiotic prophylaxis was not infused before the incision; the nurse can work with anesthesia personnel to ensure that required medications are given in a timely manner. Perhaps aseptic practices require review and improvement. Standards of care related to asepsis and other practices may require revision; additional standards can be created to reflect newer technologies and clinical trends.[22] Interviewing the patient and family postoperatively also can provide insights into the perceived quality of and satisfaction with the care received. Patient feedback is especially helpful for refining future patient teaching.

Interventions or patient goals that require revision also may be identified. Efforts directed toward improving interventions may reflect a quality improvement initiative or evidence-based changes in practice. Revising patient goals can be achieved by communicating with the patient throughout the perioperative experience, soliciting concerns and recommendations, ensuring that the patient has sufficient information for decision making, and incorporating patient/family suggestions into the plan of care whenever feasible.

Reassessment

Competency to continuously reassess all components of patient care based on new data. Patient care is a dynamic process that is changing continually as the patient's status changes. Diseases of the cardiovascular system are associated with sudden hemodynamic changes, and nurses need to respond to those changes promptly and effectively in a collaborative manner. In patients who have had previous cardiac surgery via a median sternotomy, anticipate dense adhesions between the sternum and pericardium (seen in the lateral chest x-ray film). These adhesions are dissected sharply to free the heart from the surrounding adherent pericardium. Although there tends to be some bleeding from small epicardial blood vessels, be alert to sudden, severe hemorrhage from myocardial tears or lacerations and work collaboratively with the surgeon to achieve hemostasis.

Nurses must be adaptable, flexible, and creative problem solvers in the cardiac OR where changes in the patient's health status are common. Nurses are important partners with surgeons, anesthesia providers, perfusionists, and other members of the cardiac team; joint problem solving, frequent communication, and collaborative working relationships facilitate optimal outcomes.

REFERENCES

1. Association of periOperative Registered Nurses: Competency statements. In *AORN standards, recommended practices & guidelines,* Denver, Colo, 2005 2006, The Association.
2. Beyea SC: *Perioperative nursing data set: the perioperative nursing vocabulary,* ed 2, Denver, Colo, 2002, The Association.
3. Adams DH, Filsoufi F, Antman EM: Medical management of the patient undergoing cardiac surgery. In Zipes DP, Libby P, Bonow RO, Braunwald E, editors: *Braunwald's heart disease,* ed 7, Philadelphia, 2005, Elsevier Saunders.
4. Seifert PC: *Cardiac surgery: perioperative patient care,* St Louis, 2002, Mosby.
5. Eagle KA, Guyton RA, Davidoff R, et al: ACC/AHA 2004 Guideline update for coronary artery bypass graft surgery: a report of the American College of Cardiology/American Heart Association Task Force on Practice Guidelines. *Circulation* 2004; 110(14) 340-437.
6. Norton C: The family's experience with critical illness. In Morton PG, Fontaine D, Hudak CM, Gallo BM, editors: *Critical care nursing: a holistic approach,* ed 8, Philadelphia, 2005, Lippincott Williams & Wilkins.
7. Association of periOperative Registered Nurses: Perioperative patient outcomes. In *AORN standards, recommended practices & guidelines,* Denver, Colo, 2005 2006, The Association.
8. Kouchoukos N, Blackstone EH, Doty DB et al: *Kirklin/Barratt-Boyes cardiac surgery,* vol 1, ed 3, Philadelphia, 2003, Churchill Livingstone.
9. Waldhausen JA, Pierce WS, Campbell DB: *Surgery of the chest,* ed 6, St Louis, 1996, Mosby.
10. Tatoulis J, Buxton BF, Fuller JA: Patencies of 2217 arterial to coronary conduits over 15 years, *Ann Thorac Surg* 77:93-101, 2004.
11. Buxton B, Frazier OH, Westaby S, editors: *Ischemic heart disease: surgical management,* London, 1999, Mosby.
12. Mordiffi SZ, Tan SP, Wong MK: Information provided to surgical patients versus information needed, *AORN J* 77(3):546-561, 2003.
13. Fogg DM: Infection prevention and control. In Rothrock JC, editor: *Alexander's care of the patient in surgery,* ed 12, St Louis, 2003, Mosby.
14. Lafreniere R, Berguer R, Seifert PC et al: Preparation of the operating room. In Souba WW, Fink MP, Jurkovich GJ et al, editors: *ACS surgery: principles & practice 2004,* New York, 2004, WebMD.
15. Subramanian VA, Patel NU, Patel NC et al: Robotic assisted multivessel minimally invasive direct coronary artery bypass with port-access stabilization and cardiac positioning: paving the way for outpatient coronary surgery? *Ann Thorac Surg* 79:1590-1596, 2005.
16. American Nurses Association: *Code of ethics for nurses with interpretive statements,* Washington, DC, 2001, The Association.
17. Association of periOperative Registered Nurses: Explications for perioperative nursing. In *AORN standards, recommended practices & guidelines,* Denver, Colo, 2005 2006, The Association.
18. Orringer MB: STS database activities and you: "What's in it for me?" *Ann Thorac Surg* 72:1, 2001.
19. National Quality Forum: *National voluntary consensus standards for cardiac surgery,* Washington, DC, 2004, The Forum.
20. Roques F, Nashef SA, Michel P et al: Risk factors and outcome in European cardiac surgery: analysis of the EuroSCORE multinational database of 19030 patients, *Eur J Cardiothorac Surg* 15:816-822, 1999.
21. Toumpoulis IK, Anagnostopoulis CE, Toumpoulis SK et al: EuroSCORE predicts long-term mortality after heart valve surgery, *Ann Thorac Surg* 79:1902-1908, 2005.
22. Stephens-Lesser D: *Cardiac surgery manual for nurses: orientation, policy, and procedures,* Boston, 2007, Jones and Bartlett Publishers.

■■■■ c h a p t e r **24**

Nurses in Outpatient Clinics

Sara Paul

CHAPTER ABBREVIATIONS

APN   advanced practice nurse
CNS   clinical nurse specialist
NP   nurse practitioner

The role of nurses in outpatient settings goes back to the early 20th century when visiting nurses provided health care to patients in their homes. In the 1960s, advanced practice nurses (**APN**s) began to have a role in outpatient clinics with nurse practitioners (**NP**s) who diagnosed and treated patients in an ambulatory setting.[1] Initially, NPs cared for the underserved population: persons living in rural settings, low-income and minority populations, and uninsured patients.[2] In recent years the role of the NP and other APNs (such as clinical nurse specialists [**CNS**s]) has expanded to include acute care, long-term care, and a more independent outpatient care role.

Physicians are increasingly busy performing procedures and managing complex patients in the hospital, and nurses are assuming the outpatient management of cardiovascular diseases. In outpatient settings, it is common for an APN's practice to include inpatient activities such as patient rounds, case management, and discharge planning, as well as responsibility for medical management of clinic patients.

Because nurses emphasize disease prevention, health promotion, and comprehensive care, they are well suited to manage patients who are at high risk for disease progression or poor clinical outcomes. Patients with cardiovascular disease fall into this category and require close and frequent follow-up. Clinical conditions that require close monitoring, frequent follow-up, and in-depth patient and family education are well served by nurses. Research shows that outcomes are improved in certain populations when patients are enrolled in outpatient nurse-managed clinics or programs.[3,4]

In addition to direct care, nurses have an important role in educating patients and families about their disease. Our holistic approach includes the assessment of financial and community resources and individual and family issues. In outpatient cardiovascular clinics, nurses often manage programs such as lipid, anticoagulation, heart failure, and transplant clinics (Box 24-1). In this chapter, the many roles of nurses in outpatient cardiovascular clinics are discussed.

SCOPE OF ADVANCED PRACTICE NURSING

There are approximately 120,449 registered NPs and 69,017 registered nurses who have the education and credentials to practice as CNSs in the United States (Figure 24-1).[5,6] The term *advanced practice nurse* encompasses the roles of NP, CNS, nurse-midwife, and nurse anesthetist; however, NP and CNS are the advanced practice roles most involved in managing patients with cardiovascular disease in outpatient clinics. For the purpose of this chapter, the term *advanced practice nurse* (or the abbreviation) will refer to NPs and CNSs. The American Nurses Association defines an NP as a "skilled health care provider who utilizes critical judgment in the performance of comprehensive health assessments, differential diagnosis, and the prescribing of pharmacologic and non-pharmacologic treatments in the direct management of acute and chronic illness and disease."[7] The CNS is defined as "an expert clinician in a specialized area of nursing practice." The specialized area may be defined in terms of a patient population (e.g., pediatrics or geriatrics), a setting (e.g., critical care or emergency room), a disease or medical subspecialty (e.g., cardiovascular or neurosurgery), a type of care (e.g., psychiatric or rehabilitation), or a type of problem (e.g., diabetes, pain, or wounds).[5]

The scope of APN practice usually involves all or some of the following: formulating differential diagnoses, managing acute and chronic illness, promoting health and wellness, and applying clinical reasoning skills.[8,9] APNs with different educational backgrounds and variable individual expertise may operationalize their roles in a variety of ways in the ambulatory setting. For instance, NPs traditionally have been direct care providers, whereas CNSs usually focus on one aspect of care, such as managing a foot clinic, diabetes education, weight management,[8] or working with staff nurses to effect change in a specific population.[10] Regardless of the role, advanced nursing practice has been described as "the deliberate, purposeful and integrated use of expanded nursing knowledge, research and clinical practice expertise, grounded in the profession's values of holistic, patient-centered care."[11,12] APNs are academically prepared at the master's or doctoral level and practice under their own nursing license. In contrast to APNs, physician assistants do not possess a nursing (or even necessarily a health care) background and practice primarily in a medical model of care under a physician's license.

303

BOX 24-1   ■ ■ ■
EXAMPLES OF NURSE-MANAGED SUBSPECIALTY
CARDIOVASCULAR CLINICS AND PROGRAMS

- Anticoagulation clinic
- Amiodarone clinic
- Heart failure clinic
- Lipid clinic
- Device clinic
- Rehabilitation
- Prevention programs
- Patient support groups
- Patient/family education programs
- Clinical investigational trials

ESSENTIAL NURSE COMPETENCIES IN OUTPATIENT CARDIOVASCULAR CLINICS

Competencies may be described as "a cluster of knowledge, attitudes, and skills that affects a major part of one's job, correlates with performance on the job, and can be measured against well-accepted standards."[13] The National Council of State Boards of Nursing regards competency as knowledge application with interpersonal decision-making and psychomotor skills, as used in the context of public health, welfare, and safety and applied within the nurse's practice role.[14] The Canadian Nurses Association defines competencies as "the specific knowledge, skills, judgment and personal attributes required for a registered nurse to practice safely and ethically in a designated role and setting."[15]

The American Nurses Credentialing Center describes the staff nurse role in ambulatory care as providing "direct and indirect care in a defined ambulatory care setting to individual patients/clients, families and communities."[16] Competencies of staff nurses include the assessment, planning and delivery of care, and the evaluation of the patient's response to that care. Staff nurses in outpatient clinics assist patients in promoting wellness, preventing illness, and managing their disease. These nurses also ensure the smooth flow of patients through the outpatient clinic by setting up systems to organize patient care. Competencies for staff nurses are summarized in Box 24-2.

The competencies involved in advanced nursing practice differ from basic nursing in that an APN has a "greater depth and breadth of knowledge, a greater degree of synthesis of data, and complexity of skills and interventions."[7] According to Hamric and Hanson,[17] core APN competencies include expert clinical practice, coaching and guidance, consultation, research, leadership, collaboration, and ethical decision making. Competencies that an APN may need in outpatient management of cardiovascular disease are listed in Box 24-3.

The scope of practice for an APN is defined by each state as those actions that are legally allowed in the Nurse Practice Act or Advanced Nursing Practice Act of that state. According to the American Nurses Association, the APN scope of practice is to "provide comprehensive health assessments and demonstrate a high level of autonomy and expert skill in the diagnosis and treatment of the complex human responses of individuals, families, or communities to actual or potential health problems."[7]

The role of the APN in outpatient cardiovascular clinics varies, depending on the setting and the institution.

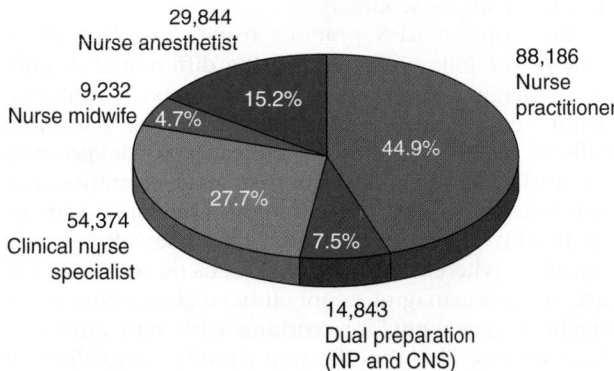

Registered Nurses Prepared for Advanced Practice, March 2000

FIGURE 24-1 ■ Advanced practice nurses include clinical nurse specialists, nurse anesthetists, nurse-midwives, and nurse practitioners. It is estimated that 196,279 registered nurses, or 7.3 percent of the registered nurse population, were prepared to practice in at least one of these advanced practice roles in March 2000. The largest group of advanced practice nurses was nurse practitioners, followed by clinical nurse specialists. These two groups together, including those with dual preparation of nurse practitioner and clinical nurse specialist, make up an estimated 80 percent of all advanced practice nurses. (Data from National Sample Survey of Registered Nurses, compiled by U.S. Department of Health and Human Services, Health Resources and Service Administration, Bureau of Health Professions, Division of Nursing, 2000.)

BOX 24-2   ■ ■ ■
STAFF NURSE COMPETENCIES IN AN OUTPATIENT
CARDIOVASCULAR CLINIC

- Controls the flow of patients through the clinic
- Communicates effectively, respectfully, and compassionately with patients and their families
- Obtains vital signs and other information using appropriate technique, such as using appropriately sized blood pressure cuff, counting apical heart rate for 1 minute, placing electrocardiogram electrodes in correct anatomical positions, performing thorough examination of all peripheral pulses, and auscultating for arterial bruits
- Notifies health care provider immediately of any abnormal findings in vital signs, history, or physical assessment
- Records and maintains a list of current and past patient medications at each visit
- Obtains or schedules laboratory studies or procedures as prescribed by the physician or advanced practice nurse
- Assists with in-office procedures
- Performs procedures such as electrocardiogram, ankle/brachial index, blood draws, assessing oxygen saturation
- Assesses patient and caregiver's knowledge of skills necessary to care for the cardiovascular patient at home
- Reinforces information as provided by the physician or advanced practice nurse
- Obtains medical records as needed
- Appreciates the influence of attitudes, roles, language, culture, race, religion, gender, and lifestyle on how families provide care to patients with cardiovascular disease
- Encourages patients to prepare advance directives for medical care
- Continues to expand one's own current knowledge of health care through continuing education

BOX 24-3
ADVANCED PRACTICE NURSE COMPETENCIES IN AN OUTPATIENT CARDIOVASCULAR CLINIC

- Demonstrates knowledge of the cardiovascular system and the pathophysiological process of cardiovascular diseases and vascular diagnoses
- Demonstrates knowledge of diagnosis, management, and complications for various cardiovascular diseases and conditions
- Conducts a thorough client-centered history and physical examination focusing on the cardiovascular system
- Conducts a pharmacological assessment, including polypharmacy, drug interactions, over-the-counter and herbal product use, ability to purchase medications, and safely and correctly self-administer medications
- Orders, collects, and interprets appropriate laboratory and diagnostic tests on patients
- Develops a plan of treatment with goals and actions to achieve the best outcomes possible for patients
- Prescribes appropriate pharmacological agents, treatments, and nonpharmacological therapies in order to manage and treat cardiovascular conditions
- Assesses patient's and caregiver's ability to execute plan of care
- Assesses patient's response to therapy through interim history, physical examination, laboratory data, and appropriate diagnostic testing in the outpatient clinic
- Reviews treatment options and facilitates decision making with the patient, family, and other caregivers
- Consults with other disciplines and specialties as needed to make sure comorbidities are addressed appropriately
- Educates patients and families about the cardiovascular disease process, treatment strategies, and expectations of outcomes
- Emphasizes health promotion and maintenance, as well as risk factor reduction for cardiovascular disease prevention
- Assesses the ability of the individual and family to manage lifestyle changes, resilience, and coping strategies
- Uses an ethical framework to address individual and family concerns about caregiving, management of the patient's disease, lifestyle changes, and end-of-life issues
- Coordinates care with home health providers and other community resources, with special attention to chronic or end-of-life needs
- Uses telephone contact with patients to monitor for early recognition of potential problems, and to follow-up on response to treatment, test results, and more
- Uses adult learning principles in patient, family, and caregiver education, such as educational level of instructions, adequate time to learn and respond, need for individualized instruction, integration of information, and use of multiple strategies of communication
- Facilitates access to hospice and palliative care to maximize a peaceful, pain-free, and compassionate death for patients with end-stage cardiovascular disease
- Disseminates the knowledge required to care for cardiovascular patients to other health care workers through peer education, staff development, and preceptor experiences
- Provides leadership skills in directing others in patient care activities
- Continues to expand own knowledge of health care through continuing education
- Performs or coordinates research studies as appropriate; utilizes research data in improving patient care

Some APN practices incorporate inpatient activities such as patient rounds, case management, clinical care, and discharge planning, in addition to outpatient clinic responsibilities. This offers a seamless continuum of care from the inpatient setting to the outpatient clinic and home management. Specific competencies are summarized next.

Encouraging Self-Care and Behavioral Change

Preparing patients to manage their disease, condition, or symptoms at home is an important responsibility of nurses in outpatient clinics. Cardiovascular diseases require patients or caregivers to engage in self-care activities such as recognizing a change in signs or symptoms and taking action to implement a self-care treatment strategy in response to those signs or symptoms. Examples include increasing a diuretic dose when swelling occurs in those with heart failure or using a sublingual nitroglycerin tablet for angina in the presence of coronary artery disease. Health maintenance behaviors of self-care involve healthful lifestyle practices such as eating a low-fat or low-sodium diet, getting adequate rest and exercise, and adhering to the prescribed medication regimen.[18]

Patients can perform self-care activities only if they are educated about signs and symptoms that signal a potential problem that requires them to take action. They must be taught the appropriate actions to take, and they must be able to evaluate the effectiveness of their action and whether they need to contact their health care provider or seek emergency care. Nurses directly teach self-care information or collaborate with other disciplines that also educate patients, such as dietitians and pharmacists.

Patients vary considerably in their level of readiness to make lifestyle changes. Prochaska and colleagues[19] proposed six stages of readiness for behavior change, ranging from being unaware that a change is necessary (precontemplation) to engaging consistently in a desired behavior (maintenance). They proposed that individuals be evaluated to determine their level of readiness to change. The processes used by clinicians to encourage change should be tailored to the appropriate level of readiness.[20] Assessing and intervening with patients, based on their stage of readiness to change, is a core competency of nurses working in outpatient clinics. See Chapter 83 for a complete discussion of the stages of change model.

Facilitating Collaborative Relationships

Patients with cardiovascular disease often have comorbidities (e.g., diabetes, obesity, or renal disease) that complicate their disease and combine to increase risk for poor outcomes. Nutritional counseling benefits these patients by teaching them the appropriate dietary choices to control their disease and reduce the risk of worsening their condition. In turn, control of comorbidities can improve risk factors and reduce complications. Examples of collaborative relationships for outpatient management of patients with comorbidities and complex management needs are listed in Box 24-4.

The development and maintenance of collaborative relationships with other disciplines and community agencies is an essential core competency of nurses in outpatient clinics. For example, nurse-physician collaboration in primary care has been shown to improve diabetic patients' blood sugars, blood pressure, quality of life, and self-care efficacy.[21]

BOX 24-4 ■ ■ ■
IMPORTANT COLLABORATIVE RELATIONSHIPS FOR OUTPATIENT MANAGEMENT OF CARDIOVASCULAR DISEASE

- Cardiac rehabilitation specialist
- Nutritionist/dietitian
- Endocrinologist
- Diabetic nurse educator
- Weight management center
- Smoking cessation program
- Lipid management specialist
- Primary care physicians
- Nephrologist
- Outpatient infusion unit
- Anticoagulation clinic staff
- Lipid clinic staff
- Inpatient hospital advanced practice nurses

FRAMEWORK FOR OUTPATIENT CARDIOVASCULAR CLINICS

The care of cardiovascular patients in the ambulatory setting is a dynamic and long-term process because cardiovascular disease is rarely "cured." Nurses in outpatient clinics care for patients throughout the spectrum of their illness, continuing to support and educate them at various phases of their disease. Continuity of care is a benefit of working in outpatient clinics. APNs based solely in an outpatient clinic generally have a little more time to spend with patients because they are not expected to perform complex procedures and do not have inpatient responsibilities that consume their time. To achieve optimal outcomes, the structure of the clinic and the process in which patients receive care must be integrated successfully.[22] (See Figure 24-1.)

Structure

The structure that supports an outpatient clinic is made up of the practice environment where patients receive their care, the population that is being served, and the health care system in which the outpatient clinic is based. The practice environment of the clinic may be a hospital-based outpatient setting, a private cardiology office, vascular surgery clinic, primary care practice, or a nurse-run clinic. The environment must be adequate to provide service to the population of patients in a timely manner, and patient privacy must be paramount. Parking should be readily available without a long or uphill walk into the clinic building. An appropriately sized waiting room and an adequate number of examination rooms are needed to avoid having the patients wait for long periods. The tools needed to examine patients should be readily available to the provider, such as blood pressure cuffs, portable Doppler ultrasound, and emergency equipment.

The structure is designed to support the patient population being served. The physical location of the clinic building may determine the patient population that attends the clinic, or the clinic may be placed in a location near the desired patient population, such as in an urban setting or adjacent to a hospital. Patients may come from a mixed-payer group, or they may be uninsured. The latter patients may require assistance in obtaining medications, and it may be necessary to employ someone to oversee the drug card or pharmaceutical assistance application process. If there is a large ethnic population with poor English language skills, signage, interpreters, or at least a language line such as that available from AT&T *(www.languageline.com/)* are important for communication. A highly educated patient population may be open to printed patient teaching materials, but patients who have difficulty reading require creative teaching techniques such as videos or picture books. An important competency of nurses working in outpatient clinics is knowledge of these issues and the skill to assess them. (See the Evidence-Based Practice feature.)

The health care system that supports the outpatient clinic will have an important influence on the APN's role and may determine whether the APN can bill for professional services. If the APN's salary is paid by a hospital, and the clinic is operated as an outpatient hospital clinic, the APN may have difficulty being reimbursed for services. In a private practice setting, such as a cardiology practice, an APN can bill for services, although rules governing the reimbursement process for APNs vary from state to state. In all states, NPs bill insurance companies directly for their services in outpatient clinics; however, most states require the NP to have a formal collaborative relationship with a physician and an APN license in order to practice. CNSs may bill for

■ EVIDENCE-BASED PRACTICE

PATIENT EDUCATION

An important role of nurses in outpatient clinics is patient education. Nurses now recognize that a huge number of persons are unable to learn the important information nurses teach them because of problems with health literacy. Health literacy is defined as the degree to which individuals have the capacity to obtain, process, understand, and act on basic health information and services needed to make appropriate health decisions. Between 60 and 70 percent of older adults perform at the lowest two (of five) levels of literacy, which translates to reading at approximately an eighth-grade level or lower. Problems with health literacy are not isolated in poor or immigrant communities. Even in affluent communities, a significant number of persons have difficulty comprehending written health care information. Further, when individuals are ill, their usual reading and comprehension abilities may decline because of stress, lack of energy, or medication side-effects.

Evidence-based practice includes preparing materials at the appropriate reading level. Avoid medical jargon (such as "take medicine TID"). Be aware of the issue of low health literacy, and assess your patients if you suspect that this is a problem. Patients are unlikely to take medicines according to directions, adhere to prescribed regimens, follow directions, make health-related decisions, participate actively in self-care, access health care, or understand their rights if they do not understand the directions.

Bibliography

Institute of Medicine: *Health literacy: a prescription to end confusion,* Washington, DC, 2004, National Academies Press.

Schwartzberg J, VanGeest J, Wang C: *Understanding health literacy: implications for medicine and public health,* Chicago, 2005, American Medical Association Press.

some aspects of care, such as patient education or wound care.

Caring for patients in a health maintenance organization may impose restrictions as to the medications, laboratory studies, and procedures that can be prescribed. These restrictions may limit the APN's ability to refer patients to other collaborative disciplines, such as a diabetic educator or a rehabilitation program. A university-based health care system may have more programs available to support patient care, such as dietary consultation, diabetes management programs, smoking cessation programs, or subspecialty consultation. In a private practice setting, the APN may have to search for community-based programs to meet patients' needs. Physician support and a strong referral base from other physicians and community practices contribute to long-term success and operation of the clinic.

Process

Process refers to the way in which nurses in an outpatient clinic execute their roles.

Staff Nurses

The staff nurse in an outpatient clinic is often the first person that patients encounter. The staff nurse obtains a brief history, assesses vital signs, and usually evaluates the patient's current medications. This information sets the foundation for the care that is to follow. If the vital signs are inaccurate or if the medication list is incorrect, inappropriate and potentially harmful therapies may be prescribed.

Maintenance of the patient's record is an important role of the clinic nursing staff. During the patient's initial entry into the clinic, the staff nurse updates the patient's current medication list and obtains pertinent records from other clinics or physician offices. In some settings, the staff nurse role consists of strictly technical support, such as obtaining vital signs or an electrocardiogram. The patient care staff in an outpatient clinic may consist of paraprofessionals or assistants who have been trained to perform patient care tasks.

Staff nurses may be accountable for educating patients about their disease, medications, and needed lifestyle changes and providing written or audiovisual materials that reinforce education. After the patient has left the clinic, the staff nurses may follow-up on laboratory results to ensure that the provider has received a copy and the patients are notified of results. The nurses also may have responsibility for contacting patients to follow-up with medication changes and to reinforce patient education. Staff nurses help patients maneuver the application process for pharmaceutical assistance programs when they cannot afford expensive medications.

Nurse Practitioners

The majority of an NP's time usually is spent in clinical care. NPs often manage a population of patients with a specific diagnosis, such as heart failure. The NP job description may include traditional nursing responsibilities, but with some aspects of the medical model, such as taking a history, conducting a physical examination, making a diagnosis, and prescribing treatments. The NP role often includes elements that traditionally have been outside the scope of nursing practice, such as ordering and interpreting diagnostic and laboratory tests, and prescribing pharmacological and nonpharmacological therapies.

Patient and family education continues to be an important component of the NP's care. Patient-centered care, as opposed to disease-centered care, is what differentiates the NP from a completely medical model of practice. Integration of a nursing paradigm with medical practice creates a holistic approach to patient care. NPs use critical thinking and reflection—building on a strong foundation in nursing obtained from their introductory programs—to keep a nursing focus to their practice, rather than being subsumed by the medical model.

Clinical Nurse Specialists

The CNS role traditionally has four dimensions of practice, composed of expert clinician, consultant, educator, and researcher. In outpatient clinics, the CNS as clinician may titrate medications or manage an aspect of patient care such as dyslipidemia according to a set of protocols. As consultant, the CNS may oversee patient support groups or counsel patients about needed lifestyle changes. As educator, the CNS can influence the patient's disease process, improve symptoms, and modify risk factors by imparting information in a manner that is easily understood by patients and family members. As a researcher, the CNS may lead nursing studies, collaborate with others, or coordinate investigational studies involving the patient population. The CNS has in-depth knowledge of the learning and change processes and is able to maximize the patient's understanding of his or her illness, medications, symptoms, and necessary lifestyle changes to modify outcomes. The CNS often is responsible for educating the nursing staff as well.

The CNS role often includes educating patients, reinforcing information, and overseeing outpatient activities such as support groups, newsletters, health fairs, and community educational programs. An APN might supervise a clinic that manages a condition or a type of medication, such as a lipid clinic, an anticoagulation clinic, a pacemaker clinic, or an infusion clinic. In this setting, the APN usually makes decisions about patient management using a set of predetermined protocols.

Outcomes

Patient outcomes are measured in terms of hospital readmissions, quality of life, functional status, and mortality. Practice outcomes may be measured by the number of patients who are on appropriate medical therapy based on current standards, such as angiotensin-converting enzyme inhibitors or beta blockers in heart failure, statin or aspirin therapy in coronary artery disease, and anticoagulation therapy in atrial fibrillation. Practice outcomes also may be measured by the number of patients who have achieved a specified goal, such as blood pressure reduction, lowered lipid levels, anticoagulation within appropriate parameters, or improved walking distance. Patient satisfaction with care is also an important outcome to measure, particularly as hospitals, clinics, and private practices become more competitive and patients have more provider options from which to choose.

Financial outcomes are important to measure, especially for nurses who must justify their salary. Care by APNs is cost-effective, with lower direct costs of care and favorable cost-saving outcomes.[3,4,23] The cost of an office visit to a NP or physician assistant is less than the cost for comparable primary care provided by a physician.[24] NPs are particularly cost-effective in preventive care because of expertise in counseling, patient and family education, and case management. Patient outcomes, patient satisfaction, and health services utilization have been found to be comparable between physicians and NPs practicing in outpatient clinics.[25] Because of the nursing perspective, APNs as a group have interpersonal communication skills that may enhance quality and continuity of care.

SUMMARY

Nurses play a key role in outpatient cardiovascular clinics. In a staff role, nurses guide the flow of patients through the clinic and perform the preliminary evaluation of patients coming into the clinic for care. Staff nurses triage most telephone calls and contribute in important ways to patient education that prepares patients to engage in self-care. APNs may play a direct role in the medical management and follow-up of patients, or they contribute to patient care through programs that support patient care. As cardiovascular care continues to subspecialize and the number of patients with cardiovascular diseases continues to rise, the nurse's role in outpatient clinics will continue to evolve. One author summarized the value of nursing in the outpatient as follows: "Nursing's focus is on people. Its blend of medical, behavioral and social science expertise and its commitment to caring, teaching, counseling and supporting patients are the characteristics of nursing that make nurses so uniquely qualified to provide advanced practice and primary care services to the public."[12] These qualities make nurses valuable contributors to outpatient clinics.

REFERENCES

1. Brown M, Draye M: Experiences of pioneer nurse practitioners in establishing advanced practice roles, *J Nurs Scholarsh* 35: 391-397, 2003.
2. Office of Technology Assessment: *Nurse practitioners, physicians assistants and certified nurse midwives policy analysis,* Washington, DC, 1986, The Office.
3. Paul S: Impact of a nurse-managed heart failure clinic: a pilot study of outcomes, *Am J Crit Care* 8:140-146, 2000.
4. Phillips CO, Wright SM, Kern DE et al: Comprehensive discharge planning with postdischarge support for older patients with congestive heart failure: a meta-analysis, *JAMA* 291:1358-1367, 2004.
5. National Association of Clinical Nurse Specialists: FAQS. What is a Clinical Nurse Specialist? Retrieved November 29, 2006 from www.nacns.org/faqs.shtml
6. Pearson L: The Pearson Report: a national overview of nurse practitioner legislation and healthcare issues, *American Journal for Nurse Practitioners* 9:9-136, 2005.
7. American Nurses Association: *Scope and standards of advanced practice registered nursing,* Washington, DC, 1996, American Nurses Publishing.
8. Burgener S, Moore S: The role of advanced practice nurses in community settings, *Nurs Econ* 20:102-108, 2002.
9. Donagrandi M, Eddy M: Ethics of case management: implications for advanced practice nursing, *Clin Nurse Spec* 14:241-249, 2000.
10. Guido B: The role of a nurse practitioner in an ambulatory surgery unit, *AORN J* 79:606-615, 2004.
11. Patterson C, Hezekiah J: What makes nursing practice advanced? In Patterson C, editor: *Nurse practitioners . . . the catalyst of change,* Troy, Canada, 2000, Newrange Press.
12. Donnelly G: Clinical expertise in advanced practice nursing: a Canadian perspective, *Nurse Educ Today* 23:168-173, 2003.
13. Parry S: The quest for competencies, *Training* 33:48-56, 1996.
14. National Council of State Boards of Nursing: *Assuring competence: a regulatory responsibility,* Chicago, 1996, National Council of State Boards of Nursing.
15. Canadian Nurses Association: *Promoting continuing competence for registered nurses.* Retrieved November 29, 2006 from http://cna-aiic.ca/CNA/documents/pdf/publications/PS77_promoting_competence_e.pdf
16. American Nurses Credentialing Center: *Ambulatory care nursing certification.* Retrieved November 29, 2006 from http://nursingworld.org/ancc/cert/eligibility/AmbCare.html
17. Hamric A, Hanson C: Educating advanced practice nurses for practice reality, *J Prof Nurs* 19:262-268, 2003.
18. Carlson B, Riegel B, Moser D: Self-care abilities of patients with heart failure, *Heart Lung* 30:351-359, 2001.
19. Prochaska J, Norcross J, DiClemente C: *Changing for good: a revolutionary six-stage program for overcoming bad habits and moving your life positively forward,* New York, 1994, Avon Books.
20. Paul S, Sneed N: Strategies for behavior change in patients with heart failure, *Am J Crit Care* 13:305-313, 2004.
21. Taylor K, Oberle K, Crutcher R, Norton P: Promoting health in type 2 diabetes: nurse-physician collaboration in primary care, *Biol Res Nurs* 6:207-215, 2005.
22. Micevski V, Korkola L, Sarkissian S et al: University Health Network framework for advanced nursing practice: development of a comprehensive conceptual framework describing the multidimensional contributions of advanced practice nurses, *Nurs Leader* 17:52-64, 2004.
23. Brooten D, Naylor M, York R et al: Lessons learned from testing the quality cost model of advanced practice nursing transitional care, *J Nurs Scholarsh* 34:369-375, 2002.
24. Roblin D, Howard D, Becker E et al: Use of midlevel practitioners to achieve labor cost savings in the primary care practice of an MCO, *Health Serv Res* 39:607-626, 2004.
25. Mundinger M, Kane R, Lenz E et al: Primary care outcomes in patients treated by nurse practitioners or physicians, *JAMA* 283:59-68, 2000.

■■■ chapter 25

Interdisciplinary Team in Cardiac Rehabilitation

Martha Biddle
Meg Gulanick
Kathy Berra

CHAPTER ABBREVIATIONS

AACVPR American Association of Cardiovascular and Pulmonary Rehabilitation

AHA American Heart Association

CR cardiac rehabilitation

ECG electrocardiogram

RD registered dietitian

In the 1960s, a cardiac rehabilitation (**CR**) program was designed to occupy 4 to 6 months after a cardiac event and was reserved primarily for survivors of an uncomplicated myocardial infarction.[1] In the early 1970s, the need for lifestyle modification as an adjunct to medical treatments produced further developments in CR. Programs began to include aerobic exercise, weight management, smoking cessation, and dietary counseling interventions.[2] Currently, CR programs may be initiated within days of an event and commonly are extended to a broad range of patients. There is a call for all CR programs to ensure integration of secondary prevention into a comprehensive cardiac treatment plan. Today's patients are more likely to be older and to have complex illnesses and comorbid conditions. These changes have direct implications for the team staffing today's CR programs.

CORE COMPONENTS

As discussed in Chapter 80, the CR programs of today are designed to reduce physiological and psychological effects of cardiac disease, stabilize the atherosclerotic process, promote regression, and enhance self-care strategies. The American Heart Association (**AHA**) and the American Association of Cardiovascular and Pulmonary Rehabilitation (**AACVPR**) advocate that all CR programs contain specific core components intended to optimize cardiovascular risk reduction, foster healthy behaviors and compliance to these behaviors, reduce disability, and promote an active lifestyle for patients with cardiovascular disease.[3] These core components include baseline physical assessment, aggressive risk factor management, counseling for nutrition, physical activity, vocation and psychosocial issues, and exercise training (Table 25-1).[4] Programs are structured around these core components where staff assist participants to meet their overall goals. The challenge for staff is to do so in progressively shorter intervals.

Traditional CR programs were divided into three phases (Table 25-2). Phase I included rehabilitation while still in the hospital with exercises such as walking in the hallway and bedside stretching. Reduced hospital length of stay has made this phase of CR almost obsolete. Phase II, or Early Outpatient, lasts 1 to 3 months. Aerobic exercise is performed under close supervision of an interdisciplinary and skilled team and with electrocardiogram (**ECG**) monitoring. Modern programs begin emphasizing secondary prevention interventions during this phase. Phase III, or Maintenance, lasts 6 to 12 months and is usually a home exercise program, one offered in a community setting, or a virtual Internet program. Phase III typically is unsupervised, is self-directed, and is not reimbursed by insurance.[4] Secondary prevention is essential during this phase. Different staff skills are required for each of these phases.

STAFFING REQUIREMENTS

An interdisciplinary CR team typically administers exercise training, education, and counseling on risk factors of heart disease to the participant and the family. CR staff members also provide counseling that addresses the recovery process after an acute cardiac event and coping with a chronic disease process. This staff, directed by a supervising physician, may include any combination of the professionals shown in Box 25-1.[4]

CR programs employ a multitude of qualified professionals, licensed and nonlicensed, to implement the interdisciplinary treatment plan. The team member responsible for day-to-day patient management is usually a registered nurse or an exercise specialist. This professional performs the ECG and monitors vital signs and the response to exercise, addressing educational needs. The staffing ratio recommendations provided by the AACVPR are 5:1 for early outpatient programs and 15:1 for maintenance programs.[4] Each facility selects the appropriate combination of staff that ensures safe patient care to all participants.

PROFESSIONAL ROLES

The AACVPR recognizes specific qualifications inherent to the positions of the medical director and program director (Box 25-2). Although one health care provider may provide administrative leadership, additional health care professionals often are hired from a variety of specialty areas, which increases the interdisciplinary team's ability to meet the needs of individual participants. The clinical expertise, knowledge, and skill of the professional staff collectively enable interdisciplinary team management (see Chapter 19). The combined expertise of the professional staff should include a comprehensive understanding of cardiovascular physiology, emergency procedures, ECG interpretation, nutrition, and second-

■ ■ ■

TABLE 25-1   CORE COMPONENTS OF CARDIAC REHABILITATION/SECONDARY PREVENTION PROGRAMS

STEP	ACTION

Patient Assessment

Evaluate	• *Medical history:* Include cardiovascular (including peripheral vascular and cerebrovascular) diagnoses and prior cardiovascular procedures (including assessment of left ventricular function), comorbidities, symptoms of cardiovascular disease, risk factors for atherosclerotic disease progression, and medications and medication compliance. • *Physical examination:* Include vital signs, cardiovascular and pulmonary examination, postprocedure wound sites, and joint and neuromuscular examination. • *Testing:* Obtain resting electrocardiogram; assess quality of life using standard questionnaires (e.g., Medical Outcomes Study SF-36).
Plan	• Develop short-term (i.e., weeks or months) and long-term (i.e., years) goals and strategies to reduce disability and subsequent cardiovascular disease risk.
Communicate	• Compose written records that reflect the patient evaluation and contain a patient care plan with detailed priorities for risk reduction and rehabilitation. • Actively communicate this plan to the patient and the primary health care provider. • Generate a written summary of patient outcomes on completion of the program and provide it to the patient and to the primary and referring health care providers. Written summaries should identify specific areas that require further intervention and monitoring.

Nutritional Counseling

Evaluate	• Obtain estimates of total daily caloric intake and dietary content of fat, saturated fat, cholesterol, sodium, and other nutrients. • Assess eating habits, including number of meals, snacks, frequency of dining out, and alcohol consumption. • Assess target areas for nutrition intervention, addressing the core components of weight, hypertension, and diabetes, as well as other comorbid illnesses.
Intervene	• Prescribe specific, individualized dietary modifications (e.g., American Heart Association Step II diet). • Educate and counsel patient (and family members) regarding dietary goals and how to attain them, incorporating behavior-change models and compliance strategies. (See Chapters 83 and 84.)

Lipid Management

Evaluate	• Obtain fasting lipid measures. (See Chapter 77.) In those with abnormal levels, as per National Cholesterol Education Program, obtain a detailed history to identify other factors affecting lipid levels. • Assess current treatment and treatment adherence. • Repeat lipid profiles 4 to 6 weeks after hospitalization and 2 months after initiation of or change in lipid-lowering medications.
Intervene	• Provide nutritional counseling and weight management training as indicated. • Address other risk factors (e.g., lack of exercise and smoking) that accentuate risk. • Provide and/or monitor drug treatment in concert with primary provider.

Hypertension Management

Evaluate	• Measure resting blood pressure on at least two visits. • Assess current treatment, comorbid conditions that may change blood pressure goals (e.g., heart failure, diabetes, and renal failure). Assess current treatment adherence.
Intervene	• If indicated, counsel on lifestyle modifications that will facilitate blood pressure control (e.g., exercise, weight management, sodium restriction, alcohol moderation, and smoking cessation). • Provide and/or monitor drug therapy in concert with primary provider.

Smoking Cessation

Assess	• Assess and document smoking status (i.e., never smoked, former smoker, current smoker, including those who have quit in the last 6 months). Specify the amount (packs per day) and duration of smoking (number of years). Assess use of cigar smoking, pipe smoking, and chewing tobacco and exposure to secondhand smoke. (See Chapter 33.) • Assess for confounding psychosocial issues and readiness to change. • Update records of smoking status at each visit during first 2 weeks of cessation and periodically thereafter for at least 6 months.
Plan	• See Chapter 33 for specific intervention approaches. • Encourage physician, staff, and family support for cessation efforts. • Provide and/or monitor pharmacological support as needed in concert with primary physician. • Support success, prevent relapse with follow-up visits or telephone contact for at least 6 to 12 months.

Weight Management

Assess	• Measure weight, height, and waist circumference. Calculate body mass index.
Plan	• In patients with body mass index greater than 25 kg/m² and/or waist greater than 40 inches in men (102 cm) and greater than 35 inches (88 cm) in women, establish reasonable, individualized short-term and long-term weight goals, aiming for an energy deficit of 500 to 1000 kcal/d. (See Chapter 36.) • Develop a combined diet, exercise, and behavioral program designed to reduce total caloric intake, maintain appropriate intake of nutrients and fiber, and increase energy expenditure. • Refer to specialized, validated nutrition weight loss programs if weight goals are not achieved.

TABLE 25-1   CORE COMPONENTS OF CARDIAC REHABILITATION/SECONDARY PREVENTION PROGRAMS—cont'd

STEP	ACTION

Diabetes Management

Assess
- Identify diabetic patients by initial history. Note medication type, dose, and regimen; type and frequency of glucose monitoring; and history of hypoglycemic reactions.
- Obtain fasting plasma glucose measurements in all patients and hemoglobin A_{1c} in diabetic patients to monitor therapy.

Plan
- Develop a plan to control blood sugar levels with dietary adherence, weight control, exercise, oral hypoglycemic agents, and/or insulin therapy. Carefully control other risk factors.
- Provide and/or monitor drug therapy in concert with primary provider.
- Monitor glucose levels before and/or after exercise sessions. Educate regarding identification and treatment of postexercise hypoglycemia. Limit or prohibit exercise if blood glucose is ≥300 mg/dl.
- Refer patients without known diabetes whose fasting glucose is greater than 110 mg/dl to their primary provider for further evaluation and treatment.

Psychosocial Management

Assess
- Using interview and/or standardized measurement tools, identify psychological distress as indicated by clinically significant levels of depression, anxiety, and anger or hostility; social isolation; sexual dysfunction/maladjustment; and substance abuse (alcohol or other psychotropic substances).

Plan
- Offer individual and/or small group education and counseling sessions to promote adjustment, stress management, and lifestyle change. Include family members/significant others whenever possible.
- In concert with primary provider, refer patients with clinically significant psychosocial distress to appropriate mental health specialists for further evaluation and treatment.
- Promote the development and maintenance of appropriate community resources (e.g., Alcoholics Anonymous).

Physical Activity

Assess
- Assess current physical activity level and determine domestic, occupational, and recreational needs and interests, including activities relevant to age, gender, and daily life (e.g., driving, sexual activity, sports, gardening, and household tasks).
- Assess readiness to change behavior, self-confidence, barriers to increase physical activity, and social support in making positive changes.
- Consider simulated work testing for patients with heavy labor jobs.

Plan
- Provide advice, support, and counseling about physical activity needs on initial evaluation and in follow-up.
- Set goals to increase physical activity that include 30 minutes per day of moderate physical activity on 5 days per week. (See Chapters 38 and 80.) Suggest ways to incorporate increased activity into usual routines.

Exercise Training

Assess
- Obtain an exercise test (or other standard measure of exercise capacity) before participation (including heart rate and rhythm, response to exercise, and exercise capacity). Repeat as changes in clinical condition warrant.
- Assess patient understanding of safety issues during exercise.

Plan
- Develop an individualized exercise prescription for aerobic and resistance training that is based on evaluation findings, risk stratification, patient and program goals, and resources. Specify frequency (F), intensity (I), duration (D), and modalities (M). (See Chapters 38 and 80.)
- Stress importance of warm-up, cooldown, and flexibility exercises in each exercise session. Provide updates to the exercise prescription routinely and as changes in patient condition warrants.
- Plan structured outpatient or home-based program. Supplement the formal exercise regimen with at-home activity guidelines. Caloric expenditure of at least 1000 kcal/wk should be a specific exercise program objective.
- Advise low-impact aerobic activity to minimize risk of injury. Recommend gradual increases in intensity over weeks.

Balady GJ, Ades PA, Comoss P et al: *Circulation* 102:1069-1073, 2000.

■ ■ ■

TABLE 25-2   CARDIAC REHABILITATION PROGRAM PHASES

PHASE	ACTIVITIES
I: Inpatient	Progressive activity, walking, and stretches
	Education focused on postdischarge priorities; recognition of signs and symptoms, medication instructions, and home activity levels
II: Early outpatient	May start within 1 to 4 weeks after the event
	Aerobic exercise, risk factor stratification, lifestyle, and behavioral modification
	Secondary prevention interventions
	Encouragement of self-care behaviors and strategies for chronic disease management
III: Maintenance	Starts within 2 to 3 months after event
	Self-directed fitness plans, at home, in the community, or continued at the rehabilitation facility
	Self-monitoring with periodic evaluation by rehabilitation staff or primary care provider
	Self-directed lifetime commitment to heart-healthy lifestyle and physical activity

BOX 25-1   ■ ■ ■
POSSIBLE MEMBERS OF THE INTERDISCIPLINARY CARDIAC REHABILITATION TEAM

- Advanced practice nurses
- Registered nurses
- Exercise specialist
- Registered dietitian
- Mental health professional
- Health educator
- Physical therapist
- Vocational/occupational rehabilitation counselor
- Pharmacist
- Physician

BOX 25-2   ■ ■ ■
MINIMUM QUALIFICATIONS FOR MEDICAL
AND PROGRAM DIRECTORS

Medical Director
- Cardiologist, internist, or other physician with interest and experience in cardiac rehabilitation
- Experience with exercise testing, prescription, and counseling
- Successful completion of an advanced cardiac life support course

Program Director
- Bachelor's degree in an allied health field, such as exercise physiology, or licensure as a registered nurse or physical therapist
- Advanced knowledge of exercise physiology, nutrition, risk-factor modification strategies, counseling techniques, administration of educational programs/technologies as applied to cardiac rehabilitation and secondary prevention services
- Experience in staff coordination and delivery of secondary prevention services
- Successful completion of basic and advanced cardiac life support
- Certification, experience, and training equivalent to those specified for an exercise specialist by the American College of Sports Medicine, certification through the American Nurses Credentialing Center, or the advanced specialty in cardiopulmonary rehabilitation of the American Physical Therapy Association

Williams MA: *Guidelines for cardiac rehabilitation and secondary prevention programs: American Association of Cardiovascular and Pulmonary Rehabilitation,* ed 4, Champaign, Ill, 2004, Human Kinetics.

---

ary prevention guidelines for coronary artery disease, behavioral modification counseling skills, pharmacology, and exercise physiology.[4]

The role of the registered nurse in a CR program is multifaceted. Primary nursing care often is associated with the case management model of care delivery.[6] The nurse is responsible for coordinating the treatment plan and the team's services. The treatment plan is individualized and organized with the AHA/AACVPR core components in mind. The nurse, in conjunction with the other team members, assesses, plans, implements, and evaluates the care provided to each participant.

The role of the exercise specialist on the interdisciplinary team is to plan, supervise, and counsel CR participants in safe and effective exercise activities. The exercise specialist works with the medical and program director in developing the exercise prescription and implementing a treatment plan designed to modify risk factors related to physical activity. The exercise specialist also conducts individual and group aerobics, strength and flexibility exercises, and observes participants during exercise activity for any signs of stress or difficulty. The exercise prescription is used to guide exercise on a variety of equipment such as treadmills, stationary bikes, step climbers, and rowers. The professional in this role also may perform physical assessments such as body fat composition, orthopedic ability, and oxygen consumption.[7] Minimum qualifications for an exercise specialist is a bachelor's degree in exercise science or an equivalent of the exercise specialist certification of the American College of Sports Medicine.[4]

The role of the registered dietitian (**RD**) in the outpatient CR setting is delineated in practice guidelines. Nutritional therapy is an integral part of the wellness approach to secondary prevention of heart disease. RDs have standardized education, clinical training, and national credentials that allow them to provide the education and counseling required of CR participants. The RD performs nutritional evaluations, one-on-one counseling sessions, group nutrition classes, cooking demonstrations, and professional support for individuals attempting weight loss. Prescriptions for specific dietary modifications, individualized diet plans, behavioral change models, and compliance strategies are a few of the interventions the RD uses in providing nutritional counseling to CR patients.

Staff competency guidelines are set forth by certifying and professional organizations and by government agencies. Individual programs are responsible for ensuring competent clinical practice and ongoing continuing education activity by all members of the interdisciplinary team.

CORE COMPETENCIES
Exercise Prescription and Supervision

Until recently, aerobic exercise was viewed as the central component of CR. Historically, traditional programs focused on supervised, ECG-monitored exercise sessions performed 3 times per week at an intensity of 70 to 85 percent of the maximal safe heart rate achieved on the entrance exercise stress test. Regular physical activity continues to be an important therapy, especially for patients who are deconditioned or disabled, those with chronic heart failure, angina, after heart transplant, and for elderly patients.[8] Thus, a core competency is the ability to prescribe and monitor exercise intensity, duration, frequency, mode, and site for exercise, as described in Chapter 29. Research demonstrating that similar benefits in functional capacity are achieved with low- versus high-intensity exercise, and intermittent- versus single-bout sessions has caused a paradigm shift in prescribing exercise. Current exercise guidelines are more creative and flexible to suit the abilities and interests of each patient.

Most patients who participate in a formal exercise program abandon exercise within a year's time.[9] Thus a lifestyle approach to exercise, based on the need for adults to accumulate 30 to 60 minutes of moderate-intensity physical activity on most, preferably all, days of the week is taken.[5] This is comparable to walking at 3 or 4 mph for most healthy adults, walking 2 miles in 30 to 40 minutes, or expending approximately 200 calories in exercise each day. This dose of activity can be divided into intermittent bouts during the day.

Team members are being challenged to work with patients to reach a weekly threshold for physical activity of at least 1000 kcal.[10] Efforts are focused on identifying opportunities for everyday physical activities, such as walking the dog, doing yard work, achieving 10,000 steps per day on a pedometer, and using stairs instead of elevators. Staff also need to ensure that clients can gauge the intensity of their physical efforts safely. Ratings of perceived exertion (Figure 25-1) generally are used as a guide, with a goal of 3 to 5 reflecting moderate exercise.[11] Self-monitoring tools such as pedometers or calendars that track walking time should be encouraged to improve adherence. Because regular physical activity may be a new behavior for many, reducing barriers, increasing self-efficacy, and finding activities that are enjoyable are ways to increase long-term adherence.

Strength training also should be incorporated into physical activity prescriptions. This can be done with resistance exercises using weight training equipment in an exercise facility, lifestyle strength training performed at home with dumbbells or wrist weights, or home-based strength training by lifting a bag of groceries from a chair to a table and back to the chair. The exercise specialist on the CR team needs to consider the unique physical profile, skill set, motivation level, and performance goals for each patient to optimally determine the appropriate exercise program. Refer to Chapters 6 and 38 for further information.

Physiological Monitoring

A key role of the CR staff is to anticipate and recognize adverse responses to exercise activity. Participants often wear ECG monitors during the early outpatient phase, and nurses are responsible for maintaining competency in ECG rhythm interpretation. A thorough understanding of physiological responses and adaptations to exercise also is required of the registered nurse and the exercise specialist. A large number of patients have implanted devices such as pacemakers and implanted cardioverter-defibrillators; all program staff must have a working knowledge of these devices so that if problems occur or the device fires, the situation is handled capably and expeditiously. Hemodynamic, hypoglycemic, and ischemic responses are a few of the adverse responses that CR staff must be able to manage quickly and efficiently. Standardized protocols and template/guidelines for the management of these adverse reactions are provided by professional organizations such as AACVPR and AHA.

Actually, exercise-related coronary events are rare, which has eased the need for ECG-monitored and even medically supervised exercise sessions.[12] Thus, initiation of an exercise program is attainable for more patients, with home- and community-based sites as options. Box 25-3 provides criteria for risk-stratifying patients for car-

---

BOX 25-3 ■ ■ ■
STRATIFICATION OF RISK FOR A CARDIAC EVENT DURING EXERCISE

Lowest Risk*
Exercise Findings
- Absence of complex ventricular dysrhythmias during exercise testing and recovery
- Absence of angina or other significant symptoms (e.g., unusual shortness of breath, light-headedness, or dizziness during exercise testing and recovery)
- Normal hemodynamics during exercise testing and recovery (i.e., appropriate increases and decreases in heart rate and systolic blood pressure with increasing workloads and recovery)
- Functional capacity = 7 metabolic equivalents (METs)

Nonexercise Findings
- Ejection fraction 50 percent or greater at rest
- Uncomplicated myocardial infarction or revascularization procedure
- Absence of complicated ventricular dysrhythmias at rest
- Absence of heart failure
- Absence of signs or symptoms of postevent/postprocedure ischemia
- Absence of clinical depression

Moderate Risk†
Exercise Findings
- Presence of angina or other significant symptoms during exercise testing or recovery (e.g., unusual shortness of breath, light-headedness, or dizziness occurring only at high levels of exertion [7 METs or greater])
- Mid to moderate level of silent ischemia during exercise testing or recovery (ST segment depression less than 2 mm from baseline)
- Functional capacity less than 5 METs

Nonexercise Testing Findings
- Ejection fraction 40 to 49 percent at rest

High Risk†
Exercise Findings
- Presence of complex ventricular dysrhythmias during exercise testing or recovery
- Presence of angina or other significant symptoms (e.g., unusual shortness of breath, light-headedness, or dizziness at low levels of exertion [less than 5 METs] or during recovery)
- High level of silent ischemia (ST segment depression = 2 mm from baseline) during exercise testing or recovery
- Presence of abnormal hemodynamics with exercise testing (e.g., chronotropic incompetence or flat or decreasing systolic blood pressure with increasing workloads) or recovery (i.e., severe postexercise hypotension)

Nonexercise Testing Findings
- Ejection fraction less than 40 percent at rest
- History of cardiac arrest or sudden death
- Complex dysrhythmias at rest
- Complicated myocardial infarction or revascularization procedure
- Presence of heart failure
- Presence of signs or symptoms of postevent/postprocedure ischemia
- Presence of clinical depression

Williams MA: *Cardiol Clin* 19:415-431, 2001.
*All characteristics listed must be present for patient to remain at lowest risk.
†Any one or more of these characteristics establishes the patient's risk.

Borg Scale for Rating Perceived Exertion

6	No exertion at all
7.5	Extremely light
8	
9	Very light
10	
12	Light
13	Somewhat hard
14	
15	Hard (heavy)
16	
17	Very hard
18	
19	
20	Extremely hard
21	
	Maximal exertion

© Gunnar Borg. Reproduced with permission

FIGURE 25-1 ■ Borg scale for rating perceived exertion. For correct usage of the Borg scale, follow the administration and instructions given in Borg G: *Borg's perceived exertion and pain scales,* Champaign, Ill, 1998, Human Kinetics.

diac events during exercise participation. Box 25-4 provides recommendations for intensity of supervision and ECG monitoring based on each of these levels of risk. These recommendations underscore the need to consider the individual profile of each patient when designing an exercise prescription and program.

Depending on the amount of cardiac muscle involved, myocardial ischemia may impair the oxygen transport system and diminish exercise capacity. Impaired oxygen transport may cause adverse exercise responses such as blunted heart rate response and lower stroke volume. Not all CR participants with prior myocardial ischemia have compromised oxygen transport. However, in any patient with coronary artery disease, an acute episode of exercise may induce a release of catecholamines sufficient enough to produce vasoconstriction of diseased coronary arteries and cause

exercise-induced ischemia. The release of endothelin, a potent vasoconstrictor, can occur with acute exercise and in patients with diseased coronary arteries.[13]

The most common abnormal hemodynamic response to exercise seen in CR is systolic hypotension. Participants who have an exercise systolic blood pressure lower than their preexercise systolic blood pressure are at increased risk for a cardiac event. These patients are monitored closely by the CR staff. It has been speculated that this adverse exercise response is related to neurogenic reflex vasodilatation involving mechanoreceptors in the myocardium.[14]

Hypoglycemic responses to exercise can occur in the diabetic population of CR participants. Blood glucose levels taken before and after exercise are monitored consistently upon entry into the CR program. The consistent monitoring of blood glucose levels serves two purposes: it provides the patient with immediate feedback as to the effects of exercise on blood glucose and minimizes the risk of hypoglycemic reactions (Box 25-5).[4]

Facilitating Behavioral Change

Another core skill of CR staff is the knowledge and skill to facilitate behavioral change and lifestyle modification. Teaching has always been a core role for nurses, and nowhere is this more evident than in CR. Along with dramatically shortened hospital stays, learning needs and readiness to learn vary greatly in CR participants. The "one size fits all" approach is ineffective, and education designed to meet unique needs is needed.

A thorough knowledge of adult learning theory is important, as is an ability to assess readiness to learn. Adult learners bring a complex and varied set of experiences, attitudes, and skills that influence their ability to accept new knowledge and behaviors and/or change old ones (Box 25-6). Patient education begins by assessing patients' baseline understanding, determining a desire for information, providing scientific evidence, involving the interdisciplinary team, developing a plan with the patient and family members or support per-

---

BOX 25-4 ■ ■ ■
RECOMMENDED INTENSITY OF SUPERVISION AND MONITORING DURING EXERCISE

Patients at Lowest Risk During Exercise
- Direct staff supervision of exercise should occur for at least 6 to 8 exercise sessions or 30 days after the event or procedure, beginning with continuous electrocardiogram (ECG) monitoring and decreasing to intermittent ECG monitoring as appropriate (e.g., at 6 to 12 sessions).
- For a patient to remain at lowest risk, ECG and hemodynamic findings must remain normal, no abnormal signs and symptoms should develop during or outside of the exercise program, and progression of the exercise regimen should be appropriate.

Patients at Moderate Risk During Exercise
- Direct staff supervision of exercise should occur for at least 12 to 24 exercise sessions or 60 days after the event or procedure, beginning with continuous ECG monitoring and decreasing to intermittent ECG monitoring as appropriate (e.g., at 12 to 18 sessions).
- For a patient to move to the lowest category, ECG and hemodynamic findings during exercise should be normal, no abnormal signs and symptoms should develop during or outside of the exercise program, and progression of the exercise regimen should be appropriate.
- Abnormal ECG or hemodynamic findings during exercise, the development of abnormal signs and symptoms during or outside of the exercise program, or the need to decrease exercise levels significantly may result in the patient remaining in the moderate-risk category or even moving to the high-risk category.

Patients at Highest Risk During Exercise
- Direct staff supervision of exercise should occur for at least 18 to 36 exercise sessions or 90 days after the event or procedure, beginning with continuous ECG monitoring and decreasing to intermittent ECG monitoring as appropriate (e.g., at 18, 24, or 30 sessions).
- For a patient to move to the moderate-risk category, ECG and hemodynamics findings during exercise should be normal, no abnormal signs and symptoms should develop during or outside of the exercise program, and the progression of the exercise regimen should be appropriate.
- Abnormal ECG or hemodynamic findings during exercise, the development of abnormal signs and symptoms during or outside of the exercise program, or significant limitations in the patient's ability to participate in the exercise regimen may result in discontinuation of the exercise program until appropriate evaluation, and intervention if needed, can take place.

Williams MA: *Cardiol Clin* 19:415-431, 2001.

BOX 25-5 ■ ■ ■
GUIDELINES FOR FINGERSTICK EVALUATION OF FASTING BLOOD GLUCOSE LEVELS

1. Patients with diabetes who are taking an oral hypoglycemic agent or who use insulin to control their diabetes will have a fingerstick test of their blood glucose level before and after exercising for six exercise sessions to establish the patient's level of glucose control and subsequent response to exercise. Pre- and post-exercise fingerstick tests will continue if the patient's glucose level is less than 90 mg/dl or 300 mg/dl or above.
2. A dietitian will be alerted when patients are in poor diabetic control to facilitate reinforcement of dietary aspects of self-care.
3. When patterns of diabetes control show change (improvement or worsening), a staff member will contact the patient's physician to provide data so that the primary care physician or endocrinologist can adjust medications as needed.

Williams MA: *Guidelines for cardiac rehabilitation and secondary prevention programs: American Association of Cardiovascular and Pulmonary Rehabilitation*, ed 4, Champaign, Ill, 2004, Human Kinetics.

sons, and contracting. Most important of these principles is the concept of "remind, repeat, and reinforce" all educational content provided.[15]

Global risk factor reduction requires an awareness of personal risks factors. Patients need clear directions and strategies for risk reduction. As described in Chapter 83, a variety of teaching formats should be used to address the patient's preferred learning style. Culturally sensitive materials are essential, as are those with an appropriate language and reading level, and those that address the special needs of elders.

Making and sustaining changes in health behavior usually require acknowledging the need for change. CR staff are skilled at facilitating successful changes in behavior in collaboration with the patient by determining realistic goals and workable treatment plans. Realistic goals include making small changes over time, with a focus on what participants *can* do rather than what they *cannot* do. Behavioral change is facilitated by positive reinforcement and encouragement. Researchers and clinicians alike acknowledge that an active and critical ingredient of CR programs is the process of strengthening patients' resolve and confidence to make lifestyle changes (Box 25-7).[16]

Promoting Problem Solving and Coping

Using a problem-centered approach, patients are taught to master "survival skills": recognizing warning signs and symptoms, assessing chest pain and other impor-

tant symptoms, and learning when to call for help, how to take and refill medications, when to progress activity, and when to return to work. Emphasis is placed on problem solving and rehearsing how to handle emergency situations. Family and friends should be included in these educational sessions whenever possible.

Adjustment to illness and changing unhealthy habits are challenging. Recurring themes in recovery literature include depression, anxiety, frustration with unrealistic expectations for lifestyle changes, a sense of powerlessness to stop disease progression, and concerns about the uncertainty of the future.[17] Depression may be the best single predictor of cardiac events during the first 12 months after acute myocardial infarction.[18] Depression is also a strong risk factor for lower functional status after coronary artery bypass grafting.[19] Thus, another integral skill of CR staff is in brief counseling interventions—that is, providing advice, support, and consultation as needed.

Questions such as these serve to open the door to honest communication:

- "How has this experience changed you?"
- "How do you deal with . . . ?"
- "What kinds of emotions have you been feeling?"
- "What role changes have occurred since your cardiac event?"
- "How do you feel about resuming sexual activity or returning to work?"

Staff use active listening to focus on what the patient is saying (and not saying) that involves listening for and reflecting on the underlying emotions behind the factual statements. Patients participating in CR benefit from repeated exposure to staff and other patients who help them verbalize concerns and normalize fears. Staff members provide anticipatory guidance as they navigate through the early weeks of recovery. Individual coping skills vary; however, all coping strategies require that one confront reality, solve problems, and maintain functional capacity. Coping strategies may include perception, performance, appraisal, correction, followed by additional activity, and then a specific motivated behavior (Figure 25-2).[16]

Usually, brief interventions are sufficient to reduce distress and promote coping. Staff members often use evaluation tools to assess the presence of clinically significant depression or anxiety (e.g., Medical Outcomes Study SF-36 questionnaire, the Geriatric Depression Questionnaire, the Beck Depression Scale, or the Profile of Mood States). See Chapter 15 for more information about how to obtain these tools and others. Patients with clinically significant depression should be referred for more intensive counseling to improve psychosocial outcomes.

The key to cost-effective CR is the provision of interventions based on each client's unique needs, interests, and skills. The staff are challenged to assess each client and select only those services needed to achieve maximal risk reduction. Box 25-8 provides a sample listing of the range of services available in contemporary programs. The following vignettes demonstrate how this "menu of services" approach can be individualized for each patient.

BOX 25-6 ■ ■ ■
CORE PRINCIPLES OF ADULT LEARNING

- Individuals develop through interacting with their environment.
- Development follows a cycle of differentiation and integration.
- Within individuals, development is a variable, not uniform, process.
- The ability to reframe experience serves as a marker of development.

Taylor K, Marienau C, Fiddler M: *Developing adult learners,* San Francisco, 2000, Jossey-Bass.

BOX 25-7 ■ ■ ■
ADDRESSING ISSUES OF HEALTH BEHAVIOR

1. Make sure that patients understand the reasons for addressing health behavior.
2. Discuss the ways you can work as partners in addressing their health issues.
3. Explore their health-related behaviors, and identify risk factors.
4. Explore attitudes toward key risk factors.
5. Explore experiences with trying to address key risk factors.
6. Explore factors that may support and obstruct their efforts to change.
7. Try to facilitate a commitment to making positive changes.
8. Help establish realistic goals.
9. Help develop workable plans for achieving their goals.
10. Monitor progress.
11. Schedule follow-ups after goals are achieved, especially those that are difficult to sustain.

Coping Strategies

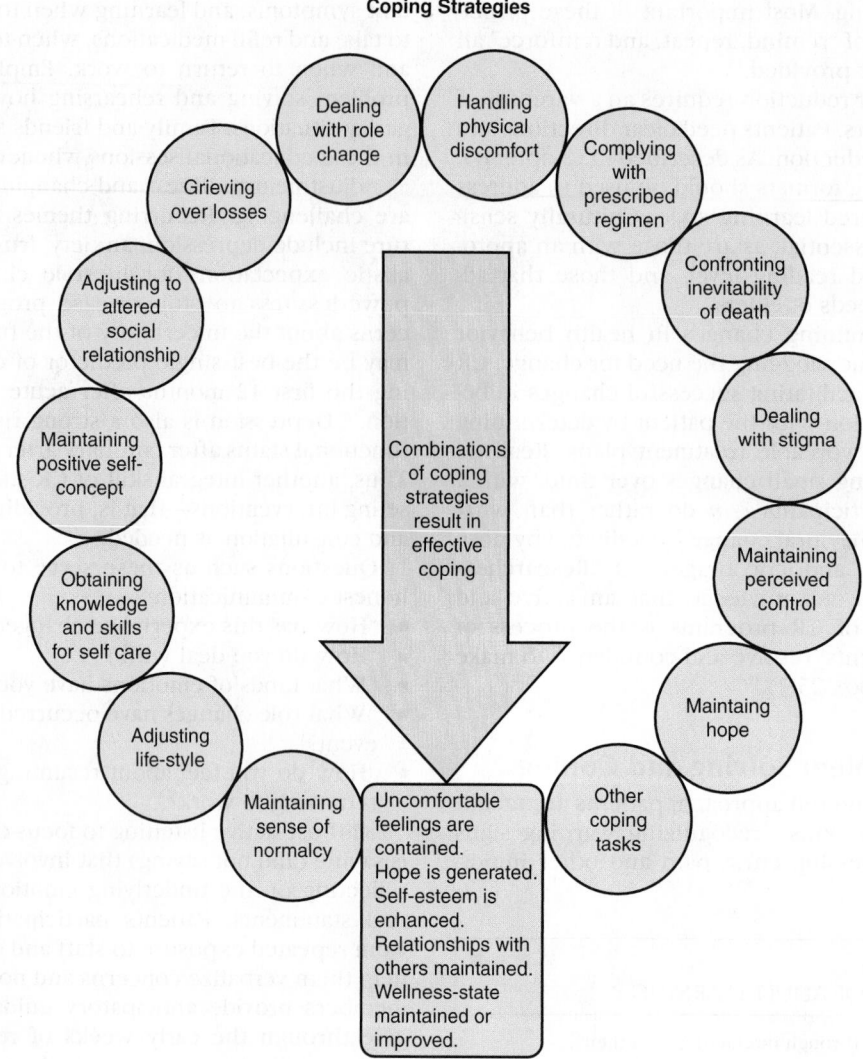

Dealing with role change

Handling physical discomfort

Complying with prescribed regimen

Grieving over losses

Confronting inevitability of death

Adjusting to altered social relationship

Dealing with stigma

Maintaining positive self-concept

Combinations of coping strategies result in effective coping

Maintaining perceived control

Obtaining knowledge and skills for self care

Maintaing hope

Adjusting life-style

Maintaining sense of normalcy

Uncomfortable feelings are contained. Hope is generated. Self-esteem is enhanced. Relationships with others maintained. Wellness-state maintained or improved.

Other coping tasks

FIGURE 25-2 ■ A model for coping with chronic illness. (From Miller JF: *Coping with chronic illness,* Philadelphia, 2000, FA Davis.)

Vignette 1

H.S. is a 60-year-old, nondiabetic, normotensive female business executive under significant work-related pressure. She has been married for 30 years. Recently, she and her husband have been experiencing marital problems, partly related to the stress of moving her parents into an assisted-living environment. She has little time for social friends and activities. She has smoked a pack of cigarettes per day for 30 years and feels that it helps her to relax and maintain her weight (body mass index is 24). She does not exercise regularly. Her blood pressure "varies" between 145/90 and 130/85 mm Hg. Recent laboratory results were as follows: total cholesterol of 220 mg/dl, low-density lipoprotein cholesterol of 145 mg/dl, high-density lipoprotein cholesterol of 45 mg/dl, and triglycerides of 150 mg/dl. Recently, she had an acute episode of chest pain and shortness of breath with an abnormal thallium stress test. On angiography, she was found to have triple vessel disease. She is recovering from an unexpected coronary artery bypass surgery (three bypasses) and becomes tearful whenever she views her scar.

Key initial interventions included stress management with counseling to improve her psychosocial status and quality of life, smoking cessation (medical therapies and support), class-based exercise therapy to provide physiological and psychological benefits as well as social support to assist in coping, and ongoing education regarding the use of medications known to improve outcomes. Adjusting to a new life free of smoking and one that includes regular medical therapies, medical visits, and a new lifestyle are part of the rehabilitation process.

Vignette 2

M.L. is a 56-year-old married man with a history of type 2 diabetes, dyslipidemia, and hypertension. He has been very physically active, participating in weekly racquetball and bicycling on the weekend. He suffered a large anterior wall myocardial infarction, experiencing severe shortness of breath and fatigue before coming to the hospital. He delayed seeking medical care for 10 hours because he did not appreciate his "high risk for heart disease." He has not adhered to his diabetic diet in the past, saying that it "never helped anyway." He does

BOX 25-8 ■ ■ ■
MENU OF CARDIAC REHABILITATION SERVICES

Psychosocial
- Stress management
- Anger management
- Coping skills for living with chronic illness
- Biofeedback
- Mind-body approaches
- Guided imagery
- Massage
- Sexual activity and concerns
- Support groups
- Mended Hearts Groups

Physical Activity
- Exercise prescription
- Aerobic exercise program
  - Supervised/electrocardiogram monitored
  - Community based
- Resistance/strength training program
- Tai chi/yoga/flexibility
- Beginning a home exercise program
- Telemetry monitoring exercise training

Education
- Understanding anatomy and function of heart
- Development of heart disease
- Understanding specific cardiac diseases
- Understanding diagnostic procedures
- Understanding interventional procedures
- "Survival skills" after the event/procedure
- Treating chest pain
- Guidelines for resumption of home activities
- Return to work assessments
- DASH (Dietary Approaches to Stop Hypertension) diet
- Complementary therapies

Counseling and Behavioral Change Services
- Smoking cessation
- Lipid management
- Hypertension management
- Weight reduction
- Diabetes management
- Overall medication management
- Compliance monitoring
- Vocational counseling

not self-monitor blood glucose or blood pressure. His body mass index is 34. M.L. was recovering psychologically; however, his wife was very scared and requested information on "survival" strategies should his symptoms reoccur. She voiced concerns about resuming sexual activity and requested instructions on how she will know when her husband can return safely to his usual level of activities.

Intervention, as part of the CR program, included an education program for couples. This program addressed intimacy, physical activity, monitoring for symptoms, nutrition, and weight loss. In addition, diabetic education was offered emphasizing blood glucose monitoring and medications and foot care. After 6 weeks in the exercise program, M.L. developed symptoms consistent with ischemia and was referred to his cardiologist for further evaluation. He subsequently underwent further cardiovascular testing and had a stent placed in his left anterior descending artery. Following a short recovery, he resumed participation in CR.

Vignette 3

J.P. is a 70-year-old woman with systolic heart failure and hypertension who complained of shortness of breath with minimal activity and difficulty with activities of daily living, especially those requiring arm exercises. She admits to being more sedentary and isolated since her dog died because she no longer needs to walk him. Her ejection fraction is stable at 25 percent, with a volume of oxygen of 18 ml/kg/min. She is on an optimal heart failure and blood pressure medication regimen, but she does not adhere to the regimen. In addition, she does not follow a low-salt diet and does not weigh herself regularly. She lives alone and wants to maintain her independence.

J.P. was referred for 3 months of supervised exercise to increase her aerobic fitness, range of motion, and musculoskeletal strength. In addition, she was referred for weight, blood pressure and symptom monitoring, nutrition evaluation and management, and medication supervision. Participation in CR made her feel less socially isolated and increased her self-efficacy for activities of daily living.

In summary, these vignettes illustrate the variety of skills needed by the nurse in CR. Beyond symptom monitoring, these expert clinicians can identify the reasons for poor coping and lack of treatment adherence. They prescribe interventions such as education, exercise, and nutrition counseling. They know the importance of social support and when intervention with the family is more important than that with the patient. Coping, quality of life, control of morbid illnesses, and survival are the key outcomes of a quality CR program. Achieving these outcomes requires a competent, qualified interdisciplinary team that works in collaboration with physicians, patients, and families to achieve these outcomes.

REFERENCES

1. Liehr P, Leaverton R, Yepes A et al: Addressing current challenges to cardiac rehabilitation care, *AACN Clin Issues* 14:13-24, 2003.
2. Aldana SG, Whitmer WR, Greenlaw R et al: Cardiovascular risk reductions associated with aggressive lifestyle modification and cardiac rehabilitation, *Heart Lung* 32:374-382, 2003.
3. Balady GJ, Ades PA, Comoss P et al: Core components of cardiac rehabilitation/secondary prevention: a statement for healthcare professionals from the American Heart Association and the American Association of Cardiovascular and Pulmonary Rehabilitation, *Circulation* 102:1069-1073, 2000.
4. Williams MA: *Guidelines for cardiac rehabilitation and secondary prevention programs: American Association of Cardiovascular and Pulmonary Rehabilitation*, ed 4, Champaign, Ill, 2004, Human Kinetics.
5. Cardiac Core Competencies Working Group (Southard DR, Certo C, Comoss P, et al): Core competencies for cardiac rehabilitation professionals, *J Cardiopulm Rehabil* 14:87-92, 1994.
6. Ehrman JK, Gordon PM, Visich PS, Keteyian SJ: *Clinical exercise physiology*, Champaign, Ill, 2003, Human Kinetics.
7. Fletcher GF, Balady GJ, Amsterdam EA et al: Exercise standards for testing and training: a statement for healthcare professionals from the American Heart Association, *Circulation* 104:1694-1740, 2001.
8. Wenger NK, Froelicher ES, Smith LK et al: *Cardiac rehabilitation as secondary prevention*, Clinical practice guideline #17, AHCPR Pub No 96-0672, Rockville, Md, 1995, US Department of Health and Human Services, Public Health Service, Agency for

Health Care Policy and Research, and the National Heart, Lung, and Blood Institute.

9. US Department of Health and Human Services: *Physical activity and health: a report of the Surgeon General,* Pittsburgh, 1996, President's Council on Physical Fitness and Sports.

10. Schairer JR, Keteyian SJ, Ehrman JK et al: Leisure time physical activity of patients in maintenance cardiac rehabilitation, *J Cardiopulm Rehabil* 23:260-265, 2003.

11. Williams MA, Balady GJ, Carlson JJ et al: *AACVPR guidelines for cardiac rehabilitation and secondary prevention programs,* ed 4, Champaign, Ill, 2004, Human Kinetics.

12. Franklin BA, Bonzheim K, Gordon S et al: Safety of medically-supervised outpatient cardiac rehabilitation exercise therapy: a 16-year follow-up, *Chest* 114:902-906, 1998.

13. Squires RW: *Exercise prescription for the high-risk cardiac patient,* Champaign, Ill, 1998, Human Kinetics.

14. Krieger EM, Brum PC, Negrao CE: State-of-the-art lecture: influence of exercise training on neurogenic control of blood pressure in spontaneously hypertensive rats, *Hypertension* 34: 720-723, 1999.

15. Gibbons RJ, Abrams J, Chatterjee K et al: ACC/AHA 2002 guideline update for the management of patients with chronic stable angina—summary article: a report of the American College of Cardiology/American Heart Association Task Force on practice guidelines (Committee on the Management of Patients with Chronic Stable Angina). *J Am Coll Cardiol* 41:159-168, 2003.

16. Evon DM, Burns JW: Process and outcome in cardiac rehabilitation: an examination of cross-lagged effects, *J Consult Clin Psychol* 72:605-616, 2004.

17. Miller JF: *Coping with chronic illness: overcoming powerlessness,* ed 3, Philadelphia, 2000, FA Davis.

18. Toobert DJ, Glasgow RE, Radcliffe JL: Physiologic and related behavioral outcomes from the Women's Lifestyle Heart Trial, *Ann Behav Med* 22:1-9, 2000.

19. Mallik S, Krumholtz HM, Lin ZQ et al: Patients with depressive symptoms have lower health status benefits after coronary artery bypass surgery, *Circulation* 111:271-277, 2005.

chapter 26

Nurses and Home Care

Marianne Roncoli
Marie Raia
Patricia S.A. Sparacino

CHAPTER ABBREVIATIONS

ADL   activities of daily living

CMS   Centers for Medicare and Medicaid Services

OASIS   Outcome and Assessment Information Set

OBQI   outcome-based quality improvement

Home care can be an integral aspect of care for all patients with chronic illness, particularly those with heart disease. In the home is where the patient lives with family, is accessible to the community, and manages his or her own care. Home is where caring and self-caring are defined; it is where not only the heart but also the true self resides. Patients survive illness in a hospital; they recover and live with illness in their homes. Patients are cared for in the hospital by doctors, nurses, and therapists; patients care for themselves, with the help of family and the health care team, in their own homes. (See the Conundrum feature.)

■■■ CONUNDRUM

BECOMING SUCCESSFULLY ILL

The term *successfully ill* means that a person is managing a chronic disease well. You might compare it, like Tim Brookes does, to "fixing one's own car: with each breakdown we learn more about our car, about cars in general; we're less thrown off stride next time. . . . Instead of sending our bodies to the dealer . . . we discover what goes on under the hood, we love tinkering and tuning, we hear the first sound of the engine running rough early enough to prevent anything serious from going wrong, we enjoy the challenge of keeping ourselves running efficiently. We become, perhaps, less apprehensive . . . more impressed by our own interior design."[1]

The structure of home care is changing to accommodate the patient as provider. The agency model of home care is being replaced with a consumer model. Unlike the agency model that determines service hours, hires and supervises the providers, handles reimbursement and payment, and determines the types of providers the patient needs, the consumers take on these tasks themselves. Consumer-driven models of home care have the patient with varying degrees of independence determining how much, what kind, and how long home care service is needed. Consumers also take over the personnel and financial matters, such as hiring persons and managing third-party reimbursement. Nurses need to be prepared to work with and test these models of home care as they become more widely available.

Reference

1. Brookes T: *Catching my breath: an asthmatic explores his illness*, New York, 1994, Time Books. P 279.

PATIENT AS PROVIDER

One of the national aims for quality improvement in health care is for care to be patient-centered, where the patient's authority and choices are respected and followed. If this aim is to be achieved, the patient must be in control, becoming his or her own primary provider. The purpose of this chapter is to describe how the nurse in home care—typically a generalist—works with patients to engage them in self-care.

When the patient learns to manage all the routine problems, doctors, nurses, and therapists become specialists with whom the patient consults when an unfamiliar problem arises. In this model, the patient does not follow orders but instead considers options and makes informed decisions.

There are barriers, however, to patients taking over the management of their own care. The cost of health care can be burdensome. As of 2001, 95 percent of patients older than age 65 were paying some portion of their health care out of pocket because third-party payers did not cover the cost.[1-3]

The elderly receive the greatest amount of home care, and they take the greatest number of medications, which can absorb 12 to 19 percent of household income.[1] With this added expense, there is a tendency for patients to take and keep medications, regardless of our instructions to discard them, even though prescriptions and dosages change. Even with the new prescription drug plan, universally available in 2006,[4] Medicare-eligible patients still need to pay a monthly premium in addition to co-payments for medications—payments that persons on fixed incomes are wary of or unable to make.

Increasing disability or lack of self-care ability,[5] decreased cognitive status, depression, and caregiver burnout[6] make it difficult for patients to adhere to treatment regimens even with the best of intentions. Furthermore, of those over age 65, 10 to 15 percent smoke, 15 to 38 percent are obese, nearly 75 percent are overweight, and less than 25 percent engage in regular physical exercise.[7] These high-risk behaviors present formidable challenges to self-care and to the caregivers who promote it.

COMPETENCIES HOME CARE NURSES NEED TO PROMOTE RECOVERY

In order to deliver home care effectively, home care nurses must know how the home care industry is financed and regulated by the Centers for Medicare and Medicaid Services, the primary payer of home care.

Within the confines of finite resources, nurses must function autonomously but collaboratively with providers, patients, and families in helping patients recover from illness and understand what impairs that recovery.

Knowledge of Home Care Service Delivery
Medicare as Primary Payer

Although the percentage of Medicare funds spent on home care is small, Medicare is the primary source of payment for home care services for Medicare-eligible patients. Of all money spent for health care, the Centers for Medicare and Medicaid Services (**CMS**) reported in 2001 that 4 percent of Medicare funds was spent on basic home care services provided by freestanding home care service agencies.[8] With the addition of hospital-based home care agencies, skilled nursing facility–based home care service agencies, and other types of government and private sources of home care, Medicare spent $7.9 billion in 2001[9]; Medicare was the primary source of payment for 85 percent of Medicare-eligible patients receiving home care.[10]

Medicare is not the only source of payment for home care in the United States, and Medicare-eligible patients are not the only ones receiving home care. In 2000, for instance, when all payment sources such as private insurance, out-of-pocket expenditures, Medicaid, and other types of payment were considered, Medicare paid only 29 percent of home care expenses for patients who received service, regardless of whether they were Medicare-eligible.[8] Medicare, then, is a primary source of payment for home care services, but only for those who are Medicare-eligible.

Medicare Reimbursement for Home Care

Home care is paid for as part of hospital insurance (Part A) and as part of supplemental medical insurance (Part B) from Medicare. This insurance includes skilled nursing services, home health aid services, and rehabilitative care. Medicare also pays for durable medical equipment, supplies, laboratory services, and other services used in the home through Part B.[4] In 2001, durable medical equipment and supplies amounted to 7 percent or $16 billion of total Medicare expenditures.[8]

Services not covered by Medicare are paid by the beneficiaries themselves or by a third party such as an employer-sponsored retiree health plan. Beneficiaries also may purchase Medigap insurance, private insurance that pays for most of the services not covered by Medicare Part A and Part B within certain limits.

Medicare beneficiaries may be covered by a fee-for-service plan, where the beneficiary is responsible for services not covered by Part A and Part B, or they may choose to enroll in a Medicare Advantage plan (Part C), which includes managed care plans such as health maintenance organizations, preferred provider organizations, or other private fee-for-service plans where beneficiaries pay premiums for coverage of services, many of which are not covered by Medicare Part A and Part B. Services such as long-term nursing care, custodial care, and health care needs such as dentures and dental care, eyeglasses, and hearing aids, which are not covered by Medicare, may be covered by Medicare Advantage plans.

The Medicare Prescription Drug Improvement and Modernization Act of 2003 (Public Law 108-173) established a fourth part of Medicare: a prescription drug benefit (Part D). In 2006, this program began providing access to prescription drug insurance coverage on a voluntary basis to individuals entitled to Part A or enrolled in Part B. Given that the patients most likely to receive home care are those with multiple prescribed medications, this benefit will influence the management of patients receiving home care.

Medicaid Reimbursement for Home Care

In addition to Medicare, patients receiving home care may be dually eligible for Medicaid reimbursement. Individual states have the option to provide services for those who would be eligible if institutionalized in a nursing home, for example, but receive care under home- and community-based waivers. For patients who meet criteria for eligibility based on available resources and medical need, states provide services that would not be provided by Medicare in the patient's home through Medicaid. In 2001, CMS provided approximately 2.2 percent Medicaid expenditure for home care.[8]

Medicare Conditions of Participation

CMS specifies the conditions of participation with which home care agencies must comply in order to receive reimbursement. These conditions detail how agency services are organized, administered, and evaluated. They include the required qualifications of personnel, the content of patient assessment, how it should be documented, and other details. They also specify how to transmit data to the state electronically for monitoring and evaluation.[11]

The conditions from CMS also include the type of patient for whom home care is administered. The patient must be homebound, but not necessarily bedridden. The patient may leave home infrequently for short duration, usually to receive outpatient medical treatment. Although patients may hire their own services to provide 24-hour care, Medicare offers intermittent, part-time care in the form of skilled nursing services, home health aides, and rehabilitation and social work services.[12]

OASIS Data and Outcome-Based Quality Improvement

Since October 2000 in the United States, Medicare-certified home care agencies have routinely collected nationally standardized assessment data as a condition of participation in and reimbursement from Medicare. These data are collected in the Outcome and Assessment Information Set (**OASIS**), which represent core elements of a comprehensive assessment.

These elements, developed by a panel of home care experts and thoroughly tested for validity and reliability, are considered essential to the management and evaluation of home care at different points in time during an episode of care. OASIS assessments measure patient status for the purposes of reimbursement and improvement of outcomes through a process of outcome-based quality improvement (**OBQI**).

On a quarterly basis, agencies receive case mix reports that compare aggregate statistics on various patient characteristics such as demographics, health, or functional status at start of care with those of a reference group of patients. Based on this comparison, a risk-adjusted outcome report is created that identifies the performance of the agency relative to the reference group on 41 OASIS measures of functional, physiological, emotional/behavioral status, and utilization outcome measures at the start of care, at the end of each 60-day episode of care, and at discharge from home care.

When an outcome in an agency is significantly worse than the reference group, it is targeted for improvement. Agency clinical staff investigate the care provided and devise a plan to enhance and then evaluate care processes. Over time the target outcome is expected to show improvement in the quarterly risk-adjusted outcome reports as care is monitored for improvement and is adjusted accordingly.

This process of quality improvement is expected to take place in a matter of weeks and to be continuous and ongoing. Because the plans of action are expected to be evidence-based, the OBQI process is essentially a research-utilization process with standardized outcomes. Multiyear demonstration trials involving New York and 27 other U.S. states compared two target outcomes—acute care hospitalizations and one other clinical outcome of the agency's choice—of agencies that used the OBQI process and those that did not. A statistically significant decline was found in hospitalization rates of 22 and 24 percent, respectively in the national and New York state demonstration trials.[13]

At this time, Medicare is the only third-party payer that requires this process of care improvement. However, other payers customarily follow Medicare policies. Thus, it is anticipated that this quality improvement process will become standard in the future.

When the Medicare prospective payment system was implemented in 2000, fixed reimbursement for home care was predetermined based on patient diagnosis and the number of services the patient was expected to receive. Agencies were free to provide whatever services they deemed necessary within this fixed revenue and to keep whatever revenue they did not spend. With the OBQI process in place, quality care is assured in a system designed to encourage agencies to generate a profit in the service of cost containment, regardless of the care delivered.

In January 2003, CMS launched *Home Health Compare,* a publication of data on 11 outcomes measures from the OASIS assessment. This publication makes outcome data from all Medicare-certified home care agencies available to the public. In February 2005, the National Quality Forum endorsed a revised list of quality measures (Box 26-1) that was implemented in the fall 2005.[14]

In 2006, CMS began using outcome data as a measure of quality and a basis for reimbursement. The system, called *Pay-for-Performance,* is being investigated not

---

BOX 26-1 ■ ■ ■
QUALITY OUTCOME MEASURES

1. Improvement in ambulation/locomotion
2. Improvement in bathing
3. Improvement in transferring
4. Improvement in management of oral medication
5. Improvement in pain interfering with activity
6. Acute care hospitalizations
7. Emergent care
8. Discharge to the community
9. Improvement in dyspnea
10. Improvement in urinary incontinence

Centers for Medicare and Medicaid Services: *Overview: home health quality initiatives.* Retrieved November 28, 2006 from www.cms.hhs.gov/HomeHealthQualityInits/

---

only for home care but also for hospitals, practice offices, nursing homes, ambulatory care, and dialysis facilities[15]—wherever CMS pays for health care. Given that Medicare is a prominent payer for home care, the Pay-for-Performance system promises to have profound impact on service delivery.

Telehealth and Technology in the Home

Most home telehealth approaches incorporate some intervention by nurses and physicians through traditional home care visitation with follow-up telephone monitoring, videoconferencing, Internet communication, or e-mail from ambulatory sites. Telehealth systems that allow patients to communicate with the provider are as effective as traditional monitoring systems.[16]

The overall effectiveness and practicality of telehealth devices in the home is still under investigation and appears to depend on the features of the device itself, the abilities of the patient, and the integration of technology into the operations of home care service delivery. The patient's ability to use a device is an important consideration that may depend more on the features of the device itself and less on factors such as patient age and education. For example, in one study, persons older than age 65 retained information as well as younger persons if they viewed a video instead of reading an instruction manual.[17]

Elderly patients can use a web-based home welfare and care services support system successfully with wireless Internet mobile phone and Internet client computers. Even elders with serious disabilities were able to call for home support using a pen-like image sensor that requested items identified with no more that eight Roman alphabet characters on a computer screen.[18] In a study of a home-based telemedicine system tested with diabetic Medicare patients, skill with numbers and mathematics was required, as were certain psychomotor skills, but age was not necessarily a factor in successful performance. Literate, motivated, older persons demonstrated remarkable adaptability when faced with home monitoring equipment, if provided the necessary instruction.[19]

The use of telehealth technology in the home also affects the productivity of home care service delivery. The Pennsylvania Homecare Association demonstrated that telehealth improved retention of nurses and enabled them to manage more patients more effectively on a daily basis.[20]

In the next section of the chapter, we describe the factors that nurses consider routinely when working with patients in the home care setting. Many of these factors are considered in depth in other chapters, but in this chapter we briefly outline the routine assessment parameters to illustrate the breadth of knowledge that home care nurse generalists must know when caring for cardiac patients.

Knowledge of Factors That Impair Recovery
Inadequate Knowledge of Regimen

Physicians and nurses do not always know best, as far as the patient is concerned. Patients do not necessarily want to know what health care professionals think they should know. Because patients may not care to know as much about their medications as nurses think they should know, especially when they are overwhelmed, nurses need to collaborate with them about the feasibility and acceptability of the medical regimen rather than simply instructing patients about medicines. Furthermore, differences in education determine what kinds of knowledge patients want to know. The nurse needs to find out whether a patient with little formal education wants to know about the disease itself. More educated persons may know about the disease already and, instead, want to know how it is progressing.

How patients experience their heart disease informs home care decisions about priorities. Men and women experience illness differently. In women, depression has been shown to interfere with self-care. When faced with chronic illness, persons make transitions—from being overwhelmed with the diagnosis and the extraordinary nature of the illness to being able to cope with the heart disease in everyday ordinary terms.[21] Determining where the patient is in terms of this normal process determines how the nurse intervenes.

Nurses need to know of patient education materials that are available in different languages and media. Although the Internet can be an invaluable source of information, the quality of information on a website about medications, treatments, and disease processes needs to be determined. Government websites (such as the National Library of Medicine and the National Institutes of Health) and websites of major nonprofit health care organizations (such as the American Heart Association, the American Lung Association, the American Red Cross, and the American Cancer Society) provide objective, unbiased, accurate information about health and disease. The Heart Failure Society of America has an educational booklet that instructs patients on "How to Evaluate Claims of New Heart Failure Treatments and Cures." The booklet is free from their website: *www.hfsa.org.* State and local health departments also provide excellent sources of free information on health and safety. The materials on government sites are usually free with unlimited access. However, the educational materials of nonprofit health care organizations, which often can be accessed from government websites, can be copied for individual use only, for the ma-

terials are copyrighted. Free print copies can be requested.

Although the National Guideline Clearinghouse, a central source of evidence-based practice guidelines, does not provide specific guidelines for home care, it does provide guidelines for the management of cardiovascular, respiratory, and muscular diseases, which are common to home care patients. The National Guideline Clearinghouse is also a source of clinical practice guidelines useful in home care, such as the guidelines for assessment and prevention of falls,[22] assessment of capacity for activities of daily living (**ADL**) in older adults,[23] and discharge planning for the older adult.[24]

Engaging in Self Care

In assessing a person's capacity for self-care, data suggest that nurses should understand that illness beliefs inform self-care.[25] Questions to consider asking in the assessment of patients include the following: What does the patient think caused their heart disease? How do patients see heart disease changing their lives? What do they see as the relationship they need with caretakers?

Self-care requires financial, educational, and personal resources. Without these resources, individuals are least likely to cope. Although there is a wealth of information on the Internet, there may be enormous barriers to patients' abilities to access and use health information because of cultural differences, language proficiency, and knowledge of and access to information technology.[26]

Beliefs about self-efficacy differ and may not reflect true abilities. Does your patient use problem-oriented or affective-oriented coping strategies? Does the person try to effect specific outcomes, such as maintaining a low blood glucose level or watching for early signs of fluid retention of heart failure? Or does the person "put faith in God" or "pray," actions that facilitate coping but probably do not directly affect a health outcome?[27] Understanding patients' beliefs allows the nurse to collaborate in setting realistic health care goals, creating a workable plan of action, and devising a method to assess success.[28]

Depression, Anxiety, and Lack of Social Support

Anxiety, depression, and lack of social support influence and are influenced by chronic illness. This relationship appears to be mediated by many factors, including age, race, and socioeconomic status. Older adults with social isolation, medical comorbidities, and physical impairment are more likely to be depressed and less able to seek treatment than elders without these characteristics.[29] Patients with poor cognitive function and depressive symptoms have mortality rates three times higher than those with better cognitive function and low depression scores.[30]

The home is an ideal place to assess emotional state. The signs and symptoms of depression include low mood, lack of interest in life, thoughts of death, and difficulties eating and sleeping.[31] These can be attributed easily to illness or aging and can be overlooked, but if these symptoms appear nearly every day, depression should be considered. Although the diagnosis of depression is considered when sleep disorders are reported, sleep disorders are the least likely symptom of depression. Depressed mood, anhedonia, and thoughts of suicide are more likely to indicate depression.[32]

Management of depression includes psychopharmacology. One in five elderly persons living in the community is prescribed an antidepressant, anxiolytic, or other psychotropic drug.[33] A search for potential medical causes of depression is important before prescribing antidepressants. The antidepressants sertraline, fluoxetine hydrochloride, paroxetine, and alprazolam were among the most frequently used prescription drugs nationwide.[34] These drugs are generally safe, but they can interact with foods and other drugs that patients are taking. For example, grapefruit juice may increase the plasma concentrations of sertraline, which is a substrate of the CYP450 3A4 isoenzyme.[35] It appears that certain compounds present in grapefruit inhibit CYP450 3A4-mediated first-pass metabolism in the gut wall. Although the extent and clinical significance of the interaction are unknown, patients who regularly consume grapefruit and grapefruit juice should be monitored for adverse effects.

Enzymes of the cytochrome P-450 enzyme system, responsible for the metabolism of many medications, such as beta blockers, affect and are affected by antidepressants. The herb *Hypericum perforatum*, St John's wort, may be effective against mild depression, but it should not be used for major depressive illness.[36]

The side effects of antidepressants include nausea, dizziness, dry mouth, constipation, agitation, sleep and dream difficulties, and sexual dysfunction, although side effects vary within and among different medicines. The selective serotonin reuptake inhibitors and the drugs that affect norepinephrine and dopamine reuptake inhibitors are generally better tolerated than the older tricyclic antidepressants. A careful review of all medications that patients are taking is essential, especially when patients are prescribed antidepressants.

Results of completed and ongoing clinical trials suggest that when used with antidepressants, nonpharmacological home-based therapy can improve outcomes from depression. Help with problem solving, physical and social activity, and social support effectively relieves depressive symptoms, improves quality of life, and prevents exacerbations of chronic illness.[29,37,38]

Social isolation, such as living alone, lacking instrumental and emotional support, and being unable to share personal experiences with someone can increase morbidity and mortality from heart disease.[39] Social isolation affects men and women equally, and it is especially prevalent in persons with lower incomes, less education, older age, and in ethnic or racial minority groups where there is a high incidence of cardiovascular disease.[40]

In persons with a limited social network, studies have shown that a home-based one-on-one peer support or community-based support groups effectively improve self-care.[40] Instrumental support for ADL such as physical care and help with shopping and housekeeping is helpful; however, emotional support appears to be more important than instrumental support in terms of morbidity outcomes. Human beings need someone in whom they can confide. A lack of meaningful emotional support is associated with increased morbidity and mortality.[39]

Anxiety, depression and social isolation are covered in depth in Chapters 15, 16, 40, 41, and 42.

Knowledge of Factors That Promote Healing
Physical Fitness

The home is a place where observation of the limits of endurance and the capacity for ADL can be assessed accurately and enhanced. The nurse can teach patients how to economize on energy expenditure by helping patients organize daily routines to include frequent rest periods between strenuous activities. Survey kitchens, bathrooms, and living rooms, and recommend energy-saving devices such as electronic can openers, lightweight vacuum cleaners, raised toilet seats, and bathtub safety devices such as tub chairs and grab bars that improve safety while conserving energy.

Physical activity has emerged as the primary predictor explaining more of the variance in health outcomes than any other risk factor for heart disease, including smoking, hypertension, hyperlipidemia, and comorbid conditions such as diabetes.[41] Muscle strength predicts independence in performance of ADL. An elderly, independent person who has limited handgrip, elbow flexion, knee extension, and trunk extension is likely to be dependent in some way within 5 years.[42] Lower extremity strength can be lost in older persons before upper extremity strength, and women have a greater risk of developing disability.[43]

After assessing lower extremity strength and the ability to get in and out of bed and up and down from a chair, help the patient to embark on a strength-training program, if needed, to prevent further decline. A program lasting 12 weeks can improve functional performance significantly.[44] No special equipment is needed; lifting 1-lb food cans over the head in a thoughtful and slow manner several times each day can increase upper body strength significantly.

Convenience and social support influence whether persons continue with an exercise program.[45] Home-based programs can eliminate the inconvenience factor. An exercise program designed around the home environment can increase aerobic capacity and endurance. Most homes have built-in step aerobics equipment (e.g., the stairs into and out of a home) that can be used effectively with the right supervision and instruction.

Lack of social support limits willingness to maintain exercise routines, and social support is likely to be greater in a home exercise program. Further, the pleasantness of exercise is greater in home-based than hospital-based exercise programs. Spouses, children, home health aides, and personal care workers can help tailor the exercise program to the specific home environment, encourage the patient to adhere to the program, and serve as the local cheering section in the home training room.

Sleep and Rest

Difficulties with sleeping have been associated with aging, chronic illness, depression, medication use, primary sleep apnea, dyspnea, and heart disease—especially heart failure. No one cause or any specific combination of causes is identified consistently. What is experienced universally is that persons with chronic heart disease are more likely to have sleep disorders than persons who are healthy.

Two-thirds of persons with heart failure perceive that they sleep too much or sleep too little. If what hospitalized patients report is accurate about sleeping at home, they have problems sleeping flat, falling sleep, and staying asleep. They experience daytime sleepiness and early morning awakening, and these difficulties decrease quality of life.[46] What effect recent illness or concern about heart disease may have on perceptions of sleep is not known.

Although cardiovascular drugs are said to cause sleeping disorders, most of these data are anecdotal or from case reports. Beta blockers, beta agonists, and antidysrhythmic drugs are reported to interfere with sleep.[47] Aging has been linked to sleep disorders, sleep apnea, nocturia, and chronic pain. Nocturia increases with age, independent of medical condition or medication use. But depression should be considered in anyone with disordered sleep.

Because patients may be taking many medications already, adding a hypnotic should be the option of last resort. Sleep hygiene measures are detailed in Chapter 17. Alcohol and caffeine-containing food and drink (e.g., cola) should be limited before bedtime. If hypnotics are to be used, short-term use of zolpidem (Ambien) has been shown to be safe and effective for sleep disturbances in older persons with comorbidities.[48]

Nutrition

Assessment of the patient's diet begins before the nurse enters the home. The neighborhood supermarkets, delicatessens, drug stores, and vitamin and dietary supplement stores illustrate what is available to the patient. Public transportation also determines the foods available. When assessing diet, note the use of herbs, vitamins, and dietary supplements. In assessing the drug regimen, the nurse may be the first to note the potential for adverse interactions among diet, drugs, and complementary or alternative medicines. For a full discussion of nutrition, see Chapter 12.

Complementary and alternative medicines are used by 64 percent of cardiovascular patients. Fish oil and vitamin K can increase the anticoagulant effects of warfarin.[49, 50] The most common dietary supplements—garlic preparations, *Ginkgo biloba,* and chondroitin—also may interact with anticoagulants.[51] Iron supplements can correct anemia in the elderly and increase weight, ejection fraction, and resting energy metabolism.[52] Iron supplements also have been shown to decrease the incidence of cough associated with angiotensin-converting enzyme inhibitors.[53]

The major comorbidity of persons with heart disease is diabetes. When adjusting the diet to maintain stable blood glucose levels—the most desirable outcome—the patient must be aware that diuretics such as furosemide and many psychotropic drugs can raise blood glucose levels irrespective of diet. The dietary supplement chondroitin has been reported to do the same.[51]

Foods such as grapefruit and grapefruit juice interact with several categories of drugs used to treat chronic cardiovascular illness, including statins, calcium channel blockers, angiotensin II receptor blockers, antidysrhythmics, beta and alpha blockers, phosphodiesterase type 5 inhibitors, and tricyclic antidepressants. The metabolism of these drugs is mediated by the cytochrome P-450 enzymes system which, as described above, inhibit or induce therapeutic drug reactions.[35]

There is a greater *potential* for, rather than actual occurrence of, interactions among drugs, herbs, and dietary supplements. The primary conclusion to draw from available data is that when drug treatment or diet therapy fails to achieve the expected results, then drug or food interactions should always be suspected.

Obesity is epidemic in the population. Between 1999 and 2002, more than one-third (36 percent) of persons ages 65 to 74 were obese, and 55 percent were overweight.[7] However, many patients with heart disease are underweight and not eating well because of poor appetite, nausea, depression, or lack of availability of food. A well-balanced diet that is rich in essential nutrients and low in salt and fat is ideal, but supplementation, including minerals such as potassium and calcium, may be needed to ensure optimal health.[54]

A salt intake greater than 113.6 mmol/d is associated with left ventricular hypertrophy in the overweight,[55] suggesting that a high-salt diet predicts heart failure, independent of weight. The National Nutrition Guidelines 2005 recommend the Dietary Approaches to Stop Hypertension (DASH) diet for persons with hypertension.[56] These guidelines include diet plans with 1500 to 2400 mg of sodium per day and include recipes to make the recommendations operational. These types of tools are helpful in home care nursing practice.

The new food pyramid[57] recommends that everyone eat a diet low in animal and *trans*-saturated fats and simple sugars; this is a diet that everyone, including patients with heart disease, should follow. The guidelines, including the recommendations of 25 to 30 g of fiber per day are difficult to achieve, and often require supplementations beyond the resources or inclinations of elders with chronic heart disease.

Hygiene

Good hygiene practices prevent the spread of microorganisms that cause infections, improve appearance and comfort, and protect the skin from breakdown. Infections that used to be confined to the hospital, such as methicillin-resistant *Staphylococcus,* now are appearing in the community with alarming regularity.[58] Hospitals are recognized as a source of drug-resistant bacteria, but there is little research on the surveillance, prevention, and control of infection in the home care setting.

In the absence of evidence, the guidelines for hand hygiene in the hospital can be transferred to the home and recommended to the patient and family. The transmission of microorganisms via the hands is well documented. The latest guidelines from the Centers of Disease Control and Prevention include washing hands that are visibly dirty with soap and water. Alcohol-based hand rub that contains 60 to 95 percent ethanol or isopropanol[59] should be used for other contact with fomites on contaminated surfaces. Because the hands are themselves contaminated, hand washing and hand disinfection with alcohol-based rub should be frequent and thoughtful. Teaching patients and family members good hygiene practices is basic to any community health nursing practice.

In matters of personal hygiene, how well a patient can get on and off a toilet seat and in and out of a bathtub depends on the physical features of the bathtub and the toilet. Therefore, raised toilet seats, shower chairs, and bathtub grips are essential for good personal hygiene in the debilitated, homebound patient. Upper body strength training may help as well.

Oral Health

Approximately 30 percent of persons older than age 65 have no permanent teeth. The risk of dental caries is greater for persons older than age 70 because of reduced saliva flow, inadequate oral hygiene, frequent sugar intake, and the presence of partial dentures.[60] Poor oral hygiene places chronically ill older adults at risk for malnutrition.

Although most persons can explain the importance of brushing their teeth, keeping teeth clean to prevent gum disease is not as widely known. Home health nurses educate persons about good dental hygiene, encouraging the use of electric toothbrushes, dental floss, and dietary supplements of calcium and vitamin D.

Whether older persons seek dental care may depend on their ability to pay using discretionary income. The Agency for Healthcare Quality and Research reported that 13 percent of the out-of-pocket health care expenditures of persons age 65 and over were for dental services in 2001.[1] Unless one is enrolled in a Medicare Advantage program, a Medicare-managed care program requiring additional premium payment by the Medicare-eligible patient, there is no health coverage for dental services offered by Medicare.[4]

Safety

The major safety concern of older cardiac patients living in the community is the risk of falls. The home should be assessed for damage to carpeting or flooring and clutter in hallways, passageways, and stairways. The best fall prevention strategy, however, is ensuring that the patient is as strong, balanced, and flexible as possible. Physical conditions that predict falling include cognitive, sensory, and motor impairments. Specific neurological and musculoskeletal limitations to monitor include poor balance requiring contact guarding, a slow get-up-and-go test[61] (Figure 26-1), inadequate depth perception and contrast sensitivity, [62] ankle dorsiflexion delay, [63] gait asymmetry, and decreased quadriceps strength.

Other threats to safety in the community for homebound patients are crime, abuse, and environmental threats. Crime is ubiquitous in poor neighborhoods, and the elderly and infirm are easy targets.

Abuse and neglect in the home can take many forms—physical, sexual, emotional, and financial. In 90 percent of cases, the perpetrator is a family member such as a child or spouse. The factors associated with abuse are low income, lack of social support, increasing age, functional and cognitive impairment, substance use, nonwhite race, and emotional distress.[64] The home care nurse considers these when evidence of injury or neglect appears. Although there are no reliable, valid instruments to measure abuse and neglect in the home, there are clinical practice guidelines for prevention, [65] identification, and management of abuse.[66] (See the Evidence-Based Practice feature.)

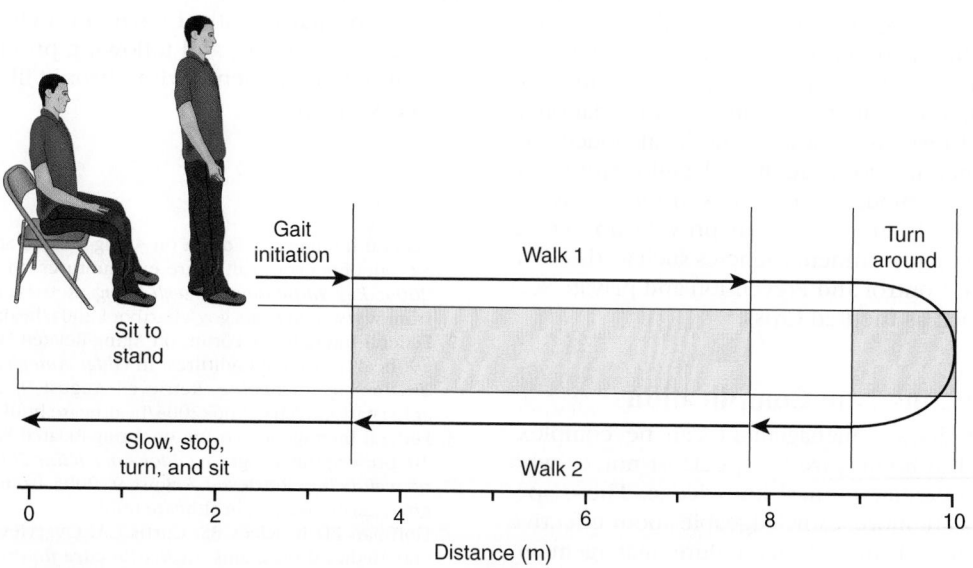

FIGURE 26-1 ■ The expanded timed get-up-and-go test. Timed tasks include sit-to-stand; gait initiation; walk 1; turnaround; walk 2; and slow, stop, turn, and sit. The tasks take place over a 10-meter distance. Elderly persons at risk for a fall completed the entire test in 18.14 ± 4.604 seconds compared with other elderly persons, who completed the test in 7.74 ± 0.851 seconds. The time it takes to complete walk 1 and walk 2 may be more predictive of a fall than any other task. Further investigation is needed, however. (From Wall JC, Bell C, Campbell S et al: *J Rehabil Res Dev* 37:109-114, 2000.)

Environmental threats can be seasonal, such as extremes of weather and outbreaks of communicable diseases such as the flu; they can be local, such as fire and hurricanes; or, they can be national or international, such as acts of terrorism. Besides the local police and fire departments and local adult and child protective services, other community resources are available by telephone or the Internet that can provide up-to-date information from government agencies such as the Centers for Disease Control and Prevention and private-sector agencies such as the Red Cross.

Skill in Detecting Late Complications

Because heart disease management can be complex, there is a need in home care for specialist nurses who have advanced cardiac clinical knowledge. These specialized nurses are more knowledgeable about effective interventions for chronic heart failure management, improved patient outcomes, and reduced risk of rehospitalization.[67]

The most common causes of preventable hospitalization of patients cared for at home include lack of adherence to the prescribed drug and diet regimen and failure to seek early intervention for escalating symptoms.

Further, poor discharge planning, haphazard follow-up visits with the provider, and failure to address patient characteristics (such as cognitive impairment, depression, and multiple comorbidities) place the patient at risk for rehospitalization. These patients need regular home visits by the same nurse to ensure consistency of assessment and interventions. Those who receive close nursing and medical supervision experience substantially fewer rehospitalizations and improved quality of life, even when few actual home visits occur.[67]

WORKING AUTONOMOUSLY ON A MULTIDISCIPLINARY TEAM

The community health nurse is basically alone with the patient when home care decisions are made. No colleague is available to check a questionable vital sign, nor is the physician down the hall available for consultation. It can be tedious and time consuming to contact a social worker, a surgeon, or a nurse practitioner who may be unavailable when needed. The physician-nurse relationship is not unlike the community health nurse–patient relationship; they are perfect strangers to each other, collaborating for the first time around a specific problem.

The home care nurse needs expert clinical skills in problem solving, critical thinking, and clinical assessment. In addition, logistical skills[68] are needed to manage time around patient schedules, bad weather, parking restrictions, traffic delays, reimbursement limitations, documentation details, and arcane state, federal, and Joint Commission on Accreditation of Healthcare Organizations regulations.

After 2 years of home care practice, the typical nurse has developed the skills to work autonomously. Having developed a reputation as an expert, the nurse now can collaborate effectively and efficiently with physicians and other providers. Moreover, this nurse now can collaborate primarily with the patient, defining problems, setting patient goals, and following progress in the service of helping patients with chronic illnesses become "successfully ill."

REFERENCES

1. Federal Interagency Forum on Aging-Related Statistics: Indicator 32: out-of-pocket health care expenditures. In *Older Americans 2004: key indicators of well-being*. Retrieved August 9, 2005 from www.agingstats.gov/chartbook2004/healthcare.html

2. Federal Interagency Forum on Aging-Related Statistics: Indicator 29: health care expenditures. In *Older Americans 2004: key indicators of well-being*. Retrieved August 9, 2005 from www.agingstats.gov/chartbook2004/healthcare.html

3. Federal Interagency Forum on Aging-Related Statistics: Indicator 30: prescription drugs. In *Older Americans 2004: key indicators of well-being*. Retrieved August 9, 2005 from www.agingstats.gov/chartbook2004/healthcare.html

4. Hoffman ED Jr, Klees BS, Curtis CA: Overview of the Medicare and Medicaid programs. In *Health care financing review Medicare and Medicaid statistical supplement, 2003*, Office of Research and Development, Centers for Medicare and Medicaid Services. Retrieved September 28, 2006 from www.cms.hhs.gov/apps/review/supp/2003/

5. Shyu YI, Lee HC: Predictors of nursing home placement and home nursing services utilization by elderly patients after hospital discharge in Taiwan, *J Adv Nurs* 38:398-406, 2002.

6. Covinsky KE, Newcomer R, Fox P et al: Patient and caregiver characteristics associated with depression in caregivers of patients with dementia, *J Gen Intern Med* 18:1006-1014, 2003.

7. Federal Interagency Forum on Aging-Related Statistics: Health risks and behaviors. In *Older Americans 2004: key indicators of well-being.* Retrieved August 9, 2005 from www.agingstats.gov/chartbook2004/healthrisks.html

8. Office of Research and Development and Information III Medicare Program Information C. *Medicare Program Spending 2002.* Centers for Medicare and Medicaid Services. Retrieved November 26, 2006 from www.cms.hhs.gov/TheChartSeries/downloads/sec3c_p.pdf

9. Centers for Medicare and Medicaid Services: Table 50: Number of providers, persons served, visits, and program payments for Medicare home health agency services, by type of agency: calender year 2001. In *Health care financing review medicare and medicaid statistical supplement, 2003.* Retrieved August 9, 2005 from www.cms.hhs.gov/apps/review/supp/2003/

10. Federal Interagency Forum on Aging-Related Statistics: Indicator 33: sources of payment for health care services. In *Older Americans 2004: key indicators of well-being.* Retrieved November 26, 2006 from www.agingstats.gov/chartbook2004/healthcare.html

11. National Archives and Records Administration: *CFR Title 42, Public health: conditions of participation: home health aide services.* Retrieved August 8, 2005 from www.access.gpo.gov/nara/cfr/waisidx_99/42cfr484_99.html

12. Centers for Medicare and Medicaid Services: Home Health Services, Ch 7, *Medicare Benefit Policy Manual,* (Pub# 100-02) Retrieved November 27, 2006 from www.cms.hhs.gov/Manuals/iom/itemdetail.asp?filterType=none&filterByDID=-99&sortByDID=1&sortOrder=ascending&itemID=CMS012673&intNumPerPage=10

13. Shaughnessy PW, Hittle DF, Crisler KS et al: Improving patient outcomes of home health care: findings from two demonstration trials of outcome-based quality improvement, *J Am Geriatr Soc* 50:1354-1364, 2002.

14. Centers for Medicare and Medicaid Services: *Overview: home health quality initiatives.* Retrieved November 28, 2006 from www.cms.hhs.gov/HomeHealthQualityInits/

15. Office of Public Affairs, Centers for Medicare and Medicaid Services: *Medicare "pay for performance (P4P)" initiatives.* Retrieved August 8, 2005 from www.cms.hhs.gov/media/press/release.asp?Counter=1343

16. Goldberg LR, Piette JD, Walsh MN et al: Randomized trial of a daily electronic home monitoring system in patients with advanced heart failure: the Weight Monitoring in Heart Failure (WHARF) trial, *Am Heart J* 146:705-712, 2003.

17. Mykityshyn AL, Fisk AD, Rogers WA: Learning to use a home medical device: mediating age-related differences with training, *Hum Factors* 44:354-364, 2002.

18. Ogawa H, Yonezawa Y, Maki H et al: A Web-based home welfare and care services support system using a pen type image sensor, *Biomed Sci Instrum* 39:199-203, 2003.

19. Kaufman DR, Patel VL, Hilliman C et al: Usability in the real world: assessing medical information technologies in patients' homes, *J Biomed Inform* 36:45-60, 2003.

20. Pennsylvania Homecare Association, Penn State University: *Telehealth project evaluation: year 2—impact of telehealth on nursing workload & retention,* Lemoyne, Pa, 2004, Pennsylvania Homecare Association.

21. Koch T, Kralik D: Chronic illness: reflections on a community-based action research programme, *J Adv Nurs* 36:23-31, 2001.

22. National Guideline Clearinghouse: *Clinical practice guideline for the assessment and prevention of falls in older people.* Retrieved November 28, 2006 from www.guideline.gov/summary/summary.aspx?doc_id=6118&nbr=3968&string=home+AND+health+AND+care

23. National Guideline Clearinghouse: *Assessment of function: of critical importance to acute care of older adults.* Retrieved August 9, 2005 from www.guideline.gov/summary/summary.aspx?doc_id=3504&nbr=2730&string=home+AND+health+AND+care

24. National Guideline Clearinghouse: *Discharge planning for the older adult.* Retrieved August 9, 2005 from www.guideline.gov/summary/summary.aspx?doc_id=3517&nbr=2743&string=home+AND+health+AND+care

25. King R: Illness attributions and myocardial infarction: the influence of gender and socio-economic circumstances on illness beliefs, *J Adv Nurs* 37:431-438, 2002.

26. Cashen MS, Dykes P, Gerber B: eHealth technology and Internet resources: barriers for vulnerable populations, *J Cardiovasc Nurs* 19:209-214, 2004.

27. St Louis L, Robichaud-Ekstrand S: Knowledge level and coping strategies according to coagulation levels in older persons with atrial fibrillation, *Nurs Health Sci* 5:67-75, 2003.

28. Von Korff M, Gruman J, Schaefer J et al: Collaborative management of chronic illness, *Ann Intern Med* 127:1097-1102, 1997.

29. Ciechanowski P, Wagner E, Schmaling K et al: Community-integrated home-based depression treatment in older adults: a randomized controlled trial, *JAMA* 291:1569-1577, 2004.

30. Mehta KM, Yaffe K, Langa KM et al: Additive effects of cognitive function and depressive symptoms on mortality in elderly community-living adults, *J Gerontol A Biol Sci Med Sci* 58:M461-M467, 2003.

31. American Psychological Association: *Diagnostic and statistical manual of mental disorders,* ed 4, Washington, DC, 1994, The Association.

32. Roberts RE, Shema SJ, Kaplan GA et al: Sleep complaints and depression in an aging cohort: a prospective perspective, *Am J Psychiatry* 157:81-88, 2000.

33. Aparasu RR, Mort JR, Brandt H: Psychotropic prescription use by community-dwelling elderly in the United States, *J Am Geriatr Soc* 51:671-677, 2003.

34. Kaufman DW, Kelly JP, Rosenberg L et al: Recent patterns of medication use in the ambulatory adult population of the United States: the Slone survey, *JAMA* 287:337-344, 2002.

35. Flockhart DA, Tanus-Santos JE: Implications of cytochrome P450 interactions when prescribing medication for hypertension, *Arch Intern Med* 162:405-412, 2002.

36. Hypericum Depression Trial Study Group: Effect of *Hypericum perforatum* (St. John's wort) in major depressive disorder: A randomized, controlled trial, *JAMA,* 287:1807-1814, 2004.

37. Berkman LF, Blumenthal J, Burg M et al: Effects of treating depression and low perceived social support on clinical events after myocardial infarction: the Enhancing Recovery in Coronary Heart Disease Patients (ENRICHD) randomized trial, *JAMA* 289:3106-3116, 2003.

38. van den Brink RH, van Melle JP, Honig A et al: Treatment of depression after myocardial infarction and the effects on cardiac prognosis and quality of life: rationale and outline of the Myocardial Infarction and Depression-Intervention Trial (MIND-IT), *Am Heart J* 144:219-225, 2002.

39. Moser DK, Worster PL: Effect of psychosocial factors on physiologic outcomes in patients with heart failure, *J Cardiovasc Nurs* 14:106-115, 2000.

40. Stuart-Shor EM, Buselli EF, Carroll DL, Forman DE: Are psychosocial factors associated with the pathogenesis and consequences of cardiovascular disease in the elderly? *J Cardiovasc Nurs* 18:169-183, 2003.

41. Myers J, Prakash M, Froelicher V et al: Exercise capacity and mortality among men referred for exercise testing, *N Engl J Med* 346:793-801, 2002.

42. Rantanen R, Avlund K, Suominen H et al: Muscle strength as a predictor of onset of ADL dependence in people aged 75 years, *Aging Clin Exp Res* 14:10-15, 2002.

43. Jagger C, Arthur AJ, Spiers NA et al: Patterns of onset of disability in activities of daily living with age, *J Am Geriatr Soc* 49:404-409, 2001.

44. Alexander NB, Galecki AT, Grenier ML et al: Task-specific resistance training to improve the ability of activities of daily living-impaired older adults to rise from a bed and from a chair, *J Am Geriatr Soc* 49:1418-1427, 2001.

45. Franklin BA, Swain DP, Shephard RJ: New insights in the prescription of exercise for coronary patients, *J Cardiovasc Nurs* 18:116-123, 2003.

46. Katz DA, McHorney CA: The relationship between insomnia and health-related quality of life in patients with chronic illness, *J Fam Pract* 51:229-235, 2002.

47. Parker KP, Dunbar SB: Sleep and heart failure, *J Cardiovasc Nurs* 17:30-41, 2002.

48. Cotroneo A, Gareri P, Lacava R et al: Use of zolpidem in over 75-year-old patients with sleep disorders and comorbidities, *Arch Gerontol Geriatr Suppl*, pp 93-96, 2004.

49. Buckley MS, Goff AD, Knapp WE: Fish oil interaction with warfarin, *Ann Pharmacother* 38:50-52, 2004.

50. Kurnik D, Lubetsky A, Loebstein R et al: Multivitamin supplements may affect warfarin anticoagulation in susceptible patients, *Ann Pharmacother* 37:1603-1606, 2003.

51. Wold RS, Lopez ST, Yau CL et al: Increasing trends in elderly persons' use of nonvitamin, nonmineral dietary supplements and concurrent use of medications, *J Am Diet Assoc* 105:54-63, 2005.

52. Vaisman N, Silverberg DS, Wexler D et al: Correction of anemia in patients with congestive heart failure increases resting energy expenditure, *Clin Nutr* 23:355-361, 2004.

53. Lee SC, Park SW, Kim DK et al: Iron supplementation inhibits cough associated with ACE inhibitors, *Hypertension* 38:166-170, 2001.

54. Gorelik O, Almoznino-Sarafian D, Feder I et al: Dietary intake of various nutrients in older patients with congestive heart failure, *Cardiology* 99:177-181, 2003.

55. He J, Ogden LG, Bazzano LA et al: Dietary sodium intake and incidence of congestive heart failure in overweight US men and women: first National Health and Nutrition Examination Survey Epidemiologic Follow-up Study, *Arch Intern Med* 162:1619-1624, 2002.

56. National Heart, Lung, and Blood Institute, National Institutes of Health, US Department of Health and Human Services: *Your guide to lowering your blood pressure with DASH*, NIH Pub No 06-4082, Bethesda, Md, 2006, The Department. Retrieved November 28, 2006 from www.nhlbi.nih.gov/health/public/heart/hbp/dash/

57. US Department of Health and Human Services, US Department of Agriculture: *Dietary guidelines for Americans 2005*, Washington, DC, 2005, The Departments. Retrieved August 17, 2005 from www.healthierus.gov/dietaryguidelines/

58. Fridkin SK, Hageman JC, Morrison M et al: Methicillin-resistant *Staphylococcus aureus* disease in three communities, *N Engl J Med* 352:1436-1444, 2005.

59. Boyce JM, Pittet D: Guideline for hand hygiene in health-care settings: recommendations of the Healthcare Infection Control Practices Advisory Committee and the HICPAC/SHEA/APIC/IDSA Hand Hygiene Task Force, Society for Healthcare Epidemiology of America/Association for Professionals in Infection Control/Infectious Diseases Society of America, *MMWR Recomm Rep* 51:1-45, 2002.

60. Anusavice KJ: Dental caries: risk assessment and treatment solutions for an elderly population, *Compend Contin Educ Dent* 23:12-20, 2002.

61. Gunter KB, White KN, Hayes WC et al: Functional mobility discriminates nonfallers from one-time and frequent fallers, *J Gerontol A Biol Sci Med Sci* 55:M672-M676, 2000.

62. Lord SR, Dayhew J: Visual risk factors for falls in older people, *J Am Geriatr Soc* 49:508-515, 2001.

63. Kemoun G, Thoumie P, Boisson D et al: Ankle dorsiflexion delay can predict falls in the elderly, *J Rehabil Med* 34:278-283, 2002.

64. Nelson HD, Nygren P, McInerney Y et al: Screening women and elderly adults for family and intimate partner violence: a review of the evidence for the US Preventive Services Task Force, *Ann Intern Med* 140:387-396, 2004.

65. National Guideline Clearinghouse: *Elder abuse prevention*. Retrieved August 9, 2005 from www.guideline.gov/summary/summary.aspx?doc_id=6829&nbr=4196&string=abuse

66. National Guideline Clearinghouse: *Screening for family and intimate partner violence: recommendation statement*. Retrieved August 9, 2005 from www.guideline.gov/summary/summary.aspx?doc_id=4427&nbr=3341&string=abuse

67. Stewart S, Horowitz JD: Home-based intervention in congestive heart failure: long-term implications on readmission and survival, *Circulation* 105:2861-2866, 2002.

68. Neal LJ: *On becoming a home health nurse: practice meets theory in home care nursing*, Washington, DC, 2000, Home Care University.

■ ■ ■ chapter **27**

Palliative Care

Patricia Davidson
Cheryl Hoyt Zambroski

CHAPTER ABBREVIATIONS

SUPPORT   Study to Understand Prognosis and Preferences for Outcomes and Risk of Treatment

The sickest patients are not necessarily the ones who die first.[1]

Heart disease has reached global epidemic proportions. Within the next two decades, cardiovascular disease will become the leading cause of death and disability worldwide.[2] It is estimated that the number of deaths will increase to more than 20 million each year.[3] In the United States alone, heart disease is an escalating public health problem, largely because it is age-related, and the fastest growing segment of the U.S. population is over 85 years.

Death for those diagnosed with heart disease may be sudden, as from a cardiac dysrhythmia, or drawn out, as experienced by many with the multiple sequelae of heart failure. Whatever the precise cause of death, dying from heart disease often is preceded by periods of lingering chronic illness with disabling symptoms including dyspnea and pain that greatly diminish quality of life.[1,4] Clearly, as the number of patients who experience significant disability and die from heart disease continues to rise, there is an urgent need to improve end-of-life care for patients with these life-threatening and life-altering conditions.[5,6]

Although predominantly associated with care of patients with cancer, patients with heart failure and their families are prime candidates for palliative care.[7] Advocates of palliative care for patients with noncancer diagnoses stress that clinicians must move beyond traditional models of care to include the goals of enhancing quality of life for patients and their families, improving decision making, and optimizing function.[8] To do so, multidimensional and interdisciplinary approaches must be used to meet the physical, psychological, social, and spiritual needs of patients and their families.

In the past, palliative care was not a focus of scholarly and research activity by cardiovascular nurses. This has changed rapidly as nurses strive to meet the growing needs of patients and their families who are faced with a wide range of medical and surgical approaches to care. New pharmacological therapies, heart transplantation, biventricular pacing, automated implantable cardiac devices, and ventricular assist devices are only a few of the therapeutic options for patients with advanced heart disease. Yet despite these therapeutic advances, clinicians, patients, and their families grapple with issues related to access and appropriateness of these interventions.

As discussed in Chapters 64 and 82, heart failure is the final common pathway for many cardiovascular diseases that result in ventricular dysfunction. Therefore, discussion of palliative care is framed within the context of living with and dying from heart failure. According to the consensus statement for palliative and supportive care in advanced heart failure,[9] advanced heart failure is "a state in which patients have significant cardiac dysfunction with marked symptoms of dyspnea, fatigue, or symptoms related to end-organ hypoperfusion at rest or with minimal exertion despite maximal medical therapy" (p. 201). By the time patients reach the stage of advanced heart failure, they face significant disability that requires additional interventions beyond traditional medical therapy.[10]

The purpose of this chapter is twofold: (1) to identify key competencies needed to provide palliative care for advanced heart failure patients and their families, and (2) to recommend strategies to improve palliative care for patients with advanced heart disease such as heart failure.

CORE COMPETENCIES

There are several core competencies necessary for nurses caring for patients with advanced heart failure. First, it is critical to recognize the conceptual differences between active and palliative care. Second, expertise is essential in assessment and management of the complex symptoms experienced by patients with advanced heart failure. Third, skill is needed in communicating about key issues facing patients with life-threatening illness and their families. Fourth, sensitivity and responsiveness to the influence of cultural factors on beliefs and values influencing patients with life-threatening illnesses is essential. Finally, nurses who work in these settings must demonstrate understanding of legal and ethical issues relating to palliative care.

Active Versus Palliative Care

A conceptual difference exists between active and palliative care. Active (often called *curative*) care is directed specifically toward disease modification. Palliative care is directed toward symptom management. In general, as the disease progresses, the emphasis on active care diminishes and the importance of palliative care increases (see Figure 82-1). Differentiation between active and palliative care may be more complex in patients with noncancer diagnoses than in those with cancer diagnoses. For patients with cancer, active treatment, such as surgery or radiation, typically is effective for a certain time. With some cancers, at some point, these treatments lose their ability to modify the disease. Interventions then become distinctively palliative with a focus on prevention and relief of suffering to support the best quality of life for the patient and family.[8] Although palliative care may be delivered regardless of the specific stages of a disease, for patients with cancer there generally is a more definitive point of transition. For patients with cancer, the criteria for admission to hospice are fairly clear within the relatively predictable cancer illness trajectory.

For patients with noncancer diagnoses such as heart failure, active treatment of the illness may be effective until death. Active disease-modifying agents such as diuretics for pulmonary edema or opioids for dyspnea provide both active and palliative symptom management.[11] No clearcut point exists between active treatment and palliation. The test of palliative care versus active care is that the expected outcome of palliative care is relief of distressing symptoms, elimination of pain, and/or enhancement of quality of life rather than modification of the disease itself.[12] For example, pacemaker insertion, which might be considered an active treatment, may be palliative if the expected outcome is relief of symptomatic dysrhythmias. Technological intervention is not necessarily precluded, as some erroneously believe. For patients with heart failure, palliative care can be delivered concurrently with active life-prolonging care.[8,11]

Palliative care nurses must be willing to initiate aggressive palliative care for patients with heart failure who will have an uncertain illness trajectory, regardless of the setting. According to the National Consensus Project for Quality Palliative Care,[8] implementation of palliative care interventions should occur at diagnosis of any life-threatening or debilitating illness and follow the patient through death and the family through the bereavement period.

The precise timeframe defining end of life remains unclear. Yet clinicians recognize that heart failure does reduce life expectancy. Integration of palliative care concepts into heart failure care ensures that patients and their families receive holistic care designed to meet multiple needs across a variety of settings and the full continuum of health.[8] Even following the patient's death, palliative care concepts warrant that the family is not abandoned and ensure the availability of bereavement support. (For a more thorough discussion of palliative and hospice care, see Chapter 82.)

Assessing and Managing Complex Symptoms

A critical competency in palliative care is the comprehensive assessment and management of complex symptoms.[8] Before beginning a plan of care, assessment includes identification of the cause of heart failure, presence of comorbidities, use of prescribed and over-the-counter medications, nutritional status, and factors that exacerbate symptoms.[13]

Regular, ongoing assessment of physical, social, psychological, cultural, and spiritual status using instruments validated for patients with advanced heart failure allows for a thorough examination of the impact of heart disease on the patient (Table 27-1). Physical and psychological symptoms such as pain, dyspnea, anxiety, or depression should be assessed for level of distress, response to medications, resulting functional impairment, and meaning to the patient and family. Psychological symptoms should be assessed in patients and their families specifically related to their understanding of the illness, coping strategies, grieving, and stress responses. Assessment of the cultural beliefs and spiritual status with regard to end-of-life issues is fundamental to providing holistic care.

■ ■ ■

TABLE 27-1 ASSESSING PATIENTS WITH ADVANCED HEART FAILURE DURING PALLIATIVE CARE

ASPECT OF CARE	ASSESSMENT
Physical	Pain*
	Dyspnea†
	Nausea
	Anorexia
	Functional impairment‡
	Bowel and bladder function: continence and constipation
	Edema
	Adverse medication effects (e.g., digoxin toxicity)
Social	Financial status
	Role change
	Capacity for self-care§
	Adherence to lifestyle recommendations
	Fear for dependents
	Caregiver burden
	Place of death
	Current advance directives
Emotional/psychological	Depression‖
	Reflection on life and events
	Delirium§
	Confusion
	Coping strategies§
	Fear and anxiety§
	Concerns for future
	Quality of life‖
Cultural	Cultural significance of death and dying
	Cultural requirements for management of death
Spiritual/existential	Meaning of death
	Preparedness for death
	Religious beliefs and desires for burial

*The World Health Organization three-step analgesic ladder is useful in assessment and management of pain or discomfort.
†A visual analogue scale is a valid and reliable strategy to monitor levels of dyspnea.
‡Consider using anchors or reference points, such as walking to the bathroom, to determine deterioration in functional status.
§Where possible, use validated measures for patient-reported outcomes, such as depression, anxiety, stress, functional status, edema, pain, and quality of life. This facilitates not only empirical clinical decision making but also communication across health care sectors and teams.
‖Sequential measurements of standardized measures over time can be useful in monitoring prognosis and functional status.
Data from Pitorak EF: *Am J Nurs* 103:42-53, 2003; Alla F, Briancon S, Guillemin F et al: *Eur J Heart Fail* 4:337-343, 2002; and Pitorak FBM: Pain assessment and management. In Sherman D, editor: *Gerontologic palliative care nursing*, St Louis, 2004, Mosby.

Significant efforts are being made nationally to improve symptom management for patients with advanced heart failure.[9,11] A recent consensus conference was convened to define the current state and important gaps in knowledge and needed research on palliative and supportive care in advanced heart failure. As a result, the Consensus Statement on Palliative and Supportive Care in Advanced Heart Failure was published in 2004. This statement serves as a basis for building the science of symptom management in palliative care for patients with heart failure.

In palliative care, symptom management strategies emphasize relief of suffering. Fundamental to all symptom management strategies for heart failure is the optimization of medications according to current guidelines. It is insufficient to judge the true burden of heart failure symptoms if the patient is inadequately or inappropriately managed pharmacologically. Once therapy is optimized, palliative care strategies can be recommended above and beyond medications.

Although it is beyond the scope of this chapter to address each of the symptoms that may occur for patients with heart failure at the end of life, the symptoms often reported in the literature include dyspnea, pain, fatigue, depression, difficulty sleeping, confusion, and gastrointestinal symptoms.[4,7,10,14,15] Key management strategies are summarized in Table 27-2. Inherent in all symptom management strategies is the judicious appraisal of risks. For example, if the patient has syncope, the risk of falls must be weighed against the potential benefits of neurohormonal blockade.

The most common symptoms of advanced heart failure are dyspnea, pain, and fatigue. Dyspnea is a distressing symptom for most patients with heart failure. Beyond dyspnea with minimal exertion or at rest, patients may experience paroxysmal nocturnal dyspnea, orthopnea, and trepopnea (inability to lie in a left lateral position).[13] A thorough history and physical examination including assessment of lung sounds, presence of jugular venous distention, weight, and increases in the intensity of the S_3 heart sound during respiration can help determine whether fluid overload is present. If so, modification of diuretic therapy may help to relieve dyspnea. Daily weighing should be continued as long as feasible. Dietary sodium and fluid restrictions may be beneficial for these patients and should not be abandoned as they may reduce symptom burden. Effective fluid management can decrease the risk of distressing respiratory symptoms.

If, however, the patient is euvolemic, other strategies may be beneficial in relieving dyspnea. A recent study demonstrated that oxygen therapy was the most common pharmacological intervention in hospice, used by 92 percent of the heart failure patients.[15] Recent consensus reports, however, do not support the use of oxygen as an effective symptom management strategy for breathlessness in patients with heart failure.[9,16] Furthermore, oxygen use may pose additional risks, including restriction of activity, cost, and fire hazard. Also, oxygen masks or cannulas may contribute to impaired communication between patient and family.[16] Therefore, oxygen should be used only in specific situations when clear benefit can be documented.

■ ■ ■

TABLE 27-2 PALLIATIVE CARE STRATEGIES FOR MAJOR SYMPTOMS IN ADVANCED HEART FAILURE

SYMPTOM	STRATEGY
Dyspnea*	Optimal heart failure pharmacotherapy (see Box 64-8)
	Continuous positive airway pressure for sleep-disordered breathing
	Opioids as tolerated
	Positioning and comfort
	Exercise as tolerated
	Fluid and sodium restriction
Anxiety	Support and reassurance
	Meditation, relaxation, and cognitive behavioral therapy
	Massage and breathing exercises
	Music therapy
	Promotion of control (e.g., action plan)
	Benzodiazepines
	Neuroleptics
Depression	Support and reassurance
	Meditation, relaxation, and cognitive behavioral therapy
	Pharmacotherapy with selective serotonin reuptake inhibitors
Fatigue*	Optimal heart failure pharmacotherapy (see Box 64-8)
	Energy conservation techniques and equipment (e.g., shower chair)
	Support and reassurance
	Organization of social supports
	Psychostimulants
	Erythropoietin, transfusions to treat fatigue from anemia
	Exercise as tolerated
	Promotion of optimal nutrition
Anorexia	Encourage eating of favorite foods
	Small, frequent meals
	Dietary supplements
Nausea	Encourage eating of easily digestible food
	Diuretics for right ventricular heart failure
	Assess and manage adverse drug effects
	Take medications with food where possible
	Antiemetics when necessary
Edema*	Optimal heart failure pharmacotherapy (see Box 64-8)
	Flexible diuretic regimen
	Addition of metolazone
	Combination of loop and thiazide diuretics
	Parenterally administered diuretics as needed
	Compression stockings for peripheral edema
	Support for scrotal edema when present
	Care of exudative edema to prevent infection, ulceration, and discomfort
	Advise sodium and fluid restriction
	Repositioning to prevent decubitus ulcers
	Avoidance of nonsteroidal antiinflammatory drugs
Pain	Nitrates for anginal pain
	Analgesia according to the World Health Organization three-step ladder and ability to take oral medications
	Nonpharmacological strategies such as massage and application of heat packs
Confusion	Treat reversible causes such as hypoxia
	Consider potential for delirium caused by reversible factors such as urinary tract infection
	Provide reassurance, support, and orientation to surroundings

*In severe cases, inotropic therapy may be considered, but the costs, place of care, venous access, and increased risk of sudden cardiac death have to be weighed carefully against potential benefit. Often, management of palliative care/hospice patients with inotropes is reserved for those unable to be weaned in the acute setting.

Opioids may benefit patients with dyspnea resulting from heart failure.[17] Opioids decrease sympathetic tone, increase venous capacitance, and suppress centers in the midbrain responsible for the subjective sensation of dyspnea.[11] An advantage of opioids is that they are available for administration through a variety of routes including oral, intravenous, subcutaneous, and rectal suppository. In general, opioid doses should be adjusted according to symptomatic response. Frequent bolus doses may be more effective than slow-release formulations or continuous infusions.[18]

A common concern among cardiovascular clinicians is a fear that opioids may cause significant respiratory depression. As with any pharmaceutical agent, the risks and benefits must be weighed carefully. The advice to *start low and go slow* is useful. Opioids should be adjusted to the level of symptoms and can be used without causing significant respiratory depression or excessive drowsiness.

Various other strategies may be used for managing dyspnea in patients with advanced heart failure. Posture, relaxation techniques, and maintaining a flow of air across the face (from a fan or an open window) also may provide symptomatic relief. It is unclear whether the symptomatic relief is related to changes in temperature or to the mechanical effect of the airflow to mechano-receptors in the upper airway and face.[19] Anxiolytics may decrease the sensation of dyspnea but should not be used as the default medication for treating dyspnea. Therapy should be tailored to improve the patient's subjective sensation rather than to correct abnormal parameters.

A key finding of the Study to Understand Prognosis and Preferences for Outcomes and Risks of Treatment (SUPPORT) was that patients with heart failure experience significant increases in severe pain in the later stages of the syndrome.[4] Similarly, Nordgren and Sorenson[14] found that 75 percent of patients had pain during the last 6 months of life. Before intervention, it is essential to assess thoroughly the quality, frequency, severity, and distress of the pain. Treatment varies with whether the pain is cardiac or noncardiac in origin. Nonsteroidal antiinflammatory drugs should be avoided because they increase sodium and water retention as a result of prostaglandin inhibition.[20]

Fatigue is a common and debilitating symptom that commonly worsens as heart failure progresses.[21] Like dyspnea and pain, fatigue is a multidimensional construct and may occur from a range of causes that should be assessed. The goal of care is to "reverse the reversible."[22] For example, fatigue resulting from anemia may be amenable to treatment. Anemia often is associated with a poor prognosis and higher rates of hospitalization,[23] but erythropoietin and iron supplementation may reduce anemia and signs and symptoms in patients with heart failure.[24] Transfusions generally are reserved for severe symptomatic anemia as they can precipitate acute fluid overload. Other potentially reversible sources of fatigue are dehydration, overmedication, and infection.

Additional interventions for fatigue include energy conservation techniques, promotion of adequate sleep, control of symptoms that may contribute to fatigue, and improved nutritional status.[25] Use of psychostimulants is a potentially fruitful area for study in treatment of fatigue in patients with advanced heart failure.[9]

In a study of persons with heart failure during their last week of life, nearly half were confused at least some of the time.[15] The nurse must be able to differentiate among delirium, dementia, and depression because assessment of the cause of confusion dictates interventions. As the patient approaches death, agitation or restlessness may be treated with pharmacological agents such as haloperidol or midazolam. Prevention of injury is vital for patients who are confused.

Gastrointestinal symptoms such as nausea or vomiting, anorexia, and constipation can be managed with medication, dietary modifications, and nonpharmacological interventions. Thorough assessment of medication side effects, fluid balance, and symptom patterns provides a basis for treatment. If the patient is euvolemic, antiemetics or prokinetic agents may be helpful to minimize nausea and vomiting. Preventing constipation is a priority at the end of life. Patients commonly require a stool softener or stimulant, particularly if they are receiving opioids. As the illness trajectory progresses, anorexia becomes a more pronounced symptom. Often more distressing for caregivers than for patients, loss of appetite is common in advanced heart failure. It is important that family members be told that loss of appetite is common at the end of life and that forcing food can increase the patient's distress significantly.

Sleep-disordered breathing is common in patients with heart failure.[26] Of those with sleep-disordered breathing, most have central sleep apnea and the minority have obstructive sleep apnea.[27] Continuous positive airway pressure may provide symptomatic relief, improve dyspnea and fatigue, and optimize cardiovascular function.[9] These disorders and management strategies are discussed in depth in Chapter 17.

Peripheral edema is a common sign of decompensated heart failure. Caution should be used, however, because edema is generally nonspecific. Edema may result from elevated right ventricular pressure, increased sodium resorption, low serum albumin, reduced lymphatic drainage, or incompetence of the venous valves.

Thorough assessment of edema is needed, whether the patient is obviously edematous or appears cachectic. As patients become more debilitated, cachexia may mask dependent edema in the sacral and scrotal areas. The presence of edema can be assessed by placing gentle pressure over a bony prominence. When severe, edema may be associated with serous exudate, requiring attentive nursing care to prevent trauma to the skin and breakdown. Elevation of the legs when resting or sleeping can improve the degree of edema to a limited extent.

Edema can extend to the intestinal wall. Bowel edema may inhibit absorption of medications, particularly diuretics. Edema may be aggravated by hypoperfusion of the gut and intestinal hypomotility from inadequate cardiac output. In this instance, administration of intravenous instead of oral diuretics needs to be explored.[20]

Absolute freedom from peripheral edema is not a treatment goal because it may result in dehydration and hypovolemia. Although peripheral edema commonly is believed to be an indicator of fluid overload, it is generally less reliable in end-stage heart failure, so treatment of edema requires a thorough assessment of fluid status before automatic treatment with diuretics.

For elderly patients and those needing large doses of diuretics, urinary incontinence can be a source of discomfort and distress to patients and families. Urinary incontinence may be managed by changing the timing of diuretic doses, scheduled fluid intake and toileting, incontinence pads or briefs, or external collection devices. For patients with chronic urine retention, intermittent or indwelling catheters may be needed.[28] In the event of incontinence, diligence in skin care assumes even greater importance.

Beyond physical and psychological symptoms, it is essential to assess the patient's and family's socioeconomic status because their financial situation influences the capacity for self-care, caregiver burden, and access to health care resources. Each of these factors affects quality of life.

Communication

At no other time is effective communication more essential than with patients and families facing the uncertainty of living with advanced heart failure.[29, 30] Effective communication must occur among patients, families, and the health care community.

Clear communication is as powerful an intervention as any invasive medical procedure.[31] In general, patients value honesty, straightforwardness, willingness to discuss death and dying, listening, and sensitivity when they are ready to talk about dying.[32] They value balanced sensitivity and honesty when talking about prognosis.

The P-SPIKES approach, summarized in Table 27-3, can be used to enhance communication for patients and families with life-threatening illness, including heart failure.[31] This approach emphasizes the need to provide for context and content of communication when delivering bad news. The main goals are to gather information from the patient and family, provide accurate information, and reduce the emotional impact and isolation experienced by the recipient.[33] This approach also should assist the provider in developing a treatment strategy by building a relationship with the patient and family.

There is no simple script for establishing care goals in palliative care. Ritualistic communication can lead to undertreatment or overtreatment of symptoms, anxiety, confusion, and a lack of clarity in the goals of care (Table 27-4). For example, use of jargon or extensive detail may be a barrier to understanding and may overwhelm patients and their families. Emphasis on "we should be positive" can lead to a lack of preparation for death, guilt, missed opportunities, and isolation of patient and family. This is particularly true for patients with heart failure, who are vulnerable to sudden death.[34]

Examining the patient's and family's values and decisions is vital to the philosophy of palliative care.[12] Assessment of the patient's wishes and clarification of treatment goals are essential in order to deliver effective and appropriate palliative care. A major opportunity for determining patient wishes is through advance care planning. Advance care planning provides information that could guide families and providers in making decisions should the patient be unable to do so.

The major mechanism for advance care planning is through the advance directive. Tilden and colleagues[35] noted that advance directives not only offer a mechanism of promoting patient autonomy but also a valuable adjunct to decreasing family members' stress. An advance directive includes documents such as a living will and the appointment of a surrogate with health care power of attorney. Of note in the United States, the Patient Self-Determination Act, passed by Congress in 1991, mandated that institutions receiving Medicare and Medicaid funding inform patients about advance directives.

Strategies used to discuss advance directives are described in Table 27-5. Providing information about resuscitation, likely outcomes, and sequelae assists patients and families in this aspect of decision making. Patients and their families should be reassured that they can change their minds as conditions change. Dracup and colleagues[36] have demonstrated, in studies of families of patients at risk for sudden death, that most family members can learn cardiopulmonary resuscitation and are not significantly distressed by conversations about sudden death and learning resuscitation skills.

Communicating the absolute risk of therapies and interventions to patients and their families helps them make informed choices. They commonly need assistance as they change their goals of care from prolongation of life to an emphasis on improving quality of life by maximizing comfort and dignity. Clinicians need to discuss the level of intervention appropriate and desirable during this phase so that unnecessary and potentially traumatic interventions are avoided. Providing information within a context of *"hoping for the best, while planning for the worst"* may assist patients with advanced heart failure to process information and plan for the future.[9]

Sensitivity to Culture

Cultural disparities can occur in every level of health care, including palliative care.[37] According to the National Consensus Project for Quality Palliative Care,[8] competent palliative care requires that clinicians thoroughly assess and attempt to meet specific cultural needs of patients and their families as they approach the end of life. Components of culture such as age, ethnicity, and spirituality influence vital issues such as patient and family responses to the illness, decision making, nutrition, pain management, attitudes toward advance directives, and mourning rituals.[37-39] To meet these needs, cultural competence is essential.

Cultural competence refers to the dynamic, ongoing process of gaining the ability to work with culturally diverse groups and communities.[40] Essential to cultural competence is the need for awareness, specific knowledge, refined skills, and respect for cultural attributes

■ ■ ■

TABLE 27-3 COMMUNICATING BAD NEWS: THE P-SPIKES APPROACH

ACRONYM	STEPS	AIM OF THE INTERACTION	PREPARATIONS, QUESTIONS, OR PHRASES
P	Preparation	Mentally prepare for the interaction with the patient and/or family.	Review what information needs to be communicated. Plan how you will provide emotional support. Rehearse key steps and phrases in the interaction.
S	Setting the interaction	Ensure the appropriate setting for a serious and emotionally charged discussion.	Ensure that patient, family, and appropriate social support are present. Devote sufficient time. Do not squeeze in a discussion. Ensure privacy and prevent interruptions by persons or beeper. Bring a box of tissues.
P	Patient's perception and preparation	Begin the discussion with establishing a baseline and whether the patient and family can grasp the information. Ease tension by having the patient and family contribute.	Start with open-ended questions to encourage participation. Possible phrases to use are these: *What do you understand about your illness?* *When you first had symptom X, what did you think it might be?* *What did Dr. X tell you when he sent you here?* *What do you think is going to happen?*
I	Invitation and information needs	Discover what information needs the patient and/or family have and what limits they want regarding the bad information.	Possible phrases to use are these: *If this condition turns out to be something serious, what do you want to know?* *Would you like me to tell you the full details of your condition? If not, then to whom would you like me to talk?*
K	Knowledge of the condition	Provide the bad news or other information to the patient and/or family sensitively.	Do not just dump the information on the patient and family. Interrupt and check that the patient and family are understanding. Possible phrases to use are these: *I feel bad to have to tell you this, but . . .* *Unfortunately, the tests showed . . .* *I'm afraid the news is not good . . .*
E	Empathy and exploration	Identify the cause of the emotions (e.g., poor prognosis). Empathize with the patient and/or family's feelings. Explore by asking open-ended questions.	Strong feelings in reaction are normal. Acknowledge what the patient and family are feeling. Remind them that such feelings are normal even if frightening. Give them time to respond. Remind patient and family that you will not abandon them. Possible phrases to use are these: *I imagine this is very hard for you.* *You must be upset. Tell me how you are feeling.* *I wish the news were different.* *I'll do whatever I can to help you.*
S	Summarizing and strategic planning	Delineate for the patient and the family the next steps, including additional tests or interventions.	It is the unknown and uncertain that increases anxiety. Recommend a schedule with goals and landmarks. Explain your rationale for the patient and/or family to accept or reject. If the patient and/or family are not ready to discuss steps, schedule a follow-up visit.

Adapted from Buchman R: *How to break bad news: a guide for health care professionals,* Baltimore, 1992, Johns Hopkins University Press.

(similar and dissimilar).[41] Cultural competence should diminish the risk of poor health care outcomes based on stereotypes, biases, and poor communication.

For those who deliver palliative care, cultural competence begins with developing awareness of one's own attitudes, belief, and practices surrounding death and dying. Articulation of these beliefs can decrease the risk of ethnocentrism in working with patients and families from diverse cultures.

An effective approach is to identify and learn about the main cultures in the community.[37] Knowledge can be gained through literature, contacts in the community, and most importantly from the patient and family. Although many authors warn against stereotyping from literature-based sources, there often are common themes discussed in the literature that can provide a platform for understanding individuals and their families. The key to using the literature is to obtain an

■ ■ ■

TABLE 27-4 COMMUNICATION TRAPS WHEN ESTABLISHING GOALS FOR PALLIATIVE CARE

COMMUNICATION TRAP	EVIDENCE OF TRAP	CONSEQUENCES OF TRAP
"We all understand each other."	Lack of explicit discussion of treatment goals	Confusion Anger Inconsistent treatment Mistrust
"Let's be polite."	Avoidance of conflict Superficial conversations Short conversations	Indirect methods of communication used Conflicts Potential for guilt later
"We should be positive."	Incomplete information shared Dishonest communication Cheerful manner Avoidance of detailed discussions of illness	Isolation of patient/family Lack of preparation for advancing illness Loneliness Guilt Frustration Missed opportunities
"More of the same."	Repeated explanations Focus on same plan of care despite lack of success or resolution	Inappropriate treatment plans False hope Avoidance of in-depth discussion of treatment goals
"Can we be clear?"	Confrontation Seeking blame Questioning approach	Premature focus on palliative care goals Rebound reactions to patient, family, and health team Regret

From Kristjanson LJ: Establishing goals: communication traps and treatment lane changes. In Ferrell BF, Coyle N, editors: *Textbook of palliative care,* New York, 2001, Oxford University Press.

■ ■ ■

TABLE 27-5 STEPS IN ADVANCE CARE PLANNING

STEP	GOALS TO BE ACHIEVED AND MEASURES TO COVER
Introduce advance care planning.	Ask what the patient knows about advance care planning and whether he or she has completed an advance care directive already. Indicate that you as a clinician have completed advance care planning. Indicate that you try to do advance care planning with all patients regardless of the prognosis. Explain the goals of the process as empowering the patient and ensuring that you and the proxy understand the patient's preferences. Provide the patient with relevant literature including the advance directive that you prefer to use. Recommend that the patient identify a proxy decision maker who should attend the next meeting. *Useful phrases or points to make* "I'd like to talk with you about something I try to discuss with all my patients. It's called advance care planning. In fact, this is such an important topic, I have done this myself. Are you familiar with advance care planning or living wills?" "Have you thought about the type of care you would like to have if you ever become too ill to speak for yourself? That is the purpose of advance care planning." "There is no change in your health that we have not discussed. I am bringing this matter up now because it is sensible for everyone. No matter how well or ill, young or old." Have copies of advanced directives available, including in the waiting room for patients and families.
Structure discussion of scenarios and patient preferences.	Affirm that the goal of the process is to follow the patient's wishes if the patient loses decision-making ability. Elicit the patient's overall goals related to health care. Elicit the patient's preferences for specific interventions in a few salient and common scenarios. *Useful phrases or points to make* Use a structured worksheet with typical scenarios. Begin the discussion with persistent vegetative state and consider other scenarios, such as recovery from an acute event with serious disability, asking the patient about his or her preferences regarding specific interventions such as ventilators, nasogastric feedings, and cardiopulmonary resuscitation, proceeding to less invasive interventions such as blood transfusions and antibiotics.
Review the patient's preferences.	Help define the threshold for withdrawing and withholding interventions. Define the patient's preference for the role of the proxy. After the patient has chosen interventions, review them to make sure they are consistent and that the proxy is aware of them and willing to uphold them. Document the patient's preferences. Formally complete the advance care directive and have the appropriate number of witnesses sign it. Provide a copy for the patient and the proxy. Insert a copy into the patient's medical record. Update the directive. Periodically and with major changes in health status, review the directive with the patient and make any modifications needed. Apply the directive. The directive goes into effect only when the patient becomes unable to make medical decisions for himself or herself. Reread the directive to be sure of its content. Discuss your proposed actions based on the directive with the proxy.

Data from Emanuel LL, Bonow RO: Care of patients with end-stage heart disease. In Zipes DP, Bonow RO, Braunwald E, editors: *Braunwald's heart disease: a textbook of cardiovascular medicine,* ed 7, Philadelphia, 2005, Elsevier.

■ ■ ■

TABLE 27-6 SUMMARY OF THE DOMAINS OF CULTURE

DOMAIN	DESCRIPTION
Ethnic identity	Country of origin, ethnicity/culture with which the group identifies, current residence, reasons for migration, degree of acculturation/assimilation, and level of cultural pride
Communication	Dominant language and any dialects, usual volume/tone of speech, willingness to share thoughts/feelings/ideas, meaning of touch, use of eye contact, control of expressions and emotions, spokesperson/decision maker in family
Time and space	Past, present, or future time orientation; preference for personal space and distance
Social organization	Family structure; head of household, gender roles, status/role of elderly; roles of child, adolescents, husband/wife, mother/father, extended family; influences on the decision-making process; importance of social organization and network
Workforce issues	Primary wage earner, impact of illness on work, transportation to clinic visits, health insurance, financial impact, importance of work
Health beliefs, practices, and practitioners	Meaning/cause of cancer and illness/health, living with life-threatening illness, expectations and use of Western treatment and health care team, religious/spiritual beliefs and practices, use of traditional healers/practitioners, expectations of practitioners, loss of body part/body image, acceptance of blood transfusions/organ donations, sick role and health-seeking behaviors
Nutrition	Meaning of food and mealtimes, preferences and preparation of food, taboos/rituals, religious influences on food preferences and preparation
Biological variations	Skin/mucous membrane color, physical variations, drug metabolism, laboratory data, and genetic variations/specific risk factors and differences in incidence/survival/mortality of specific cancers
Sexuality and reproductive fears	Beliefs about sexuality and reproductive/childbearing activities, taboos, privacy issues, interaction of cancer diagnosis/treatments with beliefs about sexuality
Religion and spirituality	Dominant religion; religious beliefs, rituals, and ceremonies; use of prayer, meditation or other symbolic activities; meaning of life; source of strength
Death and dying	Meaning of dying, death and the afterlife; belief in fatalism; rituals, expectations, and mourning/bereavement practices

From Oncology Nursing Society: *Oncology Nursing Society multicultural outcomes: guidelines for cultural competence*, Pittsburgh, 1999, The Society.

opening to further study rather than a generalization that hinders investigation.

Cultural skill can be developed through repeated interactions and evaluation of those interactions. Expertise is needed in collecting cultural data, conducting a culturally appropriate physical assessment, and clear intercultural communication (Table 27-6). As skill improves, so does the ability to recommend culturally sensitive interventions. For example, for patients with heart failure, accurate assessment of cultural dietary preferences aids in individualizing patient teaching.

Truth telling and informed consent are key components of palliative care.[37] Western cultures typically value patient autonomy in decision making at the end of life. Other cultures may view autonomy as burdensome.[40] Some cultures value truth telling; others prefer nondisclosure.[41] Certain cultures may allow advance directives or do-not-resuscitate orders, whereas others do not. Whatever the values and beliefs, the role of the family and community in decision making should be assessed thoroughly, and preferences should be honored. Box 27-1 offers helpful websites.

It is impossible to underestimate the importance of spiritual and existential care in patients with advanced conditions.[42] Physical and psychological elements often are intertwined with reflections on life passed and hopes and desires for the future. Concerns relate not only to religious and cultural beliefs and expectations but also to reflection on past life events. Ongoing assessment of spiritual and existential needs should be provided, including patients' and families' contacts with spiritual communities, hopes and fears, and meanings about death and dying (Box 27-2).[8,42] Use of an interdis-

ciplinary approach can help to ensure that skillful and systematic responses to patient and family needs are based on best available evidence.

Ethics and Legality

End-of-life care is administered within a context of accepted legal, ethical, and governance procedures.[43] These procedures may be specific to the country, state, and type of institution. Nurses must function within their regulated scope of practice and professional code of ethics, readily seeking assistance from legal officers and ethics committees at their institutions should they perceive a need for moderation and intervention.

Patient and Family Support

Additional competencies needed to ensure patient and family support during palliative care include strong interpersonal skills, excellent coping skills, sensitivity to the feelings of others, the ability to work collaboratively, and the ability to work in dynamic clinical circumstances. Caring for those with advanced heart failure can be a time of personal struggle and reflection, not only for patients and their families but also for clinicians. Not only do nurses empathetically experience the suffering of patients and their families, but also they reflect on their own mortality and personal losses. As health care systems increasingly are stretched fiscally and are short of skilled personnel, bedside clinicians are vulnerable to stress and burnout. Thus, there is a need for expert clinical supervision and support of nurses across all care settings.

BOX 27-1
HELPFUL WEBSITES

American Academy of Pediatrics
Palliative Care for Children: Policy statement pertaining to palliative care, including minimum standards, working with children and their parents, and providing support for caregivers.
   http://aappolicy.aappublications.org/cgi/reprint/pediatrics;
106/2/351.pdf

American Academy of Hospice and Palliative Medicine
Organization website that provides information on a variety of peer-reviewed educational resources and position statements on issues related to end-of-life care.
   www.aahpm.org/

American Nurses Association
Includes American Nurses Association position statements on key issues for end-of-life care, including nursing care and the do-not-resuscitate order, assisted suicide, and forgoing nutrition and hydration.
   www.nursingworld.org/readroom/position/ethics/

Center to Advance Palliative Care
Supported by the Robert Wood Johnson Foundation to provide health care professionals with tools, professional development, and technical assistance needed to build palliative care programs in diverse settings.
   www.capc.org/

End of Life/Palliative Education Resource Center
Provides a variety of educational resources for health care professional educators and providers. Includes clinical topics such as device deactivation, delivering bad news, discussing hospice with patients and families, and responding to patient emotions. Helpful "Fast Facts" are free to download and distribute for educational purposes.
   www.eperc.mcw.edu/

Ethnomed
Contains medical and cultural information on a variety of immigrant and refugee groups. Although it contains information about groups particularly in the Seattle area, it provides a range of culturally specific information, including such topics as food and nutrition, religious beliefs and practices, interpersonal relationships, and beliefs about death.
   www.ethnomed.org/

Promoting Excellence in End-of-Life Care
Includes collection of tools to improve care of dying patients and their families. Although written primarily for clinicians and researchers, it also is available to the extended health care community, grantees, peer workshop participants, and the general public. Tools are available to improve clinical assessment and research, education, and evaluation.
   www.promotingexcellence.org

National Consensus Project for Quality Palliative Care
Result of a major initiative to improve delivery of palliative care. The site provides access to the *Clinical Practice Guidelines for Quality Palliative Care.*
   www.nationalconsensusproject.org/

The Provider's Guide to Quality and Culture
Provides a general overview of information to enhance cultural competence, including information on patient provider interactions, health disparities, and common beliefs and cultural practices.
   http://erc.msh.org/mainpage.cfm?file=1.0.htm&module=provider&language=English

BOX 27-2
SPIRITual INTERVIEW

S   Spiritual belief system (religious affiliation)
P   Personal spirituality (beliefs and practices of affiliation that patient/family accepts)
I   Integration with a spiritual community (role of the religious/spiritual group; individual role in that group)
R   Ritualized practices and restrictions (health care activities that patient's or family's faith encourages or forbids)
I   Implications for medical care (beliefs that health care providers should remember during care)
T   Terminal events planning (impact of beliefs on advance directives; contacting clergy)

From Highfield MEF: *Clin J Oncol Nurs* 4:115-120, 2000.

STRATEGIES TO IMPROVE PALLIATIVE CARE

Palliative care often has been considered synonymous with hospice care. Although hospices do specialize in expert palliative care, nurses can develop palliative care expertise in any setting. Nurses must recognize their own lack of knowledge and clinical expertise in caring for dying patients.[44,45] For example, palliative care teams can be created within the acute care setting to guide nurses as they help patients and families who are facing important end-of-life issues. Nurses have demonstrated their capacity to lead these clinical teams and coordinate care.

Schools of nursing can incorporate didactic and clinical experiences within palliative care settings. Mentoring relationships can be developed for nurses in acute care, who traditionally have been immersed in a culture of cure, with nurses in hospice who have been immersed in palliative care. Also important is to reach out to palliative care colleagues who have substantial expertise in managing symptoms in order to augment nursing knowledge, develop nursing scholarship, and explore collaborative, integrated, and consultative models of care.[46] In cardiovascular care, there is no clearcut point between active and palliative care. Illness-specific interventions for patients with advanced heart disease need not be abandoned in favor of the traditional cancer model of palliative care.

Advanced heart disease can cause significant physical, psychological, and existential distress manifested by decreased quality of life, poor functional status, increasing dependence, and hospitalizations. Age and co-morbid conditions typically complicate the care of patients with heart failure. Research is needed to develop and evaluate models of care that provide effective and efficient palliative care for patients with advanced heart disease.

Clearly, a palliative care team approach needs to be individualized to meet the values, needs, and beliefs of the patient and family.[47] Tailoring the individual care plan according to the patient's wishes requires an astute and comprehensive assessment and use of advanced clinical competencies in physical, social, psychological, and existential domains. Nurses are privileged to be present with patients and their families in the most emotional and poignant life events. No doubt novel therapies will assist patients to live longer, but death is part of life's journey, albeit not always expected and desired. The challenge to nurses is to ensure that aggressive caring, whether active or palliative in nature, is truly provided across the life span.

REFERENCES

1. Fox E, Landrum-McNiff K, Zhong Z et al: Evaluation of prognostic criteria for determining hospice eligibility in patients with advanced lung, heart, or liver disease: SUPPORT investigators—Study to Understand Prognoses and Preferences for Outcomes and Risks of Treatments, *JAMA* 282:1638-1645, 1999.
2. Kelly D: Our future society: a global challenge, *Circulation* 95:2459-2464, 1997.
3. Mackay J, Mensah G: *Atlas of heart disease and stroke,* Geneva, 2004, World Health Organization and US Centers for Disease Control and Prevention. Retrieved April 4, 2005 from www.who.int/cardiovascular_diseases/resources/atlas/en/print.html
4. Levenson JW, McCarthy EP, Lynn J et al: The last six months of life for patients with congestive heart failure, *J Am Geriatr Soc* 48(5 suppl):S101-S109, 2000.
5. National Institutes of Health: *National Institutes of Health State-of-the-Science Conference Statement on improving end-of-life care.* Retrieved March 1, 2005 from http://consensus.nih.gov/2004/2004EndOfLifeCareSOS024html.htm
6. Lynn J, Nolan K, Kabcenell A et al: Reforming care for persons near the end of life: the promise of quality improvement, *Ann Intern Med* 137:117-122, 2002.
7. Gibbs JS, McCoy AS, Gibbs LM et al: Living with and dying from heart failure: the role of palliative care, *Heart* 88(suppl 2):ii36-ii39, 2002.
8. National Consensus Project for Quality Palliative Care: *Clinical practice guidelines for quality palliative care: executive summary,* May 2004. Retrieved February 17, 2005 from www.nationalconsensusproject.org/summary.pdf
9. Goodlin SJ, Hauptman PJ, Arnold R et al: Consensus statement: palliative and supportive care in advanced heart failure, *J Card Fail* 10:200-209, 2004.
10. Pantilat SZ, Steimle AE: Palliative care for patients with heart failure, *JAMA* 291:2476-2482, 2004.
11. Stuart B: Palliation in noncancer disease. In Forman WB, Kitzes JA, Anderson RP, Sheehan DK, editors: *Hospice and palliative care: concepts and practice,* ed 2, Sudbury, Mass, 2003, Jones and Bartlett.
12. National Association of Hospice and Palliative Care: *An explanation of palliative care.* Retrieved February 8, 2005 from www.nhcpo.org/i4a/pages/index.cfm?pageid=3657
13. Davis MP, Albert NM, Young JB: Palliation of heart failure, *Am J Hosp Palliat Care* 22:211-222, 2005.
14. Nordgren L, Sorensen S: Symptoms experienced in the last six months of life in patients with end-stage heart failure, *Eur J Cardiovasc Nurs* 2:213-217, 2003.
15. Zambroski CH, Moser DK, Roser LP et al: Patients with heart failure who die while in hospice, *Am Heart J* 149:558-564, 2005.
16. Booth S, Wade R, Johnson M et al: The use of oxygen in the palliation of breathlessness: a report of the Expert Working Group of the Scientific Committee of the Association of Palliative Medicine, *Respir Med* 98:66-77, 2004 [erratum in *Respir Med* 98:476, 2004].
17. Johnson MJ, McDonagh TA, Harkness A et al: Morphine for the relief of breathlessness in patients with chronic heart failure: a pilot study, *Eur J Heart Fail* 4:753-756, 2002.
18. Enck R: The role of nebulized morphine in managing dyspnea, *Am J Hosp Palliat Care* 16:373-374, 1999.
19. Manning HL, Schwartzstein RM: Mechanisms of disease: pathophysiology of dyspnea, *N Engl J Med* 333: 1547-1553, 1995.
20. Davidson P, Macdonald P, Paull G et al: Diuretic therapy in chronic heart failure: implications for heart failure nurse specialists, *Aust Crit Care* 16:59-69, 2003.
21. Abbey S: Psychiatric aspects of fatigue in the terminally ill. In Breitbart H, editor: *Handbook of psychiatry in palliative medicine,* New York, 2002, Oxford University Press.
22. McKinnon S: Fatigue. In Kuebler KK, Berry PH, Heidrich DE, editors: *End-of-life care: clinical practice guidelines,* Philadelphia, 2002, WB Saunders.
23. Shlipak M, Massie B: The clinical challenge of cardiorenal syndrome, *Circulation* 110:1514-1517, 2004.
24. Silverberg DS, Wexler D, Iaina A: The role of anemia in the progression of congestive heart failure: is there a place for erythropoietin and intravenous iron? *J Nephrol* 17:749-761, 2004.
25. Renier-Berg DM: General issues: fatigue, dyspnea, and constipation. In Forman WB, Kitzes JA, Anderson RP, Sheehan DK, editors: *Hospice and palliative care: concepts and practice,* ed 2, Sudbury, Mass, 2003, Jones and Bartlett.
26. Köhnlein T, Welte T, Tan L et al: Central sleep apnoea syndrome in patients with chronic heart disease: a critical review of the current literature, *Thorax* 57:574-554, 2002.
27. Roux F, D'Ambrosio C, Mohsenin V: Sleep-related breathing disorders and cardiovascular disease, *Am J Med* 108:396-402, 2000.
28. Gray M, Campbell FG: Urinary tract disorders. In Ferrell BF, Coyle N, editors: *Textbook of palliative nursing,* New York, 2001, Oxford University Press.
29. Boyd K, Murray S, Kendall M et al: Living with advanced heart failure: a prospective, community based study of patients and their careers, *Eur Heart J* 6:585-591, 2004.
30. Murray S, Boyd K, Kendall M et al: Dying of lung cancer or cardiac failure: prospective qualitative interview study of patients in the community, *Br Med J* 325:929-934, 2002.
31. Emanuel LL, Bonow RO: Care of patients with end-stage heart disease. In Sipes DP, Libby P, Bonow RO, Braunwald E, editors: *Braunwald's heart disease: a textbook of cardiovascular medicine,* ed 7, Philadelphia, 2005, Elsevier.
32. Wenrich MD, Curtis JR, Shannon SE et al: Communicating with dying patients within the spectrum of medical care from terminal diagnosis to death, *Arch Intern Med* 161:868-874, 2001.
33. Baile WF, Buckman R, Lenzi R et al: SPIKES: A six-step protocol for delivering bad news—application to the patient with cancer, *Oncologist* 5:302-311, 2000.
34. Narang R, Cleland J, Erhardt L et al: Mode of death in chronic heart failure: a request and proposition for more accurate classification, *Eur Heart J* 1390-1403, 1996.
35. Tilden VP, Tolle SW, Drach LL et al: Out-of-hospital death: advance care planning, decedent symptoms, and caregiver burden, *J Am Geriatr Soc* 52:532-539, 2004.
36. Dracup K, Heaney DM, Taylor SE et al: Can family members of high-risk cardiac patients learn cardiopulmonary resuscitation? *Arch Intern Med* 149:61-64, 1989.
37. Kemp C: Cultural issues in palliative care, *Semin Oncol Nurs* 21:44-52, 2005.
38. Mazanec P, Tyler MK: Cultural considerations in end-of-life care: how ethnicity, age, and spirituality affect decisions when death is imminent, *Am J Nurs* 103:50-59, 2003.
39. Searight HR, Gafford J: Cultural diversity at the end of life: issues and guidelines for family physicians, *Am Fam Physician* 71: 515-522, 2005.
40. Mazanec P, Kitzes J: Cultural competence in hospice and palliative care. In Forman WB, Kitzes JA, Anderson RP, Sheehan DK, editors: *Hospice and palliative care: concepts and practice,* Sudbury, Mass, 2003, Jones and Bartlett.
41. Suh EE: The model of cultural competence through an evolutionary concept analysis, *J Transcult Nurs* 15:93-102, 2004.
42. Westlake C, Dracup K: Role of spirituality in adjustment of patients with advanced heart failure, *Prog Cardiovasc Nurs* 16: 119-125, 2001.
43. Tarzian A, Schwarz J: Ethical and legal aspects of dying and health resource allocation. In Sherman D, editor: *Gerontologic palliative care nursing,* St Louis, 2004, Mosby.
44. Davidson P, Introna K, Daly J et al: Cardiorespiratory nurses' perceptions of palliative care in nonmalignant disease: data for the development of clinical practice, *Am J Crit Care* 12:47-53, 2003.
45. Kirchhoff KT, Spuhler V, Walker L et al: Intensive care nurses' experiences with end-of-life care, *Am J Crit Care* 9:36-42, 2000.
46. Davidson PM, Paull G, Introna K et al: Integrated, collaborative palliative care in heart failure: the St. George Heart Failure Service experience 1999-2002, *J Cardiovasc Nurs* 19:68-75, 2004.
47. Rabow MW, Dibble SL, Pantilat SZ et al: The comprehensive care team: a controlled trial of outpatient palliative medicine consultation, *Arch Intern Med* 164:83-91, 2004.

chapter 28

Nurse's Role in the Cardiac Catheterization Laboratory

Joann Eastwood

CHAPTER ABBREVIATIONS

CA   coronary angiogram

GP IIb/IIIa   glycoprotein IIb/IIIa

IV   intravenous

PSA   pseudoaneurysm

PTCA   percutaneous transluminal coronary angioplasty

RCN   radiocontrast-induced nephropathy

In the past two decades, the number of cardiac catheterizations performed annually has increased 341 percent in the United States.[1] Thousands of patients undergo diagnostic or therapeutic cardiac procedures annually on an outpatient basis because it has been determined to be safe, effective, and cost-efficient. This chapter focuses on the pivotal role nurses play in patient assessment, safety, support, and education throughout the precatheterization, intracatheterization, and postcatheterization experience.

Attempts at heart catheterization began as early as 1923 with the ability to inject a substance into an antecubital vein and observe it flow into the right side of the heart and out into the pulmonary circulation. Many technical advances were made, and in the 1940s Andre Cournand and colleagues began comprehensive and systematic investigations of cardiac function using right-heart catheterization. A special needle that could be inserted percutaneously in the brachial or femoral artery for long periods was designed and put into widespread use.[2] By 1947, Zimmerman and colleagues performed simultaneous catheterization of the right and left sides of the heart. In 1953, Seldinger used a percutaneous approach to introduce catheters for either right- or left-heart catheterization. By 1960, catheters that were practical for left-heart catheterization were introduced. Catheters specifically designed to break down soft plaque were used in the early 1960s. In 1977, Andreas Gruentzig refined earlier catheters using a balloon approach to decrease plaque and dilate the coronary arteries, which is known today as a percutaneous transluminal coronary angioplasty (**PTCA**).[3] In 2002, approximately 1.5 million diagnostic cardiac catheterizations and more than 1 million angioplasty procedures were performed.[1]

INDICATIONS AND USES FOR CARDIAC CATHETERIZATION

Categorized as a minimally invasive procedure, more than a million cardiac catheterizations are performed each year.[1] A radiopaque catheter is guided fluoroscopically into the heart, usually through the radial, brachial, or femoral artery. With the ability to gain access to the beating heart, the catheter can be used for diagnostic purposes, to assess blood supply to the heart and function of the left ventricle, and/or to perform therapeutic interventions to correct problems. The need for cardiac catheterization is based on an appropriate risk-benefit ratio. The procedure is indicated when it is clinically important to define the presence or severity of suspected cardiac lesions that cannot be evaluated by a noninvasive method. The risk of major complications is minimal, less than 1 percent, with a mortality of less than 0.08 percent.

A cardiac catheterization may include checking cardiac output, intracardiac pressures, and oxygen saturation; visualizing anatomical structural defects; viewing the aorta and coronary arteries (coronary angiogram [**CA**]); and dynamic visualization of left ventricular performance (left ventriculogram). The two most common reasons for ordering cardiac catheterizations are (1) to help diagnose suspected cardiac problem, most commonly coronary artery disease, and (2) to determine whether the patient is a good candidate for revascularization, an interventional procedure, or surgery.

The components of cardiac catheterization may include right-heart catheterization, left-heart catheterization, CA, and ventriculogram. A right-heart catheterization usually is performed when patients have dyspnea, a history of heart failure, or pulmonic or tricuspid valvular disease. Studies of the left side of the heart are performed to evaluate the mitral valve, the aortic valve, and left ventricular function.

Coronary angiography remains the gold standard for determining the presence, extent, localization, and severity of coronary artery disease. Coronary angiography permits analysis of the distal coronary vessels and provides an index of the area at risk of infarction distal to coronary stenosis and the results of reperfusion therapy (estimates of coronary blood flow), whether achieved pharmacologically or mechanically. Coronary collaterals, intracoronary thrombus, congenital anomalies of the coronary arteries, and coronary artery spasm are also visible. Using the cardiac catheter to assess the influence of drugs such as glycoprotein IIb/IIIa (**GP IIb/IIIa**) inhibitors on the microcirculation and identifying skip areas of radiation effect attributable to brachytherapy have extended the application of this procedure as technological advances evolve. Intravascular ultrasound, velocity probes, gene probes, and drug-eluting stents are among the newer intracoronary devices used in the catheterization laboratory.[3]

Guidelines for Diagnostic Coronary Angiography were established by a collaborative task force from the American Heart Association and the American College of Cardiology. These guidelines include critically ill patients and ambulatory patients. Indications for cardiac catheterization are shown in Box 28-1.

BOX 28-1
INDICATIONS FOR CORONARY ANGIOGRAPHY   ■ ■ ■

Asymptomatic or Stable Angina
Class I
1. Evidence of high risk on noninvasive testing.
2. Canadian Cardiovascular Society (CCS) class III or IV angina on medical treatment.
3. Patients resuscitated from sudden cardiac death or with sustained monomorphic ventricular tachycardia (VT) or nonsustained polymorphic VT.

Class IIa
1. CCS class III or IV angina that improves to class I or II on medical therapy.
2. Serial noninvasive testing showing progressive abnormalities.
3. Patient with disability or illness that cannot be stratified by other means.
4. CCS class I or II with intolerance or failure to respond to medical therapy.
5. Individuals whose occupation involves safety of others (e.g., pilots and bus drivers) with abnormal stress test results or high-risk clinical profile.

Nonspecific Chest Pain
Class I
High-risk findings on noninvasive testing.

Class IIa
None.

Unstable Coronary Syndromes
Class I
1. High or intermediate risk for adverse outcome in patients with unstable angina refractory to initial adequate medical therapy or recurrent symptoms after initial stabilization. Emergent catheterization is recommended.
2. High risk for adverse outcome in patients with unstable angina. Urgent catheterization is recommended.
3. High- or intermediate-risk unstable angina that stabilizes after initial treatment.
4. Initially low, short-term–risk unstable angina that is subsequently high risk on noninvasive testing.
5. Suspected Prinzmetal's variant angina.

Class IIa
None.

Patients with Postrevascularization Ischemia
Class I
1. Suspected abrupt closure or subacute stent thrombosis after percutaneous revascularization.
2. Recurrent angina or high-risk criteria on noninvasive evaluation within 9 months of percutaneous revascularization.

Class IIa
1. Recurrent symptomatic ischemia within 12 months of coronary artery bypass graft surgery.
2. Noninvasive evidence of high-risk criteria occurring at any time postoperatively.
3. Recurrent angina inadequately controlled by medical means after revascularization.

During the Initial Management of Acute Myocardial Infarction (Myocardial Infarction Suspected and ST Segment Elevation or Bundle Branch Block Present)
Coronary Angiography Coupled with the Intent to Perform Primary Percutaneous Coronary Intervention
Class I
1. As an alternative to thrombolytic therapy in patients who can undergo angioplasty of the infarct-related artery within 12 hours of the onset of symptoms or beyond 12 hours if ischemic symptoms persist, *if performed in a timely fashion by individuals skilled in the procedure and supported by experienced personnel in an appropriate laboratory environment.*

2. In patients who are within 36 hours of an acute ST elevation Q or new left bundle branch block myocardial infarction who develop cardiogenic shock, who are younger than 75 years, and in whom revascularization can be performed within 18 hours of the onset of the shock.

Class IIa
As a reperfusion strategy in patients who are candidates for reperfusion but who have a contraindication to fibrinolytic therapy, if angioplasty can be performed as outlined earlier in class I.

Early Coronary Angiography in the Patient with Suspected Myocardial Infarction (ST Segment Elevation or Bundle Branch Block Present) Who Has Not Undergone Primary Percutaneous Coronary Intervention
Class I
None.

Class IIa
Cardiogenic shock or persistent hemodynamic instability.

Early Coronary Angiography in Acute MI (MI Suspected but No ST Segment Elevation)
Class I
1. Persistent or recurrent (stuttering) episodes of symptomatic ischemia, spontaneous or induced, with or without associated ECG changes.
2. The presence of shock, severe pulmonary congestion, or continuing hypotension.

Class IIa
None.

Coronary Angioplasty During the Hospital Management Phase (Patients with Q Wave and Non-Q Wave Infarction)
Class I
1. Spontaneous myocardial ischemia or myocardial ischemia provoked by minimal exertion, during recovery from infarction.
2. Before definitive therapy of a mechanical complication of infarction such as acute mitral regurgitation, ventricular septal defect, pseudoaneurysm, or left ventricular aneurysm.
3. Persistent hemodynamic instability.

Class IIa
1. When myocardial infarction is suspected to have occurred by a mechanism other than thrombotic occlusion at an atherosclcerotic plaque (e.g., coronary embolism, arteritis, trauma, certain metabolic or hematological diseases, or coronary spasm).
2. Survivors of acute myocardial infarction with left ventricular ejection fraction less than 0.40, heart failure, prior revascularization, or malignant ventricular arrhythmias.
3. Clinical heart failure during the acute episode, but subsequent demonstration of preserved left ventricular function (left ventricular ejection fraction greater than 0.40).

During the Risk Stratification Phase (Patients with All Types of Myocardial Infarction)
Class I
Ischemia at low levels of exercise with ECG changes (greater than or equal to 1-mm ST segment depression or other predicators of adverse outcome) and/or imaging abnormalities.

Class IIa
1. Clinically significant heart failure during the hospital course.
2. Inability to perform an exercise test with left ventricular ejection fraction less than or equal to 0.45.

ECG, Electrocardiogram.
From Scanlon PJ, Faxon DF, Auden AM et al: *J Am Coll Cardiol* 33:1756, 1999.

Continued

BOX 28-1
INDICATIONS FOR CORONARY ANGIOGRAPHY—cont'd

■ ■ ■

Perioperative Evaluation Before (or After) Noncardiac Surgery
Class I: Patients with suspected or known coronary artery disease
1. Evidence for high risk of adverse outcome based on noninvasive test results.
2. Angina unresponsive to adequate medical therapy.
3. Unstable angina, particularly when facing intermediate- or high-risk noncardiac surgery.
4. Equivocal noninvasive test result in high clinical risk patient undergoing high-risk surgery.

Class IIa
1. Multiple intermediate clinical risk markers and planned vascular surgery.
2. Ischemia on noninvasive testing but without high-risk criteria.
3. Equivocal noninvasive test result in intermediate clinical risk patient undergoing high-risk noncardiac surgery.
4. Urgent noncardiac surgery while convalescing from acute myocardial infarction.

Patients with Valvular Heart Disease
Class I
1. Before valve surgery or balloon valvotomy in an adult with chest discomfort, ischemia by noninvasive imaging, or both.
2. Before valve surgery in an adult free of chest pain but with many risk factors for coronary artery disease.
3. Infective endocarditis with evidence of coronary embolization.

Class IIa
None.

Patients with Congenital Heart Disease
Class I
1. Before surgical correction of congenital heart disease when chest discomfort or noninvasive evidence is suggestive of associated coronary artery disease.
2. Before surgical correction of suspected congenital coronary anomalies such as congenital coronary artery stenosis, coronary arteriovenous fistula, and anomalous origin of the left coronary artery.
3. Forms of congenital heart disease frequently associated with coronary artery anomalies that may complicate surgical management.
4. Unexplained cardiac arrest in a young patient.

Class IIa
Before corrective open heart surgery for congenital heart disease in an adult whose risk profile increases the likelihood of coexisting coronary artery disease.

Patients with Congestive Heart Failure
Class I
1. Heart failure caused by systolic dysfunction with angina or with regional wall motion abnormalities and/or scintigraphic evidence or reversible myocardial ischemia when revascularization is being considered.
2. Before cardiac transplantation.
3. Heart failure following postinfarction ventricular aneurysm or other mechanical complications of myocardial infarction.

Class IIa
1. Systolic dysfunction with unexplained cause despite noninvasive testing.
2. Normal systolic function, but episodic heart failure raises suspicion if ischemically mediated left ventricular dysfunction.

Other Conditions
Class I
1. Diseases affecting the aorta when knowledge of the presence of extent of coronary artery involvement is necessary for management (e.g., aortic dissection or aneurysm with known coronary artery disease).
2. Hypertrophic cardiomyopathy with angina despite medical therapy when knowledge of coronary anatomy might affect therapy.
3. Hypertrophic cardiomyopathy with angina when heart surgery is planned.

Class IIa
1. High risk for coronary artery disease when other cardiac surgical procedures are planned (e.g., pericardiectomy or removal of chronic pulmonary emboli).
2. Prospective immediate cardiac transplant donors whose risk profiles increase the likelihood of coronary artery disease.
3. Asymptomatic patients with Kawasaki disease who have coronary artery aneurysms on echocardiography.
4. Before surgery for aortic aneurysm/dissection in patients without known coronary artery disease.
5. Recent blunt chest trauma and suspicion of acute myocardial infarction, without evidence of preexisting coronary artery disease.

NURSING MANAGEMENT

Cardiac catheterization has evolved into an outpatient procedure that has significant implications for nursing management and patient and family education. Nurses must be vigilant in identifying patients at high risk, detecting problems, and anticipating complications. Laboratory and other diagnostic testing are needed in advance of the procedure to assist with the evaluation process. Discharge typically occurs within six hours of the procedure, allowing limited time for patient and family education regarding postprocedure patient care and methods to maintain patient safety in the immediate postprocedure period at home.

Before Heart Catheterization
Preparation and Assessment

To ensure good outcomes, proper planning, assessment, and evaluation of patients preparing to undergo cardiac catheterization are essential. Whether a patient comes in for preadmission paperwork and laboratory work or on an emergent basis, the nursing responsibilities are similar. The patient's medical condition and overall health can be evaluated during this process. Preparing patients and their families decreases anxiety and promotes cooperation that can only enhance their capacity for understanding. This time also provides an opportunity to address patient concerns, educate, and establish a trusting nurse-patient relationship.

Verifying that the interventionalist has explained the procedure and its risks and benefits in a way that the patient understands is imperative. Before obtaining informed consent, review the following: (1) what the patient will experience before, during, and after the procedure, and (2) the possible treatment modalities that may be implemented, such as angioplasty with the deployment of a stent, rotablator procedure, and/or intravascular ultrasound measurements. Consent for coronary artery bypass surgery in the event of a life-threatening emergency also is obtained. Laboratory values are obtained, assessed for abnormalities, and reported to the interventionalist. Important tests to be performed before the procedure include a complete blood count, platelet count, serum creatinine, electrolytes, fasting blood glucose level, prothrombin time, international normalized ratio, and partial thromboplastin time.

Radiographic contrast media is nephrotoxic. Therefore, it is imperative to check the blood urea nitrogen and serum creatinine levels on all patients and specifically to scrutinize the results in patients who are diabetic and taking angiotensin-converting enzyme inhibitors or diuretics. This particular subset of patients is more likely to have increases in creatinine level (Box 28-2).

Verify that the patient has had nothing by mouth for 8 to 12 hours before the procedure. Nausea and vomiting are untoward side effects of contrast medium. Additionally, in the event of severe cardiovascular disease, the patient may go directly to surgery. Leaving dentures, glasses, and hearing aids in place facilitates communication and helps the patient follow instructions during the procedure. A detailed medication and drug history should be obtained, including any over-the-counter and herbal supplements. Unless specifically questioned, many patients will not mention such products.[4]

A head-to-toe assessment is critical just before the procedure. Obtain an accurate weight. Document the amplitude of arterial pulses in both legs distal to the planned insertion site. The baseline status of the femoral, dorsalis pedis, and posterior tibial pulses should be established at baseline so that comparisons can be made when monitoring for hematoma after the procedure. Confirm that the information on the patient identification band and allergy band is accurate. Establish patent intravenous (IV) access before the procedure for administration of fluids, sedation, and emergency medication.

During the physical preparation of the patient, obtain a concise and targeted medical history. Specifically, request information about signs and symptoms of gastrointestinal bleeding, stroke, and intolerance to aspirin or thienopyridine derivatives, such as clopidigrel and ticlopidine. With any patient, it is important to obtain a complete history of allergies, but requesting information regarding past procedures and whether there was an allergic reaction to contrast media or latex is essential in this context. Asking whether the patient is allergic to iodine or shellfish is a common question, although a history of shellfish allergy does not predispose a patient to contrast media reaction.[2]

When alerted to the fact that a patient may develop anaphylaxis to contrast media, inform the interventionalist immediately. Oral and intravenous prophylaxis should be administered as soon as possible before the procedure. Prednisone 60 mg or hydrocortisone 100 mg may be administered intravenously along with cimetidine as a histamine antagonist and diphenhydramine (Benadryl). Obtain informed consent before diphenhydramine administration.

Gather information on prior procedures, catheterizations, percutaneous coronary interventions, general surgery, or cardiac surgery. Noting chronic conditions such as renal insufficiency, peripheral vascular disease, chronic obstructive pulmonary disease, and current anticoagulation status may affect the medical or nursing care administered during the procedure. Oral anticoagulants, except aspirin, are discontinued. The recommendation is an international normalized ratio of less than 1.8. Metformin should be discontinued the morning of the procedure and preferably withheld for at least 48 hours after use of iodinated contrast media. Patients taking metformin for diabetes are at risk for severe lactic acidosis after injection of iodinated contrast media. The drug can be resumed safely when the serum creatinine level returns to baseline and remains stable 48 hours after the procedure.[5]

With the insertion of a good intravenous line, hydration should be established as soon as possible. Although 1 liter of normal saline solution is recommended, the amount of hydration is individualized according to renal status and cardiac function. Intravenous access enables the nurse to titrate small amounts of medication throughout the procedure to maintain sedation because general anesthesia is not required for routine catheterization. Record a baseline set of vital signs, including oxygen saturation by pulse oximetry. In addition to the head-to-toe assessment, ask whether the patient has any skin or musculoskeletal condition that caregivers should be aware of because the patient will be on a hard, flat table during the procedure, and the extremity used for the procedure will be immobilized for some time afterward.

BOX 28-2 ■ ■ ■

RELATIVE CONTRAINDICATIONS FOR CORONARY ANGIOGRAPHY

- Active endocarditis
- Acute renal failure
- Decompensated congestive heart failure
- Digitalis toxicity
- Ongoing stroke
- Previous contrast reaction (no pretreatment with corticosteroids)
- Severe active bleeding
- Severe anemia (hemoglobin less than 8 g/dl)
- Severe intrinsic or iatrogenic coagulopathy (international normalized ratio greater than 2.0)
- Severe electrolyte imbalance
- Uncontrolled systemic hypertension
- Unexplained fever
- Untreated infection

From Bashore TM, Bates ER, Berger PB et al: *J Am Coll Cardiol* 37:2170-2214, 2001.

Education

Undergoing a cardiac catheterization arouses anxiety in most patients. Anxiety has been reduced effectively in studies on psychological preparation using sensory-perceptual and modeling preparatory techniques.[6] When patients are scheduled for an elective cardiac catheterization, many times written instructions are given by the physician's office staff. Alternately, many institutions contact patients once the procedure is scheduled. Reinforcement of instructions on preprocedure fasting, medications, and postoperative care enhance patient compliance because this is a stressful time when the patient's ability to understand and remember information is compromised. Patients should be reminded to leave valuables at home and, if they wear contact lenses, to take them out and wear their eyeglasses. Explaining to patients why they need to arrive well before the procedure time is important so that paperwork can be completed, results of laboratory tests can be obtained, and last minute details can be managed. If a delay arises, patients need to be informed and given an explanation, which will help relieve anxiety.

Before the procedure, procedural and sensory information should be given to reduce anxiety. Explain that the patient will be transferred onto a hard table necessary for radiographic films. Also mention that the room will be cold. After describing the shaving and preparing of the inguinal area, explain that the interventionalist will inject a local anesthetic into the area to anesthetize the nerve endings and prevent pain. An introducer sheath will be inserted, and the patient will feel pressure. The purpose of the introducer sheath is to facilitate passage of tiny catheters used to inject contrast media to visualize the artery by fluoroscopy. Let the patient know that vital signs, oxygen level, and heart rhythm will be monitored throughout the procedure; the automated blood pressure monitor will feel tight. Assure the patient that intravenous sedation will be given for relaxation, and explain that the patient will be awake throughout the procedure in order to follow directions and to report any discomfort.

Before the procedure, teach the patient to report pain on a scale of 0 to 10. Patients commonly report a warm flush or warm sensation in their chest when the contrast medium is injected. If the patient is having a PTCA, mention that inflation of the balloon may cause a brief moment of pain.

Just before leaving the admitting unit, the patient should void. Let the patient know that an indwelling urinary catheter may be inserted during the procedure.

Support

While waiting for the coronary angiogram, patients commonly are quite anxious. In a recent qualitative study by De Jong-Watt and Arthur,[7] participants identified sources of anxiety as (1) the need for angiography; (2) the actual test; and (3) the eventual diagnosis and possibility of heart surgery. Anxiety can affect the cardiovascular system by stimulating cardiac irritability and increasing basal metabolic rate, bronchodilatation, blood pressure, catecholamine release, myocardial oxygen demand, and platelet aggregation.[8]

Proper preparation of the patient scheduled to undergo a cardiac catheterization procedure can optimize patient care, comfort, and satisfaction. Procedural and sensory information decreases anxiety and increases coping with invasive medical procedures; however, one study suggested that a 10-minute massage just before heart catheterization was insufficient to promote relaxation and decrease stress related to the procedure.[9]

During Heart Catheterization

A great deal of technology, nursing skill, and judgment are required to provide an environment that is safe and comfortable for the patient in the catheterization laboratory. Having a critical care background, certification in advanced cardiac life support, and knowledge of sophisticated equipment such as the intraaortic balloon pump are additional areas of expertise required to care competently for patients undergoing invasive cardiac procedures.

Upon receiving the patient in the catheterization laboratory, the registered nurse identifies the staff to the patient and provides a brief explanation of the personnel and their roles:

- The x-ray technologist is present because fluoroscopy will be used.
- The cardiovascular technician will scrub in and assist the physician.
- The registered nurse will monitor the patient, administer drugs, and circulate as needed.

Although it may seem repetitive, at this time it is also necessary to gather a brief history and verify nothing-by-mouth status and neurological and cognitive status. With repetitive questioning, patients under stress may remember and divulge different pieces of information. Critical information to obtain includes allergies, whether the patient is diabetic, the results of the most recent blood glucose level, if the patient is taking metformin (which combined with contrast medium can impair renal function), and if so, when the last dose was administered. Additionally, question the patient about medicines that have anticoagulant properties such as clopidigrel, aspirin, enoxaparin (Lovenox), and warfarin. Verification that the patient has discontinued warfarin before the procedure according to the physician's instructions is important.

Customarily, the circulating nurse in the procedure area reviews all laboratory data and confirms that the patient can state his or her name and the procedure. A brief head-to-toe assessment is conducted at this time. Assess for the following signs of potential difficulty rescuing from conscious sedation: thick neck, history of snoring, or history of adverse outcomes with anesthesia. Assessment of the patient's ability to take a deep breath is important. During the procedure, the patient will be asked to take a deep breath, which increases visualization by causing the diaphragm to descend and taking the shadow off the heart. Check the intravenous site for patency. Place a pulse oximetry probe on the patient (Figure 28-1), and start oxygen before medication is given for conscious sedation.

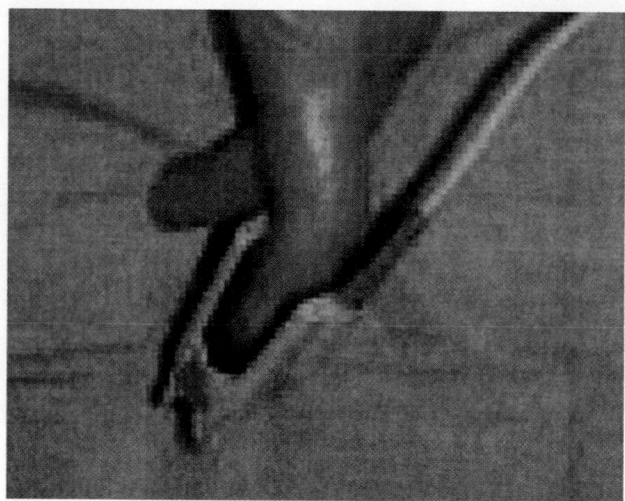

FIGURE 28-1 ■ A pulse oximetry device.

As the catheter insertion site is prepared and shaved, communicate continually with the patient to provide support and reassurance and to decrease anxiety. Both femoral access sites are prepared in case access is impaired on the right side. Baseline dorsalis pedis and posterior tibial pulses are recorded. The entire body from the neck down is covered with a sterile drape, and the patient is instructed to refrain from touching these areas. If the designated site is the brachial or radial site, the arm is stabilized on an arm board and aseptically draped to the shoulder. Because the patient will be conscious and anxiety levels are likely to be high during the

entire procedure, continual communication, along with reassurance and support, is central to providing optimal care.[10]

Administration of Conscious Sedation

"Sedation and analgesia describes a state that allows patients to tolerate unpleasant procedures while maintaining adequate cardiorespiratory function and the ability to respond purposefully to verbal command and/or tactile stimulation"[11] (p. 460). Evidence-based practice protocols for providing conscious sedation have not been established as yet, and individual patient responses vary widely and can be unpredictable. Cardiac or respiratory depression from excessive sedation or analgesia must be rapidly recognized and appropriately managed. The goal is to avoid the risk of hypoxia, which can lead to brain damage, cardiac arrest, or even death. Conversely, a lack of cooperation or adverse physiological response to stress because of inadequate sedation or analgesia may result in undue patient discomfort or injury. Sedated patients should never be left unattended. Reversal agents should always be available. Although naloxone for the reversal of opioids and flumazenil for the reversal of benzodiazepines are readily available to reverse respiratory depression, it is recommended that patients be treated initially with supplemental oxygen. Acute pharmacological reversal may result in pain, hypertension, tachycardia, or pulmonary edema[11] (Table 28-1).

Femoral, brachial, and radial vessels generally are accessed percutaneously. Inform the patient that the physician will inject a local anesthetic such as lidocaine under the skin at the insertion site and that it will feel

■ ■ ■

TABLE 28-1   DRUGS GIVEN AS PART OF HEART CATHETERIZATION

DRUG	DOSAGE	ADMINISTERED	ACTION
Aspirin	81-325 mg PO	Periprocedure	Decreases platelet aggregation
Bivalirudin	1.0 mg/kg bolus 2.5 mg/kg/hr infusion	Periprocedure	Brachial or radial access
Cimetidine (Tagamet)	300 mg IV	Preprocedure	Histamine blocker for potential anaphylaxis to contrast medium
Diazepam (Valium)	2.5-10 mg PO	1 hour before procedure	Relaxation
Diphenhydramine (Benadryl)	25-50 mg PO	1 hour before procedure	Sedation
	25-50 mg IV	Periprocedure	Additional sedation and mitigation of allergic reaction
Fentanyl	25-50 mcg IV	Periprocedure	To promote sedation
Flumazenil (Romazicon)	IV bolus	Periprocedure	Benzodiazepine antagonist
Heparin	2000-5000 units IV	Periprocedure	For patients at increased risk for thromboembolic complications or brachial or radial access
Methylprednisolone (Sterapred or Sterapred DS Prednisone) see above	60 mg PO	Night before and 2 hours before procedure	For potential anaphylaxis to contrast medium
Midazolam (Versed)	0.5-2 mg IV	Periprocedure	To promote relaxation
Nitroglycerin*	0.3 mg sublingual 50-100 mcg intracoronary 10-25 mcg/min IV	Before, during, and after the procedure	Periprocedural ischemia (BP greater than 100 mm Hg systolic)
Naloxone (Narcan)	IV bolus	Periprocedure	Opioid antagonist
Oxygen	2-4 L/min nasal	Periprocedure	To prevent hypoxemia during conscious sedation
Protamine	1 mg/100 units heparin	Periprocedure	Reversal agent for heparin

IV, Intravenous; *PO,* by mouth.

*Not for patients who use NPH insulin, who have a history of unstable angina, or who have coronary angiography by radial or brachial access.

Data from Baim D, Grossman W: Complications of cardiac catheterization. In Baim D, Grossman W, editors: *Grossman's cardiac catheterization, angiography, and intervention,* ed 6, Philadelphia, 2000, Lippincott Williams & Wilkins.

much like a bee sting before becoming numb. Advise the patient that insertion of the sheath or cannula will cause a sensation of pressure but should not cause pain. Tell the patient to report any pain so that additional anesthetic can be administered (Figure 28-2).

Once the catheter is positioned correctly, the contrast medium is injected. Immediately after, the cameras will move around the patient. Warn the patient about the proximity of the camera to the face and that it is necessary to film the heart and arteries from several different angles. The patient will be instructed where to move the arms and face and when to hold the breath for each picture.

The contrast agent is injected after pressure and volume measurements have been taken. A consequence of contrast medium directly after injection is myocardial depression. The contrast medium displaces oxygen-rich blood in the coronary arteries, which may cause the heart rate to decrease. At this point, the patient is instructed to cough to help clear the contrast medium and stimulate a return to baseline heart rate. Assess the left ventricular end-diastolic pressure before continuing with the contrast infusion. If the left ventricular end-diastolic pressure is elevated, the patient should be assessed for congestive heart failure. An ejection fraction of less than 30 percent or a pulmonary capillary wedge pressure greater than 25 mm Hg is an early warning sign of congestion that precedes frank pulmonary edema. Diuretics or vasodilators may be administered (Table 28-2).

During the procedure, vital signs, oxygen saturation, and electrocardiogram are monitored and recorded at regular intervals according to institution policy. All hemodynamic data are recorded for the left and right sides of the heart. The level of care required after the procedure is anticipated at this point, with disposition based on diagnosis, therapy, and outcome of the procedure. Communicate with the intensive care unit or operating suite in the event of an unexpected interventional pro-

TABLE 28-2   NORMAL HEMODYNAMIC PARAMETERS

PARAMETER	NORMAL MEASURE
Ejection fraction	60%-65%
Cardiac output	4-8 liter/min
Cardiac index	2.5-4 liter/min/m²
Pulmonary artery pressure	*Systolic:* 20-30 mm Hg
	Diastolic: 8-15 mm Hg
Pulmonary artery capillary wedge pressure	*Mean:* 4-12 mm Hg
Right atrial pressure	*Mean:* 2-6 mm Hg
Right ventricular pressure	*Systolic:* 20-30 mm Hg
Left atrial pressure	*Diastolic:* 2-8 mm Hg
	Mean: 4-12 mm Hg
Left ventricular pressure	*Systolic:* 100-140 mm Hg
	Diastolic: 4-12 mm Hg
Left ventricular end diastolic pressure	*Mean:* 4-12 mm Hg
Aortic pressure	*Systolic:* 120-140 mm Hg
	Diastolic: 60-80 mm Hg
	Mean: 70-90 mm Hg

Data from Grossman W: Blood flow measurement. In Baim D, Grossman D, editors: *Grossman's cardiac catheterization, angiography, and intervention,* ed 6, Philadelphia, 2000, Lippincott Williams & Wilkins.

cedure or an unstable diagnostic catheterization. The progressive care unit receives stable patients after intervention.

Patient safety during a procedure is critical. Fluid spills are monitored throughout the procedure. Electrical safety measures are followed. Guidelines for prevention of catheterization laboratory infections are based on standard precautions for preventing infection in surgical wounds. Sterile precautions should be more vigorous for cutdown than percutaneous procedures. The nurse monitors the environment to ensure appropriate cleaning, limited traffic, and maintenance of adequate ventilation. To ensure proper catheterization technique, appropriate use of sterile equipment, and disposal of contaminated equipment is within the nursing scope of practice. A well-stocked emergency cart with defibrillator within proximity to the patient area is critical.

An authorized clinician, nurse, or physician can remove the sheath postprocedure. Before the sheath is removed, the anticoagulant effects of unfractionated heparin should be dissipated (activated clotting time less than 150 to 180 seconds). Manual pressure is applied for 15 to 20 minutes until there is no evidence of bleeding. The pressure should be applied firmly, but the distal pulse should remain palpable. The insertion site is covered with a small bandage after hemostasis is confirmed.

Careful attention and assessment for bleeding are imperative, particularly when the physician orders a pressure dressing and the puncture site cannot be visualized directly. The nurse is responsible for checking for hemostasis, distal circulation, and peripheral pulses. Verify voiding, and assess for abdominal distention before the patient is transferred to the designated recovery area. Remind the patient to keep the affected extremity straight and, if applicable, explain the type of closure device used (collagen plug or suture closure). Administer an intravenous antibiotic, if warranted.

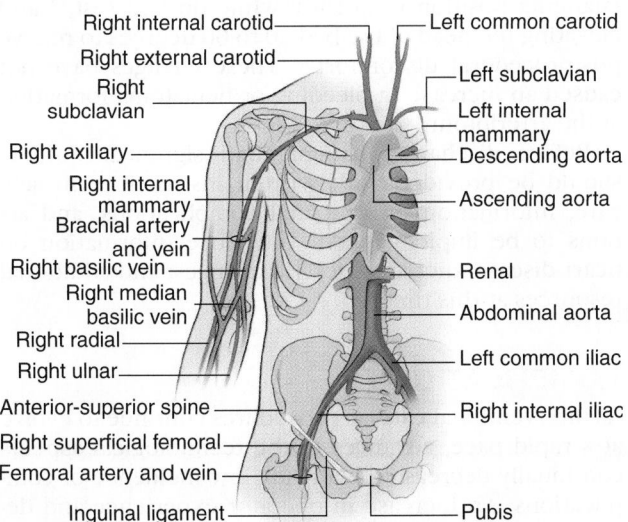

FIGURE 28-2 ■ Principal arteries used for access during cardiac catheterization. Only the superficial veins are shown on the forearm. (Modified from Thibodeau GA, Patton KT, editors: *Anthony's textbook of anatomy and physiology,* ed 17, St Louis, 2002, Mosby.)

Evidence-Based Practice for Femoral Sheath Removal

Removal of femoral sheaths has become a routine part of nursing practice. The American Association of Critical-Care Nurses surveyed members and reported that 91 percent of postcardiac catheterization sheaths and 83 percent of postangioplasty sheaths are removed by critical care nurses.[12]

Several techniques exist for sheath removal; these range from manual to mechanical compression devices. Techniques vary within and between hospitals. Mechanical compression devices include belt devices with a compression arch and translucent dome positioned over the femoral insertion site and a C-clamp with a translucent pressure pad positioned proximal to the femoral insertion site.[13] Studies have been conducted to compare compression devices to manual pressure,[13,14] but few of these studies were randomized controlled trials. Benson and colleagues[15] compared three methods of sheath removal, with groin complications such as hematoma, bleeding, pseudoaneurysm, and arteriovenous malformation as the outcome variables. Patients who had manual pressure after sheath removal experienced fewer complications than those who received mechanical compression.

Technology is evolving because of a cost-conscious health care system. Arterial puncture closing devices are being developed at a rapid rate to reduce manual compression time and promote earlier discharge.[16] The Syvek Patch (Marine Polymer Technologies) is a polymer poly-N-acetyl glucosamine vascular closure device that is isolated from microalgae and accelerates clot formation and vasoconstriction. The patch is used with a manual hold and requires only 6 minutes of manual pressure for diagnostic procedures, allowing earlier ambulation and discharge.[17] Collagen plugs with or without an anchor (Angioseal or Vasoseal), balloon-positioning catheters combined with bovine microfibrillar collagen and thrombin (Duett), and a suture-like stitch placed around the femoral artery (Perclose) now are being used in half of patients undergoing percutaneous coronary intervention.[18] Newer closure devices are being developed that will decrease equipment requirements and promote quicker discharge to increase cost savings. However, the possibility of vascular complications should be considered at least as seriously in patients treated with vascular closure devices as in those treated with manual compression.[19,20]

After Heart Catheterization

In the recovery area, the patient is assessed every 15 minutes for the first hour, every 30 minutes for the second hour, and every hour until discharge. In addition to vital signs and cardiac monitoring, catheter entry site, peripheral pulses, and neurovascular function are monitored for complications such as bleeding, arterial occlusion, and hematoma formation.

After the procedure, hydration by intravenous fluids and oral intake is essential to ensure optimum renal clearance of the contrast agent. Careful monitoring of urine output is important. Patients are encouraged to

---

> **BOX 28-3** ■ ■ ■
> RISK FACTORS FOR COMPLICATIONS AFTER FEMORAL ARTERIOTOMY
>
> - Age
> - Gender (Women had more complications in some studies but not in others.)
> - Large catheter size
> - Length of time catheter is in place
> - Peripheral vascular disease

Data from McCabe PJ, McPherson LA, Lohse CM et al: *Am J Crit Care* 10:330-340, 2001; and Christensen B, Manion R, Iacarella C: *Nurs Res* 47:51-53, 1998.

---

empty the bladder using a urinal or bedpan because a distended bladder will cause increased pain or pressure. Remind the patient not to lift the head because doing so requires abdominal muscle contraction, which might disturb the clot at the insertion site. To prevent hematoma formation, caution the patient not to bend, hyperextend, or lie on the affected extremity. Instruct the patient how to apply pressure to the site in the event of a cough or a sneeze. If the site feels wet or warm, the nurse should be alerted immediately. A regular diet may be resumed.

When the sedation and analgesia used during the procedure start to wear off in the recovery area, patients often complain of discomfort. Mobilization varies with each interventionalist and facility protocol. If the radial or brachial route were used, the patient may ambulate immediately with the affected limb on an arm board.[21] Traditionally, patients who have a femoral arteriotomy were placed on bed rest for up to 6 hours, which often aggravated preexisting musculoskeletal disorders. This inconvenience prompted research on reducing immobilization time. When the femoral approach is used, the patient is usually out of bed at 4 hours, assisted to ambulate, and discharged 5 hours after the procedure.[22] Research supports eliminating the use of sandbags to compress the arteriotomy site,[23] changing position frequently while on bed rest,[24] and elevating the head of the bed 30 to 60 degrees to relieve postprocedural discomfort.[22] These changes have not caused an increase in bleeding or hematoma formation at the arteriotomy site (Box 28-3).

Before discharge, patients and significant others should be provided with written instructions in self-care, information on potential complications, and actions to be implemented.[10] Introduce information on heart disease, diet and lifestyle changes, and additional resources at this time.

COMPLICATIONS

As interventional cardiac procedures continue to evolve at a rapid pace, advances in the technological aspects continually decrease the already low incidence of complications. An increase in operator experience and development of lower-profile diagnostic catheters, puncture closure devices, and low-osmolar contrast media have been credited with reducing complications in this population.[25] The current mortality rate is less than 1 percent.

BOX 28-4   ■ ■ ■

CRITERIA FOR THE DIAGNOSIS OF RADIOCONTRAST-INDUCED NEPHROPATHY

- Sudden reduction in renal function quantified by an absolute increase in serum creatinine level of more than 0.5 mg/dl or a relative increase of more than 25 percent of the level before administration of contrast medium
- Manifestation of impaired renal function up to 5 days after administration of contrast medium
- Exclusion of other causes of renal failure

Data from Gami A, Garovic V: *Mayo Clin Proc* 79:211-219, 2004.

Radiocontrast Nephropathy

Radiocontrast-induced nephropathy (**RCN**) is a serious complication of coronary procedures that includes intravascular infusion of iodinated contrast medium. Contrast medium is the source of this iatrogenic disease.[26] Patients who are elderly, are diabetic, and have preexisting renal insufficiency or heart failure are at increased risk for RCN. At least 5 percent of patients are estimated to have at least a 1-mg/dl increase in serum creatinine following cardiac catheterization (Box 28-4).

Findings are inconsistent regarding the efficacy of orally administered acetylcysteine, an antioxidant, in reducing the incidence of RCN.[27-29] Currently, the most effective method of reducing the likelihood of nephropathy is saline hydration 12 hours before and 12 hours after the procedure. Discontinuance of diuretics, angiotensin-converting enzyme inhibitors, and nonsteroidal antiinflammatory drugs 1 or 2 days before the procedure also is recommended.[26] Attention to baseline renal function is critically important because the most important predictor of RCN is renal insufficiency at baseline.[30] It is important to remind patients to see their physicians 2 days after the procedure before restarting metformin therapy in order to verify the return to baseline creatinine levels.

Pharmacological Complications

GP IIb/IIIa inhibitors may be given to patients with acute coronary syndrome.[31] This relatively new family of agents blocks the final common pathway mediating platelet aggregation—the fibrinogen or GP IIb/IIIa receptor.[32] These drugs prevent the formation of blood clots and subsequent infarcts during angiogram and help to prevent restenosis after angioplasty, stenting, or atherectomy procedures.[33] When angioplasty with stenting is needed or anticipated, abciximab (ReoPro), the first GP IIb/IIIa inhibitor to be developed, is frequently the drug of choice.[31,33] However, tirofiban (Aggrastat) or eptifibatide (Integrilin) may be used instead if the need for coronary artery bypass surgery is anticipated.[31]

Researchers currently are studying the use of GP IIb/IIIa inhibitors with thrombolytics to treat acute coronary syndromes. Although showing clinical benefit, the potent antiplatelet effects of these agents have been associated with an increased risk of bleeding (3 to 4 percent). Bleeding was the most common side effect in the CAPTURE,[34] PURSUIT,[35] PRISM,[18] and PRISM-PLUS[36] studies. The potential exists for bleeding at all venous and arterial puncture sites and high-risk sites (e.g., gastrointestinal, genitourinary, retroperitoneal, and brain).[32] Additionally, bruising, stomach irritation, or an allergic reaction may occur.[18,34-36] If uncontrollable bleeding occurs, infusion of a GP IIb/IIIa inhibitor and any concomitant therapy should be discontinued immediately.

Puncture Site Complications

One of the primary aims of nursing assessment of patients immediately following a cardiac procedure is the detection of puncture site-related complications. Only vague definitions of these local complications are found in the literature because there is a tendency to report only those complications that result in medical or surgical interventions.[25] Vigilant nursing assessment averts these more serious complications.

A few prospective observational studies of postprocedure bleeding complications have been done; most studies have relied on retrospective chart data, so some complications may be underreported.[16,25] This lack of evidence has resulted in few changes in practice over the last 20 years.[25]

Venous oozing can be continuous for many hours, which can be a source of distress for patients and nurses. Bleeding usually resolves when the partial thromboplastin time becomes less than 30 seconds. Changing the dressing, applying pressure, and encouraging the patient to drink additional fluids are effective nursing interventions.

Femoral puncture site bleeding can occur from 1 to 12 hours after the procedure. This variation makes it difficult to develop evidence-based observation protocols.[25] External bleeding is seen and managed easily. However, bleeding into the leg or groin results in a hematoma that is not readily visible. Factors associated with bleeding are use of anticoagulants, female gender, increased age, low body weight, and morbid obesity.[13] Some hematomas are the direct result of sheath removal. Vital sign measurement is not a reliable indicator of bleeding. Alerting patients to the signs and symptoms of a spontaneous bleed—i.e., sharp knife-like pain, or wet and warm sensations at the groin site—helps them warn the nurse if bleeding is detected. Frequent puncture site observation is critical and overshadows the importance of frequent taking of vital signs.[25]

After arterial cannulation, pseudoaneurysm (**PSA**) is the most common vascular complication. The common femoral artery is the usual site of sheath insertion. The superficial and deep femoral arteries have smaller and thinner walls, making them more susceptible to injury when they are punctured. Bleeding occurs into the tissue surrounding the artery through a small track and forms a wall around the artery that continues to enlarge. As the blood-filled cavity enlarges, it pulsates with the flow of arterial blood. The mass is pulsatile to all points of palpation and should be auscultated to detect a systolic bruit near the insertion site. Reassess the pedal pulses. Differential diagnosis of a PSA should be verified by vascular ultrasound. Treatment for PSA can be performed using ultrasound-guided compression, ultrasound-guided thrombin injection, or surgical repair.[37]

A retroperitoneal hematoma is a rare but serious complication because the retroperitoneal cavity can hold a large amount of blood. The resultant pressure on the femoral nerve can cause a palsy that affects the leg or foot. The only symptom the patient may report is leg or flank pain until hypovolemic shock occurs. A common error is the assumption that the patient's shock symptoms are from a cardiac source rather than hypovolemia. The diagnostic criteria that distinguish retroperitoneal hematoma include a rapidly falling hematocrit and blood pressure.

Most retroperitoneal hematomas are treated conservatively. Immediate discontinuation or reversal of anticoagulation and anticoagulation and antiplatelet therapy is instituted with blood transfusion, if necessary. Surgical intervention is indicated with a persistent drop in hematocrit despite transfusion and with femoral neuropathy.

Neuropathy is a rare complication but can occur after a large hemorrhage or PSA around the nerve that causes pressure and irritability. Permanent damage such as foot drop, paresthesia, chronic pain, or other neurological sequelae can occur. Early detection and management of an expanding hematoma or PSA is the best way to control neuropathy that may result from compression of the femoral nerve.

Essential nursing interventions for patients with groin complications are close monitoring of the circulation to the extremity, hematocrit, condition of the groin, and hemodynamic status. In the event of excessive bleeding, fluids and blood administration, bed rest, sedation and pain relief, and management of the surgical wound aid successful patient recovery.

Periprocedural Ischemia

Several factors can induce angina during an angiographic procedure, including tachycardia, hypertension, contrast agents, coronary spasm, vagal responses, microembolization, and platelet aggregation. In this situation, keeping the systolic blood pressure greater than 100 mm Hg is critical before administration of nitroglycerin, be it sublingual (0.3 mg), intracoronary (50 to 200 mcg), or intravenous (10 to 20 mcg/min). Intravenously administered metoprolol (2.5 to 5 mg) or propranolol (1 to 4 mg) can be given to patients without contraindications to beta blockers. For those in cardiogenic shock or refractory pulmonary edema, adjunctive therapy such as intraaortic balloon counterpulsation is needed.[38]

Bacteremia

Little is known about infections acquired during cardiac catheterization.[28] In recent studies, clinically insignificant bacteremia was correlated with the duration of the procedure, multiple skin punctures, and obesity. Clinically significant bacteremia is rare, but the infection rate is greater with repeated use of the same groin site or a procedure in which the catheter has been passed through a femoral graft.[39]

SUMMARY

Cardiac catheterization has evolved over the last six decades to a highly specialized discipline for diagnostic purposes and an expanding repertoire of therapeutic advances to treat many problems. Because of the increasing numbers of outpatient heart catheterizations, nurses play a pivotal role in patient assessment, safety, support, and education. To deliver optimal care, nurses need to prepare the patient adequately both physically and emotionally. Adequate assessment and monitoring throughout the precatherization, intracatheterization, and postcatheterization experience are paramount in avoiding complications and ensuring successful outcomes.

REFERENCES

1. *Heart disease and stroke statistics—2005 update,* Dallas, 2005, American Heart Association.
2. Davidson C, Bonow R: Cardiac catheterization. In Zipes DP, Libby P, Bonow RO, Braunwald E, editors: *Braunwald's heart disease: a textbook of cardiovascular medicine,* ed 7, Philadelphia, 2005, Saunders.
3. Ryan TJ: The coronary angiogram and its seminal contributions to cardiovascular medicine over five decades, *Circulation* 106:752-756, 2002.
4. Tsen L, Segal S, Pothier M, Bader AM: Alternative medicine use in presurgical patients, *Anesthesiology* 93:148-151, 2000.
5. Maddox T: Adverse reactions to contrast material: recognition, prevention, and treatment, *Am Fam Physician* 66:1229-1234, 2002.
6. Harkness K, Morrow L, Smith K et al: The effect of early education on patient anxiety while waiting for elective cardiac catheterization, *Eur J Cardiovasc Nurs* 2:113-121, 2003.
7. De Jong-Watt W, Arthur H: Anxiety and health-related quality of life in patients awaiting elective coronary angiography, *Heart Lung* 33:237-248, 2004.
8. Arthur H, Daniels C, McKelvie R et al: Effect of a preoperative intervention on preoperative and postoperative outcomes in low-risk patients awaiting elective coronary artery bypass grafting and percutaneous transluminal coronary angioplasty, *Eur Heart J* 17:51-61, 2000.
9. Okvat H, Oz M, Ting W, Namerow PB: Massage therapy for patients undergoing cardiac catheterization, *Altern Ther Health Med* 8:68-72, 2002.
10. Carroll D: Capacity for direct attention in patients undergoing percutaneous coronary intervention: the effects of psychological distress, *Prog Cardiovasc Nurs* 20:11-16, 2005.
11. Practice Guidelines for Sedation and Analgesia by Non-anesthesiologists: a report by the American Society of Anesthesiologists Task Force on Sedation and Analgesia by Non-Anesthesiologists, *Anesthesiology* 84:459-471, 1996.
12. Petula S, Hudacek S: The Femostop compression device: utilization guidelines for the critical care nurse, *Dimens Crit Care Nurs* 5:259-264, 1995.
13. Jones T, McCutcheon H: Effectiveness of mechanical compression devices in attaining hemostasis after femoral sheath removal, *Am J Crit Care* 11:155-162, 2002.
14. Nikolsky E, Mehran R, Halkin A et al: Vascular complications associated with arteriotomy closure devices in patients undergoing percutaneous coronary procedures: a meta-analysis, *J Am Coll Cardiol* 44:1200-1209, 2004.
15. Benson L, Wunderly D, Perry B et al: Determining best practice: comparison of three methods of femoral sheath removal after cardiac interventional procedures, *Heart Lung* 34:115-1121, 2005.
16. Koreny M, Riedmuller E, Nikfardjam M et al: Arterial puncture closing devices compared with standard manual compression after cardiac catheterization: systematic review and meta-analysis, *JAMA* 291:350-357, 2004.

17. Palmer B, Gantt S, Lawrence M et al: Effectiveness and safety of manual hemostasis facilitated by the Syvek patch with one hour of bed rest after coronary angiography using six-French catheters, *Am J Cardiol* 93:96-97, 2004.

18. A comparison of aspirin plus tirofiban with aspirin plus heparin for unstable angina, *N Engl J Med* 338:1498-1505, 1998.

19. Baim D, Grossman W: Complications of cardiac catheterization. In Baim D, Grossman W, editors: *Grossman's cardiac catheterization, angiography, and intervention,* ed 6, Philadelphia, 2000, Lippincott Williams & Wilkins.

20. Levine GN, Kern MJ, Berger PB et al: Management of patients undergoing percutaneous coronary revascularization, *Ann Intern Med* 139:123-136, 2003.

21. Nickolaus MJ, Gilchrist IC, Ettinger SM: The way to the heart is all in the wrist: transradial catheterization and interventions, *AACN Clin Issues* 12:62-71, 2001.

22. McCabe PJ, McPherson LA, Lohse CM et al: Evaluation of nursing care after diagnostic coronary angiography, *Am J Crit Care* 10:330-340, 2001.

23. Christensen B, Manion R, Iacarella C: Vascular complications after angiography with and without the use of sandbags, *Nurs Res* 47:51-53, 1998.

24. Chair SY, Taylor-Piliae RE, Lam G et al: Effect of positioning on back pain after coronary angiography, *J Adv Nurs* 42:470-478, 2003.

25. Botti M, Williamson B, Steen K: Coronary angiography observations: evidence-based or ritualistic practice? *Heart Lung* 30: 138-145, 2001.

26. Gami A, Garovic V: Contrast nephropathy after coronary angiography, *Mayo Clin Proc* 79:211-219, 2004.

27. Tepel M, van der Giet M, Schwarzfeld C et al: Prevention of radiographic-contrast-agent-induced reductions in renal function by acetylcysteine, *N Engl J Med* 343:180-184, 2000.

28. Kay J, Chow WH, Chan TM et al: Acetylcysteine for prevention of acute deterioration of renal function following elective coronary angiography and intervention: a randomized controlled trial, *JAMA* 289:553-558, 2003.

29. Briguori C, Manganelli F, Scarpato P et al: Acetylcysteine and contrast agent-associated nephrotoxicity, *J Am Coll Cardiol* 40:298-303, 2002.

30. Erdogan A, Davidson CJ: Recent clinical trials of iodixanol, *Rev Cardiovasc Med* 4(suppl 5):S43-S50, 2003.

31. Braunwald E, Antman EM, Beasley JW, et al. ACC/AHA guideline update for the management of patients with unstable angina and non-ST-segment elevation myocardial infarction—2002: summary article: a report of the American College of Cardiology/American Heart Association Task Force on Practice Guidelines (Committee on the Management of Patients With Unstable Angina), *Circulation* 106:1893-1900, 2002.

32. Koller C: The role of glycoprotein IIb/IIIa inhibition in the management of acute coronary syndromes, *Heart Lung* 30:321-331, 2001.

33. Topol EJ, Moliterno DJ, Herrmann HC et al: Comparison of two platelet glycoprotein IIb/IIIa inhibitors, tirofiban and abciximab, for the prevention of ischemic events with percutaneous coronary revascularization, *N Engl J Med* 344:1888-1894, 2001.

34. Randomized Placebo-Controlled Trial of Abciximab Before and During Coronary Intervention in Refractory Unstable Angina: the CAPTURE study, *Lancet* 349:1429-1435, 1997.

35. Inhibition of platelet gylcoprotein IIb/IIIa with eptifibatide in patients with acute coronary syndromes, *N Engl J Med* 339: 436-443, 1998.

36. Inhibition of the platelet glycoprotein IIb/IIIa receptor with tirofiban in unstable angina and non-Q wave myocardial infarction, *N Engl J Med* 338:1488-1497, 1998.

37. Samal AK, White CJ: Percutaneous management of access site complications, *Catheter Cardiovasc Interv* 57:12-23, 2002.

38. Popma J: Coronary angiography and intravascular ultrasound imaging. In Zipes DP, Libby P, Bonow RO, Braunwald E, editors: *Braunwald's heart disease: a textbook of cardiovascular medicine,* ed 7, Philadelphia, 2005, WB Saunders.

39. Banai S, Selitser V, Keren A et al: Prospective study of bacteremia after cardiac catheterization, *Am J Cardiol* 92:1004-1007, 2003.

Nurse's Role in Exercise Testing and Noninvasive Imaging

Kristine Anne Scordo

CHAPTER ABBREVIATIONS

AACUPR American Association of Cardiovascular and Pulmonary Rehabilitation

ACC American College of Cardiology

ACSM American College of Sports Medicine

AHA American Heart Association

CAD coronary artery disease

DTS Duke Treadmill Score

EBCT electron beam computed tomography

ECG electrocardiogram; echocardiographic

MET metabolic equivalent

MRI magnetic resonance imaging

RPP rate-pressure product

SBP systolic blood pressure

SPECT single-photon emission computed tomography

TEE transesophageal echocardiography

Exercise testing and noninvasive imaging are widely used procedures that provide diagnostic, prognostic, and functional information in a variety of populations. As an important component of cardiovascular nursing practice, detailed knowledge of how to use and interpret these tests is required. The purpose of this chapter is to acquaint the reader with the intricacies of each noninvasive test. Before this discussion, however, it is important to understand the concepts of sensitivity, specificity, and predictive value. A basic understanding of these concepts can lead to cost-effective care with less patient anxiety over misdiagnosis from a false-positive test.

SENSITIVITY AND SPECIFICITY

To choose an appropriate diagnostic test requires knowledge of the ability of the test to predict the presence of heart disease (posttest probability).[1] This prediction or probability depends on the likelihood that an individual has heart disease (pretest probability) and is based on Bayes' theorem. Bayes' theorem, a fundamental mathematical law that governs the process of logical inference, states the relationship between the results of a diagnostic test and prevalence of a disease in a population. For example, the presence of 2-mm ST segment depression on a graded exercise stress test in a 72-year-old man with multiple cardiovascular risk factors adds little; he already has a high probability that the test will be positive. Conversely, a finding of 1-mm ST segment depression in a 35-year-old woman with atypical chest pain (less than 5 percent pretest probability of coronary artery disease [**CAD**]) is unlikely to change her posttest probability (Table 29-1).[2] Thus, an exercise stress test for the sole purpose of diagnosing CAD in this woman will yield little and is an unnecessary expense. In situations, however, where a women's pretest probability is intermediate, further noninvasive testing is useful.

The predictive value of a diagnostic test also depends on its sensitivity and specificity. Sensitivity measures the number of persons who truly have the disease who test positive (true positives/true positives + false negatives), whereas specificity measures the number of persons who do not have the disease who test negative (true negatives/true negatives + false positives).[1]

Two possibilities for a test result to be correct are true positive and true negative, and two possibilities for a result to be incorrect are false-positive and false-negative (Figures 29-1 and 29-2). A patient who does not have CAD and who has a positive test for ischemia has a false-positive test—a measure of specificity. Conversely, a patient with CAD who has a negative test for ischemia has a false-negative test—a measure of sensitivity. The higher the sensitivity and specificity of a test, the more reliable the test is in the determination of presence or absence of CAD. Thus sensitivity and specificity, along with clinical experience and a thorough history and physical examination, can help determine the most cost-effective test to diagnose CAD. Further information about sensitivity and specificity is discussed with each test.

EXERCISE TESTING
Indications, Uses, and Contraindications

Graded exercise testing is a widely popular, relatively low-cost cardiovascular test that uses treadmill, bicycle, or arm exercise along with electrocardiographic (**ECG**) and blood pressure monitoring. This test frequently is used to determine the probability and extent of CAD, assess prognosis and functional capacity, evaluate the efficacy of therapy, aid in the selection of patients for cardiac transplantation, risk stratify patients after a myocardial infarction, and determine exercise capacity and safety for an exercise prescription or a disability. Additional techniques such as metabolic gas analysis, radionuclide imaging and echocardiography, myocardial perfusion imaging, magnetic resonance imaging, or metabolic measurements provide further information required in selected patient populations. Progressive graded exercise can produce ECG changes along with dysrhythmias and abnormal hemodynamics, such as elevated blood pressure, not present at rest. Hemodynamic responses postexercise, in particular heart rate

■ ■ ■

TABLE 29-1 PRETEST PROBABILITY OF CORONARY ARTERY DISEASE BY AGE, GENDER, AND SYMPTOMS

AGE* (YEARS)	GENDER	TYPICAL/DEFINITE ANGINA PECTORIS	ATYPICAL/PROBABLE ANGINA PECTORIS	NONANGINAL CHEST PAIN	ASYMPTOMATIC
30-39	Men	Intermediate	Intermediate	Low	Very low
	Women	Intermediate	Very low	Very low	Very low
40-49	Men	High	Intermediate	Intermediate	Low
	Women	Intermediate	Low	Very low	Very low
50-59	Men	High	Intermediate	Intermediate	Low
	Women	Intermediate	Intermediate	Low	Very low
60-69	Men	High	Intermediate	Intermediate	Low
	Women	High	Intermediate	Intermediate	Low

*No data exist for patients younger than age 30 or older than age 69, but it can be assumed that coronary artery disease prevalence increases with age. In a few cases, patients with ages at the extremes of the decades listed may have probabilities slightly outside the high or low range. High indicates greater than 90%; low, less than 10%; and very low, less than 5%.
From Gibbons RJ, Balady GJ, Bricker J et al: ACC/AHA 2002 guideline update for exercise testing: summary article—a report of the American College of Cardiology/ American Heart Association Task Force on Practice Guidelines (Committee to Update the 1997 Exercise Testing Guidelines), *J Am Coll Cardiol* 40:1531-1540, 2002.

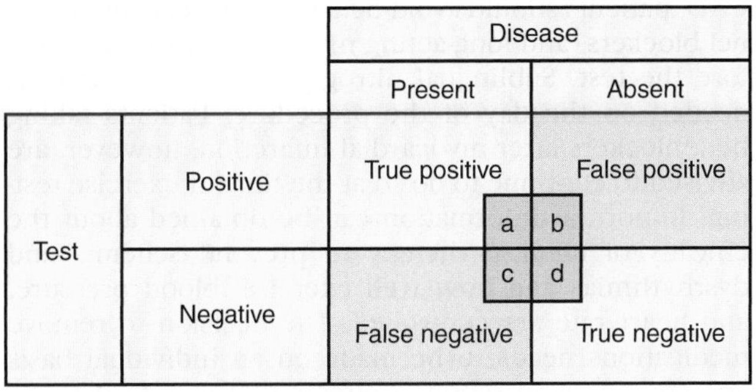

FIGURE 29-1 ▨ The relationship between a diagnostic test result and the occurrence of disease.

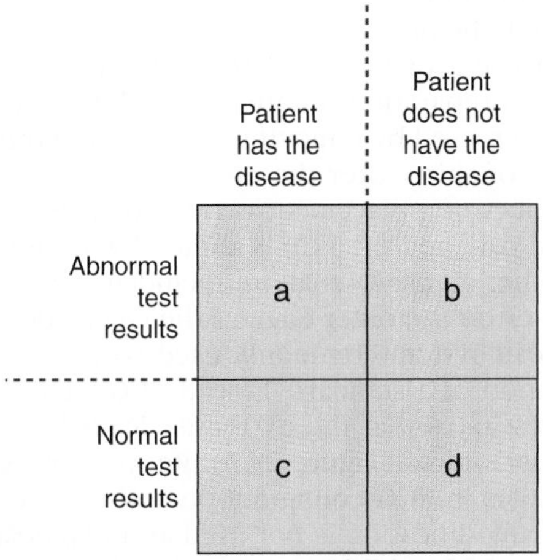

FIGURE 29-2 ▨ Value of a diagnostic test:
• *Negative predictive value* = d/c + d (probability that those with a negative test result do not have the disease)
• *Positive predictive value* = a/a + b (probability that those with positive test results have the disease)
• *Sensitivity* = a/a + c (proportion of those with disease who will yield positive test results)
• *Specificity* = d/b + d (proportion of those without disease who will yield negative test results)

recovery, also can provide valuable information regarding mortality risk.[3]

Exercise testing in men without prior myocardial infarction demonstrates a mean overall sensitivity for the detection of CAD of 76 percent and specificity of 72 percent, whereas women have a higher rate of false-positive results with a reported sensitivity and specificity of 61 and 70 percent, respectively. Although there is no universally accepted explanation, the lower sensitivity noted in women may be related to lower ECG voltage, inadequate exercise duration, a lower prevalence of multivessel CAD, a digitalis-like effect of hormone replacement therapy, or a higher incidence of mitral valve prolapse in women with associated repolarization changes.[4,5] Women, who have a negative exercise test at a maximally predicted heart rate, have a high specificity for the absence of significant CAD in all age groups, whereas women with significant ST segment depression should be considered high risk until proved otherwise.[1]

Exercise testing is generally a safe procedure. Myocardial infarction and death have been reported to occur in less than 1 per 10,000 tests.[1] Guidelines from the American College of Sports Medicine (**ACSM**), the American Heart Association (**AHA**), the American College of Cardiology (**ACC**), and the American Association of Cardiovascular and Pulmonary Rehabilitation (AACVPR) standardize the test to improve its safety. Formalized education and training, such as certification from the ACSM, is strongly advised for nurses, physicians, technologists, nurse practitioners, physician assistants, and exercise physiologists who supervise exercise testing.[2]

Although the AHA/ACC guidelines state that exercise testing should be supervised by an appropriately trained physician, investigators have demonstrated the safety of having trained nurses, exercise physiologists, and technicians perform exercise stress tests.[6] Nurses are excellent candidates to supervise exercise testing and have distinct advantages over other health professionals. Nurses, particularly those with advanced education such as nurse practitioners or clinical nurse specialists, are knowledgeable about patient assessment, patient education, pharmacological intervention, and emergency care, including the ability to initiate and administer emergency medications and perform advanced life support measures. Additionally, advanced practice nurses who supervise exercise stress testing are able to bill for their services. Advanced practice nurses who bill Medicare for the technical component of the test must adhere to federal law, which requires nurse practitioners and clinical nurse specialists to be nationally certified and have a collaborative relationship with a physician.

The ACC/AHA/American College of Physicians–American Society of Internal Medicine Task Force on Clinical Competence states that individuals who perform exercise testing must be aware of "the indications for and contraindications to the test, recognize normal endpoints and abnormal responses or complications that may require that the test be discontinued, manage complications of the test, and interpret the test results"[7] (p. 3). Competencies are outlined and include a recommendation that an individual participate in at least 50 stress tests during training and continue to perform at least 25 procedures per year. Personnel should be trained in advanced cardiac life support, and resuscitative equipment including a portable defibrillator should be readily available.

Awareness of contraindications to testing is imperative (Box 29-1). Patients with unstable angina, uncompensated or severe heart failure, severe symptomatic aortic stenosis or a recent myocardial infarction are at a high-risk for complications during the test. Therefore, exercise testing should be avoided in these patients. Patients with acute illnesses may not be able to complete the procedure; thus there is little benefit in attempting exercise testing in such patients. Severe elevated resting blood pressure poses an unnecessary risk to the patient and also may be associated with false-positive results. Patients should return for testing when their blood pressure is controlled.

Patient Preparation

To identify contraindications and to determine the objective of the test, the patient must undergo a complete history and physical examination with attention to any recent history of medical conditions or current symptoms that might preclude performing the test. Information about signs or symptoms the patient normally experiences during activity should be obtained. For instance, if a patient states that he notices palpitations with strenuous exertion, the operator would want to simulate the activity by exercising the patient to a perception of his symptom. In addition, the practitioner should review the patient's current list of medications and verify medications that were withheld before the test.

Before the test, patients are instructed to consume only light meals, preferably limited to liquids, and to avoid stimulants, caffeinated beverages, and smoking for 3 hours before testing. If the test is in the morning, instruct the patient to avoid breakfast. Also, advise against creams or body lotions. Instruct the patient to bring or wear comfortable walking clothes and shoes. If the purpose of the test is to determine the presence of CAD, patients should avoid beta blockers, calcium channel blockers, and long-acting nitrates for 1 to 2 days before the test. Sublingual nitroglycerin can be used as needed on the day of the procedure. Patients taking beta blockers after myocardial infarction, however, are advised to continue to do so at the time of exercise testing. Important information can be obtained about the efficacy of medical therapy to prevent ischemia and dysrhythmias and how well exercise, blood pressure, and heart rate are controlled. The decision to remove medications needs to be made on an individual basis and should avoid rebound effects that may lead to accelerated angina and hypertension.[8] The procedure should be explained in detail, and written consent that includes the purpose, risks, and benefits of the procedure should be obtained.

To ensure a quality ECG throughout the test, thorough skin preparation is imperative. The signal-to-noise ratio is decreased by removing skin oils and the superficial layer of skin. After the chest hair is removed, the area of electrode placement is rubbed with an alcohol-saturated pad, and the skin is abraded with fine sandpaper or other abrasives that are included in the preparation kits or on the outer edge of the electrode.

The lead system commonly used is the Mason-Likar modification of a standard 12-lead ECG.[1] This lead system necessitates that the extremity leads be moved to the patient's torso (Figure 29-3). Because of axis shifts and changes in ECG configuration and voltage, the Mason-Likar modification is not used as a diagnostic ECG. Although a 12-Lead ECG can be printed during the test, three leads commonly are monitored: II, V_1, and V_5. The majority (90 percent) of ST segment depression can be detected by the lateral precordial leads (V_4 to V_6). Cables are attached to the electrodes; cables should allow for ample length between the patient and the ECG machine. Many laboratories have customized belts that secure the common connector of the cable wires in place. This belt stabilizes the connector and portion of the electrode wiring and helps to minimize motion artifact.

Patients unfamiliar with treadmill testing should be given a demonstration of how to walk properly on the treadmill. The test is initiated by having the patient

---

BOX 29-1   ■ ■ ■
CONTRAINDICATIONS TO EXERCISE TESTING

Absolute
- Acute myocardial infarction (within 2 days)
- High-risk unstable angina
- Uncontrolled cardiac dysrhythmias causing symptoms or hemodynamic compromise
- Symptomatic severe aortic stenosis
- Uncontrolled symptomatic heart failure
- Acute pulmonary embolus or pulmonary infarction
- Acute myocarditis or pericarditis
- Acute aortic dissection

Relative*
- Left main coronary stenosis
- Moderate stenotic valvular heart disease
- Electrolyte abnormalities
- Severe arterial hypertension (systolic blood pressure of greater than 200 mm Hg and/or diastolic blood pressure of greater than 110 mm Hg)
- Tachydysrhythmias or bradydysrhythmias
- Hypertrophic cardiomyopathy and other forms of outflow tract obstruction
- Mental or physical impairment leading to inability to exercise adequately
- High-degree atrioventricular block

*Relative contraindications can be superseded if the benefits of exercise outweigh the risks.

straddle the belt and allow them to "pedal" the belt with one foot before stepping on the treadmill. Because many patients have difficulty understanding what to do, bathtub appliqués of small feet can be placed on either side of the treadmill belt close to the front end. Patients put their foot on each foot appliqué and then test the belt speed with one foot. After patients become comfortable, they are asked to begin to take long strides. Patients are encouraged to hold lightly onto the bar in front or rails on the side of the treadmill. Many persons have a tendency to grip the bar tightly. This increases ECG artifact and also decreases myocardial oxygen consumption. Patients should stand upright and look straight ahead (Figure 29-4). Encouragement is given throughout the test, and patients are made aware of their progress. Information is given before any change in grade or

intensity of the exercise equipment. Complaints of claudication may indicate peripheral vascular disease, a finding often noted in combination with CAD. Patients must be assessed continuously for symptoms and perception of effort and are encouraged to report any uncomfortable feelings experienced during and after exercise. Dyspnea and chest discomfort, two commonly reported symptoms, usually are assessed on a four-point scale (Table 29-2). Exercise-induced ST segment depression accompanied with chest discomfort significantly increases the likelihood of significant CAD.

It is helpful for the practitioner to talk to the patient during the test. Often this helps decrease patient anxiety and gives patients a sense that they have some control over the situation. Patients are encouraged to continue exercising until they perceive that they can no

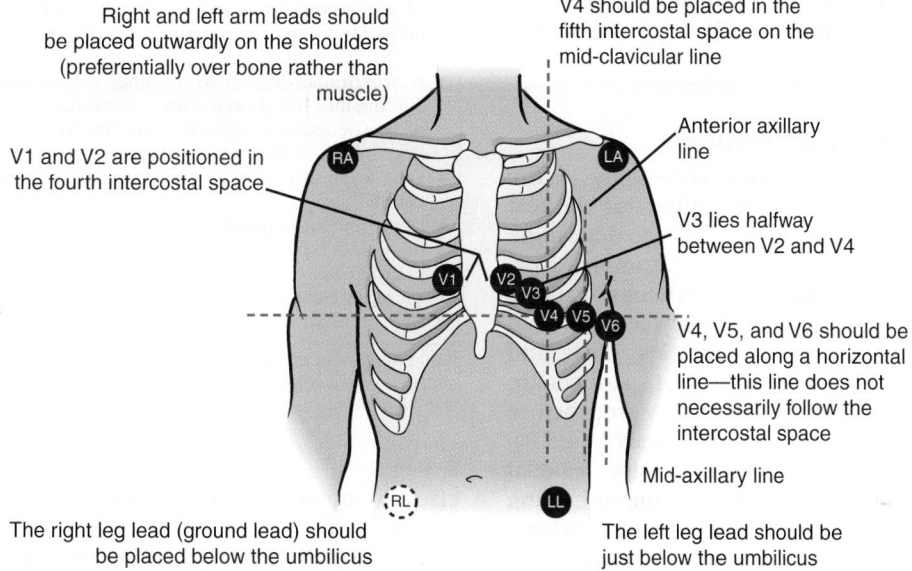

FIGURE 29-3 ■ Mason-Likar simulated 12-lead electrocardiogram electrode placement. *LA,* Left arm; *LL,* left leg; *RA,* right arm; *RL,* right leg. (From Fletcher GF, Balady GJ, Amsterdam EA: *Circulation* 104:1694-1740, 2001.)

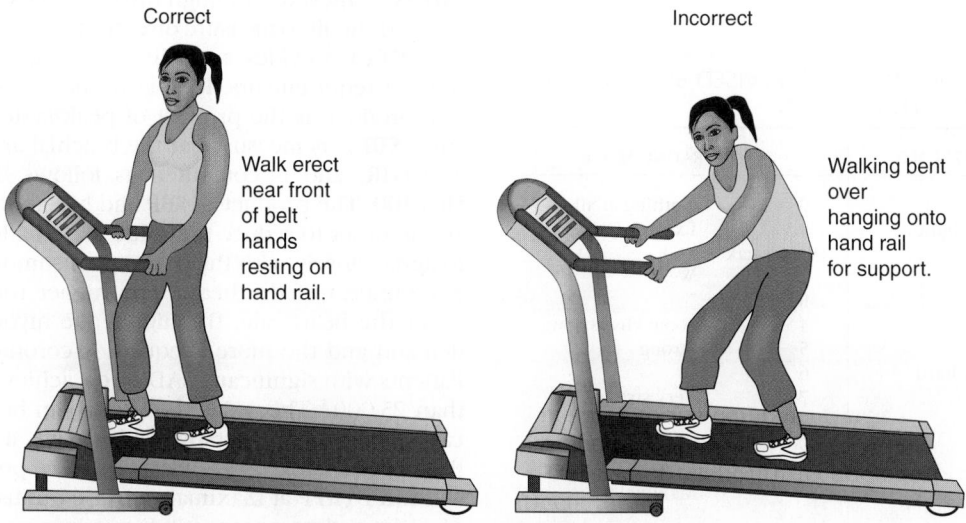

FIGURE 29-4 ■ Correct and incorrect posture for treadmill walking. (From Ellestad M: *Stress testing: principles and practice,* ed 5, New York, 2003, Oxford University Press.)

■ ■ ■

TABLE 29-2   ANGINA AND DYSPNEA SCALES

MEASURE	ANGINA SCALE	DYSPNEA SCALE
1+	Onset of discomfort	Mild; noticeable to patient but not observer
2+	Moderate, bothersome	Mild; some difficulty, noticeable to observer
3+	Moderately severe	Moderate difficulty, but can continue
4+	Severe; most pain ever experienced	Severe difficulty; patient cannot continue

longer continue. Commonly used criteria to terminate the exercise test is attainment of a predetermined endpoint such as 85 percent of age-predicted heart rate or perceived exertion of greater than "hard" on the Borg scale (Table 29-3). However, there are numerous other reasons for termination of the test. These are detailed in Box 29-2.

Exercise Modalities and Protocols

Although treadmill testing is used commonly in the United States, consideration of indications for the test along with patient capabilities is necessary to determine the appropriate mode of exercise. For example, a patient with an arthritic hip may have difficulty walking but may be able to perform on the bicycle. Although this mode of exercise is less expensive, less noisy, and produces less upper body motion artifact, patients are often unfamiliar with the bicycle and may stop before they reach a predetermined maximal heart rate. Patients who have suffered a stroke and have residual weakness that precludes them from walking or cycling may need pharmacological testing. For patients whose occupational activity is mainly upper extremity work, evaluation for job performance would be most appropriate with arm ergometry. Regardless of the mode of exer-

■ ■ ■

TABLE 29-3   ORIGINAL AND REVISED BORG RATING SCALES OF PERCEIVED EXERTION

ORIGINAL RATING SCALE		NEW RATING SCALE	
6		0	Nothing at all
7	Extremely light	0.5	Extremely weak
8	1		Very weak
9	Very light	2	Weak
10	3		Moderate
11	Fairly light	4	Somewhat strong
12		5	Strong
13	Somewhat hard	6	
14		7	Very strong
15	Hard	8	
16		9	
17	Very hard	10	Extremely strong
18	Extremely hard		Maximal
19			
20			

■ ■ ■

BOX 29-2
INDICATIONS FOR TERMINATING EXERCISE TESTING

Absolute Indications
- Drop in systolic blood pressure of greater than 10 mm Hg from baseline blood pressure despite an increase in workload, when accompanied by other evidence of ischemia
- Moderate to severe angina
- Increasing nervous system symptoms (e.g., ataxia, dizziness, or near syncope)
- Signs of poor perfusion (cyanosis or pallor)
- Technical difficulties in monitoring electrocardiogram or systolic blood pressure
- Subject's desire to stop
- Sustained ventricular tachycardia
- ST elevation (1.0 mm or more) in leads without diagnostic Q waves (other than V_1 or aVR)

Relative Indications
- Drop in systolic blood pressure of (10 mm Hg or more from baseline blood pressure despite an increase in workload, in the absence of other evidence of ischemia)
- ST segment or QRS complex changes such as excessive ST segment depression (more than 2 mm of horizontal or downsloping ST segment depression) or marked axis shift
- Dysrhythmias other than sustained ventricular tachycardia, including multifocal premature ventricular contractions, triplets of ventricular ectopic beats, supraventricular tachycardia, heart block, or bradydysrhythmias
- Fatigue, shortness of breath, wheezing, leg cramps, or claudication
- Development of bundle branch block or intraventricular conduction delay that cannot be distinguished from ventricular tachycardia
- Increasing chest pain
- Hypertensive response*

*In the absence of definitive evidence, the committee suggests systolic blood pressure of greater than 250 mm Hg and/or a diastolic blood pressure greater than 115 mm Hg.

cise, the main objective is to increase myocardial oxygen demand.

The overall hemodynamic response to exercise depends on the amount of muscle mass involved, exercise efficiency, conditioning, and exercise intensity. Maximal exercise capacity may be expressed in terms of myocardial oxygen consumption or in metabolic equivalents (**METs**) achieved. Although myocardial oxygen consumption is difficult to measure directly, the rate-pressure product (**RPP**) provides an indirect measure of myocardial oxygen requirements. RPP, also known as the pressure-rate product, is the product of peak systolic blood pressure (**SBP**), as measured at the brachial artery, and heart rate (HR) and is computed as follows: RPP = (SBP × HR)/100. The product of SBP and heart rate is divided by 100 in order to reduce the value to a smaller number and to agree closely with the oxygen consumption (milliliters per minute) of the heart. The higher the SBP and the faster the heart rate, the higher the myocardial oxygen demand and the more adequate is coronary blood flow. Patients with significant CAD rarely achieve a RPP greater than 25,000.[1] This value, however, can be influenced by cardioactive drug therapy. Additionally, a low RPP (less than or equal to 217,000) has a negative prognostic value, and dRPP (RPP at maximal exercise minus RPP at rest) is an independent prognostic factor in post–myocardial infarction patients.[9]

A MET is the amount of oxygen consumed while sitting at rest and is equal to 3.5 ml oxygen per kilogram of body mass times minutes. Exercise duration, or functional capacity, expressed in METs, provides a simple and practical method to express the estimated energy cost of physical activities as a multiple of the resting metabolic rate. For example, a 3-MET activity requires 3 times the metabolic energy expenditure of sitting quietly. METs can be estimated from treadmill speed and grade (Figure 29-5). For instance, completing stage I on the Bruce protocol (1.7 mph at a 10 percent grade) is roughly equivalent to 4 to 5 METs. Charts that detail general physical activities as defined by METs are widely available from many organizations, such as ACSM.

Maximal oxygen consumption is influenced by age, sex, exercise habits, heredity, and cardiovascular status. Exercise duration correlates poorly with left ventricular function. Exercise duration expressed as METs, however, is a strong predictor of mortality in males and females across all age groups and in the presence or absence of CAD. An exercise capacity of 5 METs or less is associated with a poor prognosis post–myocardial infarction, whereas achievement of 10 METs or higher is associated with excellent survival rates irrespective of findings on imaging studies or extent of CAD on angiography.[10] In individuals without established CAD, achievement of less than 6 METs is an independent predictor of all-cause mortality, whereas a 1-MET increase in exercise capacity is associated with an 11 percent reduction in annual mortality.[11]

The Duke Treadmill Score (DTS) allows for further risk assessment and risk prediction in symptomatic patients and is included in the recommended screening algorithms in the ACC/AHA guidelines for exercise testing.[2] The DTS is a score based on the combination of exercise time, ST segment deviation, and the presence of angina during treadmill testing. The DTS effectively can stratify men and women into diagnostic and prognostic risk categories. The DTS, however, is less predictive in patients age 75 or older.[12] The DTS is calculated using the following formula:

$$DTS = \text{Exercise time} \frac{-5 \times \text{ST segment deviation}}{-4 \times \text{treadmill angina}}$$

Exercise time is minutes on the treadmill, ST segment deviation is the largest net deviation of depression or elevation in any lead except aVR, and treadmill angina is graded using the following scale:

- 0 = no angina during exercise
- 1 = nonlimiting angina during exercise
- 2 = exercise-limiting angina

A DTS score ranges from −25, which indicates the highest risk for CAD, to +15, the lowest risk for CAD.

Although there are a variety of treadmill protocols, the most widely used is the Bruce protocol. The treadmill speed starts at 1.7 mph with a 10-degree slope and increases every 3 minutes until a predetermined endpoint is achieved.[1] This protocol is appropriate for active and younger patients but can rapidly tire older, deconditioned, or ill patients. Patients can be started on a modified Bruce protocol that starts with 0-degree slope and then progresses to 5 degrees in 3 minutes. When testing physically fit individuals, often an accelerated Bruce protocol with 2-minute stages can be used to

NYHA Functional class	Clinical status		O₂ cost mL/kg/min	METs	Bicycle ergometer	Treadmill protocols					METs
						Bruce modified 3 min Stages		Bruce 3 min Stages		Naughton	
						MPH	%GR	MPH	%GR		
					1 WATT = 6.1 Kpm/min	6.0	22	6.0	22		
						5.5	20	5.5	20		
					FOR 70 KG body weight Kpm/min	5.0	18	5.0	18		
Normal and I	Healthy, dependent on age, activity		56.0	16							16
			52.5	15							15
			49.0	14							14
			45.5	13	1500	4.2	16	4.2	16		13
			42.0	12	1350						12
			38.5	11	1200					2 min Stages MPH %GR	11
			35.0	10	1050	3.4	14	3.4	14		10
		Sedentary healthy	31.5	9	900						9
			28.0	8	750					2	17.5	8
			24.5	7		2.5	12	2.5	12	2	14.0	7
II			21.0	6	600						6
		Symptomatic	17.5	5	450					2	10.5	5
III		Limited	14.0	4	300	1.7	10	1.7	10	2	7.0	4
			10.5	3	150	1.7	5			2	3.5	3
			7.0	2		1.7	0			2	0	2
IV			3.5	1						1	0	1

FIGURE 29-5 ■ Estimating metabolic equivalents from treadmill speed and grade. *%GR*, Percent grade; *kpm*, kilopond meters; *mph*, miles per hour; *NYHA*, New York Heart Association. (From Fletcher GF, Balady GJ, Amsterdam EA: *Circulation* 104:1694-1740, 2001.)

achieve a maximal workload. The Balke protocol uses a constant treadmill speed at 2 to 3 mph with modest increments in the grade. A modified Naughton protocol, with 2-minute stages at 1 to 2 mph and gradual increases in grade, frequently is used with chronic heart failure patients who have limited exercise capacity.

Ramp protocols, designed to overcome the limitations of multistage exercise tests, use a gradual and uniform increase in the speed and grade of the treadmill. They are designed to replace the "staging" of other treadmill protocols and allow for a steady increase in cardiopulmonary and hemodynamic responses, and they offer better estimation of functional capacity.[2] These protocols also are used with bicycle and arm ergometry.

Bicycle test protocols can be intermittent or continuous with a mechanically or electrically braked cycle. Workloads are calibrated in watts or kilogram meters. Supine or upright tests are done. Ischemia is more likely to result with supine bicycling than upright pedaling. With arm ergometry, patients perform arm cranking while seated with their feet flat on the floor. Because most patients are unaccustomed to arm ergometry and a smaller muscle mass is used, fatigue is a common problem. An artifact-free ECG is difficult to obtain, therefore, ECGs often are obtained during brief pauses between stages. Blood pressure is measured by having the individual continue to crank with one arm and hold the other arm still or are taken while the ECG is done during a brief rest period. Both methods are problematic.

Exercise protocols are submaximal or symptom-limited. Symptom-limited tests are terminated when the patient develops signs or symptoms that necessitate discontinuing the test, whereas submaximal protocols have a predetermined endpoint, such as a heart rate of 120 beats/min, or 70 percent of the predicted maximum heart rate, or a peak MET level of 5. Although submaximal protocols frequently are used in the post-myocardial infarction setting, symptom-limited testing appears safe and may yield a greater incidence of ischemia.[2] ACC/AHA guidelines recommend submaximal testing as early as day 3, and symptom-limited testing at day 5 after myocardial infarction.[13]

Interpretation of Findings

Based on the presence or absence of ST segment changes, an exercise stress test traditionally is interpreted as positive or negative for ischemia. Most cases of ischemia can be detected in the lateral precordial leads (V_4, V_5, and V_6), whereas ST segment depression in the inferior leads (II, III, and aVF) has a high false-positive rate.[1,2] ST segment changes are measured relative to the P-Q junction (Figure 29-6), ideally in three consecutive beats.[2] A test is considered positive for ischemia if there is horizontal or downsloping ST segment depression of greater than or equal to 0.10 mV (1 mm) 80 msec from the J point.[1,2] Using less stringent criteria increases the number of false-positive tests and decreases the number of false-negative tests. Previously, an exercise treadmill test was considered positive at 2 mm of ST segment depression 80 msec from the J point. However, this criterion was noted to be too stringent. Upsloping ST segments are

considered abnormal if the segment is 1.5 mm below the baseline of the P-Q junction 80 msec after the J point.[1]

ST segment depression noted early during low workloads, and those that remain late into recovery, usually are associated with significant CAD.[1] Late-onset ST segment depression that is noted at high workloads and quickly resolves after exercise was thought to constitute a false-positive test. Not all patients, however, with rapid resolution of ST segment depression have normal coronary arteries. ST segment depression noted only during the recovery phase and ST segment depression appearing during exercise yield similar diagnostic and prognostic information. In patients with non–Q wave myocardial infarction and suspected myocardial ischemia, exercise-induced normalization of previously negative T waves is associated with a higher prevalence of ischemia compared with patients with persistent T wave inversion during exercise.

ST segment elevation in leads without a Q wave can occur in patients with a very high-grade proximal left anterior descending artery stenosis or a high-grade stenosis of a large right coronary artery.[1] Less commonly, ST segment elevation in leads without a Q wave can be due to coronary artery spasm, or Prinzmetal angina, and may be accompanied by dysrhythmias. ST segment elevation in leads V_2 to V_4 usually signifies involvement of the left anterior descending coronary artery. Elevation in the lateral leads signifies involvement in the left circumflex and diagonal coronary arteries. Elevation in the inferior leads (II, III, aVF) indicates involvement of the right coronary artery. Exercise-induced ST segment elevation in leads V_1 and aVR with ST segment depression in lead V_5 may signify significant left anterior descending coronary artery stenosis or significant left anterior descending coronary artery stenosis and stenosis in the left circumflex artery. Exercise-induced ST segment elevation in lead aVr and ST segment depression in lead V_5 without elevation in lead V_1 may be associated with significant left anterior descending coronary artery and right coronary artery stenoses.[14]

False-Positive and False-Negative Tests

A variety of causes exist for false-positive and false-negative tests (Box 29-3). A common cause for false-negative results is failure to achieve a predetermined heart rate. Although this may be due to medication effect from beta blockers or certain calcium channel blockers, it may be that the person is unable to complete the test because of other conditions that limit exercise capacity, such as severe arthritis or emphysema. Prior knowledge of such limitations will avoid prescribing inappropriate testing. Also, patients with ECGs uninterpretable because of preexcitation, digitalis effect, electronically paced rhythm, left bundle branch block, or other situations that would cause a false-positive or false-negative test may require imaging studies.

Blood Pressure and Heart Rate Responses

In addition to ECG information, the exercise test provides other valuable information essential to the interpretation of the test. With increasing workloads, SBP

ABNORMAL

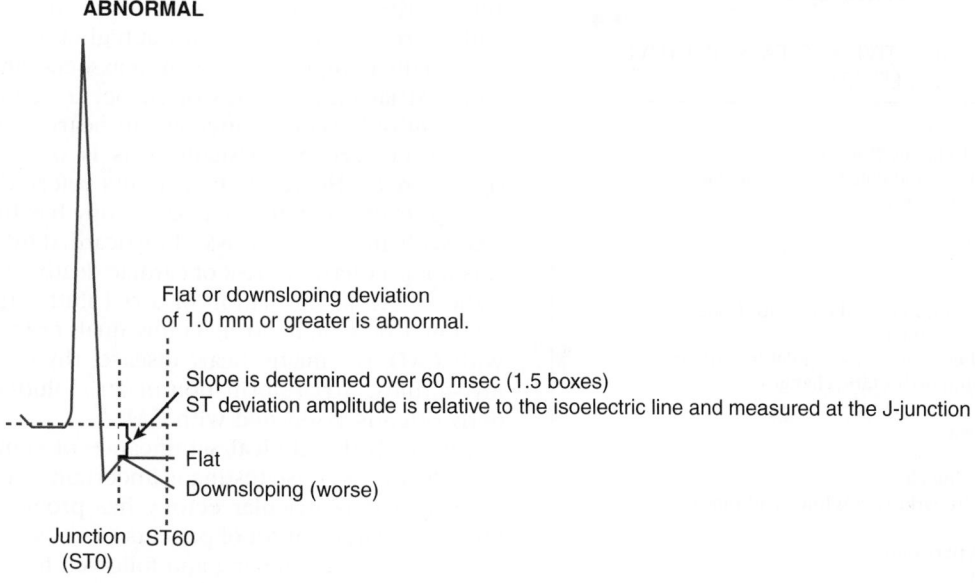

BORDERLINE

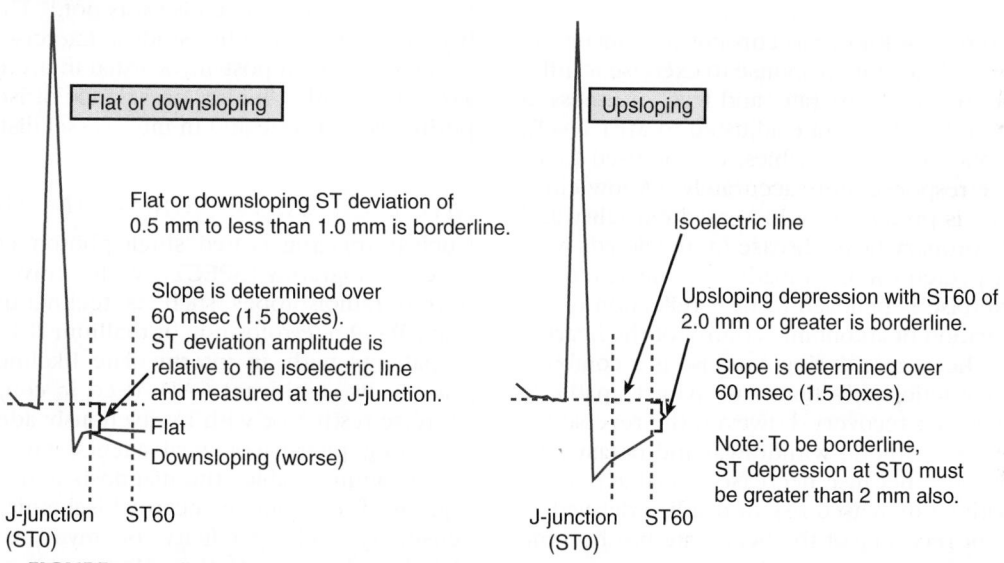

FIGURE 29-6 ▪ Measuring ST segment changes relative to the P-Q junction. (From Fletcher GF, Balady GJ, Amsterdam EA: *Circulation* 104:1694-1740, 2001.)

gradually elevates with little change in diastolic blood pressure and returns to normal during recovery.[1] An exaggerated or hypertensive response occurs when SBP is greater than 200 mm Hg at peak exercise and/or diastolic blood pressure is greater than 100 mm Hg. Exercise-induced hypertension in the setting of a normal resting blood pressure is associated with the future development of clinically significant hypertension in men and women but has not been shown to be an independent predictor of mortality.[15]

Conversely, exercise-induced hypotension, or an inadequate rise in SBP (less than 20 to 30 mm Hg), in association with evidence of ECG ischemia is associated with a poor prognosis and commonly is associated with left main or triple-vessel disease.[1,2] Exercise-induced hypotension also may result from aortic outflow obstruction, severe left ventricular dysfunction, myocar-

dial ischemia, and medications such as antihypertensives and peripheral vasodilators. Caution should be exercised when determining the presence of exercise-induced hypotension. Many individuals at the beginning of exercise are anxious and may have a sudden rise in blood pressure for the first 1 or 2 minutes. As they become more accustomed to the test, their blood pressure will stabilize, and this phenomenon should not be interpreted as hypotension. During immediate recovery, because of blood volume changes, there is a lowering of blood pressure. This might be interpreted incorrectly as a hypotensive response. A substantial decrease in blood pressure frequently is accompanied by light-headedness, dizziness, skin pallor, cool skin, and reduced vitality.[1]

During progressive exercise, there is a linear increase in heart rate. Failure of the heart rate to accelerate nor-

> **BOX 29-3** ■ ■ ■
> CAUSES OF FALSE-NEGATIVE AND FALSE-POSITIVE
> EXERCISE STRESS TEST RESULTS
>
> **False-Negative**
> - Failure to achieve ischemic threshold
> - Single vessel disease; good collateral circulation
> - Technical or observer error
>
> **False-Positive**
> - Digitalis
> - Hypokalemia
> - ST segment depression in only the inferior leads
> - Improper computer averaging
> - Increased sympathetic tone (vasoregulatory asthenia)
> - Hyperventilation and orthostatic changes
> - Short PR interval
> - Mitral valve prolapse
> - Female sex
> - Left bundle branch block
> - Preexcitation (Wolff-Parkinson-White syndrome)
> - Anemia
> - Left ventricular hypertrophy
> - Pericardial disease

mally with exercise is known as chronotropic incompetence.[1,2] Because heart rate response to exercise is influenced by age, resting heart rate, and level of fitness, a chronotropic index (heart rate adjusted to MET level), which accounts for these variables, can be used to assess heart rate response more accurately.[16] A low chronotropic index is predictive of increased mortality and incidence of coronary heart disease in individuals with known or suspected CAD. An inadequate heart rate response to exercise is believed to be a reflection of abnormal modulation of autonomic control of the heart.[1]

The rise in heart rate during exercise is a combination of sympathetic activation and parasympathetic withdrawal. During recovery, however, the reverse occurs: there is sympathetic withdrawal and parasympathetic reactivation. Because decreased vagal activity is associated with an increased risk of death, a delayed or reduced rate of recovery of the heart rate has become an important prognostic marker. Reduced heart rate recovery is defined as a decrease of fewer than or equal to 12 beats/min from peak exercise to heart rate within the 2 minutes. Reduced heart rate recovery is a predictor of overall mortality, independent of workload in individuals with or without significant CAD, and in patients with heterozygous familial hypercholesterolemia.[17] Patients who have a poor exercise capacity (less than 5 METs) and an abnormal heart rate recovery response have a particularly poor prognosis.

Dysrhythmias

In addition to ECG, blood pressure, and heart rate changes, alterations in cardiac rhythm frequently occur with exercise. Information about the type of dysrhythmia, frequency, whether the dysrhythmia is sustained or nonsustained, whether it occurs at low or high level workloads or subsides with an increase in heart rate are important in understanding an individual's symptoms and providing predictive information about mortality

and morbidity. Dysrhythmias occur more frequently with increasing age, especially at higher workloads, and are usually benign unless seen in association with ischemia. Atrial extrasystoles often occur at lower workloads, subside with an increase in heart rate and reappear after recovery. Usually, this is of little clinical significance.[1] However, in patients referred for stress testing, exercise-induced atrial ectopy has been associated with an increased risk of myocardial infarction but was not predictive of risk of cardiac death or revascularization.[18] Atrial fibrillation or atrial flutter that is transient may be seen in normal individuals or in association with CAD, rheumatic heart disease, thyrotoxicosis, or myocarditis. Atrial fibrillation or atrial flutter in the elderly often is associated with CAD.[1]

Although the clinical significance of ventricular ectopy during exercise testing is uncertain, recent studies suggest that ventricular ectopy has prognostic importance. In a large cohort of patients ($n = 29,244$) referred for exercise stress testing and followed for 5 years, frequent ventricular ectopy during recovery was a strong predictor of death from all causes, whereas ventricular ectopy only during exercise was not.[19] This finding has been confirmed in other studies. Exercise-induced ventricular ectopy in post–myocardial infarction patients is associated with a higher prevalence of ischemia in the periinfarction zone and in multivessel distribution.[20]

MYOCARDIAL PERFUSION IMAGING

Nuclear imaging (gated single-photon emission computed tomography [**SPECT**]) with intravenously administered radioisotopes such as technetium-99m sestamibi, Tc-99m tetrofosmin, or thallium-201 is most useful in patients with an intermediate likelihood of angiographically significant CAD. Used in conjunction with exercise testing or with intravenously administered vasodilating pharmacological agents, myocardial perfusion imaging enables the diagnosis and localization of regions of reversible myocardial ischemia or infarction. Sensitivity and specificity of myocardial perfusion SPECT to detect more than 50 percent coronary artery stenosis in males and females is significantly higher than exercise ECG, with reported values averaging 87 and 73 percent, respectively. Pharmacological tests have an average sensitivity of 89 percent and specificity of 75 percent.[21]

Regardless of the radioisotope used, the principle of perfusion imaging is the same. A small amount of a radioisotope is injected intravenously and is absorbed by the myocardium. A scintillation camera (gamma camera) detects the radiation (gamma rays) emitted by the isotope. A computer then collects and processes the data. Gated SPECT myocardial perfusion imaging combines ECG and image data that depict the myocardium in motion in multiple planes and gives additional information about left ventricular ejection fraction, regional wall motion, and wall thickness assessment. The use of gated SPECT enhances the detection of CAD and provides additional prognostic information.

The amount of the radiopharmaceutical given to a patient is just sufficient to obtain the required information before its decay, thus the radiation dose received is medically insignificant. Although infrequent, reported adverse events include headache, chest pain/angina, ST segment changes, nausea, and abnormal taste and smell. Acute severe allergic events of angioedema and urticaria are rare. Pregnant women should not have a nuclear test because the potential effects on the unborn fetus have not been determined conclusively. Additionally, these radioisotopes can be excreted in human milk. Therefore, formula should be substituted for breast milk until the isotopes have cleared from the body of the nursing woman.

Thallium-201 myocardial perfusion imaging has been available for more than 20 years, and therefore there are substantial data regarding its diagnostic and prognostic value in CAD. Thallium is a potassium analog that is taken up by viable myocardial cells via active transport (sodium/potassium pump) and has a half-life of 73 hours. Thallium is injected at peak exercise, and stress images are obtained within 5 to 10 minutes. Because thallium-201 redistributes over time, delayed images are obtained 3 to 4 hours later and reflect the "resting" state of myocardial perfusion. The image quality obtained with thallium-201 is less optimal than the quality obtained with Tc-99m agents, and Tc-99m is recommended for the evaluation of women.[22] Thallium-201 testing is less likely to provide diagnostic-quality images in large or morbidly obese patients. Patients who undergo thallium-201 testing must remain fasting before the test and until the test is completed. As a consequence, this 1-day test may not be optimal for a diabetic person. If 1-day testing is necessary, diabetic patients should avoid taking antiglycemic medicines the day of the test.

Technetium-99m sestamibi and Tc-99m tetrofosmin are lipophilic monovalent cations (isonitrile compounds). Both agents act by entering the cell via passive diffusion across plasma and mitochondrial membranes. Advantages of the technetium agents over thallium-201 are a shorter half-life (approximately 6 hours) and higher count rates with improved image resolution. Because there is clinically insignificant redistribution with these agents, separate stress and rest injections are required. A 2-day protocol is best in which an exercise image is obtained 1 day, followed the next day by a resting image. If the exercise stress study is normal, the rest study is not necessary.

Because a 2-day study is often impractical, single-day protocols have become common. The first study is performed with low doses of the isotope, and the second study is performed with a dose approximately 3 times the initial dose. To allow for decay of the first injection, the second set of images usually is obtained 3 to 4 hours after the initial set of scans. Exercise images can be obtained within 15 minutes after the Tc-99m tetrofosmin injection and 30 to 90 minutes after the Tc-99m sestamibi. Thus, study time is approximately 30 minutes shorter with Tc-99m tetrofosmin. A 2-day protocol may be preferable for a diabetic patient. Also, these agents are more suited for obese individuals or those with thick chest walls. In the dual-isotope protocol, a resting injection of thallium-201 is given, followed by imaging within 15 minutes. The patient then is stressed, and an injection of Tc-99m sestamibi or Tc-99m tetrofosmin is

given at peak exercise. Gated SPECT scanning is done 15 to 45 minutes after the injection. The entire test can be completed in 90 minutes and thus has a major advantage over single agent use. This protocol, however, is less likely to provide diagnostic-quality images in large or morbidly obese patients, who also will be limited to planar imaging if their weight exceeds safety limits of the SPECT imaging table (350 lb). A 2-day protocol using Tc-99m sestamibi or Tc-99m tetrofosmin is preferred for morbidly obese individuals.

Pharmaceutical Agents

Patients with functional impairments who cannot walk on a treadmill can undergo pharmacological stress imaging using intravenously administered dipyridamole, adenosine, dobutamine, or arbutamine in combination with the radioisotope.[21] These agents are used in place of treadmill or bicycle exercise and often are used with echocardiographic scanning.

Adenosine

Adenosine is a naturally occurring substance produced in small amounts during normal cellular metabolism. With the exception of renal afferent arterioles and hepatic veins where it produces vasoconstriction, adenosine acts as a potent vasodilator in most vascular beds. Adenosine exerts negative chronotropic, dromotropic, and inotropic effects on the heart. At higher (bolus) doses, adenosine is associated with transient bradycardia and decreased atrioventricular conduction, thus its use in terminating supraventricular tachycardias. After the administration of adenosine, normal coronary vessels dilate with a resultant increase in myocardial blood flow. In stenotic or diseased coronary arteries, vasodilatation is attenuated, thus a relative zone of hypoperfusion develops distal to the stenotic lesion. This leads to a "steal" of blood flow away from myocardium perfused by diseased coronary artery. This regional flow abnormality creates a perfusion defect detected during radionuclide imaging.

Because of its negative chronotropic effect, adenosine is contraindicated in patients with second-degree (Mobitz I and II) or third-degree block without a functioning artificial pacemaker, in sick sinus syndrome, or symptomatic bradycardia. Because of the potential for bronchoconstriction, adenosine should be avoided in bronchoconstrictive or bronchospastic lung disease. Because of the potent vasodilatory effects of adenosine, patients with low SBP (less than 90 mm Hg) should not undergo adenosine stress testing. Dipyridamole and methylxanthines (e.g., caffeine and aminophylline) compete with adenosine at the receptor level and potentially can decrease or attenuate the vasodilatory effects of adenosine. Therefore, patients should refrain from ingesting caffeine in any form at least 24 hours before adenosine administration. This includes caffeine-containing medications such as extra-strength Excedrin, NoDoz Tablets, and Anacin, as well as foods containing chocolate such as cookies, pies, chocolate bars, frosting, cocoa, candies, ice cream, chocolate milk, and chocolate-flavored yogurt. Because many caffeine-free coffees contain small amounts of caffeine, patients should avoid all types of coffee products. Additionally, patients should withhold dipyridamole, theophylline, or theophylline-containing products such as Primatene, Constant-T, Quibron, Slo-Phylline, or Theo-Dur at least 24 hours before the test.

Adenosine is given over 4 to 6 minutes at 140 mcg/kg/min via an infusion pump with the injection of the radioisotope at 3 minutes. Images are taken from 20 to 60 minutes postinjection. Care must be taken to inject the radiopharmaceutical slowly; forceful injection gives a bolus of adenosine that can lead to significant atrioventricular block. ECG monitoring is required throughout the test. Common side effects include headache, flushing, chest pain, and shortness of breath. The half-life of adenosine is approximately 10 seconds, and therefore these side effects quickly resolve when the infusion is discontinued. Early termination of the adenosine infusion is necessitated by severe hypotension, symptomatic Mobitz II second-degree or third-degree block, bronchospasm, severe chest pain associated with greater than 2 mm ST segment depression, or any ST segment elevation in a non–Q wave lead.[21]

ST segment depression with adenosine myocardial perfusion imaging is a marker of angiographically significant CAD in men and women and often is associated with left main and three-vessel CAD. For patients with minimal functional impairments, adenosine can be combined with low-level treadmill exercise (2.0 to 3.5 METs), or bicycle ergometry (25 to 60 W). Combining exercise with adenosine infusion is associated with a decrease in side effects, improved safety, and patient tolerance.[23]

Dipyridamole (Persantine)

Dipyridamole was the first agent approved for pharmacological tests. Dipyridamole causes coronary vasodilatation by inhibiting the cellular uptake of adenosine.[21] Similar to adenosine, dipyridamole causes nondiseased coronary arteries to undergo greater vasodilatation, creating a coronary steal phenomenon. Contraindications and precautions to dipyridamole testing are similar to adenosine. Common side effects of dipyridamole infusion are chest pain, headache, dizziness, nausea, and flushing. Dipyridamole is infused at 0.56 mg/kg over 4 minutes to a maximum total dose of 60 mg. Radioisotope is injected 3 to 4 minutes after completion of the infusion or earlier if the patient has evidence of ischemia by symptoms or profound ECG changes. Intravenously administered aminophylline, up to a maximum of 240 mg, can be administered if the patient has evidence of severe ischemia or intolerable side effects. To maintain maximal coronary vasodilatation and extraction of the radiopharmaceutical, if the patient is clinically stable, every effort should be made to wait at least 1 to 2 minutes after radiopharmaceutical injection before reversing the effects with aminophylline.

Dobutamine

Dobutamine is a synthetic catecholamine that primarily increases myocardial demand by its positive chronotropic and inotropic effects.[24] As a stressor, dobutamine is more comparable to physical exercise. The increase in coronary blood flow with dobutamine is less than that seen with dipyridamole or adenosine stress.[21] When dobutamine is combined with atropine, myocardial blood flow is similar to that seen with dipyridamole in healthy volunteers. Dobutamine generally is used for patients with contraindications to dipyridamole and adenosine. Low-dose dobutamine generally is reserved for echocardiographic studies to assess the inotropic reserve of severely dysfunctional myocardium. Dobutamine is started at 5 mcg/kg/min while observing for a biphasic response in regions with baseline wall motion abnormalities. Beta blockers, because they reduce the inotropic and chronotropic effects of dobutamine and thus the sensitivity of the test, are withheld 48 hours before the test.

Dobutamine is given intravenously with an infusion pump starting at 10 mcg/kg/min and is increased by 10 mcg/kg/min every 3 minutes to a maximum of 40 to 50 mcg/kg/min. Patients who do not achieve their predetermined maximal heart rate are given atropine up to 2 mg to increase the heart rate. Common side effects include nausea, headache, anxiety, palpitations, angina, dysrhythmias, and hypotension. Hypotension is more common in elderly patients. The test is terminated if the patient develops severe chest pain, significant ST segment depression or elevation, significant ventricular or supraventricular dysrhythmias, hypertension, or SBP decrease of more than 40 mm Hg. Side effects can be reversed by giving metoprolol (1 to 5 mg) or esmolol (0.5 mg/kg) intravenously.[25] Contraindications for dobutamine testing are noted in Box 29-4.

Patient Preparation and Safety

It is imperative to ask female patients who are postmenarchal and premenopausal about pregnancy and breast-feeding before giving any radiopharmaceutical. If the patient is uncertain, a pregnancy test should be performed. Additionally, inquire about any testing that required radioisotopes within the last 1 to 2 days. Computed tomography scans, magnetic resonance imaging, upper gastrointestinal series, lung scans, or other tests that use technetium require waiting a full 24 hours before a cardiac Tc-99m sestamibi and Tc-99m tetrofosmin or thallium-201 scan can be done. Studies using

---

BOX 29-4 ■ ■ ■
CONTRAINDICATIONS TO DOBUTAMINE AND ATROPINE TESTING

Contraindications to Dobutamine
- Acute coronary syndrome
- Severe aortic stenosis
- Hypertrophic obstructive cardiomyopathy
- Uncontrolled hypertension
- Uncontrolled atrial fibrillation
- Uncontrolled heart failure
- Known severe ventricular dysrhythmias

Contraindications to Atropine
- Narrow-angle glaucoma
- Myasthenia gravis
- Obstructive uropathy
- Obstructive gastrointestinal disorders

isotopes with a longer half-life (gallium) require a longer delay. Following all regulatory guidelines (Occupational Safety and Health Administration, Nuclear Regulatory Commission, and state) at all times is mandatory.

In addition to standard preparation for an exercise test, an intravenous catheter is inserted in a peripheral vein, capped, and flushed with heparin or saline. A two- or three-way stopcock is advisable. The procedure must be explained in detail, and patients must be informed about common side effects. Often patients hear the word nuclear and become anxious. Reassure patients that the dose they are given is safe and is relatively short-lived and that they will not emit harmful radiation. Radionuclides emit gamma rays and are sensed by Geiger counters used by airport security and to monitor workers in nuclear power plants. Therefore, patients who will be traveling within a few days of undergoing a myocardial perfusion scan or who work in a nuclear power plant are given written information to alert airport security or their employers. As with exercise testing, continuous ECG monitoring is needed along with periodic blood pressure measurements during and after the test. To minimize the radiation dose to the bladder, patients should be encouraged to void when the examination is completed and as often thereafter as possible. Adequate hydration should be encouraged to promote frequent voiding.

Interpretation of the Test

Intravenously injected radiopharmaceuticals normally distribute throughout the myocardium, and uptake of these agents generally indicates viable cellular functioning. Therefore, images taken at rest and exercise should show homogeneous uptake of radioactivity. The location of the defect is noted and described according to standardized myocardial segmentation (Figures 29-7 and 29-8). In general, patients with obstructive CAD

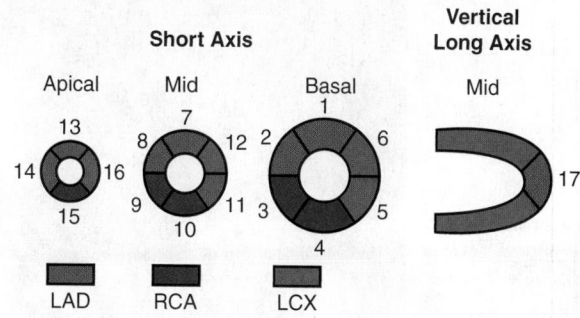

FIGURE 29-7 ■ Assignment of the 17 myocardial segments to the territories of the left anterior descending *(LAD)*, right coronary artery *(RCA)*, and the left circumflex coronary artery *(LCX)*. (From Cerqueira M, Weissman N, Dilsizian V et al: *Circulation* 105:539-542, 2002.)

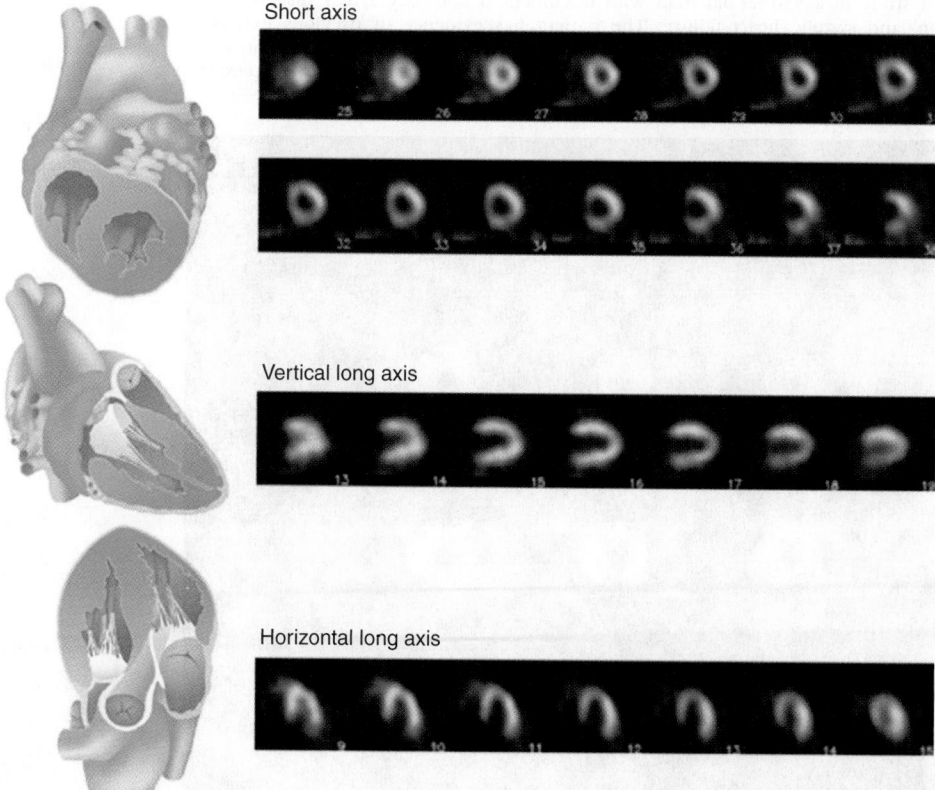

FIGURE 29-8 ■ Normal exercise single-photon emission computed tomography (SPECT) myocardial perfusion images. The display of SPECT myocardial perfusion imaging is standardized. The short-axis slices are presented from apex to base, the vertical long-axis slices are displayed from septum to lateral wall, and the horizontal long-axis slices are displayed from inferior to anterior. The radiotracer uptake is homogeneous in each of the slices. (From Dilsizian V, Narula J, Braunwald E, editors: *Atlas of nuclear cardiology* [CD-ROM], Philadelphia, 2003, Current Medicine.)

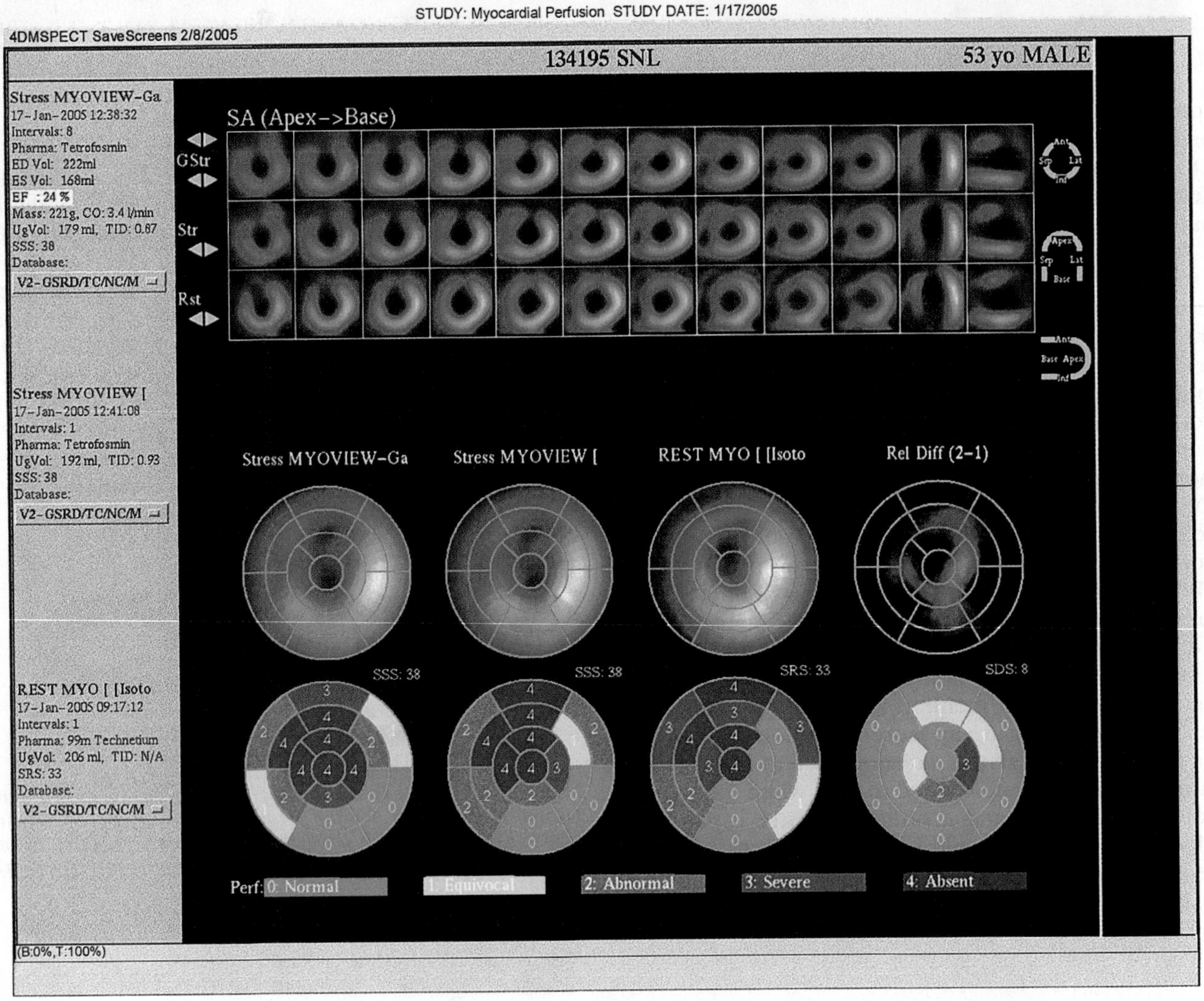

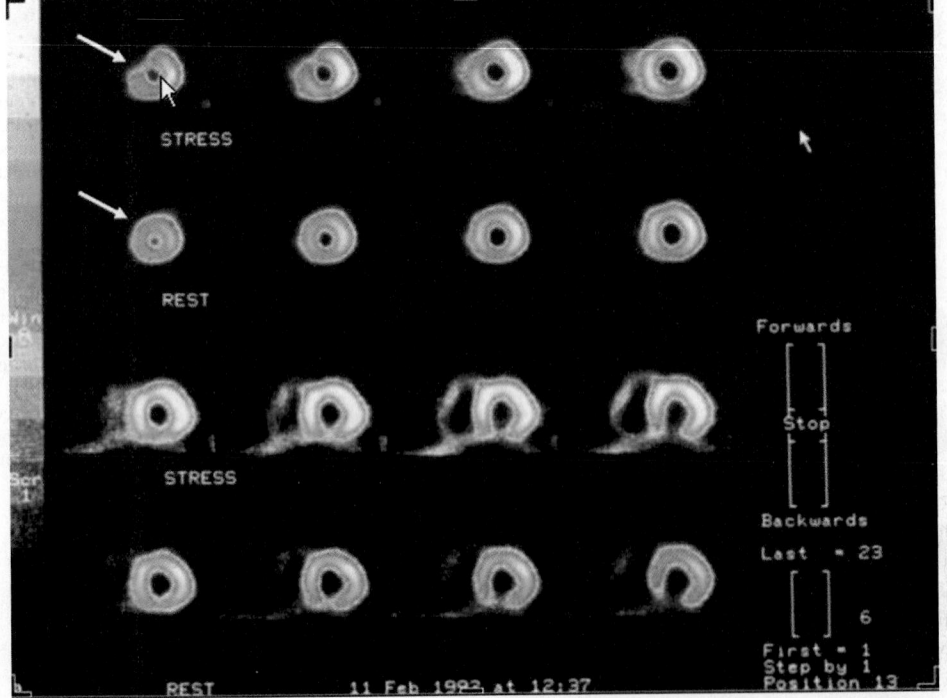

STUDY: Myocardial Perfusion STUDY DATE: 1/17/2005
4DMSPECT SaveScreens 2/8/2005
134195 SNL
53 yo MALE
Stress MYOVIEW-Ga
17-Jan-2005 12:38:32
Intervals: 8
Pharma: Tetrofosmin
ED Vol: 222ml
ES Vol: 168ml
EF : 24 %
Mass: 221g, CO: 3.4 l/min
UgVol: 179 ml, TID: 0.87
SSS: 38
Database:
V2-GSRD/TC/NC/M
SA (Apex->Base)
GStr
Str
Rst
Stress MYOVIEW [
17-Jan-2005 12:41:08
Intervals: 1
Pharma: Tetrofosmin
UgVol: 192 ml, TID: 0.93
SSS: 38
Database:
V2-GSRD/TC/NC/M
Stress MYOVIEW-Ga
Stress MYOVIEW [
REST MYO [[Isoto
Rel Diff (2-1)
REST MYO [[Isoto
17-Jan-2005 09:17:12
Intervals: 1
Pharma: 99m Technetium
UgVol: 206 ml, TID: N/A
SRS: 33
Database:
V2-GSRD/TC/NC/M
SSS: 38
SSS: 38
SRS: 33
SDS: 8
Perf: 0: Normal
1: Equivocal
2: Abnormal
3: Severe
4: Absent
(B:0%,T:100%)

FIGURE 29-9 ■ Abnormal exercise stress gated single-photon emission computed tomography myocardial perfusion study in a 53-year-old man with documented coronary artery disease, prior myocardial infarction, and systolic heart failure. The patient has evidence of previous extensive anterior-anteroseptal-septal-anteroapical transmural wall myocardial infarction, marked left ventricular dilatation with severely depressed systolic function, and a calculated ejection fraction of 24 percent. (Bull's-eye polar maps are noted on the lower half of the figure.) © KAScordo.

STRESS
REST
Forwards
Stop
STRESS
Backwards
Last = 23
6
First = 1
Step by 1
Position 13
REST
11 Feb 1993 at 12:37

FIGURE 29-10 ■ Exercise-rest single-photon emission computed tomography myocardial perfusion imaging with Tc-99m sestamibi in a patient with anterior wall reversible ischemia. © KAScordo.

without prior myocardial infarction demonstrate a "cold" spot on the exercise films, but not on the resting films (Figures 29-9 and 29-10). This is considered a reversible defect and suggests myocardial ischemia. A fixed defect noted on both scans represents an area of fibrosis from a previous infarct. In addition to the number and extent of myocardial perfusion defects, evidence of extensive abnormalities such as radiopharmaceutical lung activity and transient stress-induced left ventricular dilatation cavity enlargement are noted. These findings relate to the severity or extensiveness of CAD and indicate a poor prognosis. Lung uptake of thallium-201 or Tc-99m sestamibi on postexercise or pharmacological stress images indicates stress-induced diffuse left ventricular dysfunction.[21]

ECHOCARDIOGRAPHY

The echocardiographic examination is based on detection of echoes produced by a beam of very-high-frequency sound (ultrasound) transmitted into the heart. Transthoracic two-dimensional echocardiography (TTE) with Doppler echocardiography is a common diagnostic procedure for patients with cardiovascular disease. Indications for TTE with Doppler include diagnosing and guiding treatment for CAD, valvular heart disease, heart failure, hypertensive heart disease, congenital abnormalities, complications of pulmonary disease, tumors or masses, cardiac trauma, pericardial disease, and others.

M-Mode

Early echocardiography used an M-mode or motion technique in which the ultrasound beam transmitted and received an ultrasound signal along only one line, giving an "ice pick" view of the heart (Figure 29-11). Images are transformed electronically into gray scale images on a TV screen and are printed on paper: high echo reflection is white, less reflection is gray, and no reflection is black. Depending on the angulation of the transducer, M-mode recordings give measurements of cardiac structures and analysis of motion patterns of various structures in the heart. M-mode also allows for simultaneous analysis with ECG, heart sounds, and pulse tracings.

Two-Dimensional

Recent developments led to the use of techniques that rapidly scan the ultrasound beam across the heart to produce two-dimensional tomographic images. A two-dimensional echocardiogram is an effective method for evaluating the structure and function of the heart, providing images of the heart, paracardiac structures, and the great vessels (Figures 29-12 to 29-17). The addition

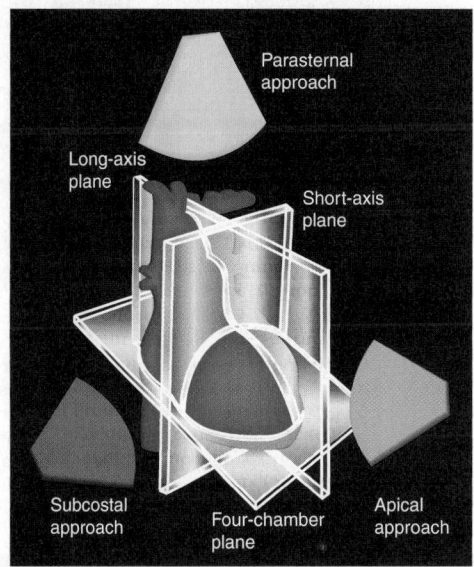

FIGURE 29-12 ■ Two-dimensional echocardiographic imaging planes.

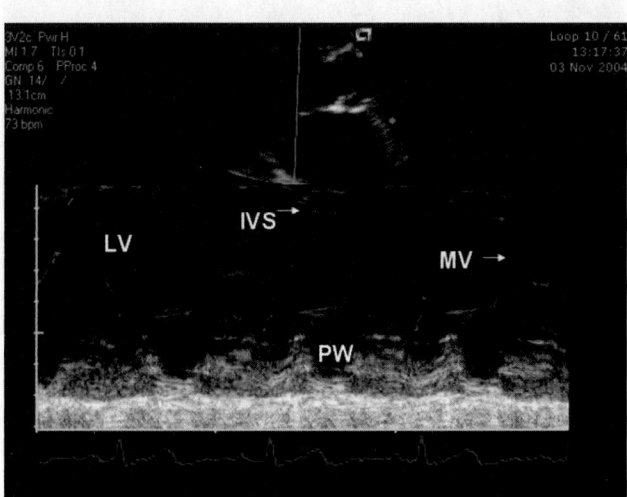

FIGURE 29-11 ■ M-mode echocardiogram depicting the M-mode beam through the mitral valve. Note the M-shaped opening pattern of the mitral valve. *IVS,* Intraventricular septum; *LV,* left ventricle; *MV,* mitral valve; *PW,* posterior wall.

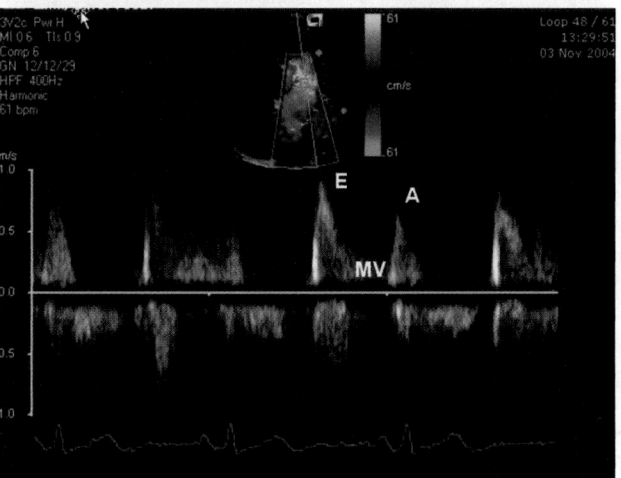

FIGURE 29-13 ■ Pulsed Doppler recording of normal flow through the mitral valve *(MV)* orifice into the left ventricular inflow tract. The first phase of flow occurs in early diastole *(E)* and the second after atrial systole *(A).* Normally, the peak velocity is greater with the early diastolic flow, and thus the E wave is higher than the A wave.

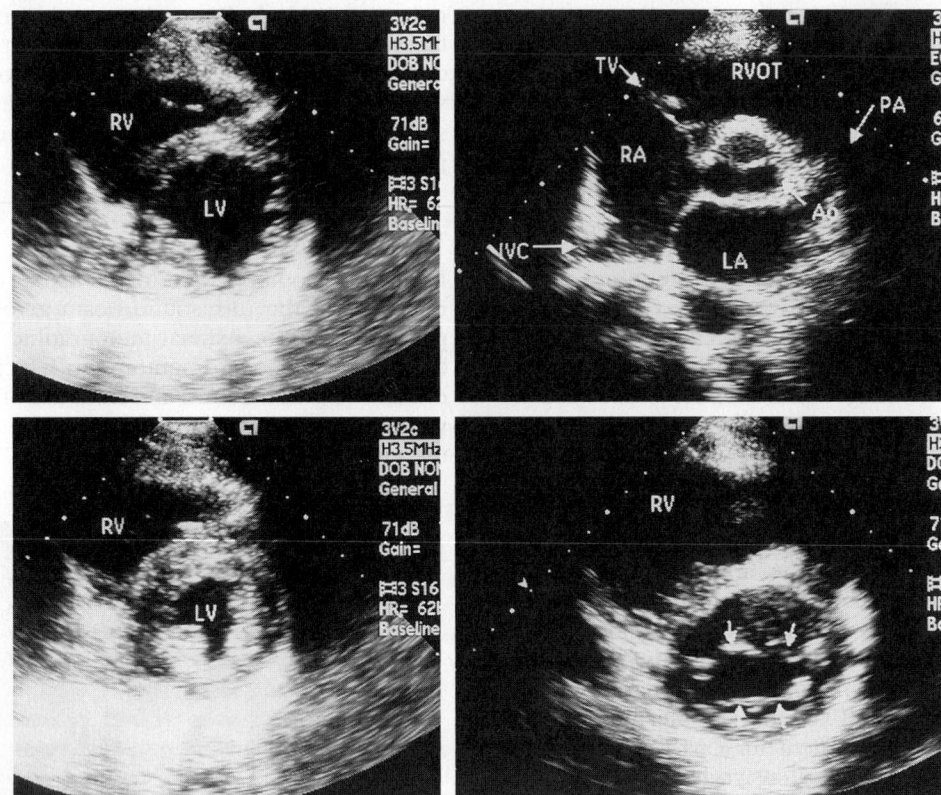

FIGURE 29-14 ■ Short-axis two-dimensional echocardiograms. The two left panels are recorded at the level of the papillary muscles in diastole *(top)* and systole *(bottom)*. Note the symmetrical thickening of the myocardium and inward motion of the endocardium representing normal ventricular function in systole. The *top right* panel is recorded at the level of the aortic valve, and the *bottom right* panel is recorded at the level of the mitral valve in diastole. *A,* Aorta; *IVC,* inferior vena cava; *LA,* left atrium; *LV,* left ventricle; *PA,* pulmonary artery; *RA,* right atrium; *RV,* right ventricle; *RVOT,* right ventricular outflow tract; *TV,* tricuspid valve. (From Zipes DP, Libby P, Bonow RO, Braunwald E, editors: *Braunwald's heart disease,* ed 7, Philadelphia, 2005, Elsevier Saunders.)

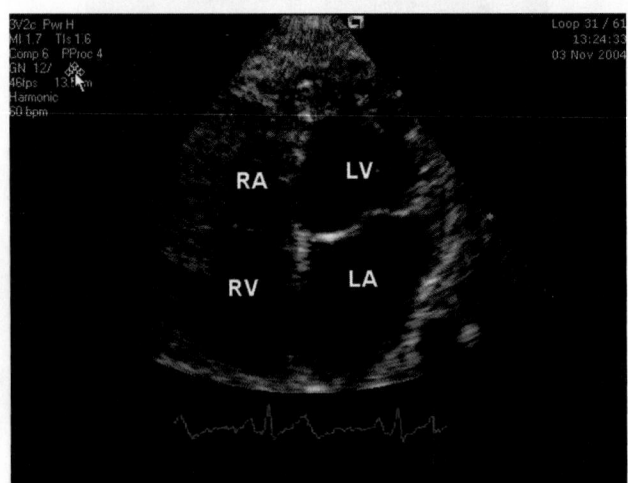

FIGURE 29-15 ■ Apical four-chamber view of the left and right ventricles and left and right atria. *LA,* Left atrium; *LV,* left ventricle; *RA,* right atrium; *RV,* right ventricle.

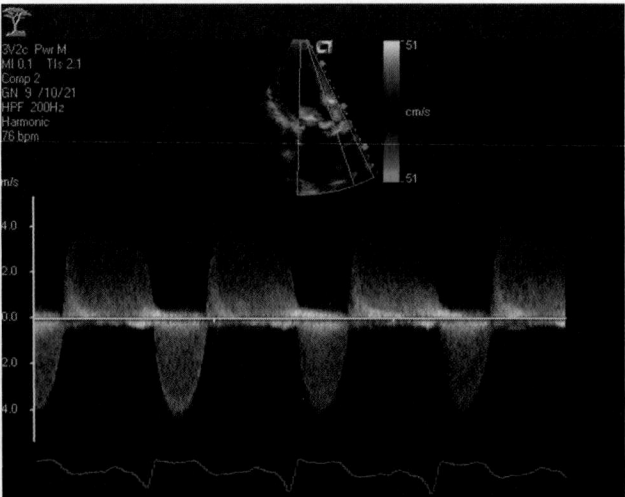

FIGURE 29-16 ■ Doppler echocardiogram of the aortic outflow tract and aortic insufficiency.

of Doppler echocardiography, which records changes in frequency of sound waves, further extends the use of echocardiography.

Doppler echocardiography is a method to detect the direction and velocity of moving blood within the heart. Red blood cells moving through the heart and great ves-

sels also reflect ultrasound waves at an altered frequency. By using specialized Doppler instrumentation, the frequency shift is used to estimate blood flow velocity. The changing frequencies are converted into audible sounds that are emitted from speakers within the echo machine. The frequency shift can be converted to a

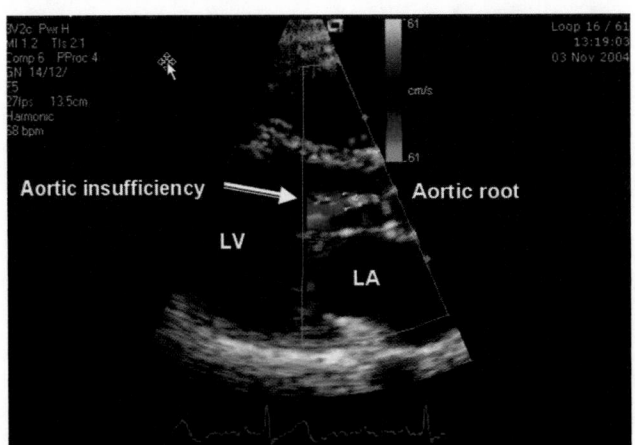

FIGURE 29-17 ■ Parasternal long-axis view with color flow Doppler demonstrating a jet of aortic insufficiency *(arrow)*. *LA,* Left atrium; *LV,* left ventricle.

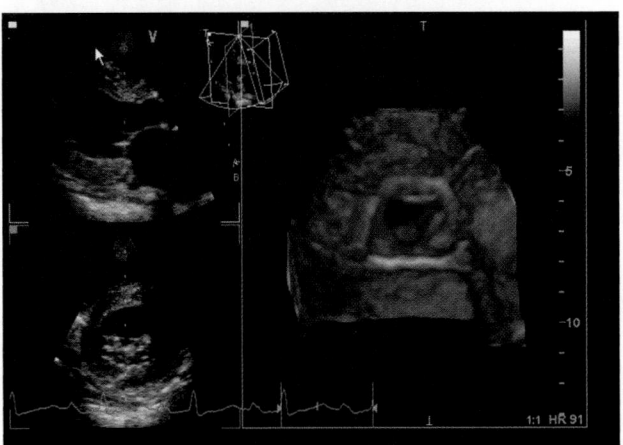

FIGURE 29-18 ■ Three-dimensional echocardiogram.

color scheme. Laminar flow is displayed in primary colors of blue and red. Flow away from the transducer is blue; flow toward the transducer is red. The intensity of the color reflects the velocity of blood flow. Lighter colors indicate higher velocity, while darker colors indicate slower velocity. Turbulent blood flow can be displayed as multiple colors that indicate multiple velocities or by shades of green. Doppler color flow imaging is helpful to detect and evaluate valvular insufficiency and stenosis, along with normal and abnormal flow states. Doppler imaging also provides quantitative data essential in the clinical decision-making process.

Three-Dimensional

Three-dimensional echocardiography was developed to provide for more realistic visualization and reproducible computerized reconstruction of the heart (Figure 29-18). Three-dimensional echocardiography allows for acquisition and processing of spatially dense image data sets that allow structures to be visualized using three-dimensional display formats. In contrast to two-dimensional echocardiography, which relies on geometrical assumptions to estimate ventricular volumes, three-dimensional echocardiography can determine ventricular volumes accurately. This becomes particularly important when evaluating disease-distorted hearts. Other advantages to three-dimensional echocardiography include more accurate measurements of ejection fraction, estimation of infarct size, determination of pericardial effusion and aneurysm volume, and more accurate quantitative analysis of valvular function.

Nurse's Role in Two- and Three-Dimensional Echocardiography

Nurses assist in providing patient education and reassurance. The procedure is virtually painless, does not require sedation, has no known risks, and usually is performed by a sonographer. Depending on imaging difficulty, preliminary findings, information needed, and patient cooperation, an examination generally lasts between 30 and 60 minutes. Patients often are asked to inhale deeply, exhale, and hold their breath. This allows

for better acquisition of images. Experienced sonographers are able to perform interrogations specific to preliminary findings noted on the echocardiographic examination, thus providing valuable information that aids in diagnosis and treatment. These individuals have advanced knowledge of cardiac anatomy and physiology and the pathophysiology of cardiac diseases, along with knowledge of the physics and mechanics of the procedure. Specific competencies for echocardiographic sonographers and physician readers are addressed in the guidelines from the ACC/AHA/American College of Physicians-American Society of Internal Medicine Task Force.[26]

Contrast Echocardiography

Contrast echocardiography is based on the use of gas microbubbles. Initial imaging studies were done by injecting microbubbles, generated by hand-agitated saline. Ten milliliters of normal saline was drawn into a syringe along with a small amount of air. The syringe was rapidly agitated to create microbubbles and then quickly injected into a peripheral vein. Today's contrast agents have revolutionized clinical echocardiography: they last longer and provide brighter echoes. Contrast echocardiography is used to enhance left ventricular endocardial border definition, augment the detection of intracardiac shunts, assess right-sided valvular insufficiency, and aid in the diagnosis of complex congenital heart defects and pulmonary arteriovenous fistulas. Spontaneous echo contrast, or a swirling "smoke-like cloud," may be seen in the left ventricle in patients with dilated ventricles and with apical aneurysms and may represent stasis of blood within the cavity.

Nurse's Role in Contrast Echocardiography

Initial preparation of the patient includes an explanation of the test and obtaining written consent. When contrast echocardiography is performed in combination with exercise, the use of contrast medium frequently is incorporated into the standard consent form for stress echocardiography. Albumin-based contrast agents should not be administered to patients with allergies or hypersensitivity to blood, blood products, or albumin. Therefore, it is important that any history of transfusion reaction be noted. Resuscitation equipment should be readily available. Inform patients of possible side effects that may occur during contrast medium administration. These include headache, nausea and/or vomiting, warm sensation or flushing, and dizziness.

Contrast echocardiography requires intravenous access with a 20-gauge or larger angiocatheter into a large antecubital or forearm vein attached to a three-way stopcock. If the patient will be scanned in a left lateral position, the intravenous access should be inserted into the patient's right arm, and visa versa. The nurse, sonographer, or physician must be familiar with the package insert for contrast medium storage and shelf-life information, such as the need for refrigeration. Contrary to what usually is done when drawing fluid from a vial, air should *not* be injected into the vial. Instead, vent the vial with a large-bore needle, and then draw the agent into the syringe. Inspect the appearance of the contrast agent for complete resuspension; the solution should appear opaque and milky white. Do not aspirate blood back into the syringe containing the contrast agent; this may promote the formation of a blood clot within the syringe. A starting dose of 0.5 ml is followed by a 5- to 10-ml flush of saline that is stopped when contrast agent is seen in the right ventricle. The injection rate should not exceed 1 ml/sec. If use of a contrast agent is combined with exercise echocardiography, communication with the nurse, physician, sonographer, and patient is imperative. Patients need to instruct the sonographer approximately 30 seconds before they anticipate reaching their exercise limit. This allows for injection of the contrast agent before acquiring images. Contrast agent also can be used with dobutamine echocardiography.

Exercise/Stress Echocardiography

Echocardiography combined with physical or pharmacological stress is an effective method for assessing regional and global ventricular function in men and women and has been described as better than exercise treadmill testing or similar to exercise thallium or sestamibi testing in identifying coronary heart disease in women.[27] A normal response to exercise or to pharmacological stress is a global increase in ventricular contractility and hyperdynamic wall motion with reduction in systolic cavity size. Hypokinetic or dyskinetic wall motion relative to other regions suggests regional ischemia or scarring. If the wall abnormality is present at rest and with exercise, it is considered a fixed defect. In contrast echocardiography, if the wall abnormality is seen only with exercise, it is suggestive of reversible ischemia. The location of the wall motion abnormality helps determine which coronary artery is involved, and the extent and severity of the wall motion abnormality correlates with the degree of myocardial ischemia.

Although stress echocardiography is highly accurate in detecting significant CAD, false-positive and false-negative tests do occur. The diagnostic sensitivity and specificity of stress echocardiography is 86 and 79 percent, respectively, and for dobutamine echocardiogra-

phy, 75 and 86 percent, respectively.[28] Meta-analysis demonstrates that the diagnostic accuracy of dobutamine and dipyridamole echocardiography is similar, with a higher sensitivity of dobutamine in single-vessel disease and a higher specificity of dipyridamole in patients with normal coronary arteries. Initial reports revealed that dobutamine stress echocardiography was frequently negative in women with single-vessel disease and in women with chest pain without angiographic coronary stenosis.[29] False-negative exercise echocardiographic studies may occur with continued antianginal therapy, poor image quality, delayed postexercise imaging, and in patients with microvascular or valvular disease. False-positive studies may be seen in patients with nonischemic cardiomyopathy and by overinterpretation of suboptimal echocardiographic images.

Nurse's Role in Exercise/Stress Echocardiography

The procedure for stress echocardiography is similar to that of exercise testing with the addition of preechocardiographic and postechocardiographic imaging (Figure 29-19). Imaging commonly is performed during upright or supine bicycle exercise or more commonly, immediately after treadmill exercise. Because ischemia-induced wall motion abnormalities may quickly resolve, images must be acquired immediately (within 2 minutes) after exercise. Therefore, communication between patients and staff is imperative. Multiple images, obtained from the parasternal long axis and short axis and apical two- and four-chamber views, enable evaluation of each myocardial region supplied by one of the major coronary arteries. Acquired digitized images allow rest and stress images to be viewed side-by-side in a continuous loop format for comparison.

Pharmacological stress testing, commonly with dobutamine, is used for patients with functional impairments making them unable to exercise (Figure 29-20). With pharmacological stress echocardiography, images are obtained at rest, at incremental stages throughout the test, and at peak stress. Patient preparation is similar to that described under myocardial perfusion imaging.

Transesophageal Echocardiography

Whereas two-dimensional echocardiography is noninvasive, transesophageal echocardiography (**TEE**), is a semi-invasive procedure that involves esophageal intubation with a TEE probe. As previously noted, echocardiography uses high-frequency ultrasound to obtain images of the heart and surrounding structures. Ultrasound beams obey the basic laws of physics, including the laws of reflection and refraction. As such, the medium through which the ultrasound beam travels influences the images obtained. Ultrasound travels poorly through a gaseous medium. Penetration is also poor when the beam encounters dense substances, such as bone, calcium, or metal. Therefore, routine echocardiography images are difficult to obtain in patients with chronic obstructive lung disease with large air-filled lungs, in thin patients with narrow rib spaces, in obese patients, or patients with thick chest walls. Other situations that can result in poor-quality images include pa-

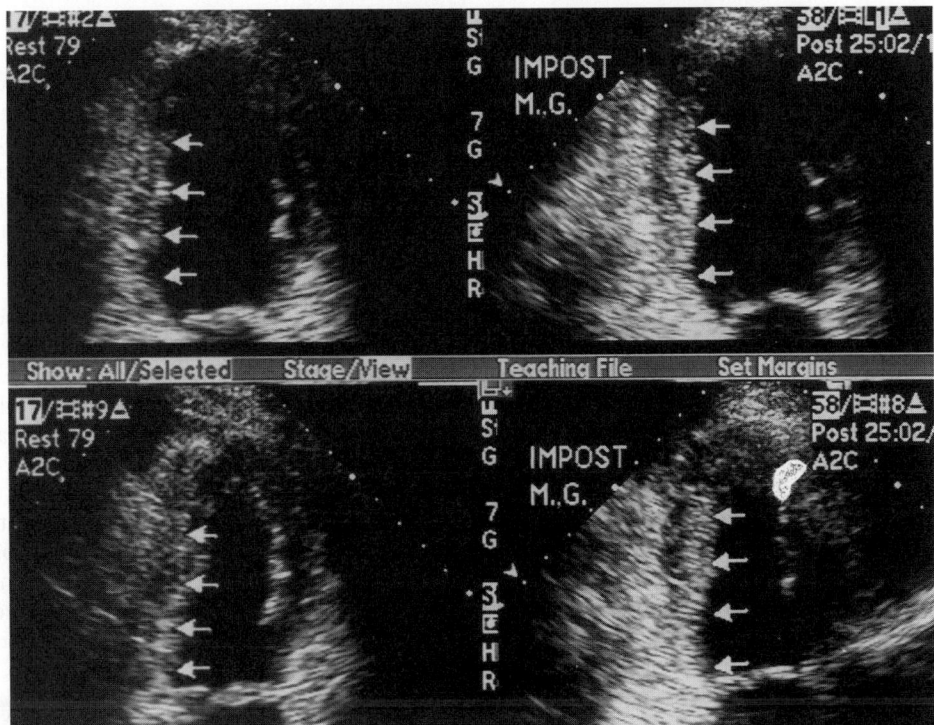

FIGURE 29-19 ■ Exercise echocardiogram in a patient with disease of the right coronary artery. The *two left panels* were recorded at rest, and the *two right panels* were recorded immediately after treadmill exercise. The *top panels* show diastole and the *bottom panels* show systole. In each panel, the *arrows* note the location of the inferior wall endocardium at end diastole. At rest there is appropriate thickening and inward motion of the inferior wall that can be seen to move inward through the body of the arrows. Immediately after exercise, the proximal inferior wall *(lower two arrows)* becomes frankly dyskinetic, and the mid and diastole portion of the inferior wall is akinetic (From Braunwald E, Zipes DP, Libby P, editors: *Heart disease,* ed 6, Philadelphia, 2001, WB Saunders.)

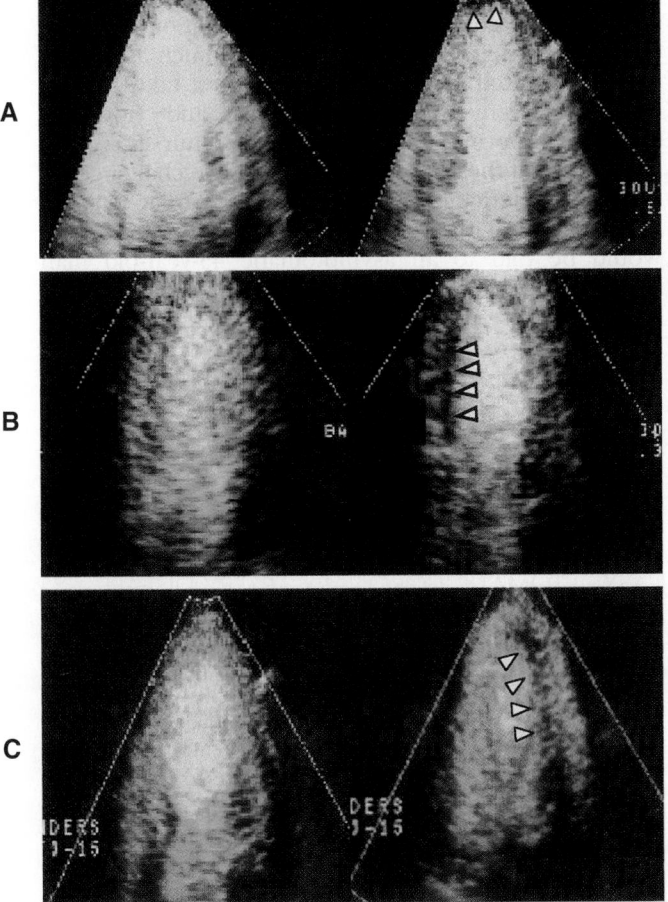

FIGURE 29-20 ■ Myocardial contrast medium at rest *(left)* and during dobutamine stress *(right)* in three different patients with significant coronary artery disease in three different coronary artery territories. **A,** Inducible anteroseptal and apical defect. **B,** Inducible inferior perfusion defect. **C,** Inducible lateral wall contrast defect. Coronary angiography showed that all patients had greater than 50 percent narrowing in the **(A)** left anterior descending artery, **(B)** right coronary artery, and **(C)** left circumflex artery. (From Otto C: *The practice of clinical echocardiography,* ed 2, Philadelphia, 2002, WB Saunders.)

tients on ventilators, patients who cannot be turned laterally, patients who have subcutaneous emphysema, and those with incisions and/or surgical bandages that limit access to a precordial or apical window.

Transesophageal echocardiographic images are not, however, limited by these circumstances. With TEE, the transducer is mounted on a flexible endoscope and is passed into the esophagus and stomach. The proximity of the esophagus to the heart and great vessels eliminates interference from structures such as air-filled lungs and ribs. This provides an excellent window with potentially high-quality images generally better than those obtained from TTE. In general, TTE is used as the initial diagnostic investigation. Common indications for TEE are listed in Box 29-5. This semi-invasive procedure, although generally safe, is not without discomfort and risks. Complications usually result from esophageal intubation and include pharyngeal and esophageal trauma, with rare esophageal perforation, hypoxemia, dysrhythmias, aspiration, and rare vasovagal reactions. Complications also can occur from intravenous sedation, topical anesthesia, or drying agents (glycopyrrolate) used.

Nurses' Role in Transesophageal Echocardiography

The nurses' role varies depending on where the TEE is performed. If the TEE is performed in the operating room, nurses likely will assume additional responsibilities. In general, TEE is performed using moderate sedation. Thus all personnel must be trained in the use and precautions of these medications, and resuscitative equipment must be immediately available. Written consent is obtained, and an intravenous line is secured. To avoid the potential for vomiting and aspiration, patients should be fasting for 4 to 6 hours before the procedure. Urgent procedures, however, can be performed if patients have only clear fluid up to 2 hours before. Similar preparation and precautions apply if the TEE is done in combination with dobutamine. Contraindications for TEE include esophageal spasm, esophageal stricture, esophageal laceration, esophageal perforation, active gastrointestinal bleeding, and perforated viscus. Esophageal diverticulum is considered a relative contraindication to TEE. The TEE often is performed in critically ill patients in the intensive care unit or emergency department. As needed, patients with unstable cardiopulmonary status should be intubated and should be ventilated during TEE. Patients with severe limitation of flexion of their necks present a relative contraindication to the procedure. Anticoagulation therapy, per se, is not a contraindication for TEE.

Before insertion of the TEE probe, the oropharynx is anesthetized with a topical agent, such as Cetacaine spray (benzocaine, butamben, and tetracaine hydrochloride), which suppresses the gag reflex. The patient is placed in a left decubitus position, and the neck is flexed slightly forward. The patient is asked to swallow the probe; this facilitates insertion of the TEE probe. After the probe is positioned properly, to prevent damage to the probe, a bite guard may be placed in the patient's mouth. Images are acquired, and the probe is quickly removed. Patients are monitored and are given clear fluids after the return of a gag reflex.

COMPUTED TOMOGRAPHY AND MAGNETIC RESONANCE TECHNIQUES

During the past decade, the development of noninvasive imaging techniques such as electron beam computed tomography, electron beam angiography, magnetic resonance imaging, and magnetic resonance angiography has resulted in significant advances in diagnostic technology. These tests provide a way to image the heart and visualize the lumen of the coronary artery without the risks and economic burden of cardiac catheterization. Cardiac nurses provide education and reassurance and help to answers questions such as, "What will the test tell me?" "How long does it take?" "Do I have to take any special precautions?" and "How reliable is the information?" To do so, these nurses require knowledge of these noninvasive tests. The challenge for advanced practice nurses who care for cardiac patients is what to do with the information. For instance, what would be told to an asymptomatic 45-year-old man whose father died from a myocardial infarction at age 46, who referred himself for ultrafast computed tomography and now has abnormal calcium scores? (See the accompanying Conundrum feature.) To answer this question and others that clinical practice poses, advanced practice nurses must be aware of the evidence

---

BOX 29-5 ◼◼◼
COMMON INDICATIONS FOR TRANSESOPHAGEAL ECHOCARDIOGRAPHY

- Nondiagnostic transthoracic echocardiogram
- Assessment of native valve disease
- Assessment of prosthetic valves
- Assessment of ineffective endocarditis
- Assessment of a suspected cardioembolic event
- Assessment of cardiac tumors
- Assessment of atrial septal abnormalities
- Assessment of aortic dissection intramural hematomas and aortic rupture
- Evaluation of congenital heart disease
- Detection of anatomical coronary artery disease
- Stress echocardiography
- Evaluation of pericardial disease
- Evaluation of critically ill patients
- Intraoperative monitoring
- Monitoring during interventional procedures
- Used in concert with cardiac catheterization to limit the quantity of radiographic contrast material

---

◼◼◼ CONUNDRUM
ASYMPTOMATIC CORONARY ARTERY DISEASE

An asymptomatic 46-year-old man recently underwent electron beam computed tomography testing. The family history of premature coronary artery disease (father died at age 49 from an acute myocardial infarction) alerted the patient to the possibility of premature disease in himself. Electron beam computed tomography scores were high and indicated elevated levels of coronary calcification that reflects coronary atherosclerosis. He has had hypertension for 7 years. His total cholesterol is 255 mg/dL, low-density lipoprotein cholesterol 156 mg/dL, and high-density lipoprotein 33 mg/dL. The patient is taking a calcium channel blocker (diltiazem). Should the patient be referred for further testing? What treatment measures would be appropriate?

and the limitations of the technology and know when to apply and when not to apply these tests in the investigation and management of CAD.

Electron Beam Computed Tomography

Electron beam computed tomography (**EBCT**) and the newer generation of multislice computed tomography scanners allow for high-resolution visualization of the beating heart and coronary arteries (Figure 29-21). EBCT is a highly sensitive, accurate technique that detects and quantitates coronary artery calcium that occurs with atherosclerosis.[30] A focused beam of electrons allows for visualization of coronary calcium and enables the noninvasive detection and localization of coronary artery plaques. Atherosclerosis is the only known process that results in the deposition of calcium in the arterial wall; therefore, any calcium in the coronary vasculature is diagnostic of coronary atherosclerosis. The amount of coronary calcium is related to the extent of coronary plaque disease, which has substantial diagnostic and prognostic implications. This noninvasive test is being used to screen asymptomatic individuals at high-risk of developing CAD, to screen symptomatic individuals at low to moderate risk of coronary events, and to assess progression or regression of CAD.

The test results are reported as a calcium score—an amalgamation of total size and density of the calcium deposits found throughout the coronary vasculature. The coronary calcium score provides a quantitative evaluation of the extent of atherosclerotic plaque burden but does not give information about the severity or

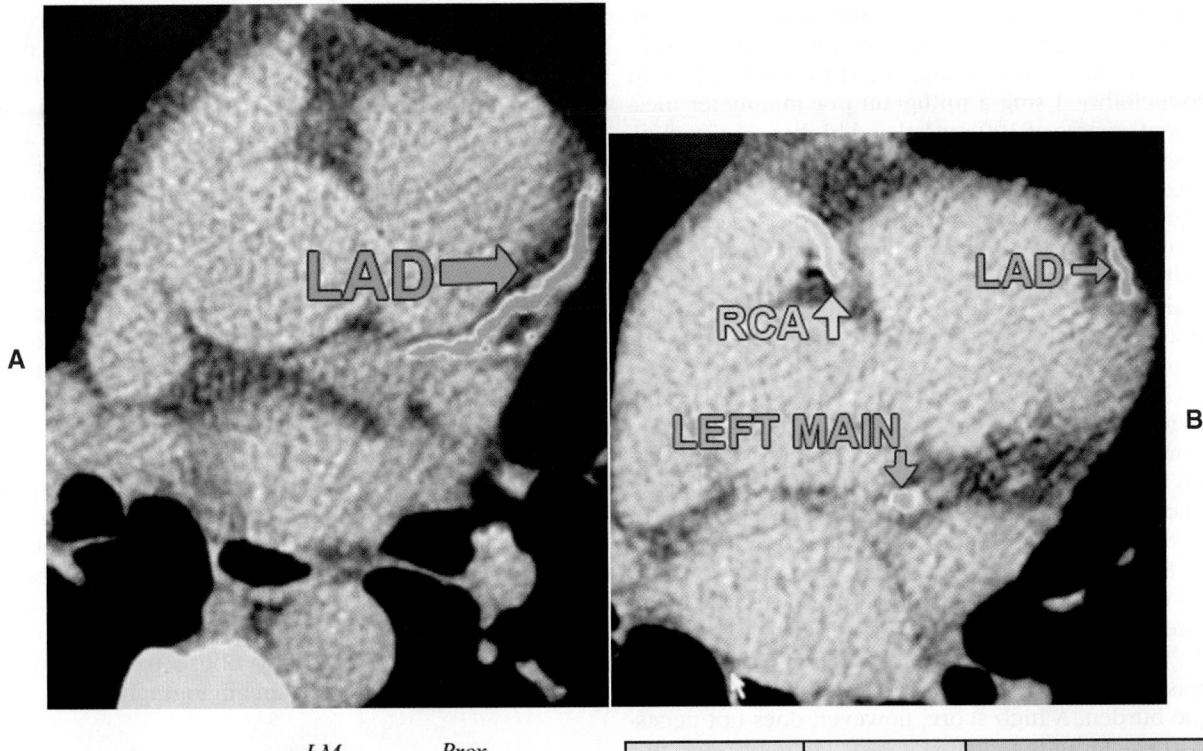

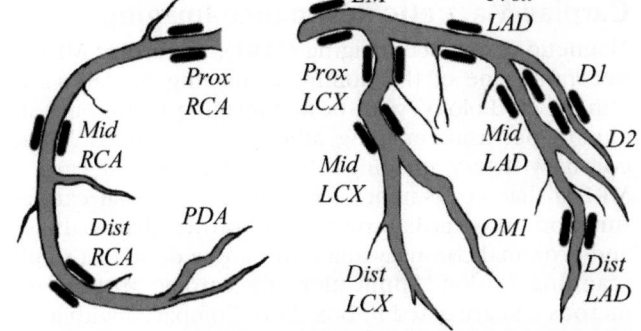

Artery	# plaques	Plaque Burden	
		Volume (mm³)	Calcium score
Left main	2	95	120
Left anterior descending	8	709	926
Left circumflex	7	451	581
Right coronary	24	1351	1795
Total	41	2607	3424

FIGURE 29-21 ■ Results of electron beam tomography showing (**A, B**) calcium lesions, (**C**) the locations of calcium plaque in the patient's coronary arteries, and (**D**) the patient's calcium score, which is high. The patient, a 43-year-old man, smoked one to two packs of cigarettes daily, had a family history of coronary artery disease, and had hypertension, for which he took verapamil. He had a body mass index of 31.5 kg/m². At 1 year after the test, the patient had stopped smoking and had begun exercising most days of the week. *D1/D2*, Diagonal branch; *Dist*, distal; *LAD*, left anterior descending artery; *LCX*, left circumflex artery; *LM*, left main; *OM1*, obtuse marginal 1; *PDA*, posterior descending artery; *Prox*, proximal; *RCA*, right coronary artery. (Courtesy Midwest Imaging & Prevention, LLC, St Louis, Mo. Retrieved February 28, 2006 from www.purescan.com/Case%20Studies.html)

degree of arterial luminal narrowing.[30] Scoring is frequently based on a scoring algorithm in which the area of individual calcified lesions is evaluated in sequential images (Agatston score). A threshold of 130 H commonly is used for identification of a calcified lesion. An Agatston score is calculated by multiplying the lesion area by a density factor derived from the maximal Hounsfield units in this area. Separate scores are derived for the left main, left anterior descending, circumflex, and right coronary arteries. A score of 0 indicates no calcium, whereas a score greater than 400 indicates a high likelihood of at least one significantly obstructed coronary artery.

Although commonly used, the Agatston method is not without limitations. In addition to variations up to 30 percent in reproducibility, the Agatston score does not use scientific units and is based on noncalibrated machine images that are open to variations in physician interpretation. Newer scoring systems use volumetric quantification algorithms and provide volume, mass, and density of calcified plaques and promise improved reproducibility. Using a milligram per millimeter measurement, scores of 100 mg/ml and higher signify clinically significant calcified plaque. Total time for EBCT is approximately 10 to 15 minutes. No special preparation is required. Radiation exposure from the test is minimal. For best results, patients must remain still; a 30-second breath hold usually is required. Thus, patients who are unable to lie supine and motionless and who cannot hold their breath may not be candidates for EBCT.

EBCT has a relatively high sensitivity for CAD ranging from 85 to 100 percent, a lower specificity (41 to 76 percent), and an overall predictive accuracy of approximately 70 percent.[31] EBCT is accurate in diagnosing significant CAD (greater than 50 percent stenosis) in women with an overall reported sensitivity and specificity at 88 and 49 percent, respectively.[32] Low calcium scores (less than 10 for Agatston scoring) have the greatest predictive value for low risk for development of CAD.[33] High calcium scores are associated with a 10-fold increased risk for heart disease and indicate a high plaque burden. A high score, however, does not necessarily translate into a critical lesion. Therefore, the use of calcium scores to predict the need for percutaneous coronary intervention or coronary artery bypass surgery is limited.

EBCT does not detect noncalcified, lipid-laden vulnerable plaque.[30] Calcium scores can be used to modify the Framingham Global Risk Score. By using a weighted factor based on the patient's individual calcium score percentile, a higher Framingham Score is given to those with high calcium scores and a lower one to those with lower calcium scores. The addition of calcium scoring, however, remains controversial. EBCT often is not covered by insurance companies. Centers that promote EBCT for the general public do not require a referral. The challenge is to define the appropriate management of asymptomatic patients with abnormal calcium scores. Thus far, there is no clear-cut evidence that supports invasive investigations in an asymptomatic patient with abnormal calcium scores.

Electron Beam Angiography

Electron beam angiography has the potential to overcome some of the limitations inherent in EBCT. Coronary artery electron beam angiography was first introduced in 1995 as a noninvasive diagnostic procedure for visualization of the coronary anatomy and was approved by the Food and Drug Administration in November 1999. Contrast-enhanced, ECG-triggered, three-dimensional electron beam angiography produces luminal views of long coronary artery segments that are comparable to those obtained from standard cardiac arteriography (Figures 29-22 and 29-23). Electron beam angiography can be used to identify lesions greater than 50 percent with a sensitivity of 74 to 92 percent, specificity of 79 to 100 percent, and accuracy of 81 to 93 percent. The accuracy for detecting coronary stenosis is highest in the left main artery and left anterior descending artery and lowest in the circumflex artery. The electron beam angiography study is limited in that distal coronary arteries are not as well visualized as proximal arteries, and collateral arteries cannot be seen. The technology is improving rapidly, and many expect a rapid implementation of 64-slice scanners over the next few years. Small vessel size is the main determinant of false-positive electron beam angiography test results.[34] Because vein grafts are large and have little cardiac motion, electron beam angiography has value in determining the patency of coronary artery bypass grafts.[35] Compared with coronary angiography, electron beam angiography of saphenous vein grafts demonstrates a sensitivity of 92 to 100 percent and specificity of 91 to 100 percent, whereas electron beam angiography of left internal mammary artery has sensitivity of 80 to 100 percent and specificity of 82 to 100 percent.[34] Approximately 150 ml of iodinated contrast medium is administered via a peripheral vein, and images are obtained during a single breath hold. The procedure can be done within 15 minutes. Patients who are unable to hold their breath for at least 25 seconds, those with significant dysrhythmias, and morbidly obese patients are poor candidates for electron beam angiography.

Cardiac Magnetic Resonance Imaging

Magnetic resonance imaging (**MRI**), or cardiac MRI, is becoming one of the dominate imaging modalities in clinical cardiology, with newer imaging techniques including perfusion imaging, atherosclerosis imaging, and coronary artery imaging.[36] One advantage of cardiac MRI is that assessment of global and regional cardiac function, myocardial perfusion, myocardial viability, and proximal coronary anatomy can be done in a single scanning session. Applications for cardiac MRI are numerous and are listed in Box 29-6. Compared with angiography or radionuclide scintigraphy, perfusion cardiac MRI with adenosine and dipyridamole (Persantine) has a sensitivity of 67 to 83 percent, specificity of 75 to 100 percent, and with dobutamine stress, sensitivity up to 91 percent and specificity of 80 percent.[37] When combined with adenosine, cardiac MRI can predict accurately the presence of significant CAD (greater than 70

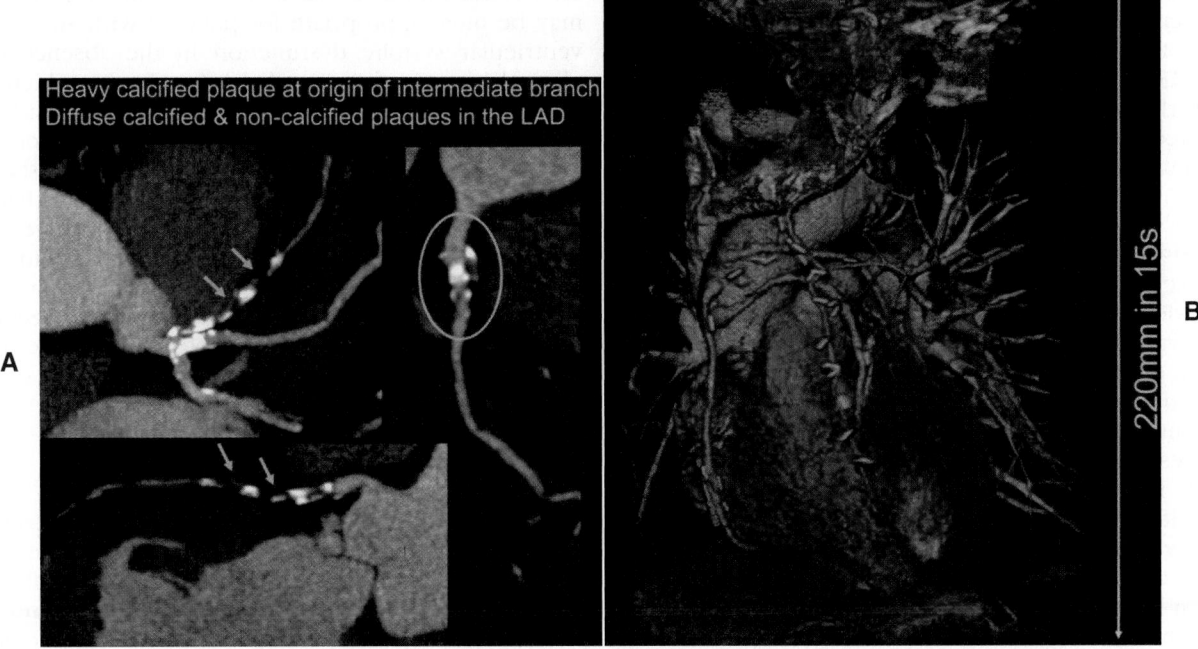

FIGURE 29-22 ■ **A,** Cardiac computed tomography angiogram *(CTA)* showing heavily calcified plague at the origin of the intermediate branch and diffuse calcified and noncalcified plaques in the left anterior descending artery. **B,** Cardiac CTA showing left internal mammary artery bypass. *LAD,* Left anterior descending artery. (**A** courtesy Mayo/Siemens Medical Innovations Center, Rochester, NY. **B** courtesy University of Erlangen, Department of Radiology and Institute of Medical Physics, Nuremberg, Germany.)

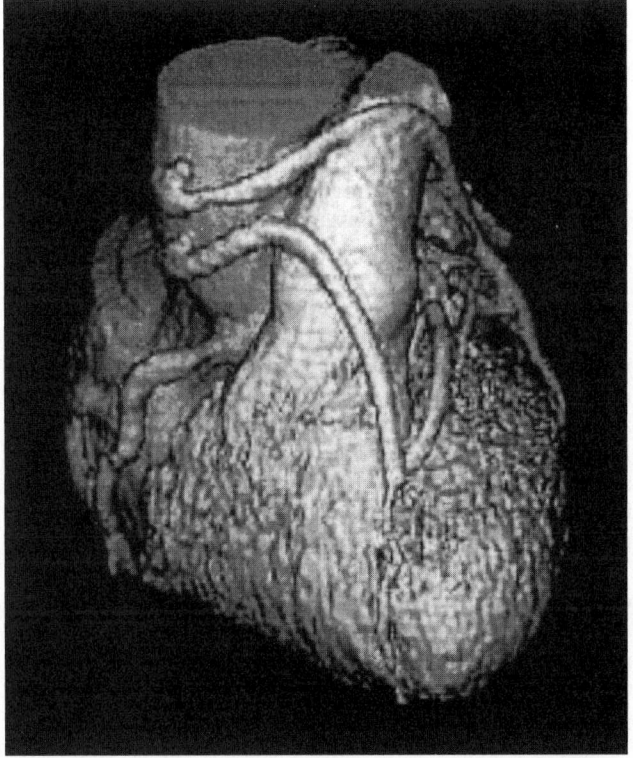

FIGURE 29-23 ■ Three-dimensional electron beam angiography showing bypass grafts.

BOX 29-6 ■ ■ ■
APPLICATIONS OF MAGNETIC RESONANCE IMAGING IN CARDIOVASCULAR MEDICINE

Current Clinical Applications
- Assessment of right and left ventricular function, volumes, and mass
- Assessment of myocardial viability
- Assessment of different cardiomyopathies
- Dilated cardiomyopathy
- Hypertrophic cardiomyopathy
- Arrhythmogenic right ventricular dysplasia
- Restrictive cardiomyopathy
- Sarcoidosis
- Amyloidosis
- Hemochromatosis
- Endomyocardial fibrosis
- Evaluation of pericardial diseases
- Evaluation of cardiac and paracardiac masses
- Benign
- Malignant
- Evaluation of congenital heart disease including shunts
- Evaluation of valvular heart diseases
- Evaluation of aortic diseases
- Aortic dissection
- Aortic aneurysm
- Congenital disorders (coarctation of aorta and Marfan syndrome)
- Evaluation of pulmonary veins

Emerging Applications
- Assessment of myocardial perfusion and ischemia
- Atherosclerotic plaque imaging
- Coronary artery angiography and vessel wall imaging
- Therapeutic magnetic resonance imaging for electrophysiology and interventional procedures

From Lima J, Desai M: *J Am Coll Cardiol* 44:1165, 2004.

percent) in patients who have non–ST segment elevation acute coronary syndromes, with a reported sensitivity of 96 percent and a specificity of 83 percent. Cardiac MRI is also more sensitive and accurate than the TIMI (thrombolysis in myocardial infarction) risk score to detect acute coronary syndrome and the need for revascularization.[38]

Cardiac Magnetic Resonance Angiography

Cardiac magnetic resonance angiography provides a three-dimensional morphological depiction of the coronary arterial tree and allows for the noninvasive visualization of the major epicardial coronary arteries.[39] This technique was developed to overcome the limitations of conventional coronary angiography, which frequently underestimates the true burden of atherosclerosis.

The initial response to endothelial injury and development of atherosclerosis is vessel enlargement with preservation of the lumen of the coronary artery. The atheroma primarily grows outward from the lumen and, at least initially, does not encroach on the lumen. Later in the course of atherosclerotic disease, the atheroma begins to narrow the lumen and result in coronary stenosis. Coronary angiography assesses luminal vessel diameter but does not provide direct information about the characteristics of an atherosclerotic plaque. Although intravascular ultrasound does allow for direct imaging of coronary plaque, the technique is invasive, expensive, and not appropriate for routine screening. Coronary magnetic resonance angiography, however, not only can determine plaque burden but also has the ability to characterize the composition of plaques and thus identify vulnerable plaques.[34,40] Newer techniques allow for quantification of velocity and flow in coronary arteries. Initial techniques required patients to hold their breath repeatedly, a task that many patients are unable to perform or tolerate. Newer technology, referred to as "non–breath holding" or "free breathing" does not require breath holding during image acquisition.[34]

Coronary magnetic resonance angiography is most accurate in detecting stenosis in the proximal and midportion of coronary arteries,[39] but it is unable to clearly visualize the distal coronaries and branch clearly.[41] A prospective multicenter study of male and female patients referred for a first elective coronary angiogram showed that coronary magnetic resonance angiography, compared with x-ray coronary angiography, has an accuracy of 72 percent in identifying CAD (greater than 50 percent stenosis).[39] Recent meta-analysis comparing coronary magnetic resonance angiography to conventional x-ray angiography reported sensitivity of 73 percent and specificity of 86 percent for detection of CAD. Currently, clinical applications for coronary magnetic resonance angiography include imaging of known or suspected coronary anomalies, imaging of patients with coronary artery aneurysms and Kawasaki disease, imaging of native coronary arteries, and imaging of the patency of bypass grafts. Assessment of coronary stent placement is limited by artifacts created by metal stents. Coronary magnetic resonance angiography is not recommended for those with a low likelihood of CAD[41] and may be most appropriate for patients with severe left ventricular systolic dysfunction in the absence of a clinical history of myocardial infarction in which the underlying process is nonischemic cardiomyopathy or severe multivessel CAD.[39] Coronary magnetic resonance angiography has the potential to eliminate a substantial percentage of the negative invasive angiograms that occur in 20 to 40 percent of all diagnostic invasive x-ray coronary angiograms done today and therefore may be most beneficial in patients with atypical chest pain and equivocal stress test results. As the technology becomes more sophisticated, it becomes necessary to determine which population groups will achieve the greatest benefit from these noninvasive studies.

Patient Preparation

Because the strong magnetic field used for coronary MRI will attract any iron-containing object in the body, patients with a cardiac pacemaker, implanted defibrillator, or other implanted electronic device cannot be scanned. The test is safe in patients with joint replacements, coronary stents, atrial septal defect/patent foramen ovale closure devices, sternal wires, and most prosthetic heart valves. Patients should be questioned about a history of ferro-magnetic (iron, nickel, and cobalt) foreign object penetration (e.g., bullets). Magnetic resonance capability with the object will need to be ascertained. Similarly, sheet metal workers and persons with potential exposure to small metal fragments should be screened for the possibility of metal shards in the eyes using x-ray films of the skull. Although the test should be avoided in pregnant women, if the risk outweighs the benefits, consideration is given to performing the test during pregnancy.[42] Patients who are uncertain as to whether they are pregnant are required to have a screening urine or blood pregnancy test. Intravenous contrast medium usually is contraindicated in pregnant patients. The contrast medium gadolinium-DTPA (diethylenetriamine pentaacetic acid) is non-iodine-based and therefore can be used in patients with iodine or shellfish allergies.

Similar preparation to that previously described is needed if the test is combined with pharmaceutical agents (adenosine, dipyridamole [Persantine], or dobutamine.) With the exception of the standard food and medication restrictions associated with pharmaceutical agents, there are no food or medication restrictions. Most patients tolerate the procedure without sedation, although severely claustrophobic patients may need to be sedated. Earphones are worn by patients to minimize noise perception.

The radio frequency fields generated during imaging can induce electrical currents to flow and can result in skin burns. Therefore, before the test, patients need to remove all readily removable metal personal belongings and devices (e.g., zippers, watches, jewelry, pagers, cell phones, body piercings, metallic drug delivery patches). Warn patients who have skin staples or superficial metal sutures that they may experience warmth or even burning along the distribution line.[42] Have them immediately alert the technician if they experience warmth or burning sensations during the study. When needed, cold compresses, can be placed on the area. Other external devices that may cause skin burns include pulse oximetry and ECG cables. Radio frequency also can heat areas of extensive or dark tattoos, including tattooed eyeliner. Cold compresses may be needed in this situation. Additionally, patients with tattoos that have been placed within 48 hours should be advised of the potential for smearing or smudging of the edges. The length of the test depends on the reason for the test; assessment of ventricular function requires approximately 15 to 20 minutes, whereas imaging for complex congenital heart disease or coronary artery visualization may require 60 to 70 minutes.

■■■ TECHNOLOGY: IMAGING

- Molecular imaging to detect atherosclerosis and vascular vulnerability[142]
- Improved motion compensation techniques and novel imaging sequences (steady state free precession) for coronary magnetic angiography

---

In summary, this chapter has reviewed the exercise testing and noninvasive imaging procedures widely used to provide detailed information about cardiac function for diagnostic, prognostic, and functional purposes. The knowledge garnered from studying this chapter can assist in using and interpreting these tests.

REFERENCES

1. Ellestad M: *Stress testing: principles and practice,* ed 5, Oxford, 2003, Oxford University Press.
2. Fletcher GF, Balady GJ, Amsterdam AE et al: Exercise standards for testing and training: a statement for healthcare professionals from the American Heart Association, *Circulation* 104:1694-1740, 2001.
3. Nishime E, Cole C, Blackstone E et al: Heart-rate recovery and treadmill exercise score as predictors of mortality in patients referred for exercise ECG, *JAMA* 284:1392-1398, 2000.
4. Tecce M, Dasgupta I, Doherty J: Heart disease in older women: gender differences affect diagnosis and treatment, *Geriatrics* 58:33-39, 2003.
5. Mora S, Redberg R, Cui Y et al: Ability of exercise testing to predict cardiovascular and all-cause death in asymptomatic women: a 20-year follow-up of the lipid research clinics prevalence study, *JAMA* 290:1600-1607, 2003.
6. Zecchin RP, Chai YY, Roach KA et al: Is nurse-supervised exercise stress testing safe practice? *Heart Lung* 28:175-185, 1999.
7. Rodgers GP, Ayanian JZ, Balady G et al: American College of Cardiology/American Heart Association Clinical Competence statement on stress testing: a report of the American College of Cardiology/American Heart Association/American College of Physicians-American Society of Internal Medicine Task Force on Clinical Competence, *J Am Coll Cardiol* 36:1441-1453, 2000.
8. Gibbons RJ, Balady GJ, Bricker J et al: ACC/AHA 2002 guideline update for exercise testing: summary article—a report of the American College of Cardiology/American Heart Association Task Force on Practice Guidelines (Committee to Update the 1997 Exercise Testing Guidelines), *J Am Coll Cardiol* 40:1531-1540, 2002.
9. Villella M, Villella A, Barlera S et al: Prognostic significance of double product and inadequate double product response to maximal symptom-limited exercise stress testing after myocardial infarction in 6296 patients treated with thrombolytic agents, *Am Heart J* 137:443-452, 1999.
10. Dominguez H, Torp-Pedersen C, Koeber L et al: Prognostic value of exercise testing in a cohort of patients followed for 15 years after acute myocardial infarction, *Eur Heart J* 22:300-306, 2001.
11. Spin JM, Prakash M, Froelicher VF et al: The prognostic value of exercise testing in elderly men, *Am J Med* 112:453-459, 2002.
12. Kwok JM, Miller TD, Dodge DO et al: Prognostic value of the Duke treadmill score in the elderly, *J Am Coll Cardiol* 39:1475-1481, 2003.
13. Antham E, Anbe DT, Armstrong PW et al: ACC/AHA guidelines for the management of patients with ST-elevation myocardial infarction: a report of the American College of Cardiology/American Heart Association Task Force on Practice Guidelines (Committee to Revise the 1999 Guidelines for the Management of patients with acute myocardial infarction), *J Am Coll Cardiol* 44:E1-E211, 2004.
14. Michaelides A, Psomadaki ZD, Aigyptiadou MN et al: Significance of exercise-induced ST changes in leads aVR, V5, and V1: discrimination of patients with single- or multi-vessel coronary artery disease, *Clin Cardiol* 26:226-230, 2003.
15. Ellis K, Pothier CE, Blackstone EH et al: Is systolic blood pressure recovery after exercise a predictor of mortality? *Am Heart J* 147:287-292, 2004.
16. Lauer MS, Okin PM, Larson MG et al: Impaired heart rate response to graded exercise: prognostic implications of chronotropic incompetence in the Framingham Heart Study, *Circulation* 93:1520-1526, 1996.
17. Cole CR, Blackstone EH, Pashkow FJ et al: Heart-rate recovery immediately after exercise as a predictor of mortality, *N Engl J Med* 341:1351-1357, 1999.
18. Bunch TJ, Chandrasekaran K, Gersh BJ et al: The prognostic significance of exercise-induced atrial arrhythmias, *J Am Coll Cardiol* 43:1236-1240, 2004.
19. Frolkis JP, Pothier JC, Blackstone EH et al: Frequent ventricular ectopy after exercise as a predictor of death, *N Engl J Med* 348:781-790, 2003.
20. Elhendy A, Bax JJ, Geleijnse ML et al: Relation among exercise-induced ventricular arrhythmias, myocardial ischemia, and viability late after acute myocardial infarction, *Am J Cardiol* 86:723-729, 2000.
21. Klocke FJ, Baird MG, Lorrell BH et al: ACC/AHA/ASNC guidelines for the clinical use of cardiac radionuclide imaging: a report of the American College of Cardiology/American Heart Association Task Force on Practice Guidelines (ACC/AHA/ASHC Committee to Revise the 1995 Guidelines for the Clinical Use of Radionuclide Imaging), *J Am Coll Cardiol* 42:1318-1333, 2003.
22. Hansen CL, Crabbe D, Rubin S: Lower diagnostic accuracy of thallium-201 SPECT myocardial perfusion imaging in women: an effect of smaller chamber size, *J Am Coll Cardiol* 28:1214-1219, 1996.
23. Gulati M, Pratap P, Kansal P et al: Gender differences in the value of ST-segment depression during adenosine stress testing, *Am J Cardiol* 94:997-1002, 2004.
24. Kim C, Kwok Y, Heagerty P et al: Pharmacologic stress testing for coronary disease diagnosis: a meta-analysis, *Am Heart J* 142:934-944, 2001.
25. Yoshinga K, Morita K, Yamada S et al: Low-dose dobutamine electrocardiograph-gated myocardial SPECT for identifying viable myocardium: comparison with dobutamine stress echocardiography and PET, *J Nucl Med* 42:838-844, 2001.
26. Douglas P, Foster E, Gorcsan J et al: ACC/AHA clinical competence statement on echocardiography: a report of the American College of Cardiology/American Heart Association/American College of Physicians-American Society of Internal Medicine Task Force on Clinical Competence, *J Am Coll Cardiol* 41:687-708, 2003.
27. Agency for Healthcare Research and Quality: *Results of systematic review of research on diagnosis and treatment of coronary heart disease in women: summary,* Evidence Report/Technology Assessment: Number 80, AHRQ Pub No 03-E034, Rockville, Md, 2003, The Agency.
28. DeCara J: Noninvasive cardiac testing in women, *J Am Med Womens Assoc* 58:254-263, 2003.
29. Picano E, Bedetti G, Varga A et al: The comparable diagnostic accuracy of dobutamine-stress and dipyridamole-stress echocardiographies: a meta-analysis, *Coron Artery Dis* 11:151-159, 2000.
30. Schmermund A, Mohlenkamp S, Erel R: Coronary artery calcium and its relationship to coronary artery disease, *Cardiol Clin* 21:521-534, 2003.

31. Haber R, Becker A, Leber A et al: Correlation of coronary calcification and angiographically documented stenoses in patients with suspected coronary artery disease: results of 1,764 patients, *J Am Coll Cardiol* 37:451-457, 2001.

32. Devries S, Wolfkiel C, Fusman B et al: Influence of age and gender on the presence of coronary calcium detected by ultrafast computed tomography, *J Am Coll Cardiol* 25:76-82, 1995.

33. Forrester J, Douglas P, Faxon D et al: American College of Cardiology/American Heart Association expert consensus document on electron-beam computed tomography for the diagnosis and prognosis of coronary artery disease, *J Am Coll Cardiol* 36:326-340, 2000.

34. Budoff M, Achenbach S, Duerinckx A: Clinical utility of computed tomography and magnetic resonance techniques for noninvasive coronary angiography, *J Am Coll Cardiol* 42:1867-1178, 2003.

35. Achenbach S, Moshage W, Ropers D: Noninvasive, three-dimensional visualization of coronary artery bypass grafts by electron beam tomography, *Am J Cardiol* 79:856-861, 1997.

36. Lima J, Desai M: Cardiovascular magnetic resonance imaging: current and emerging applications, *J Am Coll Cardiol* 44:1164-1171, 2004.

37. Nagel E, Lehmkuhl H, Bocksch W et al: Noninvasive diagnosis of ischemia-induced wall motion abnormalities with the use of high-dose dobutamine stress MRI: comparison with dobutamine stress echocardiography, *Circulation* 99:763-770, 1999.

38. Paetsch I, Gebker R, Fleck E et al: Cardiac magnetic resonance (CMR) imaging: a noninvasive tool for functional and morphological assessment of coronary artery disease: current clinical applications and potential future concepts, *J Interv Cardiol* 16:457-463, 2003.

39. Kim W, Danias P, Stuber M et al: Coronary magnetic resonance angiography for the detection of coronary stenoses, *N Engl J Med* 345:1863-1869, 2001.

40. Yuan C, Kerwin W: MRI of atherosclerosis, *J Magn Reson Imaging* 19:710-719, 2004.

41. Danias P, Roussakis A, Ioannidis J: Diagnostic performance of coronary magnetic resonance angiography as compared against conventional x-ray angiograph: a meta-analysis, *J Am Coll Cardiol* 44:1867-1876, 2004.

42. Kanal E, Borgstede J, Barkovich A et al: American College of Radiology white paper on MR safety: 2004 update and revisions, *AJR Am J Roentgenol* 182:1111-1114, 2004.

■■■ chapter **30**

Contributions of Clinical Pharmacists

Wendy Gattis Stough

CHAPTER ABBREVIATIONS

ACE   angiotensin-converting enzyme

CI   confidence interval

INR   international normalized ratio

PharmD   doctor of pharmacy

PHARM   Pharmacist Assessment Recommendation and Monitoring (Study)

V_d volume of distribution

Pharmacotherapy management in patients with cardiovascular disease is a complex process. Focus must be placed on ensuring that cost-effective, evidence-based therapies are prescribed and monitored appropriately. Medication errors and adverse effects can occur because of unrecognized pharmacodynamic and pharmacokinetic alterations.

Pharmacists are uniquely qualified to focus on the appropriate use of drugs in challenging clinical scenarios. These professionals can be extremely helpful in selecting and monitoring drug regimens, as well as providing focused patient education. Clinical pharmacy is defined as the area of pharmacy concerned with the science and practice of rational medication use.[1] This chapter reviews the role of the clinical pharmacist in the care of patients with cardiovascular disease.

Studies of the contributions of clinical pharmacists to interdisciplinary cardiovascular team management programs illustrate the important contributions made in the care of patients with heart failure, hypertension, hyperlipidemia, coronary artery disease, and diabetes.[2,3] Hypertension, hyperlipidemia, and coronary artery disease intervention programs in which pharmacists have been included have focused on long-term care and regular follow-up. In these programs, the care provided by pharmacists has emphasized teaching of self-management skills during pharmacist-managed clinics and by automated provider notices.

Programs involving the management of persons with heart failure and diabetes are typically more complex, multifaceted programs, probably because of the nature and severity of these diseases. In these programs, clinical pharmacists provide patient and physician education, promote intensive drug therapy and lifestyle modifications, and provide close patient monitoring. Multidisciplinary heart failure programs have been studied the most, so heart failure is used as the primary example in this chapter.

IMPACT ON PATIENT OUTCOMES: HEART FAILURE AS AN EXAMPLE

A multidisciplinary approach to managing heart failure has been shown to reduce rehospitalization and all-cause mortality.[4,5] Although most studies evaluated a nurse-directed multidisciplinary intervention, a few studies also have evaluated the value of adding a clinical pharmacist to the heart failure team. These studies have been conducted in long-term outpatient settings; however, the contributions of pharmacists are also evident in the acute care setting.

The Pharmacist Assessment Recommendation and Monitoring (**PHARM**) Study was the first randomized trial to evaluate the effect of including a clinical pharmacist on the heart failure team.[6] The investigators randomized 192 patients to pharmacist intervention or usual care. For patients randomized to the intervention arm, a pharmacist reviewed their medical regimen and current symptoms, recommended changes in pharmacotherapy to the attending cardiologist, provided patient education, and contacted the patient by telephone to identify new symptoms and side effects and to reinforce education principles. Patients in the usual care arm received standard follow-up, but the pharmacist was not involved in their care. The primary endpoint of the study was all-cause mortality and hospitalization or emergency department visit for heart failure. Secondary endpoints included an evaluation of angiotensin-converting enzyme (**ACE**) inhibitor use and dose prescribed.

Patients randomized to the intervention group had a lower rate of death or hospitalizations for heart failure compared with the usual care group (odds ratio, 0.22; 95 percent confidence interval [**CI**], 0.07 to 0.65; $p = 0.005$). A decrease in rehospitalization was the main contributor to this combined outcome. Additionally, patients in the intervention group were closer to the target ACE inhibitor dose compared with the usual care group ($p < 0.001$).[6]

In a similar study,[7] all patients hospitalized for heart failure during a 1 year period were evaluated for inclusion. Patients were assigned randomly to a control group or to an intervention group. Patients in the control group received routine care and discharge procedures, and a nurse reviewed their diet and medications. The intervention group received the same care; however, for these patients, the pharmacist also reviewed their medication regimen, recommended changes to their physicians, and provided education. The primary endpoint of this study was death or hospital readmission for heart failure within 1 year following discharge.

With only 38 patients, the study was too small to be adequately powered. Nonetheless, the readmission rate was more than twice as high in the control group (58.8 percent) compared with the intervention group (23.5 percent, $p < 0.05$). The combined endpoint of death or readmission occurred in 82.3 percent of the control group and 29.4 percent of the intervention group ($p < 0.01$).

Bucci and colleagues[8] conducted a study in patients with heart failure to determine the effect of a pharmacist on appropriate medication use. In addition, these investigators evaluated the pharmacist's effect on education and goal setting. In this study, 80 patients were randomized to an intervention group that received pharmacy services or to a usual care group that did not include a pharmacist. Patients were assessed at baseline and at 1 month follow-up. Medication appropriateness was assessed using the validated Medication Appropriateness Index. Although the change in the Medication Appropriateness Index score from baseline to 1 month was greater for the pharmacist intervention group, this difference did not reach statistical significance. However, the patients in the pharmacist intervention group had a significantly greater improvement in scores on a survey assessing patient education and goal setting principles ($p < 0.001$).

Bouvy and colleagues[9] evaluated the effect of a pharmacist intervention on adherence to diuretic therapy in heart failure patients. In this study, 152 patients were randomized to a pharmacist-led intervention or to usual care. Pharmacists discussed medication history and adherence issues with patients in the intervention group. Patients were contacted by the pharmacist every month for 6 months. The primary endpoint of the study was medication adherence over the study period. A medication event monitoring system was used to evaluate adherence with diuretic therapy. Nonadherence was defined as the number of days that the loop diuretic was not taken when the prescription was at least once daily. Patients in the intervention group had fewer days without diuretics compared with the usual care group. The relative risk for nonadherence with therapy was 0.33 (CI, 0.24 to 0.38). Failing to take diuretic therapy for 2 days or more was also lower in the intervention group, with a relative risk for nonadherence of 0.32 (CI, 0.19 to 0.55). Further analyses demonstrated that being in the intervention group was the only variable associated with higher adherence after adjustment for age, gender, New York Heart Association functional class, comorbidity, and being enrolled in a heart failure clinic.

Together, these studies illustrate that the addition of a clinical pharmacist to the multidisciplinary team can increase medication adherence and decrease rehospitalization and death, at least for persons with heart failure. Research among other patient populations shows similar positive results.[2,3]

Ongoing studies will provide more data on the role of the pharmacist in the care of heart failure patients. Murray and colleagues[10] are conducting a study in elderly heart failure patients with low health literacy to determine whether pharmacist intervention will improve medication adherence in this vulnerable population. In this study, patients are randomized to a pharmacist intervention consisting of verbal and written education, icon-based labeling of medication containers, and therapeutic monitoring. The pharmacist identifies barriers to appropriate drug use and designs strategies for the patient and the primary physician on how to overcome these barriers. The study is ongoing, but once completed, will provide important information on a high-risk group of patients.

KEY ROLES FOR PHARMACISTS

Pharmacists play several key roles in the management of patients with cardiovascular disease. First, pharmacists provide a clinical service in terms of designing an optimal drug regimen. This role encompasses cardiovascular and noncardiovascular therapy. Pharmacists can play a major role in ensuring that evidence-based therapies (statins, ACE inhibitors, angiotensin receptor blockers, beta blockers, aldosterone antagonists, antihypertensive therapies) are prescribed and dosed appropriately. In addition, some of these agents have similar pharmacodynamic effects, and the pharmacist can be useful in providing recommendations to minimize side effects related to pharmacodynamic interactions. Pharmacists also can review medication regimens for therapies that counteract other aspects of the treatment regimen. For example, nonsteroidal anti-inflammatory drugs may increase fluid retention in patients with heart failure. Assessment of drug interactions is also a key component of a pharmacist's drug regimen assessment, as is evaluation of hepatic or renal function to ensure any required dosage adjustments have been made. Pharmacists can be a core resource for patients and care providers on the safe use of herbal products.[11]

Patients have more access to pharmacists than to any other health care provider. With this easy access, a pharmacist may be the first provider asked about symptoms or possible adverse effects of medications. Pharmacists are also a useful resource in the development of educational materials used in inpatient, outpatient, home health, and retail settings.[12,13] Pharmacists are important collaborators in provider education. Diagnostic and management barriers exist for busy clinicians working in primary care settings, so pharmacists may be helpful in selecting and monitoring appropriate medications.[14]

In acute care and other institutional settings, pharmacists are important to include on quality improvement teams. Their expertise in evaluating drug use is helpful in establishing how systems can be improved to ensure that evidence-based medicines are prescribed.[15] Once deficiencies have been defined, pharmacists can work with other team members to develop medication protocols and care maps to ensure that all patients who are candidates for evidence-based therapies receive them.[16] Areas where the pharmacist's expertise can be particularly useful in the management of patients with cardiovascular disease are detailed in Table 30-1.

■ ■ ■

TABLE 30-1   AREAS OF PHARMACIST EXPERTISE IN PATIENT MANAGEMENT

MANAGEMENT AREA	EXPERTISE
Drug selection	Pharmacological properties of drugs differ, even among drugs in the same class. Pharmacists can help select the right drug for specific patients, for example, by avoiding or adjusting a renally excreted drug in a patient with renal failure or selecting a beta$_1$-selective beta blocker in a patient with pulmonary disease. This approach minimizes side effects and improves drug tolerability.
Dose initiation and adjustment	Pharmacists can ensure appropriate dosages by accounting for patient-specific characteristics, comorbid conditions, concurrent medications, and patient response to therapy.
Pharmacokinetic drug interactions	The risk of drug interactions is high in patients who take several drugs, and interactions may occur with cardiac and noncardiac drugs. Many cardiac patients take digoxin, amiodarone, and warfarin, all of which have a high potential for drug interactions. The pharmacist can predict interactions and offer suggestions to avoid or minimize them.
Pharmacokinetic alterations	Pharmacokinetics may be altered in certain patients, such as those with heart failure, because of changes in absorption, distribution, metabolism, and excretion. Because pharmacists understand the potential for these changes, they can help select appropriate drugs and doses.
Pharmacodynamic interactions	Heart failure patients receive multiple drugs with similar pharmacodynamic effects. For example, angiotensin-converting enzyme (ACE) inhibitors, beta blockers, and diuretics all lower blood pressure. ACE inhibitors, aldosterone antagonists, potassium supplements, and salt substitutes can cause hyperkalemia. Diuretics can increase activation of the renin-angiotensin-aldosterone system that already exists in persons with heart failure, making them more sensitive to hypotensive effects of ACE inhibitors and beta blockers. Pharmacists can develop strategies for the timing of drug administration or make other recommendations, as for needed laboratory tests, to minimize the risk of pharmacodynamic interactions.
Comorbidities	Patients with chronic cardiovascular disease commonly have comorbid conditions, such as diabetes, ischemic heart disease, pulmonary disease, arthritis, or other conditions that increase the difficulty of managing their cardiovascular disease. The pharmacist can help select and monitor drugs such as beta blockers in patients with diabetes or pulmonary disease. In patients with arthritis and heart failure, the pharmacist can suggest alternatives to nonsteroidal antiinflammatory drugs. The pharmacist can monitor fluid retention and weight gain in the diabetic patient treated with thiazoidlinediones. In addition, the pharmacist can help manage adverse effects and develop a care plan to minimize adverse drug effects and improve tolerability and compliance.
Patient education	Patient education is a key component of successful disease management. Patients need to know more than their ACE inhibitor or beta blocker is "a heart pill." Educating patients about the uses and expected outcomes of their medications, how to take them properly (such as taking diuretics in the morning to avoid nocturia), and how to identify drug-related side effects is critical to successful disease management.
Patient assistance	Most cardiovascular patients are over age 65, and many do not have prescription coverage except for the new Medicare Part D drug plan, which may limit coverage for those who cannot pay the deductible. Thus identifying cost-effective regimens and applying for pharmaceutical company–sponsored patient assistance programs is a valuable contribution that the clinical pharmacist can make to patient care.
Process implementation	In health care systems, implementing processes and pathways is a successful approach that ensures evidence-based therapies. Pharmacists can help write drug protocols and standard orders and can participate on quality improvement teams to ensure that patients receive the best care.
Clinical research	Pharmacists may be involved in clinical trials throughout drug development. They may help coordinate study sites. They may assume responsibility for drug packaging in a double-blind clinical trial. They also address drug adherence to make sure clinical trial results reflect drug efficacy rather than patient adherence.

Data from Struthers AD, Anderson G, MacFadyen RJ et al: Nonadherence with ACE inhibitors is common and can be detected in clinical practice by routine serum ACE activity, *Congest Heart Fail* 7:43-46, 2001.

CLINICAL PHARMACIST'S ROLE IN MONITORING DRUG THERAPY

Cardiovascular diseases can influence drug absorption, distribution, metabolism, and excretion. Heart failure is used as an example of the mechanisms by which the syndrome affects pharmacokinetics.

Absorption

The absorption of medications in patients with heart failure can be altered by several mechanisms. These alterations typically result in lower systemic bioavailability. As heart failure progresses, cardiac output is reduced, leading to organ hypoperfusion. Blood flow is redirected to vital organs such as the brain and kidneys. Some organ systems, such as the gastrointestinal tract, may remain hypoperfused, and drug absorption may be reduced as a result. Reduced gastrointestinal motility and delayed gastric emptying also may contribute to

reduced absorption, which may be responsible for the gastrointestinal discomfort reported by many patients with advanced heart failure. Intestinal edema is another factor that can contribute to lower absorption and bioavailability of drugs. Intestinal edema particularly may affect lipophilic compounds.

The efficacy of oral loop diuretics often declines in patients with advanced or decompensated heart failure. Clinicians often observe worsening heart failure symptoms despite increasing diuretic doses. Reduced absorption results in lower systemic bioavailability of loop diuretics, and this process may be responsible for the inadequate diuretic response that commonly occurs in this population.

Heart failure also may affect the absorption of topical drugs because peripheral perfusion may be compromised in patients with low cardiac output. Thus, oral administration may be favored in these patients. For example, oral isosorbide dinitrate or isosorbide mononitrate may be preferable to nitroglycerin patches.

The effect of heart failure on drug absorption is likely most important for drugs that have low bioavailability. Drug absorption has not been well studied in patients with advanced heart failure, but decreased absorption should be considered as a possible cause of inadequate response to drug therapy in these patients.

Distribution

The volume of distribution (V_d) for drugs can be altered (increased or decreased) in persons with heart failure. Most commonly, V_d is reduced in central and peripheral compartments, which may be from reduced cardiac output. Theoretically, the V_d may be increased for hydrophilic drugs in patients with volume overload and preserved cardiac output because these drugs may be widely distributed in the periphery. Conversely, V_d may be reduced for lipophilic drugs in these patients. Studies of changes in V_d for drugs commonly used to treat heart failure patients are greatly needed.

Protein binding can affect V_d for highly protein-bound drugs such as phenytoin. As heart failure progresses, patients may become cachectic. The decreased albumin may affect drugs that are highly protein bound, and result in a higher free fraction of active drug. The clinical significance of this has not been well described in the literature. Drugs with a narrow therapeutic index that are highly protein bound should be monitored closely in persons with heart failure.

Metabolism

Drugs that are highly protein bound may be affected by the heart failure state as well. Hepatic metabolism may decrease because of volume overload and hepatic congestion. Hepatic metabolism also may be reduced by low cardiac output because of decreased perfusion. In these scenarios, decreased metabolism, higher levels of free drug, and long drug half-lives may occur. Patients treated with drugs such as warfarin, beta blockers, amiodarone, and phenytoin, among others, should be monitored closely. Patients receiving warfarin for anti-coagulation may have significant elevations in international normalized ratio (**INR**) during episodes of acute heart failure. The exact reactions to pharmacokinetic alterations are difficult to predict, and close monitoring is needed.

Excretion

Patients with acute decompensated heart failure also may experience changes in the excretion of drugs, particularly those excreted by the kidney. In the low-output state, renal perfusion may be decreased, resulting in a decline in renal function. In addition, high doses of diuretics given to patients with decompensated heart failure also may worsen renal function. Thus, serum creatinine level should be monitored closely, and doses of drugs that are excreted renally should be adjusted. This focused monitoring approach may be particularly important with drugs such as digoxin, aldosterone antagonists, aminoglycosides, and other renally eliminated drugs that patients with heart failure may be receiving.

Clinical Pharmacist Recommendations for Drug Monitoring

The clinical importance of potential pharmacokinetic alterations should be assessed for each drug. In addition, the need for each drug should be evaluated. Patients may be taking drugs that are unnecessary or that could worsen their state. If such drugs are identified, they should be discontinued.

For drugs with narrow therapeutic indices in which a pharmacokinetic alteration is expected, drug levels should be obtained if indicated. For example, obtaining a digoxin level would be appropriate in a patient—particularly an elderly patient—with new or worsening renal insufficiency. Drug doses should be adjusted as indicated to account for significant alterations in absorption, distribution, metabolism, and excretion, as well as the presence of other interacting drugs.

Therapies also should be adjusted once symptoms of congestion have been resolved in patients who have episodes of decompensated heart failure. Often patients are discharged with higher doses of diuretics than necessary because they were receiving higher doses during a heart failure hospitalization. Similarly, if doses of other drugs were decreased (such as warfarin) because of hepatic congestion or decreased metabolism, they may need to be increased to the dose the patient was taking before admission. For therapies such as warfarin, the INR should be monitored and the dose adjusted as indicated.

REQUIRED COMPETENCIES OF CLINICAL PHARMACISTS

The doctoral degree is required for entry into clinical practice for pharmacists. In 1997, the doctor of pharmacy (**PharmD**) became the sole professional practice degree for pharmacy in the United States when the Accreditation Council of Pharmacy Education adopted new accreditation standards and guidelines.[17] The implementation timeline for the new standards required transition for students who were enrolled in accredited baccalaureate pharmacy programs already. Further, collaborative health care practice legislation now exists in more than 40 states, which specifies an expanded patient care role for pharmacists.

For pharmacists making rounds on inpatient teams or participating in disease management programs (e.g., heart failure clinics and diabetes programs), advanced clinical training is needed. This training could include postgraduate residency training, cardiology pharmacy fellowships, or certification in pharmacotherapy through the Board of Pharmaceutical Specialties with additional qualifications in cardiology (*www.bpsweb.org/default. shtml*). Training also may include working with an interdisciplinary, specialized team to become familiar with the clinical data supporting treatment approaches in the population. It is imperative that pharmacists assessing medical regimens and making recommendations to optimize therapy are aware of the latest clinical trial data supporting treatments in the population. Pharmacists educated by an accredited school of pharmacy will be knowledgeable regarding the pharmacokinetic and pharmacodynamic considerations discussed. However, they may benefit from a refresher course on disease pathophysiology and the current guidelines regarding patient management, especially in settings where pharmacists may have prescriptive authority, as in Veterans Administration facilities.

Pharmacists in other outpatient or retail settings have the knowledge foundation required to provide patient education on specific drug therapies. Ambulatory care pharmacists can help support continuity of care and act as a bridge between inpatient and outpatient care settings. However, these professionals also may benefit from focused educational sessions to learn the most recent information on epidemiology, pathophysiology, disease progression, and guidelines for recommended therapy.

CONCLUSION

Cardiovascular diseases are complex with unique medication management issues. Having a health care provider with specialized knowledge in pharmacology and therapeutics can be extremely helpful to the successful management of these patients. Clinical pharmacists can play an important role as members of interdisciplinary care teams. Their unique expertise regarding drug therapy can influence multiple components of care. Programs that truly use their pharmacists' talents have them involved assessing patients and disease states, evaluating current medication therapy, recommending changes to current and new drug therapy, creating a monitoring plan for the patient's disease state and overall pharmacotherapy, and constantly evaluating the medical literature. Pharmacists are an easily accessible resource to patients and colleagues.[18]

REFERENCES

1. American College of Clinical Pharmacy: *Clinical Pharmacy Defined.* Retrieved December 10, 2006. www.accp.com/clinical_pharmacy.php.
2. Ara S: A literature review of cardiovascular disease management programs in managed care populations, *J Manag Care Pharm* 10:326-344, 2004.
3. Clifford RM, Davis WA, Batty KT et al: Effect of a pharmaceutical care program on vascular risk factors in type 2 diabetes: the Fremantle Diabetes Study, *Diabetes Care* 28:771-776, 2005.
4. McAlister FA, Stewart S, Ferrua S et al: Multidisciplinary strategies for the management of heart failure patients at high risk for admission: a systematic review of randomized trials, *J Am Coll Cardiol* 44:810-819, 2004.
5. Holland R, Battersby J, Harvey I et al: Systematic review of multidisciplinary interventions in heart failure, *Heart* 91:899-960, 2005.
6. Gattis WA, Hasselblad V, Whellan DJ et al: Reduction in heart failure events by the addition of a clinical pharmacist to the heart failure management team: results of the Pharmacist in Heart Failure Assessment Recommendation and Monitoring (PHARM) Study, *Arch Intern Med* 159:1939-1945, 1999.
7. Rainville EC: Impact of pharmacist interventions on hospital readmissions for heart failure, *Am J Health Syst Pharm* 56: 1339-1342, 1999.
8. Bucci C, Jackevicius C, McFarlane K et al: Pharmacist's contribution in a heart function clinic: patient perception and medication appropriateness, *Can J Cardiol* 19:391-396, 2003.
9. Bouvy ML, Heerdink ER, Urquhart J et al: Effect of a pharmacist-led intervention on diuretic compliance in heart failure patients: a randomized controlled study, *J Card Fail* 9:404-411, 2003.
10. Murray MD, Young JM, Morrow DG et al: Methodology of an ongoing, randomized, controlled trial to improve drug use for elderly patients with chronic heart failure. *Am J Geriatr Pharmacother* 2:53-65, 2004.
11. Amabile CM, Spencer AP: Keeping your patient with heart failure safe: a review of potentially dangerous medications, *Arch Intern Med* 164:709-720, 2004.
12. Fradette M, Bungard TJ, Simpson SH et al: Development of educational materials for congestive heart failure patients, *Am J Health Syst Pharm* 61:386-389, 2004.
13. Patel K, Sansgiry SS, Miller L: Pharmacist participation in home health heart failure programs, *Am J Health Syst Pharm* 60: 2259-2260, 2003.
14. Bennett AA, Brien JE, Macdonald PS: Barriers to diagnosing and managing heart failure in primary care, *Med J Aust* 182:309, 2005.
15. Pearson GJ, Cooke C, Simmons WK et al: Evaluation of the use of evidence-based angiotensin converting enzyme inhibitor criteria for the treatment of congestive heart failure: opportunities for pharmacists to improve patient outcomes, *J Clin Pharm Ther* 26:351-361, 2001.
16. Struthers AD, Anderson G, MacFadyen RJ et al: Nonadherence with ACE inhibitors is common and can be detected in clinical practice by routine serum ACE activity, *Congest Heart Fail* 7: 43-46, 2001.
17. Accreditation Council for Pharmacy Education: *Implementation procedures for accreditation standards and guidelines for the professional program in pharmacy leading to the doctor of pharmacy degree.* Retrieved February 26, 2006 from www.acpe-accredit.org/standards/standards2.asp
18. Gonzalez LS: What are pharmacists, and what do they do? *Am J Health Syst Pharm* 62:2039-2040, 2005.

■ ■ ■ chapter 31

Role of the Cardiac Health Psychologist: Expanding Opportunities

Varda Konstam

CHAPTER ABBREVIATIONS

CBT cognitive-behavioral therapy
CHD coronary heart disease

"In the narrative of every human life and every family, illness is a prominent character."[1]

Coronary heart disease (**CHD**) involves a range of cardiac problems including angina, myocardial infarction, heart failure, dysrhythmias, syncope, and sudden cardiac death. As the leading cause of death and disability in the United States (494,384 deaths in 2002), CHD consumes a large portion of the nation's health budget. The number of persons diagnosed with CHD will continue to increase, in part due to technological and medical advances that prolong life.[2]

Compelling data link behavioral and psychological factors with the onset and progression of CHD.[3] Evidence suggests that psychosocial and behavioral risk factors such as smoking, diet, types A and D behavior, lack of social support, stress, self-efficacy, depression, anxiety, and hostility can influence medical outcomes in patients with CHD. The health psychologist is positioned to influence medical outcomes by providing expertise, in collaboration with related personnel, to reduce the harmful impact of psychological and behavioral factors.[3,4]

Concerted efforts are being made to implement integrated, cost-effective health care services that bring together the expertise and diverse perspectives of the cardiologist, internist, nursing staff, health psychologist, social worker, and others. For example, billing practices recently have changed to reflect this shift in perspective, creating fewer impediments to collaborative practice. The current climate provides exciting opportunities for health psychologists to become full partners in cardiac care.[3,4] This chapter focuses on the dynamic role of the health psychologist in providing integrated quality care to patients with CHD and their support networks. A brief historical perspective is provided, followed by a discussion of the role of the health psychologist, including education and training issues. A case study is used to demonstrate possibilities regarding role functioning, followed by a discussion of assessment and intervention strategies.

HISTORICAL PERSPECTIVE

Provision of health care services has been guided by mind-body dualism, an orientation that tends to limit possibilities and restrict patient care. Recently, there has been movement toward holistic approaches that acknowledge the convergence of biological, psychological, and social factors that more closely approximate human lived experiences. Health care systems have become increasingly cognizant of the potential benefits resulting from collaboration between behavioral health providers and medical providers.[5]

Linkage between mind and body can be traced to the Huang Ti, the "Yellow Emperor" (2697 to 2597 BCE) who observed that "when the minds of the people are closed and wisdom is locked out they remain tied to disease."[6] With respect to matters of the heart, Sir William Osler, the father of internal medicine, in 1897 linked atherosclerosis with excesses of behavior, stating that excesses are "the Nemesis through which Nature exacts retributive justice for the transgression of her laws."[3] Focus on the relationship between behavioral and psychological factors and onset and progression of CHD has further solidified the field of cardiac psychology. Allan[3] states that "The most compelling data in behavioral medicine today are to be found in cardiac psychology." Fisher[7] concludes that "the benefits to individuals and society from an organized and integrated cardiac care approach cannot be minimized. Cardiac psychology is fundamental to complete cardiac care."

Research demonstrating the medical cost offset of cardiac psychology is in its infancy. The beneficial effects of an organized, integrated approach to patients with CHD need far more study. Clearly, however, lifestyle choices, difficulty with treatment adherence, and affective states such as depression and anxiety are associated with increased costs. For example, up to $5 billion of the total $20 billion cost associated with heart failure may be associated with depression.[8]

One large-scale study revealed significant medical-surgical cost savings in response to implementation of a behavioral health care system.[9] Components of the intervention included the following:

- Training psychotherapists in quality assurance
- Training psychotherapists in development and implementation of empirically derived treatment protocols
- Targeting 15 percent of the most highly utilized health services
- Providing an aggressive outreach program

Pallak and Cummings[10] report significant reduction of medical-surgical days and a decrease in inpatient treatment with immediate identification of psychiatric problems, in conjunction with appropriate referrals.

Recent reviews of cost-offset literature with respect to behavioral psychology are difficult to interpret given serious methodological shortcomings. These include poorly matched treatment and comparison conditions, failure to control for severity of illness, failure to randomize subjects to experimental and comparison conditions, failure to report whether therapists adhered to operationally defined treatment protocols, and confusion between interventions that target managing costs instead of managing care. Studies suggest, however, that the cost offset is greater in organized settings where behavioral health and medical care are integrated and where standardized treatment procedures are used that involve training and monitoring.[11]

THEORETICAL FRAMEWORK

The biopsychosocial model is the theoretical framework most closely associated with health psychology. The model emphasizes the interconnectedness among biological, psychological, social, and community factors in determining health and disease. The biopsychosocial model addresses the importance of how these factors inform one another and provides a framework for clinical application.[12,13] This approach is in harmony with existing clinical and research efforts that address issues related to optimal care within a cost-conscious economic climate and mirror the complexity of human experiences. This approach also acknowledges the importance of collaboration among the various disciplines and systems organized to deliver care to the patient with CHD and his or her family.[14]

Rolland[12,13] offers an empowering and useful approach in working with patients with CHD and their families. He proposes a framework that emphasizes the "integration of the illness, the individual, and family cycles within a multigenerational perspective. . . . Rather than apply a decontextualized idea about family pathology, [Rolland defines] function and dysfunction in terms of the fit over time between the psychosocial demands of a disorder and the strengths and vulnerabilities of a family."[13] This perspective resonates with clinicians who have observed this exact phenomenon in their patients.

The three major phases of illness—crisis, chronic, and terminal—inform treatment approaches and strategies. The health psychologist, in assessing and intervening with the patient and family, needs to understand the following[13]:

- The psychosocial demands of the illness, in the context of the illness trajectory
- The patient's and family's multigenerational experience with illness and loss
- The convergence of phase of illness with the family life cycle
- Each individual's developmental needs and family belief systems

No clear distinction is made by health psychologists between psychoeducation and counseling.

THE CARDIAC HEALTH PSYCHOLOGIST: RESPONSIBILITIES AND POSSIBILITIES

Cardiac health psychologists contribute in myriad ways, often working in multidisciplinary settings that require the ability to function as generalist and specialist. The role of the cardiac health psychologist has progressed from a traditional model focused on the at-risk patient with a possible psychopathological condition to one that requires a proactive stance. Prevention and early intervention are central. Given the goal of improving medical outcomes, cardiac health psychologists are well grounded in developmental, biopsychosocial, and systemic theory and are sensitive to the contexts in which they work (e.g., community-based and academic health centers, independent practices, and health maintenance organizations). They also understand the unique medical and psychological needs of the populations they serve.

The health psychologist, in general, is called upon to demonstrate expertise in the following:

- Assessment and intervention
- Application and individualization of cutting-edge behavioral health research findings to cardiac patient care, including conducting and participating in original and multicenter research endeavors when appropriate
- Prevention and rehabilitation in the service of improving medical outcomes

All of these responsibilities are embedded within a collaborative framework that recognizes and utilizes the expertise of medical and related personnel, as well as that of patients and their supporters.

The cardiac health psychologist serves an important role in contextualizing established evidence-based practices, resulting in a more nuanced approach that reflects the needs and experiences of CHD patients and their families.[12] For example, without addressing religious, cultural, and situational variations, the work of the cardiac health psychologist is likely to be disconnected from patients' experiences, compromising quality and relevance of care. The psychologist is positioned to provide coherence to patient care by offering the patient and family assistance in coordinating care among multiple practitioners.[13] Inclusion of the patients' significant relationships in the treatment is critical. "Interventions focused on the intimate relationships of patients [with CHD] hold the promise of improving both the quality and length of life."[12] An important note is that this model of care is consistent with demands for efficient cost-effective care based on optimal effect on health status.[14-16]

Teaching, dissemination, and research activities are critical to the collaborative stance of the cardiac health psychologist. These activities facilitate opportunities for reflection and can mitigate feelings of burnout.[16] Teaching other providers interventions grounded in theory and research is integral to the functioning of the cardiac health psychologist. Reflection and dialog provide opportunities for gaining further clarity regarding the specific issues raised in day-to-day clinical work. These integrated activities are likely to improve services and outcomes for the CHD patient and family.

The role of the cardiac health psychologist continues to evolve, informed in part by innovations and medical advances that have occurred in the field. Results across the spectrum of CHD suggest that prevention is a key component to ensuring patient longevity and health-related quality of life. Screening and intervention programs that address the unique needs of the patient population can be implemented in human service delivery systems that are collaborative, inclusive, and respectful of the individual's and supporters' needs.[16] The cardiac health psychologist serves on multidisciplinary clinical teams designed to address issues related to reducing the risk of mortality and morbidity, such as designing and implementing psychosocial interventions that change behaviors associated with increased risk, such as tobacco use.

With respect to CHD, opportunities and challenges exist in terms of meeting and incorporating the needs of individuals currently underserved and at risk.[16-18] Evidence suggests that individuals in the lower socioeco-nomic classes are 3 times more likely to die of CHD than those in the highest class. They are more likely to smoke, have trouble with weight management, and experience loss of control over their lives, resulting in a magnified sum effect greater than its parts.[19] Delivery of services needs to be embedded in public health and social policy initiatives that actively address health inequalities.[20] The cardiac health psychologist works with providers and communities to forward the agenda of decreasing health disparities. The role of the cardiac health psychologist incorporates a holistic strength-based approach designed to improve medical outcomes and influence policies that address individual and public health goals.

The expertise of patients with CHD and their families needs to be acknowledged and better integrated in CHD service delivery models.[21,22] In keeping with the need to honor the expertise of CHD patients and their families, Child[23] notes that "Patients [and their families] can contribute enormously both in planning optimal

---

BOX 31-1
CASE EXAMPLE   ■ ■ ■

The case of Mr. C. illustrates how a cardiac health psychologist adds to patient care. This case raises issues related to assessment and intervention, specifically how to best proceed in establishing a working alliance that effectively will address concerns related to adherence, lifestyle choices, and affective states (depression, anxiety, and hostility). Cardiac health psychologists can make significant inroads in providing services that are individually tailored to the needs and motivation levels of their patients. This case highlights the challenges of providing psychological care that strives toward responsible evidence-based practice designed to improve medical outcomes. This approach is consistent with current medical approaches to cardiac patient care:

We must continually remind ourselves that we practice medicine on single patients, and we seek an individual response that may not match the mean effect of an intervention in a large trial. The challenge . . . is to combine the data from these trials with other therapeutic and patient related insights . . . to manage the care of a single person.[24]

Description
Mr. C., a 74-year-old black retired widower diagnosed with heart failure and diabetes mellitus, was referred by his cardiologist because of concerns regarding adherence with his medications and recommended diet. He has one daughter, Mrs. D., a 55-year-old divorced publishing executive with two adolescent children. Mr. C. reports feeling depressed and, at times, anxious. He significantly disengaged from his support system after his wife died 2 years ago.

Mr. C. has been struggling with finding meaning since his wife's death and admits to being too depressed at times to take his medicines. He is a meticulous man and has found it physically and emotionally difficult to maintain a household. He states that he misses his wife, particularly her good cooking and overall competence in providing a home that "ran smoothly." Mr. C. was hesitant to follow through on his cardiologist's recommendation for psychotherapy, but he reluctantly agreed.

Therapist Approach
The therapist, Dr. D., used life-review therapy initially, an approach that allowed Mr. C. to look back and reflect on his life and to develop a therapeutic working alliance with Dr. D.[25] Simultaneously, Dr. D. made a referral for evaluation for psychotropic medication based on his observation of depression and anxiety. He also recommended short-term group therapy with a focus on adaptation to chronic illness.

Through the process of reminiscing, Dr. D. facilitated discussion of decisions and choices made by Mr. C. For example, Mr. C. shared that he felt guilty in relation to Mrs. C. and questioned his adequacy as a caretaker during her illness with breast cancer. Dr. D. helped Mr. C. acknowledge what he was able to do for Mrs. C., not only during her illness but also during their 46 years of marriage. Mr. C. also was able to articulate what he wished he could have done differently in his relationship with his wife, and he worked toward acceptance of himself.

Dr. D. elicited the richness of Mr. C.'s life narrative and acknowledged nuance and complexity when possible. He empathized with the difficult choices that Mr. C. had faced and worked toward helping him understand and accept choices made, not only related to his wife's illness but also his own illness. Past positive encounters between Mr. and Mrs. C. that provided Mr. C. with meaning were reinforced.[26] Mr. C. was evaluated for psychotropic medication in the initial stages of the therapy.

Issues related to adherence were explored. Mr. C. was urged to view adherence as a relative term rather than an all-or-nothing dichotomy. Triggers for difficulties with adherence were identified, and alternative strategies were generated, including a plan for lapses. Efforts were made to identify relationships and activities that provided meaning and purpose to Mr. C. in the past.

Patient Response
Mr. C. responded well to medication for depression and anxiety. Though Mr. C. politely rejected Dr. D.'s recommendation for group therapy, Mr. C. did not rule out considering it in the future. The patient reconnected with his church, a place that previously provided him with comfort. Mr. C. resumed his volunteer role, providing assistance to the church on matters related to budget. He also resumed attending church services regularly.

Dr. D. recommended weekly meetings with his daughter using a family systems approach. Initially, Mr. C. was reticent about family meetings; however, after several meetings, he was able to share his frustration with what he experienced as her overbearing yet caring manner. As an outgrowth of the family meetings, Mr. C. reconnected with his grandchildren, serving as an additional resource in assisting them with school work on an as-needed basis.

Dr. D. was able to work effectively with Mr. C., initially a reluctant participant, offering him renewed hope and acceptance, which in turn provided a vehicle for Mr. C. to reinvest and reengage with previous meaningful activities.

service delivery models to suit their needs, and also in service delivery by contributing their enormous body of experience and expertise in the support and education of other patients. This can be implemented . . . by involving patients who have CHD, who have experienced recovery from an acute episode and adaptation to life with a chronic disease or have experienced lifestyle changes." The health psychologist is positioned optimally to propel this agenda.

Compelling data exist regarding the benefits of cardiac rehabilitation. Linden and colleagues,[22] based on the findings of a meta-analysis, reported that the addition of psychosocial interventions to rehabilitation programs significantly reduced mortality by approximately 40 percent 2 years postintervention. Child[23] presents promising cardiac rehabilitation delivery service models, embedded within a continuum of services designed to meet the individual needs of patients and their families. She observes that programs are "moving towards a menu-driven approach, where the patient chooses the components that are most relevant, and is supported in this decision-making by the healthcare team. This can include a range of interventions in different settings, delivered by a range of [health care professionals]." The cardiac health psychologist, in collaboration with nurses and other team members, is skilled to implement such programs. What is needed is a flexible approach that offers patients with CHD choices based on perceived needs and existing levels of motivation (Box 31-1). More recently, technological advances have resulted in the cardiac health psychologist using technology as a resource in enhancing functioning and health-related quality of life for patients with CHD. For example, therapy consultations have been provided by telephone and e-mail.

EDUCATION AND TRAINING

Many pathways are available to becoming a health psychologist. Given the expanding role of the health psychologist, guidelines have been developed to ensure quality in education and training. As early as 1983, the Arden House Working Conference on Education and Training in Health Psychology developed guidelines specifying that psychologists first be trained as generalists and then as specialists.[27] The consensus is that didactic and experiential components are critical to the training of a health psychologist. The American Psychological Association Council of Representatives (1993) established board certification in clinical health psychology as a distinct specialty. Those individuals who wish to demonstrate expertise in health psychology may apply for board certification. Competencies developed for primary care psychologists can serve as a model for future development and refinement of the role of the health psychologist. Papas and colleagues[27] provide a more thorough discussion of the educational opportunities available for health psychologists. The Division of Health Psychology (Division 38) of the American Psychological Association provides directories of educational and training opportunities at the doctoral, internship, and postdoctoral levels.

ASSESSMENT AND INTERVENTION

The process of assessment, particularly when it is linked to intervention, is critical to ensuring optimal medical and psychosocial outcomes.[7] Assessment includes thorough understanding of the unique contributions of the historical and cultural experiences of CHD patients and their families.[1,28-32] The practice of good therapy, when linked to the process of assessment, in part emerges from the "resonance" between the therapist, the patient, and the patient's support network. Successful linkage results in the patient discovering new and more satisfying responses to challenges presented by the illness. Kathy Cole-Kelly,[29] a therapist who works with chronically ill patients states, "my job is to listen for the uniqueness of each tale and to understand the intersection of the medical and the psychosocial issues. In the end, I hope I offer each family ways to work with their situation that maximize their priorities, give new possibilities to their struggles, and acknowledge their valor."

Illness tends to be isolating.[30] In the context of better understanding how to balance one's illness with competing nonillness demands, sharing of feelings and thoughts within a safe and nonblaming milieu provides patients and their families a powerful venue for affirming commonalities and humanity with others.[25,26] Steinglass[30] states that "Part of 'living with illness' includes relating to professionals who seem reluctant to look squarely and honestly at the downside of the lives they have 'created' through their technologies and treatments." Group work provides a vehicle for the health psychologist to address the dehumanization that often occurs despite best intentions on the part of medical personnel.

In my own work, I have found the themes of "putting the illness in its place" and "redesigning and/or refining the dream" helpful and empowering as well.[31,32] The health psychologist can convey a message of hope, inspired by a conviction that patients and their families can find and affirm positive aspects of their lives when facing illness. The case of Mr. C. (Box 31-1) illustrates the need to acknowledge, honor, and respect lived experience. Mr. C. was not amenable to the idea of participating in time-limited group therapy. Dr. D. respected Mr. C.'s judgment but did not rule out the possibility of participation in the future.

Cardiac health psychologists often are asked to assist in the assessment and treatment of depression, anxiety, and less frequently, hostility, which are risk factors associated with the onset and progression of CHD.[33,34] Collaborative efforts with related medical personnel are key in ensuring effective patient care. Nurses are particularly well positioned to work collaboratively with cardiac health psychologists. Data-driven guidelines are needed to inform practitioners how to proceed optimally with CHD patients who have anxiety, depression, or hostility. Questions remain about the optimal timing of psychosocial and pharmacological interventions (i.e., the juncture at which pharmacological interventions should be considered in addition to cognitive behavioral interventions).[35]

Building on existing knowledge to inform future direction in clinical care is an important agenda for the health psychologist. For example, features of cognitive-behavioral therapy (**CBT**) have been identified as key to positive outcomes in depression, and they appear to be applicable to anxiety as well.[35] These features include the following:

- Providing rationale for treatment
- Providing highly structured and clear plans for change, including the provision of a sense of control
- Providing feedback and support so that patients can receive support and attribute improvement to their own abilities and efforts
- Teaching skills that increase personal effectiveness and independence

Patients with CHD can be helped with identifying cognitive and bodily cues, as well as patterns of interactions that exacerbate, maintain, and/or improve their emotional states and overall well-being.[35] Teaching relaxation and cognitive coping skills such as cognitive restructuring of negative cognitions can be helpful and empowering to patients adapting to CHD and are within the purview of the health psychologist. The health psychologist can make significant contributions in systematically applying principles of CBT that address and respect lived experiences, informed in part by stage and severity of illness.

A need exists to acknowledge relapse rates when working with emotional states such as depression and anxiety in patients with CHD, particularly given the interplay between the episodic nature of emotional states such as depression and the episodic exacerbations of CHD. Relapse prevention and planning, in the context of assessment and intervention, is an important contribution of the health psychologist.

In the case of Mr. C. (Box 31-1), Dr. D. determined that a life-review approach would be helpful initially, followed by more traditional CBT approaches to address depression, anxiety, and issues related to treatment adherence. Mr. C. responded well to medication for depression and anxiety. Mr. C.'s case shows that approaches should be tailored to address individual motivation levels and unique circumstances, including stage of illness. Working through issues related to the loss of his wife enabled Mr. C. to engage in behaviors that were critical to his self-care.

An important resource in coping with CHD is social support.[36,37] Social support provides a vehicle by which patients can experience a sense of well-being and counteract avoidance coping behaviors such as denial and behavioral disengagement behaviors associated with poor health outcomes for patients with CHD. Bohachick and colleagues[38] suggest that successful psychosocial interventions should focus not only on reinforcing personal control but also on building and maintaining networks of helpfulness and attachments. Although there is an extensive literature that reinforces the importance of social support with cardiac patients, little is known about how to intervene effectively with patients at risk with respect to social support. Dr. D. was able to mobilize natural social networks that previously sustained Mr. C. The cardiac health psychologist acknowledged and worked with Mr. C.'s religious/spiritual life. Based on current trends, future training efforts, rather than fragmenting or isolating the religious/spiritual dimension, increasingly will focus on integrating patients' psychological and religious/spiritual lives.

CONCLUSIONS

The current health care climate provides health psychologists exciting opportunities to make continuing inroads in improving cardiac patient medical outcomes. The cardiac health psychologist is well positioned to collaborate with multidisciplinary team members to design and implement programs to improve medical outcomes. Health psychologists, in collaboration with nurses and others, can assist with critical issues such as treatment adherence and assist in implementing integrated prevention and intervention programs designed to improve medical outcomes.

Although there is increasing emphasis on a quick fix without adequate acknowledgment of the complexity of patients' experiences in adapting to illness, assessment and intervention practices are becoming increasingly collaborative, using the expertise of nurses, other personnel, and the patients' significant relationships. Tensions exist within a cost-effective climate, and attempts are being made to integrate the combined expertise of multiple disciplines servicing the patient with CHD and the patient's family. Practitioners are questioning "one size fits all" practices and are exploring tailored interventions that reflect the complexity and nuanced experiences of patients and families.

Emphasis on the perspective of the patient, who may or may not be motivated or prepared to make the prescriptive changes needed, is being acknowledged. Efforts are being made to incorporate and work with, whenever possible, the belief systems of patients and families, who are not always positioned or motivated to make needed changes. Tensions related to other domains in the patient's life may interfere with adherence; these domains increasingly are being addressed when designing interventions. Relapse prevention and planning are neglected areas of study and practice with CHD patients, areas that deserve more attention.

The health psychologist serves a critical role in contextualizing established practices, resulting in care that is nuanced and that reflects the needs of cardiac patients and their families. Looking to the future, strength-building interventions, advocated by the positive psychology movement[39-41] are expected to generate further discussion and development. Health psychologists anticipate an increased focus on prevention and early intervention, with emphasis on health-enhancing behaviors, especially with respect to underserved populations.[41] The cardiac health psychologist increasingly will use technology as a tool to enhance patient care. Teaching and dissemination of expertise will continue to be integral to the collaborative stance of the cardiac health psychologist.

In summary, health psychology is fundamental to an integrated approach to the patient with CHD and the patient's support network. There continues to be a need to focus clinical intervention and research efforts in a direction that incorporates and is consistent with the complexities and realities of patients adapting to CHD. Incorporating the influences of religion, culture, socioeconomic status, and situational variations will decrease the likelihood that assessment and treatment efforts are disconnected from the experience of living with CHD.

REFERENCES

1. McDaniel SH, Hepworth J, Doherty WJ: The shared emotional themes of illness. In McDaniel SH, Hepworth J, Doherty WJ, editors: *The shared experience of illness: stories of patients, families, and their therapists,* New York, 1997, Basic Books.
2. Thom T, Haase N, Rosamond W, et al. Heart disease and stroke statistics—2006 update: a report from the American Heart Association Statistics Committee and Stroke Statistics Subcommittee. *Circulation* 113:e85-151, 2006.
3. Allan R: Introduction: the emergence of cardiac psychology. In Allan R, Scheidt S, editors: *Heart and mind,* Washington, DC, 1996, American Psychological Association.
4. Bray JH, Frank RG, McDaniel SH, Heldring M: Education, practice, and research opportunities for psychologists in primary care. In Frank RG, McDaniel SH, Bray JH, Heldring M, editors: *Primary care psychology,* Washington, DC, 2004, American Psychological Association.
5. Wilson PG: The air force experience: integrating behavioral health providers into primary care. In Frank RG, McDaniel SH, Bray JH, Heldring M, editors: *Primary care psychology,* Washington, DC, 2004, American Psychological Association.
6. Straus MB: *Familiar medical quotations,* Boston, 1968, Little, Brown.
7. Fisher J: Is there a need for cardiac psychology? The view of a practicing cardiologist. In Allan R, Scheidt S, editors: *Heart and mind,* Washington, DC, 1996, American Psychological Association.
8. Sullivan M, Simon G, Spertus J et al: Depression-related costs in heart failure care, *Arch Intern Med* 162:1860-1866, 2002.
9. Cummings NA, Dorken H, Pallak MS et al: Managed mental health care, Medicaid, and cost-offset: the impact of psychological services in the Hawaii-HCFA-Medicaid project. In Cummings NA, Dorken H, Pallack MS, Henke CJ, editors: *Medicaid, managed behavioral health and implications for public policy,* vol 2, *Healthcare and utilization cost series,* San Francisco, 1993, Foundation for Behavioral Health.
10. Pallak MS, Cummings NA: Inpatient and outpatient psychiatric treatment: the effect of matching patients to appropriate level of treatment on psychiatric and medical-surgical hospital days, *Applied and Preventive Psychology: Current Scientific Perspectives* 1:83-87, 1992.
11. Cummings NA: Behavioral health in primary care: dollars and sense. In Cummings NA, Cummings JL, Johnson JN, editors: *Behavioral health in primary care: a guide to clinical integration,* Madison, Conn, 1997, Psychosocial Press (International University Press).
12. Rolland JS: *Families, illness and disability: an integrative treatment model,* New York, 1994, Basic Books.
13. Rolland JS: A journey with hope, fear, and loss: young couples with cancer. In McDaniel SH, Hepworth J, Doherty WJ, editors: *The shared experience of illness: stories of patients, families, and their therapists,* New York, 1997, Basic Books.
14. Rankin-Esquer LA, Deeter A, Taylor Barr C: Coronary heart disease and couples. In Schmaling KB, Sher TG, editors: *The psychology of couples and illness: theory, research and practice,* Washington, DC, 2000, American Psychological Association.
15. Ruddy NB, McDaniel SH: Couple therapy and medical issues: working with couples facing illness. In Gurman AS, Jacobson NS, editors: *Clinical handbook of couple therapy,* ed 3, New York, 2002, Guilford Press.
16. McDaniel SH, Hargrove DS, Belar CD et al: Recommendations for education and training in primary care psychology. In Frank RG, McDaniel SH, Bray JH, Heldring M, editors: *Primary care psychology,* Washington, DC, 2004, American Psychological Association.
17. Westen D, Novotny CM, Thompson-Brenner H: The empirical status of empirically supported psychotherapies: assumptions, findings and reporting in controlled clinical trials, *Psychol Bull* 130:631-663, 2004.
18. Baum A, Perry NW, Tarbell S: The development of psychology as a health science. In Frank RG, Baum A, Wallander JL, editors: *Handbook of clinical health psychology: models and perspectives in health psychology,* Washington, DC, 2004, American Psychological Association.
19. Bor R, Miller R: HIV/AIDS, families, and the wider caregiving system. In McDaniel SH, Lusterman D, Philpot CL, editors: *Casebook for integrating family therapy: an ecosystemic approach,* Washington, DC, 2001, American Psychological Association.
20. Baggott R: *Public health, policy and politics,* Basingstoke, England, 2000, Palgrave Macmillan.
21. Baum A, Revenson TA, Singer A: *Handbook of health psychology,* Mahwak, NJ, 2001, Lawrence Erlbaum Associates.
22. Linden W, Stossel C, Maurice J: Psychosocial interventions for patients with coronary artery disease: a meta-analysis, *Arch Intern Med* 15:745-752, 1996.
23. Child A: Cardiac rehabilitation: goals, interventions and action plans, *Br J Nurs* 13(12):734-738, 2004.
24. Cohn JN: Chronic heart failure and the quality of life, *New Engl J Med* 340:1511-1512, 1999.
25. Lewis MI, Butler RN: Life review therapy: putting memories to work in individual and group psychotherapy, *Geriatrics* 29:165-169, 1974.
26. Hardy KV, Laszloffy TA: Couple therapy using a multicultural perspective. In Gurman AS, Jacobson NS, editors: *Clinical handbook of couple therapy,* New York, 2002, Guilford Press.
27. Papas RK, Belar CD, Rozensky RH: The practice of clinical health psychology: professional issues. In Frank RG, Baum A, Wallander JL, editors: *Handbook of clinical health psychology: models and perspectives in health psychology,* Washington, DC, 2004, American Psychological Association.
28. Elkaïm M: *If you love me, don't love me: constructions of reality and change in family therapy,* New York, 1990, Basic Books.
29. Cole-Kelly K: Two families, two stories: courage and chronic illness. In McDaniel SH, Hepworth J, Doherty WJ, editors: *The shared experience of illness: stories of patients, families, and their therapists,* New York, 1997, Basic Books.
30. Steinglass P: Coping with an insoluble problem: renal failure. In McDaniel SH, Hepworth J, Doherty WJ, editors: *The shared experience of illness: stories of patients, families, and their therapists,* New York, 1997, Basic Books.
31. Gonzalez S, Steinglass P, Reiss D: Putting the illness in its place: discussion groups for families with chronic medical illnesses, *Fam Process* 28:69-87, 1998.
32. Konstam V, Turbett A, Konstam M: A group intervention for cardiac transplantation recipients and their families, *J Appl Rehabil and Counsel* 26:33-35, 1995.
33. Konstam V, Moser DK, DeJong MJ: Depression and anxiety in heart failure, *J Card Fail* 11:455-463, 2005.
34. Moser DK, Dracup K, Doering L et al: Depression, anxiety, hostility and perceived control in elderly cardiac patients: comparison of prevalence in heart failure, myocardial infarction, coronary artery bypass graft surgery, and healthy elders (in review).
35. Seligman L: *Selecting effective treatments: a comprehensive systematic guide to treating mental disorders,* San Francisco, 1998, Jossey-Bass.
36. Murberg TA, Bru E: Social relationships and mortality in patients with congestive heart failure, *J Psychosom Res* 51:521-527, 2001.
37. Martin PD, Brantley PJ: Stress coping and social support in health and behavior. In Boll TJ, Roczynski JM, Leviton LC, editors: *Handbook of clinical health psychology,* Washington DC, 2004, American Psychological Association.
38. Bohachick P, Taylor MV, Sereika S et al: Social support, personal control, and psychosocial recovery following heart transplantation, *Clin Nurs Res* 11:34-51, 2002.
39. Tsay SL, Chao YF: Effects of perceived self-efficacy and functional status on depression in patients with chronic heart failure, *J Nurs Res* 10:271-278, 2002.
40. Seligman M: *Authentic happiness: using the new positive psychology to realize your potential for lasting fulfillment,* New York, 2002, Free Press.
41. Johnson NG: Psychology and health: taking the initiative to bring it together. In Rozensky RH, Johnson NG, Goodheart CD, Hammond WR, editors: *Psychology builds a healthy world: opportunities for research and practice,* Washington, DC, 2004, American Psychological Association.

Risk Factor Modification in Primary, Secondary, and Tertiary Prevention

BARBARA RIEGEL and DEBRA K. MOSER

Nurses have a long history in health promotion and disease prevention. In fact, the metaparadigm—content areas core to the discipline of nursing—includes health as one of those central components. This attention to preventing illness is illustrated beautifully in this section of the book.

The chapters in this section focus on primary and secondary prevention of disease. Primary prevention refers to activities undertaken to prevent the onset of disease. Primary prevention topics addressed include smoking and promoting childhood health. Taking a uniquely nursing perspective, topics such as stress, anxiety, depression, and social support are included in this section because of the accumulating data showing the risk of negative emotions and social isolation. Because successful primary prevention can avoid much of the suffering, cost, and burden associated with disease, it often is considered the most cost-effective form of health care.

Secondary prevention refers to activities undertaken to identify and treat asymptomatic persons who already have developed risk factors or preclinical disease but in whom the condition is not yet clinically apparent. Chapters in this section address hyperlipidemia, hypertension, and novel risk factors—all conditions with a significant latency period. That is, although these risk factors are known to be significant predictors of cardiovascular disease, there typically is a relatively long lag time between identification of the risk and manifestation of the disease. With screening and early case finding, the natural history of cardiovascular disease may be altered.

A theme of this section is the need to motivate behavioral change in persons who need to modify risk factors for a disease that is not yet evident. In recent years, nurses have come to recognize that patient education is necessary but not sufficient to help individuals incorporate these recommendations into their lives. Nurse clinicians have been innovators in developing ways to work with patients and families to change behavior. Now, nurse scientists are actively studying these approaches and documenting the effectiveness of innovative tactics that work in practice. Research from nursing and from other disciplines is highlighted in these chapters that summarize the known risk factors for cardiovascular disease.

Risk Factor Modification in Primary, Secondary, and Tertiary Prevention

Primary Prevention in Childhood

Laura L. Hayman

CHAPTER ABBREVIATIONS

AHA American Heart Association

ATP Adult Treatment Panel

BMI body mass index

CDC Centers for Disease Control and Prevention

CATCH Child and Adolescent Trial for Cardiovascular Health and Healthy Start

CHD coronary heart disease

CHIC Cardiovascular Health in Children

CVD cardiovascular disease

DBP diastolic blood pressure

HDL-C high-density lipoprotein cholesterol

LDL-C low-density lipoprotein cholesterol

LRC Lipid Research Clinics

NANA National Alliance for Nutrition and Physical Activity

NCEP National Cholesterol Education Program

NHANES National Health and Nutrition Examination Survey

PDAY American Pathobiological Determinants of Atherosclerosis in Youth

PE physical education

SBP systolic blood pressure

Cardiovascular disease (**CVD**) is a major cause of morbidity and premature mortality in women and men in the United States and is becoming increasingly important as a cause of mortality worldwide.[1] Accumulated data indicate that atherosclerotic-CVD processes begin early in childhood and are influenced over the life course by genetic and potentially modifiable, established risk factors and environmental exposures. Taken together, these data argue convincingly for individual and public health approaches to primary prevention beginning in childhood. This chapter summarizes the research that informs and guides approaches to CVD prevention and presents current recommendations for assessment and management of CVD risk factors in childhood and adolescence.

EVIDENCE FOR CHILDHOOD PREVENTION

Evidence-based guidelines for primary and secondary prevention of CVD in adults are informed by the results of randomized controlled trials. Taken together, the existing evidence, discussed in this chapter, argues convincingly for prevention of CVD beginning in childhood. An important emphasis, however, is that there are

no data from randomized controlled trials comparing the effect of risk reduction in childhood on the subsequent development of atherosclerotic CVD. Similarly, no long-term longitudinal studies have been conducted to determine the absolute levels of risk factors measured in childhood that predict CVD in adult life. However, laboratory, clinical, epidemiological, and family research provide convincing evidence of the need for primary prevention of CVD in childhood. These studies have prompted and informed existing guidelines for children and adolescents.

Laboratory Studies

Autopsy studies, particularly the American Pathobiological Determinants of Atherosclerosis in Youth (**PDAY**) Study, a multicenter study of black and white adolescents and young adults provides important information about risk factors. These studies demonstrate associations between modifiable risk factors including hypertension, tobacco use, obesity, atherogenic lipids (non-high-density lipoprotein cholesterol [**HDL-C**]), and the presence and extent of atherosclerotic lesions in the aorta and coronary arteries.[2,3] The PDAY study quantified risk factors by analyses of postmortem blood samples obtained at autopsy from approximately 3000 persons ages 15 to 34 who died from external, non-CVD causes including accidents and homicide. Autopsies were conducted in forensic laboratories within 48 hours after death. Risk factor–lesion associations observed in PDAY were consistent with observations made in the pathological component of the Bogalusa Heart Study, a community-based, epidemiological landmark study of risk factors for CVD in children and young adults.[4] Building on and extending early observations made during the Korean War[5] that atherosclerotic plaques are present in about 15 percent of individuals by age 20, data from PDAY and Bogalusa indicate that the presence of modifiable risk factors during adolescence contributes to early-onset plaques and the total atherosclerotic burden observed during young adult life.[6]

In Vivo Clinical Studies

More recently, noninvasive studies have been used to examine the association of CVD risk factors with vascular structure and function in childhood and adolescence and with atherosclerosis in young adult life. Investigators from the Muscatine Study, a longitudinal, epidemiological study of CVD risk factors in children and youth, used carotid ultrasound in adults ages 33 to 42 and found that carotid intima-media thickness was associated positively with levels of total serum cholesterol and body mass index (**BMI**) measured in childhood.[7] Similar results were observed in Bogalusa: childhood measures of low-density lipoprotein cholesterol (**LDL-C**) and BMI predicted increased carotid intima-media thickness in adulthood.[8] A recent report from the Young Finns Study reaffirms the link between risk factor exposures (including LDL-C, BMI, cigarette smoking, and systolic blood pressure) in 12- to 18-year-old adolescents and preclinical atherosclerosis in adulthood. Results from this population-based prospective cohort study conducted at five centers in Finland among 2229 young adults ages 24 to 39 are particularly noteworthy because risk factor profiles assessed in adolescence predicted adult common carotid intima-media thickness independently of contemporaneous risk factors.[9] Consistent with these results are data from other noninvasive studies of adolescents and young adults indicating that intraindividual clustering of multiple risk factors adversely affects carotid intima-media thickness during this developmental period.[10,11]

Taken together, the results of laboratory and pathological studies and more recent noninvasive studies provide convincing evidence of the link between established modifiable risk factors and accelerated atherosclerotic processes in adolescence and adulthood. Clearly, these results support the need for primary prevention early in life.

Epidemiological Studies

Since the 1970s, extensive cross-sectional and longitudinal observational studies have been conducted in the United States. Of particular importance to primary prevention are observations on the distribution, tracking (i.e., maintenance of percentile rank over time), and determinants of major modifiable risk factors for CVD, including lipids and lipoproteins and systolic and diastolic blood pressure. The impact of overweight and obesity on CVD risk factors in childhood and adolescence and the independent contribution of obesity to accelerated atherosclerotic processes in adult life also have been investigated extensively. These results have implications for individual high-risk and public health approaches to reducing childhood obesity as part of CVD risk reduction.

Lipids and Lipoproteins

Data from several sources illustrate changes observed in the lipid profile with growth and maturation. Gender and racial differences have been demonstrated in the distribution of lipids and lipoproteins in childhood and adolescence. The determinants of tracking of lipids and lipoproteins have been described.

In black and white males and females, serum lipids and lipoproteins change dramatically during the first 2 years of life and during sexual maturation.[12-14] Although similar population-based data are not available for children from other ethnic groups, scattered data suggest that changes in components of the lipid profile are influenced by the physiological changes of infancy and adolescence.[15,16] Lipid and lipoprotein levels increase

throughout the first 2 years of life and reach young adult levels by age 2.[12] Based on these data, the National Cholesterol Education Program (**NCEP**) issued the first guidelines for assessing the lipid profile as part of CVD risk in children and recommended selective screening for high-risk children after age 2. NCEP also established values for acceptable, borderline, and high total cholesterol levels and LDL-C (Table 32-1).[17]

Nationally representative data from the most recent National Health and Nutrition Examination Survey (**NHANES** III) indicate that mean, age-specific values for total cholesterol peak at 171 mg/dl just before puberty at age 9 to 11. Females had significantly higher mean total cholesterol and LDL-C levels than males. Compared with non-Hispanic white and Mexican American children and adolescents (ages 4 to 19), those classified as non-Hispanic black had higher LDL-C and cardioprotective HDL-C levels.[18] Similar differences in black and white youth were observed in the population-based Cardiovascular Health in Children (**CHIC**) study; however, gender differences were not as pronounced.[19] Consistent with temporal trends observed in adults, mean total cholesterol levels in 12- to 17-year-olds decreased by 7 mg/dl from 1966 to 1970 in the most recent survey. Figure 32-1 illustrates trends in mean total cholesterol observed in the NHANES surveys.[18]

Epidemiological and clinical studies have documented a precipitous decline in total cholesterol and LDL-C levels at the onset of puberty, with a

■ ■ ■

TABLE 32-1 EVALUATING CHOLESTEROL LEVELS

EVALUATION	TOTAL CHOLESTEROL LEVEL (mg/dl)	LOW-DENSITY LIPOPROTEIN LEVEL (mg/dl)
Acceptable	Less than 170	Less than 110
Borderline	170-199	110-129
High	Greater than 200	Greater than 130

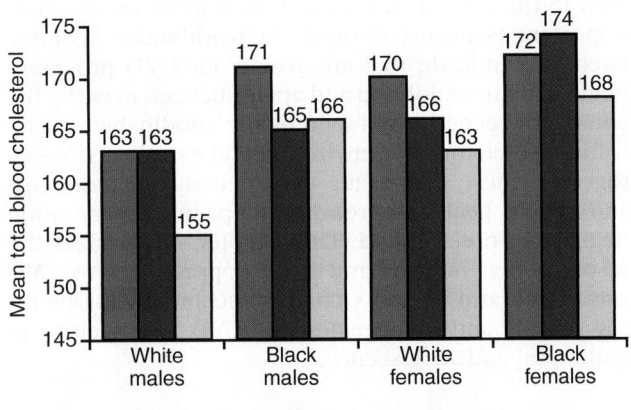

■ NHES III ■ NHANES I □ NHANES III

NHES III, NHANES I AND NHANES III:
1966-70, 1971-74, 1988-94

FIGURE 32-1 ■ Trends in mean total blood cholesterol among adolescents ages 12 to 17 by sex, race, and survey. *NHANES*, National Health and Nutrition Examination Survey; *NHES*, National Health Examination Survey. (From Hickman TB, Briefel RR, Carroll MD et al: *Prev Med* 27:879-890, 1998.)

gradual increase during adolescence and young adulthood.[12-14,17,18,20] Data indicate more pronounced and adverse maturational changes in the lipid profile in white males compared with their black and white female counterparts.[14,21] Together, these data have prompted a reexamination of current recommendations for lipid screening and follow-up of children and adolescents. Current single total cholesterol cutoff points for children ages 2 to 19, recommended by NCEP[17] and endorsed by the American Heart Association (**AHA**)[22] and the American Academy of Pediatrics,[23] fail to consider gender, race, ethnicity, and stage of sexual maturation. These factors have been shown to influence lipid levels and the sensitivity and specificity of screening. For example, because black children have higher levels of total cholesterol and HDL-C, sensitivities will be higher and specificities lower for a given total cholesterol level than in white children.

Maintenance of percentile rank from childhood to young adulthood or tracking of lipids and lipoproteins, particularly total cholesterol and LDL-C, has been observed in males and females from diverse racial and ethnic groups. Persistence of lipid levels over time is particularly evident at the upper and lower extremes of the distribution. This finding indicates that children who have total cholesterol and LDL-C levels at the 95th percentile during the school-age years are likely to have elevated levels in adulthood. Data from Bogalusa indicate that 45 percent of children with serum total cholesterol levels in the uppermost quintile at baseline remained there 12 years later, and another 26 percent moved to the fourth quintile (60th to 80th percentile) at follow-up.[24] Thus, more than 70 percent of those with elevated total cholesterol levels in childhood tended to retain them as adults. In Muscatine, 75 percent of children ages 5 to 18 at baseline with total cholesterol levels above the 90th percentile had elevated levels (= 200 mg/dl) at age 20 to 25.[25,26] From the perspective of primary prevention of CVD, this tracking phenomenon is important because of the potential for identifying children at risk for future CVD. In addition, total serum cholesterol measured early in adult life has been strongly related to CVD in midlife.

Blood Pressure

Epidemiological studies, particularly recent results from NHANES, support the need for individual and public health approaches to assessment and management of blood pressure as part of childhood CVD prevention.[27] Specifically, compared with NHANES III (1988 to 1994),[28] results from the most recent survey (1999 to 2000) of 5582 black, Hispanic, and white children ages 8 to 17 indicate substantial increases in systolic blood pressure (**SBP**) and diastolic blood pressure (**DBP**) for all age, race/ethnicity, and sex subgroups investigated.[27] In 1988 to 1994, the mean SBP of children was 104.6 mm Hg and mean DBP was 58.4 mm Hg.[28] In 1999 to 2000, the mean SBP of children was 106 mm Hg and mean DBP was 61.7 mm Hg. Adjusting for differences in age, race, and sex, mean SBP and mean DBP increased 1.4 mm Hg and 3.3 mm Hg, respectively. Further adjustments for the BMI distribution in 1988 to 1994 and 1999

to 2000 reduced the increases in SBP and DBP by 29 and 12 percent, respectively.[27] These results suggest that increases in BP in children and adolescents are partially attributable to the documented increases in the prevalence of overweight.

The clinical significance of these trends is emphasized in research indicating that, for each 1- to 2-mm Hg rise in SBP, children have a 10 percent greater risk of developing hypertension in young adulthood.[29] Evidence also suggests that even modest elevations in blood pressure levels in childhood have an adverse effect on vascular structure and function with target organ damage (left ventricular hypertrophy) observed in hypertensive children and adolescents.[30,31]

In childhood, primary hypertension usually is characterized by mild or stage 1 hypertension and often is associated with a family history of hypertension or CVD.[32,33] Accumulated data, including NHANES, indicate that overweight and obesity (as measured by BMI) are associated strongly with elevated blood pressure levels in childhood and adolescence; that is, children with primary hypertension commonly are overweight.[34,35] Data from school health screening programs reaffirm the positive association between BMI and blood pressure in adolescents and indicate a progressive increase in the prevalence of hypertension with increases in BMI.[35,36] Approximately 30 percent of overweight children in one school-based study met the criteria for hypertension.[36] Other recent data indicate a clustering of CVD risk factors, including components of the insulin resistance syndrome (high triglyceride level, low HDL-C level, hyperinsulinemia, truncal obesity), in overweight children with high blood pressure.[37,38]

Taken together, these results have prompted and informed new guidelines for clinical practice with emphasis on comprehensive assessment of the CVD risk factor profile in children and adolescents with elevated SBP, DBP, or both.[39]

Overweight, Obesity, and Metabolic Syndrome

Obesity is well recognized as a major risk factor for CVD in adulthood. The increasing prevalence of overweight and obesity in children and adolescents in the United States has become a major public health issue and has prompted the attention of the pediatric cardiovascular community.[40,41] Paralleling the trend observed in U.S. adults, the prevalence of childhood overweight tripled over the past two decades. For children in the United States, the Centers for Disease Control and Prevention (**CDC**) age- and sex-specific nomograms are used to define overweight and obesity in children and adolescents. Based on cross-sectional data acquired from sequential evaluations of representative samples of U.S. children, cutoff points (by age and sex) are defined as follows[42]:

- Normal weight—BMI above 5th percentile and below 85th percentile
- At-risk for overweight—BMI 85th to 95th percentile
- Overweight—BMI at 95th percentile or above

Emphasizing the importance of prevalence and trend data and obesity-adverse health outcome data, the recent Institute of Medicine report classifies children with a BMI at or above the 95th percentile as obese.[43] Thus, the terms *overweight* and *obesity* often are used interchangeably in pediatric patients.[44]

Using the 95th percentile of BMI values to define overweight/obesity, gender and race/ethnic group differences have been observed in representative samples of school-aged children and adolescents.[40,45,46] As illustrated in Figure 32-2, an excess prevalence of overweight/obesity is notable among non-Hispanic blacks and among Hispanics (particularly girls).[46] Other data (not shown) indicate a very high prevalence of overweight/obesity in Native American youth.[47]

The determinants and correlates of overweight/obesity in childhood and adolescence have been examined extensively and remain to be fully explicated. Particularly important from a CVD-prevention perspective are data documenting the CVD-related comorbidities associated with obesity in childhood. These include atherogenic dyslipidemia, hypertension, left ventricular hypertrophy, insulin resistance, and the clustering of risk factors into what is termed the *metabolic syndrome*.[48,49] More data exist on metabolic syndrome in adults, and controversy exists regarding the specific components and cutoff points for defining this syndrome in children and youth. However, recent epidemiological and clinical studies have attempted to estimate prevalence rates using Adult Treatment Panel (**ATP**) III criteria adapted for pediatric populations.[50-52] Accordingly, a report from NHANES III estimated that 1 million U.S. adolescents meet the ATP III criteria for metabolic syndrome.[50] Based on these data, the estimated prevalence of metabolic syndrome in the adolescent population is 4 percent. In overweight children and adolescents, prevalence estimates range from 30 to 50 percent.[53]

The negative impact of multiple risk factor clustering that characterizes the metabolic syndrome is well-documented. CVD risk increases in adolescents and young adults with these risk factors. Previously cited laboratory and clinical studies[2-4,6-9] indicate that multiple risk factor clustering increases the presence and extent of atherosclerotic lesions. In addition, there is

evidence of tracking of the factors associated with metabolic syndrome. The correlation between BMI measured during adolescence (age 13) and BMI in young adulthood (age 22) was 0.67 ($p = 0.0001$). The correlation between BMI at age 13 and glucose utilization at age 22 was -0.50 ($p = 0.006$).[54] Bogalusa results also demonstrate tracking of multiple risk factors consistent with metabolic syndrome from adolescence to young adulthood.[55] A recent report by Sinaiko and colleagues[56] extends prior research and suggests that insulin resistance (alone and interacting with body fatness) has a significant role in the development of CVD risk factors associated with metabolic syndrome during adolescence. Taken together, these results illustrate the importance of primary prevention of overweight as part of a comprehensive profile approach to CVD risk reduction in childhood.[44]

Obesity and Type 2 Diabetes Mellitus

The increase observed in the prevalence of obesity and metabolic syndrome in youth is associated with an increase in type 2 diabetes mellitus.[57] In 1990, type 2 diabetes accounted for 3 percent of all new onset/incident cases in children and adolescents. A recent report that combined population-based studies and clinical case series conducted in North America, the Asian-Pacific region, and Europe documents a global spread of type 2 diabetes in adolescents, with type 2 diabetes accounting for 45 percent of incident cases of diabetes. Patterns observed by geographic region and ethnic and cultural groups indicate a close relation between rates of type 2 diabetes in adults and the eventual appearance of this chronic condition in adolescents, suggesting that attention to the epidemiology of diabetes in adults may be helpful in predicting incident type 2 diabetes in youth.[58] The patterns and trends observed also reaffirm the association between obesity and type 2 diabetes documented in prior U.S. research, including clinical and population-based studies.[59-62]

Type 2 diabetes in adults now is recognized as a coronary artery disease risk equivalent; however, no prospective data exist regarding the impact of type 2 diabetes in adolescence on CVD in adult life. In the pediatric health care community, however, there is an increased awareness of type 2 diabetes in youth and the need for more aggressive approaches to prevention and management of CVD risk factors in these young patients.[63]

Cigarette Smoking

Substantial data provide unequivocal evidence indicating that cigarette smoking is a major independent risk factor for CVD in adults (as discussed in Chapter 33). The influence of smoking on CVD risk factors in childhood and adolescence is similar to that observed in adults. Smoking initiation in childhood and adolescence is multifaceted and includes individual, family, and society influences.[64-69] Of concern, from the perspective of prevention, are prevalence and trend data indicating that more than half of new smokers in the United States are younger than age 18. Approximately 80 percent of those who use tobacco start before age 18, with early adolescence (age 14 to 15) the most common starting age.[64,65]

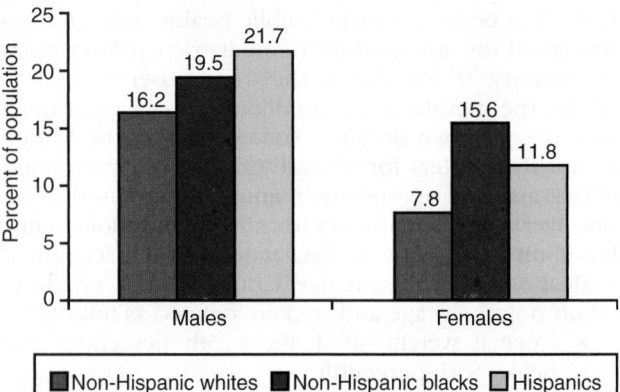

FIGURE 32-2 ■ Prevalence of overweight among students in grades 9 to 12 by sex and race/ethnicity (Youth Risk Behavior Surveillance, 2003).[46] Overweight is defined as a body mass index in the 95th percentile or higher by age and sex of the Centers for Disease Control and Prevention 2000 growth chart. (From *MMWR* 53(SS-2):May 21, 2004.)

Recent CDC data also reveal gender and race/ethnic differences in tobacco use in U.S. youth. Among high school students the prevalence of current cigarette use was higher among black males (19.3 percent) and white females (26.6 percent) than black females (10.8 percent).[66] A consistent observation across recent CDC and NHANES surveys is higher prevalence rates for whites (24.9 percent) compared with their non-Hispanic black (15.1 percent) and Hispanic (18.4 percent) counterparts. An analysis of NHANES data suggests that socioeconomic status is an important predictor of tobacco use in 18- to 24-years-olds, with higher prevalence rates observed among youth of lower socioeconomic status.[70] Other data emphasize the important role of social-ecological influences and multilevel policies, including statewide tobacco control programs, in preventing smoking initiation in youth. For example, from 2002 to 2004, overall state spending on tobacco-prevention and control programs declined by 28 percent in the United States.[69] State program cuts exceeded 75 percent in some states, including Minnesota, where program reductions were associated with reduced awareness of the state antitobacco campaign and a substantial increase in youth smoking susceptibility.[71]

These data indicate the need for individual and population-based efforts to prevent the initiation of smoking in youth and to assist with smoking cessation among those who have acquired the habit.

Physical Activity

Substantial evidence (presented in Chapter 38) underscores the cardiovascular benefits of physical activity during adult life. Data indicate that physically active children and adolescents have more favorable cardiovascular health profiles than their sedentary counterparts.[72,73] Based on a recent comprehensive review of the effects of physical activity on health and behavior outcomes, an expert panel recommended that school-age youth should participate daily in 60 minutes or more of moderate to vigorous physical activity.[74] Data from the CDC (Figure 32-3),[75] supported by other population-based studies, suggest that this goal is not being realized. Across studies, gender, age, and ethnic differences in physical activity participation have been observed. As assessed by self-report, females and black and Hispanic youth are less likely to be active than their male and white counterparts.[66,75] Consistent with results from several surveys, a recent population-based longitudinal study of black and white girls documented a precipitous decline in physical activity during the school-age–adolescent transition. By age 16 or 17, 56 percent of black girls and 31 percent of white girls reported no habitual leisure-time activity. Noteworthy is that a higher BMI was associated with a greater decline in activity among girls of both races. Cigarette smoking was associated with a decline in activity among white girls, whereas pregnancy was associated with a decline in activity among black girls.[76]

Recent CDC data indicate that only 55.7 percent of students nationwide were enrolled in physical education (**PE**) classes on 1 day or more of an average school week. Enrollment in daily PE declined from 1991 to

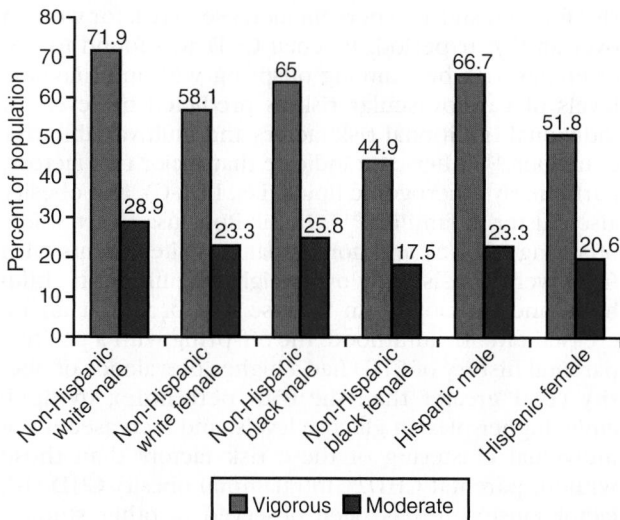

FIGURE 32-3 ■ Prevalence of students in grades 9 to 12 who participated in sufficient vigorous or moderate physical activity during the past 7 days by race/ethnicity and sex (Youth Risk Behavior Surveillance, 2003).[75] Note that "vigorous activity" is defined as activity causing sweating and hard breathing for at least 20 minutes on 3 or more of the 7 days. "Moderate activity" is defined as activities such as walking or bicycling lasting for at least 30 minutes on 5 or more of the 7 days. (From *MMWR* 53(SS-2):May 21, 2004.)

1995 (41.6 to 25.4 percent) and then increased from 1995 to 2001 (25.4 to 32.2 percent). CDC data indicate that (on average) 28.4 percent of students nationwide are enrolled in daily PE with variability across state surveys (range: 8.2 to 37.2 percent).[75] The epidemic of overweight and obesity in U.S. children and youth has prompted a reexamination of school policies and multiple efforts to mandate daily PE in schools. For example, several states, including Arkansas and New York, have introduced legislation to increase PE and physical activity in public schools statewide.

Family Studies

A family history of premature coronary heart disease (**CHD**) is considered a major nonmodifiable risk factor for cardiovascular events.[77,78] Familial aggregation of CHD and attendant risk factors is well documented, particularly in non-Hispanic white families. An early report from Glueck and colleagues[79] indicated that 31 percent of children with a parent who had a documented myocardial infarction before age 50 had elevated total cholesterol (greater than 230 mg/dl; 5.9 mmol/liter), LDL-C (greater than 170 mg/dl; 4.40 mmol/liter), and/or triglyceride levels (greater than 140 mg/dl; 1.6 mmol/liter). Subsequent reports have been consistent in showing an increased prevalence of dyslipidemia in children with a family history of premature CHD.[80-82]

Recent results from the Framingham Offspring Study indicate occurrence of parental CHD as an independent predictor of offspring cardiovascular events in middle-aged men and women (mean age 44 years). After adjustment for other risk factors, premature CHD in at least one parent was associated with a significant doubling of risk for men and a 70 percent increase in risk for women over an 8-year period. Parental CHD was found to discriminate risk best among offspring with intermediate levels of cardiovascular risk as predicted by levels of individual traditional risk factors and multivariable risk equations.[83] Other data indicate that major risk factors, particularly atherogenic lipids (i.e., LDL-C), and obesity also cluster in families.[84,85] In the Bogalusa Heart Study, offspring of black and non-Hispanic white parents with CHD were consistently overweight beginning in childhood and developed an adverse risk profile at an increased rate. In adulthood, the offspring with a positive parental history of CHD had a higher prevalence of obesity (BMI greater than the 85th percentile), dyslipidemia, higher plasma glucose levels, and increased intraindividual clustering of these risk factors than those without parental CHD.[86] Intrafamilial obesity-CHD risk factor clustering has been observed in other studies, including the Delaware Valley Twin Family Study and the Princeton Lipid Research Clinics (**LRC**) Study, with results implicating shared genes and shared common family environments, including health-related lifestyle behaviors.[87-89]

Patterns of dietary intake, physical activity, and tobacco use, recognized as potential modifiable determinants of CHD, demonstrate intrafamilial associations. In the biracial Princeton LRC Study, parental nutrient intake explained a significant portion of the variance in children's intake, with multiple R^2 ranging from 0.23 (cholesterol) for the total sample to 0.97 for total carbohydrates in black fathers over age 40 and their children.[90] Reports from the Framingham Children's Study and reports of white and Mexican-American parent-child dyads provide additional evidence of familial aggregation of macronutrients and micronutrients relevant to CHD.[91,92] Similarly, numerous studies (using family and twin study designs) have demonstrated familial resemblance of patterns of physical activity in white, black, and Hispanic families.[92,93] Finally, studies of diverse racial/ethnic groups have demonstrated familial associations of tobacco use (particularly cigarette smoking) with results implicating genetic and environmental factors in the initiation, persistence, and cessation of smoking.[94-96]

As discussed before, familial aggregation of CVD is attributed to shared genes and shared family-environmental factors. In some families, however, monogenic (single-gene) disorders account for the clustering of premature CVD. In childhood, the most commonly recognized and well-characterized disorder of lipoprotein metabolism is familial hypercholesterolemia. An autosomal dominant monogenetic condition, homozygous familial hypercholesterolemia is rare with an occurrence of 1:1,000,000; however, heterozygous familial hypercholesterolemia is the most common monogenic disorder in North America and Europe with an estimated incidence of 1:500. The genetic defect is characterized by numerous mutations affecting the production and processing of cell-surface LDL receptors resulting in impaired clearance of circulating LDL particles, exceedingly high serum levels of LDL-C (600 to 1000 mg/dl), functional and structural vascular abnormalities, and

clinical CHD in homozygotes beginning in the first decade of life.[97] Children and adolescents with heterozygous familial hypercholesterolemia are usually asymptomatic at diagnosis and have total cholesterol and LDL-C levels above the 95th percentile.[98] In addition, these children often have a family history of premature CHD, parents with dyslipidemia, or both.[99-101]

Based on this evidence, current (individual) primary prevention guidelines emphasize family-based approaches to identification and management of cardiovascular risk factors in children and adolescents. The NCEP, for example, suggests a high-risk approach to identifying children at risk for CHD based on family history of premature CHD and/or parental dyslipidemia.[17] Similarly, AHA guidelines support and extend this approach to include early identification and vigilant follow-up of children with family history of CHD and other established risk factors including hypertension and obesity.[22]

INTERVENTION APPROACHES

As applied to children and youth, prevention of CVD includes and encompasses individual and population-based strategies. Central to both approaches is the acquisition and maintenance of healthful lifestyle behaviors. In the pediatric health care community, as reflected in guidelines and scientific statements issued by the AHA, the American Academy of Pediatrics, and numerous expert panels, emphasis is placed on healthful lifestyle training to promote cardiovascular health in childhood and to reduce the risk and burden of CVD in adult life.[22,23,102] Primordial prevention, defined as prevention of the development of the risk factor in the first place, has been emphasized in recent guidelines for population-based and individual approaches to CVD prevention in childhood and adolescence.[102] The term *primordial prevention* is used interchangeably (in guidelines and scientific statements) with *cardiovascular health promotion*. Concomitantly, social-ecological models are being applied in research and practice initiatives designed to promote the development and maintenance of healthy patterns of behavior (i.e., dietary intake, physical activity, and tobacco-free lifestyle) with the ultimate goal of improving health and quality of life for individuals and diverse populations.[43] Research reviewed in this chapter (and elsewhere in this book) provides convincing evidence of the critical role of environmental and social factors and influences and regulatory policies (defined on multiple levels) in the development and maintenance of healthful lifestyle behaviors across the life span.

The epidemic of childhood obesity exemplifies the importance of the ecological approach and has called attention to the potential impact of schools, communities (including the built environment), the food industry, and the media in preventing the development of overweight in childhood (primordial prevention). The AHA, American Academy of Pediatrics, and Institute of Medicine advocate for prevention approaches that address these multiple levels of influence as applied to overweight and obesity in childhood and adolescence.[41,43,103] As discussed next, across health care and community settings, pediatric professionals are reminded to consider these multiple levels of influence in the "practice of prevention" with children and youth.

Population-Based Approaches to CVD Prevention

By definition, population-based approaches are designed to shift the distribution of risk factors (and risk for CVD) to more desirable levels. Complementary to the individual/clinical approach to CVD prevention, population-based strategies normally involve interventions at the community level, such as the CVD prevention trials implemented in the United States and Sweden during the 1970s. These resource-intensive trials showed that concerted efforts to organize and mobilize targeted communities, media, direct health education, risk factor screenings, and environmental changes through local programs and policies can change CVD-related health behaviors.[104] Schools (and preschools) have been popular venues for implementing population-based strategies with children and adolescents. As detailed in reviews on the topic,[103,105,106] school-based interventions have been effective in improving knowledge, attitudes, and CVD-related health behaviors. However, the impact of multicomponent interventions on physiological risk factors for CVD has been less promising and variable across studies. Lessons learned from methodologically rigorous, school-based, randomized controlled trials are similar to those learned from community-based prevention trials.

As exemplified in the Child and Adolescent Trial for Cardiovascular Health and Healthy Start (**CATCH**), interventions effective in changing behaviors at the individual (student) level must target the environmental factors that influence these behaviors.[107] For effective school-based strategies, this involves modifying the food and physical activity environments, as suggested in recent recommendations by numerous child health and advocacy groups. **NANA**, the National Alliance for Nutrition and Physical Activity, a 270-member coalition that advocates national policies and programs to promote healthful eating and physical activity across the life span, has been particularly instrumental in advocating for multilevel policies needed to enable healthful behaviors in school environments.[108] Most recently, NANA has recommended that federal, state, and/or local governments; schools; and school districts enact policies to ensure that foods sold from vending machines, school stores, fund-raisers, a la carte, and other venues outside of school meal programs make positive contributions to children's diets.

Although the U.S. Department of Agriculture sets the nutrition standards for school meals (for schools participating in the national school lunch or school breakfast programs), standards for foods and beverages sold outside those meals are not as regulated. Results of a recent NANA survey,[108] combined with other data, underscore the importance of policies in modifying the school food environment. The NANA survey of 1420 vending machines in 251 schools (middle, junior, and high schools) selected from urban and rural areas in the United States

indicate that the majority of options available to children are high in calories and of minimal nutritional value. Specifically, 75 percent of beverage options and 85 percent of snacks were of poor nutritional quality. As documented by Nestle and others,[109] the food industry is capitalizing on the financial challenges of schools by offering incentives to sell low-nutrition foods in the school environment. Noteworthy is that several states including Pennsylvania, California, Minnesota, and Maine have replaced soda with healthful beverages and have not lost revenue. Although the details of these successes are beyond the scope of this chapter, selected strategies outlined in Box 32-1 were incorporated with other state-specific initiatives designed to improve the food and physical activity environments of schools. As outlined by AHA, these strategies currently are being implemented in many locales and are applicable nationwide.[110]

Population-based approaches are recommended as the principal strategy for prevention of CVD beginning in childhood. Schools and preschools have been targeted as important components of population-based efforts; however, evidence suggests the need for additional research and multilevel policy changes to optimize school environments as delivery channels for CVD risk-reduction interventions.

Individual and Clinical Approaches

Across health care settings, individual approaches to cardiovascular health promotion and risk reduction with children and youth begin with a comprehensive assessment of the total risk profile (Table 32-2). In pediatric clinical practice, cardiovascular health promotion (primordial prevention) and primary prevention (interventions designed to normalize levels of risk factors and deter atherosclerotic disease processes) frequently

---

BOX 32-1 ■ ■ ■
STRATEGIES FOR SCHOOLS

- Identify a champion in the school to coordinate healthful nutrition programs.
- Establish a multidisciplinary team that includes student representation to assess aspects of the school environment using the School Health Index (Centers for Diseases Control and Prevention) or similar assessment.
- Identify local, regional, and national nutrition programs; select those proven to be effective (*www.Actionforhealthykids. org*).
- Develop policies that promote student health, and identify nutrition issues in the school (*www.nasbe.org/Healthyschools/ healthy_eating.html*).
- Work to make predominately healthful foods available at school and school functions by influencing food and beverage contracts, adapt marketing techniques to influence students to make healthful choices, and restrict in-school availability of and marketing of poor food choices.
- Maximize opportunities for all physical activity and fitness programs (competitive and intramural sports); use coaches and teachers as role models.
- Lobby for regulatory changes that improve the ability of a school to serve nutritious food.
- Ban food advertising on school campuses.

■ ■ ■

TABLE 32-2   ASSESSMENT OF CARDIOVASCULAR RISK PROFILE

RISK FACTORS AND INDICATORS	POINTS OF CONCERN	RECOMMENDATIONS
Family history	Family history of CVD, diabetes, obesity, hypertension, dyslipidemia, or cigarette smoking	Integrate with well-child care. Update history regularly. Obtain multigenerational family history of CVD, diabetes, obesity, hypertension, dyslipidemia, and cigarette smoking.
Lipids and lipoproteins	*Total cholesterol level* Borderline: Greater than 170 mg/dl Elevated: Greater than 200 mg/dl *LDL-C level* LDL-C should be less than 100 mg/dl in children with diabetes. Borderline: Greater than 110 mg/dl Elevated: Greater than 130 mg/dl *Triglyceride level:* Greater than 150 mg/dl *HDL-C level:* Greater than 35 mg/dl	Perform targeted screening of fasting lipids in children older than age 2 with family history of premature CVD, diabetes, or dyslipidemia. Screen children with other risk factors (e.g., overweight) and children whose family history of CVD, diabetes, and dyslipidemia is unknown. Averaged results of three fasting lipid profiles guides treatment decisions.
Systolic and diastolic blood pressure	*Systolic and diastolic blood pressure:* Higher than 90th percentile for age, sex, and height	Interpret blood pressure measurements by age, sex, and height. Percentiles are available at *www.nhlbi.nih.gov/guidelines/hypertension/child_tbl.htm*[39]
Body size	*Risk of overweight:* BMI above 85th percentile *Overweight:* BMI above 95th percentile	Chart body size by BMI. Norms for BMI percentiles are available at *www.cdc.gov/growthcharts/*
Health behaviors	*Cigarette smoking:* Any *Physical activity:* Less than 30 minutes moderate to vigorous physical activity daily; more than 2 hours sedentary activities daily *Dietary intake:* Excess sugar, saturated fat, and salt; less than five servings of fruit and vegetables daily; less than three servings of dairy daily; less than six servings of whole grain and grain products daily	Assess health behaviors at every visit, including tobacco use by child, family, and peers. Advise participation in 30 to 60 minutes of moderately vigorous physical activity daily. Combine resistance training (10 to 15 repetitions at moderate intensity) with aerobic activity in an overall activity program for adolescents. Assess diet at every visit. Match energy intake with energy needs for growth and developmental processes.

BMI, Body mass index; *CVD,* cardiovascular disease; *HDL-C,* high-density lipoprotein cholesterol; *LDL-C,* low-density lipoprotein cholesterol.

are implemented in tandem. Most important, as emphasized in pediatric guidelines and recommendations[17,22,39,44] (Table 32-3), CVD-related health behaviors are the cornerstone of both approaches to prevention. Thus, pediatric health care professionals are encouraged to assess these behaviors at each well-child visit. A developmental, family-based profile approach to assessing and managing cigarette smoking, physical activity, dietary intake, family history of CVD, and physiological risk factors is recommended by AHA.[22,102] For children younger than age 2, assessment of parents' behaviors is recommended, including parental/household smoking, patterns of dietary intake and physical activity, and inquiries about parents' levels of established physiological risk factors (e.g., total cholesterol level, SBP, and DBP). In addition, a multigenerational family history of CVD and attendant risk factors (hypertension, dyslipidemia, obesity, diabetes) is recommended. Because family health histories change over time, AHA and other agencies recommend an update at each visit throughout childhood and adolescence.[17,22,39,44,102] Assessment of the cardiovascular risk profile beyond age 2 and currently recommended approaches to management of these risk factors is presented in Tables 32-2 and 32-3. As emphasized, therapeutic lifestyle change, discussed further in Chapter 77, is the cornerstone of treatment for children identi-

fied with physiological risk factors for CVD including dyslipidemia, hypertension, and/or obesity. Central to therapeutic lifestyle change is effective strategies for behavioral change. Box 32-2 presents evidence-based strategies for behavioral change with children and families that have been effective in modifying CVD-related health behaviors.[111,112]

Prescriptions for an adequate trial of dietary and physical activity modifications consider the specific risk factor(s) identified, child's age, developmental level, and presence of comorbidities.[17,22,39,44] For example, a 12-year-old boy who has dyslipidemia (LDL-C level of 160 mg/dl), BMI at the 85th age- and sex-specific percentile, no other comorbidities, and no family history of premature CVD would have a diet and physical activity prescription as suggested in Table 32-3. Like adults, children and youth have interindividual differences in response to dietary modification.[110] Thus, current recommendations suggest an adequate trial (i.e., 6 to 12 months) of therapeutic lifestyle change with dietary modifications started in conjunction with a trained dietitian.[22,23] In addition to restricting saturated fat, *trans*-fat, and cholesterol intake, other dietary options such as increasing soluble fiber may be recommended. With good dietary (and physical activity) adherence and normalization of body weight, levels of LDL-C may be reduced to goal.

■ ■ ■

TABLE 32-3   CARDIOVASCULAR DISEASE RISK REDUCTION FOR CHILDREN AND ADOLESCENTS
WITH IDENTIFIED RISK

INTERVENTION	GOALS	RECOMMENDATIONS
Blood cholesterol management	LDL-C level less than 160 mg/dl (130 mg/dl is even better) If patient has diabetes, LDL-C level less than 100 mg/dl	If LDL-C is above goals, start therapeutic lifestyle changes, including diet (less than 7% of calories from saturated fat and less than 200 mg cholesterol per day), in conjunction with a trained dietitian. Consider dietary options to lower LDL-C level in conjunction with a trained dietitian: increase soluble fiber by using age (in years) plus 5 to 10 g up to age 15, when the total remains at 25 g/d. Emphasize weight management and increased physical activity. If LDL-C is persistently above goals, evaluate secondary causes (thyroid-stimulating hormone, liver function tests, renal function tests, urinalysis). Consider drug therapy for patients with LDL-C above 190 mg/dl and no other CVD risk factors or above 160 mg/dl for those with other risk factors (blood pressure elevation, diabetes, overweight, strong family history of premature CVD). Bile acid–binding resins or statins are usual first-line agents. Pharmacological intervention for dyslipidemia should be done with a physician experienced in treating cholesterol disorders in pediatric patients.
Other lipids and lipoproteins	Fasting triglyceride level less than 150 mg/dl HDL-C level greater than 35 mg/dl	Elevated fasting triglycerides and reduced HDL-C are common in the context of overweight with insulin resistance. Therapeutic lifestyle change includes weight management, appropriate energy intake and expenditure, and decreased intake of simple sugars. If fasting triglycerides are elevated persistently, evaluate for secondary causes such as diabetes, thyroid disease, renal disease, and alcohol abuse. No drug interventions are recommended in children for isolated elevation of fasting triglycerides unless very marked. Treatment may start at levels above 400 mg/dl to protect against postprandial triglyercides of 1000 mg/dl or higher, which may be associated with an increased risk of pancreatitis.
Management of blood pressure elevation	Systolic and diastolic blood pressure less than 95th percentile for age, sex, and height If patient has comorbidities, less than 90th percentile for age, sex, and height	Promote achievement of appropriate weight. Reduce sodium in the diet. Emphasize increased consumption of fruits and vegetables. If blood pressure persistently exceeds 95th percentile, consider secondary causes (renal disease, coarctation of the aorta). Consider drug therapy for patients above 95th percentile if lifestyle modification brings no improvement and there is evidence of target organ changes (left ventricular hypertrophy, microalbuminuria, renal vascular abnormalities). Start blood pressure medication individualized to other patient characteristics (e.g., age, race, need for drugs with specific benefits) and in collaboration with specialist in pediatric hypertension.
Weight management	*BMI below 85th percentile:* maintenance *BMI 85th to 95th percentile for age and sex:* maintenance with aging to reduce to below 85th percentile *BMI that exceeds 25 kg/m²:* weight maintenance *BMI 95th percentile or above (overweight):* weight maintenance (younger children) or gradual weight loss (adolescents) to reduce percentile *BMI 30 kg/m² or above (adult obesity cutpoint):* gradual weight loss (1 to 2 kg/mo) *BMI is 95th percentile or above plus comorbidity:* gradual weight loss (1 to 2 kg/mo) and treatment of associated conditions as needed	Establish individual treatment goals and approaches based on the child's age, degree of overweight, and presence of comorbidities. Involve the family or major caregivers in the treatment. Provide assessment and monitoring frequently. Consider behavioral, psychological, and social correlates of weight gain in the treatment plan. Provide recommendations for dietary changes and increases in physical activity that can be implemented within the family environment and that foster optimal health, growth and development.

BMI, Body mass index; *CVD,* cardiovascular disease; *HDL-C,* high-density lipoprotein cholesterol; *LDL-C,* low-density lipoprotein cholesterol.
Data from Kavey RE, Daniels SR, Lauer RM et al: *Circulation* 107:1562-1566, 2003 (published simultaneously in *J Pediatr* 142:368-372, 2003); National High Blood Pressure Working Group on High Blood Pressure in Children and Adolescents: *Pediatrics* 114(suppl):555-576, 2004; and Daniels SR, Arnett DK, Eckel RH et al: *Circulation* 111:1999-2012, 2005.

If LDL-C levels persist above identified goals, if secondary causes of dyslipidemia have been evaluated and ruled out, and if the child is age 10 or older, pharmacological therapy is recommended. Such therapy currently is reserved for children with LDL-C levels of 190 mg/dl or above with no additional risk factors or children with LDL-C levels of 160 mg/dl or above if additional risk factors are present.[17,22] Four general classes of lipid-lowering agents are available and have been used to treat dyslipidemia in children and adolescents. These

---

BOX 32-2　　　　　　　　　　　　　■ ■ ■

BEHAVIORAL CHANGE PRINCIPLES AND STRATEGIES
FOR CHILDREN, ADOLESCENTS, AND FAMILIES

Basic Principles

- Simplify and tailor the prescription for behavioral change to the individual and family needs and resources.
- Ask about the behavior at every health care visit.
- Involve the parents and family as partners in the behavioral change process.
- Provide information in multiple developmentally and culturally appropriate venues.

Specific Strategies

- Assess, monitor, and document patterns of behavior change at every health care visit.
- Provide developmentally appropriate behavior-specific information tailored to the child's and family's cultural background, needs, and resources.
- Identify realistic goals for behaviors with the child and family.
- Include activities to assist families monitor behaviors targeted for change.
- Mobilize family and social supports.
- Provide self-efficacy enhancement and an atmosphere of clinical empathy.
- Develop a health-promoting reward system for positive behavior change.

---

include the bile acid sequestrants, nicotinic acid derivatives, HMG-CoA (hydroxymethylglutaryl-coenzyme A) reductase inhibitors (statins), and fibric acid derivatives.[17,113] The mechanisms of action, major therapeutic effects, and adverse reactions are similar to adults and are detailed in Chapter 77.

In the pediatric health care community, there is consensus regarding lifestyle modification to reduce lipid levels (and other CVD risk factors). Controversy exists, however, regarding the use of pharmacotherapies. For example, NCEP has recommended bile acid sequestrant as the first-line lipid-lowering agent for LDL-C level.[17] A forthcoming statement from AHA suggests HMG-CoA reductase inhibitors (statins) as first-line agents.[113] The choice of medication depends on many factors, including the age and sex of the child, specific dyslipidemia, individual tolerability, child's response to therapy, and child/family preferences and resources. Recent clinical trials have demonstrated the short-term safety, efficacy, and tolerability of statins in children and adolescents, particularly those with familial dyslipidemia.[114-116] As emphasized by NCEP and AHA, pharmacological intervention for dyslipidemia (and other CVD risk factors) should be started in collaboration with a physician experienced in treating such disorders in pediatric patients.[17,22,113]

SUMMARY

This chapter has presented evidence indicating that atherosclerotic-CVD processes begin early in childhood. These processes are accelerated by potentially modifiable risk factors and environmental exposures. Data underscore the urgent need for individual and population-based CVD prevention efforts focused on children and youth. The importance of healthful lifestyle behaviors as the cornerstone of cardiovascular health promotion and risk reduction for children and youth is emphasized in current guidelines and recommendations and illustrated in this chapter. Additional research is needed to inform and guide the most effective and efficient approaches to CVD prevention in children and youth and to improve the cardiovascular health of future generations.

REFERENCES

1. American Heart Association: *Heart disease and stroke statistics: 2004 update,* Dallas, 2005, The Association.
2. McGill HC Jr, McMahan CA, Zieske AW et al: Effects of nonlipid risk factors on atherosclerosis in youth with a favorable lipoprotein profile, *Circulation* 103:1546-1555, 2001.
3. McGill HC Jr, McMahan CA, Malcolm GT et al: Effects of serum lipoproteins and smoking on atherosclerosis in young men and women: the Pathobiological Determinants of Atherosclerosis in Youth (PDAY) Research Group, *Arterioscler Thromb Vasc Biol* 17:95-106, 1997.
4. Newman WP III, Freedman DS, Voors AW et al: Relation of serum lipoprotein levels and systolic blood pressure to early atherosclerosis: the Bogalusa Heart Study, *N Engl J Med* 314:138-444, 1986.
5. Enos WF, Holmes RH, Beyer J: Coronary disease among United States soldiers killed in action in Korea: preliminary report, *JAMA* 152:1090-1093, 1953.
6. Berenson GS, Srinivasan SR, Bao W et al, for the Bogalusa Heart Study: Association between multiple cardiovascular risk factors and the early development of atherosclerosis, *N Engl J Med* 338:1650-1656, 1998.
7. Davis PH, Dawson JD, Riley WA et al: Carotid intimal-medial thickness is related to cardiovascular risk factors measured from childhood through middle age: the Muscatine Study, *Circulation* 104:2815-2819, 2001.
8. Li S, Chen W, Srinivasan SR et al: Childhood cardiovascular risk factors and carotid vascular changes in adulthood: the Bogalusa Heart Study, *JAMA* 290:2271-2276, 2003.
9. Raitakari OT, Juonala M, Kahonen M et al: Cardiovascular risk factors in childhood and carotid intima-media thickness in adulthood: the Cardiovascular Risk in Young Finns Study, *JAMA* 290:2277-2283, 2003.
10. Knoflach M, Kiechl S, Kind M et al: Cardiovascular risk factors and atherosclerosis in young males: ARMY study (Atherosclerosis Risk-Factors in Male Youngsters), *Circulation* 108:1064-1069, 2003.
11. Sanchez A, Barth JD, Zhang L: The carotid artery wall thickness in teenagers is related to their diet and the typical risk factors of heart disease among adults, *Atherosclerosis* 152:265-266, 2000.
12. National Heart, Lung, and Blood Institute: *The Lipid Research Clinics population studies book,* vol 1, *The prevalence study,* NIH Pub No 80-1527, Bethesda, Md, 1980, US Department of Health and Human Services, Public Health Service, National Institutes of Health.
13. Berenson G, Srinivasan SR, Cresanta JL et al: Dynamic changes of serum lipoproteins in children during adolescence and sexual maturation, *Am J Epidemiol* 113:157-170, 1981.
14. Srinivasan SR, Wattigney W, Webber LS et al: Race and gender differences in serum lipoproteins of children, adolescents, and young adults: the Bogalusa Heart Study, *Prev Med* 20:671-684, 1991.
15. Belcher JD, Ellison RC, Shepard WE et al: Lipid and lipoprotein distributions in children by ethnic group, gender and geographic location: preliminary findings of the Child and Adolescent Trial for Cardiovascular Health (CATCH), *Prev Med* 22:143-153, 1993.
16. Labarthe DR, Nichaman MZ, Harrist RB et al: Development of cardiovascular risk factors from ages 8 to 18 in Project Heartbeat! Study design and patterns of change in plasma total cholesterol concentration, *Circulation* 95:2636-2642, 1997.
17. National Cholesterol Education Program: *Report of the Expert Panel on Blood Cholesterol Levels in Children and Adolescents,* NIH Pub No 91-2732, Bethesda, Md, 1991, US Department of

Health and Human Services, Public Health Service, National Institutes of Health.

18. Hickman TB, Briefel RR, Carroll MD et al: Distributions and trends of serum lipid levels among United States children and adolescents ages 4-19 years: data from the Third National Health and Nutrition Examination Survey, *Prev Med* 27:879-890, 1998.

19. Bradley CB, Harrell JS, McMurray RG et al: Prevalence of high cholesterol, high blood pressure, and smoking among elementary school children in North Carolina, *N C Med J* 58:362-367, 1997.

20. Srinivasan SR, Berenson GS: Childhood lipoprotein profiles and implications for adult coronary artery disease: the Bogalusa Heart Study, *Am J Med Sci* 310(suppl 1):S62-S67, 1995.

21. Morrison JA, Friedman LA, Sprecher DL et al: Pubertal stage affects prevalence of dyslipidemia identified by national pediatric guidelines: longitudinal evidence from two cohort studies, *Circulation* 108:IV-781, 2003.

22. Kavey RE, Daniels SR, Lauer RM et al: American Heart Association guidelines for primary prevention of atherosclerotic cardiovascular disease beginning in childhood, *Circulation* 107:1562-1566, 2003 (published simultaneously in *J Pediatr* 142:368-372, 2003).

23. American Academy of Pediatrics: Cholesterol in childhood, *Pediatrics* 101:141-147, 1998.

24. Webber LS, Srinivasan SR, Wattigney WA et al: Tracking of serum lipids and lipoproteins from childhood to adulthood: the Bogalusa Heart Study, *Am J Epidemiol* 33:884-898, 1991.

25. Lauer RM, Lee J, Clarke WR: Factors affecting the relationship between childhood and adult cholesterol levels: the Muscatine Study, *Pediatrics* 82:309-318, 1988.

26. Lauer RM, Clarke WR: Use of cholesterol measurements in childhood for the prediction of adult hypercholesterolemia: the Muscatine Study, *JAMA* 264:3034-3038, 1990.

27. Munter P, He J, Cutler JA et al: Trends in blood pressure among children and adolescents, *JAMA* 291:2107-2113, 2004.

28. National Center for Health Statistics: *Plan and operation of the Third National Health and Nutrition Examination Survey, 1988-1994*, Pub No 94-1308, Rockville, Md, 1994, US Department of Health and Human Services.

29. Ingelfinger JR: Pediatric antecedents of adult cardiovascular disease, *N Engl J Med* 350:2123-2126, 2004.

30. Daniels SR, Meyer RA, Loggie JMH: Determinants of cardiac involvement in children and adolescents with essential hypertension, *Circulation* 82:1243-1248, 1990.

31. Hanevold C, Waller J, Daniels SR et al: The effects of obesity, gender, and ethnic group on left ventricular hypertrophy and geometry in hypertensive children: a collaborative study of the International Pediatric Hypertension Association, *Pediatrics* 113:328-333, 2004.

32. Kay JD, Sinaiko AR, Daniels SR: Pediatric hypertension, *Am Heart J* 142:422-432, 2001.

33. Lauer RM, Clarke WR: Childhood risk factors for high adult blood pressure: the Muscatine Study, *Pediatrics* 84:633-641, 1989.

34. Freedman DS, Dietz WH, Srinivasan SR et al: The relation of overweight to cardiovascular risk factors among children and adolescents: the Bogalusa Heart Study, *Pediatrics* 103(6 pt 1):1175-1182, 1999.

35. Sorof J, Daniels SR: Obesity hypertension in children: a problem of epidemic proportions, *Hypertension* 40:441-447, 2002.

36. Sorof JM, Poffenbarger T, Franco K et al: Isolated systolic hypertension, obesity, and hyperkinetic hemodynamic states in children, *J Pediatr* 140:660-666, 2002.

37. Sinaiko AR, Steinberger J, Moran A et al: Relation of insulin resistance to blood pressure in childhood, *J Hypertens* 20:509-517, 2002.

38. Boyd GS, Koenigsberg J, Falkner B et al: Effect of obesity and high blood pressure on plasma lipid levels in children and adolescents, *Pediatrics* 116:442-446, 2005.

39. National High Blood Pressure Working Group on High Blood Pressure in Children and Adolescents: The Fourth Report on the Diagnosis, Evaluation, and Treatment of High Blood Pressure in Children and Adolescents, *Pediatrics* 114(suppl):555-576, 2004.

40. Ogden CL, Flegal KM, Carroll MD et al: Prevalence and trends in overweight among US children and adolescents, 1999-2000, *JAMA* 288:1728-1732, 2002.

41. Eckel RH, Daniels SR, Jacobs AK et al: America's children: a critical time for prevention, *Circulation* 111:1866-1868, 2005.

42. Centers for Disease Control and Prevention, National Center for Health Statistics: *2000 CDC growth charts: United States.* Retrieved September 12, 2005, from www.cdc.gov/growthcharts/

43. Koplan JP, Liverman CT, Kraak VI, editors: *Preventing childhood obesity: health in the balance,* Washington, DC, 2004, Institute of Medicine, National Academies Press.

44. Daniels SR, Arnett DK, Eckel RH et al: Overweight in children and adolescents: pathophysiology, consequences, prevention and treatment, *Circulation* 111:1999-2012, 2005.

45. Strauss RS, Pollack HA: Epidemic increase in childhood overweight, 1986-1998, *JAMA* 286:2845-2848, 2001.

46. US Centers for Disease Control and Prevention, National Center for Health Statistics: Prevalence of overweight among students in grades 9-12 by sex and race/ethnicity, Youth Risk Behavior Surveillance (YRBS, 2003), *Morb Mortal Wkly Rep* 53(SS-2):May 21, 2004.

47. Zephier E, Himes JH, Story M: Prevalence of overweight and obesity in American Indian school children and adolescents in the Aberdeen area: a population study, *Int J Obes Relat Metab Disord* 23:S23-S30, 1999.

48. Chen W, Srinivasan SR, Elkasabany A et al: Cardiovascular risk factors clustering features of insulin resistance syndrome (syndrome X) in a biracial (black-white) population of children, adolescents and young adults: the Bogalusa Heart Study, *Am J Epidemiol* 150:667-674, 1999.

49. Goodman E, Dolan LM, Morrison JA et al: Factor analysis of clustered cardiovascular risks in adolescence: obesity is the predominate correlate of risk among youth, *Circulation* 111:1970-1977, 2005.

50. Cook S, Weitzman A, Auinger P et al: Prevalence of a metabolic syndrome phenotype in adolescents: findings from the Third National Health and Nutrition Examination Survey, 1988-1994, *Arch Pediatr Adolesc Med* 157:821-827, 2003.

51. de Ferranti SD, Gauvreau K, Ludwig DS et al: Prevalence of the metabolic syndrome in American adolescents: findings from the Third Health and Nutrition Examination Survey, *Circulation* 110:2494-2497, 2004.

52. Lambert M, Paradis G, O'Loughlin J et al: Insulin resistance syndrome in a representative sample of children and adolescents from Quebec, Canada, *Int J Obes Relat Metab Disord* 28:833-841, 2004.

53. Weiss R, Dziura J, Burgert TS et al: Obesity and the metabolic syndrome in children and adolescents, *N Engl J Med* 350:2362-2374, 2004.

54. Steinberger J, Moran A, Hong CP et al: Adiposity in childhood predicts obesity and insulin resistance in young adulthood, *J Pediatr* 138:469-473, 2001.

55. Chen W, Bao W, Begum S et al: Age-related patterns of the clustering of cardiovascular risk variables of syndrome X from childhood to young adulthood in a population made up of black and white subjects: the Bogalusa Heart Study, *Diabetes* 49:1042-1048, 2000.

56. Sinaiko AR, Steinberger J, Moran A et al: Relation of body-mass index and insulin resistance to cardiovascular risk factors, inflammatory factors, and oxidative stress during adolescence, *Circulation* 111:1985-1991, 2005.

57. Fagot-Campagna A, Pettit D, Engelgau MM et al: Type 2 diabetes among North American children and adolescents: an epidemiologic review and a public health perspective, *J Pediatr* 136:664-672, 2000.

58. Pinhas-Hamiel O, Zeitler P: The global spread of type 2 diabetes mellitus in children and adolescents, *J Pediatr* 146:693-700, 2005.

59. Pinhas-Hamiel O, Dolan LM, Daniels SR et al: Increased incidence of non-insulin dependent diabetes mellitus among adolescents, *J Pediatr* 128:608-615, 1996.

60. Scott CR, Smith JM, Cradock MM et al: Characteristics of youth-onset noninsulin dependent diabetes mellitus and insulin-dependent diabetes mellitus at diagnosis, *Pediatrics* 100:84-91, 1997.

61. Libman I, Arslanian S: Type 2 diabetes in childhood: the American perspective, *Horm Res* 59(suppl 1):69-75, 2003.

62. Sinha R, Fisch G, Teague B et al: Prevalence of impaired glucose tolerance among children and adolescents with marked obesity, *N Engl J Med* 346:802-810, 2002.

63. Hannon TS, Rao G, Arslanian SA: Childhood obesity and type 2 diabetes mellitus, *Pediatrics* 116:473-480, 2005.

64. Best JA, Brown R, Cameron SN et al: Gender and predisposing attributes as predictors of smoking onset: implications for theory and practice, *Journal of Health Education* 26:S52-S60, 1995.

65. US Department of Health and Human Services: *Reducing tobacco use: a report of the Surgeon General,* Atlanta, 2000, US Department of Health and Human Services, Centers for Disease Control and Prevention, National Center for Chronic Disease Prevention and Health Promotion, Office on Smoking and Health.

66. Grunbaum JA, Kann L, Kinchen S et al: Youth Risk Behavior Surveillance: United States, 2003, *J Sch Health* 74:307-324, 2004.

67. US Centers for Disease Control and Prevention, National Center for Health Statistics: Tobacco use, access, and exposure to tobacco in media among middle and high school students: United States, 2004, *MMWR Morb Mortal Wkly Rep* 54:297-301, 2005.

68. Emery S, Wakefield MA, Terry-McElrath Y et al: Televised state-sponsored anti-tobacco advertising and youth smoking beliefs and behavior in the United States, 1999-2000, *Arch Pediatr Adolesc Med* 159:639-645, 2005.

69. US Centers for Disease Control and Prevention, National Center for Health Statistics: Estimated exposure of adolescents to state-funded anti-tobacco television advertisement: 37 states and the District of Columbia, 1999-2003, *MMWR Morb Mortal Wkly Rep* 54:1077-1080, 2005.

70. Winkleby MA, Robinson TR, Sundquist J et al: Ethnic variation in cardiovascular disease risk factors among children and young adults: findings from the Third National Nutrition Examination Survey, 1988-1994, *JAMA* 281:1006-1113, 1999.

71. Sly DF, Arheart K, Dietz N et al: The outcome consequences of defunding the Minnesota youth tobacco-use prevention program, *Prev Med* 41:503-510, 2005.

72. US Department of Health and Human Services: *Healthy People 2010: understanding and improving health,* ed 2, Washington, DC, 2000, US Government Printing Office.

73. Cavill NS, Biddle S, Sallis JF: Health enhancing physical activity for young people: statement of the United Kingdom expert consensus conference, *Pediatric Exercise Science* 13:12-25, 2001.

74. Strong WB, Malina RM, Blimkie CJ et al: Evidence-based physical activity for school-aged youth, *J Pediatr* 146:732-737, 2005.

75. US Centers for Disease Control and Prevention, National Center for Health Statistics: Youth Risk Behavior Surveillance (YRBS, 2003), *Morb Mortal Wkly Rep* 53(SS-2):May 21, 2004.

76. Kimm S, Glynn N, Kriska A et al: Decline in activity in black girls and white girls during adolescence, *N Engl J Med* 347:709-715, 2002.

77. Khaw K, Barrett-Connor E: Family history of heart attack, *Circulation* 74:239-244, 1982.

78. Myers RH, Kiely DK, Cupples A et al: Parental history is an independent risk factor for coronary artery disease: the Framingham Study, *Am Heart J* 960-963, 1990.

79. Glueck CJ, Fallat RW, Tsang R et al: Hyperlipidemia in progeny of parents with myocardial infarction before age 50, *Am J Dis Child* 127:70-75, 1974.

80. Morrison JA, Khoury P, Laskarzewski PM et al: Familial associations of lipids and lipoproteins in families of hypercholesterolemic probands, *Arteriosclerosis* 2:151-159, 1982.

81. Shear CL, Webber LS, Freedman DS et al: The relationship between parental history of vascular disease and cardiovascular disease risk factors in children: the Bogalusa Heart Study, *Am J Epidemiol* 122:762-771, 1985.

82. Genest JJ, Martin-Munley SS, McNamara JR et al: Familial lipoprotein disorders in patients with premature coronary artery disease, *Circulation* 85:2025-2033, 1992.

83. Lloyd-Jones DM, Nam BH, D'Agostino RB: Parental cardiovascular disease as a risk factor for cardiovascular disease in middle aged adults: a prospective study of parents and offspring, *JAMA* 291:2204-2211, 2004.

84. Iannotti RJ, Zuckerman AE, Rifai N: Intrafamilial relations of cardiovascular disease risk factors in African-Americans: longitudinal results from DC SCAN, *Prev Med* 28:367-377, 1999.

85. Allen JK, Young DR, Blumenthal RS et al: Prevalence of hypercholesterolemia among siblings of persons with premature coronary heart disease, *Arch Intern Med* 156:1654-1660, 1996.

86. Bao W, Srinivasan AR, Valdez R et al: Longitudinal changes in cardiovascular risk from childhood to young adulthood in offspring of parents with coronary artery disease, *JAMA* 278:1749-1754, 1997.

87. Hayman LL, Meininger JC, Gallagher PR et al: Familial resemblance and tracking of the lipid profile from childhood to adolescence: a longitudinal twin-family study, *Circulation* 90:590, 1995.

88. Hayman LL, Meininger JC, Gallagher PR et al: Nongenetic influences of obesity on risk factors for cardiovascular disease during two phases of development, *Nurs Res* 44:277-283, 1995.

89. Morrison JA, Kelly KA, Horvitz R et al: Parent-offspring and sibling lipid and lipoprotein associations during and after sharing of household environments: the Princeton School District Family Study, *Metabolism* 31:158-166, 1982.

90. Laskarzewski P, Morrison JA, Khoury P et al: Parent-child nutrient interrelationships in school children, ages 6-19 years: the Princeton School District Study, *Am J Clin Nutr* 33:2350-2355, 1980.

91. Oliveria SS, Ellison RC, Moore LL et al: Parent-child relationships in nutrient intake: the Framingham Children's Study, *Am J Clin Nutr* 56:593-598, 1992.

92. Sallis JF, Nader PR: Family determinants of health behaviors. In Gochman DS, editor: *Health behavior: emerging research perspectives,* New York, 1997, Plenum Press.

93. Klesges RC, Malott JM, Boschee PF et al: The effects of parental influences on children's food intake, physical activity, and relative weight, *International Journal of Obesity* 5:335-346, 1986.

94. Heath AC, Cates RC, Martin NG et al: Genetic contribution to risk of smoking initiation: comparisons across birth cohorts and across cultures, *J Subst Abuse* 5:221-226, 1993.

95. Boomsma DI, Koopmans JR, van Doormen L et al: Genetic and social influences on starting to smoke: a study of Dutch adolescent twins and their parents, *Addiction* 89:219-226, 1994.

96. Carmelli D, Swan GE, Robinette D et al: Genetic influence on smoking: a study of male twins, *N Engl J Med* 327:881-883, 1992.

97. Goldstein JL, Brown MS: Familial hypercholesterolemia. In Scriver CL, Beaudet AI, Sly WS, Valle D, editors: *The metabolic basis of inherited disease,* ed 6, New York, 1989, McGraw-Hill.

98. Cortner JA, Coates PM, Gallagher PR: Prevalence and expression of familial combined hyperlipidemia in childhood, *J Pediatr* 116:514-519, 1990.

99. Hopkins PN, Heiss G, Ellison C et al: Coronary artery disease risk in familial combined hyperlipidemia and familial hypertriglyceridemia: a case-control comparison from the National Heart, Lung, and Blood Institute—Family Heart Study, *Circulation* 108:519-523, 2003.

100. Becker DM, Yook YM, Moy TF et al: Markedly high prevalence of coronary risk factors in apparently healthy African-American and white siblings of persons with premature coronary heart disease, *Am J Cardiol* 82:1046-1051, 1998.

101. Mora S, Yanek LR, Moy TF et al: Interaction of body mass index and Framingham risk score in predicting incident coronary disease in families, *Circulation* 111:1871-1876, 2005.

102. Williams CL, Hayman LL, Daniels SR et al: Cardiovascular health in childhood: a statement for health professionals from the committee on Atherosclerosis, Hypertension, and Obesity in the Young (AHOY) of the Council on Cardiovascular Disease in the Young, American Heart Association, *Circulation* 106:143-160, 2002.

103. Hayman LL, Williams CL, Daniels SR et al: Cardiovascular health promotion in the schools: a statement for health and education professionals and child health advocates from the Committee on Atherosclerosis, Hypertension, and Obesity in Youth (AHOY) of the Council on Cardiovascular Disease in the Young, American Heart Association, *Circulation* 110:2266-2275, 2004.

104. Stone EJ, Pearson TA, editors: Community trials for cardiopulmonary health: directions for public health practice, policy, and research, *Ann Epidemiol* S7:S1-S124, 1997.

105. Resnicow T, Robinson TN: School-based cardiovascular disease prevention studies: review and synthesis, *Ann Epidemiol* S7:S14-S31, 1997.

106. Meininger JC: Primary prevention of cardiovascular disease risk factors: review and implications for population-based practice, *Adv Prac Nurs Q* 3:70-79, 1997.

107. Luepker RV, Perry CL, McKinlay SM et al: Outcomes of a field trial to improve children's dietary patterns and physical activity: the child and adolescent trial for cardiovascular health (CATCH), *JAMA* 275(10):768-776, 1996.

108. National Alliance for Nutrition and Activity: *Dispensing junk: how school vending undermines efforts to feed children well,* Washington, DC, 2004, The Alliance.

109. Nestle M: *Food politics: how the food industry influences nutrition and health,* Berkeley, 2002, University of California Press.

110. Gidding S, Dennison BA, Birch LL et al: Dietary recommendations for children and adolescents: a guide for practitioners, *Circulation* 112:2061-2075, 2005.

111. Hayman LL, Reineke PR: Preventing coronary heart disease: the implementation of healthy lifestyle strategies for children and adolescents, *J Cardiovasc Nurs* 4:294-301, 2003.

112. Ockene IS, Hayman LL, Pasternak RC et al: Adherence issues and behavior change: achieving a long-term solution, *J Am Coll Cardiol* 40:630-640, 2002.

113. McCrindle B, Urbina EM, Dennison BA et al: Drug therapy of lipid abnormalities in children and adolescents: scientific statement from the AHOY Committee, Council on Cardiovascular Disease in the Young, American Heart Association, *Circulation* (in press).

114. Stein EA, Ilingworth DR, Kwiterovich PO Jr et al: Efficacy and safety of lovastatin in adolescent males with heterozygous familial hypercholesterolemia: a randomized controlled trial, *JAMA* 281:137-144, 1999.

115. De Jongh S, Ose L, Szamosi T et al: Efficacy and safety of statin therapy in children with familial hypercholesterolemia, *Circulation* 106:2231-2237, 2002.

116. Wiegman A, Hutten BA, deGroot E et al: Efficacy and safety of statin therapy in children with familial hypercholesterolemia: a randomized controlled trial, *JAMA* 292:331-337, 2004.

chapter 33

Smoking

Nancy Houston Miller

CHAPTER ABBREVIATIONS

CB1 cannabinoid-1

CHD coronary heart disease

CI confidence interval

COMMIT Community Intervention Trial for Smoking Cessation

NRT nicotine replacement therapy

PVD peripheral vascular disease

OR odds ratio

RR relative risk

Smoking contributes to the high rate of cardiovascular disease in the United States and worldwide. The annual death toll in the United States from smoking-related illnesses approaches 440,000, with more than 4.8 million deaths occurring globally.[1] Moreover, smoking cuts the life span of males by 13.2 years and females by 14.5 years.[2] The World Health Organization projects that by 2030 smoking will kill at least 10 million persons annually, making cigarette smoking the world's leading cause of death.[3] Effective methods to address this chronic and potentially addictive condition will contribute substantially to a decline in cardiovascular disease and in overall morbidity and mortality from other diseases such as cancer and chronic obstructive pulmonary disease.

Smoking in the United States declined by 47 percent from 1965 to 2004. Based on data from the Centers for Disease Control and Prevention, National Center for Health Statistics, in 2002, 22.5 percent of adults 18 and older (48.5 million persons) were smoking cigarettes.[4] However, this grossly underestimates the risk of smoking-related illnesses from all forms of tobacco use and secondhand smoke. Moreover, the average age of smoking initiation is 11 to 12 years, subjecting children to a high lifetime addiction risk. If current smoking patterns continue, it is likely that 6.4 million persons who start smoking before age 18 will die prematurely from tobacco-related illnesses. In 2002, the National Household Survey on Drug Abuse indicated that 71.5 million Americans over age 12 (30.4 percent) reported using some form of tobacco in the past month.[5] Among those smoking, 61.1 million (26.6 percent) reported smoking cigarettes; 12.5 million (5.4 percent) smoked cigars; 7.8 million (3.3 percent) used smokeless tobacco; and 1.8 million (0.8 percent) smoked pipes. Although the largest number of smokers smoke cigarettes, smokeless tobacco and cigars and pipes also have significant medical consequences, including lung, esophageal, laryngeal, and oral cancers.

Tobacco use creates a heavy economic burden to society. Direct medical costs and lost productivity costs associated with smoking are estimated to approach $155 billion per year.[4] Many strategies for prevention and intervention are needed in order to combat an aggressive tobacco industry that spent $11.2 billion in 2001 on advertising and tobacco promotion in the United States alone.[6]

SMOKING AND ITS ADDICTIVE PROPERTIES

Smoking cigarettes and other forms of tobacco is highly addicting. The addictive drug in tobacco is nicotine, which reaches the brain within 4 seconds. In addition, the pharmacological and behavioral processes that determine tobacco addiction are similar to drugs such as heroin and cocaine. As a result of the addiction associated with tobacco products, smoking causes physiological and psychological dependence. Common characteristics of addictions such as tobacco dependence include the following[2]:

- Predictable withdrawal symptoms
- Physical dependence and tolerance for the substance
- An immediate sense of gratification
- Use of the drug despite social or medical disapproval and harm to physical, social, psychological, or economic well-being
- Use of the drug to restore physical and psychological comfort

Thus, interventions need to include pharmacological aids and behavioral strategies.

GENDER- AND ETHNIC-SPECIFIC DIFFERENCES

The prevalence of smoking in the United States has always been lower in women than in men. As shown in Table 33-1, the percentage of Americans over age 18 who smoke is higher in men than women. The percentage of teens in grades 9 to 12 reporting current tobacco use in 2003 was 30.3 percent of male students and 24.6 percent of females, just a 5 percent difference.[7] However, the percentage of females ages 12 to 17 who reported using tobacco in the month before taking the Youth Risk Behavioral Surveillance Survey was higher than that of males (14.2 percent versus 13.3 percent).[4] This is a frightening trend in gender parity.

The 600 percent increase in lung cancer rates since 1950 most certainly reflects the increase in smoking rates in women in the United States. Smoking rates for women in the United States now rank in the highest

■ ■ ■

TABLE 33-1   PREVALENCE OF CIGARETTE SMOKING
IN U.S. ADULTS AGE 18 AND OLDER

POPULATION GROUP	PREVALENCE, 2002
Total population	48,500,000 (22.5%)
Total males	(25.2%)
Total females	(20.0%)
White males	25.2%
White females	20.7%
Black or African American males	27.0%
Black or African American females	18.5%
Hispanic or Latino males	23.2%
Hispanic or Latino females	12.5%
Asian-only males	21.3%
Asian-only females	6.9%
American Indian or Alaska Native males	32.0%
American Indian or Alaska Native females	36.9%

Abstracted data 1999-2001, Centers for Disease Control/National Center for
Health Statistics.

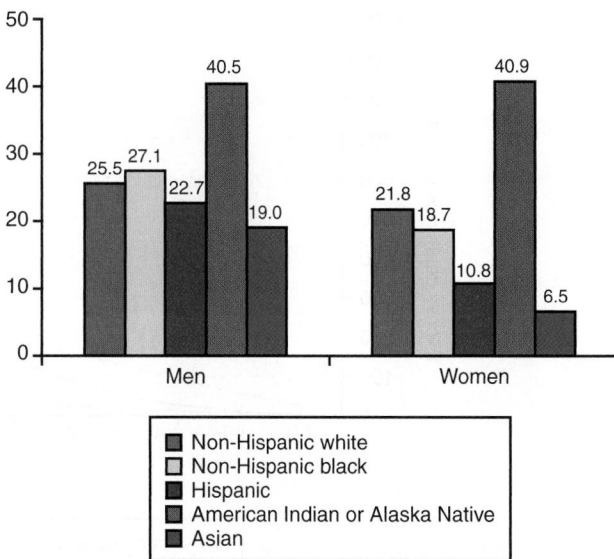

FIGURE 33-1 ■ Centers for Disease Control and Prevention:
Cigarette smoking among adults—United States 2002. (*Morbidity
and Mortality Weekly Review.* May 28, 2004; 53: 427-431.)

third for women worldwide.[8] Moreover, the decline in
smoking has occurred primarily in men, with women
showing a much slower rate in quitting. Vigilant efforts
are needed to reduce the smoking prevalence in women
in the United States and globally.

Because of the adverse synergy of oral contraceptives
and smoking, young female smokers who take oral contraceptives have a particularly high risk of premature
coronary heart disease and stroke, peripheral vascular
disease (**PVD**), and detrimental effects from phlebitis
and pulmonary embolism.[9] In addition, smoking during
pregnancy has numerous negative effects, including
low birth weight of the child, increased risk of neonatal
death, premature birth, spontaneous abortion, and potential growth-retarding effects on the fetus that affect
long-term growth and intellectual development. These
issues make a reduction in smoking prevalence imperative. The World Health Organization estimates that the
number of women smokers will almost triple over the
next generation to more than 500 million smokers,[10] of
whom 200 million will die prematurely from smoking-
related diseases. Women report significantly more barriers to quitting and more withdrawal symptoms than
men, which underscores the need to prevent the start
of tobacco use by women.

As shown in Figure 33-1, ethnicity influences smoking prevalence. Among adults age 18 and older, the
prevalence is highest in American Indians and Alaska
Natives (40.9 percent for each group), and lowest in
Asian women (6.5 percent).[11] Different smoking rates in
various populations are attributed to many factors, including socioeconomic status, cultural characteristics,
acculturation, stress, targeted advertising, the price of
cigarettes, parental and community disapproval, and
the capacity of communities to launch effective tobacco
control programs.

Non-Hispanic black adults have prevalence rates similar to non-Hispanic whites. However, it is important to
note that coronary heart disease (**CHD**) mortality rates
are much higher in non-Hispanic blacks, especially at
younger ages. In addition, black men are 50 percent

more likely to develop lung cancer than white men.
Black men are also twice as likely to suffer from a
stroke.[12]

SMOKING AND CARDIOVASCULAR RISK

Smoking significantly increases the risk of CHD, PVD,
aortic aneurysm, and stroke. The relative risk is highest
for those with PVD and lowest for stroke, with intermediate relative risk for CHD and aortic aneurysm.[13] In
addition, smoking increases the risk of coronary thrombosis and sudden cardiac death.

Coronary Heart Disease Risk

Smoking increases CHD risk at all levels of cigarette
smoking, including less than five cigarettes per day. Although smoking causes excess mortality from CHD,
lung cancer, cerebrovascular disease, and chronic obstructive pulmonary disease, excess mortality from
CHD is evident earliest in life. Under age 45, CHD is the
main cause of increased mortality caused by cigarette
smoking[13] (Figure 33-2).

In addition to CHD mortality, smoking is associated
with significant CHD morbidity in those currently using
tobacco. Yusuf and colleagues[14] found that the risk of
myocardial infarction in 30,000 subjects across 52 countries was more than doubled in smokers. Although a
combination of nine risk factors accounted for more
than 90 percent of the risk of a myocardial infarction in
all age groups, and in men and women in the INTER-
HEART study, smoking and lipids carried the greatest
attributable risk of overall cardiovascular disease (Table
33-2). Smoking also carries a higher risk of myocardial
infarction in women, especially in those younger than
age 45.[15]

The benefits of quitting occur relatively soon after
giving up tobacco. In fact, after 1 year of abstinence

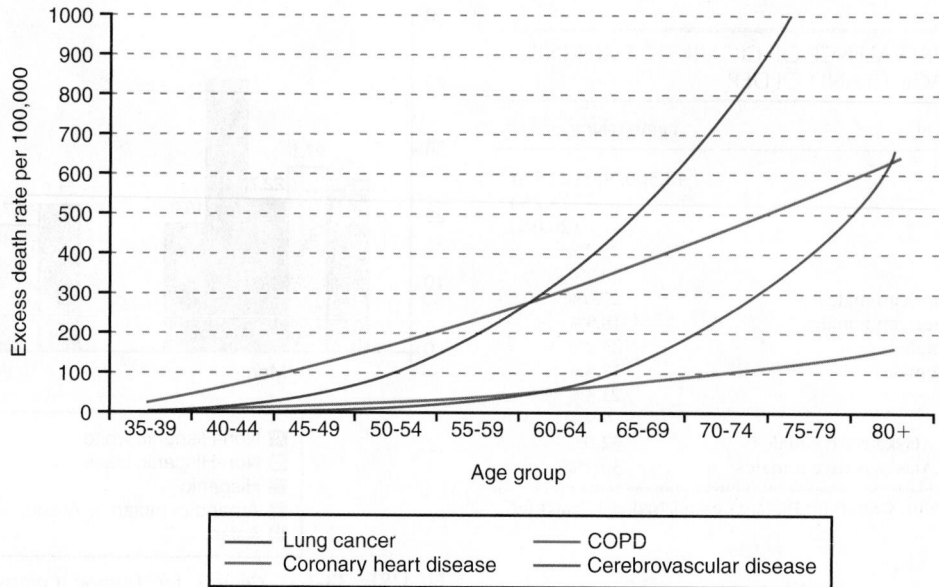

FIGURE 33-2 ■ Cause-specific death rates by age in male smokers. *COPD,* Chronic obstructive pulmonary disease. (From Thun MJ, Heath CW Jr: Changes in mortality from smoking in two American Cancer Society Prospective Studies since 1959, *Prev Med* 26(4):422-426.)

■ ■ ■

TABLE 33-2 INTERHEART STUDY: RISK OF ACUTE MYOCARDIAL INFARCTION ASSOCIATED WITH RISK FACTORS IN THE OVERALL POPULATION

RISK FACTOR	% CONTROLS	% CASES	Population Attributable Risk 1 (99% CI)	Population Attributable Risk 2 (99% CI)
APO B/APO A-I (5 v 1)	20.0	33.5	54.1 (49.6 to 58.6)	49.2 (43.8 to 54.5)
Currently smoking	26.8	45.2	36.4 (33.9 to 39.0)	35.7 (32.5 to 39.1)
Diabetes	7.5	18.5	12.3 (11.2 to 13.5)	9.9 (8.5 to 11.5)
Hypertension	21.9	39.0	23.4 (21.7 to 25.1)	17.9 (15.7 to 20.4)
Abdominal obesity (3 v 1)	33.3	46.3	33.7 (30.2 to 37.4)	20.1 (15.3 to 26.0)
Psychosocial	—	—	28.8 (22.6 to 35.8)	32.5 (25.1 to 40.8)
Vegetables and fruits daily	42.4	35.8	12.9 (10.0 to 16.6)	13.7 (9.9 to 18.6)
Exercise	19.3	14.3	25.5 (20.1 to 31.8)	12.2 (5.5 to 25.1)
Alcohol	24.5	24.0	13.9 (9.3 to 20.2)	6.7 (2.0 to 20.2)
Combined	—	—	**90.4 (88.1 to 92.4)**	**90.4 (88.1 to 92.4)**

APO, Apolipoprotein; *CI,* confidence interval.
From Yusuf A, Hawken S, Ounpuu S et al: *Lancet* 364(9438):937-952, 2004.

from smoking, the excess risk of CHD related to smoking is cut in half, and it gradually continues to decline over time. After 15 years of abstinence, a former smoker has achieved a risk level similar to that of a person who never smoked.[16]

What about the benefits of quitting smoking in older individuals? In a longitudinal follow-up of 2674 individuals ages 65 to 74, Jajich and colleagues[17] showed lower death rates from CHD within 1 to 5 years of quitting compared with elders who continued to smoke. Results from the Coronary Artery Surgery Study (CASS) also revealed that those over age 65 who quit smoking within 1 year before their diagnosis had lower rates of myocardial infarction and CHD death than those who continued to smoke.[18] This benefit was similar in older and younger individuals.

Stroke and Peripheral Vascular Disease Risk

Smoking also is associated with an increased risk of ischemic stroke in men and women. A 20-year prospective study in which all cardiovascular risk factors were controlled demonstrated that cigarette smoking increased the risk of mortality from stroke; risk also was associated with the amount smoked.[19] These findings are illustrated further in a meta-analysis that shows an overall risk ratio of 1.5 for stroke associated with cigarette smoking.[20] Recent prospective evidence has linked cigarette smoking to elevated risk of hemorrhagic stroke, including intracranial hemorrhage and subarachnoid hemorrhage. Again, risk was associated with amount smoked.[9]

Similar to CHD, giving up smoking significantly decreases the risk of stroke. In a 12-year follow-up of the

Nurses Health Study, the risk ratio for stroke in current smokers was 2.58, declining to 1.34 in former smokers. After 2 to 4 years of cessation, the excess risk among former smokers was no different from those who had never smoked.[21]

Although many of the classic risk factors such as dyslipidemia and diabetes are associated with PVD, smoking accounts for 75 percent of the risk of developing PVD.[22] This risk is strongly dose-dependent, is related to the number of cigarettes smoked, and with the number of years smoked. Cigarette smoking also has been linked to progression of PVD over a 4-year period.[23] Similar to stroke, the risk declines in those who have quit smoking and approaches normal in those who quit smoking more than 5 years previously.

Risk of Sudden Cardiac Death

Smoking is associated with a twofold to fourfold increased risk of sudden cardiac death, which has important implications for young women.[24] In young women smokers, smoking is the primary risk factor for sudden death compared with the traditional risk factors associated with sudden death in older women: diabetes, hypertension, and dyslipidemia. Smoking cessation has significant benefits in lowering risk and in reducing dysrhythmic death in patients with left ventricular dysfunction after myocardial infarction and those surviving out-of-hospital cardiac arrest.[25]

PATHOPHYSIOLOGY OF SMOKING AND VASCULAR DISEASE

Smoking has important adverse pathophysiological effects on the vascular system. Most of the toxic effects of smoking are found in the 4000 compounds in cigarettes. Although carbon monoxide and nicotine often are thought to be the worst culprits associated with smoking, toxins cause adverse effects that contribute to vascular disease.[22] Systems affected are the following:

- Endothelial system
- Lipoprotein metabolism
- Blood coagulation
- Platelets
- Oxygen supply-demand

Nicotine disrupts lipid metabolism, which results in a reduction in high-density lipoprotein and an increase in low-density lipoprotein and very low-density lipoprotein cholesterol.[26] These effects impair endothelial function and plaque stability. Cigarette smoking also is prothrombotic because of increased levels of fibrinogen, factor VII, and other factors such as a decrease in plasminogen.[27] Smoking causes spontaneous platelet aggregation, increased monocyte adhesion to endothelial cells, and adverse alterations in endothelium-derived fibrinocytic and antithrombotic factors, including plasminogen activator and tissue pathway factor inhibitor.[9]

The relationship between myocardial oxygen supply and demand is affected strongly by smoking. Nicotine stimulates the central and peripheral nervous systems, creating a hyperadrenergic state that increases myocardial contractility and vasoconstriction. This increases myocardial oxygen demand. Because carbon monoxide binds to hemoglobin, it interferes with the oxygen-carrying capacity of red blood cells. This reduces the amount of hemoglobin available to bind with oxygen and impedes oxygen release from hemoglobin.[28] Standard pulse oximetry monitors cannot distinguish carbon monoxide from oxygen in the blood. Thus, smokers may have a falsely high oxygen saturation level.

EFFECTS OF SMOKING ON OTHER DISEASES

Tobacco use accounts for at least 30 percent of all cancer deaths and 87 percent of lung cancer deaths.[29] In 1985 the International Agency for Research on Cancer identified the following cancer sites associated with tobacco smoke: lung, urinary tract, upper digestive tract, larynx, and pancreas.[30] In 2004 in a follow-up report, they added evidence that tobacco was associated with cancers of the nasal cavity, nasopharynx, paranasal sinuses, stomach, liver, kidney, and uterus and was a cause of myeloid leukemia.[31]

Secondhand Smoke

Nonsmokers exposed to environmental tobacco smoke suffer a 30 percent increased risk of ischemic heart disease. Based on measurements of urinary cotinine, the National Research Council estimates that environmental tobacco exposure is equivalent to actively smoking 0.1 to 1.0 cigarettes per day.[32] An estimated 35,000 ischemic heart disease deaths annually are believed to be due to the effects of environmental tobacco exposure.[33] Secondhand smoke is especially hazardous in children, causing approximately 150,000 to 300,000 respiratory infections annually.[4]

Exposure to environmental tobacco smoke occurs in two ways. Sidestream smoke comes from a burning cigarette, whereas mainstream smoke comes from a smoker's exhalation. Most of the hazardous effects of environmental tobacco smoke result from exposure to sidestream smoke. Moreover, many of the toxins such as carbon monoxide are concentrated in sidestream smoke. For example, carbon monoxide is 8 to 11 times more concentrated in sidestream smoke than in mainstream smoke.[34] The toxins associated with sidestream smoke account for much of the increased risk of fatal CHD caused by exposure to passive smoke by nonsmokers. A dose-related relationship exists between exposure to environmental tobacco smoke and death from ischemic heart disease. In a review of six studies of women, exposure to smokers who smoked fewer than 20 cigarettes per day resulted in a risk ratio of 1.13 (1.02 to 1.24). The relative risk was 1.18 (1.04 to 1.33) in those exposed to smokers who smoked more than 20 cigarettes per day.[35]

Others have reviewed the causal association between environmental tobacco smoke and ischemic heart disease and have demonstrated that exercise tolerance is reduced in those exposed to environmental tobacco smoke.[36] This decrease in exercise tolerance is due to an increase in myocardial oxygen demand, platelet aggregation, and oxidative stress, which lead to endothelial damage and a reduction in coronary flow.

OTHER FORMS OF TOBACCO CONSUMPTION
Smokeless Tobacco

The oldest form of tobacco use is smokeless tobacco in the form of a plug or snuff placed in the oral cavity. In the United States, moist snuff and chewing tobacco are the most popular forms of smokeless tobacco. Although peak concentrations of nicotine are similar for cigarette smokers and for smokeless tobacco users, the total amount of nicotine absorbed is much higher with smokeless tobacco: 4.5 mg for chewing tobacco and 3.6 mg for moist snuff compared with 1 mg for one cigarette.[37] In addition, smokeless tobacco users swallow a large amount of nicotine and absorption continues for up to 30 minutes after the plug is removed from the mouth.[28] Thus, exposure to nicotine is greater in those using smokeless tobacco.

Smokeless tobacco use declined considerably after the mass production of cigarettes in the early 20th century. However, consumption tripled in the United States from 1972 to 1991 and has remained stable since then. Approximately 7.8 million individuals (3.3 percent of total tobacco users) over the age of 12 in the United States who reported tobacco use in the past month used smokeless tobacco. Although this is lower than those who presently smoke cigars (5.4 percent of total smokers), the proportion of persons using smokeless tobacco daily is higher than those who use cigars.[5] Smokeless tobacco use is anticipated to rise because of the increase in settings where smoking is forbidden.

In those age 12 or older, the prevalence of smokeless tobacco use is higher in males (6.4 percent) than in females (0.4 percent). The rate of smokeless tobacco use in the past month is 8.5 percent among American Indians and Alaska Natives compared with 4.2 percent in whites. Blacks, Native Hawaiians or other Pacific Islanders, and Asians each have rates less than 2.0 percent.[5] Consumption of smokeless tobacco is highest in the South and in rural areas, among those with a high school education or less, and among those who use cigarettes or drink heavily. In fact, nearly a quarter (22.9 percent) of all those who use smokeless tobacco also use cigarettes.[38] Thus, careful assessment of cigarette smoking status is indicated in those who consume smokeless tobacco products.

Detrimental health effects of smokeless tobacco include an increased risk of oral cancer, tooth decay, and periodontal disease.[39] However, the associated risk of smokeless tobacco on cardiovascular risk has been less studied. Like other tobacco products, smokeless tobacco increases heart rate and blood pressure to a degree similar to cigarette smokers. These effects are related to the amount of nicotine absorbed. Whether the effects of smokeless tobacco are more detrimental is less known, for only small observational studies have been conducted on this topic. These studies are limited by failure to control confounding variables (smoking and alcohol use) and poor measurement approaches.[37]

One large, well-designed study in Sweden of 6297 Swedish construction workers found an increased risk of CHD events among smokeless tobacco users.[40] Users had an increased risk of death (risk ratio [**RR**] 1.4; 95 percent confidence interval [**CI**] 1.3 to 1.8). In individuals ages 35 to 54, the mortality of users was twice that of nontobacco users (RR 2.1; 95 percent CI 1.4 to 2.9). Smaller Swedish studies have suggested a possible increase in cardiovascular risk, but the results may not generalize to other countries.[39]

Cigar and Pipe Smoking

Many individuals appear to be unaware of the risks of using cigars or pipe tobacco. Because both of these products contain the same toxic products found in cigarette smoke, there is no reason to expect a difference in risk between comparable exposures to cigar smoke, pipe smoke, and cigarette smoke. However, the exposure in terms of number of cigars or pipefuls of tobacco is most often lower in individuals who use these products, and most do not inhale them.

Based on data from the National Household Survey on Drug Abuse in 2001, the prevalence of individuals aged 12 and older who smoked cigars in the previous month was 5.4 percent. Cigar smoking is more prevalent in males than in females.[5] In the largest prospective study conducted to date looking at risk associated with cigar smoking, the American Cancer Society Prevention Study II, 121,278 men aged 30 and older were followed from 1982 to 1991. Data showed an increased risk of death among younger men who currently smoked cigars, with no increased risk among current cigar smokers age 75 or older or among former cigar smokers of any age. The age-adjusted risk ratio for CHD mortality among current cigar smokers was 1.37.[41]

In 1990, the prevalence of pipe smoking in the United States had decreased from 14.4 percent in 1965 to 2.0 percent.[42] Pipe smoking was rare in U.S. women (0.1 percent in 1991).[43] Most often, men switch from cigarettes to pipes or smoke pipes in combination with cigarettes or cigars.[42]

In the American Cancer Society Prevention Study, researchers showed an increased risk of CHD (RR 1.3), stroke (RR 1.27), lung cancer (RR 5.5), and chronic obstructive pulmonary disease (RR 2.98) among current pipe smokers compared with those who never used tobacco.[41] This increase in the risk of CHD mortality among pipe smokers is similar to the risk in cigar smokers described before. In a prospective study of 7735 men ages 40 to 59 who were followed for a mean of 21.8 years in the United Kingdom, pipe and cigar smokers, compared with those who never smoked, showed significantly higher risk of major CHD events (RR 1.69), stroke events (RR 1.62), and a combination of cardiovascular, noncardiovascular events, and total mortality (RR 1.49).[44]

INTERVENTIONS TO REDUCE SMOKING

Various methods have been used to prevent smoking onset and to help individuals to quit smoking. Interventions have been undertaken in school sites, work sites, and community settings. Multiple legislative and policy initiatives have been aimed at reducing tobacco smoking and encouraging cessation by raising tobacco taxes and mandating indoor clean air policies. Raising tobacco taxes has had a major influence in many states, with taxes raised as much as $2.00 per pack in some states. The high cost of cigarettes can have a major effect on youth initiating smoking. In addition, a few states have banned smoking in all public places, including work sites, restaurants, and bars. Others have imposed at least partial restrictions on smoking.[6] Mass media campaigns have been used to focus the public's attention on the significant risks associated with tobacco use.

Community Education

Community education initiatives to reduce smoking prevalence have included mass media campaigns (print, radio, and television). Individualized approaches (self-help approaches, telephone counseling) also have been used to help reduce smoking prevalence. In the 1990s, the National Heart Lung and Blood Institute funded three large community-wide health education projects to reduce the risk of cardiovascular disease. These included the Stanford Five City Project,[45] the Minnesota Heart Health Program,[46] and the Pawtucket Heart Health Program.[47] Each of these 5- to 8-year programs used multifactorial campaigns of education and risk reduction that focused on the education of health professionals, instruction of the public through the media and personal contact, and community organization to foster institutional and environmental support.[48] Interventions to decrease smoking prevalence emphasized mass media campaigns at Stanford and community organizations in Pawtucket.

All of these community-wide health education projects reported modest but significant improvements in knowledge and risk factors. In addition, all three reported favorable changes in smoking in the intervention communities. The greatest effects were seen among lower socioeconomic groups. During the study period, no changes in cardiovascular disease morbidity or mortality were found in intervention communities compared with controls, but the follow-up period may have been too short for such changes to be seen.[48]

The largest community trial for smoking cessation in the United States is the Community Intervention Trial for Smoking Cessation (**COMMIT**).[49] This matched-community randomized controlled study was designed to reduce the prevalence of smoking among men and women who smoked 25 or more cigarettes per day. The COMMIT study used community-based task forces within communities for public education, health care providers, work sites, and community resources to design interventions addressing multiple channels, including mailings, quit contests, self-help materials, and smoking resources guides. Smoke-free policies also were promoted at multiple sites. Smoking prevalence rates did not differ for heavy smokers after 5 years in the intervention and comparison communities. However, smoking prevalence was significantly lower among light to moderate smokers in the intervention communities.[49]

A recent Cochrane review suggests that community education and intervention is less promising than other interventions.[50] Changes in smoking prevalence from 27 studies resulted in a net decline in smoking prevalence of only −1.0 to −3.0 percent in men and women combined. The authors suggest that the community approach is an important part of health promotion activities, but that planners of such interventions need to take into account the scale and resources that must be devoted to move such large projects forward.

Work Site Interventions

Work sites have been used to reach large numbers of smokers to encourage cessation. Methods used in work sites have included strong advice from health care professionals, individual and group counseling, self-help materials, contests, and pharmacotherapy. Tobacco policies and bans also have been widely implemented within work sites. A meta-analysis of work site intervention programs showed limited success of these approaches, however. Failure was attributed to the limited number of randomized, controlled trials, lack of follow-up, and the heterogeneity of studies.[51]

Work sites afford the opportunity to reach a large number of smokers. Unfortunately, participation in such programs is usually low. Limited evidence indicates that participation is increased through competition or employer incentives. Although multiple interventions have been tried, individual and group counseling along with use of pharmaceuticals appear to offer more benefit than self-help materials and other approaches. A review of individual counseling in a variety of settings, including 11 work site studies, demonstrated an odds ratio for successful smoking cessation of 1.62 (95 percent CI 1.35 to 1.94).[51]

Work site tobacco policies and bans have reduced exposure of nonsmoking employees to environmental smoke. These policies and bans decrease tobacco use at work, but evidence that these approaches decrease the prevalence of smoking or overall consumption is conflicting. More research is needed to determine whether work site smoking cessation programs reduce overall smoking prevalence.[51]

Counseling in Health Care Settings

Important opportunities exist for health care professionals to provide smoking cessation advice and counseling during primary care, specialty office visits, and hospitalization. In 2000, the U.S. Public Health Services recognized tobacco dependence as a chronic condition, recommending that all health care providers ask about tobacco use at every visit and advise all smokers to quit.[52] Although lack of time, training, and reimbursement often are used as reasons why this important condition is not addressed, treating smokers in routine clinical encounters could broaden the reach to patients considering a quit attempt. At least 70 percent of all smokers visit a primary care clinician annually, 70 percent of smokers report being interested in quitting, and 40 percent of smokers report making an attempt to quit each year. In a study of smokers who attended 12 primary care clinics in Wisconsin, 68 percent chose to participate in one of four smoking cessation counseling and pharmacotherapy interventions when approached by medical assistants. Blacks were as likely to accept an intervention as white patients.[53] This suggests that if patients were to be advised to quit smoking in routine clinical practice settings, the number of those quitting could be close to 3 million annually.[54]

The hospital also offers a unique opportunity to engage individuals in cessation attempts because smokers are not allowed to smoke during hospitalization, they are focused on their health, and there are multiple health care professionals at the bedside to advise and counsel them. In addition, many patients have been hospitalized because of a smoking-related illness. All major policy-making organizations, accrediting hospitals, and health maintenance organizations—including the Joint Commission on the Accreditation of Healthcare Organizations, the National Committee on Quality Assurance, and the Centers for Medicare and Medicaid Services—have developed performance measures to ensure the identification and treatment (advice, counseling, and pharmacotherapy) of all hospitalized smokers diagnosed with an acute myocardial infarction, heart failure, and community-acquired pneumonia.[55] These organizations recognize the efficacy and cost-effectiveness of smoking interventions for hospitalized patients.

Although health care settings offer a unique opportunity for counseling, one of the difficulties encountered in clinical practice settings is the prevalence of smoking among nurses, which is approximately 18 percent.[56] Nurses compose the largest health care discipline (2.6 million) available to provide smoking cessation advice and counseling. Yet more nurses smoke than any other group of health care providers. Being a current smoker can make it difficult to intervene with patients. Thus, nurses must be helped to quit smoking, which will decrease their overall risk of smoking-related diseases and make them more effective counselors helping patients to quit.

In office practice settings, advice from a physician to quit smoking results in quit rates of approximately 6 percent per year.[57] Community-based behavioral group programs of 10 to 12 weeks provide cessation rates of 30 to 40 percent. Another approach is to begin counseling in the hospital and extend it to the outpatient setting. Studies of CHD patients suggest that men and women benefit especially from interventions begun in the hospital, with higher quit rates noted than the general population.[58] Quit rates in these populations range from 20 to 70 percent, with the highest rates in those suffering a myocardial infarction.

Guidelines for Intervening in Clinical Practice

Authors of the U.S. Treating Tobacco Use and Dependence Clinical Practice Guideline reviewed more than 6000 smoking-related studies conducted from 1975 to 1999.[52] Recommendations in the guideline state that all patients should be asked whether they use tobacco, and if they do, they should be strongly advised to quit and should be assessed for their interest in quitting. Those

willing to quit should be provided with treatments known to be effective, and follow-up sessions should be arranged. Counseling and behavioral therapy advocated include problem-solving and skills training, use of social support during treatment, and social support outside of treatment. Pharmacotherapy is strong recommended.

Evidence from randomized controlled trials summarized in the guideline[52] indicates that smoking cessation is fostered by the following:

- A 3-minute message about the importance of cessation provided by multiple health care providers
- High-intensity counseling (more than 10 minutes per session, with a total duration of 30 minutes or more)
- Four or more follow-up sessions
- Provision of multicomponent interventions such as self-help materials, telephone follow-up, pharmacotherapy, and behavioral counseling

Treatments that last 8 weeks or more double quit rates.[52] Two meta-analyses conducted in the United States and Australia[59,60] lend support for these recommendations in hospitalized patients. Interventions lasting 20 minutes in duration with extended follow-up, at least five intervention contacts with strong advice and counseling, nicotine replacement therapy, and extended proactive telephone support over at least a 3-month period offer the greatest cessation rates.

How to Intervene in Clinical Practice

Health care professionals must be trained to provide strong advice skillfully to smokers in the various practice settings where they are encountered. Because nurses compose the single largest group of health care professionals in clinical practice, they are uniquely positioned to offer significant contributions to helping smokers quit. A Cochrane review of nursing interventions for smoking cessation found that interventions delivered by nurses significantly increased the odds of quitting compared with usual care (odds ratio [**OR**] 1.5, CI 1.29 to 1.73).[61] A five-step approach to intervening is found in Table 33-3.[58] Each of these steps is explained next.

Step 1: Ask about Tobacco Use

Whether in an office setting or the hospital, a systematic approach is needed to identify all smokers. Adding smoking as a vital sign is a method that may ensure better identification of smokers. Bright stickers on charts is another way of keeping track of all smokers who require intervention. Using multiple methods to identify smokers, such as vital sign stickers, electronic identification, and notes in the nursing/physician history, provides an opportunity to ensure that all the smokers have been identified. Patients who have just decided to quit may see themselves as nonsmokers upon admittance. Thus, using multiple methods to identify individuals who are admitted through a wide variety of hospital settings may reveal smokers who need interventions.

Step 2: Advise Smokers to Quit

Smokers need strong, clear, personalized messages about the hazards of smoking. Delivering this message in a clear, empathetic way by offering support to the

■ ■ ■

TABLE 33-3   BRIEF STRATEGIES TO HELP THE PATIENT WILLING TO QUIT TOBACCO USE

STRATEGY	ACTION	IMPLEMENTATION STEPS
Ask—Systematically identify all tobacco users at every visit.	Implement an office-wide system to ensure that tobacco use is investigated and documented for every patient at every clinic visit.	• Expand vital signs to include tobacco use, or use an alternative universal identification system. For example: *Vital signs* Blood pressure: Pulse: Weight: Temperature: Respiratory rate: Tobacco use (circle one): Current Former Never • As an alternative, place a sticker that displays tobacco use status on all patient charts or in electronic medical records or computer reminder systems.
Advise—Strongly urge all tobacco users to quit.	In a clear, strong, and personalized manner, urge every tobacco user to quit.	• Advice should be as follows: *Clear:* "I think it is important for you to quit smoking now, and I can help you. Cutting down is not enough." *Strong:* "As your clinician, I need you to know that quitting smoking is the most important thing you can do to protect your health now and in the future. The clinic staff and I will help you." *Personalized:* Tie tobacco use to current health/illness, its social and economic costs, motivation level/readiness to quit, and the impact of tobacco use on children and others in the household.
Assess—Determine willingness to make a quit attempt.	Ask every tobacco user if he or she is willing to make a quit attempt at this time (e.g., within the next 30 days).	• If the patient is willing to make a quit attempt at this time, provide assistance. • If the patient will participate in an intensive treatment, deliver such a treatment or refer to an intensive intervention. • If the patient clearly states that he or she is unwilling to make a quit attempt at this time, provide a motivational intervention. • If the patient is a member of a special population (e.g., adolescent, pregnant smoker, racial/ethnic minority), consider providing additional information.
Assist—Aid the patient in quitting.	Help the patient with a quit plan.	• Advise the patient to remove tobacco products from his or her environment. Before quitting, the patient should avoid smoking in places where he or she spends a lot of time (e.g., work, home, or car). • *Set a quit date:* Ideally, the quit date should be within 2 weeks. • Tell family, friends, and coworkers about quitting and request understanding and support. • Anticipate challenges to planned quit attempt, particularly during the critical first few weeks. These include nicotine withdrawal symptoms. Remove tobacco products from your environment. Before quitting, avoid smoking in places where you spend a lot of time (e.g., work, home, or car).
	Provide practical counseling (problem solving, training).	*Abstinence:* Total abstinence is essential. "Not even a single puff after the quit date." *Past quit experience:* Review past quit attempts, including identification of what helped during the quit attempt and what factors contributed to relapse. *Anticipate triggers or challenges in the upcoming attempt:* Discuss challenges/triggers and how the patient will successfully overcome them. *Alcohol:* Since alcohol can cause relapse, the patient should consider limiting/abstaining from alcohol while quitting. *Other smokers in the household:* Quitting is more difficult when there is another smoker in the household. Patients should encourage housemates to quit with them or not smoke in their presence.
	Provide intratreatment social support.	Provide a supportive clinical environment while encouraging the patient in his or her quit attempt. "My office staff and I are available to assist you."
	Recommend the use of approved pharmacotherapy, except in special circumstances.	Recommend the use of pharmacotherapies proved to be effective. Explain how these medications increase smoking cessation success and reduce withdrawal symptoms. The first-line pharmacotherapy medications include bupropion SR, nicotine gum, nicotine inhaler, nicotine nasal spray, nicotine patch, and nicotine lozenge.
	Help the patient obtain extratreatment social support.	Help the patient develop social support for his or her quit attempt in environments outside of treatment. "Ask your spouse/partner, friends, and coworkers to support you in your quit attempt."
	Provide supplementary materials.	*Sources:* Federal agencies, nonprofit agencies, or local/state health departments *Type:* Culturally/racially/educationally/age appropriate for the patient *Location:* Readily available at every clinician's workstation
	Schedule follow-up contact, either in person or via telephone.	*Timing:* Follow-up contact should occur soon after the quit date, preferably during the first week. A second follow-up contact is recommended within the first month. Schedule further follow-up within the first month. Schedule further follow-up contacts as needed. *Actions during follow-up contact:* Congratulate the patient for success. If tobacco use has occurred, review the circumstances and elicit recommitment to total abstinence. Remind the patient that a lapse can be used as a learning experience. Identify problems already encountered and anticipate challenges in the immediate future. Assess pharmacotherapy use and problems. Consider use or referral to more intensive treatment.

From Taylor CB, Miller NH, Herman S et al: *Am J Public Health* 86:1557-1560, 1996.

patient may increase their willingness to make a quit attempt. Personalizing the message by tailoring it to the patient's condition is also beneficial. For example, if a patient has just undergone coronary artery stent placement, discussing the increased rate of restenosis as a result of continued smoking can strengthen the message. Follow by asking whether the patient sees benefits to quitting such as those that relate to health or social issues.

Step 3: Determine Willingness to Quit

Assess: Determine smokers' willingness to quit smoking by asking a simple "yes/no" question such as, "Are you willing to make an attempt to quit smoking now?" If patients are willing to quit, they should be offered assistance, the next step in the quitting process. If they are not willing, it is important to determine why. Some patients may not be aware of the risks associated with tobacco use, whereas others may have had a number of failures and are not willing to attempt without support, or they may have failed because of significant problems with withdrawal, weight gain, or depression. The U.S. Treating Tobacco Use and Dependence Guideline[52] recommends giving a motivational message to those who are not willing to quit, which includes the "5 R's": (1) relevance, (2) risks, (3) rewards, (4) roadblocks, and (5) repetition. Patients are asked to self-identify the problems associated with quitting and share this with their provider. A repetitive intervention should be undertaken during every patient visit because it may move individuals along a continuum of change. Motivational interviewing is a useful technique that can be used when patients show a lack of interest in quitting[62] (see Chapter 83).

Step 4: Aid the Patient in Quitting

Aiding a patient in the quitting process may produce a more favorable outcome—long-term smoking cessation. Part of the process involves helping a patient to set a quit date normally within 2 weeks of an encounter, giving enough support so that the patient does not slip and smoke upon leaving. A behavioral contract in which the nurse signs an agreement to support the patient has been shown to be useful for those quitting during hospitalization. If practical, follow-up telephone contacts to determine how successful patients have been in the quitting process can be used to provide support. Nurses play an active role in helping patients by offering standardized educational materials on the quitting process, suggesting Internet sites that provide a planned approach for those wanting to quit, providing telephone numbers for state quit lines through which counseling and follow-up are provided, and giving a list of stop-smoking community programs for those interested in group support.[63] Nurses should be aware of the Tobacco Control programs and resources in their local community and state. Relapse prevention training and ways to assess the need for pharmacotherapy are discussed in the last section of this chapter.

The support of family and friends is essential to a smoker attempting to quit. Living with a smoker is a strong predictor of relapse,[64] defined as a return to regular use of tobacco products. Therefore, when smokers within a family can be encouraged to quit at the same time, the probability of relapse is decreased. It is useful to ask all family members and friends who smoke to support the patient who is quitting by not smoking in the patient's presence, never offering cigarettes to the patient, and making sure that cigarettes are not lying around tempting the patient. Encourage patients to make sure they obtain the support of family members and friends. This may take the form of having a "buddy" who quits at the same time.

Step 5: Arrange for Follow-up

Patients who are attempting to quit or who have quit should be offered support and encouragement, especially in the first 2 weeks after cessation when the probability of relapse is highest. A structured telephone contact that focuses on successes in coping with urges is one way to support patients. Telephone contacts enable office staff to provide advice on coping strategies to reinforce successes or to urge them to think about setting another quit date if they have started smoking again. Quit lines available in many states are another useful method of offering follow-up to individuals who are attempting to quit.

Populations Needing Special Attention

The best method of helping individuals who are not ready to quit remains unknown, though motivational interviewing (use of five R's) holds some promise. Low rates of success have been found in patients with psychiatric disorders such as severe depression and schizophrenia, those with dual addictions to drugs and alcohol, those who have a smoker in the household, and also those who have extremely low confidence in their ability to quit.[65] Experts advise longer and more intensive treatments for these populations, but further research is needed to help them with cessation.

Another population that deserves considerable attention is pregnant women. Cessation rates of 2 to 3 percent can be expected when women are counseled about the risks associated with smoking during prenatal visits.[63] These rates increase to 10 to 25 percent when multi-component interventions are used, such as self-help manuals, brief counseling, contracts with providers, a buddy system, social support, and multiple contacts over time. A key component to cessation programs for this population includes a strong, clear, personalized message about the need for cessation of tobacco use. Like the other more difficult-to-reach populations, experts believe that a stronger intervention dose is needed for those continuing to smoke during pregnancy.[66]

IDENTIFYING THOSE WHO WILL BENEFIT FROM PHARMACOTHERAPY

The U.S. Department of Health and Human Services Treating Tobacco Use and Dependence guideline recommends that all individuals expressing an interest in quitting smoking be offered not only counseling but also pharmacotherapy.[52] Special consideration must be given to those individuals who are pregnant, adolescents, those smoking fewer than 10 cigarettes per day, and those with medical contraindications such as a recent myocardial infarction or worsening angina. Although concern often has been raised about the risk associated with offering pharmacotherapy, specifically nicotine replacement products to patients after an acute myocardial infarction and those with dysrhythmias or worsening angina pectoris, nicotine replacement therapy (**NRT**) is not considered an independent risk factor for acute myocardial events. NRT has been found to be safe in those with cardiovascular disease[28] but continues to be listed as a contraindication for use in the *Physician's Desk Reference.*

Decisions about which pharmacotherapy offers the greatest benefit can be made by assessing nicotine dependence. The Fagerstrom Test of Nicotine Dependence Scale (score greater than 5)[67] is one method to test for nicotine dependence. Two questions that correlate strongly with physical dependence are the time to first cigarette in the morning (more or less than 30 minutes) and usually or always smoking when one is ill.[68] Determining which therapy is best for an individual is determined by patient preference, use of the Fagerstrom Test or two questions, and a history of previous quit attempts and use of pharmacological agents tried. If pharmacotherapy has been tried previously, assess the products used, duration, side effects, and use pattern.[69]

APPROVED PHARMACOLOGICAL TREATMENTS FOR SMOKING CESSATION

Five nicotine replacement products have been approved by the Food and Drug Administration (FDA) as first-line agents to treat tobacco dependence. The nicotine patch is the most commonly used agent. Nicotine replacement is also available through gum, inhaler, spray, and lozenge. In the United States, the patches, gum, and lozenge are available over the counter, whereas the inhaler and spray are prescription-only products. Because of concerns about nicotine toxicity, individuals should attempt to cease use of all tobacco products before starting NRT. Fast-acting agents such as the gum, inhaler, lozenge, and spray are useful in helping with the desire to smoke, including the pleasurable rewards, whereas the slower-acting agent, the nicotine patch, helps to relieve withdrawal symptoms by providing low levels of nicotine. A Cochrane Collaborative Review of 103 studies found that NRT increased the odds of quitting smoking and maintaining abstinence over 6 months by about 1.5 to 2.0 times versus placebo or non-NRT treatment.[70] Beyond NRT, the only other agent presently approved by the FDA to support smoking cessation is the antidepressant bupropion chloride (Zyban, also marketed as Wellbutrin). The exact mechanism by which it promotes smoking cessation is largely unknown, although some evidence suggests that it inhibits postsynaptic uptake of dopamine and norepinephrine.[71] Bupropion is also a nicotinic receptor antagonist, which may reduce the reinforcing effects of smoking.[72] Table 33-4 provides an overview of these medications, including appropriate administration and side effects.

Nicotine Gum

In 1984, nicotine gum in a 2-mg dose became the first pharmacological agent approved by the FDA for smoking cessation. Nicotine gum is highly effective in helping individuals to quit smoking, especially those who may need the oral gratification of something to replace cigarettes. The Cochrane Collaborative Review of NRT showed that individuals using nicotine gum were 1.5 times more likely to remain abstinent at 1 year than those receiving placebo.[70]

Since 1996, nicotine gum in 2- and 4-mg strengths has been widely available over the counter for treatment of nicotine dependence. Higher cessation rates have been noted with the 4-mg strength, especially in those who are highly dependent. For example, Sachs[73] found abstinence rates of 63.2 percent in those using 4-mg gum over 6 weeks compared with 25 percent abstinence rates in those using 2-mg gum or placebo. In addition, time to relapse was significantly longer in those using the higher strength.

Success in using nicotine gum is highly dependent on appropriate administration. This includes close attention to chewing instructions, avoidance of highly acidic drinks such as coffee, tea, soda, and most juices in the 15 minutes before and after use, and a regular schedule of administration, i.e., one piece during every waking hour.[69] It is important to "chew and park" the gum against the buccal membrane of the mouth rather than simply chewing like regular gum. The gum also can be used as an adjunct to the patch or bupropion chloride (Wellbutrin, Zyban). Nicotine gum is available in various flavors, including mint and orange.

Nicotine Patch

Multiple randomized controlled trials have shown the efficacy of the nicotine patch in improving cessation rates. In a meta-analysis of 17 studies involving more than 5000 subjects, Fiore[74] found that quit rates were more than doubled at the end of treatment (27 percent versus 13 percent) and at 6 months of follow-up (22 percent versus 9 percent). Compared with placebo, the patch also has been shown to be highly effective in reducing relapse rates in the first 2 weeks of quitting, when the rate of relapse is highest.[75]

Recent studies have focused on the benefits of doubling doses of the patch (44 mg versus 22 mg) and extending use beyond 8 weeks.[76] Neither of these approaches appears to improve smoking cessation outcomes. Further research is needed, including determining whether certain subgroups may benefit from higher doses and/or longer courses of therapy.

The nicotine patch is applied easily, offers no restrictions on activities, with local skin irritation being very mild. A small number of individuals using the 24-mg patch experience bad dreams and nightmares, which

■ ■ ■

TABLE 33-4   FOOD AND DRUG ADMINISTRATION–APPROVED MEDICATIONS FOR SMOKING CESSATION

NAME	DOSAGE	LENGTH OF USE	PRECAUTIONS	SIDE EFFECTS
Buproprion, Sustained-Release				
Wellbutrin SR, Zyban (prescription)	150 mg in morning for 3 days; then 150 mg (b.i.d.)	7 to 12 weeks, starting 1 to 2 weeks before quit date	Contraindicated for those with seizures or eating disorder and those who take another form of buproprion (Wellbutrin or Wellbutrin SR)	Insomnia, dry mouth, agitation
Nicotine Gum				
Nicorette, Nicorette DS, Nicorette Mint, Nicorette Orange (OTC)	Less than 25 cigarettes per day: 2 mg 25 or more cigarettes per day: 4 mg 1 piece per hour for waking hours	Up to 12 weeks	Use of proper chewing technique No eating or drinking for 15 minutes before and after chewing	Sore mouth or jaw, dyspepsia, hiccups
Nicotine Inhaler				
Nicotrol inhaler (prescription)	6 to 16 cartridges per day (4-mg cartridge)	Up to 6 months	No eating or drinking while using inhaler (15 minutes before and after use)	Mouth/throat irritation, rhinitis, cough
Nicotine Nasal Spray				
Nicotrol NS (prescription)	8 to 40 doses per day 1 to 2 doses per hour	3-6 months	Dependency Not recommended for severe reactive airway disease	Nasal irritation, sneezing, cough, watery eyes
Nicotine Patch				
Nicoderm CQ (OTC) generic/house brand patches (OTC and prescription)	7, 14, or 21 mg/24 hr	8 weeks	Replace patch daily	Local skin reaction, insomnia
Nicotrol (OTC)	15 mg/16 hr	8 weeks		
Nicotine Lozenge				
Commit (OTC)	1 lozenge q 1-8 hours, 2-4 mg Not to exceed 20 lozenges per day	Up to 12 weeks	Requires frequent dosing No eating or drinking while using gum (15 minutes before and after chewing)	Hiccups, dyspepsia

OTC, Over-the-counter.

requires switching to a 16-hour patch. The patches should not be cut because doing so can alter medication delivery.

Nicotine Inhaler

The nicotine inhaler has been available in prescription form since 2001. The inhaler uses a mouthpiece that looks like a cigarette holder. The patient places a pellet into the holder and sucks on the mouthpiece as one does on a cigarette or straw, allowing the vapors to remain in the cheek for absorption through the buccal mucosa into the bloodstream. The nicotine then is delivered to the brain. The nicotine inhaler has been shown to improve cessation rates by almost 50 percent compared with placebo and is designed to be used over a 6-month period.[77] The nicotine inhaler is the preferred mode of NRT among heavier smokers.[78] Although highly dependent smokers appear less likely to relapse with this form of NRT, overall compliance rates to the nicotine inhaler appear to be lower than other forms of pharmacological therapies.[79]

The nicotine inhaler is designed to be used for a period of 6 months, longer than most NRT products, with tapering beginning at 3 months. Like nicotine gum, the inhaler requires appropriate administration in order to be effective. Local throat and mouth irritation, cough-

ing, and rhinitis are noted in up to 40 percent of users.[80] These symptoms may account for the lack of compliance with this agent.

Nicotine Lozenge

The nicotine lozenge is the newest NRT product available over the counter. Like nicotine gum, the nicotine lozenge is absorbed directly into the mucosa of the mouth. However, the absorption of the nicotine lozenge is 25 to 27 percent higher than 2- or 4-mg nicotine gum, probably because of the residual nicotine retained in the gum.[81] Like the gum, the lozenge is designed to be administered every 1 to 2 hours during the first 6 weeks of administration and tapered over the following 6 weeks. Users should not drink or eat anything during the 15 minutes before or while using the lozenge to ensure appropriate absorption of nicotine. Also recommended is that persons who report smoking within the first 30 minutes of waking begin with 4-mg lozenges.

Users of the nicotine lozenge report reduced withdrawal symptoms such as difficulty concentrating, anxiety, impatience, and restlessness.[82] In a large study of those who had previously used other agents (NRT products or Zyban), the lozenge proved effective in promoting cessation.[83]

Nicotine Spray

The nicotine product most likely to mimic cigarette smoking is the nicotine spray. Peak plasma concentration of nicotine occurs within 10 minutes of using nicotine spray compared with other agents such as the gum that peak within 30 minutes.[84] However, the spray produces side effects of nasal irritation and burning and watery eyes after use, which may prevent adherence to this agent in the first week of quitting.[85] Eighty-one percent of users report nasal irritation after 3 weeks of use, although the severity is mild to moderate.[69]

At 6 and 12 months of follow-up, abstinence rates are 29 to 32 percent in those using the spray compared with placebo rates of 10 to 18 percent.[80] However, compared with other forms of NRT such as the nicotine patch, the results are mixed in terms of long-term cessation. Some early data suggest that there may be subpopulations that benefit more from the spray than other forms of NRT, including those who are obese, highly-dependent, and some minority group members, but this remains to be tested.[76]

Bupropion

Released in 1997, sustained-release bupropion (bupropion SR, Zyban) is an antidepressant that has been approved by the FDA for smoking cessation. Unlike NRT, in which smokers quit smoking before beginning NRT, bupropion is prescribed 1 week before cessation. Treatment is recommended for at least 7 to 12 weeks, with longer use suggested based on individual need. If cessation is not achieved by 4 weeks of treatment, therapy with bupropion should be discontinued.[86] Bupropion should be titrated beginning at a dose of one 150-mg tablet a day, taken in the morning for 3 days, to two tablets a day, one tablet to be taken on waking and one tablet taken 8 hours later. This regimen decreases the dose-related side effect of seizures and also the insomnia that can accompany bupropion use.

In a Cochrane review, bupropion has been shown to double the quit rates compared with controls (OR 1.97).[87] Bupropion had higher quit rates compared with the nicotine patch in a randomized controlled trial and a primary care setting when individuals chose their own treatment.[88] For example, Jorenby and colleagues[89] found higher quit rates in those assigned to bupropion compared with the nicotine patch at 6 months (24.8 percent versus 21.3 percent, respectively) and 12 months (30.3 percent versus 16.4 percent). However, when combined with the nicotine patch, the control of cravings seems to be better using bupropion plus the patch rather than either of these agents alone.

Bupropion may be especially helpful in special populations attempting to quit smoking, including women, blacks, and those with higher levels of nicotine dependence.[90] For example, in a randomized controlled trial of 893 women, use of bupropion tripled cessation rates at the end of 1 year compared with the nicotine patch or placebo.[91,92] In another study of 600 black smokers, bupropion resulted in 6-month cessation rates of 21 percent compared with 14 percent in those receiving placebo. These rates of cessation are comparable to trials in white populations.[93]

In clinical trials looking at the safety, like nicotine replacement products, bupropion has been found to be safe in cardiovascular patients, with no significant changes noted in heart rate or blood pressure. The main contraindication of use of bupropion is a history of seizures. The risk of seizure while taking bupropion is relatively low at 0.1 percent and is observed most often when the dose exceeds 450 mg/day.[94]

Other Antidepressants

Hughes and colleagues[95] conducted an analysis of antidepressants to determine their effectiveness in smoking cessation. In addition to bupropion, the tricyclic antidepressant nortriptyline also was shown to have a positive effect on those attempting to quit smoking. Five trials demonstrated longer-term abstinence rates in those taking nortriptyline compared with placebo (OR 2.8). Like bupropion, nortriptyline is started 10 to 28 days before cessation in order to reach a steady state, with duration of therapy most often 12 weeks. However, side effects may be significant, including dry mouth, blurred vision, urinary retention, and light-headedness. In addition, because of risk of dysrhythmias, this medication must be used with caution in those with cardiovascular disease. In the United States, nortriptyline is not approved as an aid for smoking cessation. It should be noted that although the selective serotonin reuptake inhibitors have been assessed to determine their benefit in smoking cessation, no significant difference in long-term abstinence has been found when patients treated with selective serotonin reuptake inhibitors were compared with controls.

Newer Medications

The new field of pharmacogenetics may play an important role in smoking cessation in the near future. This field is built around the premise that there are inherited differences in drug metabolism and that drug targets have important effects on treatment toxicity and efficacy. Work in this field has been undertaken primarily in Europe using controlled trials of bupropion. One of the first such studies included smokers of European ancestry who were treated with 300 mg of bupropion or placebo. Blood samples showed that persons with a slower metabolism had an increase in cravings following their quit date and had higher relapse rates than those with a higher metabolism.[93] Researchers suggest that the slow metabolism may be attributed to slower rates of inactivation of nicotine in the central nervous system and neuroadaptive changes that promote dependence and cravings.[96] Other studies in Europe also have tested the pharmacogenetic effects of NRT, focusing on the genetic variation in the dopamine pathway.[97]

Newer agents are being tested as aids for smoking cessation that may have combined effects. Cannabinoid-1 (**CB1**) receptor blockers are agents that block the endocannabinoid regulator system, which modulates the energy balance of the body and nicotine dependence.

Overstimulation of the endocannabinoid system may play a role in obesity and tobacco dependence, and CB1 blockers help to reduce overstimulation. In a trial of 800 men and women, those receiving recombinant a CB1 blocker had quit rates of 32 percent at the end of 10 weeks compared with 20 percent in those receiving placebo. They also had lower levels of weight gain (1.5 lb versus 6.6 lb).[98] Although future research is needed, modulating the endocannabinoid system offers promise as a new pathway for development of new pharmacotherapy.

WAYS TO PREVENT RELAPSE

Although many interventions exist to help individuals quit smoking, there is a steady attrition in overall success because of individuals returning to smoking over time, or relapse. Relapse is common in the early stages of quitting and most often occurs within the first 3 weeks. Preparing for relapse is essential to ensure long-term cessation.

The most widely applied approach to help prevent relapse is a skills approach in which smokers learn to identify high-risk situations and then are offered cognitive and behavioral strategies to cope with these situations. Marlatt's model of relapse[99] is based on the premise that most persons are in control of giving up an addictive substance such as cigarettes until they encounter a high-risk situation and experience an urge to smoke. If they are better prepared to manage the high-risk situation, the likelihood decreases that they will lapse or totally relapse back to the old behavior.

Three steps to prevent relapse are (1) helping to identify personal high-risk situations that may be triggers for smoking, (2) developing cognitive and behavioral strategies that focus on using these skills when faced with the urge to smoke, and (3) practicing these strategies so that when faced with an urge to smoke, one is pre-

---

Confidence Questionnaire

How confident are you that you can resist the urge to smoke in the 14 situations below?

Not at all Confident	Slightly Confident	Fairly Confident	Very Confident

| 0% | 10% | 20% | 30% | 40% | 50% | 60% | 70% | 80% | 90% | 100% |

1. When you feel bored or depressed _____

2. When you see others smoking _____

3. When you want to relax or rest _____

4. When you just want to sit back and enjoy a cigarette _____

5. When you are watching TV _____

6. When you are driving, or riding in a car _____

7. When you have finished a meal or snack _____

8. When you feel frustrated, worried, upset, tense, nervous, angry, anxious, or annoyed _____

9. When you want a snack, but don't want to gain weight _____

10. When you need more energy, or can't concentrate _____

11. When someone offers you a cigarette _____

12. When you are drinking coffee or tea _____

13. When you are in a situation where alcohol is involved _____

14. When you feel smoking is part of your self-image _____

FIGURE 33-3 ■ Confidence Questionnaire. (Modified from Condiotte MM, Lichtenstein E: *J Consult Clin Psychol* 49:648-658, 1981.)

pared.[99] Identifying high-risk situations is accomplished in three ways. In group-based behavior-oriented programs, high-risk situations most often are identified by having smokers self-monitor behaviors over 1 to 2 weeks. They record each time a cigarette is smoked, noting the situation, date and time, and their mood. Over the course of a few days, a pattern of smoking begins to show.

Another approach is to use a self-efficacy scale that measures one's confidence to resist the urge to smoke in a variety of situations. Self-efficacy ratings have been highly predictive of outcome.[100] When smoking is resumed, specific situations are frequently predictive of a relapse episode.[64] A 14-item self-efficacy tool shown to measure high-risk situations for smoking is shown in Figure 33-3.[101] Confidence ratings of less than 70 percent for a given item on the tool denote a potential high-risk situation requiring intervention. The goal is to focus on helping individuals develop their own cognitive and behavioral strategies to overcome the urge to smoke in specific situations (step 2 in the Marlatt's relapse model).

Various methods have been used to help with skills training around coping strategies. Taylor and colleagues[58] have incorporated a method of asking individuals to focus on self-efficacy ratings that are lowest, developing at least one cognitive strategy (self-talk or change in thoughts) and a behavioral strategy (direct change in behavior) to manage each of these situations. Tsoh and colleagues[102] have used an approach known as ACE (avoid, cope, escape). In some instances, individuals can avoid the high-risk situation until they feel ready to face it. For instance, if smoking is most common in social settings, they may be able to avoid the bar or restaurant where they usually smoke for a number of days or weeks. Coping with a situation can be accomplished through distraction, incompatible behaviors, and positive self-talk. Distraction may involve going for a walk, reading, or telephoning a friend to keep one's mind off the habit. Behaviors incompatible with smoking may include chewing gum, eating low-calorie snacks, or using one's hands for tasks such as knitting, sewing, or woodworking. Positive self-talk involves telling oneself that one can continue to remain a nonsmoker, such as, "I know I can do this." Escape, the third part of ACE, means getting out of the situation without a puff of a cigarette. Examples include socializing with nonsmokers in a party situation or even going outside while others are smoking after a meal in a restaurant. Like Taylor and colleagues[58], and Tsoh[102] recommend a combination of strategies to help with relapse. As individuals focus on relapse prevention, strategies that are realistic and achievable are essential.

In addition to developing specific strategies for relapse prevention in high-risk situations, other ways to prevent relapse include general lifestyle interventions that increase self-control. Exercise and relaxation techniques such as deep breathing and muscle relaxation or imagery are examples of global interventions used to prevent relapse. Taylor and colleagues[103] found that smokers who participated in an exercise training program while quitting smoking had greater cessation rates

and smoked significantly fewer cigarettes than those who did not participate in such a program. Exercise is a powerful intervention that helps to reduce weight gain and minimize withdrawal symptoms.

SUMMARY

The high rate of disease caused by tobacco use makes smoking interventions a global imperative. Smoking is associated with significant risk to the vascular system and other major organs. Community, work site, and health site interventions reduce smoking prevalence. Strong advice, counseling, pharmacotherapy, and relapse prevention help individual smokers quit. In particular, interventions applied by nurses within health care settings have the potential to affect the greatest cause of preventable death in the United States and abroad.

REFERENCES

1. Ezzati M, Lopez AD: Estimates of global mortality attributable to smoking in 2000, *Lancet* 362:847-852, 2003.
2. *The health consequences of smoking: a report of the Surgeon General*, Washington, DC, 2004, US Department of Health and Human Services, Centers for Disease Control and Prevention, National Center for Chronic Disease Prevention and Health Promotion, Office on Smoking and Health.
3. Quantifying selected major risks to health. In *World Health Report 2002: reducing risks, promoting healthy life,* Geneva, 2002, World Health Organization. Retrieved December 23, 2003 from www.who.int/whr/2002/Chapter4.pdf
4. American Heart Association: *Heart disease and stroke statistics: 2005 update,* Dallas, 2005, The Association.
5. Substance Abuse and Mental Health Services Administration: *Results from the 2002 National Survey on Drug Use and Health: national findings,* Pub No DHHS SMA 03-3836, NHSDA Series H-22, Rockville, Md, 2003, Substance Abuse Mental Health Services Administration, Department of Health and Human Services. Retrieved December 20, 2003 from www.oas.samhsa. gov/nhsda.htm
6. Schroeder S: Tobacco control in the wake of the 1998 master settlement agreement, *N Engl J Med* 350:293-301, 2004.
7. Centers for Disease Control and Prevention: Women and Smoking: A report of the surgeon general (Executive Summary)] *MMWR* 51: RR-12, 2002.
8. Centers for Disease Control and Prevention: Cigarette smoking among adults: United States, 2000, *MMWR Morb Mortal Wkly Rep* 51:642-645, 2000.
9. Ridker PM, Libby P: Risk factors for atherothrombotic disease. In Zipes DP, Libby P, Bonow RO, Braunwald E, editors: *Braunwald's heart disease,* ed 7, Philadelphia, 2005, Saunders.
10. Reichert VC, Seltzer V, Efferen LS et al: Women and tobacco dependence, *Med Clin North Am* 88:1467-1481, 2004.
11. Centers for Disease Control and Prevention: Cigarette smoking among adults—United States, 2002. *Morb Mortal Wkly Rep* 53: 427-431, 2004.
12. Centers for Disease Control and Prevention: Cigarette smoking among adults: United States, 1999, *MMWR Morb Mortal Wkly Rep* 50:869-873, 2002.
13. Burns DM: Epidemiology of smoking-induced cardiovascular disease, *Prog Cardiovasc Dis* 46:11-29, 2003.
14. Yusuf S, Hawken S, Ounpuu S et al: Effect of potentially modifiable risk factors associated with myocardial infarction in 52 countries (the INTERHEART study): case-control study, *Lancet* 364:937-952, 2004.
15. Njolstad I, Arenesen E, Lund-Larsen PG: Smoking, serum lipids, blood pressure, and sex differences in myocardial infarction: a 12-year follow-up of the Finnmark Study, *Circulation* 93:450-456, 1996.

16. Kawachi I, Colditz GA, Stampfer MJ et al: Smoking cessation and time course of decreased risks of coronary heart disease in middle-aged women, *Arch Intern Med* 154:169-175, 1994.

17. Jajich CL, Ostfeld AM, Freeman DH Jr: Smoking and coronary heart disease mortality in the elderly, *JAMA* 252:2831-2834, 1984.

18. Hermanson B, Omenn G, Krommel R et al: Beneficial six-year outcome of smoking cessation in older men and women with coronary artery disease: results from the CASS registry, *New Engl J Med* 319:1365-1368, 1988.

19. Hart CL, Hole DJ, Smith GD: Risk factors and 20-year stroke mortality in men and women in the Renfrew/Paisley study in Scotland, *Stroke* 30:1999-2007, 1999.

20. Shinton R, Beevers G: Meta-analysis of relation between cigarette smoking and stroke, *BMJ* 25(298):789-794, 1989.

21. Kawachi GA, Colditz MJ, Stampfer et al: Smoking cessation and decreased risk of stroke in women, *JAMA* 269:232-236, 1993.

22. Lu JT, Creager MA: The relationship of cigarette smoking to peripheral arterial disease, *Rev Cardiovasc Med* 5:189-193, 2004.

23. Palumbo PJ, O'Fallon WM, Osmundson PJ et al: Progression of peripheral occlusive arterial disease in diabetes mellitus: what factors are predictive? *Arch Intern Med* 151:717-721, 1991.

24. Bolego C, Poli A, Paoletti R: Smoking and gender, *Cardiovasc Res* 53:568-576, 2002.

25. Peters RW, Brooks MM, Todd L et al: Smoking cessation and arrhythmic death: the CAST experience—the Cardiac Arrhythmia Suppression Trial (CAST) Investigators, *J Am Coll Cardiol* 26(5):1287-1292, 1995.

26. Freeman DJ, Griffin BA, Murray E et al: Smoking and plasma lipoproteins in man: effects on low density lipoprotein cholesterol levels and high density lipoprotein subfraction distribution, *Eur J Clin Invest* 23(10):630-640, 1993.

27. FitzGerald GA, Oates JA, Nowak J: Cigarette smoking and hemostatic function, *Am Heart J* 115:(1 pt 2):267-271, 1988.

28. Benowitz NL, Gourlay SG: Cardiovascular toxicity of nicotine: implications for nicotine replacement therapy, *J Am Coll Cardiol* 29:1422-1431, 1997.

29. Sasco AJ, Secretan MB, Straif K: Tobacco smoking and cancer: a brief review of recent epidemiological evidence, *Lung Cancer* 45(suppl 2):53-59, 2004.

30. International Agency for Research on Cancer: *IARC monographs on the evaluation of the carcinogenic risk of chemicals to humans,* vol 38, *Tobacco smoking,* Lyon, France, 1986, The Agency.

31. International Agency for Research on Cancer: *IARC monographs on the evaluation of carcinogenic risks to humans: nonionizing radiation,* vol 80, *Tobacco smoke and involuntary smoking,* Lyon, France, 2004, The Agency.

32. National Research Council: *Environmental tobacco smoke: measuring exposure and assessing health effects,* Washington, DC, 1986, National Academy Press.

33. Glantz SA, Parmley WW: Passive smoking and heart disease: epidemiology, physiology, and biochemistry, *Circulation* 83:1, 1991.

34. Office of Health and Environmental Assessment, Office of Research and Development: *Respiratory health effects of passive smoking: lung cancer and other disorders,* Report No EPA/600/6-90/006F, Washington, DC, 1992, US Environmental Protection Agency.

35. Leone A, Mori L, Bertanelli F: Indoor passive smoking: its effect on cardiac performance, *Int J Cardiol* 33:247, 1991.

36. Kaur S, Cohen A, Dolor R et al: The impact of environmental tobacco smoke on women's risk of dying from heart disease: a meta-analysis, *J Womens Health* 13:888-897, 2004.

37. Ebbert JO, Rowland LC, Montori VM et al: Treatments for spit tobacco use: a quantitative systematic review, *Addiction* 98:569-583, 2003.

38. Centers for Disease Control and Prevention: Use of smokeless tobacco among adults: United States, 1991, *MMWR Morb Mortal Wkly Rep* 42:263-266, 1991.

39. Severson HH: What have we learned from 20 years of research on smokeless tobacco cessation? *Am J Med Sci* 326:206-211, 2003.

40. Bolinder GM, Ahlborg BO, Lindell JH et al: Use of smokeless tobacco: blood pressure elevation and other health hazards found in a large-scale population survey, *J Intern Med* 232:327-334, 1992.

41. Jacobs EJ, Thun MJ, Apicella LF: Cigar smoking and death from coronary heart disease in a prospective study of US men, *Arch Intern Med* 8(159):2413-2418, 1999.

42. Office of the Surgeon General and Office on Smoking and Health: *The health benefits of smoking cessation: a report of the Surgeon General,* DHHS Pub No (CDC) 90-8416, Rockville, Md, 1990, US Public Health Service, Office on Smoking and Health.

43. Nelson D, Davis R, Chrisman J: Pipe smoking in the United States, 1965-1991: prevalence and attributable mortality, *Prev Med* 25:91-99, 1996.

44. Shaper AG, Wannamethee SG, Walker M: Pipe and cigar smoking and major cardiovascular events, cancer incidence and all-cause mortality in middle-aged British men, *Int J Epidemiol* 32:802-808, 2003.

45. Farquhar JW, Fortmann SP, Maccoby N et al: Effects of community-wide education on cardiovascular risk factors: the Stanford Five-City Project, *JAMA* 264:359-365, 1990.

46. Luepker RV, Murray DM, Jacobs DR Jr et al: Community education for cardiovascular disease prevention: risk factor changes on the Minnesota Heart Health Program, *Am J Public Health* 84:1383-1393, 1994.

47. Carleton RA, Lasater TM, Assaf AR et al: The Pawtucket Heart Health Program: community changes in cardiovascular risk factors and projected disease risk, *Am J Public Health* 85:777-785, 1995.

48. Ades PA, Kottke TE, Miller NH et al: Task force #3—getting results: who, where, and how? 33rd Bethesda Conference, *J Am Coll Cardiol* 40:615-630, 2002.

49. The COMMIT Research Group: Community Intervention Trial for Smoking Cessation (COMMIT). II. Changes in adult cigarette smoking prevalence, *Am J Public Health* 85:193-200, 1995.

50. Secker-Walker RH, Gnich W, Platt S et al: Community interventions for reducing smoking among adults, *Cochrane Database Syst Rev* p CD001745, 2002.

51. Moher M, Hey K, Lancaster T: Workplace interventions for smoking cessation, *Cochrane Database Syst Rev* p CD003440, 2003.

52. Fiore MC, Bailey WC, Cohgen SF et al: *Treating tobacco use and dependence: clinical practice guidelines,* Rockville, Md, 2000, US Department of Health and Human Services, Public Health Service.

53. Fiore MC, McCarthy DE, Jackson TC et al: Integrating smoking cessation treatment into primary care: an effectiveness study, *Prev Med* 38:412-420, 2004.

54. Manley M, Epps RP, Husten C et al: Clinical interventions in tobacco control: a National Cancer Institute training program for physicians, *JAMA* 266:3171-3172, 1991.

55. Williams SC, Schmaltz SP, Morton DJ et al: Quality of care in US hospitals as reflected by standardized measures, 2002-2004, *N Engl J Med* 21(353):255-264, 2005.

56. Malone RE: Nursing, our public deaths, and the tobacco industry, *Am J Crit Care* 11:102-105, 2002.

57. Kottke TE, Brekke ML, Solberg LI et al: A randomized trial to increase smoking intervention by physicians: doctors helping smokers, round 1, *JAMA* 261:2101-2106, 1989.

58. Taylor CB, Miller NH, Herman S et al: A nurse-managed smoking cessation program for hospitalized smokers, *Am J Public Health* 86:1557-1560, 1996.

59. France EK, Glasgow RE, Marcus AC et al: Smoking cessation interventions among hospitalized patients: what have we learned? *Prev Med* 32:376-388, 2001.

60. Wolfenden L, Campbell E, Walsh R et al: Smoking cessation interventions for in-patients: a selective review with recommendations for hospital-based health professionals, *Drug Alcohol Rev* 22:437-452, 2003.

61. Rice VH, Stead LF: Nursing interventions for smoking cessation, *Cochrane Database Syst Rev* p CD001188, 2004.

62. Miller W, Rollnick S: *Motivational interviewing: preparing people for change,* ed 2, New York, 2002, Guilford Press.

63. Bialous SA, Sarna L: Sparing a few minutes for tobacco cessation, *AJN Am J Neuroradiol* 104:54-60, 2004.

64. Sivarajan Froelicher ES, Miller NH, Christopherson DJ et al: High rates of sustained smoking cessation in women hospitalized with cardiovascular disease: the Women's Initiative for Nonsmoking (WINS), *Circulation* 109:587-593, 2004.

65. Rigotti NA, Munafo MR, Murphy MF et al: Interventions for smoking cessation in hospitalised patients, *Cochrane Database Syst Rev* p CD001837, 2003.

66. Krummel DA, Koffman DM, Bronner Y et al: Cardiovascular health interventions in women: what works? *J Womens Health Gend Based Med* 10:117-136, 2001.

67. Heatherton TF, Kozlowski LT, Frecker RC, Fagerstrom KO: The Fagerstrom Test for Nicotine Dependence: a revision of the Fagerstrom Tolerance Questionnaire, *Br J Addict* 86:1119-1127, 1991.

68. Taylor CB, Miller NH, Killen JD et al: Smoking cessation after acute myocardial infarction: effects of a nurse-managed intervention, *Ann Intern Med* 13:118-123, 1990.

69. Talwar A, Jain M, Vijayan VK: Pharmacotherapy of tobacco dependence, *Med Clin North Am* 88:1517-1534, 2004.

70. Silagy C, Lancaster T, Stead L et al: Nicotine replacement therapy for smoking cessation, *Cochrane Database Syst Rev* p CD000146, 2002.

71. Ascher JA, Cole JO, Colin JN et al: Bupropion: a review of its mechanism of antidepressant activity, *J Clin Psychiatry* 56: 395-401, 1995.

72. Slemmer JE, Martin BR, Damaj MI: Bupropion is a nicotinic antagonist, *J Pharmacol Exp Ther* 295:321-327, 2000.

73. Sachs DP: Effectiveness of the 4-mg dose of nicotine polacrilex for the initial treatment of high-dependent smokers, *Arch Intern Med* 155:1973-1980, 1995.

74. Fiore MC, Smith SS, Jorenby DE et al: The effectiveness of the nicotine patch for smoking cessation: a meta-analysis, *JAMA* 271:1940-1947, 1994.

75. Kenford SL, Fiore MC, Jorenby DE et al: Predicting smoking cessation: who will quit with and without the nicotine patch, *JAMA* 271:589-594, 1994.

76. Lerman C, Kaufmann V, Rukstalis M et al: Individualizing nicotine replacement therapy for the treatment of tobacco dependence, *Ann Intern Med* 140:426-433, 2004.

77. Tonnesen P, Norregaard J, Mikkelsen K et al: A double-blind trial of a nicotine inhaler for smoking cessation, *JAMA* 269:1268-1271, 1993.

78. West R, Hajek P, Nilsson F et al: Individual differences in preferences for and responses to four nicotine replacement products, *Psychopharmacology (Berl)* 153:225-230, 2001.

79. Hajek P, West R, Foulds J et al: Randomized comparative trial of nicotine polacrilex, a transdermal patch, nasal spray, and an inhaler, *Arch Intern Med* 159:2033-2038, 1999.

80. Hjalmarson A, Franzon M, Westin A et al: Effect of nicotine nasal spray on smoking cessation: a randomized, placebo-controlled, double-blind study, *Arch Intern Med* 154:2567-2572, 1994.

81. Choi JH, Dresler CM, Norton MR et al: Pharmacokinetics of a nicotine polacrilex lozenge, *Nicotine Tob Res* 5:635-644, 2003.

82. Muramoto ML, Ranger-Moore J, Leischow SJ: Efficacy of oral transmucosal nicotine lozenge for suppression of withdrawal symptoms in smoking abstinence, *Nicotine Tob Res* 5:223-230, 2003.

83. Shiffman S, Dresler CM, Hajek P et al: Efficacy of a nicotine lozenge for smoking cessation, *Arch Intern Med* 162:1267-1276, 2002.

84. Henningfield JE, Keenan RM: Nicotine delivery kinetics and abuse liability, *J Consult Clin Psychol* 61:743-750, 1993.

85. Hurt R, Dale L, Croghan G et al: Nicotine nasal spray for smoking cessation: pattern of use, side effects, relief of withdrawal symptoms, and cotinine levels, *Mayo Clin Proc* 73:118-125, 1998.

86. Hays JT, Hurt RD, Rigotti NA et al: Sustained-release bupropion for pharmacologic relapse prevention after smoking cessation: a randomized, controlled trial, *Ann Intern Med* 135:423-433, 2001.

87. Hughes JR, Stead LF, Lancaster T: Antidepressants for smoking cessation, *Cochrane Database Syst Rev* p CD000031, 2003.

88. Gold PB, Rubey RN, Harvey RT: Naturalistic, self-assignment comparative trial of bupropion SR, a nicotine patch, or both for smoking cessation treatment in primary care, *Am J Addict* 11:315-331, 2002.

89. Jorenby DE, Leischow SJ, Nides MA et al: A controlled trial of sustained-release bupropion, a nicotine patch, or both for smoking cessation, *N Engl J Med* 340:685-691, 1999.

90. Smith SS, Jorenby DE, Leischow SJ et al: Targeting smokers at increased risk for relapse: treating women and those with a history of depression, *Nicotine Tob Res* 5:99-109, 2003.

91. Collins B, Wiley P, Patterson F et al: Gender differences in smoking cessation in a placebo-controlled trial of bupropion with behavioral counseling, *Nicotine Tob Res* 6:27-37, 2004.

92. Dalsgareth OJ, Hansen NC, Soes-Petersen U et al: A multicenter, randomized, double-blind, placebo-controlled, 6-month trial of bupropion hydrochloride sustained-release tablets as an aid to smoking cessation in hospital employees, *Nicotine Tob Res* 6: 55-61, 2004.

93. Hurt RD, Sachs DP, Glover ED et al: A comparison of sustained-release bupropion and placebo for smoking cessation, *N Engl J Med* 337:1195-1202, 1997.

94. Aubin HJ: Tolerability and safety of sustained-release bupropion in the management of smoking cessation, *Drugs* 62(suppl 2):45-52, 2002.

95. Hughes JR: New treatments for smoking cessation, *CA Cancer J Clin* 50:143-151, 2000.

96. Lerman C, Shields P, Wileyto E et al: Pharmacogenetic investigations of smoking cessation treatment, *Pharmacogenetics* 12:627-634, 2002.

97. Balfour DJ: Neuroplasticity within the mesoaccumbens dopamine system and its role in tobacco dependence, *Curr Drug Targets CNS Neurol Disord* 1:413-421, 2002.

98. Anthenelli RMDJ: Effects of recombinant in the reduction of major cardiovascular risk factors: results from the STRATUS_US trial (Smoking Cessation in Smokers Motivated to Quit). Paper presented at the American College of Cardiology 53rd Annual Scientific Meeting, New Orleans, March 9, 2004.

99. Marlatt AG: Relapse prevention: a self control program for the treatment of addictive behaviors. In Stuart RB, editor: *Adherence, compliance, and generalization in behavioral medicine,* New York, 1982, Brunner-Routledge.

100. Smith PM, Reilly KR, Miller NH et al: Application of a nurse-managed inpatient smoking cessation program, *Nicotine Tob Res* 4:211-222, 2002.

101. Condiotte MM, Lichtenstein E: Self-efficacy and relapse in smoking cessation programs, *J Consult Clin Psychol* 49:648-658, 1981.

102. Tsoh JY, McClure JB, Skaar KL et al: Smoking cessation. 2. Components of effective intervention, *Behav Med* 23:15-27, 1997.

103. Taylor CB, Houston-Miller N, Haskell WL, Debusk RF: Smoking cessation after acute myocardial infarction: the effects of exercise training, *Addict Behav* 13(4):331-335, 1988.

■■■ chapter **34**

Dyslipidemia

Suzanne Hughes

CHAPTER ABBREVIATIONS

4S   Scandinavian Simvastatin Survival Study

AFCAPS/TEXCAPS   Air Force/Texas Coronary Atherosclerosis Prevention Study

APO   apolipoprotein

ASCOT-LLA   Anglo-Scandinavian Cardiac Outcomes Trial-Lipid Lowering Arm

ATP   Adult Treatment Panel

CARDS   Collaborative Atorvastatin Diabetes Study

CARE   Cholesterol and Recurrent Events Trial

CETP   cholesterol ester transfer protein

CHD   *coronary heart disease*

CVD   cardiovascular disease

FATS   Familial Atherosclerosis Treatment Study

FCH   familial combined dyslipidemia

HDL   high-density lipoprotein

HIV   human immunodeficiency virus

HPS   Heart Protection Study

IDL   intermediate-density lipoprotein

LCAT   lecithin-cholesterol acyltranferase

LDL   low-density lipoprotein

LIPID   Long-Term Intervention with Pravastatin in Ischaemic Disease

LPL   lipoprotein lipase

LRC-CPPT   Lipid Research Clinics Coronary Primary Prevention Trial

NCEP   National Cholesterol Education Program

PROSPER   Prospective Study of Pravastatin in the Elderly at Risk

PROVE-IT TIMI 22   Pravastatin or Atorvastatin Evaluation and Infection Therapy-Thrombolysis in Myocardial Infarction 22

TNT   Treating to New Targets Trial

VA-HIT   Veterans Affairs High-Density Lipoprotein Cholesterol Intervention Trial

VLDL   very-low-density lipoprotein

WOSCOPS   West of Scotland Coronary Prevention Study

Optimization of the lipid profile is a key component of global cardiovascular risk reduction. Identification of dyslipidemias and initiation of appropriate lifestyle modification and pharmacological intervention are emerging as mainstream focuses for cardiovascular clinicians. Clinicians and researchers alike continue to learn that even the most promising technologies in the interventional laboratory do not address the disease process central to ischemic cardiovascular disease (**CVD**). "Systemic therapy"[1] with well-planned and well-executed risk factor management is needed to effect significant change in clinical practice and in population health.

This chapter reviews the epidemiological evidence linking dyslipidemia to atherosclerosis and cardiovascular risk. The incidence, prevalence, and types of dyslipidemias are presented. Genetic and environmental origins of dyslipidemias are discussed. Strategies for modifying dyslipidemias are detailed in Chapter 77.

Measurement of the novel risk factors related to lipid metabolism—lipoprotein (a), apolipoprotein (**APO**) B, low-density lipoprotein (**LDL**) particle size and density, lipoprotein-associated phospholipase A2 Lp-PLA2—is included in Chapter 43. The term *dyslipidemia* is used instead of *hyperlipidemia* because lipid abnormalities encompass low high-density lipoprotein (**HDL**) cholesterol in the presence of "normal" total plasma cholesterol levels, as well as disorders in the size and density of the lipoprotein particles. It should be noted that although the term *cholesterol* is recognizable in the lay vernacular, cholesterol is not synonymous with lipid. Cholesterol is one of the two major lipid particles; the other is triglyceride.

HISTORICAL PERSPECTIVE

The evolution of current thought regarding the role of dyslipidemia in the atherothrombotic process began early in the 20th century. In 1910, German chemist Adolph Windaus discovered that human atherosclerotic plaques contained greater than 20-fold higher concentrations of cholesterol than normal aortas. This discovery was followed by the work of Nikolai Anitschov who conducted the first recorded experimental production of atherosclerosis.[2] This Russian pathologist fed pure cholesterol to rabbits, which resulted not only in significant hypercholesterolemia, but more importantly, in marked aortic atherosclerosis.

Despite the discovery of aortic atherosclerosis, this disease process was not associated with heart disease until 1918 when Dr. James Herrick, a Chicago physician, recognized that acute myocardial infarction was not uniformly fatal. His use of the electrocardiogram to diagnose acute myocardial infarction led to the discovery that coronary artery disease was the cause of this acute syndrome.

The first scientist to describe the genetic origins of dyslipidemia and the association with coronary heart disease (**CHD**) was Carl Müller, a Norwegian physician. In the late 1930s, Müller noted that elevated blood cholesterol levels, xanthomatosis, and premature myocardial infarction occurred in several families.[3] Further study of familial hypercholesterolemia was published in the 1960s by Avedis Khachadurian, a Lebanese physician who differentiated the homozygous form of familial hypercholesterolemia from the heterozygous form.[4] Four biochemists—Konrad Bloch, Feodor Lynen, John Cornforth, and George Popják—are credited with identifying the processes involved in cholesterol synthesis.

The evolution of current epidemiological understanding of the role of elevated cholesterol as a risk factor for CHD began in 1955 with the work of Dr. John Gofman, a biophysicist at the University of California at Berkeley.[5] Dr. Gofman, working with a centrifuge, was able to separate lipoproteins by flotation. He made the following key observations: elevated cholesterol levels were associated with heart attacks; cholesterol was contained in a certain lipoprotein particle (the LDL particle); and elevated HDL appeared protective against heart attacks. This was followed by the seminal work of Dr. Ancel Keys at the University of Minnesota in the Seven Countries Study.[6] This landmark study of 15,000 men demonstrated that the incidence of heart attacks had a linear relationship to blood cholesterol levels. Additionally, by studying the dietary patterns in the diverse countries, Keys and colleagues observed that the concentration of dietary saturated fat was associated with elevated cholesterol levels.

In 1974, one of the most important discoveries in the field of cholesterol research was made by Drs. Michael Brown and Joseph Goldstein, whose work provided the basis for development of the hydroxymethylglutaryl-coenzyme A (HMG-CoA) reductase inhibitor class of dyslipidemic medications (later known as statins), which effectively revolutionized treatment of dyslipidemia. Their studies actually provided, for the first time, a molecular link between LDL cholesterol and atherosclerosis. They discovered that the role of LDL receptor, a cell-surface protein, is to control the level of LDL in the blood by binding LDL and delivering it to the cells. In the cell, the lipoprotein is degraded and used for metabolic and structural purposes. Further, they discovered that familial hypercholesterolemia is caused by a genetic defect in this LDL receptor, which prevents removal of LDL from the blood. No fewer than seven scientists who focused their study in the field of cholesterol research were awarded Nobel prizes for their work between 1928 and 1985.[7]

Framingham Heart Study

The epidemiological link between elevated cholesterol levels and coronary disease was established further by the Framingham Heart Study.[8] This study, now more than 50 years old, has provided a plethora of data regarding the relationship between total cholesterol, LDL, HDL, and triglyceride levels and coronary risk. The Framingham risk scoring system (see Chapter 77) is used by the National Cholesterol Education Program Adult Treatment Panel to quantify global risk level and corresponding treatment thresholds and goals.[9]

INTERHEART

A contemporary global epidemiological study identified nine risk factors that together account for 90 percent of the risk of acute myocardial infarction. The INTERHEART study, presented in 2004, has special significance in that it demonstrated that these classic risk factors and their associated population-attributable risk is essentially the same in almost every geographic region of the world, in every racial and ethnic population, and in men and women alike. Worldwide, it was demonstrated that the two most potent risk factors are dyslipidemia and cigarette smoking, conferring a fourfold and threefold risk, respectively. The lipid marker used in INTERHEART was the ratio of APO B to APO A. INTERHEART demonstrated unequivocally that across the globe, most populations have dyslipidemias that increase risk of myocardial infarction. This result has enormous public health implications regarding the importance of population-based strategies designed to shift lipid levels, in addition to clinical treatment of those at high risk.[10]

BASIC PHYSIOLOGY OF LIPID METABOLISM

Clinical assessment and management of patients with dyslipidemia begins with a basis in the understanding of lipoprotein metabolism. See Chapter 10 for full discussion of the pathogenesis of atherosclerosis. All lipoproteins consist of a central lipid core made up of cholesterol esters and triglycerides (Figure 34-1). Because lipids cannot travel alone in the bloodstream, the lipid core is packaged in an outer layer of phospholipids and apolipoproteins (Table 34-1).

The five classes of lipoproteins are chylomicrons, very low-density lipoprotein (**VLDL**), intermediate-density lipoprotein (**IDL**), LDL, and HDL. Three major metabolic pathways are involved in lipid metabolism: the exogenous pathway related to dietary intake, the endogenous pathway related to hepatic synthesis, and reverse cholesterol transport.

Exogenous Pathway

With the ingestion of fat from dietary sources, triglycerides and cholesterol are absorbed into chylomicrons (containing APO B-48) in the epithelial cells of the intestines (No. 7 in Figure 34-2). The chylomicrons circulate through the lymph system in the intestines and release triglyceride to the muscle cells and adipose tissue that is stored and available as energy. Chylomicrons bind to lipoprotein lipase (**LPL**). LPL hydrolyzes the triglycerides (LPL requires APO C-II). Free fatty acids are released and enter the tissue, and they are used for energy storage in the muscle or are stored as fat. The chylomicron, depleted of triglyceride, is released. These chylomicron remnants are taken up by the liver by binding APO E to the LDL receptor.[11,12] Various APO E genotypes affect the uptake of chylomicron remnants, in turn affecting LDL clearance.[13] See Chapter 43 for further discussion on the impact of various APO E genotypes on LDL levels and cardiovascular risk.

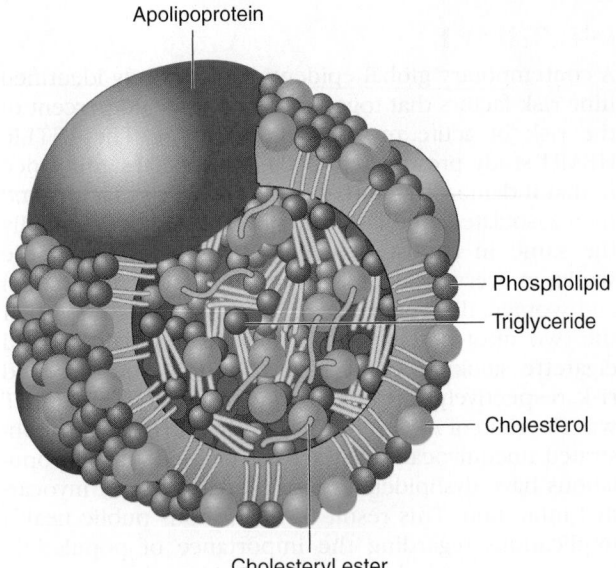

FIGURE 34-1 ■ Structure of lipoproteins. Phospholipids are oriented with their polar head toward the aqueous environment of plasma. Free cholesterol is inserted within the phospholipid layer. The core of the lipoprotein is made up of cholesterol esters and triglycerides. Apolipoproteins are involved in the secretion of the lipoprotein, provide structural integrity, and act as cofactors for enzymes or as ligands for various receptors. (From Genest J, Libby P, Gotto A: Lipoprotein disorders and cardiovascular disease. In Zipes DP, Libby P, Bonow RO, Braunwald E, editors: *Braunwald's heart disease: a textbook of cardiovascular medicine*, Philadelphia, 2005, WB Saunders.)

Endogenous Pathway

Triglyceride and cholesterol ester are produced by the liver, packaged as VLDL particles (No. 4, Figure 34-2), and released into the circulation (No. 6, Figure 34-2). The major apolipoprotein in VLDL is APO B-100. An apolipoprotein is the protein that is embedded in the outer shell of the lipoprotein and is responsible for metabolizing and transporting lipoproteins. LPL, an important regulator of lipid metabolism, hydrolyzes VLDL, forming IDLs (No. 2, hepatic pathway, Figure 34-2). IDLs then are taken up by the liver or are hydrolyzed by hepatic lipase to form LDL. LDL can be taken up by peripheral cells or by the liver. LDL is the chief carrier of circulating cholesterol and is required for cell membrane formation and synthesis of steroid hormones. A portion of the LDL is removed by a scavenger receptor mechanism, but most of the LDL particles are taken up in the liver via the LDL receptors. When LDL is taken up by the receptors, free cholesterol is released and accumulates in the cells. The action of the LDL receptors and LDL uptake controls LDL concentration in the plasma by several enzymatic mechanisms.

Reverse Cholesterol Transport

HDL cholesterol and its major protein, APO A-1, are responsible for reverse cholesterol transport, a process by which cholesterol is carried back from the tissues to the liver for excretion into the bile (Figure 34-2). Nascent HDL (a precursor to HDL), containing APO A-1, is secreted by the liver and the intestine.

Excess cholesterol and phospholipid cross the nascent HDL cell membrane, where they are converted to cholesterol ester and then to mature HDL by lecithin-cholesterol acyltranferase (**LCAT**). The esterified cholesterol subsequently is transferred from HDL to APO-B-containing proteins by cholesterol ester transfer protein (**CETP**) and then is taken up by the liver. In the liver, the nascent HDL is "regenerated" by hepatic triglyceride lipase and phospholipid transfer protein to complete the cycle. Cholesterol esters also may be taken up directly by the liver.[11,12,14]

INHERITED DYSLIPIDEMIAS

The Frederickson and Levy classification of lipid disorders has been used for many years (Table 34-2). This method of organizing dyslipidemias is arranged around the particular lipoprotein that is elevated. Over time, an evolution of the understanding of the pathophysiology and molecular basis for these disorders has led to a more practical and usable clinical approach. Overall, other than familial hypercholesterolemia, dyslipidemias based on a single gene mutation are rare. Lipid disorders, other than familial hypercholesterolemia, particularly those that contribute to atherosclerosis, typically are based on gene/environment interactions (see Chapter 13). Research into the relative contributions of genes and environment to the various dyslipidemias has dem-

TABLE 34-1   MAJOR APOLIPOPROTEINS AND ASSOCIATED LIPOPROTEIN, SOURCE, AND FUNCTION

APOLIPOPROTEIN	LIPOPROTEIN	SOURCE	FUNCTION
APO A-1	HDL	Intestine, liver	Structural protein for HDL; activates LCAT
APO A-II	HDL	Liver	Unknown
APO A-IV	HDL, chylomicrons, VLDL	Intestine	Unknown
APO B-48	Chylomicrons	Intestine	Synthesizes and secretes chylomicrons
APO B-100	VLDL, IDL, LDL, lipoprotein (a)	Liver	Synthesizes and secretes VLDL; binds to LDL
APO C-1	Chylomicrons, VLDL, HDL	Liver	Unknown
APO C-II	Chylomicrons, VLDL, HDL	Liver	Co-factor for LPL
APO C-III	Chylomicrons, VLDL, HDL	Liver	Inhibits lipoprotein binding to receptors
APO E	Chylomicrons, IDL, HDL	Liver	Binds to LDL receptor and LDL-receptor–related protein
APO (a)	Lipoprotein (a)	Liver	Unknown

HDL, High-density lipoprotein; *IDL*, intermediate-density lipoprotein; *LCAT*, lecithin-cholesterol acyltransferase; *LDL*, low-density lipoprotein; *VLDL*, very low-density lipoprotein.
From Zipes PD, Libby P, Bonow RO, Braunwald E, editors: *Braunwald's heart disease: a textbook of cardiovascular medicine*, Philadelphia, 2005, WB Saunders.

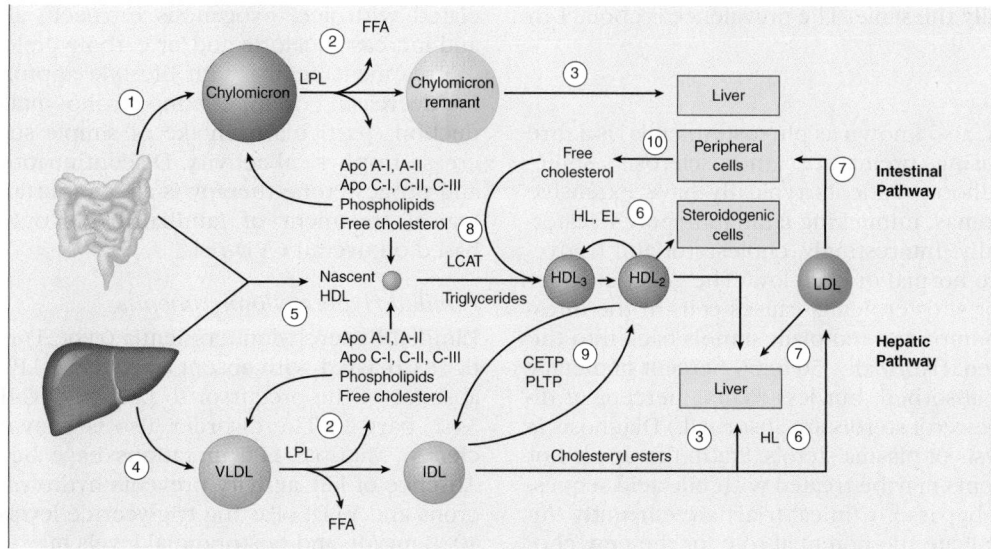

FIGURE 34-2 ■ Schematic diagram of the lipid transport system. The numbers in the circles refer to explanations in the text. *APO,* Apolipoprotein; *CETP,* cholesterol ester transfer protein; *EL,* endothelial lipase; *FFA,* free fatty acids; *HDL,* high-density lipoprotein; *IDL,* intermediate-density lipoprotein; *LCAT,* lecithin-cholesterol acyltransferase; *LDL,* low-density lipoprotein; *LPL,* lipoprotein lipase; *PLTP,* phospholipid transfer protein; *VLDL,* very low-density lipoprotein. (From Genest J, Libby P, Gotto A: Lipoprotein disorders and cardiovascular disease. In Zipes DP, Libby P, Bonow RO, Braunwald E, editors: *Braunwald's heart disease: a textbook of cardiovascular medicine,* Philadelphia, 2005, WB Saunders.)

onstrated that heritability varies across the different components of the lipid profile.[15]

Low-Density Lipoproteins
Familial Hypercholesterolemia

Familial hypercholesterolemia is associated with autosomal dominant inheritance of defective genes from one parent (heterozygous familial hypercholesterolemia) or both parents (homozygous familial hypercholesterolemia).[16] The research of Drs. Joseph Goldstein and Michael Brown directed toward understanding this genetic defect led to the discovery of the role of the LDL receptor, which subsequently became the basis for the development of the HMG-CoA reductase inhibitor class of lipid-lowering agents. Homozygous familial hypercholesterolemia is associated with the absence of LDL receptors. LDL elevations in the realm of 500 mg/dl are typical. Homozygous familial hypercholesterolemia is exceedingly rare (1 in 1 million), and this condition often is associated with cardiovascular or cerebrovascular mortality before age 20. Heterozygous familial hypercholesterolemia occurs in 1 in 500; LDL concentrations are typically 250 to 500 mg/dl. Triglycerides are usually normal.

Those with familial hypercholesterolemia can be identified by the following clinical features: family history of premature (age 20s and 30s in men, approximately 10 years later in women) CVD; corneal arcus; tendinous xanthomas over extensor tendons; and xanthelasmas.[16]

Familial Defective Apolipoprotein B

Mutations in the APO B gene cause APO B to have reduced affinity for the LDL receptor, which slows LDL clearance from plasma. Clinically, this disorder closely resembles familial hypercholesterolemia, and the treat-

■ ■ ■

TABLE 34-2   GENETIC LIPOPROTEIN DISORDERS

DISORDER	GENE	FIGURE 34-2
LDL Particles		
Familial hypercholesterolemia	LDL-R	7
Familial defective apo B-100	Apo B	7
Autosomal dominant hypercholesterolemia	PCSK9	
Abetalipoproteinemia	MTP	
Hypobetalipoproteinemia	Apo B	
Familial sitosterolemia	ABCG5/ ABCG8	
Lipoprotein(a)		
Familial lipoprotein(a) hyperlipoproteinemia	Apo (a)	
Remnant Lipoproteins		
Dysbetalipoproteinemia type III	Apo E	3
Hepatic lipase deficiency	HL	6
Triglyceride-Rich Lipoproteins		
Lipoprotein lipase deficiency	LPL	2
Apo CII deficiency	Apo CII	2
Familial hypertriglyceridemia	Polygenic	
Chylomicron retention disease	?	
Familial combined hyperlipidemia	Polygenic	
HDL Particles		
Apo AI deficiency	Apo AI	
Familial HDL deficiency/Tangier disease	ABCA1	10
Familial LCAT deficiency syndromes	LCAT	8
CETP deficiency	CETP	9
Niemann-Pick disease types A and B	SMPD1	

CETP, Cholesteryl ester transfer protein; *HDL,* high-density lipoprotein; *LCAT,* lecithin cholesterol acyltransferase; *LDL,* low-density lipoprotein.

ment is basically the same. The prevalence is about 1 in 500.[16]

Sitosterolemia

Sitosterolemia, also known as phytosterolemia, is a rare condition causing premature atherosclerosis, sometimes in childhood. Patients typically have extensive tendon xanthomas, mimicking familial hypercholesterolemia clinically. Interestingly, cholesterol and triglyceride levels are normal or even low. The genetic defect responsible for sitosterolemia causes cells in the intestinal wall to pump ingested plant stanols back into the intestinal lumen. (Normally, 50 to 60 percent of dietary cholesterol is absorbed, but less than 1 percent of dietary noncholesterol sterols are absorbed.) Diagnosis is made by analysis of plasma sterols. Statin therapy is not effective. Patients may be treated with bile acid sequestrants or ileal bypass.[17] Clinical trials are currently under way to evaluate the potential role for the new cholesterol absorption inhibitors for this disorder.[18] Research on the effect of the plant sterol margarine products on persons with sitosterolemia has been inconclusive; at this time it generally is recommended that persons with sitosterolemia avoid plant sterol margarine products.[19]

Remnant Lipoproteins

Dysbetalipoproteinemia

Dysbetalipoproteinemia also is known as type III hyperlipoproteinemia or broad beta disease, which is described in the next section.

Hepatic Lipase Deficiency

Hepatic lipase hydrolyzes triglycerides and phospholipids in VLDL remnants and IDL, promoting their conversion to LDL. It follows that a deficiency of hepatic lipase leads to an accumulation of VLDL remnants in the plasma. Hepatic lipase also promotes the conversion of HDL_2 to HDL_3, so that a deficiency of hepatic lipase results in a moderate elevation of HDL and larger HDL particles. Despite the increase in the HDL level, hepatic lipase deficiency is associated with premature atherosclerosis.[13]

Triglyceride-Rich Lipoproteins

Familial Hypertriglyceridemia

In familial hypertriglyceridemia (also known as type IV under the Fredrickson and Levy classification system), plasma triglycerides, VLDL cholesterol, and VLDL triglycerides are elevated, sometimes considerably. The prevalence of familial hypertriglyceridemia ranges from 1 in 100 to 1 in 50. An inconsistent relationship with atherosclerosis has been seen. The fasting triglyceride level is typically in the range of 200 to 500 mg/dl; postprandial levels may exceed 1000 mg/dl. Total cholesterol may be normal or elevated, depending on the VLDL cholesterol, and LDL and HDL are usually low. The expression of this familial disorder, although seen in first-degree relatives, depends greatly on gene/environment interaction. Triglyceride elevation is associated with age, exogenous estrogen, alcohol intake, and increased caloric and/or carbohydrate intake.[16]

Treatment begins with lifestyle approaches, including decreasing or eliminating alcohol intake, calorie reduction (particularly intake of simple sugars), and increase in physical activity. Discontinuation of estrogen and progesterone therapy is also important. Pharmacological treatment of familial hypertriglyceridemia is based on overall CVD risk.

Familial Hyperchylomicronemia

Familial hyperchylomicronemia (type 1) is a rare disorder associated with absent or reduced LPL, or possibly, absence of the precursor to LPL, APO C-II. (See Figure 34-2, part 2.) The disorder also is known as LPL deficiency. Multiple LPL mutations have been identified. Absence of LPL activity prevents hydrolysis of chylomicrons and VLDL. Fasting triglyceride levels may exceed 1000 mg/dl, and postprandial levels may exceed 10,000 mg/dl. Clinically, these patients have eruptive xanthomas and experience recurrent episodes of pancreatitis. They also may exhibit memory loss and neurological abnormalities.[16,20]

Type III Hyperlipoproteinemia

Type III hyperlipoproteinemia also is known as dysbetalipoproteinemia or "broad beta" disease. Patients with type III disease have the APO E-2/2 phenotype, although only 1 percent of those with the E-2/2 phenotype have dysbetalipoproteinemia. These patients have increased total cholesterol and triglyceride levels and low HDL levels. Clinically, they typically have tuberous xanthomas and palmar striated xanthomas and an increased risk of CVD. The lipid abnormalities associated with this disorder respond well to dietary modification and management of diabetes and obesity. Fibrates and statins also are effective.[16]

Familial Combined Hyperlipidemia

Familial combined dyslipidemia (**FCH**) is a genetic dyslipidemia that typically is not expressed until adulthood; the expression appears to be related to increased central adiposity.[21] The prevalence of FCH in the general population is estimated at 1 to 2 percent, but it may account for 11 percent of premature deaths from CVD.[22] The prevalence of FCH (type IIB phenotype) may be as high as 20 percent in younger (younger than age 60) patients with CVD. The diagnosis of FCH is suggested by an elevated total cholesterol and triglyceride measurement in multiple family members. Typically, those with FCH have an elevated APO B level, low HDL cholesterol level, and small, dense LDL particles. Clearly, there is great overlap between FCH and the metabolic syndrome. Secondary causes of FCH are discussed subsequently.

High-Density Lipoproteins

Apolipoprotein A-I Gene Defects

APO A-I participates in the synthesis and metabolism of HDL cholesterol. In patients with a complete deficiciency of APO A-I, there are very low levels of HDL and associated premature atherosclerosis.[23] Multiple mutations can affect the structure of APO A-I, and they are associated with low HDL levels. Patients with certain of these mutations present with CVD, whereas others do not.[16] See Chapter 43 for further discussion of APO A-I Milano.

Tangier Disease and Familial High-Density Lipoprotein Deficiency

Tangier disease is a genetic cholesterol transport disorder characterized by extremely low HDL levels. The name was derived from the island of Tangier, off the coast of Virginia, the home of the child in whom this disorder was first described. Tangier disease is caused by a mutation in the adenosine triphosphate–binding cassette transporter 1 (ABCA1) gene, which interferes with the first step in reverse cholesterol transport, that is, the transfer of unesterified cholesterol and phospholipids to lipid-poor apolipoproteins. Persons with Tangier disease are not able to eliminate cholesterol from the cells, leading to an accumulation of cholesterol in the reticuloendothelial system, which results in abnormalities of the intestinal mucosa, hepatosplenomegaly, and enlarged, orange-colored tonsils.[24] Although those with Tangier disease carry an increased risk of atherosclerosis, the risk is not proportionate to the level of HDL, suggesting that the associated low LDL levels may afford some protection.[15]

Lipoprotein Transport Genes
Lecithin-Cholesterol Acyltransferase Deficiency

Two types of LCAT deficiency occur: complete, or classic familial LCAT deficiency, and partial deficiency, which is also called fish eye disease. The features seen in familial LCAT deficiency are hypertriglyceridemia, extremely low HDL levels, clouding of the corneas, hemolytic anemia, and renal disease. Patients with fish eye disease have corneal clouding and low HDL levels. The HDL levels in both groups may be less than 10 mg/dl. Both groups have reduced levels of APO A-I and A-II.[25] Neither type of deficiency typically is associated with increased risk of premature atherosclerosis.

Cholesterol Ester Transfer Protein Deficiency

CETP is secreted chiefly by the liver and circulates in the plasma, bound to HDL. CETP facilitates the transfer of cholesterol esters from HDL to APO B–containing lipoproteins (VLDL, VLDL remnants, IDL, and LDL). A deficiency of CETP is associated with an increased HDL level and a decreased LDL. Secondarily, CETP facilitates transformation of HDL_2 to HDL_3, a process that normally augments reverse cholesterol transport. However, CETP inhibition also has been shown to promote reverse cholesterol transport and is associated with an increased HDL.[26] Observational studies of the effect of CETP inhibition caused by genetic mutations have produced mixed results; the effect may depend on the overall metabolic context, particularly on the triglyceride level. A promising pharmacological agent under study—torcetrapib, a CETP inhibitor—had been shown to increase levels of HDL cholesterol.[27] Clinical trials of torcetrapib were stopped, however, due to an increase

in mortality noted in the group taking torcetrapib with a statin compared to the group taking a statin alone.[28]

Niemann-Pick Disease

Several types of Niemann-Pick disease occur. The condition is a lipid storage disease that is an inherited type of metabolic disorder. Types A and B are associated with low HDL cholesterol and are due to a mutation at the sphingomyelin phosphodiesterase-1 gene. Patients with type A may have neurological abnormalities and mental retardation. Whether these persons have an increased risk for atherosclerosis is not clear. Patients with type C have a defect in intracellular cholesterol transport.[29]

SECONDARY CAUSES OF DYSLIPIDEMIA

Various disease processes are associated with dyslipidemia; measurement of the lipid profile sometimes can lead to a previously undiscovered clinical disorder (Table 34-3).

Metabolic Causes

By far the most common metabolic abnormality underlying dyslipidemia is the metabolic syndrome. As described in Chapter 37, the constellation of hypertension, hypertriglyceridemia, low HDL cholesterol level, abnormal glucose level, and increased abdominal adiposity affects nearly one-quarter of the adult population in the United States; at ages 60 to 69, the prevalence rises above 40 percent.[30] Although the various underlying pathophysiological conditions are debated, it appears that insulin resistance is probably a central mechanism. Meeting the criteria for metabolic syndrome by having

■ ■ ■

TABLE 34-3   SECONDARY CAUSES OF DYSLIPOPROTEINEMIAS

BODY SYSTEM/OTHER	SECONDARY CAUSES
Metabolic	Diabetes
	Lipodystrophy
	Glycogen storage disorders
Renal	Chronic renal failure
	Glomerulonephritis
	Nephrotic syndrome
Liver	Obstructive liver disease
	Cirrhosis
Hormonal	Estrogens
	Progesterones
	Growth hormone
	Thyroid disorders (hypothyroidism)
Lifestyle	Physical inactivity
	Obesity
	Diet rich in fats, saturated fats
	Alcohol intake
Medications	Immunosuppressive agents
	Corticosteroids
	Retinoids
	Highly active antiretroviral therapy
	Thiazides
	Beta-adrenergic blockers

From Zipes DP, Libby P, Bonow RO, Braunwald E, editors: *Braunwald's heart disease: a textbook of cardiovascular medicine*, Philadelphia, 2005, WB Saunders.

three of these five characteristics effectively doubles the risk for CVD and is often a precursor to type 2 diabetes. Recognition and aggressive treatment of this clinical syndrome is critical to reducing cardiovascular risk. Less common metabolic conditions that may have associated lipid abnormalities are familial lipodystrophy and glycogen storage disorders, both of which may be associated with increased triglyceride levels.[16]

Renal Causes

Dyslipidemia frequently is associated with kidney disease. Elevation of triglyceride and LDL levels may be seen in patients with nephrotic syndrome. The LDL levels may become greatly elevated. Elevated triglyceride levels and low HDL often are noted in those with chronic renal failure.[31] These patients typically have a high risk for CVD and require aggressive treatment for dyslipidemia. Immunosuppressive therapy after renal transplant raises triglycerides and lowers HDL. Concomitant administration of lipid-lowering medications and cyclosporine requires judicious monitoring for myopathy.

Hepatic Causes

Primary biliary cirrhosis and other obstructive liver diseases may be associated with hypercholesterolemia, which may be extreme.[32] Xanthomas may appear on the palms and face. High levels of an abnormal lipoprotein called *lipoprotein-x,* which is produced in patients with bile duct obstruction and is made up of nonesterified cholesterol and phospholipids, appear in the serum. Several studies of patients with primary biliary cirrhosis did not show high rates of cardiovascular mortality despite hypercholesterolemia. Late stages of the disease are associated with decreased intestinal absorption of lipids, which in part may overcome the hypercholesterolemia associated with longstanding chronic cholestasis.[33]

Hormonal Causes

Hypothyroidism may be associated with elevation of LDL cholesterol level, triglyceride level, or both. Measurement of the level of thyroid-stimulating hormone aids in identifying hypothyroidism as a secondary cause. Lipid abnormalities are generally reversible with correction of hypothyroidism. Hyperglycemia may be associated with a significant increase in triglyceride levels. Evaluation of a patient with elevated triglyceride levels should include measurement of the fasting blood glucose.

Lifestyle Causes

Unhealthful lifestyle habits may affect lipid levels. The increased prevalence of the metabolic syndrome-associated dyslipidemias are related closely to the epidemic of overweight and obesity in industrialized countries. Imbalance between excess calories consumed in the diet and too few calories expended in physical activity affect the cholesterol levels in a population, as does a diet high in saturated fats and/or simple sugars. Additionally, excessive alcohol intake can increase triglyceride levels in susceptible persons.

Drugs with Unintended Lipid Effects

Several drugs are known to affect lipid levels adversely. Thiazide diuretics can cause an increase in triglyceride levels. Beta blockers can increase triglyceride and lower HDL levels. This is particularly true for the nonselective beta blockers. Isotretinoin, used for severe acne, may cause dyslipidemia and features consistent with metabolic syndrome. Interestingly, it was found that this secondary hypertriglyceridemia confers later risk for dyslipidemia in the patient and the parents.[34] Anabolic steroids, sometimes abused by athletes, are associated with low HDL levels.[35] This should be considered when evaluating for a secondary cause of low HDL.

Highly active antiretroviral therapy prescribed for those with human immunodeficiency virus (**HIV**) infection may be associated with significant abnormalities in the lipid profile, a syndrome resembling metabolic syndrome (including diabetes), and physical characteristics of lipodystrophy. Up to 50 percent of patients taking protease inhibitors develop insulin resistance. Abnormalities in the lipid profile also have been noted in patients with HIV infection who are not taking these culprit agents. Clearly, the benefits of these agents outweigh the risks, but treatment of the associated metabolic abnormalities with lifestyle and pharmacological strategies is encouraged.[36] Some evidence indicates that HIV infection and highly active antiretroviral therapy may be associated with increased CVD risk.[37]

Estrogen

Historically, the perceived benefit of postmenopausal hormone therapy on CVD risk was attributed in part to the HDL-raising effect seen in the observational trials examining the impact of hormone therapy on CVD. Randomized controlled trials subsequently failed to show benefit of exogenous estrogen in primary[38] or secondary prevention[39] of CVD. In striving to understand the unexpected findings of these trials, researchers have found that oral postmenopausal hormone therapy is associated with an increase in certain inflammatory factors, including C-reactive protein.[40] Also, it has been demonstrated that an increase in the acute-phase reactant, serum amyloid A, content of HDL is associated with postmenopausal hormone therapy.[41,42] The increase in serum amyloid A may alter the function of HDL, diminishing its role in reverse cholesterol transport, thus increasing CVD risk even in the presence of a rise in the HDL cholesterol level.

The various hormone therapy preparations are associated with different effects on the lipid profile; transdermal estrogen exerts less effect (favorable and unfavorable) on the lipids. Estrogen alone and estrogen with progesterone are associated with a rise in HDL and triglycerides and a decrease in LDL and lipoprotein (a). The increase in triglycerides varies widely and may be significant. Evidence indicates that the triglyceride in-

■■■ CONUNDRUM

POSTMENOPAUSAL HORMONE THERAPY

Postmenopausal hormone therapy has well-demonstrated positive effects on the lipid profile, raising high-density lipoprotein and lowering low-density lipoprotein levels, as well as lowering the lipoprotein (a) level. These effects on the lipid profile contributed to the hypothesis that postmenopausal hormone therapy had cardioprotective effects. Until the results of randomized controlled trials in primary[45] and secondary prevention[35] showed that the positive effect on the lipid profile and presumed beneficial effects on the vasculature did not translate into clinical benefit, postmenopausal hormone therapy was considered a reasonable strategy to reduce cardiovascular disease risk in women. Although postmenopausal hormone therapy may be prescribed for relief of menopausal symptoms, at this time it is not recommended as a strategy to reduce cardiovascular risk.

Mosca L, Appel LJ, Benjamin EJ: Evidence-based guidelines for cardiovascular disease prevention in women, *Circulation* 109:672-693, 2004.

crease associated with postmenopausal hormone therapy may depend on abdominal adiposity and the presence of diabetes.[43] In fact, the third-generation oral contraceptives are associated with a slight increase in the HDL. Although oral contraceptives increase the risk of myocardial infarction and stroke, this risk apparently is not mediated by a negative effect on the lipid profile but rather is mediated via thrombosis, a particular risk for women smokers.[44] (See the accompanying Conundrum feature.)

CLINICAL TRIALS OF CHOLESTEROL LOWERING

Lipid Research Clinics Coronary Primary Prevention Trial

Studies of the benefits of cholesterol lowering can be divided into those done before the availability of HMG-CoA reductase inhibitors and those done afterward. The Lipid Research Clinics Coronary Primary Prevention Trial, commonly known as **LRC-CPPT**, was a landmark trial conducted over a 10-year period between 1973 to 1983 and involving approximately 4000 middle-aged hypercholesterolemic men. The trial provided the first conclusive evidence that reduction of total cholesterol and reduction of LDL reduces the incidence of CHD and myocardial infarction.[46] The group randomized to cholestyramine and low cholesterol diet had a 19 percent greater reduction in the risk of coronary death and heart attack than the group randomized to diet and placebo. Treatment with cholestyramine was associated with an 8.5 percent greater reduction in total cholesterol levels and a 12.6 percent greater reduction in LDL levels.

Helsinki Heart Study

In the Helsinki Heart Study, investigators evaluated a fibrate, gemfibrozil, in a group of 4081 men with elevated baseline lipid levels. Gemfibrozil lowered triglyceride levels by 35 percent and raised HDL cholesterol by 11 percent. LDL cholesterol was reduced by 11 percent. At the end of the 6-year follow-up period, there was a 34 percent reduction in cardiovascular events in the treatment group compared with the placebo group, although no difference in mortality was shown.[47]

Familial Atherosclerosis Treatment Study

The Familial Atherosclerosis Treatment Study (**FATS**), an angiographic study, was an examination of the effect of aggressive lipid-lowering on coronary atherosclerosis in a group of men at high CVD risk (who were found to have coronary atherosclerosis at baseline) with elevated APO B levels. One hundred twenty subjects completed the study, which included before and after coronary arteriography. Several lipid-lowering agents were used, including lovastatin, colestipol, or niacin/colestipol. Aggressive lipid lowering was associated with decreased progression of coronary disease, increased frequency of regression, and a reduction in the cardiovascular event rate.[48]

St. Thomas' Atherosclerosis Regression Study

In the St. Thomas' Atherosclerosis Regression Study (STARS), an angiographic trial, investigators measured the effect of dietary modification (alone or with cholestyramine) to lower cholesterol in progression of coronary disease. Although the changes in the lipid profiles were modest, there was a decrease in progression and an increase in the rate of regression of obstructive coronary disease.[49]

Scandinavian Simvastatin Survival Study

The Scandinavian Simvastatin Survival Study (**4S**) was a landmark trial in which investigators evaluated the benefit of a statin versus placebo in secondary prevention.[50] The study included 4444 patients, men and women, with angina or history of myocardial infarction. After 5.4 years of treatment, cardiovascular mortality decreased 42 percent in the simvastatin group and total mortality decreased 30 percent. The 4S trial was the first of many statin trials that have provided the basis for more aggressive cholesterol treatment guidelines through the National Cholesterol Education Program, discussed subsequently.

West of Scotland Coronary Prevention Study

In the West of Scotland Coronary Prevention Study (**WOSCOPS**) investigators studied 6595 men ages 45 to 64 with elevated baseline LDL cholesterol levels (155 to 232 mg/dl) who had no history of myocardial infarction. The sample was randomized to pravastatin 40 mg or placebo and was followed for 4.9 years. LDL cholesterol levels declined by 26 percent in the pravastatin-treated group and were unchanged in the placebo group. The statin-treated group had a 31 percent reduction in heart attacks compared with the placebo group, and a 32 percent reduction in cardiovascular death.[51]

Lyon Diet Heart Study

In a secondary prevention trial, the Lyon Diet Heart Study, researchers compared a Mediterranean-type diet to a prudent Western diet in a group of approximately 600 subjects who had a history of myocardial infarction. Those in the experimental group were instructed on a Mediterranean diet, that is, a diet high in fruits, vegetables, whole-grain cereals, nuts, and legumes, olive oil, fish, and poultry in low to moderate amounts; low consumption of red meat; and moderate consumption of wine. The major fat source is olive oil. Those in the control group were advised to consume a prudent diet, essentially an American Heart Association Step-1 low-fat diet. After 27 months, researchers concluded that those following the Mediterranean diet had lower rates of primary (death, myocardial infarction) and secondary (unstable angina, stroke, heart failure) endpoints. The benefit continued at the 4-year follow-up mark. The Mediterranean diet is rich in alpha-linoleic acid (omega-3 family) and is high in antioxidant-containing fruits and vegetables.[52]

Cholesterol and Recurrent Events Trial

In the Cholesterol and Recurrent Events (**CARE**) Trial investigators explored the effect of cholesterol lowering on recurrent cardiovascular events in those who had a history of myocardial infarction and who had "average" cholesterol levels. This trial included 4159 participants (3583 men and 576 women) and lasted 5 years. The group treated with pravastatin 40 mg had 24 percent fewer fatal events than the placebo group. In CARE, it was noted that the risk reduction was greater in those with higher baseline levels.[53] This led to some skepticism regarding the value of treating moderately elevated LDL levels, which was later challenged by the Heart Protection Study, discussed subsequently.

Air Force/Texas Coronary Atherosclerosis Prevention Study

The Air Force/Texas Coronary Atherosclerosis Prevention Study (**AFCAPS/TexCAPS**) was a randomized trial in which lovastatin 20 to 40 mg daily was compared with placebo for the prevention of first major coronary event in a group of 5608 men and 997 women without manifest CVD.[54] The group had baseline levels of total cholesterol and LDL that were considered average and below-average HDL cholesterol levels. At the conclusion of an average of 5.2-years follow-up, the risk of first cardiac events in the lovastatin-treated group was reduced by 36 percent compared with the placebo group. AFCAPS/TexCAPS is considered an important trial because it was the first primary prevention trial that enrolled a significant number of women who had moderate LDL elevation and slightly low HDL levels. In this trial, those with the lowest HDL levels showed the largest benefit reduction in morbidity and mortality.

Long-Term Intervention with Pravastatin in Ischaemic Disease

The Long-Term Intervention with Pravastatin in Ischaemic Disease (**LIPID**) trial included men and women with recent myocardial infarction or unstable angina who were randomized to a statin or placebo.[55] This trial was terminated early, at 5 years, because of a significant benefit in the treatment group in multiple endpoints including coronary artery disease death and need for bypass surgery. The greatest risk reduction was noted in those at highest global risk.[56]

Veterans Affairs High-Density Lipoprotein Cholesterol Intervention Trial

The Veterans Affairs High-Density Lipoprotein Cholesterol Intervention Trial (**VA-HIT**) is one of the few studies in which the benefit of raising the HDL cholesterol level was explored.[57] A secondary prevention trial, VA-HIT enrolled 2531 patients (LDL level less than 140 mg/dl, HDL level 40 mg/dl or above, and triglyceride level 300 mg/dl or below) and randomized them to gemfibrozil or placebo. Those randomized to gemfibrozil had a relative risk reduction of 22 percent. It should be noted that the population studied in this trial had elevated triglyceride levels in addition to low HDL, and as expected, the group randomized to gemfibrozil had a decrease in triglyceride levels in addition to an increase in HDL.

Heart Protection Study

The Heart Protection Study (**HPS**) is the largest ever placebo-controlled statin trial, the goal of which was to assess the effect of cholesterol-lowering with a statin in a wide range of those at high risk for CVD.[58] The HPS investigators enrolled 20,536 men and women and randomized them to treatment with simvastatin 40 mg daily or placebo. This trial provided strong evidence that those with normal or low cholesterol who are at high CVD risk benefit from statin therapy. The HPS also showed the benefit of statins for the elderly and for those with diabetes. Overall, allocation to the treatment group reduced all-cause mortality by 14 percent, vascular deaths by 17 percent, and first nonfatal myocardial infarction or coronary death by 25 percent. Most notably, the benefits were seen across all baseline cholesterol levels. From this trial came the thinking that clinicians should "treat risk—not cholesterol level."[59]

Anglo-Scandinavian Cardiac Outcomes Trial-Lipid Lowering Arm

In the Anglo-Scandinavian Cardiac Outcomes Trial-Lipid Lowering Arm (**ASCOT-LLA**), a primary prevention trial, investigators evaluated those with average cholesterol levels, randomizing more than 10,000 persons to atorvastatin or placebo. This trial was halted early when a significant benefit in cardiovascular events, procedures and stroke, was seen in the treatment group.[60]

Collaborative Atorvastatin Diabetes Study

In the Collaborative Atorvastatin Diabetes Study (**CARDS**), investigators studied the effect of atorvastatin in patients with diabetes (and no manifest CVD), enrolling 3000 patients with average or high LDL and triglyceride levels along with a current smoking habit, hypertension, albuminuria, or retinopathy. The trial was stopped early when the atorvastatin-treated group had a 36 percent reduction in coronary events, 31 percent reduction in revascularization, 48 percent stroke reduction, and 27 percent reduction in all-cause mortality.[61]

Reversal of Atherosclerosis with Aggressive Lipid Lowering Trial

In the Reversal of Atherosclerosis with Aggressive Lipid Lowering Trial, investigators sought to discover the effect(s) of intensive lipid-lowering therapy versus moderate lipid-lowering therapy on coronary artery atheroma burden and progression.[62] The groups were randomized to atorvastatin 80 mg or pravastatin 40 mg. At the end of the 18-month study period, 502 patients had intravascular ultrasound follow-up examinations. The pravastatin group showed progression in the atherosclerotic measures, whereas the atorvastatin group had no progression demonstrating the effectiveness of aggressive lipid lowering therapy; this was associated with on-treatment average LDL levels of 110 and 79 mg/dl, for the pravastatin and atorvastatin groups respectively.

Pravastatin or Atorvastatin Evaluation and Infection Therapy

In the Pravastatin or Atorvastatin Evaluation and Infection Therapy-Thrombolysis in Myocardial Infarction 22 (**PROVE-IT TIMI 22**), investigators studied 4162 patients hospitalized for acute coronary syndrome within the previous 10 days. The subjects received moderate lipid-lowering with pravastatin 40 mg or intensive lipid lowering with atorvastatin 80 mg. After a 2-year follow-up period, the mean LDL levels were 95 and 62 mg/dl, respectively. The atorvastatin-treated group had 16 percent reduction in the primary endpoint, which was a composite of death from any cause, myocardial infarction, documented unstable angina requiring rehospitalization, and revascularization.[63]

Treating to New Targets Trial

The Treating to New Targets Trial (**TNT**) was designed to test the "lower is better" hypothesis. In the TNT, investigators randomized 10,001 patients with stable coronary disease and baseline LDL levels less than 130 mg/dl to a standard or a maximum dose of a potent statin (atorvastatin 10 mg versus 80 mg) and followed them for 4.9 years, measuring safety and efficacy. The mean LDL levels achieved in the atorvastatin 80-mg group versus the 10-mg group were 77 mg/dl versus 101 mg/dl, respectively. The intensive lipid lowering was associated with a 22 percent reduction in the primary composite endpoint of death from CHD, nonfatal myocardial infarction, resuscitation after cardiac arrest, and fatal or nonfatal stroke compared with the group taking 10 mg.[64]

NATIONAL CHOLESTEROL EDUCATION PROGRAM

The National Heart, Lung, and Blood Institute launched the National Cholesterol Education Program (**NCEP**) in November 1985. The goal of the NCEP is to decrease illness and death from CHD in the United States by reducing the percentage of Americans with high blood cholesterol.[9] The purpose of the NCEP is to address the growing body of evidence regarding the role of cholesterol lowering in the prevention of CVD. The evolution of the guidelines issued by the NCEP Adult Treatment Panel (**ATP**) follows the results of epidemiological trials, angiographic outcomes trials, and finally randomized controlled trials.

Adult Treatment Panel I

The NCEP ATP issued its first set of guidelines in 1988.[65] In this document, the authors prescribed a strategy for preventing CVD in those with high cholesterol levels. These guidelines focused on primary prevention. LDL was identified as the primary target of treatment, and those individuals with high levels of LDL were specifically targeted.

Adult Treatment Panel II

In 1993, the second report of the NCEP, ATP II, was published.[66] This second set of guidelines reinforced the importance of LDL lowering in preventing CVD. Importantly, ATP II emphasized for the first time the intensive management of elevated LDL cholesterol in those with known CVD. A more aggressive LDL goal, 100 mg/dl or less, was established for this population.

Adult Treatment Panel III

In May, 2001, the NCEP ATP III clinical guidelines were released. This document continues the previous emphasis on secondary prevention and adds important new features (Box 34-1).

BOX 34-1 ■ ■ ■
NEW FEATURES IN THE NCEP ATP III CLINICAL GUIDELINES

- Recommendation of a full lipoprotein profile as the initial test
- Use of the Framingham 10-year risk scoring tool to assess global risk
- Increased aggressiveness in treatment of those at risk
- Reestablished cutoff points for low high-density lipoprotein as a major cardiovascular disease risk factor
- Increased attention to treating elevated triglyceride levels
- Recognition of the metabolic syndrome—a cluster of factors that together increase risk
- Recommendation for therapeutic lifestyle change

ATP, Adult Treatment Panel; *NCEP*, National Cholesterol Education Program.

Addendum to ATP III

In July 2004, based on the results of five important lipid-lowering trials published since the ATP III report in 2001, the NCEP ATP III panel issued a document reviewing these studies and issuing recommendations as a footnote to the current recommendations. These recommendations include an optional LDL goal of less than 70 mg/dl for very high-risk individuals and an optional goal of less than 100 mg/dl for those at moderate risk. Other recommendations are as follows:

- Addition of a fibrate or nicotinic acid to LDL-lowering therapy for hypertriglyceridemia or low HDL level
- Emphasis of therapeutic lifestyle changes (TLC) for all persons at risk who have lifestyle-related risk factors
- Recommendation that LDL-lowering therapy should begin with doses of medications sufficient to achieve at least a 30 to 40 percent reduction in LDL-C levels[67] See Chapter 77 for treatment of dyslipidemias.

SPECIAL POPULATIONS
The Elderly

Evidence regarding the benefit of pharmacological dyslipidemia management in older adults is derived from subanalyses of large clinical trials. Because mortality rates in older persons are higher, the absolute risk reduction associated with lipid lowering is greater.[68] Benefit was shown with lipid lowering in those over 65 in the 4S study,[47] the CARE study,[69] the Prospective Pravastatin Pooling Project,[70] and the Heart Protection Study.[71]

In the Prospective Study of Pravastatin in the Elderly at Risk (**PROSPER**), in which investigators enrolled high-risk patients age 70 and older, a reduction in CHD mortality rates and nonfatal myocardial infarction was shown, but not in stroke risk. Subanalysis showed no benefit in primary prevention.[72]

Women

The *Evidence-Based Guidelines for Cardiovascular Disease Prevention in Women*,[73] issued by the American Heart Association in 2004, reinforces the need for aggressive CVD risk reduction in women, including management of dyslipidemia. Women have been underrepresented in lipid-lowering trials; nevertheless, there is abundant evidence that lipid lowering has clear benefit in women. The Framingham Heart Study and others have demonstrated that high triglyceride and low HDL levels confer greater risk in women. Overall, HDL levels in women are approximately 10 mg/dl higher than in men. NCEP ATP III guidelines use an HDL level of 50 mg/dl as a cutoff for metabolic syndrome criteria in women, compared with 40 mg/dl in men.[9] The 2004 American Heart Association guidelines for women recommend raising HDL levels to 50 mg/dl.

FUTURE DIRECTIONS

Since the late 1980s, an enormous body of evidence has been amassed regarding the clinical benefit of treating abnormal blood lipids. Three iterations of the NCEP ATP are testament to the evolution of the understanding of the role of dyslipidemia in atherosclerosis and the potential clinical benefits of dyslipidemic therapy in primary and secondary prevention. Nurses have a formidable array of tools to reduce LDL levels and promising therapies to raise HDL levels. Research on targeted genetic therapies is evolving rapidly. Parallel to this are alarming statistics about the epidemic of metabolic syndrome with its associated dyslipidemias. The groundswell of interest in modifying lifestyles in an atherogenic environment needs to gather significant support from the clinical, public health, and research communities before large scale behavior change can be expected.

REFERENCES

1. Libby P, Theroux P: Pathophysiology of coronary artery disease, *Circulation* 111(25):3481-3488, 2005.
2. Anitschkow N, Chalatow S: On experimental cholesterin steatosis and its significance in the origin of some pathological processes, 1913; reprinted in *Arteriosclerosis* 3:178-182, 1983.
3. Müller C: Angina pectoris in hereditary xanthomatosis, *Arch Intern Med* 64:675-700, 1939.
4. Khachadurian AK: The inheritance of essential familial hypercholesterolemia, *Am J Med* 37:402-407, 1964.
5. Gofman JW, Lindgren F: The role of lipids and lipoproteins in atherosclerosis, *Science* 111:166-171, 1950.
6. Ancel Keys: *Seven Countries: a multivariate analysis of death and coronary heart disease*, Cambridge, Mass, 1980, Harvard University Press.
7. Brown M, Goldstein J: Nobel lecture, Dec 9, 1985.
8. Wilson PW, D'Agostino RB, Levy D et al: Prediction of coronary heart disease using risk factor categories, *Circulation* 97:1837-1847, 1998.
9. National Heart, Lung, and Blood Institute; National Institutes of Health; US Department of Health and Human Services: *Third report of the National Cholesterol Education Program (NCEP) Expert Panel on Detection, Evaluation, and Treatment of High Blood Cholesterol in Adults (Adult Treatment Panel III)*, Bethesda, Md, 2001, US Department of Health and Human Services, Public Health Service, National Institutes of Health, National Heart, Lung and Blood Institute.
10. Yusuf S, Hawken S, Ôunpuu S et al; INTERHEART Study Investigators: Effect of potentially modifiable risk factors associated with myocardial infarction in 52 countries (the INTERHEART study): case-control study, *Lancet* 364(9438):937-952, 2004.
11. Kingsbury KJ, Bondy G: Understanding the essentials of blood lipid metabolism, *Prog Cardiovasc Nurs* 18:13-18, 2003.
12. Gotto A, Pownall H: *Manual of lipid disorders: reducing the risk of coronary disease*, ed 2, Baltimore, Md, 1999, Williams & Wilkins.
13. Dammerman M, Breslow JL: Genetic basis of lipoprotein disorders, *Circulation* 91:505-512, 1995.
14. Rader DJ: Regulation of reverse cholesterol transport and clinical implications, *Am J Cardiol* 92(4A):42J-49J, 2003.
15. Hayman LL: Abnormal blood lipids: is it environment or is it genes? *J Cardiovasc Nurs* 14:39-49, 2000.
16. Genest J, Libby P, Gotto A: Lipoprotein disorders and cardiovascular disease. In Zipes DP, Libby P, Bonow RO, Braunwald E, editors: *Braunwald's heart disease: a textbook of cardiovascular medicine*, Philadelphia, 2005, WB Saunders.
17. Salen G, Patel S, Batta AK: Sitosterolemia, *Cardiovasc Drug Rev* 20:255-270, 2002.
18. Salen G, von Bergmann K, Lutjohann D et al; Multicenter Sitosterolemia Study Group: Ezetimibe effectively reduces plasma plant sterols in patients with sitosterolemia, *Circulation* 109:966-971, 2004.
19. Berger A, Jones PJH, Abumweis SS: Plant sterols: factors affecting their efficacy and safety as functional food ingredients, *Lipids Health Dis* 3:5, 2004. Retrieved October 20, 2005 from www.lipidworld.com/content/3/1/5

20. Merkel M, Eckel RH, Goldberg IJ: Lipoprotein lipase: genetics, lipid uptake, and regulation, *J Lipid Res* 43:1997-2006, 2002.

21. de Graaf J, van der Vleuten G, Stalenhoef AFH: Diagnostic criteria in relation to the pathogenesis of familial combined hyperlipidemia, *Semin Vasc Med* 4:229-240, 2004.

22. Goldstein JL, Schrott HG, Hazzard WR et al: Hyperlipidaemia in coronary heart disease. II. Genetic analysis of lipid levels in 176 families and delineation of a new inherited disorder, combined hyperlipidaemia, *J Clin Invest* 52:1544-1568, 1973.

23. Rader DJ: Regulation of reverse cholesterol transport and clinical implications, *Am J Cardiol* 92(4A):42J-49J, 2003.

24. Oram JF, Lawn RM: ABCA1: the gatekeeper for eliminating excess tissue cholesterol, *J Lipid Res* 42(8):1173-1179, 2001.

25. Santamarina-Fojo S, Lambert G, Hoeg JM, Brewer HB Jr: Lecithin-cholesterol acyltransferase: role in lipoprotein metabolism, reverse cholesterol transport and atherosclerosis, *Curr Opin Lipidol* 11:267-275, 2000.

26. Forrester JS, Makkar R, Shah PK: Increasing high-density lipoprotein cholesterol in dyslipidemia by cholesteryl ester transfer protein inhibition: an update for clinicians, *Circulation* 111:1847-1854, 2005.

27. Brousseau ME, Schaefer EJ, Wolfe ML et al: Effects of an inhibitor of cholesteryl ester transfer protein on HDL cholesterol, *N Engl J Med* 350:1505-1515, 2004.

28. U.S. Food and Drug Administration: Pfizer stops all torcetrapib clinical trials in interest of patient safety. Retrieved January 14, 2006 from www.fda.gov/bbs/topics/NEWS/2006/NEW01514.html.

29. Genest J: Lipoprotein disorders and cardiovascular risk, *J Inherit Metab Dis* 26:267-287, 2003.

30. Ford ES, Giles WH, Dietz WH: Prevalence of the metabolic syndrome among US adults: findings from the third National Health and Nutrition Examination Survey, *JAMA* 287:356-359, 2002.

31. Joven J, Villabona C, Vilella E et al: Abnormalities of lipoprotein metabolism in patients with the nephrotic syndrome, *N Engl J Med* 323:579-584, 1990.

32. Kaplan MM, Gershwin ME: Primary biliary cirrhosis, *New Eng J Med* 353:1261-1273, 2005.

33. Longo M, Crosignani A, Battezzati PM et al: Hyperlipidaemic state and cardiovascular risk in primary biliary cirrhosis, *Gut* 51:265-269, 2002.

34. Rodondi N, Darioli R, Ramelet AA et al: High risk for hyperlipidemia and the metabolic syndrome after an episode of hypertriglyceridemia during 13-cis retinoic acid therapy for acne: a pharmacogenetic study, *Ann Intern Med* 136:582-589, 2002.

35. Wu FC, von Eckardstein A: Androgens and coronary artery disease, *Endocr Rev* 24:183-217, 2003.

36. Armstrong W, Calabrese L, Taege AJ: HIV update 2005: origins, issues, prospects, complications, *Cleve Clin J Med* 72:73-78, 2005.

37. Stein JH: Managing cardiovascular risk in patients with HIV infection, *J Acquir Immune Defic Syndr* 38:115-123, 2005.

38. Writing Group for the Women's Health Initiative Investigators: Risks and benefits of estrogen plus progestin in healthy postmenopausal women: principal results from the Women's Health Initiative randomized controlled trial, *JAMA* 288:321-333, 2002.

39. Hulley S, Grady D, Bush T et al: Randomized trial of estrogen plus progestin for secondary prevention of coronary heart disease in postmenopausal women: Heart and Estrogen/Progestin Replacement Study (HERS) Research Group, *JAMA* 280:605-613, 1998.

40. Skouby SO, Gram J, Andersen LF et al: Hormone replacement therapy: estrogen and progestin effects on plasma C-reactive protein concentrations, *Am J Obstet Gynecol* 186:969-977, 2002.

41. Abbas A, Fadel P, Wang Z et al: Contrasting effects of oral versus transdermal estrogen on serum amyloid A (SAA) and high-density lipoprotein-SAA in postmenopausal women, *Arterioscler Thromb Vasc Biol* 24:e164-e167, 2004.

42. Herrington DM, Parks JS: Estrogen and HDL: all that glitters is not gold, *Arterioscler Thromb Vasc Biol* 24:1741-1742, 2004.

43. Kuller LH: Hormone replacement therapy and risk of cardiovascular disease: implications of the results of the Women's Health Initiative, *Arterioscler Thromb Vasc Biol* 23(1):11-16, 2003.

44. Rosendaal FR, Helmerhorst FM, Vandenbroucke JP: Female hormones and thrombosis, *Arterioscler Thromb Vasc Biol* 22:201-210, 2002.

45. Rossouw JE, Anderson GL, Prentice RL et al, for the Writing Group for the Women's Health Initiative Investigators: Risks and benefits of estrogen plus progestin in healthy postmenopausal women: principal results from the Women's Health Initiative randomized controlled trial, *JAMA* 288:321-333, 2002.

46. Lipid Research Clinics Program: The Lipid Research Clinics Coronary Primary Prevention Trial Results. II. The relationship of reduction in incidence of coronary heart disease to cholesterol lowering, *JAMA* 251:365-374, 1984.

47. Frick MH, Elo O, Haapa K et al: Helsinki Heart Study: primary prevention trial with gemfibrozil in middle aged men with dyslipidemia—safety of treatment, changes in risk factors, and incidence of coronary heart disease, *N Engl J Med* 317:1237-1245, 1987.

48. Brown G, Albers JJ, Fisher LD et al: Regression of coronary artery disease as a result of intensive lipid-lowering therapy in men with high levels of apolipoprotein B, *N Engl J Med* 323:1289-1298, 1990.

49. Watts GF, Lewis B, Brunt JN et al: Effects on coronary artery disease of lipid-lowering diet, or diet plus cholestyramine, in the St Thomas' Atherosclerosis Regression Study (STARS), *Lancet* 339:563-569, 1992.

50. Randomised trial of cholesterol lowering in 4444 patients with coronary heart disease: the Scandinavian Simvastatin Survival Study (4S), *Lancet* 344(8934):1383-1389, 1994.

51. Shepherd J, Cobbe SM, Ford I et al: Prevention of coronary heart disease with pravastatin in men with hypercholesterolemia, West of Scotland Coronary Prevention Study Group, *N Engl J Med* 333:1301-1307, 1995.

52. de Lorgeril M, Salen P, Martin JL et al: Mediterranean diet, traditional risk factors, and the rate of cardiovascular complications after myocardial infarction: final report of the Lyon Diet Heart Study, *Circulation* 99:779-785, 1999.

53. Sacks FM, Pfeffer MA, Moye LA et al: The effect of pravastatin on coronary events after myocardial infarction in patients with average cholesterol levels: Cholesterol and Recurrent Events Trial investigators, *N Engl J Med* 335:1001-1009, 1996.

54. Downs JR, Clearfield M, Weis S et al: Primary prevention of acute coronary events with lovastatin in men and women with average cholesterol levels: results of AFCAPS/TexCAPS—Air Force/Texas Coronary Atherosclerosis Prevention Study, *JAMA* 279:1615-1622, 1998.

55. Prevention of cardiovascular events and death with pravastatin in patients with coronary heart disease and a broad range of initial cholesterol levels: the Long-Term Intervention with Pravastatin in Ischaemic Disease (LIPID) Study Group, *N Engl J Med* 339:1349, 1998.

56. Simes RJ, Marschner IC, Hunt D et al: Relationship between lipid levels and clinical outcomes in the Long-term Intervention with Pravastatin in Ischemic Disease (LIPID) Trial: to what extent is the reduction in coronary events with pravastatin explained by on-study lipid levels? *Circulation* 105:1162-1169, 2002.

57. Rubins HB, Robins SJ, Collins D et al: Gemfibrozil for the secondary prevention of coronary heart disease in men with low levels of high-density lipoprotein cholesterol: Veterans Affairs High-Density Lipoprotein Cholesterol Intervention Trial Study Group, *N Engl J Med* 341:410-418, 1999.

58. Heart Protection Study Collaborative Group: MRC/BHF Heart Protection Study of cholesterol lowering with simvastatin in 20,536 high-risk individuals: a randomised placebo-controlled trial, *Lancet* 360:7-22, 2002.

59. *Heart experts call for urgent action to implement new findings on cholesterol-lowering treatment* [press release, July 5, 2002]. Retrieved May 15, 2005 from www.ctsu.ox.ac.uk/~hps/press_release.shtml

60. Sever PS, Dahlof B, Poulter NR et al: Prevention of coronary and stroke events with atorvastatin in hypertensive patients who have average or lower-than-average cholesterol concentrations, in the Anglo-Scandinavian Cardiac Outcomes Trial—Lipid Lowering Arm (ASCOT-LLA): a multicentre randomised controlled trial, *Lancet* 361:1149-1158, 2003.

61. Colhoun HM, Betteridge DJ, Durrington PN et al: Primary prevention of cardiovascular disease with atorvastatin in type 2 diabetes in the Collaborative Atorvastatin Diabetes Study (CARDS): multicentre randomised placebo-controlled trial, *Lancet* 364:685-696, 2004.

62. Nissen SE, Tuzcu EM, Schoenhagen P et al; REVERSAL Investigators: Effect of intensive compared with moderate lipid-lowering therapy on progression of coronary atherosclerosis: a randomized controlled trial, *JAMA* 291:1071-1080, 2004.

63. Cannon CP, Braunwald E, McCabe CH et al; Pravastatin or Atorvastatin Evaluation and Infection Therapy-Thrombolysis in Myocardial Infarction 22 Investigators: intensive versus moderate lipid lowering with statins after acute coronary syndromes, *N Engl J Med* 350:1495-1504, 2004.

64. LaRosa JC, Grundy SM, Waters DD et al; Treating to New Targets (TNT) Investigators: Intensive lipid lowering with atorvastatin in patients with stable coronary disease, *N Engl J Med* 352: 1425-1435, 2005.

65. Report of the National Cholesterol Education Program Expert Panel on Detection, Evaluation, and Treatment of High Blood Cholesterol in Adults: the Expert Panel, *Arch Intern Med* 148: 36-69, 1998.

66. Summary of the second report of the National Cholesterol Education Program (NCEP) Expert Panel on Detection, Evaluation, and Treatment of High Blood Cholesterol in Adults (Adult Treatment Panel II), *JAMA* 269:3015-3023, 1993.

67. Grundy SM, Cleeman JI, Merz CN et al; National Heart, Lung, and Blood Institute; American College of Cardiology Foundation; American Heart Association: Implications of recent clinical trials for the National Cholesterol Education Program Adult Treatment Panel III guidelines, *Circulation* 110:227-239, 2004.

68. Hanna IR, Wenger NK: Secondary prevention of coronary heart disease in elderly patients, *Am Fam Physician* 71:2289-2296, 2005.

69. Lewis SJ, Moye LA, Sacks FM et al: Effect of pravastatin on cardiovascular events in older patients with myocardial infarction and cholesterol levels in the average range: results of the Cholesterol and Recurrent Events (CARE) trial, *Ann Intern Med* 129:681-689, 1998.

70. Sacks FM, Tonkin AM, Shepherd J et al: Effect of pravastatin on coronary disease events in subgroups defined by coronary risk factors: the Prospective Pravastatin Pooling Project, *Circulation* 102:1893-1900, 2000.

71. Collins R, Armitage J, Parish S et al: Effects of cholesterol-lowering with simvastatin on stroke and other major vascular events in 20536 people with cerebrovascular disease or other high-risk conditions, *Lancet* 363:757-767, 2004.

72. Shepherd J, Blauw GJ, Murphy MB et al: Pravastatin in elderly individuals at risk of vascular disease (PROSPER): a randomised controlled trial, *Lancet* 360:1623-1630, 2002.

73. Mosca L, Appel LJ, Benjamin EJ et al: Evidence-based guidelines for cardiovascular disease prevention in women, *Circulation* 109:672-693, 2004.

Hypertension as a Risk Factor

Jennifer Dungan
Carolyn B. Yucha
Nancy T. Artinian

CHAPTER ABBREVIATIONS

ADR alpha-adrenergic receptor

AIM ancestry informative marker

BMI body mass index

BP blood pressure

CVD cardiovascular disease

DASH Dietary Approaches to Stop Hypertension

DBP diastolic blood pressure

ESRD end-stage renal disease

JNC Joint National Committee on Prevention, Detention, Evaluation, and Treatment of High Blood Pressure

LVH left ventricular hypertrophy

MI myocardial infarction

NHANES National Health and Nutrition Examination Survey

SBP systolic blood pressure

EPIDEMIOLOGY
Incidence and Prevalence

The annual rate of hypertension development, or incidence, is difficult to determine because hypertension goes undiagnosed in so many cases. Prevalence rates reflect the actual number of persons with hypertension at a given time. Figure 35-1 compares the incidence versus prevalence rates in British Columbia but reflects worldwide patterns. Hypertension increases with age, rising rapidly after age 50 in men and women. With the aging of the population, hypertension will continue to be a major health issue.

The estimated global prevalence of hypertension for the year 2000 was 26.4 percent or 972 million adults worldwide. The national prevalence rate for the United States is similar at 28.7 percent of adults (approximately 65 million persons), based on findings from the National Health and Nutrition Examination Survey for 1999-2000.[1] Similarly, the *Seventh Report of the Joint National Committee on Prevention, Detection, Evaluation, and Treatment of High Blood Pressure*[2] (commonly called **JNC**-VII) estimates that about 1 in 5 persons in the United States (1 in 3 adults) has hypertension. Table 35-1 displays prevalence rates by gender, race/ethnicity, and age for the United States from 1999 to 2002. This table also highlights the problem of diagnosis in that only 63 percent of those with hypertension are aware that they have it, and more than half are un-

treated. Of those treated, hypertension is controlled in only about one-third.

Morbidity

Hypertension is a complex, multifactorial disease process. As a result, morbidity can be "measured" in a number of ways. Typically, the focus on reducing morbidity is on reduction in blood pressure (**BP**) itself. Historically, diastolic BP (**DBP**) was viewed as the more important measure to control, but recent information shows that systolic BP (**SBP**) is the stronger predictor of total mortality and adverse cardiovascular events in a number of large, comprehensive clinical trials, including the Framingham Heart Study[3] and the Systolic Hypertension in Europe (Syst-Eur) Trial.[4]

Morbidity also can be indicated by the severity of target organ damage resulting from hypertension. Target organ damage in the heart, blood vessels, kidneys, brain, or eyes complicates the disease process and worsens the patient's prognosis. Typically, the focus of target organ damage in hypertensive patients is left ventricular hypertrophy (**LVH**), carotid wall thickening or plaques, and renal dysfunction.

Increased pressure or volume overload (as caused by high BP) can cause LVH. Hypertrophy of the left ventricle is a risk factor for cardiovascular morbidity and premature mortality; this increase in LVH is preceded even by mild hypertension.[5] Health care professionals now know that LVH may be reversible with long-term BP reduction and that reduced LVH (vis-à-vis reduction in BP) is associated with reduction in adverse cardiovascular events.[6]

Target organ damage that involves atherosclerosis, particularly carotid and coronary artery intima media thickness and/or presence of plaques, increases morbidity and mortality risk in those with hypertension because it predisposes them to stroke and myocardial infarction (**MI**). Hypertension can contribute directly to this disease process, for chronic constriction of the blood vessels in a narrowing or nearly occluded artery significantly increases the risk of untoward events. Similarly, hypertensive persons with concomitant peripheral arterial disease have an increased risk of MI and stroke.[7]

Renal impairment is another form of target organ damage monitored in persons with hypertension. Although it is still unclear exactly how renal dysfunction contributes to increased cardiac risk, it is hypothesized that glomerular filtration rates can trigger metabolic al-

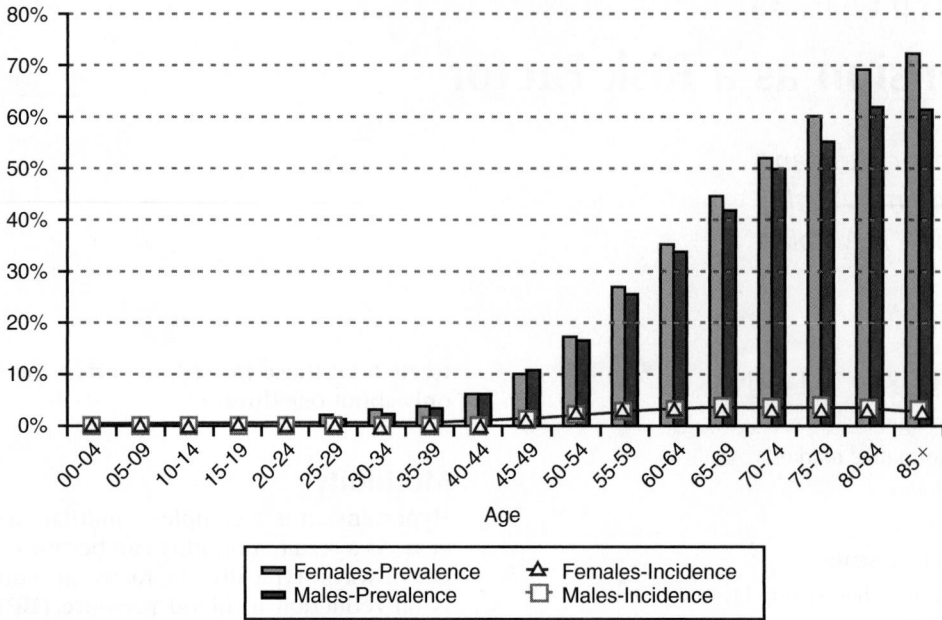

FIGURE 35-1 ▓ Hypertension incidence and prevalence, age-specific rates, by gender, in British Columbia, 2001/2002. The case definition is met if the patient received at least one hypertension-related hospital visit (ICD-9 401 to 405 or ICD-I10 to I15), as recorded in any of the diagnostic code fields, or two hypertension-related Medical Service Plan (MSP) services (ICD-9 401 to 405) within 365 days. Rates are calculated based on 2001/2002 British Columbia population, PEOPLE 27. Note that incidence rates nearly equal prevalence rates until ages 45 to 49. After age 45, new cases of hypertension continue to be identified at roughly 5 percent in each age group; yet the rate of new and previously identified hypertensive persons (prevalence) increases sharply. (With permission from British Columbia Intellectual Property Program, Ministry of Management Services.)

■ ■ ■

TABLE 35-1   PERCENTAGE OF NONINSTITUTIONALIZED U.S. ADULTS WITH HYPERTENSION* AND, AMONG THOSE WITH HYPERTENSION, ESTIMATED PERCENTAGE OF PERSONS WHO ARE AWARE OF,† TREATED FOR,§ AND IN CONTROL OF¶ THEIR CONDITION, BY SEX, RACE/ETHNICITY, AND AGE GROUP—UNITED STATES, 1999-2002

CHARACTERISTICS**	HYPERTENSION PREVALENCE		AWARENESS OF CONDITION		UNDER CURRENT TREATMENT		CONDITION CONTROLLED	
	%	(95% CI††)	%	(95% CI)	%	(95% CI)	%	(95% CI)
Sex								
Men	27.8	(24.9-29.7)	59.4	(55.8-63.1)	45.2	(40.9-49.6)	27.5	(23.7-31.3)
Women	29.0	(27.3-30.8)	69.3	(61.7-77.0)	56.1	(29.2-63.1)	35.5	(28.4-42.7)
Race/Ethnicity								
White, non-Hispanic	27.4	(25.3-29.5)	62.9	(57.3-68.5)	49.6	(44.1-53.1)	29.8	(25.7-34.0)
Black, non-Hispanic	40.5	(39.2-42.9)	70.3	(64.9-75.9)	55.4	(51.2-59.6)	29.8	(25.2-34.5)
Mexican American	25.1	(23.1-27.1)	49.8	(40.4-59.2)	34.9	(27.5-42.3)	17.3	(10.7-23.8)§§
Age Group (Years)								
20-39	6.7	(5.3-8.2)	48.7	(38.8-58.7)	28.1	(20.1-36.1)	17.6	(11.6-23.7)
40-59	29.1	(25.9-32.4)	73.5	(69.1-77.9)	61.2	(57.1-65.2)	40.5	(36.4-44.5)
≥60	65.2	(62.4-68.0)	72.4	(70.0-74.7)	65.6	(61.9-69.3)	31.4	(28.7-34.2)
Total¶¶	28.6	(26.8-30.4)	63.4	(59.4-67.4)	45.3	(45.3-52.8)	29.3	(26.0-32.7)

*Had a blood pressure measurement greater than or equal to 140 mm Hg systolic or greater than or equal to 90 mm Hg diastolic or took antihypertensive medication.
†Told by a health-care professional that blood pressure was high.
§Took antihypertensive medication.
¶Hypertension levels less than 140 mm Hg systolic and less than 90 mm Hg diastolic.
**All characteristic estimates (excluding age group) are age adjusted.
††Confidence interval.
§§Estimate should be used with caution; relative standard error is 20% to 29%.
¶¶Total population estimates (inlcuding sex and age group) include only non-Hispanic whites, non-Hispanic blacks, and Mexican Americans.
From Racial/ethnic disparities in prevalence, treatment, and control of hypertension: United States, 1999-2002, *MMWR Morb Mortal Wkly Rep* 54:7-9, 2005.

terations that lead to systemic atherogenesis.[8] Leoncini and colleagues[8] investigated the relationship between renal function and preclinical target organ damage in 934 untreated persons with primary hypertension. In this study, those with normal renal function had statistically less LVH and intima-media thickness and a lower prevalence of LVH and carotid plaque compared with those with mild renal dysfunction (glomerular filtration rate less than 60 ml/min, increased urinary albumin excretion, or both). In persons with diabetes and hypertension, another important physiological marker is microalbuminuria. Microalbuminuria is characterized by urinary excretion of albumin in small amounts (30 to 300 mg in 24 hours) and represents an early indicator of nephropathy. A positive linear association between microalbuminuria and hypertension exists, and antihypertensive therapy subsequently can reduce microalbuminuria.

Persu and De Plaen[9] recently reviewed a number of novel concepts in target organ damage caused by hypertension. These include expression of plasma brain natriuretic peptide, coronary calcifications in the heart, silent lacunar infarcts, advanced deep white matter lesions, and microbleedings in the brain, and carotid intima-media thickness, pulse wave velocity, augmentation index, and increased plasma levels of adhesion molecules for various levels of vascular target organ damage. These markers can serve as endophenotypes for target organ damage and could be helpful in the clinical assessment of such damage in patients with hypertension in the future.

Mortality

Hypertension was responsible for the death of 49,707 Americans in 2002, making the overall death rate from hypertension 17.1 percent. Males had a higher mortality rate (32 percent) than females (27.1 percent). Death rates also varied by race; the mortality rates were 14.4 percent for white males versus 49.6 percent for black males and 13.7 percent for white females versus 40.5 percent for black females.[10] Hypertension was listed as a primary or contributing cause of death in about 261,000 U.S. deaths in 2002. Mainous and colleagues[11] conducted survival analyses to determine the differences in relative risk for all-cause and cardiovascular disease mortality in a subcohort of Americans ages 30 to 74 who participated in the National Health and Nutrition Examination Survey (**NHANES**) II and NHANES II Mortality studies. After adjusting the model for age, race, gender, current smoking status, body mass index, exercise, total cholesterol, and having any other cardiovascular disease (**CVD**) risk factors (i.e., diabetes, heart failure, heart attack, or stroke), the authors concluded that "patients with HTN [hypertension] at baseline (including borderline HTN) retained a significantly elevated adjusted relative risk of both all-cause and CVD mortality over patients with normal BP" (p. 1499). The authors also examined the relative risk for prehypertension, and found that after adjusting for age, race, gender, and one or more additional risk factors (as identified by JNC-VII), prehypertension was not associated independently with increased mortality (all-cause and CVD).

This reiterates the importance of screening and prevention; even maintaining BP at prehypertensive levels compared with hypertensive levels can reduce risk of mortality significantly.

The association between CVD and mortality is depicted by the J curve phenomenon. Those with higher BP or cholesterol levels are more likely to die from CVD; those at the lowest end of the curve (with very low BP or low cholesterol levels) also have higher CVD mortality. When these levels are plotted on the horizontal axis and mortality is on the vertical axis, the curve forms a J shape. Persons who contribute to the lowest end of this curve tend to have special population differences that are likely to explain the unexpected increase in mortality.[10] This phenomenon emphasizes the importance of maintaining BP and cholesterol levels at optimal levels to reduce complications.

CAUSES OF HYPERTENSION

The cause of 90 to 95 percent of hypertension cases is unknown. This represents primary hypertension, or the multifactorial type with unknown cause. Primary hypertension has genetic and environmental influences. It is also likely that not everyone's hypertension is caused by the same insults; interindividual genetic and environmental combinations may produce the same outcome (see Chapter 13). A number of major hypotheses have been proposed for the pathophysiological mechanisms involved in the initiation of essential hypertension. These hypotheses incorporate altered homeostasis via the autoregulatory, neurohumoral, renal, transport, and hemodynamic mechanisms that link the heart, vessels, kidney, brain, and endocrine system.

Current research has focused on breaking down these factors into subcomponents, comparing genetic and physiological markers with possible modifiable factors (such as stress and sodium intake) that may contribute to the overall picture of the disease process. For example, a great deal of literature exists regarding hypertension and the following potential physiological mechanims: vasomotion (nitric oxide, endothelins, angiotensin II), fluid balance (the sodium/potassium/calcium exchange, atrial natriuretic peptide, renal tubule reabsorption), the sympathetic nervous system (environmental stress, adrenergic receptors, baroreflexes), and prostaglandins (cyclooxygenase-2). To date, most of these factors have a gene (or genes) associated with them, and a number of association studies examining polymorphisms of the genes in normotensive and hypertensive animal strains and human beings have saturated the literature with variable and conflicting results. This line of research is promising in that genetic screening for disease-specific alleles would strengthen clinical screening. Gene therapy could be developed as alternate or even "tailored" treatment options. Knowledge of protective variants of certain genes could lead to better prevention. Research on gene expression has become popularized by technological advances in high-throughput measures of transcription so that the function of the large panel of genes implicated in hypertension can be studied. This has led to advances in proteomics, whereby translation of the genes to proteins is providing even more insight into the biological processes of disease.

Genetic Basis

The remaining 5 to 10 percent of cases of hypertension are secondary, meaning that they arise from another known cause, such as a familial genetic mutation; renal, vascular, endocrine, or neurological disorder; pregnancy; stress; or a reaction to drug therapy. (See the accompanying Genetics feature.) Typically, these increase peripheral vascular resistance and/or cardiac output and produce systemic disease leading to hyper-

■■■ GENETICS

FAMILIAL HYPERTENSION

Autosomal dominant forms of hypertension—Individual has a *heterozygous* genotype (two different alleles) at the location of the hypertension-causing gene; transmitted by at least one affected parent.

Glucocorticoid-remediable Aldosteronism (most common form)	Disorder of hyperaldosteronism with high incidence of early hemorrhagic stroke caused by chimeric gene formed from portions of the 11B-hydroxylase gene and the aldosterone synthase gene. Responsive to dexamethasone. Short arm of chromosome 8 is implicated (OMIM #202010).
Bilginturan syndrome	Disorder characterized by brachydactyly (shortened tubular bones in hands and feet), short stature, and hypertension. Full penetrance is reported. The suspected gene map locus is on the short arm of chromosome 12 (OMIM #112410).
Gordon syndrome	Hypertension associated with hyperkalemia with possible relation to chromosome 1, 12, or 17, depending on the subtype of the disorder (OMIM #145260, #605232, or #601844)
Liddle syndrome	High blood pressure, low plasma renin and aldosterone levels, and hypokalemia. Possible mutation in the amiloride-sensitive distal renal epithelial sodium channel (beta or gamma subunits of the gene), located on the short arm of chromosome 16 (OMIM #177200). Treated by inhibiting the distal renal epithelial sodium channel via amiloride.

Autosomal recessive form of hypertension—Individual has a *homozygous* genotype (two copies of the same allele) at the location of the hypertension-causing gene; transmitted by two asymptomatic carrier parents.

Apparent mineralcorticoid excess	A salt-sensitive form monogenic form. Mutations in the gene that encodes 11a-hydroxysteroid dehydrogenase (on long arm of chromosome 16, OMIM #218030), a kidney enzyme that allows normal circulating concentrations of cortisol (which are much higher than those of aldosterone) to activate the mineralcorticoid receptors, producing high blood pressure.

From *OMIM™ Online Mendelian Inheritance in Man™*, Johns Hopkins University and National Center for Biotechnology Information. Retrieved March 1, 2005 from www.ncbi.nlm.nih.gov/entrez/query.fcgi?db=OMIM

tension. As a rule, if the causative insult or associated pathological mechanism is corrected, the hypertension subsides; however, the onset of hypertension still can promote target organ damage if uncorrected.

Pedigree, twin, and sibling studies have demonstrated that the heritable portion of essential hypertension is approximately 30 percent.[12] This means that up to 30 percent of the variability in hypertension could be related to the genetic variability that contributes to the phenotype. Body weight is one of the most well-known factors in hypertension, and weight is likely to have a substantial genetic component, as many studies of familial aggregation of weight phenotypes suggest. A dozen gene map loci and many polymorphisms for obesity are being studied (OMIM #601665).[13] As weight increases, so does BP; however, the exact mechanisms of their connection is unclear. Newer research in this area is expected to focus on gene loci in obesity and the presence of visceral fat.

Ethnic and Racial Differences

Ethnic differences in regard to hypertension typically are discussed in relation to prevalence, risk factors, and treatment response. It is likely that the cause of essential hypertension also could be different across racial groups. This is based on differences in the stratification of risk factors, potential pathophysiological variations, and distinctions in pharmacological response. Most commonly, differences between black/African American cohorts and white cohorts are reported in relation to distinct differences in hypertension prevalence (as shown in Table 35-1), morbidity, and mortality.

In general, blacks develop hypertension earlier, have worse target organ damage, more comorbidities, poorer rates of control, and higher death rates from hypertension than any other ethnic group.[2] Blacks or persons of African origin tend to have lower plasma renin levels and higher sensitivity to salt. In addition, a number of pharmacological differences exist in persons of African origin, involving drug disposition, receptor density and affinity, and side effects experienced related to many antihypertensive and cardiovascular medications.

Racial/ethnic differences in cardiovascular reactivity to stress, and pharmacological response to antihypertensive drugs have been demonstrated. As one example, race-specific differences in vascular reactivity may be related to increased alpha-adrenergic receptor (**ADR**) vasoconstrictor activity and/or decreased beta-ADR mediated vasodilatation.[14] These differences in ADRs may be due to homozygosity of the Gln27 allele (of the beta2-ADR gene), which confers less vasodilatory response.[15] Certain racial/ethnic factors (e.g., body mass index [**BMI**], physical inactivity, cultural dietary nuances, socioeconomic status, genetic factors, and access to health care) also may contribute to the differences in the hypertensive disease process.

RISK FACTORS

A number of nonmodifiable and modifiable risk factors increase the chance of developing hypertension (Table 35-2). Nonmodifiable risk factors include the effects of

■ ■ ■

TABLE 35-2   NONMODIFIABLE AND MODIFIABLE RISK FACTORS FOR HYPERTENSION

RISK FACTOR	COMMENTS
Nonmodifiable	
Age and aging	In general, the older one gets, the greater one's chance of developing hypertension. Hypertension occurs most often in persons older than age 35. Men tend to develop it between age 35 and 55. Women tend to develop it after menopause.
Gender	Before age 55, hypertension is more prevalent among men. After age 55, it becomes more prevalent in women.
Heredity	If your parents or other close blood relatives have hypertension, you are more likely to develop it.
Race	Blacks develop hypertension more often than whites, and it tends to occur earlier and to be more severe.
Modifiable	
Obesity	Persons with a body mass index of 30.0 or higher are more likely to develop high blood pressure.
Increased dietary sodium intake	A high sodium intake increases blood pressure in some persons.
Increased alcohol consumption	Heavy and regular use of alcohol can increase blood pressure dramatically.
Lack of physical activity	An inactive lifestyle makes it easier to become overweight and increases the chance of high blood pressure.
Stress	Stress often is mentioned as a risk factor, but stress levels are difficult to measure, and responses to stress vary from person to person.

age and aging, gender, heredity, and race. Modifiable risk factors include obesity, increased dietary sodium and alcohol consumption, sedentary lifestyle, and stress.

Although BP control is important for prevention of target organ damage, risk factors are most important in preventing mortality. Even when BP is lowered, morbid event rates increase with increased risk stratum.[16]

Nonmodifiable Risk Factors

Age and Aging

The direct relationship between age and hypertension is so well documented (Figure 35-1 and Table 35-1) that most studies in which hypertension is investigated control for age as a major covariate. Recent data from the Framingham Health Study suggest that individuals who are normotensive at age 55 have a 90 percent lifetime risk for developing hypertension.[17] Hypertension has its own specific age-related phenotype, isolated systolic hypertension. Affecting most persons age 60 or older, this form of hypertension is defined as an SBP of 140 mm Hg or higher with a DBP less than 90 mm Hg, creating a widened pulse pressure. This phenotype is attributable to reduced elasticity and increased stiffness in the aorta and is generally more resistant to antihypertensive treatment. With the aging of the U.S. population, the prevalence of hypertension and the societal burden of hypertension are expected to increase further, unless broad and effective preventive measures are implemented.

Hypertension control rates are poorest in older persons, mainly from inadequate SBP control. In those over age 50, systolic hypertension is a more important CVD risk factor than DBP. The Coordinating Committee of the National High Blood Pressure Education Program recently recommended a paradigm shift urging that SBP become the major criterion for diagnosis, staging and therapeutic management of hypertension, particularly among older Americans.[18] Clinical benefits of treatment of systolic hypertension include reduction in stroke, MI,

heart failure, kidney failure, and overall CVD morbidity and mortality. Because most persons with hypertension, especially those over age 50, will reach DBP goals once SBP is at goal, the JNC-VII[2] recommends that the primary focus should be achieving the SBP goals.

Analysis of data from the NHANES III reveals statistics similar to those shown in Table 35-1. In addition, these data showed shocking information about the elderly. Although persons age 65 or older represented only 19 percent of the total NHANES III sample, they constituted 45 percent of those unaware of their hypertension, 32 percent of those who were aware but not treated, and 57 percent of those who had treated but uncontrolled hypertension. Among persons who were being treated, hypertension was controlled in 65 percent of those age 25 to 44, 52 percent of those age 45 to 65, and only 34 percent of those age 65 and older.[19]

Twenty years ago, hypertension was regarded as normal in the elderly, and treatment frequently was regarded as unnecessary or even potentially dangerous. Since that time, numerous trials have shown reduction in morbidity and mortality in elderly adults who are treated with antihypertensives. Current treatment for this group follows the same principles as those for the general public and is described fully in Chapter 78.

Gender

Globally, men have a slightly higher prevalence of hypertension (26.6 percent) than women (26.1 percent).[20] In the United States, men typically have a higher prevalence rate of hypertension until about age 55, when women develop higher prevalence rates.[10] The female hormones (estrogen and progestin) are thought to be cardioprotective because the incidence of hypertension increases in postmenopausal women. However, the JNC-VI reported that women taking oral contraceptives were 2 to 3 times more likely to have hypertension, especially women who are older and obese.[21] This suggests that naturally occurring levels of gonadal hormones may provide benefits, but having excess hormones may be detrimental. Alternatively, androgens may affect vascular tone less prominently than female hormones. Orshal and Khalil[22] recently tackled this debate and summarized the potential benefits of hormones on the vascular system (Table 35-3). In addition, they cite possible links to these hormones and the renin-angiotensin system. This is perhaps the most promising factor to explain the gender differences in hypertension to date.

Heredity

Heredity typically is considered an unmodifiable risk factor. However, the current state of the science in genetics and genomics research raises questions about the ways in which our hereditary makeup can be altered by our own environmental influences and/or by new gene therapies. As a result, the paradigm may soon shift to one in which heredity is recognized as a modifiable risk. Genetics plays an integral role as a Mendelian factor and interacts with environment. Heredity plays a stronger role in the younger stages of life. With increasing age, environmental factors exert a stronger influence on the development of hypertension.[23] Family history alone affects risk. The recurrence risk (likelihood that a trait present in one family member will occur in a subsequent generation) for hypertension increases as the number of diagnosed parents increases, so that someone with two normotensive parents has a 4 percent chance of developing hypertension, while having one hypertensive parent confers a 10 to 20 percent risk, and having two hypertensive parents confers the greatest risk at 25 to 45 percent.[24] As genomic research becomes more popular and more feasible, many aspects of the genetic influence on BP regulation and hypertensive phenotypes are being elucidated.

Racial and Ethnic Factors

Race and ethnicity are the most widely debated risk factors in the cardiovascular literature. The racial/ethnic group with the highest risk for hypertension is the black/African American cohort, with an overall 41.8 percent prevalence in men and 45.4 percent prevalence in women.[10] Moreover, blacks were more likely than whites or Mexican Americans to be treated, but less likely to have controlled BP.[1] Figure 35-2 provides the age-adjusted prevalence by race/gender in the United States. The significance of this health disparity lies in the morbidity and mortality for blacks. Compared with whites, blacks have a 1.8 times greater rate (not risk, but rate) of fatal stroke, 1.5 times greater rate of death from

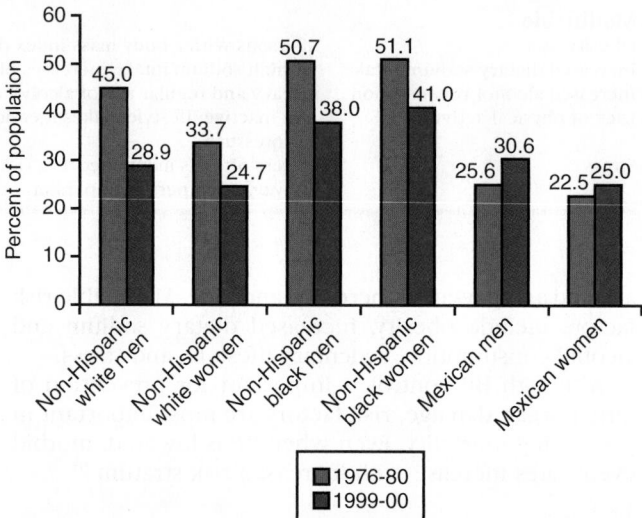

FIGURE 35-2 ■ Age-adjusted prevalence trends for high blood pressure, ages 20 to 74 by race/ethnicity, sex, and survey (NHANES 1976 to 1980, 1988 to 1994, and 1999 to 2002). Data based on single measure of blood pressure. Although overall prevalence of hypertension has decreased for all groups since the first NHANES trial (1976 to 1980), non-Hispanic black or black men and women continue to have higher prevalence rates than any other group over the past 36 years. (With permission from the American Heart Association: *Heart disease and stroke statistics: 2004 update*, Dallas, 2003, The Association.)

TABLE 35-3   BENEFICIAL VASCULAR EFFECTS AND POSSIBLE CLINICAL APPLICATIONS OF SEX HORMONES

HORMONE	ENDOTHELIAL EFFECTS	SMOOTH MUSCLE EFFECTS	OTHER VASCULAR EFFECTS	CLINICAL APPLICATIONS
Estrogen	Promotes proliferation and migration Promotes release of EDRFs Inhibits release of EDCFs	Inhibits proliferation and migration Vascular smooth muscle relaxation and vasodilatation	Anti-atherosclerotic Antioxidant Decreases LDL and increases HDL levels Inhibits lipoprotein oxidation Decreases plasma homocysteine level Increases antiplatelet aggregation factors; decreases platelet adhesion Decreases vascular collagen	Coronary artery disease Postmenopausal hypertension Thromboembolic events
Progesterone	Promotes release of EDRFs Inhibits release of EDCFs	Inhibits proliferation and migration Facilitates the vascular inhibitory effects of estrogen Acute vascular relaxation	Antiatherosclerotic Decreases LDLs and increases HDLs	Coronary artery disease Thromboembolic events
Testosterone	Promotes release of EDRFs	Inhibits proliferation Acute vascular relaxation Hyperpolarization Coronary vasodilatation	Antiatherosclerotic	Reduction of myocardial ischemia in men with coronary artery disease

EDCF, Endothelium-derived contracting factor; *EDRF*, endothelium-derived relaxing factor; *HDL*, high-density lipoprotein; *LDL*, low-density lipoprotein.
From Orshal JM, Khalil RA: *Am J Physiol Regul Integr Comp Physiol* 286:R233-R249, 2004. With permission from the American Physiological Society.

heart disease, and 4.2 times greater rate of end-stage kidney disease.[12]

Although the disparities in prevalence rates are apparent, the cause of racial/ethnic disparities is not well understood. Some associated factors were implied in an analysis of the NHANES II (1988 to 1994) data study by Collins and Winkleby.[25] They reported the following for blacks:

- Those with the highest rates of hypertension are more likely to be middle-aged or older, less educated, overweight or obese, physically inactive, and have diabetes.
- Those with the lowest rates are more likely to be younger but are also overweight or obese.
- Those with uncontrolled high BP who are not on antihypertensive medication tend to be male, younger, and have infrequent contact with a physician.

Recent studies[26,27] have reported increasing prevalence and risks in Hispanics/Mexican Americans and Chinese, often implicating the influence of Westernized culture. Most scholars argue that race alone is not a real risk factor in disease but rather that factors associated with ethnicity and culture are the culprit risks . Some of these factors include socioeconomic status, health behaviors, environmental exposures, and access to health care.

Another proxy of race is ancestry. The generic form of ancestry, noting regions of familial origins, often can provide insight into a number of sociocultural factors that may paint a more accurate picture of a person's individual or familial risk. However, the development of ancestry informative markers (AIMs) has reified ancestry as a biological stamp of sorts, supposedly identifying the percentage of one's racial makeup (for example, that an individual is X percent Northern European, Y percent African, and Z percent Asian). Although marketed as such, the AIMs procedure is really meant to group persons according to levels of ancestral similarity based on a large panel of genetic markers for which certain ones are more common to particular regions. For most, the focus is on improving health disparities in underserved populations that tend to show higher prevalence and worse prognosis. This likely will mean paying close attention to all of the possible racial/ethnic/cultural influences that make an individual, rather than a group, at risk.

Modifiable Risk Factors

Modifiable risk factors for hypertension include overweight and obesity, high dietary sodium, alcohol use, lack of physical activity, and stress.

Obesity

One of the most influential inherited and modifiable factors involved in hypertension is body weight. BMI (body weight in kilograms divided by height in meters squared) is associated positively with BP and is an independent predictor of hypertension.[27] As much as 65 to 75 percent of the risk for essential hypertension is accounted for by excess weight.[28] Weight-loss studies indicate that BP can be reduced by 5 to 20 mm Hg for every 10 kg (~ 4.5 lb) of weight loss.[2] The heritability estimate for

BMI is about 24 percent, and large population studies have implicated certain genes contributing specifically to BMI.[29] Familial aggregation of BP also can be explained by similarities in weight and incidence of obesity in family members. An increasing prevalence of obesity in urbanized and urbanizing cultures, concomitant with the increasing prevalence of hypertension in these same regions, also supports the dietary impact of obesity as it relates to high BP.

Dietary Sodium

Research on increased dietary salt and hypertension was so compelling that a targeted diet was developed as a prevention/management strategy. The Dietary Approaches to Stop Hypertension (DASH) diet is promoted by the American Heart Association. The focus of the DASH diet is not actually reducing dietary salt intake, but rather increasing fruits, vegetables, and low-fat dairy products that ultimately promote salt excretion. In a study of 375 adults with varied stages from normal to high BP, the DASH diet was shown to increase urinary sodium excretion via natriuresis (not via preglomerular vascular resistance) and reduce BP, with the most beneficial result in the intermediate sodium intake group (100 mmol/d with a 2100 kcal/d DASH diet).[30] Similar to other studies, this study also found that the effects of the DASH diet were greater in hypertensive persons than normotensive persons, in blacks than other races, and in older than younger persons. With the backing of this and other studies, the JNC VII[2] recommends the DASH diet as the most important nonpharmacological measure to control BP.

Alcohol Consumption

The relationship between heavy alcohol consumption and elevated BP was documented nearly 30 years ago in the Kaiser Permanente Multiphasic Health Examination study.[31] The strong positive association between increased alcohol consumption and increased BP is present even when age, weight (BMI), sodium and potassium intake, cigarette smoking, and education are accounted for and is reported across races. Cushman[32] delineates the possible mechanisms behind this relationship, which include stimulation of the sympathetic nervous system, inhibition of vascular relaxing factors, calcium, magnesium depletion, increased intracellular calcium/other electrolytes in vascular smooth muscle, and increased acetaldehyde.

A recent study of the European Project on Genes and Hypertension[33] examined 926 Europeans for the Pro-12Ala polymorphism of the peroxisome proliferator-activated receptor (PPAR)-γ gene. Compared with Pro12 homozygotes, Ala12 allele carriers (Ala/Ala or Ala/Pro genotype) had higher serum total and HDL cholesterol levels if they regularly consumed alcohol, with the opposite trend occurring in nondrinkers (Figure 35-3). This genotype-by-alcohol interaction was due to alcohol intake per se, independent of the type of alcoholic beverage, and was more pronounced in moderate than heavy drinkers. Statistically significant reductions in SBP and DBP have been reported with various drinking cessation and reduction interventions.[34]

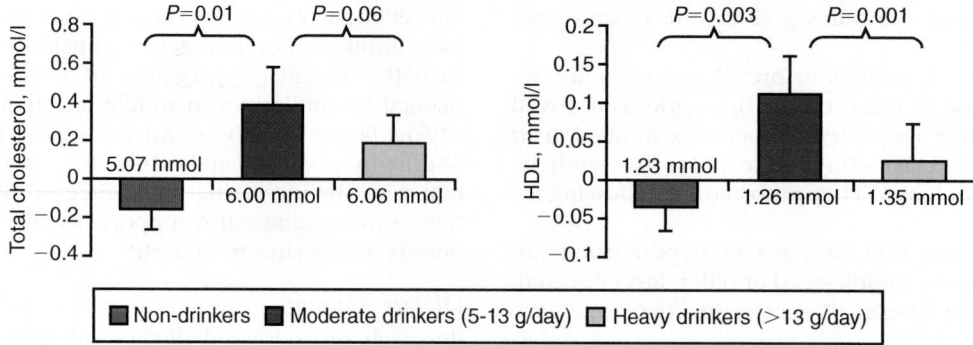

FIGURE 35-3 ■ Differences in total (left panel) and HDL (right panel) cholesterol associated with the PPAR-γ2 12Ala allele compared with Pro12 homozygotes. Reference levels in Pro12 homozygotes are given along the horizontal axis. Having the 12Ala allele conferred increased total and high-density lipoprotein cholesterol in moderate and heavy drinkers compared with having the homozygote genotype Pro/Pro at codon 12. The greatest effect of genotype-by-drinking interaction was with moderate drinkers. Having the 12Ala allele and not drinking showed lower total and high-density lipoprotein cholesterol levels. (With permission from Brand-Herrmann SM, Kuznetsova T, Wiechert A et al: *J Lipid Res* 46:913-919, 2005.)

The possible cardioprotective effects of alcohol consumption may be related to subsequent increases in high-density lipoprotein and apolipoproteins A-I and A-II, antioxidant effects, decreases in fibrinogen, and reduced platelet aggregation.[35] A commonly held belief is that fewer than two 4-oz servings of alcohol per day can be less damaging, if not cardioprotective.

Physical Activity

A sedentary lifestyle is another risk factor for increased morbidity and mortality and promotes maintaining or increasing body fat. A recent study examined the mortality risk of sedentary activity across CVD risk groups in 9611 pre–retirement age individuals. Researchers[36] found that after adjusting for age, sex, race, smoking, obesity, cancer, health status, income, and CVD risk, regular moderate to vigorous physical activity was significantly positively associated with reduced overall mortality compared with sedentary individuals. In addition, those with high CVD risk accounted for 64 percent of deaths attributable to sedentary lifestyle. Finally, those with the highest CVD risk appeared to have the greatest benefit from being active via occasional/light or regular/moderate levels of activity.

Stress

Perhaps the least well-defined risk factor for hypertension and CVD is stress. Animal and human studies have confirmed the importance of chronic stress in the pathophysiology of hypertension. Chronic stress in the form of work-related stressors, such as job strain and exposure to noise or personal stressors such as marital conflict, fear of terror, internal rumination, and exposure to violence have been associated with poor outcomes. In a study evaluating cardiovascular reactivity in 103 men, positive family history of hypertension and/or heart disease together with high cardiovascular stress reactivity significantly increased the relative risk of change in BP status (from normal to marginally elevated after a 10-year follow-up). An additional finding of the study was the prediction of higher clinic SBP levels at

10-year follow-up in those subjects with higher stress responder status and positive family history of hypertension. Although this study did not include females and was made up predominantly of whites, it does support the hypothesis that stress reactivity plays a role in hypertension and suggests the possibility of another pathophysiological hypothesis, the "gene- and environment-modulated stress responsivity hypothesis," integrating biological and environmental paradigms in stress and CVD.[37] See Chapter 39 for further discussion of chronic stress.

Novel/Potential Risk Factors

Some novel potential risk factors for hypertension in the recent literature address modifiable and nonmodifiable variables, such as smoking, access to health care, and even the number of nephrons at birth. Active smoking is a risk factor for CVD in that it adversely affects the vasculature, promoting atherosclerosis. Smoking itself significantly increases the risk of stroke, a comorbidity associated with hypertension. Even passive smoking has been associated with endothelial dysfunction and altered lipid profile, compared with nonsmokers.[38]

Some researchers have examined socioeconomic status as a direct risk factor, but it has been argued that socioeconomic status (as measured by income and education) affects health behaviors that are considered true risk factors, such as diet, activity, alcohol intake, and smoking. In a study of American women, income and education significantly predicted the prevalence of hypertension by ethnicity (Figure 35-4) in a model that included other widely known risk factors.[39] Other cofactors of socioeconomic status, such as lack of access to health care services and resources and insufficient attention by health care providers, also are suspected risk factors for ineffective prevention and poor control of hypertension.[40]

Novel research has examined the possibility of nephron endowment as a potential risk factor for hypertension, proposing that fewer nephrons at birth may lead

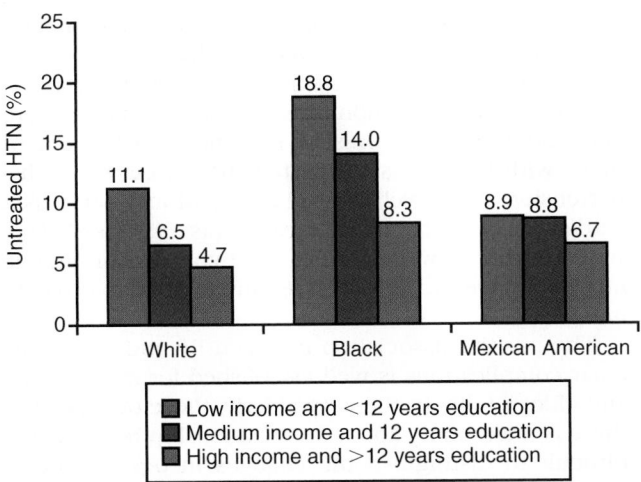

FIGURE 35-4 ■ Combined effect of income and education on predicted prevalence of hypertension in U.S. women by ethnic group. In all three female groups, as income and education declined, prevalence of untreated hypertension increased. This interaction between income and education most affected non-Hispanic black females, who maintained higher rates of untreated hypertension in each income/education bracket compared with non-Hispanic white and Mexican American women. (With permission from Bell CA, Adair LS, Popkin BM: *Soc Sci Med* 59:275-283, 2004.)

to salt-sensitive hypertension. Renal filtration surface area depends on nephron number, size of the glomeruli and length of the capillaries, and on the surface area of the glomerular capillaries; therefore, fewer nephrons would be expected to reduce renal function, contributing to the development of hypertension.

LINKS TO OTHER CARDIOVASCULAR DISEASES

Early diagnosis and treatment of hypertension are important because hypertension is a major risk factor for other vascular diseases, in particular MI, heart failure, stroke, and renal disease. Hypertension leads to arteriosclerosis—structural changes in small arterioles and large arteries. Small vessel arteriosclerosis is believed to be responsible for most of the target organ damage. The high pressure also accelerates large vessel atherosclerosis, leading to the predominantly systolic hypertension so common among the elderly. Vascular damage involves three mechanisms: pulsatile flow, endothelial cell changes, and remodeling and growth of smooth muscle cells. Together, these result in the development of different types of vascular lesions:

- Hyperplastic arteriosclerosis: proliferative reaction of the vessel wall
- Hyaline arteriosclerosis: thickening and hyalinization of the intima and media, causing vessel narrowing
- Miliary aneurysms in small cerebral arterioles
- Atherosclerosis: plaques where thrombi form that may lead to ischemia and infarction of organs

These vascular changes are responsible for the specific organ damage that accompanies sustained hypertension. The higher the BP and the longer it remains elevated, the greater the morbidity and mortality. The risk of CVD beginning at 115/75 mm Hg doubles with each elevated increment of 20/10 mm Hg.[41] The proportional difference in the risk of vascular death associated with a given absolute difference of 20/10 in usual BP is about the same. That is, a rise in SBP from 160 to 180 mm Hg provides the same proportional increase in death from CVD as does an increase from 120 to 140 mm Hg. Stated another way, throughout middle and old age, the relationship between CVD and BP is continuous without any evidence of a threshold. Therefore, any reduction in BP decreases CVD risk and suggests that continual efforts to maintain BP within the normal range are warranted.

After hypertension onset, cardiovascular events are more likely to occur before other noncardiovascular causes of death. The most common first cardiovascular events are angina and claudication in men and women, followed by coronary heart disease in men and stroke in women.[42] Another strategy used to examine complications of primary hypertension is examining the percentage of deaths from various complications. Table 35-4 presents combined data collected between 1903 and 1983 in 10 different studies. Interestingly, the overall causes of death are not different in treated and untreated hypertensive persons, although the age of death has increased markedly. Of course, some of these data are old, having been collected before newer classifications of hypertensive medications were available.

The complications of hypertension can be divided into two categories, hypertensive or atherosclerotic. Hypertensive complications are a direct consequence of increased BP and include conditions such as cerebral hemorrhage, LVH, congestive heart failure, renal insufficiency, and aortic dissection. Atherosclerotic complications have multiple causes with hypertension playing a role and include conditions such as cerebral thrombosis, MI, coronary artery disease, and claudication syndromes.

■ ■ ■

TABLE 35-4   CAUSES OF DEATH IN PRIMARY HYPERTENSION

	PERCENTAGE OF DEATHS			
	HEART DISEASE	STROKE	RENAL FAILURE	NONVASCULAR
Untreated (*n* = 1574)	40%	18%	17%	25%
Treated (*n* = 1582)	40%	19%	17%	24%

Data from Kaplan NM: *Clinical hypertension*, ed 8, Baltimore, 2002, Lippincott Williams & Wilkins.

Heart Disease

Hypertension more than doubles the risk of symptomatic coronary disease, including acute MI and sudden death, and more than triples the risk of heart failure. In response to the increased afterload imposed by hypertension, LVH develops. LVH starts out being compensatory for the increased afterload. After a certain point, however, LVH is a powerful predictor of CVD. LVH is identified by electrocardiography in 5 to 10 percent of hypertensive persons but is found in about half of untreated hypertensive by echocardiography.[43] LVH lowers the threshold for MI by the following mechanisms:

- Increasing the demand for blood flow to the larger muscle mass
- Reducing the ability of the coronary circulation to vasodilate
- Shifting the lower range of coronary flow autoregulation upward

These alterations make the heart vulnerable to ischemia when demand increases or when perfusion pressure is reduced (as represented by the J curve).

Hypertension is also the major risk factor for MI. Myocardial ischemia reflects an imbalance between myocardial oxygen supply and demand. Hypertension reduces the supply and increases demand and therefore greatly increases the incidence of MI. Contributing factors include the following:

- Atherosclerotic narrowing of coronary arteries
- High resistance of coronary microvasculature
- Impaired endothelium-dependent vasodilatation
- Limited coronary reserve

These changes make those with hypertension more susceptible to coronary ischemia, MI, and sudden death.

Hypertension is also a leading cause of heart failure. Along with obesity, diabetes, smoking, and dyslipidemia, hypertension contributes to LVH and MI. Both LVH and MI cause systolic and diastolic dysfunction, which lead to heart failure and death.

Stroke

Hypertension is the premier risk factor for stroke (cerebral infarction and hemorrhage); the risk of stroke increases in proportion to increases in BP. Smoking significantly increases this risk in hypertensive persons. In the elderly, the risk of stroke is related more clearly to SBP than to DBP. Treatment of hypertension reduces stroke incidence.

Renal Disease

The relationships between kidneys and BP are interesting in that nephropathy leads to hypertension and hypertension leads to renal disease. Approximately 90 percent of persons with end-stage renal disease (**ESRD**) have a history of hypertension.[44] The consistency and strength of the association of BP with ESRD are remarkable in that men who have high-normal BP have a twofold increased risk of developing ESRD compared with men who have optimal BP. Stage 4 hypertension imparts a 22 times greater risk of developing ESRD.

Recent evidence suggests that microalbuminuria contributes to the prediction of CVD risk in hypertension. Microalbuminuria is present in almost 40 percent of those with hypertension, particularly those whose hypertension is not well controlled,[45] and may serve as a marker of renal damage or cardiovascular risk.[8] This suggests that new guidelines for hypertension assessment may need to include measurement of microalbuminuria.

The positive association between BP and cardiovascular complications is well established for middle-aged and older adults. In the very elderly, those over age 80, there is uncertainty about this relationship because it is difficult to distinguish the changes in organ systems caused by hypertension from those of aging. O'Sullivan and colleagues[46] compared normotensive and hypertensive persons over the age of 80. They found that hypertension was associated with some target organ damage in the renal, cerebral, and (in men) cardiac systems. Nevertheless, the benefit of antihypertensive treatment for this age group remains controversial.

In summary, "a direct positive relationship between blood pressure and cardiovascular risk has long been recognized. It is strong, continuous, graded, consistent, independent, predictive, and etiologically significant for those with and without coronary heart disease; it has been identified in both men and women, younger and older adults, different racial and ethnic groups, and different countries, and applies to those with high-normal blood pressure as well as those with HTN."[47] The relationship between increasing SBP, DBP, and cardiovascular risk is confounded by the fact that SBP rises throughout adulthood, whereas DBP peaks at around age 50 in men and 70 in women, and falls gradually thereafter.[48]

PREVENTING HYPERTENSION
Primary Prevention

As stated earlier, any reduction in BP decreases CVD risk. This suggests that efforts at maintaining BP within the normal range are warranted and are the basis of prevention. Approaches to dealing with hypertension can be organized into primary, secondary, and tertiary prevention; tertiary prevention is addressed in Chapter 78. Primary prevention focuses on increasing awareness of hypertension and its complications, and taking social steps to decrease controllable risks in the population.

Persistent and effective therapy of established hypertension is difficult to accomplish and, even if accomplished, probably will not reduce the CVD risk in hypertensive patients to that of normotensive patients. Therefore, prevention of hypertension is preferred. Preventive measures are important for everyone, but especially for those carrying a genetic predisposition or having a family history of hypertension. Healthful lifestyles, as outlined subsequently, may prevent or at least delay the onset of hypertension. These involve a combination of weight loss, moderation of sodium and alcohol intake, regular physical activity, and stress management.

Primary prevention of hypertension also involves public health approaches and community education. Public health approaches include reducing calories, saturated fat, and salt in processed foods, and increasing community and school opportunities for physical activity. Together these efforts can reduce BP and the associated cardiovascular complications in the population. This is critical considering the epidemic rise in obesity. Primary prevention is especially important among children and adolescents because they are in the process of establishing health behaviors.[49] Prehypertensive children and adolescents should receive weight management counseling if overweight and should be encouraged to engage in physical activity and diet management. Family involvement and community efforts are critical for adaptation of these behavioral changes.

Despite current recommendations to consume no more than 2400 mg of sodium daily, the average American diet includes 4000 mg of sodium daily. Because most of this sodium comes from salt in processed foods, the American Public Health Association[50] has recommended that food manufacturers and restaurants reduce sodium by 50 percent over the next decade. Gradually reducing the amount of sodium added during manufacturing and commercial preparation of food is the single most effective means of decreasing sodium intake. Such strategies accompanied by those addressing racial, ethnic, cultural, linguistic, religious, and social factors related to food are critical. Much of the recent work on hypertension has focused on active and aggressive treatment with antihypertensive drugs. Many believe that a more effective strategy would be to lower the BP level of the entire population by the simple reduction of sodium intake. It has been estimated that lowering the entire distribution of BP by 2 to 3 mm Hg through reduction of sodium intake would be as effective in reducing the overall risks of hypertension as prescribing current antihypertensive drug therapy for all persons with definite hypertension.[43]

The large number of hypertensive persons who do not know that they have hypertension or are treated inadequately may lead to complications during the treatment of seemingly minor conditions. For example, epinephrine is used widely in local anesthetics to improve the depth and duration of the anesthesia and to reduce bleeding in the operative field. However, the effect of epinephrine on cardiovascular and hemodynamic factors makes its use in hypertensive persons in dentistry controversial. The use of epinephrine in minor procedures may increase the probability of acute hypertensive crisis, angina pectoris, MI, or cardiac dysrhythmias. A systematic review of literature in this area revealed that hypertensive persons undergoing a tooth extraction experience increases in SBP of 11.7 mm Hg, DBP of 3.3 mm Hg, and heart rate of 4.7 beats/min.[51] These increases were higher in hypertensive than in normotensive persons. When a local anesthetic containing epinephrine was used, SBP increased 4 mm Hg higher, and heart rate increased 6 beats/min higher. No adverse events were associated with the use of epinephrine in these studies.

In summary, primary prevention requires a comprehensive program of lifestyle interventions. These interventions are outlined in Box 35-1.[47] Such a program, involving public education, professional education, and patient education, can be successful only through a collaborative effort of health care professionals, policy makers, industry, media, and other opinion makers to mount a sustained campaign targeting all sections and age groups.

Secondary Prevention
Diagnosis

Given the proliferation of opportunities for BP measurement, one would think that identifying those persons with prehypertension would be easy. Pharmacies and supermarkets contain simple-to-use BP instruments, and BP screenings are included in all health fairs. Nevertheless, a large percentage of the population has undiagnosed hypertension or prehypertension, possibly because true diagnosis requires three consecutive elevated readings, and documentation of BP levels from health fairs and personal recordings is often poor.

The continuous relationship between the level of BP and cardiovascular risk makes any numerical definition and classification of hypertension arbitrary. Nevertheless, classification of BP levels is useful for clinicians who must make treatment decisions and for researchers who set inclusion and exclusion criteria. The classifications recommended by JNC-VII are shown in Chapter 78. Those with an SBP of 130 to 139 mm Hg are twice as likely to develop hypertension as those with lower values.[2] Therefore, secondary prevention is focused on those with prehypertension because lifestyle modifica-

---

> **BOX 35-1**   ■ ■ ■
> LIFESTYLE MODIFICATIONS FOR PRIMARY PREVENTION OF HYPERTENSION
>
> ---
>
> - Engage in regular aerobic physical activity, such as brisk walking (at least 30 minutes per day, most days of the week).
> - Maintain a normal body weight for adults (body mass index 18.5 to 24.9 kg/m^2).
> - Limit alcohol consumption to no more than 1 oz (30 ml) ethanol (e.g., 24 oz [720 ml] of beer, 10 oz [300 ml] of wine, or 2 oz [60 ml] 100-proof whiskey) per day in most men and to no more than 0.5 oz (15 ml) of ethanol per day in women and lighter-weight persons.
> - Reduce dietary sodium intake to no more than 100 mmol per day (approximately 2.4 g of sodium or 6 g of sodium chloride).
> - Maintain adequate intake of dietary potassium (more than 90 mmol [3500 mg] per day).
> - Consume a diet rich in fruits and vegetables and in low-fat dairy products with a reduced content of saturated and total fat (Dietary Approaches to Stop Hypertension [DASH] eating plan).

From *Summary report: National High Blood Pressure Program (NHBPEP); National Heart, Lung, and Blood Institute (NHLBI); and American Heart Association (AHA) Working Meeting on Blood Pressure Measurement,* Bethesda, Md, 2002, National Institutes of Health. Retrieved August 27, 2003 from www.nhlbi.nih.gov/health/prof/heart/hbp/bpmeasu.pdf

tions may prevent or delay the development of hypertension later in life.

Using these cutoffs, approximately 60 percent of American adults have prehypertension or hypertension, and some groups, such as blacks, older persons, those in low-socioeconomic groups, and overweight persons are disproportionately affected.[52] This creates a serious challenge for preventing and managing hypertension, especially when one considers that the awareness and appropriate management of hypertension among hypertensive persons remain low. Using the latest NHANES data, collected in 1999 and 2000, and the new classification guidelines, Wang and Wang[52] estimated that 31 percent of persons with hypertension were not aware they have it, only 66 percent were told by health care professionals to modify their lifestyles or take medications to control their hypertension, and only 31 percent had their hypertension under control.

The situation is no better in the rest of the world and is even worse in developing countries. For example, less than 10 percent have their hypertension under control in countries such as Cameroon, China, and India.[53] As life expectancy increases in developing countries, the cause of death from CVD is rising, while death from communicable diseases is falling. Thus prevention, detection, and management of hypertension are critical to prevent worldwide CVD.

Despite the established cutoff levels for hypertension, the real threshold for hypertension must be considered flexible, being higher or lower based on the total CV risk profile of each person (Table 35-5).

Intervention Approaches

Efforts aimed at secondary prevention involve intervention approaches to reduce those risks that are controllable. These interventions are essentially the same as those involving prevention and treatment of hypertension, except that the latter includes antihypertensive medications. However, there are numerous actions patients can take that will lower their risk of developing hypertension or at least postpone its devel-

opment. These include weight control, physical activity, adapting healthful eating habits (including lowering salt intake), stopping cigarette smoking, moderating alcohol intake, and general stress reduction techniques, as outlined in Box 35-1. These approaches can be used alone to treat mild hypertension or as adjuncts to medications, and they may decrease the need to take antihypertensive medications. Specific recommendations of the JNC-VII and the expected BP reduction associated with these approaches are discussed in Chapter 78.

Weight Control

More than 25 percent of American children are considered clinically obese, with weight that is 20 percent above ideal body weight. The highest rates of obesity are found among black and Latino youth.[54] This is of particular concern because overweight in childhood has been linked to increased rates of hypertension, hyperlipidemia, type 2 diabetes, and early atherosclerotic lesions. Rosner and colleagues[55] pooled data from eight large U.S. epidemiological studies involving more than 47,000 children to describe BP differences in relation to body size. Irrespective of race, gender, or age, the risk of elevated BP was significantly higher for children in the upper compared with the lower decile of BMI. Sorof and colleagues[56] recently reported a 3 times greater prevalence of hypertension in obese compared with non-obese adolescents in a school-based hypertension and obesity screening study.

Although the specifics of the transition from risk factors in childhood to adult diabetes and CVD are unclear, compelling evidence suggests that lifestyle modification and weight control in childhood and adolescence could reduce the risk of type 2 diabetes and CVD in adulthood.[57] The *American Heart Association Guidelines for Primary Prevention of Atherosclerotic Cardiovascular Disease Beginning in Childhood*[58] cite health promotion goals in diet, physical activity, and smoking.

Numerous diets are currently available that promote health. *Dietary Guidelines for Americans,* jointly is-

■ ■ ■

TABLE 35-5 STRATIFICATION OF RISK TO QUANTIFY PROGNOSIS

OTHER RISK FACTORS AND DISEASE HISTORY	BLOOD PRESSURE (mm Hg)				
	NORMAL SBP 120-129 or DBP 80-84	HIGH-NORMAL SBP 130-139 or DBP 85-89	GRADE 1 SBP 140-159 or DBP 90-99	GRADE 2 SBP 160-179 or DBP 100-109	GRADE 3 SBP ≥180 or DBP ≥110
No other risk factors	Average risk	Average risk	Low added risk	Moderate added risk	High added risk
One or two risk factors	Low added risk	Low added risk	Moderate added risk	Moderate added risk	Very high added risk
Three or more risk factors or TOD or diabetes	Moderate added risk	High added risk	High added risk	High added risk	Very high added risk
Associated clinical conditions	High added risk	Very high added risk	Very high added risk	Very high added risk	Very high added risk

DBP, Diastolic blood pressure; *SBP,* systolic blood pressure; *TOD,* target organ disease.
From *Summary report: National High Blood Pressure Program (NHBPEP); National Heart, Lung, and Blood Institute (NHLBI); and American Heart Association (AHA) Working Meeting on Blood Pressure Measurement,* Bethesda, Md, 2002, National Institutes of Health. Retrieved August 27, 2003 from www.nhlbi.nih.gov/health/prof/heart/hbp/bpmeasu.pdf

sued by the U.S. Department of Agriculture and U.S. Department of Health and Human Services present 10 general guidelines for dietary health.[59] The Department of Agriculture Food Guide Pyramid is the only official set of guidelines that recommends a certain number of servings from each food group based on energy intake. This guide recommends a certain number of servings from each food group based on three levels of energy intake. Unfortunately, the size of a serving is likely to be overestimated, and fruit, vegetables, and dairy are often underconsumed while meat and carbohydrates are often overconsumed. The American Heart Association *Guidelines for Primary Prevention of Atherosclerotic Cardiovascular Disease Beginning in Childhood* advocate consumption of a variety of fruits, vegetables, whole grains, dairy products, fish, legumes, poultry, and lean meat. Limiting foods high in saturated fats (less than 10 percent of calories per day), cholesterol (less than 300 mg per day), and *trans*-fatty acids, and limiting salt intake also are recommended.

Physical Activity

Similar interventions are needed to promote exercise among children, adolescents, and adults. This is challenging with the increase in sedentary activities such as television viewing, computing, and video games, especially if safe areas for outdoor recreation are not easily accessible. Again, changes are required in the home, school or workplace, and community to promote more physical activity. Adolescents and their families should be encouraged to plan regular periods of exercise and to engage in shared family activities. Schools and places of business can offer opportunities that promote regular activity. For example, some health departments are promoting a walking program that involves encouraging the use of stairs rather than elevators. Americans are fast approaching an epidemic of CVD as increasing numbers of obese, hypertensive, diabetic, or hyperlipidemic adolescents become young adults.

Cigarette Smoking

Cigarette smoking and exposure to second-hand smoke should be eliminated in children and adolescents as much as possible.[58] Starting at age 10, children need to receive clear, strong, informed, and personalized counseling against smoking and exposure to second-hand smoke at home, with friends, at school, or at work.[49]

Relaxation Techniques

Relaxation techniques, such as biofeedback and meditation, and cognitive therapy also have helped some patients to lower their BP. In a meta-analysis of 23 studies examining the effect of biofeedback-assisted relaxation training in hypertension, SBP dropped an average of 6.7 mm Hg and DBP dropped an average of 4.8 mm Hg.[60] Although this effect is not large, some patients were able to lower their BP by much larger amounts. A number of studies have attempted to explore the characteristics of these persons. In general, those with higher sympathetic basal tone (that is higher BP and heart rate and lower skin temperature) or with greater sympathetic activation during stress, appear to be most likely to benefit from biofeedback-assisted relaxation training.[61]

Motivating Behavioral Change

A major challenge in attempting to reduce hypertension and to control the complications of hypertension is the difficulty in getting patients to adhere to or comply with health and treatment recommendations. Adherence rates in most chronic diseases are poor; in hypertension they are especially poor because high BP levels usually are not sensed. Therefore, there is little immediate feedback to patients to follow their prescribed regimens, unless they are routinely monitoring their own BP.

The JNC-VII[2] recognizes the seriousness of poor adherence and suggests the following reasons for nonadherence:

- Misunderstanding of condition or treatment
- Denial of illness because of lack of symptoms or perception of drugs as symbols of ill health
- Lack of patient involvement in the care plan
- Unexpected adverse effects of medications
- Cost of medications
- Complexity of care

Lifestyle modification adherence is even lower than medication adherence because the regimens are more behaviorally demanding. The provider and the patient should develop a plan together whereupon they agree upon BP goals, agree upon the length of time needed to reach the goal, and alter the plan if BP goal is not achieved. More specific ways of promoting behavioral change to prevent hypertension are discussed in Chapters 83 and 84.

In an effort to tailor individual strategies to improve adherence, Weir and colleagues[62] developed four adherence subgroups among those with hypertension. Hypertensive persons fell into one of four groups:

- Those who strive to control BP through medications and lifestyle
- Those who rely almost exclusively on medications to control their BP
- Those who rely almost exclusively on medications to control their BP but are more likely to forget to take medications
- Those who are not afraid of hypertension and do not believe that not taking medications is a threat to their health

Using this framework, group one needs little encouragement; group two needs education and assistance with lifestyle modifications; group three needs help incorporating their medications into their daily routine, as well as information about lifestyle modifications; and those in group four are a great challenge to health care professionals.

When primary and secondary prevention efforts are not successful, hypertension is likely to occur. Tertiary prevention efforts are aimed at reducing the morbidity and mortality that result from hypertension by reducing BP to normal levels. Treatment of hypertension is discussed in Chapter 78.

REFERENCES

1. Hajjar I, Kotchen TA: Trends in prevalence, awareness, treatment, and control of hypertension in the United States, 1988-2000, *JAMA* 290:199-206, 2003.
2. Joint National Committee on Prevention, Detection, Evaluation, and Treatment of High Blood Pressure: The seventh report of the Joint National Committee on Prevention, Detection, Evaluation and Treatment of High Blood Pressure: the JNC 7 report, *JAMA* 289:2560-2572, 2003.
3. Kannel W, Sorlie P, Gordon T: Labile hypertension: a faulty concept? The Framingham Study, *Circulation* 61:1183-1187, 1980.
4. Cushman WC: The clinical significance of systolic hypertension, *Am J Hypertens* 11:182S-185S, 1998.
5. Lauer MS, Anderson KM, Levy D: Influence of contemporary versus 30-year blood pressure levels on left ventricular mass and geometry: the Framingham Heart Study, *J Am Coll Cardiol* 18:1287-1294, 1991.
6. Okin PM, Devereux RB, Jerk S et al: Regression of electrocardiographic left ventricular hypertrophy during antihypertensive treatment and the prediction of major cardiovascular events, *JAMA* 292:2343-2349, 2004.
7. Clement DL, De Buyer ML, Dupers DA: Hypertension in peripheral arterial disease, *Curr Pharm Des* 10:3615-3620, 2004.
8. Leoncini G, Viazzi F, Parodi D et al: Mild renal dysfunction and cardiovascular risk in hypertension patients, *J Am Soc Nephrol* 15:S88-S90, 2004.
9. Persu A, De Plaen JF: Recent insights in the development of organ damage caused by hypertension, *Acta Cardiol* 59:369-381, 2004.
10. American Heart Association: *Heart disease and stroke statistics: 2004 update,* Dallas, 2003, The Association.
11. Mainous AG, Everett CJ, Liszka H et al: Prehypertension and mortality in a nationally representative cohort, *Am J Cardiol* 94:1496-1500, 2004.
12. Ambler SK, Brown RD: Genetic determinants of blood pressure regulation, *J Cardiovasc Nurs* 13:59-77, 1999.
13. *OMIM™: Online Mendelian Inheritance in Man™* (OMIM #601665). Johns Hopkins University and National Center for Biotechnology Information. Retrieved March 1, 2005 from www.ncbi.nlm.nih.gov/entrez/query.fcgi?db=OMIM
14. Stein CM, Lang CC, Singh I et al: Increased vascular adrenergic vasoconstriction and decreased vasodilatation in blacks: additive mechanisms leading to enhanced vascular reactivity, *Hypertension* 36:945-951, 2000.
15. Wood AJ: Variability in beta-adrenergic receptor response in the vasculature: role of receptor polymorphism, *J Allergy Clin Immunol* 110:S318-S321, 2002.
16. Zanchetti A, Hansson L, Dahlof B et al: Effects of individual risk factors on the incidence of cardiovascular events in the treated hypertensive patients of the Hypertension Optimal Treatment Study, *J Hypertens* 19:1149-1159, 2001.
17. Vasan RS, Beiser A, Seshadri S et al: Residual lifetime risk for developing hypertension in middle-aged women and men: the Framingham Heart Study, *JAMA* 287:1003-1010, 2002.
18. Izzo JL Jr, Levy D, Black HR: *Hypertension primer,* ed 2, Baltimore, 2003, Lippincott Williams & Wilkins.
19. Hyman DJ, Pavlik VN: Characteristics of patients with uncontrolled hypertension in the United States, *N Engl J Med* 345:479-486, 2001.
20. Kearney PM, Whelton M, Reynolds K et al: Global burden of hypertension: analysis of worldwide data, *Lancet* 365:217-223, 2005.
21. Joint National Committee on Prevention, Detection, Evaluation, and Treatment of High Blood Pressure: The sixth report of the Joint National Committee on Prevention, Detection, Evaluation, and Treatment of High Blood Pressure, *Arch Intern Med* 157:2413-2446, 1997.
22. Orshal JM, Khalil RA: Gender, sex hormones, and vascular tone, *Am J Physiol Regul Integr Comp Physiol* 286:R233-R249, 2004.
23. Hong Y, Faire U, Heller DA et al: Genetic and environmental correlations among serum lipids and apolipoproteins in elderly twins reared together and apart, *Am J Hum Genet* 55:1255-1267, 1994.
24. Lucassen, A: Genetics of multifactorial diseases. In *Practical Genetics for Primary Care* by P.Rose and A.Lucassen. Oxford, 1999, Oxford University Press pp.145-165.
25. Collins R, Winkleby MA: African American women and men at high and low risk for hypertension: a signal detection analysis of NHANES III, 1988-1994, *Prev Med* 35(4):303-312, 2002.
26. Kramer H, Han C, Post W et al: Racial/ethnic differences in hypertension and hypertension treatment and control in the Multi-Ethnic Study of Atherosclerosis (MESA), *Am J Hypertens* 17:963-970, 2004.
27. Sanchez-Castillo CP, Velasquez-Monroy O, Lara-Esqueda A et al: Diabetes and hypertension increases in a society with abdominal obesity: results of the Mexican National Health Survey 2000, *Public Health Nutr* 8:53-60, 2005.
28. Wofford MR, Hall JE: Pathophysiology and treatment of obesity hypertension, *Curr Pharm Des* 10:3621-3637, 2004.
29. Hunt SC, Hopkins PN, Lalouel JM: Hypertension. In King RA, Rotter JI, Motulsky AG, editors: *The genetic basis of common disease,* ed 2, New York, 2002, Oxford Press.
30. Akita S, Sacks FM, Svetkey LP et al: Effects of the Dietary Approaches to Stop Hypertension (DASH) diet on the pressure-natriuresis relationship, *Hypertension* 42:8-13, 2003.
31. Klatsky AL, Friedman GD, Siegelaub AB, Gerard MJ: Alcohol consumption and blood pressure: Kaiser-Permanente Multiphasic Health Examination data, *N Engl J Med* 296:1194-2000, 1977.
32. Cushman WC: The burden of uncontrolled hypertension: morbidity and mortality associated with disease progression, *J Clin Hypertens* 5(3 suppl 2):14-22, 2003.
33. Brand-Herrmann SM, Kuznetsova T, Wiechert A et al: Alcohol intake modulates the genetic association between HDL cholesterol and the PPAR-gamma 2 Pro12Ala polymorphism, *J Lipid Res* 46(5):913-919, 2005.
34. Xin X, He J, Frontini MG et al: Effects of alcohol reduction on blood pressure: a meta-analysis of randomized controlled trials, *Hypertension* 38:1112-1117, 2001.
35. Cushman WC, Cutler JA, Hanna E et al: The Prevention and Treatment of Hypertension Study (PATHS): effects of an alcohol treatment program on blood pressure, *Arch Intern Med* 152:1197-1207, 1998.
36. Richardson CR, Krista AM, Lantz PM, Hayward RA: Physical activity and mortality across cardiovascular disease risk groups, *Med Sci Sports Exerc* 36:1923-1929, 2004.
37. Light KC, Girdler SS, Sherwood A et al: High stress responsivity predicts later blood pressure only in combination with positive family history and high life stress, *Hypertension* 33:1458-1464, 1999.
38. Holay MP, Paunikar NP, Joshi PP et al: Effect of passive smoking on endothelial function in healthy adults, *J Assoc Physicians India* 52:114-117, 2004.
39. Bell AC, Adair LS, Popkin BM: Understanding the role of mediating risk factors and proxy effects in the association between socio-economic status and untreated hypertension, *Soc Sci Med* 59:275-283, 2004.
40. Centers for Disease Control and Prevention: Racial/ethnic disparities in prevalence, treatment and control of hypertension: United States, 1999-2002, *MMWR Morb Mortal Wkly Rep* 54:7-9, 2005.
41. Lewington S, Clarke R, Qizilbash N et al: Age-specific relevance of usual blood pressure to vascular mortality: a meta-analysis of individual data for one million adults in 61 prospective studies, *Lancet* 360:1903-1913, 2002.
42. Lloyd-Jones DM, Leip EP, Larson MG et al: Novel approach to examining first cardiovascular events after hypertension onset, *Hypertension* 45:39-45, 2005.
43. Kaplan NM: *Clinical hypertension,* ed 8, Baltimore, 2002, Lippincott Williams & Wilkins.
44. Izzo JL Jr, Levy D, Black HR: *Hypertension primer,* ed 2, Baltimore, 1999, Lippincott Williams & Wilkins.
45. Segura J, Trollope M, Radicchio JL: Microalbuminuria, *Clin Exp Hypertens* 26:701-707, 2004.
46. O'Sullivan C, Duggan J, Lyons S et al: Hypertensive target-organ damage in the very elderly, *Hypertension* 42:130-135, 2003.
47. *Summary report: National High Blood Pressure Program (NHBPEP); National Heart, Lung, and Blood Institute (NHLBI); and American Heart Association (AHA) Working Meeting on Blood Pressure Measurement,* Bethesda, Md, 2002, National Institutes of Health. Retrieved August 27, 2003 from www.nhlbi.nih.gov/health/prof/heart/hbp/bpmeasu.pdf

48. Guidelines Committee: European Society of Hypertension, European Society of Cardiology guidelines for the management of arterial hypertension, *J Hypertens* 21:1011-1053, 2003.
49. Calderon KS, Yucha CB, Schaffer SD: Obesity-related cardiovascular risk factors: intervention recommendations to decrease adolescent obesity, *J Pediatr Nurs* 20:3-14, 2005.
50. American Public Health Association: *Reducing sodium content in the American diet,* 2002. Retrieved March 2, 2005 from www.apha.org/legislative/policy/2002/2002-4-sodium.pdf
51. *Cardiovascular effects of epinephrine in hypertensive dental patients,* Summary, Evidence Report/Technology Assessment No 48, AHRQ Pub No 02-E005, Rockville, Md, 2002, Agency for Healthcare Research and Quality. Retrieved March 1, 2005 from www.ahrq.gov/clinic/epcsums/ephypsum.htm
52. Wang Y, Wang Q: The prevalence of prehypertension and hypertension among US adults according to the new Joint National Committee guidelines, *Arch Intern Med* 164:2126-2134, 2004.
53. Erdine S, Aran SN: Current status of hypertension control around the world, *Clin Exp Hypertens* 26:731-738, 2004.
54. Williams CL, Hayman LL, Daniels SR et al: Cardiovascular health in childhood: a statement for health professionals from the Committee on Atherosclerosis, Hypertension, and Obesity in the Young (AHOY) of the Council on Cardiovascular Disease in the Young, American Health Association, *Circulation* 106:143-160, 2002.
55. Rosner B, Prineas R, Daniels SR, Loggie J: Blood pressure differences between blacks and whites in relation to body size among US children and adolescents, *Am J Epidemiol* 151:1007-1019, 2000.
56. Sorof JM, Poffenbarger T, Franco K et al: Isolated systolic hypertension, obesity, and hyperkinetic hemodynamic states in children, *J Pediatr* 140:660-666, 2002.
57. Steinberger J; Daniels SR; American Heart Association Atherosclerosis, Hypertension, and Obesity in the Young Committee (Council on Cardiovascular Disease in the Young); American Heart Association Diabetes Committee (Council on Nutrition, Physical Activity, and Metabolism): Obesity, insulin resistance, diabetes, and cardiovascular risk in children: an American Heart Association scientific statement from the Atherosclerosis, Hypertension, and Obesity in the Young Committee (Council on Cardiovascular Disease in the Young) and the Diabetes Committee (Council on Nutrition, Physical Activity, and Metabolism), *Circulation* 107(10):1448-1453, 2003.
58. Kavey RW, Daniels SR, Lauer RM et al: American Heart Association guidelines for primary prevention of atherosclerotic cardiovascular disease beginning in childhood, *Circulation* 107:1562-1566, 2003.
59. US Department of Agriculture: *Nutrition and your health: dietary guidelines for Americans, 2000,* Washington, DC, 2000, US Department of Health and Human Services.
60. Yucha CB, Clark L, Smith M et al: The effect of biofeedback in hypertension, *Appl Nurs Res* 14:29-35, 2001.
61. Yucha CB, Tsai P, Calderon KS, Tian L: Biofeedback assisted relaxation training for essential hypertension: who is most likely to benefit? *J Cardiovasc Nurs* 20:198-205, 2005.
62. Weir MR, Maibach EW, Bakris GL et al: Implications of a health lifestyle and medication analysis for improving hypertension control, *Arch Intern Med* 160:481-490, 2000.

Obesity

Melanie T. Warziski
Jina Choo
Jessica Novak
Lora E. Burke

CHAPTER ABBREVIATIONS

BMI   body mass index

CHD   coronary heart disease

CVD   cardiovascular disease

LDL   low-density lipoprotein

NHANES   National Health and Nutrition Examination Survey

PDA   personal digital assistant

SOS   Swedish Obese Subjects

VLCD   very low-calorie diet

WHR   waist-to-hip ratio

Obesity is an excessively high proportion of body fat, a condition that increases one's risk for comorbid conditions and premature death.[1] Usually, persons are classified as obese when body fat content surpasses 30 percent in women or 25 percent in men. Obesity is a chronic disorder that involves a complex interaction among environmental, cultural, psychosocial, metabolic, and genetic factors.[2,3] Moreover, obesity is a stigmatizing disease with a prevalence that is reaching epidemic proportions in the industrialized world and is undergoing rapid increases in developing nations. Body mass index (**BMI**), the relationship between weight and height, provides a classification system for body weight. A BMI of 18.5 to 24.9 kg/m² is considered normal, between 25.0 and 29.9 overweight, and over 30 obese. The obese category is subdivided further into obesity I (BMI of 30.0 to 34.9 kg/m²), obesity II (BMI of 35.0 to 39.9 kg/m²), and obesity III (BMI of 40 kg/m² or above), also known as extreme obesity.[2,4]

EPIDEMIOLOGY OF OBESITY

The prevalence of obesity has increased greatly in the past two decades in industrialized and nonindustrialized countries. Global estimates are more than 1 billion overweight adults, with at least 300 million of these being obese.[4] The latest National Health and Nutrition Examination Survey (**NHANES**) data for 1999 to 2002 show that among U.S. adults age 20 and older, 65.1 percent are overweight or obese, 30.4 percent are obese, and 4.9 percent are extremely obese (Figures 36-1 and 36-2). The prevalence of overweight and obesity exceeds 50 percent in almost every age and racial/ethnic

group.[5] The prevalence of obesity is particularly high among ethnic minority groups in the United States (e.g., black, Mexican American, Native American). Outside of the United States the prevalence rates are lower but still alarming. In the United Kingdom and in Europe, 15 percent of men and 30 percent of women are obese. In Asia, obesity is rapidly increasing; in Samoa, obesity has overtaken malnutrition as a health problem.[6]

MORBIDITY AND MORTALITY

Rates of morbidity and mortality increase with an increasing BMI. The BMI classification system for weight status provides a mechanism for identifying patients who are at increased risk for having or developing obesity-related complications. Obesity-related diseases, such as hypertension, coronary heart disease (**CHD**), and diabetes begin to increase at BMI values within the normal range (18.5 to 24.9 kg/m²). However, other factors affect adiposity-related risk for disease and increased mortality. These factors include the distribution of body fat, weight gain since young adulthood, degree of physical fitness, and ethnicity. Complications of obesity include an extensive list of diseases that lead to disorders in metabolism and endocrine function, negatively affect multiple systems, and may lead to reduced function and quality of life.[2,7] Table 36-1 lists comorbid conditions related to excess adiposity.

Evidence indicates that obesity profoundly affects life expectancy. For example, a 40-year-old nonsmoking woman who is *overweight* will have lost 3.3 years of life expectancy, whereas the same woman who is *obese* will have lost 7.1 years; male counterparts would have lost 3.1 and 5.8 years of life expectancy, respectively.[8] The absolute mortality risk associated with an elevated BMI increases with age up to age 75; in persons over 75 years of age, obesity has less of an impact on mortality.

RISK FACTORS

There are many obesity-related risk factors. Nonmodifiable factors include genetic predisposition. Studies of twins, adopted children, and families have shown that genetic factors play a significant role in the pathogenesis of obesity.[9] Although susceptibility to obesity is determined in part by genetic factors, the current obesogenic environment is required for the expression of the obesity phenotype. NHANES III data show that the prevalence of obesity is 2 times as high in families of

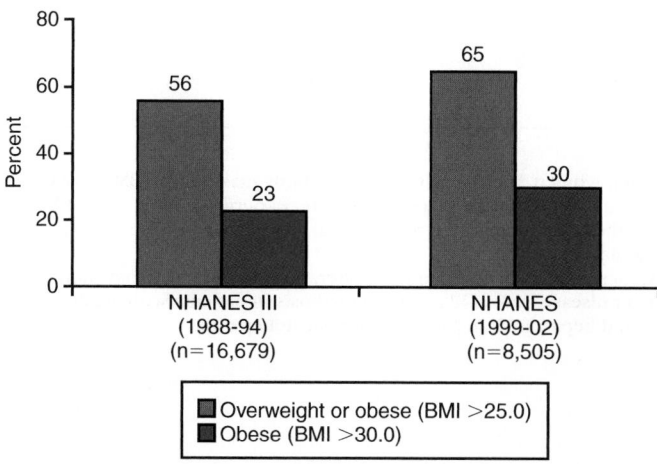

*Age-adjusted by the direct method to the year 2000 U.S. Bureau of the Census estimates using the age groups 20-39, 40-59, and 60 years and over.

FIGURE 36-1 ■ Age-adjusted prevalence of overweight and obesity among U.S. adults, ages 20 to 74. *BMI,* Body mass index; *NHANES,* National Health and Nutrition Examination Study. (From NHANES III. Retrieved November 28, 2005 from www.cdc.gov/nchs/products/pubs/pubd/hestats/obese/obsefig1.GIF)

obese individuals, whereas the risk for extreme obesity (BMI over 45 kg/m^2) is 7 to 8 times higher among individuals in families whose members are extremely obese.[10] The marked increase in the prevalence of obesity is not due to a shift in the gene pool but rather to the lifestyle in Westernized countries that provides an abundant food supply and reduces need for physical activity.

Bray and Bouchard[11] list several etiological or risk factors that may lead to obesity, some of which may be modifiable by treatment or by alterations in lifestyle or the environment. These factors include neuroendocrine disorders, such as hypothalamic obesity, Cushing syndrome, hypothyroidism, polycystic ovary disease, and growth hormone deficiency; drug-induced weight gain, particularly the psychoactive agents and hormones; smoking cessation; and sedentary lifestyle. Also included in the list are nutrition-related factors (e.g., consumption of fat and binge eating disorder) and psychological and social factors (e.g., socioeconomic status and ethnicity). Congenital and genetic disorders such as a deficiency in leptin or a defect in the leptin receptor, or Prader-Willi syndrome complete the list of potential etiological factors. Conversely, risk for obesity later in life can be reduced if a child is breast-fed or if the mother is not overweight at the time of conception.[12]

DIFFERENCES ACROSS GENDER, AGE, AND ETHNIC GROUPS

Variations occur in the development and prevalence of obesity across gender, age, and ethnic groups. Most adult women gain their excess weight following adolescence. Women experience increased risk for weight gain during certain periods of life, e.g., pregnancy and menopause. The decline in estrogen following menopause alters fat cell biology that may lead to increased central fat deposition.[11] Men gradually increase their weight in the third decade, when they assume a more sedentary lifestyle; this gain lessens in the fifth decade

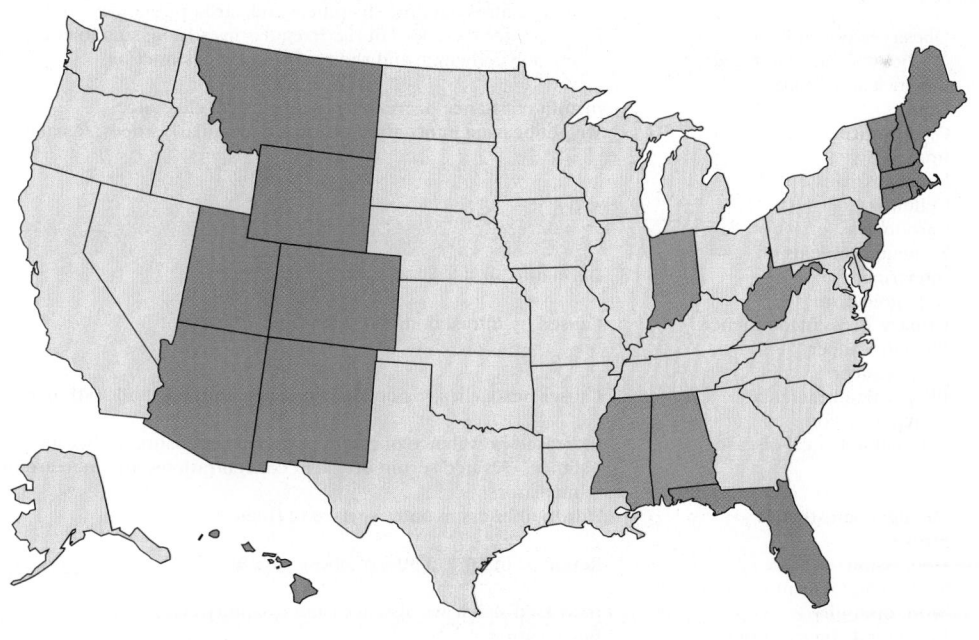

Obesity = *BMI ≥30, or ~ 30 lbs overweight for 5′ 4″ person

☐ No Data   ☐ <10%   ■ 10%-14%   ■ 15%-19%   ☐ 20%-24%   ■ ≥25%

FIGURE 36-2 ■ Obesity trends among U.S. adults: Behavioral Risk Factor Surveillance System, 2005. *BMI,* Body mass index. (Retrieved December 13, 2006 from http://www.cdc.gov/nccdphp/dnpa/obesity/trend/maps/)

■ ■ ■

TABLE 36-1 OBESITY-RELATED COMPLICATIONS AND COMORBIDITIES

SYSTEM	COMORBID CONDITION	NOTES
Gastrointestinal	Gastroesophageal reflux disease	
	Gallbladder disease (cholelithiasis)	Higher risk among women, increases linearly with body mass index (BMI). Incidence of new gallstones 25% to 35% in obese who experience rapid weight loss
	Pancreatitis	Fat deposited in the peripancreatic retroperitoneal spaces may predispose to peripancreatic fat necrosis
	Liver disease	Hepatomegaly, increased liver function tests, alterations in liver histology, nonalcoholic fatty liver disease, risk of fibrosis and cirrhosis in patients with alcoholic liver disease and hepatitis C, hepatic stenosis, steatohepatitis
	Colon cancer	
	Pancreatic cancer	
	Gallbladder cancer	
	Esophageal cancer	
	Hernias	
Endocrine/ reproductive	Metabolic syndrome	Insulin resistance, associated with abdominal obesity
	Glucose intolerance	
	Type 2 diabetes mellitus	Risk increases as BMI exceeds 22
	Dyslipidemia	Hypertriglyceridemia, increase in serum total and low-density lipoprotein cholesterol concentrations
		Decreased high-density lipoprotein cholesterol
	Amenorrhea	May be associated with infertility
	Cushing syndrome	
	Hypothyroidism	
	Polycystic ovary syndrome	
	Breast cancer	Weight gain after age 18 increases risk
	Uterine cancer	
	Cervical cancer	
Cardiovascular	Coronary heart disease	Presence of abdominal fat increases risk; mediated by obesity-related increases in risk factors, e.g., hypertension, dyslipidemia, impaired glucose tolerance/diabetes, and metabolic syndrome
	Cerebrovascular and thromboembolic disease	Increased risk of ischemic stroke, venous stasis and varicose veins, deep venous thrombosis, pulmonary embolism
	Hypertension	Blood pressure above 140/90 mm Hg, odds ratio = 2.0
Respiratory	Obstructive sleep apnea	Associated with BMI above 30, abdominal fat distribution and large neck girth; increased weight on chest wall and thoracic cage decreases respiratory compliance, causes daytime sleepiness and cardiopulmonary dysfunction
	Obesity-hypoventilation syndrome (Pickwickian syndrome)	PCO_2 greater than 50 mm Hg; irregular breathing, somnolence, cyanosis, secondary polycythemia, and right ventricular dysfunction
	Dyspnea and fatigue	
Musculoskeletal	Gout	Insulin resistance decreases renal uric acid clearance
	Osteoarthritis	Weight-bearing joints affected most, particularly knees; females affected more
	Immobility	
	Low back pain	
Integumentary	Cellulitis	
	Carbuncles	
	Hygiene problems	
	Intertrigo	Dermatitis in skinfolds
Genitourinary	Hypogonadism	
	Urinary stress incontinence	Caused by intraabdominal pressure
	Prostate cancer	
	Renal cancer	
Neurological	Idiopathic intracranial hypertension	Causes headaches, vision abnormalities, tinnitus, and sixth nerve paresis
	Ophthalmological disease	Increased prevalence of cataracts and cataract surgery because of insulin resistance, elevated serum uric acid concentrations, and increase in inflammatory mediators
	Meralgia paresthetica	Pain/numbness in outer surface of thigh
	Stroke	
Psychosocial	Depression	Reported in 20% to 30% of obese patients
	Social/employment discrimination	
	Work disability	Increased sick leave absences and disability claims
	Behavioral abnormalities	Binge eating
	Impaired quality of life	

PCO₂, Partial pressure of carbon dioxide.
From Klein S, Wadden T, Sugerman HJ: *Gastroenterology* 123:882-932, 2002.

and is followed by a gradual loss of weight in the later years. NHANES data show a gender discrepancy in prevalence rates, with females having a higher prevalence of obesity at all ages. For example, at ages 40 to 59, 33.2 percent of women are obese compared with 27.6 percent of men.

These same data show continuing disparities between racial/ethnic groups. For all age groups, non-Hispanic blacks have a significantly higher prevalence of overweight and obesity than non-Hispanic whites.[5] The relative risk for obesity decreases with advanced age. Although an elevated BMI has less impact on mortality among the elderly, excessive weight may affect an elderly person's quality of life.

SIGNIFICANCE OF THE PROBLEM WORLDWIDE

Over the last 25 years, obesity has reached epidemic proportions with significant difference in the geographic distribution[13] (Figures 36-1 and 36-2). The prevalence of overweight and obesity has increased dramatically also in European countries, with higher rates in central and eastern Europe (Figure 36-3). The highest prevalence is among minority populations in the United States followed by countries in the former eastern block of Europe. Asian Americans have median BMI levels similar to or substantially lower than those of blacks and whites, but as the time spent in the United States increases, so does BMI.[14]

Among South American countries, there is a wide range of prevalence of obesity. In Mexico, recent increases have resulted in 35 percent being overweight and 24 percent obese; the prevalence is higher in other South American countries, where rates range from 30 to 50 percent. Another part of the world with increasing rates of obesity is the Middle East and North Africa; among Egyptian women, overweight affects 31.7 percent and obesity another 23.5 percent. Asian countries, most recently China, have been going through numerous economic transitions; these changes are reflected in the increase in fat consumption and increasing rates of overweight and obesity in rural and urban areas.[14]

An index of the severity of this health problem is the increasing health care costs associated with obesity. Figure 36-4 shows the costs of health care for two levels of obesity compared with normal weight. As the BMI increases from the 30 to 34 range to 35 and above, all health care costs increase, especially those for drugs, laboratory tests, and inpatient services.[15] Figure 36-5 shows the increasing risk of cardiovascular disease (**CVD**) as one moves from a normal BMI to a BMI 40 or above; the relative risk for CVD rises to nearly 3.0.[16]

CAUSAL OR CONTRIBUTING MECHANISMS

To maintain a balance, the brain tracks the availability of food in the environment and the available energy stores in the body and adjusts the consumption of en-

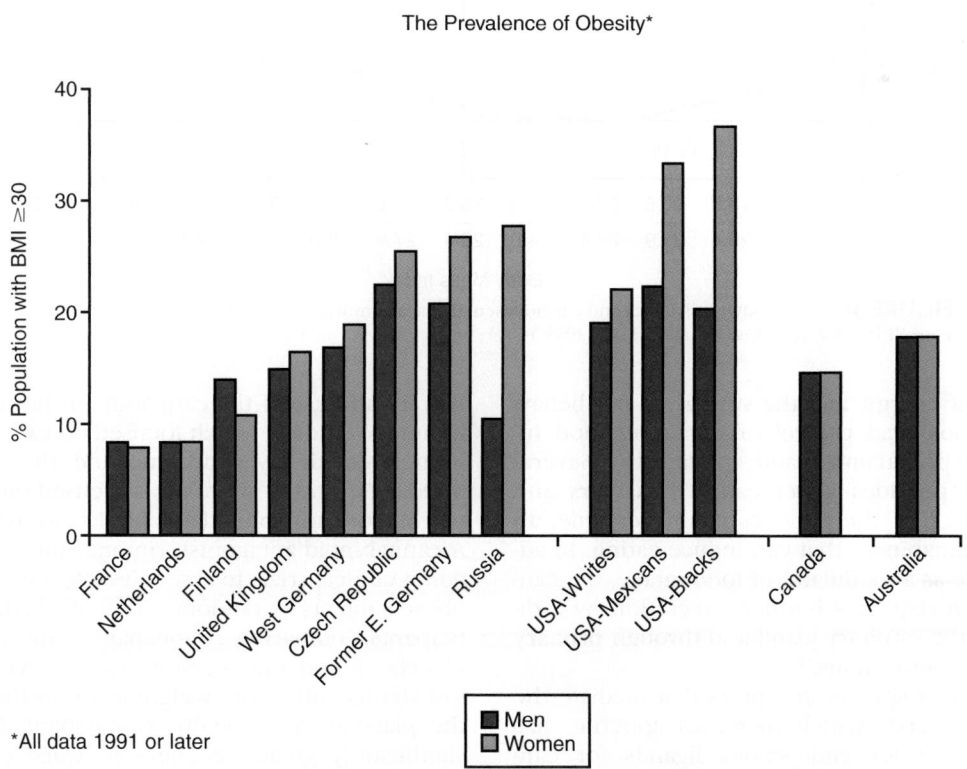

FIGURE 36-3 ■ Prevalence of obesity worldwide. *BMI,* Body mass index. (Retrieved November 28, 2005 from www.iuns.org/features/obesity/tabfig.htm#Figure%201)

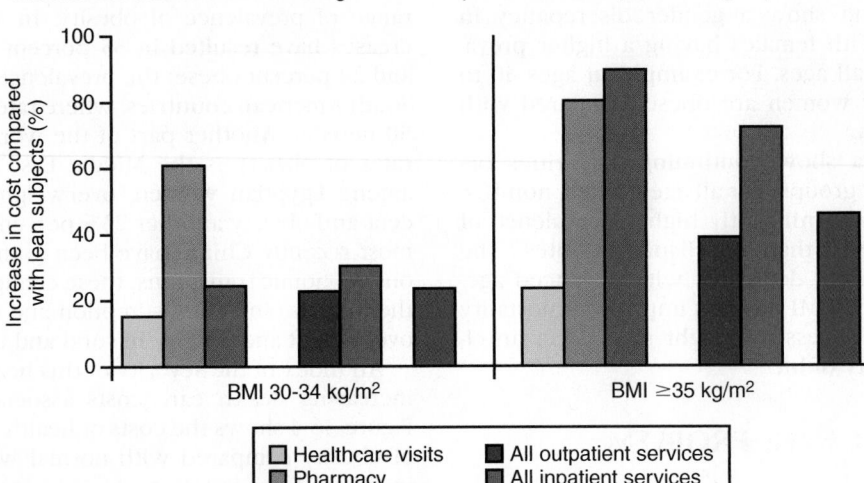

FIGURE 36-4 ▪ Health care costs by body mass index (BMI). (From Quesebberry CJ, Caan B, Jacobson A: *Arch Intern Med* 158:466-472, 1998.)

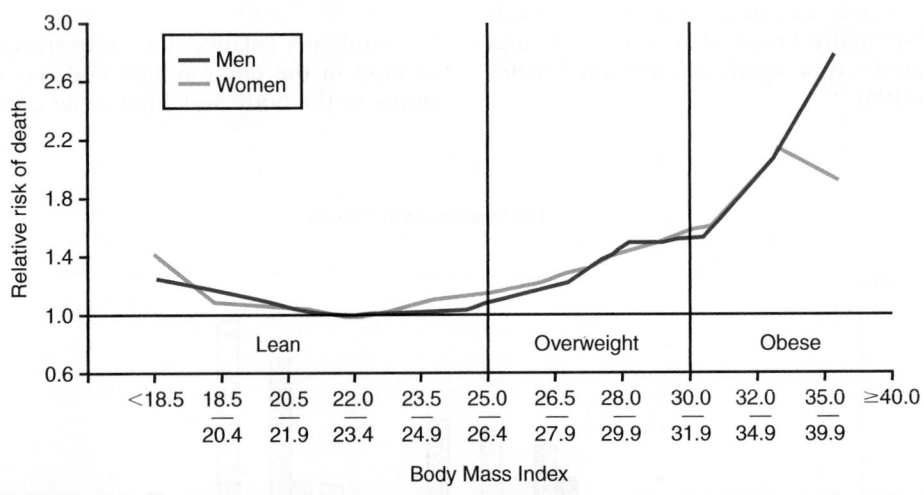

FIGURE 36-5 ▪ Body mass index and cardiovascular disease mortality. (From Calle EE, Thun MJ, Petrelli JM: *N Engl J Med* 341:1097-1105, 1999.)

ergy, the use of energy, and the storage of fat. Behavioral and physiological control of obtaining food involves the hypothalamus and pituitary.[17] Several hormones and peptides affect eating behaviors and body weight. One of the peptides is amandamide, an endogenous cannabinoid that can induce eating. In addition to its role as a modulator of food intake, the cannabinoid system regulates hormone secretion by a direct action on the pituitary gland and through primary action on the hypothalamus.[18]

The presence of specific receptors that mediate the actions of marijuana, which increases appetite, has driven the search for endogenous ligands for cannabinoid receptors. The first endogenous cannabinoid, amandamide, was identified in 1992 and was able to reproduce most of the effects of marijuana.[19] Recently,

therapeutic use of the cannabinoids has been explored in human studies, which focused on cancer or acquired immunodeficiency syndrome and the associated anorexia. Currently, attention is focused on the therapeutic role for cannabinoid antagonists for treating obesity. A cannabinoid antagonist, rimonabant, has been undergoing clinical trials to assess its effect on weight loss in obese subjects. A randomized clinical trial of 1507 participants comparing rimonabant 5 mg and 20 mg to placebo found that persons treated with rimonabant lost significantly more weight at 1 year than those given the placebo. Additionally, rimonabant 20 mg yielded significantly greater changes in waist circumference, triglyceride level, high-density lipoprotein (HDL) cholesterol level, and insulin resistance compared with placebo.[20] Another trial of 1036 dyslipidemic overweight or obese individuals found, in comparison to placebo, that those receiving 20 mg of rimonabant experienced significantly greater weight loss, decrease in waist circumference and triglyceride level, and rise in HDL cholesterol after 1 year.[21] This cannabinoid antagonist also has been found to subdue the euphoric properties of drugs such as cocaine, heroin, nicotine, and alcohol in laboratory animals and potentially could play a role in the treatment of drug addiction.[22] Although the study of the cannabinoid system is relatively new, this system appears to have the potential to direct the development of new agents that may be of use in the pharmacological treatment of obesity.[23]

OTHER CONTRIBUTING FACTORS

The discovery of leptin increased the understanding of energy storage regulation. A cytokine-like peptide, leptin is produced by fat cells (adipocytes) and controls the intake of food through its activation of the hypothalamus. The amount of adipose tissue present influences the production of leptin, and leptin informs the brain of the level of fat stores, which ultimately inhibits food intake.[24] Other hormones that are involved in the short-term control of energy intake include ghrelin, an appetite stimulant; insulin, an anorexic hormone; and cholecystokinin, another anorexic. Ghrelin, primarily produced in the stomach, stimulates food intake and is thought to oppose the signal of satiety by leptin.[25] Detailed discussion of these novel physiological factors is beyond the scope of this chapter.

SOCIETAL AND LIFESTYLE FACTORS

Recent dietary patterns reveal an overconsumption of calories related to increased availability of convenient, low-cost, energy-dense foods served in large portions.[26] The enormous investment by the food industry on promotion and advertisements influences consumer buying and eating behaviors, such as frequent eating outside the home. Healthful foods including fruits, vegetables, and other products are more costly than unhealthful foods, which may contribute to the high rate of obesity among individuals in lower socioeconomic levels.[27] Moreover, the Centers for Disease Control and Prevention reported that approximately 62 percent of American adults do not participate in vigorous physical activity (see Chapter 38).[13] Society has evolved to incorporate into daily life, technological advances, increased computer and automobile use, television viewing, and video game playing resulting in less energy expenditure.

GENETIC INFLUENCES

Obesity is well understood today to be a complex polygenic disorder that represents the interaction between an obesogenic environment and multiple genes. Monogenic forms of obesity, which result from mutations in genes involved in the central pathways of food intake regulation, are rare.[24] In most cases, the genetic susceptibility is polygenic, with each gene contributing a small

part. Twin and familial clustering studies have reported that heritability measures account for between 36 and 44 percent of obesity and BMI.[28]

Two approaches to identifying susceptibility genes are related to obesity: 1) detecting chromosomal regions showing linkage with obesity in large samples of nuclear families, or 2) identifying candidate genes. Leptin is a candidate gene for the regulation of food intake. However, results from association studies have been inconsistent in identifying the role of leptin in obesity. Candidate genes for the regulation of metabolism include insulin, which is considered an adiposity signal for the brain. Other genes are those involved in the pathways of energy expenditure and lipid and adipose tissue metabolism, such as beta-adrenergic receptors (beta$_2$ and beta$_3$). An increasing number of association studies among children are showing that candidate genes may play a minimal role in early onset obesity and that similar to the adult populations, genetic factors should be considered as only part of the contributing factors.[9] Therefore, addressing lifestyle components that lead to excess body weight is critical; behavioral and environmental change is necessary to sustain any improvement in body weight.

OBESITY AND CARDIOVASCULAR DISEASE

Obesity is strongly associated with CVD, especially stroke, ventricular dysfunction, dysrhythmias, and chronic heart failure. Obesity is associated with many of the risk factors for CHD but also is an independent risk factor for CHD. The risk of CVD mortality in obese persons with a BMI of 35 kg/m^2 or more is 2 to 3 times the risk of a lean person (BMI of 18.5 to 24.9 kg/m^2). Even though these values are within the normal range for BMI, the risk of CHD begins to increase for men at a BMI of 23 kg/m^2 and for women at 22 kg/m^2.[29] CHD mortality rate increases 30 percent for every 5-unit increment of BMI.[30]

Obesity is closely associated with traditional (dyslipidemia) and nontraditional (inflammation) risk factors. The constellation of conditions referred to as the metabolic syndrome, abdominal obesity, high fasting glucose level and triglyceride level, low HDL cholesterol, and elevated blood pressure[31] is associated with an increased risk of developing CVD and type 2 diabetes (see Chapter 37).[32] Additionally, abdominal adiposity is related to a higher risk for developing hypertension, CHD, and premature death,[33] whereas subcutaneous peripheral adiposity measured by skinfold thicknesses have not been shown to be associated with ischemic heart disease risk.[31,32]

Obesity also is associated with increased coagulability, endothelial dysfunction, and inflammation. Adipose tissue is active metabolically and secretes various proteins including tumor necrosis factor-alpha, interleukin-6, and plasminogen activator inhibitor-1, all of which may mediate the development of atherosclerosis that leads to CHD. The proinflammatory cytokines, tumor necrosis factor-alpha and interleukin-6, also regulate the production of C-reactive protein, an acute-phase protein produced by hepatocytes in response to inflammation. Evidence suggests that C-reactive protein is related to insulin resistance, the metabolic syndrome, and markers of endothelial dysfunction. Abdominal adiposity also is correlated with plasminogen activator inhibitor-1 activity, which leads to development of atherosclerosis and increased risk of CVD.[34]

Obesity affects cardiac structure and function, which may lead to ventricular dysfunction and chronic heart failure. Even in the absence of hypertension, cardiac structure also may be damaged by chronic fluid overload related to increased cardiac output, which may lead to ventricular dilatation and eccentric hypertrophy. Concentric and eccentric left ventricular hypertrophy increase the risk of systolic and diastolic ventricular dysfunction. Diastolic dysfunction from eccentric hypertrophy and systolic dysfunction from excessive wall stress result in an obesity-related cardiomyopathy. Heart failure is a frequent complication of severe obesity and a major cause of death; duration of obesity is a strong predictor of heart failure.[2] Increased left ventricular end-diastolic volume often is accompanied by decreased ejection fraction in the chronically obese, putting them at risk for heart failure and cardiac dysrhythmia.[35]

Weight loss in overweight or obese individuals can ameliorate or prevent development of several obesity-related risk factors for CHD. Weight loss can improve cardiac function and can prevent development of comorbid conditions.[30] Therefore, it is important for nurses to understand the clinical effects of weight gain and weight loss, know how to assess the overweight patient, develop an appropriate weight management program for the patient, and guide and support the patient in the implementation of the program. The first line of management of overweight and obese patients is identification of the degree to which the person is overweight or obese using standardized methods.

CLINICAL ASSESSMENT
Methods to Measure Overweight and Obesity

BMI, a calculation based on height and weight, is not gender-specific.[2] BMI provides an approximation of total body fat for monitoring trends or changes in body fat during weight management. Height and weight should be measured with the person in light clothes and no shoes. A wall-mounted stadiometer with measures in increments of 0.1 cm should be used to measure height. The two formulas for BMI calculation are shown in Box 36-1. A second and simpler approach to determining BMI is to use a standard BMI chart, which is displayed in Figure 36-6.[2]

Bioelectrical impedance analysis is a method of assessing body composition (lean and fat mass). Scales with bioelectrical impedance analysis capability are available for clinical use today where the individual stands with both feet aligned on the metal plates of the base. Values including weight, percent of body fat, and percent fat-free mass appear on the screen and paper printout.

Dual-energy x-ray absorptiometry is an accurate measurement of total body fat and lean mass. This measurement procedure uses two very low-energy x-ray beams through the body. The beams are weakened to differing degrees by tissues with dissimilar density, allowing delineation between lean body mass, fat, and minerals.[36]

BOX 36-1 ■ ■ ■
FORMULA TO CALCULATE BODY MASS INDEX

$$\text{Metric conversion formula} = \frac{\text{weight (kilograms)}}{\text{height (meters)}^2}$$

$$\text{Nonmetric conversion formula} = \frac{\text{weight (pounds)}}{\text{height (inches)}^2} \times 703$$

Body Mass Index Chart

Weight (lb)

Height (in)	120	130	140	150	160	170	180	190	200	210	220	230	240	250	260	270	280	290	300	320	340	360	380	400
60	23	25	27	29	31	33	35	37	39	41	43	45	47	49	51	53	55	57	59	63	66	70	74	78
62	22	24	26	27	29	31	33	35	37	38	40	42	44	46	48	49	51	53	55	59	62	66	70	73
64	21	22	24	26	28	29	31	33	34	36	38	40	41	43	45	46	48	50	52	55	58	62	65	69
66	19	21	23	24	26	27	29	31	32	34	36	37	39	40	42	44	45	47	49	52	55	58	61	65
68	18	20	21	23	24	26	27	29	30	32	34	35	37	38	40	41	43	44	46	48	52	55	58	61
70	17	19	20	22	23	24	26	27	29	30	32	33	35	36	37	38	40	42	43	46	49	52	55	57
72	16	18	19	20	22	23	24	26	27	29	30	31	33	34	35	37	38	39	41	43	46	49	52	54
74	15	17	18	19	21	22	23	24	26	27	28	30	31	32	33	35	36	37	39	41	44	46	49	51
76	15	16	17	18	20	21	22	23	24	26	27	28	29	30	32	33	34	35	37	40	41	44	45	49

FIGURE 36-6 ■ Body mass index chart. (From NHLBI Obesity Education Initiative Expert Panel on the Identification Evaluation and Treatment of Overweight and Obesity: *Obes Res* 6[suppl 2]:51S-209S, 1998.)

Dual-energy x-ray absorptiometry and underwater weighing are considered the gold standard for assessment of body composition; however, neither one is used for routine clinical assessment.

Methods to Measure Central Adiposity

Waist circumference is the most practical method for assessing abdominal fat or visceral adipose tissue. Waist-to-hip ratio (**WHR**) is the ratio of a person's waist circumference to hip circumference. For most persons, central adiposity increases health risks more than fat distributed around their hips or thighs. A WHR of 1.0 or more is associated with an increased risk of heart disease.[1] A recent case-control study of 27,000 persons in 52 countries found that increasing WHR was highly significantly associated with myocardial infarction even after adjusting for other risk factors, such as BMI.[37] The procedure for measuring waist and hip circumference and calculating WHR is described in Box 36-2, and a diagram for positioning the measuring tape is shown in Figure 36-7.

Computed tomography is an accurate and optimal technique for measurement of abdominal fat, including visceral and subcutaneous fat. However, it is often cost prohibitive, and the weight limitation of the computed tomography scanner table usually does not accommodate a person weighing more than 300 lb. (See the accompanying Conundrum feature.)

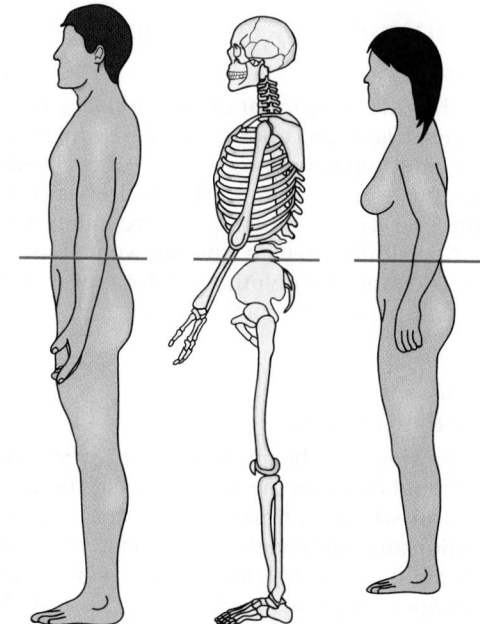

FIGURE 36-7 ▥ Measuring tape positioning for waist circumference. (From NHLBI Obesity Education Initiative Expert Panel on the Identification Evaluation and Treatment of Overweight and Obesity: *Obes Res* 6[suppl 2]:51S-209S, 1998.)

BOX 36-2   ■ ■ ■
MEASUREMENT PROCEDURE FOR WAIST CIRCUMFERENCE AND WAIST-TO-HIP RATIO

Waist
- The patient should be dressed in only undergarments or an examination gown.
- Standing to the right of the patient, palpate the upper hip bone to locate the right iliac crest.
- With a marking pen, draw a horizontal mark just above the upper border of the iliac crest (see Figure 36-7).
- Cross the line with a vertical mark on the midaxillary line.
- Place the measuring tape parallel to the floor around the abdomen at the level of the marked point and hold the tape snug to the skin, but not compressing it. If possible, use a flexible, intact fiberglass tape measure that has a tension meter indicator to ensure consistency in the tautness of the tape (Gullick II tape measure).
- Take the measurement during a normal exhalation.
- If it is difficult to identify a waist narrowing, the smallest horizontal circumference in the area between the last rib and iliac crest should be measured.
- Measure 2 times. Take a third measurement if the first two measures differ by more than 2 cm.
- Average the two values that are within 2 cm of each other.

Hip
- With the patient standing erect, arms at the sides, and feet together, measure the hip circumference at the point yielding the maximum circumference around the buttocks.
- The tape measure should be held in a horizontal plane touching the skin but not compressing the tissue.
- If the patient has a pendulous abdomen reaching the level of the hip, place the tape underneath the abdomen and measure around the buttocks horizontally.

Waist-to-Hip Ratio
- WHR = waist (in centimeters)/hip (in centimeters)

■ ■ ■ CONUNDRUM

MAKING MEASUREMENTS

Body mass index	Very muscular persons may fall into the "overweight" category.
	May underestimate body fat in the elderly who have lost muscle mass.
Waist circumference	Racial and age differences exist.
	In older persons and among Asians, abdominal fat is linked more to obesity-related disease risk than body mass index.
Waist-hip ratio	Racial/ethnic differences may exist: blacks may have smaller hips, resulting in a higher waist-to-hip ratio.
Skinfold thickness	Becomes increasingly inaccurate as obesity increases.
	Requires training and experience for accuracy.
Bioelectrical impedance analysis	May be inaccurate because of changes in ambient temperature or medical conditions such as dehydration, edema, or electrolyte imbalance.
Dual-energy x-ray absorptiometry	Accuracy declines in persons weighing more than 100 kg.
Magnetic resonance imaging or computed tomography	Most accurate way to measure abdominal or visceral fat, but these approaches are relatively expensive for routine use.
	Not available for individuals weighing more than 300 lb.

Data from NHLBI Obesity Education Initiative Expert Panel on the Identification Evaluation and Treatment of Overweight and Obesity: *Obes Res* 6(suppl 2):51S-209S, 1998; World Health Organization: *Global Strategy on Diet, Physical Activity, and Health,* Geneva 1997, The Organization. Retrieved May 30, 2005 from www.who.gov; and Pi-Sunyer FX: *Proc Nutr Soc* 59:505-509, 2000.

CLASSIFICATION OF OVERWEIGHT AND OBESITY

The World Health Organization developed a classification of overweight and obesity by BMI, which was accepted by the United States in 1998. BMI is classified as underweight, normal, overweight, and obesity I, obesity II, and obesity III.[2] When waist circumference with sex-specific cutoffs in men and in women is added, there are categories for defining risk for type 2 diabetes, hypertension, and CVD[2] (Table 36-2).

INTERVENTION APPROACHES
Primary Prevention

Primary prevention, the prevention of overweight or obesity, should focus on the health benefits of maintaining healthful weight. Primary prevention begins with identification and modification of risk factors for becoming overweight. These risk factors may be viewed in an epidemiological framework of vectors, host, and environmental factors. *Host factors* include genotype and unhealthful behavioral patterns of excessive energy intake and insufficient physical activity. Genotype (or biology) currently is an unmodifiable factor, but behavioral factors can be managed if appropriate education and interventions are provided. *Vectors (vehicles)* are devices and activities that contribute to reduced energy expenditure (e.g., the ubiquitous presence of automobiles, computers, television, computer games) and consumption of energy-dense foods in large portions. *Environmental factors* include the physical, economic, and sociocultural factors that can be addressed through policy changes and legislative action.[38] Vector, and environmental factors are closely interconnected with unhealthful behaviors and, therefore, understanding of their interaction with host factors is necessary before developing strategies for primary obesity prevention.

Home Setting

Primary prevention needs to begin with children. Children who become overweight are much more likely to be overweight or obese as adults. Food preferences formed in childhood are influenced mainly by parental food choice. These preferences may lead to habits that later require change.[39] Parents' nutrition knowledge and attitudes toward food can predict children's consumption of fruits, vegetables, and confectionery. Parental use of food as rewards may influence children's high preference for some food.[40] Time spent watching television is correlated with physical inactivity and increased food consumption. Television also exposes children to food advertising (e.g., fast food, snacks, and soft drinks).[41] In addition, parents' activity patterns can determine children's activity patterns; children whose parents are physically active have 6 times higher levels of physical activity compared with those whose parents are not physically active.[42] The importance of parental modeling of a physically active and healthful dietary lifestyle needs to be emphasized.[38] Thus, strategies for obesity prevention in the home should include basic educational counseling of parents on how to increase their children's physical activity, reduce sedentary behaviors, and encourage healthful food choices.[43]

School Setting

Schools, preschools, and after-school programs are important forums where a healthful environment can be created. Most randomized clinical trials for school-based interventions report a favorable impact on eating and physical activity behaviors, but they do not produce significant changes in body size or reduce obesity prevalence.[44] Fitzgibbon and colleagues[45] reported effectiveness of a culturally proficient dietary and physical activity program for preschool children that reduced subsequent increases in body fat. Making It Happen! School Nutrition Success Stories is a joint project of several governmental agencies in which innovative strategies were implemented to improve the nutritional quality of foods and beverages sold outside of federal meal programs in 32 schools.[46] These schools demonstrated that students would purchase healthful foods and beverages when given the opportunity.

Workplace Setting

Prevention in a workplace can reach a diverse adult population. Industrial or workplace settings can implement programs that teach or model healthful eating

■ ■ ■

TABLE 36-2   NATIONAL HEART, LUNG, AND BLOOD INSTITUTE DISEASE RISK CLASSIFICATION OF OVERWEIGHT AND OBESITY BY BODY MASS INDEX AND WAIST CIRCUMFERENCE

	CLASS	BODY MASS INDEX (kg/m²)	WAIST CIRCUMFERENCE	
			MEN: 102 cm (40 inches) OR LESS WOMEN: 88 cm (35 inches) OR LESS	MEN: MORE THAN 102 cm WOMEN: MORE THAN 88 cm
Underweight		Less than 18.5		
Normal		18.5-24.9		
Overweight		25.0-29.9	Increased	High
Obesity	I	30.0-34.9	High	Very high
	II	35.0-39.9	Very high	Very high
Extreme obesity	III	≥40	Extremely high	Extremely high

Disease risk for type 2 diabetes, hypertension, and cardiovascular disease.
Increased waist circumference also can be a marker for increased risk even in persons of normal weight.
NHLBI Obesity Education Initiative Expert Panel on the Identification Evaluation and Treatment of Overweight and Obesity: *Obes Res* 6(suppl 2):51S-209S, 1998.

patterns and various forms of physical activity. Employers can alter the environment to promote healthful behaviors. Studies using work-based interventions, especially centered in the cafeteria, showed mixed results with either no impact or significant effects on dietary intake and food sale indicators. However, not dissimilar to other studies, these approaches have had difficulty achieving a significant impact on BMI.[40]

Communities

Several community-based movements for public education and obesity prevention on a population-based level exist, e.g., creating walking trails, working with restaurants to increase the number of healthful food choices, and encouraging a healthful way of life among people of color (e.g., Sisters Together).[47] However, most community initiatives have not had a significant impact because of the competing interests of the food industry. Among the large-scale community intervention projects, the North Karelia project stands out for its success. North Karelia, a city in Finland, undertook a major community initiative to reduce the high prevalence of CVD in its population. Results showed a significant reduction in CVD risk but no reduction in BMI.[48]

Secondary Prevention

Secondary prevention requires that health care professionals engage in identification and assessment, recognize obesity as a chronic disorder, and address weight management. The Centers for Disease Control and Prevention reported that 58 percent of obese patients have never received weight loss counseling,[49] possibly because obesity often is not considered a serious medical condition. This lack of attention to weight also may reflect a bias or discomfort that the clinician feels about the obese patient[50] or a lack of knowledge about how to assist patients manage weight loss. Health care professionals receive limited education pertaining to nutrition and behavior change counseling and express discomfort managing these types of clinical situations.[51]

Clinical Evaluation

Clinical evaluation of the patient who is overweight or obese needs to include an assessment of the severity of overweight, presence of comorbid conditions (e.g., osteoarthritis, sleep apnea, or gallstones), and assessment of CVD risk factors (See Tables 36-1 and 36-2). This assessment includes a medical and weight history: How long have you been overweight? How many times have you lost and regained weight? Physical measurements include the conventional physical examination, plus height, weight, and waist circumference measurement. BMI and waist circumference should be used to estimate relative risk of disease compared with a normal-weight person.

Lifestyle Assessment

Asking a person to keep a diary of usual foods eaten and typical physical activity for 3 to 5 days provides an excellent source of information about usual behavior and also increases the person's awareness of his or her own behaviors. Questionnaires are available to assess eating behavior, such as the Connor Diet Habit Survey, which assesses the amount of dietary cholesterol and fat consumed, as well as other nutrients. This survey can be administered while the person is in the clinic and can be scored quickly.[52]

A website created by the federal government, *www.mypyramid.gov*, is an interactive site that can be used to individualize the former food pyramid guide for nutritional intake. The site provides an estimate of individual food intake needs based on age, gender, and physical activity level. An additional link geared toward children accesses a computer game showing how activity and food selections fit into the recommendations.[53] Wearing a pedometer to assess the usual number of steps taken in a day is a convenient method to assess usual physical activity, although it is limited to walking and thus does not measure other activities such as swimming or bicycling.

Intervention Opportunities

Weight loss is recommended for individuals with a BMI of 30 kg/m² or above. Weight loss also is recommended for those with a BMI of 25 to 29.9 kg/m² or a high waist circumference, especially if they have two or more comorbidities. The National Cholesterol Education Program recommends beginning therapeutic lifestyle changes—including weight control, nutrition management, and increased physical activity—if low-density lipoprotein (**LDL**) cholesterol is elevated.[31] Prevention of weight gain is needed in any individual with a BMI above 25 kg/m², even without comorbidities. Figure 36-8 depicts the algorithm to follow in the assessment and subsequent treatment decisions of an overweight or obese patient.[2]

The goals of intervening to promote weight loss are to improve health, reduce CVD risk, and improve quality of life and physical appearance. Current treatment options include dietary interventions, which are built on decreasing energy consumption, increasing energy expenditure through increased physical activity, pharmacotherapy, and surgery. Behavior modification needs to be included in all treatment options because drug and surgical therapies still require a change in eating and activity behaviors.[2,30]

The recommended initial weight loss goal is 10 percent of baseline weight, a weight loss that can be maintained for at least a year or longer. The rate of loss should be approximately 0.5 to 1 lb per week for the moderately obese and 1 to 2 lb per week in the severely obese. This loss can be accomplished by reducing the total daily calorie intake to 500 calories less than what is needed for metabolism, on an individual basis, yielding a weight reduction of 1 to 2 lb per week.

Mutual agreement on a plan of action for the short and long term will enhance the probability of a positive outcome. Providers need to emphasize the beneficial clinical health outcomes resulting from a 10 percent weight loss and assist each individual to develop a realistic goal for weight loss outcomes.[2,30] Frequent provider follow-up is imperative to assist the patient achieve weight loss goals. The CPT (Current Procedural Termi-

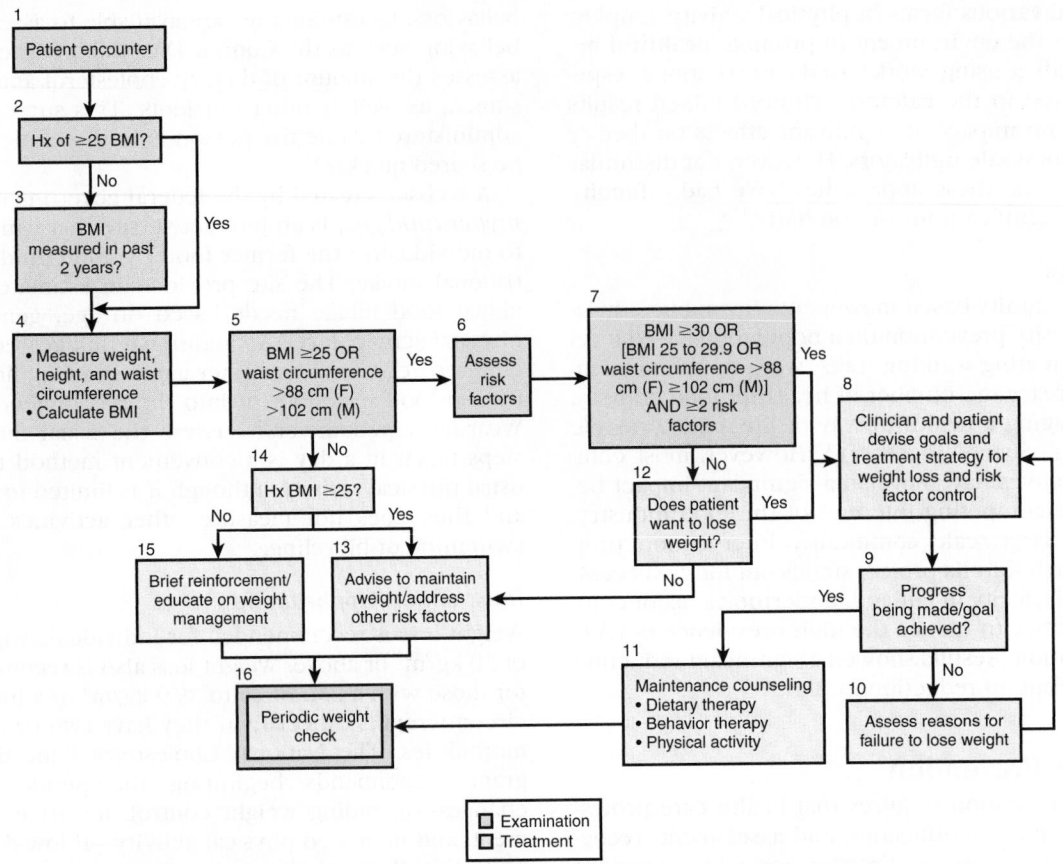

This algorithm applies only to the assessment for overweight and obesity and subsequent decisions based on that assessment. It does not include any initial overall assessment for cardiovascular risk factors or diseases that are indicated.

FIGURE 36-8 ■ Obesity treatment algorithm. *BMI,* Body mass index; *F,* female; *Hx,* history; *M,* male. (From NHLBI Obesity Education Initiative Expert Panel on the Identification Evaluation and Treatment of Overweight and Obesity: *Obes Res* 6[suppl 2]:51S-209S, 1998.)

nology) codes, including Unspecified Obesity (278.00) and Morbid Obesity (278.01), can be used for reimbursement for these visits; a new subcode that appears in the new ICD-9 for 2006 is Overweight (278.02).[54]

Patient Motivation

In addition to medical and lifestyle history and physical measures, nurses need to consider factors that may influence behavior change before recommending a weight loss program. These factors include attitude toward weight loss, prior treatment experiences, support system, willingness to initiate change, self-efficacy for achieving weight loss, time commitment, barriers to change, and financial issues. If an individual is not motivated to lose weight, a plan of weight gain prevention may be appropriate at this point. If the individual remains uninterested in treatment, management of coexisting risk factors should begin.[2]

Clinical Outcomes

A modest weight loss, defined as 5 percent of initial body weight, results in metabolic improvements and reduction in CHD risk factors.[30] Moderate weight loss has been linked to decreased need for glucose-lowering drugs and improvement in the comorbid conditions related to type 2 diabetes.[55] Reductions of 2.28 mg/dl in

serum cholesterol, 0.91 mg/dl in LDL cholesterol, and 1.54 mg/dl in triglycerides have been noted with as little as a 1-kg weight loss.

Behavior Modification

The goal of lifestyle or behavior therapy is to use behavioral strategies to facilitate and reinforce modification of lifestyle habits, specifically eating and physical activity habits. Although behavioral therapies can be delivered through group sessions or individual meetings, the group format is more economical and provides cohesiveness and support among group members. In one study, group therapy resulted in greater weight losses than individual therapy, even among participants who stated a preference for individual therapy.[56] Group sessions are held regularly, e.g., weekly initially with a gradual reduction in frequency to monthly or bimonthly; duration varies with programs.

Because significant behavior change is required for successful weight loss and maintenance and recidivism rates are high, clinical programs are increasing in duration and lasting up to 2 years, whereas commercially developed programs are available on a lifetime basis. Numerous clinical trials have validated the use of behavioral treatment for weight loss.[57] Behavioral weight loss studies from 1996 to 1999 were reviewed by Wing,[58] who found the average weight loss during treatment to be a little more than 10 percent with an average 18-month follow-up weight loss of 8.6 percent. More recent studies have yielded comparable results.[59-61] Table 36-3 shows the commonly used behavioral strategies to improve weight management.

Self-monitoring increases awareness of food consumption and physical activity through systematic observation and recording of target behaviors. Self-monitoring is performed commonly using food diaries or physical activity logs. By fostering an atmosphere of responsibility, this strategy can promote adherence to behavior, partly through self-reinforcement; the individual sees the progress being made and is motivated to continue to work toward the ultimate goal. The therapist or group leader provides written feedback to participants regarding their recorded behaviors in the weekly diaries. In a primary care setting, the practitioner can provide this feedback orally at each visit.

Burke and colleagues[62] used recent technological advances to study patterns of self-monitoring and found a significant relationship between self-monitoring and success in weight loss. Commercial and research-use only software programs are available today for self-monitoring with a personal digital assistant (PDA). These programs (Balance-Log) and a noncommercial program (DietMate Pro) include food and nutrient databases so the individual need only enter the foods eaten in the PDA, which eliminates the need to look up each food in a calorie counter booklet.[63]

Today, Internet-based programs also are available for one to self-monitor lifestyle habits (e.g., *www.ediets.com*). Additionally, studies have reported using the Internet for education alone, Internet combined with behavioral counseling, and supplementing the Internet with e-mail–delivered counseling.[64,65] The amount of weight loss achieved in these programs was related to how adherent the participants were to logging on to the website and submitting their diaries. Weight Watchers offers an Internet-based program *(www.weightwatchers.com/plan/www/online)* for individuals who are unable or who do not wish to attend the group sessions.

Dietary Intervention

An effective dietary strategy for weight loss is use of a moderate reduction in caloric intake (500 to 1000 kcal/d) along with intake of a macronutrient composition that reduces the risk of CVD (e.g., lower fat intake). This level of caloric deficit results in weight loss of approximately 1 to 2 lb/wk.[2,30] Three basic dietary interventions for weight loss include very low-calorie diets (VLCD), low-calorie diets, and low-fat diets. Despite the fact that VLCDs (less than 800 kcal/d) can result in a 15 to 20 percent weight loss in 4 months, this approach typically is not recommended because there is poor long-term weight loss maintenance, medical supervision is required, and nutritional deficits along with side effects such as hypokalemia, dehydration, and gallstones can occur. During rapid weight loss, the risk of developing gallstones is increased because of bile supersaturation and diminished gallbladder contractility.[66] Low-calorie diets (800 to 1500 kcal/d) typically result in an 8 percent loss of body weight and a decrease in abdominal fat at 6 months. Using a low-calories diet, weight loss at 1 year is no different from VLCD.

Low-fat diets (less than 25 percent of calories from fat) are effective for long-term maintenance and can result in greater reductions in triglyceride and LDL cholesterol levels.[2] A diet low in fat, saturated and *trans*-fat specifically, is of particular importance because of the increased risk of CHD associated with intake of these dietary fats.[67] However, besides restriction of fat consumption, calories also need to be restricted to achieve

■ ■ ■

TABLE 36-3   BEHAVIORAL STRATEGIES TO IMPROVE WEIGHT MANAGEMENT

STRATEGY	COMMENTS
Self-monitoring	Uses paper or electronic diary for monitoring diet (e.g., amounts and times of eating) and physical activity (e.g., frequency and duration)
	Example: interactive food pyramid *(www.mypyramidtracker.gov)*
Goal setting	Establishes short-term, achievable goals to allow for gradual improvement in eating habits and physical activity; has daily goals
Stimulus control	Pinpoints triggers for unhealthful eating and inadequate activity
	Develops strategies to sever connections to undesirable behaviors
Problem solving	Explores situations precluding a healthful lifestyle; identifies problem and possible solutions; tests and evaluates potential solutions
Relapse prevention	Provides awareness that "slips" will occur; can start over next day
	Uses methods for recovery in specific situations (e.g., vacations)
Cognitive restructuring	Identifies and replace thoughts that undermine weight control (e.g., negative thoughts, rationalization, and comparisons with others)
Stress management	Reduces mental stress to prevent inappropriate eating; uses coping strategies and relaxation techniques instead of eating to cope
Contingency management	Uses incentives (concrete or verbal) when a certain goal is achieved or to promote execution of desired behaviors
Social support	Identifies support system (e.g., family, friends, or colleagues) to enhance adherence to lifestyle change in several settings
Ongoing contact	Continues visits, telephone calls, and communication
	Refers to commercial or self-help programs (e.g., Weight Watchers)

From Klein S, Burke LE, Bray GA et al: *Circulation* 110:2952-2967, 2004.

weight loss.[68] In addition to restriction of fat, other dietary approaches, i.e., low-carbohydrate diets, are addressed under Fad Diet. Box 36-3 lists the components that need to be addressed when providing educational counseling for dietary modification.

Various commercial programs, including Jenny Craig, Weight Watchers, L.A. Weight Loss, and NutriSystem are popular methods for weight loss. Jenny Craig offers a comprehensive weight management plan emphasizing a low-fat, low-cholesterol, high-fiber diet.[69] In the Weight Watchers program, a POINTS plan is offered that assigns a point value to foods based on calories, fat grams, and fiber content; clients are assigned a point limit based on their weight. This program also offers the opportunity to attend weekly group meetings for social support and incorporates accountability at weigh-in.[70] L.A. Weight Loss uses customized meal plans based on personal preferences and individual one-on-one counseling sessions.[71] The NutriSystem Nourish meal plan features low-glycemic index foods and specific amounts of protein to help regulate blood sugar levels. Their meal plan necessitates that foods be purchased from NutriSystem.[72] The effectiveness of these treatments, however, is largely testimonial. A review of the existing literature on commercial programs found that weight losses were generally less than those seen in academically based settings.[73]

Physical Activity

Physical activity enhances weight loss through increased energy expenditure; however, physical activity alone has a minimal effect on achieving weight loss. Moderate-intensity physical activity (e.g., brisk walking) for 45 to 65 minutes 4 times per week for up to 1 year usually induces a weight loss of a few kilograms. The recommended minimal dose of physical activity for an overweight or obese individual is at least 30 minutes of moderate-intensity physical activity on most days of the week (i.e., at least 150 minutes of moderate intensity physical activity per week). Moderate intensity normally is defined as 40 to 59 percent of heart rate reserve (55 to 70 percent of maximal heart rate).[74] Jakicic and colleagues[75] reported that participants who accumulated less than 150 minutes per week of physical activity had a mean weight loss of 4.7 percent, whereas those who accumulated at least 200 minutes per week lost on average 13.6 percent of their body weight.

Physical activity is essential for weight maintenance after loss has been achieved. Subjects who reported exercising regularly maintained their weight losses significantly better than those who did not.[76] The recommended amount of physical activity for weight maintenance is approximately 2500 kcal/wk, which can be expended with moderate activity for approximately 60 to 75 minutes per day or with more vigorous activity for 30 minutes.[30] Box 36-4 addresses the strategies to promote long-term adherence to physical activity.

Tertiary Prevention

Tertiary prevention consists of reducing or eliminating long-term impairments and CVD risk factors that are associated with obesity, and facilitating adjustment to limitations that the condition has imposed. Therefore, this effort must focus on stabilization and prevention of further weight gain and adequate management of associated conditions such as hypertension and dyslipidemia. For the individual who is obese or overweight with several comorbid conditions and who has been unsuccessful in achieving weight loss through a behavioral management program that includes dietary modification and physical activity, adjunctive therapy may be indicated. Adjunctive therapy options are limited but include pharmacotherapy and surgical approaches.

Pharmacotherapy

Pharmacotherapy is indicated for patients with a BMI of 30 kg/m² or above or with a lower BMI (27 to 29.9 kg/m²) and comorbid conditions such as diabetes or hypertension. Drug therapy should always be considered adjunctive to comprehensive weight management, which

---

BOX 36-3 ■ ■ ■
THE EDUCATIONAL COMPONENTS OF A HEALTHFUL DIETARY APPROACH

- Learn energy densities of macronutrients (e.g., 9 calories/g of fat, 4 calories/g of carbohydrate, 4 calories/g of protein).
- Learn how to read nutrition labels to determine calorie content and food composition.
- Acquire new purchasing routines and a preference for low-calorie foods.
- Learn healthful cooking methods that avoid high-calorie ingredients (e.g., fats and oils).
- Avoid overconsumption of foods by reducing portion sizes.
- Maintain adequate water intake, and limit alcohol intake.
- Practice eating in social situations and ordering in restaurants.
- Maintain frequent contact with professional counselors to reinforce learning and development of new skills.

From NHLBI Obesity Education Initiative Expert Panel on the Identification Evaluation and Treatment of Overweight and Obesity: *Obes Res* 6(suppl 2):51S-209S, 1998.

BOX 36-4 ■ ■ ■
STRATEGIES TO PROMOTE ADHERENCE TO PHYSICAL ACTIVITY

- Assess readiness to adopt a physical activity program.
- Use five *A*'s (assess, advise, agree, assist, arrange).
- Provide written exercise prescription.
- Use physical activity logs and provide feedback.
- Use pedometers to provide feedback on progress in reaching activity goals.
- Multiple short bouts (e.g., two 15-minute bouts or three 10-minute bouts a day).
- Use home exercise equipment (e.g., treadmill, put equipment in front of the television to help reduce boredom often associated with this type of home activity).
- When home equipment is not available and weather does not permit outdoor activity, use a straight chair for balance and walk in place. Encourage use of indoor setting in inclement weather, e.g., malls.
- Partner with a friend in an exercise program to encourage and support each other.

Information from Jakicic JM, Otto AD: *Psychiatr Clin North Am* 28:141-150, 2005; Jacobson DM, Strohecker L, Compton MT et al: *Am J Prev Med* 29:158-162, 2005; and Jakicic JM, Winters C, Lang W et al: *JAMA* 282:1554-1560, 1999.

includes behavior modification, counseling for dietary change, and development of regular physical activity.[30] The clinician needs to be mindful that the patient who requires pharmacotherapy for the management of weight is likely to be taking other prescriptive medications. This factor increases the complexity of the medication regimen, which may affect adherence, particularly when one considers the coordination of timing for medication-taking that is required when a drug such as orlistat is added.[30] A limited number of medications are approved by the Food and Drug Administration for treating obesity. Table 36-4 includes a summary of the evidence for clinical efficacy of these agents and provides information on their side effects and their effects on the cardiovascular system.

Dietary Supplements and Herbal Products

Millions of Americans use dietary supplements daily. Although the Food and Drug Administration regulates supplements, it does not oversee manufacture of these agents, and does not require manufacturers to provide evidence of safety and efficacy before they market the supplements. Table 36-5 provides a systematic review[77] of the latest evidence for the use of dietary supplements and herbal products that have been studied; however, it should be noted that the reported studies had small samples and were not able to demonstrate efficacy or safety in their short-term trials.

Bariatric Surgery

For individuals who are extremely obese (BMI of 35 to 39.9 kg/m² and have one or more severe obesity-related comorbidities such as type 2 diabetes, heart failure, and obstructive sleep apnea) or for those whose BMI exceeds 40 kg/m², surgical therapy is an approved consideration.[2,30] The Swedish Obese Subjects (SOS) study reported 2-year ($n = 4047$) and 10-year ($n = 1703$) follow-up rates for their participants who underwent gastric surgery or were matched contemporaneously for conventional nonsurgical treatment.[78] At 2 and 10 years, the control group had gained 0.1 and 1.6 percent, respectively, whereas the surgery group had lost 23.4 and 16.1 percent, respectively, of their weight. Significant differences occurred in the incidence rates of diabetes, hypertriglyceridemia, and hyperuricemia; however, there were no differences in the rates of hypercholesterolemia and hypertension. Table 36-6 lists the five common weight-loss surgeries and the approximate initial weight loss associated with each procedure.[66]

Fad Diets

Even though many fad diets lack credibility, the use of these popular diets is highly prevalent across all groups of society. One study that compared four popular diets—the Atkins, Ornish, Weight Watchers, and Zone diets—found no significant difference between them.

■ ■ ■

TABLE 36-4 PHARMACOTHERAPY FOR WEIGHT LOSS

GENERIC DRUG NAME (ACTION)	CLINICAL EFFICACY	SIDE EFFECTS	EFFECTS ON CARDIOVASCULAR SYSTEM
Sibutramine (Blocks reuptake of norepinephrine and dopamine)	Based on three high-quality systematic reviews of 29 trials, average weight loss was 4.3 kg more (4.6%) compared with placebo; also maintained more weight loss.	Besides effects on BP and HR, drug may cause insomnia, dry mouth, nausea and constipation.	Increases systolic and diastolic BP and HR. Improves serum total cholesterol, HDL-C, LDL-C, and triglyceride levels related to magnitude of weight loss.
Orlistat (Binds to intestinal lipases and thus blocks the digestion and absorption of dietary fat)	Based on two reviews, mean weight loss was 2.8 to 4.5 kg more than placebo group. Weight regain occurred when therapy stopped. Adding orlistat after weight loss helps maintain loss.	Fifteen percent to 30% of patients had gastrointestinal effects, including oily stools or oily spotting, fecal urgency, fecal incontinence, reduced levels of fat-soluble vitamins (A, D, and E). Drug may interfere with absorption of lipophilic drugs; therefore, one needs to take orlistat at least 2 hours before or after lipophilic drugs and needs to follow plasma concentration to ensure correct dosage.	Improves all CVD risk factors via weight loss action, including BP and insulin sensitivity. Evidence that LDL-C is lowered independent of weight loss, possibly is due to blocked absorption of dietary cholesterol and triglycerides. Is less effective in reducing triglycerides because of increased absorption of energy being derived from carbohydrates.
Phentermine (Stimulates release of norepinephrine and dopamine)	Not FDA approved for long-term use. Only one review of six trials. Overall, those taking phentermine lost 0.6 to 6.0 kg more than the placebo group.	Dry mouth, constipation, and insomnia are side effects.	Drug may increase BP and HR, but these effects are uncommon in presence of adequate weight loss.

BP, Blood pressure; CVD, cardiovascular disease; FDA, Food and Drug Administration; HDL-C, high-density lipoprotein cholesterol; HR, heart rate; LDL-C, low-density lipoprotein cholesterol.

Data from Klein S, Burke LE, Bray GA et al: *Circulation* 110:2952-2967, 2004; Arterburn DE, Crane PK, Veenstra DL: *Arch Intern Med* 164:994-1003, 2004; McTigue KM, Harris R, Hemphill B et al: *Ann Intern Med* 139:933-949, 2003; Padwal R, Li SK, Lau DC: *Int J Obes* 27:1437-1446, 2003; Jain A: *BMJ* 1-62, 2004; and Haddock CK, Poston WS, Dill PL et al: *Int J Obes* 26:262-273, 2002.

■ ■ ■

TABLE 36-5 DIETARY SUPPLEMENTS FOR WEIGHT LOSS

DIETARY SUPPLEMENT (ACTION)	CLINICAL EFFICACY	SIDE EFFECTS
Conjugated linoleic acid (Inhibits lipoprotein lipase and thus breaks down fat for storage and enhances breakdown of stored fat)	No changes in weight or body mass index found in three trials; reported significant decreases in waist circumference, body fat mass, and percent body fat.	Mild gastrointestinal symptoms
Ephedra, ephedrine, ma huang	Meta-analysis of 22 studies that used ephedrine alone or with caffeine or herbs reported weight loss of 0.6 to 1.0 kg/mo, compared with placebo, 5% to 11% weight loss at 4 months.	Risk for adverse event is increased with ephedra, including high blood pressure, palpitations, and autonomic, psychiatric, and gastrointestinal symptoms. Even though it is effective for weight loss, it is not considered safe. Over-the-counter sale of ephedra-containing products has been banned.
Chitosan (Claims to inhibit fat absorption)	Two studies reported conflicting results for weight loss.	None known at present.
Pyruvate (Claims to increase fat metabolism)	Five clinical trials showed weight loss of 0.05 to 1.1 kg short-term (3 weeks) to 2.5 kg at 6 weeks.	Gastrointestinal symptoms may occur at higher doses.

Data from Lenz TL, Hamilton WR: *J Am Pharm Assoc (Wash DC)* 44:59-67, 2004; and Shekelle PG, Hardy ML, Morton SC et al: *JAMA* 289:1537-1545, 2003.

■ ■ ■

TABLE 36-6 EXPECTED WEIGHT LOSS FROM FOUR COMMONLY PERFORMED GASTRIC SURGERY PROCEDURES

PROCEDURE	APPROXIMATE 2-YEAR WEIGHT LOSS (% OF INITIAL BODY WEIGHT)
Gastric banding	20 to 35
Gastroplasty	20 to 25
Gastric bypass	25 to 30
Biliopancreatic diversion ± duodenal switch	35 to 40

From Klein S, Wadden T, Sugerman HJ: *Gastroenterology* 123:882-932, 2002.

What mattered was self-reported adherence to the diet. The four diets lowered the ratio of LDL cholesterol to HDL cholesterol ratio by approximately 10 percent without a significant effect on blood pressure or glucose at 1 year. Each of the diets resulted in modest weight loss and reduction in CHD risk, with greater adherence associated with greater weight loss and risk reduction. Adherence to the diets ranged from 50 percent for the Ornish diet, and 53 percent for Atkins to 65 percent for Weight Watchers and the Zone diet.[79] A randomized trial evaluating a low-carbohydrate diet compared with a standard, low-calorie, low-fat diet found that individuals assigned to the low-carbohydrate diet lost more weight than those on the standard diet at 3 and 6 months, but there was no significant difference between the two groups at 1 year.[80]

Why Some Persons Lose Weight on Their Own

A survey of 155 adults with a history of prior weight loss treatment found that 92 percent reported that losing weight "on their own" was their favorite approach.[81] Reasons given for why this was their favorite strategy were that all foods were permitted, it was realistic, and it gave them a sense of control and achievement. Although nearly one-third of those seeking weight loss report wanting quick results, a smaller percent report

that they are more satisfied if the program, such as doing it on their own, is feasible to do and to maintain. Motivation is an obvious consideration for one to lose weight without the support of a structured program; however, the literature is inconsistent regarding the importance of pretreatment motivation and weight loss.[82]

Ways to Maintain Behavioral Changes

An important principle of behavior change is setting a realistic goal and then striving to reach this goal through small incremental changes in behavior. Self-monitoring one's eating and activity behaviors is a highly effective strategy initially and for the long term. Ongoing contact and reinforcement to individuals as they try to manage this chronic disorder are essential for long-term adherence. Enrollment in commercial programs such as Weight Watchers could augment periodic clinic visits.

Data from the National Weight Control Registry of individuals who were successful at losing and maintaining the weight loss indicate that the most common behaviors reported included eating breakfast every day, following an eating plan that was low in fat and high in carbohydrates, monitoring eating behaviors and body weight regularly, and engaging in high levels of physical activity.[83]

SUMMARY

Today obesity is recognized as a chronic disorder and a major public health problem. Moreover, obesity is an independent risk factor for CVD. Treatment goals are to reduce body weight by 5 to 10 percent and reduce obesity-related risk factors. Evidence-based guidelines are available for the identification and treatment of obesity, as is an ever-growing body of literature on the efficacy of various treatment approaches.

During a routine examination, medical advice to lose weight has a significant impact on subsequent weight loss. Compared with individuals who had not received advice, women who had been advised to lose weight were approximately 6 times more likely to report attempting to lose weight, and men were about 10 times more likely to try to lose weight.[84]

Health care professionals need to be aware of the message they are sending to patients by their example. The Physicians' Health study recently reported that among male physicians in the United States, 44 percent are overweight and 6 percent are obese.[85] Investigators of the Nurses' Health Study II examined weight change in the cohort between 1993 and 2001 and found that the average weight gain was 11 lb, but 10 percent of the women gained more than 30 lb.[86]

Practitioners need to become informed about obesity, which has implications for the treatment and management of most acute and chronic disorders. Nurses are in an ideal position to take the lead in addressing this major health problem by educating themselves and their fellow clinicians about this chronic disorder and in serving as role models. It is much easier for the patient to be able to effect change when there is a perception that the provider lives the message as well.

REFERENCES

1. National Heart, Lung, and Blood Institute: *Guidelines on overweight and obesity: electronic textbook*. Retrieved November 28, 2005 from www.nhlbi.nih.gov/guidelines/obesity/e_txbk/index.htm
2. NHLBI Obesity Education Initiative Expert Panel on the Identification Evaluation and Treatment of Overweight and Obesity: Clinical guidelines on the identification, evaluation, and treatment of overweight and obesity in adults: the evidence report, *Obes Res* 6(suppl 2):51S-209S, 1998.
3. World Health Organization: *Preventing and managing the global epidemic of obesity: report of the World Health Organization Consultation of Obesity*, Geneva, 1997, The Organization.
4. World Health Organization: Global strategy on diet, physical activity and health.Retrieved December 30, 2006, from www.who.int/dietphysicalactivity/publications/facts/obesity/en/
5. Hedley AA, Ogden CL, Johnson CL et al: Prevalence of overweight and obesity among US children, adolescents, and adults, 1999-2002, *JAMA* 291:2847-2850, 2004.
6. Kopelman PG: Obesity as a medical problem, *Nature* 404:635-643, 2000.
7. Aronne LJ: Classification of obesity and assessment of obesity-related health risks, *Obes Res* 10:105S-115S, 2002.
8. Peeters A, Barendregt JJ, Willekens F et al: Obesity in adulthood and its consequences for life expectancy: a life-table analysis, *Ann Intern Med* 138:24-32, 2003.
9. Loos RJF, Bouchard C: Obesity: is it a genetic disorder? *J Intern Med* 254:401-425, 2003.
10. Lee JH, Reed DR, Price RA: Familial risk ratios for extreme obesity: implications for mapping human obesity genes, *Int J Obes* 21:935-940, 1997.
11. Bray GA, Bouchard C: *Handbook of obesity: etiology and pathophysiology*, ed 2, New York, 2004, Marcel Dekker.
12. Salsberry PJ, Reagan PB: Dynamics of early childhood overweight, *Pediatrics* 116:1329-1338, 2005.
13. Centers for Disease Control and Prevention: Summary health statistics for U.S. adults: National Health Interview Survey, 2004. Retrieved May 30, 2005, from http://www.cdc.gov/nchs/data/series/sr_10/sr10_228.pdf.
14. York DA, Rossner S, Caterson I et al: Prevention Conference VII: obesity, a worldwide epidemic related to heart disease and stroke: Group I—worldwide demographics of obesity, *Circulation* 110:e463-e470, 2004.
15. Quesebberry CJ, Caan B, Jacobson A: Obesity, health services use, and health care costs among members of a health maintenance organization, *Arch Intern Med* 158:466-472, 1998.
16. Calle EE, Thun MJ, Petrelli JM et al: Body-mass index and mortality in a prospective cohort of US adults, *N Engl J Med* 341:1097-1105, 1999.
17. Leibowitz SF, Hoebel BG: Behavioral neuroscience and obesity. In Bray GA, Bouchard C, editors: *Handbook of obesity: etiology and pathophysiology*, ed 2, New York, 2004, Marcel Dekker.
18. Munro S, Thomas KL, Abu-Shaar M: Molecular characterization of a peripheral receptor for cannabinoids, *Nature* 365:61-65, 1993.
19. Devane WA, Hanus L, Breuer A et al: Isolation and structure of a brain constituent that binds to the cannabinoid receptor, *Science* 258:1946-1949, 1992.
20. Van Gaal LF, Rissanen AM, Scheen AJ et al: Effects of the cannabinoid-1 receptor blocker rimonabant on weight reduction and cardiovascular risk factors in overweight patients: 1-year experience from the RIO-Europe study, *Lancet* 365:1389-1397, 2005.
21. Despres J-P, Golay A, Sjostrom L et al: Effects of rimonabant on metabolic risk factors in overweight patients with dyslipidemia, *N Engl J Med* 353:2121-2134, 2005.
22. Carai MA, Colombo G, Gessa GL: Rimonabant: the first therapeutically relevant cannabinoid antagonist, *Life Sciences* 77:2339-2350, 2005.
23. Cota D, Marsicano G, Lutz B et al: Endogenous cannabinoid system as a modulator of food intake, *Int J Obes* 27:289-301, 2003.
24. Clement K, Ferre P: Genetics and the pathophysiology of obesity, *Pediatr Res* 53:721-725, 2003.
25. Ueno H, Yamaguchi H, Kangawa K et al: Ghrelin: a gastric peptide that regulates food intake and energy homeostasis, *Regul Pept* 126:11-19, 2005.
26. Hayman LL, Hughes S: Obesity: focus on prevention and policy, *J Cardiovasc Nurs* 19:217-218, 2004.
27. Caballero B: Obesity prevention in children: opportunities and challenges, *Int J Obes* 28(suppl 3):S90-S95, 2004.
28. Rice T, Perusse L, Bouchard C et al: Familial aggregation of body mass index and subcutaneous fat measures in the longitudinal Quebec family study, *Genet Epidemiol* 16:316-334, 1999.
29. Caterson I, Hubbard V, Bray G et al: Obesity, a worldwide epidemic related heart disease and stroke: Group III—worldwide comorbidities of obesity, *Circulation* 110:e476-e483, 2004.
30. Klein S, Burke LE, Bray GA et al: Clinical implications of obesity with specific focus on cardiovascular disease: a statement for professionals from the American Heart Association Council on Nutrition, Physical Activity, and Metabolism, *Circulation* 110:2952-2967, 2004.
31. National Cholesterol Education Program Expert Panel on Detection Evaluation and Treatment of High Blood Cholesterol in Adults (Adult Treatment Panel III): Third report of the National Cholesterol Education Program (NCEP) Expert Panel on Detection, Evaluation, and Treatment of High Blood Cholesterol in Adults (Adult Treatment Panel III) final report, *Circulation* 106:3143-3421, 2002.
32. Kip KE, Marroquin OC, Kelley DE et al: Clinical importance of obesity versus the metabolic syndrome in cardiovascular risk in women: a report from the Women's Ischemia Syndrome Evaluation (WISE) study, *Circulation* 109:706-713, 2004.
33. Prineas RJ, Folsom AR, Kaye SA: Central adiposity and increased risk of coronary artery disease mortality in older women, *Ann Epidemiol* 3:35-41, 1993.
34. Rutter MK, Meigs JB, Sullivan LM et al: C-reactive protein, the metabolic syndrome, and prediction of cardiovascular events in the Framingham Offspring Study, *Circulation* 110:380-385, 2004.
35. Garrett K, Lauer K, Christopher BA: The effects of obesity on the cardiopulmonary system: implications for critical care nursing, *Prog Cardiovasc Nurs* 19:155-161, 2004.
36. Pi-Sunyer FX: Obesity: criteria and classification, *Proc Nutr Soc* 59:505-509, 2000.
37. Yusuf S, Hawken S, Ounpuu S et al: Obesity and the risk of myocardial infarction in 27000 participants from 52 countries: a case-control study, *Lancet* 366:1640-1649, 2005.
38. Mullis RM, Blair SN, Aronne LJ et al: Prevention Conference VII: obesity, a worldwide epidemic related to heart disease and stroke: Group IV—prevention/treatment, *Circulation* 110:e484-e488, 2004.

39. Skidmore PM, Yarnell JW: The obesity epidemic: prospects for prevention, *QJM* 97:817-825, 2004.
40. Swinburn BA, Caterson I, Seidell JC et al: Diet, nutrition and the prevention of excess weight gain and obesity, *Public Health Nutr* 7:123-146, 2004.
41. Flodmark CE, Lissau I, Moreno LA et al: New insights into the field of children and adolescents' obesity: the European perspective, *Int J Obes Relat Metab Disord* 28:1189-1196, 2004.
42. Fitzgibbon ML, Stolley MR, Dyer AR et al: A community-based obesity prevention program for minority children: rationale and study design for Hip-Hop to Health Jr, *Prev Med* 34:289-297, 2002.
43. Dietz WH, Robinson TN: Clinical practice: overweight children and adolescents, *N Engl J Med* 352:2100-2109, 2005.
44. Sahota P, Rudolf MC, Dixey R et al: Randomised controlled trial of primary school based intervention to reduce risk factors for obesity, *BMJ* 323:1029-1032, 2001.
45. Fitzgibbon ML, Stolley MR, Schiffer L: Two-year follow-up results for Hip-Hop to Health Jr: a randomized controlled trial for overweight prevention in preschool minority children, *J Pediatr* 146:618-625, 2005.
46. National Center for Chronic Disease Prevention and Health Promotion: Making it happen: school nutrition success stories. In *Healthy Youth!* Silver Spring, Md, 2005, Centers for Disease Control and Prevention.
47. Sisters Together Coalition. American Obesity Association- Community Programs. Retrieved December 27, 2006 www.hsph.harvard.edu/sisterstogether/
48. Pietinen P, Nissinen A, Vartiainen E et al: Dietary changes in the North Karelia Project (1972-1982), *Prev Med* 17:183-193, 1988.
49. Centers for Disease Control and Prevention, National Center for Chronic Disease Prevention and Health Promotion, Physical Activity and Good Nutrition: *Essential elements to prevent chronic disease and obesity: at a glance 2001*, [Atlanta], 2001, Centers for Disease Control and Prevention.
50. Schwartz MB, Chambliss HO, Brownell KD et al: Weight bias among health professionals specializing in obesity, *Obes Res* 11:1033-1039, 2003.
51. Burke L, Fair J: Promoting prevention: skills sets and attributes of health care providers who deliver behavioral intervention, *J Cardiovasc Nurs* 18:256-266, 2003.
52. Burke LE, Dunbar-Jacob J, Orchard TJ et al: Improving adherence to a cholesterol-lowering diet: a behavioral intervention study, *Patient Educ Couns* 57:134-142, 2005.
53. US Department of Agriculture: *Steps to a healthier you*. Retrieved November 23, 2005, from www.mypyramid.gov
54. American Medical Association: *International classification of diseases, 9th revision, clinical modification: hospital ICD-9-CM, 2005*, Chicago, 2004, AMA Press.
55. Vidal J: Updated review on the benefits of weight loss, *Int J Obes* 26:S25-S28, 2002.
56. Renjilian DA, Perri MG, Nezu AM et al: Individual versus group therapy for obesity: effects of matching participants to their treatment preferences, *J Consult Clin Psychol* 69:717-721, 2001.
57. Foster GD, Makris AP, Bailer BA: Behavioral treatment of obesity, *Am J Clin Nutr* 82(suppl):230S-235S, 2005.
58. Wing RR: Behavioral weight control. In Wadden T, Stunkard AJ, editors: *Handbook of obesity treatment*, New York, 2002, Guilford.
59. Ramirez EM, Rosen JC: A comparison of weight control and weight control plus body image therapy for obese men and women, *J Consult Clin Psychol* 69:440-446, 2001.
60. Melin I, Karlström B, Lappalainen R et al: A programme of behaviour modification and nutrition counseling in the treatment of obesity: a randomised 2-y clinical trial, *Int J Obes* 27:1127-1135, 2003.
61. Jeffery RW, Wing RR, Sherwood NE et al: Physical activity and weight loss: does prescribing higher physical activity goals improve outcome? *Am J Clin Nutr* 78:684-689, 2003.
62. Burke LE, Sereika S, Choo J et al: Ancillary study to the PREFER trial: a descriptive study of participants' patterns of self-monitoring—rationale, design and preliminary experiences, *Contemp Clin Trials* 27:23-33, 2006.
63. Burke LE, Warziski M, Starrett T et al: Self-monitoring dietary intake: current and future practices—report of a pilot study using an electronic diary, *J Ren Nutr* 15:281-290, 2005.
64. Tate DF, Wing RR, Winett RA: Using Internet technology to deliver a behavioral weight loss program, *JAMA* 285:1172-1177, 2001.
65. Tate DF, Jackvony EH, Wing RR: Effects of Internet behavioral counseling on weight loss in adults at risk for type 2 diabetes: a randomized trial, *JAMA* 289:1833-1836, 2003.
66. Klein S, Wadden T, Sugerman HJ: AGA technical review on obesity, *Gastroenterology* 123:882-932, 2002.
67. Oh K, Hu FB, Manson JE et al: Dietary fat intake and risk of coronary heart disease in women: 20 years of follow-up of the nurses' health study, *Am J Epidemiol* 161:672-679, 2005.
68. Harvey-Berino J: The efficacy of dietary fat vs total energy restriction for weight loss, *Obes Res* 6:202-207, 1998.
69. Jenny Craig: [Title]. Retrieved December 5, 2005 from www.jennycraig.com
70. Weight Watchers: *Your lifestyle, your choice*. Retrieved December 5, 2005 from www.weightwatchers.com/plan/turnaround/index.aspx
71. LA Weight Loss:*The LA Plan*. Retrieved December 5, 2005, from www.laweightlosscenters/LAplan.aspx.com
72. NutriSystem: *NutriSystem® Nourish™Programs*. Retrieved December 5, 2005 from www.nutrisystem.com/shop/main.cfm?action=catalog/displaydefault
73. Womble LG, Wang SS, Wadden TA: Commercial and self-help weight loss programs. In Wadden T, Stunkard AJ, editors: *Handbook of obesity treatment*, New York, 2002, Guilford Press.
74. Jakicic JM, Otto AD: Physical activity recommendations in the treatment of obesity, *Psychiatr Clin North Am* 28:141-150, 2005.
75. Jakicic JM, Marcus BH, Gallagher KI et al: Effect of exercise duration and intensity on weight loss in overweight, sedentary women, *JAMA* 290:1323-1330, 2003.
76. Wing RR, Hill JO: Successful weight loss maintenance, *Annu Rev Nutr* 21:323-341, 2001.
77. Lenz TL, Hamilton WR: Supplemental products used for weight loss, *J Am Pharm Assoc (Wash DC)* 44:59-67, 2004.
78. Sjostrom L, Lindroos A, Peltonen M et al: Lifestyle, diabetes, and cardiovascular risk factors 10 years after bariatric surgery, *N Engl J Med* 351:2683-2753, 2004.
79. Dansinger ML, Gleason JA, Griffith JL et al: Comparison of the Atkins, Ornish, Weight Watchers, and Zone diets for weight loss and heart disease risk reduction: a randomized trial, *JAMA* 293:43-53, 2005.
80. Foster GD, Wyatt HR, Hill JO et al: A randomized trial of a low-carbohydrate diet for obesity, *N Engl J Med* 348:2082-2090, 2003.
81. Burke LE, Steenkiste A, Music E et al: A descriptive study of individuals' past experiences with weight loss treatment, *Ann Behav Med* (under review).
82. Teixeira PJ, Palmeira AL, Branco TL et al: Who will lose weight? a reexamination of predictors of weight loss in women, *Int J Behav Nutr Phys Act* 1:12, 2004.
83. Wyatt HR, Grunwald GK, Mosca CL et al: Long-term weight loss and breakfast in subjects in the National Weight Control Registry, *Obes Res* 10:78-82, 2002.
84. Bish CL, Blanck HM, Serdula MK et al: Diet and physical activity behaviors among Americans trying to lose weight: 2000 Behavioral Risk Factor Surveillance System, *Obes Res* 13:596-607, 2005.
85. Ajani UA, Lotufo PA, Gaziano JM et al: Body mass index and mortality among US male physicians, *Ann Epidemiol* 14:731-739, 2004.
86. Field AE, Manson JE, Taylor CB et al: Association of weight change, weight control practices, and weight cycling among women in the Nurses' Health Study II, *Int J Obes* 28:1134-1142, 2004.

■ ■ ■ c h a p t e r **37**

Insulin Resistance, Diabetes, and Cardiovascular Disease

Cindy Lamendola

CHAPTER ABBREVIATIONS

ADMIT Arterial Disease Multiple Intervention Trial

BMI body mass index

CAD coronary artery disease

CARE Cholesterol and Recurrent Events (trial)

CHD coronary heart disease

CVD cardiovascular disease

DAIS Diabetes Atherosclerosis Intervention Study

DCCT Diabetes Control and Complications Trial

EGIR European Group for the Study of Insulin Resistance

FFA free fatty acid

GLUT-4 an insulin-dependent glucose transporter

HDL high-density lipoprotein

HOT Hypertension Optimal Treatment (trial)

HPS Heart Protection Study

LDL low-density lipoprotein

MI myocardial infarction

MRFIT Multiple Risk Factor Intervention Trial

NCEP ATP III National Cholesterol Education Program Adult Treatment Panel III

NHANES National Health and Nutritional Examination Survey

PPAR peroxisome proliferator-activated receptor

PPS Paris Prospective Study

SSPG steady-state plasma glucose

UKPDS United Kingdom Prospective Diabetes Study

VA-HIT Veterans Affairs High-Density Lipoprotein Cholesterol Intervention Trial

VLDL *very low-density lipoprotein*

WHO World Health Organization

EPIDEMIOLOGY OF INSULIN RESISTANCE

Insulin action is quantified as the ability of insulin to take up glucose by muscle. Decreased tissue sensitivity to the action of insulin leads to a compensatory increase in insulin secretion, resulting in hyperinsulinemia to maintain glucose homeostasis. Resistance to insulin-stimulated glucose uptake varies widely from person to person but is associated closely within families. Insulin resistance and hyperinsulinemia play a significant role in the development of several clinical syndromes and diseases.[1-3]

There is wide individual variability in insulin-mediated glucose disposal. Figure 37-1 shows the range of insulin sensitivity in 490 healthy nondiabetic volun-

teers. Insulin sensitivity was determined by a modification of the insulin suppression test, described in Box 37-1. The higher the level of the steady-state plasma glucose (**SSPG**), the more insulin resistant the subject. As seen in Figure 37-1, there is approximately sixfold to eightfold variability in insulin-mediated glucose disposal among individuals.

Compensatory hyperinsulinemia resulting from insulin resistance may delay or prevent type 2 diabetes in most persons with insulin resistance, but it is not without consequences. The cluster of abnormalities associated with insulin resistance and investigated over the past 30 years, includes some degree of glucose intolerance, atherogenic dyslipidemia (increased triglyceride and low high-density lipoprotein [**HDL**] cholesterol levels), hypertension, hyperuricemia, endothelial dysfunction, increased prothrombotic state, and increased inflammatory markers (Figure 37-2).[1,3]

These abnormalities, when clustered together in an insulin-resistant person, are referred to by several names, insulin resistance syndrome and metabolic syndrome being the two most common.[3] It has been generally accepted that the clinical consequences of the abnormalities associated with this syndrome increase the risk for type 2 diabetes, cardiovascular disease (**CVD**), or both. Continuing research in this field has expanded the list of clinical syndromes associated with insulin resistance and hyperinsulinemia (Figure 37-3) to include polycystic ovary syndrome, nonalcoholic fatty liver disease, and possibly certain forms of cancer and sleep apnea.[3-5] This chapter specifically discusses insulin resistance and its relationship to CVD and type 2 diabetes.

Identification Criteria

In 1988, Reaven[1] designated the clustering of abnormalities associated with insulin resistance and compensatory hyperinsulinemia as syndrome X. The original clustering of abnormalities associated with insulin resistance has been referred to by several different names over the years but most frequently is described as the metabolic syndrome or the insulin resistance syndrome. Because of the concern for increased risk of poor clinical outcomes, especially CVD, guidelines have been written for identifying these individuals. The World Health Organization (**WHO**) in 1998 was one of the first groups to establish guidelines for identifying persons at risk for this clustering of abnormalities. WHO researchers referred to it as the metabolic syndrome, recognizing CVD as an outcome, and insulin resistance as a required component of the criteria.[6,7] In 1999, the European Group for

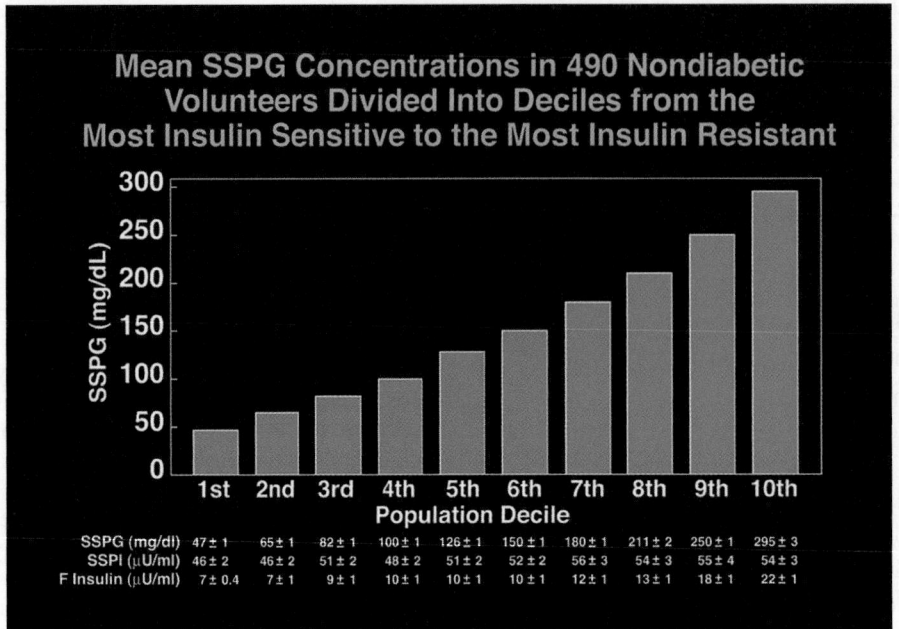

FIGURE 37-1 ■ Mean steady-state plasma glucose concentrations in 490 nondiabetic volunteers divided into deciles from the most insulin sensitive to the most insulin resistant. (From Yeni-Komshian H, Carantoni M, Abbasi F et al: *Diabetes Care* 23:171-175, 2000.) *SSPG,* Steady-state plasma glucose; *SSPI,* steady-state plasma insulin.

the Study of Insulin Resistance (**EGIR**) developed criteria to define the syndrome, which they named insulin resistance syndrome, with insulin resistance as the central feature.[8] In 2001, the National Cholesterol Education Program Adult Treatment Panel III (**NCEP ATP III**)[9] recognized the CVD risk associated with this clustering of abnormalities and called it metabolic syndrome. Unlike the WHO or EGIR, who agreed that insulin resistance was the underlying cause of this syndrome, the authors

of the NCEP ATP III reconvened to discuss management of this syndrome and felt there were three theories of underlying causes as components of what they referred to as the metabolic syndrome: obesity and disorders of adipose tissue, insulin resistance, and a constellation of independent factors that may mediate other components of the syndrome.[10,11]

Recently, the American Association of Clinical Endocrinologists and the American College of Endocrinology

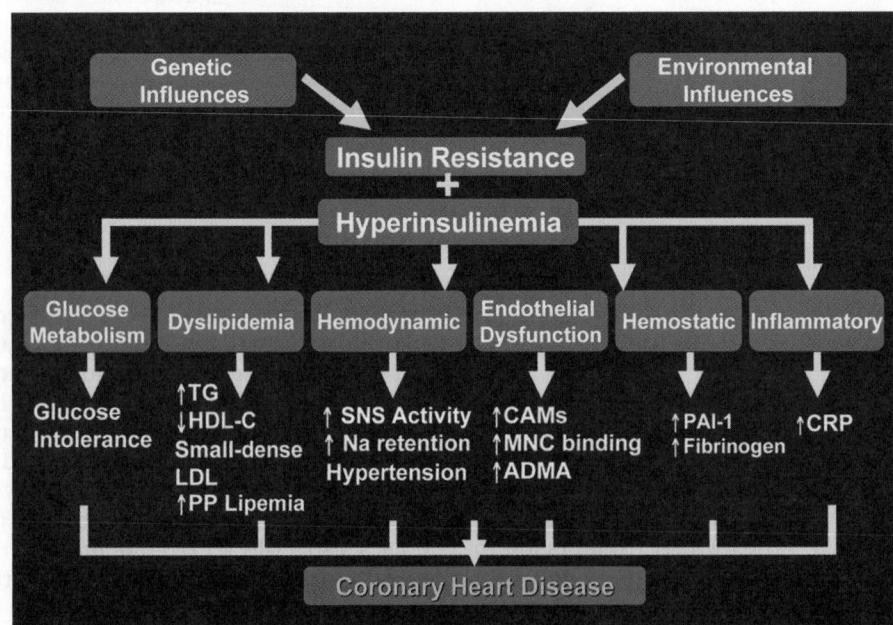

FIGURE 37-2 ■ Proposed role of insulin resistance and hyperinsulinemia in coronary heart disease. (From Reaven G: *Physiol Rev* 75:473-486, 1995.) *ADMA,* Asymmetric dimethylarginine; *CAM,* cellular adhesion molecules; *CRP,* C-reactive protein; *HDL-C,* high-density lipoprotein cholesterol; *LDL,* low-density lipoprotein; *MNC,* mononuclear cell; *Na,* sodium; *PAI-1,* plasminogen activator inhibitor-1; *PP,* postprandial; *SNS,* sympathetic nervous system; *TG,* triglycerides.

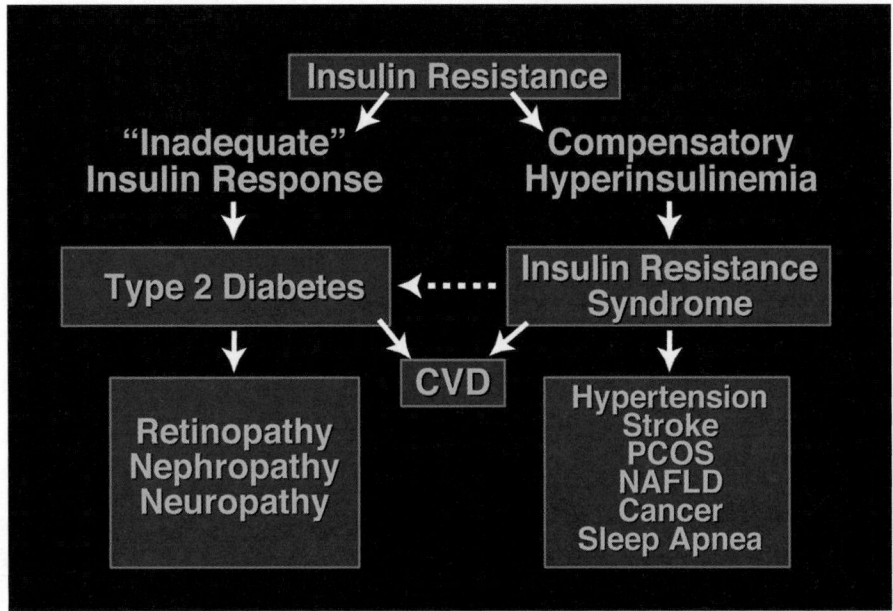

FIGURE 37-3 ■ Differentiation between the insulin resistance syndrome and type 2 diabetes. (From Einhorn D, Reaven GM, Cobin RH et al: *Endocr Pract* 9[S2]:5-21, 2003.) *CVD,* Cardiovascular disease; *NAFLD,* non-alcoholic fatty liver disease; *PCOS,* polycystic ovarian syndrome.

BOX 37-1 ■ ■ ■
MODIFIED INSULIN SUPPRESSION TEST

In the insulin suppression test, after an overnight fast, the study subject receives a 180-minute IV infusion of octreotide acetate (to inhibit endogenous insulin), insulin, and glucose. Blood samples are obtained throughout the study and every 10 minutes in the last 30 minutes. The average of the last four samples determines the steady-state plasma insulin and steady-state plasma glucose (SSPG) levels for each person. The steady-state plasma insulin concentrations are similar for all subjects, and the SSPG concentration gives a direct measure of the ability of insulin to mediate disposal of the infused glucose load. The higher the level of the SSPG, the more insulin resistant the subject.

From Pei D, Jones CN, Bhargava R et al: *Diabetologia* 27:843-845, 1994.

also defined the clustering of abnormalities as insulin resistance syndrome, with insulin resistance as the underlying pathophysiology.[3] In 2005, the International Diabetes Federation felt these different definitions created too much confusion for clinicians attempting to identify individuals with this syndrome. They convened a task force to review previous information and formulate a new worldwide definition of what they called the metabolic syndrome. They also stated that abdominal obesity was common to all the components of this syndrome.[12] Table 37-1 lists the components of these five definitions.

Incidence and Prevalence of Insulin Resistance/Metabolic Syndrome

Defining the population at risk for insulin resistance can be difficult because of the differing identification criteria. Applying the ATP III criteria to identify individuals with metabolic syndrome, Ford and colleagues[13] found that approximately one-quarter of the American population (25.8 percent) would be identified as having meta-

bolic syndrome using National Health and Nutritional Examination Survey (**NHANES**) III data (1988 to 1994) for adults ages 40 to 74 (excluding self-reported diabetes or a fasting glucose of 126 mg/dl or greater). For the population age 20 or older, it was 23.7 percent. In this same population (age 20 or older), in males the prevalence was 24.8 percent for whites, 16.4 percent for blacks, and 28.3 percent for Mexican Americans. For women, it was 22.8 percent for whites, 25.7 percent in blacks, and 35.6 percent in Mexican Americans.

The American College of Endocrinology/American Association of Clinical Endocrinologists criteria for insulin resistance syndrome were applied to the same NHANES III population (ages 40 to 74) and included data from oral glucose tolerance test results. Using two or more of the abnormalities listed in their criteria, 39.8 percent were identified as having insulin resistance syndrome: 43.7 percent men and 36.1 percent women. The prevalence of insulin resistance syndrome was higher for men and women in Mexican Americans compared with whites, blacks, or others.[14] Applying the ATP III criteria to the year 2000 NHANES III data, approximately 47 million persons in the United States could be identified as having metabolic syndrome.[13]

A recent report compared the WHO criteria and ATP III criteria for metabolic syndrome using data from NHANES III (1988 to 1994). From a representative sample of 20,050 participants of NHANES III, 8608 persons were recruited for this survey. In those age 20 and older, the age-adjusted prevalence of metabolic syndrome was 23.9 percent using the ATP III definition and 25.1 percent using the WHO criteria. Although these two definitions resulted in similar percentages, differences were found in certain ethnicities. The largest difference was noted in black men. The ATP III criteria identified 16.5 percent with metabolic syndrome, and

■ ■ ■

TABLE 37-1   DEFINITIONS OF INSULIN RESISTANCE, METABOLIC SYNDROME, AND RELATED CONCEPTS

ORGANIZATION	YEAR ESTABLISHED	NAME	PRESENCE OF INSULIN RESISTANCE	OBESITY		DYSLIPIDEMIA	GLUCOSE	OTHER
WHO	1998	Metabolic syndrome	IFG, IGT, type 2 DM and/or insulin resistance and two or more of the following:	Waist/hip ratio: Greater than 0.90 in men Greater than 0.85 in women *and/or* BMI greater than 30 kg/m²	≥140/90 mm Hg	Triglycerides ≥150 mg/dl (1.7 mmol/liter) and/or HDL less than 35 mg/dl (0.9 mmol/liter) in men or less than 39 mg/dl (1.0 mmol) in women	IGT, IGF, or type 2 DM	Urinary albumin excretion rate ≥20 mcg/min albumin-to-creatinine ratio ≥30 mg/g
EGIR	1990	Insulin resistance syndrome	Presence of insulin resistance or fasting hyperinsulinemia (highest 25%) and two or more of the following:	Waist circumference: ≥94 cm men ≥80 cm women	≥140/90 mm Hg or treated hypertension	Triglycerides ≥180 mg/dl (2 mmol/liter) HDL-C ≤40 mg/dl (1.0 mmol/liter) or treated dyslipidemia	≥110 mg/dl (≥6.1 mmol/liter) IGF or IGT but not diabetic	
NCEP III	2001/2005	Metabolic syndrome	None Must have three of the following:	Waist circumference: ≥102 cm men (≥40 inches) ≥88 cm women (≥35 inches)	≥130 or ≥85 mm Hg or on treatment	Triglycerides ≥150 mg/dl (1.7 mmol/liter) or on treatment HDL less than 40 mg/dl (0.9 mmol/liter) in men or less than 50 mg/dl (1.0 mmol) in women or on treatment	≥100 mg/dl	

ACE/AACE	2003	Insulin resistance syndrome	Acknowledges insulin resistance as underlying pathophysiology High-risk persons (see Other); have two or more of following:	See Other	Greater than 130/85 mm Hg Based on 2001 ATP III Guidelines	Triglycerides greater than 150 mg/dl Based on 2001 ATP III Guidelines HDL less than 40 mg/dl (0.9 mmol/liter) in men or less than 50 mg/dl (1.0 mmol) in women Based on 2001 ATP III Guidelines	110-125 mg/dl or 120 minutes after glucose load 140-200 mg/dl	High-risk persons: Family history of type 2 DM, hypertension, CVD; non-white ethnicity; history of glucose intolerance or gestational DM; BMI greater than 25 kg/m² or waist circumference greater than 40 inches men or greater than 35 inches women (10%-15% lower for non-white); sedentary lifestyle; age greater than 40 years; acanthosis nigricans; PCOS; NAFLD; CVD; hypertension
IDF	2005	Metabolic syndrome	No measurement of insulin resistance - must have central (abdominal) obesity Acknowledges both central obesity and insulin resistance as part of pathophysiology	Must have Central Obesity Population specific criteria for European, Asian, or Japanese: Europeans defined as ≥94 cm in men ≥80 cm in women Asians ≥ 90 cm men ≥80 cm in women Japanese ≥ 85 cm men ≥ 90 cm in women	≥130/≥85 or Rx HTN	TG ≥ 150 mg/dl (1.7mmol/L) or on Rx HDL <40 mg/dl (1.03mmol/) in men 50 mg/dl (1.29 mmol) in women or on Rx	> 100 mg/dl includes diabetes	(5.6 mmol/L) or previously diagnosed with type 2 diabetes

ACE/AACE, American College of Endocrinology/American Association of Clinical Endocrinologists; *BMI*, body mass index; *CVD*, cardiovascular disease; *DM*, diabetes mellitus; *EGIR*, European Group for the Study of Insulin Resistance; *HDL*, high-density lipoprotein; *HDL-C*, HDL cholesterol; *HTN*, hypertension; *IDF*, International Diabetes Foundation; *IFG*, impaired fasting glucose; *IGT*, impaired glucose tolerance; *NAFLD*, nonalcoholic fatty liver disease; *NCEP ATP III*, National Cholesterol Education Program Adult Treatment Panel III; *PCOS*, polycystic ovary syndrome; *TG*, triglyceride; *WHO*, World Health Organization.

the WHO criteria identified 24.9 percent of black men. Prevalence of self-reported myocardial infarction (**MI**) in this cohort was 4.5 percent among those meeting the ATP III criteria for metabolic syndrome and 2.9 percent without the syndrome; it was 5.1 percent among those meeting the WHO criteria for metabolic syndrome and 2.6 percent without the defined syndrome. Confidence intervals overlapped, suggesting the prevalence was similar in each group.[15]

Agreement on one definition is needed to determine the prevalence of insulin resistance/metabolic syndrome and the associated comorbidities more accurately. There continues to be ongoing debate among professional groups about the definition and the importance of identifying these individuals.

The NCEP ATP III criteria for diagnosis and management of the metabolic syndrome were updated recently to provide more definitive guidelines to help identify this population. Authors of the criteria still argue that individuals with insulin resistance/metabolic syndrome are at increased CVD risk and recommend that they be identified and treated accordingly.[16] A recent joint statement released from the American Diabetes Association and the European Association for the Study of Diabetes stated that more research is needed before health care professionals can understand how to identify this population accurately.[17] Although insulin resistance clearly plays an important role in CVD, more research is needed to understand the complex pathophysiology better. Does being insulin resistant or having metabolic syndrome automatically put persons at higher CVD risk?

Authors of the joint statement suggest that once those persons with diabetes and heart disease are removed from the group identified as having metabolic syndrome, others may not be at any higher risk than those with a clustering of CVD risk factors. Their position is that the evidence is currently not strong enough to conclude that identifying this population is more important than simply assessing patients for CVD risk factors and determining their appropriate treatment goals. Lifestyle intervention is strongly recommended as initial therapy for both groups.

It is well accepted that type 2 diabetes is a serious consequence of insulin resistance, but it is important to note that most individuals identified as having insulin resistance will be able to maintain the needed compensatory hyperinsulinemia to keep normal or near normal glucose tolerance. Yet this compensatory mechanism is not without its consequences. Health care professionals need to recognize that these individuals, whether referred to as having metabolic syndrome or insulin resistance, will remain at increased risk for a clustering of metabolic abnormalities and clinical outcomes such as CVD. Treatment of these abnormalities is essential to reduce the incidence of this poor outcome.[3,4]

Morbidity and Mortality in the Insulin-Resistant Person

Even with differing criteria for identifying individuals with the insulin resistance/metabolic syndrome, attempts have been made to look at the associated risk for

CVD and stroke. A recent study applying the ATP III criteria to subjects from NHANES III—after adjusting for age, sex, race, and cigarette smoking—found the metabolic syndrome was significantly associated with self-reported MI, stroke, and a combination of the two.[18] When the data were analyzed separately for patients with and without diabetes, there remained a strong relationship with CVD, even in the absence of diabetes.

The 22-year follow-up study of Helsinki policemen, using factors associated with insulin resistance/metabolic syndrome (mean blood pressure and triglyceride levels, body mass index [**BMI**], areas under the glucose and insulin curve ratio during a glucose tolerance testing, and subscapular skinfold measurements), found insulin resistance/metabolic syndrome to be an independent predictor of risk for coronary artery disease (**CAD**) and stroke.[19]

A prospective study using subjects from NHANES II evaluated the impact of insulin resistance/metabolic syndrome on mortality from coronary heart disease (**CHD**) and CVD. The metabolic syndrome was a strong predictor of CHD, CVD, and total mortality. Again, when individuals with diabetes were separated out of the population, there was still an increased risk for CHD, but not for overall mortality.[20]

RISK FACTORS
Hyperinsulinemia

Elevated insulin levels are highly correlated with insulin resistance,[1] yet it is not clear if the relationship with CVD is related specifically to insulin resistance/hyperinsulinemia, the clustering of metabolic abnormalities, or both. Many studies, but not all, suggest a strong relationship between insulin resistance/hyperinsulinemia and CVD.[21-26] Even if future research confirms fasting insulin level to be an independent risk factor for CVD or a good measure to identify those with insulin resistance, there is currently no standardized method for measuring or reporting insulin levels. Laboratory standardization and more data are needed for insulin levels to be useful in clinical practice.

Genetics

Risk factors for insulin resistance are thought to have modifiable and nonmodifiable influences, with approximately 50 percent genetic and 50 percent coming from environmental factors.[3] Studies evaluating the influence of heredity on insulin resistance have used measurements of fasting insulin levels, 1-hour insulin levels after a glucose load, or direct measures of insulin resistance, such as the SSPG method or euglycemic clamp. Because most individuals with type 2 diabetes are insulin resistant, many investigators have evaluated offspring and first-degree nondiabetic relatives of individuals with type 2 diabetes.

Figure 37-1 demonstrates that insulin resistance can vary sixfold to eightfold from person to person. Studies evaluating variability of insulin resistance within families with a history of type 2 diabetes found less variability within families than between families. Other studies measuring insulin resistance in nondiabetic relatives of persons with diabetes found them to be more insulin resistant than nondiabetic controls.[27]Although there are limitations to these studies, there appears to be strong evidence of a genetic influence on insulin resistance or hyperinsulinemia. Insulin resistance is complex and clearly polygenic. Researchers continue to evaluate genes thought to be responsible for insulin resistance.

Ethnic and Gender Differences in Insulin Resistance and Type 2 Diabetes

As noted before, in the populations more frequently identified as having insulin resistance or metabolic syndrome, ethnicity plays an important role in identifying those at increased risk. Although not free from risk, relatively speaking, white populations have the lowest prevalence of type 2 diabetes, and Pima Native Americans have the highest prevalence of insulin resistance and type 2 diabetes.[28]

More than a 10-fold variation occurs in the prevalence of type 2 diabetes between high-and low-risk populations. Interestingly, in populations at high risk for insulin resistance, there are differences in risk factors associated with insulin resistance and insulin resistance syndrome. For example, West African men have lower plasma triglyceride and higher HDL cholesterol levels than European men. This same pattern is found in West African and European older women when the data are adjusted for fat mass and visceral fat. In the United States, when comparing Europeans and black Americans with similar socioeconomic status, CHD mortality was lower in black American men despite a higher prevalence of type 2 diabetes and hypertension. Differences in the lipid pattern have been thought to offer some explanation for this finding.[28]

Patterns of obesity and physical activity also play a significant role in risk for diabetes and CHD within these ethnic groups. The Pima Native Americans have a 6 times higher incidence of type 2 diabetes than the Pima Natives living in rural Mexico. One of the main differences noted between these two groups was the level of physical activity and BMI. Those in the rural area were more active and had a mean BMI of approximately 8 kg/m² less than those in the urban setting.

South Asians also have a higher level of insulin resistance and type 2 diabetes than other ethnic/racial groups and, in many areas, high risk for CHD. Some studies suggest that South Asians also have increased central obesity compared with Europeans. Relative risk for CHD mortality varies by location, being no higher in the United States than in Europe. Rates of CHD prevalence are higher in urban areas and lower in rural areas of South Asia. Some groups of South Asians share many of the same risks noted in the insulin resistance syndrome, which may account for their increased risk for CHD.[28]

It is well established that Mexican Americans have a high prevalence of insulin resistance and type 2 diabetes. In comparison to non-Hispanic Europeans, the distribution of central obesity is higher in Mexican Americans, and there is an accompanying elevated level of plasma triglycerides and lower HDL cholesterol. Interestingly, age-standardized CHD mortality is 20 percent lower in Mexican American men in Texas than in non-Hispanic European men. CHD mortality, however, is similar in Mexican American women compared with non-Hispanic European women. One contributing factor explaining this conundrum may be an increased incidence of obesity.[28]

Age

The age at which a person is at increased risk for insulin resistance and type 2 diabetes is 40 to 45 years for both genders.[3,29] Age itself has been shown to influence insulin resistance, but aging also is associated with an increase in body weight and a decrease in physical activity. Both of these factors contribute to insulin resistance and type 2 diabetes as persons age. A recent review of studies evaluating the impact of age, physical activity, and body weight on glucose tolerance evaluated studies of men and women ages 17 to 92.[30] When adjusting for differences in physical activity and weight, age had little or no significant impact on the variability of plasma glucose response in men or women.

However, it has been reported that with increasing age there is a decrease in glucose-stimulated insulin secretion independent of abdominal circumference.[31] In another study, there was a decrease in the insulin secretory response at any given level of glucose infusion in older persons.[32] Although aging per se influences glucose tolerance, it is clear that physical activity and body weight have an even greater impact than age.

Increasing rates of overweight and obesity and decreases in physical activity in the adolescent population and the population at large are sure to decrease the age at which insulin resistance and type 2 diabetes and potentially CVD develop. We need to continue to be aggressive with lifestyle management and prevention of type 2 diabetes and CVD in all populations and ages.

Modifiable Risk Factors

As discussed before, physical activity and weight influence insulin resistance. Increased physical activity and weight loss enhance insulin sensitivity by improving insulin action.

Physical Activity

Physical activity increases insulin sensitivity, although the mechanisms are not well understood. Stimulation of glucose transport in the muscle is impaired in insulin resistance.[1] Peripheral insulin resistance involves skeletal muscle, and several steps in the process of insulin-mediated glucose uptake in tissue may be involved in the pathogenesis. These steps involve glucose transport by the insulin-dependent glucose transporter **GLUT-4**, phosphorylation (hexokinase II), and glycogen synthase.[33,34] In one study, physical training increased insulin sensitivity through stimulation of insulin-mediated glycogen synthesis in the muscle.[35] Although rates of muscle glycogen synthesis went up with exercise, they were lower than in the insulin-sensitive subjects after exercise, suggesting that other defects were not overcome or corrected with exercise.

GLUT-4, located primarily in muscle cells and adipoctyes, is the main insulin-responsive glucose transporter. When not stimulated by insulin or other stimuli such as exercise, GLUT-4 is intracellular. Exercise is thought to stimulate the movement of GLUT-4 from intracellular storage to the plasma membrane, allowing for glucose transport into the muscle cell.[36] Others have suggested that there also may be an increase in GLUT-4 content in the muscle with exercise.[37] Studies show that varying amounts and intensity of exercise increase insulin sensitivity, ranging from one bout to 6 weeks and with frequent nonvigorous or vigorous activity.[35,36] These changes were observed in a large group of culturally and ethnically diverse men and women with normal glucose levels, impaired glucose tolerance, and mild type 2 diabetes.

Weight Loss

Weight gain and loss also influence insulin resistance. A linear relationship exists between BMI and insulin resistance in nondiabetic healthy adults, yet it is important to note that not all obese individuals are insulin resistant.[38] In one study of the distribution of BMI according to tertiles of insulin resistance measured by SSPG, only 36 percent of the most insulin-resistant tertile of healthy nondiabetic individuals were obese, 43 percent were moderately overweight, and 16 percent were normal weight.[39]

Some theorize that elevated levels of insulin in insulin-resistant persons cause weight gain. In a review of five studies of adult men and women from different ethnic populations,[40] whites, Hispanics, and Pima Indians were divided into insulin-resistant versus insulin-sensitive groups. Insulin resistance was identified by fasting insulin levels, 2-hour insulin levels after an oral glucose tolerance test, insulin levels in response to oral and intravenous glucose tolerance tests, or by a euglycemic clamp study. Participants were followed for 3½ to 14 years. Results showed either no difference in weight gain between the insulin-resistant and insulin-sensitive individuals or, in some cases, less weight gain in the groups with highest insulin resistance.

Insulin-resistant overweight or obese individuals are able to lose comparable amounts of weight. Interestingly, with weight loss, only the insulin-resistant individuals become more insulin sensitive, but they do not reach the same level of insulin sensitivity as the equally overweight insulin-sensitive group. Other benefits of moderate weight loss unique to nondiabetic insulin-resistant individuals were improvements in elevated daylong plasma glucose, free fatty acid (**FFA**) levels, insulin levels, and plasma triglyceride levels.[41,42] Furthermore, C-reactive protein levels, a marker of vascular inflammation, were elevated only in the insulin-resistant obese individuals. C-reactive protein levels decreased with weight loss but did not reach the same level as those in the equally overweight insulin-sensitive subjects.[43] What is now clear is that insulin-resistant overweight and obese individuals can make significant improvements in many CVD risk factors with moderate weight loss.

HISTORICAL PERSPECTIVE

In 1939, Himsworth presented his theory regarding mechanisms of diabetes mellitus to the Royal College of Physicians of London. He reported that not all diabetes resulted in a lack of insulin and that there might be two different causes: one a primary deficiency of insulin, now known as type 1 diabetes mellitus, and the other an inefficiency or insensitivity of insulin action, now known as type 2 diabetes.[44] Type 1 diabetes is not the most common form but is more severe than type 2 diabetes. Many years later, in 1988, Reaven reported the consequences of this insensitivity to the action of insulin.[1]

Prediabetes

Prediabetes is a relatively new term used to define those with impaired fasting glucose or impaired glucose tolerance. Impaired fasting glucose is diagnosed with fasting glucose levels of 100 to 125 mg/dl. Impaired glucose tolerance is diagnosed with 2-hour glucose levels between 140 and 199 mg/dl 2 hours after a 75-g oral glucose challenge. Persons with prediabetes have an increased risk of developing type 2 diabetes. Of those predisposed to diabetes, approximately 7 percent will go on to develop type 2 diabetes each year.[45] One must remember, as described earlier and seen in Figure 37-2, that high-risk individuals who do not go on to develop type 2 diabetes share many of the same risk factors as those who develop type 2 diabetes.

In a 10-year study in which investigators following more than 7000 men with impaired glucose tolerance, the Paris Prospective Study (**PPS**), mortality from CAD was significantly increased in persons with impaired glucose tolerance, newly diagnosed diabetes, and known diabetes compared with normoglycemic individuals.[46] In another epidemiological study (DECODE) in which more than 22,000 men and women were followed for a mean of 8.8 years, impaired glucose tolerance was associated with increased risk of CAD death, CVD death, and all-cause mortality.[47] Multivariate-adjusted hazard ratios for these events were 1.28, 1.34, and 1.40, respectively. In analyzing data from 3174 individuals who underwent an oral glucose tolerance test in the period from 1976 to 1980 and were followed until 1992 by the U.S. Second National Health and Nutrition Examination Survey (NHANES II) Mortality Study, similar findings of increased mortality were reported in those with impaired glucose tolerance. The multivariate-adjusted relative risks were 1.42 for all-cause mortality and 1.15 for CVD mortality.[48]

CONNECTION BETWEEN INSULIN RESISTANCE AND TYPE 2 DIABETES

Insulin resistance exists to a similar degree in normal glycemic populations and in those with mild and severe type 2 diabetes. The ability of pancreatic beta cells to compensate for insulin resistance plays an important role in determining the degree to which glucose homeostasis can be maintained. Hyperglycemia of varying degrees results when a sufficient level of compensatory hyperinsulinemia cannot be maintained. A relatively small decrease in daylong insulin levels also affects other metabolic functions regulated by insulin. These functions, discussed subsequently, also play an important role in contributing to the development of hyperglycemia.[1]

Free Fatty Acids

Plasma FFA concentrations are tightly regulated by insulin levels. FFA concentrations can be half maximally suppressed at a plasma insulin level of ~20 μM/ml.[1,2] Normally, higher insulin levels result in lower plasma FFAs. Along with a defect in the ability of insulin to mediate glucose uptake in the muscle, persons with insulin resistance also have a defect in the ability of insulin to suppress plasma FFA concentrations (insulin resistance in the adipose tissue).[1,49] Because plasma FFA concentrations can be reduced by relatively small increases in insulin levels, the chronic compensatory hyperinsulinemia is able to regulate plasma FFA so that they are only moderately elevated.

When the pancreatic beta cell can no longer secrete the amount of insulin needed to maintain normal glucose homeostasis, hyperglycemia results. Because hyperglycemia occurs with a relative decrease in insulin levels, the FFA level also increases.[1,2] The increase in FFA levels to the liver is thought to stimulate FFA oxidation, stimulating hepatic glucose production, resulting in a further increase in plasma glucose concentrations.[50] In addition, beta cell secretory function is compromised further as plasma glucose increases.

In summary, a small decrease in insulin levels (caused by an inability of the beta cell to maintain the needed hyperinsulinemia) may decrease glucose uptake in the muscle resulting in hyperglycemia and increase FFA concentrations, which in turn stimulates hepatic glucose production. In addition, these elevations of plasma glucose and FFA levels further compromise beta cell function. These mechanisms contribute to the development of hyperglycemia.[1,2]

Prevalence of Diabetes

In 2005, it was estimated that 20.8 million persons, or 7 percent, of the U.S. population had diabetes.[51] Of those, approximately 90 to 95 percent have type 2 diabetes[29] (Box 37-2). Individuals age 65 or older make up approximately 40 percent of the total diagnosed with diabetes.[52] Blacks, Hispanics, and Native Americans have a prevalence of diagnosed diabetes at least 2 times higher than the majority of populations (Figure 37-4).[51,52] There was a fourfold to eightfold increase in the number of persons diagnosed with diabetes between 1958 and 2000. These increases occurred in all sex, race, age, and ethnicity categories, and the prevalence among adults increased in all states in the United States[53] (Figure 37-5). See Box 37-3 for key facts about diabetes.

In data collected between 1990 and 2001, the largest relative increases in diagnosed diabetes were found in persons between ages 30 to 39 and 40 to 49 years. Interestingly, according to the NHANES data, the number of

> **BOX 37-2** ■ ■ ■
> ### ADULT PREVALENCE OF DIABETES IN THE UNITED STATES
>
> *Total:* 20.8 million persons (7 percent of the population)
> *Diagnosed:* 14.6 million persons
> *Undiagnosed:* 6.2 million persons
> *Men:* 10.9 million (10.5 percent)
> *Women:* 9.7 million (8.8 percent)
> *Age:* 20.9 percent of persons age 60 or older
>
> **Race/Ethnicity**
> *Non-Hispanic whites:* 13.1 million (8.7 percent)
> *Non-Hispanic blacks:* 3.2 million (13.3 percent)
> *Hispanic/Latino Americans:* 2.5 million (9.5 percent)
> *American Indians and Alaska Natives who receive care from the Indian Health Service:* 118,000 (15.1 percent)

From Centers for Disease Control and Prevention: *National diabetes statistics fact sheet: general information and national estimates on diabetes in the United States, 2005,* Atlanta, 2005, US Department of Health and Human Services, Centers for Disease Control and Prevention.

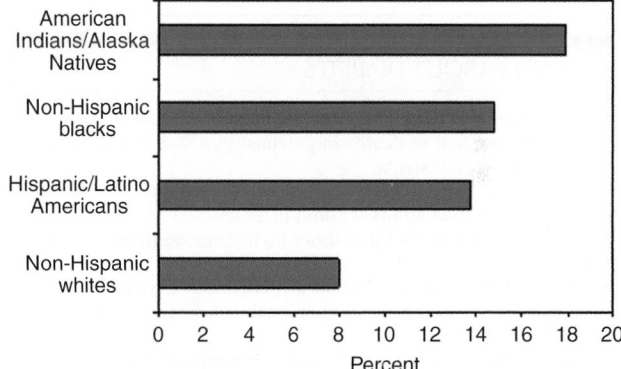

FIGURE 37-4 ■ Age-adjusted total prevalence of diabetes in persons age 20 and older by race/ethnicity, United States, 2002. (From 1999-2001 National Health Interview Survey and 1999-2000 National Health and Nutrition Examination Survey estimates projected to year 2002; and 2002 outpatient database of the Indian Health Service.)

undiagnosed diabetes (about one-third of all persons with diabetes) has not changed.[54] Some explanations for the dramatic increase in diagnosed diabetes include changes in diagnostic criteria, improved detection, decreasing mortality, an aging population, increases in overweight and obesity, decreases in physical activity, and growth in minority populations.[55] The prevalence of diabetes in U.S. adults is estimated almost to double by 2025. Worldwide, an estimated 170 million persons have diabetes. The prediction is that there will be a 50 percent increase by 2010, with the greatest increase seen in the developing countries of Africa, Asia, and South America.[56]

Genetics
Type 2 Diabetes Mellitus

A positive family history can increase one's risk for type 2 diabetes twofold to fourfold. Having a first-degree relative with type 2 diabetes leads to a 15 to 25 percent higher risk of developing impaired glucose tolerance or diabetes.[57] The underlying genetic causes of type 2 diabetes have a multifactorial pathogenesis including poly-

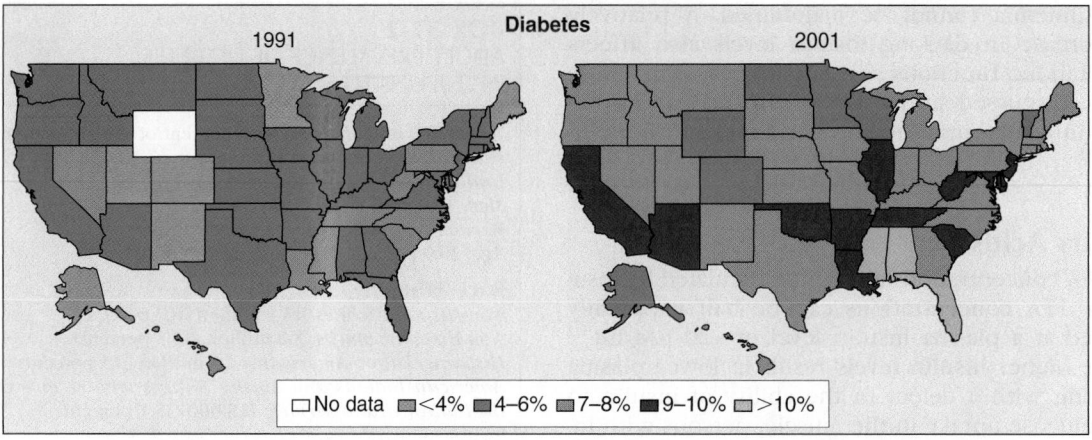

FIGURE 37-5 ■ Map of the United States illustrating the increase in diabetes between 1991 and 2001. (From Beckman JA, Libby P, Creager MA: Diabetes mellitus, the metabolic syndrome, and atherosclerotic vascular disease. In Zipes DP, Libby P, Bonow RO, Braunwald E, editors: *Braunwald's heart disease,* ed 7, Philadelphia, 2005, Elsevier.)

BOX 37-3   ■ ■ ■
KEY FACTS ABOUT DIABETES

- Heart disease is the leading cause of diabetes-related deaths.
- Sixty-five percent of deaths in persons with diabetes is due to heart disease and stroke.
- Adults with diabetes have heart disease death rates 2 to 4 times higher than adults without diabetes.
- The risk for stroke is 2 to 4 times higher among persons with diabetes.
- Seventy-three percent of adults with diabetes have blood pressure of 130/80 mm Hg or higher, or they take prescription medications for hypertension.
- Diabetes is a coronary heart disease risk equivalent.

Data from Centers for Disease Control and Prevention: *National diabetes statistics fact sheet: general information and national estimates on diabetes in the United States, 2005,* Atlanta, 2005, US Department of Health and Human Services, Centers for Disease Control and Prevention; and Third Report of the National Cholesterol Education Program (NCEP) Expert Panel on Detection, Evaluation, and Treatment of High Blood Cholesterol in Adults (Adult Treatment Panel III) final report, *Circulation* 106:3143-3421, 2002.

BOX 37-4   ■ ■ ■
CRITERIA FOR TESTING FOR DIABETES
IN ASYMPTOMATIC ADULTS

1. Testing for diabetes should be considered in all individuals at age 45 and older, particularly in those with a body mass index of 25 kg/m[2]* or higher. If results are normal, the test should be repeated at 3-year intervals.
2. Testing should be considered at a younger age or be performed more often in individuals who are overweight (body mass index of 25kg/m[2]* or above) and have additional risk factors, as described next:
   - Habitual physical inactivity
   - First-degree relative with diabetes
   - High-risk ethnic population (e.g., black, Latino, Native American, or Asian American and Pacific Islander)
   - Delivered a baby weighing more than 9 lb or diagnosed with gestational diabetes
   - Hypertensive (140/90 mm Hg or above)
   - High-density lipoprotein cholesterol lower than 35 mg/dl (0.90 mmol/liter)
   - Triglyceride level above 250 mg/dl (2.82 mmol/liter)
   - Polycystic ovary syndrome
   - Personal history of prediabetes (impaired fasting glucose or impaired glucose tolerance)
   - Other clinical conditions associated with insulin resistance (acanthosis nigricans)
   - History of cardiovascular disease

*May not be correct for all ethnic groups.
From American Diabetes Association: *Diabetes Care* 29(suppl 1):S4-S42, 2006.

---

morphisms of several genes. Although several mechanisms have been suggested relating to insulin resistance and beta cell dysfunction and several genes for peroxisome proliferator-activated receptor-gamma, insulin receptor substrate-1, and others have been identified, there are currently no definitive answers to the underlying pathophysiology.[58] Research continues to unravel this complex disease. A small subset of individuals diagnosed with type 2 diabetes has a monogenic form of diabetes. These are maturity-onset diabetes of the young, mitochondrial diabetes, and late-onset autoimmune diabetes of the adult, a late-onset type 1 diabetes.[29]

Type 1 Diabetes Mellitus
Type 1 diabetes, accounting for 5 to 10 percent of this population, results from cell-mediated autoimmune destruction of the beta cells from the pancreas. Islet cell antibodies, autoantibodies to insulin, autoantibodies to glutamic acid decarboxylase, and autoantibodies to the tyrosine phosphatases 1A-2 and 1A-2 beta are markers of the immune destruction of the beta cell. One or more markers are present in 85 to 90 percent persons when

they exhibit fasting hyperglycemia. Type 1 diabetes also is associated with the gene HLA, with linkage to the genes DQA and DOB; HLA is influenced by DRB genes.[29]

SCREENING AND DIAGNOSIS OF DIABETES
Criteria for testing asymptomatic adults for diabetes are shown in Box 37-4. Table 37-2 presents the current criteria for the diagnosis of diabetes, which were revised in 1997. The revision was made to promote early diagnosis and treatment in hopes of decreasing the microvascular and macrovascular complications associated with diabetes. As described before, the new term *pre-*

■ ■ ■

TABLE 37-2   CRITERIA FOR DIAGNOSIS OF DIABETES MELLITUS

	FASTING PLASMA GLUCOSE (AT LEAST 8 HOURS)	ORAL GLUCOSE TOLERANCE TEST (2-HOURS AFTER GLUCOSE)
Normal	Less than 100 mg/dl (less than 5.6 mmol/liter)	Less than 140 mg/dl (7.8 mmol/liter)
Impaired glucose tolerance (prediabetes)	100 to 125 mg/dl (5.6 to 6.9 mmol/liter)	140 to 199 mg/dl (7.8 to 11.0 mmol/liter)
Diabetes	≥126 mg/dl (7.0 mmol/liter)	≥200 mg/dl (11.1 mmol/liter)
Symptoms of diabetes (polyuria, polydipsia, unexplained weight loss)	Casual plasma glucose ≥200 mg/dl (11.1 mmol/liter)	NA

In the absence of unequivocal hyperglycemia, a diagnosis of diabetes must be confirmed by repeat testing on a different day by measurement of fasting plasma glucose, 2-hour plasma glucose, or random plasma glucose (if symptoms are present). The fasting plasma glucose test is preferred.
From American Diabetes Association: *Diabetes Care* 29(suppl 1):S4-S42, 2006.

diabetes was introduced at that time. Recently, the lower diagnostic level of fasting plasma glucose was decreased to 100 mg/dl. These changes were made to identify those at risk for developing type 2 diabetes who would benefit from lifestyle change interventions.

LIFESTYLE INTERVENTION APPROACHES
Primary Prevention

The effectiveness of addressing increased weight and physical inactivity in reducing insulin resistance and the risk for type 2 diabetes has been well documented in three recent diabetes prevention trials.[45,59,60] One study conducted in Da Qing, China, included men and women with impaired glucose tolerance from 33 health care clinics. Each clinic was randomized to one of three intervention groups or a control group and followed for 6 years. Participants received individual and group counseling in diet, exercise, or diet plus exercise. The diet intervention group received a diet in which 55 to 60 percent of calories came from carbohydrates, 10 to 15 percent from proteins, and 25 to 30 percent from fats. Participants with a BMI of 25 mg/kg² or greater were given diet instructions to achieve a weight loss of 0.5 to 1.0 kg/month with a goal of achieving a BMI of 23 kg/m². Those assigned to exercise were instructed to increase their leisure physical activity by one unit of exercise per day and two if possible. A unit of exercise could range from 30 minutes of mild activity to 5 minutes of very strenuous activity. Those in the diet and exercise group were given the combined diet and exercise information. Results showed a significant reduction in the rate of progression to type 2 diabetes in all intervention groups (31 percent in the diet group, 42 percent in the diet and exercise group, 46 percent in the exercise group) compared with the control group.[60]

In 2001 a similar Finnish trial was reported. The intervention group received intensive individual counseling to help them reduce total body weight by 5 percent or more, decrease total fat intake to less than 30 percent of energy consumed with less than 10 percent as saturated fat, increase fiber intake to 15 g per 1000 calories, and exercise 30 minutes each day at moderate intensity. The rate of developing diabetes was reduced overall by 58 percent in the intervention group compared with controls.[59]

The Finnish and U.S. studies were similar in design, but the U.S. study compared results in men and women, in different age groups, and in ethnically and culturally diverse populations. Investigators for the U.S. trial hypothesized that lifestyle modification or metformin 850 mg twice daily could prevent or delay the onset of type 2 diabetes in persons with impaired fasting glucose plus impaired glucose tolerance. The original design included a third treatment arm with randomization to troglitazone, but this arm was discontinued when troglitazone was removed from the market because of serious side effects of liver toxicity. The lifestyle interventions were similar to those in the Finnish trial, with a goal weight loss of at least 7 percent of initial body weight and moderate physical activity for a minimum of 150 minutes each week. Interestingly, the results in the lifestyle group were the same as those reported in the Finnish study: a 58 percent reduction in the rate of progression to type 2 diabetes compared with controls. The metformin group had a 31 percent reduction compared with the placebo group. The lifestyle group had a 39 percent lower rate of developing diabetes compared with the metformin group. Most importantly, there were no significant differences in treatment effects in age, sex, race, or ethnic subgroups.[45]

Dietary Intervention

Although it is clearly established that a diet low in saturated fat will reduce low-density lipoprotein (**LDL**) cholesterol, there is no consensus on what isocaloric dietary macronutrient composition is best suited for insulin-resistant individuals with or without diabetes. Those with insulin resistance have the same risk as the general population of having elevated cholesterol, but the dyslipidemia most highly correlated with insulin resistance is elevated triglycerides and low HDL.[1-4] The recommendation regarding what should replace the saturated fat content of the diets of persons with this atherogenic lipid abnormality remains unclear.

There was concern that all fats might raise LDL cholesterol levels, but several studies in men and women have shown that saturated fat, not total fat, was associated with increases in LDL cholesterol level.[61] Isocaloric diets higher in carbohydrates and lower in fat have been shown to increase fasting and daylong insulin secretion.

This in turn increases very low-density lipoprotein (**VLDL**)–triglyceride synthesis and secretion from the liver, resulting in an increase in fasting and postprandial triglyceride levels. This increase in fasting and daylong plasma triglycerides and triglyceride-rich lipoproteins is associated with an increase in small dense LDL cholesterol and a decrease in HDL cholesterol. This atherogenic profile increases the risk for CVD. Diets relatively lower in carbohydrates with higher levels of monosaturated and polyunsaturated fats do not increase insulin, triglyceride, or LDL cholesterol levels. Such diets have a favorable effect on moderately elevated triglycerides and the insulin-resistant atherogenic profile.[61,62]

Although all might not agree on the percentage of fat to recommend in this population, the ATP III dietary guidelines for persons with moderately elevated triglycerides recommend a diet containing 30 percent of calories from fat with low saturated fat (7 percent) and 55 percent of calories from complex carbohydrates.[9] The American Diabetes Association recommends that nutritional goals for persons with diabetes be individualized to help achieve the treatment goals. Recommendations on dietary composition include an intake of less than 7 percent of total calories as saturated fat, and a statement that diets restricting carbohydrates to less than 130 g/d is not recommended.[29]

BEYOND LIFESTYLE INTERVENTION

Nondiabetic insulin-resistant individuals share many of the same risk factors for CVD as those with type 2 diabetes. Except for treatment of hyperglycemia in those with diabetes, pharmacological treatments for related CVD risk factors do not differ, though the intensity of treatment varies depending on treatment goals.

Benefits of Glucose Lowering

Achieving glycemic control is essential in management of patients with diabetes and is associated with sustained decreases in rates of microvascular disease: retinopathy, nephropathy, and neuropathy. This benefit was well documented in two prospective randomized trials: the Diabetes Control and Complications Trial (**DCCT**) for patients with type 1 diabetes and the U.K. Prospective Diabetes Study (**UKPDS**) for patients with type 2 diabetes. Reducing the average hemoglobin A_{1c} levels to approximately 7 percent was associated with fewer long-term microvascular complications. Intensive control also was associated with episodes of severe hypoglycemia and weight gain. Therefore, careful monitoring of blood glucose levels is essential.

The DCCT study documented a mean hemoglobin A_{1c} of 9.1 percent in the conventionally treated group versus 7.3 percent in the intensive treated group. In long-term follow-up, the initial intensive glucose control group continued to have less progression of microvascular complications than the conventionally treated group. Benefit was greatest when intensive treatment was started early.[63] The reduction of risk for microvascular complications was maintained at 7 years irrespective of the fact that differences in the hemoglobin A_{1c}

between the two formerly randomized groups were not maintained. The authors concluded that intensive treatment should be started as soon as safely possible to maintain a hemoglobin A_{1c} goal of 7 percent or less to reduce the risk of microvascular complications.[64]

The benefits of intensive glucose control in terms of reducing macrovascular diseases were supported in a recent meta-analysis, although statistically significant reductions were not demonstrated in past randomized controlled trials.[65] A recent report supports the benefits of intense glycemic control on CVD.[66] In the DCCT follow-up study, carotid ultrasound 1 to 2 years after the follow-up study began and again 6 years later revealed significantly less progression of carotid intima-media thickness in the former intensively treated group compared with those in the conventionally treated group. Although glycemic control may not be the only goal in attempting to reduce CVD, it remains important. The following is a brief description of agents used for this purpose.

Glucose-Lowering Agents

Some patients diagnosed with type 2 diabetes may be able to control their blood glucose levels with lifestyle changes (i.e., exercise, diet, and weight loss). At some point, however, most will need to add oral antihyperglycemic agents to their regimen for glucose control. This loss of glucose control is related to several mechanisms, including lack of adherence or inability to maintain lifestyle changes that enhance insulin resistance. Other disease-related causes of a loss of glucose control include the progressive nature of type 2 diabetes. Insulin secretory defects in type 2 diabetes manifest in a 30- to 60-minute delay in meal-mediated insulin secretion and a deficiency of the amount of insulin secretion; over time, there is a progressive loss of beta cell function.[67] Beta cells progressively fail over time, and this failure has not been altered by treatment with diet, metformin, sulfonylureas, or insulin. Therefore, when one treatment fails, a second agent must be added.[68]

Oral Agents

Four categories of oral antihyperglycemic agents are now available for persons with type 2 diabetes (Table 37-3).

Insulin Secretagogues

Sulfonylurea drugs, the first class of oral medications used to treat type 2 diabetes, have been available for more than 50 years. These drugs stimulate the beta cells and increase basal and meal-stimulated insulin release. They also decrease overproduction of hepatic glucose and partially reverse the postreceptor defect in insulin action at the muscle and adipose levels. Improvements in glycemic control also decrease the metabolic effects of glucose toxicity. Monotherapy with this class of drugs may be effective for 4 to 5 years after the onset of type 2 diabetes.[67]

Biguanides

Currently, the only biguanide available is metformin. Although its exact mechanism of action is unclear, one known mechanism is suppression of hepatic glucose

■ ■ ■

TABLE 37-3   ORAL ANTIHYPERGLYCEMIC AGENTS*

GENERIC (BRAND) HOW SUPPLIED	DOSE INITIAL (Init) MAXIMUM (Max)	COMMENTS/POTENTIAL ADVERSE EFFECTS
Sulfonylureas		
Stimulate insulin release. Doses should be titrated carefully in the elderly and in those with renal or hepatic impairment. Monitor fasting plasma glucose (FPG) in 2 weeks/hemoglobin A_{1c} (HbA$_{1c}$) 3-6 months. HbA$_{1c}$ ↓ 1%-2%		
First-Generation (Long Half-Life)		
Tolazamide (Tolinase) 100, 250, 500 mg	*Init:* 100-250 mg once daily *Max:* 1000 mg	Initial dose depends on glucose level Daily with breakfast or first main meal Doses greater than 500 mg/d, divide into b.i.d. doses Hypoglycemia, weight gain
Tolbutamide (Orinase) 500 mg	*Init:* 250 mg once daily *Max:* 3 g	1-2 times daily 30 minutes before a meal Hypoglycemia, weight gain
Chlorpropamide (Diabinese) 100, 250, 500 mg	*Init:* 100-250 mg/d *Max:* 750 mg/d	With breakfast or first main meal Hypoglycemia, weight gain Very long-acting; use lower doses and with caution in elderly or in those with renal impairment
Second-Generation (Half Maximum Dose Typically Provides Most of Benefit)		
Glimepiride (Amaryl) 1, 2, 4 mg	*Init:* 1-2 mg once daily *Max:* 8 mg once daily	With breakfast or first main meal Hypoglycemia, weight gain May be preferred in elderly
Glipizide (Glucotrol) 5, 10 mg	*Init:* 2.5-5 mg once daily *Max:* 40 mg in two divided doses	30 minutes before breakfast or first main meal Doses greater than 15 mg/d, divide into b.i.d. doses Hypoglycemia, weight gain May be preferred in elderly
Glipizide extended release (Glucotrol XL) 2.5, 5, 10 mg	*Init:* 5 mg once daily 2.5 mg once daily (elderly) *Max:* 20 mg once daily	With breakfast or first main meal Hypoglycemia, weight gain
Glyburide micronized (Glynase) 1.5, 3, 4.5, 6 mg	*Init:* 0.75-3 mg once daily *Max:* 12 mg once daily or two divided doses	With breakfast or first main meal Hypoglycemia, weight gain
Glyburide (Micronase/DiaBeta) 1.25, 2.5, 5 mg	*Init:* 1.25-5 mg once *Max:* 20 mg/d or two divided doses	With breakfast or first main meal Doses greater than 10 mg/d, divide into b.i.d. doses Hypoglycemia, weight gain
Meglitinides and Phenylalanine Derivatives (Short-Acting Secretagogues)		
Monitor FPG in 2 weeks, HbA$_{1c}$ 3-6 months HbA$_{1c}$ ↓ 1.7%-1.9% primary therapy		
Repaglinide (Prandin) 0.5, 1, 2 mg	*Init:* 0.5 mg t.i.d. in newly treated, elderly, or HbA$_{1c}$ less than 8% 1-2 mg t.i.d. in previously treated or HbA$_{1c}$ greater than 8% *Max:* 16 mg/d	15-30 minutes before each meal Hypoglycemia
Nateglinide (Starlix) 60-120 mg	*Init:* 120 mg t.i.d. *Max:* 120 mg t.i.d.	15-30 min before each meal Hypoglycemia
Biguanides		
Decrease hepatic glucose production; exact mechanism unclear Start with initial dose and titrate up—maximum effective dose, 2 g/d Serum creatinine at initiation, periodically Monitor FPG in 2 weeks, HbA$_{1c}$ in 3-6 months HbA$_{1c}$ ↓ 1%-2%		
Metformin (Glucophage) 500, 850, 1000 mg	*Init:* 500 mg b.i.d. or 850 mg q AM *Max:* 2550 mg in two-three doses	With meals Gastrointestinal effects: abdominal cramping, diarrhea; dose related; titrate dose slowly
Metformin long acting (Glucophage XR) 500 gm	*Init:* 500 mg each evening *Max:* 2000 mg once daily	Lactic acidosis
Metformin liquid (Riomet) 500 mg/5 ml	*Init:* 500 mg once daily *Max:* 2550 mg 2-3 times in divided doses	Discontinued before surgery or studies with contrast agent Contraindicated: Serum creatinine ≥1.5 mg/dl in men, 1.4 mg/dl in women History of liver disease, heart failure with drug prescription, metabolic acidosis, alcohol abuse (binge drinker)

*Consult guidelines for comprehensive review of indications, use, and clinical follow-up recommendations.
Data from Spratto GR, Woods AL: *PDR nurses drug handbook,* Clifton Park, NY, 2004, Thomson Delmar Learning; American Association of Clinical Endocrinologists: *Guidelines pocketcard: managing diabetes mellitus type 2,* version 3.1, 2005; and Lebovitz HE: Med Clin North Am 88:847-863, 2004.

Continued

■ ■ ■

TABLE 37-3 ORAL ANTIHYPERGLYCEMIC AGENTS—cont'd

GENERIC (BRAND) HOW SUPPLIED	DOSE INITIAL (Init) MAXIMUM (Max)	COMMENTS/POTENTIAL ADVERSE EFFECTS
Thiazolidinediones Insulin sensitizers Decrease in glucose may take 4 weeks; maximum efficacy of dose may take 4-6 months Alanine transaminase (ALT) at baseline, q 2 months × 1 year, then periodically HbA_{1c} ↓ 0.7%-1.75% (pioglitazone—baseline then annually)		
Rosiglitazone (Avandia) 2, 4, 8 mg	*Init:* 4 mg/d or 2 mg b.i.d. *Max:* 8 mg/d or 4 mg b.i.d.	May be taken without regard to meals Monitor for weight gain/edema Contraindicated in New York Heart Association (NYHA) class III or IV congestive heart failure (CHF)
Pioglitazone (Actos) 15, 30, 45 mg	*Init:* 15 or 30 mg once daily *Max:* 45 mg once daily	Contraindicated when ALT greater than 2.5 times upper limits of normal, hepatic disease, alcohol abuse
Combination Drugs		
Glyburide + metformin (Glucovance) 1.5/250, 2.5/500, 5/500 mg Glipizide + metformin (Metaglip)	*Init:* 1.25/250 mg once daily or b.i.d. *Max:* 20/2000 mg daily in divided doses *Init:* 2.5/250 mg once daily or b.i.d. *Max:* 20/2000 mg daily in divided doses	Starting doses should not exceed daily doses of either drug already taken; increase dose at 2-week intervals Gastrointestinal effects: abdominal cramping, diarrhea; titrate dose slowly Lactic acidosis Discontinued before surgery or studies with contrast agent Contraindicated: Serum creatinine ≥1.5 mg/dl in men, 1.4 mg/dl in women Hypoglycemia
Rosglitazone + metformin (Avandamet) 1/500, 2/500, 4/500, 2/1000, 4/1000 mg Pioglitzone + metformin (Actoplus Met) 15/500, 15/850	*Init:* 2/500 mg b.i.d. *Max:* 4/1000 b.i.d. *Init:* One once daily or b.i.d. *Max:* 45/2550 daily in divided doses	The selection of the dose should be based on the patient's current doses of glitazone and/or metformin Check serum creatinine and ALT initially Weight gain, edema Contraindicated with NYHA class III or IV CHF Contraindicated when ALT greater than 2.5 times upper limit of normal, liver disease, alcohol abuse Gastrointestinal effects: abdominal cramping, diarrhea; titrate dose slowly Lactic acidosis: discontinue before surgery or studies with dyes Contraindicated: Serum creatinine ≥1.5 mg/dl in men, 1.4 mg/dl in women
Alpha-Glucosidase Inhibitors Inhibit starch breakdown, attenuate postprandial hyperglycemia. Start with low dose and titrate slowly Monitor HbA_{1c} 3-6 months HbA_{1c} ↓ 0.5%-1.0%		
Acarbose (Precose) 25, 50, 100 mg	*Init:* 25 mg t.i.d. (begin once daily for 2 weeks; then b.i.d., then t.i.d.) *Max:* 100 mg t.i.d.; 50 mg t.i.d. if greater than 60 kg	With first bite of each main meal Gastrointestinal: abdominal discomfort, flatulence; diarrhea decreases over time Titrate dose slowly May ↑ ALT/aspartate transaminase–dose related Oral glucose (dextrose) must be used for treatment of hypoglycemia (may occur if Precose used with sulfonylurea or insulin)
Miglitol (Glyset) 25, 50, 100 mg	*Init:* 25 mg t.i.d. Increase dose as tolerated over 3 weeks *Max:* 100 mg t.i.d.	Gastrointestinal: abdominal discomfort, flatulence, diarrhea; abdominal pain and diarrhea decrease over time. Titrate dose slowly Oral glucose (dextrose) must be used for treatment of hypoglycemia (may occur if miglitol is used with sulfonylurea or insulin)

ALT, Alanine transaminase.

production. Reducing circulating FFAs is thought to be another mechanism of action. Reduction in weight or no additional weight gain with improved glucose control and a decrease in elevated plasma triglycerides and LDL cholesterol are additional benefits noted with this drug.[68,69]

Thiazolidinediones

Thiazolidinediones are a new class of drugs known to increase insulin sensitivity by decreasing peripheral insulin resistance and improving insulin action. The mechanism of action is through activation of nuclear receptors called peroxisome proliferator-activated receptors (**PPAR**). The three subtypes of these receptors are PPAR-α, PPAR-γ and PPAR-δ. Data suggest that the thiazolidinediones bind and activate the PPAR-γ subtype.[70] When PPARs are activated, they increase gene transcription for the specific PPAR subtype. Maximum benefit on glucose metabolism may not be seen until 3 to 6 weeks after starting treatment because of their mechanism of action. In addition to glucose lowering, other benefits associated with this class of drugs include improved lipid profile and endothelial function.[71-73] Results of ongoing long-term trials will determine whether benefits of treatment with thiazolidinediones will affect CVD events in the insulin-resistant person with or without type 2 diabetes.

Alpha-Glucosidase Inhibitors

Alpha-glucosidase inhibitors delay carbohydrate absorption in the small intestine and digestion, resulting in lower postprandial glucose elevations. Because of their mechanism of action, they should be taken within the first 15 minutes of a major meal. Starting therapy with low doses can help diminish the gastrointestinal side effects of flatulence and diarrhea. Doses should be adjusted slowly each week based on tolerance and the 1-hour postprandial plasma glucose result.

A recent study comparing the alpha-glucosidase inhibitor arcabose to placebo in a sample with impaired glucose tolerance demonstrated a significant 36 percent reduction in the rate of type 2 diabetes development, even after adjusting for weight loss. Other changes observed in this study were a decrease in hypertension and cardiovascular complications.[74]

Synthetic Analog of Human Amylin

Amylin, a naturally occurring 37-amino acid peptide discovered in 1987, is located in the beta cells of the pancreas (Table 37-4). Normally, amylin works with insulin to suppress postprandial glucagon secretion. In patients with advanced type 2 diabetes or type 1 diabetes, the beta cells in the pancreas are damaged or destroyed, resulting in reduced secretion of insulin and amylin after meals. The synthetic analog of human amylin has several mechanisms of action, including modulation of gastric emptying, prevention of postprandial rise in plasma glucagons, and satiety leading to a decrease in caloric intake and potential weight loss. This new therapy is used for treatment of type 1 or type 2 diabetes.[75]

Glucagon-like Protein 1

The hormone glucagon-like protein 1, naturally found in the gut, enhances insulin secretion from beta cells in the pancreas associated with oral caloric intake (Table 37-5). Glucagon-like protein 1 also moderates glucagon secretion and lowers serum glucagon concentrations during periods of hyperglycemia. These effects decrease hepatic glucose output and insulin demand but do not impair the normal glucagon response to hypoglycemia. Another mechanism of action is the slowing of gastric emptying and related satiety, resulting in reduced food intake and potential weight loss. Current use is in patients with type 2 diabetes as adjunctive therapy to metformin, a thiazolidinedione, or a combination of metformin and a sulfonylurea or metformin and a thiazolidinedione when glycemic control has not been achieved.[76]

■ ■ ■

TABLE 37-4   SYNTHETIC ANALOG OF HUMAN AMYLIN

Pramlintide Acetate Injection (Symlin)
For use in patients with diabetes treated with insulin.
Give separately; cannot be mixed with insulin.
When starting Symlin, reduction in initial insulin dose is required

Mechanism of action	Modulation of gastric emptying
	Prevention of postprandial rise in plasma glucagon
	Satiety, leading to decreased caloric intake and potential weight loss
Adverse effects	Severe hypoglycemia, generally seen 3 hours after injection
	Nausea (may decrease with time)
Type 2 diabetes mellitus	Initial dose is 60 mcg subcutaneously, increased to 120 mcg as tolerated.
	Reduce preprandial, rapid-acting, or short-acting insulin doses, including fixed-mix insulins by 50%.
	Monitor blood glucose frequently including before and after meals and bedtime.
	Refer to Symlin drug administration for dosing information, precautions, and safety information.
Type 1 diabetes mellitus	Initial dose is 15 mcg subcutaneously.
	Before major meals, titrate gradually: 30, 45, or 60 mcg as tolerated.
	Monitor blood glucose frequently including before and after meals and bedtime.
	Reduce preprandial, rapid-acting, or short-acting insulin doses, including fix-mix insulins by 50%.
	Refer to Symlin drug administration for dosing information, precautions, and safety information.

Adapted from Amylin Pharmaceuticals: *Symlin (pramlintide acetate)*. Retrieved April 22, 2005, from www.amylin.com/pipeline/symlin.cfm

---

■ ■ ■

TABLE 37-5   INCRETIN MIMETIC AGENT

Exenatide Injection (Byetta)
For an adjunctive therapy for type 2 diabetes mellitus in patients who are taking metformin, a sulfonylurea, or a combination of both and are not achieving glycemic control.

Mechanism of action	Enhances glucose-dependent insulin secretion from the beta cells
	Moderates glucagon secretion and lowers serum glucagon concentrations during periods of hyperglycemia, leading to decreased hepatic glucose output and decreased insulin demand
	(Does not impair the normal glucagon response to hypoglycemia)
	Slows gastric emptying
	Reduces food intake
Adverse effects	Hypoglycemia (moderate to mild) in patients treated with Byetta and a sulfonylurea or a combination of sulfonylurea and metformin
	Rare in combination with metformin alone (similar to placebo and metformin)
	Nausea—mild to moderate and dose dependent, decreasing over time in most patients
Dosage	Subcutaneous injection in thigh, abdomen, or upper arm
	Initial dose is 5 mcg b.i.d. at any time within a 60-minute period *before* the morning and evening meals. Do not administer *after* a meal.
	May increase dose to 10 mcg b.i.d. after 1 month of therapy
	When Byetta is added to metformin, the current metformin dose does not need to be adjusted.
	When Byetta is added to a sulfonylurea, the sulfonylurea dose may need to be decreased to reduce risk of hypoglycemia.

Adapted from Amylin Pharmaceuticals: *Byetta exenatide injection*, 2006. Retrieved June 30, 2005, from http://pi.lilly.com/us/byetta-pi.pdf

Dipeptidyl Peptidase-4 Inhibitor

This new class of drugs is felt to inhibit the enzyme dipeptidyl peptidase-4 and thereby slow the inactivation of the incretin hormones such as the glucagon- like protein 1 and the glucose-dependent insulinotropic polypeptide. Concentrations of these incretin hormones are then enhanced and their action prolonged resulting in increases insulin release and decreases in glucagon levels in the circulation in a glucose –dependent manner. These actions reduce glucose levels in patients with type 2 diabetes. Currently this drug is approved for use either as monotherapy, or as combination therapy when added to either metformin or a thiazolidinedione.[77]

Human Insulin and Insulin Analogs

Pharmacological therapy with exogenous insulin is essential for those with type 1 diabetes but also can be used in those with type 2 diabetes who have not achieved recommended glucose goals with oral therapy. Insulin has been available since the 1920s, but in the past several years, there has been an increase in different formulations (Table 37-6). These formulations may allow better glucose control with fewer episodes of hypoglycemia. The commonly available insulins range from rapid-acting to long-acting forms. Because hypoglycemia is the most common side effect of insulin therapy, self-monitoring of glucose level and knowledge of the signs and symptoms of hypoglycemia and treatment are crucial in this patient population.[78] (See the accompanying Conundrum feature.)

With the availability of human insulin, there are fewer problems with insulin allergies and resistance, but these problems still exist in a small population of persons with diabetes. The most likely cause is an immunological reaction with antibodies produced from the insulin.[79]

BEYOND GLUCOSE CONTROL: INTERACTION OF CARDIOVASCULAR RISK FACTORS

The major cause of death in persons with diabetes is CVD; 65 percent of deaths are from heart disease and stroke. Adults with diabetes have heart disease death rates 2 to 4 times higher than adults without diabetes (Figure 37-6). These data were instrumental in changing diabetes from a risk factor to a CHD risk equivalent in the third report of the NCEP ATP III guidelines.[9,80]

In the Multiple Risk Factor Intervention Trial (**MRFIT**), after 12 years of follow-up, even when adjusting for known CVD risk factors, men with diabetes had an absolute risk of CAD death 3 times greater than those without diabetes. This was true for all age groups and ethnic backgrounds.[81] Women typically develop CAD approximately 10 years after men, but this gender differ-

---

■■■ CONUNDRUM

DOES STRICT GLUCOSE CONTROL LEAD TO HYPOGLYCEMIA UNAWARENESS?

The challenge faced by patients with diabetes, particularly those who manage their diabetes with insulin, is the difficulty of maintaining blood glucose within normal levels on a minute-to-minute basis. This complicated balancing act involves an interaction between dietary intake (particularly carbohydrate intake), insulin dose, and physical activity that modulates insulin sensitivity.

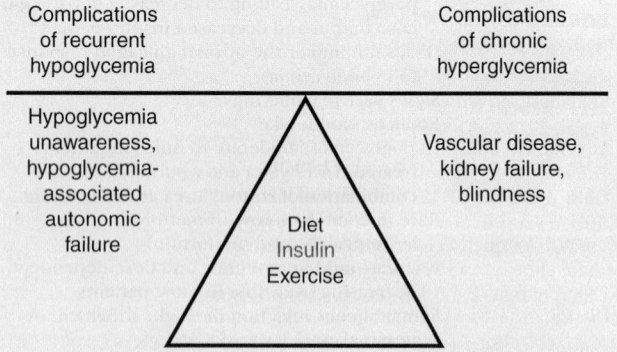

Complications of recurrent hypoglycemia — Complications of chronic hyperglycemia

Hypoglycemia unawareness, hypoglycemia-associated autonomic failure — Vascular disease, kidney failure, blindness

Diet Insulin Exercise

Among providers, there is little recognition of the complications of recurrent hypoglycemia that patients experience when adhering to intensive insulin therapy for diabetes. For example, in the DCCT, patients randomized to the intensive management group had 3 times as many episodes of severe hypoglycemia as patients in the control group. The phenomenon of hypoglycemia-associated autonomic failure is observed in many patients using insulin therapy to achieve good glycemic control. Presumably because of recurrent episodes of hypoglycemia, these patients have reduced autonomic and endocrine responses to hypoglycemia. Successive episodes of hypoglycemia provoke less and less epinephrine secretion, sweating, palpitations, hunger, and other hypoglycemic warning symptoms. For this reason, many patients with insulin-managed diabetes develop hypoglycemia unawareness because of loss of the autonomically mediated warning signs of hypoglycemia. This condition is worsened in patients who develop diabetic autonomic neuropathy.

Over time, patients drop to lower and lower levels of blood glucose before symptoms occur and, in some cases, a patient's hypoglycemic episode is identified by a family member or coworker rather than the patient himself or herself. The specter of hypoglycemia unawareness can lead to a fear of hypoglycemia that represents a significant barrier to treatment adherence with optimal diabetes management. Patients with fear of hypoglycemia may maintain higher than recommended glucose levels in order to avoid hypoglycemia, even though they understand the serious long-term consequences of chronic hyperglycemia.

Current research on mechanisms of hypoglycemia-associated autonomic failure includes the use of animal models of recurrent hypoglycemia. This research shows that after exposing a rat to even a single episode of hypoglycemia, the rat has blunted epinephrine secretion to a second episode of hypoglycemia 2 to 3 days later. Additional findings from this research indicate that the initial hypoglycemic episode causes the death of a small number of cells, apparently neurons, in a region of cerebral cortex that is associated with autonomic control and visceral perception. Thus, the defect of hypoglycemia unawareness may be caused by actual loss of neurons that are specialized to sense the peripheral signals produced by hypoglycemia and to alert the patient to seek food.

Bibliography
Tkacs NC, Dunn-Meynell AA, Levin BE: Presumed apoptosis and reduced arcuate nucleus neuropeptide Y and pro-opiomelanocortin mRNA in non-coma hypoglycemia, *Diabetes* 49:820-826, 2000.

Tkacs NC, Pan Y, Raghupathi R et al: Cortical Fluoro-Jade staining and blunted adrenomedullary response to hypoglycemia after noncoma hypoglycemia in rats, *J Cerebral Blood Flow Metab* 25:1645-1655, 2005.

(Courtesy of Nancy Tkacs, University of Pennsylvania.)

■ ■ ■

TABLE 37-6   HUMAN INSULIN AND INSULIN ANALOGS

INSULIN TYPE	ONSET	PEAK (hour)	DURATION (hour)
Rapid-Acting			
Lispro (Humalog)	5-15 minutes	1	4-5
Aspart (Novolog)	5-15 minutes	1	4-5
Glulisine (Apidra)	5-15 minutes	1	4-5
Short-Acting			
Regular	30-60 minutes	2-4	6-10
Intermediate-Acting			
NPH	1-3 hours	5-7	10-20
Long-Acting, Basal			
Glargine (Lantus)	1-2 hours	Flat	~24
Detemir (Levemir)	2-4 hours	6-14	~20-24
Combinations			
Aspart-protamine 70/30	15 minutes	2-4	10-16
NPH/regular 70/30	30-60 minutes	Dual	14-18
Lispro pen (lispro protamine suspension) 75/25	Less than 15 minutes	Dual	10-16

Time of action may vary in patients or at different times in same patient. Lente, ultralente, and animal source insulin are no longer available in the United States.

Glargine should not be mixed with other insulins.

If Levemir is mixed with other insulin preparations, the profile of action of one or both individual components will change. Mixing Levemir with a rapid-acting insulin analog should be avoided. (See *Levemir: European Public Assessment Report.* Retrieved July 13, 2005, from www.emea.eu.int/humandocs/Humans/EPAR/levemir/levemir.htm)

Data from American Association of Clinical Endocrinologists: *Guidelines pocketcard: managing diabetes mellitus type 2,* version 3.1, 2005; Lebovitz H: Cleve Clin J Med 69:809-820, 2002; and Insulins commonly used in the United States [table], *Diabetes Care* Jan 2005. Retrieved April 22, 2005, from www.diabetes.org/uedocuments/rg05insulins.pdf

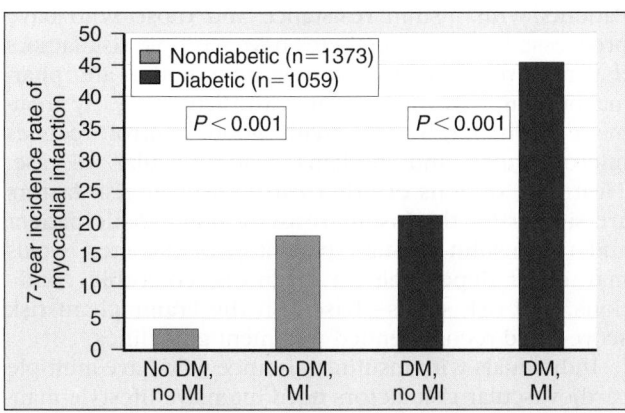

FIGURE 37-6 ■ Increased risk for myocardial infarction in those with diabetes. *DM,* Diabetes mellitus; *MI,* myocardial infarction. (From Beckman JA, Libby P, Creager MA: Diabetes mellitus, the metabolic syndrome, and atherosclerotic vascular disease. In Zipes DP, Libby P, Bonow RO, Braunwald E, editors: *Braunwald's heart disease,* ed 7, Philadelphia, 2005, Elsevier.)

ence is not true in women with diabetes. Women with type 2 diabetes have a relatively greater risk of CVD than men. The risk ratio for increased mortality is 2.4 for men with diabetes and 3.5 for women with diabetes. But the absolute rates of CVD are higher in men than women and increase with age.[82] The absolute risk for CVD appears to vary in different ethnic groups with diabetes. Mexican Americans appear to have a slightly lower absolute risk for CVD compared with the general U.S. population. Compared with non-Hispanic white Americans, blacks have similar rates of CVD.[83]

In all forms of CVD—MI, cerebrovascular disease, peripheral vascular disease, and heart failure—the prevalence, incidence, and mortality are increased in persons with diabetes compared with nondiabetic persons. Women with diabetes appear to have an increase in risk of stroke and a higher mortality versus men with diabetes.[84] As seen in Figure 37-2, risk factors for CVD in the patient with diabetes go beyond glucose control. Other major risk factors include atherogenic dyslipidemia, hypertension, prothrombotic state, smoking, obesity, and physical inactivity. A healthful lifestyle is the cornerstone of therapy for persons with diabetes, but most will need adjunct pharmacotherapy to decrease their elevated risk for CVD.

Dyslipidemia

The cause of the atherogenic lipid and lipoprotein abnormalities associated with diabetes and insulin resistance—high triglycerides, low HDL, remnant lipoproteins, and small dense LDL—is complex. Insulin resistance plays a role, with the inability of muscle to take up glucose and an inhibition of lipolysis in adipose tissue. The increase in ambient insulin and FFA levels increases hepatic production of VLDL and increases the pool size of plasma triglycerides.[85,86] Some investigators speculate that in the presence of insulin resistance, besides an increase in triglyceride pool size, there is a problem with clearance of these particles.[87] A low HDL level is almost always associated with elevated triglycerides mediated by the cholesterol ester transfer protein exchanging cholesterol from HDL to VLDL in exchange for triglycerides.[86]

Pharmacotherapy

Large clinical trials using 3-hydroxy-3-methylglutaryl-coenzyme A reductase inhibitors (statin drugs), which included persons with diabetes, have shown that lowering the LDL cholesterol level reduces CVD risk even better in diabetic populations than in nondiabetic populations. For example, in the Scandinavian Simvastatin Survival Study, there was a 43 percent reduction in total mortality among diabetic persons compared with a 29 percent reduction in the nondiabetic cohort. MI was reduced by 55 percent in the diabetic population versus 32 percent in the nondiabetic population.[88] The Cholesterol and Recurrent Events (**CARE**) trial reported that among 586 individuals with diabetes there was a significant relative risk reduction (25 percent) in coronary events.[89] The absolute risk of coronary event was greater (8.3 percent) in this population versus the nondiabetic population using pravastatin therapy (5.2 percent). Most recently the Heart Protection Study (**HPS**), the largest lipid trial to date, which included almost 6000 subjects with diabetes, found that treatment with 40 mg of simvastatin, regardless of the baseline level of LDL, decreased risk of CHD death, nonfatal MI, stroke, or revascularization by 25 percent in the diabetic group. Even those individuals with LDL levels less than 100 mg/dl had a similar risk reduction benefit.[90]

The HPS trial was instrumental in changing the American Diabetes Association guidelines for the treatment of dyslipidemia in persons with diabetes.[29] The HPS was also one of the trials that prompted an update to the NCEP ATP III guidelines. For patients with diabetes and CHD, an LDL cholesterol level less than 70 mg/dl is now an optional goal in these very high-risk individuals.[91] Besides lowering LDL cholesterol level, statins also lower remnant lipoproteins in the diabetic population and the nondiabetic insulin-resistant population.[92]

Fibrates also influence CVD risk. The Veterans Affairs High-Density Lipoprotein Cholesterol Intervention Trial (**VA-HIT**) using gemfibrozil for treatment of low HDL (typical of the atherogenic dyslipidemia accompanying elevated triglycerides in type 2 diabetes) was associated with a statistically significant 24 percent risk reduction for MI in those with diabetes.[93] In the Diabetes Atherosclerosis Intervention Study (**DAIS**) using fenofibrate, there was a decrease in progression of CAD lesions, although the decrease did not reach statistical significance because of the small sample size.[94]

Niacin, used to increase HDL cholesterol level, lower triglyceride level, and modestly lower LDL cholesterol level, would appear to be the ideal therapeutic treatment in this population. One precaution is that niacin may worsen insulin resistance and increase glucose levels. In the Arterial Disease Multiple Intervention Trial (**ADMIT**), lipid abnormalities were improved with niacin therapy in persons with diabetes. Although glucose levels did increase, the increase did not reach statistical significance. Glucose levels were managed with adjustments to glucose-lowering medications.[95] Many patients need combination therapy to reach treatment goals.

Hypertension

One possible mechanism responsible for hypertension in the insulin-resistant person is the impact of chronic hyperinsulinemia on certain insulin-sensitive tissues such as the kidney and the sympathetic nervous system. The hyperinsulinemic state is thought to increase sympathetic nervous system activity, which in turn can increase heart rate, cardiac output, vascular resistance, and sodium retention. These mechanisms increase the risk of developing hypertension.[96]

Hypertension affects 20 to 60 percent of persons with diabetes and adds to their increased risk for CVD and nephropathy. In type 1 diabetes, hypertension may be a result of nephropathy. Achieving blood glucose control may be instrumental in preserving renal function, which in turn may contribute to better blood pressure control.[97] Numerous trials in hypertensive patients with diabetes confirm the importance of reducing elevated blood pressure to lower CVD risk. The UKPDS and Hypertension Optimal Treatment (**HOT**) trials provided evidence that lowering blood pressure decreases the rate of CVD complications compared with moderate control of blood pressure.[98,99]

Blood pressure control reduces CVD events and diabetes deaths and is imperative in this patient population. Current guidelines from the *Seventh Report of the Joint National Committee on Prevention, Detention, Evaluation, and Treatment of High Blood Pressure* for hypertensive patients without diabetes or kidney disease specify a goal of less than 140/90 mm Hg. For persons with diabetes, the recommended blood pressure is less than 130/80 mm Hg.[29] The choice of medication for controlling blood pressure in the patient with diabetes may not be as important as once thought. Use of low-dose diuretics, beta blockers, angiotensin-converting enzyme (ACE) inhibitors, angiotensin II receptor blockers (ARBs), or calcium channel blockers has been found to be effective and safe in lowering blood pressure.[98,100] Most patients with diabetes will need three or more medications to reach treatment goals.[98,100] Recommendations are to begin with a diuretic and then add an ACE inhibitor, ARB, beta blocker, or calcium channel blocker as needed.[101] Initiating therapy with an ACE inhibitor or ARB is recommended when microabuminuria is present.[29]

Antiplatelet Therapy

In individuals without diabetes, the general recommendation is to prescribe aspirin when the CHD risk is greater than 10 percent, provided blood pressure is controlled.[102] Unless contraindicated, aspirin is recommended in the person with diabetes and CHD. Specific recommendations and treatment goals for those with diabetes but without CHD are provided in Table 37-7.

CONCLUSION

Patients with insulin resistance and those who have progressed to type 2 diabetes have multiple risk factors that require aggressive lifestyle intervention and pharmacotherapy. In the patient with diabetes, early treatment of hyperglycemia with good control reduces microvascular and perhaps macrovascular disease. Treatment options of other cardiovascular risk factors are similar for the insulin-resistant nondiabetic patient and the insulin-resistant patient with diabetes. Goals may differ depending on diagnosis, comorbid conditions, and risk status—based on the Framingham risk score—and recommended treatment guidelines.

Individuals with insulin resistance who have multiple cardiovascular risk factors need intensive lifestyle management and, most likely, pharmacotherapy. Those who progress to type 2 diabetes increase their CVD risk status to a coronary heart risk equivalent. Management of these individuals is complex and involves multiple disciplines. Patients must overcome many psychological, social, and economic burdens. Providers must overcome time barriers in an attempt to help patients understand the health problems associated with insulin resistance and diabetes and the importance of achieving treatment goals.

Using a team approach in caring for these complex individuals has worked well in the diabetes commu-

■ ■ ■

TABLE 37-7   RISK FACTORS AND THERAPEUTIC GOALS FOR ADULTS WITH DIABETES

RISK FACTORS	GOALS FOR ADULTS WITH DIABETES
A. Hemoglobin A_{1c}	Less than 7%
Glycemic control	Less than 6% considered on individual basis
Capillary plasma glucose	Preprandial: 90-130 mg/dl (5-7.2 mmol/liter)
	Postprandial: less than 180 mg/dl (less than 10.0 mmol/liter)
	1-2 hours after beginning a meal
Antiplatelet agents	
Aspirin	75-162 mg daily for those with CVD or increased risk of CVD (over age 40 or additional risk factors such as hypertension, smoking, dyslipidemia, albuminuria, or family history of CVD)
B. Blood pressure	Blood pressure less than 130/80 mm Hg
	All patients with diabetes and hypertension should be treated with an angiotensin-converting enzyme inhibitor or angiotensin II receptor blocker.
C. Cholesterol	
Dyslipidemia	LDL less than 100 mg/dl (less than 2.6 mmol/liter)
	HDL greater than 40 mg/dl (greater than 1.1 mmol/liter)
	Consider greater than 50 mg/dl in women.
	Triglycerides less than 150 mg/dl (less than 1.7mmol/liter)
	Non-HDL: 30 mg/dl higher than LDL goal
	In patients older than age 40 without CVD, begin statin therapy to achieve 30%-40% decrease in LDL regardless of baseline LDL.
	In patients younger than age 40 without CVD but with CVD risk factors or increased duration of diabetes, treat to LDL goal of less than 100 mg/dl.
	In patients with overt CVD, treat with lifestyle and statin to reduce LDL 30%-40%. An LDL goal of less than 70 mg/dl using high-dose statin is an option.
D. Diet	Individualized nutritional assessment, recommendations, and instruction by registered dietitian.
	Low-carbohydrate diets (restricting total carbohydrates to less than 130 g/d) are not recommended.
	Cholesterol less than 300 mg/d (less than 200 mg/d if LDL cholesterol is 100 mg/dl or more)
Weight loss	Weight loss recommended for BMI of 25 kg/m² or higher
E. Exercise	A regular physical activity program adapted for complications. If able, at least 150 min/wk, moderate intensity, distributed over 3 to 7 d/wk
S. Smoking	Complete cessation

CVD, Cardiovascular disease; *LDL,* low-density lipoprotein; *HDL,* high-density lipoprotein; *BMI,* body mass index.
Adapted from American Diabetes Association: *Diabetes Care* 29:S4-S42, 2006.

nity.[29] Using outside referral resources such as dietitians (if not available in an office setting), community health facilities, or cardiac rehabilitation programs can enhance the care provided. Providing patients with realistic lifestyle goals, follow-up visits to monitor risk factors, and contracts for behavior modification can be useful. Achieving treatment goals early helps patients with diabetes avoid complications and assists them in achieving better health outcomes.

Future studies and newer medications will pave the way to new treatments and, hopefully, better outcomes. Although promising, new data will not guarantee treatment goals unless health care professionals overcome the many barriers that are present. Even now, with current pharmacopeias, health care professionals cannot reach treatment goals. Trials such as the diabetes prevention trials should continue to motivate providers to persevere on lifestyle intervention in conjunction with pharmacotherapy. The message to patients must be caring, consistent, and receptive to their needs, working cooperatively with them as part of the team for risk factor management and prevention of CVD.

REFERENCES

1. Reaven G: The Banting Lecture: the role of insulin resistance in human disease, *Diabetes* 37:1596-1607, 1988.
2. Reaven G: Pathophysiology of insulin resistance in human disease, *Physiol Rev* 75:473-486, 1995.
3. ACE position statement on the insulin resistance syndrome, *Endocr Pract* 9(S2):5-21, 2003.
4. Reaven G: The metabolic syndrome or the insulin resistance syndrome? different names, different concepts, and different goals, *Endocrinol Metab Clin North Am* 33:283-303, 2004.
5. Furberg A-S, Veierød MB, Wilsgaard T et al: Serum high density lipoprotein cholesterol, metabolic profile, and breast cancer risk, *J Natl Cancer Inst* 96:1152-1160, 2004.
6. Alberti KG, Zimmet PZ: Definition, diagnosis and classification of diabetes mellitus and its complications. Part 1. Diagnosis and classification of diabetes mellitus provisional report of a WHO consultation, *Diabet Med* 15:539-553, 1998.
7. World Health Organization: *Definition, diagnosis and classification of diabetes mellitus and its complications. Part 1: Diagnosis and classification of diabetes mellitus,* Geneva, 1999, Department of Noncommunicable Disease Surveillance.
8. Balkau B, Charles MA: Comment on the provisional report from the WHO consultation: European Group for the Study of Insulin Resistance (EGIR), *Diabet Med* 16:442-443, 1999.
9. Adult Treatment Panel III: Executive summary of the Third Report of the National Cholesterol Education Program (NCEP) Expert Panel on Detection, Evaluation, and Treatment of High Blood Cholesterol in Adults, *JAMA* 285:2486-2497, 2001.
10. Grundy SM, Brewer HB Jr, Cleeman JI et al, for Conference Participants: Definition of metabolic syndrome: report of the National Heart, Lung, and Blood Institute/American Heart Association conference on scientific issues related to definition, *Circulation* 109:433-438, 2004.
11. Grundy S, Hansen B, Smith S et al, for Conference Participants: Clinical management of metabolic syndrome: report of the American Heart Association/National Heart, Lung, and Blood Institute/American Diabetes Association conference on scientific issues related to management, *Circulation* 109:551-556, 2004.
12. The International Diabetes Federation consensus worldwide definition of the metabolic syndrome. Retrieved 4/16/07. http://www.idf.org/webdata/docs//MetSyndrome_FINAL.pdf.

13. Ford ES, Giles WH, Dietz WH: Prevalence of the metabolic syndrome among US adults: findings from the Third National Health and Nutrition Examination Survey, *JAMA* 287(3):356-359, 2002.

14. Ford E: Insulin resistance syndrome: the public health challenge, *Endocr Pract* 9(S2):23-25, 2003.

15. Ford E, Giles W: A comparison of the prevalence of the metabolic syndrome using two proposed definitions, *Diabetes Care* 26:575-581, 2003.

16. Grundy S, Cleeman J, Daniels S et al; American Heart Association; National Heart, Lung, and Blood Institute: Diagnosis and management of the metabolic syndrome: an American Heart Association/National Heart, Lung, and Blood Institute scientific statement, *Circulation* 112:2735-2752, 2005.

17. Kahn R, Buse J, Ferrannini E et al: The metabolic syndrome: time for a critical appraisal, *Diabetes Care* 28:2289-2304, 2005.

18. Ninomiya J, L'Italien G, Criqui M et al: Association of the metabolic syndrome with history of myocardial infarction and stroke in the Third National Health and Nutrition Examination Survey, *Circulation* 109:42-46, 2004.

19. Pyörälä M, Miettinen H, Halonen P et al: Insulin resistance syndrome predicts the risk of coronary heart disease and stroke in healthy middle-aged men: the 22 year follow-up results of the Helsinki Policemen Study, *Arterioscler Thromb Vasc Biol* 20:538-544, 2000.

20. Malik S, Wong N, Granklin S et al: Impact of the metabolic syndrome on mortality from coronary heart disease, cardiovascular disease, and all causes in United States adults, *Circulation* 110:1245-1250, 2004.

21. Fontbonne A, Charles MA, Thibult N et al: Hyperinsulinemia as a predictor of coronary heart disease mortality in a healthy population: the Paris Prospective Study, 15 year follow-up, *Diabetologia* 34:356-361, 1991.

22. Moller LF, Jespersen J: Fasting serum insulin levels and coronary heart disease in a Danish cohort: 17-year follow-up, *J Cardiovasc Risk* 2:235-240, 1995.

23. Despres JP, Lamarche B, Mauriege P et al: Hyperinsulinemia as an independent risk factor for ischemic heart disease, *N Engl J Med* 334:952-957, 1996.

24. Pyörälä M, Miettinen H, Laakso M et al: Hyperinsulinemia predicts coronary heart disease risk in healthy middle-aged men: the 22-year follow-up results of the Helsinki Policemen Study, *Circulation* 98:398-404, 1998.

25. Yip J, Facchini FS, Reaven GM: Resistance to insulin-mediated glucose disposal as a predictor of cardiovascular disease, *J Clin Endocrinol Metab* 83:2773-2776, 1998.

26. Ferrara A, Barrett-Connor EL, Edelstein SL: Hyperinsulinemia does not increase the risk of fatal cardiovascular disease in elderly men or women without diabetes: the Rancho Bernardo Study, 1984-1991, *Am J Epidemiol* 140:857-869, 1994.

27. Stern M, Mitchell B: Genetics of insulin resistance. In Reaven G, Laws A, editors: *Insulin resistance: the metabolic syndrome X,* Totowa, NJ, 1999, Humana Press.

28. McKeigue P: Ethnic variation in insulin resistance and risk for type 2 diabetes. In Reaven G, Laws A, editors: *Insulin resistance: the metabolic syndrome X,* Totowa, NJ, 1999, Humana Press.

29. American Diabetes Association: Clinical practice recommendations, *Diabetes Care* 29(suppl 1):S4-S42, 2006.

30. Reaven GM: Age and glucose intolerance, *Diabetes Care* 26:539-540, 2003.

31. Iozzo P, Beck-Nielsen H, Laasko M et al: Independent influence of age on basal insulin secretion in nondiabetic humans: European Group for the Study of Insulin Resistance, *J Clin Endocrinol Metab* 84:863-868, 1999.

32. Jones CNO, Pei D, Sturis J et al: Identification of age-related defect in glucose-stimulated insulin secretion in non-diabetic women, *Endocrinol Metab* 4:193-200, 1997.

33. Shepherd P, Kahn B: Glucose transporters and insulin action-implications for insulin resistance and diabetes mellitus, *N Engl J Med* 341:248-257, 1999.

34. Rothman DL, Magnusson I, Cline GW et al: Decreased muscle glucose transport/phosphorylation is an early defect in the pathogenesis of non-insulin-dependent diabetes mellitus, *Proc Natl Acad Sci U S A* 92:983-987, 1995.

35. Perseghin G, Price T, Petersen KF et al: Increased glucose transport-phosphorylation and muscle glycogen synthesis after exercise training in insulin resistant subjects, *N Engl J Med* 335:1357-1362, 1996.

36. Mayer-Davis EJ, D'Agostino R Jr, Karter A et al, for the IRAS Investigators: Intensity and amount of physical activity in relation to insulin sensitivity, *JAMA* 279:669-674, 1998.

37. Dela F, Ploug T, Handberg A et al: Physical training increases muscle GLUT-4 protein and mRNA in patients with NIDDM, *Diabetes* 43:862-865, 1994.

38. Abbasi F, Brown BW, Lamendola C et al: Relationship between obesity, insulin resistance, and coronary heart disease risk, *J Am Coll Cardiol* 40:937-943, 2002.

39. McLaughlin T, Allison G, Abbasi F et al: Prevalence of insulin resistance and associated cardiovascular disease risk factors among normal weight, overweight, and obese individuals, *Metabolism* 53:495-499, 2004.

40. McLaughlin T: Insulin resistance syndrome and obesity, *Endocr Pract* 9(suppl 2):58-62, 2003.

41. McLaughlin T, Abbasi F, Kim HS et al: Relationship between insulin resistance, weight loss, and coronary heart disease risk in healthy, obese women, *Metabolism* 50:795-800, 2001.

42. McLaughlin T, Abbasi F, Lamendola C et al: Metabolic changes following sibutramine-assisted weight loss in obese individuals: role of plasma free fatty acids in the insulin resistance of obesity, *Metabolism* 50:819-824, 2001.

43. McLaughlin T, Abbasi F, Lamendola C et al: Differentiation between obesity and insulin resistance in the association with C-reactive protein, *Circulation* 106:2908-2912, 2002.

44. Reaven GM: Why syndrome X? from Harold Himsworth to the insulin resistance syndrome, *Cell Metab* 1:9-14, 2005.

45. Knowler WC, Barrett-Conner E, Fowler SE et al: Reduction in the incidence of type 2 diabetes with lifestyle interventions or metformin, *N Engl J Med* 346:393-403, 2002.

46. Eschwege E, Richard JL, Thibult N et al: Coronary heart disease mortality in relation with diabetes, blood glucose and plasma insulin levels: the Paris Prospective Study, ten years later, *Horm Metab Res* 17(suppl):41-46, 1995.

47. The DECODE Study Group, on behalf of the European Diabetes Epidemiology Group: Glucose tolerance and cardiovascular mortality: comparison of fasting and 2-hour diagnostic criteria, *Arch Intern Med* 161:397-404, 2001.

48. Saydah SH, Loria CM, Eberhardt MS et al: Subclinical states of glucose intolerance and risk of death in the US, *Diabetes Care* 24:447-453, 2001.

49. Reaven G: The pathophysiology consequence of adipose tissue insulin resistance. In Reaven G, Laws A, editors: *Insulin resistance the metabolic syndrome X,* Totowa, NJ, 1999, Humana Press.

50. Leahy JL, Cooper HE, Deal DA et al: Chronic hyperglycemia is associated with impaired glucose influence on insulin secretion, *J Clin Invest* 77:908-915, 1986.

51. Centers for Disease Control and Prevention: *National diabetes fact sheet: general information and national estimates on diabetes in the United States, 2005,* Atlanta, 2005, US Department of Health and Human Services, Centers for Disease Control and Prevention.

52. Centers for Disease Control and Prevention: *Diabetes surveillance system,* Atlanta, 2003, US Department of Health and Human Services.

53. Mokdad AH, Ford ES, Bowman BA et al: Prevalence of obesity, diabetes, and obesity-related health risk factors, 2001, *JAMA* 289:76-79, 2003.

54. Harris Mi, Flegal KM, Cowie CC et al: Prevalence of diabetes, impaired fasting glucose, and impaired glucose tolerance in US adults: the Third National Health and Nutrition Examination Survey, 1988-1994, *Diabetes Care* 21:518-524, 1998.

55. Engekgay M, Geiss L, Saadine J et al: The evolving diabetes burden in the United States, *Ann Intern Med* 140:945-950, 2004.

56. Zimmet P, Alberti KG, Shaw J: Global and societal implications of the diabetic epidemic, *Nature* 414:782-787, 2001.

57. Pierce M, Keen H, Bradley C: Risk of diabetes in offspring of parents with non-insulin dependent diabetes, *Diabet Med* 12:6-13, 1995.

58. Stumvoll M, Goldstein B, van Haeften TW: Type 2 diabetes: principles of pathogenesis and therapy, *Lancet* 365:1333-1346, 2005.

59. Tuomilehto J, Lindström J, Eriksson JG et al: Prevention of type 2 diabetes mellitus by changes in lifestyle among subjects with impaired glucose tolerance, *N Engl J Med* 344:1343-1350, 2001.

60. Pan XR, Li GW, Hu Y et al: Effects of diet and exercise in preventing NIDDM in people with impaired glucose tolerance: the Da Quing IGT and Diabetes study, *Diabetes Care* 20:537-544, 1999.

61. Knopp RH, Walden CE, Retzlaff BM et al: Long-term cholesterol lowering effects of 4 fat-restricted diets in hypercholesterolemic and combined hyperlipidemic men: the Dietary Alternatives Study, *JAMA* 278:1509-1515, 1997.

62. Abbasi F, McLaughlin T, Lamendola C et al: High carbohydrate diets, triglyceride-rich lipoproteins, and coronary heart disease risk, *Am J Cardiol* 85:45-48, 2000.

63. Diabetes Control and Complications Trial Research Group: The effect of intensive treatment of diabetes on development and progression of long-term complications in insulin-dependent diabetes mellitus, *N Eng J Med* 329:977-986, 1993.

64. Writing team for the Diabetes Control and Complications Trial/Epidemiology of Diabetes Interventions and Complications Research Group: Effect of intensive therapy on the microvascular complications of type 1 diabetes mellitus, *JAMA* 287:2563-2569, 2002.

65. Selvin E, Marinopoulos S, Berkenblit G et al: Meta-analysis: glycosylated hemoglobin and cardiovascular disease in diabetes mellitus, *Ann Intern Med* 141:421-431, 2004.

66. Nathan DM, Lachin J, Cleary P et al; Diabetes Control and Complications Trial; Epidemiology of Diabetes Interventions and Complications Research Group: Intensive diabetes therapy on carotid intima-media thickness in type 1 diabetes mellitus, *N Eng J Med* 348:2294-2303, 2003.

67. Lebovitz HE: Insulin secretogogues: sulfonylureas, meglitinides and phenylalanine derivatives. In LeRoith D, Taylor SI, Olefsky JR, editors: *Diabetes mellitus: a fundamental and clinical text,* ed 3, Philadelphia, 2004, Lippincott Williams & Wilkins.

68. United Kingdom Progressive Diabetes Study Group: Overview of 6 years therapy of type 2 diabetes: a progressive disease (UKPDS), *Diabetes* 44:1249-1258, 1995.

69. DeFronzo R: Pharmacologic therapy for type 2 diabetes mellitus, *Ann Intern Med* 131:281-303, 1999.

70. Bailey CJ: Metformin. In Lebovitz H, editor: *Therapy for diabetes mellitus and related disorders,* ed 4, Alexandria, Va, 2004, American Diabetes Association.

71. Lebovitz HE: Oral antidiabetic agents: 2004, *Med Clin North Am* 88:847-863, 2004.

72. Lebovitz H: Thiazolidinediones. In Lebovitz H, editor: *Therapy for diabetes mellitus disorders,* ed 4, Alexandria, Va, 2004, American Diabetes Association.

73. Chu JW, Abbasi F, Lamendola C et al: Effect of rosiglitazone treatment on circulating vascular and inflammatory markers in insulin-resistant subjects, *Diab Vasc Dis Res* 3:37-41, 2006.

74. Chiasson JL, Josse RG, Gomis R et al: Acarbose treatment and the risk of cardiovascular disease and hypertension in patients with impaired glucose tolerance: the STOP-NIDDM trial, *JAMA* 290:486-494, 2003.

75. Young AA: Amylin's physiology and its role in diabetes, *Current Opinion in Endocrinology and Diabetes* 4:282-290, 1997.

76. Uwaifo GI, Ratner RE: Novel pharmacologic agents for type 2 diabetes, *Endocrinol Metab Clin North Am* 34:155-197, 2005.

77. Adapted from Merck & Co., Inc Pharmaceuticals prescribing information issued October 2006.

78. Skyler J: Insulin treatment. In Lebovitz H, editor: *Therapy for diabetes mellitus and related disorders,* ed 4, Alexandria, Va, 2004, American Diabetes Association.

79. Holcombe J, Fineberg E: Insulin allergy and insulin resistance. In Lebovitz H, editor: *Therapy for diabetes mellitus and related disorders,* ed 4, Alexandria, Va, 2004, American Diabetes Association.

80. Centers for Disease Control and Prevention: *National diabetes fact sheet: general information and national estimates on diabetes in the United Sates, 2002,* Atlanta, 2003, US Department of Health and Human Services, Centers for Disease Control and Prevention.

81. Stamler J, Vaccaro O, Neaton JD et al: Diabetes, other risk factors, and 12-year cardiovascular mortality for men screened in the Multiple Risk Factor Intervention Trial, *Diabetes Care* 16:434-444, 1993.

82. Hu FB, Stampfer MJ, Solomon CG et al: The impact of diabetes mellitus on mortality from all causes and coronary heart disease in women: 20 years of follow-up, *Arch Intern Med* 161:1717-1723, 2001.

83. Howard B, Rodiguez B, Bennet P et al: Prevention Conference VI, Diabetes and Cardiovascular Disease Writing Group I: epidemiology, *Circulation* 105:e132-e137, 2002.

84. Grundy S, Garber A, Goldberg R et al: AHA Prevention VI: diabetes and cardiovascular disease—Writing Group IV: lifestyle and medical management of risk factors, *Circulation* 105:e153-e158, 2002.

85. Abbasi F, McLaughlin T, Lamendola C et al: Insulin regulation of plasma free fatty acid concentrations is abnormal in healthy subjects with muscle insulin resistance, *Metabolism* 49:151-154, 2000.

86. Reaven GM: Compensatory hyperinsulinemia and the development of an atherogenic lipoprotein profile: the price paid to maintain glucose homeostasis in insulin-resistant individuals, *Endocrinol Metab Clin North Am* 34:49-62, 2005.

87. Krauss R, Siri P: Metabolic abnormalities: triglyceride and low-density lipoprotein, *Endocrinol Metab Clin North Am* 33:405-415, 2004.

88. Pyörala K, Pedersen TR, Kjekshus J et al: Cholesterol lowering with simvastatin improves prognosis of diabetic patients with coronary heart disease: a subgroup analysis of the Scandinavian Simvastatin Survival Study (4S), *Diabetes Care* 20:614-620, 1997.

89. Goldberg RB, Mellies MJ, Sacks FM et al: Cardiovascular events and their reduction with pravastatin in diabetic and glucose-intolerant myocardial infarction survivors with average cholesterol levels: subgroup analyses in the cholesterol and recurrent events (CARE) trial—the Care Investigators, *Circulation* 98:2513-2519, 1998.

90. Collins R, Armitage J, Parish S et al: MRC/BHF Heart Protection Study of cholesterol-lowering with simvastatin in 5963 people with diabetes: a randomized placebo-controlled trial, *Lancet* 361:2005-2016, 2003.

91. Grundy G, Cleeman C, Bairey Mertz N et al: Implications of recent clinical trials for the National Cholesterol Education Program Adult Treatment Panel III guidelines, *Circulation* 110:227-239, 2004.

92. Lamendola C, Abbasi F, Chu JW et al: Comparative effects of rosuvastatin and gemfibrozil on glucose, insulin, and lipid metabolism in insulin-resistant, nondiabetic patients with combined dyslipidemia, *Am J Cardiol* 95:189-193, 2005.

93. Rubins HB, Robins SJ, Collins D et al: Gemfibrozil for the secondary prevention of coronary heart disease in men with low levels of high-density lipoprotein cholesterol: Veterans Affair High-Density Lipoprotein Cholesterol Intervention Trial study group, *N Engl J Med* 341:410-418, 1999.

94. Effect of fenofibrate on progression of coronary-artery disease in type 2 diabetes: the Diabetes Atherosclerosis Intervention Study—a randomised study, *Lancet* 357:905-910, 2001.

95. Elam MG, Hunninghake DB, Davis KB et al: Effect of niacin on lipid and lipoprotein levels and glycemic control in patients with diabetes and peripheral arterial disease: the ADMIT study—a randomized trial, *JAMA* 284:1263-1270, 2000.

96. Facchini FS, DoNascimento C, Reaven GM et al: Blood pressure, sodium intake, insulin resistance, and urinary nitrate excretion, *Hypertension* 33:1008-1012, 1999.

97. Shin J, Goldburt V, Sowers J et al: Antihypertensive therapy. In Lebovitz H, editor: *Therapy for diabetes mellitus and related disorders,* ed 4, Alexandria, Va, 2004, American Diabetes Association.

98. UK Prospective Diabetes Study Group: Tight blood pressure control and risk of macrovascular and microvascular complications in type 2 diabetes: UKPDS 38, *BMJ* 317:703-713, 1998.

99. Hansson L, Zanchetti A, Carruthers SG et al, for the HOT Study Group: Effects of intensive blood-pressure lowering and low-dose aspirin in patients with hypertension: principal results of the Hypertension Optimal Treatment (HOT) randomised trial, *Lancet* 351:1755-1762, 1998.

100. The ALLHAT Officers and Coordinators for the ALLHAT Collaborative Research Group: Major outcomes in high-risk hypertensive patients randomized to angiotensin-converting enzyme inhibitor or calcium channel blocker vs diuretic: the Antihypertensive and Lipid-Lowering Treatment to Prevent Heart Attack Trial (ALLHAT), *JAMA* 238:2981-2997, 2002.

101. Chobanian AV, Bakris Gl, Black HR et al: The Seventh Report of the Joint National Committee on Prevention, Detection, Evaluation, and Treatment of High Blood Pressure, *Hypertension* 42:1206-1252, 2003.

102. Pearson T, Blair S, Daniels S et al: Consensus panel guide to comprehensive risk reduction for adult patients without coronary or other atherosclerotic vascular disease: AHA guidelines for primary prevention of cardiovascular disease and stroke—2002 update, *Circulation* 106:388-391, 2002.

Sedentary Lifestyle

Barbara Fletcher
Lynne T. Braun

EPIDEMIOLOGY

The Industrial Revolution, known for the use of power-driven machinery and manufacturing, began in the late 17th century and accelerated throughout the 18th century. The development of electrical power and inexpensive steel after 1850 added to the mechanized world, firmly providing an environment conducive to a sedentary lifestyle. Sedentary lifestyle, defined as the expenditure of only small amounts of daily physical activity, has been identified as a risk factor for coronary heart disease (**CHD**) and other conditions since the early 1970s.[1] Two landmark epidemiological studies demonstrated a greater incidence of CHD[2] and first myocardial infarction[3] in subjects who were sedentary compared with those participating in more vigorous physical activity.

Many epidemiological investigations examining the impact of sedentary lifestyle have added to these original works. Later studies have included diverse populations with regard to sex, ethnicity, age, social composition, and geographic locations. These studies have helped confirm evidence supporting the negative impact on cardiovascular health of a sedentary lifestyle.[4]

SEDENTARY LIFESTYLE

Four in 10 U.S. adults report never engaging in any physical activity during their leisure time. Women (43.2 percent) are more likely to be sedentary than men (36.5 percent), and this holds true for every age group (Figure 38-1).[5] Between 1997 and 2002, the percentage of Americans classified as sedentary decreased from 40 to 38 percent; not enough to make a positive impact on public health. Adults classified as engaging in "no physical activity" increased in a linear fashion with each increasing age group from 18 to 24 years to 75 years and over. A similar trend was found in the percentage of persons age 65 and over who are obese.[6]

Sixty-five percent of students in grades 9 through 12 engage in vigorous physical activity (73 percent males; 57 percent females). Of note is that the proportion of students engaging in vigorous physical activity decreases

with each grade.[6] Children aged 9 to 13 years old engage in free-time physical activity (77.4 percent) more than in organized sports (38.5 percent). Non-Hispanic black and Hispanic children are significantly more sedentary than non-Hispanic white children.[7]

Regardless of gender, black and Hispanic adults are more sedentary than white adults (Figure 38-2).[5] In 2002, the breakdown for sedentary lifestyle for adults by race and ethnicity from the least sedentary to the most sedentary are whites, Asian, American Indian, blacks, and Hispanics.[6] When examining sedentary lifestyle and educational levels, 72 percent of adults who did not attend high school are sedentary. This percentage declines to 45 percent for high school graduates and further to 24 percent for those adults attaining graduate degrees (Figure 38-3).[5] Populations in most states do not achieve the recommended amount of physical activity (Figure 38-4).

In summary, sedentary lifestyle trends have remained relatively flat since 1986, and only in the last 4 to 5 years has there been a slight decrease in sedentary lifestyle (Figure 38-5).[8]

PHYSICAL ACTIVITY, EXERCISE, AND FITNESS

The definitions of *physical activity* and *exercise* differ. *Physical activity* is defined as bodily movement that is produced by contraction of skeletal muscle and that increases energy expenditure above the resting level. Categories of physical activity include occupational, household, and leisure-time. *Exercise* is a subclass of physical activity and is defined as planned, structured, and repetitive bodily movement performed specifically to improve or maintain physical fitness.[9]

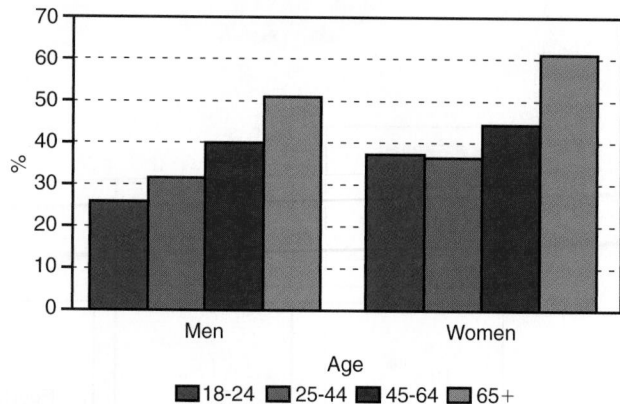

FIGURE 38-1 ■ Prevalence of sedentary leisure-time behavior among adults by sex and age, 1997.

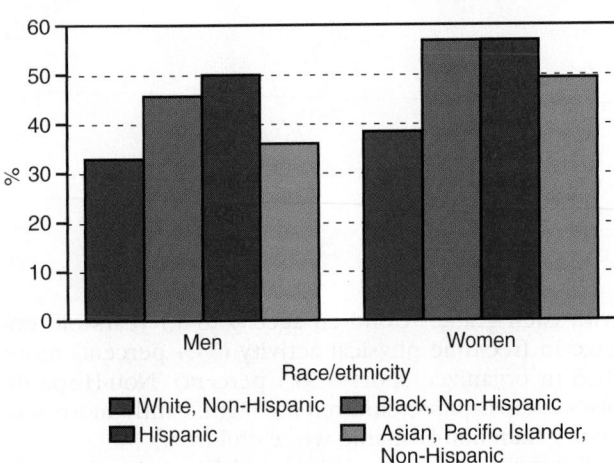

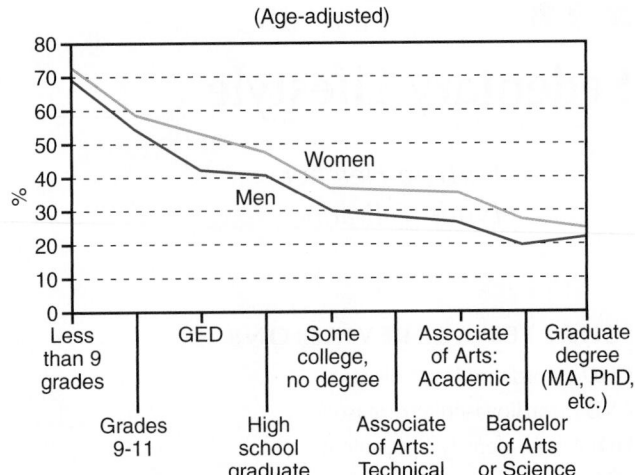

FIGURE 38-2 ■ Age-adjusted prevalence of sedentary leisure-time behavior among adults by sex, race, and ethnicity, 1997.

FIGURE 38-3 ■ Age-adjusted prevalence of sedentary leisure-time behavior among adults by sex and education, 1997. *GED,* General equivalency diploma; *MA,* Masters degree; *PhD,* Doctorate degree.

Physical activity and exercise can be estimated in terms of metabolic equivalents (**METs**), which is the metabolic energy expenditure (oxygen consumption) of a given activity. One MET approximates the resting metabolic rate of 3.5 ml O_2/kg/min, the oxygen consumption of an adult at rest. Moderate-intensity physical activity, the goal for all sedentary individuals, is activity performed at 3 to 6 METs. This is equivalent to brisk walking at 3 to 4 miles per hour, cycling for pleasure, household cleaning, and moderate-effort swimming.[10] The 1995 recommendation from the surgeon general

indicated that every adult should accumulate 30 minutes or more of moderate-intensity physical activity on most, preferably all, days of the week. In 2002, the Institute of Medicine recommended a more ambitious physical activity goal. The Institute recommended that adults and children should engage in activities equivalent to a total of 60 minutes of moderate-intensity activity throughout each day.[11]

A useful way of determining the volume of walking or jogging activity performed during the course of an entire day is with a pedometer, which is worn at the

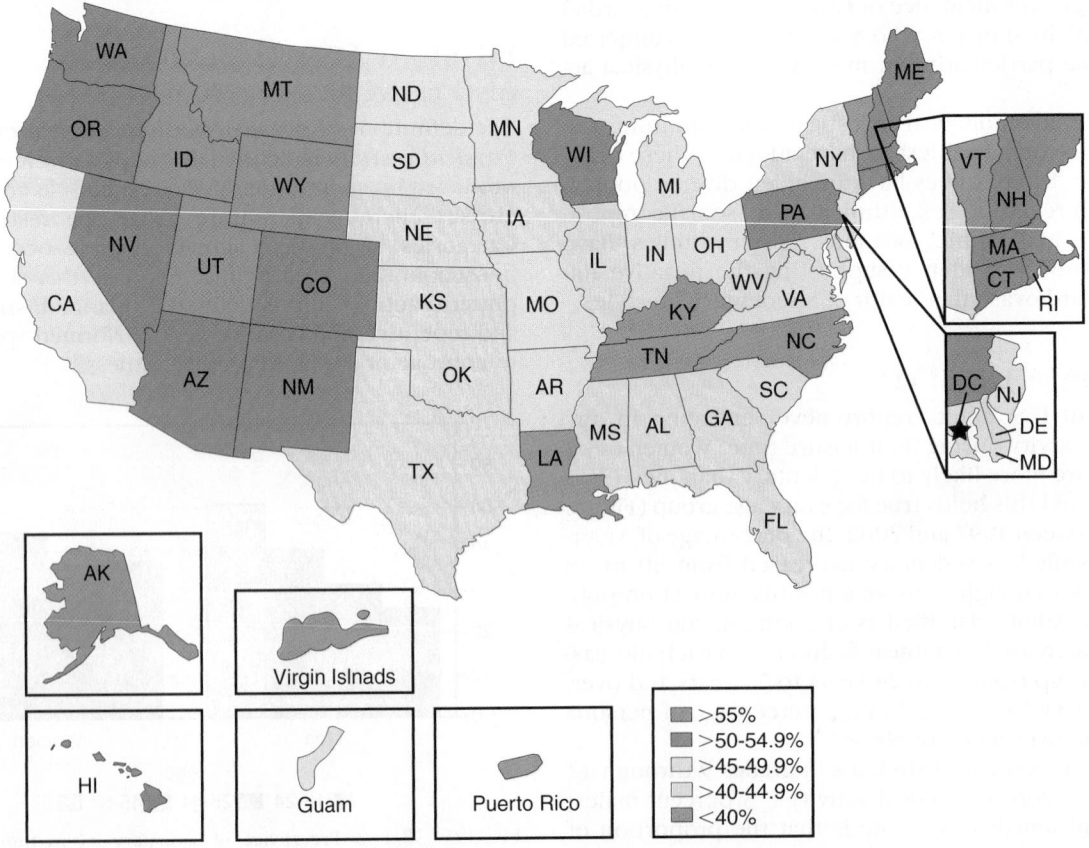

FIGURE 38-4 ■ Prevalence of recommended physical activity by state.

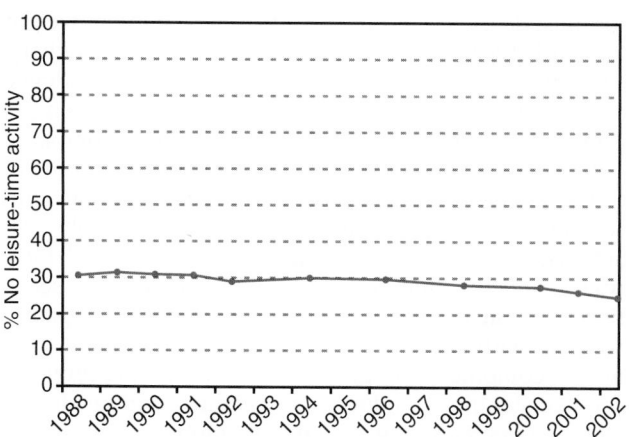

FIGURE 38-5 ■ U.S. physical activity statistics, 1988-2002: percent of adults, no leisure-time physical activity trend chart.

waist and counts steps. The goal for a moderately active lifestyle is to accrue 10,000 steps each day,[12] estimated to be equivalent to walking 4 to 5 miles per day.

Physical fitness is defined as a set of attributes that persons have or achieve that relates to the ability to engage in physical activity.[9] Physical fitness includes cardiorespiratory endurance, muscular strength, flexibility, agility, and body composition. Cardiorespiratory endurance is the health-related element of fitness that refers to the ability of the heart, vascular system, and lungs to supply oxygen to skeletal muscles during sustained physical activity. Most of the cardiovascular benefits of exercise are derived from aerobic activities, such as brisk walking, biking, or swimming, performed at a moderate intensity on a regular basis.

CARDIOVASCULAR BENEFITS OF EXERCISE

Exercise has beneficial effects on the incidence of CHD, mortality from CHD and all-cause mortality, and risk factors for CHD. These benefits are summarized in Box 38-1.

Protective Effect of Exercise and Fitness on Coronary Heart Disease Incidence and Mortality

Numerous prospective observational studies have demonstrated that regular exercise protects against the development of CHD in men and women.[13-18] Physical ac-

---

BOX 38-1   ■ ■ ■
CARDIOVASCULAR BENEFITS OF EXERCISE

Coronary Heart Disease Incidence and Mortality
- Decreased risk of coronary heart disease
- Decreased cardiovascular mortality
- Decreased all-cause mortality

Risk Factors
- Decreased incidence of hypertension
- Reduction in systolic and diastolic blood pressure
- Increase in high-density lipoprotein cholesterol and decrease in triglycerides; some studies show a decrease in cholesterol
- Improved glucose control and insulin sensitivity
- Reduction in body weight and body fat

---

tivity and health were assessed in 12,516 middle-aged and older male Harvard alumni over the course of 17 years.[13] Men who expended 4200 kJ/wk engaging in physical activity had a reduced CHD risk compared with less active men. A subgroup analysis showed that length of exercise session was unrelated to CHD risk.[14] Higher levels of energy expenditure were related inversely to CHD risk, including the accumulation of shorter sessions of physical activity. In the Health Professionals' Follow-up Study,[15] a cohort of 44,452 men was followed at 2-year intervals for 13 years. CHD risk factors, newly diagnosed cases of CHD, and levels of leisure-time physical activity were assessed. Similar to the Harvard Alumni Study, physical activity was associated inversely with CHD risk. Men who ran for an hour or more per week had a 42 percent risk reduction, whereas men who engaged in brisk walking for 30 minutes per day had an 18 percent reduction in CHD risk.

Similar results have been demonstrated in women. The Nurses' Health Study[16] consisted of 72,488 women between the ages of 40 and 65 years who were free of cardiovascular disease at baseline and were followed for 8 years. A strong, graded, inverse association was observed between physical activity and the risk of CHD events. Women who walked briskly 3 hours or more per week had a multivariate relative risk of 0.65 compared with women who walked infrequently. In the Women's Health Initiative Observational Study,[17] walking and vigorous exercise were associated with a reduced incidence of cardiovascular disease events in 73,743 postmenopausal women irrespective of race or ethnicity. Finally, a cohort study of almost 40,000 female health professionals aged 45 years or older showed that even light to moderate activity was associated with lower CHD rates; at least 1 hour of walking per week predicted a lower risk of CHD.[18]

Regular exercise not only reduces the incidence of CHD but also reduces cardiovascular and all-cause mortality.[19-21] In the Harvard alumni study,[20] men who engaged in moderately vigorous sports activity had a 23 percent lower risk of death than those who were less active. This effect was an additive survival benefit to other lifestyle measures, such as cessation of smoking, maintaining a normal blood pressure, and avoiding obesity.

In addition to regular exercise, the degree of cardiovascular fitness, as determined by treadmill exercise test performance, also is associated with a lower mortality risk in men and women.[22-26] In a prospective study, Blair and colleagues[22] evaluated 9777 men with two clinical examinations (mean interval between examinations, 4.9 years) to assess the association of change in fitness with mortality during a mean 5.1-year follow-up period after the second examination. The age-adjusted all-cause death rate was 3 times higher in men who were unfit at examinations (122.0/10,000 man-years) compared with those who were fit at both examinations (39.6/10,000 man-years). Men who improved from unfit to fit between examinations had a 44 percent lower mortality risk compared with men who remained unfit at both examinations.

In a cohort of 5721 asymptomatic women who underwent baseline examinations in 1992 and were followed through 2000, Gulati and colleagues[26] showed that risk of death, adjusted for Framingham Risk Score, was related inversely to exercise capacity. For every 1-MET increase in exercise capacity, mortality risk decreased by 17 percent. These findings demonstrated that exercise capacity is an important predictor of death in asymptomatic women.

Physical Activity Reduces Coronary Heart Disease Risk Factors

Engaging in physical activity prevents or helps treat many CHD risk factors, including hypertension, elevated triglycerides and low levels of high-density lipoprotein (**HDL**) cholesterol, insulin resistance and glucose intolerance, and obesity. The magnitude of the exercise effect depends on the characteristics of the exercise intervention, individual variation, and whether exercise also is associated with weight reduction.[27]

Physical activity and fitness are linked to reduced incidence of hypertension in white men; however, studies in white women and black subjects did not show significant relationships.[28] In a meta-analysis of randomized controlled trials of the effect of aerobic exercise training on blood pressure,[29] systolic and diastolic blood pressure decreased an average of 2.6 and 1.8 mm Hg in normotensive subjects and 7.4 and 5.8 mm Hg in hypertensive subjects, respectively. No relationship was found between training frequency, session duration, or intensity of exercise training and the magnitude of blood pressure reduction.

A review of the effects of at least 12 weeks of aerobic exercise training on blood lipids showed primarily an increase in HDL cholesterol with reductions in total cholesterol, low-density lipoprotein (**LDL**) cholesterol and triglycerides that were observed less frequently.[30] These results typically occurred with moderate to high-intensity exercise training. The Health, Risk Factors, Exercise Training and Genetics (HERITAGE) Family Study[31] evaluated the lipid effects of 20 weeks of exercise training in a sample of 200 men with various lipid disorders. Men with isolated low HDL cholesterol had a nonsignificant increase in HDL cholesterol with exercise. However, men with high triglycerides and low HDL cholesterol demonstrated a 4.9 percent increase in HDL cholesterol and a 15 percent decrease in triglycerides with exercise. In this subgroup, a 10.6 percent reduction in abdominal subcutaneous adipose tissue was associated with the increase in HDL cholesterol. An exploration of changes in fat mass and lipid changes induced by exercise training in a larger cohort of the HERITAGE study (428 white and 185 black, 46 percent men) showed that greater fat loss was associated with a greater blood lipid response to exercise (increase in HDL and decreases in LDL, triglycerides, and total cholesterol).[32]

Exercise improves glucose control and insulin sensitivity and may prevent the onset of type 2 diabetes in high-risk individuals.[33-35] The Diabetes Prevention Program[33] compared an intensive lifestyle intervention with medication (metformin 850 mg twice daily) and placebo in 3234 nondiabetic subjects with elevated fasting and postload plasma glucose concentrations. Program goals for lifestyle intervention were at least a 7 percent weight loss and at least 150 minutes of weekly physical activity. After the 2.8 year follow-up period, diabetes incidence was reduced 58 percent in the lifestyle intervention group and 31 percent in the metformin group compared with placebo. In a multicultural epidemiological study of the association between physical activity and insulin sensitivity, increased participation in overall physical activity, as well as vigorous and nonvigorous activities, was associated significantly with higher insulin sensitivity.[34] A small intervention study of postmenopausal women with type 2 diabetes[35] who underwent a 4-month combined strength and aerobic training program showed significant reductions in glucose and insulin, as well as a decrease in glycated hemoglobin.

Physical activity is an important component in weight loss regimens. Moderate-intensity exercise, such as brisk walking, results in reduced body weight and body fat in overweight men and women.[36,37] In the National Weight Control Registry,[38] more than 3000 individuals lost an average of 30 kg and maintained their weight for 5½ years; for 91 percent, regular physical activity was the mechanism for maintenance of weight loss. In this registry, women and men reported expending 2445 and 3298 kcal weekly, respectively, in activities such as walking, cycling, weight lifting, aerobics, running, and stair climbing.

LINK BETWEEN SEDENTARY LIFESTYLE AND OTHER CARDIOVASCULAR DISEASES

Sedentary lifestyle enhances development of CHD, stroke, hypertension, obesity, and non–insulin-dependent diabetes, as well as other conditions such as some cancers, negative psychological behaviors, and disabilities of aging. A sedentary lifestyle has negative effects regardless of age, gender, body mass index, smoking status, presence or absence of hypertension, or abnormal lipoprotein profile.[4] An integrative review of research methodology and results over a 10-year period showed an increase in cardiovascular disease (**CVD**) mortality and CVD risk factors in those characterized as having a sedentary lifestyle.[39]

Over the past 25 years, the prevalence and incidence of type 2 diabetes have dramatically escalated worldwide and across all age, gender, and race/ethnic groups. In accord with this increase, recent clinical and observational studies have demonstrated the adverse effects of obesity and sedentary lifestyle in relation to type 2 diabetes and the metabolic syndrome.[40,41] European Union data indicate that less than 50 percent of its citizens are involved in regular physical activity and that the increasing prevalence of obesity is associated with a sedentary lifestyle.[42] Studies also have linked sedentary lifestyle to depressive symptoms, increased blood pressure, and higher C-reactive protein levels.[43-46]

Gender/Ethnic/Racial Differences

Migration to cities appears to increase CVD risk factors in developing countries. In Guatemalan adults, rural and urban women had similar sedentary lifestyles (83 percent), whereas urban men were more sedentary (79 percent) compared with rural men (27 percent). Migration to a city was shown to increase their sedentary behavior.[47] Among Danish young adults, women are significantly more sedentary if over the age of 25, poorly educated, and smokers. Sedentary lifestyle in the young Danish men was associated negatively with high levels of parental physical work.[48]

South Asian countries have a high prevalence of CHD, and this varies with socioeconomic status. In both adult sexes, the prevalence of sedentary lifestyle is higher among higher socioeconomic groups.[49]

Barriers to physical activity, explored in a group of sedentary Native American women, demonstrated the need for programs that were compatible with the role expectations of their families and communities. Additionally, the desire for acceptance of exercise and encouragement to be physically active from their families, community, and tribal leaders was necessary.[50]

No differences in death and reinfarction rates were found between Mexican American and non-Hispanic white men and women after a first myocardial infarction. Sedentary lifestyle was related to increased rate of reinfarction and death in both groups.[51]

The Women and Physical Activity Survey (part of the Women's Cardiovascular Health Network)[52] identified personal, social, environmental, cultural, and physical environmental factors associated with physical inactivity status among a diverse group of women. Investigators from seven universities studied factors that influenced physical activity among white, black, Latina, and Native American women residing in rural, suburban, and urban environments. Younger age, good general health, and high self-efficacy were the personal correlates of physical activity. Socially knowing persons who exercise and attending religious services were associated with higher levels of physical activity across populations. Safety from crime was the physical environmental factor related to physical activity. A total of 45 to 64 percent of participants were classified as insufficiently active or inactive.[53-56]

Current health campaigns to reduce obesity and type 2 diabetes focus on increasing exercise rather than decreasing sedentary behaviors, whereas more emphasis on decreasing sedentary activities could affect cardiovascular health positively. Activities such as time spent watching television are associated positively in women with the risk of obesity (23 percent) and increase in type 2 diabetes (14 percent). Every 2 hours per day spent in a sitting position is associated with an increase in obesity of 5 to 7 percent in diabetic persons.[57]

Television viewing may represent a modifiable cause of childhood and adolescent obesity. Overall, 43 percent of high school students watch television for more than 2 hours on an average school day, but more black (74 percent) and Hispanic (52 percent) than white (34 percent) students watch more than 2 hours of television per day. Watching television more than 2 hours per day is associated with being overweight and sedentary among white females and with being overweight among Hispanic females. Television watching was associated with being overweight in white males, and no associa-tion was found in Hispanic males. To the contrary, television watching was associated with more physical activity in black males.[58]

Age-Related Changes in Exercise Tolerance

Studies from childhood through adolescence can provide insight into the prediction of future CVD. When following children in prepuberty or early puberty for 5 years, changes in muscular strength were associated with changes in systolic blood pressure, whereas changes in aerobic fitness were associated with changes in the various cholesterol levels (total cholesterol, HDL, and LDL). Combined changes in aerobic fitness and muscular strength were associated with alterations in overall adiposity and abdominal adiposity.[59]

Muscle strength declines with aging. Quantitative loss of muscle mass is the most significant factor accounting for this decline. However, qualitative changes in muscle fibers and tendons also account for age-related decline in muscle function. These changes include selective atrophy of fast-twitch fibers, reduced tendon stiffness, and neural changes such as lower activation of the agonist muscles and higher coactivation of the antagonist muscles. Single fibers of older muscles containing myosin heavy chains of type I and II show slower tension and shortening velocity compared with young muscles. Although specific exercise programs can improve muscle strength, power, and function in older adults, a sedentary lifestyle can enhance the decline seen with age in muscle strength and function.[60,61]

An objective for Healthy People 2010 is to increase to 30 percent the proportion of adults who perform 2 days per week of resistance training. Unfortunately, 2001 National Health Interview Survey data indicate that only 12 percent of persons aged 65 to 74 years and 10 percent of those above 75 years met the resistance exercise objective, and women were less likely than men to meet this objective.[62]

A reduction in compliance of the cardiothoracic (central) arteries is seen with advancing age. This reduced central artery compliance is an independent risk factor for the development of CVD. Regular exercise increases central arterial compliance, whereas a sedentary lifestyle promotes decreased central arterial compliance.[63]

Elderly individuals experience burdens from CVD in part because of global changes that occur with aging. A sedentary lifestyle is recognized to enhance many of these age-related changes in the cardiovascular system, and physical activity can retard these changes. Cardiovascular aging changes include the following[64]:

- Loss of myocytes with hypertrophy of those remaining
- Calcification involving the conduction and valvular apparatus
- Loss of arterial compliance contributing to systolic hypertension and left ventricular hypertrophy
- Slowing of myocardial relaxation
- Elevation of blood catecholamine levels that contribute to desensitization to noradrenergic stimulation leading to a decline in maximal achievable heart rate

■ Changes in the baroreception reflux function causing decreased sodium conservation leading to postprandial hypotension

The benefits of overcoming a sedentary lifestyle are overwhelming; so why are older individuals continuing their sedentary lifestyle? Barriers to physical activity in the elderly include poor health, lack of time, aging, and adverse environments.(Add ref 65 here) Persons continue to be interested in physical activity as they age but also continue to have misconceptions about physical activity.[50]

INTERVENTION APPROACHES
Primary Prevention

Primary prevention is the provision of services intended to prevent the onset of a given condition. In the case of CVD, this may refer to the prevention of modifiable risk factors, such as hypertension, smoking, hypercholesterolemia, diabetes, obesity, and sedentary lifestyle (also called "primordial prevention"[66]). Although these risk factors have independent associations with CVD, they often are interrelated and observed in the same individual. An intervention, such as regular physical activity, which often is coupled with other healthful behaviors, may prevent multiple CVD risk factors, such as hypertension, dyslipidemia, and diabetes.

The nation's health agenda, as documented in Healthy People 2010,[67] includes specific objectives to increase the proportion of adults and children who engage in moderate-intensity and vigorous physical activities. One decade ago, the Centers for Disease Control and Prevention and the American College of Sports Medicine reviewed the physiological, epidemiological, and clinical evidence on the relationship between physical activity and health. A public health recommendation was made that every adult should accumulate 30 minutes or more of moderate-intensity physical activity on most, preferably, all days of the week.[10] This recommendation is incorporated in the primary prevention guidelines of the American Heart Association.[68] Furthermore, the American Cancer Society, the American Diabetes Association, and the American Heart Association incorporated this same recommendation in a joint scientific statement on preventing cancer, CVD, and diabetes.[69]

Community Level Interventions

Community prevention trials show that organized efforts centered on mass and direct education, along with environmental change through local programs and policies, can change behavior.[70] The American Heart Association recently published a guide of a comprehensive approach for community-based prevention of heart disease and stroke.[71] Strategies and goals focus on general, school and youth, and work site education; community organization and partnering; ensuring personal health services; environmental change; and policy change. Specific recommendations are the following:

■ Mass and local media should emphasize the importance of lifestyle behaviors and risk factors on cardiovascular health.
■ Television shows for children should promote physical activity during commercial breaks.

■ Physical education should be required at least 3 times a week in kindergarten to grade 12, with an increasing emphasis on lifetime sports/activities.
■ Work sites should promote increased physical activity in the day's work (e.g., stair climbing).
■ Physical education programs should be supported within the school curricula and within community centers.
■ Every community should commit to providing safe and convenient means for walking and bicycling as a means of transportation and recreation.
■ Buildings should be designed so that stairwells are visible, convenient, and comfortable to use. Use of stairwells should be promoted through signs.
■ Work sites should provide employer-sponsored physical activity and fitness programs.
■ Schools should provide access to their physical activity space for all persons outside of normal school hours.

A mass media physical activity intervention to promote and maintain walking was instituted among sedentary 50- to 65-year-old residents of Wheeling, West Virginia.[72] During the planning phase, community members were mobilized to assist with campaign development and implementation and to address policy and environmental changes. Other strategies included television, radio, and print advertising, kickoff events, and an organized walking clinic. Telephone surveys of a probability sample followed cohorts at baseline and at 3, 6, and 12 months. Following the intervention, sedentary Wheeling residents reported significantly higher rates of walking compared with baseline. Among the most sedentary adults, a 14 percent difference in active walkers at 3 months and 12 months was observed between the intervention and comparison communities. Researchers attributed the success of the intervention to attention to three elements of behavior change: message targeting, exposure, and policy/environmental change.

A local health department, the Los Angeles County Department of Health Services, collaborated with community agencies to increase physical activity levels among black residents.[73] Community agencies participated in one or more interventions, which focused on modeling the behaviors promoted ("walking the talk") and incorporating physical activity into routine practice. Interventions included the following:

■ Incorporating fitness breaks in longer meetings and events
■ Provision of personal training to organizational leaders to promote their "leading by example" and strengthen their commitment to changes within their sites
■ Work site and organizational wellness education offered to staff and clients of local agencies
■ Small grants program to train residents for the purpose of initiating or expanding physical activity programs in targeted areas

This feasibility study of a collaborative, multisectoral, community-based model demonstrated a high level of support among community agencies to share the "cost" of physical activity engagement in black communities where the risk of obesity and other chronic diseases is high.

School-Based Approaches

Because atherosclerosis has been observed in the aorta and coronary arteries of deceased children, primary prevention of CVD must begin in childhood through population-based approaches to health promotion and risk reduction. The prevalence of overweight, obesity, and diabetes is increasing in children and adolescents, and dietary and physical activity behaviors are suboptimal among American youth. Physical activity data from the Youth Risk Behavior Surveillance showed that the proportion of students who attend daily physical education classes decreased from 41.6 percent in 1991 to 29.1 percent in 1999.[74] Therefore, population-based approaches must modify the food and physical activity environments of children. Research has shown that school-based health programs have the potential to benefit the cardiovascular health of children and adolescents.[75] In middle school children, a 2-year physical education intervention, which consisted of curricular materials, staff development, and on-site follow-up, showed an 18 percent increase in moderate to vigorous physical activity among intervention schools.[76]

Following a review of research-based interventions for promoting cardiovascular health in schools by a committee of the American Heart Association Council on Cardiovascular Disease in the Young, a scientific statement provided the following recommendations related to physical activity: the incorporation of CVD risk factor content in school curricula, as well as research-based content on effective behavior-change methods; the requirement of 3 times per week physical education classes in kindergarten through grade 12; 150 minutes of physical education per week for elementary school students and at least 225 minutes per week for middle school students; and the incorporation of physical activity into after-school programs.[75]

Secondary Prevention

For the purposes of this chapter, secondary prevention refers to the identification and treatment of asymptomatic individuals with risk factors or preclinical disease but in whom the condition is not yet clinically apparent.[77]

Intervention Opportunities

Blood pressure, cholesterol, and diabetes screenings serve to identify a mass of individuals with risk factors and provide the opportunity for counseling on health care and risk-reduction strategies. Brief physical activity questionnaires may be added to screenings to identify sedentary individuals and to relate lifestyle modifications to the reduction of other risk factors. In addition to mass screenings, clinician office visits serve as opportunities to identify risk factors and initiate preventive care. Unfortunately, there are no recommendations for the frequency of preventive health encounters for asymptomatic adults, and preventive measures often are discussed briefly during acute and chronic illness encounters. Current clinical practice guidelines for hyper-

cholesterolemia, hypertension, and diabetes address lifestyle modifications as interventions for these risk factors.[78-80] For example, regular physical activity is recommended by the *Seventh Report of the Joint National Committee on Prevention, Detention, Evaluation, and Treatment of High Blood Pressure*[79] for the management of prehypertension and hypertension.

Motivating Behavioral Change

Behavioral counseling interventions often occur during routine office visits and may continue outside of office visits. For example, a clinician may continue counseling through telephone contacts or personalized mailings of self-help materials. Behavioral counseling interventions differ from screening interventions in that they address complex behaviors that are integral to daily living. Behavioral counseling interventions vary in intensity and scope for each patient. They require repeated involvement of patients and clinicians, and they are influenced by the patient's environment (family, peers, school, work site, and community). Patients must be actively engaged in self-management practices in order to make and maintain behavior changes.[81]

The U.S. Preventive Services Task Force[77] recommends using the five *A*'s construct to target any behavior change:

- Assess: Ask about or identify risk factors that may be influenced by behavior change.
- Advise: Provide clear, specific, and personalized behavior change advice, including information about personal harm/benefits.
- Agree: Together with the patient, choose treatment goals and methods based on interest and willingness to change behavior.
- Assist: Using behavior change methods (self-help and counseling), help the patient achieve agreed-upon goals by acquiring the skills, confidence, and social/environmental supports for behavior change.
- Arrange: Schedule follow-up contacts (office visits or by telephone) to provide continual assistance/support and to adjust treatment plan as needed.[81]

Following the identification of risk factors—for example, type 2 diabetes and sedentary lifestyle—the clinician should give specific and personalized behavior change advice: "Mr. Jones, your hemoglobin A_{1c} is still elevated; therefore, we will need to increase your medication dose again. You have expressed that you don't like to take so many medications. If you start and continue a regular physical activity program, your diabetes will be easier to control without as much medication. In addition, regular physical activity will help with blood pressure control and weight loss, and in the long term, help to prevent heart disease." Following the personalized advice, a treatment goal is agreed upon by the patient and clinician. Such a goal might be a 15-minute walk during each lunch hour at work and a 30-minute walk on Saturdays. The clinician uses behavior change techniques to assist the patient in meeting this goal, e.g., instructing the patient to discuss the goal with coworkers and invite them to walk with him, giving the patient a pedometer and instructions for use, and asking the patient to record daily steps in a log. Finally, follow-up contacts are arranged.

Behavior change strategies are identified as integral to successful weight loss maintenance. Analysis of data from the National Weight Control Registry[38] and the Diabetes Prevention Program[82] shows that successful weight loss maintenance occurred in individuals who (1) engaged in self-monitoring of weight, dietary parameters (e.g., fat grams consumed each day), and minutes of physical activity per day, and (2) met physical activity goals, e.g., 150 min/wk of moderate-intensity walking. Technology is also an important adjunct for successful behavioral change interventions, allowing for passive or interactive use of telephones, videos, CD-ROMs, and the Internet.[81] The American Heart Association *(www. americanheart.org)* offers two web-based physical activity programs, *Just Move* and *Choose to Move.* These programs include an educational component, an exercise diary to track daily progress, and weekly inspirational e-mails.

Tertiary Prevention

Tertiary prevention refers to the care of established disease for the purpose of restoring an individual to highest function and avoiding complications. The American Heart Association and the American College of Cardiology have published guidelines for preventing heart attack and death in patients with established CVD.[83] The physical activity component of these guidelines begins with assessing exercise risk. An exercise test is recommended, not only to assess risk but also to guide the exercise prescription. The guidelines follow the public health recommendation for physical activity[10]: a minimum of 30 to 60 minutes of activity, preferably daily, or at least 3 or 4 times per week (walking, jogging, cycling, or other aerobic activity) supplemented by an increase in daily lifestyle activities. Moderate- to high-risk patients should first enroll in a medically supervised cardiac rehabilitation program.

A recent meta-analysis of 48 randomized trials comparing exercise-based cardiac rehabilitation with usual care[84] showed that exercise-based cardiac rehabilitation was associated with a 20 percent reduction in total mortality and a 26 percent reduction in cardiac mortality. Favorable trends also were observed for nonfatal myocardial infarction and revascularization procedures in cardiac patients who received exercise-based rehabilitation. Exercise training in patients with coronary atherosclerosis has numerous cardioprotective effects, including the following: improved endothelial function associated with greater synthesis and release of nitric oxide; antiinflammatory effects identified by reduced C-reactive protein levels; favorable modification of CHD risk factors; increase in the threshold for myocardial ischemia; and antithrombotic effects, including reduced blood viscosity, decreased platelet aggregation, and enhanced thrombolytic ability.[85]

Exercise Adherence in Patients with Coronary Artery Disease

Because a rapid dropout rate (50 percent) occurs within the first 3 to 6 months of exercise involvement among cardiac patients, researchers have investigated the significant predictors of exercise adherence according to the stages of change model.[86] The five stages of change in exercise adherence are as follows:

1. Precontemplation: currently not exercising with no intention to begin exercising
2. Contemplation: currently not exercising but thinking about starting to exercise in the future
3. Preparation: starting to participate in limited or inconsistent amounts of exercise
4. Action: less than 6 months of regular exercise (3 or more times per week for at least 20 minutes each time)
5. Maintenance: more than 6 months of regular exercise

Interventions should help an individual progress from precontemplation or contemplation into action and maintenance. Significant predictors of exercise adherence in cardiac rehabilitation participants are perceived self-efficacy, perceived benefits of exercise, perceived barriers to exercise, and interpersonal support for exercise.[86] Self-efficacy in low- and moderate-risk patients attending cardiac rehabilitation programs may be increased by educational methods and weaning patients from direct medical supervision to allow patients to monitor their own activity levels and tolerance.[87]

In summary, there is unquestionable scientific evidence to support that a sedentary lifestyle is linked to CHD and many of its related risk factors. This is true regardless of gender, race, age, or ethnicity. Sedentary lifestyle now is considered a worldwide public health problem requiring urgent attention. Like all diseases and associated risk factors, sedentary lifestyle greatly affects the health care dollar. Similarly to populations within the United States, about two-thirds of Canadians are sedentary, to which is attributed the $2.1 billion or 2.5 percent of the total direct health care costs in Canada.[88]

This chapter details the CVD problems associated with sedentary existence and conversely the benefits of incorporating physical activity in this population. The challenge belongs to the health professional and the sedentary public to overcome this unacceptable lifestyle.

REFERENCES

1. Friis RH, Sellers TA: *Epidemiology for public health practice,* ed 3, Sudbury, Mass, 2004, Jones and Bartlett.
2. Morris JN, Heady JA, Raffle PAB et al: Coronary heart disease and physical activity of work, *Lancet* 2:1053-1057, 1953.
3. Paffenbarger RS Jr, Wing AL, Hyde RT: Physical activity as an index of heart attack risk in college alumni, *Am J Epidemiol* 108:161-175, 1978.
4. Paffenbarger RS Jr, Blair SN, Lee IM: A history of physical activity, cardiovascular health and longevity: the scientific contributions of Jeremy N Morris DSc, DPH, FRCP, *Int J Epidemiol* 30:1184-1192, 2001.
5. Centers for Disease Control and Prevention, National Center for Health Statistics: *Prevalence of sedentary leisure-time behavior among adults in the United States.* Retrieved December 27, 2006 from www.cdc.gov/nchs/products/pubs/pubd/hestats/3and4/sedentary.htm
6. Progress Review - Physical Activity and Fitness; Healthy People 2010; US Department of Health & Human Services; April 14, 2004. Retrieved January 25, 2005 from www.cdc.gov/nchs/about/otheract/hpdata2010/focusareas/fa22-paf.htm

7. Centers for Disease Control and Prevention: Physical activity levels among children aged 9-13: United States, 2002, *MMWR Morb Mortal Wkly Rep* 52(33):785-788, 2003.

8. Centers for Disease Control and Prevention: *Nutrition & physical activity.* Retrieved December 27, 2005 from www.cdc.gov/nccdphp/dnpa/obesity/state_programs/index.htm ••

9. American College of Sports Medicine: *ACSM's guidelines for exercise testing and prescription,* Philadelphia, 2000, Lippincott Williams & Wilkins.

10. Pate RR, Pratt M, Blair SN et al: Physical activity and public health: a recommendation from the Centers for Disease Control and Prevention and the American College of Sports Medicine, *JAMA* 273:402-407, 1995.

11. Institute of Medicine: *Dietary reference intakes for energy, carbohydrate, fiber, fat, fatty acids, cholesterol, protein, and amino acids,* 2002. Retrieved August 3, 2005, from www.iom.edu/Object.File/Master/4/154/0.pdf

12. Thompson DL, Rakow J, Perdue SM: Relationship between accumulated walking and body composition in middle-aged women, *Med Sci Sports Exerc* 36:911-914, 2004.

13. Sesso HD, Paffenbarger RS, Lee IM: Physical activity and coronary heart disease in men: the Harvard Alumni Health Study, *Circulation* 102:975-980, 2000.

14. Lee IM, Sesso HD, Paffenbarger RS: Physical activity and coronary heart disease risk in men: does the duration of exercise episodes predict risk? *Circulation* 102:981-986, 2000.

15. Tanasescu M, Leitzmann MF, Rimm EB et al: Exercise type and intensity in relation to coronary heart disease in men, *JAMA* 288:23-30, 2002.

16. Manson JE, Hu FB, Rich-Edwards JW et al: A prospective study of walking as compared with vigorous exercise in the prevention of coronary heart disease in women, *N Engl J Med* 341:650-658, 1999.

17. Manson JE, Greenland P, LaCroix AZ et al: Walking compared with vigorous exercise for the prevention of cardiovascular events in women, *N Engl J Med* 347:716-725, 2002.

18. Lee IM, Rexrode KM, Cook NR et al: Physical activity and coronary heart disease in women: is "no pain, no gain" passé? *JAMA* 285:1447-1454, 2001.

19. Leon AS, Connett J, Jacobs DR et al: Leisure-time physical activity levels and risk of coronary heart disease and death: the Multiple Risk Factor Intervention Trial, *JAMA* 258:2388-2395, 1987.

20. Paffenbarger RS, Hyde RT, Wing AL et al: The association of changes in physical activity level and other lifestyle characteristics with mortality among men, *N Engl J Med* 328:538-545, 1993.

21. Andersen LB, Schnohr P, Schroll M et al: All-cause mortality associated with physical activity during leisure time, work, sports, and cycling to work, *Arch Intern Med* 160:1621-1628, 2000.

22. Blair SN, Kohl HW, Barlow CE et al: Changes in physical fitness and all-cause mortality: a prospective study of healthy and unhealthy men, *JAMA* 273:1093-1098, 1995.

23. Laukkanen JA, Lakka TA, Rauramaa R et al: Cardiovascular fitness as a predictor of mortality in men, *Arch Intern Med* 161:825-831, 2001.

24. Myers J, Prakash M, Froelicher V et al: Exercise capacity and mortality among men referred for exercise testing, *N Engl J Med* 346:793-801, 2002.

25. Mora S, Redberg RF, Cui Y et al: Ability of exercise testing to predict cardiovascular and all-cause death in asymptomatic women: a 20-year follow-up of the lipid research clinics prevalence study, *JAMA* 290:1600-1607, 2003.

26. Gulati M, Pandey DK, Arnsdorf MF et al: Exercise capacity and the risk of death in women: the St James Women Take Heart Project, *Circulation* 108:1554-1559, 2003.

27. Thompson PD, Buchner D, Pina IL et al: Exercise and physical activity in the prevention and treatment of atherosclerotic cardiovascular disease: a statement from the Council on Clinical Cardiology (Subcommittee on Exercise, Rehabilitation, and Prevention) and the Council on Nutrition, Physical Activity, and Metabolism (Subcommittee on Physical Activity), *Circulation* 107:3109-3116, 2003.

28. Pescatello LS, Franklin BA, Fagard R et al, for the American College of Sports Medicine: American College of Sports Medicine position stand: exercise and hypertension, *Med Sci Sports Exerc* 36:533-553, 2004.

29. Fagard RH: Exercise characteristics and the blood pressure response to dynamic physical training, *Med Sci Sports Exerc* 33(6 suppl):S484-S492, 2001.

30. Leon AS, Sanchez OA: Response of blood lipids to exercise training alone or combined with dietary intervention, *Med Sci Sports Exerc* 33(6 suppl):S502-S515, 2001.

31. Couillard C, Depres JP, Lamarche B et al: Effects of endurance exercise training on plasma HDL cholesterol levels depends on levels of triglycerides: evidence from men of the Health, Risk Factors, Exercise Training and Genetics (HERITAGE) Family Study, *Arterioscler Thromb Vasc Biol* 21:1226-1232, 2001.

32. Ardern CI, Katzmarzyk PT, Janssen I et al: Race and sex similarities in exercise-induced changes in blood lipids and fatness, *Med Sci Sports Exerc* 36:1610-1615, 2004.

33. Knowler WC, Barrett-Connor E, Fowler SE et al: Reduction in the incidence of type 2 diabetes with lifestyle intervention or metformin, *N Engl J Med* 346:393-403, 2002.

34. Mayer-Davis EJ, D'Agostino R, Karter AJ et al: Intensity and amount of physical activity in relation to insulin sensitivity: the Insulin Resistance Atherosclerosis Study, *JAMA* 279:669-674, 1998.

35. Tokmakidis SP, Zois CE, Volaklis KA et al: The effects of a combined strength and aerobic exercise program on glucose control and insulin action in women with type 2 diabetes, *Eur J Physiol* 92:437-442, 2004.

36. Irwin ML, Yasui Y, Ulrich CM et al: Effect of exercise on total and intra-abdominal body fat in postmenopausal women, *JAMA* 289:323-330, 2003.

37. Slentz CA, Duscha BD, Johnson JL et al: Effects of the amount of exercise on body weight, body composition, and measures of central obesity, *Arch Intern Med* 164:31-39, 2004.

38. Wing RR, Hill JO: Successful weight loss maintenance, *Annu Rev Nutr* 21:323-341, 2001.

39. Houde SC, Melillo KD: Cardiovascular health and physical activity in older adults: an integrative review of research methodology and results, *J Adv Nurs* 38:219-234, 2002.

40. Mayer-Davis EJ, Costacou T: Obesity and sedentary lifestyle: modifiable risk factors for prevention of type 2 diabetes, *Curr Diab Rep* 1:170-176, 2001.

41. Lakka TA, Laaksonen DE, Lakka HM et al: Sedentary lifestyle, poor cardiorespiratory fitness, and the metabolic syndrome, *Med Sci Sports Exerc* 35:1279-1286, 2003.

42. Giannuzzi P, Mezzani A, Saner H et al: Physical activity for primary and secondary prevention, *Eur J Cardiovasc Prev Rehabil* 10:319-327, 2003.

43. Brummett BH, Babyak MA, Siegler IC et al: Effect of smoking and sedentary behavior on the association between depressive symptoms and mortality from coronary heart disease, *Am J Cardiol* 92:529-532, 2003.

44. Blumenthal JA, Sherwood A, Gullette EC et al: Exercise and weight loss reduce blood pressure in men and women with mild hypertension: effects on cardiovascular, metabolic, and homodynamic functioning, *Arch Intern Med* 160:1947-1958, 2000.

45. Pihl E, Zilmer K, Kullisaar T et al: High-sensitive C-reactive protein level and oxidative stress-related status in former athletes in relation to traditional cardiovascular risk factors, *Atherosclerosis* 171:321-326, 2003.

46. Pearson TA: Education and income: double-edged swords in the epidemiological transition of cardiovascular disease, *Ethn Dis* 13 suppl 2:S158-S163, 2003.

47. Torun B, Stein AD, Schroeder D et al: Rural to urban migration and cardiovascular disease risk factors in young Guatemalan adults, *Int J Epidemiol* 31:218-226, 2002.

48. Osler M, Clausen JO, Ibsen KK, Jensen GB: Social influences and low leisure-time physical activity in young Danish adults, *Eur J Public Health* 11:130-134, 2001.

49. Reddy KK, Rao AP, Ready TP: Socioeconomic status and the prevalence of coronary heart disease risk factors, *Asia Pac J Clin Nutr* 11:98-103, 2002.

50. Thompson JL, Allen P, Cunningham-Sabo L et al: Environmental, policy, and cultural factors related to physical activity in sedentary American Indian women, *Womens Health* 36:59-74, 2002.

51. Steffen-Batey L, Nichaman MZ, Goff DC Jr et al: Change in level of physical activity and risk of all-cause mortality or reinfarction: the Corpus Christi Heart Project, *Circulation* 102:2204-2209, 2000.

52. Eyler AA, Matson-Koffman D, Young DR et al: Quantitative study of correlates of physical activity in women from diverse racial/ethnic groups: the Women's cardiovascular health network project summary and conclusions, *Am J Prev Med* 25(3 suppl 1):93-103, 2003.

53. Wilbur J, Chandler PJ, Dancy B et al: Correlates of physical activity in urban Midwestern Latinas, *Am J Prev Med* 25(3 suppl 1):69-76, 2003.

54. Evenson KR, Sarmiento OL, Tawney KW et al: Personal, social, and environmental correlates of physical activity in North Carolina Latina immigrants, *Am J Prev Med* 25(3 suppl 1):77-85, 2003.

55. Voorhees CC, Rohm YD: Personal, social, and physical environmental correlates of physical activity levels in urban Latinas, *Am J Prev Med* 25(3 suppl 1):61-68, 2003.

56. Wilbur J, Chandler PJ, Dancy B et al: Correlates of physical activity in urban Midwestern African-American women, *Am J Prev Med* 25(3 suppl 1):45-52, 2003.

57. Hu FB, Li TY, Colditz GA et al: Television watching and other sedentary behaviors in relation to risk of obesity and type 2 diabetes mellitus in women, *JAMA* 289:1785-1791, 2003.

58. Lowry R, Wechsler H, Galuska DA et al: Television viewing and its associations with overweight, sedentary lifestyle, and insufficient consumption of fruits and vegetables among US high school students: differences by race, ethnicity, and gender, *J Sch Health* 72:413-421, 2002.

59. Janz KF, Dawson JD, Mahoney LT: Increases in physical fitness during childhood improve cardiovascular health during adolescence: the Muscatine Study, *Int J Sports Med* 23(suppl 1):S15-S21, 2002.

60. Macaluso A, DeVito G: Muscle strength, power and adaptations to resistance training in older people, *Eur J Appl Physiol* 91:450-472, 2004.

61. Taaffe DR, Marcus R: Musculoskeletal health and the older adult, *J Rehabil Res Dev* 37:245-254, 2000.

62. Centers for Disease Control and Prevention: Strength training among adults aged = 65 years, United States, 2001, *MMWR Morb Mortal Wkly Rep* 53(2):25-28, 2004.

63. Tanaka H, Dinnenno FA, Monahan KD et al: Aging, habitual exercise, and dynamic arterial compliance, *Circulation* 102:1214-1215, 2000.

64. Pugh KG, Wei JY: Clinical implications of physiological changes in the aging heart, *Drugs Aging* 18:263-276, 2001.

65. Grossman MD, Stewart AL: "You aren't going to get better by just sitting around": physical activity perceptions, motivations, and barriers in adults 75 years of age or older, *Am J Geriatr Cardiol* 12:33-37, 2003. (Cited onpage 9 , 3rd line above "Intervention Approaches")

66. Fletcher GF, Balady JB, Vogel RA et al: 33rd Bethesda Conference: preventive cardiology—how can we do better? *J Am Coll Cardiol* 40:579-651, 2002.

67. US Department of Health and Human Services: *Healthy People 2010: understanding and improving health*, ed 2, Washington, DC, 2000, US Government Printing Office.

68. Pearson TA, Blair SN, Daniels SR et al: AHA guidelines for primary prevention of cardiovascular disease and stroke: 2001 update, *Circulation* 106:388-391, 2002.

69. Eyre H, Kahn R, Robertson RM et al: Preventing cancer, cardiovascular disease, and diabetes: a common agenda for the American Cancer Society, the American Diabetes Association, and the American Heart Association, *Circulation* 209:3244-3255, 2004.

70. Pearson TA, Wall S, Lewis C et al: Dissecting the "black box" of community interventions: lesions from community-wide cardiovascular disease prevention programs in the US and Sweden, *Scand J Public Health* 29:69-78, 2001.

71. Pearson TA, Bazzarre TL, Daniels SR et al: American Heart Association guide for improving cardiovascular health at the community level: a statement for public health practitioners, healthcare providers, and health policy makers from the American Heart Association Expert Panel on Population and Prevention Science, *Circulation* 107:645-651, 2003.

72. Reger-Nash B, Bauman A, Booth-Butterfield S et al: Wheeling walks: evaluation of a media-based community intervention, *Fam Community Health* 28:64-78, 2005.

73. Yancey AK, Lewis LB, Sloane DC et al: Leading by example: a local health department-community collaboration to incorporate physical activity into organizational practice, *J Public Health Manag Pract* 10:116-123, 2004.

74. Grunbaum JA, Kann L, Kinchen SA et al: Youth risk behavior surveillance: United States, 2001, *MMWR Surveill Summ* 51:1-62, 2002.

75. Hayman LL, Williams CL, Daniels SR et al: Cardiovascular health promotion in schools: a statement for health and education professionals and child health advocates from the Committee on Atherosclerosis, Hypertension, and Obesity in Youth (AHOY) of the Council on Cardiovascular Disease in the Young, American Heart Association, *Circulation* 110:2266-2275, 2004.

76. Mckenzie TL, Sallis JF, Prochaska JJ et al: Evaluation of a two-year middle-school physical education intervention: M-SPAN, *Med Sci Sports Exerc* 36:1382-1388, 2004.

77. US Preventive Services Task Force: *Guide to clinical preventive services*, ed 2, Baltimore, 1996, Williams & Wilkins.

78. Adult Treatment Panel III: Executive summary of the Third Report of the National Cholesterol Education Program (NCEP) Expert Panel on Detection, Evaluation, and Treatment of High Blood Cholesterol in Adults, *JAMA* 285:2486-2497, 2001.

79. Chobanian AV, Bakris GL, Black HR et al: The Seventh Report of the Joint National Committee on Prevention, Detection, Evaluation, and Treatment of High Blood Pressure, *JAMA* 289:2560-2572, 2003.

80. American Diabetes Association: Standards of medical care in diabetes, *Diabetes Care* 28(suppl 1):S4-S36, 2005.

81. Whitlock EP, Orleans CT, Pender N, Allan J: Evaluating primary care behavioral counseling interventions: an evidence-based approach, *Am J Prev Med* 22:267-284, 2002.

82. Diabetes Prevention Program Research Group: Achieving weight and activity goals among diabetes prevention program lifestyle participants, *Obes Res* 12:1426-1435, 2004.

83. Smith SC, Blair SN, Bonow RO et al: AHA/ACC guidelines for preventing heart attack and death in patients with atherosclerotic cardiovascular disease: 2001 update—a statement for healthcare professionals from the American Heart Association and the American College of Cardiology, *Circulation* 104:1577-1579, 2001.

84. Taylor RS, Brown A, Ebrahim S et al: Exercise-based rehabilitation for patients with coronary heart disease: systematic review and meta-analysis of randomized trials, *Am J Med* 116:682-697, 2004.

85. Leon AS, Franklin BA, Costa F et al: Cardiac rehabilitation and secondary prevention of coronary heart disease: an American Heart Association scientific statement from the Council on Clinical Cardiology (Subcommittee on Exercise, Cardiac Rehabilitation, and Prevention) and the Council on Nutrition, Physical Activity, and Metabolism (Subcommittee on Physical Activity), in collaboration with the American Association of Cardiovascular and Pulmonary Rehabilitation, *Circulation* 111:369-376, 2005.

86. Hellman EA: Use of the stages of change in exercise adherence model among older adults with a cardiac diagnosis, *J Cardiopulm Rehabil* 17:145-155, 1997.

87. Carlson JJ, Norman GJ, Feltz DL et al: Self-efficacy, psychosocial factors, and exercise behavior in traditional versus modified cardiac rehabilitation, *J Cardiopulm Rehabil* 21:363-373, 2001.

88. Katzmarzyk PT, Gledhill N, Shephard RJ: The economic burden of physical inactivity in Canada, *CMAJ* 163:1435-1440, 2000.

Stress

Connie B. Scanga

CHAPTER ABBREVIATIONS

ACTH   adrenocorticotrophic hormone

CRH   corticotropin-releasing hormone

ECG   electrocardiographic

ERI   effort-reward imbalance

HPA   hypothalamic-pituitary-adrenocortical

IL   interleukin

MI   myocardial infarction

SAS   sympathoadrenomedullary system

TABP   type A behavior pattern

Stress is defined as a state of threatened homeostasis provoked by a psychological, environmental, or physiological stimulus. The provoking stimulus, called a stressor, may be psychological (e.g., anger or fear) or physical (e.g., surgery or physical trauma).[1] The physiological stress response is characterized by an increased secretion of stress hormones, elevated heart rate and respiration rate, increased blood pressure and hemodynamic changes, and alterations in energy metabolism. The stress response is innate, rather than acquired, and historically has been viewed as an adaptive response necessary for survival, especially in animals living in environments rife with physical danger. However, there is mounting evidence that chronic or excessive stress has a negative impact on physical health, playing a direct contributing role in conditions such as cardiovascular disease, compromised cognitive function, metabolic syndrome, and affective disorders.[1-3] In this chapter the fundamentals of stress theory, the relationship between stress and cardiovascular disease, and a range of stress management techniques are discussed.

HOMEOSTASIS AND NEUROENDOCRINOLOGY OF THE STRESS RESPONSE

The contemporary understanding of stress and homeostasis traces its roots to the ancient Greeks. Approximately 2500 years ago, Heraclitus proposed that the static state is not a natural condition and that the capacity to undergo change is intrinsic to life. Building on this concept, the philosopher Empedocles proposed that matter consists of elements and qualities that are in dynamic opposition to or in alliance with one another and that balance or harmony is a necessary condition for the survival of living organisms. Hippocrates (circa 400 BC) equated health with the harmonic balance of elements

and proposed that illness and disease stem from the systematic disharmony of these elements.[1]

Walter Cannon[4] introduced the term *homeostasis* to describe the concept of internal dynamic equilibrium. Borrowing the concepts of "stress" and "strain" from the fields of physics and engineering, he discussed various stressful stimuli that induce physiological strain and introduced the concept of critical stress, i.e., stress sufficient to induce breaking strain in homeostatic mechanisms. Cannon[5] was also first to describe the fight-or-flight reaction, which he described as the response of the body to aggression. He demonstrated that the response can be evoked by emotional and physical factors that could arise internally or externally and that the physiological response was dependent on activation of the sympathetic nervous system and catecholamine secretion by the adrenal gland.[4]

Hans Selye is considered by many to be the "father of stress" because of his pioneering work in the field and his comprehensive conceptualization of the stress response. In 1936, Selye[6] reported that "various nocuous agents" (e.g., excessive heat or cold, forced immobilization or exercise, or chemical agents) elicit a predictable, nonspecific response characterized by activation of a secretory cascade involving corticotropin-releasing hormone (**CRH**), adrenocorticotrophic hormone (**ACTH**), and adrenal corticosteroid hormones. Selye[7] believed that positive and negative stressors induced essentially the same nonspecific pattern of response, and he introduced the terms *eustress* and *distress,* respectively, to distinguish the two. He postulated that eustress was ultimately the less damaging to the organism.

Selye[6] called the stress response the general adaptation syndrome, which he conceived as being a three-stage response consisting of the alarm reaction, the resistance stage, and exhaustion. The alarm reaction, equivalent to the fight-or-flight response, is the initial response to a stressor. Activation of the sympathoadrenomedullary system (**SAS**) during this stage induces widespread physiological effects and allows the organism to mount a speedy response to the stressor. The alarm reaction is associated with activation of norepinephrine-secreting neurons in a brain stem nucleus called the locus ceruleus. Neuronal pathways radiate throughout the central nervous system from the locus ceruleus, innervating regions of the cerebrum, hypothalamus, cerebellum, brain stem, and spinal cord. When activated by novel stimuli, the sensory cortex relays input to the locus ceruleus, eliciting an increased rate of norepinephrine secretion by locus ceruleus neurons that results in increased alertness or awareness. If the stimulus is perceived as harmful or threatening, locus ceruleus activation is more intense or prolonged and results in activation of the SAS and peripheral release of epinephrine and norepinephrine by the adrenal medulla.[1] The alarm response is characterized by an increased heart rate and cardiac output, increased blood pressure, bronchodilatation, increased liver glycogenolysis and resulting release of glucose to the blood, and hemodynamic changes (i.e., decreased blood flow to digestive organs, kidneys, and skin; and increased blood flow to skeletal muscle, heart, and brain).[8]

The second phase of the general adaptation syndrome, the resistance stage, is a period during which the body attempts to adapt to a stressor and restore homeostasis. This phase, which is mediated by the hypothalamic-pituitary-adrenocortical (**HPA**) axis, is induced by the central release of CRH. CRH circulates in the hypothalamo-hypophysial portal system to the anterior pituitary gland, where it causes enhanced secretion of ACTH. ACTH in turn causes increased secretion by the adrenal cortex of glucocorticoids and, to a lesser extent, mineralocorticoids. Selye[6] reported that three major organic changes were observed consistently during this stage: adrenal enlargement, gastrointestinal ulcers, and thymolymphatic atrophy.

The second component of the stress response, CRH, regulates the HPA axis and causes its activation during a stress response. In nonstressful circumstances, CRH is secreted in a pulsatile, circadian fashion with a frequency of two to three secretions per hour and with levels normally peaking in the morning near the time one arises. The normal pattern of CRH secretion is disrupted by environmental, physical, and psychosocial stress.[9] Activation of the HPA axis results in increased release of CRH and arginine vasopressin (also known as antidiuretic hormone) from the paraventricular nucleus of the hypothalamus. CRH is the primary hypothalamic stimulus for ACTH secretion; arginine vasopressin acts synergistically with CRH to enhance ACTH secretion. Secretion of ACTH by the anterior pituitary gland elicits a species-specific glucocorticoid and, to a lesser extent, mineralocorticoid (e.g., aldosterone) secretion by the adrenal cortex. Circulating glucocorticoids (specifically, cortisol in human beings and nonhuman primates and corticosterone in rodents) provide negative feedback, slowing CRH secretion, which helps to prevent excessive blood glucocorticoid levels. Glucocorticoids enhance lipid and protein catabolism, increase blood glucose levels, and suppress the immune and inflammation responses. As part of an acute stress response, glucocorticoid effects are beneficial. Chronic or intense activation of the HPA axis and prolonged glucocorticoid elevation, however, induces the pathogenesis described by Selye's general adaptation syndrome.

The paraventricular nucleus usually is considered to be a focal point for interaction and regulation of the stress system. Efferent CRH pathways radiate from the paraventricular nucleus to the median eminence of the hypothalamus, where CRH is released into the hypophysial portal network for delivery to the anterior pituitary gland.[10] CRH efferent pathways also pass to regions of the brain stem (including the locus ceruleus)

and spinal cord involved with sympathetic and parasympathetic function.[11] Neurons of the paraventricular nucleus receive afferent input from various parts of the brain and brain stem, including the locus ceruleus/norepinephrine system. The CRH and locus ceruleus/norepinephrine systems participate in reciprocal positive feedback loops; as a result, activation of one system activates the other.[12-17]

In addition to interactions with the locus ceruleus/norepinephrine system the HPA axis interacts, directly or indirectly, with the immune and metabolic systems and with the growth and gonadal axes (Figure 39-1).

According to Selye,[18] initial symptoms of stress diminish or disappear as the body makes optimal adaptation to the stressor during the resistance phase. He postulated that adaptation to a stressor and the return to homeostasis require the expenditure of adaptation energy, an innate and finite resource that is distinct from caloric energy. If exposure to a stressor is prolonged or if the stressor is sufficiently intense, adaptation cannot be achieved or maintained and the body enters into the third phase of the general adaptation syndrome, exhaustion. Exhaustion results from depletion of adaptation energy and may be permanent or reversible. Selye hypothesized that physical decompensation in the exhaustion stage played a role in the cause or exacerbation of various diseases, including peptic ulcers and hypertension.

ALLOSTASIS AND THE NATURE OF STRESS

Selye's concepts and newly developed laboratory technologies (e.g., immunoassays) stimulated numerous stress- and endocrine-related studies in the 1950s and 1960s. In reviewing his own and others' research from this period, John Mason[19,20] presented convincing evidence that psychological influences were among the most potent natural stimuli affecting pituitary-adrenal cortical activity. The brain now generally is recognized to evaluate or filter stimuli, and as a result, individual differences in perception and responsiveness to any particular situation can be expected. The cognitive activation theory of stress, which integrates stress-related findings from the fields of physiology, psychology, and endocrinology, proposes that stress is a general alarm system that operates when there is an uncomfortable gap between one's expectation(s) and one's reality. That is, cognition and psychological factors mediate the neuroendocrine response to a situation. Stressful adaptations occur when one perceives a threatening lack of control or inability to cope with a challenge.[1,21,22]

Central to stress research has been Cannon's concept of homeostasis, the understanding that in response to a stressor, adaptive cascades are evoked that help maintain a normal range of internal conditions and ensure survival. Beginning with Selye's work, there also has been recognition of the damage to the body that potentially can be induced by adaptive physiological mechanisms. Allostatic load recently has been proposed as a construct for conceptualizing how stress-induced physiological mechanisms, over long-term intervals, can promote disease and increase morbidity and mortality.[23,24]

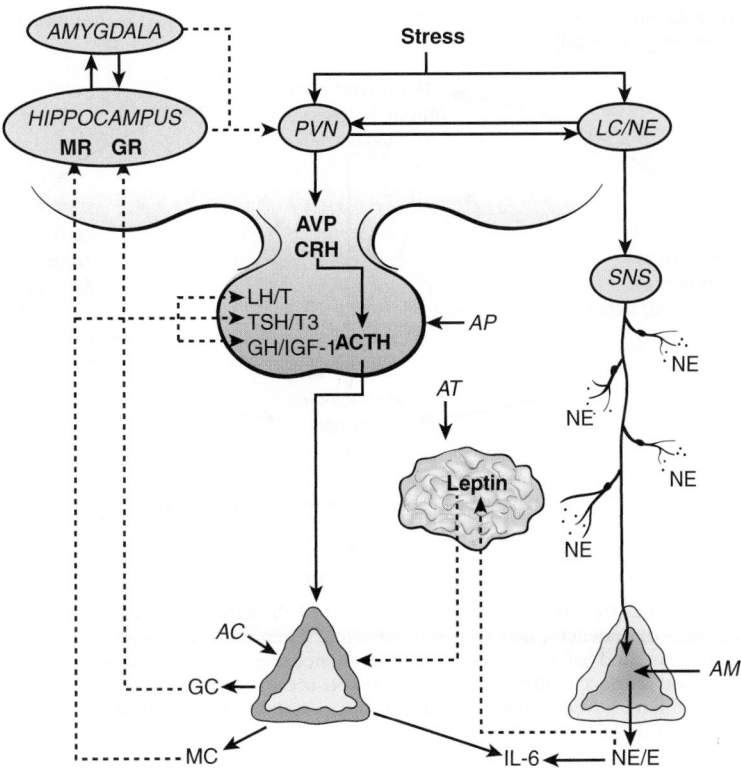

FIGURE 39-1 ▦ A schematic representation of the stress response system. Stress stimuli activate the reciprocally innervated hypothalamus-pituitary-adrenal (HPA) axis and sympathoadrenal system (SAS). Activation of the HPA axis involves release of corticotropin-releasing hormone (CRH) and arginine vasopressin (AVP) from the paraventricular nucleus (PVN) of the hypothalamus, generating increased secretion of adrenocorticotropic hormone (ACTH) by the anterior pituitary (AP) gland. ACTH stimulates increased secretion of glucocorticoids (GC) and mineralocorticoids (MC) from the adrenal cortex (AC). GC and MC modulate HPA axis activity via negative feedback effects mediated by binding to receptors (GR and MR, respectively) in the hippocampus, as well as in other parts of the stress response system. Activation of the SAS (locus ceruleus [LC]/norepinephrine [NE]/sympathetic nervous system [SNS]) causes increased release of NE from sympathetic nerve terminals, and of catecholamines (epinephrine [E] and NE) from the adrenal medulla (AM). Activation of the HPA axis leads to suppression of the growth hormone/insulin-like growth factor-1 (GH/IGF-1), luteinizing hormone/testosterone (LH/T), and thyrotropin/triiodothyronine (TSH/T$_3$) axes. Activation of the SAS results in increased interleukin-6 (IL-6) secretion. Leptin, from adipose tissue (AT), directly inhibits secretion of GC, whereas increased NE and E secretion tends to reduce serum leptin levels. Chronic increases in GC, catecholamines, and IL-6 and chronic suppression of the GH/IGF-1, LH/T, and TSH/T$_3$ axes provide a hormonal milieu that is conducive to the development of central obesity, hypertension, atherosclerosis, osteoporosis, and immune dysfunction. *CRH,* Corticotropin-releasing hormone; *GR,* glucocorticoid; *MR,* mineralocorticoid. (From Chrousos GP: *Int J Obes Relat Metab Disord* 24[suppl 2]:S50-S55, 2000.)

Allostasis, defined as the process of achieving stability through change,[23] is a concept first proposed by Sterling and Eyer[25] to denote the changes in cardiovascular function that support homeostasis as the body moves between the resting and active states. The concept was expanded subsequently to encompass physiological responses induced by changes in physical state (e.g., sleep, wakefulness, or postural changes) and by stressful situations (e.g., danger, extreme environmental temperature, or psychosocial challenge).[24] Allostasis is achieved through the integrated activity of the primary allostatic mediators, i.e., the SAS, the HPA axis, and cytokines. In response to stressors and the challenges of daily living, these systems are activated and thereby induce adaptive physiological responses, which allow bodily systems to function within optimal, homeostatic ranges (Figure 39-2).

Allostatic load is a cumulative measure of the biological strain produced by repeated cycles of allostatic activity, the changes in metabolism, and the "wear and tear" induced on tissues and organs by allostasis. Allostatic load results not only from excessive activity but also from dysregulation or inefficiency of the allostatic systems, and it may be exacerbated by genetic risk, developmental events, and behavioral and lifestyle choices.[23,24] Investigators have used a variety of parameters representing functioning across physiological systems to measure allostatic load. These parameters include blood pressure, glycosylated hemoglobin, serum lipid levels, body mass index, waist-to-hip ratio, markers of inflammation (e.g., fibrinogen and C-reactive protein), and overnight urinary cortisol and catecholamine secretion. Higher levels of allostatic load, especially of long-term duration, have been linked to increased cardiovascular disease, cognitive impairment, and mortality.[26-28]

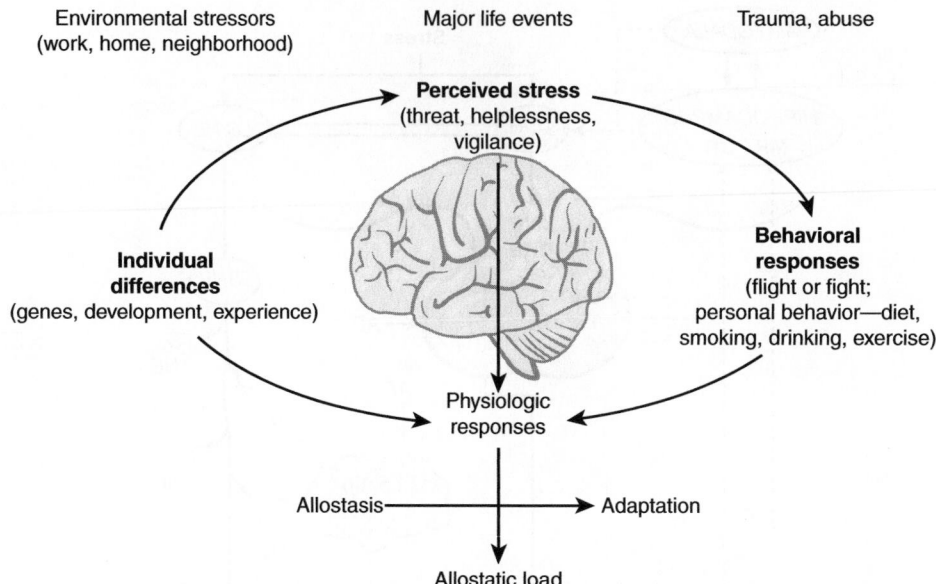

Environmental stressors
(work, home, neighborhood)

Major life events

Trauma, abuse

Perceived stress
(threat, helplessness,
vigilance)

Individual
differences
(genes, development, experience)

Behavioral
responses
(flight or fight;
personal behavior—diet,
smoking, drinking, exercise)

Physiologic
responses

Allostasis ⟶ Adaptation

Allostatic load

FIGURE 39-2 ▦ The stress response and development of allostatic load. The perception of stress is influenced by one's experiences, genetics, and behavior. When the brain perceives an experience as stressful, physiological and behavioral responses are initiated, leading to allostasis and adaptation. Over time, allostatic load can accumulate, and the overexposure to mediators of neural, endocrine, and immune stress can have adverse effects on various organ systems, leading to disease. (From McEwen BS: *N Engl J Med* 338:171-179, 1998.)

STRESS AND CARDIOVASCULAR DISEASE

The role of heredity and traditional risk factors (e.g., hypercholesterolemia, smoking, obesity, and sedentary lifestyle) for cardiovascular disease is well-established. Recently, chronic stress exposure has been recognized as an important nontraditional risk factor for the development of cardiovascular disease, playing a role in the etiology and pathophysiology of essential hypertension, atherosclerosis and coronary artery disease, and myocardial infarction (**MI**).[3,29]

Hypertension

The autonomic nervous system plays a key role in blood pressure regulation. Autonomic imbalance characterized by sympathetic hyperactivity and parasympathetic underactivity has been shown to be important in the etiology and pathology of essential hypertension.[30,31] Stress exposure and a resulting activation of the SAS, both in laboratory settings and in daily life, is one avenue through which transient or prolonged blood pressure elevations may be induced. The SAS, acting through catecholamine-induced constriction of vascular smooth muscle and increased cardiac output, is the primary mediator of blood pressure elevation during acute stress responses.[32] Parasympathetic underactivity also may contribute to acute blood pressure elevations during acute and prolonged stress responses.[33,34] Additionally, sympathetic activation directly stimulates renin release from juxtaglomerular cells of the kidney, resulting in increased angiotensin II activity and aldosterone secretion by the adrenal cortex (i.e., the renin-angiotensin-aldosterone system). Angiotensin II increases blood pressure by its direct vasoconstrictive effects and by

potentiating adrenergic activity at sympathetic synapses. Circulating angiotensin II, acting via circumventricular organs outside of the blood-brain barrier, increases peripheral sympathetic nervous system activity and elicits a pressor effect.[35,36] Aldosterone increases tubular sodium reabsorption, facilitating water retention and increasing blood volume and blood pressure.[37] Thus, complex interactions between the SAS and the renin-angiotensin-aldosterone system promote and sustain the blood pressure reactivity to stress and play a role in exacerbating prehypertensive and hypertensive pathological conditions.

Maintenance of normal blood pressure responses involves interaction between the autonomic nervous system and vascular endothelium and depends on the balance between the generalized vasoconstricting effects of sympathetic innervation and the localized modulating effects of endothelial-derived mediators. Endothelial damage caused by acute blood pressure elevation has been shown to alter the normal balance of endothelial production of nitric oxide and endothelin-1, local vasodilator and vasoconstrictor agents, respectively. Acute exposure to stressors in laboratory settings (e.g., mental arithmetic, video games, and cold pressor challenges) result in increased endothelin-1 release and decreased nitric oxide effectiveness, leading to an increase in total peripheral resistance and blood pressure.[38-40] Vascular remodeling, which also results in increased peripheral resistance, is an additional consequence of prolonged sympathetic hyperactivity. Vascular changes induced by excess sympathetic drive include rarefaction (reduction in capillary density) and decreased lumen diameter,[41] changes in wall-to-lumen ratio, and hyperresponsiveness to vasoconstrictor substances.[42]

Stress exposure also is known to disrupt the normal diurnal pattern of glucocorticoid secretion, leading to significantly increased levels of circulating cortisol.[2] Excess glucocorticoid activity may contribute to the etiology of hypertension by potentiating the vasoconstrictive effects of norepinephrine and angiotensin II through receptor upregulation and also may enhance endothelin-1 activity.[43]

Atherosclerosis and Coronary Artery Disease

Atherosclerosis has a multifaceted pathophysiology that is initiated by loss of endothelial integrity and function. This is followed by lipid insudation (accumulation) in the vascular wall, as well as migration and proliferation of smooth muscle cells and blood leukocytes (i.e, monocyte-derived macrophages and lymphocytes) in the vascular intima, inflammation of subendothelial tissue, and formation of fibrofatty plaques that slowly and progressively occlude the vascular lumen. The pathogenesis of coronary artery atherosclerosis and the role of traditional risk factors and lifestyle behaviors (e.g., heredity, diet, smoking, and sedentary lifestyle) associated with the etiology and progression of coronary artery disease are discussed in previous chapters of this text. However, traditional risk factors and adverse health behaviors do not explain fully the variations in coronary artery disease incidence. Increasing evidence indicates that psychological and psychosocial stressors also contribute to the progression of coronary artery disease and its clinical manifestations, transient ischemia and MI.[3,44]

Cardiovascular reactivity, defined as the magnitude or pattern of change in heart rate and blood pressure responses, frequently is employed to assess the physiological effects of a discrete psychological or psychosocial stressor. A well-documented dose-response relationship exists in human and animal studies between cardiovascular reactivity to behavioral and psychosocial stressors and the progression and severity of atherosclerosis[44-46] and cardiovascular disease.[47] Rapid heart rate has been shown to cause coronary atherosclerosis directly in experiments with nonhuman primates (i.e., cynomolgus monkeys),[48] an effect likely caused by the higher coronary shear forces elicited by tachycardia.[49] Large prospective studies have demonstrated that excessive cardiovascular reactivity in normotensive white and black American subjects is a consistent independent predictor of essential hypertension when long-term (20 years or more) follow-up is conducted.[50,51] Cardiovascular reactivity in borderline hypertensive subjects is also independently predictive of future essential hypertension in short-term (10 years or less) follow-up.[52] Although it is not yet clear to what extent cardiovascular reactivity and coronary artery disease share a causal relationship or common cause, research into stress-provoked cardiovascular reactivity has confirmed that there are individual differences in autonomic responsiveness to stressful stimuli. High cardiovascular reactivity may be best used as a reliable marker for long-term development of essential hypertension and coronary artery disease.

Frequent or prolonged exposure to psychosocial stressors has been shown to induce endothelial damage directly in cynomolgus monkeys, an effect mediated by beta$_1$-adrenoceptor activation.[53,54] As noted previously, a consequence of endothelial damage is alteration in the synthesis and activity of endothelial-derived mediators—such as nitric oxide, tissue plasminogen activator, and platelet-derived growth factor—that result in increased platelet aggregation, reduced fibrinolysis, and proliferation of vascular smooth muscle and connective tissue, respectively.[55] Psychosocial stress also has been shown to increase platelet aggregation and activation directly, effects that may be mediated at least partially by epinephrine.[56,57] Platelet aggregation and activation then may contribute further to vascular injury or lesion development. Gender differences have been demonstrated in the effects of psychosocial stress on progression of atherosclerosis. Estrogen exerts positive effects on vascular integrity and function by favoring a shift in autonomic tone toward parasympathetic activity.[58,59] Estrogen also increases nitric oxide release and inhibits endothelin-1 activity.[60]

Elevated blood viscosity is correlated with increased severity of coronary artery stenosis[61] and the risk of coronary events.[62] Acute mental and environmental stress elicits transient hemoconcentration and increased blood viscosity in normal[63-65] and hypertensive[66] subjects. The magnitude of stress-induced hemorheological changes correlated with the magnitude of cardiovascular reactivity observed during the stress response.[64,67] It has been proposed that stress-mediated hemoconcentration and increased blood viscosity may exacerbate atherogenesis at low pressure sites proximal to arterial bifurcation by further decreasing the pressure and increasing the exposure time of hemoconcentrated atherogenic substances to a developing lesion.[68]

The stress-induced increase in HPA axis activity also may contribute to the pathophysiology of atherosclerosis and coronary artery disease. High glucocorticoid tone is associated with increased severity of coronary artery disease risk factors, including adverse alterations in lipid metabolism, insulin resistance and hyperglycemia, and increased visceral adiposity.[69] High glucocorticoid tone also may contribute to oxidative stress and endothelial dysfunction.[70,71]

Glucocorticoids have a recognized antiinflammatory and immunosuppressive effect, which would suggest an antiatherogenic role. However, glucocorticoid therapy in patients with rheumatoid arthritis was associated with carotid plaque and arterial incompressibility, independent of cardiovascular risk factors,[72] suggesting complex vascular, inflammation, and glucocorticoid interactions in the initiation and progression of atherosclerosis. Acute glucocorticoid exposure attenuates various mediators of vascular lesion including expression of vascular adhesion molecules, monocyte and lymphocyte adherence and activation, low-density lipoprotein oxidation, and smooth muscle proliferation. When glucocorticoid exposure is prolonged, these beneficial effects are reduced substantially. It has been proposed that low levels of glucocorticoid activity exert permissive effects that promote an early and successful response to a stressor, intermediate levels (e.g., levels at unstressed diurnal peak periods) promote defensive immune responses, and high levels of glucocorticoid activity (e.g., levels observed during major stress events) have suppressive or antiinflammatory effects.[73,74] For example, glucocorticoids exert permissive or suppressive effects on the acute-phase response triggered by injury or infection.[75] This effect is dose and timing dependent. Preexposure to glucocorticoids enhances release of the proinflammatory cytokines tumor necrosis factor-alpha, interleukin-1 (**IL**-1), and IL-6, although glucocorticoid administration at the time of challenge or injury suppresses this response[76] and acute administration of glucocorticoids in a clinical setting is associated with decreased levels of circulating IL-6 and C-reactive protein.[77] It has been suggested that IL-6 is a primary mediator of the acute-phase reaction[78] and of stress-induced atherogenic effects.[79] During periods of prolonged stress, adipose tissue[80] and the adrenal gland[81] secrete IL-6 and contribute to its elevated level in the circulation. Circulating IL-6 directly stimulates the HPA axis, resulting in increased secretion of CRH, ACTH, and cortisol in human beings.[82] Plasma IL-6 levels are elevated in individuals with melancholic depression[83] and in those living in urban versus rural settings in India.[84] Recently, it was reported that stress-induced increases in IL-6 and fibrinogen independently predicted ambulatory blood pressure increases at a 3-year follow-up.[85] It may be that psychosocial or environmental stressors induce reciprocal interactions between IL-6 and the HPA axis that promote hypertension, hyperlipidemia, visceral adiposity, and insulin resistance, thus potentiating the effects of glucocorticoid excess.

Ischemia and Myocardial Infarction

Clinical manifestations of coronary artery disease appear after decades of progressive lesion development. Ischemia occurs when there is an imbalance between myocardial oxygen supply and demand. Ischemia commonly is caused by occlusion of coronary arteries by advanced lesions and can be exacerbated transiently by vasoconstriction of the coronary arteries. Advanced atherosclerotic lesions may rupture, initiating thrombus formation and vasospasm that further impede blood flow. Severe or prolonged ischemia may result in MI or sudden cardiac death.[86]

Epidemiological research has demonstrated a link between mental or life stress and the occurrence of adverse cardiovascular events. Several retrospective studies have examined spouse or informant reports of life stress in the hours[87] or months to years[88-90] preceding sudden cardiac death. Each demonstrated higher levels of informant-reported life stress during the retrospective period preceding sudden cardiac death. Unfortunately, the studies did not include control groups[88,90] or the control data could not be interpreted precisely.[87,89] Subsequent controlled retrospective studies have demonstrated a high prevalence of loss events (e.g., death of spouse or close family member) in the 6 months preceding sudden cardiac death in women with no history of coronary artery disease[91] and a significant relationship

between major life events in the preceding 1 year and the first episode of coronary heart disease.[92] An investigation using a case-crossover design, which compared each patient's pre-MI activities to his or her usual level of activities, reported an increased relative risk of MI onset within the 2 hours after episodes of anger. The relative risk was significantly lower among regular users of aspirin than among nonusers, and there were nonsignificant trends toward lower relative risk in men than in women and among regular users of beta-adrenergic antagonist users than nonusers.[93] The effects of acute stress also are thought to contribute to the increased frequency of cardiac events following large-scale crises and environmental disasters, such as war[94] and missile attacks,[95,96] earthquakes,[97-99] and blizzards[100] and extreme winter weather.[101]

Mental stress and negative emotions also have been shown to evoke myocardial ischemia in laboratory and ambulatory research models. An early study using positron emission tomography to measure altered myocardial perfusion during a stressful mental arithmetic task demonstrated reduced perfusion in 75 percent of coronary heart disease patients.[102] More recently, in studies using radionuclide ventriculography to demonstrate wall motion abnormalities as an indicator of ischemia, 58 percent[103] and 59 percent[104] of coronary artery disease patients with exercise-induced ischemia also manifested ischemia during periods of mental stress. A personally relevant and emotionally arousing speech task induced a magnitude of cardiac dysfunction greater than that observed in less specific cognitive tasks and similar to that induced by exercise.[104] Patients who exhibit mild to moderate depression are more likely than nondepressed patients to exhibit myocardial ischemia during mental stress testing and daily living.[34]

Ambulatory electrocardiographic (**ECG**) monitoring is used in combination with diaries of physical and mental activity and emotional state to assess the incidence of out-of-hospital ischemia in patients. These studies have demonstrated a relationship between the occurrence of ischemia and the intensity of physical and mental activities. Ischemia occurred most often during physical and mental activities of moderate[105] or high intensity[106] and among patients with high emotional responsivity (i.e., exhibit relatively large variations of self-reported tension).[107] Among smokers, ischemia was more than 5 times more likely when they were smoking than when they were not.[105] Strenuous physical activity and negative emotions (e.g., intense anger, tension, frustration, or sadness) were potent triggers of ischemia, and mental and emotional stress appear to be as likely to trigger ischemia as physical activity.[105,106,108] In recent studies, coronary artery disease patients with exercised-induced ischemia who experienced mental stress-induced ischemia had significantly higher rates of subsequent fatal and nonfatal cardiac events,[109-111] suggesting prognostic importance for mental stress testing in the clinical setting.

Mental and emotional stress contribute to ischemia by eliciting an increase in heart rate and contractility, an effect that is mediated by the SAS in healthy and coronary artery disease populations. Mental stress-induced ischemia is usually "silent" and occurs at a lower heart rate than exercise-induced ischemia. Although comparable systolic blood pressure elevations are induced by mental and exercise stress tests, the double product (systolic blood pressure × heart rate) at onset of ischemia is significantly less during mental stress testing than during exercise testing.[104] Because heart rate commonly is considered an index of myocardial oxygen demand, these results suggest that mental stress may reduce myocardial oxygen supply. Evidence from human and animal studies has demonstrated that one mechanism responsible for reduced myocardial blood flow is coronary artery constriction or spasm caused by endothelial dysfunction. During a mental stress test, significant vasoconstriction occurred in coronary artery disease patients at lesion sites but did not occur in nondiseased coronary segments. The vasomotor response correlated with the extent of atherosclerosis in the artery and with the endothelium-dependent response to an infusion of acetylcholine, demonstrating that the abnormal vasoconstriction was caused by a local failure of endothelium-dependent dilatation during mental stress.[112] These results were replicated in an investigation of emotional stress (i.e., recall of an anger-evoking event) in patients with ischemic heart disease.[113] It also has been reported that the coronary microvasculature dilates in response to mental stress in patients with normal coronary angiograms but fails to dilate in response to mental stress in coronary artery disease patients resulting in increased coronary vascular resistance.[114] In a canine model, an anger-like behavioral state evoked a significant decrease in coronary blood flow in a partially occluded artery,[115] significantly reducing the electrical stability of the heart and increasing the susceptibility to dysrhythmia.[116] Beta-blockade reduces the incidence of dysrhythmia evoked by anger, suggesting that this effect is at least partially mediated by the sympathetic nervous system.[117]

Abnormal platelet aggregation, activation, and procoagulant responses may contribute to the progression of coronary artery disease and predispose patients for ischemia or thrombosis. Acute mental stress elicits an increase in platelet aggregation[118,119] and activation,[119,120] platelet-dependent thrombin generation,[121] and increased fibrin turnover.[122,123] The stress-induced hypercoagulable response is correlated with increased plasma catecholamine activity,[124] but not with the degree of stress hemoconcentration,[125] and is attenuated by beta-antagonist, but not aspirin, therapy.[121] Mental and psychosocial stress-induced changes in platelet function, fibrinolytic activity, and hemoconcentration may contribute to acute coronary events such as plaque rupture and thrombosis.[118]

TYPES OF STRESSORS

During the course of daily life, individuals experience a wide variety of stressors. These range from daily hassles (e.g., traffic congestion, environmental noise and pollution, and chance occurrences) to less routine challenges (e.g., natural disasters, death of a spouse, and change of job). Although any stressor can contribute to allostatic load, certain dimensions of stress seem to be related directly to the cause and onset of coronary heart disease. This section concentrates on the four categories of stressors that share a strong link to coronary heart disease: psychological, psychosocial, socioeconomic status, and occupational.

Psychological Stress

The relationships between psychological stress (e.g., depression, anxiety, or type A behavior pattern) and physiological stress responses are well documented. Depression is the most common psychiatric illness in the general population.[126] Patients with coronary artery disease are at risk for subsequent depression,[127] and a significant number of patients who enter cardiac rehabilitation programs are clinically depressed.[128] Patients with mild to moderate depressive symptoms are more likely than patients with low depressive symptoms to exhibit ischemia during mental stress testing and daily living.[129] Depression increases the relative risk of cardiac death, MI, and all-cause mortality in healthy[130-132] and coronary artery disease[133,134] populations. Prospective studies have reported an independent, gradient relationship between coronary heart disease and negative emotion[135] and depression.[136] A positive, but not strictly linear, relationship exists between the level of depression and the incidence of angina and coronary heart disease.[130,131,137]

Individuals who experience depressive symptoms in the absence of a diagnosed incidence of major depression are also at greater risk of an acute cardiac event.[130,138] Vital exhaustion,[139] a psychological syndrome characterized by sustained fatigue, irritability, and demoralization, as well as hopelessness[130] (a depressive symptom), also is associated with increased relative risk of fatal and nonfatal coronary heart disease.

Depression may affect health directly through pathophysiological mechanisms and indirectly through health behaviors. Pathophysiological links between depression and coronary heart disease may involve neuroendocrine dysregulation and/or immunological dysregulation. Autonomic dysfunction is a possible mechanism and is evidenced in individuals with depression by reduced heart rate variability,[140,141] decreased vagal activity,[142,143] reduced baroreflex cardiac control,[142] elevated 24-hour urinary norepinephrine excretion,[144] and delayed plasma epinephrine recovery after acute psychological stress.[145] Hypercortisolemia[146] and hyperactivity of the HPA axis[147,148] are associated with depression. In otherwise healthy adults, depression also is associated with elevated plasma levels of IL-6 and C-reactive protein, proinflammatory mediators implicated in the pathogenesis of coronary heart disease.[149,150] Evidence of elevated platelet activation and reactivity[151-153] and decreased nitric oxide production[154] in depression also exists. Together, hypercortisolemia, altered platelet function, and elevated proinflammatory mediators could provide a milieu that supports progression of coronary artery disease and first ischemic events in previously healthy individuals.[104,130,149] Depression and coronary heart disease also are linked indirectly through unhealthful lifestyle behaviors, including unhealthful diet, decreased physical activity,[155] smoking,[156] and poor patient compliance.[157,158] Additionally, depression is correlated with cardiovascular risk factors, e.g., central obesity[159,160] and hypertension[161] (Figure 39-3).

Although depression has been the most studied negative affective state, there is also substantial evidence linking anxiety and coronary heart disease. Interestingly, although anxiety disorders are more common in women, the association between anxiety and coronary heart disease mainly has been studied in men.[162] Two studies have linked anxiety and progression of atherosclerosis in healthy individuals. A 20-year prospective investigation of healthy individuals found that self-reported worry increased the relative risk of nonfatal MI.[163] Stable trait anxiety was correlated with increased common carotid intima-media thickness in men and women and higher risk of plaque occurrence in men during a 4-year prospective study.[164]

Phobic anxiety,[165,166] generalized anxiety,[167] and panic disorder[168] are associated with increased relative risk of sudden and nonsudden cardiac death in populations free of coronary heart disease at baseline. It has been suggested that ventricular dysrhythmia, attributable to autonomic dysregulation, may be the pathological mechanism underlying cardiac events among individuals with anxiety disorders.[3] This hypothesis is supported by reports of decreased heart rate variability,[169] alterations in cholinergic versus adrenergic responsiveness,[170] and reduced baroreflex cardiac control in those with anxiety disorders.[171] However, evidence obtained in a 48-hour ambulatory ECG study involving coronary artery disease patients with and without panic disorder revealed that coronary artery disease patients with comorbid panic disorder exhibit lower sympathetic modulation during daily life experience.[172] It also should be noted that prospective studies of anxiety involving coronary heart disease patients have offered equivocal findings, with reports of an increase[173,174] or no increase in risk of cardiac morbidity[175] or mortality.[176,177] Further, a study that examined ambulatory ECG changes during panic attacks in 10 otherwise healthy women with panic disorder found no evidence of ischemia during periods of tachycardia, whether or not the tachycardia was triggered during panic attacks.[178] These findings suggest that pathological alterations in autonomic regulation may not account fully for the relationship between anxiety and cardiac death.

In 1959, Friedman and Rosenman[179] identified the type A behavior pattern (**TABP**)—characterized by irritability, a sense of time urgency, achievement striving, and pervasive hostility—as a potential risk factor for coronary artery disease. Subsequent studies validated the TABP as an independent risk factor for coronary heart disease,[180-182] although there are a number of studies showing no effect of the behavior pattern.[183-185] Friedman[186] attributed discrepancies to misdiagnosis of the behavior pattern through self-report questionnaires rather than structured clinical interview. Others examined individual components of TABP for "toxicity," identifying hostility[182] and social dominance[187] as significant coronary-prone facets of TABP. Hostility is a multidimensional psychological construct that encompasses an emotional component involving anger, contempt and scorn, a behavioral component marked by verbal and physical aggression, and a cognitive component charac-

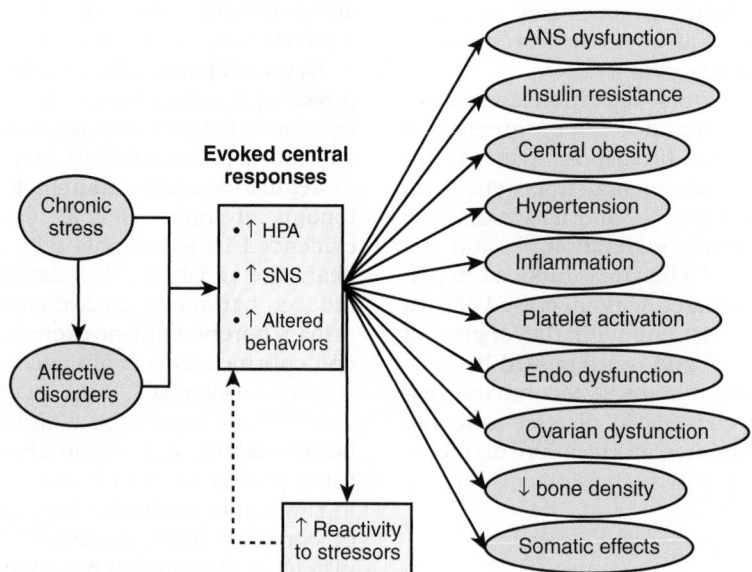

FIGURE 39-3 ■ Pathophysiological mechanisms by which chronic stress and affective disorders, such as depression, appear to promote atherosclerosis. These stressors activate the hypothalamic-pituitary-adrenal (HPA) axis and the sympathetic nervous system (SNS) and affect behaviors. Multiple adverse peripheral effects can ensue from this neuroendocrine, sympathetic, and behavioral activation, as shown. The neuroendocrine and neuroplastic changes emanating from these stressors also can induce a state of heightened physiological responsivity to acute stress that may interact with chronic stressors to cause more adverse effects. *ANS,* autonomic nervous system; *Endo,* endothelial. (From Rozanski A, Blumenthal JA, Davidson KW et al: *J Am Coll Cardiol* 45:637-651, 2005.)

terized by cynicism, mistrust, and a tendency to interpret the actions of others as having aggressive intent.[86] Despite inconsistencies in the literature, recent meta-analyses have concluded that behavioral ratings and self-reports of hostility are associated positively with coronary heart disease and all-cause mortality in healthy and coronary artery disease populations,[3,188] are predictive of the development of hypertension,[189] and are associated with elevated body mass index and physical inactivity in women.[190,191] An 11-year population-based, prospective study using a large sample of black and white young men and women reported that hostility and time urgency/impatience were associated independently with a dose-response increase in the risk of hypertension.[192]

Insomnia, the most prevalent sleep disorder, is characterized by difficulty initiating and maintaining sleep and results in daytime impairments in cognitive, psychological, physical, and social functioning. Approximately 30 percent of the U. S. adult population experiences occasional insomnia, and 9 percent suffers chronic insomnia.[193] Evidence suggests that insufficient sleep may have an adverse effect on physical and psychological health. In a cross-sectional population study, poorer sleep was associated with depression and anxiety, self-reported ill health, and pain.[194] It has been reported that all-cause mortality over 25 years was greater in working men and women who reported sleeping fewer than 7 hours daily over a prolonged period than in those sleeping 7 to 8 hours daily.[195] Among women and men the frequency of episodes of angina and/or cardiac dysrhythmia was greater in those who reported sleeping poorly than in those who slept well.[196] In a 3-year longitudinal investigation, a subjective sleep complaint was found independently to increase the likelihood of a first MI in older adults who were free of overt coronary heart disease at baseline.[197] Impaired nighttime sleep is associated with elevated evening and nocturnal plasma cortisol levels,[198] as well as elevated 24-hour IL-6 levels.[199] Alterations in HPA axis activity and plasma IL-6 may be contributing factors in maintaining disturbed sleep and progression of coronary heart disease.

In the last decade, increasing emphasis has been placed on the impact on coronary heart disease development and progression of psychological factors, not as individual entities but as elements that tend to cluster in the same persons and groups.[200,201] Negative affect, defined as a general disposition chronically to experience anxiety, sadness, guilt, anger, irritability, and other negative emotions, is conceptualized as a higher-order construct that subsumes all negative emotions. Negative affect adversely affects health via pathophysiological mechanisms (e.g., neuroendocrine dysregulation, immunological dysregulation, reduced heart rate variability, increased reactivity to acute stressors and increased expression of metabolic syndrome in nondiabetic individuals, and sleep disturbances) and lifestyle behaviors (e.g., smoking).[201] Conversely, positive affect is correlated inversely with cortisol output during a workday or day of leisure, independently of age, gender, body mass index, and other covariates. The physiological response to laboratory mental stress, as measured by plasma fi-

brinogen responses[202] and the duration of heart rate elevation,[203] were reduced substantially in happier individuals. Williams and colleagues[200] propose that there is no single biobehavioral pathway through which psychological factors influence the development and progression of coronary artery disease. They have proposed that it may be more accurate to conceptualize gene-environment interactions as influencing which, among various potential biobehavioral pathways, promotes disease development in a particular individual.

Psychosocial Stress

More than three decades of epidemiological research consistently has demonstrated an association between social factors and risk of coronary heart disease. Psychosocial investigations have focused primarily on social isolation, social support, and social dominance as major sources of chronic psychosocial stress.

Dating from 1979, a series of population-based studies has examined the influence of social factors on coronary heart disease and other aspects of physical health, repeatedly confirming the association between low levels of perceived social support and increased risk of coronary heart disease and all-cause mortality in healthy[204,205] and patient populations.[206-208] A lack of social support is associated with an average twofold to threefold increase over time in the relative risk of incident coronary heart disease.[3] A variety of instruments has been used to evaluate social support, ranging from those describing quantitative aspects of social network characteristics and activities (e.g., marital status, membership in organizations and voluntary associations, frequency of interaction with others in the social network) to those describing qualitative characteristics of the support (e.g., type and amount of resources provided by the social network including economic, informational, emotional, and instrumental support and perceptions of adequacy of available support). Network size and the quality of interaction within the network are likely to contribute to one's perceived level of social support. For example, although marriage (or cohabiting with a partner) confers reduced risk of premature mortality[209] and improved 7-year survival following a first MI in men,[210] there are inconsistent findings regarding health benefits of marriage for women.

Overall, men and women seem to derive equal benefit from social networks, although women derive less benefit from marriage and suffer fewer health consequences of separation and/or bereavement. One explanation for these findings is that women experience a lower perceived level of social support from the marital relationship than men. Gender differences in the efficacy of social support were examined by assessing responsiveness to a laboratory stressor. It was reported that support from a man did not reduce stress-induced cardiovascular reactivity in men or women, but that support from a woman attenuated the cardiovascular response to a stressor. In a 4-year prospective study, older women (ages 60 to 72) living independently were not socially isolated and were at lower risk of decline in mental health and vitality than married women living with a spouse.[211] Thus, it has been suggested that because men are less effective than women in providing social support, women do not benefit as much from marriage or suffer as much with its termination.[212,213]

Quality of the marital relationship affects coronary heart disease progression and outcomes. Evidence of a higher frequency of subclinical atherosclerosis and threefold acceleration of coronary artery disease progression over time in healthy women reporting marital dissatisfaction suggests that marriage confers cardiovascular health benefits for women only when marital satisfaction is high.[214,215] In fact, strain from problematic spousal relationships is an independent predictor of poor prognosis in women with coronary heart disease.[215] Similarly, a low level of marital conflict was associated with 4-year survival in a population of male and female patients with congestive heart failure, many of whom had experienced a prior MI.[216] Marital transitions (i.e., entry into marriage or termination of marriage through death or divorce) also have been shown to have adverse effects on health behavior[217,218] and on cardiac death and all-cause mortality in men.[219]

The demands of caregiving within a family can be a source of psychosocial stress. A 4-year prospective study of caregiving and coronary heart disease reported that compared with women providing no child care, women caring for non-ill children 21 hours or more per week and those caring for non-ill grandchildren 9 hours or more per week had an increased relative risk of coronary heart disease. Little difference in relative risk was found between caregivers who worked outside the home and those who did not.[220] Similarly, high levels of caregiving burden for ill spouses increased the risk of incident coronary heart disease in a population free of diagnosed coronary heart disease at baseline.[221] A prospective, population-based study of all-cause mortality in elderly spousal caregivers reported that caregivers who provided support to their spouse and reported caregiving strain were 63 percent more likely to die within 4 years than noncaregivers.[222] It has been suggested that unhealthful lifestyle habits may contribute to adverse health outcomes among caregivers.[220] The greater prevalence of loneliness and depression among caregivers also may contribute to the increased morbidity and mortality associated with the chronic strain of caregiving.[223,224]

The effect of social instability also has been examined. As reviewed by Rozanski and colleagues,[3] acculturation in human beings and social disruptions in animal groups independently influence coronary artery disease development. For example, 3809 Japanese Americans in California were classified according to the degree to which they retained a traditional Japanese culture. The most traditional group of Japanese Americans had a coronary heart disease prevalence as low as that observed in Japan, whereas the group that was most acculturated to Western culture had a threefold to fivefold excess in coronary heart disease prevalence. The difference in coronary heart disease rate between groups could not be accounted for by differences in major coronary risk factors.

Social dominance, an attribute of the TABP that expresses itself in social competitiveness and the tendency to control others, may be a risk factor for coronary heart disease. Dominance has been assessed through speech patterns or questionnaire. Dominating-competitive speech is characterized by short response latencies, rapid speech, frequent interruptions, and simultaneous speech (allows one to retain or retake "the floor"), contrasting with angry-hostile speech that is characterized by loud, explosive speech, a quickening pace, muscular tension, and marked hostility. Dominant and hostile speech patterns were independent predictors of coronary heart disease in 8½-year follow-up examinations[181] of the Western Collaborative Group Study and at 22-year follow-up[225] independently predicted coronary heart disease and all-cause mortality. A subsequent study involving men and women found a significant relationship between dominance and coronary heart disease in men only.[226]

Cynomolgus monkeys frequently are used in nonhuman primate investigations because not only do they resemble human beings in the pathophysiology of atherosclerosis, but also they exhibit social behaviors similar to those of human beings (e.g., elaborate patterns of affiliative and supportive social interactions, well-defined social status, and coronary-prone behaviors such as aggressiveness). Thus, investigations involving cynomolgus monkeys can provide additional insight into the effects of psychosocial stress in human beings. Studies with male monkeys suggest that atherosclerosis is exacerbated in dominant individuals, i.e., those that are habitually successful in their aggressive encounters with social strangers. The increased risk of atherosclerosis in dominant monkeys experiencing unstable social conditions is mediated in part by the SAS.[227] Female monkeys respond differently than do males to the challenges of status and group instability. Specifically, atherosclerosis progression was exacerbated in subordinate females and was attenuated in dominant females.[228] The exacerbation of atherosclerosis in subordinate females was associated with estrogen deficiency and ovulatory impairment. When subordinate females received oral contraceptive treatment, their rate of lesion development was similar to that of dominant females.[44]

As with psychological stress, the effects of psychosocial stress are mediated in part through health behaviors (e.g., physical inactivity, smoking, and diet). Lack of social support is likely to exert atherogenic effects through SAS influences on heart rate, blood pressure, cardiovascular reactivity, and platelet function, as well as through HPA axis–supported proliferation of smooth muscle.[3] Oxytocin, which is secreted in response to physical touch and appears to inhibit SAS activity, also may contribute to the protective effects of social support.[229]

Socioeconomic Status Stress

Socioeconomic stress is a multidimensional construct encompassing education level, occupation, economic resources (i.e., earned income and wealth), and social status. Longitudinal studies provide substantial evidence of an inverse gradient between socioeconomic stress and coronary heart disease[230] and all-cause mortality[231] in Westernized countries. The gradient persists into old age,[232] and socioeconomic stress-related differentials in healthful life expectancy and total life expectancy in the United States appear to have increased since 1970.[233] The prevalence of unhealthful lifestyle behaviors (i.e., smoking and low physical activity)[234] and coronary risk factors (i.e., hypertension and diabetes mellitus)[226] is associated inversely with socioeconomic stress. However, these factors account for no more than half of the socioeconomic stress–coronary heart disease gradient.[234]

It has been suggested that the chronic stress associated with low socioeconomic status may contribute to poor health outcomes.[24,235,236] The chronic stress of low socioeconomic status is embedded within daily life and is expressed, for example, in lower social status, constraints imposed by limited financial resources (e.g., poorer housing conditions and unsafe neighborhoods), and less favorable working conditions.[237] Although correlations between biological risk factors and low socioeconomic status are well established, Seeman and colleagues[236] have proposed that there is potential value in considering the biological mediation of the socioeconomic status–health relationship from a broad, multisystems viewpoint. This broader approach would better encompass the wide range of disease processes, encompassing multiple sources of dysfunction, and causes of death associated with low socioeconomic status. The concepts of allostasis and allostatic load provide a multisystems model that helps explain the cumulative physiological toll exacted on individuals of lower socioeconomic status. As noted previously, the primary allostatic mediators are the SAS, the HPA axis, and cytokines. Allostatic load is associated with four conditions: frequent stress; failure to adapt to repeated stressors of the same type; dysregulation or failure to inactivate allostatic systems after a stress is terminated; compensation by one allostatic mediator for inadequate responses by other mediators (e.g., when stress-induced cortisol secretion is inadequate, secretion of proinflammatory mediators increases and an enhanced inflammatory response occurs).[24] The chronic stress of low socioeconomic status adds to the cumulative burden of allostatic load, resulting in physiological "wear and tear," which ultimately can affect health because of the cumulative effect of dysregulation across multiple physiological systems. Thus, a substantial portion of socioeconomic status effects on health may be attributed to the inverse relationship between socioeconomic status and chronic stress.[23,235]

Occupational Stress

Occupational stress contributes to employee absenteeism and reduced productivity. An accumulating body of evidence from prospective studies links workplace psychosocial stress with cardiac disease progression and with cardiac and all-cause mortality.[238-240] Investigations of occupational stress have focused on the occupation component of socioeconomic status or, alternatively, have used work satisfaction, work load, and self-reports of medical symptoms to assess the impact of occupational stress. In recent decades, two models have guided most investigations into the adverse health effects of occupational stress: the job strain and the effort-reward imbalance models.

The job strain model, originally formulated by Karasek,[241,242] postulates that work stress results from the combined effect of two factors, job demands (i.e., workload, work pace, and conflicting job demands) and job control (i.e., decision latitude). These two factors are cross-classified to create four work stress states: low job strain (low demands × high control), active work (high demands × high control), passive work (low demands × low control), and high job strain (high demands × low control). A wide range of methodologies has been used to investigate the association between job strain and cardiovascular disease. Most have found a significant association between job strain and coronary artery disease risk,[242] an association that is more predictive of coronary heart disease risk in lower occupational classes (i.e., semiskilled and unskilled) than in higher occupational classes (i.e., executive and professional).[242,243] Low job control has been linked more consistently to coronary artery disease than high job demands.[244] Johnson and Hall[245] extended the demand-control model to include the factor of workplace psychosocial support. Low levels of emotional and instrumental support coupled with high demand/low control work was identified as the "iso-strain" work stress state. Isostrain work is associated with greater risk of coronary heart disease and poorer health status than high job strain, underscoring the importance of psychosocial factors in the work environment.[245,246]

Gender differences in the effect of work stress have been reported. For example, the effect of active job strain was associated with the 10-year incidence of coronary heart disease in women, but not men, participating in the Framingham Offspring Study. Women reporting active job strain were nearly 3 times more likely to develop coronary heart disease than those reporting high job strain. The authors suggest that the increased risk could derive from higher levels of decision latitude associated with the active versus high strain work state. They also note that the study was conducted during the 1980s when social transitions were providing greater opportunities for women to hold positions of authority, autonomy, and control. It was suggested that the social pressures associated with new social roles may have contributed to the increased coronary heart disease risk.[247] Sex discrimination and the combined effect of work and family responsibilities also have been identified as factors that contribute to gender differences in work stress.[248]

The effort-reward imbalance (**ERI**) model of work stress, originally formulated by Siegrist,[249] postulates that lack of reciprocity between efforts expended and rewards received (i.e., high-cost/low-gain condition) elicits a state of emotional distress with high propensity to autonomic arousal and neuroendocrine responses. This model incorporates the extrinsic/situational (e.g., demands and obligations) and intrinsic/individual (e.g., coping characteristics and need for control) qualities of high effort. The sources of rewards are money, esteem, and status control (e.g., job security and promotion prospects). Siegrist suggested that it is psychologically less costly to adapt cognitively to a low level of task control (as per the demand-control model) than to a low level of status control, essentially because the former is perceived as less threatening. It also has been noted that the emphasis of the ERI model on status control reflects the growing emphasis of global labor market realities, in which job instability, fragmented careers and redundancy, and forced occupational mobility have become increasingly common. ERI is likely to be experienced as more distressing by employees who exhibit the cognitive and motivational coping style defined as overcommitment. Overcommitted persons tend to underestimate the demands at work and overestimate their own capacities and coping resources.[240] Prospective studies have provided evidence supporting the impact of ERI and/or overcommitment on coronary heart disease[250] and self-reported health.[251] A study that examined biological correlates of ERI and overcommitment to work reported a strong association between ERI and ambulatory systolic blood pressure, heart rate, and heart rate variability over the workday in men, but not women.[252] The differential effects of the extrinsic (effort/reward ratio) and intrinsic (overcommitment) components of the ERI model also has been noted. Specifically, the link between coronary heart disease risk and ERI was greater in those exhibiting overcommitment.[250] Overcommitment was more likely to be linked to a higher ratio of total/HDL cholesterol and hemostatic risk factors,[253] and ERI was more likely to be linked to hypertension in men.[250]

The emphasis of the two theoretical formulations of job stress is on different characteristics of the work experience. The job strain model concentrates on extrinsic (situational) factors, whereas the ERI model encompasses intrinsic (individual) and extrinsic factors. Originators of the demand-control model and the ERI model of work stress have proposed that combining elements of the two models may enhance and improve coronary heart disease risk estimation.[242,254] Indeed, one such prospective investigation found that the imbalance between personal efforts (competitiveness, work-related overcommitment, and hostility) and rewards (poor promotional prospects and a blocked career) was associated with a 2.15 times greater risk of new coronary heart disease. Job strain and high job demands were not related to coronary heart disease in this model, but low job control was highly associated with new coronary heart disease.[254] Results of a subsequent case-control study support the findings of this prospective study and provide insight into gender-specific effects of work stress.[240] Specifically, this study reported that job strain was associated with increased risk of acute MI in men and, to a lesser extent, in women. However, the two components of the ERI model were associated with MI risk according to gender. Although the situational component of the model (effort/reward ratio) contributed to MI risk in men and women, the intrinsic (overcommitment) component contributed to risk estimation only in women.

Work stress may affect cardiovascular health by pathophysiological mechanisms, such as altered autonomic control of cardiac function,[255] elevated arterial blood pressure,[256,257] and hypercoagulability.[258] Higher work stress also has an adverse effect on health-related behavior, including smoking[259] and leisure time physical activity.[260] In a cross-sectional examination of adverse psychosocial work characteristics and allostatic load, a significant association was found between allostatic load score and job demands, but not social support or decision latitude. The association was age-dependent, becoming significant only in participants older than age 45. Individual factor analysis of allostatic load indicated that blood pressure elevation, increased inflammatory activity, increased cortisol levels, and cortisol-induced leukocyte trafficking may help explain the pathophysiological coronary heart disease effects of work stress.[261]

STRESS MANAGEMENT

As previously discussed in this chapter, psychological and psychosocial stress are linked to the development of coronary artery disease and acute cardiac events. Further, psychological and psychosocial stressors tend to cluster together (e.g., anxiety and depression, low socioeconomic stress, and occupational stress) and to cluster with other cardiovascular risk factors (e.g., depression and sedentary lifestyle). The term *stress management* encompasses a variety of biobehavioral and cognitive strategies aimed at enhancing skills necessary for coping with the stresses of daily life as a means of preventing or reversing adverse effects of stress on health. Coping, which is the cognitive and behavioral efforts one makes to manage a stressful situation, is aimed at dealing with a problem that is causing distress and with regulating the stressful emotions generated by the transaction. Problem-focused coping is characterized by direct action taken to alter or master a situation, e.g., seeking more information, confronting, or holding back from impulsive action. Whether or not the action is successful in mitigating a perceived threat, the action itself causes a reappraisal of the person-environment relationship. Emotion-focused coping aims to reduce the affective and/or somatic disturbances that are generated by the encounter, e.g., seeking social support, accepting responsibility, substance abuse (e.g., alcohol or sleeping pills), or relaxation.

Cognitive theories of stress and coping underlie many of the stress management strategies promoted in the literature. According to cognitive theory, the relationship between an individual and the environment is dynamic and bidirectional. A stressful encounter is experienced as one in which the environment is appraised as taxing or exceeding one's resources and as threatening one's well-being. Cognitive coping theories conceptualize two processes as mediating stressful individual-environment encounters and influencing their immediate and long-term outcomes: cognitive appraisal and coping.

Cognitive appraisal, a two-stage process, begins with a primary evaluation or appraisal of what stakes, if any, are involved in the encounter. Personality characteristics, e.g., values, commitments, and beliefs about oneself and the world, help define the stakes that are relevant to well-being in any given situation. During secondary appraisal, one evaluates what can be done to prevent harm or improve the prospects for benefit in a situation. Together, primary and secondary appraisals help to determine whether the person-environment encounter is regarded as important for well-being, and if so, whether it is primarily threatening (holding possibility of harm or loss) or challenging (holding possibility of benefit or mastery).[262,263] Regardless of the outcome of an encounter, appraisal and coping may affect physical health by contributing to allostatic load and/or by promoting unhealthful lifestyle behaviors (e.g., smoking, substance abuse, or overeating).

Epidemiology

Stress management is a frequently recommended preventive health strategy and often is incorporated into comprehensive cardiac rehabilitation programs. Studies have reported efficacy of stress management interventions for a wide range of chronic medical conditions, e.g., tinnitus, asthma and allergies, migraine, insomnia, hypertension, and coronary heart disease. Most stress management techniques fall under the mind-body interventions (as defined by the National Center for Complementary and Alternative Medicine) umbrella and can be classified into three broad categories: arousal reduction approaches (also known as emotion regulation); cognitive-behavioral skills training; and systems approaches (Table 39-1).

In spite of the many studies evaluating the effectiveness of stress management, variability in the operational definition of the term makes meaningful comparisons of stress management interventions difficult. Recently, Ong and colleagues[264] reviewed 153 papers, representing original investigations involving stress management or stress reduction, published in the period 1990 to 2000. Although more than 225 different stress management techniques were used in the papers, a large majority of the studies endorsed a cognitive-behavioral approach to coping skills training or arousal reduction approaches. The modal number of techniques used was six per study, making it difficult to draw conclusions about a specific technique. Only 14 percent of the studies used a single stress management approach. This is

■ ■ ■

TABLE 39-1 MIND-BODY STRESS MANAGEMENT INTERVENTIONS

MODALITY	DESCRIPTION	CONTRAINDICATIONS/COMMENTS
Autogenic training (AT)	Developed in the early 1900s by Johannes H. Schultz, a German psychiatrist, AT combines features of self-hypnosis, relaxation, and meditation. AT consists of a series of simple mental exercises designed to focus attention on bodily sensations associated with relaxation (e.g., warmth and heaviness in the limbs) as a means of quieting the sympathetic nervous system. Central to AT is passive concentration, i.e., maintenance of a nonjudgmental, meditative-like state during AT sessions.	AT exercises are taught by qualified instructors and can be learned in 8 to 10 weeks. Without regular practice, AT is not likely to be effective. AT could increase the risk of adverse emotional and/or physical outcomes in individuals with preexisting conditions (e.g., anxiety, diabetes mellitus, coronary artery disease). AT should not replace conventional treatments or therapies.
Biofeedback	Biofeedback is a technique through which individuals learn to control physiological functions (e.g., respiration, heart rate, blood pressure, muscle tension, and skin temperature). Electronic biofeedback instruments connected to surface electrodes display continuous information (feedback) to a patient about the nature of a response to be learned; through practice, individuals learn to alter the signal by taking control of bodily functions. Modalities frequently used for stress management are electromyogram muscle biofeedback, temperature biofeedback, and galvanic skin response.	Training is tailored to individual needs based on psychophysiological assessment at first session. Home exercises are assigned to reinforce learning between formal sessions. Biofeedback generally is considered a safe therapy. Self-training is possible, although equipment can be relatively expensive.
Cognitive behavioral stress management (CBSM)	Pioneered by psychologists Aaron Beck and Albert Ellis in the 1960s, cognitive behavioral therapy is one of the more traditional and more widely used stress management interventions. CBSM stipulates that thoughts (cognitive processes) shape affective and behavioral experience and that maladaptive behaviors and negative emotions result from inappropriate and irrational thought patterns (i.e., automatic thoughts). The goal of CBSM interventions is to help patients identify and unlearn maladaptive, unwanted reactions, replacing them with less stressful alternatives.	CBSM is an action-oriented, rational approach and may not be suitable for all patients, e.g., those who are cognitively impaired. Typically CBSM is used in combination with other stress management interventions.
Guided imagery	Guided imagery involves the use of visualization or imagination to evoke a pleasant, peaceful image. Guided imagery typically is more effective when multiple senses are engaged (e.g., *seeing* the ocean and sand dunes, *smelling* the salt air, *hearing* the waves crash and sea gulls cry). Objectives may be to evoke a psychophysiological state of relaxation or a specific, desired outcome (e.g., preexperiencing achievement of a successful endeavor to build self-confidence).	Sessions may be self-guided or guided by a practitioner/leader. Guided imagery often is combined with physical relaxation techniques (e.g., progressive muscle relaxation).

Continued

■ ■ ■

TABLE 39-1　MIND-BODY STRESS MANAGEMENT INTERVENTIONS—cont'd

MODALITY	DESCRIPTION	CONTRAINDICATIONS/COMMENTS
Massage therapy	Massage is the manual manipulation of the soft tissues of the body (i.e., muscles, skin, and connective tissue). Massage usually is performed to relieve muscle tension, spasms, or cramps; to increase mobility; to improve circulation; or to relieve tension and promote well-being.	Massage therapy, when provided by a trained and qualified body-worker, generally is considered to be a safe treatment. Massage is contraindicated in those with acute inflammation, redness, swelling, marked breathing difficulty, fever, skin rash, and/or varicose veins. Many states in the United States do not currently require licensure for massage therapists.
Meditation	Meditation is the self-regulation of attention, the act of allowing the mind to become calm and focused on a specific aspect of one's internal or external experience. Although most religions include ritual meditation with the goal of spiritual growth and/or personal transformation, meditation itself does not need to be a religious or spiritual activity. The two general types of meditation are concentrative meditation and mindfulness meditation. In concentrative meditation techniques, the mind is kept closely focused on a particular word, sound, image, or physical sensation of the breath and breathing. Most prominent examples in the clinical setting are transcendental meditation, developed in India by Maharishi Mahesh Yogi and brought to the United States in the 1960s, and the relaxation response, developed in the 1970s by Herbert Benson. Mindfulness meditation techniques involve the notion of nonjudgmental observation of thoughts, emotions, and sensations as they arise moment by moment to one's conscious awareness. This technique is best represented in clinical medicine by mindfulness-based stress reduction, a program developed by Jon Kabat-Zinn in 1979 to introduce patients to mindfulness practice in the context of their illness. Mindfulness practice is also integral to yoga, tai chi, and walking meditation practices, all of which use physical discipline and movement to focus the mind.	Studies of meditation have reported its positive effects on physical health (e.g., cardiovascular health, chronic pain, irritable bowel syndrome, and insomnia), as well as its ability to promote relaxation and psychological well-being. Precaution: Adverse effects of meditation have been reported. These include uncomfortable kinesthetic sensations, panic, anxiety, and psychosis-like symptoms (especially with long periods of contemplative meditation in susceptible persons). Beginners should be moderate in their practice.
Relaxation therapy	Relaxation therapies are techniques designed to teach individuals voluntarily to release muscle tension and elicit a psychophysiological state of relaxation or hypoarousal. The most prominent examples are diaphragmatic breathing and progressive muscle relaxation (PMR). Diaphragmatic breathing (sometimes called abdominal breathing) is a conscious activity that allows a person to counteract the stress-induced pattern of shallow breathing and hyperventilation and to slow the heart rate. Diaphragmatic breathing is characterized by a pattern of slow, deep breaths taken through the nostrils, which fill the entire lungs. PMR, originally developed by Edmund Jacobson in 1938, is based on the premise that mental relaxation naturally would follow muscle relaxation. PMR involves alternating periods of tension production and relaxation in a muscle group, followed by intentional awareness of the sensation of relaxation in the targeted muscle group. Muscle groups are targeted in a progressive manner, beginning with the muscles of the lower extremities and ending with those of the torso and face.	Most forms of relaxation therapy are considered safe in healthy adults. As with other mind-body interventions, relaxation therapy may increase anxiety in some persons. Precaution: PMR and similar techniques that involve tension production should be used with caution by those with coronary artery disease, hypertension, or musculoskeletal injuries.

consistent with previous reports of greater effect size associated with multicomponent stress management interventions.[265]

A 1996 meta-analysis of 23 randomized controlled trials involving 2024 subjects, which evaluated the additional impact of psychosocial treatments (e.g., relaxation, group and individual therapy, type A behavior modification, and stress management) to standard cardiac rehabilitation, reported a 41 percent reduction in all-cause mortality and a 46 percent reduction in nonfatal cardiac events at a 2-year follow-up.[266] Psychosocial interventions were associated with improvements in quality of life and reductions in psychological distress

(e.g., anxiety and depression), and in lowered heart rate, systolic blood pressure, and cholesterol levels. The effects of psychoeducational interventions (e.g., health educational and stress management) were evaluated in a meta-analysis of 37 studies (9699 subjects, all had experienced a cardiac event in the 6 months before the start of the treatment).[267] The authors found a positive treatment effect, reporting a 34 percent reduction in cardiac mortality and a 29 percent reduction in MI recurrence at 2- to 10-years' follow-up and significant positive effects on risk factors and related behaviors (e.g., blood pressure, cholesterol, body weight, diet and exercise habits, and smoking behavior) at 6 weeks to 2-

years' follow-up. In a recent prospective study, patients with coronary artery disease[268] were assigned randomly to 4 months of aerobic exercise training (3 times per week) or a weekly stress management class teaching group cognitive-behavior approaches plus relaxation training. Stress management was associated with a significant reduction in clinical coronary artery disease events relative to usual care at 2- and 5-year follow-ups. In their 2003 meta-analysis, Astin and colleagues[269] found strong evidence that mind-body therapies that focus on the development of self-regulation skills (e.g., relaxation and management of anger, hostility, and general stress reactivity) should be included as part of cardiac rehabilitation in post-MI patients.

The efficacy of psychosocial interventions on hypertension is equivocal. A meta-analysis of 26 randomized controlled trials (1264 subjects) evaluating the effect of stress management on hypertension found significant blood pressure reductions in stress management versus usual care or wait list groups, but no difference between stress management intervention and placebo or sham controls.[270] Consistent with this report, a prospective investigation of the effects of stress management intervention for the primary prevention of hypertension reported no main effect of the 18-month stress management treatment. However, adherence subgroup analysis revealed a significant reduction in diastolic blood pressure in patients who completed at least 61 percent of the intervention sessions.[271] In contrast, several randomized trials have reported beneficial effects of stress management interventions and support the efficacy of such interventions. In one study, 24-hour ambulatory blood pressure was reduced significantly at 6-months' follow-up in patients who received 10 hours of individualized cognitive-behavioral stress management training.[272] A 16-hour group stress management program that included instruction in emotional refocusing and restructuring resulted in a significant reduction in systolic blood pressure at 3-months' follow-up, as well as improvements in individual well-being, organizational effectiveness, and levels of anxiety and depression.[273] Randomized trials of transcendental meditation reported reductions in systolic and diastolic blood pressure after 3 months,[274] and reductions in carotid intima-media thickness after 6 months,[275] in hypertensive blacks.

Mind-body interventions generally are regarded as free of adverse side effects. However, recent meta-analysis demonstrated rates of relaxation-induced anxiety from 17 to 38 percent for relaxation and 53.8 percent during meditation. The most frequently reported problems patients encountered were intrusive thoughts (15 percent), fear of losing control (9 percent), disturbing sensory experiences (4 percent), and muscle cramps and spasms (4 percent). The authors note that evaluating patients before applying mind-body therapies can help minimize negative effects of therapy.[269]

Coping Strategies

During an evening spent scanning self-help books or Internet sites (or, for those so inclined, reading scientific papers), one could learn about hundreds of stress management strategies and techniques that could be categorized broadly as lifestyle modifications, action-oriented, emotionally oriented, or acceptance-oriented.

Lifestyle modifications, sometimes called self-care behaviors, include smoking cessation, maintaining a healthful diet, limiting caffeine and alcohol intake, exercising regularly, incorporating enjoyable leisure time activity into one's schedule, and adequate restorative sleep. As described throughout this text, these behaviors have a direct and positive benefit for physical health. Additionally, they enhance coping abilities by contributing to mental clarity, self-efficacy, and self-esteem.

Action-oriented approaches to stress management are those that improve mastery or modify the person-environment relationship. These include development and application of skills, e.g., time management, communication, assertiveness, problem solving, decision making, and negotiation.

Emotion-oriented approaches to stress management are aimed at limiting distressful affective and somatic responses to situations that are perceived as challenging or threatening. As noted previously, seeking social support, and practicing relaxation or meditation are beneficial strategies for bolstering emotional resilience. Research also shows that laughter generates positive emotions and that positive thoughts and emotions contribute to psychological and physical well-being.[276] For example, older men who exhibited high levels of optimism had a significantly lower incidence of fatal and nonfatal coronary heart disease during a 10-year period.[277] Refuting negative thoughts and reframing ("cognitive restructuring") are two cognitive-based strategies that promote positive emotion and empowerment. Reframing, i.e., thinking about and interpreting the person-environment relationship from a different perspective and thereby changing its meaning, is especially useful in helping distressed individuals devise better ways of coping.

Acceptance-oriented approaches are useful when an individual's goals or expectations are not met and he or she has minimal to no power to change the situation (e.g., death of a spouse). In such a situation, the most effective strategy may be to acknowledge intentionally that a goal or expectation cannot be met, thereby freeing oneself to cope constructively with the present reality.

Practical Considerations

Recognizing that stress is a risk factor for chronic diseases such as coronary heart disease, nurses and other health care providers should be prepared to help patients recognize and manage psychosocial stress. Rozanski and colleagues[237] present four compelling reasons for incorporating psychosocial risk management into cardiac practice: psychosocial risk factors are highly prevalent within cardiac populations; psychological distress commonly presents as symptoms of cardiac disease in clinical practice; psychosocial risk factors can affect adherence to treatment adversely; acute psychological stress shapes the course of cardiac disease in negative and positive fashion (e.g., exacerbating pathophysiological processes and transforming perspective, attitudes and lifestyle behaviors, respectively).

Professionals should be prepared to educate patients about the impact of acute and chronic stress on physical and psychological health. It may be advantageous to explore with patients the difficulties and benefits of lifestyle change, to help patients identify the barriers and solutions to change, and to assist the patient in assembling a supportive social network. Because of the recognized comorbidity of anxiety, depression, and coronary heart disease, it is possible that not only stress management interventions but also a more general psychological intervention aimed at reducing affective symptoms would be useful. Finally, the health care professional needs not only to provide encouragement and advocacy for, but also to role model, a healthful lifestyle and coping behaviors.

REFERENCES

1. Chrousos GP, Gold PW: The concepts of stress and stress system disorders: overview of physical and behavioral homeostasis, *JAMA* 267:1244-1252, 1992.
2. Chrousos GP: The role of stress and hypothalamic-pituitary-adrenal axis in the pathogenesis of the metabolic syndrome: neuroendocrine and target tissue-related causes, *Int J Obes Relat Metab Disord* 24(suppl 2):S50-S55, 2000.
3. Rozanski A, Blumenthal JA, Kaplan J: Impact of psychological factors on the pathogenesis of cardiovascular disease and implications for therapy, *Circulation* 99(16):2192-2217, 1999.
4. Cannon WB: Stresses and strains of homeostasis, *Am J Med Sci* 189:1-14, 1935.
5. Cannon WB: The influence of emotional states on the functions of the alimentary canal, *Am J Med Sci* 137:480-487, 1909.
6. Selye H: A syndrome produced by diverse nocuous agents, *Nature* 138:32, 1936.
7. Selye H: *Stress without distress*, Philadelphia, 1974, Lippincott Williams & Wilkins.
8. Boone JL, Anthony JP: Evaluating the impact of stress on systemic disease: the MOST protocol in primary care, *J Am Osteopath Assoc* 103:239-246, 2003.
9. Tsigos C, Chrousos GP: Hypothalamic-pituitary-adrenal axis, neuroendocrine factors and stress, *J Psychosom Res* 53:865-871, 2002.
10. Pacak K: Stressor-specific activation of the hypothalamic-pituitary-adrenocortical axis, *Physiol Res* 49(suppl 1):S11-S17, 2000.
11. Swanson LW, Sawchenko PE, Lind RW: Regulation of multiple peptides in CRF parvocellular neurosecretory neurons: implications for the stress response, *Prog Brain Res* 68:169-190, 1986.
12. Calogero AE, Gallucci WT, Chrousos GP et al: Catecholamine effects upon rat hypothalamic corticotropin-releasing hormone secretion in vitro, *J Clin Invest* 82:839-846, 1988.
13. Calogero AE, Gallucci WT, Gold PW et al: Multiple feedback regulatory loops upon rat hypothalamic corticotropin-releasing hormone secretion: potential clinical implications, *J Clin Invest* 82:767-774, 1988.
14. Valentino RJ, Foote SL: Corticotropin-releasing hormone increases tonic but not sensory-evoked activity of noradrenergic locus coeruleus neurons in unanesthetized rats, *J Neurosci* 8:1016-1025, 1988.
15. Valentino RJ, Foote SL, Aston-Jones G: Corticotropin-releasing factor activates noradrenergic neurons of the locus coeruleus, *Brain Res* 270:363-367, 1983.
16. Valentino RJ, Foote SL, Page ME: The locus coeruleus as a site for integrating corticotropin-releasing factor and noradrenergic mediation of stress responses, *Ann N Y Acad Sci* 697:173-188, 1993.
17. Valentino RJ, Wehby RG: Corticotropin-releasing factor: evidence for a neurotransmitter role in the locus ceruleus during hemodynamic stress, *Neuroendocrinology* 48:674-677, 1988.
18. Selye H: The nature of stress, *Basal Facts* 7:3-11, 1985.
19. Mason JW: A re-evaluation of the concept of "non-specificity" in stress theory, *J Psychiatr Res* 8:323-333, 1971.
20. Mason JW: A review of psychoendocrine research on the pituitary-adrenal cortical system, *Psychosom Med* 30(suppl):576-607, 1968.
21. Ursin H: The psychology in psychoneuroendocrinology, *Psychoneuroendocrinology* 23:555-570, 1998.
22. Lazarus RS: Psychological stress and coping in adaptation and illness, *Int J Psychiatry Med* 5:321-333, 1974.
23. McEwen BS, Seeman T: Protective and damaging effects of mediators of stress: elaborating and testing the concepts of allostasis and allostatic load, *Ann N Y Acad Sci* 896:30-47, 1999.
24. McEwen BS: Protective and damaging effects of stress mediators, *N Engl J Med* 338:171-179, 1998.
25. Sterling P, Eyer J: Allostasis: a new paradigm to explain arousal pathology. In Fisher S, Reason J, editors: *Handbook of life stress, cognition and health,* New York, 1988, John Wiley.
26. Seeman TE, McEwen BS, Rowe JW et al: Allostatic load as a marker of cumulative biological risk: MacArthur studies of successful aging, *Proc Natl Acad Sci U S A* 98:4770-4775, 2001.
27. Sapolsky RM, Krey LC, McEwen BS: The neuroendocrinology of stress and aging: the glucocorticoid cascade hypothesis, *Endocr Rev* 7:284-301, 1986.
28. Seeman TE, Singer BH, Rowe JW et al: The price of adaptation-allostatic load and its health consequences: MacArthur studies of successful aging, *Arch Intern Med* 157:2259-2268, 1997.
29. Kamarck TW, Jennings JR: Biobehavioral factors in sudden death, *Psychol Bull* 109:42-75, 1991.
30. Jennings GL: Noradrenaline spillover and microneurography measurements in patients with primary hypertension, *J Hypertens* 16(suppl 3):S35-S38, 1998.
31. Somers VK, Anderson EA, Mark AL: Sympathetic neural mechanisms in human hypertension, *Curr Opin Nephrol Hypertens* 2:96-105, 1993.
32. Johnson CD, Coney AM, Marshall JM: Roles of norepinephrine and ATP in sympathetically evoked vasoconstriction in rat tail and hindlimb in vivo, *Am J Physiol Heart Circ Physiol* 281:H2432-H2440, 2001.
33. Brosschot JF, Thayer JF: Anger inhibition, cardiovascular recovery, and vagal function: a model of the link between hostility and cardiovascular disease, *Ann Behav Med* 20:326-332, 1998.
34. Jiang W, Hayano J, Coleman ER et al: Relation of cardiovascular responses to mental stress and cardiac vagal activity in coronary artery disease, *Am J Cardiol* 72:551-554, 1993.
35. Shepherd JT, Mancia G: Reflex control of the human cardiovascular system, *Rev Physiol Biochem Pharmacol* 105:1-99, 1986.
36. DiBona GF: Peripheral and central interactions between the renin-angiotensin system and the renal sympathetic nerves in control of renal function, *Ann N Y Acad Sci* 940:395-406, 2001.
37. Gordon RD, Kuchel O, Grant WL et al: Role of the sympathetic nervous system in regulating renin and aldosterone production in man, *J Clin Invest* 46:599-605, 1967.
38. Noll G, Wenzel RR, Schneider M et al: Increased activation of sympathetic nervous system and endothelin by mental stress in normotensive offspring of hypertensive parents, *Circulation* 93:866-869, 1996.
39. Treiber FA, Jackson RW, Davis H et al: Racial differences in endothelin-1 at rest and in response to acute stress in adolescent males, *Hypertension* 35:722-725, 2000.
40. Stefano GB, Murga J, Benson H et al: Nitric oxide inhibits norepinephrine stimulated contraction of human internal thoracic artery and rat aorta, *Pharmacol Res* 43:199-203, 2001.
41. Noon JP, Walker BR, Webb DJ et al: Impaired microvascular dilatation and capillary rarefaction in young adults with a predisposition to high blood pressure, *J Clin Invest* 99, 1997.
42. Folkow B: Hypertensive structural changes in systemic precapillary resistance vessels: how important are they for in vivo hemodynamics? *J Hypertens* 13:1546-1549, 1995.
43. Ullian ME: The role of corticosteroids in the regulation of vascular tone, *Cardiovasc Res* 41:55-64, 1999.
44. Kaplan JR, Manuck SB: Status, stress, and atherosclerosis: the role of environment and individual behavior, *Ann N Y Acad Sci* 896:145-161, 1999.
45. Matthews KA, Owens JF, Kuller LH et al: Stress-induced pulse pressure change predicts women's carotid atherosclerosis, *Stroke* 29:1525-1530, 1998.

46. Kamarck TW, Everson SA, Kaplan GA et al: Exaggerated blood pressure responses during mental stress are associated with enhanced carotid atherosclerosis in middle-aged Finnish men: findings from the Kuopio Ischemic Heart Disease Study, *Circulation* 96:3842-3848, 1997.

47. Treiber FA, Kamarck T, Schneiderman N et al: Cardiovascular reactivity and development of preclinical and clinical disease states, *Psychosom Med* 65:46-62, 2003.

48. Kaplan JR, Manuck SB, Clarkson TB: The influence of heart rate on coronary artery atherosclerosis, *J Cardiovasc Pharmacol* 10(suppl 2):S100-S102, 1987.

49. Brook RD, Julius S: Autonomic imbalance, hypertension, and cardiovascular risk, *Am J Hypertens* 13:112S-122S, 2000.

50. Wood DL, Sheps SG, Elveback LR et al: Cold pressor test as a predictor of hypertension, *Hypertension* 6:301-306, 1984.

51. Matthews KA, Woodall KL, Allen MT: Cardiovascular reactivity to stress predicts future blood pressure status, *Hypertension* 22:479-485, 1993.

52. Falkner B, Kushner H, Onesti G et al: Cardiovascular characteristics in adolescents who develop essential hypertension, *Hypertension* 3:521-527, 1981.

53. Skantze HB, Kaplan J, Pettersson K et al: Psychosocial stress causes endothelial injury in cynomolgus monkeys via beta1-adrenoceptor activation, *Atherosclerosis* 136:153-161, 1998.

54. Strawn WB, Bondjers G, Kaplan JR et al: Endothelial dysfunction in response to psychosocial stress in monkeys, *Circ Res* 68:1270-1279, 1991.

55. Harris KF, Matthews KA: Interactions between autonomic nervous system activity and endothelial function: a model for the development of cardiovascular disease, *Psychosom Med* 66:153-164, 2004.

56. Larsson PT, Hjemdahl P, Olsson G et al: Altered platelet function during mental stress and adrenaline infusion in humans: evidence for an increased aggregability in vivo as measured by filtragometry, *Clin Sci* 76:369-376, 1989.

57. Levine SP, Towell BL, Suarex AM et al: Platelet activation and secretion associated with emotional stress, *Circulation* 71:1129-1134, 1985.

58. Du XJ, Riemersma RA, Dart AM: Cardiovascular protection by oestrogen is partly mediated through modulation of autonomic nervous function, *Cardiovasc Res* 30:161-165, 1995.

59. Kaplan JR, Manuck SB: Ovarian dysfunction, stress, and disease: a primate continuum, *ILAR J* 45:89-115, 2004.

60. Schwertz DW, Penckofer S: Sex differences and the effects of sex hormones on hemostasis and vascular reactivity, *Heart Lung* 30:410-426, 2001.

61. Lowe G, Drummond MM, Lorimer AR et al: Relation between the extent of coronary artery disease and blood viscosity, *Br Med J* 87:673-674, 1980.

62. Lowe GD, Lee AJ, Rumley A et al: Blood viscosity and risk of cardiovascular events: the Edinburgh Artery Study, *Br J Haematol* 96:168-173, 1997.

63. Bachen EA, Muldoon MF, Matthews KA et al: Effects of hemoconcentration and sympathetic activation on serum lipid responses to brief mental stress, *Psychosom Med* 64:587-594, 2002.

64. Patterson SM, Krantz DS, Gottdiener JS et al: Prothrombotic effects of environmental stress: changes in platelet function, hematocrit, and total plasma protein, *Psychosom Med* 57:592-599, 1995.

65. Ross AE, Flaa A, Hoieggen A et al: Gender specific sympathetic and hemorrheological responses to mental stress in healthy young subjects, *Scand Cardiovasc J* 35:307-312, 2001.

66. Kitahara Y, Imataka K, Nakaoka H et al: Hematocrit increase by mental stress in hypertensive patients, *Jpn Heart J* 29:429-435, 1988.

67. Veldhuijzen van Zanten JJ, Ring C, Burns VE et al: Mental stress-induced hemoconcentration: sex differences and mechanisms, *Psychophysiology* 41:541-551, 2004.

68. Allen MT, Patterson SM: Hemoconcentration and stress: a review of physiological mechanisms and relevance for cardiovascular disease risk, *Biol Psychol* 41:1-27, 1995.

69. Brindley DN: Role of glucocorticoids and fatty acids in the impairment of lipid metabolism observed in the metabolic syndrome, *Int J Obes Relat Metab Disord* 19(suppl 1):S69-S75, 1995.

70. Iuchi T, Akaike M, Mitsui T et al: Glucocorticoid excess induces superoxide production in vascular endothelial cells and elicits vascular endothelial dysfunction, *Circ Res* 92:81-87, 2003.

71. Girod JP, Brotman DJ: Does altered glucocorticoid homeostasis increase cardiovascular risk? *Cardiovasc Res* 64:217-226, 2004.

72. del Rincon I, O'Leary DH, Haas RW et al: Effect of glucocorticoids on the arteries in rheumatoid arthritis, *Arthritis Rheum* 50:3813-3822, 2004.

73. Munck A, Naray-Fejes-Toth A: The ups and downs of glucocorticoid physiology: permissive and suppressive effects revisited, *Mol Cell Endocrinol* 90:C1-C4, 1992.

74. Sapolsky RM, Romero LM, Munck AU: How do glucocorticoids influence stress responses? integrating permissive, suppressive, stimulatory, and preparative actions, *Endocr Rev* 21:55-89, 2000.

75. Jensen LE, Whitehead AS: Regulation of serum amyloid A protein expression during the acute-phase response, *Biochem J* 334:489-503, 1998.

76. Barber AE, Coyle SM, Marano MA et al: Glucocorticoid therapy alters hormonal and cytokine responses to endotoxin in man, *J Immunol* 150:1999-2006, 1993.

77. Arvidson NG, Gudbjornsson B, Larsson A et al: The timing of glucocorticoid administration in rheumatoid arthritis, *Ann Rheum Dis* 56:27-31, 1997.

78. Black PH: The inflammatory response is an integral part of the stress response: implications for atherosclerosis, insulin resistance, type II diabetes and metabolic syndrome X, *Brain Behav Immun* 17:350-364, 2003.

79. Yehuda R, McEwen BS: Protective and damaging effects of the biobehavioral stress response: cognitive, systemic and clinical aspects: ISPNE XXXIV meeting summary, *Psychoneuroendocrinology* 29:1212-1222, 2004.

80. Mohamed-Ali V, Goodrick S, Rawesh A et al: Subcutaneous adipose tissue releases interleukin-6, but not tumor necrosis factor-alpha, in vivo, *J Clin Endocrinol Metab* 82:4196-4200, 1997.

81. Yudkin JS, Kumari M, Humphries SE et al: Inflammation, obesity, stress and coronary heart disease: is interleukin-6 the link? *Atherosclerosis* 148:209-214, 2000.

82. Ross R: Atherosclerosis: an inflammatory disease, *N Engl J Med* 340:115-126, 1999.

83. Maes M, Bosmans E, De Jongh R et al: Increased serum IL-6 and IL-1 receptor antagonist concentrations in major depression and treatment resistant depression, *Cytokine* 9:853-858, 1997.

84. Yudkin JS, Yajnik CS, Mohamed-Ali V et al: High levels of circulating pro-inflammatory cytokines and leptin in urban, but not rural, Asian Indians: a potential explanation for increased risk of diabetes and coronary heart disease, *Diabetes Care* 22:363-364, 1999.

85. Brydon L, Steptoe A: Stress-induced increases in interleukin-6 and fibrinogen predict ambulatory blood pressure at 3-year follow-up, *J Hypertens* 23:1001-1007, 2005.

86. Smith TW, Ruiz JM: Psychosocial influences on the development and course of coronary heart disease: current status and implications for research and practice, *J Consult Clin Psychol* 70:548-568, 2002.

87. Myers A, Dewar HA: Circumstances attending 100 sudden deaths from coronary artery disease with coroner's necroscopies, *Br Heart J* 37:1133-1143, 1975.

88. Rissanen V, Romo M, Siltanen P: Premonitory symptoms and stress factors preceding sudden death from ischaemic heart disease, *Acta Med Scand* 204:389-396, 1978.

89. Rahe RH, Bennett L, Romo M et al: Subjects' recent life changes and coronary heart disease in Finland, *Am J Psychiatry* 130:1222-1226, 1973.

90. Rahe RH, Lind E: Psychosocial factors and sudden cardiac death: a pilot study, *J Psychosom Res* 15:19-24, 1971.

91. Cottington EM, Matthews KA, Talbott E et al: Environmental events preceding sudden death in women, *Psychosom Med* 42:567-574, 1980.

92. Rafanelli C, Roncuzzi R, Milaneschi Y et al: Stressful life events, depression and demoralization as risk factors for acute coronary heart disease, *Psychother Psychosom* 74:179-184, 2005.

93. Mittleman MA, Maclure M, Sherwood JB et al: Triggering of acute myocardial infarction onset by episodes of anger: Determinants of Myocardial Infarction Onset Study Investigators, *Circulation* 92:1720-1725, 1995.

94. Miric D, Giunio L, Bozic I et al: Trends in myocardial infarction in Middle Dalmatia during the war in Croatia, *Mil Med* 166:419-421, 2001.

95. Kark JD, Goldman S, Epstein L: Iraqi missile attacks on Israel: the association of mortality with a life-threatening stressor, *JAMA* 273:1208-1210, 1995.

96. Meisel SR, Kutz I, Dayan KI et al: Effect of Iraqi missile war on incidence of acute myocardial infarction and sudden death in Israeli civilians, *Lancet* 338:660-661, 1991.

97. Leor J, Poole WK, Kloner RA: Sudden cardiac death triggered by an earthquake, *N Engl J Med* 334:413-419, 1996.

98. Kario K: Does earthquake-induced cardiovascular disease persist or is it suppressed after the major quake? *J Am Coll Cardiol* 32:553-554, 1998.

99. Kloner RA, Leor J, Poole WK et al: Population-based analysis of the effect of the Northridge earthquake on cardiac death in Los Angeles County, California, *J Am Coll Cardiol* 30:1174-1180, 1997.

100. Glass RI, Zack MMJ: Increase in deaths from ischaemic heart-disease after blizzards, *Lancet* 1:485-487, 1979.

101. Gorjanc ML, Flanders WD, VanDerslice J et al: Effects of temperature and snowfall on mortality in Pennsylvania, *Am J Epidemiol* 149:1152-1160, 1999.

102. Deanfield JE, Shea M, Kensett M et al: Silent myocardial ischemia due to mental stress, *Lancet* 2:1001-1004, 1984.

103. Stone PH, Krantz DS, McMahon RP et al: Relationship among mental stress-induced ischemia and ischemia during daily life and during exercise: the Psychophysiologic Investigations of Myocardial Ischemia (PIMI) study, *J Am Coll Cardiol* 33:1476-1484, 1999.

104. Rozanski A, Bairey CN, Krantz DS et al: Mental stress and the induction of silent myocardial ischemia in patients with coronary artery disease, *N Engl J Med* 318:1005-1012, 1988.

105. Gabbay FH, Krantz DS, Kop WJ et al: Triggers of myocardial ischemia during daily life in patients with coronary artery disease: physical and mental activities, anger and smoking, *J Am Coll Cardiol* 27:585-592, 1996.

106. Barry J, Selwyn AP, Nabel EG et al: Frequency of ST-segment depression produced by mental stress in stable angina pectoris from coronary artery disease, *Am J Cardiol* 61:989-993, 1988.

107. Carels RA, Sherwood A, Babyak M et al: Emotional responsivity and transient myocardial ischemia, *J Consult Clin Psychol* 67:605-610, 1999.

108. Gullette EC, Blumenthal JA, Babyak M et al: Effects of mental stress on myocardial ischemia during daily life, *JAMA* 277:1521-1526, 1997.

109. Sheps DS, McMahon RP, Becker L et al: Mental stress-induced ischemia and all-cause mortality in patients with coronary artery disease: results from the Psychophysiological Investigations of Myocardial Ischemia study, *Circulation* 105:1780-1784, 2002.

110. Krantz DS, Santiago HT, Kop WJ et al: Prognostic value of mental stress testing in coronary artery disease, *Am J Cardiol* 84:1292-1297, 1999.

111. Jiang W, Babyak M, Krantz DS et al: Mental stress-induced myocardial ischemia and cardiac events, *JAMA* 275:1651-1656, 1996.

112. Yeung AC, Vekshtein VI, Krantz DS et al: The effect of atherosclerosis on the vasomotor response of coronary arteries to mental stress, *N Engl J Med* 325:1551-1556, 1991.

113. Boltwood MD, Taylor CB, Burke MB et al: Anger report predicts coronary artery vasomotor response to mental stress in atherosclerotic segments, *Am J Cardiol* 72:1361-1365, 1993.

114. Dakak N, Quyyumi AA, Eisenhofer G et al: Sympathetically mediated effects of mental stress on the cardiac microcirculation of patients with coronary artery disease, *Am J Cardiol* 76:125-130, 1995.

115. Verrier RL, Hagestad EL, Lown B: Delayed myocardial ischemia induced by anger, *Circulation* 75:249-254, 1987.

116. Kovach JA, Nearing BD, Verrier RL: Anger-like behavioral state potentiates myocardial ischemia-induced T-wave alternans in canines, *J Am Coll Cardiol* 37:1719-1725, 2001.

117. Verrier RL, Lown B: Behavioral stress and cardiac arrhythmias, *Annu Rev Physiol* 46:155-176, 1984.

118. Strike PC, Magid K, Brydon L et al: Exaggerated platelet and hemodynamic reactivity to mental stress in men with coronary artery disease, *Psychosom Med* 66:492-500, 2004.

119. Grignani G, Pacchiarini L, Zucchella M et al: Effect of mental stress on platelet function in normal subjects and in patients with coronary artery disease, *Haemostasis* 22:138-146, 1992.

120. Wallen NH, Held C, Rehnqvist N et al: Effects of mental and physical stress on platelet function in patients with stable angina pectoris and healthy controls, *Eur Heart J* 18:807-815, 1997.

121. Kawano TA, Aoki N, Homori M et al: Mental stress and physical exercise increase platelet-dependent thrombin generation, *Heart Vessels* 15:280-288, 2000.

122. Von Kanel R, Dimsdale JE, Adler KA et al: Effects of depressive symptoms and anxiety on hemostatic responses to acute mental stress and recovery in the elderly, *Psychiatry Res* 126:253-264, 2004.

123. von Kanel R, Mills PJ, Fainman C et al: Effects of psychological stress and psychiatric disorders on blood coagulation and fibrinolysis: a biobehavioral pathway to coronary artery disease? *Psychosom Med* 63:531-544, 2001.

124. Von Kanel R, Mills PJ, Ziegler MG et al: Effects of beta2-adrenergic receptor functioning and increased norepinephrine on the hypercoagulable state with mental stress, *Am Heart J* 144, 2002.

125. Zgraggen L, Fischer JE, Mischler K et al: Relationship between hemoconcentration and blood coagulation responses to acute mental stress, *Thromb Res* 115:175-183, 2005.

126. Kiecolt-Glaser JK, McGuire L, Robles TF et al: Emotions, morbidity, and mortality: new perspectives from psychoneuroimmunology, *Annu Rev Psychol* 53:83-107, 2002.

127. Lespérance F, Frasure-Smith N: Depression in patients with cardiac disease: a practical review, *J Psychosom Res* 48:379-391, 2000.

128. Todaro JF, Shen BJ, Niaura R et al: Prevalence of depressive disorders in men and women enrolled in cardiac rehabilitation, *J Cardiopulm Rehabil* 25:71-75, 2005.

129. Jiang W, Babyak MA, Rozanski A et al: Depression and increased myocardial ischemic activity in patients with ischemic heart disease, *Am Heart J* 146:55-61, 2003.

130. Anda R, Williamson D, Jones D et al: Depressed affect, hopelessness, and the risk of ischemic heart disease in a cohort of US adults, *Epidemiology* 4:285-294, 1993.

131. Everson SA, Goldberg DE, Kaplan GA et al: Hopelessness and risk of mortality and incidence of myocardial infarction and cancer, *Psychosom Med* 58:113-121, 1996.

132. Pratt LA, Ford DE, Crum RM et al: Depression, psychotropic medication, and risk of myocardial infarction: prospective data from the Baltimore ECA follow-up, *Circulation* 94:3123-3129, 1996.

133. Denoillet J, Brutsaert DL: Personality, disease severity, and the risk of long term cardiac events in patients with a decreased ejection fraction after myocardial infarction, *Circulation* 97:167-173, 1998.

134. Hermann C, Brand-Driehorst S, Kaminsky B et al: Diagnosis groups and depressed mood as predictors of 22-month mortality in medical patients, *Psychosom Med* 60:570-577, 1998.

135. Todaro JF, Shen BJ, Niaura R et al: Effect of negative emotions on frequency of coronary heart disease (the Normative Aging Study), *Am J Cardiol* 92:901-906, 2003.

136. Rowan PJ, Haas D, Campbell JA et al: Depressive symptoms have an independent, gradient risk for coronary heart disease incidence in a random, population-based sample, *Ann Epidemiol* 15:316-320, 2005.

137. Sesso HD, Kawachi I, Vokonas PS et al: Depression and the risk of coronary heart disease in the Normative Aging Study, *Am J Cardiol* 82:851-856, 1998.

138. Glassman AH, Shapiro PA: Depression and the course of coronary artery disease, *Am J Psychiatry* 155:4-11, 1998.

139. Prescott E, Holst C, Grønbæk M et al: Vital exhaustion as a risk factor for ischaemic heart disease and all-cause mortality in a community sample: a prospective study of 4084 men and 5479 women in the Copenhagen City Heart Study, *Int J Epidemiol* 32:990-997, 2003.

140. Carney RM, Blumenthal JA, Stein PK et al: Depression, heart rate variability, and acute myocardial infarction, *Circulation* 104:2024-2028, 2001.

141. Stein PK, Carney RM, Freedland KE et al: Severe depression is associated with markedly reduced heart rate variability in patients with stable coronary heart disease, *J Psychosom Res* 48:493-500, 2000.

142. Watkins LL, Grossman P: Association of depressive symptoms with reduced baroreflex cardiac control in coronary artery disease, *Am Heart J* 137:453-457, 1999.

143. Hughes JW, Stoney CM: Depressed mood is related to high-frequency heart rate variability during stressors, *Psychosom Med* 62:796-803, 2000.

144. Hughes JW, Watkins L, Blumenthal JA et al: Depression and anxiety symptoms are related to increased 24-hour urinary norepinephrine excretion among healthy middle-aged women, *J Psychosom Res* 57:353-358, 2004.

145. Gold SM, Zakowski SG, Valdimarsdottir HB et al: Higher Beck depression scores predict delayed epinephrine recovery after acute psychological stress independent of baseline levels of stress and mood, *Biol Psychol* 67:261-273, 2004.

146. Deuschle M, Weber B, Colla M et al: Effects of major depression, aging and gender upon calculated diurnal free plasma cortisol concentrations: a re-evaluation study, *Stress* 2:281-287, 1988.

147. Jiang HK, Wang JY, Lin JC: The central mechanism of hypothalamic-pituitary-adrenocortical system hyperfunction in depressed patients, *Psychiatry Clin Neurosci* 54:227-234, 2000.

148. Kunzel HE, Binder EB, Nickel T et al: Pharmacological and non-pharmacological factors influencing hypothalamic-pituitary-adrenocortical axis reactivity in acutely depressed psychiatric in-patients, measured by the Dex-CRH test, *Neuropsychopharmacology* 28:2169-2178, 2003.

149. Miller GE, Stetler CA, Carney RM et al: Clinical depression and inflammatory risk markers for coronary heart disease, *Am J Cardiol* 90:1279-1283, 2002.

150. Miller GE, Freedland KE, Carney RM et al: Pathways linking depression, adiposity, and inflammatory markers in healthy young adults, *Brain Behav Immun* 17:276-285, 2003.

151. Musselman DL, Tomer A, Manatunga AK et al: Exaggerated platelet reactivity in major depression, *Am J Psychiatry* 153:1313-1317, 1996.

152. Laghrissi-Thode F, Wagner WR, Pollock BG et al: Elevated platelet factor 4 and beta-thromboglobulin plasma levels in depressed patients with ischemic heart disease, *Biol Psychiatry* 42:290-295, 1997.

153. Walsh MT, Dinan TG, Condren RM et al: Depression is associated with an increase in the expression of the platelet adhesion receptor glycoprotein Ib, *Life Sci* 70:3155-3165, 2002.

154. Chrapko WE, Jurasz P, Radomski MW et al: Decreased platelet nitric oxide synthase activity and plasma nitric oxide metabolites in major depressive disorder, *Biol Psychiatry* 56:129-134, 2004.

155. Bonnet F, Irving K, Terra JL et al: Depressive symptoms are associated with unhealthy lifestyles in hypertensive patients with the metabolic syndrome, *J Hypertens* 23:611-617, 2005.

156. Cassidy K, Kotynia-English R, Acres J et al: Association between lifestyle factors and mental health measures among community-dwelling older women, *Aust N Z J Psychiatry* 38:940-947, 2004.

157. Carney RM, Freedland KE, Eisen SA et al: Major depression and medication adherence in elderly patients with coronary artery disease, *Health Psychol* 14:88-90, 1995.

158. Reis M, Aberg-Wistedt A, Agren H et al: Compliance with SSRI medication during 6 months of treatment for major depression: an evaluation by determination of repeated serum drug concentrations, *J Affect Disord* 82:443-446, 2004.

159. Lee ES, Kim YH, Beck SH et al: Depressive mood and abdominal fat distribution in overweight premenopausal women, *Obes Res* 13:320-325, 2005.

160. Rosmond R, Lapidus L, Marin P et al: Mental distress, obesity and body fat distribution in middle-aged men, *Obes Res* 4:245-252, 1996.

161. Meyer CM, Armenian HK, Eaton WW et al: Incident hypertension associated with depression in the Baltimore Epidemiologic Catchment area follow-up study, *J Affect Disord* 83:127-133, 2004.

162. Fleet RP, Beitman BD: Cardiovascular death from panic disorder and panic-like anxiety: a critical review of the literature, *J Psychosom Res* 44:71-80, 1998.

163. Kubzansky LD, Kawachi I, Spiro AI et al: Is worrying bad for your heart? a prospective study of worry and coronary heart disease in the Normative Aging Study, *Circulation* 95:818-824, 1997.

164. Paterniti S, Zureik M, Ducimetiàre P et al: Sustained anxiety and 4-year progression of carotid atherosclerosis, *Arterioscler Thromb Vasc Biol* 21:136-141, 2001.

165. Haines AP, Imeson JD, Meade TW: Phobic anxiety and ischemic heart disease, *Br Med J* 295:297-299, 1987.

166. Kawachi I, Colditz GA, Ascherio A et al: Prospective study of phobic anxiety and risk of coronary heart disease in men, *Circulation* 89:1992-1997, 1994.

167. Kawachi I, Sparrow D, Vokonas PS et al: Symptoms of anxiety and risk of coronary heart disease: the Normative Aging Study, *Circulation* 90:2225-2229, 1994.

168. Weissman MM, Markowitz JS, Ouellette R et al: Panic disorders and cardiovascular/cerebrovascular problems: results from a community survey, *Am J Psychiatry* 147:1504-1508, 1990.

169. Kawachi I, Sparrow D, Vokonas PS et al: Decreased heart rate variability in men with phobic anxiety (data from the Normative Aging Study), *Am J Cardiol* 75:882-885, 1995.

170. Yeragani VK, Pohl R, Berger R et al: Decreased heart rate variability in panic disorder patients: a study of power-spectral analysis of heart rate, *Psychiatry Res* 46:89-103, 1993.

171. Watkins LL, Grossman P, Krishnan R et al: Anxiety and vagal control of heart rate, *Psychosom Med* 60:498-502, 1998.

172. Lavoie KL, Fleet RP, Laurin C et al: Heart rate variability in coronary artery disease patients with and without panic disorder, *Psychiatry Res* 128:289-299, 2004.

173. Frasure-Smith N, Lesperance F, Talajic M: The impact of negative emotions on prognosis following myocardial infarction: is it more than depression? *Health Psychol* 14:388-398, 1995.

174. Denollet J, Brutsaert DL: Personality, disease severity, and the risk of long-term cardiac events in patients with a decreased ejection fraction after myocardial infarction, *Circulation* 97:167-173, 1998.

175. Legault SE, Joffe RT, Armstrong PW: Psychiatric morbidity during the early phase of coronary care for myocardial infarction: association with cardiac diagnosis and outcome, *Can J Psychiatry* 37:316-325, 1992.

176. Welin C, Lappas G, Wilhelmsen L: Independent importance of psychosocial factors for prognosis after myocardial infarction, *J Intern Med* 247:629-639, 2000.

177. Mayou RA, Gill D, Thompson DR et al: Depression and anxiety as predictors of outcome after myocardial infarction, *Psychosom Med* 62:212-219, 2000.

178. Lint DW, Taylor CB, Fried-Behar L et al: Does ischemia occur with panic attacks? *Am J Psychiatry* 152:1678-1680, 1995.

179. Friedman M, Rosenman RH: Association of specific overt behavior pattern with blood and cardiovascular findings: blood cholesterol level, blood clotting time, incidence of arcus senilis, and clinical coronary artery disease, *JAMA* 169:1286-1296, 1959.

180. Kahn JP, Kornfeld DS, Blood DK et al: Type A behavior and the thallium stress test, *Psychosom Med* 44:431-436, 1982.

181. Rosenman RH, Brand RJ, Jenkins D et al: Coronary heart disease in Western Collaborative Group Study: final follow-up experience of 8 1/2 years, *JAMA* 233:872-877, 1975.

182. Hecker MH, Chesney MA, Black GW et al: Coronary-prone behaviors in the Western Collaborative Group Study, *Psychosom Med* 50:153-164, 1988.

183. Dimsdale JE, Gilbert J, Hutter AMJ et al: Predicting cardiac morbidity based on risk factors and coronary angiographic findings, *Am J Cardiol* 47:73-76, 1981.

184. MacDougall JM, Dembroski TM, Dimsdale JE et al: Components of type A, hostility, and anger-in: further relationships to angiographic findings, *Health Psychol* 4:137-152, 1985.

185. Case RB, Heller SS, Case NB et al: Type A behavior and survival after acute myocardial infarction, *N Engl J Med* 312:737-741, 1985.

186. Friedman M: Type A behavior: a frequently misdiagnosed and rarely treated disorder, *Am Heart J* 115:930-936, 1988.

187. Houston BK, Chesney MA, Black GW et al: Behavioral clusters and coronary heart disease risk, *Psychosom Med* 54:447-461, 1992.

188. Smith TW, Glazer K, Ruiz JM et al: Hostility, anger, aggressiveness, and coronary heart disease: an interpersonal perspective on personality, emotion, and health, *J Pers* 72:1217-1270, 2004.

189. Rutledge T, Hogan BE: A quantitative review of prospective evidence linking psychological factors with hypertension development, *Psychosom Med* 64:758-766, 2002.

190. Siegler IC, Peterson BL, Barefoot JC et al: Hostility during late adolescence predicts coronary risk factors at midlife, *Am J Epidemiol* 136:146-154, 1992.

191. Thomas SP, Donnellan MM: Correlates of anger symptoms in women in middle adulthood, *Am J Health Promot* 5:266-272, 1991.

192. Yan LL, Liu K, Matthews KA et al: Psychosocial factors and risk of hypertension: the Coronary Artery Risk Development in Young Adults (CARDIA) study, *JAMA* 290:2138-2148, 2003.

193. Ancoli-Israel S, Roth T: Characteristics of insomnia in the United States: results of the 1991 National Sleep Foundation Survey. I, *Sleep* 22(suppl 2):S347-S353, 1999.

194. Nordin M, Knutsson A, Sundbom E et al: Psychosocial factors, gender, and sleep, *J Occup Health Psychol* 10:54-63, 2005.

195. Heslop P, Smith GD, Metcalfe C et al: Sleep duration and mortality: the effect of short or long sleep duration on cardiovascular and all-cause mortality in working men and women, *Sleep Med* 3:305-314, 2002.

196. Asplund R: Sleep and cardiac diseases amongst elderly people, *J Intern Med* 236:65-71, 1996.

197. Schwartz SW, Cornoni-Huntley J, Cole SR et al: Are sleep complaints an independent risk factor for myocardial infarction? *Ann Epidemiol* 8:384-392, 1998.

198. Rodenbeck A, Hajak G: Neuroendocrine dysregulation in primary insomnia, *Rev Neurol (Paris)* 157:S57-S61, 2001.

199. Vgontzas AN, Zoumakis E, Bixler EO et al: Adverse effects of modest sleep restriction on sleepiness, performance, and inflammatory cytokines, *J Clin Endocrinol Metab* 89:2119-2126, 2004.

200. Williams RB, Barefoot JC, Schneiderman N: Psychosocial risk factors for cardiovascular disease: more than one culprit at work, *JAMA* 290:2190-2192, 2003.

201. Suls J, Bunde J: Anger, anxiety, and depression as risk factors for cardiovascular disease: the problems and implications of overlapping affective dispositions, *Psychol Bull* 131:260-300, 2005.

202. Steptoe A, Wardle J, Marmot M: Positive affect and health-related neuroendocrine, cardiovascular, and inflammatory processes, *Proc Natl Acad Sci U S A* 102:6508-6512, 2005.

203. Brosschot JF, Thayer JF: Heart rate response is longer after negative emotions than after positive emotions, *Int J Psychophysiol* 50:181-187, 2003.

204. Berkman LF, Syme SL: Social networks, host resistance, and mortality: a nine-year follow-up study of Alameda County residents, *Am J Epidemiol* 109:186-204, 1979.

205. Orth-Gomer K, Johnson JV: Social network interaction and mortality: a six-year follow-up study of a random sample of the Swedish population, *J Chronic Dis* 40:949-957, 1987.

206. Woloshin S, Schwartz LM, Tosteson AN et al: Perceived adequacy of tangible social support and health outcomes in patients with coronary artery disease, *J Gen Intern Med* 12:613-618, 1997.

207. Angerer P, Siebert U, Kothny W et al: Impact of social support, cynical hostility and anger expression on progression of coronary atherosclerosis, *J Am Coll Cardiol* 36:1781-1788, 2000.

208. Wang HX, Mittleman MA, Orth-Gomer K: Influence of social support on progression of coronary artery disease in women, *Soc Sci Med* 60:599-607, 2005.

209. House JS, Robbins C, Metzner HL: The association of social relationships and activities with mortality: prospective evidence from the Tecumseh Community Health Study, *Am J Epidemiol* 116:123-140, 1982.

210. Pfiffner D, Hoffmann A: Psychosocial predictors of death for low-risk patients after a first myocardial infarction: a 7-year follow-up study, *J Cardiopulm Rehabil* 24:87-93, 2004.

211. Michael YL, Berkman LF, Colditz GA et al: Living arrangements, social integration, and change in functional health status, *Am J Epidemiol* 153:123-131, 2001.

212. Christenfeld N, Gerin W: Social support and cardiovascular reactivity, *Biomed Pharmacother* 54:251-257, 2000.

213. Glynn LM, Christenfeld N, Gerin W: Gender, social support, and cardiovascular responses to stress, *Psychosom Med* 61:234-242, 1999.

214. Gallo LC, Troxel WM, Kuller LH et al: Marital status, marital quality, and atherosclerotic burden in postmenopausal women, *Psychosom Med* 65:952-962, 2003.

215. Orth-Gomer K, Wamala SP, Horsten M et al: Marital stress worsens prognosis in women with coronary heart disease, *JAMA* 284:3008-3014, 2000.

216. Coyne JC, Rohrbaugh MJ, Shoham V et al: Prognostic importance of marital quality for survival of congestive heart failure, *Am J Cardiol* 88:526-529, 2001.

217. Lee S, Cho E, Grodstein F et al: Effects of marital transitions on changes in dietary and other health behaviours in US women, *Int J Epidemiol* 34:69-78, 2005.

218. Eng PM, Kawachi I, Fitzmaurice G et al: Effects of marital transitions on changes in dietary and other health behaviours in US male health professionals, *J Epidemiol Community Health* 59:56-62, 2005.

219. Matthews KA, Gump BB: Chronic work stress and marital dissolution increase risk of posttrial mortality in men from the Multiple Risk Factor Intervention Trial, *Arch Intern Med* 162:309-315, 2002.

220. Lee S, Colditz GA, Berkman LF et al: Caregiving to children and grandchildren and risk of coronary heart disease in women, *Am J Public Health* 93:1939-1944, 2003.

221. Lee S, Colditz GA, Berkman LF et al: Caregiving and risk of coronary heart disease in US women: a prospective study, *Am J Prev Med* 24:113-119, 2003.

222. Schulz R, Beach SR: Caregiving as a risk factor for mortality: the Caregiver Health Effects Study, *JAMA* 282:2215-2219, 1999.

223. Kiecolt-Glaser JK, Dura JR, Speicher CE et al: Spousal caregivers of dementia victims: longitudinal changes in immunity and health, *Psychosom Med* 53:345-362, 1991.

224. Beeson R, Horton-Deutsch S, Farran C et al: Loneliness and depression in caregivers of persons with Alzheimer's disease or related disorders, *Issues Ment Health Nurs* 21:779-806, 2000.

225. Houston BK, Babyak MA, Chesney MA et al: Social dominance and 22-year all-cause mortality in men, *Psychosom Med* 59:5-12, 1997.

226. Siegman AW, Townsend ST, Civelek AC et al: Antagonistic behavior, dominance, hostility, and coronary heart disease, *Psychosom Med* 62:248-257, 2000.

227. Kaplan JR, Manuck SB, Clarkson TB et al: Social status, environment, and atherosclerosis in cynomolgus monkeys, *Atherosclerosis* 2:359-368, 1982.

228. Shively CA, Clarkson TB: Social status and coronary artery atherosclerosis in female monkeys, *Atheroscler Thromb* 14:721-726, 1994.

229. Knox SS, Uvnäs-Moberg K: Social isolation and cardiovascular disease: an atherosclerotic pathway? *Psychoneuroendocrinology* 23:877-890, 1998.

230. Strand BH, Tverdal A: Can cardiovascular risk factors and lifestyle explain the educational inequalities in mortality from ischaemic heart disease and from other heart diseases? 26-year follow-up of 50,000 Norwegian men and women, *J Epidemiol Community Health* 58:705-709, 2004.

231. Steenland K, Hu S, Walker J: All-cause and cause-specific mortality by socioeconomic status among employed persons in 27 US states, 1984-1997, *Am J Public Health* 94:1037-1042, 2004.

232. Breeze E, Fletcher AE, Leon DA et al: Do socioeconomic disadvantages persist into old age? self-reported morbidity in a 29-year follow-up of the Whitehall Study, *Am J Public Health* 91:277-283, 2001.

233. Crimmins EM, Saito Y: Trends in healthy life expectancy in the United States, 1970-1990: gender, racial, and educational differences, *Soc Sci Med* 52:1629-1641, 2001.

234. Marmot MG, Bosma H, Hemingway H et al: Contribution of job control and other risk factors to social variations in coronary heart disease incidence, *Lancet* 350:235-239, 1997.

235. Baum A, Garofalo JP, Yali AM: Socioeconomic status and chronic stress: does stress account for SES effects on health? *Ann N Y Acad Sci* 896:131-144, 1999.

236. Seeman TE, Crimmins E, Huang MH et al: Cumulative biological risk and socio-economic differences in mortality: MacArthur studies of successful aging, *Soc Sci Med* 58:1985-1997, 2004.

237. Rozanski A, Blumenthal JA, Davidson KW et al: The epidemiology, pathophysiology, and management of psychosocial risk factors in cardiac practice: the emerging field of behavioral cardiology, *J Am Coll Cardiol* 45:637-651, 2005.

238. Amick BC III, McDonough P, Chang H et al: Relationship between all-cause mortality and cumulative working life course psychosocial and physical exposures in the United States labor market from 1968 to 1992, *Psychosom Med* 64:370-381, 2002.

239. Kivimaki M, Leino-Arjas P, Luukkonen R et al: Work stress and risk of cardiovascular mortality: prospective cohort study of industrial employees, *Br Med J* 325:857-862, 2002.

240. Peter R, Siegrist J, Hallqvist J et al: Psychosocial work environment and myocardial infarction: improving risk estimation by combining two complementary job stress models in the SHEEP Study, *J Epidemiol Community Health* 56:294-300, 2002.

241. Karasek RA: Job demands, job decision latitude, and mental strain: implications for job redesign, *Adm Sci Q* 24:285-308, 1979.

242. Theorell T, Karasek RA: Current issues relating to psychosocial job strain and cardiovascular disease research, *J Occup Health Psychol* 1:9-26, 1996.

243. Wamala SP, Mittleman MA, Horsten M et al: Job stress and the occupational gradient in coronary heart disease risk in women: the Stockholm Female Coronary Risk Study, *Soc Sci Med* 51:481-489, 2000.

244. Strike PC, Steptoe A: Psychosocial factors in the development of coronary artery disease, *Prog Cardiovasc Dis* 46:337-347, 2004.

245. Johnson JV, Hall E: Job strain, workplace support, and cardiovascular disease: a cross-sectional study of a random sample of the Swedish working population, *Am J Public Health* 78:1336-1342, 1988.

246. Amick BCr, Kawachi I, Coakley EH et al: Relationship of job strain and iso-strain to health status in a cohort of women in the United States, *Scand J Work Environ Health* 24:54-61, 1988.

247. Eaker ED, Sullivan LM, Kelly-Hayes M et al: Does job strain increase the risk for coronary heart disease or death in men and women? the Framingham Offspring Study, *Am J Epidemiol* 159:950-958, 2004.

248. Swanson NG: Working women and stress, *J Am Med Womens Assoc* 55:76-79, 2000.

249. Siegrist J: Adverse health effects of high-effort/low-reward conditions, *J Occup Health Psychol* 1:27-41, 1996.

250. Peter R, Siegrist J: Psychosocial work environment and the risk of coronary heart disease, *Int Arch Occup Environ Health* 73(suppl):S41-S45, 2000.

251. Niedhammer I, Tek ML, Starke D et al: Effort-reward imbalance model and self-reported health: cross-sectional and prospective findings from the GAZEL cohort, *Soc Sci Med* 58:1531-1541, 2004.

252. Steptoe A, Siegrist J, Kirschbaum C et al: Effort-reward imbalance, overcommitment, and measures of cortisol and blood pressure over the working day, *Psychosom Med* 66:323-329, 2004.

253. Vrijkotte TG, van Doornen IJ, de Geus EJ: Work stress and metabolic and hemostatic risk factors, *Psychosom Med* 61:796-805, 1999.

254. Bosma H, Peter R, Siegrist J et al: Two alternative job stress models and the risk of coronary heart disease, *Am J Public Health* 88:68-74, 1998.

255. Hanson EKS, Godaert GLR, Maas CJM et al: Vagal cardiac control throughout the day: the relative importance of effort-reward imbalance and within-day measurements of mood, demand and satisfaction, *Biol Psychol* 56:23-44, 2001.

256. Cesana G, Sega R, Ferrario M et al: Job strain and blood pressure in employed men and women: a pooled analysis of four north-ern Italian population samples, *Psychosom Med* 65:558-563, 2003.

257. Fauvel JP, Quelin P, Ducher M et al: Perceived job stress but not individual cardiovascular reactivity to stress is related to higher blood pressure at work, *Hypertension* 38:71-75, 2001.

258. Frimerman A, Miller HI, Laniado S et al: Changes in hemostatic function at times of cyclic variation in occupational stress, *Am J Cardiol* 79:72-75, 1997.

259. Kouvonen A, Kivimäki M, Virtanen M et al: Work stress, smoking status, and smoking intensity: an observational study of 46,190 employees, *J Epidemiol Community Health* 59:63-69, 2005.

260. Kouvonen A, Kivimäki M, Elovainio M et al: Job strain and leisure-time physical activity in female and male public sector employees, *Prev Med* 41:532-539, 2005.

261. Schnorpfeil P, Noll A, Schulze R et al: Allostatic load and work conditions, *Soc Sci Med* 57:647-656, 2003.

262. Folkman S, Lazarus RS, Dunkel-Schetter C et al: Dynamics of a stressful encounter: cognitive appraisal, coping, and encounter outcomes, *J Pers Soc Psychol* 50:992-1003, 1986.

263. Folkman S, Lazarus RS, Gruen RJ et al: Appraisal, coping, health status, and psychological symptoms, *J Pers Soc Psychol* 50:571-579, 1986.

264. Ong L, Linden W, Young S: Stress management: what is it? *J Psychosom Res* 56:133-137, 2004.

265. Nunes EV, Frank KA, Kornfeld DS: Psychologic treatment for the type A behavior pattern and for coronary heart disease: a meta-analysis of the literature, *Psychosom Med* 48:159-173, 1987.

266. Linden W, Stossel C, Maurice J: Psychosocial interventions for patients with coronary artery disease: a meta-analysis, *Arch Intern Med* 156:745-752, 1996.

267. Dusseldorp E, van Elderen T, Maes S et al: A meta-analysis of psychoeducational programs for coronary heart disease patients, *Health Psychol* 18:506-519, 1999.

268. Blumenthal JA, Babyak M, Wei J et al: Usefulness of psychosocial treatment of mental stress-induced myocardial ischemia in men *Am J Cardiol* 89:164-168, 2002.

269. Astin JA, Shapiro SL, Eisenberg DM et al: Mind-body medicine: state of the science, implications for practice, *J Am Board Fam Pract* 16:131-147, 2003.

270. Eisenberg DM, Delbanco TL, Berkey CS et al: Cognitive behavioral techniques for hypertension: are they effective? *Ann Intern Med* 118:964-972, 1993.

271. Batey DM, Kaufmann PG, Raczynski JM et al: Stress management intervention for primary prevention of hypertension: detailed results from phase I of Trials of Hypertension Prevention (TOHP-I), *Ann Epidemiol* 10:45-58, 2000.

272. Linden W, Lenz JW, Con AH: Individualized stress management for primary hypertension: a randomized trial, *Arch Intern Med* 161:1071-1080, 2001.

273. McCraty R, Atkinson M, Tomasino D: Impact of a workplace stress reduction program on blood pressure and emotional health in hypertensive employees, *J Altern Complement Med* 9:355-369, 2003.

274. Schneider RH, Staggers F, Alexander CN et al: A randomized controlled trial of stress reduction for hypertension in older African Americans, *Hypertension* 26:820-827, 1995.

275. Castillo-Richmond A, Schneider RH, Alexander CN et al: Effects of stress reduction on carotid atherosclerosis in hypertensive African Americans, *Stroke* 31:568-573, 2000.

276. Tugade MM, Fredrickson BL, Barrett LF: Psychological resilience and positive emotional granularity: examining the benefits of positive emotions on coping and health, *J Pers* 72:1161-1190, 2004.

277. Kubzansky LD, Sparrow D, Vokonas P et al: Is the glass half empty or half full? a prospective study of optimism and coronary heart disease in the normative aging study, *Psychosom Med* 63:910-916, 2001.

chapter 40

Impact of Depression on Cardiac Disease

Lynne Doering
Rebecca Cross

CHAPTER ABBREVIATIONS

ANS   autonomic nervous system

CABG   coronary artery bypass grafting

CBT   cognitive-behavioral therapy

CHD   coronary heart disease

CI   confidence interval

CRP   C-reactive protein

DISH   Diagnostic Interview and Structured Hamilton

DSM-IV   Diagnostic and Statistical Manual of Mental Disorders, 4th edition, text revision

ECT   electroconvulsive therapy

ENRICHD   Enhancing Recovery in Coronary Heart Disease

HPA   hypothalamic-pituitary-adrenal

HRV   heart rate variability

5-HT   5-hydroxytryptamine (serotonin)

IL   interleukin

IPT   interpersonal therapy

MAO   monoamine oxidase

MDD   major depressive disorder

MI   myocardial infarction

RR   relative risk

SCD   sudden cardiac death

SCID   Structured Clinical Interview for DSM-IV

SNS   sympathetic nervous system

SSRI   selective serotonin reuptake inhibitor

TCA   tricyclic antidepressant

TNF   tumor necrosis factor

Depression is a phenomenon that occurs across a wide spectrum of human experience. As a normal emotion or mood, depression is universal and can serve an adaptive function in social signaling, behavioral regulation, and goal setting. Depression can appear as a response to stress, trauma, or normal life events. Depression is related intimately to grief, mourning, and bereavement. Depression often is a normal response to the onset or worsening of medical illnesses. As a clinical syndrome, depression occurs across a continuum of severity from conditions associated with mild symptoms of short duration (such as adjustment disorders) to conditions involving severe, prolonged, or unremitting symptoms that cause functional impairment (such as major depressive disorder [**MDD**]).

As integrative theories of health and wellness that include biological, psychosocial, and behavioral perspectives have gained acceptance, the relationship of depression to physical illness and disease has been the topic of intense interest among researchers and clinicians. Because coronary heart disease (**CHD**) is pervasive and the leading killer of Americans, questions regarding how depression mediates or moderates the development and exacerbation of atherosclerosis have been investigated and debated. The purpose of this chapter is to evaluate current literature regarding the role of depression in CHD, consider potential biobehavioral mechanisms that can explain the role of depression in CHD, and present recommendations for assessment and management of clinical depression in cardiac patients.

DEPRESSION IN CARDIAC PATIENTS

In the general population, major depression will affect approximately 5 percent of adult Americans in the next 12 months. Across their lifetimes, more than 10 percent of adults in the United States will be affected by major depression.[1] When direct costs, mortality from suicide, and workplace costs are considered, the economic burden of depression in the United States is estimated at $83.1 billion.[2] In cardiac patients, depression exceeds the rate found in the general population, with reported prevalence of nearly 17 to 27 percent.[3] More generally, depressive symptoms and subsyndromal depression have been reported to reach 40 to 65 percent across a wide spectrum of cardiac patients.[4]

More is known about special populations of cardiac patients, especially those having myocardial infarction (**MI**) or revascularization, those with heart failure, and those undergoing heart transplantation. The incidence of depression after MI ranges from 17 to 27 percent. Variables associated with post-MI depression are degree of functional impairment, overall medical burden, family history of a psychopathological condition, and low levels of perceived social support.[3] A majority of patients with MDD are likely to have persistent depressive symptoms at 3-month follow-up compared with patients with milder baseline symptoms.[5] Persistence of symptoms, consistent with MDD rather than a transient adjustment disorder, is associated with a history of prior psychiatric morbidity and lack of social support after MI.[3]

Depressive symptoms have been reported to be common before and after coronary artery bypass grafting (**CABG**). Prevalence reports range from 32 to 65 percent for preoperative symptoms within 1 week before surgery, and 20 to 46 percent for postoperative symptoms measured up to 6 months after surgery.[6] Clinical depression has been described rarely, with reports documenting postoperative major depression in 17 to 20 percent of CABG patients, minor depression in an additional 27 percent of patients, and overall clinical depression in 35 percent of patients within the first 6 months after CABG.[7] With approximately 314,000 patients undergoing CABG annually in the United States,[8] nurses can expect more than 62,000 of them to suffer MDD and as many as 84,780 to experience minor depression annually.

In heart failure patients, researchers evaluating the incidence of MDD have reported that 14 to 36 percent of patients meet the criteria laid out in the *Diagnostic and Statistical Manual of Mental Disorders,* fourth edition, text revision (**DSM-IV**)[9,10] compared with the 5 to 7 percent seen in community samples.[1] Studies looking at depressive symptoms (not using DSM-IV criteria) have found that up to 60 percent of heart failure patients experience moderate to severe depression.[11] In heart transplant recipients, 19 percent have a lifetime history of at least one episode of MDD before transplant; cumulative prevalence climbs to 25.5 percent 3 years posttransplant.[12]

DEFINING DEPRESSION IN CARDIAC PATIENTS

Clinical or Syndromal Depression

Research on the relationship between depression and cardiac disease has focused on the diagnosis of clinical disorders, such as MDD or dysthymia, and depressive symptoms. The distinction between dysthymia and depressive symptoms is an important one. In cardiac patients, as in other individuals, clinical syndromes of depression are defined by the DSM-IV. The classifications reflect a current consensus of evolving knowledge in mental health[13] and serve as a guideline for making clinical diagnoses. In general, classifications for depressive disorders include a general description, associated features and disorders, specific factors (e.g., culture, age, and gender), and specific diagnostic criteria. Classification criteria for key depressive conditions are summarized in Table 40-1.

MDD is the most severe form of clinical depression. MDD is characterized by the presence of at least one of the two cardinal symptoms of depression: low mood or anhedonia (loss of pleasure in activities that were formerly enjoyable). In addition, a total of five somatic, affective, and/or cognitive symptoms, including low mood or anhedonia, must be present. Taken together, these symptoms must last at least 2 weeks, must occur most of the time on most days, and must be severe enough to impair usual social or functional daily activities. Other conditions, such as dysthymic disorder or adjustment disorder with low mood, are characterized by fewer or less severe symptoms or symptoms that can be traced to a specific cause, such as a known stressor, a medication, or a general medical condition.

Usually, clinical depressive syndromes are established by in-depth clinician interviews and observations. The preeminent format assessment tool is the Hamilton Rating Scale for Depression, an observer-rated scale requiring clinical expertise. The scale was originally designed in 1961 as an unstructured interview to be used by experienced clinicians as a means of measuring symptom severity in psychiatric patients in whom a diagnosis of depression already had been made. Since that time, the scale has been used widely in research and clinical practice and is accepted in community samples, psychiatric patients, and medical patients.

Other diagnostic interviews that require more limited clinical expertise have been developed. These instruments have been used primarily for research, are consistent with current DSM-IV criteria, and rely on structured or semistructured approaches. In structured interviews, the rater asks a question and then codes the respondent's answer based on preassigned values for symptom intensity and duration. In semistructured interviews, open-ended probes allow the rater more latitude in exploring symptom characteristics. The most commonly used instruments are summarized in Table 40-2. Of note, a semistructured interview to identify clinical depression specifically in cardiac patients was developed for the recent Enhancing Recovery in Coronary Heart Disease (**ENRICHD**) study. The Diagnostic Interview and Structured Hamilton (**DISH**) was designed to diagnose depression in cardiac patients, who require an approach that is flexible, sensitive, and likely to foster trust, rapport, and disclosure. The DISH includes assessment of symptom severity on an embedded version of Williams' Structured Interview Guide for the Hamilton Depression scale. In validation studies, the DISH and Structured Clinical Interview for DSM-IV (**SCID**) resulted in 88 percent agreement (K = 0.86). Interrater reliability has been established, 93 percent agreement between diagnosis by trained interviewers and clinicians, and with diagnostic agreement across symptom clusters (K = 0.75).[14]

Subsyndromal Depression

Subsyndromal depression is the presence of depressive symptoms that fall below the threshold of those involved in recognized depressive syndromes. Although such symptoms are common and can be clinically important, they are referred to as subsyndromal because they have not been measured or evaluated against specific diagnostic criteria or because they are considered to fall within the range of normal emotional valence. Multiple self-report and assessment instruments designed for research and clinical practice are available to measure depressive symptoms. Most often, these instruments are not consistent with DSM-IV criteria. They include a varying range of symptoms and have been developed for use in a variety of otherwise healthy and medically ill patients. Although many such instruments have established cutoff points for depression, it is more appropriate to use them as indicators of symptom frequency. Many such self-report instruments are used frequently as screening instruments. Commonly used instruments are summarized in Table 40-3.

Differentiating Cardiac Symptoms and Depression

Many somatic symptoms experienced by cardiac patients, such as fatigue, pain, and insomnia, overlap considerably with somatic symptoms experienced by

TABLE 40-1   SUMMARY OF CLASSIFICATION CRITERIA FOR KEY DEPRESSIVE DISORDERS

DISORDER	DIAGNOSTIC CRITERIA

Major depressive episode (MDE)	A. Five or more of the following, including at least one of the first two symptoms:
	  1. Depressed mood
	  2. Anhedonia
	  3. Significant weight change (more than 5%/month) or significant change in appetite
	  4. Sleep disturbance
	  5. Psychomotor agitation or retardation
	  6. Fatigue
	  7. Feelings of worthlessness or excessive guilt
	  8. Indecisiveness or decreased concentration
	  9. Recurrent suicidal ideation
	B. Symptoms cause clinically significant distress or functional impairment most of the day, nearly every day.
	C. Symptoms are not due to the direct physiological effects of a substance or a general medical condition (i.e., hypothyroidism).
	D. Symptoms are not better accounted for by bereavement.

Major depressive disorder (MDD)	A. Presence of a single MDE B. MDE not better accounted for by other depressive disorders. C. There has never been a manic, mixed, or hypomanic episode.

Dysthymic disorder (DD)	A. Depressed mood most of the day, more days than not, for at least 2 years.
	B. Presence of one or more of the following:
	  1. Poor appetite or overeating
	  2. Sleep disturbance
	  3. Low energy or fatigue
	  4. Low self-esteem
	  5. Poor concentration or difficulty making decisions
	  6. Feelings of hopelessness
	C. During the 2-year period, symptoms are not absent more than 2 months at a time.
	D. No MDE is present during the first 2 years of the disturbance.

Adjustment disorder with depressed mood	A. Development of emotional or behavioral symptoms in response to an identifiable stressor occurring within 3 months of stressor onset. B. Symptoms or behaviors clinically significant by marked distress in excess of what would be expected or by significant impairment in social or occupational functioning. C. Symptoms do not meet criteria for another specific disorder. D. Symptoms are not consistent with bereavement. E. Once the stressor is terminated, symptoms do not persist more than 6 months.

Mood disorder due to a general medical condition	A. Prominent and persistent mood disturbance characterized by either or both of the following:
	  1. Depressed mood or marked anhedonia in all, or almost all, activities
	  2. Elevated, expansive, or irritable mood
	B. There is evidence from the history, physical examination, or laboratory findings that the disturbance is the *direct* physiological consequence of a medical condition.
	C. Symptoms are not better accounted for by another mental disorder.
	D. Symptoms do not occur exclusively during the course of a delirium.
	E. Symptoms cause clinically significant distress or functional impairment.

Substance-induced mood disorder	A. Same as for mood disorder due to a general medical condition, EXCEPT the following:
	B. There is evidence from the history, physical examination, or laboratory findings of either of the following:
	  1. Symptoms developed during, or within a month of, substance intoxication or withdrawal
	  2. Medication use is etiologically related to the disturbance.

From American Psychiatric Association: *Diagnostic and statistical manual of mental disorders*, ed 4, Washington, DC, 2000, The Association.

■ ■ ■

TABLE 40-2   INSTRUMENTS FOR MEASUREMENT OF CLINICAL DEPRESSION

INSTRUMENT	FORMAT	TIME	POPULATION	DATA SOURCES
Structured Clinical Interview of DSM (SCID)	Open-ended probes, then closed-ended Coded responses (22 pages)	45-60 minutes	Medical or psychiatric adult patients	Respondents, medical records, other knowledgeable informants (i.e., family, significant others, or other health care providers)
Diagnostic Interview Schedule (DIS)	Designed for use by lay interviewers Closed-ended questions only No additional probes (263 items)	45-75 minutes	Clinical and community respondents	Respondents only
Composite International Diagnostic Interview (CIDI)	Fully structured interview designed to be used by lay personnel with specialized in-depth training		Community samples	Respondents only
Diagnostic Interview and Structured Hamilton (DISH)	Open- and closed-ended probes Coded responses Hamilton Rating Scale for Depression imbedded	30-60 minutes	Coronary heart disease patients, specifically post-myocardial infarction patients	

■ ■ ■

TABLE 40-3   SCREENING INSTRUMENTS FOR DEPRESSIVE SYMPTOMS

INSTRUMENT	LITERACY LEVEL; TIME	CHARACTERISTICS	TIME FRAME FOR QUESTIONS	RANGE USUAL CUT-POINTS	WEB SOURCE
Beck Depression Inventory (BDI) and BDI-II	Easy; 5-10 minutes	Developed for use in psychiatric populations, but used widely in medically ill patients Most widely established reliability and validity	Past week including today	0-63 Mild: greater than 10 Moderate: ≥20 Severe: ≥30	www.psychcorp center.com
Center for Epidemiologic Studies Depression Scale (CES-D)	Easy; 5-10 minutes	Widely used for screening in elderly and in primary care settings	Past week	0-60 Depressed: greater than 16	
Hospital Anxiety and Depression Scale (HADS)	Average; 2-5 minutes	Developed for use in hospitalized, medically ill patients Omits somatic symptoms, hopelessness, guilt, low self-esteem	Past week	Depression subscale: 0-21 Normal: ≤7 Borderline: 8-10 Clinical depression: greater than 10	www.nfer-nelson. co.uk/health_and_ psychology/ resources/hospital_ anxiety_scale/ hospital_anxiety_ scale.asp?css=1
Zung Self-Rating Depression Scale (Zung SDS)	Easy; 2-5 minutes	Developed in ambulatory patients, but used in medically ill, especially oncology, patients	Recently	25-100 Mild: 50 Moderate: 60 Severe: 70	www.medalreg.com/ qhc/index.html
Primary Care Evaluation of Mental Disorder (PRME-MD) Patient Health Questionnaire (PHQ-9)	Average; 2-5 minutes	Designed for screening in primary care	Past 2 weeks	0-27 Minimal: ≤4 Mild: 5-9 Moderate: 10-14 Moderately severe: 15-19 Severe: ≥20	www.depression-primarycare.org/ clinicians/toolkits
Geriatric Depression Scale (GDS)	Easy; 2-5 minutes	Designed for assessment of symptoms in elderly Commonly used to measure symptom severity and treatment outcomes 15-item version available	Past week	0-30 No depression: ≤9 Mild depression: 10-19 Severe depression: ≥20	www.gericareonline. net/tools/eng/ depression/index. html

otherwise healthy persons with depression. Key symptoms of depression mentioned frequently by cardiac patients are fatigue, change in appetite, and sleep disturbance. The question of how to handle somatic symptoms in medically ill patients, especially cardiac patients, always comes up when depression is considered. It remains a difficult and confounding question. (See the accompanying Conundrum feature). One solution is to eliminate consideration of these symptoms. Another solution is to dichotomize depressive symptoms as "somatic" or "affective-cognitive" and then to evaluate symptom number and severity separately. A third approach is simply to consider all symptoms as relevant for a diagnosis of depression. Each approach has advantages and disadvantages. The more narrowly symptoms are ascribed to depression, the more likely that true cases of depression will be missed (false negative). The more broadly symptoms are ascribed to depression, the more likely that some individuals without true depression may be categorized as depressed (false positive). The right decision depends on the characteristics of the individual patient, the particular circumstances in which the evaluation is taking place, the risks of missing a true case of depression, and the consequences of wrongly attributing symptoms to a depressive cause. In general, a conservative approach regarding the evaluation of somatic symptoms in the assessment of depression in cardiac patients calls for the inclusion, rather than the exclusion, of these symptoms. The most compelling argument for their inclusion is that it is often impossible to determine the precise cause of symptoms.

■ ■ ■ **CONUNDRUM**

SHOULD SOMATIC SYMPTOMS IN CARDIAC PATIENTS BE CONSIDERED IN ASSESSING DEPRESSION?

Arguments Against Inclusion of Somatic Symptoms

Elimination of somatic symptoms in the assessment of depression may result in greater specificity and internal consistency. Because it is often difficult, if not impossible, to tease out whether somatic symptoms—such as fatigue, appetite and sleep disturbance—result from depression or from cardiovascular disease, nurses may have more confidence that they are really dealing with a psychiatric problem or mood disorder if such symptoms are not considered.

Arguments for Inclusion of Somatic Symptoms

If nurses omit somatic symptoms, they run the risk of missing real cases of depression. Somatic complaints are an integral part of depressive syndromes. Somatic symptoms are so intertwined with depression that the cause of the symptoms does not really matter. Disregarding somatic symptoms assumes a dichotomy between mind and body that is not supported by current evidence.

DEPRESSION AS A PREDICTOR OF CARDIAC DISEASE
New-Onset Cardiac Disease

Depression alone is associated with high use of medical care, amplification of somatic symptoms and disability, poor self-care and adherence to medical regimens, and increased morbidity and mortality from medical illness.[15] Given the link between depression and medical comorbidity, it should be no surprise that depression is associated with cardiac disease.[8] Traditional cardiac risk factors—such as obesity, sedentary lifestyle, smoking, hypertension, diabetes mellitus, age, and family history—do not explain all cardiac disease. More than 200 risk factors for CHD have been identified, including various forms of stress and distress.[16] New evidence suggests that depression is an independent risk factor for the development of CHD.

To date, depression and/or depressive symptoms as risk factors for development of CHD have been evaluated in at least 16 population and case-control studies.[17] Only one study failed to find an association of depressive symptoms to new-onset CHD.[18] Two others reported contradictory findings related to gender differences; one study reported that preexisting depressive symptoms were predictive of incident CHD in women but not men,[19] whereas the other reported a positive finding for men but not for women.[20] On balance, these studies included community populations with unspecified CHD status or individuals with no known disease and used epidemiological and case-control methods. Most of these studies measured depressive symptoms, not clinical depression. They revealed increases in adjusted relative risk (**RR**) of new onset CHD in the presence of depressive symptoms of approximately 1.5 to 2.0. Follow-up ranged from 4 to 40 years, and endpoints included CHD diagnosis, MI, and cardiac mortality. Most studies controlled for standard cardiac risk factors, but inconsistencies in age groups across studies may have accounted for some of the differences in findings.

Two meta-analyses confirmed the overall predictive value of depression and/or depressive symptoms for incident CHD.[17,21] Both of these studies concluded that depression constitutes a significant independent risk for the onset of CHD, with a level of risk similar to that conferred by smoking. Clinical depression (RR, 2.69; 95 percent confidence interval [**CI**] 1.63 to 4.43, $p < 0.001$) was found to be a stronger predictor of CHD than depressive symptoms alone (RR, 1.49; 95 percent CI 1.16 to 1.92, $p = 0.02$).[17] The relative risks of depression and/or depressive symptoms for incident CHD associated with depression are summarized in Figure 40-1.

Only one study has evaluated the effect of depression on incident heart failure in a community sample. In a 14-year follow-up of 2500 elderly (age 65 and older) individuals, investigators found that women suffered from a significant effect of depressive symptoms on the likelihood of developing heart failure, whereas men did not.[22] Although gender differences have been reported in the prevalence of depression in other cardiac populations, this study was the first to suggest that depression might play a differentially independent role in women compared with men.

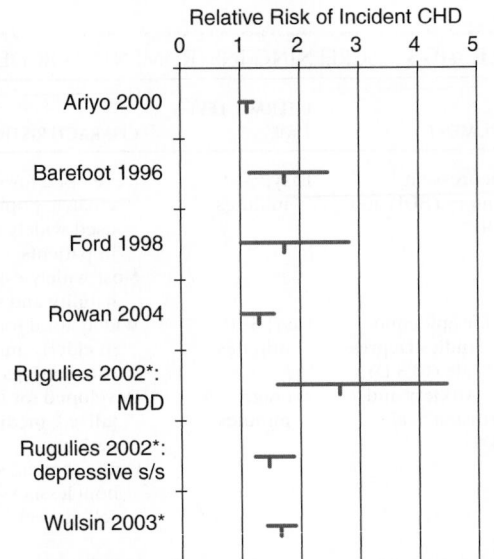

FIGURE 40-1 ■ Relative risk of new-onset coronaryr heart disease in depressive individuals. *CHD*, Coronary heart disease; *MDD*, major depressive disorder; *S/S*, signs and symptoms.

Health Outcomes in Preexisting Cardiac Disease

In patients with known cardiac disease, the relationship of depression to CHD prognosis has been studied extensively. The strongest focus has been on patients recovering from acute MI, but other studies have examined patients with heart failure and those recovering from CABG.

In post-MI and CHD patients, the majority of studies have reported a positive association between depression and/or depressive symptoms and poorer health outcomes, particularly mortality. Several studies suggest that the presence of depression and/or depressive symptoms during or shortly after hospitalization for acute MI confers 2 to 3 times the risk for subsequent mortality.[23] The risks associated with depressive symptoms were robust and persisted after the investigators controlled for other predictors of mortality. As severity of depressive symptoms increased, so too did the risk of overall mortality.[24] The impact of major depression on mortality was as strong as that of left ventricular dysfunction (Killip Class) and history of previous MI.[25] In addition to all-cause mortality, depression after acute MI is associated positively with cardiac mortality and with nonfatal cardiac events.[26]

Two recent meta-analyses support these positive associations of depression and/or depressive symptoms to adverse health outcomes in post-MI patients.[27,28] Both studies found a negative effect for depression on long-term and short-term follow-up after acute MI. Although the effect of depression and/or depressive symptoms was stronger in short-term follow-up studies, the positive finding for long-term follow-up underscores the significance of the relationship. Although the studies differentiated between findings obtained by self-report questionnaires and by diagnostic interview, both assessment methods were prognostic of poorer outcomes and were equally useful for epidemiological purposes.

Fewer studies have found negative or null associations of depression and cardiac outcomes in acute MI patients.[29] These studies do not appear to share common methodological differences with studies showing positive results. However, it is possible that assessment criteria or inconsistencies in the adjustment for mediating variables, such as traditional cardiac risk factors or history of mental illness, across studies could account for the differing findings.

Following initial studies of depression and CHD, investigators turned their attention to the role of depression in heart failure prognosis. Positive associations of depression or depressive symptoms with poor prognosis in heart failure patients have been documented consistently.[30,31] The studies included hospitalized patients and outpatients. Depression was evaluated by symptom frequency and severity and by diagnostic interview. Reported in all but one study, follow-up ranged from 3 months to 5 years. After controlling for mediating variables such as age and disease severity, patients with depression were more than twice as likely to die from heart failure than were their nondepressed counterparts.[30] In addition, there was a graded association between severity of depressive symptoms and the rate of functional decline or death.[32]

In CABG patients, depression rates are particularly high before and immediately after surgery.[33,34] Nonetheless, there are relatively few prospective studies regarding the prognostic effect of depression and/or depressive symptoms on mortality and cardiac events after CABG. Methodological approaches have involved the assessment of preoperative and postoperative depression, with follow-up periods from 1 year to more than 5 years. To date, all studies of CABG patients have shown a positive association of depression or depressive symptoms to mortality or to adverse cardiac events.[7,33,34] In the largest study of 817 patients followed for an average of 5.2 years, depression diagnosed before surgery and depression that persisted for more than 6 months after surgery were related to higher postoperative mortality rates.[7] In a study using DSM-IV criteria for clinical depression, the presence of MDD more than doubled the risk of adverse cardiac events—including heart failure, angina, and MI or revacularization—in the first year after surgery (RR, 2.31; 95 percent CI 1.17 to 4.56, $p = 0.01$).[35]

Diversity and the Predictive Value of Depression

Research regarding the effect of diversity in age, gender, or race and ethnicity on the predictive value of depression for incident CHD or CHD prognosis is scarce. To date, no one has investigated the possibility that age, gender, or race and ethnicity interact directly with depression to affect the onset or progression of CHD. Regarding age and gender, higher rates of depression have been reported in otherwise healthy younger populations and in women. A few reports have found these same relationships in cardiac patients. In heart failure patients, women were more likely to be depressed than men, and depressed patients were younger than nondepressed patients.[36] In the ENRICHD trial, female pa-

tients reported higher levels of depression and distress than male patients, with the greatest differences observed among younger women.[37]

Only a few studies have addressed racial or ethnic differences in psychosocial factors related to CHD. Preliminary evidence indicates that racial or ethnic differences in the prevalence of depression exist in the general population, in medically ill patients, and in some cardiac populations.[36,38] Some studies have shown equivocal evidence regarding the rates of depression between community-dwelling minorities, specifically blacks and whites. However, more recent work indicates that minorities (including Hispanics, blacks, and American Indians) exhibit greater depressive symptoms and have a marginally higher prevalence of MDD than do whites.[38] Greater difficulty meeting basic needs and lower household income mediate the relationship between minority status and depressive symptoms. Among medically ill minority patients, few differences in the rates of depression after adjustment for gender and income have been reported. However, among depressed patients with medical illnesses, blacks and Hispanics were significantly younger, more likely to be single and female, and had lower incomes and educational levels than depressed white patients. After sociodemographic adjustment and despite comparable levels of depressive symptoms, Asian Americans had a lower prevalence of MDD and dysthymic disorder.[39] In cardiac patients, rates of depression across race and ethnicity appear to be equivalent.[37] However, an initial study indicates that gender and ethnicity may influence response to treatment of depression.[40] These findings indicate that clinical evaluation for depression is important for all patients, regardless of race or ethnicity, and underscore the need for further study with representative samples of minorities across racial and ethnic groups.

POSSIBLE LINKS BETWEEN DEPRESSION AND CARDIAC DISEASE

Several biobehavioral mechanisms describing the relationship between depression and cardiac disease have been proposed. For simplicity, they can be broken down into two main categories: biobehavioral mechanisms and biological mechanisms, though in reality, it is most likely that both mechanisms work in concert.

Biobehavioral Mechanisms

High-risk health behaviors associated with clinical depression may contribute to the onset of CHD because they affect biological processes inherent in the CHD pathology. Depressed patients are more likely to be overweight or obese, use tobacco products, lead sedentary lifestyles, and fail to adhere to a healthful diet than are those who have never experienced a depressive episode.[15,41] These high-risk behaviors are attributed to hopelessness and anhedonia, prominent symptoms of clinical depression. Unfortunately, they are known contributors to the development of CHD.

Additionally, those suffering from clinical depression tend to have a poorer social support network than those without depression.[42] Social support refers to the number of persons in one's social network and the quality of those relationships. Low social support has been linked to recurrent cardiac events in post-MI patients[43] and increased mortality in heart failure patients.[44] The underlying mechanism for this relationship between social support and cardiac disease is unknown but is hypothesized to be associated with increased stress.

The increased incidence of morbidity and mortality observed in cardiac patients with comorbid depression may be due in part to nonadherence to recommended medical regimens.[44] Those with a clinical depression are less likely to adhere to medical treatments than are those without depression,[45] which may increase the probability of an adverse outcome.

Putative biobehavioral pathways linking depression with coronary artery disease and with heart failure are displayed in Figures 40-2 and 40-3, respectively.

Biological Mechanisms

Although behavioral factors may play a role in the development and progression of CHD in depressed patients, they certainly do not explain the full picture. Currently, researchers are investigating biological mechanisms that may explain why clinical depression is an independent risk factor for developing future cardiac disease and why those with preexisting CHD are more likely to become clinically depressed than persons without CHD. Dysfunction in the following biological networks is thought to be related to the development and/or progression of CHD in patients with a clinical depression: the hypothalamic-pituitary-adrenal (**HPA**) axis, the autonomic nervous system (**ANS**), the serotonergic (5-hydroxytryptamine [**5-HT**]) system, and the proinflammatory cytokine network.

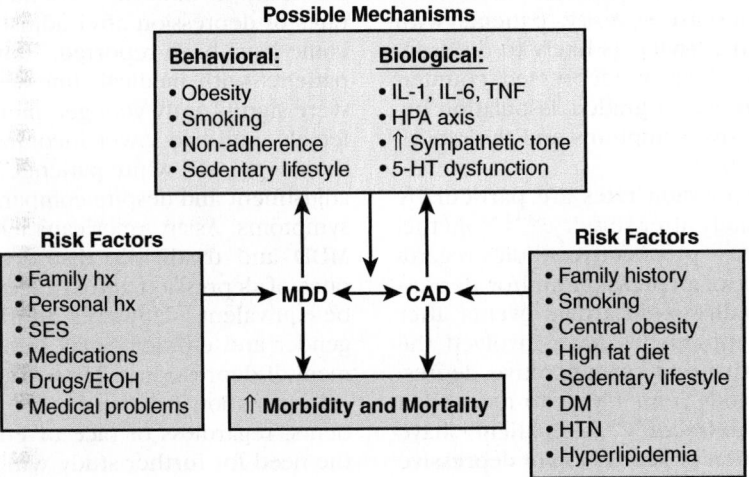

FIGURE 40-2 ■ Biobehavioral pathways linking depression and coronary heart disease.
CAD, Coronary artery disease; *DM,* diabetes mellitus; *ETOH,* alcohol; *5-HT,* 5-hydroxytryptamine (serotonin); *HTN,* hypertension; *hx,* history; *IL,* interleukin; *MDD,* major depressive disorder; *SES,* socioeconomic status.

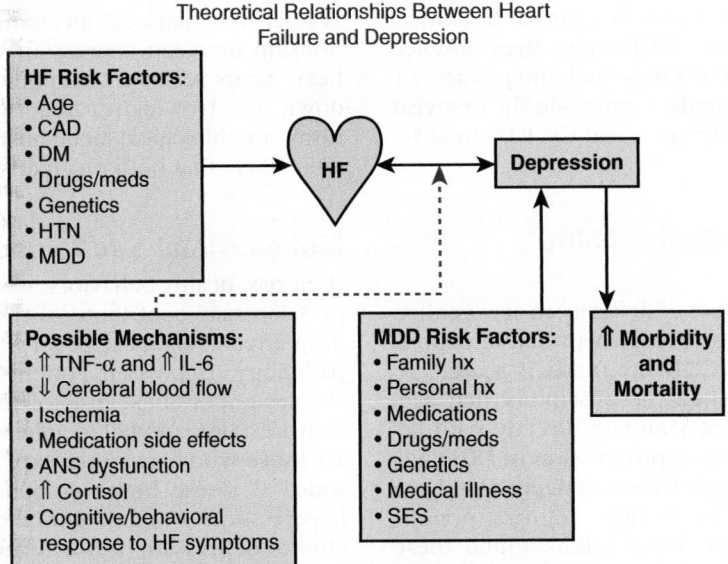

FIGURE 40-3 ■ Biobehavioral pathways linking depression and heart failure.
ANS, Autonomic nervous system; *CAD,* coronary artery disease; *DM,* diabetes mellitus; *HF,* heart failure; *hx,* history; *HTN,* hypertension; *IL,* interleukin; *MDD,* major depressive disorder; *TNF,* tumor necrosis factor.

Hypothalamic-Pituitary-Adrenal Axis Dysfunction

The HPA axis is a neuroendocrine system in which the hypothalamus produces corticotropin-releasing hormone, which stimulates the anterior pituitary gland to produce adrenocorticotropic hormone, signaling the adrenal cortex to release cortisol. Under normal circumstances, a negative feedback loop exists in which cortisol is a strong inhibitor of corticotropin-releasing hormone and adrenocorticotropic hormone.[46] In the presence of MDD, there is a dysfunction in this feedback system, resulting in persistently elevated levels of cortisol (Figure 40-4). Chronic hypercortisolemia, as is commonly seen with MDD, can contribute to the development of insulin resistance, visceral obesity, coagulation changes, increased lipid levels, and hypertension. Each of these changes is known to contribute to the development of CHD.

Autonomic Nervous System Dysfunction

The ANS is part of the peripheral nervous system. The ANS is responsible for the involuntary regulation of numerous organs and systems, including the smooth muscle lining vessel walls and cardiac muscle. ANS dysfunction includes increased sympathetic and/or decreased parasympathetic nervous system (SNS) tone. Measurements of the ANS include heart rate variability (HRV) and norepinephrine, among others.

Evidence suggests that ANS dysfunction plays a role in the relationship between clinical depression and CHD. ANS dysfunction is characteristic of patients with MDD. Specifically, persons with MDD have decreased HRV and altered plasma and urine levels of norepinephrine, signs of increased SNS tone.[47] These alterations in the ANS increase one's risk for ventricular tachycardia, ventricular fibrillation, and sudden cardiac death (SCD). In elderly persons with depressive symptoms compared with those

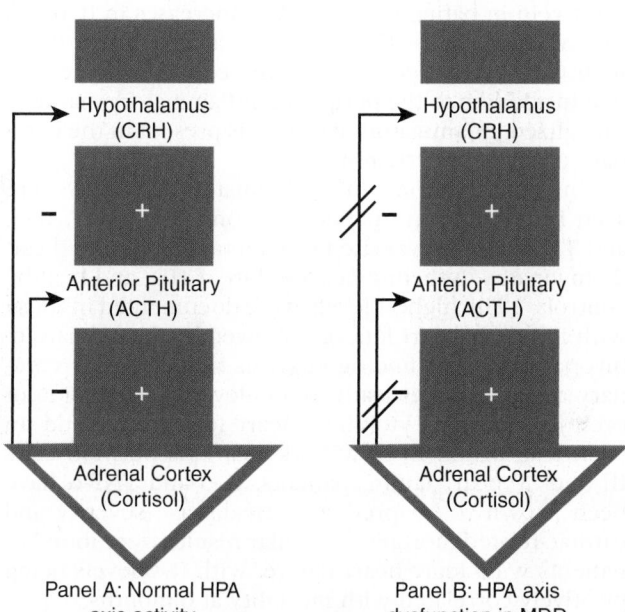

FIGURE 40-4 ■ Hypothalamic-pituitary-adrenal axis (HPA) dysfunction in clinical depression. *ACTH,* Adrenocorticotropic hormone; *CRH,* corticotropin-releasing hormone; *MDD,* major depressive disorder.

without symptoms, one study found an increased incidence of SCD, defined as death within 1 hour of symptom onset.[48] No difference was found in non-SCD between the two groups; this finding suggests that the dysrthymic properties of ANS dysfunction are responsible for increased depression-associated mortality.

In post-MI patients, HRV is to be an independent predictor of mortality. In comparing 380 depressed and 424 nondepressed acute MI patients who had 24-hour ambulatory electrocardiographic monitoring following hospital discharge, researchers found that four indices of HRV were lower (indicating higher sympathetic activity) in the depressed patients.[49] This study again suggests that ANS dysfunction is at least one of the mechanisms linking depression to increased cardiac-related mortality in post-MI patients. Similarly, findings that link decreased HRV to increased mortality are present in the heart failure literature.[50]

Serotonergic System Dysfunction

It is well accepted that levels of 5-HT, a monoamine, are altered in MDD. This observation is supported by the effectiveness of selective serotonin reuptake inhibitors (SSRIs),[51] decreased 5H1AA (a 5-HT metabolite) levels in the cerebral spinal fluid of depressed patients,[52] and in postmortem studies, which have documented higher levels of 5-HT receptors in the brains of suicide victims.[53]

In the periphery, 5-HT is found primarily on platelets. 5-HT has vasoactive properties that contribute to its involvement in thrombogenesis and platelet activation, both of which can contribute to the development of CHD. In a study looking at medically healthy subjects with and without MDD, researchers found that those with MDD had 41 percent greater procoagulant activity at rest and 24 percent increased platelet activity after an orthostatic challenge than controls.[54] In a more recent study, researchers found elevated 5-HT levels in the periphery of depressed post-MI patients compared with those who were not depressed.[55] Serebruany and colleagues[56] used an in vitro design to investigate the effect of the SSRI sertraline on platelet function. Whole blood and plasma from healthy controls and patients with CHD was used. The authors found that therapeutic levels of sertraline had a direct inhibitory effect on human platelets. Thus, the alterations in the serotonergic system seen in MDD may help to explain why MDD is an independent predictor for CHD and for mortality following MI.

Proinflammatory Cytokines

Cytokines are proteins that function as powerful mediators of immune and inflammatory reactions. They are secreted centrally and peripherally by a variety of cells, including monocytes, macrophages, endothelial cells, and glial cells, after coming in contact with antigens and a variety of other molecules.[57] Proinflammatory cytokines (i.e., those are involved in the global reaction to infection or injury called the acute-phase response) provide the most compelling link between clinical depression and cardiac disease.

Once activated, proinflammatory cytokines interact with various aspects of the central nervous system, including the HPA axis, ANS, and serotonergic systems

(Figure 40-5). These interactions are based on a bidirectional communications network between cells of the immune system and the brain, in which the brain indirectly modulates immune activity via the SNS and the HPA axis,[58] and cells of the immune system modulate brain activity directly via vagal fibers[59] and indirectly via neuroendocrine changes.[58] In the simplified model presented in Figure 40-5, depression may be elicited by the effects of internal or external psychological stress on norepinephrine, dopamine, and 5-HT activity in hypothalamic and limbic brain regions.[60] Changes in the brain alter HPA and SNS regulation, which in turn increase circulating cytokines.[58] Proinflammatory cytokines, particularly interleukin-6 (**IL**-6), IL-1β, and tumor necrosis factor-alpha (**TNF**-α), further stimulate the HPA axis and induce hepatic changes that result in production of acute phase proteins, such as C-reactive protein (**CRP**).[61] Alternately, depression may be elicited by systemic or physiological stress, which induces alterations in circulating cytokines.[13,60,62,63] Cytokines signal the brain directly via vagal stimulation and indirectly via HPA activation.[62,64] In the brain, alterations in neurotransmitters, intracerebral cytokines, and prostaglandins induce behavioral changes consistent with depression.[62,65]

Cytokines and Depression

In patients with depressive disorders, elevations in proinflammatory cytokines, as well as other inflammatory parameters, have been documented consistently. Specifically, IL-1β, IL-6, IL-1 receptor antagonist, TNF-α, and more recently CRP were found to be elevated.[60,66]

Cytokines have received recent interest among depression researchers because they are associated with a wide range of behavioral changes in animal and human models. The observation that depression and cytokines are related closely is supported by four main areas of research:

- Animals and human beings injected with IL-1β, TNF-α, or lipopolysaccharide, a bacterial endotoxin, exhibit sickness behavior and symptoms similar to those seen in depression.[65]
- In human beings, depression is one of the main, and often dose-limiting, side effects of immunotherapy using IL-2 and/or interferon-gamma (used to treat various malignancies and viruses).[67] Typically, depressive symptoms begin shortly after immunotherapy is started and resolve when treatment is stopped. The use of antidepressant medication attenuates the depressive symptoms.[68]
- Cytokines induce changes in neuroendocrine and central neurotransmitters similar to those believed to occur in depression. IL-1β has been shown to activate the HPA axis, which is accompanied by stimulation of cerebral noradrenaline and 5-HT metabolism.[69] IL-6 and TNF-α also share HPA-activating ability, although they are less potent than IL-1β.[70]
- Patients with diseases known to increase proinflammatory cytokines have higher rates of MDD. Many noninfectious conditions, such as autoimmune diseases, stroke, trauma, Alzheimer's disease and other neurodegenerative diseases are associated with chronic activation of the immune system and secretion of cytokines. The increase in proinflammatory cytokines precedes development of depression, which suggests a causal link related to immune activation.[63]

Cytokines and Cardiac Disease

Proinflammatory cytokines are known to be elevated in CHD and heart failure. A recent study comparing patients with acute coronary syndrome and documented CHD to healthy controls found elevations in plasma CRP, IL-1 receptor antagonist, and IL-6. IL-6 also is thought to be a marker of severity of myocardial dysfunction in patients with documented CHD.[71] More recently, elevations in inflammatory markers have been documented locally. Specifically, IL-6 and CRP have been measured directly via the left coronary artery and great vein in patients with CHD.[72] Increases in IL-6 and CRP were found in the coronary vasculature of those with CHD compared with healthy controls, suggesting that in addition to the peripheral inflammatory markers, a localized inflammatory pathway is present in the coronary circulatory system itself.

Similar alterations in inflammatory pathways are seen in heart failure patients. In one study CRP, IL-6, and TNF-α were evaluated in patients with dilated cardiomyopathy, ischemic heart failure, CHD, and healthy controls.[73] The highest levels were documented in those with ischemic heart failure, followed by dilated cardiomyopathy. Such a finding suggests that although coronary atherosclerosis leads to an elevated expression of proinflammatory cytokines, heart failure may add an additional insult. In New York Heart Association class III and IV heart failure patients, IL-6 and TNF-α have been shown to be predictors of disease severity and cardiac-related mortality.[74] Similar results were found in patients with acute heart failure, with IL-6 levels being positively correlated with mortality at 6 months.[75]

The elevated levels of CRP, IL-1β, IL-6, and TNF-α that are seen in clinical depression could be responsible for the future development of cardiac disease. Findings from

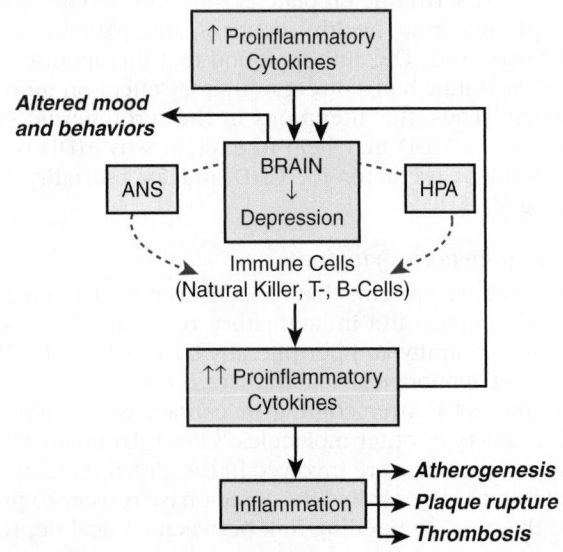

FIGURE 40-5 ■ Simplified model of brain-immune interactions in depression. *ANS,* Autonomic nervous system; *HPA,* hypothalamic-pituitary adrenal.

research investigating this hypothesis have supported such theories. Elevated levels of IL-6 in 14,916 otherwise healthy men were found to be a predictor of MI during the 6-year follow-up period.[76] These findings were replicated in postmenopausal women, in whom researchers noted that elevated levels of CRP and IL-6 were independent predictors of future vascular events.[77]

Likewise, the elevation in proinflammatory cytokines seen in CHD and heart failure may explain the increased incidence of clinical depression in these populations. In heart failure patients, TNF-α is related significantly to depressive symptoms.[78,79] Additionally, in patients with CHD 2 months after acute coronary syndrome, the diagnosis of MDD was related to increased levels of CRP, when controlling for the use of statins,[80] and patients undergoing coronary angioplasty who were depressed had higher levels of IL-1β and TNF-α than those who were not depressed/exhausted.[81]

The precise cause linking clinical depression and cardiac disease has yet to be deciphered and is likely to be multifactorial, including behavioral and biological mechanisms. Behaviors associated with clinical depression increase the risk for cardiac disease to develop and progress, and there are many shared biological underpinnings in depression and cardiac disease. Proinflammatory cytokines, and their subsequent actions in the periphery and the central nervous system, provide the most compelling link to date and are worthy of further investigation.

MANAGEMENT OF DEPRESSION
Screening for Depression

Because most depressed patients seek care first in primary care settings, the effects of screening for depression by primary care providers have been tested frequently. Although some early studies found that screening for depression did not improve patient outcomes,[82] researchers using meta-analytical techniques have concluded recently that screening for depression by primary care providers improves case finding by 10 to 47 percent.[83] When the focus of study moves from case finding to evaluation of patients outcomes, screening appears to have differential effects. Screening is most successful in settings that have integrated programs with feedback to providers, including treatment recommendations and/or access to case management or mental health care.[84] Although studies that provide feedback to providers regarding only the results of depression screening showed modest improvement in depression treatment, the few clinical trials that have combined integrated recognition and management programs with screening showed much larger treatment benefits.[83] To date, no studies have addressed the effects of screening for depression on case finding or treatment outcomes in specific populations of cardiac patients.

Despite the lack of research in this area, screening for depression in the cardiac population deserves more attention and should involve nurses with expertise in cardiology. For such a screening to be effective, nurses need adequate training in this area, particularly regarding the signs and symptoms of depression. Ideally, this training should take place during the formal training in academic programs and through continuing education.

An efficient way to screen for the presence of depression includes the use of well-known instruments. Many screening instruments are available for use in primary care and other outpatient settings (Table 40-3). Most instruments have relatively good sensitivity (i.e., the proportion of true positives), from 80 to 90 percent, but only fair specificity (i.e., the proportion of true negatives), from 70 to 85 percent.[85]

Recent studies suggest that asking two simple questions about the presence and duration of mood and anhedonia may be as effective as using longer instruments.[86] The questions can be as simple as "How would you say your mood has been?" and "Have you lost interest in doing things that you normally enjoy doing?" According to the U.S. Preventive Services Task Force, about 24 to 40 percent of patients who screen positive with these questions will have MDD. Some patients with false-positive results on screening may have dysthymia or subsyndromal depression that may benefit from treatment or closer monitoring; others may have other comorbid mood disorders or psychiatric problems, such as anxiety disorder, substance abuse, panic disorder, posttraumatic stress disorder, or grief reactions. A portion may have no mental health problems.[84]

All positive screening tests should trigger full diagnostic interviews that use standard diagnostic criteria consistent with current DSM-IV standards. In addition, clinicians should evaluate the patient for comorbid psychological problems and for other risk factors for depression (e.g., female sex, family history, chronic medical illness, and current life stress). Before a diagnosis of MDD, depression caused by a general medical condition, adjustment disorders, and grief should be ruled out. (See the accompanying Evidence-Based Practice feature).

■ EVIDENCE-BASED PRACTICE

SCREENING FOR DEPRESSION

Compared with usual care, screening for depression:
- Improves detection and diagnosis of depression
- May improve the proportion of patients receiving effective treatment, although study results are mixed
- Is likely to be more effective in improving patient outcomes if it is linked to treatment protocols and access to mental health resources

Screening instruments:
- Generally have good sensitivity (80 to 90 percent) but only fair specificity (70 to 85 percent)
- May not be better at detecting depressed patients than simply asking questions about depressed mood and anhedonia
  Sample screening questions include the following:
- "In the past two weeks, have you felt depressed or sad most of the time?"
- "In the past two weeks, have you lost interest or pleasure most of the time in doing things that you used to enjoy?"

Maintain a high index of suspicion in persons with the following:
- Family or personal history of depression or suicide attempts
- Recent stressful life events and lack of social supports
- Chronic illnesses, chronic pain, or unexplained somatic complaints
- Current alcohol or substance abuse

General Treatment Considerations

Many persons with syndromal depressive disorders experience a chronic, relapsing course even with treatment. For MDD, 20 to 30 percent of individuals suffer relapse or recurrence. Among those being treated for the first time, approximately 50 percent have a reduction in symptoms but continue to have more than minimal symptoms. Of those, only another 50 percent progress to complete remission—no longer meeting syndromal criteria with no or minimal symptoms. Given the nature of most depressive disorders, treatment is aimed at achieving remission, which is associated with the best functional status and prognosis, and preventing relapse.[87]

Treatment of depression is based on the diagnosis and the severity of symptoms and should be individualized according to history, past response, and comorbidities. One of the most important considerations in the selection of treatment is the patient's preference. Social and cultural biases may influence what treatment alternatives are acceptable to individual patients. Because the most common cause of treatment failure is nonadherence by patients, clinicians must ensure that the treatment they offer is acceptable to the patient.

In general, three types of therapies have proven efficacy for depressive disorders: pharmacotherapy, psychotherapy, and electroconvulsive therapy (**ECT**).[88] ECT is reserved for the most severe, retractable forms of MDD, including those involving psychosis. Modern ECT includes brief-pulse electrical stimulation, anesthesia, oxygenation, and continuous physiological monitoring. In selected cases, reported symptomatic response rates (up to 75 percent) and remission rates after 6 weeks of therapy (34 percent) have been higher than or similar to those reported for pharmacotherapy in less severe cases.[89] These findings are impressive, for ECT patients are typically refractory to standard depression treatment. Thus despite the stigma associated with ECT, it continues to be useful for treating severe, resistant depression. On the basis of these encouraging findings, researchers believe that ECT should be considered earlier in treatment protocols for MDD. The use of ECT in the future may be influenced by the development of newer technologies. (See the accompanying Technology feature).

Principles of Pharmacotherapy

Pharmacotherapy is the treatment of choice for severe MDD. SSRIs are now the mainstay of pharmacotherapy. Despite comparable efficacy with other classes of antidepressants such has tricyclic antidepressants (**TCAs**) and monoamine oxidase inhibitors (**MAO**), SSRIs have a more benign side effect profile and are believed to be better tolerated.[88] In clinical trials, discontinuation rates were lower with SSRIs than with TCAs.[90] Additionally, SSRIs are thought to be a safe choice for patients with CHD.[91] In general, there is no consensus on guidelines for the selection of specific antidepressants for first-line treatment in primary care. The characteristics of the most common antidepressants are shown in an accompanying

---

■ ■ ■ TECHNOLOGY

NOVEL TREATMENTS FOR DEPRESSION

Vagal Nerve Stimulation
- Developed after successful use in treatment-resistant epileptics
- Analogous to pacemaker technology, with electrode placement in the neck and generator pack placed in the chest
- Impulses delivered for 30 seconds every 5 minutes around the clock
- Thought to affect locus coreleus and limbic system
- No serious side effects
- Efficacy not yet established:
  - Only open-label pilot studies available
  - Placebo effect could be a factor
  - Approved for treatment in European Union countries

Repetitive Transcranial Magnetic Stimulation
- Not invasive
- Magnetic pulses are delivered directly to the scalp via hand-held stimulating coil
- Depolarizes neurons via magnetic pulses that pass unimpeded through the skull and induce an electrical current in the underlying tissue
- Aimed at the dorsolateral prefrontal cortex
- Can be delivered relatively painlessly to conscious patients without sedation
- Uncertainty exists regarding the following:
  - Therapeutic delivery (frequency, intensity, duration of pulses, and days of treatment)
  - Efficacy compared with sham procedures

Pharmacology feature. Suggested protocols for antidepressant management usually include at least two separate trials of antidepressant monotherapy, followed by repeated trials of combination therapy and ECT if these steps fail to provide adequate symptom relief.[92] A typical approach for pharmacological management is summarized in Figure 40-6. In general, once symptomatic response is achieved, therapy should continue for at least 12 months, with regular assessment of symptoms.[93]

No specific protocols have been reported for cardiac patients. However, recommendations for geriatric patients are probably the most applicable to cardiac patients. It should be noted that TCAs can cause orthostatic hypotension and dysrhythmias. In general, TCAs should be avoided in those with a history of dysrhythmia or ischemic heart disease and should be used with caution in the elderly and all cardiac patients.[91] Additionally, monoamine oxidase inhibitors have a relatively high side effect profile and are prescribed judiciously, typically by a psychiatrist. Recommendations for antidepressant use in cardiac patients are summarized in an accompanying Pharmacology feature.

Psychotherapy

Psychotherapy or combination therapy with antidepressants and psychotherapy is appropriate for mild to moderate MDD.[94] The forms of psychotherapy that have been evaluated most often are cognitive-behavioral therapy (**CBT**) and interpersonal therapy (**IPT**). For mild to moderate MDD, psychotherapy, particularly CBT, is as effective as antidepressants in achieving symptom response and remission.[95] Some studies show that psychotherapy is associated with more enduring effects on quality of life and on relapse prevention than

■■■ PHARMACOLOGY

CHARACTERISTICS OF COMMON ANTIDEPRESSANTS BY CLASS

DRUG EXAMPLES	CHARACTERISTICS	SIDE EFFECTS
Monoamine Oxidase (MAO) Inhibitors		
phenelzine (Nardil) tranylcypromine (Parnate)	Nonselective inhibition of monoamine oxidase prevents catabolism of serotonin and norepinephrine	Hypotension, drug and food interactions, malignant hypertension, multiple medication interactions
Tricyclic Antidepressants		
amitriptyline (Elavil) imipramine (Tofranil)	Inhibit presynaptic uptake of serotonin and norepinephrine; lethal in overdose	Dizziness, drowsiness, dry mouth, constipation, headache, orthostatic hypotension
Selective Serotonin Reuptake Inhibitors		
citalopram (Celexa) fluoxetine (Prozac) paroxetine (Paxil) sertaline (Zoloft)	Selective pharmacological effects ending in inhibition of serotonin reuptake at synaptic cleft	Nausea, diarrhea, headache, serotonin syndrome, sexual dysfunction, weight gain, withdrawal syndrome
Serotonin-Norephinephrine Reuptake Inhibitors		
venlafaxine (Effexor)	Dual serotonin and norepinephrine uptake inhibition	Blurred vision, headache, sexual dysfunction
Atypical Antidepressants		
bupropion (Wellbutrin)	Imprecise norepinephrine and dopamine reuptake actions	Agitation, anxiety
mirtazapine (Remeron)	Multiple neurotransmitter effects	Constipation, dizziness, drowsiness, dry mouth, weight gain

■■■ PHARMACOLOGY

RECOMMENDATIONS FOR ANTIDEPRESSANT USE IN CARDIAC PATIENTS

RECOMMENDATION	RATIONALE
Start treatment with citalopram.	Citalopram has limited drug-drug interactions. It is not associated with discontinuation syndrome. It causes limited central nervous system activation. It has the least cytochrome P450 interaction of similar selective serotonin reuptake inhibitors.
Establish target dose based on patient's age; modify as needed based on individual patient characteristics.	Recommended doses for geriatric patients may be appropriate for patients with multiple medical comorbidities.
Adjust up to the target dose over the first week of therapy.	Initial adjustment allows careful evaluation of adverse reactions.
Consider switching to another antidepressant or augmenting therapy with a second antidepressant only after 12 weeks of treatment.	Older patients and those with comorbidity experience a slower reduction of their symptoms than younger patients. Shorter trials of treatment are associated with higher nonresponse rates.
Educate patients about antidepressant therapy:	
Onset of symptom relief	Usually it takes 2 to 6 weeks for symptoms to improve.
Likely duration of treatment	For first episodes, treatment usually lasts 6 to 12 months, even if remission occurs earlier. For patients with suicide attempts or prior episodes, treatment may be longer.
Need to report side effects promptly	Most side effects can be managed effectively.
Need to avoid abrupt cessation of treatment	Abrupt cessation can lead to serious side effects. In all cases, patients should be encouraged to speak with their care providers.

antidepressants.[94] For severe MDD, the combination of SSRIs and psychotherapy provide the best outcomes, including reduced symptom severity, quicker remission, and better recovery.[96]

Cognitive-Behavioral Therapy

CBT, pioneered by Beck in the 1960s, is a present-oriented, problem-focused approach that has been tested extensively in group and individual formats.[97] Based on collaboration between patient and therapist, CBT is focused on examining the way in which one construes current situations and events, attitudes toward self and others, and skills and activities by which one interacts with the world. The aim of CBT is to reframe dysfunctional cognitions or thoughts by helping patients recognize them and consider alternative, more balanced interpretations of their interactions with others. A key process of CBT is the discovery and analysis of the thought processes used in relevant situations, elicited in the context of self-monitoring, guided discovery, Socratic questioning, and role playing.[98] Treatment, which usually lasts 8 to 12 weeks, has been standard-

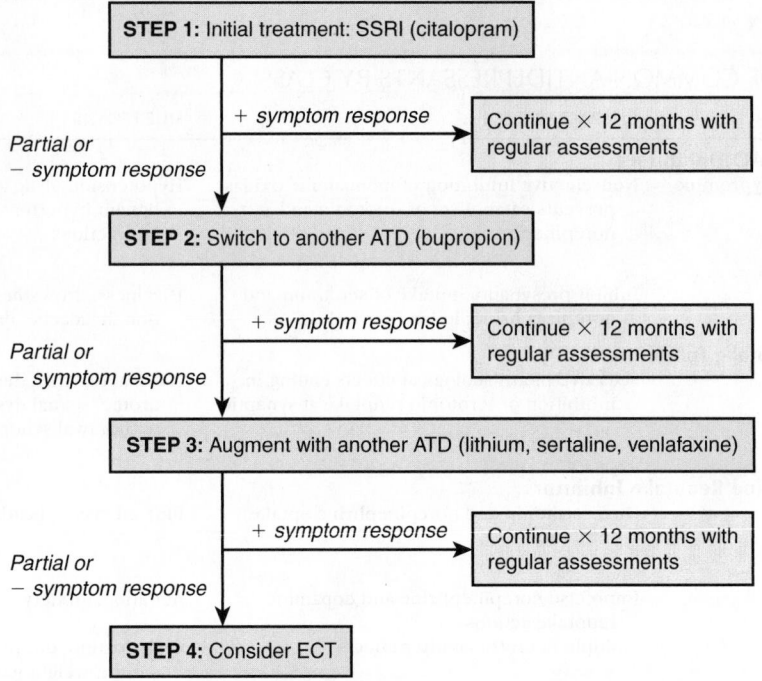

FIGURE 40-6 ■ Sample algorithm for pharmacological treatment of depression in cardiac patients. *ATD,* Atypical antidepressant; *ECT,* electroconvulsive therapy; *SSRI,* selective serotonin reuptake inhibitor.

ized and includes socialization to the therapy, weekly mood checks, joint agenda setting, analysis of dysfunctional thoughts, problem solving, mutual goal setting, homework assignments, and feedback (Table 40-4).[99]

Regarding the treatment of depressive symptoms, CBT is supported best by clinical evidence comparing it with other forms of psychotherapy. However, the largest and most rigorously designed trials of psychotherapy for depression have been conducted in psychiatric patients without medical comorbidities. In the National Institute of Mental Health Treatment of Depression Collaborative Research Program, CBT was more effective than placebo plus clinical management and nearly as effective as imipramine in reducing mild to moderate depression.[100] Compared with psychiatric patients receiving pharmacotherapy, patients who received CBT experienced lower rates of depression relapse up to 1 year after treatment.[101] In addition, CBT combined with antidepressants achieves greater symptom reduction than either therapy alone, especially in the elderly.[102] Only one study has tested CBT in cardiac patients. In the ENRICHD study, which involved post-MI patients with clinical depression or low social support, CBT reduced depressive symptoms and improved psychosocial outcomes compared with usual care.[103]

CBT is especially promising as a nursing intervention because it is well matched to the typical psychosocial problems commonly observed in cardiac patients. For example, typical themes during CBT in cardiac patients include desensitizing of health-related fears, such as return to work or resumption of sexual activity; making typical posthospitalization phenomena less catastrophic,

such as fatigue and memory loss; and redefining problems to focus on aspects of recovery, such as diet and activity that can be controlled. In addition, CBT is a relatively brief, goal-oriented, interactive, and emotionally supportive form of treatment that is compatible with other nursing interventions and generally well accepted by cardiac patients.[104]

Interpersonal Therapy

IPT, developed in the 1980s by Klerman and Weisman, is a brief and highly structured manual-based psychotherapy that addresses interpersonal issues in depression. In IPT, depression is viewed as having three components: symptom formation, social functioning, and personality contributors. IPT is based on the assumption that depression occurs in a social and interpersonal context and that the course of the disease, as well as the outcome of treatment, is based on the interpersonal relations between the depressed individual and significant others. The goals of IPT are to reduce psychological symptoms, restore morale, improve self-esteem, and improve the quality of psychosocial adjustment and interpersonal relations.[105] Usually therapy is limited to 12 weekly sessions divided into three phases of treatment, which are outlined in Table 40-5. Treatment centers on four common problem areas: grief, interpersonal role disputes, role transition, and interpersonal deficits.[106] Key to treatment is the building of a positive therapeutic relationship, which serves as a testing ground to evaluate everyday communication skills and behavior and as a model relationship to emulate.[107]

■ ■ ■

TABLE 40-4 TYPICAL WEEKLY SCHEDULE FOR COGNITIVE-BEHAVIORAL THERAPY

WEEK	AGENDA
1	*Focus: Establishment of therapeutic relationship* Establish rapport. Discuss patient expectations about therapy and recovery. Check mood. Socialize patient to therapy. Describe cognitive model of depression and explain strategies, with emphasis on rationale for behavioral assignments and homework. Provide summary and elicit feedback from patient.
2	*Focus: Behavioral activation and active problem solving* Check mood. Inquire about effects of first session. Discuss problems and accomplishments since previous session. Schedule activities for next session and focus on problems to be discussed. Inquire about reaction to this session. Administer Automatic Thoughts Questionnaire and Dysfunctional Attitudes Scale.
3	*Focus: Automatic thoughts* Prepare agenda. Inquire about effects of second session. Review homework assignments. Instruct patient in identifying negative automatic thoughts. Elicit automatic thoughts, specifically in relation to homework assignments. Prepare homework assignments, and elicit feedback about today's session.
4-6	*Focus: Automatic thoughts and self-therapy* Follow same format as above. Continue to identify negative automatic thoughts. Continue to work on rational responses to automatic thoughts. Give additional homework assignments. Discuss concept of basic assumptions.
7-8	*Focus: Automatic thoughts, self-therapy, and relapse prevention* Prepare patient for termination of therapy. Emphasize need to continue practicing strategies after termination. Delineate anticipated problems, and rehearse coping strategies. Introduce and practice self-therapy techniques. Provide closure and elicit feedback from patient. Administer Automatic Thoughts Questionnaire and Dysfunctional Attitudes Scale (week 8).

■ ■ ■

TABLE 40-5 PHASES OF INTERPERSONAL THERAPY

PHASE	ACTIVITIES
Early phase (Weeks 1-3)	Diagnostic assessment of patient's social relationships and interpersonal functioning Identification of acute life crises, e.g., recent loss, interpersonal conflict, and life transition Psychoeducation about depression with the message, "It's not your fault." Examination and prioritization of problem focus areas: • Grief or loss • Interpersonal or role disputes • Role transitions • Interpersonal deficits
Middle phase (Weeks 4-9)	Solving specific interpersonal problems based on results of early phase analysis with application of focus-specific strategies and goals Sample goals • Grief or loss: Facilitate mourning • Role disputes: Identify dispute, choose action plan, and reassess expectations and communication • Role transitions: Accept loss of old role, restore self-esteem, and establish positive approach to new role • Interpersonal deficits: Review past relationships, role play social situations, and identify correctable communication deficits
Termination phase (Weeks 10-12)	Consolidate treatment gains Foster sense of independence and competence Develop relapse prevention skills

IPT has been tested in multiple clinical trials. Its efficacy has proved to be superior to placebo, similar to antidepressants, and comparable to CBT.[108] In a recent pilot study, IPT was tested in patients with CHD. More than 50 percent of patients experienced a therapeutic (50 percent) reduction in symptoms and/or met criteria for remission after 12 weeks of therapy.[109] The findings of this "open-label" study, in which some patients received antidepressants in addition to IPT, suggest that this kind of therapy may be beneficial, alone or as an adjunct to antidepressants, in depressed patients with CHD. Further testing of IPT and CBT in cardiac patients as an alternative or an adjunct to pharmacotherapy is warranted.

TREATING DEPRESSION IN CARDIAC PATIENTS

To date, there are no systematic assessment or treatment guidelines aimed specifically at depression in cardiac patients. Aside from the obvious need to consider cardiac effects of antidepressants, experts have provided little guidance regarding this high-risk population. Reasonable principles applicable to cardiac patients are summarized in Table 40-6.

SUMMARY

Depression is a common finding among patients with cardiac disease. In addition to the deleterious effect depression can have on quality of life, depression is an independent risk factor for increased morbidity and mortality in those with CHD. For most cardiac patients, depression is a treatable condition. Thus, all clinicians should screen patients with CHD regularly for symptoms of depression and should refer patients as appropriate for further evaluation and treatment. To this end, cardiac nurses must be trained properly in screening, diagnosing, and managing depression in this population.

■ ■ ■

TABLE 40-6   GENERAL PRINCIPLES FOR DEPRESSION CARE IN CARDIAC PATIENTS

PRINCIPLE	RATIONALE
Maintain a high index of suspicion for depression in cardiac patients.	Syndromal and subsyndromal depression are common in cardiac patients. Depression is not a normal part of aging; it is common in the elderly, who constitute a large segment of the cardiac patient population. Men, who make up at least two-thirds of the cardiac population, are more likely to discount or hide depressive symptoms than women, so it is easier to overlook or miss depression in men.
Routine screening for depression is appropriate in primary care settings that serve cardiac patients and in specialty cardiac settings.	Screening improves case-finding. It may improve patient outcomes if appropriate resources are available.
Base treatment on preferences of the patient and mutual agreement between patient and clinician.	Nonadherence is the main reason for failure to reach symptom response in depression treatment.
Do not hesitate to discuss suicidal thoughts.	Patients rarely volunteer suicidal thoughts. No evidence indicates that asking about suicide precipitates suicidal thinking. Risk factors for suicide include hopelessness, substance abuse, and prior attempts.
Whenever appropriate and reasonable, combine pharmacotherapy and psychotherapy.	Combination therapy is associated with greater functional improvements and longer remission.

Refer for psychiatric assessment and/or management as needed.	Refer if the patient has the following:
	    Complex, unclear presentation
	    Suicidal thoughts
	    Psychotic depression or depression with dementia or severe anxiety
	    Bipolar disorder
	    Known substance abuse
	    Poor response, no response, or inability to tolerate first-line therapy.

REFERENCES

1. Kessler RC, Berglund P, Demler O et al: The epidemiology of major depressive disorder: results from the national comorbidity survey replication (NCS-R), *JAMA* 289:3095-3105, 2003.
2. Greenberg P, Kessler R, Birnbaum H et al: The economic burden of depression in the United States: how did it change between 1990 and 2000? *J Clin Psychiatry* 64:1465-1475, 2003.
3. Rudisch B, Nemeroff CB: Epidemiology of comorbid coronary artery disease and depression. *Biol Psychiatry* 54:227-240, 2003.
4. *The numbers count: mental disorders in America 555*, Bethesda, Md, 2001, National Institute of Mental Health.
5. Schleifer S, Macari-Hinson M, Coyle D et al: The nature and course of depression following myocardial infarction, *Arch Intern Med* 149:1785-1789, 1989.
6. McCrone S, Lenz E, Tarzian A, Perkins S: Anxiety and depression: incidence and patterns in patients after coronary artery bypass graft surgery, *Appl Nurs Res* 14:155-164, 2001.
7. Blumenthal JA, Lett HS, Babyak MA et al: Depression as a risk factor for mortality after coronary artery bypass surgery, *Lancet* 362:604-609, 2003.
8. American Heart Association: *Heart disease and stroke statistics: 2005 update*, Dallas, 2005, The Association.
9. Jiang W, Alexander J, Christopher E et al: Relationship of depression to increased risk of mortality and rehospitalization in patients with congestive heart failure, *Arch Intern Med* 161:1849-1856, 2001.
10. Wolf OT, Convit A, de Leon MJ et al: Basal hypothalamo-pituitary-adrenal axis activity and corticotropin feedback in young and older men: relationships to magnetic resonance imaging-derived hippocampus and cingulate gyrus volumes, *Neuroendocrinology* 75:241-249, 2002.
11. Havranek EP, Spertus JA, Masoudi FA et al: Predictors of the onset of depressive symptoms in patients with heart failure, *J Am Coll Cardiol* 44:2333-2338, 2004.
12. Dew MA, Kormos RL, DiMartini AF et al: Prevalence and risk of depression and anxiety-related disorders during the first three years after heart transplantation, *Psychosomatics* 42:300-313, 2001.
13. American Psychiatric Association: *Diagnostic and statistical manual of mental disorders*, ed 4, Washington, DC, 2000, The Association.
14. Freedland KE, Skala JA, Carney RM et al: The depression interview and structured hamilton (DISH): rationale, development, characteristics, and clinical validity, *Psychosom Med* 64:897-905, 2002.
15. Katon W, Sullivan MD: Depression and chronic medical illness, *J Clin Psychiatry* 51(suppl):3-11, 1990.
16. Castelli WP: Lipids, risk factors and ischaemic heart disease, *Atherosclerosis* 124:S1-S9, 1996.
17. Rugulies R: Depression as a predictor for coronary heart disease: a review and meta-analysis, *Am J Prev Med* 23:51-61, 2002.
18. Vogt T, Pope C, Mullooly J et al: Mental health status as a predictor of morbidity and mortality: a 15-year follow-up of members of a health maintenance organization, *Am J Public Health* 84:227-331, 1994.
19. Mendes de Leon CF, Krumholz HM, Seeman TS et al: Depression and risk of coronary heart disease in elderly men and women: New Haven EPESE, 1982-1991, *Arch Intern Med* 158:2341-2348, 1998.
20. Hippisley-Cox J, Fielding K, Pringle M: Depression as a risk factor for ischaemic heart disease in men: population based case-control study, *BMJ* 316:1714-1719, 1998.
21. Wulsin LR, Singal BM: Do depressive symptoms increase the risk for the onset of coronary disease? a systematic quantitative review, *Psychosom Med* 65:201-210, 2003.
22. Williams SA, Kasl SV, Heiat A et al: Depression and risk of heart failure among the elderly: a prospective community-based study, *Psychosom Med* 64:6-12, 2002.
23. Lesperance F, Frasure-Smith N, Talajic M, Bourassa MG: Five-year risk of cardiac mortality in relation to initial severity and one-year changes in depression symptoms after myocardial infarction, *Circulation* 105:1049-1053, 2002.
24. Bush DE, Ziegelstein RC, Tayback M et al: Even minimal symptoms of depression increase mortality risk after acute myocardial infarction, *Am J Cardiol* 88:337-341, 2001.
25. Frasure-Smith N, Lesperance F, Talajic M: Depression following myocardial infarction: impact on 6-month survival, *JAMA* 270:1819-1825, 1993.
26. Lett HS, Blumenthal JA, Babyak MA et al: Depression as a risk factor for coronary artery disease: evidence, mechanisms, and treatment, *Psychosom Med* 66:305-315, 2004.
27. Barth J, Schumacher M, Herrmann-Lingen C: Depression as a risk factor for mortality in patients with coronary heart disease: a meta-analysis, *Psychosom Med* 66:802-813, 2004.

28. van Melle JP, de Jonge P, Spijkerman TA et al: Prognostic association of depression following myocardial infarction with mortality and cardiovascular events: a meta-analysis, *Psychosom Med* 66:814-822, 2004.

29. Lane D, Carroll D, Ring C et al: In-hospital symptoms of depression do not predict mortality 3 years after myocardial infarction, *Int J Epidemiol* 31:1179-1182, 2002.

30. de Denus S, Spinler S, Jessup M, Kao A: History of depression as a predictor of adverse outcomes in patients hospitalized for decompensated heart failure, *Pharmacotherapy* 24:1306-1310, 2004.

31. Sullivan MD, Levy WC, Crane BA et al: Usefulness of depression to predict time to combined end point of transplant or death for outpatients with advanced heart failure, *Am J Cardiol* 94:1577-1580, 2004.

32. Vaccarino V, Kasl SV, Abramson J, Krumholz HM: Depressive symptoms and risk of functional decline and death in patients with heart failure, *J Am Coll Cardiol* 38:199-205, 2001.

33. Baker RA, Andrew MJ, Schrader G et al: Preoperative depression and mortality in coronary artery bypass surgery: preliminary findings, *Aust N Z J Surg* 71:139-142, 2001.

34. Saur C, Granger B, Mulbaier L et al: Depressive symptoms and outcome of coronary artery bypass grafting, *Am J Crit Care* 10:4-10, 2001.

35. Connerney I, Shapiro PA, McLaughlin JS et al: Relation between depression after coronary artery bypass surgery and 12-month outcome: a prospective study, *Lancet* 358:1766-1771, 2001.

36. Gottlieb SS, Khatta M, Friedmann E et al: The influence of age, gender, and race on the prevalence of depression in heart failure patients, *J Am Coll Cardiol* 43:1542-1549, 2004.

37. Mendes de Leon C, Dilillo V, Czajkowski S et al: Psychosocial characteristics after acute myocardial infarction: the ENRICHD pilot study (Enhancing Recovery in Coronary Heart Disease), *J Cardiopulm Rehabil* 21:353-362, 2001.

38. Plant E, Sachs-Ericsson N: Racial and ethnic differences in depression: the roles of social support and meeting basic needs, *J Consult Clin Psychol* 72:41-52, 2004.

39. Jackson-Triche ME, Greer Sullivan J, Wells KB et al: Depression and health-related quality of life in ethnic minorities seeking care in general medical settings, *J Affect Disord* 58:89-97, 2000.

40. Schneiderman N, Saab PG, Catellier DJ et al: Psychosocial treatment within sex by ethnicity subgroups in the Enhancing Recovery in Coronary Heart Disease clinical trial, *Psychosom Med* 66:475-483, 2004.

41. Ciechanowski PS, Katon WJ, Russo JE: Depression and diabetes: impact of depressive symptoms on adherence, function, and costs, *Arch Intern Med* 160:3278-3285, 2000.

42. Spijker J, de Graaf R, Bijl RV et al: Determinants of persistence of major depressive episodes in the general population: results from the Netherlands Mental Health Survey and Incidence Study (NEMESIS), *J Affect Disord* 81:231-240, 2004.

43. Dickens CM, McGowan L, Percival C et al: Lack of a close confidant, but not depression, predicts further cardiac events after myocardial infarction, *Heart* 90:518-522, 2004.

44. Murberg TA: Long-term effect of social relationships on mortality in patients with congestive heart failure, *Int J Psychiatry Med* 34:207-217, 2004.

45. Lin EHB, Katon W, Von Korff M et al: Relationship of depression and diabetes self-care, medication adherence, and preventive care, *Diabetes Care* 27:2154-2160, 2004.

46. de Kloet ER, Vreugdenhil E, Oitzl MS et al: Brain corticosteroid receptor balance in health and disease, *Endocr Rev* 19:269-301, 1998.

47. Yeragani VK, Rao KAR, Smitha MR et al: Diminished chaos of heart rate time series in patients with major depression, *Biol Psychiatry* 51:733-744, 2002.

48. Luukinen H, Laippala P, Huikuri HV: Depressive symptoms and the risk of sudden cardiac death among the elderly, *Eur Heart J* 24:2021-2026.

49. Carney RM, Blumenthal JA, Stein PK et al: Depression, heart rate variability, and acute myocardial infarction, *Circulation* 104:2024-2028, 2001.

50. Hadase M, Azuma A, Zen K et al: Very low frequency power of heart rate variability is a powerful predictor of clinical prognosis in patients with congestive heart failure, *Circ J* 68:343-347, 2004.

51. Steffens DC, Krishnan KR, Helms MJ: Are SSRIs better than TCAs? comparison of SSRIs and TCAs: a meta-analysis, *Depress Anxiety* 6:10-18, 1997.

52. John Mann J, Malone KM: Cerebrospinal fluid amines and higher-lethality suicide attempts in depressed inpatients, *Biol Psychiatry* 41:162-171, 1997.

53. Escriba PV, Ozaita A, Garcia-Sevilla JA: Increased mRNA expression of alpha$_{2A}$-adrenoceptors, serotonin receptors and *mu*-opioid receptors in the brains of suicide victims, *Neuropsychopharmacology* 29:1512-1521, 2004.

54. Musselman DL, Tomer A, Manatunga AK et al: Exaggerated platelet reactivity in major depression, *Am J Psychiatry* 153:1313-1317, 1996.

55. Schins A, Hamulyak K, Scharpe S et al: Whole blood serotonin and platelet activation in depressed post-myocardial infarction patients, *Life Sci* 76:637-650, 2004.

56. Serebruany VL, O'Connor CM, Gurbel PA: Effect of selective serotonin reuptake inhibitors on platelets in patients with coronary artery disease, *Am J Cardiol* 87:1398-1400, 2001.

57. Janeway C, Travers P, Walport P, Schlomshik M: *Immunobiology: the immune system in health and disease*, ed 5, New York, 2001, Garland Publishing.

58. Maier SF, Watkins LR: Cytokines for psychologists: implications of bidirectional immune-to-brain communication for understanding behavior, mood, and cognition, *Psychol Rev* 105:83-107, 1998.

59. Maier SF, Goehler LE, Fleshner M et al: The role of the vagus nerve in cytokine-to-brain communication, *Ann N Y Acad Sci* 840:289-300, 1998.

60. Anisman H, Merali Z: Cytokines, stress, and depressive illness, *Brain Behav Immun* 16:513-524, 2002.

61. Connor TJ, Leonard BE: Depression, stress and immunological activation: the role of cytokines in depressive disorders, *Life Sci* 62:583-606, 1998.

62. Maier SF: Bi-directional immune-brain communication: implications for understanding stress, pain, and cognition, *Brain Behav Immun* 17:69-85, 2003.

63. Yirmiya R, Pollak Y, Morag M et al: Illness, cytokines, and depression, *Ann N Y Acad Sci* 917:478-487, 2000.

64. Anisman H, Merali Z: Cytokines, stress and depressive illness: brain-immune interactions, *Ann Med* 35:2-11, 2003.

65. Dantzer R: Cytokine-induced sickness behavior: where do we stand? *Brain Behav Immun* 15:7-24, 2001.

66. Danner M, Kasl SV, Abramson JL et al: Association between depression and elevated C-reactive protein, *Psychosom Med* 65:347-356, 2003.

67. Bonaccorso S, Marino V, Biondi M et al: Depression induced by treatment with interferon-alpha in patients affected by hepatitis C virus, *J Affect Disord* 72:237-241, 2002.

68. Capuron L, Neurauter G, Musselman DL et al: Interferon-alpha-induced changes in tryptophan metabolism: relationship to depression and paroxetine treatment, *Biol Psychiatry* 54:906-914, 2003.

69. Dunn AJ, Wang J, Ando T: Effects of cytokines on cerebral neurotransmission: comparison with the effects of stress, *Adv Exp Med Biol* 461:117-127, 1999.

70. Dunn AJ: Cytokine activation of the HPA axis, *Ann N Y Acad Sci* 917:608-617, 2000.

71. Nijm J, Wikby A, Tompa A et al: Circulating levels of proinflammatory cytokines and neutrophil-platelet aggregates in patients with coronary artery disease, *Am J Cardiol* 95:452-456, 2005.

72. Date H, Imamura T, Sumi T et al: Effects of interleukin-6 produced in coronary circulation on production of C-reactive protein and coronary microvascular resistance, *Am J Cardiol* 95:849-852, 2005.

73. Tentolouris C, Tousoulis D, Antoniades C et al: Endothelial function and proinflammatory cytokines in patients with ischemic heart disease and dilated cardiomyopathy, *Int J Cardiol* 94:301-305, 2004.

74. Gwechenberger M, Hulsmann M, Berger R et al: Interleukin-6 and B-type natriuretic peptide are independent predictors for worsening of heart failure in patients with progressive congestive heart failure, *J Heart Lung Transplant* 23:839-844, 2004.

75. Chin BS, Conway DS, Chung NA et al: Interleukin-6, tissue factor and von Willebrand factor in acute decompensated heart failure: relationship to treatment and prognosis, *Blood Coagul Fibrinolysis* 14:515-521, 2003.

76. Ridker PM, Rifai N, Stampfer MJ et al: Plasma concentration of interleukin-6 and the risk of future myocardial infarction among apparently healthy men, *Circulation* 101:1767-1772, 2000.

77. Pradhan AD, Manson JE, Rossouw JE et al: Inflammatory biomarkers, hormone replacement therapy, and incident coronary heart disease: prospective analysis from the women's health initiative observational study, *JAMA* 288:980-987, 2002.

78. Ferketich AK, Ferguson JP, Binkley PF: Depressive symptoms and inflammation among heart failure patients, *Am Heart J* 150:132-136, 2005.

79. Parissis JT, Adamopoulos S, Rigas A et al: Comparison of circulating proinflammatory cytokines and soluble apoptosis mediators in patients with chronic heart failure with versus without symptoms of depression, *Am J Cardiol* 94:1326-1328, 2004.

80. Lesperance F, Frasure-Smith N, Theroux P et al: The association between major depression and levels of soluble intercellular adhesion molecule 1, interleukin-6, and C-reactive protein in patients with recent acute coronary syndromes, *Am J Psychiatry* 161:271-277, 2004.

81. Appels A, Bar FW, Bar J et al: Inflammation, depressive symptomatology, and coronary artery disease, *Psychosom Med* 62:601-605, 2000.

82. Gilbody SM, House AO, Sheldon TA: Routinely administered questionnaires for depression and anxiety: systematic review, *BMJ* 322:406-409, 2001.

83. Pignone MP, Gaynes BN, Rushton JL et al: Screening for depression in adults: a summary of the evidence for the US Preventive Services Task Force, *Ann Intern Med* 136:765-776, 2002.

84. US Preventive Services Task Force: Screening for depression: recommendations and rationale, *Ann Intern Med* 136:760-764, 2002.

85. Williams JW Jr, Noel PH, Cordes JA et al: Is this patient clinically depressed? *JAMA* 287:1160-1170, 2002.

86. Corson K, Gerrity MS, Dobscha SK: Screening for depression and suicidality in a VA primary care setting: 2 items are better than 1 item, *Am J Manag Care* 10:839-845, 2004.

87. Rush AJ, Trivedi M, Fava M: Depression, IV: STAR*D treatment trial for depression, *Am J Psychiatry* 160:237, 2003.

88. Snow V, Lascher S, Mottur-Pilson C: Pharmacologic treatment of acute major depression and dysthymia: clinical guideline, part 1, *Ann Intern Med* 132:738-742, 2000.

89. Husain M, Rush A, Fink M et al: Speed of response and remission in major depressive disorder with acute electroconvulsive therapy (ECT): a Consortium for Research in ECT (CORE) report, *J Clin Psychiatry* 65:485-491, 2004.

90. DeVane C, Grothe D, Smith S: Pharmacology of antidepressants: focus on nefazodone, *J Clin Psychiatry* 63:10-17, 2002.

91. Roose SP, Miyazaki M: Pharmacologic treatment of depression in patients with heart disease, *Psychosom Med* 67:S54-S57, 2005.

92. Trivedi MH, Rush AJ, Crismon ML et al: Clinical results for patients with major depressive disorder in the Texas Medication Algorithm Project, *Arch Gen Psychiatry* 61:669-680, 2004.

93. Mulsant BH, Alexopoulos GS, Reynolds CF 3rd et al: Pharmacological treatment of depression in older primary care patients: the PROSPECT algorithm, *Int J Geriatr Psychiatry* 16:585-592, 2001.

94. Hollon SD, Jarrett RB, Nierenberg AA et al: Psychotherapy and medication in the treatment of adult and geriatric depression: which monotherapy or combined treatment? *J Clin Psychiatry* 66:455-468, 2005.

95. Thase ME: When are psychotherapy and pharmacotherapy combinations the treatment of choice for major depressive disorder? *Psychiatr Q* 70:333-346, 1999.

96. DeRubeis RJ, Hollon SD, Amsterdam JD et al: Cognitive therapy vs medications in the treatment of moderate to severe depression, *Arch Gen Psychiatry* 62:409-416, 2005.

97. Clark D, Beck AB: *Foundations of cognitive theory and therapy of depression,* New York, 1999, John Wiley & Sons.

98. Deckersbach T, Gershuny BS, Otto MW: Cognitive-behavioral therapy for depression: applications and outcome, *Psychiatr Clin North Am* 23:795-809, 2000.

99. Beck J: *Cognitive therapy: basics and beyond,* New York, 1995, Guilford Press.

100. Elkin I, Shea MT, Watkins JT et al: National Institute of Mental Health Treatment of Depression Collaborative Research Program: general effectiveness of treatments, *Arch Gen Psychiatry* 46:971-982, 1989.

101. Blackburn IM, Moore RG: Controlled acute and follow-up trial of cognitive therapy and pharmacotherapy in out-patients with recurrent depression, *Br J Psychiatry* 171:328-334, 1997.

102. Karel MJ, Hinrichsen G: Treatment of depression in late life: psychotherapeutic interventions, *Clin Psychol Rev* 20:707-729, 2000.

103. Writing Committee for the ENRICHD Investigators: Effects of Treating depression and low perceived social support on clinical events after myocardial infarction: the Enhancing Recovery in Coronary Heart Disease Patients (ENRICHD) randomized trial, *JAMA* 289:3106-3116, 2003.

104. Dunbar SB, Summerville JG: Cognitive therapy for ventricular dysrhythmia patients, *J Cardiovasc Nurs* 12:33-44, 1997.

105. Judd F, Weissman M, Davis J et al: Interpersonal counselling in general practice, *Aust Fam Physician* 33:332-337, 2003.

106. Markowitz J: Interpersonal psychotherapy for chronic depression, *J Clin Psychol* 59:847-858, 2003.

107. Interpersonal psychotherapy: crises and changes in personal relationships are the chief concern of an increasingly popular therapeutic technique, *Harv Ment Health Lett* 21:1-3, 2004.

108. de Mello MF, de Jesus Mari J, Bacaltchuk J et al: A systematic review of research findings on the efficacy of interpersonal therapy for depressive disorders, *Eur Arch Psychiatry Clin Neurosci* 255:75-82, 2005.

109. Koszycki D, Lafontaine S, Frasure-Smith N et al: An open-label trial of interpersonal psychotherapy in depressed patients with coronary disease, *Psychosom* 45:319-324, 2004.

■■■ c h a p t e r **41**

Impact of Anxiety on Cardiac Disease

Marla J. DeJong

CHAPTER ABBREVIATIONS

AMI   acute myocardial infarction

BNST   bed nucleus of the stria terminalis

CHD   coronary heart disease

DSM-IV   Diagnostic and Statistical Manual of Mental Disorders, fourth edition

LVEF   left ventricular ejection fraction

SNS   sympathetic nervous system

Anxiety is a complex, powerful, and distressing emotion that individuals experience in response to real or imagined dangers. As such, there is no disputing that anxiety is a normal life experience. For some, however, anxiety is an all-consuming emotion. Numerous anxiety disorders such as generalized anxiety disorder, panic disorder, and obsessive-compulsive disorder have been recognized and are diagnosed using the *Diagnostic and Statistical Manual of Mental Disorders,* fourth edition (**DSM-IV**), criteria. Nonetheless, of primary interest to cardiovascular clinicians is subsyndromal anxiety—anxiety reactions that do not meet DSM-IV criteria for an anxiety disorder[1] but which are common, distressing, and debilitating among patients with cardiac disease.

Patients throughout the world with cardiac disease experience high anxiety, and culture itself does not explain variations in reported anxiety.[2] As many as 70 percent of patients with acute myocardial infarction (**AMI**) or heart failure are anxious.[3,4] Anxiety is also common for patients who undergo cardiac procedures such as cardiac catheterization or coronary artery bypass grafting.[5,6] Remarkably, some of these patients are more anxious than patients with neuropsychiatric disorders.[2] Anxiety reactions often are not transient but rather continue for months to years after diagnosis of cardiac disease or hospitalization for an acute event.[7] Even after controlling for demographic, clinical, and other emotions, high anxiety independently predicts increased health care consumption.[8]

Among individuals with cardiac disease, female gender,[9-12] younger age,[11] higher social class,[13] and lower income[10] are associated with anxiety. Single men reported higher anxiety than married or widowed men. In contrast, married women were more anxious than single or widowed women.[9]

Anxiety has psychological, physiological, behavioral, and cognitive manifestations. As a normal reaction to a real or perceived danger, anxiety can be protective and can motivate healthful behaviors. Cardiac patients who are anxious about their health, for example, may be more inclined to take their medications as ordered, exercise or participate in a cardiac rehabilitation program, report troublesome symptoms to their health care provider in a timely manner, or adhere to a prescribed diet. In one study, although those with mild to moderate anxiety performed more physical activity, patients with high anxiety were significantly less active.[14]

Persistent anxiety, however, is often counterproductive or even harmful. Anxiety may impede psychosocial adaptation to cardiovascular disorders, hinder physical rehabilitation, contribute to nonadherence, worsen health-related quality of life, cause greater symptom burden and disability, and interfere with patients' self-care, work, and leisure activities.[1,15,16] In addition, patients who are overly anxious may be unable to learn or act on new information about necessary lifestyle changes. More favorable findings indicated that perceived control, social support, and religiosity may moderate perceptions of anxiety.[17,18]

In many respects, it is not surprising that patients with cardiac disease are anxious. Potential sources of anxiety include progressive and debilitating physical symptoms, multifaceted treatment regimens, recurring hospitalization, perceived hopelessness and loss of control, failure of accustomed coping mechanisms, isolation from family and friends, frustrations with a complicated health care system, financial worries, and fear of death.[7] Positive correlations between patient anxiety and spousal anxiety also have been reported.[19]

ANXIETY AS A PREDICTOR OF CARDIAC DISEASE

Healthy Individuals

Accumulating evidence suggests that anxiety is related to the development of cardiac disease. Table 41-1 presents results of studies showing that healthy individuals with various anxiety disorders were more likely to develop cardiac disease than patients with lower levels of anxiety. The strength of these relationships is enhanced by prospective study designs, adjustments for recognized cardiac risk factors, and "hard" endpoints such as documented mortality or AMI. In addition, a dose-response effect was noted, meaning that increasing levels of anxiety were associated correspondingly with greater risk for cardiac disease. Interestingly, anxious cardiac patients were more likely than nonanxious patients to believe that anxiety contributed to development of their heart disease. Furthermore, men were more likely than women to attribute heart disease to anxiety.[26]

■ ■ ■

TABLE 41-1   LARGE PROSPECTIVE STUDIES OF HEALTHY INDIVIDUALS REGARDING ANXIETY AND THEIR RISK FOR CARDIAC DISEASE

AUTHORS	PARTICIPANTS	CARDIAC OUTCOME TESTED	ADJUSTMENTS	RESULTS
Haines et al., 1987[20]	1457 community-dwelling men; 10-year follow-up	Fatal and nonfatal CHD	Age, smoking, social class, systolic blood pressure, factor VII activity, fibrinogen level, cholesterol level	Men with higher anxiety were 3.8 times more likely to develop fatal CHD and 1.3 times more likely to develop nonfatal CHD.
Weissman et al., 1990[21]	3838 community-dwelling men and women; follow-up period not reported	AMI	Age, gender, marital status, race, socioeconomic status	Patients with panic disorder were 4.5 times more likely to develop AMI than persons without a psychiatric disorder.
Kawachi et al., 1994[22]	2280 community-dwelling men; 32-year follow-up	Fatal CHD; SCD	Age, BMI, smoking, blood pressure, cholesterol level, family history of CHD, alcohol use	Men who reported two or more anxiety symptoms were 1.9 times more likely to develop fatal CHD and 4.5 times more likely to experience SCD.
Kawachi et al., 1994[23]	33,999 male health professionals; 2-year follow-up	Fatal CHD; SCD	Age, BMI, smoking; history of hypertension, diabetes mellitus, hypercholesterolemia, family history of CHD, alcohol use, physical activity	Men with higher anxiety were 2.5 times more likely to develop fatal CHD and 3.1 times more likely to experience SCD.
Eaker et al., 1992[24]	749 community-dwelling women; 20-year follow-up	AMI or fatal CHD	Age, systolic blood pressure, BMI, diabetes, smoking, educational level, occupation	Homemakers with higher anxiety were 7.8 times more likely to develop AMI or fatal CHD.
Albert et al., 2005[25]	72,359 female registered nurses; 12-year follow-up	SCD and fatal CHD	Age, smoking, BMI, alcohol use, menopausal status, postmenopausal hormone use, parental history of AMI, and usual aspirin and valium use	Nurses with higher anxiety were 1.6 more likely to develop SCD and 1.3 times more likely to develop fatal CHD.

AMI, Acute myocardial infarction; *BMI,* body mass index; ***CHD,*** coronary heart disease; *SCD,* sudden cardiac death.

Patients with Cardiac Disease

Patients with known heart disease are vulnerable to anxiety. Table 41-2 shows that for patients with AMI or heart failure, many,[3,27,29-31] but not all investigators,[34,35] reported that independent of demographic and clinical variables, anxiety predicted future cardiac events (i.e., reinfarction, unstable angina, dysrhythmias, and mortality) during a long follow-up period. Anxiety also predicts other important outcomes such as functional status, quality of life, symptoms, and use of health care resources.[15]

RELATIONSHIP BETWEEN ANXIETY AND OUTCOMES

The mechanisms by which anxiety may be associated with cardiac disease outcomes are not entirely clear. Nonetheless, physiological and behavioral pathways appear to link anxiety with adverse outcomes (Figure 41-1).[38,39]

Physiological Mechanisms
Sympathetic Nervous System Activation

Physiological and psychological stressors such as anxiety activate the sympathetic nervous system (**SNS**), causing the release of two major catecholamines, epinephrine and norepinephrine. Short-term, this response enables individuals to activate internal resources and counteract threats to well-being.

Although the literature is complex, evidence suggests that anxiety and mental stress, often considered as an anxiety equivalent, activate the SNS. Positive correlations between plasma epinephrine levels and changes in heart rate, systolic blood pressure, rate-pressure product, and cardiac output have been noted for cardiac patients who underwent mental stress testing.[39] Patients with a history of AMI and elevated anxiety or prolonged stress had higher plasma norepinephrine levels than healthy volunteers, and those who developed adverse cardiovascular events had higher plasma catecholamine levels and more exaggerated blood pressure responses to mental stress than patients without complications. In addition, patients undergoing cardiac catheterization manifested higher norepinephrine, but not epinephrine, levels during mental stress testing.

Excessive SNS activation is related to increased morbidity and mortality for patients with cardiac disease. Cardiac norepinephrine spillover rates and plasma norepinephrine levels are important predictors of mortality for patients with heart failure. After AMI, persistently elevated plasma norepinephrine, aldosterone, and renin levels are noted in patients who develop recurrent cardiac events or die in subsequent months.

■ ■ ■

TABLE 41-2   STUDIES OF ANXIETY IN PATIENTS WITH KNOWN CARDIAC DISEASE

AUTHORS	PARTICIPANTS	CARDIAC OUTCOME TESTED	ADJUSTMENTS	RESULTS
Frasure-Smith et al., 1995[27]	222 patients with AMI; 1 year follow-up	Recurrent cardiac events: reinfarction, admission for unstable angina, arrhythmic deaths, survived cardiac arrests	Previous AMI, prescription for angiotensin-converting enzyme inhibitor at discharge, depression	Patients with higher anxiety were 2.5 times more likely to develop recurrent cardiac events.
Moser and Dracup, 1996[3]	86 patients with AMI; in-hospital study	In-hospital complications: recurrent ischemia, reinfarction, malignant ventricular dysrhythmias, cardiac death	Age, gender, Killip classification, worst chest pain level, thrombolytic therapy, anxiety	Patients with higher anxiety were 4.9 times more likely to develop in-hospital complications.
Konstam et al., 1996[28]	5025 patients with heart failure; 36.5-month follow-up	Heart failure–related hospitalization, all-cause mortality	LVEF, age, treatment, New York Heart Association classification, health-related quality of life	Anxiety was not associated with rehospitalization or mortality.
Thomas et al., 1997[29]	348 patients with AMI and ventricular dysrhythmias; 4-month follow-up	All-cause mortality	LVEF, diabetes, anger, past life events, expectations about future life events	Patients with higher anxiety were 1.1 times more likely to die.
Denollet and Brutsaert, 1998[30]	87 patients with AMI with an LVEF ≤50%; 7.9-year follow-up	Cardiac death, nonfatal AMI	LVEF, three-vessel disease, exercise tolerance, previous AMI, depression, type B behavior, type D personality	Patients with higher anxiety were 3.4 times more likely to experience cardiac death or nonfatal AMI.
Herrmann et al., 1998[31]	454 patients with medical conditions (274 with cardiological or pneumological disorders); 1.9-year follow-up	All-cause mortality	N/A	Patients with high anxiety were 2.5 times more likely to die.
Ketterer et al., 1998[32]	144 men with a positive diagnostic coronary angiogram	All-cause mortality, new AMI, revascularization	None	Patients with one or more events reported less anxiety.
Herrmann et al., 2000[33]	5057 patients referred for exercise testing (49% CHD); 5.7-year follow-up	All-cause mortality	Age, gender, history of cardiac disease, exercise performance	For every 1 standard deviation increase in anxiety in patients with CHD, survival improved 19%.
Welin et al., 2000[34]	275 patients with AMI; 10-year follow-up	All-cause mortality, nonfatal recurrent infarction	None	Trait anxiety was not associated with mortality or reinfarction.
Mayou et al., 2000[7]	344 with AMI; 18-month follow-up	All-cause mortality	Significant univariate predictors of mortality (not further specified)	Anxiety was not associated with mortality.
Lane et al., 2001[35]	288 patients with AMI; 1-year follow-up	Cardiac and all-cause mortality	None	Anxiety was not associated with mortality.
Frasure-Smith and Lesperance, 2003[36]	896 patients with AMI; 5-year follow-up	Cardiac mortality	Age, gender, education level, smoking, previous AMI, thrombolytic therapy, Q wave AMI, Killip Class, revascularization, LVEF, and prescription of hypoglycemic agents (for diabetics) and beta blockers at discharge	When adjusting for age and gender, patients with higher anxiety were 1.2 times more likely to die. When adjusting for cardiac disease severity, anxiety was not associated with mortality.
Strik et al., 2003[8]	318 men with AMI; 3.4-year mean follow-up	Cardiac death or recurrent AMI	Age, LVEF	Patients with high anxiety were 2.8 times more likely to die or experience recurrent AMI.
Grace et al., 2004[37]	913 patients with AMI or unstable angina; 1-year follow-up	Recurrent cardiac events: unstable angina, AMI, dysrhythmias, heart failure, stroke, blocked coronary artery, coronary artery bypass grafting, percutaneous coronary intervention, thrombolysis, death	Age, gender, income, Killip Class, diabetes, smoking, family history of cardiovascular disease, depression	Elevated anxiety was an independent predictor of recurrent coronary events.

AMI, Acute myocardial infarction; *CHD,* coronary heart disease; *LVEF,* left ventricular ejection fraction.

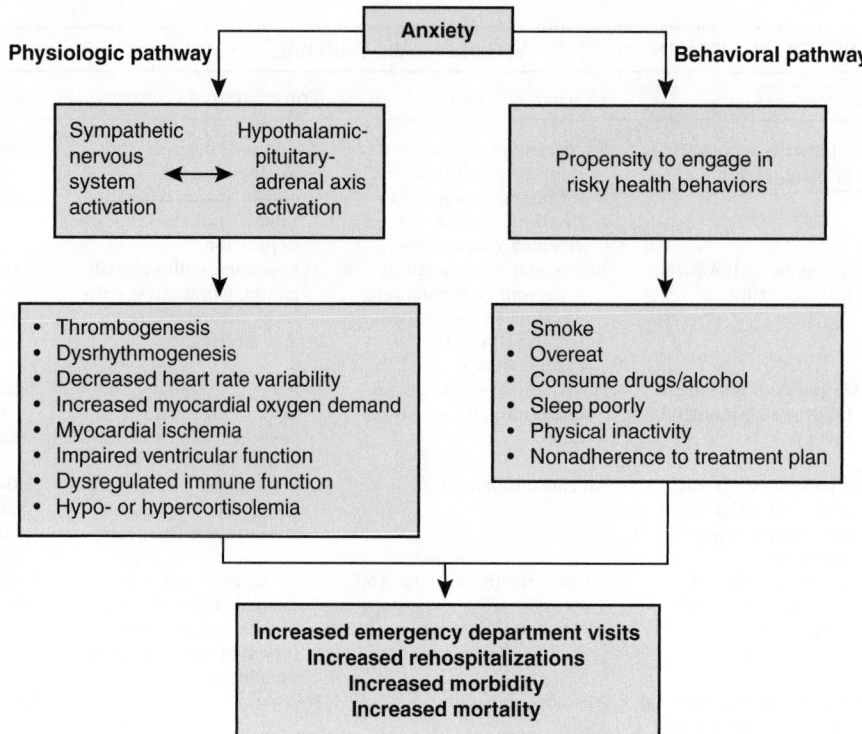

FIGURE 41-1 ▦ Physiological and behavioral pathways that may appear to link anxiety with adverse outcomes.

Parasympathetic withdrawal allows sympathetic activity to predominate. As a feature of heart failure, parasympathetic withdrawal is present already in the early phases of heart failure, and may be important in the stress response.[40]

Baroreceptor dysfunction is common for patients with heart disease and also contributes to unrestrained sympathetic outflow. Indeed, there is an important relationship between baroreflex sensitivity, and morbidity and mortality for patients with cardiovascular disease. Only recently has anxiety been associated with impaired baroreflex sensitivity in cardiac patients. Baroreflex control for patients with AMI and high anxiety was about 20 percent lower than for those with lower anxiety.[41]

By activating the SNS, anxiety triggers catecholamine production, increases heart rate and blood pressure, promotes systemic vasoconstriction, decreases plasma volume, constricts coronary arteries; and increases myocardial contractility, cardiac workload, platelet activity, coagulation, and inflammation. As a result, anxious patients are vulnerable to thrombogenesis, dysrhythmogenesis, decreased heart rate variability, increased myocardial oxygen demand, myocardial ischemia, impaired ventricular function, and dysregulated immune function.

Thrombogenesis

Endothelial dysfunction and reduced fibrinolysis are consequences of SNS activation that, in concert with platelet aggregation, promote thrombus formation.[42] Evidence suggests that epinephrine and norepinephrine function as platelet agonists and that epinephrine

accelerates hemostasis.[43] Mental stress–induced catecholamine release causes hemostasis by activating the beta$_2$-adrenergic receptor. Cardiac patients who underwent mental stress testing experienced increased platelet aggregation, formed more circulating platelet aggregates, and developed higher plasma and serum thromboxane B$_2$ levels than healthy controls.

Dysrhythmogenesis

Sympathetic stimulation is one cause of cardiac dysrhythmias for patients with cardiac disease. Anxiety and mental stress can produce cardiac electrical instability and lethal ventricular dysrhythmias.[44-46] New evidence suggests that stress-induced asymmetrical activation of the midbrain is associated with asymmetrical neural input to the heart that disrupts repolarization and predisposes patients to dysrhythmias.[47] Patients with an implantable cardioverter-defibrillator who underwent mental stress testing did not become ischemic; however, norepinephrine levels increased significantly, ventricular tachycardia cycle length shortened, ventricular tachycardia was induced 5 times faster, and it was more difficult to terminate dysrhythmias.[48] Others found an association between high anxiety and indices of repolarization that may place patients at higher risk for lethal cardiac dysrhythmias.[49]

Decreased Heart Rate Variability

Heart rate is not static but varies in response to physical and mental demands. Heart rate variability refers to the beat-to-beat variation in the RR interval and is a marker of autonomic nervous system activity. It is well established that high sympathetic activity contributes to decreased heart rate variability in patients with cardiac disease. Reduced heart rate variability is a powerful and independent predictor of short- and long-term mortality for cardiac patients.[50,51] Higher levels of anxiety are associated with reduced heart rate variability.[52]

Increased Myocardial Oxygen Demand

Mental stress increases heart rate and upsets the balance between myocardial oxygen supply and demand.[53] For patients with atherosclerosis, a catecholamine surge can cause increased myocardial oxygen demand and subsequent myocardial ischemia.[54] Vascular resistance increased when patients with heart disease were exposed to mental stress but decreased in normal controls.[55] Remarkably, patients with heart disease exhibited larger increases in systemic vascular resistance during mental stress than during exercise. When comparing mental stress–induced ischemia with exercise-induced ischemia, mental stress–induced ischemia often is associated with a sudden onset, smaller heart rate elevation, higher blood pressure, and lower double product (heart rate × systolic blood pressure).[39]

Myocardial Ischemia

Anxiety and mental stress are potent triggers of myocardial ischemia because they can produce vasoconstriction of coronary arteries, decrease coronary flow velocity, and cause rapid changes in blood pressure with ensuing atherosclerotic plaque rupture.[56-58] Mental stress can induce ischemia at lower levels of cardiac demand than exercise[59] and has caused complete coronary artery occlusion,[60] AMI,[61] and severe left ventricular dysfunction.[62] Of concern is that patients with stress-induced myocardial ischemia are usually asymptomatic.[63] Importantly, for patients with heart disease and exercise-induced ischemia, stress-induced ischemia was associated with a 2.8 times increase in mortality even when controlling for clinical risk factors.[56]

Impaired Ventricular Function

Mental stress affects systolic and diastolic ventricular function because catecholamines are toxic to cardiac myocytes and directly affect myocardial contractility. Patients with existing left ventricular dysfunction seem particularly susceptible to stress-induced ischemia.[64] When patients with heart disease and exercise-induced wall motion abnormalities were exposed to a mental stressor, 72 percent demonstrated stress-induced wall motion abnormalities that were similar to exercise-induced wall motion abnormalities.[65] In addition, 36 percent of these patients had a 5 percent or greater drop in their left ventricular ejection fraction. Yet 83 percent of these ischemic patients were asymptomatic and thus were unaware of their worsened condition. Similarly, others reported wall motion abnormalities or decreased left ventricular ejection fraction with mental stress.[66] In another study, patients with coronary disease experienced diastolic dysfunction and increases in blood pressure, heart rate, and rate pressure product during a mental stressor.[67] Diastolic dysfunction was accompanied by neither systolic dysfunction nor ST segment changes. The effects of mental stress extend beyond research settings. Patients with cardiac disease routinely experience stressful situations during the course of everyday life. Patients who developed ischemia and wall motion abnormalities in response to mental stress in a laboratory setting are more likely to experience ambulatory ischemia.[39]

Dysregulated Immune Function

Immune cells receive signals from the neuroendocrine system, and catecholamines and corticotropin-releasing hormone appear to modulate the immune response to anxiety. Anxiety enhances the production of proinflammatory cytokines, including tumor necrosis factor-alpha, interleukin-1beta, and interleukin-6.[68] In heart failure, overexpression of proinflammatory cytokines is associated with left ventricular remodeling and dysfunction, pulmonary edema, endothelial dysfunction, anorexia, cachexia, fetal gene expression, and other biological effects that likely contribute to disease progression.[69] Elevated cytokines predicted increased cardiovascular morbidity and mortality for patients who survived an acute coronary event. Cytokines also can activate the hypothalamic-pituitary-adrenal axis (discussed next) directly or indirectly through catecholaminergic pathways.

Hypothalamic-Pituitary-Adrenal Axis Activation

Anxiety activates the hypothalamic-pituitary-adrenal axis.[70] Despite an incomplete understanding, anxiety is thought to cause the hypothalamus to secrete corticotropin-releasing hormone, which in turn causes the anterior pituitary gland to secrete adrenocorticotropic hormone. In response to increased adrenocorticotropic hormone, the adrenal cortex releases increased amounts of cortisol. Hypercortisolemia may contribute to obesity, increased fatty acids, insulin resistance, and diabetes, which are known risk factors for cardiac disease and its complications. Normally, high cortisol levels function in a negative feedback loop to decrease secretion of corticotropin-releasing hormone. Repeated episodes of acute stress, however, may lead to upregulation of glucocorticoid receptors, increased negative feedback, and chronic hypocortisolemia. Anxiety-induced norepinephrine and cytokine release also can activate the hypothalamic-pituitary-adrenal axis.

Stress increases corticotropin-releasing hormone in the basolateral amygdala, a structure located in the temporal cortex of the brain, which contains corticotropin-releasing hormone receptors and nerve endings. Stress-induced release of corticotropin-releasing hormone in the basolateral amygdala results in anxiogenic effects.[71] The basolateral amygdala is thought to regulate anxiety and other emotions by filtering sensory information and sending output to its surrounding, specialized target areas. The lateral bed nucleus of the stria terminalis (**BNST**) is the area most relevant to the autonomic and motor responses associated with anxiety.[72] The BNST projects to other noradrenergic neurons and target areas within the hypothalamus and brain stem that mediate behavioral, autonomic, and electrophysiological consequences of anxiety. In addition, interactions between corticotropin-releasing hormone and catecholamines within the BNST may be important in the anxiety response.

Behavioral Mechanisms

Experts have hypothesized that health behavioral mechanisms are another link between anxiety and poor outcomes for patients with cardiac disease. Compared with nonanxious individuals, those with high anxiety may be more likely to smoke, overeat, consume drugs or alcohol, sleep poorly, and be physically inactive.[73] These risky health behaviors can provoke physiological changes, such as altered immunity and endocrine changes,[74] and are associated with the incidence and progression of cardiac disease. For example, smoking and alcohol use have long been recognized as threats to cardiovascular health.

Although most evidence is not conclusive, anxiety also may contribute to poor treatment adherence. Post-AMI, patients with anxiety and depression exercised less and smoked more.[7] In one study, mental health, which included anxiety, predicted overall, dietary, and exercise adherence rates for patients with heart failure.[75] In general, though, little is known about potential behavioral mechanisms linking anxiety with adverse cardiac outcomes, and research in this area is ongoing.

ASSESSING ANXIETY IN PATIENTS WITH CARDIAC DISEASE

Despite the high prevalence of anxiety in cardiac patients and strong evidence that anxiety is linked to poor outcomes, clinicians routinely and systematically fail to assess patients for anxiety.[76,77] Rather, a somewhat more common approach is for clinicians to use their clinical judgment to determine whether a patient is anxious.[77] This practice is problematic because patient-generated and clinician-generated ratings of patient anxiety are incongruent,[76,77] emphasizing the need to use an anxiety assessment instrument when assessing anxiety.

More than 200 instruments have been developed to assess anxiety; however, many of these were designed to assess specific anxiety disorders or anxiety associated with a certain noncardiac diagnosis or a particular anxiety-provoking stimulus. In contrast, Box 41-1 lists several valid and reliable self-report anxiety assessment instruments that have been used for patients with cardiac disease. Clinicians without formal psychiatric training can administer and interpret these instruments eas-

ily, and patients usually can complete them in 1 to 10 minutes. It is essential that clinicians identify patients with high anxiety so that interventions can be initiated.

INTERVENTIONS FOR PATIENTS WITH ANXIETY

A great diversity exists in the interventions used to treat anxiety in patients with cardiac disease. Likewise, treatment approaches used in clinical trials are sometimes dissimilar from those used in everyday clinical practice. Data, as previously presented in this chapter, suggest that intense and prolonged anxiety in patients with cardiac disease needs to be treated. Interventions are administered with the goal of reducing anxiety and severing linkages between anxiety and poor outcomes.

Pharmacological Therapy

Pharmacological therapy for anxiety includes use of anxiolytics and hypnotics. Benzodiazepines are the most widely used group of anxiolytics for patients with cardiac disease and have minimal adverse effects. Although it is recommended that anxiolytics be given on a scheduled basis,[78] it is unknown whether benzodiazepines reduce cardiac morbidity and mortality. Only one randomized trial of anxiolytic drugs for patients with AMI or heart failure has been conducted.[79] In this dated study, men with AMI were assigned randomly to receive diazepam or placebo every 6 hours. No difference in patients' self-assessed anxiety levels was found, but patients who received diazepam were drowsier than patients who received the placebo. Only males were enrolled into this study, and care for patients with AMI has changed dramatically over the years; nevertheless, this finding suggests that pharmacological interventions may be less effective than thought in decreasing anxiety in acutely ill cardiac patients.

Nonpharmacological Therapy

Music therapy, education interventions, home-based psychosocial nursing interventions, cardiac rehabilitation, cognitive-behavioral therapy, biofeedback-relaxation training, and other nonpharmacological therapies have been found to reduce anxiety in patients with cardiac disease.

Music Therapy

Music therapy has the potential to influence psychological and physiological processes. For example, patients in an intensive care unit after AMI were assigned randomly to music therapy, quiet rest, or usual care. Immediately after a 20-minute music therapy session, patients had more significant declines in state of anxiety, heart rate, respiratory rate, and myocardial oxygen demand than did the usual care group. The reduced heart rate and respiratory rate were maintained for 1 hour after the intervention. Patients in the music therapy and quiet rest groups also had higher heart rate variability immediately after the intervention.[80] In a similar study,

---

BOX 41-1   ■ ■ ■
ANXIETY ASSESSMENT INSTRUMENTS USED FOR PATIENTS WITH CARDIAC DISEASE

State-Trait Anxiety Inventory
Anxiety Subscale of the Brief Symptom Inventory
Anxiety Subscale of the Hospital Anxiety and Depression Scale
Profile of Mood States
Beck Anxiety Inventory
Symptom Checklist 90 Revised
Faces Anxiety Scale

post–open heart surgery patients were assigned randomly to receive sedative music, scheduled rest, or usual care during 30 minutes of chair rest on postoperative day 1. Although patients in both treatment groups were significantly less anxious than control patients, the sedative music group was less anxious than the chair rest group.[81]

Educational Interventions

Clinicians generally believe that patient and family education are effective means to reduce anxiety; however, evidence supporting this belief is not conclusive. Patients and their partners who received a structured nursing support and education intervention were less anxious than those who received usual care.[82] In a randomized clinical trial, patients waiting for cardiac catheterization received a nurse-delivered 1-hour education intervention or usual care. The intervention was associated with a 23 percent reduction in anxiety.[5] In contrast, patients undergoing coronary artery bypass grafting who were randomized to receive a preoperative education intervention had similar levels of postoperative anxiety as patients in the control group.[83]

Home-Based Psychosocial Nursing Interventions

Given short inpatient lengths of stay, home-based cardiac care has become increasingly important. The Montreal Heart Attack Readjustment Trial (known as M-HART) was a randomized trial of home-based psychosocial nursing interventions.[84] Patients with elevated psychological distress, including anxiety, received at least two home visits, during which a nurse completed a comprehensive stress assessment and initiated various psychosocial interventions. Patients whose psychological distress scores normalized after two visits were less anxious at 1 year and less likely to be readmitted or die of a cardiac cause. Home-based interventions may be more effective than hospital-based ones, considering that cardiac patients were more anxious and had more problems with distraction and memory during hospitalization than 6 weeks after discharge.[85] In spite of these favorable findings, others reported that home-based psychosocial nursing interventions were not associated with improved survival.[86] Further research may shed light on the characteristics of home-based interventions that benefit patients with cardiac disease.

Cardiac Rehabilitation

Cardiac rehabilitation programs typically offer psychosocial interventions. Patients with cardiac disease who completed cardiac rehabilitation had a 56 percent reduction in the prevalence of anxiety and a 69 percent reduction in the prevalence of high anxiety.[87] In the same study, highly anxious patients manifested striking improvements in weight, percent fat, body mass index, exercise capacity, lipid levels, and quality of life. In a review paper, Linden[88] concluded that psychosocial interventions offered as part of cardiac rehabilitation can improve survival and reduce recurrent AMI for patients with emotional distress; however, Linden cautioned that these effects may not apply to females and older patients.

Cognitive-Behavioral Therapy and Biofeedback-Relaxation Training

Cognitive therapy is a structured form of psychotherapy that emphasizes how thinking affects emotions. Patients are taught to unlearn dysfunctional thoughts, problem solve, and practice techniques that replace negative thinking with more desirable thoughts and emotions. Biofeedback is a noninvasive process whereby patients use electronic instruments to learn how to manage physiological processes such as blood pressure, heart rate, and anxiety. Relaxation therapy focuses on teaching patients techniques such as breathing, responding to mental or verbal cues, or contracting and relaxing muscles, which are intended to reduce tension.

Patients with heart failure who were randomized to a 6-week biofeedback-relaxation training program were less anxious, had better quality of life, and had less SNS arousal than patients in the control group.[89] Furthermore, patients in the control group were hospitalized more often. In other randomized trials, a nonpharmacological intervention, which included relaxation training, was associated with significant reductions in anxiety,[90] and patients randomized to biofeedback-relaxation training program had lower norepinephrine levels and better cardiac output and heart rate variability at 6 weeks and 6 months than control patients.[91] Finally, in a recent meta-analysis of 27 studies involving cardiac patients, relaxation and cognitive therapy was associated with profound favorable outcomes, including lowered resting heart rate, increased heart rate variability, improved exercise tolerance, increased high-density lipoprotein cholesterol levels, decreased state of anxiety and depression, fewer episodes of dysrhythmias and angina, fewer cardiac events, and lower cardiac mortality.[92] Greater benefits were realized when patients received full or expanded therapy rather than abbreviated therapy, meaning that a dedicated therapy program with intensive supervised training is advantageous.

Other Nonpharmacological Therapies

Other nonpharmacological therapies also have reduced anxiety successfully. Women randomized to a mindfulness-based stress reduction program reported a lower state of anxiety than control patients.[93] Other cardiac patients received routine care or completed audiovisual relaxation training that encompassed deep breathing, exercise, muscle relaxation, guided imagery, and meditation. Over the next year, patients in the relaxation training group had a lower state of anxiety than patients in the control group.[94] Interventions to improve perceived control also may be useful; however, randomized clinical trials are needed to appraise their worth.

Integration of Interventions into Clinical Practice

Despite the favorable evidence that interventions reduce anxiety, patients with cardiac disease and anxiety are very rarely offered psychosocial interventions. This might be the case for several reasons. First, as mentioned, clinicians infrequently assess patients for anxiety, thus failing to recognize the high prevalence of anxiety. Indeed, only 38 percent of cardiac patients in a recent study had been assessed for anxiety.[37] The reluctance to assess anxiety may stem from confusion about the nature of anxiety, inconsistent measurement of anxiety, and limited data about the mechanism(s) by which anxiety contributes to cardiovascular outcomes. Further impedances to anxiety assessment include short patient appointments and insurance providers' disinclinations to reimburse for psychosocial care. Second, some view studies of anxiety and other psychological constructs as "soft" or less scientific than biological measures. Often, clinicians rush to use new diagnostic or therapeutic equipment. Clinicians, for example, quickly integrated pulmonary artery catheters, drug-coated coronary stents, and biventricular pacemakers into practice. In contrast, clinicians seem reluctant to adopt the assessment and treatment of anxiety. Third, patients with repressive tendencies may not recognize or report anxiety and thus may downplay the effects of anxiety.[95] Clinicians who are inclined to repudiate anxiety and its impact are unlikely to further assess and treat anxiety in these patients. Fourth, most clinicians seem to underappreciate the dangerous complications associated with anxiety, possibly because formal education programs and clinical practice guidelines have not emphasized anxiety or other emotions. Fifth, some clinicians believe that anxiety is a normal time-limited response to illness and undeserving of special attention.

Sixth, others assume that other emotions (e.g., depression) or factors (e.g., culture, values, and beliefs) correlate highly with anxiety, making it difficult to isolate the unique effects of anxiety. Finally, clinicians perceive that other specialized health care professionals should address the patient's psychosocial needs.

Evidence provided in this chapter emphasizes the need for clinicians to assess and treat anxiety. Just as clinicians would consider it unethical not to treat a low cardiac output or hypotension, so it should be considered unethical to fail to assess for and treat anxiety. During the anxiety assessment process, clinicians should consider whether the anxiety may be related to an immediate physiological disturbance such as hypoxia or an adverse medication reaction. Once such disturbances are ruled out, it is necessary to provide interventions designed to alleviate anxiety. Figure 41-2 is a treatment algorithm that can help clinicians identify potential interventions while considering the nature of the patient's anxiety, clinician's ability to deliver intervention, and potential for effectiveness.

Before new strategies can be designed to combat cardiac disease, it is crucial that investigators further explicate the physiological mechanisms by which anxiety produces adverse outcomes. Research is needed, for example, to delineate the effect of anxiety on neurohormonal responses, myocyte and ventricular function, atherosclerotic plaque integrity, hemostasis, endothelial function, cognitive function, and adherence to treatment regimens. Achieving optimal results will require

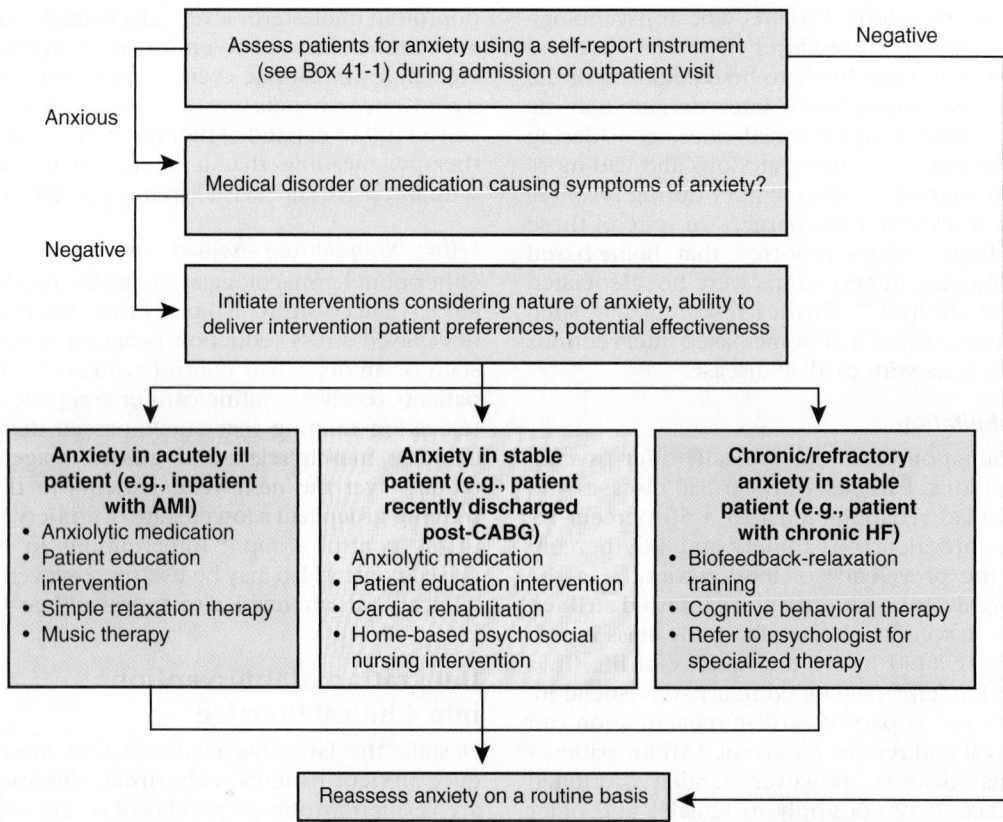

FIGURE 41-2 ■ Treatment algorithm for anxiety. *AMI*, Acute myocardial infarction; *CABG*, coronary artery bypass grafting; *HF*, heart failure

collaboration by scientists from multiple disciplines—nursing, medicine, psychoneuroendocrinology, biology, behavioral science, and neuropsychology.

REFERENCES

1. Sullivan MD, LaCroix AZ, Baum C et al: Functional status in coronary artery disease: a one-year prospective study of the role of anxiety and depression, *Am J Med* 103:348-356, 1997.
2. De Jong MJ, Chung ML, Roser LP et al: A five-country comparison of anxiety early after acute myocardial infarction, *Eur J Cardiovasc Nurs* 3:129-134, 2004.
3. Moser DK, Dracup K: Is anxiety early after myocardial infarction associated with subsequent ischemic and arrhythmic events? *Psychosom Med* 58:395-401, 1996.
4. Lainscak M, Keber I: Patient's view of heart failure: from the understanding to the quality of life, *Eur J Cardiovasc Nurs* 2:275-281, 2003.
5. Harkness K, Morrow L, Smith K et al: The effect of early education on patient anxiety while waiting for elective cardiac catheterization, *Eur J Cardiovasc Nurs* 2:113-121, 2003.
6. Rymaszewska J, Kiejna A, Hadrys T: Depression and anxiety in coronary artery bypass grafting patients, *Eur Psychiatry* 18:155-160, 2003.
7. Mayou RA, Gill D, Thompson DR et al: Depression and anxiety as predictors of outcome after myocardial infarction, *Psychosom Med* 62:212-219, 2000.
8. Strik JJ, Denollet J, Lousberg R et al: Comparing symptoms of depression and anxiety as predictors of cardiac events and increased health care consumption after myocardial infarction, *J Am Coll Cardiol* 42:1801-1807, 2003.
9. An K, De Jong MJ, Riegel BJ et al: A cross-sectional examination of changes in anxiety early after acute myocardial infarction, *Heart Lung* 33:75-82, 2004.
10. Kim KA, Moser DK, Garvin BJ et al: Differences between men and women in anxiety early after acute myocardial infarction, *Am J Crit Care* 9:245-253, 2000.
11. Moser DK, Dracup K, McKinley S et al: An international perspective on gender differences in anxiety early after acute myocardial infarction, *Psychosom Med* 65:511-516, 2003.
12. Riedinger MS, Dracup KA, Brecht M-L, for the SOLVD Investigators: Quality of life in women with heart failure, normative groups, and patients with other chronic conditions, *Am J Crit Care* 11:211-219, 2002.
13. Chiou A, Potempa K, Buschmann MB: Anxiety, depression and coping methods of hospitalized patients with myocardial infarction in Taiwan, *Int J Nurs Stud* 34:305-311, 1997.
14. De Jong MJ, Moser DK, Chung ML: Predictors of health status for heart failure patients, *Prog Cardiovasc Nurs* 20:155-162, 2005.
15. Clarke SP, Frasure-Smith N, Lesperance F et al: Psychosocial factors as predictors of functional status at 1 year in patients with left ventricular dysfunction, *Res Nurs Health* 23:290-300, 2000.
16. Sullivan MD, LaCroix AZ, Spertus JA et al: Five-year prospective study of the effects of anxiety and depression in patients with coronary artery disease, *Am J Cardiol* 86:1135-1138, 2000.
17. Dracup K, Westlake C, Erickson VS et al: Perceived control reduces emotional stress in patients with heart failure, *J Heart Lung Transplant* 22:90-93, 2003.
18. Hughes JW, Tomlinson A, Blumenthal JA et al: Social support and religiosity as coping strategies for anxiety in hospitalized cardiac patients, *Ann Behav Med* 28:179-185, 2004.
19. Moser DK, Dracup K: Role of spousal anxiety and depression in patients' psychosocial recovery after a cardiac event, *Psychosom Med* 66:527-532, 2004.
20. Haines AP, Imeson JD, Meade TW: Phobic anxiety and ischaemic heart disease, *Br Med J* 295:297-299, 1987.
21. Weissman MM, Markowitz JS, Ouellette R et al: Panic disorder and cardiovascular/cerebrovascular problems: results from a community survey, *Am J Psychiatry* 147:1504-1508, 1990.
22. Kawachi I, Sparrow D, Vokonas PS, Weiss ST: Symptoms of anxiety and risk of coronary heart disease: the Normative Aging Study, *Circulation* 90:2225-2229, 1994.
23. Kawachi I, Colditz GA, Ascherio A et al: Prospective study of phobic anxiety and risk of coronary heart disease in men, *Circulation* 89:1992-1997, 1994.
24. Eaker ED, Pinsky J, Castelli WP: Myocardial infarction and coronary death among women: psychosocial predictors from a 20-year follow-up of women in the Framingham Study, *Am J Epidemiol* 135:854-864, 1992.
25. Albert CM, Chae CU, Rexrode KM et al: Phobic anxiety and risk of coronary heart disease and sudden cardiac death among women, *Circulation* 111:480-487, 2005.
26. Day RC, Freedland KE, Carney RM: Effects of anxiety and depression on heart disease attributions, *Int J Behav Med* 12:24-29, 2005.
27. Frasure-Smith N, Lesperance F, Talajic M: The impact of negative emotions on prognosis following myocardial infarction: is it more than depression? *Health Psychol* 14:388-398, 1995.
28. Konstam V, Salem D, Pouleur H et al, for the SOLVD Investigators: Baseline quality of life as a predictor of mortality and hospitalization in 5,025 patients with congestive heart failure, *Am J Cardiol* 78:890-895, 1996.
29. Thomas SA, Friedmann E, Wimbush F et al: Psychological factors and survival in the cardiac arrhythmia suppression trial (CAST): a reexamination, *Am J Crit Care* 6:116-126, 1997.
30. Denollet J, Brutsaert DL: Personality, disease severity, and the risk of long-term cardiac events in patients with a decreased ejection fraction after myocardial infarction, *Circulation* 97:167-173, 1998.
31. Herrmann C, Brand-Driehorst S, Kaminsky B et al: Diagnostic groups and depressed mood as predictors of 22-month mortality in medical inpatients, *Psychosom Med* 60:570-577, 1998.
32. Ketterer MW, Huffman J, Lumley MA et al: Five-year follow-up for adverse outcomes in males with at least minimally positive angiograms: importance of "denial" in assessing psychosocial risk factors, *J Psychosom Res* 44:241-250, 1998.
33. Herrmann C, Brand-Driehorst S, Buss U et al: Effects of anxiety and depression on 5-year mortality in 5,057 patients referred for exercise testing, *J Psychosom Res* 48:455-462, 2000.
34. Welin C, Lappas G, Wilhelmsen L: Independent importance of psychosocial factors for prognosis after myocardial infarction, *J Intern Med* 247:629-639, 2000.
35. Lane D, Carroll D, Ring C et al: Mortality and quality of life 12 months after myocardial infarction: effects of depression and anxiety, *Psychosom Med* 63:221-230, 2001.
36. Frasure-Smith N, Lesperance F: Depression and other psychological risks following myocardial infarction, *Arch Gen Psychiatry* 60:627-636, 2003.
37. Grace SL, Abbey SE, Irvine J et al: Prospective examination of anxiety persistence and its relationship to cardiac symptoms and recurrent cardiac events, *Psychother Psychosom* 73:344-352, 2004.
38. Kubzansky LD, Kawachi I: Going to the heart of the matter: do negative emotions cause coronary heart disease? *J Psychosom Res* 48:323-337, 2000.
39. Rozanski A, Blumenthal JA, Davidson KW et al: The epidemiology, pathophysiology, and management of psychosocial risk factors in cardiac practice: the emerging field of behavioral cardiology, *J Am Coll Cardiol* 45:637-651, 2005.
40. Gevirtz R: The physiology of stress. In Kenny DT, Carlson JG, McGuigan FJ, Sheppard JL, editors: *Stress and health: research and clinical applications,* [Sydney], Australia, 2000, Harwood Academic Publishers.
41. Watkins LL, Blumenthal JA, Carney RM: Association of anxiety with reduced baroreflex cardiac control in patients after acute myocardial infarction, *Am Heart J* 143:460-466, 2002.
42. von Kanel R, Mills PJ, Fainman C et al: Effects of psychological stress and psychiatric disorders on blood coagulation and fibrinolysis: a biobehavioral pathway to coronary artery disease? *Psychosom Med* 63:531-544, 2001.
43. von Kanel R, Mills PJ, Ziegler MG et al: Effect of beta$_2$-adrenergic receptor functioning and increased norepinephrine on the hypercoagulable state with mental stress, *Am Heart J* 144:68-72, 2002.
44. Kop WJ, Krantz DS, Nearing BD et al: Effects of acute mental stress and exercise on T-wave alternans in patients with implantable cardioverter defibrillators and controls, *Circulation* 109:1864-1869, 2004.
45. Fries R, Konig J, Schafers H-J et al: Triggering effect of physical and mental stress on spontaneous ventricular tachyarrhythmias in patients with implantable cardioverter-defibrillators, *Clin Cardiol* 25:474-478, 2002.

46. Dunbar SB, Kimble LP, Jenkins LS et al: Association of mood disturbance and arrhythmia events in patients after cardioverter defibrillator implantation, *Depress Anxiety* 9:163-168, 1999.
47. Critchley HD, Taggart P, Sutton PM et al: Mental stress and sudden cardiac death: asymmetric midbrain activity as a linking mechanism, *Brain* 128:75-85, 2005.
48. Lampert R, Jain D, Burg MM et al: Destabilizing effects of mental stress on ventricular arrhythmias in patients with implantable cardioverter-defibrillators, *Circulation* 101:158-164, 2000.
49. Lampert R, Shusterman V, Burg MM et al: Effects of psychologic stress on repolarization and relationship to autonomic and hemodynamic factors, *J Cardiovasc Electrophysiol* 16:372-377, 2005.
50. Stein PK, Domitrovich PP, Huikuri HV et al: Traditional and nonlinear heart rate variability are each independently associated with mortality after myocardial infarction, *J Cardiovasc Electrophysiol* 16:13-20, 2005.
51. Aronson D, Mittleman MA, Burger AJ: Measures of heart period variability as predictors of mortality in hospitalized patients with decompensated congestive heart failure, *Am J Cardiol* 93:59-63, 2004.
52. Carney RM, Freedland KE, Stein PK: Anxiety, depression, and heart rate variability, *Psychosom Med* 62:84-87, 2000.
53. Kop WJ, Krantz DS, Howell RH et al: Effects of mental stress on coronary epicardial vasomotion and flow velocity in coronary artery disease: relationship with hemodynamic stress responses, *J Am Coll Cardiol* 37:1359-1366, 2001.
54. Krantz DS, Kop WJ, Santiago HT et al: Mental stress as a trigger of myocardial ischemia and infarction, *Cardiol Clin* 14:271-287, 1996.
55. Jain D, Shaker SM, Burg M et al: Effects of mental stress on left ventricular and peripheral vascular performance in patients with coronary artery disease, *J Am Coll Cardiol* 31:1314-1322, 1998.
56. Sheps DS, McMahon RP, Becker L et al: Mental stress-induced ischemia and all-cause mortality in patients with coronary artery disease: results from the Psychophysiological Investigations of Myocardial Ischemia study, *Circulation* 105:1780-1784, 2002.
57. Kim CK, Bartholomew BA, Mastin ST et al: Detection and reproducibility of mental stress-induced myocardial ischemia with Tc-99m sestamibi SPECT in normal and coronary artery disease populations, *J Nucl Cardiol* 10:56-62, 2003.
58. Kubzansky LD, Kawachi I, Weiss ST et al: Anxiety and coronary heart disease: a synthesis of epidemiological, psychological, and experimental evidence, *Ann Behav Med* 20:47-58, 1998.
59. Kop WJ: Chronic and acute psychological risk factors for clinical manifestations of coronary artery disease, *Psychosom Med* 61:476-487, 1999.
60. Papademetriou V, Gottdiener JS, Kop WJ et al: Transient coronary occlusion with mental stress, *Am Heart J* 132:1299-1301, 1996.
61. Gelernt MD, Hochman JS: Acute myocardial infarction triggered by emotional stress, *Am J Cardiol* 69:1512-1513, 1992.
62. Wittstein IS, Thiemann DR, Lima JA et al: Neurohumoral features of myocardial stunning due to sudden emotional stress, *N Engl J Med* 352:539-548, 2005.
63. Strike PC, Steptoe A: Systematic review of mental stress-induced myocardial ischaemia, *Eur Heart J* 24:690-703, 2003.
64. Akinboboye O, Krantz DS, Kop WJ et al: Comparison of mental stress-induced myocardial ischemia in coronary artery disease patients with versus without left ventricular dysfunction, *Am J Cardiol* 95:322-326, 2005.
65. Rozanski A, Bairey CN, Krantz DS et al: Mental stress and the induction of silent myocardial ischemia in patients with coronary artery disease, *N Engl J Med* 318:1005-1012, 1988.
66. Kuroda T, Kuwabara Y, Watanabe S et al: Effect of mental stress on left ventricular ejection fraction and its relationship to the severity of coronary artery disease, *Eur J Nucl Med* 27:1760-1767, 2000.
67. Okano Y, Utsunomiya T, Yano K: Effect of mental stress on hemodynamics and left ventricular diastolic function in patients with ischemic heart disease, *Jpn Circ J* 62:173-177, 1998.
68. Gershenfeld HK, Philibert RA, Boehm GW: Looking forward in geriatric anxiety and depression: implications of basic science for the future, *Am J Geriatr Psychiatry* 13:1027-1040, 2005.
69. Mann DL: Inflammatory mediators and the failing heart: past, present, and the foreseeable future, *Circ Res* 91:988-998, 2002.
70. Boyer P: Do anxiety and depression have a common pathophysiological mechanism? *Acta Psychiatr Scand* 102:24-29, 2000.
71. Davis M, Whalen PJ: The amygdala: vigilance and emotion, *Mol Psychiatry* 6:13-34, 2001.
72. Walker DL, Toufexis DJ, Davis M: Role of the bed nucleus of the stria terminalis versus the amygdala in fear, stress, and anxiety, *Eur J Pharmacol* 463:199-216, 2003.
73. Sirois BC, Burg MM: Negative emotion and coronary heart disease: a review, *Behav Modif* 27:83-102, 2003.
74. Kiecolt-Glaser JK, McGuire L, Robles TF et al: Emotions, morbidity, and mortality: new perspectives from psychoneuroimmunology, *Annu Rev Psychol* 53:83-107, 2002.
75. Evangelista LS, Berg J, Dracup K: Relationship between psychosocial variables and compliance in patients with heart failure, *Heart Lung* 30:294-301, 2001.
76. Frazier SK, Moser DK, O'Brien JL et al: Management of anxiety after acute myocardial infarction, *Heart Lung* 31:411-420, 2002.
77. O'Brien JL, Moser DK, Riegel B et al: Comparison of anxiety assessments between clinicians and patients with acute myocardial infarction in cardiac critical care units, *Am J Crit Care* 10:97-103, 2001.
78. Shah SU, Iqbal Z, White A et al: Heart and mind: (2) psychotropic and cardiovascular therapeutics, *Postgrad Med J* 81:33-40, 2005.
79. Dixon RA, Edwards IR, Pilcher J: Diazepam in immediate post-myocardial infarct period: a double blind trial, *Br Heart J* 43:535-540, 1980.
80. White JM: Effects of relaxing music on cardiac autonomic balance and anxiety after acute myocardial infarction, *Am J Crit Care* 8:220-230, 1999.
81. Voss JA, Good M, Yates B et al: Sedative music reduces anxiety and pain during chair rest after open-heart surgery, *Pain* 112:197-203, 2004.
82. Thompson DR: A randomized controlled trial of in-hospital nursing support for first time myocardial infarction patients and their partners: effects on anxiety and depression, *J Adv Nurs* 14:291-297, 1989.
83. Shuldham CM, Fleming S, Goodman H: The impact of pre-operative education on recovery following coronary artery bypass surgery: a randomized controlled clinical trial, *Eur Heart J* 23:666-674, 2002.
84. Cossette S, Frasure-Smith N, Lesperance F: Clinical implications of a reduction in psychological distress on cardiac prognosis in patients participating in a psychosocial intervention program, *Psychosom Med* 63:257-266, 2001.
85. Carroll DL: Capacity for direct attention in patients undergoing percutaneous coronary intervention: the effects of psychological distress, *Prog Cardiovasc Nurs* 20:11-16, 2005.
86. Frasure-Smith N, Lesperance F, Prince RH et al: Randomised trial of home-based psychosocial nursing intervention for patients recovering from myocardial infarction, *Lancet* 350:473-479, 1997.
87. Lavie CJ, Milani RV: Prevalence of anxiety in coronary patients with improvement following cardiac rehabilitation and exercise training, *Am J Cardiol* 93:336-339, 2004.
88. Linden W: Psychological treatments in cardiac rehabilitation: review of rationales and outcomes, *J Psychosom Res* 48:443-454, 2000.
89. Moser DK, Kim KA, Baisden-O'Brien J: Impact of a nonpharmacologic cognitive intervention on clinical and psychosocial outcomes in patients with advanced heart failure, *Circulation* 100:I-99, 1999 (abstract).
90. Kostis JB, Rosen RC, Cosgrove NM et al: Nonpharmacologic therapy improves functional and emotional status in congestive heart failure, *Chest* 106:996-1001, 1994.
91. Moser D, Nelson S: Impact of biofeedback-relaxation training on hemodynamics, neuroendocrine function and rehospitalization in advanced heart failure, *Am J Crit Care* 8:202, 1999 (abstract).
92. van Dixhoorn J, White A: Relaxation therapy for rehabilitation and prevention in ischaemic heart disease: a systematic review and meta-analysis, *Eur J Cardiovasc Prev Rehabil* 12:193-202, 2005.
93. Tacon AM, McComb J, Caldera Y et al: Mindfulness meditation, anxiety reduction, and heart disease: a pilot study, *Fam Community Health* 26:25-33, 2003.
94. Tsai SL: Audio-visual relaxation training for anxiety, sleep, and relaxation among Chinese adults with cardiac disease, *Res Nurs Health* 27:458-468, 2004.
95. Frasure-Smith N, Lesperance F, Gravel G et al: Long-term survival differences among low-anxious, high-anxious and repressive copers enrolled in the Montreal heart attack readjustment trial, *Psychosom Med* 64:571-579, 2002.

chapter 42

Relationship Between Social Support and Cardiac Disease

Kathryn M. King
Tracey J.F. Colella

CHAPTER ABBREVIATIONS

CABG coronary artery bypass grafting

CAD coronary artery disease

ENRICHD Enhancing Recovery in Coronary Heart Disease Patients

HPA hypothalamic-pituitary-adrenal

MI myocardial infarction

SES socioeconomic status

SOLVD Study of Left Ventricular Dysfunction

SOCIAL SUPPORT

In the broadest sense, the term *social support* may encompass any process through which social relationships promote coping and thereby enhance psychological and physical health and well-being.[1,2] Generally, social support is a resource provided by others that can take the form of emotional support (provisions of confidant support or attachment); instrumental aid (provision of tangible support or material aid); information (provision of advice, guidance, appraisal, and problem solving); and positive feedback as to one's importance, capabilities, or self-worth (validation, integration, and feedback).[3] The broad term *social support* often is linked to other terms such as *social capital* (associated with available personal and community resources),[4] *social participation* (associated with activity), *social networks* (associated with breadth and depth of available social contact), and *social relationships* (associated with the quality of social contacts). Little consensus exists about how social support should be defined or measured, and difficulties arise in designing methodologically sound studies of social support interventions. Despite the diversity of how social support is conceptualized and concerns regarding methodological issues, reviews of the relevant literature to date consistently reveal a positive association between having social support and more healthful outcomes.[5-7] In general, interventions designed to alter social networks and reap enhanced social support have been successful in facilitating psychological adjustment, aiding in recovery from traumatic experiences, and even extending life for persons with serious chronic disease.[2]

The presence of high levels of social support is known to promote psychological and physical well-being, whereas low levels of social support have been identified as threatening health. The importance of social relationships in the maintenance of health and well-being and through the trajectory of disease has drawn attention across a large number of behavioral science and health disciplines. As a discipline that values a holistic perspective, nursing has had a long historical interest in the refinement of the concept, its measurement, and undertaking of studies of social support interventions.[8] For the purpose of this work, "social support" is considered in the broadest sense and captures some of these other related terms.

A variety of models exist to explain the role and influences of social support on health. In this chapter, the stress-buffering model is used as a basis for identification of and description of the mechanisms by which social support contributes to cardiovascular health outcomes (Figure 42-1). The stress-buffering model depicts social support as protecting persons from potentially harmful external influences from stressful events or determining individual responses to potentially stressful events.[1] The stress-buffering model is guided by the work of Lazarus and Folkman[9] in which coping involves the changing of cognitive and behavioral efforts to manage specific external environmental and/or internal demands that are appraised as exceeding the resources of the person. The coping process incorporates the dual goals of problem-resolution and emotion-regulation while using affective, cognitive and behavioral responses.

According to Cohen and colleagues,[1] receipt of social support may influence a person's appraisal of a stressor through responses to direct action such as the provision of information about the nature of the stressor or active effort to alleviate or diminish it. Social support also may influence a person's appraisal of a stressor through responses to indirect action, such as those involving social comparison. In this case, "normalization" of the feelings associated with the stressor can be enhanced when one compares oneself to others in similar situations. Supportive actions (direct) are thought to enhance coping performance, whereas perceptions of available support (indirect) lead to appraisal of threatening situations as less stressful. Founded on this mutual identification, shared experience, and sense of belonging, this is the theoretical basis that suggests that social support positively affects psychological and physical health outcomes.

Social support may buffer the effect of an objective stressor such as a myocardial infarction (**MI**) or coronary artery bypass grafting (**CABG**) surgery on outcomes such as anxiety and depression.[7] In a study of patients in cardiac rehabilitation, social support contrib-

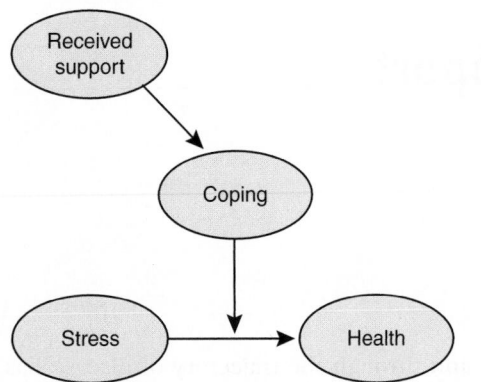

FIGURE 42-1 ■ The stress-buffering model. (From Cohen S, Underwood L, Gottlieb B: *Social support measurement and intervention: a guide for health and social scientists,* New York, 2000, Oxford University Press.)

uted to health outcomes not only directly but also indirectly through the mediation of less engagement in detrimental coping and lower depressive symptoms.[10] Cardiac rehabilitation patients who had higher levels of optimism and social support achieved better physical recovery that was not explained by demographic, health-related, or other psychosocial characteristics. The authors' conclusions supported the stress-buffering model as they concluded that social support and higher optimism likely mediate maladaptive coping and prevent depression.

Stress experiences can be short- or long-term (see Chapter 39), the effects of which can be modulated by, and in turn can influence, the availability of social support. For example, acute stressors can serve to mobilize social support networks. However, having chronically ill health can erode support networks (i.e., through less reciprocity in relationships) or access to support.[2,11] Pederson and colleagues,[11] for example, found that post-MI patients reported that social support significantly decreased over a 9-month period. The authors identified a concern regarding the potential negative consequences associated with support not being endlessly available. However, subjects' satisfaction regarding the social support received did not decrease significantly. These findings raise the question of timing (i.e., when is social support most needed) and dose (i.e., how much social support is needed) of social support interventions.

Social support can be a relatively accessible and low-cost intervention or resource for persons to reduce stress and enable maintenance of health. Holahan and colleagues[12] suggested that active coping was enhanced in a more supportive social context. A person's capacity for involvement in social networks (a source of social support) varies based on particular demographic characteristics. Persons who have higher levels of education and income are more likely to have higher levels of social support than those of lower socioeconomic status **(SES).** Men tend to have more broad social networks, whereas women have more intense social relationships. Women typically report having less social support than their male counterparts. Further, as persons age, they can have more available time to engage in social activi-

ties and reap social support. Conversely, social networks can decrease in size and social participation can be reduced as infirmity associated with age increases.[13] Moreover, culturally embedded customs of conduct also can influence the quality and receipt of social support. As yet unpublished data from Kathryn King support that certain ethnocultural groups value putting forward a particular image to others, which limits authentic and effective communications and relationships from which social support can be reaped.

Receipt of social support also can be technologically bound as technological contexts (i.e., access and competence) influence how social support can be offered and received.[8] For example, social support has been offered by telephone and Web-based access in a number of studies from a variety of health disciplines. Nursing studies undertaken largely in the 1980s and 1990s (e.g., Beckie[14]) typically revealed that telephone interventions by nurses, aimed at offering education and support, enhanced knowledge and reduced anxiety and depression in persons following an illness or event. Indeed, telephone support interventions have been used successfully in major clinical trials in cardiac patients.[15,16] Recently, Samarel and colleagues[17] revealed that telephone contact was as effective as in-person social support interventions.

As interest in peer support interventions has thrived (i.e., Colella and King[18]; Weinhert and colleagues[19]) and technological advances have been made, studies involving computer-based social support interventions have proliferated. Weinhert and colleagues[19] contend that computer-based technology offers a "new frontier" for developing and providing interventions and that "illness prevention, promotion of optimal self-management, and successful adaptation to illness can be enhanced by appropriate utilization of telecommunication technology" (p. 8). However, in a recent systematic review of "electronic support" studies, Eysenbach and associates[20] found that most studies to date have investigated complex interventions (including peer support, behavioral therapy, and education), making it difficult to draw specific conclusions regarding the relationship between particular electronic support interventions and outcome. Overall, these issues related to study design, which led the authors to conclude that there was no empirical evidence to suggest that electronic support interventions produce a benefit. Conceptually, these interventions have promise to enhance the capacity to offer and receive social support. However, in the "real world," having and successfully using telecommunication resources (i.e., telephone and computers) depends and relies ultimately on persons having financial resources to afford the hard (equipment) and soft (Internet connection) costs; technological competence; and capacity to communicate (language, typing ability/skill). Thus, these mechanisms for support may be limited by their access to persons who may need social support the most—those with lower socioeconomic and education status.

As identified before, one of the more difficult issues when considering the influence of social support on outcomes such as cardiovascular health and illness is to determine how social support is conceptualized and measured. The conceptualization of social support and its influencing factors were captured previously in this chapter. Important issues arise when measuring social support; the most fundamental issues are that the mechanism for measurement is consistent with the theoretical basis and appropriate for the group under study. For example, men tend to have more broad social networks, whereas women have more intense social relationships. Thus, an important factor in the study of men and women's social support would be whether it is the number of social contacts, their quality, or both that is being measured. The mechanism for measurement then could be objective (counting of the number of interactions) or subjective (reporting perceptions of quality) and could include measures of what activities or interactions a person has available to them, what activities or interactions in which they actually partake, or the perceptions of support received when partaking in some social activity. Important data would be missing for one or the other gender if breadth and quality of networks were not considered.

Though there are many well-documented benefits to the receipt of social support, there are less well-documented costs to those providing the support. Caring about others can be costly. One study revealed that "women seem emotionally more vulnerable to events that happen to members of their social networks"[2] (p. 66). In follow-up of 54,412 nurses enrolled in the Nurses' Health Study, Lee and colleagues[21] revealed that after adjusting for usual covariates (e.g., age, smoking, exercise, alcohol intake, body mass index, hypertension, and diabetes), the strain of caring for an ill or disabled spouse (but not parents or others) was associated with a nearly twofold increase in risk for the development of coronary artery disease **(CAD)** over a 4-year period. Having obligations to others can produce stressful demands, which in turn can be linked to the development of CAD.

LOW SOCIAL SUPPORT AND PSYCHOSOCIAL STRESSORS

Having low social support is but one of several interrelated psychosocial stressors that has been associated with the development of heart disease, ongoing morbidity, and mortality. These psychosocial stressors can be conceptualized in two general categories: emotional factors (i.e., major depression, anxiety disorders, hostility, and anger) and chronic stressors (i.e., low social support, low SES, work stress, marital stress, and caregiver strain). Psychosocial stressors usually do not occur in isolation; they often cluster. In turn, increase in heart disease risk and detrimental outcomes may be affected substantially because of the potential synergistic interaction among the stressors or with the conventionally considered risk factors.[7]

Studies have revealed the reciprocal and dynamic associations between psychosocial stressors. For example, the link between depression, an emotional factor, and low social support, a chronic stressor, has been the focus of intense investigation.[15,22-27] Depression has been

identified as a risk factor for heart disease independent of the classic coronary risk factors in patients with established CAD and in previously healthy persons.[28-31] Thus, it is imperative that depression be treated in at-risk persons. However, it is possible that depression is a marker of a broader phenomenon encompassing related behavioral and psychosocial stressors such as lack of social support, anger expression, hostility, negative emotions, and anxiety.[30] Social isolation or low perceived social support, as well as depression, confers an increased likelihood of engaging in high-risk behaviors such as smoking, eating a high-fat diet, and consuming excessive amounts of alcohol.[7] Further, depressed persons commonly experience problematic social experiences that in turn reinforce a depressive state and that can lead to an ongoing cycle of psychosocial risk.[32] Thus, determining where the focus of interventions should begin can be complex.

In a study of 2472 healthy persons, Brummett and colleagues[27] found that social support was more strongly inversely associated with depression in persons with lower income than those with higher income. Rapheal[13] recently concluded that low income and resulting poor social conditions pose the greatest risk for determining whether persons develop cardiovascular disease through the process of "social exclusion," which in turn causes excessive psychosocial stress. Indeed, SES is a powerful determinant of CAD incidence and outcomes.[29] Lower SES has been associated with lesser capacity to engage in self-care (less social activity, increased financial strain, stressful life events, and lower self-esteem) and increased exposure to chronic long-term psychosocial stress. Persons who have lower SES (i.e., lower income and education) are disproportionately susceptible to negative emotions, cognitions, and related disorders.[33] Though it is important to identify those at risk for a lack of social support, many of the purported root causes and associated psychosocial stressors may not be possible to "treat" by traditional mechanisms and can be modulated only through more broad initiatives such as social and political action.

LOW SOCIAL SUPPORT AND DEVELOPMENT OF CARDIAC DISEASE

Epidemiological evidence suggests that having high levels of social support and perceptions of social support are protective for the development of CAD in previously healthy persons. In seminal work, Berkman and Syme[34] revealed that having greater social support is associated with a reduction in all-cause mortality and, in particular, mortality from heart disease. The most important indicator of 9-year survival was the degree to which a person's social network and contacts were developed. Later, in frequently cited work, Berkman and colleagues[35] reported that having social support was a consistent predictor of survival 6 months following an MI, even when compared with sex, age, comorbidities, previous MI, and ventricular tachycardia. As outlined before, there is a theoretical and empirical link between low levels of actual and perceived social support and higher levels of psychological distress and stress.[12]

Stress plays a key role in the physiology of developing CAD, as explained later in this chapter.

Rozanski and colleagues[7] undertook an impressive review of the literature focusing on the relationship of psychosocial factors to the development of CAD. They summarized findings of studies (including those of Berkman and Syme[34] and Berkman and colleagues[35]) in which the influence of social support on the development of CAD was examined in previously healthy persons (average follow-up of 2.4 to 17 years). These authors identified that early studies focused on the "quantitative" aspects of social support (i.e., presence of spouse, number of friends, and extent of social participation) and that more recently, researchers have expanded their attention to the "qualitative" aspects of social support (i.e., the perception of support). Rozanski and colleagues[7] concluded that having a relatively small social network is associated with having on average a "2- to 3-fold increase in the incidence of CAD over time. Similarly, low levels of perceived emotional support confer an even greater increased risk for future cardiac events" (p. 2197). These findings are consistent across age groups, including the study of persons over the age of 65 years. More recently, following a 10-year prospective study of 6900 Swedish men and women, Sundquist and colleagues[4] found—after controlling for age, sex, education, housing tenure (i.e., home ownership), and smoking habits—that persons who had low social participation exhibited an almost 70 percent increased risk for developing CAD.

LOW SOCIAL SUPPORT AND CARDIAC EVENTS

A number of observational and interventional studies have been undertaken in persons with CAD that were aimed at examining and reducing the morbidity and mortality risk associated with low social support. For the most part, the focus of study has been on persons following MI. A recent systematic review of relevant epidemiological studies revealed that the lack of a social support network is associated with increased morbidity and mortality (2 to 3 times) in post-MI patients, which is independent of other known predictors of CAD morbidity and mortality (i.e., hypertension, reduced cardiac function, smoking, previous MI, age, and female sex).[5] Yet there is a body of research that suggests that this association does not exist or at least may not be direct. As indicated before, there is an interrelationship between social support and other psychosocial factors. One of the most frequently examined interrelationships investigated in patients with cardiac disease is social support and depression. Conflicting findings likely represent the dynamic associations between psychosocial stressors referred to before, the methodological issues associated with conceptualizing and measuring social support, and potentially a bias in selection of subjects and study participation—persons of lower SES groups and minority ethnocultural groups are less likely to participate in studies.[36,37] It is beyond the scope of this work to report exhaustively on the multitude of studies

in this domain. Thus, the following discussion is based on a sample of the most salient research to date.

In a study of 896 men and women following MI, Frasure-Smith and Lesperance[23] found that depression and negative affectivity, and not low social support (measured as perceived social support, as well as number of close friends and relatives) were associated directly with 5-year mortality. In a secondary analysis of data from 887 post-MI patients who were followed for a period of 1-year, Frasure-Smith and colleagues[24] found that only depression predicted cardiac mortality, but the strength of this relationship was reduced by increasing social support. Moreover, they found that persons who were depressed at baseline but who had high levels of social support were more likely to experience improvement in depression over a period of 1 year follow-up. After further analysis, Lesperance and colleagues[26] concluded that having perceived social support was associated with improvement in depression scores of persons who were mildly but not severely depressed at baseline. Thus, having higher levels of perceived social support appears to buffer the effect of lower levels of depression on 1-year mortality post-MI.[24] Yet in a large ($n = 583$) representative sample of patients admitted to a United Kingdom hospital following MI, the absence of a close confidant, and not depression, predicted further cardiac events within the first year. In this study, investigators focused on "the degree of intimacy" associated with the social relationships as opposed to the number of social contacts.[38]

Investigators are examining the effects of treating low levels of social support with an aim to reduce the potential detrimental association with cardiac morbidity and mortality. Two major trials with this aim have been undertaken in patients following MI; neither had an effect on mortality. Frasure-Smith and colleagues[16] hypothesized that a nurse who administered home-based supportive and educative intervention for post-MI patients would reduce mortality 1-year following hospital discharge. Patients ($n = 1376$) were assigned randomly to receive usual care or a protocol-driven, but individually tailored, intervention offered through monthly home visits over a period of 1 year. The interventions focused on the provision of emotional support, reassurance, education, and practical advice. This study revealed no positive effect of the intervention on cardiac and all-cause mortality. However, the most controversial findings were that women assigned to the intervention group had a higher mortality rate than women in the control group, and there was no evidence of any effect of the intervention on men. Though there were greater reductions in depression and anxiety scores in persons assigned to the intervention group, the investigators declared that these differences were "far from clinically significant" (p. 477). The investigators concluded that despite the "intuitive appeal" of offering psychosocial interventions, the outcomes may not be positive.

Subsequently, the Enhancing Recovery in Coronary Heart Disease Patients (**ENRICHD**)[15] trial revealed that treating low perceived social support and/or depression with cognitive behavioral therapy did not increase event-free survival in post-MI patients. This study was the largest of its kind to date (n = 2481). The trial investigators treated low perceived social support and/or depression with cognitive behavioral therapy and group therapy (when able) and supplemented this with antidepressant medication when indicated. Though the social support and depression scores improved significantly over time in the treatment group, there were no effects on morbidity or mortality in these patients.

Several reasons are possible for why these studies produced neutral (and negative) results. The investigators attempted to enroll subjects who were representative of the post-MI population at large; they were not, on the whole, suffering from depression or low levels of social support. Important subject recruitment issues with the trial undertaken by Frasure-Smith and colleagues[16] limited the number of women recruited into the study. Though the interventions in both studies were protocol-driven, they could not be standardized given their often "tailored" nature. Further, it is virtually impossible to appreciate what "dose" of the intervention was administered—rendering a concern that the "dose" was insufficient to produce the desired outcome. Finally, as indicated by the authors,[16] social support may be linked to mortality through only mild to moderate depression and thus may be less amenable to interventions in the general post-MI population.

Persons recovering from CABG surgery and those with heart failure have been underrepresented in psychosocial stress research. This may be in part because of the influence of the dynamic nature of recovery (i.e., early profound fatigue postoperatively that improves over time) and illness trajectories (i.e., reduced function and fatigue) on outcomes of interest such as depression.

Nonetheless, there is some beginning study of the influence of having social support on CABG surgery outcomes. Lindsay and colleagues[39] followed a cohort of 183 postoperative patients for a mean term of 16.4 months. Persons who had lower preoperative social network scores were less likely to have symptom relief than those who had higher social network scores. The authors concluded that social support may influence CABG surgery outcome. Conversely, Contrada and colleagues[40] found that independently, social support was unrelated to outcomes in a study of 142 post–CABG surgery patients. However, social support indeed was associated with the main variable of interest, stronger religious beliefs, which was associated with fewer postoperative complications and shorter hospital stays.

Through an extensive review of the literature, MacMahon and Lip[41] confirmed that the psychosocial stressors depression and anxiety are well investigated in the heart failure population but that there is a paucity of literature regarding the role of social support in morbidity and mortality from heart failure. In a substudy of 2992 subjects from the Study of Left Ventricular Dysfunction (**SOLVD**) Prevention and Treatment trials, Clarke and colleagues[42] found that patients with low ejection fractions and who were not well socially integrated, had high levels of anxiety or depressed mood or a low level of vigor, had low SES, and were non-white had a higher likelihood of experiencing serious limitations to activities of daily living 1 year later.

In another secondary analysis of data, Frasure-Smith and colleagues[24] identified that advanced Killip Class in post-MI patients leads to "more depression symptoms at 1 year than expected at baseline" (p. 1922). In a much smaller study of heart failure patients, the influence of social relationships (i.e., perceived social support and perceived social isolation) on mortality was examined. After controlling for depression, severity of heart failure, age, and functional status, Murberg and Bru[43] found that social isolation was a predictor of mortality over a period of 24 months.

Riegel and Carlson[44] undertook the only social support intervention study in this patient group; a trial of peer support intervention in heart failure patients. They encountered extraordinary difficulties in enrolling subjects rendering an underpowered study and basically neutral findings. The issues that lead to implementation difficulties with this study were similar to those in other previously cited psychosocial intervention studies: recruiting and maintaining subjects, managing the intervention, and determining the dose of the intervention. Notable is that recruitment was slow because the intervention did not appeal to the heart failure patients to whom it was offered.

LOW SOCIAL SUPPORT AND CARDIAC OUTCOMES
Physiological Mechanisms

Several biophysical mechanisms are sensitive to the effects of psychological and social stressors on myocardial perfusion, autonomic system regulation, platelet activation, hypothalamic-pituitary-adrenal (**HPA**) axis activity, and inflammatory processes. Recent studies provide clear and consistent evidence that psychosocial stressors contribute greatly to the pathogenesis and manifestations of CAD.[6] Compared with the traditionally considered CAD risk factors (i.e., smoking, dyslipidemia, hypertension, elevated body mass index, diabetes, and family history), the identification and role of psychosocial stressors (i.e., low social support, depression, anxiety, hostility/anger, low SES, and marital/work/caregiver strain) as risk factors now are gaining much recognition. The increased risk contributed by psychosocial stressors is of similar order to the more traditional risk factors that account for between 58 percent and 75 percent of cases of CAD.[45] Many of the biophysical mechanisms that lead to development of CAD may be triggered by psychosocial stressors, including low social support. "The relative risk of developing CAD owing to a lack of social support is 2- to 3-fold, even after controlling for conventional risk factors and social and behavioral demographic risk factors"[28] (p. 340).

Although the physiological correlates of emotion and stress can be protective, when prolonged or if occurring with excessive frequency and intensity, damage to bodily systems may occur, thereby resulting in health concerns.[46] Emotional strain and chronic stress can have a profound effect on the central nervous system, including increased output from the sympathetic nervous system and the HPA axis. See Chapter 39 for a complete discussion of the HPA axis and other physiological effects of stress.

Behavioral Mechanisms

DiMatteo[47] argued that obtaining improved health outcomes is mediated by the effect that social support has on adherence to treatment and health recommendations. Lack of adherence to lifestyle and therapeutic recommendations presents health care providers with challenges in primary and secondary cardiac risk prevention. In an early study of social support, Conn and colleagues[48] revealed that persons with low social support had more difficulty in undertaking some health-enhancing behaviors following MI. More recently, Thoits[2] contended that social "supporters can encourage (or sometimes sabotage) individuals' attempts to control their eating, drinking, smoking, or exercise behaviors; actively monitor and regulate a target's health-related behaviors; model or be co-participants in health-related activities; and urge medical treatment-seeking, among other possibilities" (p. 65). Husak and colleagues[49] examined the influence of social support on cardiac rehabilitation attendance in 944 patients who underwent first-time CABG surgery. Surprisingly, after adjustment for known correlates of social support (i.e., age, sex, and SES), they concluded that social support did not influence cardiac rehabilitation attendance.

Yet when undertaking a meta-analysis of 122 studies of the influence of social support on treatment adherence, DiMatteo[47] concluded that patient adherence is influenced strongly by the magnitude of adequate functional and structural social support. Further, the analysis revealed that functional measures of social support (i.e., practical, emotional, and family cohesiveness) more highly related to adherence than structural measures of social support (i.e., marital status and living arrangements of adults).

Health care providers need to be aware of the important relationship between social support and adherence to treatment recommendations. In the clinical setting, knowledge, skill, and time are required to screen persons for psychosocial stressors such as low social support or the potentially negative impact that a person's social environment may have. Health care providers need to be aware of the theoretical and clinical foundations of social support and its association to other psychosocial stressors and need to have the capacity to put this knowledge into action by effectively communicating with the at-risk person. Little clear evidence is available regarding the best approach to manage issues related to social support clinically. What is recognized with more certainty is that many psychosocial interventions are difficult and time consuming for health care providers to administer consistently. Nonetheless, when health care providers can assist patients to set beginning (i.e., ability to use knowledge to identify issues and communicate effectively), "micro," and realistic goals

for their health care (including enhancing social networks); offer feasible and practical suggestions and options to patients (which includes awareness of accessible community-based programs); and provide ongoing follow-up to monitor successes and challenges (which is supportive itself), patients' treatment adherence will be more successful.[7]

INTERVENTIONS TO ENHANCE SOCIAL SUPPORT

Despite the fact that key prospective cohort studies have revealed a consistent positive association between social support and health (including heart health) outcomes,* studies of social support interventions have rendered inconsistent outcomes.[14,16,20,23,50-59] (See the accompanying Conundrum feature.) In particular, what remains unclear is what kind of social support (i.e., functional, structural, or emotional) interventions are best, by whom it is best delivered (i.e., professional, peer, or family member), by which mechanism (i.e., in-person, by telephone, or through the Internet), or how often the intervention should be delivered to best meet the needs of the cardiac patient population. Moreover, patient needs may vary by the cardiac diagnosis and treatment received, as well as the patient's gender, age, and ethnicity.

Though questions remain regarding social support and its association with positive heart health outcomes, health care professionals must play a central role in the assessment of social support adequacy and identification of potential resources for patients and families in the hospital and community settings. Unfortunately, there is no gold standard mechanism to assess social support to determine a need or threshold at which to intervene, the best kind of social support for the need, or to assess potential benefits of an intervention. Nonetheless, as patient advocates, it is essential that nurses remain informed regarding the supportive networks that are readily available to patients and families experiencing cardiac events.

---

*References 4, 5, 21, 27, 34, 35.

■ ■ ■ CONUNDRUM

WHY DON'T ALL STUDIES SHOW AN IMPACT OF LOW SOCIAL SUPPORT?

- Problems exist in extracting or "teasing out" the influence of social support from the influences of other psychosocial stressors such as depression, socioeconomic status, level of education, and hostile personality.
- Social support is not well defined or measured.
- Social support is often not a stable construct. It can change, and a person's access to it can change over time.
- There is no evidence regarding the correct "dose" of social support that is needed.
- There is no clear evidence of the population for whom a social support intervention will have the most impact.
- The implementation of social support interventions and perceptions of social support will vary based on genders and cultural groups.

Various programs currently are available to cardiac patients and their families. For example, peer visitation programs such as Mended Hearts (in the United States and Canada; see *www.mendedhearts.org*) and Zipper Club (in the United States see *www.zipperclub. com*) offer in-hospital support and encouragement to cardiac patients and their families. Family and spousal support programs, often offered through individual institutions, also can offer education and support-based information for family members living with cardiac disease. Cardiac rehabilitation programs also have been shown successfully to offer a variety social supports to cardiac patients and families.[60] Moreover, innovative community-based programming also is being offered. One such program, the American Heart Association "Search Your Heart" program (see *www. americanheart.org*), is a faith-based (church) program for heart health and stroke prevention among communities of color. This program is aimed specifically at reducing heart disease in blacks and Latino/Hispanic American populations.

Based on the limited available evidence to date, to guide practice regarding social support, the following strategies may be helpful.

- Examine current social support networks to identify those patients who may be at higher risk for poor health outcomes. Ask patients about their social networks.[7,60]
- Work with current social support networks to increase their effectiveness. Help family members or others who offer social support to understand and enact supportive behaviors.
- Become aware of local resources (including mechanisms for travel). Refer patients to peer/social support groups within the hospital or local community settings.
- Reinforce the importance of cardiac rehabilitation and the excellent social support benefits that may be experienced by being a part of such a dynamic program (refer the patient to a local cardiac rehabilitation program).

CONCLUSION

Though the evidence is not consistent, having low levels of social support appears to place previously healthy persons and those who already have CAD at risk for morbidity and mortality. The challenge for researchers is to tease out the influence of other psychosocial stressors on health outcomes. The challenge for health care providers is to assist persons to modify factors that reduce their capacity to reap social support. There appears to be a threshold at which the improvement of social support affects health outcomes. Thus the challenge is to identify correctly those for whom the benefit of an intervention will be realized. Further, there is no clear evidence, as yet, regarding the nature or benefit of administering interventions in an attempt to modify social support. Though intuitively inconsistent, the major (i.e., large sample) trials[15,16] to date have shown no benefit, and in fact one[16] had findings suggestive of some harm.

The key to furthering an understanding of the linkage between psychosocial and conventional risk factor modification is ongoing investigation. Because some forms of psychosocial stress (i.e., depression) are subject to clinical modification, their contribution to the underlying development of disease may be reduced by interventions designed to treat such factors. The potential protective effect of psychosocial interventions designed to optimize an individual's social environment merit considerable attention. "There are many reasons why it is important to help people feel more loved, connected, and emotionally supported. It is no longer possible to be certain, however, that this will help them live longer"[61] (p. 414).

REFERENCES

1. Cohen S, Underwood L, Gottlieb B: *Social support measurement and intervention: a guide for health and social scientists,* New York, 2000, Oxford University Press.
2. Thoits PA: Stess, coping and social support processes: where are we? what next? *J Health Soc Behav* Spec Issue, pp 53-79, 1995.
3. House JS, Kahn RL: Measures and concepts of social support. In Cohen S, Syme SL, editors: *Social support and health,* Orlando, Fla, 1985, Academic Press.
4. Sundquist K, Lindström M, Malmström M et al: Social participation and coronary heart disease: a follow-up study of 6900 women and men in Sweden, *Soc Sci Med* 58:615-622, 2004.
5. Mookadam F, Arthur HM: Social support and its relationship to morbidity and mortality after acute myocardial infarction, *Arch Intern Med* 164:1514-1518, 2004.
6. Rozanski A, Blumenthal JA, Kaplan J: The impact of psychological factors on the pathogensesis of cardiovascular disease and implications for therapy, *Circulation* 99:2192-2217, 1999.
7. Rozanski A, Blumenthal JA, Davidson KW et al: The epidemiology, pathophysiology, and management of psychosocial risk factors in cardiac practice, *J Am Coll Cardiol* 45:637-651, 2005.
8. Stewart MJ, Tilden VP: The contributions of nursing science to social support, *Int J Nurs Stud* 32:535-544, 1995.
9. Lazarus RS, Folkman S: *Stress, appraisal and coping,* New York, 1984, Springer.
10. Shen B-J, McCreary CP, Myers HF: Independent and mediated contributions of personality, coping, social support, and depressive symptoms to physical functioning outcome among patients in cardiac rehabilitation, *J Behav Med* 27(1):39-62, 2004.
11. Pedersen SS, VanDomburg RT, Larsen ML: The effect of low social support on short-term prognosis in patients following a first myocardial infarction, *Scand J Psych* 45:313-318, 2004.
12. Holahan TK, Moos RH, Holahan CK et al: Social context, coping strategies and depressive symptoms: an expanded model with cardiac patients, *J Pers Soc Psychol* 72(4):918-928, 1997.
13. Raphael D: *Social justice is good for our hearts: why societal factors—not lifestyles—are major causes of heart disease in Canada and elsewhere,* Toronto, Ontario, Canada, 2002, CSJ Foundation for Research and Education.
14. Beckie T: A supportive-educative telephone program: impact on knowledge and anxiety after coronary artery bypass surgery, *Heart Lung* 18:46-55, 1989.
15. ENRICHD Study Investigators: Effects of treating depression and low perceived social support on clinical events after myocardial infarction: the Enhancing Recovery in Coronary Heart Disease Patients (ENRICHD) randomized trial, *JAMA* 289:3106-3116, 2003.
16. Frasure-Smith N, Lesperance F, Prince RH et al: Randomised trial of home-based psychosocial nursing intervention for patients recovering from myocardial infarction, *Lancet* 350:473-479, 1997.
17. Samarel N, Tulman L, Fawcett J: Effects of two types of social support and education on adaptation to early-stage breast cancer, *Res Nurs Health* 25:459-470, 2002.

18. Colella TJF, King KM: Peer support: an under-recognized resource in cardiac recovery, *Eur J Cardiovasc Nurs* 3:211-217, 2004.

19. Weinhert C, Cudney S, Winters C: Social support in cyberspace: the next generation, *Comput Inform Nurs* 23(1):7-15, 2005.

20. Eysenbach G, Powell J, Englesakis M et al: Health related virtual communities and electronic support groups: systematic review of the effects of online peer to peer interactions, *BMJ* 328:1116-1122, 2004.

21. Lee S, Colditz GA, Berkman LF, Kawachi I: Caregiving and risk of coronary heart disesase in US women: a prospective study, *Am J Prev Med* 24:113-119, 2003.

22. ENRICHD Study Investigators: Enhancing recovery in coronary heart disease (ENRICHD) study intervention: rationale and design, *Psychosom Med* 63:747-755, 2001.

23. Frasure-Smith N, Lesperance F: Depression and other psychological risks following myocardial infarction, *Arch Gen Psychiatry* 60:627-636, 2003.

24. Frasure-Smith N, Lesperance F, Gravel G et al: Social support, depression, and mortality during the first year after myocardial infarction, *Circulation* 101:1919-1924, 2000.

25. Frasure-Smith N, Lesperance F, Juneau M et al: Gender, depression, and one-year prognosis after myocardial infarction, *Psychosom Med* 61:26-37, 1999.

26. Lesperance F, Frasure-Smith N, Talajic M et al: Five-year risk of cardiac mortality in relation to initial severity and one-year changes in depression symptoms after myocardial infarction, *Circulation* 105:1049-4053, 2002.

27. Brummett BH, Barefoot JC, Vitaliano PP et al: Associations among social support, income, and symptoms of depression in an educated sample: the UNC Alumni Heart Study, *Int J Behav Med* 10(3):239-250, 2003.

28. Gallacher JE, Sweetnam PM, Yarnell JW et al: Is type A behavior really a trigger for coronary heart disease events? *Psychosom Med* 65:339-346, 2003.

29. Strike PC, Steptoe A: Psychosocial factors in the development of coronary artery disease, *Prog Cardiovasc Dis* 46:337-347, 2004.

30. Lett H, Blumenthal JA, Babyak M et al: Depression as a risk factor for coronary artery disease: evidence, mechanisms and treatment, *Psychosom Med* 66:305-315, 2004.

31. Ford DE, Mead LA, Chang PP et al: Depression is a risk factor for coronary artery disease in men, *Arch Intern Med* 158:1422-1426, 1998.

32. Gallo LC, Bogart LM, Vranceanu AM et al: Socioeconomic status, resources, exposure and emotional reactivity to stress: a test of the reserve capacity model, *J Pers Soc Psychol* 88:386-399, 2005.

33. Gallo LC, Matthews KA: Understanding the association between socioeconomic status and physical health: do negative emotions play a role? *Psychol Bull* 129:10-51, 2003.

34. Berkman LF, Syme SL: Social networks, host resistance and mortality: a 9 year follow-up study of Alameda County residents, *Am J Epidemiol* 109:198-204, 1979.

35. Berkman LF, Leo-Summers L, Horwitz RI: Emotional support and survival after myocardial infarction: a prospective, population-based study of the elderly, *Ann Intern Med* 117:1003-1009, 1992.

36. Gilliss CL, Lee KA, Gutierrez Y et al: Recruitment and retention of healthy minority women into community-based longitudinal research, *J Womens Health Gend Based Med* 10(1):77-85, 2001.

37. Lindenberg CS, Solorzano RM, Vilaro FM, Westbrook LO: Challenges and strategies for conducting intervention research with culturally diverse populations, *J Transcult Nurs* 12(2):132-139, 2001.

38. Dickens CM, McGowan L, Perciaval C et al: Lack of a close confidant, but not depression, predicts further cardiac events after myocardial infarction, *Heart* 90:518-522, 2004.

39. Lindsay GM, Smith LN, Hanlon P et al: The influence of general health status and social support on symptomatic outcome following coronary artery bypass grafting, *Heart* 85:80-86, 2001.

40. Contrada RJ, Goyal TM, Cather C et al: Psychosocial factors in outcomes of heart surgery: the impact of religious involvement and depressive symptoms, *Health Psychol* 23:227-238, 2004.

41. MacMahon KMA, Lip GYH: Psychosocial factors in heart failure, *Arch Intern Med* 162:509-516, 2002.

42. Clarke SP, Frasure-Smith N, Lesperance F et al: Psychosocial factors as predictors of functional status at 1 year in patients with left ventricular dysfunction, *Res Nurs Health* 23:290-300, 2000.

43. Murberg TA, Bru E: Social relationships and mortality in patients with congestive heart failure, *J Psychosom Res* 51:521-527, 2001.

44. Riegel B, Carlson B: Is individual peer support a promising intervention for persons with heart failure? *J Cardiovasc Nurs* 19: 174-183, 2004.

45. Beaglehole R, Magnus P: The search for new risk factors for coronary heart disease: occupational therapy for epidemiologists? *Int J Epidemiol* 31:1117-1122, 2002.

46. McEwen B, Lasley EN: Allostatic load: when protection gives way to damage, *Adv Mind Body Med* 19:28-33, 2003.

47. DiMatteo MR: Social support and adherence to medical treatment: a meta-analysis, *Health Psychol* 23:207-218, 2004.

48. Conn VS, Taylor SG, Hayes V: Social support, self-esteem, and self-care after myocardial infarction, *Health Values* 16:25-31, 1992.

49. Husak L, Krumholz HM, Lin ZQ et al: Social support as a predictor of participation in cardiac rehabilitation after coronary artery bypass graft surgery, *J Cardiopulm Rehabil* 24:19-26, 2004.

50. ENRICHD Study Investigators: Enhancing recovery in coronary heart disease patients (ENRICHD): study design and methods, *Am Heart J* 139:1-9, 2000.

51. Gilliss CL, Gortner SR, Hauck W et al: A randomized clinical trial of nursing care for recovery from cardiac surgery, *Heart Lung* 322(2):125-133, 1993.

52. Parent N, Fortin F: A randomized, controlled trial of vicarious experience through peer support for male first-time cardiac surgery patients: impact on anxiety, self-efficacy expectation and self-reported activity, *Heart Lung* 29(6):389-400, 2000.

53. Halfmann SM: Peer support with a nurse-managed intervention and compliance after a cardiac event, doctoral dissertation, Denton, TX], 2000, Texas Women's University.

54. Roebuck A: Telephone support in the early post-discharge period following elective cardiac surgery: does it reduce anxiety and depression levels? *Intensive Crit Care Nurs* 15(3):142-146, 1999.

55. Thoits P, Hohmann AA, Harvey MR, Fletcher B: Similar-other support for men undergoing coronary artery bypass surgery, *Health Psychol* 19(3):264-273, 2000.

56. Hartford K, Wong C, Zakaria D: Randomized controlled trial of a telephone intervention by nurses to provide information and support to patients and their partners after elective coronary artery bypass graft surgery: effects of anxiety, *Heart Lung* 31(3): 199-206, 2002.

57. Gallagher R, McKinley S, Dracup K: Effects of a telephone counseling intervention on psychosocial adjustment in women following a cardiac event, *Heart Lung* 3279-3287, 2003.

58. Harkness K, Smith KM, Taraba L et al: Effect of a postoperative telephone intervention on attendance at intake cardiac rehabilitation after coronary artery bypass graft surgery, *Heart Lung* 34(3):179-186, 2005.

59. Weaver LA, Doran KA: Telephone follow-up after cardiac surgery, *Am J Nurs* 101(5):24OO-24TT, 2001.

60. Prior P, Cupper L: Behavioural, psychosocial and vocational issues in cardiovascular disease. In Stone JA, editor: *Canadian guidelines for cardiac rehabilitation and cardiovascular disease prevention,* ed 2, Winnipeg, Manitoba, Canada, 2004, Canadian Association of Cardiac Rehabilitation.

61. Barr TC: Social support for patients after myocardial infarction, *J Cardiopulm Rehabil* 23:413-414, 2003.

chapter 43

Novel and Emerging Risk Factors for Coronary Heart Disease

Lorraine Frazier
Suzanne Hughes

CHAPTER ABBREVIATIONS

APO   apolipoprotein

ATP   Adult Treatment Panel

CHD   coronary heart disease

HDL   high-density lipoprotein

hs-CRP   high-sensitivity C-reactive protein

ICAM   intracellular adhesion molecule

LDL   low-density lipoprotein

Lp(a)   lipoprotein (a)

Lp-PLA2   lipoprotein-associated phospholipase A2

MACE   major adverse coronary event

VCAM   vascular cell adhesion molecule

Currently known risk factors that independently predict coronary heart disease (**CHD**) do not account for all disease cases. Of particular concern is that not all individuals with the traditional risk factors have an event, and health care professionals are unable to predict firmly which patients with diagnosed CHD will go on to have an event. The search is under way for novel risk factors that will enable clinicians to do the following accurately:

- Detect early disease in asymptomatic patients
- Predict which individuals with CHD will go on to develop a major adverse coronary event (**MACE**)
- Direct interventions and lifestyle changes to individuals at the greatest risk

The quest for risk factors that are specific and sensitive for coronary vascular outcomes has led to aggressive research on biomarkers of underlying pathophysiological processes such as inflammation and coronary plaque burden. Systemic biomarkers in healthy individuals and individuals diagnosed with CHD are being studied for their ability to predict future cardiac events. These novel biomarkers of cardiovascular risk include protein molecules in the plasma, genetic markers, and patterns of plaque that can be detected using new radiological technologies (Figure 43-1). These markers are being studied along the disease continuum for association with disease pathology, response to clinical interventions, and outcomes after adjusting for other accepted coronary risk factors.

DEFINITION OF A RISK MARKER

CHD studies designed to measure risk are typically non-experimental because ethically it is not possible to assign a CHD risk factor randomly to a group of study participants. Moreover, novel risk markers of CHD could not be assigned randomly because they are usually genetic or plasma biomarkers. However, biomarkers can be measured in relation to interventions or events. For example, biomarker level samples can be drawn during a particular window of time after a patient complains of chest pain or receives an intervention, such as a coronary stent. Plasma marker levels before and after the intervention, or the change in biomarker levels, may be associated with disease outcomes.

A risk factor is determined in research by studying a group of individuals but is applied on an individual basis. If a large number of the group that has the risk factor in consideration develops the disease compared with the group that did not have the risk factor, the risk factor is determined to be a marker of the group at increased risk. The association, however, does not determine whether the marker is a cause of disease, and this is an important distinction. The novel biomarkers discussed in this chapter are technically not risk factors, but risk markers of disease. They may not cause the disease, but they may be associated with a confounding or associated factor that causes disease. Experimental intervention studies would be necessary to suggest that any of these markers are a cause of CHD.

EMERGING AND NOVEL RISK FACTORS
Inflammation

The atherosclerosis process is inflammatory, and inflammation is believed to be the main contributor to plaque rupture.[1] The infiltration of macrophages into the coronary artery is one of the most important events associated with the rupture of coronary plaque, coronary plaque erosion in acute myocardial infarction, and sudden cardiac death.[2]

The endothelium is thought to be the source of inflammation in the coronary system. The development of atherosclerosis involves the recruitment of leukocytes to the endothelium by the adhesive interaction with leukocytes. During the inflammatory process, circulating leukocytes express adhesion molecule receptors that allow leukocytes to bind to the endothelial cell ad-

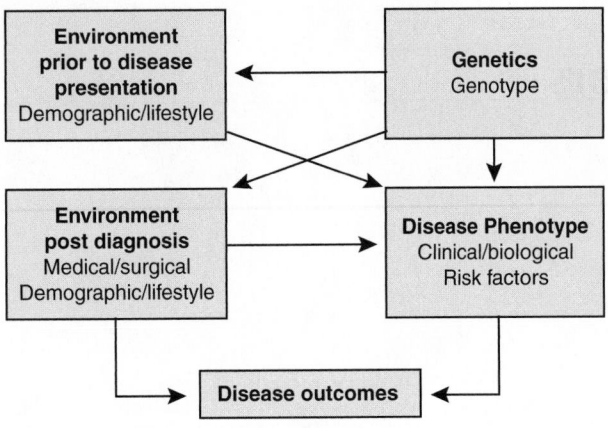

FIGURE 43-1 ■ Model of disease risk.

hesion molecules such as intracellular adhesion molecule (**ICAM**) 1 and vascular cell adhesion molecule (**VCAM**) on the endothelial surface.[3] These adhesion molecules recruit monocytes from the peripheral blood supply to the site of endothelial injury in the coronary wall. Selectins (E-selectin and P-selectin) then mediate the rolling and adhesion of the monocytes across the endothelium and the ability of the monocytes eventually to transect the vessel wall. The monocytes that are recruited to the endothelium migrate into the arterial wall with the help of the protein molecules, chemoattractant cytokines, and monocyte chemoattractant protein 1.[4] Monocyte chemoattractant protein 1 can be produced by normal arterial endothelial cells when stimulated by inflammatory mediators.

Once inside the coronary artery, the monocytes differentiate into macrophages and become major players in the inflammation process through the production of cytokines and the activation of the immune response. The uptake of modified lipoproteins by the macrophages is regulated by cytokines as part of the immune response of the host.

Markers of inflammation are present in stable and unstable coronary disease. They may *initiate* atherosclerosis and the development of an acute coronary event from coronary plaque rupture. Bursts of increased markers are present during periods of plaque rupture (Figure 43-2). These more novel markers are being studied currently for their influence on cardiovascular outcomes. More studies are needed before these markers can be

used in the clinical setting. The role of inflammation in cardiac disease is covered in detail in Chapter 9.

Inflammatory Markers

Novel markers of inflammation currently are being reported in the literature as risk factors of future coronary events in healthy individuals and in patients with CHD. Some of the markers available for use in clinical practice include leukocytes, high-sensitivity C-reactive protein (**hs-CRP**), homocysteine, and lipoprotein (Figure 43-3).

The leukocyte count, although a commonly used laboratory test, has been shown in retrospective cohort studies and in case-control studies to be an independent predictor of CHD after adjusting for other independent risk factors.[5] Although the test is inexpensive and reliable and is performed routinely in most patients, more research is needed to understand the impact of a high white blood cell count. Leukocytosis affects CHD by mediating the inflammation process causing proteolytic and oxidative damage to the coronary arteries.[6] This process may obstruct the blood flow in the microvasculature of the heart and cause infarct expansion by plugging capillaries.

Selectins and Vascular Adhesion Molecules

Selectins and adhesion molecules have been shown to vary during CHD pathology and clinical interventions and to be predictive of future MACE. For example, plasma ICAM and VCAM levels increase with ventricular reperfusion dysrhythmias that occur after coronary angioplasty[7] and after administration of tissue plasminogen activator.[8] The increase in inflammatory markers after coronary interventions may persist from 72 hours[9] up to 6 months. After acute coronary plaque rupture, VCAM and ICAM remain elevated for a 6-month period.[10]

Comorbidities that cause inflammation influence individual levels of inflammatory markers in patients with CHD. Elevations of cellular adhesion molecules (ICAM and VCAM), platelet adhesion molecule (P-selectin),[11] and endothelial-leukocyte adhesion molecule (E-selectin) during coronary insults vary with diabetes,[12] hypercholesterolemia,[13] and sepsis related to infections.[14]

Selectins and vascular adhesion molecules are not recommended as clinical tests for treatment in CHD at this time. They are part of a group of many inflammatory markers that are being studied to determine disease pathways and their influence on disease and disease outcomes. Future technology of the measurement of in-

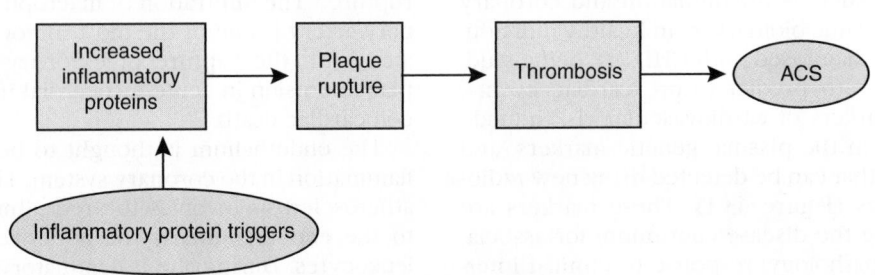

FIGURE 43-2 ■ Increased proinflammatory cytokines in acute coronary syndrome. *ACS,* Acute coronary syndrome.

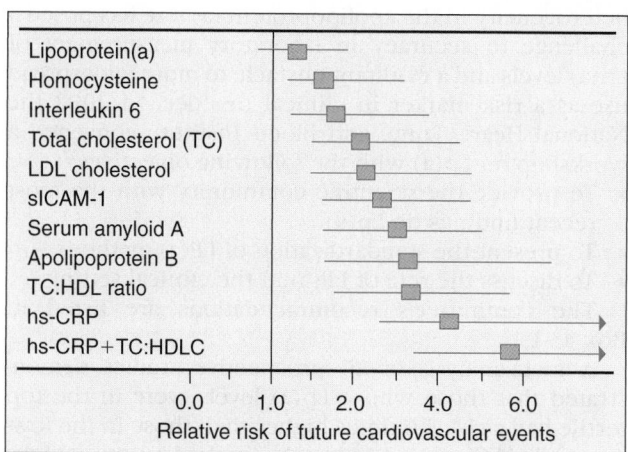

FIGURE 43-3 ▪ Relative risks of future myocardial infarction among apparently healthy women according to baseline levels of lipoprotein (a), homocysteine, interleukin-6, total cholesterol, low-density lipoprotein *(LDL)* cholesterol, soluble intercellular adhesion molecule-1 *(sICAM-1)*, serum amyloid A, apolipoprotein B, the ratio of total cholesterol to high-density lipoprotein cholesterol *(TC: HDLC)*, high-sensitivity C-reactive protein *(hs-CRP)*, and the combination of hs-CRP with the TC:HDLC. (From Ridker PM: *Circulation* 107:363, 2003.)

dividual protein expressions of the proteome in response to CHD and clinical interventions will allow the measurement and the identification of the known, the novel, and the unknown proteins and markers of disease.

C-Reactive Protein

CRP is an acute-phase reactant that increases in response to acute and chronic infection such as arthritis, smoking, diabetes, and obesity. Less than 2 percent of the population has levels that indicate a clinical condition (greater than 1.5 mg /dl).[15] CRP elevations also may contribute to the development of further inflammation/atherosclerosis by inducing the increase of other inflammatory markers such as adhesion molecules.[16]

CRP levels have been shown to reflect systemic inflammation and to be prognostic of future cardiovascular events independent of other cardiovascular disease risk factors. Elevated CRP levels (CRP levels higher than 3 mcg/ml) are associated with increased risk of future coronary events.[17] Hs-CRP should be used for risk prediction. In the Women's Health Study, nonfasting hs-CRP identified individuals with cardiovascular disease who were at higher risk of further CHD events.[18] The study used the CRP cutoff points endorsed by the American Heart Association and Centers for Disease Control and Prevention, which are less than 1 mg/dl (low risk), 1 to 3 mg/dl (medium risk), and greater than 3 mg/dl (high risk).

Although hs-CRP levels predict CHD prognosis and outcomes, typically investigators have excluded patients with chronic or acute comorbidities of inflammation from studies. Thus, it is unclear whether hs-CRP predicts events in CHD patients with comorbidities involving inflammation. As a general marker of inflammation in clinical practice, the clinician should consider the influence of other comorbidities on CRP levels.

National Cholesterol Education Program Expert Panel on Detection, Evaluation, and Treatment of High Blood Cholesterol in Adults (Adult Treatment Panel [ATP] III) guidelines recommend that in patients with high CRP levels, the level should be used to consider more aggressive treatment of low-density lipoprotein (**LDL**) cholesterol.[19] Although CRP explains risk of future CHD beyond the risk predicted by elevated LDL, there is no evidence to show that reducing CRP levels reduces future CHD risk.[20]

Homocysteine

Homocysteine, a sulfur-containing amino acid, is also an independent predictor of CHD. Homocysteine promotes increased thrombosis, consumption of nitric oxide, endothelial injury, and reduced thrombolysis. Homocysteine levels, like CRP levels, are elevated with smoking, aging, and chronic inflammatory disorders such as rheumatoid arthritis and lupus.[21] Plasma levels also can be influenced by renal function[22] and hyperinsulinemia.[23]

Homocysteine levels are measured through immunoassay. A fasting level is needed, and the sample needs to be frozen unless the analysis will be conducted within 24 hours.[24] A meta-analysis of 27 studies reported an increased risk of CHD (odds ratio 1.7) in patients with homocysteine levels over the 90th percentile.[25] Homocysteine levels greater than 10.2 μmol/liter are associated with a doubling of CHD risk. Levels over 20 μmol/ liter are associated with a 9.9 times increase in CHD risk compared with levels under 9 μmol/liter.[26]

Vitamin B_{12}, vitamin B_6, and folic acid are required for homocysteine metabolism.[27] Folic acid supplements reduce homocysteine levels through the conversion of homocysteine to the essential amino acid methionine. Homocysteine levels in the population have decreased since the addition of folic acid to the food supply to decrease neural tube defects. A cohort study of 2755 subjects revealed that in 1998 only 28 percent had high levels.[24] Because elevations of homocysteine usually stem from poor dietary intake of folate and folic acid supplements are inexpensive, supplements usually are recommended without screening for homocysteine levels. When homocysteine levels are elevated, the ATP III guidelines recommend that vitamin B_{12} levels be measured. If vitamin B_{12} levels are normal, increasing folate intake is recommended.

Homocysteine levels increase with age and menopause,[28] but because of the low prevalence of elevated homocysteine levels in the United States, ATP III guidelines do not recommend homocysteine screening for risk assessment in primary prevention.[19] Screening is usually only relevant for individuals with no traditional risk factors and a strong family history of CHD risk.

Lipid Markers

Low-Density Lipoprotein Particle Size and Density

LDL has a wide range of molecular sizes. The LDL level reported on a standard lipid profile test is the sum of all LDL particles in a deciliter of plasma. LDL particles vary greatly, however, in size, density, and composition.

Small, dense LDL particles are more atherogenic than larger, more buoyant LDL particles. Some lipidologists believe that measurement of LDL particle size and density provides additional data for assigning appropriate dyslipidemic therapy.

Small, dense LDLs are present in individuals with hypertriglyceridemia, central obesity, and insulin resistance.[29] Genetics and the environment influence the phenotype of small, dense LDL. For simplification, the particles have been dichotomized at a cut point of 24.5 nm that allows identification of an LDL phenotype. Phenotype A are individuals with a peak LDL diameter greater than 24.5 nm, and phenotype B are individuals with a peak LDL diameter less than 24.5 nm. Although phenotype A individuals are at a reduced risk for heart disease, phenotype B individuals are at increased risk independent of traditional risk factors. Phenotype B is associated with a twofold increase in triglyceride level.[30] The prevalence of small, dense LDL (phenotype B) differs with menopausal status and gender. The phenotype is 5 to 10 percent in males younger than age 20 and in premenopausal women, 30 to 35 percent in adult men, and 15 to 25 percent in postmenopausal women.[31] The B phenotype has been linked to a region of the LDL receptor gene locus on chromosome 19p.[32] Several genes most likely are involved with the B phenotype.[33] Environment by genotype interaction of the B phenotype and other genes may contribute to familial dyslipidemia syndromes.[34]

The size, density, and composition of the LDL particle are not measured as part of the standard lipid profile but can be measured using one of several methods. These methods are gradient gel electrophoretic measurement, nuclear magnetic resonance imaging technology, and vertical auto profile. However, because the measurement of small LDL particles is expensive and not yet standardized, the ATP III guidelines do not recommend measurement at this time. The only use of such measures at this time is in patients with metabolic syndrome or dyslipidemia in whom identification of elevations would support increased lifestyle changes. The ATP III guidelines suggest that nicotinic acid or fibric acid be considered when small LDL particles and low high-density lipoprotein (**HDL**) or high triglyceride levels are present.[19]

Lipoprotein (a)

Lipoprotein (a) [**Lp(a)**] was first described by Berg in 1963.[35] Lp(a) is composed of equal parts of apolipoprotein (a) and apolipoprotein B-100, linked by a disulfide bond. The biological function of Lp(a) is not known. Because apolipoprotein (a) is structurally similar to plasminogen and apolipoprotein B (**APO** B) is atherogenic, Lp(a) has unique potential to be atherogenic and prothrombotic. Lp(a) appears to participate in atherothrombosis by competing with plasminogen for plasma biding sites, thus inhibiting thrombolysis.[36] Additionally, there is evidence that Lp(a) contributes to foam cell formation, reduction of endothelium-dependent vasodilatation, and oxidation of LDL. The size of the apolipoprotein (a) portion of Lp(a) varies widely. Smaller particles translate into higher Lp(a) concentrations. This heterogeneity in the apolipoprotein (a) size has posed a challenge to accuracy in laboratory measurement of Lp(a) levels and a resultant obstacle to more widespread use as a risk marker in clinical practice. In 2002 the National Heart, Lung, and Blood Institute convened a workshop on Lp(a) with the following objectives[37]:

- To provide the scientific community with the most recent findings on Lp(a)
- To present the standardization of LP(a) methods
- To discuss the role of LP(a) in the clinical setting

The committee's recommendations are listed in Box 43-1.

A meta-analysis of 27 prospective studies demonstrated that those whose Lp(a) levels were in the top tertile had a risk 1.6 times higher than those in the lowest tertile.[38] Causation cannot be implied by any association noted in retrospective and cross-sectional trials because Lp(a) is an acute-phase reactant that rises in response to myocardial infarction. Niacin is the only dyslipidemic agent that lowers Lp(a), but there is no evidence that modification is associated with improved clinical outcomes.

Apolipoprotein B

Some researchers and clinicians hold that measurement of APO-B actually should replace LDL as the primary target of lipid-lowering therapy.[39] APO B-100 is the major apolipoprotein component of each of the atherogenic lipoproteins: very low-density lipoprotein, LDL, and intermediate-density lipoprotein. Patients with type 2 diabetes or with metabolic syndrome frequently have hypertriglyceridemia along with hyper-APO B. The risk conferred by this lipid abnormality may not be appreciated fully because levels of LDL may be normal or even low. The National Cholesterol Education Program ATP III guidelines name non-HDL cholesterol (actually total APO-B) as a secondary target of treatment. APO-B, which does

---

BOX 43-1 ■ ■ ■

RECOMMENDATIONS FROM THE NATIONAL HEART, LUNG, AND BLOOD INSTITUTE WORKSHOP, LIPOPROTEIN(a) AND CARDIOVASCULAR DISEASE

- Continue the standardization efforts that have been undertaken by the National Heart, Lung, and Blood Institute, such as validation of the accuracy of the analytical methods, use of the primary and secondary reference materials developed and validated under the National Heart, Lung, and Blood Institute lipoprotein(a) contract, and pursuit of a common approach to express lipoprotein(a) values in all studies.
- Promote more basic research to understand the fundamental functions and mechanism of actions of lipoprotein(a) and the mechanisms of lowering lipoprotein(a) levels.
- Encourage the development of animal models to study lipoprotein(a).
- Support large clinical and epidemiological studies performed with validated analytical methods and sound study design to establish the clinical relevance and the predictive power of lipoprotein(a).
- Establish common population-based reference values and lipoprotein(a) values for clinical decision.
- Design and implement a clinical study to evaluate the clinical usefulness of lowering lipoprotein(a) levels.

Information from Marcovina SM, Koschinsky ML, Albers JJ et al: *Clin Chem* 49:1785-1796, 2003.

not require a fasting sample, is a single marker for all of the atherogenic lipoproteins and thus might simplify risk assessment.[40]

Lipoprotein-Associated Phospholipase A2

Lipoprotein-associated phospholipase A2 (**Lp-PLA2**) is technically an inflammatory marker for atherosclerosis; however, discussion is included in the lipid section because of its association with small, dense LDL. Most of the circulating Lp-PLA2 is bound to LDL cholesterol, particularly to small, dense LDL particles. Lp-PLA2 hydrolyzes phospholipids. As with other inflammatory markers, the predictive ability of Lp-PLA2 is complicated by its association with other atherosclerotic risk factors. Epidemiological studies have shown an independent association between Lp-PLA2 and CHD, but at this time Lp-PLA2 is not measured routinely in clinical practice.[41]

Apolipoprotein E Isoforms

The APO E isoform is a genetically determined characteristic that has an impact on LDL cholesterol. APO E has three major variations: E2, E3, and E4. One copy is inherited from each parent. The distribution varies by racial and ethnic group, but E3 appears in approximately 75 percent of a normal white population, E4 in 15 percent, and E2 in 8 percent. The most common combination is E3/E3. Those carrying the intron 4 allele have a higher risk of coronary and carotid disease and stroke.[42] Evidence indicates that the intron 4 allele interacts with environmental factors, such as smoking, to increase cardiovascular risk.[43]

Apolipoprotein A-I Milano

A variant of APO A-I called APO A-I Milano was found in 40 inhabitants of a small northern Italian village. Despite low levels of HDL (mean levels were less than 20 mg/dl), these carriers exhibited longevity and relatively low levels of atherosclerosis.[44] A recombinant form of this variant apolipoprotein was developed and tested on the mouse model, and it was discovered that plaque burden was quickly reduced in mice with experimental atherosclerosis.[45] Next, the synthetic APO A-I Milano was administered to patients with acute coronary syndrome, demonstrating a 4.2 percent reduction change in atheroma burden after 5 weekly doses as measured by intravascular ultrasound.[46] This study, although small, has important implications for future studies.

Genetic Abnormalities

Cardiovascular disease results from the interplay of many genes with the environment and behavior. Genetic factors influence the expression of the CHD phenotype. Genetic factors also affect the outcomes of clinical interventions and therefore ultimately influence disease outcomes through many biological pathways that include inflammation, endothelial dysfunction, thrombosis, and vascular reactivity.

Because CHD is a common complex disease involving many disease pathways, many genes are involved. Genetic variation and gene-gene interactions in these biological pathways influence CHD along the disease continuum. To date, elevated LDL cholesterol, low HDL cholesterol, and elevated triglycerides and lipoproteins have the most significant genetic component.[47] Major monogenetic disorders of familial hypercholesterolemia also increase CHD risk by raising LDL levels. These disorders have genetic variations in the APO B/E receptor mutations that are autosomal codominant. APO B mutations for familial hypercholesterolemia are rare (1 in 1 million persons).[48] APO E variations lead to increased susceptibility to severe dyslipidemia and increases in LDL levels and CHD risk.

Results of large meta-analysis studies of heart disease indicate that specific gene polymorphisms influence disease risk (Table 43-1). Despite these results, there is still an incomplete understanding of these genetic effects on the increased risk of CHD. Plasma lipid levels represent an integrated marker of genetic and environmental influences.[50]

Genetic variation may account for the fact that plaque burden, vascular reactivity, levels of inflammation, and CHD prevalence is higher in blacks compared with the general U.S. population. Genetic variation also may account for the varied individual response to drug therapy in patients at higher risk for MACE.[51]

Periodontal Disease

The majority of studies on periodontal disease and CHD demonstrate increased CHD risk associated with periodontitis. Causality has yet to be demonstrated, and some hypothesize that the association between periodontitis and CHD may be a result of other lifestyle factors (high intake of fat, smoking, lack of exercise, stress) associated with periodontitis that contribute to CHD risk.[52]

However, a biological rationale exists for a causal association of periodontal disease and CHD that fits within the model for infection as a cause of CHD. Infection of the oral cavity certainly could precipitate a systemic infection that results in rupture of a vulnerable coronary plaque in an individual with CHD. The periodontal pocket in the oral cavity is able to harbor high numbers of gram-negative anaerobic microorganisms. The bacteria involved in oral infections have strong ad-

■ ■ ■

TABLE 43-1 GENETIC POLYMORPHISMS THAT INFLUENCE CORONARY HEART DISEASE RISK

GENE/ POLYMORPHISM	EFFECT	ODDS RATIO
Two copies of intron-4a alleles of endothelial nitric oxide synthase[49]	Moderate increase in coronary heart disease risk	1.31 (95% CI, 1.13-1.51)
Apolipoprotein B gene SpIns/Del DD[49]	Increase myocardial infarction risk	1.73 (95% CI, 1.19-2.50)
	Increase coronary heart disease risk	1.19 (95% CI, 1.05-1.35)

CI, Confidence interval.

hesive properties that may assist in their ability to adhere to the endothelial cells in the coronary arteries.

Influenza

Up to 90,000 deaths per year in the United States may be caused by fatal myocardial infarctions that were triggered by the influenza virus. Influenza is responsible for 20 million to 25 million physician visits and 52,000 deaths annually. Such outbreaks result in significant morbidity in the general population and an increase in mortality rates for high-risk patients from cardiovascular and pulmonary complications.[53]

Biological reasons for the effect of the influenza infection on CHD outcomes include the direct influence of the flu infection on the coronary plaque leading to plaque rupture and resulting myocardial infarction, or indirect exacerbation of the infection by the influenza infection. Indirect mechanisms may involve an increase in proinflammatory and prothrombotic cytokines, endothelial dysfunction, tachycardia, or hemoconcentration resulting from dehydration.[54]

A population-based case-control study of 342 cases and 549 controls to determine the effectiveness of the flu vaccination found a positive association with a reduced risk of cardiac arrests and flu vaccination. In this sample, the flu vaccination was associated with a reduced risk of cardiac arrest after adjusting for demographic, clinical, and behavioral risk factors.[55] Although there are many drugs available to treat heart disease, one of the most effective drugs may be inexpensive and readily available. In multiple case-control and cohort studies, it has been reported that the use of the influenza vaccine has a significant protective effect against cardiovascular events and decreases the incidence of these events by 20 to 70 percent.[54] Despite the fact that the vaccination is recommended for patients with heart disease, it is largely underused in these patients.

THE FUTURE

Case finding for secondary adverse coronary events is difficult with CHD. Patients who experience a cardiovascular event typically have disease and vulnerable plaque throughout the coronary tree and not in the single vessel or vessels that caused the clinical event (Figure 43-4). Long-term secondary events are linked to lesions other than the index lesion of the initial cardiac event.[56] Yet current methods of risk stratification do not allow for accurate prediction of which patients will have future MACE. Currently, the risk of recurrent myocardial infarction and unstable angina in patients with an acute initial event is determined clinically by measuring left ventricular function, angiography findings of disease, and the presence of continuing ischemia. In addition, traditional risk factors such as lipids, age, and blood pressure also are considered.[57]

Approximately 16 percent of patients with acute coronary events experience MACE within 6 months. The addition of some of the novel cardiac markers described to coronary risk assessment scores may help determine which of the patients will go on to experience future plaque rupture. The ability to stratify patients into high and low risk categories more accurately would enable clinicians to manage the patients at greatest risk more aggressively. The tests will have to be cost-effective, easy to perform in clinics, reliable, and valid.

Regarding interventions, the clinician should follow current American Heart Association and ATP III guidelines for interventions in CHD treatment and prevention.

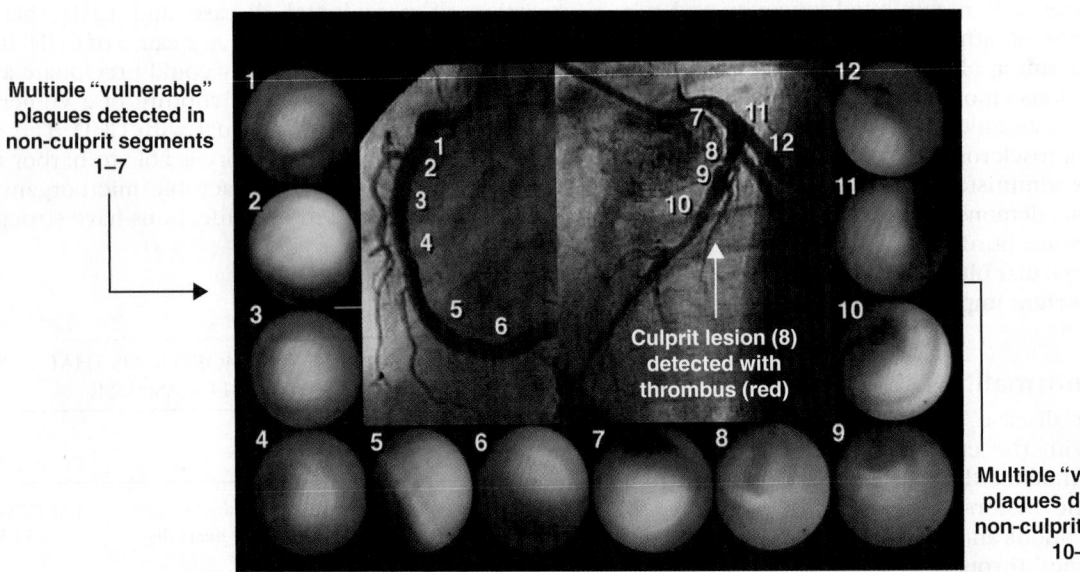

Multiple "vulnerable" plaques detected in non-culprit segments 1–7

Culprit lesion (8) detected with thrombus (red)

Multiple "vulnerable" plaques detected in non-culprit segments 10–12

FIGURE 43-4 ■ Evidence of multiple vulnerable plaques in a patient with acute coronary syndrome. Angiographic and angioscopic images of a 58-year-old man with anterior myocardial infarction are shown. The culprit lesion is seen in the proximal left anterior descending artery at site 8. However, other segments of the artery, which appear normal on the coronary angiogram, at angioscopy demonstrate the presence of vulnerable plaques (sites 10 to 12 and 1, 3, 4, and 7). (Adapted from Asakura M, Ueda Y, Yamaguchi O et al: *J Am Coll Cardiol* 37:1284, 2001.)

Most novel and inflammatory markers are still in the research phase of development and are not available for clinical use. New markers of CHD will be ready for clinical use when they are standardized and reasonable in price. However, some of the tests, like CRP, currently are recommended for use at the discretion of the clinician.

In the future, a genetic profile that adds to the Framingham risk score may be used to determine CHD risk. Until the genomic and proteomic biomarkers are available in the clinical setting, family history can be used to determine individual genetic CHD risk. Individuals and families need to understand their risk for a CHD event and the rational for family screening, mode of inheritance, and transmission risk. The health care provider needs to see beyond the individual patient and inquire about the CHD health of first-degree relatives. For example, family history of CHD in first-degree relatives is a major risk factor of CHD in most races and both genders, and the risk is increased when the affected relatives were diagnosed with CHD at a younger age. ATP III recommends that a positive family history be used in making treatment decisions relative to treating LDL.[19]

The implementation of a CHD-focused pedigree with the patient history also will open the door to the need to educate family members. On a community level, classes on CHD risk should include education on family history as a risk factor and the importance of the flu vaccination, as well as lipid control, smoking cessation, and other modifiable risk factors. Dentists and dental hygienists, who screen for and treat periodontal disease, have the opportunity to educate patients about the importance of dental hygiene to cardiovascular health.

Although there have been concerted research efforts aimed at the development of tests for novel risk factors in the diagnosis and prognosis of CHD, there has been little consensus on the use of markers in patient care. Some of the challenges are that risk markers may be different for different CHD disease processes. The same marker may be at different levels for stable versus unstable angina during an acute event. Risk markers may vary in their association with CHD outcomes. Markers that predict short-term outcomes may differ from markers that predict long-term outcomes. Some markers may be prognostics, whereas others may measure the effect of interventions.

Certain attributes make the use of new markers desirable. Markers should deliver superior clinical specificity and sensitivity, should be independent from other risk factors, and should be cost-effective.[49] A marker should be tested in different populations, and the results should be replicated. This rigor allows the generalization of the results across populations. Data on population norms of the marker also must be accumulated in order for comparisons to be made. Clinicians should be familiar with the population norms of the markers in individuals they treat. The ability to improve prediction beyond what is possible from traditional risk factors is an important aspect of clinical utility. Other considerations include difficulty of the test. Does it have to be put on ice immediately after collection? One of the most important issues is cost of the test. A test that is cost prohibitive will not be used in clinical practice.

A large body of evidence links several biomarkers to inflammation, coagulation, and fibrinolysis. A supersystem of markers may exist that can detect cardiovascular risk in individuals. Technology exists today for protein profiling in which the whole proteome can be measured at a single point in time. In the future, a combination of these markers may be used to classify cardiovascular disease risk.

REFERENCES

1. Falk E: Plaque rupture with severe pre-existing stenosis precipitating coronary thrombosis: characteristics of coronary atherosclerotic plaques underlying fatal occlusive thrombi, *Br Heart J* 50:127-134, 1983.
2. Shah PK: Insights into the molecular mechanisms of plaque rupture and thrombosis, *Indian Heart J* 1:21-30, 2005.
3. Davies MJ, Gordon JL, Gearing AF et al: The expression of the adhesion molecules ICAM-1, VCAM-1, PECAM, and E-selectin in human atherosclerosis, *J Pathol* 171:223-229, 1993.
4. Hansson GK: Immune mechanisms in atherosclerosis, *Arterioscler Thromb Vasc Biol* 21:1876-1890, 2001.
5. Madjid J, Awan I, Willerson JT et al: Leukocyte count and coronary heart disease, *J Am Coll Cardiol* 4:1945-1956, 2004.
6. Harlan JM, Killen PD, Harker LA et al: Neutrophil-mediated endothelial injury in vitro mechanisms of cell detachment, *J Clin Invest* 68:1394-1403, 1981.
7. Murohara T, Kamijikkoku S, Honda T: Increased circulating soluble intercellular adhesion molecule-1 in acute myocardial infarction: a possible predictor of reperfusion ventricular arrhythmias, *Crit Care Med* 28:1861-1864, 2000.
8. Kerner T, Ahlers O, Reschreiter H et al: Adhesion molecules in different treatments of acute myocardial infarction, *Crit Care* 5:145-150, 2001.
9. Mulvihill N, Foley JB, Ghaisas N et al: Early temporal expression of soluble cellular adhesion molecules in patients with unstable angina and subendocardial myocardial infarction, *Am J Cardiol* 83:1265-1267, 1999.
10. Mulvihill NT, Foley JB: Inflammation in acute coronary syndromes, *Heart* 87:201-204, 2002.
11. Hansson GD, Jonasson L, Seifert PS et al: Immune mechanisms in atherosclerosis, *Arteriosclerosis* 9:567-578, 1989.
12. Mulvihill N, Foley JB, Murphy RT et al: Risk stratification in unstable angina and non-Q wave myocardial infarction using soluble cell adhesion molecules, *Heart* 85:623-627, 2001.
13. Golino P, Maroko PR, Carew TE: Efficacy of platelet depletion in counteracting the detrimental effect of acute hypercholesterolemia on infarct size and the no-reflow phenomenon in rabbits undergoing coronary artery occlusion-reperfusion, *Circulation* 76:173-180, 1987.
14. Tsokos M, Fehlauer F, Puschel K: Immunohistochemical expression of E-selectin in sepsis-induced lung injury, *Int J Legal Med* 113:338-342, 2000.
15. Ridker PM: High-sensitivity C-reactive protein: potential adjunct for global risk assessment in the primary preventive of cardiovascular disease, *Circulation* 103:1813-1818, 2001.
16. Ridker PM: High-sensitivity C-reactive protein and cardiovascular risk: rationale for screening and primary prevention, *Am J Cardiol* 92(4B):17K-22K, 2003.
17. Mueller C, Buettner HJ, Hodgson JM et al: Inflammation and long-term mortality after non-ST elevation acute coronary syndrome treated with a very early invasive strategy in 1042 consecutive patients, *Circulation* 105:1412-1415, 2002.
18. Pearson TA, Mensah GA, Alexander RW et al; Centers for Disease Control and Prevention; American Heart Association: Markers of inflammation and cardiovascular disease: application to clinical and public health practice—a statement for healthcare professionals from the Centers for Disease Control and Prevention and the American Heart Association, *Circulation* 107(3):499-511, 2003.
19. *Third Report of the Expert Panel on Detection, Evaluation, and Treatment of High Blood Cholesterol in Adults (Adult Treat-*

ment Panel III), NIH Pub No 02-5215, Bethesda, Md, 2002, National Cholesterol Education Program, National Heart, Lung, and Blood Institute.

20. Ridker PM, Brown NJ, Vaughan DE et al: Established and emerging plasma biomarkers in the prediction of first atherothrombotic events, *Circulation* 109:6-19, 2004.

21. McCarty MF: Increased homocyst(e)ine associated with smoking, chronic inflammation, and aging may reflect acute-phase induction of pyridoxal phosphatase activity, *Med Hypotheses* 55:289-293, 2000.

22. Norlund L, Grubb A, Fex G et al: The increase of plasma homocysteine concentrations with age is partly due to the deterioration of renal function as determined by plasma cystatin C, *Clin Chem Lab Med* 36:175-178, 1998.

23. Giltay EJ, Hoogeveen EK, Elbers JM et al: Insulin resistance is associated with elevated plasma total homocysteine levels in healthy, nonobese subjects, *Atherosclerosis* 139:197-198, 1998 (letter).

24. Runge MS, Patterson C: *Principles of molecular cardiology,* Totowa, NJ, 2005, Humana Press.

25. Boushey CJ, Beresford SA, Omenn GS et al: A quantitative assessment of plasma homocysteine as a risk factor for vascular disease: probable benefits of increasing folic acid intakes, *JAMA* 274:1049-1057, 1995.

26. Spence JD: Patients with atherosclerotic vascular disease: how low should plasma homocyst(e)ine levels go? *Am J Cardiovasc Drugs* 1:85-89, 2001.

27. Hughes S: Novel risk factors for coronary heart disease: emerging connections, *Cardiovasc Nurs* 14:91-103, 2002.

28. Mayer EL, Jacobsen DW, Robinson K: Homocysteine and coronary atherosclerosis, *J Am Coll Cardiol* 27:517-527, 1996.

29. Festa A, D'Agostino R, Mykkanen L et al: LDL particle size in relation to insulin, proinsulin, and insulin sensitivity: the Insulin Resistance Atherosclerosis Study, *Diabetes Care* 22:1688-1693, 1999.

30. Austin MA, Breslow JL, Hennkens CH et al: Low-density lipoprotein subclass patterns and risk of myocardial infarction, *JAMA* 260:1917-1921, 1988.

31. Austin MA, King MC, Vranizan KM et al: Atherogenic lipoprotein phenotype: a proposed genetic marker for coronary heart disease risk, *Circulation* 82:495-506, 1990.

32. Nishina PM, Johnson JP, Naggert JK et al: Linkage of atherogenic lipoprotein phenotype to the low density lipoprotein receptor locus on the short arm of chromosome 19, *Proc Natl Acad Sci U S A* 89:708-712, 1992.

33. Sniderman AD, Scantlebury T, Cianflone K: Hypertriglyceridemic hyperapob: the unappreciated atherogenic dyslipoproteinemia in type 2 diabetes mellitus, *Ann Intern Med* 135:447-459, 2001.

34. Genest J, Bard JM, Fruchart JC et al: Familial hypoalphalipoproteinemia in premature coronary artery disease, *Arterioscler Thromb* 13:1728-1737, 1993.

35. Berg K: A new serum type system in man: the Lp system, *Acta Pathol Microbiol Scand* 59:369-382, 1963.

36. Loscalzo J, Weinfeld M, Fless GM et al: Lipoprotein(a), fibrin binding, and plasminogen activation, *Arteriosclerosis* 10(2):240-245, 1990.

37. Marcovina SM, Koschinsky ML, Albers JJ et al: Report of the National Heart, Lung, and Blood Institute Workshop on Lipoprotein(a) and Cardiovascular Disease: recent advances and future directions, *Clin Chem* 49:1785-1796, 2003.

38. Danesh J, Collins R, Peto R: Lipoprotein(a) and coronary heart disease: meta-analysis of prospective studies, *Circulation* 102:1082-1085, 2000.

39. Sniderman AD: Non-HDL cholesterol versus apolipoprotein B in diabetic dyslipoproteinemia: alternatives and surrogates versus the real thing, *Diabetes Care* 26:2207-2208, 2003.

40. Grundy SM: Low-density lipoprotein, non-high-density lipoprotein, and apolipoprotein B as targets of lipid-lowering therapy, *Circulation* 106:2526-2529, 2002.

41. Ballantyne CM, Hoogeveen RC, Bang H et al: Lipoprotein-associated phospholipase A2, high-sensitivity C-reactive protein, and risk for incident coronary heart disease in middle-aged men and women in the Atherosclerosis Risk in Communities (ARIC) Study, *Circulation* 109:837-842, 2004.

42. Song Y, Stampfer MJ, Liu S: Meta-analysis: apolipoprotein E genotypes and risk for coronary heart disease, *Ann Intern Med* 141:137-147, 2004.

43. Talmud PJ, Humphries SE: Gene:environment interaction in lipid metabolism and effect on coronary heart disease risk, *Curr Opin Lipidol* 13:149-154, 2002.

44. Sirtori CR, Calabresi L, Franceschini G et al: Cardiovascular status of carriers of the apolipoprotein A-I(Milano) mutant: the Limone sul Garda study, *Circulation* 103:1949-1954, 2001.

45. Shah PK, Yano J, Reyes O et al: High-dose recombinant apolipoprotein A-I Milano mobilizes tissue cholesterol and rapidly reduces plaque lipid and macrophage content in apolipoprotein e-deficient mice, *Circulation* 103:3047-3050, 2001.

46. Nissen SE, Tsunoda T, Tuzcu EM et al: Effect of recombinant ApoA-I Milano on coronary atherosclerosis in patients with acute coronary syndromes: a randomized controlled trial, *JAMA* 290(17):2292-2300, 2003.

47. Lusis AJ, Fogelman AM, Fonarow GC: Genetic basis of atherosclerosis. I. New genes and pathways, *Circulation* 110:1868-1873, 2004.

48. Chaves FJ, Real JT, Puig O et al: Familial hypercholesterolemia: molecular identification and characterization of the first compound homozygote in Spain, *Med Clin (Barc)* 110:300-302, 1998.

49. Pearson TA, Mensah GA: Markers of inflammation and cardiovascular disease application to clinical and public health practice: a statement for healthcare professionals from the Centers for Disease Control and Prevention and the American Heart Association, *Circulation* 107:499-511, 2003.

50. Humphries SE, Ridker PM, Talmud PJ: Genetic testing for cardiovascular disease susceptibility: a useful clinical management tool or possible misinformation? *Arterioscler Thromb Vasc Biol* 24:628-636, 2004.

51. Frazier L, Turner ST, Schwartz GL et al: Multilocus effects of the renin-angiotensin-aldosterone system genes on blood pressure response to a thiazide diuretic, *Pharmacogenomics J* 4:17-23, 2004.

52. Koltveit KM, Eriksen HM: Is the observed association between periodontitis and atherosclerosis causal? *Eur J Oral Sci* 109(1):2-7, 2001.

53. Dolin R: Influenza. In Jameson JL, editor: *Harrisons' principles of internal medicine,* New York, 2001, McGraw-Hill.

54. Madjid M, Awan I, Ali M et al: Influenza and atherosclerosis: vaccination for cardiovascular disease prevention, *Expert Opin Biol Ther* 5:91-96, 2005.

55. Siscovick DS, Raghunathan TE, Lin D et al: Influenza vaccination and the risk of primary cardiac arrest, *Am J Epidemiol* 152:674-677, 2000.

56. Goldstein JA, Demetriou D, Grines CL et al: Multiple complex coronary plaques in patients with acute myocardial infarction, *N Engl J Med* 343:915, 2002.

57. Pearson TA: New tools for coronary risk assessment what are their advantages and limits, *Circulation* 105:886-892, 2002.

SECTION IV

Cardiac Conditions

DEBRA K. MOSER and BARBARA RIEGEL

Chapters in this section of the book highlight the many contributions of nursing science to the improvement of cardiovascular care. Ongoing patient assessment is an underappreciated yet vital component of cardiovascular care and is the foundation for detecting and preventing complications.[1] Nurses have the major responsibility for a range of patient assessment needs, from the minute-by-minute assessment of hospitalized patients to the long-term assessment of individuals in varied outpatient settings. To fulfill these responsibilities, nurses use refined and astute assessment abilities. Several chapters in this section are devoted to providing nurses with the skills and knowledge to develop proficiency in all aspects of patient assessment.

Nurses have been the major contributors to the professional literature on electrocardiographic (ECG) and hemodynamic monitoring. They have advanced the science of monitoring in these areas to the point of providing sufficient evidence for guideline development.[2] This section contains several chapters on various aspects of ECG and hemodynamic monitoring—areas in which nursing science and practice have truly excelled.[2,3]

We now know that cardiac disease is not homogeneous between the genders and that years of failing to include women in cardiovascular studies has created a void in knowledge about cardiac disease in women.[4-9] Nurses have done much of the research examining the symptom presentation in women with acute coronary syndrome.[6,10,11] This section of the book contains a chapter dedicated solely to the unique aspects of cardiac disease in women.

We have learned that symptoms such as chest pain and fatigue are not simply indicators of cardiac pathology but are complex phenomena in themselves.[12-18] The responses of patients to symptoms are often not what health care providers consider to be logical, which contributes to the complexity of understanding cardiac symptoms.[19] To fully present the depth of the symptom phenomenon, entire chapters in this section are dedicated to specific symptoms and individuals' responses to them. These chapters were written by many of the nurses who have done and are doing the latest research in this important area.

Finally, this section of the book contains a number of chapters dedicated to optimizing the management of specific cardiac and cerebrovascular conditions. The integral role of nurses, who spend 24 hours per day with acutely ill and recovering cardiac and cerebrovascular patients, is emphasized in these chapters. The rationale behind grouping the care of patients with specific conditions and the chapters emphasizing assessment is recognition of nursing's vital role in assessment and monitoring to evidence-based and interdisciplinary care.

The state of the science regarding management of specific cardiac conditions has advanced considerably in the past two decades. Without the unique holistic perspective of nurses contributing to the science on which care is based, such advances would not be possible.

---

1. Castledine G: Patient assessment: a key requirement of nursing care, *Br J Nurs* 13:1233, 2004.
2. Drew BJ, Califf RM, Funk M et al: AHA Scientific Statement: Practice Standards for Electrocardiographic Monitoring in Hospital Settings: an American Heart Association Scientific Statement from the Councils on Cardiovascular Nursing, Clinical Cardiology, and Cardiovascular Disease in the Young: endorsed by the International Society of Computerized Electrocardiology and the American Association of Critical-Care Nurses, *J Cardiovasc Nurs* 20:76-106, 2005.
3. Drew BJ, Pelter MM, Adams MG: Frequency, characteristics, and clinical significance of transient ST segment elevation in patients with acute coronary syndromes, *Eur Heart J* 23:941-947, 2002.

4. Mensah GA, Mokdad AH, Ford ES et al: State of disparities in cardiovascular health in the United States, *Circulation* 111:1233-1241, 2005.

5. Arber S, McKinlay J, Adams A et al: Patient characteristics and inequalities in doctors' diagnostic and management strategies relating to CHD: a video-simulation experiment, *Soc Sci Med* 62:103-115, 2006.

6. McSweeney JC, Cody M, O'Sullivan P et al: Women's early warning symptoms of acute myocardial infarction, *Circulation* 108:2619-2623, 2003.

7. Mosca L, Mochari H, Christian A et al: National Study of Women's Awareness, Preventive Action, and Barriers to Cardiovascular Health, *Circulation* 113:525-534. 2006.

8. Schoenberg NE, Peters JC, Drew EM: Unraveling the mysteries of timing: women's perceptions about time to treatment for cardiac symptoms, *Soc Sci Med* 56:271-284, 2003.

9. Arber S, McKinlay J, Adams A et al: Influence of patient characteristics on doctors' questioning and lifestyle advice for coronary heart disease: a UK/US video experiment, *Br J Gen Pract* 54:673-678, 2004.

10. McSweeney JC, Lefler LL, Crowder BF: What's wrong with me? Women's coronary heart disease diagnostic experiences, *Prog Cardiovasc Nurs* 20:48-57, 2005.

11. DeVon HA, Zerwic JJ: The symptoms of unstable angina: do women and men differ? *Nurs Res* 52:108-118, 2003.

12. Goldberg R, Goff D, Cooper L et al: Age and sex differences in presentation of symptoms among patients with acute coronary disease: the REACT Trial. Rapid Early Action for Coronary Treatment, *Coron Artery Dis* 11:399-407, 2000.

13. Jurgens CY: Somatic awareness, uncertainty, and delay in care-seeking in acute heart failure, *Res Nurs Health* 29:74-86, 2006.

14. Zambroski CH, Moser DK, Roser LP et al: Patients with heart failure who die in hospice, *Am Heart J* 149:558-564, 2005.

15. Devon HA, Zerwic JJ: Symptoms of acute coronary syndromes: are there gender differences? A review of the literature, *Heart Lung* 31:235-245, 2002.

16. Schiff GD, Fung S, Speroff T, McNutt RA: Decompensated heart failure: symptoms, patterns of onset, and contributing factors, *Am J Med* 114:625-630, 2003.

17. DeVon HA, Penckofer SM, Zerwic JJ: Symptoms of unstable angina in patients with and without diabetes, *Res Nurs Health* 28:136-143, 2005.

18. Ryan CJ, DeVon HA, Zerwic JJ: Typical and atypical symptoms: diagnosing acute coronary syndromes accurately, *Am J Nurs* 105:34-36, 2005.

19. Zerwic JJ, Ryan CJ, DeVon HA, Drell MJ: Treatment seeking for acute myocardial infarction symptoms: differences in delay across sex and race, *Nurs Res* 52:159-167, 2003.

Nursing Assessment in the Inpatient Setting

Jana Glotzer

CHAPTER ABBREVIATIONS

ACS acute coronary syndrome

BP blood pressure

CAD coronary artery disease

CI cardiac index

COPD chronic obstructive pulmonary disease

DOE dyspnea on exertion

ED emergency department

H&P history and physical

HPI history of present illness

HR heart rate

JVP jugular venous pulse

PCWP pulmonary capillary wedge pressure

PMI point of maximal impulse

PND paroxysmal nocturnal dyspnea

RV right ventricular

Assessment of the acute care patient with a known or suspected cardiac condition must be quick, tailored, accurate, and ongoing.[1] The assessment must be quick because acute cardiac conditions require prompt treatment to prevent irreversible damage to organ systems. Apparently stable cardiac disease can deteriorate if not promptly recognized and properly treated. A tailored assessment is one that is designed for common diseases or conditions specific to the nursing unit and the skills of the nursing staff. Tailoring the examination to address relevant signs and symptoms to the chief complaint or diagnosis allows focus on essential information while minimizing missing assessment. An accurate cardiac assessment leads to the development of appropriate differential diagnoses, diagnostic tests, and treatment plan. The importance of an ongoing assessment cannot be underscored enough because it is vital to monitor the patient's response to the treatment, for concomitant illnesses, and for complications that may develop.

The initial inpatient assessment is called a diagnostic examination because the main objective is to find evidence (symptoms and signs) that points to the cause of the patient's condition.[2,3] Additional assessments focus on monitoring the response to treatment, on detecting concomitant illnesses, and on assessing the patient's knowledge about his or her condition. Essential to the diagnostic examination is the assessor's ability to discern the accuracy and reliability of the signs and symptoms elicited, as well as the self-care behaviors that may have contributed to the condition.

Insufficient or inaccurate assessment findings can lead to erroneous diagnoses, inadequate treatment, and poor outcomes. Acute cardiac conditions often have a multitude of signs and symptoms in almost every organ system; therefore, patients may be misdiagnosed as having noncardiac conditions. Because of fear of misdiagnosing an illness, health care providers have developed an ever-increasing reliance upon *more*: more innovative, more comprehensive, more definitive tests that unfortunately subject the patient to more risks, more unnecessary discomforts, and more costs with greater financial burden to the health care system.[4] A thorough, accurate assessment often can be as precise as some diagnostic tests and can assist in pinpointing which tests are needed and those that are not.[4,5] Consequently, it is incumbent upon nurses practicing in the acute care setting to fine tune their assessment skills continually.

Each nurse practicing in the inpatient setting can make a significant and unique contribution to comprehensive assessment. The admitting nurse may note that the prescription bottle with monthly refills has not been filled for several months. Another nurse may detect that a family member's view of the presenting symptoms or precipitating factors differs from that of the patient. The telemetry nurse responds to the call light of the patient experiencing chest discomfort and quickly assesses the likelihood of acute coronary syndrome (**ACS**) and begins definitive treatment. The experienced critical care nurse shares her knowledge and expertise with the critical care novice. The charge nurse prioritizes adequate staffing and equitable patient assignments that allow other nurses time to perform a complete assessment. Nursing managers and administrators monitor quality of care and develop assessment forms, flow sheets, and discharge forms that are disease specific and that capture important aspects of the assessment without undue overlap. The clinical nurse specialist assesses the staff's needs and arranges educational opportunities, develops nursing research protocols, and incorporates research findings into practice. The nurse practitioner is relied upon to gather a more comprehensive admission assessment, make treatment decisions, and evaluate the patient's clinical response. Clearly, quality nursing assessments at all levels can enhance patient care and outcomes.

A multidisciplinary approach is essential to caring for the acutely ill patient; however, it can appear fragmented if not done correctly and may frustrate the patient and family. A continuous barrage of essentially the same questions can become irritating, especially if the patient is in acute distress. This problem can be particularly acute in the academic setting where medical students, residents, and fellows each assess the patient in addition to the emergency department (**ED**) triage nurse, the ED nurse, then the ED physician, the admitting nurse, and the attending physician. Repetitive or overlapping questions can be interpreted as a failure to communicate information and can thereby hinder, undermine, and even fracture the patient's or family's trust in the caregivers. Consequently, it is important to delineate which areas of the assessment are best captured by each discipline to help minimize frustration. Additionally, it is helpful if each member of the team reads the information recorded from previous examiners before approaching the patient. Then the team member should preface clarifying questions with a statement such as, "I know you already told Dr. Jones the answer to this, but I need to better understand something." This approach can assure the patient that he or she is being listened to, and may help establish a trusting relationship.

The inpatient assessment is composed of the history and physical examination (**H&P**) and the analysis of diagnostic tests. From these findings, the diagnoses and plan of care are derived; therefore, desirable patient outcomes are incumbent upon a quality assessment. This chapter provides the groundwork for the essentials of the H&P, whereas the analyses of diagnostic tests are discussed specifically in the chapters involving the care of patients with specific cardiac conditions (Section IV).

HISTORY

Obtaining the history is part of the initial contact between the patient, family, and the nurse and is therefore a wonderful opportunity to develop a good relationship. Understand that each individual and family is unique, with a plethora of behavioral, psychological, and demographic variables that heavily influence their coping response to the condition, the severity of the presentation, and their readiness and willingness to report symptoms.

The artful attainment of the history requires good communication skills such as a calm, unhurried manner; active listening; establishing eye contact; and providing verbal and nonverbal affirmation.[5] These skills are essential to instill in the patient/family confidence in the nurse's ability and desire to help while developing a mutual trust, understanding, and respect between the patient, family, and caregiver. A good rapport with the nursing staff can help ease the patient's and family's stress as they experience a frightening, often painful acute cardiac condition requiring a hospitalization.[2,4] Good rapport increases the likelihood that the patient will disclose relatively more sensitive information and adhere to the treatment regimen.

Conversely, poor communications skills can undermine the relationship between the patient, family, and caregiver, and can increase the likelihood that insufficient or inaccurate data will be obtained in the history.[5] When the examiner appears hurried or distracted or repeats a question despite being given an answer the first time, the patient and the family can become concerned that they are not being heard and may be less likely to provide vital information. Poor communication skills often lead to frustration and distrust not only of the interviewer but also by transference to other care providers and of the commitment of the entire staff to the patient's well being. Therefore, the skillful attainment of an accurate history can be a challenging and exciting opportunity.

Because there is a finite amount of time that can be dedicated to the assessment process, the examiner may need to keep the history focused on obtaining relevant information. It may be necessary to redirect the patient and/or family to events pertinent to the cardiac condition. Care must be taken to affirm their less relevant concerns and to reassure them that these issues will be addressed in time. (See Box 44-1 for the components of the medical history.)

History of Present Illness

In the patient experiencing an acute cardiac condition, it is essential to obtain a comprehensive history of the present illness (**HPI**) in order to establish the proper diagnoses. The HPI begins with the chief complaint. The chief complaint is the problem that prompted the patient to seek help and may be unrelated to the underlying cardiac condition, although it may still provide insight into the patient's priorities and knowledge base. To filter out examiner bias, the chief complaint should be recorded in quotation marks.[3] The quote may include more than one complaint if the complaints are likely related and should include the duration of the problem; for example, "short of breath and weak for two weeks" or "chest pain and nausea for three hours."

Also important to the HPI is a record of past medical diagnoses likely to be associated with the chief complaint. For instance, coronary artery disease, hyperlipidemia, and diabetes mellitus should be included in the HPI of a patient who has chest discomfort, whereas allergic rhinitis would be recorded in the medical history. Then the examiner must seek out all accompanying symptoms and develop a present illness history for each.[5]

Associated Symptoms

Eliciting symptoms may be the most challenging part of the assessment. Unlike many other pathological processes, the severity of the patient's symptoms does not necessarily reflect the seriousness of the underlying cardiovascular condition, but is more often a reflection of the onset of the illness[5]. Patients who have an acute cardiac condition present in obvious distress, whereas

---

BOX 44-1   ■ ■ ■
COMPONENTS OF THE MEDICAL HISTORY

- History of the present illness
- Medical history
- Personal and social history
- Family history
- Review of systems

patients with chronic diseases who have had sufficient time to adapt physiologically to their cardiac condition often appear, to the untrained examiner, too well to require a hospitalization. Just envision the 65-year-old woman who comes to the coronary care unit in acute pulmonary edema. She is in acute distress, sitting bolt upright on a stretcher grasping her 100 percent non-rebreather mask in one hand and the stretcher side rail with the other (a positive "white-knuckle" sign). Her respiratory rate is often greater than 30 breaths/min, and her anxiety is proportionate. Compare this to the 35-year-old man who was diagnosed with chronic heart failure 3 years prior. He too is sitting with the head of the bed elevated as high as it can go but is in no apparent distress. His acute presentation may be so blunted by his body's chronic adaptation to his illness that only the experienced examiner will readily see the severity of his illness.

Another reason that eliciting accurate symptomatology can be challenging is that the patient may not report the symptoms accurately. This is not done deliberately to deceive providers but as a coping mechanism. Denial can be particularly strong in young individuals who value their physical capabilities. A chronic heart condition may produce a cognitive dissonance and prevent acceptance of the symptoms. Additionally, the patient with a chronic cardiac condition may be intentionally skilled at hiding symptoms out of fear. Fear of job loss,[6] insurance loss, or of losing a significant other are a few reasons to hide symptoms. Sometimes the patient may hide symptoms to avoid the scrutiny of a concerned family member. Therefore, it is important to observe family members' responses to the patient's answers.[5] Understand, though, that the family's response may be exaggerated because of the anxiety caused by the patient's denial. Somewhere in between, a more accurate history of presenting symptoms can be obtained.

Chest Discomfort

Chest pain or discomfort, discussed in more detail in Chapter 53, is one of the most common symptoms associated with ACS.[4-7] However, chest discomfort may be related to other nonischemic cardiac conditions.

The location of the discomfort is often helpful in determining its cause. Ask the patient to point to the location of the discomfort. Typically, if the discomfort is due to ACS, the patient will use the entire palm of his hand to indicate a region over the sternum and left side of the chest. The patient may also describe a radiation to the neck, left side of the jaw, shoulder, and left arm. The patient often will use a finger to pinpoint the exact location of the radiation down the ulnar portion of the left arm. If the patient uses a finger to point to a specific region on the chest wall, the discomfort is less likely to be due to angina pectoris. As discussed in Chapter 52, women may present with a different symptom pattern.

The quality of the discomfort in ACS often is described as pressure, burning, tightness, strangling, or choking and seldom is described as sharp. The amount of time the chest discomfort has lasted is also an indicator of the cause of the pain. Be as precise as possible when documenting the start time and date. Have the patient quantify the discomfort using the 1-to-10 pain scale. Always assess for any precipitating factors, as they often provide a strong clue to the origin of the chest discomfort. Angina pectoris typically is brought on by exertion, emotion, heavy meals, and/or cold weather, whereas pain precipitated by deep inspiration is less likely caused by ACS.

Accompanying symptoms also may suggest the cause of the discomfort. Diaphoresis could indicate ACS, pulmonary embolism, or aortic dissection. Dyspnea, nausea, and vomiting are also accompanying symptoms of an ACS. Also important ascertainment of measures that the patient has found to be helpful to alleviate symptoms. Anginal chest pain, attributed to a limited blood supply to the coronary arteries, usually is relieved within 1 to 5 minutes by rest and/or sublingual nitroglycerin.[4]

Dyspnea

Dyspnea, discussed in detail in Chapter 54, is defined simply as difficult or labored breathing. Because dyspnea is a major symptom of cardiac and pulmonary disease, a careful assessment to elicit other symptoms of cardiac or pulmonary disease is helpful in determining the cause.[4,8]

A well-obtained history, focused on precipitating and alleviating factors and other signs or symptoms of cardiac disease, is important to establishing the cause of dyspnea. Acute onset suggests an acute event such as acute pulmonary edema, pulmonary embolism, an acute myocardial infarction, pneumonia, pneumothorax, hyperventilation, or airway obstruction, and in the patient with a history of stable mitral valve disease could represent new onset atrial fibrillation.[4,5,7,8]

Chronic dyspnea may be present in heart failure, obesity, pulmonary disease, pregnancy, pleural effusions, anemia, sedentary lifestyle, and more. In chronic cardiac conditions such as heart failure, the onset may be so gradual that the patient subconsciously alters his level of activity to avoid dyspnea until it occurs at rest. The patient may insist the onset was sudden, but a thorough history, taken by a skilled examiner, can establish a history of a gradual reduction in activity over time. Although dyspnea most often is attributed to pulmonary congestion, in case of end-stage heart failure, dyspnea may be related to hypoperfusion of the lungs because of a very low cardiac index (**CI**).

When questioning the patient about dyspnea, observe the family member when the patient answers; often the family member will provide clues to a more realistic picture. Understand, though, that the patient is not trying to deceive or misguide the examiner but has adapted to the chronicity of the illness so that he or she only notices being short of breath when the work of breathing cannot be increased enough to relieve the air hunger.

When assessing dyspnea on exertion (**DOE**), it is normal for the healthy active person to experience dyspnea with exercise or maximal exertion. Also normal is for a sedentary person to experience dyspnea with moderate exertion. However, when dyspnea occurs at an inappropriate level of activity, then it is abnormal.[6] Therefore, it is important to assess activity given the patient's age, lifestyle, and body habitus. DOE as the chief complaint should be considered an anginal equivalent.

Dyspnea at rest may indicate acute conditions such as pneumonia, pulmonary embolism, pulmonary edema, pulmonary infarct, ACS, and chronic conditions such as heart failure, chronic obstructive pulmonary disease (COPD), and asthma. Anxiety, breathlessness, and distress may limit a comprehensive assessment; therefore, some of the assessment may need to be deferred until some symptom relief is achieved.

Paroxysmal nocturnal dyspnea (PND) is a common, sensitive symptom of left-sided heart failure with congestion. PND frequently occurs 2 to 4 hours after going to sleep in a recumbent position. The patient awakens with tightness in the throat, dyspnea, and/or extreme breathlessness. PND can be accompanied by diaphoresis, coughing, and wheezing. PND is relieved by sitting with legs dependent or standing upright for about 15 to 30 minutes. Then the patient usually is able to return to the recumbent position for sleep.[5,9] This differs from COPD, which also wakens the patient at night but from a fairly violent cough to relieve airway obstruction from secretions. Then breathlessness follows.[6]

Orthopnea is when the patient cannot breathe comfortably while lying flat. The presence of orthopnea is a sensitive and specific symptom of elevated filling pressures of the right side of the heart.[10] In the patient experiencing an acute cardiac condition, orthopnea can be a dramatic symptom and is therefore easy to assess. However, with chronic cardiac illness, the patient often will attribute multiple pillow use to a "habit." If the patient simply is asked "how many pillows do you sleep on?" the answer may not reflect an accurate description of the orthopnea. The patient may use one pillow to sleep but has a hospital bed and keeps the head elevated to 45 degrees, or the one pillow is a wedge pillow that elevates the head 30 degrees. Also, the patient may use one pillow when sleeping in bed but mostly sleeps in a recliner. A more clear representation of the degree of orthopnea a patient is experiencing can be obtained best by having the patient demonstrate with the hospital bed about how high the patient keeps his or her head elevated. An unusual presentation of orthopnea is the patient who denies orthopnea because he or she sleeps on the "stomach" but does so by kneeling by the bed with the anterior thorax flat on the bed.

Cough

All too often in the patient with chronic heart failure, a cough is attributed to a medication class. Angiotensin converting enzyme-inhibitors may cause buildup of bradykinin, which can result in a cough; however, a dry cough in the patient with heart failure is more likely due to pulmonary congestion and is a dyspnea equivalent. Therefore, a cough should be assessed just as one would assess dyspnea. If the cough occurs at night after a period of 2 to 4 hours of lying down, then it is a PND equivalent. The cough that occurs at night while one is supine and is relieved by elevating the head of the bed is an orthopnea equivalent. A cough that occurs with exertion is a DOE equivalent. An upper respiratory in-fection should be suspected if the cough is productive of colored sputum. A cough producing pink frothy sputum is indicative of acute pulmonary edema.

Syncope

Syncope is a sudden complete loss of consciousness that is transient. Syncopal episodes are caused by an inadequate amount of oxygen delivery to the brain. Cardiac syncope may be due to life-threatening dysrhythmias such as complete atrioventricular block, ventricular tachycardia, or fibrillation. Therefore, any patient complaining of a blackout or syncope should undergo more specific questioning in order to discern the cause of the episode.

Regardless of the chief complaint, every patient hospitalized for a suspected cardiac condition should be asked whether he or she has ever experienced a blackout, because it can be a symptom of a preventable life-threatening event. Cardiac syncope is sudden, usually is unassociated with position, and has a rapid recovery without drowsiness or a depressed sensorium.[4] A history of a myocardial infarction or cardiomyopathy places the patient at high risk for cardiac syncope because of nonsustained ventricular tachycardia.

If a syncopal episode is preceded by dizziness and occurs immediately upon or momentarily after assuming an upright position, it is suspicious for postural hypotension. Hypovolemia is a major cause of postural hypotension. Presyncope is dizziness that does not result in a complete blackout and may be referred to as a brownout. Beta blockers blunt the ability of the sympathetic nervous system to respond to rapid position changes and are more likely to cause presyncope rather than syncope. Other medications that may cause presyncope are antihypertensives, angiotension converting enzyme-inhibitors, angiotensin receptor blockers, and diuretics. Therefore, it is important to inquire about the relationship of these episodes with the timing of medication administration.[4]

Aortic stenosis can be a cause of syncope, often in association with exertion. Syncope caused by hypertrophic obstructive cardiomyopathy typically occurs immediately after exertion.[6] Syncope caused by seizures often is preceded by an aura or prodrome and usually is associated with a prolonged period of unconsciousness accompanied by loss of bladder or bowel control and is followed by a slow return to consciousness.

Fluid Retention

A cardinal symptom of cardiac insufficiency is fluid retention. Therefore, it is important to determine whether there is a history of weight gain or edema. Fluid retention may not always be perceived by the patient; therefore, specific questions may assist the patient in recognizing changes over time. To determine whether the patient is experiencing edema, ask specific questions such as "Are your shoes fitting tighter?" or "Are you more comfortable in your slippers instead of shoes?" and "Is your belt getting tighter?" or "Have you started wearing pants with elastic waist bands?"

If the patient has chronic heart failure and routinely limits dietary sodium intake the majority of the time, then a single dietary indiscretion often is the cause of fluid retention, particularly when it is rapid or overnight. Conversely, those patients who seldom limit their sodium intake may gain several pounds a week while adapting to the symptoms or limiting their activity to avoid symptoms until they can no longer adapt. These patients may have as much as a 25- to 50-lb. weight gain and appear unaware or even surprised by the amount of weight gain.

A common misconception is that removing the salt shaker from the table equates to a low-sodium diet. Many are unaware of the high sodium content in fast foods, canned soups and vegetables, and processed meats and cheeses (see Chapter 64). Therefore, in addition to the teaching the nursing staff will perform, it is important to request a dietary consult for low sodium diet teaching while the patient with heart failure is hospitalized.

When taking a history from a patient with symptoms of fluid retention, be sure to assess for noncardiac causes of edema (Box 44-2). Weight gain can be expected with the treatment of diabetes mellitus with insulin and oral agents. As much as a 12-lb weight gain can be seen with combination therapy (Table 44-1). The literature is unclear; however, whether this weight gain is actually harmful to the patient by producing circulatory overload or whether the fluid just remains in the tissues. Therefore, it is important to assess symptoms that accompany the weight gain.

Excessive Fatigue

Excessive fatigue is one of the more frequent complaints associated with unstable angina and heart failure, but it is neither sensitive nor specific to either cardiac condition. Fatigue more often is associated with depression, anemia, and deconditioning. Even if the patient attributes the cause of fatigue to "laziness", it is up to the examiner to explore all likely possibilities. Fatigue in heart failure may be due to a low cardiac output state and shunting of blood flow away from the musculoskeletal system to other organ systems. Fatigue in heart failure also is likely compounded by anemia of chronic disease. See Chapter 55 for a more in-depth review of

---

BOX 44-2
NONCARDIAC CAUSES OF EDEMA

Conditions
- Hypoalbuminemia
- Deep venous thrombosis
- Deep venous insufficiency
- Saphenous vein graft harvest
- Lymphedema
- Nephrotic syndrome
- Trauma
- Fluid resuscitation after trauma

Medications
- Insulin
- Sulfonylureas
- Thiazolidinediones
- Calcium channel blockers
- Nonsteroidal anti-inflammatory drugs
- Cyclo-oxygenase-2 inhibitors

■ ■ ■

TABLE 44-1 WEIGHT GAIN ASSOCIATED WITH HYPOGLYCEMIC AGENTS

CLASS	MEDICATION AND DOSE	WEIGHT GAIN (kg)
Sulfonylurea	Glyburide, 7.5 mg	1.9
Thiazolidinediones	Rosiglitazone, 4 mg daily	1.9
	Rosiglitazone, 8 mg daily	2.9
	Pioglitazone, 15 mg	0.9
	Pioglitazone, 30 mg	1.0
	Pioglitazone, 45 mg	2.6
Insulin	Not specified	1.0
Sulfonylureas and thiazolidinediones	Glyburide and rosiglitazone	1.8
	Metformin and rosiglitazone	1.8
Insulin and thiazolidinediones	Rosiglitazone 4-8 & Insulin 70 units/day	4.1-5.4
	Pioglitazone 15 mg and insulin	2.3
	Pioglitazone 30 mg and insulin	3.6

Adapted from Nesto RW, Bell D, Bonow RO et al:Thiazolidinedione use, fluid retention, and congestive heart failure: A consensus statement from the American Heart Association and American Diabetes Association. *Circulation* 2003, 108:2941-2948.

---

fatigue. When assessing fatigue, it is important to determine whether the patient is able to keep up with persons close to his or her own age. Also, determine whether the fatigue is affecting activities of daily living.

Medication History

The admitting nurse is optimally positioned to get the most accurate medication history from the patient and his family. First, medication allergies are an important part of this assessment and should be recorded along with the reaction that occurred when the medication was taken. Then assess all medications being taken by the patient, along with the dosages and frequencies. Information about vitamin supplements, herbal remedies, and over-the-counter pain relief is also important to attain.

Using a list of medications provided by the patient may not provide accurate data because the list can be transcribed inaccurately or may not be updated with recent changes. Medication lists obtained from other medical providers may not reflect how the patient actually is taking the medications or include medications prescribed by other health care providers. Therefore, the most accurate way to get a medication history is by reviewing the medications with the patient. If the patient did not bring his medications, use of the list is sufficient for an initial assessment, but request that a family member bring in the medication containers and update the medication history at that time.

The patient may not be taking the medication as printed on the prescription label; therefore, it is not enough simply to record the instructions. The patient may not recognize the medication by its pronunciation of the generic or trade name, and therefore the only way a medication is identified accurately is visually by size, shape, and color. Therefore, having the prescription bottle enables the patient to look at the pill. Open the bottle and show the patient the pill and ask how many and how often the patient is taking the medication.[11]

Medication bottles also can provide information about medication adherence. By looking at the number of pills remaining in the bottle and the date the prescription was filled, the examiner should be prompted to probe about issues of nonadherence. However, if the pill bottle is empty, do not rush to judgment, for the patient may have already prepared pill-dispensing boxes for the next week, or sometimes a patient will empty the pill bottles before going to the hospital for fear that the medications might be taken away. Remember, if a patient is unjustly deemed nonadherent with taking medications, not only will the teaching focus of the hospitalization be on the wrong track, but also the patient can be frustrated by the lack of trust from the healthcare providers. Conversely, if medication nonadherence is an overlooked reason for the decompensation, an excellent opportunity to affect future decompensations and readmissions will be lost.

Medical History

Based on what was learned from the HPI, the nurse now should focus on the elements of the medical history that are pertinent to the current suspected or real cardiac condition for which the patient is hospitalized. The medical history can provide important pieces to the puzzle leading to the cause of the current condition.

With all cardiac conditions, it is important to assess behaviors that put the patient at high risk. Tobacco and cocaine use put the patient at risk for coronary artery disease **(CAD)**. Long periods of heavy alcohol consumption can be a cause of heart failure or hypertension. Intravenous drug abuse, recent trauma, or renal dialysis may be the reason for endocarditis, myocarditis, or pericarditis.

Previous diagnoses of asthma, COPD, obstructive sleep apnea, renal disease, liver disease, diabetes mellitus, peripheral vascular disease, and rheumatic heart disease can put the patient at risk for many cardiac conditions. A medical history of cardiovascular conditions such as CAD, hypertension, and dyslipidemias increases the probability that the chest discomfort is due to ACS. A history of gastroesophageal reflux disease may point to a possible cause of chest pain. Additionally, it is important to assess the patient's family history, focusing on hereditary cardiac conditions such as hypertension, CAD, hypertrophic cardiomyopathy, heart failure, and cerebrovascular accidents (Table 44-2).

Personal and Social History

Assess the patient's perception of his or her condition and their role in its management. If the patient feels completely helpless and believes the disease controls him or her, then the patient is less likely to comply with the therapeutic regimen. A major part of patient education should be focused on the fact that the disease can be controlled if healthy habits are developed such as routine exercise, eating a heart-healthy diet, taking medications as prescribed, and keeping clinic appointments. Alcohol and tobacco use should be assessed at admission because withdrawal can greatly affect the patient's adjustment to hospitalization. When the illness becomes less acute, it is important to assess and encourage alcohol or smoking cessation and other health-promoting behaviors.

The patient's psychological adaptation can greatly affect the development of and recovery from cardiac illnesses, as well as compliance to the medical regimen.[12,13] Depression (see Chapter 40) and anxiety (see

■ ■ ■

TABLE 44-2   REVIEW OF CARDIAC-RELATED MEDICAL HISTORY

HISTORY	COMMENTS
General health	Health-promoting behaviors (diet, exercise, vaccines), baseline activity level, weight, and strength
Previous diagnoses	Addison's disease, arthritis, asthma, blood transfusions, coronary artery disease, chronic renal insufficiency or failure, congenital heart defects, connective tissue disorders, chronic obstructive pulmonary disease, Cushing syndrome, diabetes mellitus, dialysis, dysrhythmias (atrial flutter/fibrillation, heart blocks, nonsustained ventricular tachycardia, sudden cardiac arrest), gout, heart failure, human immunodeficiency virus, hyperlipidemia, hypertension, hyperthyroidism, hypothyroidism, myocardial infarction, obstructive sleep apnea, proteinuria, recent flu syndrome, renal failure requiring dialysis, rheumatic fever, rheumatic heart disease
Interventional/surgical/ device history	Bi-V pacemaker, carotid endarterectomy, congenital corrective surgery, coronary artery bypass grafting surgery, home inotropic therapy, implantable cardioverter/defibrillator (with or without an atrial pacing lead), percutaneous coronary interventions (angioplasty, stent, endarterectomy), peripheral vascular interventions, renal artery stents, right ventricular pacemaker, transplant listed/status, valve repair or replacement, ventricular assist device
Social history	Alcohol use, employment, illicit drug use, marital status, sexual history and behaviors, social support, tobacco use
Family history	Alcohol abuse, congenital heart disease, coronary artery disease, diabetes mellitus, heart failure, hypertension, hypertrophic cardiomyopathy, myocardial infarction, sudden cardiac death
Obstetric history	Cardiac diagnoses within 1 year of pregnancies, dyspnea with pregnancies, menarche, menopause, pregnancy-induced hypertension, use of oral contraceptives
Medication history	Current medications, financial burden for each prescription, how prescriptions are paid for, medication allergies with associated reaction, prior in-hospital intravenous vasoactive substance treatments and their success or failure

Chapter 41) have each been implicated in the development of CAD and an increase in disease-related mortality. Hopelessness is defined by Dunn[13] as "a psychological response to a physical illness" that is associated with feelings of helplessness and negative expectations about the future. Healthy men and women who exhibited the hopelessness trait were found to have higher fatal and nonfatal events than those without the trait.[14] High anxiety levels can affect the patient's ability and capacity to learn and therefore must be recognized.

The social history is important to ascertain and should include an assessment of the patient's support systems by asking about marital status, living arrangements, and other family members and their availability to help out if needed. Adequate social support (see Chapter 42) is important to adherence and coping (see Chapter 39). In the acute care setting, it is particularly important to get contact names with accurate telephone numbers of more than one family member. This information rarely is obtained by any other discipline and is essential, particularly if the patient's condition deteriorates. Also vital is to note whether the patient has an advanced directive and to ensure that a copy of it is in the chart.

Review of Systems

The review of systems is a systematic assessment of the signs and symptoms the patient is experiencing in each organ system. Although it is often the physicians, nurse practitioners, and physician assistants who most often are relied upon to obtain this portion of the assessment, it is the nurse who can augment the assessment with vital information that the patient remembers later. Also,

■ ■ ■

TABLE 44-3   REVIEW OF SYMPTOMS: CARDIAC-RELATED SIGNS AND SYMPTOMS IN BRIEF

SYSTEM	COMMENTS
Constitutional	Fevers, chills, sweats, sleeping patterns
Head, eyes, ears, nose, and throat	Visual color changes
Cardiovascular	Chest pain/discomfort, palpitations, cardiac awareness, presyncopal or syncopal episodes
Pulmonary	Wheezing, orthopnea, paroxysmal nocturnal dyspnea, dyspnea on exertion, cough, chest pain associated with respiration, hemoptysis
Endocrine	Polyuria, polydipsia, polyphagia, temperature intolerance
Gastrointestinal	Anorexia, cachexia, early satiety, nausea, emesis, bloating, diarrhea, constipation, abdominal pain, bloody diarrhea (hematochezia)
Renal	Polyuria, nocturia, oliguria, anuria
Musculoskeletal	Gout, leg muscle cramping upon exertion, weight loss, weight gain, fatigue (unable to keep up with peers), cachexia, swollen joints
Neurological	Transient ischemic attack, cerebrovascular attack, memory loss, depression, insomnia, hypersomnia
Psychological	Depression, anxiety, bipolar disorder

during daily care activities the nurse and patient often discover valuable pieces of missing information together, and it is up to the nurse to ensure that the new information is disseminated. The review of systems generally is broken up in this manner but may be different in each institution: constitutional; head, eyes, ears, neck, and throat; cardiac; pulmonary; endocrine; gastrointestinal; renal; musculoskeletal; neurological; and psychological. Table 44-3 gives symptoms that may be associated with cardiac conditions.

PHYSICAL EXAMINATION

The physical examination can elucidate further whether the patient truly is experiencing symptoms caused by a cardiovascular condition by the presence or absence of accompanying signs. Rarely can one symptom or one sign point to the cause, but it is often a unique combination of symptoms and signs that gives the clearest picture of the cause of the condition.[6] Each assessment in the acute care setting must be tailored to the severity of the condition; therefore, a focused physical examination should take no longer than 10 minutes.[15] Performing the physical examination in a methodical routine is important so as not to overlook any portion of the assessment. The spotlight of the physical examination should be on the assessment of the adequacy of the ability of the heart to perfuse organ systems, the circulatory volume status, the cause of the cardiac dysfunction, and the compensatory (and sometimes decompensatory) mechanisms the body has recruited in order to adapt. Box 44-3 gives a suggested sequence of the physical examination.

The physical examination actually begins when the nurse and the patient first meet.[11] Essential to the examination is a quick assessment of the patient's work of breathing. Prompt measures must be taken to provide symptomatic relief of dyspnea and to decrease the cardiac burden. Simply administering supplemental oxygen is a relatively harmless yet vital intervention to minimize the work of breathing and thereby rest the heart while awaiting the effects of additional interven-

---

BOX 44-3   ■ ■ ■
A SUGGESTED SEQUENCE OF THE ADMISSION PHYSICAL EXAMINATION

1. Measure height and weight.
2. Attach cardiac monitor.
3. Obtain blood pressure.
4. Count respiratory rate.
5. Obtain temperature.
6. Palpate precordium.
7. Auscultate precordium.
8. Examine sclera and oral mucous membranes.
9. Assess jugular venous pulsation.
10. Assess abdominal jugular reflux.
11. Assess for hepatomegaly.
12. Assess for ascites.
13. Auscultate posterior breath sounds.
14. Inspect extremities for color.
15. Palpate extremities for temperature, edema, pulses, and capillary refill.

tions, such as administration of diuretics. Oxygen administration must be ordered by a physician, nurse practitioner or physician's assistant and usually is started at 2 liters/min. via nasal cannula. If the patient is being transported from the ED and is receiving oxygen and does not appear dyspneic, then administer oxygen in the manner used during transport. If the patient is still apparently dyspneic despite oxygen therapy, a stronger method of oxygen administration is indicated. If the patient is still dyspneic using a 100 percent non-rebreather mask, then have the intubation equipment, a ventilation bag, and oral suction on standby in case of the need for intubation. Another safety measure is notifying the respiratory therapy department of the possible need for a ventilator or noninvasive positive pressure ventilation. If the patient does not appear in distress and is not receiving oxygen, then proceed with assessment of vital signs.

In patients with an acute cardiac condition that requires treatment in an intermediate or critical care unit, it is routine policy to monitor continuous oxygen saturations by pulse oximetry. Pulse oximetry is helpful in assessing the adequacy of oxygenation, especially in patients who are bordering on decompensation. A patient whose oxygen saturation is fine on room air when resting but drops when talking should receive oxygen so as not to stress the heart with minimal activity.

Generalities about the patient's condition—such as the distress level, functional level, body habitus, hygiene, speech, motor abilities, and interactions between family members—can be assessed simultaneously while getting the HPI and vital signs. This is a good time to assess functional capacity by observing the patient during routine admission activities such as getting weighed and getting into bed. (See Box 45-3 for the New York Heart Association functional classification system.)

General Appearance

A focused head-to-toe physical examination should include a search for signs that typically are associated with the real or suspected cardiac condition and the differential diagnoses associated with the condition. Just as with the history taking, the rapidity and focus of the examination depends on the severity of the real or suspected cardiac condition. The cardiac examination should be performed from the patient's right side and, in the inpatient setting, usually begins with the patient in the supine position.

The initial impression is important in the acute care setting. A quick inspection of the patient's coloring can tell a great deal about cardiovascular perfusion. Pale, ashen, or cyanotic coloring and cool or cold extremities often are indicative of a hypoperfusion state in acute heart failure caused by an acute myocardial infarction, acutely decompensated heart failure, or restrictive cardiac diseases—all of which can spiral into cardiogenic shock. Conversely, flushed, warm, or even hot skin may indicate an infectious state, such as acute pericarditis or viral myocarditis.[16] Peripheral cyanosis is present in most cardiac conditions that cause a low cardiac output state. Jaundiced skin color and icteric sclera can occur because of hepatic congestion in right-sided heart failure, hemolytic anemia, or primary liver disease. Perfusion status can be ascertained quickly by feeling the warmth of all four extremities. Cool and cold extremities can indicate a high systemic vascular resistance. (Table 44-4 gives general signs and symptoms suggestive of congestion or low cardiac output.)

Height and Weight

Upon admission, it is important to get an accurate height and weight. This should not be done by simply asking the patient; both values should be measured directly. If the patient is too ill to stand, then a stated height will do temporarily but should be recorded in quotes and measured when stability is achieved. Stated height may be inaccurate for many reasons. Being tall is considered a desirable attribute in the male; therefore, men may overstate their height. The elderly tend to get shorter as they age and are often unaware of the change. Obtaining an accurate height and weight in the patient with a cardiac condition helps establish a baseline for evaluating the effectiveness of therapy in treating edema, assists in hemodynamic calculations done according to body surface area, and aids in accurately prescribing intravenous therapies based on weight.

Erroneous weights often are obtained from scales that are built into the patient's bed because the amount

■ ■ ■

TABLE 44-4   SIGNS OF CONGESTION VERSUS LOW CARDIAC OUTPUT*

CONGESTION		LOW CARDIAC OUTPUT	
SYMPTOMS	SIGNS	SYMPTOMS	SIGNS
Excessive thirst	Ascites	Bloating	Cheyne-Stokes respirations
Exertional cough	Elevated jugular venous pressure	Decreased mentation	Hypotension
Expanding abdominal girth	Increased international normalized	Early satiety	Increasing creatinine level
Edema	ratio	Excessive fatigue	Low core body temperature
Nocturnal cough	Increased liver function tests	Fatigue at rest	Low mean arterial pressure
Orthopnea	Increased liver span	Nausea, vomiting, or constipation	Low proportional pulse pressure
Paroxysmal noctural dyspnea	Jaundice	Sleeping more than 14 hr/day	(less than 0.25 mm Hg)
	Peripheral edema		Narrow pulse pressure (less
	Pleural effusions		than 30 mm Hg)
	Rales		

*Congestion may be the cause of low cardiac output. Low cardiac output is a syndrome, a constellation of signs and symptoms.

of linens on the bed varies. If this is the method used to obtain weights, then a concerted effort must be made to ensure that the bed is zeroed with exactly the same amount of linens on the bed with each weight. A good general rule is to obtain admission weights with a standing scale if the patient is able to stand; document it as such. Realizing this is not always reasonable in the acutely decompensated patient, a bed weight may be the best option for an initial weight. A standing scale weight may need to be deferred until stability is achieved. In patients with heart failure being treated for fluid volume overload, standing scale weights around the same time each day will help control for accuracy.

Heart Rate, Regularity, and Rhythm

Heart rate (**HR**), regularity, and rhythm should be assessed upon admission to the nursing unit, either simultaneously or after a cursory assessment of airway and breathing. Most intensive care units ensure that several nurses admit an acutely ill patient, which makes the exact sequence unimportant but ensures that the baseline information is assessed concurrently. Place every patient on a cardiac monitor, via telemetry or a bedside monitor, to ensure the capture of any dysrhythmias that may occur. If the patient is being monitored by remote telemetry, proceed with assessing the HR and its regularity, and then proceed to the telemetry unit to assess the rhythm when the assessment is completed. Always auscultate the precordium while feeling a pulse when obtaining a HR, for ectopic atrial and ventricular beats will make a palpated pulse alone inaccurate. A blood pressure (**BP**) should be obtained immediately following the HR.

A 12-lead electrocardiogram should be obtained within 10 minutes of admission, especially if the patient is admitted with the diagnosis of suspected or real ACS.[17] However, it is a good practice to establish a baseline for all patients admitted to a coronary care unit.

As a general rule, while performing the physical examination of most organ systems, the following sequence should be followed: inspection, palpation, percussion, and auscultation. Additionally, in the acute care setting, time is limited, so the precordial examination should remain focused on essentials needed to establish a diagnosis or those that help determine the diagnostic tests most likely to confirm (sensitive) or deny (specific) a cardiac condition. Thus, palpation is abbreviated and percussion is usually unnecessary because the findings often are duplicated by more routine, equivocal diagnostic tests. For instance, percussing the precordium yields information about the size of the heart, which can be obtained more accurately by a routine chest radiograph. This diagnostic test is easy, noninvasive, and essential to rule out concomitant illness that may confound or exacerbate the underlying cardiac condition.

Blood Pressure

A BP is a simple, quick determination of hemodynamic stability and therefore should be taken soon after admission to the nursing unit. Important to an accurate reading is the proper size of the BP cuff in relation to the arm. Too large a cuff will give a falsely low BP reading, whereas too small a cuff will give a falsely high reading. If there is not a large enough cuff for the upper arm of an obese patient, a regular size cuff may be used around the forearm, and the stethoscope should be placed over the radial artery to obtain the BP.[15] The arm should be positioned horizontally, level to the right atrium (the phlebostatic axis) and should not be allowed to be dependent. The patient and the nurse should not talk while the BP is being taken. Initial BP readings should be taken in both arms. If there is a significant variation in the readings, then the BP should be taken in the same arm throughout the hospitalization.

The pulse pressure is a noninvasive reflection of the patient's cardiac output. Pulse pressure is the result of interplay between three hemodynamic parameters: stroke volume, stroke velocity, and systemic vascular resistance.[3,5,15] This measurement is obtained simply by subtracting the diastolic BP from the systolic BP. For example, a diastolic BP of 60 mm Hg subtracted from a systolic BP of 110 mm Hg would yield a pulse pressure of 40 mm Hg. A normal pulse pressure is between 30 and 50 mm Hg.[18] Additionally, a predictor of a CI range can be estimated by measuring the proportional pulse pressure. The proportional pulse pressure is calculated by dividing the pulse pressure by the systolic BP. A BP of 90/70 mm Hg would give a pulse pressure of 20 mm Hg, which if divided by the systolic BP of 90 mm Hg would give a proportional pulse pressure of 0.22. If the patient's proportional pressure is less than 0.25, there is an 88 percent chance that the CI is less than 2.2 liters/min/m^2.[2,18]

Postural Vital Sign Measurements

In a healthy state, somewhere between 300 and 800 ml of blood can pool in the lower extremities upon standing.[19,20] The decreased venous return to the heart causes a temporary drop in the BP, which is sensed by baroreceptors that trigger the sympathetic nervous system to increase the HR and stimulate peripheral vasoconstriction. A normal response is a modest drop in systolic BP of less than 10 mm Hg and an increase in the diastolic BP of 2 to 3 mm Hg. Orthostatic hypotension is defined as a drop in systolic BP of more than 20 mm Hg or in the diastolic BP of more than 10 mm Hg within 3 minutes of standing from the supine position.[21]

Although this definition lacks a HR requirement, HR is an important part of the cardiac assessment and should not be overlooked. This is particularly true in the cardiac patient, for many cardiovascular conditions, medications, and concomitant illnesses can cause postural changes in vital signs. An increased HR may cause enough of a compensatory response that the systolic BP does not strictly meet the criteria of more than 20 mm Hg yet still can signify some degree of hypovolemia. Details about how to obtain postural vital signs are described in Box 44-4.

A simple, noninvasive measurement of postural vital signs can detect changes in BP and HR with position changes. Specific to cardiac conditions, circulatory volume derangements, left ventricular systolic dysfunc-

BOX 44-4
POSTURAL VITAL SIGN MEASUREMENTS   ■ ■ ■

- Supine BP and heart rate must always be checked first, followed by the standing blood pressure and heart rate.
- The supine measurements should be taken after the patient is resting a minimum of 5 minutes in this position, followed by the upright vital sign measurement after a minimum of 3 minutes.
- As a safety precaution, have the patient sit with legs dependent between the supine and standing position.
- Orthostasis is defined as a drop in systolic BP by greater than 20 mm Hg or the diastolic BP of greater than 10 mm Hg within 3 minutes of standing from the supine position. Symptoms of positive orthostasis are dizziness, weakness, nausea, emesis, blurred vision, gray vision, or syncope.
- Hyperstasis is when the patient's systolic BP increases more than 20 mm Hg when standing and is accompanied by a drop in heart rate. This can occur when the patient is fluid volume overloaded and has an impaired left ventricular systolic dysfunction.
- Some signs of hyperstasis are inability to lie flat, a reflexive sitting up, requesting the head of the bed to be raised, and an increased respiratory rate in the supine position. Upon standing, the patient gradually may appear symptom free.

BP, Blood pressure.

TABLE 44-5   CAUSES OF ORTHOSTATIC HYPOTENSION

CAUSE	EFFECTS
Left ventricular systolic dysfunction	Aortic stenosis
	Bradydysrhythmias/tachydysrhythmias
	Chronic heart failure
	Hypertrophic obstructive cardiomyopathy
	Myocardial infarction
	Myocarditis
	Pericarditis
Intravascular volume depletion	Alcohol consumption
	Diabetes insipidus
	Diuretics
	Hemorrhage
	Hyperglycemia
	Inadequate oral intake
	Vomiting or diarrhea
Venous pooling	Heat (ambient, hot shower, bath, or sauna)
	Sepsis
	Varicose veins
Peripheral neuropathy	Alcoholic peripheral neuropathy
	Amyloidosis
	Autonomic failure
	Diabetic peripheral neuropathy
	Multiple sclerosis
	Prolonged bed rest (as little as 24 hours)
	Prolonged standing
Central neuropathy	Brain tumor
	Parkinson's disease
Medications	Sympathetic blocking agents
	Alpha blockers
	Beta blockers
	Diuretics
	Vasodilators
	Nitrates
	Inodilators
	Angiotensin converting enzyme-inhibitors
	Angiotensin receptor blockers

tion, neurohormonal blockade medications for hypertension and heart failure, and diuretics may adversely affect adaptation to postural changes. Therefore, obtaining orthostatic vital signs is an important assessment tool for any patient with a cardiac disease, real or suspected.

If, after a period of adjustment to the upright position change, there is a drop in BP accompanied by a compensatory rise in HR, then the patient is deemed orthostatic, or has "positive orthostasis." This can indicate hypovolemia. Symptomatic postural hypotension occurs when there is light-headedness, blurred vision, or if severe, a syncopal episode after standing. Conversely, if after a period of adjustment upon assuming the upright position, the BP rises and the HR drops, this condition is termed *hyperstasis* and can indicate excess circulatory volume compromising a dysfunctional left ventricle.

Many other clinical conditions, cardiac and noncardiac, and medications also can produce postural hemodynamic changes unrelated to volume status. Many concomitant illnesses closely associated with cardiac disease also can cause orthostatic hypotension (Table 44-5). Therefore, this assessment finding, as with all assessment findings, must be considered within the entire picture.

The ever-increasing reliance on noninvasive BP monitoring has some drawbacks. This is particularly true in the case of dysrhythmias and pulsus alternans. Dysrhythmias such as atrial fibrillation and frequent premature ventricular contractions may cause the noninvasive BP machine to record inaccurate HR and BP readings. In the coronary care unit, the HR often is recorded from the electrocardiogram monitor, so this is usually not a problem. However, when nurse assistants are taking and recording all the patient's vital signs, there is danger that they may not be familiar enough with the patient to recognize the disconnect. Therefore, it is up to the nurse who reviews the vital signs and the telemetry readings to ensure that the vital signs are obtained and recorded accurately.

Cardiac Examination

To determine the size and location of the left ventricular apex, inspect and palpate the apical impulse. A visible pulsation may be seen with the patient in the supine position, using tangential lighting. The normal apical impulse is located at the midclavicular line in the 4th or 5th intercostal space. The point of maximal impulse **(PMI)** is often representative of the left ventricular apex. However, in pathological states the PMI can be produced by the right ventricle, the pulmonary artery, or the aorta. The PMI will be displaced laterally in cardiomegaly and medially in COPD. The pulsation may not be visible in obese patients, weight lifters or patients with large breasts.

Next, assess for the PMI by palpating the precordium. The PMI is normally a quick impulse that occurs in a short portion of systole. Palpate to either side of the impulse along the intercostal space, and it is normally palpable for approximately 1 cm. Anything greater than 2 cm may indicate left ventricular hypertrophy or left ventricular dilatation. Palpating the precordium also can help assess right ventricular (**RV**) status and provide input about RV filling pressures and RV function. The RV is not normally palpable. Palpating a systolic pulsation over the parasternal region suggests RV hypertrophy or RV dilatation. A sustained upward thrust in the left parasternal region, often termed an *RV heave,* indicates not only RV hypertrophy but also with high pulmonary pressures. A heave can occur in RV failure or with pulmonary stenosis.[7]

A comprehensive review of cardiac auscultation is provided in Chapter 45. This chapter addresses some tips in learning how to become proficient in cardiac auscultation. First, listen intently while lightly palpating the pulse. The carotid pulse is most closely timed to the central aortic outflow tract[7]; however, the brachial pulse is close enough in timing and often more comfortable to assess by the examiner and patient. Simultaneous palpation of the pulse while auscultating the heart helps the examiner more easily distinguish sounds that occur in systole from those that occur in diastole.

First, listen for normal heart sounds such as S_1 and S_2. S_1 occurs immediately at the beginning of the pulsation, and S_2 occurs at the end of the pulsation. Then note whether there are any adventitious sounds heard. By timing the sounds with the pulse, one can discern easily whether the abnormal sound is systolic or diastolic. Many heart sound assessment tools are available that are good resources; however, they can be very advanced and relatively intimidating to the novice. Therefore, a great way to become proficient in the assessment of heart sounds is to seek other sources to confirm or deny findings. An experienced critical care nurse is a great resource; ask him or her to listen to the patient and relay the findings. The echocardiograph and right heart catheterization findings, if recent, are other good sources for confirming heart sound assessment. Reading the H&P will determine what the admitting physician heard initially. Although these are good methods, there are several caveats to consider. First, mild valvular regurgitation present on echo is not always loud enough to be auscultated. Also, the intensity of mitral regurgitation changes proportionally with intravascular volume; therefore, mitral regurgitation grading can vary from assessment to assessment. Also, an S_3 can disappear when the patient becomes normovolemic and can reappear with elevated filling pressures. So one should trust one's own judgment before deferring to results from a previous assessment.

Respiratory Rate and Rhythm

Tachypnea, often defined as a respiratory rate greater than 20 breaths/min., can reflect a compensatory response to inadequate tissue perfusion in the patient with an acute myocardial infarction, acute pulmonary edema or in heart failure. Detecting a rate and rhythm that demonstrates periods of apnea alternating with tachypnea (Cheyne-Stokes) can be a sign of end-stage circulatory collapse.[18] When the patient is not overtly dyspneic, it is important to make a careful assessment of the work of breathing, particularly in the patient with a chronic cardiac condition such as heart failure. Often the signs of dyspnea are subtle; therefore, the skilled examiner will detect a slight opening of the mouth on inspiration with slight closure on expiration (sometimes referred to as "guppy" breathing) or decreased pulse oximetry saturation or tachycardia while talking. Dyspnea avoidance may be noted by the patient responding to questions with yes-or-no answers. In these cases, ask more open-ended questions and closely observe for breathlessness. Sometimes, the patient will talk in spurts, and when closely observed, tachypnea and/or deep sighs will occur between the phrases.

Breath Sounds

Rales reflect elevated cardiac filling pressures. The presence of rales has an 87 percent positive predictive value for the presence of a pulmonary capillary wedge pressure (**PCWP**) greater than 20 mm Hg.[18] However, the absence of rales is far less likely (approximately 60 percent of the time) to indicate that the PCWP is less than 20 mm Hg.[18] A rationale for this "negative predictive value" is that with chronically elevated pulmonary pressures, the lymphatic system adapts and becomes efficient in clearing lung water from the alveoli but not the interstitium. Thus, the absence of rales does not reflect the absence of pulmonary congestion, but the absence of alveolar congestion. Interstitial edema still compromises carbon dioxide and oxygen movement into and out of capillaries. Another sign of pulmonary edema is pleural effusion, which yields unilateral or bilateral diminished breath sounds. A pleural effusion is dull to percussion.

Temperature

Abnormal temperatures are found in a variety of cardiac conditions. Abnormally low temperatures often are found in low perfusion states such as those associated with acute or chronic heart failure. Temperature elevation reflects immune competence, so an increase of 2 degrees above a patient's baseline (or an absolute temperature of 100°F) should alert the nurse to search for a source of inflammation. Cardiac sources include endocarditis, myocarditis and pericarditis, pericardial effusion, and status post an acute myocardial infarction. Also, concomitant or nosocomial infections such as pneumonia, cystitis, and line sepsis should be suspected. Note that elderly patients may have bacteremia with little or no fever. Older adults with bacteremia have fewer symptoms or signs than younger adults with bacteremia, so fever alone is an unreliable predictor of bacteremia in elders.[22]

Obtaining a temperature upon admission and routinely during the hospitalization can avoid overlooking such complications. The frequency of temperature measurements should vary with severity of the underlying condition. In the coronary care unit, invasive monitoring is more likely, and therefore the unit standard should minimally be every 4 hours, whereas a telemetry unit may have every 8 or 12 hours as a standard for temperature measurement.

Jugular Venous Pulse

The presence of an elevated jugular venous pulse (**JVP**) is one of the most specific indicators of elevated filling pressures (see Chapter 45)[18] Normally, venous blood is not pulsatile, but the pressure and flow changes caused by the right atrium and ventricle are transmitted up into the central venous system. Therefore, the measurement of the top of the pulsation reflects the right atrial pressure. Jugular venous distention, however, is not synonymous with JVP because the vein can be distended when filling pressures are normal and may not show any signs of distention when the right atrial pressures are markedly elevated.[5]

Because the right internal jugular vein is in the most direct line to the right atrium, it is the preferable jugular vein to assess for an elevated pulse pressure, although the external jugular vein also maybe used.[5-8,15] The internal jugular vein lies below the sternocleidomastoid muscle and therefore is not directly visible; however, its pulsations usually are transmitted to the skin of the neck.[5,23] The external jugular vein may be seen readily because it lies superior to the sternocleidomastoid muscle and can be made more prominent by compressing it at the clavicle. (Box 44-5 gives the sequence used to examine the JVP in a hospitalized patient.)

Although when invasively monitored and recorded, the pulsation of the central venous pressure has three positive waves, when one is examining the patient's pulse, usually just two waves are discernible. A normal patient may have a central venous pressure as high as 9 cm H_2O.[5,8,9,23] The right atrium is usually about 5 cm below the sternal angle; therefore, the measured height of JVP of 2 to 4 cm above the sternal angle can be considered normal.[5,7,8,23] (Table 44-6 offers help to differentiate the carotid from the internal jugular vein). Elevated JVP is present in hypervolemic states, RV failure, pulmonary hypertension, RV infarction, pulmonary or tricuspid stenosis, tricuspid insufficiency, constrictive pericarditis, cardiac tamponade, and obstruction of the superior vena cava.[5,7,8]

Abdominal Jugular Reflux

Performing the abdominal jugular reflux examination is of value when RV failure is suspected but not confirmed by the JVP examination.[5,23] Using the palm of the hand, press firmly in the periumbilical region of the abdomen for a minimum of 10 seconds, which increases venous return to the right side of the heart. The normal patient's JVP will be unchanged or have a minimal increase in the height of the pulsation (2 to 3 cm) for less than 10 seconds. In the face of a failing right ventricle, unable to adjust to the increased venous return, JVP can elevate more than 4 cm and either stay elevated until the abdominal pressure is released or partially decline slowly until the pressure is released.[5,21] Positive abdominal jugular reflux can reflect elevated filling pressures or elevated PCWP. This can be due to pure RV failure, biventricular failure, or tricuspid regurgitation.

Hepatomegaly

Assessment for hepatomegaly is an important part of the cardiac examination. See Chapter 45 for the explanation of how to examine the liver by percussion and palpation. An enlarged liver can indicate RV failure with elevated filling pressures leading to hepatic congestion. The liver is actually maintained in place by the abdominal muscles and the diaphragm and can rotate on two axes: the anteroposterior and the transverse axes. Hence, any condition that lowers the diaphragm (e.g., COPD) may make the liver palpable below the coastal

---

BOX 44-5   ■ ■ ■
SEQUENCE FOR ASSESSING JUGULAR VENOUS PULSE

- Ensure the patient is lying comfortably, with the head of bed elevated high enough that the peak of the pulsation is visible.
- The patient's head should be on a pillow that does not cause hyperextension or hyperflexion of the neck.
- Have the patient turn his or her head slightly to the left.
- Encourage the patient to relax the neck muscles.
- Shine a light tangentially across the neck in order to visualize the pulsation more easily.
- In a patient with normal right atrial pressure, the pulsation may be seen with the head of bed at 15 to 30 degrees.
- The head of bed should be increased 15 degrees until a pulsation is visualized.
- If there is no pulsation noted with the patient in the horizontal position, the patient's right atrial pressure is likely to be below normal.
- The higher the patient's filling pressures, the higher the head must be elevated in order to visualize the peak of the pulsation.
- In patients with a cardiac condition this is usually 45 degrees. However, the patient in right ventricular failure may have jugular venous distention at lower elevation levels.
- Examine the patient from the right side and have an additional source of light available (pen light, flashlight, lamp).
- The patient with normal filling pressures may not have any JVP evident at 30 degrees.
- To estimate the right atrial pressure, place a ruler at the sternal angle and hold it straight up. Draw a line horizontally from the peak pulsation of the jugular vein perpendicular to the ruler and measure the cm. Then add 5 cm[15] (the estimate of the central venous pressure below the sternal angle to the right atrium) to the measurement . A normal JVP is ≤9 cm.[15]

JVP, Jugular venous pulse.

■ ■ ■

TABLE 44-6   JUGULAR VENOUS PRESSURE: HOW TO DIFFERENTIATE VENOUS FROM ARTERIAL PULSATION

TRAIT OR METHOD	VENOUS PULSATION	ARTERIAL PULSATION
Palpable	Rarely	Yes
Visible	Yes	Not usually
Inspiration and head of bed elevation	Decreases with inspiration and head of bed elevation	Unchanged
Compression just superior to clavicle	Eliminates visibility	Unchanged
Abdominal pressure	May raise meniscus or make jugular venous pressure more prominent	Unchanged

margin. Loss of abdominal wall muscle strength also may allow the liver to rotate and be palpable below the costal margin. Therefore, a normal-sized liver may be palpable below the costal margin and an enlarged liver may not be palpable. The best method for assessing the liver is to determine the upper liver border by percussion and the lower liver border by palpation upon deep inspiration. If the liver edge is basically parallel to the right costal margin and is palpated far below it, then hepatomegaly is likely.[24]

Ascites

It can be difficult to assess for ascites in the patient with a protuberant abdomen. However, assessing for a "shifting dullness" often makes ascites discernible from adipose tissue. The air in the intestines and stomach causes them to float if there is free fluid in the abdomen. Therefore the highest point of the abdomen will be tympanic to percussion, and the dependent areas will be dull to percussion. After percussing the abdomen in the supine position, have the patient turn on his or her left side for at least 1 minute. Then percuss the abdomen again. The level of dullness will have "shifted" to a higher level on the left side and will be lower on the right.[24]

Edema

Edema caused by left ventricular and or RV failure[6] often begins in the lower extremities, is bilateral, and as the fluid retention progresses, moves upward to the knees, thighs, genitalia, and then into the abdomen.[4] In the average-size person, peripheral edema may not be detectable on examination until a 10–pound weight gain occurs.[4,5] Edema caused by a cardiac condition is pitting (Figure 44-1), and the edema is graded by the amount of pitting present (see Box 45-6). Constrictive pericarditis also may cause bilateral lower extremity edema and ascites. Generalized edema including that of the face and upper extremities is called anasarca and rarely is seen in heart failure except when severe. Hypo-albuminemia, liver failure, and nephrotic syndrome are other possible causes of anasarca. (See Box 44-2 for the noncardiac causes of edema.)

Unilateral peripheral edema should cause one yield a high suspicion for a deep venous thrombosis or it may be due to a saphenous vein graft harvest for a coronary artery bypass surgery. Calcium channel blockers and agents that belong to the antidiabetic class of thiazolidinediones can cause bilateral lower extremity edema. (See Table 44-1 for expected weight gain associated with diabetic agents.) Care should be taken to avoid treating lower extremity edema in patients taking these agents if there are no other symptoms of fluid volume overload, as treatment could cause intravascular volume depletion and renal insufficiency.

CONCLUSION

Because an accurate inpatient assessment is essential to the establishment of a precise diagnosis and a proper treatment plan, every member of the inpatient team can make an essential contribution to good outcomes in the patient experiencing an acute cardiac condition. Therefore, as nurses, it is incumbent upon us to refine our skills continuously in obtaining an accurate history and performing a thorough, focused, and precise physical examination.

REFERENCES

1. National Panel for Acute Care Nurse Practitioner Competencies: *Acute care nurse practitioner competencies, 2004,* Washington, DC, 2004, National Organization of Nurse Practitioner Faculties.
2. Le Blond R, De Gowin R, Brown D, editors: *Degowin's diagnostic examination: the complete guide to assessment, examination, & differential diagnosis,* ed 8, New York, 2004, McGraw-Hill.
3. Seidel H et al. The history and interviewing process. In Seidel H, Ball JW, Dains JE, Benedict GW, editors: *Mosby's guide to physical examination,* ed 5, St Louis, 2003, Mosby.
4. Braunwald E: The history. In Zipes DP, Libby P, Bonow RO, Braunwald E, editors: *Heart disease: a textbook of cardiovascular medicine,* ed 7, Philadelphia, 2005, Elsevier Saunders.
5. O'Rourke R, Silverman E, Shaver J: The history, physical exam and cardiac auscultation. In Fuster V, Alexander RW, O'Rourke RA et al, editors: *Hurst's the heart,* ed 11, New York, 2004, McGraw-Hill.
6. Willerson J: Introduction to cardiac signs and symptoms. In Willerson J, Cohn J, editors: *Cardiovascular medicine,* New York, 1995, Churchill Livingstone.
7. Braunwald E, Perloff JK: The physical examination of the heart and circulation. In Zipes DP, Libby P, Bonow RO, Braunwald E, editors: *Heart disease: a textbook of cardiovascular medicine,* ed 7, Philadelphia , 2005, Elsevier Saunders.
8. Topol E. The history. In Topol E, Califf RM, Isner J et al, editors: *The textbook of cardiovascular medicine,* ed 2, Philadelphia, 2002, Lippincott Williams & Wilkins.
9. Givertz M et al: Clinical aspects of heart failure, pulmonary edema, high output heart failure. In Zipes DP, Libby P, Bonow RO, Braunwald E, editors: *Heart disease: a textbook of cardiovascular medicine,* ed 7, Philadelphia , 2005, Elsevier Saunders.
10. Grady K, Dracup K, Kennedy G et al: Team management of patients with heart failure: a statement for healthcare professionals from the Cardiovascular Nursing Council of the American Heart Association—AHA scientific statement. *Circulation* 102:2443-2456, 2000.
11. Paul S: History taking in the cardiovascular patient. In Davis L, editor: *Cardiovascular nursing secrets,* St Louis, 2004, Elsevier Mosby.

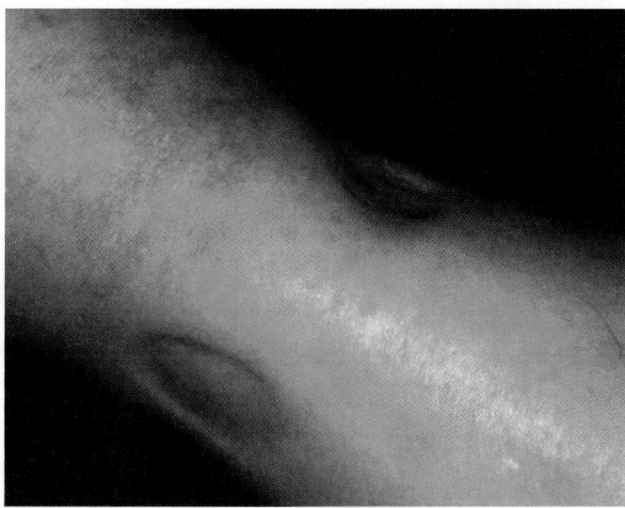

FIGURE 44-1 ■ Pitting edema. (Photo courtesy Jason R. Swanson and Jeffrey L. Melton, MD, Loyola University, Chicago.)

12. Moser D, Worster P: Effect of psychological factors on physiologic outcomes in patients with heart failure, *J Cardiovasc Nurs* 4:106-115, 2000.
13. Dunn SL: Hopelessness as a response to physical illness, *J Nurs Scholarsh* 37:148-153, 2005.
14. Anda R, Williamson D, Jones D et al: Depressed affect, hopelessness and the risks of ischemic heart disease in a cohort of US adults, *Epidemiology* 4:285-294, 1993.
15. Levine B, Motzer S: History taking and physical exam. In Woods S, Froelicher E, Motzer S, editors: *Cardiac nursing,* ed 4, Philadelphia, 2000, Lippincott Williams & Wilkins.
16. McNeill M: Pericardial, myocardial, and endocardial disease. In Woods S, Froelicher E, Motzer S, editors: *Cardiac nursing,* ed 4, Philadelphia , 2000, Lippincott Williams & Wilkins.
17. Miller C: Acute coronary syndromes. In Davis L, editor: *Cardiovascular nursing secrets,* St Louis, 2004, Elsevier Mosby.
18. Young J: Assessment of heart failure. In Colucci W, Braunwald E, editors: *Atlas of heart failure: cardiac function and dysfunction,* ed 2, Philadelphia , 1999, Current Medicine.
19. Sclater A, Alagiakrishnan K: Orthostatic hypotension: a primary care primer for assessment and treatment, *Geriatrics* 59:22-27, 2004.
20. Bradley J, Davis K: Orthostatic hypotension, *Am Fam Physician,* 68:2393-2398, 2003.
21. Consensus statement on the definition of orthostatic hypotension, pure autonomic failure, and multiple system atrophy: the Consensus Committee of the American Autonomic Society and the American Academy of Neurology, *Neurology* 46:1470, 1996.
22. Mouton CP, Bazaldua OV, Pierce B et al: Common infections in older adults, *Am Fam Physician* 63:257-268, 2001.
23. Garg N, Garg N: Jugular venous pulse: an appraisal, *Journal, Indian Academy of Clinical Medicine* 1(3):260-269, 2000.
24. LeBlond R, DeGowin R, Brown D, editors: *Degowin's diagnostic examination: the complete guide to assessment, examination, differential diagnosis,* ed 8, New York, 2004, McGraw-Hill.

chapter 45

Nursing Assessment in the Outpatient Setting

Sharon Josephson-Keeven
Sue Wingate

Cardiac patients who are treated for stable and chronic conditions in the outpatient setting require an approach different from that used for acutely ill patients in the hospital setting. Additionally, as length of stay decreases and the level of severity of the patient's condition increases, the need is intensified for nurses in the outpatient setting to have keen cardiovascular assessment skills.

To that end, this chapter provides an in-depth review of the essential components of outpatient nursing assessment of the cardiac patient. Obtaining the patient's complete medical and psychosocial history is reviewed first. This is followed by a detailed explanation of pertinent aspects of the physical examination.

HISTORY

The patient's history sets the stage for the provider's understanding of how a cardiac problem fits into the context of the patient's life. The history is a critical feature in the evaluation of a suspected cardiovascular disorder. The history includes information about the present illness, past illnesses including coronary heart disease (CHD) risk factors, and the patient's family history as it pertains to cardiovascular disease. Other important information included in the history is the social history, psychological history, sexuality concerns, sleep patterns, spirituality, and nutritional status. The patient's medication history also is obtained.

Chief Complaint

The chief complaint is the statement in the patient's own words about the reason for seeking treatment. The chief complaint or complaints are documented within quotation marks in the order of importance to the patient. Next, explore the details of the chief complaint from the time of onset to the present time. This is called the *history of the present illness.* For each symptom the patient reports, ask the eight questions that are noted in Box 45-1.

A thorough cardiac history should include eight cardinal symptoms: chest pain, dyspnea, edema, fatigue, palpitations, syncope, hemoptysis, and cyanosis. Refer to Box 45-2 for sample questions for each of these symptoms. Listen to the patient. Allow the patient to tell his or her story. Whenever possible, the nurse should question not only the patient but also relatives or close friends to obtain their perspective on the patient's symptoms—if that is acceptable to the patient and is within confidentiality guidelines.

Medical History
Personal

In the personal history, determine any history of CHD, with or without previous myocardial infarction (MI), cardiac murmurs, valvular disease, congenital heart defects, rheumatic heart disease, chronic obstructive pulmonary disease (COPD), systemic lupus erythematosus, dysrhythmias, thyroid disease, or exposure to cardiotoxins such as doxorubicin or cocaine. Ask the patient if he or she has a history of, or treatment in the past or present for, anemia or bleeding disorders, cardiac arrest (including presence of internal cardiac defibrillator), aneurysms, cancer, kidney disease, stroke, seizure disorder, gout, or claudication.

The personal history should include a focused assessment of risk factors for CHD (even if the patient has a preexisting diagnosis of CHD, these factors should still be assessed). Check for a history of smoking (current and past) and exposure to second-hand smoke. Determine the existence of hypertension, dyslipidemia, and/or diabetes mellitus, and if present, evaluate whether these conditions are controlled adequately. (Detail on each of these risk factors is provided in other chapters.) Ask the patient whether any members of the immediate family (parent or sibling) have had an MI, CHD/angina, percutaneous coronary intervention, coronary artery bypass grafting surgery, or sudden cardiac death. Note the age of onset of the relative's cardiac illness/procedure. Coronary disease is considered to be of premature onset if a first-order (parent, sibling) male relative develops CHD before age 55 and/or if a first-order female relative develops CHD before age 65.

Several tools are available to quantify a person's potential risk for CHD based on their risk factor profile. One of the most common tools is the 10-year Risk Estimate, based on data from the Framingham Heart Study (Tables 45-1 and 45-2).

Explore the patient's psychological history. Is there a recent or distant history of depression, anxiety, or other mental health problems? Depression and anxiety are common illnesses in cardiac patients, and a focused assessment of their presence and impact on the patient/family is a key component of the history. A detailed dis-

---

BOX 45-1 ■ ■ ■
QUESTIONS TO ASK FOR SYMPTOMS

When did the symptom start?
Where is the location? Ask the patient to point to it.
What does the symptom feel like?
What precipitates the onset of the symptom?
How long does the symptom last?
Are there any aggravating or relieving factors?
Are there any associated symptoms?
What are the patient's perceptions of what the symptoms mean?

---

cussion of assessment for these problems is given in other chapters.

Determine whether the patient has had prior surgeries or serious injuries. Focus especially on whether the patient has undergone prior cardiac diagnostics and treatments (e.g., noninvasive imaging, cardiac catheterization, percutaneous coronary intervention, coronary artery bypass grafting surgery, or valve repair or replacement).

Verify the patient's immunization status, especially influenza and pneumococcal vaccines. Determine allergies to medications and to environmental allergens and foods. Review the patient's current medications, including prescription medications, over-the-counter medications, vitamins, and herbal products. Make a list of all current medications, including purpose, strength, dosage, and frequency of administration. It is important to ascertain the method the patient uses to remember when and how to take medications (e.g., pill boxes, lists, or family member administering pills). Also helpful is to assess whether the patient knows why he or she is taking each medication and whether the medications are being filled and refilled in accordance with the most current prescription.

Family

As noted before, family history of CHD is a critical part of the patient's history. Other aspects of family history also should be assessed, such as the occurrence of diabetes, hyperlipidemia, stroke, hypertension, arrhythmias, heart failure, and renal disease. Note whether any genetic diseases (e.g., hypertrophic cardiomyopathy, Marfan syndrome, or sickle cell anemia) exist in the family, and elicit the pattern of occurrence if present. Determine the cause and age of death of parents, siblings, and children.

BOX 45-2 ■ ■ ■
SAMPLE QUESTIONS FOR CARDINAL SYMPTOMS

Chest Pain
- How would you describe the pain: burning, pressing, stabbing, crushing, dull, squeezing, aching, sharp, constriction?
- Where is the pain located?
- Are there any associated symptoms: arm/neck/jaw discomfort, dyspnea, fatigue, faintness, dizziness, nausea?
- What brings on the pain? Is there a pattern with exercise, effort, meals, bending over, rest, or position change of arms?
- How long does the pain last?
- How long have you had the pain? When was the last time you had the pain?

Dyspnea
- How long have you experienced shortness of breath? Did your shortness of breath come on suddenly or gradually? Have your symptoms been stable or progressively worsening?
- What type of activities provoke shortness of breath: stairs, inclines, level ground?
- How far can you walk without stopping? Why do you stop: fatigue, chest pain, shortness of breath?
- How many pillows do you sleep on at night? Do you awaken at night with difficulty breathing?
- Do you experience fluid accumulation in your ankles? Have you recently had a weight gain?

Syncope
- How long have you been experiencing faintness? When was the last time you fainted?
- What were you doing when you passed out: turning your head, coughing, urinating, swallowing, sitting to standing?
- Has anyone witnessed these events? Have you ever lost consciousness?
- Was there anything that seemed to provoke fainting: chest pain, nausea, irregular heart beat, pain?

Palpitations
- How long have you had palpitations?
- Describe your palpitations. Are the palpitations fast or slow, regular or irregular, skipping or missing a beat? Did you count your pulse?
- What are you doing when the palpitations come on: exercise, rest, stress?

- What stops the rhythm: coughing, bearing down, drinking water?
- Are there any associated symptoms: chest pain, dizziness, shortness of breath, exercise intolerance?
- Do you have a history of thyroid problems or anemia?
- How much caffeine do you have per day? What over-the-counter medications or new medications have you taken lately? Do you smoke or use recreational drugs?

Edema
- How long have you had leg swelling: gradual or sudden? Is it one or both legs?
- Is the swelling worse in the morning or evening? What makes it better: elevation, stockings?
- Have you noticed any weight changes?
- Have you noticed the presence of shortness of breath?
- Have you noticed pain in the legs?
- Do you have abdominal bloating? Is it harder to fasten your belt?
- [For men] Have you had scrotal swelling?

Fatigue
- How long have you experienced fatigue: gradual or sudden?
- What activities or situations provoke fatigue?
- Are you fatigued in the morning, evening, all day?
- What makes you better? What makes you worse?
- Do you have a history of thyroid disease or anemia?

Hemoptysis
- How long have you been coughing up blood? Was the onset sudden or gradual?
- How often do you cough blood?
- How much blood have you noticed: quantify?

Cyanosis
- How long have you experienced blue color of the lips or fingers?
- Under what circumstances have you noticed the blue color?
- Did the symptoms occur gradually or suddenly?
- Do you know of anyone in your family with this same problem?
- Do you experience cough or chest pain with these symptoms?

■ ■ ■

TABLE 45-1   ESTIMATE OF 10-YEAR RISK FOR MEN

(FRAMINGHAM POINT SCORES)

AGE	POINTS
20-34	−9
35-39	−4
40-44	0
45-49	3
50-54	6
55-59	8
60-64	10
65-69	11
70-74	12
75-79	13

	POINTS				
TOTAL CHOLESTEROL	AGE 20-39	AGE 40-49	AGE 50-59	AGE 60-69	AGE 70-79
Less than 160	0	0	0	0	0
160-199	4	3	2	1	0
200-239	7	5	3	1	0
240-279	9	6	4	2	1
≥280	11	8	5	3	1

	POINTS				
	AGE 20-39	AGE 40-49	AGE 50-59	AGE 60-69	AGE 70-79
Nonsmoker	0	0	0	0	0
Smoker	8	5	3	1	1

HDL (mg/dl)	POINTS
≥60	−1
50-59	0
40-49	1
Less than 40	2

SYSTOLIC BP (mm Hg)	IF UNTREATED	IF TREATED
Less than 120	0	0
120-129	0	1
130-139	1	2
140-159	1	2
≥160	2	3

POINT TOTAL	10-YEAR RISK %
Less than 0	Less than 1
0	1
1	1
2	1
3	1
4	1
5	2
6	2
7	3
8	4
9	5
10	6
11	8
12	10
13	12
14	16
15	20
16	25
≥17	≥30
	10-year risk _____%

HDL, High-density lipoprotein; *BP,* blood pressure.

■ ■ ■

TABLE 45-2   ESTIMATE OF 10-YEAR RISK FOR WOMEN

(FRAMINGHAM POINT SCORES)

AGE	POINTS
20-34	−7
35-39	−3
40-44	0
45-49	3
50-54	6
55-59	8
60-64	10
65-69	12
70-74	14
75-79	16

	POINTS				
TOTAL CHOLESTEROL	AGE 20-39	AGE 40-49	AGE 50-59	AGE 60-69	AGE 70-79
Less than 160	0	0	0	0	0
160-199	4	3	2	1	1
200-239	8	6	4	2	1
240-279	11	8	5	3	2
≥280	13	10	7	4	2

	POINTS				
	AGE 20-39	AGE 40-49	AGE 50-59	AGE 60-69	AGE 70-79
Nonsmoker	0	0	0	0	0
Smoker	8	5	3	1	1

HDL (mg/dl)	POINTS
≥60	−1
50-59	0
40-49	1
Less than 40	2

SYSTOLIC BP (mm Hg)	IF UNTREATED	IF TREATED
Less than 120	0	0
120-129	1	3
130-139	2	4
140-159	3	5
≥160	4	6

POINT TOTAL	10-YEAR RISK %
Less than 9	Less than 1
9	1
10	1
11	1
12	1
13	2
14	2
15	3
16	4
17	5
18	6
19	8
20	11
21	14
22	17
23	22
24	27
≥25	≥30
	10-year risk _____%

HDL, High-density lipoprotein; *BP,* blood pressure.

Personal and Social History
Personal Status

Ask the patient where he or she was born and raised and whether he or she identifies with a particular ethnic or cultural group. If appropriate, determine the patient's preferred language for communication and what systems are available to facilitate language interpretation if needed. What education level has been attained, and is the patient able to read and understand any health materials given to him or her? Determine the marital status (or partner status, as appropriate) and the ages and health of any children. Also try to elicit whether there are other social support systems in place for the patient (e.g., friends, extended family, work colleagues, or confidant).

Habits
Nutrition

What does the patient eat in a "normal" day (or 3 days)? Is the patient adhering to a particular eating plan (e.g., for diabetes) or diet restriction: calories, sodium, fats/cholesterol, proteins, carbohydrates? Numerous diet plans? What is the pattern for meals, who prepares the meals, and are meals often eaten out?

Patients with heart failure should be questioned about their fluid intake. What is their daily fluid intake, and what types of fluid are ingested? Has the patient ever been advised to restrict fluid intake, and if so, what type of restriction was imposed and how has the patient adhered to it? Does the patient have hyponatremia? More detail on nutritional assessment is provided in Chapter 12.

Sleep Patterns

What is the patient's usual sleep pattern, including naps? Does the patient or family member perceive that there are sleeping problems such as insomnia, frequent awakenings, sleeping too much, snoring, or some other type of sleep-disordered breathing? What has the patient tried thus far to remedy any sleep problem (pharmacological and nonpharmacological)? Sleep disturbances are common in cardiac patients and can complicate the treatment regimen and cause undue fatigue and daytime sleepiness. More detail on sleep assessment is provided in Chapter 17.

Activity and Exercise

How active (or inactive) is the patient in a "normal" day? What type of work (physical work) and home (e.g., house and yard work) activities are done? Does the patient perform exercise routinely, sporadically, or not at all? How are activity and exercise routines tolerated?

These questions are part of assessing the patient's functional capacity. Initial and serial assessments of functional capacity are key to detecting changes in the patient's status. Generally, functional status is determined by asking the patient about the level of activity that can be performed without symptoms of breathlessness, chest pain, or fatigue. The New York Heart Association classification is the most commonly used classification system for functional capacity (Box 45-3);

BOX 45-3 ■ ■ ■
NEW YORK HEART ASSOCIATION FUNCTIONAL CLASSIFICATION

Class I: No limitation of physical activity. Ordinary activity does not cause undue fatigue or dyspnea.
Class II: Slight limitation of physical activity. Comfortable at rest, but ordinary physical activity results in fatigue or dyspnea.
Class III: Marked limitation of physical activity. Comfortable at rest, but less than ordinary activity causes fatigue or dyspnea.
Class IV: Unable to carry out any physical activity without symptoms. Symptoms occur at rest. If any physical activity is undertaken, symptoms are increased.

BOX 45-4 ■ ■ ■
THE CANADIAN CARDIOVASCULAR SOCIETY FUNCTIONAL CLASSIFICATION OF ANGINA PECTORIS

Class I: Ordinary physical activity does not cause angina, such as walking and climbing stairs. Angina occurs with strenuous, rapid, or prolonged exertion at work or recreation.
Class II: Slight limitation of ordinary activity. Angina occurs on walking or climbing stairs rapidly, walking uphill, walking or stair climbing after meals, or in cold, or in wind, or under emotional stress, or only during the few hours after awakening. Angina also occurs with walking more than two blocks on the level and climbing more than one flight of ordinary stairs at a normal pace and in normal condition.
Class III: Marked limitations of ordinary physical activity. Angina occurs on walking one to two blocks on the level and climbing one flight of stairs in normal conditions and at a normal pace.
Class IV: Inability to carry on any physical activity without discomfort—anginal symptoms may be present at rest.

From Campeau L: *Circulation* 54:522-523, 1976 (letter).

---

however, it is subjective and is often difficult to use in patients with comorbidities that also affect their activity levels.[1] For patients with angina, the Canadian Cardiovascular Society Functional Classification of Angina Pectoris (Box 45-4) can be used. Note that this classification system has not been found to correlate with the angiographic severity of underlying coronary artery disease, except for left main coronary artery disease.[2] Further, the prognostic significance of the grading system, although this is not its primary goal, may be inadequate.[3]

Several other methods are available to assess functional capacity objectively, such as exercise stress testing and cardiopulmonary exercise testing. These tests require specialized equipment and trained personnel to perform and interpret the tests and also require that the patient be able physically to walk on a treadmill or ride a bicycle. Another test that provides objective evidence of functional capacity requires minimal equipment and personnel training and that can be performed by most patients is the 6-minute walk test (Box 45-5). This procedure can be incorporated easily into the outpatient nursing assessment.

Stimulants and Alcohol

Ask about the extent of use of caffeine products such as coffee, tea, and colas. Obtain a detailed description of the patient's current and past use of alcohol. Inquire, as appropriate, about any use of illicit drugs.

BOX 45-5
SIX-MINUTE WALK TEST

Equipment
- Timer or stopwatch
- Cones/markers for the turnaround points
- Chair

Location
- Indoors along a long, flat, straight corridor
- Course is 30 meters in length; mark off each 3 meters.

Patient Preparation
- Comfortable clothing, appropriate shoes
- Patient should use usual walking aid (walker, cane).
- Patient should not have exercised vigorously for 2 hours before the test.

Procedure
- Let patient rest in a chair at the starting position for 10 minutes; measure vital signs.
- Instruct patient to do the following:
  The object of test is to walk as far as possible in 6 minutes. You will walk back and forth in the hallway between these markers.
  You may slow down or stop and rest as needed and then resume walking when you are able.
  You may lean against the wall when you rest if needed.
  When you are done, I will measure the distance you walked.
- Set timer or stopwatch and ask patient to begin walking.
- Do not walk with the patient. Watch the patient closely while he or she is walking. Inform the patient when each minute has passed. Do not use words of encouragement.
- If patient stops before 6 minutes are done, or if the examiner thinks the patient should not continue, provide a chair for the patient and note that the test is completed.
- When 15 seconds are left, advise the patient you will soon tell him or her to stop.
- When the 6 minutes are done, tell the patient to stop; mark the spot where the patient stopped. Provide a chair if needed.
- Record the total distance covered in meters, rounding to the nearest meter.

From American Thoracic Society: *Am J Respir Crit Care Med* 166:111-117, 2002.

Sexual History

Sexuality problems are common in cardiac patients, and the nurse should purposely elicit concerns in this area because patients are frequently reluctant to introduce the topic. Are there concerns about sexual feelings or performance? Does the patient relate these concerns to particular illnesses or medications? Does the patient's partner have concerns also? What has the patient/partner tried to alleviate any problems? More detail on sexuality assessment is provided in Chapter 18.

Home Environment

What type of living arrangements does the patient have (e.g., home, apartment, or homeless)? Can the patient physically navigate the home (e.g., steps)? How many persons live with the patient (if any)? Are there pets in the home? Does the patient have transportation to appointments?

Occupation

What does the patient consider to be his or her occupation (e.g., work outside the home, retired, housewife/husband)? Does he or she work full time or part time? What type of physical activity is involved at work, and

is the patient able to perform this? Are there environmental hazards at work? Will the patient's current illness affect his or her work status?

Religion and Spirituality

Does the patient/family have a specific religious or spiritual preference? Do accommodations need to be made in the health care environment to meet these religious preferences? Does the religious preference dictate certain aspects of the patient's medical care (e.g., Jehovah's Witness and blood products)?

Financial Issues

Each patient situation is unique in terms of financial issues. However, it may be important to determine whether patients have concerns about their finances as related to their health care. Do they have health insurance? Does it provide adequate coverage? Are they able to afford their medications?

PHYSICAL EXAMINATION

Important information is obtained by a careful and deliberate physical examination. A physical examination typically is done upon initial presentation and then each subsequent time the patient is seen in the outpatient setting. The physical examination of the heart and circulation involves the following: physical appearance or general inspection; the arterial and jugular venous pulses; blood pressure; and inspection, palpation, and auscultation of the heart. Examination of the chest, abdomen, and extremities also may reveal abnormalities of cardiovascular disease.

The examiner should develop an orderly, systematic manner for performing the examination the same way each time. Consider the following in setting up the appropriate environment for the examination. The examination should take place in a quiet room that is well-lit (tangential lighting). The provider and the patient should be comfortable, and the provider's hands and instruments should be warm. The patient's upper body should be elevated 30 to 45 degrees, and the patient's clothing should be removed from the neck and thorax with the patient appropriately draped for privacy. A recommendation is that the examiner stand at the patient's right side so that he or she is able to move freely about the patient and the examination table without hindrance.

General Appearance

The assessment of the patient's general appearance begins at the time the history is being obtained. For general appearance, note the patient's toleration of walking into the examination room and sitting up on the examination table. Assess the patient's level of distress; that is, does the patient look acutely or chronically ill or well? Note the general build of the patient, skin color and temperature, and presence of shortness of breath, orthopnea, and distention of the neck veins. If the patient is in pain, is he or she sitting quietly (typical of angina pectoris), moving about to find a more comfortable position (typical of acute MI), sitting upright (heart failure), or leaning forward (pericarditis)? Does the body shake with each heartbeat, and are bounding pulses (Corrigan pulses) present in the neck (as in severe aortic regurgitation)?[4]

Assess the patient's overall nutritional state (e.g., cachectic), and look for clues as to the presence of comorbidities (e.g., barrel chest of COPD). The patient's level of consciousness should be noted (e.g., alert and oriented), as well as the patient's demeanor (e.g., anxious).

Extracardiac manifestations of heart abnormalities may provide clues to conditions that affect the cardiovascular system. In sequential order, particularly note the patient's body habitus, face, ears, eyes, extremities, skin, chest, and abdomen. Table 45-3 gives more detailed information about this aspect of the examination.

■■■

TABLE 45-3 EXTRACARDIAC FINDINGS IN CARDIAC DISEASE

	DESCRIPTION	CONDITION
Stature	Tall associated with long extremities	Marfan syndrome
	Sparse subcutaneous fat	Mitral valve prolapse
		Aortic dilatation/dissection
	Tall with long extremities	Klinefelter syndrome
	Tall stature with thick extremities of acromegaly	Hypertension
		Cardiomyopathy
		Conduction defects
	Short stature, webbed neck, low hairline, small chin, wide-set nipples, sexual infantilism of Turner syndrome	Coarctation of the aorta
		Pulmonic stenosis
	Dwarfism	Atrial septal defects
		Common atrium
	Truncal obesity associated with thin extremities, moon face, buffalo hump	Hypertension with Cushing syndrome
	Mesomorphic, overweight, tense, balding, middle-aged patient	Coronary heart disease
Face	Hypertelorism, pigmented moles, webbed neck, wide-set eyes of Turner syndrome	Coarctation of the aorta
		Pulmonic stenosis
	Premature aging of Werner syndrome and progeria	Premature coronary heart disease and systemic atherosclerotic disease
	Elfin face (small chin, malformed teeth, wide-set eyes, patulous lips, baggy cheeks, blunt and upturned nose), hypercalcemia, mental retardation	Congenital pulmonary artery stenosis
		Supravalvular aortic stenosis
	Tightening of the skin and mouth, scattered telangiectasias, hyperpigmentation or hypopigmentation of scleroderma	Pulmonary hypertension
		Pericarditis
		Myocarditis
	Round, chubby face	Congenital valvular pulmonic stenosis
	Flushed cheeks and cyanotic lips	Mitral stenosis (acrocyanosis)
Eyes	Stare and proptosis	Increased central venous pressure
	Blue sclera of osteogenesis imperfecta	Aortic regurgitation
	Icteric sclerae	Cardiac cirrhosis
	Enlarged lacrimal glands	Sarcoidosis
		Restrictive cardiomyopathy Conduction defects
		Possibly cor pulmonale
Nails	Systolic flushing of nailbeds (Quincke sign)	Aortic regurgitation
	Osler nodes (small, tender, purple erythematous lesions occurring most often in pads of fingers or toes and in palms of the hand and soles of the feet)	Infected microemboli of bacterial endocarditis
	Janeway lesions (slight raised nontender erythematous or hemorrhagic lesions of palms or soles)	Bacterial endocarditis
	Raynaud phenomenon of scleroderma	Pulmonary hypertension
		Myocardial disease
		Pericarditis
		Valvulopathy
	Hyperextendable joints of osteogenesis imperfecta	Aortic regurgitation
	Nicotine stains of smoker	Coronary heart disease
	Mainline track lines of intravenous drug abusers	Tricuspid regurgitation
		Septic emboli
		Endocarditis
Thorax	Ankylosing spondylitis	Aortic regurgitation
		Heart block
	Thoracic bulges	Atrial or ventricular septal defects
	Loss of thoracic kyphosis or straight back syndrome	Mitral valve prolapse
	Right upper quadrant pulsation	Tricuspid regurgitation
Skin	Cyanosis	Congenital heart disorder
	Mainline track lines of intravenous drug abusers	Tricuspid regurgitation
		Septic emboli
		Endocarditis
	Furuncle	Source septicemia

Head

The examination of the head includes facial characteristics, color, temperature, eyes, and ears. Examination of the face may reveal, for example, myxedema. In myxedema, the face is dull and expressionless and is associated with periorbital puffiness, loss of lateral eyebrows, large tongue, and dry, sparse hair. Bobbing of the head coincident with each heartbeat (*de Musset sign*) is characteristic of severe aortic regurgitation. Facial edema may be present in patients with tricuspid valve disease or constrictive pericarditis.[4] The earlobes may pulsate in the patient with tricuspid regurgitation, or the presence of an earlobe crease may suggest the possibility of CHD. Facial pallor may indicate anemia.

Eyes

Exophthalmos, lid lag, and stare occur not only with hyperthyroidism—which can cause high-output heart failure, supraventricular tachyarrhythmias, and angina—but also in advanced heart failure.[4] Corneal arcus, a light gray ring around the iris, is normal in the older adult but is associated with hypercholesterolemia in persons under the age of 40 years. Xanthelasmas are yellowish raised plaques in the skin that appear along the nasal side of one or both eyelids and are suggestive of hypercholesterolemia. Subconjunctival petechiae and hemorrhages of the upper and lower eyelids are seen in endocarditis.

Extremities

Various congenital and acquired cardiac malformations are associated with characteristic changes in the extremities. Inspect the extremities for overall size, shape, and position. The patient with Turner syndrome, for example, may have characteristic cubitus valgus (elbow/forearm is bent or twisted outward away from the midline). Fifty to 70 percent of these patients have clinically significant aortic coarctation. Patients with Holt-Oram syndrome (i.e., atrial septal defect with skeletal deformities) often have a thumb with an extra phalanx or radius and ulna deformities.[4]

Observe the patient's extremities for central and peripheral cyanosis. Central cyanosis, seen in lips, mouth, and conjunctivae, indicates poor arterial circulation. Peripheral cyanosis (acrocyanosis), seen in lips, ear lobes, and nail beds, indicates peripheral vasoconstriction.

Check the fingers for clubbing. Clubbing is associated with pulmonary and cardiovascular disease. Clubbing is noted when the distal tips of the fingers become bulbous, and the angle of the base of the nail and skin next to the cuticle increases from the normal 160 to 180 degrees or more, and the nail bed feels soft and spongy. Inspect the fingernails for the presence of subungual splinter hemorrhages of bacterial endocarditis. Last, if there is an alternating flushing and paling of the nail bed, specifically at the nail border (pink and white interface), this may be the Quincke sign of moderate to severe aortic regurgitation.

Pallor may suggest anemia. Sudden pallor associated with pain and coldness in the extremities may suggest peripheral embolization. Jaundice may suggest hepatic congestion that is associated with right ventricular overload.

Observe the skin, noting the color, temperature, hair distribution, and moistness because these are subtle clues about the patient's perfusion status. Assess capillary refill time by putting slight pressure on a nail bed until it blanches and then quickly releasing the pressure. When circulation is adequate, nail color returns to baseline in less than 2 seconds. Conversely, a pale nail bed with delayed capillary refill may indicate decreased peripheral perfusion. If indicated by the patient's history, test for *Homans sign*. This is done by flexing the patient's knee slightly with one hand, and with the other hand, dorsiflexing the patient's foot. The complaint of calf pain with this maneuver is a positive sign and usually indicates thrombosis.[5]

Evaluate the patient for edema, especially in the lower extremities. Edema also occurs in other dependent areas such as the sacrum and scrotum. Press the index finger over a bony prominence such as the tibia for several seconds; a depression that does not rapidly refill and resume its original shape indicates orthostatic, or pitting, edema. Edema that is accompanied by thickening and ulceration of the skin usually is associated with deep venous obstruction or valvular incompetence.[5] A scale to grade edema is shown in Box 45-6. The patient should be weighed at every office visit, and each weight should be compared with the baseline (or dry) weight. If the weight has increased since the last visit and is accompanied by edema, this could indicate decompensated heart failure.

Arterial Pulse

Evaluate the pulses in the upper extremities: brachial, radial, and ulnar. In the lower extremities, evaluate the femoral, popliteal, dorsalis pedis, and posterior tibial areas (Figure 45-1). Using the first two fingers, compare the strength of the pulse bilaterally. Note the presence and intensity of the pulses. By comparing bilateral pulses, one can detect asymmetries that may be suggestive of embolic, atherosclerotic, dissecting, or extrinsic occlusion. Ordinarily, the femoral pulse is stronger than the radial pulse. If this is reversed or if the femoral pulsation is absent, suspect coarctation of the aorta. If the radial pulse is delayed relative to the brachial pulse, this may indicate severe aortic stenosis. If an extremity does not have a palpable pulse, try using a Doppler probe to obtain the pulse. If a pulse is not discernible with the Doppler, alert the appropriate provider.

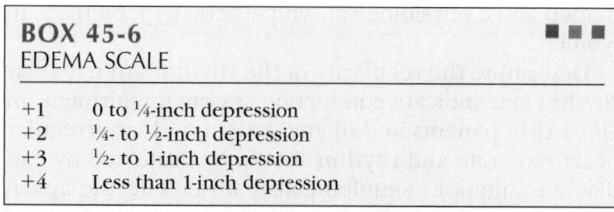

BOX 45-6 ■ ■ ■
EDEMA SCALE

+1	0 to ¼-inch depression
+2	¼- to ½-inch depression
+3	½- to 1-inch depression
+4	Less than 1-inch depression

From Stillwell SB: *Quick critical care reference*, St Louis, 1990, Mosby.

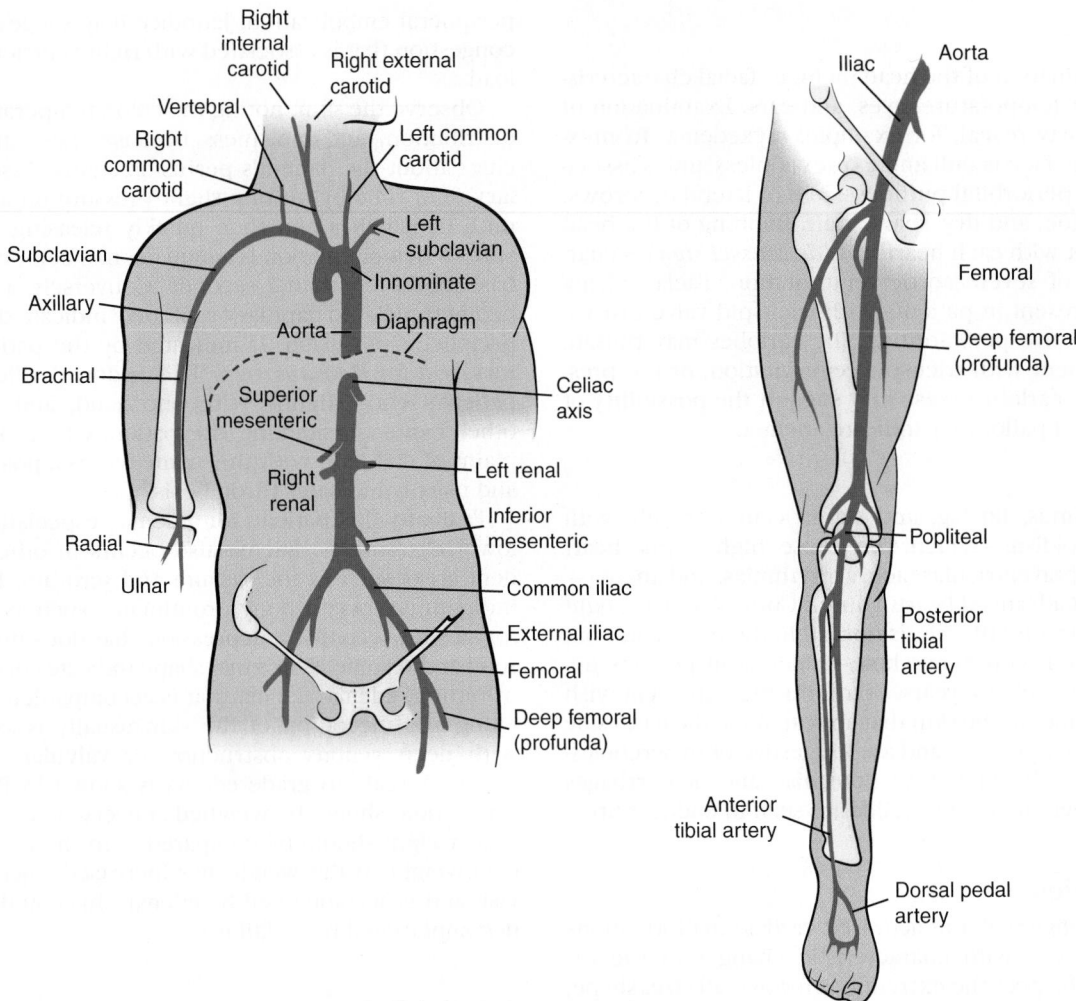

FIGURE 45-1 ■ Arterial tree. (From Price SA, Wilson LM: *Pathophysiology: clinical concepts of disease,* ed 4, St Louis, 1992, Mosby.)

The information to be gained from palpation of the arterial pulse includes information about the pulse rate and rhythm, the amplitude and contour of the pulse wave, any obstructions to arterial blood flow, and conditions associated with alterations in the arterial pulse.

Pulse Rate and Rhythm

The heart rate typically is taken at rest via the radial artery. Check the heart rate by counting the pulsation. With the pads of the index and middle fingers, compress the radial artery until maximal pulsation is detected. The normal heart rate at rest is between 60 to 100 beats/min. A rate slower than 60 beats/min is considered *bradycardia,* and a rate faster than 100 beats/min, *tachycardia.* Women have a higher resting heart rate than men because of a higher parasympathetic tone in men and a physiological sympathetic hyperactivity in women.[6]

Determine the regularity of the rhythm. An irregular rhythm may indicate conduction system impairment. In all cardiac patients and in any patient with an irregular heart rate, rate and rhythm should be evaluated by cardiac auscultation. Simultaneously auscultate the apical heart rate and palpate the radial artery (*apical-radial*

rate) for a minute, and then compare the two numbers. Normally, the numbers are the same, indicating that the heart is perfusing the peripheral tissue adequately with each beat. An abnormal finding is a difference between the apical and radial heart rate. This finding may indicate inadequate perfusion, as in the case of atrial fibrillation.

Pulse Amplitude and Contour

Because of their proximity to the heart, the carotid arteries or more specifically the right carotid artery provides the most accurate assessment of the arterial waveform and cardiac function. The carotid arteries are the largest palpable vessels and are closest to the aortic valve. The distal arteries have a palpable delay between ventricular contractions, thus making the pulses in the arms and legs unsuitable for timing cardiac events.[7] Figure 45-2 demonstrates that the arterial wave contour changes as the distance from the aortic valve increases.

The carotid arteries are located in the neck, just medial to and below the angle of the jaw (Figure 45-3). First observe the presence of visible and abnormal pulsations, which often are seen in patients with aortic re-

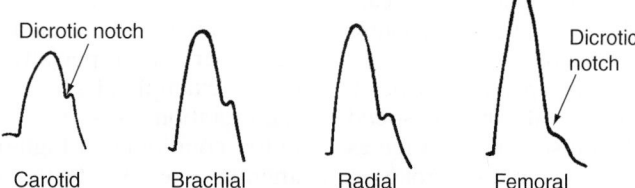

FIGURE 45-2 ■ The contour of the arterial pulse wave changes as the distance from the aortic valve increases (From Abrams J: *Synopsis of cardiac physical diagnosis,* ed 2, Woburn, Mass, 2001, Butterworth Heinemann.)

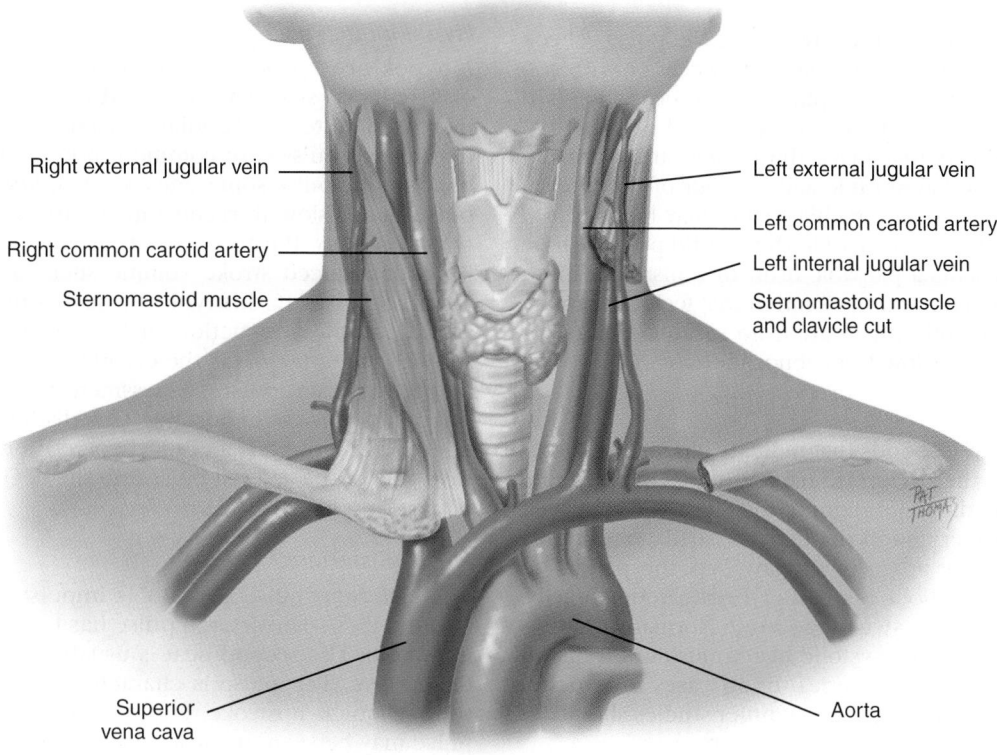

NECK VESSELS

FIGURE 45-3 ■ Neck vessels. (From Jarvis C: *Physical examination and health assessment,* ed 4, Philadelphia, 2004, WB Saunders.)

gurgitation. The palpation technique involves the use of the first two fingers palpating the lower third of the right neck. You also may use the thumb. Use light pressure and palpate only one carotid artery at a time to avoid compromising arterial blood flow to the brain. To prevent vagal stimulation, avoid compressing the carotid sinus located high in the neck.

Normally, the left ventricle ejects blood into the aorta to the arterial system. A pulse is generated when the pressure wave moves rapidly through the arterial system.[5] The first part of the central aortic pulse wave reflects the ejection of blood into the aorta (Figure 45-4). The later systolic component (*tidal wave*) includes the peak or crest of the pulse wave. A notch or change in slope of the early pulse contour is called the *anacrotic notch.* Diastole is initiated by an abrupt negative wave called the *dicrotic notch.* The dicrotic notch indicates aortic valve and pulmonic valve closure. Normally, only the systolic

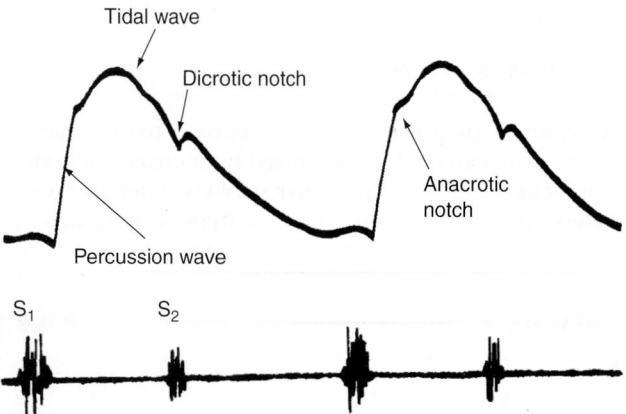

FIGURE 45-4 ■ Normal arterial pulse. (From Abrams J: *Synopsis of cardiac physical diagnosis,* ed 2, Woburn, Mass, 2001, Butterworth Heinemann.)

peak is palpable. The anacrotic and dicrotic notches cannot be felt when examining the arterial pulse because the pulse is not palpable during diastole.[8]

Pulse contour usually refers to the speed of the pulse wave upstroke, the duration of its peak, and the speed of its downstroke. Normally, the pulse contour is felt as a forceful wave that is smooth with rapid upstroke on the ascending part of the wave, becoming domed, less steep, and slower on the descending part. The contour of the arterial pulse should not be examined in peripheral vessels such as the radial artery. It is best to use the peripheral vessels for subtle findings, such as pulsus alternans.

Amplitude refers to the strength of the pulse. Check for variation in amplitude from beat to beat or with respiration. A scale to describe pulse amplitude is shown in Box 45-7. Some patients may have carotid obstruction, kinking, or thrills that make the carotid artery unsuitable for assessing amplitude and contour of the arterial pulse. In this case, the brachial artery may be used. On occasion, a shudder or *thrill* in the carotid pulse will be felt and represents a palpable bruit or transmitted murmur. A thrill is a humming vibration that feels like a purring cat. Most carotid thrills are from vascular disease or left ventricular outflow tract abnormalities.

Bruits

Bruits are arterial sounds that indicate blood flow turbulence (e.g., artherosclerotic narrowing). To auscultate for bruits, use the diaphragm of the stethoscope placed behind the upper end of the thyroid cartilage to immediately below the angle of the jaw. Ask the patient to exhale and then hold his or her breath momentarily. Listen for a blowing, swishing sound. Normally, there is no sound. Sometimes systolic heart murmurs transmit sounds to the carotid arteries. In all cases in which a carotid bruit is heard, carotid Doppler studies should be performed to check for an obstruction.

Bruits noted in the femoral arteries may suggest partial obstruction to blood flow to the legs. Bilateral bruits heard in the femoral arteries may indicate an abdominal aortic aneurysm. A patient seen in the office after cardiac angiography should be evaluated postprocedure for femoral bruits, which may indicate a pseudoaneurysm.

Alterations in Arterial Pulse
Hyperkinetic Pulse

A hyperkinetic pulse contour is represented by a larger than normal arterial pulse caused by increased left ejection velocity or left ventricular stroke volume or an elevated arterial blood pressure. A hyperkinetic arterial pulse may be present in mitral regurgitation and also in patients with decreased arterial compliance, such as elderly persons, especially if they are hypertensive. A classic example of a hyperkinetic pulse occurs in aortic regurgitation as a result of widened pulse pressure. Other conditions of high-output states such as anxiety, anemia, exercise, fever, or hyperthyroidism also can cause a hyperkinetic pulse.

Corrigan or Water-Hammer Pulse

Corrigan pulse is a bounding pulse of aortic regurgitation characterized by a rapidly rising and collapsing pulse.

Hypokinetic Pulse

A hypokinetic pulse has diminished amplitude because of a reduced stroke volume and ejection fraction and increased systemic vascular resistance. These weak or diminished pulses are common in low output states. A hypokinetic pulse sometimes is called *pulsus parvus*. A pulse that is slow in rising and late in peaking is called *pulsus tardus*. Pulsus parvus typically occurs in conditions of reduced stroke volume such as heart failure, whereas pulsus tardus typically occurs in conditions of aortic outflow obstruction such as aortic stenosis. *Pulsus parvus et tardus* is the carotid pulse characterized by both types of pulses. Assessment of the rise of a hypokinetic pulse is important. This distinction is important because there is a clinical correlation between the slow rise of the arterial pulse and the degree of severity of aortic stenosis.

Pulsus Bisferiens

The bisferious pulse is a double impulse during systole (Figure 45-5). The arterial pulse has two palpable beats in systole. The second beat is usually equal in strength to the first. The pulse is characterized by large amplitude, a quick upstroke, and a rapid downstroke. The pulse may be seen in aortic regurgitation (with or without aortic stenosis) or in normal individuals without aortic disease during high-output states such as exercise, anemia, or hyperthyroidism.

Pulsus Alternans

Pulsus alternans is the presence of alternating strong and weak arterial pulses in a patient in sinus rhythm. The presence of pulsus alternans usually indicates severe left ventricular dysfunction. The alternating amplitude of pulsus alternans is best assessed in peripheral arteries, such as the brachial or radial artery, using light palpating pressure with two fingers. The proximal finger should vary the pressure in an attempt to obliterate the second (weaker) pulse. Pulsus alternans should not be confused with bigeminal, premature beats. In bigeminy, every other pulse is diminished and early, whereas pulsus alternans has a regular rhythm.

Pulsus Paradoxus

Pulsus paradoxus is reduced pulse amplitude on inspiration. Pulsus paradoxus is defined further as a marked and exaggerated decrease in blood pressure associated with inspiration. This is a common finding in pericardial tamponade. Typically, a fall in inspiratory pressure

---

BOX 45-7 ■ ■ ■
PULSE AMPLITUDE SCALE

4+	Normal
3+	Slightly impaired
2+	Moderately impaired
1+	Markedly impaired
0	Absent, not palpable

DESCRIPTION	**ASSOCIATED WITH**

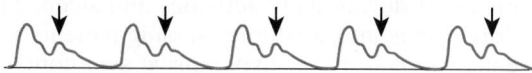

Weak "Thready" Pulse—1+
Hard to palpate, need to search for it, may fade in and out, easily obliterated by pressure

Decreased cardiac output; peripheral arterial disease; aortic valve stenosis

Full Bounding Pulse—3+ or 4+
Easily palpable, pounds under your fingertips

Hyperkinetic states (exercise, anxiety, fever), anemia, hyperthyroidism

Water-Hammer (Corrigan's) Pulse—4+
Greater than normal force, then collapses suddenly

Aortic valve regurgitation; patent ductus arteriosus

Pulsus Bigeminus
Rhythm is coupled, every other beat comes early, or normal beat followed by premature beat. Force of premature beat is decreased due to shortened cardiac filling time

Conduction disturbance, e.g., premature ventricular contraction, premature atrial contraction

Pulsus Alternans
Rhythm is regular, but force varies with alternating beats of large and small amplitude

Left-sided congestive heart failure

Inspiration   Expiration   Inspiration

Pulsus Paradoxus
Beats have weaker amplitude with inspiration, stronger with expiration. Best determined during blood pressure measurement: *reading decreases* (>10 mm Hg) during inspiration and increases with expiration

Cardiac tamponade; constrictive pericarditis

Pulsus Bisferiens
Each pulse has two strong systolic peaks, with a dip in between. Best assessed at the carotid artery

Aortic valve stenosis plus regurgitation

FIGURE 45-5 ■ Variations in arterial pulse. (From Jarvis C: *Physical examination and health assessment,* ed 4, Philadelphia, 2004, WB Saunders.)

of 10 to 12 mm Hg characterizes pulsus paradoxus. Other conditions that may be associated with pulsus paradoxus are asthma, emphysema (because of large fluctuations in intrathoracic pressure), marked obesity, severe heart failure, and constrictive pericarditis. Pulsus paradoxus is evaluated best with a sphygmomanometer. Box 45-8 details how to evaluate for pulsus paradoxus.

Blood Pressure

Normal physiology of the arterial blood pressure has two components: the systolic arterial pressure and the diastolic arterial pressure. The systolic component is related to the cardiac factors of stroke volume, left ventricular ejection, and the elasticity of the blood vessels. Thus, an increase in stroke volume and/or a decrease in arterial wall compliance results in an elevated blood pressure. The diastolic component is related to resistance and arterial compliance. For more detail about the regulation of blood pressure, see Chapter 7.

Korotkoff sounds are sounds produced by the turbulence of blood flow within the artery while the artery is occluded partially by the blood pressure cuff. The Korotkoff sounds are heard with the diaphragm of the stethoscope placed over the brachial artery just below the lower edge of the cuff. Five Korotkoff sounds are heard. Phase I is the first sound detected as the systolic blood pressure. Phase II is initiated by a murmur-like sound. Phase III sounds are easily heard. In Phase IV there is an abrupt dampening or muffling sound. In Phase V the Korotkoff sounds disappear completely when the arterial flow is no longer occluded by the blood pressure cuff. An *auscultatory gap* is a temporary silent interval that occurs between phase I and phase II. To avoid the auscultatory gap, palpate the brachial artery, then inflate the cuff until the arterial pulsation is obliterated, and then proceed to inflate the cuff 20 to 30 mm Hg beyond that point.

Proper measurement of the blood pressure by cuff sphygmomanometry is an important part of the cardiovascular examination. The recommended approach is to palpate the brachial artery and place the diaphragm of the stethoscope over it. Be sure that the patient's arm is placed at the level of the heart. The true blood pressure will be underestimated if the arm is above or below the level of the heart. The cuff should be long enough to wrap comfortably around the upper arm with the edge of the cuff positioned just at the antecubital crease. A loosely applied cuff or a cuff not long enough for a fat, large arm will result in falsely high readings. See Chapter 78 for a detailed description of the proper manner of blood pressure measurement.

The blood pressure should be measured at every outpatient visit and recorded. It is recommended that the blood pressure be taken with the patient in the supine position before upright maneuvers after the patient has been resting for at least 5 minutes. If the patient reports dizziness, syncope, or postural symptoms (often seen in the elderly), measure the blood pressure lying, sitting, and standing, waiting 1 to 3 minutes before taking each positional blood pressure. A drop of more than 12 to 15 mm Hg in the systolic pressure in the standing position accompanied by a pulse increase greater than 10 percent is called *orthostatic* or *postural hypotension* and may occur in volume depletion, in those patients on bed

rest, or in the elderly. Often, however, such hypotension may be due to the actions of medications such as antihypertensive medications. Always ensure patient safety and be prepared to return the patient to the examination table should the patient become symptomatic with position changes.

Inherently, there will be challenges to taking an accurate blood pressure in cardiac patients. Many cardiac patients have irregular rhythms such as atrial fibrillation and premature ventricular contractions. Additionally, in some patients the blood pressure in the office setting will be higher than the blood pressure taken in the patient's home, an effect labeled the "white coat phenomenon." In this situation, continuous ambulatory blood pressure measurement may be helpful in evaluating the patient's blood pressure. For this procedure, the patient wears a blood pressure monitoring device for 24 hours, with multiple blood pressure measurements therefore provided during daily activities and sleep. This procedure also is indicated for assessing patients with apparent drug resistance, hypotensive symptoms with antihypertensive medications, episodic hypertension, and autonomic dysfunction.[9]

Bilateral arm blood pressures should be taken in both arms at the first visit unless contraindicated (e.g., mastectomy, renal fistula, or shunt). Normally, there is no more than a 5- to 10-mm Hg discrepancy in systolic pressure between the arms. A pressure difference greater than 10 to 15 mm Hg may suggest arterial compression or obstruction on the side with the lower pressure. Also, calculate the pulse pressure (difference between systolic and diastolic pressures, for example, a systolic blood pressure of 140 mm Hg and a diastolic blood pressure of 60 mm Hg equals a pulse pressure of 80 mm Hg). A widened pulse pressure is greater than 50 percent of the systolic blood pressure, is suggestive of increased stroke volume and decreased peripheral resistance, and may be seen in aortic regurgitation, fever, anemia, or exercise. A narrowed pulse pressure is less than 25 percent of the systolic blood pressure and may be seen in patients with aortic stenosis, rapid tachycardias in an impaired left ventricle, heart failure, shock, or cardiac tamponade.[9]

Measuring the leg blood pressures is indicated if there is suspicion of coarctation of the aorta or in patients with peripheral vascular disease. (Box 45-9 lists a procedure for obtaining a blood pressure measurement in the leg.) Systolic blood pressure in the legs is normally higher than that in the arms. Diastolic blood pressure is the same. Blood pressure that is lower in the leg than in the arm suggests coarctation of the aorta or dissecting aortic aneurysm. If the difference exceeds 20 mm Hg, with the right arm blood pressure higher than the left arm blood pressure, this may indicate coarctation of the aorta as well.

Venous Pulse

Venous Hum

A venous hum is an innocent murmur caused by flow in the internal jugular vein. A venous hum commonly is heard in children. A venous hum can be differentiated from a carotid bruit in that the venous hum is loudest in diastole, whereas the carotid bruit is heard best in systole. To detect a venous hum, place the patient in a sitting position with the patient's head turned away from the side of auscultation and tilted slightly upward. Place the stethoscope at the medial end of the clavicle and anterior border of the sternocleidomastoid muscle. Venous hums diminish when the patient is supine, when the ipsilateral jugular vein is compressed, or when the patient performs a Valsalva maneuver.[9]

Jugular Venous Pulse

Inspection of the jugular venous pulse (**JVP**) reveals important information about hemodynamics of the right side of the heart. Evaluating the JVP is a skill that takes much practice to learn but provides valuable information regarding the patient's volume status.[1] The internal jugular vein, specifically the right, is best for examination of the JVP because hemodynamics of the right side of the heart are transmitted more directly to the right rather than to the left jugular vein. The right internal jugular vein is located lateral to the carotid artery beneath the sternocleidomastoid (sternomastoid) muscle (Figure 45-3). The patient should be lying comfortably in a 45-degree angle with the head resting on a pillow. If it is difficult to see the pulse (such as with the obese patient or the patient with a short, thick neck), gradually raise the head of the examining table so that the venous waveform is elicited. Moreover, it is easy to miss severely elevated venous pressures by failing to elevate the patient's head adequately; thus, it may be necessary to have the patient sit upright. Elevate the patient's chin and slightly rotate the head to the left, gently stretching the skin of the right lower neck and supraclavicular area. Inspect the jugular vein from different angles. Shine a penlight tangentially across the neck and observe for venous undulations in the neck: focus on skin movement rather than actual pulsations. The sternal angle of Louis, found at the junction of the manubrium and sternum at the level of the second rib, is used as the standard reference point for determining venous pressure.[10] To estimate jugular venous distention, identify the highest level of pulsations in the jugular vein (meniscus). Determine the vertical distance between the sternal angle and meniscus and add 5 cm (the sternal angle is 5 cm above the right atrium). Jugular venous distention greater than 10 cm reflects volume overload (Figure 45-6).

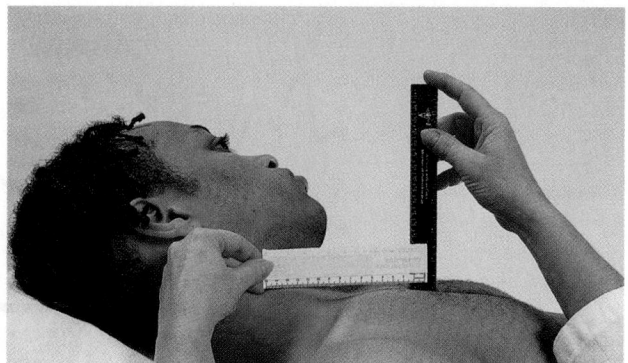

FIGURE 45-6 ■ Measurement of jugular venous pressure. (From Jarvis C: *Physical examination and health assessment,* ed 4, Philadelphia, 2004, WB Saunders.)

Observe the amplitude and the timing of the JVP. To differentiate JVP from carotid pulse, palpate the left carotid pulse while simultaneously visually inspecting the jugular veins of the right side. Alternatively, JVP is analyzed in concert with auscultation of the heart.[10] Other techniques for differentiating JVP from the carotid pulse are listed in Table 45-4.

Hepatojugular (Abdominojugular) Reflux

Creation of hepatojugular reflux is a maneuver to evaluate right ventricular failure. The technique involves applying sustained compression to the periumbilical area for 30 to 60 seconds and observing the JVP. The venous neck pulses will become more prominent, and their level will ascend in the neck. A positive hepatojugular reflux test is a rise in the jugular venous pressure by 1 cm or more that persists throughout the time pressure is applied. This is a characteristic sign of congestion in heart failure and of constrictive pericarditis, cardiac tamponade, severe tricuspid regurgitation, and massive pulmonary embolus. In patients with heart failure and hepatic congestion, avoid compression over the liver because this may cause discomfort to the patient. Important to note is that the hepatojugular reflux has no value in a patient with an already elevated JVP.

■ ■ ■

TABLE 45-4   DIFFERENTIATION OF JUGULAR AND CAROTID PULSATIONS

	INTERNAL JUGULAR VEIN	CAROTID ARTERY
Location	Low in the neck	Deep in the neck
Character	Undulant, not palpable	Brisk, easily felt
Respiration	Level of pulse wave decreased on inspiration and increased on expiration	No effect
Position	Level of the pulsation changes with position, dropping as patient becomes more upright	No effect
Compression	Gentle pressure easily eliminates the pulse wave	No effect
Abdominal pressure	May see increase in pulse pressure	No effect

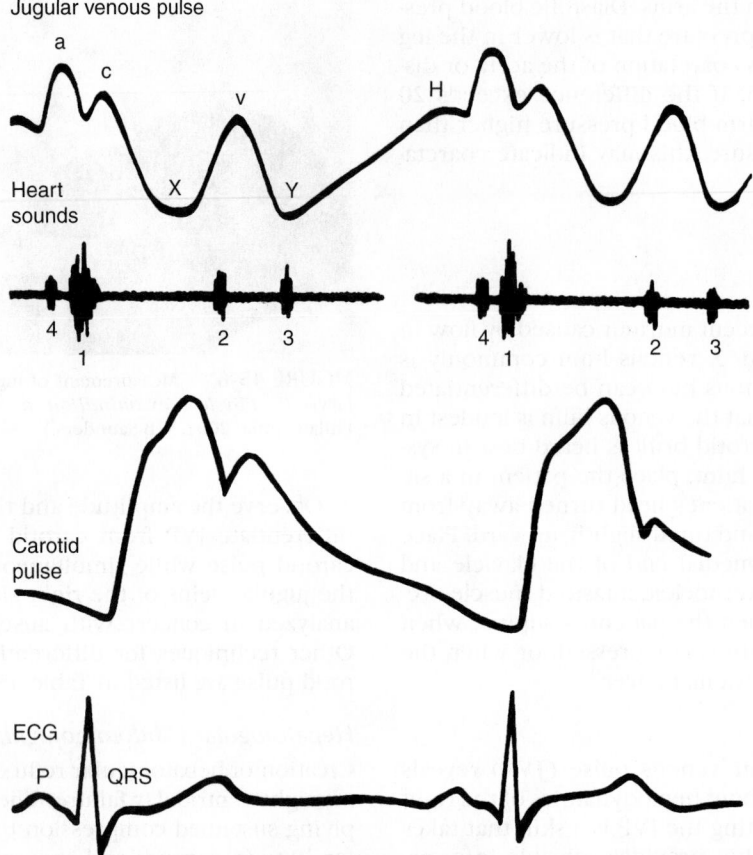

FIGURE 45-7 ■ Normal jugular venous pulse. *ECG,* Electrocardiogram. (From Abrams J: *Synopsis of cardiac physical diagnosis,* ed 2, Woburn, Mass, 2001, Butterworth Heinemann.)

Jugular Venous Pulsations

The JVP reflects the relationship between venous tone, the volume of blood in the venous system, and hemodynamics of the right side of the heart. During the cardiac cycle, there are three positive wave forms if the patient is in a normal sinus rhythm. Jugular venous pulsations occur because of the steady flow of venous return by the contraction and relaxation of the right atrium and ventricle. Because of the fluctuations of the waves, the jugular pulse can be recorded easily, but the pulse is difficult to appreciate at the bedside. At the bedside, the normal JVP consists of two visible (peaks) waves (A wave and V wave) and two visible (troughs) descents (*x* descent and *y* descent; Figure 45-7). Neither the C wave nor the *x* descent is visible (the C wave is usually lost in the A wave, and the *x* descent is merged). In general, descents are easier to detect than ascents. In general, it is easier to time the pulse by using the *x* and *y* descents instead of the A and V waves.[9] The physiological background for these waveforms is presented in Box 45-10.

Abnormalities of the Jugular Venous Pulse

The A wave is absent in atrial fibrillation and atrial flutter. Some conditions can result in prominent or large/giant A waves. The most common cause of a large A wave is when there is strong atrial resistance against an increased ventricular resistance such as obstruction to the tricuspid valve (tricuspid stenosis) or there are clots or tumors in the right ventricle. If the atrium contracts against a closed tricuspid valve, this will result in cannon A waves. Cannon A waves have more of a flickering motion than do prominent A waves. A waves can be regular or irregular. Certain forms of paroxysmal tachycardias have regular cannon waves, as do ventricular paced beats. Irregular cannon waves occur during complete heart block or with premature ventricular contractions. The x descent abnormalities are seen in cardiac tamponade. The *x* descent becomes deeper because of vigorous ventricular contractions.

The V wave is prominent in tricuspid regurgitation. Giant V waves may cause bobbing of the ear lobes and undulant venous pulsations in the neck.

The *y* descent is exaggerated in patients with increased venous pressure from any cause such as constrictive or restrictive heart disease. The striking descent of the *y* wave often is referred to as *Friedreich's sign* and often is accompanied by an S_3.[9]

Last, visually inspect jugular venous pulsations during inspiration and expiration. Normally, JVP should decrease with inspiration and increase with expiration. Elevation of JVP with inspiration is called *Kussmaul sign*. This is caused by restriction in filling of the right ventricle and therefore is seen in patients with constrictive pericarditis. Table 45-5 summarizes disease processes that can be identified by analyzing jugular venous pulsations.

THE HEART

Examination of the heart has three components: inspection, palpation, and auscultation. The examination of the precordium yields information about ventricular hypertrophy and ventricular dilatation. For most of the examination of the heart, the patient should be supine with an exposed thorax with the upper body raised to 30 degrees. During some aspects of the examination, the patient is repositioned from the supine position to the left lateral recumbent position.

■ ■ ■

TABLE 45-5 ABNORMALITIES OF JUGULAR VENOUS PULSE WAVE

WAVEFORM	POSSIBLE ABNORMALITY
Prominent A wave	Diastolic dysfunction
	Tricuspid stenosis
	Pulmonary hypertension
	Pulmonary stenosis
	Hypertrophic cardiomyopathy
	Clots or tumors in the right ventricle
Cannon A wave	Arrhythmias
	Complete heart block
Diminished or absent A wave	Atrial fibrillation
Prominent V wave	Tricuspid regurgitation
Prominent x descent	Cardiac tamponade
Decreased x descent	Atrial fibrillation/flutter
Prominent y descent	Constrictive pericarditis

Inspection

To start the examination, stand to the patient's right side and inspect the anterior chest. Inspect the chest for size and symmetry. Note any scars from cardiac surgery or an implantable device such as a pacemaker. Observe for any pulsations and/or exaggerated lifts or heaves of the chest. On rare occasions, a patient will have an apical impulse on the right side. This is called *dextrocardia*, which means the heart is situated on the right side. Increased pulsation in the sternoclavicular area may signify a possible aneurysm. A *heave* or *lift* is a sustained forceful thrusting of the ventricle during systole. It occurs with ventricular hypertrophy and is seen at the sternal border or the apex.[9] Normally there is an absence of movement except in the mitral area, where the *apical impulse* may be seen. When visible, the apical impulse occupies the 4th or 5th intercostal space at or inside the midclavicular line. Last, inspect the epigastric area for significant pulsations that may indicate possible aneurysm.

Palpation

Palpation confirms the findings noted on inspection. Further, palpation detects pulsatile movements that are not visible. The technique of palpation requires the knowledge of the four valvular landmarks. These landmarks are named for the heart valves and do not correlate anatomically with valve position but rather relate to the valvular outflow tracts. The areas shown in Box 45-11 should be palpated systematically. Knowledge of the locations of underlying cardiac and vascular structures that produce the movements is necessary in order to interpret the significance of the abnormality.

To palpate the pulsations of the heart and great vessels, the examiner should palpate the four cardiac landmarks gently using the base of the fingers. The base of the fingers is more sensitive than the finger tips in detecting pulsations. Alternate between light and heavy pressure so that high-pitched sounds (e.g., ejection sounds, opening snaps, and clicks) or low-pitched sounds (e.g., S_3 and S_4) can be appreciated. Note the presence of pulsations or movements in terms of their location, amplitude, and duration, making specific reference to thrills, lifts, or heaves. As noted, a thrill is a palpable vibration and has been described as feeling like the throat of a purring cat. Thrills are easier to detect with the palm of the hand. A heave or a lift is a sustained forceful thrust of the ventricle during systole that occurs with ventricular hypertrophy and is detected best with firm application of the hand to the chest.

BOX 45-11 ■ ■ ■
CARDIAC PALPATION AREAS

Aortic	2nd right intercostal space
Pulmonic	2nd left intercostal space
Tricuspid	5th intercostal space, lower left sternal border
Mitral	5th intercostal space, left midclavicular line
Erb's point	3rd left intercostal space

Identify the apical impulse on the thorax. The apical impulse normally is felt as a gentle nonsustained tap that is 1 cm in diameter at the 4th or 5th intercostal space medial to the midclavicular line. An area greater than 2 to 2.5 cm in diameter in the supine position or 3 cm in the left lateral decubitus position is abnormal and suggests left ventricular enlargement. Cardiomegaly, for example, displaces the apical impulse laterally and downward. The duration of the apical impulse is short, normally occupying the first half of systole. If the apical impulse lasts longer or is sustained, this is always abnormal and suggests a pressure-overloaded left ventricle such as in aortic stenosis or hypertension. The force of the impulse is also important. A hyperdynamic impulse that lifts the fingers is pathological and reflects left ventricular hypertrophy with good systolic function. The normal contour of the apical impulse is brief, early systolic, and nonsustained.[9] The apical impulse coincides with S_1 and the carotid impulse. The apical impulse may not be felt easily in the supine position in some patients, especially women with large breasts, or in some obese or very muscular patients. In these patients, locate the apical impulse by shifting the patient's position to the left side, which will move the heart closer to the chest wall. The apical impulse is generally not palpable in older individuals, patients with emphysema (because of the hyperinflation of the lungs), obese persons, or persons with increased anteroposterior diameter of the chest.

The left parasternal area is palpated next to evaluate the presence of the right ventricular impulse. The right ventricle lies underneath the anterior precordium adjacent to the lower sternal edge. Normally the right ventricle does not produce visible or palpable chest wall movements except in young or thin persons. Precordial palpation for detection of parasternal or right ventricular activity is done by using firm downward pressure with the palm or heel of the hand with the wrist cocked upward while the patient's breath is held in end-expiration.[10] A palpable right ventricular impulse is referred to as a *right ventricular heave* or *lift* and is usually a clinical sign of right ventricular hypertrophy; however, conditions such as mitral regurgitation can displace the right ventricle anteriorly and cause a right ventricular heave as well. Volume loading of the right ventricle exaggerates the amplitude of the right ventricular impulse, whereas pressure overloading exaggerates the duration of the impulse.[11]

Normally there are no precordial movements in the aortic area. Patients with an aortic aneurysm or a dilated aorta may have movement felt at the right parasternal area. The pulmonic area normally does not generate impulses; however, palpation may reveal vibrations caused by pulmonic stenosis.

Body habitus can affect the ability to assess precordial abnormalities. For example, movements may be more pronounced in someone with a thin chest than in someone with a muscular or obese chest. The precordial abnormalities described are specific but not very sensitive.

Abnormal Precordial Movements

In compensated *aortic stenosis,* the apical impulse is sustained with a left ventricular lift with little or no leftward displacement. The duration and the force of the left ventricular impulse is increased because of the increased left ventricular mass, increased ventricular pressure, and obstruction to the ventricular flow.[10]

Precordial motion in *aortic regurgitation* varies depending on the severity of aortic regurgitation. In mild to moderate aortic regurgitation, the apical impulse is normal in size and hyperkinetic, but there is no displacement of the apical impulse. In severe aortic regurgitation, the apical impulse becomes a sustained, prominent hyperkinetic impulse, and the apex is displaced inferolaterally.

Precordial motion in *mitral regurgitation* varies depending on the chronicity of the disease. Findings in chronic mitral regurgitation are described as a hyperkinetic apical impulse with a lateral downward displacement. A left ventricular heave, thrill, parasternal lift, or palpable S_3 may be present. In acute mitral regurgitation, the apical impulse is hyperkinetic without lateral downward displacement. A left ventricular heave, thrill, parasternal lift, or palpable S_3 may be present.

In patients with *mitral stenosis,* S_1 and S_2 may be palpable. The opening snap is often palpable too, and a diastolic thrill may be felt in the left lateral decubitus position over the apex.[10] The apical impulse is typically nonsustained and decreased in amplitude.

In *hypertrophic cardiomyopathy,* the apical impulse is sustained, forceful, and palpable, particularly in the left decubitus position. Abnormal precordial left ventricular activity in persons with hypertrophic cardiomyopathy is characterized by the presence of a palpable S_4 accompanied by a late systolic apical heave, thrust, or bulge. The combined presence of a palpable S_4, early systolic impulse, and a late systolic bulge may produce a triple contour to the apical impulse called the *triple ripple.*[10]

In patients with *CHD* with angina pectoris who have no history of MI, the apical impulse usually is normal. S_4 may be palpable. Examination of all patients with suspected or proven CHD in the left lateral decubitus position is important for optimal palpation.[10] In patients with prior MI, the apical impulse may be normal or *ectopic* impulses may be present, suggesting a left ventricular aneurysm or left ventricular dyskinesia.[9]

Epigastric and Abdominal Palpation

The last areas of palpation are the epigastric and abdominal areas. The normal aorta is slightly palpable, and the pulse should be in the anterior direction. A prominent pulsating mass may be caused by an aneurysm. Sometimes the right ventricular impulse can be palpated over the epigastric area, which may be related to tricuspid regurgitation.

Percussion

Percussion is used to determine the size of the heart; however, in usual practice, palpation maneuvers generally have replaced percussion for the estimation of heart size. If done, cardiac percussion is performed at the 3rd, 4th, and 5th intercostal spaces from the left and right axillary lines. The examiner places the passive hand firmly over the area to be percussed and strikes the distal interphalangeal joint of the middle finger of that hand with the middle finger of the opposite hand. Normal cardiac percussion should show dullness to percussion from the sternum to approximately 6 cm lateral to the left sternum. Left ventricular enlargement displaces the cardiac border to the left.

Auscultation

Auscultation is the last yet probably the most important component of the cardiac examination. To perform auscultation properly, it is important to use a good stethoscope. A stethoscope should have a bell to hear low-pitched sounds and a diaphragm to hear high-pitched sounds. Newer stethoscopes combine the bell and diaphragm; therefore, one should use alternating light to firm pressure in order to hear heart tones when using these new devices. The stethoscope tubing should be no longer than 12 inches. Ear pieces should point toward and fit snuggly into the external ear canal. The patient should be examined in a quiet area and in multiple positions, supine and left lateral, upright and leaning forward, as well as during inspiration and expiration. Use of maneuvers such as standing to squatting can be useful in differentiating murmurs with similar patterns. Be aware that older or debilitated patients may need time between position changes to rest.

The primary auscultatory areas of the heart are featured in Figure 45-8. It is recommended not to limit auscultation to the four discrete areas, but rather to inch the stethoscope from the base of the heart to the apex in a Z pattern; or, proceed in the same pattern from the apex to the base of the heart. Perform auscultation in the same manner each time noting the following:

- S_1 and S_2
- S_1 and S_2 separately
- Extra heart sounds
- Murmurs

Normal Heart Sounds

S_1 and S_2 are the first identifiable heart sounds with S_1 preceding S_2 and the sequence described as sounding like "lub-dub." The "lub" or S_1 reflects closure of the mitral and tricuspid valves and is loudest at the apex. It marks the beginning of systole. The "dub" or S_2 reflects closure of the pulmonic and aortic valves and is loudest at the base of the heart. It marks the end of systole. The normal S_2 has two components: the sound of aortic valve closure (A_2) and the sound of pulmonic valve closure (P_2). The acronym MTAP is a helpful way to remember the order of valve closure during the cardiac cycle.

Splitting of S_2 is physiological at the end of inspiration. Splitting of S_2 is due to the effect of respiration on the heart; that is, inspiration causes the aortic valve to close a fraction of a second before the pulmonic valve closes. Physiological splitting is absent during expiration because the aortic and pulmonic sounds fuse together. A split S_2 is heard only in the pulmonic valve area at the 2nd left interspace and has been described as "lub-T-dup."

Splitting of S_2 can be *paradoxical splitting, wide splitting,* and *fixed wide splitting.* Paradoxical splitting occurs because A_2 is delayed. Paradoxical splitting occurs in conduction delays such as left bundle branch block or right ventricular pacing and aortic stenosis. Wide splitting S_2 occurs when P_2 is delayed on expiration. On inspiration, the P_2 becomes further delayed, and the splitting increases. Wide splitting occurs with pulmonic stenosis, right bundle branch block, severe hypertension, and severe right ventricular systolic failure.[12] Wide fixed splitting occurs when P_2 is delayed, and there is no inspiratory variation. A wide fixed split S_2 is a diagnostic clue to atrial septal defect because there is no inspiratory variation because of the left-to-right shunt through the atrial septal defect.[10] One way

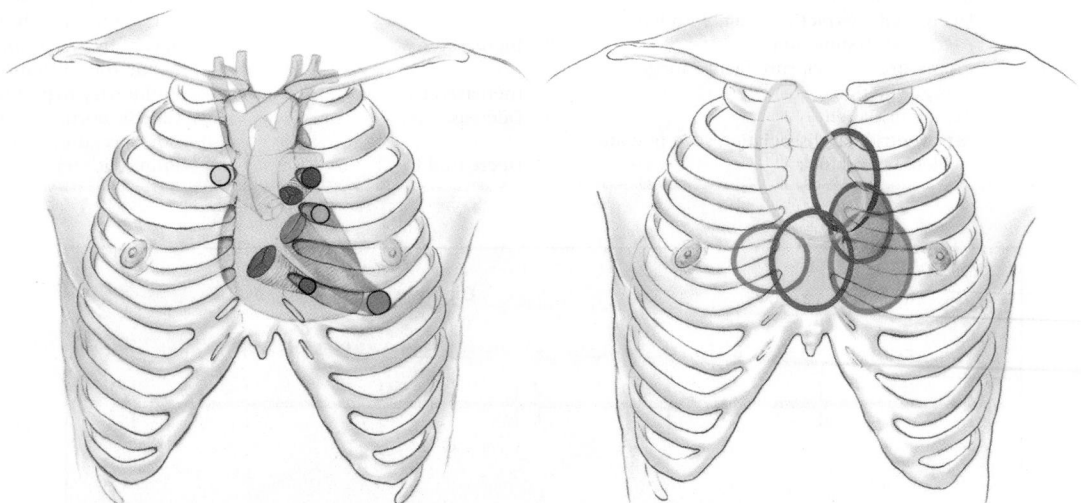

FIGURE 45-8 ■ Auscultatory areas of the heart. (From Jarvis C: *Physical examination and health assessment,* ed 4, Philadelphia, 2004, WB Saunders.)

to determine whether a split S_2 is fixed or not is to have the patient stand. A fixed split S_2 will not change appreciably with standing, whereas a widely split S_2 will become less split or disappear when the individual stands.[12]

Tables 45-6 and 45-7 summarize abnormalities related to the first and second heart sounds.

Abnormal Heart Sounds

The third and fourth heart sounds are low-frequency vibrations heard best at the cardiac apex during diastole, and they occur because of blood entering a noncompliant ventricle. S_3 is a normal finding in children and adolescents and in pregnancy. The pathological S_3 is found in congestive heart failure. Pathological S_3 is usually louder, constant in intensity, and is heard best at the left ventricular apex with the bell of the stethoscope. S_3 occurs immediately after S_2 in the cardiac cycle and sounds like "Ken-tuc-KEY."

The fourth heart sound, like the third heart sound, is also a ventricular filling sound and is heard in late diastole as a result of atrial contraction. S_4 occurs because of blood entering a stiff ventricle such as in hypertension. S_4 precedes S_1 and is heard best at the apex, with the patient lying in the left lateral position. The sound produced with S_4 sounds like "TEN-ne-see." The occurrence of S_3 and S_4 is called a *summation gallop* and resembles the sound of a galloping horse.

Opening snaps are high-pitched, snapping sounds in early diastole produced by the opening of a stenotic (calcified) mitral valve, such as in mitral stenosis (Figure 45-9). Opening snaps are best heard between the apex of the heart and the left sternal border with the diaphragm of the stethoscope.

An *ejection click* is an extra systolic sound occurring shortly after S_1 and is produced by the aortic or pulmonic valve or prosthetic valves (Figure 45-10). Normally, opening valve sounds are not heard. Aortic clicks typically occur more often than pulmonic ejection clicks. The sounds are brief, sharp, and high-pitched. The aortic ejection sound is heard at the aortic area and at the apex and is heard best with the diaphragm. Ejection sounds commonly are heard in conditions in which the aortic valve integrity is abnormal, such as aortic stenosis (Figure 45-11) or aortic regurgitation (Figure 45-12). The pulmonic ejection sounds are heard best at the pulmonic area and may radiate to the xyphoid process. Pulmonic sounds are heard in patients with pulmonic valve abnormalities or dilatation of the pulmonary artery caused by pulmonary hypertension.

Mid to late systolic clicks are associated with mitral valve prolapse (Figure 45-13) and may or may not be associated with a murmur at the apex. The Valsalva, or the squatting to standing maneuver causes the click to move closer to S_1 and will lengthen the murmur if one is present. *Ejection sounds* may accompany the open-

■ ■ ■

TABLE 45-6 ABNORMALITIES OF THE FIRST HEART SOUND

FINDING	CONDITION
Increased intensity	Mitral stenosis
	Short PR interval
	Hyperkinetic states
	Physiologically normal in children, young adults, and patients with a thin chest wall
Decreased intensity	Mitral regurgitation
	Long PR interval
	Decreased contractility seen with left ventricular dysfunction
	Premature valve closure (acute aortic regurgitation)
Variable intensity	Atrial fibrillation
	Atrioventricular dissociation seen in complete heart block

■ ■ ■

TABLE 45-7 ABNORMALITIES OF THE SECOND HEART SOUND

FINDING	CONDITION
Wide splitting (increase with inspiration)	Right bundle branch block
	Left ventricular ectopic beats
	Pulmonic stenosis
	Mitral regurgitation
	Large ventricular septal defect
Wide fixed splitting (no change with inspiration)	Atrial septal defect
Paradoxical splitting	Left bundle branch block
	Right ventricular pacing
	Severe aortic stenosis
	Left ventricular dysfunction
Increased A_2	Severe hypertension
	Aortic root dilatation
Increased P_2	Pulmonary hypertension
Decreased A_2	Calcific aortic stenosis
	Aortic regurgitation
Decreased P_2	Pulmonic stenosis

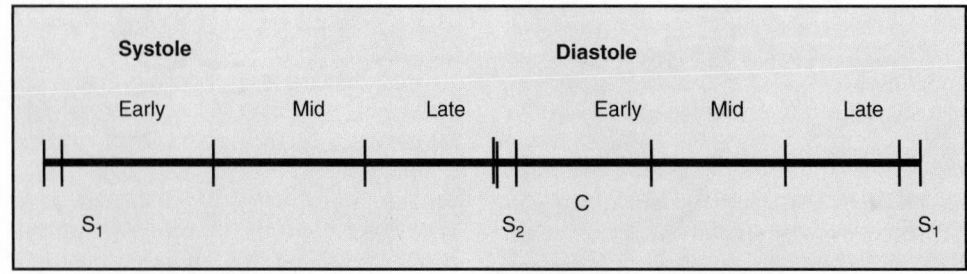

FIGURE 45-9 ■ Opening snap of mitral stenosis. High-frequency, early diastolic sound associated with mitral stenosis.

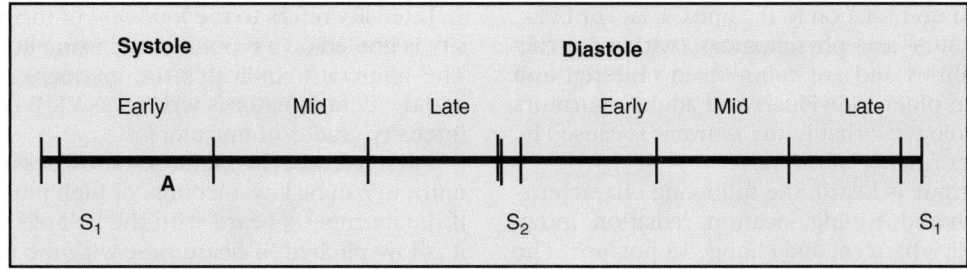

FIGURE 45-10 ■ Ejection click. High-frequency sound in early systole associated with an aortic or pulmonic disorder of the associated great artery.

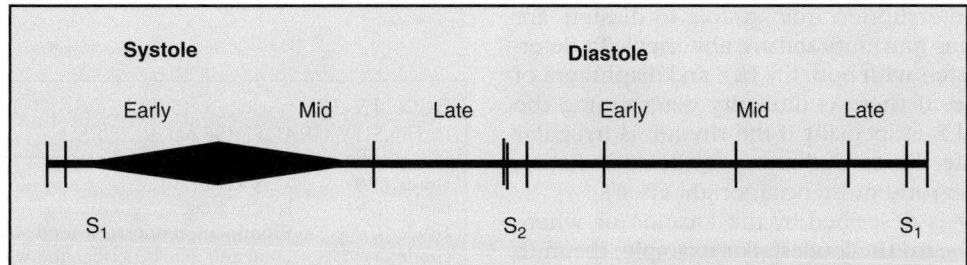

FIGURE 45-11 ■ Aortic stenosis. Harsh, late-peaking systolic murmur, crescendo-decrescendo.

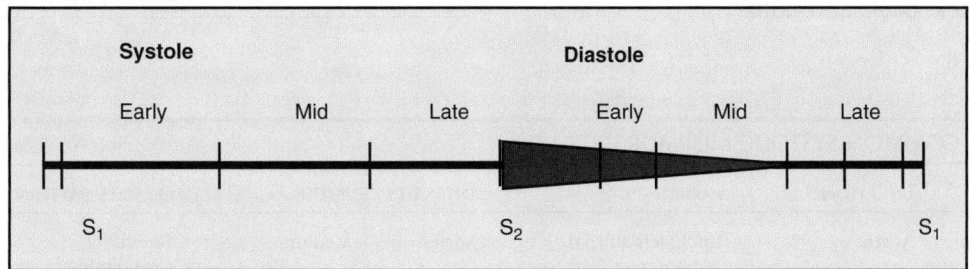

FIGURE 45-12 ■ Aortic regurgitation. High-frequency, blowing, decrescendo murmur beginning in early systole.

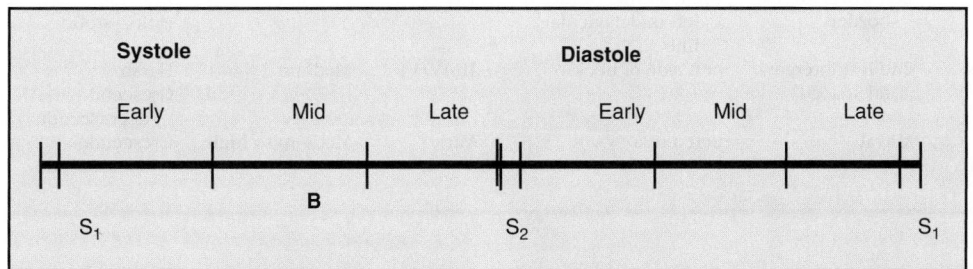

FIGURE 45-13 ■ Midsystolic click of mitral valve prolapse.

ing movement of a prosthetic valve. No ejection sound occurs with a porcine (tissue) valve.

A *pericardial friction rub* is a scratchy, grating, high-pitched sound caused by the inflammation of the parietal and visceral layers of the pericardium during cardiac movement. A pericardial friction rub is typically triple phased and encompasses midsystole, mid-diastole, and late diastole. Pericardial friction rubs may occur following a transmural MI, coronary artery by-pass grafting, or infection. Pericardial friction rubs are best heard with the diaphragm of the stethoscope at the apex of the heart and the sternum with the patient leaning forward or in a supine position.

Murmurs

Heart murmurs are produced by turbulent blood flow through the heart valves. Murmurs are caused by regurgitation (backward flow through a valve) or stenosis (obstruction of flow through a narrow orifice). Murmurs can be innocent or functional. The innocent murmur is systolic, soft, short, of medium pitch, vibratory, altered by position, and best heard at the left lower sternal border, with no radiation to the apex, base, or back. Innocent murmurs are physiological (without structural) abnormalities and are common in children and young adults. In older individuals and adults, murmurs tend to be pathological; that is, the murmur is caused by a structural abnormality of the valve.

When a murmur is heard, the following characteristics should be noted: timing, location, radiation, intensity, pitch, quality/pattern, and change in posture. The murmur should be described by its timing in the cardiac cycle. A murmur heard after S_1 and before S_2 is a systolic murmur (Table 45-8). Diastolic murmurs occur after S_2 and before the next S_1 (Table 45-9). Murmurs that proceed without interruption from systole to diastole are called continuous murmurs and are abnormal. To determine timing, listen with both the bell and diaphragm of the stethoscope. If there is difficulty determining the sound of S_1 and S_2, especially if the rhythm is irregular or rapid, palpate the carotid artery while auscultating the heart. The carotid pulse occurs right after S_1.

The murmur is described by the location or where the murmur is heard the loudest. For example, the murmur of aortic stenosis is best heard in the aortic area, the 2nd intercostal space to the right of the sternum. Sometimes a murmur can radiate to other parts of the precordium, neck, back, and axilla.

Intensity refers to the loudness of the murmur. Intensity is graded on a 6-point scale, using Roman numerals. The numerator indicates the loudness of the murmur and the denominator is written as VI. Box 45-12 lists the intensity grades of murmurs.

Pitch refers to the highness or lowness of the sound. A murmur can be low, medium, or high pitched. Generally, if the murmur is heard with the bell of the stethoscope, it is low pitched; if heard best with the diaphragm, it is high pitched; and if it sounds the same with both the bell and diaphragm, it is medium pitched.

Quality identifies the murmur by a familiar sound such as musical, blowing, harsh, or rumbling. The pat-

---

BOX 45-12   ■ ■ ■
INTENSITY GRADES OF MURMURS

Grade I/VI	Very faint
Grade II/VI	Soft, audible
Grade III/VI	Prominent, moderately loud
Grade IV/VI	Loud and may be associated with a thrill
Grade V/VI	Louder and with a thrill; may be heard with the stethoscope partially off the chest
Grade VI/VI	Very loud; may be associated with a thrill; audible with stethoscope removed from the chest

---

■ ■ ■

TABLE 45-8   COMMON SYSTOLIC MURMURS

MURMUR	LOCATION	RADIATION	INTENSITY	PITCH	QUALITY/PATTERN	CHANGES
Aortic stenosis (see Figure 45-11)	Aortic	Neck; left sternal border	Varies	Medium	Harsh Crescendo-decrescendo	Sitting Supine Squatting Holding breath
Mitral regurgitation (see Figure 45-14)	Apex	Left axilla	I-V/VI	High	Blowing Holosystolic	Increases with squatting
Tricuspid regurgitation	Left lower sternal border	Right sternal border to left midclavicular line	I-V/VI	Medium	Blowing Holosystolic	Increases with respiration
Pulmonic stenosis	2nd left intercostal space	Left side of neck	III-IV/VI	Medium	Harsh Crescendo-decrescendo	Increases with respiration
Mitral valve prolapse (see Figure 45-13)	Mitral	Left axilla	Varies	Medium to high	Crescendo-decrescendo	Supine Left lateral Squatting

---

■ ■ ■

TABLE 45-9   COMMON DIASTOLIC MURMURS

MURMUR	LOCATION	RADIATION	INTENSITY	PITCH	QUALITY/PATTERN	CHANGES
Mitral stenosis (see Figure 45-9)	Mitral	Minimal	I-II/VI	Low	Rumbling Crescendo	Increases in left lateral position, exercise
Tricuspid stenosis	4th left intercostal space	Apex	I-II/VI	Low	Rumbling Crescendo-decrescendo	Increases with inspiration
Aortic regurgitation (see Figure 45-12)	Aortic 2nd right intercostal space	left sternal border; apex	I-VI/VI	High	Decrescendo	Increases with leaning forward and exhalation
Pulmonic regurgitation	Pulmonic	Apex	Varies	High	Decrescendo	Increases with respiration

tern of the murmur refers to the progression of the sound produced by the murmur. A *crescendo* murmur starts softly and then grows louder, and the sound can be described as coarse. A *decrescendo* murmur starts loudly and then becomes soft, and the sound can be described as blowing. A combination of the two, the *crescendo-decrescendo* murmur, starts softly, becomes louder, and becomes soft again. The sound is described as harsh or coarse. *Holosystolic (pansystolic)* murmurs occur throughout systole.

Last, the murmur is described by changes in position. Some murmurs are affected by changes in respiration, position, special maneuvers, and medication. Placing the patient in the left lateral decubitus position brings the apex nearer to the heart wall and makes the detection of the third and fourth heart sounds and apical diastolic rumbles easier. Placing the patient sitting up and leaning forward with the breath held in expiration brings the heart nearer to the chest and allows the examiner to hear the soft murmur of aortic regurgitation or a pericardial friction rub.

Heart murmurs of the right side such as tricuspid regurgitation or pulmonic stenosis can be enhanced with inspiration. This maneuver increases ventricular volume because of increased blood return.

The Valsalva maneuver involves forced expiration that increases intrathoracic pressure resulting in decreased venous return and stroke volume. The fall in stroke volume tends to accentuate the murmur of hypertrophic cardiomyopathy, moves a systolic click of mitral valve prolapse closer to S_1, and/or brings out a late murmur of mitral regurgitation (Figure 45-14) in patients with mitral valve prolapse. The standing-to-squatting maneuver reduces left ventricular volume because of reduced venous return. This maneuver is helpful in the diagnosis of hypertrophic obstructive cardiomyopathy. A sustained, strong isometric handgrip may reduce the murmur of aortic stenosis and increase the murmurs of aortic regurgitation and mitral regurgitation. This maneuver increases systemic vascular resistance and thus makes the murmur louder because of increased backward pressure.

LUNGS
Inspection
Begin by observing the respiratory rate, depth, and rhythm. Normally, the respiratory rate is less than 16 breaths/min and the rhythm is regular. *Tachypnea* describes rapid, shallow respirations and may be noted in patients with heart failure, pain, or anxiety. *Cheyne-Stokes respirations* are characterized by a regular periodic pattern of breathing, with intervals of apnea followed by a crescendo-decrescendo sequence of respiration. This may be seen in patients with severe left ventricular failure. The patient's chest wall movement during respiration should be symmetrical without apparent use of accessory muscles. Note the presence of a cough with or without sputum production.

During inspection, look for scars and other obvious abnormalities. The shape of the chest may reveal *pectus carinatum* (pigeon chest), *pectus excavatum* (funnel chest), or the barrel chest of COPD.

Palpation
Palpate the thorax, feeling for pulsations, areas of tenderness, and respiratory excursion. To evaluate for respiratory excursion during respiration, stand behind the patient and place your thumbs alongside the spinal processes at the level of the 10th rib, with the palms lightly in contact with the posterolateral surfaces. As the patient inhales deeply, evaluate depth and symmetry by observing the movement of the thumbs. Normally, the thumbs should diverge bilaterally.

Fremitus is the palpable vibration of the chest wall that results from speech. Fremitus is best felt parasternally at the 2nd intercostal space with the palmar surface of the fingers or with the ulnar aspect of a clenched fist while the patient repeats the word "ninety-nine." Start over the lung apices and palpate from one side to the other. The vibrations should feel the same in all areas. Fremitus is most prominent between the scapulae and decreases as you progress down the chest. Absent fremitus is caused by excess air in the lungs in conditions such as emphysema, pneumothorax, or pleural effusion. Increased fremitus occurs in the presence of fluids or a solid mass in the lungs such as lobar pneumonia.

Percussion
The percussion technique was described previously under percussion of the heart. Percuss all areas across the back bilaterally. Start at the shoulders and then continue at 5-cm intervals making side-to-side comparisons all the way down the lung region. Avoid the scapulae

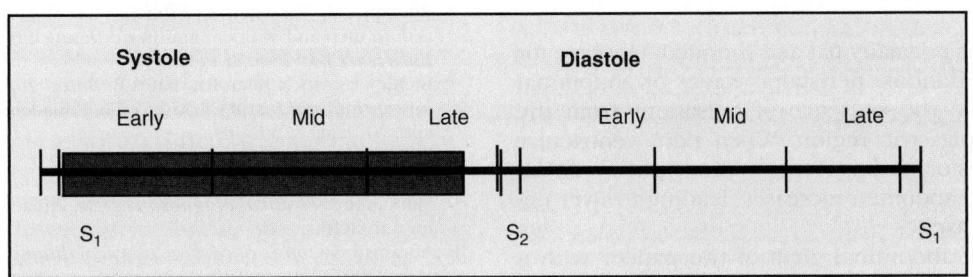

FIGURE 45-14 ■ Mitral regurgitation. High-frequency, holosystolic murmur.

and ribs. Normal lung tissue produces resonance. Hyperresonance is found when too much air is present, as in emphysema or pneumothorax. Dullness or flatness suggests atelectasis, pleural effusion, pneumothorax, or asthma.

Diaphragmatic excursion can be measured by percussion. The patient holds a deep breath while the examiner percusses the lower border (the point marked by a change from resonance to dullness) and notes the location of this border. Then, the patient exhales and the examiner percusses up from the marked location to the point where dullness changes to resonance, and the examiner marks that location. The distance between these two locations is termed the diaphragmatic excursion and it measures about 3 to 5 cm in the adult. The same technique then is performed on the other side of the chest; the diaphragmatic excursion should be equal bilaterally.

Auscultation

The diaphragm of the stethoscope is placed firmly on the skin with the patient sitting erect. Ask the patient to breathe slowly and deeply through the mouth and then systematically listen to the pitch, intensity, and quality of the breath sounds from side to side and downward from the apex to the base.

The three breath sounds heard are bronchial, bronchovesicular, and vesicular. Bronchial breath sounds are heard over the trachea and are high pitched in intensity. Bronchovesicular breath sounds are heard over the major bronchi and are typically moderate in pitch and intensity. Vesicular breath sounds are low-pitched sounds heard over healthy lung tissue.

Adventitious sounds are abnormal sounds superimposed over normal lung sounds. *Rales* or *crackles* are brief, inspiratory sounds that suggest fluid in the alveoli. Rales may be found in conditions such as heart failure or atelectasis associated with the postoperative patient. *Wheezes* are continuous, high-pitched, musical sounds heard in inspiration and expiration. Wheezes are caused by rapid air movement through constricted airways. Wheezing is found in conditions such as heart failure or COPD. *Pleural friction rub* is a dry, crackly, grating sound heard in inspiration and expiration. A friction rub in the lungs is caused by inflamed surfaces rubbing together. The patient generally complains of pain with breathing.

ABDOMEN
Inspection

The abdomen is normally flat and rounded. Observe for asymmetry, pulsations, peristaltic waves or abdominal distention. Note the presence of pulsations from the aorta at the epigastric region. When right ventricular failure develops or venous return is diminished, venous pressure in the abdomen increases, leading to liver enlargement and ascites.

Measure the abdominal girth of the patient with a tape measure. This is an important measure when evaluating the patient for abdominal adiposity and risk for metabolic syndrome and diabetes.

Auscultation

Auscultation is performed before percussion and palpation because these maneuvers can increase or diminish bowel sounds. Firmly place the diaphragm of the stethoscope on the skin and begin listening over all quadrants for bowel sounds or vascular sounds (bruits).

Percussion

Percuss lightly in all four quadrants. Evaluate the liver span by measuring the height of the liver in the right midclavicular line. Percuss upward along the midclavicular line to determine the lower border of the liver. The area of liver dullness usually is heard at the costal margin. A lower margin of more than 2 to 3 cm below the costal margin may indicate liver enlargement. To determine the upper liver border, percuss downward until the percussion tone is dull. The upper border begins at the 5th to 7th intercostal space. Measure the distance between the upper and lower measurements to estimate the vertical span. A span greater than 12 cm suggests liver enlargement.

Palpation

To palpate the liver to determine its size, place the left hand under the patient's back, parallel to the 11th and 12th ribs, and slightly lift up to support the abdomen. Place the right hand on the right upper quadrant. The patient takes a deep breath while the examiner pushes deeply down and under the right costal margin. The liver edge should come down to meet the fingers. Normally, the liver edge feels smooth and is nontender to palpation. In the patient with right ventricular failure, the liver will be enlarged, firm, smooth, and tender.

REFERENCES

1. Gramsky C, Josephson S, Langford M et al: Outpatient management of chronic heart failure, *Crit Care Nurs Clin North Am* 15:501-509, 2003.
2. Sangareddi V, Chockalingam A, Gnanavelu G et al: Canadian Cardiovascular Society classification of effort angina: an angiographic correlation, *Coron Artery Dis* 15(2):111-114, 2004.
3. Campeau L: The Canadian Cardiovascular Society grading of angina pectoris revisited 30 years later, *Can J Cardiol* 18(4):371-379, 2002.
4. Braunwald E, Perloff JK: Physical examination of the heart and circulation. In Zipes DP, Libby P, Bonow RO, Braunwald E, editors: *Heart disease: a textbook of cardiovascular medicine*, ed 7, Philadelphia, 2005, Elsevier Saunders.
5. Seidel HM, Ball JW, Dains JE, Benedict GW et al, editors: *Mosby's guide to physical examination*, ed 6, St Louis, 2006, Mosby.
6. Buonanno C, Vassanelli C, Arbustini E et al: Left ventricular function in men and women: another difference between the sexes, *Eur Heart J* 3:525-528, 1982.
7. Bickley LS, Hoekelman RA, Bates B: *Bates' guide to physical examination and history taking*, ed 6, Philadelphia, 1995, Lippincott Williams & Wilkins.
8. Stillwell SB: *Quick critical care reference*, St Louis, 1990, Mosby.
9. Mangione S: *Physical diagnosis secrets*, Philadelphia, 2000, Hanley and Belfus.
10. Abrams J: *Synopsis of cardiac physical diagnosis*, ed 2, Woburn, Mass, 2001, Butterworth-Heinemann.
11. Karnath B, Thorton W: Precordial and carotid pulse palpation, *Hosp Physician* pp 20-24, 2002.
12. Etchells E: Cardiac murmurs, *Clinical Advisor* 7/8:49-50, 2000.

Electrocardiography: Normal Electrocardiogram

Michele M. Pelter

CHAPTER ABBREVIATIONS

AV   atrioventricular
ECG   electrocardiogram
SA   sinoatrial

In 1902, the first recorded electrocardiogram **(ECG)** was published by a Dutch physiologist, Willem Einthoven.[1] Over the course of a century, this noninvasive and relatively inexpensive measure of the electrical activity of the heart has stood the test of time. Today, the standard 12-lead ECG is considered the noninvasive gold standard for identifying normal cardiac rhythm, diagnosing dysrhythmias, and discovering myocardial ischemia. The ECG is used widely in outpatient and inpatient settings and can be used to obtain static, serial, or continuous information about the status of the heart. Because this diagnostic tool is used so widely, clinicians in all medical specialties must be able to interpret ECG findings. In this chapter, the normal ECG is discussed.

NORMAL CARDIAC PHYSIOLOGY

The heart is a mechanical organ that functions to pump deoxygenated blood from the right ventricle to the lungs for reoxygenation and oxygenated blood from the left ventricle to the rest of the body. The pumping action, or myocardial contraction, follows electrical activation, or depolarization of the heart. In other words, the electrical events of the heart precede the mechanical events. The ECG is used to measure the electrical activity of the heart and serves as a valuable tool to determine normal and abnormal electrical events of the heart.

The origin of a cardiac cycle begins at the cellular level where there is a shift of charged particles, or ions, across the cellular membrane resulting in depolarization. The speed of depolarization varies depending on the cell type. For example, depolarization is slow in pacemaker cells, and very fast in atrial and ventricular cells.

Repolarization begins immediately after depolarization when the ions shift back across the cellular membrane, and the cell returns to its resting state. During this period, there is a balance in the movement of ions inward and outward across the cell membrane that maintains electrical equilibrium. The result is a plateau phase with the cell eventually returning to its resting state. This plateau allows for a refractory period, a time during which a cardiac cell cannot be reactivated. This is an important period when the cells return to their normal ionic state so that they can react to another stimulus. During the latter part of repolarization, a stimulus that is greater than that generated during normal depolarization can evoke an action potential. This period is called the relative refractory period. Different cell types have different refractory periods. For example, the bundle branches have an "all-or-none" response, so that if they respond to another stimulus, they will respond to their full capacity.[2] Whereas other tissues (e.g., the atrioventricular node) show a gradual as opposed to abrupt response to a stimulus over a relatively long time.

Automaticity is the ability of specialized myocardial cells, called pacemaker cells, to depolarize spontaneously to form new impulses. In the normal heart, the sinoatrial **(SA)** node functions to pace the heart at a rate of 60 to 90 beats/min. Secondary pacemaker cells exist in the bundle of His and the His-Purkinje system in the event the SA node fails.

The process of depolarization and repolarization evokes an action potential, which represents the electrical activity of a single heart cell. Electrical (voltage) differences across the cell membrane, or the "membrane potential," are measured by comparing the intracellular voltage to the extracellular voltage. In a normal membrane potential, the extracellular space is considered the reference point; hence, the voltage is set at 0 mV. Under normal conditions, the membrane potential for a resting cardiac cell is −90 mV, which means the inside of the cell is −90 mV compared with the reference or outside voltage of the cell, which is 0 mV.

The action potential is composed of five phases (Figure 46-1). A graphic representation of an action potential can be obtained by introducing a microelectrode into a single myocardial muscle cell. The five phases of ventricular action potential, which reflect particular electromechanical events, are described next.

Phase 0: Depolarization

The abrupt upstroke portion of the action potential represents depolarization of the myocardial cell. Under normal conditions, depolarization of ventricular myocardial cells depends on a stimulus, which comes from the pacemaker cells of the SA node. The arrival of the stimulus to the ventricular cell causes a sudden voltage change in the cellular membrane that opens fast Na^+ channels, causing a rapid influx of Na^+ into the cell. The resting membrane potential becomes less negative and shifts from −90 mV to approximately −70 to −65 mV.[3] When the myocardial cell membrane potential reaches −70 to −65 mV, the cell is said to have reached a "threshold," at which point Na^+ channels open and Na^+ rushes rapidly into the cell.[4] Chemical forces draw Na^+ into the cell because the inside of the cell has a low

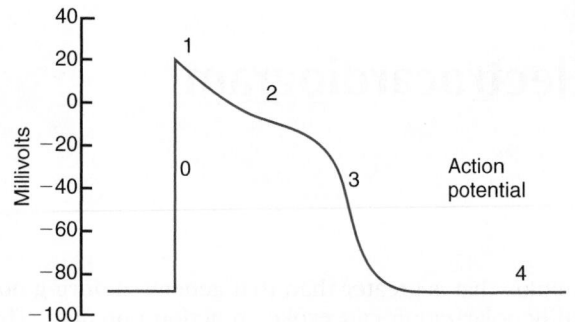

FIGURE 46-1 ■ The five phases of a ventricular action potential.

concentration of Na$^+$ ions compared with the outside. During this phase, slow Ca^{++} channels are also open, allowing Ca^{++} from the extracellular space to flow into the cell.[5] Ultimately, the inside of the cell shifts from a negative to a positive environment.

Phase 1: Early Rapid Repolarization

When the rapid influx of Na$^+$ is terminated, brief partial repolarization occurs. During this phase there is slight repolarization of the myocardial cell, causing the action potential millivolt value to decrease to approximately +20 to 0 mV. This slight repolarization develops from the activation of K$^+$ channels, resulting in the outward movement of this ion.[6,7] The outward movement of K$^+$ is due to chemical-activated (intracellular Ca^{++}) and voltage-activated forces, the latter being regulated by neurotransmitters.[8,9] The outward movement of K$^+$ ions is brief, at which point K$^+$ channels close and phase 2 begins.

Phase 2: Plateau

The plateau phase represents the longest phase of the action potential, lasting for several hundred milliseconds. The membrane potential remains between 0 and +20 mV during the plateau phase. The plateau phase results from continued slow inward movement of Ca^{++}, through L-type Ca^{++} channels, also called "long-lasting" Ca^{++} channels, into the cells of the atrium, His-Purkinje, and ventricular muscle cells.[9,10] Simultaneously, there is an outward movement of K$^+$ ions, which functions to balance the inward movement of Ca^{++}.[8]

Phase 3: Final Rapid Repolarization

Phase 3 is named the "rapid repolarization phase" and results from inactivation of L-type Ca^{++} channels so that the inward movement of Ca^{++} decreases. Simultaneously, there is an increase in outward movement of K$^+$.[10] The intracellular environment becomes increasingly negative and continues to do so until the cells return to their resting membrane potential of −90 mV, at which point phase 4 begins and the process repeats itself.

Phase 4: Resting Phase

The resting phase of the action potential coincides with the resting or diastolic phase of the cardiac cycle. K$^+$ is the major ion that determines the resting potential of

the myocardial cell and is the predominant ion inside the cell, whereas Na$^+$ is the predominant ion outside the cell. The distribution of these ions is the result of the Na$^+$-K$^+$ pump, which functions to pump Na$^+$ out of the cell against its electrical and chemical gradient and simultaneously pumps K$^+$ into the cell against its chemical gradient.

During the resting phase, the cellular membrane is permeable to K$^+$. In contrast, the cell membrane is impermeable to Na$^+$; thus, this ion remains outside of the cell. Because the outside of the cell has a low concentration of K$^+$ ions compared with the inside of the cell, K$^+$ is compelled to move down its concentration gradient, or from the inside of the cell to the outside of the cell. The movement of K$^+$, a positively charged ion, to the outside of the cell leaves the inside of the cell progressively more negative until the forces attracting K$^+$ to leave the cell equal the forces attracting K$^+$ to remain inside of the cell, and there is no net movement of K$^+$ in or out of the cell. At this point, the cell is said to be in a "polarized state" where the cell interior measures about −90 mV with respect to the exterior of the cell.

RELATIONSHIP OF ACTION POTENTIAL TO ELECTROCARDIOGRAM

The phases of the action potential are measured by inserting a microelectrode into a single myocardial cell. This is an important technique in the laboratory setting to study cellular electrical activity; however, in the clinical setting it is more important to analyze the summation of the electrical activity of the heart from the body surface to diagnose cardiac rhythm, myocardial ischemia, conduction disturbances, and structural abnormalities of the heart. The ECG measures the summation of action potentials of the heart noninvasively. The mechanical events of the heart are preceded by electrical events at the cellular level, which under normal conditions occur in a rhythmic and repetitive sequence called the cardiac cycle. Each cardiac cycle is composed of an activation or depolarization phase, termed *systole*, and a recovery or repolarization phase, termed *diastole*. The waveforms of the ECG complex include the P wave,

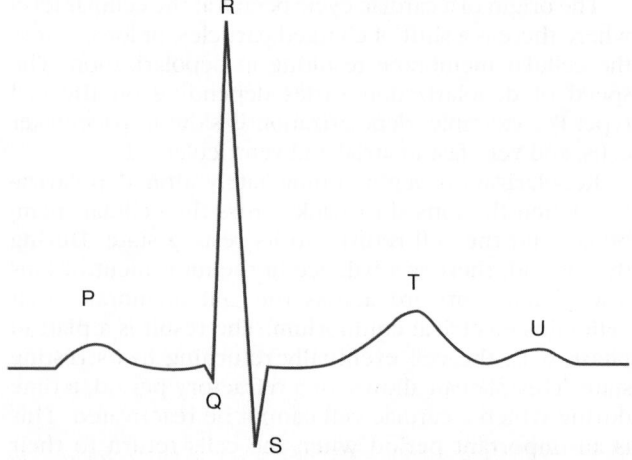

FIGURE 46-2 ■ Normal electrocardiographic waveforms including the P, Q, R, S, T, and U waves.

the QRS complex, the ST segment, the T wave, and possibly a U wave (Figure 46-2).

In ventricular myocardial cells, the QRS complex of the ECG waveform correlates with phase 0 of the action potential and thus myocardial depolarization. The ST segment correlates with phase 2 of the action potential, which is the early and slow phase of repolarization. The normal ST segment is "isoelectric," neither above nor below the baseline waveform of the PR interval, although slight upsloping, downsloping, or horizontal depression of the ST segment can be a normal variant. The T wave correlates with phase 3 of the action potential, the more rapid and terminal portion of repolarization. Thus, the QRS complex waveform represents ventricular depolarization, and the ST segment and T and U waves combined represent ventricular repolarization. The relationship of these specific waveforms with the five phases of a ventricular action potential is illustrated in Figure 46-3.

CARDIAC IMPULSE FORMATION

In the normal heart, specialized pacemaker and conduction cells generate an electrical impulse (pacemaker cells) and carry the electrical impulse (conduction pathway) to strategic anatomical locations within the heart. The initiation of an electrical impulse in a normal heart originates in the SA node. The SA node is located in the upper right atrium near its junction with the superior vena cava. Activation of the atrium spreads rapidly from the SA node in the right atrium in a rightward and anterior direction, followed by activation in the left atrium in

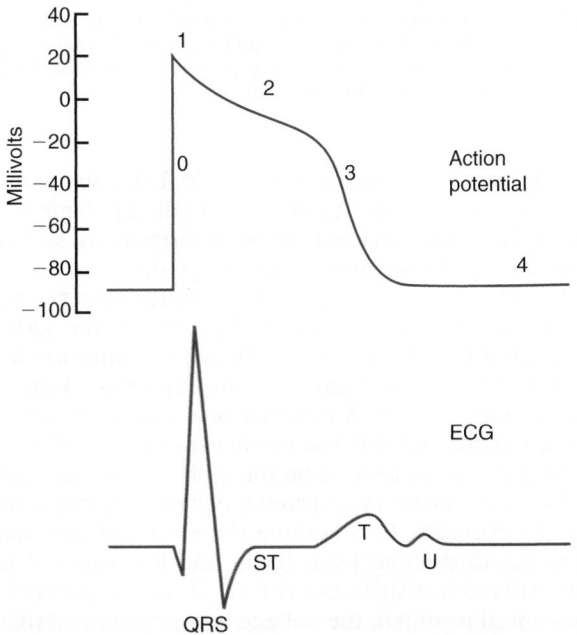

FIGURE 46-3 ■ The *top figure* illustrates the five phases of a ventricular action potential. The *bottom figure* illustrates the relationship of the electrocardiographic complex (QRS complex, ST segment, T wave, and U wave) to the five phases of the ventricular action potential. Because this is a ventricular action potential, the P wave, which is the waveform of atrial depolarization, is not shown. In a normal cardiac cycle, the P wave would be in front of the QRS complex.

a leftward and posterior direction. Conduction through the atria to the next part of the conduction pathway (atrioventricular node) occurs via three specialized tracts that contain Purkinje fibers: the anterior, middle, and posterior internodal pathways. The Bachmann bundle is a pathway connecting the right and left atria.[11]

From the SA node, the impulse arrives at the atrioventricular (**AV**) node, located low in the right atrium. The function of the AV node is to act as a gatekeeper and delay the conduction of the electrical impulse in order to allow the atria time to contract and pump blood into the ventricles. In a normal heart, the AV node is the only pathway for an electrical impulse to travel from the atria to the ventricles.

Ventricular depolarization is a complex process that requires a highly specialized conduction pathway, made up of bundle branches and fascicles in order to achieve the most efficient pumping action possible. For example, it is essential that activation of the heart proceed from the apical region of the heart to the base (i.e., pulmonary and aortic outflow valves) in order to maximize stroke volume and thus cardiac output. The ventricular conduction pathway is made up of a common bundle called the bundle of His, which connects the AV node to the right and left bundle branches. This common bundle then branches into the right and left bundle branches, which travel along the septum to their respective ventricle. The right bundle branch divides into smaller branches and eventually into Purkinje cells that are embedded in the endocardial tissue of the right ventricle. The left bundle branch divides into two fascicles, the anterior and posterior fascicle. The fascicles further divide into Purkinje cells, which are embedded in the endocardial tissue of the left ventricle. The Purkinje cells, also named the Purkinje network, function as pacemaker cells and are responsible for moving the electrical impulses rapidly into the ventricles. From the ventricles, the impulse proceeds from the endocardium (innermost aspect of the heart) to the epicardium (outermost aspect of the heart).

Basis of the 12-Lead Electrocardiogram

The standard 12-lead ECG is considered the noninvasive gold standard for diagnosis of normal cardiac rhythm, dysrhythmias, and myocardial ischemia. The electrocardiograph produces a 12-lead ECG, which is a graphic representation of the direction, magnitude, and duration of electrical activity of the heart from 12 different viewpoints. A single ECG complex represents one complete cardiac cycle. The 12-lead ECG can be used to diagnose abnormalities (see Chapter 47) and provide information about the type, location, extent, and in some cases, the coronary artery responsible for myocardial ischemia.

ELECTROCARDIOGRAPHIC LEADS

An ECG *lead* records the difference in electrical potential between a negative and positive skin electrode placed at specific locations on the body surface. The standard 12-lead ECG is composed of six limb leads, designated as I, II, III, aVR, aVL, and aVF. The six limb leads are derived from placing an electrode on each of the four limbs. The remaining six leads designated as leads V_1, V_2, V_3, V_4, V_5, and V_6 are the six chest or precordial leads. The precordial leads are obtained by placing electrodes at specific locations over the anterior chest wall overlying the heart. The limb leads view the frontal plane of the body, and the precordial leads view the transverse or horizontal plane of the body.

An essential part of understanding normal and abnormal findings on the ECG is conceptualizing the lead locations and their relationship to the anatomical parts of the heart. Figures 46-4 and 46-5 illustrate the location of the limb and precordial leads and their relationship to the myocardial structures.

The first three leads that make up the 12-lead ECG (leads I, II, and III) are termed *bipolar limb leads* because they measure the difference between two points. For each bipolar limb lead, one electrode is designated negative and one is designated positive. The electrical forces generated between the two leads are recorded using the electrocardiograph. The ECG is a printout of the waveforms of myocardial activity. Bipolar leads record from the negative to the positive lead.

Three bipolar limb leads (I, II, and III), first introduced in 1902 by Willem Einthoven, form the Einthoven triangle. For lead I the right arm electrode serves as the negative electrode, and the left arm electrode serves as the positive electrode. For lead II the right arm electrode serves as the negative electrode, and the left leg electrode serves as the positive electrode. For lead III, the left arm electrode serves as the negative electrode and the left leg electrode serves as the positive electrode. Figure 46-6 illustrates the location of the three bipolar

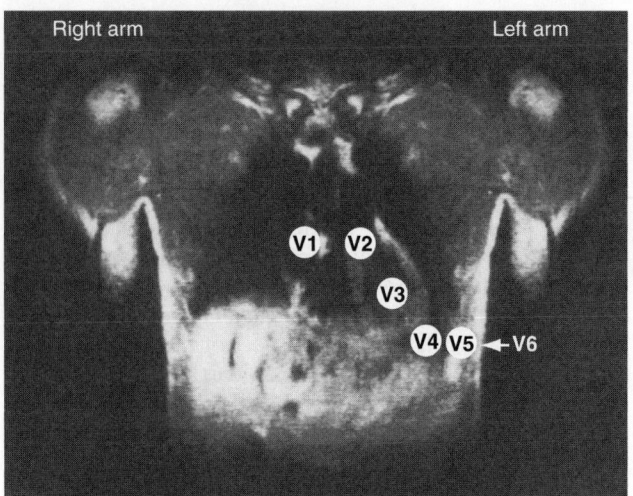

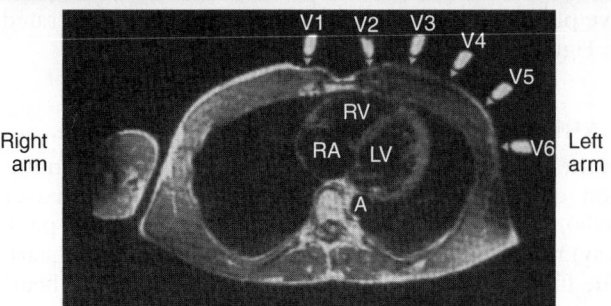

FIGURE 46-5 ■ The *top figure* illustrates the location of the six precordial leads on the torso of the chest. The *bottom figure* is a horizontal plane view (looking up toward the head from the patient's feet), illustrating the relationship between the six precordial leads (i.e., leads V_1, V_2, V_3, V_4, V_5, and V_6) and the structures of the myocardium. *A*, aorta; *RA*, right atrium; *RV*, right ventricle; *PA*, pulmonary artery; *LV*, left ventricle. (From Califf R, Mark D, Wagner G: The 12-lead ECG and the extent of myocardium at risk of acute infarction: cardiac anatomy and lead locations, and the phases of serial changes during acute occlusion. In *Acute coronary care in the thrombolytic era*, Chicago, 1988, Year Book Medical.)

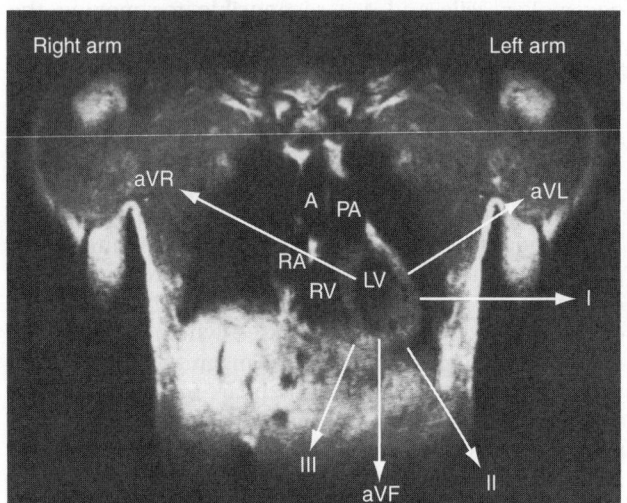

FIGURE 46-4 ■ This magnetic resonance image of the torso from the frontal plane view illustrates the relationship between the six limb leads (i.e., leads I, II, III, aVR, aVL, and aVF) and the structures of the myocardium. *A*, aorta; *RA*, right atrium; *RV*, right ventricle; *PA*, pulmonary artery; *LV*, left ventricle. The *arrows* indicate the "view" that each of the leads has to the myocardium. (From Califf R, Mark D, Wagner G: The 12-lead ECG and the extent of myocardium at risk of acute infarction: cardiac anatomy and lead locations, and the phases of serial changes during acute occlusion. In *Acute coronary care in the thrombolytic era*, Chicago, 1988, Year Book Medical.)

limb leads and the Einthoven triangle. Because the electrical forces of the heart normally are directed inferiorly (downward) and leftward, the waveforms in these three leads are predominantly upright, or positive.

In 1934, Wilson and coworkers[2] introduced the unipolar lead, which is designated by a "V" on the 12-lead ECG recording. Unlike a bipolar lead, a unipolar lead records the electrical forces at one exploring electrode on the body surface. A unipolar or V lead is created by using a central terminal as the negative pole and an exploring electrode located on the limb as a positive pole. Wilson and coworkers created a negative central terminal electronically by summing the electrical potentials from the three limb leads (right and left arm and left leg). Although, a small electrical voltage is registered at the central terminal, the voltage is nearly zero so that a negative reference point is created electronically. The waveform created on the ECG tracing measures the electrical potential at the site of the exploring (positive) electrode.

The same three limb electrodes (right and left arm and left leg) also are used to generate the unipolar limb leads, which are designated as aVR, aVL, and aVF. In

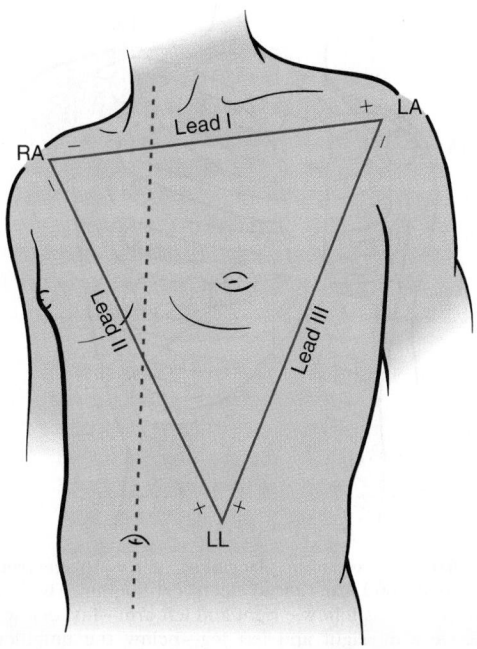

FIGURE 46-6 ■ The Einthoven triangle formed by leads I, II, and III. For lead I the left arm electrodes serves as the positive electrode, and the right arm electrode serves as the negative electrode. For lead II the left leg electrode serves as the positive electrode, and the right arm electrode serves as the negative electrode. For lead III the left leg electrode serves as the positive electrode, and the left arm electrode serves as the negative electrode. *LA,* Left arm; *LL,* left leg; *RA,* right arm.

1942 Goldberger[12] modified Wilson's central terminal in order to increase the recorded voltages of the unipolar limb leads. The resultant lead was "augmented" or amplified by 50 percent. The letter "a" is added to the designated lead to signify this modification. The remaining letters R, L, F refer to the respective extremity where the exploring electrode is recording: "R" refers to the right arm, "L" the left arm, and "F" the left foot. Figure 46-7 illustrates how the unipolar limb leads are generated. The right arm electrode serves as the positive pole for lead aVR, the left arm electrode serves as the positive electrode for lead aVL, and the left leg electrode serves as the positive electrode for lead aVF.

The final six leads that make up the standard 12-lead ECG are designated as the precordial leads. As mentioned before, these leads view the transverse plane, or the anterior-posterior axis. Their location across the torso allows these leads a direct view of the right and left ventricles. The precordial leads are unipolar leads. The limb leads are used to generate the negative central terminal, and the exploring (positive) electrodes labeled V_1 through V_6 serve as the recording (positive) electrode. Because of the proximity of the precordial leads to the heart, they do not require augmentation, hence there is no "a" designation.

Lead Placement

A valid and reliable ECG depends on accurate placement of the skin electrodes on the body surface. The location of the 10 skin electrodes used to record a standard 12-lead ECG are as follows: right and left arm—placed on the respective wrist; right and left leg—placed on the respective ankle. Location of the precordial leads is as follows: V_1—4th intercostal space right of sternum; V_2—4th intercostal space left of sternum; V_3—midway between V_2 and V_4; V_4—5th intercostal space midclavicular line; V_5—straight line from V_4 anterior axillary line; V_6—straight line from V_4 midaxillary. Correct placement of the precordial skin electrodes can be challenging in women because of breast tissue or in obese individuals. In this situation, the skin electrodes often are placed under the breast tissue, or protuberant adipose tissue, in a location below the accepted location. Studies show that R wave amplitude can be altered when the electrodes are placed under the breast tissue compared with placing the skin electrode on top of the tissue.[13,14] This may be an important issue when diagnosing anterior myocardial infarction (MI). In this situation, it is recommended that the skin electrodes be placed on top of the breast or adipose tissue as opposed to below the tissue in order to maintain accurate recording of the ECG waveform.

Modification of the limb lead locations, termed the *Mason-Likar lead configuration,*[15] is applied commonly for continuous recording of the 12-lead ECG in hospital-

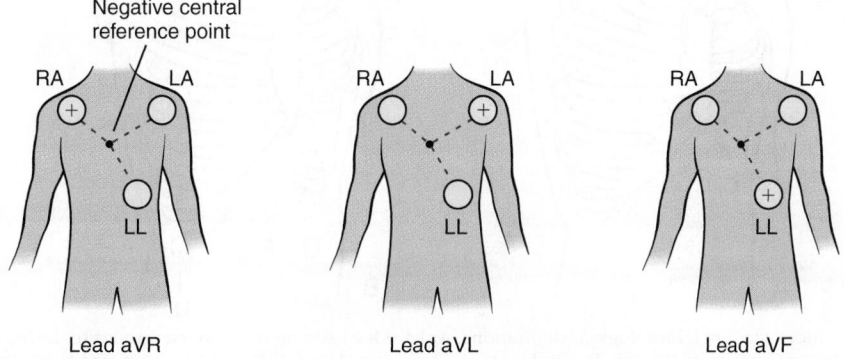

FIGURE 46-7 ■ How the unipolar limb leads designated aVR, aVL, and aVF are generated. These leads record the electrical potential between the central terminal (shown at the center of the chest) and the positive limb electrode located at the right arm (lead aVR), left arm (lead aVL), and the left leg electrodes (lead aVF). *LA,* Left arm; *LL,* left leg; *RA,* right arm. (From Lipman B, Cascio T: ECG electrodes and leads. In *ECG assessment and interpretation,* Philadelphia, 1994, FA Davis.)

ized patients in order to maintain patient comfort and reduce artifact. In the Mason-Likar configuration, the right and left arm leads are moved from the wrist locations and are placed laterally just below the clavicle. The right and left leg electrodes are placed on the lower torso below the umbilicus (Figure 46-8). Studies show ECG waveforms can be altered by moving the limb electrodes from the wrist locations to the torso. For example, placement of the limb electrodes on the torso can result in a rightward shift in QRS axis, lower R wave amplitudes in leads I and aVL; higher R wave amplitude in leads II, III, and aVF; and alterations in the R wave amplitude in the precordial leads.[16,17] Jowett and coworkers[16] showed that torso lead locations generated ECG abnormalities suggestive of heart disease in more than 30 percent of patients with normal standard 12-lead ECGs and made possible acute MI appear and disappear in patients with abnormal standard ECGs. In addition, small (less than 1 mm) differences in ST segment deviation also may be altered by moving the standard limb locations to the torso.[18] Because ECG waveforms and ST amplitude changes can occur between the standard versus the Mason-Likar lead configuration, documentation on the recorded ECG should indicate which lead placement configuration was used when the ECG was recorded. This allows clinicians to make an accurate diagnosis from the ECG. (See the Technology feature.)

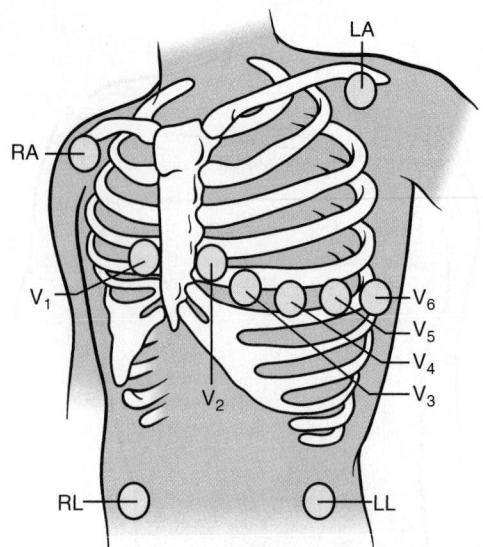

FIGURE 46-8 ■ Accurate placement of the 10 electrodes that make up the Mason-Likar 12-lead electrocardiogram. The location of the electrodes are as follows: right and left arm—just below clavicle of respective arm; right and left leg—below the umbilicus; lead V_1—4th intercostal space right of sternum; lead V_2—4th intercostal space left of sternum; lead V_3—midway between leads V_2 and V_4; lead V_4—5th intercostal space midclavicular line; lead V_5—straight line from lead V_4 anterior axillary line; lead V_6—straight line from lead V_4 midaxillary line. *LA,* Left arm; *LL,* left leg; *RA,* right arm; *RL,* right leg.

■ ■ ■ TECHNOLOGY

REDUCED LEAD SETS

Although the standard 12-lead electrocardiogram (ECG) is considered the noninvasive gold standard for diagnosis of normal cardiac rhythm, dysrhythmias, and myocardial ischemia, maintaining all 10 electrodes on the body surface is challenging for continuous monitoring. For example, the chest electrodes across the precordium (leads V_1 to V_6) interfere with defibrillation, auscultation, chest radiographs, and echocardiography. As a result, these electrodes often are moved to inaccurate locations on the torso, which significantly alters the validity and reliability of the recorded ECG. So, how can clinicians have access to multilead ECG information with-

out having to apply electrodes to locations on the torso that interfere with important tests and procedures? Over the past decade, researchers have been evaluating "reduced lead set technology" to address this problem. With this technology, the 12-lead ECG is derived, or estimated, by using only five or six skin electrodes on the body surface (see figure). Although studies show that 12-lead ECGs obtained from reduced lead set technology are *comparable* to standard 12-lead ECGs, they are not identical. Hence, when making serial comparisons in an individual patient, clinicians should not mix the two methods.

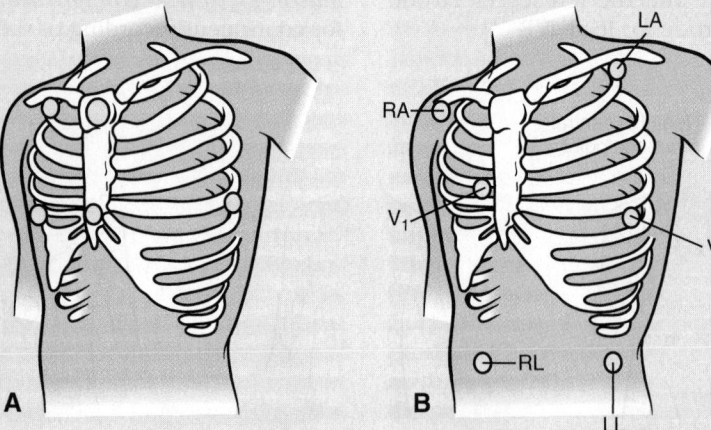

Two reduced lead set technology configurations. **A,** EASI lead system uses five electrodes to derive a 12-lead electrocardiogram (Philips Medical Systems, Andover, Mass.). **B,** The 12-RL (reduced lead) system uses six electrodes, four placed on the limbs in the modified 12-lead locations and the remaining two at lead locations V_1 and V_5. The remaining precordial leads (V_2, V_3, V_4, and V_6) are "interpolated" from the six leads (General Electric Medical Systems, Milwaukee, Wis.) *LA,* Left arm; *LL,* left leg; *RA,* right arm; *RL,* right leg.

PRESENTATION OF THE STANDARD 12-LEAD ELECTROCARDIOGRAM

Most ECG machines can be formatted to present the standard 12-lead ECG in a variety of formats. A common format selected is a 3 × 4 format with a 10-second rhythm strip, as illustrated in Figure 46-9. This format groups the frontal plane leads in columns of three in the chronological order in which they were developed, the first three leads (I, II, and III) are the original limb leads, the three augmented leads (aVR, aVL, and aVF) follow, and the remaining six leads display the transverse leads in order of their sequence V_1 to V_6.

The majority of ECG machines generate computerized heart rate, waveform interval measurements, waveform amplitudes, and axis information. Computer-generated measurements are accurate and reliable if the skin electrodes and lead wires are applied correctly and the recording is free of artifact. This offers important advantages for clinicians because computer measurements are free of human bias, they are more precise that human beings are, and they are immediately available for real-time analysis, which is ideal for clinical decision making. For example, in one study, computer-generated measurements of ST segment deviation (elevation or depression) during acute myocardial ischemia were more precise and of higher amplitude compared with measurements made with the human eye.[19] This is an important point because ST segment changes indicative of acute ischemia can be subtle, as small as 1 mm. Hence, clinicians should use computer-generated measurements when available if a reliable and valid ECG was recorded (i.e., skin electrodes and lead wires were applied correctly and the recording is free of artifact).

ELECTROCARDIOGRAPHIC WAVEFORMS

Normal myocardial depolarization spreads downward from the atria to the ventricles in a slightly leftward direction. With this in mind, ECG electrodes are placed at strategic locations on the body surface in order to record the normal activation sequence so that dysrhythmias, as well as depolarization and repolarization abnormalities, can be identified. ECG waveforms are described as positive where the waveform is predominantly upright; negative; or biphasic, where the waveform has a positive and a negative deflection.

The location of the negative and positive lead in relation to the electrical current of the heart determines the waveform morphology. As illustrated in Figure 46-10, in a heart with normal conduction, a negative electrode placed on the right shoulder and a positive electrode placed on the left leg will record a predominantly upright, or positive, ECG complex. A negative waveform is generated when the electrical current is moving away from the positive electrode. Lead aVR is an example of a negative waveform recorded on the 12-lead ECG. For example, as seen in Figure 46-4, the positive pole of lead aVR is located in the right arm position; because conduction of the heart proceeds in a downward and leftward direction away from this electrode, a predominantly negative waveform is recorded. A biphasic waveform is generated when the positive lead is perpendicular to the electrical current. In this situation, the electrical forces cancel each other out, resulting in a small biphasic (equally positive and negative) waveform. It is important to reiterate that the ECG waveforms only represent electrical activation rather than mechanical events.

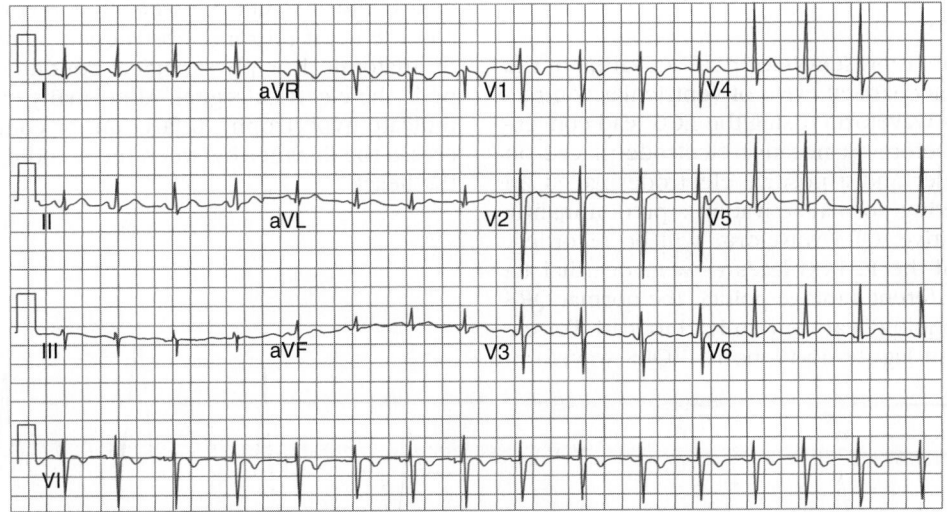

FIGURE 46-9 ■ Shows the most common printed format for displaying the standard 12-lead electrocardiogram. This format groups the frontal plane leads in columns of three in the order in which they were developed. Leads I, II, and III are the original limb leads described by Einthoven; the next three leads aVR, aVL, and aVF are the augmented limb leads introduced by Wilson. The remaining six leads display the transverse leads in order of their sequence V_1 to V_6. (From Rimmerman CM, Jain AK: *Interactive electrocardiography,* Philadelphia, 2001, Lippincott Williams & Wilkins.)

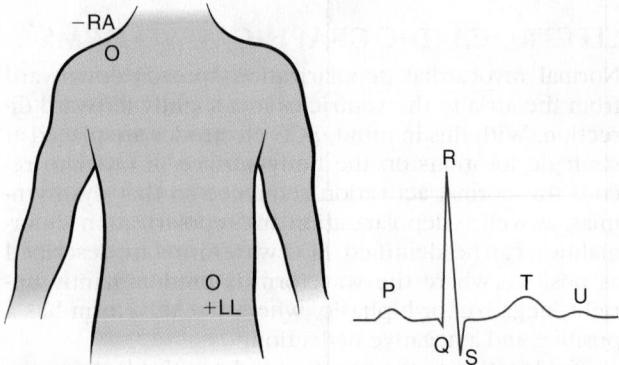

FIGURE 46-10 ■ Normal myocardial activation spreads from the atria to the ventricles in a slightly leftward direction. A negative electrode placed on the right shoulder and a positive electrode placed on the left leg *(left figure)* will record a predominantly upright, or positive, electrocardiographic waveform *(right figure)*. *LL,* Left leg; *RA,* right arm.

P Wave

The initial waveform of the cardiac cycle is the P wave, which represents atrial activation. The end of the P wave denotes that the right and left atria have been activated. Although initial activation of the AV node occurs during the middle portion of the P wave, progression of the impulse to the ventricles is delayed in order to allow the atria time to contract and pump blood into the ventricles. Recall that the P wave represents electrical activation, thus mechanical events of atrial contraction occur following the P wave.

The duration of the P wave is normally less than 0.128 second. Because the walls of the atrium are relatively thin and the body surface electrodes are located some distance from the atria, the normal amplitude of the P wave on the ECG recording is relatively small, fewer than 2.5 mm in all 12 ECG leads.[20] The P wave may be normally upright, inverted, or biphasic depending on the lead recorded.

QRS Complex

The QRS complex represents electrical activation of the ventricles; the mechanical event of ventricular contraction follows this waveform. Using the ECG lead convention discussed before—a negative electrode placed on the right shoulder and a positive electrode placed on the left leg—during normal activation a predominantly upright, or positive, QRS waveform will be recorded. Because some of the 12 ECG leads view myocardial activation from different vantage points, the normal QRS waveform morphology varies from lead to lead. For example, as seen in Figure 46-11, normal QRS waveform

deflections may be monophasic (one), biphasic (two), or triphasic (three). Nomenclature to describe these waveform variations has been developed.

If the initial deflection of the QRS complex waveform is a downward, or negative, waveform, then it is labeled a Q wave. Narrow Q waves (less than 0.30 second in duration) normally are seen in leads I, II, V_5, and V_6 because these leads capture left-to-right septal depolarization. The first upright or positive deflection is labeled an R wave. The next downward or negative waveform that follows the R wave is labeled an S wave. Large waveform deflections are labeled with a capital letter, and small deflections are labeled with a lowercase letter. A waveform with only a positive deflection is labeled an R wave, whereas a negative deflection is labeled as a QS complex. Finally, a second positive deflection that follows an RS complex is labeled R′ (pronounced "R prime"), and a second negative deflection that follows an RSR′ is labeled S′ (pronounced "S prime"). Figure 46-12 illustrates the various QRS complexes and the nomenclature used to identify QRS complex waveforms.

The duration of the QRS complex ranges from 0.07 to 0.116 second.[20] A QRS complex duration of greater than 0.11 second indicates QRS complex prolongation that may be due to bundle branch block (right or left), ventricular enlargement, drug effect, or an impulse conduction outside of the normal conduction pathway. Amplitude of the QRS complex varies widely by ECG lead, ranging from 0.13 mm to 12 mm. Because of the position of the precordial leads across the chest and the activation of the heart from the thin muscle of the right ventricle to thick muscle mass of the left ventricle, the R wave amplitude typically begins as a small complex in lead V_1 and increases in amplitude to lead V_4 or V_5.

Abnormal QRS voltage is present when the R wave amplitude is less than 5 mm in any one of the six limb leads and the absolute height is no more than 10 mm in any of the precordial leads. Causes of small-amplitude R waves include fascicular block and conditions that increase the distance between the recording electrode and the heart (chronic obstructive pulmonary disease) or anatomical or physiological conditions that can impede the electrical signal. Abnormally tall R waves may indicate hypertrophy, infarction, or conditions that decrease the distance between the recoding electrode and the heart.

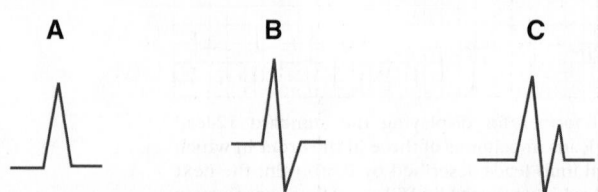

FIGURE 46-11 ■ Shows different QRS complex waveform deflections: **(A)** monophasic, **(B)** biphasic, and **(C)** triphasic.

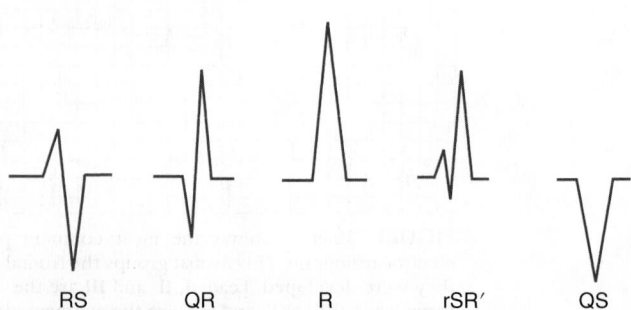

FIGURE 46-12 ■ Various QRS complexes and the nomenclature used to identify Q complex waveforms.

ST Segment

The next portion of the cardiac cycle is the ST segment. The ST segment begins at the J point, which marks the end of the QRS complex and extends to the beginning of the T wave. The ST segment corresponds with phase 2 of the action potential, when there is no movement of ions across the cell membrane and a period when the ventricles remain in the depolarized or active state. During this portion of the ECG complex, the ventricles contract. The length of ventricular activation can affect the duration of the ST segment.

Normally, the ST segment is isoelectric, meaning the ST segment is neither above nor below a stable reference point. Typically, the PR segment serves as the isoelectric reference point from which to measure ST segment deviation. ST segment deviation is measured by the number of millimeters the ST segment is deviated (i.e., elevated or depressed) from the PR segment and typically is measured at one of three sites: (1) the J point, (2) the J point + 60 msec past the J point, or (3) the J point + 80 msec past the J point. The J point marks the end of the QRS complex and beginning of the ST segment (Figure 46-13). Although the normal ST segment is isoelectric, normal variations of the ST segment include slight upsloping, downsloping, or horizontal depression. Additionally, it is considered a normal variant to see ST elevation caused by early repolarization (Figure 46-14). This condition is seen more often in young persons,[21] males,[22] athletes,[23] cocaine users,[24] obstructive hypertrophic cardiomyopathy, and defects and/or hypertrophy of the intraventricular septum.[25]

Drew and coworkers[26] reported that the ST segment was deviated (elevation or depression) in more than 60 percent of hospitalized patients with known coronary artery disease. Causes of ST segment deviation included drug effects (digitalis), hypertrophy, bundle branch block, and ventricular pacemaker. Therefore, it is unusual for the ST segment to be isoelectric. This means that a careful history and physical examination should be considered when deciding whether the ST segments are normal or abnormal, and if possible, a prior ECG should be obtained for comparison.

Myocardial ischemia should be considered if the 12-lead ECG meets the following criteria: (1) ST segment elevation at the J point in two or more contiguous leads with cutoff points of 2 mm in leads V_1, V_2, and V_3 and 1 mm in the remaining leads (contiguous leads in the limb leads are defined by the following sequence: aVL, I, aVR, II, aVF, and III); (2) new or presumed new ST segment depression in two or more contiguous leads; or (3) new or presumed new T wave inversion of greater than 1 mm in two or more contiguous leads.[27]

T Wave

The next waveform of the cardiac cycle is the T wave, which represents repolarization, or recovery of the ventricles and occurs during phase 3 of the action potential. During depolarization, electrical activation flows from the endocardium to the epicardium. During repolarization in the normal heart, cells of the epicardial layer of the heart repolarize earlier than cells in the endocardium.[28] However, the flow of electrical current

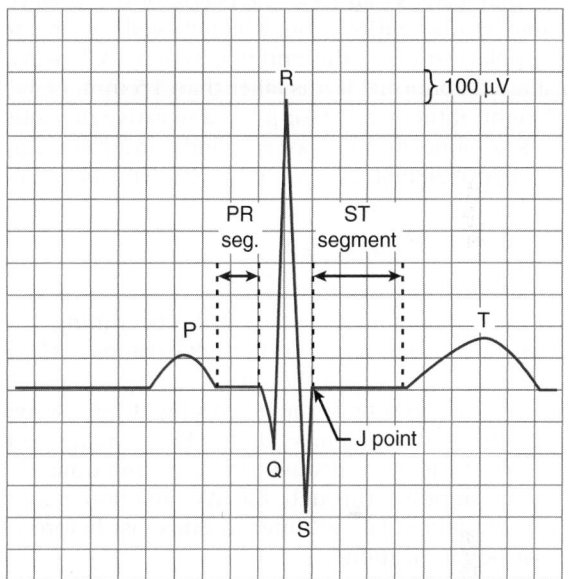

FIGURE 46-13 ▨ Normal electrocardiographic complex (one cardiac cycle) made up of P, Q, R, S, and T waves. Also shown are the PR segment, ST segment, and J point, which marks the end of the QRS complex and the beginning of the ST segment. ST segment deviation is measured by the number of millimeters or microvolts (1 mm = 1 μV) the ST segment is deviated (i.e., elevated or depressed) from the PR segment and typically is measured at one of three locations: (1) the J point, (2) J point + 60 msec past the J point, or (3) J point + 80 msec past the J point.

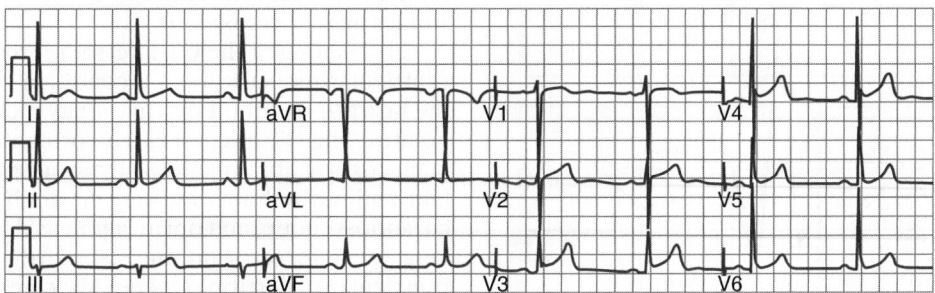

FIGURE 46-14 ▨ This standard 12-lead electrocardiogram shows an ST pattern of early repolarization. Note the ST elevation in leads V_3 to V_5. Note also in these same ECG leads the notched waveform where the QRS complex ends and the ST segment begins (J point). This is considered a normal variant and does not represent ST elevation indicative of myocardial ischemia. This condition is seen more often in young persons, males, athletes, cocaine users, obstructive hypertrophic cardiomyopathy, and defects and/or hypertrophy of the intraventricular septum.

still moves toward the epicardium. A positive electrode on the body surface will record a positive waveform in the same direction as the QRS complex. Hence, the normal deflection of the T wave should be in the same direction as the QRS complex. The reverse is true for a predominately negative complex (i.e., QS complex); the T wave also should be negative. The amplitude or height of the normal T wave should not exceed 5 mm in any of the limb leads, or 10 mm in the precordial leads. Alterations in the T wave may indicate ischemia, recovery following acute MI, drugs, dysrhythmias, or electrolyte imbalances.

U Wave

One final waveform of the cardiac cycle that may be seen after the T wave is the U wave. The U wave can be a normal or abnormal finding and is best seen in the precordial leads V_2 and V_3. The origin of the U wave is not understood entirely, but it is believed to represent late repolarization of the Purkinje system. A U wave is considered abnormal if it is taller than 1.5 mm, equal to the height of the T wave, or it has a negative deflection. Causes of abnormal U waves include antidysrhythmic drugs, hypokalemia, and acute myocardial ischemia.

ELECTROCARDIOGRAPHIC INTERVALS
PR Interval

The PR interval is measured from the beginning of the P wave to the beginning of the QRS complex (Figure 46-15). The beginning of the QRS complex is marked by the Q wave if present or the beginning of the R wave if there is no Q wave. Included in the PR interval is depolarization of the atria (P wave) and traveling time of the electrical impulse through the AV junction and the bundle branches. The PR interval ends just before ventricular depolarization.

The normal duration of the PR interval in adults ranges from 0.12 to 0.20 second.[20] The duration of the PR interval varies with heart rate, lengthening during slow heart rates and shortening with rapid heart rates.

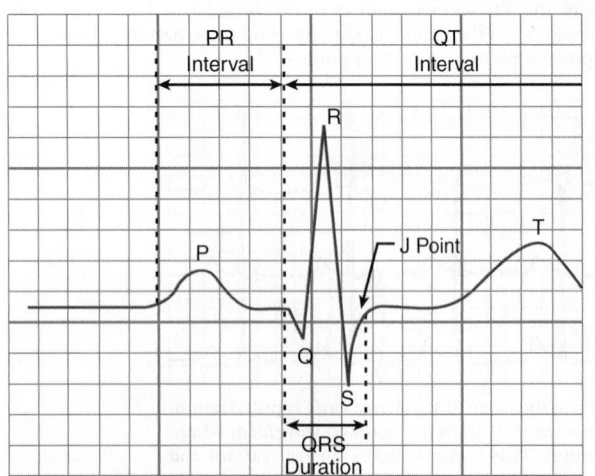

FIGURE 46-15 ▪ Cardiac intervals of the electrocardiographic complex.

Abnormal shortening of the PR interval can occur in patients with an additional conduction pathway, or accessory pathway, and in patients taking certain drugs (e.g., steroids).[29] Abnormal lengthening of the PR interval can occur because of conduction or depolarization abnormalities in the atria caused by the effects of drugs, or structural changes of the atria (e.g., hypertrophy or dilatation). The sources of PR lengthening also can occur in the AV junction because of drugs (including digitalis, beta blockers, and calcium channel blockers), aging, and MI.

QRS Interval

The QRS interval is measured from the beginning of the first waveform of the QRS complex, which might be a Q wave or an R wave, and ends at the last waveform, which might be an R, S, R′, or S′ waveform, or the J point, which marks the end of the QRS complex and the beginning of the T wave (Figure 46-15). The QRS interval is the time it takes the right and left ventricles to depolarize. The normal QRS duration ranges from 0.07 to 0.116 second.[20] On the standard 12-lead ECG, it is normal for the duration of the QRS complex to vary slightly from lead to lead. For example, the QRS complex duration may be slightly longer in the precordial leads V_1 to V_6 compared with the limb leads as the result of septal depolarization. A wide QRS complex occurs when conduction is delayed in any part of the ventricular conduction pathway (bundle branches, fascicles, or Purkinje network). Delayed conduction can occur because of hypertrophy, dilatation, or abnormal impulse conduction in the ventricular portion of the heart.

QT Interval

The QT interval is measured from the beginning of the QRS complex to the end of the T wave (Figure 46-15). This interval represents the summation of depolarization and repolarization of the ventricles. Under normal conditions, the QT interval shortens with increases in heart rate and lengthens as the heart rate slows. The QT interval may be short in individuals with acute or chronic hypercalcemia. In this condition, because the T wave merges into the QRS complex, acute ischemia may be diagnosed falsely. Additional causes of a short QT interval include endogenous or exogenous catecholamines and thyrotoxicosis.

Lengthening of the QT interval represents prolonged ventricular repolarization, a condition that predisposes the heart to reentrant dysrhythmias such as torsades de pointes. The QT interval can be prolonged as the result of electrolyte abnormalities (hypocalcemia), drugs (certain antidysrhythmic, anticancer, antibiotic, antimalarial, antipsychotic, and opiate agonists drugs), congenital long QT interval syndromes, bradydysrhythmias, left ventricular hypertrophy, acute MI, cerebral vascular accidents (typically subarachnoid hemorrhage), and hypothermia.

The QT interval should be measured in the lead in which the T wave offset is defined most clearly. This is typically lead V_2 or V_3. A major source of error when measuring the QT interval is determining at which point the T wave ends, which can be challenging when a U wave is present or when the P wave merges with the T wave during rapid heart rates. If a U wave is present, it is not included in the QT interval measurement. Because the QT interval changes with tachycardia or bradycardia, it is corrected for heart rate and is labeled as QT_C. Bazett[30] developed a formula to correct for heart rate when measuring the QT interval. Recent modifications have been made to the formula[24] as follows:

$$QT_C = QT + 1.75 \text{ (ventricular rate} - 60)$$

A QT_C of greater than 0.44 second using Bazett's formula is considered abnormal. The QT_C can vary with gender (slightly longer in women compared with men) and age (increases with age).

Normal Cardiac Rhythm

For every 12-lead ECG, a systematic approach to interpretation should be used in order to determine normal from abnormal findings. The following 10 features should be evaluated: (1) heart rate and regularity of beats, (2) P wave morphology, (3) PR interval, (4) QRS complex morphology, (5) QRS interval, (6) QT interval, (7) ST segment morphology, (8) T wave morphology, (9) U wave (if present) morphology, (10) rhythm, and (11) QRS axis.

Typically, heart rate, regularity of beats, and rhythm are interpreted together. To determine these features, it is important to understand the grid printed on the ECG paper (Figure 46-16). The grid is standardized so that there are thin lines every 1 mm and a thick line every 5 mm. The vertical lines of the grid are used to measure time, such as heart rate and waveform intervals. The typical paper speed programmed into the ECG machine

is 25 mm/sec, hence the thin lines are at 0.04 second (40 msec), and the thick lines at 0.20 second (200 msec). The horizontal lines are used to measure waveform amplitudes. Typically, the ECG machine is calibrated at 10 mm/mV; hence the thin lines are at 0.1-mV increments and the thick lines are at 0.5-mV increments.

Heart rate can be calculated easily when the rhythm is regular (equal spacing between the QRS complexes) by counting the number of large squares between QRS complex cycles. If possible, select a QRS complex that falls on a thick line, and then count each successive thick line moving from the left or the right of the identified QRS complex. Each thick line from the reference beat represents a time interval, with the first thick line representing 300 beats/min; the next, 150 beats/min; and so on for 100, 75, 60, 50, 43, 37, and 33 beats/min, respectively. In other words, divide the number of thick lines into 300. By memorizing these numbers, one can calculate heart rate quickly and easily during a regular rhythm. Figure 46-17 illustrates this methodology.

Another method of calculating heart rate during a regular heart rate is to count the number of small squares (0.04 second) between two R waves and divide by 1500. Although this method requires a calculator, it is more accurate than the "300 rule" and is helpful for very rapid heart rates.

If the rate is irregular, the average heart rate can be calculated by counting the number of cardiac cycles over a particular time interval. For example, many ECG machines record a mark on the ECG printout at

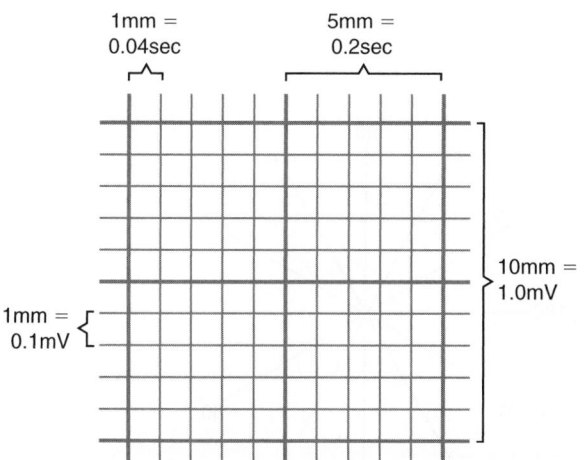

FIGURE 46-16 ■ The grid on electrocardiographic paper is standardized so that there are thin lines every 1 mm, and a thick line every 5 mm. The *vertical lines* of the grid are used to measure time, such as heart rate and waveform intervals. The typical paper speed programmed into the electrocardiogram machine is 25 mm/sec; hence the thin lines are at 0.04 second (40 msec), and the thick lines are at 0.20 second (200 msec). The *horizontal lines* are used to measure waveform amplitudes. Typically the electrocardiogram machine is calibrated at 10 mm/mV; hence the thin lines are at 0.1-mV increments and the thick lines are at 0.5-mV increments.

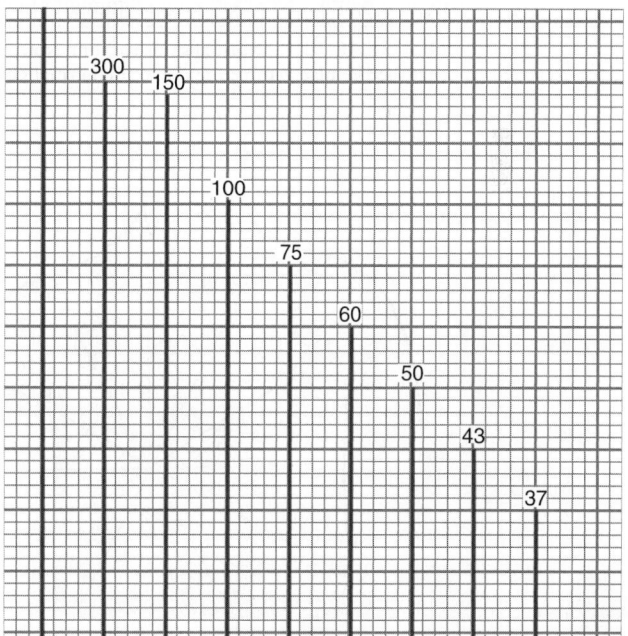

FIGURE 46-17 ■ A heart rate that is regular (equal spacing between the QRS complexes) can be calculated by counting the number of large squares between QRS complex cycles. If possible, select a QRS complex that falls on a thick line, and then count each successive thick line moving from the left or the right of the identified QRS complex. Each thick line from the reference beat represents a time interval, with the first thick line representing 300 beats/min; the next line, 150 beats/min; and so on for 100, 75, 60, 50, 43, and 37 beats/min, respectively.

3-second intervals. To calculate heart rate, count the number of cardiac cycles in a 6-second period (two 3-second tick marks) and multiply by 10.

A normal cardiac rhythm is called *sinus rhythm* because the impulse originates in the SA node and proceeds down the normal conduction pathway, as described in the preceding sections of this chapter. The rate of normal sinus rhythm is between 60 and 90 beats/min. Sinus rhythm at a heart rate below this limit is termed *sinus bradycardia,* and sinus rhythm at a heart rate that exceeds this limit is termed *sinus tachycardia.* Figure 46-18 is an example of normal sinus rhythm, there is a P wave in front of every QRS complex, and the heart rate is regular at 75 beats/min.

QRS Axis

QRS axis represents the average of all the electrical current of the heart. Although axis determination can be calculated for other ECG waveforms (P, ST, and T waves), this is not done routinely. Rather, QRS axis is a standard determination used to assess the direction of ventricular depolarization. Abnormal QRS axis may indicate structural abnormalities, coronary artery disease,

hypertrophy, heart disease caused by hypertension, MI, valvular heart disease, or cardiomyopathy. QRS axis is used to identify dysrhythmias and distinguish supraventricular tachycardia from ventricular tachycardia with aberrancy. The normal QRS axis in adults ranges from −30 to +90 degrees.[31] Most current ECG machines calculate P wave, T wave, and QRS axis.

Graettinger and coworkers[32] introduced the hexaxial reference system as a way of visualizing the relationship of the six frontal limb leads as they relate to ventricular activity of the heart. The hexaxial reference system applies a visual representation to the frontal plane of the torso similar to the face of a clock, whereby the six limb leads are separated by angles 30 degrees apart (Figure 46-19).

Lead I is used as the 0-degree reference point. Positive lead designations move from this reference point in a clockwise direction at 30-degree increments to +180 degrees. Negative lead designations move in a counterclockwise direction to −180 degrees. The positive poles for leads II, aVF, and III are located at +60, +90, and +120 degrees, respectively; lead aVL at −30 degrees; and lead aVR, designated as "minus aVR," at −150 degrees. The hexaxial reference system also can be used

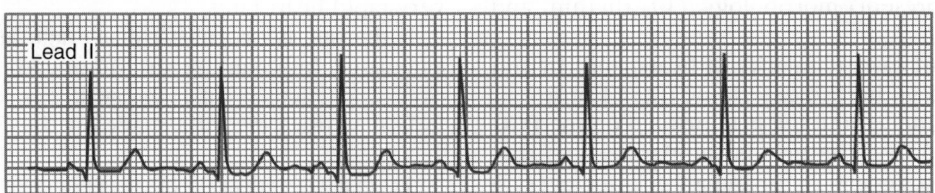

FIGURE 46-18 ■ Normal sinus rhythm. Note that a P wave precedes every QRS complex, indicating that the impulse is traveling down the normal conduction pathway.

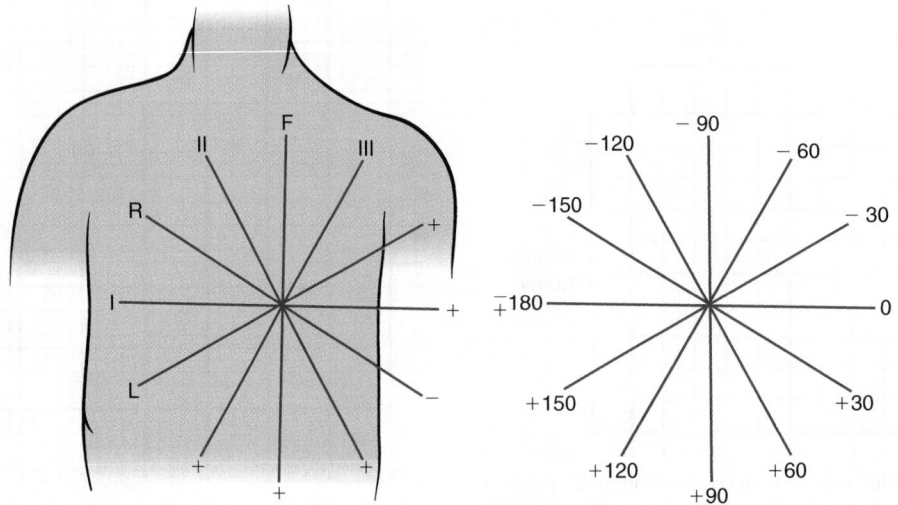

FIGURE 46-19 ■ These illustrations show the hexaxial reference system, which applies a visual representation to the frontal plane of the torso similar to the face of a clock. The six limb leads are separated by angles 30 degrees apart. Lead I is used as the 0-degree reference point; positive lead designations move from this reference point in a clockwise direction at 30-degree increments to +180 degrees, and negative lead designations move in a counterclockwise direction to −180 degrees. The positive poles for leads II, aVF, and III are located at +60, +90, and +120 degrees, respectively; lead aVL at −30 degrees; and lead aVR, designated as "minus aVR," at −150 degrees.

to localize the limb leads based on their view of the heart. For example, if one were to apply the hexaxial reference system to the anterior torso, the positive poles of leads I (0 degrees) and aVL (−30) would view the lateral myocardial activity; hence, these leads are designated lateral limb leads.

The positive poles of leads II (+60 degrees), III, (+120 degrees), and aVF (+90 degrees) view the bottom or inferior portion of the heart; hence, these three limb leads are termed the *inferior limb leads.* To differentiate normal QRS axis from abnormal QRS axis, the hexaxial reference system is divided further and is labeled into four quadrants: (1) normal axis (−30 to +90 degrees), (2) right axis deviation (+90 to +180 degrees), (3) left axis deviation (−90 to −30 degrees), (4) right superior axis deviation (−180 to −90 degrees). Also possible is to have an indeterminate axis, which is present when all the limb leads are isoelectric.

A simple and quick method for determining normal versus abnormal QRS axis is by assessing leads I and aVF (Figure 46-20). If the predominant QRS direction in both of these leads is positive (upright), then the axis is considered normal. One exception to this rule is right bundle branch block; in this instance, only the first 60 msec of the QRS complex are used to determine axis.[33] If the net QRS complex in lead I is positive and in lead aVF it is negative, left axis deviation is present. If the net QRS complex in lead I is negative and in lead aVF it is positive, right axis deviation is present. If the net QRS complex in lead I is negative and in lead II it is negative, indeterminate axis deviation is present. In addition, if the QRS area is isoelectric (not positive and not negative), then an indeterminate axis is present.

The actual degrees of QRS axis also can be determined. The method requires assessment of the six limb leads. QRS axis is directed toward the lead with the tallest positive or negative waveform. The QRS axis is directed perpendicular to the lead with the smallest or most biphasic (equally positive and negative) waveform. To determine the actual degrees of axis, do the following:

1. Assess the QRS complex in all of the six limb leads. Identify the QRS complex with the tallest positive or negative deflection. If the QRS complex is predominantly positive, then the axis points toward the positive pole of that lead. If the QRS complex is predominantly negative, then the axis points toward the negative pole of that lead.

2. Next, identify the limb lead with the smallest or most biphasic QRS complex. The QRS axis is directed perpendicular, or at a 90-degree angle, to this lead. The lead selected in step 1 determines toward which side the complex points: the positive or negative pole. See the example in Figure 46-21.

3. The QRS axis can be refined even further by assessing the most biphasic lead selected in step 2. If the QRS complex in this lead is slightly more positive than negative, then the axis is shifted slightly toward the positive pole of the perpendicular axis. Conversely, if the QRS complex in this lead is slightly more negative than positive, then the axis is shifted slightly toward the negative pole of the perpendicular axis.

Axis deviation may be a normal variant (i.e., aging), or pathological (i.e., acute MI). Nonpathological causes include lead misplacement. Causes of right axis deviation include conditions that affect the right ventricle, including pulmonary hypertension, pulmonic stenosis, and acute pulmonary edema. Additional causes of right axis deviation include right ventricular hypertrophy, congenital heart disease, MI (lateral), and left posterior fascicular block. This may be a normal variant in young persons or in tall, slender adults.

Causes of left axis deviation include left ventricular enlargement, left ventricular hypertrophy, MI (inferior), left anterior fascicular block, and ventricular pacing. This may be a normal variant in older persons.

Finally, causes of right superior axis deviation, also called "no man's land" include right ventricular hypertrophy, apical MI, ventricular tachycardia, and hyperkalemia.

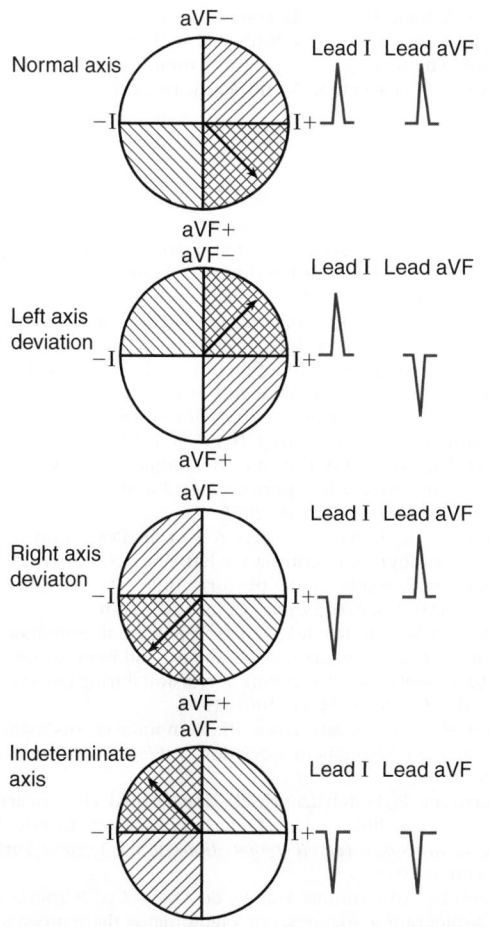

FIGURE 46-20 ■ This figure illustrates a simple and quick method for determining normal versus abnormal QRS axis by assessing leads I and aVF. (From Lipman B, Cascio T: ECG electrodes and leads. In *ECG assessment and interpretation,* Philadelphia, 1994, FA Davis.)

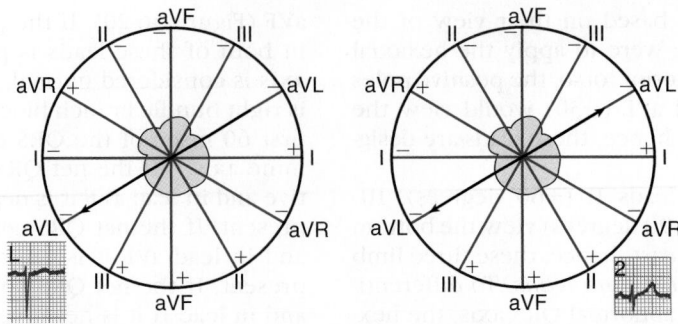

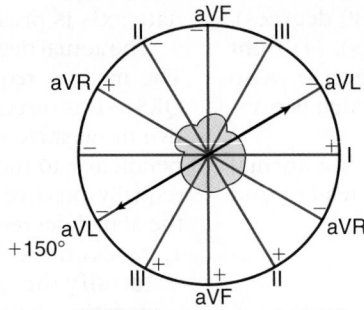

Deepest deflection = Lead aVL
(axis should point toward negative end of aVL)

Most biphasic deflection = Lead II
(axis is perpendicular to II)

Right axis deviation (+150°)
Axis points toward negative end of lead aVL

FIGURE 46-21 ■ Actual degrees of QRS axis can be calculated. Identify the QRS complex with the tallest positive or negative deflection—lead aVL in this example. Next, identify the limb lead with the smallest or most biphasic QRS complex—lead II in this example. The final QRS axis in this example is 150 degrees, or right axis deviation. (From Lipman B, Cascio T: ECG electrodes and leads. In *ECG assessment and interpretation*, Philadelphia, 1994, FA Davis.)

REFERENCES

1. Einthoven W: *Galvanometrische registratie van het menschilijk electrocardiogram*, Leiden, Netherlands 1902.
2. Wilson F, Macloed A, Barker P: The interpretation of the initial deflections of the ventricular complex of the electrocardiogram, *Am Heart J* 6:637-664, 1931.
3. Fozzard HA, Lee PJ, Lipkind GM: Mechanism of local anesthetic drug action on voltage-gated sodium channels, *Curr Pharm Des* 11:2671-2686, 2005.
4. French RJ, Zamponi GW: Voltage-gated sodium and calcium channels in nerve, muscle, and heart, *IEEE Trans Nanobioscience* 4:58-69, 2005.
5. Kamishima T, Quayle JM: Ca2+-induced Ca2+ release in cardiac and smooth muscle cells, *Biochem Soc Trans* 31:943-946, 2003.
6. Nabauer M: Tuning repolarization in the heart: a multitude of potassium channels and regulatory pathways, *Circ Res* 88:453-455, 2001.
7. Lopatin AN, Nichols CG: Inward rectifiers in the heart: an update on I(K1), *J Mol Cell Cardiol* 33:625-638, 2001.
8. Mangoni ME, Couette B, Marger L et al: Voltage-dependent calcium channels and cardiac pacemaker activity: from ionic currents to genes, *Prog Biophys Mol Biol* 90:38-63, 2005.
9. Franzini-Armstrong C, Protasi F, Tijskens P: The assembly of calcium release units in cardiac muscle, *Ann N Y Acad Sci* 1047:76-85, 2005.
10. Dhamoon AS, Jalife J: The inward rectifier current (IK1) controls cardiac excitability and is involved in arrhythmogenesis, *Heart Rhythm* 2:316-24, 2005.
11. Wittig JH, Stark J: Intraoperative mapping of atrial activation before, during, and after the Mustard operation, *J Thorac Cardiovasc Surg* 73:1-13, 1977.
12. Goldberger E: A simple, indifferent, electrocardiographic electrode of zero potential and a technique of obtaining augmented, unipolar, extremity leads, *Am Heart J* 23:483-492, 1942.
13. Colaco R, Reay P, Beckett C et al: False positive ECG reports of anterior myocardial infarction in women, *J Electrocardiol* 33(suppl):239-244, 2000.
14. Rautaharju PM, Park L, Rautaharju FS et al: A standardized procedure for locating and documenting ECG chest electrode positions: consideration of the effect of breast tissue on ECG amplitudes in women, *J Electrocardiol* 31:17-29, 1998.
15. Mason RE, Likar I: A new system of multiple-lead exercise electrocardiography, *Am Heart J* 71:196-205, 1966.
16. Jowett NI, Turner AM, Cole A et al: Modified electrode placement must be recorded when performing 12-lead electrocardiograms, *Postgrad Med J* 81:122-125, 2005.
17. Malmqvist K, Kahan T, Eriksson S et al: Evaluation of various electrocardiographic criteria for left ventricular hypertrophy in patients with stable angina pectoris: influence of using modified limb electrodes, *Clin Physiol* 21:196-207, 2001.
18. Krucoff MW, Loeffler KA, Haisty WK Jr et al: Simultaneous ST-segment measurements using standard and monitoring-compatible torso limb lead placements at rest and during coronary occlusion, *Am J Cardiol* 74:997-1001, 1994.
19. Pelter MM, Adams MG, Drew BJ: Computer versus manual measurement of ST-segment deviation, *J Electrocardiol* 29(suppl): 78-82, 1996.
20. Macfarlane P, Veitch Lawrie T: The normal electrocardiogram and vectorcardiogram. In Macfarlane P, Veitch Lawrie TD, editors: *Comprehensive electrocardiology*, vol 1, New York, 1989, Pergamon Press.
21. Lazzoli JK, Annarumma Mde O, de Araujo CG: [Criteria for electrocardiographic diagnosis of vagotonia: is there a consensus in the opinion of specialists?] *Arq Bras Cardiol* 63:377-381, 1994.
22. Mehta MC, Jain AC: Early repolarization on scalar electrocardiogram, *Am J Med Sci* 309:305-311, 1995.
23. Bjornstad H, Storstein L, Dyre Meen H et al: Electrocardiographic findings according to level of fitness and sport activity, *Cardiology* 83:268-279, 1993.

24. Hollander JE, Lozano M, Fairweather P et al: "Abnormal" electrocardiograms in patients with cocaine-associated chest pain are due to "normal" variants, *J Emerg Med* 12:199-205, 1994.

25. Vorob'ev LP, Gribkova IN, Petrusenko NM et al: [The clinico-electrocardiographic classification of the early ventricular repolarization syndrome], *Ter Arkh* 64:93-97, 1992.

26. Drew BJ, Wung SF, Adams MG et al: Bedside diagnosis of myocardial ischemia with ST-segment monitoring technology: measurement issues for real-time clinical decision making and trial designs, *J Electrocardiol* 30(suppl):157-165, 1998.

27. Alpert JS, Thygesen K, Antman E et al: Myocardial infarction redefined: a consensus document of the Joint European Society of Cardiology/American College of Cardiology Committee for the redefinition of myocardial infarction, *J Am Coll Cardiol* 36: 959-969, 2000.

28. Yan GX, Antzelevitch C: Cellular basis for the normal T wave and the electrocardiographic manifestations of the long-QT syndrome, *Circulation* 98:1928-1936, 1998.

29. Lipman B, Cascio T: *ECG assessment and interpretation,* Philadelphia, 1994, FA Davis.

30. Bazett H: An analysis of the time relations of electrocardiograms, *Heart* 7:353-370, 1920.

31. Willems JL, Robles de Medina EO, Bernard R et al: Criteria for intraventricular conduction disturbances and pre-excitation: World Health Organizational/International Society and Federation for Cardiology Task Force Ad Hoc, *J Am Coll Cardiol* 5:1261-1275, 1985.

32. Graettinger J, Packard J, Graybiel A: A new method of equating the presenting bipolar and unipolar extremity leads on the electrocardiogram: advantages gained in visualization of their common relationship to the electric field of the heart, *Am J Med* 11:3-25, 1951.

33. Evans G: *ECG interpretation cribsheets,* ed 4, Corte Madera, Calif, 1999, Ring Mountain Press.

■■■■ chapter 47

Electrocardiography: Abnormal Electrocardiogram

Laurie G. Futterman

CHAPTER ABBREVIATIONS

ARVD arrhythmogenic right ventricular dysplasia

AV atrioventricular

BER benign early depolarization

CAD coronary artery disease

COPD chronic obstructive pulmonary disease

ECG electrocardiogram

LAD left arterior descending

LAH left anterior hemiblock

LBBB left bundle branch block

LCX left circumflex

LPH left posterior hemiblock

LQTS long-QT syndrome

LQTS2 congenital long-QT syndrome

LV left ventricular

LVA left ventricular aneurysm

LVH left ventricular hypertrophy

MI myocardial infarction

PE pulmonary embolism

QTC rate-corrected QT interval

QTd QT dispersion

RBBB right bundle branch block

RCA right coronary artery

RV right ventricular

RVI right ventricular infarction

SCD sudden cardiac death

S1Q3T3 prominent S wave in lead I, ST segment elevation in lead II, and new or increasing Q waves and T wave inversion in lead III

STD ST segment depression

STE ST segment elevation

VT ventricular tachycardia

WPW Wolf-Parkinson-White

The modern electrocardiogram (ECG) is an indispensable tool used to help identify alterations of cardiac rhythm and conduction; the influence of metabolic, electrolyte, and drug effects; and other electrophysiological and pathophysiological footprints. ECG pattern recognition can help in the differentiation of ischemic and nonischemic conditions, often before serum cardiac marker or functional testing results are available. Although the majority of abnormal ECGs result from some form of electrophysiological derange-

ment, many result from physiological or adaptive processes. To appreciate the implication of an abnormal ECG waveform, it is essential to understand the genesis of what lies beneath the electronic facade of the surface ECG tracing. The normal ECG is described in detail in Chapter 46.

An abnormal ECG waveform is a compilation of physiological, biological, electrical, and pathophysiological interactions that in some way alter the formation or transmission of the cardiac electrical impulse. The presence and influence of pathological factors in each stage of impulse formation and transmission form the basis of abnormal waveform production. From the origin of the transmembrane potential to the arrival of its electrical signal at the skin surface, the interactions of five factors determine the outcome of the baseline ECG tracing: (1) cellular factors (ionic or electrolyte concentrations, the function of the conducting ion channel, and intracellular/extracellular resistance factors); (2) cardiac factors (impulse propagation within the myocardial fiber, degree of connective tissue present between fibers); (3) extracardiac factors (intracavitary elements and structures); (4) physical factors (anteroposterior positioning of the heart within the chest cavity, orientation of cardiac chambers in respect to anterior chest leads, and proper electrode placement); and (5) electromechanical factors (lead system electronics and programming, and external interference).[1]

Pathological factors such as ischemia, ion channel dysfunction, or electrolyte imbalance, can slow or speed the movement of Na^+, K^+, or Ca^{++} ions. Alterations in ion movements or ion concentrations can affect the resting membrane potential and the uniformity, speed, and duration of cardiac cell depolarization and repolarization. Altered ion activity may cause the cell to become more (or less) responsive to further depolarization. Changes in the depolarization-repolarization process may affect some cardiac cell types more so than others. This heterogeneic response results in a loss of electrophysiological uniformity among the different cardiac cell types, causing dysrhythmias.

Depending on the causative factor, alterations in ion concentration or flow patterns can abbreviate or delay depolarization or repolarization activity. *Delays* in transmission are reflected by *wider* intervals and more prolonged waveform complexes (e.g., ischemia delays repolarization and increases the QT interval), whereas *abbreviation* manifests in *narrowing* or *shortening* of these intervals and waveforms (e.g., hypercalcemia abbreviates repolarization and shortens the QT interval). Body habitus and disease can affect the height or amplitude of the QRS complex as underlying forces increase or decrease impulse transmission.

With the electrical impulse formed, the current is propagated through the cardiac tissue via the myocardial fibers. Impulse transmission is affected by the direction of its flow within the myocardial fiber. Current flow is more rapid traveling the length of the fiber than in transverse propagation. As a result, recording electrodes oriented to the long axis of a cardiac fiber display a greater electrical potential than a lead oriented along the transverse axis. The degree of fibrous tissue within the myocardial fibers also can disrupt impulse propagation by reducing the transmitting ability (electrical coupling) of the myocardial fibers. The more nonconductive tissue present (e.g., fibrosis from previous myocardial infarction, or fat in arrhythmogenic right ventricular dysplasia [**ARVD**]), the greater is the impedance to electrical flow, and a wider, more fractionated waveform is recorded. The activating vectors or wavefronts also affect the formation of the ECG waveform. Although the currents responsible for normal myocardial activation (Figure 47-1) occur in a multiphase wave, primary conduction abnormalities, infarction, heart position, electronic pacing, or other physical properties can affect the cardiac vectors, changing the net effect of the depolarizing wavefront.

NONCARDIAC CAUSES OF ELECTROCARDIOGRAPHIC ABNORMALITIES

Alterations in the normal ECG tracing are the result of a direct or indirect process that affects myocardial physiology. Depending on the clinical circumstances, this process may be considered either physiologic or pathologic. In this section, discussion will focus on ECG change caused by extra-cardiac events (e.g., normal variants, electrolytes, systemic conditions).

Normal Variants:

Due to physiologic differences within the population, several waveform alterations in the ECG are considered to be normal. When physiologic exaggerations occur in response to an activity or event, and are not associated with symptoms or physical abnormalities, these ECG changes are considered variants of normal.

Early Repolarization

In most situations, ST segment elevation (**STE**) is a marker of myocardial ischemia and is the basis upon which thrombolysis or primary angioplasty is initiated. However, numerous nonischemic conditions are associated with STE, each with its own ECG footprint (Table 47-1).

Generally, STE is not present on the resting ECG. In certain instances, however, a characteristic form of minimal STE can be found as a normal variant and is not associated with any underlying pathological condition. This variant is referred to as early repolarization or benign early repolarization.[4,5] Although considered idiopathic and innocent, the presence of STE can be confused with the ischemic ST segment patterns of acute myocardial infarction (**MI**), pericarditis, or intraventricular conduction disturbances, especially when the STE is accompanied by chest pain.[2,6]

The J point is the approximate reference point marking the end of depolarization and the beginning of repolarization, and it is located where the QRS complex joins the ST segment. When the J point becomes significantly deviated from the baseline, a notch-like waveform can occur. This waveform is referred to as a J wave. Several clinical conditions such as benign early repolarization, hypothermia, and ischemia can produce J waves or J point elevation.[7]

Benign early repolarization is characterized by J point elevation, or a small J wave on the downsloping portion of the QRS complex, where it meets the ST segment. The J wave in this condition is followed by a high takeoff of an upwardly concave ST segment—usually 0.1 to 0.2 mV in height. The STE is typically concordant with the QRS complex and is associated with large-amplitude T waves, upright in the leads displaying the elevation. Another defining feature of benign early repolarization is its localization to the mid and left precordial leads (V_2 to V_5), with prevalence in lead V_4 and less prominence in limb leads II, III, and aVF and reciprocal ST segment depression in lead aVR. These features are important when one is trying to distinguish benign and pathological causes of STE.[8]

Only recently has the electrophysiological basis of the J wave and benign early repolarization been defined.[9] The hallmark J wave represents the voltage gradient that occurs during ventricular activation when an action potential notching occurs in the epicardium, but not in the endocardium. Discordant transmural repolarization occurs when the repolarization phases of epicar-

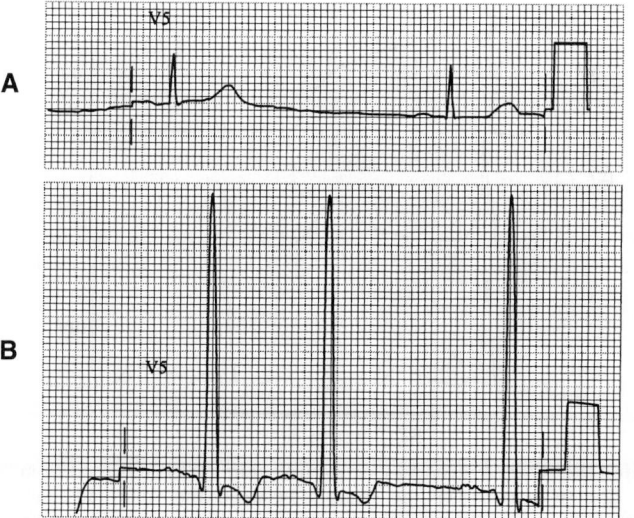

FIGURE 47-1 ■ Role of body habitus and disease on the amplitude of the QRS complex. **A,** *Top:* Low-amplitude complexes in an obese woman with hypothyroidism. **B,** *Bottom:* High-amplitude complexes in a hypertensive man. (From Meek S, Morris F: *BMJ* 324:415-418, 2002.)

■ ■ ■

TABLE 47-1 CHARACTERISTICS OF ST SEGMENT ELEVATIONS IN CARDIAC AND NONCARDIAC CONDITIONS[2,3]

CONDITION	DEFINING CHARACTERISTIC
Normal variant (male pattern)	90% incidence in healthy male population, concave ST segment elevation (STE) greater than 0.1-0.4 mV in leads V_2-V_5, most marked in V_2, with notched J point, fishhook appearance; reciprocal ST segment depression does not occur
	Increased prevalence in blacks and Hispanics
	T waves may be peaked or inverted
	Abbreviated QTC interval with increased QRS complex voltage may be seen in athletes
Early repolarization variant	Upwardly concave ST segment less than 0.2 mV that appears lifted off the isoelectric line, notching or slurring in terminal QRS complex (J point), symmetrical and concordant T waves
Acute pericarditis	PR segment depression
	Diffuse concave STE, $\geq$0.5 mV, not limited to areas of anatomical blood supply; STE typically observed in leads I-III, lead aVF, and precordial leads; ST remains concave; reciprocal changes seen in lead aVR, possibly in lead V_1
Acute myocarditis	Diffuse, nonspecific ST-T wave changes, STE (usually less than 0.5 mV) and Q waves
Ischemia	Convex or flat ST segment elevation greater than 0.1 mV, reciprocal ST segment depression
Coronary artery spasm	STE in leads associated with involved vessel
Long QT syndrome/Brugada syndrome	Coved or saddleback STE in leads V_1-V_3, prolonged QT interval, rSR' in lead V_1
Left ventricular aneurysm	STE that persists beyond 4 weeks after myocardial infarction; STE is localized over infarcted-aneurysm region
Left bundle branch block	Concave, discordant ST elevation associated with wide QRS complex greater than 12 msec
	STE usually seen in leads V_1-V_4
	Concordant STE in left bundle branch block is suggestive of acute myocardial infarction
Left ventricular hypertrophy	Concave STE in precordial leads; increased QRS complex voltage consistent with hypertrophy; poor R wave progression can be seen in leads V_1-V_3
Hypertrophic cardiomyopathy	Q wave formation, occasionally persistent STE
Hyperkalemia	Downsloping STE, associated with widened QRS complex, low amplitude P waves
Pulmonary embolism	Anteroseptal and inferior STE associated with T wave inversion in the right precordial leads
Transthoracic cardioversion	Transient (1-3 minutes) STE greater than 1 mV, occurring immediately following direct current countershock to the precordium
Intracranial hemorrhage	Diffuse STE, correlate with central nervous system symptoms

dial and endocardial action potentials become asynchronous, causing an electrical gradient to occur. The gradient results in the formation of the notch in the terminal QRS complex (Figure 47-2). The appearance of a prominent J wave also is associated with hypothermia, hypercalcemia, and the life-threatening dysrhythmia syndromes of Brugada syndrome and idiopathic ventricular tachycardia (VT).

Benign early repolarization occurs more often in men than in women, as does a difference in the degree of STE—generally 0.1 mV in men and less than 0.1 mV in females. A noticeable incidence of STE is encountered in young black men, ages 20 to 40, with a range of 0.1 to 0.4 mV. This normal variant differs slightly in that the STE is accompanied by inverted T waves and it appears coved.[6,9]

Because physiological variations in the ST segment meet the criterion for thrombolytic therapy under the American Heart Association/American College of Cardiology AMI guidelines,[10] a subcommittee of the American College of Emergency Room Physicians changed the existing indications for thrombolytic therapy.[11] Qualifications for thrombolysis now exclude STE characteristic of early repolarization, hyperkalemia, or pericarditis or characteristics stemming from repolarization abnor-

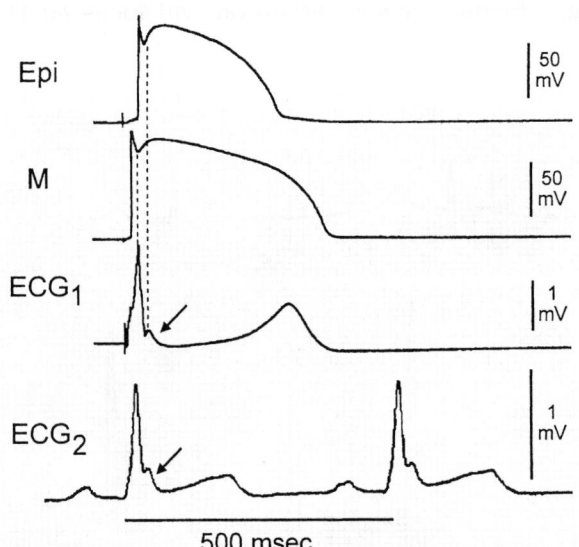

FIGURE 47-2 ■ Lead V_5 electrocardiogram (ECG) recorded from a dog in vivo shows the relation between the spike-and-dome morphology of the epicardial action potential (AP) and the appearance of the J wave. Second transmural ECG recorded across the arterially perfused left ventricular wedge isolated from the heart of the same dog. Both ECGs display a prominent J wave at the R-ST junction (*arrows*). (From Yan GX, Antzelevitch C: *Circulation* 93[2]:372-379, 1996.)

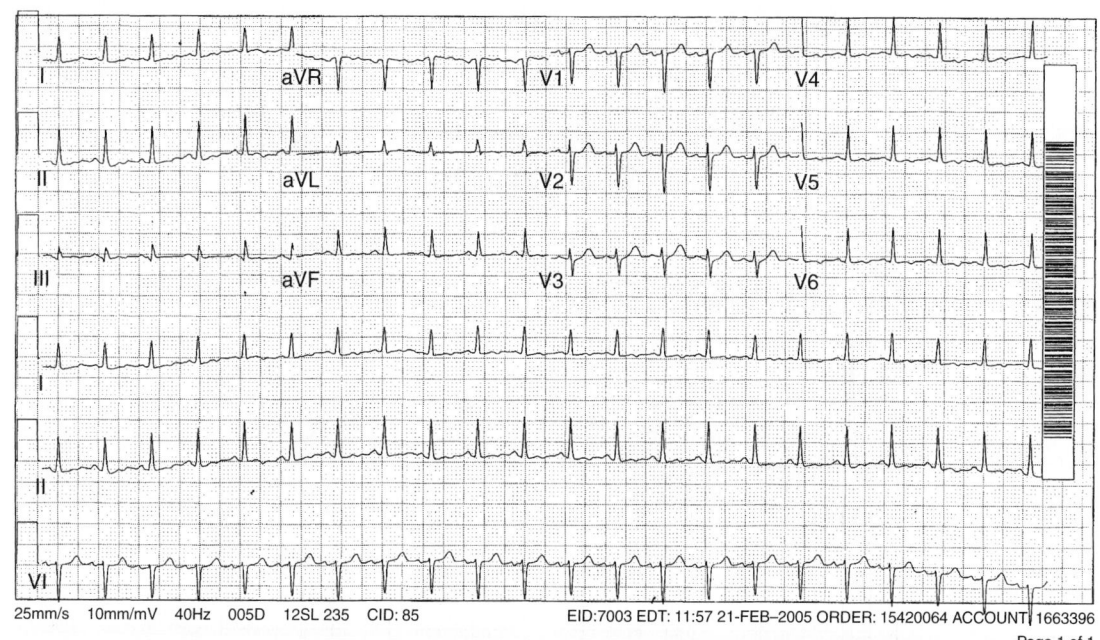

25mm/s 10mm/mV 40Hz 005D 12SL 235 CID: 85   EID:7003 EDT: 11:57 21-FEB–2005 ORDER: 15420064 ACCOUNT 1663396

Page 1 of 1

FIGURE 47-3 ■ Sinus tachycardia with nonspecific ST-T wave changes. Note the borderline, flat ST segment associated with minimal T wave inversion in the limb leads and in precordial leads V₄ to V₆.

malities of left ventricular hypertrophy **(LVH)** or preexisting bundle branch block.[6] New, or presumed new left bundle branch block **(LBBB)** is considered a criterion for thrombolysis.

Nonspecific ST-T Wave Changes

Transient and nonspecific ST-T wave changes (less than 0.1 mV ST segment depression or STE) can be found on the routine ECG and can be concerning, especially when the patient has chest pain (Figure 47-3). Transient ST-T wave changes can occur with physiological activities, such as changing position, drinking cold water, eating, hyperventilation, or following the Valsalva maneuver.[1,12]

Athlete's Heart

The cardiovascular system of endurance-trained athletes undergoes numerous physiological adaptations in response to the hemodynamic demands of regular intense exercise. These adaptations can produce varying degrees of ECG abnormalities. This syndrome, referred to as "athlete's heart" or "athlete's heart syndrome," is considered benign in most cases.[13,14] Physiological adaptations of the athlete's heart must be differentiated from similar patterns associated with cardiomyopathies of hypertrophy or of ARVD, both of which are associated with sudden cardiac death **(SCD)** in athletes. With continued training, ventricular mass and dimension increase and heightened vagal tone dominates the autonomic state. As a result, alterations in heart rate, QRS complex voltage, and repolarization occur. The majority of athletes with significant abnormalities on the ECG are found to have the greatest increase in left ventricular **(LV)** and left atrial **(LA)** cavity dimensions.

Changes on the athlete's ECG vary (Figures 47-4 and 47-5) but typically demonstrate resting sinus bradycardia and sinus dysrhythmia. Junctional rhythm can appear during the slow phase of sinus dysrhythmia. The type of sporting discipline, gender, and age of the athlete tends to have the greatest impact on the degree of ECG variation. Depending on the intensity of training, most conditioned athletes have a resting bradycardia. As many as 10 to 33 percent of conditioned athletes have first-degree atrioventricular **(AV)** conduction delay, and

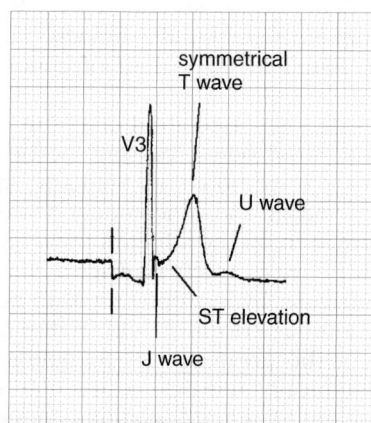

FIGURE 47-4 ■ Young athletic heart. Early repolarization changes; most prominent in leads V₅ and V₆, concave upward, minimally elevated ST segment, relatively tall, symmetrical T waves, prominent midprecordial U waves, prominent, but narrow q waves in the left precordial leads, sinus bradycardia, voltage criteria for left ventricular hypertrophy. (From Jenkins D, Gerred S: *ECGs by example*, ed 2, Edinburgh, 2005, Churchill Livingstone.)

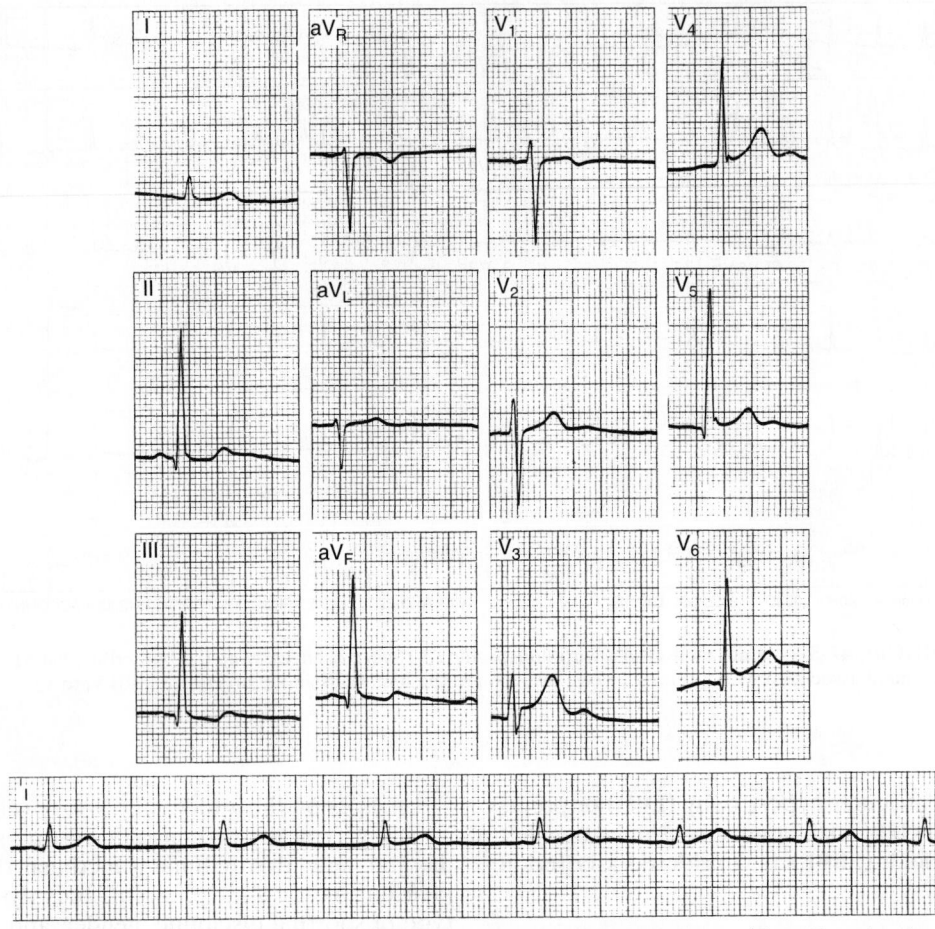

FIGURE 47-5 ■ A 12-lead electrocardiogram from a 20-year-old endurance athlete. Note the sinus bradycardia of less than 50 beats/min in the slowest part of his sinus arrhythmia and the vertical QRS axis. The early repolarization pattern is seen in the left precordial leads with ST segment elevation in leads V_3 and V_4 and J point elevation in leads V_4 to V_6. (From Conover MB: *Understanding electrocardiography,* ed 8, St Louis, 2003, Mosby.)

40 percent demonstrate second-degree Mobitz I AV block. Incomplete right bundle branch block (RBBB) patterns are found in up to half of conditioned athletes.

In the athlete, increased atrial mass can delay transmission of the atrial signal, causing increased P wave amplitude, or P wave notching. Similarly, increases in QRS complex voltage and concomitant T wave changes commonly are seen on the athlete's ECG, reflecting hypertrophy or increase in left ventricular mass. The severity of ventricular hypertrophy tends to be related to the type of training performed, with endurance athletes demonstrating the greatest wall thickness. The QRS frontal axis typically remains between 0 and 90 degrees. J point and ST segment changes compatible with benign early repolarization are common in athletes, with the STE typically normalizing with exercise.[14]

Although variations of impulse and conduction activity may be found on the athlete's ECG, abnormal patterns such as second-degree Mobitz II AV block, complete AV block, ST segment depression, and intraventricular conduction delays greater than 12 msec rarely are seen in the athlete and should be considered markers for an underlying pathological condition.

Electrocardiographic Artifacts

Erroneous ECG electrode placement, exaggerated body movements, electromagnetic interference, and poor skin-electrode contact can simulate serious dysrhythmias or abnormal waveform patterns. Misinterpretation of erroneous tracings can lead to inaccurate ECG diagnoses and can place patients at unnecessary risk when secondary diagnostic testing is recommended.[1,2,15]

Incorrect placement or connection of ECG electrodes is a common cause of ECG misinterpretation (Figure 47-6). Particular lead misplacements can create conduction patterns that simulate abnormal cardiac conditions. Reversal of the arm leads can create an ECG pattern similar to dextrocardia (technical dextrocardia). In contrast, the reversal of precordial leads can alter R wave progression, mimicking injury or infarction patterns[16,17] (Figure 47-7).

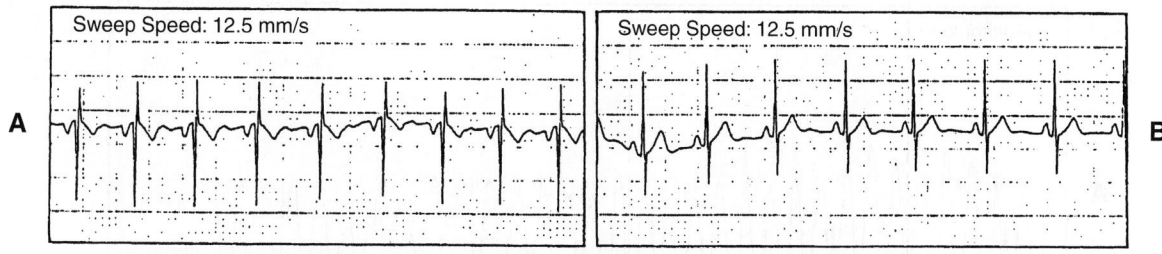

FIGURE 47-6   **A,** Initial tracing with incorrect lead connections noted at hub of the electrocardiogram (ECG) cable. Dextrocardia was suspected, but auscultation did not support this. **B,** ECG tracing after ECG leads were connected properly to ECG hub. (From Shimizu T: *Anesth Analg* 96:1232, 2003.)

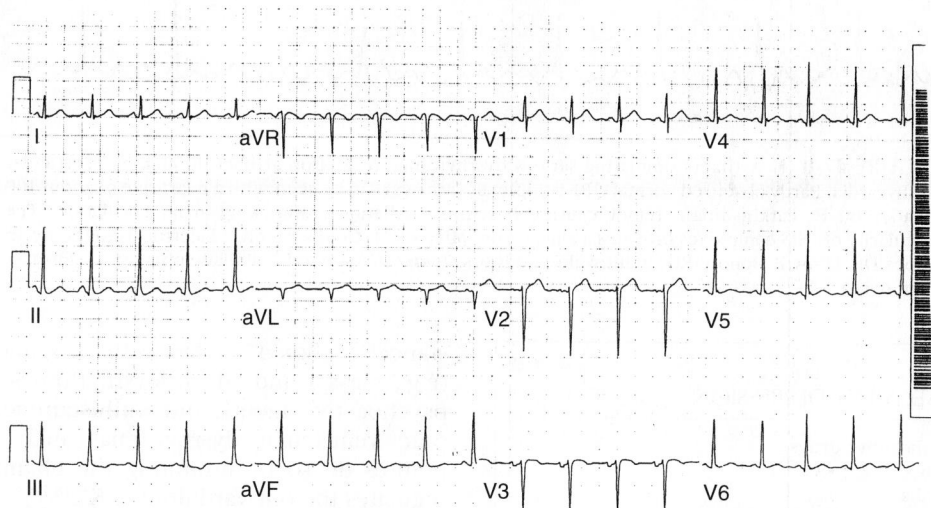

25mm/s   10mm/mV   100Hz   003A–003B   12SL4   CID: 1

FIGURE 47-7   ECG mistakenly interpreted as evidence of prior anterior myocardial infarction because of the poor R wave progression in lead V_3. This backward R wave progression and the isolated T wave flattening in lead V_3 suggest that leads V_1 and V_3 have been reversed. An even stronger clue is the presence of a biphasic P wave in lead V_3. Inverted or biphasic P waves are common in lead V_1 but are rare in the other precordial leads in the absence of an ectopic rhythm. (From Mattu A, Brady WJ, Perron AD, Robinson DA: *Am J Emerg Med* 19[6]:504-513, 2001.)

Excessive and repetitive body movements (e.g., brushing teeth, tremors, and shivering) and poor skin-electrode contact can produce flutter-like waveforms that resemble VT or atrial flutter (Figure 47-8). In monitored settings, a perfect replication of VT ("toothbrush tachycardia") often can be observed while a standing patient brushes his or her teeth. Motion activity often can be distinguished from true VT by the presence of an unstable baseline and by extrapolating QRS complexes that "march through" the artifactual tachycardia.

Toxins: Drugs and Chemicals

Medications, in therapeutic and toxic ranges, can produce ECG pattern changes. In most cases, the ST segment, QT interval, and T wave are affected, but conduction disturbances and serious dysrhythmias also may occur.

Drugs: K+-ATP Pump Inhibitors

Although numerous clinical situations can lead to ST segment depression **(STD)**, digitalis is the most common medication known to cause STD[18] (Box 47-1). The shortened QT interval and the distinct asymmetrical "sagging" or "scooping" of a downsloping concave ST-T wave complex (Figure 47-9) can be appreciated on the ECG of a patient receiving digitalis, regardless of the digitalis blood concentration. Prominent U waves also may be present.[1,17] Although the short QT interval that accompanies digitalis administration is the result of abbreviated ventricular action potential, the mechanism behind the STD is still not understood fully.

Drugs: Ion Channel Inhibitors

The length of the QT interval or, more precisely, the JT interval correlates with the depolarization and repolar-

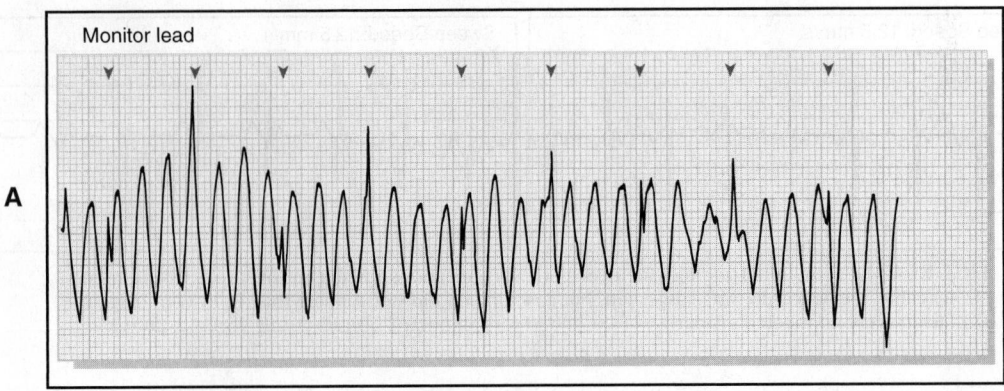

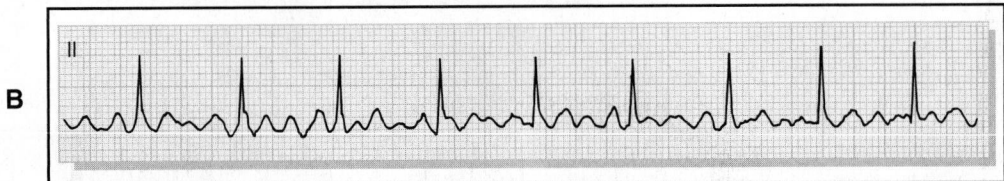

FIGURE 47-8 ■ Artifacts simulating serious dysrhythmia. **A,** Motion artifact mimicking ventricular tachycardia. Partly obscured normal QRS complexes (arrows) can be seen with a heart rate of about 100 beats/min. **B,** Parkinsonian tremor causing baseline oscillations mimicking atrial fibrillation. The regularity of QRS complexes provides a clue. (From Mirvis DM, Goldberger AL: Electrocardiography. In Zipes DP, Libby P, Bonow RO, Braunwald E, editors: *Heart disease,* ed 7, Philadelphia, 2005, Elsevier Saunders.)

BOX 47-1 ■ ■ ■
CAUSES OF ST SEGMENT DEPRESSION

Digitalis, other cardioactive drugs
Electrolyte imbalance (• K$^+$, • Ca^{++})
Sustained tachycardia
Ischemia (reciprocal changes)
Left ventricular strain
Hypothermia
Central nervous system events: subarachnoid bleeding, stroke

---

ization periods of the ventricular action potential. When estimating QT interval duration, a rate-corrected QT interval (QTc) is used to adjust for certain physiological factors that normally affect QT interval duration (e.g., age, gender, circadian rhythms, and resting heart rate). Prolongation of the QT interval correlates with delays in the action potential. In conditions in which the physiological QTc interval is greater than 440 msec, long-QT syndrome **(LQTS)** may be present. LQTS in acquired or congenital forms is characterized by a prolonged QTc interval, increased QT dispersion (**QTd,** a measurement of QT variability throughout the myocardium), and T and U wave abnormalities. LQTS also is associated with a high incidence of dysrhythmia and SCD (Box 47-2). Congenital LQTS is discussed later in this chapter.[19]

Acquired LQTS typically is associated with the use of specific medicinal and nonmedicinal agents, electrolyte abnormalities, central nervous system disorders, nutritional disorders, and myocardial ischemia. In this form of LQTS, the ion channel functions that regulate K$^+$, Na$^+$, or Ca^{++} flows are altered by an offending sub-

stance[18,19] (Box 47-3). Drugs that commonly cause LQTS (e.g., class I and III antidysrhythmics, antimicrobials, psychoactive agents, and antihistamines) and polymorphic ventricular dysrhythmias such as torsades de pointes do so by inhibiting the channel protein that regulates the outward flow of K$^+$.[18,20]

In general, alteration of K$^+$ ion flow can lead to lengthening of the action potential and QT interval prolongation. Most drug-induced QT prolongation is related to altered K$^+$ ion flow.[21] Drug-induced repolarization delays appear to have a greater effect on one myocardial cell type more than the others. Of the three myocardial cell types (endocardial, midmyocardial or M cells, and epi-

---

BOX 47-2 ■ ■ ■
CONDITIONS ASSOCIATED WITH QT PROLONGATION

Congenital Long QT Syndrome
Brugada syndrome, Ramono-Ward syndrome, and Jervell and Lange-Nielsen syndrome
Female gender

Acquired
Bradycardia induced
Drug induced: single agent, combined drug effects, organ failure causing decreased clearance
Electrolyte imbalance: • K$^+$, • Ca^{++}, • Mg^{++}
Metabolic conditions (renal disease, diabetes mellitus, hyperaldosteronism, cirrhosis)
Myocardial ischemia and inflammation
Hypothermia
Cardiotoxins: organophosphates, venom, metals
Recreational substances: cocaine
Neurological events: stroke, subarachnoid bleeding, thalamic insults

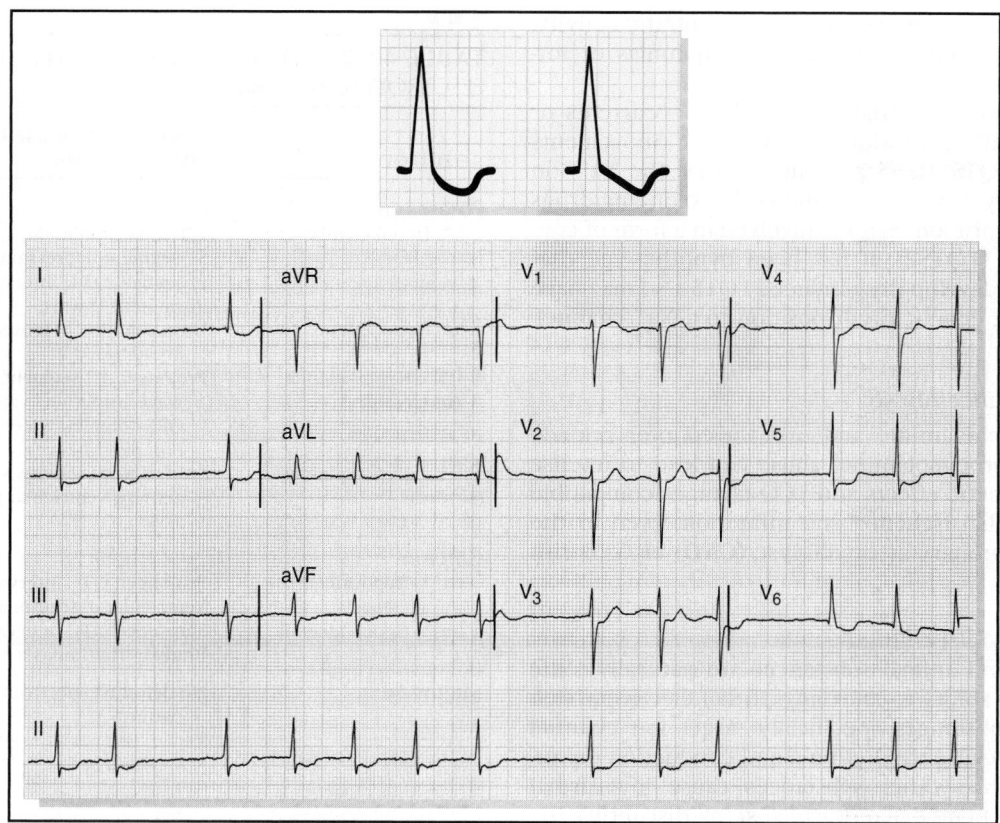

FIGURE 47-9 ■ Digitalis effect. *Top:* Digitalis glycosides characteristically produce shortening of the QT interval with a "scooped" or downsloping ST-T wave complex. *Bottom:* Digitalis toxicity. The underlying rhythm is atrial fibrillation. A "group beating" pattern of QRS complexes with shortening of the R-R intervals consistent with nonparoxysmal junctional tachycardia with exit (atrioventricular Wenckebach) block. ST segment depression and "scooping" (lead V6) are consistent with digitalis effect, although ischemia cannot be excluded. Findings were strongly suggestive of digitalis excess, and the serum digoxin level was greater than 3 ng/ml. Digitalis effect does not necessarily imply digitalis toxicity. (From Mirvis DM, Goldberger AL: Electrocardiography. In Zipes DP, Libby P, Bonow RO, Braunwald E, editors: *Heart disease,* ed 7, Philadelphia, 2005, Elsevier Saunders.)

BOX 47-3   ■ ■ ■
COMMONLY USED DRUGS ASSOCIATED WITH QT PROLONGATION

Cardioactive Agents: Antidysrhythmics
Class IA: dispopyramide, procainamide, quinidine
Class III: amiodarone, flecainide, propafenone (Rhythmol), sotalol (Betapace)

Antimicrobials
Amantadine
Azole-antifungal agents
Macrolides
Pentamadine
Quinolones
Trimethoprim-sulfamethoxazole

Psychotropic Drugs
Citalopram
Haloperidol (Haldol)
Phenothiazines
Thorazine
Tricyclic antidepressants: amitriptyline (Elavil)

Other Agents
Antihistamines: clemastine (Tavist), citirizine (Zyrtec), loratadine (Claritin)
Arsenic trioxide
Fludrocortisone (Florinef)
Inotropic agents: Amrinone (Inocor)
Tacrolimus (Prograf)

cardial), drug-induced alterations of repolarization and refractoriness impart a further increase in M cell potentials, whereas the potentials of the epicardial and endocardial cells remain largely unaffected. The resulting difference in electrical potentials between the three myocardial cell layers prolongs the QT interval and can transform a normally uniform electrical substrate into a multiphased wave of electrical recovery[22] (Figure 47-10). The drug-induced asynchrony of ventricular recovery

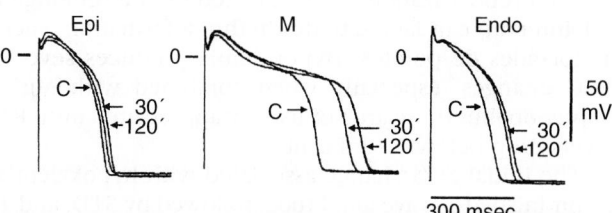

FIGURE 47-10 ■ Time course effects of erythromycin (Ery) on transmembrane activity recorded from epicardial (epi), endocardial (endo), and deep subepicardial (M region) sites in a transmural strip of canine left ventricle. Each panel shows superimposed action potentials recorded before and after 30 and 120 minutes of exposure to erythromycin (50 mcg/ml). **C,** Control tracing. (From Antzelevitch C, Sun ZQ, Zhang ZQ, Yan GX: *J Am College Cardiol* 28[7]:1836-1848, 1996.)

periods facilitate the formation of reentrant activity, such as polymorphic ventricular dysrhythmias or torsades de pointes.

Mechanisms that enhance inward Ca^{++} currents or inhibit normal inactivation of inward Na^+ movements can lead to LQTS. In 45 percent of cases, the Na^+ ion channelopathy caused by QT interval–prolonging drugs is also the culprit ion channel involved in a form of congenital LQTS (LQTS2). It has been hypothesized that patients who develop drug-induced LQTS also may have an underlying genetic predisposition to a Na^+ channelopathy.[18-20]

Drugs: Substance Abuse

Cocaine, amphetamine, and over-the-counter remedy (e.g., phenylpropanolamine) abuse can lead to intense sympathomimetic effects and ECG changes compatible with myocardial ischemia and infarction, even in the absence of coronary artery disease (CAD) or CAD risk factors.[23]

Toxins and Electrolytes

Many plant and animal substances are naturally toxic and have the ability to alter myocardial electrophysiology. Some substances specifically target ion channel function and cause dysrhythmia and conduction disturbances, whereas other substances cause myocardial ischemia and hemodynamic collapse by disrupting the balance of sympathovagal activity. Animal sources of cardiotoxins include arthropod venoms (spiders, scorpions, wasps/bees); centipede, snail, and toad venoms; and fish carrying toxins (e.g., barracuda/ciguatoxin and puffer fish/tetrodotoxin).[24-26]

Much of the function of the body depends on electrolytic homeostasis. The accumulation or loss of extracellular cations (K^+, Ca^{++}, and Mg^{++}) can cause abnormal ion gradients and altered action potentials that result in profound cardiac conduction delays[27,28] (Table 47-2).

Electrolyte Imbalance: Potassium

Hypokalemia. Hypokalemia can occur through increased renal excretion, gastrointestinal K^+ loss, transmembrane shifts, or from poor dietary K^+ intake. Hypokalemia increases the resting membrane potential, which makes the myocyte more vulnerable to abnormal stimuli. Hypokalemia also prolongs overall repolarization by lengthening phase 3 of the action potential. Increased repolarization time, reflected by the prolonged QT interval, can facilitate dysrhythmia formation, such as torsades de pointes. Hypokalemia produces several ECG changes, especially when combined with Mg^{++} depletion, but these are not usually appreciated until K^+ levels drop below 2.7 mEq/liter.

The initial ECG change associated with hypokalemia is diminished T wave amplitude, followed by STD, and T wave inversion. As K^+ levels continue to decline, the QT interval lengthens as U waves appear with increasing amplitude as K^+ levels continue to drop (Figure 47-11). Hypokalemic-induced STD can resemble myocardial ischemia or even hyperkalemia, when the T-U complex is misinterpreted as a hyperacute T wave; although hy-

■ ■ ■

TABLE 47-2   ELECTROCARDIOGRAPHIC EFFECTS OF ELECTROLYTE ABNORMALITIES[29]

ELECTROLYTE	ELECTROCARDIOGRAPHIC MANIFESTATIONS
Potassium	
↓ K^+, Hypokalemia	↓ T wave amplitude, T wave inversion ST segment depression Prolonged QT-U interval Prominent U wave
↑ K^+, Hyperkalemia (mild)	Large amplitude, tented T waves, broad-based
↑↑ K^+, Hyperkalemia (moderate)	Prolonged PR segment, decreased P wave amplitude, vanishing P wave QRS complex widening, conduction disturbances
↑↑ K^+, Hyperkalemia (severe)	Loss of atrial activity, sinoventricular activity, ventricular fibrillation, asystole
Calcium	
↓ Ca^{++}, Hypocalcemia	Prolonged QTC interval Ventricular dysrhythmias
↑ Ca^{++}, Hypercalcemia	Shortened QTC interval Bradydysrhythmias
Magnesium	No definitive electrocardiographic pattern

perkalemic T waves typically have a narrow base and often are accompanied by a widened QRS complex.[27]

Hyperkalemia. Hyperkalemia is one of the more common acute life-threatening emergencies, and the treatment depends on prompt and accurate ECG analysis. As serum and extracellular K^+ levels rise, the cell membrane becomes more permeable, allowing K^+ ions to pass into the cell. The influx increases K^+ concentration, decreases the resting membrane potential, and slows the velocity of phase 0 of the action potential, which reduces the speed of cell-to-cell current transmission. ECG pattern changes of hyperkalemia typically begin to appear when serum K^+ levels rise above 5.5 mEq/liter, although the actual level that triggers ECG change varies from patient to patient.[27] Hyperkalemia often occurs in the setting of decreased renal excretion (e.g., renal failure, medication effects, and metabolic conditions), intracellular to extracellular redistribution (e.g., burns, coronary bypass, and hypertonic glucose administration), and increased K^+ loads (e.g., oral/parental supplementation, gastrointestinal bleeding, and massive hemolysis). The earliest ECG changes associated with hyperkalemia are tall, peaked T waves. These T waves are best seen in leads II, III, and V_2 to V_4. Hyperkalemic T waves increase in amplitude until they become large, symmetrically "tented" T waves. T wave "tenting" typically begins when serum K^+ exceeds 6 mEq/liter (Figure 47-12). Hyperkalemia should always be suspected when the T wave amplitude is greater than or equal to that of the R wave in more than one ECG lead.[27,30]

In mild to moderate hyperkalemia (6.5 to 7.5 mmol/liter), Na^+ channel function becomes dysfunctional,

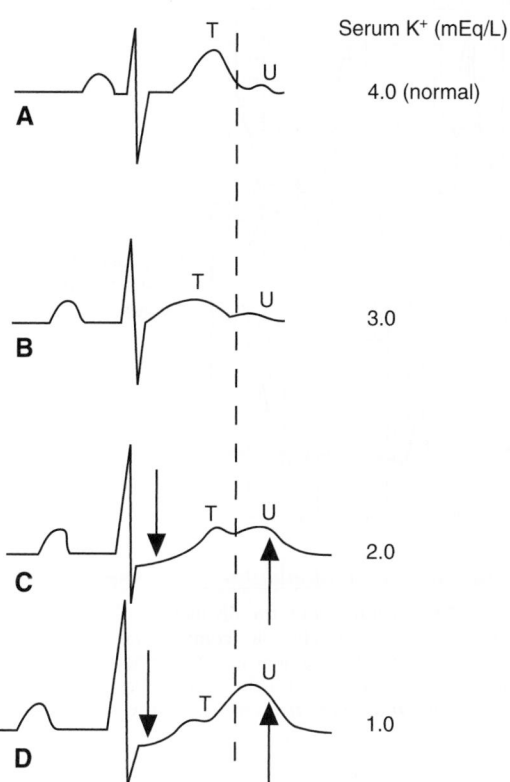

Hypokalemia

Serum K$^+$ (mEq/L)

4.0 (normal)

3.0

2.0

1.0

FIGURE 47-11 ■ T wave, U wave, and ST segment changes in progressive hypokalemia. **A,** At a normal serum concentration of 4 to 5.5 mEq/liter the amplitude of the T wave is appreciably greater than that of the U wave. **B,** By the time the serum potassium level has dropped to 3 mEq/liter, the T wave amplitude had decreased and the U wave increased, approaching the height of the T wave. **C** and **D,** With a further drop in potassium, the amplitude and duration of the QRS complex and the P wave increase, the PR interval may lengthen slightly, the ST segment becomes depressed (↓), and the U wave begins to tower over (↑) and fuse with the T wave. (From Conover MB: *Understanding electrocardiography,* ed 8, St Louis, 2003, Mosby.)

causing further depression of atrial and ventricular action potentials. As dromotropic functions deteriorate, myocardial tissue becomes less responsive to electrochemical stimuli. Changes can be seen in the PR interval and P wave; the P wave flattens, and the PR interval lengthens with eventual disappearance of the P wave. With continued increases in K$^+$ levels (7 to 8 mmol/liter), the QRS complex widens. The wide QRS complex of hyperkalemia differs from the wide QRS complex in bundle branch blocks in that all portions of the hyperkalemic QRS complex (medial and terminal) are affected. Direct sinoventricular conduction occurs as the atrial conduction tissue retreats into a toxic quiescence. In the latter phases of hyperkalemia (greater than 8 mEq/liter), sinoatrial and AV conduction become suppressed until the widened QRS complex fuses with the T wave to form a "sine-wave" (Figure 47-13). This and other morphologies of ventricular rhythms are indicative of imminent termination of organized electrical

activity. Ventricular fibrillation, pulseless idioventricular rhythm, or asystole is usually the final event in untreated hyperkalemia.

Electrolyte Imbalance: Calcium

Abnormal Ca^{++} levels predominantly alter the duration of the action potential, either by the shortening or prolongation of certain repolarization phases.[27]

Hypocalcemia. Hypocalcemia impairs myocardial contractility by prolonging the ventricular action potential (phase 2). With prolongation of repolarization, the QT$_C$ interval lengthens. Low levels of serum Ca^{++} typically are observed in the setting of functional parathyroid hormone deficiency or metabolic conditions that result in low Ca^{++} levels. Although hypocalcemia delays repolarization and can cause early after-potential-triggered dysrhythmias, life-threatening dysrhythmias are not usually common.[1,27]

Hypercalcemia. Mild hypercalcemia is most often chronic and well tolerated, although several factors (e.g., excess Ca^{++} or vitamin D intake, neoplastic processes, or hyperparathyroidism) can potentiate acute elevations in Ca^{++} greater than 14 mg/dl. On the ECG, hypercalcemia results in shortening of phase 2 of the action potential, which is reflected by abbreviation of the QTc interval. Hypercalcemia can appear with diminished, notched, or inverted T waves and sometimes produces a high takeoff of the ST segment in leads V$_1$ and V$_2$. A notching in the terminal portion of the QRS complex, also referred to as an Osborn wave, can be seen in some cases of hypercalcemia.[28] Dysrhythmias generally are not associated with hypercalcemia, although bradycardias may occur.

Electrolyte Imbalance: Magnesium

Mg^{++} is an intracellular ion that is critical for the maintenance of ionic balance and for numerous enzymatic and hormonal processes. Alterations in Mg^{++} levels generally do not manifest specific ECG change, although severe hypermagnesemia (greater than 15 mEq/liter) can cause AV conduction disturbances. Hypomagnesemia frequently may coexist with hypokalemic and hypocalcemic states and can facilitate the development of torsades de pointes associated with QT interval prolongation.[27] Magnesium sulfate bolus remains the first-line pharmacological intervention in advanced cardiac life support for torsades de pointes. Hypomagnesemia is often due to decreased Mg^{++} intake (syndromes of malabsorption, malnourished states/chronic alcohol abuse), increase in Mg^{++} loss (metabolic conditions, drug effects), or altered intracellular/extracellular Mg^{++} distribution (following administration of glucose or parenteral nutrition).

Metabolic Disorders
Thyroid Disorders

The cardiovascular system is sensitive to increases in circulating thyroid hormones. In hyperthyroid states, there is usually ECG evidence of accelerated sinus and AV node activity (sinus tachycardia, short PR interval), as well as increased QRS complex voltage. In some pa-

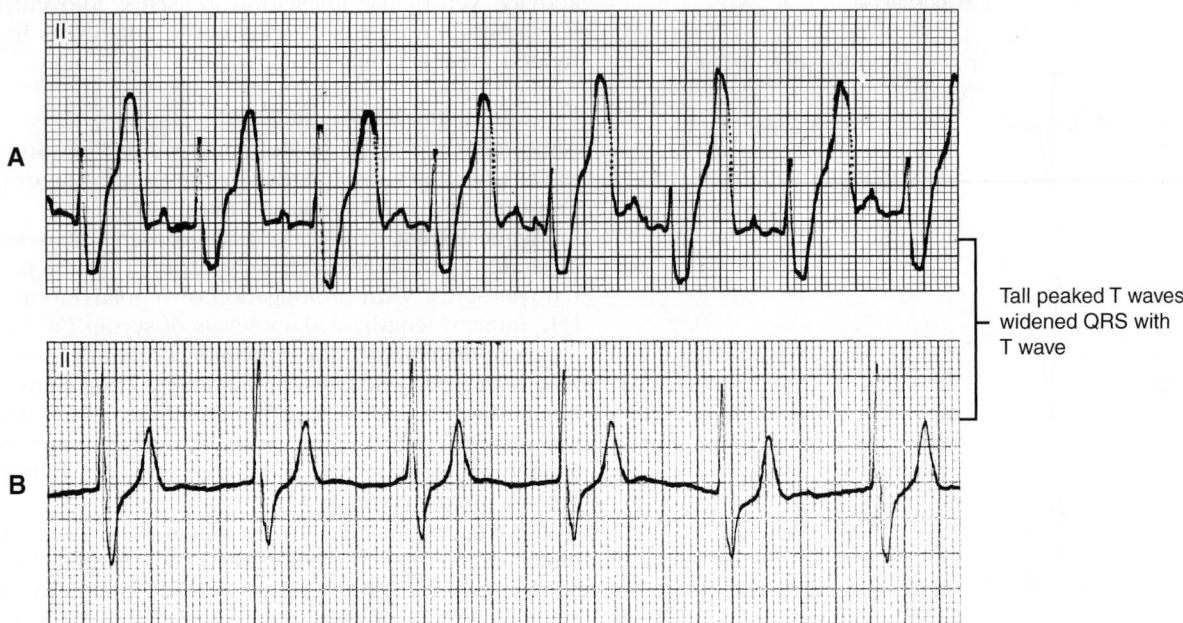

Tall peaked T waves widened QRS with T wave

FIGURE 47-12 ■ Hyperkalemia. **A,** Serum potassium level of 7.3 mEq/liter. Note the distinctive ST segment as it loses itself in the tall, tented T wave. The P wave is still intact. The QRS complex has widened to 0.20 second. **B,** Serum potassium 8.3 mEq/liter. Although the ST segment is still distinct from the tall, tented T wave, the QRS complex has broadened to 0.16 second and the P wave has disappeared. (From Conover MB: Potassium derangements. In *Understanding electrocardiography,* ed 8, St Louis, 2003, Mosby.)

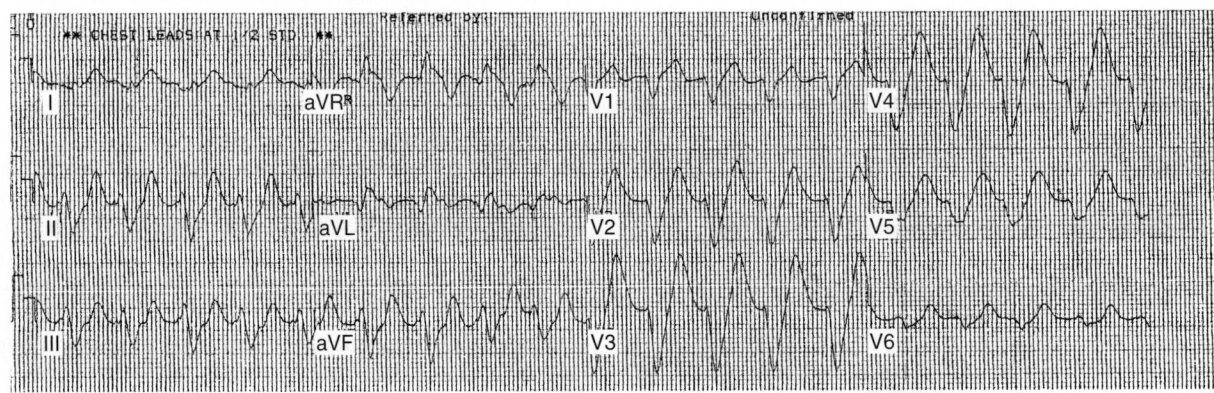

FIGURE 47-13 ■ Wide complex tachycardia compatible with a "sine-wave" appearance on the 12-lead electrocardiogram in a patient with serum K+ level of 8.1 mg/dl. (From Diercks DB, Shumaik GM, Harrigan RA et al: *J Emerg Med* 27[2]:153-160, 2004.)

tients, atrial fibrillation occurs because of the hypersensitivity of the atria to triiodothyronine. Because hypokalemia commonly is observed with elevated thyroid levels, STD, decreased T wave amplitude, and U wave formation may be seen.[31]

Hypothyroidism slows metabolism and cardiac impulse conduction. On the ECG, hypothyroidism can produce bradycardias, decreased QRS complex voltage, QT interval prolongation, and ST-T wave abnormalities (flat or inverted T waves).[30] Patients who suffer from hypothyroidism are especially prone to dysrhythmias associated with digitalis toxicity.

Eating and Nutritional Disorders

Eating disorders and fasting states, as in anorexia nervosa, have long been associated with cardiac complications, including sudden dysrhythmic death.[32] Numerous ECG derangements have been observed in the anorexic patient, the most significant being QTc interval prolongation and increased QT dispersion.

Obesity

Obesity is known to produce changes in cardiac morphology and electrocardiography.[33] Common ECG findings in this population include a leftward axis shift, LV and LA abnormalities, low QRS complex voltage, and T wave flattening in the inferior leads. A left axis shift is due to the horizontal displacement of the heart resulting from abdominal adipose tissue–induced diaphragmatic restriction, from LVH, or from a combination of the two entities. Excessive chest wall and epicardial fat can impede transmission of QRS complex signal, resulting in decreased voltage recording on the ECG.

In contrast, substantial weight loss in a previously obese patient can cause favorable hemodynamic and structural changes in the heart. In addition to decreased systemic demands, reduction of blood pressure, LV end-diastolic stress, and LVH, resolution of previous ECG patterns associated with obesity has been observed. Weight loss reduces abdominal fat, induces regression of LVH, and normalizes the P wave, QRS, and T wave axes. Weight loss also is associated with a gain in QRS complex voltage because the reduction of chest wall fat permits the transmission of a higher-voltage signal.[33]

Temperature and Electricity

Hypothermia, defined as a core body temperature less than 35°C (95°F), can alter impulse formation and conduction patterns in all cell types.[34] Hypothermia may occur in terminal metabolic conditions, from therapeutic temperature manipulations to protect vulnerable tissue from ischemia, or from environmental causes. Classic ECG manifestations of hypothermia include the presence of a prominent J wave or notch in the terminal portion of the QRS complex (Figure 47-14), multiinterval prolongations (PR interval, QRS complex, QTc), and atrial and ventricular dysrhythmias.[35] Although terminal

QRS complex notching in hypothermia originally was described by Tomasjewski in 1938, it was later explained by Osborne in 1953 during evaluation of hypothermia for cardiac surgery. Thus in the presence of hypothermia, the J wave often is referred to as an Osborne wave.

The cellular mechanism behind J wave formation generally involves the loss of synchrony between epicardial and endomyocardial action potential domes. Similar to benign early repolarization, the heterogenic response between the epicardial and endomyocardial cell types in hypothermic conditions produces a transmural voltage gradient that manifests as a notched formation on the terminal portion of the QRS complex.[9] J waves usually are seen when core body temperatures drop below 32°C and gain amplitude with continued decreases in temperature.

Hypothermia causes prolongation of the PR interval with eventual sinus bradycardia, junctional rhythms, and varying degrees of AV block. In mild hypothermia, alterations in the depolarization-repolarization phases of the action potential cause a widening of the QRS and QTc intervals, and the P wave amplitude diminishes. Atrial fibrillation with slow ventricular response may be seen in up to half of affected patients in this stage. With progressive hypothermia (temperature less than 30°C [86°F]), ventricular myocardial tissue becomes irritable, precipitating spontaneous ventricular fibrillation; below 25°C (77°F) there is electrical shut down and asystole. After rewarming, QTc prolongation may continue to be seen, although J wave amplitude typically diminishes as the patient becomes normothermic. J waves

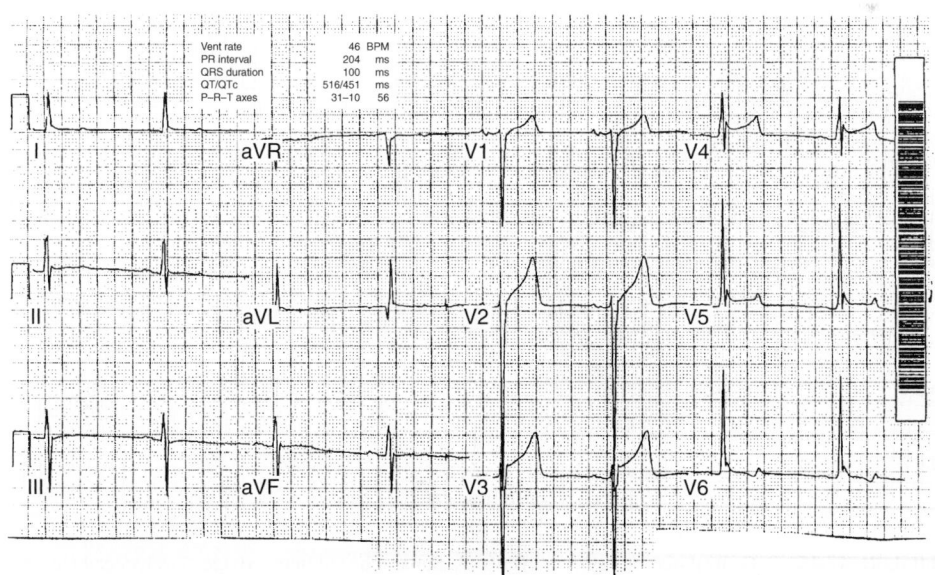

FIGURE 47-14 ■ Hypothermia. Marked sinus bradycardia with a rate of 46 beats/min and a first-degree atrioventricular block. QRS interval is slightly prolonged. Voltage criteria present for left ventricular hypertrophy. ST segment elevation exists in the precordial leads. The ST segment elevation presumed to be the result of acute myocardial infarction but later is attributed to J waves after a rectal temperature was found to be 30.9°C. (From Mattu A, Brady WJ, Perron AD: *Am J Emerg Med* 20[4]:314-326, 2002.)

also can be found in normothermic conditions such as ischemia, benign early repolarization, Brugada syndrome, hypercalcemia, and Chagas disease.

Neurological Conditions and Events

Strong evidence supports a relationship between brain injury and cardiac physiology. Central nervous system events, such as thromboembolic stroke or intracerebral and subarachnoid hemorrhage, often are associated with ECG evidence of abnormal repolarization that include ST segment, T wave, QTc interval, and U wave changes.[36,37]

Although ST-T wave changes are seen with a variety of central nervous system disorders, ECG changes associated with a subarachnoid bleed are most common. In subarachnoid bleeding, diffuse and often deep T wave inversions (up to 1.5 mV), STE or STD, QTc prolongation, and U waves may be present in the mid to lateral precordial leads (Figure 47-15). The T wave is typically asymmetrical with an ascending outward bulge. The presence of STE and abnormal Q waves in two or more leads has been shown to be predictive of myocardial dysfunction and early mortality.[37] Because hemorrhagic or ischemic central nervous system events can cause

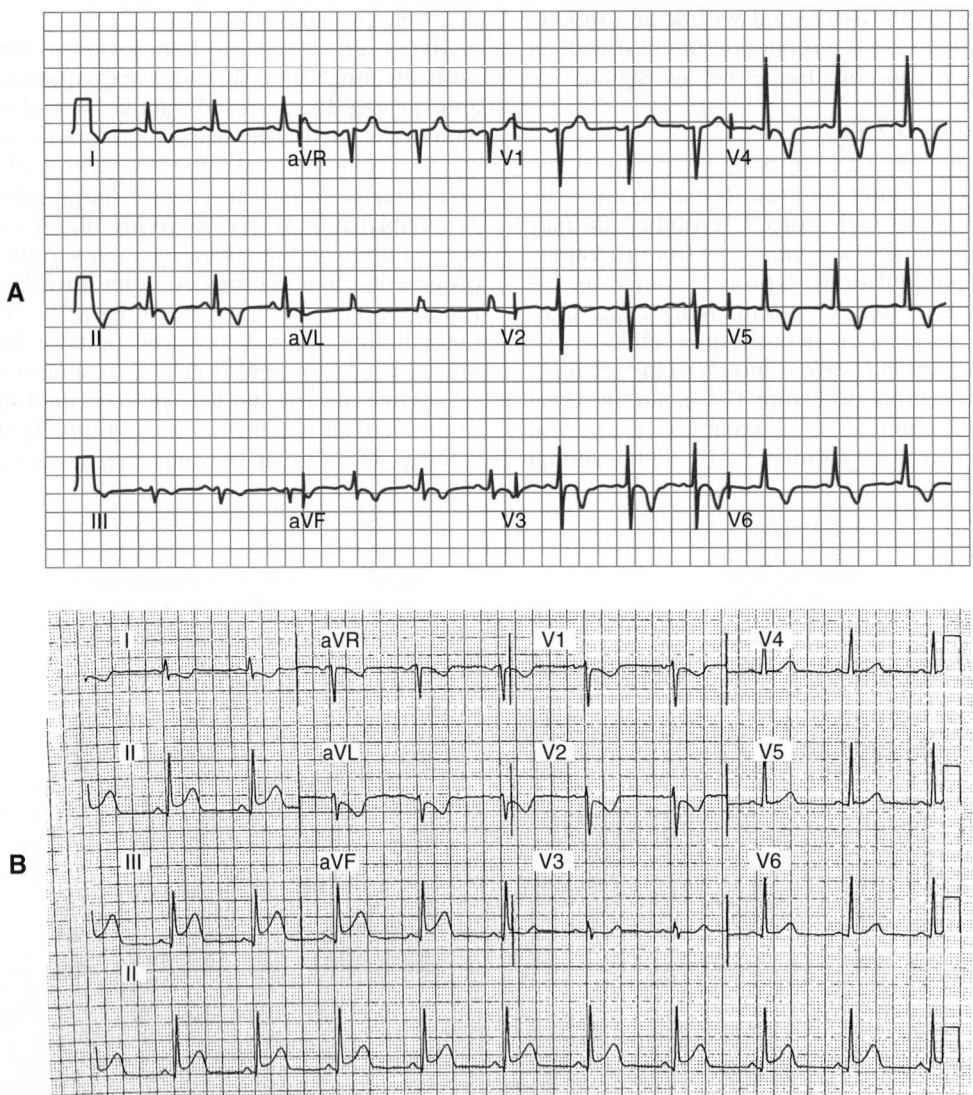

FIGURE 47-15 ■ Central nervous system events. **A,** Subarachnoid hemorrhage. Twelve-lead electrocardiogram (ECG) showing sinus rhythm with inverted T waves in inferior, anterior, and lateral distribution. Anterolateral T wave changes prominent with deep inversion. No evidence of myocardial injury was found. **B,** Pontine hemorrhage. Twelve-lead ECG with an acute injury pattern in the inferior and posterior leads with accompanying ST segment depression in the lateral distribution. ECG changes strongly suggestive of an inferoposterior acute myocardial infarction with lateral reciprocal changes. No evidence of myocardial ischemia or infarction clinically and at autopsy. (From Perron A, Brady WJ: *Am J Emerg Med* 18[6]:715-720, 2000.)

myocardial damage and dysfunction, ECG change also may be observed in this setting.

Inflammation and Infection

Pericarditis. In acute pericarditis, inflammation of the pericardium triggers atrial and ventricular tissue repolarization abnormalities and classic ECG changes of acute myopericarditis.[29] These ECG patterns can evolve over several weeks. The initial stage, seen in most patients, lasts about 2 weeks. A generalized ventricular repolarization abnormality occurs that is characterized by widespread, upward concave STE (less than 0.5 mV), seen particularly on the ST upslope, where a distinct J point is formed. Reciprocal STD can be seen in leads aVR and V_1. PR segment depression, occurring as the result of altered atrial repolarization, is diffuse throughout the ECG, except for leads aVR and V_1. PR segment depression may be the earliest and most specific ECG sign of pericarditis. See Chapter 75 for further discussion.

Thoracic and Pulmonary Conditions

Acute pulmonary embolism **(PE)** is a potentially fatal disorder that is often underdiagnosed.[38] The severity of the hemodynamic and ischemic effects of the pulmonary occlusion usually determines the degree of ECG change. In some PEs, ECG manifestations are significant, whereas in many cases there is no observable change. The classic finding of a prominent S wave in lead I, STE in lead II, and new or increased Q waves and T wave inversion in lead III, known as **S1Q3T3,** was considered pathognomonic for PE-induced right ventricular "strain," or acute cor pulmonale. This pattern, however, is found in only 10 percent of patients with PE, and several other ECG changes have since been added to the criteria (Box 47-4).[12,38]

An ECG suggestive of PE typically demonstrates three or more the following ECG changes: RBBB with associated STE or T wave inversion in lead V_1, prominent S waves in leads I and aVL, transition zone shift to lead V_5, Q waves in leads III and aVF, inferior or superior right axis deviation, low QRS complex limb lead voltage, or T wave inversions in leads III, aVF, or V_1 to V_4.

Pulmonary emphysema or chronic obstructive pulmonary disease (COPD) produces several anatomical changes that can alter the ECG. Hyperinflation of the lungs insulates the conductive wavefront, and causes a downward displacement of the diaphragm and heart and a superior and rightward frontal plane axis shift

(+70 degrees). With the heart in a lower position in relation to the standard chest wall positions of the precordial leads, the R wave transition zone shifts leftward, creating a persistent rS pattern through leads V_5 or V_6. This poor R wave progression pattern can simulate AMI. As the heart becomes more vertical, prominent P waves evolve in leads II, III and aVF, resulting in a rightward migration of the P wave axis. Low voltage is characteristic of chronic pulmonary conditions because the increased air space of the hyperinflated lungs is a poor electrical conductor and impedes the transmission of the ventricular signal[42].

CARDIAC CAUSES OF ELECTROCARDIOGRAPHIC ABNORMALITIES

Alterations of ECG patterns that result from direct myocardial involvement (e.g., coronary ischemia, myocardial infarction, myocardial hypertrophy) will be discussed in the following section.

Myocardial Underperfusion
Injury, Infarction, and Ischemia

Although angiography is the current gold standard for assessing coronary anatomy, the ECG is considered a more sensitive marker of cardiac physiology, especially in the presence of ischemia.[43] The contrast in diagnostic properties of the angiogram and the ECG make it possible for a patient to have a critical coronary artery obstruction on angiography and a normal ECG; and conversely, there may be persistent STE on the ECG despite angiographic restoration of epicardial blood flow.

In the patient with acute MI, ECG patterns can vary according to the location of the infarct and surrounding tissues at risk, the duration of the ischemia, the extent of injury (transmural versus nontransmural; Figure 47-18), and confounding or comorbid factors (bundle branch block, ventricular pacing) that can alter classic injury-infarction patterns. Because the morphologies of STE vary, the characteristics of the ST segment often can provide clues as to the cause of ECG change.

Under normal conditions the ECG baseline is generally isoelectric, and uniform depolarization and repolarization predominates throughout the tissues. In the presence of ischemia and infarction, the ECG undergoes a well-established temporal evolution and becomes a substrate of electrical disarray (Figure 47-16).[44] Ischemia disrupts normal electrophysiological functions of the myocardial cells in several ways: the resting membrane potential is reduced (becomes less negative), and the cardiac action potential of ischemic cells becomes shortened with a slowing of phase 0 (depolarization). These changes, somewhat similar to that of benign early repolarization and hypothermia, lead to asynchronized repolarization between the myocardial cells in the physiological and ischemic zones. Lack of uniform repolarization between these two zones causes a voltage gradient, which is the basis of the injury current that manifests in STE or depression on the surface ECG.

BOX 47-4 ■ ■ ■
COMMON ELECTROCARDIOGRAPHIC PATTERNS ASSOCIATED WITH PULMONARY EMBOLISM[39-41]

Complete or incomplete right bundle branch block
S1Q3T3 pattern
PR segment displacement
T wave inversion
Axis deviation to right greater than 20 degrees
Low-voltage QRS complex in limb leads
Q waves in leads III and aVF or in lead III alone

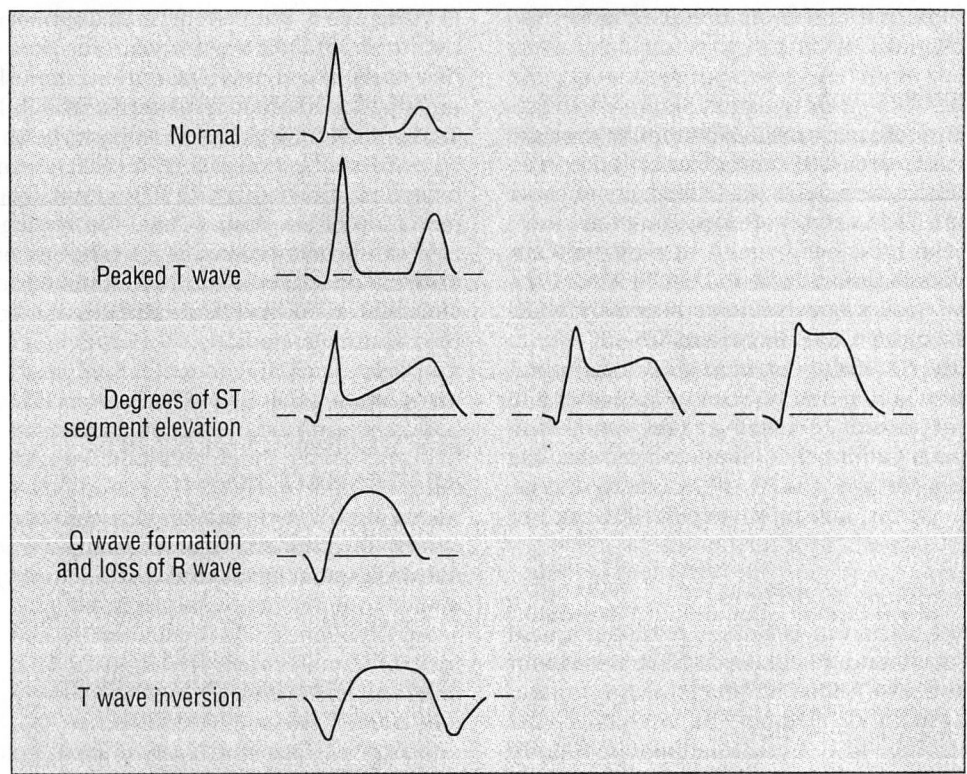

FIGURE 47-16 ■ Sequence of changes seen during evolution of myocardial infarction. (From Morris F, Brady WJ: *BMJ* 324:831-833, 2002.)

In transmural ischemia, injury currents move away from the ischemic zone, toward the epicardial or outer myocardial layers. This movement produces STE and hyperacute T waves in leads directly over the ischemic regions. Simultaneously, ECG leads opposing the injured surface(s) manifest STD as a reflection of the same injury current in the contralateral surface. Localized subendocardial ischemia causes an injury current that flows toward the inner or endocardial layer, and leads oriented toward the inner ventricular (septal wall) layer (leads V_1 to V_3) demonstrate STD, whereas lead aVR demonstrates STE.[1]

Waveform Change in Acute Myocardial Infarction
The ST Segment

Although changes in T wave morphology can occur in ischemic and nonischemic conditions, the earliest ECG signs of acute MI are so subtle that they often are missed. In leads oriented to the affected regions, early ischemia produces an increase in T wave amplitude. Although the morphology of ischemic or hyperacute T waves varies, broad-based forms can be seen as early as 30 minutes following coronary occlusion and transmural infarction but are short-lived, evolving into STE within minutes to hours[43-45] (Figure 47-17).

The ST segment represents the plateau phase (phase 2) of the cardiac action potential. In the presence of uniform electrical activity, no voltage gradient forms and the ST segment remains isoelectric with a concor-

dant T wave. In the presence of ischemia, however, the resting membrane potential becomes less negative (less than 60 mV) in ischemic cells, whereas in the unaffected myocardial cells, it remains unchanged. The greater number of injured myocardial cells plus the severity of the ischemia serve only to increase this voltage difference and the degree of resulting STE.

STE is often the earliest recognized sign of AMI and can manifest in various morphologies (Box 47-5). Because ST segment change can be found in numerous conditions other than acute MI, the evaluation of the ST segment and concurrent factors (e.g., analysis of the ST

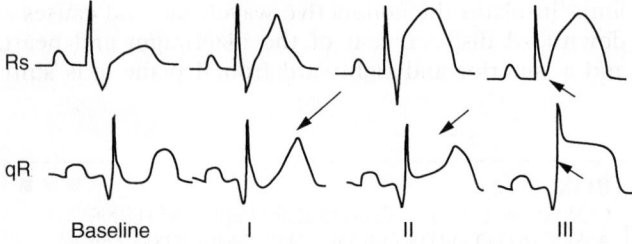

FIGURE 47-17 ■ Grades of ischemia/injury in leads with usual Rs configuration (leads V_1 to V_3): grade I, tall symmetrical T wave without ST segment elevation (STE); grade II, STE without distortion of the terminal portion of the QRS complex; grade III, STE with distortion of the terminal portion of the QRS complex (no S waves in leads V_1 to V_3; *arrow*). In leads with usual qR configuration: grade I, tall symmetrical T wave without STE; grade II, STE with J point/R wave ratio less than 0.5; grade III, STE with J point/R wave ratio of 0.5 *(arrow)*. (From Birnbaum Y: *Postgrad Med J* 79:490-504, 2003.)

slope, coexisting ECG features, clinical setting, notation of the leads in which STE is most pronounced, and an awareness of conditions with similar ECG patterns) can be crucial in determining the cause of the STE[6,45,46] (Figure 47-18).

Early in ischemia the ST segment may lose the ST-T wave slope and appear straight. Then, as the T wave broadens and the ST segment rises, the segment loses its concave form and becomes upwardly convex with elevations up to 0.1 mV or more.

Associated ECG changes that support the relationship of STE to probable Q wave acute MI are presence of nonconcave STE of 0.1 mV in two or more contiguous limb leads, evolving Q wave development (usually within 24 hours), and reciprocal STD. Diminution of R waves in leads V_4 to V_6 (often referred to as "poor R wave progression") also may be observed.[47]

Patients who have chest pain, cardiac enzyme elevation, and STD (0.1 mV in more than two contiguous leads) usually are diagnosed with a non-STE acute MI (formerly referred to as a non–Q wave MI; Figure 47-19). In the presence of negative cardiac enzymes, repeat samples should be drawn between 6 and 12 hours. The patient then can be stratified further according to the troponin level.

Reciprocal STD can be particularly useful in validating the presence and clinical significance of STE associated with acute MI (Figure 47-20) and helping approximate the infarction extension zone, a coexisting area or remote ischemia.[45] Reciprocal STD commonly is seen in the majority of large inferior wall MIs and to a lesser extent in anterior wall MIs. STD of reciprocal change is typically downsloping or horizontal.

BOX 47-5   ■ ■ ■
CONDITIONS ASSOCIATED WITH ST SEGMENT ELEVATION

Ischemic
Acute myocardial infarction
Coronary spasm
Wellen syndrome
Left main and triple-vessel coronary artery disease
Ventricular aneurysm*

Nonischemic
Acute pulmonary embolism
Acute pericarditis
Benign early repolarization
Electronic artifact
Bundle branch block

*Complication of myocardial infarction.[2]

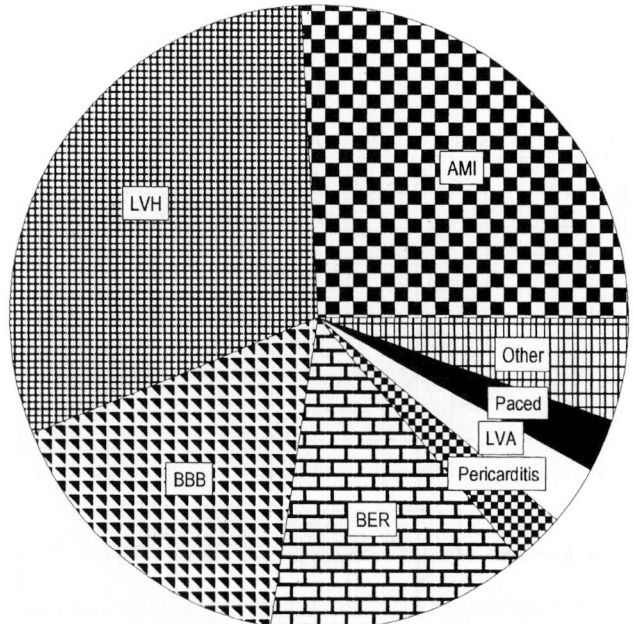

FIGURE 47-18 ■ Causes of electrocardiographic ST segment elevation among 212 patients. *AMI,* Acute myocardial infarction; *BBB,* bundle branch block; *BER,* benign early repolarization; *LVA,* left ventricular aneurysm; *LVH,* left ventricular hypertrophy. (From Brady WJ, Perron AD, Ullman EA et al: *Am J Emerg Med* 20:609-612, 2002.)

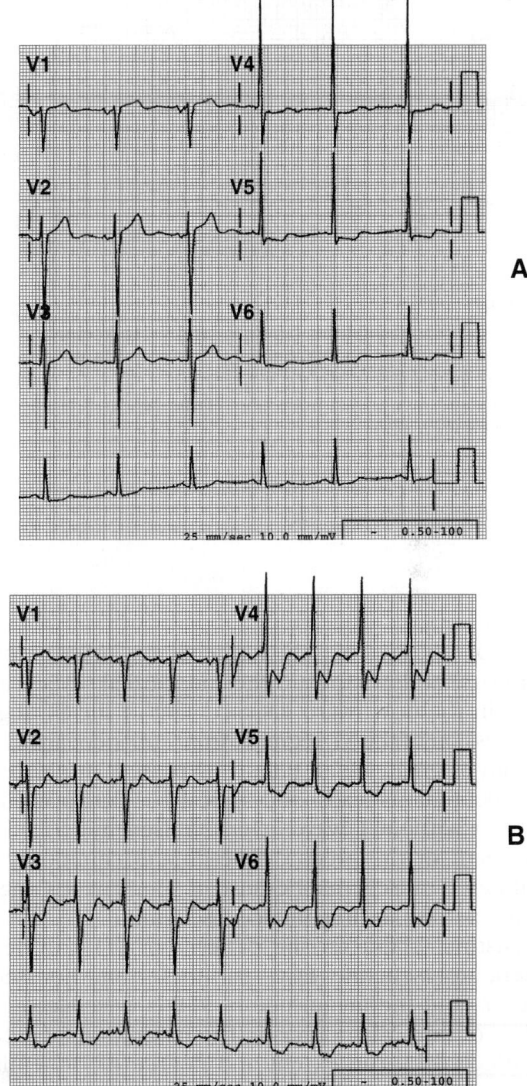

FIGURE 47-19 ■ **A,** Normal electrocardiogram (ECG) tracing. **B,** Same patient's ECG 18 hours later, showing a non-Q wave infarction (acute subendocardial infarction). The patient had a clinical picture of infarction and increased creatine kinase MB. note widespread ST-T depression but no associated Q waves. (From Khan MG: *Rapid ECG interpretation,* ed 2, Philadelphia, 2003, WB Saunders.)

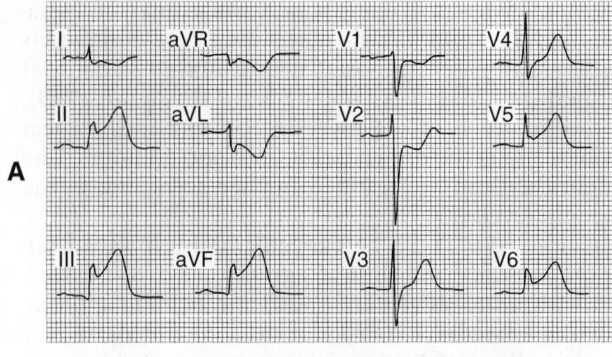

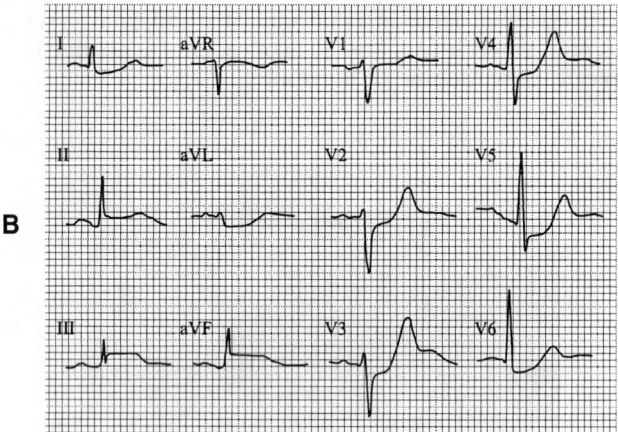

FIGURE 47-20 ■ **A,** Inferolateral myocardial infarction with reciprocal changes in leads I, aVL, V$_1$, and V$_2$. **B,** Reciprocal changes: presence of widespread ST segment depression in the anterolateral leads strongly suggest that the subtle inferior ST segment elevation is due to acute myocardial infarction. (From Morris F, Brady WJ: *BMJ* 324:831-833, 2002.)

forms with an acute rise time. The tombstone ST segment is convexed upward with the zenith of the ST segment ascending higher than the preceding R wave that is often obscured by the degree of STE. The convex ST segment then merges with the ascending limb of the following T wave. The gross STE is actually the manifestation of a prolonged R wave that results from marked ischemia-induced transmural conduction delays across the ventricular wall. Intense or prolonged ischemia causes a loss of the epicardial action potential dome but not endocardial dome that causes a voltage gradient that manifests as STE[50] (Figure 47-21).

Tombstone STE is associated with reperfusion dysrhythmias and pervasive ischemic myocardial damage caused by proximal left anterior descending **(LAD)** artery occlusion with right coronary artery **(RCA)** or left circumflex **(LCX)** artery involvement.[48]

The QRS Complex

Generally, Q waves are considered pathological if the measured width is greater than 3 msec or more than one-fourth the height of the R wave. Wide Q waves may appear normally in leads III, aVR, and V$_1$, and varying degrees of normal are acceptable in leads aVL (less than 0.04 mV, up to 0.7 mV deep in persons older than 30, up to 1 mV in children) and leads II, aVF (Q wave is 3 msec and less than 0.4 mV deep), and lead I (Q wave no greater than 0.15 mV in persons older than 30). A small q wave in V$_6$ (3 msec) also is seen in the majority of the population. In contrast, abnormal Q waves may be found in MI (Figure 47-21) and in various nonischemic conditions (i.e., acute PE, infiltrative processes [amyloidosis, ARVD], intraventricular conduction abnormali-

STD indicative of ischemia generates an injury current pattern that flows toward the endocardial surface and results in the downward displacement of the ST segment. Depression of the ST segment from subendocardial injury usually is greater than 0.1 mV, is present in greater than two contiguous leads, and typically is flat to horizontal, with or without T wave inversion. Ischemic STD is most prevalent in the precordial leads and commonly is encountered in ischemia because of spontaneous angina or from exercise or drug-induced ischemia.

Distinct characteristic patterns of STE can help differentiate ischemic ECG patterns from nonischemic causes, and the magnitude of STE is a well-known correlate of post-MI prognosis. The magnitude of elevation is affected by the extent and degree of ischemia, the amount of myocardial mass affected, and location of the electrode with respect to the ischemic tissue. Noncardiac factors, such as size and shape of the chest wall, also affect the characteristics of STE.

An extreme form of STE is referred to as tombstone STE.[48,49] In tombstone STE, a tall, convex ST segment

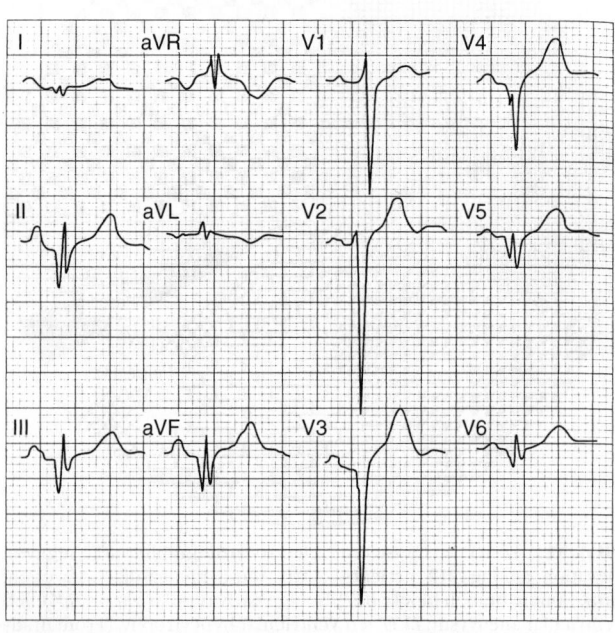

FIGURE 47-21 ■ Pathological Q waves in interior and lateral leads. (From Morris F, Brady: *BMJ* 324:831-833, 2002.)

ties [Wolff-Parkinson-White {**WPW**} syndrome (Figure 47-22), bundle branch blocks]), or in ventricular hypertrophy. In rare circumstances, Q wave MI can occur in the absence of CAD. Cocaine abuse, Kawaski disease, and severe coronary artery spasm are known to cause AMI in the absence of CAD.

Substantial areas of necrosis can manifest in Q wave formation or in diminished R wave amplitude within 2 to 24 hours of ischemic symptoms. Q waves evolve in necrotic areas and in the surrounding injury zones where ischemia-induced conduction delays are present. Q wave formation reflects the electrophysiologically silent areas in the myocardial tissues that lie beneath the recording electrodes of the affected area.

The presence of large Q waves once was considered a marker of finite necrosis, and an indicator of a large infarct size and ischemic zone. Recent information, however, suggests that Q wave formation is no longer a reliable sign of irreversible damage. Early Q wave development (less than 6 hours from symptom onset) in leads with concomitant STE may be transient and should not preclude attempts to revascularize.[43,45] Infarction Q waves, abnormal STE and T wave inversion may persist for several years after MI, with the Q waves gradually diminishing over time.

R Wave Progression. Although poor or reverse R wave progression across the precordial leads may be seen with acute anteroseptal wall MI, poor R wave progression also is found in a large number of patients with noninfarct conditions. For example, LBBB, LVH, WPW-B syndrome, severe COPD, and left anterior hemiblock **(LAH)** decrease the amplitude of anteriorly directed forces and alter the typical upright progression of the R wave pattern across the left side of the chest. Improper lead placement (reversed leads V_2 and V_3) has been associated with benign R wave transition abnormalities and in some women under 30 years of age, R wave abnormality is a normal variant.[47] Because of the absence of direct posterior leads on the standard 12-lead ECG, inverted images of anterior injury currents can be used to approximate activity in the posterior region. In patients with posterior wall MI, increased R wave amplitude often seen in precordial leads V_1 and V_2 reflects inverse ischemic activity in the contralateral posterior surface of the LV.

QT Interval and QT Dispersion. Ischemia, drugs, metabolic and ion channel abnormalities, and bradycardia can prolong repolarization phases of the ventricular action potential, resulting in QT interval prolongation. Some myocardial cell types demonstrate a greater vulnerability to elements that have the potential to alter repolarization. When ischemia or drug effects alter repolarization in some cells and not in others, erratic cellular recovery fosters a dysrhythmogenic substrate that can facilitate reentrant circuit loops and ventricular dysrhythmias. In this setting of disparate and delayed repolarization the QT interval is prolonged.

The QT interval recorded from a single lead transmits the electrical forces from that corresponding myocardial region. Interlead differences between the longest and shortest QT interval are referred to as QT dispersion (QTd). The degree of QTd corresponds with underlying repolarization heterogeneity and risk for reentrant dysrhythmia formation. The association of increased QTd and dysrhythmic SCD risk is well established, and countless cardiac and noncardiac entities now list in-

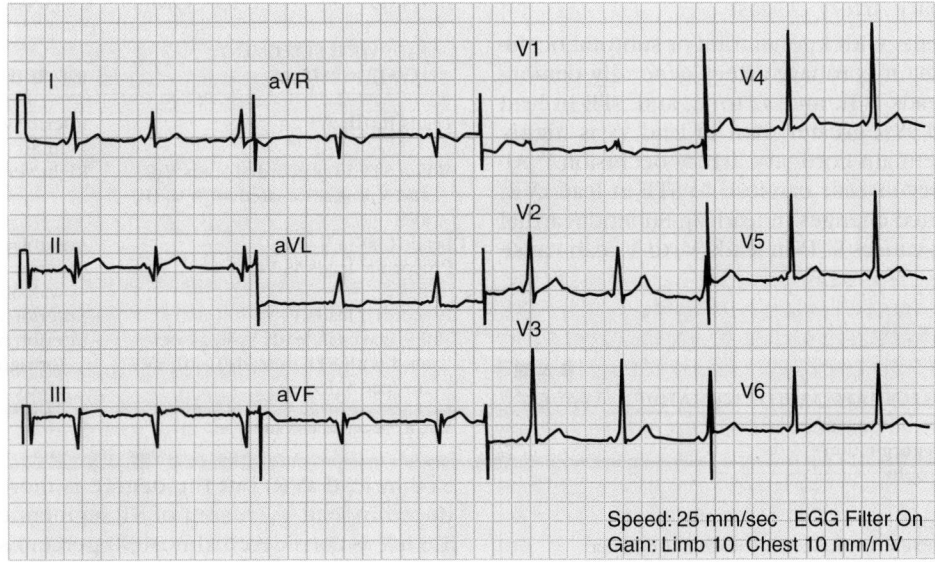

FIGURE 47-22 ■ Wolff-Parkinson-White syndrome. Deep Q waves in leads II, III, and aVF mimic inferior wall myocardial infarction. (From Khan MG: *Rapid ECG interpretation,* ed 2, Philadelphia, 2003, WB Saunders.)

creased QTd among their pathological findings.[39,40] Because of the methodological difficulties in determining and reproducing accurate and consistent QT measurements, widespread clinical use of QTd has not yet been realized.[39]

The U Wave. Under normal conditions the U wave is an upright waveform, but often is elusive, When visible, the U wave can be found between the T wave and the following P wave on a technically perfect ECG tracing.[41] The U wave is considered inverted when it manifests in an opposite direction from the corresponding T wave. U wave negativity appears to be a transient process of function rather than structure, influenced by fluctuations in cardiovascular hemodynamics (Box 47-6). In many cases, a negative or inverted U wave is associated with cardiac pathological conditions such as ischemia (Figure 47-23) or LVH with "strain."[53]

Localizing the Infarcted Region on the Electrocardiogram

The area(s) of ECG change recorded during MI can help to localize the myocardial region affected and the approximate site of coronary occlusion.[54] Location of the infarcted region can be determined by the leads in which STE is found (Table 47-3).

Proximal coronary occlusions generally produce a greater area of ischemia and more pronounced ECG abnormalities than do distal occlusions. LAD coronary artery lesions typically produce anteroseptal infarctions; RCA and distal circumflex artery lesions are the major causes of inferior wall infarctions; and proximal circumflex artery lesions lead to lateral wall infarctions (leads I, aVL, and V_5 to V_6).[45] Infarction of the RV often may go undetected because the standard 12-lead ECG has no direct markers of RV activity; however, certain subtle ECG changes (e.g., STE in lead III greater than in lead II) can suggest RV involvement (see Right Ventricular Infarction).

Left Main Coronary Artery Disease

The ECG of patients with known total or subtotal occlusion of the left main coronary artery generally demonstrates STD in leads I, II, and V_4 to V_6 and STE in lead aVR. STE in lead aVR greater than in lead V_1 is highly suggestive of left main coronary artery occlusion.[53] Although LCX artery disease can lead to STE in lead aVR, it does not produce changes in lead V_1. Subendocardial injury or MI that causes STD in leads V_4 to V_6 can cause

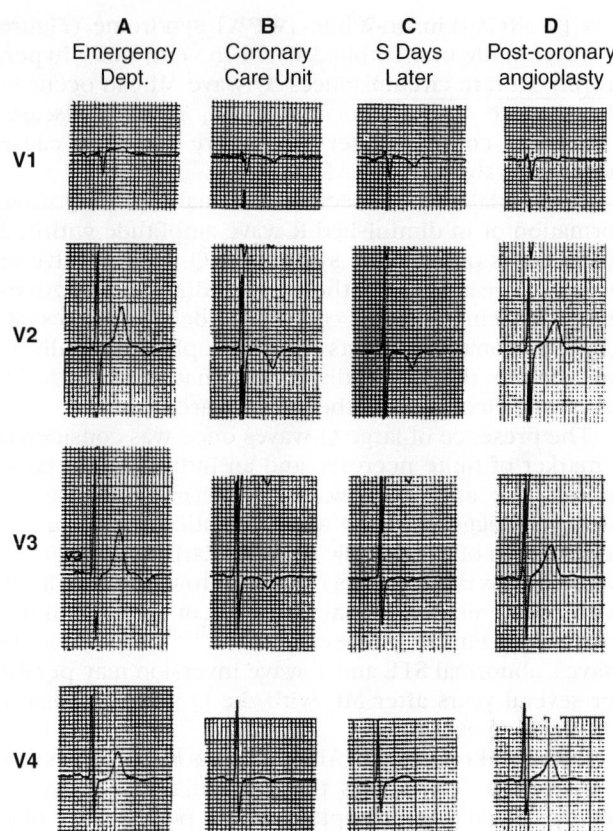

FIGURE 47-23 ■ **A,** Serial electrocardiograms obtained in emergency department show new inverted precordial U waves. **B,** Tracing after admission to coronary care unit several hours later shows resolution of previously inverted U waves, and the emergence of deep T wave inversions. **C,** Five days later, despite negative sequential cardiac enzymes, inverted precordial T waves persist. **D,** After successful coronary angioplasty, electrocardiogram normalized. (From Jaffe ND: *Am Heart J* 129:1028-1030, 1995.)

■ ■ ■

TABLE 47-3 LOCALIZATION OF MYOCARDIAL INFARCTION BY LEAD COMPLEX CHANGE[55,56]

LEADS WITH ST SEGMENT ELEVATION (STE)	INFARCTED AREA
Leads II, III, aVF	Inferior wall myocardial infarction (MI)
When STE in precordial leads V_3R and V_4R is associated with II, III, aVF	Right ventricular infarction
Leads I, aVL, V_5-V_6	Anterolateral wall MI
Precordial leads V_1-V_3	Anteroseptal or anteroapical wall MI
Precordial leads V_3-V_6	Anterior wall MI
Tall R waves in leads V_1-V_2 associated with STE in leads II, III, aVF (or lead V_4R)	Inferior, posterior wall MI (or right ventricular infarction)

STE, ST segment elevation.

STE in lead aVR, but the degree is more than that produced in lead V_1. A sum of ST segment change equal to 1.8 mV is considered almost 90 percent sensitive for left main coronary artery disease (Figure 47-24).

Wellen syndrome is a preinfarction ECG pattern that often is associated with critical left CAD caused by se-

---

BOX 47-6 ■ ■ ■
CONDITIONS ASSOCIATED WITH NEGATIVE U WAVES

Aortic and mitral regurgitation*
Myocardial hypertrophy
Hypertension*
Dilated cardiomyopathy
Coronary disease; exercise-induced myocardial ischemia*
Vasospastic angina
Provocative pharmacological testing

*Most common diagnoses with negative U wave.[51,52]

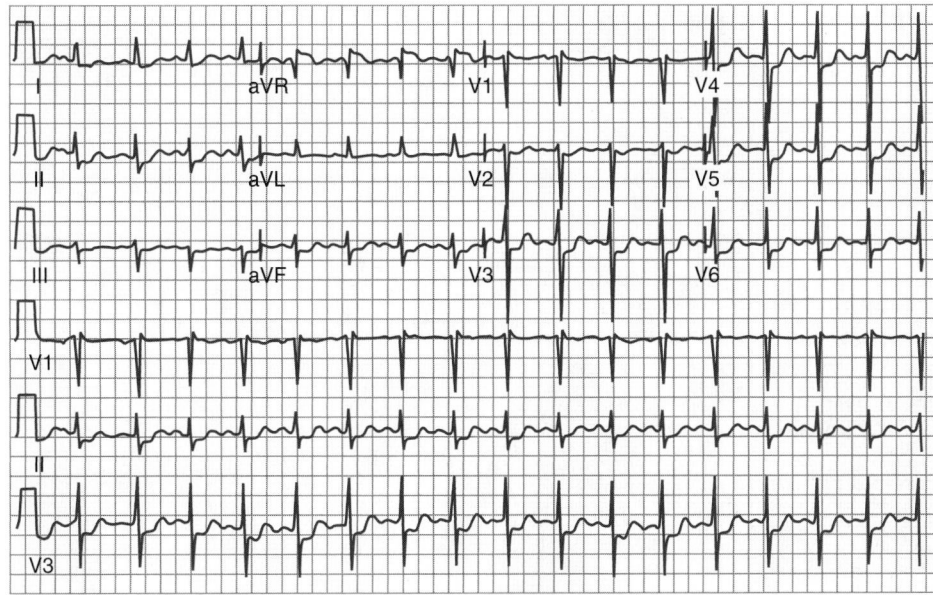

FIGURE 47-24 ▪ Electrocardiogram from patient with chest pain and left main disease. ST depression is present in leads I, II, and V₄ to V₆. (From Sgarbossa EB, Birnbaum Y, Parrillo JE: *Am Heart J* 141:507-517, 2001.)

vere, proximal LAD artery obstruction.[57] Wellen syndrome most commonly occurs in the absence of angina and consists of deeply inverted (or less commonly biphasic) T waves in anterior chest leads V_2 to V_4 (Figure 47-25). Immediate intervention usually is required in these patients to prevent significant loss of myocardial tissue when the critical stenosis evolves into a total occlusion of the proximal vessel. Because of the tenuous nature of critical proximal coronary disease, Wellen syndrome must be differentiated from other ischemic conditions before any provocative stress testing to avoid acute coronary occlusion and massive myocardial infarction.

Anterior, Anterolateral, Anteroseptal Wall Myocardial Infarction

The most common artery involved in acute MI is the LAD artery followed by the RCA and LCX arteries. Occlusion of the LAD artery most often results in STE of 0.1 mV in leads V_2 to V_5 and aVL, with the maximum STE observed in leads V_2 to V_3 (Figure 47-26). The majority of patients with anteroseptal wall MI will not demonstrate STE in the right paraseptal lead V_1. In many patients, the septum is perfused from that LAD artery and RCA branches. This dual blood supply spares the septal region in the event of an LAD artery occlusion. RV infarction **(RVI)** resulting from proximal RCA occlusion can cause precordial changes similar to those of anteroseptal wall MI. In RVI, however, STE in lead V_1 is distinctly greater than in lead V_2, and there is STE in

the right precordial leads, V_3R and V_4R. Occlusion of the LCX artery or distal diagonal branch also can cause precordial patterns similar to anteroseptal wall MI, but these are distinguished by isolated STE in the left precordial leads (V_4 to V_6), without STE in leads V_1 to V_3.[43]

In LAD artery occlusions, localization of the lesion can help determine clinical outcome. Proximal occlusion of the LAD artery is associated with an unfavorable prognosis because of the extent of myocardium exposed to injury.[58] An occlusion proximal to the diagonal or first septal perforator usually is accompanied by STE in leads I and aVL and STD in leads II, III, and aVF. The magnitude of reciprocal STD in the inferior leads often is associated with the degree of STE of leads I and aVL. Elevation of the ST segment in lead aVR, STD in precordial lead V_5, disappearance of normal septal q waves in the lateral leads, and the evolution of RBBB are associated with mid-LAD artery occlusions at the level of the first septal perforator.[59] Diminished or absent inferior lead STD, more moderate STE in precordial leads V_2 to V_3, new Q waves in V_4 to V_6, and R wave amplification in lead V_2 are predictive of distal LAD artery occlusions distal to the first septal and first diagonal arteries.[43]

Extensive anterolateral changes (STE in leads V_1 to V_6) may be observed in the setting of a long LAD artery lesion where the magnitude of injury extends from the anterosuperior region to distal anterolateral and apical regions. An extensive, high anterolateral infarction usu-

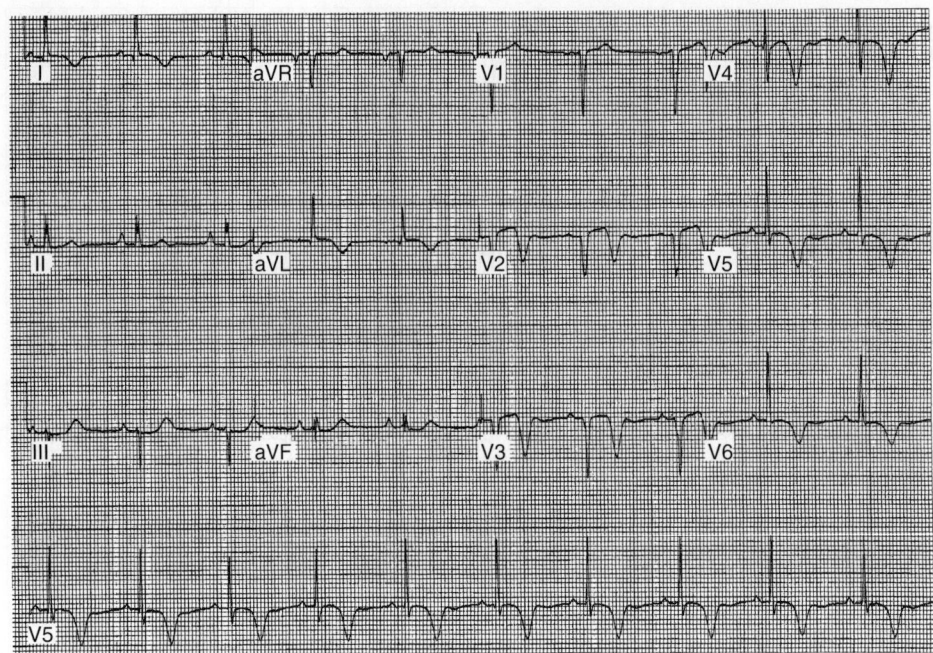

FIGURE 47-25 ■ A patient with Wellen syndrome. Normal sinus rhythm with inverted T waves in leads V_2 to V_6; T waves are deeply inverted. Note the abrupt angle of the descending limb of the T wave, accounting for its marked negative amplitude (i.e., deeply inverted). Also note the minimal ST segment elevation in leads V_2 to V_4 with a convex contour. (From Rhinehardt J: *Am J Emerg Med* 20:638-643, 2002.)

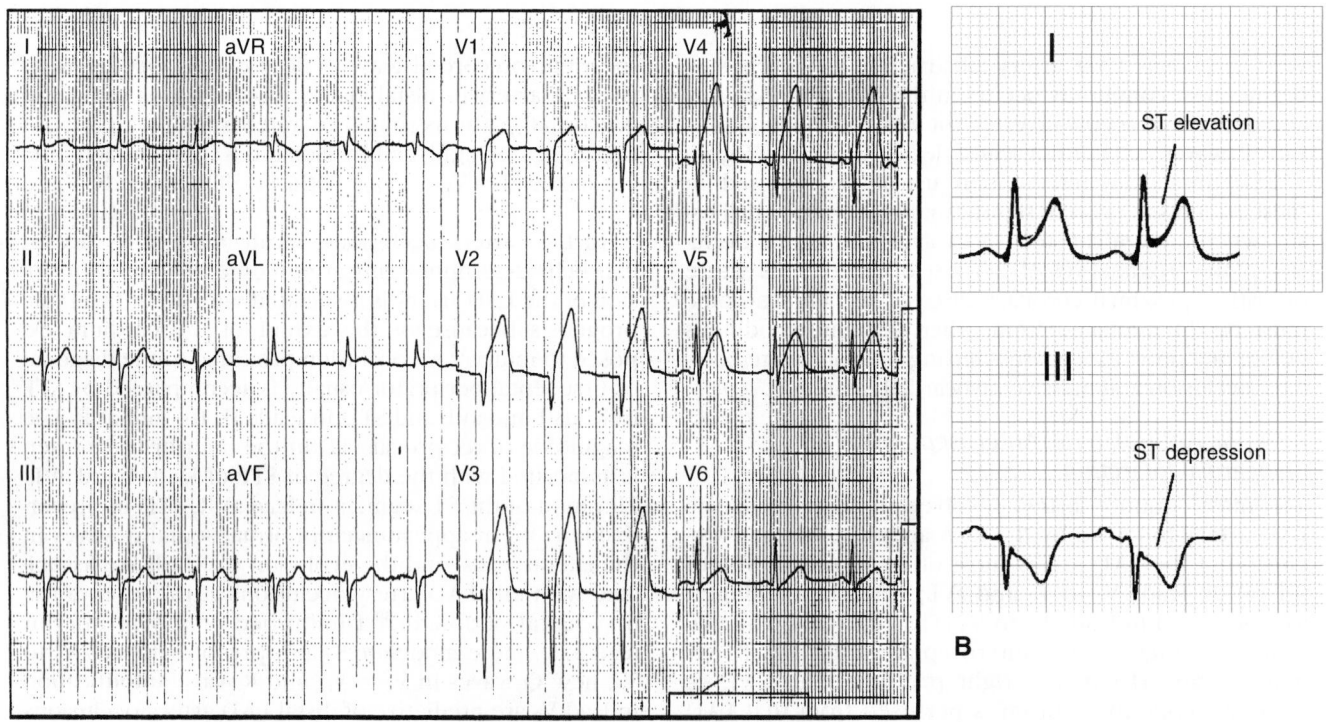

FIGURE 47-26 ■ **A,** Acute anterior myocardial infarction. Normal sinus rhythm with prominent T waves in the anterolateral distribution. The T waves are broad and symmetrical, consistent with the hyperacute T wave of early acute myocardial infarction. **B,** Acute high lateral myocardial infarction. Sinus tachycardia (108 beats/min), normal QRS axis, acute injury pattern in lead I (top; upsloping ST segments, tall T waves), reciprocal changes in the inferior lead III. (**A** from Somers MP: *Am J Emerg Med* 20:243-251, 2002. **B** from Jenkins D, Gerred S: *ECGs by example,* ed 2, Edinburgh, 2005, Churchill Livingstone.)

ally occurs when a coronary artery occlusion occurs in the proximal portion of LAD artery, before the first diagonal branch. Whereas STE in leads I and aVL and STD in leads II, III, and aVF signify an LAD artery occlusion proximal to the first diagonal branch, the presence of STD in lead aVL during an anteroseptal wall MI suggests an occlusive lesion distal to the first diagonal branch. Exceptions to these findings can occur when there is (1) isolated occlusion of the first diagonal artery without LAD artery involvement (STE in leads I, aVL, and V_2; isoelectric or depression of ST segments in leads V_3 to V_4) or (2) if the LAD artery extends around the cardiac apex (wraparound LAD artery) and the occlusion causes concomitant injury to both inferoapical and anterolateral regions (no STE in leads I and aVL or in leads II, III, and aVF). In this case, the opposing electrical forces cancel each other out.[43]

Septal Wall Myocardial Infarction

STE in precordial leads V_1 to V_3 generally has been associated with LAD artery occlusion and septal wall infarct, although echocardiographic evidence of septal hypokinesia is found more frequently in patients who have STE in leads V_3 and V_4. An anteroseptal pattern of STE in leads V_1 to V_3 is related to an obstructive lesion in a short LAD artery or in the ramus intermedius branch—both of which supply the anteroseptal region. Isolated STE in leads V_4 to V_6 is usually reflective of a LCX artery or a distal LAD artery occlusion.[60]

Inferior Wall Myocardial Infarction

Infarction of the inferior wall accounts for approximately half of all MIs, following those due to LAD artery occlusions. Although patients with inferior wall MI tend to have better survival than those with anteroseptal wall MI, certain subgroups of inferior wall MI (concomitant RVI and posterior wall infarction, very proximal RCA disease, and multivessel involvement) have higher mortality rates.[55]

In inferior wall MI, the ECG leads reflecting the greatest magnitude of STE are leads II, III, and aVF, with reciprocal STD in lead aVL. Because lead aVL is the only lead that directly opposes the inferior wall, STD in this lead reflects the injury current in the contralateral inferior region. The RCA supplies the RV and, in the majority of persons, the posterior LV septum and inferior wall. As a result, 80 to 90 percent of inferior wall MIs are usually due to occlusion of the RCA. The LCX artery is responsible for inferior and posterior blood supply in the remaining 10 to 20 percent of the population, and in these cases, inferoposterior infarctions typically are caused by LCX artery occlusion. Several ECG clues can help to differentiate the site of occlusion in inferior wall MI. The use of right ventricular and posteriorly placed ECG leads can provide additional information (Figure 47-27). Because the RV is supplied by the RV branch of the proximal RCA, the presence of STE of 0.1 mV in the right precordial leads V_3R and V_4R, plus STE in leads II, III, and aVF, provides ample evidence of RCA occlusion. Other limb lead changes that support RCA-related inferior wall MI are STE in lead III being greater than in lead

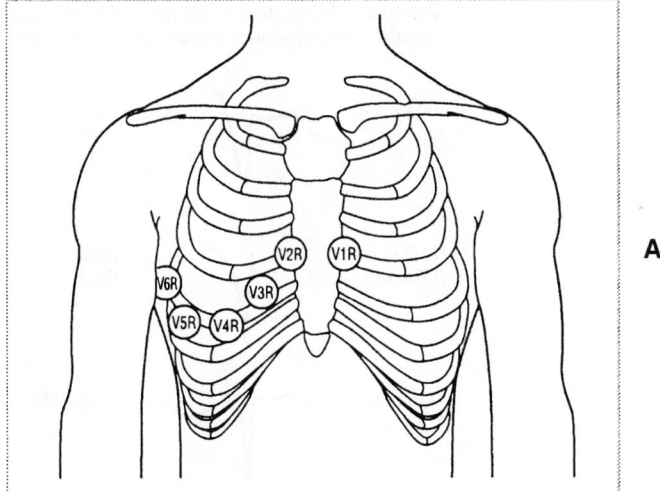

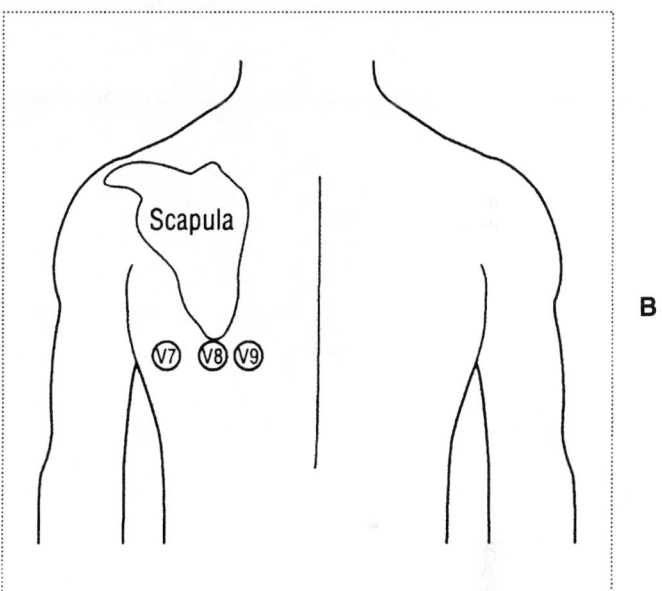

FIGURE 47-27 ■ **A,** Placement of right precordial chest leads. **B,** Placement of posterior chest leads. (From Morris F: *BMJ* 324:831-833, 2002.)

II, STD in aVL being greater than in lead I, and increased S:R ratio of greater than 3 in lead aVL.[43,60]

The LCX artery usually supplies a small area of ventricular myocardium. For this reason, an LCX artery occlusion produces less STE in the majority of cases. In an LCX artery-induced inferior wall MI, there is usually absent or minimal reciprocal STD demonstrated in lead aVL and a presence of precordial STD, and the S:R ratio in lead aVL is equal to 3, compared with ECGs of inferior wall MIs resulting from an occluded RCA. The presence of STE in leads V_7 to V_9 with STD in lead V_4R typically is associated with LCX artery disease. STE in leads II, III, and aVF, when accompanied by STE in leads V_5 and V_6, is the result of inferior wall MI with ischemic extension to the lateral region (Figure 47-28).[43,60]

Value of ST-T segment changes in lead V$_{4R}$ in acute inferoposterior myocardial infarction

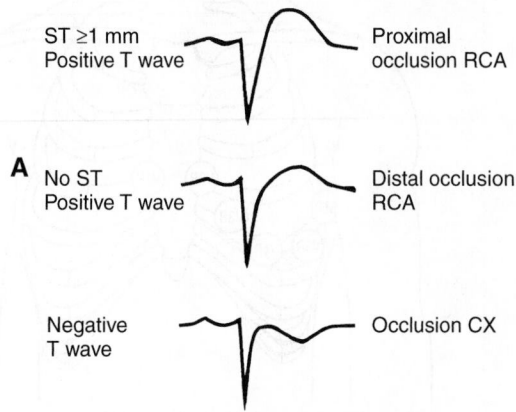

ST ≥1 mm
Positive T wave — Proximal occlusion RCA

A

No ST
Positive T wave — Distal occlusion RCA

Negative
T wave — Occlusion CX

FIGURE 47-28 ■ **A,** Different anatomical sites produce three distinctly different patterns in lead V$_4$R during the early hours of acute inferior myocardial infarction. **B,** Sinus rhythm with ST segment elevation in leads II, III, and aVF (inferior) and in leads V$_4$ to V$_6$ (lateral). ST segment depression seen in leads I, aVL, and V$_2$. Findings consistent with an inferolateral wall myocardial infarction with reciprocal changes in the high lateral area. *CX,* Circumflex artery; *RCA,* right coronary artery. (**A** from Conover MB: *Understanding electrocardiography,* ed 8, St Louis, 2003, Mosby. **B** from Ferguson JD, Brady WJ, Perron AD et al: *Am J Emerg Med* 21:136-142, 2003.)

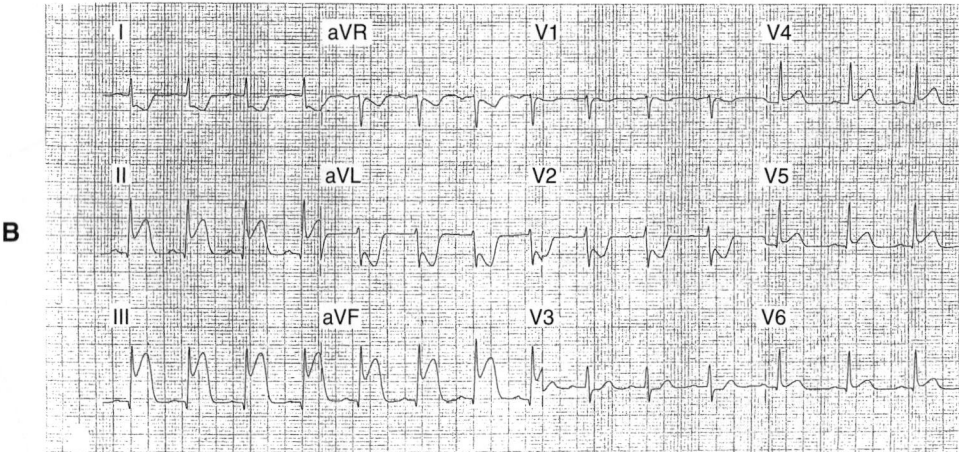

B

Right Ventricular Infarction

RVI initially was identified on autopsy and later as a clinical syndrome of hemodynamic instability in the presence of clear lung fields and accompanying inferior wall MI. The incidence of RVI varies according to the method of diagnosis but complicates up to 20 percent of all MI cases, most (about half) of which are inferior wall MI or anterolateral wall MI (10 to 15 percent).[61,62] In the rare event of an isolated RVI (3 percent incidence), there is underlying RV hypertrophy, or chronic lung disease, and the RV injury pattern is revealed as a single lead (V$_1$) STE on the standard 12-lead ECG.[55]

RVI can be caused by lesions in the RCA, LCX artery, or LAD artery but most commonly is associated with RCA occlusions proximal to the RV marginal branches. RVI resulting from proximal RCA occlusions is associated with higher incidence of complications. Occlusions of the LCX or LAD arteries are less common. RVI often is diagnosed clinically in inferior wall MI patients when right-sided hemodynamic compromise is evident, although the majority of patients with RVI do not display hemodynamic compromise and go undetected. The finding of isolated STE in lead V$_1$, in the setting of chest pain and/or inferior wall MI can be the initial indicator of RV involvement, although the right precordial chest lead tracings (leads V$_3$R to V$_5$R) should be used routinely in all patients with inferior wall MI to confirm RVI.[3,61-63] The ECG demonstrating STE and Q waves in lead III greater than in leads II and aVF plus STE in leads V$_3$R to V$_6$R is highly suggestive of RVI. Other ECG findings associated with a high incidence of RVI is the presence of RBBB and STE in lead V$_2$ greater than the STD in lead aVF. Recall that STE in lead V$_1$ is highly specific for proximal RCA occlusion.

Posterior Wall Myocardial Infarction

Infarction of the posterobasal wall of the left ventricle represents approximately 20 percent of all acute MIs and occurs in up to 53 percent of all inferior wall MIs.[64] Infarction in this area occurs as a result of extensive injury arising from an RCA or LCX artery occlusion. Although isolated posterior wall MI does occur, it most often is found in conjunction with adjacent inferior or lateral wall infarction and is associated with a higher rate of dysrhythmic complications.[55]

Similar to RV regions, there are no direct leads on the standard 12-lead system that directly record posterior wall activity. As a result, posterior wall changes are seen indirectly in the inverse images of leads V_1 to V_3, which face the contralateral endocardial surface of the LV posterior wall. Because these leads record from an opposite, rather than direct, view over the infarct site, the changes of posterior wall MI are inverted in these leads and from the typical patterns of acute transmural MI. The evolution of dominant R waves, STD, and upright T waves observed in the anterior leads V_1 to V_3, when inverted, reveal deep Q waves, STE, and T wave inversion. Although inferior and anterior LV walls are well represented on the ECG, lateral, posterior, septal, and apical regions of the LV remain relatively silent on the ECG.

Infarction of the posterior wall is likely when there are tall and wide R waves in leads V_1 and V_2, an R:S ratio greater than 1 in lead V_2, horizontal rather than downsloping STD equal to 0.1 mV in the right precordial leads (V_1 to V_3), and tall upright T waves in leads V_1 and V_2. Flat or horizontal ST segments on the right precordial leads of patients with posterior wall MI can help to differentiate downsloping STD patterns of reciprocal activity in other ischemic regions. The presence of a concurrent infarction pattern, such as inferior wall MI or lateral wall MI combined with STD in leads V_1 to V_3 and prominent R wave in lead V_1, also indicates posterior wall MI, for extension of ischemia from other re-

gions is a common observation. R wave characteristics should be analyzed carefully because numerous causes and pathological mechanisms can generate a prominent R wave in lead V_1 (Table 47-4).[16]

Posterior precordial lead recordings from leads V_7, V_8, and V_9 (placed at the left posterior axillary line, left scapular tip, and halfway between left scapular tip and left paraspinal muscles, respectively) can offer pivotal information and constitute the 15-lead ECG[63] (Figure 47-29). The addition of posterior chest leads increases the sensitivity, specificity, and prognostic capability of the ECG, especially when trying to confirm the presence of a posterior wall MI. Generally, the 15-lead ECG should be obtained when there is evidence of inferior wall MI, lateral wall MI, or unexplained STD in leads V_1 to V_3, findings suggestive of RVI (RBBB; STE in lead V_2 less than 50 percent the magnitude of STD in lead aVF) or hemodynamically compromised inferior wall MI. STE of greater than 0.1 mV in the posterior chest leads is considered more sensitive than the inverse images of STD in leads V_1 to V_3 on the standard 12-lead ECG.[61]

Confounding Factors Affecting the Electrocardiogram During Acute Myocardial Infarction

Certain coexisting ECG abnormalities, such as LBBB, LVH, and left ventricular pacing, may obscure classic ECG patterns of acute MI, reducing the utility of the ECG to detect changes associated with ischemia (Figure 47-30). Patients with acute MI have altered electrophysiology. The electrical derangements of LBBB further compound ventricular activation and recovery abnormalities

■ ■ ■

TABLE 47-4   CAUSES OF A PROMINENT R WAVE IN LEAD V_1[21]

CAUSE	MANIFESTATION
Right bundle branch block	Tall R wave in lead V_1 (rSR'), terminal delay, QRS complex greater than 12 msec Broad S wave in lead V_6
Ventricular tachycardia	Tall R wave in lead V_1 (Rsr'), tall R wave in leads V_1-V_3 with R wave greater than 4 msec with associated ST segment depression Upright tall T waves in leads V_1-V_3
Posterior wall myocardial infarction	Q waves and ST segment elevation in leads V_7-V_9
Right ventricular hypertrophy	Tall R wave in lead V_1 (greater than 0.7 mV), plus electrocardiographic criteria for right ventricular hypertrophy (R:S ratio in lead V_1 greater than in lead I, R:S ratio in lead V_5 or V_6 less than in lead I; no ST segment elevation Right atrial enlargement, secondary ST-T wave changes, leads V_7-V_9 normal
Ventricular septal hypertrophy	Q waves in septal leads, left ventricular hypertrophy
Acute pulmonary embolism	Tall R wave in lead V_1, incomplete or complete RBBB, large S wave in lead I, Q wave in lead III, nonspecific ST-T wave changes
Wolff-Parkinson-White syndrome type A (left-sided accessory pathway)	Tall R waves in right precordial leads, Q waves in the inferior leads, short PR interval, QRS complex greater than 11 msec delta wave, discordant ST-T waves
Hypertrophic cardiomyopathy	Tall R wave in lead V_1 (Rs); deep, narrow Q waves in the lateral leads (I, aVL, V_5-V_6); no ST segment elevation; upright T waves in the right precordial leads
Duchenne muscular dystrophy	Tall R wave in lead V_1; deep, narrow Q waves in lateral leads
Mirror-image dextrocardia	Tall R wave in lead V_1; decreasing QRS complexes across the precordium; inverted P wave and QRS complex in lead I; leads aVR and aVL are reversed, with an upright QRS complex in lead aVR and a negatively deflected QRS complex in lead aVL; QRS complex in leads II and III also is reversed
Lead misplacement	Substitution of lead V_1 with any precordial lead causes tall R wave in lead V_1, reverse R wave progression in leads V_1-V_3, isolated T wave inversion in lead V_3
Normal variant	Tall R wave in lead V_1

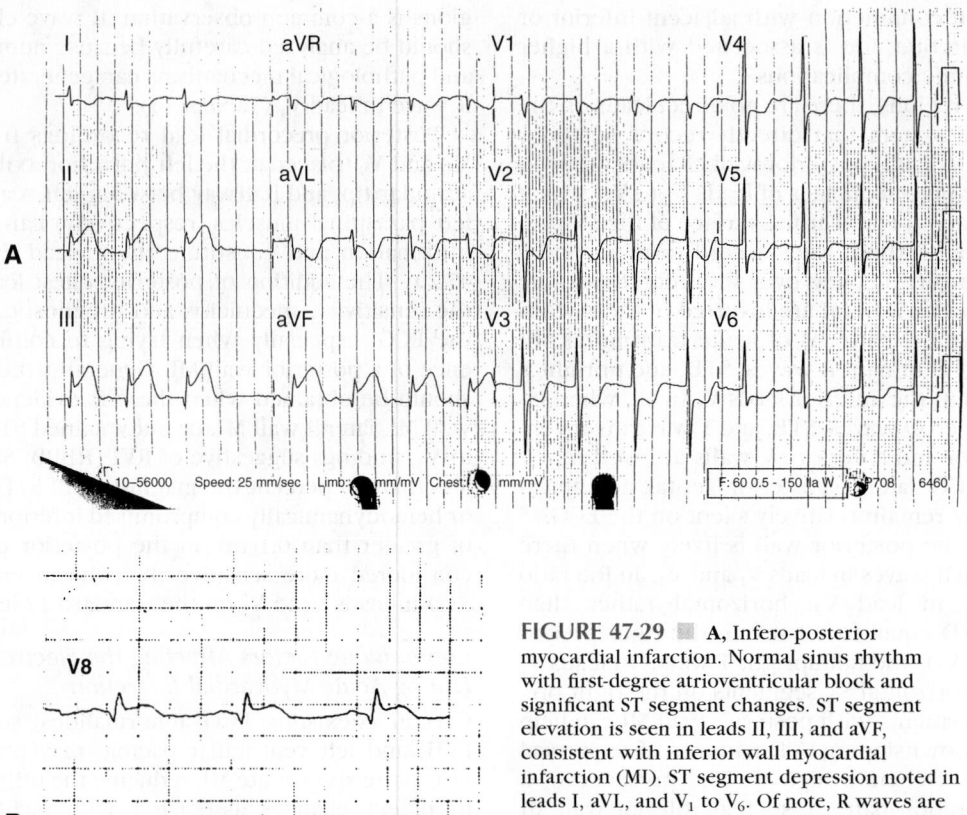

FIGURE 47-29 ▪ **A,** Infero-posterior myocardial infarction. Normal sinus rhythm with first-degree atrioventricular block and significant ST segment changes. ST segment elevation is seen in leads II, III, and aVF, consistent with inferior wall myocardial infarction (MI). ST segment depression noted in leads I, aVL, and V_1 to V_6. Of note, R waves are prominent in leads V_2 and V. The ST depression in conjunction with the prominent R waves in the right precordial leads suggests posterior wall MI. **B,** Posterior leads V_8 and V_9 reveal ST segment elevation consistent with posterior wall MI. Note the relatively minor degree of ST segment elevation. (From Brady WJ, Erling B, Pollack M, Chan TC: *J Emerg Med* 20:391-401, 2001.)

of acute MI, reducing the diagnostic power of the ECG. Independent signs of acute MI during LBBB can be scored according to the following schedule: (1) STE equals 0.1 mV in leads with concordant QRS complexes (5 points); (2) STD equals 0.1 mV in precordial leads V_1 to V_3 (3 points); and (3) STE equals 0.5 mV in leads with discordant QRS complexes (2 points). A total score of 3 or more suggests the presence of acute MI. Ventricular pacing also alters normal conduction patterns and can compound the difficulty of ECG interpretation in the presence of acute MI. Temporary reduction of the pacing rate may allow observation of intrinsic depolarization and repolarization waveform and intervals. Additional STE observed in leads with negatively deflected QRS complexes may suggest acute MI.[2,60,65]

Left Ventricular Aneurysm

Unlike the noninfarct syndrome of Tako-Tsubo syndrome[66] in which transient apical asynergy occurs in the presence of little or no CAD, dyskinetic left ven-

tricular function, or left ventricular aneurysm **(LVA)**, typically result from a localized area of infarcted myocardium. Postinfarct LVA develops in approximately 3 to 15 percent of acute MI cases, the majority of which are large anteroseptal wall MIs (total occlusion of the LAD artery), followed by less common inferoposterior wall MIs.[68] Aneurysm of the LV also can occur following blunt chest trauma. Although varying degrees of STE can be observed in the leads directly facing the aneurysm, concave STE is seen most often. Because the majority of LVAs develop in the anterolateral region, STE in LVA is seen most commonly in leads I and aVL and precordial leads V_1 to V_6. Less extensive lead involvement is seen in some LVAs, as in Figure 47-31. Inferoposterior LVAs manifest STE in leads II, III, and aVF and STD in leads V_1 and V_2. STE can be convex or concave and usually is associated with a wide distribution of infarct Q waves and poor R wave progression. In LVA, STE is from injury current emanating from still viable tissue in the infarct zone or from wall stress caused by traction on

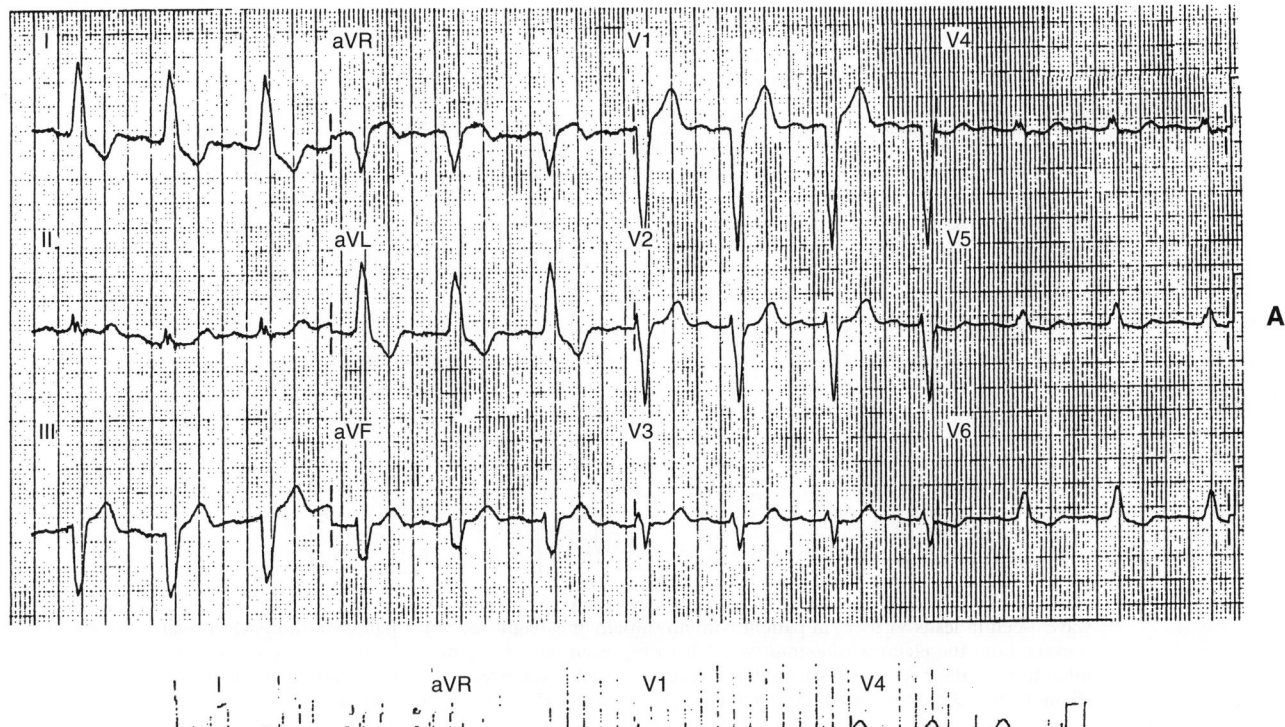

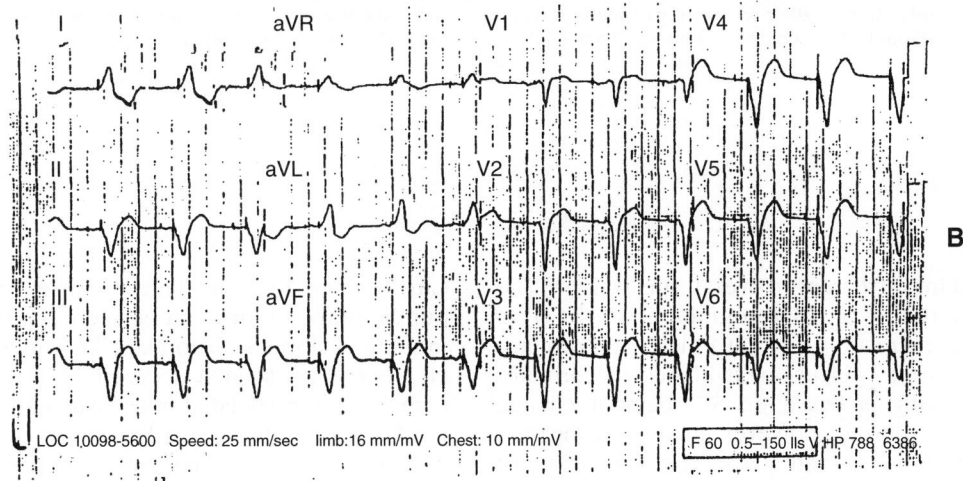

FIGURE 47-30 ▨ Confounding factors affecting the electrocardiogram in myocardial infarction. **A,** Normal sinus rhythm and left bundle branch block. The expected ST-T wave configurations are discordant. Leads with QS or rS complexes (partially or entirely negative in deflection) may have greatly elevated ST segments, mimicking myocardial infarction (MI). Leads with a large monophasic R wave demonstrate ST segment depression. T wave, especially in the right to midprecordial leads, has a convex upward shape of a tall, vaulting appearance, similar to the hyperacute T wave of early MI. The T waves in leads with the monophasic R wave frequently are inverted. **B,** Ventricular paced rhythm demonstrating lateral acute MI. Leads I and aVL demonstrate concordant ST segment depression that is not appropriate for ventricular paced rhythm. (From Brady WJ, Chan TC, Pollack M: *J Emerg Med* 18:71-78, 2000.)

normal, adjacent myocardial tissue. Post-MI, persistent STE can be observed for up to several weeks.[68]

Pseudoinfarction Patterns

Pseudoinfarction patterns and variations of STE can occur in nonischemic conditions such as in LVH, LBBB, benign early repolarization **(BER)**, acute pericarditis, hyperkalemia, acute PE, LV aneurysm, myocarditis, cardiac tumors, and hypothermia, any of which can cause misdiagnosis. In addition to clinical presentation and differences in ST segment waveform morphologies as-

sociated with ischemic versus nonischemic conditions (convex or obliquely straight ST segment upslope and concave upslope, respectively), characteristics such as the degree of STE or STD, and concordance of STE with QRS complex also can help to differentiate acute ischemic syndromes from nonischemic syndromes.[2]

Reperfusion and Coronary Artery Patency

Prompt restoration of normal epicardial blood flow and tissue perfusion results in smaller infarct size, preserved myocardial function, prevention of LV remodeling and

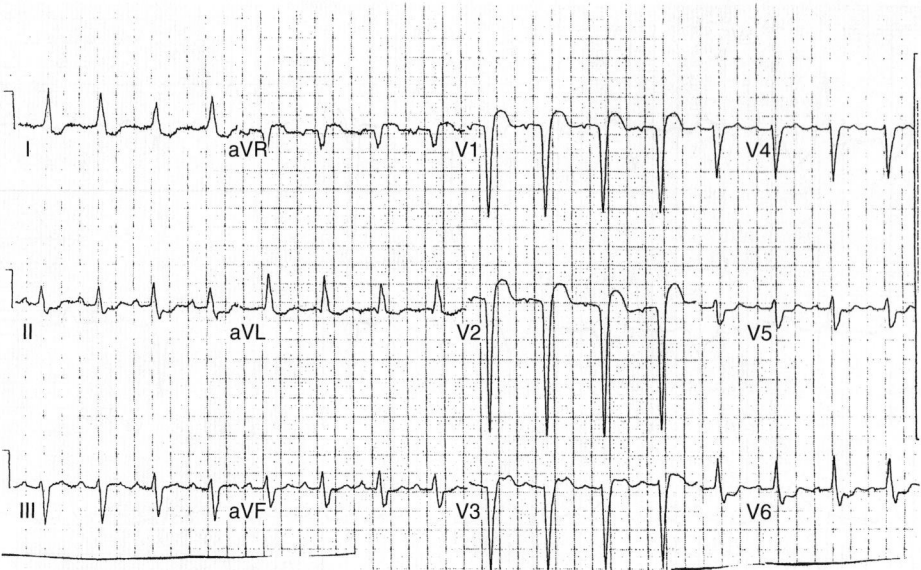

FIGURE 47-31 ■ Left ventricular aneurysm. Pronounced ST segment elevation with significant Q waves seen in leads V_1 to V_3 in patient with an initially misdiagnosed chest pain syndrome. On initial presentation, the electrocardiogram was felt to represent an ST segment elevation acute myocardial infarction. Further review of past medical records revealed the presence of left ventricular aneurysm. (From Engel J, Brady WJ, Mattu A, Perron AD: *Am J Emerg Med* 20:238-242, 2002.)

dilatation, and improvement in overall survival.[42,69] The magnitude and timing of STE resolution on the ECG remains a strong correlate of patent epicardial coronary flow and myocardial perfusion. Evidence of coronary reperfusion usually is based on ST segment change within a 72-hour period; however, many investigators report that ST segments and T wave patterns may not stabilize fully until 7 to 10 days post-MI. Correlation of STE resolution with long-term cardiac function appears to be similar in patients evaluated immediately after revascularization and those evaluated 72 hours post-MI.[51,69]

Atrial Infarction

Atrial infarction can occur concomitantly with ventricular acute MI. ECG manifestation of atrial infarction includes PR segment elevation greater than 0.05 mV in the left precordial leads V_5 and V_6 and in lead I, with PR segment depression in leads V_1 and V_2 and in limb leads II and III. The P wave becomes irregularly notched, with morphology similar to a "W" or "M" shape. Because PR segment change also is associated with atrial enlargement, pericarditis, and increased atrial pressure load, these entities must be differentiated clinically.[8,45]

Heart Failure

The ECG is usually abnormal in heart failure; several asynchronous dysrhythmias and ECG changes can be observed. Regional STE and abnormal Q wave formation

can be seen in heart failure caused by MI and LVA; bundle branch block can be seen as a result of CAD or interstitial fibrosis. Secondary ECG changes from drug effects also are seen. A decrease in heart rate variability commonly is associated with heart failure and has been used to predict future cardiac events. ECG changes suggestive of chamber enlargement and axis shift are common ECG findings as the cardiac structure remodels. Abnormal repolarization patterns (QT interval prolongation and increased QTd) remain independent predictors of adverse outcomes (dysrhythmic death) in heart failure.[52]

Congenital Disorders

Inherited disorders of ion channel, mitochondrial, and metabolic functions and inherited disorders affecting cardiac structure can produce a wide variety of ECG abnormalities.

Ventricular fibrillation is the usual cause of SCD in structural cardiac disease and ischemia, yet a small number of patients who experience SCD have no demonstrable physical pathological condition. Dysrhythmic events in this population usually result from primary torsades de pointes. In LQTS, torsades de pointes has been known to occur during vigorous exercise, stress, febrile states, and in some cases, during sleep. On the ECG, baseline QTc interval prolongation is often the common thread among patients with episodes of torsades de pointes–induced SCD[70] (Figure 47-32). LQTS is

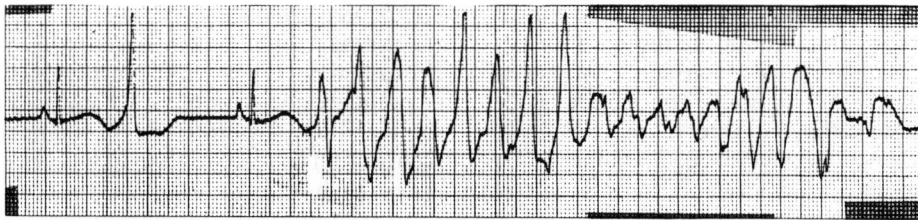

FIGURE 47-32 ■ Torsades de pointes. A short-long-short sequence of beats followed by an episode of torsades de pointes. The QT interval in the sinus beat immediately preceding the torsades de pointes is 600 msec. (From Khan IA: Clinical and therapeutic aspects of congenital and acquired long QT syndrome, *Am J Med* 112:58-66, 2002.)

■ ■ ■

TABLE 47-5   LONG QT SYNDROME GENOTYPES, ELECTROCARDIOGRAM PHENOTYPES, AND AFFECTED ION CHANNEL[71,72]

GENOTYPE	ASSOCIATED SYNDROME	ELECTROCARDIOGRAM PHENOTYPE	GENE/CHROMOSOME	ION CHANNEL AFFECTED
LQT1*	Jervell and Lange-Nielsen syndrome Romano-Ward syndrome	Prolonged T wave duration QTC 490 ± 40 msec	KCNQ1/11	Slowly activating K⁺
LQT2*	Long QT syndrome (LQTS)	Lower T wave amplitude in limb leads, bifid T waves QTC 470 ± 30 msec Auditory trigger	HERG/7	Rapidly activating K⁺
LQT3	LQTS, Brugada syndrome	Late-onset T waves (peaked) preceding a long, isoelectric ST segment QTC 470 ± 30 msec	SCN5A/3	Voltage-dependent Na⁺
LQT4	LQTS	None specified	Unknown/4	Unknown
LQT5	LQTS	None specified	KCNE1/21	Slowly activating K⁺
LQT6	LQTS	None specified	KCNE2/21	Rapidly activating K⁺
LQT7	LQTS	None specified	Unknown	Unknown

*Most common genotypes.

composed of a group of genetic mutations responsible for Na⁺ or K⁺ flow and regulation of cardiac repolarization (Table 47-5).

Ion Channel Disorders

The majority of familial patterns associated with idiopathic SCD are linked to some form of ion channel dysfunction.[56] Under normal conditions, transmembrane ions (Na⁺, K⁺, or Ca⁺⁺) flow through their respective ion channels during specific phases of the cardiac electrical cycle that form the cardiac action potential. Specific encoded proteins that dictate the properties and function of the ion channels regulate the physiological flow of these ions. Mutations of channel proteins interfere with normal ion flow patterns, which in turn disrupt cellular repolarization. In the presence of disturbed and unbalanced repolarization, the cardiac cell becomes vulnerable to serious dysrhythmia formation.

Congenital Long QT Syndrome

Channelopathic-induced transmural voltage differences and action potential gradients contribute to the characteristic ECG abnormalities observed in several clinical conditions. Action potential gradients form as a result of intrinsic (congenital; genetic ion channel alteration [LQTS]) or extrinsic factors (acquired; drug effect or electrolyte imbalance). Loss of uniform ventricular action potential domes occurs when the plateau phase of the M cell diverges from the plateau phase of the epicardial and endocardial action potentials, prolonging or shortening repolarization. On the ECG, altered repolarization manifests as lengthened or abbreviated QT_C intervals and heightened, biphasic, or flattened T waves. Divergence of the endocardial, M cell, and action potentials also may produce T wave notching in the descending limb of the T wave. The T wave in LQTS is typically broad, or biphasic, with prominent U waves following the T wave. In LQTS, it has been suggested that the prominent T-U complex is a manifestation of a prolonged and interrupted repolarization and that the U wave observed is actually a secondary T waveform, rather than a true U wave.[56]

The majority of patients with congenital LQTS demonstrate a QT_C interval greater than 440 msec, although many have QTc intervals within the normal range of up to 440 msec (6 to 12 percent) and about one-third have a QTc interval of 460 msec. As a result, there is a considerable increase in QTd throughout the myocardium.

The QT_C interval maintains a constant relationship with ventricular refractory periods. The length of the refractory period, with the QT_C interval, is considered an important marker of dysrhythmogenic vulnerability at the ventricular and atrial levels. Although certain physiological and pathological factors are known to cause QTc interval shortening (increased heart rate, hyperthermia, elevated serum K^+ or Ca^{++} levels, acidosis, or altered autonomic tone), a specific population recently has been identified to have short QT intervals, with no demonstrable cause.[73] See the Genetics feature.

Brugada syndrome, another ion channel disorder, is characterized by right precordial lead STE and high risk of SCD in the absence of ischemia or structural heart disease. Brugada syndrome is a familial disease transmitted in an autosomal dominant fashion and is linked to a mutation in the protein responsible for regulating Na^+ channel function. Brugada syndrome is responsible for up to 60 percent of cases previously diagnosed as idiopathic ventricular fibrillation.[76,77]

The most prominent ECG feature of this syndrome is the Brugada sign: paroxysmal right precordial STE in leads V_1 to V_3. In some cases, QTc interval prolongation and RV conduction delay patterns may or may not be present, but an increase in the PR interval (200 msec) is noted. A predilection for nocturnal polymorphic VT and ventricular fibrillation–induced SCD also occurs. Patients with Brugada syndrome typically have one of three ECG patterns or "Brugada waves" described as a "coved" convex or a "saddleback" concave upward ST segment.

The three established morphologies of Brugada waves represent the three variants of the syndrome (Figure 47-33). Differentiation among the variants requires confirmation of correct precordial lead placement. Primary Brugada waves (type 1) are triangular-coved elevations (J point elevation = 0.2 mV) that descend gradually, accompanied by inverted T waves in leads V_1 to V_3 that may or may not be accompanied by RV conduction delay. Brugada wave types 2 and 3 involve saddleback elevation (J point elevation = 0.2 mV) and subtle differences in the terminal portion of the ST segment (type 2 STE remains at 0.1 mV above baseline; type 3 STE descends to or less than 0.1 mV above baseline).[78]

In asymptomatic persons without a family history of SCD, type 2 and 3 variants of Brugada waves have been considered normal variants, whereas type 1 Brugada waves are those ST patterns found in unprovoked cases of aborted SCD in which syncope or SCD is the presenting symptom. These persons are typically young in age. In symptomatic patients or those with a positive family history, type 2 and 3 Brugada waves usually are encountered after the syndrome is unmasked by electrical or pharmacological provocation and involve persons of middle or older age groups.[79,80]

Under normal conditions, the J wave notch reflects the LV action potential (the RV action potential usually is obscured), and the ST segment remains isoelectric in the absence of any transmural voltage differences at the end of the action potential plateau. In pathological substrates, as in Brugada syndrome, repolarization is altered in the myocardial cells that span the RV wall. As a result, the RV notch becomes abnormally accentuated, and a transmural voltage gradient develops between the affected RV epicardium and unaffected RV endocardium, producing an exaggerated J wave and ST segment. When RV epicardial cell repolarization precedes RV M cell and RV endocardial cell repolarization, the T wave remains upright and the ST segment has a saddleback configuration. Further accentuation of the RV notch and epicardial action potential causes a reversal of the voltage gradient in the plateau phase, producing a coved ST segment and inverted T wave[81] (Figure 47-34).

Cardiomyopathy

Primary cardiomyopathies can be *genetic* or *acquired* and generally are categorized by the transformation that occurs in the myocardium: *hypertrophic* (thickened), *dilated* (thinning and enlarged), and *restrictive* (infiltrative).

In hypertrophic cardiomyopathy (a genetic disorder), myocytes become hypertrophied in an asymmetrical pattern, leading to marked myocardial thickening and development of abnormal Q waves in the anterolateral or inferior chest leads. Hypertrophied myocardium is particularly noted in the septal region at the level of the aortic outflow tract. Because of the abnormal Q wave morphology, these Q waves may be misinterpreted as Q waves of necrosis. Dilated cardiomyopathy causes a thinning of the ventricular walls and dilatation of the ventricular cavity, which produces patterns of LVH. However, diffuse myocardial fibrosis common in dilated cardiomyopathy often masks the increased voltage patterns. Restrictive cardiomyopathy causes low-voltage ECG waveforms and prolongation of the QRS complex because of the magnitude of infiltrative substances that replace myocytes and delay impulse conduction.[82] Refer to Chapter 72 for further discussion.

■ ■ ■ GENETICS

SHORT QT SYNDROME

Another ion channel disorder, short QT syndrome (SQTS), originally was described in 2000 and later was confirmed as an autosomal dominant familial pattern. Similar to patients with LQTS, the affected patients with SQTS typically demonstrate structurally normal hearts, a history of palpitations, atrial and ventricular dysrhythmias, sudden cardiac death, and easy inducibility of ventricular fibrillation with programmed stimulation. The electrocardiogram phenotype of SQTS typically manifests a marked and constant short QT interval (QTC = 300 msec) that correlates with shortened refractory periods and high-amplitude T waves.[74]

Several temporizing QT interval–lengthening therapies have been proposed to protect patients with SQTS from dysrhythmic death. Currently, the use of implantable defibrillators in combination with quinidine therapy is used in SQTS. Quinidine in this setting therapeutically lengthens the QTC and ventricular refractory period, minimizing the chance for dysrhythmia induction.[75]

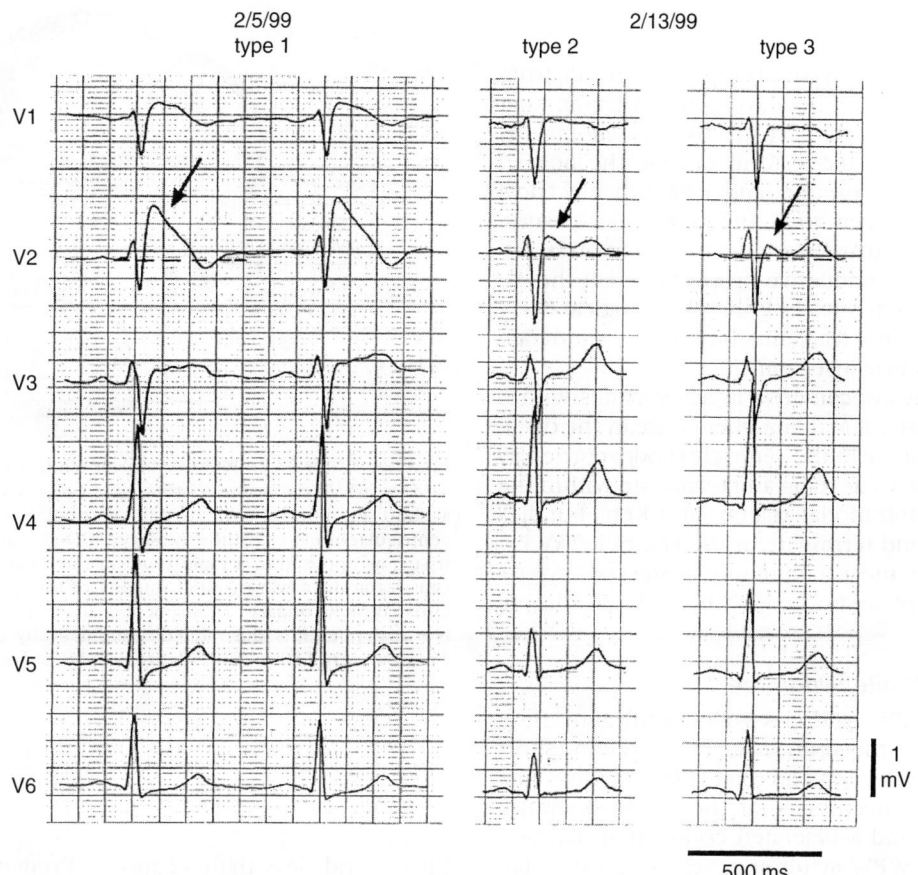

FIGURE 47-33 ▦ Brugada syndrome. Precordial leads of a resuscitated patient with Brugada syndrome. Note the dynamic electrocardiogram changes over the course of a few days. All three patterns are shown. *Left:* type 1; *middle:* type 2; *right:* type 3. (From Wilde AA, Antzelevitch C, Borggrefe M et al: *Eur Heart J* 23:1648-1654, 2002. Reproduced with permission of the European Society of Cardiology, Elsevier Science.)

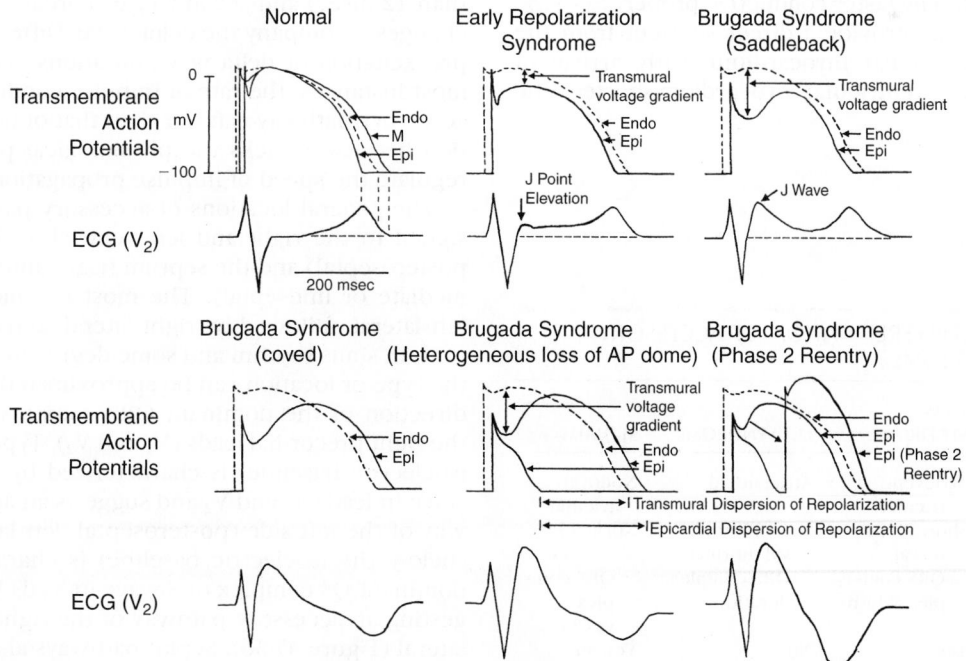

FIGURE 47-34 ▦ Schematic representation of right ventricular epicardial action potential changes proposed to underlie the electrocardiographic manifestation of early repolarization syndrome and Brugada syndrome. (From Antzelevitch C: *J Cardiovasc Electrophysiol* 12:268-272, 2001.)

Accessory Pathways

Accessory pathways or bypass tracts often result from embryological faults in the developing AV ring that separates atrial and ventricular tissue. Anomalous bridges of conductive tissue form outside the normal insulation of the AV annulus and establish electrical communication between atrial and ventricular tissues. Accessory pathways usually are derived from atrial tissue and have faster conductive properties than the AV node. Because these tissues lack the physiological delay of the AV node, impulse transmission travels unimpeded toward the ventricular insertion site.

Accessory pathways can arise in several sites within the conduction system. Mahaim fibers arise in the distal AV node and terminate in the ventricle (nodoventricular tracts), James bundles develop and terminate within the AV nodal tissue (intranodal tracts), and Kent bundles arise in the atria and terminate in the ventricle (AV bypass tracts). The most commonly observed bypass tracts typically are associated with WPW syndrome (Table 47-6).[83]

Wolff-Parkinson-White Syndrome

ECG findings of WPW syndrome reflect early activation, or preexcitation, of the ventricular myocardium (short PR interval, delta wave, and a broad QRS complex) that results from the transmission of the cardiac impulse over a secondary and accelerated conduction pathway (Figure 47-35). In WPW syndrome, ventricular depolarization is often the culmination of dual activation, partially from the physiological impulse entering the ventricle by the normal conduction pathway and partially from the impulse entering the ventricle via an accessory pathway that does not involve the AV node or His-Purkinje system. The faster conductive properties of the accessory pathway provide a direct shortcut from the atria to the ventricular myocardium. Early arrival of the impulse at the ventricular myocardium shortens the

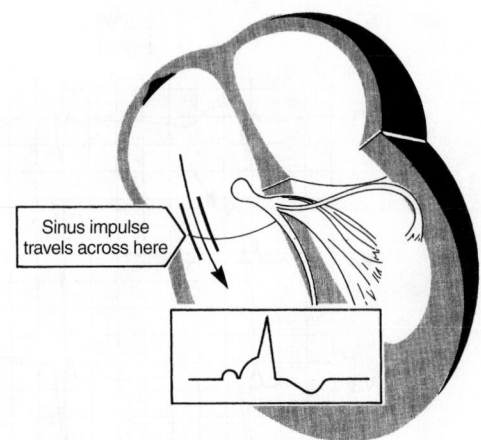

FIGURE 47-35 ▧ In Wolff-Parkinson-White syndrome the impulse arrives early in the ventricles through an accessory pathway, causing a short PR interval. The initial ventricular forces begin at the ventricular insertion of the accessory pathway, traveling in myocardial tissue, as opposed to a rapid route in the conduction system. This causes the delta wave (initial slurring of the QRS complex). There also may be secondary ST-T segment changes. The accessory pathway is a small fiber; it is illustrated diagrammatically. (From Conover MB: *Understanding electrocardiography,* ed 8, St Louis, 2003, Mosby.)

PR interval (less than 12 msec). Premature ventricular activation or preexcitation causes slurring of the initial QRS complex–delta wave, named for the resulting PQ segment deformity caused by the slow impulse propagation across the prematurely activated, nonspecialized ventricular tissue. A widened QRS complex (greater than 12 msec) and secondary discordant repolarization changes accompany the delta wave. Different degrees of preexcitation or delta wave durations may be seen. In most instances, the rate of impulse conduction over an accessory pathway is faster than that of normal conduction because it lacks the physiological properties that regulate the speed of impulse propagation.

The general locations of accessory pathways are assigned to the right and left ventricles (free walls and posteroseptal) and the septum (right anterior and intermediate or midseptal). The most common location is left lateral, followed by right lateral, and posterior septum. In sinus rhythm and some degree of preexcitation, the type or location can be approximated by noting the direction of the dominant QRS complex deflection in the right precordial leads (V_1 and V_2). Type A (above the isoelectric baseline) is characterized by a dominant R wave in leads V_1 and V_2 and suggests an accessory pathway of the left side (posteroseptal, left lateral). Type B (below the isoelectric baseline) is characterized by a dominant QS complex or S wave in leads V_1 and V_2, suggesting an accessory pathway of the right side, or right lateral (Figure 47-36). Septal pathways also are encountered, but localization depends on a QRS complex produced by maximal preexcitation. Remaining accessory pathways are considered concealed or latent.

■ ■ ■

TABLE 47-6 DIFFERENTIATION OF ACCESSORY PATHWAY SYNDROMES

	WPW SYNDROME	LGL SYNDROME	MAHAIM
Insertion site	Atrioventricular	Atrial-nodal	Nodoventricular
Electrocardiographic findings	Short PR interval, ↑ QRS complex width	Short PR interval, normal QRS complex duration	Normal PR interval, QRS complex yes/no
Delta wave	Yes	No	Yes/no
Altered repolarization	Yes	No	Yes/no

WPW, Wolff-Parkinson-White; *LGL,* Lown-Ganong-Levine.

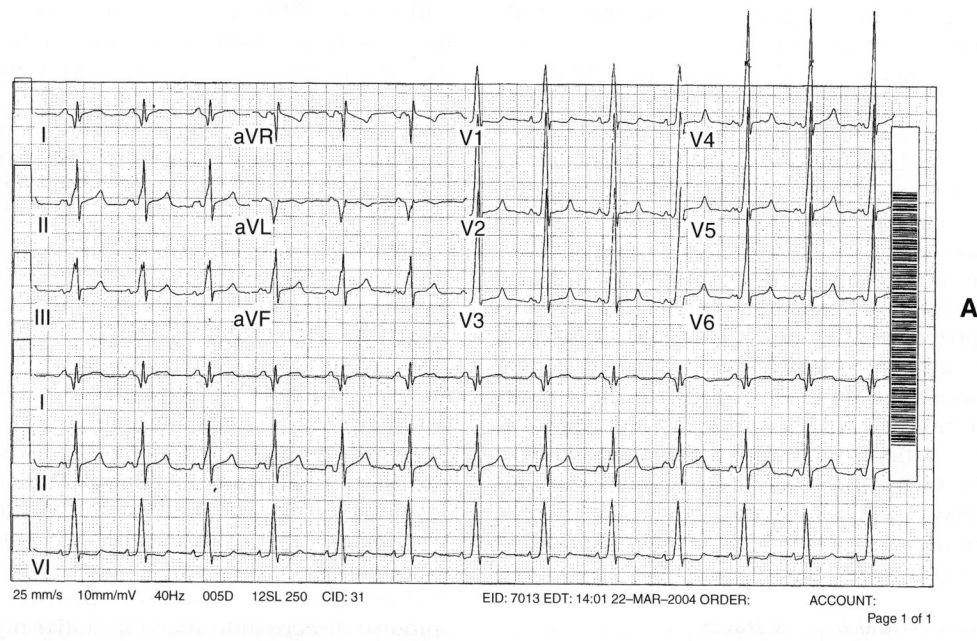

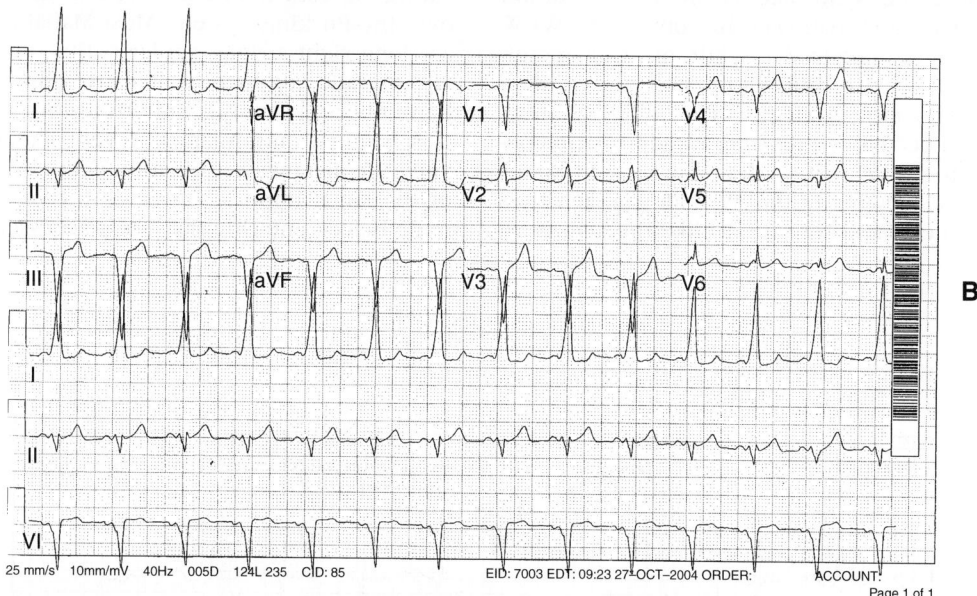

FIGURE 47-36 ▪ **A,** Wolff-Parkinson-White syndrome, type A. Left-sided accessory pathway. Impulse travels left to right, producing a positive QRS complex deflection in lead V_1. **B,** Wolff-Parkinson-White syndrome, type B. Right-sided accessory pathway. Impulse travels from right to left, away from lead V_1, resulting in a negatively deflected QRS complex.

In most accessory pathways, impulse conduction occurs in antegrade (forward) and retrograde (reverse) directions, and the presence of a secondary conduction pathway can facilitate reentrant dysrhythmia conduction. Circuitous rhythms can develop when antegrade transmission occurs over one pathway, and retrograde conduction occurs over the second. As a result, a looping or reciprocating tachycardia can develop. The most frequently occurring dysrhythmias in patients with WPW syndrome are orthodromic tachy-

cardias, which use the AV node in an anterograde fashion and the accessory pathway in a retrograde fashion, and atrial fibrillation, which is discussed in Chapter 48.

Orthodromic tachycardias manifest in narrow QRS complexes as antegrade conduction occurs over the AV node, and the accessory pathway limb transmits the impulse retrogradely back to the atria. Antidromic tachycardias have wide QRS complexes when the conduction loop functions in reverse (the accessory pathway limb conducts the antegrade impulse and the AV node provides the retrograde limb).[83,84]

Accessory pathways are not able to regulate or reduce the speed of impulses transmitted to the ventricular myocardium. As a result, the presence of atrial ectopic rhythms, such as atrial fibrillation combined with antegrade accessory pathway conduction, can be fatal when rapid atrial impulses are conducted directly into the ventricular myocardium. Because the ventricle is unable to sustain a prolonged response to the rapidly transmitted atrial impulses, the rhythm rapidly deteriorates to ventricular fibrillation. In unusual circumstances, two accessory pathways may be involved in antegrade conduction. In atrial fibrillation, this can result in the transmission of fibrillatory impulses over both pathways. Patients with WPW syndrome who have wide-complex tachycardias usually require direct current cardioversion and subsequent catheter ablation of the accessory pathway. Postablation changes are noted easily on the postprocedure ECG.

Atrioventricular Nodal Bypass Tracts

Lown-Ganong-Levine syndrome is another condition involving an accessory pathway. In contrast to WPW syndrome, Lown-Ganong-Levine syndrome is characterized by normal P wave, a short PR interval, and *normal* QRS complex morphology (Figure 47-37). The abbreviated PR interval occurs as a result of rapid impulse conduction over the accessory pathway, which bypasses the physiological slowing of the AV node and activates ventricular tissue at a faster rate. Unlike the accessory pathway of WPW syndrome that usually terminates in the ventricular myocardium and causes QRS complex distortion, the bypass tract of Lown-Ganong-Levine syndrome arises in the atria and terminates in the distal AV node or His bundle region. With this anatomy, the impulse exits the accessory pathway and reenters the normal conduction pathways, activating the ventricle in the normal fashion. As a result, the QRS complex configuration remains unaffected. The presence of this secondary conductive pathway can facilitate reentrant impulse formation and reciprocating tachycardias, similar to that of the Kent bundles in WPW syndrome.[67]

Nodoventricular or Fasciculoventricular Tracts

Another form of congenital preexcitation occurs in the presence of anomalous conductive tissue that arises in the distal AV node or His Bundle. The impulse bypasses the intraventricular fascicles and Purkinje system and terminates in a localized area of ventricular myocardium. These filamentous bypass tracts are known as Mahaim fibers. The accessory pathway propagates the impulse directly into the ventricular myocardium, activating the issue before the normal sinus impulse arrives over the Purkinje system. Most Mahaim fiber pathways are long right atriofascicular pathways capable of only anterograde conduction. Because conduction over Mahaim fibers is variable and often slow, impulse conduction results in minimal or no ventricular preexcitation, and little delta wave formation occurs. Because the path of the sinus impulse traverses the majority of the AV node before entering the nodal accessory pathway, the

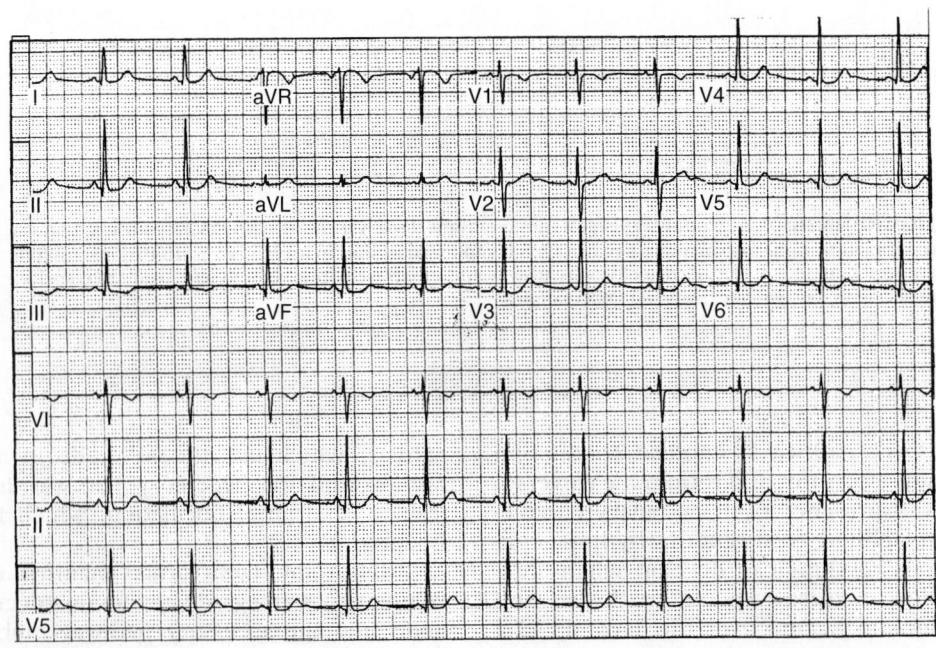

FIGURE 47-37 ■ Lowa-Ganong-Levine (LGL) syndrome. Electrocardiogram illustrating the short PR interval and normal QRS complex typical of the syndrome. (From Eichholz A, Whiting RB, Artal R: *Obstet Gynecol* 102:1393-1395, 2003.)

physiological PR interval is maintained. Mahaim fibers are suspected when narrow QRS complexes and rS patterns in lead III are found in resting ECGs of patients with known tachydysrhythmias (Figure 47-38).[67]

Arrhythmogenic Right Ventricular Dysplasia

ARVD is an inherited progressive condition that typically manifests in young adults and is associated with malignant dysrhythmias.[85] Histologically, ARVD is characterized by fibro-fatty replacement of RV myocardium. Islands of functional myocytes become surrounded by fat, which impedes the transmission of electrical current and subsequent cellular excitation. As ARVD evolves, the clinical presentation involves recurring VT, ventricular fibrillation, and SCD.

On the ECG of ARVD, precordial lead T wave inversion, QT interval prolongation, excessive ventricular ectopic complexes (more than 1000 per day), and LBBB pattern VT often are seen. The presence of fat impedes impulse transmission and causes late activation of the RV myocardium. In ARVD, delayed RV activation manifests on the ECG as a small electrical potential *(epsilon wave)* in the terminal portion of the QRS complex (Figure 47-39). The epsilon wave typically is followed by a saddle-back type of ST segment and functionally can increase the QT interval. Epsilon waves are appreciated best in the QRS complexes of precordial leads V_1 and V_2 but also can be seen in leads V_1 to V_4.

Dextrocardia

The most common form of dextrocardia, congenital malposition of the heart in the right side of the chest, is referred to as "mirror image" dextrocardia. In this form the heart is impeccably reversed, with the apex pointing toward the right, and the left atrium and left ventricle situated to the right side of the right heart chambers. Over the left precordium, starting with a tall R wave in V_1, the ECG typically demonstrates QRS complexes that decrease in amplitude, with normal R wave progression in the right precordial leads (V_4R to V_6R).[21] Several leads demonstrate reversal of normal ECG patterns. In lead I the P wave and QRS complex are negatively deflected. Lead aVR demonstrates an upright QRS complex, whereas leads aVL, II, and III are reversed with negatively deflected QRS complexes.[17] Repolarization abnormalities may be seen in dextrocardia if LVH is present. Using the ECG to determine the site of coronary artery occlusion in a patient with dextrocardia and acute MI can be challenging and usually requires reversal of lead placement to locate the culprit vessel.[86] Technical dextrocardia, the artifactual result of arm lead reversal, can be distinguished from true dextrocardia by the presence of normal R wave progression and related ECG patterns in the precordial leads (see Electrocardiographic Artifacts)[17]

Cardiac Transplant

Cardiac transplant is orthotopic (donor heart replaces the native heart) or heterotopic (donor heart is "piggybacked" onto the native heart; Figure 47-40). Originally, the surgical approach to orthotopic implantation involved the removal of the native heart, leaving remnants of right and left posterior atrial walls for anastamosis and anchoring of the donor heart. Under these circumstances, the sinus node of the recipient's remnant right atrial wall remains functional, although the impulse does not cross the suture line of the recipient and donor tissues. The sinus node of the transplanted donor heart assumes chronotropic command with its automatic rate, and as a result, it is not uncommon to see two distinct P waves and one QRS-T wave complex on the ECG in these patients. The first P wave, generated by the depolarization of the native sinus node and remnant atrial tissue, remains dissociated from the donor P-QRS-T complex. Recent adaptations in transplantation techniques now involve the total removal of the native right atrium using the inferior vena cava and superior vena cava for anastamosis but continue to leave the posterior wall of the left atrium intact for anastamosis of the left side. When the native right atrium is removed, there is usually little or no incipient sinus or atrial activity generated on the surface ECG.

Complete or incomplete RBBB patterns are seen on the transplant ECG in between 12 and 79 percent of recipients. RBBB is related to postoperative positional factors or to right ventricular damage or dysfunction. In isolated cases, WPW syndrome has been observed posttransplant as a result of a concealed bypass tract in the donor heart.[87] Although atrial and ventricular dysrhythmias commonly are found during acute cardiac allograft rejection, increased QTd is not always apparent.[88]

Heterotopic heart transplantation usually is reserved for patients with end-stage heart failure and severe, fixed pulmonary hypertension. Because the donor heart is implanted on the right side of the chest, selective analysis of donor and native heart rhythms is possible by evaluating an ECG of the right side. In this setting, right precordial chest leads more accurately reflect donor heart activity, whereas left chest leads demonstrate native heart rhythms.[89]

Intraventricular Conduction Defects

In electrocardiography, time is width and force is height. The duration or width of the QRS complex corresponds to the time required for the impulse to initiate travel over the intraventricular conduction pathways and to complete ventricular depolarization. Normal ventricular depolarization is rapid and occurs in three phases—septal wall, RV free wall, and LV free wall—although the near simultaneous depolarization of the right and left ventricular free walls is considered one phase. The resulting normal QRS complex is a narrow complex 6 to 11 msec in duration.

In the presence of RBBB, impulse conduction over the right bundle branch is functionally blocked and RV activation is delayed until after the completion of LV activation (Figure 47-41 and Table 47-7). Because RBBB does not affect septal depolarization, the initial impulse depolarizes the ventricular septum from left to right. As a result, the initial vector remains intact and the left-to-right wave current of ventricular depolarization remains

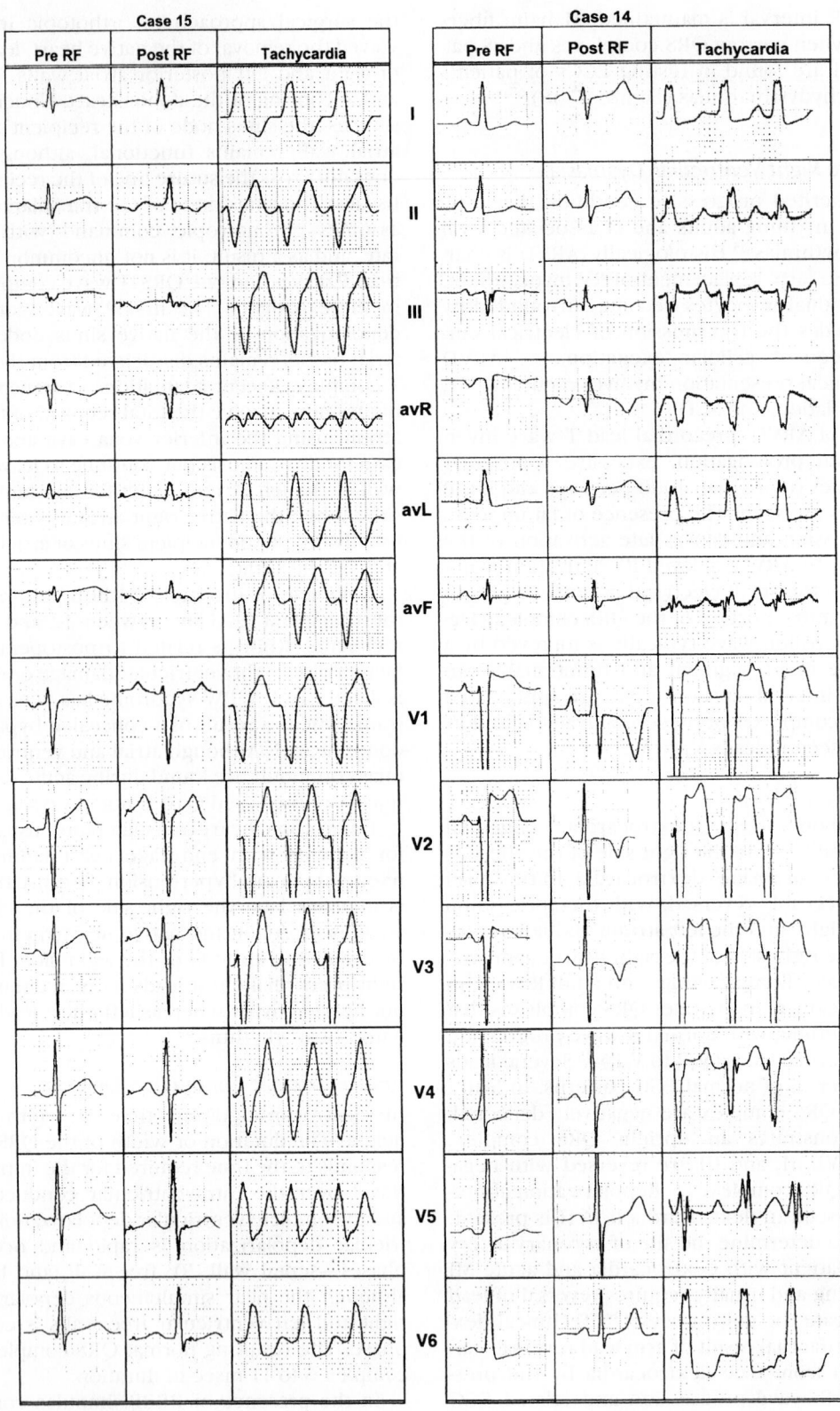

FIGURE 47-38 ■ Two patients with Mahaim fibers displaying the rS pattern in electrocardiogram lead III. *RF*, Radiofrequency ablation. (From Sternick EB: *J Am Coll Cardiol* 44:1626-1635, 2004.)

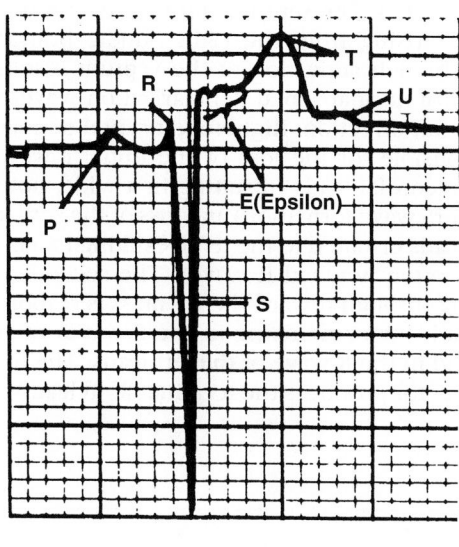

Lead V₃

FIGURE 47-39 ▥ Epsilon wave is common in patients with arrhythmogenic right ventricular dysplasia and also is seen in other diseases of the right ventricle. (From Hurst JW: *Circulation* 98[18]:1937-1942, 1998.)

unchanged. Thus leads V_1 and aVR, positioned over the RV, register an initial r wave; similarly, a q wave is formed in the leads oriented to the left (leads I, aVL, V_5, and V_6). Because the second vector normally generated by the right bundle branch does not conduct, forces are directed leftward as the LV depolarizes, and an S wave in leads V_1 and V_2 is observed. The final vector reflects late and unopposed RV depolarization. This results in a large, wide second R wave (R′), where the R′ is larger than the initial septal r wave in lead V_1 or V_2. As a result of the rSR′ configuration, the QRS complex in lead V_1 often appears as a bizarre "M" shape. In the leftward leads (I, aVL, V_5, and V_6), this terminal delay results in a slurred or widened S wave (greater than 40 msec).[90,71]

Anteroseptal wall MI causes necrotic septal tissue that is electrically silent. In anteroseptal wall MI combined with RBBB, initial forces are directed leftward, producing an initial q wave in place of the normal r wave (producing a qR pattern) in the right precordial leads. Septal q waves normally seen in the left precordial leads also are lost. RBBB itself usually does not affect the electrical axis; therefore, an axis deviation in the presence of a RBBB suggests additional pathological conditions, such as RV hypertrophy.[90,71]

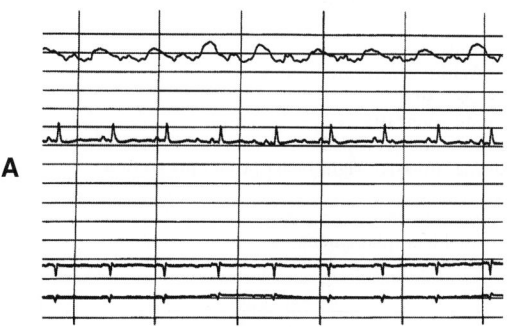

A

FIGURE 47-40 ▥ **A,** Orthotopic transplanted heart (biatrial anastamosis). Note dissociated native P waves marching through the consistent donor P-QRS-T complex and sinus rhythm. Original electrocardiogram strip. **B,** Heterotopic or "piggyback" transplanted heart. Note two separate rhythms and two separate QRS complexes. In the limb leads, the donor heart generates the narrow QRS complexes (75 beats/min) and the native heart generates the wide QRS complexes with left axis deviation and intraventricular conduction delay (80 beats/min). Each QRS complex is generated by the individual hearts. Axis deviation reflects the altered positioning of the transplanted heart.

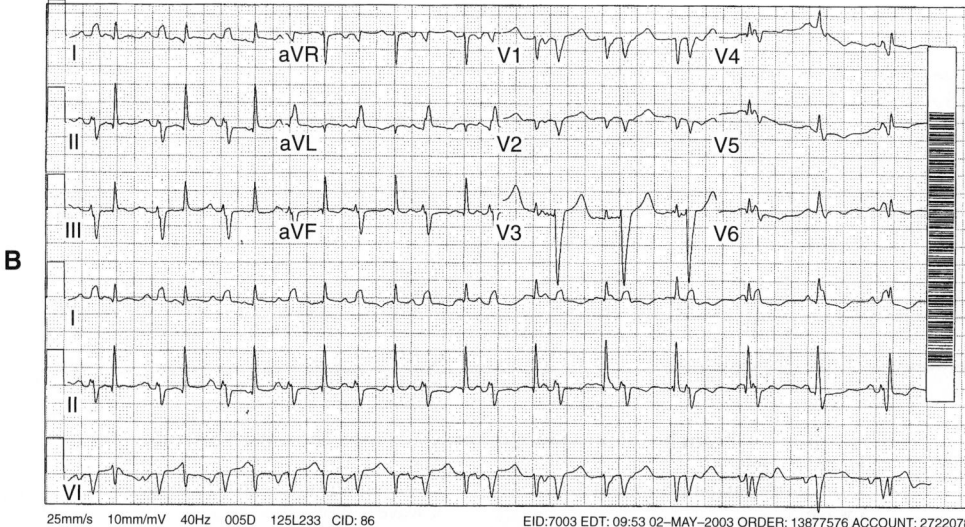

B

25mm/s   10mm/mV   40Hz   005D   125L233   CID: 86   EID:7003 EDT: 09:53 02–MAY–2003 ORDER: 13877576 ACCOUNT: 2722078
                                                                                                Page 1 of 1

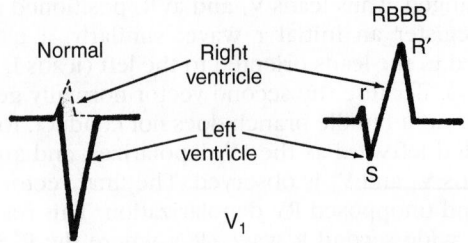

FIGURE 47-41 ▓ The ventricular complex of right bundle branch block compared with the normal complex in lead V1. The *dotted lines* indicate hidden events on the electrocardiogram. Right ventricular activation normally is obscured by left ventricular activation. *RBBB,* Right bundle branch block. (From Conover MB: *Understanding electrocardiography,* ed 8, St Louis, 2003, Mosby.)

than 12 msec). The septum and LV are activated by the impulse arising from the right bundle branch. Right bundle branch activation of the septum results in the reversal of normal septal depolarization wavefront in a right-to-left direction. Right-to-left septal depolarization is responsible for the loss of the initial r wave in the right precordial leads (resulting in a wide, notched QS wave or rS wave formation) and loss of the septal q wave in the leads oriented to the left (resulting in a monophasic and often notched R wave). The secondary vector traveling through toward the RV mass is responsible for the small slur or notching in the S waves of the right leads and in the R wave of the left leads. The final right-to-left vector produces the terminal R′ in lead V_6 (Figure 47-43).

In RBBB, the total QRS complex duration is usually greater than 12 msec with an intrinsicoid deflection of usually greater than 5 msec in the right precordial leads. Even with predetermined criteria for RBBB, there is still significant variation in the RBBB QRS complex morphologies within the general population (Figure 47-42).

In RBBB, when LV activation precedes RV activation (left-to-right depolarization), recovery patterns occur in the same general left-to-right direction. Concordant ST-T waves can be found in the leads reflecting predominant leftward forces (with upright QRS complexes in leads aVL, I, V_5, and V_6), whereas discordant ST-T waves are found in the leads that reflect predominant rightward activity (with negative QRS complexes in leads aVR, V_1, and V_2). RBBB can be found in numerous pathological conditions (Box 47-7) and in persons with no evidence of structural or functional heart disease.

When QRS complex morphology characteristics meet diagnostic criteria for RBBB, but the QRS complex duration is less than 11 msec, this usually is referred to as incomplete RBBB.

LBBB causes a delay in LV depolarization and produces medial prolongation of the QRS complex (greater

---

BOX 47-7 ▪ ▪ ▪
CONDITIONS COMMONLY ASSOCIATED WITH RIGHT BUNDLE BRANCH BLOCK

- Ischemia
- Right ventricular hypertrophy/right ventricular overload
- Cor pulmonale
- Brugada syndrome
- Cardiomyopathy
- Acute massive pulmonary embolism
- Hypertension
- Myocarditis
- Chagas disease
- Physiological (age)
- Congenital (atrial septal defect)
- Degenerative disease
- Rheumatic heart disease
- Wolff-Parkinson-White syndrome type A
- Chronic airway disease
- Orthotopic cardiac allografts
- Tricyclic antidepressant overdose
- Mechanical trauma (invasive right-heart procedures/open heart surgeries)
- Premature ectopic impulses
- Incorrect precordial lead placement
- Straight back syndrome
- Atrial septal defect

TABLE 47-7   Q-R-S DEFLECTIONS AND VENTRICULAR ACTIVATION: NORMAL AND IN BUNDLE BRANCH BLOCKS

DEFLECTION/ACTIVATION	LOCATION	
	RIGHTWARD LEADS (V_1, V_2)	LEFTWARD LEADS (aVL, I, V_5, V_6)
Normal: QRS Complex ≤0.10 Second		
Depolarization of septum (normal)	r wave	q wave
Depolarization of ventricles	S wave	R wave
Right Bundle Branch Block: QRS Complex Greater Than 0.12 Second		
Depolarization of septum (normal)	r wave	q wave
Depolarization of left ventricle	Diminished S wave	R wave
Depolarization of right ventricle	R′ wave	Slurred, wide S wave
Left Bundle Branch Block: QRS Complex Greater Than 0.12 Second		
Depolarization of septum (abnormal)	Absent r wave	Absent q wave
Depolarization of right ventricle	S wave with small positive notch	R wave with small negative notch
Depolarization of left ventricle	S wave	R wave

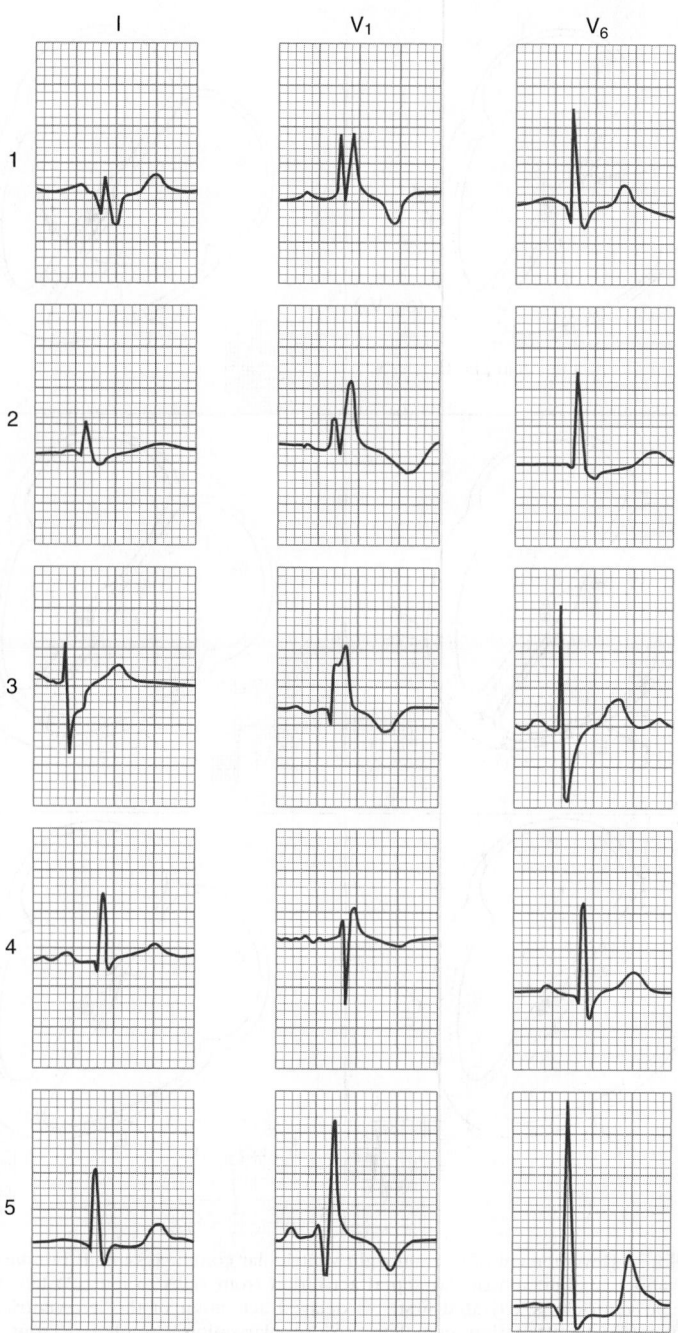

FIGURE 47-42 ▧ Electrocardiogram patterns in five patients with right bundle branch block. (From Agarwal AK: *Int J Cardiol* 71:33-39, 1999.)

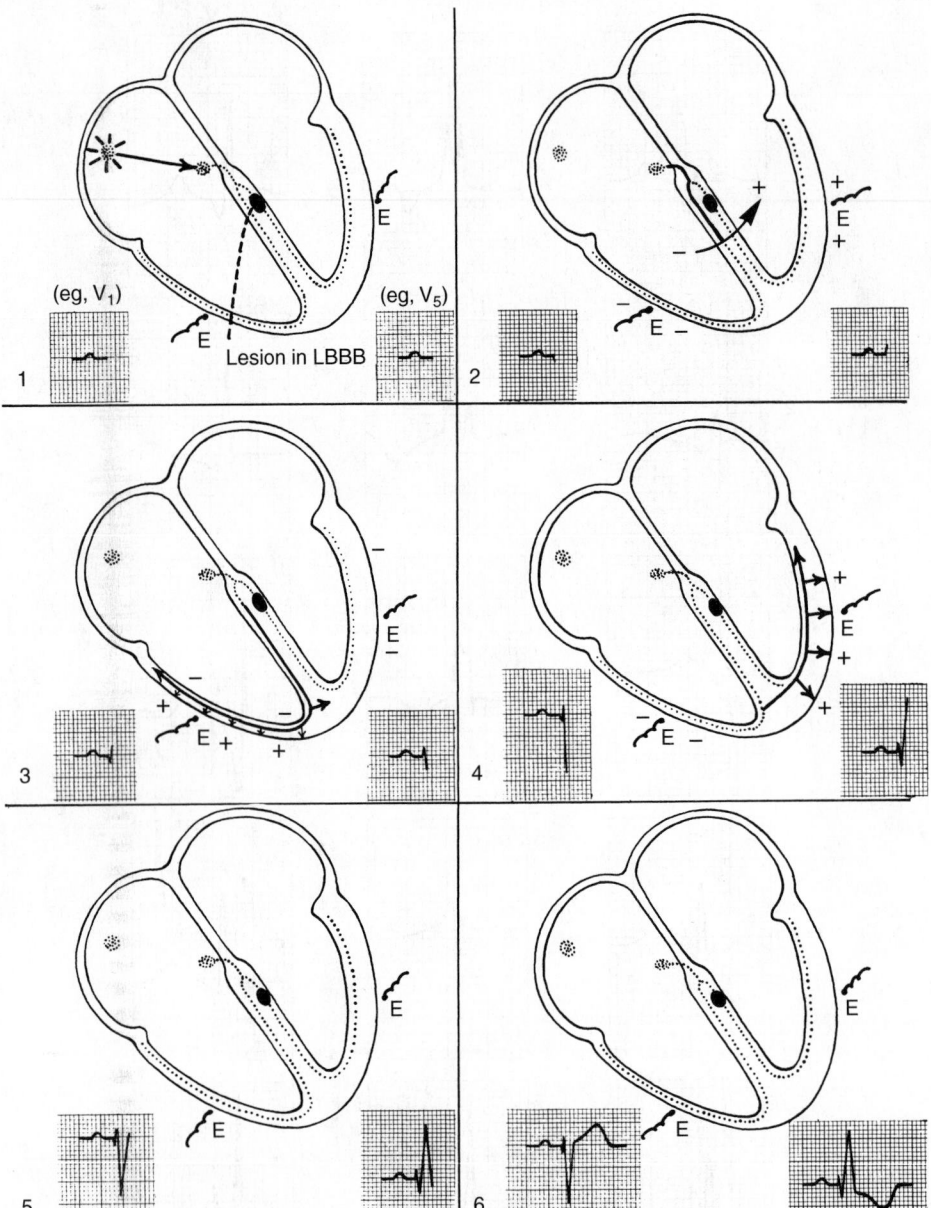

FIGURE 47-43 ■ Development of left and right ventricular complexes in left bundle branch block. (1) Atrial activation; (2) interventricular septal activation from right to left; (3) left bundle branch blocked, so right ventricle is activated first; (4) delayed activation of the left ventricle around the blocked bundle; (5) depolarization complete; (6) repolarization complete. (From Goldman MJ: *Principles of electrocardiography,* ed 10, Los Altos, Calif, 1979, Lange Publications. Reproduced with permission.)

Abnormal depolarization patterns inherent in LBBB electrophysiology result in deranged repolarization. Leads with a predominantly negative QRS complex display STE with positive T waves. Because the RV is activated first in LBBB, the repolarizing currents proceed in a right-to-left direction. As a result, ST-T wave vectors are discordant to the QRS complexes in the right and left precordial leads and in leads I and aVL. Across the right and midprecordial leads, there is usually poor R wave progression. The dominant electrical axis may remain normal or may shift leftward; in some cases, LBBB has been associated with right axis deviation.[72]

The presence of LBBB during ischemia reduces the diagnostic sensitivity of the ECG for MI because LBBB produces many of the same repolarization abnormalities (STE, STD, tall T waves). In LBBB, secondary ST-T wave changes are shifted to the opposite direction of the major QRS complex vector (discordant). In LBBB, when ST-T waves become concordant, this change is highly suggestive of concurrent AMI. Certain criteria have been suggested to help diagnose MI in the setting of LBBB, although none are reliable. These include inappropriate ST concordance (STE greater than 0.1 mV in leads with upright QRS complexes, or STD less than 0.1 mV in leads V_1 to V_3 where there is a negative predominance of the QRS complex), or extreme STE (0.5 mV) discordant to the QRS complex in lead V_1, V_2 or V_3.[71]

Incomplete LBBB produces an ECG pattern similar to that of LBBB except for a narrower QRS complex (duration usually less than 0.12 second).[71]

Nonspecific Intraventricular Conduction Delay

When a QRS complex is greater than 11 msec without satisfying criteria for RBBB or LBBB, further differentiation should be considered. A delay in impulse propagation within the inferoposterior or the anterosuperior fascicle of the left bundle causes a shift in LV activation referred to as a hemiblock. Conduction delay within the left anterosuperior fascicle is referred to as a LAH, and delay within the left inferoposterior fascicle is referred to as a left posterior hemiblock **(LPH).**

Left Anterior Hemiblock. Because of its anatomical features and single blood supply, the anterosuperior fascicle is more prone to damage from ischemia (commonly LAD artery occlusion and anteroseptal wall MI, and less often, an RCA occlusion and inferior wall MI) or fibrotic processes resulting from chronic cardiac conditions such as LVH and cardiomyopathy. In LAH, the electrically unopposed impulse exits the inferoposterior fascicle at the level of the posterior papillary muscle and inferior LV region. Because LV septal and inferior wall activation proceeds in a superior-to-inferior and left-to-right fashion, the initial q wave in the left lateral leads (I and aVL) and a small r wave (less than 0.4 mV in lead III) in the inferior leads (II, III, and aVF) are preserved. Depolarization proceeds in an upward and superior left direction where activation of the remaining anterolateral LV occurs via interconnecting Purkinje fibers distal to the lesion. Activation of the myocardium in this manner shifts the major electrical wavefront or

axis, upward and left anywhere from −45 to −90 degrees (Figure 47-44). As a result of this leftward and superior shift, a predominant negative deflection (rS pattern) is displayed in the inferior leads (II, III, and aVF), and a qR pattern is seen in the left lateral leads (I and aVL). Although other pathological conditions can lead to a superior and left axis shift (inferior wall MI, RV apical pacing), the superior-left axis shift with an rS pattern in the inferior leads is the ECG hallmark of LAH. In isolated LAH, ventricular activation remains unaffected and the QRS complex duration is in normal range; the presence of concomitant fascicular delay (RBBB) may cause an increase in ventricular activation and a widened QRS complex, which is suggestive of bifascicular conduction block (see the following discussion).[71]

When inferior wall MI occurs with LAH, the initial small r wave seen in inferior leads II, III, and aVF is lost and a QS pattern is displayed. In lead I the initial q wave is lost, resulting in the formation of an R wave. RV apical pacing also can cause an abnormal left superior axis, but a LBBB-like QRS complex pattern, preceded by pacemaker spikes, will be present on the ECG.

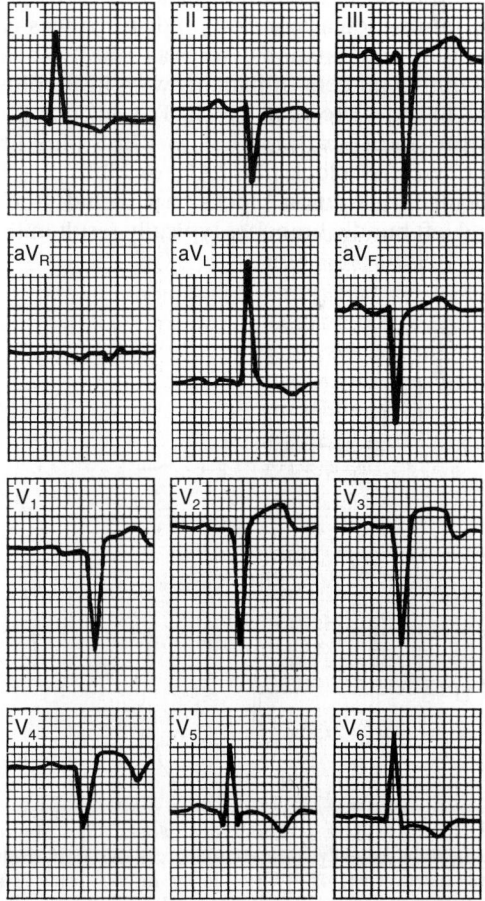

FIGURE 47-44 ■ Left anterior hemiblock in a patient with acute anterior myocardial infarction. Note the abnormal left axis deviation (greater than −30 degrees), the normal QRS complex duration, and the q waves in leads I and aVL. (From Conover MB: *Understanding electrocardiography,* ed 8, St Louis, 2003, Mosby.)

Left Posterior Hemiblock. The inferoposterior fascicle is less vulnerable to injury or insult than the anterosuperior fascicle, so LPH is rare. The diagnosis of LPH is made only after excluding RV hypertrophy and COPD, for these are the more common conditions associated with right axis deviation.

In LPH, initial LV activation occurs primarily through the anterosuperior fascicle, which first depolarizes the anterosuperior LV free wall. These initial superior and leftward forces generate an r wave in the lateral limb leads (I, aVL) and a q wave in the inferior leads (II, III, aVF). Sequential activation of the inferoposterior fascicle and inferior-posterior LV regions occurs via Purkinje fiber interconnections distal to the lesion. The resulting predominant rightward and inferior wavefront causes an axis shift ranging from +90 to +120 degrees and terminal changes in the QRS complex (S wave in lead I and aVL [rS pattern] and an R wave [qR pattern] in leads II, III, and aVF; Figure 47-45).[90-91] Because a frontal QRS axis shift of +110 degrees can encompass a broad range of related conditions (RV hypertrophy, lateral wall MI), it is difficult to ascribe LPH as the cause of the right axis shift without clinical or echocardiographic correlation.

Conduction delays that occur in more than one site are referred to as bifascicular or trifascicular blocks. Although the most common bifascicular block is RBBB plus LAH, bifascicular conduction disturbances can occur in other combinations, such as RBBB block plus LPH. About 10 percent of patients with RBBB plus LAH progress to complete heart block. Trifascicular conduction disturbances can manifest as RBBB plus first- or second-degree AV block plus LAH, or LBBB plus RBBB. Trifascicular conduction blocks that include the main right and left bundle branches typically result in the loss of AV conduction, and a ventricular escape rhythm usually is seen. Multifascicular conduction blocks generally are observed in ischemia and in chronic cardiac disease states.

Rate-related bundle branch conduction delays can occur during tachycardias or bradycardias and can involve the right bundle branch or left bundle branch. High heart rates result in bundle branch block when rapid incoming impulses arrive near or during the refractory period of the vulnerable fascicle. Physiologically, the right bundle branch is more prone to tachycardia-induced delays because of its inherently slower conduction, longer refractory period, and longer fiber length. Rate-related RBBB often manifests in an incomplete RBBB pattern. Bradycardia-related conduction delays can occur but are not common. The cause of bradycardia-induced bundle branch block is not clear, although extensive conduction system disease usually is involved.[71,90,91]

Atrial Chamber Abnormalities

Generally, changes within the atria alter the morphology, duration, and amplitude of the P wave. When right atrial wall mass or chamber size increases, the electrical force of the larger chamber predominates over the forces of the more normal LA chamber, altering the P wave morphology in a characteristic manner. Maladaptive structural or functional change of the right atria can be categorized as right atrial abnormalities (from pulmonary disease such as COPD, PE, and emphysema) and hypertrophic changes from pressure overload (tricuspid valve stenosis and regurgitation, pulmonary valve stenosis, pulmonary hypertension, RV hypertrophy, and some forms of congenital heart conditions). The degree of P wave amplitude and right axis shift, in addition to other ECG patterns of pulmonary disease (low QRS complex voltage, right axis shift, incomplete RBBB, S1Q3T3 pattern) may help to differentiate and quantify the extent of the accompanying lung disease. Characteristic P wave changes of P pulmonale may be observed transiently in acute PE.[1,72]

In right atrial abnormality, the P wave amplitude in leads II, III, and aVF typically increases (0.25 mV) to form a tall P waveform, often referred to as P pulmonale. Prominence of an upright component of the biphasic P wave in leads V_1 to V_3 (greater than 0.15 mV) is specific to right atrial hypertrophy. Although the P pulmonale patterns of lead II are not as specific for right atrial hypertrophy as the changes in the right chest leads, many conditions do not manifest changes in the right leads. In atrial abnormalities, atrial repolarization also is pronounced (Ta wave) but is obscured by the QRS complex, and the mean P wave axis shifts rightward (greater than +75 degrees).[92]

In LA abnormality, alteration of the P wave results from an increased LA wall mass or an enlarged LA chamber, an ECG finding with 40 percent sensitivity and 90 percent specificity. LA abnormality often is compounded by intraatrial conduction delays. Because the left atrium is normally last to depolarize, an increase in electrical force further broadens the P wave. LA abnormality,

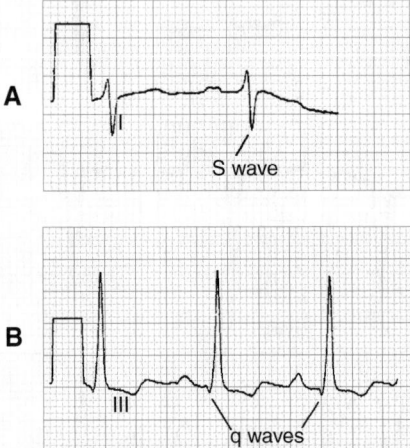

FIGURE 47-45 ▦ Left posterior hemiblock. Sinus rhythm (90 beats/min); right axis deviation +110 degrees (**A**); rS in leads I and aVL; initial negative vector (q wave) in the inferior leads II, III, and aVF (**B**) with T wave inversion; and evidence of incomplete left bundle branch block (absent small q waves in leads V5 and V6; slightly broad QRS complexes). Patient had no history of right ventricular hypertrophy or inferior wall myocardial infarction. (From Jenkins D, Gerred S: *ECGs by example*, ed 2, Edinburgh, 2005, Churchill Livingstone.)

when compounded by an intraatrial conduction delay, pushes the LA component of the P wave out further, causing a notched or double-humped M-shaped P wave with a duration of greater than 120 msec, and a shortened interval between the P wave and QRS complex. In lead V_1, the trough, or negative portion of the biphasic P wave, becomes more prominent (greater than 0.1 mV; Figure 47-46) and the mean P wave axis is shifted leftward (greater than −30 to +45 degrees). LA abnormalities are associated with conditions that cause LV enlargement or hypertrophy (systemic hypertension, mitral regurgitation, hypertrophic cardiomyopathy).[82,92]

ECG evidence of biatrial enlargement includes a large biphasic P wave in lead V_1. The positive component of this P wave is usually greater than 0.15 mV, and the terminal negative component is usually 0.1 mV in depth. The duration of the composite P wave is usually equal to 4 msec. P wave notching is evident in the left precordial leads (V_4 to V_6), and limb lead P waves demonstrate increased amplitude (0.25 mV) and duration (12 msec).

Ventricular Chamber Enlargement

Enlargement and structural alteration of the myocardium usually results from chronic states of volume or pressure overload and neurohormonal hyperactivity. ECG manifestations of systolic overload and increased LV mass are increased QRS complex voltage, STD, and T wave inversions in the left precordial leads. Chronic states of high volume (valvular regurgitation and heart failure) can cause wall stress. Constant diastolic wall stress results in dilatation, or stretching of the ventricular chamber. On the ECG, eccentric hypertrophy manifests in tall R waves in the left precordial leads.

Under normal conditions, RV activation is not appreciated on the surface ECG. In pathological states, when a significant increase in RV mass occurs, the stronger potentials of the hypertrophied myocytes generate higher QRS complex voltages that are reflected on the surface ECG. Because the increased RV mass also prolongs the impulse wavefront, the completion of RV activation occurs following completion of LV activation. This alteration in ventricular activation times causes merging of the RV activation curve with the LV curve, instead of being cancelled by it. The increase in RV mass not only alters the waveform pattern but also redirects major cardiac vectors in a rightward direction, causing right axis shift. Because of the more anterior position of the RV, the most prominent changes are appreciated in leads oriented toward the right.[1,8]

Because of the low sensitivity and high specificity of ECG change in RV hypertrophy, the diagnosis of RV hypertrophy is difficult to confirm by ECG. Although several criteria exist to help determine the presence of RV hypertrophy, not all cases of increased QRS complex voltage are considered pathological (athletes, persons younger than 30 years; Box 47-8).[42,92,93] In addition, several nonhypertrophic conditions also produce R waves in lead V_1 (WPW syndrome type A, posterior wall MI, dextrocardia, or RBBB) or right axis deviation (LPH, lateral wall MI). With a dominant R wave in lead V_1 and right axis deviation, clinical and ECG correlation is necessary to confirm the presence of RV hypertrophy or underlying pathological condition.

In minor degrees of RV hypertrophy, little to no ECG change may be seen. In more severe degrees of RV hypertrophy (pulmonary stenosis, pulmonary hypertension), large R waves can be seen in leads oriented toward the right (leads V_1, V_2, and aVR), and deep S waves and abnormally small r waves are seen in leads oriented toward the left (leads I, aVL, and V_4 to V_6).

Myocardial tissue adapts to physiological (athletic conditioning) and pathological (systemic hypertension, aortic stenosis) stress with an increase in functional myocytes and ventricular wall mass. Chronic pressure or volume overload that increases wall stress often triggers this compensatory mechanism. On the ECG, increased LV size results in higher QRS complex voltage patterns because the greater number of electrically active cells promotes a larger surface voltage potential (Figure 47-47). Hypertrophy of the LV may shift the axis leftward, but the vector shift usually remains within the normal left axis region.[93]

In addition to the increased QRS complex voltage produced by the hypertrophied myocardial cells, impulse transmission and LV activation time are delayed in LVH. Delayed LV activation manifests as a widening of the proximal portion of the QRS complex, or intrinsicoid deflection; this delay reflects the additional time required for transmission of the impulse through the thickened ventricular mass.

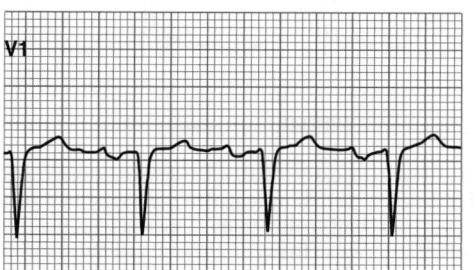

FIGURE 47-46 ■ Lead V_1 shows typical P wave pattern of left atrial enlargement. (From Khan MG: *Rapid ECG interpretation,* ed 2, Philadelphia, 2003, WB Saunders.)

BOX 47-8   ■ ■ ■
ELECTROCARDIOGRAPHIC CRITERIA SUGGESTIVE OF RIGHT VENTRICULAR HYPERTROPHY[92]

R wave (lead V_1) = 0.7 mV, and S wave (leads V_5 and V_6) = 0.7 mV
S1, Q3 pattern
Right axis shift (+90 degrees)
R:S ratio in lead V1 greater than 1, with a negative T wave
qR pattern in lead V_1 (also may be present in right bundle branch block and/or septal wall myocardial infarction)
P pulmonale

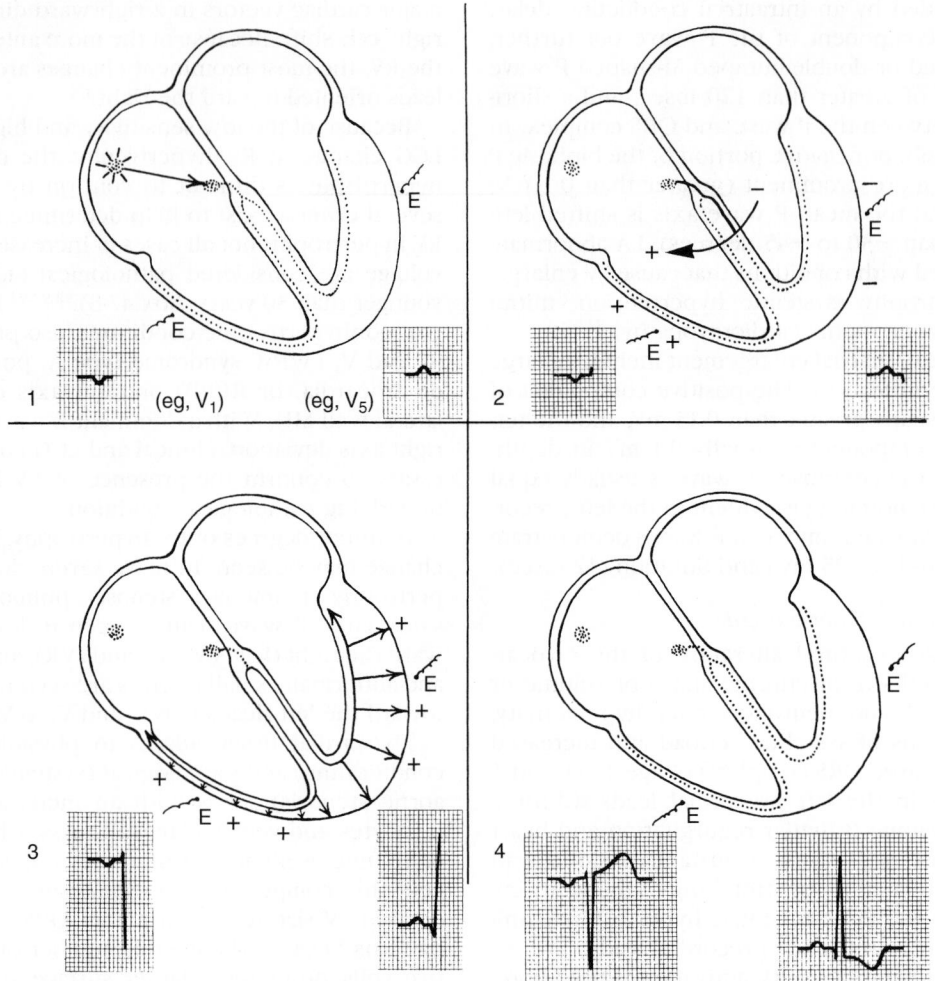

FIGURE 47-47 ■ Left ventricular hypertrophy. (1) Spread of impulse from sinoatrial node to atrioventricular node; (2) activation of interventricular septum; (3) activation of both ventricles; (4) repolarization. (From Goldman MJ: *Principles of electrocardiography,* ed 10, Los Altos, Calif, 1979, Lange Publications.)

LVH can be described by voltage or nonvoltage criteria. The most characteristic voltage pattern of LVH results from the hypertrophied LV mass that increases vector II of LV activation. The ECG pattern of LVH consists of an increase in QRS complex amplitude (tall R waves are 1.1 mV in lead aVL and greater than 2 mV in lead aVF), and deep S waves (greater than 1.4 mV) in leads aVR and V_1 or S waves in lead V_1 and R waves in lead V_5 (or V_6) equal 3.5 mV (Figure 47-48). In LVH, high-amplitude QRS complexes often are accompanied by ST-T wave changes, although the nature and degree of ST segment change vary.

Typically, the STD associated with LVH is asymmetrical and downsloping, with reciprocal STE in the right precordial leads. STD is accompanied by inverted T waves in the left precordial leads (V_4 to V_6) that descend gradually on the proximal limb and rise sharply on the ascending limb *(strain pattern)*. When strain pattern is present in a patient who has chest pain, it complicates

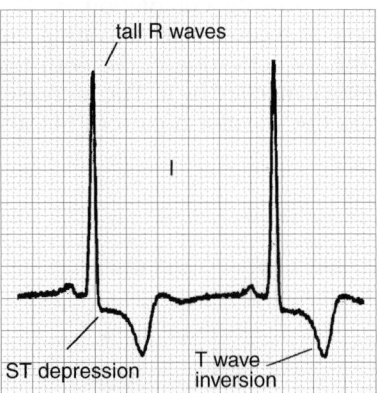

FIGURE 47-48 ■ Left ventricular hypertrophy in a patient with hypertrophic cardiomyopathy. Sinus bradycardia (54 beats/min), features of left ventricular hypertrophy (left axis shift, early electrical transition/dominant R wave in lead V_2, tall R waves in leads aVL and I and left chest leads, deep S waves in lead V_1, widespread ST depression, and T wave inversion). (From Jenkins D, Gerred S: *ECGs by example,* ed 2, Edinburgh, 2005, Churchill Livingstone.)

the ECG evaluation of ischemic ST-T wave change in AMI.[82]

LV chamber enlargement resulting from diastolic or volume overload produces tall, upright T waves and deep but narrow Q waves in the septal leads. Although several criteria and scoring systems for LVH exist, none have been accepted uniformly because of low sensitivity. It remains difficult and imprecise to use voltage criteria to diagnose LVH in individuals under 35 and in blacks because these populations often display high-amplitude QRS complexes with no underlying pathological condition.

Artificial Pacing

A complete discussion of implanted cardiac rhythm management devices is found in Chapter 61. Pacemakers are discussed in this section with respect to their effects on the surface ECG waveforms. When the preprogrammed limits of the sensing function of a pacemaker is triggered by the presence of a slow intrinsic heart rate, the device delivers an electrical current into the myocardial tissue. The ECG records this pacemaker discharge by a sharp spike or pacing artifact before the waveform of the myocardial chamber being paced (P wave, atria; R wave, ventricle). The *electrical* response of the myocardium to the discharge is referred to as capture. Capture is confirmed when the pacing artifact is followed by the presence of a wide, slurred, or notched QRS complex in the presence of ventricular pacing (Figure 47-49), a nonsinus P wave morphology in

atrial pacing, or a nonsinus P wave plus a wide QRS complex morphology in AV sequential pacing.[94]

AV sequential biventricular pacing produces a pacing artifact before atrial activation and before left and right ventricular activation. Because the time between left and right ventricular depolarization is minimal, the resulting complex is a fused biventricular complex.

Analysis of the electrical axis and QRS complex morphology can determine the origin of the dominant electrical forces and the position of the pacing source (Table 47-8). Under physiological conditions, impulses arising in the sinus node are conducted leftward and inferiorly, producing upright QRS complexes in lead I and in leads II and aVF. In contrast, a pacing wire in the RV apex activates the myocardium from the right apex, in a right-to-left and inferior-to-superior direction. As a result, superior and leftward forces produce upright QRS complexes in lead I and negative QRS complexes in leads II and aVF (Figure 47-50).

Inadvertent placement of a pacing lead wire or the migration of a preexisting pacing lead wire to a site other than the RV apex produces significant differences in the vector force and/or lead V₁. If an RV pacing lead dislodges from the apex, the lead typically floats upward into the RV outflow tract. Pacing the RV outflow area continues to activate the heart in a right-to-left direction, but the superiorly repositioned pacing lead produces a more inferior vector as the forces are directed downward toward the apex and a leftward and inferior axis shift. RBBB morphology during *temporary*

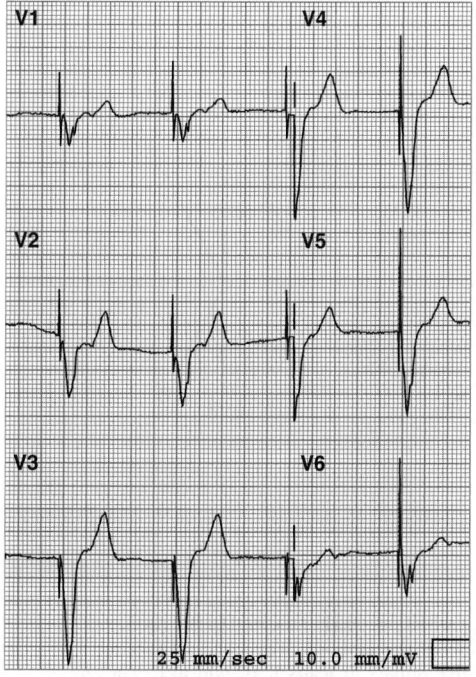

FIGURE 47-49 ■ Electronic pacemaker; ventricular capture rate is 60 beats/min. (From Khan MG: *Rapid ECG interpretation*, ed 2, Philadelphia, 2003, WB Saunders.)

TABLE 47-8 LEAD POSITION AND QRS COMPLEX MORPHOLOGY DURING PACING[94,96]

PACED LEAD POSITION	QRS COMPLEX MORPHOLOGY	ELECTRICAL AXIS
RV apex	LBBB	Superior left
RV inflow tract	LBBB	Normal
RV outflow tract	LBBB	Inferior left or slightly inferior right
Mid or high LV	RBBB	Inferior left or slightly inferior right
Inferior LV	RBBB	Superior left
Coronary sinus	RBBB	Inferior left
Cardiac veins	RBBB	Superior left

RV, Right ventricular; *LBBB,* left bundle branch block; *LV,* left ventricle; *RBBB,* right bundle branch block.

pacing may indicate a pacing wire lodged in the coronary sinus (left-to-right pacing from behind the heart), perforation of the intraventricular septum, or perforation of the venous system into the pericardium, with LV pacing.[94,95]

When LV pacing occurs via a pacing wire introduced into the middle cardiac vein, the posterior-inferior wall of the LV is activated first. Activation of the inferior wall produces a superior vector. Because a portion of the posterior wall is located spatially to the right, the vector shifts to the left. Initial posterior wall activation gener-

ates anterior forces and a positive deflection in leads V_1 and V_2. Pacing the inferolateral wall of the LV occurs when the pacing wire is introduced deep in the middle cardiac vein. This pacing orientation results in a superior right axis deviation and anterior forces causing a positive lead V_1 deflection. Specific ECG criteria (frontal axis and precordial lead transition) can help approximate the position of the pacing wire when a positive lead V_1 deflection occurs during pacing.[96,97] See Chapter 61 for assessment of pacemaker function.

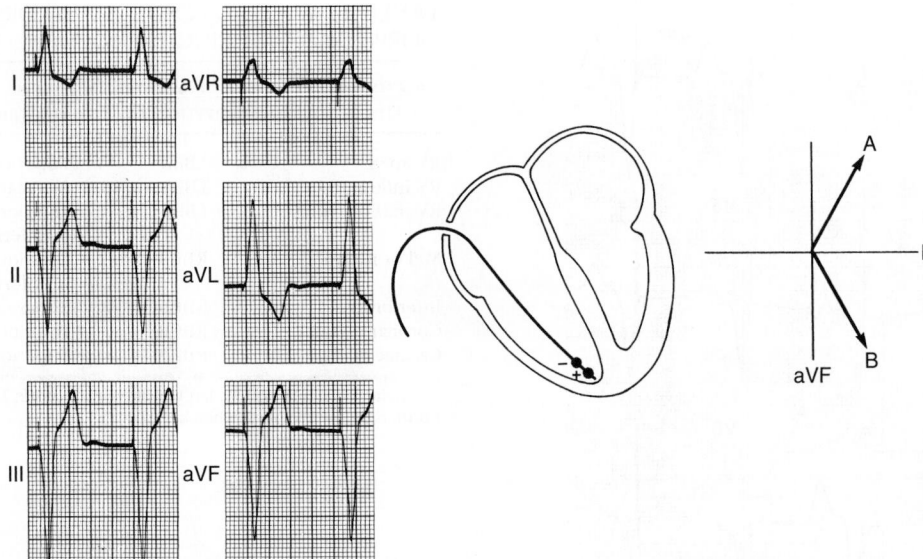

FIGURE 47-50 ▪ Diagram of a bipolar right ventricular endocardial pacemaker located in the proper apical position. Distal pole is the anode, and the proximal pole is the cathode. The pace artifact is oriented leftward and inferiorly *(arrow B),* resulting in positive spikes in leads I, II, and aVF. The myocardium is depolarized leftward and superiorly *(arrow A),* producing upright QRS complexes in leads I and aVL and negative complexes in leads II, III, and aVF. (From Goldman MJ: *Principles of electrocardiography,* ed 10, Los Altos, Calif, 1979, Lange Publications.)

REFERENCES

1. Mirvis DM, Goldberger AL: Electrocardiography. In Zipes DP, Libby P, Bonow RO, Braunwald E, editors: *Heart disease,* ed 7, Philadelphia, 2005, Elsevier Saunders.

2. Brady WJ, Perron AD, Chang T: Electrocardiographic ST-segment elevation: correct identification of acute myocardial infarction (AMI) and non-AMI syndromes by emergency physicians, *Acad Emerg Med* 8:-349, 2001.

3. Carroll R, Sharma N, Butt A et al: Unusual electrocardiographic presentation of an isolated right ventricular myocardial infarction secondary to thrombotic occlusion of a non-dominant right coronary artery: a case report and brief review of literature, *Angiology* 54:5-119, 2003.

4. Gussak I, Antzelevitch C: Early repolarization syndrome: clinical characteristics and possible cellular and ionic mechanisms, *J Electrocardiol* 33:3-299, 2000.

5. Klatsky AL, Oehm R, Cooper RA et al: The early repolarization normal variant electrocardiogram: correlates and consequences, *Am J Med* 115:11-171, 2003.

6. Wang K, Asinger RW, Marriott HJ: ST segment elevation in conditions other than acute myocardial infarction, *N Engl J Med* 349:34-2128, 2003.

7. Hurst JW: Naming of the waves in the ECG, with a brief account of their genesis, *Circulation* 98:9-1937, 1998.

8. Edhouse J, Brady WJ, Morris F: ABC of clinical electrocardiology: acute myocardial infarction—part II, *BMJ* 324:32-963, 2002.

9. Yan GX, Antzelevitch C: Cellular basis for the electrocardiographic J wave, *Circulation* 93:9-372, 1996.

10. ACC/AHA guidelines for the management of patients with ST-elevation myocardial infarction: a report of the American College of Cardiology/American Heart Association Task Force on Practice Guidelines (committee to revise the 1999 guidelines for the management of patients with acute myocardial infarction), *J Am Coll Cardiol* 44(3):E1-E211, 2004.

11. Critical issues in the evaluation and management of adult patients presenting with suspected acute myocardial infarction or unstable angina, *Ann Emerg Med* 35:3-521, 2000.

12. Van Mieghem C, Sabbe M, Knockaert D: The clinical value of the ECG in noncardiac conditions, *Chest* 125:12-1561, 2004.

13. Estes NA III, Link MS, Homoud M et al: ECG findings in active patients: differentiating benign from the serious, The *Physician and Sports Medicine* 29:2-67, 2001.

14. Pelliccia A, Maron B, Culasso F et al: Clinical significance of abnormal electrocardiographic patterns in trained athletes, *Circulation* 102:10-278, 2000.

15. Knight BP, Pelosi F, Michaud GF et al: Physician interpretation of electrocardiographic artifact that mimics ventricular tachycardia, *Am J Med* 110:11-335, 2001.

16. Mattu A, Brady WJ, Perron AD et al: Prominent R wave in lead V1: electrocardiographic differential diagnosis, *Am J Emerg Med* 19:1-504, 2001.

17. Shimizu T, Inomata S, Toyooka H: Artifactual dextrocardia associated with a defect in the ECG labeling, *Anesth Analg* 96:1232, 2003.

18. Chiang C: Congenital and acquired long QT syndrome: current concepts and management, *Cardiol Rev* 12:1-222, 2004.

19. Khan IA: Long QT syndrome: diagnosis and management, *Am Heart J* 143:14, 2002.

20. Drici MD, Barhanin J: Cardiac K channels and drug-acquired long QT syndrome, *Therapie* 55:5-185, 2000.

21. Cheng TO: Digitalis administration: an underappreciated but common cause of short QT interval, *Circulation* 109:e152, 2004.

22. Antzelevitch C, Sun ZQ, Zhang ZQ et al: Cellular and ionic mechanisms underlying erythromycin-induced long QT intervals and torsade de pointes, *J Am Coll Cardiol* 28:2-1836, 1996.

23. Gamouras GA, Monir G, Plunkitt K et al: Cocaine abuse: repolarization abnormalities and ventricular arrhythmias, *Am J Med Sci* 320:32, 2000.

24. Gueron M, Reuben I, Margulis G: Arthropod poisons and the cardiovascular system, *Am J Emerg Med* 18:1-708, 2000.

25. Alan S, Ulgen MS, Soker M et al: Electrocardiographic and echocardiographic features of patients exposed to scorpion bite, *Angiology* 55:5-79, 2004.

26. Gowda RM, Cohen RA, Khan IA: Toad venom poisoning: resemblance to digoxin toxicity and therapeutic implications, *Heart* 89:8-14, 2003.

27. Diercks DB, Shumaik GM, Harrigan RA et al: Electrocardiographic manifestations: electrolyte abnormalities, *J Emerg Med* 27:2-153, 2004.

28. Otero J, Lenihan DJ: The normothermic Osborn wave induced by severe hypercalcemia, *Texas Heart Institute Journal* 27:2-316, 2000.

29. Lange RA, Hillis LD: Acute pericarditis, *N Engl J Med* 351:35-2195, 2004.

30. Slovis C, Jenkins R: ABC of clinical electrocardiography: conditions not primarily affecting the heart, *BMJ* 324:32-1320, 2002.

31. Boccalandro C, Lopez L, Boccalandro F et al: Electrocardiographic changes in thyrotoxic periodic paralysis, *Am J Cardiol* 91:9-775, 2003.

32. Vanderdonckt O, Lambert M, Montero MC et al: The 12-lead electrocardiogram in anorexia nervosa: a report of 2 cases followed by a retrospective study, *J Electrocardiol* 34:3-233, 2001.

33. Alpert MA, Terry BE, Cohen MV et al: The electrocardiogram in morbid obesity, *Am J Cardiol* 85:8-908, 2000.

34. Mattu A, Brady WJ, Peron AD: Electrocardiographic manifestations of hypothermia, *J Emerg Med* 20:2-314, 2002.

35. Strohmer B, Pichler M: Atrial fibrillation and prominent J (Osborn) waves in critical hypothermia, *Int J Cardiol* 96:9-291, 2004.

36. Sakr YL, Lim N, Amaral ACK et al: Relation of ECG changes to neurological outcome in patients with aneurysmal subarachnoid hemorrhage, *Int J Cardiol* 96:9-369, 2004.

37. Peron D, Brady WJ: Electrocardiographic manifestations of CNS events, *Am J Emerg Med* 18:1-715, 2000.

38. Ullman E, Brady WJ, Perron AD et al: Electrocardiographic manifestations of pulmonary embolism, *Am J Emerg Med* 19:1-514, 2001.

39. Huikuri H: Dispersion of repolarisation and the autonomic system: can we predict torsade de pointes? *Cardiovasc Drugs Ther* 16:1-93, 2002.

40. Havranek S, Micek M, Paclt I et al: QT dispersion estimated from 80 body surface potential map leads and from standard 12 leads ECG in psychiatric patients treated with dosulepin, *Sb Lek* 105:10-53, 2004.

41. Ritsema Van Eck HJ, Kors JA, Van Herpen G: The elusive U wave: a simple explanation of its genesis, *J Electrocardiol* 36(suppl):133-137, 2003.

42. Harrigan R, Jones K: ABC of clinical electrocardiography: conditions affecting the right side of the heart, *BMJ* 324:32-1201, 2002.

43. Birnbaum Y, Drew BJ: The electrocardiogram in ST elevation acute myocardial infarction: correlation with coronary anatomy and prognosis, *Postgrad Med J* 79:7-490, 2003.

44. Somers MP, Brady WJ, Perron AD et al: The prominent T wave: electrocardiographic differential diagnosis, *Am J Emerg Med* 20:2-243, 2002.

45. Morris F, Brady WJ, ABC of clinical electrocardiography: acute myocardial infarction—part I, *BMJ* 324:32-831, 2002.

46. Brady WJ, Perron AD, Ullman EA et al: Electrocardiographic ST segment elevation: a comparison of AMI and non-AMI ECG syndromes, *Am J Emerg Med* 20:2-609, 2002.

47. Gami AS, Holly TA, Rosenthal JE: Electrocardiographic poor R-wave progression: analysis of multiple criteria reveals little usefulness, *Am Heart J* 148:14-80, 2004.

48. Sinha MK, Dasgupta D, Lyons JP: Tombstone ST segment elevation of acute myocardial infarction, *Postgrad Med J* 80:276, 2004.

49. Balci B, Yesildag O: Correlation between clinical findings and the "tombstoning" electrocardiographic pattern in patients with anterior wall acute myocardial infarction, *Am J Cardiol* 92:9-1316, 2003.

50. Di Diego JM, Antzelevitch C: Cellular basis for ST-segment changes observed during ischemia, *J Electrocardiol* 36(suppl):1-5, 2003.

51. Cortadellas J, Figueras J, Missorici M et al: ST segment elevation at 72 hours in patients with a first anterior myocardial infarction best correlates with pre-discharge and 1-year regional contractility and ventricular dilatation, *Eur Heart J* 25:2-224, 2004.

52. Hombach V: Electrocardiogram of the failing heart, *Card Electrophysiol Rev* 6:209, 2002.

53. Correale E, Battista R, Ricciardiello V et al: The negative U wave: a pathogenetic enigma but a useful, often overlooked bedside diagnostic and prognostic clue in ischemic heart disease, *Clin Cardiol* 27:2-674, 2004.

54. Brady WJ, Syverud SA, Beagle C et al: Electrocardiographic ST-segment elevation: the diagnosis of acute myocardial infarction by morphological analysis of the ST segment, *Acad Emerg Med* 8:961, 2001.

55. Rotondo N, Pollack ML, Chan TC et al: Electrocardiographic manifestations: acute inferior wall myocardial infarction, *J Emerg Med* 26:2-433, 2004.

56. Moss AJ: T wave patterns associated with the hereditary long QT syndrome, *Card Electrophysiol Rev* 6:311, 2002.

57. Rhinehardt J, Brady WJ, Perron AD et al: Electrocardiographic manifestations of Wellen's syndrome, *Am J Emerg Med* 20:2-638, 2002.

58. Karnath BM, Champion JC, Ahmad M: Electrocardiographic manifestations of proximal left anterior descending artery occlusion, *J Electrocardiol* 36:3-173, 2003.

59. Vasudevan K, Manjunath CN, Srinivas KH et al: Electrocardiographic localization of the occlusion site in left anterior descending coronary artery in acute anterior myocardial infarction, *Indian Heart J* 56:5-315, 2004.

60. Sgarbossa EB, Birnbaum Y, Parrillo JE: Electrocardiographic diagnosis of acute myocardial infarction: current concepts for the clinician, *Am Heart J* 141:14-507, 2001.

61. Menown IBA, Allen J, Anderson JM et al: Early diagnosis of right ventricular or posterior infarction associated with inferior wall left ventricular acute myocardial infarction, *Am J Cardiol* 85:8-934, 2000.

62. Fijewski TR, Pollack ML, Chan TC et al: Electrocardiographic manifestations: right ventricular infarction, *J Emerg Med* 22:2-189, 2002.

63. Somers MP, Brady WJ, Bateman DC et al: Additional electrocardiographic leads in the ED chest pain patient: right ventricular and posterior leads, *Am J Emerg Med* 21:2-563, 2003.

64. Brady WJ, Erling B, Pollack M et al: Electrocardiographic manifestations: acute posterior wall myocardial infarction, *J Emerg Med* 20:2-391, 2001.

65. Brady WJ, Chan TC, Pollack M: Electrocardiographic manifestations: patterns that confound the EKG diagnosis of acute myocardial infarction: left bundle branch block, ventricular paced rhythm, and left ventricular hypertrophy, *J Emerg Med* 18:1-71, 2000.

66. Kurisu S, Inoue I, Kawagoe T et al: Time course of electrocardiographic changes in patients with Tako-Tsubo syndrome: comparison with acute myocardial infarction with minimal enzymatic release, *Circ J* 68:6-77, 2004.

67. Eichholz A, Whiting RB, Artal R: Lown-Ganong-Levine syndrome in pregnancy, *Obstet Gynecol* 102:10-1393, 2003.

68. Engel J, Brady WJ, Mattu A et al: Electrocardiographic ST segment elevation: left ventricular aneurysm, *Am J Emerg Med* 20:2-238, 2002.

69. Ilkay E, Yavuzkir M, Karaca I et al: The effect of ST resolution on QT dispersion after interventional treatment in acute myocardial infarction, *Clin Cardiol* 27:2-159, 2004.

70. Meyer JS, Mehdirad A, Salem BI et al: Sudden dysrhythmia death syndrome: importance of the long QT syndrome, *Am Fam Physician* 68:6-483, 2004.
71. Conover MB: Bundle branch blocks. In Conover MB, editor: *Understanding electrocardiography,* ed 8, St Louis, 2003, Mosby.
72. Childers R, Lupovich S, Sochanski M et al: Left bundle branch block and right axis deviation: a report of 36 cases, *J Electrocardiol* 33(suppl):93-102, 2000.
73. Bellocq C, van Ginneken ACG, Bezzina CR et al: Mutation in the KCNQ1 gene leading to the short QT-interval syndrome, *Circulation* 109:10-2394, 2004.
74. Brugada R, Hong K, Dumaine R et al: Sudden death associated with short-ST syndrome linked to mutations in HERG, *Circulation* 109:10-30, 2004.
75. Gaita F, Giustetto C, Bianchi F et al: Short QT syndrome: pharmacological treatment, *JAMA* 43:4-1494, 2004.
76. Khan IA, Nair CK: Brugada and long QT-3 syndromes: two phenotypes of the sodium channel disease, *Ann Noninvasive Electrocardiol* 9:280, 2004.
77. Mattu A, Rogers RL, Kim H et al: The Brugada syndrome, *Am J Emerg Med* 21:2-146, 2003.
78. Wilde AA, Antzelevitch C, Borggrefe M et al: Proposed diagnostic criteria for the Brugada syndrome, *Eur Heart J* 23:2-1648, 2002.
79. Ahn J, Hurst JW: Worrisome thoughts about the diagnosis and treatment of patients with Brugada waves and the Brugada syndrome, *Circulation* 109:10-1463, 2004.
80. Oto A: Brugada sign: a normal variant or a bad omen? insights for risk stratification and prognostication, *Eur Heart J* 25(10):25-810, 2004.
81. Antzelevitch C: The Brugada syndrome: ionic basis and dysrhythmia mechanisms, *J Cardiovasc Electrophysiol* 12:1-268, 2001.
82. Edhouse J, Thakur RK, Khalil JM: ABC of clinical electrocardiography: conditions affecting the left side of the heart, *BMJ* 324:32-1264, 2002.
83. Nelson JA, Knowlton KU, Harrigan R et al: Electrocardiographic manifestations: wide complex tachycardia due to accessory pathway, *J Emerg Med* 24:2-295, 2003.
84. Keating L, Morris FP, Brady WJ: Electrocardiographic features of Wolff-Parkinson-White syndrome, *Emerg Med J* 20:2-491, 2003.
85. Corrado D, Basso C, Nava A et al: Arrhythmogenic right ventricular cardiomyopathy: current diagnostic and management strategies, *Cardiol Rev* 119:11-259, 2001.
86. Saha M, Chalil S, Sulke N: Situs inversus and acute coronary syndrome, *Heart* 90:e20, 2004.
87. Alexis JD, Nayak HM, Kushwaha SS et al: New pre-excitation following cardiac transplant, *Int J Cardiol* 65:6-71, 1998.
88. Eckart RE, Kolasa MW, Khan NA et al: Surface electrocardiography and histologic rejection following orthotopic heart transplantation, *Ann Noninvasive Electrocardiol* 10:1-60, 2005.
89. Vanderheyden M, de Sutter J, Goethals M: ECG diagnosis of native heart ventricular tachycardia in a heterotopic heart transplant recipient, *Heart* 82:8-323, 1999.
90. Khan MG: Bundle branch blocks. In Khan MG, editor: *Rapid ECG interpretation,* ed 2, Philadelphia, 2003, Saunders.
91. Harrigan RA, Pollack ML, Chan TC: Electrocardiographic manifestations: bundle branch blocks and fascicular blocks, *J Emerg Med* 25:2-67, 2003.
92. Khan MG: Atrial and ventricular hypertrophy. In Khan MG, editor: *Rapid ECG interpretation,* ed 2, Philadelphia, 2003, Saunders.
93. Oparil S: Pathogenesis of ventricular hypertrophy, *J Am Coll Cardiol* 5:57B-65B, 1985.
94. Wood M, Ellenbogen KA: Temporary cardiac pacing. In Ellenbogen KA, editor: *Cardiac pacing,* ed 2, Cambridge, Mass, 1996, Blackwell Scientific.
95. Berenji K, Nerheim P, Olshansky B: Inadvertent positioning of pacemaker leads in the pericardium, *Pacing Clin Electrophys* 26: e2039, 2003.
96. Trohman RG, Him MH: Cardiac pacing: state of the art, *Lancet* 364:36-1701, 2004.
97. Coman JA, Trohman RG: Incidence and electrocardiographic localization of safe right bundle branch block configurations during permanent ventricular pacing, *Am J Cardiol* 76:7-781, 1995.

■ ■ ■ c h a p t e r **48**
Dysrhythmia Monitoring and Recognition

Nancy Albert
Kathleen McCauley

MONITORING

The primary goals of monitoring are to diagnose a dysrhythmia and determine whether it will affect the patient's quality of life and mortality risk. The secondary goals are to determine the best therapeutic strategy and evaluate its safety and effectiveness based on its ability to improve patient outcome and minimize health care utilization expenditures. Monitoring can be applied externally, or patients may be monitored with an implantable device.

As the awareness of dysrhythmia morbidity and mortality increases, there is a need for new monitoring system capabilities. Currently, two types of external monitoring systems are used to collect diagnostic information: a continuous recorder that requires the application of surface electrocardiogram **(ECG)** electrodes and can be hardwire- or telemetry-driven with an intermittent recorder.

Intermittent recorders come in two forms: a loop recorder that is worn continuously and is activated by the patient when symptoms occur and an event recorder that requires patients to place a handheld device to the chest or to a wristwatch to establish contact between the skin and the recorder when symptoms occur. Intermittent recorders are activated when a patient has symptoms with a dysrhythmia; thus, these recorders

have limited efficacy in patients known to have asymptomatic dysrhythmias.

Continuous ECG monitoring in a hospital setting, when the patient is most likely to be at high risk for events, has much greater efficacy than monitoring in an outpatient setting. Patients may go for weeks without a dysrhythmic episode, or dysrhythmias may be clustered over a short time and may be missed by a continuous monitoring device if it is not programmed when events occur.

Implantable devices have the capability of extensively monitoring atrial and ventricular dysrhythmias, depending on the placement of intracardiac leads and the sophistication of the system used. See Chapter 61 for a discussion of implantable devices that monitor and treat dysrhythmias.

Nursing practice has evolved significantly since the advent of cardiac monitors.[1] Nurses practicing in areas as disparate as emergency departments, labor and delivery units, and many general medical and surgical units must be able to recognize cardiac rhythm disorders and manage the technology that supports their prompt detection. In this chapter, we review principles of cardiac monitoring, including lead selection, monitoring systems, and recognition and management of common cardiac rhythm disorders. Currently available protocols guiding practice are discussed.

MONITORING SYSTEMS AND LEAD SELECTION

Recent technological advances have included computerized dysrhythmia detection systems, multilead monitoring programs, and remote nurse notification systems. See Chapter 49 for a discussion of ST segment and ischemia monitoring and alternative lead systems for monitoring all 12 ECG leads with fewer electrodes. These advances have improved the quality of cardiac monitoring and have increased the complexity for providers (Table 48-1). Clinicians must determine not only which patients require continuous ECG monitoring but also which lead will best identify potential abnormalities given the patient's particular disease processes.

Accurate electrode placement is the first step in cardiac monitoring. For dysrhythmia monitoring, standard limb lead placement includes placing the right arm electrode in the right infraclavicular fossa near the right shoulder and the left arm electrode in the corresponding space on the left. The left leg electrode is placed on the left side of the abdomen below the level of the rib cage. A common monitoring mistake places the left leg electrode too high on the chest wall. The right leg electrode serves as the ground electrode and usually is placed on the right side of the abdomen below the rib cage. Additional leads used for ST segment monitoring—the precordial leads (V_1 to V_6)—are placed at exactly the same location as required for standard 12-lead recording (see Chapter 46). Deviation by even 1 cm can invalidate the usefulness of the lead when applying diagnostic algorithms such as Kindwall criteria in a left bundle branch morphology ventricular tachycardia (VT).[2,3] Drew et al.[2] recommend marking the chest with indelible ink to ensure that the electrodes are replaced in the same location. An alternative is to use the CardioQuick Patch (CardioQuickSys, Sharonville, Ohio) precordial overlay system that facilitates fast, accurate, and consistent 12-lead ECGs.

Factors involved in choosing the appropriate lead to monitor include clear evidence of P waves, QRS complexes, and T waves to support diagnosis of dysrhythmias and accurate rate and rhythm tracking by the computerized monitoring system. Lead II, commonly chosen for its clear waveforms, provides little diagnostic ability in differentiation of wide complex tachycardias, bundle branch blocks, and most episodes of ischemia. Lead II may be advantageous in identifying retrograde atrial conduction in certain paroxysmal atrial tachycardias, as is discussed later. Advantages of other leads include the ability to monitor ischemia (see Chapter 49) and use precordial leads V_1 and V_6 to differentiate wide complex tachycardias. Leads that promote detection of specific dysrhythmias are identified in the section of this text dealing with the rhythm disorder.

Decision Support for Electrocardiogram Monitoring

The American Heart Association recently published a scientific statement on practice standards for ECG monitoring in hospital settings, which decreased confusion over whether to initiate or continue monitoring patients with certain illnesses. An expert panel devised a three-class system for monitoring. As illustrated in Box 48-1,

■ ■ ■
TABLE 48-1 MONITORING LEAD SYSTEMS

LEAD SYSTEM	ADVANTAGES	DISADVANTAGES
Three electrodes, bipolar leads	Simple; monitors leads I, II, III and MCL1, used for portable monitors and defibrillators to record heart rate and rhythm and to track R waves for cardioversion and defibrillation	Unable to apply criteria for complex dysrhythmia monitoring (ventricular tachycardia, left and right bundle branch block) because true V lead is not achievable; inadequate for ST segment monitoring
Five electrodes; four limb leads; one precordial lead	Fairly simple, commonly used; monitors leads I, II, III, aVR, aVL, aVF, and one precordial lead (V_1 to V_6). Records true V1 lead for detection of ventricular tachycardia and bundle branch block	Cannot monitor more than one V lead; therefore inadequate for ST segment ischemia monitoring
10-electrode Mason-Likar 12-lead ECG	Obtains all 12 ECG leads via limb leads repositioned to the chest and 6 precordial leads in standard positions; capable of ST segment monitoring even on leads not displayed on monitor in some systems; capable of displaying multiple V leads simultaneously	Ten leads on the chest can interfere with care (diagnostic studies, defibrillation) Potential challenge to maintain system in patients with large breasts or chest hair
Derived 12-lead ECG with reduced lead sets: 5-electrode 12-lead system; the "EASI system"	Mathematical calculation used to derive standard 12 leads from 5 leads: 2 positioned on sternum, 1 on lateral right and left chest, and 1 ground; comparable to 12-lead system in diagnosing wide complex tachycardia and ischemia	Unconventional lead placement; caution recommended in comparing with standard 12-lead ECG
Derived 12-lead ECG with reduced lead sets: 6-electrode 12-lead system	Uses Mason-Likar limb leads and leads V_1 and V_5; other 4 precordial leads are derived; comparable to standard 12-lead ECG for diagnosing wide complex tachycardia and ischemia; uses conventional lead placement	Precordial leads have potential to interfere with diagnostic tests and defibrillation

MCL₁, Modified chest lead I; *ECG*, electrocardiogram.
From Drew BJ, Califf RM, Funk M et al: *Circulation* 110:2721-2746, 2004; Dower GE, Yakush A, Nazzal SB et al: *J Electrocardiol* 21:S182-S187, 1988; and Drew BJ, Pelter MM, Brodnick DE et al: *J Electrocardiol* 34:261-264, 2001.

BOX 48-1 ■ ■ ■

DECISION SUPPORT FOR CARDIAC MONITORING:
PATIENTS MOST LIKELY TO BENEFIT FROM
CONTINUOUS CARDIAC MONITORING

Class I: Monitoring indicated for most, if not all, patients because
of significant risk for life-threatening dysrhythmia. Patients in this
class include those who

- Have been resuscitated from cardiac arrest
- Are in the early stage of acute coronary syndromes
- Have unstable coronary syndromes with newly diagnosed
  high-risk coronary lesions
- Have undergone cardiac surgery: (1) for 48 to 72 hours for un-
  complicated patients and (2) until discharge for those at high
  risk for developing atrial fibrillation
- Are children following cardiac surgery
- Have undergone nonurgent percutaneous coronary interventions with complications such as vessel dissection, no reflow,
  or less definitive interventional outcomes
- Have had implantation of an automatic defibrillator lead or a
  pacemaker lead and are pacemaker dependent
- Have a temporary pacemaker or require transcutaneous pacing pads
- Have Mobitz II second-degree heart block, complete atrioventricular block or new bundle branch block accompanying
  acute, especially anterior, myocardial infarction
- Have Mobitz type I heart block and require monitoring until it
  is determined that the block is stable and a long-term
  condition
- Have dysrhythmias related to Wolff-Parkinson-White syndrome
  with rapid anterograde conduction via an accessory pathway
- Have long QT syndrome, torsades de pointes, or polymorphic
  ventricular tachycardia
- Require intraaortic balloon counterpulsation
- Have acute heart failure and/or pulmonary edema until resolu-
  tion of acute symptoms and absence of hemodynamically sig-
  nificant dysrhythmias for at least 24 hours
- Require care in an intensive care unit
- Are undergoing a procedure requiring conscious sedation or
  anesthesia
- Have any other hemodynamically unstable dysrhythmia
- Are children requiring further diagnosis of a dysrhythmia
- Require antidysrhythmic agents known to be proarrhythmic;
  QT prolongation should be assessed carefully
- Have received an antidysrhythmic drug known to cause tor-
  sades de pointes
- Have taken an overdose of a potentially proarrhythmic agent
- Have new onset bradydysrhythmias
- Have severe hypokalemia or hypomagnesemia

From Drew BJ, Califf RM, Funk M et al: *Circulation* 110:2722-2733, 2004.

BOX 48-2 ■ ■ ■

DECISION SUPPORT FOR CARDIAC MONITORING:
PATIENTS WHO MAY BENEFIT FROM CONTINUOUS
CARDIAC MONITORING, BUT CONTROVERSY
MAY EXIST

Class II: Monitoring indicated for some patients; not essential for
all, but may be helpful for clinical management. Patients in this
class include those who

- Are in the post–acute phase of a myocardial infarction. Monitoring may be most beneficial in those with hypertension,
  chronic obstructive pulmonary disease, previous myocardial
  infarction, higher Killip class, ST elevation, or lower systolic
  blood pressure at time of presentation
- Have chest pain syndromes consisting of chest pain without
  electrocardiogram or biomarker indications of ischemia/injury
  and who are free of dysrhythmias. Patients with low systolic
  blood pressure, pulmonary rales, and/or ischemic symptoms
  should be monitored for 12 to 24 hours until an acute myocardial infarction has been ruled out
- Have undergone uncomplicated and nonurgent percutaneous
  coronary interventions. Monitoring for 12 to 24 hours is indicated for patients not receiving coronary stents
- Have received an antidysrhythmic drug or need drug adjustment for tachydysrhythmias primarily to detect QT interval
  prolongation, assess sinus node function, determine efficacy
  of rate control in chronic atrial fibrillation/flutter, or evaluate
  hemodynamic response especially in patients with reduced
  left ventricular function
- Are nonpacemaker dependent following implantation of pacemaker lead
- Have undergone uncomplicated dysrhythmia ablation or routine coronary angiography
- Have subacute heart failure. Monitoring is indicated while
  medication and/or device therapy is being adjusted
- Are undergoing evaluation for syncope. Monitoring may be indicated if dysrhythmic cause is suspected and until it is ruled out
- Have dysrhythmias causing discomfort (e.g., shortness of
  breath or palpitations) that can be managed to reduce symptoms in patients with do-not-resuscitate orders
- Require antipsychotic or other agents with possible risk of torsades de pointes
- Have acute neurological events. Rate corrected QT interval
  greater than 0.50 second warrants continued corrected QT interval monitoring

From Drew BJ, Califf RM, Funk M et al: *Circulation* 110:2722-2733, 2004.

BOX 48-3 ■ ■ ■

DECISION SUPPORT FOR CARDIAC MONITORING:
PATIENTS WHO ARE UNLIKELY TO BENEFIT FROM
CONTINUOUS CARDIAC MONITORING

Class III: Monitoring is *not* indicated because these low-risk patients will not benefit from it. Patients in this class include those
who

- Have undergone surgery but are at low risk for dysrhythmias
- Are obstetrical patients without heart disease
- Have permanent, rate-controlled atrial fibrillation
- Are undergoing outpatient hemodialysis. Hospitalized dialysis
  patients may require monitoring based on other conditions
  (Class I or II status)
- Have chronic ventricular extrasystoles and are otherwise sta-
  ble, without serious acid-base or electrolyte abnormalities or
  myocardial ischemia

From Drew BJ, Califf RM, Funk M et al: *Circulation* 110:2722-2728, 2004.

most if not all Class I patients should be monitored.
Because these patients are at risk for life-threatening
dysrhythmias, they should be monitored continuously,
including during transport for diagnostic tests or treatments, by clinicians with the knowledge and skills to
defibrillate if necessary. Class II patients include those
with specific conditions for whom monitoring may be
beneficial but is not essential (Box 48-2). Class III patients (Box 48-3) are unlikely to derive additional benefit from cardiac monitoring.[2]

In addition to providing decision support for providers
making decisions about when to monitor individual patients, these practice standards provide support for those
making decisions about expanding monitoring systems
to general care and specialty units. They support clinicians who argue for appropriate support when patients
must travel off the monitored unit for diagnostic and
therapeutic care. Unnecessary monitoring increases the
cost of health care, diverts nursing and medical staff from
other essential duties, and may give patients an incorrect
message about their cardiac health. Thus, making decisions that are consistent with these practice standards
may optimize patient safety and system efficiency.

RECOGNITION

Dysrhythmias are labeled based on the part of the conduction system that is being assessed as malfunctioning: atrial or sinus node (pacemaker), atrioventricular (AV) or junctional node, and His-Purkinje system that consists of the His bundle, bundle branches, and Purkinje fibers. This explains why bradydysrhythmias and tachydysrhythmias are defined differently depending on the specific part of the conduction system under discussion. Generally, though, an abnormal rhythm is any cardiac rhythm that does not conform to characteristics of normal sinus rhythm at normal atrial and ventricular rates. Thus, normal sinus rhythm (NSR) is the standard against which dysrhythmias are compared.

Each dysrhythmia is described based on its distinguishing characteristics and visually is represented via ECG for recognition (refer to Table 48-2 for an overview). Management is discussed, referring the reader to other chapters, when applicable. Table 48-3 provides an overview of terms that are used to characterize common mechanisms of cardiac dysrhythmias. Reentry is the most common cause of clinical dysrhythmias.[4] When the reentrant pathway is known, drugs can be targeted to the specific tissue to interrupt the pathway and suppress the dysrhythmia (e.g., reentrant pathways in the AV node can be controlled with digoxin, calcium channel blockers, and beta blockers). When the electrophysiology of the reentrant pathway is unknown, for example, as often happens after acute myocardial infarction (MI), drugs cannot be applied. Additionally, unpredictable antidysrhythmic drug effects in abnormal myocardial substrates may not control the dysrhythmia and may even be proarrhythmic.[5] Thus, understanding the basic electrophysiological mechanisms in Table 48-3 is important, but there may be many complexities to the mechanisms of cardiac dysrhythmias that require further study, especially in damaged ventricles.

PHARMACOLOGICAL TREATMENT OVERVIEW

Antidysrhythmic agents are classified based on the Vaughan Williams classification (Table 48-4). There are four classes, each of which targets specific electrolyte channels (sodium, potassium, or calcium) or beta receptors that have electrophysiological effects. This classification system has limitations; not all drugs in the same class have identical effects, and newer drugs are complex and block more than one channel. However, this system is known widely and provides a useful approach to drug management.

Drugs that block the fast sodium channels are listed as class I agents. This class is subdivided further into three subclasses. Class IA drugs reduce the rise in action potential upstroke (phase 0) and prolong action potential duration. Class IB drugs shorten action potential duration but do not reduce the rise in action potential upstroke (phase 0). Class IC drugs reduce the rise in action potential upstroke and can prolong refractoriness. Class II drugs are those that block beta-adrenergic receptors. Class III drugs predominantly block potassium channels and prolong repolarization, and class IV drugs block the slow calcium channel.[6] Drugs are chosen based on their mechanism(s) of dysrhythmia suppression (Table 48-5), their adverse effect profile, hemodynamic and autonomic properties, type of cardiac tissue being targeted (specialized conduction fibers, atrial tissue, or ventricular tissue), and pharmacokinetic properties. In addition, it is important to know whether the cardiac tissue is normal or abnormal before selecting drugs. For example, patients with systolic left ventricular dysfunction may not tolerate some beta-adrenergic blockers that acutely and severely suppress cardiac contractility.

DYSRHYTHMIAS
Sinus Tachycardia

Sinus tachycardia refers to rapid beating of the sinus node at rates of 100 to 180 beats/min in adults (Figure 48-1). In some cases, healthy adults can have sinus tachycardia with ventricular rates beyond 180 beats/min, especially with exercise involving extreme exertion; however, maximal heart rate achieved with strenuous exercise declines with aging to less than 140 beats/min in the elderly.[7] Sinus tachycardia can occur in infants. Older nursing texts noted 160 beats/min to be the upper limit of sinus tachycardia. More recent texts, influenced by an improved understanding of electrophysiological mechanisms of narrow complex tachycardias, describe 180 beats/min as the upper limit, with even higher rates (200 beats/min) possible with extreme exertion.

At faster rates, the usual gradual onset and deceleration of sinus tachycardia help to differentiate it from paroxysmal atrial tachycardia, which starts and stops abruptly.[7,8] The usual gradual onset and termination are due to enhanced automaticity from sympathetic stimulation (fight or flight), e.g., fever, hypotension, anemia, blood loss, anxiety and other emotions, exertion, hypovolemia, thyrotoxicosis, or sudden cessation of parasympathetic restraint (vagal block) such as occurs with a sudden, loud, unexpected sound. Sinus tachycardia is often a normal physiological response to cardiovascular stressors that cause a decrease in cardiac output, such as acutely decompensated congestive heart failure, acute pulmonary emboli, acute MI, myocardial infarct extension, pericarditis, or shock. Drugs also can induce sinus tachycardia, most often catecholamines (inotropic agents dopamine and dobutamine; epinephrine, norepinephrine, and other sympathomimetic vasoconstrictors), vasodilators (nitroglycerin and nitroprusside), alcohol, nicotine, thyroid medicines, caffeine, and atropine. Because the conduction pathway in sinus tachycardia is the same as in NSR, ECG characteristics appear similar to those found in NSR. P waves may be slightly irregular in shape, reflecting a shift of the pacing site within the sinus node, or they may develop larger amplitude and become peaked. PP interval should be fixed but may vary slightly from cycle to cycle, and the PR interval shortens from shortening of AV conduction, especially when the rate is rapid. The QRS complex should appear normal, but the QT interval will shorten.[7]

TABLE 48-2 DYSRHYTHMIA CHARACTERISTICS*

TYPE OF DYSRHYTHMIA	RATE (beats/min)	P WAVES RHYTHM	P WAVES CONTOUR	RATE (beats/min)	QRS COMPLEXES RHYTHM	QRS COMPLEXES CONTOUR	TREATMENT
Sinus rhythm	60-100	Regular†	Normal	60-100	Regular	Normal	None
Sinus bradycardia	Less than 60	Regular	Normal	Less than 60	Regular	Normal	None, unless symptomatic; atropine
Sinus tachycardia	100-180	Regular	May be peaked	100-180	Regular	Normal	None, unless symptomatic; treat underlying disease
Atrioventricular (AV) nodal reentry	150-250	Very regular except at onset and termination	Retrograde; difficult to see; lost in QRS complex	150-250	Very regular except at onset and termination	Normal	Vagal stimulation, adenosine, verapamil, digitalis, propranolol Direct current (DC) shock, pacing
Atrial flutter	250-350	Regular	Sawtooth	75-175	Generally regular in absence of drugs or disease	Normal	DC shock, overdrive pacing, digitalis, quinidine, propranolol, verapamil
Atrial fibrillation	400-600	Grossly irregular	Baseline undulation, no P waves	100-160	Grossly irregular	Normal	Digitalis, quinidine, DC shock, verapamil
Atrial tachycardia with block	150-250	Regular; may be irregular	Abnormal	75-200	Generally regular in absence of drugs or disease	Normal	Stop digitalis if toxic; digitalis if not toxic; possibly verapamil
AV junctional rhythm	40-100‡	Regular	Inverted, retrograde, or absent	40-60	Fairly regular	Normal	None, unless symptomatic; atropine
Reciprocating tachycardias using an accessory (Wolff-Parkinson-White syndrome) pathway	150-250	Very regular except at onset and termination	Retrograde; difficult to see; monitor the QRS complex	150-250	Very regular except at onset and termination	Normal	See AV nodal reentry. Note: Adenosine, beta blockers, calcium channel blockers, and digitalis may be harmful if atrial fibrillation is present
Nonparoxysmal AV junctional tachycardia	60-100	Regular	Inverted, retrograde, or absent; may be difficult to see or absent	70-130	Fairly regular	Normal	None, unless symptomatic: stop digitalis if toxic

Ventricular tachycardia	60-100	Regular	Dissociated from ventricular complexes or absent	100-250 (but may be as low as 70)	Fairly regular; may be irregular	Abnormal greater than 0.12 second	Lidocaine, procainamide, DC shock, quinidine, amiodarone
Accelerated idioventricular rhythm	60-100	Regular	Dissociated from ventricular complexes or absent	50-110	Fairly regular; may be irregular	Abnormal greater than 0.12 second	None, unless symptomatic; atropine
Ventricular flutter	60-100 but rarely visible	Regular	Dissociated from ventricular complexes or absent	150-300	Regular	Sine wave	DC shock
Ventricular fibrillation	60-100 but rarely visible	Regular	Difficult to see	400-600	Grossly irregular	Baseline undulations: no QRS complex	DC shock
First-degree AV block	60-100§	Regular	Normal	60-100	Regular	Normal	None
Type I second-degree AV block	60-100§	Regular	Normal	30-100	Irregular¶	Normal	None, unless symptomatic: atropine, pacing
Type II second-degree AV block	60-100§	Regular	Normal	30-100	Irregular¶	Abnormal, greater than 0.12 second	Pacemaker
Complete AV block	60-100 but dissociated from ventricular complexes	Regular	Normal	Less than 40	Fairly regular	Abnormal, greater than 0.12 second	Pacemaker
Right bundle branch block	60-100	Regular	Normal	60-100	Regular	Abnormal, greater than 0.12 second	None
Left bundle branch block	60-100	Regular	Normal	60-100	Regular	Abnormal greater than 0.12 second	None

*In an effort to summarize these dysrhythmias in tabular form, generalizations have to be made. Acute therapy to terminate a tachycardia may be different from chronic therapy to prevent recurrence.

†P waves initiated by sinus node discharge may not be precisely regular because of sinus dysrhythmia.

‡Any independent atrial dysrhythmia may exist, or the atria may be captured retrogradely.

§Atrial rhythm and rate may vary depending on whether sinus bradycardia, sinus tachycardia, or another abnormality is the atrial mechanism.

¶Regular or constant if block is unchanging.

Modified from Olgin J, Zipes D: Specific arrhythmias: diagnosis and treatment. In Zipes D, Libby P, Bonow R, Braunwald E, editors: *Braunwald's heart disease: a textbook of cardiovascular medicine*, ed 7, Philadelphia, 2005, WB Saunders.

■ ■ ■

TABLE 48-3   COMMON TERMS THAT CHARACTERIZE THE MECHANISMS OF CARDIAC DYSRHYTHMIAS

TERM	DEFINITION	CHARACTERISTICS
1. *Triggered activity*	Pacemaker activity that results from a preceding impulse or series of impulses; thus, activity is triggered by prior stimulation • Caused by afterdepolarizations	Afterdepolarizations only trigger an impulse when they reach threshold potential. They can self-perpetuate, but not all reach threshold potential or self-perpetuate
a. Early afterdepolarizations	A form of triggered activity in which depolarization occurs before full repolarization of the fibers from the previous depolarization	Arise from a reduction in membrane potential during phases 2 and 3 of the cardiac action potential
b. Late or delayed afterdepolarizations	A form of triggered activity in which depolarization occurs after completion of repolarization	Arise from a reduction in membrane potential at or after phase 4 of the cardiac action potential when the membrane potential is more negative
2. *Block*	Impulses are blocked when the amplitude and rate of rise of phase 0 or excitability of the tissue into which the impulse is conducted is insufficient	Can occur at long diastolic intervals; with rapid pacing (overdrive suppression of conduction) More commonly occurs when there is incomplete recovery of refractoriness as seen with tachycardia or short cycle lengths
3. *Reentry* Also known as reentrant excitation, circus movement, reciprocal or echo beat, or reciprocating tachycardia	Fibers that have not been activated during the initial wave of depolarization can recover excitability in time to be discharged before the impulse dies out. These fibers serve as a link to reexcite areas that were just discharged but have recovered from the initial depolarization	A key feature of tachycardia due to reentry is entrainment. This is tested by setting a pacemaker device to increase to a faster heart rate (above the patient's intrinsic tachycardia rate) and then resuming the patient's intrinsic rate by stopping the pacemaker activity. In entrainment, pacemaker-induced activation will lead to capture or continuous resetting of the reentrant circuit of the tachycardia
a. Anatomical reentry	Anatomically defined separate pathways that have (1) an area of unidirectional block, (2) recirculation of the impulse to its point of origin, and (3) elimination of the arrhythmia by cutting the pathway	Clinical arrhythmia is more likely to have a monomorphic contour For reentry to occur continuously, the anatomical length of the circuit traveled must equal or exceed the reentrant wavelength Because the length of the pathway is fixed and determined by anatomy, reentry is promoted by conditions that depress conduction velocity or abbreviate the refractory period Reentry is hindered by prolonged refractoriness or speeding conduction velocity
b. Functional reentry	Initiation and maintenance of reentry is not related to anatomical boundaries; rather it occurs in contiguous fibers that have dispersion of excitability and/or refractoriness and anisotropic conduction distribution (elliptical pattern of activation) of intracellular resistance • Functional reentry models: — Leading circle model — Anisotropic model — Figure-of-8 model — Spiral wave model	Clinical dysrhythmia is more likely to have a polymorphic contour because of changing or drifting circuits • Leading circle reentry, important in atrial fibrillation, is a form of functional reentrant excitation • The reentrant circuit propagates around a functionally refractory core and follows a course along fibers that have a shorter refractory period so that the impulse is blocked in one direction in fibers with a longer refractory period • Anisotropic reentry is important in ventricular tachy-dysrhythmias

From Zipes DP: *Pacing Clin Electrophysiol* 26:1778-1792, 2003.

Management

Because sinus tachycardia is a normal physiological response to an underlying condition, it is treated directly. Therapies are directed toward treating or eliminating the cause of the tachycardia and may include withholding or eliminating stimulants. If sinus tachycardia is not the result of a correctable physiological stressor, beta blockers or calcium channel blockers may slow the rate of sinus node discharge. Vagal maneuvers such as forceful exhalation against a closed glottis (Valsalva), carotid sinus massage, squatting, leg elevation, and cold water in the face will slow a sinus tachycardia temporarily by stimulating activation of the vagus nerve and increasing parasympathetic tone.[7]

Sinus Bradycardia

Sinus bradycardia refers to slow beating of the sinus node at a rate slower than 60 beats/min (Figure 48-2). When hemodynamically stable, sinus bradycardia is considered a normal variant. In adults, sinus bradycardia is usually a response to vagal stimulation (e.g., carotid sinus massage) and can occur after vomiting or with ocular pressure. Sinus bradycardia is most common during sleep (normal heart rate variability as part of normal circadian variation in sinus rate) and in athletes. Sinus bradycardia can occur from decreased sympathetic tone by administration of parasympathomimetic drugs, digitalis, beta blockers, and calcium channel blockers or from anatomical changes. Disease

■ ■ ■

TABLE 48-4   ACTIONS OF DRUGS USED TO TREAT CARDIAC DYSRHYTHMIAS

| | CHANNELS | | | | | | | | CLINICAL EFFECTS | | |
| | SODIUM (Na)* | | | RECEPTORS | | | | | | | |
	FAST	MED	SLOW	Ca	K$_r$	K$_8$	β	α	LV FUNCT.	SINUS RATE	DRUG EXTRACARD.
Quinidine		●A			⊙			○	—	↑	⊙
Procainamide		●A			⊙				↓	—	⊙
Disopyramide		●A			⊙				↓	—	●
Lidocaine	○								—	—↓	○
Mexiletine	○								—	—	○
Phenytoin	○								—	—	⊙
Flecainide			●A		○				↓	—	○
Propafenone		●A			○		⊙		↓	↓	○
Moricizine	●I								↓	—	○
Propranolol	○						●		↓	↓	○
Nadolol							●		↓	↓	○
Amiodarone	○			⊙	●	⊙	⊙	⊙	—	↓	●
Bretylium					●		⊡	⊡	—	↓	○
Sotalol					●		●		↓	↓	○
Ibutilide					○				—	↓	○
Dofetilide					●				—	—	○
Azimilide					⊙	⊙		○	—	—	○
Verapamil	○			●				⊙	↓	↓	○
Diltiazem				⊙					↓	↓	○
Adenosine	Endogenous nucleoside (A$_1$ purinergic receptor)								—	↓	⊙
Digoxin	Cardiac glycoside (muscarinic receptor subtype 2; low potency) and inhibits the Na^1-K^1 ATPase: makes more Ca^{21} available for contractile proteins								↑	↓	⊙
Atropine	Belladonna alkaloid (muscarinic receptor subtype 2; high potency)								—	↑	⊙

Ca, Calcium; *K$_r$*, rapid component of delayed rectifier K$^+$ current; *K$_8$*, slow component of delayed rectifier K$^+$ current; β, beta; α, alpha; *LV funct.*, left ventricular function; *Extracard.*, extracardiac; ●, high†; *A*, activated state blocker; ⊙, moderate†; ○, low†; —, minimal effect; ↑, increase; ↓, decrease; *I*, inactivated state blocker; ⊡, agonist-antagonist.
*Fast, med (medium), and *slow* refer to kinetics of recovery from sodium channel blockade.
†Relative potency of blockade or extracardiac side effect.
Modified from Miller JM, Zipes D: Therapy for cardiac arrhythmias. In Zipes D, Libby P, Bonow R, Braunwald E, editors: *Braunwald's heart disease: a textbook of cardiovascular medicine*, ed 7, Philadelphia, 2005, WB Saunders.

processes that can cause bradycardia are inferior wall MI, reperfusion with fibrinolytic agents, cardiac fibrosis, meningitis, mediastinal tumors, myxedema, obstructive jaundice, uremia, increased intracranial pressure, glaucoma, anorexia, and sick sinus syndrome. When sinus bradycardia occurs with MI or cardiac fibrosis, it is considered beneficial because diastolic filling time is enhanced, providing greater ventricular volume for the next contraction. The slower heart rate and enhanced preload may decrease oxygen demands, minimize infarct size or expansion, and may lessen the frequency of some dysrhythmias. When sinus bradycardia occurs but does not cause hypotension in acute MI, survival may be enhanced.[7]

Because the conduction pathway in sinus bradycardia is the same as in NSR, ECG characteristics appear similar to those found in NSR. The rhythm is regular unless the bradycardia is associated with sinus arrhythmia. P waves have a consistent shape but may be slightly different from NSR P waves because of a shift of the pacing site within the sinus node. PP interval should be fixed but may vary slightly from cycle to cycle in sinus arrhythmia, and the PR interval should be 0.12 second or greater. The QRS complex should appear normal, but the QT interval will lengthen.[7]

Management

Sinus bradycardia only requires treatment in patients who become symptomatic (hypotension, confusion, or signs of other end-organ hypoperfusion, diaphoresis, chest pain, or other hemodynamic compromise) or who have syncope. The drug of choice is atropine, 0.5 to 1.0 mg intravenously. If symptomatic sinus bradycardia continues after atropine treatment, a temporary or permanent pacemaker set to provide atrial pacing may be indicated.[7] In patients with chronic heart failure, the pacemaker options for enhanced cardiac performance are atrial pacing (using normal ventricular activation) or biventricular electrical stimulation when patients meet requirements for use (see Chapter 61) rather than AV sequential pacing.[9] If the cause of bradycardia is from medications, the medications should be eliminated or withheld and reevaluated. Carotid massage should be avoided.[7]

Extrasystoles

The term *extrasystole* was first coined in the late 1800s when it was discovered that after a premature ventricular contraction (**PVC**), the next atrial impulse fell during

■ ■ ■

TABLE 48-5 CLASSIFICATION OF DRUG ACTIONS BASED ON THE MECHANISMS OF DYSRHYTHMIA INITIATION

MECHANISM	DYSRHYTHMIA	VULNERABLE PARAMETER (EFFECT)	DRUGS (EFFECT)
Automaticity			
Enhanced normal	Inappropriate ST segment	↓ in phase 4 depolarization	Beta-adrenergic blocking agents
	Some idiopathic VTs		Na$^+$ channel blocking agents
Abnormal		Maximum diastolic potential (hyper-polarization)	M$_2$ agonist
	Atrial tachycardia	↓ Phase 4 depolarization	Ca^{2+} or Na$^+$ channel blocking agents
	Accelerated idioventricular rhythms	↓ Phase 4 depolarization	M$_2$ agonist Ca^{2+} or Na$^+$ channel blocking agents
Triggered Activity			
Early after depolarization	Torsades de pointes	Action potential duration (shorten)	Beta-adrenergic agonists; Vagolytic agents (increase rate)
		Early after depolarization (suppress)	Ca^{2+} channel blocking agents; Mg^{2+}; beta-adrenergic blocking agents
Delayed after depolariza-tion (DAD)		Calcium overload (unload)	Ca^{2+} channel blocking agents
	Digitalis-induced dysrhyth-mias	Suppress DAD	Na$^+$ channel blocking agents
		Calcium overload (unload)	Beta-adrenergic blocking agents
	Right ventricular outflow tract VT	Suppress DAD	Ca^{2+} channel blocking agents; adenosine
Reentry—Na$^+$ Channel Dependent			
Long excitable gap			Type IA and IC Na$^+$ channel blocking agents
	Typical atrial flutter	Depress conduction and excitability	Type IA and IC Na$^+$ channel blocking agents
	CMT in WPW	Depress conduction and excitability	Na$^+$ channel blocking agents
	Sustained uniform VT	Depress conduction and excitability	
Short excitable gap	Atypical atrial flutter	Prolong refractory period	K$^+$ channel blocking agents
	Atrial fibrillation	Prolong refractory period	K$^+$ channel blocking agents
	CMT in WPW	Prolong refractory period	Amiodarone, sotalol
	Polymorphic and uniform VT	Prolong refractory period	Type IA Na$^+$ channel blocking agents
	Bundle branch reentry	Prolong refractory period	Type IA Na$^+$ channel blocking agents
	Ventricular fibrillation	Prolong refractory period	Type IA Na$^+$ channel blocking agents; bretylium
Reentry—Ca^{2+} Channel Dependent			
	Atrioventricular nodal reen-trant tachycardia	Depress conduction and excitability	Ca^{2+} channel blocking agents
	CMT in WPW	Depress conduction and excitability	Ca^{2+} channel blocking agents
	Verapamil-sensitive VT	Depress conduction and Excitability	Ca^{2+} channel blocking agents

Ca^{2+}, Calcium; *CMT*, circus movement tachycardia; *Mg^{2+}*, magnesium; *M$_2$*, muscarinic receptor, substrate 2, *NA$^+$*, sodium; *VT*, ventricular tachycardia; *WPW*, Wolff-Parkinson-White syndrome.
Modified from Miller JM, Zipes D: Therapy for cardiac arrhythmias. In Zipes D, Libby P, Bonow R, Braunwald E, editors: *Braunwald's heart disease: a textbook of cardiovascular medicine,* ed 7, Philadelphia, 2005, WB Saunders.

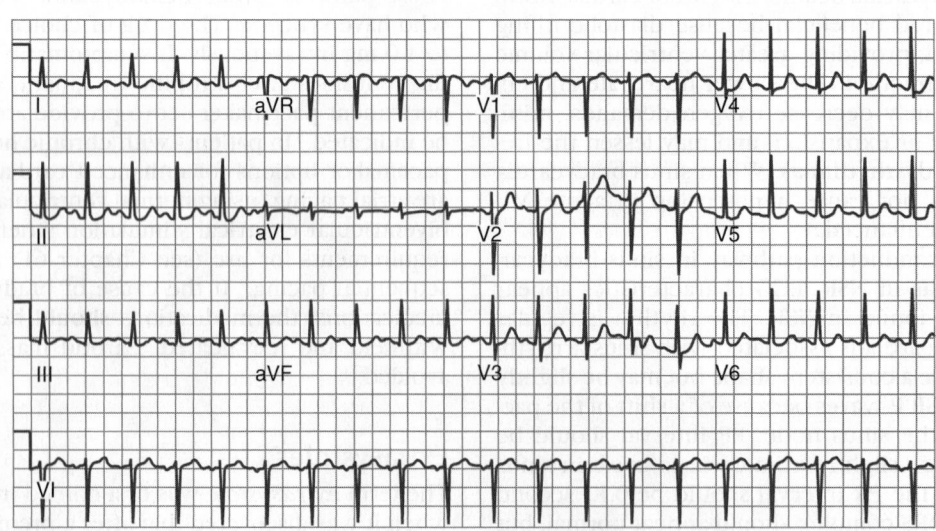

FIGURE 48-1 ■ Sinus tachycardia.

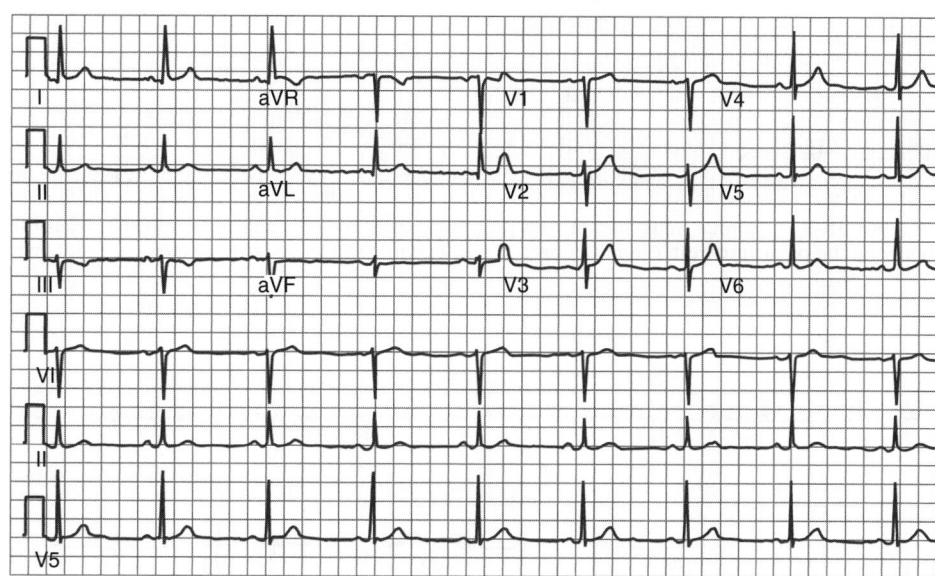

FIGURE 48-2 ■ Sinus bradycardia.

the refractory period of the PVC, making the ventricle await the next atrial stimulus. In 1904, junctional extrasystoles were discovered in venous pulse tracings, and in the early 1960s concealed ventricular extrasystoles were found in patients with bigeminy.[10]

Today, the term *extrasystole* refers to an impulse that emerges earlier than the next expected sinus beat. Essentially, extrasystoles are premature beats that arise from an ectopic focus in the atria, AV node, or His-Purkinje system. Extrasystoles can occur individually, in twos (couplets), threes (triplets), or as every other beat (bigeminy) and can result in bradycardia or can occur continuously and result in tachycardia. In most cases, extrasystoles have a fixed time relation to the previous normal depolarization. This is termed a *coupled* premature beat to signify that the premature beat is coupled to the normal sinus beat. However, extrasystoles can occur without a fixed relationship to normal beats. They may occur at a fixed interectopic interval from a *parasystolic* focus (when two pacemakers are operating simultaneously and independently; meaning that an automatic focus, protected from nonparasystolic, normal beat activations, is competing for activation of atrial or ventricular tissues).

Atrial Extrasystoles

Ectopic foci in the atria are common. Whether they are conducted to the ventricle depends on the sinus node response to the premature atrial depolarization. The sinus node response is based on the timing of the premature atrial contraction (**PAC**) in the sinus cycle and whether the premature impulse retrogradely penetrates the sinus node. Four responses are (1) impulse occurs late during diastole and fails to depolarize the sinus node because it collides with normal sinus depolarization (known as compensation; the pause created is known as a full compensatory pause because the premature beat does not disturb the regular sinus rhythm (Figure 48-3); (2) extra stimulus resets the sinus node and causes a PP interval that is of shorter duration than

a full compensatory pause (known as reset; the pause created is known as a noncompensatory pause; Figure 48-4); (3) extra stimulus, on rare occasions, does not enter the sinus node but fails to prevent conduction to the atrium of the next sinus node; thus, the atrial impulse is interpolated between two normal atrial impulses (known as interpolation; the sinus cycle length is not disturbed); and (4) the PAC, on rare occasions when it occurs early in diastole, leads to delayed entry and depolarization of the sinus node followed by sinus node reentry producing an early sinus depolarization after the PAC (known as reentry).[11]

When P waves are examined in all 12 ECG leads, the approximate site of the extrasystolic origin can be depicted. The P wave of a PAC is premature and abnormal in shape. When the focus of an atrial extrasystole P wave is close to the sinus node, the P wave resembles a normal P wave. If the focus of the abnormal beat is low in the atrium, the impulse moves away from normal electrical depolarization (downward and toward the left), so instead of an upright P wave in leads II, III, and aVF, the P wave will be negative (inversed). When an atrial extrasystole originates in the left atrial appendage or pulmonary vein area, the impulse moves toward the right instead of downward and to the left; thus, the P wave in lead I is negative.

When a PAC is followed by a ventricular complex, the PR interval may be normal or prolonged. Most PACs are conducted to the ventricle with QRS complex and T wave configurations that are the same as the surrounding conducted sinus beats; however, abnormal conduction can occur. The cycle following the atrial extrasystole is usually longer than the dominant sinus cycle, as discussed before with compensation and reset sinus node responses to the atrial extrasystole.

Not all atrial extrasystoles are conducted to the ventricles, depending on their degree of prematurity and the state of AV conduction. This is common but may be overlooked if the atrial extrasystole P wave is inconspicuous. When observing an ECG printout with an

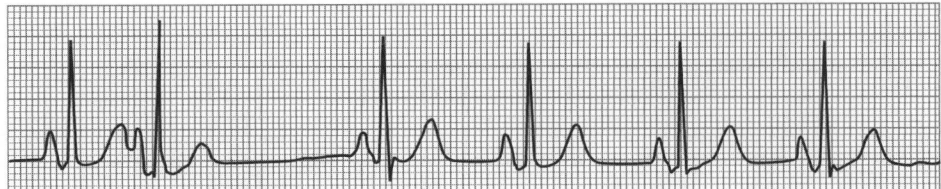

FIGURE 48-3 ▧ Normal sinus rhythm with premature atrial complex and full compensatory pause following the premature beat. (From Conover M: *Understanding electrocardiography,* ed 7, St Louis, 1996, Mosby.)

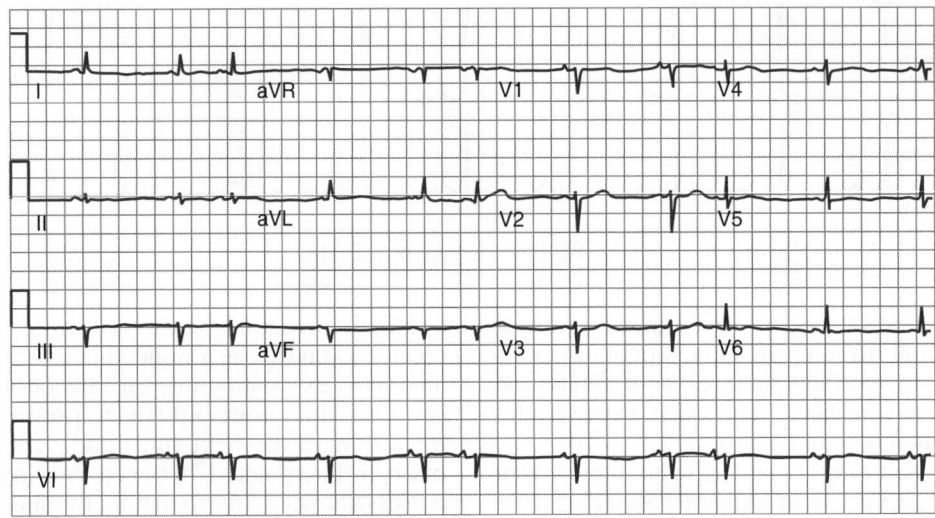

FIGURE 48-4 ▧ Normal sinus rhythm with premature atrial complex and noncompensatory pauses following each premature beat.

abruptly lengthened cycle (pause) of no apparent cause, compare the T wave of the beat immediately preceding the pause to another one. When a P wave is superimposed in the T wave, a slight distortion may occur. Nonconducted atrial bigeminy is important because it can stimulate bradycardia.

Precipitants of PACs are emotion, fatigue, alcohol, tobacco, or coffee. After MI, atrial extrasystole is reported in almost one half of all cases and can be a sign of atrial infarction. Infection, electrolyte disturbances (hypomagnesemia and hypokalemia), and hypoxia are other causes. Digitalis can lead to PACs (inhibition of sodium pump leads to decreased automaticity and increased maximum diastolic potential), and digitalis toxicity may be a forerunner to atrial tachycardia with block because toxic concentrations cause a decrease in diastolic potentials and an increase in automaticity.[12] Atrial extrasystoles can precipitate paroxysmal supraventricular tachycardias, atrial fibrillation, and atrial flutter.

Management

The incidence and significance of atrial extrasystoles are not fully known. They occur in normal adults and children; however, their incidence increases when electrical conduction abnormalities occur. In patients with complete heart block, the incidence is 30 percent, and in those with sick sinus syndrome, the incidence is as high as 88 percent.[10] Their cause should be investigated,

especially if patients are aware and bothered by their occurrence. Smoking cessation, reduction in caffeine, and restoring electrolyte balance are examples of simple interventions that may decrease occurrence. Treatment is rare and is considered only when the foci create R-on-T phenomenon leading to recurrent atrial tachycardia, flutter, or fibrillation.[13]

Atrial Tachycardia

In atrial tachycardia, impulse formation is in the atrium but outside the sinus node. The P wave precedes the QRS complex, and its polarity indicates the origin of the atrial focus. Atrial tachycardia can be *paroxysmal,* starting and stopping suddenly, or it can be *permanent* or *incessant,* defined as occurring more than 50 percent of the day.[14]

Focal atrial tachycardias, in which the impulse is formed from a discrete site, may be caused by abnormal automaticity (ischemia, electrolyte imbalance, or injury), triggered activity, or micro-reentry.[15] Atrial tachycardias can originate in the right and left atria. In the right atrium, atrial tachycardias center around the tricuspid annulus, the os of the coronary sinus, or the cristas terminalis. In the left atrium, atrial tachycardia foci tend to cluster around the ostia of the upper pulmonary veins and the mitral annulus, a similar pattern of atrial fibrillation foci.[16]

Multifocal (chaotic) atrial tachycardia is uncommon but seen most frequently in elderly, critically ill patients,

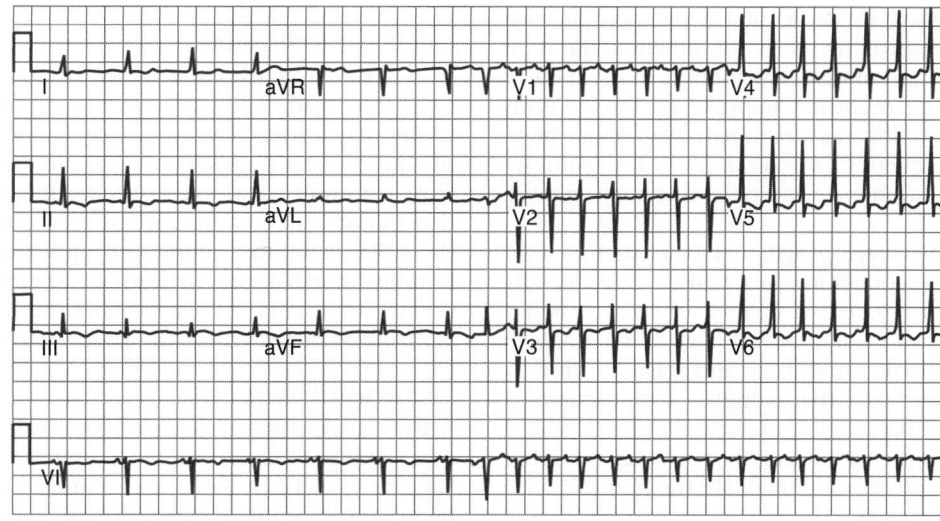

FIGURE 48-5 ▦ Normal sinus rhythm with onset of atrial tachycardia.

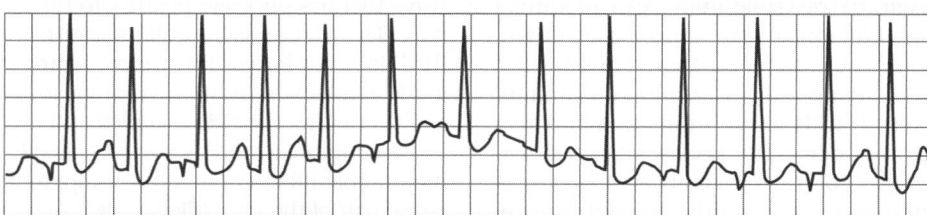

FIGURE 48-6 ▦ Macro-reentrant atrial tachycardia: multiple shaped P waves and irregular rhythm. (From Conover M: *Understanding electrocardiography,* ed 7, St Louis, 1996, Mosby.)

especially those with chronic obstructive pulmonary disease, heart failure, pulmonary infections, or pulmonary emboli. Factors associated with pulmonary disease such as hypoxia, hypercapnia, acidosis, and right atrial enlargement, as well as treatment with proarrhythmic agents such as aminophylline, contribute to development of multifocal atrial tachycardia. This tachycardia is characterized by atrial and ventricular rates greater than 100 beats/min with at least three different P wave morphologies. Given the varying focus of atrial depolarization, the atrial and ventricular rates are irregular and the PR interval is variable. Deterioration into atrial fibrillation sometimes occurs. Treatment is directed to the underlying cause, and calcium channel blockers have been used with some success.[7,17]

In autonomic atrial tachycardia, the rapid atrial rhythm speeds up after onset and slows down before termination. The atrial rate is less than 200 beats/min, and the atrial rhythm is irregular in about one half of cases. An isoelectric line between P waves, differentiating atrial tachycardia from atrial flutter, has a sawtooth pattern. AV block is often present; this only affects the ventricular rate, not the atrial rate. Intraatrial reentry is rare and is seen most commonly in congenital heart disease and in patients who had previous atrial surgery. Atrial rates are about 130 to 180 beats/min. The rhythm is usually regular, and it can be started and stopped with atrial stimulation (Figure 48-5).[7]

Macro-reentrant atrial tachycardia is rare. Foci are more likely to occur in the right atrium, and this condition is predisposed in the elderly, the critically ill, or in those with atrial incision or scar sites (e.g., a late complication after surgical repair of congenital heart disease) and is related closely to atrial flutter.[15] Macro-reentrant atrial tachycardia is characterized by multiple shapes of P waves and an irregular rhythm. Atrial rates are slower, 100 to 130 beats/min; the rhythm is irregular; P waves have three or more morphological appearances in a single ECG lead; and P waves are more likely to be conducted to the ventricles because of the slower supraventricular rate (Figure 48-6). In all forms of atrial tachycardia, the QRS complex should be normal unless there is an intraventricular conduction problem.

Implications and Management of Atrial Tachycardia

Incessant atrial tachycardia can lead to dilated cardiomyopathy.[14] Thus, a clinically significant atrial tachycardia requires therapy. In patients with focal atrial tachycardia, radiofrequency catheter ablation has a high probability of success (96 percent freedom from recurrent atrial tachycardia at 2 years) and a low risk of serious complications.[15,16] Pharmacological therapy with class III antidysrhythmic agents, calcium channel blockers, and beta blockers is the treatment of choice when multiple atrial foci are present. Class III antidysrhythmic agents might terminate ongoing reentrant excitation by blocking conduction in the reentrant pathway, at least for one beat. They prolong the action potential duration and refractory period of myocardial fibers in the reentry circuit so that the reentrant impulse no longer finds excitable tissue in the reentrant pathway. Atrial mapping and radiofrequency ablation of all foci may not be a permanent solution because new foci may emerge later.[18]

In patients who develop right atrial tachycardia after surgical repair of congenital heart disease, especially when palpitations decrease quality of life, radiofrequency ablation can be successful when all channels in and around scar tissue are isolated and ablated.[19] In multifocal atrial tachycardia that is highly symptomatic or refractory to pharmacological therapy, AV junction ablation and permanent pacemaker therapy may be more appropriate than attempting to ablate the multiple foci, especially in the elderly.[15]

Atrioventricular (Junctional) Extrasystoles

At the junction of AV tissue and the His bundle and in the His bundle itself, extrasystole impulses can spread simultaneously upward toward the atrium and downward toward the ventricles. The atria or ventricles are activated first or simultaneously depending on the rate of speed the impulse travels in each direction and also the site of the ectopic focus. The prevalence of AV extrasystole is much less common than atrial or ventricular extrasystole. In one study of healthy military personnel, only two tenths of 1 percent of adults aged 16 to over 50 years were affected.[20]

Junctional extrasystoles on an ECG strip have characteristics that are similar to junctional rhythm. An inverted P wave is found in leads II, III, and aVF, and an upright P wave is found in leads aVR and aVL. Also similar, P waves may precede the QRS complex with a shortened PR interval of less than 0.12 second, occur simultaneously with the QRS complex, or follow it (Figure 48-7). The QRS and T complex are normal unless intraventricular delays are present.

Junctional Tachycardia

In junctional tachycardia, there is usually 1:1 conduction, retrograde and antegrade to the atrium and ventricle, respectively, because the conduction systems of the atrium and ventricle are activated simultaneously.[14] Similar to junctional extrasystoles, P waves can be hidden in the QRS complex or fall on the terminal part of the QRS complex, giving the appearance of a right bundle branch block in lead V_1. Specific types of AV nodal tachycardia are discussed in the section on supraventricular tachycardias and preexcitation syndrome.

Ventricular Extrasystoles

A PVC is an extrasystole that arises from the ventricular conduction system. Ventricular extrasystoles can occur singularly, as a pair (couplet), in threes (triplet), or every other beat (bigeminy). PVCs are more likely to occur when the ventricular rate is slower. PVCs are recognized easily by their premature, wide, bizarre QRS complex (duration exceeds 120 msec), increased amplitude, and bizarre T wave that has opposite polarity to the terminal QRS complex. The rhythm is irregular because of the PVC, and the PVC does not have a P wave preceding it. Through retrograde conduction from the ventricle to the atrium, P waves can occur after the QRS complex and may be buried in the T wave. Because there is no associated P wave, there is no measurable PR interval. A full compensatory pause occurs about half of the time (Figure 48-8—compensatory pause; Figure 48-9—single PVC; Figure 48-10—couplet).

Ventricular extrasystoles are labeled by their appearance in the cardiac cycle. An end-diastolic PVC occurs late in the cardiac cycle. A P wave may immediately precede the wide, bizarre QRS complex, but it has nothing to do with the ectopic beat. Thus the PR interval is shorter than normal (Figure 48-11). In some cases, the PVC occurs closely timed to normal ventricular conduction through the His bundle. The QRS complex may begin or end normally (similar initial or late deflection of a normal QRS complex), but the ectopic activation

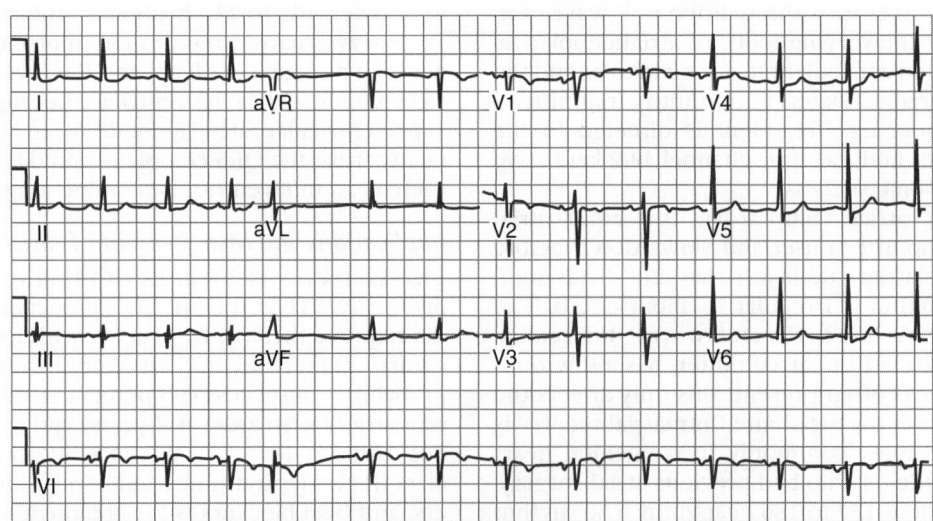

FIGURE 48-7 ■ Normal sinus rhythm with single premature junctional contraction. Note the p wave after the QRS complex (fifth impulse).

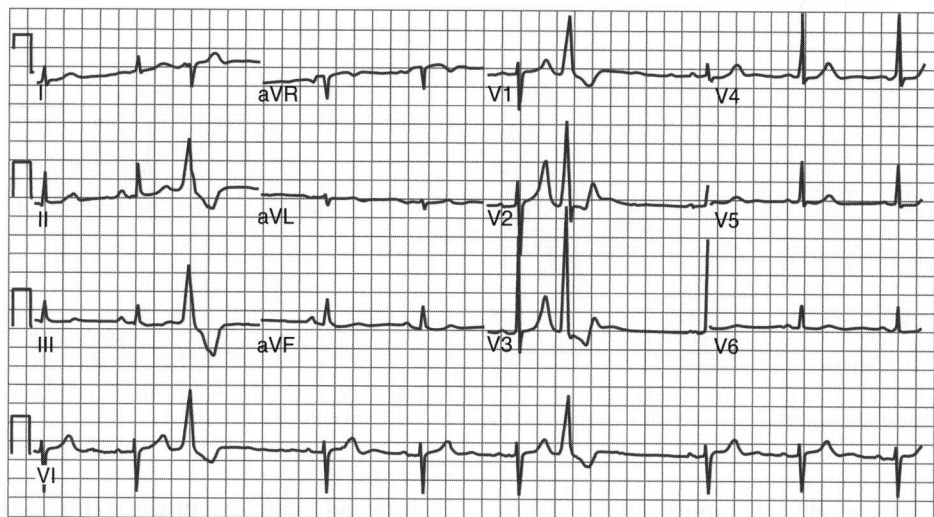

FIGURE 48-8 ▦ Sinus bradycardia with two isolated premature ventricular contractions with compensatory pauses; third and seventh QRS complexes.

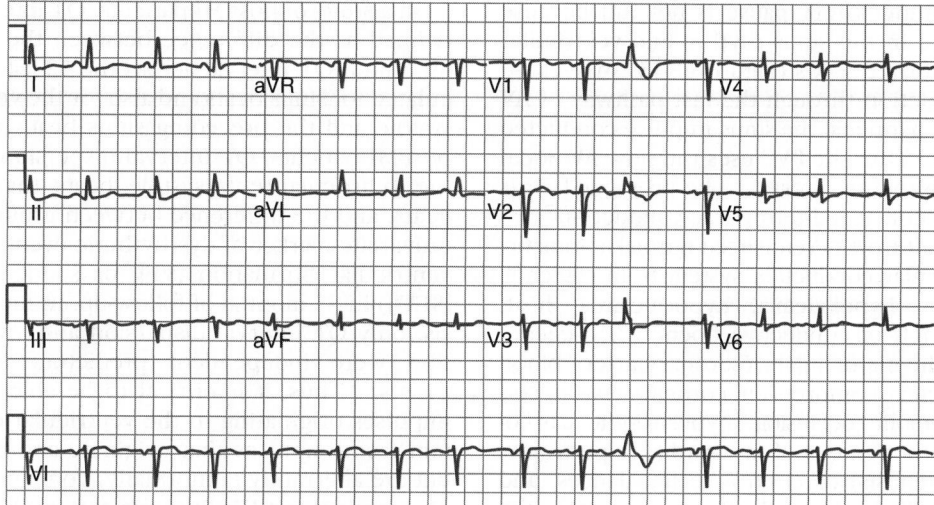

FIGURE 48-9 ▦ Normal sinus rhythm with single premature ventricular contraction. Note predominantly upright impulse in lead V_1 reflects premature ventricular impulse formation in the left ventricle.

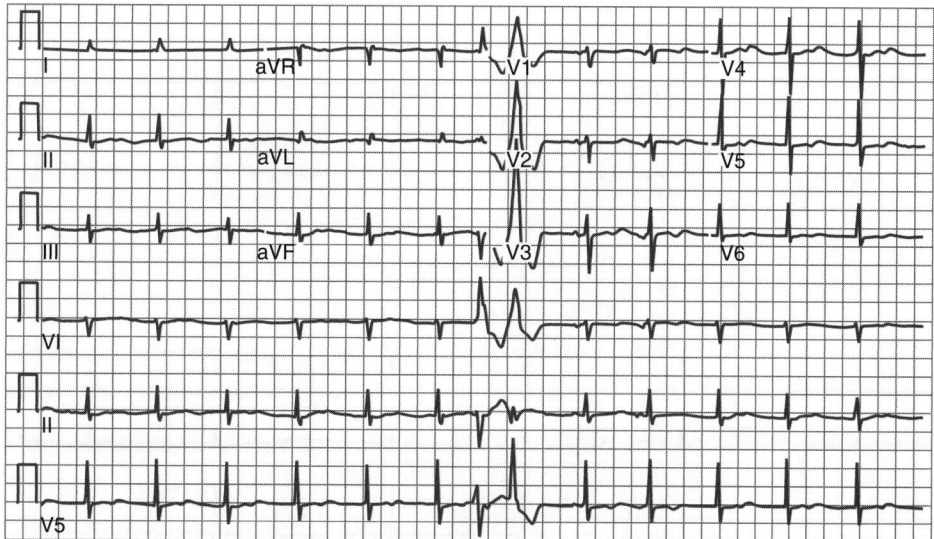

FIGURE 48-10 ▦ Accelerated junctional rhythm with premature ventricular contractions; couplet. Note that in full electrocardiogram strips (at the bottom reflecting lead V_1, II, and V_5), the different morphology of each premature ventricular contraction reflects impulse formation in different parts of the ventricles. Also note that the first two impulses after the second premature ventricular contraction are not sinus beats: the first beat has a p wave originating from the right atrium (upright in leads II, V_2, V_3, and V_5), and the second beat has a p wave originating from the left atrium (negative p wave in leads V_1 and V_2).

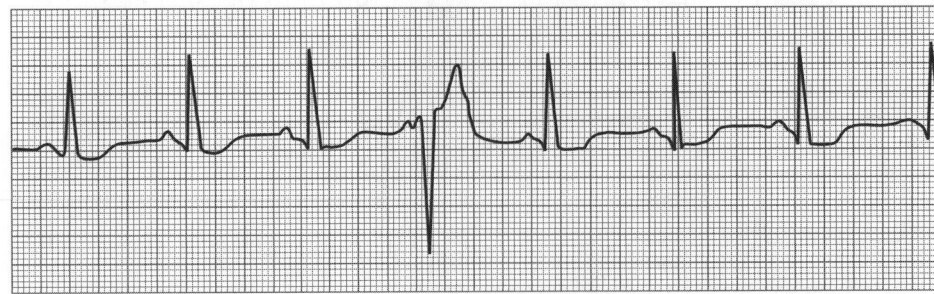

FIGURE 48-11 ■ Normal sinus rhythm with one end-diastolic premature ventricular contraction. (From Conover M: *Understanding electrocardiography,* ed 7, St Louis, 1996, Mosby.)

creates an abnormally conducted impulse (*fusion beat*) and an abnormal T wave (Figure 48-12). Ventricular extrasystoles also can be interpolated or sandwiched between two normal sinus-conducted beats. When this happens, the compensatory pause is not full because there is no pause in the sinus rhythm and ventricular response. Interpolated PVCs (Figure 48-13) may cause retrograde conduction through the fast pathway of AV node. When this happens, the sinus impulse conducted into the ventricles after the PVC uses the slow AV nodal pathway, causing the AV interval to be prolonged. This is an example of concealed retrograde conduction.[7]

A PVC can result from (1) enhanced normal automaticity in the ventricular conduction system from catecholamines, hypoxia, hypokalemia, hypocalcemia, heat, trauma, and stretch of conductive fibers; (2) triggered activity from ischemia or injury (coronary artery blood flow, coronary artery compression, coronary spasm, coronary artery embolic occlusion, hypertrophic cardiomyopathy, and other causes of myocardial hypertrophy such as aortic stenosis) or electrolyte imbalances; and (3) reentry through slowly conducting tissue within the His bundle, the bundle branches, and the Purkinje network or within the ventricular myocardium from inflammatory and infiltrative diseases (Chagas disease, arrhythmogenic right ventricular dysplasia, sarcoidosis, acute myocarditis, and muscular dystrophies), ischemia, hyperkalemia, or antidysrhythmic class IA or IC drugs.[7,14,21]

In a study of post-MI patients, QT interval dispersion, defined as the difference between the maximum and minimum QT interval across the 12-lead ECG, was calculated for sinus beats and also for the ventricular extrasystole and the preceding sinus beat. In these remote post-MI patients, QT interval dispersion was greater in the ventricular extrasystole beats than in the sinus beats, and the difference between groups was a strong univariate marker of dysrhythmic events (sustained VT, ventricular fibrillation [**VF**], or sudden cardiac death [**SCD**]) in 35 months of follow-up. In multivariate analysis, only QT interval dispersion and low ejection fraction were independent predictors of dysrhythmic events.[22] Thus, it is critical to be able to differentiate impulses originating in the ventricular conduction system from impulses that originate above the ventricles but are aberrantly (abnormally) conducted through the AV junction and His-Purkinje system, because misdiagnosis can lead to misperceptions about treatment that could affect morbidity and mortality.

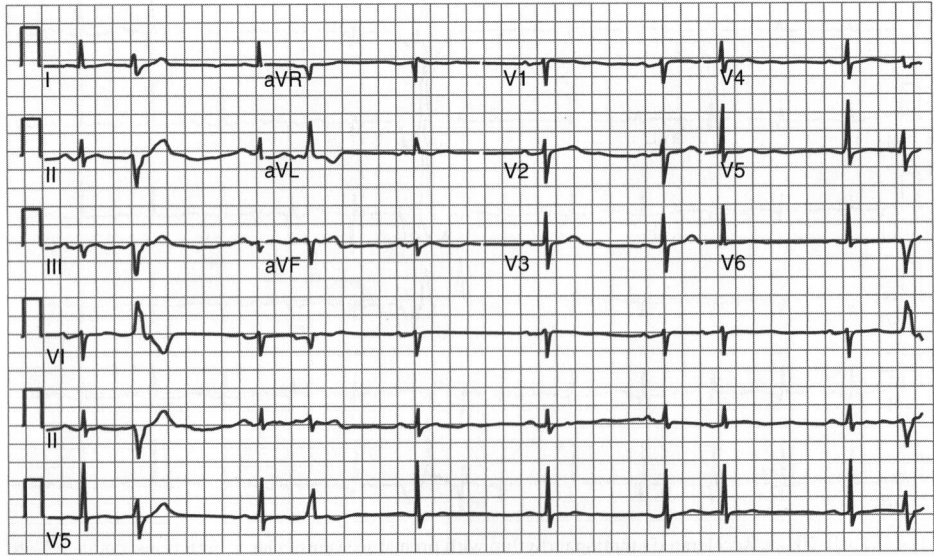

FIGURE 48-12 ■ Sinus bradycardia with first-degree atrioventricular block; one premature atrial complex (third last beat) and three premature ventricular complexes (second beat, fourth beat [fusion beat], and last beat).

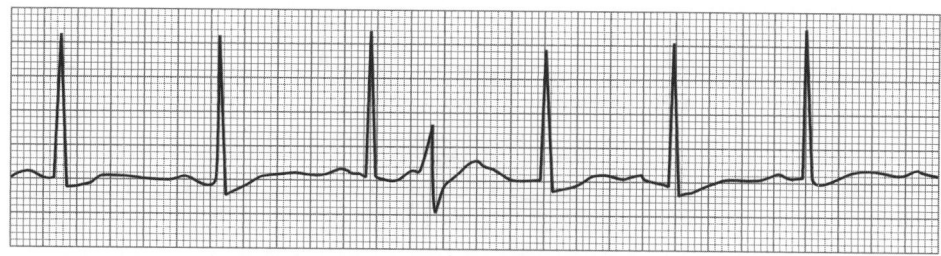

FIGURE 48-13 ■ Normal sinus rhythm with one interpolated premature ventricular contraction. (From Conover M: *Understanding electrocardiography,* ed 7, St Louis, 1996, Mosby.)

Differentiating Ventricular Extrasystole from Bundle Branch Block

To distinguish between supraventricular aberrantly conducted impulses and ventricular extrasystoles, the precordial V_1 lead should be used (lead V_6 is an alternate in patients with midsternal dressings that cover the right sternal border). In patients with a five-lead ECG monitoring system, modified chest lead 1 (**MCL$_1$**) should be used only if the V_1 lead is not an option in the monitoring system. The V_1 lead is preferred because characteristics of ventricular extrasystoles can differ in MCL$_1$ and lead V_1. Although the planes of electrical activity are different in lead V_1 (vector moves from center of body toward the lead V_1 positive electrode) and MCL$_1$ (vector moves from the negative electrode at the left clavicle to the positive electrode at the MCL$_1$ position), both have the same positive electrode placed at the right sternal border, 4th intercostal space. A ventricular extrasystole arising from the right ventricle has a wide, bizarre complex that is mainly negative (QRS complex vector created by the ectopic impulse moves away from the positive electrode; Figure 48-14). The R wave, when present, is greater than 0.04 second, and the S wave has a slurred downslope that measures 0.06 second or more from the beginning of the QRS complex to the S nadir. An ectopic impulse arising from the left ventricle has a wide, bizarre complex that is mainly positive (QRS complex vector created by the ectopic impulse moves toward the positive electrode; from left to right; Figure 48-15). Generally, the impulse is monophasic (R wave only) or biphasic (QR or Rs complex), but not triphasic.

In bundle branch blocks, the QRS complex is abnormal because impulse conduction through the ventricular conduction system is abnormal. In right bundle branch block, leads V_1 and V_6 are mainly positive but have a triphasic pattern. In lead V1, the pattern is rSR' to reflect initial normal septal depolarization (r), normal left ventricular activation (S), and delayed right bundle activation (R'; Figure 48-16). In lead V_6, there is a narrow q wave representing normal septal depolarization, an R wave representing normal left ventricular activation, and an S wave representing late right bundle activation. In left bundle branch block, lead V1 has a small, narrow R wave that measures 0.04 second or less, the downslope of the S wave is fast and without slurring or notching, and the distance from the beginning of the QRS complex to the nadir of the S wave is 0.06 second or less. In lead V6, there should be no Q or S wave (Figure 48-17).[14]

Another feature that differentiates ventricular extrasystole from aberrantly conducted supraventricular beats is *concordance*. In concordance, leads V_1 to V_6 show positive or negative QRS complexes, referred to as

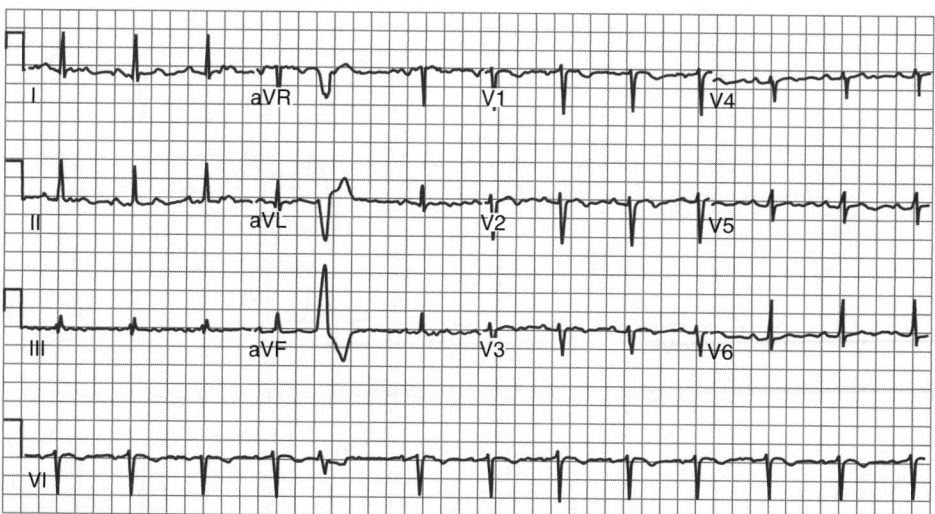

FIGURE 48-14 ■ Normal sinus rhythm with premature ventricular contraction initiated from the right ventricle; note mainly negative QRS complex with slurred S wave morphology of the fifth beat in lead V1 (bottom of figure).

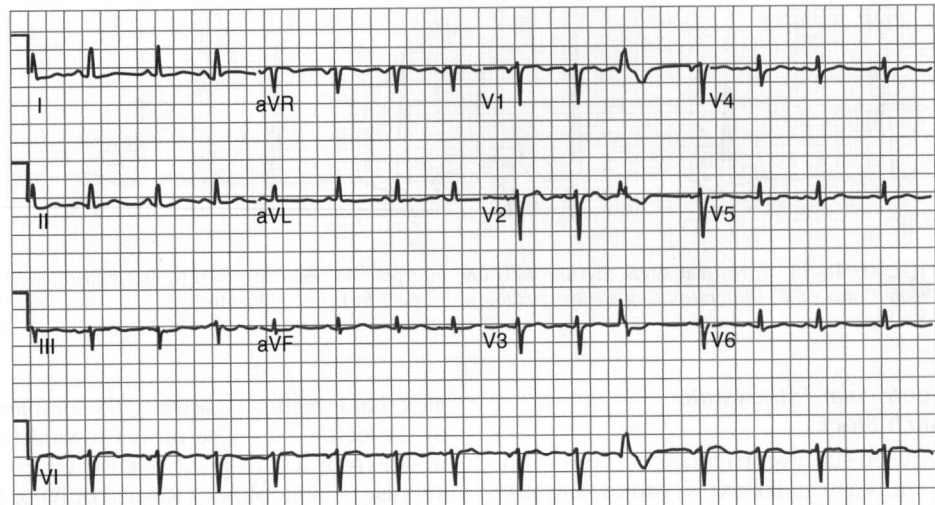

FIGURE 48-15 ■ Normal sinus rhythm with premature ventricular contraction initiated from the left ventricle; note upright QRS morphology in the eleventh beat in lead V_1 *(bottom of figure)*.

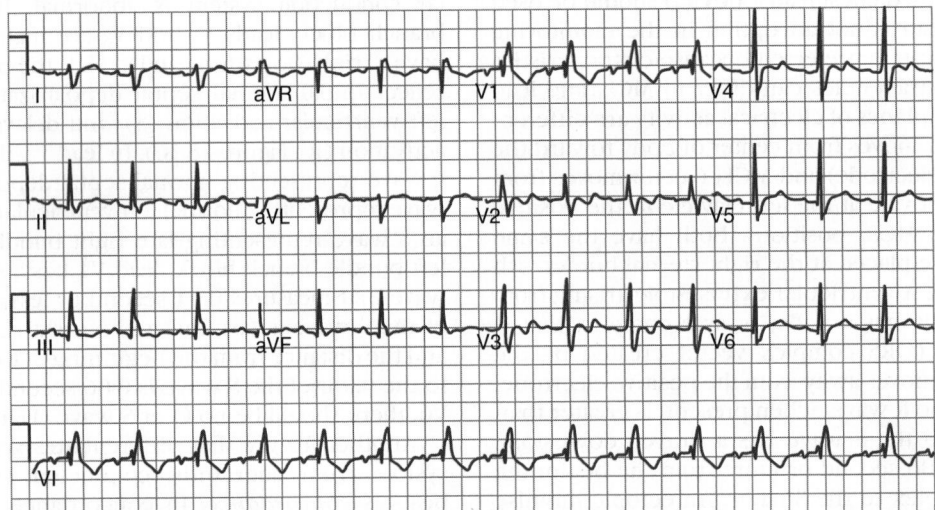

FIGURE 48-16 ■ Normal sinus rhythm with borderline first-degree atrioventricular block and right bundle branch block; note rSR′ morphology of QRS complex in lead V_1 and slurred upstroke of S wave in lead V_6.

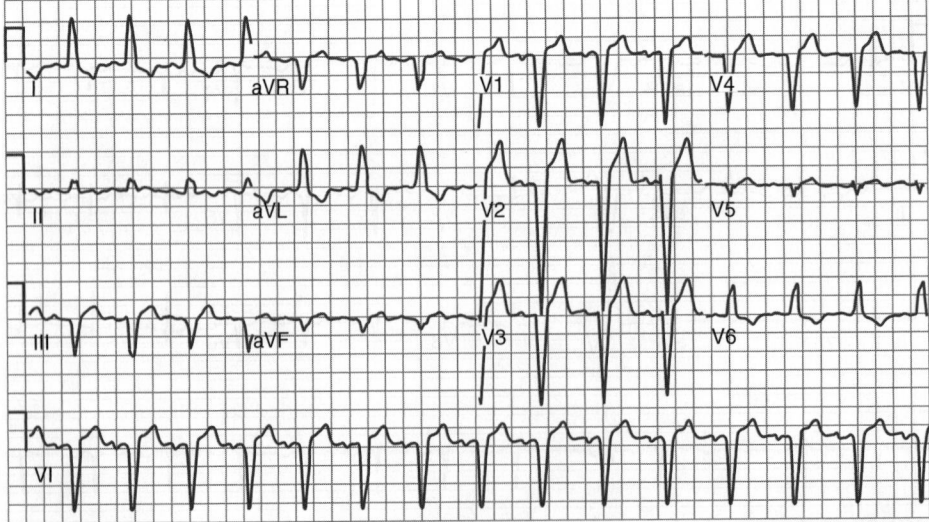

FIGURE 48-17 ■ Normal sinus rhythm with left bundle branch block; note QRS complex morphology in leads V_1 and V_6.

positive and *negative concordancy.* Although most ventricular ectopic beats are not concordant in leads V$_1$ to V$_6$, negative concordance of a wide, bizarre QRS complex impulse is diagnostic of ventricular ectopy (Figure 48-18). In positive concordance, ventricular ectopy is favored, but not absolute.[14]

Management

Management depends on the cause of the ventricular extrasystole. When PVCs are provoked by fast or slow heart rates, correction of the heart rate abolishes the dysrhythmia. Atropine, isoproterenol, or ventricular pacing can be used to speed up a slow heart rate.

In patients with left ventricular systolic dysfunction of ischemic or nonischemic origin or in post-MI and systolic left ventricular dysfunction, whether asymptomatic or symptomatic, the rate of SCD from ventricular dysrhythmias is high.[14] When PVCs are present, they are not considered benign. Amiodarone has been the drug of choice for managing ventricular tachydysrhythmias, especially in monomorphic VT, non–QT interval prolonged polymorphic VT and VF since the American Heart Association published its guidelines for cardiopulmonary resuscitation and emergency cardiovascular care in 2000.[23] Even though most of the studies were performed in hemodynamically unstable ventricular tachydysrhythmias, amiodarone is an acceptable choice in stable ventricular dysrhythmia categories as well.[24] Amiodarone is the best therapy for patients with heart failure and a low ejection fraction; however, chronic use does not improve survival.[25] (See the evidence-based practice feature.)

Atrial Fibrillation

Atrial fibrillation **(AF)** is a supraventricular tachycardia characterized by uncoordinated atrial activation. P waves are replaced by rapid oscillations or fibrillatory

waves that vary in size, shape, and timing (Figure 48-19). The ventricular response is irregular when AV conduction is intact. R-R intervals are irregularly irregular, and the ventricular rate (when not suppressed by rate lowering drug therapy) is most often greater than 100 beats/min. When AF occurs in the setting of heart block or with certain drugs, R-R intervals may be regular. The ventricular response in AF depends on AV nodal conduction properties, vagal and sympathetic tone, and drugs that affect AV nodal conduction. In addition, a permanent ventricular sensing and pacing pacemaker may produce regular R-R intervals even though the atrial rhythm is chaotic and AV conduction is not intact (Figure 48-20).[26]

AF is the most common dysrhythmia, affecting 0.4 percent of Americans, and becomes progressively more common with aging. Persons older than 65 years have a

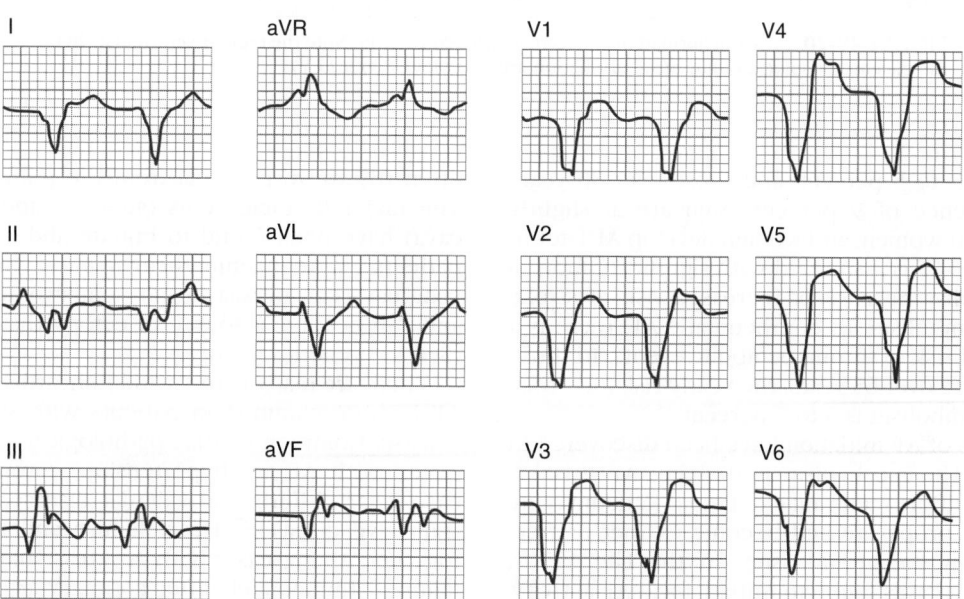

FIGURE 48-18 ■ Negative concordance in V leads favors ventricular ectopy. (From Conover M: *Understanding electrocardiography,* ed 7, St Louis, 1996, Mosby.)

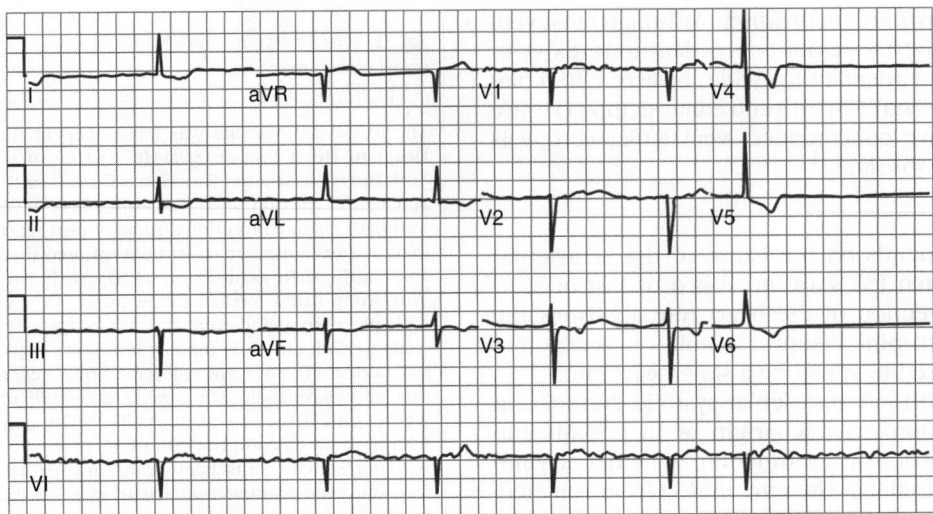

FIGURE 48-19 ▪ Course atrial fibrillation (lead V1) with slow ventricular response.

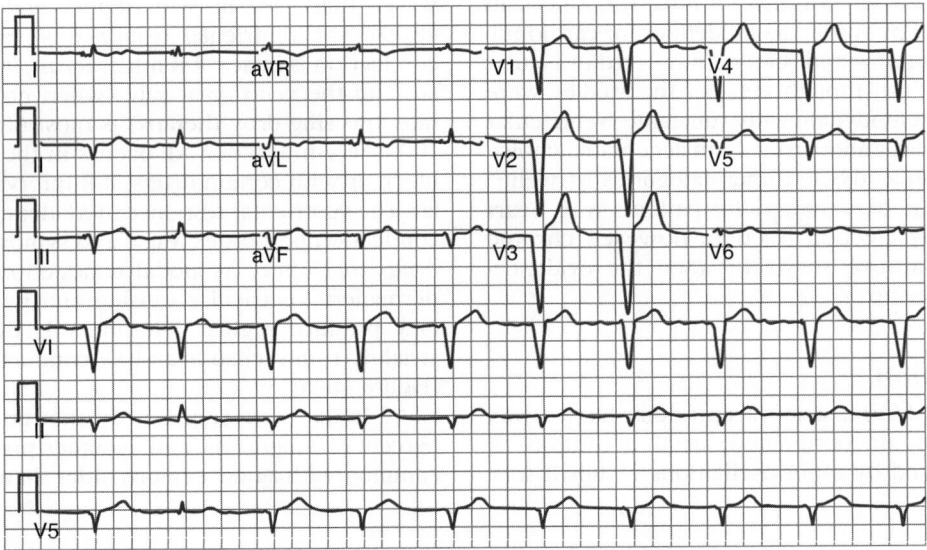

FIGURE 48-20 ▪ Atrial fibrillation in paced ventricular rhythm. Note the regular ventricular rhythm; the pacemaker spike and fine atrial fibrillation are best viewed in lead V_1.

prevalence of 3 to 5 percent, and those over 80 years have a prevalence of 9 percent. Men are at slightly higher risk than women, and women develop AF later in life than men.[27] AF is associated with significant mortality and morbidity because of increased risk of stroke and thromboembolism. In nonrheumatic AF, there is a fivefold overall risk of thromboembolic events. In those with AF who are over 65 years, the yearly risk for stroke and thromboembolism is 5 to 7 percent.[28]

The sources of AF initiation have been discovered in recent years. The mechanism underlying AF was believed to be multiple reentrant excitation. Random reentrant wavelets propagate and become extinct or fractionated within the atrial tissue. In the late 1990s, triggered activity was found to initiate focal AF activity. Researchers found that AF was initiated by a single activity or trains of ectopic activity that originated most

often (89 to 96 percent) from the pulmonary veins.[29] The major thoracic veins (superior and inferior vena cava) have been found to initiate and maintain AF. In patients with congenital heart disease, the left superior vena cava can persist despite embryonic development and can become a source of ectopy that initiates AF.[30] (See the genetics feature.)

There are many cardiac and noncardiac causes of AF. AF is more common in patients with structural heart disease. Common cardiac pathological conditions associated with AF are hypertension, coronary heart disease, heart failure, and valvular disease, especially mitral valve disease.[27] Heart failure and AF often exist together; AF increases with progression of clinical heart failure.[31] Immediately after coronary artery bypass surgery, 15 to 33 percent of patients develop AF. This compares with 38 to 64 percent of patients who develop AF

■■■ GENETICS

ATRIAL FIBRILLATION

Atrial fibrillation (AF) was thought to be caused by predominately patient factors such as white race, increasing age, hypertension, diabetes, and structural heart disease, especially left ventricular systolic dysfunction. However, new insights into the genetic basis of AF have altered this perspective. With the discovery of gene expression changes that cause electrical and structural remodeling of the atria during AF, researchers now understand that genetic factors are involved as well.[1]

In 1997, the chromosomal location of an AF gene was discovered in three families in Spain who shared common ancestry (chromosome 10q22-q24), but the culprit gene or genes were never identified.[2] This finding led to the notion that autosomal dominant AF had a genetic locus and that it might even be a single gene disorder. More recently, when studying four multigenerational families with AF, researchers determined that the locus for AF was heterogeneous.[3] In studies of families with and without documented AF, researchers mapped a novel locus for familial AF to chromosome 6q14-16 and for neonatal AF to chromosome 5p13.[4,5] Researchers now hypothesize that idiopathic or lone AF, named when AF occurs in the absence of structural heart disease and in those younger than 65, may have a genetic basis. At some point, genetic screening may become the standard in management of familial (and lone) AF in clinical practice.[1]

Can genomics play a role in nonfamilial, non-lone AF? In a study of 250 consecutive patients with a history of nonfamilial, non-lone AF and 250 controls, researchers found association between renin-angiotensin system gene polymorphisms and AF.[6] These results may provide rationale for the investigation of angiotensin-converting enzyme inhibitor or angiotensin receptor antagonist agents in the treatment of structural AF.

Learning about genes and phenotype correlations has increased the understanding of the molecular mechanisms leading to AF. This new knowledge will foster continued research in gene expression and its effect on electrical and structural remodeling of the atria, maintaining AF, and transforming paradoxical AF into persistent or permanent AF. New knowledge could have important implications for prevention, treatment with early external or implantable atrial defibrillator cardioversion, therapies aimed at reversing or modulating the remodeling process, and counseling about an optimal approach to care.[1]

References

1. Mestroni L: Genomic medicine and atrial fibrillation, *J Am Coll Cardiol* 41:2193-2196, 2003.
2. Brugada R, Tapscott T, Czernuszewicz G et al: Identification of a genetic locus for familial atrial fibrillation, *N Engl J Med* 336:905-911, 1997.
3. Darbar D, Herron KJ, Ballew JD et al: Familial atrial fibrillation is a genetically heterogeneous disorder, *J Am Coll Cardiol* 41:2185-2192, 2003.
4. Ellinor PT, Shin JT, Moore RK et al: Locus of atrial fibrillation maps to chromosome 6q14-16, *Circulation* 107:2880-2883, 2003.
5. Oberti C, Wang L, Li L et al: Genome-wide linkage scan identifies a novel genetic locus on chromosome 5p13 for neonatal atrial fibrillation associated with sudden death and variable cardiomyopathy, *Circulation* 110:3753-3759, 2004.
6. Tsai CT, Lai LP, Lin JL et al: Renin-angiotensin system gene polymorphisms and atrial fibrillation, *Circulation* 109:1640-1646, 2004.

after cardiac valvular surgery. Postoperatively, risk is highest in the elderly and in those with a previous history of AF.[27]

Researchers studied patients within the first year after isolated coronary artery bypass surgery. Those patients aged 50 to 59 and 60 to 69 years had a higher incidence of AF compared with prevalence data from the Framingham Heart Study (1.5 percent versus 0.4 percent, aged 50 to 59 years, and 3.1 percent versus 1.6 percent, aged 60 to 69 years; both $p < 0.05$); however,

the presence or absence of AF did not predict embolic events in this surgical cohort.[32] Common noncardiac factors associated with AF are alcohol (binge drinkers), fever, hyperthyroidism, electrolyte abnormalities, hypothermia, and chronic pulmonary disease.[28]

Many theories have been proposed about what causes AF to persist; however, the theory supported by high-resolution atrial mapping is the multiple wavelet hypothesis. In this hypothesis, AF persists as long as a critical number of wavelets are present in the atria. AF causes electrophysiological and structural changes in the atrial myocardium, and these changes support the initiation and maintenance of the rhythm; thus, AF begets more AF.[29]

Although the ECG is the main diagnostic tool for diagnosis, AF can be paroxysmal and is frequently asymptomatic; thus, a single ECG has limited sensitivity.[27] Holter monitors can identify the initiating mechanisms (triggers) and specific substrate of AF and the presence of other supraventricular dysrhythmias. This is important because AF can start during sinus bradycardia or tachycardia, with atrial extrasystoles or supraventricular tachydysrhythmias. Patients may alternate between atrial flutter and AF, and they may have a diurnal onset (vagal AF that has an onset at night with preceding bradycardia or adrenergic AF that has an onset during daytime or occurs with exercise). This knowledge can guide treatment modalities.[29]

AF is classified by how it terminates. *Paroxysmal* refers to episodes that terminate spontaneously within a few days of initiation. About one half of these patients have no known or obvious cause (labeled lone or idiopathic AF). *Persistent* is the term used to describe AF that does not self-terminate; it must be cardioverted to terminate and restore NSR. Persistent AF occurs less frequently than paroxysmal. *Permanent* AF is one that cannot be converted to NSR; thus, this term refers to chronic AF because a single episode of AF cannot be fully categorized. Patients with this form of AF generally have hypertension and ischemic heart disease or chronic heart failure.[33]

Atrial Flutter

Atrial flutter (**AFL**) is considered a form of supraventricular tachycardia. AFL accounts for approximately 15 percent of cases and often coexists with AF.[33] An acute disease process such as acute MI, chronic obstructive pulmonary disease exacerbation, or the effects of cardiac or pulmonary surgery can stimulate the occurrence of AFL.[17] Similar to AF, electrical remodeling of the atria can occur with AFL, and this can perpetuate the dysrhythmia.[34] AFL can be typical, originating from the right atrium, or atypical, originating from the left atrium.

In typical AFL, when atrial tissue is activated, the impulse rotates continuously in one direction (counterclockwise) through a ring of myocardium made up of septal, superior, anterior, and inferior right atrial walls. Through anisotropic conduction, the right atrium supports reentry because myocardial fibers conduct rapidly in the longitudinal direction but slowly in the transverse direction. The orifices of the superior and inferior vena cava, the tricuspid ring, and other right atrial anatomical obstacles make the virtual ring of myocardium that supports reentry in typical AFL.[35]

Flutters also can begin in the left atrium; however, these are less common. Reentry is the mechanism that begins the circuits, but the circuits tend to have large multiple macro-reentrant loops with the earliest activation neighboring the latest activation. Small reentrant circuits also have been found and are defined as those with a diameter of less than 3 cm. Loops center around the mitral annulus or in association with the pulmonary veins.[36] Loops also have been found around the left atrial septum in patients without history of cardiac surgery.[37] The stability of the single loop reentrant circuit depends on the presence of electrically silent areas or a zone of block that acts as a barrier and prevents short circuiting of the dysrhythmia. In patients who had mapping of the circuits that initiated and maintained AFL, the dysrhythmia was chronic or lasted for weeks without interruption, and maintenance was never due to a focal activity.[36]

The ECG pattern depends on the type of AFL—typical or atypical. In typical AFL, the ECG has a complex waving pattern (F, flutter wave) resembling a wood saw edge (sawtooth pattern) in leads II, III, and aVF (the inferior leads). The amplitude of atrial deflections is usually small in leads I and aVL and in the precordial leads, except for lead V1, in which discrete P wave–like positive or biphasic (but occasionally negative) deflections are seen (Figures 48-21 and 48-22).[35] In atypical left AFL, there is a clearly visible F wave; however, it may be flat in lead V1 or begin as a low-amplitude positive wave and then become negative. The amplitude of the F waves may be very low in other leads as well. Atrial rates are usually greater than 240 atrial beats/min, compared with AF atrial rates of 400 to 600 beats/min.

Management of Atrial Fibrillation and Atrial Flutter

Rate control, rhythm control, permanent pacemaker, radiofrequency ablation, or surgical ablation of AF: which is best? In the past, the notion that everyone deserved to be in NSR was acted on through strategies

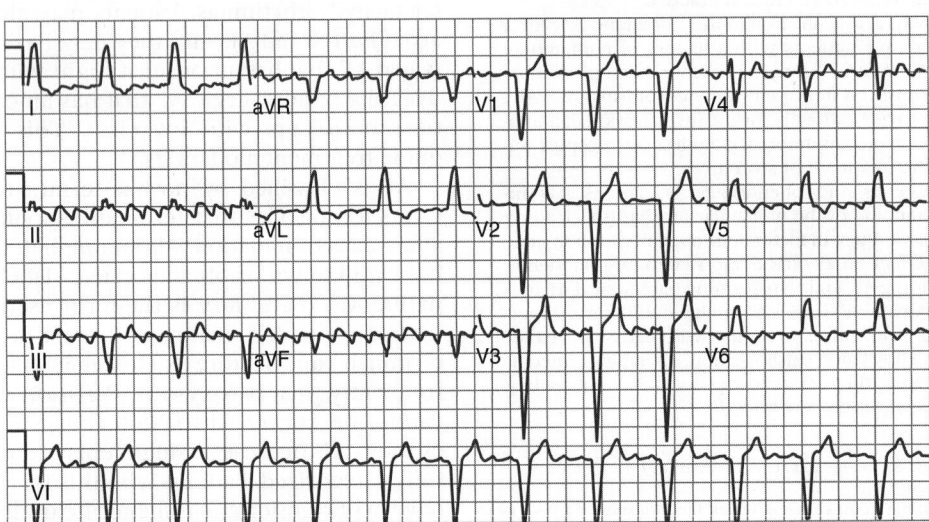

FIGURE 48-21 ▨ Atrial flutter with 4:1 atrioventricular conduction. Note left bundle branch block (leads V₁ and V₆).

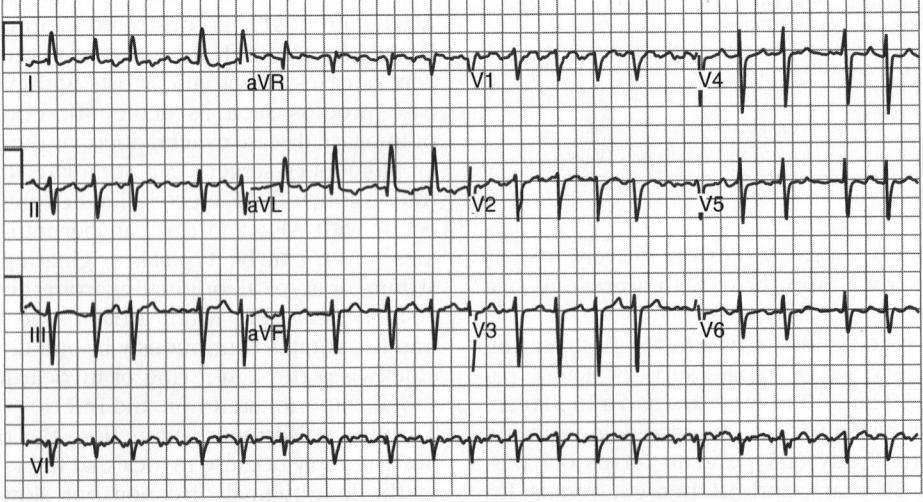

FIGURE 48-22 ▨ Atrial flutter with variable atrioventricular block; thus variable ventricular rate.

aimed at rhythm control. When rhythm was controlled, patient's symptoms were relieved and in some cases, chronic anticoagulation was no longer required. Current research data suggest that rate control is not inferior to rhythm control and that rate control is a reasonable first-line strategy in the treatment of recurrent AF, especially in patients who are asymptomatic, mildly symptomatic, or elderly. In four rate-versus-rhythm control studies, patients were generally those with persistent AF, and the mean patient age at enrollment was 60 to 69.7 years. In these studies, 59 to 74 percent of patients were male, and many had history of cardiovascular diseases. Chronic heart failure was common, but few had New York Heart Association functional Class IV symptoms. Patients were maintained on anticoagulation therapy in both arms of these studies. Compared with rhythm control, the mortality, thromboembolism, and stroke rates did not differ significantly in patients randomized to rate control.[38] Rhythm control increased hospitalizations and led to more proarrhythmias. Further research is needed to determine the benefit of rate versus rhythm control in younger patients.

Rate control drug choice depends on the presence of systolic left ventricular dysfunction. Adenosine is not recommended as a therapy of choice because the half-life is very short. In patients with preserved left ventricular function, beta-adrenergic blockers, calcium channel blockers, and digitalis can be used for rate control. Intravenously administered calcium channel blockers verapamil or diltiazem are recommended when the heart rate is greater than or equal to 120 beats/min. Intravenously administered digitalis is the least effective agent and has the slowest onset of action. Intravenously administered amiodarone (a complex drug with effects on sodium [class I], potassium [class III], calcium channels [class IV], and alpha- and beta-adrenergic blocking properties [class II]) is also effective for rate control and can be used in combination with digitalis. In heart failure with systolic dysfunction, digitalis and amiodarone are recommended. When AF has been present for greater than 48 hours, anticoagulation therapy with warfarin is recommended.[23]

The role of permanent pacing to prevent AF was summarized in a 2005 advisory report from two councils of the American Heart Association, in collaboration with the Heart Rhythm Society.[39] The role of pacing has been controversial. Ventricular pacing is associated with a higher risk of AF in patients with sinus node dysfunction; thus, if a pacemaker is needed for bradycardia, a dual-chamber or atrial pacemaker is supported, rather than a single-chamber ventricular pacemaker. In patients with dual-chamber pacemakers and intact AV conduction, the device should be programmed so that the ventricular pacemaker is activated as infrequently as possible. When a pacemaker is part of an implantable defibrillator, the rapid atrial pacing feature should be activated to terminate AF when it is sensed. Currently, permanent pacing to prevent AF is not indicated; however, the role of pacing requires further clarification and research.

When patients have AF or AFL symptoms that disrupt their quality of life or if the cause of AF is easily correct-

able, pharmacological or electrical cardioversion is warranted. Cardioversion is recommended when AF or AFL is hemodynamically unstable. Electrical cardioversion is the preferred treatment to restore sinus rhythm, but when it is not feasible, pharmacological cardioversion is recommended. If the AF has been present for more than 48 hours, anticoagulation therapy should be initiated and continued for a minimum of 3 weeks before electrical cardioversion to decrease the risk of systemic embolization. Drug treatment depends on the presence of systolic left ventricular dysfunction. Amiodarone (intravenously or orally) is recommended over other drugs when systolic dysfunction is present or in patients with preexcited AF or AFL.[23] When left ventricle function is preserved, procainamide (class IA), amiodarone (class III), flecainide (class IC), propafenone (class IC), or sotalol (class III) can be used.

Radiofrequency ablation of focal AF (using a medical or surgical approach) has been an effective form of cure in patients with drug-refractory symptomatic AF or AFL; but success rates vary by approach (22 to 86 percent for medical radiofrequency ablation and 60 to 90 percent for surgical ablation) depending on patient selection and the strategies and perioperative procedures used. Complications, although rare, are more prevalent with a surgical approach and include coronary artery damage and atrioesophageal fistula. Before medical ablation, antidysrhythmic agents and anticoagulants are discontinued. Amiodarone is discontinued 3 to 4 months before the procedure because the drug has a long half-life. Perioperative procedures include isolating all four pulmonary veins with radiofrequency ablation or identifying the critical connections between the substrate and triggers that connect electrically with the pulmonary veins using a mapping catheter and then creating discrete radiofrequency lesions to isolate these connections in addition to isolating the pulmonary veins.[40]

From a surgical approach, there has been an evolution of techniques over the last two decades. In the early 1990s the Maze procedure, which consisted of extensive surgical dissection of the right and left atria to force electrical impulses to follow a maze from the atrium to the AV node, prevented the formation and perpetuation of multiple wavelets responsible for AF maintenance.[41] This technique requires an open chest, has a long procedural time (long aortic cross clamp and extracorporeal circulation times), has a risk of bleeding, and a perioperative mortality of 1.3 to 2.1 percent. Today, simpler procedures are used surgically to dissect atrial tissue around the pulmonary veins. Different energy sources are available to create the linear lesions and include cryothermy, radiofrequency, and laser energy.[41]

In patients with symptomatic typical AFL (that originates in the right atrium), radiofrequency catheter ablation that creates a bidirectional (complete) conduction block involving the inferior vena cava and tricuspid annulus isthmus has persistent benefits in suppressing all atrial dysrhythmias in a subset of patients with AFL and AF and significantly reducing episodes of palpitations in those with AFL.[41,42] After ablation, patients still required antidysrhythmic agents because of the occurrence of late AF. These patients were maintained on oral anticoagulation therapy for the same reason. If there is no AF recurrence 3 months after the procedure, then anticoagulation therapy may be stopped.[43]

Supraventricular Tachycardias and Preexcitation Syndrome

Paroxysmal supraventricular tachycardias (PSVTs) are fairly common and frequently occur in persons with otherwise normal hearts. However, they can be highly disruptive and frightening, but fortunately, rarely fatal. Dysrhythmias caused by a reentry process within the AV node and involving the AV node and an accessory pathway are discussed. Treatment modalities such as catheter ablation have eliminated the tachycardia for many patients, enabling them to return to a full lifestyle.

Atrioventricular Nodal Reentry Tachycardia

Estimated to account for about 60 percent of all PSVT, AV nodal reciprocating tachycardia, also known as AV nodal reentry tachycardia (AVNRT) is seen in persons with no underlying heart disease and in those who because of concomitant cardiac conditions may poorly tolerate its rapid rates. More common in women, AVNRT is seen in patients with two pathways within the AV node, termed *fast* and *slow pathways*.[17] Whether these pathways are anatomically and/or functionally distinct is unclear.[8]

Commonly, the fast-conducting pathway transmits stimuli to the ventricles during sinus rhythm or following PACs that occur with longer coupling intervals. PR intervals tend to be normal and often less than 140 msec. Refractoriness of the fast-conducting pathway occurs when it is subjected to faster atrial pacing rates or a PAC with a shorter coupling interval, shifting AV nodal conduction to the slow-conducting pathway. The typical tachycardia occurs when a PAC falls at a critically early time, blocking the fast-conducting pathway but continuing to conduct via the slow-conducting pathway to the ventricles. Given the inherently slower conduction of the slow-conducting pathway, the fast-conducting pathway recovers to allow retrograde conduction to the atria, completing the reentry circuit and setting the stage for a sustained tachycardia with heart rates of 150 to 250 beats/min. Rates of 180 to 200 beats/min are common in adults and can exceed 250 beats/min in children. This pattern accounts for 85 to 95 percent of patients with AVNRT.

The QRS complex in AVNRT is narrow because conduction to the ventricles is normal. Atrial activation in the typical tachycardia occurs during or at the end of the QRS complex. P waves are therefore absent or so close to the QRS complex that in lead V1 the retrograde P wave appears as a second R wave, a "pseudo R" or r′wave, not seen during sinus rhythm. In the inferior leads (II, III, and aVF), these retrograde and inverted P waves appear as "pseudo S waves." The appearance of these P waves mimicking R or S waves during the tachycardia but absent in sinus rhythm is the most sensitive and specific factor differentiating AVNRT from other types of reentrant atrial tachycardias (Figure 48-23).[8,17]

Atypical or unusual versions of the tachycardia use the fast-conducting pathway for anterograde conduction and the slow-conducting pathway for the retrograde path (5 to 10 percent incidence), with P waves, inverted in leads III and aVF, preceding the QRS complex. A rare form uses multiple slow-conducting pathways for both arms with P waves following the QRS complex at a midway point in the cycle.[8,17]

Atrioventricular Reciprocating Tachycardia

Under normal circumstances, the only pathway for transmission of electrical impulses from atria to ventricles is through the AV node. Patients with accessory pathways have the potential for simultaneous conduction to the ventricle via the AV–His-Purkinje system and via the accessory pathway. Accessory pathways, also termed *Kent bundles,* have been located on the left and right free walls and anteroseptal, midseptal, and posteroseptal regions of the AV ring.[6] Simultaneous conduction over the AV node and accessory pathway in sinus rhythm may cause a delta wave on the ECG, indicating early ventricular muscle activation over an accessory

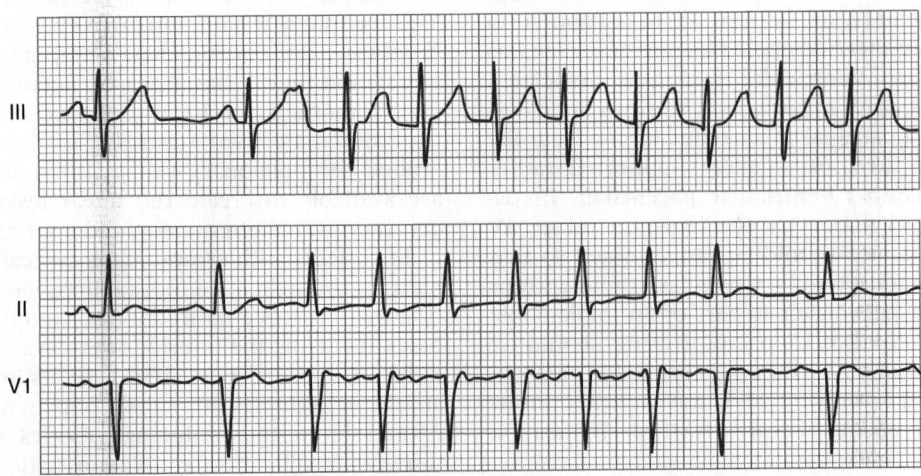

FIGURE 48-23 ■ Atrioventricular nodal reentry tachycardia. (From Conover M: *Understanding electrocardiography,* ed 7, St Louis, 1996, Mosby.)

pathway that lacks the filtering and delay characteristics of the AV node. The resulting QRS complex is a fusion of these two pathways with an initial slurred upstroke and a normal terminal portion. Some patients have accessory pathways that conduct only in the retrograde direction and therefore have no evidence of preexcitation on ECG, termed *concealed conduction*.[17]

ECG evidence of preexcitation and a reentry tachycardia is called Wolff-Parkinson-White **(WPW)** syndrome, discussed further in Chapter 47.[17] In 5 to 10 percent of patients with WPW syndrome, the tachycardia is reversed with anterograde conduction flowing via the accessory pathway and retrograde conduction via the AV node. This wide complex tachycardia shows maximal preexcitation and may resemble an exaggerated version of the delta wave–distorted sinus rhythm QRS complex. Because of the wide QRS complex, it is critical to differentiate WPW syndrome from VT. This antidromic atrioventricular reciprocating tachycardia **(AVRT)** is usually regular, although slight irregularity may occur if conduction over the left bundle branch fascicles is variable. An irregular tachycardia should prompt concern that AF may be the atrial activator with rapid conduction via the accessory pathway to the ventricles and the potential of degeneration into VF. The accessory pathway may have some role in the development of AF in these patients because they tend to be young and without evidence of structural heart disease. These patients are at risk for VF if this occurs.[8,17] Refer to Figures 48-24 to 48-27.

Another preexcitation pathway results from fibers connecting the atrium with the His bundle (atriohisian tracts) and bypassing the normal AV nodal delay. This sinus rhythm with a short PR interval, narrow QRS complex, and associated tachycardia is known as Lown-Ganong-Levine syndrome, also discussed in Chapter 47.[44] Recent evidence fails to support a specific Lown-Ganong-Levine syndrome tachycardia related to this tract.[8]

Patient Presentation

For patients who have episodes of paroxysmal, regular palpitations, AVNRT or AVRT are the most likely sources, particularly if vagal maneuvers successfully terminate the tachycardia. Associated symptoms include fatigue, dyspnea, light-headedness, chest discomfort, and polyuria resulting from release of atrial natriuretic peptide. Atrial stretch caused by repeated atrial contraction against closed AV valves stimulates release of the hormone. Presyncope may occur, but actual syncope is seen more rarely (15 percent), and the presence of causative factors such as the AF with anterograde conduction over an accessory pathway, aortic stenosis, or hypertrophic cardiomyopathy should be investigated.[17]

The most common forms of PSVT in infants and children with normal hearts are AVNRT and AVRT. Despite having structurally normal hearts, these children may develop symptoms of congestive heart failure during tachycardia because of impaired diastolic filling. In children too young to report palpitations, symptoms such as diaphoresis, vomiting, and pulmonary and intestinal congestion may mimic other disease conditions and delay accurate diagnosis. Palpitations are the dominant symptom reported by older children.[45]

Elders who have PSVT are more likely to have AVNRT because of its greater incidence in the population. Prior reports of age-related Kent bundle degeneration have been discounted somewhat by recent reports showing that accessory pathway–mediated tachycardias account for 20 percent of PSVT in those 60 to 69 years of age but fall to less than 5 percent in those over 79 years of age. Elders, however, are at greater risk because of concomitant heart disease and its effect on tachycardia tolerance; their diminished ability to feel the tachycardia, which delays treatment; greater syncope and fall risk because of vagal hypertonia following the sympathetic response; and treatment difficulties resulting from cardiac and noncardiac functional alterations.[46]

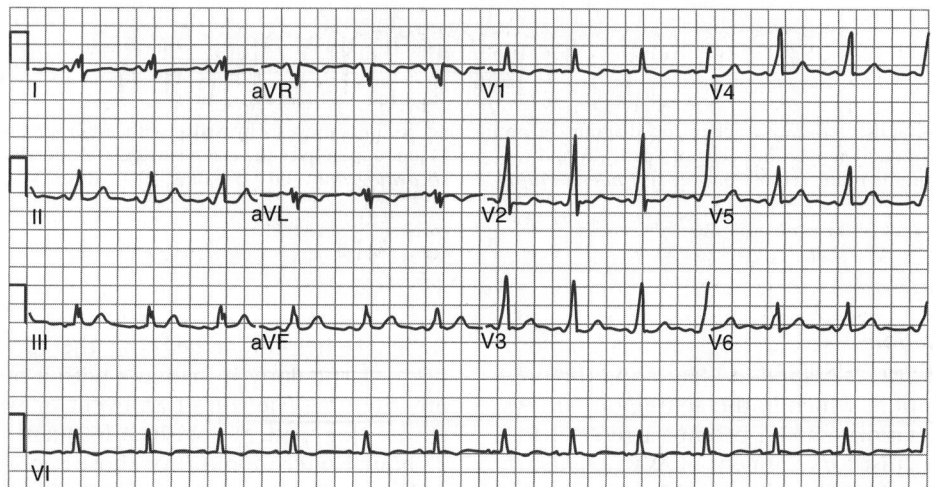

FIGURE 48-24 ■ Schematic diagram of orthodromic reciprocating tachycardia with anterograde conduction over the atrioventricular node–His bundle route and retrograde conduction over the accessory pathway. Resulting electrocardiogram shows disappearance of the delta wave and evidence of atrial activity on the ST segment. (From Conover M: *Understanding electrocardiography*, ed 7, St Louis, 1996, Mosby.)

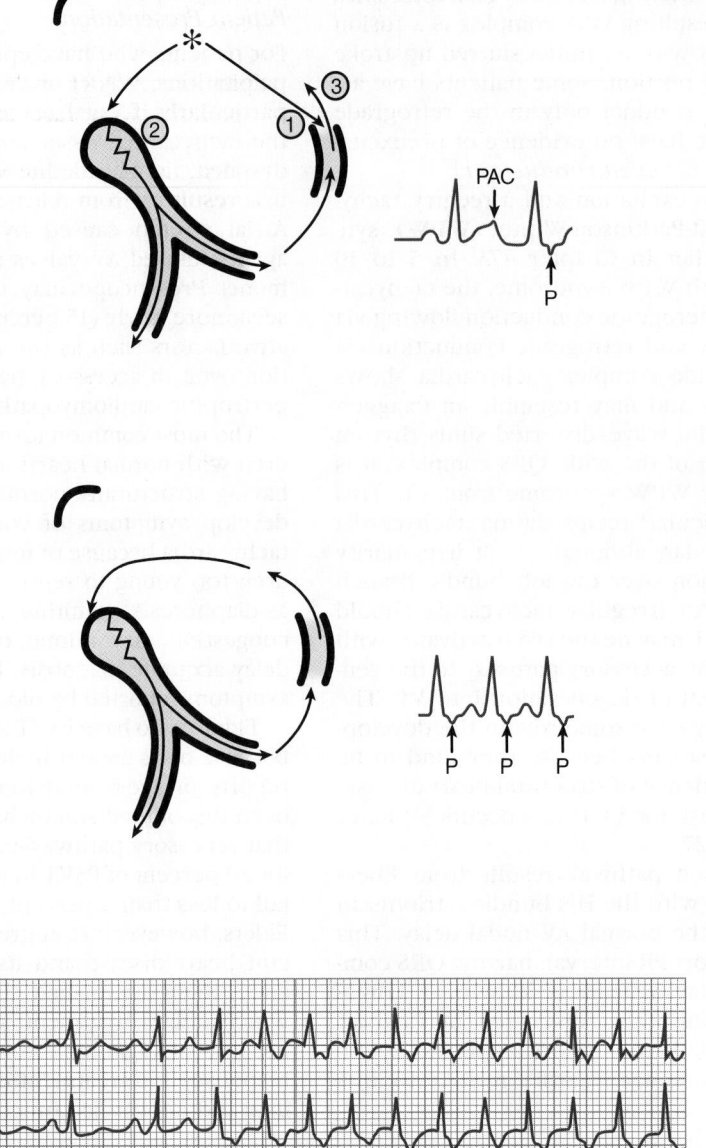

FIGURE 48-25 ■ Schematic diagram of antidromic reciprocating tachycardia with anterograde conduction over the accessory pathway and retrograde conduction over the atrioventricular node–His bundle route. (From Conover M: *Understanding electrocardiography*, ed 7, St Louis, 1996, Mosby.)

Diagnostic Evaluation

A resting 12-lead ECG is helpful in identifying the presence of preexcitation, which in the setting of paroxysmal regular palpitations should prompt a referral to a dysrhythmia specialist for treatment of AVRT. A history of irregular palpitations in patients with preexcitation warrants immediate electrophysiological evaluation because of the risk of AF and rapid ventricular conduction via an accessory pathway. A 12-lead ECG during the tachycardia, provided the patient is hemodynamically stable, is helpful in defining the tachycardia mechanism, particularly in patients with a normal ECG in sinus rhythm. The use of an event or wearable loop recorder for patients with infrequent tachycardias, a 24-hour Holter monitor for those reporting several episodes per week, or a rhythm strip from the defibrillator monitor in unstable patients may capture the tachycardia for analysis. Tachycardias associated with exercise may be recorded during exercise stress testing. ECG documentation of the response of tachycardia to vagal

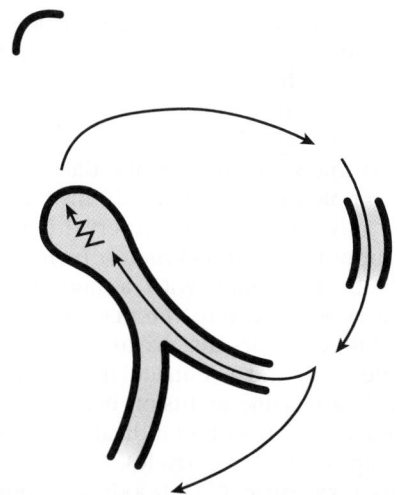

FIGURE 48-26 ■ Schematic diagram of atrial fibrillation conducting over the accessory pathway and resulting electrocardiogram. (From Conover M: *Understanding electrocardiography,* ed 7, St Louis, 1996, Mosby.)

maneuvers and its termination assists with diagnosis because AVRT and AVNRT frequently terminate with a P wave following the last QRS complex. Atrial tachycardia tends to terminate with a QRS complex.[17]

Management of Atrioventricular Nodal Reentry Tachycardia and Atrioventricular Reciprocating Tachycardia

The patient with ECG evidence of preexcitation but no tachycardia requires no electrophysiological evaluation or therapy.[8] For patients with tachycardia, vagal maneuvers such as Valsalva or carotid massage in adults and cold water facial immersion in infants may be effective

in restoring sinus rhythm, but these techniques are less effective once a sympathetic response to the tachycardia has been established. Oral administration of beta blockers or calcium channel blockers may be effective for patients with rare and well-tolerated events, although their absorption during rapid PSVT is impaired and these agents do not affect accessory pathway conduction.[8,47] Digitalis shortens the refractory period of an accessory pathway and should be avoided as a single agent in patients with AF or AFL and WPW syndrome.[8] In hemodynamically stable patients, intravenously administered adenosine is the preferred agent because of its short half-life and rapid onset. Although contraindicated in patients with severe asthma, effectiveness rates of 90 to 95 percent are reported. For patients with frequent atrial or PVCs that may serve as triggers for new episodes of PSVT, longer-acting agents such as intravenously administered calcium channel blockers (verapamil or diltiazem) or beta blockers (metoprolol) are useful.[17] Adenosine is the agent of choice for infants and neonates and patients with heart failure or severe hypotension. Verapamil may be preferable in those with poor venous access or bronchospasm but carries a hypotension risk that becomes accentuated if the tachycardia persists. The effect of these agents is predominantly on the AV node.[47] If AFL or AF is present, drug combinations that affect the accessory pathway and AV node, such as procainamide and propranolol, should be used. If rapid conversion is needed because of hemodynamic intolerance, direct current cardioversion provides the most rapid restoration of NSR.[8]

In wide complex antidromic AVRT, pharmacological agents that target the AV node or accessory pathway are effective, provided that the AV node is involved. Occasionally, patients may have two accessory pathways

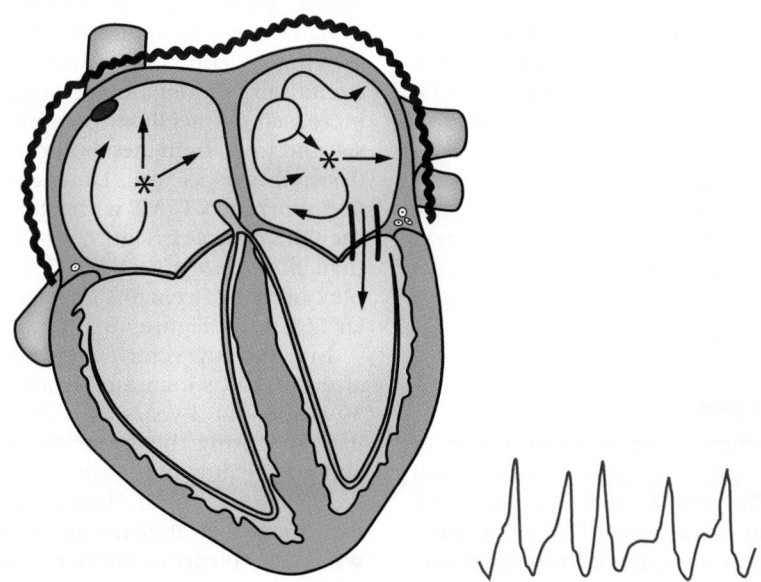

FIGURE 48-27 ■ Atrial fibrillation with conduction via a right posteroseptal accessory pathway. (From Olgin J, Zipes D: Specific arrhythmias: diagnosis and treatment. In Zipes D, Libby P, Bonow R, Braunwald E, editors: *Braunwald's heart disease: a textbook of cardiovascular medicine,* ed 7, Philadelphia, 2005, WB Saunders.)

mediating a tachycardia that excludes the AV node. Also, if the mechanism of the tachycardia is AF with anterograde conduction via the accessory pathway, treatment must target the accessory pathway. Agents such as intravenously administered ibutilide, flecainide, or procainamide are recommended.[17]

Research demonstrating effective drug therapy for long-term prophylaxis AVRT is limited to small, nonrandomized trials. Agents with some effectiveness include propafenone, flecainide, and sotalol. Amiodarone is not more effective than the other agents and is associated with significant organ toxicity when used for long-term treatment.[17]

Radiofrequency ablation applies heat at the catheter-tissue interface, creating well-demarcated lesions that permanently disrupt electrical conduction. AVNRT ablation of the slow pathway frequently cures the tachycardia while preserving normal AV nodal conduction with a normal PR interval. Success rates of 96 to 98 percent are common with low (less than 2 percent) recurrence rates and extremely low (less than 1 percent) incidence of second- or third-degree heart block or death (0.2 percent).[6,17,48]

Ablation of accessory pathways should be offered as first-line therapy for patients who have symptomatic WPW syndrome, particularly if hemodynamic instability accompanies the tachycardia. Patients with infrequent and minimally symptomatic episodes may opt for ablation if drug therapy proves ineffective or is associated with bothersome side effects or if their job, insurability, mental health, or public safety would be hindered by tachydysrhythmias.[6] Success rates of 95 percent have been reported, with slightly higher rates for ablation of left free wall accessory pathways compared with other accessory pathway locations. Complication rates are low, averaging 2 percent, and include vascular access problems, myocardial perforation, coronary dissection, heart block, and rarely, death (0.1 percent). Asymptomatic patients with preexcitation should be encouraged to seek medical attention if dysrhythmia symptoms occur. For asymptomatic patients, the benefit of electrophysiological testing to evaluate risk should be considered in light of the potential complication risk associated with catheter ablation. Patients with concealed accessory pathways do not face the risk of extreme tachycardia or VF caused by anterograde accessory pathway conduction in AF. Decreased effectiveness plus side effects associated with drug therapy have caused catheter ablation therapy to be the treatment of choice for many patients.[17,48]

Ventricular Tachycardias

Ventricular tachydysrhythmias are a major cause of SCD, and SCD is a major cause of cardiovascular death in the United States.[49] The term *ventricular tachycardia* is given to ventricular extrasystoles (ECG characteristics are described in the ventricular extrasystoles section) when three or more appear in succession. Unlike PVCs, in VT the R-R interval can be exceedingly regular or it can vary. Although many texts list the lower heart rate range of VT at 100 beats/min, it can range between 70 and 250 beats/min (depending on the type of VT),

and the onset can be sudden. VT is termed *sustained* when it lasts longer than 30 seconds or requires termination because of hemodynamic collapse. In *nonsustained* VT, the dysrhythmia terminates spontaneously in less than 30 seconds.[8]

Differentiating VT from SVT with aberrant conduction (QRS complex greater than 120 msec) may be difficult, especially when the R-R interval is regular. Features that support VT are (1) *fusion beats* (ventricular extrasystole beat collides with a normal sinus beat while being conducted into the ventricle; this creates complexes with contours that are intermediate between a normal sinus beat and a ventricular extrasystole beat), (2) *capture beats* (same as fusion beat except that the QRS complex is narrower and indicates that the normal sinus beat captured the ventricle), (3) AV dissociation, (4) compensatory pause, (5) left axis deviation, (6) QRS complex duration greater than 140 msec, and (7) specific QRS complex contours: polymorphic, as described subsequently, and concordance.[8]

VT with a negatively deflected QRS complex in lead V1 can be differentiated from a SVT with a left bundle branch block. In VT, the down stroke of the QRS complex is slurred with the time from onset to nadir exceeding 0.06 second. In left bundle branch block, the QRS complex has a sharp down stroke with the time from onset to nadir being less than 0.06 second.[3]

Most VT is due to (1) abnormal conduction of the cardiac impulse because of changes in conduction velocity, path length, and recovery of excitability (all are determinants of reentrant excitation) and (2) myocardial architecture.[50] Although reentry is the most common mechanism of VT, focal autonomic and triggered automaticity also play a role.[21]

Cardiac ischemia is a common cause of VT. During acute ischemia lasting 15 to 30 minutes or more, morphological changes in the electrophysiological structure of ventricular myocardium (such as prolonged refractoriness, shortened action potentials, electrical uncoupling of myocytes, and electrically inert cells) lead to slowing of conduction and vulnerability to reentrant excitation.[21,50] Metabolic changes during ischemia (e.g., increased extracellular potassium concentration, acidosis, and toxic lipid metabolites) can provoke ventricular dysrhythmias as well. During an acute ischemic event, *polymorphic* VT (VT with an irregularly variable axis of the QRS complex; Figure 48-28) is more likely to occur than *monomorphic* VT (VT in which each QRS complex of the VT remains constant [uniform] in a particular ECG lead; Figure 48-29).[8]

In one study, ventricular dysrhythmias were frequent after MI; PVCs increased from 29 percent at baseline to 39 percent at 2 years, and 20 to 23 percent of patients had VT during the 2-year period.[51] During the healing and posthealing phases of MI, VT can occur from microscopic architectural changes in the surviving myocardial fibers that abut the necrotic tissue and extend toward the epicardial surface.[50] In the region of the scar itself, not all fibers die, especially in the subendocardial and subepicardial layers.[21] These surviving muscle fibers can be electrically active and can generate normal-appearing action potentials. When a sufficiently premature impulse encounters a refractory region of tissue, it

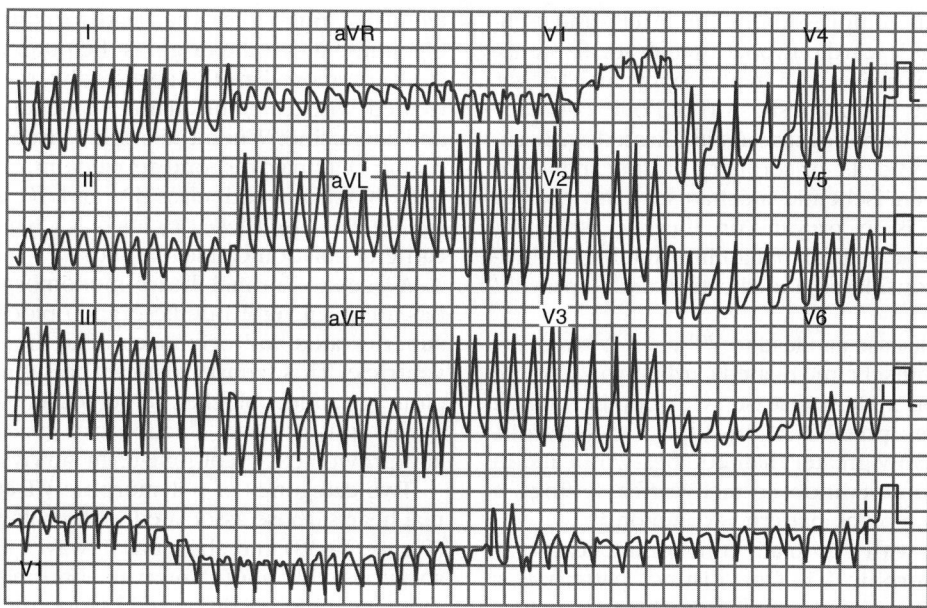

FIGURE 48-28 ■ Three recordings of polymorphic ventricular tachycardia in a patient on day 5 after an acute myocardial infarction. (From Conover M: *Understanding electrocardiography,* ed 7, St Louis, 1996, Mosby.)

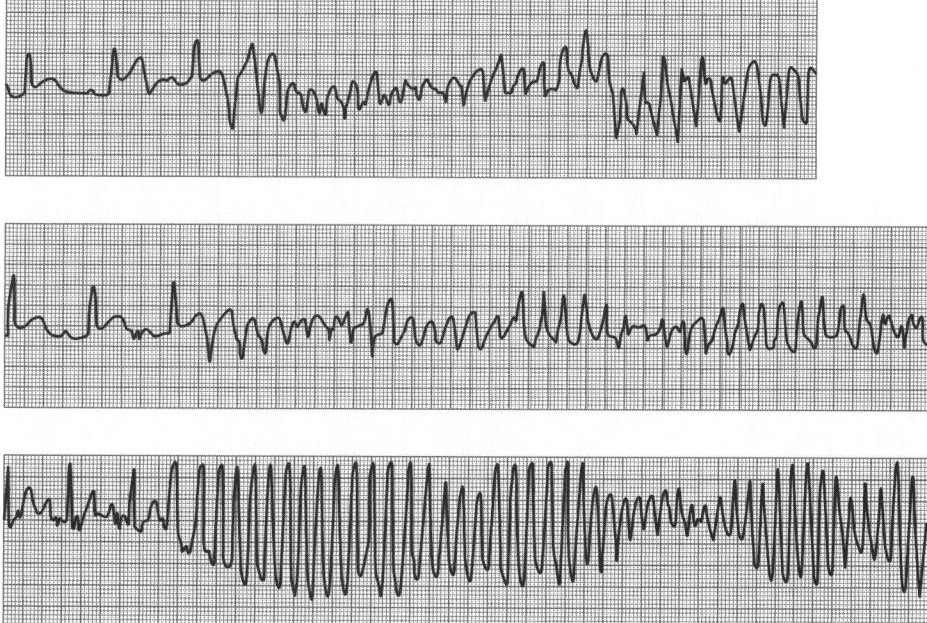

FIGURE 48-29 ■ Three recordings of monomorphic ventricular tachycardia. (From Conover M: *Understanding electrocardiography,* ed 7, St Louis, 1996, Mosby.)

circles around it to form a complete circuit of continuous reentrant excitation, producing stable monomorphic VT.[50] Because scar tissue is interwoven with these viable muscle fibers and because refractory periods may be prolonged, low amplitude and prolonged signals are common. These properties create a unidirectional block and the slow conduction necessary to sustain the reentrant wavefront.[21] In chronic ischemia, dysrhythmogenesis may arise due to slowing of conduction velocity from alterations in myocardial intracellular coupling and conduction velocity.

Thus, patients with ischemic heart disease and those who have experienced an MI have the potential for reentrant VT. Through quantitative echocardiographic assessment, researchers found that an increase in left ventricular systolic and diastolic cavity area and deteriorating left ventricle function predicted VT and PVCs greater than 10 per hour between baseline and 2 years post-MI.[51]

Other ischemic causes of VT are unrelated to coronary artery disease. Polymorphic VT and VF should be considered in athletes who have SCD. This could be due to a rare congenital abnormality such as an anomalous takeoff of a coronary artery from the wrong coronary cusp, resulting in compression of the artery and ischemia. Hypertrophic cardiomyopathy and aortic stenosis, both causes of myocardial hypertrophy, may trigger ventricular dysrhythmogenesis. An embolic coronary artery occlusion, from vegetations associated with endocarditis or blood clots, or coronary spasm can induce VT or VF from an ischemic mechanism. The goal in these situations is to prevent or alleviate ischemia. Medications may be helpful, but an implantable defibrillator should be considered if medications fail to prevent ischemia.[21]

His-Purkinje disease can lead to VT and VF. Myotonic dystrophy and nonischemic dilated cardiomyopathy can cause conduction system disease with bundle branch reentrant monomorphic VT. In this type of tachycardia, the rate is frequently greater than 200 beats/min and in clinical- and laboratory-induced tachycardia settings, a left bundle branch block pattern is common.[21]

Some patients with a normally functioning heart may develop monomorphic VT. One distinct pattern is a monomorphic VT with left bundle branch block pattern and inferior axis that originates from the outflow track regions near the aortic and pulmonic valves. Outflow track tachycardias are believed to originate from an automatic focus and may be due to depressed afterdepolarizations. These VT episodes can be exercise induced from adrenergic stimulation or by calcium loading. The dysrhythmia may begin with frequent to incessant ventricular estrasystoles that lead to constant ventricular bigeminy. When the origin is the pulmonic valve region (less common than the aortic valve region), VT can be treated with calcium channel blockers, beta blockers, and adenosine. When the origin is from the aortic valve region, VT may respond to calcium channel blockers, beta blockers, and class IA and IC antidysrhythmic agents. Because these origins of VT have a focal nature, catheter ablation can lead to cure.[21]

A second normal heart monomorphic tachycardia has a typical right bundle branch block pattern with a superior axis and originates near the apex of the left ventricle. This tachycardia can be suppressed with calcium channel blockers and other antidysrhythmic agents, but catheter ablation can cure the tachycardia and provide excellent long-term survival.[21]

Two categories of polymorphic VT can occur in normal hearts: those associated with prolonged QT interval (Figure 48-30) and abnormal T waves and those not associated with a QT interval abnormality. Unlike the monomorphic VT discussed before, these dysrhythmias are more malignant and patients may have syncope and SCD. The most common form of long QT syndrome was found to be an autosomal recessive inherited condition associated with repolarization abnormality from transmembrane ion channels abnormalities. Mutations have been found on six genes and involve multiple specific mutations that interfere with the function of the ion

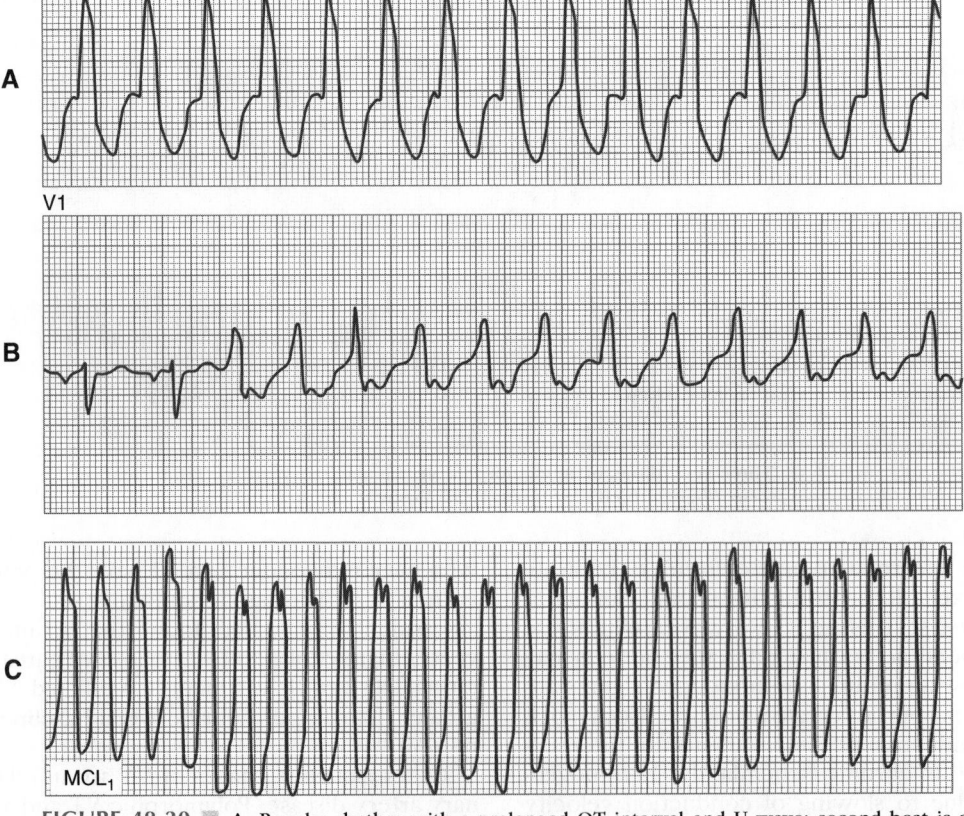

FIGURE 48-30 ■ **A,** Regular rhythm with a prolonged QT interval and U wave; second beat is a premature ventricular complex. **B,** Short run of ventricular tachycardia followed by (**C**) development of torsades de pointes. (From Conover M: *Understanding electrocardiography*, ed 7, St Louis, 1996, Mosby.)

channels. Three ECG QT interval patterns have been seen in patients with these genetic abnormalities while in NSR. The T wave is broad-based and has a robust amplitude when chromosome 11 is involved and has a low amplitude when chromosome 7 is involved. When chromosome 3 is involved, the T waves are late-initiating and late-breaking with a narrow base. Each of these patterns also has a different response to heart rate acceleration; for example, the QT interval greatly shortens in one genetic abnormality but not in another. Additionally, antidysrhythmic medications aimed at shortening the QT interval have different responses, based on the form of QT syndrome. The choice of agents that target the appropriate ion channel abnormality (i.e., agents that cause potassium loading or block sodium channels) is important to get the correct response. In addition to antidysrhythmic agents (including beta blockers), a pacemaker can prevent bradycardia, which may be a trigger for VT. High-risk patients may receive implantable cardioverter-defibrillators as a rescue device.[21]

Idiopathic VF is the label given to those with polymorphic VT or VF without prolonged QT interval, metabolic abnormalities, or cardiac ischemia. In addition, monomorphic and polymorphic VT can be induced from toxic drug reactions or electrolyte abnormalities. The malignant dysrhythmia torsades de pointes, a polymorphic VT in which the QRS axis appears to be twisting around the isoelectric line, is discussed in Chapter 47. Torsades de pointes also has been associated with hypothyroidism, electrolyte abnormalities (hypokalemia, hypomagnesemia, and hypocalcemia), bradycardia from heart block,[21] and intravenous haloperidol administration in treatment for delirium and psychosis.[52] A genetic predisposition is believed to be present in most cases because torsades de pointes seems to affect the potassium repolarization current. When QT intervals are longer than 600 msec or when the rate-corrected QT interval (**QTc**) is greater than 500 msec, the risk of torsades de pointes is high.

Because QT intervals normally vary with rate—i.e., shortening as the heart rate increases—measuring the QTC provides some compensation. Bazett's formula divides the measured QT interval by the square root of the R-R interval. A normal QTC is 460 msec for men and 470 msec for women plus 15 percent of the mean.[7] Of antidysrhythmic agents, amiodarone rarely causes torsades de pointes. Therapy is aimed at (1) preventing cardiac arrest and (2) removing the offending factors that generate the long QT interval. Temporary pacing may be needed acutely to correct bradycardia caused by sinus slowing or AV block. Raising the heart rate to 100 beats/min generally suppresses the tachycardia. Magnesium (2 g over 10 to 15 minutes) can be administered intravenously if needed.

Miscellaneous causes of VT have been identified. Although it is beyond the scope of this chapter to provide details, Box 48-4 lists these causes of VT and VF.[21]

General Management

Prevention and treatment of VT from ischemic heart disease involves use and optimal dosing of drugs known to reverse left ventricular remodeling in patients with

---

BOX 48-4 ■ ■ ■
CAUSES OF MISCELLANEOUS VENTRICULAR TACHYCARDIA AND VENTRICULAR FIBRILLATION

- Arrhythmogenic right ventricular dysplasia
- Acute myocarditis
- Tetralogy of Fallot
- Mitral valve prolapse
- Brugada syndrome
- Muscular dystrophies
- Chagas disease
- Dilated or hypertrophic cardiomyopathy

---

chronic heart failure (see Chapter 64; optimal therapy to relieve ischemia; proper use of diuretics, magnesium, and potassium supplements; and treatment with an implantable cardioverter-defibrillator (**ICD;** refer to Chapter 61). Use of amiodarone does not improve survival in patients with left ventricular remodeling,[53] but it has not demonstrated detrimental effects on cardiac tissue and may be used to decrease VT episodes in patients with an ICD. In VT from nonischemic causes, patients receiving an ICD have had better survival than those receiving antidysrhythmic drugs; however, neither strategy improved survival to that of age- and gender-matched U.S. survival rates.[54] Research results underscore the need for further improving survival and overall health in patients experiencing near-fatal ventricular dysrhythmias.

Although ICDs will terminate VT, they do not keep the dysrhythmia from occurring. When VT is frequent and incessant or when the ICD must deliver high-voltage shocks to terminate it, antidysrhythmic drugs may decrease the frequency of VT episodes. Although useful, antidysrhythmic agents are associated with cardiac toxicity (for example, many class I agents decrease contractility) and noncardiac toxicity (amiodarone can cause many noncardiac effects such as pulmonary fibrosis, hyperthyroidism or hypothyroidism, and skin discoloration). In addition, antidysrhythmic agents can increase the energy requirement for defibrillation and complicate programming of ICDs for dysrhythmia detection.[55] Saline-cooled radiofrequency catheter ablation of the ventricular dysrhythmia substrate offers an alternative method of controlling VT and may provide cure in some cases. To be successful, it is important to understand the dysrhythmia substrate and identify the ablation target. In polymorphic VT, the QRS complex morphology changes from beat to beat; therefore, there might not be a discrete substrate that can be targeted for ablation. In polymorphic VT associated with acute myocardial ischemia, catheter ablation can be used, even when the patient is not hemodynamically stable, if there is a triggered focus.[56]

Monomorphic VT is typically due to reentry, especially in patients with myocardial fibrosis. When the reentry path (circuit) can be identified and defined by the regions of conduction block, it can be interrupted by endocardial and epicardial ablation of the isthmuses supporting reentry.[57] Ablation of stable VT, guided by electroanatomical mapping of the endocardium (and epicardium), abolishes all inducible sustained monomorphic

VTs in about one third to three fourths of patients. In another 17 to 50 percent of cases, VTs were inducible but modified; and in about 10 to 20 percent of cases, ablation failed to abolish targeted inducible VT.[55] In selected patients, the risk of SCD was low and recurrences of VT were not fatal; however, an ICD provided antitachycardia pacing and a safety net for faster VTs.[55,56]

Atrioventricular Block: Overview

AV (or heart) block, first reported in human beings in 1873,[57] is divided into first, second, and third (or high-grade) degrees depending on the severity of the conduction disturbance and the direction of impulse propagation.[8] AV block can be transient or permanent based on the anatomical or functional impairment. Identifying the site of block within the AV node or His-Purkinje system can provide information about prognosis.

Atrioventricular Block: First Degree

First-degree AV block represents a prolongation of the AV conduction time, but all impulses are conducted (a QRS complex follows each P wave). PR interval is greater than 0.20 second in adults and 0.18 second in children (Figure 48-31). Prolongation of conduction time may occur from a conduction delay within the atria (not common and usually associated with congenital heart disease), AV node, His-Purkinje system, or a combination of these. When the QRS complex on the ECG is normal in contour and duration, the source of AV delay is most often in the AV node proximal to the His bundle and rarely in the His bundle. When the QRS complex displays a bundle branch block pattern, the delay may be in the AV node or the His bundle system.[8] In this case, a bundle of His electrogram can localize the site of the block.[58]

Management

First-degree AV block is considered more benign than a second- or third-degree block and generally does not progress to a more advanced conduction disturbance.

In post-MI patients, first-degree AV block is associated with inferior and right ventricular infarction, is transient, and does not require temporary pacing.[58]

Atrioventricular Block: Second Degree, Type I

Second-degree AV block occurs in two forms, type I (also known as Wenckebach block or Mobitz type I) and type II. In type I AV block, there is progressive prolongation of the PR interval until an impulse is not conducted. On ECG, an atrial impulse is not conducted into the ventricles. The PR interval immediately after the block returns to its baseline interval (may be normal or prolonged), and the cycle begins again. The typical Wenckebach pattern occurs in less than 50 percent of cases and includes these features: (1) progressive lengthening of the PR interval until an impulse is not conducted; (2) lengthening of the R-R interval at progressively decreasing increments, leading to progressive shortening of the R-R intervals; (3) a pause that contains a nonconducted P wave (the pause length is less than the sum of two consecutively conducted beats); and (4) after the block the PR interval shortens compared with the PR interval immediately before the block (Figure 48-32).

Management

For many years in the United States, Wenckebach block was considered to be benign in adults, and pacemaker insertion was considered unnecessary. In Europe, however, the British Pacing and Electrophysiology Group suggested that adults with this block should be paced if the block occurred much of the day or night, irrespective of symptoms.[59] A prospective study of this conduction disturbance in 147 subjects with chronic Mobitz type I block and without other second- or third-degree heart blocks, 90 received a pacemaker for symptoms or prophylaxis. After 5 years, unpaced patients had significantly lower survival compared with those who were paced and relative to what was expected for the normal population, even when they had no organic heart disease. There were no deaths in those 45 years or younger.

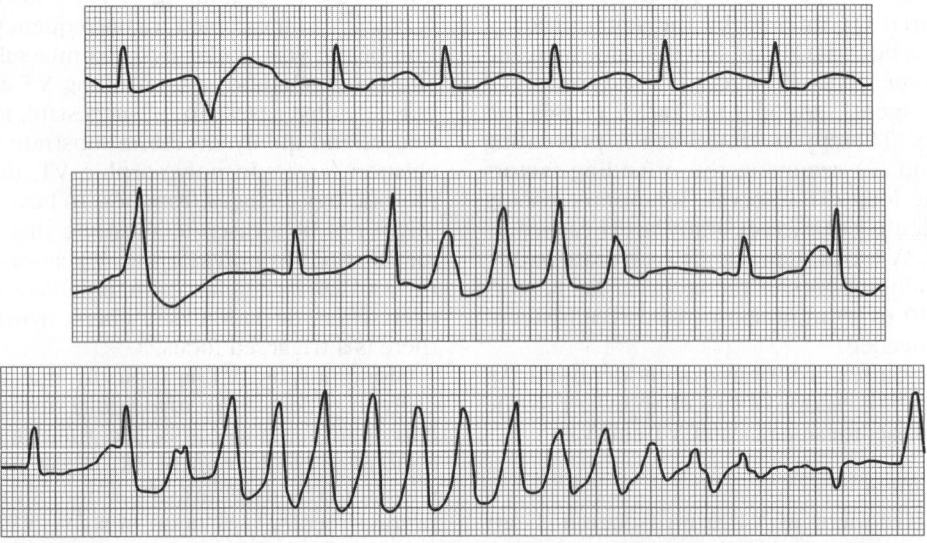

FIGURE 48-31 ■ Normal sinus rhythm with first-degree atrioventricular block (PR interval is 224 msec).

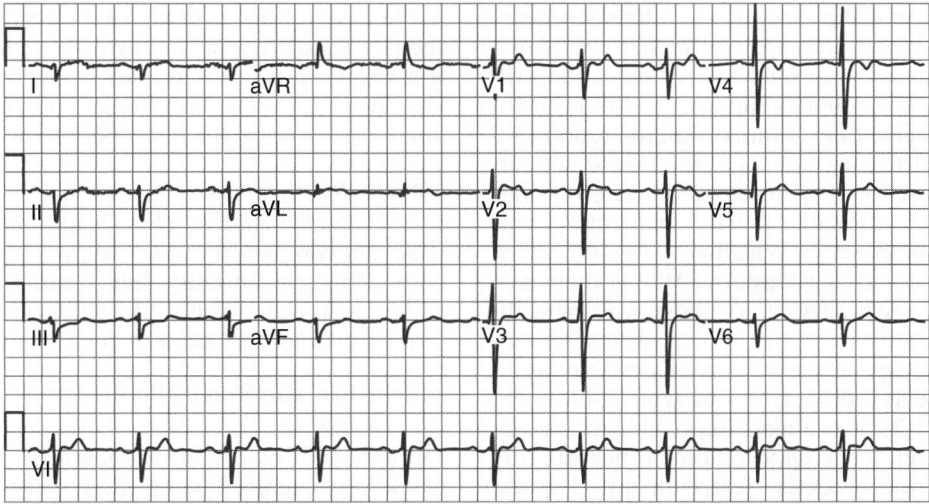

FIGURE 48-32 ▣ Normal sinus rhythm with second-degree atrioventricular block—Mobitz type I or Wenckebach. Note the long PR interval, even in the first impulse after the dropped beat.

Researchers concluded that Mobitz type I block was not benign in patients over age 45 and that pacemaker insertion should be considered, even in the absence of symptomatic bradycardia or organic heart disease.

Atrioventricular Block: Second Degree, Type II

The second form of second-degree AV block, also known as type II block or Mobitz type II, is characterized by a constant PR interval followed by a nonconducted P wave. The failure in P wave conduction to the ventricles is sudden and may be intermittent, or it can occur in regular or irregular intervals. The PP intervals remain constant, and the pause created by the blocked P wave equals two PP intervals when measured. One way to distinguish Mobitz type II block from a nonconducted PAC is by timing of the PP interval; the P wave should not occur early (Figure 48-33).[58]

Mobitz type II block usually is associated with a bundle branch block or bifasicular block, and the site of block is within or below the His bundle. Thus, when Mobitz type II block is suspected but the QRS complex is narrow, Mobitz type I block with minimal variation in PR interval should be suspected, or the cause could be a rare intrahisian block. A bundle of His electrogram can verify the site of block in Mobitz type II.[8]

As mentioned before, first-degree AV block is more common after an inferior wall MI. Of the second-degree AV blocks, type I (Wenckebach) is most common after an inferior wall MI, but it is unclear which type of MI leads to a type II second-degree AV block. Type II AV block was thought to occur more often after anterior wall myocardial infraction,[8] but in a study of 106,780 elders with acute MI complicated by heart block, second- and third-degree heart block was most common after inferior wall MI. The prevalence of second-degree type I and type II and third-degree AV block was not stated, but the overall prevalence of heart block was 4.7 percent during index hospitalization.[59] Of these patients, 3.2 percent developed the AV block during the hospitalization. Patients with heart block were slightly

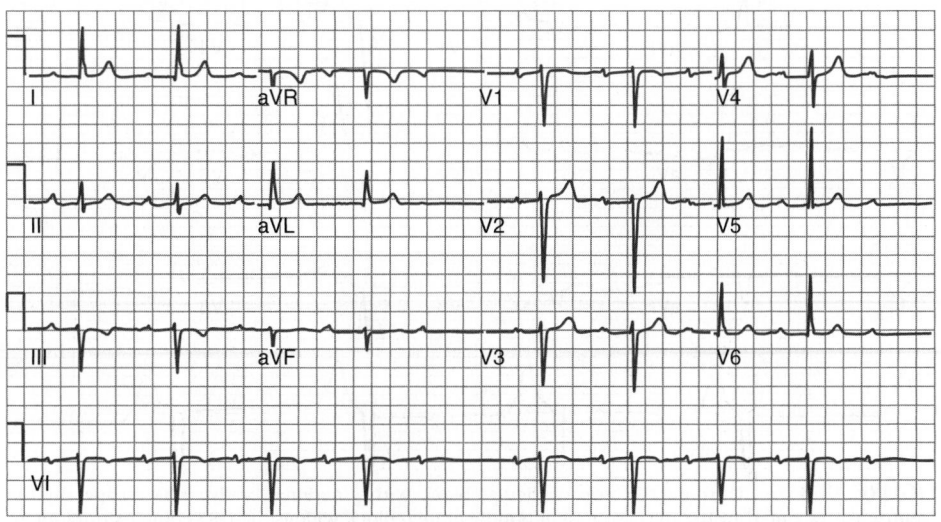

FIGURE 48-33 ▣ Normal sinus rhythm with second-degree atrioventricular block—Mobitz type II.

older, had a higher Killip class, lower admission heart rate and systolic blood pressure, and higher rate of diabetes and were more often smokers. Second- and third-degree AV block were more common after inferior infarction (7.3 percent) than anterior wall infarction (3.0 percent), and heart block was highest in those with an inferior wall infarction who received reperfusion therapy (8.3 percent).[60] After adjusting for demographic and clinical factors, heart block remained an independent predictor of in-hospital mortality after MI, but there was no difference in 1-year survival for those with or without heart block.

Some patients experience a 2:1 AV block that is difficult to diagnose as Mobitz type I or type II AV block. Using a surface ECG, it is almost impossible to classify the block; however, if the QRS complex is normal, it is most likely that the block is located in the AV node (Wenckebach). If the QRS complex is wider than normal, the block could be in the AV node or (more likely)

in the His-Purkinje system. An intracardiac recording at the His bundle region can provide definitive diagnosis. If a vagolytic drug (atropine) is given and there is no improvement in the block (e.g., a change to a 1:1 conduction), it is most likely a Mobitz type II AV block.[58]

Management

Type II block is more likely to lead to Adams-Stokes syncope and complete AV block. Type II block is associated with a higher mortality, left ventricular dysfunction, and clinical heart failure.[8] In MI, a type II block might require a temporary or permanent pacemaker.

Atrioventricular Block: Third Degree, Dissociation, and Escape

Third-degree block, also known as complete heart block, is recognized when the P waves are dissociated completely from QRS complexes (Figures 48-34 and 48-35). No atrial activity is conducted to the ventricles,

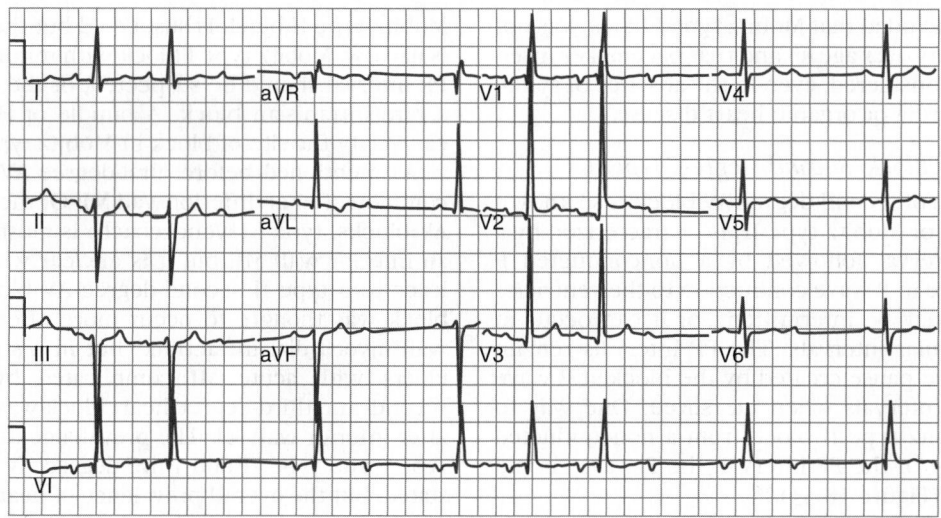

FIGURE 48-34 ■ Third-degree atrioventricular block with ventricular escape rhythm (ventricular rate of 28 beats/min). Note wide, bizarre QRS complexes and abnormal T waves.

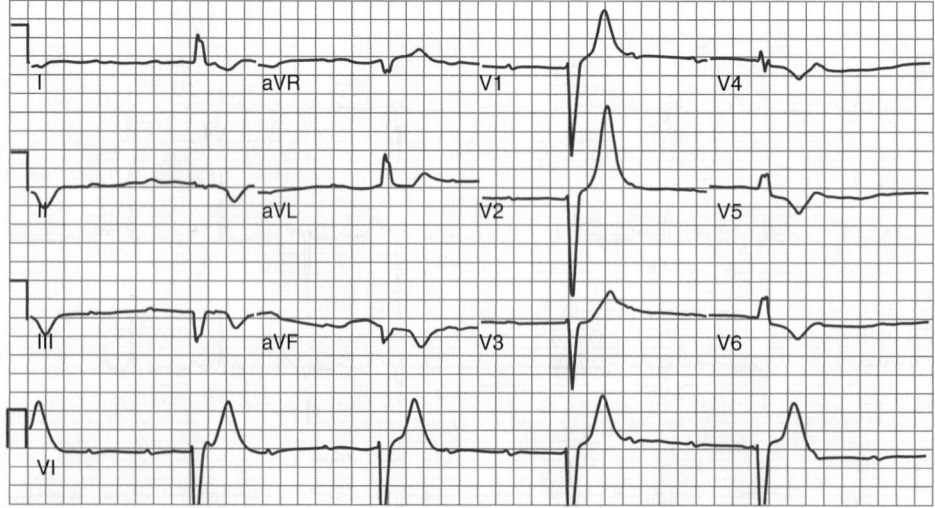

FIGURE 48-35 ■ Third-degree atrioventricular block with junctional bradycardia escape rhythm (ventricular rate of 31 beats/min). Note right bundle branch block widens the QRS complex duration to 176 msec.

even though the AV node is not physiologically refractory and the atria and ventricles are controlled by independent pacemakers, each of which fires at its own pacemaker rate. The atrial pacemaker can be sinus or ectopic atrial tachycardia, fibrillation, or flutter impulses. The atrial rate in complete AV block commonly is much faster than the ventricular or escape rate. There may be no atrial impulses; instead, there may be a junctional focus above the block that sends impulses retrogradely to the atrium, leading to atrial conduction, even though these same impulses never lead to ventricular conduction.

Escape rhythm refers to the origin of the impulses that produce the ventricular rhythm. Impulses initiated in the AV node that occur below the level of block can produce the ventricular rhythm (*junctional escape rhythm*) and can be narrow with a rate of 50 to 60 beats/min. The QRS complex morphology (narrow or wide) can provide clues about the site of the block and the rate of the escape rhythm when it originates in the ventricle (*ventricular escape rhythm*). The ventricular focus usually is located just below the region of the block and can be above or below the His bundle bifurcation. When the escape focus that controls the ventricle arises at or near the His bundle, the QRS complex may be narrow, the ventricular rhythm may appear to be more stable, and the escape rate may be faster. Alternately, the ventricular pacemaker activity can come from a distal location in the ventricular conduction system. A typical ventricular escape rate is 20 to 40 beats/min but can be faster (40 to 60 beats/min) in congenital complete heart block. The rhythm may be regular but varies in response to ventricular extrasystoles, a shift in the pacemaker site, an irregularly discharge pacemaker focus, and autonomic nervous system influences.[8] Interestingly, retrograde conduction may be intact in persons with antegrade third-degree AV block; thus, impulses initiated in the ventricle can conduct to the atrium.[58]

A third-degree AV block can be caused by many variables, including congenital heart disease and drug effects. Digitalis and beta blockers influence conduction through autonomic nervous system effects; amiodarone and calcium channel blockers directly slow AV conduction in the AV node; and type I and III antidysrhythmic drugs can affect conduction through the His-Purkinje system, especially drugs that block the sodium channels, such as flecainide.[58] Acute inferior and anterior MI (as noted before) can cause heart block, including third-degree AV blocks. Inferior wall MIs are more likely to cause a block at the level of the AV node, resulting in a junctional escape rhythm. This usually resolves in a few days and can be reversed with vagolytic drugs (atropine) or exercise. In anterior wall myocardial infraction, a third-degree block usually signifies infarction of the bundle branches. The escape rhythm is more likely to be ventricular, with a wide QRS complex because it will originate from the bundle branches or Purkinje system. This block is less likely to be reversible and may require a permanent pacemaker. Chronic coronary artery ischemic disease, progressive idiopathic fibrosis of the conduction system, calcification of the aortic or mitral valve

annulus that extends to the nearby conduction system, infiltrative cardiomyopathy, endocarditis, and collagen vascular diseases can cause third-degree AV block. In addition, electrolyte disorders, heart tumors or those that infiltrate the heart, vasovagal syncope, carotid sinus syndrome, cardiac surgery, and intracardiac catheter manipulation can produce complete heart block.[58]

Management

For patients with transient or paroxysmal block who have presyncope or syncope, an ambulatory monitor (Holter or external loop recorder) can establish the diagnosis and help determine appropriate therapy. Vagolytic drugs can be used as a temporary measure. In an emergency setting, adverse responses are uncommon, and approximately half of those treated have a partial or complete response to the therapy.[53] Because drugs that increase the heart rate cause significant side effects, a temporary or permanent pacemaker is indicated in patients with escape rhythms that are slow and produce symptoms.[8] Catecholamines, such as isoproterenol, should not be used or should be used with extreme caution in patients with acute MI. Clinical guidelines recommend that heart rate criteria are arbitrary and unnecessary as criteria for pacemaker therapy; the site of origin of the escape rhythm is the key factor determining the need for a pacemaker. Irreversible, acquired third-degree AV block is a Class I indication for pacing.[61]

Prognosis is determined by the underlying cause of the third-degree AV block and varies, even after permanent transcutaneous pacemaker therapy is established. In children with congenital complete AV block, pacemaker therapy reduced mortality and morbidity, even when the children were asymptomatic, but pacemaker system complications occurred in 42 percent of children.[62] When endomyocardial biopsies from patients with congenital AV block were studied 3 to 12 years after initiation of apical right ventricular pacing, histopathological alterations were found. Changes were thought to adversely alter myocellular growth on the cellular and subcellular level, which could diminish clinical function. The researchers recommended further research of optimized paced ventricular performance by alternative site electrode insertion and stimulus initiation.[63] In another study of pacemaker therapy in congenital complete AV block, most children, especially those who were asymptomatic, had a decrease in heart size and normalization of shortening fraction after pacemaker therapy.[64]

Adults who develop a third-degree AV block after anterior wall MI have the worst prognosis. In a study of 6317 patients, 5 percent of patients with cardiac enzymes verifying MI developed a third-degree AV block: 2.5 percent in anterior wall MI and 9.4 percent in inferior MI. In patients with anterior wall MI, left ventricular function was associated with the development of a third-degree block, and the 30-day mortality rate was significantly higher (59 percent versus 15 percent) when a block was present. Patients with inferior wall MI and third-degree AV block had a higher Killip class and greater rate of in-hospital events (cardiogenic shock, AF, and VF), but the development of block seemed unrelated to left ventricular dysfunction. Thirty-day mortality was not as high as those who developed third-degree AV heart block after anterior wall MI but was significantly higher than those without a block (24 percent versus 10 percent).[65] Those with bundle branch fibrosis but no other cardiac disease have the best prognosis.[58]

Sick Sinus Syndrome

Features of sick sinus syndrome include (1) persistent, severe, and inappropriate sinus bradycardia, (2) sinoatrial block and/or sinus arrest episodes, (3) long pauses with failure of secondary pacemakers or failure of sinus rhythm, (4) ectopic atrial or junctional pacemaker rhythm as a replacement for NSR, (5) prolonged suppression of sinus rhythm after electrical or spontaneous cardioversion from atrial tachydysrhythmias or bradycardia alternating with tachycardia, and (6) AF that may be paroxysmal, persistent, or permanent and may have a slow ventricular rate caused by permanent silence from sinus node and other AV node disease (Figure 48-36).[66]

Electrophysiological studies help establish the presence or absence of sinus node dysfunction. By establishing the diagnosis, they provide data to differentiate between mechanisms (intrinsic and extrinsic) of pathophysiological function and provide prognostic information about the severity of the disease. Symptoms are often intermittent, extremely changeable, and unpredictable. Symptoms can be subtle (fatigue, irritability, tiredness, inability to concentrate or hold interest in doing things, forgetfulness, dizziness, insomnia, aching muscles and body fatigue, and mild digestive disorders) or more obvious (congestive heart failure). Transient sinus arrest can cause syncope, near syncope, dizziness, fainting, and light-headedness. If associated with bradycardia-tachycardia syndrome, symptoms can include palpitations, angina, and congestive heart failure. In the absence of a demonstrable link between signs and symptoms, the diagnosis can be made after carefully excluding other possible causes when the following adjunct findings are present: (1) persistent diurnal bradycardia of less than 40 beats/min or second-degree AV block; (2) prolonged sinus pauses that are not associated with vagal reflex; (3) abnormal intrinsic heart rate, especially if it falls below the baseline value; (4) abnormal long (greater than 3 seconds) sinus node recovery time; and (5) severe chronotropic incompetence during standard stress testing or poor heart rate variability during 24-hour monitoring.[8,66]

The peak incidence of sick sinus syndrome is the seventh decade; however, it can occur at any age and affects men and women equally; 40 to 60 percent also have paroxysmal SVT. Because sick sinus syndrome can occur with a variety of cardiac diseases that involve the sinus node, it may be reversible and self-limiting or chronic and irreversible. In addition, drugs may produce transient sinus bradydysrhythmias.[66]

Management

The goal of treatment is to control morbidity and relieve symptoms. Because mortality is not affected by sick sinus syndrome, few persons need treatment. To control tachydysrhythmias in the bradycardia-tachycardia syndrome, antidysrhythmic drugs are used, alone or in combination with pacemaker therapy. Anticoagulation therapy is needed because of a high risk of systemic embolism, especially if it is associated with AF or heart failure. Sinus node function may be impaired by drugs commonly used to treat cardiac problems and should not be given to patients with known sinus node dysfunction: beta blockers, digitalis, class I and III antidysrhythmic drugs, and calcium channel blockers. Traditional drugs used to increase heart rate (hydralazine, belladonna, alkaloids, sympathomimetic amines, and theophylline) do not prevent syncopal recurrences. Permanent pacing is the widely accepted treatment for reducing syncopal attacks and relieving symptoms. Physiological pacing (atrial pacing or DDD pacing) is superior to VVI/R pacing in improving quality of life, lowering

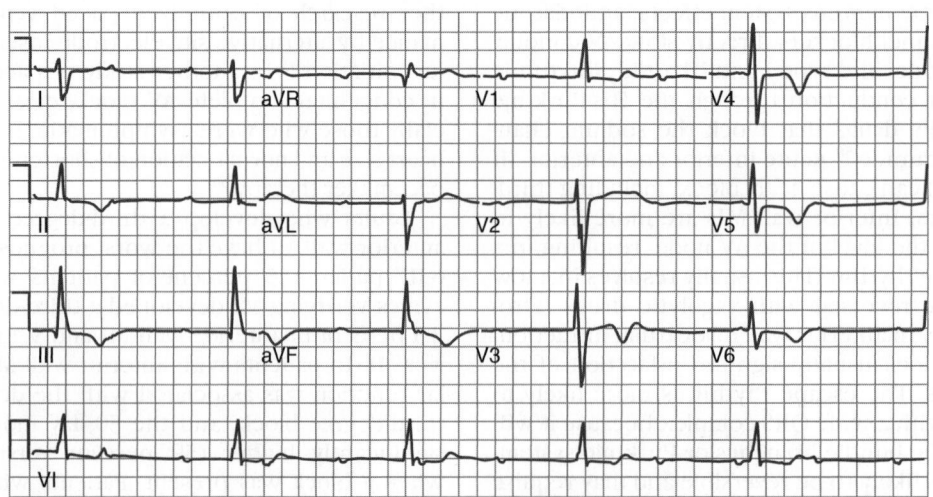

FIGURE 48-36 ■ Sinus/atrial rhythm with first-degree atrioventricular block, paroxysmal atrial tachycardia, and sinus pauses reflecting sick sinus syndrome. In lead V1, note changing morphology of atrial impulse (p wave).

the incidence of heart failure, lowering the risk of AF, and possibly lowering the risk of systemic embolisms and stroke; however, the effect of pacing mode on survival is not established.[66]

PRACTICE PROTOCOLS

Although the research supporting ECG monitoring is increasing, thanks in part to scholars such as Barbara Drew and her colleagues, monitoring practices still are driven too often by tradition. Fortunately, several practice protocols that combine research-based recommendations with the opinion of experts are available. The American Heart Association scientific statement "Practice Standards for Electrographic Monitoring in Hospital Settings"[2] was discussed previously in this chapter. In addition, the American Association of Critical-Care Nurses (AACN) has published two practice protocols. "Bedside Cardiac Monitoring" in the *AACN Research Based Practice Protocols*[67] provides a comprehensive overview of the principles of cardiac monitoring, including selection of patients most likely to benefit from it. The AACN protocol contains detailed information on skin preparation, electrode positioning for various leads, decision making for ST segment monitoring with various monitoring lead systems, setting alarm parameters, and general nursing care. This protocol will be updated soon. A more recent AACN practice protocol, "Care of the Patient with an Arrhythmia" in the *Care of the Cardiovascular Patient Series*[68] was published as part of a series of protocols dealing with the care of the cardiovascular patient. This protocol describes the defining characteristics of multiple dysrhythmias and their management. This protocol contains more detailed information on management of specific dysrhythmias than either of the previously discussed protocols. Both AACN protocols are available for purchase from *www. aacn.org*.

Finally, AACN has published a series of practice alerts. Two focus on cardiac monitoring: dysrhythmia monitoring[69] and ST segment monitoring.[70] These are clear statements about expected practice coupled with supporting research evidence and strategies to implement practice changes. These practice alerts provide succinct summaries of research-based practice and a message to alter current practice if it deviates from research recommendations. These are available free for members from the AACN website.

REFERENCES

1. Fairman J, Lynaugh J: *Critical care nursing: a history,* Philadelphia, 1998, University of Pennsylvania Press.
2. Drew BJ, Califf RM, Funk M et al: AHA scientific statement: practice standards for electrocardiographic monitoring in hospital settings, *Circulation* 110:11-2721, 2004.
3. Kindwall E, Brown J, Josephson ME: Electrocardiographic criteria for ventricular tachycardia in wide QRS complex left bundle branch block morphology tachycardia, *Am J Cardiol* 61:6-1279, 1988.
4. Zipes DP: Mechanisms of clinical arrhythmias, *Pacing Clin Electrophysiol* 26:2-1778, 2003.
5. Zipes DP, Wellens HJ: What have we learned about cardiac arrhythmias? *Circulation* 102:IV-52–IV-57, 2000.
6. Miller J, Zipes D: Therapy for cardiac arrhythmias. In Zipes D, Libby P, Bonow R, Braunwald E, editors: *Braunwald's heart disease: a textbook of cardiovascular medicine,* ed 7, Philadelphia, 2005, WB Saunders.
7. Conover M: *Understanding electrocardiography,* ed 7, St Louis, 1996, Mosby.
8. Olgin J, Zipes D: Specific arrhythmias: diagnosis and treatment. In Zipes D, Libby P, Bonow R, Braunwald E, editors: *Braunwald's heart disease: a textbook of cardiovascular medicine,* ed 7, Philadelphia, 2005, WB Saunders.
9. Gottlieb SS: The use of pacemakers as treatment for systolic dysfunction, *J Card Fail* 4:145, 1998.
10. Shapiro E: The electrocardiogram and the arrhythmias: historical insights. In Mandel WJ, editor: *Cardiac arrhythmias: their mechanisms, diagnosis and management,* ed 3, Philadelphia, 1995, Lippincott.
11. Jordan JL, Mandel WJ: Disorders of sinus function. In Mandel WJ, editor: *Cardiac arrhythmias: their mechanisms, diagnosis and management,* ed 3, Philadelphia, 1995, Lippincott.
12. Hauptman PJ, Kelly RA: Digitalis, *Circulation* 99:9-1265, 1999.
13. Shenasa H, Curry PV, Shenasa M: Atrial arrhythmias: clinical concepts and advances in mechanism and management. In Mandel WJ, editor: *Cardiac arrhythmias: their mechanisms, diagnosis and management,* ed 3, Philadelphia, 1995, Lippincott.
14. Wellens HJ: Electrocardiographic diagnosis of arrhythmias. In Topel EJ, editor: *Textbook of cardiovascular medicine,* ed 2, Philadelphia, 2002, Lippincott-Raven.
15. Morady F: Catheter ablation of supraventricular arrhythmias: state of the art, *J Cardiovasc Electrophysiol* 15:1-124, 2004.
16. Kistler PM, Sanders P, Fynn SP et al: Electrophysiological and electrocardiographic characteristics of focal atrial tachycardia originating from the pulmonary veins: acute and long-term outcomes of radiofrequency ablation, *Circulation* 108:10-1968, 2003.
17. Blomstrom-Lundqvist C, Scheinman M, Aliot E et al: ACC/AHA/ESC guidelines for the management of patients with supraventricular arrhythmias, *J Am Coll Cardiol* 42:4-1493, 2003.
18. Wit AL, Coromilas J: Role of alterations in refractoriness and conduction in genesis of reentrant arrhythmias: implications for antiarrhythmic effects of class III drugs, *Am J Cardiol* 72:3F-12F, 1993.
19. Nakagawa H, Shah N, Matsudaira K et al: Characterization of reentrant circuit in macroreentrant right atrial tachycardia after surgical repair of congenital heart disease: isolated channels between scars allow "focal" ablation, *Circulation* 103:10-699, 2001.
20. Marriott HJ, Myerburg RJ: Recognition of cardiac arrhythmias and conduction disturbances. In Hurst JW, Schlant RC, Rackley CE et al, editors: *The heart,* ed 7, New York, 1990, McGraw-Hill.
21. Tchou PJ: Ventricular tachycardia. In Topel EJ, editor: *Textbook of cardiovascular medicine,* ed 2, Philadelphia, 2002, Lippincott-Raven.
22. Dabrowski A, Kramarz E, Piotrowicz R et al: Predictive power of increased QT dispersion in ventricular extrasystoles and in sinus beats for risk stratification after myocardial infarction, *Circulation* 101:10-1693, 2000.
23. Guidelines 2000 for cardiopulmonary resuscitation and emergency cardiac care, *Circulation* 102(8 suppl):I1-I370, 2000.
24. Caron MF, Kluger J, White M: Amiodarone in the new AHA guidelines for ventricular tachyarrhythmias, *Ann Pharmacother* 35: 3-1248, 2001.
25. Bardy GH, Lee KL, Mark DB et al: Amiodarone or an implantable cardioverter-defibrillator for congestive heart failure, *N Engl J Med* 352:35-225, 2005.
26. Weiss EM, Buescher T: Atrial fibrillation: treatment options and caveats, *AACN Clin Issues* 15:1-362, 2004.
27. Crystal E, Connolly SJ: Atrial fibrillation: guiding lessons from epidemiology, *Cardiol Clin* 22:2, 2004.
28. Abusaada K, Sharma SB, Jaladi R et al: Epidemiology and management of new-onset atrial fibrillation, *Am J Manag Care* 10:S50-S57, 2004.
29. Wijffels MC, Crijins HJ: Non-invasive characteristics of atrial fibrillation: the value of holter recordings for the treatment of AF, *Card Electrophysiol Rev* 6:233, 2002.
30. Hsu LF, Jaïs P, Keane D et al: Atrial fibrillation originating from persistent left superior vena cava, *Circulation* 109:10-828, 2004.
31. Naccarelli GV, Hynes BJ, Wolbrette DL et al: Atrial fibrillation in heart failure: prognostic significance and management, *J Cardiovasc Electrophysiol* 14(suppl):S281-S286, 2003.

32. Elahi M, Hadjinikolaou L, Galinanes M: Incidence and clinical consequences of atrial fibrillation within 1 year of first-time isolated coronary bypass surgery, *Circulation* 108(suppl 2):II-207-II-212, 2003.

33. Allessie MA, Boyden PA, Camm AJ et al: Pathophysiology and prevention of atrial fibrillation, *Circulation* 103:10-769, 2001.

34. Sparks PB, Jayaprakash S, Vohra JK et al: Electrical remodeling of the atria associated with paroxysmal and chronic atrial flutter, *Circulation* 102:10-1807, 2000.

35. Cosio FG: Atrial flutter update, *Card Electrophysiol Rev* 6:-356, 2002.

36. Jaïs P, Hocini M, Weerasoryia R et al: Atypical left atrial flutters, *Card Electrophysiol Rev* 6:-371, 2002.

37. Marrouche NF, Natale A, Wazni OM et al: Left septal atrial flutter, *Circulation* 109:10-2440, 2004.

38. Anthony KK, Mauro VF: Rate versus rhythm control in atrial fibrillation, *Ann Pharmacother* 38:3-839, 2004.

39. Knight BP, Gersh BJ, Carlson MD et al: Role of permanent pacing to prevent atrial fibrillation, *Circulation* 111:11-240, 2005.

40. Saad EB, Marrouche NF, Natale A: Ablation of focal atrial fibrillation, *Card Electrophysiol Rev* 6:-389, 2002.

41. Gatia F, Riccardi R, Gallotti R: Surgical approaches to atrial fibrillation, *Card Electrophysiol Rev* 6:-401, 2002.

42. Johna R, Eckardt L, Fetsch T et al: A new algorithm to determine complete isthmus conduction block after radiofrequency catheter ablation for typical atrial flutter, *Am J Cardiol* 83:8-1666, 1999.

43. Anselme F, Saoudi N, Poty H et al: Radiofrequency catheter ablation of common atrial flutter: significance of palpitations and quality of life evaluation in patients with proven isthmus block, *Circulation* 99:9-534, 1999.

44. Lown B, Ganong W, Levine S: The syndrome of short P-R interval, normal QRS and paroxysmal rapid heart action, *Circulation* 5:-693, 1952.

45. Paul T, Bertram H, Bokenkamp R et al: Supraventricular tachycardia in infants, children and adolescents, *Paediatr Drugs* 2(3):2-171, 2000.

46. Brembilla-Perrot B: Age related changes in arrhythmias and electrophysiologic properties, *Card Electrophysiol Rev* 7:-88, 2003.

47. Ferguson J, DiMarco J: Contemporary management of paroxysmal supraventricular tachycardia, *Circulation* 107:10-1096, 2003.

48. Tracy C, Akhtar M, DiMarco J et al: American College of Cardiology/American Heart Association clinical statement on invasive electrophysiology studies, catheter ablation, and cardioversion, *Circulation* 102:10-2309, 2000.

49. American Heart Association, American Stroke Association: *Heart disease and stroke statistics: 2005 update*, Dallas, 2004, American Heart Association.

50. Peters NS, Wit AL: Myocardial architecture and ventricular arrhythmogenesis, *Circulation* 97:9-1746, 1998.

51. St John Sutton M, Lee D, Rouleau JL et al: Left ventricular remodeling and ventricular arrhythmias after myocardial infarction, *Circulation* 107:10-2577, 2003.

52. Hassaballa HA, Balk RA: Torsade de pointes associated with administration of intravenous haloperidol: a review of the literature and practical guidelines for use, *Expert Opin Drug Saf* 2:-543, 2003.

53. Brady WJ, Swart G, DeBehnke DJ et al: The efficacy of atropine in the treatment of hemodynamically unstable bradycardia and atrioventricular block: prehospital and emergency department considerations, *Resuscitation* 41:4-47, 1999.

54. Kulasingam SL, Akiyama T, Mounsey JP et al: Lowered observed versus expected (based on US age and gender specific rates) survival in patients treated for near-fatal ventricular arrhythmias, *Pacing Clin Electrophysiol* 27:2-230, 2004.

55. Soejima K, Stevenson WG: Catheter ablation of ventricular tachycardia in patients with ischemic heart disease, *Curr Cardiol Rep* 5:-364, 2003.

56. Soejima K, Stevenson WG, Sapp JL et al: Endocardial and epicardial radiofrequency ablation of ventricular tachycardia associated with dilated cardiomyopathy, *J Am Coll Cardiol* 43:4-1834, 2004.

57. Upshaw CB, Silverman ME: Alfred Lewis Galabin and the first human documentation of atrioventricular block, *Am J Cardiol* 88:8-547, 2001.

58. Wolbrette DL, Naccarelli GV: Bradycardias: sinus nodal dysfunction and atrioventricular conduction disturbances. In Topel EJ, editor: *Textbook of cardiovascular medicine*, ed 2, Philadelphia, 2002, Lippincott-Raven.

59. Shaw DB, Gowers JI, Kekwick CA et al: Is Mobitz type I atrioventricular block benign in adults? *Heart* 90:9-169, 2004.

60. Rathore SS, Gersh BJ, Berger PB et al: Acute myocardial infarction complicated by heart block in the elderly: prevalence and outcomes, *Am Heart J* 141:14-47, 2001.

61. Barold SS, Herweg B, Gallardo I: Acquired atrioventricular block: the 2002 ACC/AHA/NASPE guidelines for pacemaker implantation should be revised, *Pacing Clin Electrophysiol* 26:2-531, 2003.

62. Balmer C, Fasnacht M, Rahn M et al: Long-term follow up of children with congenital complete atrioventricular block and the impact of pacemaker therapy, *Europace* 4:-345, 2002.

63. Karpawich PP, Rabah R, Haas JE: Altered cardiac histology following apical right ventricular pacing in patients with congenital atrioventricular block, *Pacing Clin Electrophysiol* 22:2-1372, 1999.

64. Breur JM, Udink Ten Cate FE, Kapusta L et al: Pacemaker therapy in isolated congenital complete atrioventricular block, *Pacing Clin Electrophysiol* 25:2-1685, 2002.

65. Alpin M, Engstrøm T, Vejlstrup NG et al: Prognostic importance of complete atrioventricular block complicating acute myocardial infarction, *Am J Cardiol* 92:9-853, 2003.

66. Brignole M: Sick sinus syndrome, *Clin Geriatr Med* 18:1-211, 2002.

67. Jacobson C: Bedside cardiac monitoring. In Chulay M, Burns S, editors: *AACN research based practice protocols*, Aliso Viejo, Calif, 1999, American Association of Critical-Care Nurses.

68. Paul S, Dangerfield L: Care of the patient with an arrhythmia. In Chulay M, Wingate S, editors: *Care of the cardiovascular patient series*, Aliso Viejo, Calif, 2001, American Association of Critical-Care Nurses.

69. American Association of Critical-Care Nurses: Dysrhythmia monitoring practice alert, *AACN News* 21(4):4, 2004.

70. American Association of Critical-Care Nurses: ST segment monitoring practice alert, *AACN News* 21(9):4, 2004.

ST Segment Monitoring

Barbara J. Drew

Deviation of the normally isoelectric ST segment portion of the electrocardiogram (ECG) in a positive direction (ST segment elevation) or negative direction (ST segment depression) may indicate that a patient is experiencing acute myocardial ischemia (Figure 49-1). Several situations occur in which identification of ST segment changes of ischemia are valuable for clinical decision making. For example, rapid identification of ST segment *elevation* in patients who present to the emergency department with chest pain is the key to successful early reperfusion therapy for acute myocardial infarction **(MI)**. Following reperfusion therapy, rapid resolution of ST segment elevation provides evidence for a patent infarct-related artery.[1-4] In contrast, persistent ST segment elevation provides evidence of unsuccessful reperfusion. A patient with persistent ST segment elevation following fibrinolytic therapy may be a candidate for a rescue percutaneous coronary intervention.[5]

Identification of ST segment *depression* is also important in clinical practice. Transient ST segment depression in patients admitted to the hospital for acute coronary syndromes (i.e., acute MI or unstable angina) provides evidence of an inadequate treatment regimen that may warrant a more aggressive approach. Importantly, numerous studies have linked such ST segment events with adverse short- and long-term patient outcomes. A historical review of the research on this topic is summarized in Table 49-1. Moreover, because 80 to 90 percent of these ST segment events are asymptomatic ("silent" ischemia), the only practical way to detect them is with continuous ECG monitoring.

CELLULAR EVENTS PRODUCING ST SEGMENT DEVIATION

The ECG is considered the gold standard for diagnosing acute myocardial ischemia. Because ischemia *precedes* infarction, biomarkers such as troponins are not yet elevated. Thus the ECG provides critical early information about the status of the myocardium when it is still possible to reverse ischemia and prevent cell death.

ST Segment Elevation

When ischemia involves the subepicardial layer of the myocardial wall, the ECG leads facing the ischemic wall develop ST segment elevation. Sudden thrombotic occlusion of a major epicardial coronary artery causes subepicardial ischemia and, if persistent, results in cell death and ST elevation MI. As illustrated in Figure 49-2, ST segment elevation occurs because there are differences in the cellular action potential amplitude and duration between ischemic and nonischemic cells.[15] As a result, neighboring myocardial cells possess different electrical charges, and this electrical gradient creates a current flow between ischemic and nonischemic cells. Current flow occurring during electrical diastole (phase 4 of the action potential) produces a depressed T-P segment that causes the ST segment to appear elevated in comparison. Current flow occurring during electrical systole (phase 2) produces primary ST segment elevation.

The best ECG leads for detecting ST segment elevation vary depending on the coronary artery involved.[16] For right coronary artery occlusion, the inferior leads (II, III, or aVF) are most sensitive for depicting ST segment elevation. For left anterior descending coronary artery occlusion, the anterior leads (V_2 to V_4) are best. Occlusion of the left circumflex artery is not well depicted by standard ECG leads because no electrodes are placed over the posterior wall of the myocardium on the patient's back. However, mirror image reciprocal ST segment depression may be seen in ECG leads facing the opposite (anterior) myocardial wall and is best depicted in leads V_1 to V_3. Therefore, if just two ECG leads can be displayed on a bedside cardiac monitor, leads II and V_3 are reasonable to detect occlusion in any of the three main coronary arteries. Figure 49-3 illustrates how to place electrodes for obtaining the lead II and V_3 combination using routine five-electrode patient cables. Such a lead selection would be appropriate in chest pain evaluation areas of the emergency department where it is critical to identify ST segment elevation MI rapidly. Because ST segment changes can be dynamic in early MI, the routine 10-second 12-lead ECG may miss periods of ST segment elevation and appear nondiagnostic for acute MI. A case study showing the value of continuous ST segment monitoring in the emergency department setting is shown in Figure 49-4.

ST Segment Depression

When ischemia involves the subendocardial layer of the myocardial wall, the ECG leads on the body surface develop ST segment depression (Figure 49-5). When there is greater myocardial oxygen demand than supply, the subendocardial layer is especially likely to develop ischemia for two reasons. First, the subendocardial region works harder than the rest of the myocardial wall because it depolarizes first and repolarizes last. Second, the subendocardium is located at the "end of the supply

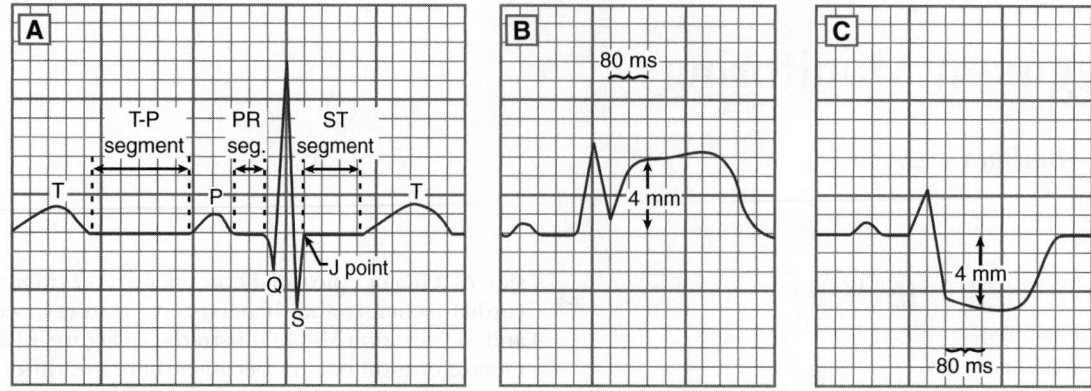

FIGURE 49-1 ▦ **A,** The normal ST segment is isoelectric; i.e., it is level with the T-P and PR segments. **B,** ST segment elevation of 4 mm measured 80 msec from the J point. **C,** ST segment depression of 4 mm. ST segment elevation and depression are indicative of acute myocardial ischemia.

▪ ▪ ▪

TABLE 49-1   PROGNOSTIC SIGNIFICANCE OF TRANSIENT MYOCARDIAL ISCHEMIA WITH ST SEGMENT MONITORING IN PATIENTS HOSPITALIZED FOR UNSTABLE ANGINA

INVESTIGATOR AND YEAR	*n*	INCIDENCE OF ISCHEMIA	SILENT ISCHEMIA	ADVERSE OUTCOME (DEATH OR MYOCARDIAL INFARCTION)
Gottlieb et al. 1986[6] 1987[7]	70	53%	90%	*30 days:* + Ischemia = 16% − Ischemia = 3% (*p* < 0.01) *2 years:* + Ischemia = 27% − Ischemia = 3% (*p* < 0.01)
Nademanee et al. 1987[8]	49	59%	91%	*3-6 months:* + Ischemia = 17% − Ischemia = 5%
Krucoff 1988[9]	282	23%	84%	*Hospital:* + Ischemia = 31% − Ischemia = 0%
Langer et al. 1989[10]	135	66%	92%	*Hospital:* + Ischemia = 16% − Ischemia = 4% (*p* < 0.05)
Larsson et al. 1992[11]	198	23%	94%	*30 days:* + Ischemia = 17% − Ischemia = 3% (*p* < 0.01)
Amanullah and Lindvall 1993[12]	43	98%	Less than 90%	*More than 3 years:* + Ischemia = 18% − Ischemia = 0%
Bugiardini et al. 1995[13]	104	93%	Unreported	*Hospital + 30 days:* + Ischemia = 38% − Ischemia = 0%
Drew et al. 2002[14]	868 (ACS + stable CAD)	20%	71%	*Hospital complications*:* + Ischemia = 41% − Ischemia = 13% (*p* < 0.0001)

ACS, Acute coronary syndrome; *CAD,* coronary artery disease.
*Hospital complications are death, myocardial infarction, cardiogenic shock, or acute pulmonary edema.

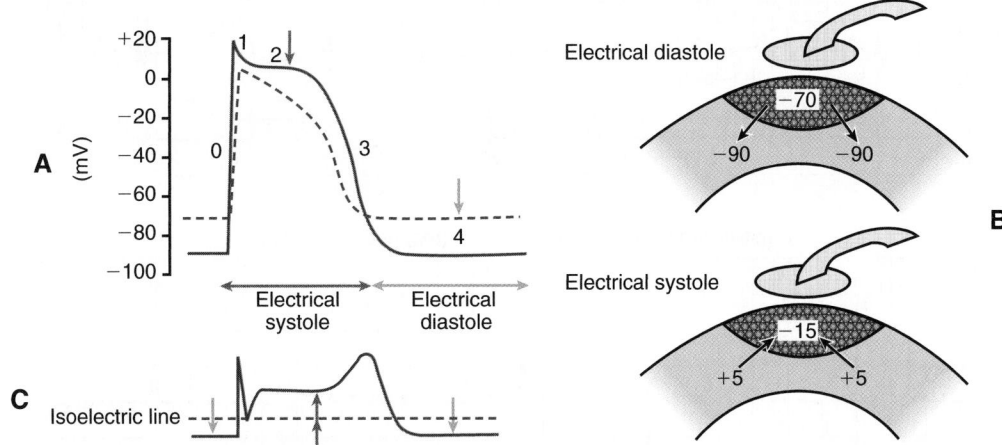

FIGURE 49-2 Cellular events producing ST segment elevation. **A,** The solid line shows the normal cellular action potential of ventricular myocardium, and the dashed line shows the abnormal action potential of ischemic cells. Differences in electrical charges between nonischemic and ischemic cells exist during electrical systole (phases 0, 1, 2, 3) and electrical diastole (phase 4). At a point during electrical diastole (orange arrow in **A**), ischemic cells have a charge of −70 mV, whereas normal cells are fully repolarized at −90 mV. **B,** Upper figure. This difference in electrical charge between ischemic (dappled area in subepicardium) and nonischemic zones of the myocardial wall during electrical diastole causes a current flow in the direction from more positive to more negative charge. Such a current flow away from the recording electrode on the body surface produces lowering of the T-P segment in the electrocardiogram (orange arrows in **C**), which makes the ST segment elevated in comparison (lower green arrow in **C**). At a point during electrical systole (green arrow in **A**), ischemic cells have a charge of −15 mV, whereas normal cells have a charge of +5 mV (**B**, lower figure), which causes a flow of current toward the electrode at the body surface, producing primary ST segment elevation (upper green arrow in **C**). Therefore in acute myocardial infarction the total ST segment elevation is a combination of T-P segment lowering and primary ST segment elevation. (Modified from Arnsdorf MF: The electrophysiologic matrix. In Gussak I, Antzelevitch C, editors: *Cardiac repolarization: bridging basic and clinical science,* Totawa, NJ, 2003, Humana Press.)

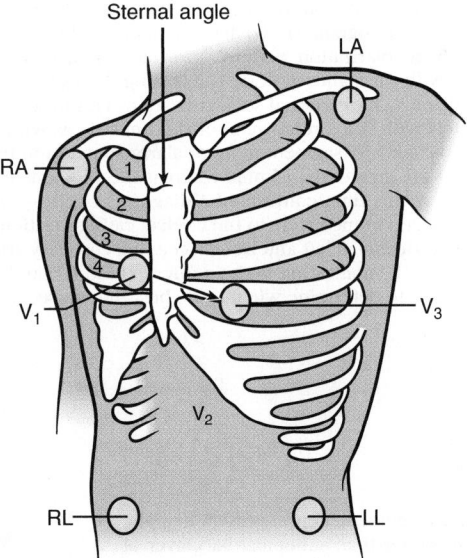

FIGURE 49-3 Electrode placement for monitoring lead II plus lead V_3 using a routine five-electrode patient cable. The four limb electrodes are placed close to where each limb joins the body torso. The chest electrode is moved from the common lead V_1 site to the lead V_3 location. *LA,* Left arm; *LL,* left leg; *RA,* right arm; *RL,* right leg.

Initial standard 12-lead ECG

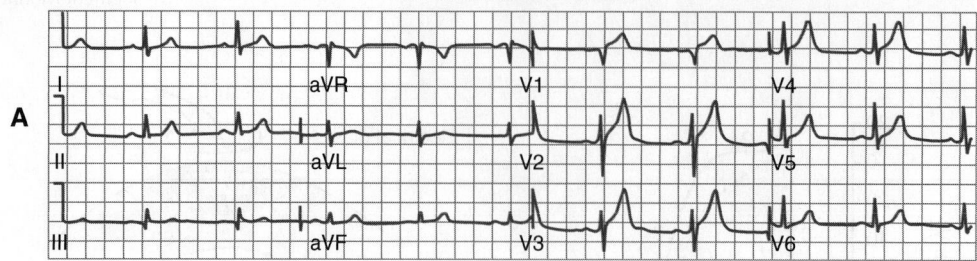

Initial cardiac rhythm strip of lead II (top) and V₃ (bottom)

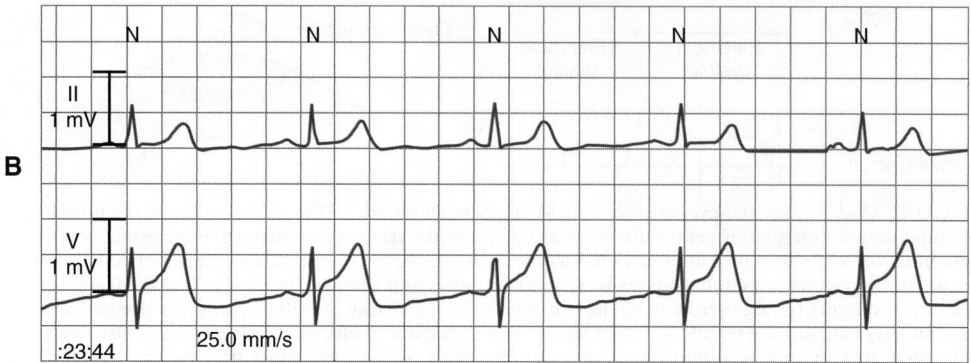

Minutes later, cardiac monitor shows striking ST elevation in Lead V₃

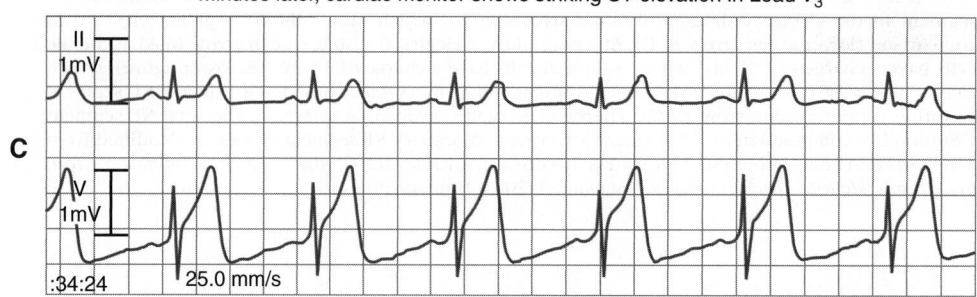

FIGURE 49-4 ▪ Value of ST segment monitoring in the emergency department for evaluation of chest pain. **A,** Initial 12-lead electrocardiogram (ECG) has a computer interpretation of "normal" and a physician diagnosis of "early repolarization pattern" (normal variant). **B,** Initial cardiac monitoring rhythm strip compares well with the standard ECG. The tracing shows the 1 mV per 10 mm calibration pulse indicating that leads II and V₃ have normal standardization. This means that ST segment amplitude can be measured as accurately with the cardiac monitor rhythm strip as with the standard 12-lead ECG. **C,** Several minutes later the bedside ST segment monitor alarm sounds and the printout shows striking ST segment elevation in lead V₃ of greater than 5 mm, whereas the ST segment in lead II remains normal. A stat 12-lead ECG recorded at this time confirms the diagnosis of ST segment elevation myocardial infarction, and the patient is taken immediately to the cardiac catheterization laboratory, where a stent is placed in the patient's totally occluded left anterior descending coronary artery. Lessons to learn from this case are the importance of (1) monitoring with an inferior lead (II) and with an anterior lead (V₃) and (2) using ST segment alarms to determine when is the best time to record a 12-lead ECG.

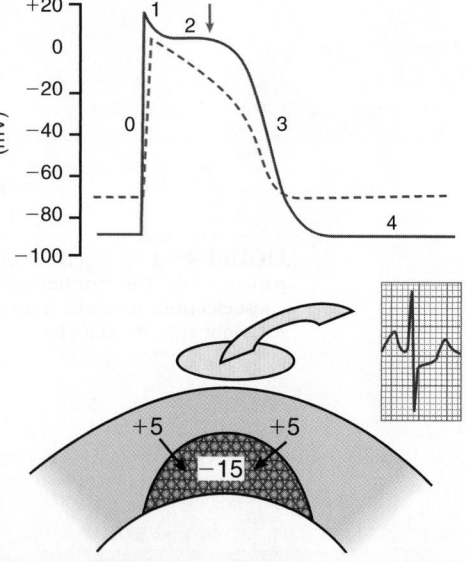

FIGURE 49-5 ▪ Cellular events producing ST segment depression. When the ischemic area is located in the subendocardial (rather than subepicardial) layer of the myocardial wall *(dappled area),* current flow during phase 2 is away from the recording electrode, which produces ST segment depression on the electrocardiogram. Such subendocardial ischemia is observed in situations in which an increased demand for myocardial oxygen (tachycardia or any condition causing arousal of the sympathetic nervous system such as exercise) cannot be met because of blood flow limitations resulting from coronary artery disease.

line," which means the small capillaries supplying blood to this region are the greatest distance from the origin of the artery in the aorta. If there are atherosclerotic narrowings along the length of the artery, the driving forces required for adequate cellular perfusion may be inadequate by the time blood reaches the subendocardium.

Clinical situations in which transient ST segment depression may be seen are conditions producing arousal of the sympathetic nervous system. The resultant increase in heart rate and blood pressure escalates the demand for oxygenated blood in the myocardium. In a patient with coronary artery disease, blood supply may not be able to match the increased demand, resulting in ischemia. Increased heart rate caused by the development of a dysrhythmia (e.g., supraventricular tachycardia) also increases the workload of the heart and may result in subendocardial ischemia and ST segment depression.

The best ECG leads for detecting demand-related ischemia are those that lie over the left ventricular apex, especially lead V_5. Such a lead selection is appropriate for detecting ischemia in areas of the hospital where patients have faster heart rates because of awakening from anesthesia (postanesthesia recovery units) or critical illness (intensive care units).[17]

ST SEGMENT MONITORING

Beginning in the mid-1980s, cardiac monitoring companies began offering special ST segment analysis software for their equipment. Because the special software may add to the cost of the equipment, hospital administrators may not choose this option, especially if clinicians do not appreciate its value. Thus even in hospitals with new cardiac monitors, the equipment may lack the capability for computerized ischemia monitoring. Also important to point out is that in most monitors with ST segment monitoring capability, the nurse must activate the software for it to work. So unlike computerized dysrhythmia monitoring, which is activated automatically when a patient is placed on a cardiac monitor, ST segment ischemia monitoring generally must be enabled manually.

In hospital units with computerized ischemia monitoring capability, ST segment monitoring is widely underused. Findings from a national random survey of 192 nurse leaders in hospital cardiac units reveal that 46 percent do not use ST segment monitoring in patients admitted with acute coronary syndromes.[18] The primary reason for nonuse is "lack of physician support." Other reasons include a high number of false ST segment alarms and lack of education about how to use the technology and what to do in response to ST segment alarms.

Who Should and Should Not Have ST Segment Monitoring?

Practice standards for ECG monitoring in hospital settings have been published recently.[19] Randomized clinical trials in the area of hospital cardiac monitoring are almost nonexistent. Thus, the practice standard is not a formal guideline with levels of evidence supported from published research but rather is expert opinions regarding the best practices.

According to the practice standard, patients with the highest priority for ST segment monitoring are those with (1) acute coronary syndromes (ST segment elevation MI, non–ST segment elevation MI, or unstable angina), (2) chest pain or an anginal equivalent who are being evaluated in the emergency department for possible acute coronary syndromes, (3) percutaneous coronary interventions with complications in the cardiac catheterization laboratory such as vessel dissection, and (4) possible variant angina caused by coronary vasospasm. Patients who should not have ST segment monitoring include those with conditions that prevent accurate assessment of the ST segment for ischemia. Such conditions include patients with (1) left bundle branch block, (2) ventricular pacing rhythm, (3) other confounding dysrhythmias that obscure the ST segment such as coarse atrial fibrillation or flutter or intermittent accelerated ventricular rhythm, and (4) agitation that produces an unacceptably noisy signal.

Best Electrocardiogram Leads for ST Segment Monitoring

In contrast to dysrhythmia detection, in which a single ECG lead is often adequate to make an accurate diagnosis, ischemia detection generally requires multiple leads. As mentioned before, to detect occlusion of any of the three main coronary arteries and to detect "demand-related" ischemia, at least three ECG leads are required. For example, the combination of leads II, V_3, and V_5 would be a valuable lead selection for ST segment monitoring. Unfortunately, many cardiac monitors do not allow for monitoring more than one precordial lead.

In response to the need for monitoring multiple ECG leads without tethering the patient to a cumbersome lead configuration, several cardiac monitoring companies have developed 12-lead ECGs that are derived from a reduced number of leads/electrodes. Reduced lead set technology is a method to derive a 12-lead ECG from a reduced number of leads/electrodes. Because derived and standard ECGs are not identical, one should not compare ST segment/T wave changes over time using both methods because ECG changes may be due to different lead systems rather than ischemia. The first such system to be introduced was the EASI 12-lead (Philips, Andover, Massachusetts), which has been investigated for dysrhythmia and ischemia diagnosis.[16,20,21] See Chapter 46 for a discussion of this technology.

Methods to Improve the Quality of ST Segment Monitoring

Because ST segment monitoring is relatively new and vastly underused, clinicians are generally less skilled in its use. Therefore, the newly published practice standard[19] reviews common problems and solutions in ST segment monitoring.

1. Identifying False Alarms Caused by Body Position Changes

Some patients have sizable changes in ST segment amplitudes when they change body position from a supine
to a right or left side-lying position.[22] Thus, a restless
patient who is turning from side to side in bed may set
off numerous ST segment alarms. Positional ST segment
changes are more difficult to distinguish from ischemia
than permanent baseline ST segment abnormalities
(e.g., fixed bundle branch block) because they, like ischemic episodes, are transient. A change in body position
is reported to be the most common cause of false ST
segment alarms in hospital units.[23] Positional ST segment changes have been a cause of unnecessary cardiac
catheterization and percutaneous coronary intervention.[24] The most likely cause of positional ST segment
changes is a slight movement in heart position relative
to the monitoring electrode.[25,26]

The best way to identify a positional ST segment
change is to observe an associated QRS complex
change as well. Transient myocardial ischemia does
not alter QRS complex size or polarity, whereas these
QRS complex variations often occur with a change in
body position. An important point is that the ST segment analysis software triggers an alarm solely based
on changes in the ST segment and does not take into
consideration what changes are occurring with the
QRS complex. Thus, the ECG rhythm strip must be
evaluated manually to distinguish true from false ST
segment alarms. To minimize possible overtreatment
in these patients, the ST segment should be evaluated
in the supine state. Therefore, when an ST segment
alarm sounds and the patient is found in a side-lying
position, the patient should be returned to the supine
position. If the ST segment deviation persists in the
supine state, it should be considered indicative of myocardial ischemia.

If a patient is agitated such that ST segment alarms
are incessant, ST segment monitoring should be disabled. However, make sure there is not another reason
for the frequent false ST segment alarms, such as poor
electrode adherence. Discontinuing ST segment monitoring in a patient with incessant false ST segment
alarms avoids the "hassle" factor, which discourages
nurses from monitoring more appropriate candidates
for ischemia, such as nonagitated patients with acute
coronary syndromes.

2. Providing Good Skin Preparation

Because the amplitudes of clinically significant ST segment changes are as small as 1 mm, a noisy signal presents a major problem for accurate diagnosis. A careful
skin preparation that includes washing the site with
soapy water is worth the extra minutes because of the
time saved in responding to false ST segment alarms.[27,28]
If a patient has a lot of hair on his chest, clipping excess
hair with a scissors is better than shaving which may
cause nicking and skin irritation.

3. Using Consistent Lead Placement

Electrodes located in proximity to the heart (i.e., those
used to record the precordial leads) are especially prone
to ST segment/T wave changes when electrodes are
moved even small distances. Marking electrode sites is
advantageous so that when electrodes are removed
(e.g., during recording of echocardiograms), they can
be replaced in the same location. If it becomes necessary to change electrode placement because of skin
breakdown or to protect a future surgical site, the
change should be documented on rhythm strips.

4. Setting ST Segment Alarm Parameters Appropriately

Most adult patients (especially elders) do not have perfectly isoelectric ST segments; therefore, if alarm parameters are set 1 to 2 mm around the isoelectric line
rather than the patient's baseline ST segment level, frequent false alarms will occur. Common causes for baseline ST segment abnormalities include (1) bundle branch
blocks, (2) left ventricular hypertrophy, (3) digitalis
therapy, and (4) cardiac dysrhythmias. The practice
standard recommends that alarm parameters be set at 1
mm above and below the baseline ST segment level in
patients at high risk for ischemia, and 2 mm in more
stable patients.[19] The wider alarm parameters may be
appropriate for most patients monitored on a telemetry
progressive care unit.

5. Understanding the Goals of ST Segment Monitoring for the Individual Patient

Determining why a patient needs ST segment monitoring is important. For example, when monitoring a patient immediately after fibrinolytic therapy for ST segment elevation MI, the goal is to document rapid
resolution of ST segment elevation, which indicates
successful reperfusion and a patent infarct-related artery.[1-4] Such resolution in ST segment elevation will
trigger alarms, which should be considered "good"
alarms. Conversely, a silent ST segment monitor after
fibrinolytic therapy indicates persistent ST segment elevation, signifying unsuccessful reperfusion.[5] In contrast to the previous MI scenario, when monitoring a
patient 48 hours later, the goal of ST segment monitoring is to detect recurrent ischemia. In this recovery
phase, an ST segment alarm should be considered a
"bad" alarm.

6. Analyzing Electrocardiogram Tracings Rather Than Just Graphic Trends

Most cardiac monitors with ST segment monitoring software provide displays of ST segment trends in a single lead or summated leads. Although such graphic trends help to identify potential ischemic events, it is important to evaluate the ECG tracing itself to confirm that ST segment changes are due to ischemia rather than a transient dysrhythmia such as an accelerated ventricular rhythm or new bundle branch block.

Role of Advanced Practice Nurses in Quality Improvement

Clinical nurse specialists, critical care educators, and nurse managers of cardiology units are in a position to promote the use and quality of ST segment monitoring.

In hospitals without ST segment monitoring capability, the local sales representative of the monitor manufacturer should be contacted to determine whether reprogramming or software upgrades are possible. In hospitals where ST segment monitoring is available but has never been used, it is best first to introduce the practice in units where patients with acute coronary syndromes are treated. These units usually include coronary intensive care and progressive care units with a predominately cardiology patient population. Patients with acute coronary syndromes stand to benefit most from ST segment monitoring. Moreover, nurses working in these units often have more expertise in ECG interpretation, which makes it more likely that physicians will trust the diagnosis of ischemic events. Once ST segment monitoring has been launched successfully in cardiac units, the practice can be introduced in other monitored units.

One technique that has been successful in moving this technology into practice is for the advanced practice nurse to partner with an influential physician on the unit who is willing to consider the potential benefits of ST segment monitoring. Physicians may be unfamiliar with ST segment analysis software and the literature regarding its use. Providing them with the recently published practice standard[19] is a good way to impress them with the recommended best practices that competing hospitals may be adopting for state-of-the-art cardiac care. A common reason for lack of physician support for ST segment monitoring is the lack of nursing expertise in evaluating ST segment deviation. Thus, physicians fear numerous calls in the middle of the night for false ST segment alarms. This fear is well founded because most hospital nurses know little about diagnosing ischemia—even nurses skilled in dysrhythmia diagnosis. Therefore the major role of the advanced practice nurse is to develop an educational program and clinical support for ST segment monitoring.

Once key physicians are identified, it is important to elicit their input regarding an ST segment monitoring protocol for the hospital unit in question. The protocol should state what patients should have ST segment monitoring, how long it should be done, which ECG leads should be used, how alarm parameters should be set, how alarm tracings should be documented in the medical record, when a stat 12-lead ECG should be recorded, and under what conditions physicians should be notified. Nurses in the expert writing group for the practice standards have recently published an executive summary that addresses how to implement the practice standards and answers common questions that arise.[29]

ST segment monitoring should not "go live" until the core nursing staff of the unit has been trained in its use. Education should involve didactic information and hands-on practice. Education should include case examples and troubleshooting of false ST segment alarms. Once ST segment monitoring has begun, assess what ongoing education is needed, and look for ways to reinforce clinicians' commitment to this practice. The best strategy for reinforcement of the practice is to present cases (formally and informally) in which ST segment monitoring has been used for clinical decision making (e.g., changing medications, transferring back to an intensive care unit, requesting a cardiology consultation, or scheduling a cardiac catheterization). Absence of ST segment events also may influence clinical decision making. For example, physicians who observe a patient ambulating on a progressive care unit without ST segment events may feel more confident about discharging the patient early. Documentation of reduced hospital length of stay following implementation of ST segment monitoring would encourage administrative support for the practice and ongoing education.

Finally, use implementation of ST segment monitoring to involve staff in a unit-based research project. Such projects can be submitted for presentation at conferences such as the National Teaching Institute of the American Association of Critical-Care Nurses or the Annual Scientific Sessions of the American Heart Association. Presentation of clinical nursing research brings

---

■ ■ ■ CONUNDRUM

WHY IS ST SEGMENT MONITORING NOT WIDELY USED?

ST segment monitoring is not used as widely as indicated for several reasons. The technology is expensive, and not all hospitals have (or use) the equipment needed to perform ST segment monitoring. Contact your local company representative to determine the cost of upgrading or expanding existing equipment. A cost-benefit analysis will help you to convince your institution of the importance of this state-of-the-art technology. To perform the cost-benefit analysis, document cases in which ST segment monitoring has been used for clinical decision making. Many of these cases have cost implications (e.g., early hospital discharge in a patient who ambulates without ST segment elevation).

Another reason that ST segment monitoring is not used more widely is that nurses are more adept at dysrhythmia monitoring than at assessing ST segments. This is content that should be added to educational curricula and hospital orientation programs to ensure that all nurses are adept in this area. The "hassle" factor is another reason; false alarms are common. This chapter describes specific techniques that can be used to decrease false alarms. Another reason that ST segment monitoring is not used widely is that physician support for the practice can be elusive. A physician champion and written standards of practice can help to get physician support.

recognition to the hospital and assists in achieving magnet status for the hospital.

CONCLUSION

Ischemia monitoring is a relatively new role for hospital nurses that is expected to improve patient outcomes, especially for patients with acute coronary syndromes. As with any new technology, the quality of its use depends largely on the knowledge and experience of the user (i.e., the nursing staff). ST segment monitoring provides an opportunity for advanced practice nurses to become leaders in improving the quality of ECG monitoring in their hospital setting.

REFERENCES

1. Veldkamp RF, Green CL, Wilkins ML et al: Comparison of continuous ST-segment recovery analysis with methods using static electrocardiograms for noninvasive patency assessment during acute myocardial infarction: Thrombolysis and Angioplasty in Myocardial Infarction (TAMI) 7 Study Group, *Am J Cardiol* 73: 7-1069, 1994.
2. Fernandez AR, Sequeira RF, Chakko S et al: ST segment tracking for rapid determination of patency of the infarct-related artery in acute myocardial infarction, *J Am Coll Cardiol* 26:2-675, 1995.
3. Klootwijk P, Langer A, Meij S et al: Noninvasive prediction of reperfusion and coronary artery patency by continuous ST segment monitoring in the GUSTO-I trial, *Eur Heart J* 17:1-689, 1996.
4. Krucoff MW, Johanson P, Baeza R et al: Clinical utility of serial and continuous ST-segment recovery assessment in patients with acute ST-elevation myocardial infarction, *Circulation* 110:e533-e539, 2004.
5. Schroder R, Dissmann R, Bruggemann T et al: Extent of early ST segment elevation resolution: a simple but strong predictor of outcome in patients with acute myocardial infarction, *J Am Coll Cardiol* 24:2-384, 1994.
6. Gottlieb SO, Weisfeldt ML, Ouyang P et al: Silent ischemia as a marker for early unfavorable outcomes in patients with unstable angina, *N Engl J Med* 314:31-1214, 1986.
7. Gottlieb SO, Weisfeldt ML, Ouyang P et al: Silent ischemia predicts infarction and death during 2 year follow-up of unstable angina, *J Am Coll Cardiol* 10:1-756, 1987.
8. Nademanee K, Intarachot V, Josephson MA et al: Prognostic significance of silent myocardial ischemia in patients with unstable angina, *J Am Cardiol* 10:11, 1987.
9. Krucoff MW: Identification of high-risk patients with silent myocardial ischemia after percutaneous transluminal coronary angioplasty by multilead monitoring, *Am J Cardiol* 61:29F-34F, 1988.
10. Langer A, Freeman MR, Armstrong PE: ST segment shift in unstable angina: pathophysiology and association with coronary anatomy and hospital outcome, *J Am Coll Cardiol* 13:1-1495, 1989.
11. Larsson H, Jonasson T, Ringqvist I et al: Diagnostic and prognostic importance of ST recording after an episode of unstable angina or non-Q-wave myocardial infarction, *Eur Heart J* 13:1-207, 1992.
12. Amanullah AM, Lindvall K: Prevalence and significance of transient—predominantly asymptomatic—myocardial ischemia on Holter monitoring in unstable angina pectoris, and correlation with exercise test and thallium-201 myocardial perfusion imaging, *Am J Cardiol* 72:7-144, 1993.
13. Bugiardini R, Borghi A, Pozzati A et al: Relation of severity of symptoms to transient myocardial ischemia and prognosis in unstable angina, *J Am Coll Cardiol* 25:2-597, 1995.
14. Drew BJ, Pelter MM, Adams MG: Frequency, characteristics, and clinical significance of transient ST segment elevation in patients with acute coronary syndromes, *Eur Heart J* 23:2-941, 2002.
15. Arnsdorf MF: The electrophysiologic matrix: equilibrium and Arnsdorf's paradox. In Gussak I, Antzelevitch C, editors: *Cardiac repolarization: bridging basic and clinical science,* Totowa, NJ, 2003, Humana Press.
16. Drew BJ, Krucoff MW, for the ST-Segment Monitoring Practice Guideline International Working Group: Multilead ST-segment monitoring in patients with acute coronary syndromes: a consensus statement for healthcare professionals, *Am J Crit Care* 8:-372, 1999.
17. Booker KJ, Holm K, Drew BJ et al: Frequency and outcomes of transient myocardial ischemia in noncardiac critically ill adults, *Am J Crit Care* 12:1-508, 2003.
18. Patton JA, Funk M: Survey of use of ST-segment monitoring in patients with acute coronary syndromes, *Am J Crit Care* 10:1-23, 2001.
19. Drew BJ, Califf RM, Funk M et al: Practice standards for electrocardiographic monitoring in hospital settings, *Circulation* 110:11-2721, 2004.
20. Drew BJ, Scheinman MM, Evans GT: Comparison of a vectorcardiographically derived 12-lead electrocardiogram with the conventional electrocardiogram during wide QRS complex tachycardia, and its potential application for continuous bedside monitoring, *Am J Cardiol* 69:6-612, 1992.
21. Drew BJ, Adams MG, Pelter MM, Wung SF: ST segment monitoring with a derived 12-lead electrocardiogram is superior to routine CCU monitoring, *Am J Crit Care* 5:-198, 1996.
22. Adams MG, Drew BJ: Body position effects on the ECG: implications for ischemia monitoring, *J Electrocardiol* 30:3-285, 1997.
23. Drew BJ, Wung SF, Adams MG, Pelter MM: Bedside diagnosis of myocardial ischemia with ST-segment monitoring technology: measurement issues for real-time clinical decision-making and trial designs, *J Electrocardiol* 30:3-157, 1998.
24. Drew BJ, Adams MG: Clinical consequences of ST-segment changes caused by body position mimicking transient myocardial ischemia: hazards of ST-segment monitoring? *J Electrocardiol* 34:3-261, 2001.
25. Feldman T, Borow K, Neumann A et al: Relation of electrocardiographic R wave amplitude to changes in left ventricular chamber size and position in normal subjects, *Am J Cardiol* 55:5-1168, 1985.
26. Sutherland DJ, McPherson DD, Spencer CA et al: Effects of posture and respiration on body surface electrocardiograms, *Am J Cardiol* 52:595, 1983.
27. Clochesy JM, Cifani L, Howe K: Electrode site preparation techniques: a follow-up study, *Heart Lung* 20:2-27, 1991.
28. Medina V, Clochesy JM, Omery A: Comparison of electrode site preparation techniques, *Heart Lung* 18:1-456, 1989.
29. Drew BJ, Funk M. Practice standards for ECG monitoring in hospital settings: Executive summary and guide for implementation. *Crit Care Nurs Clin N Am* 18:157-168, 2006.

Hemodynamic Monitoring

Susan K. Frazier

Evaluation of hemodynamic state is an integral component of the care of critically ill patients. Physical examination offers some evidence of the effectiveness of cardiovascular function, as does evaluation of indicators of end-organ system function. However, investigators have identified little relationship between clinician estimates of cardiovascular efficacy based on physical examination and invasive measures of cardiovascular function.[1-3] Ideally, clinicians gather information from a number of sources that include physical examination, diagnostic testing, and hemodynamic measurement before clinical decision making.

Historically, health care providers evaluated cardiovascular effectiveness and the adequacy of movement of blood in the cardiovascular system by physical assessment of the chest and measurement of heart rate and blood pressure. Early physicians placed their ear directly on the chest to evaluate the function of organs within the chest. However, the direct application of the ear to the chest was not always socially acceptable and not always effective in obese individuals. Because of these difficulties, Laennec developed and marketed the stethoscope in the early 1800s.[4] This tubular mechanism was used to direct sounds from the chest to the examiner for

evaluation. Binaural stethoscopes were developed in the last decade of the 19th century and supported more definitive quality of information collection.

The first report of blood pressure measurement described the technique used by Stephen Hales in the early 1700s.[5] Hales evaluated direct arterial pressure by placing a goose quill in an equine carotid artery and connecting this to a 9-foot glass column. The rise of the blood in the column indicated to this scientist that the heart generated pressure equal to the height of the arterial blood in the column. Poiseuille further developed this technique by using a column of mercury rather than the empty glass column. Even though using a mercury column provided an adequate measure of mean cardiovascular pressure, the inertia of the mercury made rapid changes in pressure during the cardiac cycle impossible to evaluate. Although these measures directly evaluated intravascular pressures, they were not useful for clinicians, and so noninvasive methods of measuring blood pressure developed over the next 100 years that were clinically suitable.

Riva-Rocci expanded the work of previous scientists to develop the noninvasive mercury sphygmomanometer in 1896.[4] With this apparatus, systolic blood pressure was determined by palpation, and in 1905, Korotkoff developed the auscultatory technique that permitted measurement of systolic and diastolic pressure using the sphygmomanometer. During the 20th century, the auscultatory technique evolved into the standard measurement used daily in clinical practice. However, this technique provides an isolated measurement in pressure, and rapid fluctuations are difficult to detect.

Lambert and Wood developed an electronic transducer with rapid response capability soon after World War II to provide beat-by-beat measurement of arterial pressure.[6] However, use of this capability was not common in patient care until the development of critical care units in the 1960s and 1970s. Since that time, hemodynamic monitoring techniques have evolved significantly to provide clinicians with important information about cardiovascular function and guide intervention.

HEMODYNAMIC MONITORING
Definition and Purpose

Hemodynamic refers to the dynamic movement of blood through the cardiovascular system. Hemodynamic monitoring is a means to evaluate the cardiovascular components that influence this movement of blood. Typical measures provide direct or indirect information about intravascular pressures, volumes, vascular resistance, and blood flow; however, the ultimate variable of interest to the clinician is cellular oxygen delivery and utilization. Unfortunately, there are no current, clinically useful, direct measures of cellular oxygen delivery and utilization. Thus, hemodynamic monitoring is used to provide information about the delivery system, and interventions are focused on improving the function of this delivery system. Clinicians use the information obtained from hemodynamic monitoring to evaluate baseline cardiovascular function, to determine the presence and degree of cardiovascular dysfunction, to guide specific interventions to promote improved cardiovascular function, and to evaluate the efficacy of these interventions.

PHYSIOLOGICAL PRINCIPLES OF HEMODYNAMICS

Using hemodynamic science, clinicians and researchers investigate and describe the cardiovascular variables that influence blood flow and oxygen delivery. These variables include volume, pressure, flow, and resistance to flow. A number of physiological principles elucidate the relationships among these factors and illustrate the importance of hemodynamic measures.

Basis of Hemodynamics
Darcy's Law of Flow

Darcy's law describes the importance of the blood pressure gradient and blood vessel resistance to forward blood flow. Flow through a simple tube depends on the pressure gradient or difference in pressure at the two ends (Figure 50-1). As the pressure gradient increases, flow increases in a linear fashion if there is no change in resistance of the tube. However, blood vessel diameter changes produce alterations in resistance to forward flow. When resistance is factored into this equation and Darcy's law is written for the cardiovascular system, it may be stated as follows:

$$CO = (MAP - CVP)/TPR$$

where **CO** is the cardiac output, **MAP** is the mean arterial pressure, **CVP** is the central venous pressure, *MAP*

− CVP is the pressure gradient for forward blood flow, and **TPR** is the total peripheral resistance. Thus, cardiac output is directly proportional to the size of the pressure gradient and inversely proportional to the degree of vessel resistance.

Poiseuille's Laws of Resistance and Flow

Once the importance of resistance to flow had been identified and described, Poiseuille studied the factors that influenced resistance. His law of resistance can be stated as follows:

$$R = 8\eta l/\pi r^4$$

where **R** is resistance, **8/π** is a proportionality constant, **η** is the viscosity of blood, **l** is tube length, and **r^4** is the radius to the fourth power. Accordingly, Poiseuille found that resistance is directly proportional to the blood viscosity and the length of the vessel and inversely proportional to the radius of the vessel. Thus, resistance increases as the blood viscosity increases, as the length of the vessel increases, and as the radius of the vessel decreases.

Poiseuille combined his resistance equation with Darcy's law of flow through a tube to describe blood flow in the cardiovascular system. This law is stated as follows:

$$Q = \pi \delta P r^4/8\eta l$$

where **Q** is blood flow, **π/8** is a proportionality constant, **δP** is the pressure gradient between the two ends of the vessel, r^4 is the radius of the blood vessel to the fourth power, η is the viscosity of the blood, and *l* is the length of the vessel. This law indicates that blood flow is directly proportional to the size of the pressure gradient and the radius of the blood vessel. Thus as these variables increase, blood flow is enhanced. However, the inverse relationship between blood viscosity and vessel length indicates that as viscosity increases and blood vessel length increases, blood flow is reduced. In the cardiovascular system, most major alterations in blood flow are due to changes in vessel radius and subsequent increases in resistance (Figure 50-2).

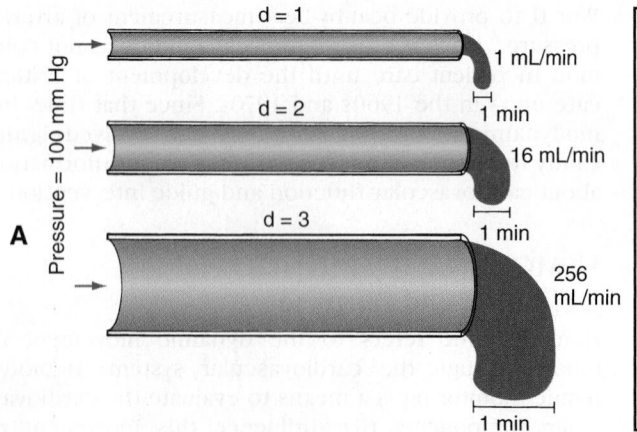
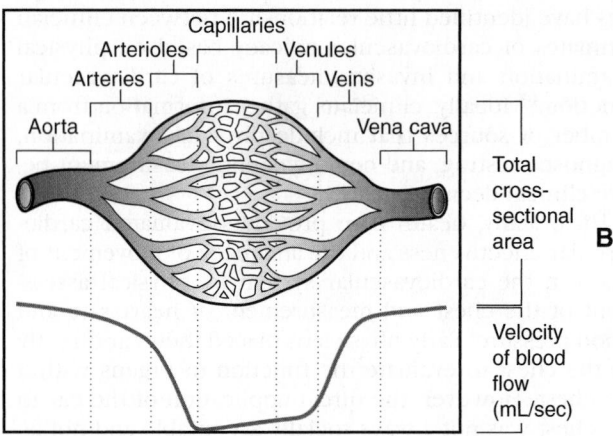

FIGURE 50-1 ■ The effect of vessel lumen diameter on blood flow (left). The association between vessel cross-sectional area and blood flow velocity (right). *d*, Diameter. (From Sole M, Klein D, Moseley M: *Introduction to critical care nursing*, ed 4, St Louis, 2005, Mosby.)

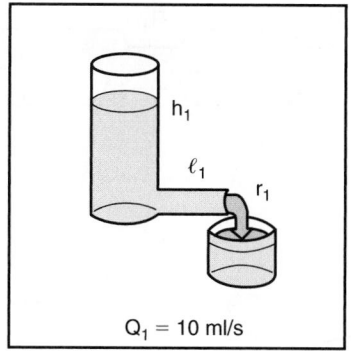

A. Reference condition: for a given pressure, length, radius, and viscosity, let the flow (V_1) equal 10 ml/s.

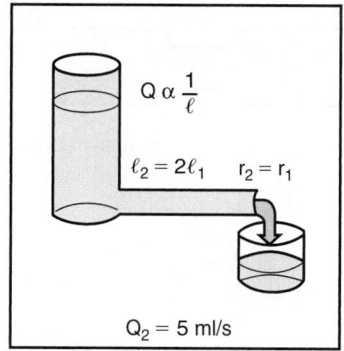

B. If tube length doubles, flow decreases by 50%.

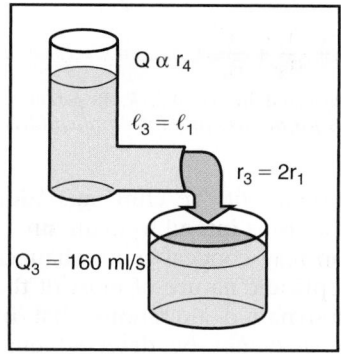

C. If tube radius doubles, flow increases 16-fold.

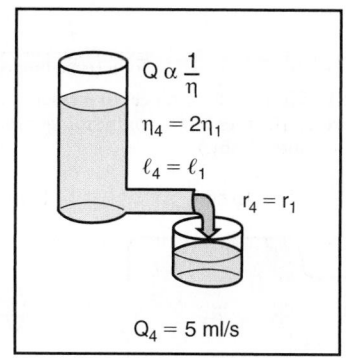

D. If viscosity doubles, flow decreases by 50%.

FIGURE 50-2 ■ **A,** Reference condition. The effect of vessel length (**B**), radius (**C**) and viscosity (**D**) on flow. Poiseuille's law. *Q,* blood flow; *h,* height; *l,* tube length; *r,* radius; *n,* blood viscosity. (From Berne R, Levy M: *Cardiovascular physiology,* ed 8, St Louis, 2001, Mosby.)

Not only does the radius of the vessels influence total resistance, but also the anatomical arrangement of the vessels in series or in parallel (Figure 50-3). For vessels arranged in series, blood flows from one vessel to the next, and the total resistance of this arrangement is the sum of the resistances of the vessels ($R_1 + R_2 + R_3$). For vessels arranged in parallel, resistance is inversely proportional to cross-sectional area; so as cross-sectional area expands, resistance is reduced. Total resistance of parallel vessels is the sum of the reciprocal of the resistance (1/R) for each of these vessels ($1/R_1 + 1/R_2 + 1/R_3$). Thus, the parallel arrangement of vessels such as capillaries significantly reduces resistance and increases flow, thus augmenting cellular oxygen delivery via the microcirculation. Cross-sectional area also is related to the velocity of blood flow in an inversely proportional fashion (Figure 50-4). As vessel cross-sectional area increases, as in the microcirculation, the velocity of blood flow decreases to provide sufficient opportunity for diffusion of gases, nutrients, and waste products.

With a clear understanding of hemodynamic principles, valid and reliable hemodynamic evaluation provides clinicians with useful data. The intent of collecting hemodynamic data is to enable clinicians specifically to target dysfunction, intervene to optimize cardiovascular function, and ultimately improve oxygen delivery with the goal of improved patient outcome.

Noninvasive Hemodynamic Evaluation

Before the development of invasive hemodynamic techniques, physical assessment and evaluation of organ function provided information about hemodynamic efficacy. Measurement of traditional vital signs including apical and peripheral pulses and auscultatory blood pressure provides information about cardiac output, vascular resistance, blood volume, and tissue perfusion. Comprehensive physical assessment, 12-lead electrocardiogram, and chest radiograph offer information about the size and location of organs (in particular the heart) and the adequacy of tissue perfusion (Box 50-1).

One must consider several factors when determining the most appropriate means to evaluate hemodynamic function. Several investigators have found poor correlation between noninvasive estimation of hemodynamic adequacy by experienced clinicians and invasive direct measurement of these variables.[1-3] Noninvasive estimates may be influenced significantly by the skill and

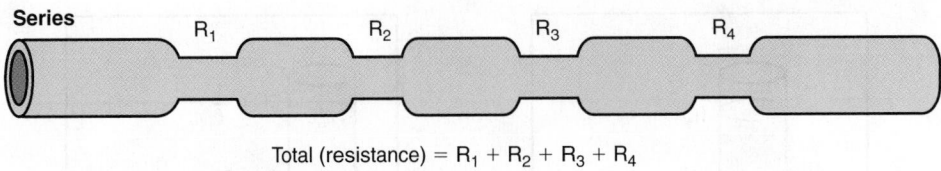

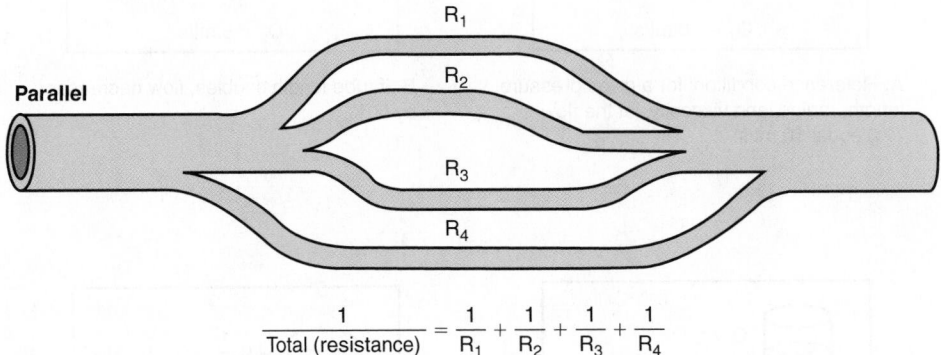

$$\frac{1}{\text{Total (resistance)}} = \frac{1}{R_1} + \frac{1}{R_2} + \frac{1}{R_3} + \frac{1}{R_4}$$

FIGURE 50-3 ■ Resistance in vessels arranged in series and in parallel. *R,* Resistance. (From McCance K, Huether S: *Pathophysiology: the biologic basis for disease in adults and children,* ed 5, St Louis, 2006, Mosby.)

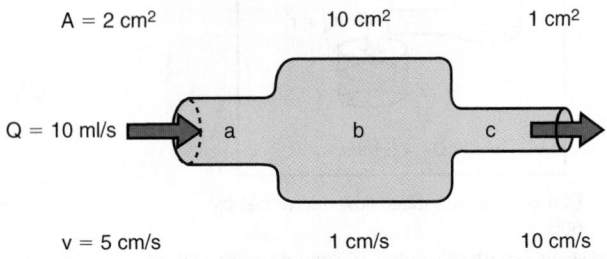

FIGURE 50-4 ■ The effect of cross-sectional area on velocity of blood flow. (From Berne R, Levy M: *Cardiovascular physiology,* ed 8, St Louis, 2001, Mosby.) *A,* Area; *v,* velocity of blood flow.

BOX 50-1

■ ■ ■

TRADITIONAL NONINVASIVE HEMODYNAMIC ASSESSMENT PARAMETERS

- Measurement of auscultatory blood pressure
- Evaluation of apical and peripheral pulses
- Assessment of precordium and point of maximum impulse
- Performance of chest percussion
- Auscultation of heart sounds and lung sounds
- Examination of 12-lead electrocardiogram and chest radiograph
- Assessment of respiratory rate and pattern
- Inspection of skin temperature, color, texture, turgor, and presence of diaphoresis
- Determination of capillary refill time
- Estimation of central venous pressure minus jugular venous pressure
- Evaluation of hepatojugular reflux
- Determination of presence of edema
- Measurement of arterial oxygen concentration and calculation of arterial oxygen content
- Measurement of urinary output, serum creatinine, and blood urea nitrogen
- Evaluation of bowel sounds
- Abdominal assessment and determination of enlargement of organs
- Assessment of neurological function

---

experience of the clinician. Additionally, homeostatic mechanisms intend to maintain stability and their activation may conceal acute changes initially. Because of the episodic nature of most of these evaluations, rapid hemodynamic alterations that influence patient outcome may not be detected quickly, and continuous measurement of the majority of these indicators is not available. Without this continuous, real-time information, effective intervention may be delayed and negatively influence patient outcome.

Invasive Hemodynamic Monitoring

Invasive hemodynamic monitoring techniques require sophisticated equipment, knowledge, and psychomotor skills for valid, reliable measurement of hemodynamic variables and appropriate selection of effective interventions. Equipment requirements for pressure monitoring include a catheter placed in a blood vessel and a fluid-filled tubing transducer system connected to an amplifier-monitor that interfaces with a printer (Figure 50-5).

Invasive pressure monitoring most commonly uses a fluid-filled system. A prepackaged tubing transducer kit is connected to and flushed with sterile solution, and then is connected securely to an intravascular catheter. In this system, pressure waves are transmitted through the blood vessel to the fluid in the system via the open catheter tip. The tubing used in this system is low compliance; it does not distend in response to this pressure wave. Thus, the pressure wave is transmitted accurately to the transducer through the tubing system.

An electronic transducer interfaces with the fluid in this system (Figure 50-6). The point of air-fluid interface is usually a thin, flexible diaphragm that is deformed by these pulsatile pressure changes. The transducer detects these deformations and converts this information

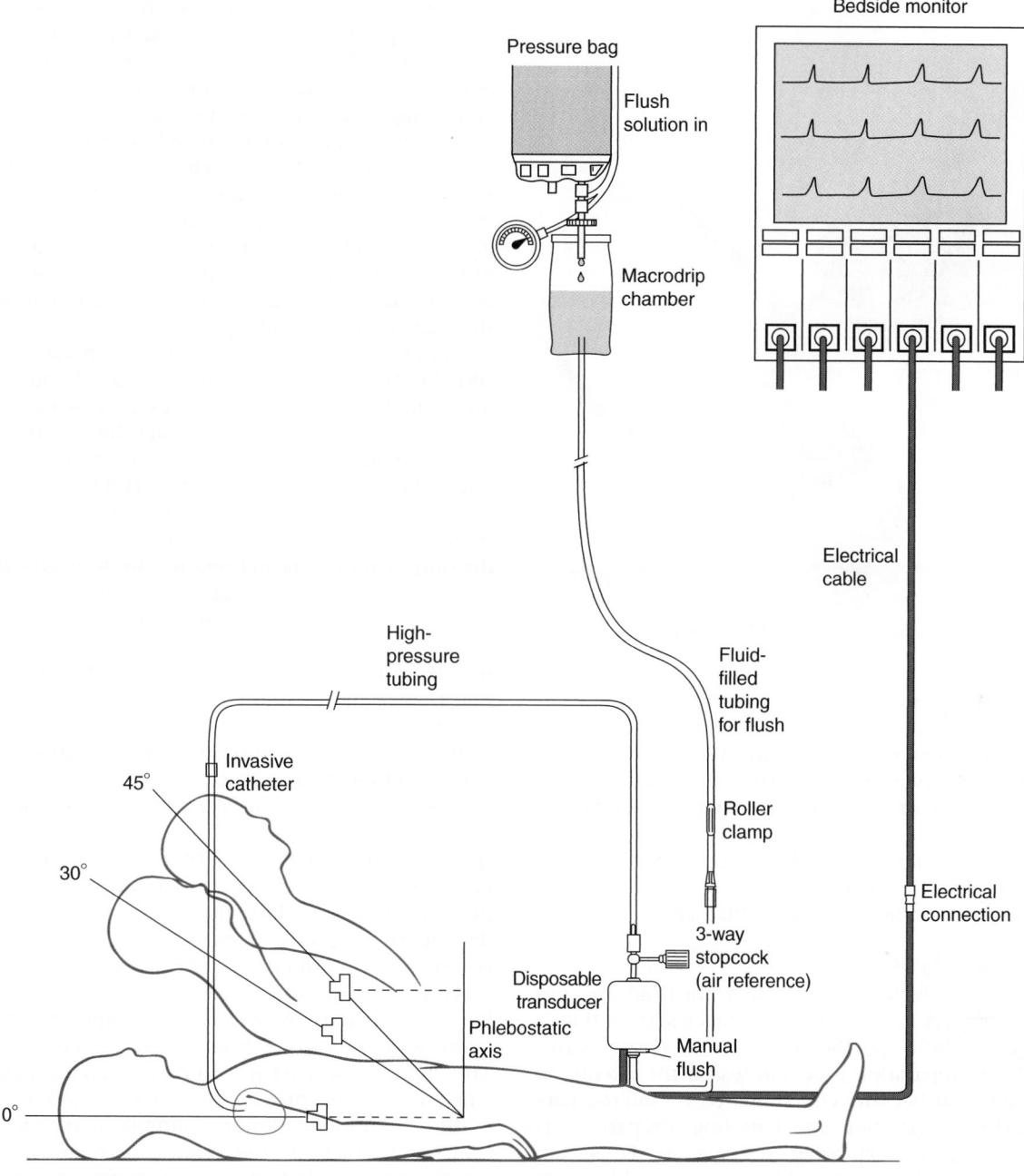

FIGURE 50-5 ■ Components of a fluid-filled monitoring system. Location of phlebostatic axis at various elevations. (From Urden L, Stacy K, Lough M: *Priorities in critical care nursing,* ed 4, St Louis, 2004, Mosby.)

into an electrical signal. The ability of a transducer to detect and produce accurate representations of pressure changes within the blood vessel is described as fidelity. Thus a high-fidelity transducer provides rapid and precise information about pressure change within a vessel.

The electronic signal is transmitted to the bedside monitor, where it is filtered and amplified or boosted in size. This process removes extraneous information and ensures that the signal is of sufficient strength for analysis. This signal then is converted and displayed as a waveform on an oscilloscope. One vital requirement of this

electronic equipment is linearity. Linearity of equipment describes the ability of the transducer and amplifier to convert the pressure signal proportionally into an accurate output. Thus for every 10-mm Hg change in intravascular pressure, there is a 10-mm Hg change in measured and displayed pressure. The bedside monitor is interfaced with a single- or multiple-channel printer/recorder so that waveforms may be documented and inspected for accurate evaluation of pressure measurements.

Reliable and valid measures are requisite for effective management of critically ill patients. To ensure that the obtained values are an accurate representation of the

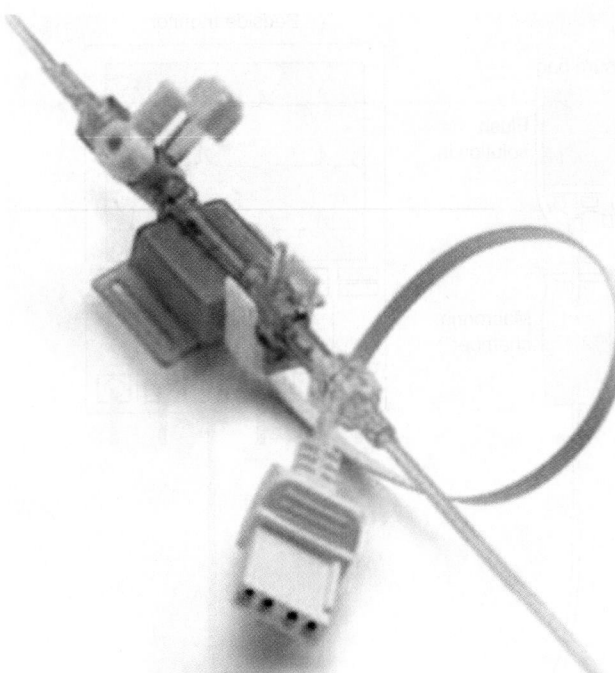

FIGURE 50-6 ■ Disposable transducer.

physiological condition of the patient, the clinician must have the ability to do the following:

- Correctly prepare and maintain this system
- Evaluate the dynamic response of the system
- Level the system to the appropriate reference point
- Zero reference this system
- Calibrate the transducer when necessary
- Troubleshoot the system
- Monitor and evaluate the data obtained

Preparation of System

Presently, most facilities purchase a one-time use, disposable, prepackaged tubing transducer system that is designed to their specifications. These cost-effective kits reduce preparation time and lessen the likelihood the system will become contaminated by microorganisms during preparation and handling. Prepared kits also ensure that monitoring systems are consistent within a unit and often a facility, which should reduce preparation error. A microdrip chamber may be included in this system to prevent administration of excess fluid volume during invasive monitoring. Another important component of this system is a continuous flush device. This mechanism is activated by the application of pressure to the fluid administration bag (usually 300 mm Hg). Consistent application of pressure ensures that this device will administer a slow infusion of solution (3 to 5 ml/hr) to maintain catheter patency. This device contains a manual trigger that also permits manual administration of rapid fluid flush to clear the catheter and maintain patency.

Aseptic technique is mandatory during preparation and management of the fluid-filled system to prevent contamination of the vascular system. Before priming the tubing, all connections should be evaluated to ensure they are secure and sterile; closed covers must be placed over all unused stopcock ports. The drip chamber is inserted aseptically into a sterile fluid bag, typically normal saline. After the drip chamber is inserted into the solution bag, all air must be removed from the solution bag and tubing by gravity. Use of the fast flush component of the system for the priming procedure produces turbulent fluid flow and results in formation of minute air bubbles, which then must be removed before monitoring. Once the tubing transducer kit has been primed, the pressure device should be placed on the solution bag and inflated to activate the continuous fluid infusion. The system then is connected to an indwelling vascular catheter for measurement of intravascular pressure.

Depending on institutional policy, heparin may be added to the solution to reduce the likelihood of thrombus formation and catheter occlusion. However, the use of heparin in flush solutions may be responsible for heparin-induced thrombocytopenia.[7] Two types of heparin-induced thrombocytopenia (**HIT**) have been described: type I and type II. Type I HIT is a mild, transient decrease in platelets that occurs 1 to 4 days after the initiation of heparin therapy.[8] Administered heparin stimulates platelet aggregation and consumption in 10 to 20 percent of patients. Thrombocytopenia is the consequence (platelet count usually greater than 100,000 platelets/μl). HIT type I usually resolves without complication or intervention even with continued heparin administration.

HIT type II is a more serious complication of heparin administration that is immune mediated. This type of HIT occurs in 1 to 5 percent of patients who receive heparin and may produce serious thrombocytopenia (platelet count less than 100,000 platelets/μl), thromboembolism (50 percent of cases), and death (25 to 30 percent of cases).[8] Thrombocytopenia occurs 5 to 14 days following initial administration of heparin. Most commonly, immunoglobulin G antibodies produce this reaction.[9] These antibodies do not bind solely with heparin; the heparin must be in a complex with platelet factor 4, a heparin-binding protein stored in platelets. The complex of heparin and platelet factor 4 produces a molecule conformation that is recognized by the antibodies.[10] Antibody binding stimulates platelet activation, degranulation, and release of platelet factor 4, which induces additional antibody binding and subsequent thrombocytopenia. Thrombosis and thromboembolism are the most common and serious complication; the consequence may be pulmonary embolus, myocardial infarction, stroke, and organ infarction. The prevalence of HIT caused by heparin flush solution or heparin-bonded catheters is currently unknown. Thus regular platelet count evaluation is necessary for patients with any exposure to heparin and especially when heparin is used in flush solutions or when the catheter used for monitoring is heparin bonded.[11,12]

Dynamic Response Testing

Dynamic response testing ensures that the pressure monitoring system will respond rapidly to pressure change and duplicate the entire pressure wave accurately. Dynamic response is evaluated by the performance of a square wave test (Figure 50-7). Several fac-

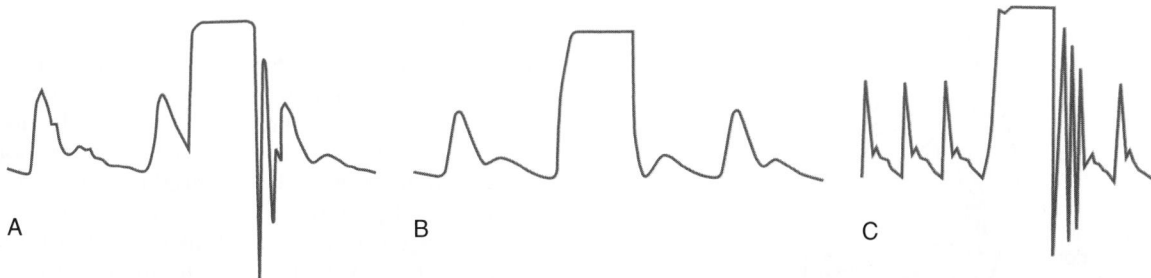

FIGURE 50-7 ■ Dynamic response testing of a fluid-filled pressure monitoring system. **A,** Optimal damping. **B,** Overdamping. **C,** Underdamping. (From Sole M, Klein D, Moseley M: *Introduction to critical care nursing,* ed 4, St Louis, 2005, Mosby.)

tors influence the dynamic response of the system (Table 50-1). To perform this evaluation, the fast flush device is activated and quickly released. This action produces a square wave response followed by several oscillations. This test provides information about the frequency response of the system and is reported as the degree of damping (optimal, overdamped, or underdamped). Damping describes the extent of loss of the pulsatile energy in the system. Pulsatile energy may be lost because of frictional resistance of the fluid or more often by absorption of this energy by some components found in the system. For example, the use of compliant tubing would produce a loss of energy, as would the presence of air bubbles in the system.

In a system with optimal damping, closure of the fast flush device produces a rapid, sharp upstroke in pressure to the maximum pressure level to produce a flat line at maximum pressure. Pressure rapidly falls below the baseline point, is quickly followed by one or two oscillations within 0.12 second with a subsequent rapid return to baseline. Pressure waveforms in an optimally damped system are reproduced accurately, and all components of the wave are visualized clearly. An overdamped system generates a square wave with a sloped or delayed rise to the maximum pressure, followed by a flat line at maximum pressure. Maximum pressure is followed by a sloped downward deflection that ends before baseline is reached. No oscillations occur after the square wave in an overdamped system, and pressure waveforms are reproduced poorly with blunted peak pressures and often loss of components of a waveform such as the dicrotic notch. Underdamped systems pro-

duce a typical square wave with several amplified oscillations detected in the flat portion of the square wave and immediately following the square wave. An underdamped system amplifies the pulsatile energy found in the system, and false pressure signals (artifact) are often present. Pressure measures in an underdamped or overdamped system are invalid.

Leveling the System

Fluid-filled systems must be leveled appropriately to ensure that measured pressures are accurate. Leveling simply ensures that the tip of the vascular catheter and the air-fluid interface of the transducer are located in the same vertical plane to remove the effects of hydrostatic pressure. Hydrostatic pressure in the system is produced by the weight of the fluid in the tubing. The phlebostatic axis or midchest position is used universally as the leveling point for vascular pressures because this is the approximate location of most vascular catheter tips.[13] The phlebostatic axis also provides a universal point for consistency of measurement between clinicians and facilities. The phlebostatic axis is located at the junction of the fourth intercostal space and the midaxillary line (Figure 50-8).

When the air-fluid interface of the transducer is above the phlebostatic axis, hydrostatic pressure is directed from the transducer to the catheter tip and artificially reduces the measured pressure (2 mm Hg less than actual for each 1 inch above the phlebostatic axis).[14] When the air-fluid interface of the transducer is lower than the phlebostatic axis, hydrostatic pressure is directed from the catheter tip to the transducer and artificially elevates

■ ■ ■

TABLE 50-1   FACTORS THAT INFLUENCE FREQUENCY RESPONSE AND THEIR MANAGEMENT

FACTOR	MANAGEMENT OF FACTORS THAT INFLUENCE DYNAMIC RESPONSE OF PRESSURE MONITORING SYSTEM
Presence of blood in catheter following blood sampling	Clear catheter immediately after blood sampling. Maintain pressure on continuous flush device at 300 mm Hg.
Presence of thrombus in catheter	Remove thrombus or replace catheter.
Air bubbles in system	Remove all air bubbles.
Tubing type and length	Use shortest length of noncompliant tubing, no longer than 4 feet.
Kinks in tubing	Use noncompliant tubing, and evaluate frequently for kinks.
Lumen size of catheter	Use largest-sized catheter appropriate for vessel.
Frequency response of bedside monitor	Use equipment with a minimum of 60 Hz frequency response.

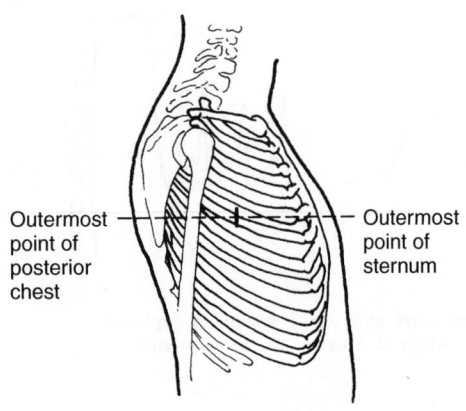

FIGURE 50-8 ■ Location of the phlebostatic axis for leveling the air-fluid interface. (From Darovic G: *Handbook of hemodynamic monitoring*, ed 2, St Louis, 2004, Saunders.)

the measured pressure (2 mm Hg greater than actual for each 1 inch below the phlebostatic axis). Once the air-fluid interface of the transducer is level with the phlebostatic axis, the effects of hydrostatic pressure are removed and measured pressures are an accurate reflection of actual vascular pressure.

Transducer leveling is performed by visual line of sight, the use of a carpenter's level, or more recently with the use of a laser level. Comparison of these methods of transducer leveling identified significant differences in transducer placement.[15,16] In one investigation,[16] the use of visual alignment produced errors that ranged from 4.6 cm above to 6.3 cm below the phlebostatic axis. The use of a carpenter's level generated errors that ranged from 2.2 cm above and 5.2 cm below the phlebostatic axis. The use of a laser level produced errors that ranged from 0.4 cm above and 0.9 cm below the phlebostatic axis. Thus, the use of a laser level to align the vertical plane was demonstrated to be the most accurate method of alignment.

Zero Referencing the System

Zero referencing the system removes the effects of atmospheric pressure from the system and ensures that the measured pressure accurately reflects intravascular pressure. The stopcock closest to the patient is turned so that the transducer diaphragm does not receive pressure from the catheter. A stopcock on the transducer then is turned to expose the transducer diaphragm to atmospheric pressure. The bedside equipment should indicate zero pressure on the oscilloscope and digital display. If positive or negative pressure is detected and displayed, the zero function on the equipment should be activated to provide the equipment with a zero pressure reference point. This procedure should be performed regularly and any time pressure measures are questionable to ensure that measured pressures are accurate. Transducer drift may occur over time and simply indicates that there is a deviation from the established zero pressure point that requires reestablishment of this neutral pressure.

Calibration of the System

Some equipment manufacturers provide a means to evaluate the equipment electronics or calibrate the equipment. Most manufacturers permit selection of a specific pressure called the sensitivity, which should be similar to that pressure being monitored (i.e., 200 mm Hg for arterial pressure). Calibration requires that the clinician trigger a mechanism, usually a button on the equipment that provides the amplifier with an electronic signal identical to a pressure signal from the transducer. Examination of the oscilloscope and digital value displayed should be equivalent to the selected pressure.

Transducers are manufacturer calibrated, industry tested, and standardized and do not require clinician calibration. Should there be any question about the validity and reliability of the pressure measures, the transducer should be replaced. The prior practice of mercury calibration of transducers is no longer considered a necessary, safe, or effective means of ensuring accuracy of pressure measures.

Troubleshooting the System

Fluid-filled monitoring systems are complex and require vigilant attention to ensure that the information obtained is accurate and clinically useful. Hemodynamic data must always be evaluated in conjunction with other data, in particular, physical assessment before the institution or alteration of an intervention such as drug therapy. Numerous errors or problems can occur that reduce the accuracy and reliability of pressure measurements (Table 50-2). Thus, hemodynamic monitoring requires an educated, technically sophisticated clinician to ensure that the data are usable. Once the fluid-filled system is prepared correctly, leveled appropriately, and zeroed and has optimal damping and the electronics have been evaluated, monitoring of hemodynamic pressures may begin.

Central Venous Pressure Monitoring

Although central venous pressure initially was measured in military trauma patients in World War II, the clinical utility of this technique was not well understood and commonly practiced until the 1960s and 1970s with development of the pulmonary artery catheter and the advent of critical care units.[17-19] Central venous pressure measurement provides a direct measure of the pressure in the large thoracic veins. The underlying assumptions of this measurement are that central venous pressure is equivalent to right ventricular pressures and that changes in venous pressure are directly equivalent to changes in right ventricular end-diastolic volume and pressure. However, a number of investigators have found poor correlation between central venous pressure and adequacy of ventricular volumes in normal individuals[20] and in heterogeneous patient populations.[21-24]

An integral relationship exists between central venous pressure and cardiac output. Central venous pressure often is used as a measure of preload of the heart,

■ ■ ■

TABLE 50-2   TROUBLESHOOTING FLUID-FILLED PRESSURE MONITORING SYSTEMS

COMMON PROBLEMS	POTENTIAL SOLUTION
Absence of a pressure waveform	Re-zero system, recalibrate equipment.
	Ensure that selected pressure range on equipment is appropriate.
	Tighten all connections in the system.
	Ensure that all stopcocks are turned appropriately.
	Evaluate catheter patency (aspirate to evaluate blood return).
	Make sure all air has been removed.
Overdamped waveform	Remove all air bubbles from system.
	Evaluate catheter and tubing patency (aspirate catheter, inspect tubing for presence of blood/thrombus or kinks).
	Flush catheter once blood/thrombus has been removed to prevent emboli.
	Replace long pieces of tubing with sh orter ones.
	Catheter may require repositioning (tip against vessel wall).
Inaccurate values: too high or too low	Re-zero and recalibrate.
	Evaluate transducer for correct level with phlebostatic axis.
	Ensure that all connections are secure and stopcocks are turned appropriately.
	Evaluate square wave test to ensure optimally damped system.
Flush system inoperable	Evaluate patency of the catheter (aspirate).
	Ensure that pressure device is transmitting 300 mm Hg pressure to the device.
	Ensure that all stopcocks are turned appropriately.
	Catheter may require repositioning (tip against vessel wall).
Waveform artifact	Secure catheter to prevent excessive movement.
	Evaluate patient for need for analgesia or sedation.
	Evaluate square wave test to ensure optimally damped system.
	Obtain biomedical engineering evaluation for electrical leakage from other equipment.
	Ensure that other equipment is not physically impinging on the system.

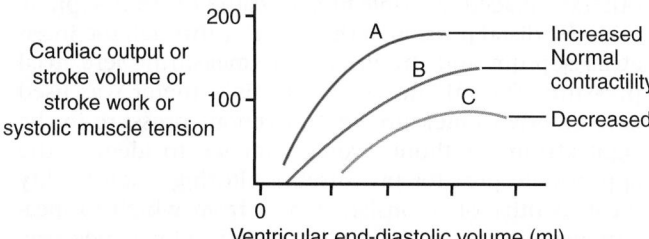

FIGURE 50-9 ▦ Association between end-diastolic volume (sarcomere length) and stroke volume (systolic tension). Frank-Starling law of the heart. (From McCance K, Huether S: *Pathophysiology: the biologic basis for disease in adults and children,* ed 5, St Louis, 2006, Mosby.)

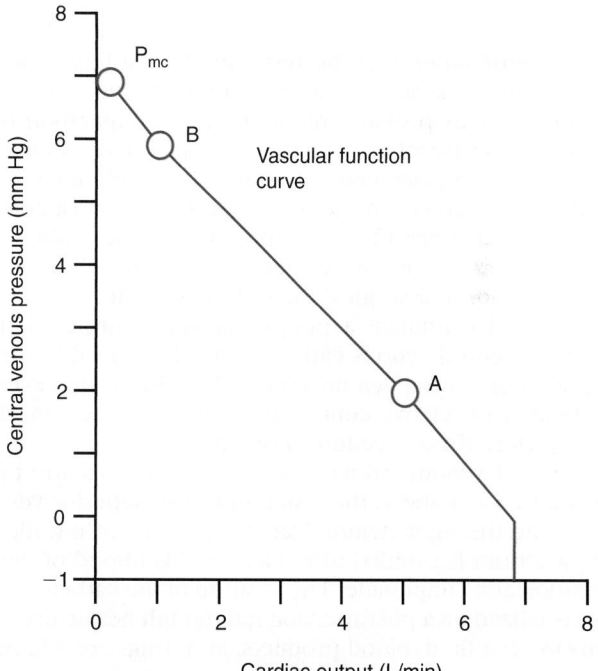

FIGURE 50-10 ▦ Association between cardiac output and central venous pressure. *A,* venous pressure when cardiac output is 1 liter/minute; *B,* venous pressure when cardiac output is 5 liters/minute. P_{mc}, circulatory pressure. (From Berne R, Levy M: *Cardiovascular physiology,* ed 8, St Louis, 2001, Mosby.)

the stretch of the ventricle at end-diastole. Cardiac output directly depends on preload as described by the Frank-Starling relationship. Accordingly, as preload increases, cardiac output increases because of an augmentation in contractility in response to greater myocardial fiber stretch (Figure 50-9). However, because of specific vascular characteristics, central venous pressure also depends on cardiac output in an inverse fashion (Figure 50-10). This relationship may be described by a vascular function curve, so as cardiac output decreases, central venous pressure increases. The specific vascular characteristics that influence this relationship include vascular resistance and compliance and the volume of blood in the vessels. Thus, central venous pressure measurements are a global index of complex cardiovascular relationships and should be used along with other data for optimal decision making.

Placement of a Central Venous Catheter

Central venous catheters typically are placed at the bedside for a variety of indications (Box 50-2). Catheters may be single lumen or multilumen; selection depends on the indications for placement. For example, rapid

BOX 50-2
INDICATIONS FOR CENTRAL VENOUS CATHETER PLACEMENT

- Intravenous fluid administration
  - Large-volume resuscitation required
  - Inadequate peripheral venous access
- Intravenous medication administration
  - Vasoactive medications
  - Highly irritating or phlebitic medications
- Intravenous nutritional intake
- Hemodynamic monitoring
  - Central venous pressure monitoring
  - Pulmonary artery pressure monitoring
- Therapeutic intervention
  - Hemodialysis
  - Transvenous pacemaker

BOX 50-3
CENTRAL VENOUS CATHETER PLACEMENT SITES

Central Placement
- Internal jugular vein
- Subclavian vein
- Femoral vein
- Axillary vein

Peripheral Placement
- Cephalic vein
- Basilic vein
- External jugular vein

BOX 50-4
CONTRAINDICATIONS TO PLACEMENT OF CENTRAL VENOUS CATHETER

- Alteration in coagulation
  - Thrombolytic or anticoagulant therapy
  - Serious thrombocytopenia
  - Other significant coagulopathies
- Infection or loss of protective integument
  - Infection at or near site of planned placement
  - High potential for infection near site of planned placement (tracheostomy)
  - Burn trauma at site of planned placement
- Inability to locate landmarks
  - Obesity
  - Trauma
- Questionable vascular patency
  - Thrombosis
  - Vena caval filter placed (femoral insertion)
  - Trauma
- High potential for pneumothorax
  - Administration of high levels of positive end-expiratory pressure or continuous positive airway pressure
  - Obstructive lung disease
- Other difficulties
  - Combative, uncooperative patient
  - Lack of skill in placement

fluid resuscitation may be performed via a large-bore, single-lumen catheter, whereas a patient who requires central venous pressure monitoring, administration of continuous vasoactive drug therapy and blood products likely requires placement of a multilumen catheter. Central venous catheter placement is performed most commonly using a percutaneous approach by the Seldinger technique or the use of a catheter over the needle. Much less commonly, a surgical incision may be necessary to locate and cannulate a peripheral vein (surgical cutdown). Central venous catheters may be placed by peripheral or central venous access (Box 50-3). However, a number of relative contraindications must be considered before this procedure (Box 50-4).

Central venous catheters are placed so that the tip lies 2 to 5 cm above the junction of the superior vena cava and the right atrium. Placement in the thin-walled right atrium is avoided to reduce the likelihood of perforation and tamponade. The location of the catheter tip is visualized on a postinsertion radiograph before use to ensure that fluid, blood products, and drugs are administered intravenously and that pressure measurements are made appropriately. The catheter is connected to a fluid-filled monitoring system for continuous evaluation of venous pressure. No current, evidence-based recommendation is available about the appropriate lumen for hemodynamic monitoring for those patients with a multilumen catheter. Scott and others[25] found significant differences in the venous pressure measures obtained from the three ports. Blot and Laplanche[26] used only the distal port of triple-lumen catheters to measure central venous pressure in their study of the utility of implanted

ports and tunneled single- and multilumen catheters for measurement of central venous pressure. Ceyran and others[27] placed a triple-lumen catheter transseptally with the distal portion of the catheter through the interatrial septum and the distal port measuring left atrial pressure. The middle lumen of this catheter was used consistently to measure central venous pressure in the right atrium. Without strong evidence to identify the appropriate port for pressure monitoring, each facility must identify one consistent port from which to measure venous pressure to ensure consistency in measurement, and this information should be communicated clearly.

Central Venous Pressure Measurement

The central venous pressure waveform contains three separate waves (Figure 50-11).[28,29] The *a* wave is a small increase in pressure produced by atrial systole; the pressure decline of the *a* wave is termed the *x* descent. The *a* wave is usually the dominant wave and follows the P wave on the electrocardiogram by approximately 80 to 100 msec. The *a* wave is followed by the *c* wave, an increase in pressure produced by the closure of the tricuspid valve just before ventricular systole. The peak of the *c* wave occurs as the pulmonic valve opens to permit ventricular ejection. The *c* wave immediately follows the QRS complex on the electrocardiogram. The *a* and *c* waves occur at a time interval identical to the PR interval on the electrocardiogram. The *v* wave is produced by ventricular systole. Although the tricuspid valve is closed, ventricular systole produces a bulging of the tricuspid valve toward the atrium and produces a small pressure wave. The decline of the *v* wave, the *y* descent, occurs when the tricuspid valve opens and ventricular filling begins. The peak of the *v* wave occurs during the T wave on the electrocardiogram.

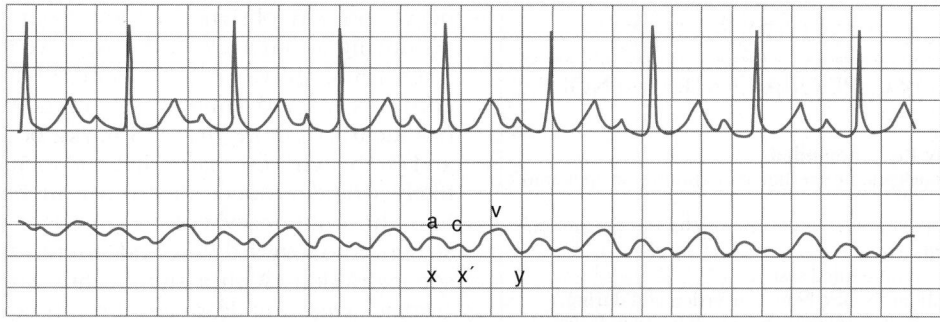

FIGURE 50-11 ▒ Morphology of central venous pressure waveform. *a, c, x, xi, v, y,* (From DeVault AO: *Pocket guide to critical care monitoring,* ed 2, St Louis, 1996, Mosby.)

Central venous pressure is the average pressure in the venous system and normally ranges from 2 to 8 mm Hg in the adult. The central venous pressure measurement is the mean of the *a* wave. Ideally, the central venous waveform is documented simultaneously with the electrocardiogram to enable the clinician to identify the low-amplitude *a, c,* and *v* waves. The ventilatory cycle produces significant alterations in venous pressure. Normal inspiration lowers central venous pressure by 2 to 3 mm Hg, thus the measurement is taken at end-expiration to reduce this influence and obtain an accurate measure of pressure (Figure 50-12). Low central venous pressure measures suggest hypovolemia, whereas elevations in central venous pressure measures suggest hypervolemia or ventricular dysfunction.

Complications of Central Venous Pressure Monitoring

Complications that may occur with placement of a central venous catheter include pneumothorax, nosocomial infection, cardiac dysrhythmias, vascular erosion or perforation and hemorrhage, and venous air embolus. Pneumothorax may occur in 0.5 to 6 percent of patients and may be related to the degree of experience and expertise of the clinician.[30] Catheter placement in the subclavian and internal jugular veins using a percutaneous technique, particularly in the patient with high levels of positive end-expiratory pressure (**PEEP**), may increase the likelihood of pneumothorax.

Nosocomial infection is a serious complication of central venous catheterization. Bacteria may enter the vascular system along the outside of the catheter from the overlying skin, although entry through the catheter lumen via stopcocks and ports is also possible. Bacteria adhere to the catheter and multiply or colonize the catheter and may be the source for systemic infection. Evidence-based guidelines for the prevention of intravascular catheter-related infections should be adopted and used to reduce the likelihood of catheter-related infection. (See the evidence-based practice feature Guidelines for Care of a Central Venous Catheter.)[31]

Central venous catheters may migrate into the right atrium or right ventricle, which can produce cardiac dysrhythmias. Should the catheter tip float freely in the ventricle, a change in patient position or alteration in

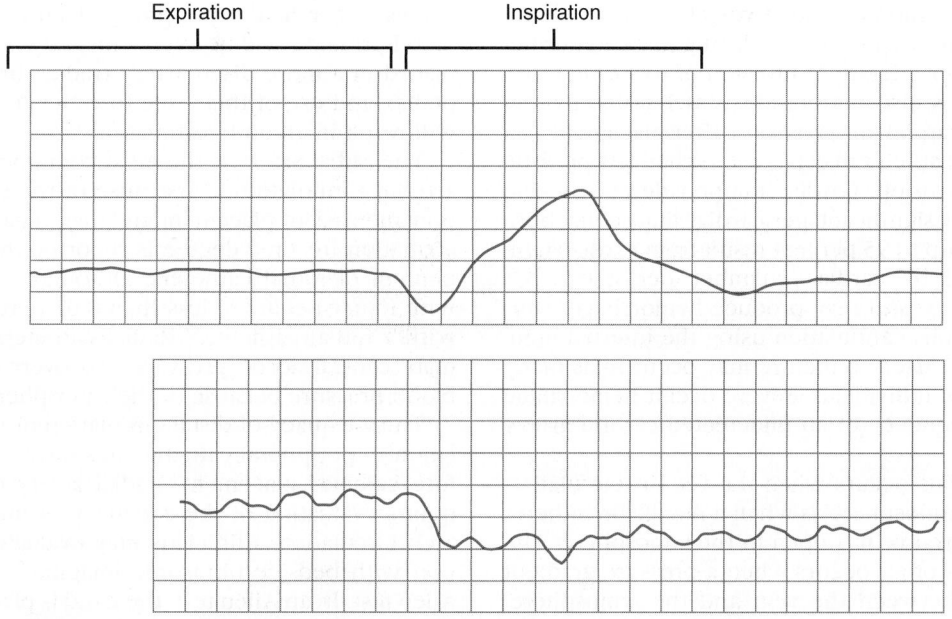

FIGURE 50-12 ▒ Effect of spontaneous ventilation on central venous pressure waveform. (From DeVault AO: *Pocket guide to critical care monitoring,* ed 2, St Louis, 1996, Mosby.)

intrathoracic pressure (as from coughing) may produce irritation of the endocardial wall of the ventricle. Premature ventricular contractions and ventricular tachycardia are the most common results. Withdrawal of the catheter to the appropriate position will obliterate these rhythm disturbances.

Perforation of thoracic blood vessels or heart chambers of the right side may occur during insertion or because of catheter migration. Infusion of irritating intravenous solutions also may erode vessel walls. A new pleural or pericardial effusion soon after placement of a central venous catheter may be due to chamber perforation or vessel erosion. Cardiac tamponade may be the consequence of significant pericardial fluid collection. Mortality rates up to 95 percent result from cardiac tamponade caused by cardiac chamber perforation.[32,33] Perforation of a vessel may produce hemorrhage. During central venous cannulation using the internal jugular vein, carotid artery puncture may occur in as many as 10 percent of individuals. Severe occult hemorrhage can be a consequence of an undetected carotid artery puncture.

An air embolus occurs when the venous circulation is open to the atmosphere as when a needle or catheter placed in a central vein is open to the atmosphere. The entry of a bolus of air occurs when a pressure gradient is established between the vein and the atmosphere. Gas follows this pressure gradient and enters the circulation. The bolus of air moves into the right side of the heart and may obstruct outflow from the ventricle by producing an air lock in the right ventricular outflow tract. Although the exact volume of air that produces clinical signs and symptoms is unknown, animal study has identified more than 1.8 ml/kg body mass as fatal, and Orebaugh[34] estimates that 300 to 500 ml in an adult likely would produce death. An air bolus that moves into the pulmonary vessels produces mechanical obstruction to forward flow and stimulates pulmonary vasoconstriction. With a significantly large air embolus, cardiac arrest and death are the consequence.

Arterial Pressure Monitoring

Continuous arterial pressure monitoring commonly is used in the management of critically ill patients. This type of hemodynamic monitoring is capable of providing a continuous measure of systolic, diastolic, and mean arterial pressure in those patients who are hemodynamically unstable, those who have a high likelihood of serious complication (e.g., postoperative cardiovascular surgery or trauma), and those who require this type of monitoring for intervention (e.g., vasoactive medication administration or intraaortic balloon counterpulsation). Placement of an arterial catheter is also useful when serial arterial blood gas measures are required for patient management.

Placement of an Arterial Catheter

Arterial catheter placement site is selected after consideration of the indication for placement, evaluation of global patient condition, determination of length of time monitoring may be required, and review of the advantages and disadvantages of potential sites (Table 50-3). Clinicians also must consider that there are significant physiological changes that occur as the pressure wave moves from the aorta to the peripheral arteries.[35] The wave narrows, the size of the dicrotic notch decreases, systolic pressure increases, and the pulse pressure becomes wider in the periphery (Figure 50-13). Systolic blood pressure will be overestimated when a catheter is placed in a more distal artery (radial, brachial, dorsalis pedis), and use of this value to estimate aortic pressure will result in an underestimation.[36,37]

The radial artery is the most commonly used site for arterial cannulation[37,38] because of the superficial location and ease of placement and maintenance. Thrombus formation to some degree is reported in as many as 75 percent of radial catheters, although serious ischemia with injury occurs in less than 0.01 percent of patients with a radial catheter.[38] Radial catheters do underestimate central aortic pressure and overestimate systolic blood pressure because of their peripheral location.[36,37]

The adequacy of distal circulation or collateral circulation in peripheral catheter sites must be evaluated before catheter placement. Radial artery cannulation requires evaluation of the adequacy of ulnar and palmar arch circulation. Clinicians may evaluate ulnar circulation with bedside ultrasonic imaging or the use of an Allen test. In an Allen test, the hand is placed in a neutral position, and the clinician compresses the radial and ulnar arteries simultaneously. The hand and fingers blanch

■ ■ ■

TABLE 50-3   ADVANTAGES AND DISADVANTAGES OF ARTERIAL CATHETER PLACEMENT SITES

SITES	ADVANTAGES	DISADVANTAGES
Radial	Visible and accessible Readily immobilized Easily cannulated by percutaneous technique Immobilization not uncomfortable for patient	Maximum catheter size restricted (20 gauge or less) Thrombus formation and occlusion more likely Neurovascular injury possible with subsequent permanent disability Frequency response may be altered by catheter size
Brachial	Visible and accessible Easily cannulated by percutaneous technique Able to use larger size of catheter Frequency response improved	Difficult to immobilize Uncomfortable for patient Neurovascular injury possible with subsequent permanent disability
Axillary	Most accurate representation of aortic pressure Able to use larger size of catheter Sufficient collateral blood flow	Catheter insertion technically difficult Immobilization difficult and uncomfortable Serious occult hemorrhage possible Brachial neurovascular sheath injury possible with subsequent permanent disability
Femoral	Visible and accessible Easily cannulated by percutaneous technique Able to use larger size of catheter Frequency response improved	Immobilization difficult and uncomfortable Serious occult hemorrhage possible Embolus of atherosclerotic plaque possible during insertion Peritoneal perforation possible
Dorsalis pedis	Visible and accessible	Immobilization difficult and uncomfortable Poorest reflection of aortic pressure Small maximum catheter diameter Thrombus formation and occlusion likely Inaccurate reflection of mean arterial pressure

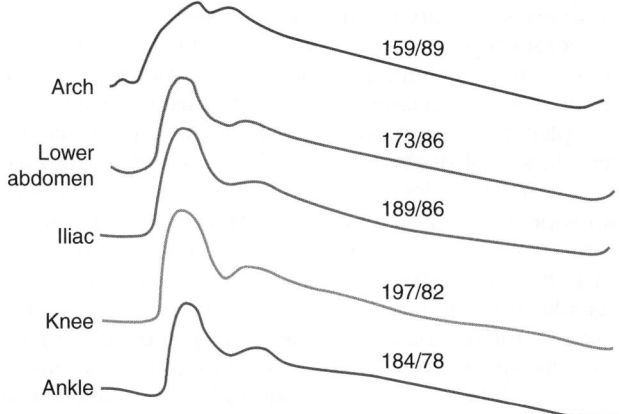

FIGURE 50-13 ■ Change in arterial waveform morphology at various anatomical sites. (From Berne R, Levy M: *Cardiovascular physiology,* ed 8, St Louis, 2001, Mosby.)

from reduced arterial flow. The clinician releases pressure on the ulnar artery; normal color should return within 7 seconds if ulnar flow is adequate. Inadequate ulnar flow is indicated by sluggish return of hand color (more than 14 seconds). A number of investigators question the predictive value of this test.[39,40] Clark and others[41] found that 14 percent of patients evaluated had a false-positive Allen test that indicated adequate collateral circulation when flow was actually inadequate as determined by ultrasound. Ultrasound evaluation should always be used when Allen test results are equivocal.

Following local anesthesia and skin preparation, arterial catheters typically are placed percutaneously using sterile technique and a catheter over the needle. Once placed in the vessel and connected to the fluid-filled system, the catheter should be sutured to reduce catheter movement and decrease the likelihood of accidental removal. Following placement of a sterile dressing,

the insertion site should be secured to prevent catheter movement in the vessel with subsequent damage to the intimal lining, to reduce the likelihood of catheter kinks developing, and to prevent accidental displacement of the catheter. Thus, joints near a catheter insertion site must be placed in a neutral position and secured.

Arterial Pressure Measurement

The morphology or shape of the arterial waveform depends on the velocity of ventricular ejection, the force generated by the ventricle, the stroke volume, arterial compliance, and the rate of forward runoff of arterial blood. Blood vessel resistance primarily determines runoff of blood. Each arterial wave consists of four sections: the anacrotic element, the peak systolic element, the dicrotic notch, and the diastolic element (Figure 50-14).

The anacrotic portion of the arterial waveform occurs when the aortic valve opens and the ventricle

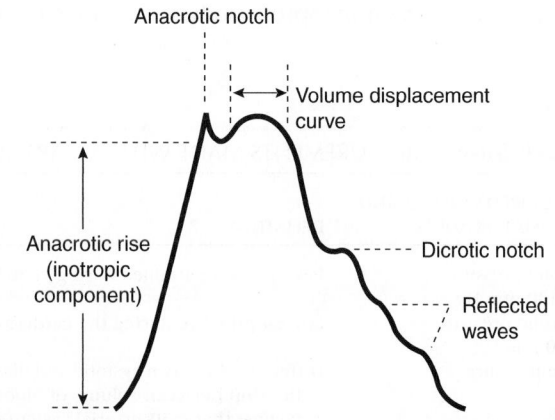

FIGURE 50-14 ■ Morphology of an arterial waveform. (From Darovic G: *Handbook of hemodynamic monitoring,* ed 2, St Louis, 2004, Saunders.)

ejects blood into the arterial tree. Ejection occurs at a rate that exceeds forward runoff of blood, and only 20 to 30 percent of ejected blood moves forward at this point. Up to 70 percent of ejected blood distends the aorta and large arteries. A sharp rise in arterial pressure occurs, and the rate of rise in pressure ($\delta P/\delta T$) may be used as an indication of ventricular contractility. The peak systolic element follows the anacrotic portion of the wave. As ventricular ejection slows, arterial pressure attains a maximum value, the peak systolic pressure. This pressure occurs when the ventricular ejection rate is equivalent to the forward runoff of blood. The period of equality between ejection and runoff is transient. Once forward runoff exceeds the ejection rate, pressure declines. The dicrotic notch is located on the descending portion of the waveform. This small indentation is produced by closure of the aortic valve. As the compliant aorta recoils, a majority of blood moves forward; however, a small portion of blood flows backward toward the aortic valve. Valve closure prevents further backflow and generates a small secondary rise in pressure, which forms the dicrotic notch. As blood continues to move forward because of elastic recoil of arterial walls, pressure continues to decline until it reaches the nadir point or the diastolic element. A number of hemodynamic values may be measured from an arterial catheter. These values include systolic and diastolic pressures, pulse pressure, and mean arterial pressure (Table 50-4).

Complications of Arterial Pressure Monitoring

Arterial catheters are used frequently in critical care settings and are the second most common vascular catheter placed (most common is intravenous).[38] Although placement of an arterial catheter provides important information and ease of blood sampling, it is not without the potential for serious complications. Complications include hemorrhage, infection, and vascular insufficiency to tissue distal to the catheter or the skin over the catheter.

Hemorrhage into surrounding tissues may occur if the needle used during catheter placement punctures the posterior wall of the vessel or if the catheter becomes displaced after insertion. Hemorrhage also occurs if the fluid-filled system becomes disconnected or a stopcock is turned inappropriately. Alterations in coagulation (e.g., from coagulopathy, thrombolytic, or anticoagulation medication administration) increase the likelihood of hemorrhage. Because a majority of arterial catheters are placed in the radial artery, good visualization of the insertion site is possible. Hematoma formation may compress nerves and vessels, obliterate blood flow to distal tissue, and alter nerve function if not recognized and managed (compartment syndrome). Catheters placed in the axillary and femoral sites are more difficult to visualize, and occult bleeding may occur without overt evidence. For example, hemorrhage of 1 to 1.5 liters from the femoral site can collect in the retroperitoneal space before clinical signs are obvious to the clinician.[38]

Bacteria may invade the arterial system from the skin by migration along the outer surface of the catheter or by migration along the inner surface from the fluid-filled system. The most common source of intraluminal bacterial invasion appears to be the catheter hub.[42] The likelihood that bacterial colonization of an arterial catheter will occur is associated with the length of time the catheter is in place and the number of entries into the system.[38] Evidence-based guidelines are available to guide the clinician in the care and maintenance of arterial catheters. (See the evidence-based practice feature Guidelines for Care of an Arterial Catheter.)

Factors reported to increase thrombotic risk include larger catheter lumen, hypotension, use of a small-lumen vessel, necessity for multiple arterial sticks before placement, duration of catheter placement, female gender, site of placement, and the concurrent administration of vasoactive medications (vasopressors, positive inotropes).[30,35] Catheters that completely fill the lumen of the vessel obstruct forward blood flow. The result is stasis of blood with potential thrombus formation and vascular obstruction. Puncture of the vessel stimulates homeostatic mechanisms designed to protect the organism. Vasospasm and vessel constriction intend to reduce bleeding. The release of endothelial cytokines and those produced and released by platelets intend to prevent bleeding and initiate the healing process. Some degree of thrombosis is reported in as many as 75 percent of radial artery catheters; however, less than 0.01 percent of patients experience serious ischemic injury.[38] The prevalence of radial artery thrombus formation is described as greater in women because of the

■ ■ ■

TABLE 50-4 MEASUREMENTS MADE WITH AN ARTERIAL CATHETER

MEASURED VARIABLE AND NORMS FOR ADULTS	DEFINITION	MEANING OF ALTERATIONS
Systolic pressure 100-130 mm Hg	Peak pressure attained during ventricular ejection	A change in stroke volume, ejection velocity, or arterial compliance
Diastolic pressure 60-90 mm Hg	Lowest pressure during the cardiac cycle	Change in vascular tone or resistance to flow; aortic valve dysfunction
Pulse pressure	Difference between systolic and diastolic pressure; reflects the relationship between volume of blood ejected into arterial system and volume that exits arterial system simultaneously	Change in stroke volume or vascular resistance
Mean arterial pressure 70-105 mm Hg	Average driving pressure of the blood during the cardiac cycle; relatively constant value regardless of measurement site	Alterations in tissue perfusion

smaller intraluminal dimension of their vessels. A low incidence of thrombus formation occurs in catheters placed in the femoral artery because of the large vessel lumen and the greater velocity of blood flow. Small arterial branches that supply the skin over the catheter insertion site may become obstructed with thrombus or embolus and produce necrosis of the overlying skin. This is more common with radial artery catheters because of the superficial location. Rapid flush of catheters with thrombus may generate emboli that obstruct flow distal to the catheter. In extreme instances, inadequate blood flow to the distal extremity can result in loss of the extremity.

Pulmonary Artery Pressure Monitoring

Pulmonary artery catheterization, first performed in the 1940s, was used exclusively for diagnostic purposes in the cardiac catheterization laboratory until the 1970s.[43] The flow-directed pulmonary artery catheter[19] developed for bedside insertion was adopted rapidly with the assumption that the use of hemodynamic information derived from this catheter would improve patient outcome. Randomized clinical trials were not conducted to evaluate this assumption. In 1976, when the Federal Food, Drug, and Cosmetic Act was amended to require the Food and Drug Administration to ensure the safety and effectiveness of medical devices, the pulmonary artery catheter was not required to undergo testing because clinicians were convinced of its significant benefit.[44]

The safety and utility of pulmonary artery catheters came into question in the late 1980s and early 1990s when investigators reported higher mortality in patients with acute myocardial infarction who received a pulmonary artery catheter.[45,46] These findings were discounted because of study design and the admonition that those patients who received a catheter were sicker and thus would be expected to have a higher mortality rate.[47] In 1996, Connors and others[48] reported increased mortality in a large sample ($n = 5735$) of critically ill medical-surgical patients in a case-matched, multisite study, and this publication initiated the expression of serious concern from clinicians and the general public. In response, the National Heart, Lung, and Blood Institute and the Food and Drug Administration held the Pulmonary Artery Catheterization and Clinical Outcomes Workshop in 1997.[44] This group of experts recommended the development and dissemination of a standardized educational program and randomized clinical trials to evaluate mortality in particular in specific patient populations that included patients with congestive heart failure, acute respiratory distress syndrome, septic shock, and elective, low-risk surgical coronary revascularization. Several trials are currently in progress,[49,50] and the Pulmonary Artery Catheter Educational Program is currently available for clinicians (*www.pacep.org*).

More recently, Vieillard-Baron and others[51] reported the use of pulmonary artery catheters in patients with acute respiratory distress syndrome. These investigators found no difference in mortality between those who received a catheter and those who did not and suggested that failure to take into account the degree of hemodynamic support influenced the prognostic effect of catheter use. Polanczyk and others[52] found no evidence to support the use of pulmonary artery catheters perioperatively in a group of noncardiac surgery patients. They concluded that use of a pulmonary artery catheter was not associated with improved outcomes in this population and was associated with the occurrence of postoperative congestive heart failure (odds ratio 2.9) and major noncardiac morbidity (odds ratio 2.2). Rhodes and others[53] compared outcomes of critically ill patients managed with a pulmonary artery catheter ($n = 95$) to those who were not ($n = 106$) and found no significant difference in mortality between the groups. However, the group managed with a pulmonary artery catheter did receive significantly more fluids in the first 24 hours after insertion and exhibited a significantly greater incidence of thrombocytopenia and renal failure. Sandham and others[54] reported the results of a randomized clinical trial performed with a group of high-risk surgical patients aged 60 years and older ($n = 1994$). Half of the subjects received goal-directed therapy guided by a pulmonary artery catheter; the other half received standard care. No differences in mortality or median hospital stay was found between the groups, but there was a higher incidence of pulmonary embolus in the catheter group. These investigators concluded that although there was no increase in mortality, there was also no benefit to goal-directed therapy guided by a pulmonary artery catheter in this type of patient.

Other clinical trials are currently under way in specific patient populations to provide more definitive information about the safety and efficacy of the pulmonary artery catheter in specific patient populations.[44,49] The ESCAPE trial investigators[55] found that use of a pulmonary artery catheter did not increase mortality or hospitalizations in New York Heart Association (**NYHA**) Class IV heart failure patients. All subjects in this study reported symptom improvement and greater exercise tolerance; the group whose management was guided by the catheter reported greater improvement in the value of their daily existence. The use of hemodynamic monitoring with a pulmonary artery catheter was termed *neutral* (without a positive or negative effect), but these results may have been influenced by the variability in the use of hemodynamic information to guide treatment. In their most recent guidelines, the Task Force on Acute Heart Failure of the European Society of Cardiology currently does recommend the use of a pulmonary artery catheter in hemodynamically unstable patients who do not respond predictably to standard treatments and in patients who have simultaneous hypoperfusion and congestion.[56] The American College of Cardiology/American Heart Association guidelines for the care of heart failure patients also recommend use of therapy guided by a pulmonary artery catheter in refractory end-stage heart failure.[57]

Placement of a Pulmonary Artery Catheter

Pulmonary artery catheters commonly are placed through the internal jugular or subclavian vein, although the femoral or brachial site also may be used. An introducer is inserted by modified Seldinger technique to provide access to the central venous circulation. The introducer has a safety seal device and usually a side arm that contains an additional port for fluid and medication administration or measurement of central venous pressure. The safety seal device protects the patient from venous air embolus and permits introduction of the catheter into the central circulation without backflow of blood. Once the introducer is placed and secured, the pulmonary artery catheter may be inserted.

Pulmonary artery catheters are polyvinyl chloride catheters with a small latex balloon located at the distal tip. These are multi-lumen catheters that range in size from 4 to 8 French and in length from 60 to 100 cm. These catheters may be bonded with heparin to reduce

> **BOX 50-5** ▪ ▪ ▪
> ## TYPES OF PULMONARY ARTERY CATHETERS
>
> - Double-lumen catheter
> - Quadruple-lumen thermodilution catheter
> - Five-lumen thermodilution catheter—additional right atrial port
> - Thermodilution ejection fraction catheter—provides measures of right ventricular end-diastolic volume and ejection fraction
> - Position monitoring thermodilution catheter—proximal lumen 10 cm from tip to assist with maintenance of appropriate catheter position
> - Fiberoptic thermodilution catheter—continuous mixed venous oxygen saturation measures
> - Pacemaker thermodilution catheter—contains atrial and ventricular pacing electrodes or provides one or two ports to permit introduction of pacing wires
> - Continuous thermodilution cardiac output catheter
> - Continuous thermodilution cardiac output and ejection fraction catheter

thrombus formation. A number of pulmonary artery catheters are commercially available, and many have sophisticated features that provide additional information about patient condition (Box 50-5). The quadruple-lumen catheter is the most commonly used pulmonary artery catheter (Figure 50-15).

The quadruple-lumen catheter consists of a distal lumen that opens at the catheter tip and, once correctly placed, that monitors pulmonary artery pressure. The proximal lumen (30 cm from tip) opens into the right atrium and may be used for pressure measurement, fluid administration, and administration of injectate volume for cardiac output measurement. When cardiac output measures are not required, this lumen may be used for vasoactive drug administration. The thermistor lumen contains a wire that terminates in a small temperature-sensitive bead located approximately 5 cm from the distal end of the catheter. This thermistor provides a constant measure of blood temperature when interfaced with a cardiac output computer, which is necessary for determination of thermodilution cardiac output. The balloon lumen permits inflation of the balloon to assist with placement of the catheter and for intermit-

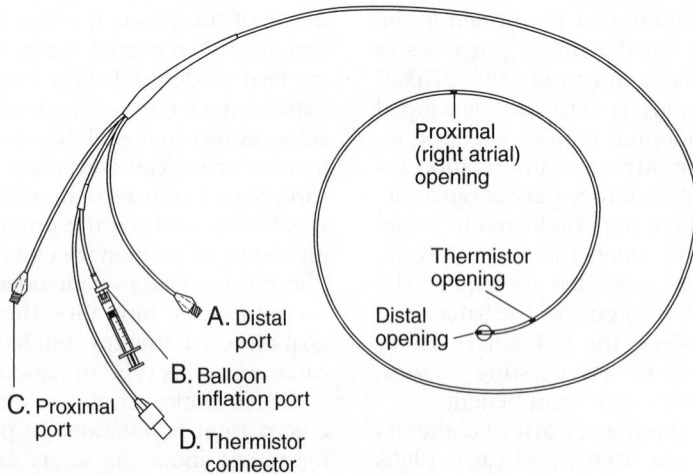

FIGURE 50-15 ▪ Components of a quadruple-lumen pulmonary artery catheter. (From Darovic G: *Handbook of hemodynamic monitoring,* ed 2, St Louis, 2004, Saunders.)

tent measurement of occlusion pressure. Balloon integrity must be evaluated before catheter insertion by submerging the distal catheter in sterile solution, inflating the balloon to the recommended volume and observing for the escape of small air bubbles. Once balloon integrity is confirmed, the balloon should be deflated passively to prevent damage to the latex balloon that would result in subsequent rupture.

Before insertion, the distal lumen of the selected catheter is flushed with solution and connected securely to a prepared fluid-filled monitoring system (leveled, zero referenced, calibrated) so that pressure waveforms may be evaluated during insertion. The proximal lumen also is flushed with solution to prevent entry of air into the central circulation and may be connected to a pressure transducer system to measure central venous pres-

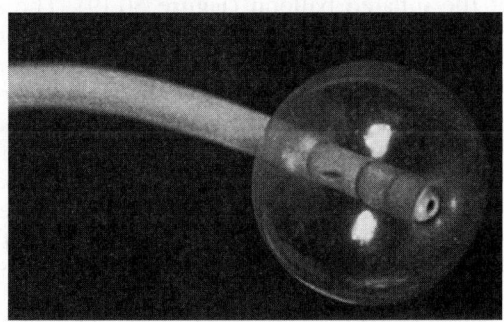

FIGURE 50-16 ■ Pulmonary artery catheter balloon correctly inflated to protect cardiovascular structures. (From Darovic G: *Handbook of hemodynamic monitoring,* ed 2, St Louis, 2004, Saunders.)

sure. Once flushed and connected to the transducer system, the catheter is wiped gently with sterile solution to facilitate catheter movement through the introducer into venous circulation. The catheter also should be placed through a sterile, transparent sleeve to reduce the likelihood of later bacterial contamination.

The pulmonary artery catheter is inserted gently through the safety seal device on the introducer and into the venous circulation. As the distal catheter enters the central venous circulation, the venous pressure waveform becomes visible (*a, c,* and *v* waves). The balloon then is inflated using the recommended volume of air, so the balloon extends over the tip of the catheter to protect vessel intima and cardiac structures during insertion (Figure 50-16). Once the balloon is fully inflated, the catheter is advanced. Blood flow will direct the forward movement of the inflated balloon into the heart (flow-directed capability).

The pressure waveform will change abruptly as the catheter tip moves through the tricuspid valve and into the right ventricle (Figure 50-17). The right ventricular pressure wave consists of a sharp increase in pressure 2 to 3 times greater than the central venous pressure followed by a rapid decrease in pressure. Right ventricular diastolic pressure is normally equivalent to central venous pressure. As the catheter is carried by forward blood flow through the pulmonic valve and into the pulmonary artery, a dicrotic notch can be visualized on the downslope of the wave, and there is a change in the diastolic pressure caused by pulmonic valve closure. Pulmonary artery peak systolic pressure is usually equivalent to right ventricular peak systolic pressure;

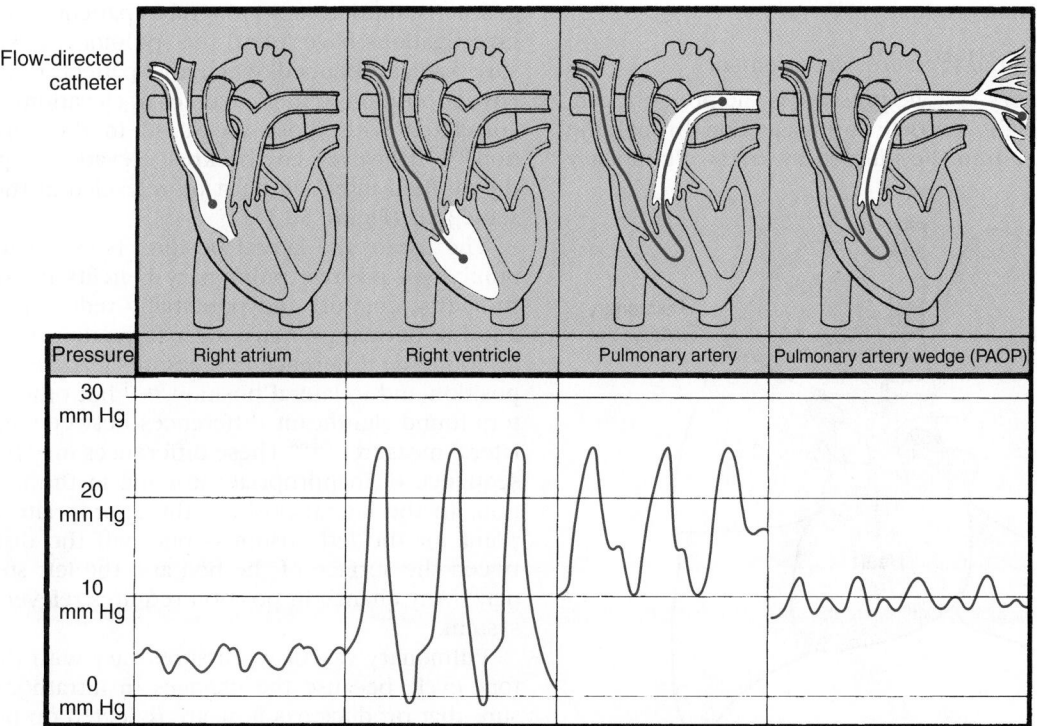

FIGURE 50-17 ■ Location of catheter tip and waveforms obtained during insertion of pulmonary artery catheter. *PAOP,* Pulmonary artery occlusion pressure. (From Urden L, Stacy K, Lough M: *Priorities in critical care nursing,* ed 4, St Louis, 2004, Mosby.)

pulmonary artery diastolic pressure is higher than right ventricular diastolic pressure.

The catheter is carried by the forward blood flow into smaller pulmonary vessels until it reaches a vessel with a diameter smaller than the inflated balloon. In this position with the balloon inflated, the pressure measured at the distal lumen is a reflection of left atrial pressure. The visualized waveform changes abruptly and significantly to a low-amplitude waveform. The *a* and *v* waves may be distinguishable; the *a* wave is generated by left atrial systole and the *v* wave by left atrial filling during ventricular systole. The catheter should not be left in the occlusion or "wedge" position for more than 15 seconds, and the balloon should be passively deflated. Deflation induces a slight withdrawal of the distal catheter tip from the pulmonary branch, and the pulmonary artery waveform should be visualized. Reinflation of the balloon will again carry the catheter tip to the occlusion position.

For valid pulmonary artery pressure measures, the catheter tip should be located in a zone III lung area where pulmonary arterial pressure is greater than venous pressure, which is greater than alveolar pressure (described fully in Chapter 8; Figure 50-18). This type of lung zone is located at or below the level of the left atrium in most individuals.[58] Once the desired catheter position is established, the introducer and sterile transparent sleeve may be connected to maintain catheter sterility. The sleeve ensures that a portion of the catheter remains sterile should manipulation of the catheter be required later. Once secured and dressed, catheter position should be evaluated postinsertion by a lateral chest radiograph to ensure that measured values are accurate. The introducer insertion site is managed similar to a central venous catheter site.

Pulmonary Arterial Pressure Measurement

Pulmonary artery systolic pressure is the pressure generated by the right ventricle during ejection through the pulmonic valve into the pulmonary artery. Pulmonary

vessel resistance and compliance, right ventricular function, and downstream pressure from the left side of the heart influence pulmonary systolic pressure. Diastolic pressure, normally 1 to 4 mm Hg higher than left atrial pressure, often mirrors the occlusion pressure and when closely correlated with the occlusion pressure may be used as an indicator of left ventricular preload when the occlusion value is not available. The mean pulmonary artery pressure is the average driving pressure of blood in pulmonary vessels and is measured by selecting a waveform at end-expiration, bisecting the waveform, and determining the pressure at that point.[59]

The pulmonary artery occlusion pressure, also known as the wedge pressure, provides an estimate of pressures of the left side of the heart. The occlusion position produces a static column of blood on the distal side of the inflated balloon (Figure 50-19). The static column of blood begins at the tip of the catheter and extends through the pulmonary veins to the left atrium. Pressure changes in this static column are measured at the catheter tip. Because the mitral valve is open during diastole, the pressure obtained also is used to estimate left ventricular end-diastolic pressure. A number of technical and pathological conditions influence the relationship between the occlusion pressure and left ventricular end-diastolic pressure and thus the validity of this estimation (Box 50-6).

The supine position is the gold standard for all hemodynamic measures including occlusion pressure. Unfortunately, pain and dyspnea may preclude this position in a number of individuals. Additionally, repositioning each time measures are required would disrupt rest and sleep, induce pain, worsen dyspnea, and increase oxygen consumption in a vulnerable patient. A number of investigations have found that pulmonary artery pressure values obtained when the patient is in a semi-Fowler position (0 to 30 degrees of elevation) are highly correlated with those measured in the supine position.[60-63] However, any backrest elevation requires that the air-fluid interface must be releveled at the phlebostatic axis (Figure 50-5).

The use of the lateral position is associated with a number of positive pulmonary benefits in addition to providing comfort and potentially reducing the likelihood of dermal pressure ulcer formation. Several studies found no difference in measures made in the supine position and in lateral position,[64,65] but other investigators found significant differences between supine and lateral measures.[66-68] These differences may be the consequence of inappropriate leveling in the lateral position. In the lateral position the appropriate reference point for the left atrium is one half the distance between the surface of the bed and the left sternal border.[69] Any change in position requires releveling of the system.

Pulmonary vascular pressures vary with the ventilatory cycle because the changes in intrathoracic pressure that produce gas flow are reflected on pulmonary blood vessels (Figure 50-20). To provide consistency, all pulmonary artery pressures are measured at end-expiration, a point in the ventilatory cycle when intra-

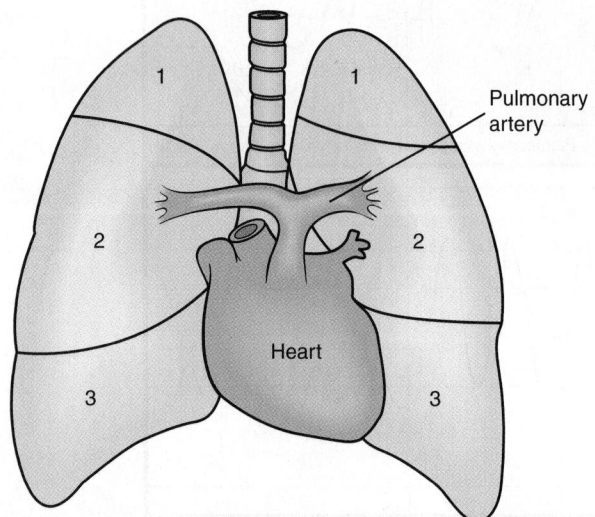

FIGURE 50-18 ■ Approximate location of lung zones in upright adult. (From DeVault AO: *Pocket guide to critical care monitoring,* ed 2, St Louis, 1996, Mosby.)

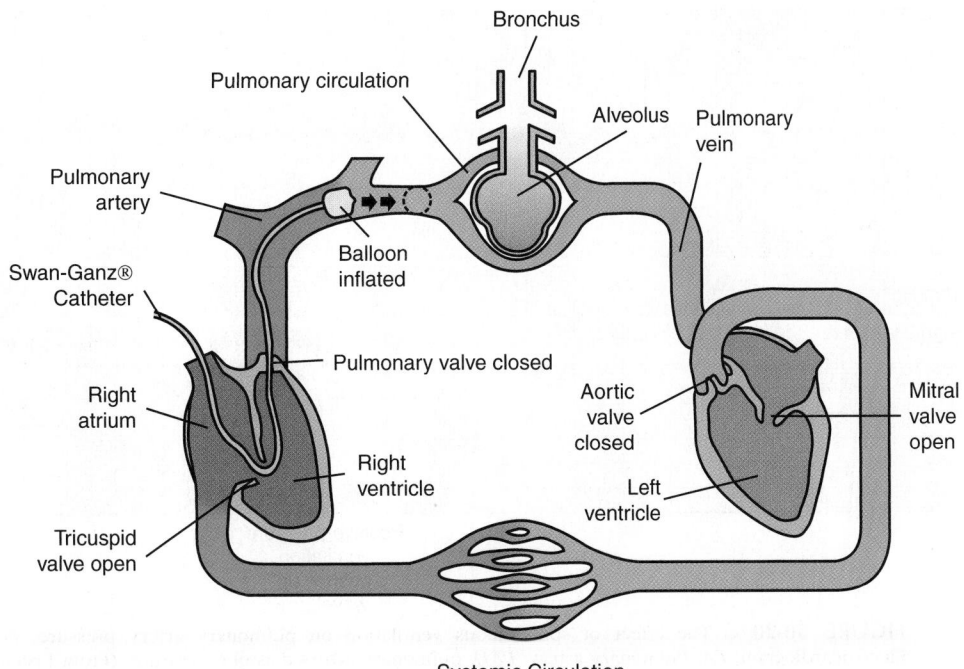

FIGURE 50-19 ■ Measurement of pulmonary artery occlusion pressure. Association between occlusion pressure and left ventricular end-diastolic pressure. (From DeVault AO: *Pocket guide to critical care monitoring,* ed 2, St Louis, 1996, Mosby.)

BOX 50-6   ■ ■ ■

FACTORS THAT INFLUENCE THE CORRELATION BETWEEN PULMONARY ARTERY PRESSURE AND LEFT VENTRICULAR END-DIASTOLIC PRESSURE

Physiological
- Chronic obstructive pulmonary disease
- Hyperdynamic circulation
- Left atrial myxoma
- Left ventricular dysfunction
- Mitral and aortic valve abnormalities
- Pneumonectomy
- Pulmonary venous thrombotic disorders
- Tachycardia

Mechanical/Technical
- Administration of positive end-expiratory pressure greater than 10 cm H_2O
- Catheter fling
- Distal catheter placed in lung zone other than type III

---

thoracic pressure is equal to atmospheric pressure. The presence of significant respiratory variations in pulmonary artery pressure waves requires the clinician use care to determine the end-expiratory point for appropriate, accurate measurement of pressure using a graphic method rather than simply using the values provided on the digital monitor display.

During spontaneous ventilation, the diaphragm contracts, the thoracic cavity enlarges, and intrathoracic pressure decreases to generate a pressure gradient for gas flow into the lungs. During expiration, the diaphragm relaxes, the thoracic cavity decreases in size, and intrathoracic pressure rises, which generates a pressure gradient for gas flow out of the lungs. In a sponta-

neously ventilating individual, pulmonary artery pressures decrease with spontaneous inspiration and increase with expiration. Positive pressure mechanical ventilation produces an increase in pulmonary artery pressure during inspiration followed by a decrease with expiration.

The use of PEEP further complicates the measurement of pulmonary vascular pressures because of its effect on intrathoracic pressure. Lung and chest wall compliance influence the degree of effect that PEEP has on vascular pressures. Reduced lung compliance and increased chest wall compliance result in less transmission of intrathoracic pressure to the pulmonary vessels. PEEP of 10 cm H_2O pressure or less usually has a negligible effect on the relationship between pulmonary pressures and left atrial pressure.[70] Those individuals who receive more than 10 cm H_2O PEEP may realize a significant influence on pulmonary artery pressures (Figure 50-21). Although there are methods used to correct for PEEP, normal lung and chest wall compliance are required for validity, and this may be uncommon in many patients who require ventilation and hemodynamic monitoring.[59] Consistency in the approach to measurement of pulmonary artery pressures is the key to valid and reliable measures. Thus a correction factor must be used consistently, and measurement without correction must consider the use of PEEP.

Complications of Pulmonary Artery Pressure Monitoring

The use of a pulmonary artery catheter may be associated with greater morbidity and mortality, as discussed before. Complications directly related to catheter use are those inherent to placement of a central venous

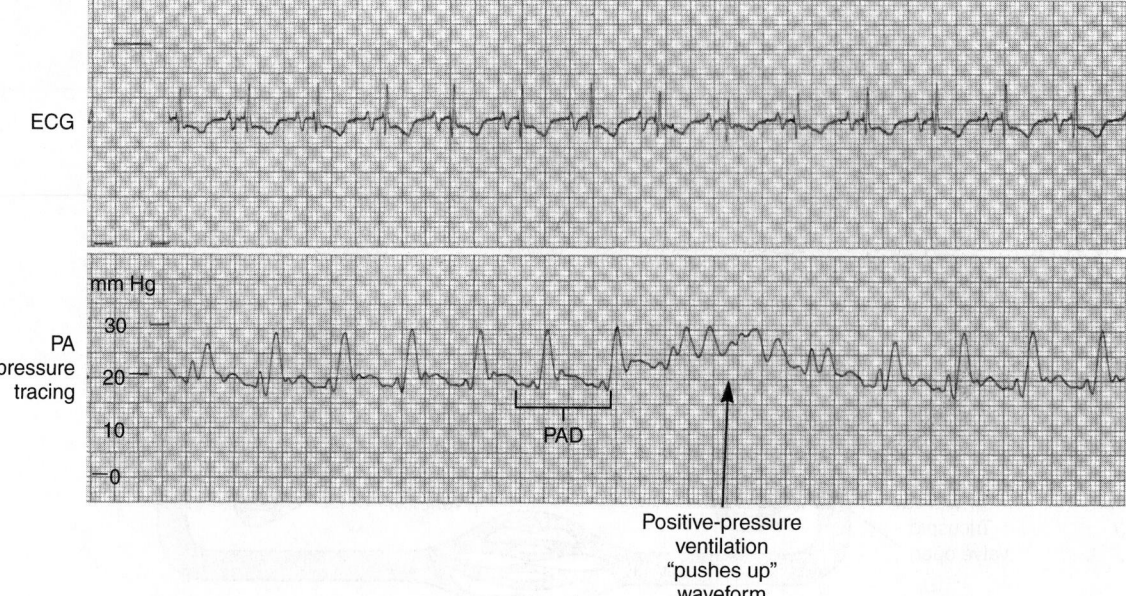

FIGURE 50-20 ■ The effect of spontaneous ventilation on pulmonary artery pressure. *ECG,* Electrocardiogram; *PA,* Pulmonary artery; *PAD,* pulmonary artery diastolic pressure. (From Urden L, Stacy K, Lough M: *Priorities in critical care nursing,* ed 4, St Louis, 2004, Mosby.)

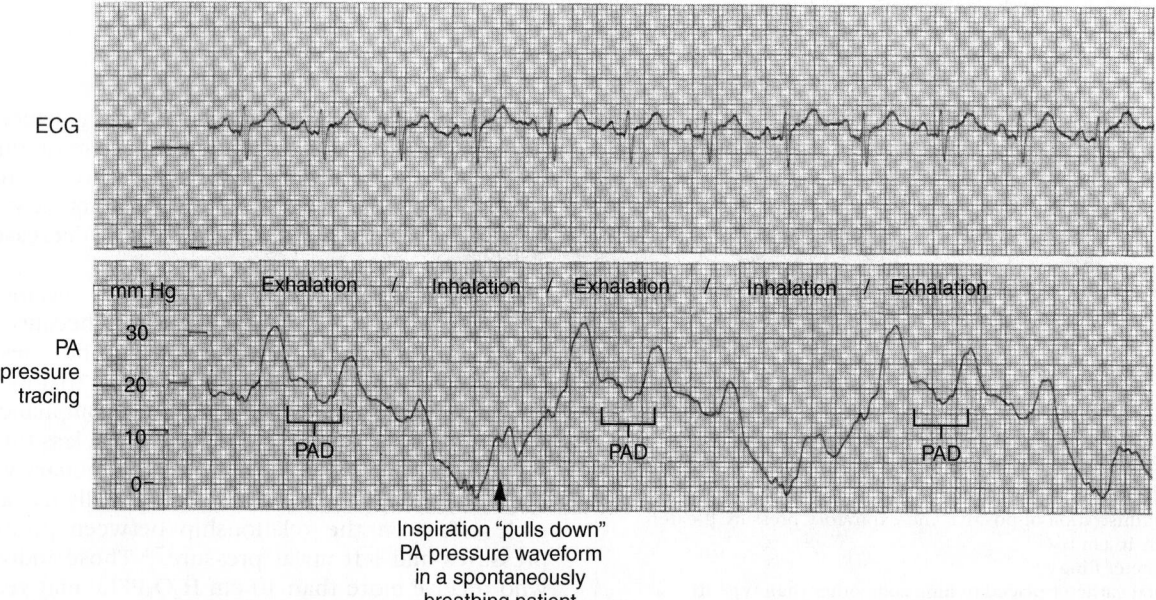

FIGURE 50-21 ■ The effect of positive pressure mechanical ventilation on pulmonary artery pressure. *ECG,* Electrocardiogram; *PA,* Pulmonary artery; *PAD,* pulmonary artery diastolic pressure. (From Urden L, Stacy K, Lough M: *Priorities in critical care nursing,* ed 4, St Louis, 2004, Mosby.)

catheter and include pneumothorax, nosocomial infection, cardiac dysrhythmias, vascular erosion or perforation and hemorrhage, and venous air embolus. Additional complications specific to right-heart catheterization include cardiac dysrhythmias and bundle branch blocks, pulmonary ischemia and/or infarctions, and pulmonary artery rupture.

The most common complication of catheter insertion is cardiac dysrhythmias.[30] Mechanical irritation of the endocardium during insertion and flotation of a pulmonary artery catheter produces ventricular ectopy in as many as 70 percent of patients.[71] Risk factors associated with dysrhythmias include shock of any type, hypoxemia and aci-

dosis, electrolyte imbalances such as hypokalemia, presence of myocardial ischemia, and increased circulating catecholamines. Premature ventricular contractions are typically transient and resolve once the catheter is advanced into the pulmonary artery. Ventricular tachycardia is less common (20 percent of cases) and is usually transient. The occurrence of ectopy during catheter insertion has not been found to be predictive of patient outcome.

The right bundle branch is located superficially inferior to the tricuspid valve, which increases the likelihood of trauma during catheter insertion or edema related to catheter placement. A new right bundle branch block caused by pulmonary artery catheter placement has not been found to be associated with prior cardiac disease and usually resolves within a 24-hour period.[72] A more serious situation occurs in the presence of an existing left bundle branch block. In this instance, complete heart block results, and a ventricular pacemaker may be required.[73]

Pulmonary ischemia or infarction may be caused by thrombus, emboli, or persistent occlusion of a blood vessel. Persistent occlusion of a vessel obstructs blood flow to that region, which may result in ischemia or infarction if the catheter is not repositioned. Additionally, blood distal to the occlusion stagnates, and thrombus formation is more likely. Thrombus formation also may occur at the catheter insertion site or intravascular and intracardiac sites where the catheter contacts the vessel intima or the endocardium and produces irritation or damage that initiates the clotting cascade. Complications resulting from thromboembolism may occur in up to 11 percent of patients.[30]

Pulmonary artery rupture is a serious complication of pulmonary artery catheter placement, with a 70 percent mortality rate.[30] Based on retrospective review, investigators estimate occurrence at 0.125 to 0.034 percent; however, other investigators believe this may be underestimated.[74] Vessel rupture may be produced by inflation of the balloon or perforation of the vessel by the catheter tip. Cardiac surgical patients have a greater risk for pulmonary vessel rupture because of changes in blood flow inherent to the use of extracorporeal circulation, manipulation of the heart, and hypothermia that stiffens the catheter. Newer surgical techniques performed without extracorporeal circulation reduce this risk. Other risk factors include pulmonary hypertension, older age (older than age 60), steroid use, anticoagulant use, and forceful flushing of the catheter.

Cardiac Output Measurement

Cardiac output, the volume of blood ejected by the heart in 1 minute, is the product of the stroke volume and heart rate. Stroke volume, the volume of blood ejected in one beat, is determined by the preload, afterload, and degree of contractility of the myocardium. Cardiac output is influenced by gender, age and body size, body position, and metabolic demand.

Bedside measurement of cardiac output may be performed by invasive or noninvasive techniques. Several techniques use the Fick principle. In 1870, Fick offered the idea that in an organ, the uptake or release of an indicator substance is the product of the arterial-venous concentration of this substance and the blood flow to the organ. Using oxygen as the indicator substance, this may be stated mathematically as follows:

$$CO = VO_2/(CaO_2 - CvO_2)$$

where CO is cardiac output, VO_2 is oxygen consumption, CaO_2 is the arterial concentration of oxygen, and CvO_2 is the venous concentration of oxygen. A number of substances have been used as the indicator, including oxygen, carbon dioxide, indocyanine green dye, and lithium. A number of invasive and noninvasive techniques are used to measure cardiac output, and several use this principle as the basis for the technique.

Thermodilution Cardiac Output

The thermodilution cardiac output technique became widely recognized and clinically accepted with the advent of the thermodilution pulmonary artery catheter in the 1970s. This technique uses blood temperature change as the indicator. The placement of a quadruple-lumen pulmonary artery catheter is necessary for this technique. This catheter contains a thermistor located near the distal tip, which continuously measures pulmonary blood temperature. When this catheter is interfaced with a cardiac output computer, changes in blood temperature are used to calculate cardiac output. Thermodilution measures may be obtained intermittently by bolus technique or continuously.

To measure cardiac output using the bolus technique, solution with a temperature less than blood temperature is injected into the proximal lumen of the pulmonary artery catheter, becomes mixed with blood, and lowers the blood temperature (Figure 50-22). The cooler blood is ejected into the pulmonary artery, and the thermistor located near the distal tip of the pulmonary artery catheter detects the change in blood temperature. This information is transmitted to the computer, and a thermal curve is engineered with the change in blood temperature plotted over time. Cardiac output is determined by analysis of the area under this thermal curve. An inverse relationship exists between the area under the thermal curve and cardiac output, so as cardiac output decreases, the area under the curve increases.

Measures of cardiac output initially used 10 ml of iced or very cold bolus injectate solution, typically 5 percent dextrose in water, to maximize the signal-to-noise ratio. A number of subsequent investigations demonstrated that room temperature injectate solution provided adequate temperature change in most patients.[75-78] Other investigators found that cardiac output measures made with room temperature injectate were not equivalent to those made with iced injectate, particularly in patients with high or low cardiac output.[79,80] Thus, iced injectate should be used in those patients with high or low cardiac output to maximize signal-to-noise ratio and increase precision. Room temperature injectate pro-

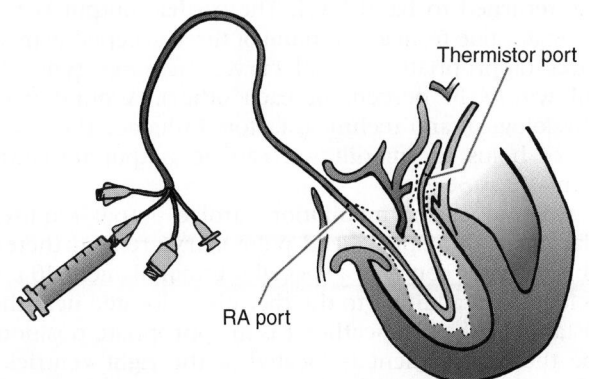

FIGURE 50-22 ■ Location of solution injection for thermodilution cardiac output measurement. *RA,* Right atrial. (From Sole M, Klein D, Moseley M: *Introduction to critical care nursing,* ed 4, St Louis, 2005, Mosby.)

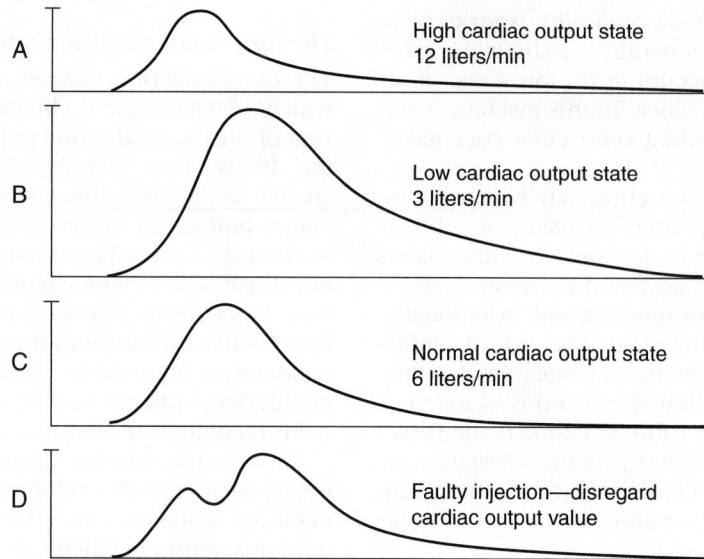

FIGURE 50-23 ■ Thermodilution cardiac output curves. (From Darovic G: *Handbook of hemodynamic monitoring,* ed 2, St Louis, 2004, Saunders.)

duces precise measures for patients with cardiac output in the normal range. The temperature of the injectate should be documented and consistent to ensure valid and reproducible measures. The use of a smaller volume of injectate (5 ml) was not found to produce significantly different measures of cardiac output compared with the 10-ml injection.[81] However, patients with low ejection fraction demonstrated greater variability of measures. The conclusion of these investigators was that the larger volume of solution should be used to maximize the signal-to-noise ratio unless the patient requires fluid restriction.

Solution should be injected in less than 4 seconds at end-expiration to reduce the influence of ventilation on pulmonary blood volume and temperature and to provide consistency across measures. The thermal curve must be inspected to determine the validity of the measure. The curve should have a smooth upstroke followed by a smooth, gradual downstroke (Figure 50-23). Abnormal curves or the presence of artifact indicates the measure should be discarded. Three measures should be made with a minimum of 1 minute between measures to ensure that pulmonary blood temperature has returned to basal level. The cardiac output is the average value from a minimum of three acceptable measures (appropriate thermal curve, measures typically fall within 10 percent of each other). A number of physiological and technical factors influence the validity of bolus thermodilution cardiac output measurements (Box 50-7).

Continuous thermodilution cardiac output requires placement of a specialized pulmonary artery catheter. This catheter contains a special thermal filament 10 cm in length, in addition to the thermistor located near the distal tip. When the catheter is in appropriate position, the thermal filament is located in the right ventricle. When interfaced with the companion cardiac output computer, the thermal filament emits 7.5 W of thermal energy into the surrounding blood, the thermistor detects changes in blood temperature, and the computer

---

BOX 50-7 ■ ■ ■
FACTORS THAT INFLUENCE THE VALIDITY OF BOLUS THERMODILUTION CARDIAC OUTPUT MEASUREMENT

Physiological
- Point in the ventilatory cycle when measure is made
- Presence of cardiac dysrhythmias
- Presence of intracardiac shunt
- Presence of low cardiac output (less than 2.5 liters/min)
- Thrombus formation over thermistor site
- Tricuspid regurgitation
- Rewarming after use of extracorporeal circulation

Technical
- Incorrect information in computer: size and type of catheter, volume and temperature of injectate solution, computation constant
- Incorrect technique for injection of solution
- Position of the pulmonary artery catheter
- Signal-to-noise ratio inadequate because of solution temperature or volume

---

plots thermal curves for calculation of cardiac output. The small amount of thermal energy is not harmful to erythrocytes or to endocardial tissue.

The association between measures made using bolus thermodilution and continuous thermodilution is adequate. Comparisons have been made in patients with low and high cardiac output,[82,83] fever,[84] and dysrhythmias,[85] and the two measures were within 1.5 liters 95 percent of the time.[86] Clinicians and investigators have identified a slow response time for detection of acute hemodynamic alterations[87,88]; the delay, between 5 and 15 minutes, may limit effectiveness.

Right ventricular end-diastolic volume and right ventricular ejection fraction also may be measured using the thermodilution technique. Bolus measures and continuous thermodilution measures may be made; however, each requires placement of specialized pulmonary artery catheters with interface to specialized computers. The measurement of these hemodynamic values appears to be most useful in the management of volume state.[89]

Carbon Dioxide Rebreathing

The carbon dioxide rebreathing technique uses a variation of the Fick equation, the indirect Fick equation, which uses carbon dioxide as the indicator substance. The indirect Fick equation is stated as follows:

$$CO = VCO_2/(CvCO_2 - CaCO_2)$$

where *CO* is the cardiac output, **VCO$_2$** or volumetric **CO$_2$** is the clearance of CO_2, **CvCO$_2$** is the mixed venous oxygen concentration of CO_2, and **CaCO$_2$** is the arterial concentration of CO_2. Volumetric CO_2 is calculated as the difference between CO_2 content in expired and inspired gas as measured by infrared spectography. End-tidal CO_2 is used as the measure of arterial CO_2 and the partial rebreathing technique eliminates the need for measurement of venous CO_2.

For this measurement, an additional volume of dead space (150 ml), a rebreathing circuit, is placed between the endotracheal tube and the ventilator circuit. At regular intervals (~3 minutes), exhaled gas is diverted from the endotracheal tube to the rebreathing circuit, and the patient rebreathes this gas for about 50 seconds. During this time, CO_2 elimination is reduced. Cardiac output is calculated by evaluating the change in CO_2 elimination during normal ventilation and rebreathing. This technique requires that an estimation of the degree of intrapulmonary shunt be added to the measurement to obtain total cardiac output. Estimates may be obtained using information provided about the fraction of inspired oxygen and oxygen saturation from pulse oximetry.

Although the relatively noninvasive nature of the measure is attractive, the reliability and validity of the measure are influenced by a number of factors. With this technique, small errors in measurement of associated variables produce large inaccuracies in cardiac output.[90] Also, the assumed relationships between variables are only valid if the PaCO$_2$ is greater than 30 mm Hg. Any alteration in ventilation pattern can influence this measure significantly. Additionally, the necessity for estimation of volume of intrapulmonary shunting provides opportunity for significant error in calculation.

Some investigators have found good association between partial rebreathing measures of cardiac output and thermodilution measures.[91,92] Others have found little relationship between these measures.[93-95] With the current technology, this method provides a better estimation of cardiac output in stable patients without pulmonary shunt who have controlled ventilation. CO_2 rebreathing has been found to have the best association with thermodilution when used to monitor patients in the operating room.[90-92]

Echocardiography

Echocardiography, a common method of cardiac imaging, is used to evaluate cardiovascular structure and valvular and ventricular function.[96] Cardiac output measurements using echocardiography are based on spatial imaging or Doppler-based methods. With spatial imaging technique, measurements of ventricular size are made at end-systole and end-diastole. Stroke volume is estimated based on this change in area. This technique may be limited by resolution. Two-dimensional echocardiography resolution ranges from 0.3 to 1.5 mm, and one group of investigators found that a 10 percent change in volume produced only a 0.7-mm change in ventricular area.[97] Thus, degree of resolution could produce significant errors in estimation of cardiac output. The use of spatial techniques for estimation of cardiac output has been demonstrated to underestimate cardiac output and stroke volume and have low association with values obtained by thermodilution.[98,99]

Doppler techniques previously used suprasternal and transgastric approaches for assessment of blood flow. Further developments in miniature ultrasonic crystals supported the development of small Doppler probes that are ideal for use in the esophagus. The use of a transesophageal approach provides proximity to the descending aorta.[100] The probe is placed in the esophagus at about the level of the fifth to sixth thoracic vertebrae. Aortic blood flow is measured and cardiac output is estimated using this technique. Calculations are based on the principle that flow in a cylinder (aorta) is the product of the area of the cross section of that cylinder and the velocity of fluid (blood) flow in the cylinder. Because blood flow is pulsatile and there are velocity changes during the cardiac cycle, a velocity time curve is constructed, and a time-integrated velocity is obtained. Stroke volume is the product of the time-integrated blood flow velocity and the cross-sectional area of the aorta. This technique requires the use of a correction factor, for cardiac output is estimated only from blood flow in the descending aorta.

Esophageal doppler estimation of cardiac output has been correlated (r = 0.6 to 0.95) to measures made using Fick and thermodilution methods.[101-103] Clinicians must be aware that this technique assumes that the aorta is cylindrical and aortic flow is laminar, and these assumptions may not hold true in all patients. Aortic geometry is influenced by vessel compliance and pulse pressure; heart rate, red cell volume, and aortic valve structure may produce turbulent blood flow and reduce the validity of estimations.[90] Currently available technologies also vary in the determination of aortic cross section. Some use a nomogram to predict diameter, whereas others use m-mode ultrasound to measure aortic diameter.

Arterial Pulse Contour Analysis

Cardiac output estimates with the arterial pulse contour analysis technique are based on a model that assumes that the contour of the arterial pressure waveform is proportional to stroke volume. Stroke volume is determined mathematically as the integral of pressure change over time from end-diastole to end-systole divided by impedance of the aorta. The pressure waveform used for analysis may arise from a catheter placed in an artery[104] or from a noninvasive finger probe.[105] However, most validation studies were performed with pulse contours obtained from a femoral arterial catheter.[104]

This technique requires calibration before monitoring, and current technology uses transpulmonary thermodilution (PiCCO, Pulsion), transpulmonary lithium dilution (LiDCO, PulseCO), or conventional thermodilution (TNO/BMI, Modelflow) for calibration purposes. Pulse contour analysis provides a continuous, beat-by-beat estimate of cardiac output. When appropriately calibrated, pulse contour analysis has been found to be associated closely with thermodilution measures.[106,107] Some investigators found that significant alterations in systemic vascular resistance induced by drug administration reduced the association between pulse contour analysis measures and thermodilution measures and suggested that frequent recalibration occur during times of hemodynamic instability to ensure valid measurement.[106,108]

The pulse contour analysis technique also permits the estimation of global end-diastolic volume, which may be used to calculate a measure of intrathoracic blood volume and extravascular lung water. These values may be used as a proxy for measures of cardiac preload and to guide fluid management. Several investigators suggest that these estimates of preload are better indicators than pulmonary artery occlusion pressure or central venous pressure.[106,109] Mitchell and others[109] suggested that fluid management based on extravascular lung water measures decreased ventilation time and length of intensive care stay in a group of medical patients. Measurement errors may result in the presence of an aortic aneurysm, a pulmonary embolus, or an intracardiac shunt.[90]

Indicator Dilution Techniques

Indicator dilution techniques include transpulmonary thermodilution and transpulmonary lithium dilution. These techniques are based on the conventional bolus thermodilution method in which an indicator is injected and the change in concentration of the indicator over time is detected. Transpulmonary thermodilution uses temperature as the indicator. Cold solution is injected intravenously, and temperature change in the arterial system is detected. Blood temperature change is used in the Steward-Hamilton equation to calculate an estimate of cardiac output.[90] In validation studies, there is good correlation between transpulmonary thermodilution and pulmonary artery thermodilution technique,[110-112] Fick,[111,113] and continuous thermodilution technique.[111] Pauli and others[114] also found that transpulmonary thermodilution measures were equivalent to Fick measures in seriously ill children. This method of measurement is less invasive because it does not require a pulmonary artery catheter and may have less respiratory variation than conventional thermodilution.[111]

Lithium dilution cardiac output is calculated from a lithium dilution curve. An injection of lithium chloride is administered intravenously. A lithium-sensitive electrode measures lithium concentration in the peripheral arterial system. Because the electrode is located outside of the artery, a small sample of blood is required for each measure. Lithium dilution cardiac output measures have good correlation with pulmonary artery thermodilution measures[115] and with transpulmonary thermodilution measures.[116] This method also may be used to calibrate pulse contour analysis, which provides a continuous estimate of cardiac output.

Thoracic Electrical Bioimpedance

Thoracic electrical bioimpedance or impedance cardiography is the least invasive technique available to estimate cardiac output. Thoracic bioimpedance is the thoracic electrical resistance to a current flow through the thorax. The volume of thoracic fluids alters impedance in an indirectly proportional fashion. Thus as thoracic fluid increases, impedance is reduced. This technique assumes that changes in thoracic impedance are primarily due to changes in aortic volume. Changes in impedance are proportional to changes in blood volume, and this permits calculation of a value for cardiac output.

With thoracic electrical bioimpedance, emitting electrodes are placed on the neck or upper thorax and sensing electrodes on the lower thorax. A high-frequency, low-magnitude current is directed through the thorax from the emitting electrodes, and the sensing electrodes detect changes in the ability of the thoracic cavity to impede this current (Figure 50-24). The sensing electrodes also detect and capture the electrocardiogram. As the ventricle ejects, the volume of aortic blood is increased and the impedance of the thorax is altered (δZ). The computer technology captures these time-varying changes in impedance and converts the data into a waveform. The impedance waveform and the electrocardiogram are used together to define important parameters used in the computer algorithm that calculates cardiac output (e.g., $\delta Z/\delta T_{max}$, preejection time, and ventricular ejection time; Figure 50-25). Parameters that may be obtained include stroke volume, cardiac output, cardiac time intervals (systolic and diastolic time), central fluid volume state, and contractility in the form of the acceleration index.

A number of limitations to impedance cardiography exist.[90,117] The technique is sensitive to changes in electrode-skin contact and alteration of electrode position, so attention to electrode contact and consistent placement are necessary. Patient movement and excessive diaphoresis also may be problematic. Additionally, the calculation of ventricular ejection time requires detectable, constant R-R intervals, so the presence of dysrhythmias, low-voltage electrocardiographic signals, ar-

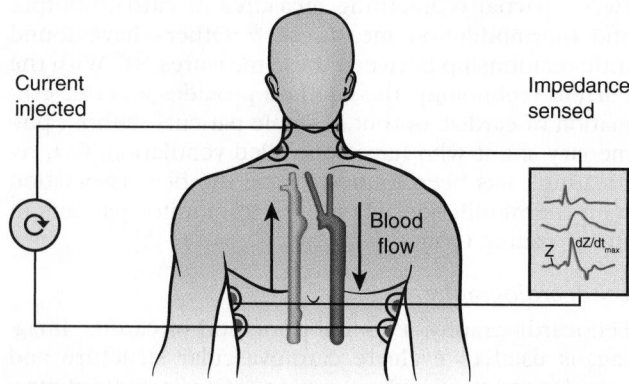

FIGURE 50-24 ■ Technique for bioimpedance cardiography. *d2/dt,* Impedance derivative or change in impedance over time; *2,* impedance; *20,* baseline impedance. (From Summers RL, Shoemaker WC, Peacock WF et al: *Acad Emerg Med* 10:669-680, 2003).

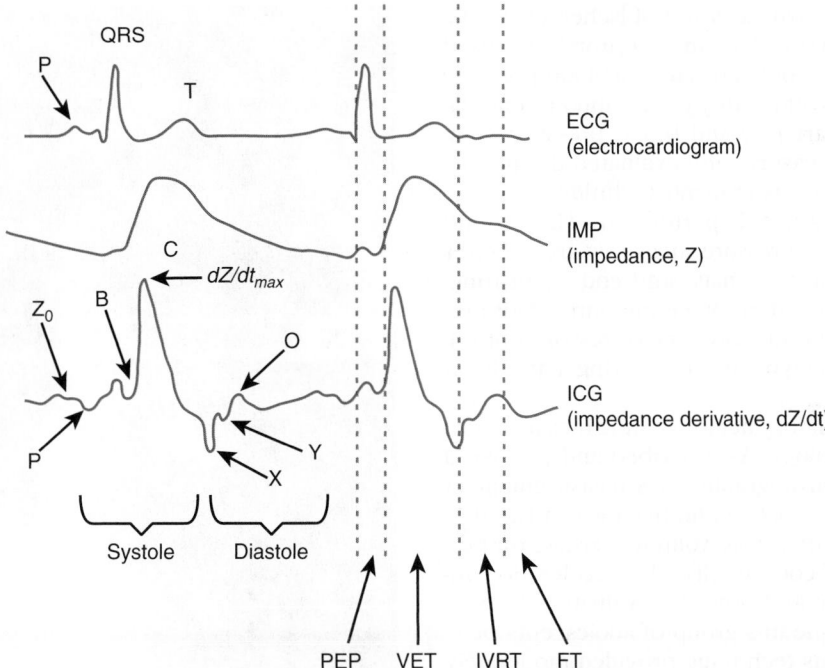

FIGURE 50-25 ■ Waveforms obtained or derived with impedance cardiography and time intervals measured. *PEP,* preejection period; *VET,* ventricular ejection time; *IVRT,* isovolumic relaxation time; *FT,* ventricular filling time. (From Summers RL, Shoemaker WC, Peacock WF et al: *Acad Emerg Med* 10:669-680, 2003.)

tifact, or signals with aberrant morphology may reduce validity. Most importantly, acute changes in thoracic fluid volume as with the development of pleural effusion or pulmonary edema can seriously reduce the validity of these measures. Excessive thoracic fluid volume reduces the signal-to-noise ratio and produces invalid measures.

The use of impedance cardiography has been reported in literally hundreds of studies.[117] A recent meta-analysis[118] included 154 studies and found correlations with invasive measures that ranged from r = 0.77 in cardiac patients to r = 0.85 in healthy subjects with repeated measures. Correlations were lower for cardiac patients with only one measurement (r = 0.66). These investigators concluded that impedance cardiography was not sufficiently accurate for diagnostic purposes but could be useful for trend analysis. Shoemaker and others[119] studied a large heterogeneous cohort of critically ill patients (*n* = 2192) and found an overall correlation of 0.85 for impedance measures compared with thermodilution. However, once patients with excessive thoracic fluid volume were excluded (8 percent of sample), the correlation between techniques was 0.93, and bias and precision were acceptable. More recently, Albert and others[120] found that impedance measures were comparable with thermodilution measures in patients with advanced, decompensated heart failure (r = 0.89, bias 0.08 liter/min, precision 1.38 liters/min). Cotter and others[121] compared a newer generation of impedance technique that used whole body bioimpedance with thermodilution measures and found the measures comparable in a wide range of cardiac clinical situations (r = 0.89, bias 0.0009 liter/min, precision 0.68 liter/min). Most investigators concluded that as this

technology continues to evolve, the reliability and validity of impedance cardiography would provide useful, noninvasive measures to guide practice.

Continuous Mixed Venous Oxygen

On average, body tissues use only 25 percent of the oxygen delivered in the arterial blood during a resting state. The remaining oxygen provides a reserve should metabolic demand increase or oxygen diffusion and supply decrease. Thus, measurement of mixed venous oxygen saturation provides information about global oxygen delivery, uptake, and cellular use. The introduction of a fiberoptic pulmonary artery catheter in 1981 offered a means to measure mixed venous oxygen saturation continuously. Several investigators proposed that measurement of mixed venous oxygen saturation might be substituted for measurement of cardiac output and provide a means for continuous evaluation rather than intermittent measurement by bolus thermodilution.[122-124] However, the relationship between cardiac output and mixed venous oxygen saturation has been inconsistent and often demonstrated poor correlation between the two variables in a variety of patient populations.[124-127] Although the continuous measurement of mixed venous oxygen saturation provides important information about the adequacy of cardiac output, this measure cannot substitute for cardiac output measures.

Ambulatory Hemodynamic Monitoring

Ambulatory continuous measurement of cardiovascular variables such as the electrocardiogram has been available in some form for several decades. Continuous electrocardiographic data have been useful in the detection of cardiac rhythm disturbances and of ischemic events. More recently, the HARVEST investigators[128,129] used ambulatory monitoring of heart rate and blood pressure to determine the reproducibility of continuous ambulatory measures of heart rate and blood pressure compared with clinical measures and evaluated the predictive power of this measurement technique for the development of sustained hypertension. They found that ambulatory blood pressure measures are a better predictor of left ventricular mass and end-organ function (renal) than intermittent office measures. More recently, invasive and noninvasive measures of continuous ambulatory hemodynamic monitoring have been evaluated.

Noninvasive ambulatory hemodynamic measures use bioimpedance technology. As described and discussed before, impedance cardiography uses measurement of changes in electrical resistance/impedance in the thoracic cavity to calculate stroke volume, cardiac output, and an indication of contractility, the acceleration index. Recently, Barnes and others[130] evaluated the reliability of this technique in a group of adolescents ($n = 35$) and found that this technique provided moderately reproducible measures over two separate 18-hour periods. Hemodynamic data were captured every 20 minutes in this study using two ambulatory monitors. Associations between the measures ranged from r = 0.43 to r = 0.82. Bias and precision were not reported. Further development of this technology likely will increase its utility in cardiovascular research and patient care.

Invasive measures of ambulatory hemodynamic monitoring require the surgical placement of a memory unit interfaced with two electrodes located in the right ventricle (Figure 50-26). The memory unit is similar in size to a pacemaker placed in a similar fashion (Chronicle IHM, Medtronic, Minneapolis, Minnesota). The electrodes are placed using a transvenous approach. One electrode contains a ratiometric reflectance oximeter and measures mixed venous oxygen saturation. The other electrode has a pressure transducer. The system has an external programmer so that monitoring format may be established or changed. Data can be downloaded and transmitted to a remote location for analysis and clinical decision making.

Ohlsson and others[131] performed a 1-year feasibility study of this technology in a group of heart failure patients ($n = 21$) over a range of time points, in a variety of body positions, during different physical activities and administration of vasoactive medications. These investigators found that the data obtained using this technique were stable, accurate, and reproducible compared with values obtained by standard right-heart catheterization. Fruhwald and others[132] used continuous hemodynamic monitoring with this technology to evaluate the hemodynamic effect of inhaled iloprost in a small group of women with pulmonary hypertension ($n = 5$). The hemodynamic measures were found to be reproducible and demonstrated that inhaled iloprost actually produced more transient alterations in hemodynamics than previously thought. Although mean pulmonary artery pressure was reduced from 68 to 49 mm Hg with drug administration, the effective treatment time

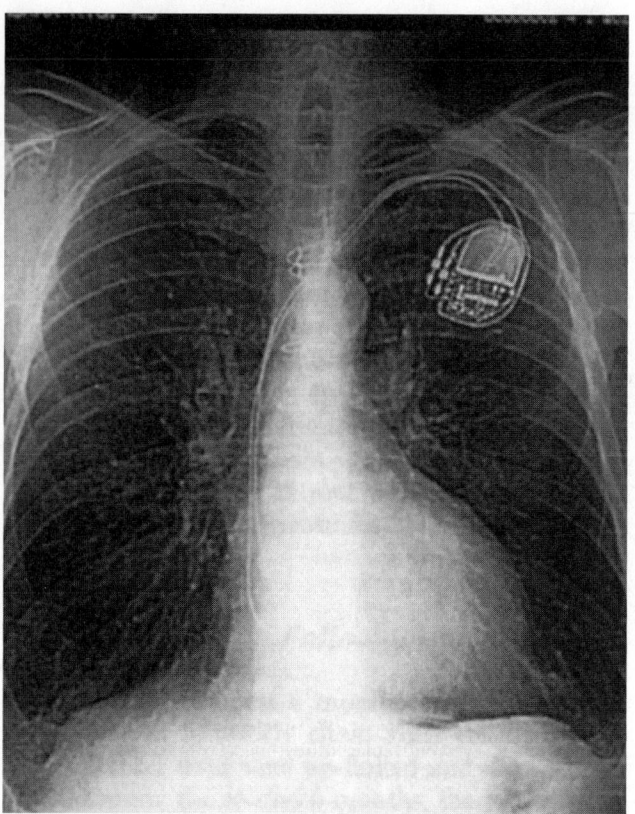

FIGURE 50-26 ■ Chest radiograph illustrating placement of the components of the implantable hemodynamic monitor. (From Ohlsson A, Kubo SH, Steinhaus D et al: *Eur Heart J* 22:942-954, 2001.)

was on average only 49 minutes with subsequent return of pulmonary hypertension.

Use of this technology for ambulatory hemodynamic monitoring with heart failure patients was reported recently to be a safe, reliable technique in the COMPASS-HF study, an investigation that included 274 patients with NYHA Class III or IV failure from 28 sites.[133] Patient management supported with the use of ambulatory hemodynamic monitoring reduced heart failure–related hospitalizations and heart failure–related emergency department and urgent care visits combined by 22 percent when hemodynamic data were evaluated regularly. For patients with NYHA Class III heart failure, there was a significant 41 percent reduction in heart failure–related hospitalizations and emergency department and urgent care visits. In the patients randomized to ambulatory hemodynamic monitoring, patient outcome was improved significantly as demonstrated by a 33 percent reduction in the proportion of patients who experienced worsening of their heart failure. This is clearly an exciting technology development that may influence the care and outcome of many patients with chronic cardiovascular and pulmonary vascular disorders.

MANAGEMENT OF PATIENTS WITH HEMODYNAMIC MONITORING

The delivery of high-quality, efficacious, cost-effective management of the patient with hemodynamic monitoring requires effective interdisciplinary communication and collaboration. Evidence supports that patient outcomes are improved with good teamwork.[134,135] Pronovost and others[135] found that the development and communication of daily goals for critically ill patients significantly improved care and reduced intensive care length of stay by 50 percent on average. The development of individualized hemodynamic goals should consider age, gender, underlying pathophysiological process, comorbidities, and prognosis. Presentation of typical hemodynamic alterations with common cardiac conditions is presented in Table 50-5. A more complete discussion that integrates hemodynamic values with pathophysiology, assessment, and management can be found in other chapters.

Critical care nurses have a comprehensive role in the management of patients who require hemodynamic monitoring (Box 50-8). The ubiquitous nature of the critical care nurse's responsibility for the patient requiring hemodynamic monitoring demands that these clinicians be sophisticated users of technology who have appropriate education about cardiovascular anatomy and physiology, pathophysiology, hemodynamic principles and equipment, and pharmacology. They must be skilled in the psychomotor activities associated with hemodynamic monitoring and appropriately educated and trained when new information, new technology, or new procedures are adopted.

A number of resources are available to ensure that critical care clinicians have sufficient knowledge to perform and use the data from hemodynamic monitoring effectively. The Pulmonary Artery Catheter Educational Program currently provides a strong foundation for clinicians responsible for critically ill patients. This program is available at *www.pacep.org*. This comprehensive education program was the result of the Pulmonary Artery Catheterization and Clinical Outcomes Workshop. The American Association of Critical-Care Nurses has published protocols for practice that include modules on arterial pressure monitoring,[136] pulmonary artery pressure monitoring,[137] and cardiac output monitoring.[127] Insufficient and inaccurate knowledge about physiology, pathophysiology, hemodynamic monitoring principles, equipment, or techniques can produce errors in equipment preparation and use, collection of invalid hemodynamic

---

BOX 50-8   ■ ■ ■
NURSES' ROLES IN HEMODYNAMIC MONITORING

Before Monitoring
- Assist with development of unit policies and procedures, preferably evidence-based, related to hemodynamic monitoring.
- Participate in appropriate educational programs to ensure adequate knowledge by all clinicians who participate in hemodynamic monitoring.
- Assist with identification of appropriate patients and risk factors for individual patients.
- Educate family and patient about procedures.
- Ensure informed consent is obtained when required.
- Collect and prepare necessary equipment and supplies.

During Placement of Intravascular Catheters
- Monitor patient during insertion of catheters.
- Support patient physically and psychologically.
- Assist with insertion of catheters.
- Document insertion and hemodynamic data.

During Monitoring of Hemodynamics
- Maintain closed fluid-filled system and catheter.
- Troubleshoot problems with hemodynamic monitoring equipment.
- Ensure that data are reliable and valid—leveling, zeroing, calibrating as needed.
- Evaluate data and respond appropriately to the obtained data.
- Document hemodynamic data and interventions used in response to changes.
- Notify appropriate team members of significant changes in hemodynamic data.
- Prevent introduction of microorganisms into system.
- Monitor patient for complications.

---

data, and inaccurate interpretation of patient hemodynamic status. Clinicians with insufficient knowledge and experience with hemodynamic monitoring may seriously compromise patient safety with erroneous clinical decisions based on invalid data.

LIMITATIONS OF HEMODYNAMIC MONITORING

Although hemodynamic monitoring is used daily in a majority of American acute care facilities, the procedures have a number of limitations. First, the measures obtained during hemodynamic monitoring are not directly providing information about the true variables of

---

■ ■ ■

TABLE 50-5   PREDICTED HEMODYNAMIC FINDINGS* WITH SOME CLINICAL CONDITIONS

CONDITION	CVP	ARTERIAL PRESSURE	PAP	PAOP	CO
Uncomplicated myocardial infarction	V	V	V	V	N/I
Myocardial infarction/cardiogenic shock	I	D	I	I	D
Hypovolemic shock with compensation	D	N	D	D	D
Septic shock—hyperdynamic	D/N	D/N	V	D/N	I
Aortic stenosis	N	N	N/I	N/I	N/D
Mitral regurgitation—acute	N/I	N/D	I	I	D
Adult respiratory distress syndrome with respiratory failure	N	N	I	N	N
Congestive heart failure	D/N	D/N	I	I	D

CO, Cardiac output; *CVP*, central venous pressure; *D*, decreased; *I*, increased; *N*, normal; *PAP*, pulmonary artery pressure; *PAOP*, pulmonary artery occlusion pressure; *V*, variable (may be increased, decreased, or normal).

*Individual patient changes in hemodynamic measures are influenced by a variety of factors that may be produced by underlying pathological conditions. These factors include blood volume, degree of vascular resistance, catecholamine levels, autonomic responses, pH, oxygen and carbon dioxide concentrations, and electrolyte concentrations. Thus, these predictions may be variable in individual patients.

interest: oxygen delivery and cellular oxygen use. Decisions about the adequacy of these variables must be inferred by examination of hemodynamic information (e.g., cardiac output and arterial pressure), physical examination (e.g., skin temperature and turgor, and heart sounds), indicators of organ function (e.g., urine output and Glasgow Coma Scale score), or laboratory analyses that evaluate organ systems (e.g., serum creatinine and cardiac and liver enzymes). Ideally, all of this information is considered during clinical decision making.

Second, the actual optimal ranges of hemodynamic variables for sick or injured populations are not clearly identified.[138-140] Normal ranges of hemodynamic values (Table 50-6) are based primarily on studies of young, healthy individuals in a resting state, and these values may not be directly applicable to individuals with pathophysiological alterations. Metabolic needs are significantly altered with injury or illness; thus the maintenance of hemodynamic values within the identified normal range for a healthy individual may provide insufficient delivery of oxygen to cells in the presence of augmented demands.

Third, clinician knowledge or lack thereof may seriously reduce the usefulness of hemodynamic data.[141-145] Clinician knowledge and psychomotor skill may be the greatest limitation to the collection and effective use of reliable and valid hemodynamic measures. A knowledge deficit can exist about normal cardiovascular anatomy and physiology, the pathophysiology of underlying disorders, the principles of hemodynamic monitoring, the appropriate preparation and use of the technology, the measurement of hemodynamic parameters, the interpretation of these data, and the selection of an intervention. The consequences of deficient and inaccurate knowledge related to any of these important areas may lead to inappropriate clinical decisions that negatively influence patient outcomes.

A fourth major limitation of hemodynamic monitoring is the lack of well-designed research studies in some areas (utility and safety of pulmonary artery catheters) and the sluggish translation of research findings in other areas into practice change.[146] The current controversy about use of pulmonary artery catheters with critically ill patients was initiated when Connors and colleagues[48] reported greater mortality and resource use in those patients whose care was managed with a pulmonary artery catheter. Prior clinical trials reported disparate findings about the efficacy of pulmonary artery catheterization and have been described as flawed because of small, widely heterogeneous samples in limited study sites and the use of subjects with greatly varying severity of illness.[147-152] The findings from current well-designed clinical trials require rapid evaluation and dissemination to clinicians. In addition, the translation of well-documented research findings into practice requires a concerted effort by national and international organizations to compile findings and disseminate them as evidence-based protocols for widespread use by clinicians. For example, the development and national promotion of evidence-based guidelines or protocols that include acceptable body positions for hemodynamic monitoring may promote greater adoption in practice. However, universal adoption likely will occur only when clinicians are well educated about research utilization and research findings are incorporated into facility policies and procedures as expected practice.

SUMMARY

Hemodynamic monitoring provides an evaluation of the components that produce dynamic movement of blood through the cardiovascular system. Clinicians use the information obtained from hemodynamic monitoring to evaluate baseline cardiovascular function, to determine the presence and degree of cardiovascular dysfunction, to guide specific interventions to promote improved cardiovascular function, and to evaluate the efficacy of these interventions. Hemodynamic evaluation may be performed noninvasively or invasively; however, the correlation between noninvasive estimates and directly measured hemodynamic variables is often low.

Invasive hemodynamic monitoring most often uses sophisticated biomedical equipment and a fluid-filled system. Reliable and valid measurement requires a clinician who is knowledgeable and adept to prepare and maintain this system correctly (evaluate dynamic response, level, zero reference, calibrate, and troubleshoot) and to monitor, evaluate, and act appropriately in response to the information obtained. Common invasive hemodynamic measures include central venous pressure, arterial pressure, pulmonary artery pressure, and pulmonary artery occlusion pressure. In addition, cardiac output may be measured invasively or noninvasively by a variety of techniques. Newer technology is now available to monitor hemodynamic state continuously in ambulatory patients and has evidence of improvement in patient management and outcomes.

■ ■ ■

TABLE 50-6   NORMAL ADULT HEMODYNAMIC MEASUREMENTS

MEASURE	VALUE
Arterial Pressure	
Systolic	100-130 mm Hg
Diastolic	60-90 mm Hg
Mean	70-105 mm Hg
Pulmonary Artery Pressure	
Systolic	15-30 mm Hg
Diastolic	5-15 mm Hg
Mean	Less than 20mm Hg
Pulmonary artery occlusion pressure	4-12 mm Hg
Right Ventricular Pressure	
Systolic	15-30 mm Hg
Diastolic	0-8 mm Hg
Other Hemodynamic Measures	
Right ventricular end-diastolic volume	100-160 ml
Right ventricular ejection fraction	40%-60%
Left atrial pressure	4-15 mm Hg
Cardiac output	4-8 liters/min
Stroke volume	60-130 ml
Cardiac index	2.5-4.5 liters/min/m²
Stroke volume index	30-65 ml/beat/m²
Systemic vascular resistance	900-1400 dynes/sec/cm⁻⁵
Pulmonary vascular resistance	100-250 dynes/sec/cm⁻⁵
Venous oxygen saturation	60%-80%

REFERENCES

1. Creed G: Can cardiac output be assessed clinically by intensive care staff? *Crit Care Med* 16:108-111, 2000.
2. Tibby SM, Hatherill M, Marsh MJ, Murdoch IA: Clinicians' abilities to estimate cardiac index in ventilated children and infants, *Arch Dis Child* 77:516-518, 1997.
3. Eisenberg PR, Jaffe AS, Schuster DP: Clinical evaluation compared to pulmonary artery catheterization in the hemodynamic assessment of critically ill patients, *Crit Care Med* 12:549-553, 1984.
4. Snellen HA: *History of cardiology: a brief outline of the 350 years prelude to an explosive growth*, Rotterdam, Netherlands, 1984, Donker Academic.
5. Hall WD: Stephen Hales: theologian, botanist, physiologist—discoverer of hemodynamics, *Clin Cardiol* 10:487-489, 1987.
6. Comroe JH: Hydrogen, balloons, and pressures, *Am Rev Respir Dis* 113:73-76, 1976.
7. Warkentin TE, Kelton JG: A 14-year study of heparin-induced thrombocytopenia, *Am J Med* 101:502-507, 1996.
8. Brieger DB, Mak KH, Kottke-Marchant K: Heparin-induced thrombocytopenia, *J Am Coll Cardiol* 31:1449-1459, 1998.
9. Amiral J, Wolf M, Fischer AM et al: Pathogenicity of IgA and/or IgM antibodies to heparin-PF4 complexes in patients with heparin-induced thrombocytopenia, *Br J Haematol* 92:954-959, 1996.
10. Visentin GP: Heparin-induced thrombocytopenia: molecular pathogenesis, *Thromb Haemost* 82:448-456, 1999.
11. Laster JL, Nichols WK, Silver D: Thrombocytopenia associated with heparin-coated catheters in patients with heparin associated antiplatelet antibodies, *Arch Intern Med* 149:2285-2287, 1989.
12. Nand S, Wong W, Yuen B et al: Heparin-induced thrombocytopenia with thrombosis: incidence, analysis of risk factors, and clinical outcomes in 108 consecutive patients treated at a single institution, *Am J Hemat* 56:12-16, 1997.
13. Kronberg GM, Quan SF, Schlobohm RM et al: Anatomic location of the tips of pulmonary artery catheters in supine patients, *Anesthesiology* 41:467, 1979.
14. Darovic GO: *Hemodynamic monitoring: invasive and noninvasive clinical application*, ed 3, Philadelphia, 2002, WB Saunders.
15. Bisnaire D, Robinson L: Accuracy of leveling hemodynamic transducer systems, *Off J Can Assoc Crit Care Nurs* 10:16-19, 1999.
16. Rice WP, Fernandez EG, Jarog D, Jensen A: A comparison of hydrostatic leveling methods in invasive pressure monitoring, *Crit Care Nurse* 20:20-30, 2000.
17. Cournand A, Ranges HA: Catheterization of the right auricle in man, *Proc Soc Exp Biol Med* 46:462, 1941.
18. Wilson JN, Grow JB, Demong CV et al: Central venous pressure in optimal blood volume maintenance, *Arch Surg* 85:563-578, 1962.
19. Swan HJC, Ganz W, Forrester JS et al: Catheterization of the heart in man with use of a flow-directed balloon-tipped catheter, *New Engl J Med* 283:447-451, 1970.
20. Kumar A, Anel R, Bunnell E et al: Pulmonary artery occlusion pressure and central venous pressure fail to predict ventricular filling volume, cardiac performance, or the response to volume infusion in normal subjects, *Crit Care Med* 32:691-699, 2004.
21. Diebel L, Wilson RF, Heins J et al: End-diastolic volume versus pulmonary artery wedge pressure in evaluating cardiac preload in trauma patients, *J Trauma* 37:950-955, 1994.
22. Buhre W, Weyland A, Schorn B et al: Changes in central venous pressure and pulmonary capillary wedge pressure do not indicate changes in right and left heart volume in patients undergoing coronary artery bypass surgery, *Eur J Anaesthesiol* 16:11-17, 1999.
23. Wagner JG, Leatherman JW: Right ventricular end-diastolic volume as a predictor of the hemodynamic response to a fluid challenge, *Chest* 113:1048-1054, 1998.
24. Tuman KJ, McCarthy RJ, March RJ et al: Effects of phenylephrine or volume loading on right ventricular function in patients undergoing myocardial revascularization, *J Cardiothor Vasc Anesth* 9:2-8, 1995.
25. Scott SS, Giuliano KK, Pysznik E et al: Influence of port site on central venous pressure measurement from triple-lumen catheters in critically ill adults, *Am J Crit Care* 7:60-63, 1998.
26. Blot F, Laplanche A: Accuracy of totally implanted ports, tunnelled, single- and multiple-lumen central venous catheters for measurement of central venous pressure, *Intensive Care Med* 26:1837-1842, 2000.
27. Ceyran H, Akcaly Y, Asgun F et al Benefit of using a triple-lumen catheter to monitor left atrial pressure, *Acta Anaesthesiol Scand* 47:430-432, 2003.
28. Sharkey SW: *A guide to interpretation of hemodynamic data in the coronary care unit*, Philadelphia, 1997, Lippincott-Raven.
29. Arnone M: Central venous/right atrial pressure monitoring. In McHale DJ, Carlson KK, editors: *AACN procedure manual for critical care*, ed 4, Philadelphia, 2001, WB Saunders.
30. Coulter TD, Wiedemann HP: Complications of hemodynamic monitoring, *Clin Chest Med* 20:249-267, 1999.
31. O'Grady NP, Alexander M, Dellinger EP et al: Guidelines for the prevention of intravascular catheter-related infections, *MMWR Recomm Rep* 51:1-29, 2002.
32. Lyew MA, Bacon DR, Nesarajah MS: Right ventricular perforation by a pulmonary artery catheter during coronary artery bypass surgery, *Anesth Analg* 82:1089-1090, 1996.
33. Maschke SP, Rogove HJ: Cardiac tamponade associated with a multilumen central venous catheter, *Crit Care Med* 12:611-613, 1984.
34. Orebaugh SL: Venous air embolism: clinical and experimental considerations, *Crit Care Med* 20:1169-1177, 1992.
35. Cousins TR, O'Donnell JM: Arterial cannulations: a critical review, *AANA J* 72:267-271, 2004.
36. Karamanoglu M, O'Rourke ME, Avolio AP, Kelly RP: An analysis of the relationship between central and aortic and peripheral upper limb pressure waves in man, *Eur Heart J* 14:160-176, 1993.
37. Dorman T, Breslow M, Lipsett PA et al: Radial artery pressure monitoring underestimates central arterial pressure during vasopressor therapy in critically ill surgical patients, *Crit Care Med* 26:1646-1649, 1998.
38. Durbin CG: Radial arterial lines and sticks: what are the risks? *Respir Care* 46:229-230, 2001.
39. Martin C, Sauz P, Papazian I, Gouin E: Long term arterial cannulation in ICU patients using the radial artery or dorsalis pedis artery, *Chest* 119:901-906, 2001.
40. McGregor AD: The Allen test: an investigation of its accuracy by fluorescein angiography, *J Hand Surg Br* 12:82-85, 1987.
41. Clarke W, Freund PR, Wasse J et al: Assessment of adequacy of arterial ulnar flow prior to radial artery catheterization, *Anesthesiology* 55:A38, 1982.
42. Raad I, Costerton W, Sabharwal U et al: Ultrastructural analysis of indwelling vascular catheters: a quantitative relationship between luminal colonization and duration of placement, *J Infect Dis* 168:7, 1993.
43. Dalen JE, Bone RC: Is it time to pull the pulmonary artery catheter? *JAMA* 276:916-918, 1996.
44. Bernard GR, Sopko G, Cerra F et al: Pulmonary artery catheterization and clinical outcomes: National Heart, Lung and Blood Institute and Food and Drug Administration Workshop Report, *JAMA* 283:2568-2572, 2000.
45. Gore JM, Goldberg RJ, Spodick DH et al: A community-wide assessment of the use of pulmonary artery catheters in patients with acute myocardial infarction, *Chest* 92:721-727, 1987.
46. Zion MM, Balkin J, Rosenmann D et al: Use of pulmonary artery catheters in patients with acute myocardial infarction: analysis of experience in 5841 patients in the SPRINT registry, *Chest* 98:1331-1335, 1990.
47. Parsons PE: Progress in research on pulmonary-artery catheters, *N Engl J Med* 348:66-68, 2003.
48. Connors AF, Speroff T, Dawson NV et al: The effectiveness of right heart catheterization in the initial care of critically ill patients, *JAMA* 276:889-897, 1996.
49. Shah MR, O'Connor CM, Sopko G et al: Evaluation study of congestive heart failure and pulmonary artery catheterization effectiveness (ESCAPE): design and rationale, *Am Heart J* 141:528-535, 2001.
50. Steinbrook R: How best to ventilate? trial design and patient safety in studies of the acute respiratory distress syndrome, *N Eng J Med* 348:1393-1401, 2003.
51. Vieillard-Baron A, Girou E, Valente E et al: Predictors of mortality in acute respiratory distress syndrome, *Am J Respir Crit Care Med* 161:1597-1601, 2000.

52. Polanczyk CA, Rohde LE, Goldman L et al: Right heart catheterization and cardiac complications in patients undergoing noncardiac surgery, *JAMA* 286:309-314, 2001.

53. Rhodes A, Cusack RJ, Newman PJ et al: A randomised, controlled trial of the pulmonary artery catheter in critically ill patients, *Intensive Care Med* 28:256-264, 2002.

54. Sandham JD, Hull RD, Brant RF et al: A randomized, controlled trial of the use of pulmonary-artery catheters in high-risk surgical patients, *New Engl J Med* 348:5-14, 2003.

55. National Institutes of Health: *No increase in deaths or hospitalizations for heart failure patients who have a pulmonary artery catheter.* Retrieved April, 27, 2005 from www.nhlbi.nih.gov/new/press/04-11-09.htm

56. Nieminen MS, Bohm M, Cowie MR et al: Executive summary of the guidelines on the diagnosis and treatment of acute heart failure: the Task Force on Acute Heart Failure of the European Society of Cardiology, *Eur Heart J* 26:384-416, 2005.

57. Hunt SA, Abraham WT, Chin MH et al: ACC/AHA 2005 guideline update for the diagnosis and management of chronic heart failure in the adult: summary article—a report of the American College of Cardiology/American Heart Association Task Force on Practice Guidelines, *Circulation* 112(12):e154-e235, 2005.

58. Glenny RW, Lamm WJ, Albert RK, Robertson HT: Gravity is a minor determinant of pulmonary blood flow distribution, *J Appl Physiol* 71:620-629, 1991.

59. Bridges EJ: Monitoring pulmonary artery pressures: just the facts, *Crit Care Nurse* 20:59-80, 2000.

60. Dobbin K, Wallace S, Ahlberg J, Chulay M: Pulmonary artery pressure measurement in patients with elevated pressures: effect of backrest elevation and method of measurement, *Am J Crit Care* 1:61-69, 1992.

61. Wilson A, Bermingham-Mitchell K, Wells N, Zachary K: Effect of back position on hemodynamic and right ventricular measurements in critically ill adults, *Am J Crit Care* 5:264-270, 1996.

62. Woods S, Grose B, Laurent-Bopp D: Effect of backrest position on pulmonary artery pressures in critically ill patients, *Cardiovasc Nurs* 18:19-24, 1982.

63. Cason C, Lambert C: Backrest position and reference level in pulmonary artery pressure measurement, *Clin Nurse Spec* 1:159-165, 1987.

64. Ross C, Jones R: Comparisons of pulmonary artery pressure measurements in supine and 30 degree lateral positions, *Can J Cardiovasc Nurs* 6:4-8, 1995.

65. Bridges EJ, Woods SL, Brengelmann GL et al: Effect of the 30° lateral recumbent position on pulmonary artery and pulmonary artery wedge pressures in critically ill adult cardiac surgery patients, *Am J Crit Care* 9:262-275, 2000.

66. Briones T, Dickenson S, Bieberitz R: Effect of positioning on SVO₂ and hemodynamic measurements, *Heart Lung* 20:297, 1991.

67. Cason CL, Holland CL, Lambert CW, Huntsman KT: Effects of backrest elevation and position on pulmonary artery pressures, *Cardiovasc Nurs* 26:1-6, 1990.

68. Groom L, Frisch S, Elliott M: Reproducibility and accuracy of pulmonary artery pressure measurements in supine and lateral positions, *Heart Lung* 19:147-151, 1990.

69. VanEtta D, Gibbons E, Woods S: Estimation of left atrial location in supine and 30° lateral position, *Am J Crit Care* 2:264, 1993.

70. Davison R, Parker M, Harrison R: The validity of determinations of pulmonary wedge pressure during mechanical ventilation, *Chest* 73:353-355, 1978.

71. Sprung CL, Pozen RG, Rozanski JJ et al: Advanced ventricular arrhythmias during bedside pulmonary artery catheterization, *Am J Med* 72:203-208, 1982.

72. Luck JC, Engel TR: Transient right bundle branch block with "Swan-Ganz" catheterization, *Am Heart J* 92:263-264, 1976.

73. Wadsworth R, Littler C: Cardiac standstill, pulmonary artery catheterization and left bundle branch block, *Anaesthesia* 51:97, 1996.

74. Fraser RS: Catheter-induced pulmonary artery perforation: pathologic and pathogenic features, *Hum Pathol* 18:1246-1251, 1987.

75. Shellock F, Riedinger M: Reproducibility and accuracy of using room-temperature vs ice-temperature injectate for thermodilution cardiac output determination, *Heart Lung* 12:175-176, 1983.

76. Vennix C, Nelson DH, Pierpont GL: Thermodilution cardiac output in critically ill patients: comparison of room-temperature and iced injectate, *Heart Lung* 13:574-578, 1984.

77. Lyons K, Dalbow M: Room temperature injectate and iced injectate for cardiac output: a comparative study, *Crit Care Nurse* 6:48-50, 1986.

78. Kiely M, Byers LA, Greenwood R, et al: Thermodilution measurement of cardiac output in patients with low output: room-temperature versus iced injectate, *Am J Crit Care* 7:436-438, 1998.

79. Wallace DC, Winslow EH: Effects of iced and room temperature injectate on cardiac output measurements in critically ill patients with low and high cardiac outputs, *Heart Lung* 22:55-63, 1993.

80. Groom L, Elliott M, Frisch S: Injectate temperature: effects on thermodilution cardiac output measurements, *Crit Care Nurse* 10:112-120, 1990.

81. McCloy K, Leung S, Belden J et al: Effects of injectate volume on thermodilution measurements of cardiac output in patients with low ventricular ejection fractions, *Am J Crit Care* 8:86, 1999.

82. Mihm FG, Gettinger A, Hanson CW et al: A multicenter evaluation of a new continuous cardiac output pulmonary artery catheter system, *Crit Care Med* 26:1346-1350, 1998.

83. Lefrant JY, Bruelle P, Ripart J et al: Cardiac output measurement in critically ill patients: comparison of continuous and conventional thermodilution techniques, *Can J Anaesth* 42:972-976, 1995.

84. Monchi M, Thebert D, Carlou A et al: Clinical evaluation of the Abbott Qvue-OptiQ continuous cardiac output system in critically ill patients, *J Crit Care* 13:91-95, 1998.

85. Boyle M, Jacobs S, Torda TA, Shehabi Y: Assessment of the agreement between cardiac output measured by bolus thermodilution and continuous methods, with particular reference to the effect of heart rhythm, *Aust Crit Care* 10:5-11, 1997.

86. Ott K, Johnson K, Ahrens T: New technologies in the assessment of hemodynamic parameters, *J Cardiovasc Nurs* 15:41-55, 2001.

87. Aranda M, Mihm FG, Garrett S et al: Continuous cardiac output catheters: delay in in vitro response time after controlled flow changes, *Anesthesiology* 89:1592-1595, 1998.

88. De Figueiredo P, Malbouisoon LM, Varicoda EY et al: Thermal filament continuous thermodilution cardiac output delayed responses limits its value during acute hemorrhagic instability, *J Trauma* 47:288-293, 1999.

89. Cheatham ML, Nelson LD, Chang MC, Safcsak K: Right ventricular end-diastolic volume index as a predictor of preload status in patients on positive end-expiratory pressure, *Crit Care Med* 26:1801-1806, 1998.

90. Chaney JC, Derdak S: Minimally invasive hemodynamic monitoring for the intensivist: current and emerging technology, *Crit Care Med* 30:2338-2345, 2002.

91. Loeb RG, Brown EA, DiNardo JA et al: Clinical accuracy of a new non-invasive cardiac output monitor, *Anesthesiology* 91:A474, 1999.

92. Watt RC, Loeb RG, Orr J: Comparison of a new non-invasive cardiac output technique with invasive bolus and continuous thermodilution, *Anesthesiology* 89:A536, 1998.

93. Gama deAbreu M, Quintel M, Ragaller M et al: Partial carbon dioxide rebreathing: a reliable technique for noninvasive measurement of nonshunted pulmonary capillary blood flow, *Crit Care Med* 25:675-683, 1997.

94. Jopling MW: Noninvasive cardiac output determination utilizing the method of partial CO₂ rebreathing: a comparison with continuous and bolus thermodilution cardiac output, *Anesthesiology* 89:A544, 1998.

95. Kuck K, Orr J, Haryadi DG et al: Evaluation of the NICO partial rebreathing cardiac output monitor, *Anesthesiology* 91:A560, 1999.

96. Brown JM: Use of echocardiography for hemodynamic monitoring, *Crit Care Med* 30:1361-1364, 2002.

97. Axler O, Tousignant C, Thompson CR et al: Comparison of transesophageal echocardiographic, Fick, and thermodilution cardiac output in critically ill patients, *J Crit Care* 11:109-116, 1996.

98. Pinto FJ, Siegel LC, Chenzbraun A et al: On-line estimation of cardiac output with a new automated border detection system using transesophageal echocardiography: a preliminary comparison with thermodilution, *J Cardiothorac Vasc Anesth* 8:625-630, 1994.

99. Greim CA, Roewer N, Laux G et al: On-line estimation of left ventricular stroke volume using transoesophageal echocardiography and acoustic quantification, *Br J Anaesth* 77:365-369, 1996.

100. Turner MA: Doppler-based hemodynamic monitoring: a minimally invasive alternative, *AACN Clin Issues* 14:220-231, 2003.

101. Madan AK, UyBarreta VV, Shaghayegh A et al: Esophageal Doppler ultrasound monitor versus pulmonary artery catheter in the hemodynamic management of critically ill surgical patients, *J Trauma* 46:607-611, 1999.

102. Valtier B, Cholley BP, Belot JP et al: Noninvasive monitoring of cardiac output in critically ill patients using transesophageal Doppler, *Am J Respir Crit Care Med* 158:77-83, 1998.

103. Cruschien J, Rivers M, Caruso J et al: A comparison of transesophageal Doppler, thermodilution, and Fick cardiac output measurements in critically ill patients, *Crit Care Med* 26(1 suppl):A62, 1998.

104. Jansen JRC, Wesseling KH, Settels JJ et al: Continuous cardiac output monitoring by pulse contour during cardiac surgery, *Eur Heart J* 11(suppl 1):26-32, 1990.

105. Harms MP, Wesseling KH, Pott F et al: Continuous stroke volume monitoring by modeling flow from non-invasive measurement of arterial pressure in humans under orthostatic stress, *Clin Sci* 97:291-301, 1999.

106. Buhre W, Weyland A, Lazmaier S et al: Comparison of cardiac output assessed by pulse-contour analysis and thermodilution in patients undergoing minimally invasive direct coronary artery bypass grafting, *J Cardiothorac Vasc Anesth* 13:437-440, 1999.

107. Zollner C, Haller M, Weis M et al: Beat-to-beat measurement of cardiac output by intravascular pulse contour analysis: a prospective criterion standard study in patients after cardiac surgery, *J Cardiothorac Vasc Anesth* 14:125-129, 2000.

108. Rodig G, Prasser C, Keyl C et al: Continuous cardiac output measurement: pulse contour analysis versus thermodilution technique in cardiac surgical patients, *Br J Anaesth* 82:525-530, 1999.

109. Mitchell JP, Schuller D, Calandrino FS et al: Improved outcome based on fluid management in critically ill patients requiring pulmonary artery catheterization, *Am Rev Respir Dis* 145:990-998, 1992.

110. Gust R, Gottschalk A, Bauer H et al: Cardiac output measurement by transpulmonary versus conventional thermodilution technique in intensive care patients after coronary artery bypass grafting, *J Cardiothorac Vasc Anesth* 12:519-522, 1998.

111. Sakka SG, Reinhart K, Wegscheider K et al: Is the placement of a pulmonary artery catheter still justified solely for the measurement of cardiac output? *J Cardiothor Vasc Anesth* 14:119-124, 2000.

112. Godje O, Peyerl M, Seebauer T et al: Reproducibility of double indicator dilution measurements of intrathoracic blood volume compartments, extravascular lung water, and liver function, *Chest* 113:1070-1077, 1998.

113. Tibby SM, Hatherill M, Marsh MJ et al: Clinical validation of cardiac output measurements using femoral artery thermodilution with direct Fick in ventilated children and infants, *Intensive Care Med* 23:987-991, 1997.

114. Pauli C, Dakler U, Genz T et al: Cardiac output determination in children: equivalence of the transpulmonary thermodilution method to the direct Fick principle, *Intensive Care Med* 28:947-952, 2002.

115. Linton R, Band D, O'Brien T et al: Lithium dilution cardiac output measurement: a comparison with thermodilution, *Crit Care Med* 25:1796-1800, 1997.

116. Linton RA, Jonas MM, Tibby SM et al: Cardiac output measured by lithium dilution and transpulmonary thermodilution in patients in a paediatric intensive care unit, *Intensive Care Med* 26:1507-1511, 2000.

117. Summers RL, Shoemaker WC, Peacock WF et al: Electrophysiologic and clinical principles of noninvasive hemodynamic monitoring using impedance cardiography, *Acad Emerg Med* 10:669-680, 2003.

118. Raaijmakers E, Raes TJ, Scholten J et al: A meta-analysis of three decades of validating thoracic impedance cardiography, *Crit Care Med* 27:1203-1213, 1999.

119. Shoemaker WC, Belzberg H, Wo CC et al: Multicenter study on noninvasive monitoring as alternatives to invasive monitoring of acutely ill emergency patients, *Chest* 114:1643-1652, 1998.

120. Albert NM, Hail MD, Li J, Young JB: Equivalence of the bioimpedance and thermodilution methods in measuring cardiac output in hospitalized patients with advanced, decompensated chronic heart failure, *Am J Crit Care* 13:469-479, 2004.

121. Cotter G, Moshkovitz Y, Kaluski E et al: Accurate, noninvasive continuous monitoring of cardiac output by whole-body electrical bioimpedance, *Chest* 125:1431-1440, 2004.

122. Edward JD: Practical application of oxygen transport principles, *Crit Care Med* 18:S45-S48, 1990.

123. Enger EL, Holm K: Perspectives on the interpretation of continuous mixed venous oxygen saturation, *Heart Lung* 19:578-580, 1990.

124. Noll ML, Fountain RL: The relationship between mixed venous oxygen saturation and cardiac output in mechanically ventilated coronary artery bypass graft patients, *Prog Cardiovasc Nurs* 5:34-40, 1990.

125. Kyff JV, Vaughn S, Yang SC et al: Continuous monitoring of mixed venous oxygen saturation in patients with acute myocardial infarction, *Chest* 95:607-611, 1989.

126. Silance PG, Simon C, Vincent JL: The relation between cardiac index and oxygen extraction in acutely ill patients, *Chest* 105:1190-1197, 1994.

127. Gawlinski A: *Cardiac output monitoring: protocols for practice,* Aliso Viejo, Calif, 1998, American Association of Critical-Care Nurses.

128. Palatini P, Mormino P, Santonastaso M et al: Ambulatory blood pressure predicts end-organ damage only in subjects with reproducible recordings: HARVEST Study Investigators—Hypertension and Ambulatory Recording Venetia Study, *J Hypertens* 17:465-473, 1999.

129. Palatini P, Winnicki M, Santonastaso M et al: Reproducibility of heart rate measured in the clinic and with 24-hour intermittent recorders, *Am J Hypertens* 13:92-98, 2000.

130. Barnes VA, Johnson MH, Treiber FA: Temporal stability of twenty-four hour ambulatory hemodynamic bioimpedance measures in African American adolescents, *Blood Press Monit* 9:173-177, 2004.

131. Ohlsson A, Kubo SH, Steinhaus D et al: Continuous ambulatory monitoring of absolute right ventricular pressure and mixed venous oxygen saturation in patients with heart failure using an implantable haemodynamic monitor, *Eur Heart J* 22:942-954, 2001.

132. Fruhwald FM, Kjellstrom B, Perthold W et al: Continuous hemodynamic monitoring in pulmonary hypertensive patients treated with inhaled iloprost, *Chest* 124:351-359, 2003.

133. King C, Lind V: *COMPASS-HF Study: Implantable hemodynamic monitor reduces heart failure hospital events for many heart failure patients.* Retrieved April 18, 2005 fromwwwp.medtronic.com/Newsroom/NewsReleaseDetails.do?itemId=1110237750252.

134. Baggs JG, Schmitt MH, Mushlin AI et al: Association between nurse-physician collaboration and patient outcomes in three intensive care units, *Crit Care Med* 27:1991-1998, 1999.

135. Pronovost P, Berenholtz S, Dorman T et al: Improving communication in the ICU using daily goals, *J Crit Care* 18:71-75, 2003.

136. Imperial-Perez F, McRae M: *Arterial pressure monitoring: protocols for practice,* Aliso Viejo, Calif, 1998, American Association of Critical-Care Nurses.

137. Keckeisen M: *Pulmonary artery pressure monitoring: protocols for practice,* Aliso Viejo, Calif, 1998, American Association of Critical-Care Nurses.

138. Pinsky MR: Hemodynamic monitoring in the intensive care unit, *Clin Chest Med* 24:549-560, 2003.

139. McKinley BA, Kozar RA, Cocanour CS et al: Normal versus supranormal oxygen delivery goals in shock resuscitation: the response is the same, *J Trauma* 53:825-832, 2002.

140. Velmahos GC, Demetriades D, Shoemaker WC et al: Endpoints of resuscitation of critically injured patients: normal or supranormal? a prospective randomized trial, *Ann Surg* 232:409-418, 2000.

141. McGhee BH, Woods SL: Critical care nurses' knowledge of arterial pressure monitoring, *Am J Crit Care* 10:43-51, 2001.

142. Iberti TJ, Daily EK, Leibowitz AB et al: Assessment of critical care nurses' knowledge of the pulmonary artery catheter: the Pulmonary Artery Catheter Study Group, *Crit Care Med* 22:1674-1678, 1994.

143. Burns S, Burns D, Shively M: Critical care nurses' knowledge of pulmonary artery catheters, *Am J Crit Care* 5:49-54, 1996.

144. Dietz B, Smith T: Enhancing the accuracy of hemodynamic monitoring, *J Nurs Care Qual* 17:30-38, 2002.

145. Johnston IG, Jane R, Fraser JF et al: Survey of intensive care nurses' knowledge relating to the pulmonary artery catheter, *Anaesth Intensive Care* 32:564-568, 2004.

146. Grap MJ, Pettrey L, Thornby D: Hemodynamic monitoring: a comparison of research and practice, *Am J Crit Care* 6:452-456, 1997.

147. Schultz RJ, Whitfield GF, LaMura JJ et al: The role of physiologic monitoring in patients with fractures of the hip, *J Trauma* 25:309-316, 1985.

148. Pearson KS, Gomez MN, Moyers JR et al: A cost/benefit analysis of randomized invasive monitoring for patients undergoing cardiac surgery, *Anesth Analg* 69:336-341, 1989.

149. Isaacson IJ, Lowdon JD, Berry AJ et al: The value of pulmonary artery and central venous monitoring in patients undergoing abdominal aortic reconstructive surgery: a comparative study of two selected, randomized groups, *J Vasc Surg* 12:754-760, 1990.

150. Joyce WP, Provan JL, Arneli FM et al: The role of central haemodynamic monitoring in abdominal aortic surgery: a prospective, randomized study, *Eur J Vasc Surg* 4:633-636, 1990.

151. Guyatt G: A randomized control trial of right-heart catheterization in critically ill patients: Ontario Intensive Care Study Group, *Intensive Care Med* 6:91-95, 1991.

152. Berlauk JF, Abrams JH, Gilmour IJ et al: Preoperative optimization of cardiovascular hemodynamics improves outcome in peripheral vascular surgery: a prospective, randomized clinical trial, *Ann Surg* 214:289-299, 1991.

Patient Delay in Seeking Treatment for Cardiac Symptoms

Mary A. Caldwell
Kathleen Dracup

CHAPTER ABBREVIATIONS

ACS   acute coronary syndrome
AMI   acute myocardial infarction
ED   emergency department
HF   heart failure

DELAY WITH SYMPTOMS OF ACUTE CORONARY SYNDROME

The importance of patient delay in seeking treatment for symptoms of acute coronary syndrome (**ACS**) and its terminal consequence, acute myocardial infarction (**AMI**), was recognized as early as the 1960s.[1] Almost two decades later and before the widespread use of revascularization therapies, the Multicenter Investigation of Limitation of Infarct Size noted the association between long delay time and increased rate of death after AMI.[2] Reperfusion therapies such as thrombolysis and angioplasty have revolutionized the treatment of ACS. However, the full potential of these therapies has not been realized because a significant proportion of patients (in some studies, greater than 30 percent) delay seeking help for longer than 6 hours.[3] Beyond this time the benefits are minimized at best, and at worst, patients are ineligible for treatment.

Delay in ACS typically is defined as the time from onset of symptoms to the time treatment is delivered. Measuring delay depends largely on what defines symptom onset, yet definitions used in reporting delay time in ACS patients are often vague or vary widely. Defining the exact time of the onset of symptoms also is made more difficult by the pattern of ACS where "stuttering" or opening and closing of an affected artery can produce intermittent symptoms. The most recent trials have used the definition of symptom onset as being the beginning of the symptoms that actually prompted the patient to take action.

Complicating the issue further, patient reports of symptom onset and the time recorded in the medical record often contain major discrepancies, with patient-reported times being significantly longer than times reported in the medical record.[4] Accurate delay times are important because they dictate whether the patient is eligible for revascularization and what type of therapy will be given. Additionally, the success of interventions aimed at reducing delay cannot be measured and compared adequately if the definition of delay is not consistent. Finally, research on the factors that influence delay is only valid if the method of measuring delay times is accurate.

Rationale for Not Delaying

The myocardium is highly dependent on oxygen for normal functioning. Under ordinary circumstances the blood flow to the heart muscle closely approximates the demand of that muscle in a variety of physiological conditions.[5] When an imbalance between supply and demand occurs as a result of the ACS disease process, a cascade of events is initiated, eventually leading to irreversible myocardial cell necrosis. Myocardial viability after a coronary occlusion is threatened and depends on the duration and severity of ischemia,[6] hence the popular phrase "time is muscle." Delay in seeking treatment is associated with increased myocardial damage and poor clinical outcomes.[7-10] More specifically, it has been shown that every 30 minutes of delay time increases the 1-year mortality risk by 7.5 percent.[7] This finding emphasizes the importance of early symptom recognition and prompt care seeking.

Extent of the Problem

Cardiovascular disease is a significant international health problem, and its major manifestation, ACS culminating in AMI, is the number one cause of death in developed countries.[11] For this reason, reducing delay time to definitive treatment could reduce death and disability substantially.

For purposes of understanding the delay process and designing interventions, total delay time often is divided into stages (Box 51-1). Significant strides have been made in the reduction of emergency medical system transport time and in hospital delay[12] because they are largely controllable by the health care system. However, the patient delay component has remained intractable. Patient delay also composes the largest component of the total delay period, making it the most visible target for interventions.

Median and mean delay times have changed little over the last two decades.[13] (Because of skewed distributions, delay time is reported most accurately as a median.) In one observational study examining temporal trends,[14] mean prehospital delay times decreased slightly (5.7 to 5.5 hours), possibly indicating that patients delaying very long periods are decreasing in number; however, median delay time (2.1 hours) did not change. In a longitudinal analysis of delay times in the

---

BOX 51-1
STAGES OF DELAY

- Patient (decision) delay = Symptom onset to first call for help
- Transport delay = Transportation time to hospital whether by self, other, or ambulance
- Hospital delay = Hospital arrival to treatment initiation (generally, angioplasty, thrombolysis, or coronary artery bypass graft surgery)

TABLE 51-1 FACTORS ASSOCIATED WITH INCREASED DELAY TIME IN ACUTE CORONARY SYNDROMES

FACTORS	COMMENTS
Sociodemographic	Older age
	Unmarried
	Lower socioeconomic status
	Some minority groups
	Diabetes
Situational factors[17-22]	Symptoms occur in the home
	Symptoms occur on weekends
	Lacking someone from whom to seek advice
	Generally more comfortable in seeking help
	Calling a physician before emergency medical services
Attitudes[17-19,23,24]	Not wanting to bother anyone
	Fear of the consequences of seeking help
	Fear of the loss of control
Symptom appraisal[17-19,22,24,25]	Gradual or intermittent onset of symptoms
	Wanting to see whether symptoms will go away
	Thinking symptoms are not serious
	Not attributing symptoms to the heart
	Low perceived risk for acute myocardial infarction
	Expectation that symptoms would be severe

GUSTO-1 and III trials from 1990 to 1997, time from symptom onset to hospital arrival remained stable.[12]

The greatest benefit from reperfusion therapies are realized when delay times are less than 1 hour.[9,12] In patients with the highest delay times (more than 4 to 6 hours) receiving reperfusion therapy, myocardial damage is indistinguishable from patients who receive no reperfusion therapy.[15] Mean and median delay times are the highest in non–ST segment elevation AMI (6.1 and 3.0 hours, respectively), followed by unstable angina (5.6 and 3.0 hours) and ST segment elevation AMI (4.7 and 2.3 hours).[3]

Internationally, delay times also remain high, although these times are difficult to compare with U.S. figures because of differences in health care systems, cultures, and protocols. One recent study reported median delay times greater than 2 hours in five diverse countries (Figure 51-1).[16]

Factors Associated with Delay

Over the last two decades, a number of factors associated with increased delay time have been identified definitely, yet others remain less clear. Table 51-1 describes some of these factors in more detail. Interestingly, it generally has been established that pain severity is not related to delay time[17,26] and that knowledge of

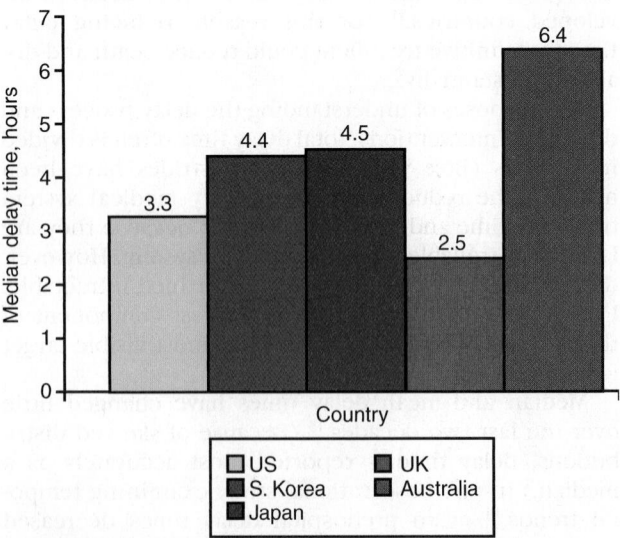

FIGURE 51-1 ■ Median prehospital delay times among patients seeking care for acute myocardial infarction in five countries. UK = United Kingdom; US = United States. (Data from Dracup K, Moser DK, McKinley S et al: *J Nurs Scholarsh* 35:317-323, 2003.)

AMI symptoms does not shorten delay.[18] Evidence as to whether lack of insurance does[12] or does not influence delay is conflicting.[27] In one study,[28] a number of community members in differing geographic regions were surveyed as to whether they would call the emergency medical response system (i.e., 911) promptly if confronted with a witnessed cardiac event. Although 89 percent said they would call promptly, in actuality only 23 percent did. It is important to understand the factors associated with patient delay in seeking treatment for cardiac symptoms and to be aware of them in clinical practice.

Although there is conflicting evidence as to whether women delay longer than men, studies have elucidated differences between genders in their symptom characteristics and how they respond to those symptoms. Women tend to have more atypical symptoms, making them more vulnerable to delay because of confusion and misidentification of the cause of the symptoms. Women more often experience vague symptoms such as unusual fatigue, sleep disturbances, shortness of breath, and weakness for the month preceding an AMI,[29] making symptom recognition difficult. More women than men experience their initial symptoms in the home and utilize emergency medical services for transport. For women, a history of a previous AMI results in shorter delay times compared with men, as does a Q wave infarction. More women than men feel that they do not want to trouble anyone, thereby increasing delay.[26] These and other gender distinctions are important and should be incorporated into the design and implementation of patient education programs by focusing on likely responses and providing anticipatory guidance to minimize delay in seeking treatment.

■ ■ ■

TABLE 51-2   INTERVENTIONS AIMED AT REDUCING DELAY TIME IN ACUTE CORONARY SYNDROME STUDIES

AUTHOR	LOCATION	YEAR	SAMPLE SIZE	RESULTS
Mitic and Perkins[31]	Eastern Canada	1982*	101 before 329 during 41 after	Delay reduction only in men
Ho et al.[32]	Washington	1986-1987	401 before 489 after	No change in patient delay
Moses et al.[33]	Midwest United States	1989*	Not stated	No change in patient delay
Herlitz et al.[34]	Sweden	1987-1988	2126 before 435 after	Delay reduced most notably in those with confirmed acute myocardial infarction; no change in ambulance use
Bett et al.[35]	Australia	1989	556 before 253 after	No change in patient delay
Gaspoz et al.[36]	Switzerland	1992-1993	1100 before 1295 after	Delay reduction only in men
Meischke et al.[37]	Washington	1991-1992	1343 control 4101 in three intervention groups	No change in patient delay
Luepker et al.[38]	20 cities/10 states	1995-1997	Reference group: 6051 before; 24,347 during Intervention group: 4582 before; 27,063 during	No change in patient delay Increased use of ambulances

*Year not stated; year given is an estimate.

Interventions to Reduce Delay

A number of studies were launched in the 1980s and 1990s that evaluated efforts to educate the public about symptoms of an AMI and the importance of seeking care quickly.[30] A wide variety of campaign methods (catchy slogans, emotional appeals, educational approaches) and media (television, radio, flyers, posters/billboards, brochures, newspapers, public speakers, mailings) targeted a variety of audiences (communities/countries, older/younger, high-risk populations). A key issue in comparing the education programs was differing "doses" of the intervention. Media campaigns ranged in duration from 1 week to 18 months, and each had differing amounts of coverage. With few exceptions, none have succeeded in reducing delay time. Few, if any, mass media campaigns to reduce delay have been launched since the late 1990s, probably owing to their lack of success. Table 51-2 describes some of the studies and their results, and the Conundrum box considers some possible reasons for failure of these programs.

Current Recommendations for Reducing Delay

What is now apparent is that mass media education campaigns have met with limited success and that more personalized education programs targeting high-risk patients (i.e., those with documented cardiovascular disease or those with two or more risk factors) might be more effective. In fact, the National Heart Attack Alert Program (designed by the National Heart, Lung, and Blood Institute of the National Institutes of Health) recommends this concept based on supporting literature.[39] Their Act in TIME campaign encourages health care providers to do the following:

- *T*alk to patients about their risk
- *I*nvestigate patients' feelings about heart attacks

■ ■ ■ CONUNDRUM

WHY HAVE DELAY-REDUCING INTERVENTIONS FAILED?

- Patient responses to symptoms of acute coronary syndrome are multifactorial, individual, and complex, making it difficult to personalize the message.
- Improving knowledge does not necessarily change behavior.
- Symptoms vary from patient to patient and from episode to episode, making it difficult to design generic education programs.
- There has been a failure to recognize the importance of prodromal symptoms and to educate the public about these symptoms.
- There has been a lack of emphasis on barriers to seeking care and how to overcome them.
- Presence of comorbidities makes it difficult for patients to evaluate symptoms.
- The use of mass media for educating the public has several limitations. Mass media are primarily for entertainment and advertising, not public health. Mass media compete with other public health causes, thereby diluting the message. Mass media are impersonal, which is counter to effective education. Evaluating the effectiveness of mass media education campaigns is difficult because of unavoidable contamination in the control group.[30]

- *M*ake a plan for action
- *E*valuate patients' understanding of AMI risks

Act in TIME targets the general public and health care providers by seeking to raise awareness about the importance of fast response to symptoms. More information may be found at *www.nhlbi.nih.gov/actintime/index.htm*. Box 51-2 lists characteristics of high-risk patients who might be targets for individualized instruction.

Significant new knowledge has been added in the last two decades regarding sociodemographic, cognitive, and psychosocial factors influencing care-seeking behavior and how these act as barriers to care. These factors must be an integral part in any education program whether individual, group, or community. Barriers to care must be addressed individually, along with definitive action plans to overcome these barriers.

Importantly, attempts at reducing delay must recognize the paradigm shift from thinking about coronary events as "heart attacks" to thinking about them as a continuous process from early vessel injury through total occlusion. New education programs need to emphasize identification and meaning of prodromal and stuttering symptoms and their importance to this continuum of disease process.

Targeted education and awareness around women's atypical symptoms should be addressed. This needs to occur with health care professionals and with women and their support networks because health care professionals can play an integral role in helping women identify and act on symptoms.

DELAY WITH SYMPTOMS OF WORSENING HEART FAILURE

Heart failure (**HF**) patients present a multifaceted, complex management challenge to health care providers. In contrast to ACS, HF is a chronic condition that requires daily self-care, monitoring, management, and timely response to symptoms in order to maintain clinical stability. However, HF patients do not perceive their symptoms as chronic, but rather as a series of acute events or exacerbations necessitating trips to the emergency department (**ED**) or the hospital for treatment of new symptom onset.[25] One study that exemplifies this problem demonstrated that most patients (more than 90 percent) presented to the ED in response to worsening symptoms rather than calling their health care provider when symptoms first emerged.[41] Therefore, symptom awareness, recognition, and timely response to worsen-

ing symptoms play a major role in preventing decompensation.

Rationale for Not Delaying

Delay in seeking treatment when HF symptoms worsen is important because prolonged periods of high cardiac filling pressure caused by fluid overload lead to increased myocardial damage and ventricular remodeling.[42] Fluid overload is a primary cause of hospital readmissions in HF patients.[25] The most common symptoms at hospital admission for HF (dyspnea and edema) are related to fluid overload. Prompt response to worsening symptoms prevents hospital readmissions, reduces cardiac remodeling, and improves survival.[43,44] Thus, a long delay time during periods of cardiac decompensation is costly to the patient's individual health status and to the health care system.

Extent of the Problem

HF is the number one cause of hospital readmission in patients over the age of 65.[45] Five million Americans are estimated to have HF, with roughly 550,000 new cases diagnosed every year. Annual hospital discharges from HF increased 175 percent for 1979 to 2004 to a total of 1,099.00.[53] Almost half of the patients discharged with a diagnosis of HF are readmitted within 6 months primarily because of exacerbation of symptoms, and this trend has not changed over the past decade.[46]

Although it has been shown that at least 20 percent of readmissions are related directly to the patient's failure to seek medical help in an appropriate amount of time,[47] few investigators have documented delay times in HF patients. Those who have documented delay times noted that patient response to worsening HF symptoms is poor. Median delay time from symptom onset to seeking care is noted consistently at 3 days[48,49] and can be longer than a week.[41,49] Delays of 8.4, 11.4, and 12.4 days have been reported when the chief symptom was dyspnea, weight gain, and edema, respectively.[41]

Despite considerable peripheral edema on admission to the ED, HF patients rarely identify weight gain as a warning sign,[25,49,50] even though HF guidelines and scientific statements recommend weighing daily. Most HF patients do not know the signs and symptoms of HF exacerbation.[41,49,50] In a study of hospitalized veterans with HF, it was found that only those with an acute onset of dyspnea responded quickly (i.e., less than 1 day).[48] Patients' inability to identify symptoms as being related to HF leads to frequent admissions to the ED, resulting in the need for costly crisis management for what might otherwise be a stable chronic condition.

Factors Associated with Delay

Although factors that affect delay in ACS patients have been studied exhaustively, there are few studies examining these characteristics in HF patients, a population that is growing exponentially in health care. The few studies to date have examined characteristics such as sociodemographic and psychosocial factors and real and perceived barriers to treatment as a reason for delay. A list of reported factors is provided in Table 51-3. Although the list is brief, it has clinical implications regarding patient education and follow-up. The ability to recognize symptoms and respond appropriately (i.e., contacting the health care provider at the onset of symptoms) is key to preventing decompensation.

Suggestions for Decreasing Delay

Some HF disease management programs may incorporate instructions about seeking care promptly; however, to date, no interventions that are aimed specifically at reducing delay in HF patients have been tested. Consequently, it is difficult to determine whether attention to this one component might be effective. Therefore, researchers, health care providers, and disease management program managers should examine factors influencing delay in HF patients so that they might be incorporated into interventions and education programs.

A first step toward reducing delay would be to gain a better understanding of the factors that influence delay and the barriers to patients seeking care. A second step would be the development and testing of HF-specific education programs that are sensitive to these influencing factors and barriers. For example, if patients are reluctant to call their physicians, they should be reassured that their physician wants to hear from them if their symptoms worsen. Additionally, helpful tools such as a script to use in speaking with the health care provider about increased symptoms could be provided that would enhance the communication and increase the chance of effecting a solution.

■ ■ ■

TABLE 51-3 FACTORS ASSOCIATED WITH INCREASED DELAY TIME IN HEART FAILURE

FACTORS	COMMENTS
Sociodemographic factors[41,48,49,51]	Unmarried
	Presence of dyspnea and edema
	Care provided by primary care provider
	Higher New York Heart Association class
	Absence of chest pain
	No previous heart failure hospital admission or newly diagnosed
	Cannot identify symptoms
Psychosocial[40]	Did not want to bother physicians, especially at night
	Did not want to be perceived as second-guessing their physician
	Feel too ill or debilitated to travel to physician's office
	No family to help identify symptoms and seek care
Perceived barriers[40]	Physicians do not return calls immediately
	Worry about waiting weeks for an appointment
	Multiple physicians make it difficult to know which one to call
	Concern that if they are not seen by the primary provider that the treatment regimens will change for the worse

Because most HF patients are cared for outside the specialty HF clinic setting, research and education programs must be adaptable to account for differences in settings, cultures, and primary care providers. Education programs should be simplified so they can be used by health care providers who are not cardiac specialists. Because HF care is multifaceted and often too complex for many patients to grasp, it is important that educational messages be distilled to the few key components that are likely to be the most beneficial to HF patients. Because of the magnitude of HF as a disease and the high rate of readmissions, self-care monitoring and prompt response to symptoms are key to successful management of this chronic condition.

SUMMARY

Delay in seeking treatment for cardiac symptoms, whether of ACS or HF, continues to be a major problem in cardiac care.[52] The problem has proved relatively intractable over the past two decades, despite an increased awareness of the problem and a variety of community-based education programs. If patients fail to seek care in a timely manner, interventions are compromised and clinical outcomes are poor. Thus, enhancing patients' ability to label cardiac symptoms accurately and seek care appropriately is an important goal for all health care professionals. One-on-one patient education in patients considered at high risk for a future cardiac event may be the most effective means of reducing delay and worthy of future research.

REFERENCES

1. Hackett TP, Cassem NH: Factors contributing to delay in responding to the signs and symptoms of acute myocardial infarction, *Am J Cardiol* 24:651-658, 1969.
2. Turi ZG, Stone PH, Muller JE et al: Implications for acute intervention related to time of hospital arrival in acute myocardial infarction, *Am J Cardiol* 58:203-209, 1986.
3. Goldberg RJ, Steg PG, Sadiq I et al: Extent of, and factors associated with, delay to hospital presentation in patients with acute coronary disease (the GRACE registry), *Am J Cardiol* 89:791-796, 2002.
4. Westbrook JI, McIntosh JH, Rushworth RL et al: Agreement between medical record data and patients' accounts of their medical history and treatment for dyspepsia, *J Clin Epidemiol* 51:237-244, 1998.
5. Lanza GA, Coli S, Cianflone D et al: Coronary blood flow and myocardial ischemia. In Fuster V, Alexander RW, O'Rourke RA, editors: *Hurst's the heart,* ed 11, New York, 2004, McGraw-Hill.
6. DeBoer LW, Rude RE, Kloner RA et al: A flow- and time-dependent index of ischemic injury after experimental coronary occlusion and reperfusion, *Proc Natl Acad Sci U S A* 80:5784-5788, 1983.
7. De Luca G, Suryapranata H, Ottervanger JP, Antman EM: Time delay to treatment and mortality in primary angioplasty for acute myocardial infarction: every minute of delay counts, *Circulation* 109:1223-1225, 2004.
8. Berger PB, Ellis SG, Holmes DR Jr et al: Relationship between delay in performing direct coronary angioplasty and early clinical outcome in patients with acute myocardial infarction: results from the global use of strategies to open occluded arteries in Acute Coronary Syndromes (GUSTO-IIb) trial, *Circulation* 100:14-20, 1999.
9. Fibrinolytic Therapy Trialists' Collaborative Group: Indications for fibrinolytic therapy in suspected acute myocardial infarction: collaborative overview of early mortality and major morbidity results from all randomised trials of more than 1000 patients, *Lancet* 343:311-322, 1994.

10. Gibson CM, Murphy SA, Kirtane AJ et al: Association of duration of symptoms at presentation with angiographic and clinical outcomes after fibrinolytic therapy in patients with ST-segment elevation myocardial infarction, *J Am Coll Cardiol* 44:980-987, 2004.

11. American Heart Association: *Heart disease and stroke statistics: 2005 update*, Dallas, 2004, The Association.

12. Gibler WB, Armstrong PW, Ohman ME et al: Persistence of delays in presentation and treatment for patients with acute myocardial infarction: the GUSTO-I and GUSTO-III experience, *Ann Emerg Med* 39:123-130, 2002.

13. Gibson CM: Time is myocardium and time is outcomes, *Circulation* 104:2632-2634, 2001.

14. Goldberg RJ, Gurwitz JH, Gore JM: Duration of, and temporal trends (1994-1997) in prehospital delay in patients with acute myocardial infarction: the second National Registry of Myocardial Infarction, *Arch Intern Med* 159:2141-2147, 1999.

15. Raitt MH, Maynard C, Wagner GS et al: Relation between symptom duration before thrombolytic therapy and final myocardial infarct size, *Circulation* 93:48-53, 1996.

16. Dracup K, Moser DK, McKinley SJ et al: An international perspective on the time to treatment for acute myocardial infarction, *J Nurs Scholarsh* 35:317-323, 2003.

17. Dracup K, Moser DK: Beyond sociodemographics: factors influencing the decision to seek treatment for symptoms of acute myocardial infarction, *Heart Lung* 26:253-262, 1997.

18. Pattenden J, Watt I, Lewin RJ, Stanford N: Decision making processes in people with symptoms of acute myocardial infarction: qualitative study, *BMJ* 324:1006-1009, 2002.

19. Burnett RE, Blumenthal JA, Mark DB et al: Distinguishing between early and late responders to symptoms of acute myocardial infarction, *Am J Cardiol* 75:1019-1022, 1995.

20. Epidemiology of avoidable delay in the care of patients with acute myocardial infarction in Italy: a GISSI-generated study—GISSI, Avoidable Delay Study Group, *Arch Intern Med* 155:1481-1488, 1995.

21. Ottesen MM, Kober L, Jorgensen S, Torp-Pedersen C: Determinants of delay between symptoms and hospital admission in 5978 patients with acute myocardial infarction: the TRACE Study Group—Trandolapril Cardiac Evaluation, *Eur Heart J* 17:429-437, 1996.

22. Johansson I, Stromberg A, Swahn E: Factors related to delay times in patients with suspected acute myocardial infarction, *Heart Lung* 33:291-300, 2004.

23. Dempsey SJ, Dracup K, Moser DK: Women's decision to seek care for symptoms of acute myocardial infarction, *Heart Lung* 24:444-456, 1995.

24. Kentsch M, Rodemerk U, Muller-Esch G: Emotional attitudes toward symptoms and inadequate coping strategies are major determinants of patient delay in acute myocardial infarction, *Z Kardiol* 91:147-155, 2002.

25. Finnegan JR, Meischke H, Zapka JG et al: Patient delay in seeking care for heart attack symptoms: findings from focus groups conducted in five US regions, *Prev Med* 31:205-213, 2000.

26. Moser DK, McKinley S, Dracup K, Chung ML: Gender differences in reasons patients delay in seeking treatment for acute myocardial infarction symptoms, *Patient Educ Couns* 56:45-54, 2005.

27. Ho PM, Rumsfeld JS, Lyons E et al: Lack of an association between Medicare supplemental insurance and delay in seeking emergency care for patients with myocardial infarction, *Ann Emerg Med* 40:381-387, 2002.

28. Brown AL, Mann NC, Daya M et al: Demographic, belief, and situational factors influencing the decision to utilize emergency medical services among chest pain patients: Rapid Early Action for Coronary Treatment (REACT) study, *Circulation* 102:173-178, 2000.

29. McSweeney JC, Cody M, O'Sullivan P et al: Women's early warning symptoms of acute myocardial infarction, *Circulation* 108:2619-2623, 2003.

30. Caldwell MA, Miaskowski C: Mass media interventions to reduce help-seeking delay in people with symptoms of acute myocardial infarction: time for a new approach? *Patient Educ Couns* 46:1-9, 2002.

31. Mitic WR, Perkins J: The effect of a media campaign on heart attack delay and decision times, *Can J Public Health* 75:414-418, 1984.

32. Ho MT, Eisenberg MS, Litwin PE et al: Delay between onset of chest pain and seeking medical care: the effect of public education, *Ann Emerg Med* 18:727-731, 1989.

33. Moses HW, Engelking N, Taylor GJ et al: Effect of a two-year public education campaign on reducing response time of patients with symptoms of acute myocardial infarction, *Am J Cardiol* 68:249-251, 1991.

34. Herlitz J, Hartford M, Blohm M et al: Effect of a media campaign on delay times and ambulance use in suspected acute myocardial infarction, *Am J Cardiol* 64:90-93, 1989.

35. Bett N, Aroney G, Thompson P: Impact of a national educational campaign to reduce patient delay in possible heart attack, *Aust N Z J Med* 23:157-161, 1993.

36. Gaspoz JM, Unger PF, Urban P et al: Impact of a public campaign on pre-hospital delay in patients reporting chest pain, *Heart* 76:150-155, 1996.

37. Meischke H, Dulberg EM, Schaeffer SS et al: 'Call fast, call 911': a direct mail campaign to reduce patient delay in acute myocardial infarction, *Am J Public Health* 87:1705-1709, 1997.

38. Luepker RV, Raczynski JM, Osganian S et al: Effect of a community intervention on patient delay and emergency medical service use in acute coronary heart disease: the Rapid Early Action for Coronary Treatment (REACT) Trial, *JAMA* 284:60-67, 2000.

39. Dracup K, Alonzo AA, Atkins JM et al: The physician's role in minimizing prehospital delay in patients at high risk for acute myocardial infarction: recommendations from the National Heart Attack Alert Program—Working Group on Educational Strategies to Prevent Prehospital Delay in Patients at High Risk for Acute Myocardial Infarction, *Ann Intern Med* 126:645-651, 1997.

40. Horowitz CR, Rein SB, Leventhal H: A story of maladies, misconceptions and mishaps: effective management of heart failure, *Soc Sci Med* 58:631-643, 2004.

41. Schiff GD, Fung S, Speroff T, McNutt RA: Decompensated heart failure: symptoms, patterns of onset, and contributing factors, *Am J Med* 114:625-630, 2003.

42. Mann DL: Mechanisms and models in heart failure: a combinatorial approach, *Circulation* 100:999-1008, 1999.

43. Happ MB, Naylor MD, Roe-Prior P: Factors contributing to rehospitalization of elderly patients with heart failure, *J Cardiovasc Nurs* 11:75-84, 1997.

44. Dracup K: *Educational strategies to prevent prehospital delay in patients at high risk for acute myocardial infarction*, Pub #97-3787, Bethesda, Md, 1997, National Institutes of Health.

45. DeFrances CJ, Hall MJ: 2002 *National Hospital Discharge Survey: advance data from vital and health statistics*, Hyattsville, Md, 2004, National Center for Health Statistics.

46. Krumholz HM, Parent EM, Tu N et al: Readmission after hospitalization for congestive heart failure among Medicare beneficiaries, *Arch Intern Med* 157:99-104, 1997.

47. Vinson JM, Rich MW, Sperry JC et al: Early readmission of elderly patients with congestive heart failure, *J Am Geriatr Soc* 38:1290-1295, 1990.

48. Evangelista LS, Dracup K, Doering LV: Treatment-seeking delays in heart failure patients, *J Heart Lung Transplant* 19:932-938, 2000.

49. Friedman MM: Older adults' symptoms and their duration before hospitalization for heart failure, *Heart Lung* 26:169-176, 1997.

50. Wright SP, Walsh H, Ingley KM et al: Uptake of self-management strategies in a heart failure management programme, *Eur J Heart Fail* 5:371-380, 2003.

51. Artinian NT, Magnan M, Sloan M, Lange MP: Self-care behaviors among patients with heart failure, *Heart Lung* 31:161-172, 2002.

52. Moser DK, Kimble LP, Alberts MJ et al: Reducing delay in seeking treatment by patients with acute coronary syndrome and stroke: A scientific statement from the American Heart Association Council on Cardiovascular Nursing and Stroke Council. *Circulation* 114:168-182, 2006.

53. Rosamund W, Flegal K, Friday G et al: Heart disease and strokes, statistics—2007 update: A report from the American Heart Association Statistics Committee and Stroke Statistics Subcommittee. *Circulation* 115(5):169-171, 2007.

Women and Cardiovascular Disease

Jean C. McSweeney
Leanne L. Lefler

CHAPTER ABBREVIATIONS

BMI	body mass index
CHD	coronary heart disease
CRP	C-reactive protein
ECG	electrocardiogram
HDL	high-density lipoprotein
HRT	hormone replacement therapy
LDL	low-density lipoprotein
MI	myocardial infarction
POS	polycystic ovarian syndrome

Cardiovascular diseases, including coronary heart disease (**CHD**), are the leading cause of death in women and claim one woman's life in the United States every minute.[1] Minority women are disproportionately at risk of developing CHD compared with their white counterparts.[1,2] Additionally, when black women experience a myocardial infarction (**MI**), they have up to a 50 percent higher rate of death than white women.[1,3] However, outcomes of MI in women of all races remain problematic because women are more likely than men (38 percent versus 25 percent) to die within 1 year of having an MI and approximately twice as likely as men to be disabled with heart failure after MI.[1,4] This trend continues up to 6 years after MI, with 35 percent of women compared with 18 percent of men experiencing another MI.[5]

Although women develop CHD approximately 10 years later than men, CHD is increasing in younger women, with more than 9000 women younger than age 45 having an MI each year.[5] Sudden death occurs more often in women than men—63 percent versus 50 percent, respectively—with death as the initial symptom of CHD.[6] In a large prospective study, 94 percent of the women experiencing sudden cardiac death had at least one modifiable risk factor for CHD.[7] This indicates that early recognition and modification of risk factors may assist in reducing sudden cardiac events in women.

Despite these alarming statistics, much of the evidence that supports current prevention, diagnosis, and treatment for CHD is extrapolated from clinical trials of primarily middle-aged male subjects.[8,9] Although women now constitute approximately 38 percent of subjects in mixed-sex CHD studies, they continue to be underrepresented in CHD diagnostic studies, thus limiting the usefulness of the findings in women.[9] Much remains to be learned about screening, diagnosing, and treating women effectively,[6] although clinicians are becoming more cognizant of the magnitude of CHD in women and the importance of early prevention.[10] Other promising works include establishing sex-related risk factors,[11] early detection of CHD,[12] and identification of women's prodromal symptoms of MI[13] and other areas.[14]

Despite recent advances, many obstacles remain that affect CHD in women. Identification of sex-specific differences is vitally important at every level, including cellular, because this may provide clues as to why diseases such as CHD and treatments may affect men and women differently. Professionals now are recognizing a multitude of sex differences. For instance, 8 of 10 prescription drugs recently removed from the market precipitated more adverse events in women than men.[5]

CHD in women is a multifaceted problem that requires a multipronged approach to eliminate the disparity in women's mortality and disability rates, treatment options, and ethnic outcomes after MI. The following brief review of obstacles affecting women shows their diverse barriers and how these barriers interfere with early detection, diagnosis, and treatment of CHD in women.

OBSTACLES TO DETECTION, DIAGNOSIS, AND TREATMENT
Lack of Perception of Risk

Many women do not appreciate their vulnerability or recognize the seriousness of CHD in women. A survey conducted in the United States indicates that women's knowledge of CHD as the leading cause of death and morbidity significantly improved from 30 percent in 1997 to 46 percent in 2003.[15] However, minority and younger women—who may benefit most from risk reduction—reported less awareness of their risk than their white, older counterparts. Although awareness increased in this sample, less than 50 percent identified CHD as women's major health problem, and only 13 percent identified CHD as their own greatest health risk. More than 90 percent of the women stated that they could discuss preventive measures comfortably with their health care providers, but only 38 percent actually had discussed CHD. Therefore, despite increasing awareness by women of CHD as their major health problem, few are personalizing the information, and providers are missing opportunities to discuss CHD prevention. If women remain unaware of their own risk for developing CHD, they are unlikely to modify behavior to decrease potential risks. One prime method to increase awareness is for providers to use every opportunity during clinical encounters to increase awareness and promote CHD risk factor modification in women.[4,15]

Health Care Issues

Lack of health care, health insurance, and access to care are problematic. The Kaiser Women's Survey reported that the most important barriers to women of all races were affordability, no insurance coverage, and inability to take time for an appointment because of caretaking and other family responsibilities.[2] These barriers resulted in up to 32 percent not seeing a clinician when they perceived a need existed and 25 percent not filling a prescription because of the cost of the medication. Women also identified lack of transportation, child care problems, access to specialists, and continuity of care with a known provider as access problems.

Health insurance rates vary by race, with uninsured rates of 16 percent for white, 20 percent for black, and 37 percent for Hispanic women.[2] Approximately 50 percent of the sampled women had employer-based health insurance, but government programs were also an important source of coverage for lower-income minority women. Thus access to health care and lack of health insurance are important barriers, especially for minority women who are most at risk for developing CHD and MI. Clearly, if at-risk women cannot access health care for preventive services, establish a personal risk profile, afford medications to control risk factors, and have little continuity with providers, it will be difficult to increase women's personal perception of CHD risk, maintain vigilance of their risk status, and take appropriate health actions. Indeed, it will be difficult to influence women's CHD status substantially unless society is able to break this trend of minorities and women being most likely to be uninsured, having inadequate access to care, and being most at risk for high rates of mortality, morbidities, and disability after MI.

Delay in Seeking Treatment

Current treatment for acute MI is reperfusion therapy, which if administered soon after onset of symptoms, is highly effective in resolving coronary occlusion and may reduce or eliminate myocardial damage. A sevenfold decrease in mortality exists in patients treated within 70 minutes of symptom onset, but most delay seeking treatment for an average of 2 to 4 hours from symptom onset. Treatment delay strongly correlates with increased mortality and disability. Numerous studies and analyses[16] indicate that women delay seeking treatment longer than men for symptoms of MI. The sociodemographic profile of those most likely to delay appears in Box 52-1.[17] A meta-synthesis identified sex-specific factors associated with women's treatment-seeking delay that included the following[16]:

- Vague atypical symptoms not perceived as serious or attributed to the heart
- Lack of knowledge regarding CHD symptoms
- Self-treating rather than seeking medical assistance

Other barriers and psychosocial factors that may influence delay in seeking treatment are discussed previously in this chapter.

BOX 52-1 ■ ■ ■

FACTORS AFFECTING PREHOSPITAL DELAY IN PATIENTS WITH SYMPTOMS OF MYOCARDIAL INFARCTION

Factors Contributing to Increased Delay
- Older age
- Female gender
- Black race
- Low socioeconomic status
- Low emotional or somatic awareness
- History of angina, diabetes, or both
- Consulting a spouse or other relative
- Consulting a physician
- Self-treatment

Factors Contributing to Decreased Delay
- Hemodynamic instability
- Large infarct size
- Sudden onset of severe chest pain
- Recognition by patient that symptoms are heart related
- Consulting a friend, coworker, or stranger

From National Heart, Lung, and Blood Institute: *Educational strategies to prevent prehospital delay in patients at high risk for acute myocardial infarction*, Pub No 97-3787, Bethesda, Md, 1997, National Institutes of Health.

Provider Bias

Although controversy exists about the extent of bias in medical research and treatment for women, most experts agree that bias does exist.[18,19] Compelling evidence exists of treatment bias for women's CHD extending for the last 10 years.[20] This is especially true in primary and secondary prevention of CHD and MI because women often are treated to suboptimal levels[21] and receive less aggressive treatment when experiencing MI.[22] In addition, providers have been less likely to evaluate women's symptoms aggressively to determine whether they are cardiac-related. Some reports indicate that women are not taken seriously by providers and that possible CHD symptoms are overlooked, misdiagnosed, or treated with antianxiety medications.[23,24] However, even when providers recommend CHD diagnostic tests, lack of specificity and sensitivity of diagnostic tests in women compound this problem. For instance, when women have chest pain and undergo routine cardiovascular diagnostic testing, they are just as likely to have CHD as not to have CHD. This increases the likelihood that clinicians may dismiss chest pain in women as insignificant and order no further evaluation. Another problem facing providers is that insurance companies and health maintenance organizations require patients to report specific symptoms, such as chest pain, before authorizing diagnostic tests. Because women often do not experience chest pain, they do not meet criteria and are not referred for further evaluation.[12] However, even among women who experience typical cardiac symptoms, men consistently are referred more frequently for cardiac imaging,[9] angiography,[25] and coronary artery bypass surgery.[20] Additionally, Sweitzer and Douglas[26] state, "Less aggressive treatment strategies in women do not represent optimal care, nor can they be attributed solely to the difficulties in diagnosing CHD in women" (p. 1956). These practice differences are attributed to bias, which must be recognized and eliminated before women may receive equal and optimal care for possible CHD symptoms.

CORONARY HEART DISEASE RISK FACTORS IN WOMEN

Women and men share common modifiable CHD risk factors. However, women have a greater number of co-occurring risk factors than men, and minority women have more risk factors than white women (Box 52-2).[27] Common CHD risk factors such as smoking and physical inactivity are well known, but only recently have researchers begun to investigate sex and racial differences. For instance, hypertension is a greater risk factor for women than men,[28] and diabetes increases CHD risk for women 3 to 7 times compared with 2 to 3 times for men.[29] Coronary risk factors also vary by age. Women older than age 65, compared with men and younger women, have more hypertension, lipid abnormalities, type 2 diabetes, obesity, and less physical activity. Therefore, risk factors in women differ by race and age and may influence CHD symptom presentation.[27,30-32]

Nurses are often in a position to gain a holistic perspective of each woman's health issues. This perspective fosters identification of each woman's risk factors associated with her various disease processes. This allows nurses to identify barriers and to tailor interventions that may help each woman make behavioral modifications to modify her CHD risk factors and to start appropriate treatment for her risk factors. Nurses are also in a prime position to provide education and counseling about CHD risk factor prevention to women's groups and communities. Earlier and more aggressive measures to control or eliminate CHD risk factors are essential to improve women's CHD outcomes.[5]

BOX 52-2   ■ ■ ■
RISK FACTORS FOR CARDIOVASCULAR DISEASE

Modifiable Risk Factors
- Smoking
- Dyslipidemia
  - Raised low-density lipoprotein level
  - Low high-density lipoprotein level
  - Raised triglyceride level
- Hypertension
- Diabetes mellitus
- Overweight and obesity
- Diet
- Physical inactivity

Nonmodifiable Risk Factors
- Older age
- Sex
  - Male with higher risk
- Heredity
  - Family history of premature coronary heart disease
  - Race

Cigarette Smoking

The leading modifiable CHD risk factor in women is cigarette smoking, which triples the risk of MI, even in premenopausal women. Currently, 21 percent of U.S. women smoke. Smoking is dose-dependent, with the more cigarettes smoked, the greater the risk, more than doubling the relative risk in women compared with 1.43 for men. On average, men are 7 years younger than nonsmokers at first MI, whereas women smokers are an astonishing 19 years younger than nonsmokers.[33] Additionally, women smokers who use oral contraceptives[34] or who are diabetic[35] have a significantly greater risk of having an MI than nonsmoking women with these characteristics, increasing their relative risk up to sevenfold. To combat the smoking problem, the U.S. Public Health Service published *Treating Tobacco Use and Dependence*[36] to provide comprehensive, clinically effective and cost-effective cessation materials for clinicians and patients. Clinicians should stress that risk of CHD events is substantially and rapidly reversible with smoking cessation.

Hyperlipidemia

Elevated serum total cholesterol, elevated low-density lipoprotein (**LDL**), and low high-density lipoprotein (**HDL**) levels are major CHD risk factors for women. Greater percentages of women than men have high total cholesterol, triglyceride, and/or LDL levels, imparting greater CHD risk and mortality for women. Research suggests that in older women (age 65 and older), low HDL and high triglyceride levels may be better indicators of CHD risk than other lipid values.[37] A recent meta-analysis indicated hypertriglycemia as an independent predictor of CHD events, especially in older women, that was independent of LDL and HDL levels.[38] Lipid-lowering therapy has been effective in improving women's lipid levels. Box 52-3 shows recommended serum lipid goals for women with and without CHD. A large evidence-based systematic review estimated that therapy could reduce women's risk of CHD mortality by 25 to 35 percent[8] and that reducing dietary fats could decrease the number of CHD events in women.[39] However, disparities persist, with women being treated less frequently than men for elevated lipid levels.[40]

Metabolic Syndrome

The National Cholesterol Education Program Adult Treatment Panel III guideline for cholesterol management defines the metabolic syndrome as the presence of three or more of the following conditions[41]:
- Abdominal obesity
- Glucose intolerance
- Hypertension
- Hypertriglyceridemia
- Low HDL level

Table 52-1 lists specific values. High triglyceride combined with low HDL cholesterol levels are hallmarks of the metabolic syndrome. This syndrome is

BOX 52-3
RECOMMENDED LIPID GOALS FOR WOMEN ■ ■ ■

Women Without Coronary Heart Disease (CHD)
- Less than two CHD risk factors: Goal is low-density lipoprotein (LDL) less than 160 mg/dl.
- Two or more CHD risk factors: Goal is LDL less than 130 mg/dl.
- Total cholesterol less than 200 mg/dl and high-density lipoprotein (HDL) greater than 45 mg/dl: Follow up in 5 years.
- Total cholesterol less than 200 mg/dl and HDL less than 45 mg/dl: Follow up with fasting lipoprotein analysis.
- Total cholesterol 200 to 239 mg/dl, HDL greater than 45 mg/dl, and less than two risk factors: Follow up in 1 to 2 years.
- Total cholesterol 200 to 239 mg/dl, HDL less than 45 mg/dl, or more than two risk factors: Follow up with fasting lipoprotein analysis.
- Total cholesterol greater than 240 mg/dl: Follow up with fasting lipoprotein analysis.

Women with Coronary Heart Disease
- LDL less than 100 mg/dl (70 mg/dl in very high-risk patients)
- HDL greater than 50 mg/dl
- Triglycerides less than 150 mg/dl
- Non-HDL less than 130 mg/dl

From Grundy SM, Cleeman JI, Merz CN et al: *J Am Coll Cardiol* 44:720-732, 2004. (Also available from www.nhlbi.nih.gov/guidelines/cholesterol/atp3upd04.htm)

■ ■ ■

TABLE 52-1 DIAGNOSIS OF METABOLIC SYNDROME*

RISK FACTOR	DEFINING LEVEL
Abdominal obesity	Waist circumference greater than 88 cm (35 inches)
Triglyceride level	150 mg/dl or higher
High-density lipoprotein cholesterol level	Less than 50 mg/dl
Blood pressure	135/85 mm Hg or higher
Fasting glucose level	110 mg/dl or higher

*Three of the following characteristics are required for diagnosis.
From Grundy SM, Cleeman JI, Merz CN et al: *J Am Coll Cardiol* 44:720-732, 2004. (Also available at www.nhlbi.nih.gov/guidelines/cholesterol/atp3upd04.htm)

highly associated with insulin resistance and increased risk of CHD independent of LDL level. Metabolic syndrome is more prevalent in older women than in men and substantially increases CHD mortality. Metabolic syndrome is associated with a greater CHD risk in women (12 percent than in men 2.2 percent).[38,42] Currently, the goals for treatment of metabolic syndrome are the same as for treating underlying conditions such as dyslipidemia and obesity.

Postmenopausal Status

In women undergoing natural menopause, the risk for CHD gradually increases. Surgical menopause causes an abrupt increase in risk. The loss of estrogen increases total cholesterol and LDL levels and decreases HDL, all of which independently increase women's CHD risk. Although exogenous hormone replacement therapy **(HRT)** previously was prescribed to decrease CHD risk, findings from the Women's Health Initiative indicate that HRT does not prevent and actually may increase the risk for a CHD event.[43] However, HRT remains beneficial in preventing osteoporosis and minimizing menopausal symptoms. Clinicians should discuss benefits and risks of HRT with each woman but stress that HRT is not indicated for primary or secondary prevention of CHD.

Physical Inactivity

Physical inactivity is a major independent risk factor for CHD in women. Unfortunately, more than 40 percent of Hispanic, 34 percent of black, and 22 percent of white women report no leisure time physical activity, with percentages increasing as women age.[1] Residents in the southern and western United States, especially in rural areas, report the highest rates of physical inactivity.[44] Hypertension, obesity, glucose intolerance, and hyperlipidemia, all more prevalent in sedentary women, exert an independent and combined increased CHD risk. Increasing physical activity is associated with a 20 to 25 percent reduction in mortality and reduces CHD events by 50 percent at the primary and secondary levels.[37,45] This reduction of CHD mortality in physically active persons is rooted biologically in the increased ability of the body to use oxygen, the antithrombotic effect of exercise through a decrease of platelet adhesiveness, a favorable modulation of autonomic balance, and improvements in endothelial function and lipid profiles.[46] Physical activity also has positive effects on other risk factors for CHD because it lowers blood pressure, reduces weight, increases HDL level, and aids in preventing type 2 diabetes. Data from a cohort of the Nurses' Health Study indicate that brisk walking and vigorous exercise are associated with similar and considerable reductions in women's CHD events if performed most days of the week.[45] Thus maintaining a regular physical activity program is a core component of effective CHD prevention.

Hypertension

The "Seventh Report of the Joint Committee on Prevention, Detection, Evaluation, and Treatment of High Blood Pressure" defines categorical hypertension as a systolic blood pressure of 140 mm Hg or greater, a diastolic pressure of 90 mm Hg or greater, or current use of antihypertensive medication.[47] Hypertension is a powerful predictor of CHD in women. The high prevalence of hypertension in women is associated with a twofold to threefold increase in risk for a CHD event. Older women, especially black women, have an increased risk for developing hypertension,[27,30] but most are unaware of their increased risk and the relationships between risk factors.[48] The relationship between blood pressure and the risk of CHD events is continuous, consistent, and independent of other risk factors in a level-dependent relationship, meaning that the higher the blood pressure, the higher the risk of CHD.[47] Treatment for hypertension yields a 20 to 25 percent reduction in incidence of MI and 50 percent in incidence of heart failure. Treatment guidelines for hypertension are similar for men and women.[47]

Obesity

In 1998, obesity was added as a major modifiable risk factor for CHD. The prevalence of overweight/obesity is increasing at epidemic proportions, with a twofold to threefold increase in the last several decades. In data released in 2005,[1] 57 percent of white, 77 percent of black, and 72 percent of Hispanic women were overweight (body mass index [**BMI**] of 25 kg/m^2 or above) with 31, 49, and 38 percent, respectively, considered obese (BMI of 30 kg/m^2 or above). Obesity has an independent and moderating effect on other conditions such as hypertension, diabetes, and dyslipidemia, and it contributes to an increased incidence of congestive heart failure, stroke, and other conditions. Prospective research data indicate that obese women have a 35 to 60 percent greater risk of developing CHD than do women of average body weight.[49] Obesity also negatively affects total cholesterol, LDL, HDL, and triglyceride levels; blood pressure; insulin resistance; and platelet aggregation. Therefore a reduction in BMI is associated with improved lipid levels across the spectrum. The Nurses' Health Study reported that a diet high in fruits, vegetables, whole grains, poultry, and fish and low in refined grains and red meats significantly lowers CHD risk and incidence of obesity.[50] Besides recommending diet modification, nurses should encourage women to increase daily activity to assist with weight reduction.

Diabetes Mellitus

Diabetes is a coronary risk equivalent, meaning that diabetic patients are in the same risk category as persons previously diagnosed with CHD. Diabetes increases one's risk of experiencing a CHD event by 5 to 7 times.[51] Regardless of weight, women age 45 and over are twice as likely as men to develop type 2 diabetes. The risk for CHD mortality is 2.6 times greater in diabetic than in nondiabetic women. Diabetes imparts a relative risk of CHD event that is twice in women what it is in men.[37] Although the primary mechanism for this sex difference is unclear, one reason may be that women have a greater number or severity of other CHD risk factors. Diabetes contributes to worsening lipid profiles and microvascular and endothelial damage and often results in hypertension. Unfortunately, more than 80 percent of diabetic patients die of CHD. Hu and colleagues[52] reported that women with CHD and diabetes were approximately 18 times more likely to die of CHD than women without the conditions. Risk-reduction strategies for diabetic women focusing on lifestyle modification and glucose management are effective in reducing CHD mortality and morbidity.

Socioeconomic Status and Education

Overall, CHD risk factors are more prevalent in those with low incomes, and they have a twofold to fourfold increased risk of a CHD event compared with those at higher socioeconomic levels.[53] In addition, women of lower socioeconomic status have a significantly higher prevalence of physical inactivity, smoking, and obesity than more affluent women. A study of middle-income women[54] found that black women had significantly more risk factors than white women, indicating that black women, regardless of socioeconomic status, continue to be more at risk for CHD. Black women and other minorities are more at risk because they have higher rates of physical inactivity, hypertension, diabetes, and obesity than white women.[27]

A low educational level carries a risk of CHD mortality comparable to traditional risk factors. Persons with fewer than 12 years of education are at higher absolute risk of death from CHD than more educated individuals.[55] The Behavioral Risk Factor Surveillance System 2005 report confirms that college graduates versus those with less than a high school education differed in presence of multiple CHD risk factors, 26 to 53 percent, respectively.[56] Additionally, household income levels also followed this prevalence pattern, indicating considerable disparities in risk factors among socioeconomic groups and racial/ethnic populations. To decrease the morbidity and mortality from CHD, public health programs are needed to identify and intervene with the most at-risk populations.

Emerging and Novel Risk Factors

Depression recently has gained attention as an emerging risk factor for CHD[57] and as a predictor of outcome after MI.[58] In a review of the literature, Bunker and colleagues[59] concluded that there was strong and consistent evidence of an independent causal relationship. One study reported that depression confers a greater risk than passive smoking (1.64 versus 1.25, respectively).[60] Although the exact association between depression and CHD is unknown, depression is associated with heightened expression of inflammatory markers such as C-reactive protein. Platelet dysfunction and autonomic dysregulation also are possible pathogenic mechanisms for end-organ damage in depressed CHD patients.[61] Chrysohoou and colleagues[28] examined sex differences in risk of MI and found a greater association between depression and CHD risk in women than in men. Others also have concluded that depression was a more important risk factor for CHD in women than in men.[28,62] In a community-based study of initially CHD-free women, Ferketich and colleagues[63] reported an adjusted relative risk of CHD incidence among depressed women at 1.73 compared with women without depression.

Preliminary evidence also suggests that polycystic ovarian syndrome may be an emerging risk factor for CHD in women.[64] Research into the association of polycystic ovarian syndrome and CHD should be a high priority, given its relative high prevalence in women.[65] (See the accompanying evidence-based practice feature.)

Novel markers of CHD risk are currently under investigation, including C-reactive protein (**CRP**), homocysteine, lipoprotein (a), apolipoproteins A-I and B, and others (Box 52-4). In response to arterial disease, CRP (an inflammatory biomarker produced in smooth muscle cells of coronary arteries) is released. CRP can be measured accurately and inexpensively. CRP may be used along with lipid profiles for risk prediction. In-

POLYCYSTIC OVARIAN SYNDROME

An emerging risk factor for coronary heart disease (CHD), poly-cystic ovarian syndrome (**POS**) affects between 5 and 10 percent of premenopausal women. POS is characterized by a decrease in insulin sensitivity similar to those with type 2 diabetes, an elevated body mass index, and dysfibrinolysis. POS is defined as an androgen excess with ovulatory dysfunction (fewer than six menstrual cycles per year), and it contributes to elevated plasma levels of tissue plasminogen activator (t-PA antigen), which is associated with disturbed fibrinolysis and endothelial dysfunction—both independently linked to risk for CHD. Based on a small study of 17 women with POS and 15 controls matched for body mass index, the POS group had significantly increased t-PA concentrations ($p = 0.013$). In other studies, high levels of t-PA antigen correlated with CHD severity as measured by angiography and with acute CHD events. The researchers conclude that because of the relatively high prevalence of POS in women, POS should be looked at closely for its link to elevated t-PA levels and increased CHD mortality seen in young women.[64]

BOX 52-4   ■ ■ ■
WOMEN'S EMERGING AND NOVEL RISK FACTORS FOR CORONARY HEART DISEASE

- Depression
- Polycystic ovarian syndrome
- C-reactive protein
- Homocysteine
- Lipoprotein (a)
- Apolipoproteins A-I and B

creased levels of serum CRP have been associated with greater risk of CHD events and independently have predicted future CHD events in men and women.[66,67] However, elevated CRP levels also predict all-cause mortality and may not be specific to CHD. Unfortunately, evidence is lacking to confirm that lowering CRP levels will lower CHD risk.[68] Elevated homocysteine levels are modest CHD predictors for men and women, although insufficient sex-related evidence is available. Elevated lipoprotein (a) levels appear to have a strong association with increased risk for CHD events, although sex-based studies have not been performed. Evidence is lacking regarding associations of apolipoproteins A-I and B to CHD risk, especially with regard to sex.

In summary, additional research is needed with emerging and novel risk factors to understand fully their influence on increasing women's CHD risk. As research evolves, important sex differences may become evident, but current findings are limited. For a more in-depth discussion of novel risk factors and their usefulness in diagnosing CHD, see appropriate chapters in this textbook.

CARDIOVASCULAR ANATOMY AND PHYSIOLOGY

Anatomical and physiological differences between men and women, as well as CHD risk factors, provide ample reasons to believe that sex differences in CHD and MI symptoms exist. Limited research had been conducted related to sex differences in the cardiovascular system,

but it was not until the Institute of Medicine released a report—*Exploring the Biological Contributions to Human Health: Does Sex Matter?*—that these differences gained widespread attention.[19] This report advised researchers and clinicians to monitor sex differences and similarities in diseases, such as CHD, at all levels—including cellular level, pathophysiology, diagnosis, treatment, and prevention. This report and others noted important sex differences in cardiovascular anatomy and physiology that may influence CHD sex differences in risk factors, symptom presentation, and response to noninvasive diagnostic tests and long-term outcomes following an event such as MI.[26,69] After the reproductive system, the cardiovascular system is most affected by sex differences.[26] For instance, women have smaller coronary arteries and more breast tissue that may interfere with CHD diagnostic scanning[70] and are more likely than men to have lower hematocrit levels, higher estrogen levels, mitral valve prolapse, and left ventricular hypertrophy, all of which may result in false positives or nonspecific electrocardiogram (**ECG**) changes.[71] Additionally, endothelial dysfunction, which appears to be associated with poor MI outcome, is influenced by sex hormones,[72,73] and sex differences exist in myocardial blood flow with women having known CHD risk factors demonstrating higher resting and hyperemic flow than men with similar risks.[74] Numerous other physiological sex differences exist,[69,70,75] such as in the renin-angiotensin system[69] and the autonomic nervous system.[76] Schwertz and Penckofer[77] formulated a review of studies focusing on sex hormones and their effect on hemostasis and vascular reactivity, which provides a wealth of information on this topic, and a 2005 review by Wu and von Eckardstein[65] focuses on androgens and CHD.

Mechanisms that lead to development of CHD in women may differ from those in men because women tend to have more metabolic syndrome and microvasculature disease, leading to angina.[26,78] Additionally, because women are typically older than men when they develop CHD, they often have more comorbidities that add to the diagnostic confusion. A meta-synthesis investigating delay in seeking treatment for MI reported that women with comorbidities delayed seeking treatment longer than women without them, indicating that comorbidities influence women's perceptions of their symptoms and also may affect clinicians' diagnosis of CHD.[16] It is well-known that women have more silent MIs than men, indicating that women may have no or very mild symptoms with MI or women mistakenly may attribute MI symptoms to their other comorbidities.

INFLUENCES ON RECOGNITION AND INTERPRETATION OF CORONARY HEART DISEASE SYMPTOMS

The media are an important source of health information to women[15] and typically have promoted MI as causing severe chest pain followed by collapse. In patients admitted for their first MI, researchers queried them regarding their prior expectation of MI symptoms.[79] They reported expecting central chest pain; radiating arm, neck, and/or shoulder pain; and collapse. Less than

7 percent identified the more atypical symptoms of dyspnea, nausea, vomiting, or dizziness as possible MI symptoms. However, in one of the most thorough studies to date, these atypical symptoms were the ones reported most frequently by women with MI.[13] Thus those who do not experience chest pain during MI often fail to recognize their other symptoms as indicative of MI and delay seeking treatment longer compared with those with chest pain.[79,80] However, the media continues to portray the primary symptom of MI as severe chest pain, and in response to this message, women delay seeking treatment when chest pain is not present. Recent lay literature for women now is including other symptoms and stating that severe chest pain may or may not be present in women experiencing MI. These updated materials may begin to help women recognize possible CHD and MI symptoms in a timelier manner.

Race and cultural interpretation are also powerful influences on symptom descriptions,[81] and if the clinician is of a different race and/or culture, women's choice of symptom descriptors may further compound the challenge of diagnosing CHD and MI.[82] Whether chest pain or atypical CHD and MI symptoms are present, race and culture also may influence women's expectations of and responses to symptoms,[83,84] as do many other factors, such as prior experience with similar symptoms, perceived risk, and socioeconomic factors.[85] For example, blacks and whites report significantly different expectations of MI symptoms and reasons for delay in seeking treatment.[83,86] Pain perception and differences between races also have been reported. In a study of black and white participants with a history of chronic pain, blacks reported significantly greater pain than whites in perceived severity of pain and pain-related disability.

Racial differences in perception of pain are especially relevant to chest pain. Klingler and colleagues[87] focused on racial differences in the perception of chest pain symptoms in black and white patients in the emergency room. Although both groups had similar symptoms, the black participants were more likely to view their symptoms as severe or life threatening. Other studies compared CHD symptoms in black and white women presenting to the emergency room and documented differences in reported symptoms, such as chest pain, shortness of breath, fatigue, and dizziness, with black women reporting more symptoms than white women.[81,88] These findings provide justification for examining racial differences in women's CHD symptoms and offer the possibility that symptoms may vary by race and/or culture. This should alert clinicians to the possibility that different cultures and races may describe or interpret CHD symptoms differently. Provider bias, as discussed before, also exerts a strong influence on interpretation of and response to women's symptoms.

CORONARY HEART DISEASE SYMPTOMS IN WOMEN

There is a paucity of research focusing on women's CHD symptoms, mainly because women essentially were excluded as participants in CHD and MI research studies before 1990.[3,89] Currently, there is an expanding body of knowledge related to women's symptoms, but controversy continues to exist about sex-specific symptoms. Some of the controversy is related to subject inclusion criteria and failure to differentiate prodromal or acute symptoms and to separate symptoms by race or sex,[90-92] whereas other problems can be attributed to lack of consistency in definitions, instruments, and study methods.[93] For instance, some studies included only persons who reported chest pain and excluded persons with atypical symptoms, those more commonly reported by women.[94] Another study reported that chest pain was the most frequent symptom in men and women diagnosed with acute coronary ischemia or MI, but they defined chest pain as any chest sensation and included tightness, heaviness, and squeezing as indicators of chest pain even if subjects never identified the sensation as pain. Some authors acknowledged that women were more likely than men to use descriptors other than pain, but because they incorporated all chest sensations into one symptom of chest pain, it confounded the reported result that chest pain was the most common symptom in both sexes.[95] However, others conclude that women are more likely to report sensations other than chest pain, even when experiencing an MI.[13]

When women are given the opportunity to differentiate between chest pain and other descriptors of chest discomfort, they most often use descriptors other than pain, such as pressure or burning.[13,79] Despite the controversy surrounding women's CHD and MI symptoms, many researchers and clinicians believe differences exist between men's and women's presentations.[26,93] Therefore, although syntheses of the research on women with CHD are increasing,[3,96-98] findings regarding women's typical CHD symptom presentation lack consistency, and no clear picture has emerged of women's typical early and acute CHD symptoms. The following sections provide the latest research on women's CHD and MI symptoms to assist clinicians in diagnosing CHD in women.

Prodromal Symptoms

McSweeney and colleagues[13,97,99,100] have conducted a series of studies that have been instrumental in identifying the early warning CHD or prodromal symptoms reported most often by women before MI. They define prodromal symptoms as those that are intermittent before MI and are of new onset or are preexisting symptoms that increase in intensity and/or frequency before MI and revert to previous levels after MI.[13] In these studies, women have reported experiencing prodromal symptoms from a month up to 2 years before MI, with most reporting symptoms for an average of 1 to 6 months. Other investigators also have reported that women may experience prodromal symptoms a month or more before MI, but they typically define prodromal symptoms as new symptoms occurring before MI.[24,97] Regardless of definition, these findings indicate that there is ample time to intervene before an MI occurs if early CHD symptoms are recognized. However, although an evidence-based list of common prodromal and acute symptoms of CHD and MI in women is beginning to emerge, this research is in its infancy.

To identify the full range of women's prodromal symptoms and symptom descriptors, McSweeney and colleagues[99-101] initially conducted qualitative interviews with women of various races and cultures. They used these findings to develop an instrument that incorporated all the identified prodromal symptoms and descriptors in women's own terms. Importantly, previous instruments primarily were developed from studies conducted with men. In their latest study, they used this instrument with 515 primarily white women. Ninety-seven percent of the women reported experiencing prodromal symptoms, which are reported in Table 52-2. Unusual fatigue, the most frequently reported prodromal symptom, was similar to vital exhaustion[102] and tiredness[103] reported as a prodromal symptom by women in other studies. Other frequently reported prodromal symptoms included sleep disturbance, shortness of breath, frequent indigestion, and fleeting feelings of anxiety. Of the 515 women in the study by McSweeney and colleagues,[13] only 30 percent of the women reported experiencing chest discomfort as a prodromal symptom. However, Sweitzer and Douglas[26] state that angina is the most common initial CHD symptom in women. Therefore the significance of chest pain in women with CHD remains problematic. Because this is the case, other prodromal symptoms in combination with risk factor evaluation may be better prognostic indicators of CHD in women than chest pain alone.

Other researchers also have reported prodromal symptoms in women before MI. For instance, Horne and colleagues[79] indicated that 58 percent of their subjects reported prodromal symptoms in the days before their MI, but the authors did not identify the specific symptoms, nor did they provide specific time frames for the appearance of symptoms. Another study compared symptoms of unstable angina in men and women and reported that even when controlling for risk factors such as age and diabetes, women had significantly more atypical prodromal symptoms (e.g., weakness, shortness of breath, and nausea) than men.[93] These symptoms were similar to those reported by women in the study by McSweeney and colleagues.[13]

Many clinicians and women continue to believe that chest pain is the hallmark symptom of CHD. Typically, cardiac evaluation is based primarily on the severity of chest pain and to a lesser extent on the presence of risk factors and the likelihood of CHD.[100] However, chest pain is often not of significant prognostic value in women[89,95,104] because it often occurs in women without identifiable CHD.[37,105]

The current practice recommendation is to complete an in-depth history on women who have possible prodromal symptoms, such as unusual fatigue. Of note is the fact that these symptoms often affect the ability of women to conduct their normal activities of daily living more so than in men.[94] Therefore an in-depth history clearly should investigate the impact of prodromal symptoms on women's daily activities. A thorough review of risk factors followed by administration of a de-

■ ■ ■

TABLE 52-2 FREQUENCY OF PRODROMAL AND ACUTE SYMPTOMS IN WOMEN

SYMPTOM	PRODROMAL FREQUENCY (%)	ACUTE FREQUENCY (%)
Discomfort/pain		
General chest	13.0	19.8
Centered high in chest	14.4	30.5
Left breast	9.3	14.8
Neck/throat	7.4	16.3
Jaw/teeth	4.5	9.5
Back/between or under shoulder blades	13.0	21.2
Top of shoulders	5.0	10.1
Both arms	5.4	12.2
Left arm/shoulder	11.8	21.7
Right arm/shoulder	2.3	4.7
Leg(s)	3.5	1.4
Cold sweat	Not asked	39.0
Hot/flushed	Not asked	32.4
Anxious	35.5	Not asked
Sleep disturbance	47.8	Not asked
Unusual fatigue	70.7	42.9
Weakness	Not asked	54.8
Cough	18.4	10.5
Heart racing	27.4	22.9
Shortness of breath	42.1	57.9
Difficulty breathing at night	19.2	Not asked
Change in taste of cigarettes	Not asked	2.9
Choking	Not asked	9.5
Loss of appetite	21.9	19.4
Indigestion	39.4	30.5
Nausea	Not asked	35.5
Vomiting	Not asked	19.0
Arms weak/heavy	24.9	34.8
Arms ache	18.8	32.4
Hands/arms tingling	21.7	21.0
Arms swollen	Not asked	4.1
Numbness/burning in both arms	5.4	7.0
Numbness/burning in right arm	1.4	1.2
Numbness/burning in left arm	7.2	8.7
Numbness in both hands	10.5	8.7
Numbness in right hand	1.9	1.0
Numbness in left hand	6.4	8.5
Dizziness	Not asked	39.0
Vision change	23.1	13.4
Headache	Not asked	15.1
Increase intensity of headaches	9.1	Not asked
Increase frequency of headaches	13.2	Not asked
Changes: thinking or memory	23.9	Not asked

From McSweeney JC, Cody M, O'Sullivan P et al: *Circulation* 108:2619-2623, 2003.

pression screen is advised because depression may produce similar symptoms, such as fatigue. Currently, researchers are investigating depression as a risk factor for CHD. This information, along with a physical examination and serum studies, such as a lipid panel, should be used to calculate a woman's risk for CHD. An excellent study by Wilson and colleagues[106] reports the effectiveness of calculating risk. Numerous risk calculators maybe downloaded free of charge. Box 52-5 offers website information.

BOX 52-5
RISK CALCULATORS AND WEBSITES
■ ■ ■

Risk assessment tool for estimating 10-year risk of developing coronary heart disease:
    http://hin.nhlbi.nih.gov/atpiii/calculator.asp?usertype=pub
    American Heart Association risk assessment:
www.americanheart.org/presenter.jhtml?identifier=3003499
International Task Force for Prevention of Coronary Heart Disease:
    http://chdrisk.uni-muenster.de/calculator.php

Clearly, health care professionals need more research to identify the full range of women's prodromal CHD symptoms. If health care professionals can determine which symptoms are most predictive of CHD in women, this will assist clinicians to make a timely diagnosis. Such information also could provide the basis for developing accurate evidence-based educational materials so that women may be knowledgeable about prodromal symptoms and seek treatment in a timely manner. This evidence could be used to modify the existing curriculum for clinicians. This dual educational approach is essential because currently, women who recognize prodromal symptoms and seek medical attention report difficulty being diagnosed with CHD and often remain untreated.[23] Further investigation is needed to determine which prodromal symptoms are most indicative of CHD, along with the influence of their timing, variation by race, cultural interpretation, and the presence of specific comorbidities.

Acute Symptoms

More research has been conducted on women's acute MI symptoms than on prodromal symptoms. Despite this fact, similar controversy continues to exist about women's most frequently reported acute symptoms.[107] Some studies have indicated that chest pain is a major symptom in women with MI,[4,71,95] whereas others report that chest pain may be a later or less significant symptom[13,97,100,108] or described differently[105] by women than by men. The significance of chest pain in women is perhaps the most controversial diagnostic problem facing clinicians. Of the more than 4 million patients who go to emergency departments for chest pain each year, only 38 percent are diagnosed with MI.[109] However, Canto and colleagues[32] reported that of 142,500 participants in an MI study, 66 percent cited chest pain (defined as any chest discomfort) as their presenting symptom, but 34 percent did not experience chest pain. Patients without chest pain were more likely to be older and female. However, Then and colleagues[90] reported that both genders have atypical presentations (no chest pain) with MI, whereas others report that exertional chest pain in older women, but not younger women, is a reliable diagnostic indicator.[78] Thus the controversy regarding chest pain may contribute to clinicians discounting chest pain as a significant symptom for women.[71]

Despite the controversy about the significance of chest pain in women with MI, clinicians are taught, continue to believe, and assess for chest pain as the primary symptom indicative of MI. In a study of 78 emergency and critical care clinicians, 85 percent of registered nurses and 66 percent of physicians stated that they primarily assessed for chest pain in patients with suspected MI.[90] Only 35 percent reported assessing for less typical symptoms, although 92 to 100 percent had previous experience with persons who had atypical symptoms. Compounding this problem, studies indicate that women often use different terms than men to describe their ischemic symptoms, such as *heaviness, tightness,* and *discomfort* to describe chest sensations, whereas men report pain high or centered in the chest.[89,105] As stated before, some investigators have classified all chest sensations, such as pressure or tightness, as chest pain.[32,95] This failure to differentiate between acute chest pain and sensations may be a significant contributing factor in the controversy surrounding chest pain in women and may lead some clinicians to indicate on emergency room medical records the presence of chest pain when women reported no pain or described other sensations.[95] Because some providers record all chest sensations as pain, retrospective studies auditing medical records may be unable to discern that chest pain was absent. Therefore, prospective studies that describe sensations in women's own terms rather than those assigned by health professionals are essential.

Many studies document other common symptoms that women report with MI, such as shortness of breath, indigestion, back or jaw discomfort, fatigue, dizziness, palpitations, cough, and nausea.* Table 52-2 contains a complete list and frequency of acute symptoms reported by the 515 women in the study by McSweeney and colleagues[13] discussed previously and allows comparison of the women's prodromal and acute symptoms.

Despite mounting evidence that women may manifest different MI symptoms, women are less likely to be diagnosed with and treated for MI when they present to the emergency department with atypical rather than classic symptoms. In a meta-synthesis of studies reporting unrecognized MIs from 1996 to 2001, the authors concluded that diagnosis bias (failure to consider and detect atypical symptoms) may be one reason women have more unrecognized MI events than men do.[110] They reported an independent association of absence of chest pain with unrecognized MI.

For these reasons and those of CHD presentation and manifestation in women, authors advocate for a sex-specific approach to increase recognition of CHD and MI in women. Vitally important is that researchers continue to investigate which symptoms are the primary predictors of CHD and MI in women because symptoms, when considered with risk factors, are important in determining which women are referred for further CHD diagnostic evaluation. Clinicians should be cognizant that women may present differently than men. Clinicians should include CHD as a differential diagnosis when women have these symptoms, especially if women have a positive risk factor profile for CHD.

---

*References 13, 26, 90, 95, 97, 100.

DIAGNOSTIC EVALUATION

Currently, women are referred less often than men for diagnostic testing, and important symptoms often are missed or ignored, thus contributing to women's high CHD mortality rates.[9] Underrecognition of women's important symptoms plus a generalized provider bias about the significance of these symptoms and CHD in women must be addressed before a significant decrease in women's mortality rates may be achieved. However, even when women are referred for additional diagnostic evaluation, they frequently encounter problems receiving a diagnosis because of sex-specific problems with diagnostic testing.

As stated before, clinicians typically base an individual's likelihood of having CHD on health history, including the presence of known cardiovascular risk factors, age, and symptom presentation, specifically chest pain. Typically, the more severe the chest pain, the faster a person seeks treatment and the more likely clinicians are to suspect CHD. This immediate symptom recognition increases the likelihood of prompt, effective treatment and a positive outcome, but because many women do not experience chest pain, they frequently are misdiagnosed.[103,104]

However, even when women have chest pain and undergo cardiac catheterization, 43 percent to 50 percent have no detectable CHD.[111,112] Despite this fact, chest pain continues primarily to drive whom clinicians refer for CHD testing and treatment.[107,113,114] Women who do not have typical chest pain often are excluded from testing,[112] perhaps contributing to the number of undiagnosed women who experience sudden cardiac death.[115] Clinicians are beginning to recognize the need for diagnostic evaluation in women who do not meet current criteria, but health insurance companies and health maintenance organizations often will not pay for additional evaluation if women do not exhibit the predetermined symptoms for referral, specifically, chest pain. Continued research is needed to develop accurate evidence-based referral guidelines for women.

Currently, diagnosing CHD in women remains challenging because cardiac diagnostic testing is less sensitive and specific in women than it is in men, resulting in a higher incidence of false-negative and false-positive results.[37] This variability in sensitivity and specificity is often attributed to physiological sex differences,[70,75] such as women having smaller coronary arteries and more breast tissue that may interfere with diagnostic scanning.[70] Other factors occur more frequently in women, such as lower hematocrit levels, mitral valve prolapse, and left ventricular hypertrophy, which may result in false-positive results or nonspecific ECG changes.[71]

The most common noninvasive CHD diagnostic test is exercise ECG.[107] Exercise is used routinely to evaluate women in an intermediate-risk category or those with symptoms and CHD risk factors. Importantly, women's lower work capacity makes it difficult to evoke myocardial ischemia during testing, and breast attenuation artifact and cyclic estrogen level differences combine to reduce the specificity and sensitivity of exercise ECG in women compared with men.[116] Clinicians must recognize these important limitations. Additionally, a higher incidence of false-positive results may cause clinicians to view a positive reading as an error, overlook disease, and delay treating women. For these reasons, stress echocardiography is often the diagnostic test of choice because it has greater specificity and accuracy than exercise ECG testing in women.[9,37] However, stress echocardiography testing also often exceeds the physical abilities of many older women.

Adding a pharmacological agent to stress the heart muscle is preferred and has shown greater sensitivity and specificity in women with ischemia, but the possibility of false-positive readings remains.[9,117] Using a combination of nuclear imaging or perfusion scans with exercise or pharmacological stress echocardiography improves sensitivity and specificity in diagnosing women, but false-positive results still may result because of small left ventricular size and breast tissue attenuation artifact.[107,118] Despite these problems, stress myocardial gated perfusion single-photon emission computed tomography imaging is considered to have high diagnostic and prognostic accuracy in women in the intermediate- to high-risk categories.[9] However, angiography remains the gold standard as the most accurate diagnostic test for CHD.[119] Importantly, women, blacks, and elders tend to be referred for angiography and other diagnostic tests less often than white males.[75,120] Other emerging diagnostic tests may be useful in diagnosing CHD in symptomatic women[121]; at this time, data are insufficient to determine efficacy, but emerging data suggest that these tests may hold promise for detecting women's CHD.[9,37,122] Emerging tests are described in Table 52-3. These promising tests, used with emerging, novel, and traditional risk factors, along with improved symptom recognition by women and clinicians, may improve earlier detection of CHD in women significantly.

To assist with the difficult task of selecting the appropriate tests for determining a woman's level of CHD risk, the American Heart Association published a consensus statement that provides specific guidance on selecting appropriate noninvasive CHD evaluation for women according to risk status.[9] This consensus statement, along with a "ACC/AHA 2002 Guideline Update for Exercise Testing"[116] offers specific guidance for enhancing appropriate referral and improving interpretation of noninvasive diagnostic tests in women. Additionally, Redberg and Shaw[107] have developed a formula for determining the probability that a woman has CHD.

■ ■ ■

TABLE 52-3   EMERGING DIAGNOSTIC TESTS FOR DETECTION OF CORONARY HEART DISEASE IN WOMEN

TEST	DETECTS OR EVALUATES
Computed tomography	Coronary calcification
Magnetic resonance imaging	Coronary blood flow
High-frequency carotid ultrasonography	Focal plaque and thickness of carotid arteries

They also include further guidelines for selecting the appropriate diagnostic tests based on women's risk and symptoms. These three publications offer a wealth of information that may assist clinicians in assessing women's risks, determining appropriate noninvasive tests, and selecting women for further diagnostic evaluation. However, as specified in these guidelines, chest pain continues to be one of the most important symptoms in calculating global risk scores that serve as a basis for referring women for additional diagnostic evaluation. This emphasizes the need for additional research into women's common CHD symptoms so that findings may serve as an evidence base to alter guidelines, if indicated, to better reflect women's common CHD symptomatology.

TREATMENT AND SECONDARY PREVENTION

Wenger[37] published a thorough meta-synthesis of women's responses, compared with men's, to the most widely accepted medical treatment modalities for CHD and MI. Importantly, many pathophysiological differences between men and women with MI can be negated with aggressive and timely treatment.[123,124] However, women often are not treated aggressively, are not treated to optimal therapeutic levels, and are not discharged on recommended secondary preventative therapies (Table 52-4).[37,125] Provider bias may be a contributing factor to these disparities and resulting diminished quality of life.[126] Results of a recent study that included

■ ■ ■

TABLE 52-4 SECONDARY PREVENTION OF CORONARY ARTERY DISEASE IN WOMEN: SUMMARY OF CURRENT DATA

STRATEGY	LEVEL OF EVIDENCE	REDUCTION IN ENDPOINTS (%)	UNDERUSED?
Lipid lowering	A	30-50	Yes
Aspirin	A	20-25	Yes
Beta blockers			
After myocardial infarction	A	20-30	Yes
With left ventricle dysfunction	A	10-40	Yes
Angiotensin-converting enzyme inhibitors			
After myocardial infarction	A	5-10*	Yes
With left ventricle dysfunction	A	25-30*	Yes
Smoking cessation	B	65	Yes
Hypertension	C	?	?
Cardiac rehabilitation	C	?	Yes
Hormone replacement therapy	A	Increase	N/A

*Although the effect is probably positive, the 95 percent confidence interval crosses 1.0.
Modified from Grady D, Chaput L, Kristof M: *Diagnosis and treatment of heart diease in women: systematic reviews of evidence on selected topics*, Evidence Report/Technology Assessment No 81, AHRQ Pub No 03-0037, Rockville, Md, 2003, Agency for Healthcare Research and Quality.

more than 10 million individual cases obtained from the National Hospital Discharge Survey compared CHD diagnosis and treatment in 1988 and 1998[20] and indicated that men were twice as likely as women with similar comorbidites to have coronary artery bypass graft surgery. Not only were bypass surgeries performed significantly less often in women, but so were angioplasty procedures. Overall treatment decisions for women were significantly more conservative than in men with similar profiles. This study concluded, "There was compelling evidence of a pernicious gender bias and a general failure to treat women in a proactive manner that extended over a decade" (p. 22). Clearly, clinicians must treat women with recommended effective treatments and ensure that therapeutic levels of medications are achieved and maintained to improve women's CHD rates.

Clinicians should monitor women closely after MI for the presence of congestive heart failure because women are more likely to develop heart failure than are men, especially as they age. After MI, women are twice as likely to be disabled from heart failure, but they often are not discharged on therapeutic levels of appropriate medications.[1,4] For secondary prevention of CHD, women should be discharged on beta blockers, angiotensin-converting enzyme inhibitors, and aspirin unless contraindicated.[4,10] Congestive heart failure is discussed further elsewhere in this book.

Strong evidence indicates that women's participation in cardiac rehabilitation programs after MI improves functional capacity, quality of life, and CHD symptom reduction.[127] Despite men and women benefiting equally from cardiac rehabilitation, women continue to be referred less often than men.[37,127] In addition, women often are discharged from the hospital after MI without adequate counseling on risk factor reduction strategies.[4] Women's age is a significant factor for referral and completion of programs, with younger women more often being referred, but less often completing programs compared with older women. The availability of resources such as transportation, distance to program, and expenses are factors that contribute to women's inability to attend and complete cardiac rehabilitation programs.[127]

SUMMARY

Overwhelming evidence indicates that cardiovascular disease in women can be prevented with appropriate attention to identifying and modifying risk factors.[10] However, women often do not have access to health care or to consistent providers who might monitor risk factor modification. When women develop CHD and MI, they typically delay seeking treatment longer than men because they may not identify themselves as being at risk for CHD and may not recognize their symptoms as being CHD related. Diagnosis of CHD in women is problematic because controversy exists about the most common prodromal and acute symptoms in women and whether they differ from men. Ample evidence indicates that women experience more atypical CHD symptoms than men. This different presentation in women and men is influenced by cellular, hormonal, anatomical, pathophysiological, and cultural differences. These evidence-based sex differences certainly support the notion that men and women are likely to have different CHD and MI symptoms. Consequently, clinicians often have difficulty diagnosing CHD in women and may delay referring women for diagnostic evaluation. Even when referred, the lack of specificity and sensitivity of CHD diagnostic tests in women adds to the diagnostic challenge. Although recommended treatments for CHD and MI and secondary prevention measures are effective in women and men, women continue to be treated less aggressively and referred less often to cardiac rehabilitation programs. Provider bias affects all aspects of CHD in women, including recognition of symptoms, delayed response to symptoms, and less aggressive treatment. Providers often do not prescribe optimal therapeutic regimens for women with known CHD, nor do they refer women as often as men to cardiac rehabilitation. Finally, health care professionals must conduct further research in order to develop sex-specific evidence-based treatment guidelines to educate and guide clinicians to facilitate recognition and treatment of CHD to combat this deadly and disabling disease in women.

REFERENCES

1. American Heart Association: *Heart disease and stroke statistics: 2006 update*, Dallas 2005, The Association.
2. Kaiser Family Foundation, Kaiser Women's Health Survey: *Racial and ethnic disparities in women's health coverage and access to care*, Report No 7018, Menlo Park, Calif, 2004, Henry J Kaiser Family Foundation.
3. Mosca L, Manson JE, Sutherland SE et al: Cardiovascular disease in women: a statement for healthcare professionals from the American Heart Association. *Circulation* 96:2468-2482, 1997.
4. Bello N, Mosca L: Epidemiology of coronary heart disease in women, *Prog Cardiovasc Dis* 46:287-295, 2004.
5. Wenger NK: You've come a long way, baby: cardiovascular health and disease in women: problems and prospects, *Circulation* 109(5):558-560, 2004.
6. Wenger NK: Coronary heart disease and women: magnitude of the problem, *Cardiol Rev* 10:211-213, 2002.
7. Albert CM, Chae CU, Grodstein F et al: Prospective study of sudden cardiac death among women in the United States, *Circulation* 107:2096-2101, 2003.
8. Agency for Healthcare Research and Quality: *Results of systematic review of research on diagnosis and treatment of coronary heart disease in women*, Report No 80, AHRQ Pub No 03-E034, Rockville, Md, 2003, US Department of Health and Human Services, Public Health Services.
9. Mieres JH, Shaw LJ, Arai A et al: Role of noninvasive testing in the clinical evaluation of women with suspected coronary artery disease: consensus statement, *Circulation* 111:682-696, 2005.
10. Mosca L, Appel LJ, Benjamin EJ et al: Evidenced-based guidelines for cardiovascular disease prevention in women, *Circulation* 109:672-693, 2004.
11. Shaw LJ, Lewis JF, Hlatky MA et al: Women's Ischemic Syndrome Evaluation: current status and future research directions—report of the National Heart, Lung and Blood Institute workshop, Oct 2-4, 2002. section 5: gender-related risk factors for ischemic heart disease, *Circulation* 109:e56-e58, 2004.
12. Maseri A: Women's ischemic syndrome evaluation: current status and future research directions—new frontiers in detection of ischemic heart disease in women, *Circulation* 109:e62-e63, 2004.
13. McSweeney JC, Cody M, O'Sullivan P et al: Women's early warning symptoms of acute myocardial infarction, *Circulation* 108:2619-2623, 2003.
14. Allen J, Szanton S: Gender, ethnicity, and cardiovascular disease, *J Cardiovasc Nurs* 20:1-6, 2005.
15. Mosca L, Ferris A, Fabunmi R, Robertson RM: Tracking women's awareness of heart disease: an American Heart Association national study, *Circulation* 109:573-579, 2004.
16. Lefler LL, Bondy KN: Women's delay in seeking treatment with myocardial infarction: a meta-synthesis, *J Cardiovasc Nurs* 19:251-268, 2004.
17. National Heart, Lung, and Blood Institute: *Educational strategies to prevent prehospital delay in patients at high risk for acute myocardial infarction*, Report No 97-3787, Bethesda, Md, 1997, National Institutes of Health.
18. Meinert CL, Gilpin AK: Estimation of gender bias in clinical trials, *Stat Med* 20:1153-1164, 2001.
19. Committee on Understanding the Biology of Sex and Gender Differences: *Exploring the biological contributions to human health: does sex matter?* Washington, DC, 2001, National Academy Press.
20. Travis CB: 2004 Carolyn Sherif Award Address: heart disease and gender inequity, *Psychology of Women Quarterly* 29:15-23, 2005.
21. Bird CE, Fremont A, Wickstrom S et al: Improving women's quality of care for cardiovascular disease and diabetes: the feasibility and desirability of stratified reporting of objective performance measures, *Womens Health Issues* 13:150-157, 2003.
22. Bhatt DL, Roe MT, Peterson ED et al: Utilization of early invasive management strategies for high-risk patients with non-ST segment elevation acute coronary syndromes, *JAMA* 292:2096-2104, 2004.
23. McSweeney JC, Lefler LL, Crowder BF: What's wrong with me? women's coronary heart disease diagnostic experiences, *Prog Cardiovasc Nurs* 20:48-57, 2005.
24. Murray JC, O'Farrell PO, Huston P: The experiences of women with heart disease: what are their needs? *Can J Public Health* 91:98-102, 2000.
25. Brieger D, Eagle KA, Goodman SG et al: Acute coronary syndromes without chest pain, an underdiagnosed and undertreated high-risk group: insights from the Global Registry of Acute Coronary Events, *Chest* 126:461-469, 2004.
26. Sweitzer NK, Douglas PS: Cardiovascular disease in women. In Zipes DP, Libby P, Bonow RO, Braunwald E, editors: *Braunwald's heart disease: a textbook of cardiovascular medicine*, ed 7, Philadelphia, 2005, Saunders.
27. Winkleby MA, Kraemer HC, Ahn DK, Varady AN: Ethnic and socioeconomic differences in cardiovascular disease risk factors: findings for women from the Third National Health and Nutrition Examination Survey, 1988-1994, *J Am Med Assoc* 280:356-362, 1998.
28. Chrysohoou C, Panagiotakos DB, Pitsavos C et al: Gender differences on the risk evaluation of acute coronary syndromes: the CARDIO2000 Study, *Prev Cardiol* 6:71-77, 2003.
29. Lee WL, Cheung AM, Cape D, Zinman B: Impact of diabetes on coronary artery disease in women and men: a meta-analysis of prospective studies, *Diabetes Care* 23:962-968, 2000.
30. Appel SJ, Harrell JS, Deng S: Racial and socioeconomic differences in risk factors for cardiovascular disease among southern rural women, *Nurs Res* 51:140-147, 2002.
31. Rosenfeld AG. State of the heart: building science to improve women's cardiovascular health. *Am J Crit Care* 15:556-567, 2006.
32. Canto JG, Shlipak MG, Rogers WJ et al: Prevalence, clinical characteristics, and mortality among patients with myocardial infarction presenting without chest pain, *JAMA* 283:3223-3229, 2000.
33. Hansen EF, Andersen LT, Von Eyben FE: Cigarette smoking and age at first acute myocardial infarction, and influence of gender and extent of smoking, *Am J Cardiol* 71:1439-1442, 1993.
34. Grodstein F, Manson JE, Stampfer MJ: Postmenopausal hormone use and secondary prevention of coronary events in the nurses' health study: a prospective, observational study, *Ann Intern Med* 135:1-8, 2001.
35. Al-Delaimy WK, Manson JE: Smoking and risk of coronary heart disease among women with type 2 diabetes mellitus, *Arch Intern Med* 162:273-279, 2002.

36. US Public Health Service: *Treating tobacco use and dependence,* 2000. Retrieved April 1, 2005, from www.surgeongeneral.gov/tobacco/smokesum.htm

37. Wenger NK: Coronary heart disease: the female heart is vulnerable, *Prog Cardiovasc Dis* 46:199-229, 2003.

38. Fruchart JC, Nierman MC, Stroes ES et al: New risk factors for atherosclerosis and patient risk assessment, *Circulation* 109S: III15-III19, 2004.

39. Summerbell HL, Higgins JPT, Thompson RL et al: Reduced or modified dietary fat for preventing cardiovascular disease, *Cochrane Database Syst Rev* 1, 2005.

40. Stein JH, McBride PE: Implementing strategies for the secondary prevention of coronary heart disease. In Douglas PS, editor: *Cardiovascular health and disease in women,* ed 2, Philadelphia, 2002, WB Saunders.

41. Grundy SM, Becker DM, Clark LT et al: *Third Report of the National Cholesterol Education Program Expert Panel on Detection, Evaluation, and Treatment of High Blood Cholesterol in Adults (Adult Treatment Panel III),* NIH Pub No 02-5215, Bethesda, Md, 2002, National Institutes of Health.

42. Gorter PM, Olijhoek JK, van der Graaf Y et al: Prevalence of the metabolic syndrome in patients with coronary heart disease, cerebrovascular disease, peripheral arterial disease or abdominal aortic aneurysm, *Atherosclerosis* 173:363-369, 2004.

43. Rossouw JE, Anderson GL, Prentice RL et al: Risks and benefits of estrogen plus progestin in healthy postmenopausal women: principal results from the Women's Health Initiative Randomized Controlled Trial, *JAMA* 288:321-333, 2002.

44. Cooper R, Cutler J, Desvigne-Nickens P et al: Trends and disparities in coronary heart disease, stroke, and other cardiovascular diseases in the United States: findings of the national conference on cardiovascular disease prevention, *Circulation* 102:3137-3147, 2000.

45. Rockhill B, Willett WC, Manson JE et al: Physical activity and mortality: a prospective study among women, *Am J Public Health* 91:578-583, 2001.

46. Giannuzzi P, Mezzani A, Saner H et al: Physical activity for primary and secondary prevention: position paper of the Working Group on Cardiac Rehabilitation and Exercise Physiology of the European Society of Cardiology, *Eur J Cardiovasc Prev Rehabil* 10:319-327, 2003.

47. Chobanian AV, Bakris GL, Black HR et al: Seventh Report of the Joint National Committee on Prevention, Detection, Evaluation, and Treatment of High Blood Pressure, *Hypertension* 42:1206-1252, 2003.

48. Behera SK, Winkleby MA, Collins R: Low awareness of cardiovascular risk among low-income African-American women, *Am J Health Promo* 14:301-305, 2000.

49. Manson JE, Willett WC, Stampfer MJ et al: Body weight and mortality among women, *N Engl J Med* 333:677-685, 1995.

50. Fung TT, Willett WC, Stamper MJ et al: Dietary patterns and the risk of coronary heart disease in women, *Arch Intern Med* 161:1857-1862, 2001.

51. Hu FB, Stamper MJ, Haffner SM et al: Elevated risk of cardiovascular disease prior to clinical diagnosis of type 2 diabetes, *Diabetes Care* 25:1129-1134, 2002.

52. Hu FB, Stampfer MJ, Solomon CG et al: The impact of diabetes mellitus on mortality from all causes and coronary heart disease in women: 20 years of follow-up, *Arch Intern Med* 161:1717-1723, 2001.

53. Wamala SP, Lynch J, Kaplan GA: Women's exposure to early and later life socioeconomic disadvantage and coronary heart disease risk: the Stockholm Female Coronary Risk Study, *Int J Epidemiol* 30:275-284, 2001.

54. Gerhard GT, Sexton G, Malinow MR et al: Premenopausal black women have more risk factors for coronary heart disease than white women, *Am J Cardiol* 82:1040-1045, 1998.

55. Fiscella K, Franks P: Should years of schooling be used to guide treatment of coronary risk factors? *Ann Fam Med* 2:469-473, 2004.

56. Centers for Disease Control and Prevention: Racial/ethnic and socioeconomic disparities in multiple risk factors for heart disease and stroke: United States, 2003, *MMWR. Morb Mortal Wkly Rep* 54:113-117, 2005.

57. Sullivan MD, LaCroix AZ, Russo JE, Walker EA: Depression and self-reported physical health in patients with coronary disease: mediating and moderating factors, *Psychosom Med* 63:248-256, 2003.

58. Wassertheil-Smoller S, Shumaker S, Ockene J et al: Depression and cardiovascular sequelae in postmenopausal women, *Arch Intern Med* 164:289-298, 2004.

59. Bunker SJ, Colquhoun DM, Esler MD et al: "Stress" and coronary artery disease: psychosocial risk factors, *Med J Aust* 178:272-276, 2003.

60. Wulsin LR, Singal BM: Do depressive symptoms increase the risk for the onset of coronary disease? a systematic review, *Psychosom Med* 65:201-210, 2003.

61. Ward HE, Tueth M, Sheps D: Depression and cardiovascular disease, *Current Opinion in Psychiatry* 16:221-225, 2003.

62. Rugulies R: Depression as a predictor for coronary heart disease: a review and meta-analysis, *Am J Prev Med* 23:51-61, 2002.

63. Ferketich AK, Schwartzbaum JA, Frid DJ, Moeschberger ML: Depression as an antecedent to heart disease among women and men in the NHANES I Study, *Arch Intern Med* 160:1261-1268, 2000.

64. Kelly CJ, Lyall H, Petrie JR et al: A specific elevation in tissue plasminogen activator antigen in women with polycystic ovarian syndrome, *J Clin Endocrinol Metab* 87:3287-3290, 2002.

65. Wu FCW, von Eckardstein A: Androgens and coronary artery disease, *Endocr Rev* 24:183-217, 2003.

66. Ridker PM, Cook N: Clinical usefulness of very high and very low levels of C-reactive protein across the full range of Framingham risk scores, *Circulation* 109:1955-1959, 2004.

67. Genest J: Preventive cardiology: move over low density lipoprotein cholesterol, hello C-reactive protein? *Can J Cardiol* 20:89B-92B, 2004.

68. Ridker PM, Brown NJ, Vaughan DE et al: Established and emerging plasma biomarkers in the prediction of first atherothrombotic events, *Circulation* 109S:IV6-IV19, 2004.

69. Fischer M, Baessler A, Schunkert H: Renin angiotensin system and gender differences in the cardiovascular system, *Cardiovasc Res* 53:672-677, 2002.

70. Sheifer SE, Canos MR, Weinfurt KP et al: Sex differences in coronary artery size assessed by intravascular ultrasound, *Am Heart J* 139:649-653, 2000.

71. Duvernoy CS, Eagle KA: Diagnosing and treating acute myocardial infarction in women, *Women's Health in Primary Care* 4:542-556, 2001.

72. Sader MA, Celermajer DS: Endothelial function, vascular reactivity and gender differences in the cardiovascular system, *Cardiovasc Res* 53:597-604, 2002.

73. Orshal JM, Khalil RA: Gender, sex hormones, and vascular tone, *Am J Physiol Regul Integr Comp Physiol* 286:R233-R249, 2004.

74. Duvernoy CS, Meyer C, Seifert-Klauss V et al: Gender differences in myocardial blood flow dynamics: lipid profile and hemodynamic effects. *J Am Coll Cardiol* 33:463-470, 1999.

75. Canto JG, Rogers WJ, Chandra NC et al: The association of sex and payer status on management and subsequent survival in acute myocardial infarction, *Arch Intern Med* 162:587-593, 2002.

76. Dart AM, Du XJ, Kingwell BA: Gender, sex hormones and autonomic nervous control of the cardiovascular system, *Cardiovasc Res* 53:678-687, 2002.

77. Schwertz DW, Penckofer S: Sex differences and the effects of sex hormones on hemostasis and vascular reactivity, *Heart Lung* 30:401-426, 2001.

78. Jneid H, Thacker HL: Coronary artery disease in women: different, often undertreated, *Cleve Clin J Med* 68:441-448, 2001.

79. Horne R, James D, Petrie K et al: Patients' interpretation of symptoms as a cause of delay in reaching hospital during acute myocardial infarction, *Heart* 83:388-393, 2000.

80. Kohlmann CW, Ring C, Carroll D et al: Cardiac coping style, heartbeat detection, and the interpretation of cardiac events, *Br J Health Psychol* 6:285-301, 2001.

81. Lee H, Bahler R, Park OJ et al: Typical and atypical symptoms of myocardial infarction among African-Americans, whites, and Koreans, *Crit Care Nurs Clin North Am* 13:531-539, 2001.

82. Balsa AI, McGuire TG: Statistical discrimination in health care, *J Health Econ* 20:881-907, 2001.

83. Finnegan JR, Meischke H, Zapka JG et al: Patient delay in seeking care for heart attack symptoms: findings from focus groups conducted in five US regions, *Prev Med* 31:205-213, 2000.

84. Goff DC, Sellers DE, McGovern PG et al: Knowledge of heart attack symptoms in a population survey in the United States: the REACT Trial, *Arch Intern Med* 158:2329-2338, 1998.

85. Meischke H, Sellers DE, Robbins ML et al: Factors that influence personal perceptions of the risk of an acute myocardial infarction, *Behav Med* 26:4-13, 2000.

86. Lee H, Bahler R, Chung C et al: Prehospital delay with myocardial infarction: the interactive effect of clinical symptoms and race, *Appl Nurs Res* 13:125-133, 2000.

87. Klingler D, Green-Weir R, Nerenz D et al: Perceptions of chest pain differ by race, *Am Heart J* 144:51-59, 2002.

88. Maynard C, Beshansky JR, Griffith JL, Selker HP: Causes of chest pain and symptoms suggestive of acute cardiac ischemia in African-American patients presenting to the emergency department, *J Natl Med Assoc* 89:665-671, 1997.

89. Cannon RO, Balaban RS: Chest pain in women with normal coronary angiograms, *N Engl J Med* 342:885-887, 2000.

90. Then KL, Rankin JA, Fofnoff DA: Atypical presentation of acute myocardial infarction in 3 age groups, *Heart Lung* 30:285-293, 2001.

91. Viejo A, Penque S, Halm M et al: Women and coronary disease: relationship between descriptors of sign and symptoms and diagnostic treatment course, *Am J Crit Care* 7:175-186, 2003.

92. Hayes SN, McBride P: Diagnosing coronary heart disease: when to use stress imaging studies, *J Fam Pract* 52:544-551, 2003.

93. DeVon HA, Zerwic JJ: The symptoms of unstable angina: do women and men differ? *Nurs Res* 52:108-118, 2003.

94. Kuster GM, Buser P, Osswald S et al: Comparison of presentation, perception, and six-month outcome between women and men > or =75 years of age with angina pectoris, *Am J Cardiol* 91:436-439, 2003.

95. Milner K, Funk M, Richards S et al: Gender differences in symptom presentation associated with coronary heart disease, *Am J Cardiol* 84:396-399, 1999.

96. Miller CL, Kollauf CR: Evolution of information on women and heart disease 1957-2000: a review of archival records and secular literature, *Heart Lung* 31:253-261, 2002.

97. McSweeney JC, Cody M, Crane PB: Do you know them when you see them? Women's prodromal and acute symptoms of myocardial infarction, *J Cardiovasc Nurs* 15:26-38, 2001.

98. DeVon HA, Zerwic JJ: Symptoms of acute coronary syndromes: are there gender differences? A review of the literature, *Heart Lung* 31:235-245, 2002.

99. McSweeney JC: Women's narratives: evolving symptoms of myocardial infarction, *J Women Aging* 10:67-83, 1998.

100. McSweeney JC, Crane PB: Challenging the rules: women's prodromal and acute symptoms of myocardial infarction, *Res Nurs Health* 23:135-146, 2000.

101. McSweeney JC, O'Sullivan P, Cody M, Crane PB: Development of the McSweeney Acute and Prodromal Myocardial Infarction Symptom Survey, *J Cardiovasc Nurs* 19:58-67, 2003.

102. Schuitemaker GE, Dinant GJ, van der Pol GA, Appels A: Assessment of vital exhaustion and identification of subjects at increased risk of myocardial infarction in general practice, *Psychosomatics* 45:414-418, 2004.

103. Hofgren C, Karlson B, Herlitz J: Prodromal symptoms in subsets of patients hospitalized for suspected acute myocardial infarction, *Heart Lung* 24:3-10, 1995.

104. Bairey-Merz CN, Johnson BD, Kelsey SF et al: Diagnostic, prognostic, and cost assessment of coronary artery disease in women, *Am J Manag Care* 7:959-965, 2001.

105. Oparil S, Robinson D, Pickeral M: *Cardiovascular disease/vascular biology: agenda for research on women's health for the 21st century—a report of the task force on the NIH women's health research agenda for 21st century,* NIH Pub No 99-4388, Bethesda, Md, 1999, US Department of Health and Human Services.

106. Wilson PWF, D'Agostino RB, Levy D et al: Prediction of coronary heart disease using risk factor categories, *Circulation* 97:1837-1847, 1998.

107. Redberg RF, Shaw LJ: Diagnosis of coronary artery disease in women, *Prog Cardiovasc Dis* 46:239-258, 2003.

108. Miller CL: A review of symptoms of coronary artery disease in women, *J Adv Nurs* 39:17-23, 2002.

109. Wischmeyer JB, Kapadia SR: Evaluation of chest pain in the emergency department. In Marso SP, Griffin BP, Topol EJ, editors: *Manual of cardiovascular medicine,* Philadelphia, 2000, Lippincott Williams & Wilkins.

110. Sheifer SE, Manolio TA, Gersh BJ: Unrecognized myocardial infarction, *Ann Intern Med* 135:801-811, 2001.

111. Sharaf BL, Pepine CJ, Kerensky RA et al: Detailed angiographic analysis of women with suspected ischemic chest pain data from the NHLBI-Sponsored Women's Ischemia Syndrome Evaluation [WISE] Study, *Am J Cardiol* 87:937-941, 2001.

112. Shaw LJ, Tarkington L, Callister T et al: The HCA National Disease Management program for coronary disease detection in women, *Am J Manag Care* 7(spec no):SP25-SP30, 2001.

113. Gibbons RJ, Abrams J, Chatterjee K et al: ACC/AHA 2002 guideline update for the management of patients with chronic stable angina: a report of the American College of Cardiology/American Heart Association Task Force on practice guidelines, *Circulation* 107:149-158, 2003.

114. Mosca L, Grundy SM, Judelson D et al: Guide to preventive cardiology for women, *Circulation* 99:2480-2484, 1999.

115. Mosca L: Epidemiology and prevention of heart disease. In Douglas PS, Foley F, editors: *Cardiovascular health and disease in women,* ed 2, Philadelphia, 2002, WB Saunders.

116. Gibbons RJ, Balady GJ, Bricker JT et al: ACC/AHA 2002 guideline update for exercise testing: a report of the American College of Cardiology/American Heart Association Task Force on Practice Guidelines, *Circulation* 106:1883-1892, 2002.

117. Kim C, Kwok YS, Heagerty P, Redberg R: Pharmacological stress testing for coronary artery disease diagnosis: a meta-analysis, *Am Heart J* 142:934-944, 2001.

118. Mieres JH, Shaw LJ, Hendel RC et al: American Society of Nuclear Cardiology consensus statement: Task Force on Women and Coronary Artery Disease—the role of myocardial perfusion imaging in the clinical evaluation of coronary artery disease in women [correction], *J Nucl Cardiol* 10:95-101, 2003.

119. Gurevitz O, Jonas M, Boyko V et al: Clinical profile and long-term prognosis of women = 50 years of age referred for coronary angiography for evaluation of chest pain, *Am J Cardiol* 85:806-809, 2000.

120. LaVeist TA, Morgan A, Artheur M et al: Physician referral patterns and race differences in receipt of coronary angiography, *Heath Serv Res* 37:949-962, 2002.

121. Pletcher MJ, Tice JA, Pignone M et al: What does my patient's coronary artery calcium score mean? Combining information from the coronary artery calcium score with information from conventional risk factors to estimate coronary heart disease risk, *BMC Med* 2:31, 2004.

122. Rumberger JA, Brundage BH, Rader DJ, Kondos G: Electron beam computed tomographic coronary calcium scanning: a review and guidelines for use in asymptomatic persons, *Mayo Clin Proc* 74:243-252, 1999.

123. Mehilli J, Kastrati A, Dirschinger J et al: Sex-based analysis of outcome in patients with acute myocardial infarction treated predominantly with percutaneous coronary intervention, *JAMA* 287:210-215, 2002.

124. Mueller C, Neumann FJ, Roskamm H et al: Women do have an improved long-term outcome after non-ST-elevation acute coronary syndromes treated very early and predominantly with percutaneous coronary intervention: a prospective study in 1,450 consecutive patients, *J Am Coll Cardiol* 40:245-250, 2002.

125. Vittinghoff E, Shlipak MG, Varosy PD et al: Risk factors and secondary prevention in women with heart disease: the Heart and Estrogen/progestin Replacement Study, *Ann Intern Med* 138:81-89, 2003.

126. Mensah GA: Eliminating disparities in cardiovascular health: six strategic imperatives and a framework for action, *Circulation* 1111:1332-1336, 2005.

127. Scott LA, Ben-Or K, Allen JK: Why are women missing from outpatient cardiac rehabilitation programs? A review of multilevel factors affecting referral, enrollment, and completion, *J Womens Health* 11:773-791, 2002.

Chest Pain

Holli A. DeVon

Chest pain is recognized by practitioners and the public alike as the hallmark symptom of coronary heart disease (**CHD**).[1,2] Although chest pain is the most common symptom during an ischemic event, it normally is not the only symptom. Usually, a cluster of associated symptoms leads a person to seek care and contributes to an accurate diagnosis and expeditious treatment.[3] Additionally, chest pain and associated symptoms occur in a number of other cardiac syndromes, presenting a considerable diagnostic challenge.

More than 5.6 million emergency department (**ED**) visits for chest pain and related symptoms occurred in 2002.[4] This accounts for 5.1 percent of the more than 110 million total visits to the ED for all causes. Approximately 35 to 40 percent of patients who present to the ED with chest pain and related symptoms are diagnosed with a coronary event.[5] The aim of the ED is to achieve the highest accuracy in the diagnosis of patients who have heart disease. This goal is attained if low-risk patients without ischemia or other cardiopulmonary diseases are discharged safely at minimal cost and those with a true diagnosis of myocardial ischemia or serious cardiopulmonary disease are admitted and treated according to American College of Cardiology (**ACC**)/American Heart Association (**AHA**) guidelines.[6] The primary goal of nurses is appropriate triage, comprehensive assessment, and administration of appropriate interventions. In the current climate of cost containment, nurses have an added responsibility of providing expert care in the most cost-effective manner. The purpose of this chapter is to describe chest pain and associated symptoms of cardiac conditions and the steps necessary to make a thorough and accurate assessment.

SYMPTOMS OF MYOCARDIAL ISCHEMIA

Myocardial ischemia is the most common and serious reason for acute chest pain or discomfort. Ischemia occurs when there is a mismatch between myocardial oxygen supply and demand. Ischemia typically results from atherosclerotic heart disease but may occur during episodes of increased coronary vascular resistance such as vasospasm. Ischemic chest pain, known as angina, may result from any process that causes partial or complete obstruction of a coronary artery.

Typical Symptoms

The AHA[7] and the National Heart, Lung, and Blood Institute[8] have published lists of the typical symptoms of myocardial infarction. These symptoms include chest discomfort in the center of the chest described as pressure, squeezing, fullness, or pain that may radiate to the arms, back, neck, jaw, or stomach and may be accompanied by shortness of breath, diaphoresis, nausea, and light-headedness (Figure 53-1). The symptoms may begin suddenly and cause collapse, but most symptoms begin slowly with mild pain or discomfort.[1] A number of investigators have described the symptoms associated with acute coronary syndrome (**ACS**) (Table 53-1). ACS is the term used to identify a spectrum of clinical syndromes that represent a progression of occlusion in the involved coronary artery.[9]

The term *acute coronary syndrome* first coined by Fuster and colleagues,[10] includes unstable angina, non–ST segment elevation myocardial infarction (**NSTEMI**), and ST segment elevation myocardial infarction (**STEMI**).[11] The most frequently reported symptoms of ACS are chest pain, diaphoresis, shortness of breath, and nausea.[12-15] If these symptoms represent what is *typical,* then one must accept the premise that there are other *atypical* symptoms. In addition, key questions must be addressed, including the following: What criteria are used to define *typical?* What populations have been sampled in order to define what symptoms are *typical* and therefore represent the dominant group norm? Is it clinically useful to label symptoms *typical* or *atypical?* Should there be a model of symptoms based on certain characteristics of the population such as age, race, or comorbid conditions? (See the Conundrum feature on p. 758.)

The labeling of symptoms as typical or atypical has been based on a male model for a number of reasons, including an historical and inaccurate belief that CHD was primarily a man's disease,[19] resistance to including women of childbearing age in clinical trials,[20] and difficulties in recruiting women and minorities into cardio-

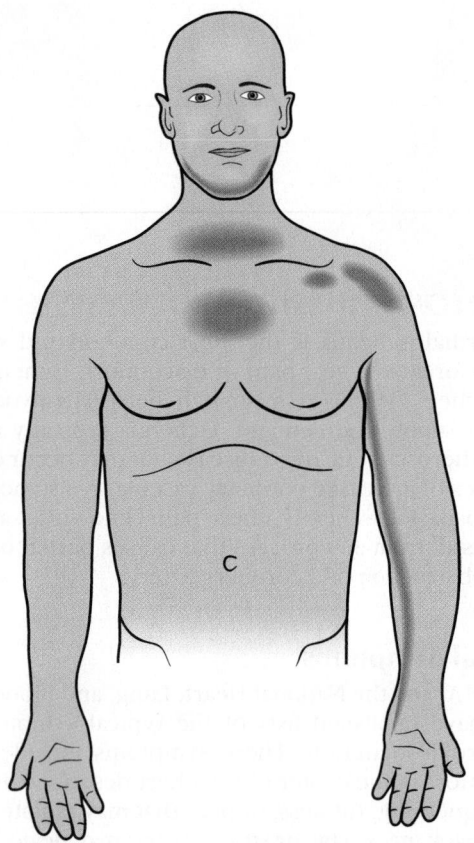

FIGURE 53-1 ■ The "pain" of myocardial infarction commonly radiates to the areas of the body shown here. (From Morris DC: "Chest pain" in patients with myocardial infarction. In Hurst JW, Morris DC, editors: *Chest pain,* Armonk, NY, 2001, Futura.)

■■■

TABLE 53-1 TYPICAL SYMPTOMS OF ACUTE CORONARY SYNDROME

TYPICAL SYMPTOMS	LOCATION	QUALITY

Discomfort or pain	Center of chest
	Radiating to the following:
	  Arms
	  Back
	  Neck
	  Jaw
	  Stomach
		Pressure
		Tightness
		Dull
		Heavy
		Aching
		Crushing
		Burning
		Squeezing
		Fullness
		Pain

Shortness of breath Diaphoresis Nausea Light-headedness		

vascular trials.[21,22] Harris and Douglas[23] found that there was no significant change in enrollment rates for women in National Heart, Lung, and Blood Institute–funded studies of cardiovascular disease from 1965 to 1998 when single-sex trials were excluded from analysis. Enrollment rates for women with CHD and hypertension were similar to the prevalence of disease in women; however, women remain underrepresented in trials of heart failure. In 1997, women represented 61.9 percent

of participants in studies funded by the National Institutes of Health. Although these data are encouraging, relying on single-sex studies does not allow for analyses of gender differences.

Atypical Symptoms

Historically, atypical symptoms have been viewed as all other symptoms not defined as typical. Atypical symptoms of ACS have included weakness, fatigue, palpitations, dizziness, indigestion, heartburn, hyperventilation, and loss of appetite (Table 53-2).[13,14,24,25] Interestingly, a number of investigators have found symptoms such as unusual fatigue and weakness to be frequent and thus not atypical. Perhaps they are not recorded in assessments because they are believed to be unimportant, vague, or not supportive of a cardiac diagnosis. Silent ischemia, or the lack of chest pain, also is considered to be atypical, although up to 30 percent of patients with ACS report no chest pain.[12,15,26-28]

■ ■ ■

TABLE 53-2 ATYPICAL SYMPTOMS OF ACUTE CORONARY SYNDROME

ATYPICAL SYMPTOMS	LOCATION	QUALITY
Dizziness	Right side of the chest	Knifelike
Hyperventilation	Right arm	Stabbing
Heartburn	Right shoulder	Sharp
Heat sensation	Left side of the chest	Tingling
Indigestion		
Loss of appetite		
Palpitations		
Unusually scared		
Weakness		
Unusual fatigue		

Braunwald and colleagues[6] list the following "atypical" descriptions of chest pain that are not attributed to myocardial ischemia:

Pleuritic pain (sharp or knifelike pain brought on by respiratory movements or cough)

- Primary or sole location of discomfort in the middle or lower abdominal region
- Pain that may be localized at the tip of one finger, particularly over the left ventricular apex
- Pain reproduced with movement or palpation of the chest wall or arms
- Constant pain that persists for many hours
- Very brief episodes of pain that last a few seconds or less
- Pain that radiates into the lower extremities

Although the majority of patients who have ACS exhibit typical symptoms, no single factor can be used to rule out those who have atypical symptoms. Determination of the urgency and level of care required depends on an assessment of symptoms, risk factors, clinical stability, risk of a life-threatening condition, and history.

A number of noncoronary conditions cause chest pain and can complicate the triage process. These conditions include vascular, pulmonary, gastrointestinal, musculoskeletal, infectious, and psychological conditions (Table 53-3).[29] The vascular syndromes of acute aortic

■ ■ ■

TABLE 53-3 COMMON CAUSES OF ACUTE CHEST PAIN

SYSTEM	SYNDROME	CLINICAL DESCRIPTION	KEY FEATURES
Cardiac	Angina	Retrosternal chest pressure, burning, or heaviness Radiating occasionally to neck, jaw, epigastrium, shoulders, or left arm	Precipitated by exercise, cold weather, or emotional stress Duration less than 2 minutes to 10 minutes
	Rest or unstable angina	Same as angina, but may be more severe	Usually less than 20 minutes; lower tolerance for exertion
	Acute myocardial infarction	Same as angina, but may be more severe	Sudden onset, usually lasting 30 minutes or longer Often associated with shortness of breath, weakness, nausea, vomiting
	Pericarditis	Sharp, pleuritic pain aggravated by changes in position Highly variable duration	Pericardial friction rub
Vascular	Aortic dissection	Excruciating, ripping pain of sudden onset in anterior of chest, often radiating to back	Marked severity of unrelenting pain Usually occurs in setting of hypertension or underlying connective tissue disorder such as Marfan syndrome
	Pulmonary embolism	Sudden onset of dyspnea and pain, usually pleuritic with pulmonary infarction	Dyspnea, tachypnea, tachycardia, and signs of right ventricular failure
	Pulmonary hypertension	Substernal chest pressure, exacerbated by exertion	Pain associated with dyspnea and signs of pulmonary hypertension
Pulmonary	Pleuritis and/or pneumonia	Pleuritic pain, usually brief, over involved area	Pain pleuritic and lateral to midline, associated with dyspnea
	Tracheobronchitis	Burning discomfort in midline	Midline location, associated with coughing
	Spontaneous pneumothorax	Sudden onset of unilateral pleuritic pain with dyspnea	Abrupt onset of dyspnea and pain
Gastrointestinal	Esophageal reflux	Burning substernal and epigastric discomfort 10 to 60 minutes in duration	Aggravated by large meal and postprandial recumbency Relieved by antacid
	Peptic ulcer	Prolonged epigastric or substernal burning	Relieved by antacid or food
	Gallbladder disease	Prolonged epigastric, right upper quadrant pain	Unprovoked or following meal
	Pancreatitis	Prolonged, intense epigastric and substernal pain	Risk factors including alcohol, hypertriglyceridemia, and medications
Musculoskeletal	Costochondritis	Sudden onset of intense fleeting pain	May be reproduced by pressure over affected joint Occasionally swelling and inflammation over costochondral joint
	Cervical disc disease	Sudden onset of fleeting pain	May be reproduced with movement of neck
Infectious	Herpes zoster	Prolonged burning pain in dermatomal distribution	Vesicular rash, dermatomal distribution
Psychological	Panic disorder	Chest tightness or aching, often accompanied by dyspnea and lasting 30 minutes or more, unrelated to exertion or movement	Patient may have other evidence of emotional disorder

From Lee TH, Cannon CP: Approach to the patient with chest pain. In Zipes DP, Libby P, Bonow R, Braunwald E, editors: *Braunwald's heart disease,* ed 7, Philadelphia, 2005, Elsevier Saunders.

dissection and pulmonary embolism are discussed in more detail in the section on differential diagnoses.

ASSESSING CHEST PAIN AND ASSOCIATED SYMPTOMS
Questions to Ask

Clinical appraisal of patients who have chest pain is based on the history, physical examination, and diagnostic testing. A number of critical questions should be asked that will aid in triage and in establishing the differential diagnosis: (1) What is the quality of the pain? (2) Where does the pain radiate? and (3) How severe was the pain at the onset of symptoms? Rosman and colleagues[30] conducted a retrospective medical record review of patients who had confirmed aortic dissection and found that if all three questions were asked, thoracic dissection was diagnosed correctly 91 percent of the time. Unfortunately, only 42 percent of conscious patients were asked all three questions.

Clinicians often ask leading or closed-ended questions, which are likely to result in a yes or no reply without eliciting any useful information. Questions such as "What brought you in today?" or "Can you describe your symptoms?" are much more valuable than asking "Do you have chest pain?" In addition, the word *pain* frequently is used by clinicians but infrequently used by patients.[31] Patients may use terms that denote less distress such as "discomfort," "sensation," or "feeling." The patient's description of pain may be related to perceptions of the attitudes of clinicians, the belief that clinicians are too busy, or the desire to be stoic and uncomplaining.[32]

Nurses frequently have used the mnemonic PQRST in performing a comprehensive assessment of chest pain and associated symptoms. "P" represents provocative and palliative features of the pain or discomfort. In other words, what activities or emotions provoke the pain, and what behaviors or interventions relieve the pain? The pain of stable angina often is induced by exertion, stress, or eating and can be treated successfully with nitrates or rest. The pain of unstable angina or NSTEMI can occur with exertion, stress, eating, or at rest. The pain usually begins gradually, takes several minutes to reach its peak intensity, and may wax and wane. The pain associated with STEMI can be provoked by exertion, stress, or eating or may begin at rest. The pain of STEMI usually lasts for more than 30 minutes and is more severe than the pain of stable angina, unstable angina, or NSTEMI.[11,33]

"Q" represents the quality of the discomfort and is best elicited from the patient without prompts. Typical quality descriptors reported in the literature for ACS include pressure, tightness, heaviness, dull, constricting, squeezing, aching, fullness, burning, and crushing. Atypical quality descriptors include knifelike, stabbing, sharp, and tingling.[13,33] The quality of pain for acute pericarditis has been described as retrosternal or precordial chest pain that is sharp or worse with inspiration.[34,35] Quality descriptors for aortic dissection include excruciating pain that may be described as ripping, tearing, shearing, knifelike, sharp, or pressure.[36-39]

"R" signifies the region or location of pain or discomfort, including radiation of pain to areas outside of the chest. Asking the patient to point to or touch the areas of pain or discomfort can aid in obtaining reliable information.

"S" describes the severity of pain or discomfort. Nurses commonly assess pain using a numeric rating scale ranging from 0 (no pain or discomfort) to 10 (the worst pain imaginable). Often patients experiencing ACS fail to seek care quickly, citing minor or moderate pain or confusion about the seriousness of the symptoms.[40] The mistaken assumption that the pain of ACS is severe can lead to failure to seek care rapidly. This delay in care can lead to irreversible myocardial damage accompanied by increased morbidity and mortality.[41-43]

"T" represents the temporal nature of symptoms. The symptoms may come and go with unstable angina or NSTEMI or may be relieved with rest. The symptoms associated with STEMI usually last longer than 30 minutes and may not be relieved with rest or nitrates.

Finally, nurses should pay particular attention to the nonverbal cues for pain that may reinforce the descriptions offered by the patient. Patients experiencing chest pain may present with Levine's sign, the classic clasped fist over the sternum (Figure 53-2) and may grimace, cry, or writhe in the bed. Cultural factors may influence how patients express their pain or discomfort. The nurse should consult with culturally competent interpreters or community members if available. The key to a positive outcome for the patient is to complete a comprehensive and reliable assessment in the shortest time possible with the goal of reducing time to treatment. Unit-specific

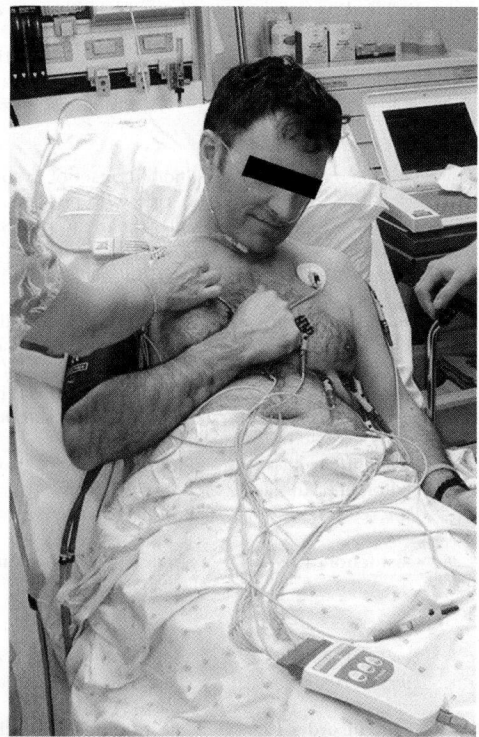

FIGURE 53-2 ■ A patient in the emergency department showing the classic Levine sign (closed fist over the sternum) reflecting the location of his chest pain.

protocols for the treatment of patient with symptoms suggestive of myocardial ischemia are useful in maintaining consistent standards of care (Table 53-4).

Examination

Diagnosis of ACS is based on the clinical presentation, history, risk stratification, physical examination, electrocardiogram (**ECG**) findings, and evaluation of cardiac markers. The ACC/AHA have formulated an algorithm for evaluating and managing patients with suspected ACS (Figure 53-3). The physical examination during an episode of ACS is frequently unremarkable unless the myocardium is seriously compromised. Vital signs, including heart rate, blood pressure in both arms, temperature, and pain assessment using a numeric rating scale of 0 to 10 should be documented. The first and second heart sounds may be diminished because of reduced myocardial contractility. An S_3 is infrequently present during an acute myocardial infarction and reflects left ventricular dysfunction. S_4 is common in patients with a long history of hypertension or chronic ischemic heart disease. An S_4 also may be heard during acute ischemia. Systolic murmurs are common and generally result from mitral regurgitation.[44] The lung fields should be auscultated. The presence of crackles may indicate the onset of pulmonary edema. Bruits may be detected in the carotid arteries. The peripheral pulses also should be palpated for pulse deficits.

■ ■ ■

TABLE 53-4 EMERGENCY DEPARTMENT NURSING PROTOCOL FOR PATIENTS WITH SUSPECTED MYOCARDIAL ISCHEMIA

A. Notify physician of patient's status immediately.
B. Undress the patient completely.
C. Place all suspected cardiac patients on a monitor. If the patient is older than age 30, obtain electrocardiogram and notify physician of results.
D. Provide continuous pulse oximetry. Document saturation without oyxgen as patient's condition allows.
E. If pain is not musculoskeletal, continue with the following:
   • Initiate intravenous capped line, draw laboratory samples.
   • Give oxygen at 2 to 4 liters/min by nasal cannula. If patient has chronic obstructive pulmonary disease, use low flow (1 to 2 liters/min).
F. Anticipate that the following may be ordered once the physician sees the patient:

LABORATORY TESTS	RADIOGRAPHS	ECG	OTHER
Complete blood count	Portable chest For pleuritic pain, posterior-anterior and lateral	Per criteria	Pulse oximetry
Metabolic panel			Arterial blood gases
Creatine kinase (CK-MB)			Nitroglycerin
Troponin			Aspirin
Prothrombin time			Beta blockers
Partial thromboplastin time			Heparin
			Morphine
Drug levels, as appropriate			Enoxaparin (Lovenox)
Urinalysis			Thrombolytics

Courtesy St. Joseph Regional Medical Center, Milwaukee, Wis.
ECG, Electrocardiogram.

Electrocardiography

The 12-lead ECG is the best tool to identify acute myocardial infarction, particularly STEMI, in the absence of left bundle branch block. A left bundle branch block may mask ST-T wave changes in acute myocardial infarction.[45] In STEMI, there is ST segment elevation in the affected leads with ST segment depression in the reciprocal leads (Figure 53-4). With NSTEMI, there is typically ST segment depression, T wave inversion, or nonspecific ST segment changes. The ECG is less useful in the diagnosis of unstable angina because there may be no changes or ST segment depression in the affected leads. The sensitivity of the ECG in correctly identifying acute myocardial infarction has ranged from 40 to 89 percent,[46,47] highlighting the limitations of the test and the importance of a comprehensive evaluation in establishing a diagnosis.

Markers of Myocardial Injury

Creatine Kinase-MB

Creatine kinase-MB (**CK-MB**), an isoenzyme released into the serum following acute myocardial infarction, was the traditional biological marker used before 2000.[48] CK-MB levels rise within 6 hours after the onset of symptoms and peak in 24 hours. Serial samples of CK-MB have a sensitivity of nearly 90 percent 3 hours after ED admission.[49] Skeletal muscle disease, overexertion of muscles, and cocaine use also can result in CK-MB elevations in the absence of myocardial injury.[50]

Cardiac Troponin

The European Society of Cardiology and the ACC have published guidelines adopting the use of troponin I or troponin T as preferred markers for detecting myocardial injury.[48] The troponins have demonstrated higher sensitivity and specificity to myocardial damage than the CK-MB isoenzyme.[51] Sensitivities ranging from 90 to 100 percent and specificities ranging from 76 to 91 percent have been reported for serial measures of troponin I and T.[49] Troponins are detectable in the serum from 3 to 6 hours after symptom onset, peak in 12 to 24 hours, and remain in the serum for 7 to 10 days following injury. Because troponin is released as a result of the disintegration of contractile proteins in the necrotic myocardium, it has a high specificity for irreversible injury.[52]

Myoglobin

Myoglobin, a hemeprotein found mainly in muscle tissue, is a reservoir for oxygen.[53] Myoglobin appears in the serum from 1 to 4 hours after the onset of symptoms, peaks in approximately 6 to 7 hours, and returns to baseline within 24 hours. Myoglobin is released more rapidly than the troponins and CK-MB and may be a useful diagnostic tool in the absence of ECG changes. For this reason, myoglobin also may be useful to detect reinfarction in the first 7 to 10 days following acute myocardial infarction, when troponin levels are still elevated.

C-Reactive Protein

C-reactive protein, a marker of inflammation, may be helpful in predicting the long-term risk for ACS.[54] Results from the Women's Health Study demonstrated a

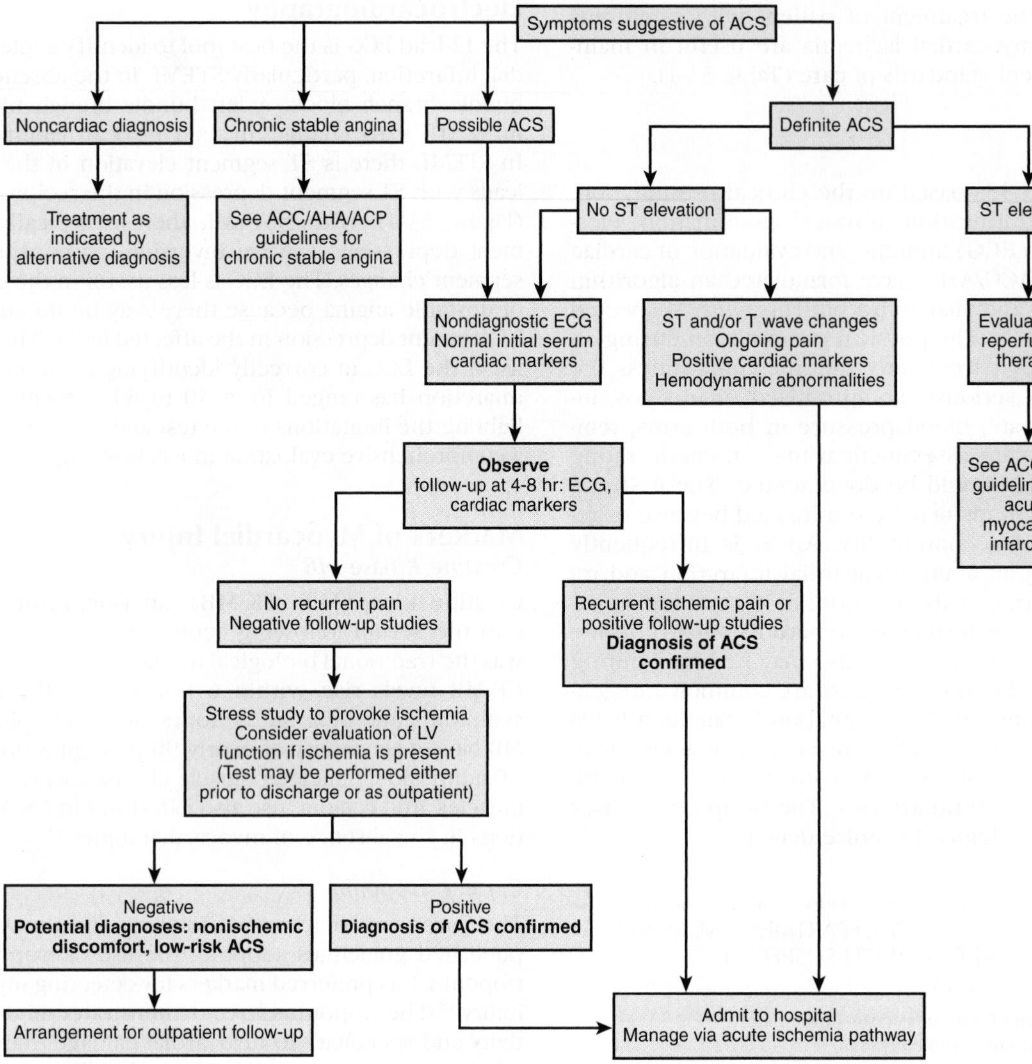

```
                            ┌──────────────────────────────┐
                            │  Symptoms suggestive of ACS  │
                            └──────────────────────────────┘
     ┌──────────────┬──────────────┬──────────────┬─────────────────────────┐
     │              │              │              │                         │
┌──────────┐ ┌─────────────┐ ┌──────────┐                          ┌────────────┐
│Noncardiac│ │Chronic stable│ │Possible  │                          │Definite ACS│
│diagnosis │ │angina       │ │ACS       │                          │            │
└──────────┘ └─────────────┘ └──────────┘                          └────────────┘
     │              │              │                 ┌──────────────┴──────────┐
┌──────────┐ ┌─────────────┐      │            ┌──────────────┐          ┌────────────┐
│Treatment │ │See ACC/AHA/ │      │            │No ST elevation│         │ST elevation│
│as        │ │ACP          │      │            └──────────────┘          └────────────┘
│indicated │ │guidelines for│     │            ┌──────┴────────────┐          │
│by        │ │chronic stable│     │       ┌──────────┐  ┌──────────────┐ ┌────────────┐
│alternative│ │angina       │     │       │Nondiagnostic│ │ST and/or T  │ │Evaluate for│
│diagnosis │ └─────────────┘      │       │ECG        │ │wave changes │ │reperfusion │
└──────────┘                      │       │Normal     │ │Ongoing pain │ │therapy     │
                                  │       │initial    │ │Positive     │ └────────────┘
                                  │       │serum      │ │cardiac      │       │
                                  │       │cardiac    │ │markers      │ ┌────────────┐
                                  │       │markers    │ │Hemodynamic  │ │See ACC/AHA │
                                  │       └──────────┘ │abnormalities│ │guidelines  │
```

(Algorithm flow chart — see figure.)

FIGURE 53-3 ■ Algorithm for evaluating and managing patients suspected of having acute coronary syndrome. *ACP,* American College of Physicians, *ACS,* acute coronary syndrome; *ECG,* electrocardiogram; *ST,* ST segment; *ACC/AHA/ACP,* American College of Cardiology/American Heart Association. (From Braunwald E, Antman EM, Beasley JW et al: ACC/AHA guideline update for the management of patients with unstable angina and non-ST segment elevation myocardial infarction: summary article 2002—a report of the American College of Cardiology/American Heart Association Task Force on Practice Guidelines [Committee on the Management of Patients with Unstable Angina], *Circulation* 106:1893, 2002.)

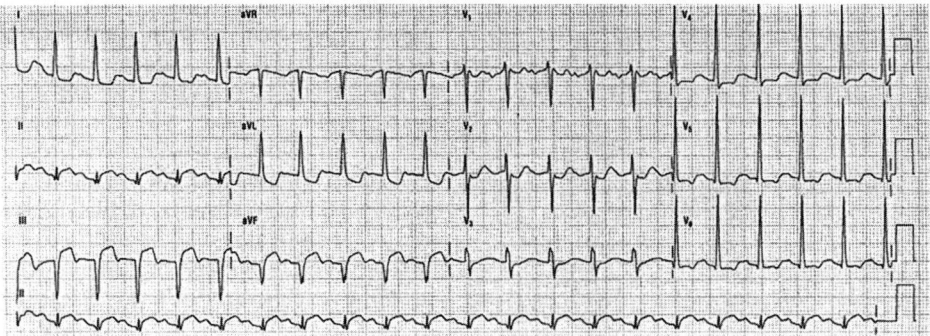

FIGURE 53-4 ■ ST segment elevation myocardial infarction. Note ST segment elevation in leads II, III, and aVF representing inferior wall myocardial infarction. Reciprocal ST segment depression is apparent in leads I, aVL, and V_4. (From Garcia TB, Holtz NE: *12-lead ECG: the art of interpretation,* Boston, 2001, Jones and Bartlett.)

direct relationship between C-reactive protein levels and risk for cardiovascular disease.[55] Other markers of inflammation and platelet aggregation, including P-selectin, are under study. No evidence exists for the utility of P-selectin in the diagnosis of ACS in the ED, but further study is warranted to address the value of these markers in risk stratification or in long-term prognosis for the development of CHD.[56]

Combinations of Cardiac Markers

Using a combination of cardiac markers increases the negative predictive value of the tests (that is, obtaining a negative test result when no injury exists). This can result in earlier discharge for those patients who do not have myocardial injury, thus reducing unnecessary treatment and costs.[57] Results from the Diagnostic Cooperative Study indicated that a combination of myoglobin and CK-MB subforms was the most sensitive marker during the early phase of acute myocardial infarction and that the combination of troponin and CK-MB was most sensitive between 8 and 12 hours after presentation.[58]

Coronary Angiography

Coronary catheterization and arteriography remain the gold standard for the diagnosis of CHD and are used in the diagnosis of ACS and stable coronary artery disease. Currently, the presence of disease is signified by more than 70 percent narrowing of the arterial lumen.[59]

Circadian Variations in Chest Pain

The onset of chest pain has been associated with biological circadian rhythms. Cannon and colleagues[60] found that participants in the Thrombolysis in Myocardial Ischemia III (TIMI) Registry had peak incidence of pain between 6 AM and 12 PM. Peak period for the onset of pain was between 8 AM and 12 PM for those with unstable angina. For those with non-Q wave myocardial infarction, the peak pain occurred between 6 and 10 AM. These data were supported by a meta-analysis of more than 83,000 patients that revealed the risk of myocardial infarction increased by 40 percent between the hours of 6 AM and 12 PM.[61] These variations in circadian rhythms have been attributed to stimulation of the sympathetic nervous system, release of catecholamines, and platelet aggregation.[62]

DIFFERENTIAL DIAGNOSES
Stable Angina

Angina is the clinical manifestation of myocardial ischemia. Stable angina is characterized by a mismatch between myocardial perfusion and demand. Typically, pain is manifested on exertion, emotional upset, or stress and is relieved with rest or nitrates. The predominant symptom of stable angina is chest discomfort, commonly perceived as pressure, burning, or heaviness. The pain of stable angina often is described as precordial tightness.[63] The pain is usually retrosternal but may radiate to the neck, left shoulder, or left arm. Equivalents of angina (i.e., symptoms other than chest discomfort) such as dyspnea, fatigue, eructation, or fainting also may be present.[59] Precipitating factors and severity distinguish stable angina from unstable angina, which is defined as angina that occurs at rest, is prolonged, or has become more severe.[64]

Examination

Extra heart sounds or murmurs may be present if there is significant left ventricular dysfunction. Splitting of the second heart sound may occur in the presence of prolonged left ventricular contraction. A third or fourth heart sound also may indicate myocardial ischemia. Early, late, or holosystolic murmurs may be present with papillary muscle dysfunction, be audible with exertion, or be audible while the patient is experiencing pain.[59] Vital signs, including heart rate, blood pressure in both arms, temperature, and pain assessment using a numeric rating scale of 0 to 10 should be documented. Examination of the eyes may reveal xanthomas, or yellowish lipid deposits, frequently found on the eyelids. This is a marker of hypercholesterolemia and often a family history of cardiovascular disease.

Noninvasive Testing
Resting Electrocardiogram

The resting ECG has little diagnostic value in stable angina. About half of all patients with coronary artery disease have a normal ECG. The most common abnormal finding in remaining patients is nonspecific ST-T wave changes. During an episode of angina, the most common finding is ST segment depression.

Noninvasive Stress Testing

Noninvasive stress testing (treadmill stress test) can be useful in making a diagnosis of stable CHD but may provide no more value than would a detailed history and physical.[65] The use of data gathered from such testing should be based on Bayes theorem, which states that the reliability and predictive accuracy of a test is determined not only by its sensitivity and specificity but also by the prevalence of disease in the population (see Chapter 29 for a complete discussion of stress testing). A general rule of thumb applicable to stress testing and to other diagnostic tests is that the test should be performed only if it will affect the treatment plan. If the results of testing will not affect the management of the disease, it is a waste of time and resources to complete the test.

Coronary Angiography

Cardiac catheterization and arteriography also are used to make a definitive diagnosis of stable coronary artery disease (see the previous discussion).

Acute Coronary Syndrome

ACS is the term used to identify a spectrum of clinical syndromes that represent progression of occlusion in the involved coronary artery.[9] The term *acute coronary syndrome* includes unstable angina, NSTEMI, and STEMI.[11] The three diagnoses represent the pathophysiological advancement from a stable to an unstable form of CHD. Occlusion usually occurs when a thrombus develops at the site of a ruptured or eroded plaque.[66]

Unstable Angina

Unstable angina is the result of a partial occlusion of a coronary artery without the presence of a cardiac marker in the serum. Braunwald[67] proposed a model for the etiology of unstable angina that includes five causes: (1) thrombosis; (2) mechanical obstruction; (3) increased myocardial oxygen consumption; (4) inflammation/infection; and (5) dynamic obstruction. The most common cause of unstable angina is thrombosis with mechanical obstruction. Prinzmetal or variant unstable angina is caused by a dynamic obstruction from intense vasoconstriction. Unstable angina represents a transition from stable angina to an unstable state. Stable angina has progressed to unstable angina when one or more of the coronary arteries is more than 60 percent obstructed and the symptoms have become more frequent, more severe, or occur at rest.[68] Patients experiencing an episode of unstable angina may have no chest pain or may experience pain or discomfort in the neck, arm, jaw, or epigastric region.[13]

Non-ST Segment Elevation Myocardial Infarction

NSTEMI results from a partial occlusion of the involved artery with a minor elevation in cardiac markers. NSTEMI in the majority of patients evolves into a non–Q wave myocardial infarction on 12-lead ECG. The pathophysiological characteristics of unstable angina and NSTEMI are so similar that the ACC/AHA guidelines recommend the same diagnostic testing and treatment for both syndromes.[64,69]

ST Segment Elevation Myocardial Infarction

STEMI occurs when a sudden and complete occlusion of the involved artery leads to acute ischemia and necrosis. The clinical scenario of most patients who have ST segment elevation on the ECG will evolve into that of Q wave myocardial infarction.[9,11]

Cocaine-Induced Acute Coronary Syndrome

Cocaine use can lead to numerous pathological processes including coronary artery vasoconstriction, tachycardia, platelet aggregation, systemic hypertension, and increased myocardial oxygen consumption.[57] Cocaine use causes acute and chronic changes. Mittleman and colleagues[70] found that the risk of acute myocardial infarction increased 24-fold in the hour following cocaine ingestion and that the increased risk remained weeks after the last use of cocaine. Although cocaine-induced myocardial infarction can occur in the absence of atherosclerotic changes, most patients with cocaine-associated myocardial infarction have some underlying atherosclerotic disease.[71]

Pericarditis

Acute pericarditis is a syndrome caused by inflammation of the pericardium. The pericardium consists of two layers; the outer or parietal layer is composed of fibrous collagen and elastin fibers, and the serous inner or visceral layer is composed of mesothelial cells and is attached to the epicardial surface of the heart. The pericardial space lies between the two layers and contains approximately 50 ml of pericardial fluid.[35,72] Pericarditis commonly is diagnosed based on a triad of findings including typical anterior chest pain, serial ECG changes, and pericardial friction rub.

Clinical Presentation and Appraisal

Acute pericarditis is the result of an inflammatory response to an infectious agent, cardiac surgery, or traumatic injury (Table 53-5).[73,74] Prodromal signs and symptoms include fever, malaise, and chest pain or discomfort. The primary presenting symptom is anterior chest pain. The pain is retrosternal or precordial; may radiate to the trapezius ridge, shoulder, arm, or epigastrium; and is often positional and aggravated with inspiration. The pain or discomfort frequently is relieved by leaning forward. The pain has been described as pleuritic but may mimic ischemic pain.[35,73-75] Associated symptoms include nausea, vomiting, palpitations, hoarseness, cough, hiccups, and dyspnea (Table 53-6). The quality of the pain has been described as sharp.[35]

Examination

A classic friction rub, representing the friction caused by contact between the visceral and parietal pericardial layers, is best auscultated over the left sternal border and is louder on expiration. The sound generated by the pericardial friction rub has been compared with rub-

■ ■ ■

TABLE 53-5 CAUSES OF PERICARDITIS

TYPE	EXAMPLES
Infectious	Viral (most common form)
	Bacterial
	Fungal
	Parasitic
Autoimmune	Dermatomyositis
	Drug-induced
	Family Mediterranean fever
	Mixed connective tissue disease
	Periarteritis nodosa
	Polyarteritis
	Postcardiotomy syndrome
	Postinfarction (Dressler syndrome)
	Reiter syndrome
	Rheumatic fever
	Rheumatoid arthritis
	Sarcoidosis
	Scleroderma
	Spondylitis ankylosans
	Systemic lupus erythematosus
	Systemic sclerosis
	Traumatic injury
Neoplastic	Primary tumors
	Secondary metastatic tumors
Metabolic	Uremia
	Myxedema
	Addison disease
Traumatic	Direct injury
	Indirect injury (irradiation)
Idiopathic	Unknown

TABLE 53-6   SYMPTOMS OF PERICARDITIS

SYMPTOM	LOCATION	RADIATION	QUALITY OF PAIN
Pain or discomfort	Retrosternal	Trapezius ridge	Pleuritic
	Precordial	Left shoulder	Ischemic
	Anterior	Left arm	Sharp
		Back	Knifelike
		Neck	
Dyspnea		Epigastrium	
Nausea			
Vomiting			
Palpitations			
Hoarseness			
Cough			
Hiccups			
Dizziness			
Light-headedness			
Anxiety			

bing hairs together or to walking on frozen snow. Typically the sound is harsh, scratching, grating, and high-pitched. The sound may be transient or may vary in intensity.[35] Pericarditis may be complicated by the accumulation of fluid in the pericardial space, restricting diastolic filling, and lead to cardiac tamponade. A reduced cardiac output associated with cardiac tamponade can result in signs and symptoms of cardiogenic shock, including a reduction in systemic systolic blood pressure on inspiration. This phenomenon, characterized by a drop of greater than 10 mm Hg in the systolic pressure, is known as pulsus paradoxus. The fact that heart sounds may be heard while a radial pulse cannot be palpated explains the "paradox." The paradoxical pulse is measured by sphygmomanometer with the patient breathing normally. The cuff should be deflated at approximately 2 to 3 mm Hg per heartbeat. Pulsus paradoxus is quantified by subtracting the value at which

the Korotkoff sound is heard with each heartbeat from the initial intermittent Korotkoff sounds heard only during expiration.[76] Nurses should anticipate the possibility of cardiac tamponade with pericarditis and assess for pulsus paradoxus.

Laboratory Tests

Slight elevations of markers of inflammation, such as white blood cell counts, erythrocyte sedimentation rate, and C-reactive protein, are common in acute pericarditis. Reports have indicated that a significant number of patients have elevated levels of CK-MB and troponin I.[77,78] This may be related to the concomitant development of myocarditis or preexisting acute myocardial infarction.

Electrocardiography

The ECG is the most important diagnostic tool in acute pericarditis (Figure 53-5). The classic findings are ST segment elevation with corresponding PR segment depression. Serial ECG changes can be delineated into four stages beginning with diffuse ST segment elevation and corresponding PR segment depression moving to T wave inversion and then return of the ST segment and T waves to preinflammatory tracings (Table 53-7).

TABLE 53-7   SERIAL ELECTROCARDIOGRAPHIC CHANGES IN PERICARDITIS

STAGE	CHANGE
Stage 1	Anterior and inferior concave ST segment elevation PR segment depression opposite of P wave polarity
Stage 2	ST segments return to baseline T waves progressively flatten and invert
Stage 3	T wave inversion
Stage 4	T wave abnormalities resolve Electrocardiogram returns to prepericarditis state

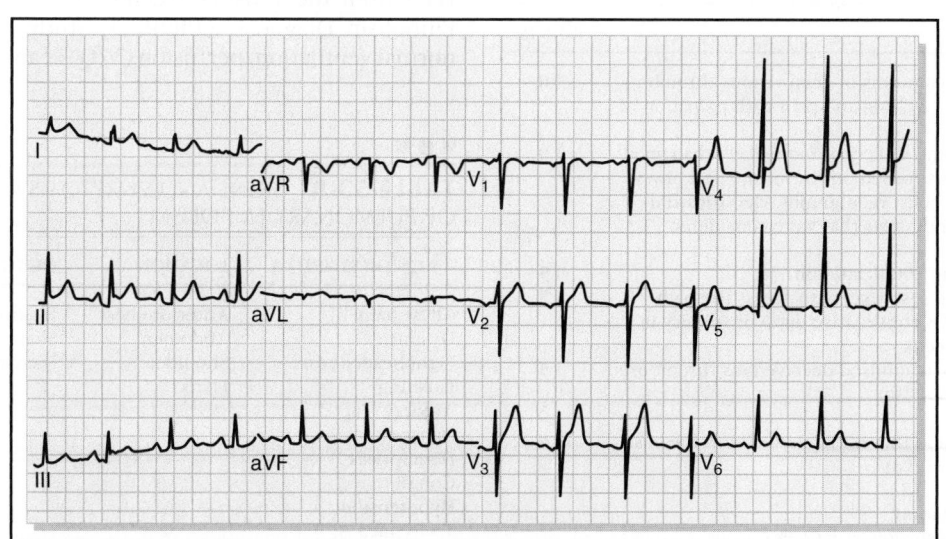

FIGURE 53-5 ■ The electrocardiogram in acute pericarditis. Note the diffuse ST segment elevation and PR segment depression. (From Le Winter MM, Kabbani S: Pericardial diseases. In Zipes P, Libby P, Bonow RO, Braunwald E, editors: *Braunwald's heart disease,* ed 7, Philadelphia, 2005, Elsevier Saunders.)

Echocardiography

Echocardiography does not contribute to a differential diagnosis of acute pericarditis but is of value in documenting pericardial effusion or cardiac tamponade, serious complications of acute pericarditis.[72]

Pulmonary Embolism

Pulmonary embolism is a formidable diagnostic challenge and an ominous emergency associated with high mortality rates. Each year, 50,000 to 100,000 deaths in the United States are attributed to pulmonary embolism.[79] Major pulmonary embolism, defined as that causing hemodynamic instability, has a mortality rate exceeding 30 percent.[80] Pulmonary embolism is ruled out in 65 to 85 percent of patients in whom it is suspected, which is a reflection of the complexities of making a differential diagnosis.[81,82] Pulmonary embolism truly presents a diagnostic conundrum; the cluster of nonspecific symptoms and the lack of sensitive and specific diagnostic tools present a challenge when a patient has suggestive symptoms. Analysis of risk factors is particularly useful in establishing a differential diagnosis. Factors including deep vein thrombosis, prolonged immobilization, or surgery in the last 4 weeks are suggestive of possible pulmonary embolism. Accuracy in diagnosis is enhanced by the use of strong predictive models based on history, presentation, blood gases, and chest x-ray films (Table 53-8).[83,84]

Clinical Presentation and Appraisal

The signs and symptoms of pulmonary embolism vary from mild to severe depending on the degree of cardiopulmonary compromise. The patient may be asymptomatic when less than 50 percent of the pulmonary vasculature is obstructed.[85] Patients have one of three syndromes: pulmonary infarction, isolated dyspnea, or circulatory collapse.[86] The classic symptoms of chest pain and dyspnea associated with pulmonary infarction are due to pleural irritation from the infarct. Because the lung has no pain fibers, pulmonary embolism only causes chest pain in the presence of peripheral parenchymal changes extending outside of the lung into the parietal pleura. Hence the term *pleuritic* chest pain.[82] Hemoptysis also may occur with this syndrome.

Patients with the syndrome of isolated dyspnea have varying degrees of shortness of breath depending on the extent of the obstruction. Syncope may be the initial symptom in the syndrome of circulatory collapse. The syncope may be transitory or progress to cardiac arrest. Syncope has been reported in 8 to 14 percent of patients with pulmonary embolism caused by obstruction of the pulmonary artery.[87] Less frequently reported symptoms of pulmonary embolism include lightheadedness, flushing, anxiety, abdominal pain, shoulder pain, and nausea.[88-90] Other quantitative data suggestive of pulmonary embolism are tachycardia, $PaCO_2$ less than 36.1 mm Hg, and PaO_2 less than 82.6 mm Hg.[86] No physical findings are uniquely suggestive of pulmonary embolism. Abnormalities in vital signs can contribute to suspicion but are not sufficient for a differential diagnosis (Table 53-9).

Laboratory Tests

D-dimer is a degradation product formed by the action of plasmin on a fibrin clot and serves as a marker for clot lysis. The plasma D-dimer assay is a test that has reported 85 percent sensitivity in identifying pulmonary embolism but has a low specificity. Because the negative predictive value is high but the positive predictive value is low, the test is valuable only in conjunction with other diagnostic modalities.

Ventilation/Perfusion Scan

Data from the Prospective Investigation of Pulmonary Embolism Diagnosis (**PIOPED**) Study indicated that a normal ventilation/perfusion (**V/Q**) scan essentially rules

■ ■ ■

TABLE 53-8   A SIMPLE CLINICAL MODEL FOR THE ASSESSMENT OF PULMONARY EMBOLISM

SYMPTOM	POINTS
Clinical signs and symptoms of deep venous thrombosis, including leg swelling and pain with palpation of the deep veins	3.0
Pulmonary embolism as likely or more likely than an alternative diagnosis (based on the history and physical examination, chest radiography, electrocardiogram, and any blood tests that were considered necessary)	3.0
Heart rate more than 100 beats/min	1.5
Immobilization (bed rest, except to access the bathroom, for at least 3 consecutive days) or surgery in the previous 4 weeks	1.5
Previous objectively diagnosed deep venous thrombosis or pulmonary embolism	1.5
Hemoptysis	1.0
Malignancy (treatment that is ongoing, within the past 6 months, or palliative)	1.0
Total points:	

Risk score interpretation:
Fewer than 2 points: low risk (2.3%)
2 to 6 points: moderate risk (16.2%)
More than 6 points: high risk (40.6%)

Adapted from Wells PS, Anderson DR, Rodger et al: *Ann Intern Med* 135:98-107, 2001.

■ ■ ■

TABLE 53-9   SIGNS AND SYMPTOMS OF PULMONARY EMBOLISM

SIGN OR SYMPTOM	LOCATION	QUALITY
Chest pain	Anterior chest	Pleuritic
Dyspnea	Abdomen	Sharp
Light-headedness	Shoulder	Increased on inspiration
Flushing	Flank	
Anxiety		
Nausea		
Hemoptysis		
Cough		
Hypotension		
Tachypnea		
Tachycardia		
Hypoxemia		
Fever		
Syncope		

out pulmonary embolism. In addition, 88 percent of subjects with a high probability for pulmonary embolism who underwent V/Q scan had the diagnosis confirmed with angiography.[91] Although the positive predictive value is excellent, the V/Q scan detects less than half of all pulmonary emboli, so it should be used in conjunction with other testing, particularly angiography.

Chest Computed Tomography

Chest computed tomography is now the imaging test of choice in the diagnosis of pulmonary embolism. The new generation of scanners have higher resolution and are able to detect smaller peripheral emboli. The scan is also valuable in examining the popliteal veins, the right ventricle, and the entire chest.[92]

Chest Radiograph

Radiographic presentation of pulmonary embolism may demonstrate abnormalities such as oligemia (decreased blood volume), pleural opacity, elevated diaphragm, or decreased pulmonary vasculature.[88] The presence of oligemia distal to the embolus is known as the Westermark sign and is considered to be the primary x-ray finding suggesting pulmonary embolus.[93]

Aortic Dissection

Aortic dissection, a tear in the intima (lining) of the aorta that results in bleeding and formation of a hematoma, is a catastrophic condition with a high mortality rate. Dissections are distinguished by location according to the Stanford classification system. Type A involves the ascending aorta regardless of the entry site, and type B involves the aorta distal to the left subclavian artery.[94] The incidence of the condition is higher in middle-aged men, blacks, individuals between ages 50 and 70, and those with a history of hypertension.[36] Aortic dissection also has occurred following cocaine ingestion as a result of catecholamine-induced profound elevation in blood pressure.[95]

Clinical Presentation and Appraisal

The majority of patients report the severe, sudden onset of pain described as tearing, sharp, ripping, or knifelike that radiates from the sternal area through to the back or interscapular area.[37,96] Two characteristics of chest pain, immediate onset and ripping quality, predicted the presence of aortic dissection in a study of 250 patients who presented to the ED with clinical suspicion of aortic dissection.[97] The pain may be accompanied by dyspnea, wheezing, sweating, chills, and nausea. Substernal pain is more typical in type A dissection, whereas back pain is more typical in type B dissection (Table 53-10).[98]

Atypical symptoms have been disclosed, including pain described as pressure, originating in the throat and radiating down the anterior chest into the abdomen and midway down the back. In addition, lower extremity pain, groin pain, and hemiplegia rarely have been reported.[99] Radiation to the shoulder or arm is also atypical compared with the typical radiation of ACS.[37,38] The sudden onset of symptoms also distinguishes aortic dissection from ACS. Generally, the patient appears in

■ ■ ■

TABLE 53-10 SIGNS AND SYMPTOMS OF ACUTE AORTIC DISSECTION

SIGN	SYMPTOM	LOCATION	QUALITY
May be normotensive	*Typical* Sudden onset of chest pain	*Typical* Anterior chest Retrosternal Radiating to back or interscapular region	*Typical* Severe Tearing Ripping Knife-like Shearing Sharp
Hypertension (with type B dissection)	*Atypical* Pain originating or radiating to other areas	*Atypical* Throat Abdomen Lower extremities Groin Flank	*Atypical* Pressure
Hypotension (with type A dissection and shock) Hematuria Oliguria *Atypical* Hemiplegia			

shock, although the blood pressure may be normal if the dissection is small or has developed slowly. Hypertension is common in type B dissection; hypotension is more typical in type A dissection. Flank pain, hematuria, or oliguria may occur with renal artery occlusion.[36]

Examination

The physical assessment should begin with vital signs. Of particular importance is the blood pressure, assessment for pulsus paradoxus, pulses on both sides of the body, and jugular venous distention.[96] Singer and Hollander[100] found that most patients who have aortic dissection had blood pressure differences greater than 10 mm Hg between arms. Von Kodolitsch and colleagues[97] reported that a blood pressure differential of more than 20 mm Hg was an independent predictor of aortic dissection. Hypotension and shock have been reported in about 25 percent of cases[37] and are caused by left ventricular dysfunction, cardiac tamponade, aortic rupture, and/or severe aortic regurgitation. Heart sounds may reveal the murmur of aortic regurgitation and an S_3 in the presence of concomitant left ventricular failure.

Diagnostic Tests

The chest x-ray is abnormal in approximately 60 to 90 percent of cases with the predominant findings of widened mediastinum and irregularities in the aortic contour.[38,96] ECG and chest radiography are not sufficient to establish a differential diagnosis of aortic dissection because of the lack of specificity in these measures. Imaging techniques useful in diagnosing aortic dissection are transesophogeal echocardiography, computed tomography scanning, magnetic resonance imaging, and angiography.

Transesophageal Echocardiography

Advantages of performing transesophageal echocardiography include ease of use at the bedside and rapid and wide availability. The test has high sensitivity and specificity and therefore is recommended in most cases when aortic dissection is suspected. The main limitations are related to inexperienced examiners and the ability to visualize only the thoracic and proximal abdominal aorta. Transesophageal echocardiography cannot be used in patients with esophageal varices.

Computed Tomography Scanning

Computed tomography is a valuable diagnostic tool for aortic dissection because it is less invasive than aortography and is widely available for emergent use. Limitations to the use of computed tomography scanning include difficulty in establishing the origin of the tear, difficulty in determining the involvement of branch vessels, and the inability to assess the degree of aortic regurgitation.[37]

Magnetic Resonance Imaging

Magnetic resonance imaging has a higher sensitivity and specificity for the detection of aortic dissection. In addition, the extent and site of dissection can be identified with precision.[37] The lack of immediate availability and longer testing time are the primary limitations of the test.

DIFFERENCES IN SYMPTOMS ASSOCIATED WITH MYOCARDIAL ISCHEMIA

Data suggest that women, the elderly, and patients with a history of stroke, heart failure, diabetes, and hypertension experience more atypical symptoms during myocardial ischemia.[13,17,101,102]

Sex

In the Worcester Heart Attack Study, women, especially women age 65 and older, were less likely than men to have a chief complaint of chest pain during acute myocardial infarction.[101] In a recent study examining sex differences in the symptoms of unstable angina, women experienced more shortness of breath, weakness, nausea, loss of appetite, discomfort in the upper back, and sharp and knifelike pain.[13] Everts and colleagues[103] also reported that women had more back pain and neck pain in a Swedish cohort of patients with suspected myocardial infarction. Results of the Rapid Early Action for Coronary Treatment Trial indicated that women with all forms of ACS experienced more nausea, back pain, neck pain, and jaw pain compared with men.[14] Preliminary reports of 935 women from the Women's Ischemia Syndrome Evaluation Study indicate that most women had chest pain but that a minority had other presenting chief complaints including exertional dyspnea.[104] Interestingly, sex differences have been reported in symptoms considered typical (shortness of breath, nausea, and jaw pain) and atypical (back pain, neck pain, and

■ ■ ■ CONUNDRUM

ARE THERE SIGNIFICANT GENDER DIFFERENCES IN CARDIAC SYMPTOMS?

Evidence indicates significant gender differences in the symptoms of acute coronary syndrome. A number of investigators sampling an array of geographic areas, racial and ethnic groups, socioeconomic groups, and age ranges have demonstrated that women experience more back, neck, and jaw pain, nausea/vomiting, dyspnea, indigestion, dizziness, fatigue, loss of appetite, and palpitations compared with men. Men have reported more chest pain and diaphoresis. In addition, results are consistent across multiple studies. These findings represent *statistical* significance, and it is unclear whether these differences are *clinically* significant. Based on available evidence, it is recommended that nurses conduct a comprehensive assessment of symptoms regardless of sex. However, it would be prudent to inform women of their risk for heart disease and to caution them that their symptoms may differ from those that have been portrayed in the mass media. Finally, women should be encouraged to seek immediate evaluation if they experience symptoms.

sharp or knifelike pain). See the accompanying conundrum feature on gender differences and Chapter 52 for a discussion of cardiovascular disease in women.

Milner and colleagues[16] hypothesized that because prior reports indicate that women with ACS have more atypical symptoms, the presence of atypical symptoms would be predictive of a diagnosis of ACS. Patients were observed in the ED and were interviewed about presenting symptoms following admission. The hypothesis was not supported, and the presence of typical symptoms (chest pain, dyspnea, diaphoresis, and arm or shoulder pain) predicted a diagnosis of ACS for women and men. Kimble and colleagues[63] studied 128 subjects with stable angina and found that women and men had more similarities than differences in chest pain characteristics; however, women were more likely to have physical limitations because of anginal pain. Friedman[105] found that women and men with heart failure had similar numbers and types of symptoms following admission to the hospital. The three most commonly reported symptoms for women and men were shortness of breath, fatigue, and weakness. No gender differences were found in eight symptoms of myocardial infarction in a study examining gender differences in the attribution of symptoms of myocardial infarction; however, women were less likely than men to attribute their prehospital symptoms to a cardiac cause.[106]

Investigators have found that women do not perceive their risk of heart disease accurately.[107] These findings are disconcerting because failure to attribute ischemic symptoms to a serious cardiac condition can cause delay in seeking emergent care or in a decision not to seek care. Mosca and colleagues,[108] in a sample of 1024 ethnically diverse women, found that awareness of the risk of heart disease has increased since 1997. In 1997, 30 percent of women surveyed identified heart disease as the leading cause of death. This increased to 46 percent by 2003. These studies serve as a reminder that nurses are

■ ■ ■

TABLE 53-11   WEB RESOURCES FOR CHEST PAIN AND WOMEN WITH CORONARY HEART DISEASE

TITLE	WEB ADDRESS
Chest Pain	www.mayoclinic.com/invoke. cfm?id=DS00016
Heart Disease and Heart Attacks: What Women Need to Know	http://familydoctor.org/287. xml?printxml
Women's Heart Foundation	www.womensheartfoundation. org
National Coalition for Women with Heart Disease	www.womenheart.org
The Heart Truth	www.nhlbi.nih.gov/health/ hearttruth/

in an excellent position to educate patients and direct them to applicable resources (Table 53-11).

Age

Older persons with ACS have reported experiencing milder and more ambiguous sensations compared with younger persons. Older persons also have more chronic disease such as diabetes, heart failure, and stroke that are associated with a higher incidence of silent ischemia.[26] Elderly persons often have the expectation that pain or discomfort are normal aspects of aging or mistakenly attribute symptoms to other minor medical conditions and therefore do not view cardiac symptoms as an emergency.[109] Differences in symptoms according to age are not limited to the symptoms of ACS. Timmons and colleagues[110] found that older patients (age 65 and older, median age 73) with pulmonary embolism experienced less pleuritic pain and more cyanosis, hypoxia, and collapse compared with patients younger than age 65 (median age 48). Although a dramatic presentation such as collapse may lead to accessing emergency services quickly and expedited diagnosis and treatment, atypical symptoms often lead to a delay in seeking treatment or to a delayed differential diagnosis.

Race/Ethnicity

Some data indicate that symptom differences exist along racial and ethnic lines. Blacks experienced significantly more shortness of breath and chest pain on the left side compared with whites when presenting to the ED with symptoms of CHD.[111] In a study of patients presenting to the ED with acute myocardial infarction, investigators found that blacks were more likely to report dyspnea and fatigue, whereas whites reported more pain in the shoulder, neck, and jaw.[112] These findings were supported in a larger study of consecutive patients presenting to the ED with acute chest pain. Blacks were less likely to experience pressure-type chest pain and diaphoresis compared with whites, who reported more radiation to the left arm, left shoulder, neck, and/or jaw.[113]

Slight variations in symptoms were found between blacks, whites, and Koreans in a study of patients experiencing acute myocardial infarction. The Korean cohort experienced more dyspnea, sweating, and palpitations compared with whites. Blacks reported more dyspnea and fatigue compared with whites. The incidence of chest pain was not significantly different between the three groups.[79] These results suggest minor variations in the typical presentation of ACS and serve as a reminder that symptoms may vary between individual patients and that the key to improving outcomes is the thorough assessment of *all* patients for typical and less typical symptoms.

Comorbid Conditions

Diabetes, heart failure, and stroke also may contribute to symptom variations during a cardiac event. An assumption has been made that patients with diabetes experience symptoms differently because of cardiac autonomic neuropathy.[114,115] Researchers have hypothesized that cardiac autonomic neuropathy involves the cardiac afferent pathways of the sympathetic nervous system, which carry pain messages from myocardial pain receptors to the cerebral cortex.[116] Dysfunction in these pathways may affect sensory and pain perceptions for patients with diabetes. In a recent large prospective study, patients with diabetes were more likely to experience weakness, cough, dyspnea, and nausea during myocardial infarction.[117] In contrast, Funk and colleagues[18] found no differences in the symptoms of CHD for those patients with or without diabetes. Patients with diabetes reported nausea less often, less squeezing and aching pain, and hyperventilation more often in a study examining the symptoms of unstable angina.[17] Other cardiac symptoms were similar between the groups. These conflicting findings are difficult to interpret and apply to clinical nursing practice. Further studies are needed to help clarify similarities and differences in symptoms. In addition, symptoms commonly associated with diabetes such as dry mouth, thirst, stomach pain, shortness of breath, and diaphoresis may mimic the symptoms of ischemia.[118,119]

The symptoms associated with heart failure can complicate the nursing assessment of symptoms during an acute cardiac event. The most common symptoms of heart failure including breathing difficulties, and fatigue are typical symptoms associated with ACS and are similar to the symptoms of chronic obstructive pulmonary disease, pericarditis, and pulmonary embolism.

A higher incidence of silent ischemia occurs during acute myocardial infarction for patients with a history of stroke.[26] The sensory losses resulting from stroke also may impair other pain sensations during myocardial infarction, especially those radiating to the affected side.

The attribution of chest pain and associated symptoms to a cardiac cause represents a great challenge to nurses. The ability to make a differential diagnosis is enhanced by an accurate and comprehensive assessment of signs and symptoms in conjunction with other clinical findings.

REFERENCES

1. American Heart Association: *Heart and stroke facts,* Dallas, 2005, The Association.

2. Greenlund KJ, Keenan NL, Giles WH et al: Public recognition of major signs and symptoms of heart attack: seventeen states and the U.S. Virgin Islands, 2001, *Am Heart J* 147(6):1010-1016, 2004.

3. Ryan CJ, Zerwic JJ: Knowledge of symptom clusters among adults at risk for acute myocardial infarction, *Nurs Res* 53(6):363-369, 2004.

4. McCaig LF, Burt CW: National Hospital Ambulatory Medical Care Survey: 2002 emergency department summary, *Adv Data* issue 340, pp 1-34, 2004.

5. Quin G: Chest pain evaluation units, *J Accid Emerg Med* 17(4):237-240, 2000.

6. Braunwald E. Antman EM. Beasley JW. Califf RM. Cheitlin MD. Hochman JS. Jones RH. Kereiakes D. Kupersmith J. Levin TN. Pepine CJ. Schaeffer JW. Smith EE 3rd. Steward DE. Theroux P. Alpert JS. Eagle KA. Faxon DP. Fuster V. Gardner TJ. Gregoratos G. Russell RO. Smith SC Jr. ACC/AHA guidelines for the management of patients with unstable angina and non–ST-segment elevation myocardial infarction. A report of the American College of Cardiology/American Heart Association Task Force on Practice Guidelines (Committee on the Management of Patients With Unstable Angina). J Amer Coll Cardiol 36(3):970-1062, 2000.

7. American Heart Association: *Heart disease and stroke statistics: 2005 update,* Dallas, 2004, The Association.

8. National Heart, Lung, and Blood Institute: *Heart attack warning signs.* Retrieved December 30, 2006 from www.nhlbi.nih.gov/actintime/haws/haws.htm

9. Fox KA: Coronary disease: acute coronary syndromes—presentation-clinical spectrum and management, *Heart* 84(1):93-100, 2000.

10. Fuster V, Steele PM, Chesebro JH: Role of platelets and thrombosis in coronary atherosclerotic disease and sudden death, *J Am Coll Cardiol* 5(6 suppl):175B-184B, 1985.

11. Cooper HA, Braunwald E: Clinical recognition of acute coronary syndromes. In Theroux P, editor: *Acute coronary syndromes: a companion to Braunwald's heart disease,* Philadelphia, 2003, Saunders.

12. Ashton KC: How men and women with heart disease seek care: the delay experience, *Prog Cardiovasc Nurs* 14(2):53-60, 1999.

13. DeVon HA, Zerwic JJ: The symptoms of unstable angina: do women and men differ? *Nurs Res* 52(2):108-118, 2003.

14. Goldberg RJ, Goff D, Cooper L et al: Age and sex differences in presentation of symptoms among patients with acute coronary disease: the REACT trial, *Coron Artery Dis* 11:399-407, 2000.

15. Milner KA, Funk M, Richards S et al: Gender differences in symptom presentation associated with coronary heart disease, *Am J Cardiol* 84(4):396-399, 1999.

16. Milner KA, Funk M, Arnold A, Vaccarino V: Typical symptoms are predictive of acute coronary syndromes in women, *Am Heart J* 143(2):283-288, 2002.

17. DeVon HA, Penckofer S, Zerwic JJ: The symptoms of unstable angina in patients with and without diabetes, *Res Nurs Health* 28(2):136-143, 2005.

18. Funk M, Naum JB, Milner KA, Chyun D: Presentation and symptom predictors of coronary heart disease in patients with and without diabetes, *Am J Emerg Med* 19(6):482-487, 2001.

19. Healy B: The Yentl syndrome, *N Engl J Med* 325(4):274-276, 1991.

20. Federal Drug Administration: *FDA plans policy change on women in clinical trials.* Retrieved December 30, 2006, from www.fda.gov/bbs/topics/ANSWERS/ANS00485.html

21. Hall WD: Representation of blacks, women, and the very elderly (aged > or = 80) in 28 major randomized clinical trials, *Ethn Dis* 9(3):333-340, 1999.

22. National Institutes of Health: *NIH policy and guidelines on the inclusion of women and minorities as subjects in clinical research.* Retrieved December 30, 2006, from http://grants.nih.gov/grants/funding/women_min/guidelines_update.htm

23. Harris DJ, Douglas PS: Enrollment of women in cardiovascular clinical trials funded by the National Heart, Lung, and Blood Institute, *N Engl J Med* 343(7):475-480, 2000.

24. McSweeney JC, Cody M, O'Sullivan P et al: Women's early warning symptoms of acute myocardial infarction, *Circulation* 108(21):2619-2623, 2003.

25. McSweeney JC, Crane PB: Challenging the rules: women's prodromal and acute symptoms of myocardial infarction, *Res Nurs Health* 23(2):135-146, 2000.

26. Canto JG, Shlipak MG, Rogers WJ et al: Prevalence, clinical characteristics, and mortality among patients with myocardial infarction presenting without chest pain, *JAMA* 283(24):3223-3229, 2000.

27. Gupta M, Tabas JA, Kohn MA: Presenting complaint among patients with myocardial infarction who present to an urban, public hospital emergency department, *Ann Emerg Med* 40(2):180-186, 2002.

28. Zucker DR, Griffith JL, Beshansky JR, Selker HP: Presentations of acute myocardial infarction in men and women, *J Gen Intern Med* 12(2):79-87, 1997.

29. Lee TH, Cannon CP: Approach to the patient with chest pain. In Zipes DP, Libby P, Bonow RO, Braunwald E, editors: *Braunwald's heart disease,* ed 7, Philadelphia, 2005, Elsevier Saunders.

30. Rosman HS, Patel S, Borzak S et al: Quality of history taking in patients with aortic dissection, *Chest* 114(3):793-795 1998.

31. Treasure T: Pain is not the only feature of heart attack, *BMJ* 317(7158):602-603, 1998.

32. Albarran J: The language of chest pain, *Nurs Times* 98(4):38-40, 2002.

33. DeVon HA, Zerwic JJ: Differences in the symptoms associated with unstable angina and myocardial infarction, *Prog Cardiovasc Nurs* 19(1):6-11, 2004.

34. Maisch B, Seferovic PM, Ristic AD et al: Guidelines on the diagnosis and management of pericardial diseases executive summary: the Task Force on the Diagnosis and Management of Pericardial Diseases of the European Society of Cardiology, *Eur Heart J* 25(7):587-610, 2004.

35. Ross AM, Grauer SE: Acute pericarditis: evaluation and treatment of infectious and other causes, *Postgrad Med* 115(3):67-70, 2004.

36. Finkelmeier BA, Marolda D: Aortic dissection, *J Cardiovasc Nurs* 15(4):15-24, 2001.

37. Khan IA, Nair CK: Clinical, diagnostic, and management perspectives of aortic dissection, *Chest* 122(1):311-328, 2002.

38. O'Gara PT, Greenfield AJ, Afridi NA, Houser SL: Case records of the Massachusetts General Hospital: weekly clinicopathological exercises. Case 12-2004: a 38-year-old woman with acute onset of pain in the chest, *N Engl J Med* 350(16):1666-1674, 2004.

39. Yee CA: Aortic dissection: the tear that kills, *Nurs Manage* 35(2):25-32, 2004.

40. Ornato JP, Hand MM: Warning signs of a heart attack, *Circulation* 104(11):1212-1213, 2001.

41. Luepker RV: Barriers to patients seeking emergency care for acute coronary heart disease, *JAMA* 284(17):2184, 2000.

42. Rosenfeld AG: Women's risk of decision delay in acute myocardial infarction: implications for research and practice, *AACN Clin Issues* 12(1):29-39, 2001.

43. Zerwic JJ, Ryan CJ, DeVon HA, Drell MJ: Treatment seeking for acute myocardial infarction symptoms: differences in delay across sex and race, *Nurs Res* 52(3):159-167, 2003.

44. Antmann AM, Braunwald E: ST-elevation myocardial infarction: pathology, pathophysiology, and clinical features. In Zipes DP, Libby P, Bonow RO, Braunwald E, editors: *Braunwald's heart disease,* ed 7, Philadelphia, 2005, Elsevier Saunders.

45. Shlipak MG, Lyons WL, Go AS et al: Should the electrocardiogram be used to guide therapy for patients with left bundle-branch block and suspected myocardial infarction? *JAMA* 281(8):714-719, 1999.

46. Fesmire FM, Hughes AD, Fody EP et al: The Erlanger chest pain evaluation protocol: a one-year experience with serial 12-lead ECG monitoring, two-hour delta serum marker measurements, and selective nuclear stress testing to identify and exclude acute coronary syndromes. Ann of Emerg Med. 40(6):595-7, 2002.

47. Savonitto S, Ardissino D, Granger CB et al: Prognostic value of the admission electrocardiogram in acute coronary syndromes, *JAMA* 281(8):707-713, 1999.

48. Alpert JS, Thygesen K, Antman E, Bassand JP: Myocardial infarction redefined: a consensus document of the Joint European So-

ciety of Cardiology/American College of Cardiology Committee for the redefinition of myocardial infarction, *J Am Coll Cardiol* 36(3):959-969, 2000.

49. Lau J, Ioannidis JP, Balk EM et al: Diagnosing acute cardiac ischemia in the emergency department: a systematic review of the accuracy and clinical effect of current technologies, *Ann Emerg Med* 37(5):453-460, 2001.

50. Hollander JE, Levitt MA, Young GP et al: Effect of recent cocaine use on the specificity of cardiac markers for diagnosis of acute myocardial infarction, *Am Heart J* 135(2 pt 1):245-252, 1998.

51. Apple FS, Falahati A, Paulsen PR et al: Improved detection of minor ischemic myocardial injury with measurement of serum cardiac troponin I, *Clin Chem* 43(11):2047-2051, 1997.

52. Jaffe AS, Ravkilde J, Roberts R et al: It's time for a change to a troponin standard, *Circulation* 102(11):1216-1220, 2000.

53. King M: "Hemoglobin" and "Role of 2,3-BPG." Retrieved March 18, 2004, from http://isu.indstate.edu/mwking/hemoglobin-myoglobin.html

54. Hamm CW: Cardiac biomarkers for rapid evaluation of chest pain, *Circulation* 104(13):1454-1456, 2001.

55. Rifai N, Buring JE, Lee IM et al: Is C-reactive protein specific for vascular disease in women? *Ann Intern Med* 136(7):529-533, 2002.

56. Hollander JE, Muttreja MR, Dalesandro MR, Shofer FS: Risk stratification of emergency department patients with acute coronary syndromes using P-selectin, *J Am Coll Cardiol* 34(1):95-105, 1999.

57. Hollander JE: Acute coronary syndrome in the emergency department: diagnosis, risk stratification, and management. In Theroux P, editor: *Acute coronary syndromes: a companion to Braunwald's heart disease,* Philadelphia, 2003, Elsevier Saunders.

58. Zimmerman J, Fromm R, Meyer D et al: Diagnostic marker cooperative study for the diagnosis of myocardial infarction, *Circulation* 99(13):1671-1677, 1999.

59. Morrow DA, Gersh BJ, Braunwald E: Chronic coronary artery disease. In Zipes DP, Libby P, Bonow RO, Braunwald E, editors: *Braunwald's heart disease,* ed 7, Philadelphia, 2005, Elsevier Saunders.

60. Cannon CP, McCabe CH, Stone PH et al: Circadian variation in the onset of unstable angina and non-Q-wave acute myocardial infarction (the TIMI III Registry and TIMI IIIB), *Am J Cardiol* 79(3):253-258, 1997.

61. Cohen MC, Rohtla KM, Lavery CE et al: Meta-analysis of the morning excess of acute myocardial infarction and sudden cardiac death, *Am J Cardiol* 79(11):1512-1516, 1997.

62. Doering LV: Pathophysiology of acute coronary syndromes leading to acute myocardial infarction, *J Cardiovasc Nurs* 13(3):1-20, 1999 (quiz, p 119).

63. Kimble LP, McGuire DB, Dunbar SB et al: Gender differences in pain characteristics of chronic stable angina and perceived physical limitation in patients with coronary artery disease, *Pain* 101(1-2):45-53, 2003.

64. Braunwald E, Antman EM, Beasley JW et al: ACC/AHA guideline update for the management of patients with unstable angina and non–ST-segment elevation myocardial infarction—2002: summary article—a report of the American College of Cardiology/American Heart Association Task Force on Practice Guidelines (Committee on the Management of Patients with Unstable Angina), *Circulation* 106(14):1893-1900, 2002.

65. Gibbons RJ, Balady GJ, Bricker JT et al: ACC/AHA 2002 guideline update for exercise testing: summary article—a report of the American College of Cardiology/American Heart Association Task Force on Practice Guidelines (Committee to Update the 1997 Exercise Testing Guidelines), *Circulation* 106(14):1883-1892, 2002.

66. Bentzon JF, Falk E: Pathology of stable and acute coronary syndromes. In Theroux P, editor: *Acute coronary syndromes: a companion to Braunwald's heart disease,* Philadelphia, 2003, Saunders.

67. Braunwald E: Unstable angina: an etiologic approach to management, *Circulation* 98(21):2219-2222, 1998.

68. Theroux P: Unstable angina. In Alexander RW, Schlant RC, Fuster V et al, editors: *Hurst's the heart,* New York, 1999, McGraw-Hill.

69. Braunwald E: Application of current guidelines to the management of unstable angina and non–ST-elevation myocardial infarction, *Circulation* 108(16 suppl 1):III28-III37, 2003.

70. Mittleman MA, Mintzer D, Maclure M et al: Triggering of myocardial infarction by cocaine, *Circulation* 99(21):2737-2741, 1999.

71. Hollander JE: The management of cocaine-associated myocardial ischemia, *N Engl J Med* 333(19):1267-1272, 1995.

72. LeWinter MM, Kabbani S: Pericardial diseases. In Zipes DP, Libby P, Bonow RO, Braunwald E, editors: *Braunwald's heart disease,* ed 7, Philadelphia, 2005, Elsevier Saunders.

73. Priori SG, Garcia AA, Blanc JJ et al: Guidelines on the diagnosis and management of pericardial diseases: executive summary, *Eur Heart J* 25:587-610, 2004.

74. Rashford S: Acute pleuritic chest pain, *Aust Fam Physician* 30(9):841-846, 2001.

75. Spodick DH: Acute pericarditis: classic electrocardiogram, *Am J Geriatr Cardiol* 12(4):266, 2003.

76. Lokhandwala KA: Clinical signs in medicine: pulsus paradoxus, *J Postgrad Med* 67(12):46-49, 2002.

77. Bonnefoy E, Godon P, Kirkorian G et al: Serum cardiac troponin I and ST-segment elevation in patients with acute pericarditis, *Eur Heart J* 21(10):832-836, 2000.

78. Brandt RR, Filzmaier K, Hanrath P: Circulating cardiac troponin I in acute pericarditis, *Am J Cardiol* 87(11):1326-1328, 2001.

79. Lee LC, Shah K: Clinical manifestation of pulmonary embolism, *Emerg Med Clin North Am* 19(4):925-942, 2001.

80. Wood KE: Major pulmonary embolism, part 1: presentation and basic diagnostic studies—rapidly recognizing the lethal signs and symptoms, *J Crit Illn* 16(9):395-405, 2001.

81. Bernard Bagattini S, Bounameaux H, Perneger T, Perrier A: Suspicion of pulmonary embolism in outpatients: nonspecific chest pain is the most frequent alternative diagnosis, *J Intern Med* 256(2):153-160, 2004.

82. Miller AC: Suspected pulmonary embolism, *Clin Med* 4(3):215-219, 2004.

83. Wells PS, Anderson DR, Rodger M et al: Excluding pulmonary embolism at the bedside without diagnostic imaging: management of patients with suspected pulmonary embolism presenting to the emergency department by using a simple clinical model and D-dimer, *Ann Intern Med* 135(2):98-107, 2001.

84. Wicki J, Perneger TV, Junod AF et al: Assessing clinical probability of pulmonary embolism in the emergency ward: a simple score, *Arch Intern Med* 161(1):92-97, 2001.

85. Riedel M: Acute pulmonary embolism 1: pathophysiology, clinical presentation, and diagnosis, *Heart* 85(2):229-240, 2001.

86. Sadosty AT, Boie ET, Stead LG: Pulmonary embolism, *Emerg Med Clin North Am* 21(2):363-384, 2003.

87. Brilakis ES, Tajik AJ: 82-year-old man with recurrent syncope, *Mayo Clin Proc* 74(6):609-612, 1999.

88. Liesching T, O'Brien A: Significance of a syncopal event: pulmonary embolism, *Postgrad Med* 111(1):19-20, 2002.

89. Schluger NW: Clearing up confusion in pulmonary embolism diagnosis: before and after diagnostic tests, give due consideration to clinical factors, *J Crit Illn* 15(11):592-598, 2000.

90. Unluer EE, Denizbasi A: A pulmonary embolism case presenting with upper abdominal and flank pain, *Eur J Emerg Med* 10(2):135-138, 2003.

91. The PIOPED Investigators: Value of the ventilation/perfusion scan in acute pulmonary embolism: results of the prospective investigation of pulmonary embolism diagnosis (PIOPED), *JAMA* 263(20):2753-2759, 1990.

92. Goldhaber SZ: Pulmonary embolism. In Zipes DP, Libby P, Bonow R, Braunwald E, editors: *Braunwald's heart disease,* ed 7, Philadephia, 2005, Elsevier Saunders.

93. Westermark N: On the roentgen diagnosis of lung embolism, *Acta Radiol* 19:357-372, 1938.

94. Daily PO, Trueblood HW, Stinson EB et al: Management of acute aortic dissections, *Ann Thorac Surg* 10(3):237-247, 1970.

95. Perron AD, Gibbs M: Thoracic aortic dissection secondary to crack cocaine ingestion, *Am J Emerg Med* 15(5):507-509, 1997.

96. Klompas M: Does this patient have an acute thoracic aortic dissection? *JAMA* 287(17):2262-2272, 2002.

97. von Kodolitsch Y, Schwartz AG, Nienaber CA: Clinical prediction of acute aortic dissection, *Arch Intern Med* 160(19):2977-2982, 2000.

98. Nauer KA: Acute dissection of the aorta: a review for nurses, *Crit Care Nurs Q* 23(1):20-27, 2000.

99. Sullivan PR, Wolfson AB, Leckey RD, Burke JL: Diagnosis of acute thoracic aortic dissection in the emergency department, *Am J Emerg Med* 18(1):46-50, 2000.

100. Singer AJ, Hollander JE: Blood pressure: assessment of interarm differences, *Arch Intern Med* 156(17):2005-2008, 1996.

101. Milner KA, Vaccarino V, Arnold AL et al: Gender and age differences in chief complaints of acute myocardial infarction (Worcester Heart Attack Study), *Am J Cardiol* 93(5):606-608, 2004.

102. Dracup K. Alonzo AA. Atkins JM. Bennett NM. Braslow A. Clark LT. Eisenberg M. Ferdinand KC. Frye R. Green L. Hill MN. Kennedy JW. Kline-Rogers E. Moser DK. Ornato JP. Pitt B. Scott JD. Selker HP. Silva SJ. Thies W. Weaver WD. Wenger NK. White SK. The physician's role in minimizing prehospital delay in patients at high risk for acute myocardial infarction: recommendations from the National Heart Attack Alert Program. Working Group on Educational Strategies to Prevent Prehospital Delay in Patients at High Risk for Acute Myocardial Infarction. *Annals of Internal Medicine.* 126(8):645-51, 1997.

103. Everts B, Karlson BW, Wahrborg P et al: Localization of pain in suspected acute myocardial infarction in relation to final diagnosis, age and sex, and site and type of infarction, *Heart Lung* 25(6):430-437, 1996.

104. Lewis JF, McGorray SP, Pepine CJ: Assessment of women with suspected myocardial ischemia: review of findings of the Women's Ischemia Syndrome Evaluation (WISE) Study, *Curr Womens Health Rep* 2(2):110-114, 2002.

105. Freidman M: Gender differences in the health related quality of life of older adults with heart failure, *Heart Lung* 35(5):320-327, 2003.

106. Martin R, Lemos C, Rothrock N et al: Gender disparities in common sense models of illness among myocardial infarction victims, *Health Psychol* 23(4):345-353, 2004.

107. Finnegan JR Jr, Meischke H, Zapka JG et al: Patient delay in seeking care for heart attack symptoms: findings from focus groups conducted in five US regions, *Prev Med* 31(3):205-213, 2000.

108. Mosca L, Ferris A, Fabunmi R, Robertson RM: Tracking women's awareness of heart disease: an American Heart Association national study, *Circulation* 109(5):573-579, 2004.

109. Berman AR, Arnsten JH: Diagnosis and treatment of pulmonary embolism in the elderly, *Clin Geriatr Med* 19(1):157-175, 2003.

110. Timmons S, Kingston M, Hussain M et al: Pulmonary embolism: differences in presentation between older and younger patients, *Age Ageing* 32(6):601-605, 2003.

111. Richards B: The sky's the limit, *Nurs Stand* 14(46):26, 2000.

112. Lee H, Bahler R, Chung C et al: Prehospital delay with myocardial infarction: the interactive effect of clinical symptoms and race, *Appl Nurs Res* 13(3):125-133, 2000.

113. Johnson PA, Lee TH, Cook EF et al: Effect of race on the presentation and management of patients with acute chest pain, *Ann Intern Med* 118(8):593-601, 1993.

114. Davidson JK: Screening for diabetes mellitus. In Davidson JK, editor: *Clinical diabetes mellitus: a problem oriented approach,* ed 3, New York, 2000, Thieme.

115. Tabibiazar R, Edelman SV: Silent ischemia in people with diabetes: a condition that must be heard, *Clinical Diabetes* 21(1):5-9, 2003.

116. Manzella, D & Paolisso, G. Cardiac autonomic activity and Type II diabetes mellitus. *Clinical Science.* 108: 93-99, 2005.

117. Culic V, Eterovic D, Miric D, Silic N: Symptom presentation of acute myocardial infarction: influence of sex, age, and risk factors, *Am Heart J* 144(6):1012-1017, 2002.

118. Bulpitt CJ, Palmer AJ, Battersby C, Fletcher AE: Association of symptoms of type 2 diabetic patients with severity of disease, obesity, and blood pressure, *Diabetes Care* 21(1):111-115, 1998.

119. Harrison Diabetes 2006

Dyspnea

Corrine Y. Jurgens

Dyspnea, or breathlessness, is a common patient complaint. Dyspnea can be acute or chronic, arise from a wide variety of physiological and pathophysiological processes and is nonspecific to a particular illness. Dyspnea most often is associated with disorders of the cardiac and pulmonary systems. Dyspnea is the most frequently reported symptom among patients with heart failure, chronic obstructive pulmonary disease (**COPD**), and lung cancer. The prevalence of these illnesses is significant with heart failure affecting 5 million Americans,[1] COPD affecting more than 9 million Americans,[2] and lung cancer affecting more than 350,000 Americans.[3] Further contributing to the pervasiveness of dyspnea are many other conditions, including acute coronary syndrome, anemia, neuromuscular disease, obesity, pneumonia, pregnancy, and poor physical conditioning (Box 54-1).

DEFINITION

Dyspnea is a multidimensional symptom with physical, affective, and cognitive components; it is inherently distressing to the patient. Dyspnea is the subjective sensation of breathlessness, which can vary in intensity and is associated with discomfort. Defined in this way, dyspnea is differentiated from a change in breathing pattern such as tachypnea or hyperventilation.[4,5] Dyspnea historically was defined by objective observations of patients with respiratory distress. A person's perception of and reaction to labored breathing also are included in the definition of dyspnea. The American Thoracic Society,[6] in a consensus statement, provides the following definition: "Dyspnea is the term used to characterize a subjective experience of breathing discomfort that is comprised of qualitatively distinct sensations that vary in intensity. The experience derives from interactions among multiple physiological, psychological, social and environmental factors, and may induce secondary physiological and behavioral responses" (p. 322).

MECHANISMS OF DYSPNEA

Understanding the mechanisms of and contributing factors to dyspnea assists the clinician in diagnosing the underlying cause and choosing the appropriate inter-

vention. The sensation of dyspnea results from complex processes involving the central nervous system (**CNS**); chemoreceptors; mechanoreceptors in the chest wall, airways, and lungs; and a sense of increased effort[6-9] (Table 54-1). Dyspnea is not merely increased effort or movement of the muscles of respiration, for the respiratory centers in the brain must be stimulated in order for dyspnea to occur.[10] Normally, receptors in the respiratory system communicate with the CNS to stimulate respiration. Dyspnea is thought to result from a mismatch between afferent feedback from these various receptors and the respiratory command center in the CNS (Figure 54-1). Hypoxia and hypercapnia stimulate peripheral and central chemoreceptors, respectively, to stimulate ventilation and maintain homeostasis. However, patients are known to experience breathlessness in the absence of hypoxia. Conversely, the presence of hypoxia does not always result in dyspnea, as seen in patients with chronic lung disease. To date, an all-encompassing explanation for dyspnea is not known.

Pathophysiology of Dyspnea

The American Thoracic Society classifies the pathophysiology of dyspnea as resulting from one or more of four different mechanisms:[6]

- Heightened ventilatory demand
- Abnormal impedance or resistance to ventilation
- Respiratory muscle weakness
- Abnormal perception of dyspnea with an increased respiratory drive

Heightened ventilatory demand may result from an increased metabolic load or increased respiratory drive that occurs with hypoxemia or acidosis. An example of abnormal ventilatory impedance is the bronchoconstriction associated with asthma or COPD. Respiratory muscle abnormalities caused by neuromuscular diseases or chronic overinflation of the lung typical in COPD result in a mismatch between central respiratory output and ventilation. Psychological and situational factors affect the potential for an abnormal perception of dyspnea. Anxiety, depression, and fatigue have been associated with dyspnea.[11-15] Medical and nursing interventions are intended to ameliorate or alleviate the underlying pathophysiological mechanisms of dyspnea.

ASSESSMENT OF DYSPNEA
History

A careful medical history and symptom analysis, physical examination, and laboratory and radiological testing guide the formulation of differential diagnoses and subsequent treatment for dyspnea.[16,17] Medical history, cur-

BOX 54-1
DIFFERENTIAL DIAGNOSIS OF DYSPNEA

■ ■ ■

Cardiac
Acute coronary syndrome
Acute myocardial infarction
Heart failure
Pericarditis
Valvular disease

Pulmonary
Chronic obstructive pulmonary disease (asthma, chronic bronchitis, emphysema)
Lung cancer
Pleural effusion
Pneumonia
Pneumothorax
Pulmonary embolism

Other
Anemia
Chest trauma
Deconditioning
Malnutrition
Neuromuscular pathology
Obesity
Psychogenic causes
Thyroid disease

rent medications, smoking history, environmental exposures (e.g., asbestos or chlorine gas), occupation, allergies, and family history are essential data to consider. The risk assessment of pulmonary embolism or an infectious process should include information about recent travel, surgery, or immobility. Analyzing dyspnea includes questions as to its onset and duration, frequency or pattern, provoking and palliative factors, quality, severity, and associated symptoms. In addition to the data generated from the history and physical examination, clinical ratings of dyspnea via scales and questionnaires are useful in the evaluation of this multidimensional subjective sensation.[18]

Making the distinction as to whether the onset of dyspnea is acute or chronic is an important initial step in symptom analysis and subsequent disposition of the pa-

tient. Acute dyspnea typically is episodic, has a limited duration, and is often severe enough to prompt medical care. Sudden acute dyspnea is associated with myocardial infarction, pulmonary edema, pulmonary embolus, pneumonia, asthma, and airway obstruction.[19] Conversely, chronic dyspnea is a more persistent shortness of breath and often has varying levels of intensity. Chronic dyspnea is associated with illnesses such as heart failure and COPD. However, patients who are chronically short of breath also can experience acute dyspnea over their baseline. In addition, baseline dyspnea can increase incrementally in severity as the underlying disease progresses. Fatigue, depression, and anxiety have been reported among patients with chronic dyspnea.[5] Patients complaining of sudden onset or acute dyspnea warrant referral for evaluation in a hospital setting.

The pattern of dyspnea may provide clues as to its cause. Is dyspnea present intermittently or chronically? What time of day does the dyspnea manifest itself or become more pronounced? Does the dyspnea disturb the patient's sleep? For example, nocturnal dyspnea is associated with asthma and heart failure.[19,20] Patients with heart failure may have paroxysmal nocturnal dyspnea (**PND**); patients report awakening with acute dyspnea 2 to 4 hours after going to sleep. The dyspnea is alleviated by sitting up for 15 to 30 minutes and may be associated with coughing. The cough associated with PND occurs *after* the onset of dyspnea. Patients with COPD also may report dyspnea awakening them from sleep; however, the cough *precedes* the dyspnea, and expectoration of sputum relieves the dyspnea.[19] Therefore, careful questioning to expose precipitating factors, associated symptoms, and the timing of dyspnea assists in determining the diagnosis.

The severity of dyspnea associated with COPD and heart failure often increases insidiously. Inquiring about current functional status and usual daily activity is valuable in assessing symptom impact and progression. Similar to the New York Heart Association scale for patients with heart failure, the American Thoracic Society developed a scale to assess the severity of chronic dyspnea (Table 54-2). Patient report of dyspnea at rest ver-

■ ■ ■

TABLE 54-1 MECHANISMS OF DYSPNEA

RECEPTOR	LOCATION	FUNCTION
Chemoreceptors	Blood and brain	Detect change in PO_2 and PCO_2 to maintain blood gas and acid-base homeostasis
Mechanoreceptors		
Upper-airway receptors	Upper airways, face	Modify dyspnea sensation
Lung receptors		
Pulmonary stretch receptors		
Large central airways		
Respond to increases in lung volume		
Irritant receptors	Epithelial cells of bronchial walls	Activated by tactile stimulation of bronchial mucosa, high rates of airflow, and increased bronchial smooth muscle tone
C fibers (also known as J fibers)	Interstitium of lung	Respond to increased pulmonary interstitial and alveolar edema pressure
Chest wall receptors	Joints, tendons, and muscles of chest	Send signals to brain for regulation of level and pattern of breathing

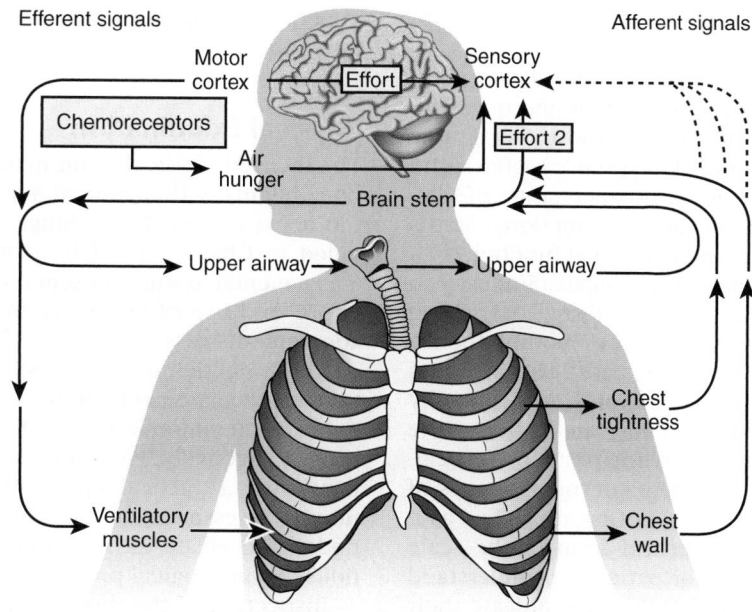

FIGURE 54-1 ■ Efferent and afferent signals that contribute to the sensation of dyspnea. (From Manning HL, Schwartzstein RM: *New Engl J Med* 333[23]:1547-1553, 1995.)

sus dyspnea precipitated by activity indicates a higher level of severity.

Identifying the factors that provoke or alleviate a patient's dyspnea is important. Dyspnea may be affected by factors such as position, activity or rest, and self-treatment with inhalers or other medications. Orthopnea, shortness of breath when lying flat, is an example of dyspnea provoked by patient position. Orthopnea is a common complaint in persons with heart failure. Patients may report using two or more pillows or sleeping in a chair to alleviate dyspnea that disturbs sleep. Furthermore, they may decrease their activity to accommodate their dyspnea and therefore decrease the likelihood of reporting dyspnea on exertion. In a study of 1091 Medicare beneficiaries admitted for heart failure, 89 percent reported dyspnea at rest; however, only 26 percent reported dyspnea on exertion.[21] Review of the general level of activity may provide this information.

The "language of breathlessness" or the way in which the quality of the dyspnea is described may assist the diagnostic process. Studies suggest that there are different descriptors of dyspnea related to particular cardio-respiratory diseases and ethnicity.[22-25] For example, asthma may be associated with "work/effort" and "tight" descriptors, whereas patients with interstitial lung dis-

ease report "work/effort" and "rapid" breathing to describe their dyspnea. Patients with COPD have described difficulty with exhalation. Heart failure patients use "shortness of breath," "gasping," and an inability to "get enough air."[22]

Differences based on race have been reported among patients with asthma. Black patients used upper airway descriptors (tight throat, voice tight), whereas white patients used lower airway and chest-wall descriptors (deep breath, out of air).[25] Others may use an associated symptom to describe dyspnea, with some patients describing the sensation of dyspnea as fatigue.[10,26,27] Dyspnea and fatigue are common correlates in patients with chronic heart failure, COPD, and advanced cancer.[11-13]

Exploring symptoms associated with dyspnea helps in differentiating cardiac, respiratory, neuromuscular, and other causes. Chest pain may indicate myocardial ischemia or may be muscular. Fever with a productive cough is associated with pneumonia and tuberculosis. Gastroesophogeal reflux disease is associated with asthma and also may precipitate complaints of chest pain. Inquiring about the presence of other symptoms explores the potential for diagnosing acute coronary syndrome, pulmonary embolism, heart failure, asthma, or pneumonia.[16,20,28]

■ ■ ■

TABLE 54-2   AMERICAN THORACIC SOCIETY DYSPNEA SCALE

GRADE	DEGREE	CRITERIA
0	None	Is not troubled with breathlessness except with strenuous activity
1	Slight	Is troubled by shortness of breath when hurrying on the level or walking up a slight hill
2	Moderate	Walks slower than most persons of the same age because of breathlessness or has to stop for breath when walking at own pace on the level
3	Severe	Stops for breath after walking 100 yards or after a few minutes walking on level ground
4	Very severe	Too breathless to leave the house or breathless when dressing/undressing

From Brooks SM: *American Thoracic Society News* 8:12-16, 1982.

Dyspnea Scales

Dyspnea, a subjective and multidimensional symptom, also can be assessed by self-report scales and questionnaires. Available instruments include those that simply measure patient perception of respiratory effort and distress and those that assess a broader range of constructs such as symptom impact on functional status and quality of life, fatigue, and emotional function.

Unidimensional tools measuring dyspnea intensity in relation to distress or effort include the visual analog scale (VAS),[29] the Borg scale,[30] the modified Borg scale,[31] and the oxygen cost diagram.[32] The VAS and modified Borg scale, the most commonly used, are easy to use and have acceptable reliability and validity. The VAS is a 100-mm line that can be horizontal or vertical. The scale is anchored by statements of "no shortness of breath" at one end and "shortness of breath as bad as it can be" on the other. The vertical form of the scale has been reported as easier for patients to understand and use to rate their dyspnea.[29] Patients indicate their perceived effort or perceived distress by marking a point on the scale. The point then is measured in millimeters with higher distress or effort corresponding with higher scores. In addition to quantifying distress numerically on a 0-to-10 scale, the modified Borg scale uses word descriptions ranging from 0 (nothing at all) to 10 (maximal dyspnea). (See Chapter 25 and Chapter 29, Table 29-3.)

The modified Borg scale is a satisfactory, brief, easy-to-use instrument that correlates well with clinical parameters such as peak expiratory flow ratings and oxygen saturation. The modified Borg scale has been used successfully in emergency triage of COPD and asthmatic patients with acute bronchospasm.[33] Patients reported that the modified Borg scale adequately expressed their subjective dyspnea. Acutely dyspneic patients may be unable to speak in full sentences; therefore, a brief interview scale that limits the need to talk and accurately captures level of distress is clinically useful. Similar to the VAS and modified Borg scale, the oxygen cost diagram is a one-item vertical line scale, 100 mm long, with a range of daily activities that correspond to oxygen requirements. The scale ranges from 0 to 100 with a score of 100 indicating no impairment resulting from dyspnea.[32]

Several multidimensional instruments include various measures of functional impairment, fatigue, emotional function, frequency of shortness of breath, and quality of life in patients with respiratory disease.[34-36] The baseline dyspnea index and transitional dyspnea index measure functional impairment, magnitude of task (difficulty of physical activity), and magnitude of effort (degree of exertion) at baseline and over time. The instruments correlate with lung function and exercise capacity.[34,36] Although developed for and most frequently used among patients with COPD, the baseline dyspnea index also has been used in studies of patients with heart failure.[37,38] Measurement instruments for dyspnea specific to the cardiac population are limited to the chronic heart failure questionnaire. This questionnaire, a quality of life measure, contains a dyspnea com- ponent in addition to assessing fatigue and emotional function.[39]

Physical Examination

The focused physical examination for evaluation of dyspnea begins with a general survey and examination of the neck, thorax, heart, lungs, and extremities, as detailed in Chapter 45.[9] Observation of general appearance, mental status, presence of cyanosis, respiratory effort, and use of accessory muscles assesses oxygenation and distress.

Abnormalities of the neck specific to dyspnea include tracheal deviation and jugular venous distention, which indicate pneumothorax and fluid overload (heart failure), respectively. Pleural effusion and atelectasis also may cause a tracheal shift.[16] Included in the examination is assessment of the thyroid glands and lymph nodes to evaluate the potential for an endocrine, infectious, or oncological process.

Inspection of the thorax may reveal a different configuration among patients with dyspnea. The anterior-posterior diameter, normally ranges from a 1:2 to 5:7 ratio. In patients with longstanding COPD, the anterior-posterior diameter is increased to 1:1 with a more horizontal orientation of the ribs. However, similar changes also can occur from aging.[16] A sudden onset of dyspnea associated with asymmetrical chest movement may indicate pneumothorax as the source of dyspnea.

Rales or crackles, rhonchi, or a friction rub upon auscultation suggest fluid overload, an infectious process, or pulmonary embolism as the source. Fine rales or crackles associated with heart failure are auscultated during inspiration and have a soft, high-pitched popping quality. Coarser rales or crackles are heard in pneumonia, COPD, and late pulmonary edema.[40,41] Crackles and friction rubs resulting from pulmonary venous embolism are nonspecific and depend on the size and number of emboli. Further testing is warranted for persons determined to be at risk.[41]

The cardiac examination is used to assess for cardiac causes of dyspnea such as fluid overload, right or left ventricular heart failure, and valvular disease. Auscultation for the presence of murmurs is important because insufficiency or stenosis of the aortic or mitral valve may lead to heart failure. Auscultation of a ventricular gallop (S_3) may indicate volume overload or heart failure.

The extremities are examined for edema, clubbing, and cyanosis. Bilateral edema of the lower extremities is suggestive of heart failure, whereas unilateral edema suggests thromboembolism. Clubbing, or a bulbous fingertip with a nail angle of greater than 180 degrees, is associated with many processes including chronic cyanosis and lung cancer.[10,16,42]

Laboratory and Radiological Testing

The laboratory and radiological test of choice for analyzing dyspnea is based on the probability of a particular diagnosis. Initial testing for the underlying cause of dyspnea likely will include tests for anemia, a chest radiograph, an electrocardiogram, pulmonary function tests, and pulse oximetry or arterial blood gas analysis. A chemistry panel may be useful to rule out dyspnea resulting from diabetic ketoacidosis. A risk factor assessment for various illnesses will assist in this determination (Figure 54-2).[43]

Differential Diagnoses

Acute Coronary Syndrome

In addition to complaints of chest pain, dyspnea is common with acute coronary syndrome and is believed to arise from left ventricular dysfunction.[42,44] Gender differences in symptoms at presentation have been reported. Women cite more throat, neck, jaw, and back pain than men. In addition to citing differences in pain location, women reported breathlessness more often than men.[45-47]

Heart Failure

Dyspnea is the most common symptom of heart failure, which ranges in severity from that induced only with activity to breathlessness at rest.[19,48] However, dyspnea is nonspecific to the syndrome. In a study of 1058 patients assessed in a primary care setting, clinical signs and symptoms were determined to be of little value when used alone. The more severe dyspnea symptoms (PND, orthopnea, and dyspnea on exertion) were associated with a diagnosis of heart failure.[49] Similarly, breathlessness was not associated significantly with left ventricular dysfunction (45 percent or less) among patients with risk factors for heart failure. Echocardiographic screening is recommended for patients with comorbid risk factors.[50]

Among patients presenting emergently with acute dyspnea, B-type natriuretic peptide, combined with clinical assessment, is useful in diagnosing or excluding heart failure, limits time to discharge, and reduces cost of treatment.[51-53] The clinical signs of jugular venous distention and auscultation of a ventricular gallop (S_3) have prognostic value for heart failure progression and adverse outcomes.[54]

Chronic Lung Disease

Chronic lung disease encompasses the diagnoses of chronic bronchitis, emphysema, and asthma. Although the pathological processes underlying the diagnoses differ, dyspnea and an increased sense of effort to breathe are held in common. Degree of reversibility of airflow obstruction, persistence of symptoms, and smoking history are variables that assist in differentiating asthma from chronic bronchitis and emphysema (COPD). Asthma is characterized by "variable airflow obstruction that is *often reversible* either spontaneously or with treatment."[55] The American Thoracic Society and the European Respiratory Society defines COPD as a "preventable and treatable disease state characterized by airflow limitation that is *not fully reversible*"[56] (p. 933). The dyspnea associated with asthma is often intermittent versus the more chronic and persistent dyspnea of chronic bronchitis and emphysema.[10] COPD is more common among those with a history of smoking.[57]

Asthma is characterized by inflammation and hyperresponsiveness of the tracheobronchial tree, resulting in dyspnea. Abnormalities in the inspiratory muscles contribute to the sensation of dyspnea. Hyperinflation shortens the muscles, impeding their ability to overcome the resistance of secondary bronchoconstriction.[58] Other symptoms associated with asthma include coughing, wheezing, and chest tightness. The sensation of chest tightness associated with asthma is thought to result from stimulation of the irritant receptors in the large airways.[7] Exposure to allergens, exercise, and respiratory infection can trigger an exacerbation. A higher incidence of gastroesophogeal reflux symptoms also has been reported in asthmatics.[20] Pulmonary function testing is used to evaluate the presence of reduction of expiratory flow.[6]

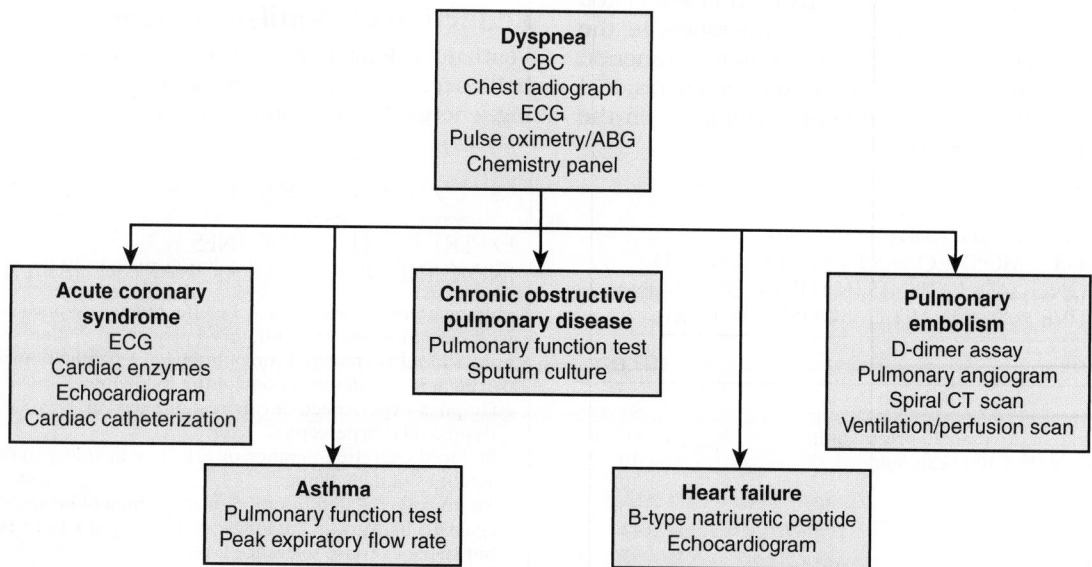

FIGURE 54-2 ■ Laboratory and radiological testing for dyspnea. *CBC,* Complete blood count; *CT,* computed tomography; *ECG,* electrocardiogram.

The mechanisms of dyspnea in COPD are similar to those of asthma. In addition, hypoxia and hypercapnia may modestly stimulate the chemoreceptors and the sensation of dyspnea. The relative absence of dyspnea in the presence of chronic hypercapnia in COPD raises some doubt about its actual contribution to the experience of breathlessness.[58]

Pulmonary Embolism

Chest pain that is pleuritic and is associated with dyspnea or hemoptysis potentially indicates pulmonary embolism. Additional symptoms may include syncope, cough, and palpitations[28,59] (Table 54-3). The clinical presentation of pulmonary embolism varies with the size, number, and location of emboli and with age. Patients age 65 and older reported pleuritic pain less often and were cyanotic and hypoxic more often than younger persons.[60] Therefore the diagnostic work-up is based on the assessment of risk together with the history and physical and results of the chest radiograph, electrocardiogram, and arterial blood gas analysis.

The initial data determine the pretest probability of pulmonary embolism and divide patients into low, moderate, and high probability groups. The simplified Wells scoring system can provide additional data to aid in assessing probability of pulmonary embolism[61] (see Table 53-8). Follow-up testing based on this probability includes D-dimer assays, pulmonary angiography, and spiral computed tomography.[28,62]

Obesity

With nearly 65 percent of Americans overweight, obesity is one of several other factors that have been reported to be associated with dyspnea.[63-66] Patients with a body mass index of 28 kg/m² or above were found to be at increased risk of being diagnosed with asthma.[64] Results from the Third National Health and Nutrition Examination Survey reported the most obese patients had the greatest risk of self-reported asthma, bronchodilator use, and dyspnea with exertion. However, there was a lack of evidence of airway obstruction associated with obesity.[66] More commonly, breathlessness in the obese is on exertion. Reduction of respiratory function has been explained by a reduced functional residual capacity from the effect of the obese abdomen on the position of the diaphragm.[67]

■ ■ ■

TABLE 54-3 MOST COMMON SYMPTOMS AND SIGNS AMONG 2454 PATIENTS IN THE INTERNATIONAL COOPERATIVE PULMONARY EMBOLISM REGISTRY

SYMPTOM OR SIGN	PERCENT
Dyspnea	82
Respiratory rate more than 20 breaths/min	60
Heart rate more than 100 beats/min	40
Chest pain	49
Cough	20
Syncope	14
Hemoptysis	7

Adapted from Goldhaber SZ, Visani L, DeRosa M: *Lancet* 353(9162):1386-1389, 1999.

Thoracic Trauma

Dyspnea resulting from thoracic trauma arises from pulmonary and cardiac origins. Most commonly, blunt chest trauma sustained in motor vehicle accidents is associated with pulmonary contusion, pneumothorax, hemothorax, flail chest, or cardiac tamponade.[68] (See Chapter 68 for further information.)

Other Factors

Dyspnea is associated with a variety of other factors such as anemia, pregnancy, poor physical condition, and psychogenic sources. A heightened ventilatory demand occurs in pregnancy and anemia. In pregnancy, dyspnea is thought to arise from a hormonally mediated increase in respiratory demand, whereas in anemia, dyspnea results from a lack of oxygen-carrying capacity.[69] Exercise testing can evaluate unexplained chronic dyspnea potentially related to physical deconditioning or psychogenic origins.[9] Psychogenic dyspnea is a diagnosis of exclusion after organic causes are ruled out.

TREATMENT

Whether acute or chronic, dyspnea is a subjective sensation that affects quality of life by limiting activities of daily living, inducing fatigue and psychological distress. An appreciation of the multidimensional aspects of dyspnea directs treatment options, which include nursing, medical, and pharmacological management and other strategies. Education, smoking cessation, social support, desensitization, and relaxation therapy are some examples of other modalities used beyond the medical regimen. Treatment choice is based on the underlying cause and the mechanisms of dyspnea that include ventilatory demand, ventilatory impedance, inspiratory muscle function, and central perception of dyspnea. An overview of the aims of treatment is provided. Refer to the cited references for more extensive treatment information.

Reduction of Ventilatory Demand

Ventilatory demand can be reduced by decreasing metabolic needs and central respiratory drive. Exercise training, energy conservation, oxygen, and pharmacological

---

■ **EVIDENCE-BASED PRACTICE**

EXPERT PANEL GUIDELINES
INDICATIONS FOR PULMONARY REHABILITATION

Pulmonary rehabilitation may be effective for dyspnea associated with certain forms of respiratory impairment. Patients with dyspnea should be referred for pulmonary rehabilitation when impairment is manifested as one of the following:
■ Dyspnea experienced during rest or exertion
■ Hypoxemia, hypercapnia
■ Reduced exercise tolerance or a decline in ability to perform activities of daily living
■ An unexpected deterioration or worsening of symptoms against a background of longstanding dyspnea and a reduced but stable exercise tolerance level

From American Association for Respiratory Care. AARC clinical practice guideline: pulmonary rehabilitation, *Respir Care* 2002: 47(5): 617-625.

■■■ CONUNDRUM

SUPPLEMENTAL OXYGEN VERSUS AIRFLOW FOR RELIEF OF DYSPNEA

Which patients will benefit from airflow and which need supplemental oxygen therapy is unknown. Studies examining the use of supplemental oxygen during rehabilitation have shown increased exercise tolerance and improved dyspnea with supplemental oxygen. Other investigators have reported improvement without oxygen. Interestingly, delivery of airflow (versus oxygen) by fan or nasal cannula also has decreased dyspnea in some patients. At this point, health care professionals remain unsure which patients need oxygen therapy.

Bibliography
Ambrosino N, Strambi S: New strategies to improve exercise tolerance in chronic obstructive pulmonary disease, *Eur Respir J* 24:313-322, 2004.
Gallagher R, Roberts D: A systematic review of oxygen and airflow effect on relief of dyspnea at rest in patients with advanced disease of any cause, *J Pain Palliat Care Pharmacother* 18(4):3-15, 2004.

■■■ TECHNOLOGY

INVESTIGATIONAL THERAPY FOR AIRFLOW LIMITATION

Inflammatory mediators have been implicated in the pathogenesis of asthma and chronic obstructive pulmonary disease. As a result, corticosteroids and phosphodiesterase inhibitors are antiinflammatory pharmacological agents presently in use. Interleukin-8 is one of several inflammatory mediators implicated in increasing airflow limitation. Monoclonal antibodies, which block interleukin-8, are being investigated in patients with asthma and COPD. Safety and efficacy studies of monoclonal antibodies have shown monoclonal antibodies to decrease dyspnea and show promise as a new approach to inflammation in these populations.

Bibliography
Mahler DA, Huang S, Tabrizi M et al: Efficacy and safety of a monoclonal antibody recognizing interleukin-8 in COPD: a pilot study, *Chest* 126:926-934, 2004.

therapy are options. Exercise reduces dyspnea by desensitization and improved physical conditioning in patients with chronic lung disease and heart failure.[6,70] (See the accompanying evidence-based practice feature.) Teaching patients to pace activities to conserve energy is also effective in reducing the metabolic demand on breathing. Oxygen is useful to decrease dyspnea at rest and with exercise in select patients. (See the accompanying conundrum feature.) Opioids modulate dyspnea but also can cause respiratory depression, which has limited their widespread use.[6] A meta-analysis of 18 clinical trials of opioids for dyspnea management supports the continued use of the oral and parenteral forms, which had a positive effect on breathlessness.[71]

Reduction of Ventilatory Impedance

Minimizing ventilatory impedance improves breathing mechanics by decreasing resistance to airflow. Depending on the underlying cause, options include surgical lung volume reduction, continuous positive airway pressure, and pharmacological therapy. Bronchodilator therapy using inhaled beta$_2$-agonists, inhaled anticholinergics, and oral sustained-release theophyllines has improved dyspnea in patients with COPD and asthma.[6,55] Inhaled or systemic corticosteroids are also useful in asthma management.[55] (See the accompanying technology feature.)

Improving Inspiratory Muscle Function

Fatigue is a common symptom associated with cardiac- and respiratory-induced dyspnea.[12,13,72] In COPD, hyperinflation impedes efficient function of the respiratory muscles. Patients with heart failure have abnormal skeletal muscle function leading to fatigue and decreased exercise tolerance.[73] In addition to muscle dysfunction, the work of breathing among these patients can increase metabolic demands and increase muscle weakness and fatigue. Therefore, nutritional supplementation can be beneficial.[10] Other treatments include optimal body positioning for breathing. Typically, sitting up and leaning forward improves use of the diaphragm and decreases the use of accessory muscles to breathe.[6,10]

Altered Central Perception

The conscious awareness of and subsequent affective response to dyspnea is a result of cognitive, emotional, and behavioral factors in addition to the physiological demand to breathe. Cognitive-behavioral strategies, education, desensitization, and pharmacological therapy are options to assist patients to improve self-management of dyspnea. Distraction and relaxation training are two strategies that may modify the perception of the intensity of the symptom. In select patients, the use of opioids or anxiolytics to decrease the perception of dyspnea can be considered.[6,10]

Dyspnea management involves a comprehensive assessment and treatment plan. Because dyspnea is a multidimensional symptom, it is important to include assessment of the patient's response. In addition to medical and pharmacological therapy, inclusion of complementary strategies tailored to the patient will promote effective self-management of dyspnea (Box 54-2).

BOX 54-2   ■■■
COMPLEMENTARY THERAPIES FOR DYSPNEA

Patients with chronic illness resistant to traditional treatment commonly try alternative therapies such as cognitive-behavioral therapy, relaxation exercises, acupuncture, and acupressure. Studies of these therapies generally have had small sample sizes, limiting the degree to which results can be generalized. However, patients have reported a decrease in dyspnea and the associated emotional responses, such as anxiety, when they use these interventions. Confirmatory research with long-term follow-up is needed to validate these therapies.

Bibliography
Pan CX, Morrison RS, Ness J et al: Complementary and alternative medicine in the management of pain, dyspnea, and nausea and vomiting near the end of life: a systematic review, *J Pain Symptom Manage* 20:374-387, 2000.
Wu H, Wu S, Lin J et al: Effectiveness of acupressure in improving dyspnea in chronic obstructive pulmonary disease, *J Adv Nurs* 45(3):252-259, 2004.

REFERENCES

1. American Heart Association: *American Heart Association heart disease and stroke statistics: 2004 update,* Dallas, 2005, The Association.
2. U.S. Department of Health and Human Services: *Summary health statistics for US adults: National Health Interview Survey, 2002,* Hyattsville, Md, 2004, National Center for Health Statistics.
3. American Lung Association: Trends in lung cancer morbidity and mortality. In *Epidemiology and statistic unit, research and program services,* 2005. Retrieved January 10, 2007, from http://www.lungusa.org/atf/cf/%7B7A8D42C2-FCCA-4604-8ADE-7F5D5E762256%7D/LCFINAL06.PDF
4. Comroe J: Some theories of the mechanisms of dyspnea. In Howell J, Campbell E, editors: *Breathlessness,* Oxford, England, 1966, Blackwell Scientific.
5. McCarley C: A model of chronic dyspnea, *J Nurs Scholarsh* 31(3):231-236, 1999.
6. American Thoracic Society: Dyspnea: mechanisms, assessment, and management—a consensus statement, *Am J Respir Crit Care Med* 159(1):321-340, 1999.
7. Manning HL, Schwartzstein RM: Mechanisms of disease: pathophysiology of dyspnea, *New Engl J Med* 333(23):1547-1553, 1995.
8. Spector N, Klein D: Chronic critically ill dypneic patients: mechanisms and clinical measurement, *AACN Clin Issues* 12(2):220-233, 2001.
9. Mahler DA, Fierro-Carrion G, Baird JC: Evaluation of dyspnea in the elderly, *Clin Geriatr Med* 19:19-33, 2003.
10. Carrieri-Kohlman V, Stulbarg M: Dyspnea. In Carrieri-Kohlman V, Lindsay AM, West C, editors: *Pathophysiological phenomenon in nursing: human responses to illness,* ed 3, Philadelphia, 2003, Saunders.
11. Bruera E, Schmitz B, Pither J et al: The frequency and correlates of dyspnea in patients with advanced cancer, *J Pain Symptom Manage* 19(5):357-362, 2000.
12. Gift AG, Pugh LC: Dyspnea and fatigue, *Nurs Clin North Am* 28:373-384, 1993.
13. Friedman MM, King KB: Correlates of fatigue in older women with heart failure, *Heart Lung* 24(6):512-518, 1995.
14. Tanaka K, Akechi T, Okuyama T et al: Factors correlated with dyspnea in advanced lung cancer patients: organic causes or what else? *J Pain Symptom Manage* 23(6):490-500, 2002.
15. O'Neill ES: Illness representations and coping of women with chronic obstructive pulmonary disease: a pilot study, *Heart Lung* 31(4):295-302, 2002.
16. Bickley LS, Szilagyi PG: *Bates' guide to physical examination and history taking,* ed 8, Philadelphia, 2003, Lippincott Williams & Wilkins.
17. Mahler DA: Diagnosis of dyspnea. In Mahler DA, editor: *Dyspnea,* New York, 1998, Marcel Dekker.
18. Nguyen HQ, Altinger J, Carrieri-Kohlman V et al: Factor analysis of laboratory and clinical measurements of dyspnea in patients with chronic obstructive pulmonary disease, *J Pain Symptom Manage* 25:118-127, 2003.
19. Zipes DP, Libby P, Bonow RO, Braunwald E, editors: *Braunwald's heart disease: a textbook of cardiovascular medicine,* ed 7, Philadelphia, 2005, Elsevier Saunders.
20. Sontag SJ, O'Connell S, Miller TQ, Bernsen M: Asthmatics have more nocturnal gasping and reflux symptoms than nonasthmatics, and they are related to bedtime eating, *Am J Gastroenterol* 99:789-796, 2004.
21. Ahmed A, Allman RM, Aronow WS, DeLong JF: Diagnosis of heart failure in older adults: predictive value of dyspnea at rest, *Arch Gerontol Geriatr* 38:297-307, 2004.
22. Caroci A, Lareau SC: Descriptors of dyspnea by patients with chronic obstructive pulmonary disease versus congestive heart failure, *Heart Lung* 33:102-110, 2004.
23. Mahler DA, Harver A, Lentine T et al: Descriptors of breathlessness in cardiorespiratory diseases, *Am J Respir Crit Care Med* 154:1357-1363, 1996.
24. Michaels C, Meek PM: The language of breathing among individuals with chronic obstructive pulmonary disease, *Heart Lung* 33:390-400, 2004.
25. Hardie GE, Janson S, Gold W et al: Ethnic differences: word descriptors used by African-American and white asthma patients during induced bronchoconstriction, *Chest* 117:935-943, 2000.
26. Meek PM, Lareau SC: Critical outcomes in pulmonary rehabilitation: assessment and evaluation of dypsnea and fatigue, *J Rehabil Res Dev* 40:13-24, 2003.
27. Janson-Bjerklie S, Carrieri VK, Hudes M: The sensations of pulmonary dyspnea, *Nurs Res* 35:154-159, 1986.
28. Chunilal SD, Eikelboom JW, Attia J et al: Does this patient have pulmonary embolism? *JAMA* 290:2849-2858, 2003.
29. Gift AG: Dyspnea assessment guide, *Crit Care Nurse* 9:79-87, 1989.
30. Borg G: Perceived exertion as an indicator of somatic stress, *Scand J Rehabil Med* 2:92-98, 1970.
31. Borg G: Psychophysical bases of perceived exertion, *Med Sci Sports Exerc* 14:377-381, 1982.
32. McGravin CR, Artvinli M, Naoe H: Dyspnoea, disability, and distance walked: comparison of exercise performance in respiratory disease, *BMJ* 2:241-243, 1978.
33. Kendrick KR, Baxi SC, Smith RM: Usefulness of the modified 0-10 Borg scale in assessing the degree of dypsnea in patients with COPD and asthma, *J Emerg Nurs* 26:216-222, 2000.
34. Mahler DA, Guyatt GH, Jones PW: Clinical measurement of dyspnea. In Mahler DA, editor: *Dyspnea,* New York, 1998, Marcel Dekker.
35. Guyatt GH, Berman LB, Townsend M et al: A measure of quality of life for clinical trials in chronic lung disease, *Thorax* 42:773-778, 1987.
36. Mahler DA, Weinberg DH, Wells CK, Feinstein AR: The measurement of dyspnea: contents, interobserver agreement, and physiologic correlates of two new clinical indexes, *Chest* 85:751-758, 1984.
37. Duncan K, Pozehl B: Effects of an exercise adherence intervention on outcomes in patients with heart failure, *Rehabil Nurs* 28:117-122, 2003.
38. McParland C, Krishnan B, Wang Y, Gallagher CG: Inspiratory muscle weakness and dypsnea in chronic heart failure, *Am Rev Respir Dis* 146:467-472, 1992.
39. Guyatt GH, Nogradi S, Halcrow S et al: Development and testing of a new measure of health status for clinical trials in heart failure, *J Gen Intern Med* 4:101-107, 1989.
40. Gillespie ND, McNeill G, Pringle T et al: Cross sectional study of contribution of clinical assessment and simple cardiac investigations to diagnosis of left ventricular systolic dysfunction in patients admitted with acute dyspnoea, *BMJ* 314:936-940, 1997.
41. Tierney LM, McPhee SJ, Papadakis MA et al: *Current medical diagnosis & treatment 2005,* ed 44, New York, 2004, McGraw-Hill.
42. Woods SL, Froelicher ES, Motzer SA, Bridges EJ, editors: *Cardiac nursing,* ed 5, Philadelphia, 2005, Lippincott Williams & Wilkins.
43. Kasper DL, Braunwald E, Fauci AS et al, editors: *Harrison's principles of internal medicine,* ed 16, New York, 2005, McGraw-Hill.
44. Clark A, Poole-Wilson P: Breathlessness in heart disease. In Adams L, Guz A, editors: *Respiratory sensation,* New York, 1996, Marcel Dekker.
45. McSweeney JC, Cody M, O'Sullivan P et al: Women's early warning symptoms of acute myocardial infarction, *Circulation* 108:2619-2623, 2003.
46. Granot M, Goldstein-Ferber S, Azzam ZS: Gender differences in the perception of chest pain, *J Pain Symptom Manage* 27:149-155, 2004.
47. Philpott S, Boynton PM, Feder G, Hemingway H: Gender differences in descriptions of angina symptoms and health problems immediately prior to angiography: the ACRE Study, *Soc Sci Med* 52:1565-1575, 2001.
48. Schiff GD, Fung S, Speroff T, McNutt RA: Decompensated heart failure: symptoms, patterns of onset, and contributing factors, *Am J Med* 114:625-630, 2003.
49. Fonseca C, Morais H, Mota T et al: The diagnosis of heart failure in primary care: value of symptoms and signs, *Eur J Heart Fail* 6:795-800, 2004.
50. Baker DW, Bahler RC, Finkelhor RS, Lauer MS: Screening for left ventricular systolic dysfunction among patients with risk factors for heart failure, *Am Heart J* 146:736-740, 2003.

51. McCullough PA, Nowak RM, McCord J et al: B-type natriuretic peptide and clinical judgment in emergency diagnosis of heart failure: analysis from Breathing Not Properly (BNP) Multinational Study, *Circulation* 106:416-422, 2002.

52. Maisel AS, Krishnaswamy P, Nowak RM et al: Rapid measurement of B-type natriuretic peptide in the emergency diagnosis of heart failure, *N Engl J Med* 347:161-167, 2002.

53. Mueller C, Scholer A, Laule-Kilian K et al: Use of B-type natriuretic peptide in the evaluation and management of acute dyspnea, *New Engl J Med* 350:647-654, 2004.

54. Drazner MH, Rame JE, Dries DL: Third heart sound and elevated jugular venous pressure as markers of the subsequent development of heart failure in patients with asymptomatic left ventricular dysfunction, *Am J Med* 114:431-437, 2003.

55. National Institutes of Health: *Global strategy for asthma management and prevention,* 2004. Retrieved January 9, 2007, from http://www.ginasthma.com/GuidelineItem.asp?intId=60

56. Celli BR, MacNee W, Force AET: Standards for the diagnosis and treatment of patients with COPD: a summary of the ATS/ERS position paper, *Eur Respir J* 23:932-946, 2004.

57. National Heart, Lung, and Blood Institute: *Global strategy for the diagnosis, management, and prevention of chronic obstructive pulmonary disease,* NIH Pub No 2701. Retrieved January 10, 2007 , from http://goldcopd.com/Guidelineitem.asp?l1=2&l2=1&intId=989

58. Manning HL, Mahler DA: Pathophysiology of dyspnea, *Monaldi Arch Chest Dis* 56:325-330, 2001.

59. Goldhaber SZ, Visani L, DeRosa M: Acute pulmonary embolism; clinical outcomes in the International Cooperative Pulmonary Embolism Registry (ICOPR), *Lancet* 353(9162):1386-1389, 1999.

60. Timmons S, Kingston M, Hussain M et al: Pulmonary embolism: differences in presentation between older and younger patients, *Age Ageing* 32(6):601-605, 2003.

61. Wells PS, Anderson DR, Rodger M et al: Derivation of a simple clinical model to categorize patients probability of pulmonary embolism: increasing models of utility with the SimpliRED D-dimer, *Thromb Haemost* 83(3):416-420, 2000.

62. Nilsson T, Soderberg M, Lundqvist G et al: A comparison of spiral computed tomography and latex agglutination D-dimer assay in acute pulmonary embolism using pulmonary arteriography as gold standard, *Scand Cardiovasc J* 36(6):373-377, 2002.

63. Flegal KM, Carroll MD, Ogden CL, Johnson CL: Prevalence and trends in obesity among U.S. adults, 1999-2000, *JAMA* 288(14):1723-1727, 2002.

64. Guerra S, Sherrill DL, Bobadilla A et al: The relation of body mass index to asthma, chronic bronchitis, and emphysema, *Chest* 122:1256-1263, 2002.

65. Ho SF, O'Mahony MS, Steward JA et al: Dyspnoea and quality of life in older people at home, *Age Aging* 30:155-159, 2001.

66. Sin DD, Jones RL, Paul Man SF: Obesity is a risk factor for dyspnea but not for airflow obstruction, *Arch Intern Med* 162:1477-1481, 2002.

67. Gibson GJ: Obesity, respiratory function and breathlessness, *Thorax* 55(1):S41-S44, 2000.

68. Yamamoto L, Schroeder C, Beliveau C: Thoracic trauma: the deadly dozen, *Crit Care Nurs Q* 17(11):22-40, 2004.

69. Manning HL, Schwartzstein RM: Mechanisms of dyspnea. In Mahler DA, editor: *Dyspnea,* New York, 1998, Marcel Dekker.

70. Beniaminovitz A, Lang CC, LaManca J, Mancini DM: Selective low-level leg muscle training alleviates dyspnea in patients with heart failure, *J Am Coll Cardiol* 40(9):1602-1608, 2002.

71. Jennings AL, Davies AN, Higgins JP et al: A systematic review of the use of opioids in the management of dyspnoea, *Thorax* 57(11):939-944, 2002.

72. Friedman MM: Older adults' symptoms and their duration before hospitalization for heart failure, *Heart Lung* 26:169-176, 1997.

73. Coats AJS: What causes the symptoms of heart failure? *Heart* 86:574-578, 2001.

chapter 55

Fatigue

Maureen M. Friedman
Sharon A. Stephens

CHAPTER ABBREVIATIONS

AMI   acute myocardial infarction
NYHA   New York Heart Association
POMS   Profile of Mood States

Fatigue is a subjective sensation with the common symptoms being extreme and persistent tiredness, lack of energy, or exhaustion.[1,2] Some authors distinguish the everyday experience of normal fatigue, which is relieved easily by rest, from unusual fatigue, which is more incapacitating and not completely relieved by rest. Unusual fatigue is what accompanies many illnesses and interferes with the ability to function normally.

Fatigue commonly is experienced in a variety of illnesses as the precursor to an acute episode, such as acute coronary syndrome, or as an ongoing symptom of a noncardiac condition such as chronic fatigue syndrome, chronic obstructive pulmonary disease, cancer, multiple sclerosis, rheumatoid arthritis, anemia, or acquired immunodeficiency syndrome. A number of cardiac conditions, including acute coronary syndrome, heart failure, and stroke, have fatigue as a common symptom. Fatigue can be incapacitating for some cardiac patients, making them unable to perform normal activities of daily living. Some patients may reduce their normal activities in an effort to diminish the fatigue.

In a study by Ekman and Ehrenberg,[3] the authors administered a scale to measure fatigue and its severity—the fatigue severity instrument—to subjects with chronic heart failure who were age 65 or older. The authors elicited descriptions about the fatigue experience and subjects' strategies for coping. Subjects included men (n = 92) and women (n = 66), most with New York Heart Association (NYHA) Class III heart failure. The most common response that subjects used to describe their fatigue was "feeling feeble," which meant not being able to complete normal daily activities. Other descriptions for fatigue included feeling listless and feeling a need to rest. Women in the sample rated their fatigue as more severe than men did, although the percent of men and women in each class of the NYHA classifications were similar. These data confirm that the common definition of fatigue as feeling a general lack of energy and inability to complete usual daily activities is consistent with the description given by patients with a chronic cardiac illness.

DIFFERENTIATING FATIGUE AND RELATED CONCEPTS

Weakness

Weakness and fatigue are two distinct symptoms that may occur simultaneously in the same person. Weakness may result from a loss of muscle strength or limited endurance. Inactivity is a common cause of weakness in cardiovascular patients. Disuse leads to muscle atrophy, causing generalized weakness. Patients recovering from cardiac surgery often experience generalized weakness during their hospitalization. During the first few weeks after surgery, weakness usually subsides in response to progressively increasing daily walking and exercise; however, for some persons, postoperative fatigue can linger for several months.[4]

Weakness has been reported as a symptom of unstable angina, with women reporting significantly more weakness than men.[5] Isolated weakness occurs in an extremity or involves the entire side of the body because of a stroke. Patients recovering from a stroke commonly suffer from a combination of weakness and fatigue.[6] Finally, patients may develop an acute and profound weakness during a drop in cardiac output because of myocardial ischemia or a cardiac dysrhythmia. These symptoms improve when normal cardiac output is restored.

Daytime Sleepiness

Daytime sleepiness and fatigue are closely related concepts that inadvertently may be assessed as the same phenomenon.[7] Excessive daytime sleepiness is not a manifestation of fatigue. Fatigue is a subjective sensation that is not observable. Excessive daytime sleepiness, or "drowsiness," is directly observable, although a patient may deny its presence. Daytime sleepiness often is the result of disrupted sleep, as occurs with sleep-disordered breathing. In addition, excessive daytime sleepiness is the hallmark symptom of narcolepsy.[8] Sleep-disordered breathing is a common comorbidity in patients with cardiovascular disease, so it follows that excessive daytime sleepiness is a prevalent symptom. Treatment consists of management of sleep disorders and use of psychostimulants. Secondary sleepiness caused by sedation will respond to withdrawal of sedating medications such as narcotics, hypnotics, and anxiolytics. See Chapter 17 for a discussion of sleep and sleep disorders.

Vital Exhaustion

Appels' research group in the Netherlands has explored the concept of fatigue and accompanying psychological concepts of loss of energy, increased irritability, and feelings of demoralization as a risk factor for myocardial infarction.[9] Appels labeled this set of symptoms "vital exhaustion" in the 1970s. In a series of studies on men, the research team demonstrated that vital exhaustion was a precursor to acute myocardial infarction (AMI) in men.[10,11]

Although the preceding studies on vital exhaustion were done on men, in 1993 the research team demonstrated that vital exhaustion also was a precursor for AMI in women.[12] The team also found that patients who completed successful angioplasty and who were positively diagnosed with vital exhaustion experienced new coronary events in subsequent years.[13] This meant that vital exhaustion was an independent predictor of future cardiac risk.

The ultimate test was to see whether an intervention could be designed to reduce vital exhaustion and subsequent coronary events. Appels and colleagues[14] randomly assigned 710 subjects in a clinical trial intervention that consisted of small-group counseling sessions to reduce stressors and improve coping, rest, relaxation, and physical exercise. The feeling of being exhausted decreased significantly in subjects in the intervention group. However, some subjects experienced new cardiac events within 6 months before the 18-month long intervention was completed, and another subset of the intervention group who had coexisting noncardiac comorbid illnesses remained exhausted without significant improvement, in spite of the intervention.

Appels[15] suggested that subsequent research trials are needed with controls for preexisting comorbid conditions and greater intensity for the intervention. The author concluded that the concept of vital exhaustion was critical in identifying subjects at risk for subsequent myocardial infarction. The best ways to intervene to alter the risks of vital exhaustion remain to be identified.

Depression

Fatigue is a dominant symptom of depression. Because of the relationship between fatigue and depression, cardiovascular-related fatigue frequently is attributed to depression. The conceptual boundary between fatigue and depression in cardiovascular patients has not been identified. In related work, Wojciechowski and colleagues[16] were unable to demonstrate that depression and vital exhaustion were separate constructs in 143 patients, mostly men, experiencing first-time AMI. They found a high correlation between depression and vital exhaustion that led to their conclusion that vital exhaustion may be a component of depression instead of being a separate entity.

It is noteworthy that in the early studies discovering the problem of persistent fatigue following AMI and coronary artery bypass surgery[4] measures (such as the profile of mood states, or POMS[17]) designed to detect mood disturbances were used. The symptoms of fatigue

and depression often overlap; however, not all fatigued patients have a depressed mood. Similarly, treatment of depression may improve mood but not extinguish fatigue. Whether fatigue leads to depression or depression leads to fatigue remains controversial. A third possibility is that fatigue and depression have a shared cause.

Depression and heart disease often coexist, and depression is an independent predictor of recurrent cardiac events.[18] In the context of symptom management, treatment of depression is comparable to correcting anemia and is a rational approach for the patient with fatigue. Research studies on cardiovascular-related fatigue should include separate measures for fatigue and depression to avoid confounding results.[19]

FATIGUE IN PARTICULAR POPULATIONS
Gender

Fatigue is more prevalent in women than men in the general population. Although women have been underrepresented in cardiovascular research, women were more likely to be included in research that focused on fatigue associated with heart disease. In addition, there is a growing body of knowledge comparing symptoms of acute coronary syndrome between men and women. Unfortunately, women who have atypical symptoms such as fatigue may not receive a cardiovascular workup because their symptoms are considered nonspecific, and a gender bias may exist where women are viewed as being at low risk for heart disease.

Gender also plays a role in the interpretation of symptoms. McCreath[20] found that fatigue differed by gender in older adults with heart failure. Women expressed difficulty fulfilling household responsibilities and described their fatigue with the words *useless, lazy,* and *inadequate,* whereas men used the words *tired, pooped,* and *sleepy* to describe their fatigue. The effect of gender on fatigue and its interpretation needs further exploration.

Older Adults

Stephen[21] explored whether older adults attribute their fatigue to age. In a sample of 50 older men and women with heart failure, those who attributed their fatigue to their age had greater fatigue than those who did not attribute their fatigue to age. Older adults with cardiovascular disease may delay seeking help because they dismiss increasing fatigue as an age-related symptom. Response-shift bias is a concern when studying older adults because an expectation of fatigue can lead to adaptation and underreporting of the severity of symptoms.[22] Further investigation is needed to learn how age influences the reporting, interpretation, and subsequent actions taken in response to changes in fatigue.

The symptoms of heart disease are often subtle in the elderly. A family member may observe that the patient spends more time in a chair and naps throughout the day. Older adults with heart failure have been shown to restrict their activities to avoid experiencing fatigue and dyspnea. Oka and colleagues[23] measured daily activity levels in a small group of older adults with heart failure and found that study participants generally had low levels of activity below their exercise capacity documented with exercise treadmill testing. Only 16 percent of the subjects reported fatigue, and nearly half of the subjects reported no symptoms. Self-imposed activity restrictions lead to muscle atrophy, deconditioning, and physical disability, ultimately making fatigue unavoidable. Sedentary behavior in older adults has been explained by avoidance of symptoms, but it is unknown how boredom contributes to fatigue and excessive daytime sleepiness.

Culture

The symptom experience occurs within the context of one's culture. Adjustment to the limitations imposed by fatigue are affected by many variables, including work ethic, social support, role expectation, and spirituality.[24] Social factors, such as marginalization, also can influence the interpretation and response to symptoms. Black women with documented acute coronary syndrome have experienced the trivialization of their symptoms.[25] Fatigue is a symptom that easily could be viewed as trivial in a society that values hard work and stoicism. Researchers investigating fatigue associated with cardiovascular disease need to develop recruitment strategies to include underrepresented ethnic groups to ensure an accurate understanding of the symptom.

MEASURING AND ASSESSING FATIGUE

Assessing for fatigue in all cardiovascular patients is an important skill for nurses. A comprehensive fatigue assessment includes severity, temporal patterns, impact on performance of daily activities and mood, and exacerbating and relieving factors. Documenting the exact words patients use to describe their fatigue is useful for reporting the full subjective sensations. Modifications of documentation tools and policies may promote more consistent and accurate documentation of all symptoms. Implementation of the pain and symptom assessment record across 12 settings in Canada has improved the documentation of fatigue.[26]

Assessment of the patient with fatigue should include an inquiry about secondary causes of fatigue. Common conditions in cardiovascular patients that contribute to fatigue include anemia, rheumatoid arthritis, multiple sclerosis, cancer, sleep-disordered breathing, hypothyroidism, and depression. Fatigue also may be caused by medications, sleep disturbances, chronic pain, acute infection, effort-demanding mobility devices, and emotional disturbances. The health care provider will order the following laboratory studies to assist in the differential diagnosis of fatigue[20]:

- Complete blood count
- Electrolyte panel with magnesium
- Thyroid screen
- Sedimentation rate
- C-reactive protein
- Urinalysis

Dittner and colleagues[1] recently completed a comprehensive review of 30 instruments used to measure fatigue in a variety of clinical populations. The scales were described, the clinical groups in whom the scales have been used were listed, and recommendations for their use were offered. To be of clinical interest and noteworthy as a symptom of illness, fatigue usually was described as "extreme and persistent tiredness, weakness or exhaustion." The authors explained that many patients reported fatigue as their most severe symptom and the cause of significant activity restriction. The authors claimed that fatigue has been ignored in most symptom severity assessments and in outcomes for many diseases, including those with fatigue as a hallmark symptom. The result has been that many patients and clinicians do not have an adequate understanding of fatigue and know little about how to treat fatigue successfully.

Dittner and colleagues[1] excluded instruments that contained fatigue as one of the items or one of the subscales on a more comprehensive index measuring a variety of symptoms or moods. One such subscale used by many in previous research is the fatigue subscale on the POMS.[17] Dittner and colleagues[1] claimed that the fatigue subscale from scales such as the POMS "should generally not be used in isolation without validation."

Fatigue scales can be sorted into unidimensional fatigue scales with severity as the core dimension or multidimensional fatigue scales. In the multidimensional scales a variety of aspects of fatigue are measured including severity, intensity, impact, and duration. The six instruments from the review by Dittner and colleagues[1] that have been or could be used with cardiovascular patients are listed and described in Table 55-1 along with their psychometric properties.

The instrument that would be easiest for clinicians to use regularly with cardiovascular patients is the visual analog scale,[1] a simple short scale that measures fatigue. The format for the visual analog scale is similar to the visual analog scale for pain that many clinicians use regularly. With fatigue, the endpoint markers would be as follows: 0 = "little or no fatigue experienced" and 10 = "most fatigue one can imagine."

In conclusion, a variety of instruments measure fatigue, but few have been tested specifically with cardiovascular patients. Depending on the clinical or research question of interest, there are instruments with good psychometric properties that could aid clinicians and researchers in their search for optimal assessment of cardiovascular patients' fatigue.

FATIGUE IN SPECIFIC CARDIOVASCULAR DISORDERS
Acute Coronary Syndromes

A number of investigators have identified common prodromal symptoms, especially in women, for an AMI.[27-29] Although many found that chest discomfort did occur in patients while at home before their hospitalization, other symptoms such as fatigue and shortness of breath were found to begin earlier than chest discomfort.

TABLE 55-1   FATIGUE SCALES

	FATIGUE SEVERITY SCALE	RHOTEN FATIGUE SCALE	FATIGUE ASSESSMENT INSTRUMENT	FATIGUE IMPACT SCALE	MULTIDIMENSIONAL FATIGUE SYNDROME INVENTORY	VISUAL ANALOGUE SCALE-F
What is assessed?	Impact and functional outcomes	Severity	Severity, impact, and possible triggers	Impact	Severity	Severity
Number of scale items	9	1	29	40	30	18
Target population	Chronic medical	General medical	General medical	Multiple sclerosis	Cancer	General medical
Internal consistency	0.88	—	0.70-0.91	0.93	0.85-0.96	0.91-0.96
Test-retest reliability	0.84	—	0.29-0.69	—	Greater than 0.50	—
Concurrent validity	Fatigue rated on visual analog scale	—		Sickness impact profile (#)	Profile of Mood Scales (POMS-F), SF-36—Vitality	Scales correlate with Stanford Sleepiness Scale and POMS-F
Discriminant validity	Distinguished patients from healthy subjects	—	Discriminates between patients and controls	Significant difference between multiple sclerosis and hypertensive patients	Distinguished cancer and noncancer patients	
Sensitivity to change	Yes	—	—	—	—	Yes

Adapted from Dittner AJ, Wessely SC, Brown RG: *J Psychosom Res* 56:157-170, 2004. *POMS,* Profile of Mood Scales.

These other symptoms occurred for many over a period of days or weeks before the acute episode.

In McSweeney and Crane's sample of women with AMI,[27] the most frequent symptoms experienced by the majority of subjects were "unusual fatigue" and feeling "no energy." In addition, subjects reported discomfort in the shoulder blade region, chest discomfort, and/or shortness of breath. The symptoms were experienced over a number of weeks for many subjects and for some over a number of months.

In another sample of 515 women, McSweeney and colleagues[28] found that unusual fatigue was experienced as the most frequent symptom for more than a month before the AMI. The majority of subjects (70 percent) reported feeling fatigue daily or several times a week. Sleep disturbance and shortness of breath also were experienced by more than 40 percent of the women. The authors concluded that the women had failed to recognize and act on the prodromal symptoms they experienced. These results are discussed further in Chapter 52.

A recently reported study of the symptoms experienced by AMI patients included men (56 percent) and women (44 percent).[30] This group of patients reported chest pain as their most frequent symptom (89 percent), followed by fatigue (65 percent). Interestingly, fatigue was found by interview in 65 percent of the patients but was recorded in the medical record on hospital admission for only 4 percent of the patients. The authors suggested that either patients discount the significance of fatigue and do not report it on admission, or that the providers who are assessing and recording the "chief complaint" discount the significance of fatigue for AMI.

In a recent study, investigators measured fatigue in women at 6 and 12 months following AMI. Women reported moderate levels of fatigue and 67 percent reported fatigue that was unlike the fatigue they experienced before their AMI.[31] In another study, sleep disturbances were prevalent and fatigue was the most common consequence of these disturbances 1 year following percutaneous transluminal coronary angioplasty.[32] Although recovery following AMI has been the subject of many studies, few studies have focused on fatigue.

In conclusion, the symptoms of fatigue, although frequent and debilitating for patients experiencing an AMI, do not appear to prompt patients to judge their condition accurately as life threatening and in need of immediate medical attention. Better health information needs to be directed at the population at risk for AMI to help them identify the possible constellation of symptoms that they may experience. Responding to the warning of fatigue associated with acute coronary syndrome may prompt early treatment and prevention of AMI. In addition, because fatigue may continue for an extended time period following an AMI or percutaneous transluminal coronary angioplasty, clinicians should continue to assess patients for fatigue and attempt to treat it when possible.

Heart Failure

In a sample of 170 male and female heart failure patients, the majority with a history of previous acute episodes of heart failure, Friedman and Griffin[33] found that shortness of breath was the most frequent symptom reported by patients when interviewed in an open-ended format regarding the time period before their hospitalization. However, when these same subjects were asked to check the symptoms they experienced before admission on a printed checklist of 13 symptoms, more than 80 percent of the subjects checked shortness of breath and fatigue. Similar to the conclusions made by DeVon and colleagues,[30] these reporting and methodological differences indicate that subjects may discount fatigue as a significant symptom to report verbally on admission to the hospital or to health care providers unless prompted. In spite of fatigue being a critical indicator of heart failure, it is not viewed as a noteworthy symptom even in patients with a history of heart failure and may not be assessed as a critical symptom by all providers.

On a follow-up analysis of a subset of these data, Friedman[34] compared the symptoms experienced by men and women in the sample ($n = 138$) who were age 65 and older. This resulting sample had the same pattern of symptoms with some variation of frequency. At the hospitalization data point, when subjects were reporting on their acute heart failure experience with the symptom checklist, shortness of breath was the most frequent symptom identified by 94 percent of men, followed by fatigue at 84 percent. For women, shortness of breath was only slightly more frequent (88 percent) than fatigue (82 percent). By the follow-up period 6 weeks after hospital discharge, when the severity of the heart failure had diminished, the frequencies of the symptoms changed for men and women. Fatigue then was reported as the most frequent symptom by 70 percent of the subjects, whereas dyspnea decreased to 51 percent of the subjects. Although fatigue had decreased by the follow-up period, it remained a significant symptom for most subjects.

Nordgren and Sorensen[35] studied the symptoms recorded for 80 patients age 75 or older who were hospitalized in Sweden with end-stage heart failure. They found that the most common symptoms recorded for the majority of patients were breathlessness (88 percent), pain (75 percent), and fatigue (69 percent). The symptom reports were obtained by retrospective record reviews, so these data were indirect patient reports of the symptoms experienced.

In another investigation[36] of older community-dwelling persons with one of three advanced chronic diseases, chronic obstructive pulmonary disease, cancer, or heart failure, the heart failure group reported limited activity as their most frequent symptom (61 percent) and fatigue as their second most frequent symptom (47 percent). Limited activity could be considered a consequence of symptoms rather than as a unique symptom. If limited activity was treated as a consequence of symptoms experienced, then fatigue would be identified as the most frequent individual symptom in this study.

In summary, these data on heart failure patients confirm that fatigue is a significant symptom for this population during acute episodes and over the course of the illness; however, fatigue may be overlooked as significant by patients and providers. Future research should examine the patterns and clusters of symptoms that persons with heart failure experience, including fatigue, in an attempt to determine the best practices for management.

Stroke

Stroke patients suffer from significant fatigue after stroke, and little research has been directed toward this population.[6,37] Ingles and colleagues[38] found that 68 percent of stroke patients reported significant fatigue after the stroke compared with 36 percent of a similar age adults who had not had a stroke. In the stroke group, 40 percent said their fatigue was either their worst or one of the worst symptoms experienced. Each of these studies of stroke patients demonstrated that fatigue is significant in this clinical population, and all of the subjects who experienced fatigue identified it as contributing to functional impairment. De Groot and colleagues[37] suggested that the pharmacological and nonpharmacological strategies used to ameliorate fatigue in other patient populations be tested for efficacy in stroke patients because efficacy in this population is yet to be determined.

INTERVENTIONS TO TREAT FATIGUE

No research studies specific to cardiovascular patients have been done to test interventions with fatigue alone as the primary outcome. However, three interventions have been shown to reduce cancer-related fatigue: exercise, energy conservation counseling, and correction of anemia.[2,39] An intervention to improve nutrition, relieve pain and stress, and balance rest with physical activities has been shown to reduce fatigue in older adults.[40] Table 55-2 provides a list of interventions that commonly are recommended by cardiovascular nurses to reduce fatigue. The next step is to test whether these interventions are effective in reducing and preventing fatigue in cardiovascular patients. Testing fatigue-reducing interventions in persons with cardiovascular disorders is a fertile area for future research and clinical practice.

Exercise

Exercise has been explored and suggested as an intervention strategy for cardiac patients to decrease the overwhelming fatigue and improve functional ability. If skeletal muscle dysfunction accounts for the diminished strength and increased fatigue experienced by heart failure patients, then training that improves the muscle function should result in improved symptomatology.[41] A number of studies have demonstrated that moderate exercise can reduce symptoms experienced by heart failure patients and improve their quality of life.[42,43] The clinical practice guidelines for heart failure patients in NYHA Classes I to III recommend regular exercise as tolerated for heart failure patients as the strategy to improve muscle strength and exercise tolerance and to reduce symptoms.[45] The recommendations for exercise in heart failure patients were reviewed in Corra and colleagues.[41] (See the accompanying evidence-based practice feature.)

■ ■ ■

TABLE 55-2   INTERVENTIONS FOR TREATMENT OF FATIGUE WITH CARDIAC DISEASE

INTERVENTION	RATIONALE
Plan an individualized exercise program adapted to limitations.	Exercise improves symptoms in congestive heart failure[41-43] and reduces fatigue in cancer patients.[2]
Refer patient to occupational therapy for energy conservation and adaptive equipment.	An energy conservation intervention reduced fatigue in cancer patients.[39]
Correct anemia.	Symptoms of congestive heart failure are worse with anemia,[44] and erythropoietin improved energy in cancer patients.[2]
Recognize and treat depression.	Fatigue associated with depression should improve with treatment of depression.
Control chronic pain.	Chronic pain may be a correlate to fatigue. Excessive energy is required to cope with chronic pain.
Minimize sleep disturbances, and educate about sleep hygiene.	Sleep disturbance is associated with fatigue.[32]
Encourage planned rest periods. Daytime naps may be helpful in older adults.[1]	Balancing activities with rest period helps to prevent fatigue. Naps were included in an intervention to reduce fatigue.[40]
Ensure adequate daily calories with a variety of easy-to-chew and nutrient-dense foods.	Minimize work of eating, and energy is derived from daily food sources. Supplements may boost energy in elderly.[40]
Screen and treat endocrine disorders such as hypothyroidism and diabetes.[19]	Metabolic abnormalities such as hypothyroidism and hyperglycemia are associated with fatigue.
Review medication list for any drugs that may be attributing to fatigue.	Some cardiac medications have been associated with fatigue as a side effect.
Monitor electrolyte balance.	Magnesium is an important intracellular electrolyte that influences potassium and calcium.

■ **EVIDENCE-BASED PRACTICE**

PRINCIPLES FOR EFFECTIVE EXERCISE IN HEART FAILURE PATIENTS

High-intensity exercise training can be considered and tried in heart failure patients who have moderate heart failure and preserved exercise capacity if high-risk patients (those with myocardial ischemia, malignant rhythm disorders, and recent hemodynamic instability) are excluded.

Resistance training alone or in combination with an exertional program should be prescribed and individually tailored for patients with coronary artery bypass grafting and after acute myocardial infarction. The prescription for resistance training with heart failure patients is much more cautious because the effects on functional capacity and peripheral skeletal muscle response is not well documented in this population.

Bibliography

Corra U, Mezzani A, Giannuzii P, Tavazzi L: Chronic heart failure-related myopathy and exercise training: a developing therapy for heart failure symptoms, *Prog Cardiovasc Dis* 44:157-172, 2002.

In conclusion, Corra and colleagues[41] recommended that exercise training definitely be considered for heart failure patients. The results from previous studies demonstrated positive effects for short-term, relatively low-intensity exercise with the majority of stable heart failure patients. In addition, some stable heart failure patients with moderate failure actually can tolerate and benefit from more intense training. Severely impaired heart failure patients (NYHA Class IV) need careful monitoring of their exercise tolerance, and low-intensity training must be conducted with caution to determine the benefits for this population.

Energy Conservation Strategies

A referral to occupational therapy for energy conservation is indicated for patients who need help learning ways to adapt their daily activities to reduce fatigue. A randomized clinical trial of a telephone-delivered energy conservation and activity management intervention was conducted with cancer patients.[39] The intervention, which consisted of three patient contacts by an oncology nurse over a 5-week period, resulted in a reduction in fatigue in patients undergoing cancer treatment. Similar intervention trials are needed urgently in cardiovascular patients.

Correction of Anemia

Fatigue is a symptom of anemia; however, no correlation was found between hematocrit or hemoglobin and fatigue in patients with chronic heart failure.[21] In a larger study of patients with NYHA Class III and IV chronic heart failure with systolic dysfunction, there was a relationship between low hemoglobin and worse symptoms.[44] In acute blood loss anemia, a randomized, placebo-controlled trial showed no effect of iron supplementation on restoring hemoglobin in patients at 3 months of recovery from coronary artery bypass surgery.[46] In cancer patients, several trials have demonstrated that erythropoietin improves energy when used for the treatment of chemotherapy-induced anemia.[2] No evidence indicates that correcting anemia in cardiovascular patients will mitigate fatigue.

FUTURE DIRECTIONS

The mechanism of fatigue associated with cardiovascular disorders is unknown. In the future, a unifying hypothesis may explain fatigue across all chronic illnesses. The symptom of fatigue may originate in the brain because of alterations in neurochemical processes. The monoamine neuronal network regulates physical and mental energy. This energy circuit operates with a continuous "rheostat" activation of the cortex and is modulated through the hypothalamus. A neurological explanatory mechanism will have implications for pharmacological treatment for fatigue. The psychostimulant modafinil currently is being studied for the treatment of fatigue in multiple sclerosis and patients who are positive for human immunodeficiency virus.[47,48] Whether psychostimulants such as modafinil will have a safety profile acceptable for the use in cardiovascular patients for the treatment of fatigue is not known.

REFERENCES

1. Dittner AJ, Wessely SC, Brown RG: The assessment of fatigue: a practical guide for clinicians and researchers, *J Psychosom Res* 56:157-170, 2004.
2. Nail LM: Fatigue in patients with cancer, *Oncol Nurs Forum* 29:537-546, 2002.
3. Ekman I, Ehrenberg A: Fatigue in chronic heart failure: does gender make a difference? *Eur J Cardiovasc Nurs* 1:77-82, 2002.
4. King KB, Porter LA, Rowe MA: Functional, social, and emotional outcomes in women and men in the first year following coronary artery bypass surgery, *J Womens Health* 3:347-354, 1994.
5. Devon HA, Zerwic JJ: The symptoms of unstable angina: do women and men differ? *Nurs Res* 52:108-118, 2003.
6. Staub F, Bogousslavsky J: Fatigue after stroke: a major but neglected issue, *Cerebrovasc Dis* 12:75-81, 2001.
7. Pigeon WR, Sateia MJ, Ferguson RJ: Distinguishing between excessive daytime sleepiness and fatigue: toward improved detection and treatment, *J Psychosom Res* 54:61-70, 2003.
8. Chakravorty SS, Rye DB: Narcolepsy in the older adult: epidemiology, diagnosis, and management, *Drugs Aging* 20:361-376, 2003.
9. Schuitemaker GE, Dinant GJ, van der Pol GA, Appels A: Assessment of vital exhaustion and identification of subjects at increased risk of myocardial infarction in general practice, *Psychosomatics* 45:414-418, 2004.
10. Falger PRJ, Schouten EW: Exhaustion, psychological stressors in the work environment, and acute myocardial infarction in adult men, *J Psychosom Res* 36:777-786, 1992.
11. Appels A, Otten F: Exhaustion as precursor of cardiac death, *Br J Clin Psychol* 31:351-356, 1992.
12. Appels A, Falger PRJ, Schouten EGW: Vital exhaustion as risk indicator of myocardial infarction in women, *J Psychosom Res* 37:881-890, 1993.
13. Kop WJ, Appels A, Mendes de Leon CF et al: Vital exhaustion predicts new cardiac events after successful coronary angioplasty, *Psychosom Med* 56:281-287, 1994.
14. Appels A, Bar FW, Lakser J et al: The effect of a psychosocial intervention program on the risk of a new cardiac event after angioplasty: a feasibility study, *J Psychosom Res* 43:209-217, 1997.
15. Appels A: Exhaustion and coronary heart disease: the history of a scientific quest, *Patient Educ Couns* 55:223-229, 2004.
16. Wojciechowski FL, Strik JJ, Falger P et al: The relationship between depressive and vital exhaustion symptomatology post-myocardial infarction, *Acta Psychiatr Scand* 102:359-365, 2000.
17. McNair D, Lorr M, Droppleman L: *The manual for the profile of mood states*, San Diego, 1992, Educational and Industrial Testing Service.
18. Lesperance F, Frasure-Smith N, Juneau M, Theroux P: Depression and 1-year prognosis in unstable angina, *Arch Intern Med* 160:1354-1360, 2000.
19. Aaronson LS, Teel CS, Cassmeyer V et al: Defining and measuring fatigue, *J Nurs Scholarsh* 31:45-50, 1999.
20. McCreath A: Fatigue and chronic heart failure: a qualitative study, Unpublished master's thesis, Spokane, Wash, 2001, Gonzaga University.
21. Stephen SA: Correlates of fatigue in older adults with chronic heart failure, doctoral dissertation, Salt Lake City, 2000, University of Utah (Dissertation Abstracts International).
22. Breetvelt IS, Van Dam FS: Underreporting by cancer patients: the case of response-shift, *Soc Sci Med* 32:981-987, 1991.
23. Oka RK, Stotts NA, Dae MW et al: Daily physical activity levels in congestive heart failure, *Am J Cardiol* 71:921-925, 1993.
24. Allen J, Szanton S: Gender, ethnicity, and cardiovascular disease, *J Cardiovas Nurs* 20:1-6, 2005.
25. Banks AD, Malone RE: Accustomed to enduring: experiences of African American women seeking care for cardiac symptoms, *Heart Lung* 34:13-21, 2005.
26. Bouvette M, Fothergill-Bourbonnais F, Perreault A: Implementation of the pain and symptom assessment record (PSAR), *J Adv Nurs* 40:685-700, 2002.
27. McSweeney JC, Crane PB: Challenging the rules: women's prodromal and acute symptoms of myocardial infarction, *Res Nurs Health* 23:135-146, 2000.
28. McSweeney JC, Cody M, O'Sullivan P et al: Women's early warning symptoms of acute myocardial infarction, *Circulation* 108:2619-2623, 2003.
29. Miller CL: A review of symptoms of coronary artery disease in women, *J Adv Nurs* 39:17-23, 2002.
30. DeVon HA, Ryan CJ, Zerwic JJ: Is the medical record an accurate reflection of patients' symptoms during acute myocardial infarction? *West J Nurs Res* 26:547-560, 2004.
31. Crane PB: Fatigue and physical activity in older women after myocardial infarction, *Heart Lung* 34:30-38., 2005
32. Eddel-Gustafsson UM, Hetta JE: Fragmented sleep and tiredness in males and females one year after percutaneous transluminal coronary angioplasty (PTCA), *J Adv Nurs* 34:203-211, 2001.
33. Friedman MM, Griffin JA: Relationship of physical symptoms and physical functioning to depression in patients with heart failure, *Heart Lung* 30:98-104, 2001.
34. Friedman MM: Gender differences in the health related quality of life of older adults with heart failure, *Heart Lung* 32:1-8, 2003.
35. Nordgren L, Sorensen S: Symptoms experienced in the last six months of life in patients with end-stage heart failure, *Eur J Cardiovasc Nurs* 2:213-217, 2003.
36. Walke LM, Gallo WT, Tinetti ME, Fried TR: Burden of symptoms among community dwelling older persons with advanced chronic disease, *Arch Intern Med* 164:2321-2324, 2004.
37. de Groot MH, Phillips SJ, Eskes GA: Fatigue associated with stroke and other neurologic conditions: implications for stroke rehabilitation, *Arch Phys Med Rehabil* 84:1714-1720, 2003.
38. Ingles JL, Eske GA, Phillips SJ: Fatigue after stroke, *Arch Phys Med Rehabil* 80:173-178, 1999.
39. Barsevick AM, Dudley W, Sweeney C et al: A randomized clinical trial of energy conservation for patients with cancer-related fatigue, *Cancer* 100:1302-1311, 2004.
40. Robinson S, Vollmer C, Hermes B: A program to reduce fatigue in convalescing elderly adults, *J Gerontol Nurs* 29:47-53, 2003.
41. Corra U, Mezzani A, Giannuzii P, Tavazzi L: Chronic heart failure-related myopathy and exercise training: a developing therapy for heart failure symptoms, *Prog Cardiovasc Dis* 44:157-172, 2002.
42. Corvera-Tindel T, Doering LV, Woo MA et al: Effects of a home walking exercise program on functional status and symptoms in heart failure, *Am Heart J* 147:339-346, 2004.
43. Gary R, Sueta C, Dougherty M et al: Home-based exercise improves functional performance and quality of life in women with diastolic heart failure, *Heart Lung* 210-218, 2004.
44. Konstam M, Dracup K, Baker D et al: *Heart failure: evaluation and care of patients with left-ventricular systolic dysfunction*, Clinical Practice Guideline No 11, AHCOR Pub No 94-0612, Rockville, Md, 1994, U.S. Department of Health and Human Services, Agency for Health Care Policy and Research.
45. Horwich TB, Fonarow GC, Hamilton MA et al: Anemia is associated with worse symptoms, greater impairment in functional capacity and a significant increase in mortality in patients with advanced heart failure, *J Am Coll Cardiol* 39:1780-1786, 2002.
46. Crosby L, Palarski VA: Iron supplementation for acute blood loss anemia after coronary bypass surgery: a randomized, placebo-controlled study, *Heart Lung* 23:493-499, 1994.
47. Rabkin JG, McElhiney MC, Rabkin R, Ferrando SJ: Modafinil treatment for fatigue in HIV+ patients: a pilot study, *J Clin Psychol* 65:1688-1695, 2004.
48. Zifko ULA: Management of fatigue in patients with multiple sclerosis, *Drugs* 64:1295-1304, 2004.

Care of Patients with Acute Coronary Syndrome: Unstable Angina and Non–ST-Segment Elevation Myocardial Infarction

Leslie L. Davis

ACC   American College of Cardiology

ACE   angiotensin-converting enzyme

ACS   acute coronary syndrome

AHA   American Heart Association

aPTT   activated partial thromboplastin time

ASA   aspirin

BNP   plasma B-type natriuretic peptide

CABG   coronary artery bypass grafting

CAD   coronary artery disease

CCB   calcium channel blocker

CK-MB   creatine kinase-MB

ECG   electrocardiogram

ED   emergency department

ESC   European Society of Cardiology

GP   glycoprotein

LMWH   low-molecular-weight heparin

NSTE ACS   non–ST segment elevation acute coronary syndrome

NSTEMI   non–ST segment elevation myocardial infarction

NTG   nitroglycerin

OASIS-2   Organization to Assess Strategies for Ischemic Syndromes (trial)

OR   odds ratio

PCI   percutaneous coronary intervention

RRR   relative risk reduction

SADHART   Sertraline Antidepressant Heart Attack Randomized Trial

STEMI   ST segment elevation myocardial infarction

TIMI   thrombolysis in myocardial infarction

UFH   unfractionated heparin

THE SPECTRUM OF ACUTE CORONARY SYNDROME

Coronary heart disease remains the number one cause of death in the United States with one in five deaths attributed to it yearly. Approximately 1.2 million new or recurrent cases of myocardial infarction or fatal coronary heart disease events occur each year in the United States alone.[1] Further, more than 5.3 million adults present to emergency departments **(EDs)** annually with a chief complaint of chest pain or other ischemic symptom.[2] Of those, more than 1.7 million are hospitalized with unstable angina or a non–ST-segment elevation

myocardial infarction **(NSTEMI)**.[1] These two conditions collectively are referred to as non–ST-segment elevation acute coronary syndrome **(NSTE ACS)**. A third type of acute coronary syndrome **(ACS)** is ST segment elevation myocardial infarction **(STEMI)**. Figure 56-1 diagrams the three types of ACS. The remainder of this chapter focuses on NSTE ACS. Refer to Chapter 57 for care of the patient with STEMI.

ACS is a major cause of morbidity and mortality in the United States and worldwide. The event rate for death, myocardial infarction (or recurrent myocardial infarction), or recurrent ischemia early after NSTE ACS is estimated to be as high as 41 percent.[3] In an effort to standardize patient care to improve outcomes, the American College of Cardiology/American Heart Association **(ACC/AHA)** developed evidence-based treatment guidelines in 2000 for patients with unstable angina and NSTEMI.[4] These guidelines were updated in 2002 to reflect the growing body of evidence for NSTE ACS treatments.[2] Despite publication of these treatment guidelines in 2002, treatment remains suboptimal in many facilities. Subsequently, the AHA published a statement outlining the practical implementation of the ACC/AHA treatment guidelines for unstable angina and NSTEMI.[5] The scientific statement provides templates to assist ED physicians, cardiologists, and other providers to streamline care for accurate diagnosis and treatment of patients with NSTE ACS. Tools provided in the statement include an ACS risk assessment record and a standardized order template for evidence-based treatment.

DIAGNOSIS
Clinical Presentation

Similar to symptoms of STEMI, typical symptoms of NSTE ACS include substernal or left-sided chest discomfort radiating to the left arm associated with dyspnea, nausea, and/or diaphoresis. The chest discomfort typically is described as heaviness, tightness, squeezing pain, constriction, band-like pain, or fullness. Most patients describe symptoms as "discomfort" rather than "pain." The onset of ischemic symptoms typically occur gradually; however, onset in some cases may be abrupt. Symptoms most commonly occur at rest, are progressive and nocturnal, and in many cases may be of recent onset. Symptoms are typically diffuse (poorly localized) as opposed to being described as a pinprick or a needle to one specific location and typically do not increase with palpation to the area or with a deep breath or cough. ACS symptoms are more severe than stable

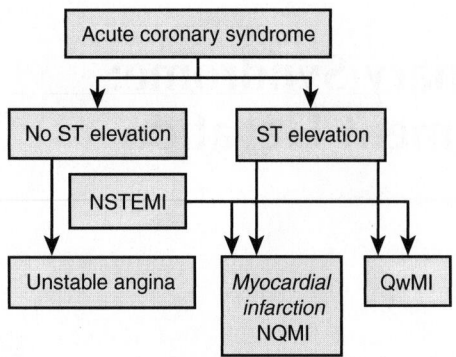

FIGURE 56-1 ■ Classification of acute coronary syndrome. *NQMI,* Non–Q wave myocardial infarction; *NSTEMI,* non–ST segment elevation myocardial infarction; *QwMI,* Q wave myocardial infarction.

chronic angina, lasting longer than 20 to 30 minutes and are not relieved promptly by nitroglycerin or rest in most cases. Prolonged episodes of symptoms usually equates with a more serious prognosis.

Atypical symptoms of ACS may include one or more of the following: neck, throat, jaw, or tooth discomfort; shoulder or arm pain; numbness or tingling in the chest or a related area; epigastric discomfort often described as indigestion; discomfort between the scapula or in the midback region; dizziness/light-headedness with or without syncope; fatigue or weakness; and/or palpitations. Atypical symptoms sometimes are referred to as the patient's *anginal equivalent.* Caution should be taken when evaluating women, persons with diabetes, and elders for suspected NSTE ACS because these subgroups are more likely to have atypical symptoms (see Chapters 52 and 53 for thorough discussions of chest pain and so-called atypical symptom presentations). Unexplained dyspnea at rest that is new in onset or worsened from baseline is a worrisome symptom, especially in elders. Refer to Box 56-1.

History and Physical Examination

Assessment typically begins in the ED where most patients with suspected NSTE ACS present for medical care. Initial assessment via the telephone or an outpatient facility is *not recommended* for patients with suspected ongoing ischemic symptoms. The patient should be transported promptly to a local ED or facility that is capable of providing a 12-lead electrocardiogram (**ECG**) with a trained provider available on site to interpret the results. For patients with a known history of coronary artery disease (**CAD**) complaining of worsening angina or a recurrence of symptoms before previous revascularization, immediate transport to a local ED that has ECG equipment and reperfusion therapy available is recommended. Emergency medical services should be called for transport unless the wait is expected to be 20 to 30 minutes, in which case a private vehicle may be used to transport the patient to the nearest facility.[2] In many cases, prehospital ECG transmission by emergency medical services is available for patients with suspected ischemia to decrease potential delays in time to ECG acquisition.

BOX 56-1   ■ ■ ■
PRESENTING SYMPTOMS SUGGESTIVE OF ACUTE CORONARY SYNDROME

Typical Chest and Associated Symptoms (Not Related to Trauma)
- Substernal or left-sided chest pain
- Chest pressure, heaviness, tightness, or squeezing in chest
- Neck/throat pain or discomfort
- Jaw pain or discomfort (not related to toothache)
- Shoulder pain or discomfort (not related to degenerative joint disease)
- Arm pain or discomfort (not related to bursitis)
- Diaphoresis
- Dyspnea (not related to preexisting pulmonary condition or renal failure)

Atypical Chest and Associated Symptoms
- Chest pain in other location
- Numbness, tingling, pricking, or stabbing chest pain
- Fullness or burning in chest
- Epigastric/indigestion-like/gas-like pain or discomfort (not related to gastrointestinal problems)
- Nausea or vomiting (not related to gastrointestinal problems)
- Upper extremity numbness or tingling (not related to stroke or carpal tunnel syndrome)
- Midback (between shoulder blades) pain (not related to degenerative joint disease or trauma)
- Pain/discomfort with deep breath or cough (not related to preexisting pulmonary condition)
- Dizziness, light-headedness, or syncope (not related to a neurological problem or hypertension)
- Fatigue or weakness (not related to a neurological problem or hypertension)
- Palpitations (new onset with no history of dysrhythmias)

Adapted from Milner KA, Funk M, Arnold A et al: *Am Heart J* 143:283-288, 2002.

Upon arrival to the ED, the priority treatment goal is to determine the likelihood that a patient has ACS caused by CAD. This assessment is based on clinical information (history and physical examination), 12-lead ECG, and cardiac biomarkers. A 12-lead ECG should be obtained immediately upon arrival to the ED. ACC/AHA guidelines call for an ECG within 10 minutes of arrival for any patient with suspected ischemia.[2,6]

Simultaneous to obtaining a 12-lead ECG, a focused history and physical examination should be conducted by trained personnel (physician, advanced practice nurse, or physician's assistant). Expertise in performing rapid risk stratification in patients with suspected NSTE ACS is essential. In addition to characteristics of the chief complaint, history also should include assessment of cardiac disease risk factors (such as age, gender, hypertension, diabetes, previous CAD including myocardial infarction, dyslipidemia, tobacco use, recent cocaine use, and family history of CAD), use of alcohol or other cardiotoxic substances and presence of other comorbidities. A thorough assessment of presenting symptoms should include ruling out other non–NSTE ACS conditions that may be life-threatening. See Box 56-2 for possible noncardiac causes of chest discomfort. The initial history also includes investigation of underlying conditions that would place the patient at high risk for side effects from the use of antiplatelet or antithrombin therapies. These conditions include the following: history of hemorrhagic stroke, intracranial tumor, any ma-

---

BOX 56-2   ■ ■ ■
POSSIBLE CAUSES OF NONACUTE CORONARY
SYNDROME CHEST PAIN

Life-Threatening
Aortic dissection
Esophageal rupture
Pulmonary embolism
Tension pneumothorax

Less-Emergent Causes
Biliary or pancreatic disease
Chest trauma
Esophageal reflux or gastric ulcer
Musculoskeletal disease
Parenchymal lung disease
Pericarditis
Psychiatric disease—depression and/or panic disorder

---

jor bleeding including gastrointestinal bleeding, aortic dissection, major surgery in the preceding 2 weeks, or any other condition that would place the patient at risk for bleeding.

Physical examination should include assessment of blood pressure in both arms; heart sounds including heart rate and rhythm; presence of adventitious lung sounds; presence of jugular vein distention or peripheral edema; peripheral pulses; presence of carotid, aortic, or peripheral bruits (to check for extracardiac vascular disease); and checking for rectal bleeding (contraindication for many ACS therapies). Physical examination findings that denote high-risk features for ACS patients include blood pressure greater than 180/100 mm Hg or less than 90 mm Hg; bradycardia, tachycardia, or an irregular heart rhythm; a new murmur, gallop (S_3 or S_4), or rub; or the presence of crackles or pulmonary edema. Assessment also should determine whether the chest discomfort is positional or reproducible by palpation, which typically indicates a low likelihood of ACS caused by CAD.

Diagnostic Procedures
Electrocardiogram

Patients in whom the ECG shows ST segment elevation of ≥1 mm (0.1 mV) in two or more anatomically contiguous leads are considered to be having a STEMI and should be considered for urgent reperfusion therapy (see Chapter 58). Patients with ST segment depression or transient ST segment elevation (less than 30 minutes) would be classified as having NSTE ACS. These patients are considered at high-risk for adverse events and should be treated aggressively. ST segment depression has been shown to be a significant independent predictor of mortality and myocardial infarction.[7] Additionally, the magnitude of the ST segment deviation (whether elevation or depression) is prognostic for poor outcomes.[2]

Posterior leads should be assessed to rule out true posterior STEMI for those patients with acute ST segment depression in the anterior and lateral leads (leads I, aVL, and V_1 to V_6) and ongoing symptoms despite initial treatment. Although infrequent, transient ST seg-

ment elevation (less than 30 minutes) during an ischemic episode in which symptoms and ECG changes resolve with rest or nitroglycerin is worrisome because there is a high likelihood of severe underlying CAD.[2] T wave inversion in two or more anatomically contiguous leads on the initial ECG is associated with about a 5 percent chance of developing an adverse event (myocardial infarction or death) in 30 days.[7] Prognosis for patients with T wave inversion is good, although the likelihood of CAD is still high.

Patients with a normal ECG at presentation are considered the lowest risk NSTE ACS subgroup. However, a normal 12-lead ECG does not rule out acute ischemia completely. Up to 6 percent of those with a normal 12-lead ECG will develop an NSTEMI by other diagnostic markers (biomarkers or anatomical findings).[5] Serial ECGs repeated at 5- to 10-minute intervals or continuous 12-lead ST segment monitoring are recommended to increase sensitivity in detecting ischemia for patients with ACS who remain symptomatic despite a nondiagnostic index ECG.[6]

Patients with new or presumably new left bundle branch block and a clinical history consistent with acute ischemia should be presumed to be having a STEMI and should be considered candidates for urgent reperfusion. Patients with ECG confounders such as previous bundle branch block, paced rhythm, or left ventricular hypertrophy should be admitted for observation and referred for additional cardiovascular diagnostic testing (i.e., serial biochemical cardiac biomarkers, echocardiography, or nuclear imaging) to determine whether the patient's symptoms are consistent with an acute ischemic process.[2,6] In these cases, initial treatment decisions are based on clinical history, physical examination, and biomarker results (Table 56-1).

Biochemical Cardiac Biomarkers

Biochemical cardiac biomarkers are the third clinical link to determining risk stratification for suspected ACS patients along with the clinical history and 12-lead ECG. Serial cardiac biomarkers (also called cardiac enzymes) confirm the diagnosis of myocardial infarction and offer information to determine treatment strategy (i.e., those patients with positive biomarkers are at more risk for poor outcomes that will necessitate more aggressive treatment). Serum biochemical tests to determine myocardial necrosis include creatine kinase (**CK-MB**), troponin T and I, and/or myoglobin. Refer to Table 56-2 for an outline of available cardiac enzyme tests and features of each.

Troponin assays, because of their increased specificity, have largely replaced CK-MB and myoglobin in most institutions. In 2000, the Joint European Society of Cardiology (**ESC**) and ACC Committee for the Redefinition of Myocardial Infarction revised the definition of myocardial infarction to include troponin measurements as evidence of cardiac necrosis consistent with myocardial infarction.[8] Blood levels of cardiac troponins are not detectable in healthy adults. Because cardiac troponins are so highly sensitive for identifying myocardial necrosis, whether from CAD or other causes, it is essential

■ ■ ■

TABLE 56-1 SIGNIFICANCE OF INITIAL ELECTROCARDIOGRAM FINDINGS IN PATIENTS WITH SUSPECTED ACUTE CORONARY SYNDROME

INITIAL ELECTROCARDIOGRAM FINDING	DIAGNOSTIC CATEGORY	TREATMENT RECOMMENDED
ST segment elevation	STEMI	Reperfusion therapy
New left bundle branch block	STEMI	Reperfusion therapy
ST segment depression	NSTE ACS	If new, treat as high-risk ACS
Transient ST segment elevation	NSTE ACS	Treat as high-risk ACS
T wave inversion	NSTE ACS	If 2.0 mV, treat as high-risk ACS
Old bundle branch block	Unclear	Need additional diagnostic testing
Permanently paced	Unclear	Need additional diagnostic testing
Normal electrocardiogram	Unclear	Treat for ACS—low risk

ACS, Acute coronary syndrome; *NSTE ACS,* non–ST segment elevation acute coronary syndrome; *STEMI,* ST segment elevation myocardial infarction.

■ ■ ■

TABLE 56-2 CARDIAC BIOMARKERS

BIOMARKER	POSITIVE VALUE	TIMING	ADVANTAGES/DISADVANTAGES
Creatine kinase (CK-MB)	Varies	Starts to rise in 3-12 hours *Peak:* 24 hours Normalizes in 48-72 hours	Readily available Bedside testing available Highly sensitive but not as specific as other tests Falsely elevated by trauma, surgery, hypothermia, diabetic ketoacidosis, seizures, intramuscular injections, stroke, or strenuous exercise
Myoglobin	Doubling of myoglobin value within 2 hours indicates myocardial infarction Negative myoglobin 4-8 hours after symptoms can rule out myocardial infarction	Starts to rise in 1-4 hours *Peak:* 6-7 hours Normalizes within 24 hours	Rises early in myocardial infarction Poor choice of tests to do for late presenters Falsely elevated in those with skeletal muscle or renal disease
Troponin T	Greater than 2.0 ng/ml*	Starts to rise within 3-12 hours after infarction *Peaks:* 12-48 hours Normalizes within 14 days	Excellent sensitivity and specificity Point of care testing available Falsely elevated by skeletal muscle disease or renal disease
Troponin I	Greater than 0.03 mcg/liter*	Starts to rise within 3-12 hours after infarction *Peaks:* 24 hours Normalizes within 5-10 days	Excellent sensitivity and specificity Point of care testing available Not influenced by skeletal muscle disease or renal disease

*May have institutional variability. *ng,* Nanograms.
Adapted from Davis L: *Cardiovascular nursing secrets: your cardiovascular questions answered by experts you trust,* St Louis, 2004, Mosby.

that the test be used in conjunction with clinical presentation and ECG findings to diagnose NSTEMI (avoiding treatment based on a false-positive troponin finding).[2,8] The ESC/ACC consensus document recommends that the cutoff value for each laboratory be defined at the 99th percentile of a normal reference population. Unfortunately, assays to meet this criterion are not uniformly consistent in facilities across the United States. The 2002 ACC/AHA guidelines for management of patients with ACS state a preference for troponin I or troponin T; however, further note that CK-MB by mass assay is an acceptable alternative.[2]

Cardiac troponin levels typically begin to rise within 3 to 12 hours after symptom onset in myocardial infarction. This time course is similar to the time for rise of CK-MB measurements. However, to reach the 99 percent cutoff for the normal population as recommended by the ESC/ACC consensus document may take between 6 and 9 hours to yield a positive result.[2]

Elevated troponin levels provide diagnostic and prognostic information for managing patients with ACS caused by NSTEMI. ACS patients with higher troponin levels have a significantly higher mortality and morbidity compared with patients with negative troponin levels. Cardiac troponins have become the standard of practice to determine which ACS patients are highest risk and therefore would receive the most benefit from therapies such as heparin, glycoprotein (**GP**) IIb/IIIa receptor inhibitors, and early invasive management (cardiac catheterization and revascularization) if indicated within the first 48 hours of symptoms onset (see the treatment section).

Testing for troponin and CK-MB levels may be done at the bedside, which may take minutes, or in the central laboratory, which may take an hour or more. Point of care (or bedside) testing may improve time to decision making in the ED; however, it should be noted that these assays are not as sensitive as those used in the central laboratory. Therefore, it is imperative that serial troponin tests (or CK-MB levels if this is the test being done via point of care) be done every 3 to 6 hours while the patient is in the ED for those ACS patients with indeterminate or normal values, especially for those patients within 6 hours of symptom onset in whom clinical suspicion remains high.[2]

Myoglobin testing is useful for those patients who present early but should not be the only marker because it has poor cardiac specificity. If, however, myoglobin testing is negative in an early presenter, it may be a good test of exclusion for myocardial infarction. Table 56-2 outlines advantages and disadvantages of each biomarker.

Risk Stratification

Once the initial clinical history, physical examination, 12-lead ECG, and cardiac biomarker results are obtained, the provider needs to determine the answer to the following two questions to determine treatment: (1) What is the likelihood of the patient having definite ACS? and (2) What is the likelihood that the patient will have a poor outcome? Using the ACC/AHA treatment guidelines for NSTE ACS, providers can use initial findings to predict the likelihood that the signs and symptoms represent an ACS caused by CAD.[2] In this schema, individuals are categorized into three groups: (1) those with a high likelihood; (2) those with intermediate likelihood; and (3) those with low likelihood of having ACS caused by CAD (Table 56-3).[2,5]

Risk stratification for the NSTE ACS patients is essential to determine which patients are at highest risk of death or recurrent myocardial infarction and who would benefit from the most aggressive therapies. Assessment of prognosis helps set the pace of treatment. Several NSTE ACS clinical trials have used multivariable regres-

sion techniques to determine high-risk indicators of poor outcomes. Data from the PURSUIT (Platelet IIb/IIIa in Unstable angina: Receptor Suppression Using Integrilin Therapy) Trial demonstrated that older age, heart rate (bradycardia or tachycardia), systolic blood pressure (hypotension), ST segment depression on initial ECG, signs of heart failure (new or worsening rales, mitral regurgitation, or S_3 gallop), positive test results for cardiac biomarkers, and presence of ventricular tachycardia were independent baseline predictors for death and recurrent myocardial infarction at 30 days.[9] In addition, the Thrombolysis in Myocardial Infarction (**TIMI**) risk scoring system tool was developed using multivariate logistic regression analysis from the TIMI 11B (Thrombolysis in Myocardial Infarction 11B) data to determine which NSTE ACS patients are at highest risk for poor outcomes.[3] Variables used in the TIMI risk scoring system include age greater than 65 years, more than three coronary risk factors, prior CAD with stenosis of greater than 50 percent, ST segment deviation, more than two angina events in the past 24 hours, use of aspirin within 7 days, or a positive cardiac biomarker. Each item is given one point to calculate a total score of 7 or less. Patients are considered high risk if they have a score of 5 or more and low risk if they have a score of 2 or less. The risk of death, infarction/reinfarction, or recurrent ischemia requiring revascularization within 14 days ranged as high as 41 percent for the high-risk individuals (score of 6 or 7) versus 5 percent for those considered at low risk (score of 0 to 1). Patients with increased TIMI risk score also receive the greatest benefit from more aggressive therapies (i.e., low-molecular-weight heparin, platelet GP IIb/IIIa receptor antagonists, and early coronary angiography).[2,10]

Three variables that stand out from these and other models to determine high risk for adverse outcomes in NSTE ACS patients are age greater than 60 years, ST seg-

■ ■ ■

TABLE 56-3   LIKELIHOOD THAT SYMPTOMS REPRESENT ACUTE CORONARY SYNDROME CAUSED BY CORONARY ARTERY DISEASE

	LIKELIHOOD		
	HIGH	INTERMEDIATE	LOW
Feature	*Any of the following:*	*Absence of high-likelihood features and presence of any of the following:*	*Absence of high- or intermediate-likelihood features but may have the following:*
History	Chest or left arm pain or discomfort as chief symptom reproducing previously documented angina Known history of coronary artery disease, including myocardial infarction	Chest or left arm pain or discomfort as chief symptom Age greater than 70 years Male sex Diabetes mellitus	Probable ischemic symptoms in absence of any of the intermediate-likelihood characteristics Recent cocaine use
Examination	Transient mitral regurgitation, hypotension, diaphoresis, pulmonary edema, or rales	Extracardiac vascular disease	Chest discomfort reproduced by radiation
Electrocardiogram	New, or presumably new, transient ST segment deviation ($\geq$0.05 mV) or T wave inversion ($\geq$0.2 mV) with symptoms	Fixed Q waves Abnormal ST segments or T waves not documented to be new	T wave flattening or inversion in leads with dominant R waves Normal electrocardiogram
Cardiac markers	Elevated cardiac troponin I, troponin T, or creatine kinase-MB	Normal	Normal

From Braunwald E, Antman EM, Beasley JW et al: *ACC/AHA 2002 guideline update for the management of patients with unstable angina and non-ST segment elevation myocardial infarction: a report of the American College of Cardiology/American Heart Association Task Force on Practice Guidelines (Committee on the Management of Patients With Unstable Angina)*, 2002. Retrieved January 22, 2007, from www.acc.org/qualityandscience/clinical/guidelines/unstable/unstable/pdf

ment deviation, and an elevated cardiac biomarker. It has been shown that the presence of two of these three high-risk features in NSTE ACS patients confer a 30-day risk of death or nonfatal myocardial infarction of between 13 and 15 percent.[11] These three variables are used most often in practice to risk stratify individuals with NSTE ACS in order to determine treatment strategies.[2,5] Table 56-4 depicts a comparison of the multivariable models discussed.

INITIAL TREATMENT

Initial therapy for all patients with suspected NSTE ACS includes (1) assessment of the ABCDs (airway, breathing, circulation, and defibrillation if needed), (2) continuous ECG monitoring, (3) supplemental oxygen to maintain arterial oxygen saturation or finger pulse oximetry ≥90 percent, (4) 12-lead ECG, (5) obtaining intravenous access, (6) obtaining laboratory work (especially cardiac biomarkers), and (7) ensuring that resuscitation equipment is available at the bedside if needed.[6] The initial goal of treatment at this point is to halt ongoing ischemia and to prevent or decrease the chance of serious adverse events (specifically death, myocardial infarction, or recurrent myocardial infarction). Thus unless contraindications exist, initial pharmacological treatment includes that of antiplatelet therapy, antiischemic therapy, and antithrombotic therapy. Each of these therapies is discussed in the pharmacological therapy section of this chapter.

Early Conservative Versus Invasive Treatment Strategies

One of the most important decisions to be made as part of risk stratification to determine treatment strategy is whether to perform coronary angiography and, if so, the timing of the procedure. An *early invasive treat-* *ment strategy* is defined by the ACC/AHA guidelines for NSTE ACS patients as undergoing cardiac catheterization and possible percutaneous coronary intervention (**PCI**), if indicated, within 48 hours of symptom onset. An early invasive strategy has a Class IA recommendation by the ACC/AHA for those NSTE ACS patients who are at highest risk. Highest risk is defined as having *one or more of the following:* recurrent angina, elevated troponin (I or T), new ST segment depression, depressed left ventricular function, hemodynamic instability, sustained ventricular tachycardia, recent PCI (within 6 months), *or* prior coronary artery bypass grafting (**CABG**). Table 56-5 outlines the ACC/AHA classification of recommendations and levels of evidence. In the absence of these high-risk findings, an early invasive *or* early conservative strategy may be used as long as the patient has no contraindication to revascularization (Class I, evidence level B). Early invasive treatment includes use of quadruple therapy: aspirin, clopidogrel (if PCI is planned with continued use for up to 12 months[12]), heparin (unfractionated heparin [**UFH**] or low-molecular-weight heparin [**LMWH**] unless CABG is planned, in which case only UFH should be used), and a GP IIb/IIIa inhibitor.[2]

An *early conservative therapy* or early noninvasive treatment strategy refers to patients *not* scheduled for planned cardiac catheterization within the first 48 hours of symptom onset. Low-risk ACS patients are treated with this strategy, which includes use of the following medical therapy: aspirin, clopidogrel for at least 1 month, heparin, and eptifibatide or tirofiban (in patients with continuing ischemia, elevated troponin levels, or other high-risk features).[2] Abciximab should be avoided unless PCI is planned. Patients treated conservatively have noninvasive testing before consideration of an invasive evaluation or treatment. If, however, a patient being treated conservatively develops recurrent symptoms of ischemia, heart failure (or tests reveal a

■ ■ ■

TABLE 56-4 PREDICTORS FOR HIGH RISK OF POOR OUTCOMES IN NON–ST SEGMENT ACUTE CORONARY SYNDROME

TRIAL	PURSUIT	TIMI RISK SCORE TIMI-11B
Number of patients	9461	1957
Predicted outcome	30-day death or recurrent myocardial infarction	14-day death, myocardial infarction, or ischemia requiring revascularization
History	Age	Age
	Recent angina	Recent angina
	Gender (male)	Family history of coronary artery disease
	Heart failure	Diabetes
		Current smoking
		Hypertension
		Previous aspirin use within 7 days
		Prior coronary artery disease with stenosis greater than 50%
Physical examination	Systolic blood pressure	
	Heart rate	
	Rales	
	Mitral regurgitation	
	S$_3$ gallop	
	Ventricular tachycardia	
Electrocardiogram	ST segment depression	ST segment elevation or depression
Cardiac biomarker	↑ Creatine kinase-MB	↓ CK-MB or troponin

TIMI, Thrombolysis in Myocardial Infarction.

■■■

TABLE 56-5 AMERICAN COLLEGE OF CARDIOLOGY/ AMERICAN HEART ASSOCIATION CLASSIFICATION OF RECOMMENDATIONS AND LEVELS OF EVIDENCE

CLASS	COMMENT
Class I	Conditions for which there is evidence and/or general agreement that a given procedure or treatment is useful and effective
Class II	Conditions for which there is conflicting evidence and/ or a divergence of opinion about the usefulness/ efficacy of a procedure or treatment
IIa	Weight of evidence/opinion is in favor of usefulness/ efficacy
IIb	Usefulness/efficacy is less well established by evidence/ opinion
Class III	Conditions for which there is evidence and/or general agreement that the procedure/treatment is not useful/ effective and in some cases may be harmful

Level of Evidence

A	Data derived from multiple randomized clinical trials
B	Data derived from a single randomized trial or nonrandomized studies
C	Consensus opinion of experts

Adapted from Braunwald E, Antman EM, Beasley JW et al: *ACC/AHA 2002 guideline update for the management of patients with unstable angina and non-ST segment elevation myocardial infarction: a report of the American College of Cardiology/American Heart Association Task Force on Practice Guidelines (Committee on the Management of Patients With Unstable Angina)*, 2002. Retrieved January 22, 2007, from www.acc.org/qualityandscience/clinical/guidelines/unstable/unstable.pdf

left ventricular ejection fraction is less than 40 percent), or a serious dysrhythmia, a change of treatment strategy may be required (i.e., cardiac catheterization sooner than previously planned). Therefore, patients being treated via the early conservative approach should be monitored closely for these signs and symptoms in the event that a more aggressive treatment approach is required.

Numerous investigators have addressed the use of an invasive versus a conservative treatment approach in managing NSTE ACS patients. Bavry and colleagues[13] published a recent meta-analysis of five trials with a combined enrollment of 6766 patients with NSTE ACS who were assigned randomly to *routine invasive* versus conservative treatment. Men and women showed improved survival with the routine invasive strategy of treatment versus conservative treatment. Males in particular showed an improved survival with *early invasive* treatment. Subgroup analyses of the TACTICS-TIMI-18 Study of NSTE ACS patients revealed that *routine early invasive* treatment strategy was associated with a 39 percent relative risk reduction (**RRR**) for those older than age 65 and a 56 percent RRR for those older than 75 years in the rate of death or nonfatal myocardial infarction at the 6 month follow-up.[14] Predictors from a meta-regression analysis that have shown increased benefit with the use of the *early invasive* treatment strategy for NSTE ACS patients include the use of aggressive therapy (triple antiplatelet therapy: aspirin [acetylsalicylic acid, or **ASA**], clopidogrel, and GP IIb/IIIa inhibitors) and intracoronary stenting. However, predictors of likelihood of bleeding with early invasive treatment include an increased number of antiplatelet and anti-

thrombin agents used concurrently for a longer period of time, unplanned revascularization, and older age.[15] One recommendation to overcome bleeding with this level of treatment is the use of a vascular closure device at the site of access for angiography.[16] Refer to Figure 56-2 for a summary algorithm of the ACC/AHA 2002 guidelines for diagnosis and treatment of patients with NSTE ACS who present to the ED.[6]

Further Diagnostic Testing

A chest x-ray film should be obtained for all NSTE ACS patients to assess for the presence of pulmonary edema, pulmonary infiltrates, cardiomegaly, or a widened mediastinum, which is suggestive of an aortic dissection. The radiograph should be done as a standing posterior-anterior and lateral view, ideally in the radiology department as opposed to using a portable chest x-ray unit, which limits the interpretation. However, the patient's hemodynamic stability should be taken into account when deciding location and views for radiography.

Echocardiography is helpful to assess for structural heart disease such as wall motion abnormalities, pericardial effusion or thickened pericardium, valvular abnormalities, left ventricular hypertrophy, or low ejection fraction. Echocardiography also can determine whether there are regional wall motion abnormalities, which may be seen within seconds or minutes of an occluded coronary artery and have very high sensitivity for ischemia. However, the specificity for ischemia is limited.

Dobutamine stress echocardiography has a higher sensitivity, specificity, and negative predictive accuracy compared with standard cardiac echocardiography. Patients with a positive predischarge dobutamine stress echocardiography were more likely at 6 months to have reached a primary endpoint of cardiac death, myocardial infarction, or rehospitalization for unstable angina.[17] Limitations of dobutamine echocardiography include cost and availability.

Exercise stress testing has a role in determining which patients have a low likelihood of coronary disease and therefore can be discharged home from observation or to chest pain units. To be eligible for exercise stress testing, patients must have a nondiagnostic ECG and negative cardiac biomarkers and must be symptom free at rest for at least 6 hours before the procedure.[5] Patients ineligible for exercise stress testing include those with acute ischemia, those unable to exercise, and those with noninterpretable ECGs (left bundle branch block, permanent paced, or left ventricular hypertrophy). Except for those patients with acute ischemia, those patients ineligible for conventional exercise testing may undergo pharmacological stress testing, such as nuclear imaging or echocardiography. If results from the stress test are strongly positive, the patient is referred for cardiac catheterization.[2] If stress testing is negative and the patient is able to complete the entire test, the patient is at very low risk and generally can be sent home with further follow-up as an outpatient.

For those patients with continued symptoms despite negative biomarkers and ECGs and in whom an ACS can-

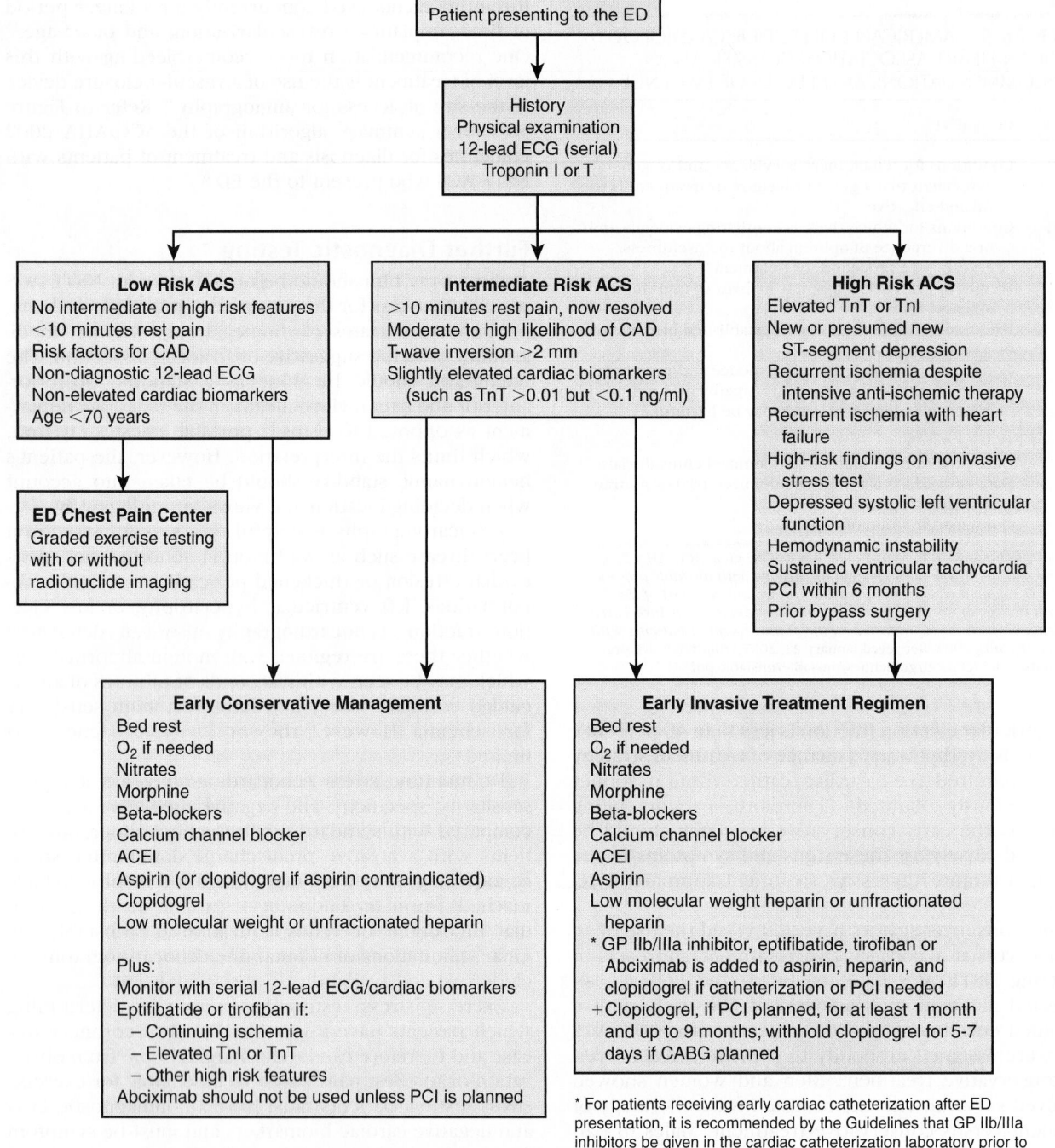

FIGURE 56-2 ■ Diagnostic and treatment strategies in the emergency department for patients with acute coronary syndrome as recommended by the 2002 American College of Cardiology/American Heart Association guidelines. *ACEI*, Angiotensin-converting enzyme inhibitor; *ACS*, acute coronary syndrome; *CABG*, coronary artery bypass grafting; *CAD*, coronary artery disease; *ECG*, electrocardiogram; *ED*, emergency department; *GP*, glycoprotein; *PCI*, percutaneous coronary intervention; *TnT*, troponin T; *TN1*, troponin-1.

not be ruled out completely, rest myocardial perfusion imaging and echocardiography are recommended. Examples include a thallium-201 or a technetium-99m sestamibi test, which can diagnose myocardial ischemia and/or dysfunction. However, there are three limitations to use of myocardial perfusion imaging: (1) patients with prior myocardial infarction may have false-positive results, (2) patients whose symptoms have resolved in 3 hours or less may have false-negative results, and (3) the

test is limited unless there is acute resting imaging available (typically within 3 hours of the last symptoms).[18] Refer to Chapter 29 for further information regarding exercise testing and noninvasive imaging.

Serum laboratory studies, in addition to cardiac biomarkers, that should be obtained in NSTE ACS patients include complete blood count (to rule out anemia or thrombocytopenia), chemistries, prothrombin time, activated partial thromboplastin time (**aPTT**), and a fasting lipid panel. Several classes of new biomarkers of inflammation may prove valuable in the future care of NSTE ACS patients. High-sensitivity C-reactive protein has been shown to predict cardiovascular risk and independently predict prognosis in ACS patients.[2,15] Myeloperoxidase, another marker of inflammation, has been shown to predict which ACS patients are at high risk for cardiovascular events independently of other biomarkers. Research is ongoing to determine how these inflammatory markers will be helpful for clinical assessment and risk stratification. In addition to markers of inflammation, three types of natriuretic peptides (plasma B-type natriuretic peptide [**BNP**], N-terminal fragment of the BNP prohormone [N-terminal pro-BNP], and Nt-pro-atrial natriuretic peptide) also have been shown to be independent predictors of mortality in NSTE ACS patients.[15] Elevation of any of these three natriuretic peptides has been associated with increased ventricular wall stress (primarily of the left ventricle).

Further research is needed to determine which combination of markers should be used (be it individual markers or classes of markers), what time frame in the course of an NSTE ACS event each should be drawn, and how to interpret results in which subgroups of patients. For example, initial studies have shown that women with ACS have a different marker combination than men. Specifically, women have been shown to have higher high-sensitivity C-reactive protein and BNP levels yet lower troponin levels in general.[15] Refer to Chapter 43 for further discussion of emerging risk factors.

Pharmacological Therapy
Aspirin (Acetylsalicylic Acid)
ASA is the cornerstone of antiplatelet therapy for patients with suspected ACS and has a Class IA recommendation by the ACC/AHA treatment guidelines.[2] Mediated through irreversible cyclooxygenase inhibition (an enzyme required to synthesize thromboxane A_2), ASA suppresses vasoconstriction and platelet aggregation, thus reducing the chance of thrombosis. Antiplatelet effects generally start within 1 hour of use and last for up to 7 to 10 days. Aspirin is generally well tolerated and inexpensive and is considered relatively safe for all patients with suspected ACS. Numerous studies have demonstrated reduction in mortality and morbidity (myocardial infarction, recurrent myocardial infarction, or recurrent ischemia) with the use of ASA. A meta-analysis of four randomized studies in patients who had unstable angina found an approximate 51 percent reduction in death at 30 days and an overall 47 percent reduction in risk of death or myocardial infarction with the use of ASA versus placebo.[4] Unfortunately, despite overwhelming evidence to treat ACS patients with ASA, ASA is underutilized. One study found that only about 75 percent of patients hospitalized for CAD received ASA, whereas only 78 to 85 percent of patients with CAD received ASA at hospital discharge.[19] Therefore, *unless absolutely contraindicated,* all patients with suspected ACS should be administered 162 to 325 mg non–enteric-coated aspirin to chew and swallow as soon as possible after symptom onset to be continued indefinitely. Many

patients may state that they have an ASA allergy, when in fact it is intolerance. True ASA allergy is rare and typically is associated with signs and symptoms of asthma, rhinitis, hives, and in severe cases, anaphylaxis. For those patients with a true ASA allergy, clopidogrel is given as a substitute. The dose of clopidogrel is a 300-mg loading dose followed by 75 mg daily. The use of clopidogrel is discussed further subsequently. Other contraindications to ASA in addition to allergy include active bleeding including gastrointestinal bleeding of any kind, severe untreated hypertension at presentation, or severe clotting disorders.

Nitroglycerin
The use of nitroglycerin (**NTG**) has a Class IC indication from the ACC/AHA treatment guidelines for NSTE ACS patients.[2] Nitrates may be beneficial in reducing myocardial oxygen demand by promoting vasodilatation in the peripheral blood vessels through vascular smooth muscle. Nitrates have not been shown to decrease mortality, nor are there randomized studies of nitrates in the setting of NSTE ACS. Nitrates act primarily on the veins with only a modest effect on arterioles. Initially, nitrates should be administered sublingually by tablet or spray at the dose of 0.4 mg for three doses at least 5 minutes apart. This should be followed by intravenously administered NTG for persistent ischemia or associated symptoms (pulmonary congestion or those with persistent hypertension). Intravenously administered NTG should be initiated at 10 mcg/min via continuous infusion followed by uptitration of 10 mcg/min every 3 to 5 minutes until symptom relief without causing hypotension.

Contraindications for nitrate use include hypotension (systolic blood pressure less than 110 mm Hg or a greater than 25 percent reduction from the baseline mean arterial blood pressure if hypertensive), bradycardia (heart rate less than 50 beats/min), tachycardia (heart rate greater than 100 beats/min), other signs of hemodynamic instability or the use of phosphodiesterase inhibitors (sildenafil [Viagra], vardenafil [Levitra], or tadalafil [Cialis] within the past 24 hours; 48 hours for tadalafil).[2,6] Extreme caution with nitrate use should be given for those patients with right ventricular infarction (typically associated with inferior infarction) or aortic stenosis because nitrate use may result in severe hypotension and hemodynamic instability.

If NTG is to be discontinued, this should be done gradually, for abrupt discontinuation may result in increased ischemia (as evident on the ECG). Intravenously administered nitrates typically are converted to oral or topical regimens within 24 hours and are continued until the patient is symptom free (from pain or ischemic ECG changes) for 12 to 24 hours.[2] A nitrate-free interval of 8 hours is needed for those patients prescribed oral or topical NTG to prevent tolerance. The nitrate-free interval is scheduled for 8 hours typically between midnight and 8 AM.

Morphine
Morphine has been shown to provide relief of persistent ischemic symptoms despite use of nitrates and/or beta blockers. Morphine has favorable venous dilatory ef-

fects, which improves myocardial contractility and ultimately decreases myocardial workload. Morphine also has a mild chronotropic effect (lowering heart rate) in addition to modestly lowering blood pressure. Patients with acute pulmonary edema, anxiety, or severe pain may benefit as well from use of morphine. Morphine is the analgesic of choice when treating pain associated with myocardial ischemia.[6] Recommended doses of morphine include an initial dose of 1 to 5 mg IV followed by 2 to 8 mg repeated every 5 to 30 minutes.[2,6] One must keep in mind that these doses must be individualized and that the use of NTG and beta blocker therapy has priority over morphine use for the treatment of NSTE ACS patients. Major adverse effects of morphine administration include hypotension (especially if the patient is volume depleted) and respiratory depression. Careful monitoring of blood pressure and symptoms is needed every 5 to 30 minutes because morphine typically is given concurrently with intravenously administered NTG and beta blockers.

Morphine has a Class IC indication for the initial treatment of NSTE ACS. However, no randomized trials have studied the effects of morphine in the setting of NSTE ACS patients. Data from the CRUSADE quality improvement initiative (Can Rapid Risk Stratification of Unstable Angina Patients Suppress Adverse Outcomes with Early Implementation of the ACC/AHA Guidelines) recently reported that NSTE ACS patients who received morphine within 24 hours of presentation ($n = 17,003$) had a higher adjusted risk of death (odds ratio **[OR]** 1.48) compared with those patients not given morphine ($n = 40,036$).[20] For patients receiving morphine and NTG the OR of death was even higher (1.50). This finding was consistent across all measured subgroups. This paper questioned the safety of morphine given within the first 24 hours of presentation for NSTE ACS patients and emphasized the need for a randomized trial to address this topic.

Antithrombin Therapy

Intravenously administered UFH is one type of antithrombin therapy receiving a Class IA indication by the ACC/AHA treatment guidelines for NSTE ACS patients when added to antiplatelet therapy (ASA and/or clopidogrel).[2] Numerous studies have demonstrated a reduction in mortality and morbidity with UFH, which has been used for more than two decades for the treatment of ACS. A meta-analysis of six clinical trials including 1353 unstable angina patients receiving UFH plus ASA versus ASA alone showed a nonsignificant ($p = 0.06$) RRR of death or myocardial infarction with the addition of UFH.[21]

Heparin suppresses coagulation indirectly by inactivating thrombin and factor Xa, which ultimately blocks the formation of fibrin. Heparin acts in conjunction with antithrombin III to inhibit clotting factor activity within minutes of administration. UFH binds nonspecifically with various plasma proteins, mononuclear cells, and endothelial cells resulting in variable responses in patients.[2] Response to the medication may be unpredictable, and frequent laboratory monitoring is required because of the narrow therapeutic margin and short half-life of UFH. UHF is administered via intravenous bolus followed by a continuous infusion. Dosing for UFH is weight based with an initial bolus of 60 to 70 units/kg, followed by initial maintenance drip of 12 to 15 units/kg/hr (maximum 1000 units/hr). The infusion then is adjusted to an aPTT 1.5 to 2.5 times control (generally between 60 and 80 seconds) to be given over 24 to 48 hours (or until time of cardiac catheterization). Lower doses of UFH should be administered to patients with hepatic or renal impairment because UFH is metabolized hepatically and is excreted renally. In addition to body weight, other factors have been associated with higher aPTT levels (age) or lower aPTT levels (smoking and diabetes).[2]

The use of LMWH is considered a Class IA recommendation for treatment of NSTE ACS patients as an alternative to intravenously administered UFH when added to the antiplatelet therapy of ASA and/or clopidogrel. ACC/AHA guidelines from 2002 conclude that *either* type of antithrombin agent (UFH or LMWH [specifically enoxaparin]) may be used for NSTE ACS patients when added to ASA and clopidogrel. However, for those patients with impaired renal function (creatinine clearance $\leq$30 ml/min), UFH is the preferred agent. LMWH is more potent than UFH and acts by inhibiting factor X by way of antithrombin. Advantages of LMWH include a dose-independent clearance, a longer half-life resulting in a more predictable response and sustained anticoagulation, no need for laboratory monitoring, and ease of administration (twice daily subcutaneous injections).[2]

Expert opinion to date indicates that LMWH (specifically enoxaparin) has similar or slightly better efficacy compared with UFH and in general is preferred for most NSTE ACS patients.[15] Regardless of which agent is used, UFH or LMWH, once an agent is initiated for a particular patient, it should *not be converted* to the other agent. Switching back and forth between agents has been shown to increase the likelihood of bleeding.[22]

As an alternative to LMWH or UFH, a third class of antithrombin therapy is available. Hirudin (lepirudin or desirudin), bivalirudin (Angiomax, formerly known as Hirulog), argatroban (Acova), and a new agent, fondaparinux, are examples of direct antithrombin agents. This class of medication differs from UFH or LMWH in that these thrombin inhibitors offer *direct* inhibition of thrombin (as opposed to UFH, which indirectly inhibits thrombin by use of antithrombin). By selectively binding to antithrombin, this class of agents neutralizes factor Xa, which interrupts the blood coagulation cascade. Thrombin formation and thrombus development are inhibited.

Initial studies of direct thrombin inhibitors were stopped prematurely because of excess bleeding in the treatment group. More recent clinical trials using bivalirudin have shown promising results with this class of medication. Specifically, lower bleeding complications have been observed with the use of direct thrombin inhibitors. In REPLACE-2, 6010 patients undergoing elective or urgent PCI were randomized to receive bivalirudin versus UFH plus a GP IIb/IIIa inhibitor.[23] For those patients randomized to the bivalirudin alone, use of bail-out GP IIb/IIIa inhibitor was permitted. Comparable results were found with both treatment arms regarding a composite endpoint of death, myocardial infarction, urgent target vessel revascularization, and major bleeding. No difference was observed in long-term efficacy. However, less bleeding was noted with bivalirudin even in the case of provisional use of GP IIb/IIIa inhibitors. In ACUITY 13,819 moderate- and high-risk patients who underwent invasive treatment were randomized to one of three groups: bivalirudin; bivalirudin plus a GP IIb/IIIa inhibitor; or heparin plus a GP IIb/IIIa inhibitor. Rates of ischemia and bleeding were similar for bivalirudin and heparin when combined with a GP IIb/IIIa inhibitor. Use of bivalirudin alone was associated with similar rates of ischemia, however significantly lower bleeding rates[24]

Contraindications for all three classes of antithrombin agents (UFH, LMWH, and direct antithrombin inhibitors) are similar and include allergy to the medication of choice, bleeding, thrombocytopenia, uncontrolled hypertension, and any other condition that places the patient at undue risk for bleeding. For patients with renal or liver impairment, lower doses are required, with studies revealing that UFH is safer and therefore is preferred over LMWH.

Platelet Glycoprotein IIb/IIIa Receptor Antagonists

The relatively new class of antiplatelet agents, platelet GP IIb/IIIa inhibitors, have greatly reduced mortality and morbidity in high-risk NSTE ACS patients. GP IIb/IIIa inhibitors act by occupying GP IIb/IIIa receptors on the surface of activated platelets. These receptors normally bind with fibrinogen to cause platelet aggregation. When occupied by GP IIb/IIIa inhibitors, platelet aggregation is inhibited. This inhibition is the final common pathway that is needed for subsequent platelet activation and ultimately platelet aggregation.[25] Examples of GP IIb/IIIa receptor antagonists include tirofiban (Aggrastat), eptifibatide (Integrilin), and abciximab (ReoPro). Tirofiban and eptifibatide are small-molecule agents, whereas abciximab is a monoclonal antibody fragment. These agents act similarly but vary in their binding site, affinity, molecular weight, half-life, and elimination. Refer to Table 56-6 for characteristics of each agent.

Platelet GP IIb/IIIa inhibitors, in addition to ASA and heparin, have a Class IA recommendation in the 2002 ACC/AHA treatment guidelines for NSTE ACS patients for whom cardiac catheterization with possible PCI is planned. Additionally, the 2002 ACC/AHA treatment guidelines indicate that these agents also may be given just before PCI if not initiated earlier in the course of treatment (Class IA).[2] This allows for those patients who may not have been started on this type of antiplatelet therapy early in their course of symptoms to receive the medication during the critical time of PCI. Most practices use triple therapy (GP IIb/IIIa inhibitors, heparin, and ASA) for patients 12 to 24 hours before cardiac catheterization with PCI (if indicated) unless the patient is having ongoing symptoms or is hemodynamically unstable, in which case the patient is taken to the catheterization laboratory sooner. Quadruple antiplatelet therapy (GP IIb/IIIa inhibitor use, heparin, ASA, and clopidogrel) is recommended for those for whom catheterization and PCI are planned (Class IIa, evidence level B per the treatment guidelines).

High-risk ACS patients (those with positive ECG readings and/or positive cardiac biomarker results) obtain the most benefit from GP IIb/IIIa inhibition when added to standard therapy with ASA and heparin.[26-28] This benefit was true for three time intervals: 48 to 96 hours, 30 days, and 6 months. The 2002 ACC/AHA treatment guidelines for NSTE ACS offer recommendations for selection of which GP IIb/IIIa inhibitor to use.[2] The guidelines indicate that eptifibatide or tirofiban should be given with ASA and heparin (UFH or LMWH) for patients *with* continuing ischemia, an elevated troponin, or other high-risk features in whom an invasive management strategy (cardiac catheterization and possible PCI within 24 to 48 hours after symptom onset) is *not* planned (Class IIaA recommendation). For patients *without* continuing ischemia who have no other high-risk features and for whom PCI in *not* planned, eptifibatide or tirofiban in addition to ASA and heparin may be used (Class IIbA recommendation). Thus abciximab *should not be used* in patients for whom PCI is *not* planned according to the 2002 treatment guidelines (Class IIIA recommendation).

■ ■ ■

TABLE 56-6   PLATELET GLYCOPROTEIN IIB/IIIA RECEPTOR ANTAGONISTS

MEDICATION	APPROVED INDICATION	HALF-LIFE	DOSE AND ADMINISTRATION	AVERAGE DURATION OF THERAPY	ELIMINATION
Tirofiban	NSTE ACS with or without PCI	4 hours	IV bolus of 0.4 mcg/kg/min for 30 minutes; plus continuous IV infusion of 0.1 mcg/kg/min	12-24 hours	Renal
Eptifibatide	NSTE ACS, thrombosis, PCI use	4 hours	IV bolus of 180 mcg/kg for 2 minutes; then continuous IV infusion of 2 mcg/kg/min	Up to 72 hours Post-PCI: 18 hours	Renal
Abciximab	Thrombosis, PCI use	Affects platelet aggregation for 12-24 hours	IV bolus 0.25 mg/kg for 10 to 60 minutes; then 0.125 mg/kg continuous IV infusion	6 hours Maximum 10 mcg/min for 12 hours Post-PCI: 12 hours	Renal, reticulo-endothelial system

NSTE ACS, Non–ST segment elevation acute coronary syndrome; *PCI,* percutaneous coronary intervention.
Adapted from Davis L: *Cardiovascular nursing secrets: your cardiovascular questions answered by experts you trust,* St Louis, 2004, Mosby. (Previously adapted from Roettig M, Tanabe P: *J Emerg Nurs* 26:6, 2000.)

Duration of use for GP IIb/IIIa inhibitor also has been studied. The TACTICS-TIMI 18 Substudy found that a shorter duration of tirofiban (less than 21 hours) started before or after PCI was associated with impaired myocardial perfusion before and after PCI.[29] Those patients who received the GP IIb/IIIa inhibitor for a longer duration (more than 21 hours) were more likely to have TIMI flow grades of 2 or 3 pre- and post-PCI. Optimal duration of eptifibatide was studied in the ESPRIT Substudy in which patients treated with eptifibatide versus placebo were assigned to five different groups based on infusion duration (16, 18, 20, 22, and 24 hours ± 1 hour).[30] Infusion duration of the eptifibatide-treated group of 16 hours or more was not associated with rebound events such as early abrupt vessel closure. Thus current recommendations by experts are for longer duration (more than 16 hours) before and after PCI for NSTE ACS patients.[15] Refer to Table 56-6 for recommended duration of GP IIb/IIIa inhibitor therapy based on agent chosen.

The most significant adverse effect from GP IIb/IIIa inhibitors is bleeding, primarily at the site of vascular access for catheterization/PCI, followed by bleeding in the gastrointestinal or genitourinary tract. Risk of bleeding is increased with concurrent use of other drugs that alter hemostasis. Because of the risk involved with use of these agents, careful patient selection and appropriate timing for use is required. Absolute contraindications to GP IIb/IIIa inhibitor use include active bleeding within the past 30 days, major surgery or trauma within the preceding 6 weeks, history of stroke within 30 days, any history of hemorrhagic stroke, intracranial mass or aneurysm, thrombocytopenia (platelet count less than 100,000 platelets/mm^3), patients who require renal dialysis, and any bleeding diathesis. Relative contraindications for GP IIb/IIIa use include concurrent warfarin therapy, use of fibrinolytic agents, renal insufficiency, age less than 18 years (all three agents) and older than 75 years (for tirofiban and eptifibatide), uncontrolled hypertension (systolic blood pressure greater than 200 mm Hg or diastolic blood pressure greater than 110 mm Hg), breast-feeding or pregnancy, or recent epidural anesthesia.[25]

Thienopyridines

Thienopyridines, such as clopidogrel and ticlopidine, irreversibly block platelet P2Y$_{12}$ receptors. Stimulation of the P2Y$_{12}$ receptor on the platelet surface leads to sustained platelet aggregation.[15] Therefore, blockade of this receptor serves as another antiplatelet treatment for ACS patients, especially those undergoing PCI. Several studies have shown the clinical benefit in thienopyridine use. This class of antiplatelet therapy is indicated for those NSTE ACS patients unable to tolerate ASA because of a true ASA allergy or gastrointestinal bleeding. Clopidogrel is preferred in these circumstances over ticlopidine because it has been shown to have a better safety profile and more rapidly reaches peak effect in platelet inhibition.[2] Thienopyridine use (specifically clopidogrel) also is indicated for management of NSTE ACS patients in addition to ASA for whom surgery is not anticipated within the following 5 to 7 days.[2]

Ticlopidine also has been used for secondary prevention of stroke and myocardial infarction to prevent stent or graft closure. Ticlopidine, however, takes about 1 week to reach steady state for antiplatelet effect. Adverse effects of ticlopidine, which also limit use, include gastrointestinal problems (such as diarrhea, abdominal pain, nausea, and vomiting), neutropenia (about 2.4 percent of patients), severe neutropenia (0.8 percent of patients), and rarely thrombotic thrombocytopenia purpura. Monitoring requires a complete blood count with a differential count every 2 weeks for the first 3 months of therapy.[2]

Clopidogrel requires about 3 to 5 days to reach steady state after a single dose of 75 mg is administered. Therefore the Food and Drug Administration–approved loading dose for clopidogrel is 300 mg to be administered with ASA.[31] Indications for clopidogrel use in NSTE ACS patients include those unable to take ASA (Class I, evidence level A), those hospitalized in whom an early intervention is *not* planned (Class I, evidence level A), and for those in whom PCI is planned and who are not at high risk for bleeding (Class I, evidence level A). Clopidogrel should be added to ASA as soon as possible after admission for NSTE ACS patients and be administered for at least 1 month, up to 12 months in duration (Class I, evidence level B).[2,12] Clopidogrel, however, should be *withheld* for patients undergoing elective CABG for 5 to 7 days preceding surgery to prevent adverse bleeding events (Class I, evidence level B).

Recent publications now question the loading dose of clopidogrel. Previous studies have shown that 40 percent of those who receive the 300-mg loading dose of clopidogrel did not achieve full antiplatelet effect within the projected 2½ hours.[15] The Antiplatelet therapy for Reduction of MYocardial Damage during Angioplasty (ARMYDA-2) study compared a loading dose of 300 mg versus 600 mg given 4 to 8 hours before PCI.[31] The higher loading dose was shown to be safe and effective. The 600-mg loading dose was associated with a reduction from 12 to 4 percent in the composite endpoint of death, myocardial infarction, or target vessel revascularization. Based on these and other data, the ESC recommended the higher loading dose (600 mg) for NSTE ACS patients undergoing immediate PCI (within 6 hours) in their recently published guidelines for PCI care.[32]

Contraindications for thienopyridines include neutropenia, thrombocytopenia, previous reaction to the agent being considered, and active bleeding. It is imperative that nurses and other health care providers monitor patients receiving these agents for bleeding, especially those patients receiving quadruple antiplatelet therapy or for those receiving multiple agents that alter hemostasis.

Other Agents
Angiotensin-Converting Enzyme Inhibitor Use

Angiotensin-converting enzyme (**ACE**) inhibitors have been shown to decrease mortality in patients with acute myocardial infarction, recent myocardial infarction with left ventricular systolic dysfunction, left ventricular systolic dysfunction in persons with diabetes, and high-risk CAD patients (with or without left ventricular dysfunction).[2] ACE inhibitors should be used for the control of hypertension (uncontrolled despite use of beta blocker and nitrate therapy) after myocardial infarction, for left ventricular dysfunction after myocardial infarction, and in ACS patients who have diabetes (Class I, evidence level B).[2,6] The guidelines also provide a Class IIa, evidence level B recommendation for use of ACE inhibitors for all post-ACS patients. The treatment guidelines for ACS patients do not indicate a preference for which ACE inhibitor. Regarding time of initiation of ACE inhibitor therapy, this class of medication may be started in the ED upon diagnosis of ACS; however, that is not absolutely necessary. For patients who are intolerant to ACE inhibitors (from a previous allergy), an angiotensin receptor blocker may be substituted.[6]

ACE inhibitors block the conversion of angiotensin I to angiotensin II, thereby preventing constriction of blood vessels and release of aldosterone. By preventing this conversion, blood vessels become dilated, fluid retention is prevented, and ultimately the workload of the heart is reduced. ACE inhibitors also attenuate ventricular remodeling, which may delay or prevent the onset of heart failure as a complication of a myocardial infarction. Contraindications to ACE inhibitor use include bilateral renal artery stenosis, aortic stenosis, pregnancy, breast-feeding, symptomatic hypotension, and hyperkalemia. Major side effects of ACE inhibitor use include chronic cough, hypotension, hyperkalemia, worsened renal insufficiency, or angioedema.

Beta Blocker Use

Most of the data to support beta blockade in the NSTE ACS patient population is extrapolated from myocardial infarction trials that have included evolving or recent myocardial infarction patients and from stable angina trials that have shown a dramatic reduction in mortality and morbidity with intravenous administration of beta blockers. The primary benefit of beta blockade in the setting of NSTE ACS includes the beta$_1$ effects of decreasing cardiac workload and myocardial oxygen demand. Slowing the heart rate helps increase time of diastole (thereby increasing coronary artery filling time). Beta blockade is indicated for high-risk ACS patients and/or those with persistent symptoms despite NTG administration. Beta blockers are administered intravenously, followed by oral administration. Choice of which beta blocker to use varies, with no evidence supporting use of one over another. In general, use of a short-acting beta$_1$ selective agent is recommended. Typical selections of beta blocker use for NSTE ACS patients include metoprolol, propranolol, or atenolol. The dose of metoprolol is 5 mg given slowly (over 1 to 2 minutes) every 5 minutes for a total of 15 mg, followed 15 minutes later by an oral dose of 25 to 50 mg every 6 hours for at least 48 hours. Thereafter the dose is 100 mg twice daily. Observing for side effects of beta blocker use includes monitoring for bradycardia, heart block, hypotension, acute heart failure, or bronchospasm. Contraindications for beta blocker use includes history of asthma, heart block (marked first-degree atrioventricular block with a PR interval of greater than 24 msec; second- or third-degree atrioventricular block), severe left ventricular dysfunction, heart rate less than 50 beats/min, and blood pressure less than 90 mm Hg. Cautious use is advised with patients with chronic obstructive pulmonary disease who are known to have a significant degree of reactive airway disease or mild wheezing at the time of presentation.[2]

Calcium Channel Blockers

Calcium channel blockers (**CCBs**) may be used for NSTE ACS patients as second- or third-line antiischemic therapy (after beta blocker and nitrate therapy have been used). Additionally, CCBs may be used sooner for patients with continued or recurrent ischemia in whom beta blocker therapy is contraindicated. This recommendation received a Class I, evidence level B rating per the ACC/AHA treatment guidelines for NSTE ACS patients.[2] To date, there are no clinical trials evaluating relative efficacy of individual CCBs in ACS patients. Data from previous studies do provide insight into which agents may do harm, as discussed next.

Nondihydropyridine calcium antagonist (such as verapamil or diltiazem) may be used as initial therapy. Long-acting oral CCBs, such as amlodipine or felodipine, may be used for recurrent ischemia (in the absence of contraindications) if beta blockers and nitrates are fully utilized before starting the therapy (Class IIa, evidence level C). The use of extended-release forms of nondihydropyridine CCBs (diltiazem or verapamil) *instead of* beta blocker therapy for treatment of ischemia is less well-established. Small studies support this recommendation, which received a Class IIb, evidence level B rating from the treatment guidelines. The use of immediate-release dihydropyridine CCB (such as nifedipine) *in the presence* of beta blocker therapy received the same level of support (Class IIb, evidence level B). However, the guidelines clearly indicate that immediate-release dihydropyridine CCB use (such as nifedipine) in the absence of beta blocker therapy *may be harmful* and should *not* be used (Class III, evidence level A). One study that was stopped prematurely because of patient safety concerns demonstrated that nifedipine treatment alone (i.e., without concurrent beta blocker therapy) increased risk of myocardial infarction or recurrent angina compared with placebo by 16 percent.[2]

Overall, CCBs act by inhibiting myocardial and vascular smooth muscle contraction, thereby causing vasodilatation. Other actions include slowing of atrioventricular conduction and sinus node automaticity. Differing degrees of vasodilatation and delayed atrioventricular conduction occur depending on agent and dose. ACS patients may benefit from CCB use because of the decrease in myocardial oxygen demand (from decreased contractility, slowing of the heart rate, and improved myocardial oxygen delivery from dilatation of the coronary arteries).[2] Major side effects from CCB use include hypotension, worsening heart failure, bradycardia, and heart block. Verapamil and diltiazem are contraindicated in patients with atrioventricular systolic dysfunction or pulmonary edema. Amlodipine and felodipine, however, have been shown to be tolerated in patients with stable chronic heart failure, but they should be used with caution. Nifedipine and amlodipine have little or no atrioventricular block or sinus node delay.

Overall trials with acute CAD have indicated that if used, verapamil or diltiazem are the preferred agents for CCB use in the absence of a contraindication.[2] In general, CCBs should not be given to patients experiencing an acute STEMI.

Nursing Management of Acute Coronary Syndrome

Patients with NSTE ACS generally are admitted to an inpatient unit and are placed on continuous ECG monitoring. Patients with ongoing ischemic symptoms or those who are hemodynamically unstable should be admitted to an intensive care unit for at least 24 hours and then remain symptom free for at least 12 to 24 hours before transferring out of the intensive care unit to a non–critical care setting. The intensive care unit setting allows for a lower nurse/patient ratio (fewer patients), which provides more frequent assessments by qualified advanced cardiac life support–certified nurses. Most often, nurses assess the patient first at the time of recurrent symptoms. Therefore, it is essential that all nurses who care for ACS patients (in the ED, intensive care unit, and other cardiac care units) be able to record and interpret a 12-lead ECG so that treatment may be initiated as soon as possible for any acute ST segment changes.

The intensive care unit setting also offers the ability to perform rapid defibrillation with all emergency supplies readily available. Continuous ECG monitoring allows for observation and rapid treatment of ventricular tachycardia or ventricular fibrillation, which are common preventable causes of sudden death early in the course of ACS. Dysrhythmia monitoring has a Class I indication for patients who are in the early phase of an ACS event.[34] Practice standards for ECG monitoring in hospital settings define a Class I indication as a treatment indicated in most, if not all, of the patients in this group. In addition ST segment ischemia monitoring has a Class I indication for all ACS patients (NSTE ACS and STEMI patients) by these same guidelines. The practice standards note that assignment of a Class I indication for ST segment ischemia monitoring was based on expert opinion, for there are no randomized clinical trials studying outcomes for patients with ongoing ST segment monitoring. However, the rationale for this technology is compelling for use with NSTE ACS patients. The recommendations indicate that NSTE ACS patients should be monitored for a minimum of 24 hours (until they are event free for at least 12 to 24 hours). Potential benefits cited for NSTE ACS patients include detection of ongoing ischemia (including infarction, reinfarction, or recurrent ischemia), transient ischemia (often asymptomatic), and subacute thrombosis if the patient underwent PCI early in the treatment.[34]

Unfortunately, although ST segment ischemia monitoring has been available clinically for nearly two and a half decades, it remains underutilized. Reasons cited for underuse include poor physician support, high number of false alarms, and lack of education on how to use the system and how to respond to the alarms. Another possible reason for underuse is that unlike dysrhythmia detection (which comes on automatically when a patient is connected to cardiac monitoring), ST segment ischemia monitoring takes action by the nurse or caregiver to enable the equipment to initiate monitoring.[34] Yet advantages outweigh disadvantages for use of ST segment ischemia monitoring if multidisciplinary support is obtained on the cardiac unit, and therefore ST segment monitoring is strongly recommended. Refer to Chapter 49 for information on how to set up an ST segment monitor including alarm settings.

Standing orders for acute ischemia, including management of dysrhythmias, often are used in intensive care unit settings. Patients should maintain complete bed rest until active ischemia has resolved, at which time they may be up to the chair or to the bedside commode if symptom free. Prolonged bed rest is associated with orthostatic hypotension when the patient resumes activity and should be avoided.

For patients admitted to an intensive care unit, transfer to a non–critical care patient setting may be initiated once symptoms have resolved, provided the patient is free of major complications for 12 to 24 hours (e.g., dysrhythmias, sustained hypotension, recurrent ischemia evidenced by ECG changes or discomfort, heart failure, shock, or a new mechanical defect such as new onset mitral regurgitation or ventricular septal defect).

For patients initially classified as having a low likelihood that symptoms represent ACS resulting from CAD, admission to an intensive care unit is not warranted. Admission to an observational unit or chest pain unit where care is provided according to preapproved protocols generally is utilized. Patient care includes continuous ECG monitoring, serial cardiac enzyme tests, serial ECGs, and in some cases noninvasive imaging to determine whether a more invasive workup is needed. Length of stay is generally less than 24 hours and in some cases less than 12 hours for stable patients not experiencing an acute myocardial infarction. Additionally, for in-patients who undergo early cardiac catheterization and who are deemed to have normal coronary arteries or nonsignificant CAD, overnight hospital stay may not be required because continued monitoring or revascularization is not needed.

Patient Education

Another important nursing role is to educate the patient and family members about secondary prevention of a subsequent cardiac event. Educational counseling should include information on smoking cessation, nutrition, weight management, physical activity recommendations, referral to cardiac rehabilitation, referral to home health (if needed), education about discharge medications, and when to return for a follow-up appointment. (Refer to Chapter 83 for more detailed information about evidence-based practice for patient education and counseling).

Smoking cessation is an important aspect of recovery for NSTE ACS patients who previously used tobacco. Patients who continue to use tobacco after an acute myocardial infarction are at high risk for adverse events such as recurrent myocardial infarction or need for repeat revascularization. (Refer to Chapter 33). Although many patients stop smoking when hospitalized for an index myocardial event, a large percentage resume tobacco use within 3 months of hospital discharge. Attebring and colleagues[35] studied smoking habits and predictors of continued smoking in 1320 patients below the age of 75 years who were admitted to a coronary care unit with ACS in Sweden. Approximately 33 percent of the patients studied were "current smokers" at hospital admission, with 51 percent of those resuming smoking within 3 months of hospital discharge. Independent predictors of continued smoking in the study included nonparticipation in cardiac rehabilitation, use of sedatives/antidepressants at the time of admission, history of cerebral vascular disease, history of previous cardiac event, history of smoking-related pulmonary disease, and cigarette consumption index. No significant differences in age, gender, or marital status were found between nonquitters and quitters. Two conclusions were drawn from this study by the authors. Either those who stopped smoking were more likely to participate in cardiac rehabilitation or perhaps cardiac rehabilitation itself influenced patients to continue smoking cessation. Because of the limitations of an observation study in one setting, more research is warranted.

Nurses should counsel hospitalized ACS patients on smoking cessation and should make referrals to cardiac rehabilitation in hope of continued reinforcement of a tobacco-free recovery. The 2002 ACC/AHA treatment guidelines for the care of ACS patients endorse the referral of patients who smoke to a smoking cessation program or outpatient cardiac rehabilitation program. Each patient should be asked about smoking exposure, firsthand or secondhand. Counseling for those who use tobacco then should include pharmacological therapy (nicotine replacement and/or bupropion) and a formal smoking cessation program (Class I, evidence level B).[2] The office of the surgeon general has dedicated a website for smoking cessation information. Recommendations for patients and providers are available at *www.surgeongeneral.gov/tobacco/default.htm.*

Dietary and weight management counseling should include information on strategies to reduce calories, low-density lipoprotein cholesterol, and total body weight (if applicable). Targets for each of these values should be discussed verbally followed by information provided in writing for patients and their family members. Inclusion of family members who are responsible for purchasing foods and those who prepare meals in the household is important. Referral to a registered dietitian (or a certified diabetes educator for patients who have diabetes) is an excellent way to ensure that comprehensive assessment and education is provided for ACS patients. Low-fat, low-cholesterol meals are beneficial for not only the post-ACS patient but in most situations for the entire family. Cardiac rehabilitation is an excellent way to reinforce this information to maintain these and other lifestyle modifications.

Weight management should include education about exercise and maintaining a lifelong healthful diet. Recommendations for activity are 30 to 45 minutes of aerobic exercise most days per week. The target body mass index should range between 18.4 and 24.9 kg/m^2. Those

patients who are starting an exercise regimen for the first time and those patients with a recent myocardial infarction should be cleared medically before initiating a new program.

Cardiac rehabilitation is an excellent strategy to continue the educational programs started in the hospital. Rehabilitation programs help motivate individuals to make long-term lifestyle modifications. Those patients who especially benefit from a cardiac rehabilitation referral include those who were previously sedentary, for there is little likelihood that inactive patients will start exercise on their own. Rehabilitation includes a comprehensive medical history and physical examination; cardiac stress testing in most circumstances; counseling on blood pressure control, smoking cessation, diabetes management, weight loss, heart-healthful diet, and physical activity; and assessment of psychosocial responses to the ACS event. A meta-analysis of 48 trials including 8940 patients found that compared with usual care, cardiac rehabilitation was associated with a reduction of all-cause mortality (OR 0.80) and cardiac related deaths (OR 0.74).[36] Greater reductions in total cholesterol levels, triglyceride levels, systolic pressure, and self-reported smoking also were found for those patients participating in cardiac rehabilitation. However, no differences were found in the incidence of nonfatal myocardial infarction, revascularization rates, or changes in high-density lipoprotein or low-density lipoprotein cholesterol levels. A subsequent meta-analysis of 63 randomized trials of 21,295 patients with CAD evaluated the effectiveness of secondary prevention programs.[37] Benefits of a secondary prevention program (with or without a structured exercise component) included reduction in all-cause mortality, myocardial infarction, or recurrent myocardial infarction. Improvement in quality of life or in functional status also was found for patients participating in the programs being reviewed, although in many cases the effect was small. Data were insufficient in the meta-analysis to determine cost-effectiveness for the programs compared with usual care. It was noted that women, the elderly, minority populations, and low-income patients frequently were underrepresented in the trials reviewed, which limits generalizability. However, despite these limitations, primary care providers and cardiologists should continue to refer patients to cardiac rehabilitation because of the clear benefit of secondary prevention programs compared with usual care.

Assessment of psychosocial status for recovering ACS patients is important. Depression has been associated with increased mortality and morbidity after an ACS event. Previous studies have shown that between 15 and 23 percent of ACS patients have clinically significant major depression after their ACS event.[38] Rumsfeld and colleagues[39] studied the relationship between depression and angina frequency, physical limitation, and quality of life in 1957 patients from 24 Veterans Affairs medical centers who had suffered an myocardial infarction or unstable angina. Nearly 27 percent of the patients had a history of depression. Multivariate analysis showed that a history of depression was more likely to be associated with more frequent angina (OR 2.40), greater physical limitation (OR 2.89), and a worse quality of life (OR 2.84) after the ACS event.

Evidence-based treatment strategies for depression after an ACS event are limited. A total of 369 patients hospitalized for an ACS event within the past 30 days who also met criteria for major depressive disorder were randomized in the Sertraline Antidepressant Heart Attack Randomized Trial **(SADHART)** to sertraline or placebo for 24 weeks.[40] At 6 months there was an improvement in depression in treatment groups (sertraline versus placebo). However, for those patients who had recurrent depression, sertraline administration resulted in greater improvement in multiple domains of quality of life and functional status. Multivariate analysis indicated that depression was a strong predictor of baseline quality of life impairment. Cardiac variables such as ejection fraction and Killip class were also independent predictors of low baseline quality of life (although not as significant as depression itself).

Steele and Wade[41] studied the relationship between optimism and depressive symptoms in ACS patients. Fifty-nine ACS patients completed self-report questionnaires at hospital discharge with 49 of these patients completing the same questionnaire 4 weeks later. At baseline the relationship between depression and optimism was related primarily to functional and symptomatic quality of life (how much the patient could do and how the patient felt). However, when analyzing which baseline variables predicted depressive symptoms at the 4-week mark, optimism was the only variable that predicted depressive symptoms (beyond the baseline level of depression). The more optimism an individual had, the less likely the individual was to be depressed at 4 weeks after hospital discharge. The authors concluded that optimism and the patient's perception of functional quality of life may be possible rehabilitation goals for this patient population. These studies and others indicate that depression is a risk marker for adverse events in ACS patients. Further research is needed to investigate which treatment strategies will prove to be effective in ACS patients who are depressed. (Refer to Chapter 40 for more information on the impact of depression on cardiac disease).

Patients and their family members also should be instructed on discharge medications including action, purpose, dose, frequency, and side effects. Discharge medications should include aspirin (75 to 325 mg daily), clopidogrel 75 mg daily (for up to 12 months), a beta blocker (unless contraindicated), a lipid-lowering agent (to achieve an low-density lipoprotein less than 70 mg/dl), and an ACE inhibitor for patients with heart failure, ejection fraction less than 40 percent, hypertension, or diabetes.[2] (Refer to Chapter 77 for further information on the management of dyslipidemia).

In addition, all ACS patients need to know what to do for subsequent angina. Instructions should include stopping any activity that possibly is causing the symptoms (rest) and then taking a NTG tablet while sitting or lying down. If symptoms persist five minutes after the first dose of NTG, the patient or family member should call 9-1-1 (or emergency medical services) then have the patient take a second NTG tablet.[6] If symptoms persist for an additional five minutes then patient should take a third NTG tablet while awaiting emergency medical services. These guidelines are different from the traditional recommendation to take up to three NTG tablets for persistent symptoms before calling 9-1-1. Patients also should be instructed to alert their provider if ischemic symptoms become more frequent or more severe.

Follow-up appointments should be scheduled within 6 weeks of hospital discharge. High-risk ACS patients should be seen by a provider within 1 to 2 weeks of discharge, whereas low-risk patients (medically treated or revascularized patients) should be seen within 2 to 6 weeks.[2] However, the timing of the follow-up visit may vary by local practice and individual patient differences.

Managing Comorbidities of Acute Coronary Syndrome: Heart Failure, Hypertension, and Diabetes

Heart failure as a comorbid condition for patients who have ACS is associated with increased morbidity and mortality. Lettman and colleagues[42] studied 298 heart failure patients who presented to their local ED with signs and symptoms suggestive of ACS. The incidence of ACS in this study population with heart failure was 32 percent. Patients with concurrent ACS and heart failure were more likely to be admitted to the hospital (97 percent versus 82 percent), to be placed in an intensive care unit (44 percent versus 13 percent), to be intubated (8 percent versus 1 percent), to have a longer length of stay (5.2 days versus 3.2 days), and to be more likely to die (15 versus 7 deaths) compared with heart failure patients without ACS.

In addition to poor short-term outcomes, heart failure in ACS patients also has been associated with worse long-term outcomes. Eagle and colleagues[43] developed a bedside tool that predicted all-cause mortality 6 months after discharge from an ACS event. Using the instrument, nine multivariate predictors of death were for patients with ACS. Patients with history of heart failure had twice the mortality at 6 months compared with ACS patients without heart failure. The other eight predictors of death at 6 months were advanced age, history of myocardial infarction, increased pulse rate, decreased systolic pressure, increased creatinine, higher cardiac enzyme elevation, presence of ST segment depression, and not having an in-hospital PCI performed. The Organisation to Assess Strategies for Ischemic Syndromes (OASIS-2) trial examined the incidence, predictors, and clinical outcomes in patients with NSTE ACS who developed heart failure.[44] Of the 10,141 patients enrolled into the **OASIS-2** Trial, 501 (4.9 percent) developed heart failure within the first week, with 643 (6.3 percent) developing heart failure within 6 months. Independent predictors as determined by multivariate analysis for the development of heart failure included older age, female sex, diabetes, prior myocardial infarction, and NSTEMI at presentation.

Despite worse outcomes for NSTE ACS patients with heart failure, those patients with ACS who develop heart failure are less likely to receive evidence-based therapies and interventions.[45] Treatment of heart failure in ACS patients begins with timely diagnosis of the heart failure. Therefore, it is essential that left ventricular function be evaluated during the initial hospitalization for NSTE ACS to determine whether ACE inhibitor and beta blocker use are indicated long term. Preferably, ejection fraction should be measured at the time of cardiac catheterization. Otherwise, echocardiography or nuclear ventriculography is an acceptable method. If an ACS patient has heart failure, ACE inhibition should be initiated. Beta blocker therapy also should be initiated as soon as possible, in the setting of euvolemia. Careful monitoring for fluid volume status is required if starting or uptitrating beta blocker therapy in the setting of ACS. (Refer to Chapters 63 and 64 for further discussion of care of patients with heart failure).

Hypertension is another frequent comorbid condition, either as a preestablished chronic condition or newly diagnosed state. Majahalme and colleagues[46] studied the difference between hypertensive and normotensive consecutive patients who had suspected ACS. Approximately two thirds (64.4 percent) had hypertension. This was not exclusive to older patients, for even the youngest third of patients (those less than 56 years of age) had a high prevalence of hypertension (45.9 percent). In the study, patients with hypertension were more likely to be older (66.6 years versus 59.9 years), female (38.7 percent versus 26.9 percent), and have more comorbid conditions such as prior myocardial infarction (47.9 percent versus 33.8 percent), heart failure (25.7 percent versus 12.0 percent), and diabetes (36.9 percent versus 17.8 percent). Not surprisingly, at admission to the facility, hypertensive patients had higher systolic pressure yet had fewer ischemic changes on their ECGs (67.9 percent versus 76.3 percent) and fewer ruled-in for myocardial infarction (70.7 percent versus 76.1 percent) than their normotensive counterparts. Those patients with hypertension had more invasive procedures (CABG and PCI) and received more cardiovascular medications.

One hypothesis as to why the hypertensive patient group had a lower rate of myocardial infarction was that these patients may have benefited from long-term medication therapy, interventions, and evaluations from previous care as a hypertensive patient. However, of those with hypertension, the patients with the highest systolic blood pressure at admission were more likely to have a myocardial infarction compared with hypertensive patients with systolic blood pressures in the medium range.

In a multicenter retrospective cohort study, 1247 patients admitted for myocardial infarction or unstable angina were followed for 6 months to investigate the impact of controlling hypertension before hospital discharge.[47] At hospital discharge, 411 patients (32.9 percent) had uncontrolled hypertension. In a multivariate analysis, age, ejection fraction, and hypertension (OR 1.9) were associated with poor outcomes (death or nonfatal myocardial infarction).

Implications for practice include ensuring that ACS patients have blood pressure controlled at hospital discharge with timely and appropriate follow-up to make sure blood pressure meets the target treatment goal. The ACC/AHA treatment guidelines for the care of NSTE

ACE patients give a Class IA recommendation for the blood pressure goal of less than 130/85 mm Hg.[2]

Diabetes is another comorbid condition of ACS that is associated with increased mortality and morbidity. Cardiovascular disease is more extensive and more labile or unstable for those patients with diabetes compared with CAD patients without diabetes. Patients with both conditions (CAD and diabetes mellitus) have more comorbidities in general and have worse outcomes from revascularization (particularly PCI). The Diabetic Patients with Acute Myocardial Infarction (DIGAMI) Study showed that tighter glycemic control (hemoglobin A_{1c} less than 7.0 percent) for ACS patients with diabetes during and after myocardial infarction was associated with decreased short-term and long-term (1 year) mortality.[48] The ACC/AHA treatment guidelines for NSTE ACS patients therefore recommend tight control of hyperglycemia in diabetic patients (Class IB).[2] Tighter control of lipids also is recommended for diabetic patients.

The presence of hyperglycemia increases the risk for the ACS patient at admission. The majority of those with ACS have unrecognized abnormal glucose tolerance. One study found that 66 percent of those who had recent myocardial infarction had undiagnosed impaired glucose tolerance or diabetes.[49] Thus timely diagnosis of impaired glucose tolerance and diabetes is imperative for patients with ACS.

ACUTE CORONARY SYNDROME IN HIGH-RISK GROUPS
Gender Differences

No large-scale prospective studies have been done to examine gender disparities for patients with NSTE ACS. Previous literature has suggested that acute ischemia is more likely to be missed in women because of the atypical nature of ACS symptoms. In a review of 12 studies, Devon and Zerwic[50] reported conflicting data as to whether women with ACS have more atypical symptoms compared with men. Much of the previous research was done retrospectively, with varying study designs and with small numbers. Authors concluded that *both* men and women do have chest pain associated with ACS; however, women are more likely to report atypical symptoms associated with chest pain. Emphasis was placed on addressing the totality of symptoms in order to make an accurate diagnosis.

Since the review by Devon and Zerwic was published, Granot and colleagues[51] reported significant gender differences in perception of chest pain for patients with ACS. In this study, 29 women and 32 men were interviewed using a semiopen questionnaire assessing chest pain intensity (0-to-10 numerical rating scale), location and characteristics of chest pain, complaints following the pain, precipitating and relieving factors, and whether the symptoms were related to heart disease. More than half (58.8 percent) of the subjects had a history of heart disease or unstable angina. Women scored pain intensity higher than men and related their chest discomfort to their heart. Men described pain as being more in the chest, whereas women located pain more in the stomach, chin, and back, *as well as the chest*. Many more women (84 percent) described the pain as "pressure" compared with men (37 percent). No differences were found regarding precipitating or relieving factors associated with symptoms. Both sexes reported dyspnea as the most frequent associated symptom. Women had a significantly higher number of associated symptoms compared with men.

Research also has been done to determine the relationship between typical versus atypical symptom presentation and determination of an ACS diagnosis by the provider. In a study done by Milner and colleagues,[52] 246 women and 276 men seen in an ED with symptoms suggestive of ACS were observed directly with subjective symptoms being documented verbatim. In total, 89 (36 percent) women and 124 (45 percent) men were diagnosed with ACS. Women reporting *typical* symptoms (chest pain or discomfort, dyspnea, diaphoresis, and arm or shoulder pain) more often were diagnosed with ACS than men. Further, atypical symptoms in men (specifically dizziness or faintness) were related inversely to the diagnosis of ACS. The authors concluded that typical symptoms remain the strongest predictors of ACS in women, as in men, and that these are an important aspect in diagnosing ACS. Yet until more research is available addressing differences in symptom presentation for men and women with NSTE ACS, providers need to remain diligent about fully evaluating women who have atypical symptoms suggestive of ACS. (Refer to Chapter 52 for further information on women and heart disease).

Gender disparities in treatment and outcomes for NSTE ACS patients also have been reported in the literature. The CRUSADE National QI initiative examined 35,875 NSTE ACS patients and found that women with NSTE ACS tend to be older (median age 73 versus 65 years) and are more likely have concurrent comorbidities such as diabetes and hypertension compared with their male counterparts.[53] In this report, women smoked less often and were less likely to have dyslipidemia or a family history of CAD compared with men. Fewer women had a history of myocardial infarction, PCI, or CABG. More women, however, had a history of heart failure upon presentation with ACS. Women were less likely to have high-risk features such as positive cardiac biomarker test results or transient ST segment elevation, yet they were more likely to have ST segment depression than men.

Women were less likely to have an ECG performed within 10 minutes of hospital presentation (25.2 percent versus 29.3 percent) and were less likely to be cared for by a cardiologist during an inpatient admission (53.4 percent versus 63.4 percent). Treatment also differed for men and women in regard to medication use (both early—within 24 hours—and at discharge). Women were less likely to receive heparin and ACE inhibitors early in their hospitalization. Also, regardless of cardiac biomarker results, women were less likely to receive GP IIb/IIIa inhibitors. Upon discharge, women were also less likely to receive ASA, ACE inhibitors, and statin agents than men. Women were more likely to undergo stress testing compared with men, who were more likely to undergo diagnostic catheterization. Re-

vascularization was also less likely for women compared with men. However, of those who underwent diagnostic cardiac catheterization, similar rates of PCIs were performed in men and women. Lastly, women were found to have worse outcomes (in-hospital death, reinfarction, heart failure, stroke, and red blood cell transfusion) than males. However, after adverse events were adjusted in the analysis, only the risk of red blood cell transfusion was higher in men than women. Possible explanations provided by the authors as to why women may have been undertreated included diagnostic uncertainty for women and delays in symptom recognition for women.

Differences in management and outcomes for men and women with ACS also were studied by the CURE trial group in which 4836 women and 7726 men were enrolled.[54] In general, women in the study were older, had more comorbidities at the time of presentation, and were less likely to undergo cardiovascular procedures. Women were less likely to have an invasive procedure (cardiac catheterization, PCI, or CABG) compared with men (47.6 percent versus 60.5 percent; $p = 0.0001$). Of those who underwent angiography, men were more likely to have triple vessel disease or left main disease (44.7 percent versus 34.9 percent; $p = 0.00001$) than women. Similarly women were more likely to have no diseased vessels (26.7 percent versus 13.2 percent; $p = 0.00001$) than men. However, when grouped by risk, of the high-risk ACS patients, women had a similar proportion of "significant" disease compared with men (60.8 percent versus 59.4 percent; $p = 0.68$), with revascularization rates being similar (64.9 percent versus 65.1 percent; $p = 0.97$). Thirty-day outcomes (cardiovascular death, myocardial infarction, stroke) were similar for men and women. However, women were more likely to have refractory angina or be rehospitalized for chest pain than men (23.9 percent versus 15.3 percent; $p = 0.0001$). Conclusions made by the authors support all high-risk ACS patients (men and women) receiving optimal medical management, including angiography with possible revascularization, if needed. These conclusions are the same as those from the ACC/AHA treatment guidelines for the care of NSTE ACS patients, which recommend that women with NSTE ACS be managed similarly to men (Class I, evidence level B).[2] The guidelines further state that women, like men, should be given ASA and clopidogrel, as well as receiving noninvasive and invasive procedures similarly. More research is needed, however, to examine differences in treatment and outcomes based on gender.

Age Differences

The ACC/AHA treatment guidelines for NSTE ACS patients define "elderly" as those patients greater than 75 years of age. However, many clinical trials have used age cutoffs of 65 or 70 years; therefore, data from trials need to be reviewed carefully when making comparisons. Elderly patients with ACS are more likely to have atypical symptoms, more comorbidities, and ECGs that are more challenging to interpret. Outcomes for the elderly are less favorable, which primarily can be attributed to the presence of comorbid conditions. Yet elderly patients can achieve greater absolute benefit from evidence-based therapies including revascularization.[2]

Halon and colleagues[55] conducted a registry of 449 consecutive patients examining differences in presentation and outcomes for two groups of elderly ACS patients. The patient population was divided into those between 70 and 79 years of age ($n = 251$) and those older than 80 years ($n = 198$). At admission for the index ACS event, the older group was more likely to have an acute myocardial infarction (35 percent versus 9.7 percent), heart failure (33.3 percent versus 19.4 percent), or renal dysfunction (21.6 percent versus 12.3 percent); however, they were less likely to undergo coronary angiography (29.3 percent versus 43.8 percent). Revascularization rates were similar in both age groups for all those who had diagnostic catheterization. However, survival at 24 months was worse (67.4 percent versus 83.5 percent) in the older cohort. Repeat revascularization rates at 24 months were similar in both age groups.

De Servi and colleagues[56] studied 1581 NSTE ACS patients in Italy as part of a registry in which 564 subjects were 75 years or older. The older patients were more likely to be female (42 percent versus 27 percent); to have hypertension (70 percent versus 59 percent), prior myocardial infarction (41 percent versus 29 percent), prior angina (18 percent versus 13 percent), prior use of ASA (49 percent versus 39 percent), and ST segment depression (54 percent versus 43 percent). The older patients also were more likely to have a positive troponin result (66 percent versus 59 percent) compared with those patients less than 75 years. Elderly patients were less likely to receive GP IIb/IIIa inhibitors and less likely to undergo interventional procedures within 4 days. The elderly patients also had worse 30-day outcomes such as higher mortality (6.4 percent versus 1.7 percent), acute myocardial infarction (7.1 percent versus 5 percent), and stroke (1.3 percent versus 0.5 percent). A conservative strategy (OR 2.31) and a diagnosis of a non–Q wave myocardial infarction (OR 2.27) were found to be independent predictors of the poor 30-day outcomes.

The CRUSADE national quality improvement initiative reviewed data from 443 U.S. hospitals between January 2001 and June 2003 to compare use of ACC/AHA guideline-recommended treatment for 56,963 NSTE ACS patients across four age groups (less than 65, 65 to 74, 75 to 84 and older than 85 years).[57] Multivariate analysis was done to determine treatment and outcome differences. Thirty-five percent of the population was ≥75 years old, with 11 percent being ≥85 years of age. Treatment with antiplatelet and antithrombin therapy within the first 24 hours was less likely in older than younger patients. As in previous studies, the elderly were also less likely to undergo early catheterization or revascularization. Discharge medications were similar with all age groups, with the exception of clopidogrel and lipid-lowering agents being used less often as age increased. Although in-hospital mortality and complications rose with increased age, those elderly patients receiving guideline-recommended care had lower mortality than those not treated accordingly.

The ACC/AHA treatment guidelines for the care of NSTE ACS patients recommend that treatment be based on the elderly patient's general health condition, including consideration of comorbidities, cognitive status, and life expectancy (Class I, evidence level C).[2] Intensive medical and interventional management may be undertaken according to the guidelines with close monitoring for adverse effects of the treatment (Class I, evidence level B).

Racial Differences

Little research has been done to examine racial differences in treatment and outcomes for patients with NSTE ACS. Previous work has reported that black patients are less likely to undergo coronary interventions compared with white patients. The CRUSADE quality improvement project examined differences between black and white patients from 400 hospitals in the United States.[58] A total of 43,317 patients were studied (37,813 of whom were white and 5504 black). Black patients were younger (median age 61 versus 70 years); more likely to be female (47.7 percent versus 39.6 percent); more likely to have hypertension, diabetes, heart failure, and renal insufficiency; and less likely to have insurance coverage or to have primary care provided by a cardiologist during their hospital stay. Similar rates of ASA, beta blocker, and ACE inhibitor use were found in both groups; however, black patients were less likely to receive GP IIb/IIIa inhibitors acutely and were less likely to receive clopidogrel and statin therapy at discharge. Blacks were also less likely to receive diagnostic catheterization, revascularization, or smoking cessation counseling. Adjusted outcomes were similar in both groups. The authors emphasized the need to look at longitudinal studies to investigate racial differences in outcomes.

Race and outcomes for NSTE ACS patients also were examined by the TACTICS-TIMI 18 trial in which 1722 white patients and 461 nonwhite patients were studied.[59] Similar to the CRUSADE study, nonwhite patients were younger, more likely to be female, and more likely to have hypertension, diabetes, and a higher serum creatinine level. History of CAD or rates of previous cardiac procedures were similar, except for history of CABG (which was twice as likely in white patients). Basic medications were administered at about the same rate with the exception of a trend toward higher use of ACE inhibition and lower statin use in the nonwhite group. ST segment deviation on the ECG was more frequent in the white patient population. Use of angiography and revascularization was similar in both groups. Nonwhites, however, were less likely to be taking their cardiac medications at follow-up (OR 0.59). Less procedural success was found after PCI for nonwhite patients (hazard ratio 0.85).

The influence of race on long-term outcomes such as mortality and quality of life has been studied in ACS patients as well. Spertus and colleagues[60] followed patients for 1 year using a prospective registry of 1159 ACS patients treated between February 2000 and October 2001. Mortality rates were similar at 1 year between blacks and whites. However, blacks had a higher prevalence of angina (43.4 percent versus 27.1 percent), worse quality of life, and poorer physical functioning than white patients. Further research is needed to document why differences in outcomes (mortality, morbidity, and quality of life) may exist according to race.

Using Acute Coronary Syndrome Guidelines in Clinical Practice

Although clinical treatment guidelines for the care of NSTE ACS patients have been published, evidence-based therapies continue to be underutilized for this patient population. Several quality improvement initiatives are under way to address the challenge of changing provider behavior and improving patient outcomes. Table 56-7 provides examples of various quality improvement initiatives being conducted in the United States. The focus of each of these initiatives is to have multidisciplinary teams design ways to improve patient care in their individual facilities. Each facility tracks adherence to guidelines as practice changes occur. Many of the quality improvement projects provide individualized quarterly reports to the facility to provide feedback on progress toward goals.

It has been shown that those institutions that provide care based on the ACC/AHA treatment guidelines have improved patient outcomes compared with those hospitals providing care less well aligned with the guidelines. The CRUSADE registry studied inpatient outcomes in high-performing hospitals compared with low-performing hospitals and found that the odds of dying decrease (OR 0.89) for every 10 percent increase in composite guideline adherence.[61]

SUMMARY

ACS continues to be a major cause of mortality and morbidity in the United States. Patient care begins with answering two basic questions: What is the likelihood of the patient having a definite ACS event? and What is the likelihood of the patient having a poor outcome? Treatment strategy then is selected based on answers to these important triage questions. Patients with positive cardiac biomarker test results *or* ST segment deviation are considered high-risk and should be evaluated for early invasive therapy. Additionally, unless contraindications exist, initial pharmacological therapy includes that of antiplatelet therapy, antischemic therapy, and antithrombotic therapy.

Treatment guidelines have been published by the ACC/AHA and providers are challenged to ensure that evidence-based treatments are implemented. Quality improvement initiatives provide an excellent opportunity to monitor adherence to practice guidelines, which ultimately will improve patient outcomes. More research is needed to provide insights into reasons for suboptimal care and ways to overcome these hurdles in order to decrease morbidity and mortality from this condition.

■ ■ ■

TABLE 56-7 QUALITY IMPROVEMENT INITIATIVES TO PROMOTE ADHERENCE TO AMERICAN COLLEGE OF CARDIOLOGY/AMERICAN HEART ASSOCIATION GUIDELINES

QUALITY IMPROVEMENT PROJECT	ACRONYM	SPONSOR OF PROJECT
Guidelines Applied in Practice	GAP	Michigan
Erlanger Project	—	Erlanger Medical Center, Chattanooga Tennessee
Cardiovascular Hospitalization Atherosclerosis Management Program	CHAMP	University of California in Los Angeles
Baptist Health Systems	—	Baptist Health Systems
Can Rapid Risk Stratification of Unstable Angina Patients Suppress Adverse Outcomes with Early Implementation of the ACC/AHA Guidelines	CRUSADE	Duke Clinical Research Institute
Get with the Guidelines	GWTG	American College of Cardiology/ American Heart Association

REFERENCES

1. Heart Association Statistics Committee and Stroke Statistics Subcommittee Heart Disease and Stroke Statistics—2007 Update. A Report From the American Heart Association: Dallas, 2007, http://circ.ahajournals.org/cgi/content/short/CIRCULATIONAHA.106.179918
2. Braunwald E, Antman EM, Beasley JW et al: ACC/AHA 2002 guideline update for the management of patients with unstable angina and non-ST segment elevation myocardial infarction: summary article: a report of the American College of Cardiology/American Heart Association Task Force on Practice Guidelines (Committee on the Management of Patients with Unstable Angina),Retrieved January 22, 2007, from www.acc.org/qualityandscience/clinical/guidelines/unstable/unstable.pdf
3. Antman EM, Cohen M, Bernink PJ et al: The TIMI risk score for unstable angina/non-ST segment elevation MI: a method for prognostic and therapeutic decision making, *JAMA* 284:835-842, 2000.
4. Braunwald E, Antman E, Beasley J et al: ACC/AHA guidelines for the management of patients with unstable angina and non-ST segment elevation myocardial infarction: a report of the ACC/AHA Task Force on Practice Guidelines, *J Am Coll Cardiol* 36:970-1062, 2000.
5. Gibler WB, Cannon CP, Blomkalns AL et al: Practical implementation of the guidelines for unstable angina/non-ST-segment elevation myocardial infarction in the emergency department: a scientific statement from the American Heart Association Council on Clinical Cardiology (Subcommittee on Acute Cardiac Care), Council on Cardiovascular Nursing, and Quality of Care and Outcomes Research Interdisciplinary Working Group, in collaboration with the Society of Chest Pain Centers, *Circulation* 111: 2699-2710, 2005.
6. Antman EM, Anbe DT, Armstrong PW et al: ACC/AHA guidelines for the management of patients with ST-segment elevation myocardial infarction-executive summary: a report of the ACC/AHA Task Force on Practice Guidelines (Writing Committee to Revise the 1999 Guidelines for the Management of Patients with Acute Myocardial Infarction), Retrieved January 22, 2007 from www.acc.org/qualityandscience/clinical/guidelines/stemi/Guideline1/index.pdf

7. Savonitto S, Ardissino D, Granger CB et al: Prognostic value of the admission electrocardiogram in acute coronary syndromes, *JAMA* 281:707-713, 1999.

8. Alpert JS, Thygesen K, Antman E et al: Myocardial infarction redefined: a consensus document of the Joint European Society of Cardiology/American College of Cardiology Committee for the Redefinition of Myocardial Infarction, *J Am Coll Cardiol* 36:959-970, 2000.

9. Boersma E, Pieper KS, Steyerberg EW et al: Predictors of outcome in patients with acute coronary syndromes without persistent ST-segment elevation: results from an international trial of 9461 patients—the PURSUIT Investigators, *Circulation* 101:2557-2567, 2000.

10. Garcia S, Canoniero M, Peter A et al: Correlation of TIMI risk store with angiographic severity and extent of coronary artery disease in patients with non–ST-elevation acute coronary syndromes, *Am J Cardiol* 93:813-816, 2004.

11. Ohman E, Granger C, Harrington R: Risk stratification and therapeutic decision making in acute coronary syndromes, *JAMA* 284:876-878, 2000.

12. Grines CL, Bonow RO, Casey DE, Jr. et al. Prevention of premature discontinuation of dual antiplatelet therapy in patients with coronary artery stents: a science advisory from the American Heart Association, American College of Cardiology, Society of Cardiovascular Angiography and Intervention, American College of Surgeons, and American Dental Association, with representation from the American College of Physicians. www.acc. org/qualityand science/clinical/pdfs/Final_Dual_Antiplatelet_ Statement_010507.pdf Retrieved Jan. 22, 2007.

13. Bavry AA, Kumbhani DJ, Quiroz R et al: Invasive therapy along with glycoprotein IIb/IIIa inhibitors and intracoronary stents improves survival in non–ST-segment elevation acute coronary syndromes: a meta-analysis and review of the literature, *Am J Cardiol* 93:830-835, 2004.

14. Bach RG, Cannon CP, Weintraub WS et al: The effect of routine, early invasive management on outcome for elderly patients with non–ST segment elevation acute coronary syndromes, *Ann Intern Med* 141:186-195, 2004.

15. Giugliano RP, Braunwald E: The year in non–ST-segment elevation acute coronary syndromes, *J Am Coll Cardiol* 46:906-919, 2005.

16. Exaire JE, Dauerman HL, Topol EJ et al: Triple antiplatelet therapy does not increase femoral access bleeding with vascular closure devices, *Am Heart J* 147:31-34, 2004.

17. Bholasingh R, Cornel JH, Kamp O et al: Prognostic value of pre-discharge dobutamine stress echocardiography in chest pain patients with a negative cardiac troponin T, *J Am Coll Cardiol* 41:596-602, 2003.

18. Gibbons RJ: Chest pain triage-another step forward, *JAMA* 288:2745-2746, 2002.

19. Califf RM, DeLong E, Ostbye T et al: Underuse of aspirin in a referral population with documented coronary artery disease, *Am J Cardiol* 89:653-661, 2002.

20. Meine TJ, Roe MT, Chen AY et al: Association of intravenous morphine use and outcomes in acute coronary syndromes: results from the CRUSADE Quality Improvement Initiative, *Am Heart J* 149:1043-1049, 2005.

21. Oler A, Whooley MA, Oler J et al: Adding heparin to aspirin reduces the incidence of myocardial infarction and death in patients with unstable angina, *JAMA* 276:811-815, 1996.

22. Ferguson J, Califf R, Antman E et al; SYNERGY Trial Investigators: Enoxaparin vs unfractionated heparin in high-risk patients with non–ST-segment elevation acute coronary syndromes managed with an intended early invasive strategy: primary results of the SYNERGY randomized trial, *JAMA* 292:45-54, 2004.

23. Lincoff AM, Kleiman NS, Kereiakes DJ et al: Long-term efficacy of bivalirudin and provisional glycoprotein IIb/IIIa blockade versus heparin and planned glycoprotein IIb/IIIa blockade during percutaneous coronary revascularization: REPLACE-2 Randomized Trial, *JAMA* 292:696-703, 2004.

24. Stone GW, McLaurin BT, Cox DA et al. Bivalrudin for patients with acute coronary syndromes. *N Engl J Med* 355: 2203-2216, 2006.

25. Atwater BD, Roe MT, Mahaffey KW: Platelet glycoprotein IIb/IIIa receptor antagonists in non–ST-segment elevation acute coronary syndromes: a review and guide to patient selection, *Drugs* 65(3):313-324, 2005.

26. Hamm C, Heeschen C, Goldmann B et al: Benefit of abciximab in patients with refractory unstable angina in relation to serum troponin T levels: c7E3 Fab Antiplatelet Therapy in Unstable Refractory Angina (CAPTURE) Study Investigators, *N Engl J Med* 340:1623-1629, 1999.

27. Newby L, Ohman M, Christenson R et al: Benefit of glycoprotein IIb/IIIa inhibition in patients with acute coronary syndromes and troponin T-positive status, *Circulation* 103:2891-2896, 2001.

28. Kong DF, Califf RM, Miller DP et al: Clinical outcomes of therapeutic agents that block the platelet glycoprotein IIb-IIIa integrin is ischemic heart disease, *Circulation* 98:2829-2835, 1998.

29. Gibson CM, Singh KP, Murphy SA et al: Association between duration of tirofiban therapy before percutaneous intervention and tissue level perfusion (a TACTICS-TIMI 18 substudy), *Am J Cardiol* 94:492-494, 2004.

30. Rebeiz AG, Dery JP, Tsiatis AA et al: Optimal duration of eptifibatide infusion in percutaneous coronary intervention (an ESPRIT substudy), *Am J Cardiol* 94:926-929, 2004.

31. The CURE Investigators: Effects of clopidogrel in addition to aspirin in patients with acute coronary syndromes without ST-segment elevation, *N Engl J Med* 345:494-502, 2001.

32. Patti G, Colonna G, Pasceri V et al: Randomized trial of high loading dose of clopidogrel for reduction of periprocedural myocardial infarction in patients undergoing coronary intervention: results from the ARMYDA-2 (Antiplatelet Therapy for Reduction of MYocardial Damage during Angioplasty) Study, *Circulation* 111:2099-2106, 2005.

33. Silber S, Albertsson P, Aviles FF et al: Guidelines for percutaneous coronary interventions: the task force for percutaneous coronary interventions of the European Society of Cardiology, *Eur Heart J* 26:804-847, 2005.

34. Drew BJ, Califf RM, Funk M et al: Practice standards for electrocardiographic monitoring in hospital settings: an American Heart Association scientific statement from the Councils on Cardiovascular Nursing, Clinical Cardiology, and Cardiovascular Disease in the Young: endorsed by the International Society of Computerized Electrocardiography and the American Association of Critical-Care Nurses, *Circulation* 20:76-106, 2005.

35. Attebring MF, Hartford M, Hjalmarson A et al: Smoking habits and predictors of continued smoking in patients with acute coronary syndromes, *J Adv Nurs* 46:614-623, 2004.

36. Taylor RS, Brown A, Ebrahim S et al: Exercise-based rehabilitation for patients with coronary heart disease: systematic review and meta-analysis of randomized controlled trials, *Am J Med* 116:682-692, 2004.

37. Clark AM, Hartling L, Vandermeer B, McAlister FA: Meta-analysis: secondary prevention programs for patients with CAD, *Ann Intern Med* 143:659-672, 2005.

38. Jiang W, Krishnan RR, O'Connor CM: Depression and heart disease: evidence of a link, and its therapeutic implications, *CNS Drugs* 16:111-127, 2002.

39. Rumsfeld JS, Magid DJ, Plomondon ME et al: History of depression, angina, and quality of life after acute coronary syndromes, *Am Heart J* 145:493-499, 2003.

40. Swenson JF, O'Connor CM, Barton D et al, for the SADHART Investigators: Influence of depression and effect of treatment with sertraline on quality of life after hospitalization for acute coronary syndrome, *Am J Cardiol* 92:1271-1276, 2003.

41. Steele A, Wade TD: The contribution of optimism and quality of life to depression in an acute coronary syndrome population, *Eur J Cardiovasc Nurs* 3:231-237, 2004.

42. Lettman NA, Sites FD, Shofer FS et al: Congestive heart failure patients with chest pain: incidence and predictors of acute coronary syndrome, *Acad Emerg Med* 9:903-909, 2002.

43. Eagle KA, Lim MJ, Dabbous OH et al: A validated prediction tool predicted all-cause mortality 6 months after discharge for the acute coronary syndrome, *ACP J Club* 141:80-83, 2004.

44. Mehta SR, Eikelboom JW, Demers C et al: Congestive heart failure complicating non–ST-segment elevation acute coronary syndrome: incidence, predictors, and clinical outcomes, *Can J Physiol Pharmacol* 83:98-103, 2005.

45. Goswami R, Chen AY, Riba AL et al: Sub-optimal care for non–ST-elevation acute coronary syndrome patients presenting with congestive heart failure is associated with higher mortality. Presented at the AHA Scientific Sessions 2004, *Circulation* 110(suppl III):518, 2004 (abstract 2427).

46. Majahalme SK, Smith DE, Cooper JV et al: Comparison of patients with acute coronary syndrome with and without systemic hypertension, *Am J Cardiol* 92:258-263, 2003.

47. Amar J, Chamontin B, Ferrieres J et al: Hypertension control at hospital discharge after acute coronary event: influence on cardiovascular prognosis—the PREVENIR Study, *Heart* 88:587-591, 2002.

48. Malmberg K, Ryden L, Efendic S et al: Randomized trial of insulin-glucose infusion followed by subcutaneous insulin treatment in diabetic patients with acute myocardial infarction (DIGAMI study): effects on mortality at 1 year, *J Am Coll Cardiol* 26:57-65, 1995.

49. Norhammar A, Tenerz A, Nilsson G et al: Glucose metabolism in patients with acute myocardial infarction and no previous diagnosis of diabetes mellitus: a prospective study, *Lancet* 359: 2140-2144, 2002.

50. Devon HA, Zerwic JJ: Symptoms of acute coronary syndromes: are there gender differences? A review of the literature, *Heart Lung* 31:235-245, 2002.

51. Granot M, Goldstein-Ferber S, Azzam ZS: Gender differences in perception of chest pain, *J Pain Symptom Manage* 27:149-155, 2004.

52. Milner KA, Funk M, Arnold A, Vaccarino V: Typical symptoms are predictive of acute coronary syndromes in women, *Am Heart J* 143:283-288, 2002.

53. Blomkalns AL, Chen AY, Hochman JS et al: Gender disparities in the diagnosis and treatment of non–ST-segment elevation acute coronary syndromes: large scale observations from the CRUSADE National Quality Improvement Initiative, *J Am Coll Cardiol* 45:832-837, 2005.

54. Anand SS, Xie CC, Mehta S et al: Differences in management and prognosis of women and men who suffer from acute coronary syndromes, *J Am Coll Cardiol* 46:1845-1851, 2005.

55. Halon DA, Adawi S, Dobrecky-Mery I et al: Importance of increasing age on the presentation and outcome of acute coronary syndromes in elderly patients, *J Am Coll Cardiol* 43:346-352, 2004.

56. De Servi S, Cavallini C, Dellavalle A et al: Non–ST-elevation acute coronary syndrome in the elderly: treatment strategies and 30-day outcomes, *Am Heart J* 147:830-836, 2004.

57. Alexander KP, Roe MT, Chen AY et al: Evolution in cardiovascular care for elderly patients with non–ST-segment elevation acute coronary syndromes: results from the CRUSADE National Quality Improvement Initiative, *J Am Coll Cardiol* 46:1479-1487, 2005.

58. Sonel AF, Good CB, Mulgund J et al: Racial variations in treatment and outcomes of black and white patients with high-risk non–ST-elevation acute coronary syndromes: insights from CRUSADE, *Circulation* 111:1225-1232, 2005.

59. Sabatine M, Blake GJ, Drazner MH et al: Influence of race on death and ischemic complications in patients with non–ST-segment elevation acute coronary syndromes despite modern, protocol-guided treatment, *Circulation* 111:1217-1224, 2005.

60. Spertus J, Safley D, Garg M et al: The influence of race on health status outcomes one year after an acute coronary syndrome, *J Am Coll Cardiol* 46:1838-1844, 2005.

61. Peterson ED, Roe MT, Lytle BL et al: The association between care and outcomes in patients with acute coronary syndromes: national results from CRUSADE—abstract presented at ACC Scientific Sessions, 2004, *J Am Coll Cardiol* 43:406A, 2004.

Care of Patients with Acute Coronary Syndrome: ST Segment Elevation Myocardial Infarction

Debra K. Moser
Barbara Riegel

CHAPTER ABBREVIATIONS

ACC American College of Cardiology

ACE angiotensin-converting enzyme

ACS acute coronary syndrome

AHA American Heart Association

ARB angiotensin II receptor blocker

CK creatine kinase

CMS Centers for Medicare and Medicaid Services

ECG electrocardiogram

ED emergency department

EMS emergency medical services

GRACE Global Registry of Acute Coronary Events

INR International normalized ratio

JCAHO Joint Commission on Accreditation of Healthcare Organizations

Non-STEMI non–ST segment elevation myocardial infarction

PCI percutaneous coronary intervention

STEMI ST segment elevation myocardial infarction

Acute coronary syndrome (**ACS**) is the umbrella term for a group of thrombotic coronary artery disease conditions that result from myocardial ischemia. Conditions that fall under the ACS umbrella include unstable angina, ST segment elevation myocardial infarction (**STEMI**), and non–ST segment elevation myocardial infarction (**non-STEMI**). This chapter focuses on the care of patients suffering from STEMI. Care for patients with unstable angina or non-STEMI is covered in Chapter 56.

The American College of Cardiology/American Heart Association (**ACC/AHA**) developed and regularly updates comprehensive evidence-based guidelines for the management of patients with the varied manifestations of ACS. Although much of the management of non-STEMI and STEMI is similar, there are important differences to consider. The guideline for management of patients with STEMI is the basis for the therapy described in this chapter.[1] The 1996 version of this guideline was one of the first guidelines to include a nurse on the writing group, and these STEMI guidelines have included some discussion of nursing management ever since.

The emphasis of this chapter is on the quality of care provided to patients with STEMI—an issue that nurses influence each day. Following a brief overview of the epidemiology and treatment of STEMI, measures of STEMI care quality and outcomes are discussed. Throughout the chapter the reader is referred to other parts of the book where in-depth explanations and specific important issues affecting care quality are developed further (e.g., inflammation, symptom presentation in women, and delay in response to symptoms).

EPIDEMIOLOGY

The American Heart Association estimates that there will be 700,000 new and 500,000 recurrent myocardial infarctions this year.[2] Approximately 30 to 45 percent of these myocardial infarctions will be STEMI. The proportion of persons diagnosed with non-STEMI compared with STEMI has increased, probably because of reperfusion therapy. A decline in STEMI incidence and in mortality rate from STEMI has occurred.[3] The decline in mortality from STEMI that has been observed over the past decades is likely due to a decrease in incidence of myocardial infarction and a decrease in mortality when an infarct does occur. Nonetheless, mortality remains substantial, and of those patients suffering STEMI, about one third will die within 24 hours of onset, and about half of these will die before reaching the hospital. About 10 percent of all deaths related to STEMI occur in the hospital and another 10 percent occur within 1 year of the infarct. Within 6 years of experiencing an infarct, 18 percent of men and 35 percent of women will have another myocardial infarction, 6 to 7 percent of men and women will suffer sudden death, 22 percent of men and 46 percent of women will develop heart failure, and 8 percent of men and 11 percent of women will have a stroke.[2]

Prevention

Given the high risk for morbidity and mortality once infarction develops, the prevention of myocardial infarction should be a major goal for health care providers. Risk factors for STEMI are outlined in Box 57-1. A number of well-designed clinical trials have demonstrated clearly that primary (prevention of coronary heart disease) and secondary (prevention of cardiac events or recurrent cardiac events in patients who have coronary heart disease) prevention are possible with effective management of modifiable risk factors. Despite beliefs by many health care providers to the contrary, at least 90 percent of those who die from coronary heart disease have one or more of the three major modifiable risk factors: hypertension, dyslipidemia, or smoking.[4] The ACC/AHA guidelines for STEMI advocate for the steps outlined in Box 57-2 to increase identification of patients at risk for STEMI to increase preventive efforts.[1] Because of their many daily patient contacts, nurses are in a unique position to identify and counsel individuals at risk for STEMI. Section III of this book contains multiple chapters that address specific risk-reduction strategies that nurses can use to manage primary, secondary, and tertiary (rehabilitation) prevention in their patients.

PATHOPHYSIOLOGY

STEMI (sometimes called Q wave myocardial infarction, although not every STEMI ends in a Q wave presentation) is most often the consequence of occlusion of an epicardial coronary artery by a thrombus formed when a vulnerable atherosclerotic plaque ruptures. When plaque rupture occurs, exposing the vascular basement

---

BOX 57-1 ■ ■ ■
RISK FACTORS FOR ST SEGMENT ELEVATION MYOCARDIAL INFARCTION

- Chronic kidney disease
- Depression
- Diabetes
- Dyslipidemia
- Hypercholesterolemia
- Hypertension
- Increasing age
- Occupational stress
- Peripheral vascular disease
- Prior cerebrovascular accident
- Smoking
- Social isolation

BOX 57-2 ■ ■ ■
STEPS IN THE IDENTIFICATION OF INDIVIDUALS AT RISK FOR ST SEGMENT ELEVATION MYOCARDIAL INFARCTION

- Evaluation by primary care providers, every 3 to 5 years, for existence of cardiac risk factors
- Evaluation by primary care providers of the level of control of cardiac risk factors
- Calculation of 10-year risk* for development of coronary heart disease for anyone who has two or more major risk factors to determine need for primary preventive strategies
- Secondary preventive strategies for any patient with known coronary heart disease
- Preventive attention at the same level afforded those with known coronary heart disease for any patient with a coronary heart disease equivalent: diabetes, chronic kidney disease, peripheral vascular disease, or 10-year risk* greater than 20 percent

*10-year risk is calculated using equations based on the Framingham database; the risk calculator can be found at *http://hp2010.nhlbibin.net/atpiii/calculator.asp?usertype=prof* and includes data on age, gender, total cholesterol level, high-density lipoprotein level, systolic blood pressure, and use of any medication to reduce blood pressure in the calculation.
Antman EM, Anbe DT, Armstrong PW et al: *Circulation* 110(5):e82-e293, 2004.

---

membrane, a cascade of effects begins that includes platelet aggregation, fibrin accumulation, thrombus formation, bleeding into the plaque, and vasospasm. The consequence is vessel occlusion and myocardial ischemia that progresses to necrosis if the myocardium is not reperfused within 4 to 6 hours. These pathophysiological events form the basis for early reperfusion therapy in STEMI. Other rarer causes of STEMI include the following: coronary vasospasm, such as that seen in variant angina or cocaine and amphetamine abuse; coronary emboli; vasculitis; severe chest trauma; and hemorrhage that causes severe oxygen supply/demand imbalance.

Recognition of another major pathophysiological change after myocardial infarction, ventricular remodeling, forms the basis for additional therapy in STEMI. Ventricular remodeling refers to changes in the cardiac architecture after infarction that affect infarcted and noninfarcted areas of the heart. In the area of the infarct, dilatation and ventricular wall thinning occur that result in increased wall stress on the healthy myocardium. The increased demand results in hypertrophy. Remodeling can set the stage for the development of heart failure, and thus use of renin-angiotensin-aldosterone system inhibitors after STEMI is important to reduce remodeling and ultimately prevent the progression to heart failure.

PREHOSPITAL ISSUES

The sooner a patient arrives at the hospital after the onset of ACS symptoms and definitive treatment is started, the better the outcome. Two prehospital factors determine how quickly a patient will arrive at the hospital: (1) how long it takes the patient to come to the decision to seek care and (2) how long it takes to transport the patient to the hospital. In most cases, transport time is minimal. Unfortunately, patient decision time is substantial; most patients delay longer than 2 hours before seeking treatment, and patient delay in seeking treatment for ACS symptoms is a worldwide problem.[5,6]

The problem of patient delay in seeking treatment for symptoms of ACS is so persistent and deleterious to patient outcomes that a number of federal agencies and specialty organizations have programs specifically targeted to this problem.[7,8] Given the extent of the problem of patient delay, an entire chapter of this book is dedicated to the topic. (See Chapter 51 for a thorough discussion of factors contributing to delay and interventions to decrease delay.) Patient education recommendations from the ACC/AHA guidelines designed to decrease patient delay are summarized in Box 57-3. Nurses provide the bulk of patient education and are positioned perfectly to influence patient outcomes positively by educating every patient and their family members about the need to respond urgently to acute cardiac symptoms.

Special mention should be made of use of emergency medical services (**EMS**) in response to acute cardiac symptoms. All patients and their family members should be educated about the importance of using the EMS in cases of acute cardiac symptoms that persist longer than

BOX 57-3
EDUCATION RECOMMENDATIONS TO REDUCE PATIENT DELAY IN SEEKING TREATMENT FOR ACUTE CARDIAC SYMPTOMS

1. Those with symptoms of ST segment elevation myocardial infarction should be taken to the hospital by ambulance and should not drive themselves or be transported by family or others.
2. Health care providers should educate patients and their families about the following:
   ■ Patient's heart attack risk
   ■ How to recognize symptoms of ST segment elevation myocardial infarction
   ■ The importance of calling 911 if cardiac symptoms occur and are unrelieved within 5 minutes, while disregarding fear of embarrassment or feelings of uncertainty
3. Health care providers should educate patients who have nitroglycerin prescribed to take one dose in response to chest discomfort and then to activate the emergency medical system if the discomfort is not relieved.

Antman EM, Anbe DT, Armstrong PW et al: *Circulation* 110(5):e82-e293, 2004.

5 minutes. Unfortunately, using EMS is rarely the patient's first response to symptoms (Table 57-1), and at any time, fewer than 50 percent of all patients experiencing acute cardiac symptoms take the appropriate step of calling 911 to be transported to the hospital for treatment. Use of EMS is associated with greater use of reperfusion therapies and faster time to fibrinolytic therapy and primary percutaneous coronary intervention (**PCI**).[9] These findings have clear implications for educating patients and their families about the importance to outcomes of using EMS. Part of the educational process must involve addressing patients' barriers to calling 911: embarrassment if the symptoms do not turn out to be cardiac; concerns about cost; attribution of symptoms to other causes; fear of troubling others; and waiting for symptoms to go away.[6] Unfortunately, the health care system presents another barrier in those situations in which an insurance plan encourages patients to go to urgent care instead of a hospital emergency department. These issues need to be addressed at the national level.

DIAGNOSIS
Presentation

The diagnosis of STEMI is made based on patient history and presentation and the results of serial electrocardiograms (**ECGs**) and cardiac enzyme levels. The so-called typical myocardial infarction presentation is one that includes chest pain/discomfort, whereas an atypical presentation is considered one without chest pain/discomfort. Other symptoms considered typical include radiation of pain to arms, back, neck, jaw, or epigastrium; shortness of breath; weakness; sweating; nausea; and light-headedness.

Although chest pain or discomfort is present in most individuals who have STEMI, as many as 20 to 30 percent of patients do not have this symptom. In a study of 2096 patients suffering a first confirmed myocardial infarction, 20.2 percent had no chest pain.[10] Patients without chest pain were older, more often women (55 percent versus 35 percent), and more likely to have a history of heart failure (18 percent versus 7 percent) than patients with chest pain. In the multinational Global Registry of Acute Coronary Events (**GRACE**), of 20,881 ACS patients, 8.4 percent did not have chest pain. The most common symptoms in the patients not having chest pain were dyspnea (49 percent), diaphoresis (26 percent), nausea/vomiting (24 percent), or presyncope/syncope (19 percent).[11] Individuals most likely not to have chest pain were women, older persons, those with diabetes or a history of heart failure, and those of nonwhite race.[12] A full discussion of the evaluation of chest pain in cardiac patients and of gender differences in ACS presentation can be found Chapters 53 and 52, respectively.

A presentation without chest pain is not benign. Patients with and without chest pain are equally likely to

TABLE 57-1   ACUTE MYOCARDIAL INFARCTION PATIENTS' (*n* = 913) FIRST RESPONSE TO SYMPTOMS

	FIRST RESPONSE OF PATIENT (%)				
	UNITED STATES (*n* = 192)	SOUTH KOREA (*n* = 127)	JAPAN (*n* = 136)	ENGLAND (*n* = 141)	AUSTRALIA (*n* = 317)
Wished or prayed symptoms would go away	14.9	25.5	15.8	10.7	9.2
Tried to relax	21.3	7.8	16.5	15.0	20.6
Pretended nothing was wrong	7.4	—	0.7	3.6	12.4
Tried not to think about it	4.3	—	0.7	2.9	4.4
Took medication	17.6	15.7	17.3	30.7	16.8
Called doctor	1.6	1.0	2.2	5.0	1.6
Tried self-help remedy	12.2	20.6	23.7	3.6	2.2
Told someone nearby	12.8	7.9	10.1	13.5	22.5
Called EMS	3.7	5.9	4.3	7.9	1.6
Transported self to the hospital without EMS	3.2	15.7	3.6	6.4	—
Drove to doctor's office or clinic	1.1	—	2.9	0.7	0.3
Other action	—	—	2.2	—	8.3

EMS, Emergency medical services.
From Dracup K, Moser DK, McKinley S et al: *J Nurs Scholarsh* 35(4):317-323, 2003.

have ischemic ECG changes.[11] Appropriate diagnosis commonly is delayed in patients without chest pain. Additionally, they are less likely to receive appropriate therapy and have higher 30-day and 1-year mortality than those who have chest pain.[10,11] All clinicians need to be aware of the frequent presentation of STEMI without chest pain and to have a high index of suspicion for STEMI when the elderly, women, diabetic persons, minorities, and those with a history of heart failure present with dyspnea, diaphoresis, nausea, or syncope/presyncope.

Electrocardiogram

Any patient with chest discomfort or other symptoms suggestive of ACS should have a 12-lead ECG done immediately on arrival to the emergency department (ED), and equally important, this ECG should be read by an experienced clinician. The ACC/AHA recommends that both of these activities should be completed within 10 minutes of a patient's arrival at the ED. In addition to identifying patients suffering from STEMI, the 12-lead ECG provides essential data about patients most likely to benefit from reperfusion therapy. Patients with ST segment elevation receive the most benefit from reperfusion.[1] Table 57-2 presents ECG signs associated with ischemia related to the specific coronary arteries, along with data about the sensitivity and specificity of these ECG changes for diagnosis of ACS, including STEMI. Detailed information about the ECG, dysrhythmia monitoring, and ST segment monitoring can be found in Chapters 46 to 49.

Cardiac Biomarkers

Serum cardiac biomarkers including creatine kinase (CK), CK-MB, and troponins are helpful in diagnosing myocardial infarction, estimating infarct size, evaluating prognosis, and providing information about infarct timing. It is not essential, however, to wait for confirmation from biomarkers to initiate reperfusion therapy. The ACC/AHA guideline recommends that in patients with symptoms suggestive of STEMI and with ST segment elevation on the 12-lead ECG, reperfusion therapy should be initiated as soon as possible without waiting for serum cardiac biomarkers.[1]

The various biomarkers of cardiac damage are summarized in Table 57-3. The troponins are considered by most experts to be the preferred biomarker for diagnosing myocardial infarction, given their high specificity for myocardial tissue damage and their sensitivity.[13] In patients in whom the greater need is diagnosis of reinfarction or detecting evidence of reperfusion noninvasively, CK-MB is the preferred biomarker.[1] Other laboratory studies that should be done in the evaluation of suspected STEMI are complete blood count, electrolytes, magnesium, blood urea nitrogen, creatinine, glucose, serum lipids, activated partial thromboplastin time, and international normalized ratio (INR).

MANAGEMENT
Nursing Management

Nurses have a number of responsibilities in the ED and in-hospital phases of care and can have a substantial impact on the quality of care received by cardiac patients suffering acute cardiac events. The goals of nursing care in the ED setting and during the in-hospital phase of care are similar:

- Perform independent and collaborative activities that limit infarct size
- Manage chest pain/discomfort
- Detect and prevent complications
- Promote optimal short- and long-term recovery
- Provide ongoing education and support for the patient and family

In-depth discussion of strategies for meeting each of these goals is provided in other chapters in this book, but Table 57-4 provides an overview.

TABLE 57-2   ELECTROCARDIOGRAM FINDINGS FOR THE DIAGNOSIS OF ACUTE CORONARY SYNDROME

ELECTROCARDIOGRAM FINDINGS	LESION	SENSITIVITY (%)	SPECIFICITY (%)	POSITIVE PREDICTIVE VALUE (%)	NEGATIVE PREDICTIVE VALUE (%)
ST segment elevation greater in lead III than in lead II plus ST segment depression of greater than 1 mm in lead I, lead aVL, or both	Right coronary artery	90	71	94	70
Absence of the above findings plus ST segment elevation in leads I, aVL, V$_5$, and V$_6$ and ST segment depression in leads V$_1$, V$_2$, and V$_3$	Left circumflex coronary artery	83	96	91	93
ST segment elevation in leads V$_1$, V$_2$, and V$_3$ plus any of the features below:					
ST segment elevation of greater than 2.5 mm in lead V$_1$, right bundle branch block with Q wave, or both	Proximal LAD coronary artery	12	100	100	61
ST segment depression of greater than 1 mm in leads II, III, and aVF	Proximal LAD coronary artery	34	98	93	68
ST segment depression of ≤1 mm or ST segment elevation in leads II, III, and aVF	Distal LAD coronary artery	66	73	78	62

LAD, Left anterior descending.
Data from Achar SA, Kundu S, Norcross WA: Am Fam Physician 72(1):119-126, 2005.

■ ■ ■

TABLE 57-3   CHARACTERISTICS OF SERUM CARDIAC MARKERS FOR THE DIAGNOSIS OF ACUTE MYOCARDIAL INFARCTION*

SERUM CARDIAC MARKER	TEST FIRST BECOMES POSITIVE (HOURS)	PEAK LEVEL (HOURS)	SENSITIVITY (%)	SPECIFICITY (%)	POSITIVE PREDICTIVE VALUE (%)†	NEGATIVE PREDICTIVE VALUE (%)†
Creatine Kinase						
Single assay	3-8	12-24	35	80	20	90
Serial assays			95	68	30	99
Creatine Kinase-MB						
Single assay	4-6	12-24	35	85	25	90
Serial assays			95	95	73	99
Troponin I and T						
Measured 4 hours after onset of chest pain	4-10		35	96	56	91
Measured 10 hours after onset of chest pain		8-28	89	95	72	98

*ST segment elevation myocardial infarction or non–ST segment elevation in patients presenting to emergency departments with chest pain.
†Given a 12.5 percent overall likelihood of acute myocardial infarction.
Data from Achar SA, Kundu S, Norcross WA: *Am Fam Physician* 72(1):119-126, 2005.

■ ■ ■

TABLE 57-4   NURSING GOALS IN THE MANAGEMENT OF PATIENTS WITH ST SEGMENT ELEVATION MYOCARDIAL INFARCTION

GOAL	STRATEGIES FOR MEETING GOAL
Perform independent and collaborative activities that limit infarct size.	Optimize patient triage and flow through the emergency department for all patients who have symptoms suggestive of cardiac ischemia to minimize time to reperfusion strategy.
	Develop and follow effective, time-efficient protocols for each reperfusion strategy.
	Administer oxygen (for 6 hours after onset and then assess for continued need using pulse oximetry); treat chest pain/discomfort.
	Provide calm, competent care, while giving support, education, and reassurance to patient and family (increased anxiety is associated with stimulation of ongoing and recurrent ischemia presumably through activation of the sympathetic nervous system).
	Monitor cardiac rhythm and ST segment elevation continuously in order to detect dysrhythmias and ischemia.
	Perform thorough assessment in order to detect potential complications.
Manage chest pain/discomfort.	Use a consistent and standardized, hospital-wide method of assessing ischemic pain/discomfort.
	Teach the patient and family the importance of reporting ischemic pain; make them aware of the benefits of reporting pain in terms of limiting infarct size or detecting and treating recurrent ischemia.
	Use nitrates and intravenous morphine sulfate as necessary to eliminate pain/discomfort on initial admission to the emergency department.
	For recurrent ischemic pain/discomfort, perform appropriate assessment for recurrence of ischemia (e.g., obtain 12-lead electrocardiogram) while treating pain with nitrates and morphine as necessary.
Detect and prevent complications.	Initiate and maintain continuous electrocardiogram monitoring using optimal lead placement.
	Assess heart and lung sounds, peripheral pulses, fluid status, neurological status, chest pain/discomfort, other pain/discomfort, anxiety and depression, patients understanding of condition, and family coping during each shift and as indicated.
Promote optimal short- and long-term recovery.	Provide frequent updates to family on patient's condition.
	Initiate patient and family education and counseling early.
	Introduce patient and family to the necessary lifestyle changes needed to manage risk factors.
	Assess for and manage patient and family anxiety, depression, and barriers to adherence.
Provide ongoing education and support for the patient and family.	Assess patient and family readiness for change; determine barriers to change and the best ways to address these.
	Determine adequacy of coping, and provide appropriate level of support.
	Explain purpose and what to expect (include sensory information) of all tests.
	Provide steadily increasing amounts of education throughout admission as patient's condition stabilizes.
	At admission to emergency department, explain diagnosis and treatment plan.
	At cardiac care unit or stepdown telemetry unit admission from emergency department, orient to unit; discuss plan of care; emphasize importance of notifying nurse for chest pain/discomfort, other symptoms, or any concerns; and begin addressing risk factor modification goals.
	Before discharge, ensure the following are covered: risk factor goals and plan, lifestyle recommendations, prescribed medications and importance of adherence, recognizing symptoms of ischemia and what to do, recommend cardiopulmonary resuscitation training for family, refer to cardiac rehabilitation, and ensure that follow-up appointments are arranged.

Emergency Department Management

The effectiveness of all definitive therapies for STEMI is time-limited. Thus once an individual arrives at the ED, all efforts should be made to avoid in-hospital delays and ensure that the patient is diagnosed and treated rapidly. To achieve this goal, the ACC/AHA guideline recommends that hospitals set up multidisciplinary teams (including primary care physicians, ED physicians, cardiologists, nurses, and laboratory technicians) that develop evidence-based protocols for the ED triage and management of patients with symptoms suggestive of STEMI.[1]

Drug Therapy

Initial therapy for patients in the ED includes placement of an intravenous line and low-flow oxygen to keep arterial oxygen saturation above 90 percent and to reduce ischemia. Aspirin should be administered if not already taken by the patient at home or administered by the paramedics. Nitroglycerin and morphine are given to relieve ischemic pain. Simultaneously, a 12-lead ECG should be done and continuous ECG monitoring should be implemented. While considering the options for reperfusion, beta-adrenergic blocking agents are given if the patient has tachycardia or hypertension; otherwise, beta blockers should be administered beginning on day 2 post-STEMI. New data on intravenous beta blockers suggest that they should no longer be routinely administered immediately to all STEMI patients. A recent study demonstrated an increase in the risk of cardiogenic shock with early intervention beta blocker administration.[11] Oral angiotensin-converting enzyme (**ACE**) inhibitors are indicated within the first 24 hours of STEMI, particularly in patients with left ventricular dysfunction, anterior myocardial infarction, or pulmonary congestion.[1]

Aspirin

The use of aspirin early in the course of STEMI is associated with improved outcomes. As such, patients should be taught to chew 162 to 325 mg of aspirin while awaiting EMS arrival in response to acute cardiac symptoms.[1] Patients who have not taken an aspirin before EMS arrival should be given a dose of 162 mg for the antithrombotic effects of aspirin, unless hypersensitivity or true allergy to aspirin exists. Hypersensitive and allergic patients may receive clopidogrel or ticlopidine.

Nitroglycerin

Nitroglycerin is used for management of persistent chest discomfort of ischemic origin unless the patient's blood pressure is lower than 90 mm Hg systolic or substantially (more than 30 mm Hg) lower than the baseline blood pressure, if known. Use of nitroglycerin also should be avoided in patients who have taken phosphodiesterase inhibitors for erectile dysfunction within the previous 48 hours. Nitroglycerin is administered sublingually at a dose of 0.4 mg every 5 minutes to a total of three doses, after which time intravenous administration should be considered if ischemic pain is unrelieved. In addition to its ability to relieve ischemic coronary pain, nitroglycerin is a preload and afterload reducer

because of its venous and arterial dilating properties. This action is helpful in patients with heart failure.

Morphine Sulfate

Morphine sulfate (2 to 4 mg IV repeated every 5 to 15 minutes) is the drug of choice for managing STEMI pain. Morphine has analgesic, antianxiety, and vasodilating effects that are beneficial in STEMI, particularly acutely when increased sympathetic activity can produce a number of negative effects, including lowering the fibrillation threshold and promoting further plaque rupture.[1] Adequate pain relief is imperative in the appropriate management of STEMI.

Beta-Adrenergic Blocking Agents

The exceptionally large ($n = 45,852$) Chinese COMMIT trial was published,[14] recently and showed that metoprolol administered immediately after hospital admission did not significantly reduce in-hospital mortality.[14] Further, there was a dramatic increase in the risk of cardiogenic shock, especially when the drug was administered during the day of admission and on day 1. When beta blocker therapy (200 mg controlled-release metoprolol once daily) was started on day 2 of hospitalization when the hemodynamic condition had stabilized, the risk of reinfarction and ventricular fibrillation were reduced. These agents exert their beneficial effects after STEMI by reducing myocardial oxygen demand, augmenting coronary artery perfusion, and reducing the occurrence of ventricular dysrhythmias. These results are consistent with those from prior studies illustrating that beta-blocking agents can reduce infarct size and mortality in patients with STEMI.[15,16] Beta blocker therapy should be continued long term following discharge in patients with STEMI who are without contraindications.[1]

Fibrinolytic Therapy and Percutaneous Coronary Intervention

The ACC/AHA guidelines strongly emphasize the importance of reperfusion therapy.[1] Every patient with STEMI needs to be evaluated immediately upon admission to the ED for reperfusion therapy so that the appropriate strategy (i.e., fibrinolysis or PCI) can be initiated. A detailed discussion of these two reperfusion strategies and associated therapies can be found in Chapter 58.

Angiotensin-Converting Enzyme Inhibitors

A number of randomized controlled trials in which more than 100,000 patients have been enrolled have demonstrated clearly the survival benefit of treating STEMI patients with oral ACE inhibitors within the first 24 hours.[17] Therapy with oral ACE inhibitors (or angiotensin II receptor blockers [**ARBs**] for those intolerant of ACE inhibitors) is indicated within 24 hours of STEMI onset in patients who have pulmonary congestion, left ventricular dysfunction (ejection fraction less than 40 percent), or anterior myocardial infarction and who are not hypotensive.[1] Intravenous use is not recommended within the first 24 hours because hypotension can occur that abolishes the benefits of ACE inhibition.

Hospital Management

During the hospital phase of care for STEMI patients, the focus shifts to the following:

- Preventing, monitoring for, and treating recurrent ischemia and dysrhythmias (see Chapters 46 to 49), and complications of reperfusion (Chapter 58) or of STEMI (Chapter 59)
- Establishing appropriate drug therapy
- Beginning the rehabilitation phase (Chapter 80)

To optimize care and ensure that all patients receive evidence-based management, care should be structured based on protocols developed using consensus guidelines.[1] Box 57-4 provides an overview of orders typical for patients with STEMI.

Nurses should take advantage of their training and ability to make decisions based on individual patient needs for the necessity of treating pain and anxiety, both of which activate the sympathetic nervous system, increase myocardial oxygen demand, and potentially stimulate ongoing and recurrent ischemia. In a prospective study of the association between anxiety, perceived control, and subsequent in-hospital complications among patients ($n = 536$) hospitalized for acute myocardial infarction, Moser and colleagues[18] demonstrated that higher levels of anxiety were associated with sig-

---

BOX 57-4 ■ ■ ■

TYPICAL HOSPITAL ADMISSION ORDERS FOR PATIENTS WITH ST SEGMENT ELEVATION MYOCARDIAL INFARCTION

- Maintain intravenous line at a "keep open" rate using normal saline or 5 percent dextrose in water
- Continuous electrocardiogram monitoring for the presence of ST segment changes and dysrhythmias
- Performance of vital signs every 30 minutes until stable and then every 4 hours
- Bed rest until stable and then progress to bedside commode (usually within 12 to 24 hours) and activity
- Oxygen at 2 liters by nasal cannula with continuous pulse oximetry for 6 hours; after 6 hours if patient is stable and oxygen saturation exceeds 90 percent, discontinue oxygen
- Nothing by mouth with sips of water until stable; NCEP ATP III Therapeutic Lifestyle Changes diet: low cholesterol (less than 200 mg/d), low saturated fat (less than 7 percent of total daily calories from saturated fats), and increased omega-3 fatty acids
- 2-g sodium diet, in addition, for patients with hypertension or heart failure
- Medications
- Nitroglycerin sublingual 0.4 mg every 5 minutes for chest pain/discomfort
- Aspirin daily 75 to 162 mg
- Oral beta blocker beginning immediately only for tachydysrhythmia or hypertension
- Oral angiotensin converting enzyme inhibitor (or angiotensin II receptor blocker if patient is intolerant of ACE inhibitor for patients with anterior infarction, pulmonary congestion, or left ventricular ejection fraction less than 40 percent, as long as patient is not hypotensive
- Intravenous morphine sulfate 2 to 4 mg every 5 to 15 minutes as needed for chest pain/discomfort
- Stool softener daily
- Anxiolytic as needed

NCEP ATP III, National Cholesterol Education Program Adult Treatment Panel III.

---

nificantly more episodes of ventricular tachycardia, ventricular fibrillation, reinfarction, and ischemia (all $p < 0.01$). Patients' anxiety levels were high (i.e., double that of the published mean from the norm reference group) and 27 percent of patients experienced one or more in-hospital complications. These results have important implications for nurses working in acute care settings because patients with higher levels of perceived control had substantially lower anxiety ($p < 0.01$). Interventions that increase patient control are important, but it should be noted that research is needed to test such approaches. Also, the combination of high anxiety and low perceived control is associated with the highest risk of complications, so detecting these patients early is particularly important.

Nurses caring for STEMI patients must be adept at monitoring for dysrhythmias and ST segment changes indicative of ischemia. (Chapter 49 includes a discussion of all aspects of ST segment monitoring.) During hospitalization, nurses are responsible for the progressive activity of STEMI patients. Given the hazards of immobility, bed rest is not indicated for more than 12 to 24 hours in patients who are hemodynamically stable and symptom free, and progressive ambulation with monitoring for ischemia is started early. Even among patients with hemodynamic instability or continued ischemia, a bedside commode is allowed after 12 to 24 hours.

Regarding drug therapy, aspirin and beta blocker therapy should continue (both for use long-term), and beta blocker therapy should be used in adequate doses. Oral ACE inhibitors should be started and used long-term in patients with anterior myocardial infarction, pulmonary congestion, or left ventricular dysfunction. In those appropriate patients who are intolerant of ACE inhibitors, ARBs can be used.

In addition to the general care applicable to all patients with STEMI, there are specific situations that require additional attention in patient subgroups. Patients who are diabetic need attention to stringent control of blood glucose, particularly in the first 48 hours after STEMI when marked sympathetic nervous system activation produces a cascade of events that seriously deranges glucose metabolism.[1] Attention to strict glucose control can improve patients' response to reperfusion therapy.[19] Patients who are suffering from a magnesium deficiency or who have episodes of torsades de pointes ventricular tachycardia should receive magnesium.[1,20] There are no other indications for the use of magnesium in STEMI patients. Although calcium channel blockers (e.g., verapamil or diltiazem) are appropriate for the management of ongoing ischemia or control of rapid ventricular response to atrial fibrillation in patients who cannot take beta blockers, their use is contraindicated in patients with STEMI and left ventricular dysfunction or heart failure. Nifedipine is contraindicated in STEMI because it causes sympathetic nervous system activation.[1]

EDUCATION

Patient and family education about living with the chronicity of cardiac disease is probably the most important nursing role in the care of patients with STEMI, yet it is among the least appreciated. As hospital stays become shorter, patient acuity becomes higher, and the reality of the nursing shortage becomes acute, the education role of nursing is often the first to be neglected.

Ultimately, patients and their families must assume lifelong responsibility for managing cardiac disease, and this responsibility means adhering to prescribed medications; undertaking risk factor modification that for many means making considerable, difficult lifestyle changes; monitoring for recurrent ischemia; taking appropriate and timely action in case of ischemic symptoms; managing emotional distress; integrating management of any comorbidities they may have; and negotiating return to work, sexual activities, or other activities and roles. Families need to do all this, plus figure out how to be supportive without being overprotective or overcritical and to learn what to do in case of an emergency. Given the enormity of this task, patient and family education must be a priority for nurses during all phases of care—ED, hospital, cardiac rehabilitation, and other outpatient settings.[1] Specific education needs of STEMI patients are similar to those of non-STEMI patients and are outlined in Chapter 56.

Quality of Care

The Joint Commission on Accreditation of Healthcare Organizations (JCAHO) developed indicators of the care provided to patients with STEMI in acute care hospitals in the United States. These nine indicators, shown in Box 57-5, have been standardized in coordination with the Centers for Medicare and Medicaid Services (CMS), adopted by the Hospital Quality Alliance, and endorsed by the National Quality Forum. These indicators are used widely to track hospital performance, although they have been found to explain only 6 percent of the variance in hospital-level variation in risk adjusted, 30-day mortality.[21]

Early in 2006 the ACC/AHA published STEMI/NSTEMI clinical performance measures derived from the ACC/AHA STEMI clinical guidelines and expert discussion. Proposed measures were chosen based on usefulness in improving patient outcomes (i.e., evidence-based, interpretable, and actionable), measure design, validity, reliability, measure implementation (e.g., feasibility, effort, cost, and time), and overall assessment. The performance measures chosen by the ACC/AHA committee are similar to those tracked by CMS/JCAHO except for the addition of low-density lipoprotein cholesterol assessment and lipid-lowering therapy at discharge. The ACC/AHA measures also emphasize exclusion criteria, which represents an important step forward in performance measurement. Most performance measurement reports exclude certain patients from analyses, but not routinely and not uniformly.

The ACC/AHA clinical performance measures also include a new reperfusion therapy measure meant to capture the percentage of patients eligible for reperfusion who are reperfused. They advocate reporting median rather than mean time to fibrinolytic therapy or PCI, which is appropriate because mean is notoriously skewed. Finally, they establish the time-to-PCI standard at 90 minutes rather than the 120-minute standard used by CMS/JCAHO.

Institutions across the United States are concerned about the change in the PCI time standard because a recent study demonstrated no substantial improvement in hospital performance in time to PCI between 1999 and 2002.[22] At baseline, 35 percent of STEMI patients in the study were treated with PCI within 90 minutes. By 2002, performance had improved to only 37 percent. Although most delay is due to patients not arriving at the hospital in a timely fashion, as discussed before, door-to-balloon time is an important component of this quality indicator. In this study the adjusted mean door-to-balloon time was 108 minutes over the 3-year study duration. This indicator of performance is discussed further subsequently.

Quality of Care Performance

In the past few years, clinical investigators across the world have begun building registries of ACS patients so that they can monitor their progress in improving the care provided to patients with STEMI. A recent study using the Hospital Quality Alliance data from 3558 U.S. hospitals revealed that care for STEMI was superior to that for heart failure or pneumonia.[23] The median quality of care score was at least 90 percent on four of five performance measures for STEMI in the vast majority of U.S. hospitals. Interestingly, substantial gaps were found within the same hospital in typical performance measures for the three conditions. That is, patients with STEMI might be treated more effectively at a particular hospital than someone with pneumonia is treated at that same hospital. Teaching hospitals, not-for-profit hospitals, and hospitals in the Midwest and Northeast United States outperformed others in STEMI care.

Other studies have demonstrated poorer quality of care for certain subgroups of patients. Analysis of data from the Second National Registry of Myocardial Infarction confirmed that patients whose STEMI is complicated by congestive heart failure are at greatly increased risk for poor in-hospital outcomes. Despite their in-

---

BOX 57-5   ■ ■ ■
CMS/JCAHO QUALITY INDICATORS FOR ACUTE MYOCARDIAL INFARCTION

- Aspirin given upon arrival at the hospital
- Aspirin prescribed at discharge
- Angiotensin-converting enzyme inhibitor or angiotensin receptor blocker for patients with left ventricular systolic dysfunction prescribed at discharge
- Smoking cessation advice/counseling
- Beta blocker given within 24 hours after arrival*
- Beta blocker prescribed at discharge
- Inpatient mortality
- Percutaneous coronary intervention received within 120 minutes of hospital arrival
- Fibrinolytic agent received within 30 minutes of hospital arrival

CMS/JCAHO, Centers for Medicare and Medicaid Services/Joint Commission on Accreditation of Healthcare Organizations.
*Note: This indicator may need to be revised based on recent data.

creased risk, patients with acute myocardial infarction who have congestive heart failure are less likely to be treated with reperfusion therapies and life-saving medications such as beta blockers and aspirin. Such patients are older and more likely to be female, to have history of diabetes or hypertension, and to have a longer time to hospital presentation.[24]

Aspirin

In studies of aspirin administration, worldwide administration rates vary from 82 percent[25] to 93 percent.[26] In one study that broke out the admission and discharge aspirin administration rates, 88 percent of eligible STEMI patients received aspirin on admission and 89 percent were prescribed aspirin at discharge.[27] One factor found to delay aspirin administration upon arrival at the hospital is delay in the diagnosis of acute myocardial infarction.[28] In a study of the effect of organizational infrastructure on therapy for STEMI, aspirin was more likely to be administered to patients in hospitals that specify aspirin administration in their admission order sets (odds ratio 1.57, confidence interval 1.01 to 2.48).[29] Being at a teaching hospital and treatment by a cardiologist were associated with increased rates of aspirin administration in another study.[26]

Angiotensin-Converting Enzyme Inhibitors

Studies of the rates at which ACE inhibitors or ARBs are administered to STEMI patients with left ventricular systolic dysfunction at hospital discharge illustrate that rates vary widely. In hospitals across the United States, ACE inhibitor therapy was the only performance indicator on which the median quality score was below 90 percent.[23] In New Zealand, Ellis and colleagues[25] found that ACE inhibitors were prescribed only 43 percent of the time, and Tang and colleagues[30] documented a rate of 55 percent of patients on hospital discharge. In three separate hospitals in Switzerland, an ACE inhibitor was prescribed at discharge in 68, 75, and 91 percent of cases.[31] In Mexico, only 64 percent for STEMI patients were prescribed ACE inhibitors.[32] In Portugal, 69 and 66 percent of patients hospitalized for STEMI received an ACE inhibitor during hospitalization or at discharge, respectively.[33] Clearly, efforts to improve the rate at which STEMI patients receive ACE inhibitors are needed.

Smoking Cessation Counseling

Counseling of smokers hospitalized for STEMI has not been studied as extensively as other quality of care indicators. In a study conducted in Oklahoma, documentation of smoking cessation counseling actually decreased between 1994 and 1998.[34] In a recent study from 12 hospitals and health care systems in rural Alberta, Canada, only 13 percent of patients who were smokers and were hospitalized for STEMI received smoking cessation counseling. In a study of 53,417 patients in the National Registry of Myocardial Infarction 4, 28.3 percent of hospitalized STEMI patients were current smokers,[27] but only 56 percent of these smokers were counseled regarding the importance of quitting. An important caveat to the interpretation of these data is that documentation may be more of an issue than actual counseling rates.

That is, clinicians may be telling patients the importance of quitting but failing to note that they did so in the records.

An interesting recent study documented a poor correlation between individual performance indicators.[21] In particular, smoking cessation counseling and time to reperfusion therapy were poorly associated ($r < 0.40$), illustrating that staff at hospitals may be concentrating on some indicators more than others.

Beta Blocker Therapy

Beta blockers were administered early during hospitalization in 73 percent of STEMI patients and on discharge in 74 percent in patients hospitalized in Connecticut.[28] Comparable rates (77.8 percent) were found in patients from the National Registry of Myocardial Infarction-4 who were telephoned between 1997 and 1999 for data collection.[27] Rates were higher in a study from a Veterans Affairs Medical Center, where 93 percent of patients received a beta blocker.[35] In another study from the National Registry of Myocardial Infarction-4 between 2000 and 2002, however, the rates were lower and far more variable. Bradley and colleagues[36] found the mean hospital-specific beta blocker rate to be 60.2 percent but the range was 19.4 to 89.3 percent and quality improvement efforts varied widely as well. In one study the factors found to be associated with higher rates of beta blocker administration were inclusion in an ED protocol or pathway, commitment by the administration to quality of STEMI care, and a physician champion.[29]

In the GRACE registry of patients with ACSs from 94 hospitals in 14 countries, beta blocker use in the first 24 hours (before the new data from the huge Chinese COMMIT study) varied from 65 to 89 percent across hospitals.[26] High-risk patients (e.g., elders, those with congestive heart failure) were least likely to receive aspirin and beta blocker therapy. Region of the world was a strong predictor of beta blocker use during the first 24 hours. Twice the rate of failure to use beta blockers occurred in Europe, Australia, New Zealand, and Canada, and a 1.75 times higher failure rate occurred in Argentina and Brazil compared with the United States. For beta blockers at discharge, region of the world, older age, and undergoing coronary bypass surgery during hospitalization were associated with lower rates of beta blocker use. Being at a teaching hospital and undergoing coronary angioplasty during hospitalization were associated with higher rates of beta blocker use. Hopefully, these same factors will be associated with a rapid change in practice based on the new COMMIT data.

Inpatient Mortality

Mortality is tracked by CMS/JCAHO as a crude measure of hospital performance, but few studies of this indicator have been published. Studies that report mortality typically report in-hospital rather than 30-day mortality rates. In a study from the National Registry of Myocardial Infarction 4 conducted between 2000 and 2002, mortality in patients hospitalized for STEMI was 14.3 percent.[27] In the GRACE registry of patients from 14 countries, in-hospital mortality was 4.1 percent in the top-performing hospitals and 5.6 percent in the bottom

quartile.[26] In the study from Portugal, in-hospital mortality was 10.2 percent in STEMI patients.[33] More study of this specific indicator would be useful.

Primary PCI has been shown to be associated with significantly lower in-hospital mortality.[37] Noting incontrovertible evidence of the effectiveness of primary PCI, volunteers representing the AHA recently published a statement encouraging establishment of systems of care that increase the number of STEMI patients with timely access to primary PCI.[8] They advocated the guiding principles listed in Box 57-6.

Reperfusion Therapy

Performance indicators with a strict time element such as PCI and fibrinolytic therapy—discussed together in this section—have been particularly difficult for hospitals to influence. Some hospitals have achieved enviable outcomes in this area, however. When the top-performing hospitals were examined using data from the National Registry of Myocardial Infarction collected between 2001 and 2002, the top 20 percent of hospitals had significantly shorter times in nearly all of the intervals after adjusting for clinical characteristics.[38] The top-performing hospitals achieved a mean door-to-ECG time of 6.8 minutes (SD = 1.7) and a mean ECG-to-fibrinolytic drug time of 18.7 minutes (SD = 3.5).

Institutions engaged in a quality improvement process realize the need for a multifaceted coordinated effort specific to the institution. However, identification of those factors associated with improvement at other institutions (i.e., benchmarking) can be useful by helping to identify where data collection is needed. No hospital characteristic was associated with an improvement in PCI over time (other than location in New England), although PCI volume was associated with improvement.[22]

Others have noted that most PCI patients are treated in off-hours when performance is the poorest. Magid and colleagues[39] found that door-to-balloon times were substantially longer during off-hours (116.1 minutes) than regular hours (94.8 minutes). During regular hours,

47 percent of patients received PCI treatment within the recommended time frame, whereas only 25.7 percent received it on time during off-hours. Door-to-balloon times exceeded 120 minutes 41.5 percent of the time during off-hours compared with 27.7 percent during regular hours. Poorest performance occurred during weekday nights. The most common source of increased door-to-balloon time was a delay in time from ECG to arrival in the catheterization laboratory.

Geographical variation in the use of PCI has been noted, with 39.5 percent of patients in the United States, 34.6 percent of those in Europe, 33.5 percent of patients in Argentina/Brazil, and 25.0 percent in Australia/New Zealand/Canada receiving PCI.[40] The use of PCI is greater in hospitals with an on-site catheterization laboratory compared with hospitals without these facilities, and PCI facilities are currently available in fewer than 25 percent of acute care hospitals in the United States. Thus many STEMI patients are transferred from one hospital to another. A study of STEMI patients transferred between 1999 and 2002 found the median door-to-balloon time to be 180 minutes; only 4.2 percent of patients were treated within 90 minutes. Only about 15 percent of transfer patients receive PCI within a 2-hour period.[41]

Beliefs of the General Public about Quality of Care

Even though the JCAHO makes standardized hospital performance data available to the general public through its website (*www.qualitycheck.org*), these data appear to be underused by the general public. Instead, popular media sources are used widely by the public. For example, the *US News & World Report* issue "America's Best Hospitals" is in its 16th edition, reaching at least 2 million online users each month with increases of 200 to 600 percent when an issue such as the one on hospital performance is released. Results from this publication also often are discussed in local newspapers.

Hospitals rated as among the top 50 heart hospitals by *US News & World Report* need to have an annual minimum rate of 770 medical discharges and to offer open-heart surgery or PCI. They also must be members of the Council of Teaching Hospitals, have a medical school affiliation, or have a minimum score on a hospital-wide Key Technology Index. Examples of elements used to calculate this index score include cardiac catheterization laboratory, cardiac intensive care beds, magnetic resonance imaging, open-heart surgery, and ultrasound. *US News & World Report* then calculates an index score using factors such as a survey of physicians, nurse staffing ratios, magnet hospital status, and community services offered.

Over the years, investigators have assessed the validity of the rankings of hospitals promoted by *US News & World Report*. In 1999, Chen and colleagues[42] reported that hospitals ranked high in the *US News & World Report* issue had lower 30-day acute myocardial infarction mortality rates and higher rates on process measures addressing aspirin and beta blocker use. In 2002, Krumholz

---

BOX 57-6 ■ ■ ■

GUIDING PRINCIPLES FOR INCREASING THE USE OF EVIDENCE-BASED RECOMMENDATIONS IN THE CARE OF PATIENTS WITH ST SEGMENT ELEVATION MYOCARDIAL INFARCTION

1. Patient-centered care as the top priority
2. High-quality care that is safe, effective, and timely
3. Stakeholder consensus on systems infrastructure
4. Increased operational efficiencies
5. Appropriate incentives for quality, such as "pay for performance," "pay for value," or "pay for quality"
6. Measurable patient outcomes
7. An evaluation mechanism to ensure quality of care measures reflect changes in evidence-based research, including consensus-based treatment guidelines
8. A role for local community hospitals so as to avoid a negative impact that could eliminate critical access to local health care
9. A reduction in disparities of health care delivery, such as those across economic, education, racial/ethnic, or geographic lines

From Jacobs AK, Antman EM, Ellrodt G et al: *Circulation* 113(17):2152-2163, 2006.

and colleagues[43] reported that hospitals graded highly performed slightly better on several measures of quality and outcome but noted that the ratings did a poor job of distinguishing between any two individual hospitals.

Most recently, Williams and colleagues[44] compared 774 hospitals, include 41 of the *US News & World Report* top 50 heart and heart surgery hospitals on six acute myocardial infarction performance measures. As a group, the *US News & World Report* hospitals performed statistically better than their peers (86 percent versus 83 percent on an aggregate performance measure ($p < 0.05$). Individually, however, only 23 of the *US News & World Report* hospitals were statistically significantly better than average, and 9 performed significantly worse. Many hospitals (167 of 774 hospitals studied) routinely implemented evidence-based heart care 90 percent of the time or more.

DIRECTIONS FOR THE FUTURE

A number of factors, such as publication of the Institute of Medicine report on the *Quality Chasm,* have coalesced to bring the issue of health care quality to the forefront. Taken as a whole, it is clear that improvement still is needed, especially in the areas of ACE inhibitor or ARB administration and smoking cessation counseling. More data are needed on 30-day mortality. Studies testing the relationships between individual indicators and those describing the quality of care provided by certain hospitals to specific patient groups would be useful.

A new trend in performance measurement is the all-or-none measurement approach.[45] With this approach, the percentage of patients receiving all the appropriate discrete elements of care is calculated. No partial credit is given, which yields a very different picture from the item-by-item measurement of quality typically used. Advantages are that all-or-none measurement reflect the interests of patients, who want total quality care, not just pieces of good care. It fosters a systems perspective by encouraging the design of whole sequences of care and handoffs, not only parts. And, it offers a more sensitive scale for assessing improvements. As noted above, 90 percent of hospitals were found to routinely implement evidence-based heart care when item-by-item analyses were performed.[44] When all-or none assessments are performed, this ceiling effect is sure to drop. It should be noted that the CMS has adopted the all-or-none approach in their 8th Scope of Work.[46] Thus nationwide movement towards this new approach to quality measurement should be adopted widely in the near future.

As this review has illustrated, there is a worldwide effort to describe and improve the care provided to patients hospitalized with acute myocardial infarction. The AHA and the ACC have led the effort, first with their efforts to develop clinical guidelines and then with their *Get with the Guidelines* (AHA) and *Guidelines in Applied Practice,* or GAP, (ACC) initiatives. Readers interested in exploring these initiatives in greater detail are encouraged to visit these websites: *www.american-heart.org/presenter.jhtml?identifier=1165* and *www.acc.org/qualityandscience/gap/gap.htm.*

REFERENCES

1. Antman EM, Anbe DT, Armstrong PW et al: ACC/AHA guidelines for the management of patients with ST-elevation myocardial infarction: a report of the American College of Cardiology/American Heart Association Task Force on Practice Guidelines (Committee to Revise the 1999 Guidelines for the Management of Patients with Acute Myocardial Infarction), *Circulation* 110(5): e82-e293, 2004.
2. Thom T, Haase N, Rosamond W et al: Heart disease and stroke statistics: 2006 update—a report from the American Heart Association Statistics Committee and Stroke Statistics Subcommittee, *Circulation* 113(6):e85-e151, 2006.
3. Furman MI, Dauerman HL, Goldberg RJ et al: Twenty-two year (1975 to 1997). trends in the incidence, in-hospital and long-term case fatality rates from initial Q-wave and non-Q-wave myocardial infarction: a multi-hospital, community-wide perspective, *J Am Coll Cardiol* 37(6):1571-1580, 2001.
4. Mensah GA, Brown DW, Croft JB et al: Major coronary risk factors and death from coronary heart disease: baseline and follow-up mortality data from the Second National Health and Nutrition Examination Survey (NHANES II), *Am J Prev Med* 29(5 suppl 1):68-74, 2005.
5. Dracup K, Moser DK, McKinley S et al: An international perspective on the time to treatment for acute myocardial infarction, *J Nurs Scholarsh* 35(4):317-323, 2003.
6. Moser DK, Kimble LP, Alberts MJ et al: Reducing delay in seeking treatment by patients with acute coronary syndrome and stroke: a scientific statement from the American Heart Association Council on Cardiovascular Nursing and Stroke Council, *Circulation* 114(2):168-182, 2006.
7. National Heart Attack Alert Program Coordinating Committee Working Group on Educational Strategies to Prevent Prehospital Delay in Patients at High Risk for Acute Myocardial Infarction: Educational strategies to prevent prehospital delay in patients at high risk for acute myocardial infarction: a report by the National Heart Attack Alert Program, *J Thromb Thrombolysis* 6:47-61, 1998.
8. Jacobs AK, Antman EM, Ellrodt G et al: Recommendation to develop strategies to increase the number of ST-segment-elevation myocardial infarction patients with timely access to primary percutaneous coronary intervention, *Circulation* 113(17):2152-2163, 2006.
9. Canto JG, Zalenski RJ, Ornato JP et al: Use of emergency medical services in acute myocardial infarction and subsequent quality of care: observations from the National Registry of Myocardial Infarction 2, *Circulation* 106(24):3018-3023, 2002.
10. Dorsch MF, Lawrance RA, Sapsford RJ et al: Poor prognosis of patients presenting with symptomatic myocardial infarction but without chest pain, *Heart* 86(5):494-498, 2001.
11. Brieger D, Eagle KA, Goodman SG et al: Acute coronary syndromes without chest pain, an underdiagnosed and undertreated high-risk group: insights from the Global Registry of Acute Coronary Events, *Chest* 126:461-469, 2004.
12. Canto JG, Shlipak MG, Rogers WJ et al: Prevalence, clinical characteristics, and mortality among patients with myocardial infarction presenting without chest pain, *JAMA* 283(24):3223-3229, 2000.
13. Alpert JS, Thygesen K, Antman E et al: Myocardial infarction redefined: a consensus document of the Joint European Society of Cardiology/American College of Cardiology Committee for the Redefinition of Myocardial Infarction, *J Am Coll Cardiol* 36(3):959-969, 2000.
14. Chen ZM, Pan HC, Chen YP et al: Early intravenous, then oral metoprolol in 45,852 patients with acute myocardial infarction: randomised placebo-controlled trial, *Lancet* 366(9497):1622-1632, 2005.
15. Yusuf S, Peto R, Lewis J et al: Beta blockade during and after myocardial infarction: an overview of the randomized trials, *Prog Cardiovasc Dis* 27(5):335-371, 1985.
16. Randomised trial of intravenous atenolol among 16,027 cases of suspected acute myocardial infarction: ISIS-1—First International Study of Infarct Survival Collaborative Group, *Lancet* 2(8498):57-66, 1986.
17. Indications for ACE inhibitors in the early treatment of acute myocardial infarction: systematic overview of individual data

from 100,000 patients in randomized trials—ACE Inhibitor Myocardial Infarction Collaborative Group, *Circulation* 97(22):2202-2212, 1998.

18. Moser DK, Riegel B, McKinley S et al: Impact of anxiety and perceived control on in-hospital complications after acute myocardial infarction, *Psychosom Med* (in press).

19. Iwakura K, Ito H, Ikushima M et al: Association between hyperglycemia and the no-reflow phenomenon in patients with acute myocardial infarction, *J Am Coll Cardiol* 41(1):1-7, 2003.

20. Antman EM, Lau J, Kupelnick B et al: A comparison of results of meta-analyses of randomized control trials and recommendations of clinical experts: treatments for myocardial infarction, *JAMA* 268(2):240-248, 1992.

21. Bradley EH, Herrin J, Elbel B et al: Hospital quality for acute myocardial infarction: correlation among process measures and relationship with short-term mortality, *JAMA* 296(1):72-78, 2006.

22. McNamara RL, Herrin J, Bradley EH et al: Hospital improvement in time to reperfusion in patients with acute myocardial infarction, 1999 to 2002, *J Am Coll Cardiol* 47(1):45-51, 2006.

23. Jha AK, Li Z, Orav EJ et al: Care in US hospitals: the Hospital Quality Alliance program, *N Engl J Med* 353(3):265-274, 2005.

24. Wu AH, Parsons L, Every NR et al: Hospital outcomes in patients presenting with congestive heart failure complicating acute myocardial infarction: a report from the Second National Registry of Myocardial Infarction (NRMI-2), *J Am Coll Cardiol* 40(8):1389-1394, 2002.

25. Ellis C, Gamble G, French J et al: Management of patients admitted with an acute coronary syndrome in New Zealand: results of a comprehensive nationwide audit, *N Z Med J* 117(1197):U953, 2004.

26. Granger CB, Steg PG, Peterson E et al: Medication performance measures and mortality following acute coronary syndromes, *Am J Med* 118(8):858-865, 2005.

27. Roe MT, Parsons LS, Pollack CV Jr et al: Quality of care by classification of myocardial infarction: treatment patterns for ST-segment elevation vs non–ST-segment elevation myocardial infarction, *Arch Intern Med* 165(14):1630-1636, 2005.

28. Graff LG, Wang Y, Borkowski B et al: Delay in the diagnosis of acute myocardial infarction: effect on quality of care and its assessment, *Acad Emerg Med* 13(9):931-938, 2006.

29. Ellerbeck EF, Bhimaraj A, Hall S: Impact of organizational infrastructure on beta-blocker and aspirin therapy for acute myocardial infarction, *Am Heart J* 152(3):579-584, 2006.

30. Tang E, Wong CK, Wilkins G et al: Use of evidence-based management for acute coronary syndrome, *N Z Med J* 118(1223):U1678, 2005.

31. Luthi JC, McClellan WM, Flanders WD et al: Variations in the quality of care of patients with acute myocardial infarction among Swiss university hospitals, *Int J Qual Health Care* 17(3):229-234, 2005.

32. Garcia-Castillo A, Jerjes-Sanchez C, Martinez Bermudez P et al: Mexican Registry of Acute Coronary Syndromes, *Arch Cardiol Mex* 75(suppl 1):S6-S32, 2005.

33. Ferreira J, Monteiro P, Mimoso J: National Registry of Acute Coronary Syndromes: results of the hospital phase in 2002, *Rev Port Cardiol* 23(10):1251-1272, 2004.

34. Bratzler DW, Oehlert WH, Walkingstick K et al: Care of acute myocardial infarction in Oklahoma: an update from the Cooperative Cardiovascular Project, *J Okla State Med Assoc* 94(10):443-450, 2001.

35. Bansal D, Gaddam V, Aude YW et al: Trends in the care of patients with acute myocardial infarction at a university-affiliated Veterans Affairs Medical Center, *J Cardiovasc Pharmacol Ther* 10(1):39-44, 2005.

36. Bradley EH, Herrin J, Mattera JA et al: Quality improvement efforts and hospital performance: rates of beta-blocker prescription after acute myocardial infarction, *Med Care* 43(3):282-292, 2005.

37. Nallamothu BK, Wang Y, Magid DJ et al: Relation between hospital specialization with primary percutaneous coronary intervention and clinical outcomes in ST-segment elevation myocardial infarction: National Registry of Myocardial Infarction-4 analysis, *Circulation* 113(2):222-229, 2006.

38. Bradley EH, Herrin J, Wang Y et al: Door-to-drug and door-to-balloon times: where can we improve? Time to reperfusion therapy in patients with ST-segment elevation myocardial infarction (STEMI), *Am Heart J* 151(6):1281-1287, 2006.

39. Magid DJ, Wang Y, Herrin J et al: Relationship between time of day, day of week, timeliness of reperfusion, and in-hospital mortality for patients with acute ST-segment elevation myocardial infarction, *JAMA* 294(7):803-812, 2005.

40. Fox KA, Goodman SG, Anderson FA Jr et al: From guidelines to clinical practice: the impact of hospital and geographical characteristics on temporal trends in the management of acute coronary syndromes: the Global Registry of Acute Coronary Events (GRACE), *Eur Heart J* 24(15):1414-1424, 2003.

41. Nallamothu BK, Bates ER, Herrin J et al: Times to treatment in transfer patients undergoing primary percutaneous coronary intervention in the United States: National Registry of Myocardial Infarction (NRMI)-3/4 analysis, *Circulation* 111(6):761-767, 2005.

42. Chen J, Radford MJ, Wang Y et al: Do "America's Best Hospitals" perform better for acute myocardial infarction? *N Engl J Med* 340(4):286-292, 1999.

43. Krumholz HM, Rathore SS, Chen J et al: Evaluation of a consumer-oriented internet health care report card: the risk of quality ratings based on mortality data, *JAMA* 287(10):1277-1287, 2002.

44. Williams SC, Koss RG, Morton DJ et al: Performance of top-ranked heart care hospitals on evidence-based process measures, *Circulation* 114(6):558-564, 2006.

45. Nolan T, Berwick DM: All-or-none measurement raises the bar on performance. *JAMA* 295(10): 1168-1170, 2006.

46. Centers for Medicare & Medicaid Services. 8th Scope of Work (version 080105-1). Available at: www.cms.hhs.gov/QualityImprovementOrgs/Downloads/8thSOW.pdf. Accessed January 21, 2007.

■■■ c h a p t e r **58**

Care of Patients Undergoing Fibrinolytic Therapy and Percutaneous Coronary Intervention

Rose Shaffer

CHAPTER ABBREVIATIONS

ACC   American College of Cardiology

AHA   American Heart Association

CK   creatine kinase

DCA   directional coronary atherectomy

FFR   fractional flow reserve

GP   glycoprotein

IVUS   intravascular ultrasound

Non-STEMI   non–ST segment elevation myocardial infarction

PCI   percutaneous coronary intervention

PT   prothrombin time

PTCA   percutaneous transluminal coronary angioplasty

PTT   partial thromboplastin time

SCAI   Society for Cardiovascular Angiography and Interventions

STEMI   ST segment elevation myocardial infarction

TIMI   Thrombolysis in Myocardial Infarction

t-PA   tissue plasminogen activator

CORONARY ARTERY DISEASE AND ACUTE CORONARY SYNDROME

Coronary artery disease affects about 13,000,000 persons each year and is the leading cause of death in the United States. Patients who have experienced an acute myocardial infarction, unstable angina, chronic stable angina, or asymptomatic coronary ischemia may be diagnosed with coronary artery disease after undergoing coronary angiography. The term *acute coronary syndrome* refers to one of three entities: ST segment elevation myocardial infarction (**STEMI**), non–ST segment elevation myocardial infarction (**non-STEMI**), or unstable angina. Determination of the diagnosis depends on the presence or absence of ST segment elevation on the 12-lead electrocardiogram and the presence or absence of cardiac biochemical markers (creatine kinase [**CK**], the CK isoenzyme MB, and troponin) in the bloodstream.[1]

The American College of Cardiology (**ACC**) and the American Heart Association (**AHA**) developed the Task Force on Practice Guidelines in order to gather evidence-based information and to make recommendations about the diagnosis and treatment of patients with cardiovascular disease.[2] The ACC/AHA created guidelines for the management of patients with STEMI,[3,4] unstable angina/non-STEMI,[2,5] and chronic stable angina.[6] Within each of the guidelines the role of percutaneous

coronary intervention (**PCI**) is discussed. The role of fibrinolytic therapy is discussed within the ACC/AHA STEMI guideline[4] because it remains an important reperfusion strategy for this group of patients. In addition, the ACC, AHA and the Society for Cardiovascular Angiography and Interventions (**SCAI**) developed an updated evidence-based guideline for patients undergoing PCI.[7]

When a patient has chest pain, it is important to obtain a focused history and physical examination, blood work, and 12-lead electrocardiogram. If the electrocardiogram demonstrates 0.1 mV or greater of ST segment elevation in two or more contiguous leads (0.2 mV or greater in leads V_1 to V_3), a new left bundle branch block, or a true posterior myocardial infarction, the evidence suggests that the patient is experiencing STEMI.[8] STEMI is caused by an occlusive thrombus in a coronary artery. Blood work may demonstrate the presence of cardiac biochemical markers, which are released into the bloodstream when myocardial necrosis occurs. Aside from the standard treatment for STEMI, which includes oxygen, pain relief (using nitrates and/or analgesics), and aspirin (160 mg to 325 mg), the immediate treatment for STEMI includes early reperfusion therapy with the goal of limiting infarct size and improving survival.[3,4] Reperfusion can be accomplished pharmacologically with fibrinolytic therapy or mechanically with primary PCI.[3] Primary PCI is defined as emergent coronary angiography followed by PCI without administration of fibrinolytic therapy in patients who have STEMI.[9,10]

Unstable angina and non-STEMI are caused by an imbalance between myocardial oxygen supply and demand. The imbalance may be caused by a nonocclusive thrombus that develops on an existing ruptured plaque or because of abnormal constriction of the coronary arteries. Unstable angina and non-STEMI are considered closely related conditions. The difference is based on whether the ischemia present is severe enough to cause myocardial necrosis, as evidenced by the release of cardiac biochemical markers into the bloodstream. Once biochemical marker results are obtained, the diagnosis may be delineated further as unstable angina or non-STEMI because cardiac biochemical markers are released only when a patient experiences a non-STEMI. A patient with unstable angina exhibits the typical discomfort associated with stable angina, but the episodes may be prolonged, more frequent, and more severe and may occur at rest or with less effort than usual. In addition, unstable angina may be defined as new-onset angina of less than 2 months' duration.[2]

Standard treatment for unstable angina and non-STEMI includes oxygen, pain relief (using nitrates and/or analgesics) and aspirin. Immediate reperfusion therapy with fibrinolytic therapy is not recommended for unstable angina or non-STEMI.[4] The role of PCI in unstable angina and non-STEMI has been studied, and an early invasive strategy (coronary angiography within 48 hours after presentation, followed immediately by PCI, if indicated) is associated with improved outcomes compared with a conservative strategy (standard medical therapy, with coronary angiography and possible PCI, if chest pain or ischemia persists).[11-13]

Stable angina often is caused by exertion or emotional stress and is relieved with rest or sublingual nitroglycerin administration. Angina usually occurs when there is angiographic evidence of obstructive coronary plaque (≥70 percent stenosis of left anterior descending, left circumflex and/or right coronary artery or ≥50 percent stenosis of the left main coronary artery) in at least one major coronary artery on coronary angiography.[6] If there is a moderate to large area of myocardial ischemia identified on noninvasive stress testing in a patient with stable angina, PCI may benefit the patient if there is a high chance of success and a low risk of mortality and morbidity. Although coronary artery bypass graft surgery is the choice of revascularization for unprotected left main coronary artery disease (i.e., left main coronary artery disease in patients who have not undergone previous coronary artery bypass graft surgery), PCI using drug-eluting stents is a feasible option in select patients that may improve cardiovascular outcomes in patients who are not eligible to undergo coronary artery bypass graft surgery. The ACC/AHA/SCAI guideline recommends follow-up angiography after PCI of an unprotected left main coronary artery within 2 to 6 months.[7]

Asymptomatic coronary ischemia is present when a patient is without angina but has myocardial ischemia identified by noninvasive stress testing. Although pharmacological therapy and risk factor modification usually is prescribed for such patients, PCI may be performed for the same reasons as in chronic stable angina.[7]

Fibrinolytic therapy and primary PCI play an important role in the treatment of patients with STEMI. Nurses must understand the pharmacology of fibrinolytic therapy so they can provide optimal care for their patients during and after therapy. The number of primary and elective PCIs continues to grow each year. Many hospitals are building cardiac catheterization laboratories with PCI capability because the literature supports primary PCI as the preferred treatment option over fibrinolytic therapy for STEMI.[9] Nurses must be knowledgeable regarding the care of patients before and after PCI in order to deliver quality care to this patient population. The purpose of this chapter is to review the relevant literature and discuss the care of patients receiving fibrinolytic therapy and PCI.

FIBRINOLYTIC THERAPY
History of Fibrinolytic Therapy

Fibrinolytic therapy dates to 1958 when the first description of a prolonged infusion of streptokinase for patients with acute myocardial infarction was published.[14] Rentrop and colleagues[15] reported the use of intracoronary streptokinase for acute myocardial infarction in 1979. This was the dawning of the age of fibrinolytic therapy.[16] Use of intracoronary streptokinase was found to salvage ischemic myocardium, resulting in less myocardial damage and greater preservation of left ventricular function. Many trials using intravenous fibrinolytic therapy followed, demonstrating improvement in mortality after acute STEMI.

In 1980, DeWood and colleagues[17] published a paper on the prevalence of coronary artery thrombosis in acute myocardial infarction. Today, it is widely accepted that STEMI is a result of vulnerable plaque rupture (Figure 58-1). A vulnerable plaque is described as a nonobstructive plaque composed of a large lipid core covered by a thin fibrous cap.[18] Plaque rupture results in endo-

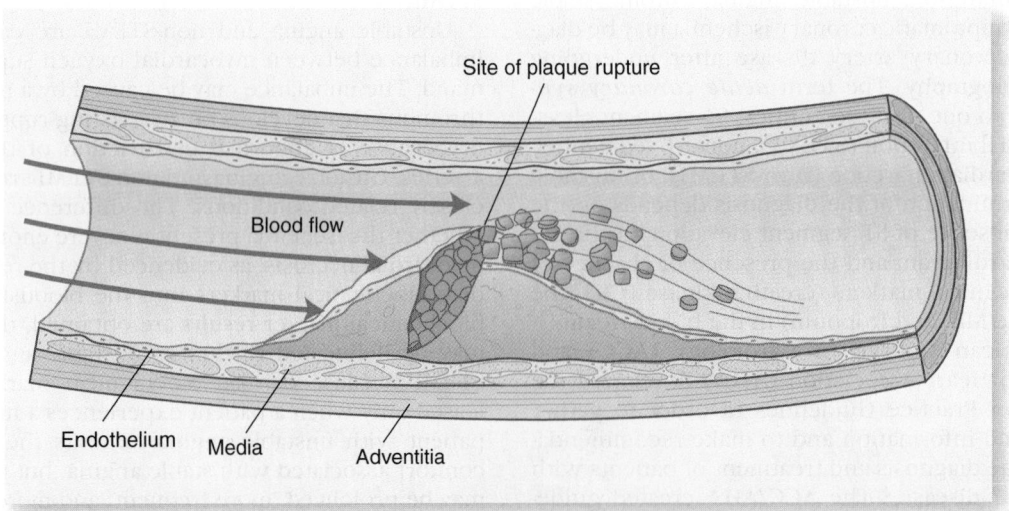

FIGURE 58-1 ■ Diagram of a ruptured vulnerable plaque responsible for ST segment elevation myocardial infarction. (From Braunwald E, Goldman L: *Primary cardiology,* ed 2, Philadelphia, 2003, Saunders.)

thelial cell injury, which causes platelet adhesion, activation, and aggregation and leads to accelerated thrombin production. Thrombin in turn converts fibrinogen to fibrin.[19] The resulting thrombus includes a high concentration of platelets ("white clots") and fibrin ("red clots").[19,20] The thin fibrin strands form a matrix, trapping more platelets and plasminogen at or near the clot surface. The body produces and breaks down physiological thrombi (those that heal a vessel) and pathological thrombi (those that occlude a vessel).[19] Fibrinolytic agents use the intrinsic thromboresistant defense mechanism of the vascular system to break down thrombi. In the presence of fibrin the endogenous tissue plasminogen activator binds to fibrin in the thrombus, converting the inactive precursor, plasminogen, to the active enzyme, plasmin. Plasmin in turn breaks down the fibrin matrix, causing lysis of the clot. Fibrinolysis (the breakdown of fibrin) also is referred to as thrombolysis (the breakdown of thrombus).[20]

Early fibrinolytic agents are referred to as fibrin nonspecific agents because they targeted not only newly formed fibrin-rich pathological thrombi but also normal physiological thrombi. This results in a systemic lytic state, which can cause serious systemic bleeding. Newer fibrinolytic agents have been developed, referred to as fibrin-specific agents, that target newly formed fibrin present in pathological thrombi while limiting the effect on physiological thrombi.[20]

Fibrinolytic therapy is indicated only for STEMI because it is caused by a complete thrombotic occlusion in a coronary artery. Coronary blood flow on angiography is measured using a scale developed by the Thrombolysis in Myocardial Infarction (**TIMI**) investigators[21] (Table 58-1). TIMI 3 flow indicates full restoration of blood flow to the myocardium. It has been reported that only 50 to 60 percent of patients achieve TIMI 3 blood flow after fibrinolytic therapy, and of these, only two thirds achieve TIMI 3 flow within 90 minutes after treatment.[21,22] Early restoration of TIMI 3 flow to the myocardium beyond the thrombotic occlusion is important to salvage myocardium, limit infarct size, and improve survival in patients with STEMI.[22,23] Over the years, limitations and complications of fibrinolytic therapy were discovered, leading to the development of newer

agents with improved efficacy and ease of administration.[16] The advantages and disadvantages of fibrinolytic therapy can be found in Box 58-1.

The most widely used first-generation fibrinolytic agent was streptokinase. Streptokinase is used infrequently today because it lacks fibrin specificity. More fibrin-specific agents have been developed. The second-generation fibrinolytic agent, tissue plasminogen activator (**t-PA** or alteplase) is more fibrin-specific than streptokinase. Alteplase activates plasmin by breaking down plasminogen at the fibrin surface where there is a high affinity for binding. Third-generation fibrinolytic agents were developed to provide safer dosing regimens and more effective therapy. Recombinant plasminogen activator (reteplase) and tenecteplase are the newest fibrin-specific fibrinolytic agents.[23] Dosing regimens for fibrinolytic agents can be found in the pharmacology feature.

■ ■ ■

TABLE 58-1   THE THROMBOLYSIS IN MYOCARDIAL INFARCTION (TIMI) FLOW SCALE

SCALE	COMMENT
TIMI grade 0	No perfusion Absence of antegrade flow beyond the point of occlusion
TIMI grade 1	Penetration without perfusion Partial penetration of contrast medium beyond the obstruction with absence of filling of the distal vessel
TIMI grade 2	Partial perfusion Patency of the vessel but with delayed filling
TIMI grade 3	Complete perfusion Normal brisk antegrade flow

Modified from The Thrombolysis in Myocardial Infarction (TIMI) trial: phase 1 findings—TIMI Study Group, *N Engl J Med* 312:932-936, 1985.

BOX 58-1   ■ ■ ■
ADVANTAGES AND DISADVANTAGES
OF FIBRINOLYTIC THERAPY

Advantages
Does not require access to catheterization laboratory facilities
Treats the underlying problem of a central occluding thrombus
Documented efficacy in large, well-controlled trials

Disadvantages
Despite widespread availability, fibrinolytic therapy is given only in approximately 30 to 40 percent of patients with acute myocardial infarction; absolute or relative contraindications are frequent
Not effective for hemodynamic instability
Early reperfusion rates range from 55 to 80 percent depending on agent used
Achievement of TIMI-3 flow in less than 50 to 60 percent of patients
Reliable assessment of reperfusion often not possible
Residual stenosis

From Califf RM: Acute myocardial infarction and other acute ischemic syndromes. In Braunwald E, editor: *Essential atlas of heart diseases,* ed 2, Philadelphia, 2001, Current Medicine.

■ ■ ■ **PHARMACOLOGY**

FIBRINOLYTIC AGENTS AND DOSES

DRUG	DOSE
Streptokinase	1.5 million units IV over 30-60 minutes
Alteplase	IV bolus 15 mg Infusion 0.75 mg/kg over 30 minutes (maximum 50 mg) Then 0.5 mg/kg not to exceed 35 mg over the next 60 minutes to an overall maximum dose of 100 mg
Reteplase	10 units IV over 2 minutes 30 minutes after first dose, give repeated dose of 10 units IV over 2 minutes
Tenecteplase	IV bolus over 10-15 seconds, based on weight, as follows: 30 mg for weight less than 60 kg 35 mg for 60-69 kg 40 mg for 70-79 kg 45 mg for 80-89 kg 50 mg for 90 kg or more

From Antman EM, Anbe DT, Armstrong PW et al: ACC/AHA pocket guideline: management of patients with ST-elevation myocardial infarction. Retrieved February 11, 2007, from *www.acc.org/qualityandscience/clinical/guidelines/stemi/index_pkt.pdf.* Based on Antman EM, Anbe DT, Armstrong PW et al: *J Am Coll Cardiol* 44:671-719, 2004.

Fibrinolytic Agents
Streptokinase
Streptokinase is a nonenzymatic protein derived from beta-hemolytic streptococci.[20] Streptokinase activates the fibrinolytic system by activating plasminogen and converting it to plasmin. Although streptokinase was the most commonly used first-generation fibrinolytic,[23] it is used rarely today for several reasons to be discussed further.

The first large mortality trial evaluating streptokinase enrolled more than 11,000 patients within 12 hours of a suspected acute myocardial infarction. Patients were randomized to receive streptokinase or standard medical therapy. In-hospital mortality was reduced significantly in patients who received streptokinase compared with patients who received standard medical therapy. An important note is that only 14 percent of patients in the study received aspirin and only 62 percent received heparin. Treatment with streptokinase reduced mortality, but the reduction was found to be time dependent. A 47 percent reduction in mortality was found for patients treated within 1 hour of the onset of symptoms, a 23 percent reduction for patients treated within 3 hours, and a 17 percent reduction for patients treated within 6 hours of the onset of symptoms. This trial demonstrated the importance of time of symptom onset to initiation of fibrinolytic therapy.[24]

Another study evaluating intravenous streptokinase enrolled more than 17,000 patients who had STEMI. Patients were randomized to receive aspirin alone, streptokinase alone, aspirin and streptokinase, or neither medication. One of the important outcomes of this trial was the synergistic effect of aspirin with streptokinase, in which there was a significant reduction in vascular mortality. Additionally, investigators noted that patients treated within 6 hours of the onset of symptoms had significantly better survival rates.[25]

In addition to the lack of fibrin specificity, streptokinase has several other problems that limit the use of the medication. Streptokinase has the potential to be antigenic, causing an allergic response (fever, pruritus, nausea, flushing, urticaria, headache, and malaise). Hypotension is common with streptokinase therapy. In addition, patients who receive streptokinase or those with a recent streptococcal infection develop antistreptokinase antibodies. Therefore, repeated use is not recommended.[23] To combat these limitations, newer fibrinolytic medications have been developed.

Tissue Plasminogen Activator
Endogenous t-PA is a serine protease.[20] Exogenous t-PA for clinical use is manufactured by recombinant DNA techniques and is referred to as t-PA or alteplase.[23] t-PA is a relatively weak enzyme in the absence of fibrin, but when fibrin is present, plasminogen activation is enhanced significantly. Plasminogen activation, with subsequent conversion to plasmin, occurs on the fibrin surface, with little plasminogen activation elsewhere in the body, making alteplase more fibrin-specific than streptokinase.[20] Alteplase is not antigenic.

Two mortality trials were undertaken to evaluate alteplase.[22,26] The investigators in one large study of more than 41,000 patients[26] found that patients receiving alteplase plus intravenously administered heparin had a significant decrease in 30-day mortality compared with the other three arms of the study (streptokinase with subcutaneously administered heparin, streptokinase with intravenously administered heparin, and a combination of alteplase and streptokinase with intravenously administered heparin). A substudy of the larger trial randomized more than 2400 patients to undergo coronary angiography at 90 minutes, 180 minutes, 24 hours, or 5 days after receiving fibrinolytic therapy. The alteplase-treated patients had significantly higher patency rates at 90 minutes and a higher incidence of TIMI 3 flow. At the other three points in time, there were no significant differences noted. Use of alteplase was associated with early opening of the occluded coronary artery and decreased mortality at 30 days posttreatment.[22]

Reteplase
Reteplase, a third-generation fibrinolytic, was one of the first mutant t-PA agents to undergo extensive clinical trials.[16] Reteplase was developed with the intent to retain plasminogen activity and fibrin specificity but with a longer half-life to permit bolus administration. Reteplase does not require weight-based dosing, making for easier administration.[23] An angiographic trial compared reteplase with alteplase in 324 patients who had STEMI. The investigators found statistically better TIMI 3 flow for patients who received reteplase compared with patients who received alteplase at 60 minutes and 90 minutes after treatment. The 35-day posttreatment mortality rate, incidence of bleeding requiring transfusion, and incidence of hemorrhagic stroke was not statistically significant between the two groups.[27] Other investigators compared reteplase with alteplase in more than 15,000 patients with STEMI. No significant differences in 30-day posttreatment mortality or stroke were found.[28] The main advantage of reteplase over alteplase is the ease of administering the fixed-dose double-bolus medication.[23]

Tenecteplase
Tenecteplase is the newest of the fibrin-specific agents. Tenecteplase is structurally identical to endogenous t-PA except for three mutations.[23] Tenecteplase has a longer half-life, which allows for a single bolus intravenous injection. Comparison of tenecteplase and alteplase was undertaken in one study in which more than 16,000 patients who had STEMI were randomized to receive alteplase or tenecteplase within 6 hours of symptom onset. Overall 30-day posttreatment mortality, as well as the rate of intracranial hemorrhage and stroke, were similar between the two groups. The rate of major noncerebral bleeding and need for transfusion was significantly lower with patients treated with tenecteplase.[29] The simple bolus dose makes this agent easier to administer.

Rationale for Bolus Dose Fibrinolytic Therapy Versus Infusion of Fibrinolytic Therapy
Overall, the clinical benefit of all of the fibrinolytic agents is well documented.[22,24-29] However, the two agents that offer bolus dosing (reteplase and te-

necteplase) have several advantages in the clinical arena. First, bolus dosing allows easier and safer administration and may facilitate more rapid treatment of STEMI. Door-to-drug time may be reduced with a simple bolus fibrinolytic agent that does not require time to perform drug calculations. Reducing door-to-drug time is critical to myocardial preservation and reduction in mortality. Second, prehospital administration may be facilitated using bolus dose therapy for the same reasons. This approach could reduce medical contact-to-drug time, again to preserve myocardium and reduce mortality. The third reason bolus dosing is more attractive is that it could decrease medication errors,[16] particularly when rapid mathematical calculations are needed in an intense situation. Decreasing medication errors is a high priority in the health care arena.[30,31]

Fibrinolytic Therapy: Contraindications and Complications

Many patients are not eligible to receive fibrinolytic therapy based on relative and absolute contraindications.[10] Box 58-2 lists the contraindications and cautions

---

BOX 58-2 ■ ■ ■
CONTRAINDICATIONS AND CAUTIONS FOR FIBRINOLYTIC THERAPY USE IN ST SEGMENT ELEVATION MYOCARDIAL INFARCTION

These are advisory guidelines for clinical decision making and may not be all-inclusive or definitive.

Absolute Contraindications
- Any prior intracranial hemorrhage
- Known structural cerebral vascular lesion (i.e., arteriovenous malformation)
- Known malignant intracranial neoplasm (primary or metastatic)
- Ischemic stroke within 3 months EXCEPT acute ischemic stroke within 3 hours
- Suspected aortic dissection
- Active bleeding or bleeding diathesis (excluding menses)
- Significant closed head or facial trauma within 3 months

Relative Contraindications
- History of chronic, severe, poorly controlled hypertension
- Severe uncontrolled hypertension on presentation (systolic blood pressure greater than 180 mm Hg or diastolic blood pressure greater than 110 mm Hg)*
- History of ischemic stroke greater than 3 months, dementia, or known intracranial pathological condition not covered in contraindications
- Traumatic or prolonged (greater than 10 minutes) cardiopulmonary resuscitation or major surgery (less than 3 weeks)
- Recent (within 2 to 4 weeks) internal bleeding
- Noncompressible vascular punctures
- For streptokinase/anistreplase: prior exposure (more than 5 days ago) or prior allergic reaction to these agents
- Pregnancy
- Active peptic ulcer
- Current use of anticoagulants: the higher the international normalized ratio, the higher the risk of bleeding

*Could be an absolute contraindication in low-risk patients.
From Antman EM, Anbe DT, Armstrong PW et al: ACC/AHA guidelines for the management of patients with ST-elevation myocardial infarction: executive summary—a report of the American College of Cardiology/American Heart Association Task Force on Practice Guidelines (Writing Committee to revise the 1999 guidelines on the management of patients with acute myocardial infarction), *J Am Coll Cardiol* 44:671-719, 2004.

---

for fibrinolytic therapy use in STEMI.[4] The main complication of fibrinolytic therapy is bleeding. Intracranial hemorrhage is the most devastating bleeding complication. The Fibrinolytic Therapy Trialists' Collaborative Group[32] reviewed nine large randomized trials and found an excess of 3.9 strokes per 1000 patients treated with fibrinolytic therapy versus placebo. Reducing the dosage of intravenously administered heparin and timing of the measurement of the partial thromboplastin time (**PTT**) decreases the risk of intracranial hemorrhage.[16] The Fibrinolytic Therapy Trialists' Collaborative Group[32] also reported a 1.1 percent incidence of major bleeding (requiring blood transfusions or bleeding considered life-threatening) in patients receiving fibrinolytic therapy compared with 0.4 percent of patients receiving placebo.

The Cooperative Cardiovascular Project[33] analyzed data from more than 31,500 patients over age 65 who received fibrinolytic therapy in 1994 and 1995. Intracranial hemorrhage occurred in 1.43 percent of patients. The authors identified several independent predictors of intracranial hemorrhage including the following: age 75 years or older, black race, female sex, history of stroke, systolic blood pressure 160 mm Hg or higher, weight 64 kg or less for women and 80 kg or less for men, international normalized ratio greater than 4 or prothrombin time (**PT**) greater than 24 seconds, and use of alteplase (versus another agent).

Nursing Care of the Patient Undergoing Fibrinolytic Therapy

Most institutions have protocols in place to provide rapid reperfusion when a patient has STEMI. Protocols usually include giving aspirin and oxygen, obtaining a 12-lead electrocardiogram and blood work, and placing the patient on a cardiac monitor. Blood work should include a complete blood count, electrolytes, blood urea nitrogen, creatinine, PT, PTT, and cardiac biochemical markers [CK, CK-MB, and troponin]. A blood type and crossmatch may be obtained because bleeding is a potential complication of fibrinolytic therapy. Obtaining a focused history and physical examination is critical. In obtaining the history, it is essential to determine the time of symptom onset. Also important is to determine whether there are any relative or absolute contraindications to fibrinolytic therapy. A list of contraindications should be readily available.

Whenever possible, all arterial and venous lines should be placed before fibrinolytic therapy is delivered in order to decrease the risk of bleeding from puncture sites. Before initiation of fibrinolytic therapy, insertion of two to three intravenous catheters is recommended.[34] One line should be dedicated to the fibrinolytic medication (especially when a fibrinolytic medication requiring a continuous infusion is used). One line should be used for concomitant intravenous heparin therapy and intravenous fluids. That line also may be used for any intravenous medications compatible with heparin. The third intravenous catheter should be connected to a saline lock and used as needed (with any intravenous medications not compatible with heparin, as a backup intravenous access, or for blood sampling). An arterial line may be placed for continuous blood pressure monitoring and for blood sampling during and after the course of fibrinolytic therapy.

Intravenous or arterial catheters should be placed at sites where firm compression can be accomplished if bleeding should occur at the insertion site (subclavian and jugular sites should be avoided because they are difficult areas to apply firm manual compression). Intramuscular and subcutaneous injections should be avoided for 24 hours after fibrinolytic therapy, if possible, to prevent hematoma formation. If venepuncture must be performed within the first 24 hours, manual pressure should be applied for 20 to 30 minutes after withdrawal of the needle followed by placement of a secure pressure dressing. The access site must be monitored closely for development of bleeding or a hematoma. Intravenous and arterial lines should not be discontinued for 24 hours after fibrinolytic therapy in order to reduce the risk of bleeding.[34]

Patients and families must be informed that bleeding and bruising are common with fibrinolytic therapy. Provide reassurance that precautions to prevent bleeding and bruising will be taken (i.e., padding side rails and limiting injections and venepunctures).[34]

Nursing care in the intensive care unit or coronary care unit includes frequent monitoring of vital signs for assessment of hemodynamic stability. The use of noninvasive blood pressure monitoring has caused concern that it may increase the risk of bruising on the extremity. One study compared the safety of using noninvasive blood cuff measurements to manual blood pressure cuff measurements during fibrinolytic therapy and 24 hours after therapy. The 96 patients in the study received streptokinase or alteplase after presenting with STEMI. The investigators found no significant difference in frequency of petechiae, ecchymosis, or hematoma formation between patients who had blood pressure measured with a noninvasive cuff and those who had blood pressure measured manually.[35]

There are several markers of successful reperfusion after fibrinolytic therapy. Ongoing evaluation of chest pain (resolution or recurrence) is one way to assess reperfusion. If fibrinolytic therapy is successful, chest pain usually improves within 90 minutes of treatment. However, analgesics or nitrates given concomitantly may mask true relief of pain from fibrinolytic therapy; therefore, other markers of reperfusion should be assessed.[36]

Serial 12-lead electrocardiograms should be performed to monitor ST segments for evidence of recurrent ischemia or extension of the STEMI. Within the first few hours after fibrinolytic therapy, a downward trend of the ST segments back to baseline in the leads facing the area of infarction is an indication of successful reperfusion of the occluded coronary artery.[36]

If the bedside monitoring system has continuous ST segment monitoring capability, it should be used to monitor for recurrent ischemia or extension of the STEMI, in addition to serial 12-lead electrocardiograms. For patients who have STEMI, the AHA practice standards recommend monitoring ST segments in the lead(s) facing the area of infarction for a minimum of 24 hours

and continuing until the patient remains event-free for 12 to 24 hours.[37]

Cardiac monitoring is used to observe for reperfusion dysrhythmias, another potential marker of successful therapy. Reperfusion dysrhythmias occur because of the sudden influx of oxygenated blood to an injured, ischemic, and irritable myocardium. This causes electrical instability and often manifests as accelerated idioventricular rhythm, ventricular tachydysrhythmias, and bradydysrhythmias. Reperfusion dysrhythmias are treated with standard therapies if the patient exhibits hemodynamic instability.[36]

Serial blood work samples should be drawn per protocol, including a complete blood count, electrolytes, magnesium, and cardiac biochemical markers (CK, CK-MB, and troponin). The complete blood count is compared with pre–fibrinolytic therapy values to assess for occult bleeding. Stool and urine should be checked for occult blood. If significant blood loss is noted, a blood transfusion may be required. If hypokalemia or hypomagnesemia is noted, the potassium and magnesium should be replaced to decrease myocardial irritability. Successful reperfusion with fibrinolysis causes a rapid rise in the CK and CK-MB (usually within 4 hours) from the sudden influx of oxygenated blood into necrotic myocardial tissue. Without reperfusion therapy, the CK and CK-MB normally peak at 24 hours after an acute myocardial infarction.[36]

Ongoing assessment of the patient's neurological status is important to assess for early signs of intracranial hemorrhage (sudden onset of a focal neurological deficit that progresses quickly, accompanied by headache, nausea, vomiting, altered level of consciousness, and elevated blood pressure[38]). If the patient's neurological status changes, consider obtaining a neurology consult and computed tomography scan of the head.

Once the acute phase of the STEMI is over, focus should turn to patient and family education about secondary prevention measures (risk factor modification and medications). A cardiac catheterization may be recommended during the index hospitalization to better assess coronary anatomy. If obstructive coronary disease is found on coronary angiography, PCI or coronary artery bypass grafting surgery may be recommended.

PERCUTANEOUS CORONARY INTERVENTION
History of Percutaneous Coronary Intervention

Percutaneous transluminal coronary angioplasty (**PTCA**) was first performed in 1977 by Andreas Gruentzig.[39] In the early days of PTCA, the procedure was limited to patients with symptomatic coronary artery disease who had discrete focal lesions in the proximal portion of a major coronary artery. PTCA was used as an alternative to coronary artery bypass grafting. The concept of catheter-based reperfusion for STEMI was first introduced in 1979, when Rentrop and colleagues[40] reported initial clinical experience with balloon angioplasty to open an occluded coronary artery in seven patients with STEMI. Their data were compared with historical controls receiving conventional therapy. The investigators found that patients in the balloon angioplasty group had improved ventricular function on follow-up angiography.

PTCA involves using a balloon catheter to stretch the coronary arterial wall and rupture the atherosclerotic plaque. Rupturing the plaque causes plaque fracturing and fissuring, creating a tear in the endothelium. Arterial injury at the PTCA site accounts for two major limitations of the procedure: acute vessel closure and restenosis.

Acute vessel closure is common with PTCA without stenting, occurring in 6.8 to 8.3 percent of cases[41-43] and often within the first 24 hours after PTCA.[42,43] Acute vessel closure may be caused by coronary artery dissection, acute platelet-mediated thrombus formation, and/or elastic recoil of the vessel.[41,43] Clinical sequelae may include myocardial infarction or death. Patients may require urgent return to the catheterization laboratory for repeat procedures or emergent coronary artery bypass grafting surgery.[42,43]

Restenosis occurs in about 30 to 50 percent of patients undergoing PTCA within the first 6 months after the procedure.[44-46] Restenosis is due to chronic vessel shrinkage (negative remodeling of the artery), smooth muscle cell proliferation, and neointimal hyperplasia.[47] Balloon inflation causes arterial injury at the PTCA site, initiating inflammation, platelet aggregation, thrombus formation, and activation of smooth muscle cells. The inflammatory response causes release of cytokines and growth factors that stimulate cell division and proliferation. Smooth muscle cells migrate from the medial layer of the coronary artery to the intimal layer through the tear in the endothelium created by the balloon inflation, where they proliferate and cause restenosis. Thrombin, released from activated platelets, activates more platelets and attracts inflammatory cells, further stimulating smooth muscle cell proliferation.[47,48] This cellular reaction, referred to as neointimal hyperplasia, is the attempt by the body to repair the artery. Restenosis often resulted in the patient returning to the cardiac catheterization laboratory for repeat interventional procedures.[49]

BOX 58-3 ■ ■ ■

THE AMERICAN COLLEGE OF CARDIOLOGY/ AMERICAN HEART ASSOCIATION/SOCIETY FOR CARDIOVASCULAR ANGIOGRAPHY AND INTERVENTIONS CORONARY LESION CLASSIFICATION SYSTEM IN THE PERCUTANEOUS CORONARY INTERVENTION STENT ERA

High-Risk Lesions
- Diffuse (length greater than 20 mm)
- Excessive tortuosity of proximal segment
- Extremely angulated segments (greater than 90 degrees)
- Total occlusions less than 3 months old and/or bridging collateral vessels*
- Inability to protect major side branches
- Degenerated vein grafts with friable lesions*

*The high risk with these criteria is for technical failure and increased restenosis, not for acute complications
Smith SC Jr. Feldman TE. Hirshfeld JW et al: ACC/AHA/SCAI 2005 guideline update for percutaneous coronary intervention: a report of the American College of Cardiology/American Heart Association Task Force on Practice Guidelines (ACC/AHA/SCAI Writing Committee to Update 2001 Guidelines for Percutaneous Coronary Intervention), *Circulation* 113:e166-286, 2006.

In the early days of PTCA, equipment was cumbersome. During the 1980s and 1990s there were dramatic improvements in equipment and operator experience. In this decade, more acutely ill patients with more high-risk lesions are treated with PCI. Coronary stenoses are classified according to anatomical risk. The ACC/AHA/ SCAI lesion classification system helps predict procedural success by differentiating high-risk lesions (Box 58-3) from non–high-risk lesions. Figure 58-2 demonstrates a high-risk lesion in a gastroepiploic artery bypass graft caused by the extremely angulated (more than 90 percent) segment.

Today, technology extends beyond balloon angioplasty to include atherectomy devices, distal protection devices, and coronary stents, to name a few. PCI is the term used to encompass the new technologies.[7]

Coronary stents, approved by the U.S. Food and Drug Administration in 1994, help prevent acute vessel closure by acting like a scaffold inside the arterial wall,

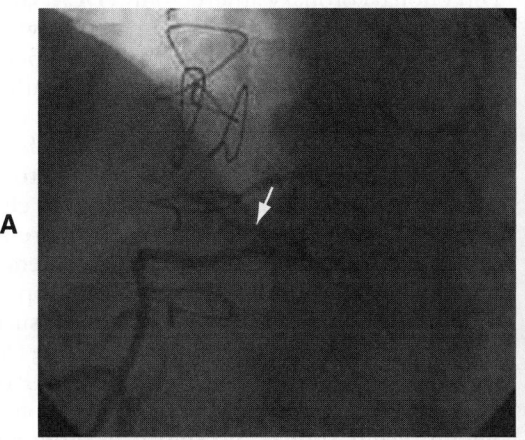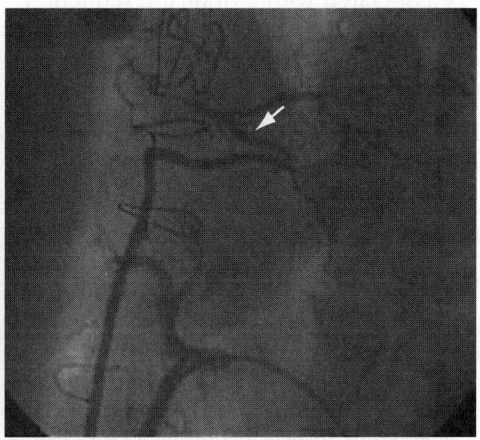

A   B

FIGURE 58-2 ■ **A,** A high-risk lesion *(arrow)* caused by the extremely angulated (greater than 90 degrees) segment in a gastroepiploic artery bypass to the distal right coronary artery. **B,** After percutaneous transluminal coronary angioplasty with stent placed *(arrow)* in the gastroepiploic artery bypass to the distal right coronary artery.

providing mechanical support to prevent elastic recoil of the artery. The original stents were not drug coated. Today these stents often are referred to as "bare metal" stents to distinguish them from drug-coated stents. Stents initially were used to "tack" down coronary artery dissection flaps. Coronary artery dissection occurs when the intimal layer of the artery separates from the medial layer of the artery (from balloon inflation) creating a false lumen for blood to enter, partially or fully obstructing blood flow through the artery.

Although the problem of acute vessel closure has been reduced with the introduction of stents, restenosis within the stent (stenosis greater than 70 percent), referred to as in-stent restenosis, continues to be a problem resulting from neointimal hyperplasia. Restenosis occurs in about 20 percent of patients in the first 6 months following bare metal stent implantation.[49,50] Treatment with repeat balloon angioplasty within the stent is associated with up to a 60 percent restenosis rate.[51] In 2000 the Food and Drug Administration approved a procedure involving intracoronary radiation, referred to as intracoronary brachytherapy, to address the issue of in-stent restenosis. This procedure is approved only for restenosis within a previously placed stent. PCI is performed to the restenosed area within the stent before delivery of a small dose of radiation inside the stent.[47,51] Brachytherapy is believed to work by inhibiting smooth muscle cell proliferation, thereby preventing neointimal hyperplasia and reducing the incidence of in-stent restenosis.[51]

Acute stent thrombosis was a major problem with early stent technology. Stent thrombosis occasionally resulted in myocardial infarction, emergent coronary artery bypass grafting surgery, and/or death. Aggressive anticoagulation with dipyridamole, aspirin, intravenously administered dextran, and heparin with crossover to warfarin did not adequately prevent acute stent thrombosis[52] and often caused hemorrhagic and peripheral vascular complications.[49,50,52] The need for better antithrombotic medications to prevent stent thrombosis, with fewer systemic side effects, led to the development of the first potent antiplatelet medication, ticlopidine (a thienopyridine). Ticlopidine, used in combination with aspirin, was associated with a dramatic reduction in stent thrombosis and vascular complications.[52]

In 2003 the U.S. Food and Drug Association approved the newest technology in stent design, the drug-eluting stent. These stents are thinner than the previous bare metal stents and have an antiproliferative medication within a polymer coating on the stent. Currently, two approved drug-eluting stents are on the market. Because of their antiproliferative properties and the slow release (elution) of the drug from the stent, the restenosis rate is less than 10 percent with drug-eluting stents.[53-56]

An estimated 657,000 PCI procedures were performed in the United States in 2002. The number of procedures increased 324 percent from 1987 to 2002. The rate of coronary stent insertion increased 147 percent between 1996 and 2000.[1] Drug-eluting stents have become a typical adjunct to PCI because they significantly reduce the rate of restenosis.

Percutaneous Coronary Interventional Technology

Percutaneous Transluminal Coronary Angioplasty

PTCA improves blood flow by expanding the lumen of the coronary artery (Figure 58-3). A sheath is inserted into the femoral, brachial, or radial artery. A guiding catheter is passed through the sheath. A guidewire then is threaded through the guiding catheter. A balloon (deflated) catheter is inserted over the guidewire and is positioned across the lesion. The balloon is inflated using a handheld inflation device. With inflation, the balloon creates a larger lumen by rupturing the plaque and stretching the arterial wall. The balloon also redistributes the plaque along the arterial wall.[57] PTCA improves ischemia by mechanically improving blood flow to the occluded coronary artery.

The advent of PTCA represented a significant advance in the treatment of coronary artery disease, but as solo therapy, it is limited by the incidence of acute vessel closure and restenosis. Balloon angioplasty is used for three purposes today: to predilate a coronary artery before stent implantation, to deploy a coronary stent, and to further expand (postdilate) a stent after deployment.[57]

Several adjunctive devices have been developed with the intent to reduce the restenosis rate. Although the devices work by different mechanisms, they were developed with the intent to debulk (ablate, shave, or cut) atheromatous plaque in order to minimize vessel injury and thereby reduce the incidence of restenosis. A meta-analysis of randomized trials comparing PTCA (with or without stenting) to special adjunctive devices (atherectomy, cutting balloon atherectomy, and laser angioplasty) did not reveal a significant reduction in mortality or restenosis with the use of these devices compared with PTCA. The analysis also revealed that adjunctive devices were associated with an increase in periprocedural myocardial infarction. The authors concluded that the routine use of adjunctive devices is not recommended.[58] Today, these devices are used only in patients with specific types of coronary lesions.

Directional Coronary Atherectomy

Directional coronary atherectomy (**DCA**; Guidant, Santa Clara, California) consists of a catheter with a cutting mechanism inside of a collection chamber and a low inflation pressure balloon that forces atherosclerotic plaque into the chamber during balloon inflation (Figure 58-4). The balloon is positioned within the lesion and is inflated. The plaque is shaved with the cutting mechanism and is stored in the collection chamber. The procedure may be repeated to shave more plaque. The device with the collection chamber is removed at the end of the procedure.[59] In theory, this approach would debulk the plaque, leaving a "smoother" surface, rather than the irregular jagged surface resulting from the ruptured plaque after balloon inflation with PTCA.[60] However, this did not prove true in one randomized trial in which results showed no statistical difference in restenosis on repeat coronary angiography between DCA-treated patients and PTCA-treated patients at 6 months post-PCI. Performing PTCA after DCA was discouraged

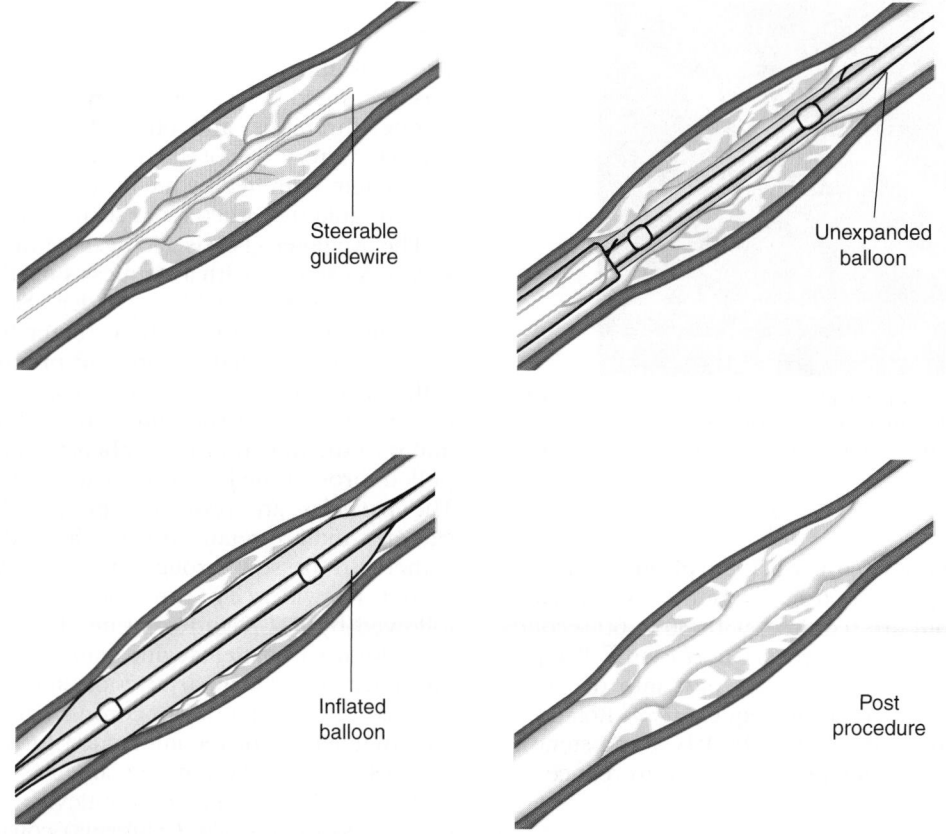

FIGURE 58-3 ▪ Illustration of percutaneous transluminal coronary angioplasty procedure. (Courtesy the Cordis Corporation.)

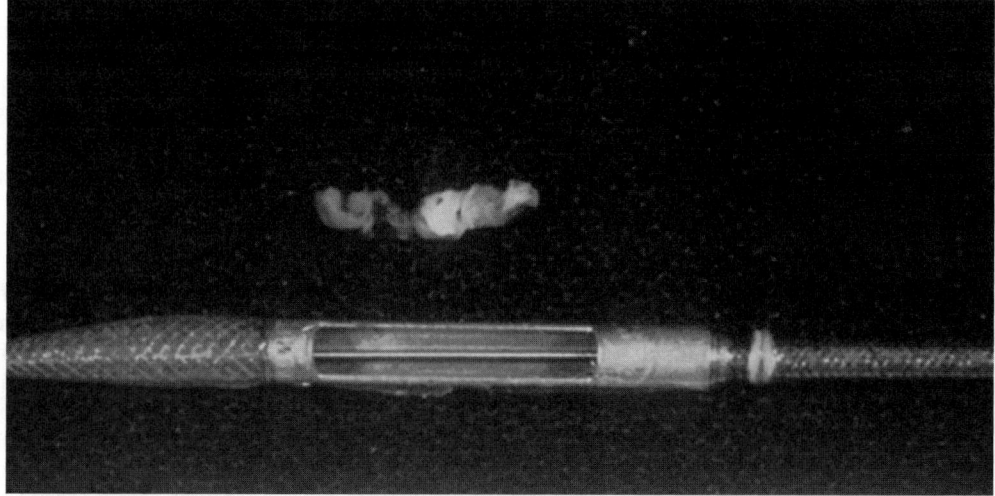

FIGURE 58-4 ▪ Directional coronary atherectomy device with resected tissue. (From Zipes DP, Libby P, Bonow RO, Braunwald E, editors: *Braunwald's heart disease: a textbook of cardiovascular medicine,* ed 7, Philadelphia, 2005, Saunders.)

in the study because there was concern over influencing the restenosis rate.[61] Two subsequent studies[62,63] evaluated DCA followed by PTCA and found that this strategy resulted in a lower restenosis rate. Use of DCA has decreased with the advancement in stent technology but is still used in specific types of lesions.[59]

Rotational Atherectomy

The rotational atherectomy device or Rotoblater (Boston Scientific, Natick, Massachusetts) is indicated for patients with heavily calcified plaques, lesions occurring at the opening of a coronary artery (ostial lesions), certain bifurcation lesions, and lesions that cannot be dilated with a balloon catheter.[57] The rotational atherectomy device uses a high-speed rotating elliptical bur coated with diamond chips to form an abrasive surface (Figure 58-5). With the rotational atherectomy catheter positioned at the proximal end of the plaque, rotation is initiated and the catheter is advanced through the plaque. When the abrasive surface revolves at very high

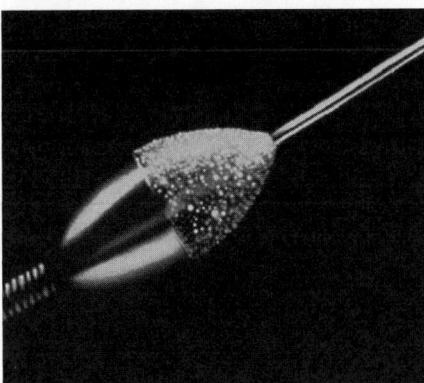

FIGURE 58-5 ■ Rotational atherectomy device. (From Zipes DP, Libby P, Bonow RO, Braunwald E, editors: *Braunwald's heart disease: a textbook of cardiovascular medicine,* ed 7, Philadelphia, 2005, Saunders.)

speeds, it pulverizes hard, calcified plaque while deflecting soft plaque away from the bur.[59] Several passes of the rotating bur are required, with 30 to 60 seconds between passes to allow coronary perfusion.[57] The pulverized particles are so tiny, they pass into the distal circulation without clinical sequelae.[57,59] Rotational atherectomy usually is followed by PTCA and stenting for a better final angiographic result and to reduce the risk of restenosis.[57]

Cutting Balloon

The cutting balloon (Boston Scientific) is a balloon with three or four microscopic blades designed to make sharp, linear incisions in the coronary lesion during balloon inflation, leaving the lesion segments intact. Theoretically, linear incisions in the plaque reduce the force needed to inflate the balloon and may reduce the incidence of flow-limiting dissections in the coronary artery. The Cutting Balloon Global Randomization Trial compared cutting balloon technology with PTCA and found no significant reduction in the angiographic restenosis rate at 6 months post-PCI. The authors concluded that the cutting balloon should be reserved for difficult lesions (i.e., lesions resistant to PTCA alone or in-stent restenotic lesions) in which controlled dilatation may provide a better initial outcome.[64]

Laser-Assisted Angioplasty

Laser (light amplification by stimulated emission of radiation) angioplasty is the process of creating a high-energy, coherent beam of light to ablate atherosclerotic plaque. Currently, two laser systems are available: the XeCl excimer laser coronary angioplasty (ELCA) system and the holmium:yttrium aluminum garnet (Ho:YAG) laser system. Laser angioplasty is used today in a specific group of patients with high-risk lesions (i.e., patients with in-stent restenosis, especially in saphenous vein grafts) that are not amenable to therapy with other PCI devices. Laser angioplasty should be used with caution in patients with thrombus or severe coronary calcification. In most cases, successful laser therapy is followed by PTCA and stenting to achieve a better final angiographic result and decrease the risk of restenosis.[57]

Thrombectomy Devices

The transluminal extraction catheter (Boston Scientific) was developed to treat lesions by cutting and aspirating plaque, thrombus, and other debris from within the coronary artery. Use of the transluminal extraction catheter system is limited by the need for a large-diameter (9 French) guiding catheter and stiffness of the device.[57]

The Angiojet (Possis Medical, Minneapolis, Minnesota) is a catheter with a stainless steel tip connected to a high-pressure flexible cylinder. Saline is ejected through the distal tip of the catheter from high-speed jets that are directed toward the proximal end of the catheter. Venturi suction is created at the tip of the catheter, forcing the surrounding blood, thrombus, and saline into the lumen of the catheter. As the thrombus is pulled through the jets, it is broken into small particles. The particles are propelled proximally through the catheter and are removed from the body. The Angiojet catheter is passed through the coronary artery until there is no evidence of thrombus on angiography and is followed by PTCA and stenting. The Angiojet is indicated for use in patients with a moderate to large thrombus in native coronary arteries or saphenous vein grafts. Because of the potential for coronary artery perforation, the Angiojet is not recommended for use in coronary arteries less than 2.0 mm in diameter.[57]

The X-SIZER thrombectomy device (EndiCOR Medical Inc., San Francisco, California) consists of a helical cutter enclosed within a protective housing attached to a double-lumen catheter. One lumen contains the guidewire, and the other lumen is used for vacuum and extraction. The device is used for thrombus in native coronary arteries or saphenous vein grafts. The X-SIZER device was evaluated in one study in which investigators found that thrombectomy with the X-SIZER device followed by PTCA and stenting reduced the extent of myocardial necrosis, but did not improve mortality, compared with stenting alone.[65]

Distal Embolic Protection Devices

Distal embolization is a frequent complication of PCI in old, diseased saphenous vein grafts, often resulting in elevation of CK-MB.[57,66,67] Embolization may result in TIMI 0 to 1 flow, which is associated with increased mortality and acute myocardial infarction.[68] Devices have been developed to keep atheroembolic material from passing into the distal circulation during PCI.[57] The PercuSurge GuardWire (Medtronic Vascular, Santa Rosa, California) balloon occlusion system (Figure 58-6) is designed to provide protection of the distal microcirculation during PCI. The balloon temporarily occludes the distal vessel during the procedure, facilitating aspiration of dislodged atheromatous and thrombotic material before it reaches the microcirculation.[68]

A feasibility study demonstrated the safety and effectiveness of the PercuSurge balloon occlusion system for patients undergoing elective PCI with stenting in saphenous vein graft lesions (mean age of the vein grafts was 8.9 ± 4.0 years).[68] A larger trial followed the feasibility trial.[69] More than 800 patients with saphenous vein graft lesions were randomized to the PercuSurge Guard-

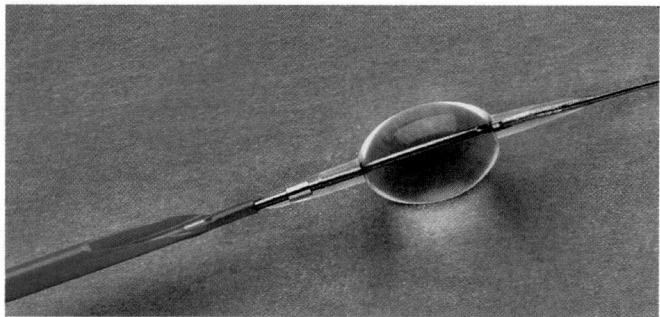

FIGURE 58-6 ■ PercuSurge GuardWire. (From Topol EJ: *Textbook of interventional cardiology,* Philadelphia, 2003, Saunders.)

Wire (median vein graft age was 10.4 years) or conventional PTCA (median vein graft age was 10.9 years). The incidence of death, myocardial infarction, emergent coronary artery bypass grafting surgery, or percutaneous revascularization of the treated vein graft was significantly less in the PercuSurge device group at 30 days post-PCI. This study demonstrated the value of distal protection in preventing major adverse cardiac events in patients with older, diseased saphenous vein grafts lesions.

The FilterWire EX (Boston Scientific) (Figure 58-7) consists of a distal polyurethane filter on a steerable guidewire that is capable of capturing dislodged atheroembolic particles in saphenous vein grafts, preventing distal embolization without occluding the distal vessel.[70] One study compared the PercuSurge Guard-Wire balloon occlusion system with the FilterWire EX distal protection filter system. The investigators found similar rates of death, myocardial infarction, or revascularization of treated saphenous vein bypass grafts at 30 days post-PCI, demonstrating the safety and effectiveness of the FilterWire EX distal protection device.[71]

Coronary Stents

Stents have changed the practice of interventional cardiology by significantly reducing the incidence of acute vessel closure and restenosis. Figure 58-8 illustrates coronary stent placement. Two landmark studies published in 1994[49,50] demonstrated a significant reduction in restenosis on coronary angiography with placement of a bare metal stent compared with PTCA in first-time coronary artery lesions. The investigators reported an increase in bleeding and vascular complications in the stent group compared with the PTCA group. This was attributed to the aggressive use of anticoagulants to reduce the incidence of stent thrombosis. Another trial evaluated the effectiveness of stenting in saphenous vein grafts.[72]

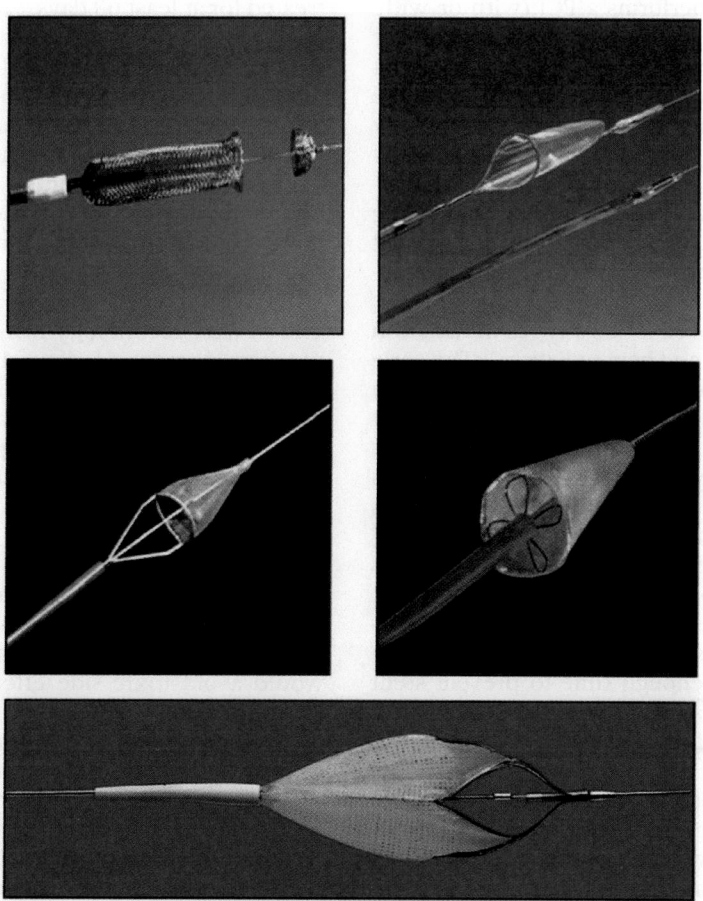

FIGURE 58-7 ■ FilterWire. (From Topol EJ: *Textbook of interventional cardiology,* Philadelphia, 2003, Saunders.)

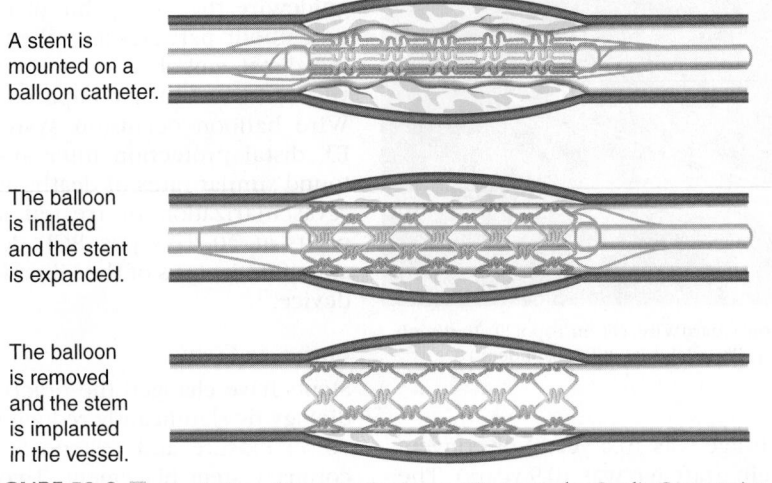

A stent is mounted on a balloon catheter.

The balloon is inflated and the stent is expanded.

The balloon is removed and the stem is implanted in the vessel.

FIGURE 58-8 ▓ Illustration of stent implantation. (Courtesy the Cordis Corporation.)

Intracoronary Brachytherapy

Local intracoronary radiation, referred to as intracoronary brachytherapy, has been shown to reduce the incidence of in-stent restenosis. When a patient has in-stent restenosis requiring brachytherapy, members of two different disciplines (interventional cardiology and radiation oncology) perform the procedure. First, the interventional cardiologist performs a PCI (with or without adjunctive devices) within the stent to improve blood flow to the coronary artery and expose the stent struts. After completion of the PCI, a member of the radiation oncology team delivers local radiation therapy within the stent through a special catheter placed by the interventional cardiologist. The radiation is withdrawn from the catheter after a specified time, and the catheter is removed. Local radiation within the stent inhibits smooth muscle proliferation and delays endothelialization.[51,73]

Brachytherapy is approved for two types of radiation sources: gamma radiation and beta radiation.[51] The early gamma radiation trials reported a significant decrease in in-stent restenosis but noted a high incidence of stent thrombosis, especially in patients who received a new stent at the time of brachytherapy.[74-76] Stent thrombosis was believed to stem from delayed endothelialization as a result of local radiation. In one gamma radiation trial,[75] antiplatelet therapy (aspirin and a thienopyridine) was used for 1 month after brachytherapy, which was the standard post-PCI course of therapy without brachytherapy. It was later discovered that 1 month of antiplatelet therapy was not enough time to prevent stent thrombosis because of delayed endothelialization within the stent. Further research examined the extended use of antiplatelet medicine for prophylaxis against late stent thrombosis after brachytherapy.[76,77] Extending the use of aspirin and clopidogrel to 12 months after brachytherapy (with or without a new stent) demonstrated a reduction in death, myocardial infarction, revascularization rates of the treated vessel, and late stent thrombosis.[77]

The second radiation source for brachytherapy is beta radiation. One pivotal trial[78] demonstrated that beta radiation was just as effective as gamma radiation to prevent recurrence of in-stent restenosis. Based on information from the gamma radiation trials, placement of a new stent was avoided as much as possible at the time of brachytherapy. The majority of patients were treated for at least 60 days with antiplatelet medications. Restenosis within the stent was significantly reduced in patients who received brachytherapy with beta radiation compared with placebo.[78] Today, antiplatelet therapy is prescribed for 1 year after brachytherapy, as it is for all PCI procedures. The increased use of drug-eluting stents has limited the use of intracoronary brachytherapy because of the lower incidence of restenosis (compared with bare metal stents).

Drug-Eluting Stents

The newest technology in interventional cardiology is the development of drug-eluting stents. The original bare metal stents were not designed to deliver medications. Heparin-coated stents, introduced in the 1990s, represented an attempt at placing medication onto a stent.[79] Heparin-coated stents help prevent thrombus formation, the first phase of restenosis, but do not prevent neointimal hyperplasia, the later phase of restenosis. The next logical step to prevent restenosis was to coat a stent with a medication that would interfere with the process of neointimal hyperplasia. It was hypothesized that low-dose local drug delivery at the stent site would avoid toxic side effects that could occur with systemic administration of the same medications.[48]

Drug-eluting stents are not just about the drug used to coat the stent. Drug-eluting stents have three important components: the stent design, the coating design, and the medication on the stent. The ideal drug-eluting stent designs should have a larger metallic surface area with minimal gaps between the struts and should be able to maintain flexibility, radial support, and a low profile.[79]

Medications applied directly onto the metallic stent surface have not shown promise because much of the drug is lost during delivery of the stent.[80] A polymer coating system containing the medication can be applied to the stent. This is the most successful design thus far, which is used by the two currently approved drug-eluting stents. The polymer coating ensures that the drug stays on the stent during delivery and controls drug release (elution).[79]

The third component of the drug-eluting stent is the medication on the stent itself. The ideal drug should have potent antiproliferative effects and still preserve vascular healing. The drug must allow local therapeutic concentrations without toxic effects, allow uniform diffusion of the drug, and not cause thrombosis or inflammation.[79]

Two early European trials demonstrated that two different drug-eluting stents dramatically reduced the incidence of in-stent restenosis.[53,56] The first drug-eluting stent approved by the Food and Drug Administration was the Cypher sirolimus stent (Cordis, Warren, New Jersey; Figure 58-9). Sirolimus is a potent immunosuppressive agent with antimitotic properties.[79] Sirolimus inhibits smooth muscle cell proliferation, a major component of in-stent restenosis. In 1999, the Food and Drug Administration approved sirolimus to prevent renal transplant rejection.[79] The sirolimus drug-eluting stent was approved in 2003 based on results from the U.S. Multicenter Trial, the SIRolImUS (SIRIUS) Trial.[54] This trial compared the sirolimus polymer coated Bx-Velocity stent with the bare metal Bx-Velocity stent in more than 1000 patients with first-time native coronary artery lesions. This study confirmed that the sirolimus drug-eluting stent significantly reduced in-stent restenosis to less than 10 percent. All patients were pretreated with aspirin 325 mg and were given a loading dose of clopidogrel of 300 mg to 375 mg 24 hours before implantation of the drug-eluting stent. Clopidogrel 75 mg and aspirin 325 mg were continued daily for 3 months following stent implantation. Stent thrombosis was infrequent in both groups.

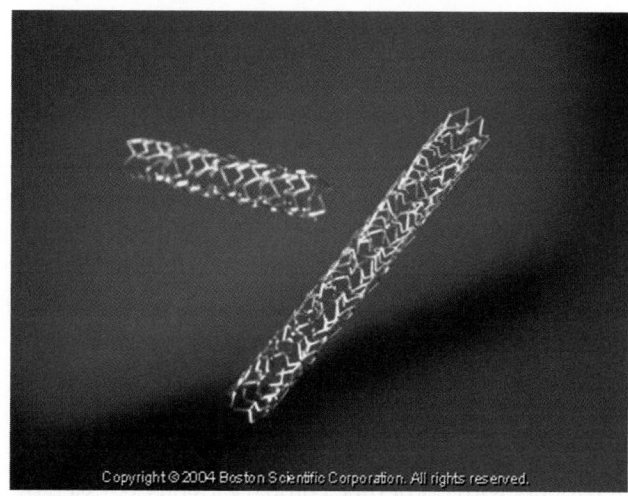

FIGURE 58-10 ▓ Taxus drug-eluting stent. (Courtesy Boston Scientific.)

The second drug-eluting stent to gain Food and Drug Administration approval was the Taxus paclitaxel stent (Boston Scientific), approved in 2004 (Figure 58-10). Paclitaxel is an antineoplastic agent capable of inhibiting cellular division, thereby reducing smooth muscle cell proliferation.[81] The U.S. study, TAXUS IV,[55] enrolled more than 1300 patients with first-time native coronary artery lesions. Patients were randomized to compare the polymer-based paclitaxel drug-eluting stent to the same bare metal stent. At 9 months post-PCI the restenosis rate was less that 10 percent in patients who received the paclitaxel drug-eluting stent. Patients were pretreated with aspirin 325 mg and clopidogrel 300 mg before implantation of the stent. Clopidogrel 75 mg and aspirin 325 mg were continued daily for 6 months after the procedure. No incidences of late stent thrombosis occurred after clopidogrel was discontinued.

Several new drug-eluting stents are being investigated (Box 58-4).

Drug-Eluting Stents for In-Stent Restenosis

Because both U.S. clinical trials with drug-eluting stents[54,55] demonstrated restenosis rates to be less than 10 percent, interest arose in using drug-eluting stents for patients with in-stent restenosis in place of intracoronary brachytherapy. One trial assessed whether the two currently approved drug-eluting stents are more effective than PTCA in preventing recurrent in-stent restenosis.[82] Three hundred patients with in-stent restenosis (restenosis within bare metal stents in native coronary

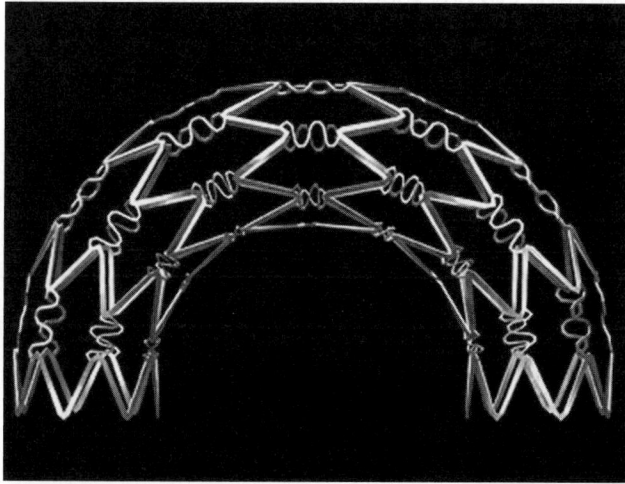

FIGURE 58-9 ▓ Cypher drug-eluting stent. (Courtesy the Cordis Corporation.)

BOX 58-4 ■ ■ ■

INVESTIGATIONAL AGENTS FOR FUTURE DRUG-ELUTING STENTS[79]

---

1. Sirolimus analog medications
   a. Evirolimus
   b. ABT-578 (zotarolimus)
2. Tacrolimus

arteries) were assigned randomly to undergo one of the following treatments: PTCA alone, PCI with a sirolimus stent, or PCI with a paclitaxel stent. All patients were pretreated with 600 mg of clopidogrel at least 2 hours before the procedure. The study showed that both drug-eluting stents were superior to PTCA for prevention of in-stent restenosis 6 months post-PCI. The investigators noted a slight decrease in restenosis rates among patients who received the sirolimus stent compared with patients who received the paclitaxel stent. Although this was not statistically significant, the investigators concluded that the sirolimus stent may be better than the paclitaxel stent for treatment of in-stent restenosis.

Devices for Quantification of Lesion Characteristics
Fractional Flow Reserve

In patients with borderline coronary lesions assessed by angiography, the concept of myocardial fractional flow reserve (**FFR**) was developed as an invasive approach to determine the functional severity of a coronary stenosis. FFR is defined as the maximal blood flow to the myocardium beyond a coronary stenosis, divided by the theoretical normal maximal flow in the same artery. FFR is derived from the ratio of the mean distal coronary artery pressure to the aortic pressure during maximal coronary vasodilatation.[83] Maximal coronary dilatation usually is achieved using intracoronary or intravenous adenosine.[84] A normal FFR value is 1.0 regardless of the coronary artery evaluated. In patients undergoing PCI, an FFR of less than 0.75 signifies a significant stenosis, representing a stenosis associated with inducible myocardial ischemia.[85] FFR during coronary angiography may be useful in determining whether a borderline coronary artery stenosis assessed on angiogram correlates to an obstructive stenosis, which may be useful in determining whether to proceed with PCI, especially when there is no other objective evidence of reversible ischemia.[7,83]

FFR also has been used after PTCA and stenting to evaluate the final angiographic result. In a registry of 750 patients, an FFR greater than 0.75 immediately after stent implantation was shown to have a strong negative predictive value with respect to death, myocardial infarction, or need for repeat revascularization of the treated coronary artery within 6 months after the PCI. The higher the FFR, the lower the event rate.[86]

Intravascular Ultrasound

Intravascular ultrasound (**IVUS**) uses a miniature transducer at the end of a flexible catheter. IVUS has evolved as a valuable adjunct to coronary angiography. Coronary angiography shows a two-dimensional silhouette of the lumen of the coronary artery when filled with contrast medium. IVUS allows precise tomographic measurement of the lumen and can evaluate plaque size, distribution, and composition. A potential application for IVUS may be to identify a vulnerable plaque before it ruptures and causes an acute event. IVUS is used in a small percentage (5 to 8 percent) of coronary interventions in the United States, mostly for optimization of coronary stent implantation.[87] IVUS also is used to evaluate brachytherapy results, quantify left main coro-

nary artery lesions, evaluate heart transplant vasculopathy, and plan which type of adjunctive debulking device to use before PTCA/stent implantation.[87,88]

Pharmacotherapy in Percutaneous Coronary Intervention
Oral Antiplatelet Therapy

Antiplatelet therapy is the cornerstone of treatment for patients undergoing PCI. Preventing acute or late thrombosis at the PTCA or stent site is of utmost importance to prevent myocardial infarction, urgent revascularization of the treated coronary artery with repeat PCI, emergent coronary artery bypass grafting surgery, and death.

Aspirin

The role of aspirin in PCI is to reduce ischemic complications.[7] Aspirin irreversibly inhibits cyclooxygenase, blocking platelet syntheses of thromboxane A_2, a humeral mediator that promotes platelet aggregation. The platelet inhibitory effects of aspirin occur within 1 hour of oral administration, and platelet inhibition lasts up to 7 days.[89] The minimum dose of aspirin in the setting of PCI has not been established[7]. The ACC/AHA/SCAI PCI guideline recommends that patients who are not on daily aspirin therapy receive a dose of 300 mg to 325 mg at least 2 hours before PCI and preferably 24 hours before the PCI. Patients already taking daily aspirin should take 75 mg to 325 mg before the PCI.[7] Aspirin is an inexpensive, relatively safe and effective antiplatelet medication.[90]

Thienopyridine Derivatives (Ticlopidine and Clopidogrel)

Adenosine diphosphate is a substance released from activated platelets that increases platelet aggregation.[90] Thienopyridine derivatives irreversibly inhibit the binding of adenosine diphosphate to its platelet receptor, thereby inhibiting platelet aggregation. Aspirin and thienopyridine derivatives have complimentary mechanisms of action. The combination of the two agents inhibits platelet aggregation more than either in isolation.[89] The two currently approved thienopyridines are ticlopidine and clopidogrel.

Two studies demonstrated that antiplatelet therapy was superior to anticoagulant therapy to prevent stent thrombosis. One randomized trial[52] compared the 30-day outcome of patients treated with two different antithrombotic regimens after placement of a coronary stent. The investigators compared antiplatelet therapy using ticlopidine plus aspirin to anticoagulant therapy (intravenously administered heparin plus a warfarin derivative and aspirin). The study demonstrated that antiplatelet therapy was associated with fewer noncardiac events (hemorrhage and peripheral vascular complications), a lower rate of cardiac events (myocardial infarction, need for repeated intervention of the treated coronary artery, and death), and a lower incidence of stent thrombosis. A later study enrolled more than 1500 patients undergoing PCI. Participants were randomized to receive aspirin 325 mg daily, aspirin 325 mg daily plus ticlopidine 250 mg twice daily for 1 month after PCI, or aspirin 325 mg daily plus warfarin for 1 month post-PCI. The investigators found that aspirin plus ticlopidine was superior to the other two regimens in preventing stent thrombosis.[91]

Ticlopidine, the first approved thienopyridine, has unfavorable side effects. The most common side effects are neutropenia and thrombocytopenia, requiring patients to undergo biweekly blood tests to monitor the white blood cell and platelet counts. In addition, the medication is dosed twice daily, compared with the newer thienopyridine, clopidogrel.[89]

Clopidogrel requires once daily administration, making it easier for patients to remember to take the medication. In addition, it has fewer side effects than ticlopidine. Clopidogrel does not cause neutropenia and rarely causes thrombocytopenia.[89] Clopidogrel has been shown to have a similar efficacy to ticlopidine in preventing stent thrombosis.[90] With a better safety profile and once daily dosing, clopidogrel has replaced ticlopidine as the thienopyridine of choice for PCI.[90,92]

Pretreatment with Clopidogrel

Many trials demonstrating the benefit of thienopyridines started the medication immediately after completion of the PCI.[89] Studies show that the platelet inhibitory effects of clopidogrel are achieved more rapidly by giving a loading dose.[92-94] One study[93] demonstrated that patients pretreated with clopidogrel up to 10 days before PCI and continued for 8 months post-PCI had better outcomes (significant reduction in cardiovascular death, myocardial infarction, and urgent revascularization of the treated coronary artery within 30 days) compared with patients who did not receive pretreatment with clopidogrel but received clopidogrel for 4 weeks post-PCI. Another group of investigators[94] also demonstrated a significant reduction in death, myocardial infarction, or revascularization of the treated coronary artery at 28 days post-PCI in patients pretreated with clopidogrel at least 6 hours before elective PCI.

Chan and colleagues[95] compared pretreatment with clopidogrel to clopidogrel given as early as possible after PCI. Pretreated patients received a one-time dose of clopidogrel 300 mg 2 to 6 hours before elective PCI (or on the catheterization table as soon as the decision to proceed with immediate PCI was made, but before initiation of a glycoprotein [GP] IIb/IIIa inhibitor). The other group of patients was given clopidogrel as early as possible after the procedure. Pretreatment with clopidogrel was associated with a reduction of death and myocardial infarction, regardless of the GP IIb/IIIa inhibitor used in the study. Based on the findings, the investigators recommend pretreatment with clopidogrel 2 to 6 hours before elective PCI.

Higher loading doses of clopidogrel are being evaluated. One trial enrolled more than 2100 patients undergoing elective PCI with the use of the GP IIb/IIIa agent abciximab.[96] All patients received clopidogrel 600 mg at least 2 hours before the procedure. About half of the patients were randomized to receive abciximab during PCI and half were randomized to placebo. Although the investigators did not assess the benefit of the higher loading dose of clopidogrel directly, they noted that pretreatment with 600 mg of clopidogrel at least 2 hours before elective PCI may have played a role in the reduction of death, myocardial infarction, and urgent revascularization of the treated coronary artery. More studies need to be done to evaluate higher-dose clopidogrel pretreatment before it can be recommended routinely.[89]

Duration of Clopidogrel Therapy after Percutaneous Coronary Intervention

Results of two trials[93,94] changed the duration of antiplatelet therapy from 1 month to 1 year post-PCI. One trial[94] randomized more than 2100 patients undergoing elective PCI. All patients received aspirin. Patients were randomized to receive a 300-mg loading dose of clopidogrel (experimental group) or placebo (control group) 3 to 24 hours before elective PCI. For the first 28 days post-PCI, patients in both groups received clopidogrel 75 mg daily. Patients in the experimental group continued to receive clopidogrel from day 29 through 1 year post-PCI, whereas patients in the control group continued to receive placebo from day 29 through 1 year. The investigators found that patients who received pretreatment with clopidogrel plus 12 months of clopidogrel post-PCI had a significant reduction in death, myocardial infarction, and stroke. The authors noted one limitation of the study: patients assigned to the placebo-loading dose were never given a true loading dose of clopidogrel after the procedure. Despite this limitation, the authors recommended that patients who undergo PCI with bare metal stents continue daily clopidogrel (plus aspirin indefinitely) for 1 year following PCI.

Important to note is that the studies looking at duration of clopidogrel therapy post-PCI[93,94] were completed before the advent of drug-eluting stents. The U.S. study with the sirolimus drug-eluting stent recommended clopidogrel 75 mg daily for a minimum of 3 months (plus aspirin indefinitely) post-PCI.[54] The U.S. study with the paclitaxel drug-eluting stent recommended clopidogrel 75 mg daily for a minimum of 6 months (plus aspirin indefinitely) post-PCI.[55] These recommendations are based on the potential for delayed stent endothelialization because of the slow release of the drug from the stent.[89] Although there are no published studies evaluating 1-year duration of daily antiplatelet therapy with drug-eluting stents, the recommendation is to continue the clopidogrel 75 mg daily (plus aspirin indefinitely) for 1 year after placement of a drug-eluting stent, if the patient is not at high risk for bleeding.[7]

There has been an increased incidence of delayed stent thombosis in patients receiving drug-eluting stents. After placement of a drug-eluting stent, sometimes patients and/or health care providers prematurely stop dual antiplatelet therapy (a thienopyridine and aspirin) before completing one year of therapy, thereby increasing the risk of stent thrombosis. Stent thombosis can lead to devastating consequences, such as an acute myocardial infarction or death. The AHA, together with the ACC, the SCAI, the American College of Physicians, the American College of Surgeons, and the American Dental Association convened an advisory panel to stress the potential complications of discontinuing thienopyridine therapy before completing one year of therapy and to make recommendations to prevent this from happening. The advisory panel determined that there seems to be an excess of delayed stent thrombosis with the use of bare metal and drug-eluting stents when used for off-label indications, compared to on-label indications. The original trials that helped gain Food and Drug Association approval of drug-eluting stents[54,55] were conducted in low-risk patients with low risk lesions. Today drug-eluting stents are placed in patients with high-risk lesions, which is associated with an increased risk of delayed stent thrombosis.[97]

Health care providers who perform invasive or surgical procedures may prematurely discontinue antiplatelet therapy because of the increased risk of bleeding. The advisory panel suggests that drug-eluting stents should not be placed in patients planning to undergo an elective invasive or surgical procedure within the next 12 months (the panel recommends placement of a bare metal stent or balloon angioplasty with provisional stent placement). Drug-eluting stents should also be avoided in patients who may not be able to comply with 12 months of thienopyridine therapy (i.e., due to cost of drug or history of bleeding). The advisory panel recommends that health care professionals reinforce the rationale for 1 year of thienopyridine therapy with patients and emphasize the risks of nonadherence with this regimen. Patients should be encouraged to contact their cardiologist before discontinuing any antiplatelet therapy, including aspirin and thienopyridines. Healthcare providers who perform invasive or surgical procedures should be encouraged to contact the patient's cardiologist to discuss optimal patient management before prematurely discontinuing any thienopyridine. For patients who receive a drug-eluting stent who must undergo an invasive or surgical procedure that requires stopping the thienopyridine, the advisory panel suggests aspirin therapy be continued if at all possible and the thienopyridine be re-started as soon as possible after the procedure to prevent stent thrombosis. The panel also made a recommendation that the health care industry, pharmaceutical industry, insurance industry, and the United Stated Congress put processes in place to ensure that the cost of thienopyridine therapy does not continue to be a factor in premature discontinuation of the medication by the patient.[97]

Glycoprotein IIb/IIIa Inhibitors

The GP IIb/IIIa receptor is the most abundant receptor on the platelet surface. Platelets cross-link through bridging of two activated GP IIb/IIIa receptor molecules on adjacent platelets with a single molecule of plasma fibrinogen. With multiple cross-linking, platelet-rich thrombi (white clots) form. Thrombin, formed by the coagulation cascade, converts fibrinogen to fibrin, forming a matrix that stabilizes the platelet-rich thrombi and traps circulating erythrocytes, forming red clots. The binding of fibrinogen to platelets by means of the GP IIb/IIIa receptor is the final common pathway of platelet-thrombus formation and can be inhibited with the use of the currently approved GP IIb/IIIa inhibitors:

abciximab, eptifibatide, and tirofiban. The three agents are potent blockers of platelet aggregation and should be considered for use in patients undergoing PCI, especially patients with unstable angina or patients with high-risk lesions. Platelet aggregation and subsequent platelet thrombus formation is prevented when more than 80 percent of the GP IIb/IIIa receptors on activated platelets are inhibited.[98] GP IIb/IIIa inhibitors are used in conjunction with other platelet inhibitors (aspirin, thienopyridines) and heparin, which may increase bleeding. The major benefit of GP IIb/IIIa inhibitors is the reduction of acute ischemic events associated with PCI.[89] See the accompanying pharmacology feature.

Abciximab

Abciximab was the first GP IIb/IIIa agent available in the United States. Several trials to evaluate the efficacy of abciximab have been published.[99,100] In one trial[99] patients who received a bolus plus infusion of abciximab had a 35 percent reduction in death, nonfatal myocardial infarction, need for revascularization, and procedural failure (requiring insertion of a coronary stent or intraaortic balloon pump) within 30 days post-PCI. Although ischemic complications were reduced with the use of abciximab, major bleeding was twice as frequent in the patients receiving abciximab, which was attributed to the use of non–weight-adjusted heparin dosing during PCI.

Another trial[100] randomized more than 2700 PCI patients to one of three treatment arms: standard-dose, weight-adjusted heparin (100 units/kg to maintain an activated clotting time of at least 300 seconds) plus placebo; standard-dose, weight-adjusted heparin (100

▪▪▪ PHARMACOLOGY

DOSING REGIMENS FOR GLYCOPROTEIN IIb/IIIa INHIBITORS USED DURING PRIMARY PERCUTANEOUS CORONARY INTERVENTION

DRUG	DOSE
Abciximab	0.25 mg/kg bolus 10 to 60 minutes before the start of percutaneous coronary intervention followed by infusion of 0.125 mcg/kg/min (maximum 10 mcg/min) for 12 to 18 hours (it is reasonable to start abciximab as early as possible before primary percutaneous coronary intervention [with or without stenting])
Eptifibatide*	Bolus of 180 mcg/kg before the start of percutaneous coronary intervention, followed by an infusion of 2 mcg/kg/min for up to 18 to 24 hours
	Give a second bolus of 180 mcg/kg 10 minutes after the first bolus
Tirofiban	Bolus of 10 mcg/kg, followed by an infusion of 0.15 mcg/kg/min for 18 to 24 hours

*For patients with serum creatinine greater that 2 mg/dl, a bolus dose of 180 mcg/kg immediately before percutaneous coronary intervention, followed by a continuous infusion of 1 mcg/kg/min. Give a second bolus of 180 mcg/kg 10 minutes after the first bolus.

From Antman EM, Anbe DT, Armstrong PW et al: ACC/AHA pocket guideline: management of patients with ST-elevation myocardial infarction. Retrieved February 11, 2007, from *www.acc.org/qualityandscience/clinical/guidelines/stemi/index_pkt.pdf*. Based on Antman EM, Anbe DT, Armstrong PW et al: *J Am Coll Cardiol* 44:671-719, 2004.

units/kg) plus abciximab; or low-dose, weight-adjusted heparin (70 units/kg to maintain an activated clotting time of 200 seconds) plus abciximab. Patients treated with low-dose, weight-adjusted heparin plus abciximab experienced reduced ischemic complications within 30 days post-PCI without increasing bleeding complications. Based on this trial, low-dose, weight-adjusted heparin should be used when GP IIb/IIIa inhibitors are used during PCI.[101]

The two previous trials evaluating abciximab[99,100] did not include patients undergoing stent implantation. A third trial[102] evaluated abciximab in patients in whom a coronary stent was placed. The investigators found a significant reduction in death and myocardial infarction within the first 30 days post-PCI.

One of the major limitations with abciximab is the effect of the medication on platelets. Thrombocytopenia is common with abciximab therapy. Platelet counts should be monitored closely. If the patient develops thrombocytopenia, the medication should be discontinued and the platelet count rechecked. In some cases, patients require platelet transfusions to normalize platelet counts.

Eptifibatide

Two landmark trials evaluated the role of eptifibatide in PCI.[103,104] The initial trial evaluated different dosing regimens of eptifibatide in patients undergoing elective or primary PCI. The investigators found no statistical difference in the two dosing regimens for the endpoints of death, myocardial infarction, unplanned coronary artery bypass grafting surgery, repeat PCI, or coronary stenting for abrupt coronary artery closure at 30-days post-PCI. They determined that the eptifibatide doses used in the study were too low to achieve adequate platelet inhibition and recommended further research.[103]

A second trial evaluated a higher dose, double-bolus dose of eptifibatide compared with placebo in more than 2000 patients undergoing elective stent implantation in a native coronary artery. The higher dose of eptifibatide in this study achieved the greater than 80 percent GP IIb/IIIa receptor blockade needed for adequate platelet inhibition. Death, myocardial infarction, and urgent revascularization of the treated coronary artery were significantly reduced in the ebtifibatide group compared with the placebo group. Major bleeding was uncommon but occurred more frequently in patients who received eptifibatide than in patients who received placebo.[104] The standard dosing of ebtifibatide used during PCI is based on the dosing regimen from this trial.[89]

Eptifibatide may cause thrombocytopenia, but to a lesser extent than abciximab. Thrombocytopenia is usually reversible with discontinuation of the medication. Eptifibatide has a shorter half-life than abciximab and must be used cautiously in patients with renal insufficiency.[105]

Tirofiban

Tirofiban is approved for use in patients with acute coronary syndromes (unstable angina and non-STEMI). Tirofiban has been studied with favorable results in pa-

tients with non-STEMI and unstable angina who undergo PCI at a later time. One trial involving patients undergoing PCI within 72 hours of presenting with an acute coronary syndrome demonstrated that at 2 days post-PCI, there was a significant reduction in cardiac events, but at 30 days post-PCI, there was no statistically significant reduction in cardiac events in patients who received tirofiban.[106] Another trial randomized patients with non-STEMI and unstable angina to an early invasive strategy (cardiac catheterization and PCI within 4 to 48 hours) or to a more conservative strategy (coronary angiography with possible PCI if chest pain or ischemia persists). All patients received pretreatment with aspirin, heparin, and tirofiban. Death, nonfatal myocardial infarction, and rehospitalization were reduced significantly at 6 months in the early invasive strategy group compared with patients treated with a more conservative strategy.[12] Tirofiban also may be used for patients undergoing elective PCI.[7]

Unfractionated Heparin

Unfractionated heparin is the most common anticoagulant used during PCI. Unfractionated heparin is used to prevent thrombus from forming on catheters, balloons, and other equipment. Unfractionated heparin is monitored in the cardiac catheterization laboratory by the activated clotting time. General recommendations for heparin dosing are as follows: in the absence of an adjunctive GP IIb/IIIa inhibitor, weight-adjusted heparin should be administered in doses of 70 to 100 units/kg with a target activated clotting time of between 250 and 350 seconds. When a GP IIb/IIIa inhibitor is used, weight-adjusted heparin should be reduced to 50 to 70 units/kg with a target activated clotting time of 200 seconds.[7] The femoral sheath can be removed safely when the activated clotting time is less than 175 seconds.[101] For patients with heparin-induced thrombocytopenia, bivalirudin or argatroban may be substituted for heparin.[7]

Low-Molecular-Weight Heparin

Low-molecular-weight heparin often is used as a replacement for intravenously administered unfractionated heparin in patients with non-STEMI and unstable angina, many of whom undergo PCI. If a patient with non-STEMI or unstable angina is to undergo a PCI within 8 hours of receiving the last dose of low-molecular-weight heparin, no further anticoagulation should be given. In the same population, if the patient is to undergo a PCI 8 to 12 hours after the last dose of low-molecular-weight heparin, an additional intravenous dose of 0.3 mg per kg should be given before the PCI. Monitoring the ACT level should not be performed with low-molecular weight heparin, because there is little effect on the ACT measurement.[7]

Direct Thrombin Inhibitors

Heparin, an indirect thrombin inhibitor, has been used as an adjunctive therapy with PCI for many years. The limitations of indirect thrombin inhibitors are the varied anticoagulant response and the risk of bleeding.[107] Newer pharmacological agents have been investigated to minimize thrombus formation and decrease the risk of bleeding in patients undergoing PCI.[108] Bivalirudin is a direct thrombin inhibitor approved for use in patients with unstable angina undergoing PCI.[107,108] Bivalirudin was first investigated in a randomized trial in the early 1990s,[109] where it was found to be as effective as heparin in preventing early ischemic events and was associated with fewer bleeding complications. Bivalirudin was not widely used until the results of a large randomized trial were published in 2003.[107] The trial involved 6010 patients undergoing urgent or elective PCI. Patients were randomized to receive intravenously administered bivalirudin with a GP IIb/IIIa inhibitor (if indicated during PCI) or heparin with planned GP IIb/IIIa inhibitor use. Both groups received aspirin and a thienopyridine for at least 30 days post-PCI. The investigators concluded that bivalirudin (with or without the use of GP IIb/IIIa inhibitors) was as effective as heparin (with planned GP IIb/IIIa inhibition) in preventing death, myocardial infarction, or repeat revascularization of the treated coronary artery within 6 months post-PCI and was associated with less bleeding. Because patients with acute myocardial infarction were excluded from the study, the effectiveness of bivalirudin in this population is unknown and use of bivalirudin is not recommended.

Bivalirudin has a rapid onset of action and a relatively short half-life. About 20 percent of the medication is cleared by the kidneys, minimizing the risk to patients with mild to moderate renal impairment. The major side effect of bivalirudin is bleeding, as with any antithrombotic agent. Bivalirudin does not cause heparin-induced thrombocytopenia and therefore is appropriate for this group of patients. Repeat exposure to bivalirudin does not increase the risk of adverse effects, nor does it decrease efficacy of the medication.[108] Bivalirudin is given as a bolus of 0.75 mg/kg before the start of the PCI, followed by an infusion of 1.75 mg/kg/hr until the end of the procedure.[107]

Percutaneous Coronary Intervention in High-Risk Groups

Percutaneous Coronary Intervention in Patients with Diabetes

Diabetes increases the risk of restenosis following PCI. Bare metal stents improved clinical outcomes of patients with diabetes, mostly because of the decreased rate of acute vessel closure.[7] The introduction of GP IIb/IIIa inhibitors and drug-eluting stents has decreased the incidence of in-stent restenosis in diabetic patients.[54,55,110,111]

One trial evaluated the use of abciximab in patients with diabetes undergoing elective PCI, predominantly with bare metal stents. The study enrolled 701 patients, all of whom received a 600-mg loading dose of clopidogrel more than 2 hours before the procedure. Three hundred fifty-one patients were assigned randomly to receive abciximab, and 350 were assigned to receive placebo during the PCI. Although the primary endpoint of death and myocardial infarction at 1 year was not supported by the results, the secondary endpoint of restenosis (defined as greater than 50 percent) on follow-up coronary angiography was significantly reduced, suggesting that abciximab may reduce the risk of restenosis in patients with diabetes.[110]

Stuckey and colleagues[111] found that patients with diabetes (especially insulin-dependent diabetes) who have STEMI are at increased risk of death, stroke, reinfarction, and urgent revascularization of the treated coronary artery within the first year after primary PCI (with bare metal stents). The researchers also found that the use of stenting in STEMI decreased restenosis in patients with diabetes, but the use of abciximab during primary PCI had no effect on mortality or restenosis.

In the sirolimus drug-eluting stent trial (SIRIUS),[54] 131 patients with diabetes received the sirolimus drug-eluting stent and 148 received a bare metal stent. A significant reduction in the rate of in-stent restenosis was found with the sirolimus group compared with the bare metal stent group. The rate of revascularization of the treated coronary artery also was reduced significantly. In the trial using the paclitaxel drug-eluting stent (TAXUS IV),[55] the risk of restenosis was reduced by more than 80 percent among patients with diabetes who received a paclitaxel drug-eluting stent. Although the trials with drug-eluting stents demonstrated a lower incidence of restenosis in patients with diabetes, more research is needed. In addition, more studies using GP IIb/IIIa inhibitors in patients with diabetes must be undertaken.

Percutaneous Coronary Intervention in Women

The effect of gender on in-hospital outcomes (death, myocardial infarction, repeat revascularization of the treated coronary artery, major vascular complications) and the 1-year outcome (death) after coronary artery stenting was analyzed in 1908 women. Women in the cohort were significantly older than men and had a higher prevalence of diabetes, hypertension, and unstable angina. They also had a smaller body habitus and a significantly lower body surface area. The investigators report that stenting in women was associated with excellent acute results. However, there was a significantly higher risk of vascular complications (access site complications requiring surgical intervention or transfusion) in women compared with men. The authors conclude that PCI is equally effective for women as for men.[112]

Procedural Complications

The ACC/AHA/SCAI PCI guideline identified six categories of procedural complications: death, periprocedural myocardial infarction, need for coronary artery bypass grafting surgery during the index hospitalization, stroke, vascular access site complications, and contrast-induced nephropathy.[7] Several of these are discussed further.

Death

Death of patients undergoing elective PCI often is due to coronary artery occlusion and most frequently occurs in patients with significant left ventricular failure. Other variables associated with increased mortality include advanced age, female gender, patients with diabetes or prior myocardial infarction, patients with a large area of myocardial ischemia on noninvasive testing, patients with preexisting left ventricular dysfunction, pre-existing renal dysfunction or post-procedure worsening renal dysfunction, patients with collateral blood flow distal to the lesion to be treated, supplying significant areas of myocardium, and patients with multivessel coronary artery disease, left main coronary artery, or equivalent disease. Primary PCI for STEMI is associated with a significantly higher mortality rate than elective PCI.[7]

Periprocedural Myocardial Infarction

After PCI, chest pain may occur in as many as 50 percent of patients. Routine post-procedure measurement of CK-MB and/or troponin I or T in all PCI patients is reasonable 8 to 12 hours after PCI. The ACC/AHA/SCAI guideline recommends serial CK-MB and/or troponin I or T measurements for all patients who have signs or symptoms suggestive of a myocardial infarction post-PCI or for patients in whom there is evidence of acute vessel closure, side branch vessel occlusion, or evidence of new or persistent slow coronary flow seen on angiography post-PCI. A clinically significant periprocedural myocardial infarction is defined as a new CK-MB or troponin I or T rise greater than 5 times the upper limit of normal. Troponin I and T are more sensitive and specific biochemical markers for the diagnosis of myocardial infarction. Minor elevations do not appear to have prognostic significance.[7]

Serial electrocardiograms should be performed for any episode of chest pain post-PCI and compared to the pre-procedure electrocardiogram, to look for evidence of ischemia. An electrocardiogram should be done routinely post-PCI, even in the absence of chest pain, to observe for "silent" ischemia (evidence of ischemia on the electrocardiogram in a patient with no symptoms of angina). If there is evidence of ischemia on the electrocardiogram, further treatment may include serial biochemical markers to rule out myocardial infarction, pharmacological therapy, return to the cardiac catheterization laboratory for repeat coronary angiography, or coronary artery bypass grafting surgery. Treatment is individualized based on the patient's hemodynamic stability, the amount of myocardium at risk, and the likelihood that the treatment will be successful.[7]

The ACC/AHA/SCAI PCI guideline defines periprocedural myocardial infarction by at least one of the following criteria: (1) the presence of newly evolving ST segment elevations, development of new Q waves in two or more contiguous electrocardiogram leads and a new (or presumably new) left bundle branch block pattern on the 12-lead electrocardiogram and/or (2) biochemical marker elevation as defined by CK-MB and/or troponin I or T more than 5 times the upper limit of normal. These criteria usually correlate with a clinically significant myocardial infarction.[7]

The AHA scientific statement on practice standards for electrocardiographic monitoring in hospital settings[37] recommends ST segment monitoring for patients with acute coronary syndromes, including patients undergoing primary PCI, to detect extension of the myocardial infarction and ongoing or recurrent myocardial ischemia. According to the practice standards, patients should be monitored for a minimum of 24 hours after primary PCI and monitoring should continue until they remain event-free for 12 to 24 hours. The practice standards state that ST segment monitoring is not mandatory for patients who undergo elective, uncomplicated PCI; however, if cardiac monitors capable of ST segment monitoring are available, ST segment monitoring is recommended for 4 to 8 hours post-PCI. For patients with suboptimal results after elective PCI, ST segment monitoring is recommended post-PCI and should be continued for 24 hours or more if ST segment changes occur.[37]

Stroke

Stroke is an uncommon but devastating complication of PCI. Stroke is defined as a loss of neurological function with symptoms lasting more than 24 hours.[7] The incidence of stroke associated with PCI was reported to be 0.38 percent in one study, with about half of those being hemorrhagic and half embolic. The authors identified several factors that increase the risk of stroke: older age, female sex, patients with non–insulin-dependent diabetes with evidence of advanced coronary artery disease, PCI on saphenous vein bypass grafts, patients with periprocedural complications (coronary artery dissection or abrupt closure of the treated coronary artery), and placement of an intraaortic balloon pump.[113]

If the patient exhibits signs and symptoms of a stroke, a neurology consult should be obtained. Diagnosis must be confirmed with a computed tomography scan or magnetic resonance imaging. If the cause is confirmed as hemorrhagic, antiplatelet therapies should be discontinued until the clinical situation warrants restarting the regimen. However, without daily aspirin and clopidogrel administration, there is a higher incidence of stent thrombosis. If the cause is confirmed as embolic, heparin may be added to the antiplatelet medication regimen with close observation for bleeding. Frequent monitoring of the complete blood count is required. Urine and stool samples should be assessed for occult blood when heparin is added to the regimen.

Vascular Access Site Complications

The aggressive antiplatelet regimen used during PCI—including aspirin, clopidogrel, heparin and GP IIb/IIIa inhibitors—increases the risk of vascular access site complications.[101] Other factors that increase access site complications include: the use of fibrinolytic therapy, pre-existing peripheral vascular disease, female gender, older age, and prolonged heparin use with delayed sheath removal.[7] Femoral vascular complications after PCI often lead to additional procedures and prolonged hospital stays. The femoral artery is the most common vascular access site for PCI; however, the radial and brachial approaches also may be used. The most common vascular access site complications are discussed further.

Bleeding

Blood loss is defined as external bleeding, an internal hematoma, or a retroperitoneal bleed. A drop in the hematocrit of greater than 5 to 6 percent post-PCI is considered significant. Significant blood loss may require a blood transfusion and prolonged hospital stay.[7]

External blood loss, which is easily recognized, is defined as blood loss at the site of arterial or venous puncture. Internal blood loss, identified as a localized hematoma (a collection of blood under the skin), may cause localized pain, lower extremity edema because of compression of the femoral vein, or lower extremity neurovascular compromise resulting from femoral nerve compression. Hematomas are identified by local swelling, fullness or tenderness in the groin, or loss of sensory or motor function in the affected extremity.[114] Ultrasound may help confirm the diagnosis. External bleeding and hematomas are controlled with manual pressure or application of a femoral artery compression device.

Retroperitoneal Bleeding

Although rare, the most serious vascular complication following PCI is retroperitoneal bleeding. Perforation of an artery or vein can result in significant blood loss. The retroperitoneal space is potential cavity that can hold a large amount of blood. A significant amount of blood can accumulate in the space before the patient becomes symptomatic. Back, abdominal, or flank pain unrelieved with analgesics and accompanied by otherwise unexplained hypotension and a rapid drop in hemoglobin and hematocrit are signs associated with retroperitoneal bleeding. The groin site itself may be undisturbed and intact. Hypovolemic shock may ensue if a rapid diagnosis is not made. Diagnosis is confirmed with a computed tomography scan. Treatment includes discontinuation of anticoagulant and antiplatelet therapy, bed rest, blood transfusions as necessary, and close monitoring of vital signs and hemodynamic status. Surgical intervention is required rarely.[114] Once the patient becomes hemodynamically stable, antiplatelet therapy should be reinstituted to prevent stent thrombosis.

Peripheral Arterial Occlusion

Total occlusion of the accessed artery is defined as obstruction by a thrombus anywhere in the artery or dissection of the artery. Arterial dissection occurs when the intimal layer of the artery separates from the medial layer, creating a false lumen, partially or fully obstructing blood flow through the artery. Total occlusion is identified by loss of palpable or Doppler distal pulses. Total occlusion often is associated with limb ischemia (alteration in sensory or motor function, alteration in skin color, or pain in the affected extremity) and requires immediate surgical intervention. Frequent monitoring of the neurovascular status of the limb, with comparison to the opposite extremity, is paramount to early recognition of this serious complication.

Pseudoaneurysm

A pseudoaneurysm is a communication between the femoral artery and the surrounding fibromuscular tissue, which results in a blood-filled cavity with a pulsatile flow. Psuedoaneurysm of the femoral artery is identified by a pulsatile mass in the groin, groin tenderness, and/or the presence of a new femoral bruit. Baseline assessment of the femoral artery for a bruit before the arterial puncture is essential for comparison post-PCI. Diagnosis is confirmed by ultrasound. If the pseudoaneurysm does not spontaneously thrombose, treatment may include ultrasound-guided compression, ultrasound-guided thrombin injection, or surgical repair.[114]

Arteriovenous Fistula

An arteriovenous fistula is communication between the femoral artery and the femoral vein resulting from sheath removal. With an arteriovenous fistula, a systolic and diastolic bruit may be auscultated.[114] Baseline assessment of the femoral artery for a bruit before the arterial puncture is essential for comparison post PCI. Diagnosis is confirmed via ultrasound. Treatment may include bed rest with close observation, ultrasound-guided compression, or surgical repair.

Vascular Complications with the Use of Arterial Closure Devices

Vascular closure devices (collagen plug devices and stitch devices) have been used to achieve hemostasis after diagnostic and interventional procedures for several years. These devices have several advantages over traditional manual compression following PCI: less time flat in bed, earlier ambulation, and improved patient comfort. Studies evaluating the effect of closure devices on vascular complications are limited. Resnic and colleagues[115] performed a retrospective analysis of more than 3027 patients who underwent PCI (1485 received a vascular closure device and 1409 received GP IIb/IIIa inhibitor therapy). Vascular complications were defined as development of arteriovenous fistula, pseudoaneurysm, large hematoma, or the need for transfusion or surgical repair. The use of vascular closure devices was associated with a significantly reduced risk of vascular complications compared with closure device-eligible patients who received conventional manual compression. This benefit was more evident in the subgroup of patients who received GP IIb/IIIa inhibitors. More studies are needed for further evaluation of arterial closure devices.

Contrast-Induced Nephropathy

Contrast-induced nephropathy is a potential complication following administration of contrast medium used during PCI and diagnostic catheterization. The ACC/AHA/SCAI PCI guideline defines contrast-induced nephropathy as an increase in serum creatinine greater than 25 percent or a greater than 0.5 mg/dl increase that occurs 48 hours after PCI (compared with preprocedure values).[7] Mehran and colleagues[116] identified several risk factors to help identify patients at risk of contrast-induced nephropathy and those at risk of requiring dialysis: age greater than 75; anemia (baseline hematocrit less than 39 percent for men and less than 36 percent for women); diabetes mellitus; hypotension (systolic blood pressure less than 80 mm Hg for at least 1 hour requiring inotropic support with medications or use of an intraaortic balloon pump within 24 hours periprocedurally); use of an intraaortic balloon pump without hypotension; chronic congestive heart failure;

acute pulmonary edema upon admission; serum creatinine greater than 1.5 mg/dl or estimated glomerular filtration rate less than 60 ml/min/1.73 m^2; and volume of contrast medium used. Preprocedure volume depletion and concomitant administration of nephrotoxic medications also have been associated with the incidence of contrast-induced nephropathy.

Care of Patients Undergoing Percutaneous Coronary Intervention

Patients and families must be educated about pre- and post-PCI procedures. Before elective PCI, patients must be hydrated because they are in a fasting state. Hydration is important because the contrast medium used during PCI is excreted through the kidneys. A baseline electrolyte panel, blood urea nitrogen level, and creatinine level should be obtained to identify abnormal values and should be used for comparison in the post-PCI period. Patients with any elevation in preprocedure creatinine levels should receive acetylcysteine[117,118] or a sodium bicarbonate drip[119] before undergoing PCI. These two medications have shown promise in decreasing the incidence of contrast-induced nephropathy. Free radicals have been suggested to mediate contrast-induced nephropathy.[117-119] In two small studies, investigators found a significant decrease in contrast-induced nephropathy with the use of acetylcysteine, a free radical scavenger. Acetylcysteine was given as a 600-mg dose by mouth twice daily the day before the procedure and twice daily on the day of the procedure, in conjunction with intravenous hydration.[117,118]

Free radicals form in an acidic environment and are inhibited by an alkaline environment.[119] Merten and colleagues[119] found that preprocedure and postprocedure hydration with sodium bicarbonate mixed in intravenous fluid was more effective in preventing contrast-induced nephropathy than sodium chloride alone. Study patients who received a sodium bicarbonate infusion (154 mEq/liter of sodium bicarbonate added to 846 ml of 5 percent dextrose and water) had a significant decrease in contrast-induced nephropathy compared with control patients who received standard hydration (154 mEq/liter of sodium chloride in 5 percent dextrose). The following protocol was used in the study. One hour before the procedure involving contrast, patients received a sodium bicarbonate infusion of 3 ml/kg/hr. Patients weighing more than 110 kg received a same initial infusion as a patient weighing 110 kg. During the procedure and for 6 hours after the procedure, the patient continued to receive the infusion at a rate of 1 ml/kg/hr. Although the sample size was small, the study was terminated early because of ethical issues. The patients receiving sodium bicarbonate infusions received such a benefit that the investigators did not want to continue to expose control patients to the higher risk of contrast-induced nephropathy.

Prevention of contrast-induced nephropathy involves obtaining a thorough history from the patient, including a history of renal disease or diabetes and history of contrast-induced nephropathy or current use of nephrotoxic medications. Consider withholding diuretic therapy on the day of the procedure. Prehydration should start as early as possible. If a sodium bicarbonate infusion is used, a second intravenous catheter should be placed because sodium bicarbonate is incompatible with many medications.

Before PCI, a baseline hemoglobin and hematocrit, platelet count, PT, and PTT should be obtained for comparison in the post-PCI period. Patients with baseline anemia, thrombocytopenia of unknown origin, or coagulopathies may need a hematological work-up before elective PCI.

Patients with previous contrast reactions must be identified and pretreated with steroids, histamine$_1$ blockers (i.e., diphenhydramine), and/or histamine$_2$ blockers (i.e., cimetidine/ranitidine).[101] Patients undergoing elective PCI should receive aspirin and clopidogrel the morning of the procedure. Box 58-5 summarizes the evidence-based recommendations regarding the use of clopidogrel in patients undergoing elective PCI.

The femoral access site should be palpated for presence and fullness of pulses and should be auscultated for a bruit before the arterial puncture (if radial or brachial artery access is planned, those sites must be assessed). The assessment provides important baseline information for comparison in the post-PCI period. Assessment of distal pulses also must be performed to provide baseline information for comparison post-PCI.

Patients with diabetes who take metformin (or combination medication containing metformin) and are exposed to contrast medium have a potential to develop lactic acidosis post-PCI. In patients with normal creatinine levels, metformin should be held the morning of the procedure (in elective cases) and should not be restarted until a stable serum creatinine is obtained, usually 48 hours post-PCI. Patients with abnormal creatinine levels who take metformin should have the elective PCI postponed if not required to be done urgently. The referring physician should be contacted about possibly discontinuing the metformin, because metformin is

---

BOX 58-5 ■ ■ ■

RECOMMENDATIONS REGARDING THE USE OF CLOPIDOGREL IN PATIENTS UNDERGOING PERCUTANEOUS CORONARY INTERVENTION

1. A loading dose of 300 mg of clopidogrel is recommended, although a 600-mg loading dose appears reasonable. More research is needed to determine the optimal loading dose.
2. Clopidogrel should be started as early as possible (more than 6 hours) before elective percutaneous coronary intervention (when the anatomy has been defined previously on diagnostic cardiac catheterization).
3. For patients undergoing cardiac catheterization with possible percutaneous coronary intervention immediately following the catheterization, clopidogrel should be given on the catheterization table before the start of percutaneous coronary intervention.
4. Glycoprotein IIb/IIIa inhibitors and clopidogrel should be used together and should be started before percutaneous coronary intervention, especially in high-risk patients.
5. Daily clopidogrel administration should be continued for up to 1 year after percutaneous coronary intervention.

Adapted from Tcheng JE, Campbell ME: Platelet inhibition strategies in percutaneous coronary intervention, *J Am Coll Cardiol* 42:1196-1198, 2003.

contraindicated in patients with significant renal insufficiency. Patients who have an abnormal creatinine, take metformin, and need to undergo primary PCI should have the risks and benefits explained before proceeding with PCI.[120]

Following PCI, nursing care should focus on monitoring the patient for the following: myocardial ischemia, vascular access site bleeding, contrast-induced nephropathy, neurovascular changes in the distal extremity, and neurological changes.

Before discharge, nurses should educate the patient and family on secondary prevention strategies (i.e., control of blood pressure, cholesterol, and blood glucose; tobacco cessation; dietary modifications; weight management; and regular exercise). Upon discharge, the importance of taking aspirin and clopidogrel daily to prevent stent thrombosis must be stressed. Aspirin 325 mg daily is continued indefinitely (dosage may be reduced at a later time). Clopidogrel 75 mg is continued daily for 1 year after a bare metal or drug-eluting stent is implanted.[7,97]

TREATMENT FOR STEMI: PRIMARY PERCUTANEOUS CORONARY INTERVENTION OR FIBRINOLYTIC THERAPY?

Three major factors result in decreased mortality in patients with STEMI: early diagnosis, immediate treatment with aspirin, and prompt reestablishment of blood flow in the occluded artery. Blood flow can be reestablished with the administration of fibrinolytic therapy or primary PCI. Despite the ease of administration with newer fibrinolytic agents, most patients who have STEMI do not receive fibrinolytic therapy because of relative or absolute contraindications. Patients who do not receive fibrinolytic therapy are disproportionately elderly, women, those with a history of myocardial infarction, multivessel coronary artery disease, or decreased left ventricular function. The majority of patients who receive fibrinolytic therapy do not regain TIMI 3 flow, which results in less myocardial preservation and poor short- and long-term survival. The clinical benefits of fibrinolytic therapy correlate with the rapid restoration of TIMI 3 flow.[10]

Primary PCI can reestablish TIMI 3 flow, which is associated with improved clinical outcomes, in 70 to 90 percent of patients with STEMI.[7] Primary PCI also provides immediate assessment of coronary anatomy and hemodynamic information, which can improve patient care and facilitate earlier hospital discharge.[10] (Refer to Figure 58-11 for a 12-lead electrocardiogram and preangiogram and postangiogram of a patient who had an acute anterior STEMI and underwent primary PTCA to reestablish coronary blood flow to the left anterior descending artery.)

A quantitative review of 23 randomized controlled trials comparing fibrinolytic therapy with primary PCI was published in 2003.[9] The review included 7739 patients randomly assigned to PCI or fibrinolytic therapy. Bare metal stents were used in 12 trials, and GP IIb/IIIa inhibitors were used in 8 trials. Studies using drug-eluting stents were not included in the review. The authors found that primary PCI was better than fibrinolytic therapy at reducing short-term and long-term major adverse cardiac events, including death, in patients with STEMI. The authors concluded that primary PCI was superior to fibrinolytic therapy regardless of the fibrinolytic agent used or if PCI was delayed because of transfer to a hospital capable of performing the procedure.

With the advent of stents, two meta-analyses of randomized trials were published comparing primary stenting (with a bare metal stent) with balloon angioplasty in patients with STEMI. The use of primary stenting with bare metal stents did not show a reduction in mortality compared with balloon angioplasty but did show a decrease in revascularization of the treated coronary artery within 12 months post-PCI.[121,122] The use of the sirolimus drug-eluting stent in primary PCI for STEMI has been investigated in two studies and has been found to be safe and effective in reducing the incidence of death and restenosis post-PCI.[123,124] Drug-eluting stents are being used frequently in primary PCI.

A limitation of primary PCI is that many patients present outside of normal working hours, so hospitals must have policies in place for prompt activation of the cardiac catheterization team.[10] Primary PCI is similar to elective PCI, except the patient is usually symptomatic and often hemodynamically unstable. Stabilization of the patient is paramount, along with quick vascular access (usually femoral; however, radial or brachial approaches may be used) in order to open the occluded vessel.

Mortality with the use of fibrinolytic therapy has been shown to be dependent on time of symptom onset to reperfusion of the occluded artery. Mortality after primary PCI appears to be less dependent on time of symptom onset to reperfusion of the occluded artery. Despite the time to reperfusion, the high rate of TIMI 3 flow after primary PCI suggests that reestablishment of blood flow to the coronary artery may be the key to survival, rather than the time to reperfusion.[125] Because primary PCI is not readily available in many community hospitals, time is required to transport a patient to a PCI-capable hospital. A meta-analysis of six randomized controlled trials compared transfer of patients for primary PCI (transfer time less than 3 hours) to patients receiving on-site fibrinolytic therapy. The meta-analysis demonstrated that emergent transfer to a PCI-capable hospital is feasible and safe and is associated with improved clinical outcomes compared with on-site fibrinolytic therapy.[126]

Because most patients do not present at a PCI-capable hospital, a trial was undertaken to evaluate the possibility of performing primary PCI for STEMI in community hospitals that did not perform elective PCI or have on-site cardiac surgery programs. In the trial, staff in 11 community hospitals in Maryland and Massachusetts were trained in primary PCI. Staff received extensive training with PCI performed by relatively high-volume interventional cardiologists from nearby communities. Four hundred fifty-one patients who had STEMI were randomized to undergo primary PCI or fibrinolytic therapy at the community hospital. Patients assigned to reperfusion with primary PCI had a lower incidence of death, reinfarction, and stroke within 30 days and

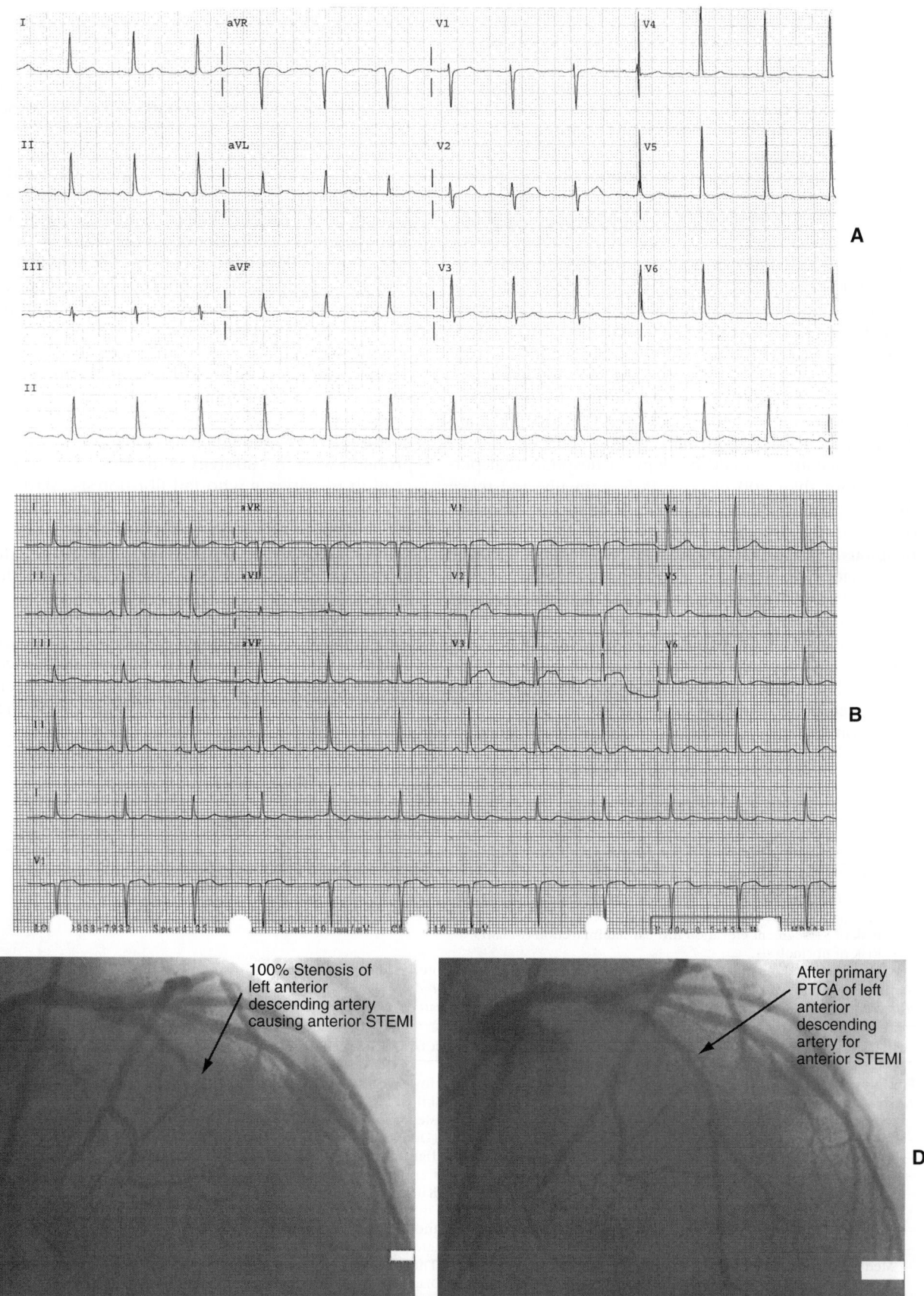

FIGURE 58-11 ■ **A,** Electrocardiogram of patient taken 1 year before presenting to the emergency room with chest pain. **B,** Electrocardiogram of patient during chest pain. Note the loss of R wave in leads V₁ and V₂ and the ST segment elevations in leads V₁ to V₃ compared with **A. C,** The patient was taken emergently to the cardiac catheterization laboratory. The left anterior descending artery was totally occluded *(arrow),* causing an anterior ST segment elevation myocardial infarction. **D,** Angiogram of patient after primary angioplasty. The left anterior descending artery was opened successfully *(arrow). PTCA,* Percutaneous transluminal coronary angioplasty.

6 months post-PCI compared with patients assigned to fibrinolytic therapy. They also had shorter hospitalizations.[127] Based on these results, many community hospitals are opening programs for primary PCI in STEMI patients. This is a concern to some authors.[128,129] PCI performed during the early phase of an acute myocardial infarction can be challenging, requiring more skill and experience than performing elective PCI. The need for an experienced interventional cardiologist and laboratory staff is essential. Having all the available equipment (catheters, guidewires, stents in various sizes), intraaortic balloon pump capability, and staff that are comfortable and skilled with the use of the equipment is of paramount importance. The ACC/AHA/SCAI guideline recommends primary PCI be performed by physicians who perform more than 75 elective PCI procedures annually, and at least 11 primary PCIs for STEMI. Ideally, these procedures should be done in hospitals that perform more than 400 elective PCIs annually and more than 36 primary PCIs annually. The guideline also recommends that primary and elective PCI be performed at hospitals with on-site cardiac surgery programs. Primary PCI performed at hospitals without elective PCI programs or those without on-site cardiac surgery programs should be restricted to those institutions with a proven plan for rapid transfer to a hospital with cardiac surgery capability, with a goal of 90 minutes from initial presentation to balloon inflation.[7] Fibrinolytic therapy is still an appropriate reperfusion strategy and is the preferred reperfusion option over primary PCI when performed by an inexperienced cardiologist in an inexperienced hospital with less experienced staff. Table 58-2 presents the ACC/AHA assessment for reperfusion options for patients who have STEMI.[4]

Facilitated PCI refers to treatment with either full-dose fibrinolytic, half-dose fibrinolytic, a GP IIb/IIIa inhibitor, or a combination of reduced-dose fibrinolytic therapy and a GP IIb/IIIa inhibitor when PCI is not immediately available and bleeding risk is low. The rationale is to provide early pharmacological reperfusion before primary PCI in order to reduce infarction size and improve outcomes.[7] Early studies have shown no benefit to facilitated PCI and actually demonstrated harm resulting from bleeding complications.[10] Newer studies will be forthcoming.[130]

Rescue PCI is defined as PCI within 12 hours of failed fibrinolysis for patients with ongoing ischemia. One problem with this strategy is the lack of accurate identification of patients who fail fibrinolysis. Markers of reperfusion (relief of chest discomfort, partial resolution of ST-segment elevation and reperfusion dysrhythmias) provide limited predictive value in identifying failed fibrinolysis. Myocardial necrosis occurs when the coronary occlusion has been present for more than 3 hours. Without early recognition of failed fibrinolysis (within 3 to 6 hours of symptom onset), salvage of the ischemic myocardium is unlikely. Given the delays common among patients presenting to the hospital after symptom onset, making the decision to proceed with fibrinolytic therapy, recognition of failed fibrinolysis, and ini-

■ ■ ■

TABLE 58-2　ASSESSMENT OF REPERFUSION OPTIONS FOR PATIENTS WHO HAVE STEMI

Step 1: Assess time and risk.
- Time since onset of symptoms
- Risk of ST segment elevation myocardial infarction (STEMI)
- Risk of fibrinolysis
- Time required for transport to a skilled percutaneous coronary intervention (PCI) laboratory

Step 2: Determine whether fibinolysis or an invasive strategy is preferred.
If presentation is less than 3 hours and there is no delay to an invasive strategy, there is no preference for either strategy.

FIBRINOLYSIS	PERCUTANEOUS CORONARY INTERVENTION
Fibrinloysis generally is preferred if:	An invasive strategy generally is preferred if:
• Early presentation (≤3 hours from symptom onset and delay to invasive strategy; see below)	• Skilled PCI laboratory*† available with surgical backup
• Invasive strategy is not an option	— Medical contact-to-balloon or door-to-balloon is less than 90 minutes
— Catheterization laboratory occupied/not available	— (Door-to-balloon) − (Door-to-needle) = Less than 1 hour‡
— Vascular access difficulties	• High risk from STEMI
— Lack of access to a skilled PCI laboratory*†	— Cardiogenic shock
• Delay to invasive strategy	— Killip class is 3
— Prolonged transport	• Contraindications to fibrinolysis, including increased risk of bleeding and intracranial hemorrhage
— (Door-to-balloon) − (Door-to-needle) = More than 1 hour‡§	• Late presentation
— Medical contact-to-balloon or door-to-balloon time is more than 90 minutes	— The symptom onset was more than 3 hours ago
	• Diagnosis of STEMI is in doubt

*Operator experience greater than a total of 75 primary PCI cases per year.
†Team experience greater than a total of 36 primary PCI cases per year.
‡Applies to fibrin-specific agents.
§This calculation implies that the estimated delay to the implementation of the invasive strategy is greater than 1 hour versus initiation of fibrinolytic therapy immediately with a fibrin-specific agent.
From Antman EM, Anbe DT, Armstrong PW et al: *ACC/AHA pocket guideline: management of patients with ST-elevation myocardial infarction.* Retrieved February 11, 2007, from *www.acc.org/qualityandscience/clinical/guidelines/stemi/index_pkt.pdf.* Based on Antman EM, Anbe DT, Armstrong PW et al: *J Am Coll Cardiol* 44:671-719, 2004.

tiation of PCI, there may be limited salvage of the ischemic myocardium. Rescue PCI is recommended only in specific circumstances.[7]

Results from studies of patients who have STEMI, non-STEMI, and unstable angina support a change in the health care system in the United States in order to provide earlier revascularization with PCI.[128] Centers of excellence for care of patients with acute coronary syndromes have been suggested.[128,129] One author makes the analogy to the emergency trauma system that exists in the United States in which there are regional centers of excellence with experienced staff 24 hours a day, 7 days a week. The number of deaths from myocardial infarction far exceed the number of deaths from trauma in the United States.[128] Cardiology centers of excellence would be responsible for delivery of high-quality care, ensuring that every patient is treated in a high-volume interventional cardiac catheterization laboratory with highly skilled physicians and nursing staff.[128,129] Centers of excellence could implement evidence-based strategies on site and in the community to improve patient care. Adherence to guidelines could be compared among the centers of excellence, potentially leading to improvement in patient outcomes. Smaller facilities could be used as triage centers with patients appropriately risk stratified for initial therapy. With a systematic approach to care, continuous quality care may be achieved and outcomes may improve.[129]

■■■ PHARMACOLOGY

CHELATION THERAPY

Chelation therapy for ischemic heart disease involves the intravenous administration of chelators, mainly ethylenediaminetetraacetic acid (EDTA).[131] EDTA injected into the blood binds heavy metals such as iron and allows them to be removed from the body. Theories as to how chelation works include liberation of calcium from plaque, causing a favorable change in the properties of the plaque; free radical scavenger function; antioxidant effects; reduction in total body iron stores; cell membrane stabilization; improvement in arterial wall elasticity; and arterial dilatation. The effectiveness of chelation therapy in patients with coronary artery disease is not proven. Chelation therapy is not approved by the Food and Drug Administration to treat coronary artery disease. Some patients undergoing chelation therapy describe an improvement in symptoms; however, it has not been studied in large randomized clinical trials. A small study published in 2002 reported no evidence to support chelation therapy in patients with coronary artery disease.[132]

In August 2002 the National Center for Complementary and Alternative Medicine and the National Heart, Lung, and Blood Institute, both of which are part of National Institutes of Health, announced a new study to evaluate chelation therapy. The Trial to Assess Chelation Therapy (TACT) will be the first large-scale, multicenter study to determine whether EDTA chelation therapy is an effective therapy for persons with coronary artery disease. This placebo-controlled, double blind study will involve more than 2300 participants age 50 years and older who have suffered a myocardial infarction. The trial will be large enough to determine whether there is any benefit to chelation therapy. About 100 sites throughout the United States will participate in the trial. Recruitment began in March 2003. Participants will receive 30 weekly intravenous treatments and then 10 bimonthly treatments over a 28-month period. They also will receive high doses of vitamins, which often are given with chelation therapy. The effect of the vitamin doses will be examined in the study. The study is estimated to take about 5 years to complete.[133]

SUMMARY

Fibrinolytic therapy and primary PCI are effective strategies to reestablish coronary blood flow and reduce mortality from STEMI. PCI is a valuable therapy for patients with unstable angina, non-STEMI, and chronic stable angina and for patients with asymptomatic coronary ischemia. PCI is a proven reperfusion strategy after coronary artery disease has presented itself but should be thought of only as palliative therapy. Even after successful pharmacological or mechanical reperfusion, coronary artery disease continues to plague the coronary vasculature, so it is imperative to discuss secondary prevention strategies with the patient and family before discharge. Patients may have difficulty understanding that coronary artery disease is a chronic disease with no known cure. Health care providers must educate the patient and family that coronary artery disease is a progressive disease but must emphasize that with secondary prevention measures, the rate of progression of the disease may be slowed. Secondary prevention measures include lifetime aspirin therapy, angiotensin-converting enzyme inhibitor therapy based on evidence-based data,[134] antianginal therapy (if the patient demonstrates small branch vessel coronary disease on angiogram not amenable to PCI or develops angina because of incomplete revascularization), beta blocker therapy, blood pressure control, cessation of tobacco use, cholesterol control, glycemic control in patients with diabetes, dietary modifications to include low-fat and low-cholesterol foods, achieving/maintaining desired weight for the individual's height, and regular cardiovascular exercise. Secondary prevention measures can reduce morbidity and mortality associated with coronary artery disease.[7]

REFERENCES

1. American Heart Association: *Heart disease and stroke statistics: 2005 update*, Dallas, 2005, The Association.
2. Braunwald E, Antman EM, Beasley JW et al: ACC/AHA guidelines for the management of patients with unstable angina and non-ST-segment elevation myocardial infarction: executive summary and recommendations—a report of the American College of Cardiology/American Heart Association Task Force on Practice Guidelines (Committee on the Management of Patients with Unstable Angina), *Circulation* 102:1193-1209, 2000.
3. Ryan TJ, Anderson JL, Antman EM et al: ACC/AHA guidelines for the management of patients with acute myocardial infarction: executive summary—a report of the American College of Cardiology/American Heart Association Task Force on Practice Guidelines (Committee on Management of Acute Myocardial Infarction), *J Am Coll Cardiol* 28:1328-1428, 1996.
4. Antman EM, Anbe DT, Armstrong PW et al: ACC/AHA guidelines for the management of patients with ST-elevation myocardial infarction: executive summary—a report of the American College of Cardiology/American Heart Association Task Force on Practice Guidelines (Writing Committee to revise the 1999 guidelines for the management of patients with acute myocardial infarction), *J Am Coll Cardiol* 44:671-719, 2004.
5. Braunwald E, Antman EM, Beasley JW et al: ACC/AHA 2002 guideline update for the management of patients with unstable angina and non-ST-segment elevation myocardial infarction: summary article—a report of the American College of Cardiology/American Heart Association Task Force on Practice Guidelines (Committee on the Management of Patients with Unstable Angina), *Circulation* 106:1893-1900, 2002.

6. Gibbons RJ, Abrams J, Chatterjee K et al: ACC/AHA 2002 guideline update for the management of patients with chronic stable angina: a report of the American College of Cardiology/American Heart Association Task Force on Practice Guidelines (Committee to Update the 1999 Guidelines for the Management of Patients with Chronic Stable Angina), Retrieved January 24, 2007, from www.acc.org/clinical/guidelines/stable/stable.pdf.

7. Smith SC Jr. Feldman TE. Hirshfeld JW et al: ACC/AHA/SCAI 2005 guideline update for percutaneous coronary intervention: a report of the American College of Cardiology/American Heart Association Task Force on Practice Guidelines (ACC/AHA/SCAI Writing Committee to Update 2001 Guidelines for Percutaneous Coronary Intervention), *Circulation.* 113:e166-286, 2006.

8. Alpert JS, Thygesen K, Antman E, Bassand JP: Myocardial infarction redefined: a consensus document of the Joint European Society of Cardiology/American College of Cardiology committee for the redefinition of myocardial infarction, *J Am Coll Cardiol* 36:959-969, 2000.

9. Keeley EC, Boura JA, Grines CL: Primary angioplasty versus intravenous thrombolytic therapy for acute myocardial infarction: a quantitative review of 23 randomised trials, *Lancet* 361:13-20, 2003.

10. Keeley EC, Grines CL: Primary coronary intervention for acute myocardial infarction, *JAMA* 291:736-739, 2004.

11. Invasive compared with non-invasive treatment in unstable coronary-artery disease: FRISC II prospective randomised multicentre study—FRagmin and Fast Revascularisation during InStability in Coronary artery disease Investigators, *Lancet* 354:708-715, 1999.

12. Cannon CP, Weintraub WS, Demopoulos LA et al: Comparison of early invasive and conservative strategies in patients with unstable coronary syndromes treated with the glycoprotein IIb/IIIa inhibitor tirofiban, *N Engl J Med* 344:1879-1887, 2001.

13. Fox KA, Poole-Wilson PA, Henderson RA et al: Interventional versus conservative treatment for patients with unstable angina or non–ST-elevation myocardial infarction: the British Heart Foundation RITA 3 randomised trial—Randomized Intervention Trial of unstable Angina, *Lancet* 360:743-751, 2002.

14. Fletcher AP, Alkjaersig N, Smyrniotis FE, Sherry S: The treatment of patients suffering from early myocardial infarction with massive and prolonged streptokinase therapy, *Trans Assoc Am Physicians* 71:287-296, 1958.

15. Rentrop KP, Blanke H, Karsch KR et al: Acute myocardial infarction: intracoronary application of nitroglycerin and streptokinase, *Clin Cardiol* 2:354-363, 1979.

16. Menon V, Harrington RA, Hochman JS et al: Thrombolysis and adjunctive therapy in acute myocardial infarction: the Seventh ACCP Conference on Antithrombotic and Thrombolytic Therapy, *Chest* 126:549S-575S, 2004.

17. DeWood MA, Spores J, Notske R et al: Prevalence of total coronary occlusion during the early hours of transmural myocardial infarction, *N Engl J Med* 303:897-902, 1980.

18. Kullo IJ, Edwards WD, Schwartz RS: Vulnerable plaque: pathobiology and clinical implications, *Ann Intern Med* 129:1050-1060, 1998.

19. Roettig ML, Tanabe P: Emergency management of acute coronary syndromes, *J Emerg Nurs* 26:S1-S42, 2000.

20. Becker RC: *Fibrinolytic and antithrombotic therapy: theory, practice, and management,* New York, 2000, Oxford University Press.

21. The Thrombolysis in Myocardial Infarction (TIMI) trial: phase I findings—TIMI Study Group, *N Engl J Med* 312:932-936, 1985.

22. The effects of tissue plasminogen activator, streptokinase, or both on coronary-artery patency, ventricular function, and survival after acute myocardial infarction: the GUSTO Angiographic Investigators, *N Engl J Med* 329:1615-1622, 1993.

23. Fowles RE: Third-generation fibrinolytics. In Bruanwald E, editor: *Harrison's advances in cardiology,* New York, 2003, McGraw-Hill.

24. Effectiveness of intravenous thrombolytic treatment in acute myocardial infarction: Gruppo Italiano per lo Studio della Streptochinasi nell'Infarto Miocardico (GISSI), *Lancet* 1:397-402, 1986.

25. Randomised trial of intravenous streptokinase, oral aspirin, both, or neither among 17,187 cases of suspected acute myocardial in-

farction: ISIS-2—ISIS-2 (Second International Study of Infarct Survival) Collaborative Group, *Lancet* 2:349-360, 1988.

26. An international randomized trial comparing four thrombolytic strategies for acute myocardial infarction: the GUSTO investigators, *N Engl J Med* 329:673-682, 1993.

27. Bode C, Smalling RW, Berg G et al: Randomized comparison of coronary thrombolysis achieved with double-bolus reteplase (recombinant plasminogen activator) and front-loaded, accelerated alteplase (recombinant tissue plasminogen activator) in patients with acute myocardial infarction: the RAPID II Investigators, *Circulation* 94:891-898, 1996.

28. A comparison of reteplase with alteplase for acute myocardial infarction: the Global Use of Strategies to Open Occluded Coronary Arteries (GUSTO III) Investigators, *N Engl J Med* 337:1118-1123, 1997.

29. Single-bolus tenecteplase compared with front-loaded alteplase in acute myocardial infarction: the ASSENT-2 double-blind randomised trial—Assessment of the Safety and Efficacy of a New Thrombolytic Investigators, *Lancet* 354:716-722, 1999.

30. Joint Commission on Accreditation of Healthcare Organizations: *2006 critical access hospital and hospital national patient safety goals.* Retrieved February 13, 2007, from www.jointcommission.org/PatientSafety/NationalPatientSafetyGoals/06_npsg_cah.htm

31. Institute for Safe Medication Practices: *ISPM's list of high-alert medications.* Retrieved February 13, 2007, from www.ismp.org/Tools/highalertmedications.pdf

32. Indications for fibrinolytic therapy in suspected acute myocardial infarction: collaborative overview of early mortality and major morbidity results from all randomised trials of more than 1000 patients: Fibrinolytic Therapy Trialists' (FTT) Collaborative Group, *Lancet* 343:311-322, 1994.

33. Brass LM, Lichtman JH, Wang Y et al: Intracranial hemorrhage associated with thrombolytic therapy for elderly patients with acute myocardial infarction: results from the Cooperative Cardiovascular Project, *Stroke* 31:1802-1811, 2000.

34. Reiss BS, Evans ME, Broyles BE: *Pharmacological aspects of nursing care,* ed 6, Albany, NY, 2002, Delmar.

35. Saul L, Smith J, Mook W: The safety of automatic versus manual blood pressure cuffs for patients receiving thrombolytic therapy, *Am J Crit Care* 7:192-196, 1998.

36. Lieberman KS: Markers of reperfusion after thrombolytic therapy for acute myocardial infarction, *J Emerg Nurs* 21:112-115, 1995.

37. Drew BJ, Califf RM, Funk M, et al: Practice standards for electrocardiographic monitoring in hospital settings: an American Heart Association scientific statement from the Councils on Cardiovascular Nursing, Clinical Cardiology, and Cardiovascular Disease in the Young—endorsed by the International Society of Computerized Electrocardiology and the American Association of Critical-Care Nurses, *Circulation* 110:2721-2746, 2004.

38. Broderick JP, Adams HP Jr, Barsan W et al: Guidelines for the management of spontaneous intracerebral hemorrhage: a statement for healthcare professionals from a special writing group of the Stroke Council, American Heart Association, *Stroke* 30:905-915, 1999.

39. Gruntzig AR, Senning A, Siegenthaler WE: Nonoperative dilatation of coronary-artery stenosis: percutaneous transluminal coronary angioplasty, *N Engl J Med* 301:61-68, 1979.

40. Rentrop KP, Blanke H, Karsch KR, Kreuzer H: Initial experience with transluminal recanalization of the recently occluded infarct-related coronary artery in acute myocardial infarction: comparison with conventionally treated patients, *Clin Cardiol* 2:92-105, 1979.

41. Detre KM, Holmes DR, Holubkov R et al: Incidence and consequences of periprocedural occlusion: the 1985-1986 National Heart, Lung, and Blood Institute Percutaneous Transluminal Coronary Angioplasty Registry, *Circulation* 82:739-750, 1990.

42. de Feyter PJ, van den Brand M, Laarman GJ et al: Acute coronary artery occlusion during and after percutaneous transluminal coronary angioplasty: frequency, prediction, clinical course, management, and follow-up, *Circulation* 83:927-936, 1991.

43. Lincoff AM, Popma JJ, Ellis SG et al: Abrupt vessel closure complicating coronary angioplasty: clinical, angiographic and therapeutic profile, *J Am Coll Cardiol* 19:926-935, 1992.

44. Holmes DR, Vlietstra RE, Smith HC et al: Restenosis after percutaneous transluminal coronary angioplasty (PTCA): a report from

the PTCA Registry of the National Heart, Lung, and Blood Institute, *Am J Cardiol* 53:77C-81C, 1984.

45. Gruentzig AR, King SB, Schlumpf M, Siegenthaler W: Long-term follow-up after percutaneous transluminal coronary angioplasty: the early Zurich experience, *N Engl J Med* 316:1127-1132, 1987.

46. Nobuyoshi M, Kimura T, Nosaka H et al: Restenosis after successful percutaneous transluminal coronary angioplasty: serial angiographic follow-up of 229 patients, *J Am Coll Cardiol* 12:616-623, 1988.

47. Morris NB: Brachytherapy: savior or tease, *Crit Care Nurs Clin North Am* 11:333-348, 1999.

48. Schwertz DW, Vaitkus P: Drug-eluting stents to prevent reblockage of coronary arteries, *J Cardiovasc Nurs* 18:11-16, 2003.

49. Fischman DL, Leon MB, Baim DS et al: A randomized comparison of coronary-stent placement and balloon angioplasty in the treatment of coronary artery disease: Stent Restenosis Study Investigators, *N Engl J Med* 331:496-501, 1994.

50. Serruys PW, de Jaegere P, Kiemeneij F et al: A comparison of balloon-expandable-stent implantation with balloon angioplasty in patients with coronary artery disease: Benestent Study Group, *N Engl J Med* 331:489-495, 1994.

51. Sapirstein W, Zuckerman B, Dillard J: FDA approval of coronary-artery brachytherapy, *N Engl J Med* 344:297-299, 2001.

52. Schomig A, Neumann FJ, Kastrati A et al: A randomized comparison of antiplatelet and anticoagulant therapy after the placement of coronary-artery stents, *N Engl J Med* 334:1084-1089, 1996.

53. Morice MC, Serruys PW, Sousa JE et al: A randomized comparison of a sirolimus-eluting stent with a standard stent for coronary revascularization, *N Engl J Med* 346:1773-1780, 2002.

54. Moses JW, Leon MB, Popma JJ et al: Sirolimus-eluting stents versus standard stents in patients with stenosis in a native coronary artery, *N Engl J Med* 349:1315-1323, 2003.

55. Stone GW, Ellis SG, Cox DA et al: A polymer-based, paclitaxel-eluting stent in patients with coronary artery disease, *N Engl J Med* 350:221-231, 2004.

56. Gershlick A, De Scheerder I, Chevalier B et al: Inhibition of restenosis with a paclitaxel-eluting, polymer-free coronary stent: the European evaLUation of pacliTaxel Eluting Stent (ELUTES) trial, *Circulation* 109:487-493, 2004.

57. Popma JJ, Kuntz RE, Baim DS: Percutaneous coronary and valvular intervention. In Zipes DP, Libby P, Bonow RO, Braunwald E, editors: *Braunwald's heart disease: a textbook of cardiovascular medicine,* ed 7, Philadelphia, 2005, WB Saunders.

58. Bittl JA, Chew DP, Topol EJ et al: Meta-analysis of randomized trials of percutaneous transluminal coronary angioplasty versus atherectomy, cutting balloon atherotomy, or laser angioplasty, *J Am Coll Cardiol* 43:936-942, 2004.

59. Senerchia CC: Highlights from the past decade of interventional device research, *Crit Care Nurs Clin North Am* 11:311-325, 1999.

60. Hinohara T, Selmon MR, Robertson GC et al: Directional atherectomy: new approaches for treatment of obstructive coronary and peripheral vascular disease, *Circulation* 81:79-91, 1990.

61. Topol EJ, Leya F, Pinkerton CA et al: A comparison of directional atherectomy with coronary angioplasty in patients with coronary artery disease, *N Engl J Med* 329:221-227, 1993.

62. Simonton CA, Leon MB, Baim DS et al: 'Optimal' directional coronary atherectomy: final results of the Optimal Atherectomy Restenosis Study (OARS), *Circulation* 97:332-339, 1998.

63. Baim DS, Cutlip DE, Sharma SK et al: Final results of the Balloon vs Optimal Atherectomy Trial (BOAT), *Circulation* 97:322-331, 1998.

64. Mauri L, Bonan R, Weiner BH et al: Cutting balloon angioplasty for the prevention of restenosis: results of the Cutting Balloon Global Randomized Trial, *Am J Cardiol* 90:1079-1083, 2002.

65. Stone GW, Cox DA, Babb J et al: Prospective, randomized evaluation of thrombectomy prior to percutaneous intervention in diseased saphenous vein grafts and thrombus-containing coronary arteries, *J Am Coll Cardiol* 42:2007-2013, 2003.

66. Lefkovits J, Holmes DR, Califf RM et al: Predictors and sequelae of distal embolization during saphenous vein graft intervention from the CAVEAT-II trial, *Circulation* 92:734-740, 1995.

67. Hong MK, Mehran R, Dangas G et al: Creatine kinase-MB enzyme elevation following successful saphenous vein graft intervention is associated with late mortality, *Circulation* 100:2400-2405, 1999.

68. Grube E, Schofer JJ, Webb J et al: Saphenous Vein Graft Angioplasty Free of Emboli (SAFE) Trial Study Group: evaluation of a balloon occlusion and aspiration system for protection from distal embolization during stenting in saphenous vein grafts, *Am J Cardiol* 89:941-945, 2002.

69. Baim DS, Wahr D, George B et al: Saphenous vein graft Angioplasty Free of Emboli Randomized (SAFER) Trial Investigators: randomized trial of a distal embolic protection device during percutaneous intervention of saphenous vein aorto-coronary bypass grafts, *Circulation* 105:1285-1290, 2002.

70. Stone GW, Rogers C, Ramee S et al: Distal filter protection during saphenous vein graft stenting: technical and clinical correlates of efficacy, *J Am Coll Cardiol* 40:1882-1888, 2002.

71. Stone GW, Rogers C, Hermiller J et al: Randomized comparison of distal protection with a filter-based catheter and a balloon occlusion and aspiration system during percutaneous intervention of diseased saphenous vein aorto-coronary bypass grafts, *Circulation* 108:548-553, 2003.

72. Savage MP, Douglas JS, Fischman DL et al: Stent placement compared with balloon angioplasty for obstructed coronary bypass grafts: Saphenous Vein De Novo Trial Investigators, *N Engl J Med* 337:740-747, 1997.

73. Waksman R, Weinberger J: Coronary brachytherapy in the drug-eluting stent era: don't bury it alive, *Circulation* 108:386-388, 2003.

74. Teirstein PS, Massullo V, Jani S et al: Three-year clinical and angiographic follow-up after intracoronary radiation: results of a randomized clinical trial, *Circulation* 101:360-365, 2000.

75. Waksman R, White RL, Chan RC et al: Intracoronary gamma-radiation therapy after angioplasty inhibits recurrence in patients with in-stent restenosis, *Circulation* 101:2165-2171, 2000.

76. Leon MB, Teirstein PS, Moses JW et al: Localized intracoronary gamma-radiation therapy to inhibit the recurrence of restenosis after stenting, *N Engl J Med* 344:250-256, 2001.

77. Waksman R, Ajani AE, Pinnow E et al: Twelve versus six months of clopidogrel to reduce major cardiac events in patients undergoing gamma-radiation therapy for in-stent restenosis: Washington Radiation for In-Stent restenosis Trial (WRIST) 12 versus WRIST PLUS, *Circulation* 106:776-778, 2002.

78. Popma JJ, Suntharalingam M, Lansky AJ et al: Stents And Radiation Therapy (START) Investigators: randomized trial of 90Sr/90Y beta-radiation versus placebo control for treatment of in-stent restenosis, *Circulation* 106:1090-1096, 2002.

79. Sousa JE, Serruys PW, Costa MA: New frontiers in cardiology: drug-eluting stents—part I, *Circulation* 107:2274-2279, 2003.

80. Teirstein PS: A chicken in every pot and a drug-eluting stent in every lesion, *Circulation* 109:1906-1910, 2004.

81. Sousa JE, Serruys PW, Costa MA: New frontiers in cardiology: drug-eluting stents—part II, *Circulation* 107:2383-2389, 2003.

82. Kastrati A, Mehilli J, von Beckerath N et al: ISAR-DESIRE Study I: sirolimus-eluting stent or paclitaxel-eluting stent vs balloon angioplasty for prevention of recurrences in patients with coronary in-stent restenosis—a randomized controlled trial, *JAMA* 293:165-171, 2005.

83. Pijls NH, De Bruyne B, Peels K et al: Measurement of fractional flow reserve to assess the functional severity of coronary-artery stenoses, *N Engl J Med* 334:1703-1708, 1996.

84. Hau WK: Fractional flow reserve and complex coronary intervention, *J Chin Med Assoc* 67:433-438, 2004.

85. Pijls NH, Van Gelder B, Van der Voort P et al: Fractional flow reserve: a useful index to evaluate the influence of an epicardial coronary stenosis on myocardial blood flow, *Circulation* 92:3183-3193, 1995.

86. Pijls NH, Klauss V, Siebert U et al: Fractional Flow Reserve (FFR) Post-Stent Registry Investigators: coronary pressure measurement after stenting predicts adverse events at follow-up—a multicenter registry, *Circulation* 105:2950-2954, 2002.

87. Nissen SE, Yock P: Intravascular ultrasound: novel pathophysiological insights and current clinical applications, *Circulation* 103:604-616, 2001.

88. Orford JL, Lerman A, Holmes DR: Routine intravascular ultrasound guidance of percutaneous coronary intervention: a critical reappraisal, *J Am Coll Cardiol* 43:1335-1342, 2004.

89. Popma JJ, Berger P, Ohman EM et al: Antithrombotic therapy during percutaneous coronary intervention: the Seventh ACCP Conference on Antithrombotic and Thrombolytic Therapy, *Chest* 126:576S-599S, 2004.

90. Jneid H, Bhatt DL, Corti R et al: Aspirin and clopidogrel in acute coronary syndromes: therapeutic insights from the CURE study, *Arch Intern Med* 163:1145-1153, 2003.

91. Leon MB, Baim DS, Popma JJ et al: A clinical trial comparing three antithrombotic-drug regimens after coronary-artery stenting: Stent Anticoagulation Restenosis Study Investigators, *N Engl J Med* 339:1665-1671, 1998.

92. Bhatt DL, Bertrand ME, Berger PB et al: Meta-analysis of randomized and registry comparisons of ticlopidine with clopidogrel after stenting, *J Am Coll Cardiol* 39:9-14, 2002.

93. Mehta SR, Yusuf S, Peters RJ et al: Effects of pretreatment with clopidogrel and aspirin followed by long-term therapy in patients undergoing percutaneous coronary intervention: the PCI-CURE study, *Lancet* 358:527-533, 2001.

94. Steinhubl SR, Berger PB, Mann JT et al: Early and sustained dual oral antiplatelet therapy following percutaneous coronary intervention: a randomized controlled trial, *JAMA* 288:2411-2420, 2002.

95. Chan AW, Moliterno DJ, Berger PB et al: Triple antiplatelet therapy during percutaneous coronary intervention is associated with improved outcomes including one-year survival: results from the Do Tirofiban and ReoProGive Similar Efficacy Outcome Trial (TARGET), *J Am Coll Cardiol* 42:1188-1195, 2003.

96. Kastrati A, Mehilli J, Schuhlen H et al: A clinical trial of abciximab in elective percutaneous coronary intervention after pretreatment with clopidogrel, *N Engl J Med* 350:232-238, 2004.

97. Grines CL, Bonow RO, Casey DE et al: Prevention of premature discontinuation of dual antiplatelet therapy in patients with coronary artery stents: A science advisory from the American Heart Association, American College of Cardiology, Society for Cardiovascular Angiography and Interventions, American College of Surgeons, and American Dental Association, with representation from the American College of Physicians, *J Am Coll Cardiol* 49:734-739, 2007.

98. Cheng JW: Efficacy of glycoprotein IIb/IIIa-receptor inhibitors during percutaneous coronary intervention, *Am J Health Syst Pharm* 59:S5-S14, 2002.

99. Use of a monoclonal antibody directed against the platelet glycoprotein IIb/IIIa receptor in high-risk coronary angioplasty: the EPIC Investigation, *N Engl J Med* 330:956-961, 1994.

100. Platelet glycoprotein IIb/IIIa receptor blockade and low-dose heparin during percutaneous coronary revascularization: the EPILOG Investigators, *N Engl J Med* 336:1689-1696, 1997.

101. Bashore TM, Bates ER, Berger PB et al: American College of Cardiology/Society for Cardiac Angiography and Interventions Clinical Expert Consensus Document on cardiac catheterization laboratory standards: a report of the American College of Cardiology Task Force on Clinical Expert Consensus Documents, *J Am Coll Cardiol* 37:2170-2214, 2001.

102. Randomised placebo-controlled and balloon-angioplasty-controlled trial to assess safety of coronary stenting with use of platelet glycoprotein-IIb/IIIa blockade: the EPISTENT Investigators—Evaluation of Platelet IIb/IIIa Inhibitor for Stenting, *Lancet* 352:87-92, 1998.

103. Randomised Placebo-Controlled Trial of effect of eptifibatide on complications of percutaneous coronary intervention: IMPACT-II—Integrilin to Minimise Platelet Aggregation and Coronary Thrombosis-II, *Lancet* 349:1422-1428, 1997.

104. ESPRIT Investigators: Enhanced Suppression of the Platelet IIb/IIIa Receptor with Integrilin Therapy: novel dosing regimen of eptifibatide in planned coronary stent implantation (ESPRIT)—a randomised, placebo-controlled trial, *Lancet* 356:2037-2044, 2000.

105. DiDomenico RJ: New antithrombotics for the intensive care unit setting: GP IIb/IIIa inhibitors, low-molecular-weight heparins, and direct thrombin inhibitors, *Crit Care Nurs Q* 22:61-74, 2000.

106. Effects of platelet glycoprotein IIb/IIIa blockade with tirofiban on adverse cardiac events in patients with unstable angina or acute myocardial infarction undergoing coronary angioplasty: the RESTORE Investigators—Randomized Efficacy Study of Tirofiban for Outcomes and REstenosis, *Circulation* 96:1445-1453, 1997.

107. Lincoff AM, Bittl JA, Harrington RA et al: Bivalirudin and provisional glycoprotein IIb/IIIa blockade compared with heparin and planned glycoprotein IIb/IIIa blockade during percutaneous coronary intervention: REPLACE-2 randomized trial, *JAMA* 289:853-863, 2003.

108. Caron MF, McKendall GR: Bivalirudin in percutaneous coronary intervention, *Am J Health Syst Pharm* 60:1841-1849, 2003.

109. Bittl JA, Strony J, Brinker JA et al: Treatment with bivalirudin (Hirulog) as compared with heparin during coronary angioplasty for unstable or postinfarction angina: Hirulog Angioplasty Study Investigators, *N Engl J Med* 333:764-769, 1995.

110. Mehilli J, Kastrati A, Schuhlen H et al: Intracoronary Stenting and Antithrombotic Regimen: Is Abciximab a Superior Way to Eliminate Elevated Thrombotic Risk in Diabetics (ISAR-SWEET) Study Investigators—randomized clinical trial of abciximab in diabetic patients undergoing elective percutaneous coronary interventions after treatment with a high loading dose of clopidogrel, *Circulation* 110:3627-3635, 2004.

111. Stuckey TD, Stone GW, Cox DA et al: Impact of stenting and abciximab in patients with diabetes mellitus undergoing primary angioplasty in acute myocardial infarction (the CADILLAC Trial), *Am J Cardiol* 95:1-7, 2005.

112. Chauhan MS, Ho KK, Baim DS et al: Effect of gender on in-hospital and one-year outcomes after contemporary coronary artery stenting, *Am J Cardiol* 95:101-104, 2005.

113. Fuchs S, Stabile E, Kinnaird TD et al: Stroke complicating percutaneous coronary interventions: incidence, predictors, and prognostic implications, *Circulation* 106:86-91, 2002.

114. Levine GN, Kern MJ, Berger PB et al: American Heart Association Diagnostic and Interventional Catheterization Committee and Council on Clinical Cardiology: management of patients undergoing percutaneous coronary revascularization, *Ann Intern Med* 139:123-136, 2003.

115. Resnic FS, Blake GJ, Ohno-Machado L et al: Vascular closure devices and the risk of vascular complications after percutaneous coronary intervention in patients receiving glycoprotein IIb-IIIa inhibitors, *Am J Cardiol* 88:493-496, 2001.

116. Mehran R, Aymong ED, Nikolsky E et al: A simple risk score for prediction of contrast-induced nephropathy after percutaneous coronary intervention: development and initial validation, *J Am Coll Cardiol* 44:1393-1399, 2004.

117. Tepel M, van der Giet M, Schwarzfeld C et al: Prevention of radiographic-contrast-agent-induced reductions in renal function by acetylcysteine, *N Engl J Med* 343:180-184, 2000.

118. Kay J, Chow WH, Chan TM et al: Acetylcysteine for prevention of acute deterioration of renal function following elective coronary angiography and intervention: a randomized controlled trial, *JAMA* 289:553-558, 2003.

119. Merten GJ, Burgess WP, Gray LV et al: Prevention of contrast-induced nephropathy with sodium bicarbonate: a randomized controlled trial, *JAMA* 291:2328-2334, 2004.

120. Heupler FA: Guidelines for performing angiography in patients taking metformin: members of the Laboratory Performance Standards Committee of the Society for Cardiac Angiography and Interventions, *Cathet Cardiovasc Diagn* 43:121-123, 1998.

121. Zhu MM, Feit A, Chadow H et al: Primary stent implantation compared with primary balloon angioplasty for acute myocardial infarction: a meta-analysis of randomized clinical trials, *Am J Cardiol* 88:297-301, 2001.

122. Nordmann AJ, Hengstler P, Harr T et al: Clinical outcomes of primary stenting versus balloon angioplasty in patients with myocardial infarction: a meta-analysis of randomized controlled trials, *Am J Med* 116:253-262, 2004.

123. Saia F, Lemos PA, Lee CH et al: Sirolimus-eluting stent implantation in ST-elevation acute myocardial infarction: a clinical and angiographic study, *Circulation* 108:1927-1929, 2003.

124. Lemos PA, Saia F, Hofma SH et al: Short- and long-term clinical benefit of sirolimus-eluting stents compared to conventional bare stents for patients with acute myocardial infarction, *J Am Coll Cardiol* 43:704-708, 2004.

125. Brodie BR, Stone GW, Morice MC et al: Stent Primary Angioplasty in Myocardial Infarction Study Group: importance of time to reperfusion on outcomes with primary coronary angio-

plasty for acute myocardial infarction (results from the Stent Primary Angioplasty in Myocardial Infarction Trial), *Am J Cardiol* 88:1085-1090, 2001.

126. Dalby M, Bouzamondo A, Lechat P, Montalescot G: Transfer for primary angioplasty versus immediate thrombolysis in acute myocardial infarction: a meta-analysis, *Circulation* 108:1809-1814, 2003.

127. Aversano T, Aversano LT, Passamani E et al: Thrombolytic therapy vs primary percutaneous coronary intervention for myocardial infarction in patients presenting to hospitals without on-site cardiac surgery: a randomized controlled trial, *JAMA* 287:1943-1951, 2002.

128. Topol EJ, Kereiakes DJ: Regionalization of care for acute ischemic heart disease: a call for specialized centers, *Circulation* 107:1463-1466, 2003.

129. Califf RM, Faxon DP: Need for centers to care for patients with acute coronary syndromes, *Circulation* 107:1467-1470, 2003.

130. Antman EM, Van de Werf F: Pharmacoinvasive therapy: the future of treatment for ST-elevation myocardial infarction, *Circulation* 109:2480-2486, 2004.

131. Quan H, Ghali WA, Verhoef MJ et al: Use of chelation therapy after coronary angiography, *Am J Med* 111:686-691, 2001.

132. Knudtson ML, Wyse DG, Galbraith PD et al: Program to Assess Alternative Treatment Strategies to Achieve Cardiac Health (PATCH) Investigators: chelation therapy for ischemic heart disease—a randomized controlled trial, *JAMA* 287:481-486, 2002.

133. *Chelation therapy:AHA recommendation* Retrieved February 6,2007,from www.americanheart.org/presenter.jhtml?identifier =4493

134. Yusuf S, Sleight P, Pogue J, et al: Effects of an angiotensin-converting-enzyme inhibitor, ramipril, on cardiovascular events in high-risk patients. The Heart Outcomes Prevention Evaluation Study Investigators, *N Engl J Med* 342:145-153, 2000.

Care of Patients with Complications of Acute Myocardial Infarction

Susan J. Appel

CHAPTER ABBREVIATIONS

AMI acute myocardial infarction

CK-MB creatine phosphate–myocardial band

ECG electrocardiogram

STEMI ST segment elevation myocardial infarction

In this chapter, complications that may occur after an acute myocardial infarction (**AMI**) are reviewed. The complications addressed in this chapter are recurrent ischemia, reinfarction, thromboembolic events, and pericarditis. Other common complications—dysrhythmias, poor psychosocial adaptation, and acute heart failure—are covered in depth in other chapters in this book and are not addressed in this chapter. Thorough knowledge of potential complications enables nurses to care competently for patients suffering from them. Vigilant monitoring is needed after AMI so that complications are recognized early to prevent serious morbid or fatal sequelae.

RECURRENT ISCHEMIA

AMI manifests as ST segment elevation myocardial infarction (**STEMI**) or non-STEMI (see Chapters 56 and 57). Recurrent ischemia after either commonly presents as postinfarction angina. Postinfarction angina includes a pattern of chest pain, usually similar to the initial ischemic pain, occurring at rest or during minimal activity within hours and up to 30 days following AMI. Among patients who have been reperfused successfully using fibrinolytic therapy, the incidence of recurrent ischemia is 20 to 30 percent.

Upon reoccurrence of chest discomfort after AMI, patients immediately should undergo thorough re-evaluation and escalation of medical therapy.[1] Evaluation should include physical examination for presence of new abnormalities, evaluation of serial cardiac enzymes, and electrocardiograms (**ECGs**), with consideration for angiography and possible percutaneous coronary intervention or coronary artery bypass grafting.

The American College of Cardiology and the American Heart Association jointly formulated guidelines for the management of STEMI (full text guideline is available at *www.acc.org* or *www.americanheart.org*) that include recommendations for the management of postinfarction ischemia (Figure 59-1).[1] Reduction of myocardial oxygen demand is the major goal of therapy, and this goal is accomplished by intensification of nitrate

and beta blocker therapy that are a part of routine AMI care. Intravenous anticoagulation therapy will probably be started if not already initiated. Nursing care for patients experiencing recurrent ischemia includes monitoring carefully for the effectiveness of therapy by assessing chest pain and hemodynamic status. Nurses also should participate in the search for, and correction of, possible secondary causes of ischemia such as dysrhythmias or anemia. Support with intraaortic balloon pumping is indicated when patients suffer recurrent ischemia accompanied by left ventricular dysfunction or hemodynamic instability.[2]

A 12-lead ECG is obtained to determine whether ST segment elevation is present. If ST segment elevation is not present and the chest pain is controlled by intensification of medical therapy, then nonemergent cardiac catheterization is used. If chest pain is not controlled with medical therapy, then urgent cardiac catheterization is indicated.[3]

REINFARCTION

Reinfarction occurs in up to 5 percent of AMI patients who have undergone fibrinolysis. Reinfarction is more common after fibrinolytic therapy than after PCI, and it is less common in patients receiving beta blockers. Reinfarction increases patients' risk of in-hospital and 1-month mortality.

In the first 24 to 48 hours after an AMI it may be difficult to identify reinfarction in a separate area of the myocardium. As multivessel coronary artery disease is common in patients experiencing AMI, reinfarction may occur in a different vessel than the original culprit vessel. Angiographic evidence of complex plaques in coronary arteries not responsible for the initial infarct is present in approximately 40 percent of patients after AMI.[4]

The diagnosis of reinfarction can be made when the ECG reveals new changes associated with a rise in cardiac enzymes. Findings from echocardiography or nuclear imaging scan can add additional information[5]; new wall motion abnormalities, larger infarct size, new area of infarction, or persistent reversible ischemic changes help to substantiate the diagnosis. Creatine myocardial band (**CK-MB**), the myocardial component of CK, is a more useful marker for tracking ongoing reinfarction than are troponins, given their shorter half-life.[6] Elevations of CK-MB greater than or equal to 50 percent more than a previous nadir are diagnostic for reinfarction. If the timing is less than 18 hours from initial AMI, diagnostic criteria include elevated enzymes, ST segment elevations, and another criterion such as chest pain or hemodynamic deterioration.

Reinfarction is associated with increased risk for mechanical complications of AMI (e.g., ventricular rupture or papillary muscle rupture) possibly leading to mitral regurgitation, ventricular failure with cardiogenic shock, ventricular aneurysm, or dynamic left ventricular outflow tract obstruction.[7,8] Repeated physical examination, compare new findings to baseline findings, is essential.

Management of reinfarction begins with escalation of medical therapy as outlined before. If the patient's condition is not appropriate for revascularization or if angiography cannot be done within 1 hour, then fibrinolytic therapy can by administered or readministered (although if streptokinase was used, it is not given again).

Coronary angiography should be performed in patients who have been stabilized with medical therapy and in whom revascularization would be possible and appropriate. Emergency angiography should be undertaken in unstable patients. Revascularization, percutaneous or surgical, is associated with improved prognosis.[9]

Figure 59-2 shows the management of patients who first were treated with an initial invasive strategy, received fibrinolytic agents, or did not undergo reperfusion therapy for STEMI. For those patients not managed by an initial invasive strategy and not high risk, their evaluation consists of using one of the noninvasive tests shown in Figure 59-2. In the presence of significant ischemia, catheterization and revascularization are indicated; when no clinically significant ischemia is detected, medical therapy is prescribed.

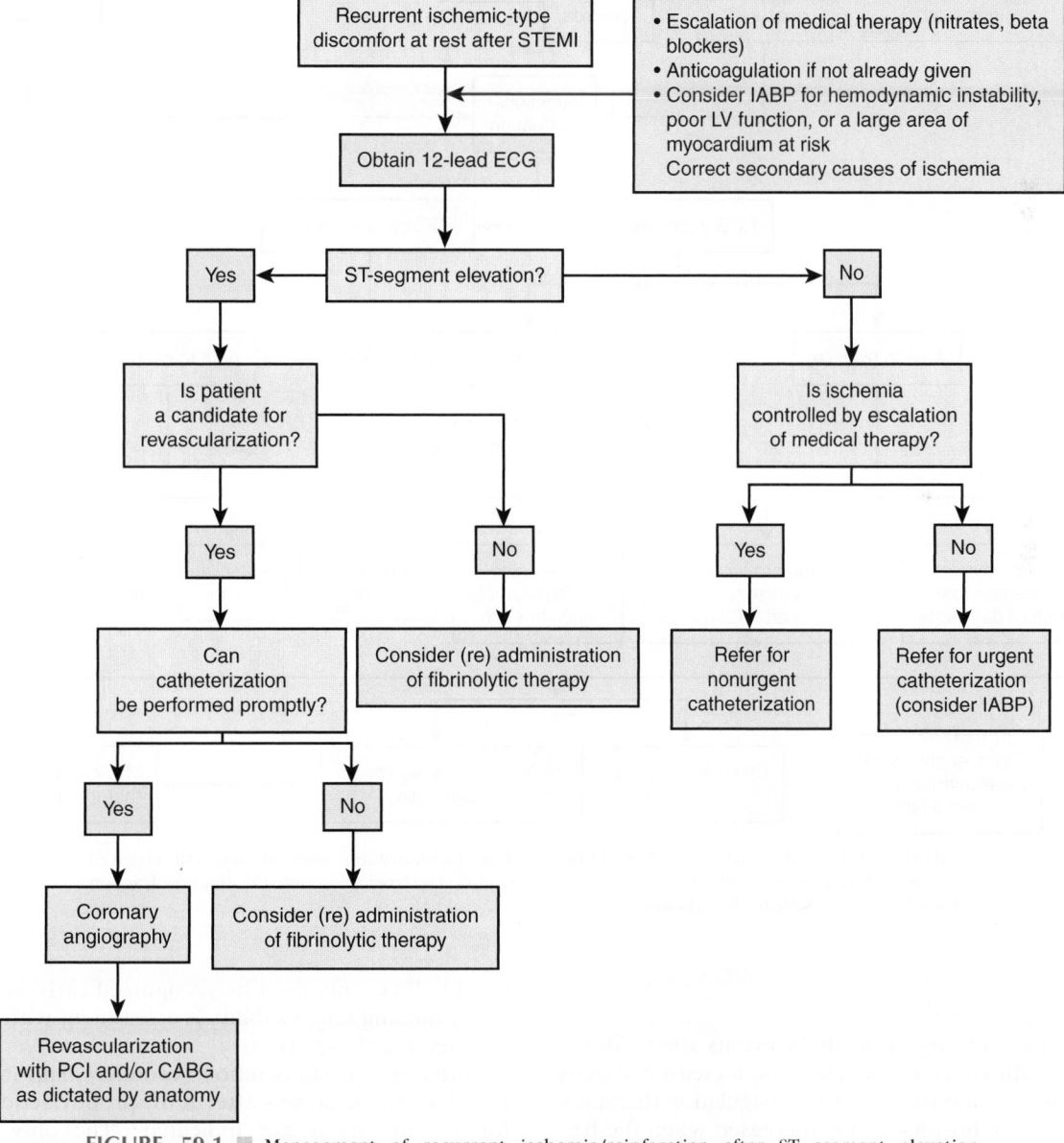

FIGURE 59-1 ▓ Management of recurrent ischemia/reinfarction after ST segment elevation myocardial infarction (STEMI). *CABG,* Coronary artery bypass grafting; *ECG,* electrocardiogram; *IABP,* intraaortic balloon pump; *LV,* left ventricular; *PCI,* percutaneous coronary intervention. (From the American Heart Association.)

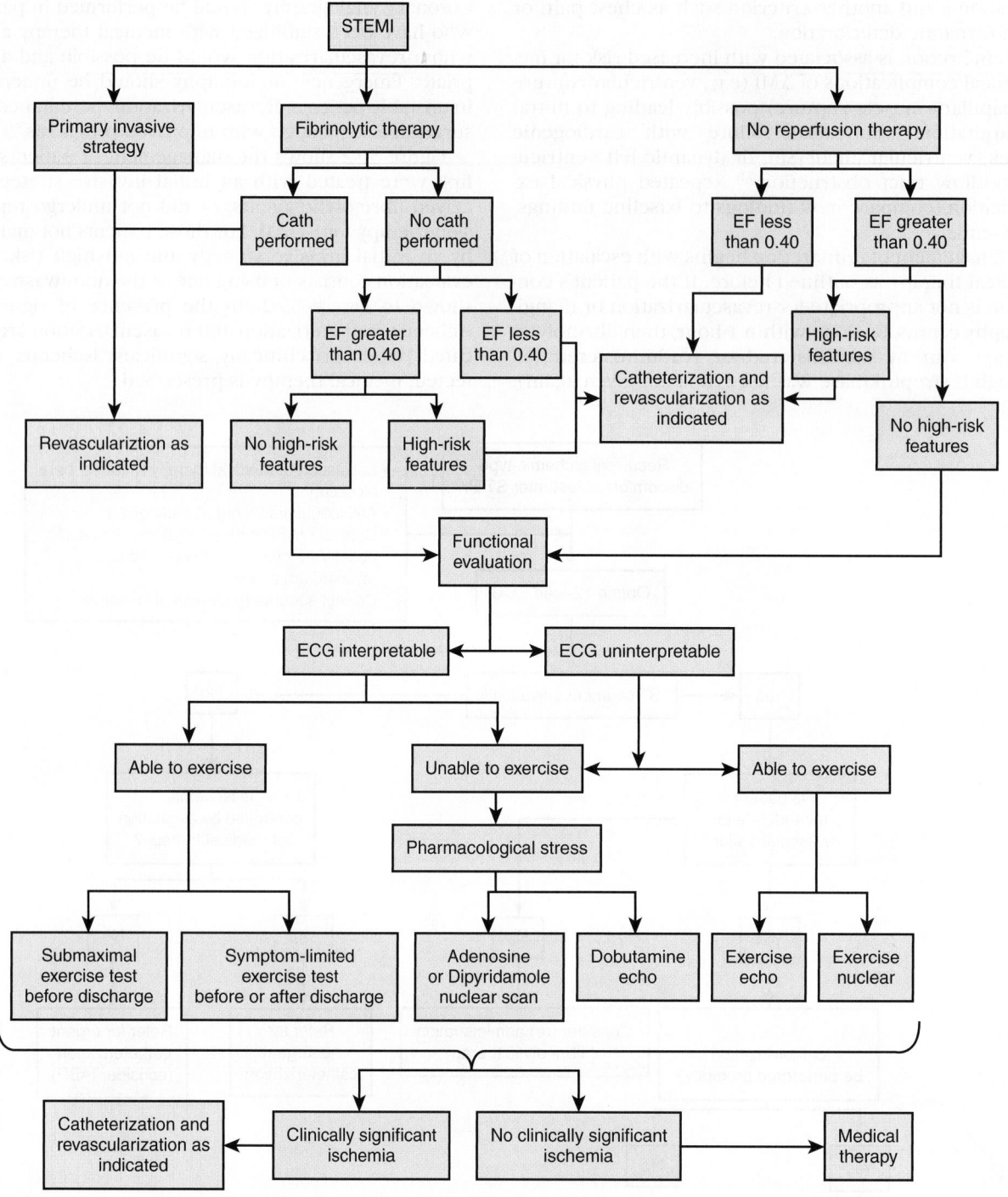

FIGURE 59-2 ■ Approach to catheterization and revascularization after ST segment elevation myocardial infarction (STEMI). *Cath,* Catheterization; *ECG,* electrocardiogram; *EF,* ejection fraction. (From the American Heart Association.)

THROMBOEMBOLIC EVENTS

The incidence of thromboembolic events after AMI has declined with shorter hospital stays, increased activity in the hospital, and the use of anticoagulation therapies. Activity during hospitalization increased when the hazards of immobility were recognized. Nonetheless, patients still may experience thromboembolic events: deep vein thrombosis and pulmonary embolus. Thromboembolic events must be recognized early, and thus a major nursing responsibility is assessment with the goal of detecting these events.

Although thromboembolic events remain important possible complications after AMI, prophylactic therapy for all patients is not indicated.[1] The only patients thought to be appropriate candidates for prophylaxis are heart failure patients with AMI who experience long hospitalizations and periods of immobility or who are at risk for deep vein thrombosis. Appropriate prophylaxis in this patient group is low-dose heparin using low-molecular-weight heparin.[1]

ISCHEMIC STROKE

The incidence of ischemic stroke after AMI is about 1 percent. Despite the advances made in reducing mortality from STEMI, the mortality from stroke suffered after AMI remains high at about 40 percent.[1] A number of risk factors for embolic stroke should stimulate increased vigilance for signs of stroke after AMI (Box 59-1). Of these, the presence of atrial fibrillation is the most prominent. The origin of ischemic stroke after AMI is left ventricular thrombi or atrial thrombi in the patient with atrial fibrillation. Ventricular akinesis or dyskinesis promote conditions that contribute to ventricular thrombus development. Even patients who have been treated with fibrinolytic therapy can develop ischemic stroke, so it is important to maintain a high index of suspicion for stroke in all AMI patients.

Development of ischemic stroke is suspected with sudden onset of neurological changes, particularly a focal neurological deficit. In patients who have had fibrinolytic therapy, intracerebral hemorrhage is a possibility. Accurate determination of the source of neurological symptoms is essential because treatment varies considerably and inappropriate treatment can have disastrous consequences. Computed tomography assists the clinician in making the distinction between intracerebral hemorrhage and ischemic stroke.[11] Once ischemic stroke has been diagnosed, the following Class I recommendations from the American College of Cardiology/American Heart Association guideline for management of STEMI are indicated to improve patient outcomes[1]:

- Obtain a neurological consultation.
- Determine the cause of the ischemic stroke using echocardiography, neuroimaging, and vascular imaging studies.
- Administer warfarin therapy to maintain an INR of 2 to 3 for life is indicated for STEMI patients with chronic atrial fibrillation and ischemic stroke.
- Administer aspirin and warfarin therapy to an INR of 2 to 3 in patients with an embolus of cardiac origin; heparin is used until warfarin reaches therapeutic level.

Frequent assessment of neurological status is essential in AMI patients who suffer ischemic stroke. Vigilant assessment can prevent complications from stroke and optimize patients' functional status. A full discussion of nursing management of ischemic stroke can be found in Chapter 76.

MECHANICAL COMPLICATIONS

The major mechanical complications of AMI include left ventricular free wall rupture, interventricular septum rupture and development of mitral regurgitation resulting from rupture of the papillary muscle or cordae tendinae, papillary muscle rupture, or left ventricular dilatation or aneurysm. Characteristics of these complications are outlined in Table 59-1. In the majority of cases, these complications are immediately life-threatening and require emergent cardiac surgery with medical support while preparing for surgery. Chapter 65 provides an extensive review of nursing care before, during, and after cardiac surgery.

PERICARDITIS

Pericarditis is inflammation of the pericardial sac surrounding the heart. The pericardial sac consists of fibrous tissue that encircles the heart and has its origin near the great vessels, where the vessels are inserted and either enter or leave the heart. A minute amount of fluid (i.e., ~30 ml) is contained within the pericardial sac and acts as a lubricant. The pericardial sac functions to prevent the heart and other organs from impinging on each other. Because the pericardial sac is attached only at the top of the heart, near the origin of the great vessels, the heart is suspended freely within the sac. Normally the heart moves without touching the pericardial sac. When inflammation is present, the heart is likely to rub against the pericardial sac. When the heart rubs against the inflamed pericardial sac as it beats, severe pain may occur along with a pericardial friction rub.

Pericarditis as a complication of AMI occurs when the infarction extends transmurally to involve the epicardium. Although pericarditis is the second most common cause of chest pain after AMI (recurrent ischemia being the first), the pain of pericarditis often has characteristics that distinguish it from ischemic pain (Box 59-2). Pericarditis usually does not occur within the first 24 hours of AMI.

In patients with pericarditis, persistently positive T waves or elevation of initially inverted T waves are evident on the ECG. The cardiac enzyme CK-MB is not elevated with pericarditis. Nonetheless, it still can be difficult to distinguish pericarditis from recurrent ischemia

---

BOX 59-1 ■■■
RISK FACTORS FOR EMBOLIC STROKE AFTER ACUTE MYOCARDIAL INFARCTION

- Atrial fibrillation—considered the most important risk factor
- Hypertension
- Prior stroke
- Older age
- Decreased ejection fraction
- Presence of multiple ulcerated plaques

BOX 59-2 ■■■
CHARACTERISTICS OF CHEST PAIN IN PERICARDITIS AFTER ACUTE MYOCARDIAL INFARCTION

- Chest pain is pleuritic.
- Positional discomfort is present (as opposed to chest pain with rest or minimal activity that is typical of ischemic pain).
- Pain may radiate to left shoulder, scapula, or trapezius.
- Pericardial rub is present (diagnostic of pericarditis).
- PR segment depression may be evident on electrocardiogram.

■ ■ ■

TABLE 59-1 CHARACTERISTICS OF MECHANICAL COMPLICATIONS AFTER ACUTE MYOCARDIAL INFARCTION[14]

	VENTRICULAR FREE WALL RUPTURE	VENTRICULAR SEPTAL RUPTURE	MITRAL REGURGITATION
Incidence	Less than 1% of all AMI patients; 14%-26% in AMI patients dying suddenly; higher in patients receiving fibrinolytic therapy	1%-3% of AMI patients	3% moderate to moderately severe mitral regurgitation in a group of AMI patients undergoing cardiac catheterization; in patients with cardiogenic shock, 39% had moderate to severe mitral regurgitation
Timing of occurrence	Within first 5 days in 50% of cases and in the first 2 weeks of AMI in 90%	Between days 3 and 5-7 after AMI	Within first week of AMI
Risk factors	Thrombolytic therapy; no history of previous AMI; ST segment elevation or Q wave on initial electrocardiogram; large transmural infarcts; age less than 70; female sex	Single-vessel disease; occlusion of wraparound left anterior descending vessel disease, extensive infarct, poor septal collateral circulation; right ventricular infarct	First AMI; poor collateral circulation; inferior wall AMI; subendocardial AMI
Clinical presentation	*Usual:* Sudden death with hemopericardium, cardiac tamponade, pulseless electrical activity *Rare:* Subacute rupture with pericardial pain, pericardial effusion, electrocardiogram suggestive of pericarditis, restlessness	Sudden hemodynamic compromise including hypotension, severe heart failure, holosystolic murmur, thrill	Sudden hemodynamic compromise, new holosystolic murmur; pulmonary congestion
Management	Very high mortality Immediate surgery with medical therapy support consisting of fluid resuscitation, inotropic support, vasopressor, pericardiocentesis, intraaortic balloon bump counterpulsation	Surgical repair with medical support of cardiogenic shock while preparing for surgery: vasodilators, inotropic agents, diuretics, and intraaortic balloon pump counterpulsation	While preparing for surgery, initiation of medical therapy for support: afterload reduction using nitrates, nitroprusside, diuretics, and intraaortic balloon pump counterpulsation Emergent surgery with papillary muscle rupture with mitral valve replacement

AMI, Acute myocardial infarction.

because troponin I elevations have been seen in patients with pericarditis and no evidence of recurrent ischemia.[11] In addition, although in up to 40 percent of cases of pericarditis a (usually hemodynamically inconsequential) pericardial effusion is present, small effusions are present in many cases of STEMI without pericarditis.[1]

Pericarditis should be monitored carefully because it may progress to cause a life-threatening effusion with tamponade if not treated in a timely manner. Detection of enlarging effusion is particularly important when a patient has been receiving antithrombotic therapy and when such therapy is continued. Although it is safe to continue antithrombotic therapy in the face of pericarditis, careful monitoring is required. Antithrombotic therapy is stopped immediately if there are signs of tamponade (cardiac tamponade is discussed in greater detail in Chapter 75).

The mainstay of treatment of postinfarction pericarditis is aspirin at doses of 162 to 325 mg per day, but doses up to 650 mg (enteric coated) every 4 to 6 hours are used if lower doses are ineffective.[1] Nonsteroidal antiinflammatory agents and corticosteroids, which are effective in the relief of pain and inflammation, are not recommended as first-line therapy because of the increased risk of myocardial scar thinning, which is associated with myocardial rupture. Nonsteroidal antiinflammatory agents, if used for pain relief, are used for short periods only. Corticosteroids are reserved as the drug of last choice if all else fails.

Dressler syndrome, autoimmune carditis that occurs after AMI, was first identified in 1965.[13] Dressler syndrome also has been referred to as the post–myocardial infarction syndrome. Clinical presentation of the syndrome occurs 2 to 3 weeks after AMI and may include fever, chest pain, pericarditis, pleurisy, and a strong propensity for reoccurrence. Although Dressler syndrome still may occur today, it is rare and its incidence is thought to be decreasing substantially in the era of reperfusion. Reasons for the decreasing prevalence of Dressler syndrome occurring over the past 25 years include (1) increased use of lytic agents and/or balloon angioplasty, which limit infarct size; (2) advent of more standardized approaches for the management of patients after an AMI, coupled with the aggressive use of efficacious medications that minimize infarct size; and (3) use of medications that may possess "immunomodulatory properties" (e.g., angiotensin-converting enzyme inhibitors and statins).[14]

SUMMARY

This chapter provided an overview of the major complications of AMI—recurrent ischemia, reinfarction, thromboembolic events, stroke, mechanical complications, and pericarditis. The other common complications of AMI are covered in other chapters. Exceptional nursing care is exemplified by anticipation of and early identification of complications so that the best possible outcomes can be achieved. Knowledge of the possible complications to consider after AMI assists in achieving that goal.

REFERENCES

1. Antman EM, Anbe DT, Armstrong PW et al: ACC/AHA guidelines for the management of patients with ST-elevation myocardial infarction: a report of the American College of Cardiology/American Heart Association Task Force on Practice Guidelines (Committee to Revise the 1999 Guidelines for the Management of patients with acute myocardial infarction), *J Am Coll Cardiol* 44: E1-E211, 2004.

2. Santa-Cruz RA, Cohen MG, Ohman EM: Aortic counterpulsation: a review of the hemodynamic effects and indications for use. *Catheter Cardiovasc Interv* 67:68-772006.

3. Scirica BM, Morrow DA: Appropriate invasive and conservative treatment approaches for patients with non-ST-elevation MI. *Curr Treat Options Cardiovasc Med* 8:13-21, 2006.

4. Timoteo AT, Fiarresga A, Feliciano J et al: Importance of complex additional stenosis after primary angioplasty for acute myocardial infarction in medium-term prognosis, *Rev Port Cardiol* 23:853-864, 2004.

5. Positano V, Pingitore A, Giorgetti A et al: A fast and effective method to assess myocardial necrosis by means of contrast magnetic resonance imaging, *J Cardiovasc Magn Reson* 7:487-494, 2005.

6. Meier MA, Al-Badr WH, Cooper JV et al: The new definition of myocardial infarction: diagnostic and prognostic implications in patients with acute coronary syndromes, *Arch Intern Med* 162:1585-1589, 2002.

7. Vargas-Barron J, Molina-Carrion M, Romero-Cardenas A et al: Risk factors, echocardiographic patterns, and outcomes in patients with acute ventricular septal rupture during myocardial infarction, *Am J Cardiol* 95:1153-1158, 2005.

8. Nishiyama K, Okino S, Andou J et al: Coronary angioplasty reduces free wall rupture and improves mortality and morbidity of acute myocardial infarction, *J Invasive Cardiol* 16:554-558, 2004.

9. Halkin A, Singh M, Nikolsky E et al: Prediction of mortality after primary percutaneous coronary intervention for acute myocardial infarction: the CADILLAC risk score, *J Am Coll Cardiol* 45:1397-1405, 2005.

10. Matchar DB, Jacobson AK, Edson RG, et al: The impact of patient self-testing of prothrombin time for managing anticoagulation: rationale and design of VA Cooperative Study #481—the Home INR Study (THINRS). *J Thromb Thrombolysis* 19:163-172, 2005.

11. Masdeu JC, Irimia P, Asenbaum S, et al. EFNS guideline on neuroimaging in acute stroke. Report of an EFNS task force. *Eur J Neuro* 13:1271-1283, 2006.

12. Mahajan N, Mehta Y, Rose M, et al: Elevated troponin level is not synonymous with myocardial infarction. *Int J Cardiol* 111:442-449, 2006

13. Bendjelid K, Pugin J: Is Dressler syndrome dead? *Chest* 126:1680-1682, 2004.

14. Laham RJ, Simons M: Mechanical complications of acute myocardial infarction, *UpToDate Online 14.2.* Retrieved July 11, 2006, from www.utdol.com/utd/content/topic.do?topicKey=chd/14697&view=outline

Care of Patients with Sudden Cardiac Death, Cardiac Arrest, and Life-Threatening Dysrhythmias

Mary Elizabeth Mancini
Rosemary S. Bubien

CHAPTER ABBREVIATIONS

ACE   angiotensin-converting enzyme

AED   automatic external defibrillator

AHA   American Heart Association

AV   atrioventricular

CAD   coronary artery disease

CAST   Cardiac Arrhythmia Suppression Trial

CPR   cardiopulmonary resuscitation

DCM   dilated cardiomyopathy

EMS   emergency medical services

HCM   hypertrophic cardiomyopathy

ICD   implantable cardioverter-defibrillator

LQTS   long QT syndrome

MET   medical emergency team

MI   myocardial infarction

PAD   Public Access Defibrillation (Trial)

NSVT   nonsustained ventricular tachycardia

NYHA   New York Heart Association

RRT   rapid response team

SCD   sudden cardiac death

SCD-HeFT   Sudden Cardiac Death in Heart Failure Trial

SPAF   Stroke Prevention in Atrial Fibrillation

SWORD   Survival with Oral d-Sotalol

VF   ventricular fibrillation

VT   ventricular tachycardia

As its name implies, sudden cardiac death (**SCD**) or sudden cardiac arrest is an unexpected death from a cardiac cause that occurs in a person who may or may not have been known to have preexisting heart disease. SCD occurs without warning because of a natural disruption in cardiovascular function. Blood flow cannot be maintained, and perfusion is inadequate to maintain consciousness. In SCD, progression from the initial disrupting event to cardiac arrest to biological death occurs rapidly. Death is related to the mechanism of the event and the presence or absence of underlying disease. The underlying causes of cardiac arrest and subsequent SCD are associated with the age at which cardiac arrest occurs.[1]

Electrical instability leading to dysrhythmias causes an estimated 88 percent of SCD episodes. The dysrhythmias most commonly causing SCD are ventricular tachycardia (**VT**) and ventricular fibrillation (**VF**), but bradycardia, asystole, and pulseless electrical activity may occur also. In up to 12 percent of cases, SCD may be precipitated by cardiac or noncardiac conditions including coronary vasospasm, anomalous coronary arteries, congenital defects, stroke, pulmonary embolism, and ruptured aneurysm. Arrest occurs in the setting of coronary artery disease (**CAD**) in about 75 percent of cases. Other causes include genetic and acquired forms of cardiomyopathy and less commonly valvular heart disease and congenital heart disease. Primary electrical diseases related to abnormal cardiac sodium and potassium ion channels caused by genetic mutations account for 1 to 5 percent of diseases associated with SCD.[1,2]

No specific tests accurately predict an individual person's risk or identify the time a cardiac arrest will occur. Nurses' knowledge of susceptibility to SCD is based on clinical manifestations that reflect the extent of the disease and are derived from observational population-based studies and, in limited instances, genetic data. As such, "risks" are population risks, not individual risks. Because the timing of cardiac arrest cannot be forecast accurately, primary prevention strategies that range from healthful lifestyle habits to medical interventions are integral to prevent SCD. For example, regular exercise, even moderate-intensity exercise such as walking or gardening, lowers risk factors and decreases the risk of cardiac arrest compared with a sedentary lifestyle.[3] The time of the arrest will not be known even if an individual is at high risk. Thus rapid deployment of interventional strategies to reverse cardiac arrest and prevent SCD is crucial to save lives. Individuals who have clinical markers that were identified in population-based studies as causing SCD benefit from implantation of the implantable cardioverter-defibrillator (**ICD**).

The availability of automatic external defibrillators (**AED**s) in areas such as airports, community centers, schools, and the workplace facilitates timely reversal of cardiac arrest in the general population whose risk is typically unknown. In the medical literature, SCD frequently is used as a synonym for cardiac arrest, whereas public education and awareness campaigns use the term *sudden cardiac arrest* to emphasize that the individual is not dead and to focus on the necessity for prompt intervention.[1] The term *sudden cardiac death* will be used in this chapter.

DEFINITIONS

The *International Classification of Diseases,* 10th revision, defines SCD as a death from any cardiac disorder or disease that occurs outside of the hospital or in the emergency department. To be classified as SCD, the death should have occurred within 1 hour after the onset of symptoms. In practice, however, SCD commonly is used to describe situations that are outside of the strict parameters of this definition. Progression from cardiac arrest to biological death with a diagnosis of SCD is related to the mechanism of cardiac arrest, underlying disease, and time-dependent resuscitation. According to the American Heart Association (**AHA**), SCD is defined as the sudden, abrupt loss of heart function in a person who may or may not have diagnosed heart disease. The time and the mode of death are always unexpected. SCD occurs instantly or shortly after symptoms appear.[4]

Using this definition, an individual who survives a cardiac arrest or a cardiovascular collapse is described as having an "aborted sudden cardiac death." Beyond this difference in definition, SCD also frequently is used to reference events that occur in the hospital setting as opposed to restricting the term to events that occur outside of the hospital or in the emergency department.

To help clarify the language and avoid what they describe as clear contradictions in terms such as "survival from cardiac death," Myerburg and Castellanos[1] developed definitions and a temporal sequence for the events associated with the concept of SCD. Table 60-1 and Figure 60-1 summarize this information.

EPIDEMIOLOGY

Incidence

SCD is a significant clinical and public health problem. SCD is the leading cause of death in the United States, Canada, and in developed countries worldwide. More persons die suddenly each year from cardiovascular disease than die from acquired immunodeficiency syndrome, breast cancer, lung cancer, and stroke combined (Figure 60-2). Estimates of cardiac arrest/SCD in the United States vary from 200,000 to 460,000 deaths per year. More recent analyses place the incidence at approximately 325,000 deaths annually or 1 death every 2 minutes.[5-7]

■ ■ ■

TABLE 60-1   DEFINITION OF TERMS RELATED TO SUDDEN CARDIAC DEATH

TERM	DEFINITION	QUALIFIERS OR EXCEPTIONS
Death	Irreversible cessation of all biological functions	None
Cardiac arrest	Abrupt cessation of cardiac pump function, which may be reversible but will lead to death in the absence of prompt intervention	Rare spontaneous reversions, likelihood of successful intervention relates to mechanism of arrest, clinical setting, and time to intervention
Cardiovascular collapse	A (sudden) loss of effective blood flow resulting from cardiac and/or peripheral vascular factors that may revert spontaneously (e.g., vasodepressor or cardioinhibitory syncope) or only with interventions (e.g., cardiac arrest)	

From Myerberg RJ, Castellanos A: Cardiac arrest and sudden cardiac death. In Zipes DP, Libby P, Bonow RO, Braunwald E, editors: *Braunwald's heart disease: a textbook of cardiovascular medicine,* ed 7, Philadelphia, 2005, Saunders.

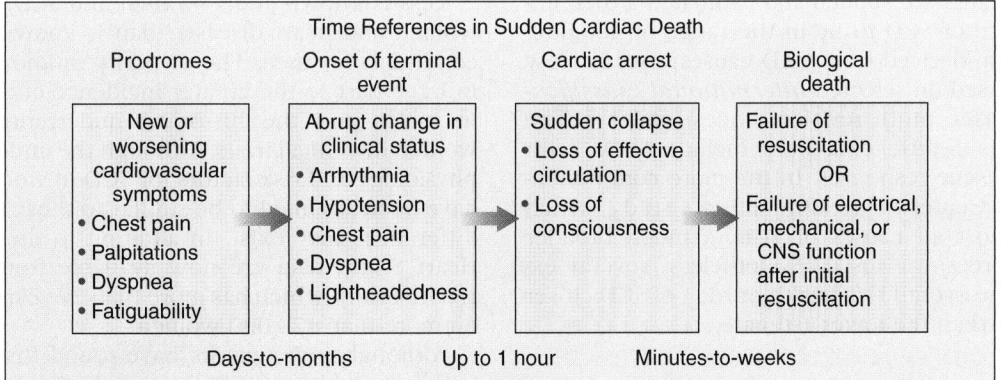

FIGURE 60-1 ■ Sudden cardiac death viewed from four temporal perspectives: (1) prodrome, (2) onset of the terminal event, (3) cardiac arrest, and (4) progression to biological death. Individual variability of the components influences clinical expression. Some victims experience no prodrome, with onset leading almost instantly to cardiac arrest; others may have an onset that lasts up to 1 hour before clinical arrest. Some patients may live days to weeks after the cardiac arrest with irreversible brain damage before biological death, often because of dependence on life support. These factors influence interpretation of the 1-hour definition. The two most relevant clinical factors are onset of the terminal event (2) and the clinical cardiac arrest itself (3); legal and social considerations focus on the time of biological death (4). *CNS,* Central nervous system. (From Myerberg RJ, Castellanos A: Cardiac arrest and sudden cardiac death. In Zipes DP, Libby P, Bonow RO, Braunwald E, editors: *Braunwald's heart disease: a textbook of cardiovascular medicine,* ed 7, Philadelphia, 2005, Saunders.)

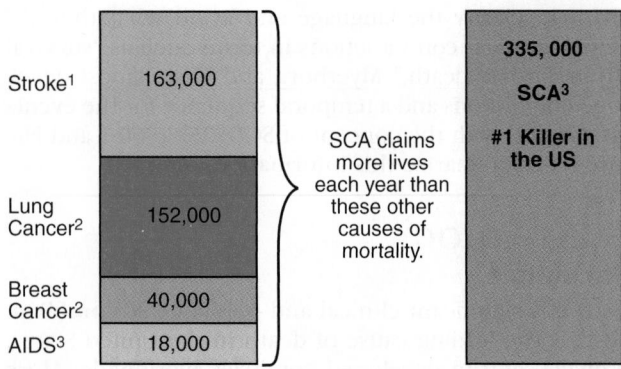

Stroke[1]	163,000
Lung Cancer[2]	152,000
Breast Cancer[2]	40,000
AIDS[3]	18,000

SCA claims more lives each year than these other causes of mortality.

335,000
SCA[3]
#1 Killer in the US

FIGURE 60-2 ■ More persons die suddenly each year from cardiovascular disease than die from acquired immunodeficiency syndrome, breast cancer, lung cancer, and stroke combined.
1. American Heart Association: *Heart disease and stroke statistics: 2005 update*, Dallas, 2004, The Association.
2. Jemel A: *CA Cancer J Clin* 53:5-26, 2003.
3. *United States Statistics Summary.* Retrieved February 7, 2007 from www.avert.org/statsum.htm (Adapted from material on Medtronic Connections, www.Medtronic.com)
AIDS, Acquired immunodeficiency syndrome; *SCA,* sudden cardiac arrest.

Myerburg and colleagues[7] attribute the range in estimates to several factors, including whether the definition of SCD used was broad and included many causes or whether SCD was defined narrowly. The population sources used also influence the incidence. Because there are no direct epidemiological studies, the incidence is calculated from observational data and is subject to bias. Retrospective death certificate analyses include assumptions about whether the cardiovascular death was sudden. The Seattle, Washington, Emergency Medical System database, extrapolated to total U.S. population numbers, calculated 184,000 cardiac arrests nationwide in the year 2000. In contrast, a death certificate–based study from the National Center for Health Statistics suggested that more than 50 percent of all cardiac deaths are sudden and estimated a total annual incidence of SCD to be in the range of 460,000. The AHA data, derived from CAD causes, uses narrow definitions based on selected *International Classification of Diseases,* ninth revision, codes (codes 410 to 414), whereas Seattle data only include SCDs with emergency rescue responses. In the more comprehensive National Center for Health Statistics study, which included almost all causes of SCD, a much broader range of sources was used. Nonetheless, several experts place the overall U.S. health burden of SCD closer to the higher than the lower estimate.

Influence of Age, Race, and Gender

No age group is exempt from SCD. The overall incidence of SCD is low in those age 21 and younger, with approximately 600 cases reported per year. SCD accounts for 19 percent of sudden death in children between ages 1 and 13 and 30 percent between ages 14 and 21. Approximately 90 percent of the time, structural cardiac abnormalities can be identified.[1,2,4]

Although SCD in the young is rare, when it does occur, it is particularly devastating because it is unexpected. The most common cause of death in persons younger than age 30 is preexisting cardiac abnormality, including hypertrophic cardiomyopathy. The incidence of SCD in children and adolescents who die from the more malignant hypertrophic cardiomyopathy (**HCM**) mutations is 4 to 6 percent per year and declines to 2 to 4 percent per year in adults and 4 to 6 percent per year in children and adolescents who die from the more malignant mutations.[4] Other preexisting structural abnormalities associated with SCD in young persons include anomalous coronary arteries and Marfan syndrome.[1,8] Electrical abnormalities caused by ion channel mutations in long QT syndrome (**LQTS**) and Brugada syndrome are also an important cause of SCD in young persons. Inherited LQTS, associated with torsades de pointes VT is the most common cause, accounting for up to 4000 SCD deaths per year with mortality approaching 50 percent over 10 years in untreated symptomatic individuals. Brugada syndrome now is recognized as the second most common cause of SCD in youth.[7,9,10]

The individual risk for cardiac arrest in the general adult population is approximately 0.1 percent per year.[4] Increasing age is the single most prominent risk factor for cardiac arrest irrespective of race or gender and parallels that of death from cardiac causes that also increase as persons age. In adults the risk of SCD increases approximately twofold to fourfold for every 10-year increase in age.[11,12] Blacks have an elevated risk for cardiac arrest and a higher mortality from CAD compared with other ethnic groups in every age group, whereas Asian Americans traditionally have had a lower risk. Survival following cardiac arrest is lower for blacks compared with whites (0.8 percent versus 2.6 percent; $p < 0.001$) even after controlling for other variables.[4,13] These findings may reflect the increased prevalence of cardiovascular risk factors in these populations.

Less is known about women and SCD, and likewise women and heart disease, than is known about these conditions for men. The disparity in knowledge is due in large part to the greater incidence of SCD and CAD in males and the historical underrepresentation of women in clinical trials. Although the underlying pathophysiology and risk factors for SCD in women generally have been assumed to be similar to those in men, some differences may exist. In addition to the Framingham Heart Study, data are now available from the Nurses Health Study, which has more than 20 years of follow-up on more than 120,000 women.

Although investigators have found that women are less vulnerable to SCD than men, the rate of SCD in women ages 38 to 45 has increased 21 percent over the past 10 years while the rate for white men in the same age group has decreased by 2.8 percent.[1,4] Women with a parent who died from SCD before age 60 have an elevated risk of SCD. Particularly worrisome is new information reporting a 30 percent increase in SCD in young women ages 15 to 34.[4] This recent trend is being monitored closely to determine possible causes and effective interventional strategies. As in men, CAD risk factors predict the risk of SCD. The risk of SCD in women with CAD, however, has been found to be only half as high as the risk in men. Likewise, SCD is usually due to dysrhythmias.

Whereas increasing age is associated with an increased risk of SCD, the percentage of cardiac deaths that are sudden in women decreases with age. The Framingham Heart Study investigators reported that in women the incidence of SCD lagged behind that of men by more than 10 years. The difference has been attributed to the benefits conferred before menopause. It also has been suggested that women who have SCD are less likely to have a history of documented heart disease and that women at any age are less likely to have a cardiac arrest.[14-16] Albert and colleagues[17] reported, based on a retrospective study of survivors of cardiac arrest who were referred for electrophysiological testing, that women survivors were less likely to have CAD than men (45 percent versus 80 percent) and were more likely to have other forms of heart disease and structurally normal hearts. Predictors of survival differ between males and females who succumb to cardiac arrest. Data from the Framingham Heart Study indicate that 50 percent of men and 64 percent of women who die from SCD had no history of heart disease.[14]

RISK FACTORS
Coronary Artery Disease

In the United States, SCD from coronary disease occurs almost 900 times per day. On autopsy, 90 percent of adult victims of SCD have significant stenosis in two or more coronary arteries. Thus the most frequent diagnosis associated with SCD remains CAD. Among adults who have one or more risk factors for CAD, the rate of SCD is 2 to 4 times that of the population at large. In patients with a previous myocardial infarction (**MI**), the rate of SCD is 4 to 6 times greater. Within 6 years after an MI, 7 percent of men and 6 percent of women will succumb to SCD. If the infarct was large, the risk of SCD is highest in the first year postinfarction and then decreases over time. In patients receiving beta blocking therapy a higher incidence of dysrhythmia events has been observed after 18 months.[1,2,4] Figure 60-3 illustrates a continuum of risk of SCD ranging from the general population to individuals deemed at high risk because of coronary events, heart failure, and survival of prior cardiac arrest.[1] This increased susceptibility places millions of Americans at an elevated risk for SCD. At any given time, approximately 13 million persons in the United States have CAD, 7.6 million of whom have had a MI; 80 to 90 percent of SCD victims have CAD. In up

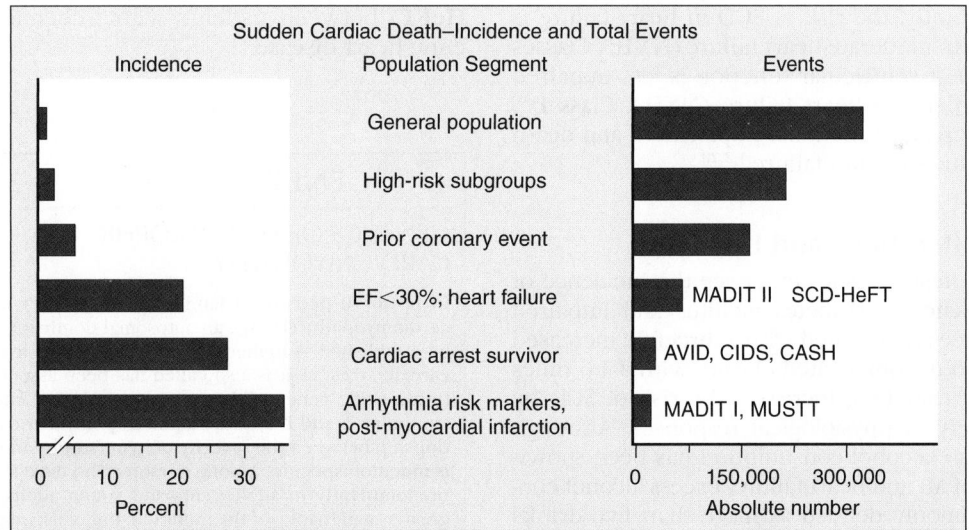

FIGURE 60-3 ■ The influence of population subgroups and time from events on the clinical epidemiology of sudden cardiac death (SCD). Estimates of incidence (percent per year) and the total number of events per year are given for the general adult population in the United States and for increasingly high-risk subgroups. With the identification of increasingly powerful risk factors, the incidence *increases* progressively, but it is accompanied by a progressive *decrease* in the total number of events represented by each group. The inverse relationship between incidence and total number of events occurs because of the progressively smaller denominator pool in the highest subgroup categories. Successful interventions among larger population subgroups require identification of specific markers to increase the ability to identify specific patients who are at particularly high risk for a future event. (Note: The horizontal axis for the incidence figures is not linear and should be interpreted accordingly.) *AVID*, Antiarrhythmics Versus Implantable Defibrillators; *CASH*, Cardiac Arrest Study-Hamburg; *CIDS*, Canadian Implantable Defibrillator Study; *EF*, ejection fraction; *MADIT*, Multicenter Automatic Defibrillator Implantation Trial; *MUSTT*, Multicenter Unsustained Tachycardia Trial; *SCD-HeFT*, Sudden Cardiac Death in Heart Failure Trial. (From Myerberg RJ, Castellanos A: Cardiac arrest and sudden cardiac death. In Zipes DP, Libby P, Bonow RO, Braunwald E, editors: *Braunwald's heart disease: a textbook of cardiovascular medicine*, ed 7, Philadelphia, 2005, Saunders.)

to one-third of these instances, SCD is the first manifestation of CAD. A previous MI can be identified in up to 75 percent of persons who die from SCD. The importance of family history and an individual's risk for SCD is moving beyond the association of CAD to recognition of the genetic variants that may affect SCD, particularly factors associated with acute coronary syndrome such as plaque stability and rupture.[1,2,7]

Left Ventricular Function

An increase in risk of 2 to 2.5 times for SCD is associated with hypertension. The presence of left ventricular dysfunction or heart failure increases the risk of SCD and overall death in men and women significantly as noted during 39 years of follow-up in the Framingham Heart Study.[18] SCD occurs 6 to 9 times more often in the setting of left ventricular dysfunction than in the general population. Currently, left ventricular function remains the single most important independent predictor for overall mortality, SCD, and cardiac mortality regardless of whether ischemic heart disease is present or absent. The greatest increase in risk for SCD occurs between ejection fractions of 30 and 40 percent with measurable changes in risk deviating from the general population beginning at 40 percent. An ejection fraction less than 30 percent, although a powerful independent predictor of SCD, is associated with a low specificity.[19]

In men, impaired left ventricular function, commonly based on the New York Heart Association (**NYHA**) classification, is the most important predictor of SCD. Importantly, the risk of SCD in heart failure is greater in mild to moderate heart failure (NYHA Classes I to III) when left ventricular function is less impaired compared with severe heart failure (NYHA Class IV) when there is greater functional impairment and death is more often due to pump failure.[1,2,20]

Metabolic Alterations and Lifestyle

Metabolic and lifestyle issues influence the incidence of SCD. The presence of diabetes mellitus and impaired glucose tolerance is associated with a threefold increased risk of SCD, and uncomplicated obesity with a 1.6 times increased risk.[21] Smoking increases the risk of SCD by altering a variety of physiological responses. Although light to moderate alcohol consumption has been shown to lower rates of MI and heart failure, excess alcohol consumption, commonly defined as more than five drinks per day, is associated with increased risk of SCD.[22] Recreational drug abuse is a significant cause of SCD even when structural heart disease is absent.[21] Strenuous exercise increases the relative risk of SCD during and up to 30 minutes after exertion. However, the absolute risk of SCD during any individual episode of exertion is extremely low (1 SCD per 1.51 million episodes).[23]

Emotional and Psychological Factors

The emotions of anxiety, anger, hostility, and depression are recognized risk factors for CAD and SCD, as are phobic disorders.[24] Recently, the Nurses Health Study reported that high levels of phobic anxiety are associated with an increased risk of fatal CAD, particularly from SCD.[25] Women are reported to have a higher frequency of generalized anxiety disorders compared with men. Adverse physiological changes occurring in depression have been linked to adverse cardiac events that also can be induced by stress (see Chapters 39 and 40). One explanation is that patients who are depressed are in a constant state of perceived stress. An increase in VT attributable to stress has been observed on Monday in ICD patients, and also has been linked with disasters such as earthquakes.[24] Others have suggested that patients who are depressed are less likely to adhere to prescribed therapies including lifestyle modifications and that depression can result from more severe pathophysiological cardiac conditions.[26]

Cardiomyopathy

The SCD risk factors for persons with cardiomyopathy have not been as well defined as those for persons with CAD. Overall, approximately 10 percent of SCD events are attributed to dilated cardiomyopathy (**DCM**) and mortality related to the severity of left ventricular dysfunction. General assumptions have been that SCD risk is increased when there is greater impairment of left ventricular dysfunction and prolongation of the QRS complex. Unexplained syncope has been associated with a high incidence of SCD.[1,2] No specific risk factors or differences were reported in the recently completed Sudden Cardiac Death in Heart Failure Trial (**SCD-HeFT**) between patients with ischemic and nonischemic heart disease.[27]

■ ■ ■ GENETICS

GENETICS OF HYPERTROPHIC CARDIOMYOPATHY

In up to 70 percent of families of someone with hypertrophic cardiomyopathy (HCM), an autosomal dominant genetic link can be established. A higher risk for sudden cardiac death or sudden cardiac arrest as it is also called has been associated with mutation-specific genes of the beta-myosin heavy chain, the cardiac troponins T and I, and the alpha-tropomyosin cohorts. The relationship between the severity of hypertrophy and the risk of SCD is mutation specific. Among persons who have HCM, SCD occurs predominantly in adolescents and young adults because of the greater malignancy of the mutation, but it also may occur in older adults. Up to 70 percent of all deaths are sudden in the setting of obstructive HCM.

Bibliography
Maron BJ, McKenna WJ, Danielson GK et al: American College of Cardiology/European Society of Cardiology Clinical Expert Consensus Document on Hypertrophic Cardiomyopathy: a report of the American College of Cardiology Foundation Task Force on Clinical Expert Consensus Documents and the European Society of Cardiology Committee for Practice Guidelines, *J Am Coll Cardiol* 42:1687-1713, 2003.
Myerburg RF, Interian A, Simmons J, Castellanos A: Sudden cardiac death. In Zipes DP, Jalife J, editors: *Cardiac electrophysiology from cell to bedside*, ed 4, Philadelphia, 2004, Saunders.
Wynne J, Braunwald E: The cardiomyopathies. In Zipes DP, Libby P, Bonow RO, Braunwald E, editors: *Braunwald's heart disease: a textbook of cardiovascular medicine*, ed 7, Philadelphia, 2005, Saunders.

SCD, Sudden cardiac death.

Clinical predictors of SCD in HCM include age of onset; family history; magnitude of ventricular mass, specifically a septal thickness greater than 3 cm; ventricular dysrhythmias; syncope; and outflow gradient in the obstructive form.[28,29] (See the accompanying Genetics feature.)

One diagnostic risk stratification tool (T wave alternans) has shown promise in predicting the risk of SCD in DCM and HCM. Beat-to-beat measurements of the amplitude and morphology of ventricular repolarization are thought to represent a reasonably reliable indicator of electrical instability.[1]

Ventricular Dysrhythmias

The significance of ventricular dysrhythmias varies depending on the underlying physiological status. In the absence of structural heart disease, premature ventricular contractions and runs of monomorphic nonsustained ventricular tachycardia (**NSVT**) are benign. The occurrence of the dysrhythmias, when a person has structural heart disease during exercise (particularly recovery), is a warning of an increased risk of SCD. NSVT in DCM identifies a higher risk of SCD.[1]

Antiarrrhythmic drugs were prescribed routinely to abolish premature ventricular contractions and NSVT and provide symptom relief before the Cardiac Arrhythmia Suppression Trial (**CAST**).[30] In that trial, Vaughn-Williams Class IC agents encainide and flecainide were shown to increase mortality rates more than 3 times that seen in the placebo group. Because moricizine was not associated initially with an increase in mortality, the trial continued as CAST II and was stopped when similar mortality outcomes became evident with moricizine.[31] Class I agents likewise were reported to increase mortality in patients with atrial fibrillation in the Stroke Prevention in Atrial Fibrillation (**SPAF**) study and in retrospective studies.[32-34] Because of the increase in mortality in the Survival with Oral d-Sotalol (**SWORD**) Study, which compared the Class III agent d-sotalol with placebo post-MI, the clinical trial was halted and the drug was not released to the market. (Sotalol is a market-released Class III antiarrrhythmic with beta-blocking properties.[35]) The common denominator in these antiarrhythmic drug trials was the effect of the drug on the risk of SCD in the setting of left ventricular dysfunction.

Conduction Abnormalities

Structural abnormalities of the anatomically continuous atrioventricular (**AV**) conduction system associated with SCD include acquired diseases of the AV node and His-Purkinje system and may be due to age-related idiopathic fibrosis, MI, and cardiac surgery. Conduction abnormalities related to a prolonged QRS complex duration include intraventricular conduction delay and left bundle branch block, as well as infrahisian block. Unlike the benign clinical course associated with AV nodal block, block within and below the bundle of His is associated with risk of SCD related to bradycardia-related VT, torsades de pointes, and an unreliable QRS complex escape rhythm.[1,2,36]

Pathophysiology

Most commonly, SCD is due to electrical instability in the setting of an abnormal myocardial substrate. The biological model of SCD (Figure 60-4) illustrates how transient alterations in function in combination with an abnormal substrate may trigger a cardiac arrest. Abnor-

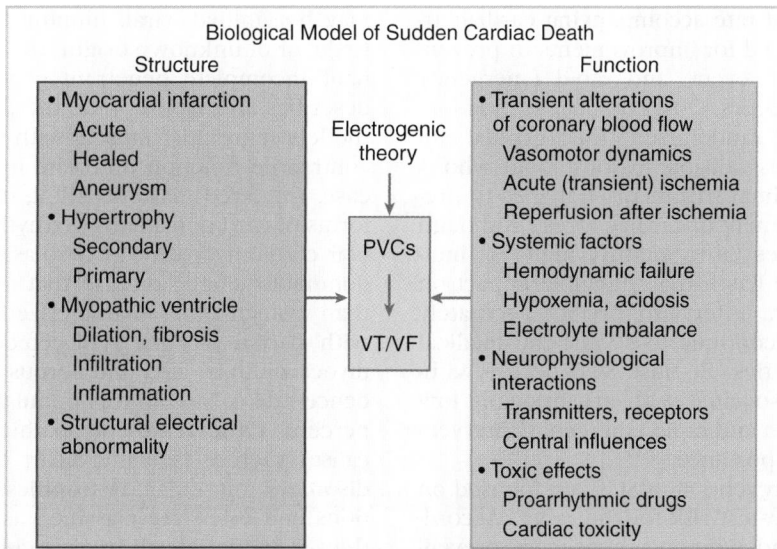

FIGURE 60-4 ■ This biological model illustrates how transient alterations in function, combined with an abnormal substrate, may trigger a cardiac arrest. Coronary heart disease, cardiomyopathies, and other structural abnormalities such as left ventricular hypertrophy produce anatomical and functional changes that alter impulse formation, excitation, and propagation. *PVCs,* Premature ventricular contractions; *VT/VF,* ventricular tachycardia/ventricular fibrillation. (From Myerberg RJ, Castellanos A: Cardiac arrest and sudden cardiac death. In Zipes DP, Libby P, Bonow RO, Braunwald E, editors: *Braunwald's heart disease: a textbook of cardiovascular medicine,* ed 7, Philadelphia, 2005, Saunders.)

mal ion channel function from inherited electrical abnormalities produces similar changes. These changes produce a substrate with an increased susceptibility to SCD. Occurrence of SCD depends on functional factors that trigger electrical instability in the substrate. See Chapters 46, 47, and 48 for further discussion of the pathophysiology underlying dysrhythmia propagation.

Dysrhythmia Presentation

In the majority of SCD instances, VT is thought to degenerate to VF. Although some reports cite VF as the first recorded rhythm, in one series of patients undergoing ambulatory monitoring at the time of their cardiac arrest, 62 percent developed VT degenerating into VF followed by asystole, whereas only 8 percent initially manifested VF. Torsades de pointes, a specific type of VT occurring in the setting of a prolonged QT interval resulting from genetic or acquired causes, accounted for 13 percent of SCD. Bradydysrhythmias accounted for the remaining 17 percent.[37] Bradycardias, including pulseless electrical activity (formerly known as electromechanical dissociation), occur more commonly in the setting of advanced heart disease. The conduction delays create disparities in tissue excitability and recovery, increasing the risk of VT and VF.[1,2,38] Several studies indicate that the incidence of VF as the initially recorded rhythm during SCD is decreasing with a higher proportion due to asystole and pulseless electrical activity. The mechanisms associated with these dysrhythmias are discussed in detail in Chapter 48.

APPROACHES TO DEALING WITH CARDIAC ARREST

Regardless of age, few persons survive cardiac arrest. Those who do survive remain at high-risk for recurrence. The low survival rate accompanying cardiac arrest underscores the need for improvements in prevention, prediction of the event, and rapid emergency intervention when it occurs. Observational population-based research studies, randomized clinical trials, and registries have taught us valuable lessons about who is at risk of SCD, the optimal treatment strategies to prevent SCD, and the treatment of cardiac arrest. Although this information enables us to identify high-risk individuals, the knowledge has had a negligible impact on the general population. Efforts to predict accurately when SCD will strike continue to stymie the medical and research communities. Because SCD occurs without warning and is associated with an abysmally low survival rate, prevention and rapid emergency interventions are of primary importance.[1,2,39]

Efforts at primary prevention of SCD are focused on identifying those at greatest risk for the event. According to Obias-Manno and Wijetunga,[16] primary prevention of SCD involves the development and implementation of strategies and interventions directed at preventing the initial occurrence of SCD. Primary prevention of SCD requires targeted interventions to identify persons at risk in the general population and a rapid response when cardiac arrest occurs. Secondary prevention of SCD is directed at preventing a recurrence of the event and implies an approach targeted to a known high-risk population subgroup. Risk stratification is the process of identifying and defining the risks for SCD within various subsets of the population.

Interventions to prevent SCD can take several forms. They can focus on community approaches to screening, risk reduction, and strengthening the chain of survival, or they can take the form of specific medical interventions for populations known to be at an increased risk for SCD. Interventions also can be designed to address organizational strategies to improve management of patients in the clinical setting.

Conditions Associated with Increased Susceptibility to Sudden Cardiac Death
Coronary Artery Disease

In persons with CAD, progression of pathophysiological processes such as sudden rupture of an unstable plaque may cause an occlusion in an artery that previously had minor narrowing. The ensuing ischemia creates electrical instability and can provoke VT/VF. Acute and chronic pathological changes to the anatomical substrate generated by MI or hypertrophy, described in Figure 60-5, may culminate in SCD via interaction with functional triggers. At the cellular level, triggering events may result in the threshold potential being attained more easily such that VT/VF is provoked (Figure 60-6).[1]

Cardiomyopathies

Cardiomyopathies account for the second largest number of sudden deaths. Approximately 15 percent of SCD victims have disorders of the heart muscle itself.[1] Cardiomyopathies commonly are grouped based on the underlying anatomical-based functional abnormalities (see Chapter 72). DCM, the most common syndrome, is characterized by systolic dysfunction. Nonischemic DCM may be familial, viral, immune, peripartum, alcoholic-toxic, or of unknown origin. HCM is an autosomal dominant incomplete penetrant genetic abnormality. HCM describes an inappropriate increase in the thickness of the left ventricular muscle with preserved or enhanced contractile function until late in the course of the disease. Impaired diastolic filling characterizes restrictive forms of cardiomyopathy. Arrhythmogenic right ventricular cardiomyopathy, or dysplasia, is also an autosomal-dominant genetic disease that affects men more often than women and is characterized by myocardial cell loss with partial or total replacement of right ventricular myocardium by fatty and fibrous tissue. The annual incidence rate of SCD in this population is approximately 2 percent. Other cardiomyopathies result from specific causes such as ischemic heart disease, neuromuscular disorders, muscular dystrophies, and peripartal conditions and often are classified as specific cardiomyopathies.[28] Sudden death in a specific cardiomyopathy generally is classified by its underlying primary cause. For example, ischemic DCM following MI is not a primary disorder of the heart muscle but a consequence of CAD.

At the cellular level, protein abnormalities linked to precipitation of dysrhythmias include cytoskeletal proteins in dilated cardiomyopathies, cell-to-cell junction proteins in arrhythmogenic right ventricular dysplasia, and contractile sarcomere proteins in HCM.[9]

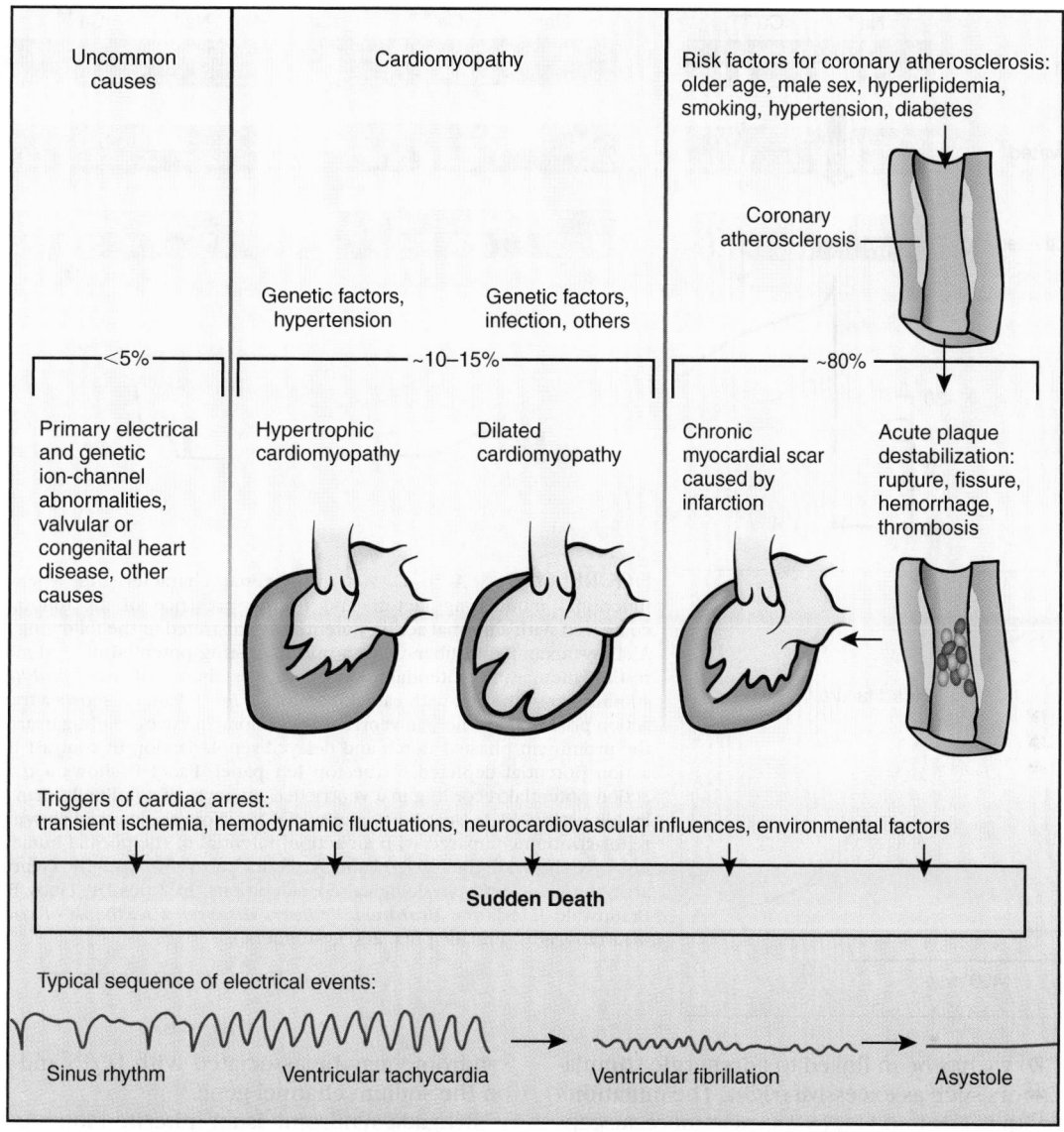

FIGURE 60-5 ▨ Acute and chronic pathological changes to the anatomical substrate that occur with myocardial infarction or hypertrophy can cause sudden cardiac death (SCD) by interacting with functional triggers. The relationship among risk factors identified in epidemiological studies of SCD from cardiac causes, the initiation of pathophysiological processes, and the influence of transient changes in function are illustrated. The cascade of events associated with SCD in the myocardial infarction and hypertrophic structural changes of the model is represented by the 80 percent of deaths attributable to coronary artery disease on the far right. Risk factors such as hyperlipidemia produce coronary atherosclerosis. Acute and chronic pathophysiological processes create structural abnormalities that increase the susceptibility of the myocardium to electrical instability. Acute plaque destabilization or rupture or a scar from a myocardial infarction may interact with ischemia or other trigger, resulting in SCD. Genetics, viruses, and a wide array of factors also may produce structural changes in the myopathy model. A schematic representation of the structural changes observed in hypertrophic and dilated cardiomyopathy that increase susceptibility to electrical instability is presented in the middle section. Cardiomyopathies represent the second largest group of SCD from cardiac causes. Ion channelopathies or primary electrical disease and other structural diseases account for the remaining 5 percent of SCD. Although persons with SCD typically have ventricular fibrillation, the initiating rhythm is thought to be ventricular tachycardia that degenerates to ventricular fibrillation and progresses to asystole. (From Huikuri HV, Castellanos A, Myerburg RJ: *N Engl J Med* 345:1473, 2001.)

Inherited Electrical Abnormalities

Primary electrical diseases related to abnormal cardiac sodium and potassium ion channels caused by genetic mutations accounts for up to 5 percent of diseases associated with SCD. Many ion currents contribute to the formation of the action potential. A defect in any ion current can alter the action potential and create the substrate for dysrhythmias. Long QT syndrome (LQTS 1 to 7) is a genetic disease caused by ion channel defects. The most common forms of LQTS (LQTS 1 and LQTS 2) are associated with potassium ion channel defects, whereas LQTS 3 is caused by a mutation in the gene that encodes the sodium channel. Transient changes caused by changes in sympathetic nerve activity can occur during a range of emotional responses including anger, excitement, stress, and depression and therefore also may

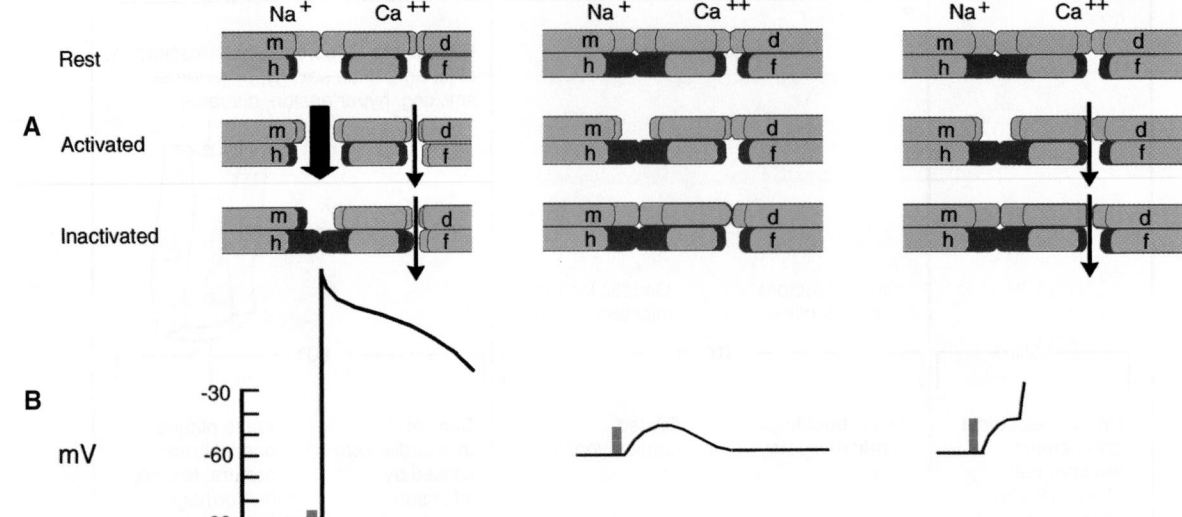

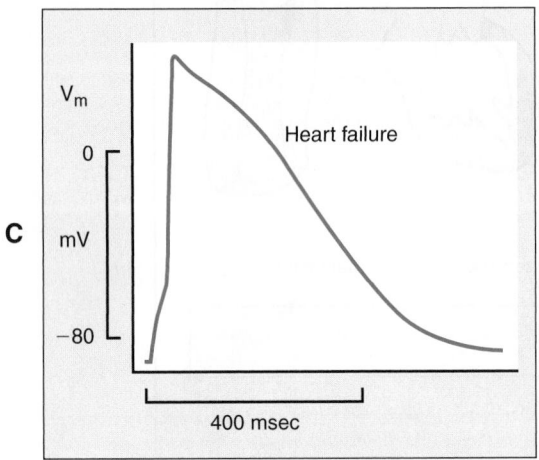

FIGURE 60-6 ■ **A** to **C,** Action potential characteristics when exposed to functional modulating factors and in the presence of an abnormal substrate compared with a normal action potential as illustrated in the following panels. Panel **A** shows example of fibers with a normal resting potential of −90 mV *(left),* with resting membrane potential reduced to less than −60 mV *(middle),* and after stimulation of the cell with catecholamines *(right).* Panel **B** shows a transmembrane action potential in a human ventricular cardiomyocyte of a failing heart. Note loss of the prominent phase 1 notch and delayed repolarization in contrast to the normal action potential depicted in the top left panel. Panel **C** shows a transmembrane action potential recording in a ventricular myocyte of a failing human heart caused by idiopathic dilated cardiomyopathy (DCM). Note the marked slowing of phase 3 repolarization compared with an action potential of the normal human ventricular myocyte shown in the *top left* Panel **A.** (From Rubart M, Zipes DP: Genesis of cardiac arrhythmias: electrophysiological considerations. In Zipes DP, Libby P, Bonow RO, Braunwald E, editors: *Braunwald's heart disease: a textbook of cardiovascular medicine,* ed 7, Philadelphia, 2005, Saunders.)

provoke SCD. VT has been linked to adrenergic stimulation from factors such as excessive fright. The mutations associated with LQTS 1 and LQTS 2 appear more susceptible to SCD in the settings of sympathetic stimulation. In particular, there is a strong association between LQTS 1 and swimming, whereas increased SCD events have been reported at rest in LQTS 3. Although varying degrees of lethality are associated with the dysrhythmias provoked by the different LQTS mutations, all are capable of inducing SCD.[7,9]

As illustrated in the risk stratification scheme in Figure 60-7, the risk of dysrhythmias varies among the types of LQTS. Because of the differences in incidence and lethality, overall mortality is approximately equivalent and is estimated at approximately 10 percent per year in pediatric patients. The range of normal QT_C intervals (QT interval corrected for heart rate) varies. As a consequence, the QT_C, although identifying persons with the phenotypic characteristics of LQTS, does not have a high degree of specificity needed to predict risk of SCD.[36] In most instances, the identity of the genetic mutation is unknown. Reliable clues to aid in discerning the type of LQTS and assist in risk stratification are based on analysis of ST-T wave morphologies and clinical presentation. T wave morphology changes have been linked to specific types of LQTS. In some instances, sudden infant death syndrome may be associated with LQTS and a mutation on the sodium channel gene.[9]

Brugada syndrome is an inherited ion channel disorder attributed to a mutation in the cardiac sodium channel gene SCN5A. As discussed in Chapter 47, its hallmark features are an accentuated J wave that appears as segment elevation in surface electrocardiogram leads V_1 to V_3 and often is followed by a negative T wave. Dysrhythmia manifestations include closely coupled extrasystoles and a rapid polymorphic VT. The abnormalities occur in the absence of ischemia, electrolyte abnormalities, or structural abnormalities. Although the genetic anomaly is on the same gene as LQTS 3, the QT interval is normal. The genetic anomaly results in rapid recovery of the sodium channel activity, which can encroach on the plateau of the action potential.

Brugada syndrome can be unmasked by Vaughn-Williams Class I antiarrhythmic compounds such as procainamide and flecainide, which block the sodium channel. Sudden unexplained death syndrome, prevalent in Southeast Asia (and occurring in the Asian population in the United States), has been shown to be phenotypically and genetically the same disorder as Brugada syndrome. Cocaine toxicity and alcohol intoxication also may unmask Brugada syndrome. Deaths attributed to Brugada syndrome have risen exponentially as the

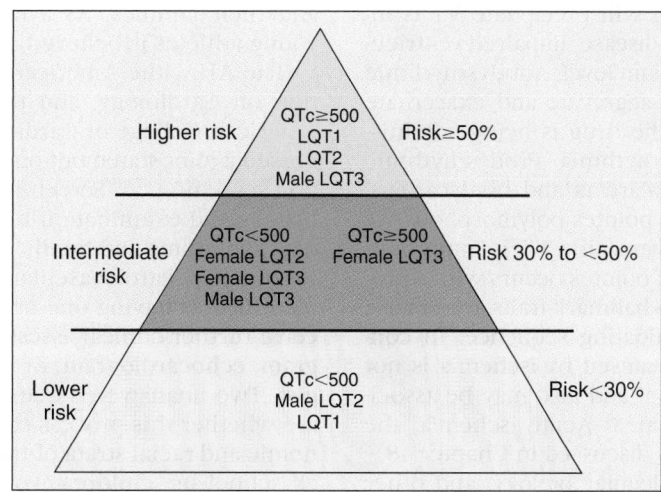

FIGURE 60-7 ■ Risk stratification in the long QT syndrome (LQTS). Shown is the risk stratification scheme for patients with LQTS according to genotype and gender. The risk groups have been defined based on the probability of experiencing a first cardiac event (syncope, cardiac arrest, or sudden death) by age 40 years. A 50 percent or higher probability of events constitutes the higher-risk subgroup, a risk between 30 and 50 percent the intermediate-risk group, and a risk less than 30 percent the lower-risk group. (From Myerberg RJ, Castellanos A: Cardiac arrest and sudden cardiac death. In Zipes DP, Libby P, Bonow RO, Braunwald E, editors: *Braunwald's heart disease: a textbook of cardiovascular medicine,* ed 7, Philadelphia, 2005, Saunders.)

syndrome has become better known. Death occurs primarily in young and otherwise healthy adults but may also occur in infants and children.[40]

Idiopathic VF is estimated to occur in 1 to 8 percent of out-of-hospital cardiac arrests. Idiopathic VF affects primarily middle-aged men and is associated with a risk of recurrence. A family history of SCD may be present.[1]

Catecholaminergic polymorphic VT is an inherited stress-induced VT occurring in children and adolescents in a structurally normal heart and normal QT interval. A family history of SCD or stress-induced syncope is present in approximately 30 percent of cases.

Wolff-Parkinson-White Syndrome

In rare instances, SCD may occur in Wolff-Parkinson-White syndrome. Because these accessory AV connections join the atria to the ventricle and bypass the physiological safety net imposed by the AV node, atrial fibrillation with conduction over the AV bypass tract may be lethal. Sudden death is more likely to occur if an AV nodal blocking agent has been administered as concealed retrograde conduction to the AV node is blocked, and more impulses may traverse the accessory pathway unimpeded to the ventricle.[41]

Transient Reversible Causes of Dysrhythmias

Modulation of function related to changes in autonomic tone, electrolytes, ischemia, pH balance, and other factors affect the excitability, automaticity, conductivity, and contractility of cardiac muscle, and favor the development of cardiac dysrhythmias. Myriad factors influence the response elicited. Likewise, the response varies by the phase of the action potential affected and tissue refractoriness encountered. Alteration in electrolytes may occur because of a decrease in intake or an increase in excretion. This may be caused by intrinsic or extrinsic factors including diuretic therapy. The in-

terplay of factors may provoke life-threatening dysrhythmias even when heart disease is absent.[1] The lethal association between black licorice and low potassium levels is one example that has gained notoriety.

Metabolic Abnormalities

Changes in the pH of the blood are capable of provoking cardiac dysrhythmias. Catecholamine levels can increase when acidemia develops. Typically, acidosis and alkalosis are associated with altered potassium and calcium concentrations.[42] In acidosis, potassium moves out of the cell. Potassium redistribution may occur during acute treatment for hyperglycemia and asthma. Sudden death related to metabolic and electrolyte abnormalities has been reported in persons on liquid protein diets and in persons with bulimia.[43] Electrolyte abnormalities commonly cause dysrhythmias.

Drug-Induced Dysrhythmias

A number of drugs are prodysrhythmic. Torsades de pointes VT, the characteristic polymorphous VT that occurs with a prolonged QT interval, may develop in response to administration of pharmacological agents that prolong repolarization. When this occurs, persons are said to have acquired LQTS. Torsades de pointes is not limited to Class I and III antidysrhythmic agents but may occur with a wide variety of agents from quinolone antibiotics to antidepressants. Often, persons who develop torsades de pointes are suspected of having LQTS syndrome despite the absence of phenotypic characteristics before drug administration. As such, administration of a pharmacological agent may be the stimulus that unmasks an underlying genetic anomaly. An increased propensity to manifest torsades de pointes may occur if several drugs use similar metabolic targets along the cytochrome P450 pathway.

The likelihood that a drug will precipitate VT is increased with structural heart disease, impaired ventricular function, and a low potassium level. Antidysrhythmic agents have the potential to aggravate and exacerbate the dysrhythmia for which the drug is being administered or provoke a new dysrhythmia. Prodysrhythmic responses may include tachycardias and bradycardias. Differentiation of torsades de pointes polymorphous VT from ischemic mediated polymorphic VT is important. Characteristically, torsades de pointes occurs with a prolonged QT interval. Among its hallmark traits are a pause dependency or long-short initiating sequence. In contrast, the polymorphous VT caused by ischemia is not limited to a prolonged interval and also may be associated with a short QT interval.[1,44] Acute ischemia, the most common cause of VT, is discussed in Chapter 48.

Advances in genetics, molecular biology, and other fields of basic science are shifting our view of CAD paradigm and its relationship to SCD. New information, from the expression of multiple elements in the cascade of lesion formation to initiation of acute syndromes, is providing insights into triggers of SCD. Genetic influences have been identified for multiple sites along the cascade from general risk factors for atherosclerosis to dysrhythmia expression. Integration between basic scientists and future applications in clinical practice offer hope of a genetic epidemiology that eventually can identify single-person probabilities for the risk of occurrence of SCD.[2,7,38]

COMMUNITY APPROACHES
Primary Prevention

Currently there is no population-based screening tool for SCD. Because approximately 80 percent of SCD is associated with coronary heart disease, traditional modifiable coronary risk factors such as diet, hypertension, obesity, smoking habits, hyperlipidemia, and sedentary life style consequently are used as surrogate markers for the risk of SCD. Primary prevention efforts therefore focus on preventing or slowing the progression of coronary heart disease. For example, after controlling for age, education, physical activity, smoking habits, alcohol consumption, body mass index, and antidysrhythmic medications, an increased intake of omega-3 fatty acids—as found in cold water fish such as salmon, tuna, and mackerel—has been shown to decrease the risk of SCD.[45] The risk reduction for SCD may be explained in part by the association between fish consumption and decreased heat rate because an increased heart rate is associated positively with the risk of SCD.[46] Moderate alcohol consumption, a consistent level of exercise, and an Indo-Mediterranean diet are associated with a reduced risk of SCD.[16] Increasing public awareness of the need for behavior modification can be an effective tool in preventing SCD and improving survival from cardiac arrest.

Changing population behaviors is a monumental challenge. Focusing on individual behaviors during each interaction with a health care provider provides an individual opportunity for discussion of risks and identification of needed behavioral changes for individuals

and their families. As a targeted group, screening of young athletes is believed to have value.

The AHA, the American Academy of Pediatrics Section on Cardiology, and the board of trustees of the American College of Cardiology have prepared and endorsed a joint statement on cardiovascular preparticipation screening.[47,48] Screening should include a thorough history and examination to look for any history of cardiac symptoms and family history of heart disease, and to identify cardiovascular abnormalities. Individuals identified as having one or more risk factors should receive further clinical assessment with an electrocardiogram, echocardiogram, or consultation with a cardiologist. Two unanswered questions related to this strategy are whether this process can be applied across the economic and racial strata of the United States and whether all school-age children would benefit from a modification of this approach.

The "Chain of Survival"

Failure to intervene in a timely and appropriate manner at the time of an unanticipated cardiac arrest can lead to SCD. Unexpected cardiac arrest can strike ostensibly healthy persons in their most productive years. The event can happen at home, school, work, shopping malls, and other public places. Prompt intervention at the time of the arrest provides an opportunity to restore a perfusing cardiac rhythm and avoid the progression from cardiac arrest to death. Recognizing the time-sensitive nature of successful resuscitation, the AHA developed a four-step process to save lives during cardiac emergencies.[49] The chain of survival is an educational metaphor emphasizing the time-sensitive sequential activities that are needed to optimize the chance of survival from cardiac arrest (Figure 60-8). Each of the four links—early access, early cardiopulmonary resuscitation (**CPR**), early defibrillation, and early advanced life support—is interrelated. Where one link is weak, the chance for survival decreases, regardless of the strength of the others.

Early Access

Early access to the emergency medical services (**EMS**) system is the first link in the chain of survival. Good evidence indicates that survival from out-of-hospital cardiac arrest is linked directly to EMS response time. Wide-

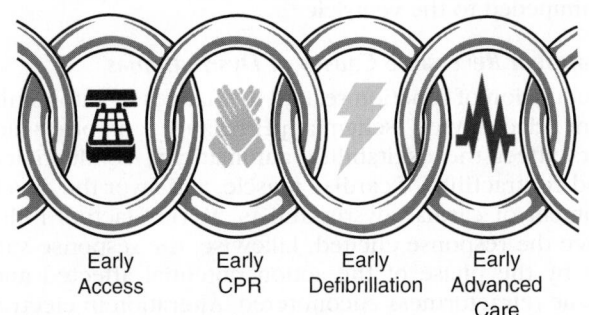

| Early Access | Early CPR | Early Defibrillation | Early Advanced Care |

FIGURE 60-8 ■ The American Heart Association's "Chain of Survival": early access, early cardiopulmonary resuscitation, early defibrillation, and early advanced life support.

spread community education on the importance of early access has resulted in the implementation of 911 systems throughout the country. Further educational efforts are focused on developing programs that maximize the likelihood that individuals indeed will respond appropriately and call 911 when they witness a cardiac emergency.

Early Cardiopulmonary Resuscitation

CPR by itself is a temporizing measure that extends the time available for a cardiac arrest victim to receive definitive treatment. When begun within 4 minutes after collapse, CPR can extend viability until therapeutic interventions such as defibrillation, medications, or pacing can occur. Bystander-initiated CPR has almost doubled the number of persons who can be discharged from the hospital alive after cardiac arrest.[50]

Millions of individuals worldwide have already been exposed to various elements of CPR or have taken courses in the techniques of CPR. However, the number of trained individuals is insufficient. Making CPR training programs more available to all citizens is a high-priority public policy agenda item for health care professionals and organizations. The epidemiology of cardiac arrest, however, indicates that mass training efforts aimed at the general population are not the most efficient intervention to ensure that CPR will be performed when a cardiac arrest occurs in an out-of-hospital setting.[51] The assessment is based on the finding that most CPR trainees are young, whereas approximately 80 percent of unexpected cardiac arrests occur in homes and almost 60 percent are witnessed, usually by older individuals well known to the victim.[52] Targeted CPR programs aimed at family members of those known to be at risk for SCD have been shown to be effective and cost-efficient.[53] (See the accompanying conundrum feature.)

Early Defibrillation

For patients in cardiac arrest with a shockable rhythm—VF or VT—every minute of delay in defibrillation is associated with a 7 to 10 percent decrease in survivability.

By 10 minutes, few patients survive. In community settings, the life-saving intervention of defibrillation historically has had to wait until the arrival of EMS personnel. Delays in notification and arrival of EMS, therefore, have been associated with decreased survival rates.

The development of AEDs has made it possible to decrease the time to first defibrillation (Figure 60-9). AEDs are easy to use, small, safe, and low-maintenance devices that allow trained lay rescuers to defibrillate patients before the arrival of professional rescuers. These devices are being placed in locations where large numbers of persons gather, such as sports arenas, court buildings, airports, casinos, schools, and shopping malls. In addition, AEDs are being placed in locations where there are known delays in the arrival of EMS, such as airplanes, high-rise buildings, and remote locations such as golf courses and manufacturing plants. The Public Access Defibrillation (**PAD**) Trial found that trained laypersons using AEDs and CPR doubled the number of survivors from cardiac arrest compared with CPR alone in public locations.[54] Based on these findings, the AHA recommends that AEDs be placed in all public locations in which one cardiac arrest occurs every 5 years, on average. Table 60-2 provides a strategy for community deployment of AEDs. As AEDs become more available in public settings, increased community awareness and training is necessary to maximize their use and improve survival from cardiac arrest.

Early Advanced Life Support

Defibrillation may not be enough to achieve and sustain a perfusing rhythm. Advanced life support interventions including endotracheal intubation, intravenous medica-

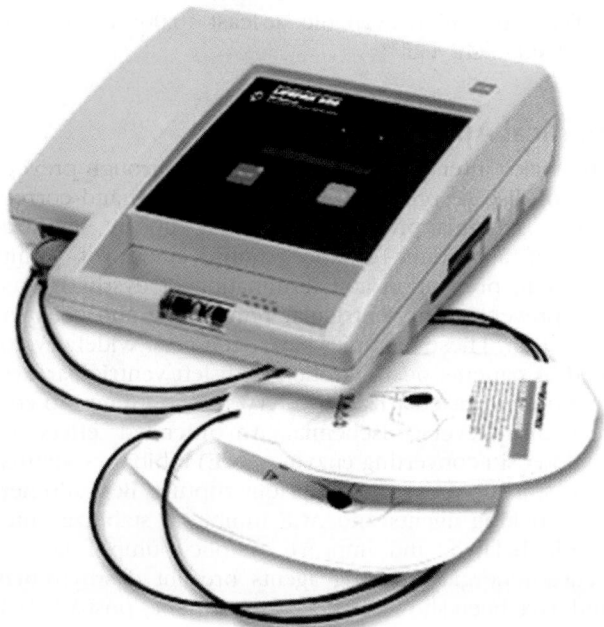

FIGURE 60-9 ■ An automatic external defibrillator (AED). The LIFEPAK 500® AED is designed to be used by first responders to cardiac emergencies. Intuitive operation makes it usable by infrequent users. The AED has clear screen messages, voice prompts, and lighted buttons to guide responders through operation. This AED weighs only 7 lb and is rugged and portable. (Courtesy Medtronic.)

■■■ CONUNDRUM

TARGETED VERSUS MASS CARDIOPULMONARY RESUSCITATION TRAINING

Most sudden cardiac deaths occur in individuals with intermediate or no known risk factors. However, the highest-risk groups—patients with previous out-of-hospital cardiac arrest, patients with ejection fractions of less than 35 percent and patients with previous myocardial infarctions, a low ejection fraction, and ventricular tachydysrhythmias—actually compose a small proportion of sudden cardiac deaths.

Primary and secondary prevention interventions in the high-risk groups have been demonstrated to be effective and relatively efficient. To affect the largest number of individuals requires focus on the low-risk general population with the largest absolute number of events. Current strategies that target this group are relatively inefficient because of the low yield of having a trained individual prepared and willing to intervene at the site of an actual cardiac arrest.

With limited resources, organizations have to determine which strategies are most effective and efficient in affecting the incidence of sudden cardiac death.

■ ■ ■

TABLE 60-2 OUT-OF-HOSPITAL CARDIAC ARREST SURVIVAL AND DEPLOYMENT STRATEGIES FOR AUTOMATIC EXTERNAL DEFIBRILLATORS*

DEPLOYMENT	EXAMPLES	RESCUERS	ADVANTAGES	LIMITATIONS
Emergency vehicles	Police cars Fire engines Ambulances	Trained emergency personnel	Experienced users Broad deployment Objectivity	Deployment time Arrival delays Community variations
Public access sites	Public buildings Stadiums, malls Airports Airliners	Security personnel Designated rescuers Random lay persons	Population density Shorter delays Lay and emergency personnel access	Low event rates Inexperienced users Panic and confusion
Multifamily dwellings	Apartments Condominiums Hotels	Security personnel Designated rescuers Family members	Familiar locations Defined personnel Shorter delays	Infrequent use Low event rates Geographic factors
Single-family dwellings	Private homes Apartments Neighborhood "Heart Watch"	Family members Security personnel Designated rescuers	Immediate access Familiar setting	Acceptance Victim may be alone One-time user; panic

*Various deployment strategies for nonconventional responders with access to automatic external defibrillators are suggested. For each example, the type of rescuer and the advantages and limitations of each strategy are provided. Any single strategy is unlikely to dominate; rather there will be a cumulative benefit from the additive effect of multiple approaches.
From Myerburg RJ, Castellanos A: Cardiac arrest and sudden cardiac death. In Zipes DP, Libby P, Bonow RO, Braunwald E, editors: *Braunwald's heart disease: a textbook of cardiovascular medicine,* ed 7, Philadelphia, 2005, Saunders.

tions, and other highly technical interventions are often necessary. Outside of hospitals, advanced life support is typically provided by EMS units staffed by paramedics acting under the authority of a medical director.

With a fully integrated system that includes timely activation of EMS, immediate bystander-initiated CPR, and the first defibrillation shock delivered within 3 to 5 minutes, successful resuscitation rates from witnessed VF have been reported as high as 48 to 74 percent. According to the AHA, if the chain of survival were maximized with bystander CPR consistently initiated and AEDs more widely available, at least 40,000 lives could be saved each year.[54]

Medical Approaches

The major interventions to reduce SCD through prevention of disease progression include reversal and correction of ischemia, prevention of plaque rupture, stabilization of autonomic balance, improvement of pump function, prevention and termination of dysrhythmias, and prevention of ventricular remodeling and collagen formation. These therapies have been most widely evaluated in patients postinfarction with left ventricular dysfunction. Revascularization interventions attempt to correct and reverse ischemia. An intended effect of angiotensin-converting enzyme (**ACE**) inhibitors, statins, and aspirin is prevention of plaque rupture. Beta-adrenergic blocking agents and ACE inhibitors stabilize autonomic balance and improve systolic pump function. Beta-adrenergic blocking agents prevent dysrhythmias and have been shown to decrease mortality post-MI. ACE inhibitors and angiotensin receptor blockers prevent ventricular remodeling. Aldosterone antagonists also reduce mortality.[55] Although these strategies have been incorporated increasingly into medical management these therapies remain underutilized and the overall incidence of SCD has changed little in the last 25 years.

More than a decade of randomized clinical trials has demonstrated unequivocally the superior efficacy of the ICD compared with optimal medical therapy and optimal medical therapy plus antidysrhythmic agents (Table 60-3). ICDs are the treatment of choice for survivors of cardiac arrest, based on the results of numerous clinical trials (secondary prevention: AVID, CIDS, CASH) and for patients with known risk factor for SCD (primary prevention: MADIT, MUSTT, MADIT II, DEFINITE, COMPANION, SCD-HeFT).[56]

The adoption of cardiac resynchronization pacing therapy to ameliorate intraventricular dyssynchrony and augment systolic function has rekindled attention on the significance of intraventricular conduction delays and its known increased risk of SCD.[15,16,23] Cardiac resynchronization therapy is used increasingly to overcome intraventricular and interventricular dyssynchrony resulting from intraventricular conduction delays and when combined with the ICD to prevent SCD and to terminate VT/VF (see Chapter 61). Figure 60-10 provides a treatment algorithm for patients resuscitated from cardiac arrest.

MANAGEMENT IN THE CLINICAL SETTING
Patients with Existing Implantable Cardioverter-Defibrillators

Despite the proven efficacy of ICDs to terminate VT/VT, it is crucial that persons with ICDs also promptly receive CPR and advanced cardiac life support. Treating the patient and not waiting for the ICD to treat the patient is of utmost importance. Because the tachycardia termination or bradycardia support therapies of the ICD depend on how the device is programmed, it is possible that the device may not detect or "see" VT/VF. In other situations the ICD may detect VT/VF when the patient is in sinus rhythm. Examples of these situations and the appropriate medical interventions are presented in Table 60-4.

TABLE 60-3 SUMMARY OF MAJOR IMPLANTABLE CARDIOVERTER-DEFIBRILLATOR TRIALS FOR PREVENTION OF SUDDEN CARDIAC DEATHS

TRIAL	STUDY GROUP	2-YEAR OUTCOMES (%)			
		CONTROL	ICDs	Rel RR	Abs RR
Secondary Prevention*					
AVID (*n* = 1061)	VF, VT-syncope, VT: EF ≤40%	25	18	−27	−7
CIDS (*n* = 659)	VF, VT-syncope, VT: EF ≤35% and CL ≤400 msec	21	15	−30	−6
CASH (*n* = 346)	Cardiac arrest survivors (VF, VT)	20 (combined)	12	−37	−8

	2-YEAR (MADIT, CABG-Patch, MADIT-2) AND 5-YEAR (MUSTT, SCD-HeFT) OUTCOMES (%)				
		CONTROL	ICDs	Rel RR	Abs RR
Primary Prevention†					
MADIT (*n* = 196)	Prior MI, EF ≤35%, NS VT, inducible VT, failed IV PA	32	13	−59	−19
MUSTT (*n* = 704)	Prior MI, EF ≤40%, NS VT, inducible VT	55	24	−58	−31
CABG-Patch (*n* = 900)	Coronary bypass surgery, EF less than 36%, SAECG (+)	18	18	0	0
MADIT-2 (*n* = 1232)	Prior MI (greater than 1 month), EF ≤30%	22	16	−28	−6
SCD-HeFT (*n* = 2521)‡	Class II-III CHF, EF ≤35%	36	29	−23	−7

*Three major randomized trials for secondary prevention among survivors of out-of-hospital cardiac arrest, or high-risk ventricular tachycardia (VT), have been completed: the Antiarrhythmics Versus Implantable Defibrillators (AVID) Trial, the Canadian Implantable Defibrillator Study (CIDS), and the Cardiac Arrest Study of Hamburg (CASH). Each used an active control, randomized design, comparing ICDs with antiarrhythmic drug (AAD) therapy, primarily amiodarone. The cumulative data, as well as the individual data from the larger studies, support the idea that the ICD is preferable to drug therapy for this high-risk population. However, the large relative benefits translated to more modest absolute benefits, with a large residual risk among the ICD-treated groups in each study.
†Four primary prevention trials among patients presumed to be at high risk but who have not had spontaneous life-threatening ventricular arrhythmias have been completed: the Multicenter Automatic Defibrillator Implantation Trial (MADIT), the Multicenter Unsustained Tachycardia Trial (MUSTT), the Coronary Artery Bypass Surgery/Implantable Defibrillator Trial (CABG-Patch), and the Multicenter Automatic Defibrillator Implantation Trial-2 (MADIT-2). MADIT showed an advantage of ICD therapy over AAD therapy, MUSTT showed superiority of electrophysiologically guided evaluation leading to ICD therapy compared with that leading to drug therapy, and CABG-Patch showed no benefit to ICDs for patients undergoing routine coronary bypass surgery. MADIT-2 showed a benefit of ICD therapy compared with usual therapy for post–myocardial infarction patients with an EF ≤30%. The other large primary prevention trial, the Sudden Cardiac Death in Heart Failure Trial (SCD-HeFT), was in progress (along with a number of smaller trials) at the time of writing.
‡Presented as a late-breaking trial at the Annual Scientific Sessions of the American College of Cardiology, March 8, 2004. No difference shown between amiodarone and control.
Abs RR, Absolute risk reduction; *CHF,* congestive heart failure; *CL,* cycle length; *EF,* ejection fraction; *EP,* electrophysiological; *ICD,* implantable cardioverter-defibrillator; *IV PA,* intravenous procainamide; *MI,* myocardial infarction; *NS,* nonsustained; *Rel RR,* relative risk reduction; *SAECG,* signal-averaged electrocardiogram; *VF,* ventricular fibrillation; *VT,* ventricular tachycardia.
From Myerburg RJ, Castellanos A: Cardiac arrest and sudden cardiac death. In Zipes DP, Libby P, Bonow RO, Braunwald E, editors: *Braunwald's heart disease: a textbook of cardiovascular medicine,* ed 7, Philadelphia, 2005, Saunders.

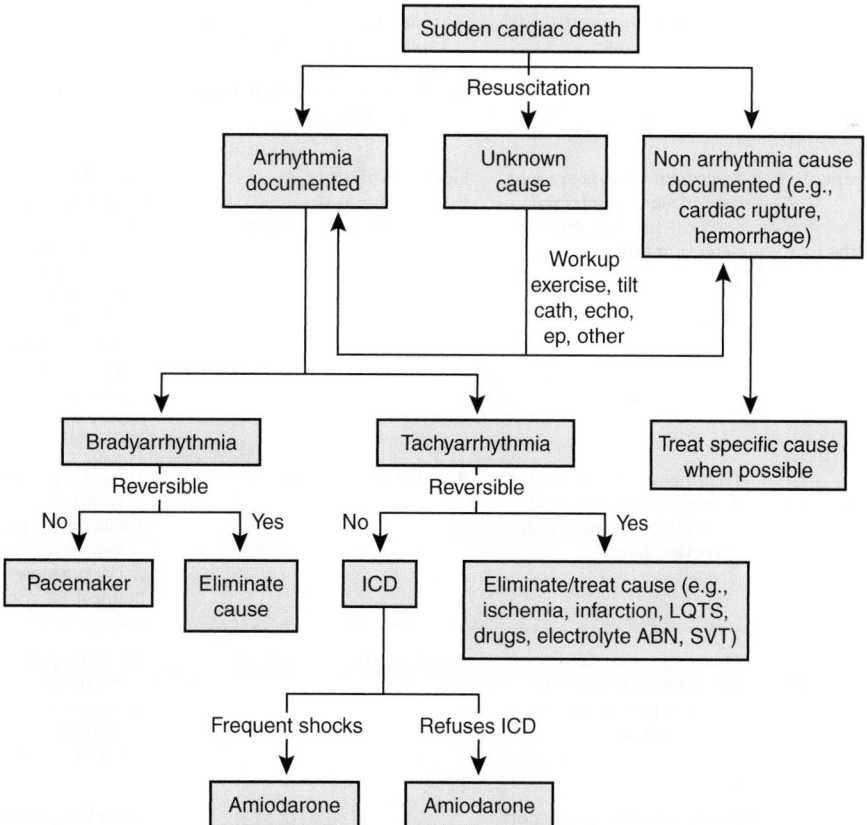

FIGURE 60-10 ■ Treatment algorithm for patient resuscitated from cardiac arrest. *ABN,* Abnormality; *Cath,* catheterization; *echo,* echocardiography; *EP,* electrophysiological study; *ICD,* implantable cardioverter-defibrillator; *LQTS,* long QT syndrome; *SCD,* sudden cardiac death; *SVT,* supraventricular tachycardia. (From Zipes D, Wellens HJJ: *Circulation* 98:2334-2351, 1998.)

TABLE 60-4 ASSESSMENT AND MANAGEMENT OF PATIENTS WITH IMPLANTABLE CARDIOVERTER-DEFIBRILLATORS

ICD THERAPY ABSENCE OF THERAPY	ICD FUNCTION	POSSIBLE CAUSES	CLINICAL INTERVENTIONS
Ventricular Tachycardia (VT) *ICD sees VT.* Rapid ventricular pacing (anti-tachycardia pacing) to terminate VT Or High-voltage stimulus artifact reflecting ICD shock	Treatment criteria are met. Rate of signals detected meets programmed detection rate.		Treat the patient according to ACLS protocol. Request electrophysiology/device evaluation and reprogramming (EP consult).
ICD does not see VT.	Treatment criteria are not met. Rate of signals detected below programmed detection rate.	The R-R interval or cycle-length of the VT has been lengthened by the start of an anti-arrrhythmic drug. Device may be turned off. There is a "new," slower VT. Worsening chamber dilatation has increased the time for VT to traverse the reentrant circuit.	
Ventricular Fibrillation (VF) *ICD Sees VF.* Large stimulus artifact Shock delivered Resumption of sinus or non-VF rhythm	Treatment criteria are met. Rate of signals detected meets programmed VF detection rate.		Treat the patient according to ACLS protocol. Request EP consult.
VF continues. Multiple large stimulus artifacts visible Multiple shocks delivered *No ICD therapies* Apparent Absence of high-voltage stimulus		Programmed voltage for shock therapy may be insufficient to terminate VF.	
ICD does not see VF.	Treatment criteria are not met. Device is not turned on. Rate of signals detected is below programmed VF detection rate.	Device may be off. For example, it may have been programmed off for surgery to prevent delivery of shock from electrical noise during cautery and not turned on after the surgery. The R-R interval or cycle-length of VF is longer.	
Normal Sinus Rhythm Patient reports multiple repetitive shocks. *ICD sees VT/VF.* High-voltage stimulus artifact appears on ECG.	Treatment criteria are met. Rate of signals detected meets programmed detection rate.	Electrical noise ICD lead fracture Procedures using cautery	Treat the patient. Obtain immediate EP consult. Magnet application with most ICDs in a continuously monitoring setting/resuscitation equipment available. If R wave synchronous beeping is audible with magnet placement, continue to hold magnet 30 seconds and withdraw when beeping changes to a continuous tone. Device is turned off.
Atrial Fibrillation *ICD sees VT/VF.* High-voltage stimulus artifact appears on ECG. Shock is delivered.	Treatment criteria are met. Rate of signals detected meets programmed detection rate.	Rapid ventricular rate	Treat the patient according to ACLS protocol. Antiarrhythmic drug (I/III) and atrioventricular nodal blocking agents (II/IV) slow ventricular response. Request EP consult.
Sinus Tachycardia *ICD sees VT/VF.* High-voltage stimulus artifact appears on ECG. Shock is delivered.	Treatment criteria are met. Rate of signals detected meets programmed detection rate.	Rapid ventricular rate	Treat the patient according to ACLS protocol. Atrioventricular nodal blocking agents (II/IV) slow ventricular response. Request EP consult.
Self-Terminating VF *ICD sees VF and sees termination.* No shock is delivered. Shock is delivered.	Treatment criteria are not met. Treatment criteria are met.		Treat the patient according to ACLS protocol. Request EP consult.

ICD, Implantable cardioverter-defibrillator; *ACLS,* advanced cardiac life support; *EP,* electrophysiological; *ECG,* electrocardiogram.

Medical Emergency Teams

Most hospitals have a cardiac arrest team that is activated after cardiopulmonary arrest occurs. Once a cardiac arrest occurs, the likelihood of successful resuscitation with survival to hospital discharge is poor—averaging only 18 percent.[57] Retrospective record reviews and prospective analyses have indicated that patients with unexpected in-hospital cardiac arrest often have abnormal clinical observations before the arrest.[57-59] In a retrospective analysis, Buist and colleagues[59] determined the predictive value of selected abnormal clinical observations for subsequent in-hospital mortality in a non–intensive care unit population. The two most common abnormal clinical events were arterial oxygen desaturation (51 percent of all events) and hypotension (17.3 percent of all events). Six clinical observations were identified as significant predictors of mortality: a decrease of 2 points in Glasgow Coma Scale score; onset of coma; hypotension (systolic pressure less than 90 mm Hg); respiratory rate less than 6 breaths/min; oxygen saturation less than 90 percent; and heart rate less than 30 beats/min. The presence of any one of the six events was associated with a 6.8 times increase in the risk of mortality.

Medical emergency teams (**METs**), sometimes called medical evaluation teams or rapid response teams (**RRTs**), encompasses a proactive response to the wide range of clinical situations that have been identified as predictive of an impending arrest. The underlying concept for METs is an early warning system for patients at higher risk of unexpected cardiopulmonary arrest. The MET response system includes planned and systematic processes that allow early identification of seriously ill patients on general hospital units and provides a comprehensive assessment of the patient by a trained team focused on prompt intervention aimed at preventing irreversible organ failure or arrest. Facilities that embrace the MET concept recognize the importance of educating the nursing staff on the critical nature of their involvement in this early warning system. Key to a successful program is empowering nursing staff to mobilize the team anytime they feel the need for additional support for patient assessment.

Although not all studies of METs have demonstrated a reduced incidence of cardiac arrest,[60] others have reported that implementing METs can decrease the incidence of cardiac arrest and in-hospital mortality from cardiac arrest. Buist and colleagues[62] reported a 50 percent reduction in non–intensive care unit arrests following MET implementation. Bellomo and colleagues[63] reported a 58 percent decrease in postoperative emergency transfers into the intensive care unit and a 37 percent reduction in deaths associated in a controlled trial. In a study to determine the effect of a critical care outreach team on survival to hospital discharge and readmission to critical care, Ball and colleagues[64] noted that the introduction of the MET improved survival to discharge by 6.8 percent and that readmission to the intensive care units decreased by 6.4 percent.

Recognizing the opportunity to save lives through specific, targeted interventions in the hospital setting, the Society of Critical Care Medicine, in conjunction with the Institute for Healthcare Improvement, developed the "100,000 Lives Campaign." One specific intervention in the campaign is the development of RRTs.[65] The role of an RRT is to assess and stabilize the patient, assist with communication between caregivers, educate and support the staff on the unit, and assist with transfer, if necessary. (See the accompanying Evidence-Based Practice Feature.) The "100,000 Lives Campaign" was so successful in achieving not only its goals for RRT but its overall patient safety goals that in December, 2006 it was expanded in scope and duration to the "5 Million Lives Campaign." The new campaign is an initiative to protect 5 million patients from incidents of harm over the next two years. [65]

In-Hospital Response to Cardiac Arrest

The goal of in-hospital resuscitation is to resuscitate the right patients and resuscitate them correctly. It is commonly believed that because of the ready availability of qualified staff and appropriate equipment, cardiac arrests in the hospital setting are well managed and patient outcomes are maximized. Despite more than 30 years of basic and advanced life support training and interventions, the overall survival rate from in-hospital cardiac arrest remains relatively stable at 15 to 18 percent.[66] The lack of improvement in the overall survival rate over time may reflect increasing patient condition severity or other patient characteristics. Another factor that may explain the lack of improvement in survival rate from in-hospital cardiac arrest is the quality of basic and advanced life support provided.

Consistent with the prehospital setting, efforts to improve outcomes from cardiac arrest should be directed at strengthening the in-hospital chain of survival. Efforts include focusing on improving the quality of CPR given by health care providers,[64] the deployment of AEDs on general patient care units and in clinics to decrease the time to first defibrillation by non–critical care nurses before the arrival of the code team,[66,67] and emphasizing the adoption and implementation of existing postresuscitation care standards such as glycemic control and induced hypothermia.[68]

■ EVIDENCE-BASED PRACTICE

CRITERIA FOR ACTIVATING THE RAPID RESPONSE TEAM

- Staff member is worried about the patient.
- Acute change in heart rate to less than 40 or more than 130 beats/min.
- Acute change in systolic blood pressure to less than 90 mm Hg.
- Acute change in respiratory rate to less than 8 or more than 28 breaths/min.
- Acute change in oxygen saturation to less than 90 percent despite oxygen administration.
- Acute change in conscious state.
- Acute change in urinary output to less than 50 ml in 4 hours.

Recommendations from the Society of Critical Care Medicine and the Institute for Healthcare Improvement.

CONCLUSION

SCD resulting from VT/VF is a leading cause of death. Many risk factors that identify an increased risk for SCD from cardiac causes such as hypertension, smoking, obesity, and glucose intolerance are related to CAD and its consequences. Unquestionably, these risk factors are useful in identifying high-risk subgroups because interventions aimed at decreasing these risk factors likely will reduce the risk of SCD. The limitation of these markers is that they primarily identify the risk of the underlying disease that may be responsible for SCD, not the risk of the event responsible for death. Whereas the risk factors for CAD are present and fairly constant over time, fatal dysrhythmias are transient, dynamic, pathophysiological events and have been likened to an "electrical accident."

Outcomes from randomized clinical trials provide evidence to identify who is at an increased risk for SCD and overall mortality. Clinical trials also inform us, through a comparison of medical management strategies, which strategy provides superior survival outcomes compared with an alternative treatment. Meta-analyses of clinical trials, particularly when an individual trial did not have enough patients to determine whether survival was influenced, facilitate evaluation of markers of increased risk and the potential benefit conferred by therapies. Initially, clinical trials may focus on populations defined by specific disease states and progress toward less well-stratified groups of individuals as has happened with those assessing the efficacy of therapies to prevent recurrence of SCD (secondary prevention) and clinical trials assessing the efficacy of therapy to prevent SCD (primary prevention). The progression of ICD clinical trials reflects this strategy.

The risk of SCD now can be predicted with some degree of precision in known high-risk groups. Despite substantial evidence from a plethora of randomized clinical trials identifying secondary and primary prevention strategies, however, it is still not possible to predict when a SCD event will occur. Until the time when cardiac arrest events can be predicted with accuracy, primary and secondary prevention efforts and strategies to strengthen the out-of-hospital and in-hospital chain of survival will continue to be important public health concerns. Collaboration among basic scientists; medical, nursing, and allied health professionals; and the public at large to prevent SCD and minimize its effects reflects the coordinated efforts required to minimize the impact to society.

REFERENCES

1. Myerberg RJ, Castellanos A: Cardiac arrest and sudden cardiac death. In Zipes DP, Libby P, Bonow RO, Braunwald E, editors: *Braunwald's heart disease: a textbook of cardiovascular medicine,* ed 7, Philadelphia, 2005, Saunders.
2. Pinto DS, Josephson ME: Sudden cardiac death. In Fuster V, Alexander RW, O'Rourke RA: *Hurst's the heart,* ed 11, New York, 2004, McGraw-Hill.
3. Lemaitre RN, Siscovick DS, Gaghunathan TE et al: Leisure-time physical activity and the risk of primary cardiac arrest, *Arch Intern Med* 159:686-690, 1999.
4. American Heart Association: *Heart disease and stroke statistics: 2005 update,* Dallas, 2004, The Association.
5. Centers for Disease Control and Prevention: State-specific mortality from sudden cardiac death: United States, 1999, *MMWR Morb Mortal Wkly Rep* 51:123-126, 2002.
6. Vaillancorte C, Stiell IG, the Canadian Cardiovascular Outcomes Research Team: Cardiac arrest care and emergency medical services in Canada, *Can J Cardiol* 20:1081-1090, 2004.
7. Myerburg RF, Interian A, Simmons J, Castellanos A: Sudden cardiac death. In Zipes DP, Jalife J, editors: *Cardiac electrophysiology from cell to bedside,* ed 4, Philadelphia, 2004, Saunders.
8. Beckerman J, Wang P, Hlatky M: Cardiovascular screening of athletes, *Clin J Sport Med* 14:127-133, 2004.
9. Antzelevitch C: Molecular genetics of arrhythmias and cardiovascular conditions associated with arrhythmias, Heart*Rhythm* 1:42C-56C, 2004.
10. Zareba W, Moss AJ, Locati EH et al: International Long QT Syndrome Registry: modulating effects of age and gender on the clinical course of long QT syndrome by genotype, *J Am Coll Cardiol* 42:103-109, 2003.
11. Rea TD, Pearce R, Ragunathan TE et al: Incidence of out-of-hospital cardiac arrest, *Am J Cardiol* 93:1455-1460, 2004.
12. Zheng Z, Croft J, Giles WH, Mensah GA: Sudden cardiac death in the United States, 1989-1998, *Circulation* 104:2158-2163, 2001.
13. Becker LB, Han BH, Meyer PM et al: The CPR Chicago project: racial differences in the incidence of cardiac arrest and subsequent survival, *N Engl J Med* 329:600-606, 1993.
14. Levy D, Brink S: *A change of heart: how the people of Framingham, Massachusetts, helped unravel the mysteries of cardiovascular disease,* New York, 2005, Knopf Publishing Group.
15. Albert CM, Chae CU, Grodstein F et al: Prospective study of sudden cardiac death among women in the United States, *Circulation* 107:2096-2101, 2003.
16. Obias-Manno D, Wijetunga M: Risk stratification and primary prevention of sudden cardiac death, *AACN Clin Issues* 15:404-418, 2004.
17. Albert CM, McGovern BA, Newell JB, Ruskin JN: Sex differences in cardiac arrest survivors, *Circulation* 93:1170-1176, 1996.
18. Kannel WB, Plehn JF, Cupples LA: Cardiac failure and sudden death in the Framingham Study, *Am Heart J* 115:869-875, 1988.
19. Bigger JT, Fleiss JL, Kleiger R et al, and the Multicenter Post-Infarction Research Group: The relationships among ventricular arrhythmias, left ventricular dysfunction, and mortality in the 2 years after myocardial infarction, *Circulation* 69:250-825, 1984.
20. Deedwania PC: The key to unraveling the mystery of mortality in heart failure: an integrated approach, *Circulation* 107:1719-1721, 2003.
21. Ganz LI: Primary prevention of sudden cardiac death, *Curr Cardiol Rep* 6:339-347, 2004.
22. Standridge JB, Zylstra RG, Adams SH: Alcohol consumption: an overview of benefits and risks, *South Med J* 97:664-672, 2004.
23. Albert CM, Ruskin JN: Risk stratifiers for sudden cardiac death in the community: primary prevention of sudden cardiac death, *Cardiovasc Res* 50:186-196, 2001.
24. Lampert R, Joska T, Burg MM et al: Emotional and physical precipitants of ventricular arrhythmias, *Circulation* 106:1800-1805, 2002.
25. Albert CM, Chae CU, Rexrode KM et al: Phobic anxiety and risk of coronary heart disease and sudden cardiac death among women, *Circulation* 111:480-487, 2005.
26. Rumsfeld JS, Ho PM: Depression and cardiovascular disease: a call for recognition, *Circulation* 111:250-253, 2005.
27. Bardy GH, Lee KL, Mark DB et al, for the Sudden Cardiac Death in Heart Failure Trial (SCD-HeFT) Investigators: Amiodarone or an implantable cardioverter-defibrillator for congestive heart failure, *N Engl J Med* 352:225-237, 2005.
28. Wynne J, Braunwald E: The cardiomyopathies. In Zipes DP, Libby P, Bonow RO, Braunwald E, editors: *Braunwald's heart disease: a textbook of cardiovascular medicine,* ed 7, Philadelphia, 2005, Saunders.
29. Maron BJ, McKenna WJ, Danielson GK et al: American College of Cardiology/European Society of Cardiology Clinical Expert Consensus Document on Hypertrophic Cardiomyopathy: a report of the American College of Cardiology Foundation Task Force on Clinical Expert Consensus Documents and the European Society

of Cardiology Committee for Practice Guidelines, *J Am Coll Cardiol* 42:1687-1713, 2003.

30. The Cardiac Arrhythmia Suppression Trial Investigators: Preliminary report: effect of encainide and flecainide on mortality in a randomized trial of arrhythmia suppression after myocardial infarction, *N Engl J Med* 321:406-412, 1989.

31. Echt DS, Liebson PR, Mitchell LB et al: Mortality and morbidity in patients receiving encainide, flecainide, or placebo: the Cardiac Arrhythmia Suppression Trial, *N Engl J Med* 324:781-788, 1991.

32. Coplen SE, Antman EM, Berlin JA et al: Efficacy and safety of quinidine therapy for maintenance of sinus rhythm after cardioversion: a meta-analysis of randomized control trials, *Circulation* 82:1106-1116, 1990 (published erratum, *Circulation* 83:7141, 1991).

33. Stroke Prevention in Atrial Fibrillation Investigators: Stroke prevention in atrial fibrillation study: final results, *Circulation* 84:527-539, 1991.

34. Levy S, Breithardt G, Campbell RW et al: Atrial fibrillation: current knowledge and recommendations for management: Working Group on Arrhythmias of the European Society of Cardiology, *Eur Heart J* 19:1294-1320, 1998.

35. Waldo AL, Camm AJ, de Ruyter H et al, for the SWORD Investigators: Effect of d-sotalol on mortality in patients with left ventricular dysfunction after recent and remote myocardial infarction, *Lancet* 348:7-12, 1996.

36. Silvert H, Amin J, Padmanabhan S, Pai R: Prognostic implications of increased QRS duration in patients with moderate and severe left ventricular systolic dysfunction, *Am J Cardiol* 88:182-185, 2001.

37. Bayes de Luna A, Coumel P, Leclercq JF: Ambulatory sudden death: mechanisms of production of fatal arrhythmia on the basis of data from 157 cases, *Am Heart J* 117:151-159, 1989.

38. Josephson M, Wellens HJJ: Implantable defibrillators and sudden cardiac death, *Circulation* 109:2685-2691, 2004.

39. Huikuri HV, Mäkikallio TH, Raatikainen P et al: Prediction of sudden cardiac death: appraisal of the studies and methods assessing the risk of sudden arrhythmic death, *Circulation* 108:110-115, 2003.

40. Antzelevitch A, Brugada P, Borggrefe M et al: Brugada syndrome: report of the second consensus conference, *Circulation* 111:659-670, 2005.

41. Klein GJ, Bashore T, Sellers TE et al: Ventricular fibrillation in the Wolff-Parkinson-White syndrome and atrial fibrillation, *N Engl J Med* 301:1080-1085, 1979.

42. Felver L: Acid-base balance and imbalance. In Woods SL, Froelicher ESS, Motzer SA, editors: *Cardiac nursing*, ed 4, Philadelphia, 2000, Lippincott.

43. Chou T, Knilans TK: *Electrocardiography in clinical practice*, ed 4, Philadelphia, 1996, WB Saunders.

44. Chiang CE: Congenital and acquired long QT syndrome: current concepts and management, *Cardiol Rev* 12:222-234, 2004.

45. Albert CM, Hennekens CH, O'Donnell CJ: Fish consumption and decreased risk of sudden cardiac death, *JAMA* 279:23-28, 1998.

46. Dallongeville J, Yarnell J, Ducimetiere P et al: Fish consumption is associated with lower heart rates, *Circulation* 108:820-825, 2004.

47. Maron BJ, Thompson PD, Puffer JC et al: Cardiovascular pre-participation screening of competitive athletes: a statement for health professionals from the Sudden Death Committee and Congenital Cardiac Defects Committee, American Heart Association, *Circulation* 94:850-856, 1996.

48. Maron BJ, Thompson PD, Puffer JC et al: Cardiovascular pre-participation screening of competitive athletes: addendum, *Circulation* 97:2294, 1998.

49. Cummins RO, Ornato JP, Thies WH, Pepe PE: Improving survival from sudden cardiac arrest: the Chain of Survival Concept, *Circulation* 85:1832-2351, 1991.

50. Cobb LA, Weaver WD, Fehrenbrush CE: Community-based interventions for sudden cardiac death: impact, limitations, and changes, *Circulation* 85(suppl I):198-102, 1992.

51. Swor R, Compton S: Estimating cost-effectiveness of mass cardiopulmonary training strategies to improve survival from cardiac arrest in private locations, *Prehosp Emerg Care* 8:420-423, 2004.

52. Eisenberg MS, Mengert TJ: Primary care: cardiac resuscitation, *N Engl J Med* 344:1304-1313, 2001.

53. Groeneveld PW, Owens DK: Cost-effectiveness of training unselected laypersons in a cardiac resuscitation and defibrillation, *Am J Med* 118:58-67, 2005.

54. Hallstrom AP, Ornato JP, Weisfeld M et al: Public-access defibrillation and survival from out of hospital cardiac arrest, *N Engl J Med* 251:637-646, 2004.

55. Pitt B, Zannad F, Remme WJ et al: The effect of spironolactone on morbidity and mortality in patients with severe heart failure, *N Engl J Med* 341:709-717, 1999.

56. AVID Investigators: A comparison of antiarrhythmic-drug therapy with implantable defibrillators in patients resuscitated from near-fatal ventricular arrhythmias: the Antiarrhythmic versus Implantable Defibrillator (AVID) Investigators, *N Engl J Med* 337:1576-1583, 1997.

57. Nanthakumar K, Epstein AE, Kay GN et al: Prophylactic implantable cardioverter-defibrillator therapy in patients with left ventricular systolic dysfunction: a pooled analysis of ten primary prevention trials, *J Am Coll Cardiol* 44:2166-2172, 2004.

58. Peperdy MA, Kaye W, Ornato JP et al: Resuscitation of adults in the hospital: a report of 1472. cardiac arrests from the National Registry of Cardiopulmonary Resuscitation, *Resuscitation* 58:297-308, 2003.

59. Buist MD, Moore GE, Bernard SA et al: Effects of a medical emergency team on reduction of incidence of and mortality from unexpected cardiac arrests in hospital: preliminary study, *BMJ* 324:387-390, 2002.

60. Hodgetts TJ, Kenward G, Vlachonikolis IG et al: The identification of risk factors for cardiac arrest and formulation of activation criteria to alert a medical emergency team, *Resuscitation* 54:125-131, 2002.

61. Subbe CP, Davies RG, Williams E et al: Effect of introducing the Modified Early Warning score on clinical outcomes, cardiopulmonary arrests and intensive care utilisation in acute medical admissions, *Anaesthesia* 58:797-802, 2003.

62. Buist M, Bernard S, Nguyen TV et al: Association between clinically abnormal observations and subsequent in-hospital mortality: a prospective study, *Resuscitation* 62:137-141, 2004.

63. Bellomo R, Goldsmith D, Uchino S et al: Prospective controlled trial of effect of medical emergency team on postoperative morbidity and mortality rates, *Crit Care Med* 32:916-921, 2004.

64. Ball C, Kirkby M, Williams S: Effect of the critical care outreach team on patient survival to discharge from hospital and readmission to critical care: non-randomized population based study, *BMJ* 327:1014, 2003.

65. 5 Million Lives Campaign. Retrieved March 31, 2007 from www.ihi.org/IHI/Programs/Campaign

66. Abella BS, Alverado JP, Mykleburst H et al: Quality of cardiopulmonary resuscitation during in-hospital cardiac arrest, *JAMA* 293:305-310, 2005.

67. Peperdy MA, Ornato JP: Post-resuscitation care: is it the missing link in the Chain of Survival? *Resuscitation* 64:135-137, 2005.

68. Abella BS, Rhee JW, Huang KN et al: Induced hypothermia is underused after resuscitation from cardiac arrest: a current practice survey, *Resuscitation* 64:181-186, 2005.

Care of Patients with Implanted Cardiac Rhythm Management Devices

Robin J. Trupp
Rosemary S. Bubien

CHAPTER ABBREVIATIONS

AF	atrial fibrillation
AV	atrioventricular
AVID	Antiarrhythmics Versus Implantable Defibrillators Trial
CARE-HF	Cardiac Resynchronization in Heart Failure Trial
CASH	Cardiac Arrest Study of Hamburg Trial
CIDS	Canadian Implantable Defibrillator Study
COMPANION	Comparison of Medical Therapy, Pacing, and Defibrillation in Heart Failure Trial
CRM	cardiac rhythm management
CRT	cardiac resynchronization therapy
CRT-D	cardiac resynchronization therapy with a defibrillator
DAVID	Dual Chamber and VVI Implantable Defibrillator Trial
ECG	electrocardiogram
f	fibrillatory (wave)
ICD	implantable cardioverter-defibrillator
LBBB	left bundle branch block
LV	left ventricular
MADIT	Multicenter Automatic Defibrillator Implantation Trial
MOST	Mode Selection Trial
MUSTT	Multicenter Unsustained Ventricular Tachycardia Trial
NYHA	New York Heart Association
RCT	randomized clinical trial
RV	right ventricular
SCD	sudden cardiac death
SCD-HeFT	Sudden Cardiac Death in Heart Failure Trial
VF	ventricular fibrillation
VT	ventricular tachycardia

Since the first pacemaker was implanted in 1958, millions of persons worldwide have experienced the benefits and life-saving therapies provided by pacemaker and defibrillation systems, now known as cardiac rhythm management (CRM) devices. Technological innovations have transformed CRM devices into versatile devices capable of meeting diverse patient needs, including supporting inappropriately slow heart rates, terminating lethal ventricular dysrhythmias, and correcting conduction abnormalities. Thus CRM device use is expected to expand. In the United States, approximately 2 million CRM devices have been implanted, and

current projections are for 300,000 pacemakers and 125,000 defibrillators annually.[1]

CRM devices are implanted to reduce cardiac mortality and to improve functional status and well-being. The mortality benefit from bradycardia support pacing was first demonstrated in patients with complete atrioventricular (AV) block. Recently, the benefits of pacing therapy to circumvent the hemodynamic sequelae caused by ventricular conduction abnormalities have been demonstrated in patients with chronic heart failure caused by systolic dysfunction. An abundance of clinical trial data describe the beneficial impact of the CRM device intervention on mortality, prevention of sudden cardiac death (SCD), and quality of life. These data provide evidence to support indications for CRM device implantation, influence device selection, and guide programming choices for pacing (including resynchronization) and defibrillation therapies.[2]

The selection of the appropriate implantable CRM device may be relatively straightforward or ambiguous. Underlying conduction abnormalities may be overt or masked. Patients who are at high risk to develop an abnormality may be better served by implantation of a device that will meet their future and immediate needs. Indications for CRM devices with defibrillation capabilities include offering implantable cardioverter-defibrillators (ICDs) as primary prevention to individuals who have a higher risk for SCD than the general population. This chapter discusses the pathophysiological basis for CRM device indications and therapies, the operation of CRM devices, and the management of patients with CRM devices.[2]

CARDIAC DYSRHYTHMIAS: RATIONALE FOR PACING AND DEFIBRILLATION THERAPY

Cardiac impulse generation and conduction from the sinus node to the atria and the AV conduction system, the physiology of the conduction system, and the electrocardiogram (ECG) characteristics of normal activation and dysrhythmias are detailed in Chapters 46 to 48. Intrinsic pacing and dysrhythmias commonly requiring CRM are briefly described in this chapter.

Effect of Pacing on the Electrocardiogram

The ECG provides information about the chamber(s) being paced and the pacing mode. Pacing occurs when a low-voltage electrical stimulus, discharged by a pacemaker or ICD, initiates electrical signals of sufficient strength to successfully "capture" the myocardial tissue in that chamber and produce depolarization. Most commonly, CRM devices are programmed to deliver electrical stimulation when the device does not detect or sense the patient's intrinsic electrical signals within a prespecified amount of time. The pacing stimulus artifact, often referred to as a "spike," precedes a P wave and/or QRS complex that has a different shape than a nonpaced or intrinsic complex. Depending on how the CRM device is configured, the stimulus artifact (particularly in the atrium) may not be visible in all ECG leads. A differently shaped P wave or QRS complex also may arise when fusion (i.e., simultaneous depolarization from the pacing impulse and the intrinsic conduction) occurs. When the intrinsic beat initiates depolarization immediately before delivery of the pacing spike, the pacing stimulus may appear embedded within the QRS complex. Often mistaken as malfunction, this indicates that the patient's intrinsic electrical signal was not detected by the CRM device within the programmed time interval and that the device discharged its stimulus to pace the heart.

Absence of capture is demonstrated when a pacing spike is not followed by a P wave or QRS complex and may herald significant problems. Ventricular depolarization from a single lead position at the right ventricular (RV) apex produces a paced complex similar to a left bundle block, with the QRS complex duration exceeding 120 msec because of slower propagation of the pacing stimulus through the nonspecialized myocardial tissue. RV pacing leads positioned at other locations, such as the bundle of His and septum, may resemble the normal QRS morphology more closely because the pacing impulse is closer to the normal conduction system.[3]

Paced complexes that represent a combination of RV and left ventricular (LV) depolarization, or cardiac resynchronization therapy (CRT), have various morphologies. Because the paced complex is derived from variable LV lead placement locations and the ECG is actually a composite of the depolarization of both ventricles, there is no single classic ECG complex pattern. A single pacing stimulus artifact preceding the onset of a QRS complex may represent RV, LV, or CRT pacing. Discerning whether someone is receiving biventricular or LV pacing is complex, often requiring comparison with the preimplant 12-lead ECG. Typically, in patients whose preimplant QRS complex duration exceeds 120 msec, the QRS complex narrows with the initiation of CRT. Loss of CRT capture and potential lead dislodgment should be suspected when the ECG complex following the pacing spike has a bundle branch block configuration and is similar to the preimplant morphology.

Dysrhythmias
Sinus Node Dysfunction
Impairment of impulse generation and propagation is present in sinus node dysfunction. Abnormalities may occur at rest or during exercise from physiological, pathological, and pharmacological causes. Although age-related fibrotic change is the most common cause of sinus node dysfunction, imbalances in autonomic tone may suppress impulse formation, delay impulse exit from the sinus node, and result in a transient, abnormally slow heart rate or an abrupt change in heart rate. Extrinsic factors, such as pharmacological agents, also may suppress impulse formation and impulse propagation. Examples of these agents include amiodarone, sotalol, beta-adrenergic blocking agents, some calcium channel blocking agents, lithium, antihypertensive agents such as clonidine, tricyclic antidepressants, and phenothiazines.[2,4,5] Sinus bradycardia and respiratory-related rhythmic variations in the P-P interval (sinus arrhythmia) are normal. Sinus bradycardia in an alert individual during activities of daily living is abnormal when it is accompanied by symptoms related to a decreased cardiac output and accompanying decreased cerebral perfusion. Typically, symptomatic sinus bradycardia occurs when the ventricular heart rate is less than 40 beats/min. Intermittent sinus pauses greater than 3 seconds' duration or failure of the sinus node to resume normal pacemaker activity following spontaneous termination or cardioversion of atrial tachydysrhythmias also reflects impairment of impulse generation and propagation indicative of sinus node dysfunction. When sinus node dysfunction is present, the heart rate may remain relatively fixed and unable to increase sufficiently to meet the metabolic needs of the body. This is known as chronotropic incompetence.[2,4,6,7]

Atrioventricular and His Bundle Conduction Abnormalities
Impaired or blocked impulse transmission through the AV node also can have physiological, pathological and pharmacological origins. Prolongation of AV conduction traditionally is described as first-degree AV block, in which conduction time is prolonged but all impulses are conducted to the ventricles. Intermittent loss of AV conduction, second-degree block, is subdivided into Mobitz I (Wenckebach) and Mobitz II block. The Wenckebach response, prolongation of the PR interval preceding a dropped beat, is a physiological response and often is observed in response to tachycardias and AV nodal block.

The anatomical location of block within the conduction system characterizes the severity of the pathological abnormality. Block is classified as suprahisian, above the bundle of His in the AV node region, and infrahisian, below the bundle of His. Usually, the anatomical location of block can be identified when there is 2:1 conduction by assessing the response to autonomic stimulation or inhibition. Fixed 2:1 AV conduction may indicate AV nodal block above or below the bundle of His. Unlike suprahisian block, AV block below the bundle of His is characterized by a wide QRS complex (QRS complex more than 120 msec), is associated with heart rates of 30 to 45 beats/min, and is not stable.[2,4,7,8]

Ventricular Conduction Abnormalities
Conduction abnormalities of the His-Purkinje system result in loss of the specialized rapidly conducting Purkinje fiber network. Impulse propagation outside the His-Purkinje system occurs inordinately slowly via the ventricular muscle. This is depicted by QRS complex

durations exceeding 120 msec. The conduction delay may be a nonspecific intraventricular conduction delay, a left bundle branch block (**LBBB**), or a right bundle branch block, which occurs less often. Intraventricular and interventricular conduction abnormalities produce contractile abnormalities. Left ventricular dyssynchrony, or discoordinated ventricular contraction, occurs as a consequence of the abnormal activation sequence and is estimated to affect 30 to 50 percent of patients with heart failure. Instead of the right and left ventricles contracting simultaneously, contraction occurs sequentially. Late activation of the LV free wall in LBBB results in the septum moving away from the LV wall during systole (paradoxical motion), producing a reduced stroke volume and elevated filling pressures in an already struggling heart. This electrical conduction abnormality is associated with poor outcomes in this population. The prolonged activation also interferes with diastole by disrupting left atrial and ventricular synchrony. Traditional RV pacing induces conduction abnormalities similar to LBBB. However, instead of normal conduction occurring in the RV with conduction to the LV via septal depolarization, conduction to both ventricles progresses from the site of RV pacing stimulation. The hemodynamic sequelae of RV pacing are nearly identical to the electromechanical dyssynchrony seen in heart failure patients with prolonged QRS complex durations.[2,8-11]

Ventricular Tachycardia and Ventricular Fibrillation

Characterized by unpredictability of onset, ventricular tachycardia/ventricular fibrillation (**VT/VF**) arises distal to the bifurcation of the His bundle and is associated with SCD (detailed discussion in Chapters 48 and 60). SCD is due to VT/VF in the vast majority of instances, with bradycardia-related deaths representing approximately 13 percent of SCD. Unlike the other pathological changes discussed, the onset of VT/VF has been compared with an "electrical accident," preceded by an abnormal substrate that perpetuates the dysrhythmia once triggered. Although short self-terminating episodes of VT and VF may occur, cardiac arrest typically ensues unless the dysrhythmia is terminated promptly. Although VT may not result in significant hemodynamic impairment, symptoms of reduced cardiac output, including syncope or chest pain, are likely to occur, particularly in the setting of LV dysfunction. VT can be classified as monomorphic or polymorphic. In general, monomorphic VT is uniform in appearance and regular. The electrical axis, superior/inferior orientation of depolarization, and bundle branch block morphology of VT are related to the site of origin or exit point on the endocardial surface and subsequent activation sequence. Monomorphic VT, particularly following myocardial infarction, is a reentrant-maintained dysrhythmia that can be terminated reliably with antitachycardia pacing techniques to be discussed later.[7,12]

Polymorphic VT is likely to be more rapid, irregular, and less stable. Polymorphic VT, when the QT interval is short, may be related to ischemia. In contrast, polymorphic VT in the setting of a long QT interval is related to ion channel repolarization abnormalities and may be due to genetic disease, such as the long QT syndrome, or may occur as a proarrhythmic response to certain pharmacological agents.

VF, in contrast to VT, is characterized by multiple wandering and colliding wavelets and totally discoordinated ventricular activity. Electrical activation propagates when excitable tissue is encountered but is extinguished when excitable tissue is not encountered. The wave fronts may split into other wavelets and thus become self-sustaining once initiated.[5]

Atrial Fibrillation

Like VT/VF, atrial fibrillation (**AF**) is produced by a trigger and is maintained by a substrate. Premature atrial contractions and ectopic foci typically initiate AF. Paroxysmal AF, which stops spontaneously, lacks the substrate to maintain AF. As the substrate becomes more entrenched in persistent AF, termination requires intervention (pharmacological agents and/or electrical therapy). In permanent AF (previously referred to as chronic), the extent of structural remodeling precludes restoration of sinus rhythm. Although AF is not immediately life threatening, it is associated with many complications, such as embolic events and stroke, and is also an independent risk factor for death. AF produces significant impairment in quality of life for patients, more so than that seen with myocardial infarction and often more so than that seen with heart failure or myocardial infarction. Symptoms resulting from AF are highly variable and are related to the decrease in cardiac output caused by the loss of AV synchrony, impaired ventricular filling, and the underlying disease pathology.[13,14]

AF is prevalent in those with structural heart disease, including hypertension, coronary artery disease, and heart failure—conditions common in those receiving CRM devices. As previously mentioned, AF also is observed in persons with sinus node dysfunction. Pacing therapy delivered from the ventricle also influences the development of AF. Regardless of the type of CRM device implanted, the occurrence and/or presence of AF presents unique management challenges.[2,6]

Specific characteristics of AF that affect CRM device therapy are the atrial rate detected by the device, the rapidity of AV nodal conduction, and the accompanying irregularly irregular ventricular rate. Atrial activity is represented by fibrillatory (**f**) waves and exceeds 350 beats/min. Unlike sinus-initiated p waves, f waves exhibit varying rate, amplitude, duration, and shape. Instead of the regular ventricular rate and 1:1 AV relationship, the ventricular rhythm is irregularly irregular, and unless AV nodal blocking agents have been administered or heart block is present, the ventricular rate is inappropriately rapid. Not uncommonly, the ventricular rate may remain rapid despite administration of AV nodal blocking agents.[15]

CARDIAC RHYTHM MANAGEMENT DEVICE INDICATIONS
The Role of Evidence-Based Guidelines

Guidelines to define appropriate indications for implantation of CRM devices were first established by the Joint Task Force from the American College of Cardiology, the American Heart Association, and the Heart Rhythm Society (HRS, formerly called the North American Society of Pacing and Electrophysiology, NASPE) in 1984.[16] As with other disciplines, each iteration of the guidelines reflects increasing evidence from large randomized clinical trials (**RCTs**). Over time, the role of RCTs in establishing clinical benefit and the subsequent development of clinical practice guidelines has surpassed treatment based solely on modifying and/or interrupting symptoms and pathophysiological processes. Today, the pathophysiological processes often serve as the premise to begin exploration and evaluation of a potential new role for CRM device therapy. Evidence from RCTs has been invaluable in differentiating the significance of pacing mode selection, establishing new indications for pacing, such as CRT (to be discussed later), and expanding the indications for ICDs.

Indications for CRM devices incorporate an evidence-based approach, and recommendations reflect demonstration of documented clinical benefit from RCTs. The level of recommendation for CRM devices is derived from the evidence supporting the benefit of the indication (see Chapter 1).[2,16]

Cardiac Pacing Nomenclature

Standardized five-letter nomenclature is used to describe cardiac pacing system operation and to indicate whether the device can provide AV synchrony and artificially increase the heart rate. Pacing literature is replete with references to the nomenclature to describe clinical trial outcomes and their therapeutic implications. Understanding why a mode of pacing may be indicated for a specific conduction abnormality or why superior outcomes may be achieved with one mode compared with an alternative mode requires understanding the nomenclature. The code is explained in Table 61-1. Pacing nomenclature relies on the letters "A," "V," and "D" to indicate operation in the *A*trium, *Ve*ntricle, and *D*ual chamber (atrium and ventricle), respectively. The response of the pacing system to an intrinsic (nonpaced) event is described in the third position as *I* or *T*. The "R," in the fourth position, indicates that an artificial sensor is used to determine the paced heart rate response independent of the intrinsic rate.

Pacing Therapy for Bradycardia Support
Sinus Node Dysfunction

Failure to initiate and conduct the impulse within the sinus node is caused most commonly by idiopathic fibrosis of the conduction system. The incidence of sinus node dysfunction increases with age. More than 50 percent of patients with sinus node dysfunction are more than 50 years of age. In children and adolescents, sinus node dysfunction may occur following surgical correction of congenital cardiac anomalies, whereas in middle-aged adults, CAD may be the causative factor. Neural-mediated changes are also an important cause of sinus node dysfunction in the elderly. Persons with sinus node dysfunction caused by idiopathic fibrosis of the conduction system also may have AV conduction abnormalities.

Typically, sinus node dysfunction is diagnosed when inappropriate heart rates are coupled with symptoms related to an inadequate cardiac output and decreased cerebral perfusion, such as fatigue or dizziness. Sinus node dysfunction also may be manifested as a tachycardia-bradycardia syndrome, commonly called sick sinus syndrome, in which episodes of sinus bradycardia and/or sinus arrest are interspersed with episodes of tachycardia (typically AF). Often, pauses are more pronounced following termination of AF or flutter before the resumption of sinus rhythm.

Correlation between sinus node dysfunction and symptoms is crucial because the pacing indication depends on establishing a causative relationship. Symptoms vary depending on physiological status, age, body position, and activity being performed at the onset of and during sinus node dysfunction. Commonly, patients report fatigue, a decrease in their ability to perform activities of daily living, and exercise intolerance. Although dizziness and shortness of breath also frequently are reported, these symptoms are often nonspecific and unrecognized as being clinically important. Additional possible complaints include listlessness, depression, altered mental acuity, heart failure, or syncope.[4,6,17]

Sinus node dysfunction is the most common indication for cardiac pacing. Pacemaker implantation for symptomatic bradycardia and other manifestations of sinus node dysfunction predates the era of RCTs. As a

■ ■ ■

TABLE 61-1 NOMENCLATURE USED TO DESCRIBE PACING THERAPIES*

POSITION	I	II	III	IV	V
Category	Chamber(s) paced	Chamber(s) sensed	Response to sensing	Rate modulation	Multisite pacing
	O = None	O = None	O = None	O = None	O = None
	A = Atrium	A = Atrium	T = Triggered	R = Rate modulation	A = Atrium
	V = Ventricle	V = Ventricle	I = Inhibited		V = Ventricle
	D = Dual (A + V)	D = Dual (A + V)	D = Dual (T + I)		D = Dual (A + V)
Manufacturer's designation only	S = Single (A or V)	S = Single (A or V)			

*See text for explanation of use of the code.
From Zipes DP, Libby P, Bonow RO, Braunwald E, editors: *Braunwald's heart disease: a textbook of cardiovascular medicine*, ed 7, Philadelphia, 2005, Saunders.

rule, in the absence of symptoms, pacing therapy is not indicated. However, pacing therapy may be appropriate if sinus node dysfunction is caused by medications deemed essential to the patient, such as amiodarone, sotalol, or other similar agents that suppress impulse formation and conduction. Clinical trials, as discussed later in this chapter, have contributed greatly to understanding the selection of the appropriate pacing mode and its effects on morbidity and mortality.[2,17]

Atrioventricular Block

AV block may be congenital or may occur because of disease. Most commonly, AV block is due to age-related idiopathic fibrosis. Other causes include disease of the coronary arteries and valves, hypertension, cardiomyopathies, and systemic rheumatological and infiltrating diseases. Acute AV conduction disturbances are typically due to myocardial infarction, AV nodal blocking agents, or cardiac surgery.[2,4,8]

Specific conduction abnormalities may occur following surgical repair of congenital defects or valve replacement. Mitral valve replacement may impair AV nodal function, whereas aortic valve replacement is associated with damage to the His bundle. Complete AV block may be created intentionally or inadvertently during electrophysiological procedures. For example, creating complete AV block by ablating the AV node to treat AF with a chronically rapid ventricular response that is refractory to drug therapy is a planned palliative treatment, whereas AV block during catheter ablation of AV node reentrant tachycardia is inadvertent and a procedure-related complication.

Stokes-Adams syndrome, recurrent sudden attacks of unconsciousness caused by impaired conduction, was the first condition for which cardiac pacing was used. In general, cardiac pacing is indicated for Mobitz II heart block, complete heart block, and bilateral bundle branch block. As with sinus node dysfunction, RCTs have provided evidence to support the selection of pacing mode and the effect of that selection on morbidity and mortality.

Neurocardiogenic Syncope

Neurocardiogenic syncope describes syncope that arises from inappropriate autonomic responses in which profound vasodilatation and bradycardia occur. Carotid sinus hypersensitivity and vasovagal syncope are the most common causes. In rare cases, this syncope may be caused by coughing, swallowing, micturition, or defecation. Several clinical trials have shown that pacemaker implantation can abort and blunt vasovagal syncope. Cardiac pacing is indicated for recurrent syncope associated with bradycardia. In general, pacing therapy may be provided after other causes have been excluded and pharmacological therapy has been optimized. Clinical trials evaluating specific pacing algorithms in dual-chamber pacing systems have been shown to alleviate symptoms associated with sudden abrupt decreases in heat rate.[2,4,7,17]

Carotid sinus hypersensitivity occurs as a result of an exaggerated physiological or pathophysiological response to stimulation of the carotid sinus. Carotid massage causes a cardioinhibitory response from the vagally mediated suppression of impulse formation and the withdrawal of sympathetic stimulation, resulting in syncope and hypotension. Sinus bradycardia, prolongation of AV conduction, and AV block may be observed. Carotid sinus massage may elicit pauses more than 3 seconds in duration. Men with arteriosclerotic heart disease are most commonly affected. The typical clinical presentation of patients with carotid sinus hypersensitivity is one of blurred vision, light-headedness, or confusion, while standing or sitting, in conjunction with head or neck movements. Characteristically, carotid sinus hypersensitivity is provoked by head turning, tight neckware, shaving, and neck hyperextension. However, unlike sinus node dysfunction and AV block, the symptoms of carotid sinus hypersensitivity are reproducible, thus facilitating diagnosis.[2,4,7]

In the absence of medications that depress sinus node function or AV conduction, pacing therapy is indicated for recurrent syncope caused by carotid sinus stimulation that induces asystole for more than 3 seconds or in the setting of a hypersensitive inhibitory response. In addition to providing bradycardia support, pacing therapy can prevent the precipitous drop in heart rate associated with the cardioinhibitory response. The efficacy of pacing to treat carotid sinus hypersensitivity, syncope, and falls in the elderly currently is being assessed in the SAFE-PACE-2 clinical trial.[2,4,17]

Implications of Pacing Mode Selection

In the absence of impaired impulse formation or conduction, the heart is able to adapt its rate in response to metabolic demands, and AV synchrony is maintained. The physiological changes resulting from sinus node dysfunction, AV block, and neurocardiogenic syncope require artificial cardiac stimulation to provide appropriate increases in heart rate and/or maintain AV synchrony. Cardiac pacing and the mode of therapy interrupt the natural history of the conduction disturbance and affects survival. CRM devices can increase heart rate by using an artificial sensor to gauge the desired heart rate while maintaining AV synchrony. Prospective RCTs, as well as retrospective observational studies, have demonstrated that pacing the atria to maintain AV synchrony provides greater benefit than simply pacing the RV alone. The major clinical trials and outcomes assessing the benefit of pacing mode are presented in Table 61-2.[2,17,18]

The standardized pacing nomenclature used to describe the pacing modes for the trials referenced are described. To facilitate understanding, the Danish Study, which compared the AAI pacing mode with the VVI pacing mode, is explained in greater detail. In this study, patients with sinus node dysfunction without AV block, pacing only the right atrium (A), sensing intrinsic atrial events (A), and not pacing the atrium when the sensed atrial intrinsic rate was equal to or greater than a predetermined rate (I) [AAI] has been shown to provide greater clinical benefit than pacing the RV (V), sensing ventricular events (V), and not pacing the RV when the sensed ventricular rate was equal to or greater than a predetermined ventricular rate (I) [VVI]. In addi-

■ ■ ■

TABLE 61-2   SUMMARY OF MAJOR PACING TRIALS AND OUTCOMES

STUDY	PATIENT INCLUSION CRITERIA	ENDPOINT(S)	TREATMENT ARMS*	KEY RESULTS*
Danish study	Sick sinus syndrome requiring pacing	Mortality Cardiovascular death AF TE events Heart failure AV block	AAI pacing ($n = 110$) vs. VVI pacing ($n = 115$)	Cumulative incidence of CV death, PAF, chronic AF, and TE events lower with AAI pacing Less severe heart failure with AAI Multivariate analysis: AAI associated with freedom from TE events, survival from CV death
PASE	Age 65 years or older Need for PPM for prevention or treatment of bradycardia	QOL All-cause mortality First nonfatal CVA or death First hospitalization for CHF AF PM syndrome	Single-blind, randomized, controlled comparison: VVIR pacing vs. DDDR pacing	QOL improved significantly, but no difference between pacing modes 26% of patients with VVIR crossover to DDDR because of PM syndrome Trends of borderline statistical significance in endpoints favoring DDDR in patients with SND
CTOPP	Initial PM Life expectancy more than 1 year Not in chronic AF	Cardiovascular mortality or stroke Paroxysmal or chronic AF Hospitalization for CHF QOL 6-minute walk	DDDR or AAIR pacing vs. VVIR pacing	No difference in QOL, VVI vs. DDD/AAI No statistically significant difference in mortality or stroke No difference in hospitalizations 24% ↓ incidence of chronic or paroxysmal AF with DDD/AAI
MOST	SND requiring PM NSR or atrial standstill at time of implantation	Stroke Health status Cost-effectiveness Total mortality CV mortality AF Heart failure score PM syndrome	DDDR vs. VVIR	Lower incidence of AF with DDDR No difference in any other endpoint
UKPACE	AV block requiring PM Age more than 70 years	All-cause mortality Composite endpoint of the following: • CV deaths • AF • HF hospitalization • CVA or events • Reoperation	DDDR vs. VVI or VVIR	No difference in any endpoint
DANPACE	Tachycardia-bradycardia syndrome with normal AV conduction	All-cause mortality CV mortality Incidence of AF and TE events QOL Cost-effectiveness	AAIR vs. DDDR	In progress

*See Table 61-1 for nomenclature used to describe pacing therapies.
AF, atrial fibrillation; *AV,* atrioventricular; *CHF,* congestive heart failure; *CTOPP,* Canadian Trial of Physiologic Pacing; *CV,* cardiovascular; *CVA,* cardiovascular accident; *DANPACE,* Danish Pacing Trial; *HF,* heart failure; *MOST,* Mode Selection Trial; *NSR,* normal sinus rhythm; *PAF,* paroxysmal atrial fibrillation; *PASE,* Pacemaker Selection in the Elderly; *PM,* pacemaker; *PPM,* permanent pacemaker; *QOL,* quality of life; *SND,* sinus node dysfunction; *TE,* thromboembolic; *UKPACE,* United Kingdom Pacing and Cardiovascular Events.
From Zipes DP, Libby P, Bonow RO, Braunwald E, editors: *Braunwald's heart disease: a textbook of cardiovascular medicine,* ed 7, Philadelphia, 2005, Saunders.

tion, the incidence of AF and thromboembolism were reduced significantly after 3 years of follow-up. Importantly, improved survival and a lower incidence of heart failure have been observed through an additional 5 years of follow-up.[2]

In trials enrolling those with AV block, the DDD pacing mode (pacing the right atrium and ventricle (D), sensing atrial and ventricular events (D), and inhibiting pacing the atrium and/or ventricle if a response is detected and delivering a pacing stimulus if the intrinsic signal was not detected within a prespecified time interval (I and T, thus D) was the basis for comparison. Single-chamber atrial pacing and dual-chamber atrial pacing, with or without accompanying ventricular pacing, maintain AV synchrony. But in general, clinical trials have demonstrated that atrial and dual-chamber pacing are more effective than ventricular pacing in delaying the progression to AF. This lower incidence is attributed to the attenuation of atrial stretch and enlargement that is associated with atrial pacing. Atrial pacing also decreases irregularities in atrial tissue that are associated with bradycardia and can suppress atrial premature beats. Although improvements in quality of life have been reported, significant differences in cardiovascular death, stroke, and total mortality have not emerged. The percentage of RV pacing and follow-up duration now are suspected to influence these data.[2,18-22]

Right Ventricular Pacing-Induced Dyssynchrony

The Dual Chamber and VVI Implantable Defibrillator (**DAVID**) Trial, comparing ventricular inhibited (VVI-40) to dual-chamber rate adaptive (DDD-R) pacing, demonstrated that RV pacing in patients with an ICD indication, LV dysfunction but no pacing indication adversely affected mortality and hospitalizations for heart failure. The mortality was 6.5 percent for the group randomized to backup VVI pacing, compared with 10.1 percent for the DDD-R group. Hospitalization for new-onset or worsening heart failure was 13.3 percent for the VVI pacing group compared with 22.6 percent for the DDDR group at 1 year. These deleterious consequences appeared early in the postimplantation course and continued throughout the study period, especially the heart failure hospitalizations. The heart failure hospitalization differences did not appear to emerge until after 6 months of follow-up in the randomized pacing mode. Because of these adverse effects, the trial was stopped early.[21] Further data analysis showed that patients randomized to the DDD-R group who received more than 40 percent RV pacing had worse outcomes compared with patients with less than 40 percent RV pacing.

Other trials involving RV pacing were reexamined in light of the DAVID trial. A substudy analysis of the Mode Selection Trial (**MOST**) recently has reported adverse effects from RV pacing on the incidence of AF and heart failure exacerbation.[22] Deleterious hemodynamic effects also have been reported in young adults (mean age 24 ± 3 years) with congenital complete heart block who received dual-chamber pacing systems. Lastly, reexamination of outcomes in the MADIT II ICD Trial provide corroborating evidence of the deleterious effects of RV pacing in the setting of LV dysfunction.[22,23]

In summary, pacing therapy improves survival and ameliorates symptoms of dizziness, near-syncope, syncope, and reduced exercise tolerance that accompany the rate-related reduced cardiac output. The benefits of pacing may be compromised when RV pacing therapy is delivered. The DAVID, MOST, Danish, and MADIT II Trials support minimizing RV pacing when possible.[12,20-23]

Pacing Therapy for Hemodynamic Improvement

Hypertrophic Cardiomyopathy

Dual-chamber cardiac pacing is not indicated for patients with hypertrophic cardiomyopathy in the absence of sinus node dysfunction or AV block. Delivery of the pacing stimulus to the RV apex alters the normal LV septal activation and depolarization, thereby reducing the LV outflow gradient. Despite reported 50 percent reductions in the gradient, the M-Pathy Trial reported no differences between pacing and no pacing in exercise capacity, peak oxygen consumption, or quality of life scores. Therefore, pacing therapy is indicated as adjunctive therapy only in selected patients who remain symptomatic despite optimal medical management.[2,17]

Cardiac Resynchronization Therapy

Ventricular conduction abnormalities, as seen in electrical abnormalities such as bundle branch blocks, have mechanical and hemodynamic consequences that adversely affect LV performance, morbidity, and mortality. As a result of LV dyssynchrony, contractility is de-

creased, diastolic filling time is reduced, and mitral regurgitation occurs. CRT, also known as biventricular pacing, restores intraventricular synchrony and left AV synchrony. Approved as a pacing indication in 2001, CRT currently is indicated for patients with symptomatic heart failure, LV ejection fraction less than 35 percent, optimal medications, and a QRS complex duration greater than 120 msec. Stringent clinical trial protocols, including the requirement for stable optimal medical therapy, blinding, and a period of no pacing therapy, were implemented to separate the effects of CRT from optimal heart failure medical therapy. Multiple RCTs, including MUSTIC, MIRACLE, DEFINITE, and the Comparison of Medical Therapy, Pacing, and Defibrillation in Heart Failure (COMPANION) Trial have shown the effects of CRT on improving a variety of endpoints including quality of life, cardiac performance, and functional capacity. Further information on the acronyms, inclusion criteria, primary endpoints, and key results for these trials can be found in Table 61-3.

The safety and efficacy of CRT was first demonstrated in cardiac pacing devices and later in ICD devices in patients with known VT/VF.[4,9,17,24,25] Similar hemodynamic effects and functional benefits were observed in patients with and without an ICD indication (Contak CD, MIRACLE ICD, InSync ICD II). Importantly, unlike positive inotropic agents, enhancements in contractility are not accompanied by increased myocardial oxygen requirements. In addition to improving well-being and functional status, CRT improves survival. A survival benefit was first shown in COMPANION and later in the Cardiac Resynchronization in Heart Failure (CARE-HF) Trial. The COMPANION Trial also demonstrated greater survival benefit for CRT combined with a defibrillator (**CRT-D**) than with CRT alone.[26]

The ability of CRT to provide symptom relief, improve functional capacity, and reduce mortality has greatly affected the adoption and use of CRT. Since receiving Food and Drug Administration approval, CRT has transitioned rapidly from a novel adjunctive therapy to a mainstream therapy of proven benefit. The IIa indication in the American Heart Association/American College of Cardiology 2001 guidelines for the treatment and management of chronic heart failure reflects the limited data then available.[27] However, in the most recent update published in 2005, CRT is now a Class Ia indication that should be given to "all patients with LV ejection fraction (LVEF) 35% or less, sinus rhythm, and NYHA functional class III or ambulatory class IV symptoms, despite recommended optimal medical therapy, and who have cardiac dysynchrony, which is currently defined as a QRS duration 120 msec or more, unless contraindicated."[28]

Despite this plethora of evidence, there are several issues that remain to be answered regarding CRT. The current selection criteria based on QRS complex duration in the presence of LV dysfunction and heart failure are less than ideal. The QRS complex duration, while easily obtained and measured at low cost, is a surrogate measure that only weakly correlates with indices of dyssynchrony. Is there a better way to determine dyssynchrony, such as through tissue Doppler ultrasonography or magnetic resonance imaging? Failure to respond to

TABLE 61-3 SUMMARY OF MAJOR TRIALS OF CARDIAC RESYNCHRONIZATION THERAPY AND DEFIBRILLATION

STUDY	PATIENT INCLUSION CRITERIA	ENDPOINT(S)	TREATMENT ARMS	KEY RESULTS
InSync	NYHA Class III or IV on stable drug regimen LVEDD greater than 60 mm, LVEF ≤ 0.35 QRS complex width ≥ 150 msec	QOL NYHA class 6-minute hall walk	Nonrandomized	Sustained improvement in all three endpoints
MIRACLE	NYHA Class III or IV on stable drug regimen LVEDD ≥ 55 mm, LVEF ≤ 0.35 QRS complex width ≥ 130 msec	QOL NYHA class 6-minute hall walk	Randomized to pacing or no pacing for 6 months and then to pacing	Sustained improvement in all three endpoints
PATH-CHF	DCM of any cause NYHA Class III or IV on stable drug regimen QRS complex ≥ 120 msec PR ≥ 150 msec	Acute maximum LV pressure derivative Aortic pulse pressure Chronic oxygen uptake Anaerobic threshold 6-minute walk	Acute hemodynamic and chronic assessment of RV pacing vs. LV pacing vs. BiV pacing	Acute BiV and LV: ↑ LV pressure derivative and aortic pulse pressure more than RV pacing Sustained chromic improvement in all endpoints
MUSTIC-NSR	NYHA Class III Refractory symptoms on stable drug therapy LVEF less than 0.35 LVEDD greater than 60 mm 6-minute walk less than 450 m NSR with QRS complex greater than 150 msec	Functional capacity QOL Metabilic exercise performance Mortality or need for transplant or LVAD Hospital admission for CHF	BiV pacing vs. No pacing with crossover	Sustained improvement in all endpoints Fewer hospital admissions with CRT
MUSTIC-AF	NYHA Class III LVEF less than 0.35 LVEDD greater than 60 mm 6-min walk less than 450 meters AF with paced QRS complex greater than 200 msec	Refractory symptoms on stable drug therapy Functional capacity QOL Metabolic exercise performance Mortality or need for transplant or LVAD Hospital admission for CHF	BiV pacing vs. No pacing with crossover	Sustained improvement in all endpoints Fewer hospital admissions with CRT
InSync-III	NYHA Class III or IV on stable drug regimen LVEDD ≥ 60 mm, LVEF ≤ 0.35 QRS complex width ≥ 130 msec	QOL NYHA class 6-minute hall walk	BiV pacing with optimized AV and VV intervals vs. No pacing with crossover	Sustained improvement in all endpoints
CARE-HF	NYHA Class III or IV on stable drug regimen LVEDD ≥ 60 mm, LVEF ≤ 0.35 QRS complex width ≥ 150 msec or greater than 120 msec with echo study	Mortality Hospitalization QOL Seconday Economic outcomes	BiV pacing vs. No pacing with crossover	Sustained improvement in all primary endpoints Enrollment completed; in follow-up phase
PACMAN	Functional NYHA Class III CHF LVEF less than 0.35 DCM of any etiology QRS complex greater than 150 msec Optimal medical management Hospitalization at least once in past 12 months	Functional capacity by 6-minute walk Secondary endpoints of QOL, adverse events, ventricular arrhythmias, hospitalizations	Observation over 1 year with randomization of patients to CRT vs. No CRT (1:1 randomization)	
VecToR	NYHA Class III or IV LVEF ≤ 0.35 QRS complex ≥ 140 msec LVEDD greater than 54 mm	QOL Mortality Echo parameters	BiV pacing vs. No pacing with crossover	In progress
ReLeVent	NYHA Class III or IV LVEF less than 0.35 QRS complex greater than 140 msec LVEDD greater than 55 mm	6-minute walk LVEDD LVESD Mortality QOL	BiV pacing vs. No pacing with crossover	In progress
PAVE	NYHA Class II or III Status post AV nodal ablation Able to complete 6-minute hall walk 3 months stable medical therapy	6-minute walk QOL LVEF	BiV pacing vs. RV pacing	Improved endpoints for BiV pacing group at 6 months
MUSTIC-II	NYHA Class III or IV AF after ablation and paced for greater than 3 months LVEDD greater than 60 mm QRS complex greater than 200 msec 6-minute walk less than 450 meters LVEF less than 0.35	Exercise tolerance QOL Hospitalization rates Modification of drug therapy	BiV pacing vs. No pacing with crossover	In progress

AF, atrial fibrillation; *BiV,* biventricular; *CARE-HF,* Cardiac Resynchronization in Heart Failure; *CHF,* congestive heart failure; *CRT,* cardiac resynchronization therapy; *DCM,* dilated cardiomyopathy; *echo,* echocardiographic; *LV,* left ventricular; *LVAD,* left ventricular assist device; *LVEDD,* left ventricular end-diastolic dimension; *LVEF,* left ventricular ejection fraction; *LVESD,* left ventricular end-systolic dimension; *MIRACLE,* Multicenter InSync Randomized Clinical Evaluation; *MUSTIC,* Multisite Stimulation in Cardiomyopathy; *NSR,* normal sinus rhythm; *NYHA,* New York Heart Association; *PACMAN,* Pacing for Cardiomyopathy: a European Study; *PATH-CHF,* Pacing Therapy in Congestive Heart Failure; *PAVE,* Left Ventricular Post-AV Nodal Ablation Evaluation; *QOL,* quality of life; *ReLeVent,* Remodeling of Cardiac Cavities by Long-Term Ventricular-Based Stimulation; *RV,* right ventricular; *VecToR,* Ventricular Resynchronization Therapy Randomized; *VV,* (see Table 61-1).

From Zipes DP, Libby P, Bonow RO, Braunwald E, editors: *Braunwald's heart disease: a textbook of cardiovascular medicine,* ed 7, Philadelphia, 2005, Saunders.

CRT occurs in approximately 30 percent of patients and is not well understood. No universal criteria are available to identify who is most likely to benefit from CRT. For example, a divergence of opinion exists within the electrophysiological community as to whether patients with right bundle branch block derive the same degree of benefit from CRT as those with an intraventricular conduction defect or LBBB. Because AF is a common comorbidity in heart failure, can CRT offer benefits to patients with chronic AF?[2,29,30] What about individuals with pacing indications who typically have been excluded from the clinical trials? Hence, ongoing research continues to obtain the empirical evidence necessary to answer these and many other questions. Trials evaluating CRT are summarized in Table 61-3. Figure 61-1 depicts lead placement in an implanted CRT device.

Rate Modulation

Rate modulation, or rate adaptive pacing, provides bradycardia support pacing via feedback from an artificial sensor that serves as a surrogate for the sinus node. The goal of rate adaptive pacing is to emulate the sinus node by providing a physiological heart rate when the sinus node response fails to increase the heart rate proportionally to meet metabolic needs. Several sensors are available in cardiac pacing systems, including activity, minute ventilation, QT interval sensing, and intraventricular impedance. Activity sensors may rely on a piezoelectric crystal to detect vibration or an accelerometer to detect motion. The pacemaker adjusts the rate of pacing in response to the level of vibration or motion detected. Minute ventilation, the product of respiratory rate and tidal volume, correlates well with metabolic demand. Derived from transthoracic impedance as measured by the pacing lead, the paced heart rate response increases as breathing excursions deepen and increase in frequency. Although activity sensors typically respond rapidly at the onset of exercise, minute ventilation pacemakers usually require a slightly longer time to increase pacing rates. For this reason, the two sensors may be combined to achieve an optimum response. The QT interval sensing and intraventricular impedance sensors are sensitive to autonomic stimulation. Because the QT interval sensor may react more slowly, it too often can be paired with an activity sensor.[31]

Rate adaptive pacing is indicated for those who require bradycardia support pacing or who have permanent AF with a slow ventricular response. Rate adaptive pacing commonly is used to manage self-terminating episodes of AF in conjunction with mode switching and can be beneficial in patients receiving pharmacological agents that impair the ability of the sinus node to generate or conduct impulses. For patients with AF who undergo AV nodal ablation, rate adaptation has been shown to improve quality of life.[2,31]

Pacing for Other Cardiac Conditions
Long QT Syndrome

Long QT syndrome is caused by genetic defects in ion channel currents that result in abnormalities in cardiac repolarization and a characteristic long-short initiating sequence or pause-dependent VT. Atrial-based rate-modulated pacing therapy, with a baseline or minimal heart rate programmed to 80 beats/min, can be used to prevent the development of the long-short initiating pauses associated with provoking torsades de pointes VT. Beta-adrenergic blocking agents also may be prescribed depending on the type of long QT syndrome present. Cardiac pacing is indicated in persons with pause-dependent VT. Increasingly, ICDs are replacing pacemakers as the device of choice, particularly in individuals who have a positive family history of SCD. In this situation, ICDs are implanted as primary prevention to provide a "safety net" because there is no guarantee that cardiac pacing will prevent VT.[2,4,7]

Pacing to Prevent and Palliate Symptoms of Atrial Fibrillation

The Framingham Heart Study has demonstrated that persons with AF have shorter life spans than those without AF. Not only does AF independently increase the risk of death, stroke, and heart failure, but it negatively affects quality of life and decreases cardiac output too. The incidence of AF increases with age and in heart failure. Because of the many complications seen, strategies to prevent AF or suppress its recurrence are highly desirable. Whether CRM devices can successfully utilize pacing techniques to do this remains under investigation. Multiple differences in trial designs—including patient populations, the techniques used, and atrial pacing sites to eliminate pauses and increase atrial pacing—may explain the mixed results. Currently, permanent pacing to prevent AF is not indicated in the absence of bradycardia.[2,32]

Management of AF can be challenging in patients with CRM devices. Despite the known advantages and benefits of ensuring AV synchrony in sinus rhythm, in patients with atrial dysrhythmias such as AF, atrial flutter, or atrial tachycardia, dual-chamber pacing modes

Achieving Cardiac Resynchronization
Leads for transvenous biventricular pacing

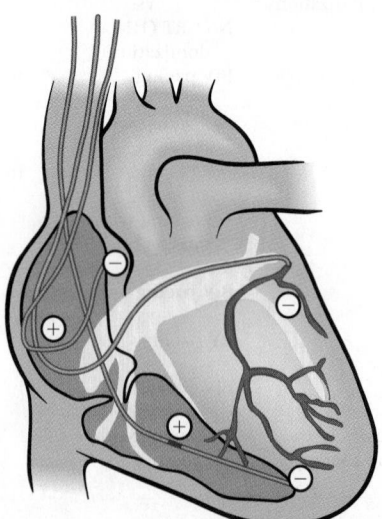

FIGURE 61-1 ■ Lead placement for cardiac resynchronization therapy. Three leads are used in cardiac resynchronization: a right atrial lead, a right ventricular lead, and a left ventricular lead that is placed in a lateral coronary vein position via the coronary sinus. (Courtesy Medtronic Inc, Minneapolis, Minn.)

can result in an inappropriately paced ventricular response (Figure 61-2). "Mode switching" is a feature that automatically changes the pacing mode upon detection of an inappropriately fast atrial rhythm to prevent conduction of the rapid atrial rates to the ventricle. In essence, when a CRM device operates in the dual-chamber pacing mode, atrial events detected by the device are "tracked" to ensure that a pacing stimulus is delivered to the ventricle for each atrial event sensed up to a predesignated upper rate limit. However, mode switching overcomes this liability by changing the pacing mode to a nontracking mode, such as DDIR or VVIR, thereby eliminating the paced response to the inappropriately rapid rate. When the rapidity of the atrial events sensed indicates the dysrhythmia is no longer present, the device automatically switches back to the original pacing mode, restoring AV synchrony. When mode switching is used in conjunction with rate adaptive pacing, rate response is provided. Control of AF is essential for the delivery and benefits of CRT.[33]

For symptomatic patients with chronic AF whose ventricular rate cannot be controlled, AV nodal ablation accompanied by permanent pacemaker implantation has been shown to improve quality of life because the intrinsic rhythm after ablation is usually less than 45 beats/min. However, as curative ablation strategies to maintain sinus rhythm have progressed, fewer AV node ablation procedures are being performed.

Implantable Defibrillator Therapy
Secondary Prevention

Because of the risk-benefit profile and ethical concerns, there are no, nor will there ever be, placebo-controlled trials evaluating the efficacy of ICD therapy in saving lives. Significant risks associated with ICD implantation during its infancy initially restricted therapy to only the 5 to 10 percent at highest risk, those who survived a cardiac arrest and had VT/VF that could be elicited during electrophysiological testing and could not be suppressed with antidysrhythmic drugs. It was not until the mid-1990s when ICD implantation evolved from an invasive surgical procedure, with epicardial defibrillation patches placed during an open heart-like operation, to a less invasive, transvenous pacemaker-like procedure that RCTs comparing ICD therapy to drug therapy were undertaken in this population (secondary prevention). Three trials, the Antiarrhythmics versus Implantable Defibrillators (**AVID**), Canadian Implantable Defibrillator Study (**CIDS**), and Cardiac Arrest Study of Hamburg (**CASH**), indicated that the ICD improved survival over antidysrhythmic drug therapy. Also important to note is that the AVID Registry revealed a decreased survival in persons with hemodynamically tolerated VT and syncope resulting from VT.[34]

Primary Prevention

Because nearly all SCD episodes occur in the setting of heart disease, most clinical trials contained a preponderance of persons with ischemic heart disease and LV dysfunction, factors known to be associated with an increased mortality.[2,35] The first trial to shed insight on the benefit of ICDs for primary prevention was the Multicenter Automatic Defibrillator Implantation Trial (**MADIT**). The Multicenter Unsustained Ventricular Tachycardia Trial (**MUSTT**) sponsored by the National Institutes of Health confirmed that impaired ventricular function in the setting of coronary disease conferred a high risk for SCD and resulted in changes in clinical practice and increased utilization of ICDs. Subsequent

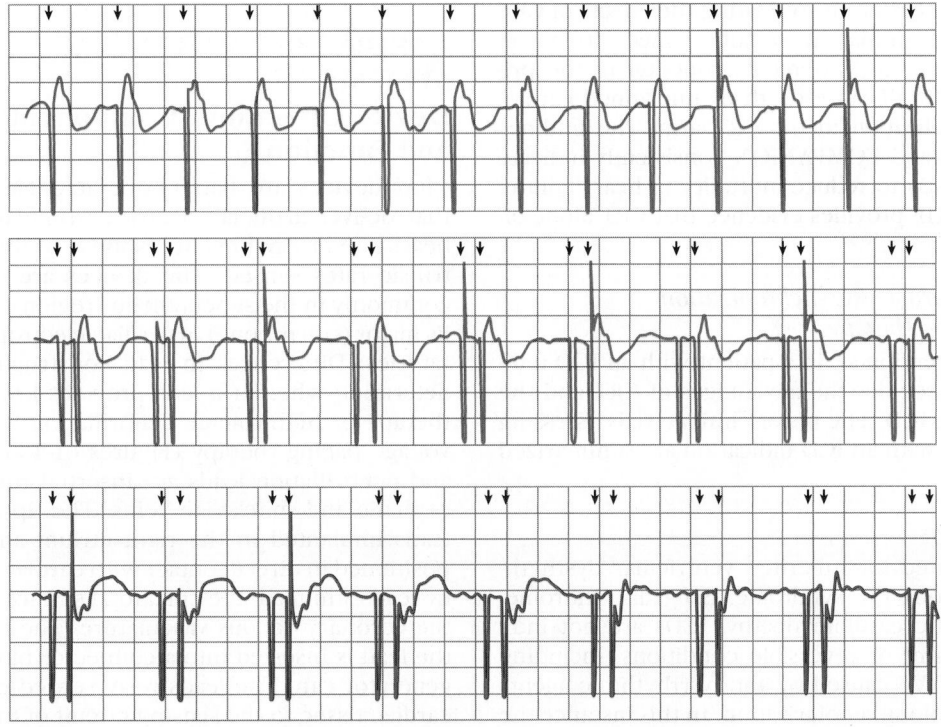

FIGURE 61-2 ■ Example of mode switching.

clinical trials have examined the efficacy of an ICD to abort SCD in broader patient populations without the requirement of electrophysiological testing. Reductions in mortality now have been replicated in multiple trials. Thus the advantage of ICDs recently has been expanded to include those with not only ischemic disease but also nonischemic conditions. A summary of these trials is provided in Table 61-3.

The role of ICD therapy in reducing mortality in heart failure has been addressed in several primary prevention trials. Most recently, the placebo-controlled Sudden Cardiac Death in Heart Failure Trial (**SCD-HeFT**) determined that a single-chamber ICD in patients without a pacing indication and receiving optimal heart failure medications awarded survival benefits superior to treatment with amiodarone. Of note, SCD-HeFT enrolled approximately equal numbers of patients with ischemic and nonischemic heart failure. Thus the survival benefit seen with ICD therapy is additive to the survival benefits seen with beta blockers, angiotensin-converting enzyme inhibitors or angiotensin II receptor blockers. Unlike other ICD trials, the New York Heart Association (**NYHA**) Class II individuals (70 percent of the subjects enrolled) manifested a greater survival benefit compared with NYHA Class III patients.

The **COMPANION** Trial evaluated whether a CRT-D system, on top of optimal heart failure medications, provided a greater survival advantage than optimal medications alone or than CRT and optimal medications. COMPANION enrolled NYHA Class III and IV patients, with ischemic and nonischemic conditions but without a pacing or ICD indication, who had been hospitalized for decompensation during the preceding 12 months. Compared with optimal heart failure pharmacological therapy, CRT pacing therapy reduced the risk of death by 24 percent and CRT-D therapy by 36 percent. The **CARE-HF** Trial, a European study evaluating the effects of CRT combined with optimal heart failure medications on mortality, reported a 37 percent reduction in the primary endpoint of all-cause death or unplanned cardiovascular hospitalization in the CRT arm. The findings from SCD-HeFT and COMPANION consistently indicate the ability of ICDs to reduce mortality in heart failure, whereas CARE-HF provides evidence that CRT alone offers survival benefits.[36-38]

Combination Cardiac Resynchronization and Defibrillator Therapy

As previously mentioned, in a patient with an ICD indication, CRT-D provides the advantages of CRT and the protection of an ICD. The major clinical trials assessing CRT in patients with an ICD indication are summarized in Table 61-3.

Other Conditions

ICDs are indicated for inherited ventricular dysrhythmias, such as long QT syndrome, Brugada syndrome, and hypertrophic cardiomyopathy. ICDs are not indicated for transient or reversible conditions, including the onset of VT/VF caused by antidysrhythmic agents or drugs that prolong repolarization. In this instance the appropriate therapy is to discontinue the agent. ICDs

also can deliver atrial defibrillation therapy, with and without accompanying ventricular defibrillation therapy, in individuals with infrequent episodes of AF. As catheter ablation therapy for AF has progressed, the perceived need for devices to treat primary AF has decreased. However, the incidence of AF as a coexisting dysrhythmia in patients with CRM devices suggests a role for atrial defibrillation in addition to ventricular defibrillation.[2]

Device Selection and Patient Management Implications

Therapeutic implications obviously are associated with device selection. In clinical practice, patients have varying combinations of CRM device indications. Frequently, patients require pacing, manifest abnormal ventricular conduction, and meet primary prevention ICD indications. An example of an algorithm used to guide device selection in patients is depicted in Figure 61-3. Data from clinical trials of pacing modes is taken into account. Ideally, following device implantation, underlying conduction abnormalities are rectified, AV synchrony is provided, and the heart rate is sufficient to meet the metabolic needs. The incidence for AF and the adverse effects associated with RV pacing also need to be factored into device selection.

Ultimately, CRM device selection is based on the patient's underlying conduction abnormality, risk of SCD, functional status, concomitant medical problems, heart rate response to activities of daily living and exercise, and the effects of the pacing mode on long-term mortality and morbidity. Regardless of the device to be implanted, a complete evaluation of the patient and the conduction system is essential before scheduling the implantation.

CARDIAC RHYTHM MANAGEMENT SYSTEMS
Device Operation: Components and Function

CRM devices are battery-operated electronic devices that deliver artificial electrical stimulation to manage heart rate or rhythms in response to the underlying intrinsic rates sensed. The devices are implanted most commonly in the subcutaneous region over the pectoralis major (collar bone) in cardiac electrophysiology laboratories. Differences in lead construction and design determine whether a lead provides low-voltage pacing therapy or high-voltage defibrillation therapy and low-voltage pacing therapy (Figures 61-4 and 61-5). Pacing and defibrillation leads are inserted routinely into the cephalic and subclavian veins. The tip or distal end of leads implanted in the right atrium and ventricle are positioned in direct contact with cardiac tissue, whereas LV leads stimulate the epicardial surface of the heart via the coronary venous vasculature. The proximal end of the lead is inserted into a connector block in the pulse generator can. The leads relay sensed events from the cardiac tissue to the sensing circuit of the pulse generator. The output computer circuits in the pulse generator

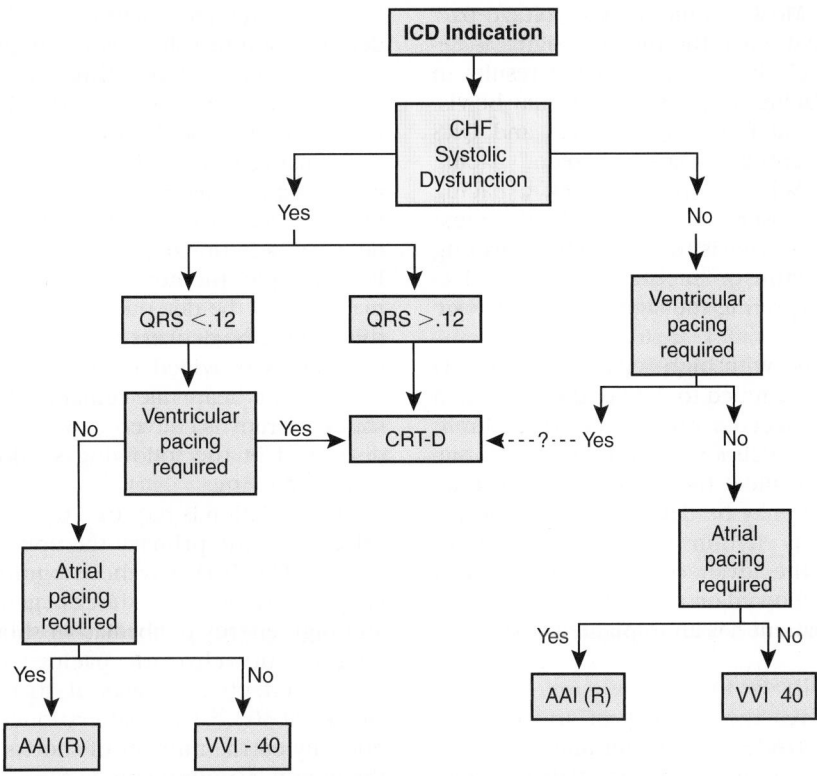

FIGURE 61-3 ■ Algorithm to assist with device selection. *AAI,* (see Table 61-1); *CHF,* Chronic heart failure; *CRT-D,* Cardiac resynchronization therapy with a defibrillator; *ICD,* implantable cardioverter-defibrillator; *QRS,* ; *VVI,* (see Table 61-1). (Courtesy G. Neal Kay, MD.)

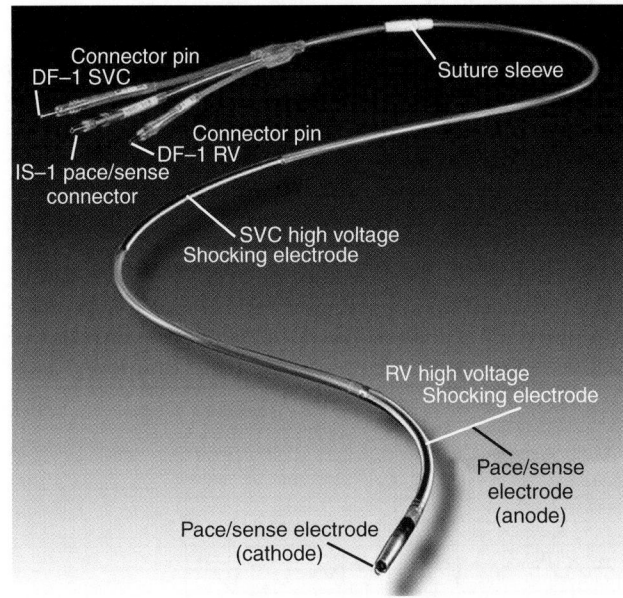

FIGURE 61-4 ■ Implantable cardioverter-defibrillator lead. *DF-1RV,* High-voltage defibrillation lead; *IS-1,* low-voltage pacemaker lead; *RV,* right ventricular; *SVC,* superior vena cava. (Courtesy Medtronic Inc, Minneapolis, Minn.)

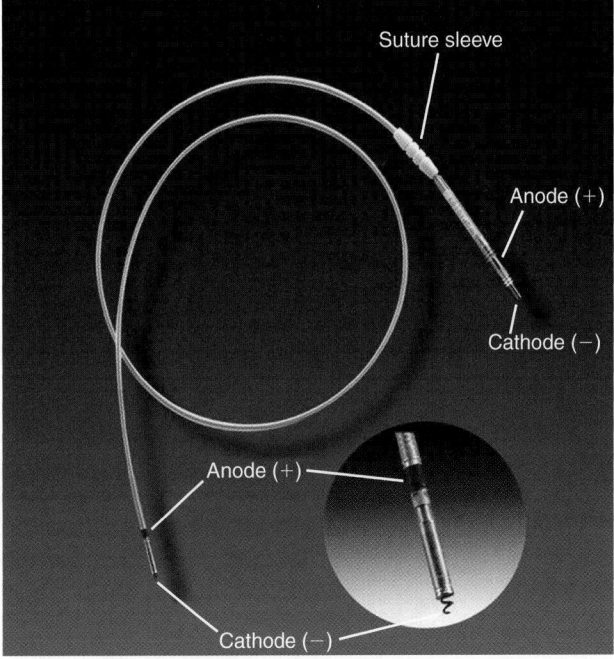

FIGURE 61-5 ■ Pacing lead.

determine whether electrical stimulation will be delivered from the battery to pace or defibrillate the heart, depending on the device implanted and its programming. In addition to containing a distal electrode to pace the heart and sense intrinsic signals, defibrillation leads also contain one or more coils to deliver high-voltage therapy to a large surface area.

Sensing

All CRM devices contain sensing circuits to enable detection of the intrinsic electrical signals of the heart. The response to signals differs between low-voltage and high-voltage devices. Most commonly, low-voltage pacing therapy is withheld when the intrinsic signal is detected. Failure to "see" the electrical signal results in delivery of therapy. Pacing stimulus artifacts may be visible before, during, and following P waves and QRS complexes. When electrical signals are "seen," pacing therapy is withheld. When pauses, without a pacing stimulus artifact, are observed on the ECG, the most likely cause is that the device is "oversensing," meaning that the device is detecting or "seeing" noncardiac electrical signals and interpreting the signal as an intrinsic heartbeat.

The converse is true with high-voltage therapy ICD devices. ICDs are programmed to deliver therapy when the detected signals exceed a prespecific upper limit. Not "seeing" VT or VF occurs when the rate of the signals detected does not meet the prespecified criteria. However, ICD therapy may be delivered when the patient is in normal sinus rhythm if the rate criteria are met. For this reason, the advanced cardiac life support protocols should be followed on telemetry units regardless of whether the patient has an implanted ICD.

Pacing Stimulation Thresholds

Cardiac pacing involves the delivery of an electrical impulse from the electrode of sufficient intensity to induce a wave of propagating action potentials to excite (pace) the heart. The pacing stimulation threshold is defined as the minimum stimulus intensity and duration to initiate and propagate the impulse reliably from the electrode-tissue interface. The strength of the output signal delivered at the electromyocardial interface is measured in volts, and the duration of the stimulus or pulse width is measured in milliseconds.[39]

Defibrillation

CRM devices with defibrillation capabilities deliver a high-voltage stimulus from a specially designed shocking lead to terminate VT and VF. Defibrillation is achieved when a critical mass of myocardium is depolarized through a critical voltage gradient throughout the ventricular tissue. The amount of energy required to defibrillate the heart successfully and terminate VF is known as the defibrillation threshold. Determining the defibrillation threshold is an integral component of ICD implantation, and the threshold is known to be increased in patients with heart failure. Therapy to terminate lethal ventricular dysrhythmias is delivered when the sensing circuits identify that the ventricular rate exceeds a prespecified rate, referred to as the detection rate. To decrease the chances of inappropriate shock delivery, additional parameters may be programmed. For example, the heart rate during exercise or anxiety may exceed the detection rate, and subsequent therapy then would be delivered to a sinus rhythm. Often, when a shock is provided in this situation, the anxiety increases, the heart rate remains elevated, and additional shock therapy is delivered. Additional parameters, to be discussed in the following sections, can prevent this from occurring.

Defibrillation is required to terminate VF and may be selected as the primary therapy delivered by the CRM device. The ICD may be programmed to deliver low-energy cardioversion shocks (generally less than 10 J) and high-energy defibrillation shocks (30 to 35 J on average) if antitachycardia pacing stimuli (discussed later) are not effective. Shocks of 10 J use less energy than shocks of 30 J.[32] Thus battery longevity depends directly not only on the number of shocks delivered but also on the energy requirements to terminate the dysrhythmia. An example of device defibrillation is provided in Figure 61-6.

Antitachycardia Pacing

Provided that the dysrhythmia is due to a reentry mechanism, VT may be terminated painlessly by delivering pacing stimuli to the ventricle at a rate faster than the rate of the tachycardia, known as antitachycardia pacing (Figure 61-7). Because a gap in tissue excitability exists within reentrant circuits, it is possible for these pacing impulses to enter the reentrant circuit during this gap, thereby activating the tissue earlier than otherwise would occur and creating a conduction block. Antitachycardia pacing success is enhanced when the gap in excitability is wider, as often occurs with slower tachycardias. Antidysrhythmic drugs commonly slow

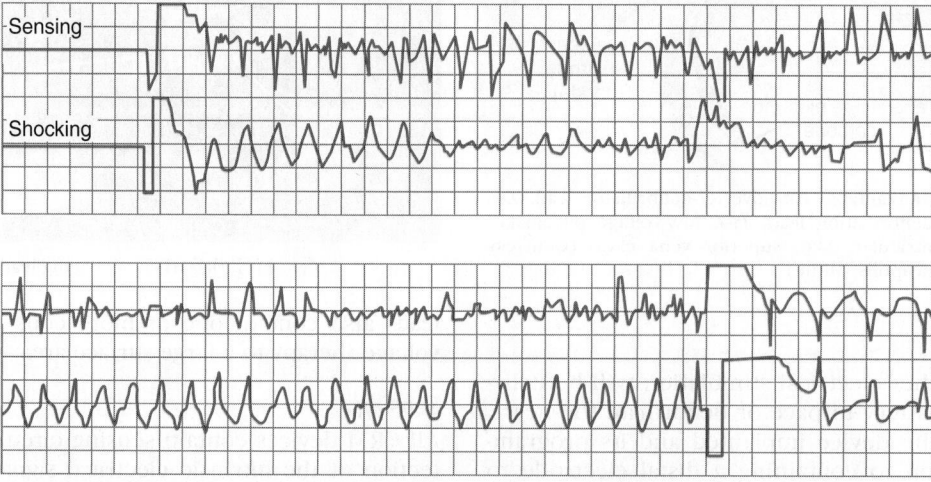

FIGURE 61-6 ■ Example of termination of ventricular tachycardia with device defibrillation.

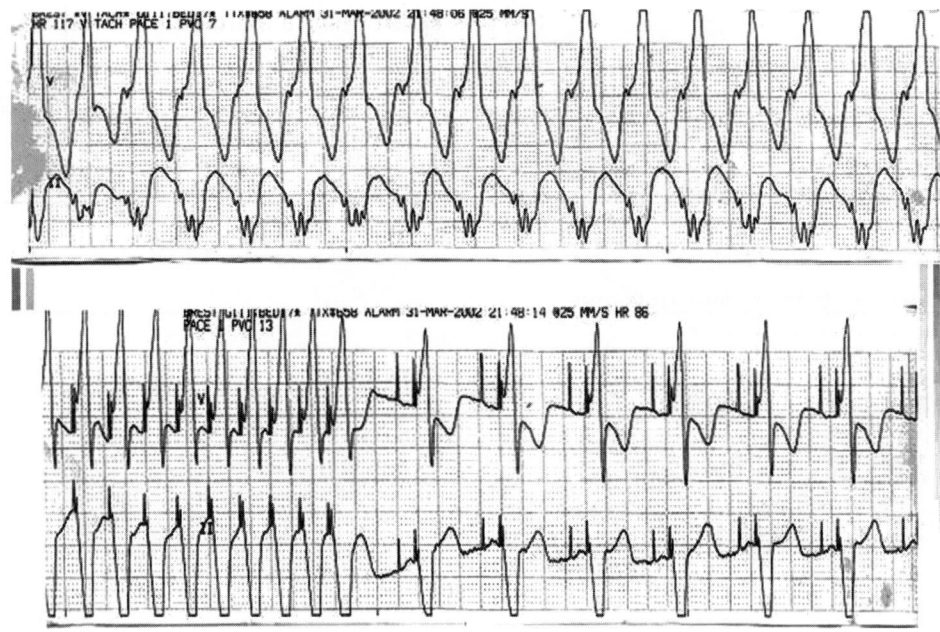

FIGURE 61-7 ■ Example of termination of ventricular tachycardia with antitachycardia pacing.

the rate of the tachycardia and increase this gap. Most CRM devices with defibrillation capabilities also offer antitachycardia pacing from the pacing tip of the high-voltage lead, which is programmed to be the first therapy delivered. If unsuccessful, defibrillation or shock therapy then ensues.[39]

Device Diagnostics
Device Integrity and Status

Device diagnostics provide important information about device function and lead integrity, atrial and ventricular dysrhythmias detected, therapies delivered, and the patient's functional status. Regardless of the type of CRM device implanted, all offer information on battery status, electrical integrity of the implanted lead systems, amplitude of the intrinsic signals of the heart, and the pacing stimulation thresholds. Device longevity, although typically in the range of 4 to 7 years, can vary widely depending on the stimulation thresholds, the frequency of pacing, and the frequency ICD therapies and energy required to defibrillate the heart.

Diagnostics Related to Therapy Delivery

All CRM devices provide detailed information about device-detected frequency of pacing and sensed events in the atrium and the ventricle. Because patients may develop concomitant AV block after implant, the status of the underlying rhythm is evaluated during all follow-up visits. When AV block is not present, attempts are made to minimize RV pacing and promote intrinsic conduction. However, for optimal CRT therapy, the amount of biventricular pacing being delivered must be as close to 100 percent as possible in order for the patient to receive the full benefit of CRT. In this instance, pacing and sensing counters and rate distribution histograms are scrutinized to determine whether CRT has been

delivered over the full range of intrinsic heart rates. In both scenarios, the device is adjusted to better meet the patient's needs. It is important to discern the possible causes for any loss of pacing, including lead dislodgment, increased pacing thresholds resulting in loss of capture, or AF with a rapid ventricular response. Assurance of pacing is particularly important in patients with AV block, who are pacer dependent and at risk for asystole if the device fails, and in patients with CRT devices as discussed before.

ICDs provide real-time intracardiac views, called electrograms, of the ventricular rhythm. At follow-up it is possible to retrieve these electrograms from the device and to evaluate whether a shock was delivered appropriately. In addition, a description of the date and time of each episode of VT and VF detected and the therapies delivered is provided. This information also can be helpful to confirm patient self-reports regarding therapy delivery and to differentiate actual episodes from phantom shocks, patient reported events that are unsubstantiated from the device.

Diagnostics Facilitating Assessment of Patient Status

Device diagnostic reports can be useful in assessing the activity status for patients. An example of one device diagnostic report is seen in Figure 61-8. Activity and trending reports are utilized routinely at follow-up visits to determine whether rate adaptation should be turned "on" and, if it is "on," to assess the appropriateness of the paced heart rate response. If the sensor is not optimized, false low or high heart rates, regardless of the level of exertion, can provide misleading information. For example, if a patient reports tiredness or difficulty getting dressed, and the report indicates the patient's heart rate did not exceed 80 beats/min, the sensitivity of the sensor should be adjusted. Conversely, if the patient reports a rapid heart rate with minimal activities,

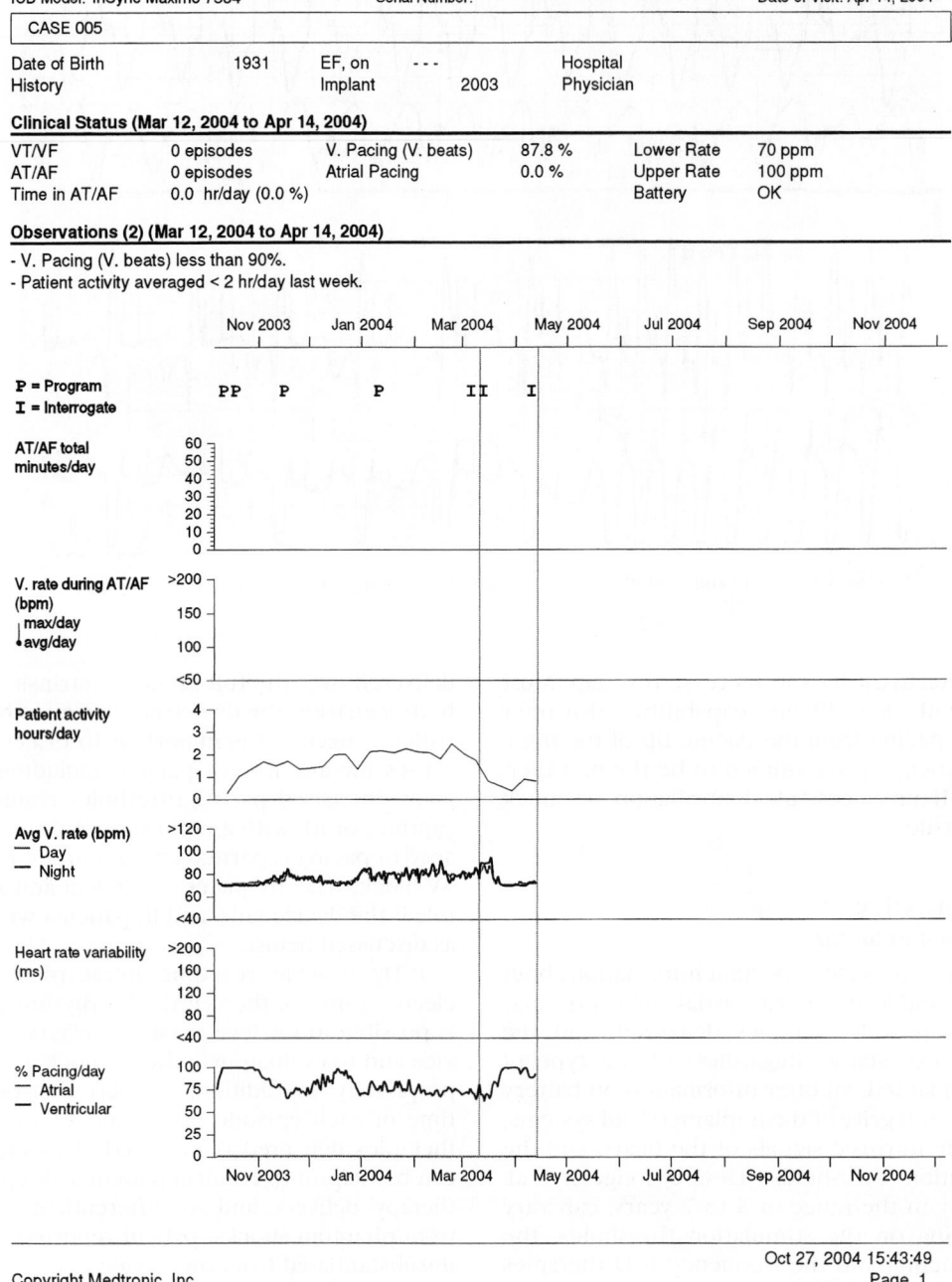

Heart Failure Management Report

ICD Model: InSync Maximo 7304   Serial Number: Date of Visit: Apr 14, 2004

CASE 005

| Date of Birth | 1931 | EF, on | - - - | Hospital |
| History | | Implant | 2003 | Physician |

Clinical Status (Mar 12, 2004 to Apr 14, 2004)

VT/VF	0 episodes	V. Pacing (V. beats)	87.8 %	Lower Rate	70 ppm
AT/AF	0 episodes	Atrial Pacing	0.0 %	Upper Rate	100 ppm
Time in AT/AF	0.0 hr/day (0.0 %)			Battery	OK

Observations (2) (Mar 12, 2004 to Apr 14, 2004)

- V. Pacing (V. beats) less than 90%.
- Patient activity averaged < 2 hr/day last week.

Oct 27, 2004 15:43:49
Page 1

FIGURE 61-8 ■ Device diagnostics report. *AT/AF,* Atrial tachydysrhythmia/Atrial fibrillation; *bpm,* beats per minute; *EF,* ejection fraction; *ICD,* implantable cardioverter-defibrillator; *ms,* milliseconds; *V,* ventricular; *VT/VF,* ventricular tachycardia/ventricular fibrillation.

and the report indicates a paced rate of 100 beats/min, the sensitivity of the sensor also should be adjusted.

To better manage AF, CRM devices provide diagnostic information on the amount of time a patient experiences atrial high rates and coinciding ventricular rates as seen in histogram reports (Figure 61-8). When correlated with other measures, such as activity trends, additional insights about the effect of AF on functional status can be obtained. Typically, activity levels decrease when AF is present. Evaluation of these diagnos-

tics can assist in determining the frequency of the atrial dysrhythmia and the amount of time spent in AF. Knowledge of the AF burden may affect medical treatment, such as the use of warfarin or antidysrhythmic drug therapy.

Specific heart failure status diagnostics, such as heart rate variability, activity levels, or fluid status, are used to better determine patient status. Heart failure patients are encouraged to remain active and to engage in regular physical exercise, such as walking. The activity trend provides an objective record of the number of hours per day that patient activity exceeded a 60- to 70-step per minute walk level. Thus the activity report can serve as a useful teaching and reinforcement tool to the patient and family about the importance and level of activity.

Heart rate variability (Figure 61-9) is a physiological marker of autonomic dysfunction in patients with heart failure and characterizes excessive sympathetic activation paired with attenuation of the parasympathetic nervous system.[40] Lower levels of heart rate variability have been associated with increased all-cause mortality risk, and thus this parameter is of clinical significance.[40] Declining heart rate variability should prompt patient assessment and evaluation as soon as possible to determine possible causes, such as heart failure decompensation or dysrhythmias. Increasing resting heart rates are indicative of increased sympathetic nervous system activity and may also reflect worsening heart failure.

The ability to use intrathoracic impedance, defined as the opposition to current flow within the chest cavity, as a surrogate marker for fluid status, or the accumulation of excess volume, is a new diagnostic feature available on some CRT-D devices. Impedance between the generator and the ICD lead is assessed multiple times throughout the day and then is plotted on a graph. Thresholds can be adjusted by the clinician based on patient symptoms. Clinical evaluation of intrathoracic impedance has demonstrated its ability to predict hospitalizations for decompensated heart failure 10 to 14 days in advance of the event.[41] The clinical challenge of exactly how to react to this information remains to be seen, especially in the absence of symptoms of congestion, yet is clinically important. Further evidence of the impact of intrathoracic fluid monitoring on outcomes is under investigation.

Device Implantation and Procedure Complications

Typically, CRM devices are implanted using intravenous sedation on the patient's nondominant side. Regardless of the procedure scheduled or the device to be implanted, all patients should be fully informed of all potential complications.[2,42] Chest x-ray films are obtained to verify lead placement following device implantation and before discharge. The risks associated with implantation of a CRM device include perforation of a vein or the heart with the lead(s), infection, bleeding/pocket hematomas, clot formation, blockage of a vein, random component failure of the device or lead(s), and death. Implantation of the LV lead is more complex and is associated with additional complications, including coronary sinus dissection, vein perforation, LV lead dislodgment, and other complications related to the introduction of multiple leads. In all cases, if an infection develops, the generator and lead may require extraction. If an opacity is observed and the infection is treated early, the existing system may be saved. Pocket erosion may occur, and the device may protrude through the skin. Lead dislodgment may occur following implantation. During ICD implantation, it is crucial to verify that the ICD system is working properly and can safely termi-

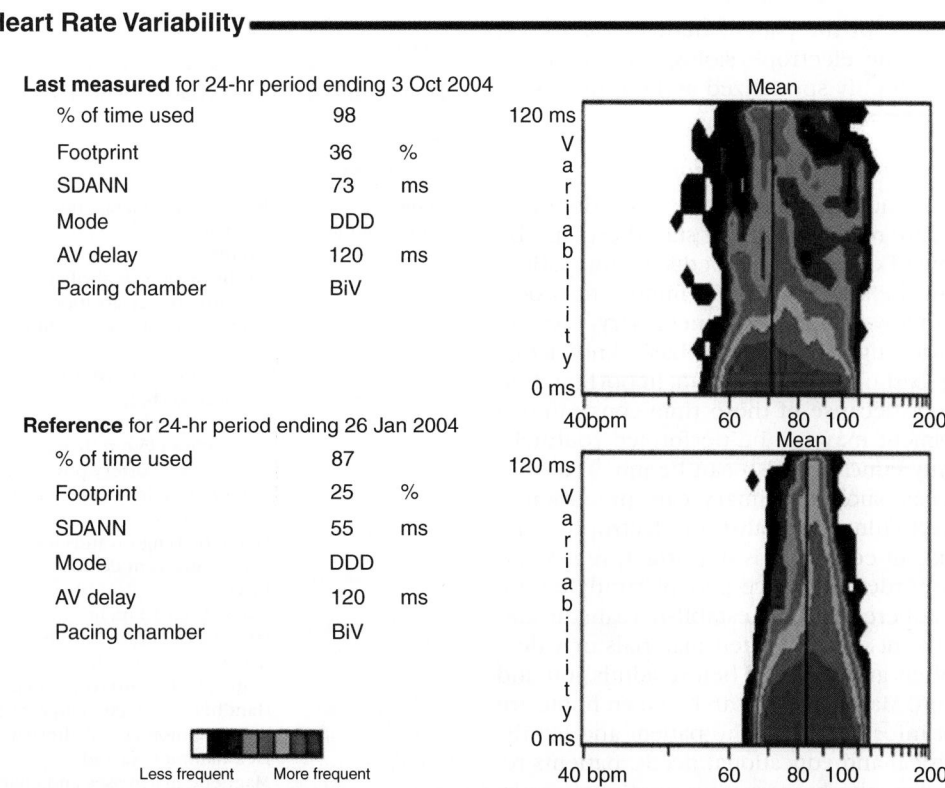

FIGURE 61-9 ■ Example of heart rate variability information. (Courtesy Guidant Inc, St Paul, Minn.) *AV,* Atrioventricular; *BIV,* biventricular; *bpm,* beats per minute; *DDD,* (see Table 61-1); *MS,* milliseconds; *SDANN,* standard deviation of sequential 5-minute R-R interval means.

nate VF through defibrillation threshold. It is also possible that the ICD may deliver inappropriate therapy because of improper sensing of signals. Regardless of the type of system implanted, the connector pins from the near or proximal end of the lead must be inserted properly into the connector block. If not properly inserted, the device will fail to recognize and/or deliver appropriate therapy.

Many device-related complications are linked directly to the experience of the implanting and following physician. Competency-based training requirements and guidelines are in place to address the physician qualifications to implant and follow CRM devices. Increasingly, as indications have broadened and the numbers of patients receiving CRM devices has dramatically increased, physicians other than electrophysiologists are implanting CRM devices. The guidelines and competency statements provide a vehicle to determine whether physicians are receiving the minimum training necessary to implant, follow, and troubleshoot these devices.

Follow-up of CRM devices is done by health care professionals who have undergone specialized training related to the operation of the device and the patient responses to device therapy. As the volume of patients expands, more specially trained nurses, engineers, and technologists provide follow-up care, and competency-based guidelines are published for nonphysicians. These guidelines are available at *www.hrsonline.org*.[43]

NURSING CARE AND MANAGEMENT OF THE CARDIAC RHYTHM MANAGEMENT PATIENT

Procedure-Related Care and Education

Intra-procedure care of the patient undergoing a CRM device implant in the electrophysiology laboratory or operating room is highly specialized and not discussed in this chapter.

Preprocedural Treatment and Education

Because of the urgency for some device indications and the short procedure-related length of stay, there may be a limited window of opportunity to educate the patient and family about the specific device, important procedural aspects, follow-up care, and necessary lifestyle modifications. Although appraisal of basic knowledge and underlying pathophysiology is an important first step in education, because of these time constraints a thorough assessment may not be performed routinely. Patient and family education also can be initiated from a variety of arenas, such as primary care practitioner, cardiologist, heart failure specialist, or electrophysiologist. Thus consistent education is important, regardless of the source, in order to reduce patient/family confusion, enhance adherence, and establish realistic and reasonable treatment goals. Written materials or videotapes (DVDs) often are provided before admission and after implantation. Materials that can be taken home are good sources of information for the patient and family. Besides the physical and educational needs, patients requiring CRM devices also have varying emotional needs. Depending on the indication (i.e., risk of SCD versus

treatment of sinus node dysfunction), emotional responses can differ significantly, especially when procedural risks are presented. Fear, anxiety, depression, anger, loss of control, or powerless are possible responses that may be encountered. Some emotions may be reduced simply by talking about them, whereas others may require referral to a counselor or psychiatrist postprocedure.

The impact of device therapy is typically more pronounced in patients with ICDs and may be related to requisite postimplant lifestyle modifications. Limitations related to driving, occupation, and/or recreational activities that place the patient or others at risk are imposed. Poor knowledge of the device functioning may cause patients to avoid performing an activity that previously resulted in the delivery of a shock.

The most common questions asked by patients and their families are whether they can continue to use their cell phone and microwave oven. Although microwave ovens have not posed a problem for well over a decade, cell phone signals actually may interfere with device operation. Patients should be instructed to use the phone on the ear opposite the device, to carry the phone on the opposite side of the body, and to maintain a minimum distance of 6 inches between the cell phone and the device. Common sources of electromagnetic interference of household appliances and medical procedures are discussed in Table 61-4. Important to remember is that these cautions apply to patients with pacemakers as well, because patients who are pacemaker dependent may have prolonged periods of asystole when pacing output is inhibited by electromagnetic interference.

■ ■ ■

TABLE 61-4   COMMON SOURCES OF ELECTROMAGNETIC INTERFERENCE

LOCATION	SOURCES
Medical environments	Magnetic resonance imaging and diathermy (avoid)
	Cautery
	Cardioversion/defibrillation
	Radiofrequency ablation
	Transcutaneous nerve stimulators
	Electrolysis
Everyday environments	Antitheft equipment (walk through briskly without lingering)
	Cellular telephones with open antenna less than 6 inches (15 cm) from device
	Chain saws, battery-powered cordless power tools and drills less than 12 inches (30 cm) from device
	Magnetic bingo wands less than 12 inches (30 cm) from device
	Lawn mowers, leaf blowers, and snow blowers less than 12 inches (30 cm) from device
	Stereo speakers and police radio antennas
	Arc welders and CB radio antennas less than 24 inches (60 cm) from device
	Handheld body fat analyzers/monitors (avoid)
	Running motors and alternators (avoid)
	Jack hammers (avoid)
	Magnetic mattresses and chairs

CB, Citizen's band.

Postprocedure Care and Follow-up

Discharge instructions on wound care, signs and symptoms of infection, activity, medications, and diet must be provided to the patient/family in verbal and written formats with time allotted for questions and answers. Mild to moderate incision pain is to be expected, and over-the-counter analgesics are prescribed routinely. Actual care of the surgical incision is practitioner-specific and highly variable, with ranges from no shower for the first 7 to 10 days to daily showers, and from occlusive to gauze dressings. Patients should be instructed to report any temperatures of 101°F or greater and any incisional redness, tenderness, or swelling. Activity instructions include limitation of arm movements on the affected side for the first 1 or 2 weeks in order to avoid lead dislodgments, weight-lifting restrictions of 10 lb for the first month, and no automobile driving for 2 to 4 weeks postoperatively. Because of dysrhythmia concerns, patients receiving an ICD for a VT/VF event typically are restricted from driving for at least 6 months, and feelings of isolation or frustration are common. Referral to a local ICD support group to assist with coping may be helpful. Physical activities that require full arm extension or shoulder rotation, such as golf, are discouraged for the first 6 months. However, patients should be encouraged to be as active as possible and engage in physical activity such as walking each day.

All patients are instructed to avoid electromagnetic fields and on the importance of carrying the identification card that specifies the device manufacturer and model. Patients with ICDs require additional instructions and information, particularly on what to do in the event of a shock and how and when to notify the physician. Patients are curious to know what a shock feels like, and recipients of device discharges usually describe it as a strong blow to the chest. Thorough instructions about what to do in the event of a shock are essential because approximately 50 percent of patients receive at least one device firing during the first year following ICD implantation.[44] Dizziness or syncope may occur before the event, and those touching the patient as the device discharges are not in danger. Typically, the patient is instructed to notify the physician of the first shock, but additional intervention is unlikely. In the event of recurring single shocks, clinical evaluation is necessary to determine the cause and to treat precipitating causes. Device reprogramming of the VT detection rate may be necessary if the shock was delivered during activity and sinus tachycardia. Cluster shocks are a medical emergency requiring immediate attention. Emergency medical services should be activated by calling 911. Numerous causes for cluster firings can occur, including electrolyte imbalances, ischemia, or lead fracture and these require prompt evaluation.[45] Regardless of the scenario, the establishment of clearly written plans to address these issues in advance of an event may assist with alleviating anxiety for the patient and family and can improve survival.

The first postprocedure visit occurs approximately 1 month after implantation. At that time the wound is examined for healing and the absence of infection. The patient is assessed, subjectively and objectively, based on the underlying disease process and for signs of response to therapy. Follow-up frequency varies depending on the type of the device implanted and the patient's needs. Frequency may range from monthly for some CRT patients requiring more aggressive monitoring, to every 3 months for those with ICD and CRT therapy, to annual follow-up for patients with traditional pacing indications. Between scheduled appointments patients with some newer CRM devices are able to transmit device information over telephone lines for review and evaluation by health care providers.

Continued optimal medical therapy is essential to prevent disease progression and should be considered an integral aspect of care. Adherence to the medical regimen, as established before device implantation, is vital unless instructed otherwise. Optimal medications are the first line to ensure a good response to CRT. Patients occasionally seek device therapy, such as CRT, as a way to avoid the need for medication, and so patients and families must understand that heart failure medications are the life-long, life-sustaining therapies. Discussion about medication regimens should take place before hospital discharge and at every follow-up visit. The dialog must include not only prescription medications but also any over-the-counter or herbal remedies taken. Patients and families also should be encouraged to call with any questions, rather than simply stopping medications because of real or perceived side effects or uncertainty.

Assessment of the Cardiac Rhythm Management System

Assessment of the CRM system functioning includes evaluation of the battery status, electrical performance of the implanted lead systems, review of device history and diagnostics, and final programming of the device. The first step is to evaluate the battery status of the device, which provides an estimation of device longevity. Based on the programmed parameters and frequency of use, longevity is approximately 4 to 7 years, which is similar across standard pacemakers, CRTs, and ICDs. Patients are scheduled for device replacement as the elective replacement indicator is approached or reached.

The next steps include evaluating lead integrity by measuring lead impedance and sensing signals. Pacemaker stimulation threshold is assessed, and parameters are adjusted to provide a safety margin in the event increased electrical current is required to capture and pace the heart. An example demonstrating loss of atrial and ventricular capture while determining thresholds is provided in Figure 61-10.

As previously discussed, many CRM devices have sensors that allow physiological rate variation, but pacing rates generally are set around 50 to 80 beats/min. The appropriateness of the overall heart rate, both sensed and paced events, is evaluated within the context of the patient's physical condition, lifestyle, and programmed parameters. The presence of an extremely low or extremely high pacing rate is an indication for immediate interrogation and investigation, especially in

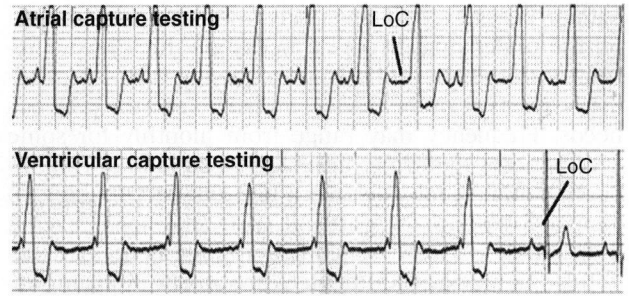

FIGURE 61-10 ■ Example of loss of atrial capture and loss of ventricular capture. *LoC,* Loss of capture.

the presence of adverse symptoms. Pacemaker mediated tachycardia, which occurs as a result of conducted P waves being sensed retrograde, may or may not produce reportable symptoms. More commonly, reports of palpitations are due to AF.

Inappropriate pacing or withholding of pacing therapy may occur because of operator programming errors or changes in the patient's condition and/or medications. As discussed before, undersensing occurs when the device does not "see" signals, whereas oversensing occurs when the device incorrectly "sees" electrical signals and interprets them as the intrinsic heart rate, thus inhibiting further pacing. Thus regardless of the intrinsic rhythm, pacing stimuli are delivered when the device does not see electrical signals and are withheld when the device sees signals. Delivery of the pacing stimulus during the vulnerable phase of the T wave may induce ventricular dysrhythmias. Reprogramming the device restores appropriate sensing and pacing.

Diagnostic information related to pacing and ICD therapy also is retrieved from the device and evaluated to confirm that therapy is being delivered as prescribed. Prevailing day and night heart rates, dysrhythmias, heart failure status, heart rate variability, and fluid volume also are evaluated and are discussed in greater detail next.

Management of CRT and CRT-D Devices

The management of CRT devices requires careful coordination between the heart failure and electrophysiology clinicians and warrants additional discussion. Regular evaluation of the CRT device can provide important insight on the device performance, including the delivery of CRT and patient status. Unfortunately, not all patients experience benefit from CRT. Table 61-5 provides some patient and device management strategies to assist with optimal outcomes.

Just as with other CRM device follow-up, the assessment of a CRT system includes evaluation of the battery status, electrical performance of the implanted lead systems, review of device diagnostics, and final program-

■ ■ ■

TABLE 61-5 STRATEGIES TO OPTIMIZE THE CARDIAC RHYTHM MANAGEMENT PATIENT AND/OR DEVICE

	NONRESPONDERS	LOST RESPONDERS	SLOW RESPONDERS
Definition	No benefit from cardiac rhythm management (CRT)	Had initial improvement from CRT	Slow improvements after CRT
Optimizing the device	Electrophysiological device evaluation every 6 months or per routine	Electrophysiological device evaluation every 6 months or per routine	Electrophysiological device evaluation every 6 months or per routine
	Perform device check to verify pacing and sensing thresholds and left ventricular (LV) capture	Perform device check to verify pacing and sensing thresholds and LV capture	Perform device check to verify pacing and sensing thresholds and LV capture
	Consider a chest x-ray film to evaluate lead position	Consider a chest x-ray film to evaluate lead position	
	Repeat echocardiogram with atrioventricular optimization	Repeat echocardiogram with atrioventricular optimization	
Optimizing the patient	Stress adherence to medical plan and nonpharmacological regimen	Stress adherence to medical plan and nonpharmacological regimen	Stress adherence to medical plan and nonpharmacological regimen
	Take medications as directed	Take medications as directed	Take medications as directed
	2-g sodium diet	2-g sodium diet	2-g sodium diet
	Daily weights	Daily weights	Daily weights
	Be alert for signs and symptoms of hypovolemia, dizziness, increased shortness of breath, orthostasis, increased blood urea nitrogen	Objectively evaluate symptoms 6-minute walk test Cardiopulmonary test Quality of life	Be alert for signs and symptoms of hypovolemia, dizziness, increased shortness of breath, orthostasis, increased blood urea nitrogen
	Encourage exercise	Encourage exercise	*Slowly* increase physical activity
	Use programmer diagnostics to determine activity	Use programmer diagnostics to determine patient activity	Use programmer diagnostics to determine patient activity
	Optimize angiotensin-converting enzyme (ACE) inhibitors and/or beta blockers	Optimize ACE inhibitors and/or beta blockers	*Slowly* optimize ACE inhibitors and/or beta blockers
	Repeat 12-lead electrocardiogram	Repeat 12-lead electrocardiogram	Outpatient surveillance weekly to monitor symptoms
	Heart failure evaluation every month	Heart failure evaluation every month	Heart failure evaluation 1-2 weeks after implant, and then every 2-3 weeks until clinical improvement
	Refer to electrophysiologist for in-depth device assessment if no improvement from above strategies	Refer to electrophysiologist for in-depth device assessment if no improvement from above strategies	

ming of the device. Additional echocardiographic evaluation also may be required to further optimize the delivery of CRT.

For CRT to be effective, the device must deliver biventricular pacing as close to 100 percent as possible, or the patient will not receive the full benefit of CRT. Therefore, it is important to evaluate the electrical performance of the RV and LV leads to ensure capture. Causes for loss of CRT to be evaluated include correctable increased LV pacing thresholds resulting in loss of capture, LV lead dislodgment requiring lead repositioning, frequent premature ventricular contractions, or AF with a rapid ventricular rate. Elevated pacing thresholds may indicate lead dislodgment. A chest x-ray film may be required to determine whether the lead has dislodged. Reported dislodgment rates for the LV lead range from 6 to 7 percent, and lead repositioning to achieve better capture and CRT delivery may be necessary.

For patients with chronic heart failure, small improvements in hemodynamics have a significant impact on symptoms. For this reason, determining an optimal AV delay in patients with a CRT system can be critical. The optimal AV delay is defined as the shortest possible AV delay that allows complete ventricular filling, thereby optimizing stroke volume and minimizing mitral regurgitation. Even though the preprogrammed device settings are effective for the majority of patients, further optimizing AV delay can be advantageous to those with minimal or no perceived benefit from CRT. The goal in programming this parameter is to prolong LV diastolic filling without shortening the atrial contribution or "kick." In the presence of interventricular conduction delay, LV activation is delayed, but atrial activation is not. Hence early passive LV filling and the atrial "kick" occur simultaneously, resulting in diminished transmitral blood flow and decreased preload of the left ventricle. By optimizing the AV delay and activating both ventricles simultaneously, the LV is able to complete contraction and begin relaxation earlier, which increases filling time and ultimately results in improved cardiac performance.[46]

Several techniques can be used to optimize the AV delay. While some newer devices use auto optimization algorithms to adjust the AV and V-V timing, traditionally echocardiography has been used to optimize this parameter. A baseline evaluation before AV optimization will demonstrate a "fused" E and A wave on Doppler echocardiogram of transmitral flow, representing the simultaneous passive LV filling and atrial kick. By reprogramming the AV delay, LV filling time will be increased with a resultant separation of the E and A wave on Doppler echocardiogram of transmitral blood flow. Results from the CRT trials demonstrate that an AV delay of 100 msec is a good initial setting.

Patients with ventricular dyssynchrony exhibit intraventricular and interventricular conduction delays. By varying the interventricular pacing interval, or V-to-V timing, additional hemodynamic benefits may be obtained. Newer-generation cardiac resynchronization devices allow biventricular pacing to be delivered simultaneously or sequentially. By either activating the LV or RV first, followed by the other ventricle, additional im-

provements in hemodynamics may be obtained, and increased response to CRT may be feasible. The response to sequential biventricular pacing is patient specific and can be optimized via echocardiography.

CRT improves hemodynamic performance, including increased cardiac output. With increased cardiac output, renal blood flow also is increased, thus the kidneys are better perfused, prompting an improved response to diuretics. Therefore, increased diuresis may occur, and patients frequently become hypovolemic. Differentiation of symptoms between hypovolemia and hypervolemia is difficult because increased fatigue, increased shortness of breath, and dizziness may be reported on either end of the fluid spectrum. Close surveillance of symptoms and weight is necessary to avoid complications related to hypovolemia and ensuing dehydration.

As discussed in Chapter 19, collaboration between those who implant and manage the device and those who manage patients with CRM devices requires a "team" approach. This is particularly true for patients who have CRT devices as traditional workflow patterns, "we've always done it that way," are transformed and revised into efficient, accommodating systems respectful of other caregivers involved and of the patient's needs. The exchange of information on patient status, device functioning and diagnostics, response to therapy, and medication changes must become routine, rather than only upon request.

Some examples of possible plans to enhance collaboration include establishing a device clinic where electrophysiological staff and other clinicians evaluate the patient and device during the same visit, produce patient educational materials for consistent information on implant or follow-up procedures, or hold conferences in which patients with current devices and those identified as needing a device can be discussed and their care coordinated. With an open mind and willingness to consider alternate methods, satisfaction and outcomes can be improved for all involved: patients, families, and staff.

SUMMARY

In less than 50 years, innovations in technology have produced CRM devices that are much smaller, safer, smarter, and capable of delivering a variety of therapies to address a variety of patient needs. As understanding of cardiovascular disease continues to evolve, the utilization of these therapies, as well as new realms for devices, will continue to advance. This chapter is intended to provide a solid background in understanding what CRM devices and therapies are available, issues that are important when considering device selection, and the management of patients with such devices.

REFERENCES

1. Bear Stearns Equity Research: *Healthcare/medical supplies and devices,* Feb 11, 2005.
2. Hayes DL, Zipes DP: Cardiac pacemakers and cardioverter-defibrillators. In Zipes DP, Libby P, Bonow RO, Braunwald E, editors: *Braunwald's heart disease: a textbook of cardiovascular medicine,* ed 7, Philadelphia, 2005, Saunders.

3. Berne RM, Levy MN, Koepen BM, Stanton BA: Electrical activity of the heart. In *Physiology,* ed 5, St Louis, 2004, Mosby.

4. Peters RW, Ellenbogen KA: Indications for permanent and temporary cardiac pacing. In Ellenbogen KA, Wood MA: *Cardiac pacing and ICDs,* ed 3, Malden, Mass, 2002, Blackwell Science.

5. Rubart M, Zipes DP: Genesis of cardiac arrhythmias: electrophysiological considerations. In Zipes DP, Libby P, Bonow RO, Braunwald E, editors: *Braunwald's heart disease: a textbook of cardiovascular medicine,* ed 7, Philadelphia, 2005, Saunders.

6. Gillis AM: Sinus node disease. In Ellenbogen KA, Kay GN, Wilkoff BL, editors: *Cardiac pacing and defibrillation,* ed 2, Philadelphia, 2000, WB Saunders.

7. Olgin JE, Zipes DP: Specific arrhythmias: diagnosis and treatment. In Zipes DP, Libby P, Bonow RO, Braunwald E, editors: *Braunwald's heart disease: a textbook of cardiovascular medicine,* ed 7, Philadelphia, 2005, Saunders.

8. Ellenbogen KA, deGuzman M, Kawanishi DT, Rahimtoola SH: Pacing for acute and chronic atrioventricular conduction system disease. In Ellenbogen KA, Kay GN, Wilkoff BL, editors: *Cardiac pacing and defibrillation,* ed 2, Philadelphia, 2000, WB Saunders.

9. Kass DA: Pathophysiology of cardiac dyssynchrony and resynchronization. In Ellenbogen KA, Kay GN, Wilkoff BL, editors: *Device therapy for congestive heart failure,* Philadelphia, 2004, Saunders.

10. Silvert H, Amin J, Padmanabhan S et al: Prognostic implications of increased QRS duration in patients with moderate and severe left ventricular systolic dysfunction, *Am J Cardiol* 88:182-185, 2001.

11. Cowburn PJ, Cleland JG, Coats AJ et al: Risk stratification in chronic heart failure, *Eur Heart J* 19:696-710, 1998.

12. Kass DA: Ventricular resynchronization: pathophysiology and identification of response, *Rev Cardiovasc Med* 4(suppl 2):S3-S13, 2003.

13. Josephson M, Wellens HJJ: Implantable defibrillators and sudden cardiac death, *Circulation* 109:2685-2691, 2004.

14. Bubien RS, Sanchez JE: Atrial fibrillation: treatment rationale and clinical utility of non-pharmacological therapies, *AACN Clin Issues* 12(1):140-155, 2001.

15. Chou T, Knilans TK: Atrial arrhythmias. In *Electrocardiography in clinical practice,* ed 4, Philadelphia, 1996, WB Saunders.

16. Gregoratos G, Abrams J, Epstein AE et al: ACC/AHA/NASPE 2002 guideline update for implantation of cardiac pacemakers and antiarrhythmia devices: summary article—a report of the American College of Cardiology/American Heart Association Task Force on Practice Guidelines (ACC/AHA/NASPE Committee to Update the 1998 Pacemaker Guidelines), *Circulation* 106:2145-2161, 2002.

17. Lee TH: Guidelines. In Zipes DP, Libby P, Bonow RO, Braunwald E, editors: *Braunwald's heart disease: a textbook of cardiovascular medicine,* ed 7, Philadelphia, 2005, Saunders.

18. Barlow MA, Kerr CR, Connolly SJ: Survival, quality of life, and clinical trials of pacemaker patients. In Ellenbogen KA, Kay GN, Wilkoff BL, editors: *Cardiac pacing and defibrillation,* ed 2, Philadelphia, 2000, WB Saunders.

19. Kerr CR, Connolly SJ, Abdollah H et al: Canadian Trial of Physiological Pacing: effects of physiological pacing during long-term follow-up, *Circulation* 109:357-362, 2004.

20. Gillis AM, Chung MK: Pacing the right ventricle: to pace or not to pace? *Heart Rhythm* 2:201-206, 2005.

21. The DAVID Trial Investigators: Dual chamber pacing or ventricular backup pacing in patients with an implantable defibrillator, *JAMA* 288:3115-3123, 2002.

22. Sweeny MO, Hellkamp AS, Ellenbogen KA et al, and the MODE Selection Trial Investigators: Adverse effect of ventricular pacing on heart failure and atrial fibrillation among patients with normal baseline QRS duration in a clinical trial of pacemaker therapy for sinus node dysfunction, *Circulation* 107:2932-2937, 2003.

23. Steinberg JG, Fisher AVI, Wang P et al: The clinical implications of cumulative right ventricular pacing in the Multicenter Automatic Defibrillator Trial II, *J Cardiovasc Electrophysiol* 16:359-365, 2005.

24. Auricchio A, Stellbrink C, Butter C et al: Clinical efficacy of cardiac resynchronization therapy using left ventricular pacing in heart failure patients stratified by severity of ventricular conduction delay, *J Am Coll Cardiol* 42:2125-2127, 2003.

25. Kadish A, Dyer A, Daubert JP et al: Defibrillators in Non-Ischemic Cardiomyopathy Treatment Evaluation (DEFINITE) Investigators: prophylactic defibrillator implantation in patients with nonischemic dilated cardiomyopathy, *N Engl J Med* 350:2151-2158, 2004.

26. Bradley DJ, Bradley EA, Baughman KL et al: Cardiac resynchronization and death from progressive heart failure: a meta-analysis of randomized controlled trials, *JAMA* 289:730-740, 2003.

27. Hunt SA, Baker DW, Chin MH et al: ACC/AHA Guidelines for the Evaluation and Management of Chronic Heart Failure in the Adult: Executive Summary A Report of the American College of Cardiology/American Heart Association Task Force on Practice Guidelines (Committee to Revise the 1995 Guidelines for the Evaluation and Management of Heart Failure). *Circ,* Dec 104: 2996 - 3007, 2001.

28. Hunt SA, Abraham WT, Chin MH et al: ACC/AHA guideline update for the diagnosis and treatment of chronic heart failure in the adult: summary article, *Circulation* 20:1-28, 2005.

29. Jessup M: Resynchronization therapy is an important advance in the management of congestive heart failure: view of an antagonist, *J Cardiovasc Electrophysiol* 4:S30-S34, 2003.

30. Auricchio A, Abraham WT: Cardiac resynchronization therapy: current state of the art—cost versus benefit, *Circulation* 109:300-307, 2004.

31. Wilkoff BL, Firstenberg MS: Cardiac chronotropic responsiveness. In Ellenbogen KA, Kay GN, Wilkoff BL, editors: *Cardiac pacing and defibrillation,* ed 2, Philadelphia, 2000, WB Saunders.

32. Knight BP, Gersh BJ, Carlson MD et al, for the AHA Writing Group: Role of permanent pacing to prevent atrial fibrillation: science advisory from the American Heart Association Council on Clinical Cardiology (subcommittee on Electrocardiography and Arrhythmias) and the Quality of Care and Outcomes Research Interdisciplinary Working Group in collaboration with the Heart Rhythm Society, *Circulation* 111:240-243, 2005.

33. Lloyd MA, Hayes DL, Friedman PA: Programming. In Hayes DL, Lloyd MA, Friedman PA, editors: *Cardiac pacing and defibrillation: a clinical approach,* Armonk, NY, 2000, Futura.

34. Gold MR: The implantable cardioverter defibrillator. In Ellenbogen KA, Wood MA: *Cardiac pacing and ICDs,* ed 3, Malden, Mass, 2002, Blackwell Science.

35. Buxton AE, Lee KL, DiCarlo L et al: Electrophysiologic testing to identify patients with coronary artery disease who are at risk for sudden cardiac death, *N Engl J Med* 342:1937-1945, 2000.

36. Bristow MR, Saxon LA, Boehmer J et al: Cardiac resynchronization therapy with or without implantable defibrillator in advanced heart failure, *N Engl J Med* 350:2140-2150, 2004.

37. Bardy GH, Lee KL, Mark DB et al, for the Sudden Cardiac Death in Heart Failure Trial (SCD-HeFT) Investigators: amiodarone or an implantable cardioverter-defibrillator for congestive heart failure, *N Engl J Med* 352:225-237, 2005.

38. Cleland JGF, Daubert J-C, Erdmann E et al, for the Cardiac Resynchronization in Heart Failure (CARE-HF) Study Investigation: the effects of cardiac resynchronization on morbidity and mortality in heart failure, *N Eng J Med* 352:1539-1549, 2005.

39. Kay GN: Basic concepts of pacing. In Ellenbogen KA, Wood MA, editors: *Cardiac pacing and ICDs,* ed 3, Malden, Mass, 2002, Blackwell Science.

40. Adamson P, Smith A, Abraham W et al: Continuous autonomic assessment in patient with symptomatic heart failure, *Circulation* 110:2389-2394, 2004.

41. Yu CM, Wang L, Chau E et al: Intrathoracic impedance monitoring in patients with heart failure: correlation with fluid status and feasibility of early warning preceding hospitalization, *Circulation* 112:841-848, 2005.

42. Hayes DL: Complications. In Hayes DL, Lloyd MA, Friedman PA, editors: *Cardiac pacing and defibrillation: a clinical approach,* Armonk, NY, 2000, Futura.

43. Curtis AB, Ellenbogen KA, Hammill SC et al: Clinical competency statement: training pathways for implantation of cardioverter defibrillators and cardiac resynchronization devices, *Heart Rhythm* 1:371-375, 2004.

44. Jacobson C, Gerity D: Pacemaker and defibrillators. In Woods S, editor: *Cardiac nursing,* Philadelphia, 2000, Lippincott Williams & Wilkins.

45. Bubien RS, Ching EA, Kay GN: Cardiac defibrillation and resynchronization therapies: principles, therapies, and management implications, *AACN Clin Issues* 15(3):340-361, 2004.

46. Trupp RJ: Cardiac resynchronization therapy: optimizing the device, optimizing the patient, *J Cardiovasc Nurs* 19(4):223-233, 2004.

chapter 62

Pathophysiology of Heart Failure

Mariann R. Piano

CHAPTER ABBREVIATIONS

ANP atrial natriuretic peptide

ATP adenosine triphosphate

BNP B-type natriuretic peptide

GFR glomerular filtration rate

HF heart failure

LV left ventricular

MI myocardial infarction

ROS reactive oxygen species

SERCA 2a sarcoplasmic reticulum-ATPase

TNF-α tumor necrosis factor alpha

Heart failure is a syndrome that is preceded by an initiating cardiovascular event such as myocardial infarction (**MI**) or longstanding hypertension. Therefore, in the continuum of cardiovascular disease, heart failure is viewed as an end event and represents the most severe manifestation of cardiovascular disease. Heart failure can arise from alterations in systolic or diastolic function, hence the more recent designation of heart failure as systolic heart failure or diastolic heart failure. Also important to note is that heart failure still is referred to by some as congestive heart failure and that congestive heart failure still is used as a diagnostic label. However, there is growing recognition that not all heart failure patients (especially those with diastolic heart failure) routinely exhibit signs and symptoms of congestion. Heart failure is the preferred term.

Systolic heart failure and diastolic heart failure are progressive syndromes that develop over the course of many years and (regardless of the cause) arise from a multitude of abnormalities in cardiomyocyte and non-myocyte function and structure. This chapter addresses the pathophysiology related to systolic heart failure and diastolic heart failure. However, it is important to note that the cell changes associated with remodeling, neurohormonal system activation, and changes in other body systems have been studied most extensively and systemically in the setting of systolic heart failure. Health professionals only recently are beginning to understand the pathophysiology of diastolic heart failure. Insight into the pathophysiological mechanisms and signals that underlie the development and progression of heart failure will provide the clinician with a background and rationale for the care and management of the heart failure patient.

DEFINITION AND CLASSIFICATION OF HEART FAILURE

In 1933, Thomas Lewis defined heart failure as "a condition in which the heart fails to discharge its contents adequately." Fifty years later, heart failure was defined as "the state of any heart disease in which despite adequate ventricular filling, the heart's output is decreased or in which the heart is unable to pump blood at a rate adequate for satisfying the requirements of the tissues with function parameters remaining within normal limits." In 1985, Poole-Wilson defined heart failure as "an abnormality of the heart and recognized by a characteristic pattern of hemodynamic, renal, neural and hormonal responses."[1] These early definitions emphasized the failure of the heart as an organ and the accompanying circulatory consequences. A more updated definition would reflect the recent advances in understanding of the pathophysiology of heart failure and ventricular remodeling and therefore include some aspect of the genetic, molecular, and cellular changes in the myocardium. This definition also would reflect how heart failure could arise from abnormalities in systolic or diastolic function. However, to date no such encompassing definition has been published. Instead (and appropriately so), committees representing the American College of Cardiology, American Heart Association, and European Society of Cardiology have focused their attention on developing diagnostic criteria for heart failure and using this to define heart failure.[2] As noted subsequently in more detail, definitions and diagnostic criteria have been proposed for systolic heart failure and diastolic heart failure.

Chronic Versus Acute Heart Failure

Heart failure is a progressive syndrome that develops over the course of many years, which qualifies it as a chronic condition. Therefore the term *chronic* often is used to denote the slow progression and continuance of the heart failure syndrome. Once individuals are diagnosed with chronic heart failure, they frequently experience exacerbations of heart failure. The latter was once designated as acute heart failure; however, experts agree that the more appropriate designation should be decompensated heart failure.[3] Decompensated heart failure is defined as new or worsening signs and symptoms of the heart failure syndrome, frequently leading to emergency room visits or hospitalization. Decompensated heart failure also can be the sudden onset of heart failure signs and symptoms that occur in a patient with no history of heart failure with previously normal cardiac function. The latter, however, represents only a small percentage of patients. Most often, patients have chronic heart failure and experience exacerbation or decompensation of their heart failure.[3,4]

Systolic Versus Diastolic Heart Failure

As highlighted before, heart failure was once previously conceptualized as a circulatory disorder resulting from poor pump function (decreased ejection fraction) or systolic dysfunction. However, it is well recognized that a large percentage of heart failure patients have a predominant abnormality in diastolic function, with a normal or preserved ejection fraction.[5] These patients are considered to have diastolic heart failure, which is defined as a clinical syndrome characterized by signs and symptoms of heart failure, a preserved ejection fraction, and abnormal diastolic function.[6,7] Patients with diastolic heart failure have abnormalities of diastolic distensibility, filling, or relaxation of the left ventricle.[7] The left ventricle is less accommodating, and normal end-diastolic volumes are associated with high end-diastolic pressures.

Systolic heart failure is defined as an inability of the left ventricle to contract against a load and eject blood volume into the aorta. Therefore a hallmark sign of systolic heart failure is a reduced stroke volume and ejection fraction.[2] It has become important to determine whether the patient has systolic heart failure or diastolic heart failure because patient outcomes, signs and symptoms, and treatment options are different between the two types of heart failure.

Heart Failure Classification

Several classification schemas for heart failure have been proposed, and these were linked to the side of the heart affected (left versus right), direction of blood flow affected (backward versus forward), or the underlying condition (abnormal cardiac muscle contraction and relaxation and/or both, excessive pressure or volume overload, or limited ventricular filling). Another classification system used by clinicians and researchers is the New York Heart Association classification (Table 62-1). The classification is subjective (based on what the patient says) and is therefore an indirect measure of functional status. Recently, the American College of Cardiology and American Heart Association have taken a new approach to the classification of heart failure and have developed a classification and staging system that highlights the evolution and progression of heart failure (Table 62-2).[2] Most importantly, this staging system identifies patients who are also at high risk of developing heart failure, such as patients with hypertension, who should be monitored more closely.[8] These patients are also those who should be considered for pharmacological treatment with agents that are known to attenuate the progression of heart failure.

VENTRICULAR REMODELING: DEFINITION AND GROSS STRUCTURAL CHANGES

Regardless of the cause of heart failure (see Chapter 3 for a discussion of the epidemiology of heart failure), the development and progression is associated with profound changes in the architecture of the myocardium or (more specifically) the process of ventricular remodeling. Ventricular remodeling occurs in response to an injury (such as MI) or longstanding pressure overload (such as hypertension) and is defined as progressive changes in the size, architecture, and shape of the myocardium.[9-11] Remodeling occurs because of changes that begin at the cellular level and involve cardiomyocytes and extracellular matrix cell types such as fibroblasts and endothelial cells. Changes that occur in the cardiomyocyte include myocyte hypertrophy and intrinsic myocyte dysfunction. In addition, there is myocyte loss caused by apoptosis or necrosis. Changes in the nonmyocytes, such as the fibroblasts, include fibroblast proliferation, interstitial fibrosis, and excessive degradation of collagen; all of the latter result in significant remodeling of the extracellular matrix.

The initial etiopathology, stage of remodeling, and area of the myocardium evaluated will affect the changes that one finds in the remodeled myocardium, not only in ventricular geometry and shape but also in the involvement of specific cell types. For example, ventricular remodeling after MI is characterized by increased ventricular dilatation and stretch, increased ventricular volume, wall thinning, increased heart size, and depressed systolic function (Figure 62-1, *left*). Patients

■ ■ ■

TABLE 62-1   NEW YORK HEART ASSOCIATION FUNCTIONAL CLASSIFICATION SYSTEM

CLASS	FUNCTIONAL CAPACITY	OBJECTIVE ASSESSMENT
I	Patients with cardiac disease but without resulting limitation of physical activity.	No objective evidence of cardiovascular disease
II	Patients with cardiac disease resulting in slight limitation of physical activity. They are comfortable at rest. Ordinary physical activity results in fatigue, palpitation dyspnea, or anginal pain.	Objective evidence of minimal cardiovascular disease
III	Patients with cardiac disease resulting in marked limitation of physical activity. They are comfortable at rest. Less than ordinary activity causes fatigue, palpitation, dyspnea, or anginal pain.	Objective evidence of moderately severe cardiovascular disease
IV	Patients with cardiac disease resulting in inability to perform any physical activity without discomfort. Symptoms of heart failure or the anginal syndrome may be present even at rest. If any physical activity is undertaken, discomfort is increased.	Objective evidence of severe cardiovascular disease

∎ ∎ ∎

TABLE 62-2 HEART FAILURE STAGING

STAGE	DESCRIPTION	EXAMPLES
A	Patients at high risk of developing heart failure (HF) because of the presence of conditions strongly associated with the development of HF. Such patients have no identified structural or functional abnormalities of the pericardium, myocardium, or cardiac valves and have never shown signs or symptoms of HF.	Hypertension, coronary artery disease, diabetes mellitus, history of cardiotoxic drug therapy or alcohol abuse, personal history of rheumatic fever, family history of cardiomyopathy
B	Patients who have developed structural heart disease that is strongly associated with the development of HF but who have never shown signs or symptoms of HF.	Left ventricular hypertrophy or fibrosis; left ventricular dilatation or hypocontractility; asymptomatic valvular heart disease; previous myocardial infarction
C	Patients who have current or prior symptoms of HF associated with underlying structural heart disease.	Dyspnea or fatigue caused by left ventricular systolic dysfunction; asymptomatic patients who are undergoing treatment for prior symptoms of HF
D	Patients with advanced structural heart diseases and marked symptoms of HF at rest despite maximal medical therapy and who require specialized interventions.	Patients who are frequently hospitalized for HF or cannot be discharged safely from the hospital; patients in the hospital awaiting heart transplantation; patients at home receiving intravenous support for symptom relief or being supported with a mechanical circulation assist device; patients in a hospice setting for the mismanagement of HF

Data from Hunt SA, Baker DW, Chin MH et al: *J Heart Lung Transplant* 21(2):190-203, 2002.

with this type of remodeling are categorized as having eccentric hypertrophy, or a myocardium that is dilated and enlarged (increased ventricular mass/weight).[11] Unfortunately, individuals who develop eccentric hypertrophy have greater risk of developing heart failure compared with those with concentric hypertrophy, which is associated with longstanding hypertension or aortic stenosis.

Concentric hypertrophy is characterized by increase in wall thickness and reductions in the intraventricular chamber (less room for filling) and diastolic dysfunction (at least in the early stages; Figure 62-1, bottom right).[11] The heart depicted in Figure 62-1, bottom right, is from an individual with longstanding hypertension, and as can be seen, because of the extreme thickening of the chamber walls, the intraventricular cavity is very small.

SYSTOLIC HEART FAILURE: PATHOPHYSIOLOGICAL FEATURES

The global pathophysiological features of systolic heart failure include a decreased ejection fraction, increased left ventricular mass, decreased relative wall thickness, increased end-diastolic volume and pressure, and increased left atrial size. During exercise, patients with systolic heart failure have a decreased exercise capacity and cardiac output augmentation. Two-dimensional echocardiography with Doppler typically reveals increased end-diastolic and end-systolic dimension, left ventricular (LV) dilatation, atrial enlargement, and regional wall motion abnormalities. Some patients also may have evidence of mitral valve inflow abnormalities.[12,13] As detailed subsequently, there are usually increases in B-type natriuretic peptide (greater than 100

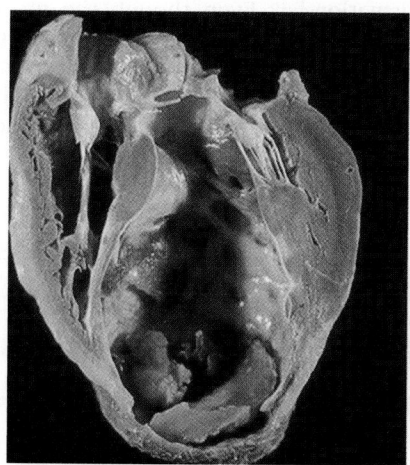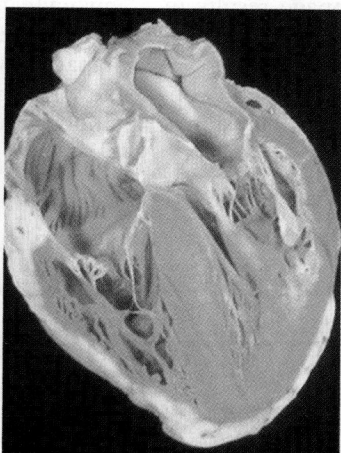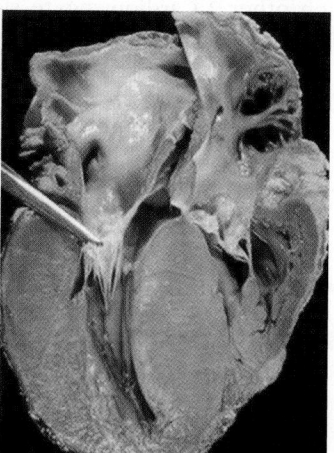

FIGURE 62-1 ∎ A normal heart *(top)* and cardiac remodeling associated with myocardial infarction *(bottom left)* and hypertension *(bottom right)*. (From Pfeffer MA, Pfeffer JM: *Circulation* 75[suppl]: IV-93–IV-97, 1987.)

pg/ml) that correlate to increased LV volume and pressure.

The most common cause of systolic heart failure is systolic dysfunction, which arises from a loss of contractile function following an MI or obstructive coronary artery disease. As detailed subsequently, the loss of contractile function or the ability to generate an adequate cardiac output arises from loss of functioning cardiomyocytes and functional changes in the cardiomyocytes. Even though diastolic heart failure occurs nearly as often as systolic heart failure, to date researchers have studied most extensively the time course and pathophysiological post-MI ventricular remodeling and systolic dysfunction. Post-MI remodeling has been divided into two phases: early (within 72 hours of infarct) and late (months to years).[11,14]

Cellular events involved in early post-MI remodeling begin in the initial hours following ischemia and cell necrosis and usually involve the area surrounding the infarct. The main changes occurring are wall thinning and stretching of the acutely infarcted area; this is referred to as infarct expansion.[15]

In the immediate hours after an MI, an inflammatory reaction is initiated through activation of the complement cascade and cytokines, such as tumor necrosis alpha (**TNF-α**) and the interleukin-1 and interleukin-6 families. This initial inflammatory response facilitates the healing process and removal of necrotic cells; however, it is detrimental to the collagen and intercalated disk connections between neighboring surviving myocytes. Numerous cell types (monocytes, macrophages, neutrophils) are activated and recruited to this region of myocardium.[14] Neutrophils release matrix metalloproteinases, which degrade the supporting fibrillar collagen network that weaves around and connects the myocytes. Release of metalloproteinases results in collagen breakdown, cardiomyocyte slippage, and ventricular wall thinning. Ventricular wall thinning occurs because of loss of myocytes and stretching of the surviving myocytes. Stretching of surviving myocytes coupled with loss of the collagen connections (struts) between the cardiomyocytes leads to speculation that there is cardiomyocyte slippage, whereby the cardiomyocytes slide across each other.[15] Cardiomyocyte slippage results in impaired contractile coordination among cardiomyocytes.

Wall thinning, however, leads to an increase in ventricular volume and wall tension because wall tension is the product of the transmural pressure times the radius of the wall divided by the wall thickness (law of Laplace). Wall thinning coupled with an increase in ventricular radius resulting from increased volume translates into an increase in wall tension and oxygen consumption. Finally, the inflammatory cell types such as the macrophages and mast cells also secrete cytokines, which stimulate fibroblasts to proliferate and synthesize collagen.[14] As noted in the subsequent section, there is extensive remodeling of the extracellular matrix with the development of fibrosis.

Over the course of months to years, there is involvement of the entire ventricle, such that the entire ventricle becomes dilated and globular (late remodeling). Usually, the LV thinning and elongation occur in the area close to the infarct, whereas the noninfarcted area of the myocardium dilates and hypertrophies (Figure 62-2).[11] Late remodeling arises from a multitude of changes that occur in the cardiomyocyte and extracellular matrix cell types, such as the fibroblasts, endothelial cells, and smooth muscle cells. Changes that occur in the cardiomyocyte include cardiomyocyte hypertrophy, intrinsic myocyte dysfunction, and myocyte loss (apoptosis/necrosis). Changes in the nonmyocytes such as the fibroblasts include fibroblast proliferation, interstitial fibrosis, excessive breakdown, or degradation of collagen and endothelial dysfunction.

The Cardiomyocyte
Hypertrophy

Myocyte hypertrophy is a key feature of the remodeling process. Myocyte hypertrophy is defined as an increased myocyte size in the absence of cell division.[16] Unlike other organs such as the liver and skeletal muscle, the myocardium has a limited ability to repair or regenerate (undergo mitosis to generate more myocytes) after muscle injury or infarction.[17] In the past, researchers thought that the inability of the myocardium to regenerate was due to the fact that the adult myocyte is a terminally differentiated cell type, which means the cell cannot divide and reproduce. More recent evidence suggests that there may be some degree of mitosis and new myocyte formation.[17,18] Even though the myocardium may have the capacity for new myocyte generation, this capacity is not enough to overcome or generate enough new myocytes after an event such as an MI. Therefore, under conditions of physiological demand, such as in-

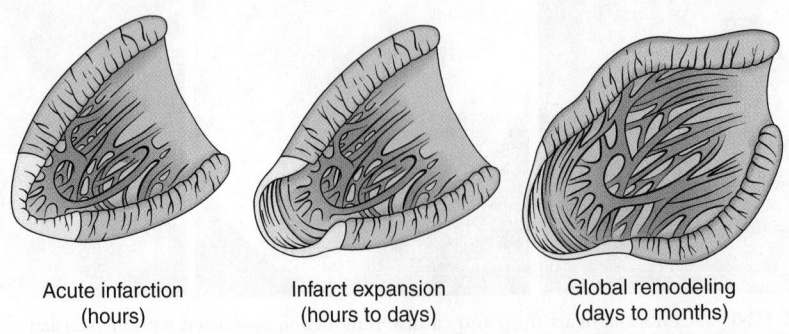

Acute infarction   Infarct expansion   Global remodeling
(hours)   (hours to days)   (days to months)

FIGURE 62-2 ▪ Ventricular remodeling post–myocardial infarction. (From Pfeffer MA, Pfeffer JM: *Circulation* 75[suppl]:IV-93–IV-97, 1987.)

creased pressure or stretch or after an injury such as an MI, surviving myocytes will hypertrophy to maintain contractile force and cardiac output.

Hypertrophy occurs because of a coordinated increase in cardiomyocyte protein synthesis that results in an increase in the size of the cardiomyocyte (Figure 62-3),[19,20] accompanied by a change in the genetic expression of certain proteins. For example, there is an increase in the amount, and altered expression of, the contractile protein myosin. In the adult human heart the predominant form of myosin is referred to as alpha-myosin heavy chain; however, in heart failure the new myosin synthesized has a slightly different amino acid structure and is referred to as beta-myosin heavy chain. Increases in the amounts of noncontractile proteins also occur, such as atrial natriuretic peptide (**ANP**) and B-type natriuretic peptide (**BNP**). As noted later, BNP is used as a marker of systolic heart failure severity and progression. Some of these changes (in particular the increased synthesis of beta-myosin heavy chain protein and increased synthesis of BNP) are referred to as activation of a fetal program because these changes are similar to what is found in the embryonic neonatal heart. Finally, within the hypertrophied cardiomyocyte, there is an increase in the number of mitochondria; the sarcoplasmic reticulum enlarges; and there are changes (increases and decreases) in many of the membrane-bound transport pumps, ion channels, and receptors.[16] For example, there is a decrease in the number of beta-adrenergic receptors and an increase in the number and activity of the sodium-calcium exchanger.

Initially, myocyte hypertrophy and some of the changes in the membrane protein transport pumps and receptors are considered adaptive and protective mechanisms. For example, downregulation of beta-adrenergic receptors allows the heart to contract less forcefully during a stressful state (e.g., in the presence of increased plasma levels of epinephrine and norepinephrine). Norepinephrine and epinephrine stimulate an increase in heart rate, speed of electrical impulse

conduction, and contractile force. All of these effects increase myocardial workload and oxygen consumption. Heart failure patients with a history of MI have limited coronary artery blood flow because of their coronary artery disease and usually have a limited ability to increase flow (due in part to endothelial dysfunction and other mechanisms). Therefore, the downregulation of beta-adrenergic receptors may have a protective effect and serve to protect against increases in heart rate and contractile force in the setting of increased adrenergic activation (e.g., stress).

Intrinsic Myocyte Dysfunction

The term *intrinsic myocyte dysfunction* refers to a multitude of alterations that include changes in components of the sarcomere and contractile proteins and intracellular events involved in excitation-contraction coupling and relaxation.[21] Intrinsic myocyte dysfunction can arise from alterations in any of the proteins or steps involved in the process of excitation contraction coupling. Excitation-contraction is a process that couples the depolarization of the plasma membrane (electrical event) to cross-bridge cycling and contraction. Many steps are involved, and the role of each protein and various steps are reviewed in Figure 62-4. In the setting of human and experimental heart failure, researchers have found many changes in the events involved in excitation-contraction coupling, for example, calcium release from the sarcoplasmic reticulum, calcium entry through the L-type channel, and calcium uptake by the sarcoplasmic reticulum-ATPase (**SERCA2a**) pump.[19,21] Alterations in the excitation-contraction process could alter the action potential duration or force generation of the myocyte and relaxation. Not surprisingly, almost every aspect of excitation-contraction coupling has been studied in relation to heart failure, and these findings along with other cell changes are summarized in Table 62-3 along with the clinical consequences of these changes.[22]

Cell Death: Apoptosis and Necrosis

In systolic heart failure, cell death or cell dropout is another important mechanism that may contribute to decreased contractility, wall thinning, and dilatation. Cell death may occur by necrosis or apoptosis.[23] Cell necrosis can occur in response to a physical or chemical injury, such as ischemia or toxins. In necrosis, there is cell swelling, clumping of the nuclear chromatin, disruption of intracellular organelles, and eventual rupture of the membrane and calcium overload, all of which occur over the course of 20 to 30 minutes. The cell contents are released into the surrounding tissue, initiating an inflammatory response.[24]

Apoptosis is a process whereby cells undergo an orderly program of suicidal and adenosine triphosphate (**ATP**)-dependent cell death. Apoptosis is a critical physiological mechanism by which cells are deleted during normal development and other stages of life to regulate cell mass and organ architecture.[25] In later stages of life, apoptosis may play a role in maintaining health by eliminating malignant, infective, or redundant cells. However, excessive and unbalanced apoptotic cell death can lead to disease or organ failure. At the whole

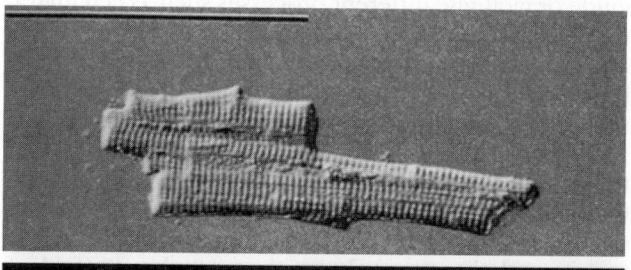
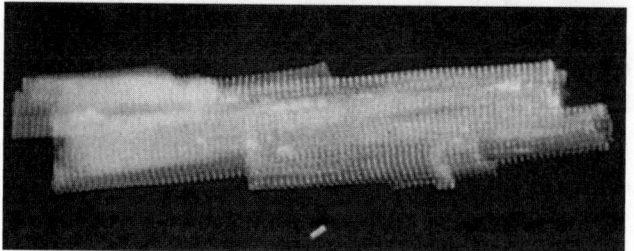

FIGURE 62-3 ▪ Myocyte hypertrophy. (From Gerdes AM, Kellerman SE, Moore JA et al: *Circulation* 86:426-430, 1992.)

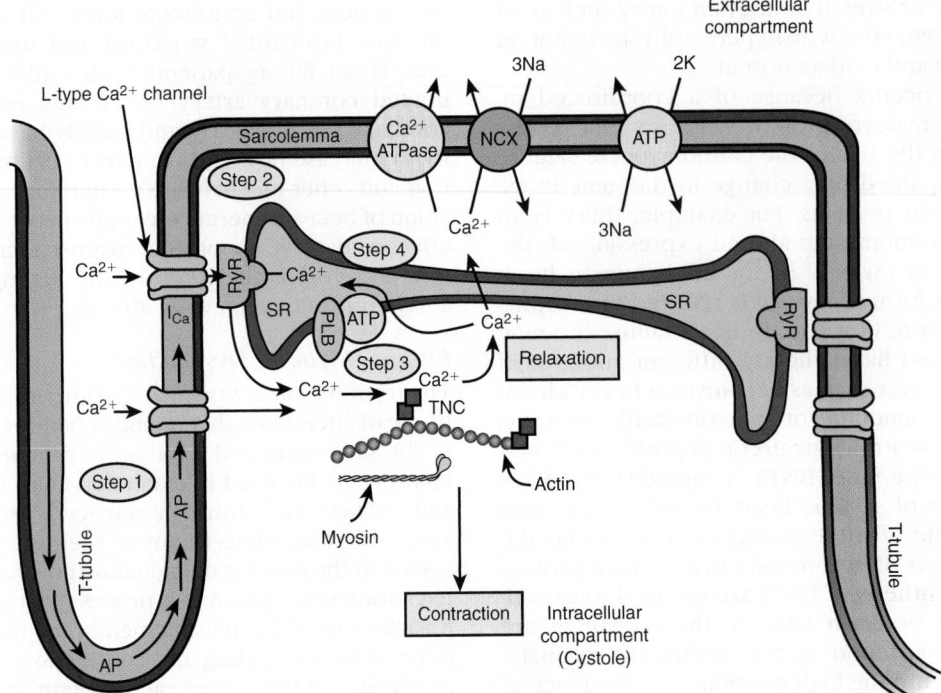

FIGURE 62-4 ▪ Electromechanical coupling. A summary of key events during the excitation-contraction coupling cycle of a myocyte. Depolarization of the membrane stimulates the opening of voltage-dependent Ca^{2+} channels and increases Ca^{2+} current (I_{Ca}; *Step 1*). Ca^{2+} entry through the L-type calcium channels stimulates the release of Ca^{2+} from the sarcoplasmic reticulum (SR) ryanodine receptor (RyR; *Step 2*). Ca^{2+} released from the SR binds troponin C (TNC), which elicits a conformational change in the actin filament that exposes the myosin binding sites (*Step 3*). This allows the strong cross-bridge formation between actin and myosin and force generation. Relaxation is an active process and is brought about by the release of Ca^{2+} and reuptake back into the SR via the SERCA2a pump. Depending on the levels of intracellular Ca^{2+}, some Ca^{2+} also is removed via the sarcolemmal Ca^{2+} ATPase pump and sodium-calcium exchanger (NCX). *ATP*, Adenosine triphosphate; *ATPase*, enzyme that catalyzes decompensation of ATP; *CA^{2+}*, calcium; *NCX*, sodium-calcium exchanger; *PLB*, phospholamban; *RyR*, ryanodine receptor; *SR*, sarcoplasmic reticulum; *TNC*, cardiac troponin C.

heart level, the functional consequences of cell death because of apoptosis or necrosis may include electrical heterogeneity, which gives rise to dysrhythmias, myocyte misalignment, and wall thinning.[22]

The Role of Nonmyocytes (Fibroblasts and Endothelial Cells)

Nonmyocytes also play a role in ventricular remodeling. These cells include fibroblasts and endothelial cells. The main function of the fibroblast is to synthesize and secrete collagen. Collagen is a critical component of the extracellular matrix, a two-dimensional extracellular scaffold-like structure that weaves around and tethers together myocytes and other cell types (Figure 62-5, panel A).[26] The major structural proteins of the extracellular matrix are type I and III collagens. In the heart, type I collagen is the most abundant of the collagens and has the tensile strength of steel. The collagen component of the extracellular matrix is important in maintaining myocyte alignment, transducing force generated by the myocytes, and preventing myocyte slippage and overstretching during the cardiac cycle.[27] Collagen is also a major determinant of myocardial compliance.

The extracellular matrix also contains important nonfibrillar collagen proteins, such as fibronectin, laminin, cell adhesion molecules, and integrins. Fibronec-

tins within the extracellular matrix serve to adhere the myocytes to collagen. Cardiac laminin is found predominately in the basal membrane (a thin sheet-like network of extracellular matrix proteins linked to the cell membrane) and also binds collagen.[28,29] Collectively, these noncollagen proteins function as anchors and also guide or facilitate different processes such as cell migration and proliferation. A loss of these noncollagen fibers could result in myocyte detachment to the basal membrane and a loss of ventricular force transmission from the myocyte to the extracellular matrix.[30] Finally, the integrins located in the cell surface are important in mediating cell-cell interactions and communication between the extracellular matrix and cytoskeleton.[29] Integrins form a physical link between the extracellular matrix and the cytoskeleton (intracellular scaffold of connective proteins).[28] Myocardial integrins also play a role in transmitting and distributing mechanical force generated by the myocyte to the extracellular matrix.[29]

In the setting of systolic heart failure caused by MI, there are specific and distinct extracellular matrix changes that occur at different times post-MI. In the early phase following MI, neutrophils release matrix metalloproteinases, which degrade the supporting fibrillar collagen network. Loss of the supporting fibrillar collagen network is shown in Figure 62-5, panel B.[26] Loss of the collagen tethers leads to myocyte slippage,

■ ■ ■

TABLE 62-3   CHANGE IN EXCITATION-CONTRACTION COUPLING

	PHYSIOLOGICAL ROLE OF SARCOLEMMAL CHANNELS/PUMPS	CHANGE IN HEART FAILURE	CLINICAL CONSEQUENCE OF CHANGE AND/OR EFFECT
Sarcolemmal			
L-type calcium channel (ryanodine receptor)	Ca^{2+} entry through these voltage-activated channels stimulates Ca^{2+} release from SR.	↓ and ↔ channel number	Potential affect on peak Ca^{2+} current, ↓ SR Ca^{2+} release: these changes could influence systolic force development
Na-Ca exchanger	Bidirectionally transports three Na^+ ions for one Ca^{2+} ion.	↑ Na-Ca protein levels and mRNA levels	May be an adaptive mechanism that permits Ca^{2+} removal during diastole ↑ mRNA indicates there is a change at the level of the gene transcription. mRNA is transcribed from the DNA (gene) and contains the genetic code for the synthesis of the Na-Ca exchanger protein/pump. mRNA is transported to the ribosomes, where protein translation occurs. An ↑ mRNA synthesis indicates an ↑ at the genetic (DNA) level for the synthesis of the protein.
Beta$_1$-adrenergic receptors	Activation of these receptors is associated with an ↑ in myocardial force, rate of relaxation, and heart rate.	Downregulation of beta receptors (desensitization)	↓ Response to catecholamines, which translates into a ↓ in myocardial reserve manifested by a ↓ in the patient's ability to exercise. Initially this may be a protective mechanism because catecholamines such as norepinephrine stimulate different aspects of the remodeling process, such as hypertrophy and apoptosis
Intracellular Organelles			
SR-CRC	The SR is the major site for Ca^{2+} storage and release. Ca^{2+} is released from the CRC.	↓ CRC number and mRNA levels	↓ Ca^{2+} release from SR occurs and ↓ in peak Ca^{2+} transients and therefore force production ↓ mRNA indicates there is a change at the level of the gene transcription. mRNA is transcribed from the DNA (gene) and contains the genetic code for the synthesis of the Na-Ca exchanger protein/pump. mRNA is transported to the ribosomes, where protein translation occurs. If there is a ↓ in mRNA, this could suggest a decrease in transcription or that there is an ↑ in the breakdown of mRNA.
SERCA2a	This is a Ca^{2+}-activated ATPase protein, which is responsible for the reuptake of Ca^{2+} into the SR and is critical for relaxation.	↓ SERCA2 levels and mRNA levels	↓ Ca^{2+} uptake into SR occurs and therefore the relaxation is impaired (rate of relaxation is slowed and less time is spent in diastole). See above for interpretation of mRNA levels.
Phospholamban	Protein co-localized with SERCA2, which regulates SERCA2a activity. Phospholamban phosphorylation increases SERCA2a activity and therefore increases Ca^{2+} uptake into SR.	↓ and ↔ in phospholamban protein and mRNA levels See above for interpretation of mRNA levels	↓ Ca^{2+} uptake into SR occurs and therefore a ↓ in the rate of relaxation occurs.

CRC, Calcium release channel; *DNA,* deoxyribonucleic acid; *mRNA,* messenger RNA; *NaCa,* sodium-calcium; *SERCA2,* sarcoplasmic reticulum Ca^{2+}-activated ATPase pump; *SR,* sarcoplasmic reticulum.
From Piano MR, Jarvis C: *J Cardiovasc Nurs* 14:1-23, 2000.

ventricular wall thinning, and enlargement. However, over the course of months to years, in areas remote to the infarct, there is a disproportionate increase in collagen type III relative to type I, and there is myocyte hypertrophy. Fibroblasts proliferate and increase their production of collagen, as well as the noncollagen proteins fibronectin and laminin. The increase in collagen synthesis, which is referred to as interstitial fibrosis, contributes to the increase in cardiac mass and size, as well as reorganization and cross-linking among collagen fibers types.[29] Various stimuli—such as angiotensin II, aldosterone, and stretch—are important stimulators of fibroblast proliferation.

Patients with systolic heart failure also exhibit abnormalities in mechanisms that regulate the tone and responsiveness of the microvasculature and midsize peripheral arteries.[31] Collectively, this abnormal micro-vascular response is referred to as endothelial dysfunction and is exemplified by an increased systemic vasoconstriction and decreased vasodilator response to exercise and vasodilator substances.[31] In the setting of heart failure, some effects may be attributable to a decrease in nitric oxide. In heart failure, there is an increase in circulating cytokines, which may increase the levels of inducible nitric oxide synthase, an enzyme that metabolizes nitric oxide, therefore decreasing basal levels of nitric oxide. In addition, the response to the vasodilators acetylcholine and bradykinin are attenuated in heart failure patients.[32] These important changes result in what is referred to as impaired endothelium-dependent vasodilatation. Impaired endothelium-dependent vasodilatation is probably an important reason why heart failure patients experience exercise intolerance and fatigue easily.[32]

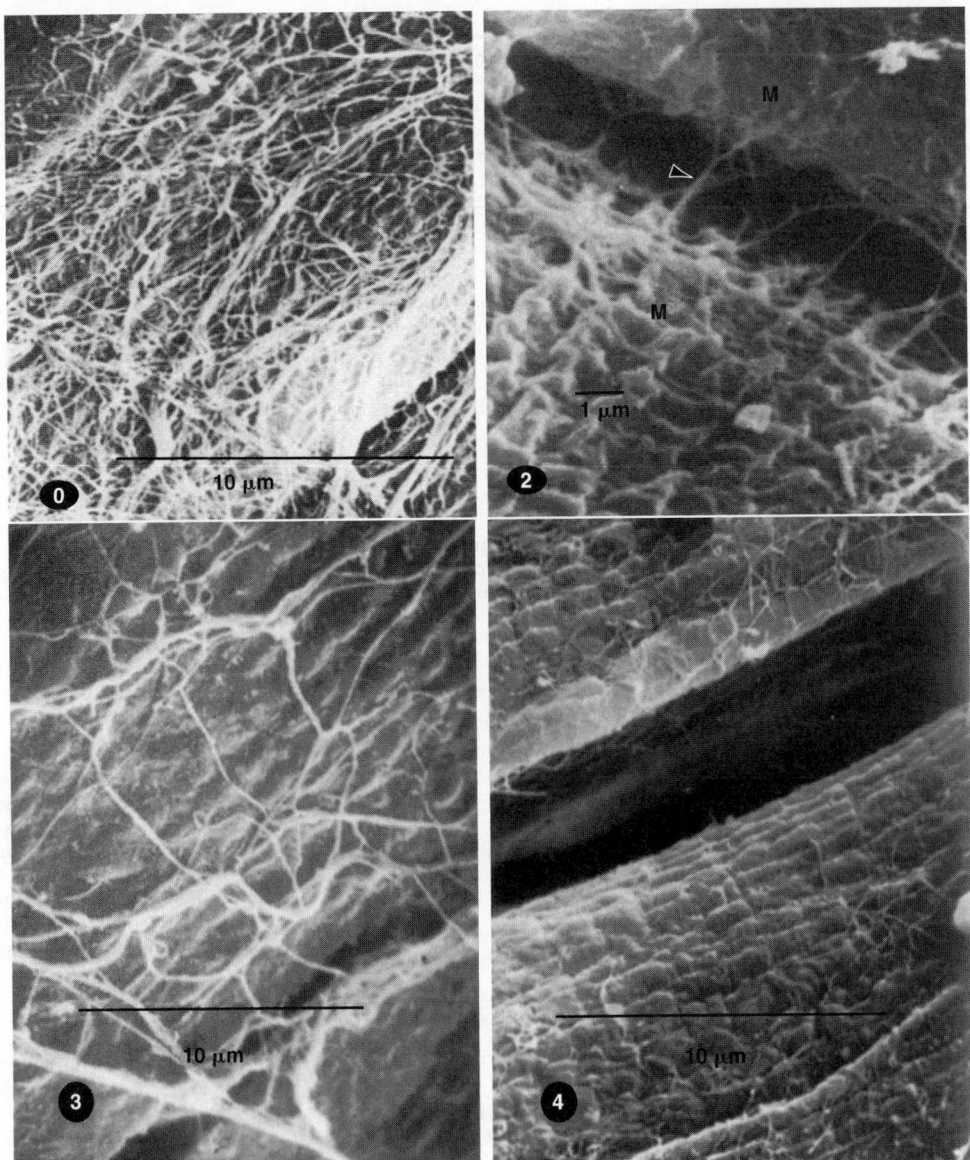

FIGURE 62-5 ■ Scanning electron micrograph at 5,200× *(left)* and 10,000× *(right)* of *normal* extra cellular matrix (ECM). As shown, the collagen fibers weave around the myocytes, and at the higher magnification, collagen struts can be seen between adjacent myocytes. Bottom (panel B) scanning micrographs of the ECM obtained after myocardial infarction: this figure shows loss of the fibrillar network and tethers between the myocytes. (From Caulfield JB, Norton P, Weaver RD: *Mol Cell Biochem* 118:171-179, 1992.)

Hemodynamic and Chemical Signals Involved in Systolic Heart Failure

In the setting of systolic heart failure, there are hemodynamic (increased afterload and volume) and chemical (neurohormones, peptides, growth factors, natriuretic peptides) signals that stimulate changes in the biology of the myocyte and nonmyocyte. Neurohormones/ peptides include norepinephrine, angiotensin II, aldosterone, and the natriuretic peptides. Many of these neuroendocrine systems are activated in response to a variety of stimuli. The neuroendocrine systems serve to regulate renal and cardiovascular compensatory mechanisms that occur in response to activities in daily life (e.g., exercise) or in the setting of acute stress (e.g., hemorrhagic shock or heart failure). Initially, activation of the mechanical/hemodynamic and chemical systems serves a compensatory role to maintain cardiac output and blood flow. Over time, however, these signals become pathogenic. Not surprisingly, the results of many prospective randomized clinical pharmacological trials have demonstrated in patients with systolic heart failure that inhibition of the renin-angiotensin-aldosterone system and beta-adrenergic blockage therapy are associated with attenuation of heart failure progression. This suggests that activation of the renin-angiotensin-aldosterone and sympathetic nervous systems are involved in the progression and development of systolic heart failure. A major aim of pharmacological therapy is to block or inhibit these signals. In the following sections, the hemodynamic and individual chemical signals are reviewed.

Hemodynamic Signals: Pressure and Stretch

The pressure/volume/stretch cycle generated by the myocardium is critical for maintaining myocardial weight and is also an important determinant of myocardial function. However, sustained or repetitive increases in pressure and stretch of the ventricle contribute to the remodeling process in many ways. Sustained increases in afterload (resulting from hypertension) and preload (resulting from LV dilatation or increased diastolic filling pressure) are considered important remodeling signals. Specifically, sustained increases in preload and afterload may stimulate increased expression of a variety of cardiac genes and proteins that are part of the myocyte hypertrophy process. In particular, stretch stimulates the release of tissue angiotensin II and growth factors, both of which stimulate myocyte hypertrophy, fibroblast proliferation, and apoptosis.[33,34]

Stretch also serves as a signal in the remodeling of the extracellular matrix. The integrins are important in communicating outside signals from the extracellular matrix into the cell, and therefore may play a role in stimulating the changes in fibroblasts. Only recently has the role of the cell surface integrins been investigated, and some data support the idea that physical stimulation of the integrins may activate intracellular signal transduction cascades that affect fibroblast and other cell type proliferation within the extracellular matrix.[34]

Chemical Signals: Neurohormones and Peptides
Norepinephrine

Many heart failure patients have increased norepinephrine levels, and increased plasma norepinephrine levels have been associated with an increased mortality rate in systolic heart failure patients.[35] In the setting of heart failure, there is increased sympathetic activity to the myocardium that results in increased norepinephrine levels in the vicinity of the myocyte and in the circulation. In systolic heart failure, the stimulus for norepinephrine secretion or sympathetic activation is a decrease in cardiac output, renal hypoperfusion, and arterial underfilling.[36] Norepinephrine stimulates a variety of cellular events in the remodeling process, such as myocyte hypertrophy, fibroblast proliferation (increased collagen production), activation of fetal-gene programs, downregulation of beta receptors, and apoptosis.[16] Norepinephrine also produces arterial vasoconstriction (increased afterload), redistribution of regional blood flow, and dysrhythmias.

Renin-Angiotensin-Aldosterone System

Two pathways for the generation of angiotensin II are a circulating pathway (Figure 62-6, top panel) and tissue-derived pathway (Figure 62-6, bottom panel). In the circulation pathway, angiotensin II is produced via angiotensin-converting enzyme–stimulated conversion of

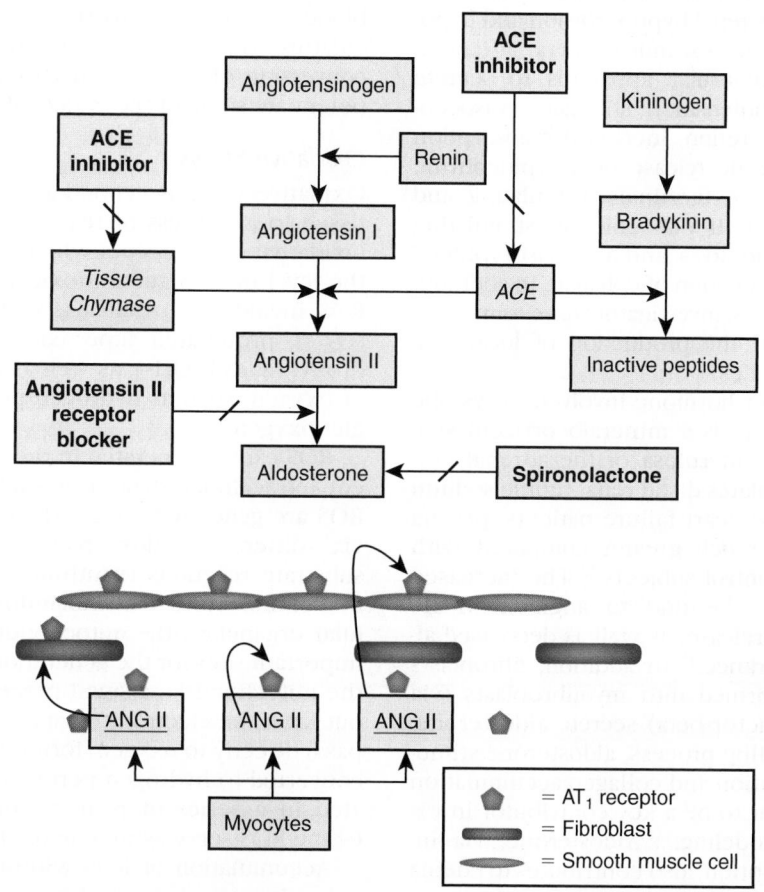

FIGURE 62-6 ■ Formation of circulating and tissue angiotensin II. *ACE,* Angiotensin-converting enzyme; *ANG II,* angiotensin II.

angiotensin I to angiotensin II. Angiotensin I is derived from angiotensinogen (renin substrate). Renin released from the kidney stimulates the conversion of angiotensinogen to angiotensin I. Angiotensin-converting enzyme (also known as kinase II) breaks down bradykinin. Bradykinin has many effects that antagonize angiotensin II, some of which include vasodilatation and antigrowth and antiapoptotic effects.[37] Therefore, more than likely the beneficial effects of angiotensin-converting enzyme inhibitors are due to a decrease in angiotensin II formation and an increase in bradykinin levels.

Angiotensin II also is produced *within* the myocardial tissue (i.e., tissue-derived), and several of the circulating components, such as renin and angiotensinogen, are involved in tissue angiotensin II formation. However, at least in the human heart, angiotensin II is formed by non–angiotensin-converting enzyme–dependent mechanisms involving different enzyme systems (e.g., cathepsin G, chymostatin-sensitive angiotensin II–generating system, and heart chymase).[38] Activation of serine proteases (enzymes) is associated with an increase in myocardial tissue angiotensinogen gene expression, and stretch resulting from increased wall stress increases the release of angiotensin II from cytoplasmic (within the cell) granules.[37] Once angiotensin II is secreted from the cell, it acts in a paracrine manner to stimulate neighboring myocytes and fibroblasts.

Similar to increased norepinephrine plasma levels, increased plasma levels of angiotensin II are correlated to increased morbidity and mortality.[39] The stimulus for angiotensin II production is renal hypoperfusion and hypotension. Norepinephrine also stimulates $beta_1$ adrenoreceptors in the juxtaglomerular apparatus to secrete renin.[40] Circulating angiotensin II stimulates vasoconstriction, aldosterone secretion, increased reabsorption of sodium, and presynaptic release of norepinephrine from postganglionic nerve terminals. Circulating and tissue-derived angiotensin II play roles in stimulating myocyte hypertrophy, apoptosis, and fibroblast proliferation with subsequent production of collagen. In addition, in other in vitro cell studies, investigators have found that angiotensin II enhanced the production of local free radicals such as superoxides.[37]

Aldosterone is another hormone involved in systolic heart failure. Aldosterone is a mineralocorticoid synthesized in the zona glomerulosa of the adrenal cortex.[41] Aldosterone stimulates distal renal tubule sodium reabsorption. In systolic heart failure patients, plasma aldosterone levels are much greater compared with age-matched healthy control subjects.[39] The increased aldosterone levels may be due to angiotensin II–stimulated aldosterone release, as well as decreased aldosterone hepatic clearance.[41] In addition, fibroblasts that have been transformed into myofibroblasts (via transforming growth factor beta) secrete aldosterone. In terms of the remodeling process, aldosterone stimulates fibroblast proliferation and collagen accumulation and is therefore thought to be a key contributor in extracellular matrix remodeling.[34] Aldosterone, via increased sodium reabsorption, also contributes to edema formation.

Cytokines

Plasma levels of cytokines such as TNF-α, are elevated in heart failure patients compared with control patients.[42,43] Cytokines are proteins released by cells such as macrophages and are important in stimulating different aspects of the immune response. For example, proinflammatory cytokines stimulate the synthesis of other inflammatory mediators such as platelet-activating factor, eicosanoids, and oxidative radicals. In the setting of heart failure the major source of plasma TNF-α is the heart itself. TNF-α contributes to the remodeling process by stimulating apoptosis, necrosis, and cell proliferation. Also, in systolic heart failure, increased cytokine levels are associated with several adverse effects such as decreased contractility, pulmonary edema, decreased peripheral organ perfusion, anorexia, and cachexia.[44]

In systolic heart failure patients, there are increased plasma levels of another cytokine-like molecule, endothelin-1. Endothelin-1 is potent vasoconstrictor released from endothelial cells. In normal or healthy conditions, there is little to no release of endothelin-1. However, significantly increased plasma levels are primarily found in patients with severe heart failure (New York Heart Association Class IV).[45] Because the major source of endothelin-1 is endothelial cells, increased endothelin-1 levels may reflect endothelial cell injury or dysfunction. Endothelin-1 is a potent vasoconstrictor, and adverse effects in the setting of heart failure may include increased blood pressure (afterload) and increased pulmonary vasculature resistance. Endothelin-1 also stimulates the conversion of angiotensin I to angiotensin II and may potentiate some of the effects of angiotensin II.[46]

Oxidative Stress

Oxidative stress is defined as the exposure of a cell or tissue to an excess of reactive oxygen species (**ROS**). Oxidative stress occurs when there is an imbalance in the level of ROS and antioxidant defense mechanisms. ROS include free radicals, such as superoxide anion ($O_2^-\bullet$), protonated superoxide anion ($HO_2\bullet$), and hydroxyl radical ($OH\bullet$), as well as partially reduced forms of oxygen, such as hydrogen peroxide (H_2O_2) and singlet oxygen ($^1O_2$).[47]

ROS can be generated in the cytosol or within different intracellular structures such as the mitochondria. ROS are generated within the cytosol or mitochondria via different redox reactions including enzyme-substrate reactions (xanthine oxidase) and autooxidation of molecules (catecholamines). In terms of intracellular organelles, the mitochondria are one of the most important sites for the generation and release of ROS. In the mitochondria, a small percentage of electrons leak out from the electron transport chain and combine (or pass) directly to oxygen, forming $HO_2\bullet$, which in turn is converted to hydrogen peroxide. Other ROS are generated in a series of primary and secondary reactions (some ROS serve as precursors for other ROS).[47]

Accumulation of ROS within the mitochondria and cytosol can cause many degrees of cell and tissue injury.

The highly reactive ROS can react with DNA, proteins, carbohydrates, and lipids in a destructive manner. Consequently, the cell and mitochondria have evolved an elaborate system of antioxidant defense mechanisms to combat oxidative stress. Even though there are several reports of elevated oxidative stress markers in patients with heart failure, the exact role of ROS in the development and progression of heart failure is not known.[48] Several clinical trials are under way to evaluate the effects of drugs believed to interfere with the formation and accumulation of free radicals.

Natriuretic Peptides

The natriuretic peptides include ANP, BNP, and C-type natriuretic peptide. This discussion is limited to ANP and BNP because these peptides are most relevant in the setting of heart failure. The nature and role of natriuretic peptides in heart failure is twofold. First, the natriuretic peptides may be involved in the pathogenesis of heart failure because, in heart failure, the physiological response to the natriuretic peptides is attenuated, and this may contribute to increased water and sodium retention. Secondly, in the setting of systolic heart failure the remodeled ventricle becomes a major source for circulating BNP; therefore, BNP has emerged as an important biomarker of LV dysfunction and development of systolic heart failure.

ANP and BNP are released from cardiac cells (atrial and ventricular cells) in response to stretch (increased preload). The major physiological actions of the natriuretic peptides are natriuresis, diuresis, and arterial and venous vasodilatation. The natriuretic and diuretic effects of the natriuretic peptides are due to renal hemodynamic and direct tubular actions.[49,50] The afferent renal arterioles are stimulated to dilate, and the efferent arterioles constrict, leading to increased pressure within the glomerular capillaries and resulting in increased glomerular filtration. Binding of the natriuretic peptides to their specific receptor subtype stimulates the formation of the second messenger, cyclic guanosine monophosphate, in renal mesangial cells, which relax the cells and ultimately increase the effective surface area for filtration.[50] In addition, ANP and BNP inhibit sodium and water transport in the proximal convoluted tubules and inhibit tubular sodium transport in the inner medullary collecting duct.[51] ANP and BNP also attenuate norepinephrine release and sympathetic activation.

Theoretically, high levels of these natriuretic peptides should serve a compensatory and not an adverse effect. However, in the setting of systolic heart failure, many of the physiological effects of the natriuretic peptides are attenuated. Some researchers have shown that there is a decreased renal response of the natriuretic peptides that may be related to natriuretic peptide receptor downregulation and/or increased ANP and BNP degradation.[52] Others have suggested that the levels of the other hormones, specifically angiotensin-II and norepinephrine, may be too high to be antagonized by the natriuretic peptides.

ANP and BNP have been used as biomarkers of heart failure onset and progression. However, BNP has emerged as the more important diagnostic marker. Under normal physiological conditions, the ventricles do not synthesize or secrete BNP. However, in the setting of systolic heart failure, the ventricle becomes the primary source of BNP. Also important to note is that the left ventricle does not store BNP in secretory granules. Instead, as the ventricle synthesizes BNP, the peptide is released via a constitutive pathway, indicating that there is no processing or storage of this peptide. In systolic heart failure, BNP plasma levels increase much more rapidly compared with ANP plasma levels, and BNP plasma levels exceed ANP plasma levels.[53]

BNP plasma levels are currently approved for the diagnosis of heart failure. BNP values (Triage BNP assay, Biosite Diagnostics, San Diego, California) for healthy persons aged 55 to 64 years of age are 26 ± 1.8 pg/ml, and values for older healthy persons (older than 75 years of age) are around 63 ± 6 pg/ml. Women tend to have somewhat higher values. Levels of BNP greater than 100 pg/ml are considered diagnostic for heart failure.[54] BNP also is used in the treatment of decompensated heart failure and exerts vasodilatory, natriuretic, and diuretic effects.[55]

DIASTOLIC HEART FAILURE: PATHOPHYSIOLOGICAL FEATURES

Diastolic heart failure is due to an isolated abnormality in diastolic function and is characterized by signs and symptoms of heart failure with a preserved ejection fraction.[6] Vasan and Levy[56] have put forth the following diagnostic criteria for diastolic heart failure: (1) definite evidence of congestive heart failure, (2) objective evidence of normal systolic function with an ejection fraction greater than 50 percent within 72 hours of an episode of congestive heart failure, and (3) objective evidence of diastolic dysfunction on cardiac catheterization. If all the criteria are present, the patient has the diagnosis of diastolic heart failure; however, if the first two criteria are present, the diagnosis is probable rather than definitive.

How is diastolic function evaluated in the clinical setting? To begin with, in healthy individuals there are four phases to diastole: (1) isovolumic relaxation, in which there is a large decrease in LV pressure at a constant LV volume; (2) the rapid diastolic filling phase, in which there is a rapid increase in LV volume with a variable and small increase in LV pressure (rate of change in LV volume [dV/dt] reaches its maximum and the peak filling rate occurs); (3) diastasis; and (4) atrial systole, in which atrial contraction fills the LV to its end-diastole volume (Figure 62-7).[57] The last three phases also collectively are referred to as the auxotonic relaxation phase. At the whole heart level, many variables can affect diastolic filling, and diastole is an active or energy-requiring process (Table 62-4).

Diastole occurs as a result of ATP-stimulated calcium uptake into the sarcoplasmic reticulum and extrusion across the sarcolemma (see Figure 62-4, step 4). In patients with diastolic heart failure, the isovolumic pressure decline is prolonged, and auxotonic relaxation is

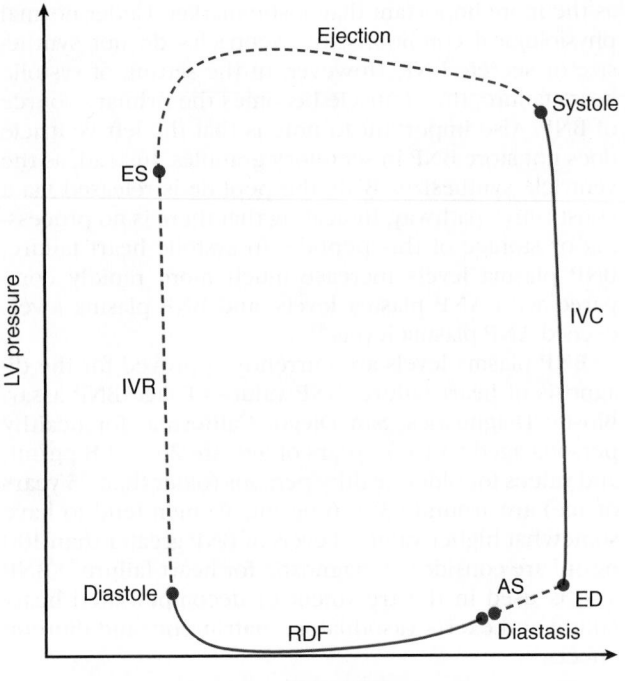

FIGURE 62-7 ■ The four phases of diastole: (1) isovolumic relaxation (IVR), in which there is a large decrease in left ventricular (LV) pressure at a constant LV volume; (2) the rapid diastolic filling (RDF) phase, in which there is a rapid increase in LV volume with a variable and small increase in LV pressure (rate of change in left ventricular volume [dV/dt] reaches its maximum and the peak filling rate occurs); (3) diastasis (D); and (4) atrial systole (AS), in which atrial contraction fills the LV to its end-diastole volume. *ED,* End diastolic; *ES,* end systolic; *IVC,* inverior vena cava. (From Apstein CS: Diastolic dysfunction: pathophysiology, clinical features and treatment. In Colucci WS, editor: *Atlas of heart failure cardiac function and dysfunction,* ed 4, Philadelphia, 2005, Current Medicine.)

■ ■ ■

TABLE 62-4 DETERMINANTS AND VARIABLES INVOLVED IN DIASTOLE

	MAJOR DETERMINANTS OF LEFT VENTRICULAR FILLING
Whole heart determinants and cellular time course of diastole	Rate and extent of left ventricular pressure decay
	Elastic recoil or restoring force of myocardium
	Small transmitral gradients
	Low-resistance mitral valve orifice gradients
	High distensibility or low passive stiffness of left ventricle
	Force of atrial contraction
	Lack of external constraint from pericardium, pleura, lungs, intrathoracic pressure
Cellular event responsible for diastole	**Early Diastole**
	Myocyte relaxation and relengthening
	Cytosolic calcium removal via sarcoplasmic calcium SERCA2a uptake
	Sarcolemmal calcium efflux via the sodium/calcium exchanger and calcium ATPase pump
	Actin-myosin cross-bridge detachment
	Expansion of compressed titin
	Left ventricular elastic recoil
	Transmitral pressure gradient from left ventricular suction
	Late Diastole
	Left ventricular passive stiffness
	Left atrial function

SERCA2, Sarcoplasmic reticulum Ca^{2+}.
Data from Apstein CS: Diastolic dysfunction: pathophysiology, clinical features and treatment. In Colucci WS, editor: *Atlas of heart failure cardiac function and dysfunction,* ed 4, Philadelphia, 2005, Current Medicine.

characterized by elevated diastolic filling pressures reflecting abnormalities in the active aspect of relaxation and the passive stiffness of the ventricle. A hallmark sign is that, during rapid diastolic filling, small increases in diastolic volume are associated with significant increases in LV pressure (Figure 62-8, panel C).[57] The latter reflects an increase in myocardial stiffness and resistance to passive diastolic filling. Therefore at near normal filling intraventricular volumes, there is an elevated pressure. Over time an increased intraventricular pressure (high diastolic pressure) can compromise coronary perfusion and increase myocardial oxygen consumption.

In the clinical setting, a combination of techniques such as cardiac catheterization (radionuclide angiocardiography), pulsed wave Doppler and M-mode echocardiography are used to assess LV geometry, LV contraction and filling patterns, and mitral and pulmonary venous flow patterns.[57,58] An important aspect of the analysis is examination of LV inflow velocity and the volume rate of LV filling. LV filling is greatest during early diastole (after opening of the mitral valve), whereas velocity and filling are low toward the end of diastole (i.e., during diastasis and atrial systole). On the Doppler echocardiogram (Figure 62-9), the tall E wave represents early LV filling velocity, and the A wave represents late diastolic filling velocity as a consequence of atrial

contraction. A normal E wave/A wave ratio is greater than 1. In diastolic heart failure the rate and amount of early diastolic LV filling is reduced, with greater filling and velocity toward the end of diastole. This is reflected in a reversal of the E wave/A wave ratio, such that the A wave is greater than the E wave (see Figure 62-9, top and bottom panels).[57] Other parameters that are altered in the setting of diastolic heart failure are noted in Table 62-5 and reflect significant abnormalities in active relaxation and passive stiffness of the ventricle.

Some heart failure specialists have challenged the notion that heart failure can be solely due to isolated abnormalities in diastolic function.[58] However, recently Ziles and colleagues,[6] using cardiac catheterization and echocardiography, prospectively evaluated patients who met the diagnostic criteria for diastolic heart failure. In all patients, the time constant of isovolumic pressure decline, as well as parameters reflecting diastolic pressure (before and after atrial contraction) and measures of diastolic stiffness (i.e., diastolic pressure versus volume measurements), were significantly different compared with patients with no evidence of cardiovascular disease. The importance of this study is that it was the first to demonstrate that patients with heart failure and a normal ejection fraction have abnormal diastolic function.

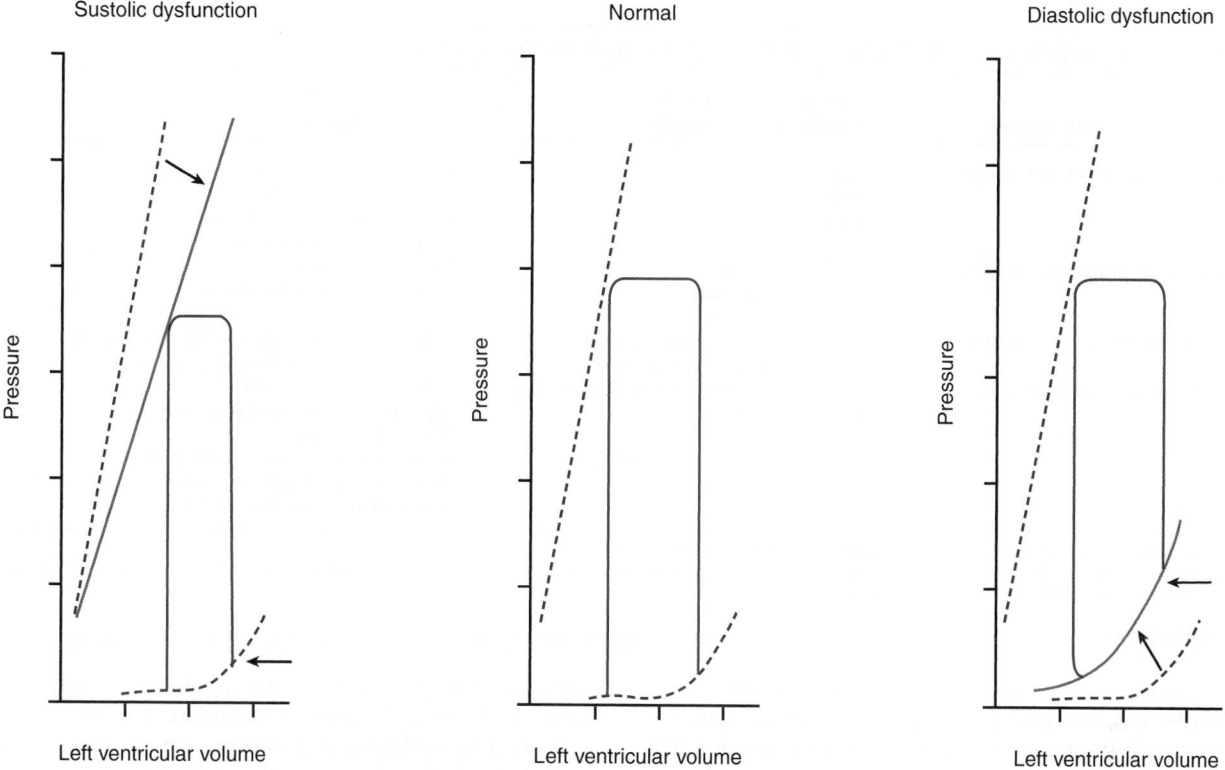

FIGURE 62-8 ■ Changes in the pressure-volume relationship with systolic and diastolic dysfunction compared with normal cardiac function. (Used with permission from Apstein CS: Diastolic dysfunction: pathophysiology, clinical features and treatment. In Colucci WS, editor: *Atlas of heart failure cardiac function and dysfunction,* ed 4, Philadelphia, 2005, Current Medicine.)

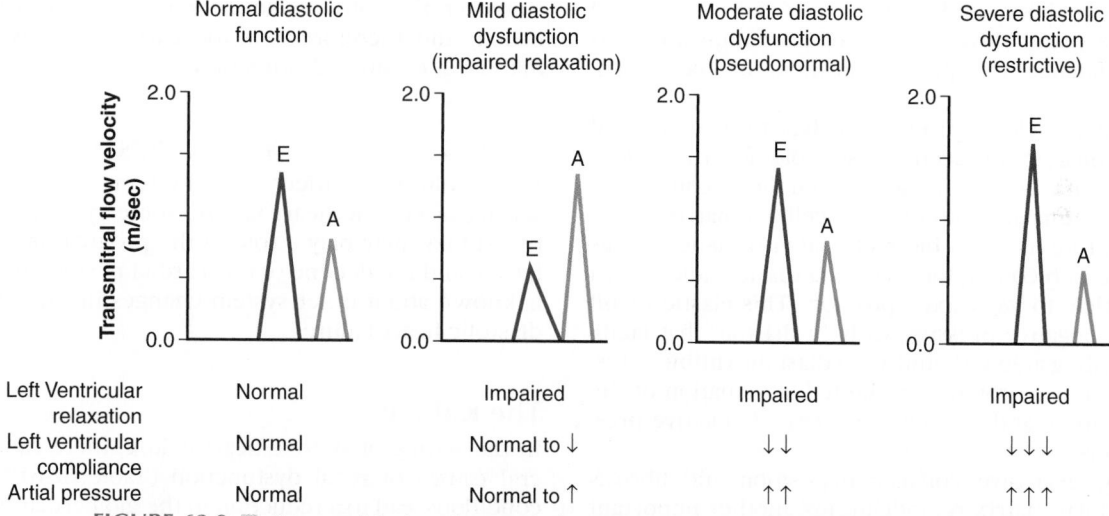

FIGURE 62-9 ■ *Top panel* depicts changes in the E wave to A wave relationship that occurs with varying forms of diastolic dysfunction. *Bottom panel* depicts a representative Doppler echocardiogram of E and A waves. (From Apstein CS: Diastolic dysfunction: pathophysiology, clinical features and treatment. In Colucci WS, editor: *Atlas of heart failure cardiac function and dysfunction,* ed 4, Philadelphia, 2005, Current Medicine.)

Cellular Mechanisms Underlying Diastolic Heart Failure

Cellular changes have been studied most extensively and systematically in the setting of systolic heart failure and only recently has attention shifted to diastolic heart failure. Theoretically, however, impaired relaxation can arise from alterations in calcium removal after systole or cross-bridge formation or from alterations in cytoskeleton and extracellular matrix proteins.[59] These potential changes are discussed next.

Relaxation is initiated by calcium removal from the cytosol, primarily by the sarcoplasmic reticulum SERCA2a pump. Prolonged calcium removal, which could occur with decreased SERCA2a activity, would greatly affect the reuptake of calcium into the sarcoplas-

■ ■ ■

TABLE 62-5 PARAMETERS AND CAUSES ASSOCIATED WITH DIASTOLIC DYSFUNCTION

PHYSIOLOGICAL ABNORMALITY	PARAMETER THAT REFLECTS THE RELAXATION ABNORMALITY	COMMON CAUSE
Delayed or incomplete relaxation	↑ Tau ↑ IVRT ↓ E wave/A wave ratio	Left ventricular hypertrophy Myocardial ischemia Left ventricular asynchrony ↑ Afterload and preload
Early diastolic filling abnormalities	↓ Peak filling rate ↓ E wave/A wave ratio ↑ Time to peak filling	Delayed relaxation Left ventricular asynchrony
Late diastolic filling abnormalities	↑ Diastolic pressure-volume relationship Normal or ↑ E wave/A wave ratio	Left ventricular chamber dilatation and thinning Restrictive/constrictive filing pattern
↑ Left ventricle passive chamber stiffness	↑ Diastolic pressure-volume relationship ↑ Stiffness constant	↑ Collagen and fibrosis Myocardial infiltration (e.g., amyloid) ↑ Vascular turgor Concentric left ventricular hypertrophy Post–myocardial infarction hypertrophy and fibrosis Left ventricle chamber dilatation

IVRT, Isovolumic relaxation time; *Tau,* time constant of isovolumic pressure decay.
Adapted from Apstein CS: Diastolic dysfunction: pathophysiology, clinical features and treatment. In Colucci WS, editor: *Atlas of heart failure cardiac function and dysfunction,* ed 4, Philadelphia, 2005, Current Medicine.

mic reticulum.[59,60] This could result in an increase in cytosolic calcium and prolongation of the systolic calcium transient, causing abnormalities in active relaxation and passive stiffness.[59] In terms of cross-bridge kinetics, calcium dissociation from the troponin complex (specifically troponin C) is critical for dissociation of the strong cross-bridge formation between actin and myosin and the cessation of cross-bridge cycling.[60] If calcium remains bound to troponin C for a prolonged time, this could slow the rate of relaxation and also could influence the passive stiffness of the ventricle.[57,59]

Many cytoskeleton proteins, such as titin, are critical in providing an intracellular scaffold for the lateral transmission of force among and from the sarcomeres to the sarcolemma and into the extracellular matrix. Some of these proteins act as bidirectional visoelastic springs that serve as recoiling forces during diastole and return the ventricle to its relaxed position. This elastic recoil creates a negative pressure early in diastole that facilitates LV filling at low LV and atrial diastolic (filling) pressures.[57] If these proteins are altered, attenuation of the recoiling force and amount of generated negative pressure occurs.

Finally, excessive collagen deposition and fibrosis (extracellular matrix remodeling) is another important cellular component affected in diastolic heart failure. Specifically, myocardial fibrosis contributes to the increase in myocardial mass, decreased myocardial compliance, and abnormalities in electrical conduction.[59]

Neurohormones

Compared with systolic heart failure, the role of neurohormones in the pathophysiology of diastolic heart failure has not been studied extensively, and diastolic heart failure patients have not been included in large-scale pharmacological trials. Angiotensin II and aldosterone more than likely are key pathophysiological chemical signals in the progression of diastolic heart failure because both neurohormones stimulate fibroblast proliferation and collagen deposition. Angiotensin II and endothelin-1 also slow the rate of relaxation, especially in hypertrophied hearts.[59]

Lubien and colleagues[61] found that serum levels of BNP correlated to increased diastolic pressures and abnormal Doppler echocardiographic filling patterns. However, the cutoff values have not been clearly established, and therefore it is too early to use BNP as a marker of diastolic dysfunction.

OTHER SYSTEM INVOLVEMENT

Heart failure can affect many systems. At least in the setting of systolic heart failure, some systems, such as the kidney, may play a role in the progression of heart failure and the decline of myocardial performance. Less is known about other system changes in the setting of diastolic heart failure.

The Kidney

In the setting of systolic heart failure, there can be several causes of renal dysfunction (Table 62-6).[62] These conditions lead to a reduction in the glomerular filtration rate (**GFR**) and may cause renal insufficiency and impaired excretion of creatinine and blood urea nitrogen. GFR in healthy young (65 years of age) individuals is defined as a 125 ml/min or 7.6 liters/hr or 180 liters/d. However, GFR is reduced with advancing age, and therefore there are ranges of normal values, which are defined according to a person's age (and sex).[63] Others have found that a GFR less than 60 ml/min is associated with an increased mortality rate in patients with heart failure.[64] Reduced renal function has important implications for dosing many pharmacological agents because many drugs are cleared by the kidney. Drugs such as aspirin, especially in patients with a history of MI, require further

■ ■ ■

TABLE 62-6 SIGNS AND SYMPTOMS OF HEART FAILURE AND DEFINITION AND UNDERLYING PATHOPHYSIOLOGICAL MECHANISMS

SIGN OR SYMPTOM	DEFINITION AND PATHOPHYSIOLOGICAL MECHANISM
*↓ Stroke volume, cardiac output/index, and ejection fraction (EF less than 40%)	Stroke volume (SV) is the amount of blood in milliliters ejected from the left ventricle (LV) into the aorta each time the heart contracts. SV is derived mathematically as follows: the end-diastolic volume (EDV; the amount of blood that fills the heart during diastole) − the end-systolic volume (amount of blood left in the LV after contraction) = SV.
	EF represents the amount of blood ejected from the LV relative to how much was delivered. EF is derived mathematically by the equation EDV/SV = EF. A normal EF should be greater than 60%.
†Tachycardia	Heart rate is increased to compensate for the decrease in SV (Cardiac output = SV × Heart rate).
*Ventricular dilatation and ↑ intraventricular volume	An increase in the entire ventricle occurs as a consequence of myocyte hypertrophy and interstitial fibrosis.
(This is usually characterized by an increase in LV end-diastolic pressure and volume and pulmonary artery occlusion pressure.)	Increase in ventricular chamber size occurs to accommodate chronic increases in preload; however, this is accompanied by an increased ventricular pressure because the heart already is stretched to the maximum part of the Starling curve.
†Peripheral and pulmonary edema (Usually characterized by elevated right atrial and pulmonary artery occlusion pressure; the goal of therapy in most patients is ≤8 mm Hg and ≤15 mm Hg, respectively)[73]	In systolic heart failure (SHF), Na^+ and H_2O retention leads to an increase in blood volume and venous hydrostatic pressure, which produces transudation of fluid into subcutaneous tissue. Additionally, there is a decrease in plasma levels of albumin because of altered liver function. ↑ Aldosterone and angiotensin II secretion in SHF.
	In diastolic heart failure (DHF), there is an increase in LV stiffness and ↑ vulnerability for pulmonary edema, rather than ↑ Na^+ retention and hormonal activation, and there is increased LV pressure with small or no change in LV volume.
†Paroxysmal nocturnal dyspnea	When a heart failure patient assumes a supine position, venous return from the peripheral extremities is increased. This "autotransfusion" of blood from the lower extremities back to the heart produces an abrupt increase in preload and left ventricular end-diastolic pressure (LVEDP), which is transmitted backward into the pulmonary circulation, leading to pulmonary alveolar edema.
†Crackles	The increased left ventricular end-diastolic volume and LVEDP are transmitted backward into the pulmonary circulation, causing an increase in pulmonary vein hydrostatic pressure. This leads to interstitial and pulmonary alveolar edema. However, many patients may not have pulmonary crackles because of a compensatory increase in pulmonary lymph flow.
†Hepatomegaly and splanchnic enlargement	Because of chronic venous congestion in the splanchnic vasculature (i.e., gastrointestinal circulation), fluid can move from the vascular compartment into the interstitial fluid compartment of various splanchnic tissues.
Liver dysfunction	Low perfusion and chronic venous congestion can lead to early stages of liver cirrhosis.
†S_3 and S_4	Early and late diastolic sounds, respectively.
	S_4—Late diastolic sound results from a forceful atrial contraction into a volume-loaded noncompliant ventricle (conditions found in ventricular hypertrophy and hypertrophic cardiomyopathy).
	S_3—Early diastolic sound caused by excessively rapid early diastolic filling and may arise because of a complex interplay of factors such as ventricular systolic dysfunction, ↑ end-diastolic and end-systolic volume, and ↓ EF; new onset in patient with history of cardiac disease may indicate volume overload and hemodynamic compromise.
†Fatigue and reduced cardiac reserve exercise capacity	In SHF, caused by a chronically low cardiac output and is limited along with skeletal muscle dysfunction.
	In DHF, one has a limited ability to use the Frank-Starling mechanism to increase SV during exercise.
†Dysrhythmias	Ventricular enlargement and fibrosis decreases conduction of cardiac impulses and increases susceptibility to reentrant impulses.
	Molecular abnormalities in ion channels (possibly L-type Ca^{2+} channel) may lead to ionic imbalances.
	Spontaneous calcium oscillations occur.
†Jugular vein distention	Increased central venous pressure caused by increases in venous blood volume.
†Cough	Cardiac asthma.
	Angiotensin-converting enzyme inhibitor therapy (caused by ↑ bradykinin levels).
†Sleep-related breathing disorders (little is known about prevalence in DHF)[68]	There are several sleep-related breathing disorders and causes[68]:
	• *Apnea:* Absence of inspiratory airflow for ≥10 seconds, and there are two types: obstructive (usually caused by upper airway occlusion) and central (caused by absence of activation of inspiratory muscles)
	• *Hypopnea:* Reduction in breathing that is ≥10 seconds in duration and results in a reduction in arterial oxyhemoglobin saturation
	In heart failure, the occurrence of these sleep-related disorders can be associated with the following: hypoxemia, hypercapnia, and hyperpnea. These in turn can contribute to a decrease in myocardial oxygen delivery, indirect activation of the sympathetic nervous system, pulmonary arterial vasoconstriction, nocturnal angina, and myocardial infarction.
	Gender specificity: Greater prevalence is found in men than in women.
†Enlarged pulmonary vessels on x-ray film and interstitial hydrothorax	Chronic pleural effusions that cause an increase in pleural capillary pressure and movement of fluid into pleural edema and cavities.

*Indicates possibility of occurring in systolic and diastolic heart failure.
†Indicates primarily systolic heart failure.
LVEDP, Left ventricular end-diastolic pressure.
Adapted from Piano MR, Bondmass M, Schwertz DW: *Heart Lung* 27:3-19, 1998.

Continued

■ ■ ■

TABLE 62-6   SIGNS AND SYMPTOMS OF HEART FAILURE AND DEFINITION AND UNDERLYING
PATHOPHYSIOLOGICAL MECHANISMS—cont'd

SIGN OR SYMPTOM	DEFINITION AND PATHOPHYSIOLOGICAL MECHANISM
†Confusion, difficulty in concentrating, impaired memory, headaches, and anxiety	Chronically decreased cerebral perfusion (caused by vascular disease or multiple microemboli), transient hypotension, low serum albumin, sodium and potassium levels, hyperglycemia, and anemia.
Blood pressure changes (↑ or ↓) (Elevated systemic vascular resistance; goal of therapy in most patients is 1000-1200 dynes-sec·cm⁻⁵)[73]	↓ Systolic and diastolic blood pressure caused by low cardiac output ↑ Blood pressure and ↑ systemic vascular resistance caused by vasoconstriction and elevated neurohormone levels.
Decreased clearance of administered medications and metabolism of hormones (e.g., aldosterone)	Chronic hepatomegaly and liver dysfunction (as described above).
†Ischemia and chest pain	↑ LV dilatation and LV volume are associated with an increase in wall stress and oxygen consumption, which usually cannot be met with an increase in flow because of coronary artery disease. Reduced coronary blood flow is caused by increases in LVEDP and impaired diffusion of oxygen in the hypertrophied myocardium. The intercapillary distance ↑ between the myocyte and capillary because of the hypertrophy and interstitial collagen accumulation. ↓ In the time the heart spends in diastole because of ↑ heart rate. If one considers the entire duration of the cardiac cycle as 100%, diastole should represent 60%-70% of that cycle and systole 30%. The majority of LV perfusion occurs during diastole; therefore, a decrease in the duration of diastole can comprise coronary artery perfusion of the LV. The right ventricle is less affected because the changes in pressure during systole are less (because of the force of right ventricular contraction and right intraventricular pressures). ↑ In ventricular filling pressures with reduced coronary perfusion pressure and ↓ blood flow gradient from the epicardium to endocardium.

LV, Left ventricular; *LVEDP,* left ventricular end diastolic pressure.

BOX 62-1   ■ ■ ■
CAUSES OF RENAL DYSFUNCTION IN HEART FAILURE

Inadequate Renal Perfusion
Hypovolemia (inadequate preload)
Inadequate cardiac output (excessive vasoconstriction)
Hypotension with normal cardiac output but low systemic vascular resistance (vasodilatory shock)
Hypotension with low cardiac output (severe pump failure, cardiogenic shock)
Abnormally high central venous pressures

Drug-Induced
Nonsteroidal antiinflammatory drugs
Cyclosporine
Angiotensin-converting enzyme inhibitors
Angiotensin receptor blockers

Intrinsic Renal Disease
Renal vascular disease
Nephron loss (diabetes, hypertension)
Diuretic resistance

Data from Heywood JT: *Heart Fail Rev* 9:195-201, 2004.

caution and as noted in Box 62-1 can be a cause of renal dysfunction. Aspirin and other nonsteroidal antiinflammatory agents inhibit prostaglandin formation. In the kidney, prostaglandins are vasodilators and usually have protective effects on renal blood flow, especially in the setting of high levels of angiotensin II and sympathetic activation.[65] Therefore, patients receiving aspirin or other nonsteroidal antiinflammatory drugs do not have the protective function of prostaglandin formation. Aspirin and nonsteroidal antiinflammatory drugs can cause sodium retention. Some experts have suggested that the adverse effects of aspirin are dose-dependent; however, this remains controversial, and even low-dose aspirin likely inhibits prostaglandin formation.[66]

Reduced renal artery perfusion is a major stimulus for renin secretion from the juxtaglomerular apparatus, increased sodium and water absorption from the renal tubules, and aldosterone release.[41] Therefore, altered renal function is an important mechanisms leading to increased fluid and water retention in heart failure. Increased sodium and water absorption from the renal tubules increases preload and stretch, activating signals involved in the remodeling process. Excessive sodium and water absorption are also responsible for the signs and symptoms of fluid overload.

Skeletal Muscle Changes

As the syndrome of heart failure progresses, patients develop skeletal muscle dysfunction, which may contribute to decreased exercise tolerance, fatigue, and an overall decline in functional capacity. The skeletal muscle dysfunction is characterized by muscle atrophy, a change in the muscle fiber type ratio (increased fast-twitch glycolytic and decreased slow-twitch oxidative fibers), decreased capillary density, and changes in muscle metabolism. Collectively, these changes affect the amount of muscle mass, muscle performance (strength and endurance), ATP production and utilization, and blood flow reserve.[67] The overall decrease in muscle mass or muscle body wasting is referred to as cardiac cachexia. The mechanisms that underlie these aspects of skeletal muscle dysfunction are not completely known but may be due to increased levels of TNF-α and interleukins. These cytokines can decrease protein synthesis and increase protein catabolism. Finally, it is important to note that many of these changes also are found in sedentary patients and are thought to be related to muscle disuse. So perhaps some of the described changes are not specific or resulting from heart failure per se but rather are a consequence of muscle disuse (lack of physical activity).[67]

Pulmonary Function Changes

Many pulmonary and diaphragmatic changes occur in heart failure, as noted in Box 62-2. Dyspnea is a common and debilitating heart failure symptom and most likely arises from a combination of the factors.[68] Some of these changes (such as ventilation/perfusion abnormalities, which may alter arterial oxygen concentrations) also may contribute to the progression of heart failure. The diaphragm, which is composed of skeletal muscle fibers similar to the peripheral skeletal muscles, develops a myopathy, most likely resulting from similar mechanisms.

Cognitive Impairment and Brain Changes

Patients with heart failure do not uncommonly experience cognitive impairment.[69] Cognitive impairment can involve or be defined as impairments in, or partial or full loss of, perception, attention, memory, judgment, thinking (particularly abstract), decision making, language, nonverbal communication, problem solving, rote learning, and generalization.[70] In the setting of heart failure, causes of cognitive impairment can be decreased cerebral perfusion (because of vascular disease or multiple microemboli) and transient hypotension. Recently, Zuccala and colleagues[69] found low serum albumin, sodium, and potassium levels; hyperglycemia; anemia; and systolic blood pressure levels were associated independently with cognitive impairment. Most importantly, normalization of glucose, potassium, and hemoglobin levels during the patient's hospital stay was associated with increased cognitive performance at discharge.[69]

Woo and colleagues[71] also have reported that some patients with heart failure may undergo loss of brain gray matter in a variety of brain areas such as the insula and basal ganglia, right cingulate gyrus, parahippocampal/fusiform gyrus, and dorsal midbrain. These investigators speculated that loss of gray matter in these areas potentially could contribute to cognitive impairment, as well as inappropriate autonomic and breathing regulation in heart failure.

CIRCULATORY CHANGES AND SIGNS AND SYMPTOMS

In heart failure, there are can be changes in many circulatory or hemodynamic parameters. At one time, heart failure was defined and conceptualized as a circulatory/hemodynamic disorder that arose because of changes in renal and neurohormonal function, manifested by decreased cardiac output, arterial underfilling, and venous and pulmonary congestion.[72] The treatment strategies primarily were aimed at reducing the signs and symptoms associated with these circulatory changes, as well as sodium and water retention. This paradigm emphasized the importance of treating increased afterload (using vasodilators) and preload (using vasodilators and diuretics) and increasing myocardial contractility (using inotropes and cardiac glycosides).[72] However, it is now realized that heart failure is not just a hemodynamic disorder. As emphasized in this chapter, the development and progression of systolic and diastolic heart failure is due to ventricular remodeling, and most treatment strategies are designed to attenuate the remodeling process. However, despite this therapeutic approach, hemodynamic alterations and their associated signs and symptoms occur in patients with systolic and diastolic heart failure. In systolic and diastolic heart failure, these signs and symptoms may arise from different mechanisms, and in both situations the patient requires treatment. Heart failure signs and symptoms and hemodynamic changes, along with their definition and underlying pathophysiological mechanisms, are listed in Table 62-6. Although beyond the scope of this chapter, some hemodynamic parameters such as resting cardiac output/cardiac index, right atrial pressure/volume, pulmonary artery diastolic pressure, pulmonary wedge pressure, and systemic vascular resistance are used for patient selection for heart transplant and to guide treatment of acute decompensated heart failure.[73]

SUMMARY

In the United States, heart failure has reached epidemic proportions. In the continuum of cardiovascular disease, chronic heart failure is an end event that can be initiated by a number of cardiovascular conditions; however, the most prevalent causes and risk factors are MI, hypertension, and diabetes mellitus. Heart failure is defined and classified as diastolic heart failure or systolic heart failure. Systolic heart failure is defined as the inability of the ventricle to contract and eject a sufficient amount of blood, whereas diastolic heart failure is defined as the inability of the ventricle to relax sufficiently and fill with blood. Systolic heart failure and diastolic heart failure arise from a number of changes in myocyte and nonmyocyte structure and function. These cell changes are stimulated by hemodynamic and chemical signals that ultimately lead to ventricular remodeling, myocardial dysfunction, and heart failure signs and symptoms. Many cellular events and signals are activated in heart failure, which makes this syndrome complex pathophysiologically. Many physiological systems are redundant; therefore, it is not unlikely that many systems must fail and/or be activated for the heart itself to fail and lose its ability to maintain cardiac output and sufficiently relax.

REFERENCES

1. Davies RC, Hobbs FDR, Lip GYH: ABC of heart failure, history and epidemiology, *BMJ* 320:39-42, 2000.
2. Hunt SA, Abraham WT, Chin MH et al: *ACC/AHA 2005 guideline update for the diagnosis and management of chronic heart failure in the adult: a report of the American College of Cardiology/American Heart Association Task Force on Practice Guidelines (Writing Committee to Update the 2001 Guidelines for the Evaluation and Management of Heart Failure).* Retrieved January 30, 2007 from http://circ.ahajournals.org/cgi/content/full/112/12/e154f
3. O'Conner CM, Gattis WA, Teerlink JR et al: Design considerations and proposed template for clinical trials in hospitalized patients with decompensated chronic heart failure, *Am Heart J* 145(2 suppl):S47-S52, 2003.
4. Felker GM, Adams KF, Konstam MA et al: The problem of decompensated heart failure: nomenclature, classification, and risk stratification, *Am Heart J* 145:S18-S25, 2003.
5. Philbin EP, Rocco TA, Lindenmuth NW et al: Systolic versus diastolic heart failure in community practices: clinical features, outcomes, and the use of angiotensin-converting enzyme inhibitors, *Am J Med* 109:605-613, 2000.
6. Zile MR, Baicu CF, Gassch WH: Diastolic heart failure: abnormalities in active relaxation and passive stiffness of the left ventricle, *N Engl J Med* 350:1953-1959, 2004.
7. Zile MR, Baicu CF, Bonnema DD, Diastolic heart failure: Definitions and terminology. Progress in Cardiovascular Diseases 47(50:307-313,2005.
8. Levy D, Larson MG, Vasan RS et al: The progression from hypertension to congestive heart failure, *JAMA* 275:1557-1562, 1996.
9. Mandinov L, Eberli FR, Seiler C, Hess OM: Diastolic heart failure, *Cardiovasc Res* 45:813-825, 2000.
10. Pfeffer MC: Cardiac remodeling and its prevention. In Braunwald E, editor: *Atlas of heart diseases: heart failure—cardiac function and dysfunction,* New York, 1995, Mosby.
11. Pfeffer MA, Pfeffer JM: Ventricular enlargement and reduced survival after myocardial infarction, *Circulation* 75(suppl):IV-93–IV-97, 1987.
12. Kass DA: Systolic dysfunction in heart failure. In Mann DL, editor: *Heart failure: a companion to Braunwald's heart disease,* Philadelphia, 2004, Saunders.
13. Kitzman DW, Little WC, Brubaker PH et al: Pathophysiologic characterization of isolated diastolic heart failure in comparison to systolic heart failure, *JAMA* 288:2144-2150, 2002.
14. Lindsey ML, Mann DL, Entman ML, Spinale FG: Extracellular matrix remodeling following myocardial injury, *Ann Med* 35:316-326, 2003.
15. Anand IS, Florea VG: Alterations in ventricular structure: role of left ventricular remodeling. In Mann DL, editor: *Heart failure: a companion to Braunwald's heart disease,* Philadelphia, 2004, Saunders.
16. Izumo S, Pu WT: The molecular basis of heart failure. In Mann DL, editor: *Heart failure: a companion to Braunwald's heart disease,* Philadelphia, 2004, Saunders.
17. Anversa P, Kajstura J: Ventricular myocytes are not terminally differentiated in the adult mammalian heart, *Circ Res* 83:1-14, 1998.
18. Nadal-Ginard B, Kajstura J, Leri A et al: Myocyte death, growth, and regeneration in cardiac hypertrophy and failure, *Circ Res* 92:139-150, 2003.
19. Houser SR, Margulies KB: Is depressed myocyte contractility centrally involved in heart failure? *Circ Res* 92:350-364, 2003.
20. Gerdes AM, Kellerman SE, Moore JA et al: Structural remodeling of cardiac myocytes in patients with ischemic cardiomyopathy, *Circulation* 86:426-430, 1992.
21. Sawyer DB, Colucci WS: Molecular and cellular events in myocardial hypertrophy and failure. In Colucci WS, editor: *Atlas of heart failure: cardiac function and dysfunction,* Philadelphia, 2005, Current Medicine.
22. Piano MR, Jarvis C: Cellular events linked to cardiac remodeling in heart failure: targets for pharmacologic intervention, *J Cardiovasc Nurs* 14:1-23, 2000.
23. Foo R S-Y, Mani K, Kitsis RN: Death begets failure in the heart, *J Clin Invest* 115:656-571, 2005.
24. Nanji AA, Hiller-Strumhofel S: Apoptosis and necrosis: two types of cell death in alcoholic liver disease, *Alcohol Health Res World* 21:325-330, 1997.
25. Anversa P, Leri A, Kajstura J: Myocardial basis for heart failure: role of cell death. In Mann DL, editor: *Heart failure: a companion to Braunwald's heart disease,* Philadelphia, 2004, Saunders.
26. Caulfield JB, Norton P, Weaver RD: Cardiac dilatation associated with collagen alterations, *Mol Cell Biochem* 118:171-179, 1992.
27. Pelouch V, Dixon IMC, Golfman L et al: Role of the extracellular matrix proteins in heart function, *Mol Cell Biochem* 129:101-120, 1994.
28. Carver W, Terracio L, Borg TK: Cell-matrix interactions: matrix receptors in the development and maintenance of the heart. In *molecular biology of collagen matrix in the heart,* Austin, Texas, 1994, RG Landes.
29. Booz GW, Baker KM: Molecular signaling mechanisms controlling growth and function of cardiac fibroblasts, *Cardiovasc Res* 30:537-543, 1995.
30. Weber KT, Sun Y, Tyagi SC et al: Collagen network of the myocardium: functional, structural remodeling and regulatory mechanisms, *J Mol Cell Cardiol* 26:279-292, 1994.
31. Drexler H, Hornig B: Role of peripheral circulation and endothelial cell dysfunction. In Mann DL, editor: *Heart failure: a companion to Braunwald's heart disease,* Philadelphia, 2004, Saunders.
32. Linder L, Kiowski W, Buhler FR et al: Indirect evidence for release of endothelium-derived relaxing factor in human forearm circulation in vivo: blunted response in essential hypertension, *Circulation* 81:1762-1767, 1990.
33. Yamazaki T, Komuro I, Yazaki Y: Molecular mechanisms of cardiac cellular hypertrophy by mechanical stress, *J Mol Cell Cardiol* 27:133-140, 1995.
34. Sadoshima J-I, Jahn L, Takahashi T et al: Molecular characterizations of the stretch-induced adaptation of cultured cardiac cells: an in vitro model of load-induced cardiac hypertrophy, *J Biol Chem* 267:10551-10560, 1992.
35. Cohn JN, Levine TB, Oivari MT et al: Plasma norepinephrine as a guide to prognosis in patients with congestive heart failure, *N Engl J Med* 311:819-823, 1984.
36. Simpson PC, Karija K, Karns LR et al: Adrenergic hormones and control of cardiac myocyte growth, *Mol Cell Biochem* 104:35-43, 1991.
37. Dzau VJ, Pratt RE: Renin-angiotensins system. In Fozzard HA, Haber E, Jennings RB, editors: *The heart and cardiovascular system,* ed 2, New York, 1992, Raven Press.
38. Simko F, Simko J: Heart failure and angiotensin converting enzyme inhibition: problems and perspectives, *Physiol Res* 48:1-8, 1999.
39. Swedberg K, Eneroth P, Kjekshus J et al: Hormones regulating cardiovascular function in patients with severe congestive heart failure and their relation to mortality (follow-up of the CONSENSUS Trial), *Am J Cardiol* 66:40D-45D, 1990.
40. Cody R: The integrated effects of angiotensin II, *Am J Cardiol* 79(5A):9-11, 1997.
41. Greenspan FS, Strewler GJ: *Basic & clinical endocrinology,* ed 5, Stamford, Conn, 1997, Appleton and Lange.
42. Torre-Amione G, Kapadia S, Benedict C: Proinflammatory cytokine levels in patients with depressed left ventricular fraction: a

report from the Studies of Left-Ventricular Dysfunction (SOLVD), *J Am Coll Cardiol* 27:1201-120, 1996.

43. Ferrari R, Bachetti T, Confortini R: Tumor necrosis factor soluble receptors in patients with various degrees of congestive failure, *Circulation* 92:1479-1486, 1995.

44. Torre-Amione G, Bozkurt B, Deswal A et al: An overview of tumor necrosis factor α and the failing human heart, *Curr Opin Cardiol* 14:206-210, 1999.

45. Wei C-M, Lerman A, Rodeheffer RJ et al: Endothelin in human congestive heart failure, *Circulation* 89:1580-1586, 1994.

46. Suresh DP, Lamba S, Abraham WT: New developments in heart failure: role of endothelin and of endothelin receptor antagonists, *J Card Fail* 6:359-368, 2000.

47. Kaul N, Siveski-Iliskovic N, Hill M et al: Free radicals and the heart, *J Pharmacol Toxicol Methods* 2:55-67, 1993.

48. Diaz-Velez CR, Garcia-Castineras S, Mendoza-Ramos E et al: Increased malondialdehyde in peripheral blood of patients with congestive heart failure, *Am Heart J* 131:146-152, 1996.

49. Levin E, Gardner D, Samson W: Natriuretic peptides, *N Engl J Med* 339:321-328, 1998.

50. Ruskoaho H: Atrial natriuretic peptide: synthesis, release, and metabolism, *Pharmacol Rev* 44:479-601, 1992.

51. Marin-Grez M, Fleming J, Steinhausen M: Atrial natriuretic peptide causes pre-glomerular vasodilatation and post-glomerular vasoconstriction in rat kidney, *Nature* 324:473-476, 1986.

52. Dillingham M, Anderson R: Inhibition of vasopressin action by atrial natriuretic factor, *Science* 231:1572-1573, 1986.

53. Troughton RW, Frampton CM, Yandle TG et al: Treatment of heart failure guided by plasma aminoterminal brain natriuretic peptide (N-BNP) concentrations, *Lancet* 351:9-13, 1998.

54. Yamamoto K, Burnett JC Jr, Burmudez EA et al: Clinical criteria and biochemical markers for the detection of systolic dysfunction, *J Card Fail* 6:194-200, 2000.

55. Colucci WS, Elkayam U, Horton DP et al: Intravenous nesiritide, a natriuretic peptide, in the treatment of decompensated congestive heart failure: Nesiritide Study Group, *N Engl J Med* 343:246-253, 2000.

56. Vasan RS, Levy D: Defining diastolic heart failure: a call for standardized diagnostic criteria, *Circulation* 101:2118-2121, 2000.

57. Apstein CS: Diastolic dysfunction: pathophysiology, clinical features and treatment. In Colucci WS, editor: *Atlas of heart failure cardiac function and dysfunction*, ed 4, Philadelphia, 2005, Current Medicine.

58. Burkhoff D, Maurer MS, Packer M: Heart failure with a normal ejection fraction: is it really a disorder of diastolic function? *Circulation* 107:656-658, 2003.

59. Zile MR, Baicu CF: Alterations in ventricular function: diastolic heart failure. In Mann DL, editor: *Heart failure: a companion to Braunwald's heart disease*, Philadelphia, 2004, Saunders.

60. Yano M, Ikeda Y, Matsuzaki M: Altered intracellular Ca^{2+} handling in heart failure, *J Clin Invest* 115:556-564, 2005.

61. Lubien E, De Maria A, Krishnaswamy P et al: Utility of B-natriuretic peptide in directing diastolic dysfunction: comparison with Doppler velocity recordings, *Circulation* 105:595-601, 2002.

62. Heywood JT: The cardiorenal syndrome: lessons from the ADHERE database and treatment options, *Heart Fail Rev* 9:195-201, 2004.

63. National Kidney Foundation: *National Kidney Foundation DOQI guidelines*, 2002. Retrieved January 30, 2007, from http://www.kidney.org/professionals/KDOQI/guidelines.cfm

64. Hillege HL, Girbes AR, de Kam PJ et al: Renal function, neurohormonal activation, and survival in patients with chronic heart failure, *Circulation* 102:203-210, 2000.

65. Burnett JC Jr, Costerllo-Boerrigter L, Boerrigter G: Alterations in the kidney in heart failure: the cardiorenal axis in the regulation of sodium homeostasis. In Mann DL, editors: *Heart failure: a companion to Braunwald's heart disease*, Philadelphia, 2004, Saunders.

66. Davie AP, Love MP, McMurray JJV: Even low-dose aspirin inhibits arachidonic acid-induced vasodilatation in heart failure, *Clin Pharmacol Ther* 67:530-537, 2000.

67. Le Jemtel T, Farr M, Moskowitz RM: Alterations in skeletal muscle in heart failure. In Mann DL, editor: *Heart failure: a companion to Braunwald's heart disease*, Philadelphia, 2004, Saunders.

68. Mancini DM, Lang CC: Alterations in pulmonary and diaphragmatic function in heart failure. In Mann DL, editor: *Heart failure: a companion to Braunwald's heart disease*, Philadelphia, 2004, Saunders.

69. Zuccala G, Marzetti E, Cesari M et al: Correlates of cognitive impairment among patients with heart failure: results of a multicenter survey, *Am J Med* 118:496-502, 2005.

70. Roman GC: Brain hypoperfusion: a critical factor in vascular dementia, *Neurol Res* 26:454-458, 2004.

71. Woo MA, Macey PM, Fonarow GC et al: Regional brain gray matter loss in heart failure, *J Appl Physiol* 95:677-684, 2003.

72. Piano MR, Bondmass M, Schwertz DW: The molecular and cellular pathophysiology of heart failure, *Heart Lung* 27:3-19, 1998.

73. Stevenson WL: Management of acute decompensation. In Mann DL, editor: *Heart failure: a companion to Braunwald's heart disease*, Philadelphia, 2004, Saunders.

chapter 63

Care of Patients with Acute Heart Failure

Sara Paul
Lisa Vollano

CHAPTER ABBREVIATIONS

ACEI   angiotensin-converting enzyme inhibitor

ADHERE   Acute Decompensated Heart Failure National Registry

ADHF   acute decompensated heart failure

ARB   angiotensin receptor blocker

BNP   B-type natriuretic peptide

IABP   intra-aortic balloon pump

LVAD   left ventricular assist device

PAOP   pulmonary artery occlusion pressure

At least 5 million persons in the United States have been diagnosed with heart failure, and approximately 550,000 new cases are diagnosed each year. Over the past two decades, the incidence of heart failure has not declined. In the United States, heart failure is the leading cause of hospitalization in persons over age 65 years, and there is no sign that another illness will overtake heart failure any time soon. The number of hospital discharges for heart failure rose 175 percent from 1979 to 2004.[1] Heart failure accounts for nearly 1 million hospitalizations each year, with an estimated direct and indirect cost of $33.2 billion in 2007. The leading cause of hospitalization for acute decompensated heart failure (**ADHF**) is exacerbation of chronic heart failure.[2] This chapter focuses on the management of acutely decompensated chronic heart failure. Acute heart failure as a complication of acute myocardial infarction is covered elsewhere.

As many as 50 percent of patients with ADHF are readmitted to the hospital within 6 months of discharge.[3] Common reasons for frequent readmissions include nonadherence to diet or medications, failure to seek medical care when symptoms arise, or receiving inappropriate therapy.[4] Patients can be readmitted if they were released from the hospital too early, before meeting appropriate discharge criteria such as stable fluid status, blood pressure, and renal function; freedom from dyspnea or dizziness; and at least 48 hours off of intravenous inotropic agents.[5] Other cardiac problems can precipitate ADHF, such as worsening ischemia, new myocardial infarction, worsened valvular function, and new onset of atrial fibrillation.[6] Noncardiac problems such as uncontrolled hypertension, pulmonary embolism, acute infection, substance abuse, renal or hepatic failure, and thyroid dysfunction also can precipitate ADHF.[6,7] Use of certain over-the-counter medications

such as nonsteroidal antiinflammatory drugs also can exacerbate heart failure and lead to ADHF.

According to the Acute Decompensated Heart Failure National Registry (**ADHERE**), the median age of patients admitted to the hospital for ADHF is about 75 years. Slightly more than half of patients are female, and most patients are white, but about 20 percent are black.[8] Medicare is the predominant payer, insuring about 72 percent of the patients. Common comorbidities in patients with ADHF include hypertension, coronary artery disease, diabetes, atrial fibrillation, obstructive pulmonary disease or asthma, and renal insufficiency. The majority of patients come to the emergency department with symptoms of ADHF, but about 20 percent are admitted directly to a hospital bed. Once admitted, 14 percent of patients are placed in an intensive care unit, whereas most are cared for on a telemetry or step-down unit. About 2 percent of patients with heart failure are admitted to the observation unit for short-term management and early discharge.[8]

ETIOLOGY

In recent years, it has become increasingly clear that heart failure is not simply a problem of poor cardiac pump function. Heart failure is a combination of factors that include decreased ventricular function (systolic or diastolic), reshaping or remodeling of the ventricle (dilatation or hypertrophy) and a confluence of hormone, cytokine, and neuroregulatory disturbances that ultimately result in decreased circulatory capability. The chief contributors to the development of heart failure are coronary artery disease and hypertension, both of which are found in 40 percent of patients with heart failure. Diabetes mellitus is also an independent risk factor for heart failure, and the incidence of diabetes has increased dramatically over the last several decades.[9,10] Other causes of heart failure include valve disorders, persistent tachydysrhythmias, inflammatory processes, toxins such as chemotherapy agents or alcohol abuse, connective tissue disorders, and thyroid abnormalities.

Regardless of the original cause of heart failure, it is a chronic condition that becomes progressively worse, culminating in the patient's premature death. Patients initially may remain asymptomatic or minimally symptomatic for months or years because of compensatory mechanisms that become activated in the presence of cardiac injury or depressed myocardial function. These compensatory mechanisms may include activation of the sympathetic nervous system, salt- and water-retaining systems, and activation of a number of vasodilatory

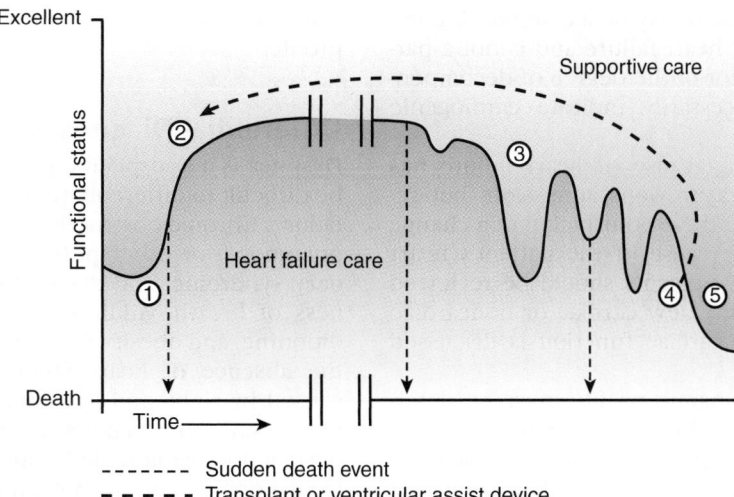

FIGURE 63-1 ■ Progression of heart failure. (From Goodlin SJ, Hauptman PJ, Arnold R et al: Consensus statement: palliative and supportive care in advanced heart failure, *J Card Fail* 10:200-209, 2004.)

molecules such as natriuretic peptides, prostaglandins, and nitric oxide. Knowledge about the full spectrum of compensatory systems in heart failure is incomplete, and much is yet to be learned.

Activation of neurohormonal and cytokine systems leads to adaptive changes in the myocardium, resulting in ventricular remodeling and represented by a change in the shape of the heart. A healthy heart is cone-shaped, like the bottom half of a football standing on end. After ventricular remodeling, the heart is more spherically shaped, like a basketball. At some point along the heart failure continuum, patients become overtly symptomatic with an accompanying increase in morbidity and mortality. The transition to symptomatic heart failure appears to occur independently of the patient's hemodynamic status. Continued activation of neurohormonal mechanisms and alterations in myocardial cell morphology and cardiac structures may explain why heart failure continues to progress over time following an index event such as myocardial infarction, despite the absence of ongoing ischemia. The neurohormonal model also may explain why the maladaptive mechanisms leading to remodeling and myocardial failure are remarkably consistent, regardless of the cause that initiated the heart failure. It should be noted that the term *neurohormonal* is a historical term, for a variety of other biologically active molecules such as norepinephrine, angiotensin II, endothelin, aldosterone, and tumor necrosis factor are produced within the heart and do not necessarily have a neuroendocrine origin.[11]

As the condition progresses, patients with chronic heart failure experience a downward trajectory of their illness over time with repeated episodes of decompensated heart failure, never fully recovering to their baseline of clinical stability after each exacerbation (Figure 63-1). "Decompensated" heart failure is defined as an abrupt worsening of New York Heart Association functional status by at least one class with evidence of fluid volume overload or increased left ventricular filling pressures.[6] Patients often are readmitted to the hospital for each episode of ADHF, contributing to soaring increases in direct and indirect health care costs. Eighty percent of hospital admissions for ADHF occur in patients with previously diagnosed heart failure.[7]

DIAGNOSIS
Clinical Presentation

Patients with ADHF often come to the hospital with symptoms indicative of fluid volume overload. The most common presenting signs and symptoms in patients with ADHF include dyspnea, rales, and peripheral edema.[8] Signs and symptoms of ADHF are listed in Box 63-1. An important note is that the absence of rales or peripheral edema in patients with chronic heart failure does not indicate an absence of fluid volume overload with elevated filling pressures in ADHF.[12] Patients usually describe rapid onset of their symptoms, from minutes to days before admission. Most patients admitted with ADHF have heart failure with systolic dysfunction, whereas heart failure with preserved systolic function accounts for about one-third to one-half of ADHF admissions.[7,13] Low blood pressure in the absence of other

---

BOX 63-1   ■ ■ ■
CLINICAL FEATURES OF ACUTE DECOMPENSATED HEART FAILURE

- Dyspnea/tachypnea
- S_3
- Jugular venous distention
- Hepatojugular reflux
- Edema of legs and/or feet
- Abdominal ascites
- Enlarged or pulsatile liver
- Tenderness to palpation in right upper quadrant
- Rales (although can be absent)
- Anxiety/apprehension

signs of decreased perfusion may be a common finding in patients with chronic heart failure and is not a particularly accurate indicator of the degree of decompensation, nor does it necessarily indicate cardiogenic shock.

Usually, the underlying cause of heart failure has been diagnosed during a previous admission, but re-evaluation is warranted if there is suspicion of a change in cardiac function. The cause of the patient's heart failure and exacerbating elements should be reviewed thoroughly to rule out any new cardiac or noncardiac problems. Evaluation of cardiac function is discussed later in this chapter.

The patient's hemodynamic profile must be determined in order to proceed along the appropriate course of therapy. Elevated filling pressures and decreased cardiac output make up the most common hemodynamic profile in decompensated heart failure. To frame the patient's hemodynamic situation in the context of being wet, dry, warm, or cold is helpful (Figure 63-2).[14] Wet or dry refers to the patient's fluid volume status, whereas warm or cold refers to the patient's cardiac output and peripheral perfusion. "Wet" patients have signs of fluid volume overload, such as dyspnea, edema, and elevated jugular venous pressure. "Dry" patients are those who do not have intravascular volume expansion or are volume depleted. "Warm" patients have adequate peripheral perfusion and adequate cardiac output. Those patients who are "cold" have poor cardiac output or decreased circulation with poor perfusion of body organs or extremities.

Of the four hemodynamic profiles, "warm and wet" is the most commonly seen in hospitalized patients. This means that the patient's perfusion is adequate (warm), but that fluid volume excess is present (wet). Patients who are admitted to the hospital with a diagnosis of ADHF but are warm and dry without volume overload or poor perfusion are probably symptomatic from some other cause besides heart failure, such as pulmonary disease. Most patients who are defined as "dry and cold" (not fluid overloaded, but perfusion is poor at the time of admission) probably are misdiagnosed and have unrecognized fluid congestion and are actually "wet and cold." Patients who are cold and wet have a worse prognosis than those who are warm and wet,[2] presumably because as they are diuresed, intravascular volume is decreased, leading to lower blood pressure and a further decrease in perfusion. The goal of therapy is to restore the patient to a warm and dry hemodynamic profile.

Differential Diagnoses

Dyspnea is a nonspecific presenting symptom that may be difficult to differentiate from causes other than heart failure. Chronic obstructive pulmonary disease, asthma, pneumonia or other pulmonary infection, acute coronary syndrome, and dysrhythmias may promote shortness of breath. Additionally, anemia, physical deconditioning, and obesity frequently cause dyspnea, even in the absence of heart failure. Ankle edema may be caused by right- and left-sided heart failure, but it also may result from venous insufficiency and pelvic vein obstruction. Fatigue, lethargy, and weakness may arise from poor perfusion, but numerous other causes also may provoke these symptoms. The strongest clinical predictor of heart failure is a known history of heart failure.[15]

Diagnostic Procedures
Pulmonary Artery Catheterization

Vascular hydrostatic and colloid osmotic pressure control fluid fluctuation between the vascular space and the interstitial space. When the pressure in the vasculature of the lungs is elevated, as in the presence of fluid volume excess, fluid is forced out of the vascular space and into the interstitial space and alveolus. This vascular pressure is reflected by the pulmonary artery occlusion pressure (**PAOP**), which is usually less than 15 mm Hg in normal patients. The lymphatic vessels are unable to clear the fluid from the interstitial space in the acute process, and fulminant pulmonary edema can occur. Patients with chronic heart failure who come to the hospital with ADHF often have greatly elevated PAOP, greater than 20 mm Hg.

The physical examination alone is a poor indicator of filling pressures and degree of cardiac function or dysfunction. Because the physical examination may be unreliable in diagnosing ADHF or may vary between practitioners, a pulmonary artery catheter may be used to assess the patient's volume status and to guide therapy during the patient's hospitalization. The hemodynamic features obtained from a pulmonary artery catheter in patients with ADHF include low cardiac index, decreased mixed venous oxygen saturation, and elevated PAOP. Pulmonary artery catheterization also is used to evaluate pulmonary pressures and reversibility of pulmonary hypertension in the evaluation for cardiac transplantation.[16]

Pulmonary artery catheterization is used to guide therapy toward the goal of achieving near-normal filling pressures. Initially, intravenously administered diuretics and vasodilators are used, and the patient then is transitioned to oral medications to achieve the same filling pressures. This is termed *tailored therapy,* indicating that the therapeutic steps are individualized for each patient. Once the patient has been diuresed, hemodynamic monitoring may be useful to guide the adjustment of the oral regimen that will be prescribed for the

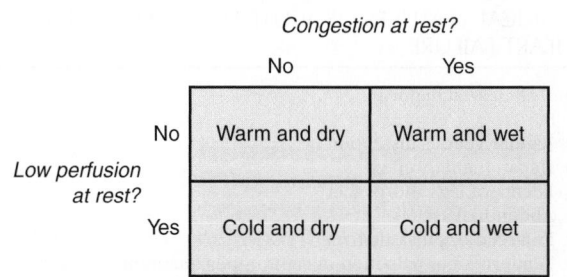

Congestion at rest?

	No	Yes
No	Warm and dry	Warm and wet
Yes	Cold and dry	Cold and wet

Low perfusion at rest?

FIGURE 63-2 ■ Hemodynamic profile in acute decompensated heart failure.

patient when discharged to home. The safety of using pulmonary artery catheters to guide therapy in ADHF has been controversial because of the increased risk of infection or complications from the catheter. The ESCAPE trial (Evaluation Study of Congestive Heart Failure and Pulmonary Artery Catheterization Effectiveness) showed that therapy guided by pulmonary artery catheter hemodynamic monitoring is as safe as treatment based on clinical signs alone, although clinical outcomes were not improved with the pulmonary artery catheter.[17]

Recently, thoracic electrical bioimpedance, also called impedance cardiography, has been used to gather information about cardiac output, cardiac contractility, and volume status in a noninvasive manner. Bioimpedance cardiography is based on technology that converts the measurement of electrical resistance of blood flow in the thoracic cavity into a variety of parameters indicating physiological functions. Hemodynamic parameters such as stroke volume, cardiac output, total peripheral resistance, and aortic compliance can be estimated, as well as central fluid volume, cardiac time intervals, and contractility. A number of authors have reported that impedance cardiography devices accurately determine cardiac output and cardiac index compared with traditional invasive methods of hemodynamic monitoring.[18]

B-Type Natriuretic Peptide Testing

In recent years, natriuretic peptides have been found to have diverse actions in the cardiovascular, renal, and endocrine systems.[19] In human beings, B-type natriuretic peptide (**BNP**) is released from the heart, predominantly the ventricles, in response to increased myocardial pressure and stretch, often associated with volume overload. Endogenous BNP causes natriuresis and vasodilatation in a compensatory effort to maintain homeostasis by overcoming intravascular fluid volume excess. Unfortunately, these effects are not adequate to overcome the adverse effects of the counterregulatory hormones of the neuroendocrine system that are activated in heart failure.

The Breathing Not Properly Study was the first large multinational prospective study using BNP levels to evaluate the causes of dyspnea. In this study, BNP levels were found to be more accurate at predicting heart failure than history, physical findings, or laboratory values. Patients with elevated BNP values were much more likely to have dyspnea caused by heart failure than patients with lower BNP levels. A BNP level greater than 100 pg/ml had a 90 percent sensitivity and 76 percent specificity for differentiating heart failure from other causes of dyspnea.[20] For this reason, BNP levels often are measured in the emergency department in patients who have dyspnea. BNP levels also are measured in patients with chronic heart failure to evaluate trends and exacerbations of their heart failure.

Elevated BNP levels do not always correlate with elevated filling pressures and increased PAOP. High BNP levels with normal filling pressures may be seen with right-sided heart failure resulting from cor pulmonale, pulmonary embolism or primary pulmonary hypertension, and acute or chronic renal failure. Conversely,

normal BNP levels and elevated filling pressures may be seen with acute mitral regurgitation or "flash" pulmonary edema, in which the increase in capillary pressure is upstream from the ventricle. However, in patients admitted with heart failure who have elevated filling pressures from fluid volume overload, high BNP levels drop dramatically with the treatment-induced decrease in PAOP. Important to note is that in patients with end-stage heart failure who are not acutely volume overloaded, BNP levels may not decline as PAOP decreases.

A BNP level usually is measured when the patient first comes to the hospital with symptoms of ADHF and again before discharge. The frequency of BNP evaluation throughout the hospitalization depends on the provider's clinical judgment. Usually, BNP levels are checked when there is any major clinical change, although some health care providers evaluate BNP after the first 24 hours of treatment.[20] If BNP levels do not fall after 24 hours of therapy, this may indicate that the patient needs more aggressive treatment.

Other Laboratory Testing

Laboratory testing in patients who have ADHF includes a complete blood count, panel of electrolytes, blood urea nitrogen, and serum creatinine (Box 63-2). Patients should be tested for diabetes mellitus, and if they are diagnosed with diabetes already, a hemoglobin A_{1c} level should be obtained. A fasting lipid panel and thyroid panel also should be obtained. These laboratory tests are helpful to evaluate comorbidities that contribute to worsening heart failure, such as anemia, diabetes, renal insufficiency, hyperlipidemia, and thyroid abnormalities. According to the ADHERE registry data, 20 percent of patients admitted for ADHF have a serum creatinine greater than 2 mg/dl, indicating some level of renal insufficiency.[15] Measurement of serum laboratory data cannot be overstated, for blood urea nitrogen greater than 43 mg/dl was the best predictor of in-hospital mortality, followed closely by serum creatinine greater than 2.75 mg/dl, and initial systolic blood pressure under 115 mm Hg.[21]

Chest X-Ray Films

The chest x-ray film is an important part of the assessment of ADHF. Despite the absence of rales on physical examination, findings of pulmonary congestion may be

---

BOX 63-2 ■ ■ ■

LABORATORY STUDIES IN ACUTE DECOMPENSATED HEART FAILURE

Complete blood count
Electrolyte panel (including glucose, magnesium, potassium, creatinine, and blood urea nitrogen)
B-type natriuretic peptide
Thyroid panel
Liver profile
Lipid panel
Cardiac enzymes if coronary syndrome suspected
If appropriate:
   Toxicology
   Coagulation studies

seen on x-ray film.[22] With elevated pulmonary venous pressure, fluid leaks from the capillary bed, and the ability of the lymphatic vessels to handle the fluid is surpassed. Fluid accumulates in the interstitium. An early sign of this process is the presence of Kerley B lines, which represent fluid accumulation in the interlobular septa.[23] The findings of cardiomegaly, pulmonary edema, or pleural effusion on the chest x-ray film are indicative of heart failure, but these findings alone cannot make the diagnosis of heart failure.[24]

Electrocardiogram

The findings on the electrocardiogram are limited when it comes to establishing a diagnosis of heart failure; however, it is helpful in determining the onset of new dysrhythmias that may precipitate ADHF, such as atrial fibrillation, bradycardia, or incessant atrial or ventricular tachycardia. The electrocardiogram should be examined for signs of myocardial ischemia or infarction and conduction abnormalities such as bundle branch block.[22]

Echocardiography

Echocardiography may provide important information to determine whether a change in the patient's myocardial performance or valvular integrity may have precipitated ADHF. Echocardiography also may give information about the presence of an acute ischemic syndrome or the status of the pericardium.[6] To obtain an echocardiogram during each admission for ADHF is not necessary if it is clear that volume overload is the cause of the patient's decompensation. Repeated assessment of left ventricular function in patients with heart failure does not affect or alter the treatment plan unless significant changes in the patient's cardiac function or clinical status have occurred.

Patients with symptoms of ADHF and a normal ejection fraction are labeled as having "diastolic heart failure" or "heart failure with preserved systolic function." A previous diagnosis of hypertension, coronary artery disease, or valve surgery can add to the suspicion of diastolic heart failure.[22] Although the diagnosis is made clinically, objective echocardiographic assessment is needed to make the definitive diagnosis of diastolic heart failure. The phases of diastolic filling are measured via Doppler interrogation of inflow across the mitral valve. Normally, early diastolic ventricular filling is greater, whereas late diastolic filling during atrial contraction contributes less to overall ventricular filling. In diastolic heart failure, early diastolic filling is diminished, whereas filling during late diastole is increased, as seen by a low E wave and an enhanced A wave on Doppler echocardiogram.[25]

Assessment of Coronary Arteries

If acute myocardial infarction or unstable coronary syndrome precipitated the patient's ADHF, it would be appropriate to proceed to the catheterization laboratory for urgent coronary angiography with percutaneous intervention and/or initiation of reperfusion therapy.[6] In elderly patients, however, it may be important to determine the patient's wishes regarding ongoing interventions to prolong life. If there is suspicion of new coronary lesions or worsening of existing lesions, but the patient is unwilling to undergo any intervention to reduce or bypass the lesions, then it is questionable as to the benefit of doing a diagnostic catheterization that has its own inherent risks. It is important to speak with the patient and to outline possible interventions before proceeding to the catheterization laboratory and to determine the patient's wishes for future therapy.

TREATMENT

Treatment of patients in ADHF is guided by a careful assessment and determination of the hemodynamic profile. Thereafter, treatment is primarily pharmacological.

Pharmacological Management
Initial Therapy

The initial goal of therapy in ADHF is to return the patient to the "warm and dry" hemodynamic profile by reducing filling pressures. Intravenous vasodilators decrease filling pressures and increase cardiac output in most patients with ADHF. Vasodilator therapy with nitroprusside or nesiritide quickly decreases neurohormonal activation, whereas intravenous diuretic therapy and intravenous nitroglycerine decrease filling pressures.[6,26,27] If diuretic therapy is used alone, without vasodilatation, the reduction in vascular volume will decrease cardiac output and will increase renin-angiotensin-aldosterone system activation. Excessive diuresis leads to hypotension and worsening azotemia, which makes initiation and uptitration of afterload-reducing agents such as angiotensin-converting enzyme inhibitors (**ACEI**) difficult later during the hospitalization. Initiation of vasodilator therapy augmented with modest doses of diuretics, usually loop diuretics such as furosemide, can quickly stabilize most patients with ADHF.[6,27]

Some patients need additional support to improve cardiac output. Modest doses of positive inotropic agents, such as dopamine, dobutamine, or milrinone, may be used until the patient is stabilized. Important to note is that use of inotropic drugs in patients with heart failure may increase the incidence of dysrhythmias and may hasten mortality in patients with chronic heart failure.[2,6] See the pharmacology feature for the vasoactive drugs used most commonly in the management of ADHF.

Overall, therapy can be summarized according to the patient's hemodynamic profile on admission. Patients who present "wet and warm" usually do well after improving diuresis. Occasionally, vasodilator therapy may speed up the relief of symptoms by enhancing forward flow from the heart. The average amount of diuresis for patients hospitalized with ADHF is 4 liters, but it may be greater than 15 liters in patients who have chronic anasarca.[28]

Patients who present as "cold and wet" usually need vasodilatation in order to increase cardiac output and decrease filling pressures before initiating diuretic therapy. The mitral regurgitant flow that is increased in the pres-

■ ■ ■ PHARMACOLOGY

COMMONLY USED VASOACTIVE DRUGS FOR THE MANAGEMENT OF ACUTE DECOMPENSATED HEART FAILURE[2,6,7,39]

| | | | HEMODYNAMIC EFFECT | | | | | |
DRUG	STARTING DOSE/ BOLUS	EFFECTIVE RANGE	CO	HR	PAOP	PVR	SVR	COMMENTS
Vasodilators								
Nesiritide	Bolus 2 mcg/kg	0.005-0.03 mcg/kg/ min	↑	✓	↓↓↓	↓	↓	Rapid onset of effect; leave infusion off for 2 hours before drawing serum BNP level; monitor for hypotension
Nitroglycerin	20 mcg/min	40-400 mcg/min	↓ ✓	↑ ✓	↓↓	↓	↓	Rapid decline of effects when stopped; headache common; requires frequent uptitration because of tolerance
Nitroprusside	10 mcg/min	30-350 g/min; less than 4 mcg/kg/min	↑	↑	↓	↓↓	↓	Protect solution from light; potential for thiocyanate toxicity; requires ICU bed ± pulmonary artery catheter
Inotropic Agents								
Dobutamine	2.5 mcg/kg/min	2-10 mcg/kg/min for vasodilatation and inotropy	↑↑	↑ ✓	↓ ✓	↓	↓	May cause tachydysrhythmias or worsen ischemia; beta blockers may decrease response to dobutamine
Dopamine	1-2 mcg/kg/min	2-5 mcg/kg/min for vasodilatation and inotropy	↑↑	↑	↑ ✓	↑	↑ ✓	
	4-5 mcg/kg/min	6-15 mcg/kg/min for vasoconstriction and inotropy	↑	↑↑	↑	↑	↑↑	May cause tachydysrhythmias or worsen ischemia; increases afterload
Milrinone	Optional bolus 50-75 mcg/kg over 10 minutes	0.10-0.75 mcg/kg/min; usual dose 0.5 mcg/ kg/min	↑	↑ ✓	↓	↓	↓	Monitor closely for hypotension; bolus often is omitted; may cause tachydysrhythmias; long half-life with elimination about 2½ hours

CO, Cardiac output; *HR,* heart rate; *PAOP,* pulmonary artery occlusion pressure; *PVR,* pulmonary vascular resistance; *SVR,* systemic vascular resistance; ↑, increase; ✓, neutral effect; ↓, decrease; *BNP,* B-type natriuretic peptide; *ICU,* intensive care unit.

ence of elevated afterload may consume up to 75 percent of total stroke volume. By unloading the ventricle and improving cardiac output, the mitral regurgitant flow may be reduced by as much as 25 percent.[29] Low doses of dopamine, dobutamine, or milrinone may help improve contractility in these patients, but at the expense of increasing risk of dysrhythmias or ischemia.[2,6]

Patients who present "cold and dry" are the most difficult to manage. They should be evaluated carefully to make sure that filling pressures are not actually elevated, and they should be managed accordingly. If, however, filling pressures are truly reduced in these patients, a cautious trial of fluid replacement may be attempted.[2] Treatment depends on the patient's clinical situation. Inotropic support may benefit the patient temporarily but may lead to further deterioration. Additional afterload reduction with vasodilators may exacerbate hypotension.

Diuretic Therapy

Diuretics do not treat the pathological changes that occur with heart failure, but they are the mainstay of symptomatic treatment to remove excess extracellular fluid. Diuretics that affect the loop of Henle, such as

furosemide, bumetanide, and torsemide, are the most commonly used in treating heart failure. Diuretics initially are given intravenously during hospitalization for ADHF, usually once or twice daily. The reduction in filling pressures that is induced by diuretics lowers the intravascular pressure, thus mobilizing edema fluid from the interstitium back into the intravascular space where it can be filtered by the kidney and excreted from the body.[30]

Loop diuretics tend to be short-acting, lasting about 6 hours. After the drug effect wears off, the renin-angiotensin system becomes activated because of a sudden decrease in sodium excretion. This can make subsequent daily doses of diuretic less effective. Concomitant use of neurohormonal blocking agents, such as ACEIs, will decrease this effect. Patients who do not respond to diuretic therapy may have "diuretic resistance," which occurs in 20 to 30 percent of patients with severe left ventricular dysfunction.[31] Suggestions to improve diuretic effectiveness in patients with diuretic resistance include doubling the dose of diuretic, using a continuous infusion of the diuretic rather than bolus dosing, or adding a thiazide or thiazide-like diuretic such as metolazone to the patient's medication regimen. The combination of a thiazide diuretic and a loop diuretic may result in electrolyte wasting, particularly potassium and sodium. Patients receiving these medications must be monitored carefully for electrolyte disturbances, and any resulting deficiencies should be corrected.[32]

The term *cardiorenal syndrome* has been coined to describe those patients in whom renal function declines progressively as diuresis relieves symptoms of ADHF. About 25 percent of patients hospitalized with heart failure have aggravated renal dysfunction, which can lead to prolonged hospitalization and increased mortality.[33] Preexisting renal insufficiency can be aggravated with diuretic therapy, use of ACEI or angiotensin receptor blockers (**ARBs**), and infusion of nesiritide.[34] The main components of cardiorenal syndrome include a rise in serum creatinine and findings of diuretic resistance, anemia, hyperkalemia, or decreased systolic blood pressure.[35]

Parameters to identify patients at risk for the development and progression of renal dysfunction include admission blood urea nitrogen level ≥43 mg/dl and serum creatinine ≥2.75 mg/dl.[36] Temporary inotropic support may improve cardiac output and improve cardiorenal syndrome, but renal function often declines once again after inotropic support has been removed. Renal function may improve over several weeks if the patient maintains a lower volume status. Discontinuation of ACEI or ARB therapy may be required, with transition to a hydralazine and nitrate combination if the serum creatinine increases by greater than 25 percent of baseline during acute exacerbation and fails to fall back to baseline, or the blood urea nitrogen remains above 80 to 100 mg/dl.[2]

A subset of patients is refractory to diuretic therapy and requires further intervention to reduce filling pressures and intravascular volume. Generally, patients should respond to diuretic therapy within 2 to 3 hours because of the rapid effect of loop diuretics. However, in patients who do not respond to maximal medical therapy, hemofiltration ultrafiltration provides another treatment option. This procedure is similar to hemodialysis in which toxic substances are removed from the blood across a semipermeable membrane; however, during ultrafiltration, only water is extracted. Blood is pumped from the patient, is anticoagulated, and is passed through a porous filter where fluid is removed. The blood then is returned to the patient without large fluctuations in electrolytes or acid-base balance.

Patients with heart failure and refractory volume overload tolerate this therapy well because it does not produce considerable swings in blood pressure when a venovenous pump is used. Usually, 100 to 200 ml/hr is removed, though 500 ml/hr has been shown to be well tolerated.[37] As short-term therapy for diuretic-refractory ADHF, hemofiltration relieves symptoms of pulmonary edema, reduces ascites and peripheral edema, and enhances the subsequent response to diuretics.[37,38] In the past, hemofiltration was not widely used in ADHF because it required the use of a central line. However, newer ultrafiltration devices allow withdrawal and infusion through catheters in peripheral arm veins.

Vasodilators
Nitroprusside

Vasodilator therapy should be initiated early in the course of treatment for patients with ADHF. Nitroprusside was the first intravenous vasodilator shown to improve cardiac output in heart failure. With a half-life of approximately 2 minutes, nitroprusside has a rapid onset and is easily titrated upward or weaned. Patients receiving a nitroprusside infusion generally are managed in the intensive care unit with a pulmonary artery catheter in place to monitor cardiac output and filling pressures invasively. Nitroprusside usually is started at 10 mcg/min and titrated up by 10 to 20 mcg/min every 10 to 20 minutes, with a goal of lowering the PAOP to 16 mm Hg without causing the systolic blood pressure to fall below 80 mm Hg. Doses usually are measured as absolute doses but also may be defined as micrograms per kilogram per minute, ranging from 0.5 mcg/kg/min to 10 mcg/kg/min. Dosage requirements vary from patient to patient. Some patients' filling pressures may improve at 50 mcg/min, whereas others require up to 400 mcg/min.

Side effects from nitroprusside include nausea, vomiting, and disorientation, particularly if the infusion continues for more than 48 hours.[39] The most serious danger of nitroprusside is cyanide toxicity, which is most likely to occur in patients with reduced hepatic or renal function. If cyanide toxicity is suspected, the infusion should be discontinued; no further treatment of the toxicity usually is required.

Nitroglycerin

Nitroglycerin is predominantly a venodilator with mild arteriolar vasodilating effects. Nitroglycerin has a rapid onset of action, usually within 3 to 5 minutes, and may be titrated rapidly to achieve specific hemodynamic goals. Nitroglycerin is most effective when used in pulmonary edema related to myocardial ischemia, but it is also an effective vasodilator in ADHF. Dosing usually is initiated at 20 mcg/min and increased by 20-mcg increments until the hemodynamic goals are achieved.[2] The most common side effect of nitroglycerin is headache, which can be treated with analgesics. Nitrate tolerance may occur after 4 to 8 hours of infusion but usually is overcome by increasing the dose. As with nitroprusside, hypotension may occur, and the patient's blood pressure should be monitored frequently.

Nesiritide

Nesiritide is an intravenous vasodilator used specifically to lower preload and afterload in the treatment of patients with ADHF. Nesiritide is a recombinant form of the BNP that is secreted by the ventricles in response to myocardial stretch. A clinical response from nesiritide is usually rapid, with significant reduction in PAOP and symptoms of dyspnea within 15 minutes of initiation of therapy.[26] Nesiritide potentiates the effect of diuretics, such that lower doses of diuretic may be used to reduce filling pressures. Nesiritide also inhibits the renin-angiotensin-aldosterone system, leading to a reduction in plasma aldosterone and norepinephrine.[40] Nesiritide has a renal effect as an efferent arteriolar vasoconstrictor that augments glomerular filtration rate and urine output and promotes sodium excretion.[41] Unlike nitroprusside or nitroglycerin, nesiritide may be infused safely in an intermediate care unit or emergency department observation unit and does not require intensive care unit admission or pulmonary artery catheter monitoring.

The recommended starting dose of nesiritide is a 2 mcg/kg bolus followed by an infusion of 0.01 mcg/kg/min until the desired hemodynamic profile is achieved. Many clinicians opt to start the infusion without a loading bolus for a more gradual onset of vasodilatation. Hypotension is rare but may occur with nesiritide, thus close blood pressure monitoring is required. The half-life is 18 minutes. If the patient becomes hypotensive, the infusion should be stopped until an adequate blood pressure is obtained. Once the blood pressure is stabilized, the nesiritide infusion may be restarted at a dose reduced by 30 percent. Nesiritide should not be infused through the same intravenous tubing as heparin or furosemide.[6]

Important to remember is that intravenous BNP infusion is basically the same BNP that is released from the ventricles in response to myocardial stretch. A serum BNP level should not be obtained while nesiritide is infusing. Additionally, because of the half life and excretion time of nesiritide, a serum BNP level should not be obtained in the first 2 hours after nesiritide is discontinued.[42] It is preferable to draw the blood from another site, other than from the same site where the nesiritide is infusing. If the blood is drawn too soon after stopping the infusion or if any of the nesiritide infusion is drawn into the blood tube, the serum BNP level will be artificially elevated and will not reflect the patient's true BNP level.

Inotropic Agents

Vasodilating drugs do not improve cardiac function directly but rather unload the heart by decreasing the pressure against which the heart must pump and by decreasing the preload volume of the ventricle. The use of nesiritide and other vasodilators in ADHF is associated with better outcomes than with the use of inotropic agents.[43] However, patients with end-stage heart failure caused by contractile dysfunction that does not support circulation may not benefit from vasodilating agents. These patients with refractory hypoperfusion may require pharmacological inotropic support or the use of an intraaortic balloon pump or other cardiac support device.

Dobutamine

Dobutamine is a beta-adrenergic–stimulating agent that exerts a potent inotropic effect, along with a peripheral and pulmonary vasodilating effect. Inotropic therapy should be used only in situations in which improved contractility is the desired endpoint and should be used for as short a duration as possible because of the increased risk of tachydysrhythmias and ischemia. Situations that may require inotropic support include profound hypotension, inadequate renal perfusion, or

multiorgan dysfunction until cardiac transplantation or left ventricular assist device insertion can be performed. Dobutamine also may be used short term following surgery or myocardial infarction.[2] Occasionally, patients may become dependent on inotropic infusion for palliative support in end-stage heart failure and may be discharged from the hospital with a permanent intravenous catheter for home infusion.

Doses usually start at 2 mcg/kg/min, with titration upward to achieve the desired hemodynamic profile. Patients who are taking beta-adrenergic blocking agents may require slightly higher doses of dobutamine; however, dosage should not exceed 10 to 15 mcg/kg/min because of the possibility of prodysrhythmia. Increased risk of premature ventricular contractions, episodes of nonsustained ventricular tachycardia, and prodysrhythmia have been seen in patients with ADHF who are receiving dobutamine compared with patients receiving nesiritide.[2] This may be related to the fact that dobutamine infusions have been shown to increase aldosterone levels significantly.[44]

Dopamine

Dopamine stimulates alpha and beta receptors in the heart and dopaminergic receptors that cause vasodilatation in the renal and peripheral vasculature. At low doses, dopamine increases blood flow to the renal, mesenteric, coronary, and cerebral beds; however, at high doses, it causes alpha receptor stimulation and peripheral vasoconstriction.[39] By increasing renal blood flow, dopamine may improve diuresis because it augments the effects of loop diuretics. The starting dose of dopamine is 0.5 to 1 mcg/kg/min and is increased until the desired effect is achieved, such as increased urine output or improved blood pressure. Up to 3 mcg/kg/min, dopamine is predominantly vasodilatory; however, when a dose of 5 mcg/kg/min is reached, alpha receptors are stimulated and it becomes a vasoconstrictor.[2] When dopamine is used as a pressor agent, weaning may have to be discontinued at 3 mcg/kg/min because lower doses may promote vasodilatation and lower blood pressure. Like dobutamine, dopamine may promote tachydysrhythmias and worsening ischemia. Extravasation of dopamine may cause sloughing, so the intravenous site should be monitored carefully for patency.

Milrinone

Milrinone is a phosphodiesterase inhibitor that increases contractility by improving sarcolemma calcium uptake. Milrinone produces positive inotropic effects in the myocardium and promotes peripheral and pulmonary vasodilatation through smooth muscle relaxation.[7] In contrast to dobutamine, milrinone does not compete for receptor sites in patients taking beta blockers. The dosage range is from 0.375 to 0.75 mcg/kg/min, titrated up to achieve the desired hemodynamic effect, usually to a dosage of about 0.5 mcg/kg/min. Hypotension may be a problem, so the patient's blood pressure should be monitored closely. If hypotension is the reason inotropic support is needed in a patient with ADHF, milrinone is not the appropriate agent to use. Similar to other inotropic agents, milrinone may increase the frequency of tachydysrhythmias and ischemic events. The elimination half-life of milrinone is long and is increased even further in the presence of renal failure. After weaning from milrinone, patients should be observed carefully for 48 hours. The effects of milrinone may linger after discontinuation of the drug, and patients may deteriorate after being discharged from the intensive care unit or from the hospital once the drug is truly cleared out of the system.

Some experts feel that the benefit of being able to use beta blockers with milrinone is an advantage. However, the recent Outcomes of a Prospective Trial of Intravenous Milrinone for Exacerbations of Chronic Heart Failure (OPTIME-CHF) trial revealed that treatment with intravenous milrinone as an adjunct to standard medical care did not reduce the average length of hospital stay or mortality rate compared with placebo. Furthermore, an increase in adverse events was seen in the patients receiving milrinone.[45] Milrinone is excreted renally, so the dose should be reduced in patients with renal insufficiency. Milrinone may be used to support patients awaiting cardiac transplantation and can be infused alone or in combination with dobutamine. Milrinone also is used as palliative care to improve symptoms and quality of life in end-stage patients with heart failure.

Other Vasoactive Agents

Occasionally, patients with ADHF require additional vasopressor agents to support hemodynamic status. In patients with worsening circulatory status and life-threatening hypoperfusion, dopamine is the initial agent for blood pressure support. If dopamine fails to improve the patient's clinical status, intravenous epinephrine infusion may be necessary for short-term therapy. Epinephrine provides profound vasoconstriction for stabilization of blood pressure until more definitive action may be taken, such as surgical intervention or insertion of a ventricular assist device. Epinephrine is given at a starting dose of 1 mcg/min and is uptitrated until the patient's hemodynamic status is stabilized. Vasopressin may be used in patients who maintain a systolic blood pressure of ≤70 mm Hg despite maximum vasopressor therapy. Vasopressin may be used for short periods at doses of 0.05 to 0.1 units/min. Obviously, such powerful vasoconstricting agents can contribute to the formation of dysrhythmias and worsening ischemia, as well as necrosis of organs and extremities.[2]

Angiotensin-Converting Enzyme Inhibitors and Angiotensin Receptor Blockers

Once the patient's hemodynamic profile is stable and the symptoms are relieved, intravenous vasoactive drugs may be weaned gradually while oral vasodilating agents are uptitrated. When hemodynamic goals have been achieved and are stable for 24 hours, PAOP ≤20 mm Hg, systemic vascular resistance ≤1200 dynes-sec·cm⁻⁵, and systolic blood pressure ≥80 mm Hg, an oral ACEI or ARB is added as the infusions are tapered off. This is known as "tailored therapy," in which the patient's fill-

ing pressures are monitored with a pulmonary artery catheter while intravenous vasoactive agents and diuretics are transitioned to an outpatient oral regimen.[46]

ACEI therapy is the mainstay of treatment for heart failure, but ARBs may be used if ACEIs are contraindicated. Numerous studies have confirmed the benefit of these agents in decreasing mortality in patients with heart failure.[47-51] The goal for dose titration should be that which was reached in the clinical trials; however, hypotension may be an issue. It is important that the patient should not be overdiuresed early in the hospitalization in order to avoid hypotension later while uptitrating oral agents. The patient may have been receiving an ACEI or ARB before admission, and this should be continued following discharge. It may be beneficial to the patient to continue with the same drug to avoid confusion and possible duplication of drugs after discharge. If the patient is intolerant to ACEI or ARB therapy because of angioedema or hyperkalemia, a combination therapy of nitrate and hydralazine may be used.

Beta Blockers

Beta blockers should be initiated in euvolemic patients with heart failure before hospital discharge, provided the patient no longer requires intravenous therapy for heart failure.[52] Beta blocker therapy should never be initiated in patients with unstable heart failure or while the patient is receiving dobutamine.[53] The effectiveness of beta agonist agents such as dobutamine is reduced if the patient is taking a beta blocker. It is important to start beta blockers at the lowest dose possible and to uptitrate the dose slowly over the course of several weeks or even months after the patient is discharged from the hospital. The IMPACT-HF trial showed that initiation of carvedilol before discharge in stabilized patients hospitalized for heart failure improved the use of beta blocker at 60 days without increasing side effects or length of stay.[52] The point in the ACEI/ARB uptitration process at which beta blocker therapy may be introduced varies among practitioners.[54,55]

In patients who come to the hospital in ADHF who are receiving beta blocker therapy, the decision to continue or discontinue the drug is up to the health care provider. If the patient is in the early phase of shock or is in cardiogenic shock, the beta blocker should be stopped immediately. If the patient is able to tolerate the beta blocker, but at a lower dose, it may be continued at a reduced dosage. The patient's clinical situation determines whether the patient may continue with beta blocker therapy during admission for ADHF. Important to note is that abrupt beta blocker withdrawal may precipitate dysrhythmias, tachycardia, or sudden death.[53] If the beta blocker is held initially but restarted once the patient is stable, it should be restarted at a low dose, to be uptitrated after discharge.

Aldosterone Antagonists

Aldosterone antagonists are adjunctive oral neurohormonal blocking agents that have been shown to further decrease mortality from heart failure when added as triple therapy in New York Heart Association functional class III or IV patients already receiving ACEI/ARB and beta blocker therapy.[56,57] Spironolactone is a potassium-sparing diuretic that has aldosterone blocking properties and currently is recommended for the management of stage C chronic heart failure.[58] Recently, a clinical trial of the aldosterone antagonist eplerenone was found to decrease mortality in patients with left ventricular ejection fraction ≤40 percent and clinical evidence of heart failure or diabetes following acute myocardial infarction.[57] Aldosterone antagonists should not be given to patients with serum potassium greater than 5.5 mEq/liter, creatinine clearance less than 30 ml/min or who are concomitantly taking CYP3A4 inhibitors.[59] Hyperkalemia can be a problem with aldosterone antagonists, so the patient's potassium level should be checked within 3 days and again in 1 week of starting the medication.

New and Future Medications for Treatment of ADHF

Levosimendan is a calcium-sensitizing agent being evaluated in clinical trials for treatment of ADHF. Levosimendan increases the intracellular calcium concentration by enhancing calcium release from the sarcolemma. This allows more calcium to bind to troponin C for better cross-bridge attachments between actin and myosin. The contractile apparatus becomes "sensitized" to calcium, unlike beta agonists and phosphodiesterase inhibitors that prompt an increase in the overall amount of intracellular calcium.[39] The end result is an increase in cardiac contractility without increasing intracellular calcium concentration. The Levosimendan Infusion vs Dobutamine (LIDO) study compared levosimendan with dobutamine in ADHF. Survival was improved, and the incidence of major events was reduced in the levosimendan group compared with dobutamine.[60] An oral form of levosimendan is currently under development.

Vasopressin is an antidiuretic hormone that is secreted from the posterior pituitary gland. Vasopressin binds to receptors in the distal or collecting tubules of the kidney and promotes reabsorption of water into the circulation, thus decreasing urine output. Concentrations of vasopressin are elevated in advanced heart failure.[61] High concentrations of vasopressin cause widespread constriction of arterioles, which leads to increased arterial pressure. Several studies supported the use of vasopressin antagonists in the treatment of ADHF because these agents increase urine flow without decreasing serum sodium concentration.[62] Patients benefit from acute changes in hemodynamics; however, there are no morbidity and mortality data yet available. Several vasopressin antagonists currently are being evaluated for potential use.

Plasma adenosine levels are elevated in patients with heart failure, causing decreased glomerular filtration and less diuresis.[63,64] Adenosine antagonists are under investigation in heart failure, both as a single agent and in combination with furosemide, to increase urine output and prevent decreased creatinine clearance, as may be seen with furosemide alone.[65]

Therapeutic Interventions
Intraaortic Balloon Pump

The intraaortic balloon pump (**IABP**) is the most widely used mechanical support device in the world today. The IABP increases blood flow to heart muscle, decreases the workload of the heart, and may be used in the presence of cardiogenic shock and ADHF caused by acute myocardial infarction.[66] A balloon in the proximal aorta inflates when the heart relaxes, thus forcing blood forward to perfuse the periphery and backward into the coronary arteries. The balloon deflates abruptly when the aortic valve opens and systolic contraction begins, thus creating a suction to "pull" the blood out of the ventricle and augment forward blood flow. This greatly reduces the workload of the myocardium by reducing afterload and oxygen consumption, thus allowing the heart an opportunity to recover. Cardiac output may be improved by as much as 40 percent, and ventricular filling pressures are lowered with IABP therapy.[67] This therapy can be used in patients as a bridge to transplant and in patients who are hemodynamically unstable. Of note, in hospitals that support use of left ventricular assist devices, use of IABP is often a bridge to left ventricular assist device insertion.

Patients with IABPs must be monitored closely in an intensive care unit. A chest x-ray film is obtained after insertion for catheter position, and daily chest x-ray films are recommended while the IABP is in place to make sure the catheter is in the correct position. Intravenously administered heparin must be started after placement to prevent clot formation. Patients must be kept supine in bed, and pedal pulses must be checked often. Removal of the balloon pump depends on several factors, including hemodynamic status of the patient, left ventricular function, and duration of therapy. Usually, patients are weaned by changing the timing of inflations to 1:2 (one inflation per every two cardiac contractions) for several hours and then to 1:3. If weaning is tolerated hemodynamically, the balloon pump can be removed. Contraindications to IABP therapy include aortic dissection, abdominal or thoracic aortic aneurysm, severe peripheral vascular disease, coagulopathy or contraindication to heparin, and moderate to severe aortic insufficiency. Disadvantages of prolonged IABP therapy include risk of infection and need for continuous bed rest.

Left Ventricular Assist Device

A left ventricular assist device (**LVAD**) is used to control acute reversible heart failure resulting in cardiogenic shock, which often is caused by acute myocardial infarction.[68] Under these conditions, mechanical support may augment the patient's circulation until the myocardium improves enough for the patient to undergo revascularization. LVAD completely unloads the left ventricle while supporting the pulmonary or systemic circulation. LVADs traditionally have been used in patients awaiting heart transplantation but are implanted now in patients with severe left ventricular dysfunction and cardiogenic shock. Candidates for assist devices typically have a low cardiac output, systolic blood pressure less than 90 mm Hg, PAOP greater than 18 mm Hg, and oliguria despite maximal medical therapy. Cardiac output, mean blood pressure, and PAOP measurements generally are improved with LVADs.[69]

Evidence suggests that LVAD support before transplantation improves hemodynamic, anatomical, and histological values and decreases levels of neurohormones such as norepinephrine.[70,71] LVAD support has been shown to reverse chamber enlargement and normalize end-diastolic pressure, decrease left ventricular mass, and increase ventricular contractility.[72] These effects are seen after long-term support, not short-term therapy.

Contraindications to the use of LVAD include severe peripheral vascular disease and severe hepatic or renal failure. In addition, many devices are large and cannot be implanted into small adults and children.[73] Complications include perioperative bleeding, malignant dysrhythmias, infections, embolic complications, and right ventricular dysfunction. In addition, patients may experience loss of appetite, swelling at the incision site, insomnia, constipation, depression, and memory loss. See Chapter 66 for further discussion of LVAD therapy.

Daily In-Hospital Care

Routine hospital care for patients with ADHF should include telemetry monitoring to watch for new onset of dysrhythmias. Patients must be weighed daily to assess fluid loss from diuresis. Intake and output of liquids are monitored to ensure that patients do not continue to retain the fluids that they consume during their hospitalization. Fluid intake should be restricted to 1500 to 2000 ml per 24 hours in order to optimize diuresis. Supplemental oxygen may make the patient breathe easier with less effort, particularly if the patient's oxygen saturation is less than 90 percent on room air. It is important for patients to ambulate, and if possible, to participate in cardiac rehabilitation. If the patient is on bed rest and unable to ambulate, subcutaneously administered low-molecular-weight heparin may be used to prevent the development of venous thrombosis.[6] Diet should be limited to 2000 mg of sodium daily. If the patient has coronary artery disease, diabetes, or renal failure, those aspects of the diet also must be addressed.

If the patient was taking an ACEI or ARB before hospital admission, it is reasonable to continue the same medications after discharge at doses that have been "tailored" to the patient's tolerance while in the hospital. The patient may have a supply of that medication at home, and prescribing a different medication will require the patient to pay money for medication needlessly. Furthermore, patients often are confused between trade names and generic names of drugs. For instance, the patient may be discharged on lisinopril who was placed on benazepril before hospitalization. This increases the possibility that the patient may end up taking both drugs after discharge, and this potentially could lead to hyperkalemia or other complications. The danger of such medication errors is increased in elderly patients who are taking numerous medications and who may become confused about their drug

regimen. Simplicity is a key element to a successful medication regimen, and if it is possible to use a drug with which the patient is already familiar, the likelihood of errors will be reduced. This message applies to beta blockers also as long as the prehospitalization agent was carvedilol, metoprolol succinate, or bisoprolol. If the patient was taking an alternative beta blocker agent, it should be changed to one of these three agents. In patients with heart failure and preserved left ventricular systolic function, alternative beta blocker agents can be used.

CRITERIA FOR DISCHARGE

Thirty to 60 percent of heart failure patients are readmitted within 3 to 6 months after discharge from the hospital.[74] Failure to meet adequate discharge criteria contributes to this readmission rate.[75] Before considering the patient for discharge, the patient should be stable on an oral regimen for 24 hours, have resolution of symptoms from fluid volume overload, and have adequate blood pressure and renal function. Discharging patients too soon, before their decompensated heart failure is resolved, generally results in another hospitalization in the near future. Box 63-3 outlines criteria for discharge from the hospital.

PATIENT EDUCATION AND FOLLOW-UP

Discharge education is critical to enhance the effects of medications, prevent the recurrence of symptoms, and teach the patient to participate in self-care management.[76] Unfortunately, discharge education is often left

---

BOX 63-3 ■ ■ ■
DISCHARGE CRITERIA FOR HOSPITALIZATION WITH HEART FAILURE

Clinical Status Goals
- Achievement of dry weight, without orthostatic hypotension
- Appropriate blood pressure range (systolic blood pressure ≥90 mm Hg if possible)
- Walking without dyspnea or dizziness
- Patient free of symptoms from fluid volume overload

Stability Goals
- 24 hours without changes in oral heart failure regimen
- 48 hours off intravenous inotropic agents, if used
- Fluid balance on oral diuretics
- Renal function stable or improving

Home Maintenance Plan
- Patient/family education about the following:
- Sodium restriction
- Fluid limitation
- Medication schedule and effects
- Exercise prescription
- When to call health care provider for problems
- Flexible diuretic plan (if appropriate for patient)
- Patient has prescriptions, preferably using previous angiotensin-converting enzyme inhibitor/angiotensin receptor blocker and beta blocker
- Scheduled call to patient within 3 days
- Clinic appointment within 10 days

Adapted from Stevenson L: Management of acute decompensation. In Mann D, editor: *Heart failure: a companion to Braunwald's heart disease*, Philadelphia, 2004, Saunders.

until the last minutes of the hospital stay, just before the patient leaves to go home. When this is the case, little of the information may be absorbed by the patient and the family. It is imperative to include the family member who assumes responsibility for cooking and/or grocery shopping when discussing dietary sodium restriction. All family members would benefit from hearing the discharge instructions so that they may support the patient in maintaining these lifestyle changes at home after discharge. The discharge information should always be given to the patient in writing, and when possible, other media forms should be used as well. Videos, computer programs, websites, compact disc recordings, and other audiovisual tools may be incorporated into the educational armamentarium.

Patients should be contacted at home via telephone by the hospital-based heart failure follow-up program in order to ensure adequate understanding and use of information given before discharge and to enhance optimal self-care. Patients should be assessed by their doctor or nurse practitioner within 10 days of discharge to continue the uptitration of heart failure medications and to assess self-care adherence and therapies. Patient admitted to the hospital for ADHF two or more times over a 12-month period should be referred to an outpatient heart failure program for closer monitoring. Active outpatient heart failure programs reduce readmissions, decrease cost of care, and improve quality of life for patients with heart failure.[77-80] These programs may be managed by advanced practice nurses who provide medical care and patient-focused aspects of care, such as ongoing education and self-care management. Advanced practice nurses are more likely than physicians to expand the patient's care to include assessment of barriers to medication use and providing some form of ongoing monitoring. Additionally, they may spend time counseling patients about psychosocial issues.

SUMMARY

Regardless of the cause of heart failure, it is a chronic illness that becomes progressively worse over time. Intrinsic compensatory mechanisms actually become harmful and contribute to worsening of cardiac function. Numerous reasons exist why patients with heart failure frequently are admitted to the hospital, but admission often is related to noncompliance with medications or diet.

The acute management of ADHF is targeted toward decreasing filling pressures with vasodilators and ensuring adequate diuresis. Diuretics are used to decrease vascular and interstitial volume. Nesiritide, nitroglycerin, nitroprusside, dobutamine, dopamine, and milrinone are intravenous vasoactive agents used to stabilize patients with ADHF. These intravenous agents are used initially, sometimes with a pulmonary artery catheter to guide therapy, but the patient is transitioned quickly to oral agents before discharge.

The impact of heart failure on health care costs is large, namely because hospitalization in heart failure is very high. Consistent use of inpatient guidelines in

ADHF[81] may decrease length of stay and improve patient outcomes, whereas better outpatient management of patients with heart failure may decrease readmission frequency.[82] The patient's preparation for discharge while hospitalized plays an important role in postdischarge morbidity. It is important that patients are adequately stable before being discharged from the hospital and have appropriate outpatient follow-up. As heart failure medications and devices improve, mortality from heart failure may decrease, but morbidity may increase as more patients are living with this disabling condition. Investigational medications are being evaluated for the management of heart failure, and perhaps the next two decades will bring improved therapies that decrease hospitalizations and mortality from this devastating condition.

REFERENCES

1. American Heart Association: *Heart disease and stroke statistics: 2007 update*, Dallas, 2006, American Heart Association. Accessed February 1, 2007 at http://circ.ahajournals.org/cgi/content/short/CIRCULATIONAHA.106.179918
2. Stevenson L: Management of acute decompensation. In Mann D, editor: *Heart failure: a companion to Braunwald's heart disease*, Philadelphia, 2004, Saunders.
3. Krumholz H, Parent E, Tu N et al: Readmission after hospitalization for congestive heart failure among Medicare beneficiaries, *Arch Intern Med* 157:99-104, 1997.
4. Vinson J, Rich M, Sperry J et al: Early readmission of elderly patients with congestive heart failure, *J Am Geriatr Soc* 38:1290-1295, 1990.
5. Stevenson L, Massie B, Francis G: Optimizing therapy for complex or refractory heart failure: a management algorithm, *Am Heart J* 135:S293-S309, 1998.
6. Young J, Mills R: *Clinical management of heart failure*, West Islip, NY, 2004, Professional Communications.
7. Greenberg B, Hermann D: *Contemporary diagnosis and management of heart failure*, Newton, Pa, 2002, Handbooks in Health Care.
8. The ADHERE Registry: *First quarter 2003 national benchmark report*, Fremont, Calif, 2003, Scios.
9. Wilhelmsen L, Rosengren A, Eriksson H, Lappas G: Heart failure in the general population of men-morbidity, risk factors and prognosis, *J Intern Med* 249:253-261, 2001.
10. Ho K, Pinsky J, Kannel W, Levy D: The epidemiology of heart failure: the Framingham Study, *J Am Coll Cardiol* 22:6A-13A, 1993.
11. Mann D: Heart failure as a progressive disease. In Mann D, editor: *Heart failure: a companion to Braunwald's heart disease*, Philadelphia, 2004, Saunders.
12. Stevenson L, Perloff J: The limited reliability of physical signs for estimating hemodynamics in chronic heart failure, *JAMA* 261:884-888, 1989.
13. Yancy C, Chang S: Clinical characteristics and outcomes in patients admitted with heart failure with preserved systolic function: a report from the ADHERE database, *J Card Fail* 9(suppl 5): S84, 2003.
14. Norhia A, Tsang S, Fang J et al: Clinical assessment identifies hemodynamic profiles that predict outcomes in patients admitted with heart failure, *J Am Coll Cardiol* 41:1797-1804, 2003.
15. Fonarow G, for the ADHERE Scientific Advisory Committee: The Acute Decompensated Heart Failure National Registry (ADHERE): opportunities to improve care of patients hospitalized with acute decompensated heart failure, *Rev Cardiovasc Med* 4(suppl 7): S21-S30, 2003.
16. Hunt S, Frazier D: Mechanical circulatory support and cardiac transplantation, *Circulation* 97:2079-2090, 1998.
17. Shah M, Stevenson L: Evaluation Study of Congestive Heart Failure and Pulmonary Artery Catheterization Effectiveness: the ES-

CAPE Trial. Paper presented at American Heart Association 2004 Scientific Sessions, Nov 7-10, 2004, New Orleans.

18. Yancy C, Abraham W: Noninvasive hemodynamic monitoring in heart failure: utilization of impedance cardiography, *Congest Heart Fail* 9:241-250, 2003.

19. Chen H, Burnett J: The natriuretic peptides in heart failure: diagnostic and therapeutic potentials, *Proc Assoc Am Physicians* 111:406-416, 1999.

20. Maisel A, Krishnaswamy P, Nowak R et al, for the Breathing Not Properly Multinational Study Investigators: Rapid measurement of B-type natriuretic peptide in the emergency diagnosis of heart failure, *N Engl J Med* 347:161-167, 2002.

21. Fonarow G, Adams K, Abraham W et al, for the ADHERE Scientific Advisory Committee, Study Group, and Investigators: Risk stratification for in-hospital mortality in acutely decompensated heart failure: classification and regression tree analysis, *JAMA* 293:572-580, 2005.

22. Francis G, Tang W: Clinical evaluation of heart failure. In Mann D, editor: *Heart failure: a companion to Braunwald's heart disease*, Philadelphia, 2004, Saunders.

23. Barron M: Radiology of the heart. In Goldman L, Ausiello D, editors: *Cecil textbook of medicine*, ed 22, Philadelphia, 2004, Saunders.

24. O'Brien T, Paul S: Chest x-ray and vascular studies. In Taylor G, editor: *Primary care management of heart disease*, St Louis, 2000, Mosby.

25. Paul S: Diastolic dysfunction, *Crit Care Nurs Clin North Am* 15:495-500, 2003.

26. Publication Committee for the VMAC Investigators: Intravenous nesiritide versus nitroglycerin for treatment of decompensated congestive heart failure: a randomized controlled trial, *JAMA* 287:1531-1540, 2002.

27. Johnson W, Omland T, Hall C et al: Neurohormonal activation rapidly decreases after intravenous therapy with diuretics and vasodilators for Class IV heart failure, *J Am Coll Cardiol* 39:1623-1629, 2002.

28. Lucas C, Johnson W, Hamilton M et al: Freedom from congestion predicts good survival despite previous Class IV symptoms of heart failure, *Am Heart J* 140:840-847, 2000.

29. Stevenson L, Brunken R, Belil D et al: Afterload reduction with vasodilators and diuretics decreases mitral regurgitation during upright exercise in advanced heart failure, *J Am Coll Cardiol* 15:174-180, 1990.

30. Paul S: Balancing diuretic therapy in heart failure: loop diuretics, thiazides, and aldosterone antagonists, *Congest Heart Fail* 8:307-312, 2002.

31. Ellison D: Diuretic drugs and the treatment of edema: from clinic to bench and back again, *Am J Kidney Dis* 23:623-643, 1994.

32. Kazanegra R, Cheng V, Garcia A et al: A rapid test for B-type natriuretic peptide correlates with falling wedge pressures in patients treated for decompensated heart failure: a pilot study, *J Card Fail* 7:21-29, 2001.

33. Krumholz H, Chen Y, Vaccarino V et al: Correlates and impact on outcomes of worsening renal function in patients ≥ 65 years of age with heart failure, *Am J Cardiol* 85:1110-1113, 2000.

34. Sackner-Bernstein J, Kowalski M, Fox M, Aaronson K: Short-term risk of death after treatment with nesiritide for decompensated heart failure: a pooled analysis of randomized controlled trials, *JAMA* 293:1900-1905, 2005.

35. The ADHERE Registry: *Acute Decompensated Heart Failure National Registry (ADHERE): management of the cardiorenal syndrome*, Orlando, Fla, 2003, ADHERE Registry and Cardiorenal Syndrome Investigators.

36. Fonarow G, Adams K, Abraham W, ADHERE Investigators: Risk stratification for in-hospital mortality in heart failure using classification and regression tree (CART) methodology: analysis of 33,046 patients in the ADHERE registry, *J Card Fail* 9(suppl):S79, 2003 (abstract).

37. Sackner-Bernstein J, Obeleniene R: How should diuretic-refractory, volume overloaded heart failure patients be managed? *J Invasive Cardiol* 15:585-590, 2003.

38. Bart B, Boyle A, Bank A et al: Ultrafiltration versus usual care for hospitalized patients with heart failure: the Relief for Acutely Fluid-overloaded Patients With Decompensated Congestive Heart Failure (RAPID-CHF) Trial. *JACC*, 46:2043-6, 2005.

39. Opie L, Gersh B: *Drugs for the heart*, ed 6, Philadelphia, 2004, WB Saunders.

40. Abraham W, Lowes B, Ferguson D et al: Systemic hemodynamic, neurohormonal, and renal effects of a steady-state infusion of human brain natriuretic peptide in patients with hemodynamically decompensated heart failure, *J Card Fail* 4:37-44, 1998.

41. Jensen K, Eiskjaer H, Carstens J, Pedersen P: Renal effects of brain natriuretic peptide in patients with congestive heart failure, *Clin Sci* 96:5-15, 1999.

42. Silver M, Maisel A, Yancy C et al, for the BNP Consensus Panel: BNP Consensus Panel 2004. a clinical approach for the diagnostic, prognostic, screening, treatment monitoring, and therapeutic roles of natriuretic peptides in cardiovascular diseases, *Congest Heart Fail* 10(suppl 3):1-30, 2004.

43. Abraham W, Adams K, Fonarow G et al, for the ADHERE Scientific Advisory Committee and Investigators: Comparison of in-hospital mortality in patients treated with nesiritide vs other parenteral vasoactive medications for acutely decompensated heart failure: an analysis from a large prospective registry database, *J Card Fail* 9(suppl):S81, 2003 (abstract).

44. Aronson D, Horton D, Burger A: The effect of dobutamine on neurohormonal and cytokine profiles in patients with decompensated congestive heart failure, *J Card Fail* 7(suppl2):28-31, 2004 (abstract).

45. Cuffe M, Califf R, Adams K et al, for the Outcomes of a Prospective Trial of Intravenous Milrinone for Exacerbations of Chronic Heart Failure (OPTIME-CHF): Short term intravenous milrinone for acute exacerbation of chronic heart failure: a randomized controlled trial, *JAMA* 287:1541-1547, 2002.

46. Stevenson L, Dracup K, Tillisch J: Efficacy of medical therapy tailored for severe congestive heart failure in patients transferred for urgent cardiac transplantation, *Am J Cardiol* 63:461-464, 1989.

47. Swedberg K, Pfeffer M, Granger C et al, for the Charm-Programme Investigators: Candesartan in heart failure—assessment of reduction in mortality and morbidity (CHARM): rationale and design, *J Card Fail* 5:276-282, 1999.

48. The CONSENSUS Trial Study Group: Effects of enalapril on mortality in severe congestive heart failure: results of the Cooperative North Scandinavian Enalapril Survival Study (CONSENSUS), *N Engl J Med* 316:1429-1435, 1987.

49. The SOLVD Investigators: Effect of angiotensin converting enzyme inhibition with enalapril on survival in patients with reduced left ventricular ejection fraction and congestive heart failure: results of the treatment trial of the Studies of Left Ventricular Dysfunction (SOLVD)—a randomized double blind trial, *N Engl J Med* 325:293-302, 1991.

50. Sutton MSJ, Pfeffer M, Plappert T et al: Quantitative two dimensional echocardiographic measurements are major predictors of adverse cardiovascular events after acute myocardial infarction, the protective effect of captopril, *Circulation* 89:68-75, 1994.

51. Cohn J, Tognoni G: A randomized trial of the angiotensin-receptor blocker valsartan in chronic heart failure, *N Engl J Med* 345:1667-1675, 2001.

52. Gattis W, O'Connor C, Gallup D et al: Predischarge initiation of carvedilol in patients hospitalized for decompensated heart failure: results of the Initiation Management Predischarge: Process for Assessment of Carvedilol Therapy in Heart Failure (IMPACT-HF) trial, *J Am Coll Cardiol* 43:1534-1541, 2004.

53. Eichhorn E, Bristow M: Antagonism of beta adrenergic receptors in heart failure. In Mann D, editor: *Heart failure: a companion to Braunwald's heart disease*, Philadelphia, 2004, Saunders.

54. MERIT-HF Group: Effect of metoprolol CR/XL in chronic heart failure: Metoprolol CR/XL Randomised Intervention Trial in Congestive Heart Failure (MERIT-HF), *Lancet* 353:2001-2007, 1999.

55. CIBIS-II Investigators and Committees: The Cardiac Insufficiency Bisoprolol Study II (CIBIS II): a randomised trial, *Lancet* 353:9-13, 1999.

56. Pitt B, Zannad F, Remme W: The effect of spironolactone on morbidity and mortality in patients with severe heart failure, *N Engl J Med* 341:709-717, 1999.

57. Pitt B, Remme W, Zannad F et al, for the Eplerenone Post-Acute Myocardial Infarction Heart Failure Efficacy and Survival Study Investigators: Eplerenone, a selective aldosterone blocker, in pa-

tients with left ventricular dysfunction after myocardial infarction, *N Engl J Med* 348:1309-1321, 2003.

58. Packer M, Cohn JN, on behalf of the Steering Committee and Membership of the Advisory Council to Improve Outcomes Nationwide in Heart Failure (ACTION-HF): Consensus recommendations for the management of chronic heart failure, *Am J Cardiol* 83(suppl):1A-38A, 1999.

59. Pfizer Pharmaceuticals: Inspra package insert prescribing information, 2003.

60. Packer M, Nieminen M, Hasenfuss G et al: Effect of intravenous levosimendan, a calcium sensitizer, on the survival of hospitalized patients with heart failure, *Circulation* 100:16-46, 1999 (abstract).

61. Goldsmith S, Francis G, Cowley A et al: Increased plasma arginine vasopressin levels in patients with congestive heart failure, *J Am Coll Cardiol* 1:1385-1390, 1983.

62. Abraham W, Oren T, Crisman T et al: Effects of an oral, non-peptide, selective V2 receptor vasopressin antagonist in patients with chronic heart failure, *J Am Coll Cardiol* 29:169A, 1997.

63. Schnermann J: Juxtaglomerular cell complex in the regulation of renal salt excretion, *Am J Physiol* 274:R263-R279, 1988.

64. Funaya H, Kitakaze M, Node K et al: Plasma adenosine levels increase in patients with chronic heart failure, *Circulation* 95:1363-1365, 1997.

65. Gottlieb S, Skettino S, Wolff A et al: Effects of BG9719 (CVT-124), an A1 adenosine receptor antagonist, and furosemide on glomerular filtration rate and natriuresis in patients with congestive heart failure, *J Am Coll Cardiol* 35:56-59, 2000.

66. Papaioannou T, Stefanadis C: Basic principles of the intraaortic balloon pump and mechanisms affecting its performance. *ASAIO Journal*, 51:296-300, 2005.

67. Jeevanandum V, Jayakar D, Anderson A et al: Circulatory assistance with a permanent implantable IABP: initial human experience, *Circulation* 106:183-188, 2002.

68. Tayara W, Starling R, Yamani M, Wazni O, Jubran F, Smedira N: Improved survival after acute myocardial infarction complicated by cardiogenic shock with circulatory support and transplantation: comparing aggressive intervention with conservative treatment. *Journal of Heart and Lung Transplantation*, 25:504-9, 2006.

69. Thiele H, Lauer B, Hambrecht R et al: Reversal of cardiogenic shock by percutaneous atrial to femoral arterial bypass assistance, *Circulation* 104:2917-2922, 2001.

70. Delgado R, Radovancevic B, Massin E et al: Neurohormonal changes after implantation of a left ventricular assist system, *ASAIO J* 44:299-302, 1998.

71. Frazier O, Benedict C, Radovancevic B et al: Improved left ventricular function after chronic left ventricular unloading, *Ann Thorac Surg* 62:675-681, 1996.

72. Birks E, Tansley P, Hardy J et al. Left ventricular assist device and drug therapy for the reversal of heart failure. *N Eng J Med* 355:1922-5, 2006.

73. Potapov E, Loebe M, Nasseri B et al: Pulsatile flow in patients with a novel nonpulsatile implantable ventricular assist device, *Circulation* 102:183-187, 2000.

74. Aghababian R: Acutely decompensated heart failure: opportunities to improve care and outcomes in the emergency department, *Rev Cardiovasc Med* 3(suppl 4):S3-S9, 2002.

75. Fonarow G, Abraham W, Albert N et al: Association between performance measures and clinical outcomes for patients hospitalized with heart failure. *JAMA*, 297:61-70, 2007.

76. Koelling T, Johnson M, Cody R, Aaronson K: Discharge education improves clinical outcomes in patients with chronic heart failure, *Circulation* 111:179-185, 2005.

77. Fonarow G, Stevenson L, Walden J et al: Impact of a comprehensive heart failure management program on hospital readmission and functional status of patients with advanced heart failure, *J Am Coll Cardiol* 30:725-732, 1997.

78. Paul S: Impact of a nurse-managed heart failure clinic: a pilot study of outcomes, *Am J Crit Care* 8:140-146, 2000.

79. Paul S, Sneed N: Patient perceptions of quality of life and treatment in an outpatient congestive heart failure clinic, *Congest Heart Fail* 8:74-79, 2002.

80. Rich M, Beckham V, Wittenberg C et al: A multidisciplinary intervention to prevent the readmission of elderly patients with congestive heart failure, *N Engl J Med* 333:1190-1195, 1995.

81. DiDomenico R, Park H, Southworth M et al: Guidelines for acute decompensated heart failure treatment, *Ann Pharmacother* 38:649-660, 2004.

82. Hunt S, Abraham W, Chin M et al: ACC/AHA 2005 guideline update for the diagnosis and management of chronic heart failure in the adult: a report from the American College of Cardiology and the American Heart Association Task Force on Practice Guidelines. Retrieved August 23, 2005, from http://www.acc.org/qualityandscience/clinical/measures/HF/HFPerfMeasFinal2[1]032726.pdf

■■■■ c h a p t e r **64**

Care of Patients with Chronic Heart Failure

Barbara Riegel
Debra K. Moser

CHAPTER ABBREVIATIONS

ACC American College of Cardiology

ACE angiotensin-converting enzyme

AHA American Heart Association

AMI acute myocardial infarction

ARB angiotensin receptor blocker

BEST Beta-Blocker Evaluation of Survival Trial

BNP B-type natriuretic peptide

CRT cardiac resynchronization therapy

DIG Digitalis Investigation Group

HOPE Heart Outcomes Prevention Evaluation

ICD implantable cardioverter-defibrillator

NYHA New York Heart Association

PRAISE Prospective Randomised Amlodipine Survival Evaluation

Heart failure is not a "disease"; rather, it is a clinical syndrome. This syndrome is the result of progressively deteriorating cardiac pumping ability that typically is manifested by vasoconstriction and fluid retention, substantial activity intolerance from dyspnea and fatigue, seriously impaired quality of life, and premature death. Heart failure is considered an epidemic because of its high incidence, prevalence, morbidity, and mortality. Despite advances in the management of heart failure, incidence and prevalence are expected to continue to rise in the United States and in other developed and developing countries. New data indicate that survival in men hospitalized for heart failure has improved in the last half of the 1990s (2000 versus 1995), but no improvement was seen in women during that same interval.[1] The Technology feature illustrates cutting-edge advancements for chronic heart failure that may stem the epidemic and improve outcomes in the future.

Given its increasing incidence and prevalence and continued high morbidity and mortality, heart failure has emerged as a major public health problem. Heart failure is the final common pathway for a number of cardiac conditions and cardiovascular risk factors. Recognition that many of these risk factors can be modified to reduce the risk of heart failure has focused attention on preventive strategies for this syndrome. The difficulties and cost of treating heart failure demand a preemptive approach.

Ventricular remodeling (Figure 64-1), discussed in detail in Chapter 62, is the process underlying the development of systolic and diastolic dysfunction. Ventricular remodeling is now understood to take years to produce significant adverse effects. Although the precise mechanisms for the transition to symptomatic heart failure have yet to be understood completely, many factors that predispose or aggravate the remodeling process and the development of cardiac dysfunction have been identified. For example, treatment of systemic hypertension with or without left ventricular hypertrophy, has a major impact on the development of heart failure in patients with this condition. Prevention of myocardial infarction is a particularly notable target for intervention, because occurrence of myocardial infarction confers an eightfold to 10-fold risk for subsequent heart failure.[2] Some factors related to risk for coronary artery disease—such as age, gender, and genetic makeup—are not modifiable. However, many other risk factors respond to interventions.[3] Nowhere is the imperative to embrace prevention more important than in efforts to stem the heart failure epidemic.

The purpose of this chapter is to describe the care of patients with chronic heart failure. The framework in which this care is discussed is the American College of Cardiology/American Heart Association **(ACC/AHA)** heart failure guideline. (See the Evidence-Based Practice feature Using Guidelines to Provide Evidence-Based Care for Patients with Heart Failure.) The ACC/AHA guideline emphasizes primary, secondary, and tertiary prevention throughout by conceptualizing heart failure in four progressive stages beginning with a stage for patients who have not yet developed heart failure but who are at risk for its development (Figure 64-2).[4] These stages do not replace but complement the New York Heart Association **(NYHA)** functional classifications (Figure 64-3).[4] Patients with heart failure are ubiquitous, and nurses care for these patients in a wide variety of settings. This chapter builds on nurses' holistic perspective to describe ways in which they can positively affect the course of heart failure in all settings in which they practice.

STAGE A HEART FAILURE

A unique aspect of the ACC/AHA guidelines is the specification of "pre-heart failure" categories. Patients in stage A do not have heart failure or even structural heart disease; rather, they are at risk for the development of heart failure or its precursors, and this is the ideal time to intervene. The goal of therapy for patients in this stage is the prevention of heart failure. This goal is met by identifying and treating individuals at high risk for developing heart failure.

Coronary artery disease and hypertension are the two most common causes of heart failure. Persons with heart failure are classified as having (1) systolic, impaired, or nonpreserved systolic function or (2) diastolic or preserved systolic function, with approximately half in each group. Coronary artery disease is the major precursor to heart failure with systolic dysfunction, whereas hypertension (also a major cause of systolic dysfunction heart failure) is the primary precur-

sor to heart failure with diastolic dysfunction. Thus, coronary artery disease and hypertension, and risk factors for them, put individuals at heightened risk for heart failure.[5] Persons at risk for developing heart failure include those with the conditions shown in Box 64-1.

Management

Current recommendations for the prevention of heart failure call for the control of hypertension, lipid disorders, diabetes, and metabolic syndrome, along with patient education and counseling directed at the avoidance of risky behaviors such as smoking, sedentary lifestyle, alcohol or drug abuse, high dietary fat consumption, and other measures to prevent atherosclerotic heart disease (Figure 64-4).[6,7] For example, appropriate treatment of hypertension can reduce a patient's risk of developing heart failure by approximately 50 percent.[7] Use of statins to control dyslipidemia reduces the risk of heart failure by about 20 percent. Once an individual develops an acute myocardial infarction **(AMI),** progression to heart failure is common and mortality is high.[8] Diabetes

---

■ ■ ■ **TECHNOLOGY**

NEW TECHNOLOGY FOR CHRONIC HEART FAILURE

- Cardiomyocyte replication
- Cloning of artificial organs
- Organ regeneration using stem cells

von Harsdorf R, Poole-Wilson PA, Dietz R: Regenerative capacity of the myocardium: implications for treatment of heart failure, *Lancet* 363:1306-1313, 2004.

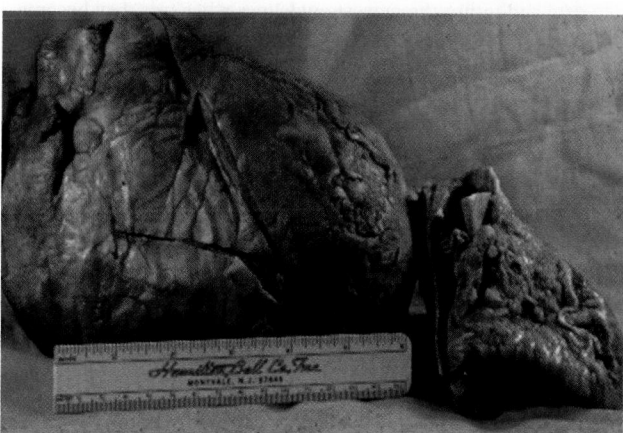

FIGURE 64-1 ■ Profound hypertrophy as a result of remodeling. The heart on the right is a normal heart. The heart on the left is from a patient who died during an episode of decompensated heart failure.

BOX 64-1   ■ ■ ■
RISK FACTORS FOR HEART FAILURE

- Atherosclerosis
- Diabetes mellitus and the metabolic syndrome
- Depression
- Dyslipidemia
- Hypertension
- Lifestyle factors
  - Chronic stress
  - Excessive alcohol intake
  - Illicit drug use
  - Obesity
  - Sedentary behavior
  - Smoking
- Myocarditis
- Some chemotherapeutic agents

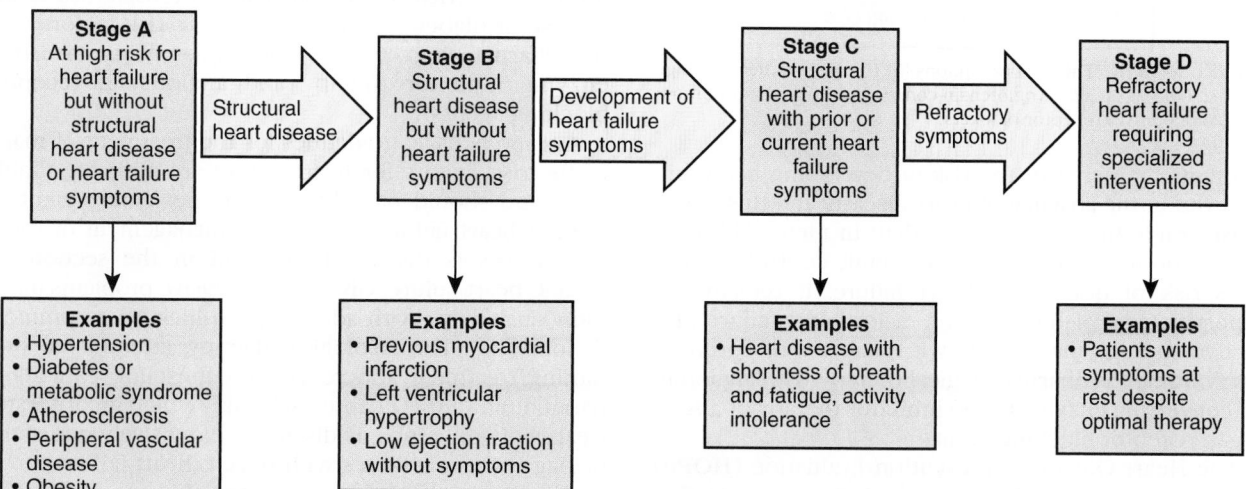

FIGURE 64-2 ■ The four stages in the development of heart failure as described by the American College of Cardiology/American Heart Association.[4] (Modified from Hunt SA, Baker DW, Chin MH et al: *J Am Coll Cardiol* 38:2101-2113, 2001.)

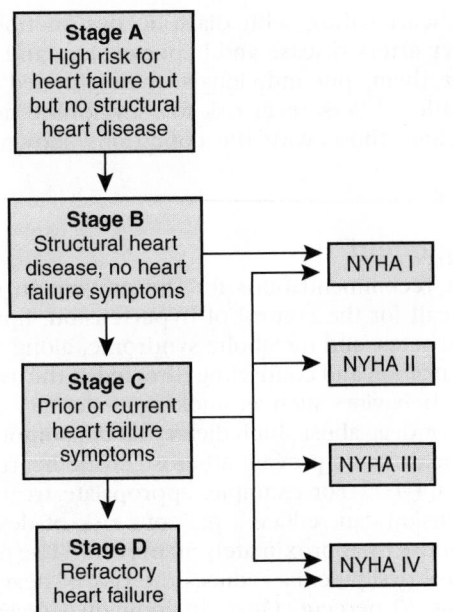

FIGURE 64-3 ■ The relationship between stages of heart failure and New York Heart Association functional classifications. *NYHA,* New York Heart Association.

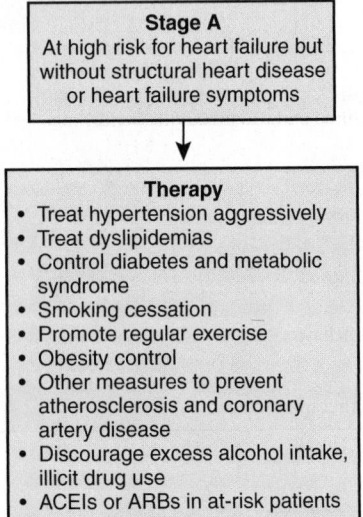

FIGURE 64-4 ■ Therapeutic options for the management of stage A heart failure. *ACEIs,* Angiotensin-converting enzyme inhibitors; *ARBs,* angiotensin receptor blockers.

substantially increases the risk of developing heart failure even in the absence of heart disease, and this risk is considerably higher in women than in men.[3] Although there is no firm evidence that glycemic control reduces one's risk of developing heart failure, it remains an important goal of therapy. The major heart failure preventive strategy for patients with diabetes or coronary artery disease is pharmacological therapy with angiotensin-converting enzyme **(ACE)** inhibitor therapy or angiotensin receptor blocking agents.

The Heart Outcomes Prevention Evaluation **(HOPE)** Study was a large, multicenter, randomized, controlled clinical trial conducted in patients age 55 or older who had coronary artery disease, peripheral vascular disease, or diabetes with one additional risk factor (i.e.,

USING GUIDELINES TO PROVIDE EVIDENCE-BASED CARE FOR PATIENTS WITH HEART FAILURE

In conditions such as heart failure with high morbidity and mortality and for which outcomes can be highly variable depending on the quality of care delivered, guidelines give practitioners needed assistance in providing optimal care. Guidelines are the result of a consensus process whereby experts in a given area review, evaluate, integrate, and summarize the review regarding care. The evidence then is presented in the form of specific recommendations about the pharmacological and nonpharmacological care of patients with the given condition. When there is insufficient evidence to make an evidence-based recommendation but care guidelines must still be provided, expert judgment and consensus about the best care is used to write the recommendation.

All nurses who care for patients with heart failure should be familiar with the latest guidelines so that they can deliver the best evidence-based care and advocate for the best medical care. A number of thorough heart failure guidelines are available to guide care. In writing this chapter, the most current guidelines available at the time were used, but it is important for nurses to remain up-to-date and to use the newest guidelines whenever they become available. Societies and organizations that produce heart failure guidelines and update them regularly include the following:

- The Heart Failure Society of America (available at *www.hfsa.org*)
- The American College of Cardiology and American Heart Association (available on the websites of organizations *www.acc.org* and *www.americanheart.org*)
- The European Society of Cardiology (available at *www.escardio.org*)

smoking, elevated total cholesterol, low high-density lipoprotein levels, hypertension, or microalbuminuria). The study demonstrated that ACE inhibitor use significantly decreased the risk of future cardiovascular events, including myocardial infarction, cardiac death, and heart failure.[2] Similarly, angiotensin receptor blockers **(ARBs)** reduce risk of heart failure in diabetic patients.[9] Thus, current pharmacological recommendations for patients in stage A heart failure call for the use of ACE inhibitors or ARBs in persons with atherosclerotic heart disease or diabetes with other cardiac risk factors (see the Pharmacology features on angiotensin-converting enzyme inhibitor therapy and angiotensin receptor blocking agents).

Comprehensive guidelines for the treatment of many of the risk factors for heart failure are available (Table 64-1) and should be followed for the management of stage A heart failure.[4,6] Complete management of these risk factors is discussed in detail in the section on stage C heart failure. Given the extensive problems many individuals have with adherence to lifestyle recommendations and pharmacological therapy, attention to promoting treatment adherence by counseling patients is paramount. In this chapter, self-care, which incorporates treatment adherence, is discussed extensively under the management of patients with stage C heart failure.

The prevention of heart failure also can be accomplished by limiting infarct size when an individual experiences acute coronary syndrome. Timely receipt of reperfusion therapies (i.e., fibrinolysis, percutaneous

■■■ PHARMACOLOGY

ANGIOTENSIN-CONVERTING ENZYME INHIBITOR THERAPY

DRUG	INITIAL DOSE	MAXIMUM DOSE	SIDE EFFECTS	COMMENTS
Captopril	6.25 mg t.i.d.	50 mg t.i.d.	Hypotension, hyperkalemia, renal insufficiency, cough, angioedema	Efforts to avoid sodium retention or depletion should be made because volume imbalance affects the effectiveness of ACE inhibitor therapy; fluid retention decreases benefits, and fluid depletion increases potential for hypotension or renal insufficiency. Nonsteroidal antiinflammatory drugs adversely affect ACE inhibitor effectiveness and should be avoided.
Enalapril	2.5 mg b.i.d.	10-20 mg b.i.d.		
Lisinopril	2.5-5 mg daily	20-40 mg daily		
Quinapril	5 mg b.i.d.	20 mg b.i.d.		
Ramipril	1.25-2.5 mg daily	10 mg daily		

ACE, Angiotensin-converting enzyme.

■■■ PHARMACOLOGY

ANGIOTENSIN RECEPTOR BLOCKING AGENTS

DRUG	INITIAL DOSE	MAXIMUM DOSES	SIDE EFFECTS	COMMENTS
Candesartan	4-8 mg daily	32 mg daily	Hypotension, hyperkalemia, worsening renal function, angioedema (less often than ACE inhibitors, but still occurs)	ACE inhibitors are the first choice renin-angiotensin system antagonism. ARBs are an alternative in those intolerant to ACE inhibitors because of refractory cough. ARBs appear to cause hypotension (worsening renal function) and hyperkalemia as often as ACE inhibitors.
Losartan	25-50 mg daily	50-100 mg daily		
Valsartan	20-40 mg b.i.d.	160 mg b.i.d.		

ACE, Angiotensin-converting enzyme; *ARB*, angiotensin receptor blocker.

■■■

TABLE 64-1   GUIDELINES AVAILABLE FOR THE MANAGEMENT OF RISK FACTORS FOR HEART FAILURE

RISK FACTOR	GUIDELINE
Hypertension	*Seventh Report of the Joint National Committee on Prevention, Detection, Evaluation, and Treatment of High Blood Pressure (JNC 7)* *www.nhlbi.nih.gov/guidelines/hypertension/jnc7full.htm*
Dyslipidemia	National Cholesterol Education Program: *Third Report on the Detection, Evaluation, and Treatment of High Blood Cholesterol in Adults (Adult Treatment Panel III)* guidelines *www.nhlbi.nih.gov/guidelines/cholesterol/atp3_rpt.htm*
Smoking	Department of Health and Human Services: *Clinical Practice Guideline: Treating Tobacco Use and Dependence* *www.surgeongeneral.gov/tobacco/treating_tobacco_use.pdf*
Sedentary lifestyle	*Exercise and Physical Activity in the Prevention and Treatment of Atherosclerotic Cardiovascular Disease: A Statement from the Council on Clinical Cardiology (Subcommittee on Exercise, Rehabilitation, and Prevention) and the Council on Nutrition, Physical Activity, and Metabolism (Subcommittee on Physical Activity)* *http://circ.ahajournals.org/cgi/reprint/107/24/3109*
Obesity	National Heart, Lung, and Blood Institute: *Clinical Guidelines on the Identification, Evaluation, and Treatment of Overweight and Obesity in Adults* *www.nhlbi.nih.gov/guidelines/obesity/ob_home.htm*
Cardiovascular disease	European Society of Cardiology: *European Guidelines on Cardiovascular Disease Prevention in Clinical Practice* *www.escardio.org/NR/rdonlyres/E2EA65FA-93EC-4C03-AB1D-1D944AFA1690/0/cvdprevention_ex_sum.pdf*
Cardiovascular disease in women	American Heart Association: *Evidence-Based Guideline for Cardiovascular Disease Prevention in Women* *http://circ.ahajournals.org/cgi/reprint/109/5/672.pdf*
Cardiovascular disease and diabetes	*Preventing Cancer, Cardiovascular Disease, and Diabetes: A Common Agenda for the American Cancer Society, the American Diabetes Association, and the American Heart Association* *http://circ.ahajournals.org/cgi/reprint/109/25/3244*
Cardiovascular disease	*AHA Guidelines for Primary Prevention of Cardiovascular Disease and Stroke: 2002 Update Consensus Panel Guide to Comprehensive Risk Reduction for Adult Patients Without Coronary or Other Atherosclerotic Vascular Diseases* *http://circ.ahajournals.org/cgi/reprint/106/3/388*

coronary intervention, coronary artery bypass surgery) during AMI can preserve ischemic myocardium, reduce infarct size, and maintain left ventricular function. Thus, ensuring that all AMI patients receive timely reperfusion therapies is an important goal for the prevention of heart failure.

The greatest impact in reducing the epidemic of heart failure likely will be made if primary prevention becomes a major focus for all health care providers. Lifestyle interventions and drug therapy to address risk factors can make a substantial impact in attenuating risk and preventing development of structural heart disease and ventricular dysfunction.

STAGE B HEART FAILURE

Like stage A, stage B is considered a "pre-heart failure" stage. Stage B occurs when an individual, often with poorly treated risk factors, progresses to develop structural heart disease but has no current or past signs or symptoms of heart failure. Examples of patients in stage B heart failure include those who have had a myocardial infarction, those with asymptomatic valvular disease, or individuals with evidence of left ventricular remodeling and low ejection fraction. In systolic heart failure, structural changes in the healthy area of the myocardium adjacent to but separate from an area of infarction are referred to as remodeling. These structural changes are caused by mechanical, humoral, and neurohormonal processes.[10] In diastolic heart failure, remodeling is due to hypertrophy that occurs in response to prolonged elevations in afterload (e.g., hypertension and aortic stenosis) and/or volume overload (e.g., aortic regurgitation). Hypertrophy of the ventricular myocytes causes regression from an adult to a fetal phenotype.[11] These large, genetically abnormal cells cannot contract as efficiently as normal myocardial cells. The result is ventricular dilatation, diastolic dysfunction, and eventual cardiac failure.

Systolic and diastolic dysfunction often occur in the same individual. One reason for this is that chronic hypertension is the primary cause of diastolic dysfunction

and one of the major risk factors for coronary artery disease (Figure 64-5). Mixed systolic and diastolic dysfunction involves chronic cardiac decompensation with impaired systolic function plus diastolic stiffness resulting from myocyte hyperplasia and collagen deposition.

Management

The patient with stage B heart failure is, by definition, without symptoms but with evidence of structural changes that reflect remodeling. Management includes all of the preventive strategies recommended for stage A patients plus additional pharmacological measures to prevent recurrent cardiac events and the progression to symptomatic heart failure (Figure 64-6).[4] The goals of therapy in stage B are to prevent progression of remodeling and prevent further ischemic or other cardiac events that damage healthy myocardium. To achieve these goals, it is vital to manage hypertension, dyslipidemia, metabolic syndrome, and diabetes aggressively. Other risk factors for coronary artery disease should be sought out and treated vigorously. As in stage A, there is a strong emphasis on lifestyle behavior change to address risk factors for coronary artery disease and heart failure. Counseling is essential to assure treatment adherence in these asymptomatic patients. (See Stage C Heart Failure for comprehensive coverage.)

Pharmacological therapy for stage B patients includes the use of ACE inhibitors or ARBs and use of beta-adrenergic blocking agents (see the Pharmacology features on ACE inhibitors, ARBs, and beta-adrenergic blocking agents) for select groups. A recent meta-analysis confirmed that aggressive blood pressure reduction is an effective way to prevent remodeling.[12] Not all antihypertension medications are equally effective in promoting regression of left ventricular hypertrophy; ACE inhibitors, beta-adrenergic blocking agents, and ARBs are preferred. All patients who have had a myocardial infarction should be treated with ACE inhibitors or ARBs and a beta-adrenergic blocking agent regardless of the age of the myocardial infarction. Any patient with a low ejection fraction, whether or not that person has had a myo-

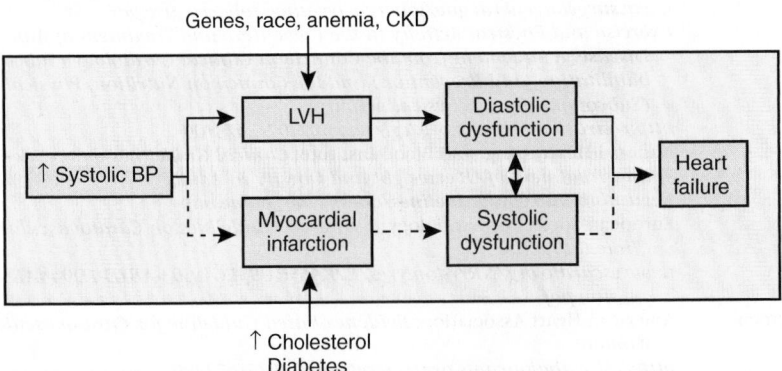

FIGURE 64-5 ■ The spectrum of hypertensive heart disease and major exacerbating conditions. Hypertensive heart disease in a spectrum of conditions *(large box)* that culminates in heart failure is not adequately treated. The major pathway *(solid arrow)* includes left ventricular hypertrophy and diastolic dysfunction. Hypertension also exacerbates coronary artery disease and myocardial infarction, which cause systolic dysfunction *(broken arrows)*. Systolic and diastolic dysfunction have a complex cause-effect relationship *(double-ended arrow)* and often coexist. *BP,* Blood pressure; *CKD,* chronic kidney disease; *LVH,* left ventricular hypertrophy. (Used by permission from Izzo JL Jr, Gradman AH: *Med Clin North Am* 88:1257-1271, 2004.)

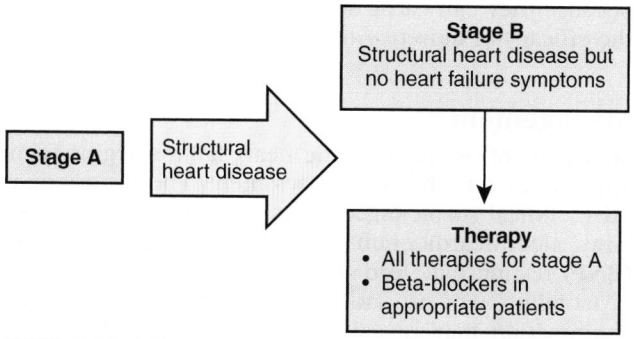

FIGURE 64-6 ■ Therapeutic options for the management of stage B heart failure.

cardial infarction, also should be treated with ACE inhibitors or ARBs and a beta-adrenergic blocking agent. In a sample of elders with a prior myocardial infarction and asymptomatic left ventricular systolic dysfunction, the combination of ACE inhibitors and beta blockers reduced new coronary events 37 percent.[13] In a recent meta-analysis of ARBs and ACE inhibitors, these classes of drugs were equally effective in decreasing all-cause mortality and hospitalizations in high-risk AMI patients.[14] Consequently, ARBs are recommended when ACE inhibitors are not tolerated. Surgical options that are considered in the prevention of progression of myocardial damage are coronary artery revascularization with percutaneous coronary intervention or coronary artery bypass and valvular repair for appropriate patients. Indications for surgery and care of patients following cardiothoracic surgery are covered in Chapter 65.

STAGE C HEART FAILURE

Patients with structural heart disease who go on to develop symptoms of heart failure or who come to the attention of a health care provider with a history of heart failure symptoms have progressed to stage C. The goals of therapy in stage C patients include prevention of further progression of heart failure, prevention of exacer-

bations of heart failure, control of symptoms, enhancement of quality of life, and improved survival. All of the lifestyle strategies recommended in stages A and B are recommended for stage C, and dietary sodium restriction is an added recommendation (Figure 64-7). Routine pharmacological therapy for patients in this stage of heart failure with nonpreserved ejection fraction consists of an ACE inhibitor (or ARB if patient is truly unable to take an ACE inhibitor), beta-adrenergic blocking agent, and diuretic. (See the Pharmacology feature on diuretic therapy.) Aldosterone antagonists, digoxin, and hydralazine/nitrates are added in appropriate patients. (See the Pharmacology feature on aldosterone antagonists.) Calcium channel blockers, even newer-generation formulations, should be avoided in heart failure

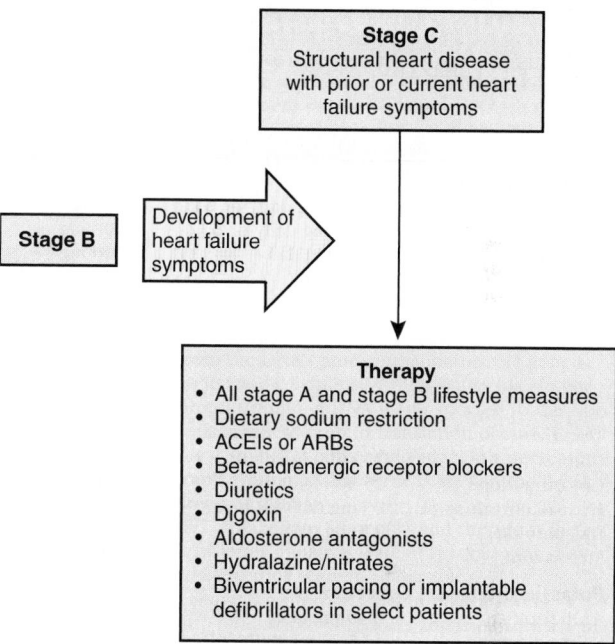

FIGURE 64-7 ■ Therapeutic options for the management of stage C heart failure. *ACEIs,* Angiotensin-converting enzyme inhibitors; *ARBs,* angiotensin receptor blockers.

■■■ PHARMACOLOGY

BETA-ADRENERGIC BLOCKING AGENTS

DRUG	INITIAL DAILY DOSE	MAXIMUM DAILY DOSES	SIDE EFFECTS	COMMENTS
Bisoprolol	1.25 mg daily	10 mg	Hypotension, bradycardia and heart block, fatigue, fluid retention, and worsening heart failure	Use with ACE inhibitors, but if hypotension is a problem, consider giving ACE inhibitor and beta-blocker at different times of day.
Carvedilol	3.125 mg b.i.d.	25 mg b.i.d. or 50 mg b.i.d. for patients greater than 85 kg		In patients with fluid overload, diuretics improve the action of beta blockers by maintaining fluid and sodium balance. These may increase fluid retention during initiation of therapy; close monitoring of fluid status by patient with daily weights is necessary.
Metoprolol CR/XL	12.5-25 mg daily	200 mg		Symptoms may take weeks to months to improve, and beta-blockers should be continued even if symptom status is unchanged because they protect against future adverse cardiac events.

ACE, Angiotensin-converting enzyme.

because they stimulate the sympathetic nervous system.[15] Some of the older, long-acting calcium channel blockers have negative inotropic and chronotropic properties, with the potential to exacerbate heart failure. Two recent trials of the newer calcium channel blockers amlodipine (the Prospective Randomised Amlodipine Survival Evaluation [PRAISE] Trial) and felodipine (V-HeFT III) in patients with heart failure suggest that these drugs may have beneficial effects, although further studies are needed. Also to be avoided in heart failure are antidysrhythmic agents (with the exception of amiodarone) because they have cardiodepressant and prodysrhythmic effects that negatively affect survival. Nonsteroidal antiinflammatory agents should be avoided because they can cause sodium retention and decrease the efficacy of diuretics and ACE inhibitors.

Management

Management of symptomatic heart failure begins with appropriate and thorough assessment. The history may raise clinical suspicion, or physical examination, chest x-ray, electrocardiogram, or B-type natriuretic peptide (BNP) testing may lead the clinician to a diagnosis of heart failure. For patients in mild heart failure, physical examination may reveal an S_4 gallop or subtle ankle edema. The chest x-ray might reveal an enlarged heart. The electrocardiogram is nonspecific for heart failure

---

■■■ PHARMACOLOGY

DIURETIC THERAPY

DRUG	INITIAL DAILY DOSE	MAXIMUM TOTAL DAILY DOSE	SIDE EFFECTS	COMMENTS
Loop Diuretics			Electrolyte depletion, hypotension, and azotemia	Diuretics cannot be used alone for the management of heart failure. By promoting fluid and sodium balance, diuretics enhance the effectiveness of other heart failure medications. Care should be taken to avoid overdiuresis and underdiuresis.
Bumetanide	0.5-1.0 mg daily or b.i.d.	10 mg		
Furosemide	20-40 mg daily or b.i.d.	600 mg		
Torsemide	10-20 mg daily	200 mg		
Thiazides			Electrolyte depletion, hypotension, and azotemia	
Chlorothiazide	250-500 mg daily or b.i.d.	1000 mg		
Chlorthalidone	25-50 mg daily	100 mg		
Hydrochlorothiazide	25 mg daily or b.i.d.	200 mg		
Indapamide	2.5 mg daily	5 mg		
Metolazone	5 mg daily	20 mg		
Potassium-Sparing Diuretics			Hyperkalemia, volume depletion (particularly when taken with other diuretics)	
Amiloride	5-10 mg daily	20 mg		
Spironolactone	12.5-25 mg daily	50 mg		
Triamterene	100 mg b.i.d.	300 mg		
Sequential Nephron Blockade				
Metolazone		2.5-10 mg once plus loop diuretic		
Hydrochlorothiazide		25-100 mg once or twice plus loop diuretic		
Chlorothiazide (IV)		500-1000 mg once plus loop diuretic		

ACE, Angiotensin-converting enzyme; *IV,* intravenous.

■■■ PHARMACOLOGY

ALDOSTERONE ANTAGONIST THERAPY

DRUG	INITIAL DAILY DOSE	MAXIMUM TOTAL DAILY DOSE	SIDE EFFECTS	COMMENTS
Eplerenone	25 mg daily	50 mg	Hyperkalemia, volume depletion (particularly when taken with other diuretics)	Used with other diuretics for management of severe symptomatic heart failure. Monitor renal function and potassium levels closely during therapy; monthly for first 3 months and then every 3 months.
Spironolactone	12.5-25 mg daily	25-50 mg		

ACE, Angiotensin-converting enzyme.

but may indicate a prior myocardial infarction or long-standing hypertension with left ventricular hypertrophy (Figure 64-8). In patients with more advanced heart failure and marked fluid overload, the most common complaint is increasing shortness of breath. Physical examination probably will reveal an S_3 gallop, lung crackles, 2+ or 3+ dependent edema, jugular venous distention, and perhaps a tender liver edge. The chest x-ray may show Kerley B lines, tiny horizontal lines at the bases that indicate fluid accumulation, as well as cardiac enlargement.

Laboratory testing should include a complete blood count, a chemistry panel, and a urinalysis to identify etiological (e.g., thyroid dysfunction) or aggravating factors (e.g., renal failure and anemia) that may require treatment or influence the choice of therapy (e.g., liver dysfunction). BNP testing can be used to rule out a suspected diagnosis of heart failure; with a BNP less than 100 pg/ml, a diagnosis of heart failure is improbable. Once diagnosed, BNP can be used to assess disease severity and the efficacy of therapy.

It is vital that reversible causes of heart failure be detected and treated (Box 64-2). Reversible causes include significant coronary artery disease, valvular stenosis, and regurgitation and chronic or recurrent dysrhythmias such as atrial fibrillation, and these are discussed in detail in other chapters.

Medical Management

As described in Chapter 62, the failing heart is thought to be energy starved,[16] with 25 to 30 percent lower levels of adenosine triphosphate available for vital functions. Key to understanding the importance of energy starvation is the realization that sustained increases in hemodynamic load cause a change in gene expression for some of the proteins involved in energy synthesis and utilization.[17] This mechanism has implications for pharmacological management and patient self-care.

Pharmacological management of the symptomatic patient continues to emphasize drugs that reduce metabolic demand such as ACE inhibitors, ARBs, and beta-adrenergic blockers. In systolic heart failure, aggressive blood pressure control is essential because the failing ventricle is exquisitely sensitive to increased cardiac afterload. Beta blockers are an important adjunctive therapy but are not considered to be helpful as the sole pharmacological therapy in heart failure. Loop diuretics improve symptoms and health-related quality of life, but not mortality.

Some standard therapies for heart failure have been questioned recently. Digitalis was found to lower the risk of worsening heart failure and hospitalization in symptomatic patients with left ventricular dysfunction; low serum digoxin concentrations (0.5 to 0.9 ng/ml) may be most effective.[18] The liberal use of diuretics has been questioned because high diuretic doses have been

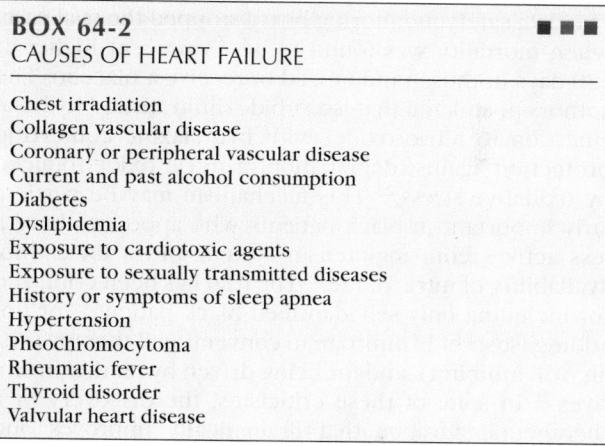

BOX 64-2   ■ ■ ■
CAUSES OF HEART FAILURE

Chest irradiation
Collagen vascular disease
Coronary or peripheral vascular disease
Current and past alcohol consumption
Diabetes
Dyslipidemia
Exposure to cardiotoxic agents
Exposure to sexually transmitted diseases
History or symptoms of sleep apnea
Hypertension
Pheochromocytoma
Rheumatic fever
Thyroid disorder
Valvular heart disease

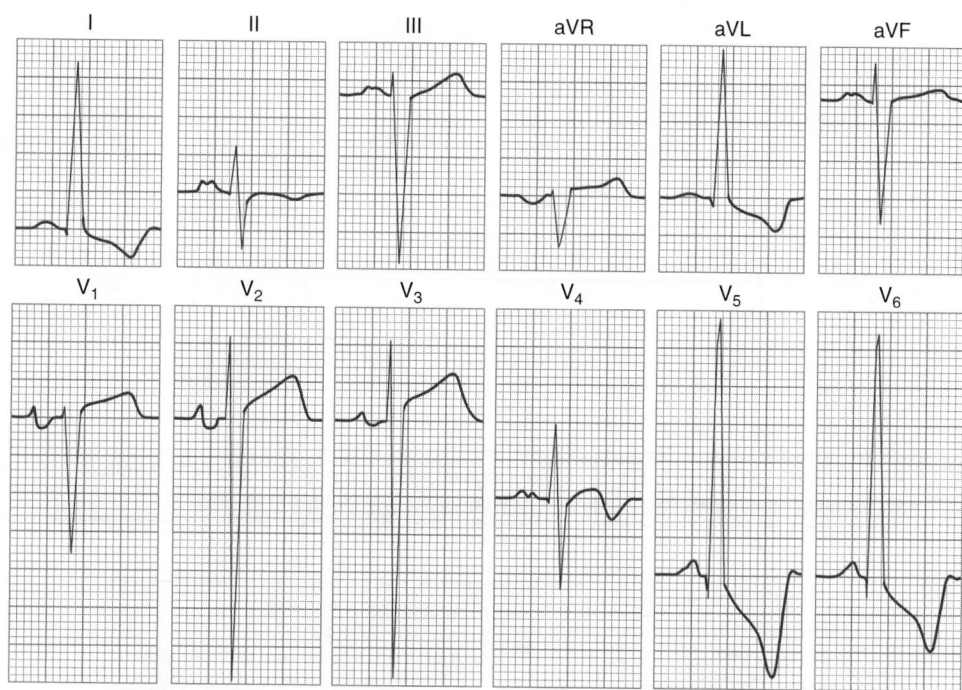

FIGURE 64-8 ■ Left ventricular hypertrophy on a 12-lead electrocardiogram.

associated independently with mortality, sudden death, and pump failure death in patients with advanced heart failure.[19] When trials of aspirin compared with warfarin were reanalyzed in a recent meta-analysis, heart failure hospitalizations were higher in patients taking aspirin.[20] Aspirin probably should be avoided in patients receiving ACE inhibitors because the symptom and survival benefits of ACE inhibitors are attributable to their effects on the circulation and the kidneys, but this benefit is cancelled by aspirin. If inhibition of platelet aggregation is necessary, glycoprotein IIb/IIIa receptor antagonists may be superior to aspirin.

A new study of heart failure pharmacotherapy was accused of leading in a "new era of race-based therapeutics."[21] A regimen of a beta blocker, a fixed dose of 37.5 mg of hydralazine hydrochloride, and 20 mg of isosorbide dinitrate 3 times daily increased to a total daily dose of 225 mg of hydralazine hydrochloride and 120 mg of isosorbide dinitrate was tested in a clinical trial of self-identified black patients with systolic heart failure and impaired functional status (NYHA Class III or IV). The data safety monitoring board stopped the trial early when mortality was found to be 43 percent higher at 180 days in those randomized to receive a placebo. The authors postulated that isosorbide dinitrate and hydralazine donate nitric oxide, with hydralazine conferring protection against degradation of nitric oxide induced by oxidative stress.[22] This mechanism may be particularly important in black patients who appear to have a less active renin-angiotensin system and a lower bioavailability of nitric oxide.[23] The trial has been criticized for including only self-identified black patients, for not adding isosorbide dinitrate to conventional therapy (i.e., an ACE inhibitor), and for being driven by market incentives.[21] In spite of these criticisms, the discovery of a therapeutic advance that dramatically improves outcomes in a segment of the population known to receive substandard care is of great interest. This is an early step toward genetically based pharmacological therapy designed for specific populations.

The pharmacological therapy for symptomatic stage C diastolic heart failure is less clear than that for systolic heart failure because patients with an ejection fraction greater than 40 percent have been included in so few clinical trials. Acute management consists of central volume reduction with loop diuretics and long-acting nitrates. The ARB candesartan was associated with a decrease of 11 percent in hospitalizations.[24] Heart rate slowing with beta blockade and nondihydropyridine calcium antagonists may improve ventricular filling. Digitalis should be used with caution for the reasons cited before. Diastolic heart failure now is appreciated as having a high death rate; 23 percent of patients enrolled in the Digitalis Investigation Group **(DIG)** trial died during a 3.1-year follow-up.[25] Predictors of death included impaired renal function, worse functional class, male gender, and older age.

For patients with systolic heart failure and an ejection fraction of 30 percent or less, an implantable cardioverter-defibrillator **(ICD)** may be placed as primary prevention of sudden death. In appropriate patients, ICD implantation can reduce mortality risk by approximately one-third in the following 2 years.[26] Cardiac resynchronization therapy **(CRT)** or biventricular pacing is another novel adjunctive therapy for patients with advanced heart failure. In those patients with a left bundle branch block or an intraventricular conduction delay that causes significant left ventricular dyssynchrony, the mortality rate is high. CRT reduces the conduction delay, optimizes the ejection fraction, and decreases mitral regurgitation and left ventricular remodeling, all of which improve symptoms. Recently, the COMPANION Trial showed a 43 percent reduction in a composite endpoint of all-cause mortality and hospitalization in patients receiving CRT and an ICD.[27] Chapter 61 describes the care of patients with implanted cardiac rhythm management devices.

Self-Care and Treatment Adherence

Self-care is an integral aspect of care at the early symptomatic stage because patients are typically not ill enough to see a provider frequently. So they need to engage in behaviors that maintain physiological stability (including treatment adherence) and to manage symptoms when they occur. In our model of self-care (Figure 64-9),[28] these behaviors of self-care maintenance and

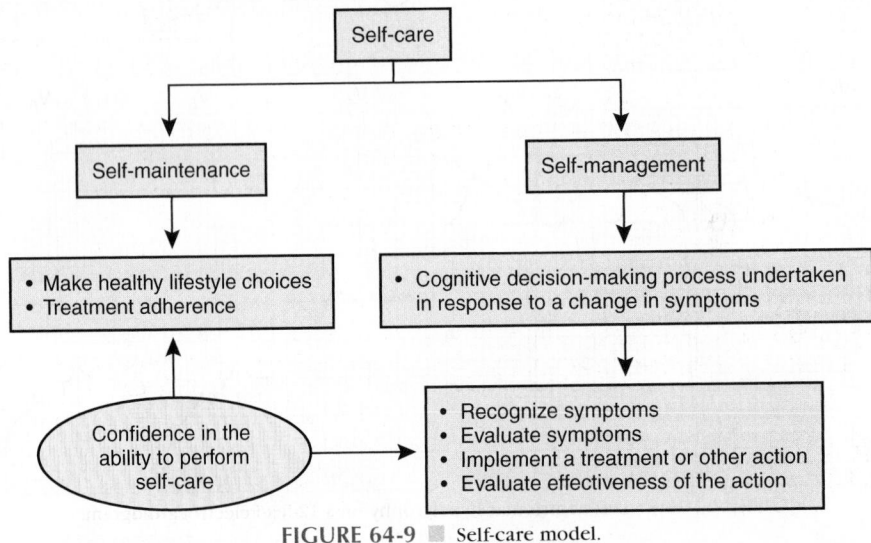

FIGURE 64-9 ■ Self-care model.

management are explored within the context of naturalistic decision making, which addresses how persons make decisions in real-world settings. Critical thinking is emphasized in formal educational programs, but naturalistic decision makers rely more on experience and acquired expertise to mentally simulate actions and anticipate how those actions will play out. Values influence how likely they are to act on symptom changes. For example, naturalistic decision makers might revise decision rules to match a particular situation. They respond differently to symptoms depending on the situation and may make snap decisions based on the information available at the moment. These inconsistent, seemingly illogical decisions frustrate clinicians but are typical of laypersons.

Self-Care Maintenance

The health promoting behaviors that keep the patient with heart failure physiologically stable are shown in Box 64-3. These behaviors do not seem difficult to clini-

---

BOX 64-3 ■ ■ ■

SELF-CARE MAINTENANCE BEHAVIORS ADVOCATED FOR PERSONS WITH HEART FAILURE

- Monitor daily weights, looking for any 2-day 3-lb weight gain or 1-week 3- to 5-lb weight gain.
- Follow a low-sodium diet.
- Take medications as prescribed.
- Prevent infections (including obtaining an annual flu vaccination and pneumonia vaccination [Pneumovax]).
- Modify unhealthy lifestyle behaviors such as smoking, inactivity, and excess alcohol intake.

■ ■ ■ **CONUNDRUM**

THE OBESITY PARADOX IN HEART FAILURE

In the general population, obesity is associated with increased risk of adverse outcomes such as hypertension and coronary artery disease. In the heart failure population, however, patients who are overweight and obese have been shown repeatedly to have better outcomes than those who are within a normal range of body mass index. This general finding has been replicated sufficiently at this point to convince the heart failure community of its validity.

The underlying mechanism of the obesity paradox is unknown, but possibilities that are being explored are (1) differences in the timing of diagnosis among those of different body weights and (2) cardiac cachexia. The possibility that these results are simply a reflection of obese patients being diagnosed with heart failure at an earlier stage than those with lower BMI has not received much support. Support is accumulating for an explanation of obesity as a countermeasure for the wasting syndrome of cardiac cachexia seen in advanced heart failure. Physiological changes such as low levels of insulin-like growth factor 1 and elevated circulating renin, catecholamines, transforming factor B (beta), and inflammatory cytokines are associated with anorexia and muscle wasting. Excess body weight may protect patients who are exposed to this physiological onslaught from excessive wasting.

More research is needed to understand the obesity paradox, but in the meantime, effort should be given to preventing malnutrition and cardiac cachexia rather than to encouraging all heart failure patients to achieve a normal body weight.

Curtis JP, Selter JG, Wang Y et al: The obesity paradox: body mass index and outcomes in patients with heart failure, *Arch Intern Med* 165:55-61, 2005. *BMI*, Body mass index.

---

cians, but study after study has demonstrated the challenge that patients face in trying to implement these behaviors. One factor currently under active debate is the value of weight loss for obesity. (See the Conundrum feature on the obesity paradox in heart failure.)

Daily Weighing

Changes in body weight represent the most sensitive indicator of fluid volume overload currently available for monitoring the general population of persons with heart failure. However, fewer than half of patients weigh themselves daily.[29,30] One reason is that the rationale behind the request that patients monitor their body weight daily is difficult for patients to understand. Most assume that daily weighing is done to monitor adipose tissue. As one patient told us, when we asked her about daily weighing, "No! That's a bad habit for anyone to get into."[31]

Dietary Sodium Restriction

Excessive dietary sodium intake contributes to volume overload and subsequent systemic edema and pulmonary congestion. Even in mild, asymptomatic heart failure, the ability to excrete sodium is impaired. A high-sodium diet increases ventricular end-diastolic and end-systolic volumes without a corresponding increase in ejection fraction or stroke volume. Reducing dietary sodium intake can produce significant hemodynamic and clinical improvement, even without other interventions. Diuretic therapy is more effective when a reduced-sodium diet is followed. Many cases of apparent refractoriness to diuretics are caused by excessive dietary sodium intake.

Despite evidence of the effectiveness of a low-sodium diet, sodium overload is one of the most common reasons for acute decompensation and recurrent rehospitalization in this population. Fewer than half of patients adequately limit dietary sodium.[32] Reasons that patients have difficulty adhering to dietary sodium restriction include (1) inadequate knowledge about food choices that are low in salt, (2) inability to apply their knowledge about salt once that knowledge is acquired (i.e., lack of skill in making food choices), (3) social discomfort related to the need to modify family meals, (4) age-related changes in smell and taste that make salt restriction especially difficult, and (5) little desire to relinquish one of their few remaining pleasures.[33]

Many patients know not to add salt to their food but have no idea of the sodium content of the foods they regularly eat, what level of daily sodium they should aim for, or how to keep track of their daily intake. Some are knowledgeable about obvious sources of sodium such as table salt but are unaware of the significant sodium content of canned foods, convenience foods, food with preservatives (sodium benzoate, sodium bisulfite), and over-the-counter medicines such as Alka-Seltzer that are made with sodium bicarbonate (baking soda). Clinicians have been shown to address the importance of dietary sodium restriction in a cursory fashion or not at all.[34] Even patients who have been hospitalized for heart failure have surprisingly poor knowledge of how to follow a low-sodium diet.[35] See Box 64-4 for specifics of prescribing a low-sodium diet.

Adhering to diet recommendations is particularly challenging for patients when dining in restaurants or attending social events where there is little control over the hidden salt content of food. An important part of the satisfaction derived from eating is the social milieu in which it occurs. Therefore, dietary interventions that are most effective are centered on the family.

Although the dietetic literature is replete with studies about age-related changes of taste and smell that alter food choices, little attention has been given to the implications of these changes for elders with heart failure. Logically, these elders may have difficulty limiting salt intake because of age-related decrements in the palatability of food. One team that investigated taste loss found a generic loss of taste with aging; older persons, and especially older men, were less sensitive to the taste of salt than the young men and women.[36] Others have argued that the decline with age is small but accentuated by health disorders, medications, oral hygiene, denture use, and environmental insults such as chronic smoking, which alter chemosensation.[37] Further research is needed to identify the contribution of aging to dietary salt indiscretions of persons with heart failure.

Medication Adherence

Medication adherence or compliance refers to the extent to which medication taking coincides with medical or health advice. The problem with this definition is that some forms of noncompliance are more problematic than others and patients are not "noncompliant" or "compliant." For example, in one study, patients chose what drugs to take when rather than simply taking ev-

ery drug in the manner in which it was ordered.[38] Others have documented that clinically important medication noncompliance is common and found in more than half of heart failure patients.[32,35]

Studies in which compliance was assessed using objective indicators usually, although not always,[38] demonstrated that poor medication compliance is associated with increased cardiovascular related-hospitalizations, longer lengths of hospital stay, and higher mortality.[39] Patients who should be screened carefully for medication nonadherence are unmarried or unsupported, taking multiple medications, and low in self-efficacy.[35,40] Those who have not had a recent hospitalization that impressed upon them the need to take their medicines and provided an opportunity for patient education may be less adherent than others. See Box 64-5 for ways to improve medication adherence.

Fluid Restriction

Fluid restriction is common during hospitalization for acute heart failure, but there is no consensus on the need for continued fluid restriction as part of outpatient therapy or evidence that stringent chronic fluid restriction is beneficial. Holst and colleagues[41] argue that fluid restriction may be detrimental because the common prescription for 1.5 liter/d is appropriate only for a 50-kg person. For someone who weighs 80 kg, a fluid intake of 1.5 liter/d would result in a 1 liter/d deficit after physiological fluid requirements are met. The resulting intracellular fluid deficiency could reduce cell function, including myocyte function. Strict fluid restriction greatly impairs quality of life and may be responsible for the dizziness reported in some samples by significantly lowering cardiac output.

Adequate symptom control with sodium restriction and drug therapy usually negates the need for rigorous fluid restriction. Counsel patients to avoid excessive (more than 2 to 2.5 liters per day) intake of fluids, but reserve stringent fluid restriction for selected patients with severe heart failure and difficult-to-control hyponatremia that may benefit from fluid restriction.

A common misconception among heart failure patients is that they should *increase* their fluid intake to "flush the system" or "cleanse the body" when they are ill or to compensate for the excessive urination caused by diuretics.[42] This misconception is so common that it should be explored with every patient and corrected early in the course of therapy.

Prevention of Infection

Heart failure is associated with compromise of the immune system, so efforts to minimize the risk of contracting a preventable infection such as influenza or pneumonia are essential. In the 1990s, approximately 36,000 deaths were attributed annually to influenza, and most of these deaths were in elders. Pneumonia remains one of the primary causes of death in the United States, with 40,000 deaths occurring each year from pneumococcal disease. One of the objectives of Healthy People 2010 is to achieve 90 percent coverage of noninstitutionalized adults aged 65 and older for influenza and pneumococcal vaccinations. Yet influenza and pneumococcal vaccination levels vary widely among states/areas and racial/ethnic populations.[43]

All patients with heart failure should receive an annual influenza vaccination, and anyone over age 2 with heart failure should receive a pneumonia vaccination. Cigarette smoking is a strong independent risk factor for invasive pneumococcal disease,[44] so vaccination for pneumonia is particularly important for any heart failure patient who is exposed to cigarette smoke. Those with comorbid renal failure should be revaccinated at 6 years. Currently available pneumonia vaccinations are safe, cost-effective, and associated with only minor side effects such as mild erythema and pain at the site of injection. The efficacy in persons with heart failure is 69 percent.[45]

Alcohol Restriction

Persons with heart failure typically are told to abstain totally from drinking alcohol because of the belief that alcohol is a myocardial depressant. The wisdom of this recommendation was questioned recently by Piano,[46] who argued that the acute effects of alcohol often are minor and transient. She reviewed research demonstrating that alcohol acutely depressed myocardial contractility, prolonged systolic time intervals, decreased ejection fraction, decreased velocity of left ventricular fiber shortening, and decreased cardiac output. In normal persons these effects were mild and probably offset by corresponding changes in other hemodynamic parameters such as afterload and systemic vascular resistance. Little is known about whether these same effects occur in persons with heart failure. Only one small study of the acute effects of alcohol consumption on cardiac performance in human beings has been conducted.[47] No significant changes were found in cardiac index, stroke volume, or any other echocardiographic parameter in that small sample of eight patients given 0.9 g/kg of 80 proof vodka. Piano's recommendations, based on the data available at this time, are summarized in Table 64-2.

Exercise

Another important goal at this stage is maintenance of functional capacity and exercise. A meta-analysis of nine studies with 801 patients revealed a survival advantage in the 395 persons randomized to exercise training.[48] A recently updated Cochrane review concluded that exercise training improved short-term exercise capacity and quality of life in persons with mild to moderate heart failure.[49] Exercise is clearly beneficial for those with mild to moderate heart failure, and ongoing studies are defining its role in patients with severe heart failure. See Box 64-6 for recommendations to assist patients in starting and maintaining an exercise program.

Self-Care Management

In addition to the self-care maintenance behaviors discussed before, persons with heart failure also must use problem-solving skill, make decisions, and address new signs and symptoms quickly—self-care *management*. Our prior research suggests that the key to self-care for the naturalistic decision maker is symptom recognition. Patients' decision-making abilities in response to

■ ■ ■

TABLE 64-2   ALCOHOL RESTRICTION RECOMMENDATIONS FOR PERSONS WITH HEART FAILURE

RECOMMENDATION	RATIONALE
Carefully consider the cause of heart failure before advising patients about the use of alcohol. Someone with ischemic left ventricular dysfunction probably can consume one standard (12 g of alcohol) drink occasionally if taken with a meal.	Evidence is accumulating that small amounts of alcohol provide some physiological benefit for persons with ischemic heart disease. Food slows absorption of alcohol and moderates the physiological effects.
Avoid alcohol if heart failure is due to nonischemic causes or alcoholic cardiomyopathy.	No data support the benefit of alcohol in someone without ischemic heart disease. There is some indication that alcohol consumption may increase hospitalization rates.
Avoid alcohol in persons with major depression, anxiety disorder, behavioral disorder, or sleep disorders.	Alcohol can interfere with the effectiveness of some antidepressants, complicate a psychiatric condition, and interfere with sleep.
Avoid alcohol in persons with recurrent dysrhythmias, a history of hypertension, and diabetes.	Dysrhythmias and high blood pressure could be accentuated. The sugar content of alcohol could complicate control of diabetes.
Women should drink less alcohol than men.	Alcohol is metabolized differently in men and women.
Always avoid intoxication, drinks high in alcohol content (greater than 60%), and those with additives.	The hemodynamic effects of alcohol are accentuated at higher doses.

Adapted from Piano MR: *J Card Fail* 8:239-246, 2002.

BOX 64-6   ▪ ▪ ▪

ASSISTING PATIENTS TO START AND MAINTAIN AN
EXERCISE PROGRAM

- Conceptualize exercise as increasing and maintaining activity, not necessarily a formal, rigorous exercise program.
- Ask about perceived advantages and disadvantages of exercise.
- Explore barriers that impede exercise (most commonly lack of time) and facilitators that would increase exercise.
- Elicit descriptions of past exercise patterns and activities of interest to the patient.
- Encourage activities with the potential for social support (e.g., mall walking or contracting with a friend or neighbor).

symptoms can distinguish those with better outcomes. The response to symptoms may translate into a more favorable physiological state or attenuate a maladaptive signal or event, which may prolong survival.

The fluid overload of heart failure causes increased and repetitive myocardial volume and stretch, which are associated with activation of different hypertrophic signaling pathways in the myocardium.[50] Although the manner in which different forms of mechanical stretch are linked to activation of hypertrophic signaling pathways is unknown, excessive and repetitive myocardial stretch is an important adverse signal involved in left ventricular remodeling and progression of heart failure.[51] A rapid and appropriate response to the symptoms of fluid overload may modulate the repetitive and prolonged stretch of the myocardium. Although speculative, involving patients in self-care may translate into a beneficial physiological response that ultimately attenuates left ventricular remodeling and the progression of heart failure.

Self-care is particularly challenging in the early symptomatic phase of the syndrome because patients and providers alike are prone to ignoring the risk of progression in these patients. From the patient's perspective, motivating behavioral change requires a perceived need to change. Without evidence of such a need, such as a significant new symptom, patients are unlikely to engage actively in self-care. Few investigators have included patients with few or early symptoms in clinical trials, but one study that did, enrolled hospitalized heart failure patients into a multidisciplinary disease management trial, regardless of their symptom history.[52] Six months later, acute care costs were highest in the patients who were asymptomatic before the acute index hospitalization and lowest in those in the early symptom stages. The investigators postulated that increased costs in asymptomatic patients might have resulted from improved access to care. That is, providers may have appropriately used the hospitalization of a previously asymptomatic heart failure patient as a signal to begin a full diagnostic work-up.

Another reason why acute care costs were higher in the asymptomatic patients in this trial[52] could be the negative impact of the intervention on previously asymptomatic patients. According to the common sense model of illness, symptom interpretation by patients is guided by their cognitive representations of the event. These representations or images incorporate symptom labels, expected timeline, causal attributions, beliefs about symptom control, and perceived consequences. For patients, images of "heart failure" may invoke memories of someone who had the syndrome years ago before treatment had advanced and include beliefs about rapid functional decline and inevitable death. Applying these concepts to the newly hospitalized, previously asymptomatic patient participating in a 6-month educational intervention, perhaps the repetitive education provided to these patients made it difficult for them to maintain denial. It would not be surprising if worried patients sought care more quickly than those who had accommodated to a chronically symptomatic state.

Patient desire to maintain denial for as long as possible was suggested by the results of a qualitative study conducted in New Zealand. Approximately four-fifths (51/62) of patients interviewed in an outpatient clinic reported not wanting more or better information about their heart failure. Reasons for the lack of desire included lack of interest or avoidance and trust in their provider.[53]

Living with Advanced Stage C Heart Failure

When heart failure progresses, symptomatic periods increase. Living with heart failure has been described as a process of navigating physical, social, and emotional turbulence.[54] Patients live with shortness of breath, fatigue, peripheral swelling, difficulty sleeping in a supine position, coughing, inability to perform normal activities of daily living, and fluid retention. Dizziness, light-headedness, and palpitations are common but worrisome symptoms that suggest dysrhythmias, dehydration, or hypotension. An unintentional weight loss may indicate cardiac cachexia, which would suggest a transition to stage D heart failure.

Social losses occur when persons are no longer physically able to perform activities of daily living and the social behaviors that previously gave them pleasure, such as social outings with friends. The practice of skipping diuretic doses is a constant source of concern and frustration to clinicians,[38] but diuretics curtail social events because of the need always to be near a bathroom. Social isolation probably contributes to emotional turbulence, but the research in this area is currently insufficient to make such a statement with confidence.[55]

The emotional burden is intense in this patient population. Depression and anxiety are most common. In the general population, 5 to 10 percent are depressed, but in persons with heart failure, rates range from 11 to 25 percent of outpatients and from 35 to 70 percent of those hospitalized.[56] A recent, carefully conducted study of the prevalence of depression in a large sample of hospitalized patients with heart failure revealed that 51 percent had significant depression on the Beck Depression Inventory (10 or greater). Of these, 20 percent met the *Diagnostic and Statistical Manual of Mental Disorders,* fourth edition, criteria for a current major depressive episode, and 16 percent for a minor depressive episode. Depression may be more common in women with heart failure and in patients with relatively worse symptoms.[57] A strong and graded association has been documented between the severity of depressive symptoms in persons with heart failure and functional decline, rehospitalization, cost, and death.[58]

Although anxiety is an important, debilitating symptom of heart failure, few investigators have studied this response. One group of investigators[59] found no significant differences in state or trait anxiety when a sample of predominately NYHA Class III heart failure patients were compared with persons admitted with other illnesses. However, a recent comparison of heart failure patients, AMI patients, coronary artery bypass patients, and healthy elders revealed that although patients with heart failure have anxiety levels similar to the other cardiac groups, they have substantially more anxiety than healthy elders.[60]

Dracup and colleagues[61] studied the relationship between perceived control and anxiety, depression, and hostility and demonstrated that heart failure patients with low perceived control were more anxious, more depressed, and more hostile than those high in perceived control. One method of increasing perceived control is by encouraging self-care.

Self-Care and Treatment Adherence

At this point in the inexorable progression of heart failure, self-care is essential because unloading the failing heart can reverse gene expression toward the normal adult phenotype,[16] which can slow the progression of disease. Behaviors associated with escalations in ventricular load and sporadic increases in myocardial stretch are those that contribute to fluid overload: dietary salt indiscretion and skipping of diuretic doses.

The importance of early symptom recognition was introduced before. Even in patients with advanced heart failure, symptoms often are initially subtle or difficult to discern from those associated with comorbid conditions. In these situations, when symptom recognition fails, a naturalistic decision maker will revert to assumption-based reasoning (e.g., "my weight will be stable today because I didn't eat much salt yesterday"). Decisions made in this way are commonly erroneous, which can cause symptom exacerbation and lead to hospital admission.

Exploring errors in decision making can assist clinicians to identify how to improve patients' decision-making performance. Errors are most likely to be due to insufficient attention and inadequate problem detection, which are aggravated by inexperience and/or inadequate training. Several investigators have explored the educational needs of patients with heart failure. In one study, the primary learning needs of patients, in order of importance, were medications, anatomy and physiology, and risk factors.[62] The top ranked learning needs were different in another study,[63] in which the most important learning needs were diet, general heart failure information, and prognosis. Another investigator reported that most patients hospitalized for heart failure in their sample lacked a clear understanding of the condition.[64] Similar results were found in a qualitative study of heart failure patients seen in a general office practice in New Zealand.[53]

It should be noted that when nurse perceptions of patient learning needs are compared with patient reports of learning needs, differences are always evident.[62,63] Two investigative teams have questioned whether hospital staff nurses have a knowledge base sufficient to teach heart failure patients. When Albert and colleagues[65] studied staff nurses, the average score on a test of basic heart failure knowledge was 76 percent even though heart failure educational offerings were available before the survey period. In a similar study of staff nurses who routinely care for heart failure patients who took the same test, the average knowledge score was 73 percent.[66] Frequently missed questions (scores less than 70 percent) addressed the use of nonsteroidal antiinflammatory drugs, use of potassium-based salt substitutes, assessment of daily weights, and physician notification of asymptomatic low blood pressure and momentary dizziness upon rising. Together, the results of these studies suggest that staff nurses—who must counsel this common patient population—could benefit from more education about heart failure.

In patients who are symptomatic, self-care management involves an active, deliberate decision-making process undertaken in response to symptoms. The self-care management process involves symptom recognition, symptom evaluation, treatment implementation, and treatment evaluation—all of which are thought to be influenced by confidence in one's ability to perform self-care. Once changes in signs and symptoms are recognized, those patients who are most successful at self-care are those who detect signs and symptoms early, know what to do about them, have the skill to respond and do so in a timely fashion.

The personal characteristics of those most likely to master heart failure self-care may be those that contribute to problem solving in other, general situations. Persons most likely to master a complex set of skills such as self-care are those who are more highly educated,[10] those with some experience with the diagnosis,[28] those who received patient education, and those with support from others. Those who see a need (i.e., have symptoms and/or were hospitalized recently)[28] are more likely to master self-care, but not those who are overwhelmed by their symptoms. Other factors that impair self-care include financial hardship, low health literacy, impaired cognition, poor functional status, and sensory impairments.[31]

Monitoring symptoms is especially difficult for patients in stage C heart failure, apparently because they become acclimated to their progressing symptoms. Investigators have demonstrated that dyspneic patients are slow to recognize their shortness of breath. Once they recognize it, only a small percentage is adventuresome in their self-care remedies. Most simply wait for their symptoms to resolve. Those who attempt self-care are often unable to evaluate the effectiveness of the strategy they tried.[67]

Provider Factors

Unfortunately, failed self-care often reflects poor care from providers who may focus more on the treatment of symptoms rather than on their prevention. Changes in the physician reimbursement system have complicated this problem. Office visits have become shorter and shorter; the average visit length in the United States is currently 15 minutes.[68] In most encounters, providers lack the time needed to explore fully the needs of patients with complex conditions. The physician in solo practice is now rare, and patients commonly see different providers when they come for follow-up. This lack of continuity in the provider-patient relationship underlies many of the current problems in poor self-care. Lack of time to obtain an adequate patient history compromises the quality of patient care. For information on patients taking herbal therapies, see the Pharmacology feature on nutraceuticals.

Several investigative teams have demonstrated a consistent failure of providers to use clinical guidelines.[69,70] A recent study of 30,228 Medicare patients hospitalized with heart failure revealed regional differences in the pattern of ACE inhibitor prescriptions, with prescribing rates varying from 56 to 87 percent.[71] Rural community hospitals without invasive cardiac capabilities and the provision of care by a physician other than a cardiologist were associated with lower rates of ACE inhibitor usage. A similar pattern was documented in a recent study from Portugal in which 58 percent of heart failure patients were prescribed an ACE inhibitor, only 7 percent were prescribed a beta blocker, but most (78 percent) were treated with diuretics.[72] Care for these patients was primarily from primary care physicians. These results reveal that failure to use evidence-based practice is a worldwide problem.

■■■ PHARMACOLOGY

NUTRACEUTICALS

Although clinicians largely ignore nutraceuticals or herbal therapies, as many as half of all heart failure patients take herbal or other dietary supplements and megavitamins in order to improve heart disease, and most do not inform their clinician. More than 50 products claim to have some benefits for cardiovascular conditions. The likelihood of an adverse reaction increases with the number of supplements taken. The safety and efficacy of these products are not well documented. In particular, combining herbal preparations with prescription medications in the setting of aged or impaired physiological condition and metabolism is not advised.

Currently, no compelling evidence exists that any herbal therapy or nutraceutical has benefits in the prevention of heart failure progression. As such, and given potential interactions with common heart failure medications, use of herbals and nutraceuticals is not recommended. Although garlic may have some benefit in lowering blood pressure, it, along with *Ginkgo biloba* and ginseng, interfere with platelet function and could increase the risk of bleeding in patients taking warfarin. Cardiotonic herbs such as hawthorn can have an added effect with digitalis or could affect digoxin levels. Licorice root can produce hypokalemia and hypertension in susceptible individuals. Ephedra or ma huang, found in herbal diet pills, can raise blood pressure.[99] These effects are not widely known, and the Food and Drug Administration does not regulate herbal remedies, so it is important that clinicians educate themselves about the properties of nutraceuticals that patients report taking.

Brace LD: Cardiovascular benefits of garlic (*Allium sativum* L), *J Cardiovasc Nurs* 16:33-49, 2002.
Awang DV, Fugh-Berman A: Herbal interactions with cardiovascular drugs, *J Cardiovasc Nurs* 16:64-70, 2002.

Prevention of Hospitalizations

The effectiveness of heart failure disease management is addressed in Chapter 79. This section addresses the influence of comorbid conditions and stability at discharge on outcomes such as hospital readmission rates and mortality.

A large proportion of the heart failure population has comorbid conditions that complicate their treatment plan and negatively affect their outcomes. A study of U.S. Medicare beneficiaries 65 years of age and older found that close to 40 percent of persons with heart failure had five or more noncardiac comorbid conditions. Those with multiple comorbid conditions had more frequent hospitalizations and a relatively higher mortality rate. Interestingly, it does not appear to be simply the number of comorbid conditions that predicts hospital readmission but the severity of those comorbid conditions. The comorbidities that were associated independently with notably poorer outcomes were chronic obstructive pulmonary disease, renal failure, diabetes, depression, and other lower respiratory diseases such as asthma.[73] Another group demonstrated that elders hospitalized for heart failure have a high incidence of diabetes (38 percent), chronic lung disease (33 percent), atrial fibrillation (30 percent), and prior stroke (18 percent).[74]

Chronic Lung Disease

Chronic obstructive lung disease, encompassing chronic bronchitis and emphysema, is the fourth leading cause of death in the United States today and is predicted to rise to third in 2020.[75] Chronic lung disease, including obstructive lung disease, asthma, and other lower respiratory tract diseases, has the highest readmission rate in the U.S. Medicare population and is the most common comorbid condition in persons with heart failure.[73] Dyspnea is the presenting symptom of chronic lung disease and heart failure, making the differential diagnosis and treatment difficult. See Chapter 54 for a full discussion of dyspnea.

Outpatient pharmacological management for patients with heart failure and lung disease can be challenging. Therapies that are particularly problematic are the use of bronchodilators, corticosteroids, loop diuretics, and digitalis. Although beta blockers, important in the care of those with heart failure, traditionally were contraindicated in persons with chronic lung disease, there is clear evidence that these drugs can be used in persons with mild to moderate chronic lung disease.[76] Bronchodilators are prescribed for chronic lung disease, but there may be an increase in mortality associated with the use of bronchodilators in patients with heart failure. Corticosteroids are important for patients with chronic lung disease, but they cause fluid retention, which is dangerous in heart failure. Digoxin can cause pulmonary vasoconstriction, decreased venous return and cardiac output, and dysrhythmias resulting from hypoxia and acidosis in persons with chronic lung disease. Loop diuretics, which are useful in heart failure, can be dangerous in those with chronic lung disease because patients with obstructive lung disease have increased minute ventilation, which can decrease respiratory drive and accentuate the risk of metabolic acidosis. Patients with heart failure and chronic lung disease should be taught to seek care immediately if dyspnea is not relieved quickly by their usual measures (e.g., extra diuretic) to avoid an acute exacerbation of their lung disease.

Renal Dysfunction

Renal dysfunction in patients with chronic heart failure, referred to as cardiorenal syndrome, is common and consistently one of the strongest predictors of death in this population; the risk becomes apparent at a serum creatinine level greater than 1.3 mg/dl.[77] When creatinine rises during hospitalization—and approximately 45 percent of hospitalized heart failure patients have a rise in serum creatinine of 0.3 mg/dl)—this is a prognostic indicator of greatly increased risk of a lengthy hospital course and increased mortality. A recent trial of nesiritide in chronic heart failure patients with worsening serum creatinine demonstrated no effective on glomerular filtration rate, renal plasma flow, urine output, or sodium excretion.[78] (See the Conundrum feature on treatment of cardiorenal disorder for more information.)

The triad of chronic renal insufficiency, anemia, and heart failure is known as the cardiorenal anemia syndrome. The three conditions form a vicious circle, in which each condition is capable of causing or being caused by the other. The role of anemia in heart failure only recently has been appreciated; anemia alone occurs in 15 to 55 percent of persons with heart failure. Anemia is recognized as associated with more symptoms, less exercise capacity, and a rise in mortality, hospitalization, and malnutrition in persons with heart failure. Chronic renal insufficiency causes anemia, which worsens renal function and increases the rapidity of progression to dialysis. In heart failure patients, rapid deterioration of renal function and development of anemia indicate that heart failure is not controlled adequately. Aggressive and appropriate pharmaceutical therapy often fails to improve heart failure if anemia is present but untreated. Conversely, when anemia is corrected with erythropoietin and iron therapy, left ventricular ejection fraction, symptoms, and exercise capacity improve.[79]

Diabetes Mellitus

Diabetes is diagnosed in 20 to 25 percent of the heart failure population, and the incidence increases with age.[80] The amount of diabetes in persons with heart failure reflects its effects on the microvascularity and macrovascularity. As discussed in Chapter 37, elevated proinsulin (the substance made in the pancreas that is converted to insulin), hyperinsulinemia, and hyperglycemia adversely affect the vascular endothelium, leading to accelerated atherosclerosis. Insulin resistance may be associated with cardiomyopathy, even in the absence of hyperglycemia, and has been linked with cardiovascular remodeling.[81] When diabetes and heart failure coexist, morbidity and mortality are significantly increased,[80] especially in heart failure patients with ischemic cardiomyopathy.[82]

The primary pharmacotherapy for heart failure is beneficial for diabetes as well. ACE inhibitors also improve glucose metabolism. Diabetes mellitus was thought to be a contraindication for beta blockers, although recent results of **BEST** (Beta-Blocker Evaluation of Survival Trial) demonstrated that in advanced heart failure patients with diabetes (36 percent of 2708 patients), compared with those without diabetes, bucindolol therapy effectively reduced death, heart failure hospitalizations, total hospitalizations, and AMI.[82] These results were confirmed by a recent meta-analysis of six large beta blocker trials that reported a mortality benefit in patients with diabetes mellitus and heart failure.[80] Compared with placebo, beta blocker therapy for heart failure was beneficial in patients with diabetes mellitus and in those without diabetes mellitus, although the risk reduction was greater in those without diabetes mellitus. Thiazolidinediones are likely to be of cardiovascular benefit in patients with diabetes and heart failure because they improve insulin sensitivity.[81] These agents may cause edema or weight gain as a result of fluid retention and fat accumulation, however, and should be used with caution. These patients also are prone to hyperkalemia when taking aldosterone inhibitors.

Depression

The prevalence of depression in the heart failure population was discussed before. Joynt and colleagues[56] have suggested that heart failure and depression share a common pathophysiology. Several shared mechanisms were suggested, and the top three compelling arguments are the following: Heart failure causes neurohormonal activation in response to increases in left ventricular filling pressure. Similar hyperactivity of the hypothalamic-pituitary-adrenal axis has been found in persons who are depressed. Hypothalamic-pituitary-adrenal hyperreactivity augments sympathetic hyperactivity in persons with heart failure and in those who are depressed. Joynt and colleagues suggest that this mechanism could explain the high rates of depression in persons with heart failure, and conversely, depression could speed the progression of heart failure in susceptible persons.

Another postulated shared mechanism is the parasympathetic activity of heart failure and depression that could increase susceptibility to dysrhythmias triggered by inadequately opposed sympathetic stimulation. Heart rate variability, a measure of sympathetic-parasympathetic imbalance, is abnormal in persons with heart failure. Similar abnormalities have been

---

■■■ **CONUNDRUM**

TREATMENT OF CARDIORENAL DISORDER

The treatment of cardiorenal syndrome is largely empirical at this time because so few clinical trials have included this patient population. Although angiotensin-converting enzyme (ACE) inhibitors are the standard of care for persons with heart failure, renin-angiotensin-aldosterone inhibitors such as ACE inhibitors may elevate serum creatinine. Should ACE inhibitors be avoided in persons with cardiorenal disorder? Or should ACE inhibitors be continued as long as renal dysfunction does not steadily deteriorate?

demonstrated in depressed persons.[83] A third important mechanism shared between heart failure and depression is inflammation. Proinflammatory cytokines such as tumor necrosis factor, interleukin-1, and the interleukin-6 family have been implicated in the pathogenesis and progression of heart failure. Interestingly, a similar proinflammatory response is seen in response to acute or chronic psychological distress.[56] Others have suggested that cytokines actually may cause depression.[84] A recent study demonstrated that depression significantly predicted increased mortality during the 1-year follow-up of a sample of patients with chronic heart failure.[85]

Sleep-Disordered Breathing

Sleep-disordered breathing is common in persons with heart failure; approximately 40 to 60 percent have sleep-disordered breathing, defined as an apnea-hypopnea index of 15 per hour or greater. In adults, sleep-disordered breathing is more common than asthma. Central sleep apnea with Cheyne-Stokes respiration is thought to be more common than obstructive sleep apnea in this population. Of those with sleep-disordered breathing, it is estimated that 75 percent have central sleep apnea and the other 25 percent have obstructive sleep apnea or a combined form of sleep-disordered breathing.[86] Most studies of sleep-disordered breathing in heart failure have included only patients with systolic heart failure, but sleep-disordered breathing is also common in those with diastolic heart failure. In one small study, 55 percent of diastolic heart failure patients had sleep-disordered breathing, and obstructive sleep apnea was the primary type.[87] Sleep disorders are discussed further in Chapter 17.

STAGE D HEART FAILURE

Stage D patients are those with advanced heart failure who remain symptomatic despite optimal therapy and whose refractory heart failure requires specialized interventions. Patients in this stage of heart failure usually have seriously impaired functional status with persistent NYHA Class III or IV symptoms and frequent rehospitalizations for heart failure exacerbations. The goal of therapy for patients in this stage of heart failure is relief of symptoms with improvement or maintenance of quality of life.

Two major management avenues for patients in stage D are (1) referral for so-called extraordinary measures, such as ventricular assist devices or cardiac transplantation, or (2) palliative care (Figure 64-10). Patients in stage D heart failure also are treated using all the measures outlined for the management of patients in stages A through C. This aspect of care is often overlooked in patients with end-stage heart failure. If the patient has not been referred already to a comprehensive heart failure disease management program, such a program should be strongly considered at this time. Despite evidence that heart failure disease management improves patient outcomes substantially compared with usual care, most patients do not receive care using these superior models of care and thus do not have access to opti-

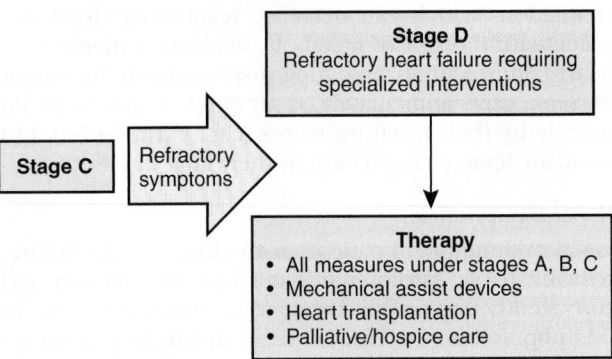

FIGURE 64-10 ■ Therapeutic options for the management of stage D heart failure.

mal management strategies. It is essential that patients considered to be in this stage of heart failure be evaluated by a cardiologist with special expertise in the care of patients with heart failure, and nurses should strongly advocate for this aspect of care. Many patients are thought erroneously to be in refractory heart failure when their medical and nonpharmacological therapy has not been optimized appropriately.

Fluid overload is common in patients with advanced heart failure, and scrupulous attention to fluid status can improve symptoms and quality of life. The incidence of malnutrition or nutritional deficiencies in patients with heart failure is high;[88,89] as many as 50 to 70 percent of hospitalized heart failure patients may suffer from malnutrition.[90] Thus, control of fluid status and attention to nutritional status require special attention in patients with stage D heart failure. Control of fluid status is covered in previous sections of this chapter. Nutritional status is covered in brief next; detailed coverage of this topic can be found in Chapter 12.

Malnutrition in Heart Failure

Chronic malnutrition is common, is associated with poor outcomes in patients with heart failure, and is an independent risk factor for mortality.[91] Nonetheless, nutritional status is not assessed routinely in patients with heart failure because clinicians underestimate the importance of nutrition in patients with heart failure. As a consequence, nutritional deficiencies and even overt malnutrition frequently are not recognized or treated. When nurses caring for patients with heart failure have an understanding of nutrition assessment and needs and malnutrition in heart failure, they can advocate for and initiate appropriate assessment and management.

Protein energy malnutrition is the most common form of malnutrition among those with chronic illnesses. Protein energy malnutrition is inadequate nutritional intake or use of protein and energy to maintain normal body tissue stores. In its most advanced stages, protein energy malnutrition in heart failure results in cardiac cachexia (Figure 64-11). As many as 35 to 50 percent of patients with advanced heart failure have cardiac cachexia. Malnutrition, particularly when associated with muscle wasting, can cause decreased functional capacity, anemia, decreased bone mass, impaired

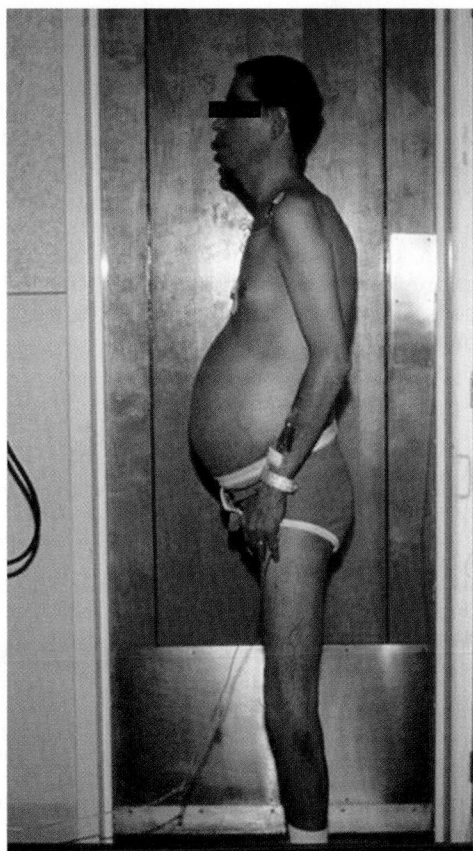

FIGURE 64-11 ■ A patient with advanced heart failure and cardiac cachexia. He has typical characteristics of cardiac cachexia: marked ascites, muscle wasting in limbs, and shrunken face with prominent cheekbones.

cognitive function, immune dysfunction, and perhaps cardiac muscle atrophy. Loss of cardiac muscle contributes to progression of heart failure and is associated with an increased risk of mortality that is additive to the high mortality seen in heart failure.[91] Causes of protein energy malnutrition and cardiac cachexia, nutrition assessment, and interventions are covered in depth in Chapter 12.

Cardiac Transplantation and Mechanical Ventricular Assist Devices

A number of factors, but most importantly the small supply of donor hearts, limits the viability of cardiac transplantation as a therapeutic option for most patients. Fewer than 2500 cardiac transplants are performed in the United States each year, and this number has not increased appreciably over the years.[92] Nonetheless, stage D patients are the most appropriate candidates for cardiac transplantation. A complete discussion of selection criteria for transplantation and preoperative, postoperative, and long-term nursing care of patients undergoing cardiac transplantation can be found in Chapter 67.

Advances in the development and use of left ventricular assist devices have made this therapeutic option useful as destination therapy and bridge therapy in selected patients with advanced heart failure. A full discussion of the care of patients who receive a left ventricular assist device can be found in Chapter 66.

Hospice and Palliative Care

Despite data suggesting that heart failure is more malignant than many common types of cancer, the most ignored aspect of heart failure management is end-of-life care. More than one-quarter million individuals die prematurely each year as a result of heart failure. Across all classes of heart failure, approximately 20 percent of individuals die within 1 year of diagnosis. The yearly incidence of death is higher in patients with the most advanced heart failure and may be near 50 percent in that subgroup. Nonetheless, patients with heart failure and their families rarely receive assistance from their physicians and nurses regarding end-of-life issues.[93] Many symptomatic patients with advanced heart failure feel unsupported by their health care providers, have poor understanding of their condition and its management, suffer poor quality of life with emotional distress, and do not receive appropriate palliation.

End-of-Life Care in Heart Failure

Most clinicians do not have a good understanding of what is meant by end-of-life care. For many, end-of-life care means giving up hope and abandoning usual care. To the contrary, end-of-life care refers to high-quality, comprehensive care delivered to provide symptom relief, comfort, and support for patients and their families as they cope with managing an illness when optimal treatments have failed to halt its progression or relieve symptoms. For patients with heart failure, optimal care, particularly drug therapy, is not necessarily discontinued.

The major component of appropriate end-of-life care is palliative care. Palliative care is an interdisciplinary care process. The goals of palliative care are improving quality of life, relieving suffering, and providing comfort for patients and families facing a life-threatening illness by promotion of psychological and spiritual well-being, improved symptom management, and support of family members. According to the World Health Organization, palliative care is appropriate early in the course of an illness in conjunction with therapies that may be intended to prolong a patient's life.

The concept and practice of palliative care have evolved beyond just treating patients with terminal cancer to managing those with illnesses that traditionally are not thought of as terminal.[94] Although palliative care openly acknowledges death, it should not be characterized by less care or withdrawal of care in the face of death. Palliative care experts advocate for use of curative and palliative therapies and suggest earlier use of palliative care in patients with illnesses likely to result in premature death, such as heart failure.

With optimal medical management, quality of life and survival can be improved for many patients with heart failure. Some patients remain symptomatic with poor functional status and are labeled, inappropriately, as end-stage when evidence-based and guideline-driven pharmacological and nonpharmacological therapies have not been delivered. Any decision to institute end-of-life care should be made only after assurance that therapy has been optimized appropriately (Box 64-7).

Although research has been done to describe symptoms and quality of life for those with advanced heart failure, efforts to better understand the impact of hospice care on patients with end-stage heart failure have lagged behind. Investigators in one of the few studies of hospice care for patients with heart failure demonstrated a decrease in hospital days and emergency room visits using cardiac protocols for symptom management in hospice.[95] Emergencies related to pain and shortness of breath were managed more effectively at home while the patient was receiving hospice care.

Future research needs to occur to address changes in the health care environment to provide the best care for patients with end-stage heart failure. Advanced heart failure is characterized by an increase in physical and emotional symptoms, decreased quality of life, poor functional status, and recurrent hospitalizations. During acute exacerbations, clinicians can take the opportunity to improve the quality of the care and improve patients' quality of life by addressing end-of-life issues. The approach taken with each patient depends on the individual's condition and preferences. However, at a minimum, clinicians should engage each patient with heart failure in a discussion about advance directives and the patient's prognosis. Such discussions do require a fine balancing act as the clinician strives to maintain hope yet provide patients with a realistic view of their condition. The benefits of such discussions far outweigh the difficulties. See Chapters 27 and 82 for a full discussion of hospice and palliative care and their use in patients with heart failure.

SUMMARY

This chapter has described heart failure as a progressive illness that could be prevented or delayed if more attention were given to risk factor modification. Once structural changes have occurred, the progression of heart failure can be attenuated by guideline-driven pharmaceutical therapy. At this stage, every effort should be made to engage patients in a process of learning about

the illness and engaging actively in self-care aimed at maintaining physiological stability. Much of this early self-care should emphasize the importance of treatment adherence. In stage C, when symptoms are common, self-care management requires that patients develop problem-solving skills that will assist them to recognize early symptoms, differentiate them from the symptoms of comorbid illnesses, and make appropriate decisions about them. Once patients reach stage D or end-stage heart failure, knowledge of the prognosis should stimulate discussions about hospice and palliative care in preparation for a good death.

REFERENCES

1. Shahar E, Lee S: Historical trends in survival of hospitalized heart failure patients: 2000 versus 1995. *BMC Cardiovascular Disorders* 7(2). Accessed January 27, 200t *http://www.biomedcentral.com/1471-2261/7/2*.
2. Arnold JM, Yusuf S, Young J et al: Prevention of heart failure in patients in the Heart Outcomes Prevention Evaluation (HOPE) Study, *Circulation* 107:1284-1290, 2003.
3. He J, Ogden LG, Bazzano LA et al: Risk factors for congestive heart failure in US men and women: NHANES I epidemiologic follow-up study, *Arch Intern Med* 161:996-1002, 2001.
4. Hunt SA, Abraham WT, Chin MH et al: ACC/AHA 2005 guideline update for the diagnosis and management of chronic heart failure in the adult: a report of the American College of Cardiology/ American Heart Association Task Force on Practice Guidelines (Writing Committee to Update the 2001 Guidelines for the Evaluation and Management of Heart Failure). Retrieved January 27, 2007 from http://content.onlinejacc.org/cgi/reprint/46/6/e1
5. Katz DL: Lifestyle and dietary modification for prevention of heart failure, *Med Clin North Am* 88:1295-1320, 2004.
6. Adams K, Lindenfelt J, Arnold J, et al: HFSA 2006 Comprehensive Heart Failure Practice Guideline. *J Card Fail*;12:e1-e122, 2006.
7. Baker DW: Prevention of heart failure, *J Card Fail* 8:333-346, 2002.
8. Hellermann JP, Jacobsen SJ, Redfield MM et al: Heart failure after myocardial infarction: clinical presentation and survival, *Eur J Heart Fail* 7:119-125, 2005.
9. Zanella MT, Ribeiro AB: The role of angiotensin II antagonism in type 2 diabetes mellitus: a review of renoprotection studies, *Clin Ther* 24:1019-1034, 2002.
10. Sutton MG, Sharpe N: Left ventricular remodeling after myocardial infarction: pathophysiology and therapy, *Circulation* 101:2981-2988, 2000.
11. Izzo JL Jr, Gradman AH: Mechanisms and management of hypertensive heart disease: from left ventricular hypertrophy to heart failure, *Med Clin North Am* 88:1257-1271, 2004.
12. Verdecchia P, Angeli F, Borgioni C et al: Changes in cardiovascular risk by reduction of left ventricular mass in hypertension: a meta-analysis, *Am J Hypertens* 16:895-899, 2003.
13. Aronow WS, Ahn C, Kronzon I: Effect of beta blockers alone, of angiotensin-converting enzyme inhibitors alone, and of beta blockers plus angiotensin-converting enzyme inhibitors on new coronary events and on congestive heart failure in older persons with healed myocardial infarcts and asymptomatic left ventricular systolic dysfunction, *Am J Cardiol* 88:1298-1300, 2001.
14. Lee VC, Rhew DC, Dylan M et al: Meta-analysis: angiotensin-receptor blockers in chronic heart failure and high-risk acute myocardial infarction, *Ann Intern Med* 141:693-704, 2004.
15. Moser M, Schocken DD, Basile JN et al: Hypertension and heart failure: roundtable discussion, *J Clin Hypertens (Greenwich)* 6:326-332, 2004.
16. Ingwall JS, Weiss RG: Is the failing heart energy starved? On using chemical energy to support cardiac function, *Circ Res* 95:135-145, 2004.
17. Park SJ, Zhang J, Ye Y et al: Myocardial creatine kinase expression after left ventricular assist device support, *J Am Coll Cardiol* 39:1773-1779, 2002.

BOX 64-7   ■ ■ ■

SPECIFIC FACTORS TO BE ADDRESSED BEFORE INSTITUTING END OF LIFE CARE FOR PATIENTS WITH HEART FAILURE

- Patient referred to clinician with expertise in the management of heart failure
- Pharmacological and nonpharmacological therapy optimized for an adequate time to realize benefit
- Reversible causes of heart failure and exacerbations treated
- Adequate patient and family/caregiver education and counseling delivered
- Reasons for persistent nonadherence determined and addressed if possible
- Depression and anxiety treated
- Social support enhanced
- Patient and family wishes identified and respected

18. Adams KF Jr, Gheorghiade M, Uretsky BF et al: Clinical benefits of low serum digoxin concentrations in heart failure, *J Am Coll Cardiol* 39:946-953, 2002.

19. Neuberg GW, Miller AB, O'Connor CM et al: Diuretic resistance predicts mortality in patients with advanced heart failure, *Am Heart J* 144:31-38, 2002.

20. Cleland JG, Ghosh J, Freemantle N et al: Clinical trials update and cumulative meta-analyses from the American College of Cardiology: WATCH, SCD-HeFT, DINAMIT, CASINO, INSPIRE, STRATUS-US, RIO-Lipids and cardiac resynchronisation therapy in heart failure, *Eur J Heart Fail* 6:501-508, 2004.

21. Bloche MG: Race-based therapeutics, *N Engl J Med* 351:2035-2037, 2004.

22. Taylor AL, Ziesche S, Yancy C et al: Combination of isosorbide dinitrate and hydralazine in blacks with heart failure, *N Engl J Med* 351:2049-2057, 2004.

23. Kalinowski L, Dobrucki IT, Malinski T: Race-specific differences in endothelial function: predisposition of African Americans to vascular diseases, *Circulation* 109:2511-2517, 2004.

24. Yusuf S, Pfeffer MA, Swedberg K et al: Effects of candesartan in patients with chronic heart failure and preserved left-ventricular ejection fraction: the CHARM-Preserved Trial, *Lancet* 362:777-781, 2003.

25. Jones RC, Francis GS, Lauer MS: Predictors of mortality in patients with heart failure and preserved systolic function in the Digitalis Investigation Group trial, *J Am Coll Cardiol* 44:1025-1029, 2004.

26. Boriani G, Biffi M, Martignani C et al: Cardioverter-defibrillators after MADIT-II: the balance between weight of evidence and treatment costs, *Eur J Heart Fail* 5:419-425, 2003.

27. Morgan JM: The MADIT II and COMPANION studies: will they affect uptake of device treatment? *Heart* 90:243-245, 2004.

28. Riegel B, Carlson B, Moser DK et al: Psychometric testing of the self-care of heart failure index, *J Card Fail* 10:350-360, 2004.

29. Hershberger RE, Ni H, Nauman DJ et al: Prospective evaluation of an outpatient heart failure management program, *J Card Fail* 7:64-74, 2001.

30. DeWalt DA, Malone RM, Bryant ME, et al: A heart failure self-management program for patients of all literacy levels: a randomized, controlled trial [ISRCTN11535170]. *BMC Health Serv Res* 6:30, 2006.

31. Riegel B, Carlson B: Facilitators and barriers to heart failure self-care, *Patient Educ Couns* 46:287-295, 2002.

32. Tsuyuki RT, McKelvie RS, Arnold JM et al: Acute precipitants of congestive heart failure exacerbations, *Arch Intern Med* 161:2337-2342, 2001.

33. Bentley B, DeJong MJ, Moser DK et al: Factors related to nonadherence to a low sodium diet in heart failure patients, *Eur J Cardiovasc Nurs* 4(4):331-336, 2005.

34. Horan M, Barrett F, Mulqueen M et al: The basics of heart failure management: are they being ignored? *Eur J Heart Fail* 2:101-105, 2000.

35. Ni H, Toy W, Burgess D et al: Comparative responsiveness of Short-Form 12 and Minnesota Living With Heart Failure Questionnaire in patients with heart failure, *J Card Fail* 6:83-91, 2000.

36. Mojet J, Heidema J, Christ-Hazelhof E: Taste perception with age: generic or specific losses in supra-threshold intensities of five taste qualities? *Chem Senses* 28:397-413, 2003.

37. Mattes RD: The chemical senses and nutrition in aging: challenging old assumptions, *J Am Diet Assoc* 102:192-196, 2002.

38. MacFadyen RJ, Gorski JC, Brater DC et al: Furosemide responsiveness, non-adherence and resistance during the chronic treatment of heart failure: a longitudinal study, *Br J Clin Pharmacol* 57:622-631, 2004.

39. Chui MA, Deer M, Bennett SJ et al: Association between adherence to diuretic therapy and health care utilization in patients with heart failure, *Pharmacotherapy* 23:326-332, 2003.

40. Evangelista LS, Dracup K: A closer look at compliance research in heart failure patients in the last decade, *Prog Cardiovasc Nurs* 15:97-103, 2000.

41. Holst M, Stromberg A, Lindholm M et al: Fluid restriction in heart failure patients: is it useful? the design of a prospective, randomised study, *Eur J Cardiovasc Nurs* 2:237-242, 2003.

42. Horowitz CR, Rein SB, Leventhal H: A story of maladies, misconceptions and mishaps: effective management of heart failure. *Soc Sci Med* 58:631-643, 2004.

43. Public health and aging: influenza vaccination coverage among adults aged 50 years and pneumococcal vaccination coverage among adults aged 65 years—United States, 2002, *MMWR Morb Mortal Wkly Rep* 52:987-992, 2003.

44. Sisk JE, Whang W, Butler JC et al: Cost-effectiveness of vaccination against invasive pneumococcal disease among people 50 through 64 years of age: role of comorbid conditions and race, *Ann Intern Med* 138:960-968, 2003.

45. Butler JC, Breiman RF, Campbell JF et al: Pneumococcal polysaccharide vaccine efficacy: an evaluation of current recommendations, *JAMA* 270:1826-1831, 1993.

46. Piano MR: Alcohol and heart failure, *J Card Fail* 8:239-246, 2002.

47. Greenberg BH, Schutz R, Grunkemeier GL et al: Acute effects of alcohol in patients with congestive heart failure, *Ann Intern Med* 97:171-175, 1982.

48. Piepoli MF, Davos C, Francis DP et al: Exercise training meta-analysis of trials in patients with chronic heart failure (ExTraMATCH), *BMJ* 328:189, 2004.

49. Rees K, Taylor RS, Singh S et al: Exercise based rehabilitation for heart failure, *Cochrane Database Syst Rev* 2004CD003331.

50. Force T, Michael A, Kilter H et al: Stretch-activated pathways and left ventricular remodeling, *J Card Fail* 8:S351-S358, 2002.

51. Calaghan SC, Belus A, White E: Do stretch-induced changes in intracellular calcium modify the electrical activity of cardiac muscle? *Prog Biophys Mol Biol* 82:81-95, 2003.

52. Riegel B, Carlson B, Glaser D et al: Which patients with heart failure respond best to multidisciplinary disease management? *J Card Fail* 6:290-299, 2000.

53. Buetow SA, Coster GD: Do general practice patients with heart failure understand its nature and seriousness, and want improved information? *Patient Educ Couns* 45:181-185, 2001.

54. Zambroski CH: Qualitative analysis of living with heart failure. *Heart Lung* 32:32-40, 2003.

55. MacMahon KM, Lip GY: Psychological factors in heart failure: a review of the literature, *Arch Intern Med* 162:509-516, 2002.

56. Joynt KE, Whellan DJ, O'Connor CM: Why is depression bad for the failing heart? a review of the mechanistic relationship between depression and heart failure, *J Card Fail* 10:258-271, 2004.

57. Freedland KE, Rich MW, Skala JA et al: Prevalence of depression in hospitalized patients with congestive heart failure, *Psychosom Med* 65:119-128, 2003.

58. Sullivan M, Simon G, Spertus J et al: Depression-related costs in heart failure care, *Arch Intern Med* 162:1860-1866, 2002.

59. Majani G, Pierobon A, Giardini A et al: Relationship between psychological profile and cardiological variables in chronic heart failure: the role of patient subjectivity, *Eur Heart J* 20:1579-1586, 1999.

60. Moser DK, Zambroski CH, Lennie TA et al: Aging with a broken heart: the effect of heart disease on psychological distress in the elderly, *Circulation* 110:416, 2004 (abstract).

61. Dracup K, Westlake C, Erickson VS et al: Perceived control reduces emotional stress in patients with heart failure, *J Heart Lung Transplant* 22:90-93, 2003.

62. Hagenhoff BD, Feutz C, Conn VS et al: Patient education needs as reported by congestive heart failure patients and their nurses, *J Adv Nurs* 19:685-690, 1994.

63. Wehby D, Brenner PS: Perceived learning needs of patients with heart failure, *Heart Lung* 28:31-40, 1999.

64. Rogers AE, Addington-Hall JM, Abery AJ et al: Knowledge and communication difficulties for patients with chronic heart failure: qualitative study, *BMJ* 321:605-607, 2000.

65. Albert NM, Collier S, Sumodi V et al: Nurses's knowledge of heart failure education principles, *Heart Lung* 31:102-112, 2002.

66. Washburn SC, Hornberger CA, Klutman A et al: Nurses' knowledge of heart failure education topics as reported in a small Midwestern community hospital, *J Cardiovasc Nurs* 20(3):215-220, 2005.

67. Carlson B, Riegel B, Moser DK: Self-care abilities of patients with heart failure, *Heart Lung* 30:351-359, 2001.

68. Bensing JM, Roter DL, Hulsman RL: Communication patterns of primary care physicians in the United States and the Netherlands, *J Gen Intern Med* 18:335-342, 2003.

69. Krumholz HM, Baker DW, Ashton CM et al: Evaluating quality of care for patients with heart failure, *Circulation* 101:E122-E140, 2000.

70. Cleland JG, Cohen-Solal A, Aguilar JC et al: Management of heart failure in primary care (the IMPROVEMENT of Heart Failure Programme): an international survey, *Lancet* 360:1631-1639, 2002.

71. Havranek EP, Wolfe P, Masoudi FA et al: Provider and hospital characteristics associated with geographic variation in the evaluation and management of elderly patients with heart failure, *Arch Intern Med* 164:1186-1191, 2004.

72. Ceia F, Fonseca C, Mota T et al: Aetiology, comorbidity and drug therapy of chronic heart failure in the real world: the EPICA substudy, *Eur J Heart Fail* 6:801-806, 2004.

73. Braunstein JB, Anderson GF, Gerstenblith G et al: Noncardiac comorbidity increases preventable hospitalizations and mortality among Medicare beneficiaries with chronic heart failure, *J Am Coll Cardiol* 42:1226-1233, 2003.

74. Havranek EP, Masoudi FA, Westfall KA et al: Spectrum of heart failure in older patients: results from the National Heart Failure project, *Am Heart J* 143:412-417, 2002.

75. Afessa B, Morales IJ, Scanlon PD et al: Prognostic factors, clinical course, and hospital outcome of patients with chronic obstructive pulmonary disease admitted to an intensive care unit for acute respiratory failure, *Crit Care Med* 30:1610-1615, 2002.

76. Aronow WS: Treatment of heart failure in older persons: dilemmas with coexisting conditions—diabetes mellitus, chronic obstructive pulmonary disease, and arthritis, *Congest Heart Fail* 9:142-147, 2003.

77. Shlipak MG, Massie BM: The clinical challenge of cardiorenal syndrome, *Circulation* 110:1514-1517, 2004.

78. Wang DJ, Dowling TC, Meadows D et al: Nesiritide does not improve renal function in patients with chronic heart failure and worsening serum creatinine, *Circulation* 110:1620-1625, 2004.

79. Paul S, Paul RV: Anemia in heart failure: implications, management, and outcomes, *J Cardiovasc Nurs* 19:S57-S66, 2004.

80. Haas SJ, Vos T, Gilbert RE et al: Are beta-blockers as efficacious in patients with diabetes mellitus as in patients without diabetes mellitus who have chronic heart failure? a meta-analysis of large-scale clinical trials, *Am Heart J* 146:848-853, 2003.

81. Giles TD: The patient with diabetes mellitus and heart failure: at-risk issues, *Am J Med* 115(suppl 8A):107S-110S, 2003.

82. Domanski M, Krause-Steinrauf H, Deedwania P et al: The effect of diabetes on outcomes of patients with advanced heart failure in the BEST trial, *J Am Coll Cardiol* 42:914-922, 2003.

83. Carney RM, Blumenthal JA, Stein PK et al: Depression, heart rate variability, and acute myocardial infarction, *Circulation* 104:2024-2028, 2001.

84. Leonard BE: The immune system, depression and the action of antidepressants, *Prog Neuropsychopharmacol Biol Psychiatry* 25:767-780, 2001.

85. Jiang W, Kuchibhatla M, Cuffe MS: et al: Prognostic value of anxiety and depression in patients with chronic heart failure, *Circulation* 110:3452-3456, 2004.

86. Javaheri S: Heart failure and sleep apnea: emphasis on practical therapeutic options, *Clin Chest Med* 24:207-222, 2003.

87. Chan J, Sanderson J, Chan W et al: Prevalence of sleep-disordered breathing in diastolic heart failure, *Chest* 111:1488-1493, 1997.

88. Lennie TA: Nutritional recommendations for patients with heart failure. *J Cardiovasc Nurs* 21:261-268, 2006.

89. Lennie TA, Moser DK, Heo S, et al: Factors influencing food intake in patients with heart failure: a comparison with healthy elders. *J Cardiovasc Nurs* 21:123-129, 2006.

90. Schwengel RH, Gottlieb SS, Fisher ML: Protein-energy malnutrition in patients with ischemic and nonischemic dilated cardiomyopathy and congestive heart failure, *Am J Cardiol* 73:908-910, 1994.

91. Anker SD, Steinborn W, Strassburg S: Cardiac cachexia, *Ann Med* 36:518-529, 2004.

92. Mahon NG, O'Neill JO, Young JB et al: Contemporary outcomes of outpatients referred for cardiac transplantation evaluation to a tertiary heart failure center: impact of surgical alternatives, *J Card Fail* 10:273-278, 2004.

93. Boyd KJ, Murray SA, Kendall M et al: Living with advanced heart failure: a prospective, community based study of patients and their careers, *Eur J Heart Fail* 6:585-591, 2004.

94. Formiga F, Espel E, Chivite D et al: Dying from heart failure in hospital: palliative decision making analysis, *Heart* 88:187, 2002.

95. Lynn J, Schuster JL, Kabcenell A: Offering end-of-life services to patients with advanced heart failure. In Lynn J, Schuster JL, Kabcenell A, editors: *Improving care for the end of life: a sourcebook for health care managers and clinicians,* New York, 2000, Oxford University Press.

Care of Patients Undergoing Cardiac Surgery

Kristen Sethares
Patricia C. Seifert
Heather Smith

CHAPTER ABBREVIATIONS

CABG   coronary artery bypass grafting

CAD   coronary artery disease

CPB   cardiopulmonary bypass

ECG   electrocardiogram

ICU   intensive care unit

IMA   internal mammary artery

LAD   left anterior descending (artery)

MI   myocardial infarction

NSAID   nonsteroidal antiinflammatory drug

OR   operating room

PCI   percutaneous coronary intervention

PTFE   polytetrafluoroethylene

Cardiac surgery has been affected by consumer demand for improved outcomes, cost-driven changes in health care, an aging population, endoscopic and distance technologies, and an expanding array of percutaneous coronary interventions. Additionally, consumer demands for less invasive procedures are reflected in the rapid growth of minimally invasive techniques for the treatment of coronary artery disease (CAD). This growing trend has not replaced the need for traditional "open" techniques; rather, it has expanded the treatment options for myocardial revascularization. Newer technologies using lasers, robots, genetic engineering, and heterograft replacement organs have increased the number of available therapeutic interventions for CAD.

Nurses care for patients throughout all phases of the cardiac surgical experience and have an important role in enhancing psychological, physiological, and functional status and self-care outcomes. As a result, knowledge of advances in cardiac surgical techniques, perioperative cardiac risks, and implementation of evidence-based interventions is essential to practice.

INDICATIONS

The American College of Cardiology/American Heart Association categorize indications for coronary artery bypass grafting (CABG) according to (1) the classification of recommendations supporting the intervention, with Class I reflecting the strongest evidence, and (2) the level of evidence supporting a treatment or proce-

dure, with level A representing the strongest level of evidence. CABG is recommended as a *Class I* and *level of evidence A* indication in patients with significant left main coronary artery stenosis or left main equivalent disease (i.e., 70 percent or greater stenosis of the proximal left anterior descending [LAD] and proximal left circumflex coronary arteries). CABG also is recommended for patients with three-vessel disease and stable or unstable angina and in patients with two-vessel disease with stable or unstable angina and severe proximal LAD artery lesions.[1] Other indications include failed angioplasty with persistent pain or hemodynamic instability, persistent or recurrent angina, post–myocardial infarction ventricular septal defect, and ischemia-related mitral valve insufficiency (e.g., papillary muscle rupture). CABG alleviates angina pectoris and prolongs life in the subsets of patients with disease of the left main and LAD coronary arteries.[2]

The impact of surgery in the growing number of patients older than age 75 is being investigated. The Trial of Invasive versus Medical therapy in Elderly patients[3] has shown that invasive revascularization in elderly patients with refractory angina is associated with a relatively low risk compared with medical therapy consisting of pharmacological intervention and lifestyle changes.

PREOPERATIVE ASSESSMENT AND CARE
Assessment

Nurses are responsible for evaluating a variety of physiological, clinical, and health history data in the preoperative phase in order to judge symptoms and risk for complications and to intervene when any potentially adverse conditions exist. Preoperative patients may display symptoms of ischemic chest pain. In this situation, the anesthesia care provider and the perioperative staff should be notified, and sublingual nitroglycerin should be offered to the patient, if transdermal patches have not been applied. Occasionally, patients present for surgery emergently after failed percutaneous coronary intervention. Although the availability of back-up surgical support remains a generally accepted standard of care, there is a growing controversy about requiring mandatory surgical back-up support. (See the accompanying Conundrum feature.)

A history of diabetes is significant because diabetes promotes arterial atherosclerosis, retards healing, and predisposes to infection. Antibiotic prophylaxis in the preoperative period can reduce the risk of postoperative infection fivefold.[1,4] In diabetic patients, a continu-

SHOULD THERE BE SURGICAL BACK-UP FOR PERCUTANEOUS CORONARY INTERVENTIONS?

Debate is ongoing about the need for surgical back-up in patients undergoing percutaneous coronary intervention (**PCI**). Akdemir and colleagues[1] reviewed 78 primary angioplasty procedures performed on patients in a mobile catheterization facility; they reported an 88.8 percent angiographic success rate (defined as postprocedural residual stenosis not exceeding 50 percent). Mortality was 4.1 percent, and no patients were referred for urgent surgery; the authors conclude that angioplasty can be performed effectively and safely in a facility without on-site surgical back-up using a mobile catheterization unit.

Conversely, Wennberg and associates[2] showed a higher risk of adverse outcomes after PCI in facilities without on-site surgical back-up. They reviewed Medicare hospital (Part A) data from 178 hospitals performing PCI without surgical back-up and 943 hospitals performing PCI with on-site cardiac surgery. They found that mortality for patients with primary/rescue PCI was similar in institutions without and with cardiac surgery; however, for the larger non–primary/rescue PCI population, the risk of post-PCI mortality was 29 percent higher in hospitals without on-site cardiac surgery. According to these authors, this increased mortality was limited primarily to hospitals performing 50 or fewer Medicare PCI procedures per year.

Although the need for emergency surgery post-PCI is small (1 percent or less), Weaver[3] notes that Wennberg and colleagues' findings[2] of a 29 percent higher mortality in patients undergoing PCIs without surgical back-up are provocative and illustrate a need for more data. As the number of PCIs rapidly increase, there will be greater scrutiny of the risk/benefit ratio for patients being treated for acute myocardial infarction.

References

1. Akdemir R, Ozhan H, Erbilen E et al: Primary angioplasty without on-site surgical back-up: the first experience with mobile catheterization facility, *J Invasive Cardiol* 16:645-648, 2004.
2. Wennberg DE, Lucas FL, Siewers AE et al: Outcomes of percutaneous coronary interventions performed at centers without and with onsite coronary artery bypass graft surgery, *JAMA* 292:1961-1968, 2004.
3. Weaver WD: Is onsite surgery backup necessary for percutaneous interventions, *JAMA* 292:2014-2016, 2004.

ous intravenous insulin infusion during surgery can reduce the incidence of postoperative deep sternal wound infection.[5] Diabetic patients also tend to have diffuse CAD, making the technical aspects of CABG more difficult.

During the preoperative assessment, vital signs (including pain) are checked. Blood pressures should be checked bilaterally. Unequal pressures in the arms may be a contraindication for the use of the internal mammary artery. The arm with a lower blood pressure is potentially a poor site for graft harvest because perfusion may not be optimal. Unequal arm blood pressures also may alert the nurse to the presence of a coarctation in the descending thoracic aorta or some other vascular anomaly. The presence of hypertension and obesity increase the workload of the heart. Obesity also may increase the risk for postoperative infection because adipose tissue is poorly vascularized.[6] Additionally, the nurse observes for shivering, which can increase endogenous catecholamine release; patients should be kept warm with blankets or an adjustment of room temperature to reduce myocardial oxygen consumption.

Chest x-ray films provide information about the size of the cardiac chambers, thoracic aorta, and pulmonary vasculature, as well as the presence of calcium in valves, pericardium, coronary arteries, and aorta. Lateral chest x-ray films of patients with a prior sternal operation can be used to identify the chest wires and the extent of pericardial adhesions. Radiographic evidence of calcium deposits in the ascending aorta is significant because manual or instrumental manipulation by the surgeon during surgery can increase the risk of calcium particulate embolization and subsequent stroke. In patients with extensive calcification of the ascending aorta, the surgeon may elect to perform CABG without the use of an aortic vascular clamp or cardiopulmonary bypass.

Echocardiography commonly is used to assess ventricular function before and immediately after the surgical intervention. Echocardiography also can identify a tumor, thrombus, or air remaining in the ventricular and/or atrial cavities after completion of the cardiac repair.

Cardiac catheterization performed preoperatively provides the most definitive information about the extent and location of ischemic heart disease. Coronary angiography can be used to evaluate coronary anatomy, obstructions, flow, and distal perfusion. Contrast dye may be injected into the ventricular cavity (i.e., ventriculography) to illustrate contractile weaknesses of the ventricles and shunting and regurgitation of blood. These studies are used to assess the degree of myocardial dysfunction and to calculate the ejection fraction.

Hematological tests include a detailed coagulation profile to uncover hemorrhagic disorders. In patients who have been taking aspirin or dipyridamole, decreased platelet activity alerts the perioperative nurse to anticipate prolonged bleeding requiring the possible infusion of replacement platelets. Clopidogrel should be withheld for 5 to 7 days before elective surgery.[1] Blood type also is determined, and an order for two to four units often is placed with the blood bank; unused bank blood is returned after surgery. Precautions are taken to test the blood for viral contamination and for cold antibodies that could produce blood agglutination during cardiopulmonary bypass when the patient is cooled to hypothermic temperatures. The priming volume (approximately 1500 ml) within the bypass circuit mixes with the patient's blood at the commencement of cardiopulmonary bypass. In individuals with a small body mass (e.g., less than 50 kg) or hemoglobin less than 12 g/dl, there is a risk of significantly lowering the oxygen-carrying capacity of the circuit volume when the patient's blood mixes with the pump prime; the perfusionist may be required to add a unit of bank blood to the pump prime in order to raise the hemoglobin. Additionally, blood glucose levels are tested and monitored closely for hyperglycemia, especially in patients with diabetes mellitus.[7]

Preoperative Education

With shortened hospital lengths of stay, patient education and preparation for home care maintenance have become even more critical for enhancing positive patient outcomes. Many patients are admitted to the cardiac service on the day of surgery; teaching sessions can be scheduled before admission in conjunction with preoperative laboratory testing. The perioperative nurse can reinforce, review, clarify, and add to important information and instructions that the patient and family need in planning for surgery, recovery, discharge, and posthospital rehabilitation. Patients may be hesitant to complain of pain and to request pain medication. The nurse can anticipate this concern and encourage the patient to request pain medication. Although patients undergoing repeat operation have had previous experience with cardiac surgery, they also have significant learning needs, and nurses can assist them to achieve optimum outcomes by sharing information about traditional and newer techniques such as minimally invasive cardiac surgery and off-pump surgery.

Specific instructions can include discussing the importance of postoperative coughing and deep breathing by using a cough pillow or splinting device. Information about postoperative lifting restrictions and body mechanics can be discussed preoperatively; postoperatively, the nurse reinforces this information, which can make the postoperative course more manageable for the patient. Required lifestyle changes also should be reviewed and the patient's feelings about these modifications elicited. Verify that the patient knows reportable signs and symptoms associated with the specific procedure and understands prescribed medications, dosages and times, potential side effects, and signs and symptoms of complications. Any misconceptions should be clarified or referred to an appropriate source.

The family or significant other's ability and willingness to assist the patient in home care maintenance should be queried; referrals to an agency for assistance at home may be required. Although these teaching interventions are provided in greater depth during the postoperative period, preoperatively, patients and families can benefit from an introduction to issues that will be important during recuperation. Special patient concerns should be reported to the critical care colleagues receiving the patient after surgery.

INTRAOPERATIVE CARE

After entry to the operating room (**OR**), the patient is transferred to the OR bed and given general anesthesia through the endotracheal tube. The choice of anesthetic agent(s) depends on the cardiovascular effects of the anesthetic and the patient's hemodynamic status and general health. Because the period of induction is one of the most critical during the procedure, close monitoring of the patient is required, especially for patients with ventricular ischemia. Anesthetic management focuses on keeping myocardial oxygen demand low and the oxygen supply high. Central lines (i.e., central venous and pulmonary artery pressure lines) are inserted before or after anesthesia induction, depending on the preference of the anesthesia care provider.

Positioning

Commonly, the patient is placed in the supine position. This allows the best exposure of the heart and great vessels, as well as access to these organs for establishing cardiopulmonary bypass. With this approach, there is also less respiratory impairment and postoperative discomfort. Dependent areas and bony prominences (occipital area, buttocks, heels, hands, and elbows) are padded with soft material to prevent skin breakdown, neurological damage, and pressure necrosis resulting from immobility, hypoperfusion, and hypothermia during bypass. Padding of these areas also assists in avoiding venous stasis ulcers, especially in the elderly, debilitated, or obese patient. Significant factors associated with the development of pressure ulcers include diabetes mellitus; lower preoperative hemoglobin, hematocrit, and serum albumin levels; and the presence of intraaortic balloon pumps.[8] The arms are positioned anatomically along the side of the body; patients with severely misshapen arthritic joints are positioned as their functional ability allows. The legs may be everted slightly to provide access to the femoral arteries for insertion of pressure lines or intraaortic balloon pump lines or to excise the saphenous vein.

Assessment

Maximal monitoring of hemodynamic and other variables is indicated during cardiac surgery. After intubation and positioning, additional pressure lines may be inserted to measure central venous pressure and pulmonary artery pressures. Peripheral and central arterial and venous pressures usually are monitored directly by means of a transducer and oscilloscope. During this period, perioperative nurses observe the electrocardiogram (**ECG**) monitors for signs of ventricular irritability such as ectopy, tachycardia, or fibrillation and are prepared to assist with defibrillation, as indicated. If the patient fibrillates and cannot be resuscitated, the chest is opened rapidly, and internal cardiac massage is performed by one team member(s) while another team member(s) cannulates the patient for cardiopulmonary bypass. Once on bypass, the patient's heart is arrested quickly to conserve myocardial energy resources. Conduits are harvested and coronary bypass grafts are attached.

Incisions
Median Sternotomy

The skin incision extends from the sternal notch to the linea alba below the xiphoid process (Figure 65-1). The sternum is divided with a saw, and a sternal retractor is inserted to spread open the bone edges. CABG conduits such as the internal mammary artery and/or the saphenous vein are harvested at this time. In repeat sternotomies, there are commonly dense adhesions formed between the sternum, the pericardium, and the heart. These adhesions must be dissected carefully in order to free the heart from the surrounding adherent tissue. The sternum may be split with a vibrating saw and the retrosternal tissue dissected from the anterior pericardium and adherent cardiac tissue. The increased risk of fibrillation from manipulation of the heart and bleeding and laceration of the ventricle alerts the perioperative nurse to be prepared to institute cardiopulmonary by-

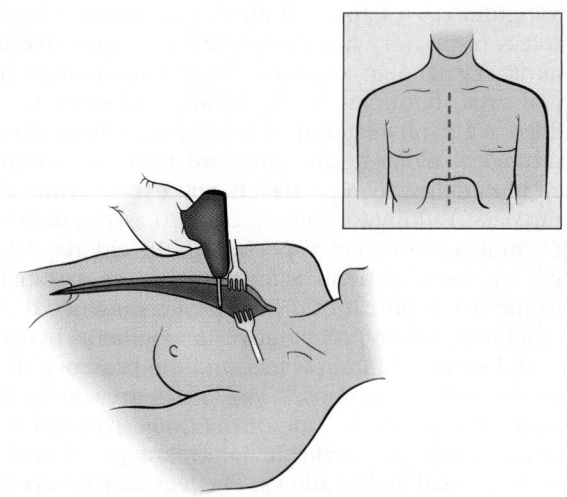

FIGURE 65-1 ▪ Median sternotomy with a power saw (*inset* shows incision line).

pass promptly. If the patient fibrillates during dissection, external defibrillator patches or sterile internal paddles are used.

Minithoracotomy

For minimally invasive cardiac procedures, a variety of smaller (up to approximately 8 cm) incisions can be used. These include anterolateral chest incisions small enough for the insertion of specially designed retractors and instruments. Increasingly, video-assisted techniques are used commonly, especially for the excision of saphenous vein conduits.

Selection of Conduits

Myocardial revascularization is accomplished by bypassing the stenotic portion of a coronary artery with a conduit attached distally to the coronary artery beyond the stenosis. The proximal portion of the conduit is attached to the ascending aorta or, in the case of in situ grafts such as the internal mammary artery (**IMA**), the proximal portion remains attached to the artery from which it branches (for example, the right and left IMA branch respectively from the right and left subclavian arteries). Usually a combination of arterial and venous grafts is required because patients often have multivessel CAD.

The most commonly used conduits are the IMA and the greater saphenous vein (Figure 65-2), described in detail next. The IMA demonstrates excellent long-term patency,[9] and this has promoted the use of arterial conduits such as the radial artery,[10] the gastroepiploic artery,[11] and the inferior epigastric artery.[12] (See the accompanying Evidence-Based Practice feature.) The saphenous vein remains an effective conduit when multiple grafts are needed. The increasing number of reoperations for CAD also has stimulated the use of alternative conduits (Box 65-1). These conduits are often a last resort spurred by the absence or previous use of more traditional bypass grafts.

Other ischemia-related disorders requiring cardiac surgery include mitral valve regurgitation resulting from ruptured papillary muscles, left ventricular aneurysm, and post–myocardial infarction ventricular septal defect. Bypass grafts to areas of the myocardium associated with the mitral regurgitation, left ventricular aneurysm, or ventricular septal defect often accompany the repair of these lesions.

BOX 65-1 ■ ■ ■
ALTERNATIVE CONDUITS

Biological Conduits
- Freeze-dried arterial conduits
- Bovine internal mammary artery
- Sheep collagen tube
- Human umbilical vein
- Cryopreserved allograft artery and vein (e.g., internal mammary artery and saphenous vein)
- Cephalic vein
- Dacron-meshed, bandaged saphenous vein
- Intercostal artery
- Subscapular artery
- Ulnar artery

Synthetic Conduits
- Dacron tube
- Polytetrafluoroethylene (PTFE) tube
- Polyglycolic acid tube

From Buxton B, Frazier OH, Westaby S, editors: *Ischemic heart disease: surgical management*, St Louis, 1999, Mosby.

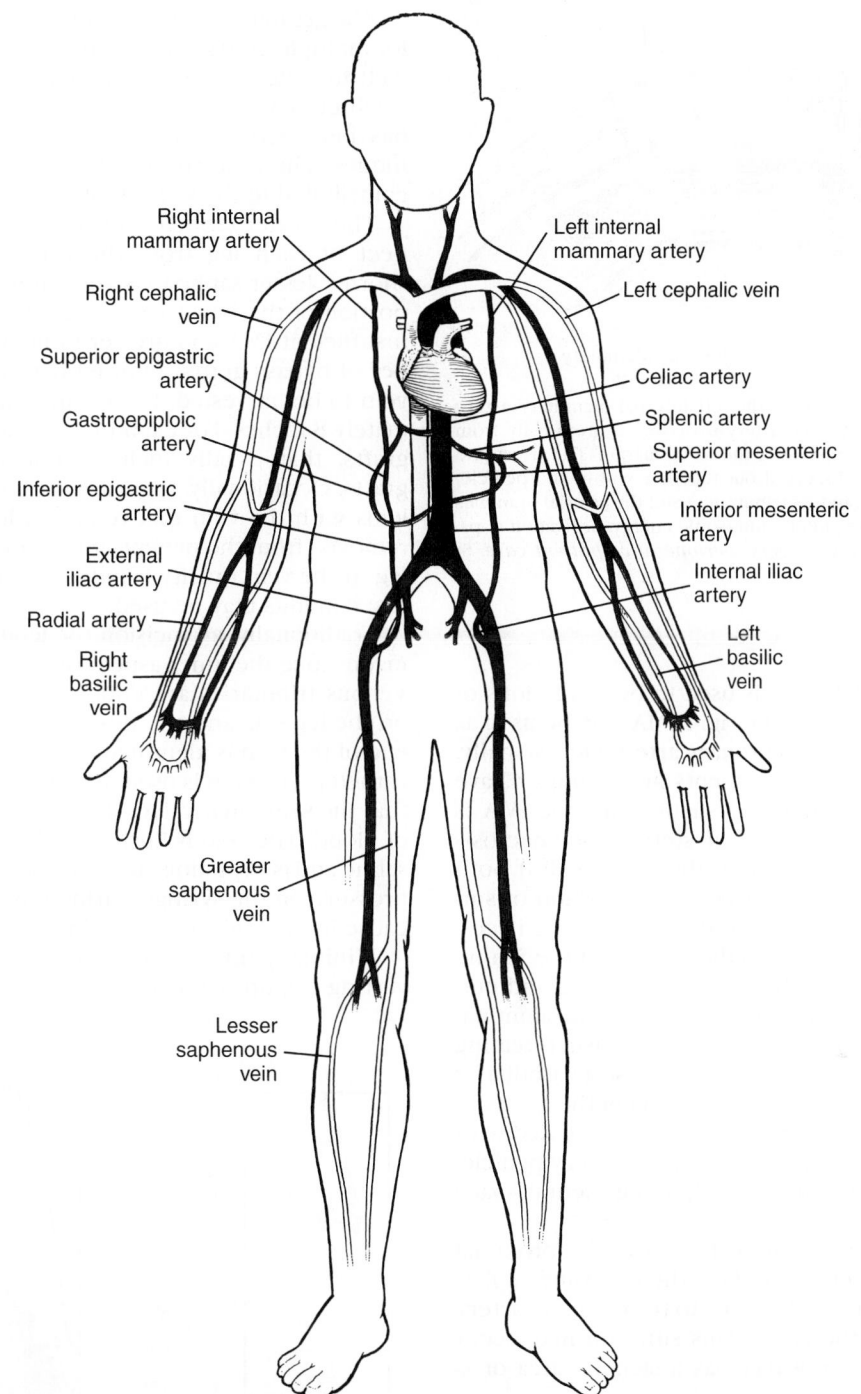

FIGURE 65-2 ■ Autologous arterial and venous conduits for coronary artery bypass grafting. (From Seifert PC: *Cardiac surgery: perioperative patient care,* St Louis, 2002, Mosby. Drawing by Peter Stone.)

Internal Mammary Artery

The excellent long-term patency of the IMA makes it a conduit of choice in most CABG patients. The excellent performance of the IMA is thought to be related to the function of its endothelial cells, which continue to produce endothelium-derived relaxation factor and prostacyclin.[12] The left and/or right IMA branches off from its respective subclavian artery and runs along the posterior portion of the left or right sternal border (Figure 65-3). The artery is dissected free from its retrosternal bed as a pedicle, in-situ graft (i.e., proximally, it remains attached to the subclavian artery). A special retractor elevates the sternal border, allowing the surgeon to visualize the artery. The right and left phrenic nerves are located near the proximal portion of the respective IMA, and the surgeon identifies the nerve to avoid injury; postoperative motor nerve injury to the diaphragm may result if the phrenic nerve is lacerated. Phrenic nerve injury can result in an elevated hemidiaphragm and compromised respiration after surgery.

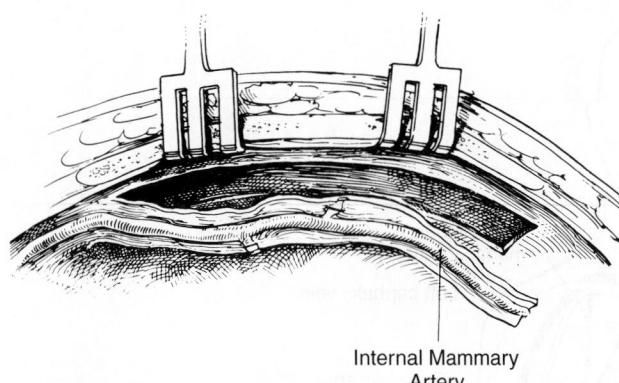

FIGURE 65-3 ■ Dissection of the left internal mammary artery from the retrosternal bed. The artery is dissected proximally from the subclavian artery and distally to the costal margin. The artery and accompanying vein are dissected out together within the pedicle; bleeding from the vein (and its tributaries) and the arterial branches is controlled with electrocautery, ultrasonic energy, or ligation clips. (From Seifert PC: *Cardiac surgery: perioperative patient care,* St Louis, 2002, Mosby.)

Internal Mammary Artery

Commonly, the left IMA is used to bypass lesions of the LAD coronary artery. The right IMA may be used as a bypass graft to the right coronary artery. Occasionally, both IMAs are used when patients are young or have few other available conduits. Usually, only one IMA is used in diabetic patients because sternal bone necrosis compromises wound healing of the chest wall if both arteries are dissected. The artery and a portion of surrounding connective tissue are dissected to the necessary length (approximately to the vicinity of the 5th intercostal space). Before the artery is clamped and cut, heparin is given systemically to prevent intraluminal thrombosis. Arterial grafts are prone to spasm (creating the potential for downstream ischemia), so a vasodilator often is injected into the distal (cut) end of the artery to reduce vasoconstriction; a small sponge moistened with papaverine may be wrapped around the artery pedicle, which then is tucked into the adjoining pleural space until it is needed.

Occasionally, the IMA must be cut at the proximal (subclavian artery) end. The IMA then becomes a *free graft* that can be attached distally to the coronary artery and proximally to the aorta. This situation may occur when a portion of the artery has a stenotic area or is injured.

Minimally invasive IMA dissection can be performed via a left anterior thoracic incision at the level of the 4th intercostal space. A lighted endoscope is used to visualize the proximal IMA. Ligation of arterial branches is performed with hemostatic metal clips and electrocoagulation.

Saphenous Vein

Because a single IMA can be used for one graft and most patients have multivessel CAD, the saphenous vein often provides the additional conduits required for complete revascularization. Multivessel CABG using only arterial conduits may not be feasible or necessary in all instances.

The greater saphenous vein provides sufficient length for multiple grafts, and the loss of this superficial vein is well tolerated by most patients. The postoperative leg swelling, pain, and infection seen with open excision has been reduced with the use of endoscopic techniques. The cosmetic results of smaller incisions have contributed to the growth of less invasive techniques.[13]

The greater saphenous vein runs along the inner aspect of each leg from the thigh to the ankle. The shorter, lesser saphenous vein runs along the posterior portion of the lower leg; it may be used when there is insufficient IMA and greater saphenous vein. The number of bypass grafts required determines the length of vein to be harvested. Each vein graft averages approximately 8 inches. For example, if a patient requires three grafts, that usually includes one IMA and two vein grafts. Occasionally, there are varicosities or other problems with the vein that require a longer section to be removed from the patient or excision from the opposite leg. If the vein quality is judged to be too poor, alternative conduits may be used.

Traditionally, an incision the length of the conduit is made along the inner aspect of the leg (Figure 65-4, *A*). Venous tributaries are doubly ligated with metal clips on the leg side and silk ties on the vein side. The distal end of the vein is identified and cannulated with a small catheter. The vein is used in an upside down position so that the semilunar valves do not interfere with the flow of blood. The vein is flushed with heparinized blood or saline and is kept moist until needed. Exerting too much pressure on the syringe during flushing of the vein can cause intimal injury and lead to early graft closure.

Minimally invasive, endoscopic saphenous vein harvesting (Figure 65-4, *B* to *D*) is achieved with one to

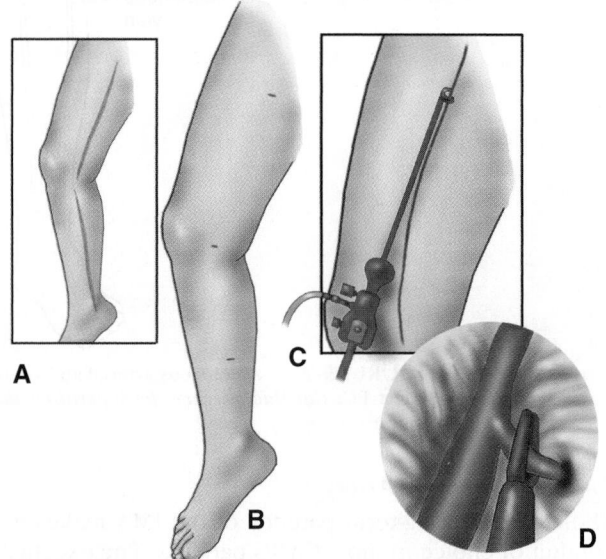

FIGURE 65-4 ■ Minimally invasive approaches to saphenous vein harvesting have significantly reduced incisional morbidity. Traditional harvesting requires long incisions (**A**) compared with less invasive videoscopic harvesting (**B**). A dissection cannula is introduced through a small incision (**C**), and branches are later divided (**D**) under videoscopic guidance. (From Zipes DP, Libby P, Bonow RO, Braunwald E, editors: *Braunwald's heart disease,* ed 7, Philadelphia, 2005, Saunders.)

three incisions over the vein at the knee and at the ankle and the inguinal area if necessary. The vein is located under direct vision. A lighted endoscope is inserted into the small knee incision, and the necessary length of vein is dissected and removed with video monitoring. To reduce postoperative tunnel dead space and minimize fluid accumulation, the leg may be wrapped with a sterile pressure bandage. Access to the posteriorly located lesser saphenous vein requires elevating the leg with a sling or bending the lower leg, making it technically more difficult to harvest.

Although early results of vein grafts are excellent, within 10 years, more than half of the grafts demonstrate some intimal hyperplasia, atheromatous irregularities, and stenoses. Whether these changes result from initial injury to the vein during harvest, the patient's own atherogenic tendencies, or the inability to modify atherogenic risk factors is uncertain.[12]

Radial Artery

The radial artery initially was proposed as a conduit in the 1970s, but early graft occlusion led to its abandonment. More recently, the radial artery has been reintroduced after the use of vasodilators to reduce spasm and less traumatic harvesting techniques.[14] Before excising the artery, it is necessary to ensure that there is adequate collateral ulnar circulation to the forearm. Doppler echocardiography is used widely to test the adequacy of circulation; the Allen test also remains a useful, albeit a less precise, testing technique (Box 65-2). In some patients for whom arterial conduits are preferred (e.g., those with two-vessel disease), the radial artery and the IMA can be used. Postoperatively, the affected forearm and hand should be monitored for ischemia.

For excision, the right (or left) arm is outstretched (palm upraised) on a narrow board. The radial artery is harvested through a longitudinal incision from about 3 cm distal to the elbow crease lateral to the biceps tendon, to the wrist crease (Figure 23-3). The artery is harvested with adjacent veins and fatty tissue. After

---

BOX 65-2
ALLEN TEST
■ ■ ■

The Allen test measures the adequacy of the collateral circulation from the ulnar artery in the forearm and hand after the radial artery has been occluded. The test measures the time of recovery of the capillary circulation in the hand following release of the ulnar artery after the forearm and hand have been rendered ischemic by exercise and manual occlusion of the radial and ulnar arteries. The normal time for blood return to the hand is less than 10 seconds, although some clinicians prefer a time of less than 6 seconds.

1. The patient clenches the affected hand into a fist to squeeze blood from the fingers and hand.
2. The radial and ulnar arteries are compressed by the clinician's thumbs.
3. The ulnar artery is released, and the time to perfusion of the hand and fingers is counted; less than 6 to 10 seconds indicates adequate collateral flow.

Modified from Buxton B, Acar C, Suma H et al: Conduits. In Buxton B, Frazier OH, Westaby S, editors: *Ischemic heart disease: surgical management*, St Louis, 1999, Mosby.

---

systemic heparinization, the artery is cut proximally and distally; papaverine is injected into the lumen to reduce spasm. The artery may be placed in a small, labeled cup until needed.

Gastroepiploic Artery

The right gastroepiploic artery travels along the greater curvature of the stomach and perfuses the lower two thirds of that portion of the stomach. The artery is dissected as a pedicle graft, with the proximal portion of the graft remaining attached to the gastroduodenal artery; gastric ischemia is rarely a problem unless there is extensive proximal dissection. Because of its vicinity to the pancreatic blood supply, pancreatitis is a rare but potential complication. Like the IMA, the gastroepiploic artery functions best when it is attached to a coronary artery with significant stenosis (greater than 70 percent). When arterial grafts are used in areas demonstrating subclinical stenosis (less than 50 percent), there is the potential that competitive flow from the native coronary artery will produce inadequate graft function and may promote graft occlusion.

The gastroepiploic artery is useful in situations in which the IMA cannot reach the posterior descending coronary artery on the back surface of the heart. To expose the gastroepiploic artery, the sternal incision is lengthened an additional 5 cm beyond the xiphoid process. An abdominal retractor is inserted to expose the peritoneum and the stomach. A nasogastric tube is especially useful to decompress and empty the stomach of its contents. The gastroepiploic artery is dissected to the necessary length, heparin is given, and the artery is cut. Papaverine is injected to reduce spasm. The artery is attached to the target coronary artery by making a small incision in the diaphragm through which the gastroepiploic artery is passed and then sewn to the heart.

Postoperatively, the patient is monitored for possible peritoneal symptoms of paralytic ileus, pancreatitis, intestinal ischemia, and other abdominal problems. Patients with a gastroepiploic artery graft can be expected to have abdominal discomfort and increased pain; aspirin may be contraindicated.

Inferior Epigastric Artery

The inferior epigastric artery is a continuation of the IMA (Figure 65-2), and the right and left inferior epigastric arteries run longitudinally within the rectus muscle. An abdominal incision is made to harvest the artery as a free graft. Postoperatively, there may be muscle weakness if both inferior epigastric arteries have been harvested because of denervation of the rectus wall.

Less information is available on the long-term effectiveness of the inferior epigastric artery compared with the IMA and saphenous vein grafts. It has been noted that in certain instances of graft narrowing or occlusion, the native arteries were not severely stenosed and may have produced competing flow with the inferior epigastric artery conduit.[12] This graft may be indicated in young patients or those in whom vein grafts should be limited or in those in whom bilateral IMAs are contraindicated.

Cryopreserved Allograft Veins

Cadaver saphenous veins that have been cryopreserved can be used when there are few autologous conduits. Their long-term patency is not as good as that of autograft veins, but cadaver saphenous veins can serve as a conduit in patients who have undergone multiple reoperations for CAD. After removal from the cadaver, the veins are tested for disease, treated with antibiotic solutions, and frozen. When needed, the vein is thawed and implanted in a manner similar to that for an autologous vein.

Prosthetic and Xenograft Conduits

Dacron, polytetrafluoroethylene (**PTFE**), and polyglycolic acid have been used as prosthetic conduits (Box 65-1). The greatest challenge for prosthetic grafts is that the size of the graft (2 to 4 mm) that would be useful in bypass surgery makes them prone to occlusion. Moreover, prosthetic grafts have no endothelium, and they tend to thrombose at the anastomotic site. In the future, prosthetic grafts probably will be able to be seeded with gene-encoded endothelial cells that form a neo-intima less conducive to thrombosis.

Bovine IMAs are available as a xenograft. Like cryopreserved saphenous veins, these conduits are useful in situations in which autologous grafts are largely unavailable. Other biological allografts, such as human umbilical vein, are available but they also tend to thrombose within the first year.

Cardiopulmonary Bypass

Bypass conduits are harvested and prepared before the institution of cardiopulmonary bypass (**CPB**) in order to minimize pump time. CPB allows the surgeon to stop the heart in order to perform the coronary attachments under direct vision in a relatively dry, motionless field. CPB also allows the surgeon to manipulate the heart without jeopardizing perfusion to the rest of the body.

In traditional CPB circuits (Figure 65-5), systemic venous return to the heart flows by gravity drainage through a cannula in the right atrium. The cannula is connected to tubing connected to the bypass machine.

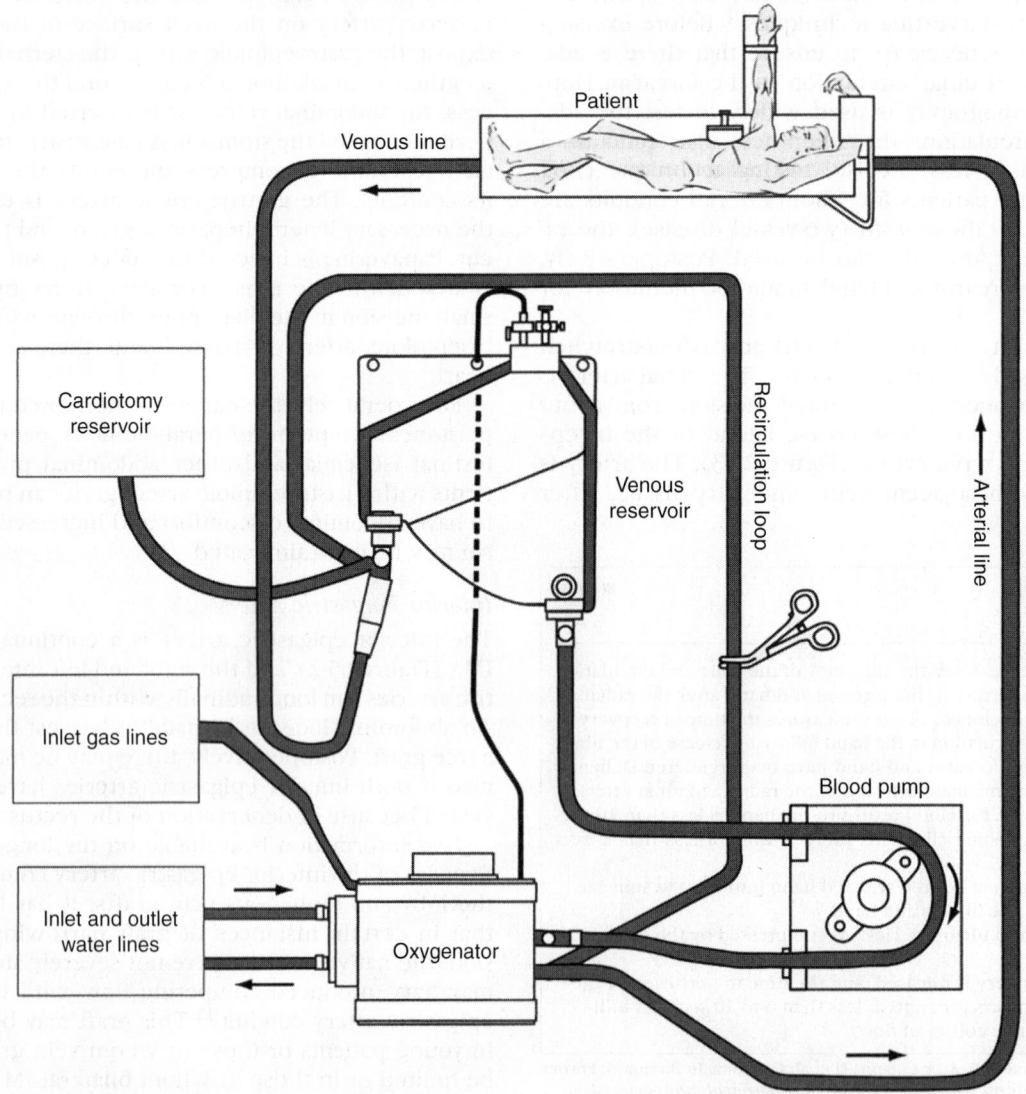

FIGURE 65-5 ■ Cardiopulmonary bypass circuit. (From Seifert PC: *Cardiac surgery: perioperative patient care,* St Louis, 2002, Mosby.)

Blood is oxygenated, filtered, warmed or cooled, and pumped back into the systemic circulation through a cannula placed in the ascending aorta (see Chapter 23 for discussion of CPB). Because blood is oxygenated by the CPB machine, the lungs do not need to function and can be deflated to provide better exposure of the mediastinal structures. By diverting blood away from the heart, CPB also decompresses the ventricles, thereby reducing myocardial wall tension, which is a significant determinant of myocardial oxygen demand. CPB also enables surgery to be performed inside the heart and on the surface of the heart. Opening the heart to repair a diseased valve, for example, would be nearly impossible without isolating and stopping the heart and using bypass to perfuse noncardiopulmonary organs.

However, there is considerable morbidity associated with the use of CPB. An inflammatory response is triggered when blood touches any surface other than autogenous endothelium. Complement, neutrophils, and monocytes are the principle mediators of the inflammatory response, which produces a wide array of cytotoxins that disrupt interstitial fluid balance and homeostasis.[15] Extracorporeal circulation causes fluid retention and intercompartmental fluid shifts, multiple organ dysfunction, showers of microemboli, inflammatory responses, and unique bleeding complications.[12,15] Attempts to minimize the inflammatory reaction have focused on modifying the activation of platelets and blood factors that play a major role in initiating the responses. These complications have stimulated the development of "beating heart" or "off-pump" techniques for myocardial revascularization that do not use CPB.

Off-Pump Coronary Artery Bypass

Early attempts to perform coronary artery surgery on a beating heart without the use of CPB and induced cardiac arrest focused on lesions in the LAD artery located on the anteroapical portion of the heart. This approach can be achieved with little manipulation of heart, therefore reducing the risk of inducing ventricular fibrillation. As surgeons grew more technically proficient in the creation of anastomoses, they expanded their targets to lesions in the lateral and posterior coronary arteries. Early results demonstrated a higher risk for graft occlusion compared with CABG performed using the CPB pump. Graft occlusion was thought to be due to the difficulty of constructing small (1.5 mm to 2.0 mm) anastomoses on a moving target. Other factors leading to less than optimal outcomes included incomplete revascularization and hemodynamic instability from manipulating the heart.[16] Off-pump coronary artery bypass became technically feasible with the introduction of coronary stabilizers (Figure 65-6), which immobilize the area of the coronary artery to be bypassed. With stabilization, the surgeon has a motionless field, allowing greater precision in attaching the conduit. The further addition of a suction cup device placed over the cardiac apex enables surgeons to retract the apical portion of the heart to expose the lateral and posterior surfaces of the heart, thereby facilitating complete revascularization. Hemodynamic instability remains a risk, and patients may have to be placed on CPB if homeostasis cannot be achieved. Patient characteristics and skill of the surgeon and surgical team remain im-

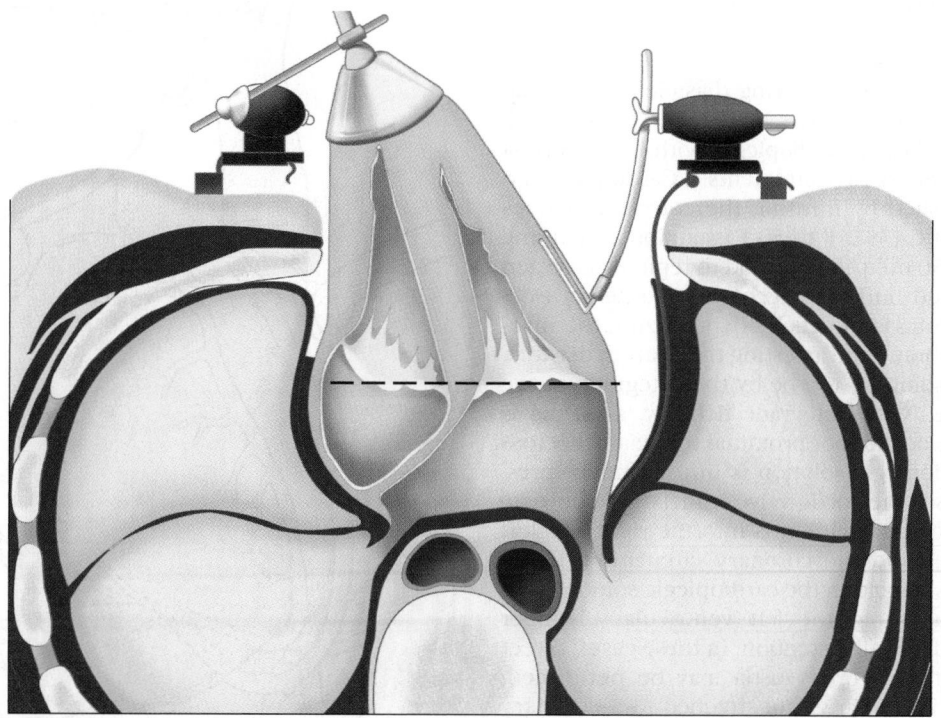

FIGURE 65-6 ■ Off-pump coronary artery bypass surgery on the beating heart has been facilitated by the development of positioning devices and stabilizer systems. Positioning devices using apical suction cups *(top left)* now allow optimal exposure of the posterolateral circulation while minimizing hemodynamic compromise. Platform stabilization systems *(top right)* provide isolated immobilization during the performance of distal anastomoses. (From Zipes DP, Libby P, Bonow RO, Braunwald E, editors: *Braunwald's heart disease*, ed 7, Philadelphia, 2005, Saunders.)

portant considerations in determining whether to use, or not use, CPB.

Myocardial Protection During Cardiopulmonary Bypass

When CPB is used, the heart itself is isolated from the CPB circuit when the aorta is occluded. Consequently, the myocardium needs to be protected from the effects of coronary circulatory interruptions, ischemia, and hypoperfusion that accompany induced cardiac arrest. Improvements in the results of cardiac surgery are due to technical proficiency in repairing a mechanical problem and to progress made in protecting the myocardium.[17] Unless measures are taken to protect the myocardium during these periods, irreversible damage can result. The two main myocardial protective strategies are cooling the heart to reduce metabolic demand and rapidly arresting the heart so that myocardial energy resources are preserved.

Hypothermia

Hypothermia is defined as the deliberate reduction of body temperature for therapeutic purposes. Moderate hypothermia (28°C [82.4°F]), used during most CABG procedures, significantly reduces oxygen consumption.[17] Systemic circulatory cooling is achieved with the heat exchanger of the heart-lung machine. Surface cooling of the heart with topical application of cold saline or continuous irrigation of the pericardial wall can be used. Large ice chips in pericardial irrigating solutions should be avoided to prevent injury to the phrenic nerve and cardiac tissue. Transmural cooling of the heart is achieved with cardioplegia.

Cardioplegic Arrest

Rapidly arresting the heart during diastole is beneficial because an arrested heart uses less energy than a fibrillating or beating heart. Cardioplegia with hypothermia further reduces energy requirements.[17] Cardioplegic arrest is accomplished by infusing the coronary arteries with a 4°C to 10°C (39.2°F to 50°F) solution containing potassium (2 to 50 mEq/liter), blood to replenish oxygen and nutrients, and buffering agents to counteract ischemic acidosis. Potassium acts by depolarizing the myocardial cell membrane and arresting the heart in diastole. Delivery of the solution may be by the antegrade or the retrograde route. With antegrade delivery, a needle is inserted into the aortic root proximal to the aortic cross clamp; the cardioplegic solution is infused under pressure, which closes the aortic valve leaflets. The only remaining route for the solution is into the right and left coronary arteries and the coronary circulation. If the aortic valve does not close, the cardioplegic solution will flow preferentially into the left ventricular chamber causing myocardial wall distention; in these cases, direct cannulation of the coronary ostia may be performed. Direct infusion into vein grafts attached to a coronary artery protects the myocardium distal to the coronary lesions and enhances transmural cooling.

Retrograde infusion is achieved with a catheter placed transatrially into the coronary sinus; the cardioplegic perfusate enters the coronary venous system and flows through the myocardial circulation, exiting through the coronary ostia. The retrograde route is especially useful in the presence of coronary artery obstructions that impede antegrade cardioplegic solution infusion and left ventricular hypertrophy. When the heart is sufficiently arrested, the ECG reflects a straight line; when electrical activity is noticed on the monitor (approximately every 15 to 20 minutes), cardioplegic solution is reinfused when continued cooling and arrest is desired. After the bypass grafts are completed (Figure 65-7), the patient is prepared for weaning from CPB. Systemic rewarming via the bypass circuit heat exchanger is begun during the attachment of the last bypass graft.

Just before the cross clamp is to be removed, a warm terminal bolus of cardioplegic solution is given to avoid reperfusion injury caused by oxygen free radicals and lactic acid buildup during arrest and by providing oxygen and other nutrients to the heart. The heart often starts to contract spontaneously; if the heart is fibrillating, internal defibrillation (5 to 10 J) is applied.

Myocardial Protection During Off-Pump Coronary Artery Bypass

Although myocardial protection strategies commonly are associated with CPB and induced cardiac arrest, off-pump coronary artery bypass procedures also have the potential

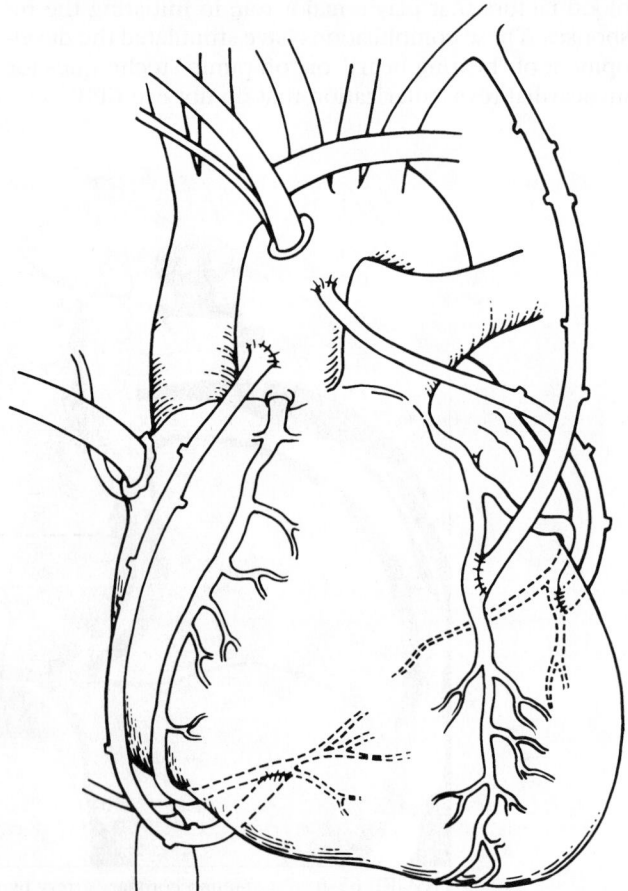

FIGURE 65-7 ■ Completed internal mammary artery and vein graft anastomosis. (From Seifert PC: *Cardiac surgery: perioperative patient care*, St Louis, 2002, Mosby.)

for myocardial injury. During the period of coronary anastomosis in the beating heart, the target coronary artery often is occluded with a small tourniquet or clamp in order to minimize blood flow through the artery from obscuring the surgical site. This period of ischemia may last between 5 and 10 minutes, depending on the cardiac anatomy and operator proficiency. Other potential injuries to the myocardium can occur from excessive pressure of the stabilizing device, manual retraction or some other technical aspect of the procedure. The importance of preparation, anticipation, vigilance, and teamwork is especially evident when the safety net of CPB is not present. Team members should have all necessary supplies, closely monitor the patient's hemodynamic status, and avoid delays that could jeopardize myocardial viability.

Other Revascularization Procedures

It is not uncommon for ancillary procedures to be performed during CABG. Left ventricular aneurysm is a ballooning, dyskinetic area of infarcted myocardium. Without excision and repair of the affected area, the heart is prone to dysrhythmias, intraventricular thrombus formation, and possible rupture. The weakened section of myocardium is removed, and a patch is sewn to the edges of the remaining viable myocardium.

Ventricular septal defect and free wall rupture are catastrophic complications of myocardial infarction and originate in the necrotic zone of myocardial tissue. These are true surgical emergencies requiring prompt repair of the defect with biological or prosthetic patch material. Adjunctive bypass grafting also is performed in post–myocardial infarction aneurysm and ventricular septal defect repairs.

Patients with chronic, severe angina who cannot be revascularized with CABG or percutaneous catheter interventions may be appropriate candidates for transmyocardial revascularization. Transmyocardial revascularization uses laser energy to create a series of left ventricular transmural channels. The current suggested mechanisms for improving anginal symptoms include denervation of the affected myocardium and laser-induced angiogenesis.[1,18]

Termination of Cardiopulmonary Bypass and Closing Procedures

When the last bypass graft is being attached, the perfusionist rewarms the patient via the CPB circuit heat exchanger. Air is evacuated from the coronary grafts with a small gauge (e.g., 27 gauge) hypodermic needle and from the proximal aorta with the needle used for antegrade cardioplegia that has been "Y"-connected to a suction line. The cross clamp is removed, whereupon the heart often converts spontaneously to sinus rhythm.

Signs of ischemia may appear in the form of ST segment elevation, dysrhythmias, and/or systemic hypotension and elevated pulmonary artery pressures. Ischemia may be due to air remaining in the grafts, incomplete revascularization, kinking of a graft, inadequate myocardial protection, reperfusion injury, myocardial distention, or preexisting impaired left ventricular func-

tion. Mechanical problems including retained air, kinked grafts, or wall distention can be treated by correcting the underlying problem. Biochemical problems may require pharmacological or mechanical support to correct the underlying intracellular derangement.

The patient may remain on CPB to keep the heart decompressed while an intraaortic balloon is inserted. Pharmacological support is instituted. When ventricular function improves, the patient can be weaned from CPB with the assistance of the balloon pump.

Two to three chest tubes are inserted to drain blood, irrigating solutions, or other fluids from the pericardium in order to avoid cardiac tamponade. If one or both pleural cavities have been entered, a chest tube is inserted into the affected pleural cavity to maintain negative pressure and facilitate lung expansion.

Temporary epicardial pacing electrodes usually are sewn to the right atrial appendage and/or the right ventricle with the wires attached to temporary external pacemaker generator. The pacemaker generator may be activated when the heart rate falls below 90 beats/min or when dual-chamber pacing is indicated for optimal cardiac output. Perioperatively, the temporary wires can be used to terminate atrial flutter with rapid atrial pacing or to treat other dysrhythmias.[19]

Chest closure of the median sternotomy is accomplished with wire sutures (Figure 65-8). The wire su-

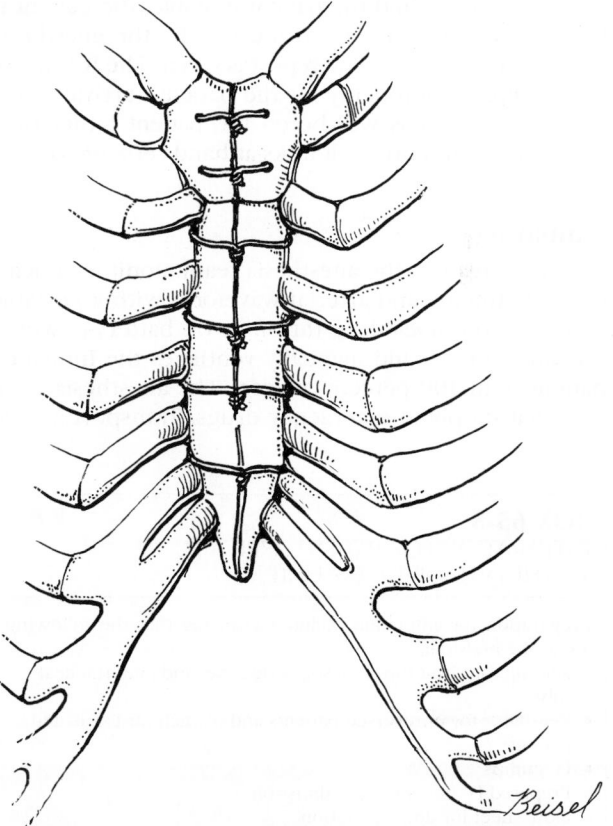

FIGURE 65-8 ■ Sternal closure with stainless steel wire. Wires may be placed around the ribs or through the sternum from the sternal notch to the xiphoid process. Twisted wire cables and other sternal closing devices are also available, depending on surgeon preference. (From Seifert PC: *Cardiac surgery: perioperative patient care,* St Louis, 2002, Mosby.)

tures are twisted, excess wire is cut, and the wire ends are buried into the sternal periosteum. Some surgeons use small metal crimpers to approximate and hold the wires.

The linea alba is closed with suture. A layer of sutures is placed to approximate the fascia over the sternum; the subcutaneous tissue and skin are closed. If metal staples are used on the skin, a staple remover should accompany the patient to the recovery area.

Before transferring the patient, the nurse telephones a report to the recovery area, usually the intensive care unit (see Table 23-8). The patient's special concerns and fears, as well as procedural information, recent laboratory results, blood and blood products used and available, and significant physiological alterations, should be communicated.

POSTOPERATIVE CARE IN THE INTENSIVE CARE UNIT
Preparation

Before the patient arrives in the intensive care unit (ICU), the OR nurse or anesthesiologist should provide the ICU nurse with the patient's medical and surgical history and an update on the operative procedure, including any complications experienced, current condition, continuous infusions, and intravenous access and hemodynamic monitoring lines in place. Once the surgery is complete and the patient is stable, the patient is transferred from the OR to the ICU by the anesthesia team, and a more detailed report is given. The ICU nurse must prepare thoroughly for the patient's arrival to ensure that the focus will be on the patient rather than solely on the multitude of tasks at hand (Box 65-3).

Transport

During transport, the anesthesia team monitors at least the ECG tracing and arterial waveform with a portable monitor, continues drug infusions on battery-powered infusion pumps, and manually ventilates the intubated patient with 100 percent oxygen. The anesthesia team carries a supply of emergency drugs. Transport should proceed quickly yet cautiously because it is a vulnerable period, and the need to respond to an untoward event in an uncontrolled environment such as an elevator or hallway is to be avoided. Potential complications during transport include hypotension, hypertension, dysrhythmias, disconnection of lines from the portable monitor, decannulation of lines from the patient, and inadvertent extubation.

Arrival

On arrival to the ICU, a team effort is necessary to provide for an immediate assessment and safe transition from portable to bedside equipment (Box 65-4). The team includes several nurses, physician assistants, or advanced practice nurses and respiratory therapy personnel. The anesthesia team remains at the bedside until hemodynamic stability is confirmed.

Early Complications

Remediation of any complications takes precedence over other admission activities. The most common problems noted on admission to the ICU are hypotension and cardiac rhythm disturbances. Disrupted ventilation, hemorrhage, rhythm disturbances, or drug infusion disruption may be the cause of hypotension and should be corrected quickly. Hypotension may be treated with volume expansion, intravenous administration of 500 mg calcium chloride, and/or pacing if related to a rhythm disturbance.[20] Infusions may need to be adjusted if they are contributing to or are not at a dose sufficient to treat hypotension. Additional vasoactive or inotropic infusions may be added to correct the hypotension.

BOX 65-3 ■ ■ ■
PREPARATION FOR PATIENT ARRIVAL TO THE INTENSIVE CARE UNIT

Preparation for admission includes ensuring that the following are at the bedside:
- Suction for chest tubes, nasogastric tube, and endotracheal tube
- Ventilator for unreversed patients and oxygen for extubated patients
- IV pumps
- Prepared IV line for fluid admission
- Flow sheet for documentation
- Report sheet
- Cardiac output equipment
- Transducers and cables for hemodynamic lines
- Warming blanket and machine
- Pulse oximeter
- Drainage collectors for emptying urine or drainage from tubes

---

BOX 65-4 ■ ■ ■
STEPS TO ENSURE A SAFE ADMISSION PROCESS

- Connect an intubated patient to the ventilator or an extubated patient to oxygen.
- Connect the patient to a pulse oximeter.
- Connect the patient to a cardiac monitor, and obtain cardiac output and index.
- Transduce and zero hemodynamic monitoring lines.
- Set up cardiac output equipment.
- Connect chest tubes to 20 cm H_2O suction.
- Assess for bleeding and urine production.
- Verify pacemaker connection and function.
- Check intravenous infusions.
- Record first set of vital signs.
- Send blood specimens for chemistry, hematology, coagulation, and arterial blood gas analysis.
- Obtain portable chest x-ray film.
- Obtain 12-lead electrocardiogram.
- Obtain detailed report from the anesthesia team:
- Height and weight
- Drugs administered, including current infusions and antibiotics
- Colloid and crystalloid solutions administered
- Whether the airway was difficult to establish
- Cross clamp and bypass times
- Allergies
- Urine output
- Estimated blood loss

A suspected rhythm disturbance should be verified by checking the arterial waveform or the patient's pulse because there is often artifact from moving wires. Suspected rhythm disturbances can be confirmed with a 12-lead ECG. The pacemaker should be used for bradycardia or asystole. Advanced cardiac life support protocols must be initiated immediately if the rhythm is ventricular fibrillation or ventricular tachycardia.

A patient should be considered to be in immediate danger of cardiac arrest if hypotension and a rhythm disturbance coexist and are unresponsive to immediate treatment. Confirmed cardiac arrest requires initiation of advanced cardiac life support protocols. The surgeon should be summoned stat to the bedside; the sternotomy cart, defibrillator, and portable bypass machine should be prepared for use, and preparation should be made for return to the OR (Box 65-5). OR staff also should be called to assist if it becomes necessary to open the chest at the bedside, but if at all possible, the chest opening should be delayed until the patient is returned to the OR.

Postoperative Assessment and Care

Nurses play a pivotal role in preventing complications in the immediate postoperative period through vigorous monitoring of hemodynamic, laboratory, and other physiological parameters. Rapid assessment and intervention for identified problems can improve patient outcomes.

Hemodynamic Monitoring

Postoperative management varies depending on the operative procedure, but all patients require vigilant and continuous nursing assessment.[21] Vital signs are recorded frequently. Hemodynamic monitoring includes continuous ECG, arterial blood pressure, central venous pressure, pulmonary artery pressure, cardiac output, cardiac index, and systemic vascular resistance monitoring. A pulmonary artery catheter is not always part of postoperative hemodynamic monitoring. Cardiac output is calculated intermittently using the thermodilution (bolus) method or continuously by an oximetric pulmonary artery catheter. Alternative methods for calculating cardiac output include the Fick calculation, thoracic bioimpedance, and Doppler methods. The most important goal of hemodynamic monitoring is to maintain adequate systemic perfusion, and values should be analyzed individually and collectively to achieve that goal.

Temperature is documented frequently postoperatively. Patients generally arrive to the ICU hypothermic, and the use of warm air blankets is common to aid gently in the return to a normothermic state. Hypothermia after CPB can have many effects, including hypotension related to vasodilatation during rewarming, increased myocardial oxygen demand, interference with coagulation, increased risk of dysrhythmias, and shivering.

Chest Tubes

Mediastinal and pleural chest tubes should be checked at least hourly for any signs of hemorrhage. Chest tubes are connected to suction of 20 cm H_2O, and all connections should be maintained tightly to ensure sterility and prevention of air leaks.[20] Autotransfusion of blood collected in chest tubes may be performed. Milking or stripping the chest tubes is not necessary to ensure patency, and suctioning the chest tubes should be avoided because of the risk of infection.

Temporary Pacemaker

The connection and function (capture and sensing) of the temporary pacemaker should be examined on arrival and then periodically as necessary. The goal of temporary pacing is hemodynamic stability. Bradycardia resulting in hemodynamic insufficiency after cardiac surgery is estimated to occur in between 0.8 and 4 percent of patients.[22] Patients may require complete dual-chamber pacing for a significant bradycardia or asystole or a back-up setting that will be initiated if the patient becomes bradycardic.

Frequent Laboratory Tests

The use of CPB can lead to sodium retention associated with potassium excretion and decreased insulin response.[23] Calcium, potassium, and magnesium have an impact on myocardial function. Serum chemistries therefore are checked frequently. The need for potassium replacement is common, especially once diuresis begins. Glucose control has become a main concern in the postoperative care of the cardiac surgery patient, and insulin resistance may result from CPB and hypothermia. Therefore, blood glucose is checked frequently, and an insulin infusion may be used to maintain normoglycemia. Hematological work is done on admission and then with daily laboratory work. Serial hemoglobin and hematocrit level samples are drawn depending on the amount of chest tube output. Coagulation tests are sent with the initial blood work and thereafter as dictated by anticoagulant use preoperatively and postoperatively and by chest tube output.

BOX 65-5 ■ ■ ■
STERNOTOMY CART CONTENTS

Contents of a sternotomy cart may include the following:
- Caps, masks, sterile gloves, sterile gowns, sterile linen
- Povidone-iodine (Betadine)
- Staple removers
- Scalpels
- Wire cutters
- Sterile pacemaker wires
- Suction equipment, sterile suction tubing, and Yankauers
- Handheld electric cautery
- Bone cutter
- Laparotomy sponges
- Bypass and sternotomy trays that contain operating room equipment for these procedures
- Sterile irrigation tray and liter bottles of normal sterile saline
- Pacemaker with battery
- Sterile sutures
- Gelfoam
- Sternal wires
- Internal defibrillator paddles
- Intraaortic balloon pump

Frequently Used Medications

Nurses administer a variety of medications in the postoperative period, including vasoactive and inotropic agents and analgesics and anxiolytics. Inotropic agents assist in the maintenance of adequate cardiac output until the myocardium is recovered. Epinephrine often is used because it causes less tachycardia than other drugs such as dopamine. Sodium nitroprusside or other vasodilators may be necessary to control blood pressure and reduce systemic vascular resistance. Morphine is the most common analgesic used and may be administered by patient-controlled analgesia pump. The patient is switched to oral analgesics when appropriate. Midazolam or propofol may be used for anxiolysis. Anticoagulation therapy is used depending on the surgical procedure, postoperative bleeding, and the patient's medical history. Other medications may be used in the postoperative setting as determined by patient age and allergies, the patient's clinical course, physician or institutional preference, and medication half-life.

Ventilator Management

Gas exchange should be assessed frequently via arterial blood gas sampling, pulse oximetry, and breath sounds. Early extubation (within 12 hours of arrival to the ICU) is a goal with nearly every postoperative cardiac surgery patient. Common ventilator settings postoperatively are assist control or synchronized intermittent mandatory ventilator mode, tidal volume between 8 and 10 ml/kg, 100 percent fraction of inspired oxygen, positive end-expiratory pressure of 5 cm H_2O, and pressure support, if appropriate, of 8 cm H_2O. Suctioning of the endotracheal tube is performed as necessary. After the initial arterial blood gas sample on arrival to the ICU, pulse oximetry and/or end-tidal carbon dioxide monitors are adequate to guide weaning. Many institutions now use weaning protocols that guide the respiratory therapist who works closely with the nurse to assess readiness for extubation. When the patient meets extubation criteria, the physician will place the order, and the respiratory therapist and nurse should collaborate on the extubation itself and on the postextubation care.

Common extubation criteria include spontaneous respiratory rate, adequate gas exchange and oxygen saturation, and recovery from anesthesia. Some institutions also may assess weaning parameters such as vital capacity and negative inspiratory force, though such parameters are considered poor predictors of successful extubation except in patients whose functional capacity was reduced preoperatively.

Other Assessment Parameters

Urinary output measurement, peripheral vascular assessment, and neurological examination should be monitored hourly in the immediate postoperative period and then as dictated by clinical condition. The patient arrives with a sternal dressing that should be checked periodically for drainage. A nasogastric tube may be present or may need to be inserted in the ICU.

The urinary catheter is removed as early as possible to prevent a urinary tract infection. Sternal dressing removal is at the discretion of the surgeon, and wound care thereafter usually consists of gentle cleansing with normal saline. The nasogastric tube is removed when the patient is extubated. The hemodynamic monitoring lines are discontinued once intensive care is no longer required, and the nurse may remove these lines. The amount of output from the chest tubes dictates when they are discontinued. Pacemaker wires are removed before the patient is discharged from the hospital.

Prevention of Early Complications after Surgery

CPB is implicated in many postoperative complications, and the best-prepared nurse fully understands how a patient may be affected by the use of CPB. For patients undergoing conventional cardiac surgery, the three major causes of complications are CPB, median sternotomy incision, and aortic manipulation.[23] For patients undergoing cardiac surgery without the use of CPB, causes of complications are temperature disturbances, perioperative ischemia, bleeding, and fluid overload. Many studies have revealed lower incidence of blood loss, renal dysfunction, and neurological complications such as alterations in cognition for patients who are not placed on CPB.[20] Other studies comparing on-pump versus off-pump cardiac surgery revealed similar postoperative complication rates in all risk groups. Although mortality rates with or without the use of CPB have not been shown to differ significantly in several studies, operative mortality in a high-risk group in one study was much higher for patients having surgery with the use of CPB. The mortality rate for cardiac operations is less than 5 percent, with higher mortality in women than in men, and morbidity postoperatively ranges between 25 and 40 percent.[24]

Cardiovascular Complications
Bleeding

All patients are expected to have some degree of mediastinal bleeding postoperatively, which usually decreases over a few hours. Chest tube output is ideally less than 100 ml/hr immediately postoperatively. Between 1 and 3 percent of patients need to return to the OR for continued bleeding.[20] Mediastinal bleeding can lead to life-threatening cardiac tamponade and therefore must be recognized and managed early and aggressively. Early intervention may prevent the need to transfuse banked blood and the problems associated with transfusion. For patients requiring reoperation for bleeding, there is an increased incidence of operative mortality, failure to wean from the ventilator, sepsis, and atrial dysrhythmias.[25]

The nurse is the first line of defense against complications from bleeding and must be vigilant in assessing chest tube output amount and characteristics. Acute awareness of hemodynamic signs of cardiac tamponade, coagulation study results, and changes in breath sounds or inspiratory pressures on the ventilator are also crucial to early identification of and intervention for bleeding. Additionally, achievement of normothermia and prevention of hypertension are important nursing interventions that may prevent bleeding.

Administration of blood products and/or medications such as protamine or aprotinin may be warranted to help control bleeding. It should be noted that no prospective randomized trial has definitively defined the hemoglobin level at which blood transfusion improves clinical outcome.[26] The desire to transfuse has decreased because of concern about the blood supply, acceptable clinical outcomes with lower hemoglobin levels, and the risk of adverse effects of transfusion including allergic reactions and infection, particularly in postoperative cardiac surgery patients. Therefore, it is recommended that signs of inadequate tissue oxygenation be used as the trigger for transfusion rather than a number based on physician preference or random criteria.[27] Institutions should establish thresholds for transfusion because this is shown to result in lower rates of transfusion.[1]

Cardiac Tamponade

Cardiac tamponade is the compression of the heart resulting from a buildup of fluid or blood around the heart and is a potentially fatal complication. Suspicion of cardiac tamponade may arise if hemodynamic monitoring reflects the inability of the myocardium to pump effectively and/or by a sudden end of chest tube output. Transesophageal or transthoracic echocardiography may be used to diagnose or confirm cardiac tamponade. Indications of cardiac tamponade must be reported immediately to the surgeon, and preparation must be made for emergency sternotomy (Box 65-6). The mortality rate associated with cardiac tamponade is 25 percent.[20]

Myocardial Infarction

The risk for perioperative myocardial infarction (**MI**) has been decreased to about 5 percent because of advances in cardiac surgery. An MI that causes hemodynamic instability is more likely to result in higher perioperative mortality. Perioperative MIs are usually mild but can be a major complication. Causes of perioperative MI include graft failure, vessel spasm, and suboptimal myocardial protection. ECG monitoring is crucial for diagnosis and early intervention. A 12-lead ECG may be necessary to confirm new Q waves, new left bundle branch block, or ST segment changes that may be indicative of MI. Because creatine kinase–myocardial band levels may be elevated postoperatively, levels in excess of 5 times the upper limit of normal define a perioperative MI.[20] Serum troponin levels also may be analyzed because they are cardiac specific and indicative of MI.[28] Low cardiac output, hypotension, tachycardia, and ventricular ectopy also may be indicative of MI.

Nursing interventions focus on ECG monitoring, optimizing cardiac function and hemodynamic stability, minimizing oxygen demand, and administration of medications such as nitroglycerin or milrinone, antidysrhythmic agents if indicated, and analgesia. Intraaortic balloon pump support may be necessary for hemodynamic support and/or prevention of ischemia.

Dysrhythmias

Atrial fibrillation is the most frequent dysrhythmia after cardiac surgery, with an incidence of up to 70 percent.[24,29] The use of overdrive pacing, or pacing the atrium at a rate higher than the intrinsic rate, may prevent postoperative atrial fibrillation.[21] Beta blockers also may be used to prevent atrial fibrillation. Treatment of atrial fibrillation may include administration of amiodarone, flecainide, ibutilide, beta blockers, and calcium channel blockers and/or cardioversion, and the main goal is rate control. If atrial fibrillation continues on the second postoperative day, the patient will need anticoagulation therapy.[1]

Although any dysrhythmia may occur postoperatively, supraventricular tachydysrhythmias are the most common.[30] To prevent these dysrhythmias, electrolyte abnormalities, especially hypomagnesemia and hypokalemia, should be avoided or treated immediately. Hypoxia, acid-base disorders, hypovolemia, or irritability from a pulmonary artery catheter must be considered as potential causes. Preparation should be made for cardioversion or defibrillation as appropriate. In addition, conduction disturbances may occur, particularly in patients who have had valvular surgery. Conduction disturbances may require use of the temporary pacemaker and ultimately implantation of a permanent pacemaker. The goal of prevention or treatment of dysrhythmias or conduction disturbances is hemodynamic stability and systemic perfusion.

Pulmonary Complications
Hemothorax and Pneumothorax

Many cardiac surgery patients have pleural chest tubes inserted in the OR. Pneumothorax or hemothorax is more likely to arise in the patient without chest tubes, but signs and symptoms must be assessed in either case. The need for a chest tube to be inserted for a new or expanding pneumothorax depends on size and whether it causes symptoms. A hemothorax is drained because blood remaining in the pleural space is a medium for bacterial growth and because moderate amounts of blood eventually become fibrous and restrict lung expansion. Existing chest tubes must be assessed for air leaks; chest tubes are not removed as long as an air leak exists.

Atelectasis

Atelectasis can contribute to impaired gas exchange postoperatively and, if left untreated, may lead to pneumonia and reintubation. Atelectasis may be caused by

---

BOX 65-6 ■ ■ ■
SIGNS AND SYMPTOMS OF CARDIAC TAMPONADE

- Increased venous pressures
- Equalization of intracardiac pressures
- Significant and/or sudden decrease or cessation of chest tube drainage, especially in patients who had a large amount of output or output consisting of clots
- Widened mediastinum on chest x-ray film
- Decreased electrocardiogram voltage
- Decreased hemoglobin levels
- Dysrhythmias
- Low cardiac output
- Hypotension
- Decreased urine output
- Muffled heart sounds

anesthesia or by factors that negatively affect the patient's respiratory effort. For intubated patients, the ventilator settings referred to before are generally adequate to prevent atelectasis in the immediate postoperative period. Ideally, to prevent atelectasis, the head of the bed should be elevated as much as possible while the patient is intubated. Once the patient is extubated, early mobilization and frequent and proper use of the incentive spirometer are the two most important lung volume expansion interventions to prevent atelectasis.[26] Chest radiographs reveal the presence of atelectasis. Breath sounds may be decreased in an atelectatic area.

Pneumonia

The incidence of pneumonia in cardiac surgery patients is about 2 to 9 percent; pneumonia is the second most common nosocomial infection after urinary tract infection.[31] Patients with chronic obstructive pulmonary disease, preoperative respiratory tract colonization, or who smoke have a higher incidence of pneumonia, so a complete health history must be obtained and communicated in the postoperative report.[24,32,33] Postoperatively, the presence of a nasogastric tube, multiple blood transfusions, dysphagia, and the need for reintubation are risk factors for pneumonia.[32] The paradigm for preventing ventilator-associated pneumonia includes strict hand washing, elevating the head of the bed, frequent and meticulous mouth care, and ensuring proper functioning of the nasogastric tube. Suctioning the endotracheal tube must be done in a sterile fashion.

Pulmonary Embolism

The incidence of pulmonary embolism is only about 1 to 2 percent in cardiac surgery patients, mainly because of heparinization during surgery and hemodilution after surgery. Compression stockings may be used after surgery to prevent a pulmonary embolism. Sequential compression devices and subcutaneously administered heparin often are not used, except for patients who have an extended hospital course or who are not mobilizing well after surgery.[20] Acute onset of chest pain and shortness of breath immediately should raise suspicion of pulmonary embolism. Particularly in the long-term or immobilized patient, assessment for these symptoms along with at least daily mobilization out of bed and range of motion exercises are important nursing interventions. In the patient with a suspected pulmonary embolism, the nurse will need to accompany the patient to radiology for a computed tomograph scan or ventilation/perfusion scan.

Failure to Wean

Respiratory insufficiency is one of the two most common postoperative complications in cardiac surgery patients.[34] Ventilator dependence that exceeds 5 days is associated with a 25 percent mortality rate. The most common reason for ventilator dependence is primary ventilatory failure caused by a disparity between ventilatory capacity and demand[20] (Box 65-7). Important nursing strategies for aiding in ventilator weaning include following a weaning protocol, aggressive pulmonary toilet, pulse oximetry monitoring, early and fre-

---

> **BOX 65-7**
> FACTORS IMPLICATED IN FAILURE TO WEAN FROM THE VENTILATOR
>
> - Congestive heart failure with pulmonary edema*
> - Advanced age
> - Hemodynamic instability
> - Chronic obstructive pulmonary disease
> - Pain or anxiety
> - Pneumonia
> - Altered mental status
> - Obesity
> - Electrolyte abnormalities
> - Fever
> - Phrenic nerve injury
>
> *The most significant independent risk factor.
> From Pezzella AT, Ferraris VA, Lancey RA: *Curr Probl Surg* 41:526-574, 2004.

quent mobilization (including while the patient remains on the ventilator), and incentive spirometry once extubated. Pain and anxiety management are also essential. Patients who fail to wean from the ventilator have a tracheostomy performed after they have spent several weeks on the ventilator.

Renal Complications

Preoperative renal insufficiency (serum creatinine level greater than 1.5 mg/dl) places patients at higher risk for postoperative complications including stroke, ventilator dependence, need for dialysis, and death. CPB has many effects on renal function. The need for dialysis postoperatively occurs in about 1 percent of patients, but the mortality rate can exceed 60 percent in this group.[31] Postoperative maintenance of adequate hemodynamics is critical to ensuring adequate renal perfusion. A decrease in urine output may be the first sign of renal insufficiency. Dopamine has not shown effectiveness as a renal protective agent in patients who had normal renal function preoperatively and in fact may exacerbate renal tubular injury.[35] Higher blood pressure may be achieved with volume rather than with vasopressors, which may decrease renal perfusion. Diuretics are used for oliguria and may be administered continuously or intermittently. Evidence is growing that early intervention with intermittent hemodialysis or continuous renal replacement therapy improves outcomes and increases survival.[20]

Gastrointestinal Complications

Complications of the gastrointestinal system occur in about 2.5 percent of patients and have a mortality rate of about 33 percent.[34] Splanchnic ischemia is considered the most common cause of all gastrointestinal complications.[20,35]

Ileus

In addition to splanchnic ischemia, an ileus may result from the use of narcotics or calcium channel blockers.[20] An ileus may continue for several days, and ongoing assessment for bowel sounds and distention is essential. The nasogastric tube should not be discontinued until bowel sounds have returned. Clear liquids are allowed after removal of the nasogastric tube, and diet progression is determined by patient tolerance.

Gastrointestinal Bleeding

Gastrointestinal bleeding is more common in patients who have had surgery without CPB, although upper gastrointestinal tract bleeding is one of the most common gastrointestinal complications after surgery with or without CPB.[20] A nasogastric tube helps differentiate upper gastrointestinal bleeding from lower gastrointestinal bleeding. Stress ulcer prophylaxis should be administered as indicated, and assessment of nasogastric tube drainage and bowel movements should be documented. Complaints of nausea also should be monitored as a potential early sign of upper gastrointestinal bleeding. Patients who continue with an anticoagulation regimen should be monitored especially closely for signs of gastrointestinal bleeding.

Neurological and Psychological Complications

The overall incidence of neurological complications is about 6 percent in the postoperative cardiac surgery patient population. Embolism is the most common cause of stroke and hypotension and also may contribute to neurological complications. The second most common cause of operative mortality is stroke.[31] Neurological examination including functional assessment identifies deficits and direct diagnostic testing and treatment.

Neuropsychiatric complications occur in up to 70 percent of postoperative cardiac surgery patients.[31] Anxiety or depression, as well as an exacerbation of a preexisting psychiatric disorder, may be observed in the cardiac surgery patient. Assessment for anxiety and depression are important, and preoperative medications should be restarted as soon as possible. The use of anxiolytics or antidepressants may be appropriate.

Neurocognitive Dysfunction

Cerebral microemboli and hypoperfusion are believed to be the causes of neurocognitive dysfunction. About 20 percent of patients experience neurocognitive dysfunction postoperatively. Patients with preexisting cognitive dysfunction, anxiety, depression, a low educational level, and those who experience complications are more likely to experience postoperative neurocognitive dysfunction.[20] However, not all patients exhibit symptoms of neurocognitive dysfunction even when it is present.

Postcardiotomy Delirium

Delirium is a disorder of consciousness that occurs in about 32 percent of cardiac surgery patients and is associated with longer lengths of stay and increased morbidity and mortality yet is often not recognized. Agitation may accompany delirium, but the assessment for delirium should focus on attention, concentration, orientation, sleep-wake cycle, and presence of delusions or hallucinations. The delirious patient often has lucid intervals. Treatment of delirium includes correcting hypoxemia or metabolic derangements, discontinuation of medications that may be contributing to confusion, reorientation as necessary, and provision of a safe environment.[36] Haloperidol (Haldol) is the preferred pharmaco-

therapy, but when it is administered, there is a risk for torsades de pointes.[35] The ultimate goal is patient safety. Delirium may resolve within a few days or may continue for several weeks. In extreme cases and if not resolved, delirium can presage irreversible neurological deterioration.[36]

Postoperative Infection

All cardiac surgery patients receive antibiotics prophylactically. Importantly, the first dose must be given before the skin incision is made in the OR. Most protocols continue administration for 24 hours, but overuse of antibiotics must be avoided. Foley catheters, chest tubes, intravenous lines, and endotracheal tubes must be removed as early as possible to prevent infection.

Mediastinitis

Sternal wound complications can be classified as uninfected dehiscence, infection without stenal instability, or deep sternal wound infection with or without dehiscence.[37] Deep sternal wound infection does not occur frequently, but when it does, it carries a mortality rate of about 25 percent. Diabetes, older age, impaired immune response, obesity, numerous blood transfusions, and prior cardiac surgery increase the risk for wound infection. Strict aseptic technique, proper administration of perioperative antibiotics, limiting blood transfusions, and tight control of blood glucose levels are strategies that help to reduce the incidence of sternal wound infection. In addition, close observation of the incision and assessment for pain and fever are important for early detection of mediastinitis. For the patient with a deep sternal wound infection, a return to the OR for débridement and muscle flap may be indicated.[20]

Nosocomial Infection

Nosocomial infections are associated significantly with multisystem organ failure and increased operative mortality. Nosocomial infection occurs in 10 to 20 percent of postoperative cardiac surgery patients and may manifest as bloodstream infection or urinary tract infection. Nosocomial infections are prevented first and foremost with proper hand cleansing. Early removal of central venous lines, Foley catheters, and chest tubes also significantly reduces the risk of nosocomial infection. Timely administration of proper antibiotics is crucial to preventing these infections, but empirical and prolonged use of antibiotics is not an effective preventive. Sepsis and septic shock are uncommon in cardiac surgery patients, but preventing nosocomial infection reduces the likelihood of this complication, which carries a significant mortality rate.[20]

Glucose Control

Aggressive management of blood glucose perioperatively has emerged as a vital method for reducing morbidity and mortality. The stress of surgery, anesthesia, CPB, hypothermia, and inotropic infusions can affect glucose metabolism and cause severe hyperglycemia.[38] Hyperglycemia can have adverse effects on the renal and neurological systems and the incidence of infection. In diabetic patients, the incidence of deep sternal wound infection is significantly reduced with the use of an insulin infusion to maintain a blood glucose level less than 200 mg/dl.[1] More and more often, nurses are responsible for titrating insulin infusions to maintain blood glucose within the range of 110 to 180 mg/dl for all patients. Care must be taken to prevent hypoglycemia in such situations. In addition, the administration of high doses of insulin while the patient is on CPB may cause profound hypoglycemia when the patient is rewarmed and the insulin begins to act, so the nurse must be prepared to identify this problem and respond appropriately.

PREPARING FOR DISCHARGE FROM INTENSIVE CARE

Most postoperative cardiac surgery patients remain in the critical care environment for 1 to 2 days and then are transferred to a general care floor or progressive care unit that specializes in cardiac patients. Some hospitals are using a universal bed or a one-stop recovery concept in which the patient remains on the same unit throughout hospitalization. Hospitals also are using fast-track programs that emphasize expeditious recovery and discharge to improve patient comfort, enhance quality of care, and ultimately decrease costs.[39]

The average hospital stay is between 5 and 7 days but may be as short as 3 days. The nurse plays a critical role in preparing the patient for discharge with education regarding wound care, driving, diet, pain management, medication use, and activity restrictions including resumption of sexual activity and hygiene. The nurse also must advise the patient on when to call a physician and about any follow-up visits with the physician. With the length of stay ever decreasing, the burden on patients and families to absorb a huge amount of new information during a stressful time presents a greater need for the cardiac surgery patient to be assisted at home after discharge by a registered nurse.

POSTOPERATIVE CARE AFTER DISCHARGE
Pain Management

Pain is the most frequently reported problem for recovering cardiac surgical patients during the first 8 weeks after surgery, and inadequate relief of pain is one of the greatest fears of this population.[40,41] Depending on the type of surgery performed, pain may occur in as few as one to as many as six sites and often in unexpected locations.[42] Although reported levels of pain decrease throughout hospitalization, moderate pain levels that are worse than expected continue to be reported by two-thirds of patients in the month following discharge.[43] In the home setting, less is known about the experience of pain because most studies explore pain in the acute and critical care settings.

Acute pain occurs because of initiation of the inflammatory response as a result of surgical trauma to affected tissues.[44] The inflammatory response triggers the release of enzymes that initiate the pain phenomenon at local nociceptive nervous tissues. Many more nociceptors are located in the skin than in deeper visceral structures, explaining the presence of increased pain in graft sites. Pain impulses travel from nociceptors through afferent fibers to the central nervous system. In the central nervous system, the limbic system plays a role in interpretation and modulation of behavioral responses to painful stimuli.[45] Previous experience with pain and the expectation of pain can affect the patient's response to this afferent fiber stimulation.

The sensation of pain is influenced by gender, age, race, and type and location of surgery performed.[46] Following cardiac surgery, older women[46,47] and nonwhites reported greater pain intensity and received less pain medication than primarily white men.[46] Persons with IMA and saphenous vein grafts report relatively more pain, even when receiving higher doses of pain medication.[42,48] The IMA requires the use of electrocautery and greater manipulation of the sternum to remove the artery from the chest wall. Removal of the saphenous vein requires large leg incisions in a location used during walking. These factors need to be considered when evaluating the pain management regimen.

Pain can prevent participation in activities necessary for recovery. Inadequate pain relief can impair mobility and increase complications in the postoperative period.[49,50] These complications include atelectasis, thrombi development, sleep disturbances, poor appetite, and psychological distress. Coughing, moving in bed, getting up to the chair, and ambulating are associated with the greatest pain during the first week after surgery.[42,49] After discharge, it is expected that mobility levels gradually will increase, and with it, the risk of increased pain.

Untreated pain also stimulates the sympathetic nervous system, which increases heart rate and blood pressure and decreases ventricular filling time and cardiac output. This combination of events can predispose the postoperative cardiac patient to ischemia and hypoxemia.[45] Therefore, adequate assessment and management of postoperative pain is critical to prevention of postoperative ischemic processes. A thorough assessment of pain levels with activity and at rest is a crucial first step to pain control. Assess the patient's perceptions of the pain, physiological and behavioral responses to pain, and self-care remedies implemented by the patient to manage pain[51]; most important is the patient's actual report of pain.

In the acute care setting, post–cardiac surgery patients frequently report inadequately treated pain. Undertreatment of pain may be due to knowledge and beliefs about pain and its management. Nurses' knowledge has been shown repeatedly to be related to pain management.[52-55] Nurses with lower knowledge scores used less pain medication than ordered because of concerns about addiction, medication side effects, and underestimation of pain.[54,56] Knowledge scores were typically lower in medication management and understanding of equianalgesic dosing than in assessment of pain, suggesting a need to include these topics in education programs. Nurses with lower knowledge scores may educate patients inadequately in postdischarge pain management strategies.

Patients do not routinely report their pain to nurses because they do not want to be perceived as a burden, they believe that pain is expected postoperatively, they fear addiction, or they doubt that the nurse believes the level of pain they report.[54] In one study, less than half of cardiac surgery patients always told the nurses that they were experiencing pain, and only one-third felt that the nurses noticed their pain.[42] In another study, nurses disagreed with patients' complaints of pain one-quarter of the time and felt that patients overestimated their pain at least 25 percent of the time.[54]

A combination of medications is needed to treat postoperative pain. Clinical practice guidelines from the American Pain Society[51] (Table 65-1) recommend nonopioids and nonsteroidal antiinflammatory drugs (**NSAIDs**) for mild to moderate postoperative pain if there are no contraindications. NSAIDs reduce the inflammatory response from tissue damage during surgery, and nonopioids have analgesic properties. When these medications are administered around the clock, they minimize the dosage of opioids needed.[44] The use of NSAIDs and opioid analgesics provides more effective pain relief than NSAIDs alone, and these are effective for moderate to severe pain. Opioids can cause constipation, urine retention, sedation, respiratory depression, nausea, and confusion, but using NSAIDs with the opioids can reduce the amount of opioids needed and minimize the side effects of opioid therapy.

Nonpharmacological approaches such as guided imagery, music, therapeutic touch, meditation, and massage can reduce pain, promote relaxation, and decrease anxiety in general surgical patients.[57] A music intervention administered twice a day in the ICU reduced heart rate and systolic blood pressure in post–cardiac surgery patients.[58] More studies of these modalities in the cardiac surgical population are needed.

Education and Counseling

The education and counseling needs of cardiac surgery patients and family members vary over time and with the type of surgery, length of hospitalization, degree of social support, personal meaning of the surgery, presence of comorbidities, and personal preferences. Despite research demonstrating the need for education and support in the recovery period, only 25 percent or less of cardiac surgery patients receive nursing home care after discharge.[59] With abbreviated lengths of hospital stays, referral of high-risk patients to home care is paramount.

Patients and caregivers consistently report a need for information about what to expect postoperatively in terms of self-care and physical and psychosocial recovery. In the immediate postdischarge phase, patients and caregivers need to know potential complications and how to improve physical function, manage physical sensations, and decrease psychological distress. Recognizing expected versus unexpected findings and knowing what to report is difficult for this group, especially when supportive others have not been included in hospital-based education.[60] Confusion about medication management is common, with lack of recognition of multiple names for medications and the risk of double dosing.

In the month after discharge, information needs often change. Concerns with mood changes, fatigue, sleep disturbances, pain, and return of appetite become relatively more pressing, especially for those without a prior cardiac diagnosis. As activity increases, pain, fatigue, and trouble sleeping become more apparent. Those who have not begun cardiac rehabilitation may not feel educated adequately to address these new concerns.

Family is the primary source of support during the early recovery phase, but many family members may not feel adequately prepared to provide the needed support.[59,61] Patients may not remember instructions given in the hospital because of stress, fatigue, and medications, which affect attention and memory.[62] Reinforcement and personalization of education is essential. Moore and Dolansky[63] developed an audiotape outlining postoperative recovery expectations and expected sensations. Concrete descriptors of problems encountered in the early postdischarge period and explanations about symptoms improved reports of physical function and movement in women and psychological distress in men.

Peer coaching is another effective method of support in the early recovery phase. Cardiac surgery patients visited by a peer within 24 hours and again 2 to 5 days after surgery had a significant reduction in anxiety and increased activity levels.[64]

■ ■ ■

Table 65-1   GUIDELINES FOR THE MANAGEMENT OF CARDIAC SURGERY PATIENTS

GUIDELINE	SOURCE	WEBSITE
General guideline	ACC/AHA Guideline Update for Coronary Artery Bypass Graft Surgery [1]	www.acc.org/qualityandscience/clinical/guidelines/cabg/index/pdf
Pain management	American Pain Society: *Principles of Analgesic Use in the Treatment of Acute Pain and Cancer Pain,* ed 5, Glenview, Ill, 2003, The Society.	*www.ampainsoc.org*
Diet	Krauss RM, Eckel RH, Howard B et al: AHA Dietary Guidelines: Revision 2000—A Statement for Healthcare Professionals from the Nutrition Committee of the American Heart Association, *Circulation* 102:2284-2299, 2000.	*http://circ.ahajournals.org/cgi/content/full/102/18/2284*
Atrial fibrillation	Fuster V, Ryden LE, Asinger RW et al: ACC/AHA/ESC Guidelines for the Management of Patients with Atrial Fibrillation, *Circulation* 104:2118-2150, 2001.	*http://circ.ahajournals.org/cgi/content/full/104/17/2118*

ACC, American College of Cardiology; *AHA,* American Heart Association.

From 2 to 6 months after discharge, patients begin to return to their presurgical levels of activity. Concerns at this phase include lingering psychological effects of surgery, adhering to risk factor modification, and reintegrating work and social activities into their lifestyle.[65] Interventions aimed at supporting a heart-healthful lifestyle include education on cooking methods, meal choices at restaurants, and exercise.

Smoking Cessation

Fewer repeat CABG surgeries are seen in smokers who quit. Most tobacco withdrawal symptoms occur within the first 2 to 3 days or during acute hospitalization. Therefore, a major emphasis of nurses after discharge from the hospital is assessment of smoking status and reinforcement of smoking cessation begun during hospitalization. Nicotine replacement therapy should be used cautiously in post–cardiac surgery patients who have severe unstable angina or serious dysrhythmias or who had an MI within 4 weeks of surgery.[66] See Chapter 33 for a more complete discussion of smoking cessation.

Diet

The major dietary recommendations for persons after cardiac surgery focus on maintaining or achieving a healthful body weight, desirable blood cholesterol levels, and blood pressure.[67] Including this information in discharge education is essential because dietary changes often do not occur after CABG.[68] Education should include family members, especially if they are responsible for food preparation or purchasing.

Resumption of Sexual Activity

Resumption of sexual activity is a concern after cardiac surgery. Risk of opening the median sternotomy incision is a concern of patients. Instruct patients to assume a dependent position initially and to take pain medication 30 minutes before sexual activity.[69] Stabilization of the median sternotomy generally occurs around the fourth week, and sexual activity in a variety of positions can be resumed safely at that time.

Sleep

Changes in the timing, quality, and duration of sleep have been reported after cardiac surgery. In the first 4 to 8 weeks, an increase in daytime sleep and reductions in nighttime sleep and rapid eye movement sleep cycles have been found, with the greatest period of sleep disturbance in the first week after surgery.[70] Impaired sleep contributes to worse physical and emotional function, but the mechanisms that are not well understood.[71] Pain, nocturia, impaired sleep cycles, difficulty finding a comfortable position, and inability to perform usual routines before bed appear to be important contributors to poor sleep after cardiac surgery.[72] Preoperative sleep quality predicts postoperative sleep pattern disturbance, suggesting that it may be beneficial to evaluate usual sleep quality before surgery.[70]

Nonpharmacological interventions such as music, therapeutic touch, and back massage have varying degrees of success in decreasing pain and anxiety and improving sleep efficiency in post–cardiac surgery patients.[73,74] These approaches should be combined with pharmacological measures for maximal effect. Further study is needed.

Later Postoperative Complications
Respiratory Complications

Respiratory complications develop in 5 to 90 percent of post–cardiac surgery patients. The most common ones are atelectasis (90 percent), pleural effusion (49 percent), and pneumonia (5 to 19 percent).[75] These complications can lead to hypoxemia, impaired wound healing, altered cognition, myocardial ischemia, and increased personal and financial cost. Further, these complications often can be prevented with nursing intervention, although the evidence is sparse and guidelines do not address how to prevent respiratory complications in post–cardiac surgery patients.

Atelectasis, closure or collapse of the alveoli that generally resolves within 48 hours after surgery, can be identified through auscultation. Suggestive evidence includes decreased lung sounds or crackles, cough, increased sputum production, and fever. Atelectasis is confirmed with radiography.[75] Atelectasis in cardiac surgery patients has been linked to diaphragmatic dysfunction caused by injury of the phrenic nerve during cold cardioplegia,[75,76] narcotic analgesics that depress respiratory drive, use of the IMA, and decreased mobility.[75] Some suggest that a median sternotomy increases postoperative respiratory complications by altering chest wall mechanics, and others refute it.[76]

Pneumonia, inflammation of the lungs caused by bacteria or viruses, is another complication that can occur after cardiac surgery. Factors implicated in pneumonia include a history of smoking, preexisting obstructive lung disease, dehydration, malnutrition, immunosuppression, increased duration of anesthesia, advanced age, narcotic use, postoperative pain, and length and orientation of the surgical incision (horizontal versus vertical).[77,78] Each of these factors increases risk of respiratory complications in isolation, but multiple factors additively increase risk. In elders, decreased muscle strength, alveolar surface area and elasticity of the alveoli, and increased pulmonary compliance and chest wall stiffness can predispose to respiratory complications in the absence of previously identified risk factors.

Nursing interventions can reduce the risk of postoperative respiratory complications in the home. Post–cardiac surgery patients who develop postoperative respiratory complications report inadequate pain relief and less participation in postoperative activities such as ambulation, sitting in a chair, deep breathing and coughing than patients without respiratory complications.[50] Therefore, teaching adequate pain management strategies before and in anticipation of activity is essential.

Ambulation promotes oxygenation and improves perfusion. Progressive increases in activity after discharge should be encouraged every day. Generally, patients are encouraged to increase walking activity by

5 minutes every day until the goal of 30 minutes a day is reached. Incentive spirometry use should be continued at home because the device serves as an external reinforcement. However, bacterial growth can occur in the spirometer after 4 weeks, and a new one should be ordered. Coughing is effective in removing secretions, but pain can decrease effort. So nurses should instruct patients in methods to splint the incision with a pillow or towel when coughing.

Postpericardiotomy Syndrome

Postpericardiotomy syndrome, an autoimmune inflammatory response, occurs in about 20 percent of patients. This syndrome may occur several months after surgery; a history of pericarditis or steroid use increases the risk of it. Symptoms include fever, lethargy, chest or joint pain, pleural effusions, and pericardial rub. Postpericardiotomy syndrome can lead to restrictive pericarditis, cardiac tamponade, or vein graft closure. Diuretics, aspirin, NSAIDs, colchicine, pericardiocentesis, and pericardectomy may be used to treat the syndrome.[20]

Wound Infection

Wound infections, reported in 0.4 to 24 percent of postoperative cardiac surgery patients, are a major cause of morbidity. Wound infections are generally a later postoperative complication that increases cost, length of stay, and unplanned rehospitalization.[79,80] The rates of wound infection vary by site with reported incidences ranging from 1 to 13 percent for saphenous vein grafts,[81] 0.4 to 5 percent for sternal wounds,[82] and 4.1 percent for radial artery wounds.[83] On average, the length of time passing before wound infection develops varies from 10 to 21 days.[84] Most wound infections are identified after discharge from the hospital, making patient education in signs and symptoms and adequate follow-up in high-risk patients a priority.[85,86]

Risk factors for the development of postoperative wound infections vary. Many patient-specific factors are not alterable. For example, women have a higher incidence of wound complications because of increased stress of the breasts on the incision line, especially in those with cup size of C or greater, and the smaller size of arteries.[81,87] Men also have a risk of wound complications because of stress on the suture line.[82] Older age,[88] cefuroxime given more than 2 hours before surgery,[86] obesity,[79,82] diabetes,[79,86,88] chronic pulmonary disease,[75] impaired immune response, New York Heart Association functional Class III or higher,[80] smoking, decreased hematocrit levels,[83] and diagnosed and previously undiagnosed peripheral vascular disease[81] have been linked to increased incidence of wound infections in post-cardiac surgery patients. Persons with type 2 diabetes have higher levels of calcium in polymorphynuclear leukocytes, which can lead to impaired phagocytosis and impaired immune response.[89] Obesity may require a greater incision depth. Decreased blood flow to adipose tissue also is associated with an increased risk of infection.[90]

Intraoperative risk factors including type of graft chosen, increased length of operative procedure,[82] increased number of grafts, and the use of Ace bandages postoperatively have been related to an increased risk of wound infection. The use of unilateral or bilateral mammary artery grafts increases the risk for deep sternal wound infection because of decreased perfusion of the sternum.[80] The location of the saphenous vein on the thigh increases the risk for wound complications because of decreased vascularity in a fatty area, as well as greater surgical manipulation to remove the vein.[83] Less invasive endoscopic techniques have been associated with a higher incidence of hematoma formation, faster closing times, and longer vein lengths harvested, with fewer incisions than with bridge techniques.[91] Endoscopic techniques also have allowed patients to ambulate sooner because of lessened pain.

Hypoperfusion, hypotension, and the use of inotropes decrease blood flow to the skin and can increase the risk of wound infection.[82] Reoperation for postoperative bleeding,[80,82,92] longer time on mechanical ventilation,[80] staples for skin closure in nonobese patients,[86] and use of an intraaortic balloon pump[81] are thought to increase the risk for wound infections, both by introducing microbes through alternate routes and potentially impairing lymphatic flow.

The most commonly identified organisms associated with wound infection are *Staphylococcus aureus* and *S. epidermidis*, normally found on the skin and in the nares.[80,84,92] Nasal carriage of *S. aureus* has been posited as a mechanism in sternal wound infection; perioperative nasal administration of mupirocin has been used to treat these infections.[84,91]

Currently, there are no standard guidelines for treatment of postoperative wounds. Alternatives to conventional wet-to-dry sterile dressings have been explored with varying degrees of success. Negative pressure therapy increases microcirculation to the wound bed through the use of suction and a porous foam dressing covered by an adhesive drape that promotes rapid progression of the wound from the inflammatory stage to the proliferation stage.[93,94] The wound is débrided before initiating this therapy. Because life-threatening limb complications can occur in those with previously undiagnosed peripheral vascular disease, it is important to assess for the presence and quality of peripheral pulses.

Psychological Complications

Adverse psychological outcomes, including anxiety, fear, and depression, have been described in the cardiac surgery population and linked to worsened morbidity, mortality, functional status, and adherence to prescribed medical regimens.[95] A more complete discussion of anxiety and depression is found in Chapters 15, 40, and 41. The development of anxiety and depression preoperatively[62,96,97] and during a 6-month follow-up[98] predicted worse health outcomes, anxiety, and depression for up to 3 years after surgery.

The pattern of anxiety and fear changes over time, with the highest levels generally reported before surgery and a steady decrease during recovery.[39,60,99] This pattern illustrates the need to evaluate emotions before surgery. Intervention is essential in an effort to improve postsurgical outcomes.

Women report more depression and anxiety than men throughout the recovery period.[100,101] Nearly half of the women in one study reported depression 4 to 8 weeks after surgery.[101] This distress has been correlated with lower functional status, undesirable cardiac events, increased pain, lower self-esteem, and ineffective coping.[95,100-102] Anxiety and depression prevent women from participating in roles in the home that lead to poor role quality and impaired home management.[99] Reframing the recovery process or educating women about what to expect postoperatively may help them to gain a sense of mastery over recovery and improve outcomes. Women typically worry more about who will help care for them when they return home, whereas men worry mostly about return to previous functional status. Role quality appears to moderate the effects of physical health and recovery.

Social support interventions have varying degrees of success in reducing psychological distress in cardiac surgical populations. Persons who are married and have spouses able to adjust to the illness may have better psychosocial functioning because there is a supportive person with whom to share their fears.[39] However, a supportive telephone intervention provided during the first 7 weeks after discharge did not significantly lower anxiety more than a control group, perhaps because anxiety levels lower naturally during the recovery period.[103]

Gastrointestinal Complications

Constipation is the most frequent complication in the later postoperative period. Constipation is not defined by stool frequency alone, but the presence of excessive straining, hard stools, and a sense of incomplete evacuation.[104] Constipation may be caused by low activity levels, medication side effects, and dietary changes. Iron supplements, anticholinergics, antidepressants, and opioids decrease peristalsis by interfering with nervous stimulation of the colon. Elders are at greatest risk for constipation because of age-related changes in the intestinal tract such as impaired reabsorption of fluid and decreased peristalsis.

Nursing interventions to prevent or minimize constipation include a thorough assessment of persons at greatest risk for constipation and education in methods to prevent it. Dietary fiber for those at risk for constipation should include 20 to 30 g of fiber daily to increase the bulk and water content of stool. Increased activity levels promote blood flow to the intestinal musculature and can improve peristalsis. Fluid intake should be increased to 2000 ml a day except for those at risk for fluid overload. Stool softeners can promote easier passage of stools, and laxatives can be used when the patient has not had a bowel movement in 3 days. Education in the proper use of laxatives for elders is especially important, for 30 percent of this population report using laxatives weekly.[105]

Although rare, gastrointestinal bleeding, paralytic ileus, or intestinal ischemia can occur after discharge. These complications have been reported in 0.2 to 2.3 percent of post–cardiac surgery patients within the first 30 days after surgery. Bleeding generally occurs because of stress from the surgery and is treated with prophylactically administered antacids, H_2-receptor antagonists, and sucralfate (Carafate).[106] Paralytic ileus can occur because of narcotics, general anesthesia, and impaired electrolyte levels. Intestinal ischemia results from emboli and thrombi that develop during cross-clamping of the aorta during surgery. Assessment of the abdomen for bowel sounds, pain, and distention should be part of routine postoperative assessment.

POSTOPERATIVE OUTCOMES
Functional Status

Impaired functional status, common in the first 6 to 8 weeks after cardiac surgery, affects quality of life and social and emotional function.[107,108] Even low-intensity exercise significantly reduces the physical, social, and emotional effects of cardiac surgery. Exercise should begin early in recovery because physical and functional status at 3 months is a primary determinant of recovery at 1 year.[109]

Reperfusion of the cardiac muscle during CABG surgery may improve physical activity by alleviating preoperative angina and dyspnea. However, symptom relief is rarely sufficient to increase activity, and deconditioning of cardiac and skeletal muscles can be improved only with exercise. Women who have a decrease in physical function have problems with role function, which may cause emotional distress when they cannot maintain the home, especially in older women who live alone. Patients over age 75 may have slower recovery of physical function than those who are younger.[107] Low to moderate levels of exercise (3 days a week for 30 minutes a day) improve physical, emotional, and social outcomes after cardiac surgery, even after controlling for the effects of age and gender.[108] Efficacy beliefs and recovery expectations may influence functional outcomes.

Atrial Fibrillation

Atrial fibrillation (see Chapter 48) is the most common complication following cardiac surgery, occurring in 8 to 70 percent of patients; this dysrhythmia is a major cause of increased morbidity and mortality.[29,110-112] Atrial fibrillation can occur at any point during recovery, but the first incidence is typically in the first week after surgery, with a peak incidence on the second or third postoperative day.[111,113] This finding could be misleading, however, because few investigators have monitored patients beyond the first few days after surgery.

Etiology

Numerous causes have been suggested for the development of postoperative atrial fibrillation in cardiac surgery patients. Atrial fibrillation leads to structural and electrical remodeling of the atria, but trigger sites also have been identified in the pulmonary veins.[114] Mechanisms implicated in the development of fibrosis and atrial remodeling include oxidative stress, contact of blood with the extracorporeal circuit during CPB, which triggers the inflammatory process, and increased atrial volume triggering the release of angiotensin II.[114,115] Oxidative stress can occur because of decreased atrial and ventricular filling times, loss of atrial kick, and rapid ventricular rates that decrease cardiac output.

Complement activation and increased C-reactive protein and interleukin-6 levels, all components of the inflammatory response, have been found in cardiac surgery patients and have been linked to the development of atrial fibrillation.[29] However, atrial fibrillation also occurs in patients undergoing minimally invasive procedures, sometimes at comparable rates, suggesting that a more complex mechanism is responsible.[116] Perhaps the magnitude of the inflammatory response rather than the presence or absence of it places the person at risk for postoperative atrial fibrillation.[29]

Atrial size may be a trigger for atrial fibrillation, but studies are inconclusive. Some have found a larger left atrial area and fibrosis in persons with atrial fibrillation, suggesting atrial remodeling,[113] whereas others have found no association between postoperative atrial fibrillation and atrial enlargement.[117] Prolonged atrial stretch leads to increased myocardial fiber length, decreased resting potential, and the development of multiple re-entry pathways, especially in the area of greatest stretch.[118,119] Larger atria delay conduction and may harbor greater numbers of wavelets, as well as disperse the wavelets throughout the atria.[114]

Autonomic nervous system activation may be another mechanism for atrial fibrillation. Norepinephrine levels are 3 times higher in the atria than the ventricles, and hypothermia can increase norepinephrine levels during the rewarming period of CPB.[115] This electrical remodeling can shorten the refractory period and increase automaticity of atrial tissue and sensitivity of catecholamines.[120] Increased atrial stroke volume has been found, suggesting increased autonomic activity.[113]

Risk Factors

The only consistent predictor of postoperative atrial fibrillation is age, with an increased incidence of 70 percent per decade. The changes in atrial size and structure found in older adults may contribute to the development of atrial fibrillation. Disease processes such as diabetes mellitus, valvular heart disease, hypertension, and heart failure, known to accelerate cardiac structural remodeling, are more common in elders.[121] This explanation is confounded, however, because these disease processes also serve as markers for CAD severity, which may independently predispose a person to atrial fibrillation.

Patients with a history of atrial fibrillation,[122] heart failure,[121] MI, valvular heart disease,[117] hypertension, rheumatic heart disease, chronic obstructive pulmonary disease,[121] renal dysfunction,[110] right coronary artery disease, and pulmonary hypertension had an increased risk of developing atrial fibrillation during hospitalization and after discharge. These conditions can change the structure of the atria because of prolonged pressure and ischemic mechanisms. The possibility of a genetic predisposition is discussed in Chapter 48.

The operative procedure itself may increase the risk for postoperative atrial fibrillation. The use of CPB with cardioplegic arrest and increased cross-clamp time are independent risk factors.[76] They may trigger myocardial damage because of ischemia during cardioplegia, with dysrhythmias during rewarming. Cross-clamping may trigger the inflammatory response.

Treatment

The choice of treatment depends on the length of time with atrial fibrillation, underlying hemodynamic status, and putative cause of atrial fibrillation. In postoperative atrial fibrillation, sotalol, either alone or in combination with other medications, effectively controls the ventricular rate.[111] Amiodorone reduced the incidence of atrial fibrillation in complex surgical cases more effectively than sotalol.[123] Magnesium, given before surgery and daily until discharge, may be effective.[116] Anticoagulation should be achieved with aspirin in low-risk patients or warfarin in higher-risk patients with therapeutic international normalized ratio between 2 and 3.[118]

SUMMARY

Recent advances in medical technologies have expanded options available to cardiac surgical patients. More rapid recovery times, noninvasive surgical techniques, and greater understanding of the risks for potential complications have led to quicker treatment and decreased mortality rates. Evidence to support nursing interventions that improve outcomes in this population has increased significantly in the past two decades. Health care professionals know more about the prevalence and cause of complications such as pain, dysrhythmias, sleep disturbances, and respiratory alterations, but evidence-based interventions are sparse. Research is greatly needed to quantify the effective dose of nursing intervention necessary to improve functional, physiological, psychological, and self-care outcomes for post–cardiac surgery patients and their families.

REFERENCES

1. Eagle KA, Guyton RA, Davidoff R et al: ACC/AHA guideline update for coronary artery bypass graft surgery, *Circulation* 110:1168-1176, 2004.
2. CABRI Trial Participants: First-year results of CABRI (coronary angioplasty versus bypass revascularization investigation), *Lancet* 346:1179-1184, 1985.
3. TIME Investigators: Trial of invasive vs medical therapy in elderly patients with chronic symptomatic coronary-artery disease (TIME): a randomized trial, *Lancet* 358:951-957, 2001.
4. Kreter B, Woods M: Antibiotic prophylaxis for cardiothoracic operations: meta-analysis of thirty years of clinical trials, *J Thorac Cardiovasc Surg* 104:590-599, 1992.
5. Furnary AP, Zerr KJ, Grunkemeier GL et al: A continuous insulin infusion reduces the incidence of deep sternal wound infection in diabetic patients after cardiac surgical procedures, *Ann Thorac Surg* 67:352-360, 1999.
6. Garrett K, Lauer K, Christopher BA: The effects of obesity on the cardiopulmonary system: implications for critical care nursing, *Prog Cardiovasc Nurs* 19:155-161, 2004.
7. Lorenz RA, Lorenz RM, Codd JE: Perioperative blood glucose control during adult coronary artery bypass surgery, *AORN J* 81:126-150, 2005.
8. Davenport J: Patient assessment: integumentary system. In Morton PG, Fontaine D, Hudak CM, Gallo BM, editors: *Critical care nursing: a holistic approach,* ed 8, Philadelphia, 2005, Lippincott Williams & Wilkins.

9. Cameron A, Davis KB, Green G et al: Coronary bypass surgery with internal-thoracic-artery grafts-effects on survival over a 15-year period, *N Engl J Med* 334:216-219, 1996.

10. Arquero OR, Navia JL, Navia JA et al: A new method of myocardial revascularization with the radial artery, *Ann Thorac Surg* 67:1817-1818, 1999.

11. Suma H, Isomura T, Horii T et al: Late angiographic result of using the right gastroepiploic artery as a graft, *J Thorac Cardiovasc Surg* 120:496, 2000.

12. Kouchoukos N, Blackstone EH, Doty DB et al: *Kirklin/Barratt-Boyes cardiac surgery,* ed 3, vol 1, Philadelphia, 2003, Churchill Livingstone.

13. Carpino PA, Khabbaz KR, Bojar RM et al: Clinical benefits of endoscopic vein harvesting in patients with risk factors for saphenectomy wound infections undergoing coronary artery bypass grafting, *J Thorac Cardiovasc Surg* 119:69-76, 2000.

14. Royce AG, Royce CF, Tatoulis J et al: Postoperative radial artery angiography for coronary artery bypass surgery, *Eur J Cardiothorac Surg* 17:294, 2000.

15. Edmunds LH: Cardiopulmonary bypass after 50 years, *N Engl J Med* 351:1603-1606, 2004.

16. Peterson ED, Mark DB: Off-pump bypass surgery: ready for the big dance? *JAMA* 291:1897-1901, 2004.

17. Buckberg GD: Overview: procedure versus protection—an impossible separation, *Semin Thorac Cardiovasc Surg* 13:29-32, 2001.

18. Bridges CR, Horvath KA, Nugent WC et al: The Society of Thoracic Surgeons practice guideline series transmyocardial laser revascularization, *Ann Thorac Surg* 77:1494-1502, 2004.

19. Adams DH, Filsoufi F, Antman EM: Medical management of the patient undergoing cardiac surgery. In Zipes DP, Libby P, Bonow RO, Braunwald E, editors: *Braunwald's heart disease,* ed 7, Philadelphia, 2005, Saunders.

20. Bojar RM: *Manual of perioperative care in adult cardiac surgery,* ed 4, Malden, Mass, 2005, Blackwell.

21. Wiegand DL: Advances in cardiac surgery: valve repair, *Crit Care Nurse* 23(2):72-90, 2003.

22. Timothy PR, Rodeman BJ: Temporary pacemakers in critically ill patients: assessment and management strategies, *AACN Clin Issues* 15:305-325, 2004.

23. Chen-Scarabelli C: Beating heart coronary artery bypass graft surgery: indications, advantages and limitations, *Crit Care Nurse* 22:44-58, 2002.

24. Pezzella T, Ferraris VA, Lancey RA: Care of the adult cardiac surgery patient: part I, *Curr Probl Surg* 41:458-516, 2004.

25. Paparella D, Brister SJ, Buchanan MR: Coagulation disorders of cardiopulmonary bypass: a review, *Intensive Care Med* 30:1873-1881, 2004.

26. Hess DR, MacIntyre NR, Mishoe SC et al: *Respiratory care: principles, and practice,* Philadelphia, 2002, WB Saunders.

27. Maglish Ehrman BL, Moore HA: Blood conservation strategies in cardiovascular surgery, *Dimens Crit Care Nurs* 23:244-252, 2004.

28. Fransen EJ, Diris JH, Maessen JG et al: Evaluation of "new" cardiac marker for ruling out myocardial infarction after coronary artery bypass grafting, *Chest* 122:1316-1321, 2002.

29. Gaudino M, Andreotti F, Zamparelli R et al: The 174G/C interleukin-6 polymorphism influences postoperative interleukin-6 levels and postoperative atrial fibrillation: is atrial fibrillation an inflammatory complication? *Circulation* 108:II-195–II-199, 2003.

30. Knotzer H, Dunser MW, Mayr AJ et al: Post bypass arrhythmias: pathophysiology, prevention, and therapy, *Curr Opin Crit Care* 10:330-335, 2004.

31. Pezzella AT, Ferraris VA, Lancey RA: Care of the adult cardiac surgery patient: part II, *Curr Probl Surg* 41:526-574, 2004.

32. Leal-Noval SR, Marquez-Vacaro JA, Garcia-Curiel A et al: Nosocomial pneumonia in patients undergoing heart surgery, *Crit Care Med* 28:935-940, 2000.

33. Carrel TO, Eisinger E, Vogt M et al: Pneumonia after cardiac surgery is predictable by tracheal aspirates but cannot be prevented by prolonged antibiotic prophylaxis, *Ann Thorac Surg* 72:143-148, 2001.

34. Mason VF, Miller KH: Optimizing outcomes: nurses caring for patients after cardiac surgery can promote early transfers, *Am J Nurs* 101(suppl):13-15, 2001.

35. Hessel EA: Abdominal organ injury after cardiac surgery, *Semin Cardiothorac Vasc Anesth* 8:243-263, 2004.

36. Segatore M, Dutkiewicz M, Adams D: The delirious cardiac surgical patient: theoretical aspects and principles of management, *J Cardiovasc Nurs* 12:32-48, 1998.

37. Douville EC, Asaph JW, Dworkin RJ et al: Sternal preservation: a better way to treat most sternal wound complications after cardiac surgery, *Ann Thorac Surg* 78:1659-1664, 2004.

38. Carvalho G, Moore A, Qizilbash B et al: Maintenance of normoglycemia during cardiac surgery, *Anesth Analg* 99:319-324, 2004.

39. Brown MM: Implementation strategy: one-stop recovery for cardiac surgical patients, *AACN Clin Issues* 11:412-423, 2000.

40. Koivula M, Tarkka M-T, Tarkka M et al: Fear and anxiety in patients at different time-points in the coronary artery bypass process, *Int J Nurs Stud* 39:811-822, 2002.

41. Miller KH, Grindel CG: Comparison of symptoms of younger and older patients undergoing coronary artery bypass surgery, *Clin Nurs Res* 13:179-193, 2004.

42. Yorke J, Wallis M, McLean B: Patients' perceptions of pain management after cardiac surgery in an Australian critical care unit, *Heart Lung* 33:33-41, 2004.

43. Mueller XM, Tinguely F, Tevaearai HT et al: Pain location, distribution, and intensity after cardiac surgery, *Chest* 118:391-396, 2000.

44. Reimer-Kent J: From theory to practice: preventing pain after cardiac surgery, *Am J Crit Care* 12:136-143, 2003.

45. Huether SE, Leo J: Pain, temperature regulation, sleep, and sensory function. In *Pathophysiology,* ed 4, St Louis, 2002, Mosby.

46. Celia B: Age and gender differences in pain management following coronary artery bypass surgery, *J Gerontol Nurs* 26:7-13, 2000.

47. Watt-Watson J, Stevens B, Katz J et al: Impact of preoperative education on pain outcomes after coronary artery bypass graft surgery, *Pain* 109:73-85, 2004.

48. El-Ansary D, Adams R, Ghandi A: Musculoskeletal and neurological complications following coronary artery bypass graft surgery: a comparison between saphenous vein and internal mammary artery grafting, *Aust J Physiother* 46:19-25, 2000.

49. Milgrom LB, Brooks JA, Qi R et al: Pain levels experienced with activities after cardiac surgery, *Am J Crit Care* 13:116-125, 2004.

50. Shea RA, Brooks JA, Dayhoff NE et al: Pain intensity and postoperative pulmonary complications among the elderly after abdominal surgery, *Heart Lung* 31:440-449, 2002.

51. American Pain Society: *Principles of analgesic use in the treatment of acute pain and cancer pain,* ed 5, Glenview, Ill, 2003, The Society.

52. Glajchen M, Bookbinder M: Knowledge and perceived competence of home care nurses in pain management, *J Pain Symptom Manage* 21:307-316, 2001.

53. Merboth MK, Barnason S: Managing pain: the fifth vital sign, *Nurs Clin North Am* 35:375-383, 2000.

54. Watt-Watson J, Stevens B, Garfinkel P et al: Relationship between nurses' pain knowledge and pain management outcomes for their postoperative cardiac patients, *J Adv Nurs* 36:535-545, 2001.

55. Vallerand AH, Hasenau SM, Templin T: Barriers to pain management by home care nurses, *Home Healthc Nurse* 22:831-838, 2004.

56. Herr KA, Kwekkeboom KL: Assisting older clients with pain management in the home, *Home Healthc Manage Pract* 15:237-250, 2003.

57. Snyder M, Lindquist R, editors: *Complementary/alternative therapies in nursing,* ed 4, New York, 2002, Springer.

58. Byers JF, Smyth KA: Effect of a music intervention on noise annoyance, heart rate, and blood pressure in cardiac surgery, *Am J Coll Cardiol* 6:183-191, 1997.

59. Rantanen A, Kaunonen M, Astedt-Kurki P, Tarkka M-T: Coronary artery bypass grafting: social support for patients and their significant others, *J Clin Nurs* 13:158-166, 2004.

60. Davies N: Patients' and carers' perceptions of factors influencing recovery after cardiac surgery, *J Adv Nurs* 32:318-326, 2000.

61. Koivula M, Paunonen-Ilmonen M, Tarkka M-T et al: Social support and its relation to fear and anxiety in patients awaiting coronary artery bypass grafting, *J Clin Nurs* 11:622-633, 2002.

62. Andrew MJ, Baker RA, Kneebone AC et al: Mood state as a predictor of neuropsychological deficits following cardiac surgery, *J Psychosom Res* 48:537-546, 2000.

63. Moore SM, Dolansky MA: Randomized trial of a home recovery intervention following coronary artery bypass surgery, *Res Nurs Health* 24:93-104, 2001.

64. Parent N, Fortin F: A randomized, controlled trial of vicarious experience through peer support for male first-time cardiac surgery patients: impact on anxiety, self-efficacy expectation, and self-reported activity, *Heart Lung* 29:389-400, 2000.

65. King KB, Rowe MA, Zerwic JJ: Concerns and risk factor modification in women during the year after coronary artery surgery, *Nurs Res* 49:167-172, 2000.

66. Charlson M, Isom W: Care after coronary-artery bypass surgery, *New Eng J Med* 384:1456-1463, 2003.

67. Krauss RM, Eckel RH, Howard B et al: AHA dietary guidelines: revision 2000—a statement for healthcare professional for the nutrition committee of the American Heart Association, *Circulation* 102:2284-2299, 2000.

68. Allen JK: Changes in cholesterol levels in women after coronary artery bypass surgery, *Heart Lung* 28:270-275, 1999.

69. Huerta-Torres V: Preparing patients of early discharge after CABG, *Am J Nurs* 98:49-51, 1998.

70. Redeker NS, Ruggeiro J, Hedges C: Patterns and predictors of sleep pattern disturbance after cardiac surgery, *Res Nurs Health* 27:217-224, 2004.

71. Redeker NS, Rugiero JS, Hedges C: Sleep is related to physical function and emotional well-being after cardiac surgery, *Nurs Res* 53:154-162, 2004.

72. Redeker NS, Hedges C: Sleep during hospitalization and recovery after cardiac surgery, *J Cardiovasc Nurs* 17:56-68, 2002.

73. Redeker NS: Sleep in acute care settings: an integrative review, *J Nurs Scholarsh* 32(1):31-38, 2000.

74. Richards K, Nagel C, Markie M et al: Use of complementary and alternative therapies to promote sleep in critically ill patients, *Crit Care Nurs Clin North Am* 15:329-340, 2003.

75. Brooks-Brunn JA: Postoperative atelectasis and pneumonia: risk factors, *Am J Crit Care* 4:340-349, 1995.

76. Wynne R: Postoperative pulmonary dysfunction in adults after cardiac surgery with cardiopulmonary bypass: clinical significance and implications for practice, *Am J Crit Care* 13:384-393, 2004.

77. Brooks-Brunn JA: Risk factors associated with postoperative pulmonary complications following total abdominal hysterectomy, *Clin Nurs Res* 9:27-46, 2000.

78. Brooks JA: Postoperative nosocomial pneumonia: nurse-sensitive interventions, *AACN Clin Issues* 12:305-323, 2001.

79. Jenney AWJ, Harrington GA, Russo PL et al: Cost of surgical site infections following coronary artery bypass surgery, *Aust N Z J Surg* 71:662-664, 2001.

80. Lu CY, Grayson AD, Jha P et al: Risk factors for sternal wound infection and mid-term survival following coronary artery bypass surgery, *Eur J Cardiothorac Surg* 23:943-949, 2003.

81. Paletta CE, Huang DB, Fiore AC et al: Major leg wound complications after saphenous vein harvest for coronary revascularization, *Ann Thorac Surg* 70:492-497, 2000.

82. Noyez L, van Druten JAM, Schroen AMA et al: Sternal wound complications after primary isolated myocardial revascularization: the importance of the post-operative variables, *Eur J Cardiothorac Surg* 19:471-476, 2001.

83. Greene MA, Malias MA: Arm complications after radial artery procurement for coronary bypass operation, *Ann Thorac Surg* 72:126-128, 2001.

84. Sharma M, Berriel-Cass D, Baran J: Sternal surgical-site infections following coronary artery bypass graft: prevalence, microbiology, and complications during a 42-month period, *Infect Control Hosp Epidemiol* 25:468-471, 2004.

85. Avato JL, Lai KK: Impact of post discharge surveillance on surgical-site infection rates for coronary artery bypass procedures, *Infect Control Hosp Epidemiol* 23:364-367, 2002.

86. Trick WE, Scheckler WE, Tokars JI et al: Modifiable risk factors associated with deep sternal site infections after coronary artery bypass grafting, *J Thorac Cardiovasc Surg* 119:108-114, 2000.

87. Lutarewych M, Morgan SP, Hall MM: Improving outcomes of coronary artery bypass graft infections with multiple interventions: putting science and data to the test, *Infect Control Hosp Epidemiol* 25:517-519, 2004.

88. Harrington G, Russo P, Spelman D et al: Surgical-site infection rates and risk factor analysis in coronary artery bypass graft surgery, *Infect Control Hosp Epidemiol* 25:472-476, 2002.

89. Alexiewicz JM, Kumar D, Smogorzewski M et al: Polymorphonuclear leukocytes in non-insulin dependent diabetes mellitus: abnormalities in metabolism and function, *Ann Intern Med* 123:919-924, 1995.

90. Wilson JA, Clark JJ: Obesity impediment to wound healing, *Crit Care Nurs Q* 26:119-132, 2003.

91. Horvath KD, Gray D, Benton L et al: Operative outcomes of minimally invasive saphenous vein harvest, *Am J Surg* 175:391-395, 1998.

92. Wang F-D, Chang C-H: Risk factors of deep sternal wound infections in coronary artery bypass graft surgery, *J Cardiovasc Surg* 41:709-713, 2000.

93. Fleck TM, Fleck M, Moidl R et al: The vacuum assisted closure system for the treatment of deep sternal wound infections after cardiac surgery, *Ann Thorac Surg* 74:1596-1560, 2002.

94. Verrillo S: Negative pressure therapy for infected sternal wounds, *J Wound Ostomy Continence Nurs* 31:72-74, 2004.

95. Connerney I, Shapiro JS, McLauglin JS et al: Relation between depression after coronary artery bypass surgery and 12-month outcome: a prospective study, *Lancet* 358:1766-1771, 2001.

96. Rymaszewska J, Kiejna A , Hadrys T: Depression and anxiety in coronary artery bypass grafting patients, *Eur Psychiatry* 18:155-160, 2003.

97. Saur CD, Granger BB, Muhlbaier LH: Depressive symptoms and outcome of coronary artery bypass grafting, *Am J Coll Cardiol* 10:4-10, 2001.

98. Peterson JC, Charlson ME, Williams-Russo P et al: New postoperative depressive symptoms and long-term outcomes after coronary artery bypass surgery, *Am J Geriatr Psychiatry* 10:192-198, 2002.

99. Plach SK, Heidrich SM: Social role quality, physical health, and psychological well-being in women after heart surgery, *Res Nurs Health* 25:189-202, 2002.

100. Ben-Zur H, Rappaport B, Ammar R et al: Coping, lifestyle changes, and pessimism after open-heart surgery, *Health Soc Work* 25:201-209, 2000.

101. McCrone S, Lenz E, Tarzian A et al: Anxiety and depression: incidence and patterns in patients after coronary artery bypass surgery, *Appl Nurs Res* 14:155-164, 2001.

102. Vaccarino V, Lin ZQ, Kasl SV et al: Gender differences in recovery after coronary artery bypass surgery, *J Am Coll Cardiol* 41:307-314, 2003.

103. Hartford K, Wong C, Zakaria D: Randomized controlled trial of a telephone intervention by nurses to provide information and support to patients and their partners after elective coronary artery bypass surgery: effects of anxiety, *Heart Lung* 31:199-206, 2002.

104. Sweeney MA: Constipation diagnosis and treatment, *Home Care Provid* 2:250-255, 1997.

105. Winney J: Constipation, *Elder Care* 10(4):26-31, 1998.

106. Halm MA: Acute gastrointestinal complications after cardiac surgery, *Am J Coll Cardiol* 5:109-118, 1996.

107. Conway DG, House J, Bandt K et al: The elderly: health status benefits and recovery of function one year after coronary artery bypass surgery, *J Am Coll Cardiol* 42:1421-1426, 2003.

108. Treat-Jacobsen D, Lindquist RA: Functional recovery and exercise behavior in men and women 5 to 6 years following coronary artery bypass surgery, *West J Nurs Res* 26:479-498, 2004.

109. Hamalainen H, Smith R, Puukka P et al: Social support and physical and psychological recovery one year after myocardial infarction or coronary artery bypass surgery, *Scand J Public Health* 28:62-70, 2000.

110. Elahi M, Hadjinikolaou L, Galinanes M: Incidence and clinical consequences of atrial fibrillation within 1 year of first-time isolated coronary bypass surgery, *Circulation* 108:II-207–II-212, 2003.

111. Forlani S, De Paulis R, de Notaris S et al: Combination of sotalol and magnesium prevents atrial fibrillation after coronary artery bypass grafting, *Ann Thorac Surg* 74:720-726, 2002.

112. Zimmer J, Pezzullo J, Choucair W et al: Meta-analysis of antiarrhythmic therapy in the prevention of postoperative atrial fibrillation and the effect on hospital length of stay, costs, cerebro-

vascular accidents, and the mortality of patients undergoing cardiac surgery, *Am J Cardiol* 91:1137-1140, 2003.

113. Leung JM, Bellows WH, Schiller NB: Impairment of left atrial function predicts postoperative atrial fibrillation after coronary artery bypass graft surgery, *Eur Heart J* 25:1836-1844, 2004.

114. Kay CN, Plumb VJ: Atrial fibrillation, atrial flutter, and atrial tachycardia. In Fuster V, Alexander RW, O'Rourke RA, Roberts R, editors: *Hurst's the heart,* ed 11, New York, 2004, McGraw-Hill.

115. Kern LS: Postoperative atrial fibrillation: new directions in prevention and treatment, *J Cardiovasc Nurs* 15:103-115, 2004.

116. Salamon T, Michler RE, Knott KM, Brown DA: Off-pump coronary artery bypass grafting does not decrease the incidence of atrial fibrillation, *Ann Thorac Surg* 75:505-507, 2003.

117. Mathew JP, Parks R, Savino JS et al: Atrial fibrillation following coronary artery bypass graft surgery, *JAMA* 276:300-306, 1996.

118. Fuster V, Ryden LE, Asinger RW et al: ACC/AHA/ESC guidelines for the management of patients with atrial fibrillation, *J Am Coll Cardiol* 38:1266i-1266ixx, 2001.

119. Allessie MA, Boyden PA, Camm AJ et al: Pathophysiology and prevention of atrial fibrillation, *Circulation* 103:769-781, 2001.

120. Prasun MA, Kocheril AG: Treating atrial fibrillation: rhythm control or rate control, *J Cardiovasc Nurs* 18:369-373, 2003.

121. Villareal RP, Hariharan R, Liu BC et al: Postoperative atrial fibrillation and mortality after coronary artery bypass surgery, *J Am Coll Cardiol* 43:742-748, 2004.

122. Deliargyris EN, Raymond RJ, Guzzo JA et al: Preoperative factors predisposing to early postoperative atrial fibrillation after isolated coronary artery bypass grafting, *Am J Cardiol* 85:763-764, 2000.

123. Mooss AN, Wurdeman RL, Sugimoto JT et al: Amiodarone versus sotalol for the treatment of atrial fibrillation after open heart surgery: the Reduction in Postoperative Cardiovascular Arrhythmic Events (REDUCE) trial, *Am Heart J* 148:641-648, 2004.

Care of Patients with Circulatory Assist Devices

Kathleen L. Grady
Julie A. Shinn

CHAPTER ABBREVIATIONS

AC alternating current

ACT activated clotting time

BSA body surface area

FDA Food and Drug Administration

INR international normalized ratio

LVAD left ventricular assist device

LVAS left ventricular assist system

MCSD Mechanical Circulatory Support Device (registry)

NYHA New York Heart Association

REMATCH Randomized Evaluation of Mechanical Assistance for the Treatment of Congestive Heart Failure

TAH total artificial heart

VAD ventricular assist device

HISTORY OF CIRCULATORY ASSIST DEVICES

Heart failure currently affects approximately 5 million Americans, with at least 500,000 new cases diagnosed each year and 300,000 deaths (as a primary or contributory cause) annually.[1] As survival from cardiovascular diseases improves and as the population ages, the incidence of heart failure continues to increase. Severe heart failure unresponsive to maximal medical therapy occurs in approximately 60,000 patients each year.[2] Two-year survival in patients categorized as New York Heart Association (**NYHA**) class IV (unable to carry on any activity without symptoms of heart failure and presence of symptoms at rest) continues to be very poor (20 to 30 percent).[3]

Heart transplantation has been a successful treatment for end-stage heart failure with 1-year survival rates of 80 percent or higher and 10-year survival rates of up to 50 percent.[4] Approximately 2000 of these procedures are performed annually in the United States, yet 500 to 1000 patients in the United States die each year while on the waiting list.[5] Patients also frequently are removed from the heart transplant waiting list because of intervening illnesses or complications of heart failure. Furthermore, many patients with end-stage heart failure are not eligible for heart transplantation because of demographic (e.g., advanced age) and medical (e.g., end-stage renal disease, complications of diabetes, and cancer) factors.[6] Interest in the development of left ventricular assist devices (**LVADs**) and total artificial hearts (**TAHs**) has been pursued because of (1) the disparity between the number of patients listed for heart trans-

plantation and actual surgeries performed[7] and (2) the number of end-stage heart failure patients not eligible for heart transplantation.

The first LVAD was implanted in a human being in 1964 in order to provide temporary postoperative support of the left ventricle,[8] and the first TAH was implanted in 1969 as a bridge to heart transplantation.[9] Development of circulatory support devices was encouraged through a grant to the Artificial Heart Program, sponsored by the National Institutes of Health, National Heart, Lung, and Blood Institute in 1964.[10] During the 1970s, several important requests for proposals from the National Institutes of Health laid the groundwork for the development of LVADs in use today.[11]

During the 1990s, successful outcomes (including acceptable morbidity and mortality rates) prompted the Food and Drug Administration (**FDA**) to approve several devices (including the HeartMate pneumatic and electric LVADs [Thoratec Corporation, Pleasanton, California], Thoratec VAD [Thoratec Corporation], and Novacor LVAD [WorldHeart, Oakland, California]) for use as bridges to heart transplantation.[12] In 2002 the HeartMate XVE LVAD was approved for use as destination therapy for patients with end-stage heart failure who are not candidates for heart transplantation.[13]

TAHs also have been tested in clinical trials, but most TAHs require further study before possible FDA approval for clinical use. The Symbion Jarvik 7-70 (subsequently renamed the CardioWest C-70 TAH [SynCardia Systems, Tucson, Arizona]) has been under study since the early 1980s.[14] This device (initially designed as a permanent artificial heart) has been studied most extensively and is the first TAH to be approved by the FDA for use as a bridge to heart transplantation. Two other fully implantable TAHs are currently under development in the United States. Clinical trials of the AbioCor TAH (ABIOMED Cardiovascular Inc., Danvers, Massachusetts) began in 2001.[15] Another totally implantable TAH, developed at Pennsylvania State University in conjunction with 3M Company, may be ready for clinical trials in the near future.[16]

By the end of 2004, approximately 500 TAHs[14] had been implanted in patients with advanced heart failure worldwide. By the end of 2006, more than 12,800 ventricular assist devices (**VADs**) were implanted (personal communications David Farrar, Thoratec Corporation and Frank Beering, WorldHeart). The purposes of this chapter are to describe indications for use of circulatory support devices, types of circulatory support devices, complications, nursing care, patient outcomes, and future directions.

USE IN PATIENTS WITH END-STAGE HEART FAILURE

VADs may be implanted in patients with severe heart failure that is unresponsive to medical therapy. These patients may have acute or chronic heart failure. Acutely, patients may require VAD support during acute myocardial infarction, acute myocarditis, or if they are unable to be weaned from cardiopulmonary bypass.[17] These patients may receive short-term VAD support and, if ventricular recovery does not occur, subsequently may be placed on long-term VAD therapy.[18] More commonly, patients who have longstanding NYHA class IV (stage D) heart failure and who are unresponsive to maximal medical management are candidates for VAD implantation.[17] These patients frequently have ischemic or dilated cardiomyopathy.

Patients who require LVAD implantation have significant hemodynamic compromise requiring inotropic and/or intraaortic balloon support, with a systolic blood pressure less than 80 mm Hg (or mean arterial pressure less than 65 mm Hg), pulmonary capillary wedge pressure greater than 20 mm Hg, cardiac index less than 2 liter/min/m^2, systemic vascular resistance greater than 2100 dynes-sec·cm^{-5}, and urine output less than 20 ml/hr (despite diuretics).[17-19] Patients who require biventricular support additionally have right atrial pressures greater than 20 mm Hg.[20] Patients with end-stage biventricular dysfunction are candidates for biventricular assist devices and TAHs. TAHs provide complete right and left ventricular support (i.e., replace the native ventricles).

In addition to hemodynamic compromise, it is important to assess other factors to maximize survival and quality of life outcomes and to minimize postoperative morbidity and mortality. Other factors requiring assessment include cardiac factors (e.g., right-sided heart function, valvular disease, and intracardiac shunt), noncardiac factors (e.g., neurological status, infection, and presence of severe pulmonary, renal, or liver disease), technical considerations (e.g., body surface area [BSA] should be greater than 1.5 m^2 for implantable LVADs, presence of prosthetic valves, and number of reoperations), and psychological factors (e.g., patient preferences, treatment compliance, and psychosocial support).[17]

VADs may be used as a bridge to heart transplantation in patients who are candidates for heart transplantation, as destination therapy, or as a bridge to recovery. LVADs were first used as bridges to heart transplantation. All patients who receive a long-term implantable LVAD or biventricular support as a bridge to heart transplantation also must meet selection criteria for heart transplantation. Selection criteria for heart transplantation may be found in Chapter 67. Since 2002, patients who are not eligible for heart transplantation may receive the HeartMate LVAD (the only LVAD approved for permanent implantation) as destination therapy. More than 550 nontransplant patients have received the HeartMate LVAD as destination therapy (personal communication, David Farrar, Thoratec Corporation). Fewer patients (who may or may not be candidates for heart transplantation) have received VADs as bridges to recovery.

The CardioWest TAH is the only TAH that is FDA approved as a bridge to heart transplantation in patients with biventricular failure. The AbioCor TAH has been implanted only in a clinical trial of patients with end-stage biventricular failure who were not candidates for heart transplantation.

TYPES OF CIRCULATORY SUPPORT DEVICES

Many types of circulatory support devices exist today that are capable of supporting ventricular function on a short-term basis (i.e., for several weeks) or long-term basis (i.e., for several months to years). Some have been designed to provide support on a permanent basis in lieu of transplantation. The type of device selected for an individual patient is determined by the urgency of the situation, anticipated length of support, transplant candidacy, whether there is the potential for recovery in the immediate future, and the overall mortality risk.

Devices typically used to support patients in cardiogenic shock after cardiotomy and acute myocardial infarction tend to be those designed for temporary support. Because of the higher mortality associated with these scenarios, these patients typically do not do as well if they are subjected to a longer implant procedure. Longer-term devices also use ventricular cannulation, which a surgeon might be reluctant to use in a patient whose ventricular function might recover. Only two widely used short-term devices—the Biomedicus pump (Medtronic, Minneapolis, Minnesota) and the BVS 5000 (ABIOMED Cardiovascular, Inc., Danvers, Massachusetts)—are included in this discussion. Another commonly used device to support patients in cardiogenic shock, the intraaortic balloon pump, is discussed elsewhere in this book.

The emphasis of this chapter is support for end-stage heart failure and the devices most likely to be used in that scenario. Commercially available LVADs, axial flow devices, and total replacement devices are addressed. The common short-term devices are described briefly. Table 66-1 lists the devices discussed and the current FDA-approved indications for their use.

■ ■ ■

TABLE 66-1 INDICATIONS FOR CIRCULATORY ASSIST DEVICES

FDA-APPROVED DEVICES	INDICATION
Postcardiotomy Support	
ABIOMED BVS 5000	LVAD, RVAD, BiVAD
Biomedicus	LVAD, RVAD, BiVAD
Thoratec VAD	LVAD, RVAD, BiVAD
Bridge to Transplant	
CardioWest TAH	Heart replacement
HeartMate LVAD	LVAD
Novacor LVAS	LVAD
Thoratec VAD	LVAD, RVAD, BiVAD
Destination Therapy	
HeartMate LVAD	LVAD

BiVAD, Biventricular assist device; *FDA,* Food and Drug Administration; *LVAD,* left ventricular assist device; *LVAS,* left ventricular assist system; *RVAD,* right ventricular assist device; *TAH,* total artificial heart; *VAD,* ventricular assist device.

Short-Term Ventricular Assist Devices

Short-term support for the postcardiotomy patient can be achieved with a Biomedicus pump (a device that provides nonpulsatile blood flow) or the ABIOMED BVS 5000 (a device that provides pulsatile blood flow). Of these pumps, the Biomedicus pump is more suitable for a short transition period following cardiopulmonary bypass because of lower cost and ease of management. The BVS 5000 is a better choice if support is needed beyond a few days. It potentially can support a patient long enough to wait for a donor heart if transplantation is an option or until elective replacement to a longer-term device can be achieved.

Biomedicus

The Biomedicus pump is a continuous flow extracorporeal pump that uses centrifugal forces to create kinetic energy that propels blood in the pump forward. The device is relatively easy to implant. A median sternotomy is required to place the cannulas that bring blood flow to and from the pump. A cannula is placed in the left atrium to divert blood flow subcostally to the extracorporeal pump. Blood from the pump is propelled back to the systemic circulation via a cannula that is anastomosed to the ascending aorta. If biventricular support is required, cannulas can be placed in the right atrium and pulmonary artery. Ventricular cannulation is avoided because the intent is to provide short-term support, assuming that the ventricles have the potential for recovery. As blood enters the pump, kinetic energy is created by the spinning of a magnet on the pump console. Magnetic force causes a coupling to the magnet inside the blood pump. As the operator sets the spin rate of the magnet (in revolutions per minute) on the console, the magnet within the pump spins at the same rate, creating the centrifugal effect on the blood. Figure 66-1 illustrates the pump housing with the magnet. Anticoagulation with heparin is required because of the blood-contacting surfaces between the blood, cannulas, and blood pump.

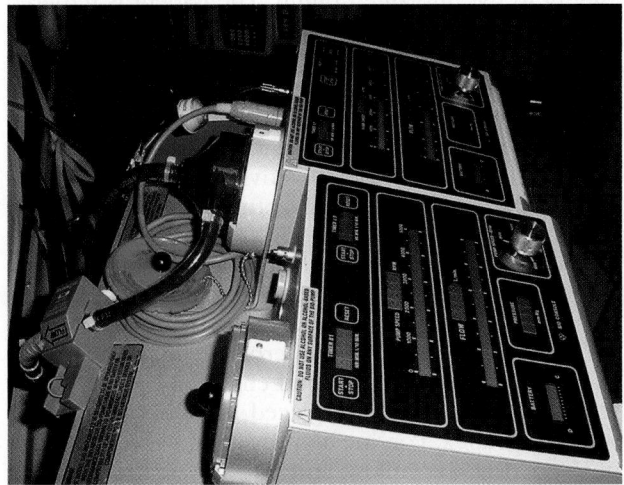

FIGURE 66-1 ■ Biomedicus pump housing with magnet. (Courtesy Medtronic, Minneapolis, Minn.)

Usually, after the Biomedicus device is placed, the sternum is left open with skin closure. As a result, the device is considered to be temporary. Lengthy support is associated with a high-risk of infection. Most patients who are successfully supported with this device are weaned from support within 3 to 4 days. If further support is required beyond that time, consideration is given to reoperation and conversion to a device that can provide longer support. The long-term disadvantage of a continuous flow pump, like the Biomedicus, is the lack of pulsatile flow.

ABIOMED BVS 5000

The Abiomed BVS 5000 is a relatively short-term, pulsatile device. Pulsatile devices have the advantage of being more physiological with respect to end-organ function. Surgical time required to place the ABIOMED pump is similar to the Biomedicus device. A sternotomy incision is required for placement of the cannulas to the extracorporeal pump. Typically, the left atrium is cannulated to bring flow to the external pump, and the ascending aorta is cannulated for the return of blood flow in left-sided support. If this form of support is chosen, the expectation is that there is potential for ventricular recovery so ventricular cannulation most often is avoided. If longer-term support and bridge to transplantation are anticipated, it is possible to cannulate the ventricle.

The ABIOMED pump is a two-chambered pneumatic system that consists of an atrial chamber that houses a blood sac passively filling with blood via gravity from the native atria. An Angioflex® trileaflet valve separates the atrial bladder or blood sac from the ventricular chamber and its blood sac (Figure 66-2). When pressure in the ventricular chamber falls below pressure in the atrial chamber, the valve opens and the ventricular blood sac fills passively. The blood pump diastole is complete when the ventricular chamber reaches full fill capacity or 100 ml. The target stroke volume for each beat is 70 to 80 ml. The capacity of the system is an output of up to 5 liters/min. Output from the pump depends totally on the patient's preload and the amount of systemic resistance. The ventricular blood sac empties with the assistance of compressed air that fills the ventricular chamber during pump systole. The compressed air causes collapse of the blood sac and the forward ejection of the stroke volume.

A second trileaflet valve positioned between the ventricular blood sac and the return cannula maintains forward flow. The top of the pump normally is positioned between 0 and 10 inches below the level of the patient's atrium and then is left in that position. Any adjustment of the height of the pump alters the rate of blood flow into the pump. The BVS 5000 can be used for right, left, or biventricular support. Patients who receive the pump must receive anticoagulation therapy with heparin for the duration of support. The usual goal is to maintain an activated clotting time (**ACT**) of 200 to 300 seconds, which may vary between institutions. The lower the flow of the pump, such as during weaning, the higher the ACT will need to be maintained to prevent thrombus formation in the pump.

Because the Biomedicus and ABIOMED pumps often require that the sternum be left open to create more

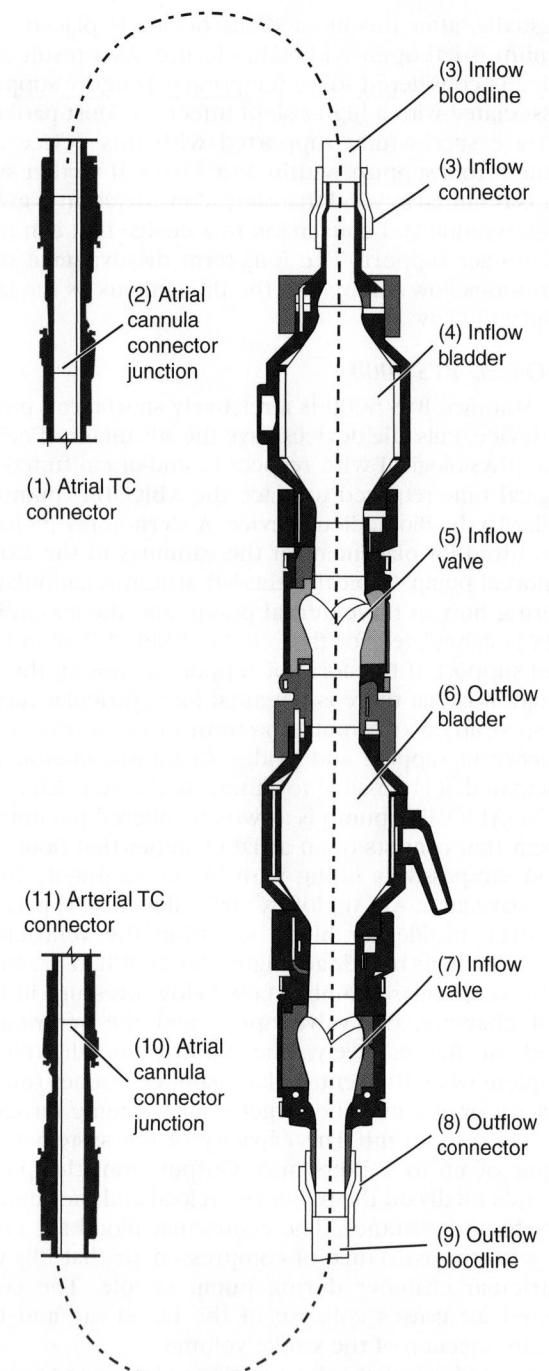

FIGURE 66-2 ■ ABIOMED BVS 5000 Blood Pump. (Courtesy ABIOMED, Inc, Danvers, Mass.) *TC,* Two chamber.

room in the chest for the cannulas, mobility is restricted. Patients are intubated and sedated during the course of support. In situations of cardiac arrest, cardiopulmonary resuscitation is limited to pharmacological and hemodynamic interventions. Chest compression cannot be performed because of the risk of dislodging the pump cannulas. The chest can be opened for internal cardiac massage.

Long-Term Ventricular Assist Devices

Several devices are available for long-term support of ventricular function. The most frequently used pumps include two implantable, electrically driven pumps: the HeartMate VE and XVE LVADs and the Novacor left ventricular assist system (**LVAS**). As previously stated, both of these devices are approved by the FDA for bridge to transplantation in the United States. In addition, the HeartMate XVE LVAD also has been approved for use as destination therapy. In Europe, both pumps are being used as destination therapy. Another frequently used long-term pump is the Thoratec VAD, which is an extracorporeal pneumatic system. Because of the external position of the blood pump, its use is limited to bridge to transplant, and it is more appropriately defined as an intermediate-term device. Other examples of pumps that can provide intermediate- to long-term support are the newer axial flow pumps currently in FDA clinical trials in this country. They include the Jarvik Heart 2000 (Jarvik Heart Inc., New York), the MicroMed-DeBakey pump (MicroMed Technology, Inc., Houston, Texas), and the HeartMate II (Thoratec Corporation, Pleasanton, California). Lastly, total heart replacement is an option for a few selected patients. Two examples of these devices are the CardioWest TAH and the AbioCor TAH. Many other devices are under investigation that are too numerous to address in detail in this chapter.

HeartMate XVE LVAD

One of the most frequently used pumps is the HeartMate XVE LVAD. The HeartMate XVE LVAD has a redesigned inflow graft but otherwise does not differ significantly from the HeartMate VE LVAD. The device is a totally implantable, pulsatile LVAD positioned in the left upper abdominal quadrant. The pump is connected to a microprocessor-based computer (referred to as an external controller) via a tunneled percutaneous driveline that exits the body at the right upper abdominal quadrant just above the waist level. This controller monitors performance of the LVAD, diagnoses and generates advisory and hazard alarms, allows for rate mode changes, brings data about pump function to an external monitor, displays battery charge levels, and carries electrical energy to the implanted pump. The patient is tethered to alternating current (**AC**) power via a power base unit or can move about freely with the use of battery power (Figure 66-3). Two fully charged batteries provide approximately 6 hours of support. When on battery power, the system is light weight and allows the patient to have almost unrestricted activity. Its portability and ease of operation allow for eventual discharge from the hospital.

Placement of the pump requires an incision from the sternal notch to the umbilicus. The pump most often is placed in a preperitoneal pocket in the left upper abdominal quadrant, or as an alternative, it can be placed in the peritoneal cavity. Blood enters the pump via an inflow cannula, which is placed directly into the left ventricular apex. Porcine bioprosthetic tissue valves are positioned at the inflow and outflow of the pump in order to provide unidirectional blood flow. An outflow

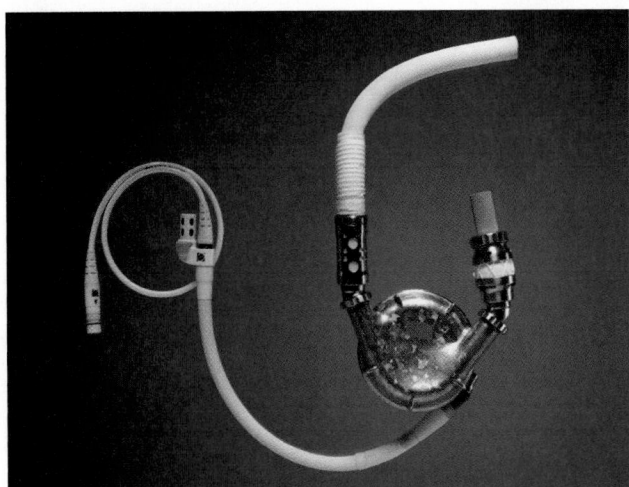

FIGURE 66-3 ■ Thoratec HeartMate XVE. (Courtesy Thoratec Corporation, Pleasanton, Calif.)

graft composed of a Dacron material is used to return blood flow to the ascending aorta. The system uses an electrical motor to drive a pusher plate that is responsible for collapsing a diaphragm inside the pump housing and causing ejection of the stroke volume. The pump has a flow rate capability of 10 liters/min and can be run in a fixed-rate or automatic mode.[21] Ejection occurs in the automatic mode when the pump reaches full fill. The automatic mode is preferred by most clinicians because it is more physiological and allows for change in pump rate and support with varying activity levels. Pump output responds to the patient's preload status. Thus as venous return to the heart increases with exercise, the pump rate increases accordingly. A fixed-rate mode provides a pump rate that is programmed and does not change under any condition. This rate commonly is used during pump start-up in the operating room.

A unique feature of the HeartMate LVAD is the textured interior surface of the blood pump, which encourages endothelial cells to adhere to the surface, thus creating a biological lining. As a result of this smooth interface with the blood, patients do not require anticoagulation with warfarin. Only antiplatelet therapy is required.

Because the blood sac is contained in a rigid titanium shell, air in the space must be displaced to allow the blood sac to fill, and air must be able to enter the space as the blood is displaced out of the pump. This air displacement is achieved via venting through the percutaneous driveline. Air continuously moves in and out of the pump housing through a filter externally located on the driveline. This vent also allows for the pump to be driven pneumatically with a hand pump or pneumatic console in the event of failure of the electrical system.

A feature common to all heart assist devices that have percutaneous leads (the HeartMate, Novacor, and Thoratec devices) is that these leads are covered with a velour-like material that encourages tissue in-growth into the material. This in-growth effectively seals the percutaneous tract and reduces the risk of infection.

Novacor LVAS

Like the HeartMate LVAD, the Novacor LVAS is also an electrically driven, pulsatile circulatory support device that is totally implantable. Pump placement of the device is similar to that of the HeartMate LVAD. The pump is placed in the left upper abdominal quadrant in a preperitoneal pocket. The inflow cannula is placed in the left ventricular apex and tunneled into the abdominal pocket. Porcine tissue valves are used with this pump as with the HeartMate LVAD. Blood is returned to the systemic circulation via a cannula that is anastomosed to the ascending aorta (Figure 66-4). Although the principles of the pump are similar to the HeartMate LVAD, the design is different. The pump uses an electromagnet that attaches to two springs that press on two pusher plates on either side of the blood sac when activated, causing compression and ejection of blood from the sac. The blood sac itself is made of a smooth polyurethane material. The pump housing is coated with a silicone material.

The Novacor LVAS has an option of running in a fixed-rate setting or in the more physiological fill-to-empty mode. The fill-to-empty mode, which is called the automatic mode, is preferred because it allows the pump rate to adjust to changes in preload with increased activity. In this mode the pump runs asynchronous to the native heart and ejects whenever it reaches full fill. The pump also can be run synchronously with the patient's native cardiac cycle by timing ejection to occur when the rate of pump filling tapers off after a native systole. The decrease in the rate of filling is the trigger for pump ejection and can be adjusted from zero to 100 percent. Delay can be added to coordinate pump activity with native

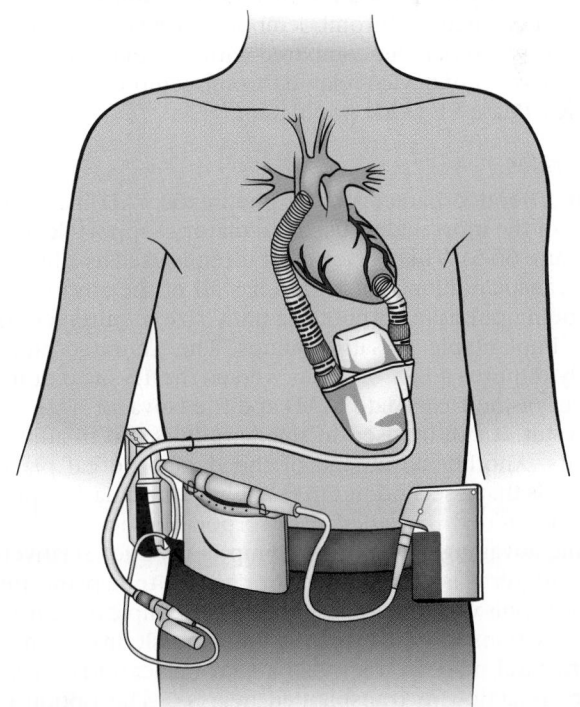

FIGURE 66-4 ■ Novacor left ventricular assist system. (Courtesy Baxter International, Deerfield, Ill.)

heart activity. This feature can be useful in the small number of patients who are potentially weanable from LVAS support.[22] A third option is to run the pump in a fixed rate, which is used in the operating room during initial operation when slow rates are desirable while the patient is still on cardiopulmonary bypass. The Novacor LVAS blood sac capacity is 70 ml with stroke volumes that are typically 60 to 65 ml. Pump flow rates of 10 liters/min are achievable with this LVAS, but most patients do not require more than 5 to 6 liters/min.

The pump can be run from AC power or battery operation. The pump is operated by a portable controller programmed to run the pump in the desired mode. Two batteries are used when the patient is untethered, and they provide support to the patient for up to 6 hours at an output of 6 liters/min.

The only back-up system for the Novacor LVAS is a fail-safe mode that is preset by selecting a preset run rate. The device goes into a fail-safe preset rate when there is any pump and controller miscommunication. The fail-safe mode is initiated automatically by the controller if there are any problems interpreting information from the pump sensors. The Novacor LVAS offers a warranty on pump durability. The pump is insured to last at least 3 years with no device malfunction. As with any machine, moving parts eventually wear out, and this pump has required valve or pump replacement in selected cases after a few years of use. Greater than 86 percent of pumps are still in service at 3 years.[23] This is a unique and important feature of this pump.

Patients who have the Novacor LVAS require anticoagulation with warfarin and antiplatelet agents. One historical problem associated with use of the Novacor pump has been its incidence of thromboembolism. Recent conversion to a different type of inflow graft has dramatically decreased the incidence of these events.[24] The incidence of thromboembolic events in a recent report was 6 percent compared with a similar incidence of 6 percent of device-related thromboembolic events in a HeartMate VE LVAD population.[24,25]

Thoratec

The Thoratec paracorporeal pneumatic VAD has been one of the most widely used circulatory support devices (Figure 66-5). This device most often is used as a bridge to transplantation. The pump has all of the advantages of being pulsatile without the body size requirement of the implantable pulsatile pumps. The Thoratec pump only requires a BSA of 1.3 m² versus the 1.5 m² requirement of the HeartMate LVAD and the Novacor LVAS. As a result, it can be used in smaller adults and in adolescents. Another advantage of the paracorporeal placement is that a second pump for right ventricular support can be added if needed. Paracorporeal placement has some advantages when the pump is used for relatively shorter-term support than bridge to transplant but where pulsatile flow is desirable. The pump can be used in situations in which recovery is a possibility, such as with viral myocarditis, postpartum myocarditis, or severe rejection in transplanted hearts.[26] The option of cannulating the atrium instead of the ventricle is desirable if recovery is possible.

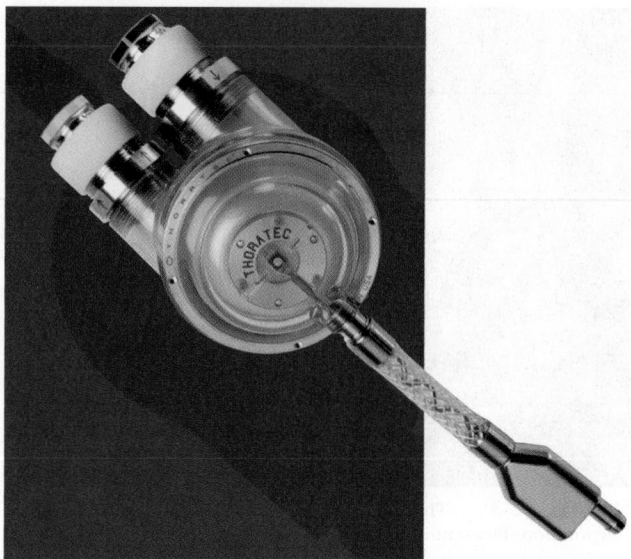

FIGURE 66-5 ▓ Thoratec ventricular assist device. (Courtesy of Thoratec Corporation, Pleasanton, Calif.)

A median sternotomy (with cardiopulmonary bypass) is required to place the pump. The inflow cannula is placed in the left atrium or left ventricle for LVAD support. Left ventricular cannulation is preferred for bridge-to-transplant patients because higher flows are achievable using this technique. If right ventricular support is required, the right atrium is cannulated. The cannula is tunneled subcostally to the external pump. Blood enters a smooth, polyurethane blood sac that is contained inside a rigid pump housing. Blood is returned to the patient via a second cannula that is anastomosed to the ascending aorta. With right-sided support, blood is returned to the pulmonary artery. Tilting disc valves are used to maintain unidirectional blood flow. The pump console or pump driver is connected to the pump housing with a pneumatic hose that delivers alternating pressure and vacuum to the chamber housing the blood sac. Pressure collapses the blood sac, causing ejection to occur. A small amount of vacuum is applied during pump diastole to create a pressure gradient that assists with pump filling.

The pump runs asynchronous to the native heart rate in a fixed rate or in a "fill to empty" mode. This mode is termed the *volume* or *automatic* mode depending on which of two available pump drivers is being used. The volume or automatic mode is essentially the same as the fill-to-empty modes used for the HeartMate or Novacor devices. The pump is triggered to eject when it becomes fully filled. The blood sac has a capacity of 65 ml; therefore the output of the pump depends on the rate of the pump. Pump rates depend on how quickly the pump is filled from the left ventricle. A patient with optimum preload can have pump flow rates of up to 7.2 liters/min.[27] The smaller stroke volumes in pediatric patients may require the use of a fixed rate setting because of the length of time it may take to reach full fill in the volume or automatic mode.

Anticoagulation is required with the Thoratec pump. Heparin is used initially until full anticoagulation with warfarin is achieved. Some centers use low-molecular-weight dextran as an alternative to heparin. The goal of anticoagulation is to maintain the international normalized ratio (**INR**) between 2.5 and 3.5.

Similar to the long-term LVADs, the cannulas are covered in velour-like material that allows for endothelial cell in-growth, which eventually seals the cannula tract from the surface of the skin. This process of sealing helps to protect the patient from the introduction of bacteria from the skin down the cannula tract to the mediastinum.

The Thoratec pump is a pneumatic system, but it also requires electricity to run the compressors that generate the alternating vacuum and pressure. The patient can be attached to a bedside driver (which is connected to electricity at all times) or to a portable driver (which runs on battery or external power). The portable driver uses two batteries at a time with each capable of supporting a single VAD for up to 80 minutes. The portable driver also can be run with a car power adapter plugged into a power socket during travel.[28] Patients who have access to portable drivers potentially can be discharged from the hospital, but the paracorporeal location does place some limits on patient mobility and use as a preferred long-term device.[21,29]

A second, smaller design of the Thoratec pump was approved for use by the FDA in August 2004. The smaller pump is essentially the same pump, with the same principles of operation. The difference is that it is contained in a titanium alloy case and is an implantable system that can be placed preperitoneally or intraabdominally. A percutaneous line carries an optic sensor that detects pump filling and a pneumatic hose that connects to the bedside or portable drive console. The Thoratec implantable ventricular assist device (IVAD) has obvious advantages for increased patient mobility and esthetics, making living outside the hospital easier and more appealing. Implanted pumps are also in a higher reimbursement category, making this choice a financial advantage for institutions choosing to use it versus the paracorporeal version of the pump.

Axial Flow Technology

LVAD axial flow technology is relatively new and currently is being evaluated in clinical trials. One of the problems with the previously described implantable LVAD is the body size requirement. Because the Heart-Mate and Novacor LVADs require a BSA of 1.5 m² or more, they are not an option for smaller male patients, the majority of female patients, and the pediatric population. The smaller, axial flow pumps are an option for many of these patient groups.

Some axial flow pumps provide continuous, nonpulsatile blood flow. They have the advantage of smaller size, lower power consumption, minimal moving parts, and no need for valves because the blood flow is nonpulsatile.[21] Instead of capturing the entire left ventricular output, they operate as true assist or booster pumps, augmenting left ventricular function rather than replacing it.[30] Unlike implantable pulsatile pumps, there is no need for venting air externally or to an internal compliance chamber. The pumps create axial flow by rotation of one or more impellers (rotating blades) that are contained in a titanium housing. Two of these devices, the MicroMed-DeBakey and the HeartMate II, receive blood from inflow cannulas implanted in the left ventricle. The pump is placed in circuit, with the return cannula anastomosed to the ascending aorta. A third device, the Jarvik Heart 2000, is placed directly into the left ventricle and has only an outflow cannula that can be placed into the ascending or descending aorta (Figure 66-6). An advantage of these positioning techniques is that the tethering of the heart in a fixed position, as with the HeartMate and Novacor devices, is avoided, which may allow for remodeling of the ventricular architecture.[31] Also, because there is no flow resistance from an inflow cannula and because of the characteristics of the Jarvik 2000 blade design, it can produce true pulsatile flow. Therefore Jarvik 2000 patients often have a palpable pulse, and their blood pressure can be measured using a standard cuff technique. The higher the flow rate of any of these pumps, the less likely pulsatile flow will be present. Under these conditions, blood pressure is not audible.

Candidates for these pumps are somewhat different from the candidates who require a pump to be the primary source of systemic circulatory support. The axial flow pumps are functioning as assist pumps and cannot replace the entire workload of the left ventricle. Patients who need total resuscitation from a pump that can take over left ventricle workload will not do as well as patients who need assistance for left ventricular dysfunction. The axial flow pumps are not presently designed for total support of the systemic circulation. In the future, the best candidates for these pumps may be more stable patients who are waiting for heart transplantation outside of the hospital and have not yet deteriorated to the point where they need to be hospitalized for inotropic support or intraaortic balloon pump ther-

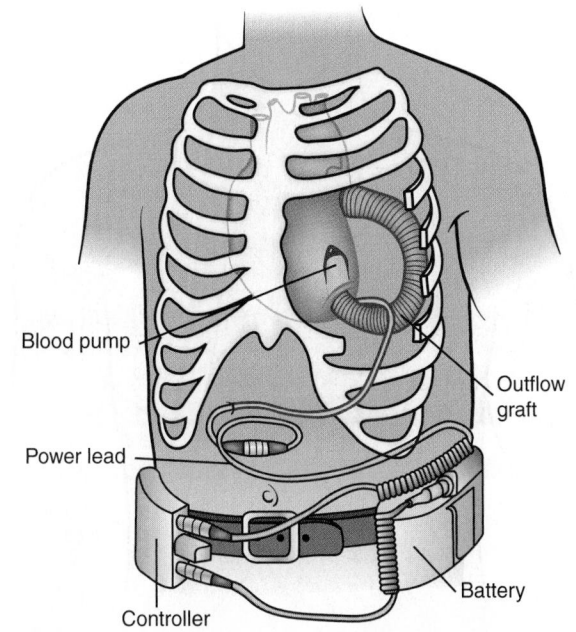

FIGURE 66-6 ■ Jarvik Heart 2000. (Courtesy Jarvik Heart, Inc, New York, NY.)

apy. Anticoagulation is required with these pumps, initially with heparin followed by conversion to warfarin. Patients can be discharged from the hospital after appropriate training to await heart transplantation.

These devices are currently in clinical trials in this country[30,32]. The surgical implant procedure for these pumps is less extensive, so it is hoped that they will be associated with less postoperative bleeding and fewer infections and other postoperative complications than are seen with the larger, implantable devices.[30]

Total Heart Replacement

TAH devices have been developed, but their use has never been widespread because of complications and the success that can be achieved with left ventricular support alone. A TAH is implanted orthotopically in the location of the native heart after the patient's ventricles have been removed. The device that has been used the longest is the CardioWest TAH. The device, successfully used as a bridge to transplant in more than 150 patients,[33] is a pneumatic system that is implanted in the chest cavity. The two artificial ventricles and their prosthetic valves are connected to the patient's atrial cuffs. Blood is returned from the TAH to the great vessels. Figure 66-7 illustrates this pump. Because of its considerable size, patients must have a BSA of 1.7 m² or more.[21]

A newer TAH design is the AbioCor totally implantable artificial heart. Like the CardioWest TAH, it is implanted in the chest cavity after excision of the native ventricles and then is anastomosed to the atrial cuffs and great vessels. Two blood pump chambers have a 60-ml stroke volume capacity and can produce a flow of up to 8 liters/min. Like the CardioWest device, the AbioCor requires considerable space in the chest cavity to house the pump. Unlike the CardioWest pump, the AbioCor does not require a percutaneous driveline for power. The pump does not require air to drive the pumping mechanism but instead uses low-viscosity oil that is

shunted back and forth between the ventricles using a rotary pump. Other implanted components include a controller, battery, and a transcutaneous energy transfer coil.[34] The pump receives electrical energy that is transmitted subcutaneously through the skin from an external power source. This pump represents a truly totally implantable TAH.

COMPLICATIONS

All circulatory assist devices have complications in common. The causes of death following device implant include multiorgan failure, right ventricular failure in the LVAD only groups, bleeding, infection, thromboembolism, and device malfunction.[21,35-37] Box 66-1 lists potential complications of this therapy. The incidence of complications reported in this chapter is from the International Society for Heart and Lung Transplantation Mechanical Circulatory Support Device (**MCSD**) registry. The incidence of complications represents an accumulation of data from all types of devices reported to the registry, including devices not discussed in this chapter.

Multiorgan Failure

Patients' preoperative condition has a significant influence on recovery following device implantation. Many preoperative conditions predispose patients to development of multiorgan failure. A low perfusion state, seen with end-stage heart failure, affects every organ system. Patients often suffer from poor nutrition because of malabsorption from the gastrointestinal tract. Inadequate renal perfusion is often present and is manifested by elevated blood urea nitrogen and serum creatinine levels. Hepatic dysfunction caused by low perfusion and liver engorgement is demonstrated by elevated bilirubin and hepatic enzymes. Some degree of pulmonary dysfunction may be present, and patients may require mechanical ventilation. The single most important risk factor for mortality in the postoperative period is mechanical ventilation in the preoperative patient.[38] Multiorgan failure accounted for 27 percent of deaths with all forms of circulatory assist devices that were reported to the MCSD registry.[35]

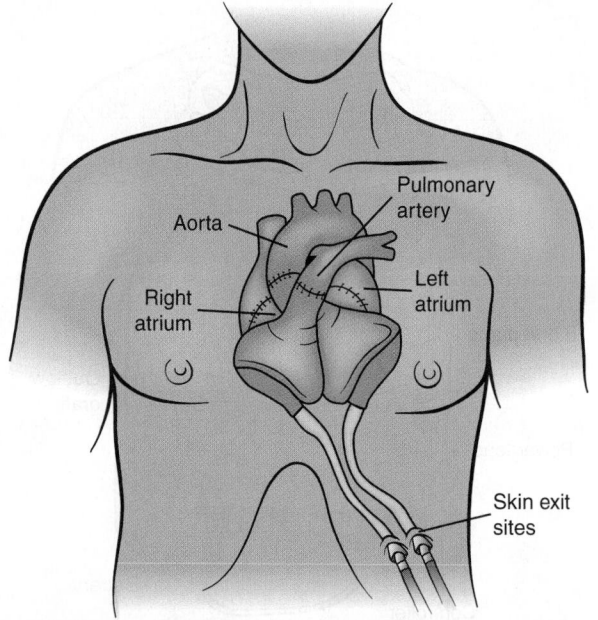

FIGURE 66-7 ■ CardioWest temporary total artificial heart. (Courtesy SynCardia Systems, Tucson, Ariz.)

> **BOX 66-1** ■ ■ ■
> ## COMPLICATIONS OF CIRCULATORY ASSIST DEVICE THERAPY
>
> Bleeding
>   Anticoagulation complication
>   Coagulopathy
>   Surgical bleeding
> Device endocarditis
> Device malfunction
> Driveline infection
> Multiorgan failure
> Neurological dysfunction
> Pump pocket infection
> Right-sided heart failure
> Tamponade
> Thromboembolism

Right Ventricular Failure

Right ventricular failure or dysfunction occurs in approximately 10 percent of patients during the postoperative period,[35] most common in those who receive LVAD support only and who have elevated pulmonary and central venous pressures preoperatively. Because the LVAD depends on the right ventricle to fill the left side of the heart and the pump, a hallmark of right ventricular failure is low pump output and a relatively empty left ventricle. Right ventricular failure is accompanied by high central venous pressure. Given time and support, the right ventricle usually recovers from the insult of surgery and normal right-sided pressures and function are restored. Pulmonary vasodilators and/or nitric oxide are used to unload the right ventricle. In addition, inotropic support of contractility may be required for several days until right ventricular dysfunction abates. Occasionally, temporary right-sided support with a circulatory assist device, such as the Biomedicus pump, is required. If a patient is deemed to be at excessively high risk for right ventricular failure postoperatively, the choice of LVAD only support might be abandoned for biventricular support using a Thoratec VAD or TAH.

Bleeding

Many factors contribute to the risk of bleeding after device implant. Patients with end-stage heart failure often are maintained on anticoagulation therapy in addition to having some inherent coagulopathy from liver dysfunction preoperatively. Some of these patients have had previous cardiothoracic surgery, which also makes them prone to bleeding because of the amount of surgical dissection that is required to expose the heart through extensive pericardial adhesions. Prolonged cardiopulmonary bypass may contribute further to postoperative bleeding. Any device requiring the creation of an abdominal pocket, such as with the HeartMate and Novacor LVADs, naturally is associated with a higher risk of bleeding because of the greater extent of the surgery. A bleeding incidence of 27.8 percent has been reported in the MCSD registry.[35] Strategies used to minimize bleeding include the administration of intraoperative fresh frozen plasma, cryoprecipitate, platelets, and vitamin K. Drugs such as aminocaproic acid (an antifibrinolytic), aprotinin (a serine protease inhibitor of plasmin), and desmopressin (which shortens bleeding time and improves platelet function) may be used to minimize bleeding.

Infection

Unfortunately, infection is a common complication in the short- and long-term circulatory assist device patient. Patients are prone to the usual postoperative infections associated with mechanical ventilation, central venous catheterization, bladder catheterization, and drain placement seen in critically ill patients.[21] In addition, infection is associated with the presence of the assist device itself and the presence of a driveline that connects the device to an external source of power and a control mechanism. These device-related infections include infections in the bloodstream, percutaneous driveline tract, pump pocket, and in the pump itself in the form of a pump endocarditis. *Candida, Enterococcus, Pseudomonas,* and *Staphylococcus* are the most common organisms seen in pump-related infections. Once established, the infection is difficult to eliminate. Patients may require chronic antibiotic therapy. Infection can be controlled but often recurs and is the cause of late mortality and morbidity in long-term assist device patients.[39] In addition to antibiotics, the ultimate treatment of a device-related infection is the removal of the device, which may be seeding the infection. Transplantation is not contraindicated as long as the organism has been identified and can be treated following the transplant. The MCSD registry reported a 32.5 percent incidence of infection, which resulted in the death of 7 percent of patients.[35]

In the Randomized Evaluation of Mechanical Assistance for the Treatment of Congestive Heart Failure (**REMATCH**) Trial, a destination therapy trial using the HeartMate LVAD, the probability of infection within 3 months of implant was 28 percent.[13] Infection was the leading cause of death. Infection is a major problem yet to be solved in long-term bridge and destination therapy patients. Infection will become a less frequent problem when VADs become totally implantable.

Thromboembolism

The artificial blood interface in all pump designs has the potential for thrombus formation and subsequent thromboembolism with the exception of the biological lining seen in the HeartMate LVAD. Low pump stroke volumes and stopping the pump for more than a few minutes also may contribute to the potential for thrombus formation in all pumps. The potential for thrombus formation is a major reason for the preferred method of allowing pumps to fill fully before triggering ejection, thus encouraging optimal washing of blood through the pump with minimal opportunity for thrombus formation. Initial anticoagulation is achieved with heparin until patients are able to take oral agents. Heparin is discontinued when patients have achieved anticoagulation at therapeutic levels with oral agents. Warfarin, antiplatelet agents, or both are required for all devices. INRs usually are maintained between 2.0 and 3.5 depending on the device and institutional preference. In patients who develop heparin antibodies, a direct thrombin inhibitor, such as argatroban, can be used initially instead of heparin. Neurological impairment following a thromboembolic event may be transient with no residual effect or may be associated with permanent impairment. Patients who have one neurological event are prone to subsequent events. Neurological dysfunction occurred in 14 percent of patients in the MCSD registry, and death from stroke resulted in 10 percent of all deaths.[35]

Device Malfunction

These devices are machines and therefore are subject to wear over time. Thus device malfunction and failure are not unexpected events. Failure of motors, wear on bearings, wear on prosthetic valves, and breakage of external components by patient wear and tear have contributed to device malfunction and failure. Continual modification of pump designs has resulted in more reliable systems with less mechanical failure compared with earlier devices.[21] Predictable signs of device wear allow for elective replacement of mechanical parts. For example, impending malfunction of the Novacor pump in long-term patients can be diagnosed at least 2 months before anticipated potential failure.[40]

PATIENT MANAGEMENT
Immediate Postoperative Care in an Intensive Care Unit

Except for the differences in drive mechanisms and device consoles, immediate postoperative care of the patient after device implant is similar regardless of the device. Issues related to vital signs, fluid volume status, right ventricular function, secondary organ function, anticoagulation, nutrition, pump maintenance, infection control, and physical therapy must be addressed in the intensive care unit. A major feature that all devices have in common is their dependence on the patient's preload status for optimal pump output. Insufficient venous return or volume status dramatically impairs the ability of the pump to maintain output and blood pressure. Maintaining adequate preload is a priority of postoperative care.

Close attention to central venous pressure correlated to pump output is required. Pulmonary artery pressure monitoring may or may not be used because most pumps are capable of sending flow rate or pump output data to the pump console display. In cases in which this does not occur, continuous cardiac output via pulmonary artery catheters capable of reading venous oxygen saturation often is used. Continuous arterial pressure monitoring is always used in the intensive care unit for blood pressure and blood gas assessment. Data from these catheters is helpful not only for preload assessment but also for weaning patients from vasoactive drugs.

Alterations in preload occur as a result of bleeding and fluid shifts that are not uncommon after cardiopulmonary bypass support. As with any cardiothoracic surgery patient, cardiac tamponade can occur and will impair filling of the heart and subsequent filling of the assist device. Tamponade should always be considered as a potential cause of low pump output in the immediate postoperative patient who is actively bleeding.

Inadequate LVAD pump filling occurs in the presence of right ventricular failure and is evident by low pump output. A fluid challenge in this situation likely will raise the central venous pressure with no improvement in pump output. An echocardiogram will reveal a relatively empty left ventricle and a dilated right ventricle with impaired contractility. As mentioned previously, right ventricular afterload reduction with nitric oxide and inotropic support with dopamine, dobutamine, and/or epinephrine may be required to support the right ventricle. Maintenance of this therapeutic approach for several days is important even in the presence of optimal pump output. Early attempts to wean inotropic support likely will cause the return of right ventricular failure. Because right ventricular failure is almost always caused by profound left ventricular dysfunction, right-sided heart performance can be expected to improve over time with the restoration of normal left-sided output via the newly implanted pump. If right ventricular failure is not present, only small amounts of inotropic support usually are required.

Because patients likely have secondary organ dysfunction, careful monitoring of liver function, serum creatinine, and blood urea nitrogen are important to determine the extent of further impairment following cardiopulmonary bypass. Many patients exhibit a rise in these laboratory indicators in the initial postoperative period because the liver and kidneys usually incur some injury during the time they were perfused at low pressure on cardiopulmonary bypass. The majority of patients experience a reversal of secondary organ dysfunction over a period of several days once optimal tissue perfusion is restored by the assist device.

Another condition that might impair optimal pump performance is hypertension. Hypertension increases the impedance to pump ejection. This impedance, which is actually afterload for the pump, might interfere with optimal pump emptying and result in smaller than desired stroke volumes. A byproduct is a notable increase in the rate of the pump when set in an automatic or "fill to empty" mode. Rates increase to accommodate the patient's preload in light of the smaller stroke volumes. Hypertension should be monitored and treated so that optimal pump performance is maintained.

Initiating anticoagulation to protect the patient from thrombus formation is a priority as soon as postoperative bleeding abates. Many institutions use dextran infusions in the first 24 hours. Other institutions begin with heparin administration after the first 24 hours or after chest tube drainage diminishes. Heparin infusions are maintained until therapeutic levels of warfarin are achieved. For the HeartMate device, antiplatelet therapy is all that is required. It is important to monitor the appropriate anticoagulation tests (e.g., INR, partial thromboplastin time, and/or ACT) regularly. The type of test and therapeutic ranges depends on manufacturer recommendations and device type. Platelet function also may be monitored, which is a new approach to titrating patient-specific doses of antiplatelet agents. Platelet aggregation is thought to have an important causative role in the thromboembolic phenomena seen in device patients. Routine inspection of the externally visible pumps should be part of nursing assessment. A flashlight can be used to inspect for thrombus formation in the externally visible ABIOMED and Thoratec pumps. Assessment usually is done every 4 to 8 hours. Thrombus formation is more likely to occur in these valved, pulsatile pumps than in the centrifugal pumps. The development of thrombus in the pump housing might require replacement of the pump to prevent sequelae of thromboembolism.

Nutritional status usually is impaired in patients preoperatively because their profound heart failure results in hypoperfusion of the gastrointestinal tract and inadequate absorption of nutrients. Anorexia and fatigue also contribute to the poor nutrition seen in heart failure patients. Following surgery, nutritional repletion is important to minimize the risk of infection and to promote wound healing. Parenteral or enteral nutrition should be started within 48 hours of implant if the patient shows signs of a potentially protracted recovery. Patients who might require parenteral or enteral nutritional support include those with secondary organ dysfunction, right-sided heart failure, or other immediate postoperative complications. Nutritional status is discussed in more detail in the postintensive care section of this chapter.

As mentioned previously, all of the pumps that have percutaneous leads or cannulas connecting to external controllers have a velour-like wrap around the lead or cannula. This wrap protects the patient from infection because it serves as a medium that stimulates endothelial cell in-growth. In-growth is not secure for approximately 10 to 14 days after implant. After healing, in-growth effectively seals the percutaneous track and reduces the risk of infection. It is crucial to keep the driveline as immobile as possible during this time to prevent disruption of the process. Care also should be taken to prevent any tension or pulling on the lead or cannula. If disruption of the process occurs, the tract may never heal completely, predisposing the patient to infection. A secure dressing that includes lead or cannula immobilization with tape, a company-designed restraining belt, or mechanical immobilizers used for other types of tubes or drains can be helpful. Another strategy to prevent excessive movement is to have the patient wear an abdominal binder at all times until healing occurs. After that, it is recommended that a binder or some type of restraining belt be used with any activity.

Patient activity is progressed much as it is after any other cardiothoracic surgery. Once a patient is hemodynamically stable and extubated, he or she can begin to dangle at the bedside or sit in a chair for short periods. Periods of activity gradually are increased. Ambulation usually does not begin until transfer out of the intensive care unit, although that depends on a particular institutional protocol and how long patients usually stay in the intensive care unit. The surgical dissection is fairly extensive for implanted pumps, so adequate pain management is a priority of care, especially because the patient is encouraged to progress in his or her activity.

Postintensive Care

After transfer from an intensive care unit to an intermediate or general care unit, the focus of nursing care changes to rehabilitation and patient/family education. Rehabilitation goals include attainment of improved nutritional and physical functional status. Patient and family education focuses on device management and troubleshooting, drive-line exit site care, home preparation, and community awareness/education in order to provide for a safe discharge.

Nutrition

Achieving adequate nutritional status begins with a dietary consult before LVAD implantation. Advanced heart failure patients are frequently cachectic, and cachexia is

an independent risk factor for mortality[41] in this patient population. Therefore, early nutritional assessment and support are important strategies in the care of advanced heart failure patients who undergo LVAD implantation. Assessment may include determination of weight change over time (including calculation of body mass index), anthropometric measurements (e.g., triceps skinfold thickness), dietary intake, gastrointestinal symptoms, functional capacity, laboratory tests (i.e., electrolytes, albumin, prealbumin, renal function, liver function, lipid profile, hematology studies, and trace elements), and energy expenditure. After intensive care, preferred nutritional support is via oral dietary intake with nutritional supplements.

The literature is replete with evidence that cachectic surgical patients are at increased risk for infection (including wound infection), respiratory failure, renal failure, gastrointestinal complications, and prolonged hospital length of stay.[42-45] In addition, unique complications of HeartMate and Novacor LVAD implantation include delayed gastric emptying, reduced motility, anorexia, nausea, a bloated feeling in the stomach, and early satiety (primarily because of placement of the pump in the left upper abdominal quadrant).[46,47] Therefore, continued nutritional follow-up postoperatively is essential.

Initiation of an oral diet plan, including nutritional supplementation, is an important nutritional goal. Because of pump placement and gastrointestinal symptoms, LVAD patients typically only tolerate small meals. Therefore a meal plan should include three small meals per day and three nutritional snacks between meals and at bedtime. Ongoing nutritional assessment and individualization of the dietary plan is critical to achievement of improved nutritional status.

Physical Function

Physical therapy after VAD implantation is critical to successful outpatient rehabilitation. After discharge, patients are encouraged to return to activities of daily living, exercise regimens, and work. Physical functional assessment should begin before VAD implantation to determine the extent of reduced exercise capacity and to formulate a plan for postoperative rehabilitation. Preoperative assessment includes determination of current physical status and muscle strength, history of performance of activities of daily living, work history, exercise capacity (as determined by prior metabolic treadmill testing), and comorbidities that adversely influence mobility.

After surgery, a progressive exercise plan is developed and tailored to meet the individual needs of each VAD patient.[48-50] Passive range of motion may be performed immediately after surgery. During postoperative days 1 to 3, patients are encouraged to be out of bed and in a chair, as tolerated. Subsequently, patients should participate in active range of motion, sit in a chair 2 to 3 times daily, and ambulate with assistance. Duration and frequency of assisted range of motion and ambulation should increase over time. Patients should progress to independence in activities as much as possible while hospitalized. After 1 week postoperatively, patient goals include independent ambulation, ambulation on stairs, and exercising on a stationary bicycle, as tolerated. From 2 weeks after surgery until discharge, patients should further increase their exercise frequency and duration. By discharge, patients should be ambulating on a flat surface independently, climbing stairs with handrails independently, and performing 20 to 30 minutes of aerobic exercise up to 5 times per week. These discharge goals must be tailored individually by age, comorbidity, and other factors that affected premorbid functional status. For example, an older patient with a history of arthritis and difficulty with ambulation and fine motor movement may require a more specialized exercise regimen and an occupational therapy consult to assist with fine hand movement (which is needed for some activities in monitoring VAD function). Jaski and colleagues[51] reported that age was an independent predictor of post-LVAD peak exercise capacity.

In addition, caveats related to rehabilitation post-LVAD implantation include ensuring that the driveline is secure and avoiding any movement or pulling at the exit site during activities, as well as ensuring that all exterior LVAD components are placed appropriately and secured in a waist pack, vest, or shoulder holster. LVAD patients need to be monitored during exercise (especially early after implantation). Monitoring of pump parameters (pump rate, pump flow, and stroke volume) and patient vital signs (heart rate and blood pressure) are important to determine hemodynamic response to exercise. Patients also should report symptoms such as fatigue and shortness of breath during exercise sessions. Lastly, patients need to bring an LVAD travel case (with extra batteries) if they exercise outside of the unit. Depending on the type of LVAD, a support person or staff nurse with training in use of a hand pump may need to accompany the patient to other units such as physical therapy. An alternative is to train members of other departments likely to see patients with implants in emergency procedures, such as hand pumping. Discharge planning includes determination of outpatient physical rehabilitation needs, which may include in-home physical therapy or referral to a cardiac rehabilitation program.

The benefits of physical rehabilitation after LVAD implantation are demonstrated in studies of exercise capacity in this patient population. Exercise capacity of LVAD patients (mean, 2.6 months after LVAD implantation) was significantly better than exercise capacity of advanced heart failure patients[52] and improved over time from 2 to 3 months postimplant[53] (as measured by maximal oxygen consumption on bicycle and treadmill exercise testing). In addition, NYHA class significantly improved after LVAD implantation.[54]

Patient and Caregiver Education

A major focus of care (which may begin in the intensive care unit and is intensified in the intermediate care unit or on the general cardiac care floor) is patient and caregiver education, home preparation, and community awareness/education. Patients with long-term VADs (HeartMate, Thoratec, and Novacor pumps) can be discharged from the hospital. To be discharged safely, patients and a caregiver must (1) learn about device man-

agement/troubleshooting and driveline exit site care and (2) have a plan for community response in the event of an emergency.

Patient and caregiver LVAD management education typically involves learning about the components of the device, how the device functions, modes of operation, daily system checks, how to change components, equipment maintenance and cleaning, warning lights and their meanings, general warnings and precautions, troubleshooting, emergency response, and telephone numbers to call for technical support or emergencies (Box 66-2). Device manufacturers frequently provide patient education booklets and videos or computer discs that can be used as teaching guides.

LVAD education should be provided in a systematic way with demonstration and return demonstration, as well as discussion and encouragement of questions. Provision of teaching based on patient and caregiver readiness and ability to learn is important. Postoperative recovery, medical comorbidities, cognitive factors (e.g., patient and caregiver educational levels and learning abilities), readiness to learn (i.e., level of anxiety and ability to cope), sessions provided at a time of day conducive to learning, and educational tools that best facilitate learning are critical to assess a priori in order to provide effective LVAD patient education. Patient education is documented in the medical record.

The caregiver also learns how to change the driveline exit site dressing. Changing the driveline exit site dressing is achieved through demonstration and return demonstration. The LVAD nurse coordinator and/or staff nurse gathers supplies, explains the procedure, prepares for the procedure, and changes the dressing while the caregiver observes. Subsequently, the caregiver changes the dressing with observation and critique by the nurse. Signs and symptoms of driveline exit site infection also are discussed, as well as a plan of action. In addition, it is emphasized that the driveline needs to be stabilized so that it does not move because movement can contribute to lack of in-growth at the driveline exit site and possible irritation and infection. Box 66-3 provides a sample driveline exit dressing change procedure for caregivers. Techniques will vary somewhat in different institutions. As previously stated,

---

BOX 66-2 ■ ■ ■
LEFT VENTRICULAR ASSIST DEVICE PATIENT AND FAMILY EDUCATION

Patient and family education typically includes learning about the following:
- Device components
- Device function
- Modes of operation
- Daily system checks
- How to change components (such as batteries and controllers)
- Equipment maintenance and cleaning
- Warning lights and their meanings
- General warnings and precautions
- Troubleshooting/emergency response
- Telephone numbers to call for technical support and/or emergencies
- Driveline exit site dressing change

BOX 66-3
LEFT VENTRICULAR ASSIST DEVICE DRIVELINE DRESSING CHANGE PROCEDURE

To be Taught to Patient and Support Person

Purpose
To provide sterile dressing change guidelines for the left ventricular assist device (LVAD) driveline exit site. The goal is to prevent LVAD driveline infection by maintaining a consistent technique by the support persons.

Supplies Needed for Each Dressing Change
1 0.9 percent normal saline bottle
1 10-sponge pack container of 4 × 4-inch gauze sponges
3 2-sponge packs of 4 × 4-inch gauze sponges
1 2-sponge pack of drain sponges
2 facemasks
1 pair clean gloves
1 pair sterile gloves
1 roll silk or paper tape

Procedure
1. Immediately before starting, wash your hands with soap and water.
2. Set up supplies:
   - Open the 10-sponge pack container of 4 × 4-inch gauze sponges and add enough normal saline to soak all 4 × 4-inch gauze sponges.
   - Open one drain sponge pack and three 4 × 4-inch sponge packs.
   - Make sure all of the supplies remain sterile by not touching anything. If at any time you contaminate any of the sterile supplies, you must replace them.
3. Wet your hands, apply soap, and wash your hands vigorously and thoroughly for approximately 3 minutes. Rinse and dry your hands thoroughly.
4. Place a facemask on yourself and the patient.
5. Put on clean gloves and remove and discard the old LVAD driveline exit site dressing.
6. Inspect the driveline exit site, and notify the LVAD coordinator of any redness or unusual or excessive drainage and/or tenderness.
7. Remove your clean gloves and put on *sterile* gloves, ensuring sterile technique.
8. If at any time you touch a nonsterile item, *you must change your gloves.*
9. Use one normal saline wetted 4 × 4-inch gauze sponge to clean the driveline exit site in a circular motion starting at the driveline exit site and working outward. Repeat this process with a second wetted 4 × 4-inch gauze sponge. Let the site dry, but do not fan the area. To assist in the drying process, you may gently pat with dry sterile 4 × 4-inch gauze sponges. If you need to touch the driveline while cleaning around the driveline exit site, use a sterile 4 × 4-inch gauze sponge to pick up the driveline gently.
10. Place a dry drain sponge around the driveline exit site.
11. Cover with a dry 4 × 4-inch gauze sponge. If the driveline exit site is draining, you may use more than one 4 × 4 gauze sponge.
12. Do not cover and occlude the LVAD vent.
13. Remove your sterile gloves and mask.
14. Use silk or paper tape to secure the dressing. The dressing should be occlusive.
15. Put the abdominal binder back on the patient. It must be worn at all times.

abdominal binders are available through device manufacturers in order to stabilize the drivelines.

After a patient and caregiver have been instructed in management of their LVAD and exit site dressing change, their skill and knowledge should be tested and documented in the medical record. Typical LVAD management testing includes written and hands-on tests. Written testing may include multiple choice, true/false, fill-in-the-blank, and open-ended questions related to the purpose of an LVAD, usual length of battery life, items to carry in one's travel bag, the meaning of different alarms, and what to do in the event of an alarm or emergency. Hands-on testing may include initiation of device self-testing, changing batteries, changing a controller, and hand pumping. Dressing change mastery is assessed through the caregiver's ability to change the dressing (as per protocol) without contamination of gloves or sterile supplies.

Discharge Planning

Patients are discharged post-LVAD implantation based on multiple criteria. These criteria include surgical recovery, medical stability; achievement of NYHA class I to II, stable LVAD function; physical functional and nutritional recovery; acceptable wound healing without signs or symptoms of infection; patient and caregiver competence in management/troubleshooting of the LVAD and driveline exit site dressing change; patient and caregiver emotional readiness; and home environment and community readiness.

When LVAD patients are ready to be discharged, they are provided with necessary equipment and supplies. A discharge checklist is helpful to ensure that patients are discharged with all necessary items (Box 66-4). A list of equipment and supplies also should be provided to the patient and support person along with the items. Patients are instructed that replacement of all LVAD-related items used at home is through the hospital or LVAD clinic, not through the device manufacturer. Thus the health care provider serves as an intermediary (between the patient and device manufacturer) for LVAD equipment and supplies. The health care provider does not need to serve as an intermediary for dressing change supplies. A written list of needed dressing supplies and company name/telephone number (per insurance company instructions) to contact for supplies are provided to patients and caregivers.

Additional discharge planning includes consideration of many other factors. Patients are provided with a medication list and prescriptions as needed. Depending on the device, the patient and family may need to be instructed on warfarin management. Patients also are discharged with a flow sheet to record vital signs and/or pump parameters, as needed (Figure 66-8). Multiple copies of an emergency contact list and a patient identification card with information on (1) where to take an LVAD patient in case of an emergency, and (2) special instructions for emergency care of LVAD patients also are provided to patients. Patients may also purchase Medic Alert bracelets.

Patients also are given information regarding the date, time, and location of their first postoperative clinic visit, usually 1 week after discharge. Some patients and their caregivers may have planned visits away from the hospital for 4 to 24 hours before discharge if needed. These visits can provide patients and families with the confidence to leave the "safety net" of the hos-

---

BOX 66-4   ■ ■ ■
SAMPLE DISCHARGE CHECKLIST FOR LEFT VENTRICULAR ASSIST DEVICE PATIENTS

Discharge planning activities for:
Patient Name: _____   **Caregiver Name:** _____
Person Responsible for Discharge: [name/title] _____

_____ Document patient training [circle all that apply]   LVAD   Dressing change   Coumadin management
_____ Document caregiver training [circle all that apply]   LVAD   Dressing change   Coumadin management
_____ Administer patient and caregiver posttest:
    _____ Patient   _____ (test result [pass/no pass])
    _____ Caregiver   _____ (test result [pass/no pass])
_____ Determine plan for emergency transfer to hospital
_____ Notify community hospital of patient's impending discharge
_____ Provide information to emergency room personnel
_____ Notify local first responders of patient's impending discharge:
_____ EMTs/Fire Department
_____ Police
_____ Ambulance Service
_____ Train local first responders:
_____ EMTs/Fire Department
_____ Police
_____ Ambulance Service
_____ Notify patient's cardiologist
_____ Notify patient's primary care physician
_____ Notify patient's private payer(s)
_____ Notify local electric company and request priority power restoration status
_____ Determine need for home health services [check all that apply]
    _____ Nursing care   _____ [date]
    _____ Dietary consultation   _____ [date]
    _____ Pharmacy consultation   _____ [date]
    _____ Cardiac rehabilitation consultation   _____ [date]
    _____ Physical therapy consultation   _____ [date]
    _____ Social services consultation   _____ [date]
    _____ Other _____
    _____ Complete home assessment by: _____
    _____ Grounded three-prong electrical outlet dedicated to powering the LVAD near the bed
    _____ Outlet not controlled by a wall switch
    _____ Cart for equipment available

Give the following information and equipment to the patient and caregiver:
Informational Materials: [check all that apply]
_____ Discharge instruction sheet[s] in folder
    _____ Written dressing change protocol
    _____ Contact telephone number to obtain dressing change supplies
    _____ List of dressing change supplies
    _____ Medication list
    _____ Flow sheet to record vital signs and pump parameters
    _____ Prescriptions
    _____ Appointment card for clinic visit
    _____ Letter to patient: no driving/flying privileges (if applicable)
    _____ Copy of letter sent to power company [with telephone number]
    _____ Wallet card with special instructions for LVAD patients
    _____ Patient LVAD handbook (and other materials as applicable)
    _____ Emergency contact list [multiple copies]
LVAD Equipment and Supplies [as ordered from the device company]

Dressing Change Supplies for Exit Site Care [e.g., abdominal binder and gauze] **for ____ Days**

Additional Materials, Equipment, or Supplies:
_____ Thermometer   _____ Abdominal binder
_____ Blood pressure cuff   _____ Other [describe] _____

LVAD, Left ventricular assist device.

pital before discharge actually is scheduled. In addition, if a patient was seeing a psychologist or psychiatrist before discharge for anxiety, depression, or difficulty coping an outpatient follow-up visit for continued psychosocial support also should be scheduled.

Patients often ask many questions about returning to daily activities after LVAD implantation. Many of these questions may have been discussed earlier during hospitalization but need to be reinforced at the time of discharge. Patients are allowed to shower, but only after their

Patient Name: _____

Date/Time	Weight	Temperature	Blood Pressure	Pump Rate	Stroke Volume	Pump Flow

FIGURE 66-8 ■ Flow sheet of vital signs and pump parameters after implantation of a left ventricular assist device.

driveline exit site has healed and with use of a special shower kit provided by the device manufacturer. Also, although exercise and cardiac rehabilitation are encouraged, certain activities are not allowed, such as contact sports and swimming. Sexual activities are allowed and usually are resumed at 6 to 8 weeks after implant. Patients and partners need to consider positioning and being careful not to cause movement or tension on the driveline.

Traveling involves extra planning. Patients need to remember to carry extra batteries, controllers, a hand pump (if applicable), and other equipment and supplies with them. In addition, if traveling by air, patients may want to carry on all LVAD-related equipment (so that it does not become lost luggage). Also important is to give patient's the name and telephone number of the LVAD center nearest the travel destination in case of an emergency and to notify the LVAD center of the patient's travel plans. Patients who travel by automobile are encouraged to sit in the back seat of cars with front seat passenger side air bags because deployment of an air bag may cause damage to the LVAD or internal bleeding.

Although LVAD center policies and state driving regulations vary, patients may be instructed not to drive (or if a pilot not to fly an airplane) after LVAD implantation. Lastly, return to work depends on a patient's health and the type of work. It is important for patients to speak with their physician about what type of work they can resume and how soon to return to work after LVAD implantation.

Two other important components of discharge planning are home safety and local community awareness/education about LVADs. Home safety includes discussion of necessary factors for an LVAD patient's safe return to the home and a home inspection if necessary. Important items to consider are the availability of one to two grounded three-prong electrical outlets dedicated to powering the LVAD. The primary electrical outlet must be near the bed. In addition, the outlet(s) should not be controlled by a wall switch. A cart also should be available to house the LVAD equipment in the patient's bedroom, near the bed. Further discussion about general safety in the home (e.g., having a telephone with emergency numbers near the bed and on the first floor of a two-story home, slip-resistant surfaces, rugs and grab bars in the shower [for patients who have shower kits]) is also important before discharge. Potential problems with electrical outlets and other safety issues should be resolved before discharge.

Community awareness begins with letters being sent to the patient's cardiologist, primary care physician, local hospital emergency room, and local first responders about the unique needs of an LVAD patient. Before discharge, an individualized plan for emergency patient return to the hospital that implanted the LVAD must be developed. This plan includes contacting community first responders and the local hospital emergency room. The LVAD coordinator and/or designate at the implanting hospital is contacted immediately for all emergencies. Air transportation may need to be arranged if patients live far from the implanting medical center. In addition, a letter is sent to the local electrical company about placing the patient on a "priority restoration list" in the event of an electrical power failure because the primary electrical power source to support the LVAD is AC power.

Patients who have been discharged from the hospital to home have experienced good outcomes. Approaches to discharge may vary somewhat by device and from center to center.[55-61] Careful planning and attention to specific LVAD patient outpatient needs can result in successful patient discharges.[62,63]

Outpatient Management

LVAD patients who have been discharged from the hospital typically are discharged home. If home health services are required, it is important to collaborate with the home health agencies well in advance of discharge to develop a plan of care, protocols, and home care orders. Ideally, development of home health plans of care are incorporated into the development of the entire VAD program. Home care staff education is also important so that the nurses and other staff are comfortable with providing care to these patients. Although VAD programs may vary in their approach, it is important to determine in advance whether home health nurses will be involved in providing VAD-related care and thus require more focused training, such as learning to change driveline exit site dressings per protocol.[58,64]

Sometimes, patients require discharge to a rehabilitation center, extended care facility, or nursing home.[65] VAD program staff and postdischarge facility staff need to meet in advance and determine whether the facility is able to provide care to VAD patients. When facilities are able to provide care to these patients, plans for staff education (including orientation, regular in-service training, and competency testing), visits from VAD center staff (possibly including obtaining staff privileges at the facility), and protocols/plans of care are central to providing safe and effective VAD care.[64]

Patients discharged home or to other facilities return to the hospital campus for regularly scheduled clinic visits. Although the frequency of clinic visits may vary, outpatients often are seen weekly for 4 weeks, biweekly for 4 to 8 weeks, and monthly thereafter.[58,66] Nonscheduled patient appointments should be available for urgent matters. Ideally, it is efficient to see patients in a clinic setting that includes all needed supplies and equipment. Clinic visits may be conducted by advanced practice nurses, physician assistants, cardiac surgeons, and/or cardiologists.[65]

Clinic visits typically include a history of symptoms, concerns, and problems since discharge or the previous clinic visit; a review of current medications; a physical examination; an assessment of vital signs and pump parameters (derived during the clinic visit and from the VAD parameters recorded by patients at home); a driveline exit site dressing change (with inspection of the driveline exit site); and a discussion about dressing change concerns (if any), needed equipment, and replacement of supplies. The following issues also are discussed[58,67,68]:

- Performance of routine LVAD care
- Alarm occurrences
- Anticoagulation status monitoring
- Activities of daily living and recreational activities
- Need for home health services
- Outpatient physical rehabilitation
- Diet
- Sleep
- Anxiety, depression, and coping (Box 66-5)

Subsequently, laboratory test samples usually are drawn (which may include a complete blood count with differential, basic or comprehensive chemistry panel, coagulation studies [if the patient is taking warfarin]), and other testing as indicated (e.g., panel reactive antibody levels every 1 to 2 months and as needed if awaiting transplantation).[68] Patients who receive an LVAD as a bridge to heart transplantation also may be scheduled for right-heart catheterizations and echocardiograms every 3 to 6 months, and as needed. In addition, patients are reminded that a member of the LVAD team can be reached 24 hours per day, 7 days per week for emergencies (including activation of the plan for emergency return to the hospital), as needed.[65] Plans for maintenance

---

BOX 66-5 ■ ■ ■
ELEMENTS OF A CLINIC VISIT

- History of symptoms and problems since discharge and/or previous clinic visit
- Review of current medications
- Assessment of vital signs and pump parameters
- Physical examination
- Driveline exit site dressing change
- Discussion about dressing change concerns, needed equipment, and replacement of supplies
- Discussion of other issues including performing routine left ventricular assist device (LVAD) care, alarm occurrence, monitoring of anticoagulation status if indicated, activities of daily living and recreational activities, need for home health services, outpatient physical rehabilitation, diet, sleep, anxiety, and coping
- Blood work (which may include a complete blood count with differential, basic or comprehensive chemistry panel, coagulation studies [if taking warfarin]), and other testing as indicated (e.g., panel reactive antibody levels every 1 to 2 months if awaiting transplant)
- Determination of the need to schedule a right-heart catheterization/echocardiogram
- Reminder about emergency contacts for LVAD-related problems
- Plans for maintenance checks on home equipment as needed
- Revised plan of care (which may include medication changes and new prescriptions, additional blood draws) and next appointment

---

checks on home equipment also may be discussed (typically scheduled once each year).

Subsequently, the revised plan of care and next appointment are given to the patient. It is strongly recommended that information be communicated in writing and verbally. Single-page written summaries of clinic visits with the following information are recommended:

- Medication changes
- Dates and times of future blood work and tests
- Date and time of the next clinic appointment
- Patient education and other instructions (including symptoms that require a telephone call to the LVAD coordinator)

OUTCOMES
Survival

Reports of survival (range, 60 to 77 percent) in LVAD patients bridged to heart transplantation have been encouraging.[69-75] Reports from the HeartMate registry and Novacor registry suggest that more than two-thirds of LVAD patients have had successful outcomes (being transplanted, having the device removed, or being supported for 1 year or longer).[76,77]

Furthermore, preimplant independent risk factors for mortality after VAD and LVAD implantation have been identified using multivariate analyses (Cox proportional hazard modeling) and have included the following variables: older than age 60, receiving mechanical ventilation, respiratory failure associated with septicemia, right-sided heart failure, prior cardiac surgery, acute postcardiotomy, acute myocardial infarction, and elevated baseline creatinine or total bilirubin levels.[40,78,79]

The REMATCH trial provided important data regarding survival after LVAD implantation as destination therapy for patients with end-stage heart failure.[13] Survival was better in patients randomized to LVAD implantation compared with optimal medical therapy (1-year survival 52 percent versus 25 percent [$p = 0.002$] and 2-year survival 23 percent versus 8 percent [$p = 0.09$].) After adjusting for date of surgery, in patients randomized to LVAD implantation, a 25 percent decline in mortality relative risk per year was demonstrated, though it was not statistically significant. Implantation of an LVAD was associated with a 48 percent relative risk reduction for death.[13]

Fewer researchers have reported survival of patients implanted with an LVAD as a bridge to recovery. Hetzer and colleagues[80] described the outcomes of 23 LVAD patients who underwent removal of their devices after cardiac recovery (7 patients had recurrent cardiac failure within 4 to 24 months [6 of these patients had transplants and 1 patient died on the waiting list]; 3 patients died of noncardiac causes; and 13 patients experienced stable cardiac recovery for 3 to 49 months).

Survival after TAH implantation has been reported recently as a bridge to heart transplantation and as destination therapy. In a recent study, 81 patients with end-stage heart failure underwent implantation of the CardioWest TAH, and their outcomes were compared with 35 retrospectively matched control subjects. Patients who received the CardioWest TAH had a significantly higher rate of survival to transplant (79 percent versus 46 percent) compared with the control group. Overall survival for the CardioWest TAH group was 70 percent versus 31 percent in the controls.[81] Overall survival on the device has been reported to be as high as 83 percent. It has been suggested that this pump be considered in patients who have biventricular failure and a large chest cavity.[21] In a clinical trial of the AbioCor TAH (a totally implantable TAH), Samuels and Dowling[82] reported that out of eight implants, five patients died within 5 months of implant and one patient was alive and had survived 1-year after implant.

Quality of Life

Limited research has been conducted on quality of life in patients after LVAD implantation, and no studies were found in the literature regarding quality of life in patients who underwent TAH implantation. Besides anecdotal reports, early studies of quality of life after VAD implantation were cross-sectional, included very small sample sizes (fewer than 12 patients), lacked preimplant data, queried patients retrospectively, and used single instruments without report of psychometric data.[83,84]

The few longitudinal studies of quality of life outcomes in patients after LVAD implantation have been primarily from patients awaiting heart transplantation. Only two research teams[85-90] have reported results from longitudinal studies of quality of life outcomes after LVAD implantation in bridge to heart transplant applications, and only Rose and colleagues[13] have reported longitudinal quality of life outcomes after LVAD implantation as destination therapy in the REMATCH trial. Results from these longitudinal studies suggest that overall, quality of life is improved after LVAD implantation.

Grady and colleagues[87] reported improved quality of life outcomes in 30 LVAD patients awaiting heart transplantation from before to 2 weeks after device insertion. Although satisfaction with life overall was fairly good and did not change over time, patients were significantly more satisfied with their health and functioning and with significant others, but less satisfied with their socioeconomic status 2 weeks after LVAD implant compared with the pre-LVAD period. Overall symptom distress and symptom distress for specific areas (cardiopulmonary, gastrointestinal, and genitourinary) decreased significantly over time. As one might expect, preimplant symptoms primarily were related to heart failure. Symptoms after device insertion were related to the surgery and postoperative recovery (i.e., insomnia, fatigue, early satiety, and incisional pain). The areas of greatest functional disability remained the same before and early after surgery: work, recreation, home management, and sleep/rest. The only significant change in functional disability detected from before to after surgery was an increase in self-care disability that may have been related to the need for patients to learn to care for their personal needs in the presence of an LVAD. For example, patients need to learn to use the special shower kit designed to protect external components of the LVAD from getting wet.

Demographic, clinical, physical, and psychosocial variables were examined as potential predictors of quality of life in 92 LVAD patients awaiting heart transplantation.[88] Predictors of greater satisfaction with overall quality of life at 1 month after LVAD implantation included being less bothered by psychological symptoms, having less psychological stress after implant, and being black. Patients also stated that they still would have decided to have an LVAD implant knowing what they knew 1 month later (76 percent definitely yes and 11 percent probably yes). Dew and colleagues[90] also reported that early after surgery, most patients would consent again to receiving a VAD and would recommend implantation of such a device to others.

Dew and colleagues[90] also reported the impact of LVAD implant on psychological status and global quality of life within a few months after surgery. In their study (n = 38) of patient perception of a VAD after implantation as a bridge to heart transplantation, responses were generally positive. However, patients described worry and concerns about device noise, driveline pain, device malfunction, possible infection, and difficulty sleeping.

Grady and colleagues[86] and Dew and colleagues[89,90] examined the impact of hospital discharge on quality of life for LVAD patients bridged to heart transplantation. Grady and colleagues[86] determined that being discharged from the hospital (n = 62) predicted increased satisfaction with socioeconomic areas of life and decreased overall stress, psychological stress, and stress related to family and friends, self-care, work, school, and finances. Additionally, she and her team determined that hospital discharge predicted decreased physical and self-care disability. Dew and colleagues[89] examined

quality of life from approximately 1 month before (n = 35) to 1 month after hospital discharge (n = 10) after LVAD implantation. After discharge, LVAD patients demonstrated improved physical function (mobility, ambulation, and self-care) and improved emotional well-being (specifically reduced depression and anxiety symptoms) compared with before discharge.

Longitudinal change in quality of life in LVAD patients through 1 year postimplant was reported by only two research teams: Grady and colleagues[85] in their study of LVAD patients bridged to heart transplant and Rose and colleagues[13] in their landmark clinical trial (REMATCH). Both groups of investigators experienced reductions in LVAD patient sample size, primarily because of heart transplantation[85] and death[13] by 1 year after LVAD insertion. Grady and colleagues[85] described fairly good and stable quality of life outcomes in patients from 1 month (n = 55) to 1 year (n = 9) after LVAD implantation. Positive and negative changes were detected in all quality of life domains after LVAD insertion.

The psychological domain of quality of life was generally good, but the social domain was more variable in Grady's longitudinal study of LVAD patients.[85] Patients reported generally good quality of life, moderate stress levels, good coping ability, and satisfaction with psychological areas of life, although symptoms of emotional distress (i.e., feeling anxious, sad, helpless, and depressed) were present at all periods. Satisfaction with significant others was ranked highest at all periods compared with other domains of quality of life, yet patient satisfaction with this area decreased significantly at 3 to 6 months after implant. Patients reported being least satisfied with usefulness to others for all periods.

Lastly, overall perception of health status in LVAD patients was described as fairly good, and satisfaction with health and functioning increased between 1 and 2 months after surgery.[85] Physical functional disability was low and remained stable through 1 year after implant. However, work, home management, and recreation continued to be ranked as the areas of greatest disability after LVAD insertion.

Rose and colleagues[13] examined change in quality of life from baseline to 1 year later in end-stage heart failure patients ineligible for heart transplantation who were randomized to optimal medical management (n = 61) or LVAD implantation (n = 68). Baseline quality of life did not differ significantly between groups. One year later, LVAD patients (n = 23) reported significantly better physical and emotional functioning and less depression compared with medically managed patients (n = 6).

Limited study of other indicators of quality of life outcomes (e.g., exercise capacity measured by treadmill testing) has been done. Mancini and colleagues[91] reported that exercise capacity was significantly better in LVAD patients (early after implant) versus end-stage heart failure patients awaiting heart transplantation. However, post-LVAD exercise capacity did not reach levels achieved by healthy individuals. Researchers also noted that LVAD patients (within 12 weeks of implant) experienced levels of exercise compatible with activities of daily living.[49,51,53,92]

Patient preference, or utility (a measure of quality of life that quantifies preferences for health state and survival) is an increasingly important outcome in studies involving patients with heart disease. Moskowitz and colleagues[93] studied 29 patients with advanced heart failure undergoing LVAD implantation as a bridge to heart transplantation. In this population, utility scores significantly improved from baseline to early after LVAD implantation and after heart transplantation. This indicates that after both surgeries, patients were less willing to trade time for better health.

Relationships between quality of life and clinical outcomes increasingly have been recognized within the research community. In Grady and colleagues[85] study of quality of life within 1 year after LVAD implantation, two items from the physical domain of quality of life (ambulation and being able to dress oneself) were associated with an increased risk of mortality while on an LVAD. Being able to walk only short distances with a need to stop or rest and being able to dress oneself, but more slowly, are classic indicators of unstable chronic heart failure.[94] In patients with LVADs, the usefulness of these items may be partly as indicators of right-sided heart failure or diminished LVAD reserve.

In summary, studies of quality of life outcomes after LVAD implantation have included the study of overall quality of life and quality of life domains such as physical function, emotional status, social interaction, and patient preferences. However, current published reports are limited. Although the reports described in this section have included appropriate designs, instruments, procedures, and statistics, results have been limited by decreased sample sizes beyond a few months after surgery. Given that LVAD implantation improves survival of patients with end-stage heart failure, it is equally important to understand whether implantation (1) improves perceived overall quality of life and quality of life outcomes and (2) affects patient preferences for health and survival.

Resource Utilization

Considerable variability in time to discharge has been reported for patients bridged to heart transplantation with means from 37 ± 22 days to 61 ± 13 days[86,89,95] and a range from 18 to 132 days.[86,89] Likewise, percent of patients discharged to home to await transplantation has been variable. Richenbacher and Seemuth[62] surveyed 24 institutions that had implanted more than 10 LVADs per year since 1998 ($n = 640$) and reported discharge rates of 27 to 93 percent (mean = 53 percent). Readmission rates after initial discharge were reported as 1.2 days/3 months with an average length of stay of 5.6 ± 10.6 days.[95] For destination therapy patients, median time spent in the hospital for LVAD implantation, median days spent out of the hospital, and median days alive were 29, 340, and 408 days, respectively.[13]

Although there have been several attempts to determine VAD implantation-related costs,[95-97] Evans[98] has provided a thoughtful and thorough discussion of costs associated with permanent cardiac assistance and replacement. Evans has suggested that based on existing data, total first-year costs associated with VAD implantation are approximately $300,000.

SUMMARY AND FUTURE DIRECTIONS

Much progress has been made in the past two decades in the field of circulatory support. The goal of device manufacturers has been to develop a durable device (with a low incidence of complications) capable of long-term support (at a reasonable cost) as an alternative to heart transplantation. The HeartMate LVAD is the first device to be approved for this indication. Subsequently, in 2003 the Centers for Medicare and Medicaid Services approved national insurance coverage for the HeartMate XVE LVAD as destination therapy. Since that time, the Centers for Medicare and Medicaid Services have made significant improvement in the base reimbursement rates for VAD therapy in general. Better reimbursement may encourage increased use of VAD therapy by institutions.

Destination therapy will stimulate much discussion on the allocation of medical resources, as did heart transplantation in its early days as a treatment option for end-stage heart failure. In addition, ventricular recovery and VAD removal require further understanding. It is important to understand better the mechanisms of ventricular recovery and identification of potentially weanable patients. If, as suggested, the total first year costs associated with VAD implantation are approximately $300,000,[98] that represents an annual expenditure of $18 billion for relatively few members of society. The onus will be on device manufacturers to reduce the costs of these pumps through design changes on existing pumps and development of new pumps with the goal of decreasing the incidence of adverse events (e.g., infection and device malfunction and failure) and developing smaller, totally implantable pumps. Better patient selection also will help to decrease costs associated with this therapy. In the future, implanted pumps may become as inconspicuous as implanted defibrillators and pacemakers and as cost-effective.

REFERENCES

1. American Heart Association, Heart Disease and Stroke Statistics—2007 Update. Accessed February 2, 2007 at http://circ.ahajournals.org/cgi/content/full/CIRCULATIONAHA.106.179918
2. Funk D: Epidemiology of end-stage heart disease. In Hogness JR, Van Antwerp M, editors: *The artificial heart: prototypes, policies, and patients,* Washington, DC, 1991, National Academy Press.
3. Schocken DD, Arrieta MI, Leaverton PE et al: Prevalence and mortality rate of congestive heart failure in the United States, *J Am Coll Cardiol* 20:301-306, 1992.
4. Taylor DO, Edwards LB, Boucek MM et al: Registry of the International Society for Heart and Lung Transplantation: twenty-third official adult heart transplant report—2006, *J Heart Lung Transplant* 25:869-879, 2006.
5. Kauffman HM, McBride MA, Schield CF et al: Determinants of waiting time for heart transplants in the United States, *J Heart Lung Transplant* 18:414-419, 1999.
6. Jessup M: Mechanical cardiac-support devices: dreams and devilish details, *N Engl J Med* 345:1490-1493, 2001.
7. Oz MC, Argenziano M, Catanese KA et al: Bridge experience with long-term implantable left ventricular assist devices, *Circulation* 95:1844-185, 1997.

8. Hall CW, Liotta D, Henly WS et al: Development of artificial intrathoracic circulatory pumps, *Am J Surg* 108:685-692, 1964.

9. Cooley DA, Liotta D, Hallman GL et al: Orthotopic cardiac prosthesis for two-staged cardiac replacement, *Am J Cardiol* 24:723-730, 1969.

10. The artificial heart program: current status and history. In Hogness JR, VanAntewerp M, editors: *The artificial heart: prototypes, policies, and patients,* Washington, DC, 1991, National Academy Press.

11. Frazier OH: Mechanical cardiac assistance: historical perspectives, *Semin Thorac Cardiovasc Surg* 12:207-219, 2000.

12. Helman DN, Rose EA: History of mechanical circulatory support, *Prog Cardiovasc Dis* 43:1-4, 2000.

13. Rose EA, Gelijns AC, Moskowitz AJ et al: Long-term use of a left ventricular device for end-stage heart failure, *N Engl J Med* 345:1435-1443, 2001.

14. Copeland JG, Arabia FA, Tsau PH et al: Total artificial hearts: bridge to transplantation, *Cardiol Clin* 21:101-113, 2003.

15. Samuels LE, Dowling R: Total artificial heart: destination therapy, *Cardiol Clin* 21:115-118, 2003.

16. Frazier OH: Future directions of cardiac assistance, *Semin Thorac Cardiovasc Surg* 12:251-258, 2000.

17. Williams MR, Oz MC: Indications and patient selection for mechanical ventricular assistance, *Ann Thorac Surg* 71:S86-S91, 2001.

18. Oz MC, Rose EA, Levin HR: Selection criteria for placement of left ventricular assist devices, *Am Heart J* 129(1):173-176, 1995.

19. Mielniczuk L, Mussivand T, Davies R et al: Patient selection for left ventricular assist devices, *Artif Organs* 28(2):152-157, 2004.

20. Scherr K, Jensen LJ, Koshal A: Mechanical circulatory support as a bridge to cardiac transplantation: toward the 21st century, *Am J Crit Care* 8:324-337, 1999.

21. Kukuy EL, Oz MC, Haka Y: Long-term mechanical circulatory support. In Cohen LH, Edmunds LH Jr, editors: *Cardiac surgery in the adult,* New York, 2003, McGraw-Hill.

22. Young JB: Healing the heart with ventricular assist device therapy: mechanisms of cardiac recovery, *Ann Thorac Surg* 71:S210-S219, 2001.

23. World Heart Corporation: *Novacor LVAS physicians' manual,* Oakland, Calif, 2004, World Heart Corporation.

24. Strauch JT, Spielvogel D, Haldenwang PL et al: Recent improvements in outcome with the Novacor left ventricular assist device, *J Heart Lung Transplant* 22:674-680, 2003.

25. Frazier OH, Rose ER, Oz MC et al: Multicenter clinical evaluation of the HeartMate vented electric left ventricular assist system in patients awaiting heart transplantation, *J Thorac Cardiovasc Surg* 122:1186-1195, 2001.

26. Korfer R, El-Banayosy AM, Arnsoglu L et al: Single-center experience with the Thoratec ventricular assist device, *J Thorac Cardiovasc Surg* 119:596-602, 2000.

27. Farrer DJ: The Thoratec ventricular assist device: a paracorpeal pump for treating acute and chronic heart failure, *Semin Thorac Cardiovasc Surg* 12:243, 2000 (Medline).

28. Thoratec Corporation: *Thoratec VAD/IVAD system clinical operation and patient management,* Pleasanton, Calif, 2004, Thoratec Corporation.

29. Shinn JA: Implantable left ventricular assist devices, *J Cardiovasc Nursing* 20(5 suppl):S22-S30, 2005.

30. Frazier OH, Meyers TJ, Gregoric ID et al: Initial clinical experience with the Jarvik 2000 implantable axial-flow left ventricular assist system, *Circulation* 105:2855-2860, 2002.

31. Westaby S, Banning AP, Saito S et al: Circulatory support for long-term treatment of heart failure: experience with an intraventricular continuous flow pump, *Circulation* 105:2558, 2002.

32. Noon GP, Morley DL, Irwin S et al: Clinical experience with the MicroMed DeBakey ventricular assist, *Ann Thorac Surg* 71:S133-S138, 2001.

33. Copeland JG: Mechanical assist; my choice: the CardioWest total artificial heart, *Transplant Proc* 32:1523, 2000 (Medline).

34. Dowling RD, Etoch SW, Stevens KA et al: Current status of the AbioCor implantable replacement heart, *Ann Thorac Surg* 71:S147, 2001.

35. Deng MC, Edwards LB, Hertz MI et al: Mechanical circulatory support device database of the International Society for Heart and Lung Transplantation: second annual report—2004, *J Heart Lung Transplant* 23:1027-1034, 2004.

36. Miller LW: Patient selection for the use of ventricular assist devices as a bridge to transplantation, *Ann Thorac Surg* 75:S66-S71, 2003.

37. Minami K, El-Banayosy A, Sezai A et al: Morbidity and outcome after mechanical ventricular support using Thoratec, Novacor and HeartMate for bridging to heart transplantation, *Artif Organs* 24:421-426, 2000.

38. Rao V, Oz MC, Flannery MA et al: Revised screening scale to predict survival after insertion of a left ventricular assist device, *J Thorac Cardiovasc Surg* 125:855-862, 2003.

39. Holman WL, Rayburn BK, McGiffin DC et al: Infection in ventricular assist devices: prevention and treatment, *Ann Thorac Surg* 75:S48-S57, 2003.

40. Deng MC, Loebe M, El-Banayosy A et al: Mechanical circulatory support for advanced heart failure: effect of patient selection on outcome, *Circulation* 103:231-237, 2001.

41. Anker SD, Ponikowski P, Varney S et al: Wasting as an independent risk factor for mortality in chronic heart failure, *Lancet* 349:1050-1053, 1997.

42. Mullen JL: Consequences of malnutrition in the surgical patient, *Surg Clin North Am* 61:465, 1981.

43. Otaki M: Surgical treatment of patients with cardiac cachexia: an analysis of factors affecting operative mortality, *Chest* 105:1347-1351, 1994.

44. Rich MW, Keller AJ, Schechtman KB et al: Increased complications and prolonged hospital stay in elderly cardiac surgical patients with low serum albumin, *Am J Cardiol* 63:714-718, 1989.

45. Rady MY, Ryan T, Starr NJ: Clinical characteristics of preoperative hypoalbuminemia predict outcome of cardiovascular surgery, *JPEN J Parenter Enteral Nutr* 21:81-90, 1997.

46. El-Amir NG, Gardocki M, Levin HR et al: Gastrointestinal consequences of left ventricular assist device placement, *ASAIO J* 42(3):150-153, 1996.

47. Grady K, Meyer P, Mattea A et al: Improvement in quality of life outcomes 2 weeks after left ventricular assist device implantation, *J Heart Lung Transplant* 20:657-669, 2001.

48. Reedy JE, Swartz MT, Lohmann DP et al: The importance of patient mobility with ventricular assist device support, *ASAIO J* 38:M151-M153, 1992.

49. Morrone TM, Buck LA, Catanese KA: Early progressive mobilization of patients with left ventricular assist devices is safe and optimizes recovery before heart transplantation, *J Heart Lung Transplant* 15:423-429, 1996.

50. Buck LA: Physical therapy management of three patients following left ventricular assist device implantation: a case report, *Cardiopulmonary Physical Therapy* 9:8-14, 1998.

51. Jaski BE, Lingle RJ, Kim J et al: Comparison of functional capacity in patients with end-stage heart failure following implantation of a left ventricular assist device versus heart transplantation: results of the experience with left ventricular assist device with exercise trial, *J Heart Lung Transplant* 18:1031-1040, 1999.

52. Mancini D, Goldsmith R, Levin H et al: Comparison of exercise performance in patients with chronic severe heart failure versus left ventricular assist devices, *Circulation* 98:1178-1183, 1998.

53. De Jonge N, Kirkels H, Lahpor JR et al: Exercise performance in patients with end-stage heart failure after implantation of a left ventricular assist device and after heart transplantation, *J Am Coll Cardiol* 37:1794-1799, 2001.

54. Kormos RL, Murali S, Dew MA et al: Chronic mechanical circulatory support: rehabilitation, low morbidity, and superior survival, *Ann Thorac Surg* 57:51-58, 1994.

55. Swartz MT, Ruzevich SA, Reedy JE et al: Team approach to circulatory support, *Crit Care Nurs Clin North Am* 1:479-484, 1989.

56. Capretta CJ, Winowich S, Pristas JM: et al: Nursing management and rehabilitation of chronic ventricular assist device (VAD) patients, *Prog Cardiovasc Nurs* 7(4):16-20, 1992.

57. Pristas JM, Winowich S, Nastala CJ et al: Protocol for releasing Novacor left ventricular assist system patients out-of-hospital, *ASAIO J* 41:M539-M543, 1995.

58. Chillcott SR, Atkins PJ, Adamson RM: Left ventricular assist as a viable alternative for cardiac transplantation, *Crit Care Nurs Q* 20(4):64-79, 1998.

59. McCafferty M, Sorbellini D, Cianci P: Telemetry to home: successful discharge of patients with left ventricular assist devices, *Crit Care Nurse* 22(3):43-51, 2002.

60. Maroney DA, Powers K: Outpatient use of left ventricular assist devices: nursing, technical, and educational considerations, *Am J Crit Care* 6:355-362, 1997.

61. Thoratec Corporation: *HeartMate LVAS community living manual,* Pleasanton, Calif, 2003, Thoratec Corporation.

62. Richenbacher WE, Seemuth SC: Hospital discharge for the ventricular assist device patient: historical perspective and description of a successful program, *ASAIO J* 47:590-595, 2001.

63. Vigano M, Scuri S, Corbelli F: Staged discharge out of hospital of the Novacor left ventricular assist system (LVAS) recipients, *Eur J Cardiothorac Surg* 11(suppl):S45-S50, 1997.

64. Seemuth S, Richenbacher W: Education of the ventricular assist device patient's community services, *ASAIO J* 47:596-601, 2001.

65. Morales D, Argenziano M, Oz M: Outpatient left ventricular assist device support: a safe and economical therapeutic option for heart failure, *Prog Cardiovasc Dis* 43(1):55-66, 2000.

66. Holman W, Ormaza S, Seemuth K et al: How to run an outpatient VAD program: overview, *ASAIO J* 47:588-589, 2001.

67. Fey O, El-Banayosy A, Arosuglu L et al: Out-of-hospital experience in patients with implantable mechanical circulatory support: present and future trends, *Eur J Cardiothorac Surg* 11(suppl):s51-s53, 1997.

68. Holmes E: Outpatient management of long-term assist devices, *Cardiol Clin* 21:93-99, 2003.

69. Ashton RC, Goldstein DJ, Rose EA et al: Duration of left ventricular assist device support affects transplant survival, *J Heart Lung Transplant* 15:1151-1157, 1996.

70. Kasirajan V, McCarthy PM, Hoercher KJ et al: Clinical experience with long-term use of implantable left ventricular assist devices: indications, implantation, and outcomes, *Semin Thorac Cardiovasc Surg* 12:229-237, 2000.

71. EL-Banayosy A, Deng M, Loisance DY et al: The European experience of Novacor left ventricular assist (LVAS) therapy as a bridge to transplant: a retrospective multi-centre study, *Eur J Cardiothorac Surg* 15:835-841, 1999.

72. Koul B, Solem JO, Steen S et al: HeartMate left ventricular assist device as bridge to heart transplantation, *Ann Thorac Surg* 65:1625-1630, 1998.

73. Oz MC, Argenziano M, Catanese KA et al: Bridge experience with long-term implantable left ventricular assist devices, *Circulation* 95:1844-1852, 1997.

74. Griffith BP, Kormos RL, Nastala CJ et al: Results of extended bridge to transplantation: window into the future of permanent ventricular assist devices, *Ann Thorac Surg* 61:396-398, 1996.

75. Argenziano M, Catanese KA, Moazami N et al: The influence of infection on survival and successful transplantation in patients with left ventricular assist devices, *J Heart Lung Transplant* 16:822-831, 1997.

76. Damme L, Heatley J, Radovancevic B: Clinical results with the HeartMate LVAD: Worldwide Registry update, *Journal of Congestive Heart Failure and Circulatory Support* 2:5-7, 2001.

77. Dagenais F, Portner PM, Robbins RC et al: The Novacor left ventricular assist system: clinical experience from the Novacor registry, *J Card Surg* 16:267-271, 2001.

78. Frazier OH, Rose EA, Oz MC: Multicenter clinical evaluation of the HeartMate vented electric left ventricular assist system in patients awaiting heart transplantation, *J Thorac Cardiovasc Surg* 122:1186-1195, 2001.

79. El-Banayosy A, Arusoglu L, Kizner L et al: Predictors of survival in patients bridged to transplantation with the Thoratec VAD device: a single-center retrospective study on more than 100 patients, *J Heart Lung Transplant* 19:964-968, 2000.

80. Hetzer R, Muller JH, Weng Y et al: Midterm follow-up of patients who underwent removal of a left ventricular assist device after cardiac recovery from end-stage dilated cardiomyopathy, *J Thorac Cardiovasc Surg* 120:843-855, 2000.

81. Copeland JG, Smith RG, Arabia FA et al: Cardiac replacement with a total artificial heart as a bridge to transplantation, *N Engl J Med* 351:859, 2004.

82. Samuels LE, Dowling R: Total artificial heart: destination therapy, *Cardiol Clin* 21:115-118, 2003.

83. Ruzevich SA, Swartz MT, Reedy JE et al: Retrospective analysis of the psychologic effects of mechanical circulatory support, *J Heart Transplant* 9:209-212, 1990.

84. Abou-Awdi NL, Frazier OH: Quality of life of patients on LVAD support. In *Quality of life after heart surgery,* Netherlands, 1992, Kluwer Academic.

85. Grady KL, Meyer PM, Dressler D et al: Longitudinal change in quality of life and impact on survival after left ventricular assist device implantation, *Ann Thorac Surg* 77:1321-1327, 2004.

86. Grady KL, Meyer PM, Mattea A et al: Change in quality of life from before to after discharge following left ventricular assist device implantation, *J Heart Lung Transplant* 22:322-333, 2003.

87. Grady KL, Meyer P, Mattea A et al: Improvement in quality of life outcomes 2 weeks after left ventricular assist device implantation, *J Heart Lung Transplant* 20:657-669, 2001.

88. Grady KL, Meyer P, Mattea A et al: Predictors of quality of life at 1 month after implantation of a left ventricular assist device, *Am J Crit Care* 11:345-352, 2002.

89. Dew MA, Kormos RL, Winowich S et al: Quality of life outcomes in left ventricular assist system inpatients and outpatients, *ASAIO J* 45:218-225, 1999.

90. Dew MA, Kormos RL, Winowich S et al: Human factors issues in ventricular assist device recipients and their family care givers, *ASAIO J* 46:367-373, 2000.

91. Mancini D, Golsmith R, Levin H et al: Comparison of exercise performance in patients with chronic heart failure versus left ventricular assist devices, *Circulation* 98:1178-1183, 1998.

92. Kormos R, Murali S, Dew MA et al: Chronic mechanical circulatory support: rehabilitation, low morbidity, and superior survival, *Ann Thorac Surg* 57:51-58, 1994.

93. Moskowitz AJ, Weinberg AD, Oz MC et al: Quality of life with an implanted left ventricular assist device, *Ann Thorac Surg* 64:1764-1769, 1997.

94. Grady KL, Dracup K, Kennedy G et al: Team management of patients with heart failure: a statement of healthcare professionals from the Cardiovascular Nursing Council of the American Heart Association, *Circulation* 102:2443-2456, 2000.

95. DiGiorgio PL, Reel MS, Thornton B et al: Heart transplant and left ventricular assist device costs, *J Heart Lung Transplant* 24:200-204, 2005.

96. Gelijns AC, Richards AF, Williams DL et al: Evolving costs of long-term left ventricular assist device implantation, *Ann Thorac Surg* 64:1312-1319, 1997.

97. McGregor M: Implantable ventricular assist device: is it time to introduce them in Canada? *Can J Cardiol* 16:629-640, 2000.

98. Evans RW: Costs and insurance coverage associated with permanent mechanical cardiac assist/replacement devices in the United States, *J Card Surg* 16:280-293, 2001.

chapter 67

Care of Patients Undergoing Cardiac Transplantation

Connie White-Williams
Kathleen L. Grady

CHAPTER ABBREVIATIONS

ALS antilymphocyte serum

ALG antilymphoblast serum

ATG antithymocyte globulin

CABG coronary artery bypass graft

CMV cytomegalovirus

DEXA dual-energy x-ray absorptiometry

DRWR donor/recipient weight ratio

FDA Food and Drug Administration

HLA human leukocyte antigen

HMG-CoA 3-hydroxy-3-methylglutaryl-CoA

IL interleukin

ISHLT International Society for Heart and Lung Transplantation

IVUS intravascular ultrasound

LVAD left ventricular assist device

NYHA New York Heart Association

OPTN Organ Procurement and Transplant Network

OBRA Omnibus Reconciliation Act

PCI percutaneous coronary intervention

PET positron emission tomography

PRA panel reactive antibody

PVR pulmonary vascular resistance

TOR target of rapamycin

TPG transpulmonary gradient

UAGA Uniform Anatomical Gift Act

UNOS United Network for Organ Sharing

VO$_2$ oxygen consumption

HISTORY OF CARDIAC TRANSPLANTATION
Development of Clinical Cardiac Transplantation

The first clinical cardiac transplantation was performed in 1964 in Jackson, Mississippi when a chimpanzee heart was transplanted into a 68-year-old man with shock.[1-3] The patient died 1 hour after surgery related to the size discrepancy between the recipient and donor; the donor heart was unable to maintain the circulatory load. In December, 1967, the first successful human heart transplant was performed by Dr. Christian Barnard in Capetown, South Africa.[4] This patient survived 18 days before subsequently succumbing to pneumonia. During the next 12 months, many cardiac surgical teams all over the world performed heart transplant operations. Most of these patients died early after the operation, and, by the end of the 1960s, only a handful of institutions persevered in their clinical efforts at heart transplantation.[1,2]

The Stanford team made many contributions to the early success of cardiac transplantation during the 1970s, including the development of the right ventricular endomyocardial bioptome to sample myocardial tissue for the surveillance of allograft rejection, a grading system for rejection detected on endomyocardial biopsy samples, use of immunosuppression for the treatment of rejection and long-term use, improved donor management and development of techniques that allowed for distant procurement, and refinement of recipient selection criteria.[1] One-year patient survival rose from 20 percent in 1969 to 60 percent to 70 percent by 1980.[1]

The discovery of the immunosuppressive properties of the fungal derivative, cyclosporin A (cyclosporine), at Sandoz Laboratories propelled solid organ transplantation into the modern era. Cyclosporine was first used in humans following renal transplantation and resulted in a 1-year graft survival rate of 86 percent. Clinical trials with cyclosporine in heart transplant recipients were begun in 1980 at Stanford. The achievement of 1-year survival rates of 80 percent[1] with this therapy contributed to the expansion of heart transplantation worldwide. While only 90 heart transplants were performed in 1981, 2437 were performed by the end of the decade at 236 centers worldwide.[5] See Box 67-1 for historical events in cardiac transplantation.

Although "double therapy" with cyclosporine and prednisone was initially used as maintenance immunosuppression, azathioprine (initially abandoned after the introduction of cyclosporine) was reintroduced in order to reduce the doses and thus minimize toxicity of each immunosuppressive agent. The widespread use of "triple therapy" (cyclosporine, prednisone, and azathioprine) continues today. Data regarding the efficacy of mycophenolate mofetil is producing a transition to triple therapy, consisting of cyclosporine, prednisone, and mycophenolate mofetil.[6]

Further advances in immunosuppression in the late 1980s and refinements in the 1990s have included (1) the development and use of monoclonal antibodies, specifically OKT3; (2) discontinuation of long-term corticosteroid use; and (3) total lymphoid irradiation and the use of methotrexate to manage rejection refractory to augmentation of conventional immunosuppression.[7,8] With these advances, recipient selection criteria have expanded. The upper age limit has increased to equal to or more than 65 years in selected patients, and the lower age limit has decreased to include newborns. Patients with comorbidities, such as insulin dependent diabetes,[9,10] prior cancer without evidence of recur-

---

BOX 67-1   ■ ■ ■
LANDMARK EVENTS IN THE EVOLUTION
OF CARDIAC TRANSPLANTATION

1905	Carrel and Guthrie transplant hearts and other organs into dogs
1908	Metchnikoff relates inflammation to immunity
1912	Stone sets forth the concepts of transplantation immunology
1933	Mann and Priestly suggest that biological events (ultimately understood as allograft rejection) limit canine cardiac heterotopic transplant experimentation
1940-1950s	Demikhov experiments with heart and heart-lung transplant models in Russia
1944	Medawar suggests that allograft rejection is an immunological process
1945	Owen reports that cell chimeras in cattle display tolerance
1951	Marcus, Wong, and Luisada speculate on therapeutic potential of heart transplantation
1953	Downie reproducibility demonstrates canine heterotopic heart transplant success
1957	Webb uses hypothermic cardiac preservation for heart transplant experiments
1958	Goldberg, Berman, and Akman perform first orthotopic canine heart transplant using cardiopulmonary bypass support
1959	Cass and Brock refine experimental orthotopic surgical techniques
1960s	Lower and Shumway report rejection to be the main challenge in canine heart transplant and suggest that long-term survival could be achieved with immunosuppression
1962	Reemstma reports prolonged survival after canine orthotopic heart transplant
1964	Hardy performs first human xenograft (chimpanzee) heart transplant
1965	Kondo and Kantrowitz suggest newborn puppies are immunologically privileged
1967	Barnard performs the first human-to-human heart transplant
1968-1971	100 to 200 heart transplants performed worldwide with limited success; moratorium established
1974	Caves develops technique of graft surveillance with endomyocardial biopsy
1980	Cyclosporine is introduced into clinical transplant arena with center proliferation

---

rence,[11,12] and peripheral vascular disease are also being successfully transplanted.

Development of Organ Allocation

The development of ethical and moral criteria for organ donation is paramount to the evolution of transplantation. During the past 30 years, legislation has been enacted to support transplantation and strengthen organ procurement activities. In 1968, the Uniform Anatomical Gift Act **(UAGA)** became law in all 50 states. The UAGA provides a legal and binding means for an individual to document his/her intent to donate organs before death. The purpose of this law is to increase the donor supply. However, this law has not seriously impacted the donor pool, and the wishes of families who openly object to organ donation, even in the presence of a previously signed document indicating intent to donate, are respected. The National Organ Transplant

Act was signed in 1984, and a task force was established to examine issues related to organ recovery and transplantation.[13-15] Recommendations to Congress included adoption of policies regarding the determination of brain death and required request by hospitals (to facilitate identification of donors) and establishment of the Organ Procurement and Transplant Network **(OPTN)** to expand organ matching and allocation.[16] In 1986, the Omnibus Reconciliation Act **(OBRA)** became law and required hospitals participating in Medicare and Medicaid programs to become members of the OPTN and abide by its rules.[16] The United Network for Organ Sharing **(UNOS)** was awarded the contract to administer and operate the OPTN. The goals of UNOS are to improve the effectiveness of organ procurement, the system for organ sharing, and the outcomes of transplantation, and to enhance the skills of professionals involved in transplantation.

The diagnosis of brain death (legally and medically) is central to the transplantation of organs. In 1980, the President's Commission Report set forth guidelines for the determination of death. For the diagnosis of brain death, there must be complete loss of cerebral and brainstem function, including lack of spontaneous respiration or response to external stimuli.[16] These conditions must exist in the absence of hypothermia, drug overdose, or other complicating metabolic situations and must be deemed irreversible.[16] Common events resulting in brain death include acute head trauma, anoxic encephalopathy, intracerebral bleed, and primary brain lesion.[16]

RECIPIENT EVALUATION AND SELECTION
Conditions Considered for Cardiac Transplantation

The majority of adult patients who undergo heart transplantation have a primary indication of either coronary artery disease (45 percent) or cardiomyopathy (45 percent).[17] Other less frequent diagnoses include valvular heart disease (3 percent to 4 percent), retransplantation (2 percent), and congenital heart disease (2 percent).[17]

The dilated nonischemic cardiomyopathies are characterized primarily by left or biventricular systolic dysfunction associated with variable degrees of diastolic dysfunction. The etiology of dilated nonischemic cardiomyopathy is unknown in more than 80 percent of cases, hence the term "idiopathic" may include a variety of hereditary or acquired disorders. An etiologic classification of the dilated cardiomyopathies includes the following common causes: (1) idiopathic, (2) inflammatory, (3) toxic, (4) metabolic, and (5) familial.[18]

The dilated cardiomyopathies with an inflammatory cause can be of an infectious or noninfectious etiology. Myocarditis has classically been defined as a process characterized by an inflammatory infiltrate of the myocardium with necrosis and/or degeneration of adjacent myocytes not typical of ischemic damage associated with coronary artery disease.[18] Although every major category of infectious organism (including bacteria, mycobacteria, parasites, rickettsia, fungi, and viruses) has been implicated in the causation of myocarditis, the most common agent in the western world is viruses. In an early study, heart transplantation of patients with active myocarditis met with limited success. O'Connell and associates,[18] in their analysis of the outcomes of 12 (predominately female) patients who were transplanted for active myocarditis, reported a 2.2-fold increase in rejection compared to age-matched control subjects. In addition, 1-year survival in the myocarditis patients was 58 percent versus 82 percent in the age-matched control subjects and 78 percent in age-matched female control subjects (*p* 0.0014) . In a larger study, survival of patients with myocarditis was not significantly different than survival of patients with other forms of dilated cardiomyopathy. It is important to point out that patients with myocarditis can also experience spontaneous remission and, therefore, may not require heart transplantation.[16,22]

The noninfectious etiologies of dilated nonischemic cardiomyopathy for which heart transplantation is a therapeutic option include peripartum cardiomyopathy and transplant rejection.[19-21] Peripartum cardiomyopathy is characterized by the development of heart failure during the last trimester of pregnancy or the first 6 months postpartum in the absence of a prior history or demonstrable cause of heart disease. In a multi-institutional study comparing posttransplant outcomes of peripartum cardiomyopathy patients (*n* = 40) with females of childbearing age transplanted for other indications (*n* = 200), similar rates of survival and rejection were found.[21] Interestingly, significantly greater cumulative rejection and a shorter time to first rejection were also found for parous versus nulliparous females or males.

Toxic causes of dilated nonischemic cardiomyopathy include ethyl alcohol and chemotherapeutic agents. At least 7 percent to 10 percent of patients with dilated nonischemic cardiomyopathy are thought to have an alcoholic etiology. Patients with moderate alcohol-induced cardiomyopathy may improve with abstinence, while patients who are diagnosed early may experience normalization of cardiac function with abstinence. Therefore observation and medical therapy as needed are warranted in select patients since some may improve spontaneously. Transplantation of patients with alcoholic cardiomyopathy who continue to drink is infrequent because of psychosocial issues that do not meet selection criteria. The cardiotoxic effect of the chemotherapeutic agent doxorubicin (Adriamycin) is dose related, and, during its use, tests of cardiac function should be monitored at a frequency depending on potential risk.[16] Doxorubicin cardiotoxicity may be irreversible and, although infrequent, can be an indication for cardiac transplantation. A thorough oncologic evaluation to assess the risk of tumor recurrence is warranted before consideration of heart transplantation.

Familial (hereditary) dilated cardiomyopathy has been reported in 20 percent to 30 percent of patients with dilated nonischemic cardiomyopathy based on the prospective study of asymptomatic as well as symptomatic relatives.[22] Transplantation of patients with familial dilated cardiomyopathy and progressive heart failure is indicated.

Retransplantation has generated much dialogue and controversy in the transplant community. Some trans-plant programs consider retransplantation in light of their commitment to a patient while others will not consider any patients for retransplantation, citing generally poor outcomes and reduced rates of survival. Most programs assess patients individually and retransplant only if the chances of a successful outcome are high. There is evidence that the condition (emergent versus elective) in which retransplantation occurs is the determinant for survival.[23,24] Radovancevic and associates[24] found that those retransplanted for early graft failure and acute rejection in an emergent situation usually had poor outcomes. Those retransplanted for coronary artery disease in an elective situation had significantly better survival.[24] Given the costs associated with retransplantation (which exceed the costs of primary transplant[25]) and the reduced rates of survival, retransplantation may best be considered only for patients with the highest likelihood of a good outcome.

Indications for Cardiac Transplantation

Cardiac transplantation is reserved for patients with advanced heart failure who are mostly likely to benefit in life expectancy and overall improvement in quality of life. Patients selected for transplant should have a predicted 2-year survival of 60 percent and/or severe limitations in quality of life not amenable to other medical or surgical therapy.[22] Patients are generally less than age 65, New York Heart Association (**NYHA**) Class III or IV, and do not have comorbid conditions that may limit life expectancy after transplant. (Box 67-2)

BOX 67-2
GENERAL INDICATION FOR CARDIAC TRANSPLANTATION

Criteria for Considerations of Heart Transplantation in Advanced Heart Failure
- Significant functional limitation (NYHA Class III-IV heart failure) despite maximum medical therapy, which includes digitalis, diuretics, and vasodilators (preferably angiotensin-converting enzyme inhibitors) at maximum tolerated doses
- Refractory angina or refractory life-threatening dysrhythmia
- Exclusion of all surgical alternatives to transplantation, such as the following:
  1. Revascularization for significant reversible ischemia
  2. Valve replacement for severe aortic valve disease
  3. Valve replacement or repair for severe mitral regurgitation
  4. Appropriate ventricular remodeling procedures

Indication for Cardiac Transplantation Determined by Severity of Heart Failure Despite Optimal Therapy
- Definite indications
  1. VO_{2max} less than 10 ml/kg/min
  2. HYHA Class IV
  3. History of recurrent hospitalization for congestive heart failure
  4. Refractory ischemia with inoperable coronary artery disease
  5. Recurrent symptomatic ventricular dysrhythmias
- Probable indications
  1. VO_{2max} less than 14 mg/kg/min
  2. NYHA Class III-IV
  3. Recent hospitalizations for congestive heart failure
  4. Unstable angina not amenable to coronary artery bypass grafting, percutaneous transluminal coronary angioplasty with left ventricular ejection fraction less than 0.25

From NYHA, New York Heart Association.

Contraindications for Cardiac Transplantation

Contraindications for cardiac transplantation are based on the evaluation of the severity and number of comorbid conditions that may affect life expectancy after transplantation. Potential contraindications, both absolute and relative, are identified during the evaluation process. See Box 67-3 for contraindications for cardiac transplantation. Many contraindications previously felt to be absolute have become more relative over the last several years, resulting in a growing United States waiting list.

Age

Although not a contraindication to cardiac transplant per se, there is no agreement on upper age limits for cardiac transplantation, and, in fact, age limits have been liberalized considerably over the last decade. Studies suggest that successful outcomes can be achieved in transplantation of selected candidates over 55 years.[26,27] Older transplant recipients have been found to have similar or fewer episodes of rejection and infection, similar survival rates, and acceptable rehabilitation as compared to younger recipients.[26-29] However, the incidence of steroid-related complications, including diabetes and osteoporosis, was significantly higher in older recipients.[26] Luciani and colleagues[28] compared recipients over 55 years who received donor hearts older than 40 years ($n = 18$) versus those who received donor hearts younger than 40 years ($n = 37$) and found no differences in survival at 1 year (88 percent versus 84 percent) and 4 years (81 percent versus 80 percent), respectively. Heroux and colleagues[29] caution that in patients older than 65 years, functional limitations are more severe than in younger patients, and comorbidities should be carefully evaluated when considering transplantation. Transplantation of older recipients, therefore, appears to be more of an ethical than medical issue because expansion of the upper age limit places a greater burden on a limited donor pool. In fact, Laks and colleagues[30] have created an "alternate recipient list" for patients who would otherwise be turned down for heart transplantation, including patients over 65 years. When compared with standard waiting list patients, no differences in survival at 1-year posttransplant were found.

Pulmonary Vascular Resistance

Pulmonary vascular hypertension was identified as an operative risk early in the heart transplant experience.[22,31] Subsequent studies have identified measures of pulmonary hypertension that may be useful in determining operative risk. Bussieres and associates[31] found that patients with an increased pulmonary vascular resistance (**PVR**) (more than 2.5 Wood units) had higher early mortality after transplant. However, a subsequent study demonstrated that patients whose baseline PVR could be reduced to less than 2.5 Wood units with sodium nitroprusside without systemic hypotension had a lower posttransplant mortality than patients whose PVR could not be reduced without hypotension.[32] Butler and associates[33] found that even with pretransplant reversible pulmonary hypertension, an increased risk of posttransplant mortality exists. An elevated transpulmonary gradient (**TPG**) (mean pulmonary artery pressure-pulmonary capillary wedge pressure) of more than 12 to 15 mm Hg was also identified as predictive of mortality within 1 year after transplant.[34] Current contraindications to heart transplantation include a PVR of more than 4 to 6 Wood units and/or a transpulmonary gradient greater than or equal to 15 mm Hg.[22] Pulmonary hypertension associated with chronic congestive heart failure may be reversible or irreversible, depending on the severity and duration of heart failure. If baseline pulmonary pressures are elevated, vasodilator therapy (nitroprusside and prostaglandin E_1) is given in an attempt to reduce pressures. Chronic vasodilator or inotropic therapy may be required in patients who do not respond to initial attempts to reduce pulmonary pressures.

BOX 67-3 ■ ■ ■
CONTRAINDICATIONS TO CARDIAC TRANSPLANTATION

General Contraindications
Presence of any noncardiac condition that would itself shorten life expectancy or increase the risk of death from rejection or complications of immunosuppression

Specific Contraindications*
Older age (more than about 65 years) (program variability)
Active infection
Active peptic ulcer disease
Severe diabetes mellitus with end-organ damage
Severe peripheral vascular or cerebrovascular disease
Coexisting active neoplasm
Morbid obesity (more than 140% predicted ideal body weight)
Creatinine clearance less than 40-50 ml/min, ERPF less than 200 ml/min†
Bilirubin greater than 2.5 mg/dl (when not due to reversible hepatic congestion), transaminases greater than 2 × normal‡
Severe pulmonary dysfunction with forced vital capacity (FVC) and forced expired volume in 1 second (FEV1), less than about 40% of predicted, especially with intrinsic lung disease
Pulmonary artery systolic pressure greater than 60 mm Hg, mean transpulmonary gradient greater than 15 mm Hg, and/or pulmonary vascular resistance greater than 5 Wood units§
Acute pulmonary thromboembolism
Active diverticulitis
History of smoking within last 6 months
High risk of life-threatening noncompliance
Inability to make strong commitment to transplantation
Cognitive impairment severe enough to limit comprehension of medical regimen
Psychiatric instability severe enough to jeopardize incentive for adherence to medical regimen
History of recurring alcohol or drug abuse
Failure of established stable address or telephone number
Previous demonstration of repeated noncompliance with medication or follow-up
Lack of independent family or social support system
History of marked depression or emotional instability

ERPE, effective renal plasma flow.
*May be relative or absolute, depending on severity or program philosophy.
†May be suitable for cardiac transplantation if inotropic support and hemodynamic management produce a creatinine less than 2 mg/dl and creatinine clearance greater than 50 ml/min. Transplantation may also be advisable as combined heart-kidney transplant.
‡Requires liver biopsy to exclude cirrhosis or other intrinsic liver disease.
§These apply only if the increased resistance is largely nonreactive (fixed).

Renal Dysfunction

Renal dysfunction has been shown in many studies to be a risk factor for mortality after cardiac transplantation.[22] A serum creatinine of 2 mg/dl or greater, a 24-hour creatinine clearance of less than 50 ml/min, a glomerular filtration rate less than 50 ml/min, and a effective renal plasma flow less than 200 ml/min are indicators of poor prognosis after transplant. One challenge is determining if renal dysfunction is due to advanced heart failure (low cardiac output) or intrinsic renal disease. Due to use of long-term nephrotoxic medications after transplantation, a combined heart/kidney transplant may be indicated in select patients.

Diabetes

Diabetes has been shown to increase morbidity and mortality in heart transplant patients. One study has shown diabetic patients ($n = 37$) who have undergone transplantation have had similar rates of rejection, infection, and survival without an increased risk of renal dysfunction or allograft arteriopathy as compared to nondiabetic patients ($n = 305$).[9] However, Radovancervic and colleagues[35] reported that absence of pretransplant diabetes predicts better long-term survival posttransplant. Most programs carefully evaluate diabetes during the transplant evaluation and exclude diabetic patients with end-organ damage (neuropathy, retinopathy, and nephropathy). Hence the presence of insulin-dependent diabetes without end organ damage is no longer considered a contraindication to heart transplantation.[36]

Malignancy

A history of prior malignancy has been shown to increase the risk of subsequent malignancy after transplantation. Two studies with small sample sizes have demonstrated preliminary success in the transplantation of patients with a history of malignant disease.[12,37] Armitage and colleagues[12] reported 100 percent survival (with a follow-up of 4 to 41 months, mean = 18 months) in 11 patients with a history of malignant disease. Goldstein and associates[37] retrospectively reviewed eight cases with primary cardiac neoplasms and reported long-term survival (14 to 78 months) after transplantation in patients ($n = 6$) with tumor-free surgical margins. The two patients with neoplastic disease at the surgical margins after cardiectomy died of metastases within 2 years of transplant. All patients should be screened thoroughly for malignancies and be malignancy-free for 5 years before transplantation should be considered.

Psychosocial Factors

A discussion of contraindications to heart transplantation often includes psychosocial issues. Psychosocial issues that might affect heart transplant outcome must be examined but are among the most difficult to quantify. Some researchers suggest that pretransplant psychological distress, anxiety, and depression do not predict posttransplant outcome.[38,39] Bunzel and Wollenek[39] found social support from one partner to be the most predictive of excellent postoperative outcomes, indicating the importance of psychosocial issues. Psychiatric diagnoses, including alcohol and/or drug abuse, antisocial personality, chronic paranoid psychosis, major depression, and borderline or low intellectual functioning, are commonly considered contraindications to transplant.[40] In a study of 17 patients with a preoperative psychiatric diagnosis (adjustment disorder, alcohol abuse, compulsive personality disorder, dementia, life circumstance problems, and antisocial personality disorder), posttransplant follow-up revealed difficulty with adjustment, conflicts with the hospital staff, and noncompliance.[40] These psychiatric problems and noncompliance can lead to increased hospital readmissions and cost of medical care.[41] Psychosocial problems in transplant candidates continue to require better definition, measurement, and management. Many centers consult social workers, psychiatrists, psychologists, or neuropsychologists to evaluate patients preoperatively.

Amyloidosis

Although studies of transplantation in patients with systemic disease processes are encouraging, they must be regarded cautiously. The need to be careful when expanding the inclusion criteria for transplantation has been aptly demonstrated for amyloidosis. Although Hosenpud and associates[42] first reported intermediate success (5/7 patients alive and rehabilitated) in the transplantation of patients with cardiac amyloidosis, a follow-up study ($n = 10$) revealed a survival of only 39 percent 4 years posttransplant with the majority of deaths due to progression of amyloidosis.[43] Clearly, expanding transplant selection criteria is performed with some risk and must be undertaken with rigorous reporting of results and awareness of the limited donor supply.

Amiodarone

Fatal pulmonary deaths have been reported in patients with the use of acute and chronic amiodarone therapy prior to cardiac transplantation. Pulmonary fibrosis, hypoxia, and pulmonary edema associated with amiodarone therapy have resulted in pulmonary dysfunction.[44] Patients on amiodarone should be monitored frequently while waiting with pulmonary function tests, right heart catheterization to ensure low artrial pressures, and serial chest radiographs.[22] It is important that patients awaiting transplant be placed on the lowest possible dose (200 to 400 mg/day), and, at the time of transplant, it should be communicated to operating room personnel to use 50 percent or less oxygen to prevent production of oxygen free radicals.

Hepatitis C

The natural history of hepatitis C in cardiac transplantation is relatively unknown. However, it does appear that recipients who are hepatitis C–positive generally have a benign course. Lake and associates[45] reported no difference in survival between hepatitis C–positive recipients and a control group. However, there was a 50 percent incidence of liver dysfunction and more liver-related deaths in the hepatitis C–positive patients.

Other contraindications include severe primary pulmonary or hepatic disease, profound neurological or neuromuscular disorders, and acquired immunodeficiency syndrome.

Certain coexistent conditions must be resolved prior to transplantation. These include active peptic ulcer disease, active diverticulitis, infection, and recent pulmonary embolization.[22] Nutritional status also requires assessment and possible intervention prior to heart transplantation. Severe cachexia may delay wound healing and contribute to increased postoperative infection while pretransplant obesity may be a risk factor for posttransplant mortality.[46]

Referral and Evaluation of Potential Candidates

Patients with advanced, persistently symptomatic heart failure despite optimal medical therapy may be referred for heart transplantation. Referral can be initiated by a primary cardiologist, internist, family practitioner, the patient, or a family member. Referral is usually made to the nearest heart transplant center but can also be influenced by the patient's medical insurance. Insurance companies have contracts with individual transplant centers that are considered "centers of excellence" and refer their clients to centers that fulfill the company's standards. Referred patients undergo extensive cardiac and noncardiac testing as inpatients or outpatients, depending on their medical condition, to determine the need and suitability for transplant. These tests are listed in Box 67-4. Whether a patient is listed for transplant depends on three major factors: (1) the severity of a patient's heart disease, (2) absence of absolute contraindications to transplantation, and (3) exclusion of other surgical therapeutic options. Standard recipient selection criteria for heart transplantation, which broadly encompass severity of illness and contraindications, are listed in Boxes 67-2 and 67-3.

Severity of heart disease should be assessed when a patient is receiving optimal medical therapy. Traditional measures of severity of heart failure include NYHA classification, hemodynamics, echocardiographic findings (ejection fraction), duration of treadmill exercise testing, and symptoms. Patients with end-stage heart failure are NYHA Class III-IV. These patients may have increased pulmonary capillary wedge pressures, a decreased cardiac output and index, and increased systemic vascular resistance.[47] Left ventricular ejection fraction is often 20 percent or less (normal = 40 percent to 65 percent).[48] Echocardiography reveals a dilated, hypokinetic left ventricle and mitral and tricuspid regurgitation. Duration of exercise on a treadmill is often limited by symptoms, ischemia, or ventricular dysrhythmias and is frequently suboptimal. Symptoms of fatigue, shortness of breath, difficulty sleeping, and overall weakness are common.[49]

More objective prognostic indicators of severe ventricular dysfunction have been identified and include oxygen consumption **(VO₂)** at maximal exercise and markers of neurohumoral activation. Although there is as yet no uniform consensus on values of maximal oxygen consumption at which survival is reduced and heart transplantation is recommended, a VO_{2max} of 10 to 14

BOX 67-4   ■ ■ ■
EVALUATION PROTOCOL FOR CARDIAC TRANSPLANTATION

General
Complete history and physical examination
Nutritional status evaluation*
Blood chemistries, including liver and renal profiles (bilirubin, SGOT [AST], alkaline phosphatase, blood urea nitrogen (BUN), creatinine, calcium, phosphorus, magnesium)
Hematology and coagulation profile (complete blood cell count, differential, platelet count, prothrombin time or international normalized ratio, partial thromboplastin time, fibrinogen)
Serum electrolytes
Lipid profile*
Urinalysis
24-hour urine for creatinine clearance (and protein if diabetic or urinalysis positive for protein)*
Nuclear renal scan with measurement of effective renal plasma flow (ERPF)
Pulmonary function testing with arterial blood gases
Ventilation-perfusion scan*
Stool for heme (×3)
Mammography*
Prostate-specific antigen (PSA)*
Abdominal ultrasound study (liver, pancreas, gallbladder, and kidney evaluation)
Carotid ultrasound
Social evaluation
Psychiatric evaluation
Neuropsychiatric evaluation (neurocognitive evaluation)*
Dental evaluation
Sinus films*

Cardiovascular
Electrocardiogram
Chest x-ray (PA and lateral)
Two-dimensional echocardiogram with Doppler study
Exercise test with oxygen consumption (peak oxygen consumption [VO₂])
Right heart catheterization with detailed hemodynamic evaluation
Shunt series*
Left heart catheterization with coronary angiography*
Myocardial biopsy
Radionuclide angiogram (grated blood pool study)*
Nuclear imaging study for myocardial viability (thallium-201 or positron emission tomography)*
Holter monitor for dysrhythmias (if ischemic cardiomyopathy)*

Immunology
ABO blood type and antibody screen
Panel reactive antibody **(PRA)** screen
Human leukocyte antigen **(HLA)** typing (if to be listed for transplantation)

Infectious Disease Screening
Serologies for: Hepatitis A, B, and C; herpes virus human immunodeficiency virus (HIV), cytomegalovirus **(CMV)**, toxoplasmosis, varicella, rubella, Epstein-Barr virus, venereal disease research laboratory (VDRL), Lyme titers,* histoplasmosis, and coccidioidomycosis complement fixing antibodies*
Throat swab for viral cultures (cytomegalovirus, adenovirus herpes simplex virus)*
Urine culture and sensitivity*
Stool for ova and parasites*
Purified protein derivative (PPD) skin test with controls (i.e., mumps, dermatophyton, histoplasmosis, and coccidioidomycosis)*

*Only performed if appropriate or indicated.

ml/kg/min portends a poorer prognosis.[50] Mancini and colleagues[50] compared patients accepted for transplant ($n = 35$) with a VO_{2max} less than or equal to 14 ml/kg/min, patients with a low VO_{2max} who were denied transplant ($n = 27$), and patients who were too stable for transplant ($n = 52$) with a VO_{2max} greater than 14 ml/kg/min. This study found that patients with VO_{2max} greater than 14 could be safely deferred from transplant.

Prior to referring a patient for cardiac transplantation, formulation of a therapeutic plan for ischemic cardiomyopathy patients should include evaluation for evidence of reversible myocardial ischemia (hibernating myocardium), which may involve the use of nuclear cardiology techniques such as positron emission tomography (**PET**) and thallium imaging or 2-D echocardiographic imaging. If significant areas of hibernating myocardium are identified, coronary revascularization should be considered. Given that we live in an era of a limited donor supply, high-risk coronary revascularization must be considered, particularly in patients with large areas of ischemic but viable myocardium.

Listing Patients for Cardiac Transplantation

Once patients have completed their evaluation for heart transplantation, the information is compiled and presented at a team meeting to determine whether or not they will be placed on the waiting list. Cardiologists, cardiothoracic surgeons, nurse coordinators, social workers, psychologists, psychiatrists, and ethicists attend "Patient Selection Committee Meetings." After a decision is made that a patient is a candidate for transplant, this is discussed with the patient, who ultimately decides if he/she wants to be placed on the waiting list for a donor organ.

Candidates for heart transplantation are listed on a national computerized waiting list maintained by UNOS, a private organization contracted by the federal government to allocate organs according to sharing policies. Listing information consists of patient name, age, sex, race, social security number, blood group, acceptable donor weight range, and whether a donor specific crossmatch will be needed at the time of transplant. In addition, the medical severity of the candidate is indicated (Box 67-5) to prioritize patients during the donor-recipient selection process.

Candidates are generally required to remain within a 2-hour drive of the transplant center. However, transplant centers may assist patients and families by making arrangements for air transportation when a donor heart becomes available; thus, allowing patients at a greater distance from the transplant center the opportunity to wait for their donor at home.

Management of Patients Awaiting Cardiac Transplantation

Patients are seen regularly by the transplant cardiologist in conjunction with their referring physician while awaiting surgery. Stable heart failure patients are managed as outpatients while unstable patients may require hospitalization until a donor heart is located. Medical

---

> ### BOX 67-5　■ ■ ■
> ### UNOS STATUS CODES FOR MEDICAL URGENCY
>
> **Status 1A.** Patient listed as Status 1A is admitted to the listing transplant center hospital and has at least one of the following devices or therapies in place:
> (a) Mechanical circulatory support for acute hemodynamic decompensation that includes at least one of the following:
> i. Left and or/right ventricular assist device implanted for 30 days or less
> ii. Total artificial heart
> iii. Intra-aortic balloon pump
> iv. Extracorporeal membrane oxygenator
> (b) Mechanical circulatory support for more than 30 days with objective medical evidence of significant device-related infection, mechanical failure, and/or life-threatening ventricular dysrhythmias
> (c) Mechanical ventilation
> (d) Continuous infusion of a single high-dose intravenous inotrope (e.g., dobutamine greater than or equal to 7.5 mcg/kg/min, or milrinone greater than or equal to 0.50 mcg/kg/min, or multiple intravenous inotropes, in addition to continuous hemodynamic monitoring of left ventricular filling pressures; qualification for Status 1A under this criterion is valid for 7 days with a one-time 7-day renewal for each occurrence for a Status 1A listing for the same patient.
> (e) Patient who does not meet the criteria specified in (a), (b), (c), or (d) may be listed as Status 1A if the patient is admitted to the listed transplant center hospital and has a life expectancy without a heart transplant of less than 7 days. Qualification for Status 1A under this criterion is valid for 7 days and must be recertified by an attending physician every 7 days to continue the Status 1A listing. A patient listed as Status 1A under this criterion shall be reviewed by the applicable UNOS Regional Review Board and the UNOS Thoracic Organ Transplantation Committee.
> **Status 1B.** Patient listed as Status 1B has at least one of the following devices or therapies in place:
> (a) Left and/or right ventricular assist device implanted for more than 30 days or
> (b) Continuous infusion of intravenous inotropes
> **Status 2.** A patient who does not meet the criteria for Status 1A or 1B is listed as Status 2.
> **Status 7.** A patient listed as Status 7 is considered temporarily unsuitable to receive a thoracic organ transplant.
>
> For all adult patients listed as Status 1A, a complete Heart Status 1A Justification Form must be received by the UNOS Organ Center within 24 hours of a patient's listing as Status 1A or continuance as Status 1A in accordance with the criteria in (d) or (e). If a completed Heart Status 1A Justification Form is not received by the UNOS Organ Center within 24 hours of a Status 1A listing, the patient shall be reassigned to his or her previous status.

UNOS, United Network for Organ Sharing.

---

management of the patient with acute and chronic heart failure, including nonpharmacological and pharmacological therapies, is discussed in Chapters 63 and 64.

If patients awaiting transplantation continue to deteriorate despite oral and intravenous infusion therapy, mechanical circulatory assistance must be considered.[51-53] While the intraaortic balloon pump may be the only mode of support available at some transplant centers, others have access to commercially available or investigational ventricular assist devices. The HeartMate pneumatic left ventricular assist device (**LVAD**), HeartMate vented electric LVAD, and the Novacor left ventricular assist system are approved to provide long-term circulatory support of patients as a bridge to transplantation. While limitations of the intraaortic balloon pump include relative immobility, increased risk of infection, and thrombocytopenia, advantages of

LVADs are stabilization of end-organ function, increased mobility, and reduced medical costs because hospitalized patients can be cared for on stepdown or general floor units and discharged to home (to await transplantation) on the "wearable" circulatory support systems. Please see Chapter 66 for a detailed discussion of ventricular assist devices.

As more patients are listed for heart transplantation (more than 3200 annually since August, 2005)[54], the wait for a new heart has become longer. Patients typically wait from 6 months to 1 year, but some can wait as long as 2 to 3 years. Patients who are waiting should be routinely assessed (every 1 to 4 months) for stability of their heart failure. Echocardiogram, right heart catheterization, and exercise testing are recommended every 4 to 6 months while a patient is waiting for a donor heart. In a study of stable patients awaiting cardiac transplant, death before transplant was due primarily to sudden unexpected death.[55] Patients with ischemic cardiomyopathy, lower ejection fraction, and higher right atrial pressure were at highest risk for cardiac death. Patients can also improve while awaiting transplantation. Stevenson and colleagues[56] found that 38/68 ambulatory transplant candidates (with initial peak O_2 uptake less than 14 ml/kg/min), who did not experience early deterioration after listing or undergo transplantation, increased their peak O_2 uptake by more than or equal to 2 ml/kg/min to a level more than or equal to 12 ml/kg/min at an average of 6 months later. Thirty-one of these patients whose clinical status also stabilized were removed from the waiting list.[104] Stevenson and colleagues[56] suggest that selected outpatients should periodically be reevaluated to determine whether transplantation remains indicated.

DONOR SELECTION AND OPERATIVE TECHNIQUES

Donor Selection

When brain death has been established, organ donation should be discussed with the patient's family. This should be done only after the family has been informed of their loved one's death and has had time to assimilate that information. Required request can be initiated by anyone designated by the hospital to act in that capacity, including a physician, nurse, social worker, or chaplain; however, many times consent is obtained by trained procurement coordinators. A private, quiet location away from the bedside provides a comfortable setting for the discussion of organ donation. An overview about the organ donation process is provided and questions are answered honestly and thoroughly. When the family consents to organ donation, the local organ procurement organization is notified by hospital personnel. Donor procurement coordinators (usually nurses) are on-call 24 hours/day to receive phone calls. The coordinator's role involves evaluation of the potential donor and donor management. Careful evaluation of donors involves assessment of demographic data, social history, medical history (including medications, surgeries, and previous illnesses), and current clinical status.[16,57] Cardiac donor criteria are listed in Box 67-6.

BOX 67-6 ■ ■ ■
CARDIAC DONOR CRITERIA

Brain death
Consent
Age generally less than 55
ABO blood type compatibility
Compatible donor-recipient weight
Absence of active infection
Absence of malignancy except primary brain tumor
Absence of preexisting heart disease or cardiac tumor
Negative serologic test for human immunodeficiency virus, hepatitis B, hepatitis C
Acceptable left ventricular function
If indicated, negative prospective crossmatch
Anticipated ischemic time less than 4 hours

Criteria for organ allocation are based on age, size, ABO blood group compatibility, medical history, and distance of the donor from the recipient hospital.[58] When the placement and recovery process begins, the procurement coordinator notifies the heart transplant team of the patient whose name is listed first as a match for that donor based on a policy for allocation of hearts that was developed by UNOS.[16,59] Geographically, organs are allocated locally first, then by increasing concentric circles of less than 500 nautical miles. Patients awaiting heart transplantation are classified by severity of illness, and a status is assigned as shown in Box 67-5. In addition, length of time on the waiting list is used for allocation of organs. Severity of illness and length of time on the waiting list are the factors considered when a donor organ becomes available; blood type and body size are used for matching of a donor to a recipient.

As the donor supply is limited, criteria for cardiac donation have been expanded to enhance the donor pool. Typically, donor weight is ± 20 percent to 30 percent of the weight of the recipient.[60] However, clinicians have reported the use of both undersized[93-95] and oversized[96] hearts. Patients with donor/recipient weight ratios (**DRWR**) as low as 0.5 (50 percent) have been successfully transplanted and have had comparable survival to patients who fell within the DRWR of .70 to .80 (20 percent to 30 percent of recipient weight).[60-63] However, Blackbourne and colleagues[63] noted an increased mortality in status I candidates who received undersized donor hearts when compared with all other patients undergoing transplant as status I.

Other criteria, including allograft ischemic time (the length of time a donor organ is without perfusion) and donor age, have also been extended. Conventionally, acceptable allograft ischemic time is 4 hours; however, studies of allograft ischemic times greater than 4 hours have reported no difference in recipient survival versus patients whose ischemic times were less than 4 hours.[61,64] Likewise, older donor age (more than 35 to 40 years) did not increase mortality compared to younger donors.[61,64] However, allograft coronary artery disease occurred more frequently in older than in younger donors in one study,[65] while rates were similar in older versus younger donors in another study.[66] A large multi-institutional study identified risk factors for death within the first year following transplant, including the following donor variables: older donor age, smaller donor body surface area, greater donor inotropic support, donor with diabetes mellitus, longer ischemic time, and diffuse donor heart wall motion abnormalities by echocardiography.[67] A thorough history, noninvasive cardiac testing (i.e., echocardiography), and coronary angiography in donors with major risk factors for coronary artery disease are recommended.[66]

The crucial importance of donor management is reflected in the fact that from 1 to 15 transplant candidates may benefit from a single donor, and poor management results in deterioration and loss of donor organs. Principles of donor management include: (1) restoration and maintenance of hemodynamic stability, (2) maintenance of adequate organ perfusion, and (3) treatment of brain death related complications.[68] Restoration of hemodynamic stability and maintenance of adequate organ perfusion involves the administration of crystalloid solutions and transfusions (only if necessary), with hemodynamic monitoring via a central venous or Swan-Ganz catheter if possible. Vasopressors (e.g., dopamine) may be used initially if necessary but should be weaned off as soon as possible. Brain death related complications also contribute to donor instability. Diabetes insipidus, changes in vasomotor tone, faulty thermal regulation, neurogenic pulmonary edema, and coagulopathy often occur and require immediate treatment.[68,69] Donors are also placed on prophylactic antibiotics after screening cultures are drawn.

Surgical Techniques

Timing and coordination of the recipient surgery with the donor cardiectomy is critical. Multiple procurement teams confer regarding scheduling of the surgery. At the same time, a candidate for heart transplantation who "matches" the donor is called from home or notified in the hospital of the availability of a heart. The final decision to proceed with heart transplantation is made by the procuring surgeon after on-site assessment of the adequacy of the donor heart. An estimate of arrival time is then given to his/her colleagues caring for the recipient and to the surgical staff.

Removal of the donor heart (cardiectomy) is completed when, after aortic cross clamp, the donor heart is removed and infused with a hypothermic preservation solution. Although different preservation solutions are used, they are generally crystalloid, cardioplegic (high potassium) solutions.[16] The donor heart is immersed in cold saline or cardioplegic solution and is placed in a cooler with ice for transport. On arrival at the recipient hospital, the donor heart is prepared for transplantation.

Standard surgical preparation of the transplant candidate is initiated, including signing of an operative consent; initiation of NPO status; assessment of vital signs and weight; type and crossmatching for blood products; and documentation of complete blood count, chemistry profile, anticoagulation profile, urinalysis, chest x-ray, and electrocardiogram. Anticoagulation is discontinued, and, when appropriate, vitamin K or fresh frozen plasma is given to reverse warfarin. Patients are given

the following medications: immunosuppressive therapy (based on the individual institutional protocol), prophylactic antibiotics, and preoperative medications per anesthesia. A central venous or Swan-Ganz catheter and arterial line are inserted in the operating room (if they are not already present) to monitor pulmonary vascular pressures, administer medications, and obtain blood samples. Peripheral intravenous lines are inserted to administer fluids and blood products. The patient is given anesthesia and intubated. A urinary catheter and nasogastric tube are placed. Subsequently, a median sternotomy is performed, and the patient is cooled and placed on cardiopulmonary bypass. An intraoperative echocardiogram may be used at some centers.

The standard surgical technique of biatrial orthotopic heart transplantation, developed by Lower and Shumway, involves excising all but the posterior aspects of the right and left atria and transecting the aorta and pulmonary artery.[2] Anastomosis of the donor heart, with a running suture, is performed in the following order: left atrial free wall, intraatrial septum, right atrium, pulmonary artery, and aorta[2] (Figure 67-1). After completion of the transplant procedure, initiation of rewarming, and establishment of an adequate cardiac rhythm (usually normal sinus rhythm), patients are slowly weaned from cardiopulmonary bypass. Mediastinal chest tubes and temporary epicardial pacemaker wires are placed before closing the chest.

An alternative technique for orthotopic heart transplantation (bicaval technique) has been developed, which involves total excision of the recipient's right atrium (leaving the origins of the superior and inferior vena cavae) and left atrium (leaving two cuffs of tissue which have the ostia of the pulmonary veins).[69,70] Implantation of the donor heart is performed by suturing the two left atrial cuffs of the recipient heart to the cor-

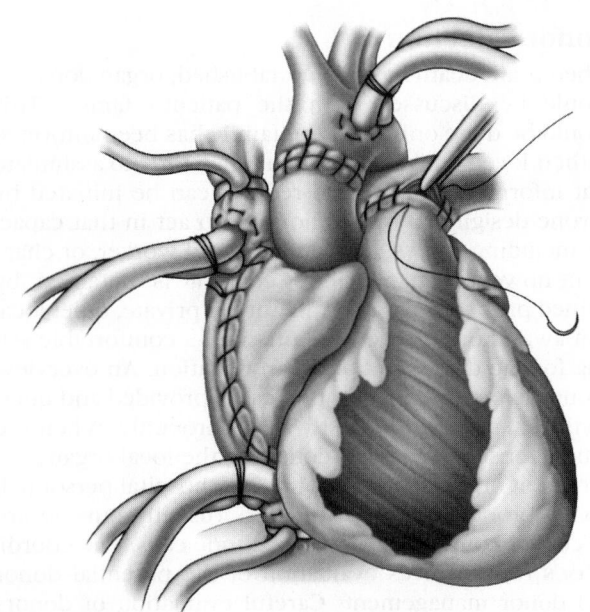

FIGURE 67-1 ■ Biatrial heart transplant operation. Completion of the aortic and pulmonary artery anastomosis. (From Kirklin J, Young J, McGiffin D: *Heart transplantation*, Philadelphia, 2002, Churchill Livingstone, p. 342.)

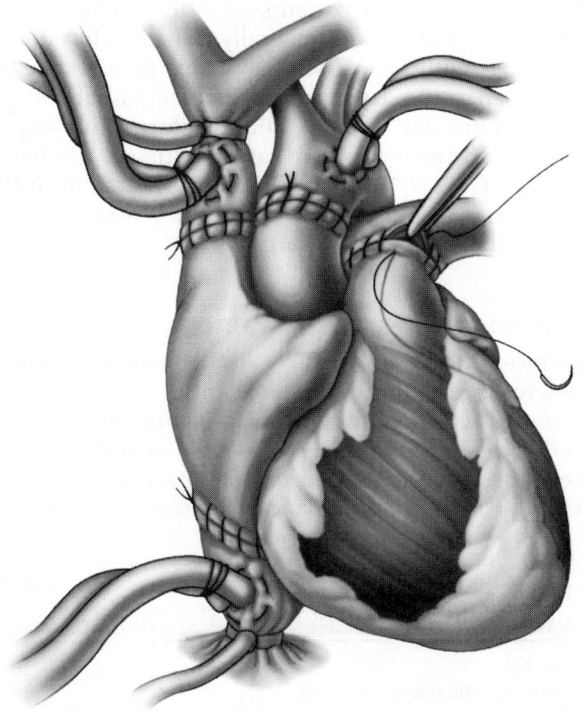

FIGURE 67-2 ■ Bicaval heart transplant operation. Completion of the bicaval transplant technique. (From Kirklin J, Young J, McGiffin D: *Heart transplantation*, Philadelphia, 2002, Churchill Livingstone, p. 344.)

responding left atrial donor structures and suturing the native inferior and superior vena cavae, end to end, to the inferior and superior vena cavae of the donor heart.[70-72] The pulmonary artery and aorta are anastomosed last in standard fashion (Figure 67-2). This surgical technique has potential physiological advantages over the standard orthotopic technique, including maintenance of the physiological size and shape of the atrial cavities and absence of mitral and tricuspid incompetence, conduction disturbances, and asynchronous atrial contraction. Two studies reported significantly decreased tricuspid regurgitation[70,71] and decreased need for pacemaker implantation for severe bradydysrhythmias early posttransplant[70] in patients in whom this surgical technique was used. It is necessary to weigh the relative benefits of this newer procedure versus the longer required ischemic time.

POSTOPERATIVE CARE AND LONG-TERM FOLLOW-UP
Physiology of the Transplanted Heart
Immediately posttransplantation, right- and left-sided filling pressures are elevated. These elevated pressures gradually normalize, possibly due to resolution of ventricular ischemia (which occurs during the recovery process and surgery), resolution of pulmonary hypertension, and improvement of diastolic function.[73] Mild-to-moderate elevations in left ventricular end-diastolic pressure may continue because of increased afterload from cyclosporine-induced systemic hypertension.[73] At rest, cardiac output and left ventricular ejection fraction are usually in the normal range.

Valvular incompetency may also occur. Mild mitral regurgitation may be seen and mild tricuspid regurgitation has also been demonstrated. Tricuspid regurgitation can be significant in patients with right ventricular dysfunction as a result of prolonged donor heart ischemic time or continued pulmonary hypertension.

Denervation
The donor heart is denervated (without autonomic nervous system control) after transplantation because the nerves are severed during surgery.[73] Therefore the sinus rate tends to be faster than normal due to the lack of parasympathetic tone. Heart rate and contractility during exercise can increase only by circulating catecholamines, which explains the slower rise of heart rate with exercise and its slower decline at rest than that observed in innervated hearts.[73] Also, the peak heart rate during exercise is lower in denervated hearts (130 to 150 beats/min) versus innervated hearts (170 to 200 beats/min). Drugs that act indirectly on the heart via autonomic stimulation are not effective in these patients. For example, atropine does not increase heart rate, and digoxin does not slow atrioventricular nodal conduction in the transplanted heart. Therefore drugs should be administered according to their direct effects, not according to those mediated through the autonomic nervous system. Isoproterenol is used for its chronotropic effect, and verapamil and beta blockers can be used to treat supraventricular dysrhythmias. Lastly, although many heart transplant patients cannot experience typical angina due to cardiac denervation, reinnervation may occur in patients about a year after transplant.[73-77] In addition, sympathetic reinnervation of the sinus node may result in a return toward normal heart rate response to exercise.[76,77]

Electrophysiology
The electrocardiogram of patients after standard orthotopic heart transplantation demonstrates two P waves, which are the result of the electrically isolated sinus node in the native, atrial remnant and the donor sinus node.[73,76] The native P wave "marches through" the P-QRS-T of the donor heart and can lead to the mistaken diagnosis of complete heart block if the donor P wave is of low amplitude. Donor sinus node or atrioventricular node dysfunction have been reported in 5 percent to 10 percent of patients early after heart transplantation, probably due to injury during procurement and implantation of the donor heart. Electrophysiological study and permanent pacemaker insertion have been indicated when bradydysrhythmias persist. Atrial dysrhythmias are common early after heart transplantation; however, ventricular dysrhythmias are not common and may be related to rejection.[73]

Immediate Postoperative Care of the Transplanted Patient
Immediately after heart transplantation, patients are taken to a surgical or transplant intensive care unit. Patients are generally admitted to a private room, and care is similar to that provided for standard open heart surgi-

cal patients. Because the donor heart generally functions well after transplant, the patient usually requires only low dose chronotropic and inotropic support with intravenous drips, commonly, isoproterenol. Additional inotropic support may be necessary with longer allograft ischemic times, hearts from marginal donors, poor preservation, or rejection.[73] If additional inotropic support is required, dobutamine (which directly stimulates cardiac beta-1 receptors) or milrinone (a phosphodiesterase inhibitor) are usually administered. These continuous intravenous medications can often be weaned and discontinued by 3 to 5 days posttransplant. Elevated pulmonary or systemic vascular resistance may be treated with sodium nitroprusside, prostaglandin E$_1$, or inhaled nitric oxide. Occasionally, patients may require an intraaortic balloon pump. Counterpulsation is often discontinued within 1 to 3 days after surgery.

Intravascular volume is assessed and replaced as needed. Postoperative mediastinal hemorrhage is a potential problem related to coagulopathies secondary to hepatic dysfunction, inadequate reversal of warfarin, or platelet dysfunction secondary to cardiopulmonary bypass.[78] Hemorrhage may be manifested through increased chest tube drainage, hemodynamic instability, a decreased hematocrit, and/or cardiac tamponade. Rewarming can also contribute to intravascular volume deficits. Once the cause of intravascular volume deficit is determined, appropriate replacement therapy can be initiated with crystalloids, colloids, and/or blood products. Further reversal of anticoagulation administered in the operating room may also be indicated. The use of aprotinin in the operating room has decreased the incidence of postoperative bleeding. Occasionally, return to the operating room is necessary for mediastinal exploration and hemostasis.

Many candidates for heart transplantation have borderline kidney function due to chronically decreased renal perfusion secondary to heart failure. Further insult to the kidneys may occur from cardiopulmonary bypass, periods of perioperative hypotension, and the administration of cyclosporine.[78] Depending on the extent of renal dysfunction, calcinurin inhibitors may be avoided in the early postoperative period. Other nephrotoxic drugs given prophylactically, such as ganciclovir and trimethoprim-sulfamethoxazole, may also be delayed or given at reduced doses. Dopamine may be administered in "renal doses" to promote adequate renal perfusion and urine output. Dialysis is rarely required if renal function and immunosuppressive drug levels are carefully monitored.

Patient recovery immediately posttransplant is often dramatic but also reflects preoperative physical and mental functional status. Ambulatory heart failure patients may recover more quickly than hemodynamically unstable patients confined to bedrest. Postoperatively, patients are generally extubated within 8 to 24 hours of surgery. Most intravenous lines, except one for administration of fluid and medications, are removed within 1 to 2 days of surgery. Chest tubes are removed 2 to 3 days postoperatively after chest tube drainage is minimal. Patients begin clear liquid diets after surgery and as bowel sounds return, advance to a general diet as toler-

ated. Given that many patients are often cachectic preoperatively, patients are generally not introduced to a low-fat diet until after discharge. Many patients are sitting in a chair the day after surgery and ambulating on the following day. By the third postoperative day, a structured exercise program can be initiated. Discharge education (Box 67-7) is completed. Discharge from the hospital to a local apartment or home is expected between 7 and 14 days after surgery.

Immunosuppressive therapies

Immunosuppressive therapy after transplantation is given to reduce the intense response of the immune system to the degree the transplanted organ is accepted and there is low incidence of toxicity. A combination of several drugs (usually two or three) are administered over the patient's lifetime and are titrated according to

---

BOX 67-7 ■ ■ ■
PATIENT AND FAMILY DISCHARGE EDUCATION

General
Members of the transplant team
When to call the transplant coordinator
Phone numbers of the transplant team

Immunosuppression
Administration of medications
Side effects of medications
Drug interactions
Rejection
Definition, signs and symptoms, diagnosis, treatment

Infection
Definition, signs and symptoms, diagnosis, treatment

Routine Care
Temperature
Weight
Skin care
Incision care
Intake and output
Pedal pulses
Clinic schedule

Diet After Transplant

Physical Activity After Transplant

Self-Care
Blood pressure
Blood sugar
Medical identification bracelet
Sun exposure
Sexual activity
Driving
Over-the-counter medications
Birth control

Routine Surveillance

Psychosocial Issues
Social support
Cost
Physical appearance
Writing the donor family
Health maintenance
Dental care
Ophthalmic examinations
Dermatologic examinations
Gynecologic examinations
Yearly evaluation of transplant

the patient's clinical history and development of toxicities. Immunosuppressive therapies are used in four situations after transplant[79]:

1. High dose initial immunosuppression with the goal of preventing rejection and producing tolerance, often referred to as *induction therapy*
2. Maintenance immunosuppression for long-term acceptance of the allograft
3. Augmented immunosuppression for the treatment of rejection episodes
4. Long-term immunosuppression therapies to prevent the development of coronary vasculopathy

Corticosteroids

Corticosteroids, generally prednisone, are also part of maintenance immunosuppressive therapy after heart transplantation. Corticosteroids inhibit initial helper T-cell activity and have direct lymphocytotoxic effects.[80] Intravenous corticosteroids, such as methylprednisolone, are usually administered preoperatively as a 500-mg single dose and intraoperatively at the same dose prior to release of the cross clamp. Immediately after surgery, patients receive methylprednisolone 125 mg intravenously every 8 hours $\times$ 3 doses. After extubation, patients are started on a rapidly tapering schedule of oral prednisone therapy. Tapering protocols are highly variable between centers. One center's protocol involves the administration of prednisone at 1 mg/kg/day for 21 days, followed by tapering to 0.1 to 0.2 mg/kg/day or off by 6 to 12 months. Side effects of corticosteroids are well known and have prompted transplant programs to investigate the use of steroid-free immunosuppressive regimens. In a retrospective review of 160 heart transplant recipients, 81 (51 percent) required maintenance corticosteroid therapy while 79 (49 percent) were successfully withdrawn.[81] While not all heart transplant recipients can be successfully withdrawn from steroids, some researchers found that those who could be withdrawn experienced similar survival rates,[80] similar or lower acute rejection rates,[81,82] no difference in allograft arteriopathy,[83] similar allograft function,[79,84] lower serum cholesterol levels,[86] less weight gain,[81] and decreased hypertension[81] versus patients requiring corticosteroid therapy up to 3 years posttransplant. Other researchers found higher rates of acute rejection in patients withdrawn from corticosteroids during the first 3 months posttransplant[84] or through 2 years posttransplant[82] and no difference in posttransplant weight gain, lipid abnormalities, and incidence of hypertension[84] compared to patients maintained on corticosteroid therapy. Furthermore, some patients who have been withdrawn from steroids have required a return to corticosteroid therapy. It appears that steroid withdrawal is safe and effective in select patients, but its long-term benefits require further study.[84]

Cyclosporine

Cyclosporine's basic immunosuppressant mechanism of action is blockade of the calcinurin pathway; thus, inhibiting the synthesis of interlukin 2, a cytokine which mediates activation of helper T lymphocytes.[79] Standard cyclosporine, Sandimmune, is supplied in oral solution, capsules, and intravenous solution. The microemulsion formulation of cyclosporine (Neoral) was developed to reduce variability in absorption, which in turn enhances bioavailability.[79,85] The U.S. Food and Drug Administration (**FDA**) approved two generic forms of Neoral, Gengraf by Abbott and EON's Cyclosporin Capsules USP Modified, which are equivalent to Neoral capsules.

Cyclosporine may be administered by mouth preoperatively and is continued postoperatively initially per nasogastric tube and then by mouth every 12 hours. Dosing of cyclosporine is usually center-specific. Cyclosporine may also be given at a decreased dose intravenously until patients are able to take fluids by mouth or if gastrointestinal absorption is poor. Cyclosporine trough blood levels are drawn beginning post-op day 1 or 2 in order to adjust subsequent doses to achieve adequate bloods levels. After consistent blood levels have been achieved, patients may be switched from the oral solution to capsules. See Box 67-8 for detailed use of cycloporine.

Two of the most frequent and serious side effects associated with cyclosporine are nephrotoxicity and hypertension. Researchers have found that with low doses of cyclosporine (an average of 5 mg/kg/day), while serum creatinine levels were higher than normal by 12 months posttransplant, there were no further increases through 5 postoperative years. Hypertension can occur as early as 1 month after transplant, whether or not patients have a history of hypertension, and usually requires more than one antihypertensive drug to achieve

---

BOX 67-8 ■ ■ ■
CYCLOSPORINE

Clinical Use
- Chronic maintenance immunosuppression, usually combined with azathioprine or mycophenolate mofetil, with or without corticosteroids

Mechanism
- Calcineurin blockade, inhibition of interleukin-2 production, inhabitation of T-cell proliferation

Dose
Adult
- Initial posttransplant infusion of 0.5-1 mg/hr continuous infusion
- Initial oral dose 25-50 mg b.i.d. and, if renal function remains normal, rapidly increase over 3-4 days to achieve whole blood trough level of 300-400 ng/ml

Pediatric
- Initial infusion of 0.25-0.5 mg/kg/day as continuous infusion while observing urine output and renal function. If renal function stable, begin PO dose at 1 mg/kg/day in three divided doses. If renal function remains normal, rapidly increase over 3-4 days to achieve target trough levels

Target Levels
- 0-3 months-350-450 ng/ml
- 12 months-100-200 ng/ml

Toxicity
- Nephrotoxicity, neurotoxicity, hypertension, hypercholesterolemia, hepatotoxicity, hyperkalemia, renal tubular acidosis, hypermagnesemia, hyperuricemia, hypertrichosis, gingival hyperplasia

Drug Interactions
- See Box 67-9

adequate blood pressure control. Other reported side effects include hyperlipidemia, tremors, gingival hyperplasia, hirsutism, paresthesias, seizures, abnormal liver function tests, hyperkalemia, and hyperuricemia.[79]

It is important to monitor all medications taken by patients who require cyclosporine. A large number of drug interactions have been identified between cyclosporine and commonly used drugs. Some are due to enhancement or inhibition of cyclosporine metabolism, which results in either subtherapeutic or toxic levels while others are due to potentiation of nephrotoxicity. Commonly used drugs that interact with cyclosporine are listed in Box 67-9. Furthermore, the side effects of other drugs can be potentiated with concomitant administration of cyclosporine. While treatment with 3-hydroxy-3-methylglutaryl CoA (HMG-CoA) reductase inhibitors (i.e., lovastatin, pravastatin, and simvastatin) have effectively lowered cholesterol levels in patients on cyclosporine, they have also contributed to acute, severe muscle damage with rhabdomyolysis and acute renal failure.[86,87] Lower doses of HMG-CoA reductase inhibitors have decreased this problem. Patients, therefore, need to be educated about contacting their heart transplant centers before taking over-the-counter medications or medications prescribed by other physicians.

Tacrolimus

Tacrolimus (Prograf), initially known as FK506, is also a calcinurin inhibitor. Similar to cyclosporine, tacrolimus blocks the calcinurin pathway by inhibiting the calcium-dependent transcription. It is different from cyclosporine in that tacrolimus binds to an FK-binding protein, producing an FKBP-12-tacrolimus complex that inhibits calcinurin. Tacrolimus was first used clinically in 1989 with liver transplantation and has been studied as primary immunosuppressive therapy in conjunction with low-dose steroids and azathioprine.[79,88,89] Tacrolimus can be administered orally in 1 mg or 5 mg capsules or in an intravenous solution. Tacrolimus is about 100 times more potent and more toxic than cyclosporine. Patients who received tacrolimus experienced rates of survival and rejection similar to those seen with cyclosporine. Less hypertension was observed with the use of tacrolimus versus cyclosporine while nephrotoxic effects were similar.[79]

Azathioprine

Azathioprine is in a class of drugs known as thiopurines. Azathioprine acts as an antiproliferative agent, which impairs DNA synthesis. Azathioprine is supplied in oral tablets or intravenous solution. The dose is administered at 1 to 2 mg/kg/day to maintain leukocyte cell count greater than 3000/ml, platelet count above 100,000, and a hematocrit of at least 27 percent. Side effects include neutropenia; thrombocytopenia; anemia; pancreatitis; gastrointestinal disturbances, including nausea and vomiting; hepatotoxicity; and increased risk of infection. Caution should be taken when azathioprine is administered concurrently with other bone marrow suppressing drugs.[79] The most important drug interaction is with allopurinol. Allopurinol impairs inactivation of azathioprine, and, therefore, the dose of azathioprine should be lowered to 25 to 30 percent of the usual dose.

Mycophenolate Mofetil

Mycophenolate mofetil, which is rapidly hydrolyzed to mycophenolic acid (MPA), inhibits the de novo pathway of purine synthesis and thereby suppresses both T and B lymphocyte function.[79,90] Mycophenolate mofetil is supplied in 250-mg capsules, 500-mg tablets, and an intravenous solution. Recent studies have shown trough whole blood levels of 2.5 to 5 ng/ml are desirable. Patients treated with mycophenolate mofetil versus azathioprine had lower 1-year mortality and a lower requirement for treatment of rejection.[79] In addition, mycophenolate mofetil may contribute to decreased cardiac allograft vasculopathy. Side effects reported thus far have been predominantly dose- related gastrointestinal symptoms, including diarrhea, soft stools, nausea, vomiting, and anorexia.[91] See Box 67-10 for quick reference.

Methotrexate

Methotrexate, a folic acid antagonist, is an antiproliferative agent that inhibits the proliferation of lymphocytes and other cells, thereby having inhibitory effects on both cellular and humoral immunity. Methotrexate can be given orally or intravenously as adjunct therapy for recurrent rejection.[8] The standard adult dose is 1 to 5 mg two or three times a day for 3 to 12 weeks. Bone marrow suppression is the major toxicity, so other myelosuppressive agents may need to be reduced or stopped and careful surveillance of leukocyte and platelet counts are warranted.

Cyclophosphamide

Cyclophosphamide (Cytoxan) is an alkylating agent that interferes with DNA replication. While both T and B cells are affected, studies suggest that cyclophosphamide has a greater specificity for B cells.[79] Hence cyclophosphamide is used when antibody-medicated rejection is suspected. Cyclophosphamide is supplied in 25 mg and 50-mg tablets and an intravenous solution. Usual dosage is titrated to 1 to 1.5 mg/kg/day with careful monitoring of the leukocyte count.

BOX 67-9 ■ ■ ■
CYCLOSPORINE DRUG INTERACTIONS

Increases Blood Levels
- Erythromycin
- Ketoconazole
- Intraconazole
- Diltiazem
- Verapamil
- Nicardipine
- Cimetidine
- Methylprednisolone
- Metoclopramide

Decreases Blood Levels
- Rifampin
- Isoniazid
- Phenobarbital
- Phenytoin
- Carbamazepine

Sirolimus

Sirolimus is a macrolide antibiotic in a class of immunosuppressants known as inhibitors of the target of rapamycin (TOR). TOR which plays a significant role in the stimulation and proliferation of lymphocytes. Thus, sirolimus, a TOR inhibitor, inhibits T-cell proliferation and differentiation, B-cell activation and proliferation, mesenchymal cell proliferation, and preserves T-cell apoptosis[92]. Sirolimus was discovered in 1988 by Morris at Stanford University and FDA approved in 1999 to be used in renal transplantation.[92] The recommended loading dose is 6 mg with a 2- to 5-mg daily maintenance dose. Therapeutic trough blood levels are between 5 to 20 ng/ml. Major toxicities include elevated blood cholesterol and triglycerides.[93] Many centers use sirolimus to reduce or eliminate the use of calcinurin inhibitors, which are associated with renal dysfunction after transplant.

Polyclonal and Monoclonal Antibodies

Polyclonal antibody preparations (antilymphocyte serum [ALS], antilymphoblast serum [ALG], antithymocyte globulin [ATG]) were the first agents used in clinical transplantation that were lymphocyte-specific. Polyclonal antibody preparations block T-cell surface receptors and, thus, destroy T lymphocytes. Polyclonal antibodies also cause B-cell depletion. Variations in the quality and potency of the preparations is the major disadvantage of the agents; however, many centers continue to use polyclonal antibodies as induction therapy and for the treatment of acute rejection.[94]

Monoclonal antibodies provide a more specific blockade of T-cell surface receptors with less variability of polyclonal preparations. Orthoclone OKT3, a anti-CD3 antibody, blocks the recognition of CD3 molecules from the T-cell surface. OKT3 is administered in a dose of 2.5 to 5 mg intravenously for 7 to 14 days. Monitoring of CD3 counts are important due ensure T-cell count depletion. Monoclonal antibodies can provide rejection prophylaxis as induction therapy or can treat recurrent or hemodynamic-compromised rejection.

The value of routine use of induction immunosuppression with anti–T-cell therapy is unclear. Small studies have reported similar survival, rates of rejection, and time to first rejection episode in heart transplant patients randomized to ATG versus OKT3, a monoclonal antibody.[94,95] OKT3 was also associated with a higher incidence of viral infections and adverse reactions.[95] Other studies have compared the use of OKT3 to no induction (i.e., only the use of triple drug therapy) in post-heart transplant patients and also found no difference in patient survival, incidence of rejection, and time to first rejection.[96,97] An increased incidence of posttransplant infection in patients receiving OKT3 was reported by one research team[96] but not by others.[97,98] Induction protocols may be most useful in patients at risk for significant rejection and patients with renal dysfunction in whom delayed initiation of cyclosporine would be beneficial.[99]

Anti-CD25 monoclonal antibodies suppress interleukin (**IL**)-2 IL-2 induced ribonucleic acid (**RNA**) synthesis. These newer antibodies were designed to suppress T lymphocytes, which attack the donor allograft, while leaving other immunity intact. These antibodies are humanized and do not exhibit the side effects seen by OKT3. Daclizumab (Zenapax) and basiliximab (Simulect) are two of the currently approved monoclonal antibodies. Basilximab is supplied in a 20-mg vial. Adult dosing is 20 mg intravenously within 2 hours of transplant and then 4 days later. The recommended dose of daclizumab is 1 mg/kg. The adult patient is given 5 doses, with the first dose given at the time of transplant and then 4 subsequent doses every 14 days. Delgado and colleagues[100] found that the use of basiliximab for induction therapy in patients with preoperative renal function may provide renal protection posttransplant.

Apheresis Therapies

The use of apheresis technology is reserved for the treatment of refractory rejection not amenable to the use of usual immunosuppression. Apheresis, which refers to extracorporeal fluid and cell separation, includes plasmapheresis and photopheresis.

Plasmapheresis involves removal of the blood from the patient, separating the plasma via centrifugation, and reconstituting the remaining blood with fresh plasma or albumin to achieve the original volume.[79] Removal of the antibodies causing the antibody-mediated rejection is believed to be the mechanism of action.[79] Extracorporeal photopheresis is a relatively new immunotherapy that involves the extracorporeal photochemotherapy of lymphocytes pretreated with 8-methoxypsoralen. The exact mechanism of action of photopheresis is unknown; however, the induction of suppressor T-cell response leading to immune modulation is theorized. Photopheresis is performed on two consecutive days about every 4 to 6 weeks for 1 year or on two consecutive days every other week for 6 months.

Total Lymphoid Irradiation

Total lymphoid irradiation is an immunosuppressive therapy for the treatment of recurrent rejection after transplantation. Low-dose irradiation targets major lymph node regions, causing deoxyribonucleic acid (DNA) damage in susceptible lymphocytes resulting in cell death.[101] Both T and B cells are susceptible to radiation injury. It is important to note that incidence of fatal acute megakaryocytic leukemia at 4 to 5 years after total lymphoid irradiation has been reported, which questions the safety of this therapy.

COMPLICATIONS OF CARDIAC TRANSPLANTATION
Cardiac Allograft Rejection

Cardiac allograft rejection is the histologic result of the immune response within the cardiac allograft. The immune system, in response to the transplanted organ, activates multiple pathways that attack the foreign organ. The success of organ transplantation is based on the ability to use immunosuppressive modalities to suppress the immune system against its attack on the transplanted heart. Rejection is classified into several categories, which include hyperacute rejection, acute cardiac rejection, and chronic rejection, also called *cardiac vasculopathy*.[102]

Hyperacute rejection is a violent immune attack on the transplanted organ as a result of preformed antidonor antibodies or ABO incompatibility.[102,103] The result is almost always loss of the graft. Histologic findings include diffuse interstitial hemorrhage, polymorphonuclear margination, and fibrin thrombi in intramural vessels.[103] These findings unfortunately are found during autopsy. In the event the patient survives, severe hemodynamic compromise accompanies hyperacute rejection. Inotropic support and mechanical circulatory assistance with biventricular assist devices or a total artificial heart may be instituted while patients are relisted for heart transplantation.

Hyperacute rejection can generally be avoided by ensuring donor-recipient ABO blood group compatibility and the absence of preformed antidonor antibodies in the recipient. Transplant programs perform panel reactive antibody (**PRA**) levels before transplant to identify the existence of preformed antibodies against a panel of donor lymphocytes representative of the most common human leukocyte antigens (**HLAs**).[104] If a transplant candidate has a PRA greater than or equal to 10 percent, a donor-specific crossmatch is performed before transplantation to ensure absence of reactivity. PRA levels are repeated after blood transfusions while patients await transplantation because transfusions can result in sensitization. In addition, patients with ventricular assist devices implanted while awaiting transplantation may also become sensitized. Thus PRA should be checked on a monthly basis on patient with an LVAD.

Treatment with plasmapheresis, intravenous immune gamma globulin, and cyclophosphamide have been successful in reducing sensitization.[105]

Acute cardiac rejection is the mononuclear inflammatory response, mediated by T lymphocytes, directed against the cardiac allograft.[102,106] Diagnosis of acute cardiac rejection is based on clinical findings with or without supporting evidence of an endomyocardial biopsy. Acute cardiac rejection can be asymptomatic or exhibit clinical signs of hemodynamic compromise. Clinical signs and symptoms can be labeled into three categories. Constitutional signs and symptoms include fatigue, fever, malaise, and flulike symptoms. Signs of cardiac irritation include tachycardia, dysrhythmias, pericardial friction rub, or pericardial effusion. Signs of cardiac dysfunction include decreased cardiac output or index, increased pulmonary capillary wedge pressure, S_3 or S_4 gallop, dyspnea, hypotension, lethargy, or diminished peripheral pulses.[102] Any clinical evidence of rejection reported by the patient should lead to an echocardiogram to evaluate cardiac systolic function and/or endomyocardial biopsy.

An endomyocardial biopsy, the gold standard for diagnosis of rejection, is an invasive procedure performed under fluoroscopy or echocardiographic guidance.[102] Informed consent is required. The procedure is performed with the patient in a fasting state without premedication. After preparation of the patient, a bioptome is passed via the right internal jugular vein through the superior vena cava and into the right heart where 4 to 7 specimens from the intraventricular septum are removed.[107] These specimens are placed in formalin and sent to pathology where they are sectioned, placed on a microscope slide, stained with hematoxylin-eosin, and visualized under a microscope for clinical interpretation. Endomyocardial biopsies are relatively safe with a complication rate of less than or equal to 3 percent.[107] Complications associated with catheter insertion have included carotid puncture, prolonged bleeding, and vasovagal reaction. During the procedure, dysrhythmias and conduction disturbances may occur. Rarely, pneumothorax and cardiac tamponade have been reported. Postprocedure, a Band-Aid is applied at the insertion site, vital signs are taken, a brief cardiopulmonary exam is performed, and patients are returned to their hospital room or discharged to home. Endomyocardial biopsies are performed frequently after transplantation (weekly for 6 weeks) and gradually tapered over time to one or two a year.

Acute rejection is manifested histologically by varying degrees of inflammatory infiltrate and myocardial damage.[102,103] The infiltrate is composed primarily of lymphocytes but may include eosinophils and neutrophils in more severe cases.[103] The intensity of cellular infiltration may range from a single focus to diffuse involvement of all pieces of tissue examined. Injury to the myocardium is referred to as "myocyte necrosis." In an attempt to standardize reporting of endomyocardial biopsy results, a cardiac biopsy grading system (Box 67-11) was developed by cardiac pathologists.[108]

The incidence of acute rejection is variable. The Cardiac Transplant Research Database has reported nearly 40 percent of patients experience one or more rejection

BOX 67-11   ▪ ▪ ▪
ISHLT STANDARDIZED ENDOMYOCARDIAL BIOPSY GRADING SCHEME

GRADE*	DESCRIPTION	NOMENCLATURE
0	No lymphocytic infiltrate	No rejection
1A	Focal (perivascular or interstitial) lymphocytic infiltrate without myocyte necrosis	Focal mild acute rejection
1B	Diffuse but sparse lymphocytic infiltrate without myocyte necrosis	Diffuse mild acute rejection
2	One focus only with "aggressive" lymphocytic infiltrate and/or focal myocyte injury	Focal moderate rejection
3A	Multifocal aggressive lymphocytic infiltrates and/or myocyte necrosis	Multifocal moderate acute rejection
3B	Diffuse, inflammatory process with myocyte necrosis	Diffuse borderline severe acute rejection
4	Diffuse, aggressive, polymorphous infiltrate with necrosis (± hemorrhage; ± vasculitis)	Severe acute rejection

Additional Information that Should be Reported
- Biopsy less than 4 pieces
- Resolving rejection—denoted by lesser grade than prior biopsy
- Humoral rejection (positive immunofluorescence, vasculitis, or severe edema in absence of cellular infiltrate)
- "Quilty" effect
  - A = No myocyte encroachment
  - B = With myocyte encroachment
- Ischemia
  - A = Up to 3 weeks after transplant
  - B = Late ischemia
- Infection present
- Lymphoproliferative disorder
- Other

From Billingham ME, Cary NRB, Hammond ME et al: A working formulation for the standardization of nomenclature in the diagnosis of heart and lung rejection, *J Heart Lung Transplant* 9:587-593, 1990.
*Biopsy graded by worst infiltrate noted on at least 3 to 5 specimens reviewed.
ISHLT, International Society for Heart and Lung Transplantation.

episodes in the first month after transplant while over 60 percent experience one or more in the first 6 months.[109] At 1 year, about one third of the patients are rejection free. Factors that increase the risk of acute rejection include younger age, female gender, PRA greater than or equal to 10 percent, positive donor-specific crossmatch, and viral infection.[110] Assessment of patients for signs and symptoms of rejection along with prompt treatment is essential to prevent important myocardial damage. Treatment of acute rejection varies, depending on the histologic severity of rejection, time after transplant, and associated clinical manifestations. Standard therapy includes the use of oral or intravenous corticosteroids and anti-T-cell therapy, including ATG, ALG, and OKT3. A variety of oral prednisone protocols with rapid or slow taper have been successfully used in the treatment of moderate acute rejection without hemodynamic compromise. More than 85 percent of acute rejection episodes (mild to severe) respond to intravenous methylprednisolone (1 g/day × 3 days).[102,111]

Acute rejection with hemodynamic compromise or recalcitrant acute rejection are generally treated more vigorously with anti-T-cell therapy. Patients have been successfully treated with intravenous polyclonal agents (ATG or ALG) for 7 to 14 days or monoclonal therapy (OKT3) for 5 to 14 days.[102] These therapies are viewed as rescue therapy and are often life-saving. However, a small subset of patients have recurrent rejection despite successful treatment with anti-T-cell therapy. The repeated use of corticosteroid therapy or anti-T-cell therapy is associated with a higher risk of infection and other drug-specific complications.

Researchers have, therefore, explored other pharmacological and nonpharmacological therapies to treat severe acute rejection and recurrent rejection. Methotrexate has been used to treat recalcitrant rejection.[8,112] In one study, methotrexate was administered orally at a dose of 2.5 to 15 mg per week over 1 to 2 days for 3 to 9 weeks.[112] Additional courses of methotrexate therapy were given for ongoing rejection. Successful reduction in the incidence of acute rejection was reported by all research groups compared to pre-methotrexate therapy. Transient leukopenia and infection were observed in patients receiving methotrexate therapy. Other drugs are also being used for the treatment of acute rejection, including conversion from cyclosporine to tacrolimus[113] and conversion from azathioprine to mycophenolate mofetil[91] or cyclophosphamide.[114] Researchers have also reported early results regarding the use of total lymphoid irradiation as adjunct therapy for reversal of early, severe acute rejection and recurrent acute rejection[116,117] and photochemotherapy for treatment of recurrent acute rejection[118,119] and as adjunct therapy for rejection prophylaxis.[119]

The risk of rejection continues throughout the lifetime of the transplant recipient. Because the risk is lower after the first year, many programs have established protocols for decreasing rejection surveillance and the frequency of endomyocardial biopsies. A sample protocol can be seen in Box 67-12. Ongoing patient and family education regarding the signs and symptoms of rejection along with reporting them to the transplant team is an important surveillance modality to ensure long-term outcome of the transplanted patient.

Microvascular or humoral rejection is a rejection process resulting from antibodies directed against donor antigens located on the coronary vasculature.[120] Although diagnosis of humoral rejection is difficult, some researchers have suggested diagnosis via endomyocardial biopsy with the use of immunofluorescence.[121] Criteria used to diagnose humoral rejection are endothelial cell selling, endothelial cell necrosis, inflammatory infiltrates, microvascular thrombosis, and interstitial edema and hemorrhage.[102,103] Humoral rejection has been most frequently observed early after heart transplantation although it has also occurred several months to years after transplant.[120,121] It is often associated with elevated PRA levels and the development of donor-specific antibodies after transplant. Symptoms of heart failure and hemodynamic compromise requiring inotropic support frequently accompany this type of rejection. Treatment of humoral rejection has included high-dose corticosteroids, plasmapheresis (to directly remove the circulating antibodies), photopheresis, and cytolytic therapy.[102,122] While short-term prognosis has been favorable in some series of patients, long-term allograft and patient survival have often been poor.

Chronic Rejection (Cardiac Allograft Vasculopathy)

Chronic rejection, also known as cardiac allograft vasculopathy, refers to the concentric narrowing or obstruction of the coronary arteries of the transplanted heart. Although chronic rejection is viewed as a long-term complication, it can be detected as early as several months after transplantation. Long-term survival after heart transplantation is limited by the development and progression of cardiac allograft vasculopathy.[123-126] The incidence of coronary vasculopathy, documented by coronary angiography, has been reported as 10 percent to 15 percent per year with a prevalence of 50 percent by 5 years after heart transplantation[124,125] (Figure 67-3). Pathologic changes in the coronary arteries involve diffuse narrowing of the entire vessel, rather than the discrete, proximal focal lesions seen in "native" coronary artery disease. The small, distal coronary vessels are the earliest to become obstructed.

The pathologic mechanisms leading to the development of coronary vasculopathy are not entirely known. A favored hypothesis is that the primary process is "injury" to endothelial cells, which then results in subsequent vascular damage.[126] Immunological and nonimmunological risk factors are believed to contribute to the development and progression of chronic rejection. Histocompatibility, frequency and severity of acute rejection, and cytotoxic B-cell antibodies have been linked to the development of coronary vasculopathy.[125] Primary cytomegalovirus (CMV) infection has also been implicated in the pathogenesis of coronary vasculopathy, given the ability of enteroviruses (especially CMV) to stimulate immunological responses.[127] Nonimmunological risk factors for the development of coronary vasculopathy include recipient age and sex, donor age and sex, obesity, hypercholesterolemia, hypertriglyceridemia, pretransplant diagnosis, and ischemic time.[124-128] Many researchers suggest a multifactorial etiology of coronary vasculopathy. However, the contributory role of any or all of the identified factors requires further study and elucidation. The immunological event is that endothelial cells function as both antigen-presenting cells and targets of the immune response, which leads to endothelial cell activation. These activated endothelial cells produce growth factors, leading to smooth muscle cell proliferation that results in progressive luminal narrowing.

Diagnosis of chronic rejection has traditionally been via coronary angiography, with angiography performed shortly after heart transplantation (to establish a baseline) and annually thereafter. Due to denervation, patients do not typically experience angina and the initial clinical manifestation of coronary vasculopathy is unfortunately acute myocardial infarction, heart failure, or sudden death. In the 1990s, intravascular ultrasound (IVUS) imaging was introduced to aid in the diagnosis.[129] Increased sensitivity for detection of transplant coronary disease, better quantification of the extent of disease, and the possibility of characterization of vessel wall morphology with the use of IVUS imaging versus coronary angiography has contributed to the earlier detection of coronary vasculopathy and may provide useful prognostic data because it shows intimal thickening before any abnormalities appear on the angiogram.[124]

While improvement in detection of transplant vasculopathy has occurred, prevention and treatment remain elusive. Prevention involves risk factor modification although no studies have conclusively demonstrated benefit.[130,131] Patients are encouraged to follow low-fat diets and control their body weight and weight gain. The use of HMG-CoA reductase inhibitors to manage hypercholesterolemia after heart transplantation is actively pursued by many transplant centers. Cyclosporine-related hypertension is also aggressively treated. There have been reports to suggest that CMV status of donor and recipient may influence chronic rejection.[132] While many transplant centers use antiplatelet therapy routinely, no controlled clinical studies have proven efficacy in the prevention of chronic rejection.[130] Promis-

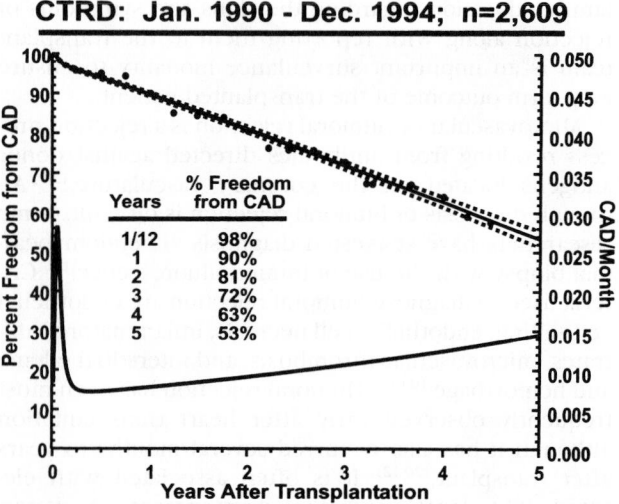

CTRD: Jan. 1990 - Dec. 1994; n=2,609

Years	% Freedom from CAD
1/12	98%
1	90%
2	81%
3	72%
4	63%
5	53%

FIGURE 67-3 ■ Coronary artery disease (CAD). Actuarial freedom from the presence of CAD. *CTRD*, Cardiac Transplant Research Database. (From Kirklin J, Young J, McGiffin D: *Heart transplantation*, Philadelphia, 2002, Churchill Livingstone, p. 642.)

ing data suggest that calcium channel blockers may prevent or retard the development of vasculopathy and induce regression of existing lesions.[124,125]

Treatment of coronary vasculopathy has involved the use of coronary artery bypass grafting **(CABG),** percutaneous coronary intervention **(PCI),** and retransplantation.[133,134] Recently, coronary stenting has shown improvement of outcome in transplant patients.[124] The diffuseness of coronary vasculopathy often contraindicates the potential effectiveness of CABG. Anecdotal case reports in the literature, however, have suggested the usefulness of CABG in patients with coronary anatomy amenable to revascularization.[133] PCI has also been performed in heart transplant recipients with angiographic success achieved in 88/95 (93 percent) lesions and 66 percent patient survival at a mean follow-up of 13 months.[134] However, the long-term effects of CABG and PCI on cardiac allograft survival remain to be determined. Currently, the only definitive therapy for coronary vasculopathy is cardiac retransplantation. However, given the reduced rates of survival, limited donor supply, and higher costs associated with retransplantation, this therapy requires careful consideration.

Infection

Infection is one of the major complications of immunosuppression after heart transplantation. A major, multi-institutional study of post-heart transplant infection reported that 69 percent of patients were free from infection during the study period (mean = 8.2 mos), 22 percent had one infection, and 9 percent had more than one infection.[135] The most frequently occurring infections were bacterial (47 percent), viral (41 percent), fungal (7 percent), and protozoal (5 percent).[136] Gram-positive organisms (53 percent) and gram-negative organisms (41 percent) were identified as the causes of bacterial infections. Miller and colleagues[135] found that staphylococcal organisms accounted for 77 percent of gram-positive infections; they further identified CMV as the most common infecting agent as it caused 26 percent of all infections. The most common sites of infection identified by the multi-institutional study group were lung (28 percent), blood (26 percent), gastrointestinal tract (17 percent), and urinary tract (12 percent). The incidence of wound infection was low (3 percent).

The risk for developing all types of infection is highest during the first month after transplantation and decreases subsequently.[136,137] Risk factors for early infection have been identified and include older recipient age, ventilator support at the time of transplant, ventricular assist device at the time of transplant, OKT3 induction therapy, donor black race, and positive donor cytomegalovirus serology.[137] Other researchers have reported that the actuarial risk of late infection (2 years after heart transplant) is only 13 percent. Bacterial and viral infections continue to be the most frequent types of infection identified late after transplant. Furthermore, actuarial freedom from fatal infection is 96 percent at 1 year and 95 percent at 3 years.[136]

Strategies to prevent infection include the use of prophylactic antiinfective therapy and other infection control practices. Donors are routinely screened for infection, and antibiotics are instituted as indicated. Heart transplant recipients receive routine surgical prophylaxis with a cephalosporin for up to 36 postoperative hours. Researchers have also shown that the prophylactic administration of intravenous ganciclovir from 2 to 8 weeks posttransplant reduces the incidence of CMV illness in seropositive and seronegative heart transplant recipients.[138,139] Therefore many transplant programs initiate ganciclovir for 2 or more weeks postoperatively, possibly followed by 3 to 6 months of acyclovir or ganciclovir to prevent CMV infection when the incidence is highest. In addition, oral trimethoprim-sulfamethoxazole has been shown to prevent *Pneumocystis jiroveci* (formerly *carinii*) pneumonia, which occurs most commonly within the first 3 to 4 months posttransplant, and is therefore administered prophylactically at least 3 days per week for at least 12 months.[136] Other prophylactic strategies include the use of clotrimazole lozenges or nystatin solution after meals and at bedtime to reduce the incidence of oral fungal infections.

Infection control practices vary among heart transplant programs. In a survey of these programs, handwashing, masks, gowns, and gloves were used by 50 percent or more of the staff. There was no correlation between number of infection control measures used and patient survival rates. Interestingly, more experienced transplant programs used significantly fewer infection control measures. However, 64 percent of patients were admitted to private rooms with limited access immediately after surgery. Also usual intensive care visitation restrictions were followed with more attention paid to visitor health status.

Other usual practices including extubation within 24 hours; removal of invasive lines and indwelling catheters within 72 hours; use of standardized protocols for dressing, tubing, bottle, and catheter change; early ambulation; pulmonary care; and optimal nutrition contribute to the prevention of infection in heart transplant patients. Also, at some centers patients receive leukodepleted blood products to reduce sensitization and the incidence of CMV infection. CMV-negative recipients who receive CMV-negative donor organs should also receive CMV-negative blood products.

At discharge, patients are instructed about the use of infection control measures in the home. These measures are based on "common sense" and usual practices to prevent the spread of infection in the community. Treatment of infection is instituted rapidly and aggressively. Assessment involves a history, thorough physical examination, and laboratory and other tests. Broad spectrum antibiotic coverage may be initiated until an infecting agent is identified. Depending on clinical status, patients may be admitted to the hospital for treatment or followed in a clinic setting with home health nurses, if needed.

Other Complications

While early graft failure, cardiac allograft rejection, infection, and coronary vasculopathy are major complications that limit survival after cardiac transplantation, there are other important complications that contribute to morbidity and mortality and warrant discussion.

Hypertension

Arterial hypertension is one of the most common and frustrating medication-induced complications after cardiac transplantation with an incidence of 40 percent to 90 percent in the first year after transplant.[140] Patients with preexisting hypertension and on cyclosporine drug regimen are the most difficult to control. Cyclosporine-induced hypertension results from three proposed mechanisms: sympathetic stimulation, neurohormonal activation, and direct vascular effects. Multiple antihypertensive agents are often needed for blood pressure control.

Hyperlipidemia

Hyperlipidemia occurs in 60 percent to 80 percent of heart transplant patients. Causes of hyperlipidemia in heart transplant patients include obesity, high fat diets, genetic predisposition, and immunosuppressive therapy, particularly the use of corticosteroids and cyclosporine.[141] Treatment of dyslipidemia includes weight loss, exercise, and lipid-lowering agents such as HMG-CoA reductase inhibitors, bile acid sequestrants, and fibric acid derivatives. In a randomized trial for heart transplant patients, pravastatin was shown to reduce cholesterol levels after transplant and lead to a reduced incidence of coronary vasculopathy, decreased rejection, and improved 1-year survival.[141,142] Thus it is currently recommended that all patients begin pravastatin early after heart transplantation.[142]

Renal Dysfunction

Renal dysfunction after heart transplantation can include both acute and chronic renal failure. Acute renal failure is thought to be drug induced and due to renal afferent arteriolar vasoconstriction. Renal function may also be impaired prior to transplantation due to low cardiac output and aggressive diuretic therapy.[143] Cardiac performance is the primary determinant of renal function after transplantation. Low-dose dopamine, delaying the administration of cyclosporine, and careful administration of diuretics may reverse early renal dysfunction.

The major risk factor for chronic renal failure after heart transplantation is chronic administration of calcinurin inhibitors (cyclosporine and tacrolimus). Chronic renal dysfunction is associated with afferent renal arteriolar lesions, glomerular sclerosis, proximal tubular atrophy, and progressive interstitial fibrosis.[136,143] The management of chronic renal dysfunction after heart transplantation includes early recognition of elevated serum creatinine (greater than or equal to 2 mg/dl), reduction of calcinurin inhibitors, treatment of hypertension, and avoiding other nephrotoxic agents. Studies have shown that using angiotensin–converting enzyme (ACE) inhibitors may reduce the renal effects of cyclosporine.[144] In the event that renal function deteriorates, chronic dialysis and renal transplantation may be necessary.

Malignancy

Other complications that require discussion include posttransplant lymphoproliferative disease and malignant neoplasia. Posttransplant lymphoproliferative disease, which involves abnormal B lymphocyte proliferation, has been acknowledged as an often fatal complication of immunosuppression. One study described the occurrence of posttransplant lymphoproliferative disease with the use of OKT3 (prophylactic and therapeutic) versus no OKT3 (9/79, 11.4 percent, versus 1/75, 1.3 percent, respectively) and further reported an increased incidence with increasing doses of OKT3.[136] Other studies have revealed a low incidence of posttransplant lymphoproliferative disease in heart transplant patients receiving induction with Minnesota ALG and augmented immunosuppression for rejection[145] or no induction and methylprednisolone pulse therapy for rejection.[146]

Armitage and colleagues[12] reported an overall incidence of posttransplant lymphoproliferative disease in heart transplant patients (n = 503) of 3.4 percent (15/503), with diagnosis from as early as 1 month to 7 years posttransplant. The most common presentation of posttransplant lymphoproliferative disease was isolated lymphadenopathy. Diagnosis involved lymph node biopsy and obtaining Epstein-Barr virus titers because Epstein-Barr virus is thought to play a role in the pathogenesis of posttransplant lymphoproliferative disease. The cornerstone of treatment has been reduction in immunotherapy. Chemotherapy and radiation have also been used. The overall incidence of heart transplant neoplasia after transplant was low and the majority of cancers were cutaneous.[146,147]

Bone Complications

Bone complications after transplantation include osteoporosis and avascular necrosis.[136,148] Osteoporosis is defined as an abnormally low bone volume for age, race, and sex. The technique of choice for measuring bone mineral density is the dual-energy x-ray absorptiometry or **DEXA** scan. Corticosteroids (well known to cause accelerated bone loss and vertebral fractures), cyclosporine, renal insufficiency, and being a postmenopausal woman are risk factors for osteoporosis.[148] Avascular necrosis is a condition that interrupts blood supply to the bone and results in death of bone and cartilage. This complication occurs in 3 percent to 6 percent of heart transplant patients, and most commonly affects the femoral head or the shoulders. Corticosteroid therapy is the major causative factor. Treatment depends on the severity of symptoms. Pain management, physical therapy, and total joint replacement may be indicated.

Gastrointestinal Complications

Gastrointestinal complications after heart transplantation may be minor or life-threatening in nature. Minor complications, such as nausea, vomiting, and diarrhea, affect about two thirds of posttransplant patients and are many times drug related. Careful reduction in corticosteroids and increasing frequency of lower dosing with mycophenolate may help to alleviate minor symptoms. About 30 percent to 50 percent of heart transplant patients develop major gastrointestinal complications in the first 3 to 5 years.[150] These major complications include peptic ulcer disease, cholelithiasis, diverticular disease, pancreatitis, and CMV gastrointestinal disease. Prompt diagnosis, aggressive treatment, and surgical intervention if indicated are essential for long-term survival.

Outcomes and Quality of Life

Overall 1-year actuarial survival after heart transplantation is 79 percent with an approximate 4 percent mortality per year for the next 13 years.[5] When 1-year survival was examined by era, improved survival was found during the most recent era versus earlier eras, showing an approximate 81 percent 1-year and 73 percent 3-year survival versus 70 percent 1-year and 60 percent 3-year survival, respectively.[5] Multivariate analyses of a large patient registry ($n = 10,782$) revealed the following as risk factors for 1-year posttransplant survival: previous heart transplantation, mechanical support before transplantation (including ventilators and circulatory assist devices), age (being very old or young), female recipient or donor, congenital heart disease, program volume of fewer than 9 transplants per year, older donor, longer ischemic time, and patients at risk for primary CMV disease. Furthermore, a large, collaborative study examined the influence of HLA compatibility on 3-year graft survival after heart transplantation and found that patients with 0 or 1 mismatch ($n = 128$) had significantly better survival than patients with 2 mismatches ($n = 439$) or 3 to 6 mismatches ($n = 7764$) (83 percent versus 76 percent versus 71 percent, p less than 0.001, respectively).[150] Knowledge of risk factors for heart transplantation can contribute to improved selection of patients and matching of recipients and donors. Unfortunately, donor ischemic time is currently a limiting factor when considering prospective HLA matching to improve posttransplant survival.

With improved survival posttransplant over the last two decades, quality of life as a posttransplant outcome has also become important. Researchers have reported decreased symptom distress,[151-153] improved functional ability (especially physical functioning),[151-154] improved health status,[152] and increased satisfaction with life and improved quality of life in heart failure patients who underwent transplantation. Furthermore, patients have reported low-to-moderate stress levels both before and after heart transplantation and were coping fairly well. After transplant, patients have experienced some symptom distress (dermatologic and gastrointestinal), work-related disability, stress related to finances, rehospitalization, self-care, and inadequate or dissatisfaction with sexual function.[154-158] Clearly, for most patients, life after heart transplantation is better than life with end-stage heart failure; however, complications, adverse effects of immunosuppression, the need to comply with rigorous

posttransplant follow-up, and vocational and financial issues underscore the chronicity of the posttransplant period.

Lastly, costs of transplantation and assumption of financial risk have become more important outcomes as "managed care" continues to expand in the United States.[159] "Transplant networks" have been established by major insurers, wherein selective contracting with transplant centers, referred to as "centers of excellence" is based on quality and price. While hospitals that join these networks are often referred to as "centers of discount," one major insurer with such a network reported major savings (reflecting reduced reimbursements to centers) with center survival rates similar to or better than national rates reported by UNOS.[159] Given health care reform and the costs associated with transplantation, it would benefit heart failure and transplant programs to examine the cost-effectiveness of their care delivery in order to provide quality care competitively.

Advances in transplantation will require new immunosuppressants and creative, new approaches to the problem of allograft rejection. Many new drugs are being evaluated for use as immunosuppressants after transplantation. Some of these drugs have been previously discussed. In addition, the field of experimental cardiac xenotransplantation is dedicated to the development of transplantation between species.[160] Transplantation between closely-related species (concordant xenografting) has made slow and steady progress.[160,161] However, human concordant xenografting would entail the use of a closely-related primate species, which is constrained by availability, small size relative to adult humans, and opposition by animal rights groups.[162] Discordant xenotransplantation (between more genetically dissimilar species such as pig to baboon or human) is currently limited by hyperacute rejection.[161] Genetic engineering of pigs is being investigated, and clinical trials of xenotransplantation may be initiated within 3 to 5 years.

Indeed, cardiac transplantation has evolved over the decades to become a successful treatment for select patients with end-stage heart disease. The future holds new and improved immunosuppression therapies (including the initiation of immune tolerance of the allograft), overcoming organ donor shortage, developing strategies to prevent long-term complications, and continuing to explore ways to improve overall quality of life.

REFERENCES

1. McGregor CG: Evolution of heart transplantation, *Cardiol Clin* 8(1):3-10, 1990.
2. Lower RR, Dong E Jr, Shumway NE: Long-term survival of cardiac homografts, *Surgery* 58:110, 1965.
3. Hardy JD, Chavez CM, Kurrus FD et al: Heart transplantation in man, *JAMA* 188:1132, 1964.
4. Barnard CN: A human cardiac transplant: an interim report of a successful operation performed at Groote Schuur Hospital, Cape Town, *S Afr Med J* 41:1271, 1967.

5. Kriett JM, Kaye MP: The Registry of the International Society for Heart Transplantation. Seventh Official Report—1990, *J Heart Transplant* 9(4):323-330, 1990.

6. Renlund DG, Gopinathan SK, Kfoury Ag et al: Mycophenolate mofetil (MMF) in heart transplantation: rejection prevention and treatment, *Clin Transplant* 10:136-139, 1996.

7. Salter SP, Salter MM, Kirklin JK et al: Total lymphoid irradiation in the treatment of early or recurrent heart transplant rejection, *Int J Radiation Oncol Biol Phys* 33(1):83-88, 1995.

8. Bourge RC, Kirklin JK, Naftel DC et al: Methotrexate pulse therapy in the treatment of recurrent acute heart rejection, *J Heart Lung Transplant* 11:1116-1124, 1992.

9. Lang C, Beniaminovitz A, Edwards N et al: Morbidity and mortality of diabetic patients following cardiac transplantation, *J Heart Lung Transplant* 22:244-240, 2003.

10. Mancini D, Beniaminovitz A, Edwards et al: Survival of diabetic patients following cardiac transplantation, *Transplantation* 20:168, 1996.

11. DiSalvo T, Naftel DC, Kasper E et al: The differing hazard of lymphoma vs. other malignancies in the current era—a multi-institutional study, *J Heart Lung Transplant*17:70, 1998.

12. Armitage JM, Kormos RL, Griffith BP et al: Heart transplantation in patients with malignant disease, *J Heart Lung Transplant* 9(6):627-630, 1990.

13. O'Connell JB, Bourge RC, Costanzo-Nordin MR et al: Cardiac transplantation: recipient selection, donor procurement, and medical follow-up, *Circulation* 86(3):1061-1079, 1992.

14. Kirklin JK, McGiffin DC, Pinderski L et al: Selection of patients and techniques of heart transplantation, *Surg Clin North Am* 84:257-287, 2004.

15. Brennan DC, Lowell JA: Pretransplant preparation of the cadaver donor/organ procurement. In Norman DJ, Suki WN, editors: *Primer of transplantation,* Philadelphia, 1998, American Society of Transplant Physicians.

16. Kirklin JK: The donor heart. In Kirklin JK, Young J, McGiffin DC, editors: *Heart transplantation,* Philadelphia, 2002, Churchill Livingstone, pp. 293-352.

17. Taylor DO, Edwards LB, Boucek M et al: The Registry of the International Society for Heart and Lung Transplantation: Twenty-first Official Adult Heart Transplant Report, *J Heart Lung Transplant* 23:796-803, 2004.

18. O'Connell JB, Breen TJ, Hosenpud JD: Heart transplantation in dilated heart muscle disease and myocarditis, *European Heart J* 16(Supp O):137-139, 1995.

19. Costanzo MR, Augustine S, Bourge RC et al: Selection and treatment of candidates for heart transplantation, *Circulation* 92(12):3593-3612, 1995.

20. Johnson MR, Costanzo-Nordin MR, Gunnar RM: Peripartum cardiomyopathy, *Progress Cardiol* 5(2):145-157, 1992.

21. Johnson MR, Naftel DC, Hobbs, RE et al: The incremental risk of female gender in cardiac transplantation: a multi-institutional study of peripartum cardiomyopathy and pregnancy, *J Heart Lung Transplant* 16(8):801-812, 1997.

22. Kirklin JK: Recipient evaluation and selection. In Kirklin JK, Young J, McGiffin DC, editors: *Heart transplantation,* Philadelphia, 2002, Churchill Livingstone, pp. 198-231.

23. Kirklin JK: Cardiac retransplantation. In Kirklin JK, Young J, McGiffin DC, editors: *Heart transplantation,* Philadelphia, 2002, Churchill Livingstone, pp. 820-826.

24. Radovancevic B, McGiffin DC, Kobashigawa JA et al: A multi-institutional study of cardiac retransplantation: incidence, risk factors for mortality and outcome, *J Heart Lung Transplant* 22:862-868, 2003.

25. Evans RW, Manninen DL, Dong EB et al: Is retransplantation cost effective? *Transplant Proc* 25(1):1694-1696, 1993.

26. Olivari MT, Antolick A, Kaye MP et al: Heart transplantation in elderly patients. *J Heart Transplant* 7(4):258-264,1988.

27. Blanche C, Takkenberg JJM, Nessim S et al: Heart transplantation in patients 65 years of age and older: a comparative analysis of 40 patients, *Ann Thorac Surg* 62:1442-1447, 1996.

28. Luciani GB, Livi U, Faggian G et al: Clinical results of heart transplantation in recipients over 55 years of age with donors over 40 years of age, *J Heart Lung Transplant* 11(6):1177-1183, 1992.

29. Heroux AL, Costanzo-Nordin, MR, O'Sullivan JE et al: Heart transplantation as a treatment option for end-stage heart disease in patients older than 65 years of age, *J Heart Lung Transplant* 12(4):573-579, 1993.

30. Laks H, Scholl FG, Drinkwater DC et al: The alternate recipient list for heart transplantation: does it work? *J Heart Lung Transplant* 16:735-742, 1997.

31. Bussieres LM, Cardella CJ, Daly PA et al: Relationship between preoperative pulmonary status and outcome after heart transplantation, *J Heart Transplant* 9(2):124-128, 1990.

32. Costard-Jackle A, Hill I, Schroeder JS et al: The influence of preoperative patient characteristics on early and late survival following cardiac transplantation, *Circulation* (Supp. III)84(5):329-337, 1991.

33. Butler J, Stankewicz M, Wu J et al: Pre-transplant reversible pulmonary hypertension predicts higher risk for mortality after cardiac transplantation, *J Heart Lung Transplant* 24:170-177, 2005.

34. Bourge RC, Kirklin JK, Naftel DC et al: Analysis and predictors of pulmonary vascular resistance after cardiac transplantation, *J Thorac Cardiovasc Surg* 101:432-445, 1991.

35. Radovancevic B, Konoralp C, Vrtovec B at el: Factors predicting 10-year survival after heart transplant, *J Heart Lung Transplant* 24:156-159, 2005.

36. Czerny M, Sahin V, Zuckerman A: Diabetes affects long-term survival after heart transplantation, *J Heart Lung Transplant* 20:245, 2001.

37. Goldstein DJ, Oz MC, Rose EA et al: Experience with heart transplantation for cardiac tumors, *J Heart Lung Transplant* 14(2)382-386, 1995.

38. Dew MA, Switzer G, DiMartini A et al: Psychosocial assessments and outcome in organ transplantation, *Progress Transplant* 10:239-259, 2000.

39. Bunzel B, Wollenek G. Heart transplantation: are there psychosocial predictors for clinical success of surgery? *Thorac Cardiovasc Surg* 43:103-107, 1994.

40. Frierson RL, Lippmann SB: Heart transplant candidates rejected on psychiatric indications, *Psychosomatics* 28(7):347-355, 1987.

41. Paris W, Muchmore J, Pribil A et al: Study of the relative incidences of psychosocial factors before and heart transplantation and the influence of posttransplantation psychosocial factors on heart transplantation outcome, *J Heart Lung Transplant* 13(3):424-430, 1994.

42. Hosenpud JD, Uretsky BF, Griffith BP et al: Successful intermediate-term outcome for patients with cardiac amyloidosis undergoing heart transplantation: results of a multicenter survey, *J Heart Transplant* 9(4):346-350, 1990.

43. Hosenpud JD, DeMarco T, Frazier OH et al: Progression of systemic disease and reduced long-term survival in patients with cardiac amyloidosis undergoing heart transplantation, *Circulation* (Suppl III)84(5):338-343, 1991.

44. Mieghem WV, Coolen L, Malysse I et al: Amiodaraone and the development of ARDS after lung surgery, *Chest* 105:1645, 1994.

45. Lake KD, Smith CI, Pritzker M et al: Outcomes with hepatitis C following cardiac transplantation—a multiinstitutional study, *J Heart Lung Transplant* 18:81, 1999.

46. Grady K, White-Williams C, Naftel DC et al: Are preoperative obesity and cachexia risk factors for post heart transplant morbidity and mortality: a multiinstitutional study of preoperative weight-height indices? *J Heart Lung Transplant* 18(8):750-763, 1999.

47. Stevenson LW, Dracup KA, Tillisch JH: Efficacy of medical therapy tailored for severe congestive heart failure in patients transferred for urgent cardiac transplantation, *Am J Cardiol* 63:461-464, 1989.

48. Ventura HO, Stapleton DD, VanMeter CH et al: Cardiac transplantation: clinical aspects of recipient selection, *Med Clin N Am* 6(5):1196-1206, 1992.

49. Grady KL, Jalowiec A, Grusk BB et al: Symptom distress in cardiac transplant candidates, *Heart Lung* 21(5):434-439, 1992.

50. Mancini DM, Eisen H, Kussmaul W et al: Value of peak exercise oxygen consumption for optimal timing of cardiac transplantation in ambulatory patients with heart failure, *Circulation* 83(3):778-786, 1991.

51. McCarty PM, Sabik JF: Implantable circulatory support devices as a bridge to heart transplantation, *Sem Thorac Cardiovasc Surg* 6(3):174-180, 1994.

52. Pennington DG, McBride LR, Peigh PS et al: Eight years' experience with bridging to cardiac transplantation, *J Thorac Cardiovasc Surg* 107(2):472-481, 1994.

53. Frazier OH, Macris MP, Myers TJ et al: Improved survival after extended bridge to cardiac transplantation, *Ann Thorac Surg* 57:1416-1422, 1994.

54. www.UNOS.org accessed 8/8/2005.

55. Moriguchi J, Kirklin JK, Stevenson L et al: Risk factors for sudden death in non-urgent (status II) patients awaiting cardiac transplantation, *J Heart Lung Transplant* 16:42, 1997.

56. Stevenson LW, Steimle AE, Fonarow G et al: Improvement in exercise capacity of candidates awaiting heart transplantation, *JACC* 25(1):163-170, 1995.

57. Bogan L, Rosson M, Peterson F: Organ procurement and the donor family, *Crit Care Clinics North Am* 12:23-33, 2000.

58. Zaroff JG, Rosengard BR, Armstrong WF et al: Consensus Conference Report: Maximizing Use of Organs Recovered from the Cadaver Donor: Cardiac Recommendations March 28-29, Crystal City, VA, *Circulation* 106:836-41, 2002.

59. United Network of Organ Sharing Polices 2005, www.UNOS.org

60. Macoviak JA: The perioperative and surgical aspects of heart transplantation, *Cardiol Clin* 8(1):73-82, 1990.

61. Menkis AH, Novick RJ, Kostuk WJ et al: Successful use of the "unacceptable" heart donor, *J Heart Lung Transplant* 10(1):28-32, 1991.

62. Jeevanandam V, Mather P, Furukawa S et al: Adult orthotopic heart transplantation using undersized pediatric donor hearts, *Circulation* 90(5):II74-II77, 1994.

63. Blackbourne LH, Tribble CG, Langenburg SE et al: Successful use of undersized donors for orthotopic heart transplantation—with a caveat, *Ann Thorac Surg* 57:1472-1476, 1994.

64. Pflugfelder PW, Singh NR, McKenzie FN et al: Extending cardiac allograft ischemic time and donor age: effect on survival and long-term cardiac function, *J Heart Lung Transplant* 10(3):394-400, 1991.

65. Schuler S, Matschke K, Loebe M et al: Coronary artery disease in patients with hearts form older donors: morphologic features and therapeutic implications, *J Heart Lung Transplant* 12(1):100-109, 1993.

66. Livi U, Bortolotti U, Luciani GB et al: Donor shortage in heart transplantation: is extension of donor age limits justified? *J Thorac Cardiovasc Surg* 107(5):1346-1355, 1994.

67. Young JB, Naftel DC, Bourge RC et al: Matching the heart donor and heart transplant recipient. Clues for successful expansion of the donor pool: a multivariable, multiinstitutional report, *J Heart Lung Transplant* 13(3):353-365, 1994.

68. Smith M: Physiologic changes during brain stem death—lessons for management of the organ donor, *J Heart Lung Transplant* 23: S217-222. 2004.

69. Blanche C, Czer LS, Valenza M et al: Alternative technique for orthotopic heart transplantation, *Ann Thorac Surg* 57:765-767, 1994.

70. Blanche C, Valenza M, Czer LSC et al: Orthotopic heart transplantation with bicaval and pulmonary venous anastomoses, *Ann Thorac Surg* 58:1505-1509, 1994.

71. Sievers HH, Leyh R, Jahnke A et al: Bicaval versus atrial anastomoses in cardiac transplantation, *J Thorac Cardiovasc Surg* 108(4):780-784, 1994.

72. Kirklin JK: The heart transplant operation. In Kirklin JK, Young J, McGiffin DC, editors: *Heart transplantation,* Philadelphia, 2002, Churchill Livingstone, pp. 339-352.

73. Kirklin JK: Physiology of the transplanted heart. In Kirklin JK, Young J, McGiffin DC, editors: *Heart transplantation,* Philadelphia, 2002, Churchill Livingstone, pp. 353-372.

74. Hosenpud JD, Shipley GD, Wagner CR: Cardiac allograft vasculopathy: current concepts, recent developments, and future direction, *J Heart Lung Transplant* 11(1):9-23, 1992.

75. Halpert I, Goldberg AD, Levine AB et al: Reinnervation of the transplanted human heart as evident from heart rate variability studies, *Am J Cardiol* 77:180-183, 1996.

76. Wilson RF, Christensen BV, Olivari ME et al: Evidence structural sympathetic reinnervation after orthotopic cardiac transplantation in humans, *Circulation* 83:1210-1220, 1991.

77. Wilson RF, McGinn AL, Johnson TH et al: Sympathetic reinnervation after heart transplantation in human beings, *J Heart Lung Transplant* 11(3):S88-S89, 1992.

78. Kirklin JK: Management of the recipient during the transplant hospitalization. In Kirklin JK, Young J, McGiffin DC, editors: *Heart transplantation,* Philadelphia, 2002, Churchill Livingstone, pp. 375-389.

79. Kirklin JK: Immunosuppressive modalities. In Kirklin JK, Young J, McGiffin DC, editors: *Heart transplantation,* Philadelphia, 2002, Churchill Livingstone, pp. 390-463.

80. Hricik DE, Almawi WY, Stomm TB et al: Trends in the use of glucocorticoids in real transplantation, *Transplantation* 57:979, 1994.

81. Price GD, Olsen SL, Taylor DO et al: Corticosteroid-free maintenance immunosuppression after heart transplantation: feasibility and beneficial effects, *J Heart Lung Transplant* 11(2):403-414, 1992.

82. Olivari MT, Jessen ME, Baldwin BJ et al: Triple-drug immunosuppression with steroid discontinuation by six months after heart transplantation, *J Heart Lung Transplant* 14(1):127-135, 1995.

83. Keogh A, Macdonald P, Mundy J et al: Five-year follow-up of a randomized double-drug versus triple-drug therapy immunosuppressive trial after heart transplantation, *J Heart Lung Transplant* 11(3):550-556, 1992.

84. Keogh A, Macdonald P, Harvison A: Initial steroid-free versis steroid-based maintenance therapy and steroid withdrawal after heart transplantation: two views of the steroid question, *J Heart Lung Transplant* 11(2):421-427, 1992.

85. Carrier M, White M, Pellerin M et al: Comparison of Neoral and Sandimmune cyclosporine for induction of immunosuppression after heart transplantation, *Can J Cardiol* 13(5):469-473, 1997.

86. Regazzi MB, Iacona I, Campana C et al: Altered disposition of pravastatin following concomitant drug therapy with cyclosporine in transplant recipients, *Transpl Pro* 25(4):2732-2734, 1993.

87. Vanhaecke J, Van Cleemput J, Van Lierde J et al: Safety and efficacy of low dose simvastatin in cardiac transplant recipients treated with cyclosporine, *Transplantation* 58:42-45, 1994.

88. Armitage JM, Kormos RL, Morita S et al: Clinical trial of FK506 immunosuppression in adult cardiac transplantation, *Ann Thorac Surg* 54:205-211, 1992.

89. Tsamandas AC, Pham SM, Saeberg EC et al: Adult heart transplantation under tacrolimus (FK506) immunosuppression: histopathologic observations and comparison to a cyclosporine-based regimen with lympholytic (ATG) induction, *J Heart Lung Transplant* 723-734, 1997.

90. Taylor DO, Ensley RD, Olsen SL et al: Mycophenolate mofetil (RS-61443): preclinical, clinical, and three-year experience in heart transplantation, *J Heart Lung Transplant* 13(4):571-582, 1994.

91. Kirklin JK, Bourge RC, Naftel DC et al: Treatment of recurrent heart rejection with mycophenolate mofetil (RS-61443): initial clinical experience, *J Heart Lung Transplant* 13(3):444-450, 1994.

92. MacDonald AS, the Rapamune Global Study Group: A worldwide, phase III, randomized controlled safety and efficacy study of a sirolimus/cyclosporine regimen for prevention of acute rejection in recipients of primary mismatched renal allografts, *Transplantation* 71:271-280, 2002.

93. Keogh A, the Sirolimus Cardiac Transplant Trial Group: Sirolimus immunotherapy reduces rates of cardiac allograft rejection: 6-month results from a phase II, open-label study, *Am J Transplant* 2(53):246, 2002.

94. Menkis AH, Powell AM, Novick RJ et al: A prospective randomized controlled trial of initial immunosuppression with ALG versus OKT3 in recipients of cardiac allografts, *J Heart Lung Transplant* 11(3):569-576, 1992.

95. Macdonald PS, Mundy J, Keogh AM et al: A prospective randomized study of prophylactic OKT3 versus equine antithymocyte globulin after heart transplantation—increased morbidity with OKT3, *Transplantation* 55(1):110-116, 1993.

96. Johnson MR, Mullen GM, O'Sullivan EJ et al: Risk/benefit ratio of perioperative OKT3 in cardiac transplantation, *Am J Cardiol* 74:361-266, 1994.

97. Stapleton DD, Ventura HO, Grundtner SE et al: Induction immunosuppression with the monoclonal antibody OKT3 after cardiac transplantation, *Am J Med Sci* 306(1):16-19, 1993.

98. Kobashigawa JA, Stevenson LW, Brownfield E et al: Does short-course induction with OKT3 improve outcome after heart trans-

plantation: a randomized trial, *J Heart Lung Transplant* 12(2):205-208, 1993.

99. Higgins R, Kirkin JK, Brown RN et al: To induce or not to induce: current assessment of perioperative immunosuppression practices and outcomes in heart transplantation, *J Heart Lung Transplant* 24:392-400 2005.

100. Delgado D, Miriuka S, Cusimano R et al: Use of baxiliximab and cyclosporine in heart transplant patients with pre-operative renal dysfunction, *J Heart Lung Transplant* 24:166-169, 2005.

101. Salter MM, Kirklin JK, Bourge RC et al: Total lymphoid irradiation in the treatment of early or recurrent heart rejection, *J Heart Lung Transplant* 11(5):902-912, 1992.

102. Kirklin JK: Cardio allograft rejection. In Kirklin JK, Young J, McGiffin DC, editors: *Heart transplantation*, Philadelphia, 2002, Churchill Livingstone, pp. 464-520.

103. Winters GL: The pathology of heart allograft rejection, *Arch Pathol Lab Med* 115:266-272, 1991.

104. Lavee J, Kormos RL, Duquesnoy RJ et al: Influence of panel-reactive antibody and lymphocytotoxic crossmatch on survival after heart transplantation, *J Heart Lung Transplant* 10(6):921-930, 1991.

105. Loh E, Bergin JD, Couper GS et al: Role of panel-reactive antibody cross-reactivity in predicting survival after orthotopic heart transplantation, *J Heart Lung Transplant* 13(2):194-201, 1994.

106. Pattison JM, Krensky AM: New insights into mechanisms of allograft rejection, *Am J Med Sci* 313(5):257-263, 1997.

107. Baraldi-Junkins C, Levin HR, Kasper EK et al: Complications of endomyocardial biopsy in heart transplant patients, *J Heart Lung Transplant* 12(1):63-67, 1993.

108. Billingham ME, Cary NR, Hammond ME et al: A working formulation for the standardization of nomenclature in the diagnosis of heart and lung rejection, Heart Rejection Study Group, *J Heart Transplant* 9(6):587-593, 1990.

109. Kubo S, Naftel D, Mills R et al: Risk factors for late recurrent rejection after heart transplantation: a multiinstitutional study, *J Heart Lung Transplant* 14:409-418, 1996.

110. Kobashigwa JA, Kirklin JK, Naftel DC et al: Pretransplant risk factors for acute rejection after heart transplantation: a multiinstitutional study, *J Heart Lung Transplant* 12:355-366, 1993.

111. Miller LW: Treatment of cardiac allograft rejection with intravenous corticosteroids, *J Heart Transplant* 9(3):283-287, 1990.

112. Hosenpud JD, Hershberger RE, Ratkovec RR: Methotrexate for the treatment of patients with multiple episodes of acute cardiac allograft rejection, *J Heart Lung Transplant* 11(4):739-745, 1992.

113. Meiser BM, Uberfuhr P, Fuchs A et al: A superior agent to OKT3 for treating cases of persistent rejection after intrathoracic transplantation, *J Heart Lung Transplant* 16:795-800, 1997.

114. Wagoner LE, Taylor DO, Olsen SL et al: Cyclophosphamide in cardiac transplant recipients with frequent rejection: a six-year retrospective review, *Clin Transplant* 10:437-443, 1996.

115. Evans MA, Schomberg PJ, Rodeheffer RJ et al: Total lymphoid irradiation: a novel and successful therapy for resistant cardiac allograft rejection, *Mayo Clin Proc* 67:785-790, 1992.

116. Salter MM, Kirklin JK, Bourge RC et al: Total lymphoid irradiation in the treatment of early or recurrent heart refection, *J Heart Lung Transplant* 11(5):902-912, 1992.

117. Keogh A, Morgan G, Macdonald P et al: Total lymphoid irradiation for resistant rejection after transplantation: only moderate success medium-term, *J Heart Lung Transplant* 15:231-233, 1996.

118. Meiser BM, Kur F, Reichenspurner H et al: Reduction of the incidence of rejection by adjunct immunosuppression with photochemotherapy after heart transplantation, *Transplantation* 57:563-568, 1994.

119. Kirklin J, Brown R, Naftel D et al: Rejection with hemodynamic compromise: objective evidence for efficacy of photopheresis, *J Heart Lung Transplant* 24:566, 2005.

120. Costanzo-Nordin MR, Heroux AL, Radvany R et al: Role of humoral immunity in acute cardiac allograft dysfunction, *J Heart Lung Transplant* 12(2):s143-s146, 1993.

121. Mills RM, Naftel DC, Kirklin JK et al: Heart transplant rejection with hemodynamic compromise: a multiinstitutional study of the role of endomyocardial cellular infiltration, *J Heart Lung Transplant* 16:813-821, 1997.

122. Hammond EH, Yowell RL, Price GD et al: Vascular rejection and its relationship to allograft coronary artery disease, *J Heart Lung Transplant* 11(3):s111-s119, 1992.

123. Ventura HO, Mehra MR, Smart FW et al: Cardiac allograft vasculopathy. Current concepts, *Am Heart J* 129:791-798, 1995.

124. Kirklin JK: Cardiac Allograft vasculopathy. In Kirklin JK, Young J, McGiffin DC, editors: *Heart transplantation*, Philadelphia, 2002, Churchill Livingstone, pp. 615-665.

125. Costanzo M, Naftel D, Pritzker M et al: Heart transplant coronary angiography: a multiinstutional study of preoperative donor and recipient risk factors, *J Heart Lung Transplant* 17:744-753, 1998.

126. Billingham ME: The pathologic changes in long-term heart and lung transplant survivors, *J Heart Lung Transplant* 11(4):S252-S257, 1992.

127. Costanzo-Nordin MR: Cardiac allograft vasculopathy: relationship with acute cellular rejection and histocompatibility, *J Heart Lung Transplant* 11(3):s90-s103, 1992.

128. Kendall TJ, Wilson JE, Radio SJ et al: Cytomegalovirus and other herpes viruses: do they have a role in the development of accelerated coronary arterial disease in human heart allografts? *J Heart Lung Transplant* 11(3):s14-s20, 1992.

129. Johnson MR: Transplant coronary disease: nonimmunologic risk factors, *J Heart Lung Transplant* 11(3):s124-s132, 1992.

130. Schroeder JS, Shao-zhou G, Hunt SA et al: Accelerated graft coronary artery disease: diagnosis and prevention, *J Heart Lung Transplant* 11(4):S58-S265, 1992.

131. Mehra MR, Ventura HO, Smart FW et al: New developments in the diagnosis and management of cardiac allograft vasculopathy, *Tex Heart Inst J* 22:138-144, 1995.

132. Luckraz H, Charman S, Wreghitt T et al: Does cytomegalovirus status influence acute and chronic rejection in heart transplantation during the ganciclovir prophylaxis era? *J Heart Lung Transplant* 22:1023-1027, 2003.

133. Fraizer OH, Vega JD, Dunsan JM et al: Coronary artery bypass two years after orthotopic heart transplantation: a case report. *J Heart Lung Transplant* 10(6):1036-1040, 1991.

134. Halle III AA, Wilson RF, Vetrovec GW: Multicenter evaluation of percutaneous transluminal coronary angioplasty in heart transplant recipients, *J Heart Lung Transplant* 11(3):S138-S141, 1992.

135. Miller LW, Naftel DC, Bourge RC et al: Infection after heart transplantation: a multiinstitutional study, *J Heart Lung Transplant* 13(3):381-393, 1994.

136. Kirklin JK: Infections after heart transplantation. In Kirklin JK, Avery R, Pappas P, editors: *Heart transplantation*, Philadelphia, 2002, Churchill Livingstone, pp. 521-583.

137. Smart FW, Naftel DC, Costanzo MR et al: Risk factors for early, cumulative, and fatal infections after heart transplantation: a multiinstitutional study, *J Heart Lung Transplant* 15:329-341, 1996.

138. Merigan TC, Renlund DG, Keay S et al: A controlled trial of ganciclovir to prevent cytomegalovirus disease after heart transplantation, *N Engl J Med* 326(18):1182-1186, 1992.

139. Macdonald PS, Keogh AM, Marshman D et al: A double-blind placebo-controlled trial of low-dose ganciclovir to prevent cytomegalovirus disease after heart transplantation, *J Heart Lung Transplant* 14(1):32-38, 1995.

140. Kirklin JK: Other long term complications. In Kirklin JK, McGiffin DC, Young J, editors: *Heart transplantation*, Philadelphia, 2002, Churchill Livingstone, 4666-4702.

141. Kobashigawa J, Kasiake B: Hyperlipidemia in solid organ transplantation, *Transplantation* 63:331-338, 1997.

142. Kobashigawa J, Katznelson, Laks H et al: Effect of pravastatin on outcomes after cardiac transplantation, *N Engl J Med* 333:621, 1995.

143. Zietse R, Balk A, Doprel M et al: Time course decline in renal function in cyclosporine-treated heart transplant recipients, *Am J Nephrol* 14:1-5, 1994.

144. Bantle J, Paller M, Boudrzau R et al: Long term effects of cyclosporine on renal function in organ transplant recipients, *J Lab Clin Med* 115:233-240, 1990.

145. Dresdale AR, Lutz S, Drost C et al: Prospective evaluation of malignant neoplasm in cardiac transplant recipients uniformly treated with prophylactic antilymphocyte globulin, *J Thorac Cardiovasc Surg* 106:1202-1207, 1993.

146. Olivari MT, Diekmann RA, Kubo SH et al: Low incidence of neoplasia in heart and heart-lung transplant recipients receiving triple-drug immunosuppression, *J Heart Lung Transplant* 9(6):618-621, 1990.

147. DeSalvo T, Naftel D, Kasper E et al: The differing hazard of lymphoma vs other malignancies in the current era, *J Heart Lung Transplant* 17:70, 1998.

148. Kerschan-Schindf K, Strametz-Juranek J, Heinze G et al: Pathogenesis of bone loss in transplant candidates and recipients, *J Heart Lung Transplant* 22:843-850, 2003.

149. Cates J, Chavez M, Laks H: Gastrointestinal complications after cardiac transplantation: a spectrum of diseases, *Am J Gastroenterol* 86:412-416, 1991.

150. Opelz G, Wujciak MS: The influence of HLA compatibility on graft survival after heart transplantation, *N Engl J Med* 330(12):816-819, 1994.

151. Mai FM, McKenzie FN, Kostuk WJ: Psychosocial adjustment and quality of life following heart transplantation, *Can J Psychiatr* 35(3):223-227, 1990.

152. Grady KL, Jalowic A, White-Williams C: Improvement in quality of life in heart failure patients who undergo transplantation, *J Heart Lung Transplant* 15(8):749-757, 1996.

153. Walden JA, Stevenson L, Dracup K et al: Heart transplantation may not improve quality of life for patients with stable heart failure, *Heart Lung* 18(5):497-506, 1989.

154. Bunzel B, Grundbock A, Laczkovics A et al: Quality of life after orthotopic heart transplantation, *J Heart Lung Transplant* 10(3):455-459, 1991.

155. Cain N, Sharples LD, England TAH et al: Prospective study comparing quality of life before and after heart transplantation, *Transplant Proc* 22(4):1437-1439, 1990.

156. Bohachick P, Anton BB, Wooldrige PJ et al: Psychosocial outcome six months after heart transplant surgery: a preliminary report, *Res Nurs Health* 15:165-173, 1992.

157. Jones BM, Taylor F, Downs K et al: Longitudinal study of quality of life and psychological adjustment after cardiac transplantation, *Med J Aust* 157:24-26, 1992.

158. Mulligan T, Sheehan H, Hanrahan J: Sexual function after heart transplantation, *J Heart Lung Transplant* 10(1):125-128, 1991.

159. Evans RW: Socioeconomic aspects of heart transplantation, *Curr Opin Cardiol* 10:169-179, 1995.

160. Aufiero TX, Reddy RC, Magovern JA et al: Alternatives to human heart replacement, *Curr Opin Cardiol* 10:218-222, 1995.

161. Minanov OP, Itescu S, Michler RE: Recent advances and the potential for clinical use of xenotransplantation, *Curr Opin Cardiol* 11:214-220, 1996.

162. Cozzi E, White D: The generation of transgenic pigs as potential organ donors for humans, *Nat Med* I:964-966, 1995.

chapter 68

Care of Patients with Cardiac Trauma

Beth Broering

INCIDENCE

Trauma is the leading cause of death in persons younger than age 45 and the fourth leading cause of death in the United States. More than 20 percent of deaths are due to thoracic trauma.[1] The majority of these injuries and fatalities are related to motor vehicle collisions. Whereas the incidence of injury to thoracic structures is high, the true incidence of cardiac injury is unknown.[2] Vague terms have been used to define blunt cardiac injury (myocardial concussion, cardiac contusion), which vary from clinically insignificant electrocardiogram (**ECG**) abnormalities to catastrophic hemopericardium or chamber wall rupture. Investigators have reported the incidence of blunt cardiac trauma to be as high as 76 percent in patients with severe thoracic or multisystem injury.[3] Penetrating cardiac injuries are highly lethal and account for an estimated 10 percent of all gunshot wounds.[2] Immediate deaths are caused by direct penetration of the heart by the wounding agent (e.g., bullet, knife), and these patients seldom reach the hospital. With advances in prehospital care and transport systems, many patients with potentially life-threatening injuries may be relatively asymptomatic. Prompt evaluation and treatment are critical.

CAUSES AND TRAUMA PATTERNS

Common causes of cardiac injury include both blunt and penetrating mechanisms (Box 68-1). Iatrogenic injuries from central line insertion, invasive procedures, such as cardiac catheterization, stenting, and thoracostomy tube insertion are much less common, but may be highly lethal if the cause of a patient's clinical deterioration is not recognized and treated quickly. Indirect cardiac insult may be seen in the critically ill or injured patient as a result of significant shock and cellular hypo-

perfusion. A patient with no prior cardiovascular disease may develop cardiac dysfunction as a result of sepsis, the systemic inflammatory response syndrome, or multisystem organ failure.

The spectrum of cardiac injury can be seen in all ages and ethnicities. Blunt cardiac injury in children is more likely related to child abuse or sports-related injuries; whereas in the remainder of the population, it is commonly related to motor vehicle collisions or falls. Men, particularly young men, are less likely to wear seat belts and therefore are at higher risk for serious thoracic injury. Young, black men have the highest incidence of penetrating injuries and are often victims of homicide related to gunshot wounds and stab wounds.[4] In the Hispanic population, motor vehicle collisions and homicide are the leading causes of death.[4] Understanding the injury trends for one's local region helps in planning and identifying opportunities for community education and injury prevention.

Blunt Cardiac Injury

Blunt cardiac injuries (**BCIs**) are most commonly due to motor vehicle collisions, falls, and direct blows to the chest wall. The mechanism of injury and kinetic energy are significant factors when determining the risk for myocardial and associated injuries. Mechanism of injury is the process by which the injury occurred (i.e., motor vehicle collision). Factors associated with mechanisms of injury include the direction, duration of force, and area of the body to which a force is applied. The forces of kinetic energy refer to the amount of energy or force transferred to the human body during the event. If forces exceed body tissue stress and strain thresholds, injury can result. In motor vehicle collisions, there are three separate collisions that occur. The first collision is when the vehicle crashes into another object. The victim's body continues in motion until it collides with the vehicle's interior structures, the second collision, and the third collision occurs when the internal organs and tissues impact against the rigid body structures.

A rapid deceleration type of injury occurs with a fall, landing on a solid surface or when a moving vehicle stops suddenly during a collision. Rapid deceleration produces shearing or traction forces on vessels, on the heart, and its supporting structures.[1] Major vessels may be sheared from their point of fixation on the myocardium resulting in rapid exsanguination. Falls from heights *greater than* 20 feet are considered significant and may be associated with a higher incidence of cardiac injury. In one study, 61 deaths were attributable to falls *greater than* 6 meters; 54 percent of victims had cardiac injury, and 76 percent had multiple cardiac injuries.[5] Pericardial tears were the most frequent finding. Myocardial hematomas, transmural tears, and ruptures of the right coronary artery were also found on autopsy and were associated with falls from heights *greater than* 15 meters (49 feet).

Direct pressure on the myocardium occurs during compressive forces as the heart is "pinned" between the sternum and thoracic spine. The right atrium and ventricle are at greatest risk for injury as a result of the anatomical location beneath the sternum. Direct force to the heart can occur from assaults or other incidents when the patient sustains a direct blow to the chest. The spectrum of injury can range from a minor bruise on the myocardium to cardiac rupture. Associated injuries include rib and sternal fractures, pulmonary contusions, and pneumothoraces. Patients who come to the emergency department after a motor vehicle collision with chest wall contusions or "seat belt signs" should be evaluated for underlying thoracic and cardiac injury.

Indirect forces, such as the hydraulic effects of severe abdominal, pelvic, or lower extremity compression, lead to increased intrathoracic and elevated venous pressures resulting in pericardial rupture.[3] This pattern of injury is less common; nonetheless, it requires a high index of suspicion when a patient with known pelvic or abdominal trauma from crush or compressive injuries has evidence of cardiac dysfunction despite aggressive resuscitation and stabilization procedures.

Penetrating Cardiac Injury

Penetrating injuries are most commonly caused by gunshot wounds and stab wounds. The location of a chest wall wound can often predict the location of cardiac injury, particularly with stab wounds. As with blunt injuries, because of the anatomical location, the right ventricle is at greatest risk for injury followed by the left ventricle.[6] More than one third of penetrating injuries involve multiple cardiac structures.[6] Gunshot wounds have a higher mortality rate than stab wounds, and victims often are in cardiac arrest. Injuries may be caused by small caliber handguns, high-energy automatic and semiautomatic weapons, or multiple pellets after shotgun injury. Shotgun pellets have the potential to embed or embolize occluding the coronary circulation. Patients may have symptoms typical of an acute myocardial infarction. Penetrating cardiac injury from fractured ribs is extremely rare and *less than* 10 cases have been reported in the literature.[7] Right and left ventricles are again at highest risk for this pattern of injury.

Iatrogenic and Other Mechanisms of Injury

Iatrogenic cardiac injuries can occur with central line insertion in the left subclavian or left internal jugular vein. Common sites of injury include the superior caval-atrial junction and the superior vena cava-innominate junction. Electrical injuries are responsible for more than 1000 deaths annually in the United States.[2] Death is a result of cardiac arrest, and more than one third of patients manifest a cardiac component with electrocution. Common ECG (electrocardiogram) changes include sinus tachycardia, nonspecific changes in the ST segment and T wave, or more serious conduction disturbances.[8]

Hemorrhage, shock, burns, sepsis, and multisystem trauma may lead to the development of the systemic inflammatory response syndrome. Cardiac dysfunction is a result of the effects of multiple inflammatory mediators on the myocardium. The exact mechanisms responsible for this dysfunction are not clearly understood. Clinical manifestations include dysrhythmias, myocardial depression, diminished response to adrenergic stimulation, and altered calcium utilization.[2]

CLINICAL PRESENTATION AND PATHOPHYSIOLOGY
Blunt Cardiac Injury

In most cases cardiac injury is minor, and patients are asymptomatic. More severe blunt injuries include septal rupture, valvular dysfunction, papillary muscle or cordae tendineae rupture, and although extremely rare, cardiac wall rupture. Myocardial rupture occurs when blood-filled chambers are compressed with enough force to generate a tear in the chamber wall or septum or to rupture a cardiac valve.

Cell membrane destruction, myocyte necrosis, tearing of muscle fibers, and microvascular hemorrhage occur in focal or diffuse areas of the myocardium. Unlike the ischemia and myocardial injury of coronary artery occlusion, the epicardium is the primary site of injury in blunt trauma. Severe contusions may extend transmurally resulting in significant cardiac dysfunction.

Patients with BCI may have a wide range of clinical signs and symptoms from being completely asymptomatic to hemodynamically unstable. It requires careful evaluation to determine if the patient's symptoms are related to cardiac injury or to other traumatic injuries, hemorrhage, and shock. The common signs and symptoms of blunt cardiac injury are relatively nonspecific. Patients complain of chest pain, dyspnea, and nausea. The pain may be anginal in nature, but is more likely related to concomitant thoracic trauma including rib and/or sternal fractures and chest wall contusions.

Electrocardiographic changes may or may not be present, but are also nonspecific (Box 68-2). Dysrhythmias are due to the increased levels of catecholamines, hypoxic areas of the myocardium, and direct damage to conduction pathways. Common dysrhythmias include sinus tachycardia, ST-segment elevation or depression, and T-wave inversion and usually resolve within several hours of presentation. Electrocardiographic changes that correspond to clinically significant cardiac injury are usually present at the time of admission and range from atrial fibrillation, atrioventricular blocks, and bundle branch blocks to ventricular tachycardia and fibrillation.

Severe cardiac dysfunction, tamponade, or hemorrhage may be seen with septal rupture, valvular dysfunction, or myocardial rupture. Hypotension and low cardiac output are present despite volume resuscitation. Early in tamponade, tachycardia, increases in ventricular filling pressure, and enhanced myocardial contractility from endogenous catecholamines result in augmentation of right ventricular diastolic filling. Clinical signs include pulsus paradoxus, Kussmaul sign (increase in jugular venous distention on inspiration), and narrowing pulse pressure. The classic findings of cardiac tamponade (Beck triad) including muffled heart sounds, jugular venous distension, and hypotension may be seen in only 10 percent of patients.[2] Patients with valvular lesions may have either systolic or diastolic murmurs.[1]

Penetrating Cardiac Injury

Any penetrating wound in the "box," (Figure 68-1) between the clavicles and subxiphoid area and between the midclavicular lines, endangers the mediastinal structures.[9] Clinical presentation may range from asymptomatic to moribund and is dependent on the size and loca-

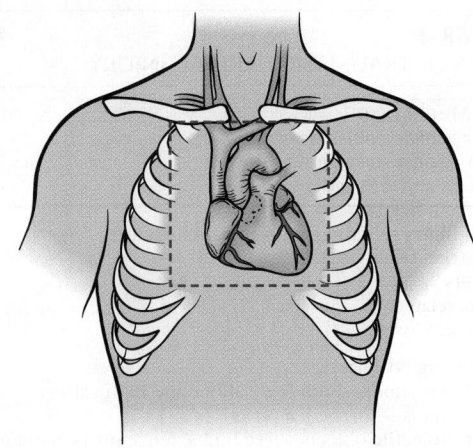

FIGURE 68-1 ■ Precordial "box" of penetrating cardiac trauma. (From Rozycki, G S et al: The role of ultrasound in patients with possible penetrating cardiac wounds: a prospective multicenter study, *Journal of Trauma* 46(4):543-552, 1999.)

BOX 68-3 ■ ■ ■
PENETRATING CARDIAC INJURIES SIGNS AND SYMPTOMS

- Severe hypotension
- Distended jugular veins
- Elevated central venous pressure
- Muffled heart sounds
- Decreased electrocardiogram voltage
- Hemothorax
- Pneumothorax

---

tion of the injury and the extent of hemorrhage (Box 68-3). More than 80 percent of patients with stab wounds have tamponade, but this is seldom present in gunshot wounds.[6] Minor injuries to the coronary arteries may have coronary occlusion and myocardial insufficiency.

Electrical Injury

The extent of myocardial damage from electrical injury is associated with the voltage and type of current. Higher voltage or alternating current is associated with more severe injury. Direct necrosis of myocardial cells may be focal or diffuse and usually consists of patchy contraction band necrosis of the myocardium, nodal tissue, conduction pathways, and coronary arteries.[10] Even low current exposure can produce rhythm disturbances that can include ventricular fibrillation. Lightning acts as a massive countershock that causes asystole or cardiac standstill. There may be a spontaneous return of sinus rhythm after lightning strike caused by the inherent cardiac property of automaticity of the heart.

Rhythm disturbances are due to the myocardial necrosis, changes in myocyte membrane permeability, and alteration in the Na^+-K^+-adenosine triphosphatase concentration.[10]

EVALUATION AND TREATMENT
Emergency/Resuscitative Phase

When caring for a patient with suspected cardiac injury, the patient's hemodynamic stability and response to initial interventions will determine the course of evalu-

---

BOX 68-2 ■ ■ ■
ELECTROCARDIOGRAPHIC FINDINGS IN BLUNT CARDIAC INJURY

Dysrhythmias
- Sinus tachycardia
- Atrial and ventricular ectopy
- Atrial fibrillation
- Ventricular tachycardia
- Ventricular fibrillation
- Sinus bradycardia
- Atrial tachycardia

Nonspecific Abnormalities
- Pericarditis-like ST segment elevation or depression
- Prolonged QT interval

Conduction Disorders
- Right bundle branch block
- Fascicular block
- AV nodal blocks

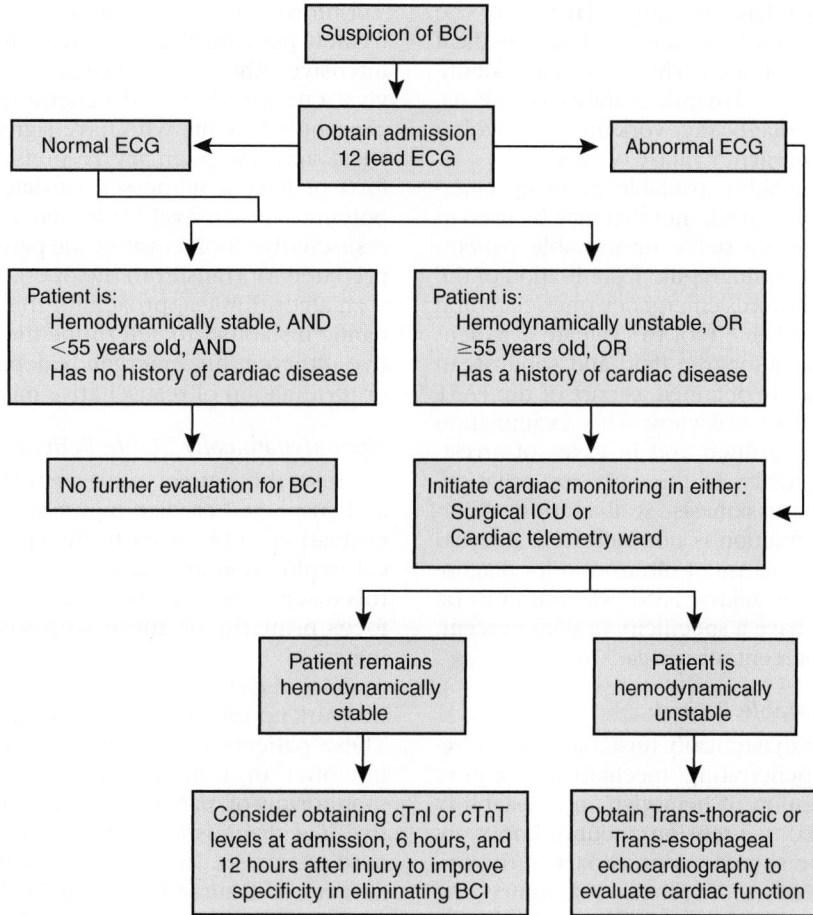

FIGURE 68-2 ▪ Evaluation of the patient with suspected blunt cardiac injury. *BCI,* Blunt cardiac injury; *cTnI,* cardiac troponin I; *cTnT,* cardiac troponin T; *ECG,* electrocardiogram; *ICU,* intensive care unit. (From Schultz, J M, Trunkey, DD: Blunt cardiac injury, *Critical Care Clinics* 20:57-70, 2004.)

ation and definitive management (Figure 68-2). In any patient with traumatic injury, a primary, secondary, and focused assessment should be performed based on advanced trauma life support guidelines (Box 68-4). All patients should receive supplemental oxygen. If the patient's airway is patent, oxygen can be administered via nasal cannula or nonrebreather mask. Endotracheal intubation should be considered in any patient who cannot protect their airway or with multisystem injury and

hemodynamic instability. Assessment of breathing should include respiratory rate, work of breathing, breath sounds, and inspection for open or sucking chest wounds. Patients with cardiac injury frequently have concomitant rib fractures, flail chests, pneumothoraces, or hemothoraces.

In patients with severe ventilatory compromise, mechanical ventilation should be considered to improve oxygenation. Fluid resuscitation with crystalloids via two large-bore intravenous catheters is the accepted standard in the trauma setting. Any patient who is hypotensive should receive an initial 2-liter bolus with ongoing resuscitation based upon patient response. Central venous access via the femoral, subclavian, or internal jugular veins allows for larger catheter and/or Cordis placement and rapid volume administration and measurement of central venous pressure. Patients with hemodynamic instability, penetrating injuries, or multisystem injuries will likely require early transfusion of blood products. Type and crossmatch should be obtained and sent for laboratory processing as early as possible after patient presentation.

Once the primary assessment is completed and life-threatening problems are corrected, a secondary survey is performed. The secondary survey is a complete head-to-toe assessment in an attempt to identify all potential

---

BOX 68-4 ▪ ▪ ▪
PRIMARY AND SECONDARY ASSESSMENT

Primary Assessment
- Airway
- Breathing
- Circulation
- Disability, neurological status

Secondary Assessment
- History, mechanism of injury, medical and surgical history, prior treatment
- Head-to-toe physical exam
- Initiate continuous cardiac monitoring

Focused Assessment
- Detailed examination of patient complaints or findings on head-to-toe examination

injuries the patient may have sustained. History of the mechanism of injury, prior treatment, and past medical and surgical history is obtained. The injuries are identified, and the overall hemodynamic stability of the patient should direct the diagnostic work-up and ongoing management in the emergency phase of care.

Ultrasonography is readily available in many emergency departments and is an adjunct that may be used in both the hemodynamically stable or unstable patient. Focused Assessment for Sonographic Examination of the Trauma Patient (**FAST**) affords emergency physicians and surgeons a rapid and reliable tool to evaluate a patient with blunt truncal injury for free fluid and solid organ injury. One view routinely obtained as part of the FAST examination is the pericardial view. This examination evaluates for hemopericardium and in cases of arrest, presence of cardiac activity. In the early resuscitation, detailed evaluation for dyskinesis, wall motion abnormalities, and ejection fraction is not indicated. Rozycki and colleagues studied the use of ultrasound for diagnosis of penetrating cardiac injury. FAST was found to be 100 percent sensitive, have a specificity of 96.6 percent, and accuracy of 97.3 percent for cardiac injury.[11]

Hemodynamically Unstable Patient

Patients who are hemodynamically unstable or in extremis from blunt or penetrating mechanisms require rapid surgical intervention. If hemodynamic instability is thought to be related to a tension pneumothorax, insertion of a chest tube should occur as part of the primary assessment. In cases of penetrating injury, the chest tube should be inserted through a separate incision and not the traumatic wound to reduce the potential for empyema. When a hemothorax is suspected or confirmed, autotransfusion should be considered. Most chest drainage systems offer prepackaged autotransfusion units. Large defects in the chest wall compromise respiration, and air preferentially passes through the wound instead of the airway.[9] If a sucking chest wound is present, the wound should be covered with an occlusive dressing taped on three sides. This serves as a flutter valve to release pleural air and prevents insufflation of outside air.

Both pericardiocentesis and thoracotomy are procedures that may be performed in the emergency department once a diagnosis of pericardial tamponade or cardiac injury with hemorrhage is established. Many emergency departments and trauma centers have sterile trays or resuscitation carts prepared and packaged specifically for these resuscitative procedures. Nurses and other personnel working in the emergency department need to be familiar with the location and setup of sterile trays and equipment for these procedures. Pericardiocentesis for hemopericardium acts as a temporizing measure and may result in a temporary improvement in a patient's vital signs and overall clinical status allowing for prompt transfer to the operating room for definitive surgical management. Once the pericardiocentesis is performed, a catheter may be left in place for repeated aspiration. This technique may be beneficial in situations where surgical capability is not readily available, and a patient must be transferred to a tertiary care facility.

Unfortunately, resuscitative thoracotomy has an extremely poor survival rate, in addition to being resource intensive. Rhee and colleagues found a combined survival rate for blunt and penetrating trauma of only 7.4 percent.[12] Patients who have signs of life (cardiac electrical activity, pupillary response, and respiratory effort) or have a witnessed cardiac arrest have a better potential for survival.[2,12] If vital signs are restored after resuscitative thoracotomy, the patient should be quickly prepared for transfer to the operating room. Figure 68-3 is an algorithmic approach for the patient with hemodynamic instability to determine the need for rapid operative intervention, emergency department thoracotomy, or termination of resuscitative measures.

Hemodynamically Stable Patient

Because the patient with penetrating thoracic injury and suspected cardiac injury will likely undergo rapid evaluation and transfer to the operating room for surgical exploration and definitive management of injuries, this discussion on hemodynamically stable patients will focus primarily on those with suspected blunt cardiac injury.

Once the secondary survey is complete, the diagnostic work-up for suspected cardiac injury is determined. These patients with suspected cardiac injury have the potential to rapidly decompensate, and continuous monitoring of patient hemodynamic status is imperative. The diagnostic criteria are vague, and no gold-standard test exists. In 1998 the Eastern Association for the Surgery of Trauma (**EAST**) published practice management guidelines for screening of blunt cardiac injury.[13]

All patients in whom BCI is suspected should have a baseline or admission ECG.[13] The ECG can provide a sensitivity of 100 percent, but a specificity of *less than* 50 percent in the detection of BCI.[3] If the admission ECG is normal, the risk for significant blunt cardiac injury is low. Positive findings on admission ECG include the presence of dysrhythmias, ischemic changes, or heart block. In most cases of suspected or confirmed blunt cardiac injury, continuous cardiac monitoring for 24 to 48 hours along with serial 12-lead ECGs every 12 hours is recommended. Admission to a unit where continuous cardiac monitoring can be provided is suggested. Admission to an intensive care unit is not necessary unless hemodynamic stability or other traumatic injuries warrant closer observation and invasive hemodynamic monitoring. Patients who have preexisting heart disease or are older than age 55 should be considered at higher risk for complications of BCI, and continuous cardiac monitoring for 24 hours despite a normal ECG is recommended.[13]

Controversy exists over the use of cardiac enzymes as a determinant of blunt cardiac injury. Trauma patients typically have some component of skeletal muscle injury with a subsequent release of creatine kinase (**CK**) making CK irrelevant in the diagnosis of BCI. CK-MB is more specific to myocardial muscle damage, but in the multiply injured patient, high concentrations of CK may result in false-positive elevations of the MB fraction. Cardiac troponins (**cTnI** and **cTnT**) are highly specific to myocardial injury and are not found in skeletal mus-

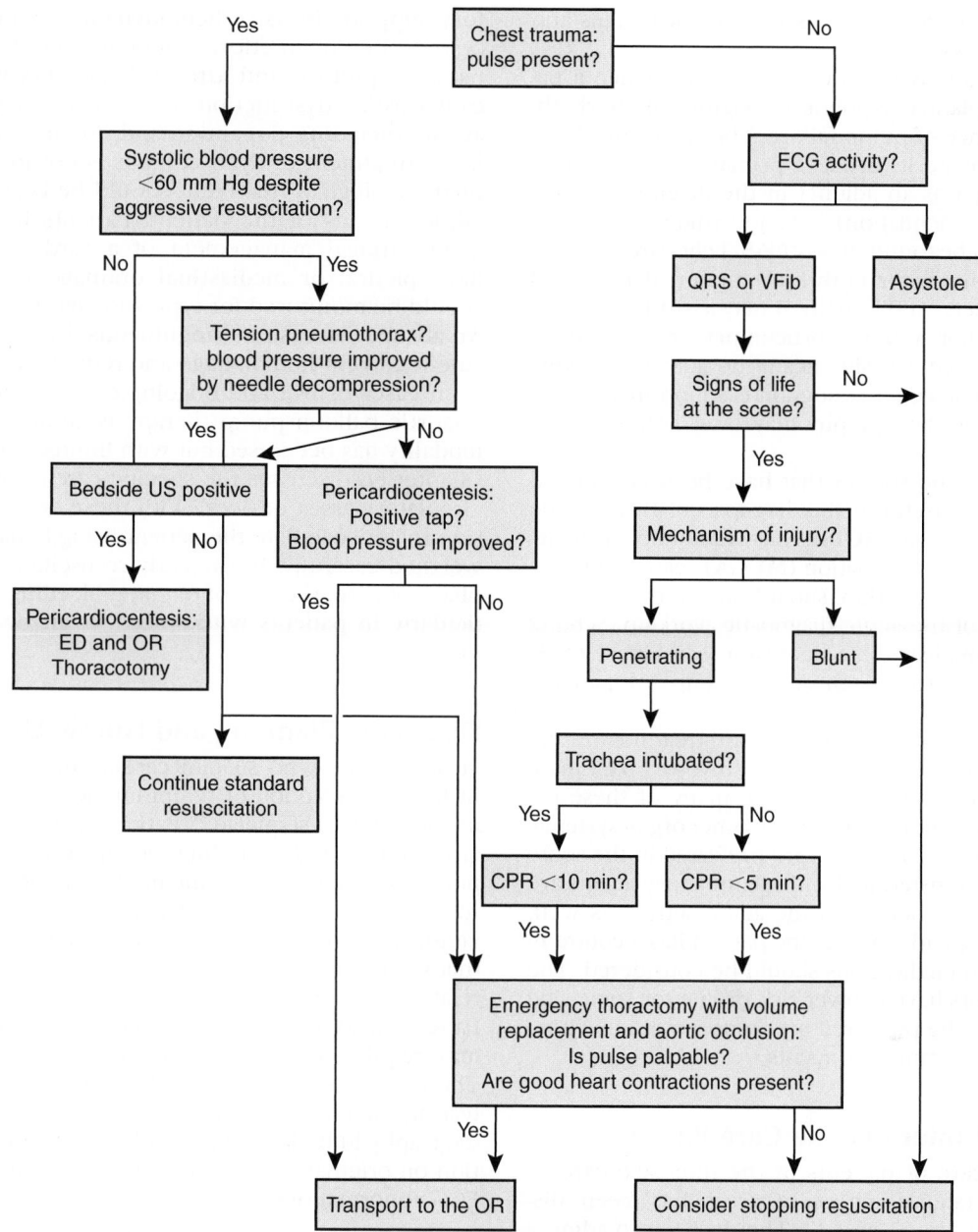

FIGURE 68-3 ▨ Algorithm for determining need for emergency thoracotomy in chest/cardiac trauma. *CPR,* Cardiopulmonary resuscitation; *ECG,* electrocardiogram; *ED,* emergency department; *OR,* operating room; *VFib,* ventricular fibrillation. (From Roberts JR, Hedges JR, editors: *Clinical procedures in emergency medicine,* ed 4, Philadelphia, 2004,WB Saunders.)

cles. The 1998 EAST guidelines reported that cardiac enzymes, including TnI, added no important clinical value in the diagnosis of BCI. More recent studies, however, have found TnI to be helpful in this diagnosis.[14,15]

Salim and colleagues recommend at least 24 hours of cardiac monitoring when a patient has both an abnormal admission ECG and elevated TnI.[15] In this study, the ECG had a positive predictive value of 28 percent and negative predictive value of 95 percent. TnI had a positive predictive value of 48 percent and negative predictive value of 93 percent. When both tests were abnormal or normal, the positive and negative predictive values increased to 62 percent and 100 percent respectively.[15] More recently Velmahos and colleagues reconfirmed this recommendation and hypothesis that if both

the admission and 8-hour follow-up TnI and ECG are normal, BCI may be safely ruled out. Those patients with abnormal results on both ECG and TnI should be monitored for 24 hours.[14]

The question remains, using objective criteria, who is at risk for clinically significant BCI? In their study, Velmahos and colleagues defined major blunt trauma as multiple rib fractures, sternal fracture, pulmonary contusion occupying more than 20 percent of the lung, hemopneumothorax requiring thoracostomy tube drainage, scapular fracture, and significant anterior thoracic seat belt marks. Therefore when assessing patients during the initial work-up, consideration of these injuries along with baseline abnormalities of ECG and TnI may represent high risk for blunt cardiac injury. Ongoing assessment and management based on clinical signs and symptoms are essential.

Echocardiography is another useful test when a patient has unexplained hypotension, significant dysrhythmias, or evidence of pump failure. The FAST guidelines do not recommend its use as a primary screening modality but rather as an adjunct in the diagnosis of BCI (level II recommendation).[13] Echocardiographic findings of BCI can be found in Box 68-5. Echocardiography evaluates the heart for both wall motion defects and structural defects. Additionally, it may assist in the diagnosis of hemothorax, blunt aortic injury, or major vessel injury. If the patient has significant thoracic wall trauma or a transthoracic echocardiogram is suboptimal, transesophageal echocardiography may offer better evaluation.

Other diagnostic studies that have been considered but that are not useful in the diagnosis of BCI include computed tomography (CT) scans, radionuclide imaging, multiple gated acquisition (MUGA) scans, and thallium scans. Therefore they should not be routinely ordered as part of the acute diagnostic work-up. Schultz and Trunkey published an algorithm (see Figure 68-3) that summarizes the diagnostic work-up for patients with suspected BCI.

Along with the diagnostic work-up, treatment of patients with suspected cardiac injury involves pain management. As previously mentioned, many of these patients will have traumatic injuries to other organ systems. Parenteral narcotic analgesics are preferred in the acute phase of care. Nonsteroidal antiinflammatory agents are useful as adjunct therapy in the acute setting as well. Risk of bleeding and whether the patient has a contraindication to oral medications should be considered. The COX-2 inhibitors have a lower risk profile for some side effects and may be preferred over more traditional nonsteroidal antiinflammatory agents.

Critical and Intermediate Care Phase

The general care of patients in the intensive care or intermediate (step-down) care areas has been discussed in Chapters 21 and 22. The decision to admit a patient to a critical care or monitored setting is often based on the patient's overall injuries and hemodynamic status. Most patients, particularly those with isolated cardiac injury, simply require close observation. Oxygenation can be maximized through ventilatory support. Invasive hemodynamic monitoring may be indicated in an effort to monitor and maximize the patient's preload and afterload. Patients with significant cardiac dysfunction may benefit from inotropic agents including dopamine and dobutamine. Prophylactic treatment of dysrhythmias is not indicated, and pharmacological treatment should be based upon the clinical status of the patient. Patients having undergone surgical management of a cardiac injury may have pleural or mediastinal drainage tubes. Output should be monitored for type and amount of drainage. An abrupt increase in sanguineous drainage may indicate recurrent hemorrhage and require reexploration.

In cases of BCI and ongoing cardiogenic shock, intraaortic balloon pump therapy is an alternative. This modality has been used but with limited effectiveness.[6] Chapter 66 discusses the specific care of patients with circulatory assist devices. With these devices, the decision to anticoagulate the patient using heparin must be weighed carefully. In the early resuscitation and acute phase of care, the risk of ongoing bleeding is high, particularly in patients with spleen, liver, or intracranial injury.

Discharge Planning and Follow-Up

Most patients who sustain cardiac injury, particularly BCI, have resolution of symptoms within 24 hours and no long-term sequelae.[3] Patient education revolves around their understanding the injury and symptoms of potential complications including fatigue, dyspnea, irregular pulse rate, or chest pain. The difficulty in providing patient education specific for cardiac injury is that many patients will have fatigue, dyspnea, and pain related to trauma, hospitalization, and other injuries. Patients who have undergone surgical repair of injuries may require teaching on wound or incision site care. There are no evidence-based guidelines for follow-up testing. Some studies recommend follow-up echocardiography in patients with evidence of cardiac dysfunction on original echocardiogram or who had persistent ECG abnormalities.[2]

Complications

Complications of traumatic cardiac injuries are uncommon, but include pericarditis, valve and/or papillary muscle rupture, intracardiac fistulas, and delayed tamponade. Pericarditis may develop days to weeks after the injury. Chest pain, fever, friction rub, and ECG changes are typical findings on physical examination. Effusion and symptoms of pericardial tamponade may also develop. Late development of constrictive pericarditis is possible, but uncommon.

Although extremely rare, valve rupture and subsequent mitral or tricuspid regurgitation from blunt trauma is a potential early or delayed complication.[16,17] The aortic valve is the most common site of lesion.[16] Evidence of a new systolic murmur, new onset of right bundle branch block, or development of congestive heart failure warrant further investigation and should be evaluated by echocardiography.

BOX 68-5 ■ ■ ■
ECHOCARDIOGRAPHIC FINDINGS OF ACUTE BLUNT CARDIAC INJURY

- Regional wall motion abnormalities
- Pericardial effusion
- Valvular lesions
- Right and left ventricular enlargement
- Ventricular septum rupture
- Intracardiac thrombus
- Aortic dissection or rupture (transesophageal echocardiography)

SUMMARY

The incidence of cardiac injury ranges from 10 percent to 75 percent for both blunt and penetrating mechanisms. Penetrating injuries are highly lethal and require rapid surgical intervention to maximize survival. Blunt cardiac injuries are more common, but the true diagnosis is difficult to make. No gold standard exists for diagnosis or management. Fortunately, most patients of both blunt and penetrating mechanisms recover without significant long-term sequelae. A multidisciplinary approach with nurses, physicians, surgeons, and allied health care providers will afford the best outcomes for these patients.

REFERENCES

1. Rosen CL, Wolfe RE: Blunt chest trauma. In Ferrara PC, Colucciello SA, Marx JA et al, editors: *Trauma management: an emergency medicine approach,* St Louis, 2001, Mosby, pp 332-358.
2. Mattox KL, Estrera AL, Wall MJ: Traumatic heart disease. In Braunwald E, Zipes DP, Libby P, editors: *Heart disease: a textbook of cardiovascular medicine,* Philadelphia, 2001, WB Saunders.
3. Schultz JM, Trunkey DD: Blunt cardiac injury, *Crit Care Clin* 20:57-70, 2004.
4. National Center for Injury Prevention and Control: *Injury Fact Book 2001-2002,* Atlanta, 2001, Centers for Disease Control and Prevention.
5. Turk EE, Tsokos M: Blunt cardiac trauma caused by fatal falls from height: an autopsy-based assessment of the injury pattern, *J Trauma* 57:301-4, 2004.
6. Ivatury RR: The injured heart. In Mattox KL, Feliciano DV, Moore EE, editors: *Trauma,* New York, 2004, McGraw-Hill, pp 555-568.
7. Patetsios P, Priovolos S, Slesinger TL et al: Laceration of the left ventricle from rib fractures after blunt trauma, *J Trauma* 49:771-773, 2000.
8. Van Mieghem C, Sabbe M, Knockaert D: The clinical value of the ECG in noncardiac conditions, *Crit Care Rev* 125:1561-1576, 2004.
9. Mosesso VN: Penetrating chest trauma. In Ferrara PC, Colucciello SA, Marx JA et al, editors: *Trauma management: an emergency medicine approach,* St Louis, 2001, Mosby, pp 259-278.
10. Koumbourlis AC: Electrical injuries, *Crit Care Med* 30:S424-S429, 2002.
11. Rozycki GS, Feliciano DV, Ochsner MG et al: The role of ultrasound in patients with possible penetrating cardiac wounds: a prospective multicenter study, *J Trauma* 46:543-552, 1999.
12. Rhee PM, Acosta J, Bridgeman A et al: Survival after emergency department thoracotomy: review of published data from the last 25 years, *J Am Coll Surg* 190:288-298, 2000.
13. Pasquale M, Fabian TC: Practice management guidelines for screening of blunt cardiac injury from the Eastern Association for the Surgery of Trauma, *J Trauma* 44:941-956, 1998.
14. Velmahos GC, Karaiskakis M, Salim A et al: Normal electrocardiography and serum troponin I levels preclude the presence of clinically significant blunt cardiac injury, *J Trauma* 54:45-50, 2003.
15. Salim A, Velmahos GC, Jinda A et al: Clinically significant blunt cardiac trauma: role of serum troponin levels combined with electrocardiographic findings, *J Trauma* 50:237-243, 2001.
16. Knobloch K, Rossner D, Struber M et al: Traumatic tricuspid insufficiency after horse kick, *J Trauma* 56:694-696, 2004.
17. Zakynthinos EG, Vassilakopoulos T, Routsi C et al: Early and late-onset atrioventricular valve rupture after blunt chest injury: the usefulness of transesophageal echocardiography, *J Trauma* 52:990-996, 2002.

chapter 69

Care of Patients with Acquired Valvular Disease

Debra Lynn-McHale Wiegand
Terry Preuss
Cynthia Hambach

CHAPTER ABBREVIATIONS

ACC   American College of Cardiology

ACCP   American College of Chest Physicians

ACE   angiotensin-converting enzyme

AHA   American Heart Association

APTT   activated partial thromboplastin time

AR   atrial regurgitation

AS   aortic stenosis

AVR   aortic valve replacement

ECG   electrocardiogram

INR   international normalized ratio

LMWH   low-molecular-weight heparin

MR   mitral regurgitation

MS   mitral stenosis

MVP   mitral valve prolapse

NYHA   New York Hospital Association

PMV   percutaneous mitral valvuloplasty

PR   pulmonary regurgitation

PS   pulmonary stenosis

TEE   transesophageal echocardiography

TR   tricuspid regurgitation

TS   tricuspid stenosis

Valvular heart disease is a common cardiovascular disorder that affects people of all ages and both sexes (Box 69-1). It can occur acutely, but is usually a chronic process that evolves over time. Valvular heart disease can lead to heart failure, sudden death, dysrhythmias, and stroke unless the course of the disease is interrupted.[1] Common causes of acquired valvular heart disease include rheumatic heart disease, degenerative disease, and infective endocarditis. Less common causes include trauma, lupus, tumors, syphilis, cancer, arthritic disease, and side effects of medications, such as appetite suppressants[2] (e.g., fenfluramine, dexfenfluramine), migraine medications[3] (e.g., methysergide, ergotamine) and Parkinson medication[4] (e.g., pergolide).

Significant advances have been made in the early assessment and management of valvular heart disease. Innovations in diagnostic tools, pharmacological developments, and surgical techniques have contributed to these advances. Cardiac catheterization, color-flow Doppler, transesophageal echocardiography, and cardiac magnetic resonance imaging have in many ways revolutionized the diagnostic approach to valvular heart disease. Pharmacology agents including diuretics, nitrates, digitalis, anticoagulants, calcium channel blockers, phosphodiesterase inhibitors, antidysrhythmics, and antibiotics have improved medical management. Balloon valvuloplasty offers select patients an invasive, yet nonsurgical option. Balloon valvuloplasty has been successful in treating mitral stenosis **(MS)** in patients without heavily calcified valves and has served as a temporizing procedure in settings of excessive surgical risk. Great strides have been made in the development of mechanical and bioprosthetic valves. In addition, sophistication in valvular repair and reconstruction has contributed to successful surgical corrections.

Despite these advances valvular heart disease remains a serious problem with a significant impact on patients' health and quality of life. Although surgery often can be delayed and the patient managed medically, delay only postpones the inevitable time that the native diseased valve is replaced by a new problem—the prosthetic valve. This chapter discusses the many challenges that still exist in the diagnosis and management of patients with valvular heart disease.

PREVALENCE

Although less information is available on the epidemiology of valvular heart disease than on that of atherosclerotic disease, approximately 98,000 patients were discharged from U. S. hospitals with diagnoses of valvular heart disease in 2002.[5] Diseases of the mitral and aortic valves are more prevalent than diseases of the tricuspid and pulmonic valves. Valvular heart disease is associated with appreciable morbidity and mortality.[5,6]

Using only hospital discharge data does not truly reflect the magnitude of the prevalence of valvular heart disease. Counting only individuals treated at hospitals reflects those with chronic progressive valvular heart disease at an advanced level and those with acute valvular heart disease. However, the majority of individuals with valvular heart disease are treated medically on an outpatient basis.

Rheumatic Heart Disease

In the United States, there has been a decrease in the incidence of rheumatic valve disease. In 1950 approximately 15,000 Americans died of rheumatic fever or rheumatic heart disease compared with approximately 3500 today.[5] From 1992 to 2002, the death rate from rheumatic fever and rheumatic heart disease fell by 23.5 percent.[5]

Although the incidence of rheumatic heart disease has decreased in the United States, the disease is far from eradicated. Rheumatic fever and its sequelae, chronic rheumatic heart disease, is the most common single cause of valvular heart disease in the world.[7] It is estimated that more than 12 million people are affected by rheumatic fever or rheumatic heart disease, and there are more than 400,000 deaths annually, mainly children and young adults.[7] Rheumatic fever continues to be prevalent, especially in developing countries, in the tropical areas of the world, and in isolated pockets of developed countries.[8] Outbreaks of rheumatic fever have been reported in the United States.[7,8]

The pathogenesis of rheumatic fever combines environmental and socioeconomic risk cofactors, group A streptococcal exposure, and individual susceptibility.[8] Reasons proposed are overcrowding, poor nutrition, and poor hygiene. The majority of affected people are of lower socioeconomic status and primarily minorities.[9] The incidence of rheumatic fever is higher in blacks, Puerto Ricans, Mexican Americans, and American Indians.[5]

The decline in the incidence of rheumatic fever in the United States is thought to be due to current antimicrobial therapy, the changing virulence of group A streptococci, changing social conditions, and improvements in health care delivery.[10] Rheumatic fever commonly affects school-age children in whom social contact is high, but involvement of adults is not rare.[10] Also affected are the elderly and immigrants from countries with limited antimicrobial therapy and poor health care.

Degenerative Valve Disease

Although the overall incidence of rheumatic heart disease is declining, no significant changes have occurred in the incidence of valvular heart disease. Two factors that influence this include the improvement in assessment of valvular disorders and the increased number of elders. Advances in Doppler echocardiography, transesophageal echocardiography, and other diagnostic tests have made diagnosis of valvular dysfunction more precise, leading to a greater number of recognized cases.[11]

The aging of the population, especially in developed countries, has increased the incidence of degenerative valve disease. During the past 90 years, the proportion of persons in U.S. society older than 65 years of age has increased steadily.[11] In 2003, 3 percent of the population was over the age of 80, and the fastest growing segment of the nation's population is those age 85 and older.[12] Symptoms of valvular heart disease may be underreported in the elderly because elders may attribute fatigue, dizziness, or decreased mobility to aging rather than a disease process.

Infective Endocarditis

The incidence of infective endocarditis is estimated to be 3 to 6 cases per 100,000.[13] Approximately 17,000 patients were discharged from U.S. hospitals in 2002 with a primary diagnosis of bacterial endocarditis.[5] Mortality rates of 26 percent to 40 percent have been reported, despite antibiotic therapy and surgical intervention.[13]

NATURAL HISTORY OF VALVE DISEASE

Valvular heart disease is most commonly a chronic, progressive disease. Cardiac compensatory mechanisms often maintain a state of equilibrium for years before the disease deteriorates to the point at which symptoms are evident and more definitive therapy is needed. The natural history of valvular heart disease has been dramatically altered during the past 40 years by medical and surgical management. The development of effective surgical treatment has obscured our understanding of its natural history. The optimal timing of intervention is directed toward prevention of the long-term consequences of valve disease including heart failure, pulmonary artery hypertension, atrial fibrillation, and thromboembolism.

Natural History of Rheumatic Heart Disease

Rheumatic fever usually occurs under age 20. The course of rheumatic fever is variable and difficult to predict, although the usual duration of a rheumatic attack is *less than* 3 months. Rheumatic heart disease becomes clinically apparent usually in the third, fourth, and fifth decades of life. One or more valves may be affected. The valves affected may develop stenosis, insufficiency, or a combination of both. In patients with rheumatic fever, if there is no evidence of carditis, very few ever go on to have any valvular problems. Among those who develop carditis, approximately half will develop valvular heart disease at some point, despite initiation of prophylactic antibiotic therapy.

Approximately 25 percent of all patients with rheumatic heart disease have pure MS, and an additional 40 percent have combined MS and mitral insufficiency. More women than men have rheumatic MS.[6] Although rheumatic heart disease was traditionally considered the preponderant cause of mitral regurgitation (**MR**), this is no longer the case as a result of a true decrease in the prevalence of rheumatic heart disease and to the recognition that many instances of pure MR that would have been classified as rheumatic before 1965 are in fact caused by mitral valve prolapse (**MVP**).

The primary cause of acquired tricuspid stenosis (**TS**) is rheumatic heart disease. Females are affected more often than males. TS occurs in 3 percent to 5 percent of cases and is usually associated with either mitral or aortic valvular disease.[14] The most common causes of acquired tricuspid regurgitation (**TR**) are rheumatic fever and endocarditis.

Aortic stenosis (**AS**) remains the most common valvular lesion in the elderly. As large numbers of elderly survive, degenerative AS has come to exceed rheumatic heart disease in frequency. Pulmonic involvement caused by rheumatic heart disease is rare.

Long-term prognosis following rheumatic fever has changed substantially over the years in Western countries, partly because the disease seems to have moderated, but also because recurrences and further carditis can be and have been prevented by antibiotic therapy. Rheumatic fever affects only a small percentage of those with epidemic streptococcal pharyngitis, yet when a patient with previous rheumatic fever develops such an infection, the risk of recurrence may approach 65 percent. Long-term antibiotic therapy is important for patients diagnosed with rheumatic fever. Prophylaxis should be started immediately after rheumatic fever is diagnosed and is continued for a minimum of 5 years if rheumatic fever does not include carditis and is continued for at least 10 years if rheumatic fever includes carditis.[10]

Natural History of Degenerative Valve Disease

Degenerative aortic valve disease represents a process of wear and tear. Although the prevalence of aortic valve disease increases with age, degenerative aortic valve disease is not simply caused by aging. Degenerative aortic valve disease is characterized macroscopically as increased leaflet thickening, stiffening, and calcification without fusion of the commissures. Although the pathogenesis of degenerative aortic valve disease is poorly understood, it is thought that a chronic inflammatory process similar to atherosclerosis damages the valve leaflets.[15] The early stages consist of fibrosis and mild calcification, referred to as aortic valve sclerosis, whereas the late stages consist of valve distortion by calcification and fibrotic thickening.[11] The presence of calcific aortic valve disease is associated with increasing age, male gender, hypertension, hyperlipidemia, smoking, and diabetes.[16]

Calcification of the mitral valve occurs less commonly than aortic valve calcification. Mitral annular calcification increases with age, particularly in women over age 70.[17] Calcification usually involves the posterior leaflet and results in MR. Although rare MS caused by annular calcification is easily distinguished from rheumatic MS because of the lack of involvement of the free edges of the leaflets.[11]

Natural History of Infective Endocarditis

Infective endocarditis is an inflammation of the endocardium induced by microorganisms. Valvular damage can occur if the infection invades the valve tissue. Vegetations, consisting of platelets, fibrin, and proteins with a high concentration of the infective organisms, form on the valve.[18] The vegetation may cause regurgitation because the valve is unable to close properly or stenosis if the valve is unable to open properly. If not treated with antibiotics, the mortality rate of infective endocarditis is near 100 percent.[1]

Predisposing risk factors for infective endocarditis include an underlying valvular disorder (e.g., bicuspid aortic valve), presence of a prosthetic valve, or history of intravenous drug use.[19] Although most patients have a predisposing risk factor, some patients have no risk factors, but still develop infective endocarditis.

Acute infective endocarditis is most commonly caused by *Staphylococcus aureus*.[19] *S. aureus* endocarditis involving the mitral or aortic valves can lead to extensive tissue destruction and a high prevalence of complications, whereas *S. aureus* endocarditis involving the tricuspid or pulmonic valves (associated with intravenous drug use) has a more benign course and usually responds to a short course of antibiotic therapy.[18] Additional organisms causing infective endocarditis include streptococci, enterococci, and fastidious gram-negative coccobacilli. The rapidity of the disease course is a function of the virulence of the causative organism and the specific cardiac structures affected by the disease process.[18]

VALVULAR DISORDERS

Nursing care for patients with valvular heart disease is based on an understanding of the structure and function of the heart valves and the causes and treatments of each disorder.

Mitral Valve Disease

The anatomy of the mitral valve is described in detail in Chapter 4, but briefly the mitral valve has a large anterior and a small posterior leaflet. The leaflets are joined at two commissures (the lateral and medial) and are supported by a subvalvular mechanism (i.e., chordae tendineae and papillary muscles). The mitral valve leaflets arise from the mitral annulus. The chordae tendineae arise from the papillary muscles and attach to the free edges and the undersurfaces of the mitral leaflets. The papillary muscle is attached to the left ventricular wall. These structures prevent the leaflets from prolapsing into the left atrium during systole, thus contributing to the competency of the mitral valve.

Mitral Stenosis

In MS, the mitral valve fails to open completely, restricting the flow of blood from the left atrium to the left ventricle. The major cause of MS is rheumatic heart disease,[20] which causes thickening and limits movement of the mitral valve leaflets with fusion of the commissures.[21] Less common causes of MS include calcification of the mitral annulus or leaflets, neoplasm, and endocardial vegetations.[22,23]

Pathophysiology

When the opening of the diseased mitral valve becomes restricted, the mitral valve area decreases. When the area is decreased from its normal valve area of 4 to 6 cm^2 to 2 cm^2 or less, the workload of the left atrium increases, and a pressure gradient is needed to propel the blood through the reduced opening.[21,24,25] When the area is further reduced to 1 cm^2 with severe MS, a pressure gradient of at least 20 mm Hg is needed to maintain a normal cardiac output at rest.[25,26] This decrease in blood flow causes a decreased cardiac output. The resulting pressure on the left atrium causes left atrial dilatation and hypertrophy, which may lead to atrial fibrillation. Left atrial blood flow becomes stagnant, which can result in clot formation and thromboembolism. An increase in left atrial pressure may cause a back pressure in the pulmonary circulation causing pulmonary hypertension, congestion, and right-sided heart failure. The left ventricular size and contractility usually remain normal in MS.[22-24]

Clinical Manifestations

MS occurs more frequently in women rather than men.[25,27,28] The interval between rheumatic disease and the onset of symptoms ranges from 10 to 20 years.[24] Symptoms are generally first experienced in the fourth or fifth decade of life.[27] A woman may remain asymptomatic until an added stress, such as pregnancy, is placed on the heart.[27,28]

The first symptom of mild disease (valve area of 1.6 to 2.0 cm^2) is dyspnea on exertion.[21] This results from pulmonary congestion, secondary to increased left atrial pressure. As the disease progresses (valve area of 1 to 1.5 cm^2), fatigue, paroxysmal nocturnal dyspnea, and atrial fibrillation can occur. When it becomes severe (valve area of 1 cm^2 or less), dyspnea on mild exertion or at rest may occur.[21]

Other symptoms of MS include cough, hoarseness, and hemoptysis. Hoarseness is caused by the enlarged left atrium impinging on the left recurrent laryngeal nerve (Ortner syndrome).[24] Hemoptysis may be due to rupture of small bronchial veins[27] or a chronic elevation in pulmonary venous pressures.[22,23]

Later in the disease process, symptoms of right-sided heart failure may occur, including jugular vein distension, hepatomegaly, ascites, and peripheral edema. The patient who develops atrial fibrillation is at risk for thromboembolism and cerebral vascular accident.

Physical Assessment

Auscultation of the patient with MS reveals a loud S$_1$, an opening snap, and a diastolic, rumbling murmur heard best at the apex of the heart in the left lateral decubitus position.[22] The S$_1$ heart sound is louder than normal because the increased pressure gradient holds the mitral valve open until the force of ventricular systole closes it.[27] The opening snap results from a sudden tensing of the valve leaflets opening to their full extent.[22,24] The murmur is caused by the turbulence of blood flow through the abnormal valve.

A lower left parasternal lift or heave may be detected secondary to right ventricular hypertrophy.[21] The decreased cardiac output can cause weak pulses upon palpation. Less frequently the patient may exhibit a malar flush, a pinkish-purple discoloration of the cheeks.[21,24] This is thought to result from peripheral vasoconstriction secondary to a decreased cardiac output.[22,24]

Diagnostic Tests

Echocardiography is the diagnostic tool of choice for evaluating the patient with MS. The echocardiogram provides information about the valve area and gradient, left ventricular ejection fraction, left atrial enlargement, evidence of mitral valve calcification, pulmonary artery pressures, and right ventricular function. Other tests include electrocardiography **(ECG),** chest x-ray, and cardiac catheterization (Table 69-1).

Management

If the patient remains asymptomatic, antibiotic prophylaxis to prevent endocarditis may be the only treatment necessary. Diuretics can be used to relieve pulmonary congestion, and beta blockers are helpful in decreasing the heart rate, thus lengthening diastolic filling time.

If atrial fibrillation develops, digoxin, beta blockers, or calcium channel blockers can be used to control the ventricular rate. Rate control is important because an increased heart rate can further decrease diastolic filling time, adding to the left atrial pressure and further decreases cardiac output. Antidysrhythmic medications, such as amiodarone or sotalol, can be used to restore normal sinus rhythm. If medications are unsuccessful, electrical cardioversion can be considered.[27] If atrial fibrillation persists, anticoagulation is necessary to prevent thromboembolism.

Medical management will only be helpful for a certain length of time. Once symptoms begin to escalate, additional interventions should be considered. These include percutaneous mitral catheter balloon valvuloplasty and mitral valve repair or replacement. Intervention also should be considered if the patient remains in atrial fibrillation or pulmonary artery hypertension develops.[27,29]

Management includes an evaluation of the patient and/or the family's understanding of the disease and the level of family support available. Patient education is the key to facilitate early recognition of symptoms, periodic monitoring, adherence to the medication regimen, and prevention of complications. Education should include

■ ■ ■

TABLE 69-1   DIAGNOSTIC TESTS FOR MITRAL STENOSIS

TEST	FINDING
12-Lead ECG	P mitrale (large notched P waves in leads II and V$_1$ seen when patient in normal sinus rhythm), which is evidence of left atrial hypertrophy
	Large R wave in V$_1$ and large S wave in V$_6$ associated with right ventricular hypertrophy
	Atrial fibrillation
Echocardiogram	Valve area and gradient
	Left ventricular ejection fraction
	Left atrial enlargement
	Evidence of mitral valve calcification
	Pulmonary artery pressures
	Right ventricular function
Chest x-ray	Straightening of left heart border secondary to left atrial enlargement, enlargement of pulmonary arteries, and interstitial edema
Cardiac catheterization	Presence or absence of coronary artery disease
	Right atrial, right ventricular, and pulmonary artery pressures
	Valve area and pressure gradient

ECG, Electrocardiogram.

information related to reducing the risk of infective endocarditis and for some patients, the importance of anticoagulation therapy. Pregnancy risks should be discussed as appropriate.

Mitral Regurgitation

In MR, the mitral valve fails to close completely, and blood is propelled backward into the left atrium during ventricular systole. The mitral valve relies on its four components—mitral annulus, valve leaflets, chordae tendineae, and papillary muscle—for effective functioning. Any disease process that affects one of these components can lead to MR. Causes of MR include MVP, rheumatic heart disease, infective endocarditis, collagen-vascular disease, cardiomyopathy, and ischemic heart disease.

Pathophysiology

MR places a strain on both the left ventricle and the left atrium. When a portion of the blood is ejected backward into the left atrium during ventricular systole, cardiac output is decreased. Later, that blood flows back into the left ventricle, causing an increased preload. The left atrium has to withstand the added volume of blood, increasing left atrial pressure, which in time will increase pulmonary pressure and cause pulmonary congestion.

In chronic MR, left ventricular hypertrophy develops, which maintains a normal cardiac output for some time. Ejecting the blood into the left atrium increases ventricular preload; however, it also causes a decrease in ventricular afterload. The combination of the two increases cardiac output; however, the left ventricle can only compensate for a certain period of time. A decrease in cardiac output into the normal range can signify ventricular dysfunction.[27] In acute MR, left ventricular hypertrophy does not have time to develop, and left atrial pressure increases rapidly, causing acute pulmonary congestion.

Clinical Manifestations

Patients with chronic MR may remain asymptomatic for years.[27,30] Initial symptoms of decompensation are those seen with left-sided heart failure: dyspnea on exertion, orthopnea, and paroxysmal nocturnal dyspnea. Additional symptoms include cough and peripheral edema. Patients also may have palpitations secondary to a new onset of atrial fibrillation.

The patient with acute MR experiences symptoms of left-sided heart failure; however, the symptoms are relatively more severe in nature. This patient experiences dyspnea secondary to pulmonary congestion and edema and tachycardia in response to a decrease in cardiac output. Increased pulmonary pressures may cause signs of right-sided heart failure.

Physical Assessment

Auscultation of the patient in MR reveals a holosystolic murmur heard best at the apex, which radiates to the axilla. The increased, rapid flow of blood into the left ventricle during diastole may produce a third heart sound. The point of maximal impulse is displaced downward and to the left as a result of the enlarged left ventricle.[31] A left parasternal lift may also be appreciated secondary to dilatation of the left atrium.[21]

In acute MR, signs of left-sided heart failure will be present. These include: tachycardia, diaphoresis, hypotension, and pulmonary crackles. Jugular vein distension, ascites, hepatomegaly, and peripheral edema will be noted as a result of right-sided congestion.

Diagnostic Tests

Echocardiography is the most helpful diagnostic tool for MR. The echocardiogram provides information about left atrial size, left ventricular size and function, pulmonary artery pressures, and the cause and degree of MR. Transesophageal echocardiography **(TEE)** may be used for further evaluation of the mitral valve anatomy and to investigate the cause of MR. The 12-lead ECG, chest x-ray, and cardiac catheterization also may be used in diagnosis (Table 69-2).

Management

Asymptomatic MR patients should be followed annually with a physical exam and an echocardiogram.[27,30] The echocardiogram is useful in assessing left ventricular function as estimated by the ejection fraction and end-systolic dimension (or volume). If symptoms develop or the echocardiogram reveals an ejection fraction *less than* 60 percent or a left ventricular end-systolic dimen-

■ ■ ■

TABLE 69-2 DIAGNOSTIC TESTS FOR MITRAL REGURGITATION

TEST	FINDING
12-lead ECG	Signs of left atrial enlargement and left ventricular hypertrophy in a patient with severe, chronic mitral regurgitation (MR)
	Ischemic changes secondary to papillary muscle dysfunction
	Signs of acute myocardial infarction seen with papillary muscle rupture
	Atrial fibrillation
Echocardiogram	Left atrial size
	Left ventricular size and function
	Pulmonary artery pressures
	Cause of MR
	Degree of MR
TEE	Evaluation of mitral valve anatomy
	Cause of MR
Chest x-ray	Pulmonary congestion and left ventricular hypertrophy if patient is in heart failure
	Left ventricular hypertrophy, left atrial enlargement, and calcification of mitral valve in chronic MR
	If heart size is normal, suggests either chronic MR of a mild nature or an acutely occurring regurgitation in which the left ventricle has yet to become enlarged
Cardiac catheterization	Degree of MR
	Presence or absence of coronary artery disease
	Left- and right-sided heart measurements
	May be used before surgical treatment of disease

ECG, Electrocardiogram; *TEE,* transesophageal echocardiography.

sion equal to 45 mm, surgical therapy, such as mitral valve repair or replacement, should be considered.[27,28] The goal of surgical therapy is to restore valve competency, decrease symptoms, and to prevent left ventricular systolic dysfunction from occurring.

Vasodilators, such as nitroprusside or angiotensin-converting enzyme **(ACE)** inhibitors, are used for patients with acute MR to decrease the ventricular afterload, thus propelling the blood forward and increasing the cardiac output. The result is a decrease in the regurgitant volume, reduced left atrial pressure, and a decrease in pulmonary congestion. Intravenous diuretics also may be used to decrease preload. If severe hypotensive and hemodynamic instability develops, an intraaortic balloon pump may be used to increase cardiac output by decreasing afterload and augmenting coronary artery blood flow.[20,27]

Patients with chronic MR may benefit from afterload reduction and diuretics as well. If atrial fibrillation develops, digoxin and beta blockers may be helpful in controlling the ventricular rate. Patients in atrial fibrillation should be anticoagulated to prevent thromboembolism.

Mitral Valve Prolapse

Mitral valve prolapse (MVP) refers to a group of conditions in which the mitral valve leaflets prolapse back into the left atrium during systole. MVP affects 2 percent to 6 percent of the U.S. population and often occurs as a clinical entity with little or no MR.[20] MVP occurs primarily in women; although when associated with severe MR, it is seen more frequently in older men.[24] The most common cause of MVP is myxomatous degeneration of the valve. Other causes include Marfan syndrome, collagen-vascular disease, and ischemia from coronary artery disease.[27]

Pathophysiology

Myxomatous degeneration of the valve leaflets causes them to enlarge and prolapse into the left atrium during systole.[21] As the valve leaflets prolapse, they pass a point where the leaflet edges are unable to coapt, which can lead to MR.[24] Constant prolapse of the valve leaflets can put a strain on the other components of the valve, primarily the chordae tendineae and papillary muscle.[21]

Clinical Manifestations

Patients with MVP are frequently asymptomatic. The most common symptoms are atypical chest pain, palpitations, dyspnea, fatigue, and dizziness. Symptoms may be secondary to an associated dysrhythmia or regurgitant blood flow.[32] Chest pain may be related to abnormal tension on the papillary muscles.[24]

Physical Assessment

Cardiac auscultation may reveal a midsystolic click and a late systolic murmur.[27,32] The click may occur as a result of the sudden tensing of the valve leaflets as they reach their limit in midsystole.[32] The late systolic murmur may result as the leaflets pass their point of coaptation, causing mitral valve incompetence.[27,32]

Diagnostic Tests

The diagnosis of MVP is based on echocardiographic findings. The mitral valve leaflets will be seen superior to the plane of the mitral annulus (revealing prolapse) during systole. The echocardiogram can also provide useful information about the morphology of the valve and the degree of MR. As with other diseases of the mitral valve, the 12-lead ECG, chest x-ray, and cardiac catheterization may be used to further the diagnosis (Table 69-3).

Management

Asymptomatic patients with MVP require no medical therapy,[21] but reassurance is extremely important. Patients with mild or no symptoms may be assured of a benign prognosis.[20] Those diagnosed with MVP associated with MR should receive antibiotic prophylaxis for infective endocarditis.[20] Beta blockers or calcium channel blockers may be used to treat patients with chest pain or palpitations.[21,27] Cessation of alcohol, tobacco, and caffeine may help to control the symptoms. Since a small percentage of patients are at risk for sudden cardiac death, patients with palpitations, syncope, or dizziness should be further evaluated for dysrhythmias.[24,32]

Patients with a thickened or redundant mitral valve on echocardiographic exam may benefit from low-dose aspirin therapy because they are at risk for thromboembolism.[27] Certain conditions involving the patient with MVP may warrant long-term warfarin anticoagulation, including a documented systemic embolic event; recurrent unexplained transient ischemic attacks despite antiplatelet medication; and atrial fibrillation.[20]

Aortic Valve Disease

The aortic valve, described in detail in Chapter 4, has three cusps or leaflets. The aortic valve, which lies between the left ventricle and the ascending aorta, does not have a subvalvular mechanism. The cusps open as pressure builds in the left ventricle and blood is propelled into the aorta. The cusps close as the pressure in

■ ■ ■

TABLE 69-3 DIAGNOSTIC TESTS FOR MITRAL VALVE PROLAPSE

TEST	FINDING
12-lead ECG	Usually normal findings Nonspecific ST segment and T-wave changes may be seen in inferior leads
Echocardiogram	Mitral valve leaflets seen superior to the plane of the mitral annulus (revealing prolapse) during systole Morphology of mitral valve Degree of mitral regurgitant (MR)
Chest x-ray	Usually normal Left atrial enlargement, left ventricular enlargement, pulmonary congestion in patient with severe MR
Cardiac catheterization	Identify if coronary artery disease is the possible cause of chest pain Degree of MR

ECG, Electrocardiogram.

the aorta becomes *greater than* the pressure in the left ventricle.

Aortic Stenosis

AS, the obstruction of blood flow across the aortic valve during systole, is the most common cardiac valve lesion in the United States.[33-35] AS may be caused by degenerative calcification, hypercholesteremia, and rheumatic valve disease.

Pathophysiology

Degenerative calcific AS results from mechanical stress on the valve and inflammatory changes. The cusps become immobilized, and stenosis is caused by calcium deposits that develop along the flexion lines at their bases (Figure 69-1). Rheumatic AS results from adhesion and fusion of the commissures and cusps leading to retraction and stiffening of the cusps (Figure 69-2). Calcific nodules develop on both surfaces, and the orifice is reduced to a small round or triangular opening. The functional area of the valve is decreased enough to cause measurable obstruction of outflow because the valve area is reduced from the normal 3 to 4 cm^2 to 1.5 to 2 cm^2.[33] Severe AS is defined as the aortic valve area *less than* 1.0 cm^2.[33,35]

Clinical Manifestations

AS is a gradually progressive disease in which patients may remain asymptomatic for decades. Symptoms, including decreased exercise tolerance, fatigue, dyspnea, angina, cough, syncope, and pulmonary edema,[36,37] are due to AS if the mean aortic valve gradient exceeds 50 mm Hg or if the aortic valve area is no larger than 1 cm^2.[33] Once symptoms occur, this is a sign of severe AS, and immediate surgical intervention is often warranted.[27,34,35] As AS progresses, a higher left ventricular systolic pressure is required to drive blood across the obstructed valve, resulting in left ventricular hypertrophy. Initially the hypertrophy is compensatory, but eventually the left ventricle becomes stiff, which causes

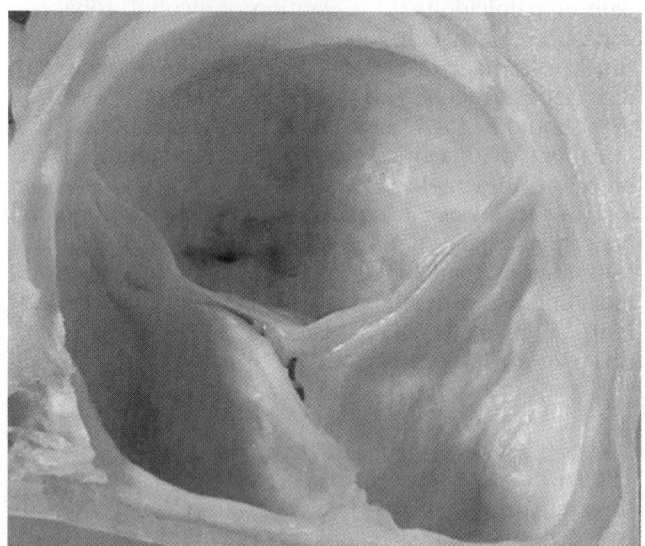
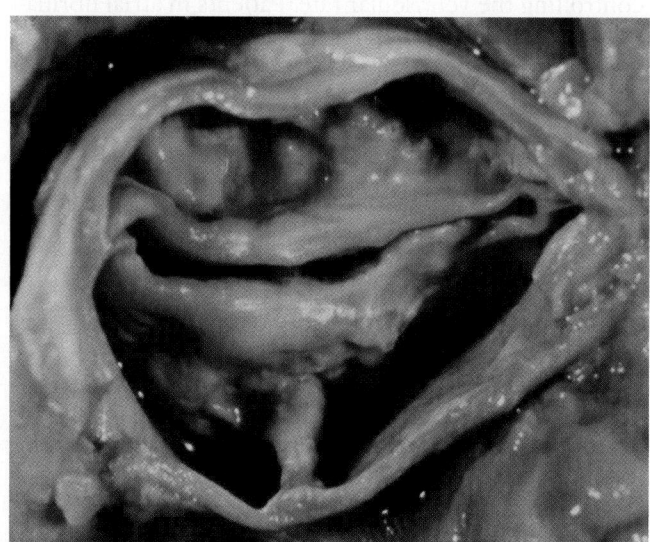

FIGURE 69-1 ■ Calcific aortic stenosis. (From Manabe H, Yutani C, editors: *Atlas of valvular heart disease,* Singapore, 1998, Churchill Livingstone, pp 131.)

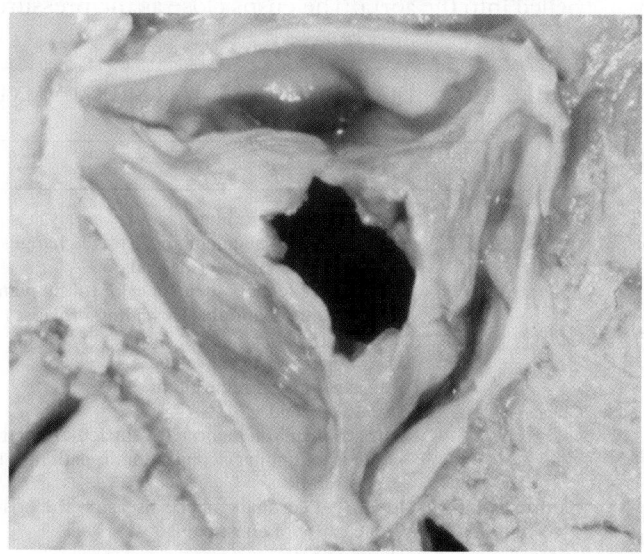
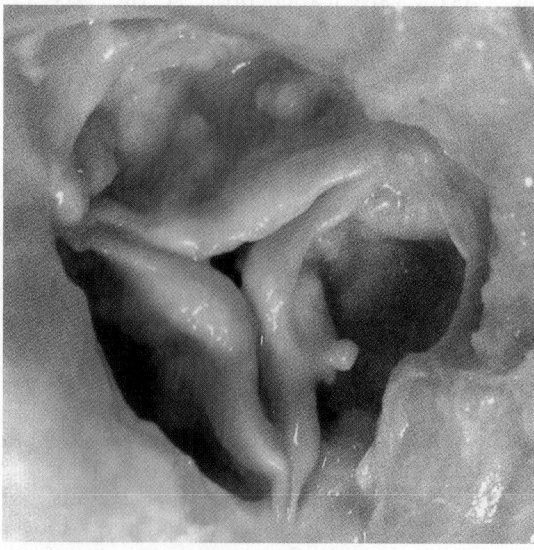

FIGURE 69-2 ■ Rheumatic aortic stenosis. (From Zipes DP, Libby P, Bonow RO, Braunwald E, editors: *Braunwald's Heart Disease,* ed 7, Philadelphia, Elsevier Saunders, 2005.

TABLE 69-4   DIAGNOSTIC TESTS FOR AORTIC STENOSIS

TEST	FINDING
12-lead ECG	Left ventricular hypertrophy found in 85% of patients with severe aortic stenosis (AS)
	May also have left atrial enlargement, left axis deviation, and left bundle branch block
Echocardiogram	Thickened valve leaflets with restricted motion
	Degree of stenosis
	Left ventricular ejection fraction
	Extent of left ventricular hypertrophy
	Degree of coexisting aortic regurgitation
	Estimation of pulmonary artery pressures
Chest x-ray	May be normal
	May demonstrate a boot-shaped heart consistent with development of left ventricular concentric hypertrophy
Stress testing	Not routine
	May be done to measure exercise capacity in asymptomatic patients
Cardiac catheterization	Not routine
	Performed in patients only when echocardiographic data are non diagnostic or not congruent with other clinical data
	Indicated to determine if anginal symptoms are due to coexisting coronary artery disease in patients with mild or moderate AS
	Valve area and pressure gradient

AR, Aortic regurgitation; *AS*, aortic stenosis; *ECG*, electrocardiogram.

high pressures in the left ventricle. When these pressures are transmitted to the lungs, dyspnea results.[27,37]

Physical Assessment

AS is generally discovered by the finding of a systolic ejection murmur at the right upper sternal border that radiates to the neck. When the murmur peaks progressively later in systole and its intensity decreases as cardiac output falls, AS is at least moderate in severity. As the stenosis worsens, valve motion is reduced, and the aortic component of the second heart sound disappears.[33]

Diagnostic Tests

Diagnostic tests assist in the diagnosis and determination of the severity of AS. Common tests include a 12-lead ECG and an echocardiogram (Table 69-4). Repeat echocardiogram is indicated for any change in clinical status and before any major noncardiac procedure or event (e.g., pregnancy).

Management

If the patient is asymptomatic, no therapy is required. Medical therapy is aimed at prevention of complications and prompt recognition of symptom onset.[38] Antibiotic prophylaxis against infective endocarditis is required before and after dental or other surgical procedures.[20] If the patient develops symptoms, surgical intervention is indicated. Nitrates, digoxin, and diuretics may be used to treat angina and heart failure in the interim between diagnosis and surgery. Nitrates should be used cautiously because of the potential for orthostatic hypotension and syncope. Digoxin and diuretics may be pre-

scribed for controlling left ventricular dysfunction and dyspnea.[27] Nursing interventions are based on each patient's response to the diagnosis of AS and focus on minimizing discomfort related to angina, dyspnea, and fatigue (see special feature: Conundrum). Research is needed to determine the effect of hydroxymethylglutaryl coenzyme A reductase inhibitors (statins) on the progression of AS.[34]

Aortic Regurgitation

The ascending aorta is 5 cm long and has two segments. The lower segment is the aortic root, which begins at the level of the aortic valve and extends to the sinotubular junction. The base of the aortic cusps are supported by the aortic root.[39]

Aortic regurgitation **(AR)** is the backflow of blood into the left ventricle during diastole. The aortic valve becomes incompetent as a result of pathological conditions of either the aortic valve cusps or the aortic root.[1,27,37] There are several causes of AR (Box 69-2), but the most common cause in developing countries is rheumatic disease, with the clinical presentation in the second or third decade of life.[1,40] Rheumatic disease is rare in Western countries, and severe AR is most frequently caused by a congenital bicuspid valve or a degenerative disease, such as annuloaortic ectasia, which typically arises in the fourth to sixth decades.[40] In annuloaortic ectasia, histological changes lead to weakening of the aortic wall, resulting in formation of a fusiform aneurysm. These aneurysms often involve the aortic root and may cause AR.[39]

■■■ CONUNDRUM

TREATMENT OF AORTIC STENOSIS

One to 2 percent of asymptomatic patients with severe aortic stenosis (AS) die suddenly or have a very rapid rate of progression to the symptomatic state and then to death.[33] Surgery for this group exposes them to risks of surgery, valve-related complications, and death, but some experts advocate this approach. Should patients with severe asymptomatic AS undergo aortic-valve replacement to prevent sudden death? The answer to this clinical conundrum is not yet known.

BOX 69-2   ■■■
CAUSES OF AORTIC REGURGITATION

Valve Cusps
Rheumatic heart disease
Infective endocarditis
Myxomatous valve
Systemic lupus erythematous
Rheumatoid arthritis
Pharmacological agents

Aortic Root
Annuloaortic ectasia
Idiopathic aortic root dilatation
Hypertension
Marfan syndrome
Aortic dissection
Syphilis
Ankylosing spondylitis

Pathophysiology

AR is a unique valvular disease with both ventricular volume overload and pressure overload.[20] The volume overload leads to compensatory adjustments, such as left ventricular hypertrophy and an increase in end-diastolic volume, permitting the ventricle to maintain a normal ejection fraction despite the elevated afterload.[20,41] Left ventricular afterload increases as the increased volume is ejected into a high-pressure chamber, the aorta. Eccentric hypertrophy (ventricular wall thickens with dilatation) occurs to accommodate for the volume overload, and modest concentric hypertrophy (ventricular wall thickens without enlargement but with diminished capacity) occurs to compensate for the pressure overload.[27] Most patients remain asymptomatic for decades during this compensated phase.[20,41] The balance between afterload excess, preload reserve, and hypertrophy cannot be maintained indefinitely, and patients commonly develop symptoms when there is a reduction in ejection fraction or left ventricular dysfunction develops.[20]

Clinical Manifestations

Signs and symptoms vary depending on the severity of the disease. Symptoms, such as fatigue, dyspnea on exertion, orthopnea, pulmonary edema, and angina are a sign that AR is severe, and immediate surgical intervention is often warranted.[42] Severe symptoms (New York Heart Association [NYHA] Class III or IV) and left ventricular dysfunction with an ejection fraction *less than* 50 percent are independent risk factors for poor postoperative survival. Surgery should be done when patients are in New York Hospital Association (NYHA) Class II before severe left ventricular dysfunction develops.[20]

Physical Assessment

AR is usually detected by the finding of a decrescendo, blowing, diastolic murmur in the 3rd or 4th intercostal space along the left sternal border. The valve lesion creates an orifice that allows regurgitant flow throughout diastole (measured as the regurgitant volume). An S_3 or S_4 may be heard depending on the degree of AR.[27,40] Other assessment findings are shown in Box 69-3.

Diagnostic Tests

Common diagnostic tests including chest x-ray, 12-lead ECG, and echocardiogram (Table 69-5) help classify the severity of regurgitation. Doppler echocardiography and color-flow Doppler imaging are used in the diagnosis and evaluation of AR. Yearly echocardiographic re-evaluation is recommended for asymptomatic patients with mild to moderate AR with stable physical signs and normal to near normal left ventricular chamber size.[20]

Management

Once the diagnosis of AR is made, medical management is directed at slowing the disease progression, preventing complications, and identifying the ideal timing of surgery.[76] Vasodilators (e.g., nifedipine) and afterload reduction therapy (e.g., nitroprusside) decrease the pressure and volume overload of the left ventricle in an effort to prevent progressive left ventricular dilatation and systolic dysfunction. Hydralazine, ACE inhibitors, and calcium channel blockers are effective in reducing afterload.[20,24,41,42] In one study of asymptomatic patients with chronic severe AR, vasodilator therapy with nifedipine reduced the rate of symptom onset and left ventricular dysfunction and was associated with a reduced need for aortic valve replacement **(AVR).**[43] Patients with AR are at risk for endocarditis, and antibiotic prophylaxis therapy is prescribed for prevention of endocarditis. In addition, antibiotic prophylaxis may be prescribed for patients with an audible AR murmur, a grade +2 or higher regurgitation by Doppler criteria, a bicuspid valve with any degree of AR, or rheumatic valvular disease.[40,42]

Nursing interventions are based on the patient's response to AR. Education related to the disease process, targeted therapy with afterload reducing agents, and antibiotic therapy is essential. Nursing interventions focus on treatment of angina, dyspnea, and orthopnea.

■ ■ ■

BOX 69-3   ■ ■ ■
ASSESSMENT FINDINGS IN AORTIC REGURGITATION

- Decrescendo diastolic blowing murmur (Austin Flint murmur), which may be accentuated by the patient sitting upright and leaning forward
- Widened pulse pressure (*greater than* 50 mm Hg)
- Systolic blood pressure in lower extremities at least 20 mm Hg higher than in the arms (Hill sign)
- Systolic and diastolic bruit heard when femoral artery is compressed by stethoscope (Duroziez sign)
- An increased volume and rate of rise of the radial pulse when the wrist is elevated perpendicular to the body of a supine patient (Corrigan pulse)
- Bobbing of the head (de Musset sign)

TABLE 69-5   DIAGNOSTIC TESTS FOR AORTIC REGURGITATION

TEST	FINDING
Chest x-ray	• Enlarged heart • Dilatation of proximal aorta
12-Lead ECG	• Left ventricular hypertrophy
Echocardiogram	• Enlarged left ventricle and degree of regurgitation
Exercise testing	• Not routine. • May be helpful when there is a discrepancy between clinical presentation and diagnostic testing occurs or indication for aortic valve replacement in asymptomatic patients
Cardiac catheterization	• Degree of aortic regurgitation • Presence or absence of coronary artery disease • Left- and right-sided heart measurements • May be performed before surgical intervention

AR, Aortic regurgitation; *ECG,* electrocardiogram.

Tricuspid Valve Disease

Similar to the mitral valve, the tricuspid valve consists of three cusps. The tricuspid valve is located between the right atrium and the right ventricle.

Tricuspid Stenosis

Tricuspid stenosis (TS), obstruction of blood flow from the right atrium to the right ventricle during diastole, is a rare disorder with 90 percent of all cases caused by rheumatic disease. Other causes include carcinoid disease, right atrial tumors, and infective endocarditis.[44] Isolated TR is uncommon and often occurs with mitral and aortic valve disease.[24]

Pathophysiology

Rheumatic inflammation of the tricuspid valve results in scarring and fibrosis of the valve leaflets with fusion of the commissures. The chordae tendineae shorten, limiting leaflet mobility, and the size of the tricuspid orifice is reduced, obstructing right ventricular filling.

Clinical Manifestations

Symptoms of TS include fatigue, dyspnea, peripheral edema, neck vein distention, hepatic congestion, and ascites, which are secondary to an elevated systemic venous pressure.[24,44]

Physical Assessment

TS is characterized by a diastolic, rumbling murmur at the left sternal border that increases in intensity with respiration. The lung fields are clear, and the patient may be comfortable lying flat despite neck vein distention and ascites. A diastolic thrill may be palpable at the lower left sternal border and becomes more prominent during inspiration.[24]

Diagnostic Tests

Diagnostic tests assist in defining the cause and severity of the stenosis. Refer to Table 69-6 for common diagnostic tests used to assess for TS.

■ ■ ■

TABLE 69-6   DIAGNOSTIC TESTS FOR TRICUSPID STENOSIS

TEST	FINDING
ECG	• Atrial enlargement (in the absence of atrial fibrillation) • Some patients may have atrial fibrillation. • Tall right atrial P waves
Chest x-ray	• Enlarged right atrium but normal pulmonary artery size • Clear lung fields
Echocardiography	• Reduction in the diameter of the orifice • Right atrial size • Right ventricular size and function • Cause of mitral regurgitation • Degree of mitral regurgitation
Cardiac catheterization	• Quantification of tricuspid stenosis with assessment of associated tricuspid regurgitation

ECG, Electrocardiogram.

Management

In the absence of symptoms, no treatment is indicated for TS although antibiotic prophylaxis to prevent infective endocarditis is indicated. Medical management may include sodium restriction and diuretic therapy to decrease the symptoms of systemic venous congestion, but may be ineffective since diuresis further reduces cardiac output. A period of diuresis may diminish hepatic congestion and improve hepatic function to diminish surgical risks.[24,44] Nursing interventions are based on each patient's individual response to TS.

Tricuspid Regurgitation

TR is the backflow of blood from the right ventricle into the right atrium during systole. The most common cause of TR is right ventricular dilation and failure.

Pathophysiology

TR is caused by both intrinsic involvement of the valve itself (primary TR) and is most often caused by right ventricular dilatation and dilatation of the tricuspid annulus causing secondary (functional) TR.[24,44] The most common cause of primary TR is infective endocarditis secondary to intravenous drug use.[27] Right ventricular dilatation in secondary TR develops from left ventricular failure, pulmonary hypertension, or both.[45,46] Mild TR is a common echocardiographic finding that is present in 80 percent to 90 percent of healthy people and is generally well tolerated in the absence of pulmonary hypertension.[24]

Clinical Manifestations

In isolated TR, patients have vague signs and symptoms because moderate to severe TR produces few overt symptoms. These symptoms include fatigue, decreased exercise tolerance (as a result of low forward cardiac output), peripheral edema, decreased appetite, and abdominal fullness. Patients may have signs and symptoms of right-sided heart failure, including neck vein distention, dyspnea, orthopnea, lower extremity edema, ascites, and hepatomegaly.[44,47,48] Since symptoms may be nonspecific and physical findings are often subtle, the diagnosis of TR is often made at the time of echocardiographic evaluation of left-sided heart disease.[27,44]

Physical Assessment

In the presence of pulmonary hypertension, a systolic, high-pitched, pansystolic murmur is loudest at the 4th intercostal space in the parasternal region, but occasionally is loudest in the subxiphoid region. In the absence of pulmonary hypertension, the murmur is usually of low intensity and limited to the first half of systole. The murmur is characteristically augmented during inspiration (Carvallo sign).[24] Hepatomegaly is present in 90 percent of patients[44] with the liver tender if right ventricular failure has been rapid in onset.[27] In patients with chronic TR and congestive cirrhosis, the liver may be firm and nontender.[24] Diagnostic tests are shown in Table 69-7.

■ ■ ■

TABLE 69-7 DIAGNOSTIC TESTS FOR TRICUSPID REGURGITATION

TEST	FINDING
12-lead ECG	• Atrial fibrillation • Right axis deviation • Incomplete right bundle branch block • Right ventricular hypertrophy
Chest x-ray	• Right ventricular enlargement • Cardiomegaly • Ascites with upward displacement of the diaphragm
Echocardiogram	• Degree of tricuspid regurgitation • Cause of tricuspid regurgitation • Pulmonary arterial pressures • Right ventricular function
CT	• Contrast in the inferior vena cava or hepatic veins indicative of tricuspid regurgitation in patients with pulmonary hypertension

CT, Computed tomography; *ECG,* electrocardiogram.

Management

The management of TR is usually aimed at treating the disease responsible for right ventricular failure. In chronic secondary TR, diuretics are the therapy of choice in reducing right ventricular overload, decreasing pulmonary pressures, and controlling peripheral venous congestion.[27,44] When antibiotic therapy is unsuccessful, diseased valvular tissue may be excised to eradicate the endocarditis and antibiotic therapy continued.[24] In patients with endocarditis, surgical intervention may be required for severe TR with annuloplasty the most common procedure performed.[20,44]

Pulmonary Valve Disease

The pulmonary valve is composed of three cusps. It is located between the right ventricle and the pulmonary artery.

Pulmonary Stenosis

Pulmonary stenosis **(PS)** is the obstruction of blood flow from the right ventricle to the pulmonary artery during systole. Most (95 percent) of cases of PS are congenital.[44] Acquired PS is rare and may be caused by rheumatic fever, cancerous valvular lesions, syphilis, endocarditis, and tuberculosis.

Pathophysiology. Inflammatory changes can occur from rheumatic fever and endocarditis causing a fibrous thickening of the pulmonic valve cusps, resulting in a decreased valvular orifice. PS leads to pressure overload in the right atrium and ventricle[49] and may cause symptoms that are due to reduced cardiac output.[44]

Clinical Manifestations. Most patients with mild or moderate PS are asymptomatic, and it is likely that some patients with severe obstruction adjust their lifestyle to prevent symptom onset.[44] The appearance of symptoms is proportional to the severity of the stenosis and includes dyspnea, fatigue, syncope, and angina.[44]

Physical Assessment. On exam patients with PS have a crescendo-decrescendo systolic murmur that is loudest at the upper left sternal border and radiates to the suprasternal notch and left neck. A loud, late-peaking murmur

suggests severe obstruction. The murmur is longer in duration than AS, so the systolic murmur extends beyond the aortic closure sound.[44] S_2 is widely split or may be absent. Diagnostic tests are shown in Table 69-8.

Management. In patients with mild PS (gradient *less than* 50 mm Hg) symptoms are uncommon, and the outcome is excellent.[44] Treatment is based on the presence of symptoms, age of the patient, and the degree of right ventricular hypertrophy. Vasodilator therapy is used to decrease the severity of pulmonary hypertension. Diuretics, digoxin, and a low-sodium diet may be used to treat symptoms of heart failure. Patients with severe PS (gradient *greater than* 80 mm Hg) may be symptomatic and have evidence of right heart failure. These patients may benefit from surgical or percutaneous procedures.[44]

Pulmonary Regurgitation

Pulmonary regurgitation **(PR)** is the backward leakage of blood from the pulmonary artery into the right ventricle during diastole. In PR the valve leaflets do not close firmly resulting in elevation of right heart pressures and hypertrophy.

Pathophysiology. Minor degrees of PR can be found in healthy people, and PR is rarely associated with progressive valve dysfunction or adverse clinical outcomes.[44] Clinically significant PR is rare. PR occurs mainly as a congenital defect with acquired PR occurring as a result of any condition that causes pulmonary hypertension, such as MS, chronic obstructive pulmonary disease, pulmonary embolism, or endocarditis. PR is a consequence of pulmonary artery hypertension.[24,44] Clinical manifestations include peripheral edema, dyspnea on exertion, and fatigue.[44]

Physical Assessment. The murmur of PR without elevated pulmonary artery pressures is an early diastolic decrescendo murmur heard best in the second-left intercostal space at the left sternal border. This murmur may increase during quiet inspiration. The murmur of PR with elevated pulmonary pressures is a high-pitched, blowing, diastolic murmur heard at the mid left sternal border. When PR is caused by infective endocarditis, patients who develop septic pulmonary emboli and pulmonary artery hypertension often exhibit severe right ventricular failure. The clinical manifestations of the

■ ■ ■

TABLE 69-8 DIAGNOSTIC TESTS FOR PULMONARY STENOSIS

TEST	FINDING
12-Lead ECG	• May be normal • With more severe lesions reveal right atrial and ventricular hypertrophy, tall P waves, marked right axis deviation, tall R wave in lead V_1
Chest x-ray	• Cardiomegaly
Echocardiography	• Visualize thickened leaflets with doming during systole • Degree of stenosis • Coexisting pulmonic regurgitation
Cardiac catheterization	• Before surgical intervention, when clinical picture and echocardiographic data are discordant

ECG, Electrocardiogram.

■ ■ ■

TABLE 69-9   DIAGNOSTIC TESTS FOR PULMONARY REGURGITATION

TEST	FINDING
12-lead ECG	• In the absence of pulmonary hypertension, reflects right ventricular diastolic overload (an rSr or rsR configuration in the right precordial leads) • Pulmonary regurgitation (PR) secondary to pulmonary hypertension shows evidence of right ventricular hypertrophy
Chest x-ray	• Pulmonary artery and right ventricle usually enlarged (nonspecific)
Fluoroscopy	• PR diagnosed by observing opacification of the right ventricle • Pronounced pulsation of the main pulmonary artery
Echocardiography	• Motion of pulmonic valve may identify cause • Right ventricular dilatation, hypertrophy, and function can be estimated • Degree of regurgitation

ECG, Electrocardiogram.

primary disease overshadow the PR, which may only be discovered by detection of the murmur.[24]

Diagnostic Tests. The most common diagnostic tests include 12-lead ECG, chest x-ray, and echocardiogram. The diagnosis of PR is often initially made by echocardiography. Additional diagnostic tests used to assess PR can be found in Table 69-9.

Management. Since the severity of PR is generally mild, there is no specific treatment needed for most adults.[44] Symptoms of right heart failure can be treated with a medical regimen of diuretics, digoxin, and a low-sodium diet. Treatment of the primary condition, such as infective endocarditis, or the cause of the pulmonary hypertension can alleviate the symptoms of PR.[24] In severe PR, with or without the onset of right ventricular systolic dysfunction, surgical intervention should be considered.[44]

MULTIVALVULAR DISEASE

Diseases that affect heart valves can occur in a variety of ways. Two separate processes can have an effect on the same valve (e.g., MS and MR), and one disease can affect two or more valves.[50] Lastly, different diseases may affect two different valves in the same patient; for example, infective endocarditis may cause AR, and ischemia may result in MR.[24] Persons with rheumatic fever may have both mitral and aortic valvular disease. Other causes of multivalvular disease include: infective endocarditis, myxomatous proliferation and prolapse, and valvular calcification in the elderly.[50]

In multivalvular disease, it is difficult to assess the severity of a specific valvular disease because the symptoms may be masked by the other diseased valve. Patients suspected of multivalvular disease should have a careful history and physical examination, echocardiography, and a cardiac catheterization. Right and left cardiac catheterization is decisive in identifying the preponderant valvular disorder and the degree of stenosis or regurgitation of the affected valves. Diagnosing multival-

vular disease preoperatively is imperative because if a valvular disorder is not corrected during surgery, mortality is increased significantly.[50]

Mitral Stenosis and Aortic Regurgitation

Patients with MS and AR generally experience dyspnea and fatigue secondary to pulmonary congestion and heart failure. They also may experience angina. On physical examination, the widened pulse pressure seen with AR may be absent.[24] Left ventricular hypertrophy may be seen on 12-lead ECG or chest x-ray. Echocardiography is specifically helpful in diagnosing MS and AR. Interventions may include a mitral valve repair or balloon valvuloplasty with an AVR if possible. Replacement of both valves is usually avoided because of the increased short-term and long-term risks.[24,51] A surgeon may consider performing a valvuloplasty first and then reassessing cardiac function. If the signs and symptoms of AR resolve, AVR may be delayed.[20]

Mitral Stenosis and Aortic Stenosis

Left ventricular hypertrophy and diminished cardiac output are usually present in patients with MS and AS. Many of the signs and symptoms associated with MS, such as pulmonary congestion, atrial fibrillation, and thromboembolism, will be seen more frequently in patients with AS as well.[24] Auscultation of the heart reveals a diastolic, rumbling, murmur and an aortic systolic murmur, which is usually loud, but may be decreased with severe MS.[50] An S_4, usually auscultated with AS, may not be present.[24] Left ventricular hypertrophy, left atrial enlargement, and atrial fibrillation may be determined by the 12-lead ECG. The chest x-ray reveals left atrial and left ventricular enlargement. Again, echocardiography is most helpful in identifying the stenosis of both valves. Mitral balloon valvuloplasty and AVR are commonly the surgical treatments of choice.[24] If the AS is mild, the valvuloplasty may be performed first and then the aortic valve may be reevaluated.[20]

Aortic Stenosis and Mitral Regurgitation

Rheumatic fever is generally the cause of these two combined disorders. AS increases the MR flow; resulting in increased left atrial and pulmonary pressures. The MR also decreases the ventricular preload needed to overcome the aortic pressure in AS, resulting in a decreased cardiac output. Cardiac auscultation reveals an apical holosystolic murmur. Left ventricular hypertrophy and atrial fibrillation are determined by the 12-lead ECG. A chest x-ray reveals cardiomegaly secondary to both left atrial and left ventricular enlargement. Surgical treatment often includes an AVR and mitral valve repair.[51]

Aortic Regurgitation and Mitral Regurgitation

This combination of valvular disorders results in left ventricular dilatation accompanied by left atrial dilatation and subsequent development of heart failure. Physical examination will show evidence of both lesions. Left atrial and left ventricular enlargement and atrial fibrillation will be seen on the ECG.

Echocardiography and cardiac catheterization can be used to evaluate the severity of each lesion. MR that occurs in patients with AR that is secondary to left ventricular dilatation may improve following AVR surgery. If MR is severe, annuloplasty is recommended to correct the MR at the time of the AVR.[24]

VALVULOPLASTY

Percutaneous balloon dilatation of stenotic valves is an alternative to surgical valve repair and replacement in select patients with valvular heart disease. Approaches for percutaneous valvuloplasty vary depending on the valve to be dilated. Mitral valvuloplasties are most commonly performed using a transvenous approach, whereas aortic valvuloplasties use an arterial approach. There are a variety of balloon-dilating devices including, double, single, and circular balloons.

PERCUTANEOUS MITRAL VALVULOPLASTY

Percutaneous mitral valvuloplasty **(PMV)** for treatment of symptomatic MS was first performed in 1984 and became a clinically approved technique in 1994.[20] Patient selection is determined by the severity of obstruction, coexisting MR, presence, and severity of other valve lesions or coronary artery disease, any comorbid conditions and patient preference for percutaneous versus surgical intervention.[29] PMV is most successful when the mitral valve leaflets are mobile and uncalcified. Contraindications include the presence of left atrial thrombus[52] and significant MR.[20]

For PMV, a transvenous or antegrade approach is most commonly used with a transseptal puncture from the right atrium into the left atrium. The balloon is then passed across the mitral valve into the left ventricle. A retrograde, transarterial approach is used less often to prevent the creation of an atrial septal defect[24] or when a transseptal approach is contraindicated or impossible.[52] A double balloon technique can be used, but most centers now use the Inoue balloon. The double-balloon method, for mitral valvuloplasty, uses a transseptal puncture with a balloon catheter advanced across the mitral valve into the left ventricle. Two long exchange wires are then positioned in the left ventricle, and the interatrial septum is dilated. Two mitral valvuloplasty balloons are advanced across the mitral valve and inflated simultaneously to split the sclerosed mitral commissures.[53]

The Inoue balloon is a self-positioning balloon that locks itself into the stenotic valve orifice and progressively dilates the orifice as the inflation pressure increases.[53] The Inoue balloon, an hour glass-shaped, low profile, single balloon (shown in Figure 69-3) is easy to maneuver,[20] creates a smaller defect in the atrial septum,[54] and allows precise control of the extent of dilatation.[13] Using the Inoue technique has resulted in less complications and comparable rates of success when compared with closed mitral commissurotomy, and long-term results are as favorable as open commissurotomy.[52,54]

Echocardiographic imaging, right atrial angiography, and cardiac catheterization are used for patient evalua-

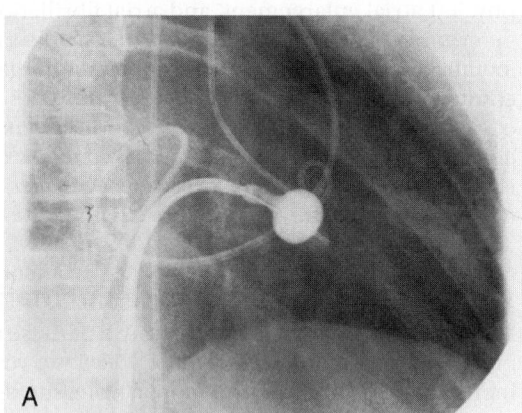
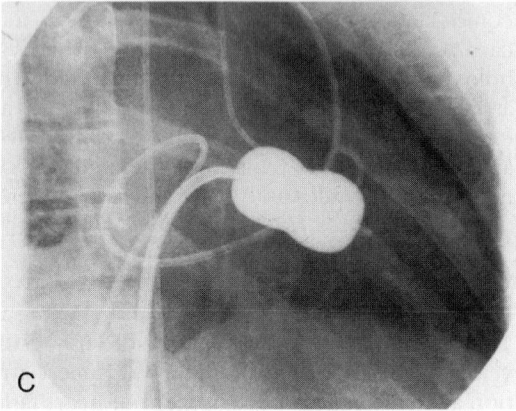
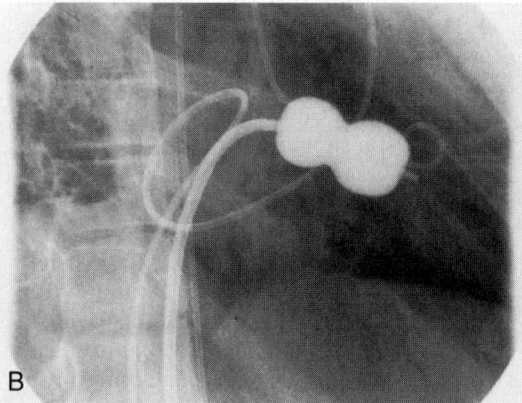

FIGURE 69-3 ■ Fluoroscopic images during a percutaneous balloon valvuloplasty using an Inoue balloon. **A,** Distal balloon inflation securing position at the valvular level. **B,** Proximal balloon inflation. **C,** Inflation of the dilating segment. (From Otto CM: Surgical and percutaneous intervention for mitral stenosis. In Otto CM, editor: *Valvular heart disease,* ed 2, Philadelphia, 2004, Saunders. pp 272-301.)

tion and guidance during the procedure.[29] A percutaneous reusable metallic device has been developed to decrease the cost of the procedure. This metallic device has been used in developing counties where there is high incidence of MS and limited financial resources.[55]

Complications include development of an atrial septal defect at the transseptal puncture site, cardiac tamponade from perforation of a guiding or dilating catheter, an increase in MR from none or mild at baseline to moderate or severe postprocedure, and systemic embolization by dislodging a left atrial thrombus.[29] Overall event free (without death, repeat PMV, or mitral valve replacement) survival ranges are from 85 percent to 72 percent at 5 to 10 years, respectively in patients with favorable mitral valve morphology.[20,56]

Nursing interventions for patients undergoing PMV focus on patient education, including explanations of the procedure and preprocedure and postprocedure care. Postprocedure acute nursing care includes monitoring vital signs, assessing heart sounds, assessing the insertion site for signs of bleeding, and assessing distal limb perfusion.

Percutaneous Aortic Valvuloplasty

Percutaneous aortic valvuloplasty was performed in the late 1980s and early 1990s, but it is now clear that there is little benefit of this procedure in adults with calcific AS or with secondary calcification of a bicuspid valve.[38] Percutaneous aortic valvuloplasty can be performed on adult patients with severe comorbidities who are not candidates for AVR or in patients as a "bridge" to surgical correction.[24] The femoral approach is most frequently used for this procedure. The aortic valve is crossed with a guidewire, and an extra stiff wire is inserted into the apex of the left ventricle to stabilize the balloon during inflation. An antegrade approach necessitates a transseptal puncture and is a more difficult procedure.[24,52]

Long-term clinical benefits of percutaneous aortic valvuloplasty for calcific AS is limited[24,33,52] with evidence that mortality is no different from that for untreated AS.[38] Long-term survival after this procedure is poor with a 1-year survival rate reported of 55 percent and a 3-year survival rate reported of 23 percent.[38] Percutaneous aortic valvuloplasty is reserved for children and young adults with congenital AS.[20,37,38]

Percutaneous Tricuspid Valvuloplasty

Percutaneous tricuspid valvuloplasty is rare and reserved for patients having a tight TS either pure or associated with mild regurgitation.[52] Severe TR is a common consequence of this procedure and is far more detrimental than TS. Results are poor when TR develops.[20] In patients with TS and MS, the TS is not corrected alone because the patient may develop pulmonary congestion or edema.[24]

Percutaneous Pulmonary Valvuloplasty

Balloon valvuloplasty is the treatment of choice for patients with severe (a gradient *greater than* 80 mm Hg) pulmonary valve stenosis.[57] Patients are likely to be symp-

tomatic and have evidence of right heart failure.[44] The procedure has been performed for acquired PS caused by carcinoid or rheumatic disease with suboptimal results when the valve is dysplastic, the cusps are excessively thickened, or the annulus is hypoplastic.[44] It is most often performed using a circular balloon, although both the double balloon and Inoue balloon techniques have been used. The circular balloon can be oversized by 20 percent to 40 percent relative to the pulmonary annulus.[44] Postprocedure, transpulmonic gradients decrease,[58] and the pulmonary trunk may reduce in size. Complications are rare, yet include PR that is typically mild, perforation with tamponade, and worsened tricuspid insufficiency as a result of right ventricular papillary muscle rupture.[44] In 10-year follow-up exams, beneficial effects are well maintained with low restenosis rates.[57,58]

CARDIAC VALVE SURGERY

In 2002, more than 90,000 surgical valve procedures were performed in the United States.[5] The timing of surgery varies based on the patient, the valve disorder, and the progression of the valve disease. Most patients are managed medically until symptoms develop or until ventricular dysfunction begins to develop. Surgical intervention for valve disorders includes valve repair or valve replacement with mechanical prostheses, biological prostheses, or homograft valves.

Cardiac Valve Repair

Although valve repair can be performed to improve the function of insufficient or stenotic valves, most surgeries are performed for valve insufficiency. Valve repair can be performed for aortic valve disease; however, it is more commonly performed for mitral valve dysfunction. The majority of nonrheumatic mitral valve disorders can be repaired.[59,60] A much smaller percentage of aortic valves can be repaired.

Mitral Valve Repair

Surgery is performed to repair damaged commissures, chordae tendineae, valve leaflets, and papillary muscles. Open mitral commissurotomy is performed when the mitral valve is stenotic as a result of fused commissures. The commissures are incised from the annulus to the center of the mitral valve in an effort to improve leaflet mobility and increase the size of the valve orifice. An open mitral commissurotomy can usually be performed if the valve has good leaflet mobility and no valvular calcification. Surgery is recommended for patients when the mitral valve area is *less than* 1.5 cm^2.[61]

Surgery for mitral insufficiency may involve repair of the mitral annulus. One technique involves suturing the enlarged annulus to reduce its size. Another technique involves insertion of a preshaped, flexible, prosthetic annuloplasty ring, which is sewn to the mitral valve annulus to reshape it (Figure 69-4). Both techniques are effective in reducing mitral valve insufficiency.

Mitral insufficiency may be due to dysfunction of the subvalvular mechanism. Elongated or detached chordae contribute to prolapse of the anterior or posterior valve leaflets resulting in mitral insufficiency. The chordae tendineae are essential in supporting the valve leaflets and preventing the leaflets from prolapsing into the left atrium during systole. If the chordae are elongated or some of them are detached, the valve leaflets often prolapse back into the left atrium during systole causing insufficiency.

Shortening or lengthening of the chordae tendineae may preserve valve leaflet function. Elongated chordae tendineae can be shortened and attached to the mitral valve leaflet or to the papillary muscle. The chordae can also be folded onto itself and then sutured to the valve leaflet or can be folded and tucked within the papillary muscle or folded and sutured to the exterior of a papillary muscle. Ruptured chordae of the anterior leaflet may be replaced by transposing chordae from the posterior leaflet.[62] Another technique, chordal replacement (Figure 69-5), involves excising the ruptured chordae and replacing the chordae with chordae made of natural or artificial materials, such as polytetrafluoroethylene

suture material.[62,63] Elongated chordae tendineae can also be repaired by excising shortened or fused chordae tendineae. Shortened chordae can be longitudinally cut to lengthen the chordae in an effort to improve support of the valve leaflets. If chordae tendineae are fused together, a triangular segment of fibrous tissue can be excised.[62]

Myxomatous and degenerative changes in the leaflet tissues, with subsequent elongation or even rupture of the chordae, can result in mitral insufficiency. Changes in the posterior or anterior leaflets can be repaired by resecting a segment of the prolapsed leaflet (Figure 69-6). A prosthetic annuloplasty ring may be inserted to provide additional support to the valve annulus after leaflet resection. Leaflets damaged by infection also may be amenable to valve repair. Excessive or redundant portions of the valve leaflet can be resected in an effort to improve valve leaflet function. The infected leaflets may be repaired with pericardial tissue. Valve leaflets can also be repaired with patches of glutaraldehyde-treated autologous or bovine pericardium.[62]

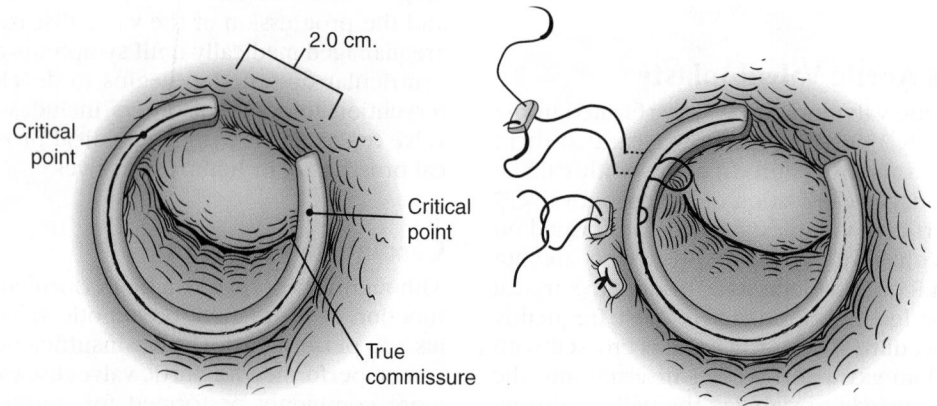

FIGURE 69-4 ■ An annuloplasty ring is sutured in place to reshape a dilated mitral valve annulus.

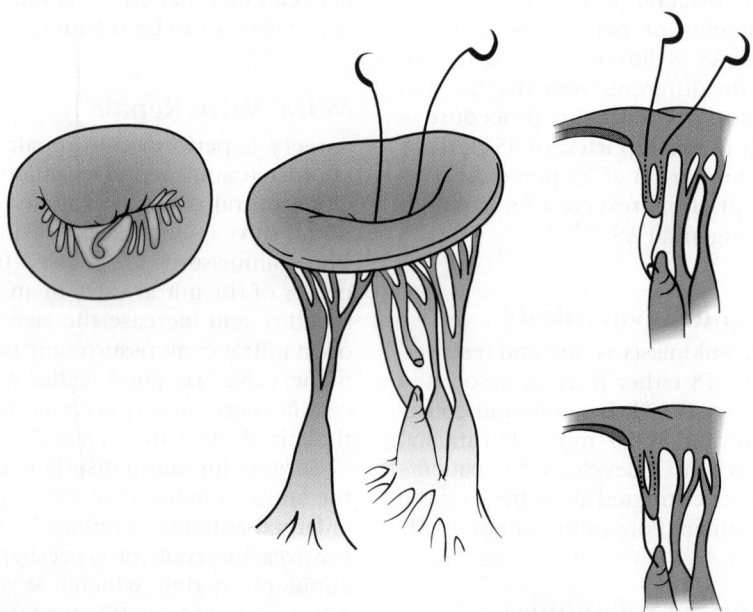

FIGURE 69-5 ■ Chordal replacement using expanded polytetrafluoroethylene sutures. (From David TE, Omran A, Armstrong S et al: Long-term results of mitral valve repair for myxomatous disease with and without chordal replacement with expanded polytetrafluoroethylene, *Thorac Cardiovasc Surg* 115:1279-1286, 1998.)

When chordae are ruptured...

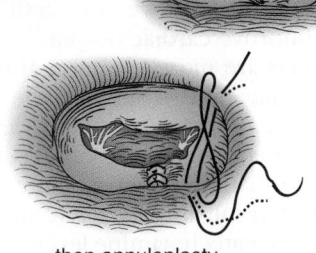

Interrupted sutures
placed to invert
valve leaflet

then annuloplasty
performed.

FIGURE 69-6 ■ Resection and repair of a prolapsed valve segment.

Myocardial ischemia can result in a tear or detachment of a papillary muscle. Repair involves reattachment of the papillary muscle to the endocardium.

Aortic Valve Repair

Repair of the aortic valve is not as common as repair of the mitral valve. Repair of a stenotic or insufficient aortic valve is more difficult than the mitral valve because the closing mechanism is more precise.[64] Open aortic commissurotomy may be performed on valves that are stenotic or fused. The commissures are incised in an attempt to open the stenotic valve. AR may be due to cusp retraction (caused by fibrosis or calcification), prolapse and perforation, or dilatation of the aortic root.[62] Cusp retraction may be treated by extension or substitution by glutaraldehyde-treated bovine or autologous pericardium.[62] A triangular section of a prolapsed aortic valve cusp can be excised to eliminate AR. Pericardial patches can be used to repair perforations in the aortic valve cusps. Another technique involves resuspending the valve to decrease or eliminate the amount of valve regurgitation caused by dilatation of the aortic valve annulus. Fibrosis of the valve cusps can contribute to aortic insufficiency. Carpentier[64] developed a technique to shave thickened valve leaflet edges in an attempt to improve or eliminate aortic insufficiency.

Cardiac Valve Replacement

The most commonly replaced valves are the mitral and aortic valves. Mitral valve replacement is indicated for patients with severe valve calcification, significant subvalvular stenosis, or MS accompanied by significant MR.[24] AVR of the native valve with a prosthetic valve is performed for severely calcified or damaged valves.[27] Valve replacement may be the primary intended surgical intervention or may be performed during surgery when valve repair is unsuccessful.

Diseased valves are replaced with mechanical or bioprosthetic valves. A prosthetic valve is selected based on the location the valve will be placed, the patient's age, lifestyle, and past medical history. The main advantage of a bioprosthetic valve is that anticoagulation usually is not required, whereas the main disadvantage is limited durability. Bioprosthetic valves are commonly used in the elderly.

Mechanical valves are very durable, yet require lifelong anticoagulation therapy. Anticoagulation therapy is contraindicated if the patient has a history of coagulopathy, bleeding disorder, hepatic disorder, or participates in contact sports. Mechanical valves are selected if a long life expectancy is likely (e.g., *greater than* 15 years) and there are no contraindications to anticoagulation.

The most common mechanical valve inserted today is the St. Jude Medical valve (Figure 69-7). The St. Jude Medical valve is a bileaflet valve. Pressure changes force the valve to open and close. For example, in the aortic position, the valve opens as pressure increases in the left ventricle and pushes open the valve discs during systole. The leaflets close as pressure decreases in the aorta and the valve discs passively close. The St. Jude Medical valve has excellent long-term durability.

Bioprosthetic or biological valves include porcine, bovine, and homograft. A porcine valve is a pig aortic valve that is mounted on a stent (Figure 69-8). A bovine valve is constructed from the pericardial tissue of calves. The pericardial tissue is used to form the valve leaflets, which are mounted on a stent (Figure 69-9). Homografts are valves retrieved from human hearts within 24 hours of cardiac arrest. More recently developed valves include stentless bioprosthetic valves, which have the advantage of improved flow and lower transvalvular gradients.[24]

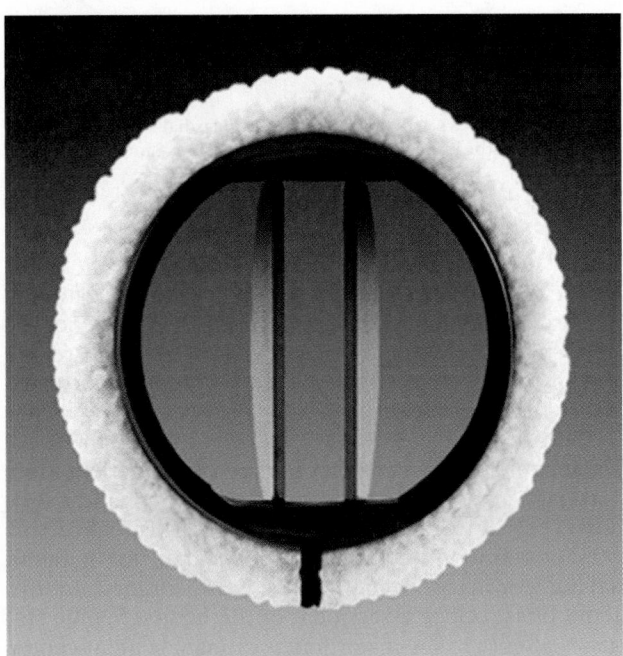

FIGURE 69-7 ■ St. Jude Medical mechanical heart valve. (Courtesy of St. Jude Medical, Inc, Saint Paul.)

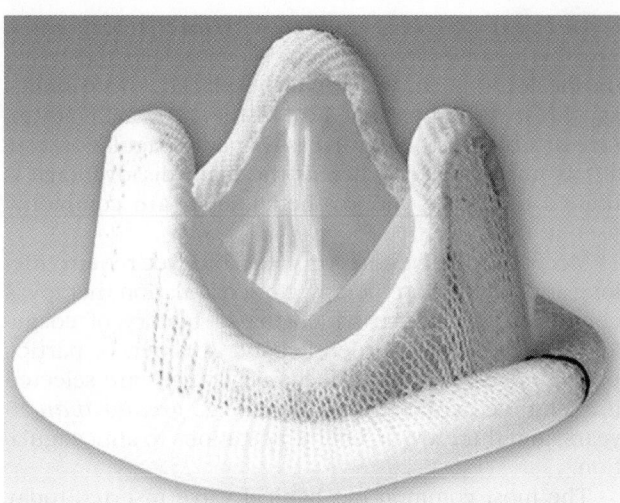

FIGURE 69-8 ■ Carpentier-Edwards porcine valve. (Courtesy of Baxter Healthcare Corp, Edwards CVS Division, Santa Ana, Calif.)

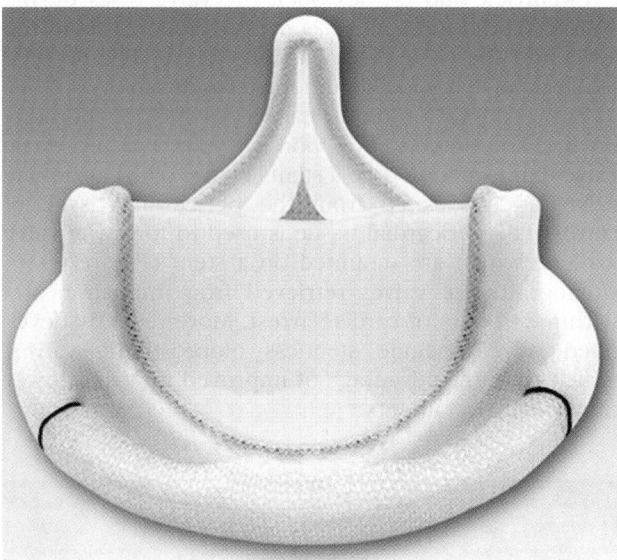

FIGURE 69-9 ■ Carpentier-Edwards pericardial valve. (Courtesy of Baxter Healthcare Corp, Edwards CVS Division, Santa Ana, Calif.)

Patient Care after Cardiac Surgery

Before cardiac valve surgery, a cardiac catheterization is performed to determine the presence or absence of stenosis of the coronary arteries. Cardiac valve repair and/or replacement surgery often accompany coronary artery bypass graft surgery.

Care of the patient after cardiac valve repair or replacement surgery is similar to care of the patient after coronary artery bypass surgery (refer to Chapter 65); however, the recovery process after cardiac valve surgery is commonly a slower process than for patients having coronary artery bypass graft surgery. In the acute phase, close assessment of the hemodynamic status is essential. The major tenets of management center on optimizing preload, enhancing contractility, and reducing afterload. Patients with valvular disorders com-

monly have increased cardiac filling pressures. Although the valve has been repaired or replaced, time is often needed for the heart to adjust to the improved hemodynamic function. Preoperative pulmonary artery pressures and hemodynamic values are useful in guiding postoperative management. Patients usually do well in the postoperative phase if fluids are adjusted based on presurgical right atrial and pulmonary artery wedge pressures. A combination of vasoactive, inotropic, and vasodilator medications are used in the immediate postoperative period to improve contractility, decrease afterload, and improve cardiac output.[65]

Dysrhythmias are more common after valve surgery than after cardiac bypass surgery and occur in more than 50 percent of patients having cardiac valve surgery.[66] The most common dysrhythmias are atrial (tachycardia, atrial fibrillation, and atrial flutter). Dysrhythmias may occur as a result of electrolyte imbalances, hypothermia, elevated catecholamine levels, inflammation, or myocardial stunning. Medications, such as digoxin, beta blockers, and calcium channel blockers are commonly used to treat atrial dysrhythmias. Beta blockade is the most effective pharmacological agent to prevent and manage atrial dysrhythmias after cardiac surgery.

Conduction disturbances are very common after cardiac valve surgery. The tricuspid, mitral, and aortic valves lie close to the conduction pathways. Conduction disturbances occur because of tissue edema or damage from surgery. Continuous ECG monitoring is essential in the postoperative period to assess for first, second, and third degree heart block. Conduction disturbances usually necessitate temporary epicardial pacing and at times even permanent pacemaker therapy.

Anticoagulation therapy is commonly initiated within 48 hours of cardiac valve replacement, but it is usually delayed until after epicardial pacing wires are removed. Anticoagulation therapy is recommended for all patients after cardiac valve surgery to decrease the incidence of thrombus and embolus formation.

ADDITIONAL CONSIDERATIONS FOR PATIENTS WITH VALVE DISORDERS

After valvular surgery, the health care team works together and with the patient to prevent bacterial endocarditis and manage anticoagulation therapy.

Bacterial Endocarditis

Patients with valve disease are at an increased risk for bacterial endocarditis because abnormal valves produce turbulent blood flow, and bacteria can adhere to the damaged or diseased valve surfaces. Antibiotic prophylactic treatment before dental and most surgical procedures decreases the risk of endocarditis. Lifelong antibiotic prophylaxis is recommended for patients with valvular disorders.[20]

Bacterial endocarditis is a serious and potentially life-threatening complication of cardiac valve surgery.[20,67] After valve repair, it is important that patients follow recommendations regarding the need for antibiotic prophylaxis before dental work, surgery, and other invasive procedures. Patients with replaced cardiac valves need lifelong prophylactic antibiotic therapy before oral, urogenital, or invasive procedures. The American Heart Association has published specific recommendations (Table 69-10) regarding prevention of bacterial endocarditis. Antibiotic prophylaxis to genitourinary and gastrointestinal procedures is no longer recommended by AHA as of April, 2007.

Anticoagulation Therapy

Thromboembolism is a major complication for patients with valvular disease and prosthetic heart valves. Systemic embolism can occur secondary to left atrial thrombus formation in patients with a dilated left atrium and a decreased flow of blood, with or without atrial fibrillation. Antithrombotic and anticoagulant medications are used to reduce the risk of thromboembolism, although they place the patient at risk for hemorrhage (Tables 69-11 and 69-12).[68]

Risk Factors

When assessing the need for antithrombotic therapy, certain risk factors increase the incidence of thromboembolism (Box 69-4). Another consideration is the type, number, and location of implanted prostheses.[68]

Patients with mechanical prosthetic valves require lifelong antithrombotic therapy because these prostheses are more thrombogenic. First-generation prosthetic valves, such as the Starr-Edwards caged-ball valve and the Björk-Shiley valve have a high thromboembolic rate. Single tilting disc valves have an intermediate risk. The newer bileaflet valves have a lower risk. As the risk of

TABLE 69-11 RECOMMENDATIONS FOR ANTITHROMBOTIC THERAPY FOR PROSTHETIC VALVE REPLACEMENT ACCORDING TO ACC/AHA GUIDELINES

INDICATION	MEDICATION	TARGET
First 3 months after valve replacement	Warfarin	INR 2.5-3.5
3 months after valve replacement		
Mechanical valve		
AVR with no risk factor*		
Bileaflet valve or Medtronic-Hall valve	Warfarin	INR 2-3
Other disc valves or Starr-Edwards valve	Warfarin	INR 2.5-3.5
AVR with risk factor*	Warfarin	INR 2.5-3.5
MVR	Warfarin	INR 2.5-3.5
3 months after valve replacement		
Bioprosthetic valve		
AVR with no risk factor*	Aspirin	80-100 mg/day
AVR with risk factor*	Warfarin	INR 2-3
MVR with no risk factor*	Aspirin	80-100 mg/day
MVR with risk factor*	Warfarin	INR 2.5-3.5

ACC/AHA, American College of Cardiology; American Heart Association; *AVR,* aortic valve replacement; *INR,* international normalized ratio; *MVR,* mitral valve replacement.
*Risk factors: atrial fibrillation, LV dysfunction, previous thromboembolism, and hypercoagulable condition.
From Bonow RO, Braunwald E: Valvular heart disease. In Zipes DP, Libby P, Bonow RO, Braunwald E, editors: *Braunwald's heart disease: a textbook of cardiovascular medicine,* ed 7, Philadelphia, 2005, Elsevier Saunders, p 1632.

thromboembolism is decreased, so is the intensity of the treatment.[68]

Bioprosthetic valves have a lower risk of thromboembolism, and these patients may require a different type of antithrombotic therapy, such as an anticoagulant, for the first 3 months followed by lifelong antiplatelet therapy. The treatment varies based on the patient's risk factors.[68] The location of the valve prosthesis also plays a key factor in determining the need for antithrombotic therapy. Prosthetic valves implanted in the mitral orifice carry a greater risk of thrombosis than those implanted in the aorta. The incidence of thromboembolism also increases with the number of prosthetic valves implanted. Double valve replacement has a higher incidence of thromboembolism when compared with single valve replacement. The risk of thromboembolism is greatest in the first 3 months after surgery.[68]

Antithrombotic Medications

Patients are usually anticoagulated with the oral medication, warfarin. The degree of anticoagulation is based upon the international normalized ratio **(INR),** a diagnostic test used to gauge the dose of the medication. Heparin may also be used on a short-term basis. Patients are usually given heparin to achieve anticoagulation until the oral anticoagulant takes effect. It is also used during short periods when the oral anticoagulant needs to be stopped, such as if surgery or an invasive procedure is needed. The dosage of heparin is prescribed according to the ac-

TABLE 69-10 AHA RECOMMENDATIONS FOR ENDOCARDITIS PROPHYLAXIS (ADULTS)

SITUATION	AGENT	REGIMEN
Dental, Oral, Respiratory Tract, or Esophageal Procedures		
Standard oral prophylaxis	Amoxicillin	2 g orally 1 hr before procedure
Unable to take oral medications	Ampicillin or	2 g IM or IV within 30 min before procedure
	Cefazolin or ceftriaxone	1 g IM or IV within 30 minutes before procedure
Oral regimen for those allergic to penicillin	Clindamycin or	600 mg 1 hr before procedure
	Cephalexin or cefadroxil*	2 g 1 hr before procedure
	Azithromycin or clarithromycin	500 mg 1 hr before procedure
Allergic to penicillin and unable to take oral medications	Clindamycin or	600 mg IM or IV within 30 min before procedure
	Cefazolin*	1 g IM or IV within 30 min before procedure

Im, Intramuscular; *IV,* intravenous; *MVP,* mitral valve prolapse.
*Cephalosporins should not be used in individuals with immediate-type hypersensitivity reaction (urticaria, angioedema, or anaphylaxis) to penicillin.

■ ■ ■

TABLE 69-12 RECOMMENDATIONS FOR ANTITHROMBOTIC THERAPY FOR PROSTHETIC VALVE REPLACEMENT ACCORDING TO ACCP GUIDELINES

INDICATION	MEDICATION	TARGET
Mechanical valve		
AVR with St. Jude Medical bileaf-let valve	Warfarin	INR 2-3
AVR with CarboMedics bileaflet valve or Medtronic-Hall tilting disc valve with normal left atrial size, in normal sinus rhythm	Warfarin	INR 2-3
AVR with risk factor*	Warfarin Aspirin	INR 2.5-3.5 80-100 mg/day
MVR with tilting disc valve or bileaflet valve	Warfarin	INR 2.5-3.5
MVR with risk factor*	Warfarin Aspirin	INR 2.5-3.5 80-100 mg/day
Caged-ball or caged-disc valve	Warfarin Aspirin	INR 2.5-3.5 80-100 mg/day
Bioprosthetic valve		
AVR—first 3 months	Warfarin Aspirin	INR 2-3 80-100 mg/day
MVR—first 3 months	Warfarin	INR 2-3
Bioprosthetic valve replacement with history of systemic embolism	Warfarin 3-12 months	
Bioprosthetic valve replacement with evidence of left atrial thrombus at surgery	Warfarin	INR 2-3
Bioprosthetic valve replacement in NSR	Aspirin	80-100 mg/day
Bioprosthetic valve replacement with AF	Long-term Warfarin	INR 2-3

AF, Atrial fibrillation; *AVR*, aortic valve replacement; *INR*, international normalized ratio; *MVR*, mitral valve replacement.
*Risk factors: atrial fibrillation, myocardial infarction, left atrial enlargement, endocardial damage, and low ejection fraction.

BOX 69-4 ■ ■ ■
RISK FACTORS FOR THROMBOEMBOLISM

Age
Smoking
Hypertension
Diabetes
Hyperlipidemia
Type and severity of valve lesion
Presence of atrial fibrillation, heart failure, or low cardiac output
Size of left atrium (more than 50 mm on echocardiography)
Previous thromboembolism
Abnormalities of coagulation system

---

tivated partial thromboplastin time **(APTT)**. An alternative to heparin is low-molecular-weight heparin **(LMWH)**. Antiplatelet medications, such as aspirin or dipyridamole, may be used for their antithrombotic effect.[68]

Native Valve Disease

Certain patients with native valve disease are candidates for antithrombotic therapy. Oral anticoagulant medications are prescribed for patients with valvular disease and atrial fibrillation.[20,68] They may also be prescribed for patients with MS who are in normal sinus rhythm, based on the following characteristics: degree of stenosis, patient's age, size of the left atrium, and echocardiographic evidence of left atrial appendage thrombus.[68] Anticoagulant medications should achieve a target INR range of 2 to 3.[68]

Patients with MVP and a thickened or redundant mitral valve on echocardiographic exam may benefit from low-dose aspirin therapy because they may be at risk for thromboembolism.[27] Patients with MVP may also require long-term warfarin anticoagulation if they have had a systemic embolism; have had unexplained transient ischemic attacks despite antiplatelet medication; or have atrial fibrillation.[20]

Valvuloplasty

Patients with MS who are scheduled to have a percutaneous balloon valvuloplasty may be given a TEE first to assess for the presence of a thrombus. If a thrombus is detected, anticoagulant therapy is usually prescribed for 2 months before the procedure, achieving an INR range of 2 to 3. If a thrombus is not found but the patient has a history of a previous thromboembolism, enlarged left atrium, or atrial fibrillation, anticoagulants also will be given for a period of 1 month.[68]

Heparin is given to the patient during the valvuloplasty and should be continued afterward for 24 hours. Oral anticoagulants are started 24 hours after the procedure in patients with the risk factors described above. Heparin is also prescribed for the patient undergoing an aortic valvuloplasty who is in normal sinus rhythm; however, these patients do not usually require long-term treatment.[68]

The most recent guidelines from the American College of Chest Physicians **(ACCP)** recommend that patients undergoing a mitral valvuloplasty should be anticoagulated with vitamin K antagonists with a target INR of 2.5 (range 2 to 3) for 3 weeks before the procedure and for 4 weeks after the procedure.[69]

Mitral Valve Repair

Patients undergoing mitral valve repair may be anticoagulated for 6 to 12 weeks following the procedure with a target INR of 2.5.[68] Long-term administration of aspirin also may be considered after surgery.[70] After 3 months, antithrombotic treatment is based on the presence or absence of risk factors, such as atrial fibrillation, heart failure, or an enlarged left atrium.[68]

Bioprosthetic Valves

Patients who receive a bioprosthetic heart valve replacement receive oral anticoagulant therapy for a period of 3 months, maintaining an INR range of 2 to 3. Patients also receive lifelong treatment with antiplatelet therapy, usually low-dose aspirin.[20,68] Lifelong anticoagulant therapy is considered for those with the following risk factors: previous thromboembolism, atrial fibrillation, and left ventricular dysfunction.[20] If thromboembolism occurs despite adequate anticoagulation, the INR target range is increased and aspirin is added to the treatment regimen.[20]

Mechanical Valves

Patients with mechanical valve prostheses require lifelong anticoagulant therapy to prevent the risk of thromboembolism. Their target INR range depends upon the valve used and the number of valves involved in replacement. As mentioned earlier, first-generation valves carry a higher risk of thromboembolism and require a higher intensity of therapy. Risk factors also are taken into consideration when prescribing anticoagulant therapy.[68] Tables 69-11 and 69-12 outline recommendations for antithrombotic therapy for patients with prosthetic valve replacement according to the guidelines of the American College of Cardiology (ACC), American Heart Association (AHA),[24] and the ACCP.[69] As with bioprosthetic valves, if thromboembolism occurs despite adequate anticoagulation, the INR target range is increased and aspirin is added.[20,69]

Heparin is administered until the oral anticoagulant medication reaches the target INR range.[68] The ACCP recommends administration of heparin or LMWH until the INR is at a therapeutic level for 2 consecutive days.[69] The dosage of heparin is adequate if the patient's APTT is twice normal.[68]

Patients Requiring a Surgical Procedure

The dosage of anticoagulant therapy may need to be adjusted if the patient needs a surgical procedure. Anticoagulant therapy may be continued in minor procedures, such as dental surgery, where the blood loss is expected to be minimal and easy to control.[20,68]

In patients requiring noncardiac surgery, warfarin is discontinued 3 to 4 days before the procedure to allow the INR to return to the normal range. A small dose of vitamin K (0.5 to 1 mg) can be given to reverse the effects of warfarin if the INR remains elevated. Once the postprocedure bleeding is controlled, warfarin is restarted.[20] If emergency surgery is necessary, the effect of warfarin can be reversed by transfusion of fresh frozen plasma. This can be administered quickly to achieve adequate clotting for the procedure.[71]

Certain patients are at high risk for developing a thromboembolism while they are off anticoagulant therapy, including patients with mitral valve prostheses, atrial fibrillation, left ventricular dysfunction, or a history of prior embolization. Intravenous heparin can be administered to these patients to maintain anticoagulation when the INR falls below 2.0. The APTT should be maintained at 55 to 70 seconds to achieve a therapeutic effect. It can be discontinued 6 hours before surgery to allow for normal clotting function. It can then be restarted within 24 hours of the procedure after bleeding is controlled and continued until the INR reaches 2.0. A 3- to 5-day overlap of heparin and warfarin is recommended.[20]

Patient Education

Patient education regarding anticoagulation therapy is extremely important. Because patients are at risk for thromboembolism and bleeding, they need frequent assessment of their INR levels. Monthly determination of the INR is necessary, and their anticoagulant medications are adjusted according to their target INR range. Patients need to report any symptoms of bleeding, such as bruising, bleeding, epistaxis, and hemoptysis.

Dietary education is important as well. Patients need to know the foods that contain vitamin K. Since these foods influence the effectiveness of the medication, consistent quantities should be ingested to help keep the INR within the targeted range.[72] Patients should avoid alcohol and specific medications, such as aspirin, that may interact with warfarin. Both can potentiate the anticoagulant effect of the medication.

Management of Therapy

Patients derive benefits from attending an anticoagulation clinic for management of long-term anticoagulation therapy. Their physician or nurse practitioner prescribes a target INR range and refers them to the clinic. The clinic interviews the patient with regard to their current medication, diet, and lifestyle. The staff initiates therapy and monitors each patient's INR at specific intervals to adjust the dosage of the medication when necessary. Patient education is an important part of the process. The team monitors for drug interactions as well.

INR self-management is a novel approach to anticoagulant management. Patients test their own INR using home testing equipment and adjust their medication dosage. Menéndez-Jándula and associates[73] compared the level of control and clinical outcomes of oral anticoagulant therapy in self-managed patients versus patients following conventional management ($n = 737$). The percentages of in-range INRs in both groups were similar (58.6 percent in the self-management group and 55.6 percent in the conventional management group). Major complications related to anticoagulant treatment were 2.2 percent in the self-management group versus 7.3 percent in the conventional management group.

Earlier work by Körtke and colleagues[74] found that self-managed patients had 80 percent of their measured INR values within therapeutic range when compared with patients managed by their family physician (62 percent). Bleeding complications were evenly distributed between the groups. In another study, Christensen's[75] research team followed 24 patients who were on self-managed oral anticoagulation therapy for up to 4 years and compared them with a control group of conventionally managed patients. The self-managed patients maintained a therapeutic INR 78 percent of the time compared with 61 percent in the control group. Self-management of anticoagulation therapy appears to be a viable alternative in the treatment of patients with valvular disease. See Box 69-5 for a summary of available guidelines for the management of valvular heart disease.

BOX 69-5 ■ ■ ■
GUIDELINES AVAILABLE FOR THE MANAGEMENT OF VALVULAR HEART DISEASE

RISK FACTOR	GUIDELINE
Valvular disease	ACC/AHA guidelines for treatment of valvular heart disease *www.americanheart.org*
Valvular disease	Heart Center Online *www.heartcenteronline.com*
Valvular disease Warfarin	Medline Plus—U.S. National Library of Medicine and National Institutes of Health *www.nlm.gov/medlineplus*

ACC/AHA, American College of Cardiology/American Heart Association.

REFERENCES

1. Otto CM: Valvular heart disease: prevalence and clinical outcomes, In Otto CM, editor: *Valvular heart disease,* ed 2, Philadelphia, 2004, Saunders, pp 1-17.
2. Teramae CY, Connolly HM, Grogtan M, Miller F: Diet drug-related cardiac valve disease: the Mayo clinic echocardiographic laboratory experience, *Mayo Clinic Proceed* 75:456-461, 2000.
3. Redfield MM, Nicholson WJ, Edwards WD, Tajik AJ: Valve disease associated with ergot alkaloid use: echocardiographic and pathologic correlations, *Ann Intern Med* 117:50-52, 1992.
4. Baseman DG, O'Suilleabhain PE, Reimold SC et al: Pergolide use in Parkinson disease is associated with cardiac valve regurgitation, *Neurol* 63:301-304, 2004.
5. American Heart Association: *Heart disease and stroke statistics—2005 update,* Dallas, 2005, American Heart Association.
6. Devereux RB: Valvular heart disease. In Douglas PS, editor: *Cardiovascular health and disease in women,* Philadelphia, 2002, WB Saunders, pp 405-425.
7. Wolfe RR: Incidence of acute rheumatic fever: a persistent dilemma, *Pediatrics* 105(6):1375, 2000.
8. Smoot JC, Korgenski EK, Daly JA et al: Molecular analysis of group A streptococcus type emm18 isolates temporally associated with acute rheumatic fever outbreaks in Salt Lake City, Utah, *J Clin Micro* 40(5):1805-1810, 2002.
9. Gordis L, Lilienfeld A, Rodriguez R: Studies in the epidemiology and preventability of rheumatic fever: I. demographic factors and the incidence of acute attacks, *J Chronic Dis* 21:645-54, 1969.
10. Dajani AS: Rheumatic fever. In Zipes DP, Libby P, Bonow RO, Braunwald E, editors: *Braunwald's heart disease: a textbook of cardiovascular medicine,* ed 7, Philadelphia, 2005, Elsevier Saunders, pp 2093-2099.
11. Otto CM: Pathology and etiology of valvular heart disease. In Otto CM, editor: *Valvular heart disease,* ed 2, Philadelphia, 2004, Saunders, pp 18-50.
12. U.S. Census Bureau: Annual estimates of the population by sex and selected age groups for the United Sates: April 1, 2000 - July 1, 2003 (NC-EST2003-02), Source: Population Division, U.S. Census Bureau.
13. Hoen B, Alla F, Selton-Suty C et al: Changing profile of infective endocarditis: results of a 1-year survey in France, *JAMA* 288:75-81, 2002.
14. Brundage BH, Rich S, Levitsky S, Shanes JG: Acquired tricuspid valve disease. In Greenberg BH, Murphy E, editors: *Valvular heart disease,* Littleton, Mass, 1987, PSG Publishing, pp 46-57.
15. Shahi CN, Ghaisas NK, Goggins M et al: Elevated levels of circulating soluble adhesion molecules in patients with nonrheumatic aortic valve disease, *Am J Cardiol* 79:980-2, 1997.
16. Boon A, Cheriex E, Lodder J, Kessels F: Cardiac valve calcification: characteristics of patients with calcification of the mitral annulus or aortic valve, *Heart* 78:472-4, 1997.
17. Silver MD, Silver MM: Valvular heart disease: conditions causing regurgitation. In Silver MD, Gotlieb AI, Schoen FJ, editors: *Cardiovascular pathology,* Edinburgh, 2001, Churchill Livingstone, pp 443-470.
18. Otto CM: Infective endocarditis. In Otto CM, editor: *Valvular heart disease,* ed 2, Philadelphia, 2004, Saunders, pp 482-521.
19. Karchmer AW: Infective endocarditis. In Zipes DP, Libby P, Bonow RO, Braunwald E, editors: *Braunwald's heart disease: a textbook of cardiovascular medicine,* ed 7, Philadelphia, 2005, Elsevier Saunders, pp 1633-1658.
20. Bonow RO, Carabello B, de Leon AC Jr et al: ACC/AHA guidelines for the management of patients with valvular heart disease: a report of the American College of Cardiology/American Heart Association task force on practice guidelines (committee on management of patients with valvular heart disease), *J Am Coll Cardiol* 32:1486-1588, 1998.
21. LeDoux D: Acquired valvular heart disease. In Woods SL, Sivarajan Froelicher ES, Adams Motzer S, editors: *Cardiac nursing,* ed 4, Philadelphia, 2000, Lippincott, pp 699-718.
22. Otto CM: Mitral stenosis. In Otto CM, editor: *Valvular heart disease,* ed 2, Philadelphia, 2004, Saunders, pp 247-271.
23. Rahimtoola SH, Enriquez-Sarano M, Schaff HV, Frye RL: Mitral valve disease. In Fuster V, Alexander RW, O'Rourke RA, editors: *Hurst's the heart,* New York, 2001, McGraw-Hill, pp 1697-1727.
24. Bonow RO, Braunwald E: Valvular heart disease. In Zipes DP, Libby P, Bonow RO, Braunwald E, editors: *Braunwald's heart disease: a textbook of cardiovascular medicine,* ed 7, Philadelphia, 2007, Elsevier Saunders, pp 1553-1621.
25. Segal BL: Valvular heart disease, part 2: mitral valve disease in older adults, *Geriatrics* 58(10):26-31, 2003.
26. Rahimtoola SH, Durairaj A, Mehra A, Nuno I: Current evaluation and management of patients with mitral stenosis, *Circulation* 106:1183-8, 2002.
27. Carabello BA: Recognition and management of patients with valvular heart disease. In Braunwald E, Goldman L, editors: *Primary cardiology,* ed 2, Philadelphia, 2003, Saunders, pp 553-573.
28. Shipton B, Wahba H: Valvular heart disease: review and update, *Am Fam Physician* 63:2201-8, 2001.
29. Otto CM: Surgical and percutaneous intervention for mitral stenosis. In Otto CM, editor: *Valvular heart disease,* ed 2, Philadelphia, 2004, Saunders, pp 272-301.
30. Otto CM: Mitral regurgitation. In Otto CM, editor: *Valvular heart disease,* ed 2, Philadelphia, 2004, Saunders, pp 336-367.
31. Scott RL: Native mitral valve regurgitation, *Postgrad Med* 110(2):57-63, 2001.
32. Otto CM: Mitral valve prolapse. In Otto CM, editor: *Valvular heart disease,* ed 2, Philadelphia, 2004, Saunders, pp 368-387.
33. Carabello BA: Aortic stenosis, *N Engl J of Med* 346:677-82, 2002.
34. Chan KL: Is aortic stenosis a preventable disease?, *J Am Coll of Cardiol* 42:593-9, 2003.
35. Rahimtoola SH: Valvular heart disease, *Circulation* 102S:IV24-IV33, 2000.
36. Kupari M, Turto H, Lommi J: Diagnosing heart failure in aortic valve stenosis, *J Intern Med* 256:381-7, 2004.
37. Nishimura RA: Aortic valve disease, *Circulation* 106:770-2, 2002.
38. Otto CM: Aortic stenosis. In Otto CM, editor: *Valvular heart disease,* ed 2, Philadelphia, 2004, Saunders, pp 197-246.
39. Isselbacher EM: Diseases of the Aorta. In Zipes DP, Libby P, Bonow RO, Braunwald E, editors; *Braunwald's heart disease: a textbook of cardiovascular medicine,* ed 7, Philadelphia, 2005, Elsevier Saunders, pp 1403-36.
40. Enriquez-Sarano M, Tajik AJ: Aortic regurgitation, *N Engl J Med* 35:1539-46, 2004.
41. Gaasch WH, Schick EC: Symptoms and left ventricular size and function with chronic aortic regurgitation, *J Am Coll Cardiol* 41:1325-8, 2003.
42. Otto CM: Aortic regurgitation. In Otto CM, editor: *Valvular heart disease,* ed 2, Philadelphia, 2004, Saunders, pp 302-335.
43. Scognamiglio R, Rahimtoola SH, Fasoli G et al: Nifedipine in asymptomatic patients with severe aortic regurgitation and normal left ventricular function, *N Engl J Med* 331:689-94, 1994.
44. Otto CM: Right-sided valve disease. In Otto CM, editor: *Valvular heart disease,* ed 2, Philadelphia, 2004, Saunders, pp 415-436.
45. Behm CZ, Nath J, Foster E: Clinical correlates and mortality of hemodynamically significant tricuspid regurgitation, *J Heart Valve Dis* 13:784-9, 2004.

46. Nath J, Foster E, Heidenreich PA: Impact of tricuspid regurgitation on long-term survival, *J Am Coll Cardiol* 43:405-9, 2004.

47. Lau GT, Tan HC, Kritharides L: Type of liver dysfunction in heart failure and its relation to the severity of tricuspid regurgitation, *Am J Cardiol* 90:1405-9, 2002.

48. Vaturi M, Shapira Y, Vaknin-Assa H et al: Echocardiographic markers of severe tricuspid regurgitation associated with right-sided congestive heart failure, *J Heart Valve Dis* 12:197-201, 2003.

49. Harrington RA, Jones K: Conditions affecting the right side of the heart, *BMJ* 324:1201-4, 2002.

50. O'Rourke RA: Tricuspid valve, pulmonic valve, and multivalvular disease. In Fuster V, Alexander RW, O'Rourke RA, editors: *Hurst's the heart,* New York, 2001, McGraw-Hill, pp 1741-1758.

51. Gillinov AM, Blackstone EH, Cosgrove DM et al: Mitral valve repair with aortic valve replacement is superior to double valve replacement, *J Thorac Cardiovasc Surg* 125:1372-87, 2003.

52. Vahanian A, Palacios IF: Percutaneous approaches to valvular disease, *Circulation* 109:1572-9, 2004.

53. Popma JJ, Kuntz RE, Baim DS: Percutaneous coronary and valvular intervention. In Zipes DP, Libby P, Bonow RO, Braunwald E, editors: *Braunwald's heart disease: a textbook of cardiovascular medicine,* ed 7, Philadelphia, 2005, Elsevier Saunders, pp 367-1402.

54. Cheng TO, Holmes DR: Percutaneous balloon mitral valvuloplasty by the Inoue balloon technique: the procedure of choice for treatment of mitral stenosis, *Am J Cardiol* 81:624-8, 1998.

55. Cribier A, Eltchaninoff H, Koning R et al: Percutaneous mechanical mitral commissurotomy with a newly designed metallic valvulotome: immediate results of the initial experience in 153 patients, *Circulation* 99:793-9, 1999.

56. Ben-Farhat M, Betbout F, Gamra H et al: Predictors of long-term event-free survival and of freedom from restenosis after percutaneous balloon mitral commissurotomy, *Am Heart J* 142:1072-9, 2001.

57. Fawzy ME, Awad M, Galal O et al: Long-term results of pulmonary balloon valvulotomy in adult patients, *J Heart Valve Dis* 10:812-8, 2001.

58. Teupe CHJ, Burger W, Schrader R, Zeiher AM: Late (five to nine years) follow-up after balloon dilatation of valvular pulmonary stenosis in adults, *Am J Cardiol* 80:240-2, 1997.

59. Braunberger E, Deloche A, Berrebi A et al: Very long-term results (more than 20 years) of valve repair with Carpentier's techniques in nonrheumatic mitral valve insufficiency, *Circulation* 104(suppl I):I-8-1-11, 2001.

60. Pomerantzeff PMA, Brandao, CMA, Faber CM et al: Mitral valve repair in rheumatic patients, *Heart Surg Forum* 3:273-276, 2000.

61. Harlan BJ, Starr A, Harwin FM: *Manual of Cardiac Surgery,* ed 2, New York, 1995, Springer-Verlag.

62. Antunes MJ: Repair for acquired valvular heart disease. In Rahimtoola SH, editor: *Atlas of heart diseases,* Philadelphia, 1997, Mosby.

63. Adams DH, Kadner A, Chen RH: Artificial mitral valve chordae replacement made simple, *Ann Thorac Surg* 71:377-379, 2001.

64. Carpentier A: Cardiac valve surgery: the "French correction," *J Thorac Cardiovasc Surg* 86:323-37, 1983.

65. Wiegand D: Advances in cardiac surgery: valve repair, *Crit Care Nurse* 23(2):72-6, 78-91, 2003.

66. Adams DH, Filsoufi, F, Antman EM: Medical management of the patient undergoing cardiac surgery. In Zipes DP, Libby P, Bonow RO, Braunwald E, editors: *Braunwald's heart disease: a textbook of cardiovascular medicine,* ed 7, Philadelphia, 2005, Elsevier Saunders, pp 1993-2020.

67. Thai HM, Gore JM: Prosthetic heart valves. In Alpert JS, Dalen JE, Rahimtoola SH, editors: *Valvular heart disease,* ed 3, Philadelphia, 2000, Lippincott Williams & Wilkens, pp 393-407.

68. Goldsmith I, Turpie AGG, Lip GYH: ABC of antithrombotic therapy: valvular heart disease and prosthetic heart valves, *BMJ* 325:1228-31, 2002.

69. Salem DN, Stein PD, Al-Ahmad A et al: Antithrombotic therapy in valvular heart disease—native and prosthetic: the seventh ACCP conference on antithrombotic and thrombolytic therapy (the seventh ACCP conference on antithrombotic and thrombolytic therapy: evidenced based guidelines, *Chest* 126(Suppl):457S-82S, 2004.

70. Hvass U, Calliani J, Nagaf I et al: Transfer of the posterior tricuspid leaflet and chordae for mitral valve repair, *Thorac Cardiovasc Surg* 110:859-861, 1995.

71. Kouchoukos NT, Blackstone EH, Doty DB et al: *Kirklin/Barratt-Boyes Cardiac Surgery,* ed 3, Philadelphia, 2003, Churchill Livingstone.

72. Cheah GM, Martens KH: Coumadin knowledge deficits: do recently hospitalized patients know how to safely manage the medication? *Home Health Nurse* 21(2):94-100, 2003.

73. Menéndez-Jándula B, Souto JC, Oliver A et al: Comparing self-management of oral anticoagulant therapy with clinic management: a randomized trial, *Ann Intern Med* 142:1-10, 2005.

74. Körtke H, Koerfer R: International standardized ratio self management after mechanical heart valve replacement: is an early start advantageous? *Ann Thorac Surg* 72:44-8, 2001.

75. Christensen TD, Attermann J, Pilegaard HK et al: Self-management of oral anticoagulant therapy for mechanical heart valve patients, *Scand Cardiovasc J* 35:107-13, 2001.

■■■ chapter 70
Care of Children with Heart Disease

Vicki L. Zeigler
Shelly Devillier

CHAPTER ABBREVIATIONS

AS   Aortic stenosis
ASD   atrial septal defect
AV   atrioventricular
AVSD   atrioventricular septal defect
BDG   bidirectional Glenn
BT   Blalock-Taussig
CAM   complementary and alternative medicine
CAVB   complete atrioventricular block
CAVSD   complete atrioventricular septal defect
CHD   congenital heart disease
CHF   congestive heart failure
CO   cardiac output
COA   coarctation of the aorta
CPR   cardiopulmonary resuscitation
CT   cardiothoracic
DORV   double outlet right ventricle
ECD   endocardial cushion defect
ECG   electrocardiogram
ECMO   extracorporeal membrane oxygenation
EST   exercise stress test
HLHS   hypoplastic left heart syndrome
ICD   implantable cardioverter-defibrillator
ICU   intensive care unit
INR   international normalized ratio
JET   junctional ectopic tachycardia
LAP   left atrial pressure
LQTS   long QT syndrome
NEC   necrotizing enterocolitis
PA   pulmonary artery
PAP   pulmonary artery pressure
PDA   patent ductus arteriosus
PFO   patent foramen ovale
PGE1   prostaglandin E1
PFO   patent foramen ovale
PLE   protein-losing enteropathy
QTc   corrected QT interval
RAP   right atrial pressure
RV   right ventricle
RVH   right ventricular hypertrophy
RVOT   right ventricular overflow tract
TA   tricuspid atresia
TAPVR   total anomalous pulmonary venous return
TEE   transesophageal echocardiography
TGA   transposition of the great arteries
TOF   tetralogy of Fallot
VSD   ventricular septal defect

Nurses and other health care professionals who refer to children with heart disease are generally speaking in terms of "congenital" heart disease **(CHD)**, yet there are specific cardiovascular conditions seen in children that are considered "acquired" (e.g., cardiomyopathy and myocarditis). Because of the wide spectrum of heart disease in neonates, infants, and children in addition to the overwhelming amount of published information on CHD, this chapter will not be all-inclusive; however, the most common congenital structural cardiac defects and some of the more commonly seen congenital dysrhythmias will be discussed.

CHD refers to "any abnormality in cardiocirculatory structure or function that is present at birth, even if it is discovered much later.[1]" The true "incidence" of CHD is elusive in that most calculations do not include bicuspid aortic valves, mitral valve prolapse, or congenital dysrhythmias, such as long QT syndrome **(LQTS)** and complete atrioventricular block **(CAVB)**; however, an analytical review of previous studies on the incidence of CHD has been reported. Accordingly the incidence of moderate and severe forms of CHD is approximately 6/1000 live births (which increases to 19/1000 live births if serious bicuspid aortic valves are included) and if all forms of CHD, including tiny muscular ventricular septal defects **(VSD)** present at birth and other trivial lesions are included in the analyses, the incidence increases to 75/1000 live births.[2]

The prevalence of CHD represents the total number of living individuals with CHD at any given time, including all survivors regardless of when they were born. This prevalence is rapidly increasing as a result of the number of survivors with CHD who are reaching adulthood, a direct result of technological advances in cardiovascular diagnostics and advances in surgical and catheter interventions. Over a period of 62 years (from 1940 to 2002), approximately one million children with simple lesions and another 500,000 with moderate and complex lesions were born in the United States.[3] Using the incidence data, annual birth rates, and survival rates for each lesion, the estimated prevalence is as follows: (a) between 400,000 (untreated) and 750,000 (treated) for *simple* lesions, (b) between 220,000 (untreated) and 400,000 (treated) for *moderate* lesions, and (c) between 30,000 (untreated) and 180,000 (treated) for *complex* lesions. Additionally, it is estimated that there are approximately 3,000,000 individuals alive with bicuspid aortic valves. Again, these estimates do not include acquired heart disease in children or those with congenital electrical abnormalities.

Patterns of recurrence, in which there is one or more affected first-degree relative, have been estimated at 2.7

percent in a recent analysis of 6640 consecutive pregnancies using detailed fetal echocardiography.[4] Although concordance rates of the different types of CHD vary, exact concordance was seen in 37 percent of cases, and group concordance was seen in 44 percent of cases. Furthermore, in families with two or more recurrences, the exact concordance rate was 55 percent, with exact concordance rates for isolated atrioventricular septal defects **(AVSD)** being particularly high (80 percent).[4]

The cause of cardiac disease in the child is primarily environmental or genetic. Such environmental factors associated with congenital cardiac disease include maternal rubella, chronic maternal alcohol abuse, and various maternal medications.[1] Briefly maternal rubella is associated with patent ductus arteriosus **(PDA)**, pulmonary valve stenosis, and atrial septal defect **(ASD)**, whereas prenatal maternal alcohol abuse is often associated with VSD in addition to other anomalies associated with fetal alcohol syndrome. Maternal connective tissue disorders are associated with an increased incidence in congenital CAVB. Medications ingested by the mother also associated with congenital cardiac malformations (e.g., lithium and tricuspid valve abnormalities, specifically Epstein anomaly).

The genetic contribution to CHD is currently being investigated; however, the process has proven challenging, requiring multiple investigative tools including linkage analyses, candidate gene studies, animal models, and molecular dissection of chromosomal rearrangements.[5] This had led to the identification of various related genes and loci specific to CHD. Most recently the 22q11 deletion syndrome has been associated with aortic arch anomalies (the most common feature), tetralogy of Fallot **(TOF)**, truncus arteriosus, and VSD.[5] Primary electrical diseases caused by mutated genes for cardiac ion channels, known as channelopathies, include the congenital LQTS, short QT syndrome, and Brugada syndrome. The majority of the existing data concerning the genetic basis of CHD has been in identifying "syndromes" in which there is a genetic cardiovascular component versus just a stand alone defect.[7]

ASSESSMENT OF THE CHILD WITH HEART DISEASE

Nurses are often the first individuals to touch babies born with CHD. These babies are often critical and may be at an increased risk for death in the first few hours of life. A prompt assessment and quick diagnosis is crucial in caring for the congenital heart patient; however, not all defects are identified at birth. The following discussion will include methods for assessing the child with known or suspected CHD, from the neonatal period through adolescence. These methods include a detailed history including a family and maternal history, a developmental history for the child, and a health status assessment of the child. The methods used for the physical assessment of the child with cardiac disease include vital signs, inspection, palpation, and auscultation.

History
Family and Maternal History

When obtaining a family and maternal history, it is important that the nurse establish a quick and detailed dialogue with parents. In the case of older children and adolescents, it is critical to always include him or her when obtaining a history. Specific questions used to obtain information about a family's history include "Are there any other family members *born* with a cardiac defect?" and "Have any family members *died suddenly* at birth or at a very young age for unknown reasons?" A maternal history can elucidate problems encountered in pregnancy, such as the use of alcohol or drugs and/or rubella exposure, conditions that are associated with multiple cardiac anomalies. Additionally, conditions, such as diabetes and lupus erythematosus, are associated with hypertrophic cardiomyopathy or transposition of the great arteries **(TGA)** and CAVB, respectively. Specific aspects of history taking in children with heart disease can be found in Box 70-1.[8]

Developmental Status

To ascertain information regarding the child's developmental milestones, questions should focus on issues such as "Is your child crawling? If so, at what age did this occur?" The nurse should be observing for these milestones while gathering information, keeping in mind that some children with cardiac disease may lag behind other children their age in reaching certain developmental milestones. Some cardiac defects are first diagnosed because the child comes to the primary care practitioner for poor weight gain and/or developmental delay.

BOX 70-1 ■ ■ ■
SELECTED ASPECTS OF HISTORY TAKING

Gestational and Natal History
Infections, medications, excessive smoking, or alcohol intake during pregnancy
Birthweight

Postnatal (or Past) History
- Weight gain, development, and feeding pattern
- Cyanosis, "cyanotic spells," and squatting
- Tachypnea, dyspnea, puffy eyelids
- Frequency of respiratory infections
- Exercise intolerance
- Heart murmur
- Chest pain
- Joint symptoms
- Neurological symptoms
- Medications

Family History
- Hereditary disease
- Congenital heart disease
- Rheumatic fever
- Sudden, unexpected death
- Diabetes mellitus, arteriosclerotic heart disease, hypertension, etc.

From Park M K: *Pediatric cardiology for practitioners,* ed 4, St louis, 2002, Mosby, p 3.

Health Status

Often, a parent's first complaint regarding their child's health is that they are not gaining weight and tire easily when feeding. Specific questioning will assist in assessing the child's eating habits (e.g., the volume of food or liquid ingested and the amount of time it takes for the child to be fed). This information can be used to calculate total volume for a 24-hour period. Also, the child's birth weight should be documented on a growth chart, with subsequent plotting of the child's height and weight at each clinic visit. Parents should be asked to voice any observations or concerns noted while feeding the baby, such as tiring with feeding, falling asleep during feeding, and/or becoming diaphoretic or cyanotic with feeding. Parents should be asked to describe their child's overall breathing pattern as well. If this is not the parent's first child, inquire about how this baby compares with the previous ones.

Activity level in babies is generally assessed by their feeding routines, whereas to determine a toddler's activity, parents are asked about their child's ability to keep up with other children their age. Older children are asked about their tolerance to exercise. It is important to ascertain if the child has experienced a syncopal or near syncopal episode. A description of any syncopal or near syncopal episode should include any and all surrounding circumstances. For example, some children with congenital LQTS will experience syncope when hearing sudden, loud noises.

Additional areas of concern for children with cardiac disease are the number of previous respiratory infections and how they were treated (i.e., were they treated for pneumonia or bronchitis and not the common cold). Children with left to right shunt lesions are prone to an increase in the incidence of lower respiratory illnesses for reasons that are poorly understood at this time. Episodes of diaphoresis are not always cardiac in nature; however, if a child has experienced diaphoresis, it is important to know when the episode occurred (e.g., during feeding, while crying, while sleeping, or with activity). Other symptoms associated with CHD include cyanosis, cyanotic spells, and squatting, most commonly seen in children with cyanotic lesions, such as TOF.

Physical Assessment

The single most important part of the physical examination of a child is the provision of a quiet, nonthreatening environment. It is important when caring for children of all ages that the physical assessment is performed while the child is in his or her "comfort zone." Communication of what will be done during the examination is crucial in gaining trust and cooperation and in alleviating stress resulting from fear of the unknown. It is always best to start with the least intrusive part of the assessment, such as history taking, which also serves to establish a relationship with the child and family. If the neonate or infant is quiet, auscultation is performed first. The child with a known or suspected cardiac defect is physically assessed using the following methods: vital signs, inspection, palpation, and auscultation.

Vital Signs

The vital signs of a child can provide clues to the presence of cardiac disease. An apical assessment of heart rate can be obtained with auscultation, and the femoral artery is often used to assess pulse rate, with a pedal pulse used to assess peripheral perfusion. Because heart and respiratory rates in children are inherently faster and blood pressure is inherently lower than their adult counterparts, smaller changes in the vital signs of a child may be more significant than in adults. A guide for normal vital signs in children can be found in Table 70-1; however, it is important that nurses realize that what may be normal for a healthy child may not be normal for the child with a cardiac defect.

The respiratory assessment of the child with a known or suspected cardiac defect should be performed when the child is quiet and preferably at rest. In addition to assessing respiratory rate, the effort of those respirations also requires astute observation. The clinician should note any nasal flaring, use of accessory muscles, and/or grunting with respiration. If the child's respiratory rate is irregular, a repeat measurement over a full minute will provide a more accurate reading. Tachypnea, coupled with tachycardia, is often an early sign of left-sided heart failure.

It is critical when measuring the blood pressure of a child that the correct sized cuff is used for the measure-

■ ■ ■

TABLE 70-1   NORMAL VITAL SIGN PARAMETERS IN CHILDREN

AGE	RESPIRATORY RATES* (breaths/min)	HEART RATES (AWAKE) (beats/min)	HEART RATES (SLEEPING) (beats/min)	BLOOD PRESSURE (SYSTOLIC) (mm Hg)	BLOOD PRESSURE (DIASTOLIC) (mm Hg)
Newborn	35	100-180	80-160	60-90	20-60
Infant	30-60	80-160	75-160	87-105	53-66
Toddler	24-40	80-160	60-90	95-105	53-66
School age	18-30	65-110	50-90	97-112	57-71
Adolescent	12-16	55-90	40-90	112-128	66-80

Data from Curley MAQ, Smith JB, Moloney-Harmon PA: *Critical care nursing of infants and children*, Philadelphia, 1996, WB Saunders.

ment and that many different sized cuffs are available when assessing the neonate, infant, child, and adolescent with a cardiac problem. The cuff width should be 40 percent to 50 percent of the circumference of the limb being measured for both upper and lower extremities.[8] Without proper cuff size, inaccurate blood pressure readings may occur, with narrow cuffs resulting in higher readings and cuffs that are too wide resulting in lower readings. It is best to obtain blood pressure measurements at the end of the physical assessment. This indirect measurement of blood pressure can be obtained using the traditional method or with an automated machine on the child's upper arm, thigh, or calf. Infants in particular do not like the automated method and may need distraction during the measurement to obtain an accurate measurement. Owing to the fact that the first blood pressure measurement is almost always elevated, two or more readings may be necessary. If this is the child's initial cardiac assessment, blood pressure measurements from all four extremities should be obtained.

Blood pressure measurements can yield lesion-specific information (e.g., the child with coarctation of the aorta **(CoA)** will have higher right upper extremity blood pressures when compared with the lower extremity measurements). For children who have undergone repair of CoA, the left subclavian artery may be transected making the blood pressure inaccurate on the left upper extremity. This requires that all future measurements be obtained from the right upper extremity.

Inspection

The inspection component of the physical assessment should begin with a head-to-toe assessment, with particular attention paid to general appearance, nutritional state, height and weight proportions, color, clubbing, and the presence of any dysmorphic features. An overall visual inspection allows the clinician to look for overt signs produced by syndromes associated with CHD because 25 percent of congenital heart defect patients will have noncardiac anomalies.[5]

Good lighting is essential during inspection, especially when assessing a child's skin color. Parents may not report cyanosis in their child because they are unable to detect it, especially if the child is dark skinned (e.g., black or Hispanic children). Assessing for cyanosis in these children is best accomplished by inspecting the mucous membranes and/or conjunctiva. It is important for those caring for children with suspected cardiac disease to realize that not all cyanosis is cardiac in nature. Should cyanosis be detected, it is important to differentiate between central and peripheral cyanosis. Central cyanosis is generally exhibited by a bluish appearance in the mouth and sclera. Acrocyanosis, a bluish-reddish discoloration of the distal peripheries and circumoral area, is a normal finding.

The child's fingers, nail beds, and toenails should be inspected for clubbing. It generally takes approximately 6 months of decreased oxygen saturations before clubbing is evident; however, it is often much later before it is detected.[8] It is imperative that clothing be removed to inspect the chest area. Any scars or pectus deformities should be documented. Bulging or pulsing of the chest may indicate cardiac enlargement. Precordial bulging is generally indicative of "chronic" cardiac enlargement. A general appearance assessment should include inspection for edema, especially around the eyelids, and an inspection of the forehead for diaphoresis. In particular, infants with CHF may exhibit a "cold sweat" coupled with edematous eyelids.

Palpation

Depending on the age of the child, palpation may be deferred until the lungs and heart have been auscultated. The trunk should be compared with the extremities when palpating the patient's skin temperature to detect any decreased peripheral circulation. Cool extremities are often present in children who have defects that produce a decrease in systemic output. When palpating peripheral pulses in children, it is important to note the following: (a) regular or irregular, (b) equal when comparing the left side with the right side of the body and the upper and lower parts of the body, and (c) the presence of threadiness, weakness, and/or a bounding pulse. Extremities should be compared for pulse strength and any noted differences. For example, a child with CoA will exhibit strong upper extremity pulses, but weak lower extremity pulses.

A capillary refill assessment is used to evaluate peripheral perfusion, with the great toe being the best location in younger children. A capillary refill of *greater than* 3 seconds may be indicative of decreased peripheral perfusion. Peripheral pulses should be palpated with documentation of a pedal pulse. Chest palpation can yield additional information pertinent to the cardiovascular assessment of the child. Any hyperactivity of the precordium and any thrills (murmurs that can be palpated) detected with the palm of the hand should be noted on the assessment. Because some children with congestive heart failure **(CHF)** can exhibit hepatomegaly, it is important to carefully palpate the edges of the liver for location.

Auscultation

Good auscultation skills are imperative in performing a cardiac examination on a child. Owing to the fact that younger patients are not always cooperative, nurses working with children should "seize the moment" when it presents itself. Auscultation should include the lungs with an emphasis on respiratory rate and the presence of any extra breath sounds. Such extra breath sounds (e.g., wheezing) may not be respiratory in nature, but may be a cardiac finding instead.

Both sides of the stethoscope are beneficial when auscultating the heart of a child. The bell is useful for detecting low-pitched sounds, whereas the diaphragm is useful for detecting high-pitched sounds. The starting location for the procedure of auscultation is irrelevant; however, each clinician should develop and consistently use a systematic approach. Things to listen for include: heart rate and regularity, heart sounds, systolic and diastolic sounds, extracardiac sounds, and murmurs. Four main areas are identified when listening to the heart: apical, left lower sternal border, aortic (right upper sternal border), and pulmonary (left upper sternal border). The clinician should always listen to the entire chest area along with the sides and back of the chest and should begin by listening for the heart sounds.

The first heart sound (S_1), indicating closure of the mitral and tricuspid valves, is best heard at the left lower sternal border. Although mitral valve closure occurs slightly before tricuspid valve closure, this heart sound is rarely heard, resulting in a single S_1 in the majority of cases. The second heart sound (S_2), indicating closure of the aortic and pulmonary valves, is best heard at the left upper sternal border. During inspiration physiological splitting of S_2 may be heard when the aortic valve closes before the pulmonary valve. Splitting of S_2 is a normal finding; however, if splitting does not occur, pulmonary hypertension is a concern. Wide fixed splitting may indicate the presence of an ASD.

Once these two heart sounds have been identified, it is then that one begins listening for murmurs, which are described according to their intensity, pitch, timing, location, and transmission. Intensity is graded on a scale of 1 to 6, with a grade 1 murmur being one that is barely audible. A grade 6 murmur can be heard without the stethoscope being placed on the chest. (Box 70-2).

Three major categories of murmurs, identified according to when they are heard in the cardiac cycle, can be present in children with cardiac disease. They include systolic (ejection-type or regurgitant-type), diastolic (early diastolic, middiastolic, or presystolic), and continuous murmurs. Murmurs occurring between S_1 and S_2 are systolic murmurs, whereas those that occur between S_2 and S_1 are known as diastolic murmurs. Continuous murmurs can be heard in systole and part or all of diastole. Murmurs may be high pitched or low pitched and with respect to timing are classified as early, mid, or late *systolic, holosystolic,* or early, mid, or late *diastolic.* The area of the chest where the murmur is heard the loudest should be noted, while continuing to listen to the entire chest to determine if and where the murmur radiates to, known as transmission.

Innocent murmurs frequently occur in children without a cardiac abnormality and are grouped into systolic and continuous and vary with positional changes (Box 70-3). Beginning around 3 to 4 years of age, 80 percent of children will have an innocent murmur of some type.[8] Most murmurs intensify with fever, anemia, or increased cardiac output **(CO)**.[9] It is also important to note that children can have severe CHD and not exhibit a murmur (e.g., neonates or infants with d-TGA).

BOX 70-2
INTENSITY GRADES FOR HEART MURMURS

Grade 1	Barely audible
Grade 2	Soft, but easily audible
Grade 3	Moderately loud, but not accompanied by a thrill
Grade 4	Louder and associated with a thrill
Grade 5	Audible with stethoscope barely on the chest
Grade 6	Audible with stethoscope off the chest

From Park M K: *Pediatric cardiology for practitioners,* ed 4, St louis, Mosby, p 23.

BOX 70-3 ▪ ▪ ▪
INNOCENT MURMURS OF CHILDHOOD

Systolic Murmurs
- Vibratory still murmur
- Pulmonary flow murmur
- Peripheral pulmonary arterial stenosis murmur
- Supraclavicular systolic murmur
- Aortic systolic murmur

Continuous Murmurs
- Venous hum
- Mammary arterial soufflé

From Pelech AN: The physiology of cardiac auscultation, *Pediatr Clin North Am* 51:1530, 2004.

DIAGNOSTIC TESTING

Many of the diagnostic tools used in adults with cardiovascular disease are also used for children who have or who are suspected of having congenital or acquired heart disease; however, this does not make them "little adults." Because many of these diagnostic tools are described in depth elsewhere in this text, this section will highlight the nuances associated with the use of each of these tools in the pediatric population. The tests that will be discussed below will include: chest radiography, electrocardiography, echocardiography, exercise stress testing **(EST)**, ambulatory monitoring, pulse oximetry monitoring, and cardiac catheterization.

Chest Radiography

The use of chest radiography as an aid in the diagnosis of congenital or acquired heart disease in children has waned over the years owing to the fact that it has been replaced with better and more accurate diagnostic tools, such as the echocardiogram. The chest radiograph can, however, provide valuable information regarding heart size and silhouette and pulmonary vascular markings. Depicted by the cardiothoracic **(CT)** ratio, cardiomegaly is indicated by a value *greater than* 0.5 (50 percent). CT ratios are not always helpful in neonates since the thymus gland can make the heart appear larger than it really is. Pulmonary vascular markings can be indicative of shunting and can be used to delineate shunt direction. In general left to right shunts will produce increased pulmonary vascular markings, whereas right to left shunts will produce decreased pulmonary vascular markings. A lung field assessment may yield information regarding which side the aortic arch is on and pulmonary venous congestion.

Electrocardiography

The normal and abnormal electrocardiogram **(ECG)** is discussed in depth in chapters 46 and 47, respectively; however, there are specific nuances pertinent to children. In contrast to adults, the right ventricle **(RV)** is thicker than the left ventricle in newborns and infants. These nuances make the ECG interpretation in a child age specific. In most cases a 15-lead ECG is performed to assess heart rate and rhythm, chamber enlargement, hypertrophy (atrial or ventricular), and ischemic changes.

The ECG is pivotal in diagnosing rhythm disorders, such as congenital LQTS and CAVB. Additionally, children who have undergone repair of certain defects may exhibit bundle branch block. For example, right bundle branch block is often seen after surgery for TOF. It is important to note that the ECG is only a *screening* tool and can result in frequent false-positive and false-negative findings.

The quality of the ECG is inversely dependent on the skill of the individual acquiring it. Owing to the fact that the assessment of heart rate, conduction intervals, axis, and hypertrophy are all age specific, the age of the child is critical for correct ECG interpretation. Equally important are factors that can affect the quality of the ECG including patient movement, incorrectly placed electrodes, lack of correct skin preparation, static or alternating current, poor signal quality, broken lead wires, and improper grounding.

Echocardiography

As a result of advances in technology, the echocardiogram has replaced many of the diagnostic cardiac catheterizations of the past that were used as the "gold standard" for diagnosing CHD. Today many types of echocardiography are used to diagnose and treat children with CHD. The following types of echocardiography are used in children with heart disease: transthoracic, transesophageal, and fetal echocardiography.

Transthoracic Echocardiography

The use of transthoracic echocardiography and color-flow Doppler has revolutionized the diagnosis and treatment of cardiac disease in children. Using high-frequency ultrasonic waves, the echocardiogram is used to identify cardiac structure and function. Two-dimensional (2-D) echocardiography records sound waves that are reflected from cardiac structures, whereas Doppler echocardiography records the velocity of moving objects (i.e., blood flow) and is useful in defining obstructive lesions. Pulsed Doppler echocardiography is used to determine the presence, timing, and direction of intracardiac shunts, pressure differences, and valve regurgitation or stenosis.

To assess function, various gradients and measurements are calculated, such as end diastolic and end systolic chamber measurements, which are the simplest measures of cardiac performance. In contrast to adult measures of cardiac function, pediatric function is measured as a shortening (versus an ejection) fraction; however, both can be used in the diagnosis of CHD. Other measures obtained by transthoracic echocardiography include diastolic function and CO. Impediments to good images include obesity, prior cardiac surgery, and chest wall deformities.

Transesophageal Echocardiography

Transesophageal echocardiography **(TEE)** is generally performed when additional and/or more detailed images of the heart are needed. Using a flexible endoscope with a high resolution ultrasonic transducer, it can be especially useful in neonates, in obese patients that have poor acoustical windows, and as an aid to device placement in the catheterization laboratory. It can also provide images of intracardiac vegetations and small tumors or clots. TEE is now being routinely performed in the operating room to allow further imaging during surgery. In 2002 Randolph and colleagues[10] assessed the impact of TEE during surgery for CHD and found that TEE had a major impact on 13.8 percent of the patients, specifically, the information obtained prompted a change in surgical course that may have resulted in an additional surgery had the information not been obtained during the initial operation.

Fetal Echocardiography

With technological improvements, fetal echocardiography has become more widely used for aid in diagnosing congenital heart defects in utero. Recently the diagnosis of congenital heart defects has shifted from neonatal life toward fetal life, with an emphasis on cardiac detection from the third trimester (24 to 40 weeks) to the second trimester (12 to 24 weeks) and perhaps even during the first trimester (transvaginal if *less than* 12 weeks).[11] Broad indications for fetal echocardiography include: (1) a previous child with CHD, (2) a mother with CHD, (3) gestational diabetes, (4) maternal connective tissue disorder, (5) the four chambers of the fetal heart cannot be visualized by obstetrical ultrasound, and (6) fetal bradycardia or tachycardia. Specific maternal and fetal indications can be found in Box 70-4.

The greatest benefit of an in utero diagnosis is the gift of time.[12] Time allows parents to gather and receive information regarding their child's diagnosis, treatment options, and available treatment centers. Arrangements can be made for delivery at or near a center that performs congenital heart surgery, and parents have time to come to a level of acceptance and grieve the loss of a "normal child."

BOX 70-4 ■ ■ ■
INDICATIONS FOR FETAL ECHOCARDIOGRAPHY

Maternal Indications
- History of congenital heart disease
- Diabetes
- Metabolic disorders (e.g., phenylketonuria)
- Teratogen exposure (e.g., lithium)
- Exposure to prostaglandin synthetase inhibitors
- Rubella infection
- Maternal autoimmune disease
- Familial inherited disorders (e.g., Marfan syndrome, Ellis-van Creveld syndrome, Noonan syndrome)
- In vitro fertilization
- Fetal Indications
- Aneuploidy (chromosomal abnormality)
- Extracardiac abnormality
- Fetal heartbeat irregularity
- Fetal hydrops
- Increased nuchal translucency (first trimester)
- Multiple gestation with suspicion of twin-twin transfusion syndrome
- Abnormal obstetric ultrasound screen

From Rychik J: Frontiers in fetal cardiovascular disease, *Pediatr Clin North Am* 51:1492, 2004.

Exercise Stress Testing

EST is used to determine a quantitative and a reproducible index of the patient's cardiorespiratory performance by illuminating the physiological changes associated with exercise. EST is frequently used to detect ischemia or cardiac dysrhythmias; however, it can be helpful in certain clinical situations. For example, an EST in a child with unrepaired aortic stenosis (**AS**) or with aortic insufficiency can reveal ST-segment or T-wave changes during exercise. These findings may be indicative of subendocardial ischemia and/or severe obstruction. In children who have undergone the arterial switch procedure for d-TGA, exercise-induced ischemia could indicate a possible stenotic coronary artery, whereas an individual who has undergone a Mustard or Senning repair for dextro-TGA (usually called d-TGA) may exhibit atrial dysrhythmias (sinus node dysfunction and/or atrial reentry tachycardia), chronotropic impairment, and a decreased exercise capacity (most often related to a decrease in right heart function).

Ambulatory Monitoring

Ambulatory monitoring is of little value in diagnosing structural cardiac defects; however, its use as a follow-up tool is invaluable. Most notably ambulatory monitoring is helpful in ascertaining the presence of dysrhythmias, the monitoring of heart rate and rhythm over a prolonged period (i.e., 24 to 48 hours), and the efficacy of various pharmacological therapies.

Pulse Oximetry Monitoring

Pulse oximetry has become a valuable clinical tool in the assessment of children with heart disease; however, it must be used properly. To verify the accuracy of the measurement, obtain a manual or auscultated pulse or heart rate and compare it with the reading displayed on the machine. If the heart rates do not correlate, the oxygen saturation is not accurate. Simultaneous placement of a probe on an upper and a lower extremity can be used to assess accuracy. The child who is agitated, crying, or moving will likely produce an inaccurate measurement. A comparison of the measurement with the child's baseline oxygen saturation should be made, and the clinician should be knowledgeable of saturations that are "acceptable" for specific lesions and clinical conditions because placement of oxygen on palliated cardiac patients with decreased oxygen saturations could be harmful.

Cardiac Catheterization

Routine cardiac catheterization is no longer performed specifically for the diagnosis of CHD. Owing to improvements and advances in pediatric echocardiography, diagnostic cardiac catheterizations are performed when: (1) actual physiological data is needed to confirm and/or complete a diagnosis, (2) precise pressure and saturation measurements are needed, and (3) in between the stages of the Fontan procedure. In some individuals with Fontan physiology, anatomy and physiology is difficult to visualize with echocardiography. In rare cases, cardiac catheterization is necessary because of a poor acoustical window, most often in the extremely obese. Divided into three categories, diagnostic, interventional, and electrophysiological, there has been a recent decrease in the number of diagnostic procedures and a rapid increase in the number of interventional and electrophysiological procedures, mostly as a result of an increase in the number of available devices, ballooning procedures, and catheter ablations. Specific interventional cardiac procedures for structural congenital heart defects can be found in Table 70-2. The nursing considerations associated with caring for children undergoing cardiac catheterization can be found in the section on caring for the child undergoing an invasive cardiovascular procedure.

SPECIFIC CONGENITAL DEFECTS AND LESIONS

There are many ways in which to classify CHD and the following categories of CHD will be used in this chapter: (1) left to right shunt lesions, (2) obstructive lesions, and (3) cyanotic lesions. Additional categories of cardiovascular disease in the child included in this chapter include congenital dysrhythmias, including LQTS and CAVB. To appreciate the complexity of CHD, nurses should be knowledgeable of normal cardiovascular anatomy and physiology of the neonate, infant, and child (Figure 70-1).

■ ■ ■

TABLE 70-2 PEDIATRIC INTERVENTIONAL CARDIAC CATHETERIZATION PROCEDURES FOR STRUCTURAL CHD

INTERVENTION	DIAGNOSIS
Balloon atrial septostomy (Rashkind)	Transposition of great arteries
Blade atrial septostomy*	atrioventricular/pulmonary valve atresia with restrictive atrial communication
Balloon angioplasty	Pulmonary artery (PA) stenosis
	Recurrent coarctation of the aorta (CoA)
	Native CoA
	Conduit stenosis
Balloon valvuloplasty	Pulmonary stenosis-valvular
	Aortic stenosis-valvular
Coil occlusion	Patent ductus arteriosus (PDA) (small to medium)
	Aortopulmonary collaterals
	Arteriovenous malformations
Device placement	Patent ductus arteriosus
	Atrial septal defect
	Ventricular septal defect
	Fenestrated Fontan
Stent placement	PA stenosis
	CoA
	Occluded inferior vena cavae
	Pulmonary veins

AS, Aortic stenosis; *ASD*, atrial septal defect; *AV*, atrioventricular; *CoA*, coarctation of aorta; *PA*, pulmonary artery; *PDA*, patent ductus arteriosus; *PS*, pulmonary stenosis; *TGA*, transposition of great vessels; *VSD*, ventricular septal defect.
*Used with thicker septa.

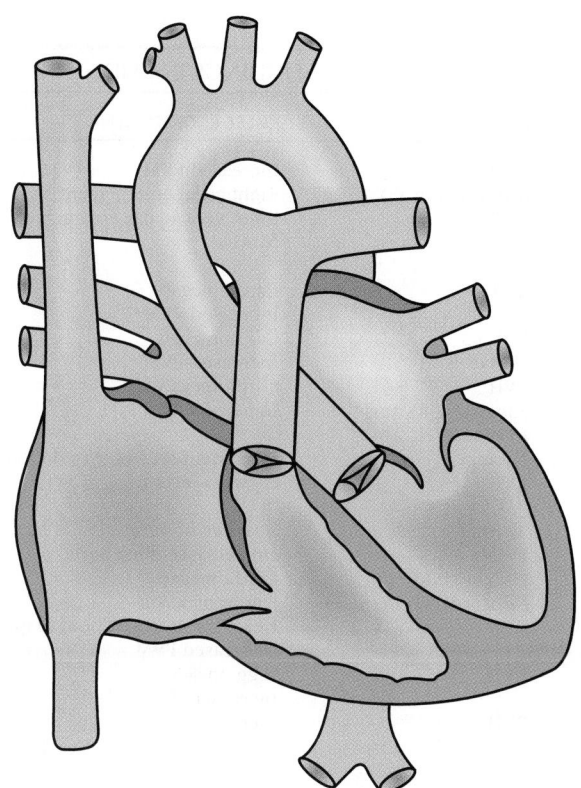

FIGURE 70-1 ▦ Normal heart. (Courtesy Scientific Software Solutions, PedCath version 7.4.3.)

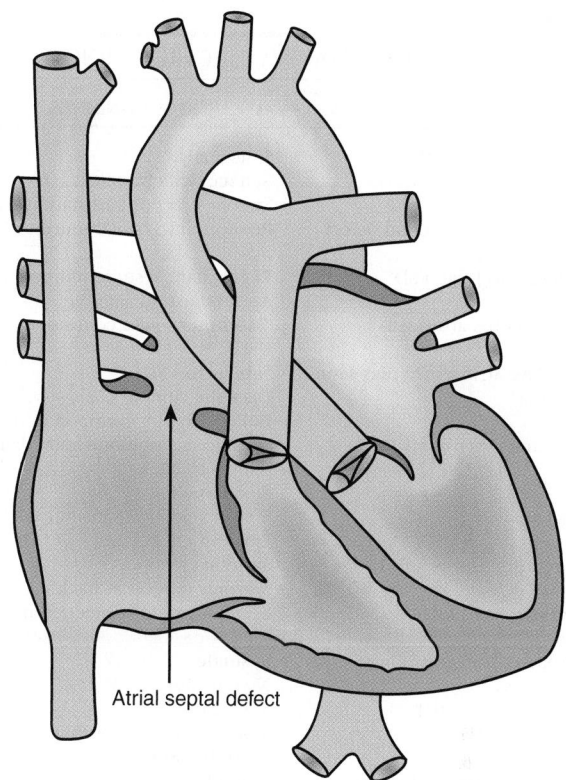

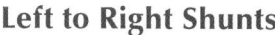

Atrial septal defect

FIGURE 70-2 ▦ An ostium secundum atrial septal defect (ASD), occurring in the center of the septum, is the most common type of ASD in children. (Courtesy Scientific Software Solutions, PedCath version 7.4.3.)

Left to Right Shunts

ASDs, VSD, PDA, and AVSD are considered lesions that produce left to right shunting. These lesions can cause an increase in pulmonary blood flow. The following discussion will include the following: a brief overview of each defect, the clinical manifestations of each defect, and the management strategies for each defect. The nursing considerations associated with caring for the child with a left to right shunt will be discussed at the end of this section.

Atrial Septal Defect

ASDs account for approximately 10 percent of all congenital heart defects.[13] An opening that occurs between the left and right atria, an ASD (Figure 70-2) produces increased pulmonary blood flow and increased work for the right side of the heart because blood is shunted from the left to the right atrium. ASDs are described according to their location and include the following: (a) sinus venosus defect, (b) ostium secundum defect, and (c) ostium primum defect. *Sinus venosus* defects are located near the upper septal region (at the level of the superior vena cava) and are almost always associated with anomalous pulmonary venous return. An *ostium secundum* defect is the most common type of ASD in which the opening occurs in the middle section of the septum and at the same location as a patent foramen ovale **(PFO).** The *ostium primum* defect, the opening of which is seen in the lower part of the septum, is less common and is often seen with complete atrioventricular septal defects **(CAVSDs).**

Clinical Manifestations

In most instances, children with an ASD are asymptomatic, and in the case of the majority of moderate openings, symptomatology does not appear until late adolescence or adulthood. Symptoms associated with larger openings and increased shunting include dyspnea and exercise intolerance. CHF is rare in children with an ASD. Over time individuals with an ASD are prone to atrial dysrhythmias caused by the increased volume to the right side of the heart. ASDs that are left untreated may result in pulmonary hypertension, although this is rare with advances in diagnostic and treatment capabilities. Auscultatory, electrocardiographic, and chest radiographic findings can be found in Table 70-3.

Management

The management of the child with an ASD is totally dependent on the symptomatology. Treatment options include outpatient follow-up, catheter intervention, or surgical intervention. Spontaneous closure of ASDs can occur and does so at a higher percentage in children with smaller defects. Catheter or surgical closure for ASDs in asymptomatic children is not recommended until the ages of 2 to 4 years, to allow spontaneous closure to occur. In rare cases, treatment of CHF requires the administration of digoxin and/or diuretics, such as Lasix. Older children with an ASD who were not diagnosed at a younger age may require cardiac catheterization to assess hemodynamics, specifically pulmonary vascular resistance, before recommendation for closure.

■ ■ ■

TABLE 70-3 AUSCULTATORY, ELECTROCARDIOGRAPHIC, AND CHEST RADIOGRAPHIC FINDINGS IN CHD

LESION	AUSCULTATORY FINDINGS	ECG	CHEST RADIOGRAPH
Atrial septal defect*	S_1 normal	RVH	Increased PVM
	S_2 fixed/widely split	RBBB (rsR in V_1)	Right atrial enlargement
	Systolic ejection murmur at ULSB	RAD	Right ventricular enlargement
Small ventricular septal defect (VSD)*	Regurgitant systolic murmur LLSB	Normal	Normal
Moderate to large VSD*	Regurgitant systolic murmur LLSB	LVH	Cardiomegaly
	Apical diastolic rumble	LAH	Increased PVM
Patent ductus arteriosus*	"Machinery"-like continuous murmur USLB	Normal	Cardiomegaly
		LVH or BVH	Increased PVM
Complete atrioventricular septal defect*	Similar to VSD	BVH	Cardiomegaly
	Diastolic rumble LLSB	Superior QRS axis	Increased PVM
	Gallop rhythm common in infants	LVH or BVH	
Pulmonary stenosis†	Systolic ejection murmur ULSB that transmits to back	Normal	Prominent PA Decreased PVM (with severe)
	Ejection click	RVH	
Atrial stenosis†	Systolic ejection murmur URSB	Normal	Absence of prominent MPA
	Ejection click	LVH	Dilated ascending aorta
Coarctation of the aorta†	Systolic ejection	LVH in children	Cardiomegaly
	Murmur loudest at back	RBB (or RVH) in infants	Figure-of-3 sign
Tetralogy of Fallot‡	S_2 single systolic ejection murmur, ULSB	RVH	Heart size normal "boot-shaped" Decreased PVM
d(dextro)-Transposition of great arteries‡	S_2 single	RVH	"Egg-on-side"
	No murmur		Increased PVM
Truncus arteriosus‡	S_2 single	BVH	Increased PVM
	Systolic ejection murmur		
	Diastolic murmur		
Total anomalous pulmonary venous return-obstructed‡	P_2 loud	RAH	Small heart
	Usually no murmur	RVH	"Ground glass" appearance
Total anomalous pulmonary venous return-unobstructed‡	S_2 widely split	RVH	Cardiomegaly
	Systolic ejection murmur, ULSB middiastolic rumble, LLSB		"Snowman sign"
Tricuspid atresia‡	S_1 single	RAH	RA and LV enlargement
		LVH	Decreased PVM
Hypoplastic left heart syndrome‡	S_2 Single and loud	RVH	Cardiomegaly
	Murmur usually absent	QR pattern in V_1	

*Left to right shunts
†Obstructive lesions
‡Cyanotic defects
BVH, biventricular hypertrophy; *LAH,* left atrial hypertrophy; *LLSB,* lower left sternal border; *LV,* left ventricle; *LVH,* left ventricular hypertrophy; *MPA,* main pulmonary artery; *PA,* pulmonary artery; *PVM,* pulmonary vascular markings; *RA,* right atrium; *RAD,* right axis deviation; *RAH,* right atrial hypertrophy; *RBBB,* right bundle branch block; *RV,* right ventricle; *RVH,* right ventricular hypertrophy; S_1, first heart sound; S_2, second heart sound; *ULSB,* upper left sternal border; *URSB,* upper right sternal border.

Closure is recommended if the pulmonary-to-systemic blood flow ratio (Qp/Qs) is equal to 1.5:1.[15]

Catheter closure of selected *secundum* ASDs can be performed with the Amplatzer septal occluder, which was approved by the U.S. Food and Drug Administration in December of 2001. Criteria for device closure includes absolute defect size, defect size related to heart size, and adequate anchoring margins.[15] Recent clinical trails have shown that transcatheter closure of selected *secundum* ASDs using the Amplatzer septal occluder when compared with surgical closure has similar success rates, shorter hospital stays, and less patient discomfort.[16,17]

ASDs that do not meet the above criteria for closure in the catheterization laboratory are referred for surgical closure. The mortality rate for surgical closure of an ASD is *less than* 1 percent; however, in small infants with increased pulmonary vascular resistance, the risk is increased.[18] The ASD can be closed using the child's own pericardium as patch material, using a patch made of synthetic material, or using sutures. Cardiopulmonary bypass is used while closing the ASD. A minimally invasive, surgical approach is being used for an ASD closure, which results in a smaller incision; however, this approach is generally used for cosmetic purposes and does not reduce pain or hospital length of stay.[14] General nursing considerations for children undergoing interventional cardiac catheterization can be found in the section of caring for the child undergoing invasive cardiac procedures. The specifics of caring for children with left to right shunts can be found at the end of this section.

Ventricular Septal Defects

VSD is the most common congenital cardiac lesion, accounting for 15 percent of all congenital heart defects. An abnormal opening between the left and RVs (Figure 70-3), VSDs are classified according to their location. The types of VSDs include *perimembranous, muscular* (specifically inlet, outlet, mid, and apical),

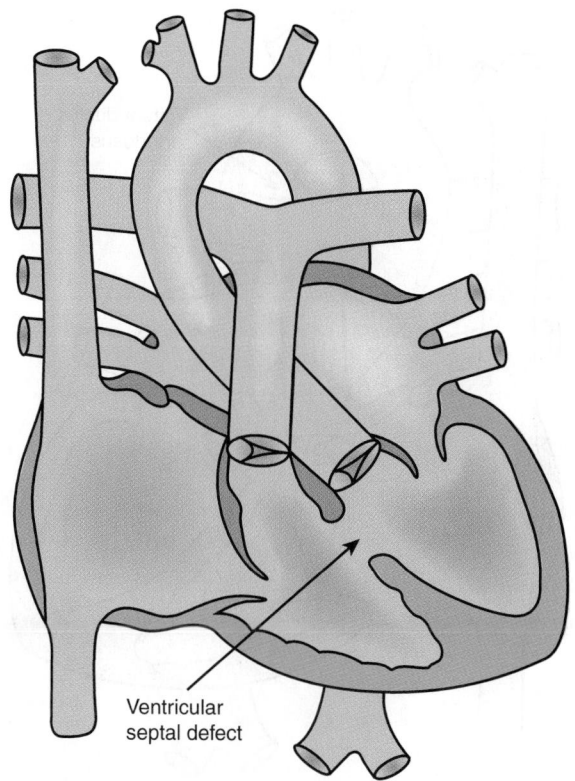

FIGURE 70-3 ■ A membranous ventricular septal defect (VSD) in which the opening is just below the aortic valve. (Courtesy Scientific Software Solutions, PedCath version 7.4.3.)

and *malalignment*. In the *perimembranous* and *muscular* regions, spontaneous closure is likely to occur. Multiple VSDs, referred to as a "Swiss cheese" septum, are often more difficult to close surgically.[19] Anomalies associated with VSD include Down syndrome and other autosomal trisomies, renal abnormalities, and other cardiac lesions.

Although not always detected immediately at or after birth, the VSD forces blood to be shunted from left to right as a result of the higher left-sided pressures. The left ventricle receives the shunted blood and assumes the workload for both ventricles because the blood is shunted in systole. Blood goes directly to the pulmonary arteries. In neonates with pulmonary hypertension, blood may also be shunted in a right to left direction.

Clinical Manifestations

Symptoms associated with VSDs vary according to the size of the VSD. Children with small VSDs may be totally asymptomatic; however, those with moderate to large VSDs, signs of CHF may be exhibited by the child. Additionally, large VSDs can produce pulmonary vascular changes that can eventually lead to pulmonary hypertension, a condition known as Eisenmenger syndrome (See Chapter 71). Children with VSDs often have poor weight gain. Because of their tachypnea and tachycardia, they are poor feeders. With increased pulmonary blood flow, an increased incidence of respiratory infections may be seen including pneumonia. Auscultatory, electrocardiographic, and chest radiographic findings can be found in Table 70-3.

Management

The clinical management of infants and children with VSDs varies according to the size and location of the defect, which is directly responsible for the signs and symptoms exhibited by the child. Children with VSDs may remain asymptomatic and simply require regular outpatient follow-up. Some will experience CHF and require aggressive medical management and diligent follow-up. Closure can occur spontaneously, with cardiovascular surgery, with interventional cardiac catheterization, or with a combined catheter-surgical approach.

Owing to the fact that small VSDs can close spontaneously in the first 4 to 6 years of life, these children require outpatient follow-up at regular intervals. In children with moderate to large VSDs, follow-up assessment should include any changes noted in the child's growth and development, which could be suggestive of increasing shunt size or early signs of pulmonary hypertension.

Children with CHF secondary to VSDs may require anticongestive medications, such as digoxin and/or diuretics, and will occasionally require afterload reduction with agents, such as enalapril. To promote weight gain in infants with failure to thrive, caloric content per ounce should be increased. Newborns may require 120 to 150 calories/kg/day to gain weight. Occasionally, nasogastric feedings are necessary to promote further weight gain.

For children with small VSDs or those that do not produce symptoms and/or early sequelae, closure may be postponed just before the school-age years. Surgical closure in infants may be required earlier if medical therapy is unsuccessful in reducing the signs and symptoms of CHF or if growth and development is impeded. Increased pulmonary pressures are also a factor when considering surgical closure. If pulmonary hypertension is suspected, a cardiac catheterization should be performed. For the child with a small VSD with a Qp/Qs *less than* 1.5:1, surgery is not recommended,[8] owing to the fact that the risk of associated complications, such as AV block, outweigh the benefits.

Device closure in children with VSDs compared with those with ASDs and PDA is more difficult because of surrounding anatomy and location.[16] Current data shows promise of the efficacy of the Amplatzer septal occluder for *perimembranous* and *muscular* types with success rates of 90 percent and 93 percent, respectively.[20,21] In a study published in 2004, Holzer and colleagues[22] assessed immediate and midterm results, using the United States registry of patients using the Amplatzer *muscular* VSD occluder. Eighty-six percent (72/83) of devices were implanted successfully; however, 8 of 75 (10.7 percent) of patients experienced major procedure-related complications, with 2 (2.7 percent) of those being procedure-related deaths. The Amplatzer muscular device has closed its clinical trials and is waiting Food and Drug Administration approval for use in children to close VSDs.

Another treatment modality for children with VSDs is a combined catheter-surgical approach.[13] The chest is opened by the cardiovascular surgeon, and a device is placed into the VSD. The benefits of this approach are that cardiopulmonary bypass is avoided, and it allows for closure in areas that the surgeon may typically have difficulties reaching.

Surgical closure of a VSD is performed on cardiopulmonary bypass with a median sternotomy incision; however, minimally invasive approaches are also possible with some VSD closures. When closing a VSD, a transatrial approach is preferred over a ventriculotomy because of concerns about postoperative dysrhythmias. Surgical closure is accomplished using a patch (or patches) or with sutures.

Children with increased pulmonary pressures before surgery often require added postoperative support. Oxygen therapy or nitric oxide may be administered. Patients that continue exhibiting the signs and symptoms of CHF and have decreased CO postoperatively may have a residual VSD. These children should be followed closely in the postoperative period for dysrhythmias, specifically atrioventricular (AV) block (perimembranous and inlet) and junctional ectopic tachycardia (JET) (as a result of proximity of His bundle). Dysrhythmias in a repaired VSD tend to occur in younger children.[23] Patients with pulmonary hypertension may exhibit cyanosis, dyspnea, and/or hypotension.

Over time if a VSD is not closed, the pulmonary pressures begin to rise causing a right to left shunt. This phenomenon is known as Eisenmenger syndrome or pulmonary hypertension (see Chapter 71).

Patent Ductus Arteriosus

The ductus arteriosus is a normal communication in utero that generally closes early in the postnatal period in the majority of newborns (i.e., closing within 10 to 14 hours after birth with full closure at around 3 weeks in term neonates). Spontaneous closure may not occur in premature neonates. Accounting for 5 percent of congenital heart defects (excluding premature infants), a PDA is located between the descending aorta and the left PA. (Figure 70-4). After birth pulmonary vascular resistance decreases, and blood is shunted from the higher-pressure aorta to the lower-pressure pulmonary artery (PA) resulting in left to right shunting, which causes pulmonary overcirculation and increased workload for the left side of the heart. In addition to prematurity, other factors known to promote ductal patency include hypoxia and first trimester maternal rubella exposure. In some cases of complex congenital (usually cyanotic) lesions, the ductus is deliberately kept patent to promote pulmonary or systemic blood flow.

Clinical Manifestations

The signs and symptoms exhibited by neonates with PDA vary according to the size of the ductal opening. Neonates and infants with small PDA are usually asymptomatic, whereas children with large PDA may exhibit signs and symptoms of CHF. These children are generally poor feeders, tachypneic, and tachycardic with bounding pulses generally noted on palpation. In contrast to children with a VSD, children with PDA exhibit symptoms shortly after birth, whereas a child with a VSD may exhibit symptoms 1 to 2 months after pulmo-

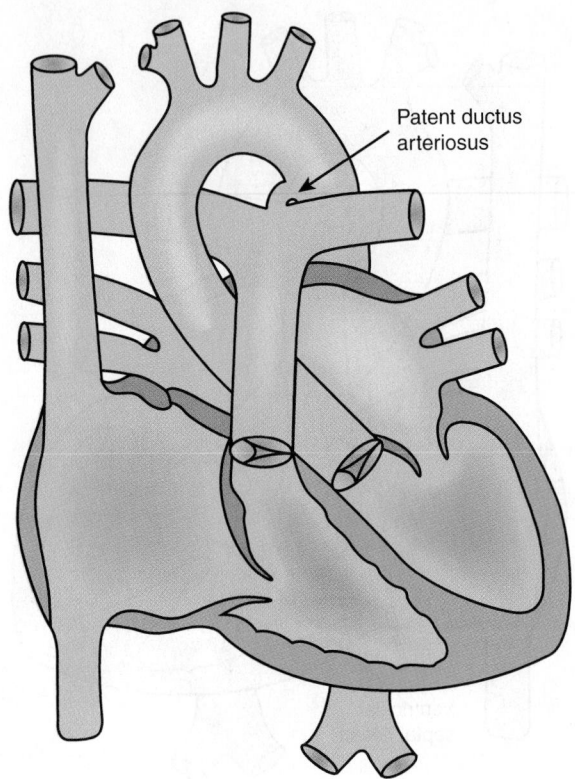

FIGURE 70-4 ■ A patent ductus arteriosus allows aortic blood to recirculate to the lungs. (Courtesy Scientific Software Solutions, PedCath version 7.4.3.)

nary vascular resistance drops. In premature neonates with PDA, the respiratory status can become more compromised over time and potentially lead to bronchopulmonary dysplasia. Auscultatory, electrocardiographic, and chest radiographic findings can be found in Table 70-3.

Management

The management of the child with a PDA is totally dependent on the symptomatology, which again is secondary to the size of the ductal opening. The treatment options include outpatient follow-up, medical management, catheter intervention, or surgical intervention. Medical therapy consists of managing the signs and symptoms of CHF and/or the administration of indomethacin, a medication that is used to stimulate ductal closure. Children with CHF are treated with anticongestive medications, most commonly digoxin and diuretics. A continuous and thorough assessment of the premature infant's respiratory status is important. In an attempt to prevent surgery, preterm infants may be given indomethacin, which is associated with a 70 percent to 90 percent success rate for ductal closure in this age group.[24] Cerebral vascular hemorrhage is a concern for neonates and infants receiving indomethacin, and the debate of administering indomethacin versus ibuprofen for ductal closure remains.

Preterm infants in whom medical management is not successful and who continue to exhibit the signs and symptoms of CHF (symptoms that are not related to the underlying condition of prematurity) require PDA closure within 48 to 72 hours of birth. Most PDA can be closed in the catheterization laboratory, with the exception of preterm infants who are extremely small in size. PDA may be closed with an Amplatzer ductal occluder or via coil occlusion technique. Length, diameter, and shape of the PDA are factors to consider in device selection. Coil occlusion is often recommended for PDA *less than* 3 mm in size,[25] whereas the Amplatzer ductal occluder is recommended for moderate to large PDA.[26] The ductal occluder works well with various shaped PDA lesions, whereas coil occlusion is not always feasible for all PDA shapes. Potential complications specific to coil occlusion include embolization and persistent residual shunt. Potential complications associated with device occlusion include embolization, device protrusion into the aorta, and left PA stenosis; however, the occurrence of complications related to either technique is low. Device closure has evolved as the preferred treatment modality for PDA because it is safer, less painful for the child, and equally effective as surgery.[25] The Amplatzer has been used successfully to close PDA, with a 92.5 percent success rate.[26] Surgical PDA closure is performed via thoracotomy without the use of cardiopulmonary bypass, using ligation or hemoclip.

Atrioventricular Septal Defect

Atrioventricular septal defect (AVSD), also referred to as endocardial cushion defect (**ECD**) or AV canal defect, accounts for 4 percent of congenital cardiac defects and occurs when the cardiac cushions fail to develop adequately during fetal cardiac development. In an AVSD, an abnormal communication exists between the atria and ventricles, which may or may not be associated with AV valve insufficiency. AVSDs are classified as complete, incomplete, balanced, and unbalanced. (Figure 70-5) A complete AVSD will have a common valve, ASD (primum), and VSD (inlet-muscular), whereas an incomplete AVSD consists of an ASD (primum) and in most cases, a cleft mitral valve. With a complete AVSD, shunting occurs left to right in both the atria and ventricles allowing free communication between all four chambers. To be considered balanced, the AVSD consists of two functioning ventricles with well-balanced AV valve tissue. In the unbalanced AVSD, only one functioning ventricle is present. In children with Down syndrome, 50 percent have some form of CHD and in more than half of those, the defect is an AVSD.[27]

Several sources of shunting can be seen with a complete AVSD, occurring through the incompetent AV valve and through the ASD and VSD, resulting in increased pulmonary blood flow and increased workload for both sides of the heart. An insufficient mitral valve can produce increased work for the left side of the heart and in combination with an ASD produces increased work for the right side as well. Because of the numerous areas of possible shunting in children with a complete AVSD, the signs and symptoms of CHF generally occur earlier when compared with children with isolated septal defects. Children with Down syndrome and a AVSD will often develop pulmonary hypertension earlier than children without Down syndrome.

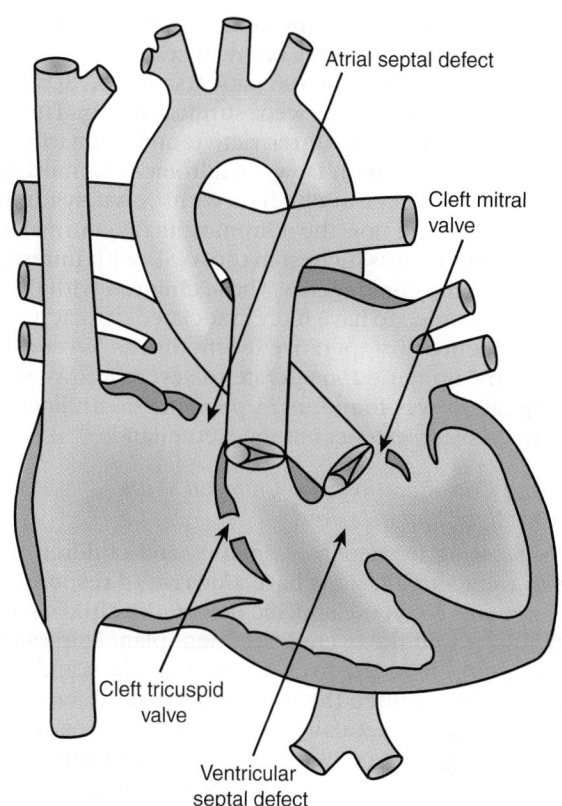

FIGURE 70-5 ■ Atrioventricular septal defect. Combination defect of the atria, ventricles, and mitral and tricuspid valves. (Courtesy Scientific Software Solutions, PedCath version 7.4.3.)

Clinic Manifestations

Symptoms associated with a complete AVSD vary according to the amount of leakage at the common AV valve (MR) and are similar to the symptoms seen in children with a large VSD. Contrary to children with the previously described left to right shunts, children with an AVSD are generally more symptomatic and critically ill. Children with a complete AVSD usually experience tachypnea, tachycardia, and diaphoresis. Failure to thrive is common with these children and as a result of the increased pulmonary blood flow, these children may be susceptible to recurrent respiratory infections. Specific auscultatory, electrocardiographic, and chest radiographic findings can be found in Table 70-3.

Management

The management of children with an AVSD is aimed directly at reducing the symptoms of CHF using inotropic agents, diuretics, and afterload reduction. Surgery is generally recommended earlier for patients that have failed medical management. Complete surgical repair is generally performed between 3 and 9 months of age, and surgery is performed with cardiopulmonary bypass via median sternotomy. In the infant with CAVSD, one or two patch repair with valve reconstruction is performed, a repair that is technically more challenging because of the common valve separation. The surgery for an incomplete AVSD consists of an ASD patch closure and a mitral cleft suture, whereas the complete repair requires ASD and VSD patch closure, and mitral and tricuspid valve repair with valve reconstruction using available tissue from the common AV valve leaflets. Mitral valve replacement is rarely necessary.

In a 10-year review of 106 patients with AVSDs,[28] 81 percent of patients underwent surgical repair. The majority of defects were unrestrictive and primarily occurred in children with Down syndrome. The mortality rate was 9.5 percent in children with Down syndrome and 14.3 percent for the chromosomally normal patients. Mortality was highest in the AVSD with unrestrictive ventricular components. Those children with Down syndrome tended to have more associated cardiac anomalies and more postoperative dysrhythmias. Over a 3.5-year follow-up period, moderate to severe left AV valve regurgitation was found in 23 percent,[28] a finding corroborated by researchers in the Netherlands.[29]

Nursing Considerations for Children With Left to Right Shunt Lesions

Nurses caring for neonates, infants, and children with left to right shunt lesions have a myriad of responsibilities, depending on the specific defect, the child's symptomatology, and the overall treatment plan. Nurses play an integral role in the lives of these children and their families and are often the individuals that interact most with the family on a daily basis. The following discussion will include general considerations and patient and family education, content that is generic to all children with cardiac defects. The general considerations for children undergoing catheter and surgical procedures can be found in the section of caring for children undergoing invasive cardiac procedures.

General Considerations

Caring for children with heart disease is quite different than caring for adults. In addition to the clinical and physical aspects of the child's care, nurses must remain cognizant of the psychosocial and developmental aspects of caring for children at different ages. In most pediatric cardiovascular care environments, the concept of family-centered care is emphasized. This model of care delivery recognizes that the family serves as a "constant" in the child's life, and cardiovascular health care providers strive to provide support, respect, encouragement, and enhancement of the family unit by empowerment and effective help giving.[30] By establishing a parent-professional partnership, cardiovascular health care providers acknowledge the parents rightful role in making decisions that are important for individual family members and the family as a whole, while supporting and strengthening their ability to nurture and promote its development.[31] Some of the demonstrated benefits of family-centered care include: (1) less stress and increased confidence and competence for the parents, (2) decreased dependency on cardiovascular caregivers, (3) decreased care costs, and (4) empowered families and health care providers, with regard to developing new skills and expertise.[32,33]

Patient and Family Education

Patient and family education is critical when caring for children with heart disease. Unlike adults, children progress through various developmental stages that cor-

relate with their understanding of illness, which must be taken into account when planning an educational session. When caring for neonates with CHD, it is crucial that the parents be allowed and encouraged to grieve for the loss of a "normal" child. Many parents, mothers especially, are concerned that something that they did during pregnancy caused the heart defect. Although there are some defects directly related to the mother's behavior (e.g., fetal alcohol syndrome in which there is a heart defect), the majority of cases are not, and the mother should be informed, even if she does not verbalize this thought. It is important that nurses caring for these children and their families be as honest as possible regarding the child's diagnosis, prognosis, and available treatment options. Because of the explosion of information that patients and parents can now retrieve from the Internet, it is important for cardiovascular nurses to be able to direct these families to reputable websites, some of which can be found in Box 70-5.

Patient and family education is difficult to provide in today's harried work environment, but remains one of the single most important facets of caring for children with heart disease. Patient and family education should take place in a quiet and relaxed atmosphere. First, what is already known by the patient and family should be assessed, keeping in mind the child's developmental level, previous hospital experience, timing, temperament, and coping styles. Parents are extremely important in this process, a process that aids in decreasing anxiety and increasing understanding of the child's heart condition. General guidelines for planning patient and family education have been published by Wong and colleagues[34] and are summarized in Box 70-6.

Lesion-Specific Postprocedural Care

The potential complications associated with interventional cardiac catheterization procedures can be found in the section on caring for children undergoing invasive cardiac procedures. Following an ASD device closure, children receive aspirin and maintain endocarditis protection for 6 months following the procedure. If no residual shunt exists at that time, prophylaxis is discontinued.

BOX 70-5 ■ ■ ■
INTERNET RESOURCES FOR FAMILIES AND CHILDREN WITH CONGENITAL HEART DISEASE

- American Heart Association
- *www.americanheart.org/presenter.jhtml?identifier=1200000*
- Cardiac Arrhythmias Research and Education Foundation (CARE)
  www.longqt.org/
- Children's Hospital of Boston
  www.childrenshospital.org
- Congenital Heart Disease—Information and Resources
  www.ltchin.org
- Patient Education for Congenital Heart Disease
  www.pted.org
- PediHeart
  www.pediheart.org/parents/index.html
- The Children's Heart Foundation:
  www.childrensheart.com

CHD, Congenital heart disease.

The potential complications associated with cardiac surgery can be found in the section on caring for children undergoing invasive cardiac procedures. Children who have undergone surgery for an ASD are prone to atrial dysrhythmias in the acute and chronic postoperative period, owing to the fact that there is atrial stretch and an atriotomy. These children are also prone to a potentially late complication know as postpericardiotomy syndrome, prompting a 14-day follow-up visit to assess for this complication. (Box 70-7).

The majority of children who have undergone surgery to repair a VSD are extubated quickly; however, children with increased pulmonary pressure before surgery often require added support in the postoperative period, specifically with oxygen or nitric oxide therapy. Continued signs of CHF in association with decreased CO may be indicative of residual shunt. Dysrhythmias commonly seen in the acute postoperative period after a VSD repair include AV block, particularly in the perimembranous and inlet types, and JET.

For the neonate or infant who has undergone surgical repair of PDA, hemorrhage, thoracotomy care, and astute pain management are the major postoperative concerns. Additional respiratory support may be necessary in premature infants with ductal closure related to their lung prematurity.

The postoperative management of the child who has undergone repair of a complete AVSD can be quite challenging as a result of the repaired valve. Volume precau-

tions are important because of the repaired valve and numerous suture lines. Afterload-reducing agents are recommended to aid in decreasing AV valve regurgitation. Inotropes may be given to help with cardiac function. Diuretics are administered, and patients are usually discharged home on them. Pressure monitoring should include left atrial and PA measures. Pulmonary hypertensive episodes should be treated, and nitric oxide has shown some benefit in treating severe postoperative pulmonary hypertension. Owing to the fact that the AV node in AVSD is not located in the normal anatomical position, AV block is a postoperative concern.

Children who have undergone repair of a CAVSD often require additional surgeries because of valve incompetence. Reoperation for the left AV valve occurs in 10 percent of the patients.[35] Valve replacement may be recommended. In a study by Lindberg and colleagues,[36] severe pulmonary hypertension was most commonly seen postoperatively in CAVSDs. The increased pulmonary blood flow with increased pulmonary venous pressures coupled with the increased number of Down syndrome patients may explain why pulmonary hypertension is often seen postoperatively in children with a CAVSD.[36]

Obstructive Lesions

The three major congenital cardiac lesions that pose obstruction to blood flow include pulmonary stenosis **(PS)**, AS, and CoA. In the child with PS, pulmonary blood flow is obstructed. In contrast children with CoA and AS experience an obstruction in systemic blood flow.

Pulmonary Stenosis

Pulmonary stenosis is responsible for approximately 10 percent of CHD and is simply a narrowing into the PA that interferes with blood flow from the RV. (Figure 70-6) This narrowing can occur at the valve level (*valvular* PS), below the valve (*subvalvular* PS), or above the valve (*supravalvular* PS). Several areas of stenosis may occur jointly. *Valvular* stenosis is the most common form of PS. The valve leaflets may be fused at the commissure, and a dysplastic valve (abnormal, thickened leaflets) may also be seen with *valvular* stenosis. Dysplastic valves are often seen with Noonan syndrome, an autosomal dominant syndrome in which children have short stature, a short webbed neck, and mild mental retardation. Fifty percent of patients with Noonan syndrome have some form of CHD.[37]

Mild *valvular* obstruction does not usually progress, whereas *subvalvular* obstruction alone usually progresses in severity. To maintain forward flow into the lungs, the RV becomes overworked and over time may produce right ventricular failure, prompting an increase in right atrial pressure **(RAP)**. Right atrial enlargement may be seen on the surface ECG. *Critical* PS is defined as a 50-mm Hg peak-to-peak systolic gradient. A mean gradient of 50 mm Hg by Doppler measurement provides a rough estimate of the right ventricular pressure. In *critical* PS, the RV pressure can be higher than 70 (20 being normal) with a normal (20) PA pressure. The

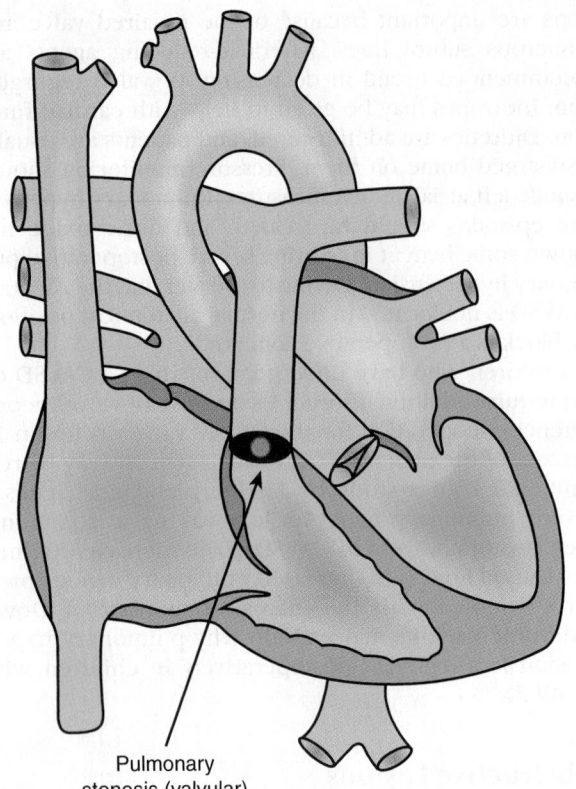

FIGURE 70-6 ■ Valvular pulmonary stenosis impedes blood flow from the right ventricle to the lungs. (Courtesy Scientific Software Solutions, PedCath version 7.4.3.)

Pulmonary
stenosis (valvular)

heart is able to compensate by maintaining a normal PA pressure until eventually failure occurs.

Subvalvular stenosis with right ventricular outflow obstruction can be seen in conjunction with TOF and double outlet right ventricle **(DORV).** The valve may also be atretic as in pulmonary atresia, a defect in which there is no communication between the RV and PA. Some atretic pulmonary valves may be amenable to transcatheter puncture using radiofrequency with balloon dilatation. Although this procedure does not alleviate the need for surgery in all patients, it has been reported as a successful alternative to surgery in patients with a well-formed tricuspid valve, with a patent infundibulum, and without an RV-dependent coronary circulation.[38]

Clinical Manifestations

The clinical signs and symptoms of PS in neonates and infants are dependent on the degree of obstruction (i.e., gradient) measured in mm Hg. Neonates or infants with *critical* PS are often tachypneic and may be cyanotic (if the PFO is open), which could progress to cardiogenic shock if adequate support is not provided. Children with mild PS may remain totally asymptomatic, whereas children with moderate to severe PS are often referred to a cardiologist for murmur evaluation rather than symptoms. These children usually remain asymptomatic, but eventually right ventricular failure can occur, and if it does, it is hard to reverse. Children with PS require close outpatient follow-up. Auscultatory, electrocardiographic, and chest radiographic findings can be found in Table 70-3.

Management

Neonates or infants with critical PS require immediate medical management with measures intended to support the circulation, which may include intubation and inotropic support. Prostaglandin E_1 **(PGE$_1$)** is administered to reopen the ductus arteriosus. Infants and children with *critical* PS are referred for balloon valvuloplasty. Patients with *valvular* PS may be candidates for balloon valvuloplasty if the right ventricular systolic pressures are *greater than* 50 mm Hg.[8] In *valvular* PS, balloon valvuloplasty has become the preferred method of treatment. Balloon valvuloplasty is performed in the catheterization lab and is considered a low-risk procedure with a high success rate. After balloon valvuloplasty, children may exhibit some associated *subvalvular* stenosis, but this usually resolves with time. Dysplastic valves are not always amenable to ballooning and may require surgical intervention.

Emergent surgery is recommended for *critical* PS if valvuloplasty is not successful. Surgical valvotomy is performed on cardiopulmonary bypass, and the narrowed pulmonary valve or fused leaflets are repaired through the PA. Some valves may not be repairable and may require complete removal. Children can tolerate the absence of a pulmonary valve for decades. Eventually the patient will need a pulmonary valve placed to preserve right ventricular function. Surgery is recommended in *supravalvular* and *subvalvular* PS as RV pressure increases. The surgical approach for PS is to widen the narrowed area with muscle resection or patch repair.

Aortic Stenosis

AS is a narrowing into the aorta and occurs in 5 percent of all CHD (Figure 70-7). This narrowing causes an obstruction to blood flow from the left ventricle (systemic) and may occur at the following levels: valvular, subvalvular, or supravalvular. *Valvular* AS is the most common type and is often associated with a bicuspid valve, but may be associated with other lesions as well. The increased stress on the left ventricle and ascending aorta results in muscular hypertrophy and aortic dilatation. *Subvalvular* AS occurs when a membrane forms below the normal anatomical location commonly resulting in aortic insufficiency. *Supravalvular* AS produces increased stress on the left ventricle, resulting in left ventricular hypertrophy. This type of AS is often associated with Williams syndrome, a genetic defect related to abnormal calcium metabolism, which is associated with distinct facial features, such as a wide mouth and thick lips, and mild to moderate mental retardation.[39] Failure of the left ventricle can cause an increase in left atrial pressure **(LAP),** and when LAPs increase, pulmonary venous pressures may also increase resulting in pulmonary congestion.

Clinical Manifestations

Symptoms associated with AS are based on the amount of obstruction. Patients with mild AS are usually asymptomatic. In neonates with *critical* AS, the following conditions may be observed: decreased perfusion, faint peripheral pulses, decreased CO, and oliguria. Circula-

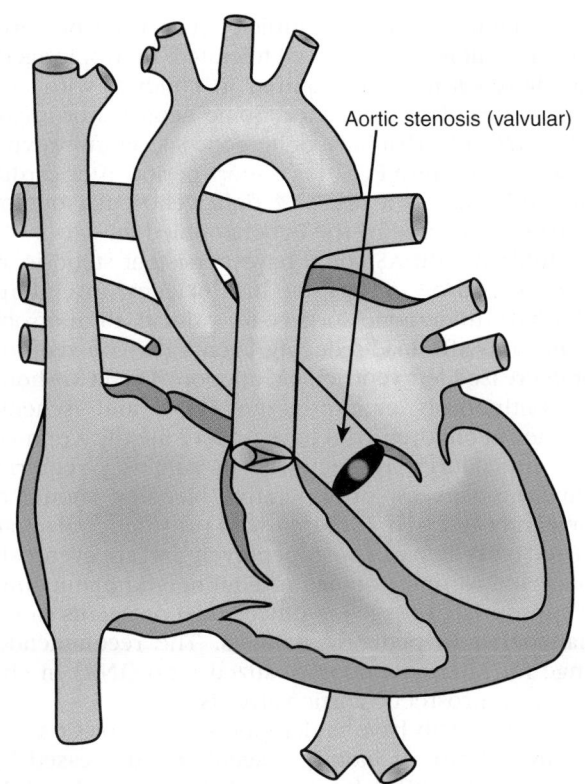

Aortic stenosis (valvular)

FIGURE 70-7 ▪ Valvular atrial stenosis impedes the flow of blood from the left ventricle to the body. (Courtesy Scientific Software Solutions, PedCath version 7.4.3.)

tory collapse can occur, and sudden death is more common than symptoms of obstruction in children with AS. In children additional symptoms may include dyspnea, exercise intolerance, chest pain, and syncope. In children with *supravalvular* AS, the right and left upper extremity blood pressures may be different. Auscultatory, electrocardiographic, and chest radiographic findings can be found in Table 70-3.

Management

The management of children with AS includes medical management, catheter intervention, and/or surgical intervention. Neonates or infants with *critical* AS should be started on PGE_1 immediately to keep the ductus open (to allow the RV to perfuse the body) usually requiring intubation and positive pressure ventilation. Metabolic acidosis should be corrected, and inotropic agents and diuretics may be administered for CHF.

Valvular AS may be treated in the catheterization laboratory with balloon valvuloplasty; however, if the valve annulus is small, surgical intervention may be necessary. An antegrade or retrograde approach may be taken when ballooning *valvular* AS. Aortic insufficiency is a possible complication with balloon valvuloplasty, and abnormal aortic valves may require surgical intervention at a later date even after successful relief of obstruction using balloon valvuloplasty.

Surgery may be performed for *critical* AS if balloon valvuloplasty is not successful. Surgery may be recommended in older children when: (1) symptoms are present, (2) the EST is abnormal (i.e., ST segment changes),

or (3) a mean gradient of at least 50 mm Hg is detected by echocardiography.[40] A surgical valvotomy requires widening the aortic valve orifice by releasing the fused leaflets with careful attention to prevent aortic insufficiency. Children that have had a successful valvotomy may require aortic valve replacement secondary to aortic insufficiency; however, if the child has recurrent stenosis, the valve can be ballooned again. A prosthetic, porcine, or aortic homograft valve may be used when replacing the aortic valve with a prosthetic valve requiring chronic anticoagulation therapy.

The Ross procedure, an alternative to the use of a prosthetic valve, involves replacing the aortic valve with the child's own pulmonary (autologous) valve with subsequent placement of an aortic or pulmonary homograft in the pulmonary valve position. The advantages of the Ross procedure are long-term growth potential of the autograft alleviating the need for chronic anticoagulation therapy. Recent data suggests that the Ross procedure is an important tool for children with AS with no autograft stenosis at a midterm follow-up of 9 years; however, autograft dilatation remains a concern.[41]

Surgical correction of *supravalvular* AS involves placing a patch to the narrowed area. A "Y" patch technique may be performed to open the narrowed area. In *subvalvular* AS, where the obstruction can be a discrete membrane or fibromuscular, the narrowed area is resected. Careful attention is taken when resecting fibrous muscle to prevent aortic valve damage or the creation of a traumatic VSD. For severe *subvalvular* AS in which the annulus is small, a Konno procedure may be performed, in which the entire area (at the valve and below) is enlarged with a patch. Additionally, combination surgical procedures can be used including the Konno procedure and a valve replacement *or* a Konno procedure and a Ross procedure.

Coarctation of the Aorta

Coarctation of the aorta is simply a narrowing of the aorta that impedes systemic blood flow and occurs in 10 percent of children with CHD. The narrowing in CoA is generally beyond the left subclavian artery at the location of the ductus arteriosus; however, it may also occur in locations proximal or distal to this site as well. Approximately 50 percent of children with CoA also have a bicuspid aortic valve. With CoA left ventricular pressures begin to rise as blood is pumped through the narrowed area, which in turn can lead to left ventricular hypertrophy. As pressures in the left ventricle rise, pressures in the left atrium will also start to rise. Pulmonary blood flow then becomes congested, and pulmonary hypertension can result (Figure 70-8).

Clinical Manifestations

The clinical manifestations of children with CoA vary; however, in infants with severe CoA and ductal closure, cardiac collapse may be seen. Some children are asymptomatic, but abnormal assessment findings may be discovered during physical examination. Differences in upper and lower extremity blood pressures may be noted, with upper extremity blood pressures being higher than the lower extremities. Older children with

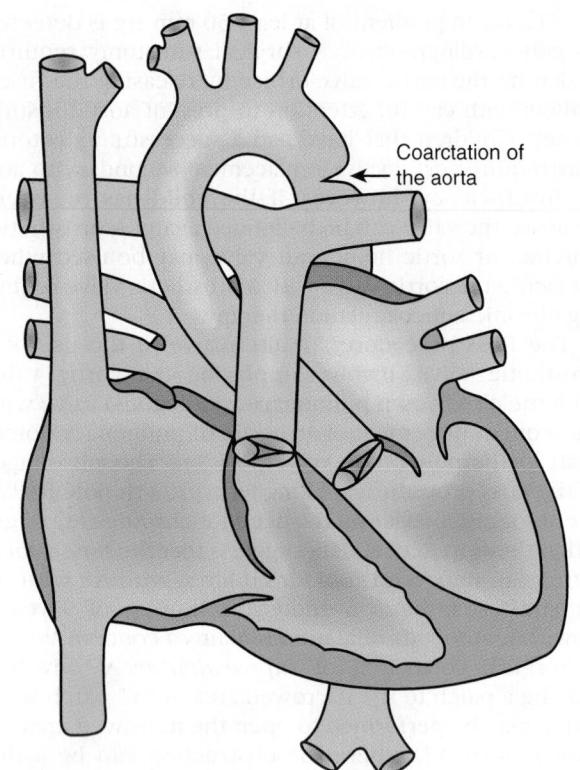

FIGURE 70-8 ■ In coarctation of the aorta, the aorta is narrowed just beyond the left subclavian artery. (Courtesy Scientific Software Solutions, PedCath version 7.4.3.)

CoA may have headaches and dizziness. Elevated blood pressures and a decreased femoral pulse may be noted on examination, and these children are at risk for strokes. Auscultatory, electrocardiographic, and chest radiographic findings can be found in Table 70-3.

Management

In neonates, PGE₁ is administered to reopen the ductus. Metabolic acidosis should be corrected, and inotropic agents may be administered. In recurrent CoA, balloon angioplasty is often recommended as the treatment of choice; however, its use in native CoA remains controversial. Stent placement in older children with near adult size aortas is being performed more often, but long-term studies remain to be performed.[42] Surgical intervention is the preferred treatment method for neonates with CoA, with elective surgery recommended between 1 and 3 years of age. Symptomatic patients with CoA are generally referred for surgery upon diagnosis. The following techniques are used to repair CoA: (1) *end-to-end anastomosis,* in which the narrowed area is resected, and the aortic ends are sewn together, (2) *subclavian flap repair,* in which the distal subclavian is divided and then used to patch the narrowed area, (3) *patch repair,* in which a patch is sewn over the narrowed area, and (4) *conduit repair,* in which a conduit is placed between the ascending and descending aorta. The various surgical techniques have been studied to determine the best approach; however, no true consensus has been reached at this time.

Nursing Considerations for Children With Obstructive Lesions. In children who have undergone surgical repair

of PS, pulmonary valve insufficiency is a postoperative concern, but is generally well tolerated. Inotropic agents and diuretics may be required in children with poor right ventricular compliance. Some neonates or infants with *critical* PS that have undergone successful valvuloplasty may require PGE₁ for a short period after cardiac catheterization as a result of right ventricular outflow obstruction caused by the hypertrophied muscle.

Children with AS could have persistent stenosis, restenosis, and/or aortic valve insufficiency. In children who have undergone surgery for critical AS, inotropic agents and afterload-reducing agents may be required for decreased left ventricular function. The ECG should be continuously monitored for CAVB and ischemic changes in children who have undergone the Konno or Ross procedures, respectively. In surgeries requiring numerous sutures, postoperative bleeding should be constantly assessed. Children with prosthetic valves are started on IV heparin postoperatively and are eventually converted to oral Coumadin. Finding and maintaining an appropriate dosage for anticoagulation agents can be challenging in pediatric patients. The recommended range for international normalized ratio **(INR)** in children with prosthetic aortic valves is 2.5 to 3.5.

Children who have undergone surgery for CoA may require the use of inotropic agents for decreased left ventricular function. If a residual CoA is noted and the child is not gradually getting better, a return to surgery may be necessary. Postoperative management is aimed at controlling blood pressure and heart rate to alleviate stress on the suture lines. Agitation should be prevented, and postoperative pain control is imperative. Upper and lower extremity blood pressures should be constantly assessed and for children who experience high blood pressure immediately after surgery, a continuous infusion with esmolol (beta blocker) or Nipride (vasodilator) may be administered. Once blood pressures have improved, these medications may be discontinued; however, some children will require antihypertensive medications at hospital discharge.

A potential complication known as postcoarctectomy syndrome may be observed in the postoperative period, more commonly in older children. The signs and symptoms include abdominal pain and/or distention, nausea, and ascites, prompting the cessation of any oral feedings until bowel sounds are noted upon auscultation. Bowel infarction can result from this complication. A rare complication, spinal cord ischemia, should be assessed by evaluating movement of the child's lower extremities. This complication and rebound hypertension occur more commonly in older children. Balloon angioplasty is an option for residual CoA and can be performed a few months after surgical intervention.

Cyanotic Defects

Congenital cardiac defects in which there is right to left shunting are considered cyanotic defects. The child with a cyanotic defect may experience increased or decreased pulmonary blood flow depending on the specific lesion. Additionally, and as a result of the physiological changes produced by a specific lesion, children may experience alternating periods of cyanosis and acyanosis. The following section will include a discussion of the following major cyanotic defects: TOF, TGA, truncus arteriosus, total anomalous pulmonary venous return **(TAPVR)**, tricuspid atresia **(TA)**, and hypoplastic left heart syndrome **(HLHS)**.

Tetralogy of Fallot

Tetralogy of Fallot is the most common cyanotic defect and accounts for 9 percent of all CHDs. The four abnormalities making up TOF are: (1) VSD (malalignment), (2) an overriding aorta, (3) PS, and (4) right ventricular hypertrophy **(RVH)**. (Figure 70-9) This defect may appear in conjunction with other abnormalities (e.g., TOF with pulmonary atresia, TOF with absent pulmonary valve, and TOF with multiple aortopulmonary collateral arteries).

In children with TOF, the right to left shunting varies with the amount of PS and the degree of right ventricular outflow obstruction, with moderate pulmonary obstruction producing elevated right ventricular pressures. This causes unoxygenated blood to be shunted from right to left through the VSD and then out of the overriding aorta. Elevated right ventricular pressures cause RVH. With mild pulmonary obstruction, minimal right to left shunting occurs, and these children are referred to as "pink" TOF. Over time the obstruction impedes progress. Auscultatory, electrocardiographic, and chest radiographic findings can be found in Table 70-3.

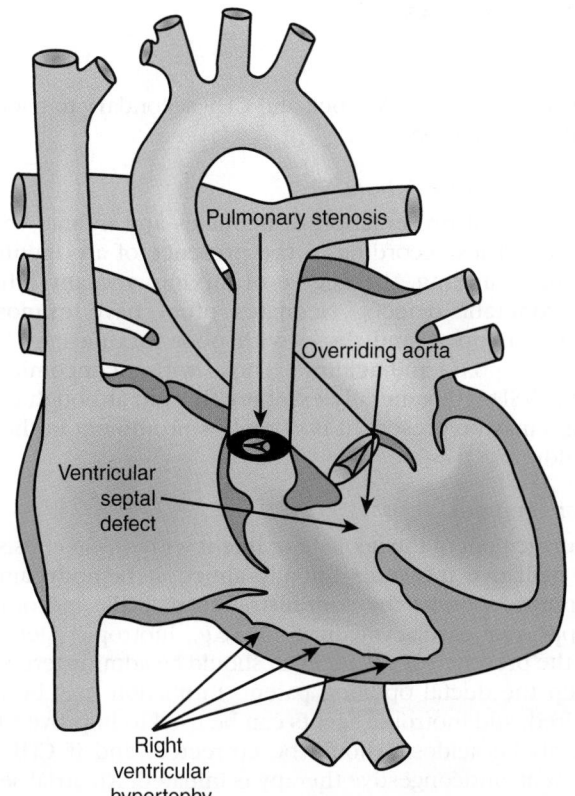

FIGURE 70-9 ■ Uncomplicated tetralogy of Fallot with the usual four defects: pulmonary stenosis an aorta that overrides the septum, a ventricular septal defect, and right ventricular hypertrophy. (Courtesy of Scientific Software Solutions, PedCath version 7.4.3.)

Clinical Manifestations

Infants and children with TOF exhibit signs and symptoms based on the amount of pulmonary obstruction and the size of the VSD. Mild obstruction may result in oxygen saturations in the 90s, with most of these patients remaining asymptomatic. As the obstruction increases, the degree of cyanosis increases. Hemodynamically, there is a decrease in pulmonary blood flow (as a result of a VSD and blood flow obstruction from the RV).

Owing to the fact that many infants now undergo surgical treatment much earlier than in the past, children with TOF rarely exhibit hypoxic episodes referred to as "tet spells"; however, those caring for children with TOF must remain aware of their potential occurrence. "Tet spells" often occur when the child is agitated, cries, or after feedings. Associated observations include hyperpnea (rapid and deep breathing), cyanosis, and syncope in rare instances. Although the exact mechanism for these hypoxic episodes remains unclear, severe brain injury or death could result from a severe episode. Causative factors for these hypoxic episodes may be contraction of the right ventricular outflow tract, increase in oxygen needs, or a decrease in systemic vascular resistance. Strategies for managing hypoxic spells in children with TOF can be found in Box 70-8.

Management

Management strategies for children with TOF are primarily surgical and include a palliative shunt procedure or complete surgical repair. Some children with TOF may undergo a palliative shunt procedure before the complete repair, which may be recommended for children with severe cyanosis, an increased propensity for hypoxic episodes, or hypoplastic pulmonary arteries. A modified Blalock-Taussig **(BT) shunt** is usually performed, at which time a gortex shunt is placed between the subclavian artery and a branch of the PA. Surgically placed shunts and their associated defects can be found in Table 70-4.

Current data suggest that total repair of TOF is being performed in younger and smaller children.[43] A complete repair consists of closing the VSD, resecting the muscle bundles, and patching the right ventricular outflow tract via the right atrium and PA. Potential advantages of early complete repair in TOF include a single operation, decreased frequency of low oxygen satura-

---

BOX 70-8   ■ ■ ■
STRATEGIES FOR MANAGING HYPOXIC SPELLS IN CYANOTIC CHILDREN

- Place infant in knee-chest position if possible.
- Administer morphine sulfate (0.1-0.2 mg/dose) IV or subcutaneously.
- Administer ketamine (1-2 mg/kg IM or 1 mg/kg IV).
- Correct acidosis.
- If severe, increase level of sedation, paralytics, and consider intubation.

IM, Intramuscular; *IV*, intravenous.

■ ■ ■

TABLE 70-4 SURGICALLY PLACED SHUNTS

BT shunt	An end-to-side anastomosis of the subclavian artery to the ipsilateral PA
Potts shunt	A creation of a window between the ascending aorta and the distal left PA
Waterston shunt	A creation of a window between the descending aorta and the proximal right PA
Modified BT shunt	A tube of prosthetic material (gortex) placed between the subclavian artery and branch PA
Central shunt	A tube of prosthetic material placed between the ascending aorta and main PA

PA, Pulmonary artery.

tions, and reduced complications resulting from long-term increasing right ventricular pressures.[43] A complete repair versus shunt palliation remains variable among institutions as does the age of the infant undergoing a total repair, with many centers performing repairs at age 1 to 4 months.

Various surgical techniques used for TOF have been modified over the years in an attempt to reduce late complications. Initially, large transannular patches were placed using a right ventriculotomy; however, this often resulted in pulmonary regurgitation.[44] This pulmonary regurgitation and the right ventriculotomy itself have resulted in adverse affects on right ventricular function and also a predilection to postoperative dysrhythmias. Currently, surgeons use smaller right ventriculotomy incisions and smaller transannular patches.

Transposition of the Great Arteries (d-TGA)

Transposition of the great arteries (**d-TGA**) is a cyanotic defect that occurs in 10 percent of children with CHD. Also known as complete transposition, with d-TGA, the aorta arises from the RV (versus the proper left ventricle), and the PA arises from the left ventricle (versus the proper RV) (Figure 70-10). The transposed great arteries result in unoxygenated blood entering the right atrium, continuing to the RV, and out of the aorta into systemic recirculation. Oxygenated blood enters the left atrium, continues to the left ventricle, and through the PA to recirculate through the pulmonary system, resulting in two separate circulations. Mixing of oxygenated blood with unoxygenated blood *cannot* occur without the presence of a VSD, an ASD, a PFO, or a PDA. A neonate or infant in whom there is no mixing will not survive. This defect can occur as an isolated lesion or in combination with other lesions.

Another version of TGA, known as corrected transposition or **levo-TGA** usually called (**l-TGA**) is a rare defect and accounts for *less than* 1 percent of all congenital heart defects, most often occurring in conjunction with other congenital heart defects. Although the PA and aorta are reversed, the anatomical ventricles are also reversed with the RV positioned on the left and the anatomical left ventricle positioned on the right, hence the term "corrected" transposition (Figure 70-11). Surgical intervention is not necessary for isolated l-TGA, but cardiac follow-up is needed to monitor for dysrhyth-

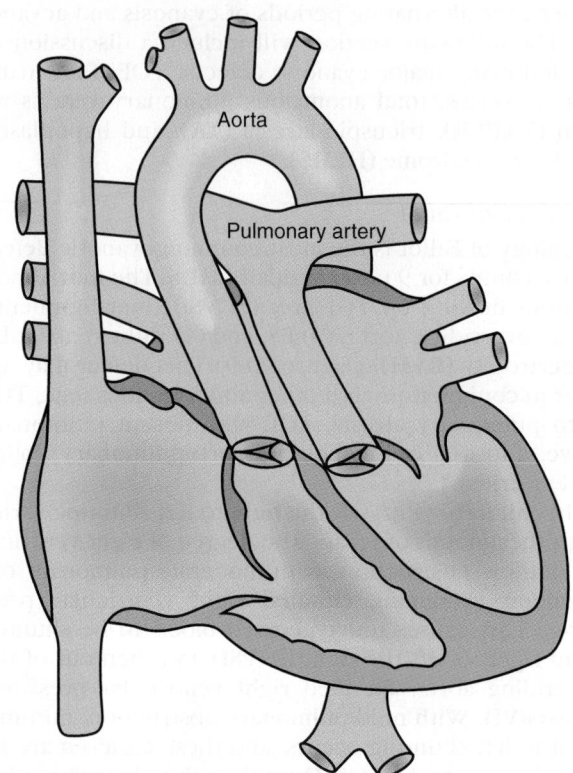

FIGURE 70-10 ■ Dextrotransposition of the great arteries (d-TGA) in which the aorta and pulmonary artery are completely reversed, resulting in two separate circulations. The aorta receives blood from the right ventricle and the pulmonary artery receives blood from the left ventricle. (Courtesy Scientific Software Solutions, PedCath version 7.4.3.)

mias, specifically AV block and CHF secondary to tricuspid regurgitation.

Clinical Manifestations

The clinical presentation of neonates and infants with d-TGA varies according to the presence of an opening to allow mixing, the degree of mixing, and any other concomitant defects. Neonates often have cyanosis and tachypnea, and those with poor mixing may become hypoxic and acidotic. Those with a concomitant large VSD will generally exhibit CHF, and although cyanosis may be present, it is often less prominent in these children.

Management

Management of the neonate or infant with d-TGA consists of palliative measures initially aimed at hemodynamic support, such as the administration of PGE$_1$ and other supportive cardiac medications (e.g., inotropic agents). In the presence of a PDA, PGE$_1$ should be administered to keep the ductal opening patent. Intubation may be required, and inotropic agents can be used to improve CO. Metabolic acidosis should be corrected, and if CHF is present, anticongestive therapy is initiated. An atrial septostomy may be necessary to aid mixing at the atrial level. This procedure may be performed at the neonate's bedside with echocardiographic guidance or in the catheterization laboratory with fluoroscopic guidance.

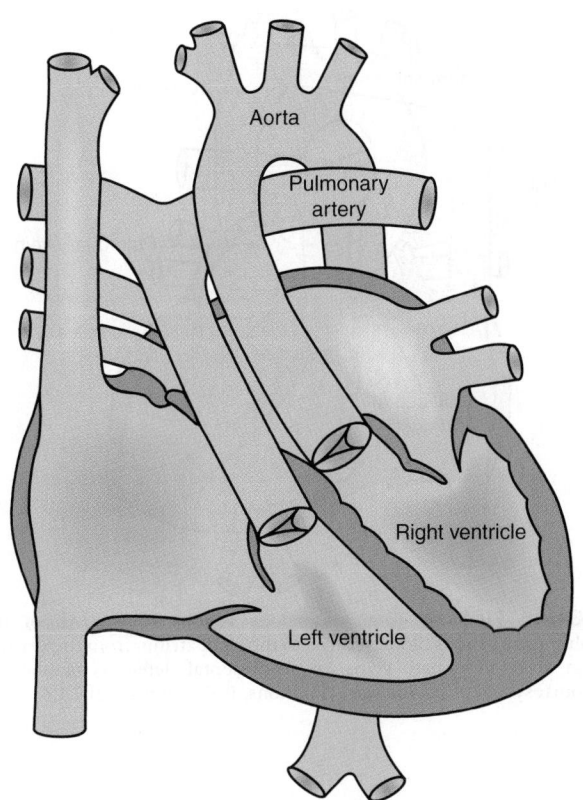

FIGURE 70-11 ▪ Levo transposition of the great arteries (l-TGA), known as corrected TGA, in which the pulmonary artery and the aorta are reversed, but so are the ventricles. (Courtesy Scientific Software Solutions, PedCath version 7.4.3.)

Once the neonate or infant has been hemodynamically stabilized, an immediate decision must be made regarding surgical intervention. The current surgery of choice for d-TGA is the *arterial* switch procedure, which provides anatomical correction of the defect. In the past, an *atrial* switch procedure, known as the Mustard or Senning procedure, was undertaken to reroute the circulation at the atrial level; however, the long-term complications associated with the operation (i.e., sinus node dysfunction, atrial tachydysrhythmias, and RV dysfunction) have rendered it extinct today. Many individuals who underwent the Mustard or Senning operation are currently still alive, prompting the need for a new specialty of adults with CHD (see Chapter 71).

In neonates with d-TGA, early surgical intervention is necessary because the left ventricle is delivering blood to the low-resistance pulmonary circulation. In cases in which there is moderate surgical delay, the left ventricle becomes pressure deconditioned, an impediment to postoperative systemic blood flow, which would require the extra step of "retraining" it before the arterial switch procedure. This is accomplished by banding the PA.

Early surgical intervention is impacted by the following variables: presence and location of VSD, degree of PS, and type of right ventricular outflow tract (RVOT) obstruction. The arterial switch procedure requires that the surgeon transect the aorta and PA above the pulmonary valve, before suturing them to the *supravalvular*

area. The coronary arteries must then be moved, usually via button technique and reattached to the aorta.

The majority of neonates and infants who have undergone the arterial switch procedure do well with a mortality rate below 5 percent.[45] Complications associated with transplanting the coronary arteries remain a concern and can be life threatening. The most frequent cause for additional intervention is *supravalvular* PS, but with improved surgical techniques, this complication has decreased.[46]

Truncus Arteriosus

Truncus arteriosus, accounting for *less than* 10 percent of all CHDs, is defined as a conotruncal defect and occurs when the conotruncal area does not divide and separate during fetal cardiac development into a separate PA and aorta; consequently a common trunk supplies arterial, systemic, and coronary artery circulation (Figure 70-12). Infants with truncus arteriosus will have a common valve referred to as a truncal valve instead of two separate pulmonary and aortic valves. This truncal valve may have one to five leaflets, with three being the most common. A perimembranous VSD is also seen with this defect. Truncal valve insufficiency becomes worse over time, which may eventually produce an increase in ventricular volume. Arterial and systemic blood is shunted through the common valve, and the amount of pulmonary blood flow is related to the amount of PS and the degree of pulmonary vascular resistance. With increased pulmonary blood flow, the

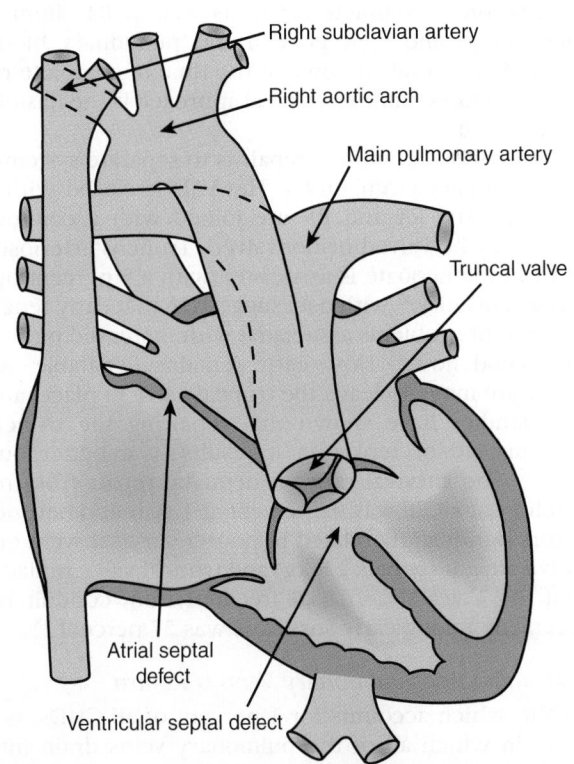

FIGURE 70-12 ▪ Truncus arteriosus, Type I with a main pulmonary artery arising from the ascending aorta and a right aortic arch. (Courtesy Scientific Software Solutions, PedCath version 7.4.3.)

lungs become congested producing the signs and symptoms of CHF.

Clinical Manifestations

The neonate with truncus arteriosus may exhibit cyanosis. As pulmonary vascular resistance decreases, the signs and symptoms of CHF may occur, and cyanosis may decrease. Infants with truncus arteriosus may also be dyspneic and poor feeders. Auscultatory, electrocardiographic, and chest radiographic findings can be found in Table 70-3.

Management

Without treatment these infants will usually die within 6 months from CHF, PA disease, or coronary artery steal. While awaiting surgical intervention, supportive measures aimed at reducing the signs and symptoms of CHF are undertaken, including digoxin, diuretics, and afterload-reducing agents. Nasogastric feeds may be implemented for those infants with failure to thrive. The treatment method of choice for infants with truncus arteriosus is early surgical intervention. Cardiac catheterization is only necessary when questions, such as visualization of coronary and pulmonary arteries, remain unanswered after echocardiography.

Some infants may undergo a palliative procedure before complete repair if the complete repair cannot be done early. This palliative procedure is referred to as PA banding, in which a band is placed around the PA in an attempt to decrease pulmonary blood flow and protect the lungs from pulmonary vascular disease. If a PA band is placed, it is removed at the time of complete repair.

Based on PA anatomy, infants may undergo a BT shunt before a complete repair as well. A BT shunt is placed to promote PA growth and pulmonary blood flow and is also taken down at the time of complete repair. The most common surgical approach is the Rastelli procedure.

The goal of a complete repair is to separate systemic and pulmonary circulations. The VSD is closed with a patch and the PA and RV are joined with a conduit, which may be valved or nonvalved. Truncus arteriosus repair in the neonate is associated with a 5 percent operative mortality,[47] with data suggesting that early repair can prevent problems associated with increased pulmonary blood flow.[47] How early remains debatable. Attempts are made to leave the truncal valve in place, and some studies have shown that repairing the truncal valve instead of replacing it results in a better outcome.[47] The survival rate for neonatal repair from researchers at UCSF was 92 percent at 1 year and beyond. Factors significantly related to poorer survival were operative weight (equals 2.5 kg) and truncal valve replacement. At 3 years, actuarial freedom from conduit replacement among early survivors was 57 percent.[48]

Total Anomalous Pulmonary Venous Return

TAPVR, which accounts for 1 percent of all CHDs, is a defect in which all of the pulmonary veins drain into the right atrium or into one of the systemic veins, instead of the left atrium (Figure 70-13). For infants with TAPVR to survive, an intraarterial communication of

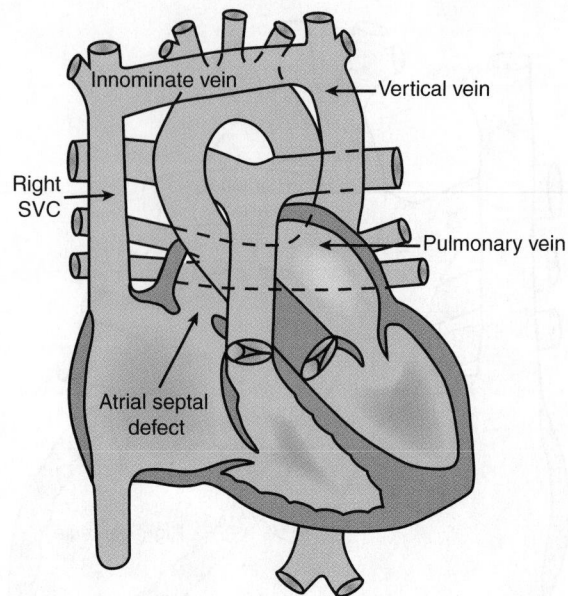

FIGURE 70-13 ■ Total anomalous venous return. All of the pulmonary venous blood returns to the right atrium from the vertical vein and innominate vein. An atrial septal defect is mandatory. (Courtesy Scientific Software Solutions, PedCath version 7.4.3.)

some sort must be present. Asplenia and polysplenia are often associated with TAPVR. TAPVR may be divided into four types: (1) *supracardiac*—from the common confluence, blood drains into the right vena cava through the left vertical vein to the left innominate vein, (2) *cardiac*—the common pulmonary confluence drains into the coronary sinus or directly into the right atrium, (3) *infracardiac (subdiaphragmatic)*—the common pulmonary confluence drains into the portal system and to the inferior vena cava, and (4) *mixed*—a combination of the previous three types. The most commonly occurring type of TAPVR is *supracardiac*.

The veins in TAPVR may be obstructed or unobstructed, with subdiaphragmatic types being more often unobstructed and cardiac and supracardiac types less likely to be obstructed. In *nonobstructive* TAPVR, pulmonary venous blood enters the right atrium with blood being shunted to the RV or left atrium. The size of the ASD and the degree of pulmonary vascular resistance contribute to the amount and direction of blood shunting. Once pulmonary vascular resistance decreases, more blood is shunted to the RV and into the lungs, producing overcirculation of blood in the lungs. In *obstructive* TAPVR, pulmonary blood flow to the right atrium is restricted making the arterial pressures in the lungs elevated. Right-sided heart pressures begin to rise. and blood is then shunted from right to left producing severe systemic hypoxemia and eventual end-organ failure.

Clinical Manifestations

The clinical manifestations associated with TAPVR depend on whether the return is obstructed or unobstructed. Children with *unobstructed* TAPVR may have mild cyanosis. CHF may be observed as a result of the increased blood flow to the lungs. Poor growth is seen as a result of feeding difficulties. Tachypnea and tachycardia may be observed, and an increase in the number of respiratory infections may be seen.

Children with *obstructed* TAPVR are very critically ill and exhibit severe cyanosis and respiratory distress (tachypnea and dyspnea) and pulmonary edema. In general these infants are acidotic and poorly perfused. Hepatomegaly is usually present, and pulmonary crackles may be heard upon auscultation. Auscultatory, electrocardiographic, and chest radiographic findings can be found it Table 70-3.

Management

Infants with TAPVR are generally hemodynamically unstable and require immediate measures for stabilization. In infants with *unobstructive* TAPVR, medical management is aimed at reducing CHF. Surgical intervention is inevitable, and in children with *obstructive* TAPVR, intubation and immediate surgery is necessary. These children may benefit from inotropic support and volume replacement. Metabolic acidosis should be corrected.

Variations in surgical technique are performed based on the location of the veins. The goal with this surgery is to attach the anomalous veins to the left atrium and close the ASD. In a study by Wang and colleagues,[49] no significant differences in surgical mortality were noted among children with obstructive and unobstructive forms of TAPVR, with an overall surgical mortality of 5 percent.[50] Restenosis of the veins can be a recurrent problem, and some surgeons use a sutureless technique for restenosed pulmonary veins.[51]

Tricuspid Atresia

TA accounts for 1 percent of all CHDs and consists of an atretic tricuspid valve and a hypoplastic RV. Communication between the right atrium and RV does not exist (Figure 70-14). This results in a right to left shunt at the atrial level. This defect can occur in conjunction with TGA, a VSD, PS, or pulmonary atresia; however, the majority of children with TA have normally related great vessels, a VSD, and PS. An opening, such as an ASD, PFO, PDA, or VSD must be present for mixing to occur. TA typically occurs an isolated defect, although additional cardiac anomalies have been reported in up to 20 percent of these patients.[52]

In the child with TA and normally related great vessels, blood from the right atrium is shunted via an ASD or PFO to the left atrium where the mixing of arterial and systemic blood occurs. The left ventricle then pumps the mixed blood out into the systemic system via the aorta; however, if a VSD is present, some of the blood will be pumped into the hypoplastic RV through the pulmonary arteries. The degree of PS and the size of the VSD help determine the amount of pulmonary blood flow. Pulmonary blood flow may increase as the pulmonary vascular resistance decreases. In children with a restrictive VSD and PS, pulmonary blood flow will not be increased. In children without a VSD, pulmonary blood flow is supplied via the PDA.

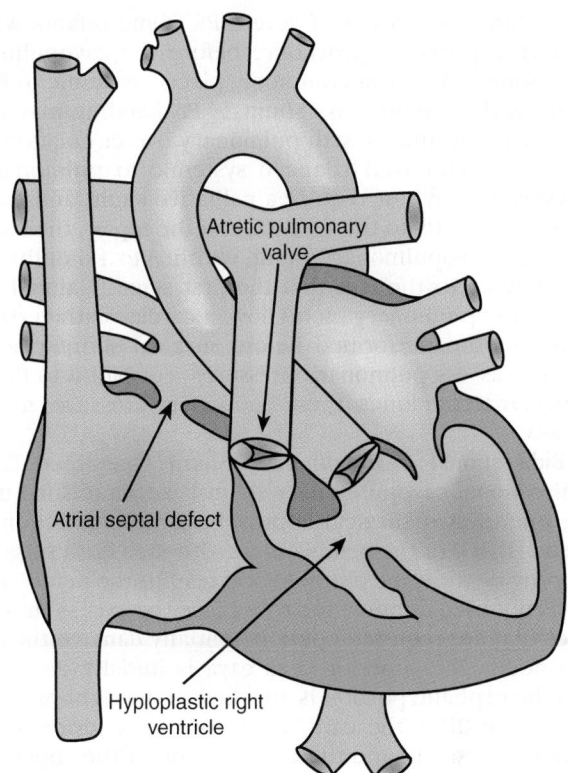

FIGURE 70-14 ■ Tricuspid atresia, in which the tricuspid valve is completely absent. A ventricular septal defect allows blood from the left ventricle to the anatomical right ventricle and pulmonary arteries. (Courtesy Scientific Software Solutions, PedCath version 7.4.3.)

Clinical Manifestations

Children generally have systemic arterial desaturations caused by some extent to the mixing of systemic and pulmonary blood. Cyanosis is usually present by 1 week of age, the degree of which varies according to the amount of pulmonary blood flow and the degree of mixing. Cyanosis is almost always observed in children with a restrictive VSD and PS. CHF may be noted in some infants with increased pulmonary blood flow. Auscultatory, electrocardiographic, and chest radiographic findings can be found in Table 70-3.

Management

The management of the child with TA depends on presenting symptomatology, which is dependent on the amount of mixing that occurs with stabilization efforts aimed at correcting acidosis, controlling hypoxia, and managing CHF. PGE_1 is initiated for severe cyanosis to keep the ductus patent, and because of associated apnea from PGE_1, intubation may be necessary. Anticongestive medications should be administered for CHF. A balloon atrial septostomy may be performed to aid systemic and pulmonary mixing when atrial blood flow is restrictive. Sometimes these children are well balanced and may not require PGE_1. Surgical intervention is mandatory if these infants are to survive.

Surgical intervention for infants with TA involves a staged approach consisting of the placement of a bidirectional cavopulmonary shunt followed by the Fontan procedure. As a result of severe PS, some infants will require a palliative procedure before the cavopulmonary shunt. The most commonly placed systemic to PA shunt is the modified BT shunt. A PA banding may be necessary for infants with pulmonary overcirculation.

Infants with well-balanced systemic to pulmonary physiology may not require a palliative shunt and may proceed directly to the first stage of the repair, the bidirectional cavopulmonary shunt, within 3 to 4 months of age. Owing to the fact that the first stage is aimed at increasing pulmonary blood flow, a cardiac catheterization must be performed before surgical shunt placement to assess pulmonary pressures. For blood to flow passively to the lungs, these pulmonary pressures must be low.

Bidirectional Cavopulmonary Shunt Operation. The bidirectional cavopulmonary shunt is accomplished using one of two surgical approaches, the bidirectional Glenn **(BDG)** or the hemi-Fontan. Although both surgeries provide the same physiological results, the hemi-Fontan is not used as much today because the excess suture lines that are required could potentially damage the sinus node. The superior vena cava is initially divided, and the cephalic portion is attached to the right branch PA. In the BDG, the cardiac end of the superior vena cava is oversewn, and the cephalic end of the superior vena cava is attached to the PA. With the hemi-Fontan, the cardiac end and the cephalic end are both attached to the PA, and a patch is placed in the right atrium occluding blood flow from the superior vena cava. This allows for systemic blood from the upper part of the body to bypass the heart and flow passively into the lungs. By alleviating extra blood flow to the heart, the overall workload of the heart is decreased. Oxygen saturations should increase after this procedure (average 85 percent) as a result of decreased mixing of unoxygenated blood with oxygenated blood. The BDG without bypass is being performed, but further studies are needed to support this approach; however, potential advantages include a reduction in neurological sequelae and earlier extubation.[53] If a previous shunt was placed, it is removed at the beginning of the surgery.

Fontan Procedure. The final stage of repair for the child with TA is referred to as the Fontan procedure and is performed from the age of 18 months to 5 years. The goal of the Fontan procedure is for all systemic blood flow to passively enter the lungs by bypassing the heart. Many variations of the original Fontan have been performed in an attempt to reduce mortality and morbidity. The two most widely used procedures are the *intraatrial* and *extracardiac* conduit. In an *intraatrial* procedure, a tunnel is constructed using a patch from the inferior vena cava to the superior vena cava. The inferior vena cava is then attached to the right PA. With an *extracardiac* procedure, a tube is placed outside the heart from the inferior vena cava to the right branch of the PA. The advantages and disadvantages of both procedures have been investigated, but no true consensus has been established as to which procedure is the optimal. One potential advantage of the *intracardiac* procedure is growth potential.[54] Some of the disadvantages include potential dysrhythmias secondary to suture lines, increased atrial pressures, and the need for cross clamping during the surgery. The *extracardiac* Fontan offers such advantages as the potential to prevent dysrhythmias caused by suture lines, stable laminar flow, and the possibility of no cross clamping during the surgery. A potential disadvantage includes possible distortion of the pulmonary arteries as a result of the large size of the conduit used in children.[54]

Some children may have a fenestration placed during the Fontan procedure. A fenestration is defined as an opening. An advantage associated with a fenestration is that it allows for a "pop off" when pulmonary pressures are high and remain high. The disadvantages include decreased oxygen saturations and the possible need for fenestration closure at a later date. which may be performed in the catheterization laboratory with a device, most commonly the Amplatzer device. To close a fenestration, pressure measurements are assessed by balloon occlusion. If the measurements are acceptable, then fenestration is closed. Increased oxygen saturations may not be observed immediately after the procedure: however, this generally occurs over time. Over the years, there has been a significant decrease in the mortality and morbidity associated with the Fontan procedure. In a study using 25 years of data, Mair and colleagues[55] reported a continuing decline in operative mortality (down to 2 percent) in children who underwent nonfenestrated Fontan procedures. Long-term survival has continued to improve, and 89 percent of these patients are in NYHA Class I or II.[55] One of the major causes of morbidity and mortality after the Fontan procedure is thromboembolic events, and currently, there is no consensus regarding the use of prophylactic anticoagulation in this patient population. The postoperative care associated with infants with TA is similar to that of neonates with HLHS and will be presented in the section on caring for children with cyanotic heart disease.

Hypoplastic Left Heart Syndrome

HLHS is a serious defect that accounts for 1 percent of all CHDs and is the most common cause of death in neonates with a CHD in the first month of life. The major defect in HLHS is a severely underdeveloped left ventricle (Figure 70-15), necessitating the presence of a PDA and ASD for survival. Common variations of HLHS include mitral atresia and/or stenosis, aortic atresia and/or stenosis, and hypoplasia of the aorta.

In HLHS, blood enters the right side as normal. From the RV, some blood goes to the lungs and some to the aorta via a right to left shunt across the PDA. Systemic blood is supplied via the PDA. Pulmonary blood enters the left atrium and is shunted across the ASD/PFO into the right atrium. When the atrial communication is restrictive, pulmonary blood flow is decreased.

Clinical Manifestations

Neonates with HLHS may not exhibit signs of distress during the first few hours of life. Poor perfusion, decreased peripheral pulses, and cyanosis can be seen once the PDA begins to close. Tachypnea and respiratory distress may be noted with increased pulmonary blood flow secondary to a decrease in pulmonary vascu-

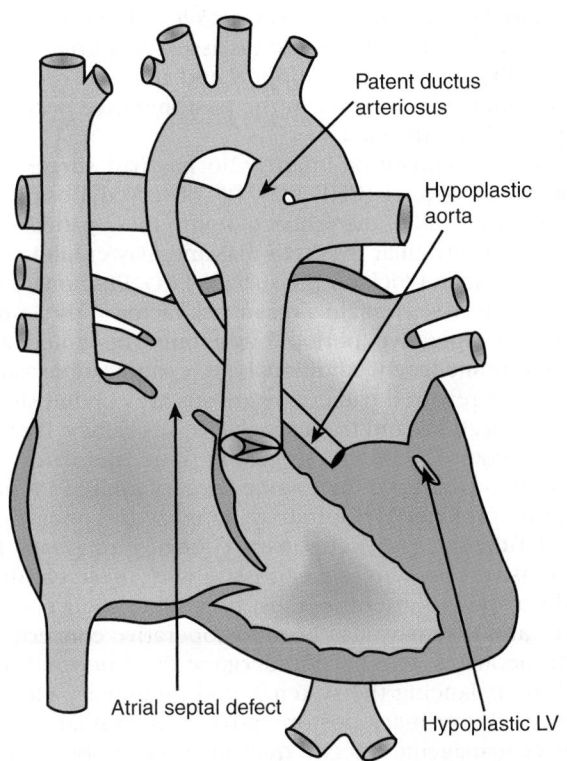

FIGURE 70-15 ■ Hypoplastic left heart syndrome. The variety of defects seen in this defect renders the left side of the heart almost nonfunctional. *HLHS;* Hypoplastic left heart syndrome. (Courtesy Scientific Software Solutions, PedCath version 7.4.3.)

(Figure labels: Patent ductus arteriosus; Hypoplastic aorta; Atrial septal defect; Hypoplastic LV)

lar resistance. As a result of increased pulmonary blood flow, there is a decrease in systemic flow resulting in an unbalanced Qp/Qs. Neonates with HLHS can quickly become critically ill and rapidly progress to cardiogenic shock.

Occasionally a neonate with HLHS may be discharged home before a diagnosis because of the absence of symptoms as a result of a PDA; however, improvements in fetal echocardiography have reduced this incidence. When the PDA starts to close, symptoms will appear including cyanosis, poor feeding, and irritability. Prompt intervention and management is critical if neonates with HLHS are to survive. Auscultatory, electrocardiographic, and chest radiographic findings can be found in Table 70-3.

Management

Neonates that are in cardiogenic shock must be intubated quickly. Inotropic infusions, PGE₁, sodium bicarbonate, and sedatives must be administered quickly to treat metabolic acidosis, respiratory difficulties, and decreased CO. These patients may undergo a head and abdominal sonogram to screen for other defects. Preoperative management is very important and has been linked to how well the patient does postoperatively.[56] Emergent intervention is needed when the ASD and/or PFO is restrictive.

To survive neonates (rarely infants) with HLHS, PGE₁ is administered immediately to maintain ductal patency. PGE₁ can cause apnea, so intubation may be necessary if patient is not intubated. Once the ductus reopens and peripheral perfusion has improved, PGE₁ may be titrated down to help decrease possible adverse reactions of the drug. Balancing the two systems (pulmonary and systemic) is important both preoperatively and postoperatively. Neonates with HLHS are very fragile and can easily decompensate if signs or symptoms are not recognized and managed. Metabolic acidosis is treated with sodium bicarbonate, and frequent assessments of perfusion are pivotal. Urine output is used to assess renal function, and diuretics may be given to increase urine output. Inotropic support may be administered for decreased CO, which can lead to brain and renal dysfunction if not promptly recognized and managed. These neonates are at a higher risk for developing necrotizing enterocolitis **(NEC),** and specific risk factors have been identified that are associated with an elevated risk of NEC: (1) premature birth, (2) diagnosis of HLHS or truncus arteriosus, and (3) episodes of poor systemic perfusion or shock.[57] Some data suggest that managing decreased CO and systemic resistance may be more beneficial than attempts at adjusting pulmonary vascular resistance.[58] Neonates with HLHS may be pulmonary overcirculated or undercirculated, with those with pulmonary overcirculation exhibiting saturations in the 90s. Subatmospheric oxygen may be used to increase pulmonary vascular resistance and thus decrease pulmonary blood flow. Supplemental oxygen should be avoided because too much oxygen can cause flooding of the lungs and "stealing" from the systemic system. Low saturations may be accepted in HLHS and may be in the 70s.

Without surgical intervention, neonates with HLHS will usually die by 1 month of age. Although palliative or end-of-life care is a treatment option for neonates with HLHS,[59] the majority of families choose between two surgical options: cardiac transplantation or a three-staged series of surgical procedures. Although cardiac transplantation has been touted as the "best" treatment option for HLHS,[60] it is not without its pitfalls. In a multicenter, national study of patients awaiting cardiac transplantation as a primary therapy for HLHS, 25 percent died while waiting for an organ.[61] In addition to a scarcity of donors, other issues associated with neonatal heart transplantation include having to transfer the infant to a transplant center necessitating family relocation as well and the lifelong need to balance preventing rejection with immunosuppressive therapy against infection. Despite these limitations, survival for cardiac transplant recipients with HLHS has improved dramatically over the years indicating that those infants who received organs before their first birthday and who survived their first year had a 95 percent survival rate of 4 years.[62] The remainder of this discussion will focus on the staged surgical repair.

Norwood Operation. The Norwood operation is the first stage of a three-staged surgical procedure and must be performed in the neonatal period. The steps of the Norwood operation are as follows: (1) the PDA is ligated; (2) the main PA is ligated and oversewn, and the proximal main PA is sewn to the aorta; (3) a shunt is placed, most commonly a BT shunt; (4) an atrial septectomy is performed; and (5) the aorta is enlarged. The shunt allows pulmonary blood flow while protecting the lungs from overcirculation. Some surgical institutions are using a right ventricular to PA shunt, with reported advantages of a stable systemic circulation, adequate pulmonary blood flow, and an improvement in coronary perfusion.[63] However, the midterm and long-term effects of a right ventricular incision and diastolic regurgitation through the conduit remain unclear.[63] In this midterm study, ventricular efficiency was the same in the systemic to PA shunt as the RV to PA conduit; however, following a BDG and/or the bidirectional cavopulmonary shunt, the contractility of the RV in patients who had an RV to PA conduit was inferior to the systemic to PA shunt.[63] The atrial septectomy allows for better mixing at the atrial level.

Before the second stage of the repair, a cardiac catheterization is performed to assess for pulmonary pressures because low pressures are necessary for passive blood flow to the lungs. This stage consists of the placement of a cavopulmonary shunt (i.e., a BDG or hemi-Fontan) as previously discussed with TA. Cardiac function is assessed before both surgical procedures. The bidirectional cavopulmonary shunt in infants with HLHS is performed at approximately 4 to 6 months of age, the surgical details of which were previously discussed in the section on TA. Before Fontan completion, stage three, a cardiac catheterization, will be performed. Angiograms of specific cardiac structures (PA, aorta) are beneficial in determining if additional surgical work should be performed at the time of the Fontan. Pulmonary pressures are assessed at this time, and low pulmonary pressures are required for the next process because passive blood low to the lungs is required. Right ventricular function is also assessed at this time. Collaterals may be coil occluded as well. Favorable cardiac catheterization data may indicate that the patient is a good candidate for Fontan completion, but it is not a guarantee that the patient will have a good outcome. Patients with less favorable data have done well after the Fontan. The Fontan procedure is performed from 18 months to 3 years of age, depending on institutional preference. The surgical details for the Fontan procedure can be found in the section on TA.

Nursing Considerations for Children with Cyanotic Heart Defects

Children with cyanotic heart disease generally require more intricate nursing care because of the complexity of the anatomy and physiology of these defects. General considerations for those undergoing cardiac catheterization and/or surgery are included in the section on children undergoing invasive procedures. Issues of concern after surgery for TOF include right ventricular dysfunction of which pulmonary insufficiency may be a contributing factor and postoperative dysrhythmias. The ECG often exhibits right bundle branch block, and ventricular dysrhythmias are the most common postoperative rhythm disturbance in these children; however, there is a risk of AV block associated with a VSD closure.

For neonates who have undergone the arterial switch operation, ischemia is a major concern because of the coronary artery transplantation. If ST-segment changes are noted on the rhythm strip, a 15-lead ECG should be obtained. Ventricular function is assessed with echocardiography and inotropic support and afterload-reducing agents may be necessary in the postoperative period to improve hemodynamics.

For the neonate or infant who has had surgery for truncus arteriosus, CHF may be observed postoperatively. As a result of the ventriculotomy, these patients are prone to ventricular dysrhythmias and may exhibit right bundle branch block on the surface ECG. Pulmonary hypertensive crises remain a major risk factor in the immediate postoperative period[64] and must be noted and treated immediately. Additional late complications often seen with repaired truncus arteriosus are conduit stenosis/calcifications and truncal valve insufficiency, both of which require additional surgery at some later date.

Infants who have undergone surgery for TAPVR may require prolonged respiratory support for poor right heart function and pulmonary edema. Pulmonary hypertensive crises are also an issue with these children and scrupulous attention must be paid to their respiratory care. CHF may also be a postoperative concern.

In neonates who have undergone the Norwood procedure, balancing the systemic and pulmonary circulations is the primary postoperative goal. Similar preoperative management techniques may also be performed postoperatively. Inotropic support may be given for low CO and afterload-reduction agents may be beneficial as well. Metabolic acidosis should be corrected, and the ECG monitored for dysrhythmias. Postoperatively, pulmonary blood flow is largely based on shunt size. Frequent arterial blood gases are necessary in assessing respiratory status, and cyanosis should be assessed using pulse oximetry. Once the child becomes hemodynamically stable, transfer to a cardiac unit for continued cardiac monitoring and additional work-up for nonrelated cardiac issues ensues. Feeding issues often prolong hospital stay, and some of these children may require a gastrobutton before discharge if intake remains inadequate despite interventions.

Central venous pressures following a cavopulmonary procedure are very important, and any increases should be of concern. Should head and neck swelling be observed, they should be elevated to promote passive blood flow to lungs. Administration of diuretics may be beneficial, and afterload-reducing agents may be administered for elevated pulmonary artery pressures (**PAP**)s. If oxygen desaturations are noted and continue or worsen, the child may need to undergo cardiac catheterization to assess for Fontan patency and microarteriovenous malformations. Anemia is a concern for these children, and their hematocrit should be *greater than* 45 percent.

Following the Fontan procedure, left and right atrial pressures are helpful when assessing Fontan function. Inotropic medications and afterload-reducing agents may be administered for low CO. Milrinone is often used because of its dual action as an inotrope and afterload reducer. Pleural effusions are a concern with Fontan patients and may include the following signs and symptoms: increased work of breathing, decreased oxygen saturations, irritability, and decreased breath sounds. If pleural effusions persist, a cardiac catheterization may be recommended to assess for Fontan patency and aortopulmonary collaterals. Strict intake and output measurements are critical because fluid replacement may be required. Sinus node dysfunction and atrial dysrhythmias are a concern because of the potential to cause a decrease in CO. Temporary cardiac pacing and antidysrhythmic medication may be required to treat these dysrhythmias, respectively. Postoperative oxygen saturations may vary, with those children with fenestrations usually exhibiting lower saturations.

One of the long-term complications associated with the Fontan operation is the development of collaterals, which may be arterial and venous. Collaterals may be closed in the catheterization laboratory with coil embolization devices. Other potential complications associated with this operation include baffle stenosis, cardiac dysrhythmias, and protein-losing enteropathy **(PLE)**. Baffle stenosis can be treated with stents, and the myriad of dysrhythmias may be treated with permanent pacing, antidysrhythmic medications, implantable cardioverter defibrillator **(ICD)**s, and often a combination of these therapies. PLE is associated with hypoproteinemia, diarrhea, peripheral edema, malaise, and ascites. Although the exact cause of PLE is unknown, it has been hypothesized that it results from increased systemic venous pressures.[65] Various treatment modalities have been used with little to no success. Some children are treated with albumin injections or infusions, corticosteroids, and heparin. When heparin and albumin therapies failed, Kim and colleagues[65] used calcium (calcium gluconate) to successfully manage a patient with PLE; however, the cause for this success has not been studied.

As previously mentioned, Fontan patients are prone to chronic postoperative dysrhythmias, included but not limited to sinus node dysfunction and atrial reentry tachycardia. In many cases, medication is ineffective in controlling the tachydysrhythmia and may even worsen the bradydysrhythmia, making more aggressive treatment necessary. These therapies include atrial overdrive pacing, catheter ablation, or various surgical approaches.[66] With varied surgical techniques (e.g., the extracardiac Fontan) the aim is to decrease the incidence of postoperative dysrhythmias, but this remains to be seen. With continuous improvements in surgical technique and more aggressive postoperative care, it is anticipated that morbidity and mortality associated with the Fontan will decline further in the future. The survival rate of children born with HLHS increases after stage I.[67]

Congenital Dysrhythmias

A child's heart may be totally normal, both mechanically and hemodynamically, yet may still have electrical abnormalities. The most common of these rhythm disturbances seen in children and that are generally accepted as congenital include congenital CAVB and the congenital form of LQTS.

Congenital Complete Atrioventricular Block

The congenital form of complete CAVB is relatively rare with an estimated prevalence of 1 in 15,000 to 1 in 20,000 live births.[68] It is associated with maternal con-

nective tissue disorder, and in utero diagnosis is commonly made by 20 and 30 weeks of gestation as a result of fetal bradycardia or a history of maternal connective tissue disease.[69,70] Although the precise cause is unknown, there is a recognized association between congenital CAVB and dilated cardiomyopathy.[71] Particularly disturbing is that there is a 43 percent mortality rate in the first two decades of life in one series of children in which 29 were diagnosed in utero; the associated risk factors were the fetal diagnosis, fetal hydrops, endocardial fibroelastosis, and delivery at 32 weeks of gestation or less.[72]

Clinical Manifestations

The clinical manifestations associated with congenital CAVB vary and are generally dependent on the junctional or ventricular escape rate and the presence or absence of structural heart disease. In some cases, the neonate is totally asymptomatic and may not exhibit symptoms until childhood or adolescence. Severe symptoms include hydrops fetalis, CHF, and low CO. Other associated symptoms include fatigue, low stamina, exercise intolerance, and cardiomegaly.

Management

Immediate management for the neonate, infant, or child with CAVB who exhibits severe symptoms (such as hydrops fetalis, CHF, or low CO) includes inotropic support and temporary pacing while awaiting placement of a permanent cardiac pacemaker. Pharmacological agents that may be helpful in this situation include atropine and isoproterenol. Temporary pacing can be accomplished transcutaneously or transvenously.[73] Despite the fact that the indications for permanent pacing vary,[74] most pediatric cardiologists would agree that a ventricular rate *less than* 50 to 55 beats per minute or *less than* 70 beats per minute in the presence of a concomitant CHD is an indication for a permanent pacemaker.

In those children who are asymptomatic, routine follow-up is necessary to monitor for symptoms that necessitate permanent pacing. Those symptoms include increasing heart size, decreased ventricular function, premature ventricular contractions, and syncope. Permanent pacemaker implantation can be accomplished by epicardial or transvenous approach and may consist of a single or dual chamber system. In most cases, dual chamber pacing is preferred because it restores AV synchrony. In a recent study,[75] epicardial pacing was associated with low morbidity and mortality, but required some type of reintervention (e.g., lead fracture, infection, or generator change for battery depletion) within 5 years. There is also a high incidence of lead failure in the pediatric population,[76] and in one study, was most commonly associated with age (*less than* 12 years), structural heart disease, and epicardial leads.[77]

Congenital Long QT Syndrome

The congenital form of long QT syndrome **(LQTS)** has been defined as a genetically determined abnormality of ventricular repolarization that results in cardiac instability that can lead to potentially life-threatening dysrhythmias and/or sudden death. It was originally characterized by Jervell and Lange-Nielsen in 1957 as a syndrome involving congenital deafness, prolonged QT and/or torsades de pointes, syncope and/or sudden death, and autosomal recessive transmission.[78] In 1963 Romano[79] and in 1964 Ward[80] described the characteristics of prolonged QT and/or torsades de pointes, syncope and/or sudden death, and an autosomal dominant pattern. More recently it has become known that the sodium and potassium ion channel abnormalities seen in patients with LQTS are caused by abnormal proteins coded by mutated genes. These genes, both dominant and recessive, have linkage to chromosome 11 **(LQT1)**, chromosome 7 **(LQT2)**, chromosome 3 **(LQT3)**, and chromosome 4 **(LQT4)**. It is pertinent to note that not all patients with prolonged QT intervals have LQTS, and perhaps more importantly, not all patients with LQTS have a prolonged QT interval at rest. Approximately 50 percent of patients with LQTS in a recent comprehensive cardiac channel gene study had an identifiable mutation.[81]

Clinical Manifestations

Many children with LQTS are frequently misdiagnosed with benign syncope or seizure disorders. The clinical presentation of patients with LQTS is varied and can include the following symptoms: syncope (associated with noise, stress, and/or exercise), presyncope, palpitations, seizures, ventricular dysrhythmias, cardiac arrest, and sudden death. Neonates with LQTS may exhibit bradycardia, most often AV block, torsades de pointes, and/or T wave alternans. The ECG criteria associated with LQTS include, but are not limited to, a prolonged corrected QT interval **(QTc)**, variations in T-wave morphology, bradycardia, and ventricular dysrhythmias, most notably torsades de pointes.

Management

The management of children with congenital LQTS has progressed over the years from secondary to primary prevention of sudden cardiac death in these children. Antidysrhythmic drug therapy is initiated with beta blockers, mexiletine, and in some cases, phenytoin. The placement of an ICD is becoming the method of choice for primary prevention. For the child who experiences torsades de pointes, defibrillation may be necessary in the event of hemodynamic compromise. Other management strategies for torsades de pointes include the administration of magnesium sulfate and/or lidocaine. Drugs that prolong the QT interval, such as procainamide and amiodarone, should be avoided. An ICD has been used in a child as young as 7 months for severe neonatal dysrhythmias unresponsive to multiple antidysrhythmic drugs.[82] It has proven to be a safe and effective treatment modality for children with congenital LQTS.[83-85]

Nursing Considerations for Children with Congenital Cardiac Dysrhythmias

Caring for children with cardiac rhythm disturbances can be quiet challenging.

In the child with CAVB who requires emergent therapy, nurses must be cognizant of the implications of the various treatment methods. When administering atropine in infants, the drug should not be given slowly be-cause this may result in paradoxical bradycardia. For the child who is being paced transcutaneously, astute attention to skin integrity is critical. Sedation is recommended because of the painful nature of this treatment modality. In the child with a temporary transvenous pacemaker, a continuous assessment for any signs and symptoms at the catheter entry site is pivotal. Pacemaker function should be documented with ECG rhythm strips.[73]

In the child with congenital LQTS, defibrillation may be necessary for sustained torsades de pointes. If administering lidocaine, monitor serum potassium concentrations because it will be more effective with higher potassium levels. The placement of an ICD requires major preoperative and postoperative nursing considerations, including site care, follow-up visits, and issues associated with device discharge. QT-prolonging agents should be avoided, with some of the more common agents being erythromycin and its derivatives, ketoconazole and its derivatives, and tricyclic antidepressants. Other issues for home care include activity restrictions, CPR training for family members, no competitive sports, prevention of dehydration and electrolyte imbalance.

CARE OF CHILDREN UNDERGOING INVASIVE CARDIAC PROCEDURES

Providing care for the neonate, infant, child, or adolescent undergoing an invasive cardiac procedure requires in-depth knowledge and understanding of cardiac disease in children. As previously discussed, it is imperative that cardiovascular caregivers make time to provide patient and family education. In 2003 and in concert with the Council of Cardiovascular Diseases of the Young, the American Heart Association Pediatric Nursing Subcommittee of the Council on Cardiovascular Nursing published a scientific statement on recommendations for preparing children and adolescents for invasive cardiac procedures.[86] All nurses who care for children with heart disease should be familiar with these recommendations.

According to the authors, there are six expected outcomes for preprocedural preparation for invasive cardiac procedures: (1) reduced anxiety for patients and families; (2) better cooperation and adjustment during and between procedures; (3) improved postprocedural recovery; (4) increased sense of mastery and self-control for patients and families; (5) enhanced trust between patients, families, and members of the health care team; and (6) improved long-term adjustments, both emotional and behavioral, in patients and families. The major focus areas suggested by the statement for preparing children and adolescents for invasive procedures include information giving/sensory experiences, cognitive behavioral interventions, and parental involvement.[86]

Diagnostic and Therapeutic Cardiac Catheterization

As previously mentioned, diagnostic procedures are on the decline, whereas therapeutic procedures are on the rise.[87] Diagnostic cardiac catheterization is performed to assess hemodynamics and angiographic evaluation and is accomplished by extracting blood and measuring oxygen saturations, measuring gradients, and injecting contrast material to assess wall motion abnormalities, valvular problems, specific anatomy, and in some cases coronary angiography using a catheter. Other diagnostic procedures performed in the pediatric catheterization laboratory include intracardiac electrophysiology studies and myocardial biopsies.

There are many therapeutic or interventional procedures that are performed in the pediatric catheterization laboratory. The American Heart Association's statement on pediatric therapeutic cardiac catheterization[88] provides detailed information on personnel requirements, facilities and equipment, and a discussion on procedures used to open atrial communications, closure devices, balloon dilatation of cardiac valves, balloon angioplasty, stent placement, coil occlusion, and endocarditis prophylaxis.

Before the Procedure

Issues to be discussed with the patient and family before cardiac catheterization include the type of sedation or anesthetic to be used, a description of the room, a description of the chain of events for the day (being careful to use age-appropriate language for the child), and to correct any misconceptions about the procedure or its process. If the child is old enough to receive conscious sedation, an explanation of the noise level, alarms, and fluoroscopy should be given to the patient. A preprocedural visit to the catheterization laboratory is appreciated by most families, although it tends to increase anxiety in others.

Cardiac catheterizations are considered low-risk procedures because the incidence of serious adverse effects is quite low. Potential risks associated with cardiac catheterization include infection, hemorrhage, hypotension, hematoma, vascular and/or arterial injury, thrombophlebitis, emboli, perforation and/or tamponade, pneumothorax, allergic reactions, intractable arrhythmia, and death. Risks increase slightly with intervention.

During the Procedure

In most cases, vascular access is not an issue; however, it can be extremely difficult in children who have undergone multiple catheterizations and/or surgeries. In most cases, the femoral vein is used; however, the brachial, cephalic, internal jugular, median antecubital, and subclavian veins may be used. Venous sheaths are used to place the catheters, most commonly in the femoral veins. Catheters come in various shapes and sizes, ranging from 4 to 8 French. Access to the left side of the heart can be accomplished via transseptal or retrograde (arterial) approach, the former of which is preferred by pediatric cardiologists. In either case, anticoagulation is necessary with close observation of activated clotting times during the procedure.

After the Procedure

The nurse assuming care for the child after diagnostic or interventional cardiac catheterization needs a report on the following information from catheterization laboratory personnel: (1) why the procedure was performed, (2) significant findings, (3) type and amount of sedation or anesthetic used, (4) any problems or complications encountered during the procedure, (5) the number and condition of the puncture site(s), and (6) dressings placed at the completion of the procedure. These sites should be inspected immediately upon arrival for presence of hemorrhage, swelling, or hematoma and the affected extremity(ies) evaluated for warmth, color, capillary refill, and palpable pulses. A Doppler measurement should be obtained in the event that a pedal pulse cannot be palpated. The child's LOC should be assessed and heart rate and rhythm, blood pressure, respiratory rate and effort, and body temperature.

The affected extremity, usually a leg, is generally kept straight for several hours following the procedure, but may be kept straight longer if anticoagulation was used during the catheterization procedure. Although a relatively rare complication, if bleeding occurs at the puncture site, have another individual contact the physician while holding firm pressure, which generally stops the bleeding. Most children are awake upon returning to the recovery area, but may remain somnolent depending on the type and amount of sedation or anesthetic used during the procedure. Diet progression can proceed as soon as the child is fully awake and alert. Any ECG changes or alterations in vital signs should be documented and reported to the child's physician. Children undergoing cardiac catheterization may be discharged the day of the procedure or the day after the procedure, with the majority of neonates and infants being monitored a little longer than older children.

Discharge instructions should be given to a parent or responsible person in a relaxed, quiet environment and in an unrushed atmosphere. Instructions should include: (1) keeping the puncture site clean and dry; (2) reporting any drainage, swelling, redness, or hematoma; and (3) maintaining a light activity level for 2 to 3 days after the procedure. Issues, such as activity levels and subacute endocarditis prophylaxis SBE, can be found in the section on home care.

Cardiovascular Surgery

Pediatric cardiovascular surgery is being performed with increasing frequency in the neonatal and infant period. Owing to this fact, most of the surgical preparation is geared toward the family; however, in the case of the older child, preparation must include and be tailored to the child's developmental status, which does not always correlate with chronological age. The principles for patient and family education discussed previously can be used to structure education for the child undergoing surgery for a CHD.

Before Surgery

Cardiovascular surgery is a major stressor for the child and family. It generally requires more preparation than cardiac catheterization and is associated with multiple medical procedures before and after surgery. In today's health care environment, children generally undergo a preoperative work-up the day before surgery is scheduled. This work-up may include venipuncture, ECG, and/or an echocardiogram. At this time. the child and family meet the anesthesia and surgical teams. Patient and family preparation should include information about anesthesia induction, the intensive care unit (ICU) environment, multiple medical procedures that will be performed postoperatively, and the estimated hospital stay. A visit to the ICU is helpful for some patients and families, but may further increase anxiety in others. Each family should be given the option, and if they choose not to visit, a description of the various lines and monitors should be provided.

During Surgery

The surgical approach used by the surgeon is dependent on the specific procedure being performed and most often includes a median sternotomy or thoracotomy. Most procedures require the use of cardiopulmonary bypass and cardioplegia in addition to astute anesthesia management, most often provided by pediatric cardiovascular anesthesiologists. The responsibilities of the surgical team are immense and require extensive expertise.

After Surgery

Complications associated with CHD surgery include CHF, hypoxia, dysrhythmias, cardiac tamponade, atelectasis, pneumonia, pulmonary edema, pleural effusions, cerebral edema, infection, hemorrhage, and death. The child's vital signs can provide information regarding the child's hemodynamic status and should include heart rate, respiratory rate, temperature, and blood oxygen saturation (SpO_2) monitoring. Owing to the fact that many of the cardiac procedures use deep hypothermia, it is equally important to note low temperatures and high temperatures, the latter of which may indicate infection. Continuous blood pressure monitoring is achieved using an intraarterial catheter, which poses the potential complications of arterial thrombosis, infection, air embolism, or blood loss from the catheter. These children will be maintained on mechanical ventilation, the duration of which is patient and procedure specific. Pain control is very important in the postoperative period.

Dysrhythmias after surgery for a CHD are not uncommon and include sinus bradycardia, second or third degree AVB, atrial tachydysrhythmias, ventricular dysrhythmias including premature ventricular contractions, ventricular tachycardia, and ventricular fibrillation, and JET. In one study, the risk factors associated with early postoperative dysrhythmias including sinus bradycardia, second or third degree AVB, and SVT included lower body weight, longer duration of cardiopulmonary bypass, and higher surgical complexity.[89] Treatment of these dysrhythmias may include antiarrhythmic drugs, temporary pacing, cardioversion, and/or defibrillation.

Intracardiac monitoring is achieved using various catheters to assess RAP, LAP, and pulmonary artery pressure (PAP). The RAP catheter is intended to monitor central venous pressures, whereas the LAP catheter is intended to monitor systemic ventricular pressures.

Failure to ensure that the transducer is properly leveled, calibrated, and zeroed has the potential to produce artifact indicating an increase or decrease in any of the aforementioned pressure measurements. Additional causes of *increased* RAP include increased right ventricular pressures (decreased right ventricular function), tricuspid valve disease (stenosis and/or regurgitation), and tachydysrhythmias. A *decreased* RAP may be indicative of inadequate preload. Potential causes of *increased* LAP include increased systemic ventricular pressures (decreased systemic ventricular function), mitral valve disease (stenosis and/or regurgitation), a large left to right shunt, and tachydysrhythmias. A *decreased* LAP may be indicative of inadequate preload. Potential causes of *increased* PAP include pulmonary defects or disease, obstruction of airway or pulmonary circulation, and an increased LAP. A *decreased* PAP may indicate severe obstruction to pulmonary blood flow.

Most children who return from the operating room after CHD surgery will have temporary pacing wires, which have a myriad of uses. The atrial wires, located on the right, can be used to pace the atrium in the event of sinus bradycardia, discern the atrial role in certain postoperative dysrhythmias, and to convert reentrant atrial dysrhythmias. The ventricular wires, located on the left, are generally used to provide ventricular rate support and AV synchrony in children with second or third degree AV block. Gloves should always be used when handling temporary wires to prevent inadvertent static electricity transfer to the patient through the wires.

Children who have undergone cardiac surgery may have pleural or mediastinal chest tubes that should be frequently assessed for patency drainage amount, drainage consistency, and drainage appearance. For example, some children who have undergone the Fontan operation may develop a chylothorax. The drainage that results from this will be characteristically thick and white in color. Fluid intake and output is extremely important in children after surgery, with a minimum urine output of 1 ml/kg/hr.

Extracorporeal membrane oxygenation (**ECMO**) is being used with increasing frequency in children who have undergone cardiac surgery. Morris[90] had 137 patients managed with ECMO in a PICU and had a 58 percent survival rate for *greater than* 24 hours after decannulation and 39 percent to hospital discharge. Mortality risk in patients who had undergone surgery for a CHD included being male, being *less than* 1 month of age, having a longer duration of mechanical ventilation before ECMO, and developing renal or hepatic failure while on ECMO.

Surgical outcomes for neonatal heart surgery have steadily improved over the last several decades. In a recent study of neonates and infants who had undergone the arterial switch operation, the 30-day surgical mortality rate was only 1.6 percent.[91] There were two deaths in the study, and the overall actuarial survival rate at 7 years was 96.3 percent. In a group of low birth weight (*less than* 2500 grams), the overall surgical mortality rate is much higher at 18 percent.[92] Although the researchers considered this acceptable, it came with the cost of considerable postoperative morbidity of 53 percent and was irrespective of age, weight, prematurity, type of surgical procedure (palliative versus complete), or use of cardiopulmonary bypass.

HOME CARE OF THE CHILD WITH A CARDIAC CONDITION

Preparing patients and families for discharge is very important in the care of the child with a heart defect. Nurses often become the gatekeepers with these families and must remain cognizant of issues of concern after the child is discharged from the health care environment. Topics to be discussed include the follow-up schedule, activity level, medications, and SBE prophylaxis. Another topic of interest that will be included in this section is the use of complimentary and alternative therapy in this patient population.

Follow-Up Schedule

The follow-up schedule for children with heart disease is based primarily on the child's age, specific defect, symptomatology, and treatment procedure. Neonates and infants are generally followed on a more frequent basis than older children because of constant changes in their growth and development and their inability to verbalize symptoms. Infants with a VSD are followed on a more frequent basis to ascertain spontaneous closure and to assess for signs of CHF and failure to thrive. Children who have undergone cardiac catheterization may not be seen for several months to a year after the procedure, whereas children who have undergone surgery generally return for a 1- to 2-week follow-up visit. In particular, children who have undergone surgical ASD closure are generally seen 14 days after surgery to assess for postpericardiotomy syndrome as previously described.

Activity Level

Activity level, activity restrictions, and sports participation are important components of the follow-up care of children with heart disease. In those children with known heart disease, sports participation is dependent on the disease process, symptoms, and the extent of residual defects. The degree of physical activity and activity restrictions are generally defect specific; however, those children with complex defects require highly individualized recommendations based on cardiac function, symptomatology, residual defects, dysrhythmias, and results of noninvasive and invasive monitoring.[93] For example, children with moderate to severe AS are instructed not to perform competitive sports.

Medications

Many children with heart disease will require some type of medication on a routine basis. Patients and families should be provided with the following information regarding each medication that the child is receiving: the intended action of the medication, potential adverse effects, dosage schedule, and instructions on what to do if a dosage is missed. Owing to the fact that children are constantly experiencing growth spurts, medication dosages require constant assessment and adjustment. The provision of any written material on the medication is a useful adjunct to oral instruction (Box 70-9).

Bacterial Endocarditis Prophylaxis

Infective endocarditis, although rare in children, occurs primarily in children with congenital heart defects. Because of the mortality and morbidity associated with infective endocarditis antibiotic prophylaxis, its importance should be emphasized at every opportunity. In a study of 205 parents of children with CHD, only 64 percent who had children at risk for endocarditis were aware of measures needed to prevent endocarditis.[94] This is a very important issue when caring for patients with a CHD. Recommendations for specific lesions requiring endocarditis prophylaxis can be found in Table 70-5.[95] For additional information on specific procedures requiring endocarditis prophylaxis and the antibiotic regimens, see the website of the American Heart Association (www.americanheart.org) under endocarditis prophylaxis information. Each patient and family should be given a copy of the SBE card before discharge and discussed at each clinic visit.

Complementary and Alternative Therapy

The use of complementary and alternative medicine (CAM) in children with heart disease has not been documented to be safe or effective, despite the fact that approximately 59 percent of adults in the United States used CAM therapies. Of particular concern to those who care for children with a CHD on a regular basis is the use of common herbs and nutritional supplements, specifically their potential adverse effects in this growing population.[96] Common herbal medicines that may be of harm to patients with a CHD include ephedra, garlic, gingko biloba, and St. John's wort. Ephedra is especially dangerous in children because of its propensity to increase blood pressure and heart rate, which could lead to palpitations, stroke, or death and should be avoided in all children with heart disease. As a result of their ability to inhibit platelet aggregation, garlic and gingko biloba can lead to increased bleeding in patients who are receiving blood thinners. Their use could also

---

BOX 70-9 ■ ■ ■
TIPS FOR COUMADIN ADMINISTRATION

- Maintain consistency in diet.
- Avoid large amounts of foods high in vitamin K (green leafy vegetables) since this could cause a decrease in effectiveness.
- Monitor for signs of bruising and bleeding.
- Growth spurts and illnesses can cause Coumadin dosages to change.
- Coumadin is contraindicated in pregnancy.
- Coumadin should be taken at approximately the same time every day.
- Continued laboratory checks for PT and INR are necessary.

INR, International normalized ratio; *PT*, prothrombin time.

■ ■ ■

Table 70-5 CARDIAC CONDITIONS IN WHICH ENDOCARDITIS PROPHYLAXIS IS/IS NOT RECOMMENDED

HIGH RISK CATEGORY	MODERATE RISK CATEGORY	NEGLIGIBLE RISK CATEGORY*
Prosthetic cardiac valves	Most other defects (other than the high risk and negligible risk)	Isolated secundum ASD
Previous bacterial endocarditis		Surgical repair of ASD, VSD, or PDA without residual beyond 6 months
Complex cyanotic disease, including single ventricle states, TGA, TOF	Acquired valvular dysfunction (rheumatic heart disease)	Previous CABG surgery
	Hypertrophic cardiomyopathy	Mitral valve prolapse without valvar regurgitation
Surgically corrected systemic pulmonary shunts or conduits	Mitral valve prolapse with valvular regurgitation and/or thickened leaflets	Physiological, functional, or innocent heart murmurs
		Previous Kawasaki disease without valvar dysfunction
		Cardiac pacemakers (intravascular and epicardial) and implanted defibrillators

*No greater risk than the general population and prophylaxis not recommended.
ASD, Atrial septal defect; *CABG,* coronary artery bypass grafting; *TGA,* transposition of the great arteries; *TOF,* tetralogy of Fallot.
From Prevention of bacterial endocarditis, American Heart Association, Dallas. Retrieved April 27, 2005 from www.americanheart.org/.

lead to an increased risk of stroke or excessive hemorrhage following cardiac surgery. Used for mild to moderate depression, St. John's wort may cause decreases in serum digoxin concentrations, decreased INR, and is associated with photosensitivity. Plotnikoff[97] recommends incorporating specific questions into each clinical interview specific to the use of CAM: (1) Are you using any herbs, vitamins, dietary supplements, and if so, what is the dose, source, how often do you take it, and why do you take it? This information should be documented on the child's medical record.

In summary caring for children with heart disease is very complex and challenging. Nurses caring for these children and their families must be knowledgeable regarding the specific congenital cardiac lesions, their associated treatments, and disease trajectories. Although intense at times, caring for these children and their families can be quite rewarding.

REFERENCES

1. Webb GD, Smallhorn JF, Therrien J et al: Congenital heart disease. In Zipes DP, Libby P, Bonow RO, Braunwald E, editors: *Braunwald's heart disease: a textbook of cardiovascular medicine,* ed 7, Philadelphia, 2005, Elsevier Saunders, pp 1489-1552.
2. Hoffman JIE, Kaplan S: The incidence of congenital heart disease, *J Am Coll Cardiol* 39:1890-900, 2002.
3. Hoffman JIE, Kaplan S, Liberthson RR: Prevalence of congenital heart disease, *Am Heart J* 147:42-39, 2004.
4. Gill HK, Splitt M, Sharland GK et al: Patterns of recurrence of congenital heart disease. An analysis of 6,640 consecutive pregnancies evaluated by detailed fetal echocardiography, *J Am Coll Cardiol* 42:923-9, 2003.
5. Goldmuntz E: The genetic contribution to congenital heart disease, *Pediatr Clinics North Am* 51(6):1721-1737, 2004.
6. McElhinney DB, Driscoll DA, Emanuel BS et al: Chromosome 22q11 deletion in patients with truncus arteriosus, *Pediatr Cardiol* 24(6):569-73, 2003.
7. Marino B, Diglio MC: Congenital heart disease and genetic syndromes: specific correlation between cardiac phenotype and genotype, *Cardiovasc Pathol* 9(6):303-15, 2000.
8. Park MK: *Pediatric cardiology for practitioners,* ed 4, St Louis, 2002, Mosby.
9. Pelech AN: The physiology of cardiac auscultation, *Pediatr Clinics North Am* 51(6):1515-1535, 2004.
10. Randolph GR, Hagler DJ, Connolly HM et al: Intraoperative transesophageal echocardiography during surgery for congenital heart defects, *J Thorac Cardiovasc Surg* 124(6):1176-1182, 2002.
11. Rychik J: Frontiers in fetal cardiovascular disease, *Pediatr Clin North Am* 51:1489-1502, 2004.
12. Jaworski A: Hypoplastic left heart syndrome: a parent's perspective. In Hennein HA, Bove EL, editors: *Hypoplastic left heart syndrome,* Armonk, NY, 2002, Futura Publishing, pp 319-338.
13. Rome JJ, Kruetzer J: Pediatric interventional catheterization: reasonable expectations and outcomes, *Pediatr Clin North Amer* 51(12):1589-1610, 2004.
14. Baskett RJ, Tancock E, Ross DB: The gold standard for atrial septal defect closure: current surgical results, with an emphasis on morbidity, *Pediatr Card* 24:444-447, 2003.
15. Harper RW, Mottram PM, McGaw DJ: Closure of secundum atrial septal defects with the Amplatzer septal occluder device: techniques and problems, *Catheter Cardiovasc Interv* 57(4):508-524, 2002.
16. Du ZD, Hijazi ZM, Kleinmann CS et al: Comparison between transcatheter and surgical closure of secundum atrial septal defect in children and adults: results of a multicenter nonrandomized trial, *J Am Coll Card* 39(11):1836-1844, 2002.
17. Berger F, Vogel M, Alexi-Meskishvili V et al: Comparison of results and complications of surgical and Amplatzer device closure of atrial septal defects, *J Thorac Cardiovasc Surg* 118(4):674-678, 1999.
18. Khairy P, O'Donnell CP, Landzberg MJ: Transcatheter closure versus medical therapy of patent foramen ovale and presumed paradoxical thromboemboli: a systematic review, *Ann Intern Med* 139:753-760, 2003.
19. Waight DJ, Bacha EA, Kahana M et al: Catheter therapy of Swiss cheese ventricular septal defects using the Amplatzer muscular VSD occluder, *Catheter Cardiovas Interv* 55:355-361, 2002.
20. Thanopoulos BD, Tsaousis GS, Karanasios E et al: Transcatheter closure of perimembranous ventricular septal defects with the Amplatzer asymmetric ventricular septal defect occluder: preliminary experience in children, *Heart* 89(8):918-22, 2003.
21. Thanopoulous BD, Rigby ML: Outcome of transcatheter closure of muscular ventricular septal defects with the Amplatzer ventricular septal defect occluder, *Heart* 91(4):513-6, 2005.
22. Holzer R, Balzer D, Cao QL et al: Device closure of muscular ventricular septal defects using the Amplatzer muscular ventricular septal defect occluder: immediate and mid-term results of a U.S. registry, *J Am Coll Cardiol* 43(7):1257-63, 2004.
23. Pfammatter JP, Wagner B, Berdat PL et al: Procedural factors associated with early postoperative arrhythmias after repair of congenital heart defects, *J Thorac Cardiovas Surg* 23(2):258-262, 2002.
24. Hammerman C, Kaplan M: Comparative tolerability of pharmacological treatments for patent ductus arteriosus, *Drug Saf* 24(7):537-51, 2001.
25. Arora R, Sengupta PP, Thakur AK et al: Pediatric interventional cardiac symposium. Device closure of patent ductus arteriosus, *J Interv Cardiol* 16(5):385-91, 2003.
26. Thanopoulos BD, Hakim F, Hiari A et al: Further experience with transcatheter closure of the patent ductus arteriosus using the Amplatzer duct occluder, *J Am Coll Cardiol* 35(4):1016-1020, 2001.
27. Burn J: The aetiology of congenital heart disease. In Anderson RH, Baker EJ, Macartney FJ, editors: *Paediatric cardiology,* ed 2, London, 2002, Churchill Livingstone, pp 141-213.
28. Dunlop KA, Mulholland HC, Casey FA et al: A ten year review of atrioventricular canal defects, *Cardiol Young* 14(1):15-23, 2004.
29. Ten Harkel AD, Cromme-Dijkhuis AH, Heinerman BC et al: Development of left atrioventricular valve regurgitation after correc-

tion of atrioventricular septal defect, *Ann Thorac Surg* 79(2):601-12, 2005.

30. Dunst CJ, Trivette C: Empowerment, effective healthgiving practices, and family centered care, *Pediatr Nurs* 22:334-337, 1996.
31. Zeigler VL, Marlow D, Gillette PC: Mechanisms, diagnostic tools, and patient and family education. In Zeigler VL, Gillette PC, editors: *Practical management of pediatric cardiac arrhythmias,* Armonk, NY, 2001, Futura Publishing pp 1-52.
32. Curley M, Wallace J: Effects of the nursing mutual participation model of care on parental stress in the pediatric intensive care unit: a replication, *Pediatr Nurs* 7:377-385, 1992.
33. Johnson BH, Jeppson ES, Redburn L: *Caring for children and families: guidelines for hospitals,* Bethesda, Md, 2002, Association for the Care of Children's Health.
34. Wong DL, Hockenberry-Eaton M, Wilson D, editors: *Whaley and Wong's nursing care of infants and children,* ed 6, St Louis, 1999, Mosby-Year Book, pp 1210-1282.
35. El-Najdawi, Driscoll DJ, Puga FJ et al: Operation for partial atrioventricular septal defect: a forty-year review, *Thorac Cardiovasc Surg* 119(5):880-9, 2000.
36. Lindberg L, Olsson AK, Jogi P et al: How common is severe pulmonary hypertension after pediatric cardiac surgery?, *J Thorac Cardiovas Surg* 123(6):1155-1163, 2002.
37. Bertola DR, Sugayama SM, Albano LM et al: Noonan syndrome: a clinical and genetic study of 31 patients, *Rev Hosp Clin Fac Med Sao Paulo* 54:147-50 1999.
38. Humpl T, Söderberg B, McCrindle BW et al: Percutaneous balloon valvotomy in pulmonary atresia with intact ventricular septum: impact on patient care, *Circulation* 108(7):826-32, 2003.
39. Neilson DE, Robin NH: Advances in the genetics of pediatric heart disease, *Contem Pediatri* 85-100, 2002.
40. Chang AC, Hanley F, Wernovsky G, editors: *Pediatric cardiac intensive care,* Baltimore, Md 1998, Williams & Wilkins.
41. Hazekamp MG, Grotenhuis HB, Schoof PH et al: Results of the Ross operation in a pediatric population, *Eur J Cardiothorac Surg* 27(6):975-9, 2005.
42. Hamdan, MA, Maheshwari S, Fahey JT et al: Endovascular stents for coarctation of the aorta: initial results and intermediate-term follow-up, *J Am Coll Cardiol* 38(5):1518-23, 2001.
43. Mulder TJ, Pyles LA, Stolfi A et al: A multicenter analysis of the choice of initial surgical procedure in tetralogy of Fallot, *Pediatr Card* 23:580-586, 2002.
44. Therrien J, Marx GR, Gatzoulis MA: Late problems in tetralogy of Fallot: recognition, management, and prevention, *Cardiol Clin* 20:395-404, 2002.
45. Prêtre R, Gendron G, Tamisier D et al: Results of the Lecompte procedure in malposition of the great arteries and pulmonary obstruction, *Eur J Cardiothorac Surg* 19(3):283-9, 2001.
46. Hutter PA, Kreb DL, Mantel SF et al: Twenty-five years' experience with the arterial switch operation, *J Thorac Cardiovasc Surg* 124(4):790-797, 2002.
47. Rodefeld, MD, Hanley FL: Neonatal truncus arteriosus repair: surgical techniques and clinical management, *Ann Semin Thoracic Cardiovas Surg* 5:212-217, 2002.
48. Thompson LD, McElhinney DB, Reddy M et al: Neonatal repair of truncus arteriosus: continuing improvement in outcomes, *Ann Thorac Surg* 72(2):391-5, 2001.
49. Wang PY, Hwang BT, Lu JH et al: Significance of pulmonary venous obstruction in total anomalous pulmonary venous return, *J Chin Med Assoc* 67(7):331-5, 2004.
50. Kirshborm PM, Myung RJ, Gaynor JW et al: Preoperative pulmonary venous obstruction affects long-term outcome for survivors of total anomalous pulmonary venous connection repair, *Ann Thorac Surg* 74(5):1616-1620, 2002.
51. Yun TJ, Coles JG, Konstantinov IE et al: Conventional and sutureless techniques for management of the pulmonary veins: evolution of indications from postrepair pulmonary vein stenosis to primary pulmonary vein anomalies, *J Thorac Cardiovas Surg* 129(1):167-174, 2005.
52. Epstein M: Tricuspid atresia. In Allen HP, Gutgesell EB, Clark DJ, Driscoll, **initials?)** editors: *Moss and Adams' heart disease in infants, children, and adolescents,* Philadelphia, 2002, Lippincott Williams & Wilkins.
53. Liu J, Lu Y, Chen H et al: Bidirectional Glenn without cardiopulmonary bypass, *Ann Thoracic Surg* 77:1349-52, 2004.

54. Galantowicz M, Cheatham JP: Fontan completion without surgery, *Ann Semin Thorac Cardiovasc Surg* 7:48-55, 2004.
55. Mair DD, Puga FJ, Danielson GK: The Fontan procedure for tricuspid atresia: early and late results of a 25-year experience with 216 patients, *J Am Coll Cardiol* 37(3):933-939, 2001.
56. Soetenga D, Mussatto KA: Management of infants with hypoplastic left heart syndrome: integrating research in nursing practice, *Crit Care Nurse* 24(6):46-8, 50, 52, 2004.
57. McElhinney DB, Hedrick HL, Bush DM et al. Necrotizing enterocolitis in neonates with congenital heart disease: risk factors and outcomes, *Pediatrics* 106(5):1080-7, 2000.
58. Tweddell JS, Litwin SB, Thomas JP Jr et al: Recent advances in the surgical management of the single ventricle patient, *Pediatr Clin North Am* 46(2):465-80, 1999.
59. Zeigler VL: Ethical principles and parental choice: treatment options for neonates with hypoplastic left heart syndrome, *Pediatr Nurs* 29(1):65-69, 2003.
60. Bailey LL: Transplantation is the best treatment option for hypoplastic left heart syndrome, *Cardiol Young* 14:109-11, 2004.
61. Chrisant MR, Naftel DC, Drummond-Webb J et al: Fate of infants with hypoplastic left heart syndrome listed for cardiac transplantation: a multicenter study, *J Heart Lung Transpl* 24(5):576-82, 2005.
62. Boucek RJ Jr, Chrisant MR: Cardiac transplantation for hypoplastic left heart syndrome, *Cardiol Young* 14:83-7, 2004.
63. Tanoe Y, Kado H, Shiokawa Y et al: Midterm ventricular performance after Norwood procedure with right ventricle to pulmonary artery conduit, *Ann Thora Surgery* 781:1965-71, 2004.
64. Brown JW, Ruzmetoz M, Okada Y et al:Truncus arteriosus repair: outcomes, risk factors, reoperation and management, *Euro J Cardiothorac Surg* 20:221-227, 2001.
65. Kim SJ, Park IS, Song JY et al: Reversal of protein-losing enteropathy with calcium replacement in a patient after Fontan operation, *Ann Thorac Surg* 77(4):456-457, 2004.
66. Balaji S, Gillette PC, Case CL, editors: *Cardiac arrhythmias after surgery for congenital heart disease,* London, 2001, Arnold.
67. Manle WT, Spray TL, Wernovsky G et al: Survival after reconstruction surgery for hypoplastic left heart syndrome: a 15-year experience from a single institution, *Circulation* 102:136-141, 2000.
68. Michaelsson M, Jonzon A, Risenfeld T: Isolated congenital complete atrioventricular block in adult life: a prospective study, *Circulation* 91:442-449, 1995.
69. Byron JP, Hiegert R, Cope J et al: Autoimmune-associated congenital heart block. Demographics, mortality, morbidity, and recurrence rates obtained from a national neonatal lupus registry, *J Am Coll Cardiol* 31:1658-1666, 1998.
70. Fukushige J, Takahashi N, Igarashi H et al: Perinatal management of congenital complete atrioventricular block: a report of nine cases, *Acta Pediatr* 40:337-340, 1998.
71. Yasuda K, Hayashi G, Ohuchi H et al: Dilated cardiomyopathy after pacemaker implantation in complete heart block, *Pediatr Int* 47(2):121-125, 2005.
72. Jaeggi ET, Hamilton RM, Silverman ED et al: Outcome of children born with fetal, neonatal, or childhood diagnosis of isolated congenital atrioventricular block. A single institution's experience of 30 years, *J Am Coll Cardiol* 39(1):130-137, 2002.
73. Zeigler VL: Pediatric cardiac arrhythmias resulting in hemodynamic compromise, *Crit Care Nurs Clin N Am* 17:77-95, 2005.
74. Gregatoros G, Abrams J, Epstein AE et al: ACC/AHA/NASPE 2002 guideline update for implantation of cardiac pacemakers and antiarrhythmia devices. Summary article: a report of the American College of Cardiology/American Heart Association task force on practice guidelines, *Circulation* 106:2145-2161, 2002.
75. Noiseux N, Khairy P, Fournier A et al: Thirty years of experience with epicardial pacing in children, *Cardiol Young* 14(5):512-519, 2004.
76. Thompson JD, Blackburn ME, Van Doorn C et al: Pacing activity, patient, and lead survival over 20 years of permanent epicardial pacing in children, *Ann Thorac Surg* 77(4):1366-1370, 2004.
77. Fortescue EB, Berul CI, Cecchin F et al: Patient, procedural, and hardware factors associated with pacemaker lead failures in pediatrics and congenital heart disease, *Heart Rhythm* 1(2):150-159, 2004.

78. Jervell A, Lange-Nielsen: Congenital deaf-mutism, functional heart disease with prolongation of the QY and sudden death, *Am Heart J* 54:59-68, 1957.

79. Romano C, Gemme G, Pongiglione R: Artmie cardiache rare dell 'eta pediatrica, *Clin Pediatr* 45:658-683, 1963.

80. Ward OC: A new familial cardiac syndrome in children, *J Irish Med Assoc* 54:103-106, 1964.

81. Tester DJ, Will ML, Haglund CM et al: Compendium of cardiac channel mutations in 541 consecutive unrelated patients referred for long QT syndrome genetic testing, *Heart Rhythm* 2(5):507-17, 2005.

82. Ten Harkel AD, Witsenburg M, deJong PL et al: Efficacy of an implantable cardioverter-defibrillator in a neonate with LQT3 associated arrhythmias, *Europace* 7(1):77-84, 2005.

83. Chatrath R, Porter CJ, Ackerman MJ: Role of transvenous implantable cardioverter-defibrillators in preventing sudden cardiac death in children, adolescents, and young adults, *Mayo Clinic Proceedings* 77:226-231, 2002.

84. Goel AK, Berger S, Pelech A et al: Implantable cardioverter defibrillator therapy in children with long QT syndrome, *Pediatric Cardiology* 25:370-78, 2004.

85. Mönig G, Köbe J, Löher A et al: Implantable cardioverter-defibrillator therapy in patients with congenital long QT syndrome: a long term follow-up, *Heart Rhythm* 2(5):497-504, 2005.

86. LeRoy S, Elixson, M, O'Brien P et al: Recommendations for preparing children and adolescents for invasive cardiac procedures. A statement from the American Heart Association pediatric nursing subcommittee of the council on cardiovascular nursing in collaboration with the council on cardiovascular diseases of the young, *Circulation* 108:2250-2564, 2003.

87. Uzark K: Therapeutic cardiac catheterization for congenital heart disease. A new era in pediatric cardiology, *J Pediatr Nurs* 16(5):300-307, 2001.

88. Allen HD, Beekman RH, Garson A Jr et al: Pediatric therapeutic cardiac catheterization. A statement for healthcare professionals from the council on cardiovascular diseases in the young, *Circulation* 97:609-625 1998.

89. Valsangiacomo E, Schmid ER, Schüpbach RW et al: Early postoperative arrhythmias after cardiac operation in children, *Ann Thorac Surg* 74(3):792-796, 2002.

90. Morris MC, Ittenback RF, Godinez RI et al: Risk factors for mortality in 137 pediatric cardiac intensive care unit patients managed with extracorporeal membrane oxygenation, *Crit Care Med* 32(4):1061-1069, 2004.

91. Dibardino DJ, Allison AE, Vaughn WK et al: Current expectations for newborns undergoing the arterial switch operation, *Ann Surg* 239(5):588-596, 2004.

92. Bové T, Francois K, DeGroote K et al: Outcome analysis of major cardiac operations in low weight neonates. *Ann Thorac Surg* 78(1):181-187, 2004.

93. Cava JR, Danduran MJ, Fedderly RT et al: Exercise recommendations and risk factors for sudden cardiac death, *Pediatr Clin N Am* 51(5):1401-1420, 2004.

94. Al-Jarrallah AS, Lardhi AA, Hassan AA: Endocarditis prophylaxis in children with congenital heart disease. A parent's awareness, *Saudi Medical Journal* 25(2):182-185, 2004.

95. Dajani AS, Taubert KA, Wilson W et al: Prevention of bacterial endocarditis - recommendations by the American Heart Association, *JAMA* 277:1794-1801, 1997.

96. Artman M: Herbal preparations may produce adverse cardiovascular complications in children, Presented at American Academy of Pediatrics meeting Oct. 23, 2001. Retrieved April 15, 2005 from www.med.nyu.pedcard/news/#herbal.

97. Plotikoff GA: Herbal medicines. In Snyder M, Lindquist R, editors: *Complementary/alternative therapies in nursing*, New York, 2002, Springer, pp 259-271.

Care of Adults with Congenital Heart Disease

Philip Moons
Mary M. Canobbio
Michelle J. Nickolaus
Amy Verstappen

CHAPTER ABBREVIATIONS

ACE   angiotensin-converting enzyme

ASD   atrioseptal defect

AV   atrioventricular

AVSD   atrial septal defect

BT   Blalock-Taussig

CoA   coarctation of the aorta

CCTGA   congenitally corrected transposition of the great arteries

IART   intraatrial reentry tachycardia

ICD   implantable cardioverter-defibrillator

MCV   mean cell volume

MRI   magnetic resonance imaging

PA-VSD   pulmonary atresia with ventricular septal defect

PFO   patent foramen ovale

PLE   protein-losing enteropathy

PDA   patent ductus arteriosus

Qp/Qs   pulmonary-to-systemic blood flow ratio

RAPA   right atrium to pulmonary artery

STD   sexually transmitted disease

SVT   supraventricular tachycardia

TEE   transesophageal echocardiogram

TGA   transposition of the great arteries

TOF   tetralogy of Fallot

VSD   ventricular septal defect

WPW   Wolff-Parkinson-White

The ongoing care of the adult survivors of congenital heart disease will be a major challenge for twenty-first century medicine and nursing. These challenges are the direct result of major triumphs of the previous century—the development of successful treatments for congenital cardiac disease. Long-term management of these complex patients requires an understanding of commonly encountered acyanotic and cyanotic congenital heart lesions, previous surgical approaches, sequelae and/or residua for both repaired and unrepaired lesions in adulthood, and psychosocial issues that might impact their quality of life.

HISTORY

Congenital heart defects are the most common birth defect and occur in approximately 8 in 1000 births.[1] Before heart-lung bypass, surgical treatment was limited to extracardiac repairs, beginning with the first successful ligation of a patent ductus arteriosus **(PDA)** in 1938, the first coarctation repair in 1944, and culminating in the Blalock-Taussig shunt **(BT).** First performed on November 29, 1944, the BT shunt involved the suturing of the oxygen-rich subclavian artery to the pulmonary artery and resulted in a dramatic improvement in oxygenation. Although the BT shunt was palliative and not reparative, its usage enabled tetralogy of Fallot **(TOF)** to become the first newly survivable complex congenital heart defect. Many recipients of these first procedures are still alive today.[2] In 1953, in the first cardiac surgery to successfully use heart-lung bypass, Dr. John Gibbon successfully closed an atrial septal defect **(ASD)** in an 18-year-old patient.[3] This procedure ushered in an ever increasing number of new surgical treatments for complex congenital heart disease.

As technology and knowledge progressed, new surgical approaches were adopted and discarded. The complexity of diagnoses, combined with the wide range of surgical strategies, has left behind a uniquely complex population of patients. This population continues to increase in complexity as more patients survive into adulthood with conditions that would have previously taken their lives in infancy. With improvements in diagnosis and intervention, it is now expected that now more than 90 percent of infants with congenital heart disease will survive to adulthood.[4,5]

Despite the common misperception that these surgeries are "curative," all survivors of congenital heart disease, with the exception of ligated and divided ductus arteriosus, have been shown to be at risk of residua and sequelae and should continue to receive cardiac care.[4] In this chapter, we will review the incidence and prevalence of congenital heart disease, access to health care, the more common defects seen in adulthood with their sequelae and residua, and common clinical problems in these patients. We will describe the counseling issues in which nurses play a pivotal role.

Congenital heart disease consists of a wide spectrum of cardiac defects with varying severity and prognosis. The American College of Cardiology task force 1 of the 32nd Bethesda conference developed a classification scheme to categorize patients according to the disease

BOX 71-1 ■ ■ ■
SIMPLE CONGENITAL HEART DISEASE

Group 1
These patients can usually be cared for in the general medical community.

Native Conditions
- Isolated congenital aortic valve disease
- Isolated congenital mitral valve disease (except parachute valve, cleft leaflet)
- Isolated PFO or small ASD
- Isolated small VSD (no associated lesions)
- Mild pulmonic stenosis

Repaired Conditions
- Previously ligated or occluded ductus arteriosus
- Repaired secundum or sinus venosus
- ASD without residua
- Repaired VSD without residua

ASD, Atrial septal defect; *PFO*, patent foramen ovale; *VSD*, ventricular septal defect.
Adapted from Warnes CA, Liberthson R, Danielson GK et al: Task force 1: the changing profile of congenital heart disease in adult life, *J Amer Coll Cardiol* 37:1170-1175, 2001.

BOX 71-2 ■ ■ ■
CONGENITAL HEART DISEASE OF MODERATE SEVERITY

Group 2
These patients should be seen periodically at regional congenital heart centers.
Aorto-left ventricular fistulae
- Anomalous pulmonary venous drainage(partial or total)
- AV canal defects (partial or complete)
- CoA
- Epstein anomaly
- Infundibular right ventricular outflow obstruction of significance
- Ostium primum ASD
- PDA (not closed)
- Pulmonary valve regurgitation (moderate to severe)
- Pulmonic valve stenosis (moderate to severe)
- Sinus of Valsalva fistula and/or aneurysm
- Sinus venosus ASD
- Subvalvar or supravalvar aortic stenosis (except HOCM)
- TOF
Ventricular septal defect with
  - Absent valve or valves
  - Aortic regurgitation
  - CoA
  - Mitral disease
Right ventricular outflow tract obstruction
- Straddling tricuspid and/or mitral valve
- Subaortic stenosis

ASD, Atrial septal defect; *AV*, atrioventricular; *COA*, coarctation of the aorta; *PDA*, patent ductus arteriosus; *TOF*, tetralogy of Fallot.
HOCM, hypertrophic obstructive cardiomyopathy
Adapted from Warnes CA, Liberthson R, Danielson GK et al: Task force 1: the changing profile of congenital heart disease in adult life, *J Amer Coll Cardiol* 37:1170-1175, 2001.

BOX 71-3 ■ ■ ■
CONGENITAL HEART DISEASE OF GREAT COMPLEXITY

Group 3
These patients should be seen regularly at adult congenital heart disease centers.
- Conduits, valved or nonvalved
- Cyanotic congenital heart (all forms)
- Double-outlet ventricle
- Eisenmenger syndrome
- Fontan procedure
- Mitral atresia
- Single ventricle (also called double inlet or outlet, common or primitive)
- Pulmonary atresia (all forms)
- Pulmonary vascular obstructive diseases

Transposition of the great arteries
- Congenitally corrected transposition of the great arteries
- Tricuspid atresia
- Truncus arteriosus/hemitruncus
- Other abnormalities of atrioventricular or ventriculoarterial connection not included above (i.e., crisscross heart, isomerism, heterotaxy syndromes)

Adapted from Warnes CA, Liberthson R, Danielson GK et al: Task force 1: the changing profile of congenital heart disease in adult life, *J Amer Coll Cardiol* 37:1170-1175, 2001.

severity; they were categorized into three classes: simple lesions, moderate lesions, and complex lesions[6,7] (Boxes 71-1, 71-2, and 71-3).

INCIDENCE AND PREVALENCE OF CONGENITAL HEART DISEASE

The overall incidence of congenital heart disease is estimated to be 0.8 percent.[1] The incidence of congenital heart disease varies, however, depending on which heart defects are included in the assessment, the patient's age at diagnosis, and the study design (population studies or patient referral studies). Hence, overall rates of congenital heart disease incidence in various studies have ranged from 4/1000 to 75/1000 live births.[1] Moderate and severe forms have an incidence of approximately 6/1000 live births. If serious bicuspid aortic valve disease is included, the incidence is approximately 19/1000 live births. If trivial lesions are included, such as a small muscular ventricular septal defect **(VSD)** present at birth, incidence increases to 75/1000 live births.[1]

Hoffman and Kaplan reviewed incidence data for the last 50 years and concluded that the overall incidence of congenital heart disease is stable and does not vary among countries.[1] The variations in reported incidence are primarily attributed to the inclusion or noninclusion of trivial lesions. Simple lesions, as defined by the 32nd Bethesda conference, are estimated to account for 51 percent of all congenital heart defects, whereas moderate and severe lesions account for 26 percent and 23 percent, respectively.[6] As a consequence of higher survival rates, the prevalence of adults with congenital heart disease will increase toward an estimated 3700 patients per million.[6] For the first time in history, there are now more adults than children living with congenital heart disease, and this population is growing by approximately 5 percent/year.[8]

HEALTH CARE FACILITIES FOR ADULTS WITH CONGENITAL HEART DISEASE

This growing patient population requires specialist care and attention. Several North American and European task forces and expert panels have been formed to develop recommendations for the management of adult patients with congenital heart disease and for best health care practice.[7,9-17] It is recommended that the care for adults with congenital heart disease be stratified into three levels: specialist care, shared care in which a specialist center is collaborating with a general adult cardiac facility, and "nonspecialist" care with access to specialized care if needed.[12] Regionalized adult congenital heart centers should be developed, and all patients with moderately complex and highly complex conditions should have their care overseen by specialized centers. These centers are not intended to replace local care, but rather to supplement care with specialized expertise and services since few community cardiologists have training and expertise in the diagnosis and management of these new and challenging patients. Hence, appropriate referral of patients to specialist centers is imperative. The specialized diagnostic, surgical, clinical, and psychological services that should be offered are also outlined in the guidelines. It is recommended that new training programs be developed to train adult congenital heart disease specialists.[18]

Currently, there is a severe international shortage of adult congenital heart specialists and clinics.[12,19,20] The Adult Congenital Heart Association, www.achaheart.org, the International Society of Adult Congenital Cardiac Disease, www.isaccd.org, and the working group on grown-up congenital heart disease of the European Society of Cardiology, www.escardio.org, offer on-line listings of specialized adult congenital heart clinics internationally.

CONGENITAL HEART DEFECTS
Simple Congenital Heart Defects

The category of simple congenital heart disease encompasses the conditions depicted in Box 71-1. These are typically conditions that involve isolated lesions and repaired conditions without residua that can be cared for by the general medical community. Exceptions are noted below.

Atrial Septal Defect

ASD represent abnormal direct communications between the left and right atria. This defect accounts for approximately 6 percent to 10 percent of all cardiac defects.[1] ASDs are two times more common in women than in men. Although there are several types of ASDs (Table 71-1), the most common type is the ostium secundum ASD, in which the defect occurs centrally at the fossa

■ ■ ■

TABLE 71-1   COMPLICATIONS AND FOLLOW-UP REQUIREMENTS AFTER REPAIR OF ATRIAL SEPTAL DEFECT

TYPE OF DEFECT	LONG-TERM COMPLICATIONS	LONG-TERM FOLLOW-UP NEEDS
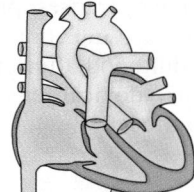 Secundum defect 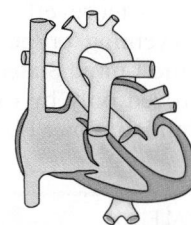 Sinus venosus defect with partial anomalous pulmonary venous connection 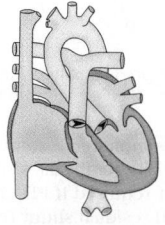 Ostium primum defect	**Relatively common:** • Dysrhythmia • Atrial flutter • Atrial fibrillation • Mitral regurgitation (primum defect) **Rare:** • Subaortic stenosis (primum) • Pulmonary vascular disease	**No cardiomegaly, normal exam and ECG:** • No specialized follow-up needed **Cardiomegaly and/or significant murmur—Assess for the following with echocardiography (use TEE if TTE not adequate):** • Residual shunt • Valvular regurgitation • Ventricular dysfunction • Pulmonary vascular disease • Cardiac catheterization if incompletely resolved and/or management is unclear **Key points:** • Dysrhythmias can occur late after either type of repair, especially when residual atrial enlargement is present (atrial fibrillation). • Endocarditis prophylaxis: None required in repaired patients unless mitral regurgitation is present (as in primum). • After percutaneous closure, current recommendations are endocarditis prophylaxis for ONLY the first 6 mo after closure; afterwards it is not necessary. • After percutaneous closure, current recommendations are for aspirin 81 mg to 325 mg daily for the first 6 mo after closure.

ECG, Electrocardiogram; *TEE,* transesophageal echocardiogram; *TTE,* transthoracic echocardiography.
Adapted from Graham TP: Long-term care of patients with repaired congenital cardiac abnormalities, *Adv Cardiovasc Med* 5:1-12, 1998 and Mullins CE, Mayer DC: *Congenital heart disease: a diagrammatic atlas,* ed. I. Jasper Burns (developed as CD-ROM) by Scientific Solutions, 1998, John Wiley and Sons, Inc.

ovalis. Although many ASDs are repaired in childhood, this defect can go unnoticed until the fourth or fifth decade of life because of trivial or absent physical examination findings.[8,21,22] In general, catheter or surgical closure for ASD is recommended if the pulmonary-to-systemic blood flow ratio (Qp/Qs) is 1.5:1 or greater.

Long-Term Survival and Complications

Long-term survival and low morbidity is reported in patients who have undergone closure of their ASD. Rates of complications in postoperative patients is dependent in part on age at closure, with those undergoing closure in infancy showing lowest rates of long-term complications. In patients with an unrepaired ASD, the continuous shunting of blood across the atrium from left to right over time produces fatigue, shortness of breath on exertion, and palpitations with normal pulse oximetry saturations. Dyspnea on exertion is seen in about 30 percent of these patients by the third decade and in 75 percent by the fifth decade. In these patients, the right atrial volume increases over time. This causes enlargement and overstretching of the right atrium, resulting in potential substrate for atrial fibrillation. These patients are also vulnerable to paradoxical embolism and stroke.[8,22-25] Pulmonary hypertension, although a rare complication, can occur in patients with unrepaired defects. Table 71-1 lists the common problems in adults with repaired ASD.

Follow-up and Management at Adult Age

Following repair, patients should have periodic cardiac follow-up to check for residual effects, such as atrial dysrhythmias. Adults with simple ASD repaired in infancy and no residual cardiac effects may be followed at the community level. Patients with the more complex forms of ASDs should be evaluated at a regional adult congenital heart disease care center. Indications for specialty care include preoperative or postoperative dysrhythmias, valvular or ventricular dysfunction, and elevated pulmonary pressures.

As in childhood, hemodynamically significant ASDs in the adult patient (Qp/Qs 1.5:1 or greater) should be closed for the best prognosis. The exception is if significant pulmonary hypertension has developed. If closure is indicated, it can be accomplished either surgically or via transcatheter approach. Percutaneous ASD closure candidates must meet criteria for closure just as surgical patients must; however, selection criteria are stricter because the defect size cannot be larger than the device and there must be adequate rim margins for anchoring. Surgical closure is achieved by either using primary suture or a pericardial or synthetic patch. Mortality rates for surgical ASD closure in the adult without pulmonary hypertension are less than 1 percent.[23] The initial data on the Amplatzer percutaneous device has been encouraging because patients experience similar success rates, shorter hospital stays, and a decreased rate of complications.[26]

Patent Foramen Ovale

A patent foramen ovale (PFO) is estimated to occur in about 30 percent of the population.[27] As with the ASD, the PFO is a communication between the atria. However, in PFO there is no structural deformity of the septum, but rather a failure of the anatomical tissue fusion of valve remnant of the septum primum (see diagram in Table 71-2). Normally after birth, when left atrial pressures exceed right atrial pressure, the flap valve of the septum primum functionally closes, and the tissue fuses together. In PFO, fusion of the tissue does not take place. Although the flap valve is functionally closed, if right atrial pressure exceeds left atrial pressure it can open and shunt blood.

Differential diagnosis between an ASD and PFO can be challenging and is typically made by transesophageal echocardiogram (TEE) with contrast injection. Most frequently PFO is diagnosed in adulthood after cryptogenic stroke associated with paradoxical embolism crossing from the right atrium to the left.

Management at Adult Age

Closure of PFO for secondary prevention of stroke is still controversial. Clinical trials to evaluate whether surgical or percutaneous closure is more efficacious than medical management in preventing cryptogenic stroke are ongoing. Currently in the United States, percutaneous device closure is approved only by exemption by the Food and Drug Administration (FDA) for

---

TABLE 71-2 COMPLICATIONS AND FOLLOW-UP REQUIREMENTS FOR PATENT FORAMEN OVALE

TYPE OF DEFECT	LONG-TERM COMPLICATIONS	LONG-TERM FOLLOW-UP NEEDS
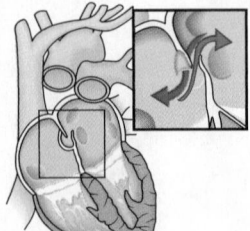 Patent foramen ovale	**If no closure recommended:** • Aspirin or warfarin should be used. However, the evidence is insufficient to determine if warfarin or aspirin is superior in preventing recurrent stroke or death, but minor bleeding is more frequent with warfarin. • Presently there is insufficient evidence to evaluate the efficacy of surgical or endovascular closure.	**After surgery closure:** • No specialized follow-up needed **After device closure:** • Periodic follow-up needed at present since long-term issues are not well-known **Key points:** • Aspirin therapy typically recommended, sometimes along with clopidogrel (Plavix) therapy as well • Endocarditis prophylaxis not required if PDA eliminated; recommended if small residual shunt remains • After percutaneous closure current recommendations: prophylaxis for ONLY the first 6 mo after closure; afterwards it is not necessary

PDA, Patent ductus arteriosus.
Adapted from *Patent foramen ovale,* Last updated October 2005, The Cleveland Clinic Foundation http://www.clevelandclinic.org/heartcenter/pub/guide/disease/congenital/pfo.htm.

patients with recurrent cryptogenic stroke caused by presumed paradoxical embolism despite optimal medical therapy with anticoagulation.

Long-Term Survival and Follow-Up

An unrepaired PFO does not appear to influence mortality. Typically, adult PFO patients are asymptomatic, although occasionally, oxygen desaturation may occur with exercise. There is a reported association between migraine headaches and PFO, but this is not clearly understood.[28,29] Right to left shunting in atrial septal aneurysm is associated with PFO in about 78 percent of patients with atrial septal aneurysm. Atrial septal aneurysm associated with cerebral embolus is more common in patients younger than age 55 years, but it has also been seen in those ages 60 to 80.

Patients who have undergone device closure for a PFO require endocarditis prophylaxis and aspirin for the first 6 months following closure (see Chapter 73). They are also encouraged to undergo periodic follow-up since long-term issues are less well known. Table 71-2 lists the common problems and recommended follow-up in adults with PFO.

Ventricular Septal Defect

Ventricular septal defects are the most common heart defects, representing about 35 percent of all congenital cardiac anomalies.[1] VSDs occur with similar frequency in boys and girls. VSDs are characterized by an abnormal opening between the left and right ventricles. There are three main categories of VSD: perimembranous (65 percent); muscular (30 percent); and malalignment or subarterial (5 percent) (see figures in Table 71-3). In the perimembranous and muscular regions, spontaneous closure occurs in 50 percent of the patients. Furthermore, VSDs are categorized as restrictive or unrestrictive. Restrictive VSDs are small, resulting in a high gradient of pressure between right and left ventricle, and nonrestrictive VSDs are large in which the pressure between right and left ventricle is equal. Unrestricted defects are typically repaired in childhood, but restrictive VSDs can be newly found in the adult. Isolated small perimembranous VSDs do not require closure as long as patients do not have problems with recurrent endocarditis.

Long-Term Survival and Complications

The patient with an unrepaired restrictive or perimembranous VSD is typically asymptomatic and has normal pulmonary pressure. The primary concern in these patients is the risk for endocarditis.

The nonrestrictive VSD or muscular VSD repaired early in childhood typically results in normal hemodynamics without residual shunt or pulmonary arterial hypertension. For patients with good left ventricular function before surgery and good functional class afterward, life expectancy is close to normal. However, residual defects, such as aortic regurgitation, right or left outflow tract obstruction, and tricuspid regurgitation, can be present. Ventriculotomy and right atrial approach through the tricuspid valve often leads to a right bundle branch block as a result of the patch being sewn into the septum. This right bundle branch block, in combination with an acquired left bundle branch block, may result in a complete atrioventricular (AV) block. Large unrestricted defects that go unrepaired in childhood often lead to Eisenmenger syndrome, discussed below.

Follow-Up and Management at Adult Age

In general isolated small VSDs can be cared for by the general medical community. Follow-up visits every 3 to 5 years are sufficient.[15] On the other hand, patients with

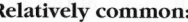

TABLE 71-3 COMPLICATIONS AND FOLLOW-UP REQUIREMENTS AFTER REPAIR OF VENTRICULAR SEPTAL DEFECT

TYPE OF DEFECT	LONG-TERM COMPLICATIONS	LONG-TERM FOLLOW-UP NEEDS
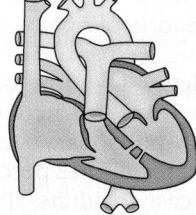 Perimembranous VSD Muscular VSD	**Relatively common:** • Residual small VSD • Mild tricuspid regurgitation • Aortic regurgitation, if present preoperatively **Rare:** • Subaortic stenosis • Infundibular PS • Double-chambered right ventricle • Right bundle branch block • Dysrhythmias • Ventricular ectopy • Ventricular dysfunction (especially with muscular VSDs that had a repair through a left ventriculotomy) • Pulmonary vascular disease	**No murmur, normal exam and chest x-ray:** • No specialized follow-up needed **Residual murmur, cardiomegaly, question of increased pulmonary artery pressure** **Should have periodic Doppler echocardiography to assess:** • Systolic murmur (VSD, tricuspid regurgitation, pulmonic stenosis, double-chambered right ventricle, subaortic stenosis) • Diastolic murmur Aorta regurgitation, pulmonary regurgitation • Pulmonary pressure increased (±Significant shunt) **Key points:** • Repeat surgery for small VSD is not recommended • Endocarditis prophylaxis required in: Unrepaired VSD Residual VSD patch leak Associated AI or pulmonary outflow tract obstruction

AR, Aortic regurgitation; *PS,* pulmonary stenosis; *VSD,* ventricular septal defect.
Adapted from Graham TP: Long-term care of patients with repaired congenital cardiac abnormalities, *Adv Cardiovasc Med* 5:1-12, 1998. and Mullins CE, Mayer DC: *Congenital heart disease: a diagrammatic atlas,* ed. I. Jasper Burns (developed as CD-ROM) by Scientific Solutions, 1998, John Wiley and Sons, Inc.

residual defects or sequelae require specialized follow-up. In VSD patients with right ventricular outflow tract obstruction, left ventricular outflow tract obstruction, aortic regurgitation that is unrepaired, and for adults with atrial or ventricular dysrhythmias, cardiac evaluation is necessary on an annual basis. When Eisenmenger physiology exists, cardiac exams also need to be undertaken at least on an annual basis, if not more frequently. Patients who had late repairs of moderate-sized or large defects should have follow-up every 1 to 2 years to assess for left ventricular dysfunction and elevated pulmonary pressures.[15]

Adult patients with a moderately restrictive VSD frequently have complaints of dyspnea or atrial fibrillation. In asymptomatic adults with a moderately restrictive VSD, VSD closure will be considered if the Qp/Qs is *greater than* 2:1. If these patients concomitantly have an elevated pulmonary pressure and dilatation of the left ventricle, closure is indicated because of diminished life expectancy. In general reoperation is required in 4 percent to 6 percent of patients with an isolated VSD.[30,31] About 4 percent of the postoperative patients need a pacemaker.[31] Repeat surgery for a small VSD is not recommended (see Table 71-3).

Simple to Moderate Congenital Heart Defects

Some congenital heart defects can be considered simple if they are isolated form, but of moderate severity if they are associated with other anomalies. Defects of moderate severity are described in Box 71-2. Here we describe congenital aortic stenosis, pulmonary stenosis, atrioventricular septal defect (AVSD), and coarctation of the aorta (CoA).

Congenital Aortic Stenosis

The incidence of congenital aortic stenosis is 0.4/1000 live births.[1] It occurs four times higher in males than in females.[8] A congenital stenosis of the aorta is characterized by an obstruction of the outflow of the left ventricle. Three types of congenital aortic stenosis can be identified: valvular, subvalvular, and supravalvular. Valvular aortic stenosis is the most common form, occurring in 3 percent to 6 percent of all congenital heart defects, and is mostly the result of a bicuspid aortic valve. In about 20 percent of the patients, the valvular aortic stenosis is associated with other heart defects, mainly with COA (see below) or PDA.

Primary subvalvular aortic stenosis comes in three varieties: hypertrophic cardiomyopathy, membranous type, and tunnel type. Hypertrophic cardiomyopathy results in a local hypertrophy of the ventricular septum in the part that forms the left ventricular outflow tract. The membranous type is characterized by a fibrous ring that encircles and therefore narrows the outflow tract of the left ventricule. The tunnel type corresponds with a relatively long and narrow outflow tract. For subvalvular aortic stenosis, there is a male preponderance of 2:1.

Supravalvular aortic stenosis is uncommon and refers to a stenosis of the ascending aorta. Three types of supravalvular stenosis have been described: hourglass, hypoplastic, and membranous. The hourglass is the variation most likely to be seen. The shape of the ascending aorta yields the name of this type. In the hypoplastic type, the entire ascending aorta is narrow, which causes a severe obstruction of the outflow. The membranous type is characterized by a fibrous ring in the ascending aorta. Supravalvular aortic stenosis occurs seldom in isolation; it is usually part of the Williams syndrome, a developmental disorder involving connective tissue and the central nervous system.

Congenital aortic stenosis is treated by balloon or surgical valvuloplasty (see Chapter 69). If valvotomy results in aortic regurgitation, aortic valve replacement may be indicated.

Long-Term Survival and Complications

The 25-year survival of patients treated for aortic stenosis is about 75 percent.[6] However, the 25-year rate of event-free survival, free from associated complications, such as infective endocarditis, heart failure, reoperation, or valve replacement, is only 25 percent to 50 percent.[6] Residual or recurrent stenosis, aortic regurgitation, elevated end-diastolic pressure, and dilated aortic root are common after aortic stenosis repair (Table 71-4). The classic symptoms of severe aortic stenosis are angina pectoris, syncope or near syncope, and heart failure.

Follow-Up and Management at Adult Age

Patients with mild and isolated aortic valve disease can be followed in the community. For patients with significant residual effects, follow-up visits in a regional adult congenital heart disease center every 1 to 2 years are recommended.[15]

Symptomatic patients should be treated aggressively because morbidity and mortality increase once symptoms appear.[8] Therefore not only patients with critical aortic stenosis, but also those with dyspnea, angina, dysrhythmias, presyncope, or syncope should undergo intervention. Valve replacement is done using the Ross procedure. In this operation, the aortic valve is replaced with the patient's own pulmonary valve, and then a pulmonary allograft is used to replace the pulmonary valve. The main advantage of the Ross operation compared with insertion of a mechanical valve is the ability to avoid lifelong Coumadin therapy. However, progressive pulmonary homograft regurgitation and neoaortic valve regurgitation make these patients prone to needing future valve replacement.

Pulmonary Stenosis

Twenty-five percent to 30 percent of all patients with congenital heart disease have one form of right ventricle outflow obstruction, which can be seen at the valvular, subvalvular, and supravalvular level. In 90 percent of the cases, right ventricle outflow tract obstruction is at the valvular level, referred to as pulmonary stenosis. This latter defect constitutes 10 percent to 12 percent of the cases of congenital heart disease in adults.[8] Pulmonary stenosis caused by a dysplastic valve is often part of the Noonan syndrome, which includes noncardiac abnormalities, such as small stature, possible mental

■■■

TABLE 71-4   COMPLICATIONS AND FOLLOW-UP REQUIREMENTS AFTER REPAIR OF CONGENITAL AORTIC STENOSIS

TYPE OF DEFECT	LONG-TERM COMPLICATIONS	LONG-TERM FOLLOW-UP NEEDS

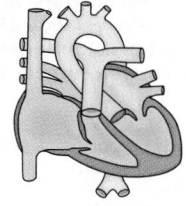
Valvular AS
 	
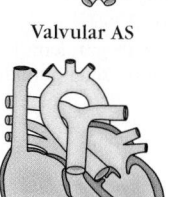
Subvalvular AS
 	
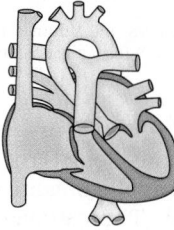
Supravalvular AS
	Relatively common:
	• Residual or recurrent stenosis
	• Aortic regurgitation
	• Elevated end-diastolic pressure
	Rare:
	• Mitral valve abnormalities
	• Heart block
	• Dysrhythmias:
	  • Ventricular tachycardia
	  • Sudden death
		Doppler echocardiography usually needed to assess:
		• LV-aortic gradient
		• Aortic regurgitation
		• Presence of mitral regurgitation
		• LV hypertrophy, ventricular size and function
		Treadmill test:
		• Presence of ischemic symptoms
		Key points:
		• ECG not extremely sensitive for LV hypertrophy
		• T-wave abnormalities can persist postoperatively despite a good hemodynamic result
		• Discrete subaortic stenosis recurs frequently
		• Endocarditis prophylaxis required in:
		  Unoperated AS
		  Postoperative or repaired AS
		  Bicuspid aortic valve

AS, Aortic stenosis; *LV,* left ventricular.
Adapted from Graham TP: Long-term care of patients with repaired congenital cardiac abnormalities, *Adv Cardiovasc Med* 5:1-12, 1998. and Mullins CE, Mayer DC: *Congenital heart disease: a diagrammatic atlas,* ed. I, Jasper Burns (developed as CD-ROM) by Scientific Solutions, 1998, John Wiley and Sons, Inc.

retardation, hypertelorism (eyes widely set), low-set ears, and webbed neck.

Supravalvular pulmonary stenosis results from the narrowing of the pulmonary trunk, its bifurcation, or its peripheral branches. This defect is often associated with other congenital cardiac abnormalities, such as valvular pulmonary stenosis, ASD, VSD, PDA or TOF.[8] Supravalvular pulmonic stenosis is a common feature of Williams syndrome. Balloon valvuloplasty is indicated in critical pulmonary stenosis or if the right ventricular systolic pressures are 50 mm Hg or greater. If balloon valvuloplasty is not successful in critical stenosis, surgery with muscle resection or patch repair is required. Sometimes the pulmonary valve is completely removed.

Long-Term Survival and Complications

Life expectancy depends on the severity of the stenosis. Patients with mild pulmonary stenosis and those who have undergone balloon valvuloplasty have an excellent survival.[32,33] They must, however, be periodically evaluated for mild residual pulmonary stenosis or for pulmonary regurgitation that can occur as a result of the valvuloplasty (Table 71-5). Moderate valvular outflow tract obstruction may progress in 20 percent of unoperated patients, especially in adults, because of valve calcification.

Follow-Up and Management at Adult Age

Patients with mild pulmonic stenosis require follow-up visits every 3 to 5 years. When moderate to severe stenosis or regurgitation is observed, follow-up should be intensified to a visit every 1 to 2 years.[15] Although survival rates are good, a substantial number of patients will require reintervention as adults. The actuarial reintervention-free rate at 10 years was 84 percent.[34] However, after 25 years, the percentage of patients who need reintervention significantly increases to 33 percent, 50 percent, and 80 percent at 30, 40, and 45 years of follow-up, respectively.[35]

Intervention is required if the combined gradient across the right ventricular outflow tract is *greater than* 50 mm Hg at rest; if symptoms, such as exertional dyspnea, angina, presyncope, or syncope, are present; if there is severe pulmonary regurgitation associated with reduced exercise capacity; or if there is evidence of deteriorating right ventricular function. Dysplastic valves are usually poorly responsive to balloon valvuloplasty. In these patients, surgical valvotomy, complete valvec-

■ ■ ■

TABLE 71-5 COMPLICATIONS AND FOLLOW-UP REQUIREMENTS AFTER REPAIR OF PULMONARY STENOSIS

TYPE OF DEFECT	LONG-TERM COMPLICATIONS	LONG-TERM FOLLOW-UP NEEDS

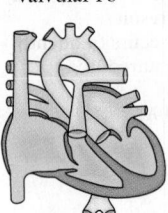
Valvular PS
 	
Branch PS
	Common:
	• Mild PS
	• Mild pulmonary regurgitation
	Rare:
	• Severe PS
	• Severe pulmonary regurgitation
	• Right ventricular dysfunction
		Most patients need Doppler echocardiography:
		• Residual gradient common (usually *less than* 25 mm Hg peak systolic): usually requires no treatment
		Balloon valvuloplasty very successful; surgery rarely needed
		Key points:
		• Dysplastic valve usually poorly responsive to balloon treatment; valvectomy may be necessary
		• Endocarditis prophylaxis:
		  • Recommended—trivial PS
		  • Required—mild to moderate PS gradient
		  • Required—after repair with residual pulmonary insufficiency

PS, Pulmonary stenosis.
Adapted from Graham TP: Long-term care of patients with repaired congenital cardiac abnormalities, *Adv Cardiovasc Med* 5:1-12, 1998. and Mullins CE, Mayer DC: *Congenital heart disease: a diagrammatic atlas,* ed. I, Jasper Burns (developed as CD-ROM) by Scientific Solutions, 1998, John Wiley and Sons, Inc.

tomy, or occasionally valve replacement may be necessary (see Chapter 69).

Atrioventricular Canal Defect

Atrioventricular septal defects, also called AV canal septal defects or endocardial cushion defects, represent 3 percent of all congenital heart diseases. Essentially, this defect is a combination of both an ASD (primum) and a VSD. In patients with a complete AVSD, the endocardial cushions do not develop, resulting in a common AV valve, a primum ASD, and a VSD. Incomplete or partial AV canal defects typically consist of a primum ASD with a cleft mitral valve without VSD. VSD, if present, is typically restrictive.[22,23] Although an AVSD can occur in those with normal chromosomes, it is much more frequently found in patients with Down syndrome.[1]

Patients with an AVSD have invariably undergone some surgical intervention in infancy or childhood for incomplete or complete AVSD repair. Incomplete repair includes an ASD patch closure and a mitral cleft suture. Complete repair includes not only ASD and VSD patch closure, but also mitral and tricuspid valve repair with valve reconstruction using available tissue from the common AV valve leaflets.

Long-Term Survival and Complications

Actuarial survival of patients with surgical correction of an AVSD after 20 years is 65 percent.[36] However, long-term survival of patients with a complete AVSD is significantly reduced compared with patients with an primum ASD.[36] Patients with an unoperated AVSD progress to cyanotic congenital heart disease accompanied by pulmonary hypertension, as discussed below.

Patients with this AVSD are at risk for developing tricuspid and mitral regurgitation, atrial or ventricular tachydysrhythmias, AV block, heart failure, and pulmonary vascular disease (Table 71-6).

Follow-Up and Management at Adult Age

Because of the risk of complications, long-term follow-up every 1 to 2 years in a regional adult congenital heart disease center is recommended.[15] The estimated incidence of reoperation in an AVSD is 25 percent over 20 years with a partial AVSD being lower at 12 percent over 20 years.[37] The most common reasons for reoperation are AV valve replacement or annuloplasty, relief of left ventricular outflow tract obstruction, residual ASD closure, and pacemaker implantation.[36,37]

Coarctation of the Aorta

Coarctation of the aorta is a relatively common heart defect, occurring in 5 percent to 9 percent of all congenital heart defects. This defect occurs twice as frequently in boys than in girls. CoA involves a discrete obstruction in the aorta, usually resulting from a sling of tissue from the ductus arteriosus, which creates a diaphragm-like ridge in the aorta. This ridge obstructs aortic blood flow within the lumen, typically just below the left subclavian artery, resulting in upper extremity hypertension and decreased blood pressure in the lower extremities (postductal type).

CoA may be diagnosed on physical exam by taking blood pressures in all four extremities. If the coarctation site is proximal to the left subclavian artery (preductal type), there will be a significant difference in the arterial pressure in the right and left arms. In some cases clinical findings are less pronounced as a result of development of significant collateral circulation. In these patients, however, atypical signs, such as hypertension, leg claudication, and rib notching on x-ray, should raise suspicion of the presence of CoA.

CoA can occur in isolated form, but it is most often associated with other cardiac defects, including PDA, VSD, mitral valve stenosis, and valvular or subvalvular

■ ■ ■

TABLE 71-6 COMPLICATIONS AND FOLLOW-UP REQUIREMENTS AFTER REPAIR OF ATRIOVENTRICULAR CANAL DEFECTS

TYPE OF DEFECT	LONG-TERM COMPLICATIONS	LONG-TERM FOLLOW-UP NEEDS

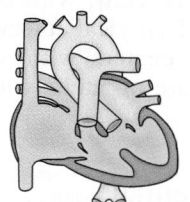
Endocardial cushion defect
(AV canal)
	Common:
	• Mild mitral regurgitation
	• Mild tricuspid regurgitation
	Rare:
	• Severe mitral or tricuspid regurgitation
	• Residual left to right shunt
	• Mitral stenosis
	• Tricuspid stenosis
	• Subaortic stenosis
	• Pulmonary vascular obstructive disease
	• Dysrhythmias:
	  • Heart block
	  • Atrial flutter
	  • Atrial fibrillation
	Sudden death
		Most patients need Doppler echocardiography and x-ray.
		If pulmonary hypertension is supposed, catheterization evaluation is usually needed.
		Key points:
		• Mitral regurgitation frequently can be treated without valve replacement; sutures placed at surgery may have pulled out.
		• Mild mitral and/or tricuspid regurgitation usually does not require treatment.
		• Endocarditis prophylaxis required for:
		  • Unrepaired
		  • Repaired with residual lesions

Adapted from Graham TP: Long-term care of patients with repaired congenital cardiac abnormalities, *Adv Cardiovasc Med* 5:1-12, 1998. and Mullins CE, Mayer DC: *Congenital heart disease: a diagrammatic atlas*, ed. I. Jasper Burns (developed as CD-ROM) by Scientific Solutions, 1998, John Wiley and Sons, Inc.

aortic stenosis.[8] In about three quarters of the patients with coarctation, the aortic valve is bicuspid, and in 3 percent to 5 percent of the patients, intracerebral aneurysms may occur. Additionally, 35 percent of the patients diagnosed with the genetic disorder Turner syndrome will have CoA.

Most patients with CoA will have undergone surgical repair in infancy or childhood. It is recommended that all patients with CoA, regardless of absent clinical symptoms, undergo repair since unrepaired patients have a lower life expectancy as a result of heart failure, cerebral hemorrhage, infective endocarditis, or dissection of the aorta.[38]

Long-Term Survival and Complications

Thirty-year survival rate after surgical correction for CoA is reported to be 72 percent to 82 percent.[39] If the repair occurred between ages 20 and 40, the 25-year survival is 75 percent.[8] The most common late-onset complications are residual or recurrent CoA, systemic hypertension, and, in the case of bicuspid aortic valve, aortic regurgitation or stenosis (Table 71-7). Less com-

■ ■ ■

TABLE 71-7 COMPLICATIONS AND FOLLOW-UP REQUIREMENTS AFTER REPAIR OF COARCTATION OF THE AORTA

TYPE OF DEFECT	LONG-TERM COMPLICATIONS	LONG-TERM FOLLOW-UP NEEDS

Endocardial cushion defect
(AV canal)
	Relatively common:
	• Residual or recurrent CoA
	• Systemic hypertension
	• Bicuspid aortic valve: aortic regurgitation or stenosis
	Rare:
	• Aneurysm (much higher incidence in prosthetic patch or angioplasty)
	• Aortic dissection
	• Intracranial Berry aneurysm
	• Mitral valve abnormalities
	• Subaortic stenosis
	• Mitral regurgitation
		If significant murmur and/or:
		• Blood pressure abnormality: Doppler echocardiography
		• Measure blood pressure in all four extremities, use pencil Doppler study
		Treadmill test if blood pressure is abnormal
		MRI if aneurysm is supposed, prepregnancy
		Catheterization when balloon dilatation and/or stent placement are being considered
		Key points:
		• Rarely, patients have aberrant right subclavian arteries arising below the coarctation and left subclavian arteries involved in coarctation anatomy or repair. In these patients. arm-leg blood pressure gradients are not useful.
		• Doppler echocardiography is helpful to assess gradients.
		• Absence of significant collateral vessels may increase risk for paraplegia with repeat operation.
		• Residual obstruction can be due to a small transverse arch.
		• Endocarditis prophylaxis required for:
		  Unrepaired
		  Repaired

COA, Coarctation of aorta.
Adapted from Graham TP: Long-term care of patients with repaired congenital cardiac abnormalities, *Adv Cardiovasc Med* 5:1-12, 1998. and Mullins CE, Mayer DC: *Congenital heart disease: a diagrammatic atlas*, ed. I. Jasper Burns (developed as CD-ROM) by Scientific Solutions, 1998, John Wiley and Sons, Inc.

monly aneurysms at the site of operation can occur. Patients should undergo regular cardiac magnetic resonance imaging (MRI) to detect potential aneurysms. Recoarctation is presumed when there is a difference in blood pressure of more than 30 mm Hg between the upper and lower extremities.

There is increasing evidence that patients with CoA are prone to arterial hypertension and subsequent coronary heart disease because of arterial wall stiffness and alterations in vascular reactivity.[40-43] Indeed both functional data and histological findings suggest a systemic vascular disease of the prestenotic arteries, even after successful surgical repair.[40,44] Coronary artery disease is the most common cause of death in patients with CoA.[45-48]

Follow-Up and Management at Adult Age

CoA is typically considered as a heart defect of moderate severity. Therefore follow-up visits should be scheduled every 1 to 2 years,[15] preferably in an adult congenital heart disease center.

Because hypertension is a common complication, aggressive risk factor management should be done for prevention of general acquired heart disease. Angiotensin-converting enzyme **(ACE)** inhibitors and beta blockers are particularly useful in the management of these patients.[22] If recoarctation or aneurysm occur, reintervention is required.

When the anatomy permits, interventional catheter therapy, with balloon angioplasty alone or with a stent, is now the preferred therapy for recurrent coarctation. Catheter-based intervention in native or unoperated CoA is less well established.[39] Aneurysms at repair sites are treated surgically or, more recently, with covered stents. Both catheter-based and surgical intervention should only be undertaken at centers with specific training and expertise in the care of adults with congenital heart disease.

Moderate to Severe Congenital Heart Defects
Tetralogy of Fallot

TOF accounts for about 10 percent of all congenital heart disease and has an equal sex distribution. The components of this cyanotic tetrad include a nonrestrictive VSD, severe pulmonary stenosis causing obstruction to pulmonary blood flow, right ventricular hypertrophy, and various degrees of overriding or dextroposition of the aorta (Table 71-8). The degree of pulmonary obstruction is a primary determinant of clinical presentation with the most severe variant being pulmonary atresia with VSD **(PA-VSD).** Most patients are diagnosed and undergo surgical repair in infancy. Occasionally, patients with mild pulmonary obstruction

■ ■ ■

TABLE 71-8   COMPLICATIONS AND FOLLOW-UP REQUIREMENTS AFTER REPAIR OF TETRALOGY OF FALLOT

TYPE OF DEFECT	LONG-TERM COMPLICATIONS	LONG-TERM FOLLOW-UP NEEDS
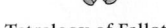 Tetralogy of Fallot	**Relatively common:** • Pulmonary regurgitation • Pulmonary artery stenosis (left *greater than* right) • Right ventricular outflow tract obstruction • Conduit or homograft stenosis (pulmonary atresia/VSD variant) **Rare:** • Pulmonary valvular stenosis • Residual VSD • Dysrhythmias: 　Heart block 　Atrial flutter 　Atrial fibrillation 　Ventricular tachycardia 　Residual aorticopulmonary shunt • Acquired left pulmonary artery atresia after Potts shunt takedown (Potts shunt: descending aorta to left pulmonary artery, side-to-side anastomosis) • Acquired pulmonary artery stenosis after Waterston shunt takedown (Waterston shunt: ascending aorta to right pulmonary artery, side-to-side anastomosis) • Aortic regurgitation • SAS	**Cardiomegaly, loud murmur, symptoms: Doppler echocardiography and cardiac catheterization to assess for:** • PS • Pulmonary regurgitation • Pulmonary artery stenosis • Residual VSD? • Right and left pulmonary artery size • Right ventricular function • Tricuspid regurgitation **Palpitations, ectopic beats: Holter monitoring, exercise stress testing, CardioMemo recorder, electrophysiology study if needed (definitely when symptomatic)** **Key points:** • Very common: systolic/diastolic murmur at ULSB; may represent only mild PS or PR. • If RV-RA conduit or homograft used for repair, significant systolic murmur and progressive obstruction relatively uncommon. • Symptomatic dysrhythmias need urgent work-up. • Left pulmonary artery stenosis and pulmonary regurgitation relatively common; usually need cardiac catheterization for complete evaluation; consideration for pulmonary artery balloon angioplasty and/or pulmonary valve replacement. • The decision to replace pulmonary valve is a difficult one: assess symptoms, exercise ability, heart size, RV function, and tricuspid regurgitation. Valve replacement should be performed before right ventricular dysfunction becomes more than mild. • Endocarditis prophylaxis required for: 　Unoperated, palliated or repaired TOF

PR, Pulmonary regurgitation; *PS,* pulmonary stenosis; *RV,* right ventricular; *SAS,* subvalvular aortic stenosis; *TOF,* tetralogy of Fallot; *ULSB,* upper left sternal border.

Adapted from Graham TP: Long-term care of patients with repaired congenital cardiac abnormalities, *Adv Cardiovasc Med* 5:1-12, 1998. and Mullins CE, Mayer DC: *Congenital heart disease: a diagrammatic atlas,* ed. I, Jasper Burns (developed as CD-ROM) by Scientific Solutions, 1998, John Wiley and Sons, Inc.

and minimal cyanosis may be seen in adulthood, but the majority will have undergone a palliative shunt procedure or total repair during childhood.

Long-Term Survival and Complications

Long-term survival after correction ranges from 86 percent to 95 percent after 30 to 35 years.[49,50] Older age at repair is associated with decreased survival. The majority of patients who undergo total correction lead full and productive lives with little to no physical restrictions.[51] However, the typical patient with unrepaired TOF has mild to moderate cyanosis, clubbing, and erythrocytosis or excess erythrocytes.

Morbidity and mortality associated with long-term postoperative TOF include heart failure, sudden death presumably caused by ventricular dysrhythmias and endocarditis. The most frequent problem encountered after TOF repair is pulmonary regurgitation as the result of surgical repair of the right ventricular outflow tract. Pulmonary regurgitation can lead to right ventricle dilatation and eventually right ventricular dysfunction.[52,53] These patients often have dyspnea or complain of effort intolerance. Patients may also have residual or recurrent right ventricular outflow tract obstruction. Ventricular dysrhythmias are associated with ventricle dilatation, repair at older age, and repair via right ventriculotomy. Long-term problems that occur less frequently are reported in Table 71-8.

Adults who have undergone palliative shunt procedures in infancy may experience distortion of the pulmonary arteries (e.g., thrombosis or occlusion) and pulmonary vascular disease when the shunt is too large. The latter creates volume overload on the ventricle and pulmonary vascular disease rendering the patient inoperable.

Follow-Up and Management at Adult Age

Follow-up visits with the cardiologist are needed every 1 to 2 years.[15] When right ventricular outflow tract obstruction and pulmonary regurgitation occur, reintervention is required. Reoperation is needed in about 7.5 percent of the TOF patients.[54] Currently, pulmonary valves are replaced with bioprosthetic or homograft valves. Percutaneous implantation of the pulmonary valve is becoming a valuable alternative for surgery in select patients.[55] Patients with transannular patches are currently not candidates for this procedure. Patients with residual or recurrent right ventricular outflow tract obstruction need either resection of infundibular muscle, pulmonary valvotomy, right ventricular outflow patch, transannular patch, or excision of the pulmonary valve. Severe obstruction or an absent pulmonary valve usually requires placement of a conduit from the right ventricle to the pulmonary artery. Patients with a residual VSD may require surgery at an adult age if the defect is of sufficient size. Adult intervention should only be undertaken at centers with specific training and expertise in the care of adults with congenital heart disease.

Complete Transposition of the Great Arteries

Complete transposition of the great arteries (**TGA**) occurs in 5 percent to 8 percent of all congenital heart diseases. There is a male preponderance in this defect,

with a sex ratio of 1:5.[56] In TGA the aorta arises from the right ventricle and is located anterior to the pulmonary artery, with the pulmonary artery arising from the left ventricle. Blood returning to the heart from the systemic circulation is ejected from the right ventricle into the aorta, sending unoxygenated blood back into the systemic circulation.

Natural survival is extremely rare, and survival into adulthood is dependent on the early use of palliative shunting procedures (atrioseptectomy, atrioseptostomy), a pulmonary artery banding to regulate pulmonary flow, and later, the atrial switch procedures known as the Mustard or Senning operations. Both of these procedures divert caval blood to the mitral valve and pulmonary venous blood to the tricuspid valve. In the Mustard procedure, venous blood is diverted to the mitral valve by means of an intraatrial baffle. In the Senning procedure, a tunnel is created within the right atrium that carries caval blood to the mitral valve. The Mustard and Senning operations have been replaced by the arterial switch operation because of complications, such as dysrhythmias, baffle obstruction, and progressive failure of the systemic right ventricle.

Long-Term Survival and Complications

The 20- and 30-year survival rates associated with the atrial switch procedures are 75 percent and 67 percent, respectively.[57] The long-term complications are significant because of the demand placed on the right ventricle to support the systemic circulation. In this respect, decreased right ventricular function and tricuspid regurgitation are common. In a 20-year postoperative course, about 40 percent of the patients experience at least one form of dysrhythmia, of which sinus node dysfunction and atrial flutter are most prevalent.[57] More details on postoperative complications and long-term follow-up needs are provided in Table 71-9.

The first patients who have undergone an arterial switch operation are now reaching adulthood. Long-term survival data associated with the arterial switch is therefore limited; however, an overall 10- to 15-year survival rate of 88 percent has been reported.[58] The majority of patients are asymptomatic, ventricular function is good, and rhythm disturbances are uncommon. The major long-term concern is the status of coronary arteries. Earlier studies reported kinking and obstruction of the reimplanted arteries resulting in myocardial ischemia and infarction. However, as the operative techniques have improved, the incidence of coronary insufficiency has been low. Survival without coronary events was 92.7 percent, 91 percent, and 88.2 percent at 1, 10, and 15 years, respectively.[59] Cardiac MRI for assessment of right ventricular function is optimal because of the documented limitations of using echocardiography in the context of a systemic right ventricle.

Follow-Up and Management at Adult Age

Follow-up at a regional adult congenital heart disease center after repair of TGA is recommended every 6 to 12 months.[15] Medical management is focused on support of a failing systemic right ventricle and treatment of dysrhythmias. Dysrhythmias are mainly treated using drugs or catheter radiofrequency ablation. Pacemakers

■ ■ ■

TABLE 71-9 COMPLICATIONS AND FOLLOW-UP REQUIREMENTS AFTER REPAIR OF TRANSPOSITION OF THE GREAT ARTERIES

TYPE OF DEFECT	LONG-TERM COMPLICATIONS	LONG-TERM FOLLOW-UP NEEDS

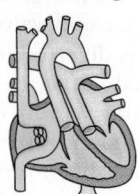
 	
Transposition of the great arteries
 	
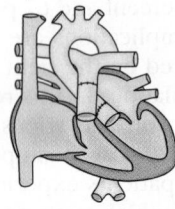
 	
Atrial switch procedure
"Mustard or Senning" baffle between atria
Baffle material:
  Mustard—pericardium
  Senning—atrial septum
 	
Arterial switch procedure—arteries are switched, and coronary buttons created
	After Mustard, Senning relatively common:
	• Right ventricular dysfunction
	• Sinus node dysfunction
	• Dysrhythmias:
	  • Bradydysrhythmias
	  • Atrial flutter, fibrillation
	  • Atrial tachycardia
	  • AV nodal tachycardia
	  • Tricuspid regurgitation
	  • Systemic venous baffle obstruction
	  • Mild LV outflow obstruction
	Rare:
	• Pulmonary venous baffle obstruction
	• Severe LV outflow obstruction; valvular or subvalvular PS, anomalous mitral valve attachment in LV outflow tract, aneurysm of the ventricular septum
	• Pulmonary vascular disease
	• Dysrhythmias:
	  Ventricular tachycardia
		Doppler echocardiography to assess:
		• RV function
		• Tricuspid regurgitation
		• LV outflow obstruction
		• Baffle obstruction
		• Pulmonary artery pressure
		Holter monitoring and/or cardiac event monitor for occurrence of symptomatic dysrhythmias
		Catheterization and stenting for symptomatic pulmonary venous obstruction
		Key points:
		• Patients with an associated VSD repair have a higher incidence of RV dysfunction and tricuspid regurgitation.
		• Symptomatic dysrhythmias require full work-up: definite incidence of late sudden death, probably related to tachydysrhythmias
		• Mild to moderate LV outflow tract obstruction well tolerated and usually does not require surgery
		• Mild to moderate systemic venous baffle obstruction without associated symptoms usually does not need treatment
		• Endocarditis prophylaxis required for:
		  Unoperated, repaired by atrial switch (Mustard, Senning) or Rastelli

LV, Left ventricular; *PS,* pulmonary stenosis; *RV,* right ventricular; *VSD,* ventricular septal defect.
Adapted from Graham TP: Long-term care of patients with repaired congenital cardiac abnormalities. *Adv Cardiovasc Med* 5:1-12, 1998. and Mullins CE, Mayer DC: *Congenital heart disease: a diagrammatic atlas,* ed. I. Jasper Burns (developed as CD-ROM) by Scientific Solutions, 1998, John Wiley and Sons, Inc.

are implanted in patients with sick sinus syndrome. The need for surgical reintervention is rather limited.[60] It is most frequently needed when baffle obstruction occurs, which has been more often observed in patients after the Mustard operation than after the Senning operation.[57] After the arterial switch operation, patients are followed for right and left ventricle outflow tract obstruction in the supravalvular areas as a result of suture line stenosis. If an outflow tract obstruction occurs, balloon angioplasty or surgical intervention with patch augmentation is the treatment of choice.

Congenitally Corrected Transposition of the Great Arteries

Congenitally corrected transposition of the great arteries **(CCTGA)** occurs in only 1 percent of all cardiac anomalies. In this form of transposed great arteries, the aorta arises from the right ventricle, and the pulmonary trunk arises from the left ventricle. However, the transposition is "corrected" by the fact that the ventricles are inverted, with the right ventricle on the left and the left

ventricle on the right. The circuit is physiologically correct, but the morphological right ventricle serves as the systemic ventricle. Since the AV valves follow the ventricles, the left-sided AV valve is the anatomical tricuspid valve, whereas the right-sided valve is the anatomical mitral valve. Also the coronary arteries mirror the normal situation.

CCTGA is frequently associated with VSD (60 percent), single-ventricle physiology (40 percent), pulmonary valve stenosis (30 to 50 percent), and with tricuspid valve regurgitation as the result of an Ebstein type of configuration (25 percent to 30 percent). Surgical intervention is only indicated to repair associated anomalies, such as a VSD or pulmonary stenosis, which if left unrepaired, can result in cyanosis or heart failure.

Long-Term Survival and Complications

In the adult setting, two groups of patients may be seen. First are patients in whom diagnosis and surgical correction occurred in infancy or childhood, but in long-term follow-up, residual VSDs or pulmonary stenosis are common. A second group of patients are those who have gone undiagnosed and are seen for the first time with clinical findings, such as dysrhythmias, systolic murmurs caused by a failing AV valve, atrial tachycardia, or AV block. Generally 20-year survival rates of 75 percent in patients with CCTGA are reported.[61]

Complications commonly seen in patients with CCTGA include right ventricular dysfunction, tricuspid regurgitation, residual left ventricle outflow obstruction, and complete heart block (Table 71-10). Heart failure occurs, most typically in the fifth decade, as the morphological right ventricle begins to fail as the systemic ventricle. Complete heart block is often present at birth; if not it is likely to develop at a rate of 2 percent per year, mainly because of the abnormal and prolonged course of the His bundle.

Follow-Up and Management at Adult Age

Because of the long-term sequelae associated with CCTGA, follow-up in a regional adult congenital heart disease center is recommended every 6 to 12 months.[15] The focus of treatment is to protect the integrity of the systemic ventricle by preventing dilatation and failure. Tricuspid valve repair or replacement may be indicated, but should only be undertaken if the right ventricular function is well preserved. Tricuspid valvuloplasty is rarely successful because of recurrent regurgitation. In patients without associated lesions, 27 percent needed a pacemaker. This percentage increased to 45 percent in patients with associated heart defects.[62]

To make the morphological left ventricle the systemic ventricle, the double switch operation has been developed. This operation consists of a combination of the atrial (Mustard or Senning) and the arterial switch operation (Jatene) or alternatively an atrial switch operation and a Rastelli operation. The Rastelli operation is a very extensive surgical procedure with high perioperative mortality and a substantial risk for developing the complications associated with both atrial and arterial switch. Moreover, a double switch operation is only feasible after training of the morphological left ventricle by surgically narrowing the pulmonary artery (arterial banding).

Single-Ventricle Physiology

The term single-ventricle physiology refers to a group of cardiac defects that share the common feature that only one of the two ventricles is of adequate functional size. Anomalies that are described as single-ventricle defects include tricuspid atresia, mitral atresia, double inlet left ventricle, AVSDs with a dominant left or right ventricle, hypoplastic left heart syndrome, univentricular heart with or without TGA, and some variations of double outlet right ventricle. Single-ventricle physiology is reported to occur in 1 percent to 2 percent of all congenital heart defects.[63] Tricuspid atresia is the most common form of single-ventricle physiology.

Most patients with a single-ventricle physiology die in infancy or early childhood unless palliative surgery is performed. Biventricular repair is usually not possible. Today all surgical approaches are either staged or pallia-

---

■ ■ ■

TABLE 71-10   COMPLICATIONS AND FOLLOW-UP REQUIREMENTS IN PATIENTS WITH CONGENITALLY CORRECTED TRANSPOSITION OF THE GREAT ARTERIES

TYPE OF DEFECT	LONG-TERM COMPLICATIONS	LONG-TERM FOLLOW-UP NEEDS
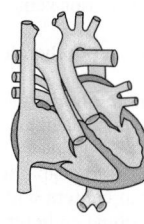 CCTGA	**Relatively common:** • Right ventricular dysfunction • Tricuspid regurgitation • Residual left ventricle outflow obstruction (left ventricle to pulmonary artery) • Dysrhythmias: 　Second-degree AV block 　Complete heart block **Rare:** • Dysrhythmias: 　Atrial flutter 　Atrial fibrillation 　Ventricular tachycardia 　Symptomatic aortic regurgitation	Doppler echocardiography to assess: • Tricuspid regurgitation • Occurrence of PS or VSD • Ventricular function Ambulatory ECG may be useful to assess heart block. **Catheterization or MRI may be useful for evaluation of RV dysfunction.** **Key points:** • Congestive heart failure occurs commonly in older adults. • Systemic AV valvular (tricuspid) regurgitation plays a role in progressive RV dysfunction. • Tricuspid valvuloplasty rarely successful • Tricuspid valve replacement frequently associated with worsening heart failure postoperatively • Mild aortic regurgitation common; virtually never severe • Some groups performing double switch (atrial and arterial) now in patients with systemic ventricular dysfunction • Endocarditis prophylaxis required for patients with: 　VSD 　Tricuspid regurgitation 　Aortic regurgitation 　Mitral regurgitation

Adapted from Graham TP: Long-term care of patients with repaired congenital cardiac abnormalities, *Adv Cardiovasc Med* 5:1-12, 1998. and Mullins CE, Mayer DC: *Congenital heart disease: a diagrammatic atlas,* ed. I, Jasper Burns (developed as CD-ROM) by Scientific Solutions, 1998, John Wiley and Sons, Inc.

tive in nature, each providing an atriopulmonary, AV, or cavopulmonary connection. The overall aim of these procedures is to direct systemic venous blood directly into the pulmonary artery via the right atrium or via an intracardiac or extracardiac conduit.

Long-Term Survival and Complications

Life expectancy after palliation for single-ventricle physiology is considerably lower than that of other congenital heart defects. It is reported that the 10-year survival rates following Fontan type of repair is about 60 percent.[64-66] Survival is, however, dependant on the type of underlying defect, with a substantially better survival rate for patients with tricuspid atresia compared with those with more complex congenital malformations.[67]

However, the long-term concerns associated with these surgical procedures persist. These include the physiological effects of persistent elevated right atrium pressure and elevated systemic venous pressure and problems with stenosis or obstruction of the conduit used in the different connections. Additional long-term complications associated with the Fontan and its modifications include a chronic low cardiac output state, development of atrial dysrhythmias, thromboembolism,

Fontan pathway obstruction, and protein-losing enteropathy **(PLE)** (Table 71-11).

Despite the often chronic problems associated with Fontan procedures, adult survivors lead a relatively normal life, are able to work, and women are able to have successful pregnancies.[68,69] However, pregnancy in these patients is associated with substantial complications and morbidity.[70]

Follow-Up and Management at Adult Age

Patients with univentricular physiology must be committed to long-term care and frequent follow-up in a regional adult congenital heart disease program.[15] Although the majority of patients with single-ventricle physiology are operated on during childhood, up to 58 percent of patients will require reoperation as adults.[71] Indications for reoperation included cyanosis, failing Fontan circulation or exercise intolerance, PLE, AV valve regurgitation, and dysrhythmias.[72] Revision or conversion of the Fontan connection is the most common reintervention.[71] In patients with a failing Fontan caused by ventricular failure or increased pulmonary resistance, heart or heart-lung transplantation becomes necessary as rescue therapy.[73]

■ ■ ■

TABLE 71-11   COMPLICATIONS AND FOLLOW-UP REQUIREMENTS AFTER REPAIR OF SINGLE VENTRICLE PHYSIOLOGY

TYPE OF DEFECT	LONG-TERM COMPLICATIONS	LONG-TERM FOLLOW-UP NEEDS

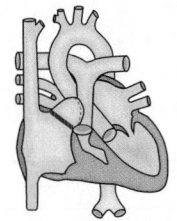
Fontan-Kreutzer in tricuspid atresia
 	
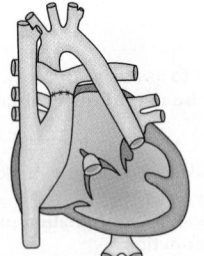
Fontan repair
 	
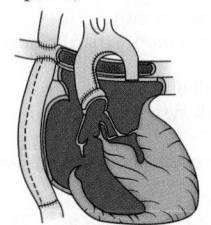
Total extracardiac conduit fontan palliation of hypoplastic left heart
	Relatively common before Fontan:
	• Ventricular dysfunction and/or congestive heart failure
	• AV valvular regurgitation
	• Atrial tachydysrhythmias
	• Pulmonary vascular disease
	After Fontan:
	• Ventricular dysfunction and/or congestive heart failure
	• AV valvular regurgitation
	• Dysrhythmias:
	  Atrial fibrillation
	    Atrial flutter
	    Sinus node dysfunction
	• Systemic venous congestion
	• Pulmonary artery stenosis
	• Thromboembolism
	Rare:
	• Arterial shunts or no operation (AR, ventricular dysrhythmia)
	• After Fontan (AR, ventricular dysrhythmia, late onset of cyanosis, dysrhythmia, pulmonary AV fistulae, systemic venous to left atrial connections, PLE, hepatic dysfunction)
		Doppler echocardiography to assess:
		• Fontan flow; ventricular function, AV valve regurgitation
		Cardiac catheterization for symptoms, check for baffle or pulmonary artery stenosis and cyanosis
		Key points:
		• PLE may respond to creation of ASD with decrease in central venous pressure and/or relief of even mild degrees of pulmonary artery stenosis or narrowed connection of right atrium and/or superior vena cava to pulmonary artery
		• Systemic AV valvular regurgitation poorly tolerated; should be treated aggressively
		• Sluggish venous flow can promote poorly tolerated thrombus formation; usually need aspirin and warfarin therapy
		• Baffle leaks with cyanosis may be amenable to percutaneous device closure of defect at centers with experience and expertise in interventional catheterization in congenital heart disease
		• Endocarditis prophylaxis required

ASD, Atrioseptal defect; *AV,* atrioventricular; *PLE,* protein-losing enteropathy.
Adapted from Graham TP: Long-term care of patients with repaired congenital cardiac abnormalities, *Adv Cardiovasc Med* 5:1-12, 1998. and Mullins CE, Mayer DC: *Congenital heart disease: a diagrammatic atlas,* ed. I, Jasper Burns (developed as CD-ROM) by Scientific Solutions, 1998, John Wiley and Sons, Inc.

Supraventricular dysrhythmias occur frequently in patients after Fontan operation. In a 15- to 20-year postoperative course, about 55 percent of the patients experience supraventricular tachycardia **(SVT)**, with the elapsed time after Fontan operation as the sole risk factor for reentrant tachycardia.[67,71] Electrophysiological ablation is the treatment of choice for these patients, with freedom from recurrent tachycardia of more than 80 percent.[67] In about 50 percent of the patients, a concomitant permanent pacemaker is also needed.[72,74]

CLINICAL PROBLEMS IN ADULT CONGENITAL HEART DISEASE

Among the challenges in caring for adult survivors of congenital heart disease are the clinical sequelae associated not only with the primary cardiac defect but also with the long-term postoperative follow-up. The most common clinical problems that require continuous monitoring and evaluation include dysrhythmias, heart failure, bacterial endocarditis, Eisenmenger complex, and hematological consequences of cyanotic heart disease. Additionally, because of the potential risk that pregnancy carries in a setting of congenital heart disease, it is now regularly addressed as a clinical issue for female patients.

Dysrhythmias

Cardiac rhythm disturbances are one of the more common problems associated with long-term survival of congenital heart disease. The clinical manifestation can vary in severity, ranging from asymptomatic dysrhythmias to sudden death. In long-term follow-up studies of common congenital heart defects (VSD, ASD, PDA, pulmonary stenosis, and CoA), it has been consistently reported that despite living normal lives, patients were at risk for developing late dysrhythmias.[75] The reported high incidence of dysrhythmia in the adult with congenital heart disease demonstrates the need for diligent follow-up in high-risk patients because recurrent or incessant dysrhythmia can lead to gradual hemodynamic and clinical deterioration.

In the postoperative patient, dysrhythmias occur as the result of irritable foci caused by abnormal pressure and/or volume changes, in addition to reentrant circuits created by septal patches and suture lines.[76] For example, patients who underwent repair for TOF in the early years of congenital heart surgery may have undergone right ventriculotomy and large right ventricular muscle resection, which predisposes them to ventricular dysrhythmias and sudden death.[77] Progressive changes in these patients may also include myocardial fibrosis of the right ventricle, with corresponding slowing of conduction (right bundle branch block) increasing the incidence of reentrant ventricular dysrhythmias.

Some patients with "older" versions of an operative procedure that has since been revised may have serious rhythm disorders. For example, about 50 percent of the Fontan patients who had an early connection of right atrium to pulmonary artery **(RAPA)** anastomosis or conduit repair are likely to develop intraatrial reentry tachycardia **(IART)** within 20 years of surgery.[67] There are no specific factors to predict who will or will not develop

dysrhythmias after surgical repair. It is generally agreed, however, that an older patient,[67,78,79] the patient repaired later in life,[79] or one with compromised hemodynamic status are more likely to develop dysrhythmias.[80]

In patients who remain unrepaired, cardiac disturbances are often the result of a complication or electrophysiological instability associated with the primary congenital defect. For example, patients with Ebstein anomaly, a defect that involves downward displacement of the tricuspid valve into the right ventricle, may have rapid heart action resulting from SVT. These rhythm disturbances, which have been reported to occur in 25 percent to 30 percent of patients, represent reentrant SVT, atrial fibrillation, and atrial flutter, and are not necessarily related to accelerated or anomalous AV conduction.[81,82] Ebstein anomaly is also associated with preexcitation patterns such as Wolff-Parkinson-White (WPW), which usually represents a right bypass tract.

Several congenital heart anomalies will show evidence of AV conduction abnormalities. For example, first-degree AV block is characteristically seen in endocardial cushion defects (as in ostium primum). Atrial fibrillation and flutter are frequently encountered in patients who develop volume overload. Lesions, such as ASD or VSD, that produce significant left-to-right shunting will, over time, develop atrial tachydysrhythmias. Ventricular dysrhythmias are characteristically seen in the setting of long-standing volume overload and/or ventricular failure and in conditions where there has been chronic pressure overload of the left ventricle as seen in aortic valve disease and palliative systemic-pulmonary shunts.

Management

Management of cardiac dysrhythmias in congenital heart disease has evolved rapidly over the past decades. Current therapies include antidysrhythmic medications, catheter- and device-based therapies and surgical interventions. Antidysrhythmic medications remain the primary treatment modality for most acute dysrhythmias; however, the long-term use of these medications has proven disappointing because of frequently severe adverse effects. For this reason, antidysrhythmic medications are increasingly used in conjunction with other forms of therapy, such as catheter ablation, implantable cardioverter-defibrillator **(ICD)** therapy, and/or pacemaker implantation.

Radiofrequency ablation has been successful for treatment of incessant atrial flutter and ventricular tachycardia and for atrial dysrhythmias originating from areas of a surgical scar. Surgical intervention is indicated in cases of refractory dysrhythmias. They have had good results in treatment of accessory pathway-mediated tachycardia and in AV node reentrant tachycardia.[83] For the best result, a combined approach of surgical revision of the original operation (e.g., Fontan procedure) with cryoablation done under intraoperative electrophysiological mapping is preferred.[84]

Heart Failure

Most congenital heart defects, operated on or not, have the potential to lead to clinical heart failure.[85] Heart failure in adults with congenital heart disease occurs as a result of excessive workload imposed by structural defects or by basic changes in myocardial performance. Excessive workload refers to a chronically pressure-overloaded systemic right ventricle (transposition after atrial correction or CCTGA) or left ventricle as a result of outflow obstruction (aortic stenosis or COA), failure of a volume-overloaded subpulmonic right ventricle (TOF with pulmonary regurgitation, Ebstein, and large left to right shunt), failure from single-ventricle physiology, or biventricular failure.[85]

Myocardial performance may be impaired either by changes in the chronotropic state of the heart, as observed with tachydysrhythmias that can arise as a result of a primary defect, or as a consequence of surgical intervention. The onset of symptoms of cardiac failure in the adult with congenital heart disease is not predictable. Therefore it is important to continue follow-up on patients with congenital heart defects who have residual effects.

Assessment

Ascertaining volume status and filling pressures in patients with congenital heart disease is difficult because of morphological abnormalities, residua, and sequelae from operations or the presence of intraatrial baffles or direct caval-pulmonary connections. Therefore symptoms of volume overload, such as paroxysmal nocturnal dyspnea, orthopnea, and abdominal distention, may be the best indicators of heart failure in the congenital population.

To date, evidence on the diagnostic and prognostic value of neurohormonal markers in congenital heart disease is increasing. It has been determined that natriuretic peptides, neurohormones, and several inflammatory cytokines, all products of the failing heart, are present in elevated concentrations in the circulation of patients with congenital heart disease of all types.[86] In some patient groups, neurohormonal activation is associated with ventricular function, cardiopulmonary exercise capacity, or functional status[87,88] and can therefore be used as a therapeutic target and to evaluate outcomes. However, determining the cause of neurohormone elevation in patients with congenital heart disease is difficult. For instance it is reported that all cyanotic congenital heart defects are associated with elevations of plasma atrial natriuretic peptide and brain natriuretic peptide levels, presumably from hypoxia.[89] Further research will guide the applicability of neurohormonal markers in congenital heart disease.

Management

In general, the standard heart failure treatment is also used for patients with congenital heart disease who experience a failing heart. However, the literature as to the appropriateness of this treatment is limited.[90] For instance few clinical trials have investigated the use of ACE inhibitors and beta blockers in patients with congenital heart disease. Future research is needed to close this knowledge gap.[90] Typical heart failure interventions are needed: educating with respect to daily weights, signs and symptoms of fluid retention, hidden sources of sodium, and self-adjustment of diuretics (see Chapter

64). These interventions are efficacious in the majority of patients with volume retention, irrespective of the underlying anatomy.[85]

Infective Endocarditis

Infective endocarditis is characterized by an inflammatory process involving the endothelial layers of the heart including cardiac valves and great vessels (see Chapter 73). In the adult patient with congenital heart disease, susceptibility to infective endocarditis is an essential concern in the management and long-term follow-up. Defects associated with high-velocity flow, or jet impact vortex shedding, present more endocarditic risk than low-pressure-high-flow lesions.[91] For example, left ventricular outflow tract lesions, such as aortic valve disease (bicuspid aortic valve or aortic stenosis), are usually found to be more at risk for endocarditis. However, in one collaborative study, 51 percent of right-sided lesions were found to have sites of infection and 46 percent of left sided lesions.[92] In surgically ligated or device-closed patent ductus, or a secundum ASD, the risk of endocarditis may be decreased or eliminated.[93]

All patients must be carefully evaluated for the presence of residual lesions or shunts that will necessitate continued measures for prevention of endocarditis. Individuals with prosthetic valves and other prosthetic material, such as conduits and shunts, should be included among those for whom lifelong prophylaxis is required.

The most common source of bacteremia is the oral cavity, with cleaning, filling, or extraction of teeth precipitating most events. These common dental procedures have been consistently associated with bacteremia and positive blood cultures in 12 percent to 85 percent of patients.[91] Additional sources of infection are found in Table 71-12. With good aseptic techniques, infection rates can be considered relatively low.

■ ■ ■

TABLE 71-12 SOURCES OF BACTEREMIA

Dental procedures	Cleaning of teeth Filling of teeth Extraction of teeth	
Surgical procedures	Open heart surgery	
	Noncardiac surgery	Gastrointestinal Genitourinary
Nails and skin	Infected acne Nail biting or picking Tattooing Body piercing IV drug use	
Invasive procedures	Obstetrical	Vaginal delivery
	Gynecological	Abortion Insertion of contraceptive device
	Genitourinary procedures in males	
	Gastrointestinal	Sigmoidoscopy Colonoscopy

Prevention and Management

In view of the serious nature of infective endocarditis, any measure that either corrects any structural congenital heart defect or lessens the risk of bacteremia will reduce the chance of acquiring endocarditis. Therefore it is imperative that long-term follow-up of at risk patients include regular discussions and counseling regarding preventive measures and signs and symptoms associated with infective endocarditis that must be reported (see below).

Eisenmenger Reaction

The incidence of Eisenmenger reaction in adults with congenital heart disease is unknown. A distinction between the terms Eisenmenger complex, Eisenmenger syndrome, and Eisenmenger reaction should be made. In 1958, Wood defined Eisenmenger complex as "pulmonary hypertension at systemic level, due to a high pulmonary vascular resistance (more than 800 dynes-sec/cm^5), with reversed or bidirectional shunting through a large ventricular septal defect (1.5 to 3 cm across).[94]" Eisenmenger syndrome was defined as any large congenital communication at the aorticopulmonary, ventricular, or atrial levels that behaved physiologically like Eisenmenger complex.[94] Finally, Eisenmenger reaction characterizes the development of Eisenmenger physiology in patients with a large congenital communication. Eisenmenger physiology is usually a consequence of delayed operation, the need for which has gone undetected until adolescence or adulthood when surgical repair is no longer possible. Although the incidence of Eisenmenger reaction is assumed to have declined in the Western world, some countries have high numbers of afflicted patients migrating from developing countries.

Eisenmenger reaction is associated with decreased oxygen saturation in the systemic circulation, cyanosis, and polycythemia, discussed below. The most common complaint is effort intolerance, including shortness of breath with exertion and fatigue. Palpitations are common and are most often caused by atrial fibrillation or flutter.[52]

Long-Term Survival and Complications

Today about half of the patients with Eisenmenger reaction can reach the fifth decade of life.[95] This rate of survival is much better than reported in previous studies.[96,97] Prognosis seems, however, to be dependent on the age at diagnosis. When diagnosis is made during adulthood, the estimated 10-year survival of patients is 58 percent.[98] Sudden death, presumably from dysrhythmias, is the usual cause of death. Other causes of death include heart failure, pulmonary infarction from arterial thrombosis, and complications of cerebral abscesses and stroke.

Although the quality of life of these patients is somewhat lower than that of patients with other congenital heart disease,[99] many patients can have a reasonably active and productive life.[100] However, pregnancy is contraindicated in females because of the high fetal and maternal mortality. Therefore counseling regarding permanent sterilization should be provided; contraceptive pills are often contraindicated because of the increased thrombogenesis.

Management

Patients with Eisenmenger reaction have uniquely complex needs, and it is essential that their care be followed closely by adult congenital heart specialists trained in the treatment of this physiology. Medical therapy is directed by the clinical presentation of the patient. The treatment of patients with Eisenmenger syndrome may include the use of supplemental oxygen, digitalis, diuretics, pulmonary vasodilator therapy, and anticoagulants.[101] Treatment of erythrocytosis is described below. Once Eisenmenger reaction has developed, closure of the systemic-to-pulmonary connection is not possible anymore because it is associated with increased mortality. The only definitive treatment is lung transplantation and repair of the congenital heart defect(s) or heart-lung transplantation.

Hematological Effects of Cyanotic Congenital Heart Disease

The hematological response to chronic hypoxemia of cyanotic congenital heart disease is a secondary erythrocytosis. Secondary erythrocytosis is an adaptive increase in red blood cell production designed to compensate for decreased systemic oxygen saturation. Because of erythropoietin production in response to tissue hypoxia, the result is an increase in the number of circulating red blood cells and expansion of whole blood volume. The increase in whole blood volume increases the oxygen-carrying capacity of the blood and maintains an adequate oxygen supply to metabolizing tissues. This hematological response, however, produces a number of adverse multisystemic physiological effects including hyperviscosity, iron deficiency anemia, bleeding diatheses, and several metabolic complications.

Clinically, patients can be divided into compensated or decompensated erythrocytosis. Patients with compensated erythrocytosis have established equilibrium in an iron-replete state where hyperviscosity symptoms are absent or mild. Hematocrit can range up to 70 percent. Decompensated erythrocytosis consists of patients who fail to establish equilibrium with rising hematocrit levels and report recurrent moderate to severe symptoms of hyperviscosity (Box 71-4) relieved only by phlebotomy.

BOX 71-4 ■ ■ ■
SYMPTOMS AND SIGNS OF HYPERVISCOSITY

- Altered mental state
- Bleeding diathesis
- Faintness, dizziness
- Fatigue
- Headache
- Impaired alertness
- Muscle weakness
- Myalgia
- Paresthesia of fingers, toes, lips
- Urate metabolism
- Visual disturbances

Hyperviscosity is associated with increased bleeding diatheses, which is attributed to platelet and coagulation-factor abnormalities. Bleeding tendencies and hemostatic problems are characterized by a number of symptoms, such as hemoptysis, epistaxis, and in some female patients, heavy menses. These problems, together with an injudicious use of phlebotomy, may lead to anemia and subsequently to iron deficiency in these patients.

Metabolic complications associated with secondary erythrocytosis may include diminished glomerular filtration rate, proteinuria, and hyperuricemia. The changes in urate metabolism can result in arthralgias and acute gouty arthritis.

Management

Therapeutic phlebotomy is reserved for patients with an elevated hematocrit (above 65 percent) who are symptomatic. If performed it should be done concomitant with isovolumic fluid replacement, particularly in patients with Eisenmenger physiology because they may experience hypotension and even sudden death. Frequent phlebotomy should be avoided because this can lead to rebound response from the bone marrow and iron deficiency anemia. Regular checks of hemoglobin, hematocrit, and mean cell volume (**MCV**) will help determine if recurring symptoms are related to increased red cell mass or iron deficiency. Attention should be paid to use of vasodilator therapy, which can cause a sudden decrease in systemic vascular resistance. Reduced stroke volume increased the right to left shunt, which can lead to increased cyanosis and tissue hypoxia.

Prophylactic administration of anticoagulants or aspirin should be avoided because neither is beneficial in prevention of thromboembolic disease and may reinforce hemostatic abnormalities and bleeding tendencies. The complex issues that encompass Eisenmenger reaction require that these patients are cared for in regional adult congenital heart disease facilities or at least under supervision of a regional center.

Pregnancy

Females born with congenital heart disease are reaching their childbearing years. Cardiac diseases complicate up to 23.5 percent of pregnancies in women with congenital cardiac abnormalities.[102] Providers must be prepared to counsel women in advance about the risk of pregnancy.

Profound hemodynamic alterations occur during pregnancy, labor and delivery, and in the postpartum period. These changes begin during the first 5 to 8 weeks of pregnancy and reach their peak late in the second trimester. Factors found to predict maternal cardiac complications include:

- Having a prior cardiac event
- Cyanosis or poor functional class
- Left heart obstruction
- Systemic ventricular dysfunction[103]

Maternal mortality is reported to be 2.7 percent in the entire population of women with congenital heart disease.[102] Specific subgroups, such as those with Eisenmenger reaction, have a 50 percent mortality risk.[104]

Physiological Changes in Pregnancy and Delivery
During Pregnancy

Blood volume increases 40 percent to 50 percent during normal pregnancy. The rise in blood volume is *greater than* the increase in red blood cell mass, contributing to a fall in hemoglobin (e.g., the "anemia of pregnancy"). Cardiac output rises 30 percent to 50 percent above baseline, peaking by the end of the second trimester, after which it reaches a plateau until delivery. The change in cardiac output is mediated by:

- Increased preload caused by the rise in blood volume
- Reduced afterload caused by a fall in systemic vascular resistance
- A rise in the maternal heart rate by 10 to 15 beats/min.

Stroke volume increases during the first and second trimesters, but declines in the third trimester because of caval compression by the gravid uterus. Blood pressure typically falls to 10 mm Hg below baseline by the end of the second trimester. The decline in blood pressure is mediated by a fall in systemic vascular resistance induced by hormonal changes and by the addition of a low-resistance circuit through the uteroplacental bed.

During Labor and Delivery

During labor and delivery, hemodynamic changes are dramatic. With each uterine contraction, 300 to 500 ml of blood is displaced into the general circulation. Stroke volume increases, with a resultant rise in cardiac output by an additional 50 percent with each contraction. Mean systemic pressure also rises, in part as a result of maternal pain and anxiety.

During Postpartum Period

During the postpartum period, hemodynamic changes are due to relief of vena caval compression after delivery. The resultant increase in venous return augments cardiac output and causes a brisk diuresis. Hemodynamic changes return to the prepregnant baseline within 3 to 4 weeks following delivery.

Risk Stratification

With respect to pregnancy risk, congenital or acquired cardiac lesions are generally classified as low, intermediate, or high risk lesions.

Low Risk Lesions

Lesions considered low risk include uncomplicated secundum type of ASD or an isolated VSD. Pregnancy is usually well tolerated with these lesions. PDA is not associated with additional maternal risk if the shunt is small to moderate and if pulmonary artery pressures are normal. These women may be followed by a community-based obstetrician. Antibiotic prophylaxis before labor and delivery is recommended for a VSD and PDA except in patients who are more than 6 months after repair.

Moderate Risk Lesions

Lesions or defects with residual effects after repair fall into the moderate risk category because they may present actual or potential risk for hemodynamic complications during pregnancy. These include COA with residual hypertension, TOF with moderate right ventricle outflow tract stenosis or residual VSD, and unrepaired TOF, ASD, or COA.

Women with residual effects or unrepaired defects should be referred to a cardiologist for evaluation before conception and ideally should undergo correction of the abnormality before becoming pregnant. Depending on the degree of residual effect and potential risk for ventricular dysfunction or dysrhythmia, it is often recommended that these women be delivered in an institution that has experience in managing high risk pregnancy, preferably one that understands the risks associated with congenital heart disease. Women who have undergone Fontan, Mustard, or Senning repair—defects for which pregnancy data are limited—even if clinically stable at the time pregnancy should be carefully followed in a regional center with clinical experience in managing complex congenital cardiac diseases. Antibiotic prophylaxis is recommended during labor and delivery.

High Risk Lesions

The high risk conditions, such as Eisenmenger physiology or severe ventricular dysfunction, are associated with increased maternal and fetal mortality. Pregnancy is not advised. If pregnancy should occur, therapeutic abortion is advised. These patients are best managed with the assistance of a cardiologist specialized in congenital heart disease.

Prepregnancy Assessment

Owing to the potential risk associated with pregnancy in congenital heart disease, patients should be advised to plan all pregnancies, particularly women who remain unrepaired or with residual effects. If discussions about pregnancy begin before becoming pregnant, time will be available for a full clinical evaluation to determine the risk associated with a pregnancy.

Genetic Transmission

The risk for genetic transmission is a concern of both male and female patients with congenital heart disease. Although transmission risk differs between the respective heart defects, it is generally accepted that the risk of heredity of the defect varies from 3 percent to 5 percent for males and from 5 percent to 8 percent for females.[105] A recent study reported a 2.7 percent risk if the mother was the one with congenital heart disease.[106] In a small number of patients, the heart defect is part of autosomal dominant syndromes (e.g., Marfan, Turner, hypertrophic cardiomyopathy, and deletion of chromosome 22q11). In these patients, recurrence risk is 50 percent. If the patient and spouse or partner are concerned about transmission risk or if the heart defect is associated with other genetic anomalies, referral for genetic counseling and screening is recommended.

COUNSELING ISSUES

Despite improved life expectancy, many patients have residua and sequelae from initial surgical or interventional procedures. These patients are prone to complications and often have social and psychological concerns. Assessment and counseling of the adult patient is imperative, particularly related to self-care.

Patient's Understanding of the Defect, Treatment, and Preventive Measures

To prevent complications and to improve overall health status, patients with congenital heart disease are expected to adopt adequate and lifelong health behaviors, using preventive measures for infective endocarditis, restricting rigorous physical activities, and adhering to prescribed medications. Self-care requires knowledge about the disease, its treatment, and essential lifestyle adaptations.

Many adult patients know little about their heart defect, the treatment, and the prevention of endocarditis. In a series of studies, only 54 percent to 68 percent of patients could name their heart defect[107-109]; 26 percent to 50 percent were able to locate the lesion on a diagram.[107,108] Knowledge of current medication regimen (78 percent to 98 percent) and former treatment modalities (53 percent to 95 percent) for the lesion were better.[107-109] Inadequate patient knowledge has been reported to be the reason for poor follow-up and symptoms of deterioration since less than half of patients could describe these aspects of self-care.[107] Some patients and families may erroneously believe that, because they were surgically corrected, their heart defect is no longer relevant and they are "cured."

Sixteen percent to 50 percent of patients could define or describe endocarditis,[107-110] but only 8 percent were aware that the most typical symptom of it was unexplained fever lasting more than 5 days.[107] Knowledge about risk factors for endocarditis varied significantly.[107,108] Dental abscesses, for instance, were correctly identified as a potential risk factor by 71 percent of patients, but poor nail and skin care was known by only 10 percent.[107,108]

Important areas for patient teaching are physical and vocational activity and reproductive issues. In one study,[107] one third did not know that they could engage in any activity that they believed they were capable of doing, but that competitive sports were prohibited.[107] In this same study, only one fourth of patients knew the rate of genetic transmission for their heart defect. Females were unaware that an intrauterine device was an inappropriate contraceptive method for them because of the increased risk of endocarditis.[107]

These data illustrate that, although these adults with congenital heart disease have lived with the condition for their entire lives, they understand it poorly. This lack of knowledge is usually because their parents assumed total responsibility for their care. Ideally, responsibility should be transferred to the patient as he or she becomes an adolescent.[111] These data demonstrate the need for a collaborative educational effort between parents, the patient, and providers. This education should begin in late childhood and continue throughout life-long follow-up. Topics to be included in structured patient education programs are discussed below.

Congenital Heart Disease and Treatment

Patients should be informed about the name and anatomy of their heart defect, using both medical and lay terms. This prepares patients to engage in discussions about their condition with health care professionals. To facilitate understanding, provide diagrams that patients can refer to at home. Even with simple heart defects, we need to illustrate and explain the type and progression of the lesion in detail; simply telling patients that they are doing well often causes misunderstanding and anxiety.[112]

Patients need to be educated about the past and current treatment options. More specifically, the type of operation performed should be explained and diagrammed so patients have full understanding of their current anatomy. They should be familiar with symptoms that require immediate reporting when they occur: dizziness, shortness of breath, palpitations, chest pain, fainting, increasing fatigue, and swollen ankles. Medication teaching should provide the name and dosing schedule, the reason or function of the drug, the most common side effects, and interactions with other drugs and foods.

Most patients will require lifelong medical follow-up, even if they are doing well. To keep patients motivated to schedule and attend outpatient visits, they must understand the purpose of follow-up. Most heart defects are operated on during childhood, but many will need reoperation during adulthood. An open discussion about the optimal timing for reoperation is critical.

Infective Endocarditis

Education on endocarditis should not be limited to anti-biotic prophylaxis.[113,114] Attention should be given to other health behaviors that decrease the risk of infection, such as good dental hygiene, regular dental visits, and careful skin and nail care. Because body piercing and tattooing are risk factors for endocarditis (see Chapter 73) and these procedures are popular among teenagers and young adults, this issue needs to be addressed during education. Although serious infection following tattooing and piercing are rare, it does occur.[115,116] For patients at risk for endocarditis because of transient bacteremia or those on an anticoagulant, tattooing should be discouraged.[117]

Patients must know how to recognize bacterial endocarditis if it occurs. Unexplained fever that persists for more than 5 days is most typical, so patients should be counseled to ask for blood cultures before antibiotics are administered.

Exercise and Activity Recommendations

Physical fitness is important for optimal physical and psychosocial development,[118] and regular exercise should be recommended for most patients with con-genital heart disease.[119] However, teach patients which activities are permitted and which are not so that both dangerous activities and inappropriate restrictions are avoided.[107]

Noncompetitive sports, such as swimming, cycling, walking, dancing, playing tennis, and soccer, are safe.[120,121] In general 30 minutes of moderate exercise each day is recommended for a heart-healthy lifestyle, and this recommendation is applicable to patients with congenital heart disease. Obviously, there is wide variability among patients, so individuals need to be able to recognize their physical limitations and to acknowledge signs of overexertion. If chest pain, shortness of breath, palpitations, or dizziness occurs, physical activity should be stopped immediately, and the cardiologist should be contacted.

Competitive sports or those that require heavy lifting (e.g., moving furniture) are prohibited for some patients, such as those with obstructive outflow lesions or pulmonary hypertension.[120,121] Sports with the risk of bodily collision (e.g., football) should be avoided by patients with a severely dilated aortic root or COA, at least during the first postoperative year. Patients taking an anticoagulant or an antiplatelet drug should avoid contact sports.[122]

Recently, task force 2 of the 36th Bethesda conference and the study group on sports cardiology of the European Society of Cardiology provided recommendations for patients with congenital heart disease who want to engage in competitive sports.[122,123] Refer to these recommendations for more details and when in doubt about the need for exercise testing.

Psychosocial Issues

Psychosocial functioning refers to a range of psychological and social issues faced by adults with congenital heart disease.

Academic Abilities

Several studies have reported that children with congenital heart disease can achieve an educational level equivalent to that of healthy peers, whereas others suggest that they have significant learning disabilities.[32,51,57,124-131] Of course these observations largely depended on whether patients with mental retardation were included. Indeed a high proportion of certain groups of patients need special education. Learning disabilities are primarily associated with either chromosomal or noncardiac syndromes or with neurological deficits resulting from extended hypoxemic periods during infancy.

Employment and Career

A significant proportion of adults with congenital heart disease have problems with employability, including those with high academic achievements. In particular, patients with complex or only partially repaired lesions are at a disadvantage in this area.[100,130,132,133,137] Education and career counseling that matches interests with physical abilities can prevent or reduce job-related problems.[132,140,141]

Insurability: Life and Health

Obtaining life insurance can be very difficult for patients with congenital heart disease, even for those in whom health status is rated as "excellent" or "good" by a cardiologist. One study estimated that about one third of patients are unable to obtain life insurance,[141] with severity of the defect as the most critical determinant.[133,142] However, a recent report indicated that even in patients with a mild congenital heart defect, more than one third are refused life insurance, a percentage equal to that of patients with a moderate or complex heart lesion.[143] Even if they are successful in obtaining coverage, insurance companies tend to charge higher premiums to patients with more severe heart lesions.[133,142,143] This same pattern applies to mortgage applications.[143]

Obtaining health insurance can be problematic as well, especially in the United States where health insurance is not mandatory.[133,144,145] Over the years, health coverage has improved, but there are still many patients with an excellent or good clinical prognosis who are without health insurance.[32] Additionally, certain policies, particularly those from private carriers, include an exclusionary clause for "preexisting" illness, which would exclude all cardiac care. Patients with cyanotic heart disease and those with complex lesions are at highest risk for being uninsured.

Advice on strategies for obtaining or maintaining health insurance is critical. Adolescents are often under their parent's policy until age 20, so advise the parents or the young adult to begin exploring other forms of coverage before the policy expires.[146] Patients who are denied insurance or offered insurance at high premiums should shop around because not all insurance companies rate the risks of congenital heart disease in the same way.[147] Advise patients to seek employment in large companies because their group policies tend to be less costly, easier to obtain, and obtainable without requiring a physical examination.[147]

Sexuality and Contraception

Parents of children with congenital heart disease may be reluctant to discuss sexuality and reproduction.[117] As a result, many teenagers and young adults enter adulthood with misconceptions and fears about their sexuality and their ability to conceive and bear children, which may influence relationships and marriage.[117] It is important to discuss these issues with adolescents and in adult settings, to assess the patient's knowledge about sexuality.[117]

Reassure patients that sexual activity is not harmful to their hearts. For females discuss contraception and childbearing. Many low-dose estrogen-based contraceptive methods may be acceptable, but for females who remain cyanotic or have residual lesions that are at risk for embolism, alternatives, such as progestin-based methods, should explored.[148] Intrauterine devices are an alternative in selected cases, but are not recommended for females with a history of or high risk for endocarditis, for females with multiple partners, or women with a history of a sexually transmitted disease **(STD)** because of the risk of endocarditis. Women with Eisenmenger physiology are advised against estrogen-containing contraceptives because they augment the risk of thromboembolic events. Permanent sterilization is recommended for these women, so alternative methods of motherhood, including adoption and surrogacy, should be explored. Contraceptives recommended for females with congenital heart disease are summarized in Table 71-13.

Marital Status

Data on social functioning and marital status are limited. Young adults with congenital heart disease tend to live at home longer than their peers. Rates of marrying

■ ■ ■

TABLE 71-13   RECOMMENDED CONTRACEPTIVE USE IN FEMALES WITH CONGENITAL HEART DISEASE

DEFECT/RESIDUA	COCs	MINI PILL	NORPLANT	DEPO PROVERA	IUD*	BARRIER
I. Surgically Repaired Defects						
A. No residua: ASD, VSD, PDA	+	+	+	+	+	+
B. Residual shunt and/or obstruction	−	+	+	+	+	+
C. Prosthetic valves, conduits, baffles	−	+	+	+	−	+
D. Residual pulmonary and/or systemic hypertension	−	+	+	+	−	+
II. Unrepaired Defects, Postoperative Residua						
A. Small VSD	+	+	+	+	+	+
B. Mild to moderate residual shunts (ASD, VSD, PDA)	−	+	+	+	−	+
C. Residual systemic or pulmonary hypertension (CoA)	−	+	+	+	−	+
D. Complex cyanotic defects (TA, SV, TR)	−	+	+	+	−	+
III. Defects Complicated By						
A. Cyanosis	−	+	+	+	−	+
B. Ventricular dysfunction	−	+/−	+/−	+/−	−	+
C. Atrial fibrillation or flutter	−	+	+	+/−	−	+
D. Eisenmenger physiology	−	+	+	+	−	+

ASD, Atrial septal defect; *CoA*, coarctation of the aorta; *COCs*, low-dose combined oral contraceptives; *IUD*, intrauterine device; *PDA*, patent ductus arteriosus; *SV*, single ventricle; *TA*, tricuspid atresia; *TR*, truncus arteriosus; *VSD*, ventricular septal defect.
*Recommend administration of antibiotic prophylaxis with insertion.
From Canobbio MM, Perloff JK, Rapkin AJ: Gynecological health of females with congenital heart disease, *Internat J Cardiol* 98:379-387, 2005.

appear to be comparable with that of the general population.[32,51,130,131] These patients may cohabitate less often, marry at a later age, and have children later.[125] These differences may reflect self-perception and body image, particularly in patients repaired at an older age, as discussed below.

Illness Experience

Certain heart lesions may disproportionately affect the daily lives of patients. The "feeling of being different" seems to be a key theme in the lived experiences of these patients.[149-152] They also may perceive that others (e.g., parents, school, and friends) see them as different. Visible signs (e.g., cyanosis, digital clubbing, and scars) may influence these perceptions.[150-152] Depending on lesion severity, physical limitations and restrictions may impede social independence.

This "feeling of being different" seems to emerge most strongly during adolescence,[149,152] a period when physical performance, bodily appearance, and peer pressure are important. In contrast young adults feel different in terms of career or relationship choices.[149] These studies reflect patients with moderate to complex heart defects; patients with mild lesions remain unstudied.

Psychopathology

Some studies of adults with congenital heart disease found favorable emotional functioning,[131,153] whereas others demonstrated that adults have more psychological distress or psychopathology compared with healthy subjects.[124,154] Depression and anxiety in particular are prevalent problems experienced by patients with congenital heart disease.[155-157]

CONCLUSION

Adults with congenital heart disease constitute a growing population of patients. Although life expectancy is increasing, these individuals may be confronted with specific medical, psychosocial, and behavioral problems throughout their lives. Specialized facilities and properly trained professionals are required for comprehensive care of this vulnerable group of patients. Nurses have a crucial role with this population since these patients face several nurse-sensitive issues, such as poor knowledge and psychosocial issues.

REFERENCES

1. Hoffman JI, Kaplan S: The incidence of congenital heart disease, *J Am Coll Cardiol* 39:1890-1900, 2002.
2. Blalock A, Taussig HB: Surgical treatment of malformation of the heart in which there is pulmonary stenosis or pulmonary atresia, *JAMA* 128:189, 1945.
3. Miller BJ, Gibbon JH, Fineberg C: An improved mechanical heart and lung apparatus; its use during open cardiotomy in experimental animals, *Med Clin North Am* 1:1603-1624, 1953.
4. Warnes CA: The adult with congenital heart disease: born to be bad? *J Am Coll Cardiol* 46:1-8, 2005.
5. Garson A Jr, Allen HD, Gersony WM et al: The cost of congenital heart disease in children and adults. A model for multicenter assessment of price and practice variation, *Arch Pediatr Adolesc Med* 148:1039-1045, 1994.
6. Hoffman JI, Kaplan S, Liberthson RR: Prevalence of congenital heart disease, *Am Heart J* 147:425-439, 2004.
7. Warnes CA, Liberthson R, Danielson GK et al: Task Force 1: the changing profile of congenital heart disease in adult life, *J Am Coll Cardiol* 37:1170-1175, 2001.
8. Brickner ME, Hillis LD, Lange RA: Congenital heart disease in adults. First of two parts, *N Engl J Med* 342:256-263, 2000.
9. Therrien J, Dore A, Gersony W et al: CCS Consensus Conference 2001 update: recommendations for the management of adults with congenital heart disease. Part I, *Can J Cardiol* 17:940-959, 2001.
10. Therrien J, Gatzoulis M, Graham T et al: Canadian Cardiovascular Society Consensus Conference 2001 update: recommendations for the management of adults with congenital heart disease. Part II, *Can J Cardiol* 17:1029-1050, 2001.
11. Therrien J, Warnes C, Daliento L et al: Canadian Cardiovascular Society Consensus Conference 2001 update: recommendations for the management of adults with congenital heart disease. Part III, *Can J Cardiol* 17:1135-1158, 2001.
12. Deanfield J, Thaulow E, Warnes C et al: Management of grown up congenital heart disease. *Eur Heart J* 24:1035-1084, 2003.
13. Foster E, Graham TP Jr, Driscoll DJ et al: Task force 2: special health care needs of adults with congenital heart disease, *J Am Coll Cardiol* 37:1176-1183, 2001.
14. Child JS, Collins-Nakai RL, Alpert JS et al: Task Force 3: workforce description and educational requirements for the care of adults with congenital heart disease, *J Am Coll Cardiol* 37:1183-1187, 2001.
15. Landzberg MJ, Murphy DJ Jr, Davidson WR Jr et al: Task Force 4: organization of delivery systems for adults with congenital heart disease, *J Am Coll Cardiol* 37:1187-1193, 2001.
16. Skorton DJ, Garson A Jr, Allen HD et al: Task force 5: adults with congenital heart disease: access to care, *J Am Coll Cardiol* 37:1193-1198, 2001.
17. Daenen W, Lacour-Gayet F, Aberg T et al: Optimal structure of a congenital heart surgery department in Europe, *Eur J Cardiothorac Surg* 24:343-351, 2003.
18. Gurvitz MZ, Chang RK, Ramos FJ et al: Variations in adult congenital heart disease training in adult and pediatric cardiology fellowship programs, *J Am Coll Cardiol* 46:893-898, 2005.
19. Gatzoulis MA, Hechter S, Siu SC et al: Outpatient clinics for adults with congenital heart disease: increasing workload and evolving patterns of referral, *Heart* 81:57-61, 1999.
20. Wren C, O'Sullivan JJ: Survival with congenital heart disease and need for follow up in adult life, *Heart* 85:438-443, 2001.
21. Canobbio MM: Congenital heart disease. In Woods S, editor: *Cardiac nursing*, ed 5, Philadelphia, 2005, Lippincott Williams & Wilkins, pp 794-806.
22. Gatzoulis MA, Swan L, Therrien J et al: *Adult congenital heart disease: a practical guide,* Malden, Mass, 2005, Blackwell Publishing Ltd.
23. Webb G, Smallhorn JF, Therrien J et al: Congenital heart disease. In Zipes DP, Libby P, Bonow RO et al, editors: *Braunwald's heart disease,* Philadelphia, 2005, Elsevier Saunders.
24. Gersony WM, Rosenbaum MS: *Congenital heart disease in the adult,* New York, 2002, McGraw-Hill.
25. Ghosh S, Chatterjee S, Black E et al: Surgical closure of atrial septal defects in adults: effect of age at operation on outcome, *Heart* 88:485-487, 2002.
26. Du ZD, Hijazi ZM, Kleinman CS et al: Comparison between transcatheter and surgical closure of secundum atrial septal defect in children and adults: results of a multicenter nonrandomized trial. *J Am Coll Cardiol* 39:1836-1844, 2002.
27. Hagen PT, Scholz DG, Edwards WD: Incidence and size of patent foramen ovale during the first 10 decades of life: an autopsy study of 965 normal hearts, *Mayo Clin Proc* 59:17-20, 1984.
28. Beda RD, Gill E Jr: Patent foramen ovale: does it play a role in the pathophysiology of migraine headache? *Cardiol Clin* 23:91-96, 2005.
29. Post MC, Thijs V, Herroelen L et al: Closure of a patent foramen ovale is associated with a decrease in prevalence of migraine, *Neurology* 62:1439-1440, 2004.
30. Nygren A, Sunnegardh J, Berggren H: Preoperative evaluation and surgery in isolated ventricular septal defects: a 21 year perspective, *Heart* 83:198-204, 2003.

31. Roos-Hesselink JW, Meijboom FJ, Spitaels SE et al: Outcome of patients after surgical closure of ventricular septal defect at young age: longitudinal follow-up of 22-34 years, *Eur Heart J* 25:1057-1062, 2004.

32. Gersony WM, Hayes CJ, Driscoll DJ et al: Second natural history study of congenital heart defects. Quality of life of patients with aortic stenosis, pulmonary stenosis, or ventricular septal defect, *Circulation* 87:I52-I65, 1993.

33. Fawzy ME, Awad M, Galal O et al: Long-term results of pulmonary balloon valvulotomy in adult patients, *J Heart Valve Dis* 10:812-818, 2001.

34. Rao PS, Galal O, Patnana M et al: Results of three to 10 year follow up of balloon dilatation of the pulmonary valve, *Heart* 80:591-595, 1998.

35. Earing MG, Connolly HM, Dearani JA et al: Long-term follow-up of patients after surgical treatment for isolated pulmonary valve stenosis, *Mayo Clin Proc* 80:871-876, 2005.

36. Boening A, Scheewe J, Heine K et al: Long-term results after surgical correction of atrioventricular septal defects, *Eur J Cardiothorac Surg* 22:167-173, 2002.

37. El Najdawi EK, Driscoll DJ, Puga FJ et al: Operation for partial atrioventricular septal defect: a forty-year review, *J Thorac Cardiovasc Surg* 119:880-889, 2000.

38. Jenkins NP, Ward C: Coarctation of the aorta: natural history and outcome after surgical treatment, *QJM* 92:365-371, 1992.

39. Webb G: Treatment of coarctation and late complications in the adult, *Semin Thorac Cardiovasc Surg* 17:139-142, 2005.

40. Vogt M, Kuhn A, Baumgartner D et al: Impaired elastic properties of the ascending aorta in newborns before and early after successful coarctation repair: proof of a systemic vascular disease of the prestenotic arteries? *Circulation* 111:3269-3273, 2005.

41. Guerin P, Jimenez M, Vallot M et al: Arterial rigidity of patients operated successfully for coarctation of the aorta without residual hypertension, *Arch Mal Coeur Vaiss* 98:557-560, 2005.

42. Vriend JW, de Groot E, Bouma BJ et al: Carotid intima-media thickness in post-coarctectomy patients with exercise induced hypertension, *Heart* 91:962-963, 2005.

43. de Divitiis M, Pilla C, Kattenhorn M et al: Vascular dysfunction after repair of coarctation of the aorta: impact of early surgery, *Circulation* 104:I165-I170, 2001.

44. Sehested J, Baandrup U, Mikkelsen E: Different reactivity and structure of the prestenotic and poststenotic aorta in human coarctation. Implications for baroreceptor function, *Circulation* 65:1060-1065, 1982.

45. Cohen M, Fuster V, Steele PM: Coarctation of the aorta. Long-term follow-up and prediction of outcome after surgical correction, *Circulation* 80:840-845, 1989.

46. Brouwer RM, Erasmus ME, Ebels T et al: Influence of age on survival, late hypertension, and recoarctation in elective aortic coarctation repair. Including long-term results after elective aortic coarctation repair with a follow-up from 25 to 44 years, *J Thorac Cardiovasc Surg* 108:525-531, 1994.

47. Toro-Salazar OH, Steinberger J, Thomas W et al: Long-term follow-up of patients after coarctation of the aorta repair, *Am J Cardiol* 89:541-547, 2002.

48. Clarkson PM, Nicholson MR, Barratt-Boyes BG et al: Results after repair of coarctation of the aorta beyond infancy: a 10 to 28 year follow-up with particular reference to late systemic hypertension, *Am J Cardiol* 51:1481-1488, 1983.

49. Murphy JG, Gersh BJ, Mair DD et al: Long-term outcome in patients undergoing surgical repair of tetralogy of Fallot, *N Engl J Med* 329:593-599, 1993.

50. Jimenez M, Espil G, Thambo JB et al: Outcome of operated Fallot's tetralogy, *Arch Mal Coeur Vaiss* 95:1112-1118, 2002.

51. Walker WT, Temple IK, Gnanapragasam JP et al: Quality of life after repair of tetralogy of Fallot, *Cardiol Young* 12:549-553, 2002.

52. Brickner ME, Hillis LD, Lange RA: Congenital heart disease in adults. Second of two parts, *N Engl J Med* 342:334-342, 2000.

53. McRae ME: Repaired tetralogy of Fallot in the adult, *Prog Cardiovasc Nurs* 20:104-110, 2005.

54. Faidutti B, Christenson JT, Beghetti M et al: How to diminish reoperation rates after initial repair of tetralogy of Fallot? *Ann Thorac Surg* 73:96-101, 2002.

55. Khambadkone S, Coats L, Taylor A et al: Percutaneous pulmonary valve implantation in humans: results in 59 consecutive patients, *Circulation* 112:1189-1197, 2005.

56. Francannet C, Lancaster PA, Pradat P et al: The epidemiology of three serious cardiac defects. A joint study between five centres, *Eur J Epidemiol* 9:607-616, 1993.

57. Moons P, Gewillig M, Sluysmans T et al: Long term outcome up to 30 years after the Mustard or Senning operation: a nationwide multicentre study in Belgium, *Heart* 90:307-313, 2004.

58. Losay J, Touchot A, Serraf A et al: Late outcome after arterial switch operation for transposition of the great arteries, *Circulation* 104:I121-I126, 2001.

59. Legendre A, Losay J, Touchot-Kone A et al: Coronary events after arterial switch operation for transposition of the great arteries, *Circulation* 108(suppl 1):II186-II190.

60. Dos L, Teruel L, Ferreira IJ et al: Late outcome of Senning and Mustard procedures for correction of transposition of the great arteries, *Heart* 91:652-656, 2005.

61. Rutledge JM, Nihill MR, Fraser CD et al: Outcome of 121 patients with congenitally corrected transposition of the great arteries, *Pediatr Cardiol* 23:137-145, 2002.

62. Graham TP Jr, Bernard YD, Mellen BG et al: Long-term outcome in congenitally corrected transposition of the great arteries: a multi-institutional study, *J Am Coll Cardiol* 36:255-261, 2000.

63. Samanek M: Children with congenital heart disease: probability of natural survival, *Pediatr Cardiol* 13:152-158, 1992.

64. Fontan F, Fernandez G, Costa F et al: The size of the pulmonary arteries and the results of the Fontan operation, *J Thorac Cardiovasc Surg* 98:711-719, 1989.

65. Driscoll DJ, Offord KP, Feldt RH et al: Five- to fifteen-year follow-up after Fontan operation, *Circulation* 85:469-496, 1992.

66. Lee JR, Choi JS, Kang CH et al: Surgical results of patients with a functional single ventricle, *Eur J Cardiothorac Surg* 24:716-722, 2003.

67. Weipert J, Noebauer C, Schreiber C et al: Occurrence and management of atrial arrhythmia after long-term Fontan circulation, *J Thorac Cardiovasc Surg* 127:457-464, 2004.

68. Saliba Z, Butera G, Bonnet D et al: Quality of life and perceived health status in surviving adults with univentricular heart, *Heart* 86:69-73, 2001.

69. Canobbio MM, Mair DD, van d V et al: Pregnancy outcomes after the Fontan repair, *J Am Coll Cardiol* 28:763-767, 1996.

70. Drenthen W, Pieper PG, Roos-Hesselink JW et al: Menstrual disorders, fertility, pregnancy and delivery after Fontan palliation, *Am J Cardiol* 2005.

71. van den Bosch AE, Roos-Hesselink JW, van Domburg R et al: Long-term outcome and quality of life in adult patients after the Fontan operation, *Am J Cardiol* 93:1141-1145, 2004.

72. Petko M, Myung RJ, Wernovsky G et al: Surgical reinterventions following the Fontan procedure, *Eur J Cardiothorac Surg* 24:255-259, 2003.

73. Kaulitz R, Hofbeck M: Current treatment and prognosis in children with functionally univentricular hearts, *Arch Dis Child* 90:757-762, 2005.

74. Kim WH, Lim HG, Lee JR et al: Fontan conversion with arrhythmia surgery, *Eur J Cardiothorac Surg* 27:250-257, 2005.

75. Silka MJ, Hardy BG, Menashe VD et al: A population-based prospective evaluation of risk of sudden cardiac death after operation for common congenital heart defects, *J Am Coll Cardiol* 32:245-251, 1998.

76. Furer SK, Gomes JA, Love B et al: Mechanism and therapy of cardiac arrhythmias in adults with congenital heart disease, *Mt Sinai J Med* 72:263-269, 2005.

77. Gatzoulis MA, Balaji S, Webber SA et al: Risk factors for arrhythmia and sudden cardiac death late after repair of tetralogy of Fallot: a multicentre study, *Lancet* 356:975-981, 2000.

78. Gelatt M, Hamilton RM, McCrindle BW et al: Risk factors for atrial tachyarrhythmias after the Fontan operation, *J Am Coll Cardiol* 24:1735-1741, 2004.

79. Law IH, Fischbach PS, Goldberg C et al: Inducibility of intra-atrial reentrant tachycardia after the first two stages of the Fontan sequence, *J Am Coll Cardiol* 37:231-237, 2001.

80. Paul T, Ziemer G, Luhmer L et al: Early and late atrial dysrhythmias after modified Fontan operation, *Pediatr Med Chir* 20:9-11, 1998.

81. Khositseth A, Danielson GK, Dearani JA et al: Supraventricular tachyarrhythmias in Ebstein anomaly: management and outcome, *J Thorac Cardiovasc Surg* 128:826-833, 2004.

82. Natterson PD, Perloff JK, Klitzner TS: Electrophysiologic abnormalities: unoperated occurrence and postoperative residua and sequelae. In Perloff JK, Child JS, editors: *Congenital heart disease in adults,* Philadelphia, 1998, WB Saunders Company, pp 316-345.

83. Deal BJ, Mavroudis C, Backer CL: Beyond Fontan conversion: surgical therapy of arrhythmias including patients with associated complex congenital heart disease, *Ann Thorac Surg* 76:542-553, 2003.

84. Mavroudis C, Deal BJ, Backer CL: The beneficial effects of total cavopulmonary conversion and arrhythmia surgery for the failed Fontan, *Semin Thorac Cardiovasc Surg Pediatr Card Surg Annu* 5:12-24, 2002.

85. Book WM: Heart failure in the adult patient with congenital heart disease, *J Card Fail* 11:306-312, 2005.

86. Bolger AP, Gatzoulis MA: Towards defining heart failure in adults with congenital heart disease, *Int J Cardiol* 97(suppl 1):15-23, 2004.

87. Norozi K, Buchhorn R, Kaiser C et al: Plasma N-terminal pro-brain natriuretic peptide as a marker of right ventricular dysfunction in patients with tetralogy of Fallot after surgical repair, *Chest* 128:2563-2570, 2005.

88. Bolger AP, Sharma R, Li W et al: Neurohormonal activation and the chronic heart failure syndrome in adults with congenital heart disease, *Circulation* 106:92-99, 2002.

89. Hopkins WE, Chen Z, Fukagawa NK et al: Increased atrial and brain natriuretic peptides in adults with cyanotic congenital heart disease: enhanced understanding of the relationship between hypoxia and natriuretic peptide secretion, *Circulation* 109:2872-2877, 2004.

90. Vonder MI, Liu P, Webb G: Applying standard therapies to new targets: the use of ACE inhibitors and ß-blockers for heart failure in adults with congenital heart disease, *Int J Cardiol* 97(suppl 1):25-33, 2004.

91. Child JS, Perloff JK, Kubak B: Infective endocarditis: risks and prophylaxis. In Perloff JK, Child JS, editors: *Congenital heart disease in Adults,* Philadelphia, 1998, W. Saunders, pp 129-143.

92. Niwa K, Nakazawa M, Tateno S et al: Infective endocarditis in congenital heart disease: Japanese national collaboration study, *Heart* 91:795-800, 2005.

93. Morris CD, Reller MD, Menashe VD: Thirty-year incidence of infective endocarditis after surgery for congenital heart defect, *JAMA* 279:599-603, 1998.

94. Wood P: The Eisenmenger syndrome or pulmonary hypertension with reversed central shunt I, *Br Med J* 46:701-709, 1958.

95. Cantor WJ, Harrison DA, Moussadji JS et al: Determinants of survival and length of survival in adults with Eisenmenger syndrome, *Am J Cardiol* 84:677-681, 1999.

96. Kidd L, Driscoll DJ, Gersony WM et al: Second natural history study of congenital heart defects. Results of treatment of patients with ventricular septal defects, *Circulation* 87:I38-I51, 1993.

97. Saha A, Balakrishnan KG, Jaiswal PK et al: Prognosis for patients with Eisenmenger syndrome of various aetiology, *Int J Cardiol* 45:199-207, 1994.

98. Oya H, Nagaya N, Uematsu M et al: Poor prognosis and related factors in adults with Eisenmenger syndrome, *Am Heart J* 143:739-744, 2002.

99. Moons P, Van Deyk K, De Geest S et al: Is the severity of congenital heart disease associated with the quality of life and perceived health of adult patients? *Heart* 91:1193-1198, 2005.

100. Daliento L, Somerville J, Presbitero P et al: Eisenmenger syndrome. Factors relating to deterioration and death, *Eur Heart J* 19:1845-1855, 1998.

101. Rosenzweig EB, Barst RJ: Eisenmenger's syndrome: current management, *Prog Cardiovasc Dis* 45:129-138, 2002.

102. Avila WS, Rossi EG, Ramires JA et al: Pregnancy in patients with heart disease: experience with 1,000 cases, *Clin Cardiol* 26:135-142, 2003.

103. Siu SC, Sermer M, Colman JM et al: Prospective multicenter study of pregnancy outcomes in women with heart disease, *Circulation* 104:515-521, 2001.

104. Lupton M, Oteng-Ntim E, Ayida G et al: Cardiac disease in pregnancy, *Curr Opin Obstet Gynecol* 14:137-143, 2002.

105. Burn J, Brennan P, Little J et al: Recurrence risks in offspring of adults with major heart defects: results from first cohort of British collaborative study, *Lancet* 351:311-316, 1998.

106. Gill HK, Splitt M, Sharland GK et al: Patterns of recurrence of congenital heart disease: an analysis of 6,640 consecutive pregnancies evaluated by detailed fetal echocardiography, *J Am Coll Cardiol* 42:923-929, 2003.

107. Moons P, De Volder E, Budts W et al: What do adult patients with congenital heart disease know about their disease, treatment, and prevention of complications? A call for structured patient education, *Heart* 86:74-80, 2001.

108. Kantoch MJ, Collins-Nakai RL, Medwid S et al: Adult patients' knowledge about their congenital heart disease, *Can J Cardiol* 13:641-645, 1997.

109. Cetta F, Warnes CA: Adults with congenital heart disease: patient knowledge of endocarditis prophylaxis, *Mayo Clin Proc* 70:50-54, 1995.

110. Vogel M, Knirsch W, Lange PE: Severe complications caused by inattention to endocarditis prevention during dental procedures in adults with congenital heart abnormalities, *Dtsch Med Wochenschr* 125:344-347, 2000.

111. Warnes C: Establishing an adult congenital heart disease clinic, *Am J Card Imaging* 9:11-14, 1995.

112. Manning JA: Congenital heart disease and the quality of life. In Engle MA, Perloff JK, editors: *Congenital heart disease after surgery: benefits, residua, sequelae,* New York, 1983, Medical Books, pp 347-361.

113. Dajani AS, Taubert KA, Wilson W et al: Prevention of bacterial endocarditis. Recommendations by the American Heart Association, *Circulation* 96:358-366, 1997.

114. Horstkotte D, Follath F, Gutschik E et al: Guidelines on prevention, diagnosis and treatment of infective endocarditis executive summary, *Eur Heart J* 25:267-276, 2004.

115. Satchithananda DK, Walsh J, Schofield PM: Bacterial endocarditis following repeated tattooing, *Heart* 85:11-12, 2001.

116. Weinberg JB: Case report of Staphylococcus aureus endocarditis after navel piercing, *Pediatr Infect Dis J* 22:94-95, 2003.

117. Canobbio MM: Health care issues facing adolescents with congenital heart disease, *J Pediatr Nurs* 16:363-370, 2001.

118. Calzolari A, Giordano U, Di Giacinto B et al: Exercise and sports participation after surgery for congenital heart disease: the European perspective, *Ital Heart J* 2:736-739, 2001.

119. Marcon F: Sports and congenital heart disease in the adult, *Arch Mal Coeur Vaiss* 95:1045-1055, 2004.

120. Koster NK: Physical activity and congenital heart disease, *Nurs Clin North Am* 29:345-356, 1994.

121. Swan L, Hillis WS: Exercise prescription in adults with congenital heart disease: a long way to go, *Heart* 83:685-687, 2000.

122. Graham TP Jr, Driscoll DJ, Gersony WM et al: Task force 2: congenital heart disease, *J Am Coll Cardiol* 45:1326-1333, 2005.

123. Pelliccia A, Fagard R, Bjornstad HH et al: Recommendations for competitive sports participation in athletes with cardiovascular disease: a consensus document from the study group of sports cardiology of the working group of cardiac rehabilitation and exercise physiology and the working group of myocardial and pericardial diseases of the European Society of Cardiology, *Eur Heart J* 26:1422-1445, 2005.

124. Brandhagen DJ, Feldt RH, Williams DE: Long-term psychologic implications of congenital heart disease: a 25-year follow-up, *Mayo Clin Proc* 66:474-479, 1991.

125. Kokkonen J, Paavilainen T: Social adaptation of young adults with congenital heart disease, *Int J Cardiol* 36:23-29, 1992.

126. Wray J, Sensky T: Congenital heart disease and cardiac surgery in childhood: effects on cognitive function and academic ability, *Heart* 85:687-691, 2001.

127. Griffin KJ, Elkin TD, Smith CJ: Academic outcomes in children with congenital heart disease, *Clin Pediatr (Phila)* 42:401-409, 2003.

128. Kirshbom PM, Myung RJ, Gaynor JW et al: Preoperative pulmonary venous obstruction affects long-term outcome for survivors of total anomalous pulmonary venous connection repair, *Ann Thorac Surg* 74:1616-1620, 2002.

129. Mahle WT, Clancy RR, Moss EM et al: Neurodevelopmental outcome and lifestyle assessment in school-aged and adolescent

children with hypoplastic left heart syndrome, *Pediatrics* 105:1082-1089, 2000.

130. Nieminen H, Sairanen H, Tikanoja T et al: Long-term results of pediatric cardiac surgery in Finland: education, employment, marital status, and parenthood, *Pediatrics* 112:1345-1350, 2003.

131. van Rijen EH, Utens EM, Roos-Hesselink JW et al: Psychosocial functioning of the adult with congenital heart disease: a 20-33 year follow-up, *Eur Heart J* 24:673-683, 2003.

132. Kamphuis M, Vogels T, Ottenkamp J et al: Employment in adults with congenital heart disease, *Arch Pediatr Adolesc Med* 156:1143-1148, 2002.

133. Celermajer DS, Deanfield JE: Employment and insurance for young adults with congenital heart disease, *Br Heart J* 69:539-543, 1993.

134. Miyamura H, Eguchi S, Asano K: Long-term results of the intra-cardiac repair of tetralogy of Fallot: a follow-up study conducted over more than 20 years on 100 consecutive operative survivors, *Surg Today* 23:1049-1052, 1993.

135. Miyamura H, Takahashi M, Sugawara M et al: The long-term influence of pulmonary valve regurgitation following repair of tetralogy of Fallot: does preservation of the pulmonary valve ring affect quality of life? *Surg Today* 26:603-606, 1996.

136. Park I, Nakazawa M, Imai Y et al: Prediction of quality of life at long-term follow-up after Fontan operation by scoring risk factors, *Jpn Circ J* 58:646-652, 1994.

137. Pressley JC, Wharton JM, Tang ASL et al: Effect of Ebstein's-anomaly on short-term and long-term outcome of surgically treated patients with Wolff-Parkinson-White syndrome. *Circulation* 86:1147-1155, 1992.

138. Stewart AB, Ahmed R, Travill CM et al: Coarctation of the aorta life and health 20-44 years after surgical repair, *Br Heart J* 69:65-70, 1993.

139. Wilson NJ, Clarkson PM, Barratt-Boyes BG et al: Long-term outcome after the Mustard repair for simple transposition of the great arteries. 28-year follow-up, *J Am Coll Cardiol* 32:758-765, 1998.

140. Nieminen H, Sairanen H, Tikanoja T et al: Long-term results of pediatric cardiac surgery in Finland: education, employment, marital status, and parenthood, *Pediatrics* 112:1345-1350, 2003.

141. McGrath KA, Truesdell SC: Employability and career counseling for adolescents and adults with congenital heart disease, *Nurs Clin North Am* 29:319-330, 1994.

142. Truesdell SC, Skorton DJ, Lauer RM: Life insurance for children with cardiovascular disease, *Pediatrics* 77:687-691, 1986.

143. Crossland DS, Jackson SP, Lyall R et al: Life insurance and mortgage application in adults with congenital heart disease, *Eur J Cardiothorac Surg* 25:931-934, 2004.

144. Kaemmerer H, Tintner H, Konig U et al: Psychosocial problems of adolescents and adults with congenital heart defects, *Z Kardiol* 83:194-200, 1994.

145. Truesdell SC, Clark EB: Health insurance status in a cohort of children and young adults with congenital cardiac diagnosis, *Circulation* 84(suppl):II, 386, 1991.

146. Hellstedt LF: Transitional care issues influencing access to health care: employability and insurability, *Nurs Clin North Am* 39:741-753, 2004.

147. Vonder Muhll I, Cumming G, Gatzoulis MA: Risky business: insuring adults with congenital heart disease, *Eur Heart J* 24:1595-1600, 2003.

148. Canobbio MM: Contraception for the adolescent and young adult with congenital heart disease, *Nurs Clin North Am* 39:769-785, 2004.

149. Tong EM, Sparacino PS, Messias DK et al: Growing up with congenital heart disease: the dilemmas of adolescents and young adults (see comment), *Cardiol Young* 8:303-309, 1988.

150. Gantt LT: Growing up heartsick: the experiences of young women with congenital heart disease, *Health Care Women Int* 13:241-248, 1992.

151. McMurray R, Kendall L, Parsons JM et al: A life less ordinary: growing up and coping with congenital heart disease, *Coronary Health Care* 5:51-57, 2001.

152. Claessens P, Moons P, de Casterle BD et al: What does it mean to live with a congenital heart disease? A qualitative study on the lived experiences of adult patients, *Eur J Cardiovasc Nurs* 4:3-10, 2005.

153. Utens EM, Bieman HJ, Verhulst FC et al: Psychopathology in young adults with congenital heart disease. Follow-up results, *Eur Heart J* 19:647-651, 1998.

154. Spurkland I, Bjornstad PG, Lindberg H et al: Mental health and psychosocial functioning in adolescents with congenital heart disease. A comparison between adolescents born with severe heart defect and atrial septal defect, *Acta Paediatr* 82:71-76, 1993.

155. Bromberg JI, Beasley PJ, D'angelo EJ et al: Depression and anxiety in adults with congenital heart disease: a pilot study, *Heart Lung* 32:105-110, 2003.

156. Popelova J, Slavik Z, Skovranek J: Are cyanosed adults with congenital cardiac malformations depressed? *Cardiol Young* 11:379-384, 2001.

157. Lip GY, Lane DA, Millane TA et al: Psychological interventions for depression in adolescent and adult congenital heart disease, *Cochrane Database Syst Rev* CD004394, 2003.

chapter 72

Cardiomyopathy and Myocarditis

Jill Howie

Most will agree that cardiomyopathy is a primary disorder of cardiac muscle causing abnormal myocardial performance.[1] It is not the result of disease or dysfunction of nonmuscular cardiac structures; therefore the definition of cardiomyopathy excludes myocardial infarction, systemic arterial hypertension, and valvular heart disease.[1] However, the classification of cardiomyopathies presents a challenge. The science of classification requires that all items within the classified domain be included and that each item have designation in only one class.[1] A clear understanding between biological systems involved with cardiomyopathies is not currently appreciated; therefore designation of classifications continues to be debated. Clinicians often use a functional classification scheme because it is based on physiology and is germane to treatment.[1] In the future, a greater understanding of the molecular genetics of myocardial disease may offer insight into a more meaningful classification scheme.[2]

The most widely used functional classification of cardiomyopathy identifies three abnormalities of function: dilatation, hypertrophy, and restriction.[1] This chapter focuses on the diagnosis and management of patients with cardiomyopathies and myocarditis, including dilated, hypertrophic, and restrictive cardiomyopathies (Figure 72-1). Care of patients with chronic heart failure, the symptomatic manifestation of many cardiomyopathies, is discussed in Chapter 64.

DILATED CARDIOMYOPATHIES

Dilated cardiomyopathies have both primary and secondary causes that are wide ranging and abundant (Table 72-1). Dilated cardiomyopathies are the most common cause of heart failure. The course of heart failure depends on the degree of left ventricular dysfunction and the ability for treatment to improve intrinsic ventricular function.[1] Although the causes of dilated cardiomyopathies are numerous, this chapter discusses only the most commonly encountered dilated cardiomyopathies. Idiopathic dilated cardiomyopathy (**IDC**) is a type of primary dilated cardiomyopathy whereas ischemic, hypertensive, valvular, anthracycline, peripartum, and alcohol-related cardiomyopathies are secondary dilated cardiomyopathies. Both primary and secondary types of cardiomyopathy are discussed in this chapter.

Common Selected Dilated Cardiomyopathies
Idiopathic Dilated Cardiomyopathy

Idiopathic dilated cardiomyopathy, a primary cardiomyopathy, has a prevalence rate of 0.04 percent and is a relatively common cause of heart failure.[3] When coronary artery disease, thyroid disease, valvular abnormalities, and infiltrative causes are excluded, the diagnosis of IDC is suspected. The incidence of IDC increases with age and is higher in males.[3] In patients with a history of hypertension or excessive alcohol intake, the cause is not typically attributed to IDC. As discussed below, a history of prolonged, sustained hypertension or alcohol intake *greater than* 80 g per day for males (40 g for females) for more than 5 years suggests a secondary cause of the cardiomyopathy, and the cause is not attributed to IDC.[1]

Data from screening of first-degree relatives suggests that as many as 50 percent of IDC cases may be familial. There is a wide range of clinical manifestations of familial IDC, which demonstrates genetic heterogeneity.[4] Recently, several chromosomal genes have been identified with autosomal dominant and X-linked inheritance patterns. The mutations of genes may involve only myocardial cell function or involve a wider range of musculoskeletal cell disease, such as with mutations in the dystrophin gene.[5-6] A greater understanding of the genetics of IDC has clinical relevance because of the opportunity for family screening and genetic counseling.[7] Early detection and therapeutic intervention can be considered in affected relatives.

Endomyocardial biopsy provides the definitive diagnosis of IDC when myocardial cell hypertrophy with varying amounts of interstitial fibrosis is found. The major cellular change is an increase in cell length without an increase in cell size; this lengthening or remodeling is what typifies IDC and various other cardiomyopathies, such as ischemic dilated cardiomyopathy (**IDM**).[8-9] Myo-

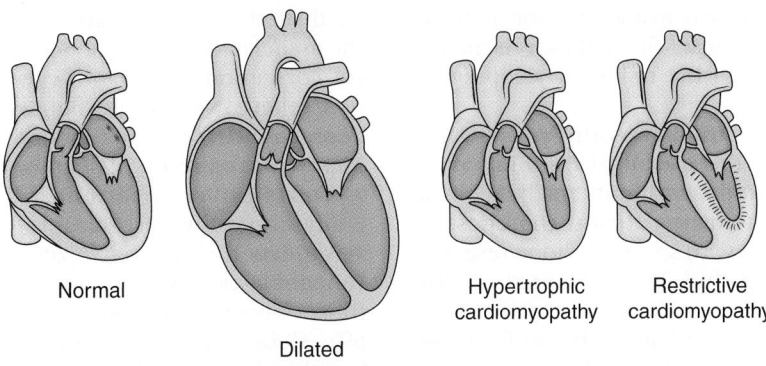

Normal

Dilated
cardiomyopathy

Hypertrophic
cardiomyopathy

Restrictive
cardiomyopathy

FIGURE 72-1 ▨ Three main types of cardiomyopathy are dilated, hypertrophic, and restrictive. In dilated cardiomyopathy, the ventricles enlarge. In hypertrophic cardiomyopathy, the walls of the ventricles thicken and become stiff. In restrictive cardiomyopathy, the walls of the ventricles become stiff, but not necessarily thickened. (Courtesy Merck Manual on-line www.merck.com/mmhe/sec03/ch026/ch026a.html, accessed 12-31-05.)

■ ■ ■

TABLE 72-1   CAUSES OF DILATED CARDIOMYOPATHY

MORE COMMON TYPES	TOXINS	METABOLIC	INFECTIOUS	SYSTEMIC	OTHERS
Idiopathic	Ethanol	Nutritional deficiencies (thiamine)	Viral	Systemic lupus erythematosus	Tachydysrhythmias
Ischemic	Anthracyclines	Endocrine (hypothyroidism and hyperthyroidism, etc.)	Rickettsial	Juvenile arthritis	Neuromuscular dystrophies
Valvular	Cobalt	Hypocalcemia	Bacterial	Polyarteritis nodosa	
Hypertensive	Antiretroviral agents	Hypophosphatemia	Myobacterial	Kawasaki disease	
Familial	Phenothiazines		Spirochetal	Collagen vascular	
	Lithium		Fungal	Hemochromatosis	
	Lead		Parasitic	Amyloidosis	
	Cocaine			Sarcoidosis	
	Mercury			Hypereosinophilic syndrome	
				Hypersensitivity myocarditis	
				Peripartum	
				Infantile histiocytoid	

Fuster V, Alexander RW, O'Rourke R: Classification of cardiomyopathies. In *Hurst's The heart,* ed 11, 2004-2005, McGraw-Hill Access Medicine.

cyte hypertrophy, large and bizarrely shaped nuclei, and interstitial fibrosis are characteristic findings of IDC.[10]

Immune regulatory abnormalities have been identified with IDC suggesting that immune defects may be important associated causative factors.[11-12] IDC also has developed in patients after resolution of viral myocarditis.[13] This observation has provided speculation that IDC may sometimes be due to subclinical viral myocarditis. Links between viral infection and genetic disorders are not yet well understood. The prognosis of IDC is generally better than that for ischemic cardiomyopathy.[14] Before angiotensin-converting enzyme **(ACE)** inhibitors were available, survival was approximately 50 percent in 5 years,[15] but is substantially better now.

Treatment of IDC includes the use of ACE inhibitors and beta blockers. The risk of thromboembolism is elevated in IDC, so treatment with anticoagulant agents is required.[1] Improvement over time of left ventricular function is often better in IDC than in patients with

IDM, either because of improved adrenergic activation or the presence of more viable myocardial tissue.[1,16]

Secondary Cardiomyopathy
Ischemic Dilated Cardiomyopathy

The most common type of dilated cardiomyopathy is ischemic cardiomyopathy.[17] Ischemic dilated cardiomyopathy occurs when coronary artery disease, or ischemic heart disease, causes remodeling of the left ventricle with an associated reduction in ejection fraction. Remodeling, the compensatory response of the ventricle to improve its function, ultimately harms the ventricular muscle, worsening stroke volume over time (see Chapter 62). Between 15 percent and 45 percent of patients who have a myocardial infarction will develop dilatation of the left ventricle with a decrease in ejection fraction. Scarring that is transmural or subendocardial may compromise up to 50 percent of the left ventricular chamber.[1,18] It is theorized that the prognosis for ischemic cardiomyopathy is worse than for nonischemic cardiomyopathy because the risk for ischemic events is compounded with the risk of developing dilated cardiomyopathy.[19]

Treatment for dilated cardiomyopathy and chronic heart failure consists of the use of ACE inhibitors in symptomatic and asymptomatic patients and beta blockers and digoxin in symptomatic patients. Diuretics are used for volume reduction with spironolactone reserved for advanced cardiomyopathy.[1] The implanted cardiac rhythm management devices used in these patients are implantable cardioverter-defibrillators (**ICDs**) for those without intraventricular conduction defects and biventricular pacing in addition to ICD for those with an intraventricular conduction defect.[20] Thromboembolic complications are a risk in patients with decreased ejection fraction, necessitating the use of anticoagulation therapy. Amiodarone may be used to prevent dysrhythmias. Maintenance of normal electrolytes levels and a digoxin level of 1.0 ng/ml or less also will help prevent dysrhythmias.[1,21] Close monitoring and frequent medication adjustment is required in these patients.

Hypertensive Dilated Cardiomyopathy

Hypertensive dilated cardiomyopathy is diagnosed when systolic function remains depressed despite adequate treatment of hypertension.[1] This cardiomyopathy is defined as myocardial systolic function that is depressed out of proportion to the increase in wall stress.[22] A sustained increase in myocardial wall stress can result in dilatation and systolic impairment but with variable increases in wall thickness. In addition, the degree of dilatation and systolic impairment also may be variable.[23] The prognosis of hypertensive cardiomyopathy is influenced by comorbid conditions, such as coronary artery disease and diabetes mellitus. Control of afterload is essential in these patients, and when achieved, prognosis is typically better than for other types of dilated cardiomyopathy.[24]

The treatment for hypertensive dilated cardiomyopathy is the same as for IDM, but afterload reduction is the most important goal of therapy.[23] Antihypertensive vasodilators, such as amlodipine or alpha-blocking agents, are used in addition to the therapies outlined under IDM.

Valvular Dilated Cardiomyopathy

Valvular dilated cardiomyopathy occurs when myocardial systolic function is depressed out of proportion to an increase in wall stress secondary to a valvular abnormality.[1] Most cases are caused by left-sided regurgitant valve disorders, such as a mitral regurgitation and aortic regurgitation; aortic stenosis is less commonly the cause.[1] Eccentric hypertrophy will develop from increased wall stress, but the distribution of wall stress is related to the type of valvular abnormality. For example, mitral regurgitation is associated with hypertrophy of the left ventricle, which may eventually progress to a dilated failing ventricular chamber. Aortic regurgitation is associated with increased wall stress in both systolic and diastolic phases of contraction and is therefore poorly tolerated.[25] The prognosis associated with valvular dilated cardiomyopathy is variable and depends on the associated valvular abnormality and timing of surgical correction. In general valve repair or replacement will relieve wall stress, but will not improve severely depressed ventricular function. However, prognosis is improved as a result of stabilized hemodynamics.[1]

Treatment for valvular dilated cardiomyopathy is generally surgical with surgical valve replacement or repair as soon as the cardiomyopathy is recognized. Catheter valvuloplasty may be an option for particular patients or those who are poor surgical candidates (see Chapter 69). Medical treatment consists of ACE inhibitors and beta blockers in addition to aggressive afterload reduction, such as with hydralazine and nitrates. In aortic regurgitation, calcium blocker therapy may be associated with improved outcomes.[26]

Anthracycline Dilated Cardiomyopathy

Anthracycline anticancer agents are commonly used, although they are known to cause a dilated cardiomyopathy. Doxorubicin and daunorubicin are associated with a cardiomyopathy that is dose related; the higher the total cumulative dose, the higher the risk for cardiomyopathy in patients without underlying cardiac problems or other risk factors.[27] A known risk for anthracycline cardiomyopathy is prior mediastinal radiation involving the heart. With this risk, cardiomyopathy may occur at relatively lower drug doses.[27]

A definitive diagnosis of anthracycline dilated cardiomyopathy is made by endomyocardial biopsy, although clinical features in a patient who has undergone anthracycline therapy may suggest the diagnosis. The mechanism by which anthracycline causes cardiomyopathy is inhibition of contractile protein synthesis, preventing compensatory dilatation and remodeling.[28] The result is very little hypertrophy; dilatation of the left ventricle occurs late in the course of the illness. The onset of symptoms is generally acute, and patients often have tachycardia. This tachycardia is an adrenergic response that occurs because a larger end-diastolic volume cannot be achieved to improve cardiac output (blunted compensatory response). These patients may be dependent on adrenergic support.[1] The prognosis is often related to the underlying health status of the patient and the patient's age, but is generally poor. Myocardial impairment takes 60 days to fully emerge,[1] so patients who are diagnosed months to years after the last anthracycline dose have a better prognosis because this delay suggests that there was less of an insult from the drug.

Treatment of anthracycline dilated cardiomyopathy consists of aggressive conventional heart failure therapies including ACE inhibitors and beta blockers, but the high adrenergic drive makes these patients challenging to manage.[29] Diuretics may be administered for fluid reduction. Cardiac transplant may be considered in patients who are refractory to treatment, when the patient's cancer is not likely to recur.

Peripartum Dilated Cardiomyopathy

Postpartum or peripartum cardiomyopathy occurs when myocardial systolic dysfunction occurs during the last trimester of pregnancy or within 6 months of childbearing.[30] This type of cardiomyopathy is most often thought of as a dilated cardiomyopathy, but it may also be "unclassified" because dilatation and remodeling may not have had time to occur. Peripartum cardiomyopathy may be heterogeneous in cause because of possible associated hypertension, familial or idiopathic cardiomyopathy, or myocarditis in the setting of increased hemodynamic load.[31] Outcomes are better with peripartum cardiomyopathy than with other causes of dilated cardiomyopathy.[24] Half of all patients who develop peripartum cardiomyopathy will recover completely, and most of the others will improve. Treatment is aggressive and consistent with that used for IDC. In a very small minority of patients, cardiac transplantation may be considered.

Alcohol-Related Dilated Cardiomyopathy

Alcohol-related cardiomyopathy is diagnosed when there is a history of sustained and heavy alcohol consumption with other causes of a dilated cardiomyopathy excluded. Males who consume more than 80 g of alcohol per day and females who consume 40 g or more per day over prolonged periods, such as several years, are at risk for dilated cardiomyopathy.[32] One drink (12 oz of beer, 5 oz of wine, or 1½ oz of hard liquor) delivers about 12 to 14 g of alcohol.[33] Lower amounts of ethanol intake may also produce cardiomyopathy in individuals with specific risks for cardiomyopathy. The toxic effects of alcohol are thought to cause the nonspecific changes in myocardial muscle cells that occur with this type of cardiomyopathy. Thiamine deficiencies are often present in persons who consume large amounts of alcohol, which can further compromise cardiac function. Prognosis depends on alcohol abstinence and the degree of myocardial impairment, but typically prognosis is somewhat better for alcohol-related dilated cardiomyopathy than for IDC.[34] Treatment of alcohol-related cardiomyopathy is the same as that for IDC, although alcohol abstinence is imperative to successful treatment.

Common Overlapping Dilated Cardiomyopathy Types

Chagas cardiomyopathy is a cause of myocarditis and therefore overlaps with the classification of dilated cardiomyopathy. The left ventricular functional abnormalities are initially segmental and progress to global impairment. More discussion can be found below in the section on Myocarditis. Amyloid cardiomyopathy is a group of diseases characterized by extracellular deposition of proteins with characteristic B-pleated sheet conformation and nonbranching fibers.[35] It is most commonly classified as a restrictive cardiomyopathy (RC), but can also be found under dilated and "unclassified" categories.[1] More discussion of amyloid cardiomyopathy can be found later in the section on Restrictive Cardiomyopathy.

Summary

Dilated cardiomyopathies are the most common cause of the syndrome of heart failure. Cardiomyopathies are a group of diseases functionally classified as dilated, hypertrophic, and restrictive. Treatment is specific to the type of cardiomyopathy, but medical therapy commonly overlaps. Genetic causes of cardiomyopathy are increasingly recognized; molecular genetic scientists will likely provide new understanding of the classification of the dilated cardiomyopathies.

HYPERTROPHIC CARDIOMYOPATHY

Hypertrophic cardiomyopathy (HCM) has been defined and redefined several times since the 1950s.[36-38] An early definition stated that HCM was myocardial hypertrophy without the presence of associated hemodynamic stress. HCM can also be defined histologically by the presence of myocyte disarray; the normal parallel pattern of myocytes is replaced by unorganized myocytes interspersed with connective tissue.[39] This pattern, however, is not specific to HCM because it is found in other disorders, such as Noonan syndrome, Friedreich ataxia, and some congenital heart disease. Furthermore, myocyte disarray is difficult to observe through biopsy, with this finding usually appreciated only on postmortem examination.

As new understanding of genomic disorders has emerged, yet another definition of HCM has been proposed. Mutations in sarcomeric protein genes are found in many patients with HCM (see the accompanying Genetics feature). Defining HCM based on genetic analysis has become an important method of understanding the widely varying phenotypic expression of the disease. However, genetic analysis is not always available to clinicians, and mutations in sarcomeric protein genes are thought to account for only 60 percent of cases of the disease.[40-42] Therefore defining HCM is practically accomplished using the definition from five decades ago: myocardial hypertrophy without the presence of associated hemodynamic stress.

■■■ GENETICS

GENETIC SARCOMERIC PROTEIN DISEASES

The majority of sarcomeric protein gene abnormalities are a result of single amino acid substitution within or close to important functional domains. This type of missense mutation is thought to be associated with reduced contractile function in patients with HCM. Some have suggested that a final common pathophysiological pathway is related to dysfunctional myocyte bioenergetics, but further study is needed.

- Chromosome 1—cardiac troponin T
- Chromosome 14—beta-myosin heavy chain
- Chromosome 11—cardiac myosin binding protein C
- Chromosome 3—essential myosin light chains
- Chromosome 12—regulatory myosin light chains
- Chromosome 19—cardiac troponin I
- Chromosome 15—cardiac actin
- Chromosome 15—alpha-tropomyosin

Titin, troponin C, and alpha-cardiac myosin heavy chain mutations are unconfirmed in three possible genes. A poorer prognosis and higher risk for sudden death are associated with certain mutations within the beta-myosin heavy chain. Troponin T mutations are associated with higher mortality even without associated hypertrophy.

Robbins M, McRae T: Hypertrophic cardiomyopathy. In Griffin B, editor: *Manual of cardiovascular medicine*, ed 2, Philadelphia, 2004, Lippincott Williams & Wilkins.

The use of M-mode echocardiography has enabled further understanding of HCM. Outflow obstruction was thought to be a hallmark for HCM. The term idiopathic hypertrophic subaortic stenosis was subsequently coined to describe a subaortic pressure gradient that was thought to accompany HCM. M-mode echocardiography allowed more complete visualization of the mitral valve, demonstrating that outflow obstruction was present in only a small percentage of patients with HCM. Most recently, genetic characterization of HCM has led to the initial understanding that particular genetic defects associated with HCM can lead to varying cardiac problems. In other words, a specific genetic defect might cause HCM in one individual or dilated cardiomyopathy in another, suggesting that both genetic and environmental factors influence the development of HCM.[43,44]

Epidemiology and Cause

HCM can occur as early as during the first year of life and is found more frequently in males than females. The annual incidence of all-cause left ventricular hypertrophy is between 0.3 and 0.5 per 100,000, [45] making it likely that HCM is the most common genetically transmitted cardiovascular disease.[46] HCM is the leading cause of sudden death in athletes younger than age 35. Between 5 percent and 10 percent of patients with HCM progress to severe systolic dysfunction associated with progressive left ventricular wall thinning and enlargement.

In children, left ventricular hypertrophy is often associated with congenital defects and rare metabolic and neuromuscular diseases.[42] In adults familial disease is more frequent and associated with an autosomal dominant pattern of inheritance.[36,45] The causes of HCM can be generally categorized as sarcomeric protein diseases, metabolic diseases, and miscellaneous causes (Table 72-2).[42] At least eight genes that encode components of the myocyte sarcomere are implicated in approximately 60 percent of cases. Other causes of HCM probably involve genetic mutations that remain to be discovered or nonsarcomeric diseases, such as metabolic disorders.

Diagnosis

HCM develops most commonly during adolescence, with hypertrophy manifesting after age 20.[47] The diagnosis is usually made by age 25; persons with a normal echocardiogram and electrocardiogram (ECG) after age 25 are unlikely to develop HCM. The clinical presentation is often made incidentally or during family screening because these patients are usually asymptomatic. If symptomatic dyspnea on exertion and chest pain are most frequently reported. The chest pain is typically associated with exercise and persists at rest. It can also be caused by large meals.[12] Syncope, present during exercise or at rest, is worrisome because it suggests an increased risk for sudden death. Palpitations may be reported with dysrhythmias, such as atrial fibrillation, bradydysrhythmias, or vasovagal episodes. The presence of myocyte disarray is thought to be associated with conduction disturbances throughout the myocardium.

Jugular venous pulsation may be associated with a prominent "a" wave secondary to decreased right ventricular compliance. Left ventricular hypertrophy may cause an S_4. The left ventricular impulse can be laterally

■ ■ ■

TABLE 72-2   CAUSES OF LEFT VENTRICULAR HYPERTROPHY IN CHILDREN AND ADULTS

SARCOMERIC PROTEIN DISEASE	METABOLIC DISEASE	SYNDROMIC HCM	MISCELLANEOUS
• β-myosin heavy chain • Cardiac myosin binding protein C • Cardiac troponin I • Troponin T • α tropomyosin • Essential myosin light chain • Regulatory myosin light chain • Cardiac α-actin • α-myosin heavy chain • Titin • Troponin C	• Glycogen storage disease II (Pompe disease) • Glycogen storage disease III (Forbes disease) • Anderson-Fabry disease • Carnitine deficiency • Phosphorylase B kinase deficiency • Infant of diabetic mother • AMP kinase (WPW, HCM, conduction disease) • Debrancher enzyme deficiency • Hurler syndrome • Hurler-Scheie disease • Hunter syndrome • Mannosidosis • Fucosidosis • Total lipodystrophy • Mitochondrial cytopathy • MELAS • MERRF • LHON	• Noonan syndrome • LEOPARD syndrome • Friedreich ataxia • Beckwith-Wiedemann syndrome • Swyer syndrome (pure gonadal dysgenesis)	• Obesity • Athletic training • Muscle LIM protein • Phospholamban promoter • Amyloidosis • Pheochromocytoma

AMP, Adenosine monophosphate; *HCM,* hypertrophic cardiomyopathy; *LEOPARD,* lentigines, electrocardiogram conduction abnormalities, ocular hypertension, pulmonary stenosis, abnormalities of genitalia, retardation of growth, deafness; *LHON,* Leber hereditary optic neuropathy; *MELAS,* mitochondrial encephalomyopathy, lactic acidosis, and stroke-like episodes. *MERRF,* myoclonic epilepsy and ragged red fibers. *WPW,* Wolff-Parkinson-White syndrome.
Elliott P, McKenna W: Hypertrophic cardiomyopathy, *Lancet* 363:1882, 2004.

displaced and sustained. In patients with obstruction, the arterial pulse has a rapid upstroke and downstroke. Also a harsh systolic murmur can be appreciated at the left sternal border upon auscultation. This murmur increases with movement and radiates to the aortic and mitral sites. Maneuvers affecting preload and afterload, such as Valsalva and standing, will increase the harshness and length of the murmur because venous return is decreased and contractility is increased.[11] Some also have mitral regurgitation and a pansystolic murmur radiating to the axilla. In addition, a paradoxically split S_2 may be heard in those with obstruction because of a prolonged ejection time. On the other hand, physical examination may be unremarkable.

Diagnostic evaluation includes echocardiography and ECG. The diagnosis of HCM is made in an adult with a thickened left ventricular wall segment *greater than* 15 mm. Most patients also have an increase in the thickness of the interventricular septum.[48] Approximately 25 percent of HCM cases are accompanied by a dynamic outflow tract obstruction in the left ventricle.[49] This obstruction is caused by an abutment between the anterior (rarely posterior) mitral valve leaflet and the interventricular septum during contraction, thereby obstructing flow from the ventricle (Figure 72-2). Other variations of anatomy can cause obstruction, such as anomalous papillary muscles, pulmonary valve abnormalities, or other rare supravalvular problems.

Echocardiography is helpful in detecting the amount of obstruction, which is usually visualized as failure of valve leaflet apposition. Systolic function is usually normal or increased at rest. The diagnosis of HCM with obstruction is based on resting gradients *greater than* 30 mm Hg or gradients *greater than* 50 mm Hg with exercise. Systolic impairment with hypertrophy warrants further investigation for amyloidosis. Diastolic abnormalities, present in the active and passive phases, affect ventricular wall compliance. In some patients, diastolic abnormalities dominate the clinical features, taking on the characteristics of RC.

Electrocardiography may provide the initial clues to HCM. Changes most frequently found include repolarization abnormalities, atrial enlargement, and pathologi-

cal Q waves. These ECG changes are usually seen in the inferior leads.[36] Giant negative T waves appearing in the midprecordial leads suggest that hypertrophy is present in the distal left ventricle. Left ventricular hypertrophy causes increased voltage, but is a nonspecific finding. Rarely a short PR interval not usually associated with Wolff-Parkinson-White syndrome may be found. Dysrhythmias include premature ventricular complexes; supraventricular tachycardia may be demonstrated on ambulatory monitoring.

Other types of testing for HCM may include cardiopulmonary exercise testing in which an abnormal or reduced peak oxygen consumption (compared with healthy normal controls) will be found, even in patients who are asymptomatic. Up to 25 percent of patients will have an abnormal blood pressure exercise response characterized by a systolic blood pressure that falls or fails to rise by more than 20 to 25 mm Hg from baseline.[50]

Diagnostic difficulties arise when evaluating athletes and when differentiating between hypertension and hypertrophy. Mild to moderate hypertension does not usually produce wall thickening *greater than* 1.5 cm, but in persons with severe hypertension, genetic testing or investigating family history of HCM may be necessary to make the diagnosis of HCM. Athletic training can result in increased left ventricular wall thickness, but this is rare and only seen in the most elite of athletes.[51] Differentiation of physiological hypertrophy is important because HCM is the most common cause of sudden death in young athletes. Athletes without HCM have increased left *and right* ventricular size, normal diastolic function, and a normal ECG.

Treatment

The management of patients with HCM is aimed at symptom relief and prevention of sudden cardiac death. Beta blockers can be effective in patients with left ventricular outflow tract obstruction who experience chest pain and dyspnea during exertion, but side effects are common. The addition of disopyramide can reduce obstruction by reducing inotropic action. Disopyramide

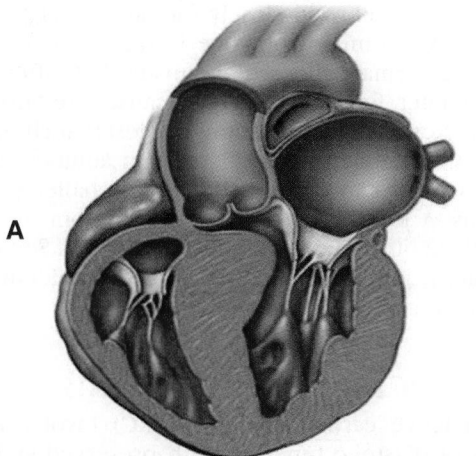
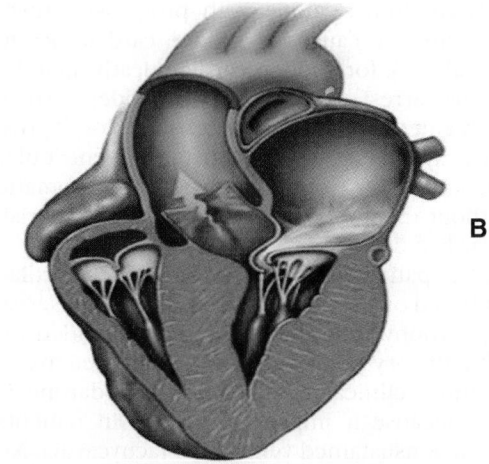

FIGURE 72-2 ■ Hypertrophic cardiomyopathy during relaxation **(A)** and contraction **(B)**.

can cause uncomfortable anticholinergic side effects, so low doses are recommended.[36] Verapamil can be effective, but is only recommended in patients with mild obstruction; outflow gradients may be worsened, resulting in hemodynamic deterioration. If symptoms persist, septal myotomy-myectomy, removal of muscle from the interventricular septum, is performed.[52] The operative mortality for septal myotomy-myectomy is between 1 percent and 5 percent.

An alternative to surgery is alcohol ablation of the interventricular septum. During this procedure, alcohol is injected into septal perforator vessels to induce localized necrosis. No randomized trial comparing surgery and alcohol ablation exists, but nonrandomized trials suggest similar improvement with the two approaches. The long-term effects of ablation—regardless of method—are not known. Atrioventricular sequential pacing has not produced the beneficial effects that caused initial enthusiasm.[36]

Patients without obstruction also may have dyspnea and chest pain because of diastolic dysfunction and myocardial ischemia. Angina during exercise may be treated with beta blockers or calcium antagonists. Nitrates may be useful in chest pain, but care is necessary to prevent excessive reductions in preload. Diuretics can also relieve dyspnea, but judicious use is also needed. Severe heart failure symptoms are rare, but develop when end-stage ventricular dilatation and systolic impairment occurs. When systolic impairment occurs, standard diuretic and vasodilator therapy is needed.

Atrial fibrillation can cause a rapid deterioration of exercise capacity or milder symptoms of exercise intolerance. In addition, atrial fibrillation is associated with a high risk of thromboembolism.[53] Restoration of sinus rhythm is optimal to reduce symptoms, but beta blockers and calcium antagonists can be used to control ventricular rate. Amiodarone is also helpful in preventing atrial fibrillation. All patients with HCM and persistent atrial fibrillation require anticoagulation.

Ventricular dysrhythmias and bradydysrhythmias associated with thromboembolism account for the majority of deaths in patients with HCM.[53] Children and adolescents have a 2 percent to 4 percent frequency of sudden death annually, with frequency decreasing to approximately 1 percent in adults with HCM. Exercise and atrial dysrhythmias, along with progressive myocyte disarray, are the causes of sudden cardiac death. Patients at high risk for sudden cardiac death include: previous cardiac arrest, family history of sudden cardiac death, unexplained syncope, hypotensive blood pressure response during exercise, nonsustained ventricular tachycardia, and severe hypertrophy.[54] Asymptomatic patients without the above risk factors have a low risk of sudden cardiac death.

Treatment of patients at high risk for sudden cardiac death is not based on randomized trials, but on observational data.[36] Prophylactic therapy is recommended for people with a history of sustained ventricular tachycardia and multiple clinical risk factors. Amiodarone is used widely because it improves survival in patients with HCM and nonsustained ventricular tachycardia. No prospective trials have compared amiodarone with ICDs

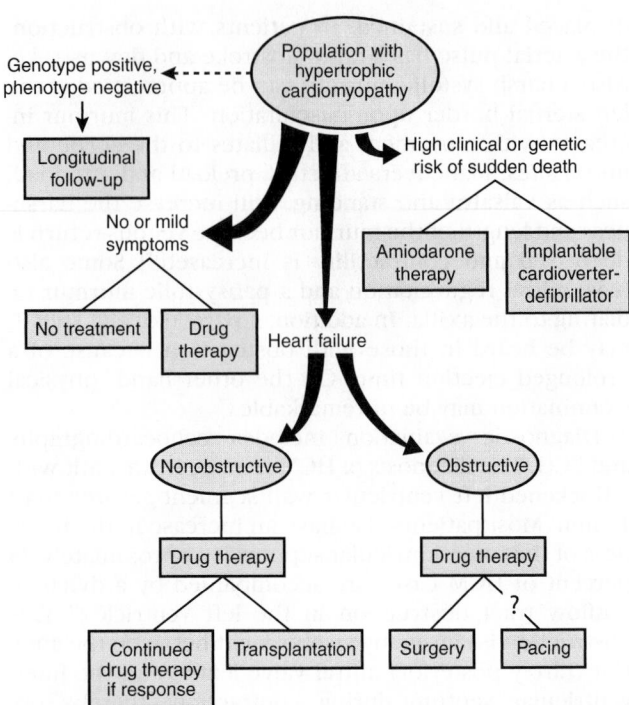

FIGURE 72-3 ■ Principal clinical presentations of HCM and corresponding treatment strategies. The *size of the arrows* indicates the approximate proportion of patients with HCM in each subgroup. The dashed arrow indicates the present uncertainties regarding the size of this subgroup, and the question mark indicates the uncertainties regarding the therapeutic efficacy of pacing. (Spirito P, Seidman CE, McKenna WJ, et al: The management of hypertrophic cardiomyopathy, *New Engl J Med* 336:775-785, 1997.)

in patients with HCM. However, the findings of several trials in patients with coronary artery disease and heart failure suggest that ICDs are better than pharmacological therapy. In view of these data, ICDs are regarded as the best current treatment for HCM patients with a history of cardiac arrest or sustained ventricular dysrhythmia and in patients with multiple clinical risk factors (Figure 72-3).

Counseling is an important part of caring for patients with HCM. Genetic testing may not always be feasible, but careful pedigree analysis can reassure members of families who are not at risk of inheriting the disease. Those found to carry the genetic features of HCM should be followed closely for early signs or symptoms of HCM. Common practice is such that relatives who have a normal echocardiogram and ECG after age 25 are no longer followed yearly because late-onset HCM is rare. New recommendations suggest that clinical screening should occur every 5 years in adults.[38] Atypical or mild cases can present diagnostic challenges for clinicians. A joint consensus document from the American College of Cardiology and the European Society of Cardiology, published in 2003, provides guidelines for the general care of patients with HCM.[38]

RESTRICTIVE CARDIOMYOPATHY

Restrictive cardiomyopathies (**RC**) involve abnormalities of diastolic function with preserved systolic function. There are primary and secondary causes of RC characterized by restrictive filling and reduced diastolic volume of either or both ventricles.[55] The noncompliant ventricle resists ventricular filling because of myocardial or endocardial involvement (dependent on cause); as the volume of the ventricle(s) increase, a steep rise in pressure ensues. Just as with HCM, investigators working with sarcomeric protein genes have now found genetic causes for RC.[56] This is a growing area of research that will provide answers to long-asked questions regarding the cause of RC. The prognosis of RC is generally poor except in reversible cases, such as hemochromatosis. Cardiac amyloidosis is the most common type of RC, and further classification is found in Figure 72-4. Approximately 5 percent to 8 percent of patients with RC die each year; prognosis is closely associated with comorbidities. One-year hospital readmission rates are approximately 50 percent.

Diagnosis

Patients with RC have symptoms of congestive heart failure. Patients report fatigue, dyspnea on exertion, and edema. An elevated jugular venous pressure, S_4, and late S_3 may be present. The ECG in amyloidosis is typically discordant with the echocardiographic findings, demonstrating low voltage and increased wall thickness.

Echocardiography should reveal the anatomical and functional abnormalities typical of RC. Diastolic heart failure is unlikely when no structural abnormalities are detected by echocardiography. Both ventricles are typi-

cally small with decreased volumes and large atria. Atrial septum and cardiac valves may be thickened, and pericardial effusion may be present. The inferior vena cava is usually dilated and does not collapse with inspiration reflecting increased right atrial pressure. In early RC, impaired relaxation may be present, whereas abnormal compliance arises at a later stage.[55] The severity of diastolic impairment reflects diagnostic and prognostic information; the restrictive filling patterns have a five-fold higher mortality risk than nonrestrictive patterns.[57] Diastolic dysfunction can be staged from I to IV, with IV representing severe RC.

It is essential to differentiate RC from constrictive pericarditis, discussed in Chapter 75, because surgical stripping may relieve constrictive pericarditis.[55] Two-dimensional echocardiography is useful in distinguishing between RC and constrictive pericarditis. Furthermore, RC must be distinguished from HCM and from left ventricular hypertrophy secondary to causes, such as hypertension. Endomyocardial biopsy is used to diagnose RC if infiltrative myocardial disease is suspected.[58]

Treatment

No treatment has been shown to be effective for diastolic heart failure, including RC. Treatment is aimed at improving symptoms and preventing tachycardias.[58] Diuretics reduce pulmonary pressure and fluid volume allowing relief of dyspnea. Nitrates can also provide relief, but

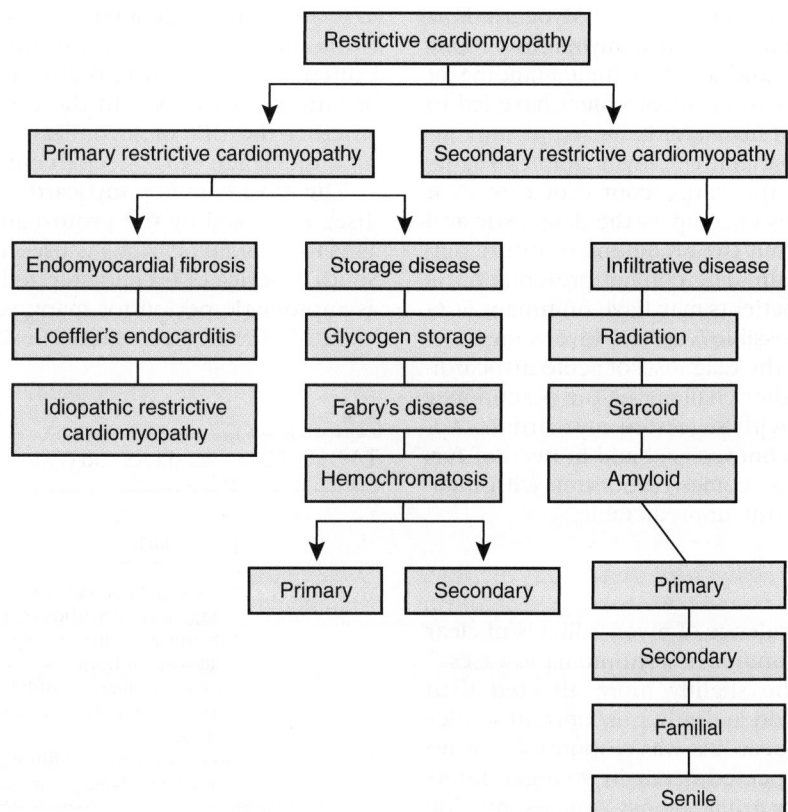

FIGURE 72-4 ▓ Classification of RC, O'Neill J, Ng K. (In Griffin B, editors: *Manual of cardiovascular medicine,* ed 2, Philadelphia, 2004, Lippincott Williams & Wilkins.)

both diuretics and nitrates reduce preload, so caution is necessary to prevent overdiuresis. Patients are advised regarding reduction of sodium intake, daily weight monitoring, and restricted water intake (see Chapter 64). ACE inhibitors and angiotensin-receptor blockers improve stroke volume and reduce myocardial oxygen demand.[58]

Controlling tachycardia is essential in patients with diastolic dysfunction because heart rate is the primary determinant of diastolic filling. Beta blockers and calcium channel blockers slow the heart and enhance diastolic filling in patients with mild diastolic dysfunction. Prolonging diastole in patients with severe diastolic dysfunction will not improve filling and may reduce cardiac output, so great caution is needed in patients with moderate to severe diastolic dysfunction. Atrial fibrillation is poorly tolerated and may cause hemodynamic collapse. Thus it is essential to restore normal sinus rhythm in these patients. Beta agonists and digoxin provide no benefit and are to be avoided.

MYOCARDITIS

Myocarditis is simply defined as inflammation of the heart muscle.[59] It was used to describe all diseases of the heart muscle (unrelated to valvular abnormalities) during the early 1800s. An appreciation for coronary artery disease was gained in the early 1900s, making the term myocarditis obsolete. However, postmortem studies performed in the latter half of the 1900s revealed myocarditis in a surprisingly large number of cases. Thus the term myocarditis reemerged. In 1995 the World Health Organization relabeled myocarditis as myocarditis with cardiac dysfunction.[60] Myocarditis is also known as inflammatory cardiomyopathy. Today endomyocardial biopsy and a better understanding of systemic diseases with cardiac involvement have led to improved recognition of myocarditis.

Management of the patient with myocarditis presents challenges throughout the entire course of care. Not only do these challenges encompass the diagnostic and therapeutic processes, but the prediction of future outcomes remains uncertain. The clinical presentation is highly variable; these patients may have fulminant ECG changes hinting at possible cardiac involvement. A "gold standard" test for the diagnosis of acute myocarditis remains elusive, further challenging the practitioner caring for the patient with suggested myocarditis. Appropriate treatment is controversial and in need of further research. Finally, outcomes of persons with myocarditis remain persistently unpredictable.

Epidemiology

The incidence and prevalence of myocarditis is unclear because of the large number of asymptomatic cases.[59] Men are thought to be slightly more affected than women.[61] In cases of sudden death, postmortem studies have demonstrated myocarditis was responsible for up to 20 percent of unexpected death in younger adults and athletes. Endomyocardial biopsy studies provide highly variable results related to patient selection, biopsy technique, and diagnostic criteria used.

In 1986, the Dallas criteria were developed to better define histological diagnostic criteria (Table 72-3).[62] Biopsies were considered diagnostic of active myocarditis if light microscopy exhibited infiltrating lymphocytes and myocardial necrosis. Although endomyocardial biopsy provides a gold standard for diagnosing myocarditis, the Dallas criteria are criticized for being too restrictive. Some authors suggest that the Dallas criteria probably underestimate the true incidence of myocarditis since the degree of intraobserver variability is large.[63] A clinicopathological classification system was proposed in 1991, but is rarely used.[64]

Causes

Myocarditis has both infectious and noninfectious causes. Often, however, the cause is unknown. Feldman and McNamara categorize the causes of myocarditis into three types: infectious, immune mediated, and toxic (Table 72-4).[59] Mason proposed six distinct forms of myocarditis: acute viral, postviral (most common form), infectious, hypersensitivity, autoimmune, and giant cell myocarditis.[65]

Infectious causes of myocarditis include bacterial, spirochetal, fungal, protozoal, parasitic, rickettsial, and viral. In North America and European nations, viruses are an important cause of myocarditis. Cardiotropic viruses (enteroviruses, adenoviruses) and human immunodeficiency virus type 1 (HIV-1) have been detected in heart tissue. Within the enterovirus group, the Coxsackie B virus is most frequently found. This type of myocarditis results from an infiltration of lymphocytes in response to a recent enteroviral infection. Enteroviral is the most common form of myocarditis found in the United States; this form is also referred to as idiopathic or viral myocarditis.[61] In the case of HIV, it is unclear whether the HIV or secondary viruses account for the high incidence (up to 83 percent) of myocarditis.

The most common myocarditis worldwide is Chagas disease, caused by the protozoan *Trypanosoma cruzi*. This form of myocarditis is present in rural Central and South America. It is characterized by acute infection, an asymptomatic period for many years, and the development of chronic heart failure in 20 percent of patients.

■ ■ ■

TABLE 72-3 DALLAS CRITERIA FOR MYOCARDITIS

	INITIAL BIOPSY	SUBSEQUENT BIOPSY
Myocarditis	Myocardial necrosis or damage or both without CAD Inflammatory infiltrates or fibrosis or both	Ongoing myocarditis or fibrosis
Borderline	Rare inflammatory infiltrates or myocyte damage not apparent	Resolving myocarditis or fibrosis
None	No inflammatory infiltrates, myocyte damage, or both	Resolved myocarditis or fibrosis

CAD, coronary artery disease.
Tang W: Myocarditis. In Griffin B, editor: *Manual of cardiovascular medicine,* ed 2, Philadelphia, 2004, Lippincott Williams & Wilkins.

■■■

TABLE 72-4   CAUSES OF MYOCARDITIS*

Infectious	**Bacterial**	Brucella, *Corynebacterium diphtheriae,* gonococcus, *Haemophilus influenzae,* meningococcus, mycobacterium, *Mycoplasma pneumoniae,* pneumococcus, salmonella, *Serratia marcescens, Staphylococcus, Streptococcus pneumoniae, S. pyogenes, Treponema pallidum, Tropheryma whippelii,* and *Vibrio cholerae*
	Spirochetal	*Borrelia* and leptospira
	Fungal	Actinomyces, aspergillus, blastomyces, *Candida, Coccidioides, Cryptococcus, Histoplasma,* mucormycosis, *Nocardia,* and *Sporothrix*
	Protozoal	*Toxoplasma gondii* and *Trypanosoma cruzi*
	Parasitic	Ascaris, *Echinococcus granulosus, Paragonimus westermani, Schistosoma, Taenia* solium, *Trichinella spiralis,* visceral larva migrans, and *Wuchereria bancrofti*
	Rickettsial	*Coxiella burnetii, Rickettsia rickettsii,* and *R. tsutsugamushi*
	Viral	**Coxsackievirus,** cytomegalovirus, dengue virus, echo virus, encephalomyocarditis, Epstein-Barr virus, hepatitis A virus, hepatitis C virus, herpes simplex virus, herpes zoster, **human immunodeficiency virus,** influenza A virus, influenza B virus, Junin virus, lymphocytic choriomeningitis, measles virus, mumps virus, parvovirus, poliovirus, rabies virus, respiratory syncytial virus, rubella virus, rubeola vaccinia virus, varicella-zoster virus, variola virus, and yellow fever virus
Immune mediated	**Allergens**	Acetazolamide, amitriptyline, cefaclor, colchicine, furosemide, isoniazid, lidocaine, methyldopa, penicillin, phenylbutazone, phenytoin, reserpine, streptomycin, tetanus toxoid, tetracycline, and thiazides
	Alloantigens	Heart-transplant rejection
	Autoantigens	**Chagas disease,** *Chlamydia pneumoniae,* Churg-Strauss syndrome, inflammatory bowel disease, giant cell myocarditis, insulin-dependent diabetes mellitus, Kawasaki disease, myasthenia gravis, polymyositis, **sarcoidosis, scleroderma, systemic lupus erythematosus,** thyrotoxicosis, and Wegener granulomatosis
Toxic myocarditis	**Drugs**	Amphetamines, **anthracyclines,** catecholamines, cocaine, cyclo phosphamide, **ethanol,** fluorouracil, hematin, interleukin 2, lithium, and trastuzumab
	Heavy metals	Copper, iron, and lead
	Physical agents	Electric shock, hyperpyrexia, and radiation
	Miscellaneous	Arsenic, azides, bee and wasp stings, carbon monoxide, inhalants, phosphorus, scorpion bites, snake bites, and spider bites

*The most common causes are shown in bold.
Feldman A, McNamara D: Myocarditis, *N Engl J Med* 343:1390, 2000.

Interestingly the heart failure syndrome is caused by activation of the immune system rather than a direct effect of the protozoan. Therefore Chagas disease is categorized as immune mediated.

Drugs and allergens are also important causes of myocarditis.[66,67] Both immune-mediated mechanisms and the direct toxic effects of drugs and allergens cause myocarditis. The most common drug causes of myocarditis are ethanol and anthracyclines, as discussed above. Cocaine is now appreciated as a cause of myocarditis. Drug-induced allergic or hypersensitivity myocarditis is often unsuspected. Patients may have a serum eosinophilia or the presence of eosinophilic myocardial infiltrates found in endomyocardial biopsy.[68]

Autoantigens are also associated with myocarditis. Chagas disease is the most common autoantigen-associated myocarditis, but other associated systemic diseases including sarcoidosis, scleroderma, and systemic lupus erythematosus also cause myocarditis. Unusual causes include physical agents, heavy metals, and insect and reptile bites.

Pathophysiology

An understanding of the pathophysiology of myocarditis is derived from animal models. Although animal models are not identical to human, insight into the cascade of events associated with myocarditis is provided using cardiotropic viruses. Kawai describes the viral infection response in three phases: the acute phase (0 to 3 days), the subacute phase (4 to 14 days), and the chronic phase (15 to 90 days).[69] These phases are described in Table 72-5.[59]

During the acute phase, myocytes are directly damaged by viral invasion. The virus replicates in the cytoplasm of the myocytes and is released into the interstitium where it undergoes phagocytosis by macrophages. Myocyte antigens and various cytokines, such as tumor necrosis factor (**TNF**) alpha, interferons, and interleukins, are released. The virus can prove lethal to some hosts at this point. In the subacute phase, the virus is cleared by antibodies, cytokines, and natural killer cells. After 2 weeks, the virus is often absent in the myocardium. Persistent cytokines, however, produce a redundant action that is both harmful and beneficial to myocytes. During the second week of acute illness, T and B lymphocytes infiltrate the myocardium. Infected myocytes are lysed, cytotoxic T cells attack viral remnants, and intercellular adhesion molecule-1, expressed on infected myocytes, stimulates the continuation of the immune response. TNF alpha activates endothelial cells, recruits inflammatory cytokines, and has significant negative inotropic effects. TNF alpha also appears necessary for the clearance of viral particles.

■ ■ ■

TABLE 72-5 PHASES OF MYOCARDITIS

PHASE	CHARACTERISTICS
Acute myocarditis (d 0-3)	Viral infection
	Myocyte damage
	Myocyte antigens released
	Cytokines released
Subacute myocarditis (d 4-14)	Infiltrating mononuclear cells
	Cytokine production
	T and B lymphocytes activated
	Neutralizing antibodies
	Viral clearance
Chronic myocarditis (d15-90)	Fibrosis
	Cardiac enlargement
	Apoptosis

Feldman A, McNamara D: Myocarditis, *N Engl J Med* 343:1388-1398, 2000.
Tang W: Myocarditis. In Griffin B, editor: *Manual of cardiovascular medicine,* ed 2, Philadelphia, 2004, Lippincott Williams & Wilkins.
Haas G: Etiology, evaluation, and management of acute myocarditis, *Cardiology in Rev* 9:88-95, 2001.

■ ■ ■

TABLE 72-6 INCIDENCE OF VARIOUS CLINICAL CHARACTERISTICS IN PATIENTS WITH MYOCARDITIS

CHARACTERISTIC	INCIDENCE
Age	42 ± 14 years
Male gender	62%
Female gender	38%
Antecedent viral illness	59%
Fever	19%
Chest pain	35%
CK-MB increase	12%
ESR increase	60%
Leukocytosis	24%
Cardiac immunoglobulin antibody titer 1:40 or greater	62%

CK-MB, isoenzyme of creatine kinase with muscle and brain subunits; *ESR,* erythrocyte sedimentation rate.
Mason JW, O'Connell JB, Herskowitz A et al: A clinical trial of immunosuppressive therapy for myocarditis. The myocarditis treatment trial investigators, *N Engl J Med* 333:270, 1995.

The chronic phase is characterized by continued myocyte injury that can lead to fibrosis and dilated cardiomyopathy or myocardial recovery. Many factors are involved in the recovery or development of chronic disease, such as host and genetic factors, age, nutritional state, and prior chest radiation.[70]

Diagnosis

Clinical features of myocarditis vary widely from symptomatic patients with ECG abnormalities to those with fulminant heart failure.[60] Approximately 60 percent of patients with viral myocarditis report a history of recent flu-like symptoms, such as fever, arthralgias, and fatigue. Investigators from the myocarditis treatment trial reported additional clinical characteristics, such as fever, chest pain, and specific laboratory findings, shown in Table 72-6.[65]

Signs and symptoms may include dyspnea, S_3 gallop, jugular venous distention, edema, and orthopnea if systolic dysfunction is experienced. Patients may also report syncope and palpitations if the myocarditis is associated with dysrhythmias. Specific findings associated with underlying systemic illnesses may also be found. Sarcoid myocarditis may include findings of lymphadenopathy, dysrhythmias, and additional organ involvement. Acute rheumatic fever is associated with erythema marginatum, polyarthralgia, chorea, and subcutaneous nodules. Hypersensitivity myocarditis may manifest a maculopapular rash along with a history of current medication and/ or drug use. Giant cell myocarditis is associated with ventricular tachycardia and rapid and progressive heart failure.

Laboratory findings may include leukocytosis, elevated sedimentation rate, eosinophilia, and elevated cardiac fraction of creatine kinase. Electrocardiographic findings may show ventricular dysrhythmias or heart block or ST-segment changes with Q waves often consistent with acute myocardial infarction. The endomyocardial biopsy remains the best approach to diagnosis despite its limited sensitivity and specificity.[61] However, investigators suggest that the diagnosis of myocarditis cannot be based on histological findings alone. It is important to include other diagnostic tests, including assays for autoimmune serum markers or histocompatibility and intercellular adhesion molecules on cardiac myocytes to identify patients with autoimmune causes of myocarditis.

Additional diagnostic testing may be required in suspected, albeit unusual, causes of myocarditis. Rheumatological testing may include antinuclear antibodies and rheumatoid factor. For suggested systemic lupus erythematosus, anti-dsANA is required. For polymyositis, Wegner granulomatosus and scleroderma, anti-Jo1, c-ANCA, and anti-SCL70, respectively, is required. Cardiac troponin I is elevated 50 percent of the time with proven myocarditis. Troponins are superior to creatine kinase testing in early and late myocarditis presentation.[61] Echocardiogram is standard to exclude alternative causes of heart failure, detect thrombi and valvular disease, and to monitor therapy. Coronary angiography may be needed to rule out coronary disease as a cause of new-onset heart failure and because myocarditis may mimic acute myocardial infarction.

Treatment

Supportive care is the first line of treatment for patients with myocarditis.[59,60] Heart failure therapies are standard (e.g., diuretics, ACE inhibitors, beta blockers, and aldosterone antagonists). Digoxin is not recommended or recommended in low doses because of its prodysrhythmic properties.[60] Anticoagulation is used to prevent thromboembolic events, especially in association with Chagas disease, atrial fibrillation, and prior embolic episodes. Inotropic therapy is reserved for severe hemodynamic compromise. Aggressive mechanical support with intraaortic balloon pump counterpulsation or a ventricular assist device may be required. Early consideration for cardiac transplantation is given to patients with progressive heart failure or giant cell myocarditis.[71]

Bed rest is advocated because of the theoretically increased risk of myocardial inflammation and necrosis, as shown in animal models. Patients are usually advised to abstain from exercise for several months. Elimination of unnecessary medication, especially in patients with eosinophilia, is recommended to reduce the possibility of hypersensitivity myocarditis.

Dysrhythmias are managed with standard therapies, such as beta blockers and amiodarone. Given the often transient nature of dysrhythmia in myocarditis and dysrhythmia resolution with left ventricular recovery, ICDs are used only for those refractory to medical therapy.[61] Permanent pacemakers are used in patients with heart block or bradydysrhythmia.

Close and consistent follow-up is required in patients with myocarditis because of the possibility that persistent chronic inflammation will lead to dilated cardiomyopathy. Initially, pharmacological and physical monitoring is done every 1 to 3 months.[60]

Controversies that remain surrounding the care of patients with myocarditis include the use of endomyocardial biopsy and immunosuppressive therapy. Routine use of endomyocardial biopsy to confirm myocarditis is unnecessary.[59,60] No difference in treatment would be undertaken unless rapid deterioration occurs. Furthermore, there is only a 10 percent incidence myocarditis with positive biopsy results in recent-onset heart failure. False-positive rates are high because of wide interobserver variability. There are some exceptions, however. In patients with rapidly progressive heart failure, despite conventional therapy, or in those with new-onset ventricular tachydysrhythmias or conduction disturbances, biopsy might provide direction for care. Also when specific causes of myocarditis are suggested, such as sarcoid, systemic lupus erythematosus and others, biopsy is indicated. The sensitivity of one biopsy is approximately 50 percent.[64]

The association between myocarditis and autoimmunity suggests that immunosuppressive therapy may be of benefit. However, results from early uncontrolled studies using immunosuppressive therapy were conflicting.[70,72] The myocarditis treatment trial ($n = 111$) is the largest randomized trial designed to explore the efficacy of immunosuppression.[65] The primary outcome measure was change in left ventricular ejection fraction **(LVEF).** Two groups received standard therapy, one of which was randomized to receive prednisone combined with either azathioprine or cyclosporine for 6 months. The results showed no difference in mean LVEF between the groups. In addition, there was no difference in survival between groups. These results suggest that there is no clinical benefit from immunosuppressive therapy in myocarditis. Routine immunosuppressive therapy is not recommended.

Currently, many practitioners still initiate immunosuppression in patients with biopsy-proved myocarditis in whom clinical deterioration has taken place, despite maximal therapy. Some argue that immunosuppressive therapy is needed in extraordinary circumstances. Immunosuppressive therapy in patients with giant cell myocarditis is an exception. These patients are treated with combination therapy. In a study using cyclospo-rine, muromonab-CD3, corticosteroids, and azathioprine patients had improved survival.[73]

Investigational therapies include immune modulatory therapy. This therapy has shown promise in a small group of pediatric patients.[74] No benefit has been established for antiviral regimens or nonsteroidal agents.

SUMMARY

Caring for patients with cardiomyopathies and myocarditis presents challenges in diagnosis, treatment, and in counseling because our understanding of the long-term outcomes of these diseases remains unclear. Genetic studies have provided a better understanding of the causes and pathophysiology of hypertrophic and restrictive cardiomyopathies than previously held. The widely varying physical presentation and difficulties in diagnosing myocarditis continue to present challenges in caring for these patients. Future research may enable identification and treatment of cardiac genetic abnormalities, which would provide hope for patients and families affected by HCM and restrictive cardiomyopathies. Heightened suspicion for, early identification of, and close monitoring of patients with cardiomyopathies and myocarditis is essential in the care of these complicated and often perplexing patients.

REFERENCES

1. Fuster V, Alexander RW, O'Rourke R et al: *Hurst's The heart,* ed 11, 2004-2005, McGraw-Hill Access Medicine.
2. Chien KR: Genome circuits and the integrative biology of cardiac diseases, *Nature* 407:227-232, 2000.
3. Codd MB, Sugrue DD, Gersh BJ et al: Epidemiology of idiopathic dilated and hypertrophic cardiomyopathy. A population-based study in Olmsted County, Minnesota, 1975-1984, *Circulation* 80:564-72, 1989.
4. Gregori D, Rocco C, Miocic S et al: Estimating the frequency of familial dilated cardiomyopathy in the presence of misclassification errors, *J Appl Statistics* 28:53-62, 2001.
5. Milasin J, Muntoni F, Severini GM et al: A point mutation in the 5′ splice site of the dystrophin gene first intron responsible for X-linked dilated cardiomyopathy, *Hum Mol Genet* 5:73-9, 1996.
6. Towbin JA, Hejtmancik JF, Brink P et al: X-linked dilated cardiomyopathy, Molecular genetic evidence of linkage to the Duchenne muscular dystrophy (dystrophin) gene at the Xp21 locus, *Circulation* 87:1854-65, 1993.
7. Mestroni L, Maisch B, McKenna WJ et al: Guidelines for the study of familial dilated cardiomyopathies. Collaborative research group of the European human and capital mobility project on familial dilated cardiomyopathy, *Eur Heart J* 20:93-102, 1999.
8. Gerdes AM, Kellerman SE, Moore JA et al: Structural remodeling of cardiac myocytes in patients with ischemic cardiomyopathy, *Circulation* 86(2):26-30, 1992.
9. Gerdes AM, Onodera T, Wang X et al: Myocyte remodeling during the progression to failure in rats with hypertension, *Hypertension* 28:9-14, 1996.
10. Rowan RA, Masek MA, Billingham ME: Ultrastructural morphometric analysis of endomyocardial biopsies. Idiopathic dilated cardiomyopathy, anthracycline cardiotoxicity, and normal myocardium, *Am J Cardiovasc Pathol* 2:137-44, 1988.
11. Caforio AL, Keeling PJ, Zachara E et al: Evidence from family studies for autoimmunity in dilated cardiomyopathy, *Lancet* 344:773-7, 1994.
12. Kawai C, Takatsu T: Clinical and experimental studies on cardiomyopathy, *N Engl J Med* 293:592-7, 1975.
13. Gilbert EM, Mason JW: Immunosuppressive therapy of myocarditis, In Engelmeier RS, O'Connell JB, editors: *Drug therapy in di-*

lated cardiomyopathy and myocarditis, New York, 1987, Marcel Dekker, pp 233-263.

14. Franciosa JA, Wilen M, Ziesche S et al: Survival in men with severe chronic left ventricular failure due to either coronary heart disease or idiopathic dilated cardiomyopathy, *Am J Cardiol* 51:831-6, 1983.

15. Fuster V, Gersh BJ, Giuliani ER et al: The natural history of idiopathic dilated cardiomyopathy, *Am J Cardiol* 47:525-31, 1981.

16. Tiret L, Rigat B, Visvikis S et al: Evidence, from combined segregation and linkage analysis, that a variant of the angiotensin I-converting enzyme (ACE) gene controls plasma ACE levels, *Am J Hum Genet* 51:197-205, 1992.

17. Richardson P, McKenna W, Bristow M et al: Report of the 1995 World Health Organization/International Society and Federation of Cardiology task force on the definition and classification of cardiomyopathies, *Circulation* 93:841-2, 1996.

18. McKay RG, Pfeffer MA, Pasternak RC et al: Left ventricular remodeling after myocardial infarction: a corollary to infarct expansion, *Circulation* 74:693-702, 1986.

19. Moss AJ, Zareba W, Hall WJ et al: Prophylactic implantation of a defibrillator in patients with myocardial infarction and reduced ejection fraction, *N Engl J Med* 346:877-83, 2002.

20. Bristow MR, Feldman AM, Saxon LA: Heart failure management using implantable devices for ventricular resynchronization: comparison of medical therapy, pacing, and defibrillation in chronic heart failure (COMPANION) trial. COMPANION steering committee and COMPANION clinical investigators, *J Card Fail* 6:276-85, 2000.

21. Rathore SS, Curtis JP, Wang Y et al: Association of serum digoxin concentration and outcomes in patients with heart failure: *JAMA* 289:871-8, 2003.

22. Levy D, Larson MG, Vasan RS et al: The progression from hypertension to congestive heart failure, *JAMA* 275:1557-62, 1996.

23. Bristow MR: Mechanisms of development of heart failure in the hypertensive patient, *Cardiology* 92(suppl 1):3-6,7-9,20-21, 1999.

24. Felker GM, Thompson RE, Hare JM et al: Underlying causes and long-term survival in patients with initially unexplained cardiomyopathy, *N Engl J Med* 342:1077-84, 2000.

25. Grossman W: Cardiac hypertrophy: useful adaptation or pathologic process?, *Am J Med* 69:576-84, 1980.

26. Plante E, Couet J, Gaudreau M et al: Left ventricular response to sustained volume overload from chronic aortic valve regurgitation in rats, *J Card Fail* 9:128-40, 2003.

27. Bristow MR, Mason JW, Billingham ME et al: Dose-effect and structure-function relationships in doxorubicin cardiomyopathy, *Am Heart J* 102:709-18, 1981.

28. Lewis W, Kleinerman J, Puszkin S: Interaction of Adriamycin in vitro with cardiac myofibrillar proteins, *Circ Res* 50:547-53, 1982.

29. Shaddy RE, Olsen SL, Bristow MR et al: Efficacy and safety of metoprolol in the treatment of doxorubicin-induced cardiomyopathy in pediatric patients, *Am Heart J* 129:197-9, 1995.

30. Pearson GD, Veille JC, Rahimtoola S et al: Peripartum cardiomyopathy. National Heart, Lung, and Blood Institute and Office of Rare Diseases (National Institutes of Health) workshop recommendations and review, *JAMA* 283:1183-8, 2000.

31. Midei MG, DeMent SH, Feldman AM et al: Peripartum myocarditis and cardiomyopathy, *Circulation* 81:922-8, 1990.

32. Maisch B: Alcohol and the heart, *Herz* 21:207-12, 1996.

33. Dietary Guidelines for Americans, U.S. Department of Agriculture, US Department of Health and Human Services. Accessed on 12 March, 2003.

34. Prazak P, Pfisterer M, Osswald S et al: Differences of disease progression in congestive heart failure due to alcoholic as compared to idiopathic dilated cardiomyopathy, *Eur Heart J* 17:251-7, 1996.

35. Jacobson DR, Buxbaum JN: Genetic aspects of amyloidosis, *Adv Hum Genet* 20:69-123,309-11, 1991.

36. Elliott P, McKenna W: Hypertrophic cardiomyopathy, *Lancet* 363:1881-1891, 2004.

37. Report of the 1995 World Health Organization/International Society and Federation of Cardiology task force on the definition and classification of cardiomyopathies, *Circulation* 93:841-842, 1996.

38. Maron BJ, McKenna WJ, Danielson GK et al: American College of Cardiology/European Society of Cardiology clinical expert consensus document on hypertrophic cardiomyopathy. A report of the American College of Cardiology foundation task force on clinical expert consensus documents and the European Society of Cardiology committee for practice guidelines, *Eur Heart J* 24:1965-1991, 2003.

39. Maron BJ, Sato N, Roberts WC et al: Quantitative analysis of cardiac muscle cell disorganization in the ventricular septum: comparison of fetuses and infants with and without congenital heart disease and patients with cardiomyopathy, *Circulation* 60:685-696, 1979.

40. Marian AJ, Roberts R: The molecular genetic basis for hypertrophic cardiomyopathy, *J Mol Cell Cardiol* 33:655-670, 2001.

41. Franz WM, Muller OJ, Katus HA: Cardiomyopathies: from genetics to the prospect of treatment, *Lancet* 358:1627-1637, 2001.

42. Richard P, Charron P, Carrier L et al: Hypertrophic cardiomyopathy: distribution of disease genes, spectrum of mutations, and implications for a molecular diagnosis strategy, *Circulation* 107:2227-2232, 2003.

43. Ackerman MJ, VanDriest SL, Ommen SR et al: Prevalence and age dependence of malignant mutations in the beta-myosin heavy chain and troponin T genes in hypertrophic cardiomyopathy: a comprehensive outpatient perspective, *J Am Coll Cardiol* 39:2042-2048, 2002.

44. Mogensen J, Kubo T, Duque M et al: Idiopathic restrictive cardiomyopathy is part of the clinical expression of cardiac troponin I mutations, *J Clin Invest* 111:209-216, 2003.

45. Lipshultz SE, Sleeper LA, Towbin JA et al: The incidence of pediatric cardiomyopathy in two regions of the United States, *N Engl J Med* 348:1647-1655, 2003.

46. Robbins M, McRae T: Hypertrophic cardiomyopathy. In Griffin B, editor: *Manual of cardiovascular medicine,* ed 2, Philadelphia, 2004, Lippincott Williams & Wilkins.

47. Maron BJ, Spirito P: Implications of left ventricular remodeling in hypertrophic cardiomyopathy, *Am J Cardiol* 1:1339-1344, 1998.

48. Klues HG, Schiffers A, Maron BJ: Phenotypic spectrum and patterns of left ventricular hypertrophy in hypertrophic cardiomyopathy: morphologic observations and significance as assessed by two-dimensional echocardiography in 600 patients, *J Am Coll Cardiol* 26:1699-1708, 1995.

49. Panza JA, Petrone RK, Fananapazir L et al: Utility of continuous wave Doppler echocardiography in the noninvasive assessment of left ventricular outflow tract pressure gradient in patients with hypertrophic cardiomyopathy, *J Am Coll Cardiol* 19:91-99, 1991.

50. Olivotto I, Maron BJ, Montereggi A et al: Prognostic value of systemic blood pressure response during exercise in a community based population with hypertrophic cardiomyopathy. *J Am Coll Cardiol* 33:2044-2051, 1999.

51. Shapiro LM, Kleinebenne A, McKenna WJ: The distribution of left ventricular hypertrophy in hypertrophic cardiomyopathy: comparison to athletes and hypertensives, *Eur Heart J* 6:967-974, 1985.

52. Schoendube FA, Klues HG, Reith S et al: Long-term clinical and echocardiographic follow-up after surgical correction of hypertrophic obstructive cardiomyopathy with extended myectomy and reconstruction of the subvalvular mitral apparatus, *Circulation* 92:II122-127, 1995.

53. Maron BJ, Olivotto I, Bellone P et al: Clinical profile of stroke in 900 patients with hypertrophic cardiomyopathy, *J Am Coll Cardiol* 39:301-307, 2002.

54. Elliott PM, Poloniecki J, Dickie S et al: Sudden death in hypertrophic cardiomyopathy: identification of high risk patients, *J Am Coll Cardiol* 36:2212-2218, 2000.

55. Asher C, Klein A: Diastolic heart failure: restrictive cardiomyopathy, constrictive pericarditis, and cardiac tamponade: clinical and echocardiographic evaluation, *Card in Rev* 10:218-229, 2002.

56. Huang X, Du J: Troponin I, cardiac diastolic dysfunction and restrictive cardiomyopathy, *Acta Pharmacol Sin* 12:1569-1575, 2004.

57. Klein AL, Hatle LK, Taliercio CP et al: Prognostic significance of Doppler measures of diastolic function in cardiac amyloidosis: a Doppler echocardiography study, *Circulation* 83:808-816, 1991.

58. O'Neill J, Ng K: Heart failure with preserved systolic function. In Griffin B, editor: *Manual of cardiovascular medicine,* ed 2, Philadelphia, 2004, Lippincott Williams & Wilkins.

59. Feldman A, McNamara D: Myocarditis, *N Engl J Med* 343:1388-1398, 2000.

60. Tang W: Myocarditis. In Griffin B, editor: *Manual of cardiovascular medicine,* ed 2, Philadelphia, 2004, Lippincott Williams & Wilkins.

61. Haas G: Etiology, evaluation, and management of acute myocarditis, *Cardiology in Rev* 9:88-95, 2001.

62. Aretz HT, Billingham ME, Edwards WD et al: Myocarditis: a histopathologic definition and classification, *Am J Cardiovasc Pathol* 1:3-14, 1987.

63. Shanes JG, Gahli J, Billingham ME et al: Interobserver variability in the pathologic interpretation of endomyocardial biopsy results, *Circulation* 75:401-405, 1987.

64. Lieberman EB, Hutchins GM, Herskowitz A et al: Clinicopathologic description of myocarditis, *J Am Coll Cardiol* 18:1617-1626, 1991.

65. Mason JW, O'Connell JB, Herskowitz A et al: A clinical trial of immunosuppressive therapy for myocarditis, *N Engl J Med* 333:269-275, 1995.

66. Billingham ME: Pharmacotoxic myocardial disease: an endomyocardial study. In Sekiguchi M, Olsen EGJ, Goodwin JF, editors: Myocarditis and related disorders: proceedings of the International Symposium on Cardiomyopathy and Myocarditis, Tokyo, 1985, Springer-Verlag, pp 278-282.

67. Feenstra J, Grobbee DE, Remme WJ et al: Drug-induced heart failure, *J Am Coll Cardiol* 33:1152-1162, 1999.

68. Morimoto S, Kubo N, Hiramitsu S et al: Changes in the peripheral eosinophil count in patients with acute eosinophilic myocarditis, *Heart Vessels* 18:193-196, 2003.

69. Kawai C: From myocarditis to cardiomyopathy: mechanisms of inflammation and cell death: learning from the past for the future. *Circulation* 99:1091-1100, 1999.

70. O'Connell JB, Mason JW: Diagnosing and treating active myocarditis, *West J Med* 150:431-435, 1989.

71. Cooper L, Berry G, Shabetai R: Idiopathic giant-cell myocarditis: natural history and treatment. Multicenter giant cell myocarditis study group investigators, *N Engl J Med* 336:1860-1866, 1997.

72. Parrillo JE, Cunnion RE, Epstein SE et al: A prospective, randomized, controlled trial of prednisone for dilated cardiomyopathy, *N Engl J Med* 321:1061-1068, 1989.

73. Rosenstein E, Zucker MJ, Kramer N: Giant cell myocarditis: most fatal of autoimmune diseases, *Semin Arthritis Rheum* 30:1-16, 2000.

74. Drucker N, Colan S, Lewis et al: Gamma-globulin treatment of acute myocarditis in the pediatric population, *Circulation* 89:252-257, 1994.

■■■ chapter 73
Care of Patients with Endocarditis

Megan White
Jill Howie

CHAPTER ABBREVIATIONS

CNS   central nervous system

CVA   cerebrovascular accident

ECG   electrocardiogram

ESR   erythrocyte sedimentation rate

IE   infective endocarditis

PCR   polymerase chain reaction

TEE   transesophageal echocardiogram

TTE   transthoracic echocardiogram

Despite impressive advances in both technological and diagnostic capabilities, the identification of infective endocarditis (**IE**) remains challenging to even the most skilled practitioner. In fact William Osler,[1] a physician-scientist investigating IE in the late 19th century, expressed a similar sentiment: "Few diseases present greater difficulties in the way of diagnosis than malignant endocarditis. . . . It is no disparagement to the many skilled physicians who have put their cases on record to say that, in fully one-half (of cases) the diagnosis was made post mortem."

Endocarditis is an infection of the endocardium, or innermost lining of the heart, caused typically by bacteria or fungus. The most common pathogens are *Staphylococcus* and *Streptococcus,* as described in detail below. The intruding pathogen typically adheres to heart valves, but may also take hold at the site of a structural defect (e.g., mitral valve prolapse, pacemaker insertion site). Intact endothelium is relatively resistant to infection. The pathogen creates solid vegetations, or masses consisting of bacteria, white blood cells, fibrin, and platelets that invade and destroy surrounding tissue (Figure 73-1).

The clinical presentation of IE is often perplexing; patients may have either a myriad of specific symptoms or vague symptoms, such as fever, chills, and myalgias. There exists no single diagnostic test to either confirm or reject the presence of endocarditis; rather diagnosis relies on the thoughtful analysis of all microbiological, technological, and clinical data. Antibiotic regimens are a mainstay of treatment today, and indeed with the advent of penicillin in the 1940s, there followed a drastic reduction in the number of IE-related deaths. However, multidrug-resistant bacteria challenge conventional therapeutic regimens. The necessity of an early diagnosis cannot be emphasized enough because the mortality rate from this disease remains high without prompt and aggressive treatment. In 2000, IE represented the fourth leading cause of life-threatening infectious disease states.[2]

CAUSES OF INFECTIVE ENDOCARDITIS

The foundation for endocardial infection is either an aortic, mitral, or less commonly, tricuspid valve that has experienced epithelial injury and thus attracts bacteria to its flawed surface. This accumulation of bacteria, fibrin, and platelets creates a thrombus, or vegetation, that stands poised to dislodge into the circulation and give rise to harmful and potentially deadly complications. Valvular damage can occur as a result of age-associated degenerative changes; structural changes, such as mitral valve prolapse; congenital defects, such as coarctation of the aorta, or bicuspid aortic valve, patent ductus arteriosus; or the presence of a prosthetic valve (Figure 73-2). Additionally, history of rheumatic heart disease—an acute febrile illness following a streptococcal infection—can result in inflammation and fibrosis of the heart valves. Each of the above conditions significantly increases the risk of developing IE.

The incidence of IE does not appear to be diminishing; estimates today range between 15,000 and 20,000 cases each year in the United States alone.[3] The median incidence was 3.6 per 100,000 population per year in a recent review of contemporary cases.[3] Twice as many men develop IE as women.

New societal factors are contributing to the high incidence of IE. Although illnesses, such as rheumatic heart disease, are less common in the industrialized world today, increases in intravenous drug use and body piercing contribute to the incidence of IE. Injection drug use increases the risk of IE seven times more than rheumatic heart disease or a prosthetic valve.[2] Body piercing has become increasingly popular and may be an important consideration in a young adult with endocarditis. One group of researchers surveyed university undergraduates and reported that 51 percent had undergone body piercing (14.7 percent of the campus enrollment).[4] Most body-piercing practitioners are unlicensed, and few states have authority over these businesses.[5] Case reports of endocarditis have emerged following oral, nasal, and nipple body piercing with both gram-positive and gram-negative organisms isolated. In addition, case reports include previously healthy adults and those known to be at risk for endocarditis, such as intravenous drug users and those with a prosthetic cardiac valve.[5,6] Although patients with underlying cardiac disease, a prosthetic valve, or intravenous drug use account for approximately 70 percent of IE cases, between 20 percent and 30 percent of patients with IE have no predisposing risk factors[7,8] (see accompanying Genetics feature on bicuspid aortic stenosis).

Implantable devices, such as pacemakers and defibrillators, can damage the endocardium, creating a suit-

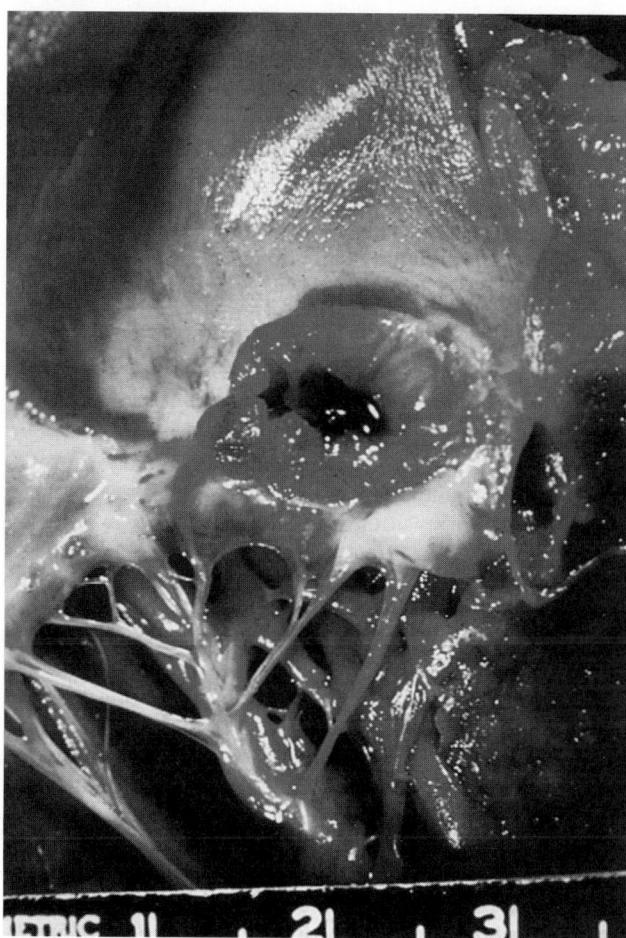

FIGURE 73-1 ■ A large, bulky vegetation on the mitral valve seen at autopsy. Clot is present centrally in the vegetation. From Karchmer AW: Infective endocarditis. (In Zipes DP, Libby P, Bonow R et al, editors: *Braunwald's heart disease: a textbook of cardiovascular medicine,* Philadelphia, 2005, Elsevier Saunders.)

▪▪▪ GENETICS

GENETIC BASIS FOR INFECTIVE ENDOCARDITIS

Bicuspid aortic valve is a structural variant associated with an increased risk of infective endocarditis. The incidence in the general population of bicuspid aortic valve is 0.9% to 2.0%. Although 54% of adults with valvular aortic stenosis have a bicuspid aortic valve, in most cases it remains undetected until infective endocarditis or calcification occurs.

Studies have established familial clustering of bicuspid aortic valve and genetic inheritance. To determine genetic heritability, Cripe and colleagues tested 50 probands with bicuspid aortic valve, obtaining a three-generation family history and echocardiograms on first-degree relatives. In all, 309 probands and their relatives participated in the study. The prevalence of bicuspid aortic valve was 24% (n = 74 individuals). The heritability of bicuspid aortic valve was 89%, suggesting that bicuspid aortic valve was almost entirely genetic in this population. The inheritance patterns are complex, with several different genes that have varying alleles, and not all occurrences of bicuspid aortic valves have the same genetic basis. There may be a number of genes involved in a given individual with bicuspid aortic valve, and the pattern may be multigenic.

Cripe L, Andelfinger G, Martin LJ et al: Bicuspid aortic valve is heritable, *J Am Coll Cardiol* 44:138-43, 2004.

Yener N, Oktar GL, Erer D et al: Bicuspid aortic valve, *Ann Thorac Cardiovasc Surg* 8:264-7, 2002.

able environment for the development of IE. Nosocomial sources have been reported to cause between 7 percent and 29 percent of all cases of IE[9]; in one series, infected intravascular devices were responsible in at least 50 percent of the cases. The placement of prosthetic valves, intravenous and arterial catheters, and pacemaker and/or defibrillator leads is associated with *Staphylococcus* infection.[2] Interestingly, *Staphylococcus* infection following hemodialysis has become more common, emerging as an important risk factor for the development of IE. In fact hemodialysis patients are two

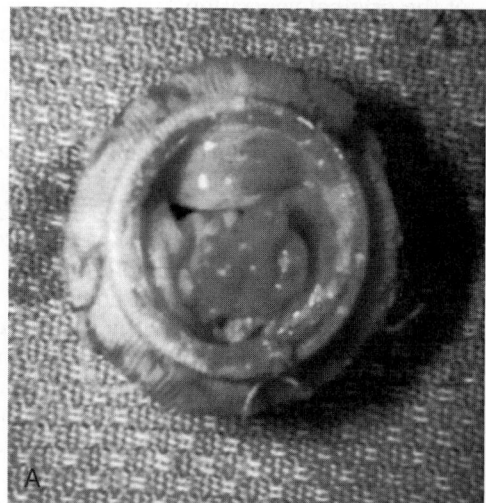
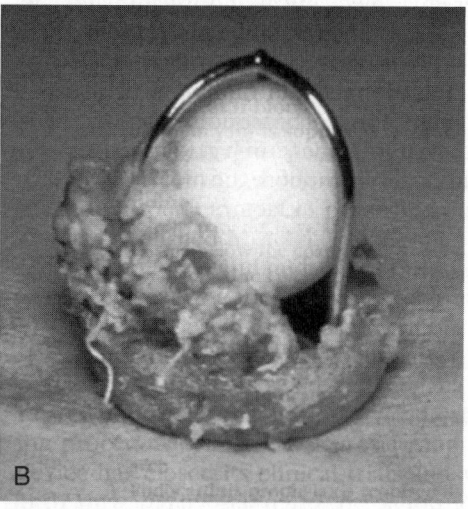

FIGURE 73-2 ■ A Starr-Edwards prosthesis removed from the aortic position, where this large vegetation related to *Aspergillus* infection partially obstructed the outflow tract, but also allowed regurgitation by preventing valve closure. (From Karchmer AW: Infective endocarditis. In Zipes DP, Libby P, Bonow R et al, editors: *Braunwald's heart disease: a textbook of cardiovascular medicine,* Philadelphia, 2005, Elsevier Saunders, p 1636, Figure 58-1B.)

to three times more likely to develop IE than peritoneal dialysis patients or the general population.[10]

In the United States, 93,000 valve procedures were done in 2002.[11] Prosthetic valve-associated endocarditis is often differentiated between early and late onset endocarditis. Early prosthetic valve endocarditis occurs within 60 days of valve surgery and is commonly caused by either *Staphylococcus aureus* or *S. epidermidis*. Late prosthetic valve endocarditis occurs more than 60 days following surgery and is typically associated with streptococci and gram-negative bacteria.

INFECTIOUS AND PATHOLOGICAL PROCESS

Staphylococci and streptococci together account for 80 percent of all cases of IE, although some previously undetected pathogens, such as *Chlamydia,* are seen increasingly.[10,12] Infection rates caused by staphylococcus species are slightly higher in patients with native valve disease. Coagulase-negative *Staphylococcus* is the most common pathogen in early prosthetic valve endocarditis.[9]

At this time, *S. aureus,* part of the normal flora of the skin, mucous membranes, and nasopharynx, is the most common cause of IE, surpassing streptococci. *S. aureus* has been closely linked to IE in injection drug users. The pathogen has been found on the right side of the heart, involving the tricuspid valve in more than 50 percent of cases.[10]

The pathogens causing IE have the unique ability to bind to the inflamed surface of damaged endothelium. They colonize the affected area and trigger vegetation formation by encouraging platelet aggregation and fibrin deposition. Once the bacteria enter the bloodstream and target the endocardium, infection follows a particularly aggressive course and is commonly associated with local endocardial tissue destruction. The exact process by which the organisms interact with the human host is complex. At the cellular level, during transient bacteremia, mechanical and inflammatory lesions promote adherence of microbes to injured endothelium. This process stimulates an inflammatory response with expression of beta 1 integrins by endothelial cells.[12] The inflammatory response facilitates adhesion of pathogens that carry fibronectin-binding surface proteins. With endothelial disruption, the microbes contact blood carrying subendothelial factors that promote coagulation. The pathogens bind to the resultant coagulum, which initiates a cycle of monocyte activation, cytokine and tissue factor production, and progressive enlargement of the infected vegetation. As the vegetation grows, it damages local tissues. Paravalvular abscesses result from extension of infection, and septic emboli are a risk. The abscesses are often resistant to antibiotic treatment and require surgical débridement.

Streptococcus species, specifically *Streptococcus viridans* and *S. bovis,* are often associated with IE in the elderly and those with poor dentition. Transient bacteremia with oral *Streptococcus,* occurring with chewing or brushing the teeth, has been linked to the development of endocarditis. The elderly represent an increasing segment of the population susceptible to IE; in fact approximately 50 percent of cases occur in persons older than age 60.[13] This fact is not surprising because increasing age is associated with degenerative or structural valve changes, which maximize the opportunity for infection. In addition, it is not uncommon for the elderly to undergo therapies likely to result in bacteremia, such as the placement of prosthetic valves, pacemakers and/or defibrillators, and urinary catheters.

Although uncommon, gram-negative bacteria, such as the HACEK group of microorganisms (*Haemophilus parainfluenzae, H. aphrophilus, Actinobacillus actinomycetemcomitans, Cardiobacterium hominis,* and *Eikenella* and *Kingella* species) can lead to endocardial infection. Fungal infection is also seen in postoperative, immunosuppressed, and intravenous drug use populations. Ten percent of all IE cases involve several newly evolving bacteria, including *Tropheryma whippelii, Coxiella burnetii, Bartonella, Chlamydia,* and *Legionella* species. These bacteria are extremely difficult to identify by conventional diagnostic methods and therefore often result in a negative blood culture.[10] Fungi documented to cause IE include *Candida, Histoplasma,* and *Aspergillus* species, and *Torulopsis glabrata.*[12]

DIAGNOSIS

IE has historically been diagnosed as either acute or subacute, reflecting the onset, severity, and progression of the disease.[9] The *acute* form of the disease progresses rapidly and is often caused by *Staphylococcus* infection, whereas *subacute* disease commonly results from *Streptococcus* or gram-negative infection and follows a slower, more prolonged course.

Manifestation of IE can range from nonspecific symptoms of fever, diaphoresis, weight loss, myalgias, and night sweats to overt complications, including cerebrovascular accident and heart failure. Characteristic signs associated with IE, such as Osler nodes, Janeway lesions, and Roth spots, are a result of microembolization of the original vegetation.

Osler nodes are *tender* and erythematous nodules on the pads of the fingers and toes, whereas Janeway lesions are *nontender* macules on the palms and soles (Figure 73-4). Roth spots are found on funduscopic examination and are oval, retinal hemorrhages with pale centers. Persons with IE may also have splinter hemorrhages beneath the fingernails (Figure 73-3) and petechiae on the conjunctivae, the oral mucosa, the neck, chest, and abdomen (see Chapter 45).

Laboratory and electrocardiographic abnormalities may also be present, but are not specific to IE. These findings may include anemia, leukocytosis, abnormal urinalysis and elevated sedimentation rate (**ESR**), and C-reactive protein level. Electrocardiographic findings of bundle or fascicular blocks suggest paravalvular invasion. A new atrioventricular block has a moderately positive predictive value for formation of myocardial abscess.[9]

The variable clinical presentation of endocarditis necessitated the establishment of diagnostic criteria that allows the clinician to effectively summarize data

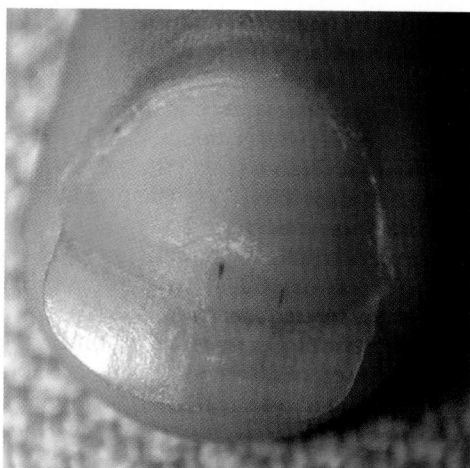

FIGURE 73-3 ■ Splinter hemorrhages beneath the fingernail. (Courtesy Chris Ha, MD and Dermatlas www.dermatlas.org).

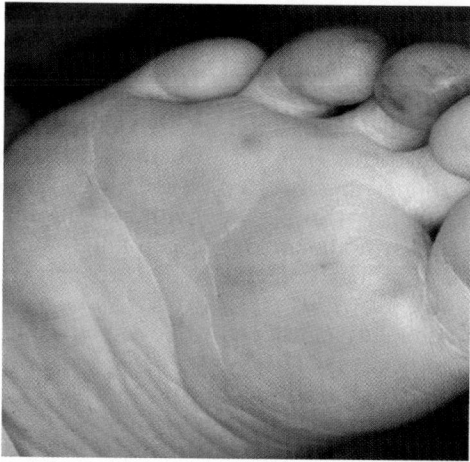

FIGURE 73-4 ■ Janeway lesions on the sole of the foot. (Courtesy Bernard Cohen, MD and Dermatlas *www.dermatlas.org*).

BOX 73-1 ■ ■ ■
MODIFIED DUKE CRITERIA FOR THE DIAGNOSIS OF INFECTIVE ENDOCARDITIS

Major Criteria
1. Positive blood culture
   A. Typical microorganisms from two separate cultures, or
   B. Persistently positive blood cultures
      ➤ Two or more positive blood samples drawn more than 12 hours apart
2. Evidence of endocardial involvement
   A. Positive echocardiogram for infective endocarditis (IE)
      ➤ Oscillating intracardiac mass on valve supporting structures, in the path of regurgitant jets, or on implanted material, or
      ➤ Abscess, or
      ➤ Dehiscence of prosthetic valve, or
   B. New valvular regurgitation (worsening or changing of preexisting murmur not sufficient)

Minor Criteria
1. Predisposing cardiac condition or intravenous drug use
2. Fever (higher than 38° C)
3. Vascular: major arterial emboli, septic pulmonary infarcts, mycotic aneurysm, intracranial hemorrhage, conjunctival hemorrhages, Janeway lesions
4. Immunologic: glomerulonephritis, Osler nodes, Roth spots, and positive rheumatoid factor
5. Microbiologic: positive blood cultures not meeting major criterion, or serologic evidence of active infection with organism consistent with IE
6. Echocardiogram consistent with IE, but not meeting major criterion

Definite Diagnosis
1. Two major criteria, or
2. One major and three minor criteria, or
3. Five minor criteria, or
4. Pathology or bacteriology of vegetations, major emboli, or intracardiac abscess specimen

Possible Diagnosis
1. One major and one minor criterion, or
2. Three minor criteria

Rejected Diagnosis
1. Firm alternate diagnosis, or
2. Resolution of IE manifestations with antibiotic therapy for 4 days, or less
3. No pathological evidence of IE at surgery or autopsy after antibiotic therapy for 4 days or less

Tak T, Reed KD, Haselby RC et al: An update on the epidemiology, pathogenesis and management of infective endocarditis with emphasis on *staphylococcus aureus*, Wisconsin Med J 2002;101:27.

---

and promptly select an appropriate treatment regimen. Investigators at Duke University established such standardized and validated criteria in 1994, appropriately named the Duke criteria, to reflect the importance of both microbiological and echocardiographic findings in endocarditis. These criteria were later refined and are today recognized as the principle standard in the recognition of IE (Box 73-1).

Although echocardiography has assumed an important role in the diagnosis of IE, positive blood cultures are highly sensitive for the presence of the disease. It is currently recommended that three sets of blood cultures be obtained within the first 12 to 24 hours of presentation. Cultures may remain negative in up to 5 percent of patients with IE.[2] This negative culture may be a result of prior antibiotic administration or the presence of bacteria that are either slow growing or difficult to culture by traditional methods. In culture-negative cases, longer incubation times or the use of alternate techniques, such as polymerase chain reaction (**PCR**), should be considered. It is obvious that blood culture-negative cases cause an unfortunate delay in the recognition of the offending bacteria and treatment of the disease. Investigators have recognized this fact and are presently considering modifications to the Duke criteria to include specific serological criteria applied to organisms traditionally difficult to culture.

For the past 20 years, echocardiography has proved essential in characterizing and diagnosing IE. It has the added benefit of enabling the clinician direct visualization of the heart, detection of the presence or absence of vegetations, and estimation of cardiac function. Although transthoracic echo (**TTE**) is rapid and noninvasive, it is limited in patients with pulmonary disease, chest wall deformities, and those who are obese; in fact TTE may be inadequate in up to 20 percent of adults. Transesophageal echo (**TEE**), superior to TTE, is highly sensitive (48 percent to 100 percent) and specific (85 percent to 98 percent) in comparison with TTE.[2,9] Although there exists some controversy with respect to the use of the two types of echo for diagnosis, TTE is presently recommended for low-risk patients with suspected IE who have native heart valves and are good candidates for imaging. On the other hand, TEE is advised in high-risk patients who have prosthetic valves, congenital disease, heart failure, history of IE, or a new heart murmur.[14]

Persons with intermediate risk for IE undergo TTE first and if negative are followed-up with TEE. Intermediate probability patients include those with unexplained bacteremia with a gram-positive coccus, catheter-associated *S. aureus* bacteremia, and injection drug user admitted with fever or bacteremia. Based on the Duke criteria, there are three echocardiographic findings that are considered major criteria in the diagnosis of IE: a mobile mass attached to the valve, endocardium, or prosthetic material; evidence of extension of the infection by detection of abscesses or fistulae; and the dehiscence of a prosthetic valve.[15]

In addition to serological criteria, future amendments of the Duke criteria may include additional laboratory and electrocardiographic criteria, such as an elevated erythrocyte sedimentation rate **(ESR)** and C-reactive protein, newly detected clubbing or splenomegaly, and microscopic hematuria on urinalysis.[14,16] In addition to the above diagnostic tests, a baseline electrocardiogram **(ECG)** should be obtained and repeated to detect a new heart block or conduction delay that could indicate extension of infection.

COMPLICATIONS

Complications of IE can involve all body systems, but most are cardiac or neurological, resulting from direct bacterial invasion or effects of systemic emboli (Box 73-2). Complications of IE are a direct result of embolic events in 22 percent to 50 percent of cases.[8,14] Embolism occurs most frequently with aortic and mitral valve infection caused by either *S. aureus, Candida* species, or organisms of the HACEK group.[14] Embolic complications follow an unpredictable course and remarkably may occur before, during, or even following antimicrobial therapy. The devastation that occurs when part or all of a vegetation breaks into the systemic circulation is striking.

The central nervous system **(CNS)** is most frequently ravaged by systemic emboli; between 60 percent and 70 percent of all embolic events involve the CNS, often the middle cerebral artery.[8] Sadly, greater than 90 percent of embolic episodes involving this artery are also the deadliest.[14] In some cases, the initial presentation of IE may be a cerebrovascular accident **(CVA).** Patients may have stroke symptoms, such as lethargy, confusion, paralysis, fever, or blindness (see Chapter 76). Another neurological manifestation of septic emboli is the formation of intracranial mycotic aneurysms, representing the spread of infection to the arterial intraluminal space and extension through the intima and vessel wall. Emboli commonly lodge at areas of vessel bifurcation, and often this is where mycotic aneurysms are found. Although such aneurysms are a rare finding, their presence should be considered in patients who have headache, delirium, or focal neurological deficits.

Embolic complications have been known to occur in other organs, including the lungs. Often associated with right-sided IE and intravenous drug use, pulmonary emboli may be misdiagnosed as pneumonia, the chest radiograph revealing multiple, scattered infiltrates.[17] Other sites of occlusion include the kidneys, joints, bone, spleen, and coronary arteries. Acute renal failure may ensue following assault to the kidney, or patients may have arthritic pain or osteomyelitis if either the joints or bones are involved, respectively. Abdominal pain may manifest in patients with splenic infarcts or abscess, and symptomatology resembling acute myocardial infarction may coincide with coronary artery involvement.

Although neurological embolic events in conjunction with IE are a relatively frequent occurrence, the most common cause of death in patients with IE is heart failure.[18] Heart failure may develop rapidly or evolve over time as the affected valve becomes increasingly dysfunctional. If, however, infection progresses to valve perforation, rupture of chordae tendineae, vegetation obstruction, prosthetic valve dehiscence, or the creation of endocardial fistulae, acute heart failure is likely to ensue. Emergent surgery is indicated in such instances where medical management alone is unlikely to succeed.

Another reason for the development of heart failure is the presence of valvular or paravalvular abscesses. These are extensions of infection to tissue surrounding the valve. In extreme instances, extension may progress into the pericardial space itself resulting in pericarditis or into cardiac conduction tissue manifesting on the ECG as atrioventricular, fascicular, or bundle branch block patterns. It is essential to stay alert to the possible presence of abscess formation, particularly in the patient with new heart block, or one in whom fever persists for longer than 14 days, despite appropriate antibiotic treatment.

TREATMENT

Antimicrobial therapy is the foundation of treatment in IE. The goal of this therapy is the eradication of endocardial vegetations and prevention, to the extent possible, of complications arising from disease progression. Long-term parenteral therapy with bactericidal antibiotics is often indicated after identification of the offending

---

BOX 73-2 ■■■
COMPLICATIONS ASSOCIATED WITH INFECTIVE ENDOCARDITIS

- Acute renal failure
- Cerebrovascular accident
- Conduction abnormalities
- Congestive heart failure
- Mycotic aneurysm
- Paravalvular abscess, perforation, or fistula
- Pericarditis
- Pulmonary emboli
- Septic arthritis
- Splenic abscess/infarct
- Systemic embolization

microorganism by microbiological assays. This latter point—long-term therapy—is essential to successful treatment. The ideal patient condition is one that grants the clinician time to determine the bacteria involved *before* commencing antibiotic therapy. However, not all clinical scenarios afford the luxury of time in designing and implementing a detailed treatment plan.

When IE is suspected, several questions arise: (1) Is the infection culture positive or negative? The accompanying pharmacology feature suggests antimicrobial therapy based on culture results for common organisms. If culture results identify a less common organism, therapy is still not adequately defined. If culture results are negative, therapy should be individualized and usually includes ceftriaxone, penicillin, vancomycin, or ampicillin along with an aminoglycoside. (2) Does the patient have a prosthetic valve or native valve? The suspected organisms will differ based on valve origin, thereby affecting treatment choice. (3) If the patient has a prosthetic valve and the culture results are negative, is the IE early or late occurring? If the IE is within the first 12 months after prosthetic valve placement, treatment must include ceftriaxone or cefotaxime to cover the HACEK organisms.

Naturally, empiric therapy is initiated immediately in patients who are either unstable or acutely ill with endocarditis or those patients with prosthetic valves. It has also been suggested that elderly patients undergo immediate empiric therapy following the retrieval of blood cultures.[13] Antibiotics effective against the most common bacterial offenders (staphylococci, *S. viridans*, and enterococci) are required. Penicillin, or vancomycin if a penicillin allergy is present, with rifampin and/or gentamicin are employed in initial therapy.[2,13] Essential in caring for elders is frequent evaluation of renal function and aminoglycoside concentrations to prevent nephrotoxicity.

Once a result has been obtained from blood cultures and susceptibility patterns determined, a treatment plan can be initiated. In patients with a prosthetic heart valve in which *S. aureus* is the causative agent, the differentiation between methicillin-sensitive *S. aureus* and methicillin-resistant *S. aureus* must be made and treatment followed accordingly.

Prosthetic valve endocarditis is treated with vancomycin plus gentamicin plus rifampin in cases of methicillin-resistant *S. aureus* and nafcillin or oxacillin plus rifampin plus gentamicin in cases of methicillin-sensitive *S. aureus*. The aggressive nature of IE caused by *S. aureus* in patients with prosthetic valves and the associated 40 percent mortality rate necessitates early and decisive treatment.

In persons with native valve endocarditis, methicillin-resistant *S. aureus* is treated with vancomycin for 6 weeks. Treatment of methicillin-sensitive *S. aureus* native valve endocarditis entails nafcillin or oxacillin with or without gentamicin for the first 3 to 5 days of therapy. Specific antimicrobial therapies for uncomplicated, penicillin-susceptible and penicillin-resistant *Streptococcus* species, in addition to right-sided endocarditis, are provided in detail in the Pharmacology feature.

Anticoagulant therapy requires careful consideration for individual needs. In patients with native valves, anticoagulants are only required for indications separate from IE. Patients with a prosthetic valve require cautious anticoagulation because anticoagulant therapy does not reduce the risk of embolization and may increase intracerebral hemorrhage risk.

Medical management is a viable option in many cases of IE; however, there are times when surgery becomes necessary. Interdisciplinary care is now the state of the science in excellent patient care and the treatment of IE is no exception. Consultation with and advice from cardiothoracic surgeons must occur early in the course of illness because surgery may be required in the event of failed antibiotic therapy or unpredicted change in patient status.

There are several indications for surgery, including persistent infection or the development of heart failure despite antibiotic therapy. Endocarditis resulting from difficult-to-treat organisms, such as fungi and vancomycin-resistant *Enterococcus,* more than one episode of systemic embolization, paravalvular abscess, fistula detected on echocardiogram, a new conduction delay on the ECG, septal perforation, vegetation greater than 1 centimeter in diameter, and prosthetic valve endocarditis caused by nonstreptococcal organisms, all require surgical therapy.[2,13,19] The optimal time for surgery is when hemodynamic status is stable; stability is the principle determinant of operative mortality. Serial echocardiograms may be used to monitor the status of valve function.

Mortality rate for persons with IE vary in relation to several factors: the organism involved, presence of complications or comorbid conditions, presence of paravalvular extension, and combination therapy using medical and surgical management.[20] Overall mortality rates for both native and prosthetic valve patients remain as high as 20 percent to 25 percent with death resulting from CNS events or hemodynamic deterioration.[21] Injection drug users generally suffer from right-sided endocarditis, and mortality is approximately 10 percent in this group.[9]

PROPHYLAXIS

Prevention of IE is essential in select at-risk patient populations and with certain interventional procedures that tend to result in transient bacteremia. Persons with a prosthetic valve, a previous history of IE, congenital and rheumatic heart disease, hypertrophic cardiomyopathy, and mitral valve prolapse with regurgitation should receive antibiotic prophylaxis (shown in the Evidence-Based Practice feature).

Procedures requiring prophylaxis in the above at-risk population are dental procedures likely to result in gingival or mucosal trauma, tonsillectomy, bronchoscopy, esophageal dilatation or sclerotherapy, gallbladder surgery, cystoscopy, urethral dilatation or catheterization, prostate surgery, gynecological procedures in the presence of infection, and the incision and drainage of infected tissue. Prophylaxis for procedures involving the oral cavity, respiratory tract, or esophagus targets or-

■■■ PHARMACOLOGY

TREATMENT FOR COMMON CAUSES OF INFECTIVE ENDOCARDITIS

PATHOGEN	NATIVE-VALVE ENDOCARDITIS	PROSTHETIC-VALVE ENDOCARDITIS
Penicillin-susceptible viridans strep, strep bovis, strep with MIC of penicillin 0.1 or less	Penicillin G or ceftriaxone for 4 weeks	Penicillin G for 6 weeks and gentamicin for 2 weeks
Relatively penicillin-resistant strep	Penicillin G for 4 weeks and gentamicin for 2 weeks	Penicillin G for 6 weeks and gentamicin for 4 weeks
Strep species with MIC of penicillin greater than 0.5, enterococcus species	Penicillin G (or ampicillin) and gentamicin for 4-6 weeks	Penicillin G (or ampicillin) and gentamicin for 6 weeks
Methicillin-susceptible staph	Nafcillin or oxacillin for 4-6 weeks, with or without gentamicin for first 3-5 days of therapy	Nafcillin or oxacillin and rifampin for 6 weeks and gentamicin for 2 weeks
Methicillin-resistant staph	Vancomycin for 6 weeks	Vancomycin and rifampin for 6 weeks and gentamicin for 2 weeks
Right-sided staph native-valve IE	Nafcillin or oxacillin with gentamicin for 2 weeks	N/A
HACEK organisms*	Ceftriaxone for 4 weeks (or ampicillin and gentamicin for 4 weeks as an alternative)	Ceftriaxone for 6 weeks (or ampicillin and gentamicin for 6 weeks as an alternative)

*A slow-growing gram-negative bacterium that is a normal component of human flora. The name is formed from the initials of included organisms: *Haemophilus, Actinobacillus, Cardiobacterium, Eikenella,* and *Kingella.*
Mylonakis EM, Calderwood SB: Infective endocarditis in adults, *New Engl J Med* 345:1325, 2001.
IE, Infective endocarditis; *MIC,* minimum inhibitory concentration; *staph,* Staphylococcus; *strep,* Streptococcus.

■ EVIDENCE-BASED PRACTICE

PROPHYLACTIC ANTIBIOTIC REGIMENS FOR INFECTIVE ENDOCARDITIS

Dental, Oral, Upper Respiratory Tract Procedures

No penicillin allergy	Amoxicillin 2 g P.O. 1 hr before procedure
	Amoxicillin or ampicillin 2 g I.V. ½ to 1 hr before procedure
Allergy to penicillin	Clindamycin 600 mg P.O. 1 hr before procedure
	Azithromycin/clarithromycin 500 mg P.O. 1 hr before procedure
	Cephalexin 2 g P.O. 1 hr before procedure
	Clindamycin 600 mg I.V. 30 min before procedure
	Cefazolin 1 g I.V. 30 min before procedure

Genitourinary or Gastrointestinal Procedures

No penicillin allergy: high risk	Ampicillin or amoxicillin 2 g I.V. plus gentamicin 1.5 mg/kg I.V. ½ to 1 hr before procedure **AND** ampicillin or amoxicillin 1 g P.O. 6 hr later
No penicillin allergy: moderate risk	Ampicillin or amoxicillin 2 g I.V. ½ to 1 hr before procedure
	Amoxicillin 2 g P.O. 1 hr before procedure
Allergy to penicillin: high risk	Vancomycin 1 g **AND** gentamicin 1.5 mg/kg I.V. or I.M. before procedure
Allergy to penicillin: moderate risk	Vancomycin 1 g before procedure

I.V., intravenous; *I.M.,* intramuscular; *P.O.,* by mouth.
Horstkotte D, Follath F, Gutschik E et al: Guidelines on prevention, diagnostic and treatment of infective endocarditis. Executive summary. The task force on infective endocarditis of the European Society of Cardiology, *Euro. Heart J* 25:270, 2004.

ganisms common to these areas, such as viridians streptococci and organisms of the HACEK group, whereas gastrointestinal and genitourinary procedure prophylaxis addresses enterococci and *S. bovis* organisms.

FUTURE DIRECTIONS

The diagnosis of IE has proven evasive and puzzling and will remain so as society today faces an increase in at-risk behaviors and newly emerging infectious causes of endocarditis. As the fourth leading cause of life-threatening infectious disease, IE remains a continuing threat. Although diagnostic criteria are updated and modified to ensure the optimal approach to disease recognition, it is paramount that IE be promptly recognized to ensure appropriate management.[22]

Nurses play an important role in the initial diagnosis of IE, maintaining an index of suspicion when working with at-risk populations. Clinical signs and symptoms of IE may be variable in their presentation, often masked by other comorbid conditions. Whether we work with the aging population or adolescents doing body piercing, it is critical that we have a heightened awareness and suspicion for IE. Staying up to date on the guidelines for prophylaxis is essential because nurses often identify persons who would benefit from antibiotic prophylaxis.

Existing treatment options for IE include antibiotic and surgical therapy, but the timing of these treatments remains challenging. Adherence to the lengthy course of antibiotics is essential, and nurses are closely involved with teaching patients and helping them overcome barriers to extended adherence. With newly evolving bacterial species, continuing research is essential to identify new approaches and therapies for this patient population.

REFERENCES

1. Prendergast BD: Diagnostic criteria and problems in infective endocarditis, *Heart* 90:611-613, 2004.
2. Tak T, Reed KD, Haselby RC et al: An update on the epidemiology, pathogenesis and management of infective endocarditis with emphasis on *Staphylococcus aureus, Wisconsin Med J* 101:24-33, 2002.

3. Moreillon P, Que Y: Infective endocarditis, *Lancet* 363:139-49, 2004.
4. Mayers LB, Judelson DA, Moriarty BW et al: Prevalence of body art piercing, *Mayo Clinic Proc* 77:29-34, 2002.
5. Akhondi H, Rahimi AR: Haemophilus aphrophilus endocarditis after tongue piercing, *Emerg Infect Dis* 8:850-851, 2002.
6. Goldrick BA: Endocarditis associated with body piercing: the implications for advanced practice nurses, *Amer J Nurs* 103:26-27, 2003.
7. Hoen B, Alla F, Selton-Suty C et al: Changing profile of infective endocarditis: results of a 1-year survey in France, *JAMA* 288:75-81, 2002.
8. Murtagh B, Frazier OH, Letsou GV: Diagnosis and management of bacterial endocarditis in 2003, *Current Opin Cardiol* 18:106-110, 2003.
9. Mylonakis EM, Calderwood SB: Infective endocarditis in adults, *New Engl J Med* 345:1318-1330, 2001.
10. Moreillon P, Que Y: Infective endocarditis, *Lancet* 363:139-149, 2004.
11. Heart disease and stroke statistics - 2005 update, 2005. Retrieved August 17, 2005 from http://www.americanheart.org.
12. Prendergast BD: The changing face of infective endocarditis, *Heart* Online first published on October 10, 2005 as 10.1136hrt.2005.067256 (later in *Heart* 92, 2005).
13. Dhawan VK: Infective endocarditis in elderly patients, *Clin Infect Dis* 34:806-812, 2002.
14. Bayer AS, Bolger AF, Taubert KA et al: Diagnosis and management of infective endocarditis and its complications, *Circulation* 98:2936-2948, 1998.
15. Horstkotte D, Follath F, Gutschik E et al: Guidelines on prevention, diagnostic and treatment of infective endocarditis. Executive summary. The task force on infective endocarditis of the European Society of Cardiology, *Europ Heart J* 25:267-276, 2004.
16. Petti CA, Fowler VG: Staphylococcus aureus bacteremia and endocarditis, *Cardiol Clin* 21:219-233, 2003.
17. Crawford MH, Durack DT: Clinical presentation of infective endocarditis, *Cardiol Clin* 21:159-166, 2003.
18. Sexton DJ, Spelman D: Current best practices and guidelines: assessment and management of complications in infective endocarditis, *Cardiol Clin* 21:273-282, 2003.
19. Devlin RK, Andrews MM, Von Reyn CF: Recent trends in infective endocarditis: influence of case definitions, *Curr Opin Cardiol* 19:134-139, 2004.
20. Eykyn SJ: Endocarditis: basics, *Heart* 86:476-480, 2001.
21. Homma S, Grahame-Clarke C: Toward reducing embolic complications from endocarditis. *JACC* 42:781-783, 2003.
22. Millar BC, Moore JE: Emerging issues in infective endocarditis. *Emerg Infect Dis* 10:1110-1116, 2004.

Care of Patients with Peripheral Vascular Disease

Sharon K. Christman

CHAPTER ABBREVIATIONS

AAA abdominal aortic aneurysm

ABI ankle brachial index

ACCP American College of Chest Physicians

AV arteriovenous

AVA American Vascular Association

CE-MRA Contrast-enhanced magnetic resonance angiography

CEA carotid endarterectomy

CN cranial nerve

CPT claudication pain time

CT computed tomography

CTV computed tomography venography

DSA digital subtraction angiography

DVT deep vein thrombosis

FDA Food and Drug Administration

HDL high-density lipoprotein

INR international normalized ratio

LDL low-density lipoprotein

MRI magnetic resonance imaging

MWT maximum walking time

PAD peripheral arterial disease

PE pulmonary embolism

PTA percutaneous transluminal angioplasty

PTS post-thrombotic syndrome

PVD peripheral vascular disease

SLP segmental limb systolic pressure measurement

TASC TransAtlantic Inter-Society Consensus

TIA transient ischemic attack

t-PA tissue plasminogen activator

USPSTF U.S. Preventative Services Task Force

VTE venous thromboembolic disease

V/Q ventilation/perfusion

V ascular disease is the major cause of death and disability in Western society. The number of people with vascular disease exceeds 25 million in the United States, and this number will continue to rise as the population ages.[1] Peripheral vascular disease (PVD) is arguably one of the most comprehensive classifications of disorders in health care today. As a result, vascular nurses must be prepared to care for patients with a multitude of disorders and educational needs including,

but not limited to: ischemic bowel disease (acute mesenteric arterial occlusion), arteriovenous (AV) fistula repair, carotid artery disease, lower extremity arterial occlusive disease, Raynaud disease, Coumadin management, abdominal aortic aneurysms (AAAs), subclavian steal phenomenon (proximal subclavian artery stenosis or occlusion), venous stasis ulcers, venous varicosities, wound management, deep vein thrombosis (DVT), and pulmonary embolism (PE). However, for the cardiac nurse, both at the bedside and in an advanced practice role, their understanding of the treatment and care of the PVD patient should be more focused, with a more in-depth knowledge of the prevalent and life-threatening peripheral vascular disorders.

The decision on which disorders to include in this chapter was determined by their relative prevalence and virulence. Virulence refers to the severity of possible sequelae and the frequency of those sequelae. The purpose of this chapter is to expound on the pertinent information that a cardiac nurse should know to provide excellent care to patients who also have PVD. Specifically, the cause of arterial and venous disease will be discussed, followed by an in-depth discussion of the four vascular disorders with the highest prevalence and virulence. These four disorders are: carotid artery disease, lower extremity peripheral arterial disease (PAD), AAA, and venous thromboembolic disease (VTE).

Stroke is the third leading cause of death and one of the leading causes of adult disability. Although stroke may be caused by a variety of disease, atherothrombosis is the most common contributing factor.[2] (Note: *Carotid artery disease: prevalence = high; virulence = high*).

Limb ischemia, both acute and chronic, is a result of a decrease or worsening in limb perfusion from arterial occlusion, causing a potential threat to limb viability (i.e., amputation). Eight to twelve million Americans are presumed to have PAD,[3] and amputation occurs in about 2 percent of these patients every year. In addition, these patients are six times more likely to die from cardiovascular causes than those without the disease.[4] (Note: *PAD: prevalence = high; virulence = high*).

AAAs are the fifteenth leading cause of death overall, with a reported 15,000 deaths from aneurysm every year.[5] The incidence of AAA in patients with PAD has a reported range of 3.2 percent to 13 percent.[6,7] In a first-degree relative of the person with an aneurysm, the incidence of AAA is 15 percent to 20 percent.[8] (Note: *AAA: prevalence = moderate; virulence = high*.)

VTE, which includes DVT and PE, represents the third most common cardiovascular disorder, affecting more than 2 million Americans annually.[9,10] PE occurs in 80 percent of patients with proximal DVT, 46 percent with calf DVT, and 10 percent with superficial venous thrombosis.[11] About 10 percent of symptomatic PE are thought to be rapidly fatal, and another 5 percent of those diagnosed and treated for PE die as a result.[12] (Note: *VTE: prevalence = high; virulence = moderate*).

In the last 20 years, significant advancements have occurred in the treatment of vascular disease through improved technology in vascular imaging, endovascular intervention, surgical techniques, and pharmacotherapy. As a result, the standard treatment of many of the peripheral vascular disorders is continually changing. However, there are a number of guidelines and publications that help guide practice. In 2001, the American Heart Association published a guideline for the prevention of stroke,[13] which was updated in 2002[14] and used to frame the discussion of cause and medical treatment of carotid artery disease. In 2000, The TransAtlantic Inter-Society Consensus **(TASC)**, with members from 16 international vascular societies, published a consensus statement on the diagnosis and treatment PAD.[15] The TASC document was used as a framework for the section of this chapter on lower extremity PAD. Although there are no guidelines for the treatment of AAA, the data from the past 10 years of open repair versus endovascular repair are now being reported.[16] As a result, clinicians are able to draw evidence-based conclusions from aggregate data rather than from small data sets or single case studies. In addition, in February 2005 the U.S. Preventive Services Task Force **(USPSTF)** published screening guidelines for AAA.[17] Finally, in 2004 an evidence-based guideline on antithrombotic therapy was published by the American College of Chest Physicians **(ACCP)** and was the primary source of information for this chapter related to the pharmacological management of VTE.[18]

There are several guidelines published on the treatment of risk factors for PVD: hypertension,[19] dyslipidemia,[20] smoking,[21] sedentary lifestyle,[22] and obesity.[23] These are the same risk factors identified for cardiac disorders, such as coronary artery disease and heart failure, and are discussed in their respective chapters. As a result, these guidelines will not be discussed in-depth here, but will be referred to as appropriate.

ARTERIAL SYSTEM
Anatomy and Physiology
A detailed description of the peripheral vasculature can be found in Chapter 4 of this text. The primary function of the arterial system is to conduct and distribute oxygen and other nutrients to the tissues of the body. Conductive arteries are relatively straight and have few branches, whereas distributive arteries arise from the conductive arteries and divide into multiple branches. Examples of conductive arteries include the common and external iliac arteries, the common and superficial femoral arteries, and the popliteal arteries, whereas examples of distributive arteries include the arteries to the abdominal viscera and the internal iliac arteries (Figure 74-1).

The arterial wall is composed of three layers, the inner intima, the middle media, and the outer adventitia. Changes that occur with aging most often affect the larger and medium-sized vessels, and primarily occur in the intima, with the elasticity decreasing and thickness and collagen content increasing.[24] As a result of intimal thickening, there is a decreased delivery of nutrients to the media, resulting in calcification and degeneration of the smooth muscle in the media. Blood flow is dependent on the resistance in the muscular arteries and arterioles and is controlled both locally and systemically. Local factors include tissue oxygen and carbon dioxide tension, potassium and lactic acid levels, prostaglandins, and endothelial cell-derived relaxing and constricting factors.[25] Systemic control involves neurohormonal control involving a delicate balance between the vasoconstricting sympathetic adrenergic system and vasodilating parasympathetic nervous system and their respective primary neurotransmitters epinephrine, norepinephrine, and acetylcholine.

Causes of Arterial Disease
Atherosclerosis is responsible for the majority of PAD. Although all arteries may be affected by atherosclerosis, the conductive arteries are most often affected, particularly at their branch points. The segments of the arterial tree most commonly affected by atherosclerosis include the carotid arteries, aortic bifurcation, iliac and common femoral arteries, femoral profunda, superficial femoral artery, and distal popliteal artery. Generally the lesions are segmental, with unaffected segments interspersed between lesions (Figure 74-2). Depending on the location of the lesion, clinical manifestations can begin to occur when the vessel is anywhere between 20 percent and 70 percent occluded.

Although the exact cause of atherosclerosis is not fully known, there are several theories (see Chapter 10). The underlying pathological condition involves smooth muscle cell migration and proliferation to a specific area of the vessel, attachment of platelets, monocytes, and lymphocytes, and the combination of macrophages and lipids to form foam cells, resulting in the presence of a lesion attached to the vessel wall. Ultimately, atherosclerosis leads to a narrowing of the vessel from gradual thickening of the intimal and medial lining and decreased blood flow distal to the narrowing. Sometimes thrombus formation occurs at the narrowing, resulting in complete occlusion of the artery, which necessitates emergency medical intervention.

Whereas atherosclerosis is the leading cause of PAD, other arterial pathological conditions can also occur including aneurysm formation. Aneurysms are diseased areas of arteries that become thinned and dilated.[26] Although the exact cause of these changes is not completely known, most of the research in the area of aneurysm formation has focused on structural changes of the middle layer of the artery, the media. The two primary structural proteins of the media, elastin and collagen, have been found in decreased quantities in aneurysms.[27] Elastin provides elasticity to the vessel, whereas collagen allows vessel distention without rupture. The

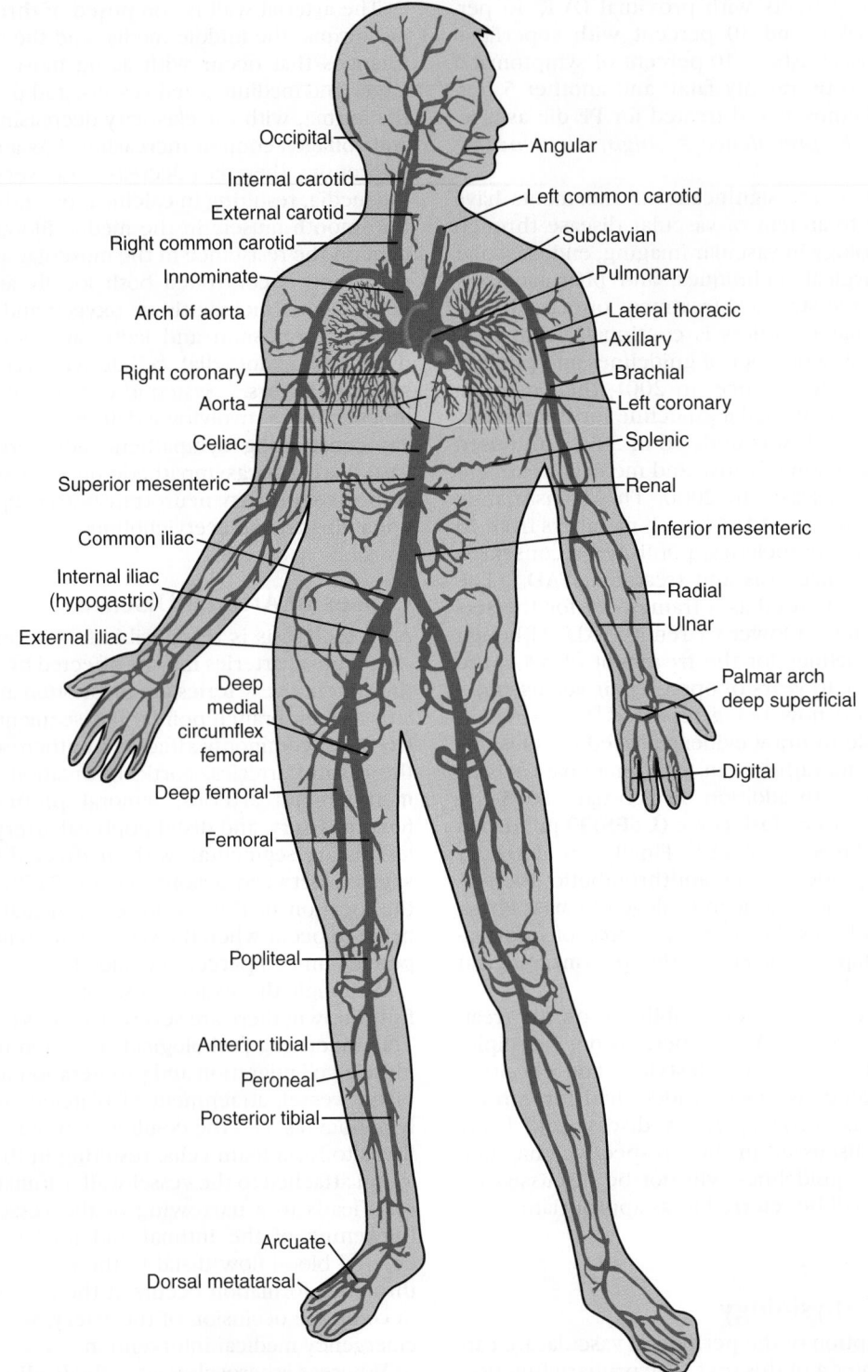

Occipital
Internal carotid
External carotid
Right common carotid
Innominate
Arch of aorta
Right coronary
Aorta
Celiac
Superior mesenteric
Common iliac
Internal iliac
(hypogastric)
External iliac
Deep
medial
circumflex
femoral
Deep femoral
Femoral
Popliteal
Anterior tibial
Peroneal
Posterior tibial
Arcuate
Dorsal metatarsal

Angular
Left common carotid
Subclavian
Pulmonary
Lateral thoracic
Axillary
Brachial
Left coronary
Splenic
Renal
Inferior mesenteric
Radial
Ulnar
Palmar arch
deep superficial
Digital

FIGURE 74-1 ■ The anatomy of the peripheral arterial system. (From Beare PG, Myers JL: *Adult health nursing,* ed 2, 1994, Mosby, Figure 29-1, p 681.)

current theory of aneurysm formation suggests that two pathophysiological changes occur: elastin fragmentation allowing the aneurysm to form and collagen deposition and degradation, which allows the aneurysm to enlarge and rupture.[27] Additional theories of aneurysm causes have been proposed, including but not limited to: (1) a genetic link; (2) atherosclerosis leading to uncontrolled compensatory dilatation; (3) an inflammatory process leading to an autoimmune response; and (4) hemodynamic changes resulting in increased wall tension, turbulence, vibration, and shear stress.[26]

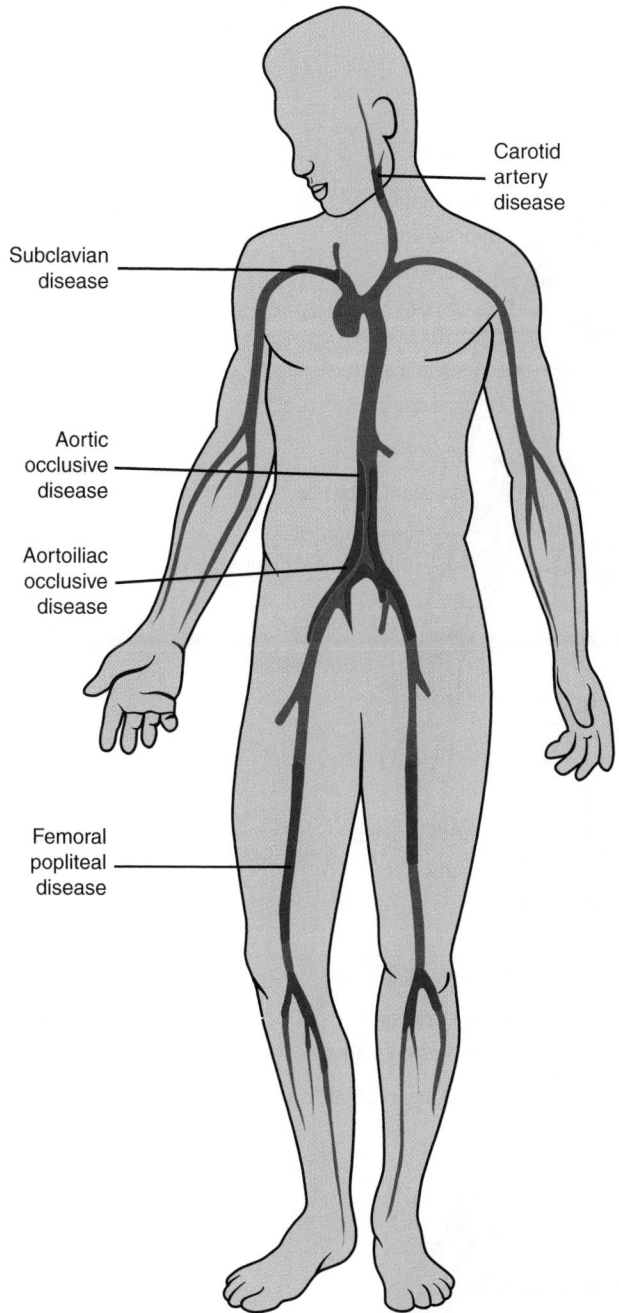

FIGURE 74-2 ■ Common anatomical locations of atherosclerotic lesions. (From Beare PG, Myers JL: *Adult health nursing,* ed 2, 1994, Mosby, Figure 30-2, p 696.)

Other, less commonly seen, PAD causes are associated with vasospasm and arteritis. The classic vasospastic disorder is Raynaud disease, which is usually a benign syndrome without demonstrable cause. Arteritis is an inflammatory process that involves the arterial wall and has been classified into four groups: Buerger disease, granulomatous or giant cell arteritides, polyarteritis nodosa group, and hypersensitivity arteritides. Although Raynaud and Buerger disease are not discussed in this chapter, pertinent clinical information can be found elsewhere.[28-30]

VENOUS SYSTEM
Anatomy and Physiology

The primary function of the venous system is to return blood to the right side of the heart. This action occurs as a result of several factors: pressure changes within the vascular bed allowing blood to flow from areas of higher pressure (arteries) to lower pressure (veins); adequate serum protein levels to maintain plasma oncotic pressure; venous distensibility and corresponding compliance; intact valves within the venous system preventing retrograde flow; phasic changes in intrathoracic and abdominal pressure increasing venous return to the heart from the thorax and upper extremities; and intermittent peripheral skeletal muscle contraction. Although there is little if any parasympathetic innervation to the veins, the superficial venous system has extensive sympathetic innervation, which allows it to play an important role in the maintenance of body temperature.

The anatomy of veins is similar to that of arteries. The primary difference between the two is found in the composition of the media, which generally is much thicker in arteries and accounts for their firmer and less distensible character. In contrast the media of the deep veins is thin and almost completely devoid of smooth muscle. It is of note, however, that the media of the superficial veins contains more smooth muscle than the deep veins. This difference allows for medial hypertrophy in response to increased intraluminal pressure, which is clinically significant when superficial veins of the forearm are used for the creation of an AV fistula, or the saphenous vein is used for an arterial bypass.[31] The superficial veins run through the subcutaneous tissue of the extremity and channel flow into the deep veins through communicating or perforating veins (Figure 74-3). The principle superficial veins of the lower extremity are the greater and lesser saphenous veins. The greater saphenous vein has clinical significance because of its length and easy accessibility and is an ideal conduit for coronary artery and lower-extremity bypass procedures.[31] In addition, the deep venous system remains intact with the surgical removal of one or several superficial veins, which decreases complications associated with this procedure.

Causes of Venous Thromboembolic Disorder

The cause of venous thromboembolic disorder is not completely understood. However, in 1859 Rudolph Virchow observed and reported the major pathogenic determinants for VTE. Today, Virchow triad is still considered the theory that best describes the cause of thrombus formation. The three factors are: stasis of venous blood flow, damage to the endothelial lining of the vein, and coagulation changes (hypercoagulability). First, venous stasis is probably the most treatable predisposing factor. Venous flow is dependent on leg muscle movement and adequate venous valves. As a result, stasis can occur with immobility or incompetent valves. Second, local venous trauma damages the endothelial lining leading to local platelet aggregation, fibrin forma-

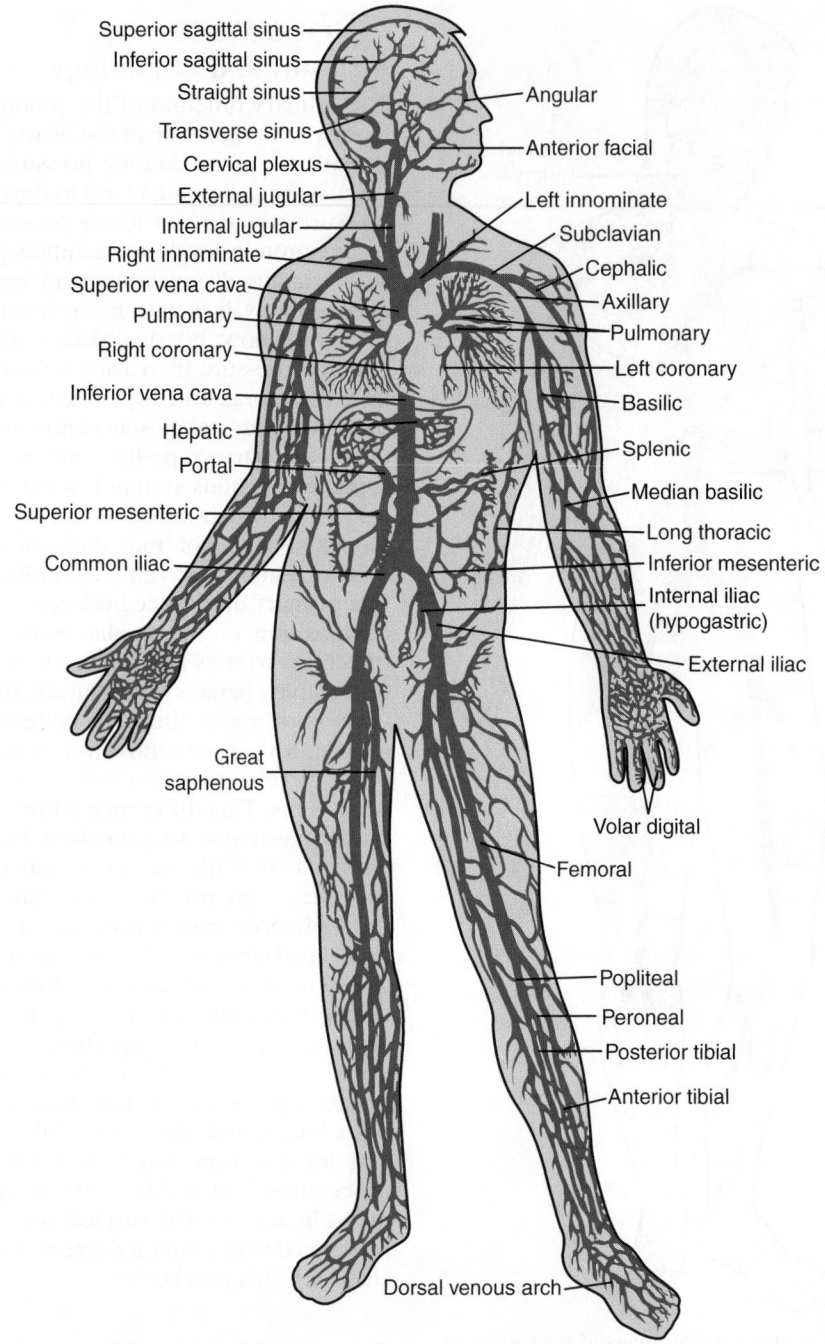

FIGURE 74-3 The gross anatomy of the systemic venous system. (From Beare PG, Myers JL: *Adult health nursing,* ed 2, 1994, Mosby, Figure 29-3, p 682.)

tion, and entrapment of white and red blood cells, resulting in thrombus formation.[32] And third, coagulation changes, whether acquired or inherited, lead to an increased risk of thrombus formation (Table 74-1).

In most cases, the natural history of VTE is gradual resolution of the occlusion and a recanalization of the lumen, allowing a return to near normal venous flow. Unfortunately, there is usually permanent damage done within the vessel as a result of a VTE, including residual webs and bands or remaining thrombosis anchored by epithelial cells. Although rare phlegmasia cerulea dolens is a near-total occlusion of venous outflow from thrombosis in the periphery. When this occurs, the rap-

idly rising venous pressure leads to obstructed arterial flow and ultimately gangrene, which requires emergency intervention.

CAROTID ARTERY DISEASE

The blood supply to the brain is provided through the carotid and vertebral arteries (Figure 74-4). The carotid arteries supply blood to the anterior portion of the brain and arise from the aortic arch (left side) and the innominate artery (right side). The common carotid artery bifurcates into the external and internal carotid arteries at about the angle of the jaw. The vertebral ar-

■ ■ ■

TABLE 74-1   RISK FACTORS FOR VENOUS THROMBOSIS

VIRCHOW TRIAD	ACQUIRED	INHERITED
Blood stasis	Increased age Obesity Pregnancy Immobility or Hospitalization Long flights Right heart failure	None
Vessel injury	Chemotherapy Hyperhomocysteinemia Vasculitis Intravascular catheters Trauma Surgery Smoking	None
Hypercoagulability	Malignancy Pregnancy Hormone replacement therapy	Protein S deficiency Protein C deficiency Factor V Leiden Prothrombin mutation

teries originate from the subclavian arteries bilaterally and provide blood to the brain stem, cerebellum, and occipital lobes. They are surgically accessible only for a short distance in the neck before entering the bony canal at the base of the skull.[33] As in other parts of the body, most atherosclerotic plaques occur at branch points, and in fact almost 40 percent of all extracranial lesions occur at the carotid bifurcation.

As a person ages, the risk of developing a carotid plaque significantly increases. The prevalence of carotid artery stenosis has been estimated from high-resolution B-mode carotid ultrasonography. In the Framingham Heart Study cohort, *greater than* 1000 subjects were studied (mean age 75 years). Of this group, about 42 percent had carotid stenoses of 0 percent to 10 percent, and 35.5 percent had carotid stenoses of 11 percent to 30 percent. Slightly more than 10 percent of the cohort had stenoses *greater than* 40 percent and most of these had lesions in the range of 41 percent to 60 percent.[34]

Not all carotid lesions are asymptomatic. There are two primary causes of symptomatic atherosclerosis: embolization and thrombosis. First, embolization occurs when ulcerated lesions along the arterial wall rupture, allowing emboli to break off the exposed cholesterol deposits and travel to the brain. Second, thrombosis can occur because of slowed blood flow across a ruptured lesion or a high-grade stenosis (*greater than* 90 percent occlusion).[33] The risk of symptomatic carotid artery disease is stroke. Approximately 85 percent of all strokes are ischemic; of these most are attributable to atherothrombotic disease. The number of strokes related to carotid atherosclerosis is less certain, but probably approaches 20 percent of all strokes.[2]

The goal of treating carotid artery disease is to prevent a stroke. However, the primary treatment for carotid artery disease is a carotid endarterectomy **(CEA)**, which carries with it the primary risk of stroke. Therefore before a treatment option is chosen, a complete evaluation of the patient and their symptoms must be completed so that the appropriate risk versus benefit ratio can be determined.

Evaluation
History

The majority of patients with carotid artery disease will be asymptomatic. However, as the size of the lesion progresses and the lumen of the artery narrows, most patients will begin to experience symptoms. Some patients with significant lesions remain asymptomatic because the remaining three blood vessels increase blood flow to accommodate the decreased blood flow in the narrowed carotid artery. It is of note that there are a

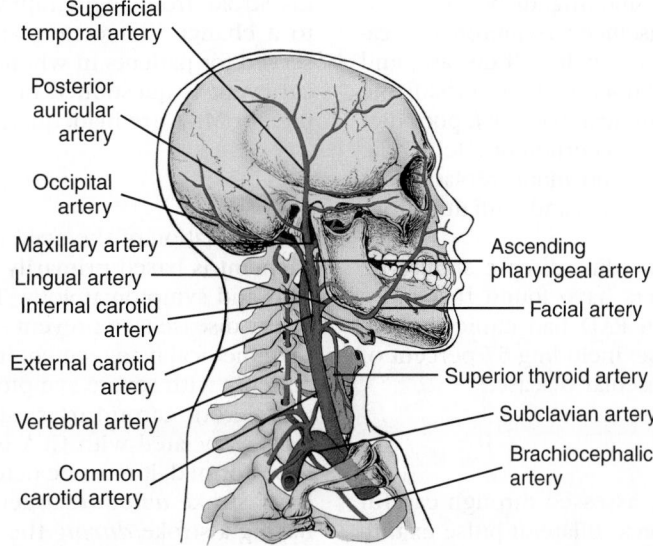

FIGURE 74-4 ■ Arteries of the head and neck: right common carotid, vertebral artery, and the internal and external carotid arteries. (From Lewis SL, Heitkemper MM, and Dirksen SR: *Medical-surgical nursing*, ed 6, 2004, Mosby, Figure 54-13, p 1475.)

certain number of patients who will experience an asymptomatic 100 percent occlusion of their carotid artery. Unless the occlusion is caught immediately, which is unlikely since the patient is asymptomatic, surgical recanalization is no longer an option. With complete occlusion, the blood distal to the plaque becomes static and clots. If the plaque were to be removed, it would be impossible to ensure removal of all the clots, and the risk of stroke would be so high as to negate the benefit of the surgery. As a result, a good symptoms history significantly contributes to the clinical decision-making process.

The symptoms of carotid artery disease can be very subtle. As a result, the ischemic event should be described in detail.[33] Specifically, subjective symptoms and findings observed by others during the event should be recorded. The patient and/or family should be questioned about such symptoms as speech difficulties, visual disturbances, motor weakness or paralysis, vertigo, syncope, confusion, and memory loss.[33] In addition, such symptoms as amaurosis fugax, headache, or difficulty chewing or swallowing may have occurred. Amaurosis fugax is defined as fleeting monocular blindness, but it may help the patient to understand if the clinician describes it as a "shade coming down over one eye." Timing of the event should include time of day, activity the patient was involved in at the time, the duration of symptoms, and the frequency of the episode. If the neurological deficit lasts *less than* 24 hours, it is termed a transient ischemic attack **(TIA),** if *greater than* 24 hours, it is called a stroke.

Risk Factors

Because atherosclerosis accounts for the majority of ischemic attacks, the patient should be evaluated for risk factors that may be modified. Nonmodifiable risk factors include age (older), sex (men), race (black and some Hispanic Americans), and family history of stroke or TIA.[13] Well-documented modifiable risk factors include hypertension, smoking, diabetes, hyperinsulinemia and insulin resistance, asymptomatic carotid stenosis, atrial fibrillation, sickle cell disease, and hyperlipidemia.[13] Less well-documented modifiable risk factors include obesity, physical inactivity, poor diet or nutrition, alcohol abuse, hyperhomocysteinemia, drug abuse, hypercoagulability, hormone replacement therapy, oral contraceptive use, and inflammatory process.[13]

Finally, any indication of cardiac disease should be carefully assessed. Researchers have found that more than half of all patients with PAD had clinically suggested coronary artery disease, including 57 percent of those evaluated for cerebrovascular disease.[35]

Physical Exam

Carotid artery disease can be assessed through careful evaluation of the head and neck. Bilateral pulse examination should include the superficial temporal and carotid arteries. The superficial temporal artery can be palpated just anterior to the ear, whereas the carotids should be palpated low in the neck to prevent dislodging plaque from the bifurcation.[33] Auscultation over the carotid arteries should be completed with the bell of the stethoscope, which is best to detect a bruit. The location of the bruit should be described as being at the angle of the jaw, in the midportion of the neck, or low in the neck. Particular attention should be paid to carotid bruits heard during both systole and diastole because they indicate severe stenosis.[33] It is of note, however, that severe stenosis may not be associated with a bruit. An ophthalmoscopic inspection should be undertaken to visualize Hollenhorst plaques, bright reflective spots seen in the retinal arteries, which represent cholesterol emboli from ulcerated plaque in the carotid or innominate arteries. The fundi should also be inspected for evidence of severe hypertension, diabetes mellitus, or extensive atherosclerosis.

In addition to the examination of the head and neck, a complete neurological exam should be performed. This includes evaluation of sensory and motor function, visual acuity, speech, memory, level of consciousness, and comprehension.[33]

Diagnostic Testing

The primary tool for evaluation of the carotid artery is the duplex ultrasound (Table 74-2). The duplex scan is noninvasive and accurate in quantifying carotid artery stenosis. As a result, many surgeons will perform surgery based solely on the duplex scan itself.[33] Computed tomography **(CT)** scan and magnetic resonance imaging **(MRI)** can be used to determine the extent of damage done if a stoke has already occurred or if a tumor, hemangioma, or intracranial vascular disease is suspected. If the duplex study is inadequate, a *contrast-enhanced* magnetic resonance angiography **(CE-MRA)** or digital subtraction angiography **(DSA)** may be performed (see Table 74-2). Although angiography used to be the conventional test before surgery would be performed, the improvement of noninvasive tests and the risk of causing stroke from angiography (up to 1 percent) have led to a change in recent years. Typically the DSA is reserved for patients in whom the cause of the neurological event is questioned or when the results of the duplex or MRA are inadequate.[33]

Treatment

Determination of the need for medical or surgical management is based primarily on the extent of the occlusion and symptomatology. The goal of treating carotid artery disease is to prevent stroke. CEA is more effective than medical management in the prevention of stroke in patients with severe symptomatic or asymptomatic atherosclerotic carotid artery stenosis.[36] Because one of the risks associated with CEA is stroke, before the surgery is performed, it must be determined that the risk of having a stroke *without* surgery is greater that the risk of having a stroke *during* the surgery. In the early 1990s, the results from two large-scale randomized prospective studies were published, which provide some guidelines for determining the need for CEA in the presence

■■■

TABLE 74-2   DESCRIPTION OF FREQUENTLY USED DIAGNOSTIC TESTS

DIAGNOSTIC TEST	DESCRIPTION
Duplex ultrasonography	Ultrasonography relies on sound waves striking a surface and being reflected back. Sound is expressed in terms of frequency, and there is a change in sound frequency in relation to a moving source, similar to the change in sound of a train whistle as the train approaches, then moves off. A Doppler transducer uses piezoelectric crystals and electrical voltage to produce sound waves that are then directed to strike moving red blood cells. The sound waves are reflected back to the transducer and recorded. The color duplex ultrasound is a method of displaying Doppler-shifted frequencies that are reflected from moving red blood cells. The image is displayed with colors that correspond to direction of the blood flow. Flow toward the Doppler transducer is displayed in red and flow away from the transducer is displayed in blue. As flow velocities increase at an area of stenosis, the colors lighten, going from red to orange to yellow or from blue to aqua to white. Poststenotic blood flow is turbulent and is represented by a mosaic pattern of all colors. The duplex ultrasound can precisely localize occlusions, provide information concerning artery wall thickness, degree of flow turbulence, vessel morphological characteristics, and changes in blood flow velocity in areas of stenosis. The specificity (accuracy) of the duplex ultrasound is very high for stenoses *greater than* 70% (94%), with an acceptable sensitivity (90%).
Contrast-enhanced magnetic resonance imaging (CE-MRA)	The CE-MRA is considered a noninvasive test and recently has evolved as an alternative to DSA (the gold standard) and the duplex ultrasound as a means of depicting the arterial tree. Using the CE-MRA, three-dimensional images of the arterial tree can be obtained with and without contrast. Sensitivity and specificity data is not available for the CE-MRA at this time. However, there is evidence that when the CE-MRA is used for diagnosis of peripheral atherosclerosis versus the duplex ultrasound, the CE-MRA is considered to be sensitive enough to determine intervention, including surgical intervention, significantly more often than the duplex ultrasound. In addition, in April 2003, Medicare announced it would expand its coverage of catheter angiography in addition to CE-MRA when clinically warranted, decreasing some clinicians hesitancy to use CE-MRA for diagnostic purposes.
Digital subtraction angiography (DSA)	DSA is considered the gold standard for the assessment of the arterial tree and is invasive with the insertion of a catheter into a major artery, usually the femoral. It is used most commonly in the presence of occlusive vascular disease in the extremities, extracranial or intracranial circulation, or visceral arteries, and sometimes for those with aneurysms of the aorta or extremities. DSA is not a screening technique. Before the DSA is performed, a patient must have undergone a thorough history and physical examination and appropriate screening with noninvasive techniques as appropriate. A DSA should be performed if vascular disease of sufficient severity is detected, the patient is considered a good candidate for surgical intervention, and other noninvasive tests do not provide sufficient evidence to proceed. The technique for performing a DSA is similar to that of a cardiac catheterization with a similar nursing role.

Rutherford RB, Krupski WC: Current status of open versus endovascular stent-graft repair of abdominal aortic aneurysm, *J Vasc Surg* 39:1129-39, 2004.

U.S. Preventive Services Task Force: Screening for abdominal aortic aneurysm: recommendation statement, *Ann Intern Med* 142:198-202, 2005.

Jahromi AS, Cina CS, Liu Y et al: Sensitivity and specificity of color duplex ultrasound measurement in the estimation of internal carotid artery stenosis: a systematic review and meta-analysis, *J Vasc Surg* 41:962-72, 2005.

Chobanian AV, Bakris GL, Black HR et al: Seventh report of the joint national committee on prevention, detection, evaluation, and treatment of high blood pressure, *Hypertension* 42:1206, 2003.

National Heart, Lung, and Blood Institute, National Institutes of Health, U.S. Department of Health and Human Services: Third report of the national cholesterol education program **(NCEP)** expert panel on detection, evaluation, and treatment of high blood cholesterol in adults (adult treatment panel III), Bethesda, Md, 2001, U.S. Department of Health and Human Services, Public Health Service, National Institutes of Health, National Heart, Lung, and Blood Institute.

of internal carotid artery stenosis (Table 74-3). Despite the presence of symptoms, for those with a 50 percent to 69 percent stenosis, CEA is only of moderate benefit. Clinically, however, if a patient is 50 percent to 69 percent stenosed and experiencing symptoms, a CEA is usually recommended, particularly if the risk of mortality and morbidity associated with the operation at that particular institution is *less than* 2 percent. In contrast the asymptomatic patient with a 50 percent to 69 percent stenosis would be carefully watched with annual or twice a year carotid duplex ultrasound examinations. For internal carotid artery stenosis of *greater than* or equal to 70 percent, CEA is recommended.

For patients not needing or not eligible for CEA, medical management has been their only option. However, in September 2004, the Centers for Medicare and Medicaid Services announced that evidence was adequate to conclude that percutaneous transluminal angioplasty **(PTA)** with carotid stent placement is reasonable and necessary when performed consistent with the Food and Drug Administration **(FDA)** approval of the carotid stent device and in an FDA-required postap-

■■■

TABLE 74-3   CLINICAL EVIDENCE OF THE NEED FOR CAROTID ENDARTERECTOMY

STENOSIS	BENEFIT FROM CAROTID ENDARTERECTOMY
Greater than 70%	Significant benefit
50-69%	Moderate reduction in risk of stroke
Less than 30%	No benefit

proval study. As a result, carotid stenting is now being performed in select locations around the Unites States

Risk Factor Modification

Instruction on risk factor modification for carotid artery disease should follow the American Heart Association recommendations for primary prevention of ischemic stroke and the recommendations' subsequent update.[13,14] See Table 74-4 for specific recommendations for modifying well-documented risk factors. In addition, detailed information on ways to modify lifestyle to achieve these

■ ■ ■

TABLE 74-4   AMERICAN HEART ASSOCIATION RECOMMENDATIONS FOR PREVENTING ISCHEMIC STROKE: WELL-DOCUMENTED MODIFIABLE RISK FACTORS

RISK FACTOR	RECOMMENDATION
Hypertension (HTN)	Regular screening for HTN (at least every 2 years in adults) and appropriate management. Goal: *less than* 140/90 mm Hg; *less than* 130/85 mm Hg if renal insufficiency or heart failure is present; or *less than* 130/80 mm Hg if diabetes is present.
Smoking	Smoking cessation for all current smokers. No exposure to environment tobacco smoke. Ask about tobacco use status at every visit. In a clear, strong, and personalized manner, advise every tobacco user to quit. Assess the tobacco user's willingness to quit. Assist by counseling and developing a plan for quitting. Arrange follow-up, referral to special programs, or pharmacotherapy. Urge avoidance of exposure to secondhand smoke at work or home.
Diabetes, hyperinsulinemia, and insulin resistance	Initiate appropriate hypoglycemic therapy to achieve near normal fasting plasma glucose or as indicated by near normal HbA1c. First step is diet and exercise. Second step therapy is usually oral hypoglycemic drugs. Third-step therapy is insulin.
Asymptomatic carotid stenosis	Endarterectomy may be considered in patients with high-grade asymptomatic carotid stenosis performed by a surgeon with *less than* 3% morbidity-mortality rate. Careful patient selection, guided by comorbid conditions, life expectancy, and patient preference, and other individual factors, including sex, and followed by a thorough discussion of the risks and benefits for the procedure is required. It is important that patients with asymptomatic carotid artery stenosis be fully evaluated for other treatable causes of stroke.
Atrial fibrillation	Antithrombotic therapy (warfarin or aspirin) should be considered for patients with nonvalvular atrial fibrillation based on an assessment of their risk of embolism and risk of bleeding complications.
Sickle cell disease (SCD)	Children with SCD should be screened with transcranial Doppler ultrasonography at 6-month intervals to determine their level of stroke risk. Those at elevated risk should be considered for transfusion therapy.
Hyperlipidemia	Primary goal: LDL-C *less than* 160 mg/kl if *less than* 1 risk factor; LDL-C *less than* 130 mg/dl if *greater than* 2, risk factors are present, and 10-year coronary heart disease (CHD) is *less than* 20%; or LDL-C *less than* 100 mg/kl if *greater than* 2, risk factors are present, and 10-year CHD risk is *greater than* 20% or if patient has diabetes. Management according to the national cholesterol education program II guidelines.

Goldstein LB, Adams R, Becker K et al: Primary prevention of ischemic stroke: a statement for healthcare professionals from the stroke council of the American Heart Association, *Circulation* 103:163-182, 2001.

Pearson TA, Blair SN, Daniels SR et al: AHA Guidelines for primary prevention of cardiovascular disease and stroke: 2002 update, *Circulation* 106:388-391, 2002.

objectives can be found in Section III of this text; specifically Chapters 33 (smoking), 34 (dyslipidemia), 35 (hypertension), 36 (obesity), 37 (diabetes), 38 (sedentary lifestyle), and 39 (stress).

Pharmacotherapies

Aspirin acts to inhibit platelet aggregation, but has no direct effect on the coagulation cascade and should not be used for treatment of active venous or arterial thrombosis. Recent research indicates that antiplatelet therapy reduces the risk of fatal and nonfatal stroke by 22 percent.[37] Aspirin specifically was found to reduce the risk of adverse cardiovascular outcomes by 23 percent. Although doses ranged from 75 to 1500 mg, there was comparable efficacy across dosages. However, others have found aspirin to have no effect on ischemic stroke or all-cause mortality over 5 years.[38] In addition, aspirin therapy was found to increase the risk for gastrointestinal bleeding and hemorrhagic stroke.[38] Although antiplatelet medication has been an established medical treatment for prevention of stroke for years, when considering whether to use aspirin chemoprevention, it is important to remember that it does not change the progression of the arterial plaque, nor is it likely to prevent thrombosis of highly stenotic lesions.[33] However, if a clinician chooses to recommend the use of aspirin, current practice is a daily dose of 325 mg or less.

Ticlopidine (Ticlid) and clopidogrel (Plavix) are both adenosine diphosphate receptor antagonists that have potent antiplatelet actions.[39] Although ticlopidine has been found to reduce cardiovascular events and mortality, the side effects of this medication make its use very limited. Bone marrow suppression (neutropenia) has been reported in 2.4 percent of patients taking this drug. In addition, thrombotic thrombocytopenia purpura occurs in about 1 out of 3000, resulting in a recommendation for frequent hematological monitoring in patients who take ticlopidine.[40] On the other had, clopidogrel provides many of the same benefits as ticlopidine, without any of the hematological complications. And in fact when compared with aspirin, clopidogrel has been found to prevent significantly more vascular events in patients with systemic atherosclerosis.[41] As a result, the recommendation is that clopidogrel can be as safely used as medium-dose aspirin (325 mg) with no significant difference in frequency of neutropenia or thrombocytopenia (Table 74-5).

Surgical Treatment

The risk of stroke during CEA is directly related to the surgeon's skill and qualifications. Because the benefit of this surgery is based on a low incidence of stroke, it is important that the surgeon have an operative stroke rate of *less than* 6 percent in symptomatic patients and *less than* 3 percent in asymptomatic patients. During surgery a skin incision is made just over the location of the branch point of the carotid artery, usually along the border of the sternocleidomastoid muscle. The dissection of the lesion must be performed gently to prevent atheroembolization, and the patient is typically given

■ ■ ■

TABLE 74-5 PHARMACOLOGY FOR PERIPHERAL VASCULAR DISEASE TREATMENT

MEDICATION	PURPOSE	DOSE	RISKS
CAROTID ARTERY DISEASE			
Aspirin	Inhibits platelet aggregation; prophylactic against thromboembolism	81 mg PO qd or 325 mg PO qd	Bleeding in patients with bleeding disorders (e.g., GI ulceration, vitamin K deficiency)
Ticlopidine (Ticlid)	Adenosine diphosphate receptor antagonist; Inhibits platelet aggregation and prolongs bleeding time	250 mg PO b.i.d. with food	Bleeding, nausea, vomiting, diarrhea; bone marrow suppression (neutropenia); thrombotic thrombocytopenia purpura
Clopidogrel (Plavix)		75 mg PO qd	Bleeding (see aspirin)
LOWER EXTREMITY PERIPHERAL ARTERIAL DISEASE			
Pentoxifylline (Trental)	Hemorheological agent that decreased blood viscosity and improves erythrocyte flexibility	400 mg PO t.i.d. with meals	Dizziness, dyspepsia, nausea, and vomiting
Cilostazol (Pletal)	Antiplatelet and vasodilatory and antiproliferative properties	50-100 mg PO b.i.d.	Headache, diarrhea, palpitations, dizziness

GI, Gastrointestinal; *b.i.d.,* twice per day; *PO,* orally; *t,i.d.,* three times per day; *qd,* every day.

heparin to prevent thrombus. After the artery is opened, the plaque, arterial intima, and portions of the media are removed. A patch of autogenous vein or prosthetic material may be used if primary closure of the carotid artery will cause narrowing of the artery or when the endarterectomy is being repeated.

Postoperative complications include stroke, cranial nerve (CN) injuries, and wound complications. Although the incidence of perioperative stroke has greatly declined over the past decade, if signs and symptoms of stroke are assessed postoperatively, the patency of the carotid artery must be determined immediately. This can be done using a duplex ultrasound or taking the patient directly back to surgery. Depending on the reason for occlusion, treatments include a return to surgery for a revision and repair of irregularities and heparin therapy.

Endovascular Treatment

Carotid angioplasty and stenting, a less invasive alternative to CEA, is in the clinical trial phase and will only be accepted as a treatment for high-grade carotid disease if it has adverse event rates similar to or lower than those associated with CEA. The primary limitation of carotid angioplasty and stenting has been the risk of distal embolization during the procedure. However, in 1990 it was proposed that cerebral protection be provided by means of temporary balloon occlusion and aspiration.[42] In the past decade, several different techniques and devices designed to prevent cerebral damage associated with embolization have been developed. The principal types of cerebral protection devices are occlusion balloons, distal filters, and reversal-of-flow mechanism. Recently, the results of a study comparing carotid angioplasty and stenting with a protection device versus CEA were reported.[36] In this group, the carotid angioplasty and stenting patients had fewer incidences of major

cardiovascular events at 1 year (death, stroke, or myocardial infarction), and carotid revascularization was repeated in fewer patients who received stents than in those who underwent CEA. These researchers concluded that carotid stenting with the use of an emboli-protection device is not inferior to CEA.

Thrombolysis

A number of randomized stroke trials and case studies have been reported in the literature to evaluate the safety and efficacy of thrombolytic therapy for the treatment of ischemic stroke.[43] These stroke trials have included intravenous, intraarterial, and combination studies, in addition to the use of mechanical devices for removal of thromboemboli and the use of neuroprotectant drugs alone or in combination with thrombolytic therapy. Currently the only therapy demonstrated to improve outcomes in ischemic stroke is thrombolysis of the clot responsible for the ischemic event.[43] One of the most important predictors of clinical success is time to treatment. Tissue plasminogen activator (t-PA) should be administered intravenously *less than* 3 hours after the event, and intraarterial thrombolysis can occur as late as 6 hours after the event.[43] However, it is not a simple correlation between opening the vessel and observed clinical benefit in all patients with ischemic stroke. Other factors influence outcomes, such as collateral circulation, the ischemic penumbra, lesion location and extent, time to treatment, and hemorrhagic conversion.[43]

Nursing Care

Appropriate nursing care of the patient after CEA is summarized in Table 74-6. Most patients will be discharged within 24 hours of surgery. They are admitted postoperatively to a step-down telemetry unit, with monitoring every hour of vital signs, oxygen saturation,

■ ■ ■

TABLE 74-6 EXAMPLE OF A CLINICAL PATHWAY AFTER CAROTID ENDARTERECTOMY

ASSESSMENT DATA	0-6 HR POSTOPERATIVELY	7-24 HR POSTOPERATIVELY
VS and O$_2$ saturation	q 1 hr	q 4 hr
Neurological checks	q 1 hr	q 4 hr
Telemetry	Continuous	Continuous until discharge
Circulation checks	q 1 hr	q 4 hr
Intake and output	q 1 hr	q 8 hr
Activity	Bedrest, HOB elevated 30°	Morning after surgery may get out of bed, ambulate in hall before discharge
Treatments	Monitor dressing, watch for signs of hematoma	Morning after surgery may discontinue: Urinary catheter Arterial line IV fluids if taking PO well Telemetry Dressing (by surgeon)
Diet	Clear liquids as tolerated	Advance as tolerated, must show tolerance to food before discharge
Tests	ECG p.r.n. Labs p.r.n. ABG p.r.n.	Morning after surgery: CBC, metabolic panel as needed: CK-MB, troponin, PTT, PT/INR, ABG, ECG
Psychosocial	Provide support	Provide support, intervene p.r.n.
Patient education	Assess family level of understanding Discuss postoperative course with family	Provide discharge teaching re: Follow-up with surgeon Activity level Incision care, signs/symptoms of infection Prescriptions Diet Signs/symptoms of stroke
Expected outcomes	VS WNL (SBP not *less than* 100 mm Hg or *greater than* 180 mm Hg) Neurologically intact No signs or symptoms of bleeding	VS WNL Neurologically intact No signs or symptoms of bleeding or infection Able to void without difficulty Able to ambulate as before surgery Tolerates regular diet Patient and family verbalize understanding of discharge instructions

ABG, Arterial blood gases; *CBC,* complete blood count; *CK-MG,* creatine-kinase-myocardial band; *ECG,* electrocardiogram; *HOB,* head of bed; *INR,* international normalized ratio; *PO,* by mouth; *PRN,* as needed; *PT,* prothrombin time; *PTT,* partial thromboplastin time; *Q,* every; *SBP,* systolic blood pressure; *VS,* vital signs; *WNL,* within normal limits.

BOX 74-1
A GUIDE TO THE BRIEF INTERVENTION

■ ■ ■

- Ask about tobacco use
- Advise to quit
- Assess willingness to make a quit attempt
- Assist in quit attempt
- Arrange for follow-up

urinary output, neurological exam, peripheral circulation, and the incision. Assessment for postoperative nerve injuries can be done with a thorough neurological examination. In addition, evaluation of specific CN function is necessary. This involves asking the patient to talk (CN XII and X), stick out their tongue (CN XII), swallow (CN X and IX), smile (CN VII), and shrug their shoulders (CN XI). Deficits in these areas are a result of traction or inadvertent transaction during surgery. Most of these deficits will resolve in time. Wound complications are relatively infrequent after CEA. However, the neck incision should be watched for bleeding and hematoma, and bleeding should be managed aggressively to prevent tracheal compression. Signs and symptoms of this complication include bleeding from the incision; increased neck circumference; swelling, bruising, and induration at the incision site; and signs or symptoms of

decreased intravascular volume (tachycardia, anxiety, restlessness, pallor, and cyanosis).

Sometimes the patient will return from surgery with an arterial line for continuous blood pressure measurement (see Chapter 50 for detailed information on arterial line management), in addition to continuous cardiac rate and rhythm monitoring via a telemetry unit. Maintaining a systolic blood pressure between 100 to 180 mm Hg (an outside range) is imperative to allow for adequate perfusion of the brain without so much pressure as to cause hemorrhage. As a part of each institution's care map for CEA, there are usually standing orders for treating hypotension (fluid bolus) or hypertension (oral beta blockers as needed or intravenous Nitroprusside).

After the first 6 hours, routine monitoring returns to every 4 hours. The morning after surgery, the care map usually contains standing orders for removal of the urinary catheter and arterial line, discontinuing intravenous fluids, ordering the patient a meal, and getting him or her out of bed. However, some surgeons will prefer to see their patients the morning after surgery before any of these things are done, so the nurse should know the routine of the floor and each surgeon's individual preferences before implementing standing orders. Usually, once all the lines and catheters are pulled and the patient is tolerating food and activity, discharge is ordered. Discharge teaching should include plans for follow-up with the surgeon; signs and symptoms of infection, bleeding, and stroke; wound care; activity level; pain management; and medication information. Most patients will be discharged home on either 325 mg of aspirin alone, or 81 mg of aspirin in addition to a second antiplatelet medication.

PERIPHERAL ARTERIAL DISEASE

Chronic arterial insufficiency of the lower extremity causes two very characteristic types of pain: intermittent claudication and ischemic rest pain. "Claudication," derived from the Latin word for "limp," has come by usage to mean a pain or discomfort associated with exercise, relieved by rest, hence the addition of the term "intermittent." The pain of intermittent claudication is determined by the level and extent of the arterial occlusive disease. Lesions in the femoral or popliteal arteries produce a cramping pain in the calf muscles.[15] More proximal (i.e., aortoiliac) occlusive lesions usually produce an aching discomfort, often associated with a sensation of weakness in the hip, buttocks, or thigh.[15] Although the term intermittent claudication is universally used to describe the pain of arterial occlusive disease, the actual terminology used to describe the disease itself has less consensus. Terms, such as lower extremity arterial occlusive disease, peripheral arterial occlusive disease, and PAD, are used interchangeably in the literature. For the purpose of clarity, the term PAD and the abbreviation PAD, will be used here exclusively as an umbrella term to describe the formation of atherosclerotic plaques in the aortic bifurcation, iliac and common femoral arteries, femoral profunda, superficial femoral, distal popliteal, and tibial arteries.

The natural progression of PAD can occur in four different ways: (1) improvement or stabilization of intermittent claudication; (2) worsening claudication not requiring intervention; (3) a need for intervention, such as surgical revascularization or angioplasty; or (4) a need for amputation. Unfortunately, PAD is chronically underdiagnosed, and treatment of atherosclerotic risk factors by medical or lifestyle management tends to be less intensive in patients with PAD versus those with coronary artery disease. Although reasons for this underdiagnosis is not completely known, experts in the field hypothesize that possible reasons may include lack of awareness of the importance of PAD among primary care clinicians, a limited understanding of the disease among the public, an assumption that exertional leg pain is a normal part of aging, inadequate understanding of appropriate office-based disease detection methods, and limited knowledge of treatment options.[44]

The goal of screening, diagnosis, and treatment of PAD is to prevent the progression of the disease, which can lead to amputation of the affected extremity. However, in most cases, the fate of the claudicant is relatively benign as regards to local disease in the leg, but is increasingly malignant in terms of fatal and nonfatal cardiovascular events. Only about 5 percent of patients with PAD need surgical or endovascular intervention over 5 years for either severe claudication or deterioration to critical limb ischemia.[15] Approximately 2 percent of PAD patients with intermittent claudication need a major amputation.[15] Nevertheless, early detection and treatment can help overall morbidity and mortality.

Evaluation
History
The chief complaint of the patient who has PAD will usually be intermittent claudication. However, pain in the buttock, thigh, or calf can be a result of many things, not just atherosclerosis. Pertinent information that can help make a differential diagnosis include the following[15]:

- The location of the pain or discomfort
- The duration of the symptoms
- Whether it is worsening or improving with time and whether conservative therapy has had any effect
- The distance the patient can walk before (a) experiencing the discomfort and (b) being forced to stop
- The elapsed time after exercise is stopped before the pain is relieved
- The type of rest or position of patient (standing at rest, sitting, or lying) necessary to relieve the pain
- Whether the pain returns after the same time and distance if exercise is then resumed

The patient with PAD will answer that the pain always occurs after the same degree of exercise, is quickly relieved with rest, that body position has no effect on the pain, and that the pain is reproducible. The only difference between patients with PAD may be the site and description of the pain: cramping pain in the calf; aching discomfort or weakness in the hip, thigh, or buttocks; or severe pain in the arch of the foot. The recommendation of the TASC is that the history of claudication as a result of chronic PAD is characteristic and reproducible enough that diagnosis can be made on the basis of interrogation alone in the majority of patients.[15]

As PAD progresses, the patient may be assessed at a point beyond uncomplicated intermittent claudication. Acute limb ischemia is any sudden decrease or worsening in limb perfusion causing a potential threat to limb viability.[15] The history should have two primary aims: asking about leg symptoms relative to the present illness (limb ischemia) and obtaining background information.[15] Information regarding suddenness and time of onset of pain, its location and intensity, and change in severity over time should all be determined. Whereas assessing the degree of leg weakness is part of the physical exam, the duration of the weakness and whether it is improving or worsening is important to the differential diagnosis. In addition, history of claudication, recent surgical intervention, cardiac catheterization, or history of atrial fibrillation should be determined.

The term critical limb ischemia should be used for all patients with chronic ischemic rest pain, ulcers, or gangrene attributable to objectively proven PAD. The term critical limb ischemia implies chronicity and is thereby distinguished from acute limb ischemia.[15] The history of critical limb ischemia is dominated by pain. Ischemic rest pain typically occurs at night, but can occur during the day when the patient is resting in a supine position. The pain is localized in the distal part of the foot and is often severe, causing the person to awaken at night to rub their foot, hang it over the bed, or get up and walk around. This pain often is relieved only by large doses of strong analgesics or opiates. In addition, ischemic rest pain usually precedes the formation of an ischemic ulcer or gangrene.

Risk Factors

PAD in the absence of risk factors is very rare. Risk factors for PAD include diabetes mellitus and impaired glucose tolerance, smoking, hypertension, hyperlipidemia, and hyperhomocysteinemia.[15] The relationship between diabetes and intermittent claudication is well documented. Overall PAD seems to be about twice as common among diabetic patients as among nondiabetic patients.[15] The relationship between smoking and PAD is strong and has been suggested to be stronger than the relationship between smoking and coronary artery disease. The severity of PAD tends to increase with the number of cigarettes smoked. In addition, a diagnosis of PAD is made up to 10 years earlier in smokers than in nonsmokers.[15] Although the link between PAD and hypertension is strongly supported in the literature, their relationship is a bit paradoxical. Hypertension elevates the central perfusion pressure, thus allowing greater circulation through narrowed arteries. As a result, it is not uncommon for a hypertensive patient to develop intermittent claudication when high blood pressure is discovered and treated.[15] Although there is some conflicting evidence regarding the relationship between high cholesterol and PAD, it appears as though the ratio of total to high-density lipoprotein (**HDL**) cholesterol is the best predictor of occurrence of arterial disease. An association between PAD and hypertriglyceridemia has also been reported, but the strength of this association remains unclear. Finally the incidence of hyperhomocysteinemia is as high as 60 percent in the vascular population, compared with 1 percent in the general population. The suggestion that hyperhomocysteinemia may be an independent risk factor for atherosclerosis has been supported by the results of several studies.[15]

Physical Examination

The TASC group[15] makes two recommendations for assessing the PAD patient with intermittent claudication: (1) In evaluating claudication, a complete examination of the patient is necessary to detect important factors that may significantly impact management and (2) pulse palpation should be correlated with claudication distance and location of pain because this assessment data can accurately predict the location and severity of the responsible arterial lesion(s). Auscultation of bruits may give additional information.

When performing the complete examination, as per the first recommendation, at the very least the circulatory system as a whole should be assessed. Specifically watch for signs or symptoms of hypertension, cardiac murmurs or dysrhythmias, carotid bruits, signs of respiratory impairment, anemia, or an AAA.[15] In addition, assess for signs of poor circulation and oxygenation to the feet and nails; skin color and temperature; swelling, ulcerations, or trophic changes, such as thin dry skin, loss of hair or subcutaneous fat; or thickened nails.

The most important part of the physical examination is the completion of the second recommendation: pulse assessment. The femoral, popliteal, posterior and anterior tibial, and dorsalis pedis pulses should be palpated. Grading of these pulses is easiest on a 0 to 2 point scale: 0 = absent; 1 = diminished, and 2 = normal. From a practical standpoint, however, most vascular clinicians just care whether the pulse is palpable or not. If not the presence of blood flow should be assessed with a Doppler and documented as Doppler signals present or not present. Assessment of the pulses is significant in that blood flow distal to the atherosclerotic narrowing is reduced, and pulses become either diminished or not palpable. Therefore the location of the narrowing can be predicted with a high degree of accuracy simply through pulse assessment.

In addition to the general vascular assessment for the patient with intermittent claudication, the physical exam of the patient with acute limb ischemia should include assessment of the six Ps: pulselessness, pain, pallor, poikilothermy (cold), paresthesia, and paralysis. Assessment of the critically ischemic leg should include all of the previous data. However, it is important to watch for some symptoms specific to critical limb ischemia, such as atrophy of the calf muscles, thickening of toenails, and dependent rubor. Dependent rubor is a deep red-purple color of the feet and lower legs when the legs are dependent. In fact the dependent toes may appear so red and may refill so rapidly after pressure application that it may be mistaken for hyperemia rather than severe ischemia. One way to differentiate between hyperemia and dependent rubor is by having the patient in a supine position with their legs elevated 30 to 45 degrees and watching for extreme pallor in the toes that were previously purple-red. In addition, the skin should be closely inspected for ulcerations. Arterial ulcerations occur at the most distal part of the extremity, usually the toes or heel. They also occur at the inner surface of the digits; not uncommonly a companion ulcer develops on the adjacent toe ("kissing ulcer").[15] Arterial ulcers usually have irregular borders with a pale base, unless inflammation or infection occurs. Gangrene usually affects the digits, but in severe cases may involve the forefoot. Gangrenous tissue, if not infected, tends to shrink and eventually mummify the affected part. Spontaneous amputation sometimes follows.[15]

Diagnostic Tests

The TASC group recommends routine tests to be performed on all patients being seen for the first time with PAD.[15] Any test that has already been performed in the previous months need not be repeated, but should be noted. These tests should be used to detect treatable risk factors or to diagnose associated diseases. Recommended laboratory *tests* include: complete blood count (hemoglobin, hematocrit, and white cell count), platelet count, fasting blood glucose or hemoglobin A1c, creatinine, fasting lipid profile, and urinalysis (for glycosuria and/or proteinuria).[15] In addition, the TASC group recommends a baseline electrocardiogram for new patients with PAD, but in the absence of family history, risk factors, or suggestive symptoms or signs, there is as yet no good evidence for routine further investigation of other circulatory problems (e.g., carotid artery disease).[15]

Of primary importance is the TASC[15] recommendation that all new PAD patients should have the ankle brachial index **(ABI)** measured in both legs. Normally, pedal blood pressures (use the greater pressure of either the dorsalis pedis or posterior tibial) are equal to or slightly higher than those in the upper extremities. In the presence of arterial disease, pressures drop distal to the occlusion, resulting in dropping pedal pulse pressures. The ABI is a comparison of the pedal pulse to the brachial pulse (highest pressure left or right) using the equation:

$$\frac{\text{Ankle pressure}}{\text{Brachial pressure (highest)}} = \text{ABI}$$

When there is no occlusive disease in the lower extremities, the ABI will equal about 1. However, as ankle pressures drop, the ABI drops as well, and an ABI of *less than* or equal to 0.9 is considered diagnostic of lower extremity PAD. Pressures are always measured using a sphygmomanometer and a 5 to 7-MHz Doppler. An ABI of *less than* or equal to 0.9 is diagnostic of PAD with 95 percent sensitivity and almost 100 percent specificity. An ABI of 0.71 to 0.90 represents mild obstruction, and practically speaking, indicates a 10 percent to 30 percent decrease in blood flow to the affected extremity. Some patients will begin to experience intermittent claudication at this point, but some may not depending on their degree of daily activity, current and past history of regular aerobic exercise, weight, smoking status, and presence of comorbidities, such as diabetes. An ABI of 0.41 to 0.70 is defined as moderate obstruction and represents a 30 percent to 60 percent decrease in blood flow to the affected extremity. At this point, all patients will begin to suffer some degree of disability. Intermittent claudication is generally the first symptom, with dependent rubor and pallor with elevation occurring as the disease progresses. An ABI of 0.00 to 0.40 represents severe obstruction, where mobility is severely limited, and patients experience distal tissue breakdown and necrosis. It is important to note that patients with calcified vessels, such as those with diabetes, will have abnormally increased pressures in their legs. It is important to take this into consideration when interpreting the results of an ABI.

Segmental limb systolic pressure measurement **(SLP)**, more commonly known as lower extremity Doppler studies, is now widely used because it accurately detects and localizes large-vessel occlusive lesions in the major arteries between the heart and the point of measurement.[15] The test is performed the same way as the ABI, only the sphygmomanometer cuff is placed segmentally along the leg (upper and lower thigh and calf), while the Doppler probe is over one of the pedal arteries, and the systolic pressure is measured at the level of the cuff. The location of the occlusive lesion is apparent from the drop in pressure between the different cuffs.[15]

The accuracy of this test alone in detecting and localizing occlusive lesions has been reported to be 85 percent against the gold standard, angiography.[45] However, limitations of SLP include missing iliac stenosis and falsely elevated pressures in diabetic patients with calcified incompressible arteries.

Functional testing, using treadmill exercise is an additional means to determine the severity of the disease. Sometimes a patient has typical intermittent claudication symptoms, but will have a normal ABI at rest. In this case a standard exercise test should be performed to determine a postexercise ABI. This test consists of walking on a treadmill for 10 minutes, at 1.5 miles/hr, at a 10° incline. A postexercise pedal pressure drop of 15 mm Hg or more is considered diagnostic for PAD. Additional measures that may be considered beneficial in determining the degree of the patient's disability are claudication pain time **(CPT)** and maximum walking time.

Claudication pain time is the time a person can walk before they begin to experience pain in their leg, whereas maximum walking time **(MWT)** is the maximum time a person can walk until the severity of their pain demands that they stop and rest. A graded, progressive treadmill exercise test initiated at 1 mph with a grade of 5 percent, increasing in speed and grade at 5-minute intervals through four stages to 2.5 mph at 10 percent grade can be used to determine CPT and MWT in minutes and seconds. In addition to determining functional ability, this information is extremely useful for helping a patient with PAD begin and adhere to an exercise program. When counseling a patient with intermittent claudication, it is imperative that the patient understand that he or she should not stop exercising when the pain in their calf begins. Although intermittent claudication could correctly be termed "angina of the leg," this pain does not do permanent damage to the muscle. In fact if the patient does not learn to walk through most of the pain (nearly to MWT), they will never see the physiological improvements associated with exercise training—specifically an increase in both capillary density and oxidative enzyme capacity of the exercised muscle. These changes in the muscle's ability to take up and use oxygen more efficiently are what allow the patient with PAD to have a 100 percent or more improvement in pain-free walking time after at least 26 weeks of regular exercise training.

The main reason to image the arteries supplying the claudicating leg is to find and define an arterial lesion that has a suitable morphology for some form of intervention, such as balloon angioplasty or bypass surgery.[15] Angiography (DSA) is the imaging technique of choice to visualize the lesion (see Table 74-2). However, MRA is becoming more popular at locations around the United States where it is available and where there are experienced radiologists who can read the results.

Treatment
Risk Factor Modification

There are seven pertinent risk factor recommendations given by the TASC group.[15] All patients with PAD should be strongly and repeatedly advised to stop smoking.

Cessation rates are likely to be enhanced by a special program. When initiating a smoking cessation program with a PAD patient, the clinical practice guidelines for treating tobacco use and dependence should be followed.[21] Principles of smoking cessation are discussed in detail in chapter 33, including a brief intervention that every nurse should complete with every patient (Box 74-1). This intervention begins by simply asking about tobacco use and advising those who use tobacco to quit. If a complete history is completed, the patient's willingness to quit should already be assessed.

Patients with diabetes and PAD should have aggressive control and normalization of blood sugar. Fasting blood sugars should range from 80 to 120 mg/dl, and postprandial sugars should be *less than* 180 mg/dl; hemoglobin A1c should be *less than* 7.0 percent. Further information about care for the diabetic patient can be found in Chapter 37.

All diabetic patients with PAD should receive special advice and regular supervision to minimize the risks of developing diabetic foot complications. Diabetic patients are also at high risk for developing ulcers on their feet because of preexisting sensory neuropathy and foot deformity. The combination of diabetes and PAD predisposes a small foot injury to progress to a large necrotic lesion very quickly.

Because of the high incidence of coexistent coronary disease and similar mortality risk to coronary patients, patients with PAD with a low-density lipoprotein **(LDL)** cholesterol level *greater than* 125 mg/dl should be placed on therapy. In the first instance, a diet should be tried. If this fails to achieve a goal of LDL *less than* 100 mg/dl, then medications should be tried. Practitioners should follow the current national cholesterol education program recommendations, discussed in detail in Chapter 77.[20] On the basis of reported trials, the use of statins would result in preventing one death per year in 640 patients treated.[46]

PAD patients with hypertension should have this risk factor controlled according to joint national committee (JNC VII) guidelines.[19] PAD patients should be advised that although treatment of their hypertension may exacerbate their symptoms of intermittent claudication, there is a more serious risk to their life from uncontrolled high blood pressure.

Patients with PAD who have hypercoagulable state and proven arterial or venous thrombosis should be anticoagulated with Vitamin K antagonists (warfarin). The only treatment for these conditions is oral anticoagulation.

A program of exercise therapy (preferably supervised) should always be considered as part of the initial treatment for patients with PAD. Principles of exercise training have already been reviewed in this chapter (see Special Feature: Evidence-Based Practice) and in Chapter 38. However, it cannot be stated emphatically enough the degree to which claudication symptoms can be managed using a regular walking program. The primary physiological change that helps to improve claudication symptoms occurs at the local level. These local changes allow more oxygen to be taken up and used. Since claudication is a symptom of muscle hypoxia, training the

affected muscle has significant benefit. In fact lower-extremity bypass surgery alone has been found to increase pain-free walking time by 100 percent, but exercise training alone, with walking as the mode of exercise, has been found to increase pain-free walking time by as much as 200 percent—without all the potential complications of surgery. In areas where a vascular rehabilitation program is provided, the Current Procedural Terminology code published by the American Medical Association for PAD rehabilitation is 93668.

Pharmacotherapies

Although there is no indication that antiplatelet therapy improves symptoms of intermittent claudication, the TASC group[15] recommends that all patients with PAD

■ **EVIDENCE-BASED PRACTICE**

Exercise is known as one of the cornerstones of managing lower extremity peripheral arterial disease (PAD). The pathology of intermittent claudication involves a lack of oxygenation to the exercising muscles, which leads to cramping muscle pain, relieved by rest. Regular, routine, aerobic exercise has been found to increase pain-free walking time in claudicants by as much as 200 percent. However, ABIs before and after exercise training have not been found to change. The reason for this significant symptom improvement does not lie then in a reversal of the atherosclerotic plaque, but is a result of an increase in the oxygen uptake ability in the muscle itself, specifically an increase in capillary density and the number of mitochondria in the exercised muscle. As a result, the four principles of exercise training must be taken into consideration when recommending an exercise program to the patient with lower extremity PAD.

First, the specificity principle states that to engage in an activity with less effort, the muscles that are used in that activity must be specifically trained. In other words, if a person wishes to be able to walk farther, then walking would be the exercise mode of choice. Second, the overload principle states that the muscle that needs to be trained must be overloaded to achieve a significant training effect. This means that if a person already spends a lot of time walking at work, they must walk at a higher intensity during exercise to see the desired training effect. Third, the individual differences principle states that each person will experience a training effect specific to their body's ability to change. In other words, although exercise training has been found to increase pain-free walking time by 200 percent, not all patients will experience such a dramatic improvement. Fourth, the reversibility principle states that once a person stops exercising, they will lose all the positive physiological changes within a few short weeks. Taking these four exercise principles into consideration, there are three critical exercise components specific to the person with intermittent claudication. In a meta-analysis conducted by Gardner and Poehlman, these three components were found to be a part of exercise regimens that provided the greatest improvement in pain-free walking time:

1. Incorporating near maximal claudication pain end point during exercise training
2. At least 26 weeks of exercise, three times per week for at least 30 min/session
3. Walking as the mode of exercise

For the claudicant, any exercise prescription should include these three components. Incorporating a near maximal claudication end point means that the patient should not stop walking as soon as the pain in their leg begins, but should continue walking until they are near maximal pain before stopping to take a break. In addition, walking is the best mode of exercise, and 30 minutes each session should be spent walking, not including rest times.

Gardner AW, Poehlman ET: Exercise rehabilitation programs for the treatment of claudication pain. A meta-analysis, *JAMA* 274:975-80, 1995.

(whether symptomatic or asymptomatic) should be considered for treatment with low-dose aspirin or another approved antiplatelet (unless contraindicated) to reduce the risk of cardiovascular morbidity and mortality. Clopidogrel (Plavix), which has already been described, is frequently prescribed to prevent thrombosis and acute total occlusion of the peripheral arteries.

Two other drugs are typically given to treat the pain of intermittent claudication. Pentoxifylline (Trental) is a hemorheological agent that for years was the only available medication to treat intermittent claudication. Although improvements in pain-free walking time were thought to be minimal (20 percent), something seemed to be better than nothing. However, recent studies have shown pentoxifylline to be of no real clinical benefit, and generally speaking, the only patients taking this medication are those who have "always taken it," and do not want to stop. The newest medication available for the treatment of intermittent claudication is *cilostazol (Pletal*—pronounced play-tall). Although the mechanism of action for this drug is known, the mechanism by which cilostazol produces improvement in pain-free walking time remains speculative.[39] For patients taking cilostazol alone, improvements in pain-free walking time can improved by as much as 20 percent for those taking 50 mg twice a day, and by 40 percent for those taking 100 mg twice a day.[47] The two side effects that most often cause patients to stop taking this medication are severe headache and diarrhea. Patients suffering from intermittent claudication should be started initially on the 50-mg dose, and increased to 100 mg as they can tolerate it (see Table 74-5).

Surgical Treatment

Lower-extremity bypass procedures, also known as arterial reconstruction, are indicated to prevent limb loss in patients with critical leg ischemia, for the treatment of chronic distal leg wounds (a nonhealing amputation or ulcers that fail to heal over time), wet or dry gangrene of the toes or forefoot, or ischemic rest pain.[48] Over recent years, arterial reconstruction has also been used selectively with those who experience severe, disabling intermittent claudication. However, surgical procedures should not be undertaken with those who develop asymptomatic PAD before risk factor modifications are attempted.

Lower-extremity bypass procedures can be classified one of two ways: those that reestablish inflow and those that provide outflow perfusion to the ischemic extremity.[48] Many patients with more severe PAD symptoms, such as ischemic rest pain or gangrene, are likely to have occlusive disease at multiple levels (refer to Figure 74-2 to note the segmented nature of PAD). Procedures that establish inflow are intended to increase the pressure in the major arteries that supply blood to the lower extremities so that there is adequate pressure to move the blood into the smaller vessels of the legs. Sometimes even when there is extensive segmental disease all through the aortoiliac, femoral, and popliteal arteries, simply establishing adequate inflow will significantly improve intermittent claudication symptoms. It is a fundamental principle that inflow should be established before outflow to the lower extremity can be repaired. Bypass procedures to establish inflow include aortofemoral artery bypass graft, axillofemoral reconstruction (for those who cannot tolerate abdominal surgery), or femoral-femoral bypass if the blood flow to the noninvolved leg is adequate (Figure 74-5).

Bypass procedures to return outflow to the distal extremity involve surgically positioning a bypass around the arterial occlusion. The location of the bypass graft will be determined by the location of the occlusion. Bypass procedures to return outflow will always originate at the femoral artery, unless attempts to reestablish inflow failed, and then inflow is established by the axillary artery. Examples of outflow procedures include: above the knee femoral-popliteal bypass with saphenous vein and femoral-tibial artery anastomoses (Figure 74-6). A variety of conduits are available for bypass grafting, with the preferred grafts being autogenous (vein) (Table 74-7).

Endovascular Treatment

The technique for transluminal angioplasty was developed in 1964, but was perfected in 1974 by the development of a balloon dilating catheter that has since been used successfully to open every major artery in the body, including those in the lower extremities.[49] In recent years, endoluminal metallic stents have been developed that are left in the artery to maintain patency and have helped improve the long-term success of angioplasty. As a result, transluminal balloon angioplasty with or without stenting has become an accepted therapy for certain iliac artery stenoses, but are used selectively in more distal arteries.[50] An effective surgical combination is the use of balloon angioplasty to restore inflow in the iliac arteries and traditional bypass surgery for the outflow procedure.

Thrombolysis

The TASC group[15] identifies thrombolysis as the treatment of choice for patients experiencing acute limb ischemia where the limb is not immediately threatened or marginally threatened, with minimal sensory loss and no muscle weakness. The recommendation states that if the decision is made to proceed with thrombolysis after arteriography, then the intrathrombus infusion should be used.[15] In addition, intravenous administration of high doses of currently available thrombolytic agents should no longer be used for the treatment of arterial occlusion of the leg.[15] With intraarterial streptokinase, t-PA, or urokinase, successful recanalization is possible in most carefully selected patients. Furthermore, after successful thrombolysis in atherosclerotic arteries, the underlying lesion should be identified, and the most appropriate endovascular or surgical treatment should be undertaken to achieve long-term patency.[15] The role of thrombolysis for treating critical limb ischemia is controversial. There is a need for studies to determine whether preliminary catheter-induced thrombolytic therapy enhances the efficacy or safety of angioplasty and stenting of chronic iliac occlusions.[15]

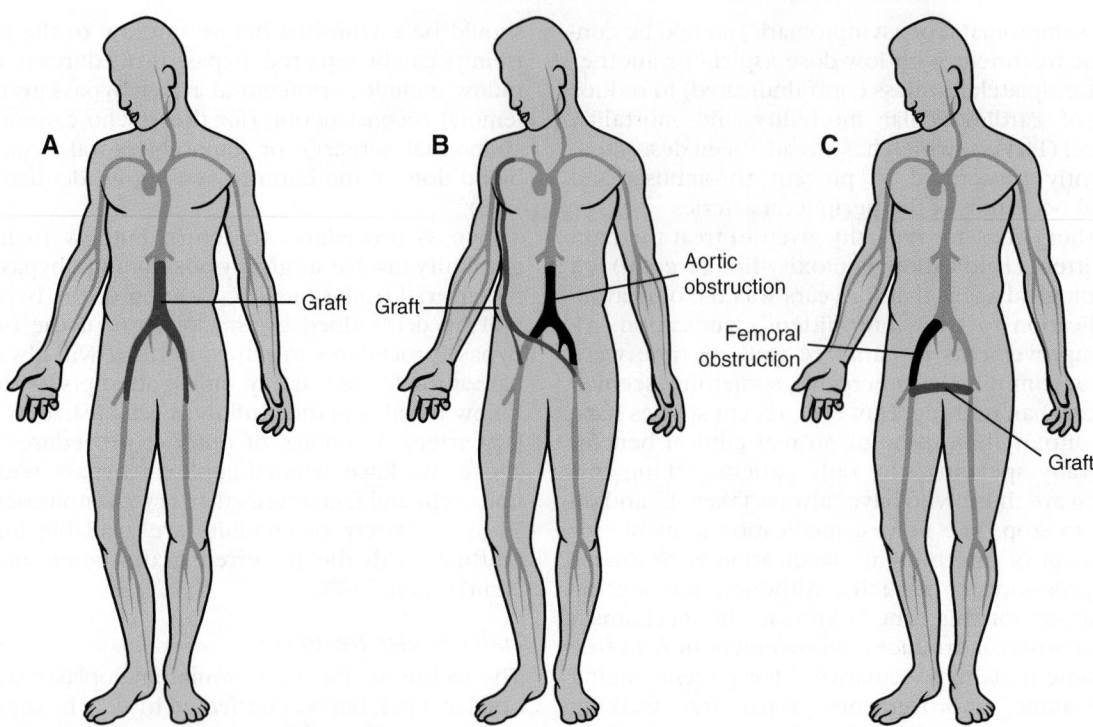

FIGURE 74-5 ■ Bypass surgery to reestablish inflow: **A,** Aortobifemoral bypass graft. **B,** Axillo-bifemoral bypass graft. **C,** Femorofemoral bypass graft. (From Beare, Myers: *Adult health nursing,* ed 2, 1994, Mosby, Figure 30-5 and 30-6, p 702.)

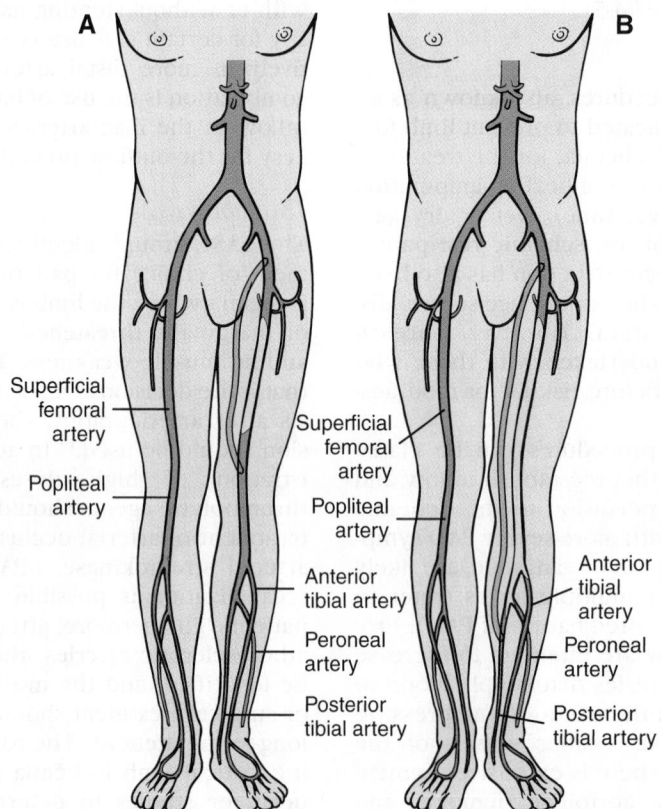

FIGURE 74-6 ■ Bypass surgery to return outflow to the distal lower extremity: **A,** Femoral-popliteal bypass graft. **B,** Femoral-posterior tibial bypass graft. (From Lewis SL, Heitkemper MM, and Dirksen SR: *Medical-surgical nursing,* ed 6, 2004, Mosby, Figure 37-6, p 923.)

■■■

TABLE 74-7 THREE PERIPHERAL BYPASS SURGERY GRAFT OPTIONS

Reversed greater saphenous vein	The saphenous vein has a series of valves allowing unidirectional blood flow. The traditional way to use the saphenous vein for bypass surgery is to surgically remove it and reverse the vein.
In situ saphenous vein	This allows the saphenous vein to be used in its natural position (without reversal). The benefit is that the venous endothelium is preserved, and the vein retains its adventitial blood supply. Valves are rendered incompetent through various techniques.
Synthetic prosthetic graft	In the absence of an adequate vein, the synthetic or Dacron prosthetic graft may be used.

Nursing Care

From a nursing perspective, all vascular recanalization procedures (e.g., angioplasty), whether cardiac or peripheral, are quite similar and require similar nursing care during and after the procedure. Chapter 28 discusses the nurse's role in cardiac catheterization procedures in depth. Chapter 58 also can be used to understand the nursing role during and after a balloon angioplasty and stent placement, with the addition of nursing care concentrating on the assessment of the treated limb and the puncture site.

Nursing care of the patient after peripheral bypass surgery primarily involves frequent assessment to ensure graft patency. This is not to say that other nursing activities are not important, such as increasing activity, promoting a healthy diet to facilitate wound healing, monitoring for wound infection, and treating comorbidities, such as hypertension and diabetes. However, the most important piece of assessment data collected after bypass surgery is the presence or absence of pedal pulses. Generally, after a bypass graft operation, the patient is returned to a telemetry progressive care or medical-surgical unit. The exception is the aorta-femoral bypass graft procedure, which requires a hospitalization similar to the open aortic aneurysm repair (discussed below).

Nursing care on the day of surgery involves frequent vital signs and pulse checks (Box 74-2). Peripheral pulse evaluation can be done with a Doppler if pedal pulses are not palpable. Doppler signals after bypass surgery are considered a normal assessment finding. However, if the pulses were palpable during the immediate postoperative period, but later can only be found with the Doppler, this is considered a significant change and should be reported to the surgeon. Intake and output should be monitored every 1 to 2 hours during the immediate postoperative period, and continuous intravenous (IV) fluids will be running between 75 to 100 ml/hr to ensure adequate intravascular volume and organ perfusion. Adequate blood pressure must be maintained to ensure graft patency, so if systolic blood pressure drops to *less than 100* mm Hg, the surgeon should be notified. Promoting lung expansion to prevent pneumonia postoperatively

BOX 74-2   ■■■
NURSING CARE AFTER PERIPHERAL BYPASS GRAFT (MAY VARY FROM INSTITUTION TO INSTITUTION)

Operative Day
- Frequent VS monitoring per postoperative routine along with pedal pulse check (q 15 min × 4, q 30 min × 4, q 1 hr × 4)
- Urinary catheter with strict I/O monitoring
- Cough and deep breath q 1 hr while awake
- Continuous IV fluids; antibiotic therapy if arterial ulcerations present
- Assess incisions for s/s of bleeding and infection q 2 hr
- Continuous cardiac rate and rhythm monitoring depending on cardiac history and risk
- Pain medication p.r.n.
- Antiplatelet therapy
- Lower extremity compression therapy to reduce swelling
- Apply sheepskin and foot cradle to the foot of the bed, wrap in between toes with lambs wool if ulcers are present
- Keep feet wrapped in warm blankets
- Bedrest
- NPO until fully awake then sips of clears
- Provide emotional support; assess patient and family understanding of postoperative course

Postoperative Day 1
- VS, pedal pulse, and incision check q 4 hr, clean incisions at least qd, apply dry sterile dressing as needed
- I/O q 8 hr (urinary catheter may or may not be discontinued)
- Cough and deep breath q 1 hr while awake
- Continuous IV fluids to maintain vascular volume to promote circulation through the graft
- Continue cardiac monitoring as needed
- Pain medication p.r.n.
- Continue antiplatelet therapy
- Continue lower extremity compression therapy, foot cradle, sheepskin, lambs wool: good skin care
- Increase activity, up to chair at least b.i.d. with legs elevated
- Advance diet as tolerated
- Begin to teach patient and family about incision care, activity level, and the importance of risk factor modification

Postoperative Days 2-5 (or until Discharge)
- VS, pedal pulse, and incision check q 4 hr, clean incisions at least qd, apply dry sterile dressing as needed
- I/O q 8 hr (Foley discontinued)
- Cough and deep breath q 1 hr while awake
- Once adequate PO intake is established, IV fluids will be discontinued
- Continue cardiac monitoring as needed
- Pain medication p.r.n., convert to PO if initially using IV
- Continue antiplatelet therapy
- Continue lower extremity compression therapy, foot cradle, sheepskin, lambs wool, and overall good skin care
- Increase activity until walking in the hall at least t.i.d.
- Continue regular diet
- Continue to reinforce teaching regarding risk factor modification and answer patient and family questions about discharge

b.i.d., Twice each day; *I/O,* intake and output; *IV,* intravenous; *NPO,* nothing by mouth; *PO,* orally; *p.r.n.,* as needed; *q,* every; *qd,* every day; *t.i.d.,* three times each day; *VS,* vital signs.

should begin immediately through incentive spirometry and coughing. Because the risk of cardiac events in patients with PAD is so high, continuous cardiac monitoring is often ordered for the entire hospital stay. Assessment of the incisions will be somewhat limited because the postoperative dressing should still be intact. However, the nurse must assess the incision sites for hematoma or bleeding. If the surgeon wants the patient to begin antiplatelet therapy, it could begin as early as the day of surgery. Pain medication should be administered as needed to provide adequate pain relief. With the return of blood flow to the affected leg after bypass surgery, edema in the operative leg is considered a normal assessment finding. In addition, the skin of the operative leg may be ruborous and very warm. However, too much swelling can compress the graft and should be prevented through the use of compression wraps or hose. Providing good skin care of the lower extremities and feet is of utmost importance. The application of sheepskin to the foot of the bed provides a softer surface for the fragile skin of the feet to rest, foot cradles keep sheets and blankets off sensitive skin, and lambs wool between toes reduces rubbing and irritation. In addition, some institutions advocate wrapping the feet in warm blankets during the first few hours after surgery to promote circulation to the feet. The patient will be on bedrest on the day of surgery. Unless the bypass includes abdominal surgery, once the gag reflex has returned the patient is permitted sips of clear liquids. The patient may be relatively sleepy the afternoon after surgery, but as needed, the nurse should be prepared to offer emotional support and teaching with the family about the expected postoperative course. In addition, risk factors for PAD should be assessed.

On the first postoperative day, the typical patient will be much more awake and alert. At this point, assessment of vital signs and pedal pulses should continue every 4 hours. In addition, if the surgeon removed the postoperative dressings, the nurse should clean the incisions at least once a day with a ½ hydrogen peroxide, ½ normal saline mixture. In addition, continue to monitor at least every 4 hours for hematoma, bleeding, or infection. Incisions in the groin area are the most likely to become infected because of the potentially moist environment. The best thing the nurse can do is keep the incisions as clean and dry as possible. A dry, sterile dressing may need to be applied to achieve this goal. Intake and output will still be monitored every 8 hours, pulmonary toilet should be continued while the patient is awake, and a continuous IV drip will remain until the patient is taking oral fluids well. Cardiac monitoring and pain medication will continue as needed and if ordered antiplatelet therapy as well. Although it is no longer necessary to wrap the feet in warm blankets, continue good skin care, sheepskin, foot cradle, and compression therapy as needed. At this point, the patient should be expected to get out of bed to the chair at least twice per day. The feet should be elevated while in the chair to promote venous return to the heart. In addition, the diet should be advanced to what is a regular diet for the patient.

The typical length of hospital stay for an uncomplicated bypass surgery is 4 to 5 days. During days 2 through 5, vital signs, pedal pulses, and incisions will continue to be monitored every 4 hours. The urinary catheter will be discontinued, although output should still be calculated every 8 hours. Pain medication should be converted to oral if IV was used initially, but should be adequate to allow the patient to increase his or her activity to ambulation at least three times a day. Good skin care is imperative, and compression therapy will continue to help control any lingering edema. During these days of recu-

peration, the nurse should take the window of opportunity to offer counseling on ways to manage the risk factors of PAD, including smoking cessation, exercise adoption, cholesterol management, blood pressure management, and strict control of diabetes.

Cardiovascular mortality is high for lower-extremity bypass surgery patients. In fact only 60 percent to 70 percent 5-year survival is reported for most surgical cases, and only about half of those who undergo limb-salvage surgery are still living 5 years later.[48] For those who do survive, the patency rates for autogenous saphenous-vein bypasses should be expected to reach 70 percent or higher at 5 years. However, patency rates significantly decrease with the use of synthetic or Dacron graft material. In fact the type of conduit, the status of arterial runoff beyond the graft, and continued cigarette smoking are the most important predictors for long-term graft patency.[51] Good patient care after bypass surgery should take long-term outcomes into consideration. Any intervention in the short-term should be done with long-term survival and graft patency as the ultimate goal.

ABDOMINAL AORTIC ANEURYSM

Aneurysm, derived from the Greek word aneurysma, means widening and can be defined as a permanent and irreversible localized dilatation of a vessel.[52] Although any aneurysm occurring in the infradiaphragmatic aorta could be termed an abdominal aortic aneurysm, common practice restricts this definition to an aneurysm of the infrarenal aorta. In 1991 two national vascular surgery groups proposed that if a widened vessel was to be termed an aneurysm, it must be 1.5 times the expected normal diameter.[52] However, AAA is conventionally diagnosed if the aortic diameter is 3 cm or more. This dilatation must affect all three layers of the artery; otherwise, it is called a pseudoaneurysm.[52]

AAAs are found in 4 percent to 8 percent of older men and 0.5 percent to 1.5 percent of older women.[53] This incidence has increased in the past two decades. As a result, the **USPSTF** published clinical guidelines for the screening of AAA.[17] Most aneurysms discovered by screening are small; however, they grow at an average of 10 percent per year.[26] In general the risk of rupture increases and the diameter increases, and the overall mortality rate for ruptured AAA is 65 percent to 85 percent.[52] Traditionally, aneurysms *less than* 4 cm are observed with periodic ultrasound surveillance. Treatment is generally recommended for symptomatic aneurysms, rapidly enlarging aneurysms, and aneurysms *greater than* 5 cm in size.[54]

Evaluation
Risk Factors

Male sex is one of the highest risk factors for AAA, along with age (*greater than* 65 years), smoking, and a first-degree relative with an aneurysm.[55,17] The incidence of AAA in chronic cigarette smokers is four times that of lifelong nonsmokers; however, the mechanism by which smoking promotes aneurysm formation is unknown.[56] The frequency of this disorder in first-degree relatives is

15 percent to 19 percent.[57] It is doubtful that familial clustering of AAA is due to chance alone, but probably to a common genetic background (see Special Feature: Genetics Box) in conjunction with environmental factors (see Chapter 13).[52] Other less common risk factors for AAA include trauma, acute infection (salmonellosis), inflammatory diseases, and connective tissue disorders (Marfan syndrome, Ehlers-Danlos type IV). In addition, although AAA is usually thought of as atherosclerotic disease, there is only a modest association between risk factors for atherosclerotic disease and AAA.[17]

Screening

The USPSTF recommends one-time screening for AAA by ultrasonography in men age 65 to 75 years who have ever smoked. However, they make no recommendation for or against screening for AAA in men age 65 to 75 who have never smoked. They recommend against routine screening for AAA in women.[17] In contrast The Society for Vascular Surgery and the Society for Vascular Medicine and Biology recommend AAA screening in all men age 60 to 85 years, women age 60 to 85 years with cardiovascular risk factors, and men and women age 50 and older with a family history of AAA.[58] In addition, they recommend no further testing if the aortic diameter is *less than* 3 cm, yearly ultrasonographic screening if the aortic diameter is 3 to 4 cm, ultrasonography every 6 months if the aortic diameter is 4 to 4.5 cm, and referral to a vascular specialist if the diameter is *greater than* 4.5 cm.

History and Physical Examination

Most patients with AAA will be asymptomatic. However, if they have symptoms, the most common complaints are abdominal, back, or flank pain. In addition, unruptured AAA may be incidentally diagnosed after the appearance of complications, such as distal embolization or acute thrombosis.[52]

Ruptured AAA presents by a clinical triad of sudden-onset pain in the midabdomen or flank, shock, and the presence of a pulsatile abdominal mass. Degree of shock will depend on the location and size of the rupture and the delay between onset of symptoms and assessment.[52]

The physical examination involves inspection of the patient's abdomen while in a supine position. The abdomen should be lightly to moderately palpated just above the umbilicus for the aortic pulse. Sensitivity of abdominal palpation for detection of AAA increases with the diameter of the lesion: 61 percent for aneurysms 3 to 3.9 cm, 69 percent for those 4 to 4.9 cm, and 82 percent for those 5 cm and larger.[52] Auscultation for bruits over the abdominal aorta can also provide beneficial assessment data.

Diagnostic Tests

The AAA diameter can be reliably measured using duplex ultrasound with a reproducibility of + or − 0.2 cm.[59] As a result, ultrasonography is a highly sensitive and specific screening tool for AAA. However, before surgery will be performed, a definitive diagnosis is always made using *CT.* In fact a CT scan is required before a decision can be made on whether the AAA can be repaired surgically or with an endovascular procedure. A high-resolution CT scan, with 3-mm or thinner cuts, is used to obtain measurements of several anatomical structures. For elective endovascular repair, a helical CT scan with dynamic radiocontrast infusion provides the best picture.[61] In rare cases, a preoperative angiography will be done out of concern for the stenoses of internal iliac, mesenteric, or renal artery branches.[60]

In addition to an evaluation of the aneurysm, before an endovascular procedure will be considered, anatomical planning must be undertaken. Anatomical planning involves two main assessment components. First, there must be adequate length of normal aorta between the renal arteries and the aneurysm (typically 15 mm). The second consideration requires assessment of the iliac artery diameter, tortuosity, calcification, and stenoses to allow passage of the delivery catheter (at least 7.5 mm). This is completed with the results from the helical CT scan.

As a result of the high prevalence of coronary artery disease, myocardial infarction remains the most frequent cause of death in patients with AAA.[59] As a result, all patients who are eligible for AAA repair should undergo evaluation of their cardiac risk. This can be done using exercise electrocardiography, Holter monitoring, dipyridamole-thallium scintigraphy, stress echocardiography, and/or coronary angiography, depending on risk factors and the cardiac practitioner's preferences.

Treatment
Risk Factor Modification

Three of the four primary risk factors are nonmodifiable: age, male sex, and family history. However, the fourth, smoking, is an area where nurses can and should intervene. As with other cardiovascular and peripheral vascular disorders, when planning and implementing a smoking cessation program, the clinical practice guidelines for treating tobacco use and dependence should be followed.[21]

Open Surgical Repair

An open AAA repair is normally approached through a long midline incision, although a transverse incision is recommended in patients with chronic obstructive pulmonary disease. Exteriorization of the small bowel is usually required, which can lead to insensible fluid loss, hypothermia, and postoperative paralytic ileus.[61] After heparinization (3000 to 5000 units IV), a proximal clamp is placed on the aorta above the aneurysm, and the common iliac arteries are clamped for distal control. The aneurysm sac is then opened and a Dacron graft is hand sewn above and below the aneurysm using a non-absorbable suture. The aorta can be reconstructed using a tube graft or a bifurcated aortobiiliac or aortobifemoral graft, depending on the anatomy and distal vessel disease.[61]

Endovascular Repair

Endovascular repair of AAA was introduced in 1991 by Parodi, using straight tubes that were placed in the normal aorta and kept in place by stainless steel or nitinol stents. Although this procedure removed arterial pressure from the aneurysm, typically, there was insufficient normal aorta above the aortic bifurcation to prevent reperfusion of the sac around the distal graft (endoleak). Since then endovascular repair has been perfected, and most repairs are done with a bifurcated graft (upside down Y shape).

Current data available on outcomes after open versus endovascular repair of intact AAA suggest that endovascular repair results in a significantly lower number of complications and deaths, a shorter hospital stay, and improved likelihood of discharge to home when compared with open repair.[62] However, there are not enough data to make the determination that endovascular repair is superior to open repair. Some researchers have shown that the failure rate of endovascular repair (by rupture or conversion to open repair) is higher in endovascular repair than open repair.[52] In addition, there is some question whether endovascular repair is appropriate for large aneurysms.

Nursing Care

The hospital stay after open AAA repair is an average of 6 days, with an initial return to the intensive care unit before transfer out to the floor after 24 hours. The nurse's job is to watch for complications and intervene early. The patient will return from surgery with a large midline abdominal incision. The nurse must watch for bleeding, and when the surgeon removes the dressing, watch for signs and symptoms of infection. The patient will go home with staples intact, and wound care will need to be taught before discharge.

Because of the close association between AAA and cardiac disease, the nurse must carefully monitor for myocardial ischemia or infarction, congestive heart failure, dysrhythmias, and atelectasis.[26] Nursing activities include monitoring vital signs, oximetry, and electrocardiogram; reviewing laboratory values, initiating appropriate diuretic medications, restarting appropriate cardiac medications; implementing analgesic medications, and anticipating early mobilization (usually by postoperative day 1). As with any peripheral vascular surgery, maintaining a blood pressure high enough to maintain perfusion through the graft, but not so high as to cause a leak or rupture, is one of the highest priorities. An outside limit for systolic blood pressure in this case is 100 to 180 mm Hg, though some surgeons prefer 110 to 150 mm Hg.

A complication of anesthetic is atelectasis, and the nurse should initiate good pulmonary toilet every hour while the patient is awake. A complication of major abdominal surgery is a prolonged ileus, and the nurse should carefully monitor nasogastric tube output, bowel sounds, and the return of bowel function (passing flatus and/or bowel movement).

During open AAA repair, the aorta and iliac arteries are cross clamped. In addition, within the lumen of the aneurysm there is extensive thrombus formation. Additional complications of open AAA repair are related to ischemia from prolonged cross clamping or embolization of peripheral arteries. As a result, it is essential to watch for renal failure, ishemic colitis, leg ischemia, and compartment syndrome. Carefully watch urine output, assess the abdomen for pain or distention, or the appearance of bloody diarrhea, assess pedal pulses, and watch the lower extremities for edema and tenderness. In addition, a neurological exam should be completed to rule out a cerebrovascular event or spinal cord ischemia.

In an uncomplicated open AAA repair, the nasogastric tube and urinary catheter are pulled the third or fourth postoperative day. A clear liquid diet is begun, and the patient is ambulated three times a day. By day 5, IV pain medicine is discontinued, oral analgesics are prescribed, and the patient is started on a soft diet. If the patient can tolerate these changes, they are usually discharged on the sixth postoperative day.

Patients undergoing endovascular repair can suffer any of the complications associated with open repair with the exception of paralytic ileus. However, special attention should be given to complications specific to endovascular repair. First, watch for hematoma at the catheter insertion site (groin) and for signs of retroperitoneal bleeding (back pain). Second, watch for signs and symptoms of thrombus including a drop in ABI and changes in neurovascular status. Third, watch for signs and symptoms of renal failure, such as oliguria and elevated serum creatinine. Finally, watch for signs of an endoleak, which is primarily manifested by an enlargement of the aneurysm on a follow-up CT scan. The typical length of stay for a patient after endovascular AAA repair varies from institution to institution, but may be as short as 1 day.

VENOUS THROMBOEMBOLIC DISEASE

Venous thromboembolic disease includes DVT and PE. A wide variety of medical conditions and surgical and interventional procedures place patients at risk for VTE. The sequelae of venous thrombosis include pulmonary or systemic embolism, post-thrombotic syndrome **(PTS),** and recurrent VTE. Reducing the burden of disease caused by VTE requires effective primary and secondary prevention, prompt diagnosis, and appropriate treatment of acute thrombosis. Fortunately, because of available prophylaxis, sensitive and specific methods of diagnosis, and effective treatment options, all nurses have the opportunity to play a significant role in reducing the morbidity and mortality associated with VTE.

Evaluation

Risk Factors and Symptom History

During the initial assessment, the nurse should carefully assess for the risk factors of VTE (see Table 74-1). Explaining the cause of the event is important for preventing VTE during hospitalization and for making treatment decisions.[63] Particularly significant risk factors include a history of VTE; cancer; familial or personal history of abnormal clotting; medications, such as estrogen replacement therapy; recent surgical history; or a recent history of travel.

The symptom history of DVT will be specific to the location of the thrombus. Distal (calf vein) DVT is usually asymptomatic and in about half of the patients resolves within 72 hours.[64] With a proximal (popliteal and thigh) DVT, the patient usually complains of pain, swelling, tenderness, and redness. About half of these patients will have a silent PE at the time of diagnosis, and 10 percent will have symptomatic PE.[65]

The symptom history of PE is directly related to the magnitude of the pulmonary circulation and obstruction caused by the clot.[32] Many symptoms are nonspecific; however, dyspnea and chest pain have been identified as the most commonly expressed symptoms. Any abrupt or unexplained episode of hypotension, chest pain, or respiratory distress should be considered suspicious of PE.

Physical Examination

Most extremities affected by acute DVT appear normal. However, if the patient is symptomatic, classic physical assessment findings include unilateral swelling of the extremity and possible tenderness with palpation (Figure 74-7). In addition, pedal pulses should be assessed to determine if the venous occlusion and edema are compromising arterial flow. If the arterial flow is compromised, the limb is at risk for gangrene. Historically a positive Homan sign (pain with forced dorsiflexion of the foot when the leg is raised) was a clinical indicator of DVT, but has since been found to have a high incidence of false-positive results and is no longer considered as part of the diagnosis of DVT.

In addition to the symptom history of PE, the severity of the event must be determined. To determine the patient's oxygenation status, visible signs of respiratory distress should be observed including tachypnea, use of accessory muscles, pallor, and cyanosis. In addition, pulse oximetry measurements and arterial blood gases are helpful in determining treatment options.

Diagnostic Tests

The venous duplex, or B-Mode ultrasound (brightness mode), is a method of processing reflected ultrasound waves to produce a two-dimensional image and is most often used in the diagnosis of VTE.[66] The B-Mode image is displayed in shades of gray; the higher the density, the brighter the color. This procedure is able to identify specific venous structures and blood flow. Venous obstruction appears as a segment of vein where there is a

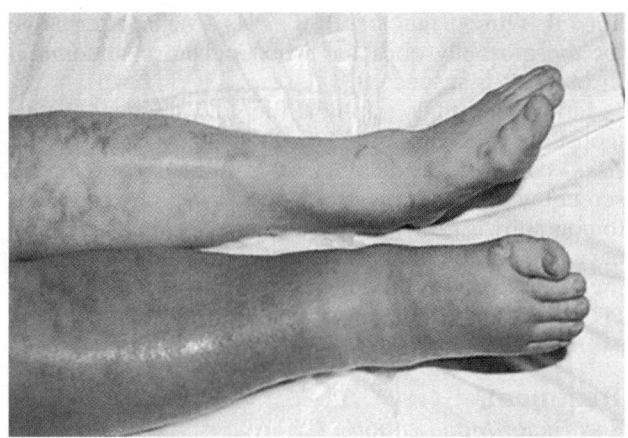

FIGURE 74-7 ■ Deep vein thrombosis. (From Lewis SL, Heitkemper MM, and Dirksen SR: *Medical-surgical nursing*, ed 6, 2004, Mosby, Figure 37-8, p 929.)

loss of flow signal. Chronic venous obstruction can be differentiated from acute venous thrombosis by the degree of wall inflammation and venous distention, which occurs with acute thrombosis. Chronic occlusion causes fibrosis of the vein so that it is smaller than normal caliber.

A ventilation/perfusion lung scan **(V/Q)** assesses airflow patterns and circulation of the lungs. In the case of PE, the V/Q scan shows pulmonary artery blood flow and any underperfused areas of the lung.[32] Although the V/Q scan is relatively specific, it is not very sensitive, with a high false-positive result rate caused by preexisting lung disease, such as atelectasis, pneumothorax, emphysema, or neoplasm.[63] The V/Q scan may be repeated in 1 to 3 days if a PE remains suspect.

Sometimes a venous duplex cannot differentiate between and old and new DVT, whereas the V/Q scan has a high incidence of false-positive results. As an adjunct, the *d-dimer* is a laboratory test ordered to help rule out VTE. A positive d-dimer test result indicates an abnormally high level of fibrin degradation products in the body. The proper interpretation of a positive d-dimer test result is that there has been significant thrombus formation and breakdown in the body, but it does not give the location or the cause. Elevated d-dimer levels can also be seen with surgery, trauma, infection, liver disease, pregnancy, eclampsia, heart disease, and some cancers. Anticoagulant therapy can cause a false-negative d-dimer test result. A normal d-dimer test result indicates less likelihood of abnormal clot formation and degradation in the body. However, in the presence of other factors that put the patient at high risk for clot formation, additional testing should still be performed. A standard reference range is not available for the d-dimer test. Because reference values are dependent on many factors, including patient age, gender, sample population, and test method, numeric test results have different meanings in different labs. As a result, the reference range should be specific to each institution.

Computed tomography venography *(CTV)* is a highly sensitive (97 percent) and specific (100 percent) test for the detection of DVT. Because of the cost of CTV, it is not a first-line diagnostic test, but is a viable alternative for the morbidly obese or when pelvic or abdominal thrombosis is suspected.[32]

Pulmonary angiography is the gold standard for establishing a diagnosis of PE. However, because of the risks, cost, and availability, it is not appropriate for screening and routine use. However, spiral computed tomography is nearly as sensitive and specific as pulmonary angiography and is expected to become increasingly popular in evaluating patients suspected of having PE, particularly in the emergency setting.[32]

Treatment

Risk Factor Modification

Many patients will experience an idiopathic VTE or VTE as a result of a nonmodifiable risk factor. However, for those VTE patients with an identified risk factor, steps should be taken to modify or reverse their risk. One of the most easily modified risk factors is inactivity. It is important to encourage patients to intersperse activity during long periods of inactivity. Examples include getting up and walking around during long plane rides, stopping to walk during long car trips, or intermittent contraction and relaxation of calf muscles when sitting for long periods.

Pharmacotherapies

The primary treatment for both DVT and PE is anticoagulation therapy. Anticoagulants do not break down clots, but inhibit clot formation through various means. Unfractionated heparin can be given subcutaneously or IV and enhances the inhibitory actions of antithrombin III on several factors essential to normal blood clotting, thereby blocking the conversion of prothrombin to thrombin and fibrinogen to fibrin. Low-molecular-weight heparin is given subcutaneously and opposes factors Xa and IIa in the coagulation cascade. Use of low-molecular-weight heparin does not require routine coagulation tests, so it is safe to have patients self-administer this medication in an outpatient setting. In contrast Vitamin K antagonists, such as warfarin, indirectly interfere with blood clotting by depressing hepatic synthesis of vitamin K-dependent clotting factors II, VII, IX, and X.

The administration of anticoagulants in the treatment of VTE should follow the guidelines from the Seventh ACCP Conference on Antithrombotic and Thrombolytic Therapy[18] (Table 74-8). For patients with a confirmed DVT or those with a high clinical suspicion of DVT, heparin therapy should begin immediately. For most patients, the preferred route of heparin administration would be subcutaneous; but for patients with renal failure, a hospital admission would be required to administer IV heparin. In either case, a vitamin K antagonist should be started on day 1, and the heparin should be continued until the international normalized ratio **(INR)** reached 2.0. At this time, the heparin can be discontinued, and the vitamin K antagonist would be continued, maintaining an INR between 2 and 3.

For the patient with a nonmassive PE, the treatment would be the same, with the exception that subcutaneous low-molecular-weight heparin is the drug of choice except in the case of renal failure, when IV unfractionated heparin would be administered. For patients with a first occurrence of DVT or PE secondary to a reversible risk factor, the vitamin K antagonist should be continued for 3 months. For the first occurrence of idiopathic DVT or PE, the vitamin K antagonist should be continued for 6 to 12 months, and indefinite anticoagulation should be considered. For two or more objectively

■ ■ ■

TABLE 74-8 ANTITHROMBOTIC THERAPY FOR VENOUS THROMBOEMBOLIC DISEASE: RECOMMENDATIONS FROM THE SEVENTH ACCP CONFERENCE ON ANTITHROMBOTIC AND THROMBOLYTIC THERAPY

RECOMMENDATION CATEGORY	DEEP VEIN THROMBOSIS	NONMASSIVE PULMONARY EMBOLISM
Initial treatment (first 5 days)	Subcutaneous low-molecular-weight heparin or IV unfractionated heparin or Subcutaneous unfractionated heparin or	Subcutaneous low-molecular-weight heparin or IV unfractionated heparin
Vitamin K antagonists	Start the first day until INR stable and *greater than* 2. For first occurrence of DVT or PE secondary to a reversible risk factor, continue vitamin K antagonist for 3 mo. For first occurrence of idiopathic DVT or PE continue, vitamin K antagonist for 6-12 mo and consider indefinite anticoagulation therapy. For two or more objectively documented occurrences of DVT or PE, continue vitamin K antagonist indefinitely.	Same
Thrombolytic therapy	Recommend against except with massive iliofemoral DVT with a risk of limb gangrene and loss	Recommend against except when hemodynamically unstable and then the infusion time should be short
Vena caval interruption	Should only be used for patients with: a contraindication for anticoagulation therapy recurrent thromboembolism despite adequate anticoagulation	Same

DVT, Deep vein thrombosis; *INR,* international normalized ratio; *PE,* pulmonary embolism.
Buller HR, Agnelli G, Hull RD et al: Antithrombotic therapy of venous thromboembolic disease: the Seventh ACCP Conference on Antithrombotic and Thrombolytic Therapy, *Chest* 126:401S-428S, 2004.

documented occurrences of DVT or PE, vitamin K antagonists should be continued indefinitely, maintaining an INR between 2 and 3.

Thrombolytic Therapy

The ACCP guidelines are very clear in their recommendation against the use of thrombolytic therapy for the treatment of DVT with one exception (see special considerations below). In addition, for most patients with PE, thrombolytic therapy is not recommended unless the patient is hemodynamically unstable with a low risk to bleed. In this case clinicians should not use local administration of thrombolytic therapy via a catheter, but should administer thrombolytic therapy systemically (IV) and for a short infusion time.[18]

Thrombectomy and Embolectomy

The ACCP guidelines do not recommend the use of venous thrombectomy except in select cases (see special considerations below). For most patients with PE, they recommend against pulmonary embolectomy, except in highly compromised patients who are unable to receive thrombolytic therapy or whose critical status does not allow sufficient time to infuse thrombolytic therapy.[18]

Vena Caval Interruption

For most patients with DVT and PE, implantation of a vena cava filter is not recommended.[18] However, vena caval interruption is recommended for patients who are unable to take anticoagulation therapy and for those with recurrent thromboembolism despite adequate anticoagulation. Filtration devices are percutaneously placed in the vena cava to "catch" clots without obstructing blood flow (Figure 74-8). Postoperative complications are rare and include insertion site thrombosis or hemorrhage, infection, development of an AV fistula, and migration of the filter more distally into the venous system. Although the filtration device may eventually become clogged with clots, this usually happens over time, giving time for collateral circulation to develop and maintain venous flow.

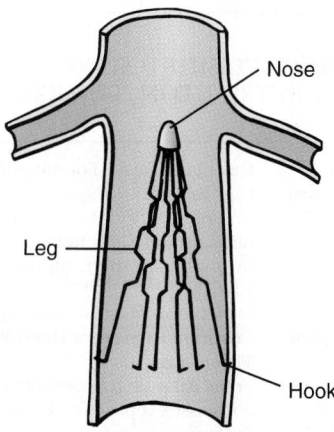

FIGURE 74-8 ■ Vena caval filter to prevent pulmonary embolus. (From Lewis SL, Heitkemper MM, and Dirksen SR: *Medical-surgical nursing,* ed 6, 2004, Mosby, Figure 37-9, p 933.)

Nursing Care

Historically, nursing care of the patient with DVT has been bedrest, bedrest, and bedrest. However, in the 2004 ACCP guidelines, the recommendation for patients with DVT is ambulation as tolerated.[18] In fact the usual care today of a patient with a DVT occurs as an outpatient. In this case the role of the nurse is to educate the patient on how to administer subcutaneous injections and how to modify risk factors for DVT. There are no activity recommendations for PE given in the ACCP guidelines. Usual practice today remains hospitalization for symptomatic PE.[18] Many clinicians will remain conservative in their activity restrictions and limit the patient's activity for at least the first 24 hours.

Additional nursing responsibilities include teaching patients about anticoagulation therapy. This includes signs of unusual bleeding from the gums or nose, excessive bruising, or blood in the urine or stool. Teaching about drug administration includes taking the medication at the same time each day, not stopping the drug unless ordered by a physician, and taking a missed dosage as soon as possible, but not doubling the dose if one is completely missed. Drugs administered by injection should be given in the abdominal subcutaneous tissue at least 2 inches from the naval, the injection site should be rotated, and the needle should be discarded in the appropriate dispenser (not the trash). Patient should limit their consumption of alcohol, vitamin E, and green tea, and should not take aspirin unless ordered by the physician. Historically, patients were advised to limit their dietary intake of vitamin K. However, this concept was challenged recently when researchers reported that short-term variability in intake of vitamin K is less important to fluctuations in the INR than has been commonly assumed and that food supplements providing 100 mg/d of vitamin K do not significantly interfere with oral anticoagulant therapy.[67]

For hospitalized patients, graduated compression stockings and intermittent pneumatic compression devices help control edema and promote venous return. They should be applied every shift, but should be removed to inspect the skin and for patient comfort. While in bed, legs should be elevated 10° to 20° above the level of the heart.

Special Considerations

Iliofemoral venous thrombosis is not common, but the sequelae are potentially devastating. About 95 percent of patients with iliofemoral thrombosis treated with anticoagulants alone exhibit severely compromised muscle function and valvular incompetency at 5 years following treatment.[68,69] In addition, because of severe edema that can occur with iliofemoral thrombosis, arterial flow can be compromised, and limb ischemia with gangrene can occur. As a result, the ACCP guidelines published in 2004 recommend IV thrombolysis for patients with massive iliofemoral DVT and catheter-directed thrombolysis for those requiring limb salvage.[18] In addition, venous thrombectomy should be considered for these patients when limb gangrene is a threatening.

PTS is characterized by chronic leg pain, swelling, venous stasis, and leg ulcers.[65] It occurs in 20 percent of patients with symptomatic DVT after 2 years.[64] To prevent PTS, the ACCP guidelines recommend the use of an elastic compressing stocking with a pressure of 30 to 40 mm Hg at the ankle for 2 years after an episode of DVT.[18] For patients with PTS and mild edema, elastic compressing stockings may be used indefinitely, and for those with severe edema, intermittent pneumatic compression may be used. In patients with mild edema caused by PTS, the administration of rutosides is recommended.[18] Rutosides are classified as a vasoprotector. Their primary pharmacological effect is a reduction of the capillary filtration rate of water and microvascular permeability to proteins. The only reported adverse reactions to this drug were skin rashes, minor gastrointestinal disturbances, headaches, and flushes. All reactions disappeared quickly when treatment was stopped. (See Special Feature on Biotechnology).

■ ■ ■ BIOTECHNOLOGY

The main problem for patients with peripheral arterial disease (PAD) is poor tissue oxygenation, which leads to limb threatening ischemia. Lifestyle modifications, pharmacological therapies, and surgical interventions are all viable options for many patients. However, there are a significant number of patients who have tried medical management, undergone surgery, or are not surgical candidates because of comorbidities who are at risk for amputation. Many of these patients have diffuse distal disease or are diabetic. Preliminary research has shown good evidence that the development of collateral circulation can slow the symptoms of PAD, aid in wound healing, and reduce rest pain. The development of new vessels (neovascularization) involves angiogenesis, arteriogenesis, and vasculogenesis. Angiogenesis is the sprouting of new capillaries from existing vascular structures usually as a result of hypoxia, whereas arteriogenesis is the increase in the size and wall thickness of collateral vessels, primarily from shear stress (as opposed to hypoxia). Vasculogenesis is the in situ formation of new blood vessels from circulating endothelial progenitor cells (EPCs). Under normal conditions, the number of circulating EPCs is relatively small, but vascular trauma or ischemia results in mobilization and proliferation of EPCs from the bone marrow. Angiogenesis is tightly regulated by proangiogenic and antiangiogenic mechanisms. Many of the proangiogenic mechanisms are growth factors released, for example, by the vascular endothelium or the platelets in response to hypoxia. Examples of factors that inhibit angiogenesis would include troponin I and endostatin. Cancer researchers are particularly interested in blocking angiogenesis to inhibit tumor growth, whereas cardiovascular researchers are interested in promoting angiogenesis to promote wound healing and decrease ischemic pain, either in the heart (angina), or in the periphery (claudication). Vascular researchers have studied ways to promote angiogenesis through local administration of recombinant proteins or genes for angiogenic growth factors or by reimplantation of EPCs harvested from the bone marrow or peripheral circulation. These studies have been conducted in animals and humans with critical limb ischemia and intermittent claudication. Although early uncontrolled studies were encouraging, more recent multicenter randomized controlled trials have had mixed results. In patients with intermittent claudication, the administration of intraarterial recombinant growth factor improved maximum walking time after 90 days, but gene transfer was ineffective. Case reports and small uncontrolled studies have shown dramatic benefits from gene transfer on critical limb ischemia, but larger controlled trials have found no changes in terms of restenosis after angioplasty, amputation rates, ulcer healing, or severity of rest pain. As a result, researchers continue to study the question of whether biotechnology can produce and effective collateral circulation.

CONCLUSION

PVD is an umbrella term that encompasses a plethora of diseases and disorders. It is pertinent for the cardiac nurse to know how to properly assess and care for patients with PVD because so many PVD patients also suffer from coronary artery disease. In an attempt to raise the awareness of vascular disease in the community, several large organizations have undertaken campaigns to encourage screening for a multitude of vascular disorders. The American Vascular Association (**AVA**) has undertaken an initiative to have more people screened for PAD. During the 2004 screening initiative, PAD was found in 10.5 percent of people screened, as compared with slightly *less than* 10 percent in 2003. Another group, the PAD coalition made up of 15 vascular organizations, is working with the National Institutes of Health to select a public relations or advertising agency that will design and carry out a national PAD awareness campaign. In addition, Legs for Life offers free screenings for those at risk for PAD at hundreds of sites across the country. In Denver Colorado, an annual event titled *Keeping in Circulation* is held at the Garden. At this event, information and presentations about vascular disease, free screenings, and a garden walk are available. Finally, at a political level, the SAAAVE Act, HR 827 and S-390, is a proposed law to provide one-time screening for AAAs.

As various organizations continue to seek ways to increase public awareness of and public education about vascular disease, other organizations work to increase clinicians' ability to conduct the screening. For example, in March 2004, the Society for Vascular Nursing provided an opportunity for its members to learn how to measure the ABI, the primary screening test for PAD. Similar educational opportunities would also be of benefit for cardiac nurses. Cardiac nursing leaders and cardiovascular nursing organizations can take the initiative to learn how to screen their patients for PVD and teach their colleagues to do the same. See Box 74-3 for a list of websites that provide further information about PVD both for professionals and patients.

BOX 74-3　■ ■ ■
LIST OF INTERNET WEBSITES FOR PROFESSIONALS AND PATIENTS INTERESTED IN PERIPHERAL VASCULAR DISEASE

www.vdf.org	Vascular Disease Foundation
www.legsforlife.org	Legs for Life
http://amputee-coalition.org	An organization that reaches out to people with limb loss to empower them through education, support, and advocacy
www.svnnet.org	Society for Vascular Nursing
www.preventdvt.org	Coalition to prevent Deep Vein Thrombosis
www.tasc-pad.org	Trans-Atlantic Intersociety Coalition. The consensus report can be accessed here for free.
www.pvss.org	Peripheral Vascular Surgery Society
www.svmb.org	Society for Vascular Medicine and Biology

REFERENCES

1. A Report of the American College of Cardiology/American Heart Association/American College of Physicians task force on clinical competence: ACC/ACP/SCAI/SVMB/SVS clinical competence statement on vascular medicine and catheter-based peripheral vascular interventions, *J Amer Coll Cardiol* 44:1-17, 2004.

2. Pasternak RC, Criqui MH, Benjamin EJ et al: Atherosclerotic vascular disease conference writing group 1: epidemiology, *Circulation* 109:2605-2612, 2004.

3. Belch JJ, Topol EJ, Agnelli G et al: Critical issues in peripheral arterial disease detection and management: a call to action, *Arch Int Med* 163:884-892, 2003.

4. Hackam DG: Cardiovascular risk prevention in peripheral artery disease, *J Vasc Surg* 41:1070-1073, 2005.

5. Fahey VA: *Vascular nursing,* ed, 4, Philadelphia, 2004, WB Saunders.

6. Taylor LM Jr, Porter JM: Abdominal aortic aneurysms. In Porter JM, Taylor LM Jr, editors: *Basic data underlying clinical decision making in vascular surgery,* St Louis, 1994, Quality Medical Publishing, pp 98-100.

7. Barba A, Estallo L, Rodrigeuz L et al: Detection of abdominal aortic aneurysm in patients with peripheral artery disease, *Eur J Vasc Endovasc Surg* 29:504-508, 2005.

8. Cronenwett JL, Krupski WC, Rutherford BR: Abdominal aortic and iliac aneurysms. In Rutherford RB, editor: *Vascular surgery,* Philadelphia, 2000, WB Saunders, pp 1246-1280.

9. Hirsh J, Hoak J: Management of deep vein thrombosis and pulmonary embolus: a statement for healthcare professionals, *Circulation* 93:2212-2245, 1996.

10. Jaff MR: Venous thromboembolic disease, *Ochsner J* 4:6-8, 2002.

11. Kennedy D, Setnik G, Li J: Physical examination findings in deep vein thrombosis, *Emerg Med Clinics No Amer* 19:869-876, 2001.

12. Lopez JA, Kearon C, Lee AYY: Deep vein thrombosis, *Hematol* 439-456, 2004.

13. Goldstein LB, Adams R, Becker K et al: Primary prevention of ischemic stroke: a statement for healthcare professionals from the stroke council of the American Heart Association, *Circulation* 103:163-182, 2001.

14. Pearson TA, Blair SN, Daniels SR et al: AHA guidelines for primary prevention of cardiovascular disease and stroke: 2002 update, *Circulation* 106:388-391, 2002.

15. Dormandy JA, Rutherford RB: Management of peripheral arterial disease (PAD). TASC Working Group: TransAtlantic Inter-society Consensus (TASC), *J of Vasc Surg* 31(1 pt 2):S1-296, 2000.

16. Rutherford RB, Krupski WC: Current status of open versus endovascular stent-graft repair of abdominal aortic aneurysm, *J Vasc Surg* 39:1129-39, 2004.

17. U.S. Preventive Services Task Force: Screening for abdominal aortic aneurysm: recommendation statement, *Ann Intern Med* 142:198-202, 2005.

18. Buller HR, Agnelli G, Hull RD et al: Antithrombotic therapy of venous thromboembolic disease: The seventh ACCP conference on antithrombotic and thrombolytic therapy, *Chest* 126: 01S-428S, 2004.

19. Chobanian AV, Bakris GL, Black HR et al: Seventh report of the joint national committee on prevention, detection, evaluation, and treatment of high blood pressure, *Hypertension* 42:1206, 2003.

20. National Heart, Lung, and Blood Institute, National Institutes of Health, U.S. Department of Health and Human Services: Third report of the national cholesterol education program (NCEP) expert panel on detection, evaluation, and treatment of high blood cholesterol in adults (adult treatment panel III), Bethesda, Md, 2001, U.S. Department of Health and Human Services, Public Health Service, National Institutes of Health, National Heart, Lung, and Blood Institute.

21. U.S. Department of Health and Human Services, Public Health Service, Fiore MC, Bailey WC, Cohen SJ et al: Treating tobacco use and dependence. Clinical practice guideline, Rockville, Md, 2000, U.S. Department of Health and Human Services, Public Health Service.

22. Thompson PD, Buchner D, Pina IL et al: Exercise and physical activity in the prevention and treatment of atherosclerotic cardiovascular disease, *Circulation* 107:3109, 2003.

23. National Heart, Lung, and Blood Institute, National Institutes of Health, The National Institute of Diabetes and Digestive and Kidney Disease: Clinical guidelines on the identification, evaluation, and treatment of overweight and obesity in adults, U.S. Department of Health and Human Services, Public Health Service, 1998. NIH Publication No. 98-4083.

24. Johnson WTM, Solanga G, Lee W et al: Arterial intimal embrittlement: a possible factor in atherogenesis, *Atherosclerosis* 59:161-171, 1986.

25. McGrath MA, Verhaighe RH, Shepherd JT: The physiology of limb blood flow. In Juergens JL, Spittell JA Jr, Fairborn JF II, editors: *Peripheral vascular diseases,* Philadelphia, 1980, WB Saunders, pp 83-105.

26. Eskandari MD, Matsumura JS, Anderson L: Surgery of the aorta. In Fahey, VA, editor: *Vascular nursing,* ed 4, Philadelphia, 2004, WB Saunders, pp 215-236.

27. Goldstone J: Aneurysms of the aorta and iliac arteries. In Moore WS, editor: *Vascular surgery: a comprehensive review,* Philadelphia, 2002, WB Saunders, pp 457-480.

28. O'Connor CM: Raynaud's phenomenon, *J Vasc Nurs* 19:87-94, 2001.

29. McGrath A: Raynaud's syndrome, *Amer J Nurs* 97:34, 1997.

30. Olin JW: Thromboangiitis obliterans (Buerger disease). *New Engl J Med* 343:864, 2003.

31. Varma S, Pappas PJ: The venous system. In Fahey, VA, editor: *Vascular nursing,* ed 4, Philadelphia, 2004, WB Saunders, pp 21-32.

32. Walsh ME, Rice K: Venous thromboembolic disease. In Fahey VA, editor: *Vascular nursing,* ed 4, Philadelphia, 2004, WB Saunders, pp 365-398.

33. Morasch MD, Pearce WH: Extracranial cerebrovascular disease. In Fahey VA, editor: *Vascular nursing,* ed 4, Philadelphia, 2004, WB Saunders, pp 365-398.

34. Fine-Edelstein JS, Wolf PA, O'Leary DH et al: Precursors of extracranial carotid atherosclerosis in the Framingham Study, *Neurology* 44:1046-1050, 1994.

35. Hertzer NR, Beven EG, Young JR et al: Coronary artery disease in peripheral vascular patients: a classification of 1000 coronary angiograms and results of surgical management, *Ann Surg* 199:223-233, 1984.

36. Yadav JS, Wholey MH, Kuntz RE et al: Protected carotid-artery stenting versus endarterectomy in high-risk patients *New Engl J Med* 351:1493-1501, 2004.

37. Antithrombotic Trialists' Collaboration. Collaborative meta-analysis of randomised trials of antiplatelet therapy for prevention of death, myocardial infarction, and stroke in high risk patients, *Brit Med J* 324:71-86, 2002.

38. Hayden M, Pignone M, Phillips C et al: Aspirin for the primary prevention of cardiovascular events: a summary of the evidence for the US preventive services task force, *Ann Intern Med* 136:161-172, 2002.

39. Kim CK, Schmalfuss CM, Schofield RS et al: Pharmacological treatment of patients with peripheral arterial disease, *Drugs* 63:637-647, 2003.

40. Prescribing information: Ticlid (ticlopidine hydrochloride) tablets. In *Physician's desk reference,* Montvale, NJ, 2000, Medical Economics Co, pp 2670-2673.

41. CAPRIE steering committee: A randomized, blinded, trial of clopidogrel versus aspirin in patients at risk for ischemic events, *Lancet* 348:1329-1339, 1996.

42. Schonholtz CJ, Uflacker R, Mendaro E et al: Techniques for carotid artery stenting under cerebral protection, *J Cardiovasc Surg* 46:201-217, 2005.

43. The technology assessment committees of the American Society of Interventional and Therapeutic Neuroradiology and the Society of Interventional Radiology: Trial design and reporting standards for intraarterial cerebral thrombolysis for acute ischemic stroke, *J Vasc Interv Rad* 14:S493-S494, 2003.

44. Treat-Jacobson D, Walsh ME: Treating patients with peripheral arterial disease and claudication, *J Vasc Nurs* 21:5-14, 2003.

45. Rutherford RB, Lowenstein DH, Klein MF: Combining segmental systolic pressures and plethysmography to diagnose arterial disease of the legs, *Amer J Surg* 138:211, 1979.

46. Freemantle N, Barbour R, Johnson R et al: The use of statins: a case of misleading priorities? *Brit Med J* 315:826-828, 1997 (editorial).

47. Regensteiner JG, Ware JE, MacCarthy WJ et al: Effect of cilostazol on treadmill walking, community-based walking ability, and health-related quality of life in patient with intermittent claudication due to peripheral arterial disease: meta-analysis of six-randomized controlled trials, *JAGS* 50:1939-1946, 2002.

48. Feinglass J, Morasch M, McCarthey WJ: Measures of success and health-related quality of life in lower-extremity vascular surgery, *Ann Rev Med* 51:101-113, 2000.

49. Vogelzang RL: Percutaneous endovascular intervention and imaging techniques. In Fahey JA, editor: *Vascular nursing,* ed 4, Philadelphia, 2004, WB Saunders, pp 97-126.

50. Fahey VA, Schindler N: Arterial reconstruction of the lower extremity. In Fahey VA, editor: *Vascular nursing,* ed 4, Philadelphia, 2004, WB Saunders, pp 251-286.

51. Myers KA, Fuller JA, Scott DF et al: Multivariate cox regression analysis of covariates for patency rates after femorodistal vein bypassing grafting, *Ann Vasc Surg* 7:262-269, 1993.

52. Sakalihasan N, Limet R, Defawe OD: Abdominal aortic aneurysm, *Lancet* 365:1577-1589, 2005.

53. Fleming C, Whitlock EP, Beil T et al: Screening for abdominal aortic aneurysm: a best-evidence systematic review for the U.S. preventive services task force, *Ann Int Med* 142:203-211, 2005.

54. Cronenwett JL: Abdominal aortic aneurysms: predicting the natural history. In Yao JST, Pearce WH, editors: *Progress in vascular surgery,* Stamford, Conn, 1997, Appleton & Lange, pp 127-138.

55. Cornuz J, Pinto CS, Tevaerai H et al: Risk factors for asymptomatic abdominal aortic aneurysm, *Eur J Publ Health* 14:343-349, 2004.

56. Vardulaki KA, Walker NM, Day NE et al: Quantifying the risks of hypertension, age, sex, and smoking in patients with abdominal aortic aneurysm, *Brit J Surg* 87:195-200, 2000.

57. Kuivaniemi H, Shibamura H, Aruthur C et al: Familial abdominal aortic aneurysms: collection of 233 multiplex families, *J Vasc Surg* 37:340-345, 2003.

58. Kent KC, Zwolak RM, Jaff MR et al: Screening for abdominal aortic aneurysm: a consensus statement, *J Vasc Surg* 39:267-269, 2004.

59. The UK small aneurysm trial participants. Mortality results for randomised controlled trial of early elective surgery or ultrasonographic surveillance for small abdominal aortic aneurysms, *Lancet* 352:1649-1655, 1998.

60. Eastridge D, Rodriguez H, Matsumura JS: Endovascular repair of aortic aneurysms. In Fahey VA, editor: *Vascular nursing,* ed 4, Philadelphia, 2004, WB Saunders, pp 237-250.

61. Daly KJ, Torella F, Ashleigh R et al: Screening, diagnosis, and advances in aortic aneurysm surgery, *Gerontology* 50:349-359, 2004.

62. Lee WA, Carter JW, Upchurch G et al: Perioperative outcomes after open and endovascular repair of intact abdominal aortic aneurysms in the United States during 2001, *J Vasc Surg* 39:491-496, 2004.

63. Haines ST, Nutuscu EA: Current and emerging treatment options for venous thrombosis: a case discussion, *Amer J Health Syst Pharm* 62:593-605, 2005.

64. Kearon C: Natural history of venous thromboembolism, *Circulation* 107:I22-I30, 2003.

65. Ho WK, Hankey GJ, Lee CH et al: Venous thromboembolism: diagnosis and management of deep venous thrombosis, *Med J Aust* 182:476-481, 2005.

66. Blackburn DR, Peterson-Kennedy L: Noninvasive vascular testing. In Fahey VA, editor: *Vascular nursing,* ed 4, Philadelphia, 2004, WB Saunders, pp 73-96.

67. Schurgers LJ, Shearer MJ, Hamulyak K et al: Effect of vitamin K intake on the stability of oral anticoagulant treatment: dose-response relationships in healthy subjects, *Blood* 104:682-2689, 2004.

68. Moh DN, Silverstei MD, Hei JA et al: The venous stasis syndrome after deep venous thrombosis or pulmonary embolism: a population based study, *Mayo Clinic Proceed* 75:1249-1256, 2001.

69. AbuRahma AF, Perkin SE, Wulu JT et al: Iliofemoral deep vein thrombosis: conventional therapy versus lysis and percutaneous transluminal angioplasty and stenting, *Ann Surg* 233:752-760, 2001.

■■■■ chapter 75

Care of Patients with Pericardial Diseases

Taletha Carter
Barbara Riegel

CHAPTER ABBREVIATIONS

AMI acute myocardial infarction

CBC complete blood count

CK creatine kinase

CT computed tomography

ECG electrocardiogram

ESR erythrocyte sedimentation rate

ESRD end-stage renal disease

HIV-AIDS human immunodeficiency virus-autoimmune deficiency syndrome

JVD jugular venous distention

MRI magnetic resonance imaging

NSAID nonsteroidal antiinflammatory drug

PT prothrombin time

PTT partial thromboplastin time

PPD purified protein derivative

PAP pulmonary artery pressure

PAWP pulmonary artery wedge pressure

RAP right atrial pressure

RVED right ventricular end diastolic

SLE systemic lupus erythematosus

TEE transesophageal echocardiogram

TB tuberculosis

The pericardium is composed of two layers, the visceral (inner) layer that adheres to the heart, and the parietal (outer) layer. Together these layers are referred to as the pericardial sac since the visceral pericardium bends back around the great vessels and becomes continuous with the parietal pericardium, creating a sac. These two layers enclose the heart, separating the walls with a space containing a thin layer of serous fluid (15 to 50 ml). This fluid lubricates cardiac motion, decreasing friction between the two layers. The pericardium itself has three functions: it attaches the heart to the mediastinum and diaphragm, thus limiting its motion; it controls dilatation as a result of sudden increases in intracardiac volume; and it serves as a barrier for infection that may occur from the adjacent lungs.[1]

Pericardial disease can be either acute or chronic in nature. Forms of acute pericardial disease include pericarditis and cardiac tamponade. Pericardial effusion and pericardial constriction are chronic forms of pericardial disease. These entities are discussed below.

PERICARDITIS

Pericarditis is an inflammation of the pericardial sac (Figure 75-1). The causes of acute pericarditis are many and varied as detailed below. The more common causes of pericarditis are listed in Box 75-1.

Pericarditis is more common in men than women and occurs most typically between the ages of 20 and 50 years. The causes of pericarditis are numerous, but viral illness is the most common cause.[2] Idiopathic pericarditis, relatively more common in developing countries, often turns out to be viral in cause.[3] In fact, the term idiopathic often is used interchangeably with viral pericarditis because of the frequency with which young individuals recover before identification of the virus. In immune-compromised patients, pericarditis can be relatively common.[4]

Viruses associated with pericarditis are listed in Box 75-2. Tuberculosis **(TB)** was once a common cause of acute infectious pericarditis before the discovery of antituberculosis drugs. Unfortunately, TB pericarditis is again on the rise as a complication of human autoimmune deficiency syndrome **(HIV-AIDS)**. Bacterial invasion of the pericardium also can occur as a result of trauma, such as a stab wound, endocarditis, pneumonia, sepsis, or contamination during thoracic or cardiac surgery. Common fungal infectious agents, listed in Box 75-2, are seen most often in the immunocompromised patient.[5]

Neoplasms are known to cause pericarditis, but primary neoplasms or tumors of the pericardium are rare. When they occur, they may be benign or malignant. Metastasis to the pericardium is usually secondary to lung or breast tumors or lymphoma.[6] Pericardial metastasis occurs in approximately 30 percent of lung cancers and is associated with hemorrhagic effusions, which can lead to cardiac tamponade.[4] Radiation therapy can also produce a local inflammatory response that results in an effusion and fibrosis. A cytology examination of the pericardial fluid is needed to distinguish radiation-induced versus tumor-induced pericarditis.

Pericarditis associated with chronic renal failure is referred to as uremic pericarditis. The cause of uremic pericarditis in chronic renal failure is unknown, but often develops in the early months after dialysis is initiated. Dialysis pericarditis is seen in end-stage renal disease **(ESRD)**. The incidence of dialysis pericarditis ranges from 2 percent to 21 percent.[4] It is important to note that patients with ESRD may have an underlying condition or receive medications that cause pericarditis.

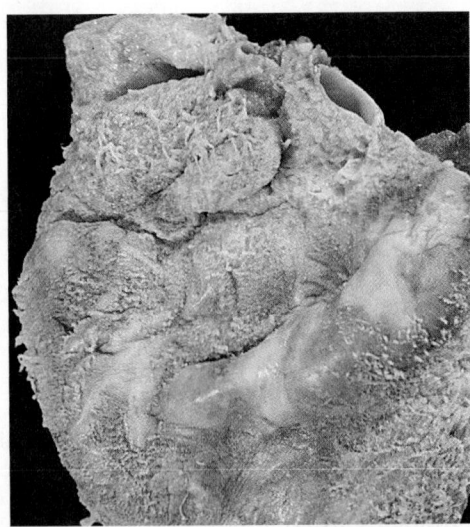

FIGURE 75-1 ■ Acute pericarditis. Note shaggy coat of fibers covering surface of heart. (From McCance KL, Huether SE: *Pathophysiology: The Biologic Basis for Disease in Adults and Children*, ed 5, St Louis, 2006, Mosby, Figure 30-27.)

BOX 75-1 ■■■
COMMON CAUSES OF PERICARDIAL DISEASES

- AMI
- Bacterial infection
- Chest trauma
- Idiopathic
- Medications
- Neoplasm
- Uremia and/or renal failure
- Viral infection

AMI, Acute myocardial infarction.

BOX 75-2 ■■■
COMMON VIRUSES AND FUNGI ASSOCIATED WITH PERICARDITIS

Fungi
- *Aspergillus*
- *Blastomyces*
- *Candida*
- *Histoplasma*

Viruses
- Coxsackie A or B
- Echovirus
- Hepatitis B
- Human immunodeficiency virus
- Influenza
- Mononucleosis
- Mumps
- Varicella

Pericarditis occurring within 2 to 7 days following acute myocardial infarction **(AMI)** is considered a pericardial inflammatory response to the underlying acute myocardial injury. Alternately, Dressler syndrome is thought to be an autoimmune response to myocardial necrosis involving both the pleura and the pericardium rather than an acute inflammatory response of the pericardium. Dressler syndrome can occur 2 weeks to several months following AMI.[6] A similar condition may develop following cardiac surgery-postcardiotomy pericarditis. Other autoimmune disorders, such as connec-

tive tissue diseases (i.e., systemic lupus erythematosus **[SLE]** and rheumatoid arthritis) also can produce inflammation of the pericardium. The autoimmune process involves SLE autoantibodies that engulf the pericardium, producing the inflammatory response.[7] Certain medications, such as procainamide (Pronestyl), hydralazine (Apresoline) and INH (isoniazid) may produce the symptoms of pericarditis seen in individuals with SLE or a lupus-like syndrome.

Clinical Presentation

Acute pericarditis can mimic AMI, with chest pain and ST-segment elevation. Distinguishing AMI and pericarditis involves careful assessment of the characteristic of the chest pain and the associated electrocardiographic **(ECG)** changes. Pericardial pain is pleuritic in nature; fever may be present or antecedent. Other symptoms include dyspnea, shortness of breath, cough, chills, and weakness.[5] Chest pain in pericarditis is often localized to the retrosternal area and the left precordium. It is typically a persistent, sharp, pleuritic type of stabbing pain that is aggravated by inspiration and coughing. With deep inspiration, the diaphragm pulls on the inflamed pericardium resulting in sharp stabbing pain radiating to the back and left trapezius muscle.[6] Relief is obtained by sitting upright and leaning forward. The pain is worse when recumbent.

Careful assessment of chest pain is essential when differentiating ischemic pain from nonischemic pain, to prevent missing AMI. To differentiate the pain of pericarditis from ischemic pain or pain of AMI, ask the patient to point to the exact location of the pain. With pericarditis, sharp, piercing pain often occurs in the area between the neck and shoulder. Dyspnea unrelated to exertion is another clinical finding in pericarditis. Instead of exertion, the dyspnea is most likely related to an inability to take deep breaths, giving the appearance of shortness of breath. True dyspnea and shortness of breath are more apparent in cardiac tamponade caused by pulmonary congestion, decreased cardiac compliance, and decreased tissue perfusion.[8]

A common physical finding in pericarditis is a pericardial friction rub. The rub is produced by the movement of the inflamed pericardial layers against one another and is best heard along the left lower sternal border (4th to 5th intercostal space) using the diaphragm of the stethoscope (see Chapter 45). Have the patient lean forward and exhale, which brings the pericardium closer to the chest wall. The rub has three components that correspond to the phases of greatest cardiac movement: ventricular contraction, ventricular relaxation, and atrial contraction.[5] Some components may be present without the others. Characteristically a pericardial friction rub is evanescent (i.e., heard only intermittently).

Diagnostic Tests

Diagnostic procedures for acute pericarditis include an ECG, chest radiography (chest x-ray), echocardiogram, and laboratory tests.

Electrocardiogram

The 12-lead ECG is the most definitive diagnostic test in acute pericarditis. It will often show diffuse ST-segment elevation in most leads except V_1 and AVR—not the localized and specific changes typical of AMI (see Chapter 47). In acute pericarditis, there are no reciprocal changes or T-wave inversion, as is typically seen in AMI. ECG changes involving the ST segment and T waves may occur in stages. During the first few days, the ST-segment changes are diffuse and have a concave appearance or "smiling face." These changes can last up to 2 weeks. The PR segment is depressed as a result of abnormal atrial depolarization resulting from inflammatory changes in the atrial wall.[9] The QRS may vary from beat to beat (electrical alternans), a phenomenon found typically in the presence of a sizeable pericardial effusion (Figure 75-2). Atrial dysrhythmias are common, with atrial fibrillation occurring in one third of patients with pericarditis.[10] These 12-lead ECG changes are not seen in all cases of acute pericarditis.

Chest Radiography

The chest x-ray is usually normal in patients with acute pericarditis. The cardiac silhouette may be enlarged (so called water bottle heart) if more than 250 ml of fluid is present.[11] However, in smaller accumulations, the heart silhouette appears normal. A pleural effusion may be associated with an underlying condition that causes pericarditis, such as SLE, chronic renal failure, infection, or lung cancer.[4]

Echocardiogram

The echocardiogram is usually normal in acute idiopathic pericarditis. An echocardiogram with Doppler studies is ordered to look for a pericardial effusion and to evaluate hemodynamic changes associated with cardiac tamponade (Figure 75-3). A transesophageal echocardiogram (**TEE**) is also helpful in evaluating the size of an effusion and whether ventricular filling is compromised.[12]

Laboratory Tests

Laboratory tests may reveal the cause of pericarditis or exclude other possible causes. Erythrocyte sedimentation rate (**ESR**) and complete blood count (**CBC**) may show nonspecific elevations. Blood chemistries, including liver function tests, prothrombin time (**PT**), and partial thromboplastin time (**PTT**) are useful. A cardiac profile that includes creatine kinase (**CK**), CK-MB, and troponin is useful to exclude AMI. Additional tests to discern the cause of pericarditis may include purified protein derivative (**PPD**) skin test for TB, HIV-AIDS screening, and rheumatoid factor and antinuclear antibodies to screen for connective tissue disorders. A computed tomography (**CT**) scan may be done to locate neoplastic lesions.

Clinical Management

The current treatment of choice for uncomplicated idiopathic pericarditis is nonsteroidal antiinflammatory agents (**NSAIDs**).[5] Indomethacin and colchicines were used extensively in the past, but NSAIDs are preferred now because of fewer side effects. Indomethacin and colchicines can be used in patients who cannot tolerate or are allergic (e.g., aspirin allergy) to NSAIDs. Some patients do not respond to NSAIDs and may require narcotic analgesia and/or a short course of corticosteroid therapy. For pericarditis after an AMI, however, corticosteroids and antiinflammatory agents should be avoided because they can cause rupture of the infarcted area. For recurrent or severe pain and connective tissue disorders, corticosteroids may be more effective. Colchicine has been shown to be effective in cases of recurrent pericarditis. If medications are the cause of the pericarditis, withdrawal of the medication is necessary. Therapy is directed at the underlying cause, if known.[6]

The vast majority of idiopathic pericarditis cases are uncomplicated. In those patients in whom complications occur, pericardial effusion, tamponade, and constrictive pericarditis can result.

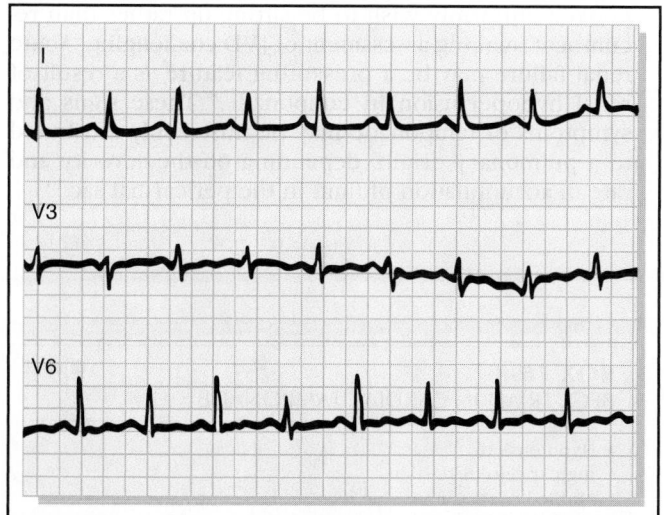

FIGURE 75-2 ■ Illustration of electrical alternans seen in a constrictive state showing alternans of the QRS complex. (From Zipes DP, Libby P, Bonow R et al: *Braunwald's heart disease,* ed 7, Philadelphia, 2005, Elsevier Saunders, p 1765, Figure 64-7.)

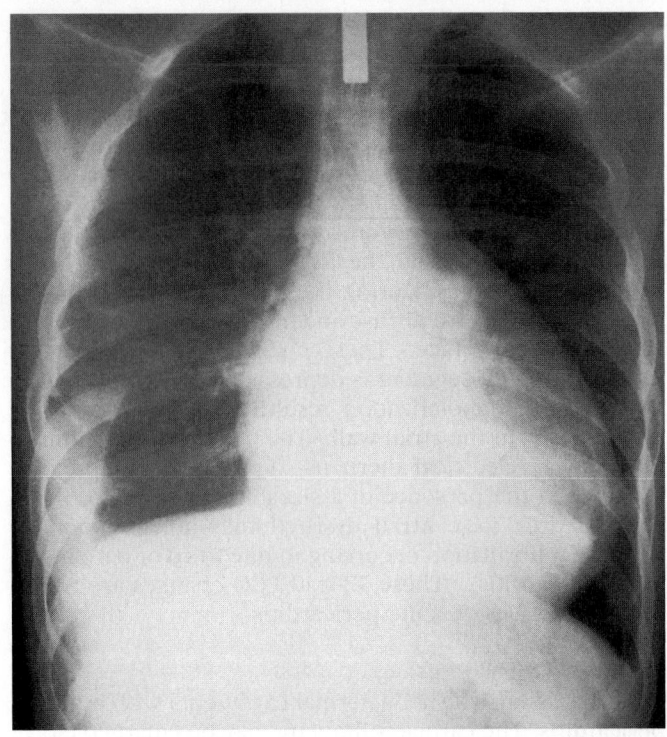

FIGURE 75-3 ■ Anteroposterior chest radiograph of a patient with a large pericardial effusion. (From Zipes DP, Libby P, Bonow R et al: *Braunwald's heart disease,* ed 7, Philadelphia, 2005, Elsevier Saunders, p 1766, Figure 64-8.)

PERICARDIAL EFFUSION AND TAMPONADE

Pericardial effusion is the accumulation of excessive fluid in the pericardial space. The pericardial sac normally holds 15 to 50 ml of fluid, but large volumes of fluid can be accommodated by the pericardium if the rate of accumulation is slow, allowing the pericardium adequate time to stretch. The rapid accumulation of pericardial fluid or buildup of a volume of pericardial fluid exceeding the pericardium's ability to expand will lead to tamponade, which compromises ventricular filling and causes a fall in cardiac output. A sudden increase of as little as 100 to 200 ml in the volume of pericardial fluid can elevate the pericardial pressure from a normal pressure of 1 to 5 mm Hg to 30 mm Hg or more. A rise of this amount reflects severe cardiac tamponade.[13]

There are many different causes of pericardial effusion, most of which are the initial causes of pericarditis (e.g., idiopathic, inflammatory, and infectious processes). Noninfectious causes include cancer, autoimmune diseases, AMI, coronary artery bypass surgery, radiation, drugs, chronic renal failure on dialysis, and hypothyroidism.[14] Heart failure also can cause small or moderate sized effusions. Other causes include blunt or penetrating chest trauma, retrograde extension of aortic dissection, and iatrogenic factors. Iatrogenic causes of pericardial effusion include complications of coronary angioplasty, venous line placement (e.g., central venous catheter), and transvenous pacemaker insertion.

Clinical Presentation

Pericardial effusions that occur slowly over time allow for a gradual stretching of the pericardium. This gradual process does not compromise ventricular filling and will thus be asymptomatic. A slowly developing effusion can remain undetected until signs and symptoms of cardiac tamponade occur.

Symptoms of pericardial effusion with tamponade include: dyspnea, dizziness, lightheadedness, weakness, and retrosternal chest pain. Signs of ensuing tamponade include tachypnea, tachycardia, cool extremities, hypotension, jugular venous distention **(JVD),** muffled heart sounds—the latter three known as Beck triad (Box 75-3). Kussmaul sign, increased central venous pressure with inspiration, is absent in tamponade. Pulsus paradoxus—a decrease of more than 10 mm Hg in systolic BP with inspiration—is usually present in tamponade (Figure 75-4).

Although the *y* descent in the jugular venous pulse is classically absent in tamponade, jugular waveforms are often difficult to discern in the tachycardic patient with imminent tamponade. Additionally, patients with tamponade uniformly wish to be sitting up rather than recumbent, making assessment of JVD challenging. Acute renal failure may be a presenting feature as a result of renal hypoperfusion in tamponade.[8] These signs and symptoms of tamponade may be mistakenly attributed to a pulmonary origin, depending on the severity and rate of accumulation of fluid in the pericardial sac.[10]

BOX 75-3 ■ ■ ■
BECK TRIAD IN CARDIAC TAMPONADE

- Hypotension
- Jugular vein distension
- Muffled heart sounds

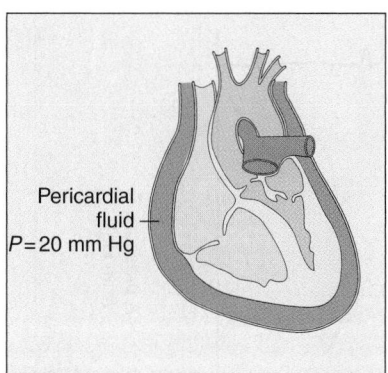

FIGURE 75-4 ■ Schematic illustration of leftward septal shift that encroaches on the left ventricular volume during inspiration (pulsus paradoxus) in cardiac tamponade. (From Zipes DP, Libby P, Bonow R et al: *Braunwald's heart disease,* ed 7, Philadelphia, 2005, Elsevier Saunders, p 1764, Figure 64-6A.)

Diagnostic Tests

Chest x-ray and ECG may reveal initial abnormalities prompting further testing. An enlarged, rounded cardiac silhouette on chest x-ray is consistent with an effusion. ECG changes may include tachycardia, premature ventricular contractions, and electrical alternans, a pattern of alternating amplitude of the P wave and QRS complex with every other heartbeat, caused by the heart swinging anteriorly and posteriorly in a large effusion. A definitive diagnosis of an effusion can be made with a two-dimensional echocardiogram, CT, or MRI.[10]

One of the echocardiographic findings diagnostic for tamponade is a leftward shift of the septum with inspiration—the occurrence of which limits left ventricular filling and subsequent cardiac output (see Figure 75-4). A Swan Ganz catheter will provide evidence of abnormally equalized right atrial **(RA)** pressure, right ventricular end-diastolic **(RVED)** pressure, and pulmonary artery wedge pressure **(PAWP)**.[15] In addition, in tamponade the RA pressure will show the absence of a *y* descent. The *y* descent normally occurs with a drop in RA pressure with tricuspid valve opening. In tamponade the rapid flow into the right ventricle does not occur.

Clinical Management

Patients with an effusion in whom tamponade is of concern are admitted to an intensive care unit for close monitoring. Vital signs are watched closely to detect early signs of cardiac tamponade. Physical assessment of the patient, looking for the distinctive changes in signs and symptoms detailed above, is critical in the detection of impending cardiac tamponade. Any decompensation in hemodynamic status must be reported immediately. A fall in blood pressure or cardiac output in the setting of pericardial effusion when impending tamponade is suspected is grounds for emergent pericardiocentesis.[8,16]

For a patient with tamponade or impending tamponade, a closed pericardiocentesis is the intervention of choice. This procedure is performed in intensive care or the cardiac catheterization laboratory following a two-dimensional echocardiogram to assess the size of the effusion. A moderate sized effusion provides an adequate target that minimizes the risk of a procedural complication. A subxiphoid pericardiocentesis can be performed quite safely in experienced hands. After removal of the effusion, hemodynamic recovery of the patient is both immediate and dramatic (Figure 75-5, *A* and *B*).

For patients with stable, chronic effusions, diagnostic closed pericardiocentesis may be done electively. Although assessment of pericardial fluid rarely provides a diagnosis, it is reasonable to obtain a sample from patients in whom the diagnosis remains unclear. In some situations, analysis is beneficial—occult infection, neoplastic implants in the pericardium, and TB. Tuberculous pericarditis is notoriously difficult to diagnose even with multiple pericardial biopsies. Analysis of pericardial fluid for adenosine deaminase levels is most helpful in diagnosing TB pericarditis, which was quite rare before the advent of HIV-AIDS.

Patients with chronic and/or recurrent effusions progress to tamponade in greater numbers than previously thought. Surgical (open) pericardiocentesis, with the creation of a pericardial window to chronically drain the pericardium into the left pleural space, is the preferred therapy for these patients. Surgical pericardiocentesis is also preferred for patients with loculated effusions that are not accessible by closed technique and to obtain samples of pericardium in patients for whom no diagnosis has been identified. Other options, at some centers, are creation of a window using thoracoscopy and percutaneous balloon dilatation of a pericardial window.

CONSTRICTIVE PERICARDITIS

Another complication of pericardial disease is constrictive pericarditis (Figure 75-6). It is important to recognize this form of pericarditis because it may be correctable if treated early. The challenge with constrictive pericarditis is that it can mimic common disorders that produce symptoms of right-sided heart failure, such as restrictive cardiomyopathy, pulmonary embolism, pulmonary hypertension, right ventricular infarction, mitral stenosis, and left ventricular systolic dysfunction.[17]

TB that led to calcification of the pericardium was the major cause of constrictive pericarditis in the early twentieth century. Now the most common cause is idiopathic.[18] Radiation therapy and open heart surgery are also frequent causes.

Constrictive pericarditis causes fibrosis and calcification of the pericardium, which inhibit normal ventricular filling while systolic contraction of the ventricles remains normal.[19] Pericardial scarring usually occurs over a period of years. Classically, the pericardial scarring is uniform involving all chambers of the heart. The restricted filling leads to equal and elevated pressures in all chambers. As blood flows from the right atrium to the right ventricle during diastole, the right ventricle expands and quickly reaches the limit imposed by the rigid, constricting pericardium. The ventricle is now unable to fill further, resulting in an increase in systemic venous pressure and signs and symptoms of right heart failure. Decreased left ventricular filling decreases stroke volume and cardiac

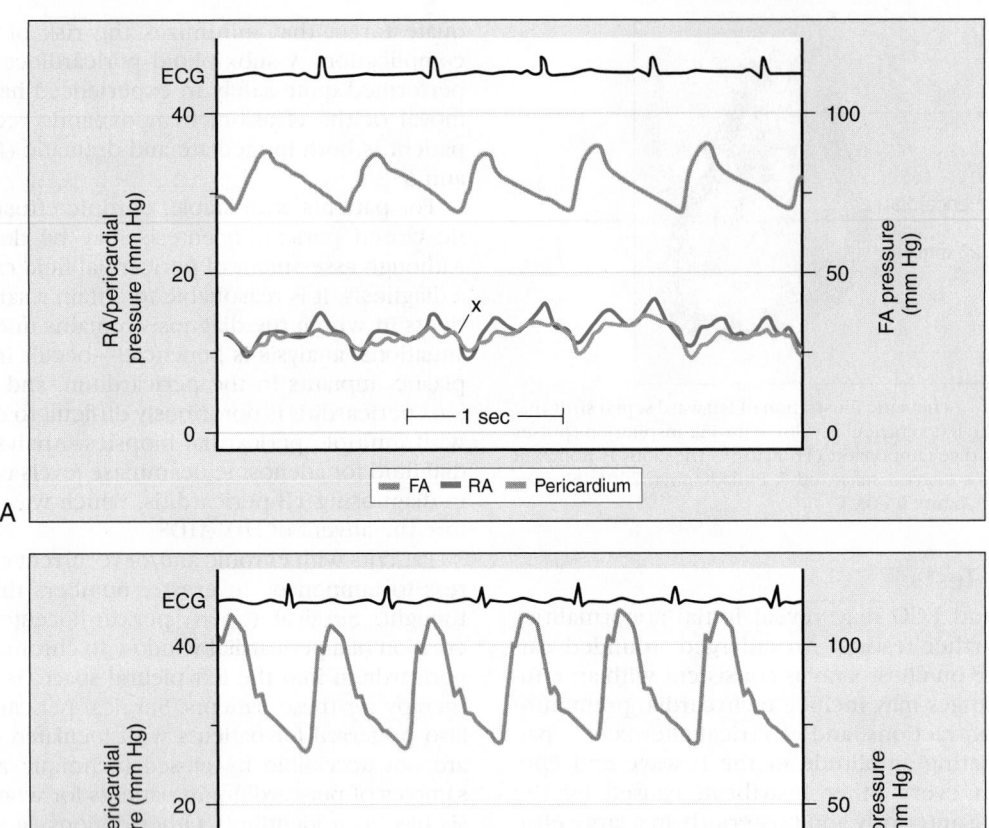

FIGURE 75-5 ■ Femoral arterial (FA), RA, and pericardial pressure before **(A)** and after **(B)** pericardiocentesis in a patient with cardiac tamponade. Both RA and pericardial pressure are about 15 mm Hg before pericardiocentesis. In this case, there was a negligible paradoxical pulse. Note presence of *x* descent but absence of *y* descent before pericardiocentesis. Pericardiocentesis results in a marked increase in FA pressure and marked decrease in RA pressure. During inspiration pericardial pressure becomes negative, there is clear separation between RA and pericardial pressure, and *y* descent is now evident and prominent, suggesting the possibility of an effusive-constrictive picture. (From Zipes DP, Libby P, Bonow R et al: *Braunwald's heart disease,* ed 7, Philadelphia, 2005, Elsevier Saunders, p 1764, Figure 64-5, *A* and *B*).

output, which leads to hypotension—similar to that seen with restrictive cardiomyopathy (see Chapter 72).[20] The differentiation between these two maladies can be very difficult, but is exceedingly important in that the treatments are quite different.

Clinical Presentation

Constrictive pericarditis can take months or years to develop. Early in the course of the disease, patients manifest signs and symptoms of right heart failure—often severe. Subsequently, they may develop signs and symptoms of left heart failure. At end stage, these patients develop cardiac cachexia with weakness, fatigue, and tissue wasting.[21]

Pertinent physical findings in constrictive pericarditis include significantly increased JVD; often Kussmaul sign, a paradoxical (jugular veins normally collapse during inspiration) increase in JVD during inspiration; and a prominent *y* descent in the jugular waveforms.[22] Lung sounds may be clear despite the presence of JVD and peripheral edema.

In contrast to the muffled heart sounds heard in cardiac tamponade, an early diastolic filling sound may be heard in constrictive pericarditis, known as a "pericardial knock." A pericardial knock is a high-pitched, sharp sound heard early in diastole at the 4th or 5th intercostal space along the left sternal border or at the apex of the heart with the patient leaning forward. The knock occurs as a result of a constrictive pericardium abruptly

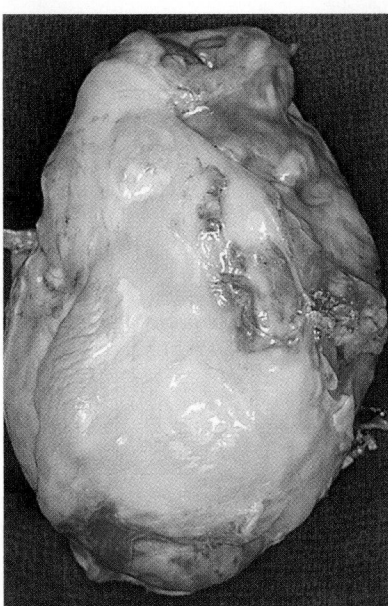

FIGURE 75-6 ■ Constrictive pericarditis. The fibrotic pericardium encases the heart in a rigid shell. (From McCance KL, Huether SE: *Pathophysiology: the biologic basis for disease in adults and children*, ed 5, St Louis, 2006, Mosby, Figure 30-28.)

limiting early rapid filling of the ventricle.[19] These signs and symptoms—except for the pericardial knock—may be mistaken for restrictive cardiomyopathy.

Diagnostic Tests

Chest X-ray may show a calcified pericardium and often RA enlargement. ECG findings of low voltage and sometimes atrial fibrillation are nonspecific. The echocardiogram may be helpful in revealing pericardial thickening, "septal bounce" during diastole, and septal shifting with inspiration.

CT is better than MRI in providing excellent resolution of the pericardium, which can detect a thickened pericardium (more than 2 mm) quite accurately. However, 20 percent of patients exhibit no signs of a thickened pericardium.[17] Cardiac catheterization may yield similar findings in both constrictive pericarditis and restrictive cardiomyopathy. Diastolic pressures in all chambers are usually equalized. Rapid *y* descent of early diastole with a rapid upswing and plateau yields the classic "square root sign," which can be present in both diseases.

One distinguishing feature of constrictive pericarditis is a pulmonary artery pressure (PAP) *greater than* 50 mm Hg on cardiac catheterization. This finding can support the diagnosis of constrictive pericarditis. Endomyocardial biopsy is most useful and may be performed to distinguish between constrictive pericarditis and restrictive cardiomyopathy. The only clinical or diagnostic findings that help to differentiate these two maladies are the following: pericardial knock in constrictive pericarditis, PAP *greater than* 60 mm Hg in restrictive cardiomyopathy, and the "septal bounce" on echocardiogram in constrictive pericarditis.

Clinical Management

Clinical management of constrictive pericarditis includes monitoring of vital signs and managing symptoms of the disease process. Early conservative management with diuretics alleviates symptoms of volume overload. Many of these patients will develop atrial fibrillation, and digoxin is appropriate for rate control. Beta blockers and calcium channel blockers should not be used in these patients because they slow the heart rate and may interfere with the compensatory tachycardia.[18]

Surgical treatment is the only effective treatment of constrictive pericarditis. A complete resection of the pericardium is performed via a median sternotomy, often without cardiopulmonary bypass. The earlier in the disease process surgical intervention is accomplished, the less ill the patient and the better the outcome. Late in the disease, removal of the pericardium may be of little benefit to a patient who is now critically ill and wasted.

CONCLUSION

Pericardial disease is typically uncomplicated and self-limiting. This is not to suggest, however, that this is a benign group of cardiovascular diseases. A minority of cases can be life threatening and must be treated expeditiously. Those conditions known to cause pericarditis must be monitored so that an early effusion is detected before it deteriorates into tamponade. Careful monitoring is a skill of the expert cardiovascular nurse that is essential to successful management of pericardial disease.

REFERENCES

1. Lilly LS: *Pathophysiology of heart disease*, Philadelphia, 2003, Lippincott Williams and Wilkins.
2. Soler-Soler J: Pericardial disease: introduction, *Heart* 90:251, 2004.
3. Permanyer-Miraldo G: Acute pericardial disease: approach to the aetiologic diagnosis, *Heart* 90:252-254, 2004.
4. Gentlesk PJ: Acute pericarditis, Retrieved April 1, 2004, from www.emedicine.com/med/topic1781.htm.
5. Goyle KK, Walling AD: Diagnosing pericarditis, *Amer Fam Physician* 66:1695-1702, 2002.
6. Spodick DH: Acute pericarditis: current concepts and practice, *JAMA* 289:1150-1153, 2003.
7. Weich HS, Burgess LJ, Reuter H et al: Large pericardial effusions due to systemic lupus erythematosus: a report of eight cases, *Lupus* 4:450-457, 2005.
8. Spodick DH: Current concepts: acute cardiac tamponade, *N Engl J Med* 349: 684-690, 2003.
9. Brady WJ: Electrocardiographic diagnosis: specific clinical syndromes, Retrieved April 12, 2004 from www.thrombosis-consult.com/articles/Textbook/58_ECG2.htm.
10. Gollapudi RR, Yeager M, Johnson AD: Left ventricular cardiac tamponade in the setting of cor pulmonale and circumferential pericardial effusion. Case report and review of the literature, *Cardiol Rev* 13:214-217, 2005.
11. Parnaet S: Pericarditis, *JAMA* 289:1194, 2003.
12. Maisch B, Ristic AD: Practical aspects of the management of pericardial disease, *BMJ Heart* 89:1096-1103, 2003.
13. Shabeti R: Pericardial effusion: haemodynamic spectrum, *Heart* 90:255-256, 2004.

14. Levy P, Corey R, Berger P et al: Etiologic diagnosis of 204 pericardial effusions, *Medicine* 82:385-391, 2003.

15. Hancock EW: A clearer view of effusive-constrictive pericarditis, *N Engl J Med* 350:435-437, 2004.

16. Hoit B: Management of effusive and constrictive pericardial heart disease, *Circulation* 105:2939-2942, 2002.

17. Nishimura, RA: Constrictive pericarditis in the modern era: a diagnostic dilemma, *BMJ Heart* 86:619-623, 2001.

18. Saad BE: Constrictive pericarditis, Retrieved March 13, 2005, from www.medstudents.com.br/cardio/cardio6.htm.

19. Skubas NJ, Beardslee M, Barzilai B et al: Constrictive pericarditis: intraoperative hemodynamic and echocardiographic evaluation of cardiac filling dynamics, *Anesthesia Analgesia* 92:1424-1426, 2001.

20. Hancock EW: Differential diagnosis of restrictive cardiomyopathy and constrictive pericarditis, *BMJ Heart* 86:343-349, 2001.

21. Anker SD et al: Cardiac cachexia, Retrieved May 5, 2005 from www.ncbi.nlm.nih.gov/entrez/query.

22. Silver MD, Gotlieb AI, Schoen FJ: The pericardium and its diseases, *Cardiovascular pathology,* Philadelphia, 2001, Churchill Livingstone.

Care of Patients with Stroke

Anne Leonard

CHAPTER ABBREVIATIONS

ABC airway, breathing, circulation assessment

aPTT activated partial thromboplastin time

ATP adenosine triphosphate

CBF cerebral blood flow

CN cranial nerve

CT computed tomography

DVT deep vein thrombosis

ED emergency department

EVD endoventricular device

ICH intracerebral hemorrhage

INR international normalized ratio

JCAHO Joint Commission on Accreditation of Healthcare Organizations

MERCI mechanical embolus removal in cerebral ischemia

MRI magnetic resonance imaging

NIHSS National Institute of Health Stroke Scale

NPO nothing by mouth

PT prothrombin time

rt-PA recombinant tissue plasminogen activator

SAH subarachnoid hemorrhage

TIA transient ischemic attack

UTI urinary tract infection

Stroke should be assessed and treated as a life-threatening emergency. Optimal early treatment of acute stroke improves long-term outcome and reduces death and disability.[1,2] Systematic and informed nursing care is an important factor both for patient survival and for favorable short- and long-term outcomes. Nursing care is the foundation of all care provided by the multidisciplinary team to the stroke patient. Positive patient outcomes depend on basic knowledge of stroke, interaction with the multidisciplinary team, and excellent execution of comprehensive nursing care.

EPIDEMIOLOGY OF STROKE

Stroke is a major public health problem. It is the third leading cause of death in the United States and the most frequent cause of adult disability. Many people who survive stroke are cared for in long-term care facilities.[3] More than 700,000 strokes occur each year in the United States; 500,000 of which are new strokes and 200,000 of which are recurrent. There are more than 4 million stroke survivors.[3] The cost of stroke is estimated at about $58 billion annually, accounting for both direct costs (hospitalization, rehabilitation) and indirect costs (lost job/wages, long-term care).

Stroke is particularly common in African Americans. African American men and women not only have higher stroke rates but also a higher death rate from stroke compared to whites. The prevalence of stroke is highest in the southeastern United States, an area dubbed "the stroke belt." The stroke belt comprises about 13 southern states.

Stroke Risk Factors

Risk factors for stroke have been classified as non-modifiable or modifiable. Non-modifiable risk factors include age, gender, race/ethnicity, personal or family history of stroke, and genetic factors. Modifiable risk factors include hypertension, diabetes, smoking, alcohol use, obesity and sedentary lifestyle, carotid stenosis, heart disease (such as atrial fibrillation), hyperlipidemia, oral contraceptive use, and illicit drug use/abuse (such as cocaine). Patient and family education should focus on prevention of stroke by modifying risk factors. Strict control of modifiable risk factors prevents initial and recurrent stroke.

Most strokes can be prevented by controlling major risk factors, such as hypertension, which is the number one risk factor for stroke because of its high prevalence in the general population. Moreover, once someone has a stroke they have a 10-fold increased risk of having another stroke, making secondary prevention an important long-term goal. Public health education should focus on public awareness of what a stroke is, prevention, signs and symptoms of stroke, and what to do if stroke is suspected.[4]

TYPES OF STROKE

Stroke is a syndrome with many different causes. Strokes are classified as either ischemic (due to cerebrovascular occlusive disease) or hemorrhagic (due to ruptured blood vessels in the brain). Approximately 85 percent of all strokes are ischemic (Figure 76-1). Of these, about 20 percent are caused by cerebral vascular atherosclerosis (large-artery atherosclerosis such as of the major extracranial and intracranial arteries), while 20 percent are caused by cardiogenic embolism (i.e., emboli from the left atrium in non-valvular atrial fibrillation, myocardial infarction, prosthetic heart valves). About 25 percent of ischemic strokes are caused by small-artery occlusive disease, which results in subcortical lacunar strokes, and about 30 percent are cryptogenic (nonspecific, etiology unknown). The remaining 5 percent are due to uncommon etiologies, for example, dissections, vasculi-

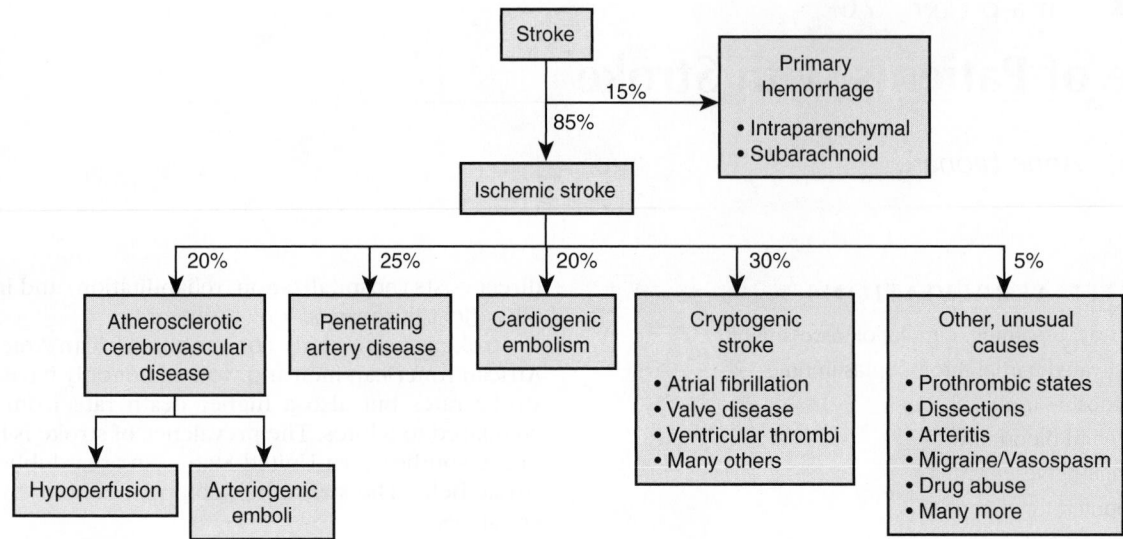

FIGURE 76-1 ▒ Ischemic and hemorrhagic stroke subtypes.

tis, prothrombotic states, migraine/vasospasm, and drug abuse.

Hemorrhagic stroke accounts for about 15 percent of all strokes. The two most common types are primary intraparenchymal hemorrhage (usually due to uncontrolled hypertension) and subarachnoid hemorrhage (most often secondary to ruptured aneurysms). Of the hemorrhagic strokes, about 10 percent are caused by intracerebral hemorrhage and about 5 percent are caused by subarachnoid hemorrhage.

Pathophysiology of Cell Death

Stroke occurs when the blood supply to the brain is disturbed by occlusion of a cerebral blood vessel or rupture with hemorrhage. Brain cells survive only about 3 to 4 minutes when totally deprived of blood and oxygen. Normal cerebral blood flow **(CBF)** is approximately 50 ml/100 g/minute. When CBF drops to 25 ml/100 g/minute, neurons become electrically silent but remain potentially viable for several hours. This region of the brain is known as the *ischemic penumbra*. The ischemic penumbra is the area of interest during reperfusion (rescue) therapy with tissue plasminogen activator. Reperfusion of the ischemic penumbra may prevent extension of the area of infarct, thus potentially decreasing the final neurological disability. If CBF falls below the critical level of 10 ml/100 g/minute, irreversible brain cell damage occurs. A cascade of metabolic and chemical disturbances follow; including lactic acidosis, glutamate release, depletion of adenosine triphosphate **(ATP),** and the entry of sodium and calcium into the cells, leading to cytotoxic edema and mitochondrial failure.

Large-Artery Atherosclerosis

Large-artery atherosclerosis usually involves diseases of the carotid artery.[5,6] These atherosclerotic plaques produce symptoms by embolization superimposed on an unstable plaque or from a flow-restricted stenosis or occlusion. The most common sites of carotid occlusion are the carotid bifurcation or the internal carotid artery. An embolus may occur when the plaque fractures, breaks off, and travels to the brain. This is sometimes referred to as *artery-to-artery embolus*. When a high-grade stenosis occurs, blood flow can be greatly reduced or flow can be shut off completely, causing stroke (Figure 76-2). Hypertension, diabetes, smoking, and possibly hyperlipidemia are risk factors for this type of stroke.

Cardioembolic Stroke

Atrial fibrillation, rheumatic heart disease, acute myocardial infarction, endocarditis, mitral valve stenosis, and prosthetic heart valves are the most common causes of cardioembolic stroke (Figure 76-3).[5,6] Non-valvular atrial fibrillation is by far the most frequent cause of cardioembolic stroke (also called *cardiogenic stroke*). Non-valvular atrial fibrillation is the most common dysrhythmia in persons age 65 and older. Stroke from an embolic source typically is associated with very large infarcts (Figure 76-4). Hemorrhagic transformation (also called *hemorrhagic conversion*) is common in cardioembolic strokes. The presumed mechanism is lysis of the embolus, with reperfusion of ischemic tissue, which becomes hemorrhagic depending on the extent of vascular ischemic injury. Hemorrhagic transformation may be asymptomatic or symptomatic with worsening of neurologic function. Clinicians may delay the use of antithrombotic therapies, especially warfarin, in persons suspected of having cardioembolic stroke, in an effort to prevent hemorrhagic conversion. Usually, patients will go home from the hospital on an appropriate antithrombotic therapy. In cases of a cardiac abnormality causing cardioembolic stroke, it is important to treat the underlying cardiac problem as well as the neurological problem. Treatment for secondary prevention depends on the specific cardiac source of stroke.

Lacunar or Subcortical Stroke

Chronic hypertension and diabetes cause lipohyalinosis of the very small cerebral arteries in the deep subcortical structures of the brain. Characteristic locations of

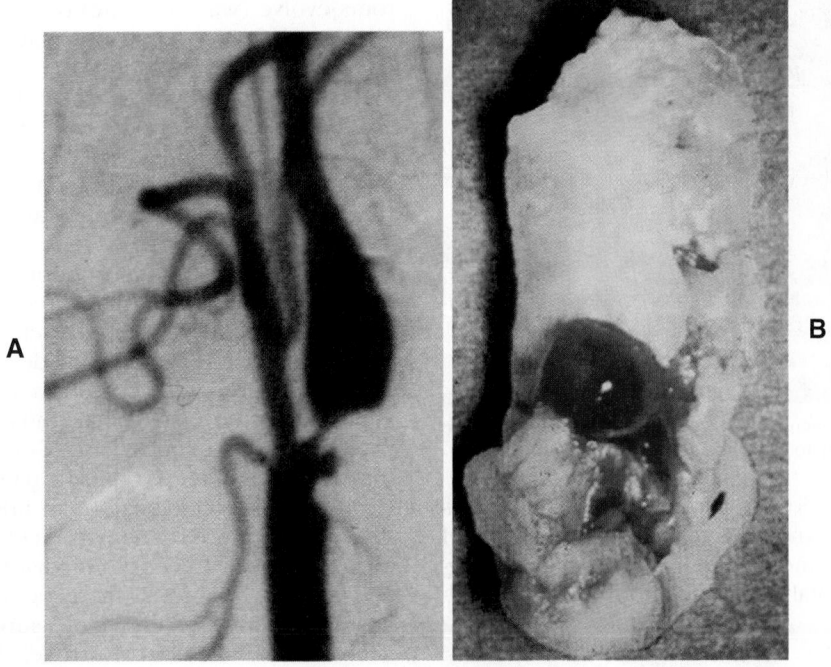

FIGURE 76-2 ■ **A,** High-grade internal carotid artery stenosis with ulceration. **B,** Neuropathological specimen of a carotid artery plaque with thrombus.

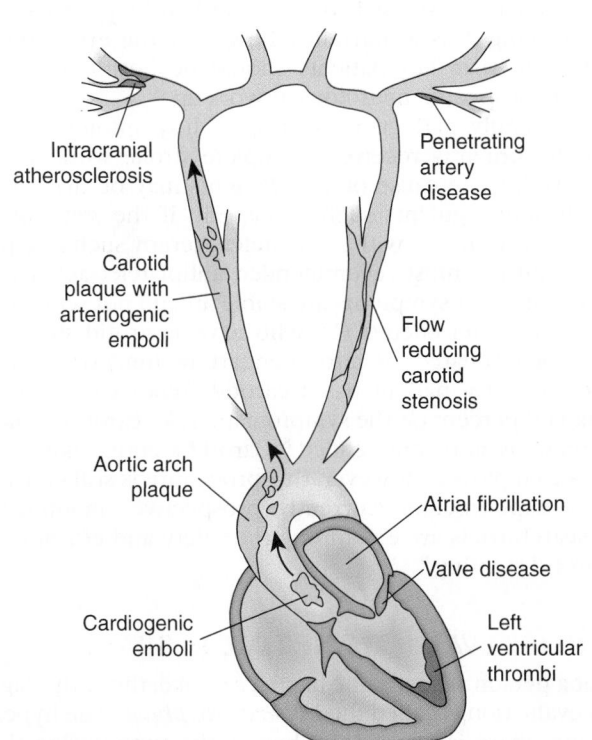

FIGURE 76-3 ■ Common sites of arterial and cardiac abnormalities that cause ischemic stroke.

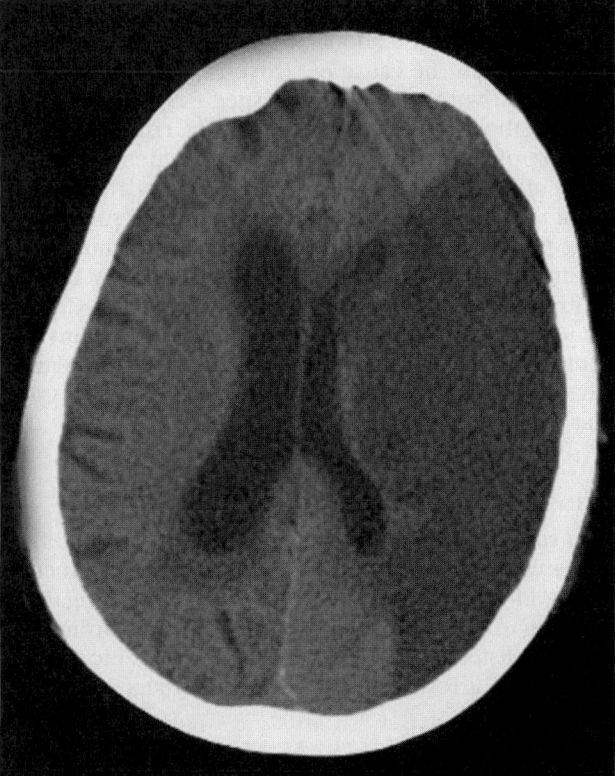

FIGURE 76-4 ■ CT scan of left middle cerebral artery stroke caused by either artheriogenic emboli or a cardioembolic source.

lacunar infarcts are the basal ganglia, subcortical white matter, thalamus, cerebellum, and brain stem.[5,6] Lacunar strokes are also known as *small vessel strokes* because they are caused by occlusive small vessel disease. The recurrence rate of these strokes is about 10- to 12-fold compared to other stroke types (Figure 76-5). This

type of stroke can cause not only physical impairment but also cognitive impairment (i.e., vascular dementia). It is common for persons with lacunar stroke to experience several small strokes, which can lead to cognitive decline and dementia over time. Antiplatelet therapies should be instituted, unless contraindicated, for second-

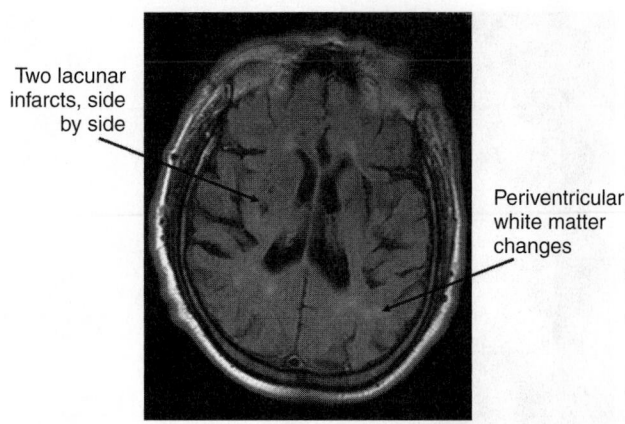

Two lacunar infarcts, side by side

Periventricular white matter changes

FIGURE 76-5 ■ Right lacunar infarct with periventricular white matter changes, secondary to uncontrolled hypertension.

ary prevention in addition to strict control of risk factors such as hypertension and diabetes. Aspirin, clopidogrel (Plavix), and dipyridamole combined with aspirin (Aggrenox) are all acceptable antithrombotics for secondary prevention.

Cryptogenic Stroke

The term *cryptogenic stroke* designates an ischemic stroke for which the cause is unknown.[5,6] Cryptogenic stroke accounts for about 30 percent of all ischemic strokes. When the cause of stroke is unknown, that is, the stroke work-up reveals no specific cause (such as cardioembolism) or the patient has no risk factors per se for stroke, the cause is cryptogenic. Often, when the cause of stroke is unknown, the stroke work-up will include tests for lower probability conditions, such as genetic prothrombotic states. This work-up might include testing for antiphospholipid antibodies, factor V Leiden, antithrombin III, protein C and S deficiency. Cryptogenic strokes can be most frustrating for clinicians, patient, and family. Prevention modalities are similar to what would be recommended for other stroke types, that is, use of antithrombotic therapy.

Unusual Causes of Stroke

This designation encompasses about 5 percent of all ischemic strokes.[5,6] These causes of stroke are uncommon and include oral contraceptive use and cigarette smoking, migraine headache, vasculitis, prothrombotic states (as listed in the section under cryptogenic stroke), dissections, arteritis, drug abuse, and others.

DEFINING STROKE AND TRANSIENT ISCHEMIC ATTACK

The hallmark of stroke is the sudden onset of focal, nonconvulsive neurological symptoms associated with interruption of blood flow to the brain (due to either a blockage of flow or hemorrhage). Ischemic stroke is also called *cerebral infarction,* or death of a focal area of brain tissue due to low blood flow. Stroke patients can present with maximal focal neurological deficits or with stroke in evolution or progression, where symptoms evolve (wax or wane) over several hours. Generally, the definition of stroke includes neurological deficits lasting 24 hours or longer.

Transient ischemic attacks **(TIAs)** are common and are defined as a focal neurological deficit lasting 24 hours or less (although most TIAs last less than 5 to 10 minutes). It has been proposed that this outdated definition be changed to a focal neurological deficit lasting 1 hour or less.[4]

Many persons with TIA go on to have a stroke with permanent deficits. In the United States, approximately 5 percent of persons who presented to the emergency room with a TIA went on to develop a stroke within 2 days; 10 percent did so within 90 days.[3] Symptoms of a TIA are often exactly like those of stroke. Unfortunately, persons experiencing TIAs often ignore symptoms because they are typically painless and short-lived. Health care professionals may miss the symptoms of TIA and therefore do not treat TIA as a potentially serious problem that needs immediate attention.

TIAs are important to recognize because, if diagnosed properly, preventive measures can be initiated to decrease the chance of stroke. TIAs are commonly caused by stenosis of the large arteries in the anterior circulation, the carotid arteries. TIAs can present as transient monocular blindness where a transient occlusion of the central retinal artery has occurred. Transient monocular blindness is often described by patients experiencing it as a "curtain falling over the eye." Some advocate that TIA patients should be hospitalized to initiate a specific neurological work-up.

Generally, patients presenting with symptoms of TIA should urgently receive a complete stroke work-up to determine the cause of TIA. Patients may be managed with anticoagulants such as heparin if the symptoms wax and wane, or with antiplatelet therapy such as aspirin (still the most recommended antiplatelet agent for prevention) if symptoms are stable and do not reoccur.[7] Persons experiencing TIA who have a carotid stenosis may be evaluated for carotid endarterectomy or carotid stenting. If a patient has a carotid stenosis of greater than 69 percent on the symptomatic side, carotid endarterectomy is recommended.[8] Carotid stenting is sometimes employed, however, this procedure is still considered experimental. Currently, prospective randomized research trials are examining the safety and efficacy of carotid stenting.[9]

INITIAL EVALUATION: TIME IS BRAIN

For a person who may be having a stroke, the early stage of evaluation is called the *hyperacute phase.* The hyperacute phase is often described as the time during the pre-hospital initiation of 911 after the onset of stroke symptoms through the time the patient is being cared for in the emergency department **(ED).** This phase consists of:

- Rapid assessment of the patient to make the diagnosis of acute stroke.
- Stabilization of the patient with initiation of the ABCs (assessment of airway, breathing, circulation) of emergency care.

- Initiation of crucial testing to determine eligibility for thrombolytic therapy.
- Rapid action to meet recommended time parameters for administration of thrombolysis within the 3-hour time window (Box 76-1).

The most important early step in evaluating a person with acute neurological changes suggestive of stroke is to rule out hemorrhagic stroke. The following assessments are done in the emergency room:

- Neurological exam, including mental status testing (level of consciousness and cognition), cranial nerve function, motor strength, sensory function, language, neglect (or hemi-inattention), coordination, and deep tendon reflexes
- Emergent computed tomography (CT) scan without contrast (magnetic resonance imaging [MRI] is sometimes done but is not the gold standard for ruling out intracerebral hemorrhage)
- 12-lead electrocardiogram
- Chest x-ray
- National Institutes of Health Stroke Scale (NIHSS)
- Review of time of onset and inclusion criteria to determine patient eligibility for recombinant tissue plasminogen activator (rt-PA)
- Maintaining systolic blood pressure equal to or less than 220 mm/Hg systolic and equal to or less than 110 mm/Hg diastolic if the patient is not a thrombolysis candidate. If a thrombolysis candidate, maintaining blood pressure less than 185 mm/Hg systolic and less than 110 mm/Hg diastolic.
- Emergent laboratory work:
  - Complete blood count (red blood cells, hemoglobin, hematocrit) with platelet count
  - Coagulation studies—prothrombin time/international normalized ratio, activated partial thromboplastin time (fibrinogen may be ordered)
  - Serum electrolytes (including renal function tests) and glucose
  - Troponin or creatine kinase CK/MB (per a cardiac protocol)
  - Urinalysis
  - Illicit drug screen (especially for patients who are unresponsive)
- Cervical films ruling out trauma (as clinically indicated)

Following this initial evaluation, other diagnostic tests may be done as indicated in Box 76-2.[1,6]

BOX 76-2
OTHER POSSIBLE TESTS AFTER INITIAL EVALUATION

- Magnetic resonance imaging with diffusion and perfusion images (sensitive to the presence and extent of ischemia)
- Transthoracic echocardiography, to screen for cardiac abnormalities suggestive of a cardioembolic source of stroke
- Arteriography, magnetic resonance imaging or computed tomographic angiography (demonstrates stenosis, occlusion, ulcerated plaques, thrombus, dissections, multiple lesions, aneurysms, arterial-venous malformations, collateral blood flow)
- Digital subtraction angiography (detects occlusion or stenosis of the extracranial [carotid, vertebral] and intracranial arteries)
- Transcranial Doppler imaging (middle cerebral artery stenosis or occlusion)
- Carotid ultrasound studies (imaging for carotid artery stenosis or occlusion)
- Transesophageal echocardiogram, especially if transthoracic echocardiography suggests a possible cardiac source of stroke
- Fasting lipid profile (done after admission to the hospital)
- Other tests for unusual causes of stroke may include: protein C or S, antithrombin III, factor IV Leiden, lupus anticoagulant (these are usually done as a part of the stroke work-up in the young [younger than age 45] or in patients without definite cause of stroke)

Early Assessments

Nurses in the ED make early assessments about the condition of the stroke patient. These assessments carry over to all other care areas during the hospital stay. The baseline characteristics of stroke observed during the ED phase will serve as a benchmark for outcomes as the stroke patient progresses through the hospital stay.

The most important early assessment is identification of stroke signs and symptoms so that early diagnosis and treatment can be initiated (Box 76-3). Toward this end, the public must be educated regarding recognition of the symptoms of stroke. The term *brain attack* has been coined to help the general public understand the urgency of stroke and to seek emergent medical care when symptoms of stroke are experienced.

In general, early assessment observations include initiating the ABCs to stabilize the patient once admitted to the ED. The head of the bed should be elevated to about 30 degrees, and the patient placed in a lateral position on the affected side to promote venous drainage, reduce cerebral edema, and help prevent aspiration. Urgent testing, as described above, is a priority after the patient arrives in the ED.

BOX 76-3
SIGNS AND SYMPTOMS OF STROKE

- Weakness or numbness of one side of the body (face, arm, leg, or any combination of these)
- Slurred speech
- Inability to comprehend what is being said
- Visual disturbance (transient loss of vision in one or both eyes [transient monocular blindness] or a visual field deficit)
- Dizziness, incoordination/ataxia, double vision, vertigo
- Nausea/vomiting
- Severe headache ("worst headache of my life")

Patients are expeditiously and systematically evaluated for eligibility for rt-PA in the ED if the patient presents within the 3-hour time window after symptoms begin. Nurses play a vital role in ensuring that tests and evaluations are accomplished within certain time parameters (see Box 76-1), so that rt-PA can be administered per protocol when appropriate.[10]

Neurological Vital Signs

Assessment of neurological vital signs in the ED includes blood pressure, pulse, respirations, temperature, pulse oximetry, level of consciousness, pupils, speech, gag reflex, motor strength, and sensory testing. The importance of this assessment cannot be overstated. Neurological vital signs should also include use of the NIHSS (or similar scale that standardizes assessment).

Intravenous Access

In patients admitted with signs and symptoms of stroke, intravenous access should be obtained immediately upon admission to the ED if not done in the pre-hospital setting. At a minimum, two intravenous sites should be obtained. A dedicated site should be used only for administration of rt-PA.

Fluid Balance

Assessment of hydration is important for proper care of the stroke patient.[5,10,11] There are several reasons that may account for dehydration after stroke: swallowing deficits, communication deficits, cognitive impairment, immobility, infection, diuretic therapy, hyperthermia, and restlessness. In addition, many elderly patients with stroke present with dehydration. Early assessment of these possible conditions contributing to dehydration is part of the stabilization process. Maintaining good fluid balance is crucial in maintaining proper hydration after stroke so that stroke symptoms do not worsen or induce electrolyte imbalances.

Dehydration after stroke can cause a reduction in blood pressure (leading to decreased CBF), which can worsen the cerebral ischemic processes. Dehydration in the initial days after stroke is frequently hyperosmolar. This state is caused by inadequate intake of water due to drowsiness or dysphagia, a reduction of thirst in general, the presence of infection, concomitant medications (such as diuretics), and poorly controlled blood glucose levels in the diabetic patient. Some studies have shown that persons who have high plasma osmolality levels on admission have a worse chance of survival at 3 months.

Avoiding intravenous fluids such as D5W and excessive fluid loading is thought to reduce the chance of the patient developing cerebral edema, especially in large cortical or lobar strokes. Isotonic fluids such as physiological saline are recommended to hydrate stroke patients. The conventional wisdom of the past indicated that the patient should be kept "slightly dry" to prevent cerebral edema, but studies have shown that administration of normal saline solution may contribute to improving functional ability in stroke patients in the long run.[10,11] Fluid disturbances can be assessed by[11]:

- Clinical observation
- Evaluation of intake and output
- Measurement of central venous pressure via a central venous line or pulmonary artery occlusion pressure using a pulmonary artery catheter
- Measurements of serum osmolarity, urine osmolarity, and serum sodium concentration

Blood Pressure and Blood Pressure Control

Transient elevations in blood pressure are common in the stroke patient. In fact, these elevations occur in about 80 percent of persons with acute stroke. This elevation has been seen as a physiological response to brain ischemia and to the stress of acute illness. A cautious approach is taken to treating hypertension unless the patient is a candidate for thrombolysis, has malignant hypertension that could cause hypertensive encephalopathy, or the patient has an intracranial hemorrhage. It is postulated that transient elevation in blood pressure may be caused by catecholamine release in response to stress.[11] Elevated blood pressure is seen in persons with both ischemic and hemorrhagic stroke. In general, reduction of blood pressure to normal levels is not recommended. Elevated blood pressure is thought to be a compensatory reflex of the brain to maintain cerebral perfusion pressure during the acute event and for some time thereafter. Reduction in blood pressure can exacerbate the lack of blood and oxygen to the ischemic penumbra, causing enlargement of the area of infarct and worsening of the neurological deficit. There is no definitive agreement of how to manage blood pressure, but gradual lowering is recommended, keeping the systolic blood pressure lower than 220 mm Hg and the diastolic lower than 110 mm Hg.[1]

Cardiac Status

Assessment of cardiac status is important so that occult heart disease or cardiac abnormalities that cause or complicate stroke can be identified. Moreover, it is essential that cardiac conditions that could complicate recovery be identified and managed.

In general, continuous cardiac monitoring is indicated for at least the first 24 to 48 hours and possibly up to 72 hours after the onset of stroke symptoms. Monitoring of cardiac dysrhythmias is important as these are potential causes of the stroke (Box 76-4). In addition, electrocardiographic changes often occur as a result of the stroke (Box 76-5). There is a strong interaction between stroke and heart disease. Patients with stroke may have had a clinically silent myocardial infarction. Cardiac dysrhythmias are particularly common as a complication of hemorrhagic stroke. Once patients with cardioembolic stroke have stabilized, heparin and then transition to warfarin therapy is instituted in anticoagulant eligible patients. See Chapter 88 for a more complete discussion of cardiac and neurological interactions.

BOX 76-4
COMMON DYSRHYTHMIAS FOLLOWING STROKE

- Atrial fibrillation
- Sinus bradycardia
- Premature ventricular contractions
- Paroxysmal supraventricular tachycardia
- Sinoatrial block
- Atrioventricular block or dissociation
- Idioventricular rhythms
- Nonsustained ventricular tachycardia
- Torsades de pointes
- Ventricular fibrillation

BOX 76-5
ELECTROCARDIOGRAPHIC CHANGES FOLLOWING STROKE

- ST-segment elevation/depression
- ST-T wave segment changes
- Pathologic Q waves
- Negative T waves
- Abnormal U waves
- Prolonged PQ or QT interval

Temperature

Temperature elevations are common during the initial acute stroke period. Temperature elevation could be a marker of stroke severity or of a concurrent infectious process. Thus, it is crucial to monitor temperature throughout the stroke hospitalization and recovery period. Temperature elevations can exacerbate the metabolic needs of an already oxygen-deprived brain and cause further neuronal damage.[11-13] Even a 1° increase (between 37° and 38° C) in temperature is associated with an increase in morbidity and mortality in stroke patients.[11,14] When the core body temperature is lowered, the systemic oxygen demand is lessened. As body temperature falls, carbon dioxide levels, plasma potassium levels, and carbohydrate metabolism decrease. Mechanisms for hyperthermia-induced brain damage may include neurotransmitter release, free radical formation, and disturbed recovery of brain metabolism.[12] The use of acetaminophen or a cooling blanket may be indicated, and early aggressive treatment and control of fever is imperative in the acute stroke patient.

Pulmonary Function

Maintenance of proper oxygenation is important in patients with acute stroke. Proper oxygenation preserves brain metabolic functions and decreases anaerobic processes that can be deleterious to the ischemic penumbra. It is important to avoid hypercapnia as this condition leads to vasodilatation of cerebral arterioles that supply healthy brain tissue, a condition that could lead to reduction of blood and oxygen to the infarct site.[12]

Knowing the baseline respiratory pattern is important because changes in the pattern can herald the onset of complications in certain types of stroke. Initially, a baseline pulse oximetry evaluation without supplemental oxygen should be done. If oxygen saturation measured by pulse oximetry is below 95 percent on room air, supplemental oxygen may be necessary.[5]

As oxygen saturation does not necessarily indicate adequate oxygenation, hypercapnia should be monitored, and arterial blood gases should be done as necessary. Hypoxia following stroke is common and results in anaerobic metabolism and depletion of energy stores, worsening brain injury. Stroke patients are at risk of hypoxia due to concurrent medical conditions such as aspiration pneumonia, hypoventilation, atelectasis, and pulmonary embolism.[15,16] Maintaining CBF is crucial to stroke patients in order to maintain cerebral oxygenation to the ischemic penumbra.

Respiratory failure in patients with acute stroke is usually caused by aspiration pneumonia, impairment of central respiratory drive (as is the case in brain stem stroke), or neurogenic pulmonary edema. Further respiratory compromise may also be caused by atelectasis or pneumonia due to immobilization or decreased level of consciousness. Mechanical ventilation should be instituted if the PO_2 drops below 60 to 70 mm Hg or the PCO_2 rises above 50 to 60 mm Hg. In general, signs of respiratory failure include tachypnea, dyspnea with the use of accessory muscles, and respiratory acidosis.[11]

Serum Glucose Level

Assessment of serum glucose level is important in the hyperacute stroke period. Approximately 20 percent to 50 percent of stroke patients are hyperglycemic on presentation, and about 20 percent of patients presenting with stroke are diabetic.[11,17] Several research studies have shown that persons with hyperglycemia tend to have poorer outcomes as compared with those that are normoglycemic. Hyperglycemia may increase infarct size and may increase the chance of hemorrhagic transformation. Elevated glucose levels have been associated with an increased hemorrhage rate in persons treated with thrombolysis. Hyperglycemia seems to increase neuronal injury. The stress of stroke in diabetic patients may exacerbate glucose levels and make glucose control more difficult. Current recommendations indicate that serum glucose levels should be kept at 144 mg/dl or less. Subcutaneous fast-acting insulin or, in difficult to control cases, intravenous insulin infusion should be instituted to meet this goal.[1] Conversely, extreme hypoglycemia can cause stroke-like symptoms referred to as *hypoglycemia hemiplegia*. This set of symptoms is commonly seen after the insulin-dependent diabetic has a change in insulin dosing and the blood sugar drops precipitously. Treatment with intravenous D_{50} will reverse symptoms almost immediately.

Aspiration Precautions

Aspiration precautions should be instituted, keeping the patient NPO until a formal swallow study rules out dysphagia or until the patient is assessed for swallowing ability.[18] Often, stroke patients cannot clear secretions and the cough and gag reflexes are impaired due to motor deficits, cranial nerve deficits, or decrease in level of consciousness. As a consequence, patients are at risk for developing pneumonia, which is a major complication and cause of mortality after stroke.

Nutrition

Nutritional status is an often overlooked part of the early care of the acute stroke patient. Nutritional status should be assessed as soon as possible after admission to hospital. Frequently, patients with stroke have abnormal low albumin levels, revealing inadequate nutritional status that potentially could affect patient outcomes. Low serum albumin levels may be associated with an increased risk of developing an infectious process. In some studies, low serum albumin levels predicted death at 3 months. It has been postulated that a hypercatabolic state due to stress reaction from the stroke modifies carbohydrate metabolism. This modification may be one explanation for the malnutrition seen.[12] For malnourished patients or alcoholic patients, supplementation with thiamine is advised. Feeding should begin as soon as possible after admission to the hospital once the patient has been cleared for risk of aspiration. If the patient cannot safely swallow, feeding may be instituted using a nasogastric approach. Otherwise in able, non-dysphagic patients, oral feedings may be instituted.[19]

POTENTIAL COMPLICATIONS FROM STROKE

There are several complications associated with stroke. These include urinary tract infection (especially from prolonged Foley catheter use), deep venous thrombosis, pneumonia, cerebral edema leading to cerebral herniation, bowel irregularities, decubitus ulcer formation, the development of stress ulcers, dysphagia, nutritional deficiencies, depression, and seizures.[5,6]

Urinary Tract Infection

Urinary tract infection (UTI) is one of the most common complications after stroke. It is not uncommon for patients to present with stroke and concurrently have a urinary tract infection, especially in the diabetic patient. Use of an indwelling catheter is an exogenous cause of infection and careful, consistent perineal care should be instituted daily. Any infectious process is potentially deleterious for the stroke patient. UTI will raise temperature and further compromise viable brain tissue in the ischemic penumbra. Early assessment of urinalysis can be crucial to long-term care of the stroke patient.

Deep Venous Thrombosis and Pulmonary Embolus

Patients with ischemic stroke are at risk of developing deep venous thrombosis (DVT). Patients at greatest risk are those with a dense hemiparesis or impaired mobility of the hemiparetic or hemiplegic leg. DVT can also form in a densely hemiplegic arm. Development of DVT is

common among stroke patients and puts them at risk for pulmonary embolus. Prevention modalities include unfractionated heparin 5000 units twice daily subcutaneously, enoxaparin (Lovenox) 40 mg to 80 mg subcutaneously once daily. Pneumatic devices may be used although their efficacy has been questionable. Thromboembolic stockings also may be used.[5]

Cerebral Herniation

Cerebral herniation due to cerebral edema is a life-threatening emergency and a common cause of early death in persons with large hemispheric strokes (usually cortical).[17] The risk of cerebral herniation reaches a peak at about 72 hours after stroke, and cerebral herniation is usually synonymous with increased intracranial pressure. Changes in level of consciousness, agitation, drowsiness, and difficulty concentrating may be some of the first symptoms of herniation. As herniation progresses, further alterations in consciousness may occur. Pupillary changes (typically pupillary asymmetry, with dilatation on the same side as the herniation), altered respiratory patterns, temperature fluctuations, and changes in reflexes (hyperreflexia, Babinski's sign or abnormal rigidity, decorticate or decerebrate posturing) may also occur.[5,6,20]

In decorticate posturing or rigidity, the arms are held tightly to the sides with the elbows, wrists, and fingers flexed; the legs are extended and internally rotated, with the feet in a plantar-flexed position. In decerebrate posturing or rigidity, the arms are held tightly to the sides but in an extensor position, adducted with the forearms pronated, the wrists and fingers flexed; the jaw is clenched; and the neck is extended. The legs are extended at the knees, and the feet are in a plantar position. This type of posturing suggests a lesion in the diencephalon, midbrain, or pons. Certain metabolic conditions, hypoxia, or hypoglycemia also can cause this type of posturing. Both types of abnormal posturing are associated with a poor prognosis, but decerebration is considered a more ominous sign.

Patients can also experience nausea and vomiting, new or progressive neurological deficits, or the loss of spontaneous venous pulsation. Hypo-osmolar intravenous fluids such as D_5W should be avoided because these fluids tend to potentiate cerebral edema under these circumstances.[8] The head of the bed should be raised about 30 degrees to promote venous drainage. Controlling fever is important as fever increases metabolic demands on the ischemic brain. Cough can increase intracranial pressure. If the patient is in pain, pain control will also help lower intracranial pressure. Pharmacological modalities commonly used to avoid cerebral herniation are mannitol 20 percent (1 g/kg over 30 minutes), diuretics (furosemide), dexamethasone, and barbiturate coma.[5,6]

Controlling blood pressure is of utmost importance in reducing the risk of herniation. Maintaining CBF is the goal, and there is a delicate balance in achieving this while avoiding hypoperfusion. Keeping blood pressure controlled also reduces the risk of rebleeding (if the patient has had an intracerebral hemorrhage) or hemorrhagic transformation in the patient with a large lobar ischemic stroke. If the signs of increased intracranial pressure or cerebral herniation are allowed to continue without intervention, decorticate and decerebrate posturing can ensue. These signs are life-threatening and require rapid medical intervention.

Seizures

Seizures can occur after a stroke. Patients with large cortical/lobar strokes are particularly susceptible.[21] The frequency of seizures reported in various studies during the first few days after stroke ranges between 4 percent and 43 percent. Seizures are most common during the first 24 hours after stroke symptoms start. Recurrent seizures develop in approximately 20 percent to 80 percent of those who have seizures. Seizures are treated with anticonvulsants, commonly phenytoin (Dilantin).

Hemorrhagic Transformation

Hemorrhagic transformation or hemorrhagic conversion occurs in about 5 percent of persons with acute ischemic stroke. A hemorrhagic transformation occurs when there is reperfusion of blood into the area of infarct, and there is a leaking of blood through the wall of blood vessels that supply the area of ischemia and the area of the infarct.[6] The occurrence of hemorrhagic transformation depends on the size, location, and etiology of the stroke. Often, large hemispheric strokes have hemorrhagic transformation. Small petechial hemorrhages are less important than larger frank hematomas. Large hematomas can cause mass effect and increase the likelihood of cerebral herniation. Hemorrhagic transformation can be either symptomatic or asymptomatic. Careful use of antithrombotic therapy is essential because of the likelihood of hemorrhagic transformation in certain strokes.

Falls

Stroke patients are particularly prone to falls. Early assessment of the patient's risk for falling is important, followed by appropriate fall-prevention strategies. Unfortunately it may be necessary to place some stroke patients in restraints, especially persons with intracerebral hemorrhage or large cortical strokes. These patients are often very confused and agitated due to irritation from blood in the cerebral spinal fluid. They also may suffer from increased intracranial pressure.

The use of chemical restraints is not recommended. Masking neurological and cognitive impairment may lead to failure to recognize an acute neurological change, such as that seen in the case of cerebral herniation. Sedative drugs are usually reserved for those patients who are receiving mechanical ventilation.[12]

TREATMENT OF ACUTE ISCHEMIC STROKE

The only approved therapy for acute ischemic stroke is rt-PA.[22] The earliest possible intervention is recommended. Careful assessment of patients potentially eli-

gible for thrombolytic therapy focuses on the inclusion and exclusion criteria shown in Box 76-6. The risk of serious bleeding related to the administration of rt-PA is decreased if inclusion and exclusion criteria are strictly used. Thrombolytic therapy with rt-PA is recommended for acute ischemic stroke, if administered within 3 hours after symptom onset. Administration of rt-PA after this time has not been shown to be beneficial. The earlier patients are treated within the 3-hour window, the better the outcome.

The recommended dose of rt-PA is 0.9 mg/kg up to a maximum of 90 mg. An initial bolus dose of 10 percent of the total dose is given over 1 minute. The remaining dose is infused over an hour. This dosing is far different than that given to patients with acute myocardial infarction. Anticoagulants and antiplatelet drugs should be avoided within 24 hours after administration of rt-PA to prevent complications.[23] Stroke severity is assessed using the NIHSS (Table 76-1).[24] Generally, rt-PA is not given if NIHSS scores are less than 4 and is given only with careful consideration in persons with scores of 22 or greater.

Cerebral hemorrhagic transformation is the most feared complication after the administration of rt-PA; the chances of hemorrhagic transformation occurring can be reduced by maintaining blood pressure less than 185 mm Hg systolic or less than 105 mm Hg diastolic. Antihypertensive treatment should be given judiciously to these patients to keep the mean arterial pressure about 130 mm Hg. The risk of hemorrhage for those receiving rt-PA is 6.4 percent compared to 0.6 percent for the placebo group. Nursing personnel must be

---

BOX 76-6
INCLUSION AND EXCLUSION CRITERIA FOR ADMINISTRATION OF TISSUE PLASMINOGEN ACTIVATOR IN ACUTE ISCHEMIC STROKE

Inclusion Criteria
- Onset of stroke symptoms less than 3 hours
- Clinical diagnosis of ischemic stroke with a measurable deficit using the National Institutes of Health Stroke Scale
- Patient older than age 18
- Computed tomography consistent with ischemic stroke

Exclusion Criteria
- Onset of stroke symptoms more than 3 hours
- Rapidly improving minor or major stroke
- Evidence of intracerebral bleed including intraparenchymal or subarachnoid hemorrhage or other pathology
- Systolic blood pressure greater than 185 mm Hg or diastolic blood pressure greater than 110 mm Hg
- Glucose level less than 50 mg/dl or greater than 400 mg/dl
- Recent myocardial infarction
- Seizure at the onset of stroke
- Active internal bleeding within 21 days
- Arterial puncture at non-compressible site
- Known bleeding diathesis, including but not limited to current use of oral anticoagulants with prothrombin time greater than 15 seconds
- Administration of heparin with 48 hours preceding the onset of stroke and an elevated activated partial thromboplastin (aPTT) time at presentation
- Platelet count less than 100,000/mm^3
- Lumbar puncture within 7 days, major surgery within 14 days

■ ■ ■

TABLE 76-1 NATIONAL INSTITUTES OF HEALTH STROKE SCALE

ITEM TESTED	TITLE/DOMAIN	RESPONSE/SCORE
1A	Level of consciousness	0 – alert 1 – drowsy 2 – obtunded 3 – coma/unresponsive
1B	Orientation	0 – answers both correctly 1 – answers one correctly 2 – answers none correctly
1C	Response/commands (two)	0 – performs both correctly 1 – performs one correctly 2 – performs none correctly
2	Gaze	0 – normal horizontal movements 1 – partial palsy 2 – complete gaze palsy
3	Visual fields	0 – no visual field defect 1 – partial hemianopia 2 – complete hemianopia 3 – bilateral hemianopia
4	Facial movement	0 – normal 1 – minor facial weakness 2 – partial facial weakness 3 – complete unilateral palsy
5	Motor function (arm) a. left b. right	0 – no drift 1 – drift before 5 seconds 2 – falls before 10 seconds 3 – no effort against gravity 4 – no movement
6	Motor function (leg) a. left b. right	0 – no drift 1 – drift before 5 seconds 2 – falls before 10 seconds 3 – no effort against gravity 4 – no movement
7	Limb ataxia	0 – no ataxia 1 – ataxia in one limb 2 – ataxia in two limbs
8	Sensory	0 – no sensory loss 1 – mild sensory loss 2 – severe sensory loss
9	Best language	0 – normal 1 – mild aphasia 2 – severe aphasia 3 – mute or global aphasia
10	Articulation (dysarthria)	0 – normal 1 – mild dysarthria 2 – severe dysarthria
11	Extinction or inattention	0 – absent 1 – mild (loss 1 sensory modality) 2 – severe (loss 2 modalities)
Total NIHSS (National Institutes of Health Stroke Scale)		Score TOTAL _____ (0–42)

From Spilker J, Kongable G, Barch C et al: Using the NIH Stroke Scale to assess stroke patients, *J Neurosci Nurs* 29(6):384-391, 1997.
NIHSS, National Institutes of Health Stroke Scale.

aware of the signs and symptoms of intracerebral hemorrhage (symptoms related to increased intracranial pressure and especially a change in level of consciousness). If intracranial hemorrhage is suspected, an emergent CT scan (no contrast) of the head is done, and if rt-PA is infusing, the infusion is stopped and fresh frozen plasma or platelets may be administered.[25] Bleeding can occur elsewhere as well, including local intravenous puncture site oozing, gastrointestinal bleeding, urinary bleeding, and retroperitoneal bleeding.

Before rt-PA is infused, all intravenous access sites needed should be obtained, catheters inserted, and, if indicated, a nasogastric tube inserted prior to administration. A repeat CT scan of the head is done about 24 hours after infusion of intravenous rt-PA looking for hemorrhagic transformation.

Recently, the mechanical embolus removal in cerebral ischemia (**MERCI**) device was approved by the Food and Drug Administration. The MERCI device is a clot retrieval apparatus that is used to extract a clot when visualized by cerebral arteriography. If the clot is accessible, a catheter is introduced into the cerebral circulation and the MERCI device is then guided through the clot where a corkscrew-like device embeds within the clot. This corkscrew-like apparatus is then deployed and the occluding clot is gently removed from the vessel. This procedure may be done up to 8 hours after the onset of ischemic stroke symptoms and is usually done by an experienced neuroradiologist or neurointerventionalist. The MERCI device may or not be used with rt-PA.[26]

TRANSITION TO INTENSIVE CARE UNIT, STROKE UNIT, OR GENERAL FLOOR

There are several reasons for admission of the stroke patient to the intensive care unit, including depressed consciousness, progressive or fluctuating symptoms, airway impairment, seizures, significant comorbid conditions, or use of rt-PA. Several complications are common in seriously ill stroke patients. These include fever, increased intracranial pressure, hypertension, pneumonia, deep venous thrombosis, pulmonary embolism, and recurrent cerebral ischemia (or worsening of the initial neurological deficit).

Continue the neurological and other assessments started in the ED. Neurological vital signs and other assessments occur more frequently in the intensive care unit. Neurological vital signs should be done in persons treated with thrombolytics every 30 minutes for the first 8 hours, then every 60 minutes for the next 16 hours. Neurological vital signs include assessment of level of consciousness and an assessment of neurological deficits, such as arm and leg weakness, and assessments of worsening or improvement of the neurological deficits. These assessments should be compared with the baseline assessments started in the ED.

Hemodynamic instability is of concern in the first hours to days after stroke. Fluid balance and electrolytes should be monitored closely and fluids delivered appropriately. Electrolyte abnormalities including hypo- or hypernatremia, hyper- or hypokalemia should be treated to avoid potential poor outcomes.

Care following an intensive care unit stay is generally focused on continuing the stroke work-up (to understand the cause of stroke), stabilizing the patient in all areas of medical management, and preparing the patient for rehabilitation. The goals of patient and family education at this point are to prepare them for secondary prevention therapies and to emphasize the importance of adherence to these therapies.

In-Hospital Strokes

Stroke is common in patients hospitalized for other reasons. Such strokes are particularly common in persons with cardiac conditions or who have undergone cardiac procedures such as cardiac catheterization. A "Code Stroke" should be developed in hospital units where there might be a higher likelihood of stroke occurring (such as cardiac care units). Patients admitted with TIA may be particularly prone to progression to stroke. The American Heart Association/American Stroke Association Advanced Cardiac Life Support, Case 10, is a good model for development of an in-hospital stroke code.[27]

HEMORRHAGIC STROKE

Intracerebral hemorrhage **(ICH)** represents about 15 percent of all strokes. The primary causes of hemorrhagic stroke are hypertension, ruptured saccular aneurysm or arteriovenous malformation, bleeding into a tumor, amyloid angiopathy, and trauma. Secondary causes of hemorrhagic stroke include over-anticoagulation, vasopressor drugs, illicit drug or alcohol abuse, leukemia, aplastic anemia, hemophilia, and liver disease. Even though ICH represents a small fraction of all strokes, the 30-day mortality is 2- to 6-fold that of ischemic stroke. The mortality rate for ICH in the first 30 days is 35 percent to 50 percent. More than half of those deaths occur within the first 2 days.[28] The primary reason for the high mortality is that the blood causes a space-occupying lesion leading to increased ICP and cerebral herniation. ICH is divided into two categories, intracerebral or intraparenchymal stroke, and subarachnoid hemorrhage.

Primary Intraparenchymal Hemorrhage

The most common type of intracranial hemorrhage is primary intraparenchymal hemorrhage (within the brain tissue), accounting for about 67 percent of ICH. The pathophysiology or the phases of intraparenchymal hemorrhage are described as follows[28]:

- Phase I: vascular rupture into the brain parenchyma (1 to 10 seconds)
  Implicated mechanism: chronic vascular changes such as lipohyalinosis, amyloid angiopathy, hypocholesterolemia)
- Phase II: hematoma formation (less than 1 hour)
  Implicated mechanism: blood pressure, coagulation abnormalities
- Phase III: hematoma expansion (1 to 5 hours)
  Implicated mechanism: blood pressure, perihematomal vascular plus tissue injury
- Phase IV: edema formation (24 to 72 hours)
  Implicated mechanism: cellular and humoral toxicity, blood degradation products)

Extravasation of blood forms an irregular circular or oval mass within the parenchyma. The extending mass displaces and compresses tissue, and fibers begin to

separate. The severity of physiological symptoms depends upon the location of the bleed.

About 50 percent of primary intraparenchymal hemorrhages occur in the putamen and internal capsule (subcortical part of the brain). Resorption of extravasated blood occurs, causing a clot. The clot undergoes fibrinolysis and liquefaction within days of the bleed. The mass can enlarge with the influx of fluid into the cavity, or edema can be present in adjacent tissue.[12]

Characteristics

Unlike subarachnoid hemorrhage, an ICH can occur with no warning or prodrome. These strokes are most commonly associated with extreme hypertension but can occur with moderately high blood pressures as well. ICH can occur in any age group and usually occurs while the person is up and active. Symptoms include headache or an abnormal sensation in the head. Focal neurological deficits include slurred speech, hemiparesis or plegia, or other symptoms of stroke. There is a rapid progression within minutes to hours, and the patient's status commonly includes progressive decline in consciousness leading to coma. The first 72 hours are the highest risk for herniation due to the potential for enlargement of the hemorrhage, midline shift, or cerebral edema. The size of the bleed usually determines the extent of neurological symptoms.

The mortality rate due to ICH is high, but those who survive usually have a good outcome. Neurosurgical intervention is sometimes considered but is reserved mainly for large bleeds that cause compression or are life-threatening. The diagnosis is made by CT scan. CT imaging will reveal a hyperintense signal from the area affected (Figure 76-6). The differential diagnosis of the cause of hemorrhage may be hypertension, drug abuse, amyloid angiopathy, or arteriovenous malformation.

General Care

Care of the person with ICH generally starts with ensuring the airway and checking blood pressure and cerebral perfusion pressure. Protection of airway and adequate oxygenation are high priorities. Intubation may be neces-

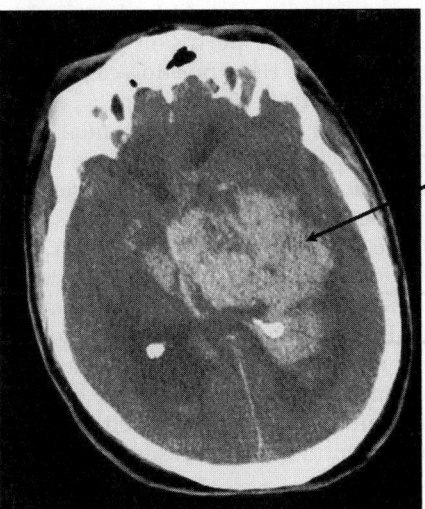

Large left intraparenchymal hematoma

FIGURE 76-6 ■ CT scan of intracerebral hemorrhage.

sary, especially in patients with decreasing level of consciousness or signs of brainstem involvement. Intubation should be guided by the clinical features of respiratory dysfunction rather than any measurement such as the Glasgow Coma Scale score. In general, parameters such as hypoxia of PO_2 less than 60 mm Hg or PCO_2 greater than 50 mm Hg, or the obvious risk of aspiration (in the presence of impairment of arterial oxygenation) are indicative of the need for intubation.[12,29] However, some literature suggests that all persons with a Glasgow Coma Scale of 8 or less should be intubated.[30]

Patients with intracerebral bleeds rarely benefit from surgical intervention, although it is sometimes attempted with clots 2 to 4 cm in diameter, to reduce the symptoms due to mass effect. Smaller hematomas in awake patients usually resolve without surgery.[30] Comatose patients with large lesions (6 cm in diameter) usually have poor outcomes, regardless of treatment. Nursing care of the patient with intraparenchymal hemorrhage is essentially the same as with ischemic stroke.

Blood Pressure Control

Blood pressure is carefully monitored in these patients to prevent recurrent hemorrhage. In general, the optimal level of blood pressure should be based on several individual indicators such as history of chronic hypertension, age, cause of the hemorrhage, and elevated intracranial pressure.[29] Elevations in blood pressure are usually treated more aggressively in patients with increased intracranial pressure. The mean arterial pressure is often maintained at 130 mm Hg in persons with known hypertension.[29] If treatment is required, blood pressure should be lowered cautiously to prehemorrhage levels. Aggressive lowering of blood pressure can compromise cerebral perfusion pressure; however, blood pressure should be brought down to prevent expansion of the hematoma. Patients are assessed for changes in level of consciousness as well as changes in neurological status.

Increased Intracranial Pressure

Increased intracranial pressure is defined as pressures greater than 20 mm Hg for 5 minutes or more. Therapeutically, intracranial pressure should be kept at less than 20 mm Hg, with cerebral perfusion pressure of greater than 60 to 70 mm Hg. Head position can make a significant difference in intracranial pressure.[12]

Patients with suspected increased intracranial pressure and deteriorating level of consciousness are candidates for invasive intracranial pressure monitoring. In this instance, if a Glasgow Coma Scale score is less than 9, monitors should be placed.[12,30] Increased intracranial pressure frequently follows ICH and is considered a major contributor to the mortality following ICH. Management for increased intracranial pressure related to ICH includes osmotherapy (mannitol and furosemide therapy), hyperventilation (producing hypocarbia) or barbiturate coma.[12,29] Barbiturate coma is reserved for situations where increased intracranial pressure cannot be controlled by other means.

Another modality used to observe and treat intracranial pressure is the placement of an endoventricular device (**EVD**) via ventriculostomy. Typically, an EVD is placed in one of the lateral ventricles and is then attached to an intracranial monitoring device. The utility of using an EVD includes drainage of cerebral spinal fluid to maintain intracranial pressure of less than 20 mm Hg or lower.[30] Nursing care of the patient with ICH can greatly influence outcomes.

CEREBRAL ANEURYSMS AND SUBARACHNOID HEMORRHAGE
Epidemiology and Pathophysiology

Subarachnoid hemorrhage (**SAH**), bleeding into the subarachnoid space, accounts for about 33 percent of hemorrhagic strokes each year. SAH has a 30-day mortality of about 45 percent, with approximately half of survivors sustaining irreversible brain damage with neuropsychiatric and functional deficits.[31,32] SAH is most often caused by a ruptured cerebral aneurysm, a saccular out-pouching of a cerebral artery. The most common site for the formation of aneurysms is the circle of Willis, involving most commonly the anterior communicating artery. The etiology of cerebral aneurysms is unclear, but some believe that there is a congenital/developmental defect in the medial and adventitial layers of an artery in the circle of Willis. It is usually accepted that there are extrinsic, genetic, and congenital factors causing the formation of aneurysms. Most patients with cerebral aneurysms are asymptomatic before rupture unless they experience a warning "leak," sometimes called a "sentinel bleed." Aneurysms commonly rupture into the subarachnoid space of the basal cisterns. Occasionally, cerebral aneurysms rupture into the ventricular system or into brain tissue.

When rupture occurs, it usually occurs at the thin-walled dome of the aneurysm, causing blood to enter into the subarachnoid space. The tissue around the ruptured aneurysm stops the bleed, and the fibrin, platelets, and fluid form a plug that seals off the site of bleeding. This clot can occlude the area or obstruct the flow of cerebral spinal fluid absorption, causing hydrocephalus. The blood released into the subarachnoid space irritates the brain substance, causing an inflammatory response that can result in cerebral edema and vasospasm. At the time of rupture, intracranial pressure can increase to the mean arterial pressure and lower cerebral perfusion pressure. These pressure changes account for altered level of consciousness.

Characterization of Aneurysms

Cerebral aneurysms are characterized by size and shape (Box 76-7).[33] Additionally, there is an aneurysmal bleeding classification known as the Hunt and Hess Classification of Subarachnoid Hemorrhage (Table 76-2). Neurosurgeons use this classification to decide on timing of surgery if this is an option for treatment.

Before rupture, a cerebral aneurysm can mimic a mass lesion and compress brain tissue, cranial nerves, and blood vessels. Immediately after the rupture, there is bleeding into adjacent tissue, and increased intracranial pressure may be focal (near the aneurysm) or global.

BOX 76-7   ■ ■ ■
CLASSIFICATION OF ANEURYSMS BY SIZE AND SHAPE

Size

Small:	Less than 15 mm
Large:	15 to 25 mm
Giant:	25 to 50 mm
Super-giant:	More than 50 mm

Shape

Berry:	Berry-shaped with a neck or stem (most common)
Charcot-Bouchard:	Microscopic formation associated with hypertension and involving the basal ganglia and brainstem
Dissecting:	Related to atherosclerosis, whereby the intimal lining is pulled from the medial layer, allowing blood between the two layers
Fusiform:	Outpouching of an arterial wall without a stem
Mycotic:	Caused by septic emboli from infections such an endocarditis (rare)
Saccular:	Any aneurysm with saccular outpouching
Traumatic:	Occurring from head trauma (not common)

■ ■ ■

TABLE 76-2   HUNT AND HESS CLASSIFICATION OF SUBARACHNOID HEMORRHAGE BLEEDING

GRADE	DESCRIPTION
I	Asymptomatic or mild headache and slight nuchal rigidity
II	Cranial nerve (CN) palsy in CN III (Oculomotor), CN VI (Abducens) Mild to moderate nuchal rigidity
III	Mild focal deficit, lethargy, or confusion
IV	Stupor, moderate to severe hemiparesis, early decerebrate posturing
V	Deep coma, decerebrate rigidity, moribund appearance

Add one grade for serious systemic disease (e.g., hypertension, chronic obstructive pulmonary disease) or severe vasospasm on angiography
From Hickey JV: *The clinical practice of neurological and neurosurgical nursing,* ed 5, Philadelphia, 2003, Lippincott Williams & Wilkins.

Symptoms

The most classic symptom of ruptured aneurysm is a complaint of "the worst headache of my life." Nausea and vomiting, photophobia, and nuchal rigidity may occur. Other potential symptoms, particularly of, as yet, unruptured aneurysms include dilated pupil (loss of light reflex; oculomotor nerve deficit), extraocular movement deficits of cranial nerve (CN) III (oculomotor), CN IV (trochlear), or CN VI (abducens), ptosis, pain above and behind the eye, and localized headache.[34,35]

Diagnosis of Cerebral Aneurysm

The CT scan without contrast is 95 percent accurate in the diagnosis of SAH.[33] In a CT scan positive for subarachnoid hemorrhage bleeding, blood will appear white in the subarachnoid space. If the CT scan is negative and SAH is still suspected, lumbar puncture may be done; the presence of red blood cells in the cerebral spinal fluid exceeding 100,000 per mm^2 is indicative of a bleed. Conventional cerebral angiography remains the gold standard for the diagnosis of cerebral aneurysm. It will show the source of the aneurysm in about 80 percent of cases as well as vasospasm (a narrowing of cerebral blood vessels seen radiographically). CT angiography is used at some institutions, and is 85 percent accurate in diagnosing SAH. CT angiography can provide a three-dimensional view of cerebral structures, but specificity and sensitivity are lower with CT than conventional angiography.

Medical and Nursing Management

SAH is a serious condition requiring immediate diagnosis and treatment. Treatment modalities will depend on several factors, including age, neurological condition, Hunt and Hess grade, size of the aneurysm, and the patient's current and previous medical history.

Complications After Rupture

After rupture of an aneurysm, the patient can experience cardiac dysrhythmias, rebleeding, hydrocephalus, seizures, and vasospasm. Neurological injury can be related to any of these events.[36]

Cardiac dysrhythmias occur as a result of stimulation of the sympathetic nervous system. Increased sympathetic tone also causes a high incidence of T wave inversion, prolonged QT intervals, and ST abnormalities.

Rebleeding is another serious problem following the initial aneurysm rupture. The mechanism of rebleeding is increased tension on the aneurysm wall. The increase in tension is due to hypertension and a sudden decrease in pressure around the aneurysm. Rebleeding can also occur from normal breakdown of the clot in 7 to 10 days following the initial bleed. Early surgical intervention is recommended to prevent rebleeding. If the patient is unstable, aminocaproic acid is administered to prevent the clot from breaking down.

SAH can impair the circulation and reabsorption of CSF. A blood clot can obstruct the flow in the ventricular system, causing an obstructive hydrocephalus. As blood enters the subarachnoid space, an inflammatory response is triggered. This inflammatory response can cause fibrosis and thickening of the arachnoid villi, which inhibits reabsorption of cerebral spinal fluid. Inhibition of reabsorption causes communicating hydrocephalus. Both obstructive and communicating hydrocephalus cause increased intracranial pressure.[33]

Seizures are another potential complication that can occur after a ruptured aneurysm. Seizures occurring within the first 12 hours after rupture are attributed to increased intracranial pressure. After the initial 12 hours (but before surgical clipping of the aneurysm), seizures are associated with rebleeding of the aneurysm. Because of the potential dangerous effects of seizures, most patients are given phenytoin to prevent seizures from occurring.

Cerebral vasospasm is a narrowing of arteries adjacent to the aneurysm, which results in ischemia and infarction of brain tissue if it is unresolved. Cerebral vasospasm is very common and is the leading cause of death after aneurysmal SAH. The usual period for vasospasm to occur is 3 to 14 days after the rupture. The exact mechanism for vasospasm is unknown, but some factors that contribute to vasospasm are structural changes in the adjacent cerebral arteries, denervation of adjacent arteries, generation of oxygen free radicals, and release of vasoactive substances (serotonin, catecholamines, prostaglandins, oxyhemoglobin) that initiate vasospasm, inflammatory response, and calcium influx.[37] Vasospasm is often treated with volume expansion (known as *triple H therapy*-hypertension, hypervolemia, hemodilution).[35-37] The goal of triple H therapy is to increase cerebral perfusion pressure. Volume expansion is achieved by administering agents such as albumin and plasma protein fraction (Plasmanate). If the patient's blood pressure becomes lower than prehemorrhage levels, hypertensive (vasoactive) infusions, such as dopamine, may need to be administered. The addition of a calcium channel blocker, nimodipine, is standard therapy for treatment of subarachnoid hemorrhage to prevent vasospasm. The recommended dosage is 60 mg every 4 hours for 21 days.

Novel therapies for the treatment of symptomatic vasospasm are the use of intraarterial papaverine and angioplasty. The frequency of clinical improvement with papaverine is approximately 70 percent.[37] Intraarterial papaverine infusion is most frequently performed at about day 8 after SAH, at the time of the appearance of symptoms of vasospasm. Papaverine increases the diameter of the vasospastic blood vessel. The effect of papaverine lasts less than 24 hours. Angioplasty has a longer-lasting effect than papaverine application alone but is associated with a risk of vessel rupture and requires anticoagulation. Recurrent vasospasm after angioplasty has been reported. Complications of angioplasty include increased intracranial pressure, transient neurological deficits, and mydriasis (asymmetric pupils).

Nursing Assessments and Interventions

A patient with a subarachnoid hemorrhage presents many challenges for nursing and medical care. When arterial blood enters the subarachnoid space, its presence is irritating to the meninges. These patients commonly experience increased intracranial pressure with alterations in CBF, hemodynamic instability, vasospasm, rebleeding, and hydrocephalus.[33] Vigilant nursing care and assessment is vital to recognizing and managing these complications.

Routine assessment includes neurological vital signs, determination of Glasgow Coma Scale, strict intake and output recording, and daily weights. Important interventions for a patient with SAH include these aneurysm precautions:

- Avoid increases in blood pressure.
- Ensure complete bedrest with the head of the bed up 30 degrees.
- Ensure a quiet environment, private room, and limited visitors.

- Decrease environmental stimulation by dimming the room lights, turning down the volume on monitors, and turning off the telephone.

Antiembolism stockings or pneumatic compression devices are used to prevent DVT development. An indwelling urinary catheter is used if the patient is incontinent, unable to void, or has a depressed level of consciousness

Surgical Interventions

For a ruptured aneurysm, early surgical intervention (within 24 hours of admission) is recommended for patients in good neurological condition when the aneurysm is surgically accessible. The goal for timing of a surgical intervention is to operate when there is minimal neurological dysfunction and before any episodes of rebleeding or vasospasm occur.

Surgery for a cerebral aneurysm consists of occlusion of the neck of the aneurysm (using a ligature or metal clip), reinforcement of the sac (wrapping the sac with muscle, fibrin foam, or solidifying polymer), or proximal ligation of a feeding vessel. If the neck of the aneurysm is narrow, using a ligature or metal clip is desirable. When the neck of the aneurysm is too broad, reinforcing the aneurysmal sac is the goal of surgery. Proximal ligation may be preferred when the aneurysm arises from the internal carotid artery.

Interventional techniques, such as endovascular treatment with Guglielmi detachable coils, are sometimes used to occlude the aneurysm.[38,39] This therapy consists of navigating a microcatheter through the femoral artery to the aneurysm, and then placing platinum coils into the aneurysm sac, producing thrombosis and occluding the aneurysm from the feeder vessel. This technique can be done with ruptured or unruptured aneurysms.

Patients with severe neurological compromise after a ruptured aneurysm may benefit from emergency ventriculostomy. The ventriculostomy assists in treating the hydrocephalus associated with the bleeding and aids in monitoring patients for increased intracranial pressure.

SECONDARY PREVENTION OF STROKE

The care that nurses provide can have a profound effect on secondary prevention of stroke. Secondary prevention of stroke will not only reduce the human costs of stroke but will reduce the huge expenditure of health care dollars spent on stroke annually in the United States. Nurses educate patients and families at the bedside while the patient is in the hospital, in the outpatient clinic, and in rehabilitation.

Secondary prevention strategies include the following:

- Assessing patient understanding of stroke and what causes stroke
- Assessing and managing individual risk factors
- Assessing patient understanding of how each risk factor can cause stroke (linking a disease process such as hypertension or diabetes with stroke pathophysiology)

- Assessing patient readiness to learn and make life-style changes
- Promoting the notion of patient self-management
- Assisting patients to understand the role of treatment adherence in long-term stroke prevention

Frequently, stroke patients will be admitted to the hospital with a stroke but may not be aware that they have hypertension, diabetes, or any other risk factor for stroke. All too often a diagnosis of "new-onset hypertension" or "new-onset diabetes" will be made at the time of admission. Patients will be reeling from the diagnosis of stroke and also have to deal with an additional new diagnosis. Patient education can be very complicated at this time. Refer to Chapters 83 and 84 for in-depth information about appropriate education and counseling and the promotion of treatment adherence.

During patient and family education and counseling, a weaving of the risk factors into the discussion of secondary prevention can create a broader picture of how these risk factors fit together and cause stroke. Frequently, patients do not understand what a risk factor is. Teaching them about "risk factors" is an important beginning in the dialog about prevention. Using pictorials to help them visualize a disease process (i.e., atherosclerosis) can help understanding. If patients understand the relationship between risk factors and stroke, they can more easily make the connection between medications used to treat these disorders and secondary prevention of stroke. Patient education can empower the patient to self reliance.

Anti-Platelet Agents

Most ischemic stroke patients should be treated with an antithrombotic agent for secondary prevention of ischemic stroke. Several large randomized trials using antiplatelet agents have shown a strong beneficial effect for prevention of stroke. Current evidence-based guidelines recommend that all patients with ischemic stroke be treated with an antithrombotic medication upon discharge from the hospital and that this therapy be continued for the long-term.[40] The only reason for a stroke patient not to be discharged from the hospital on an antithrombotic medication is the existence of a contraindication to taking one of this class of medications.

Options for treatment include one of the following:
- Aspirin (50 to 325 mg daily)
- Clopidogrel (Plavix) 75 mg daily
- Dipyridamole 200 mg plus aspirin 25 mg (Aggrenox) twice a day

Aspirin has been the staple drug treatment of choice because it is easily available, inexpensive, and well known by most people. Aspirin should be started within the first 48 hours after stroke symptoms onset. Enteric-coated aspirin is recommended to avoid the development of gastrointestinal disorders such as ulcers or gastrointestinal bleeding. Clopidogrel (Plavix) 75 mg daily may also be prescribed for secondary prevention of ischemic stroke, especially in the setting of second stroke, where the stroke has occurred while the patient was taking aspirin. The combination of aspirin plus clopidogrel has been used for secondary prevention of ischemic stroke. This combination was shown to be equivocal in secondary prevention of stroke. In the MATCH Study, there was an insignificant reduction in the rate of ischemic stroke in the combination group versus the clopidogrel group. The rate of bleeding was higher in the combination only group.[41] The combination of clopidogrel plus aspirin was compared to aspirin alone, showing no difference in treatments and a higher rate of bleeding.[42,43] The combination of clopidogrel plus aspirin is not recommended for secondary prevention of stroke. Aggrenox twice a day (the combination of dipyridamole 200 mg and aspirin 25 mg) is another antiplatelet agent used for secondary prevention of stroke.

Warfarin (Coumadin) is the recommended therapy for both primary and secondary prevention of stroke due to nonvalvular atrial fibrillation if the patient has a history of ischemic stroke, TIA, or systemic embolism; is older than age 75; or has moderately or severely impaired left ventricular systolic function, heart failure, a history of hypertension, or diabetes mellitus. The recommended INR range for warfarin is 2.0 to 3.0. If a patient has atrial fibrillation, is age 65 to 75, and has no other risk factors, the recommendation is warfarin with an INR range of 2.0 to 3.0 or aspirin 325 mg/day. If a patient is younger than age 65 and has no risk factors, aspirin 325 mg is recommended, but patients may choose to take warfarin for added protection.[44] Warfarin is also recommended for primary and secondary prevention in other major cardiac disorders that may predispose the patient to ischemic stroke.

When educating the patient and family about warfarin therapy, emphasis should be placed on treatment adherence, the need to obtain monthly INR levels to monitor anticoagulation, and drugs and foods that can interact with warfarin therapy (either inhibit or potentiate the effects of anticoagulation therapy) such as those high in vitamin K. There should be a discussion about bleeding as a potential side effect of anticoagulation therapy, how to recognize it, and what to do if bleeding is suspected.

Blood Pressure Management

Hypertension is the number one cause of both ischemic and hemorrhagic stroke. Blood pressure management is one of the single most important factors in the secondary prevention of stroke.[45] Several classes of antihypertensives are used to control blood pressure. Thiazide diuretics, beta blockers, calcium channel blockers, angiotensin-converting enzyme inhibitors, and angiotensin receptor blockers are the common classes of antihypertensive medications. Evidence-based recommendations for the control of blood pressure from the Seventh Joint National Committee on Prevention, Detection, Evaluation, and Treatment of High Blood Pressure Guidelines[46] are outlined in Chapters 35 and 78.

Patient education regarding consistently taking antihypertensive medications is very important. Educating about potential side effects may aid adherence by allowing patients to discuss side effects rather than simply discontinuing therapy. A discussion with men about the potential of impotence with some antihypertensives and the option of discussing alternative medications may prevent patients from stopping the medication without first discussing the issues with their provider.

Hyperlipidemia

Statin therapy is a potent preventive strategy in coronary artery disease, but the evidence for benefit in secondary prevention of stroke is not strong.[47] There is some evidence that use of statins might inhibit the arterial intimal inflammatory process in the atherosclerotic process seen in the carotid artery. Regardless of the limited evidence for stroke prevention, persons with diabetes, coronary artery disease, and hyperlipidemia should be treated with a statin because stroke patients often have these concurrent disease processes.[1] Encouraging lifestyle modification in addition to the statin is an important step in secondary prevention. Lifestyle changes for hyperlipidemia include exercise and following a low fat diet. Those with diabetes should follow an American Diabetic Association diet, increase physical activity, lose weight, and quit smoking. The complete management of hyperlipidemia is covered in Chapters 34 and 77. Diabetes is discussed in Chapter 37.

Special Areas of Interest
Angiotensin Receptor Blockers

There is much current interest in the role of angiotensin receptor blockers in the treatment of hypertension in persons with stroke. Systolic hypertension is considered one of the most problematic causes of stroke. Elevated systolic blood pressure is thought to be associated with a progressive structural and functional deterioration of the arterial wall, endothelial dysfunction, atherosclerosis, aortic stiffness, and increased wall stress and pulse pressure.[48] According to this model, atherosclerosis is triggered by vascular endothelial damage and mechanical strain from each stroke volume, thus playing a central role in the development of pathology of vessels. Atherosclerosis leads to replacement of elastin by collagen and other structural proteins and the buildup of calcium in the arterial wall. These processes lead to hypertrophy and fibrosis of arterial smooth muscle and the diminished capacity of arteries to dampen the pressure wave produced by ventricular contraction. There are several factors that lead to an increased risk of developing arterial stiffness, including obesity, diabetes, hypercholesterolemia, and elevated homocysteine levels. The widening pulse pressure, increased wave reflection, and systolic hypertension that these processes produce eventually contribute to the development of a spectrum of cardiovascular disorders that include cardiac and vascular hypertrophy and target organ damage including stroke.[48]

The renin-angiotensin system plays an important role in the pathogenesis of vascular hypertrophy and arterial stiffness. All of the principal biological effects of the system may be involved in the pathogenesis of systolic hypertension through several mechanisms, including decreased elastin content and increased collagen con-

tent of the arterial wall, thickening and fibrotic remodeling of the vascular intima, and proliferation of small muscle cells in the arterial wall. Pharmacological blockade of angiotensin II may have some unrecognized benefits on age-related vascular damage and provide particular benefits in stroke patients with systolic hypertension.[44,46] The current hypothesis under study is that angiotensin receptor blockade might be beneficial in changing the arterial vasculature in order to retard the atherosclerotic process. There are several studies ongoing examining this effect in secondary prevention of ischemic stroke.[48,49]

Metabolic Syndrome

Diabetes is a potent risk factor for stroke, and it is clear that there is a relationship between the metabolic syndrome and stroke. In the United States, about 22 percent of adults over age 20 have metabolic syndrome. Metabolic syndrome is known to be associated with an increased risk of cardiovascular disease, but studies have shown an association between the metabolic syndrome and stroke as well. Studies suggest that by treating persons with insulin resistance, the underlying culprit in metabolic syndrome, the risk of TIA and stroke are reduced.[50]

SPECIAL AREAS OF RESEARCH IN ACUTE STROKE
Induced Hypothermia

The notion of induced hypothermia in acute stroke as a neuroprotective agent has been a topic of interest for several years. Induced hypothermia (cooling to a core temperature of less than 35° C) has favorable effects in persons with cardiac arrest.[51] Hypothermia has been shown to be effective in animal models by inhibiting the apoptotic cell death cascade.[51,52] Currently, there are trials examining the efficacy of hypothermia in humans with acute stroke. Modalities for cooling include external cooling systems (cooling blankets or topical pads) and intravascular catheters; the target temperature is 33° C. The Cooling for Ischemic Brain Damage (called COOL AID) study showed this to be feasible, and most patients in this small cohort of study participants tolerated the modality well.[54] However, this study did not examine outcomes, and further studies are needed to determine if hypothermia improves outcomes.

Neuroprotective Agents

Neuroprotection in acute stroke has been under investigation for some time. The idea in neuroprotection is to protect or salvage brain cells in the area of the ischemic penumbra, thus preserving potentially viable cells from succumbing to cell death and avoiding more extensive neurological deficits. Over the years, several experimental agents have shown to be effective in animal models. Many experimental compounds have been shown to be safe; however, no compound to date has demonstrated efficacy in humans. The therapies tested include glutamate antagonists, free-radical scavengers, astrocyte inhibitors, and suppressors of 20-HETE.[55] Research continues in this area, in the hope of finding a neuroprotective drug that will reduce the neurological damage caused by stroke. Some agents are being tested in combination with rt-PA. Most compounds being tested today have an extended window of delivery.

Recombinant Factor VIIa Treatment

Currently, there is no specific therapy for the treatment of ICH in the early hours after hemorrhage when expansion of the hematoma occurs. Hematoma expansion is the main reason for morbidity and mortality. Recently, investigators reported results of a trial in which r-Factor VIIa, administered within 4 hours of onset of ICH, reduced hematoma enlargement, improved functional outcome, and reduced mortality.[56] Currently, a large multicenter, multinational, double-blind, randomized trial is underway in order to determine whether the results will be generalizable to a larger population.

Development of Stroke Teams and Organization of Stroke Care

Stroke teams became widely known after the results of the National Institutes of Neurological Disorders and Stroke rt-PA trial, the first hyperacute beneficial treatment for stroke patients, were published in 1995. The U.S. Food and Drug Administration approved rt-PA in 1996, and the paradigm of stroke care at hospitals nationwide began to change. Most stroke teams consist of a neurologist, neuroscience (stroke) nurse, ED physicians, and staff from the radiology department (for emergent neuroimaging). As stroke teams were developed, hospitals designed standardized order sets for the ED, clinical care pathways, and teaching was accelerated to train nursing and medical personnel to deliver new state-of-the-art stroke care.[4,6]

Another result of this paradigm shift was the development of "stroke units." Most hospitals do not offer a specific "stroke unit," but many hospitals have neuroscience units where stroke patients are admitted. Concentrating stroke patients in a single area is advised because of the additional monitoring and skilled care that is needed for the stroke patient. Nursing staff in a designated stroke unit are especially trained in preventing complications likely to occur following a stroke, leading to better patient outcomes.[57,58,59] Several studies have shown lower mortality, lower levels of dependency and or institutionalization, and reduced length of stay when care is delivered in a stroke unit.[57-59]

A European consensus statement set the goal of having all persons with acute stroke admitted to specialized treatment facilities.[60] Stroke units offer a systematic, streamlined approach to patient care, using stroke protocols, preprinted or standing orders, and pathways to facilitate this process.[61] Because stroke units are not uniformly present in the United States, all units within hospitals that admit and treat stroke patients should have clear guidelines and protocols with preprinted order sets to enable consolidated and organized care.

> **BOX 76-8**   ■ ■ ■
> JOINT COMMISSION PERFORMANCE MEASURES FOR PRIMARY STROKE CENTERS
>
> - Tissue plasminogen activator (rt-PA) considered*
> - Deep vein thrombosis prophylaxis*
> - Patients with atrial fibrillation receiving anticoagulation therapy*
> - Discharged on antithrombotic therapy*
> - Screen for dysphasia
> - Antithrombotics within 48 hours of admission to hospital
> - Lipid profile
> - Rehabilitation considered
> - Smoking cessation
> - Stroke education

*Denotes performance measures (initial standardized stroke measure set for pilot testing) that are mandatory for Joint Commission (formerly known as JCAHO) certification.

Primary Stroke Centers

In June 2000, the *Journal of the American Medical Association* published a paper outlining recommendations by the Brain Attack Coalition on designating hospitals as "Stroke Centers." These recommendations called for an organized approach to the care of stroke patients. In 2003, the Joint Commission on Accreditation of Healthcare Organizations (JCAHO, now known as the Joint Commission) developed a mechanism for hospitals to become certified as Primary Stroke Centers. The Joint Commission outlined 10 performance measures that needed consideration in order for a hospital to become certified (Box 76-8).[62] These performance measures should be a part of basic care of the stroke patient but are often neglected in routine care.

SUMMARY

Nursing care of the stroke patient is challenging and complex. Excellent nursing care can make the difference in whether or not the stroke patient has a positive outcome. Comprehensive knowledge of stroke and stroke care is essential to the multidisciplinary approach to care. Promotion of nursing care modalities can serve as a way of advocating for the stroke patient. Nursing care integrates all care areas in a way that threads the continuum of acute care of the stroke patient to long-term secondary prevention. Although researchers continue to investigate novel therapeutic modalities for treatment of acute stroke, excellent bedside nursing care remains the most important factor contributing to favorable long-term outcomes for stroke patients.

REFERENCES

1. Adams HP, Adams R, Brott T et al: Guidelines for the early management of patients with ischemic stroke. A scientific statement from the Stroke Council of the American Heart Association, *Stroke* 34:1056-1083, 2003.
2. Rapp K, Bratina P, Barch C et al: Code stroke: rapid transport, triage, and treatment using rt-PA therapy, *J Neurosci Nurs* 29(5):361-366, 1997.

3. American Heart Association: *Stroke Facts* 2006. All American, Dallas, TX, 2006, American Heart Association.

4. Manzella SM, Galante K: Establishment of stroke treatment plans: one hospital's experience, *J Neurosci Nurs* 32(6):306-310, 2000.

5. Leonard A: *Acute stroke: principles of modern management. General care after stroke, including stroke units and prevention and treatment of complications of stroke.* An unrestricted grant for continuing education, Section 6, St Paul, MN, 2002, American Academy of Neurology.

6. Rice JN, Robichaux CM, Leonard AD: Nervous system alterations: acute stroke. In Sole M, Klein DG, Moseley MJ, editors: *Introduction to critical care,* ed 4, Philadelphia, 2005, Elsevier Saunders, pp. 391-401.

7. Albers GW, Hart RG, Lutsep HL et al: Supplement to the guidelines for the management of transient ischemic attacks. A statement from the Ad Hoc Committee on Guidelines for the Management of Transient Ischemic Attacks, Stroke Council, American Heart Association, *Stroke* 30:2502-2511, 1999.

8. North American Symptomatic Carotid Endarterectomy Trial Collaborators: Beneficial effect of carotid endarterectomy in symptomatic patients with high-grade carotid stenosis, *N Engl J Med* 325(7):445-453, 1991.

9. Hobson RW: CREST (Carotid Revascularization Endarterectomy versus Stent Trial): background, design and current status, *Sem Vasc Surg* 13(2):139-143, 2000.

10. Donnarumma R, Kongable G, Barch C et al: Overview: hyperacute rt-PA stroke treatment, *J Neurosci Nurs* 29(6):351-355, 1997.

11. Castillo J, Dávalos A, Marrugat J et al: Timing for fever-related brain damage in acute ischemic stroke, *Stroke* 29:2455-2460, 1998.

12. Johnston KC, Li JY, Lyden PD et al: Medical and neurological complications of ischemic stroke: experience from the RANTTAS trial, *Stroke* 29:447-453, 1998.

13. Hilker R, Poetter C, Findeisen N et al: Nosocomial pneumonia after acute stroke: implications for neurological intensive care medicine, *Stroke* 34:975, 2003.

14. Sabin-Alverez J, Molina CA, Montaner J et al: Effects of admission hyperglycemia on stroke outcome in reperfused tissue plasminogen activator treated patients, *Stroke* 34:1235, 2003.

15. Mann G, Hankey GJ, Cameron D: Swallowing function after stroke: prognosis and prognostic factors at 6 months, *Stroke* 30:744-748, 1999.

16. FOOD Trial Collaboration: Poor nutritional status on admission predicts outcome after stroke: observational data from the FOOD trial, *Stroke* 34:1450-1456, 2003.

17. Krieger DW, Demchuk AM, Kasner SE et al: Early clinical and radiologic predictors of fatal brain swelling in ischemic stroke, *Stroke* 30:287-292, 1999.

18. Reith J, Jorgensen HS, Nakayama H et al: Seizures in acute stroke: predictors and prognostic significance, The Copenhagen Stroke Study, *Stroke* 28:1585-1589, 1997.

19. The NIH-NINDS and Stroke rt-PA Stroke Study Group: Tissue plasminogen activator for acute ischemic stroke, *N Engl J Med* 333:1581-1587, 1995.

20. Braimah J, Kongable G, Rapp K et al: Nursing care of acute stroke patients after receiving rt-PA therapy, *J Neurosci Nurs* 29(6):373-383, 1997.

21. Spilker J, Kongable G, Barch C et al: Using the NIH stroke scale to assess stroke patients, *J Neurosci Nurs* 29(6):384-391, 1997.

22. Barch C, Spilker J, Bratina P et al: Nursing management of acute complications following rt-PA in acute ischemic stroke, *J Neurosci Nurs* 29(6):367-372, 1997.

23. Gobin YP, Starkman S, Duckwiler G et al: MERCI I: a phase one study of mechanical embolus removal in cerebral ischemia, *Stroke* 35:2848-2854, 2004.

24. American Heart Association: *ACLS provider manual* (case 10), Dallas, TX, 2006, American Heart Association.

25. Bhalla A, Wolfe CDA, Rudd AG: Management of acute physiological parameters after stroke, *QJM* 94:167-172, 2001.

26. Georgiadis D, Schwab S, Hacke W: Critical care of the acute stroke patient. In Mohr JP, Choi D, Grotta J et al, editors: *Stroke: pathophysiology, diagnosis, and management,* ed 4, London, 2004, Churchill Livingstone, pp. 987-1024.

27. Ginsberg MD, Busto R: Combating hyperthermia in acute stroke: a significant clinical concern, *Stroke* 29:529-534, 1998.

28. Rincon F, Mayer SA: Novel therapies for intracerebral hemorrhage, *Curr Opin Crit Care* 10:94-100, 2004.

29. Broderick JP, Adams HP, Barson W et al: AHA Scientific Statement—Guidelines for the Management of Intracerebral Hemorrhage. A Statement for Healthcare Professionals from a Special Writing Group of the Stroke Council, American Heart Association, *Stroke* 30:905-915, 1999.

30. Greer D: Acute stroke and other neurological emergencies. In Layon AJ, Gabrielli A, Friedman WA, editors: *Textbook of neurointensive care,* Philadelphia, 2003, Saunders, pp. 397-436.

31. Kirkness CJ, Thompson JM, Ricker BA et al: The impact of aneurysmal subarachnoid hemorrhage on functional outcome, *J Neurosci Nurs* 34(3):134-141, 2003.

32. Van Gijn J, Rinkel GJE: Subarachnoid hemorrhage: diagnosis, causes and management, *Brain* 124:249-278, 2001.

33. Hickey JV: *The clinical practice of neurological and neurosurgical nursing,* ed 5, Philadelphia, 2003, Lippincott Williams & Wilkins.

34. Bederson JB, Awad IA, Wiebers DO et al: Recommendations for the management of patients with unruptured intracranial aneurysms: a statement for healthcare professionals from the Stroke Council of the American Heart Association, *Circulation* 102:2300-2308, 2000.

35. American Association of Neuroscience Nurses: *AACN core curriculum for neuroscience nursing,* ed 4, Glenview, IL, 2004, American Association of Neuroscience Nurses.

36. Galley HF: *Critical care focus 3: neurological injury,* London, 2003, BMJ Publishing Group.

37. Fisher M, Bogousslavsky J: *Current review of cerebrovascular disease,* ed 4, Philadelphia, 2001, Current Medicine, Inc.

38. Morrison SR: Guglielmi detachable coils: an alternative therapy for surgically high-risk aneurysms, *J Neurosci Nurs* 29(4):232-237, 1997.

39. Schievink WI: Intracranial aneurysms, *N Engl J Med* 336(1):28-40, 1997.

40. Albers GW, Amarenco P, Easton JD et al: Antithrombotic and thrombolytic therapy for ischemic stroke: the Seventh ACCP Conference on Antithrombotic and Thrombolytic Therapy, *Chest* 126(3Suppl):483S-512S, 2004.

41. Deiner HC, Bogousslavsky J, Brass LM et al: Aspirin and clopidogrel compared with clopidogrel alone after recent ischemic stroke or transient ischemic attack in high-risk patients (MATCH): randomized, double-blind, placebo-controlled trial, *Lancet* 364:331-337, 2004.

42. Hankey GJ: Ongoing and planned trials of antiplatelet therapy in the acute and long-term management of patients with ischemic brain syndromes: setting a new standard of care, Review, *Cerebrovascular Diseases* 17(suppl 3):11-16, 2004.

43. Bhatt DL, Keith AA, Fox MB et al: Clopidogrel and aspirin versus aspirin alone for the prevention of atherothrombotic events, *N Engl J Med* 354:1-12, 2006.

44. Singer DE, Albers GW, Dalen JE et al: Antithrombotic therapy in atrial fibrillation: the Seventh ACCP Conference on Antithrombotic and Thrombolytic Therapy, *Chest* 126(suppl 3):429S-56S, 2004.

45. Chobanian AV, Bakris GL, Black HR et al: Seventh Report of the Joint National Committee on Prevention, Detection, Evaluation and Treatment of High Blood Pressure, *Hypertension* 42(6):1206-1252, 2003.

46. Mancia G: Prevention and treatment of stroke in patients with hypertension, *Clinical Therapeutics* 26(3):631-648, 2004.

47. Third Report of the National Cholesterol Education Program (NCEP) Expert Panel on Detection, Evaluation, and Treatment of High Blood Cholesterol in Adults (Adult Treatment Panel III), *Circulation* 106:3143-3421, 2002.

48. Volpe M: Treatment of systolic hypertension: spotlight on recent studies with angiotensin II antagonists, *J Human Hypertension* 19:93-102, 2005.

49. Dahlöf B, Devereux RB, Kjeldsen SE et al: Cardiovascular morbidity and mortality in the Losartan Intervention for Endpoint Reduction in Hypertension Study (LIFE): a randomised trial against atenolol, *Lancet* 359:995-1003, 2002.

50. Kernan WN, Inzucchi SE, Viscoli CM et al : Pioglitazone improves insulin sensitivity among non-diabetic patients with a recent TIA or ischemic stroke, *Stroke* 34:1431-1436, 2003.

51. Nolan JP, Morley PT, Vanden Hock TL et al: 2003 International Liaison Committee on Resuscitation. Therapeutic hypothermia after cardiac arrest: an advisory statement by the Advanced Life Support Task Force of the International Liaison Committee on Resuscitation, *Circulation* 108:118-121, 2003.

52. Mohammad YM, Divani AA, Kirmani JF et al: Acute treatment for ischemic stroke in 2004, *Emerg Radiol* 11:83-86, 2004.

53. Hachimi-Idrissi S, Huyghens L: Resuscitative mild hypothermia as a protective tool in brain damage: is there evidence? *Euro J Emerg Med* 11:335-342, 2004.

54. De Georgia MA, Krieger DW, Abou-Chebl A et al: Cooling for acute ischemic brain damage (COOL AID): a feasibility trial of endovascular cooling, *Neurology* 63:312-317, 2004.

55. Hinkle J: Pharmacology update: neuroprotection for ischemic stroke, *J Neurosci Nurs* 35(2):114-118, 2003.

56. Mayer SA, Brun NC, Begtrup K et al: Recombinant activated factor VII for acute intracerebral hemorrhage, *N Engl J Med* 352(8):777-785, 2005.

57. Jorgensen HS: The Copenhagen Stroke Study experience, *J Stroke Cerebrovascular Diseases* 6:5-15, 1996.

58. Stroke Unit Trialists Collaboration: Collaborative systematic review of randomized trials of organized inpatient (stroke unit) care after stroke, *BMJ* 314:1151-1159, 1997.

59. Jorgensen HS, Nakayama H, Raaschau HO et al: The effect of a stroke unit. Reduction in mortality, discharge rate to nursing home, length of stay and cost, *Stroke* 26:1178-1182, 1995.

60. Abdoderin I, Verables G: Stroke management in Europe. Pan European Consensus Meeting on Stroke Management, *J Intern Med* 240:173-180, 1996.

61. Sinha S, Warburton EA: The evolution of stroke units—towards a more intensive approach? *QJM* 93:633−638, 2000.

62. Joint Commission on Accreditation of Healthcare Organizations Primary Stroke Centers. Available at: *www.jcaho.org/dscc/psc/index.htm*

Using Evidence-Based Practice to Improve Outcomes in Outpatient Settings

Barbara Riegel and Debra K. Moser

Professional nursing has undergone a major transition in practice over the past century. In the late 1800s and the early 1900s, clinical practice in a community setting was routine and the major practice setting for nurses. But, by the middle of the 20th century, professional nurses were employed primarily in hospital settings. It was not until 1965, with the growth of the nurse practitioner movement, that nurses reclaimed their pivotal role in outpatient settings. Since that time, nursing roles have flourished in the outpatient setting. Nurses have taken leadership roles, managing patients, adjusting therapy, and making autonomous decisions.[1]

In this section of the book, you will read about clinics, disease management programs, cardiac rehabilitation, home health, and hospice and palliative care settings where nurses manage the care. Historical forces, such as a decline in the number of physician general practitioners, higher education for nurses, and the rising cost of health care, have promoted these roles. These outpatient settings have evolved to showcase nursing care at its best—interdisciplinary, collaborative, responsible, and patient-focused.

Numerous studies have now documented the positive influence of nursing care on patient outcomes in outpatient settings.[2-4] One reason why nurses have been successful in improving outcomes is their willingness to use clinical guidelines in practice.[5] Several examples of nurse-run clinics in which state-of-the-science care is delivered based on clinical guidelines will be found in this section of the book. Other reasons why nursing care has been associated with positive outcomes include a holistic focus rather than an emphasis on the diagnosed disease. Also, nurses focus on the patient's perspective (e.g., quality of life), which has been shown to improve

satisfaction with care.[6] Nurses are typically proactive, seeking positive outcomes such as better health status, rather than being reactive, simply avoiding complications.

This perspective—holistic, patient-focused, proactive—is epitomized in the education, counseling, and support strategies that nurses use routinely in clinical practice. These strategies are used liberally in outpatient settings and are discussed in detail in this section. One very important aim of education and counseling is promoting self-care and treatment adherence. A recent meta-analysis of 21 studies, 13 related to cardiovascular disease and including 46,847 participants, documented the importance of treatment adherence in decreasing mortality (pooled odds ratio for mortality [good versus poor adherence]: 0.56 [95 percent, CI 0.50 to 0.63]).[7] In work by Stromberg and colleagues,[8] for example, a nurse-run clinic for persons with heart failure improved self-care and increased survival and time to first rehospitalization.

The chapters in this section illustrate the power of nurses to lead care in a direction associated with excellent patient outcomes and responsiveness to patient-centered concerns. These chapters also provide the reader with the knowledge and skills needed to emulate this high-quality care.

1. Fairman J: The roots of collaborative practice: nurse practitioner pioneers' stories, *Nurs Hist Rev* 10:159-174, 2002.
2. Laurant M, Reeves D, Hermens R et al: Substitution of doctors by nurses in primary care, *Cochrane Database Syst Rev* (2):CD001271, 2005.
3. Mundinger MO, Kane RL, Lenz ER et al: Primary care outcomes in patients treated by nurse practitioners or physicians: a randomized trial, *JAMA* 283(1):59-68, 2000.

4. Rudy EB, Davidson IJ, Daly B et al: Care activities and outcomes of patients cared for by acute care nurse practitioners, physician assistants, and resident physicians: a comparison, *Am J Crit Care* 7(4):267-281, 1998.

5. Fletcher L, Thomas D: Congestive heart failure: understanding the pathophysiology and management, *J Am Acad Nurse Pract* 13(6):249-257, 2001.

6. Brostrom A, Johansson P: Sleep disturbances in patients with chronic heart failure and their holistic consequences—what different care actions can be implemented? *Eur J Cardiovasc Nurs* 4(3):183-197, 2005.

7. Simpson SH, Eurich DT, Majumdar SR et al: A meta-analysis of the association between adherence to drug therapy and mortality, *BMJ* 333(7557):15, 2006.

8. Stromberg A, Martensson J, Fridlund B et al: Nurse-led heart failure clinics improve survival and self-care behaviour in patients with heart failure: results from a prospective, randomised trial, *Eur Heart J* 24(11):1014-1023, 2003.

■■■ chapter 77

Management of Dyslipidemia

Lynne T. Braun
Suzanne Hughes

CHAPTER ABBREVIATIONS

ALLHAT—LLT Antihypertensive and Lipid-Lowering Treatment to Prevent Heart Attack Trial—Lipid-Lowering Trial

ASCOT—LLA Anglo-Scandinavian Cardiac Outcomes Trial—Lipid Lowering Arm

ATP III Adult Treatment Panel III

BMI body mass index

CETP cholesteryl ester transfer protein

CHD coronary heart disease

CYP cytochrome P-450

DHA docosahexaenoic acid

EPA eicosapentaenoic acid

FDA Food and Drug Administration

GI glycemic index

GL glycemic load

HDL high-density lipoprotein

HMG Co-A 3-hydroxy-3-methylglutaryl coenzyme A

HPS Heart Protection Study

LDL low-density lipoprotein

MIRACL Myocardial Ischemia Reduction with Aggressive Cholesterol Lowering Trial

MONICA Multinational Monitoring of Trends and Determinants in Cardiovascular Disease

MUFA monounsaturated fatty acid

NCEP National Cholesterol Education Program

PAD peripheral arterial disease

PROSPER Prospective Study of Pravastatin in the Elderly at Risk

PROVE IT—TIMI Pravastatin or Atorvastatin Evaluation and Infection Trial—Thrombolysis in Myocardial Infarction

TLC therapeutic lifestyle changes

TNT Treating to New Targets

TSH thyroid-stimulating hormone

TZD thiazolidinedione

VA-HIT Veterans Affairs High-Density Lipoprotein Cholesterol Intervention Trial

VLDL very-low-density lipoprotein

WHO World Health Organization

As described in Chapter 34, dyslipidemia is a disorder of lipoprotein metabolism, which may include lipoprotein overproduction or deficiency. Dyslipidemias may manifest as an elevation of total cholesterol, low-density lipoprotein **(LDL)** cholesterol, triglyceride level, or a decrease in high-density lipoprotein **(HDL)** cholesterol, or a combined disorder.

Dyslipidemia, specifically hypercholesterolemia, is a major cause of coronary heart disease **(CHD).** Generally, hypercholesterolemia refers to an elevation in LDL cholesterol because, the higher the LDL cholesterol level, the greater the CHD risk.[1] Although national guidelines for cholesterol management have been in place since 1988,[2] under-diagnosis and under-treatment remain substantial health problems. Data from the World Health Organization (WHO) Multinational Monitoring of Trends and Determinants in Cardiovascular Disease (MONICA) Project,[3] conducted in adults 35 to 64 years of age in 19 countries, show that the prevalence of hypercholesterolemia varies across populations from 3 percent to 53 percent in men and from 4 percent to 40 percent in women. However, awareness of hypercholesterolemia is extremely low, ranging from 1 percent to 33 percent in men and from 0 percent to 31 percent in women. When hypercholesterolemia is identified and treated, studies[4,5] show that relatively few patients meet their guideline-suggested cholesterol target levels. In fact, patients in the highest risk category (those with known CHD) rarely meet their cholesterol target level (Figure 77-1).

The Third Report of the National Cholesterol Education Program **(NCEP)** Expert Panel on Detection, Evaluation, and Treatment of High Blood Cholesterol in Adults,[6] known as Adult Treatment Panel **(ATP) III,** provides the complete guidelines on dyslipidemia management. ATP III[6] recommends that adults age 20 or older should have a fasting lipoprotein profile (total cholesterol, triglycerides, HDL cholesterol, and LDL cholesterol) once every 5 years. If a dyslipidemia is identified, follow-up lipoprotein profiles should be performed on a more frequent basis (most likely, annually) or more often during treatment.

A COMPREHENSIVE APPROACH

Patients with dyslipidemia require a comprehensive evaluation. Manifest atherosclerotic disease, including CHD, peripheral vascular disease, cerebrovascular disease, or diabetes, changes the threshold at which treatment should be initiated as well as intensifying treatment goals.

Clinical Evaluation

Clinical evaluation includes a detailed family history with particular attention to premature cardiovascular disease, diabetes, and/or dyslipidemia. Concomitant

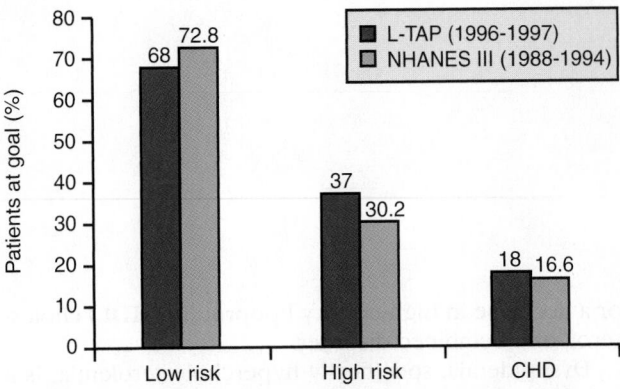

FIGURE 77-1 ■ Graph illustrating that National Cholesterol Education Program targets have not been achieved. *CHD,* Coronary heart disease. *L-TAP,* lipid treatment assessment project; *NHANES,* National Health and Nutrition Examination Survey.

risk factors such as smoking, hypertension, and diabetes should be addressed. A thorough examination includes an evaluation of physical manifestations of dyslipidemia, including xanthomas on the hands, elbows, knees, Achilles tendons, and palms. Skin tags and acanthosis nigricans can indicate insulin resistance. Height, weight, blood pressure, and waist circumference should be measured. Measurement of waist circumference is performed at the end of a normal respiration. Locate the top of the right iliac crest and wrap the tape in a horizontal plane around the abdomen at this level. The tape should be parallel to the floor and should not compress the skin.[7]

Examination should always include the eyes to look for xanthelasmas, corneal arcus (a significant finding in younger patients), and corneal opacities. As described in detail in Chapter 45, the cardiovascular exam should include an evaluation of the peripheral pulses as well as measurement of the ankle-brachial index, which provides a simple and inexpensive measure of peripheral vascular disease and a surrogate measure of generalized atherosclerosis. Depending on the choice of pharmacological therapy, baseline chemistries to evaluate renal and hepatic function prior to initiation may be indicated. Some clinicians obtain a baseline total creatine kinase level for comparison should complaints of myalgias occur on treatment. Additional laboratory tests may be done, depending on the complexity of the dyslipidemia (Box 77-1).

Risk Assessment and LDL Goal Determination

Patients with dyslipidemia often have additional risk factors and/or may have established CHD. The presence of CHD or other risk factors, as well as their magnitude, will influence treatment goals for dyslipidemia, particularly elevated LDL cholesterol. Since epidemiological, laboratory, and clinical investigations indicate that elevated LDL cholesterol is a major cause of CHD, ATP III[6] identifies LDL as the primary (first) target of dyslipidemia management. Table 77-1 displays the ATP III[6] classification of components of the standard lipoprotein profile.

BOX 77-1   ■ ■ ■
LABORATORY TESTS FOR THE DIAGNOSIS
OF COMPLEX DYSLIPIDEMIAS

Fasting lipid profile with:
- Cholesterol
- Triglycerides
- HDL cholesterol
- LDL cholesterol (calculated or directly measured)

The following tests may be helpful in making the diagnosis:
- Lipoprotein separation by ultracentrifugation
- Apo B
- Apo A-I
- Apo E genotype/phenotype
- Lipoprotein(a)

Specialized centers may measure:
- LDL particle size
- LPL assay
- LCAT assay
- Apo E levels
- Apolipoprotein separation by Pore Gradient Lipoprotein Electrophoresis System (PGGE)
- LDL-R assay
- Apo C-II, C-III

APO, Apolipoprotein, *HDL,* high-density lipoprotein; *LDL,* low-density lipoprotein; *LPL,* lipoprotein lipase; *LCAT,* lecithin-cholesterol acyl transferase; *PGGE,* polyacrylamide gradient gel.

■ ■ ■

TABLE 77-1   ATP III CLASSIFICATION OF TOTAL CHOLESTEROL, TRIGLYCERIDES, LDL CHOLESTEROL, AND HDL CHOLESTEROL

Total Cholesterol	
Less than 200 mg/dl	Desirable
200-239 mg/dl	Borderline high
240 mg/dl or greater	High
Triglycerides	
Less than 150 mg/dl	Normal
150-199 mg/dl	Borderline-high
200-499 mg/dl	High
500 mg/ld or greater	Very high
LDL Cholesterol	
Less than 100 mg/dl	Optimal
100-129 mg/dl	Near optimal/above optimal
130-159 mg/dl	Borderline high
160-189 mg/dl	High
190 mg/dl or greater	Very high
HDL Cholesterol	
Less than 40 mg/dl	Low
Greater than or equal to 60 mg/dl	High

From Expert Panel on Detection, Evaluation, and Treatment of High Blood Cholesterol in Adults: Executive Summary of the Third Report of the National Cholesterol Education Program (NCEP) Expert Panel on the Detection, Evaluation, and Treatment of High Blood Cholesterol in Adults (Adult Treatment Panel III), *JAMA* 285:2486-2497, 2001.
ATP III, Adult Treatment Panel III. *HDL,* High-density lipoprotein; *LDL,* low-density lipoprotein.

The presence of risk factors other than elevated LDL cholesterol, CHD, or other forms of atherosclerotic vascular disease, shown in Box 77-2, will modify the LDL goal. Diabetes is not included on the list because it is considered a CHD risk equivalent and carries a risk for major CHD events equal to that of established CHD (more than 20 percent in the next 10 years). Other CHD risk equivalents are clinical forms of atherosclerotic disease (peripheral arterial disease, abdominal aortic

BOX 77-2 ■ ■ ■

MAJOR RISK FACTORS (EXCLUSIVE OF LDL CHOLESTEROL) THAT MODIFY LDL GOALS

- Cigarette smoking
- Hypertension (BP greater than or equal to 140/90 mm Hg or on antihypertensive medication)
- Low HDL cholesterol (less than 40 mg/dl)
- Family history of premature CHD (CHD in male first-degree relative younger than 55 years; CHD in female first-degree relative younger than 65 years)
- Age (men 45 and older; women age 55 and older)

Note: diabetes is regarded as a CHD risk equivalent.
BP, Blood pressure; *CHD*, coronary heart disease; *HDL*, high-density lipoprotein; *LDL*, low-density lipoprotein.
From Expert Panel on Detection, Evaluation, and Treatment of High Blood Cholesterol in Adults: Executive Summary of the Third Report of the National Cholesterol Education Program (NCEP) Expert Panel on the Detection, Evaluation, and Treatment of High Blood Cholesterol in Adults (Adult Treatment Panel III), *JAMA* 285:2486-2497, 2001.

aneurysm, and symptomatic carotid artery disease) and multiple risk factors that confer a 10-year risk for CHD that exceeds 20 percent (when the Framingham risk score is calculated).

In patients without known CHD or other forms of atherosclerotic disease, ATP III[6] recommends that risk determination be performed using a two-step procedure. First, the number of risk factors is counted. Second, if an individual has two or more risk factors, a Framingham risk score is calculated to assess the 10-year risk for developing CHD. The purpose of calculating the Framingham risk score is to determine if a patient requires more intensive management of LDL cholesterol. Men and women have separate Framingham risk scoring systems (Figures 77-2 and 77-3). The risk factors included in the Framingham calculation of 10-year risk are age, total cholesterol, HDL cholesterol,

Framingham Risk Score for Men

Age Years	Points
20–34	-9
35–39	-4
40–44	0
45–49	3
50–54	6
55–59	8
60–64	10
65–69	11
70–74	12
75–79	13

Total Cholesterol (mg/dL)	20–39	40–49	50–59	60–69	70–79
<160	0	0	0	0	0
160–199	4	3	2	1	0
200–239	7	5	3	1	0
240–279	9	6	4	2	1
≥280	11	8	5	3	1

Cigarette Smoking	20–39	40–49	50–59	60–69	70–79
Nonsmoker	0	0	0	0	0
Smoker	8	5	3	1	1

Systolic Blood Pressure	Untreated	Treated
<120	0	0
120–129	0	1
130–139	1	2
140–159	1	2
≥160	2	3

HDL-C (mg/dL)	Points
>60	-1
50–59	0
40–49	1
<40	2

Score = _____
Risk _____
LDL-C goal: _____ mg/dL

CHD Risk Points	10-y Risk(%)
<0	<1
0	1
1	1
2	1
3	1
4	1
5	2
6	2
7	3
8	4
9	5
10	6
11	8
12	10
13	12
14	16
15	20
16	25
≥17	≥30

FIGURE 77-2 ■ Calculation of the Framingham Risk Score for Men. *CHD*, Coronary heart disease; *HDL-C*, high-density lipoprotein cholesterol; *CDL-C*, low-density lipoprotein cholesterol.

Framingham Risk Score for Women

Age Years	Points
20–34	-7
35–39	-3
40–44	0
45–49	3
50–54	6
55–59	8
60–64	10
65–69	12
70–74	14
75–79	16

Total Cholesterol (mg/dL)	20–39	40–49	50–59	60–69	70–79
<160	0	0	0	0	0
160–199	4	3	2	1	1
200–239	8	6	4	2	1
240–279	11	8	5	3	2
≥280	13	10	7	4	2

Cigarette Smoking	20–39	40–49	50–59	60–69	70–79
Nonsmoker	0	0	0	0	0
Smoker	9	7	4	2	1

Systolic Blood Pressure	Untreated	Treated
<120	0	0
120–129	1	3
130–139	2	4
140–159	3	5

HDL-C (mg/dL)	Points
>60	-1
50–59	0
40–49	1
<40	2

Score = _____
Risk _____
LDL-C goal: _____ mg/dL

CHD Risk Points	10-y Risk(%)
<9	<1
9	1
10	1
11	1
12	1
13	2
14	2
15	3
16	4
17	5
18	6
19	8
20	11
21	14
22	17
23	22
24	27
≥25	≥30

FIGURE 77-3 ■ Calculation of the Framingham Risk Score for Women.

systolic blood pressure and whether or not hypertension is treated, and cigarette smoking. Point values are associated with each level of risk factor, and the points are totaled. The total point value is associated with a specific 10-year risk estimation.

Although LDL cholesterol is the primary target of therapy, the Framingham scoring system uses total cholesterol in its calculation because there is a relatively larger database available for total cholesterol values. Only systolic blood pressure is used in the risk estimation. However, if a patient is on antihypertensive drug therapy, an extra point is added because treated hypertension carries a residual risk. In the Framingham scoring system, a patient is identified as a smoker if he/she has smoked in the past month.

Based on the assessment of risk factors and the presence of CHD risk equivalents, ATP III[6] identifies three categories of risk that modify a patient's LDL cholesterol goal (Table 77-2). The first category (highest risk) includes patients with known CHD or CHD risk equivalents. These are individuals who have a greater than 20 percent chance of having a CHD event in the next 10 years. Adults with diabetes are included in this category because they have a 2- to 4-times higher death rate from heart disease than adults without diabetes.[8] Thus, patients with diabetes require a more intensive approach for lowering LDL cholesterol. The LDL cholesterol goal for persons with CHD or CHD risk equivalents is less than 100 mg/dl.

The second category consists of those with two or more risk factors; however, these individuals have a 10-year risk for CHD of 20 percent or less, as estimated by the Framingham risk score.[6] The major risk factors, other than elevated LDL cholesterol (see Box 77-2), are assessed, and, if two or more are present, the LDL cholesterol goal is modified accordingly. For patients with two or more risk factors and a 10-year CHD risk of 20 percent or less, the LDL cholesterol goal is less than 130 mg/dl.

The third category consists of the lowest risk individuals, those with one or no risk factors. These patients have a 10-year CHD risk of less than 10 percent. Their LDL goal is less than 160 mg/dl.[6]

Since the publication of ATP III[6] in 2001, five major clinical trials of statin therapy and clinical end points have been published. These trials are the Heart Protection Study (HPS),[9] the Prospective Study of Pravastatin in the Elderly at Risk (PROSPER),[10] Antihypertensive and Lipid-Lowering Treatment to Prevent Heart Attack Trial—Lipid-Lowering Trial (**ALLHAT—LLT**),[11] Anglo-Scandinavian Cardiac Outcomes Trial—Lipid-Lowering Arm (**ASCOT—LLA**),[12] and the Pravastatin or Atorvastatin Evaluation and Infection Trial—Thrombolysis in Myocardial Infarction 22 (**PROVE IT—TIMI 22**).[13] These recent trials add further support for the ATP III priority of elevated LDL cholesterol.[14] Four of these trials[9,10,12,13] showed that effective LDL lowering significantly reduced CHD risk; however, in one trial,[11] treatment and

■ ■ ■

TABLE 77-2   ADULT TREATMENT PANEL III: UPDATED LDL CHOLESTEROL GOALS AND TREATMENT CUTPOINTS

RISK CATEGORY	LDL GOAL	INITIATE TLC	CONSIDER DRUG THERAPY
High Risk CHD* or CHD risk equivalents† (10-year risk greater than 20%)	Less than 100 mg/dl (optional: less than 70 mg/dl)‡	100 mg/dl or greater	100 mg/dl or greater (less than 100 mg/dl: consider drug options)
Moderately High Risk Greater than or equal to 2 risk factors§ (10-year risk 10% to 20%)	Less than 130 mg/dl (optional: less than 100 mg/dl)	130 mg/dl or greater (100-129 mg/dl: consider drug options)	130 mg/dl or greater
Moderate Risk Greater than or equal to 2 risk factors§ (10-year risk less than 10%)	Less than 130 mg/dl	130 mg/dl or greater	160 mg/dl or greater
Lower Risk 0-1 risk factor	Less than 160 mg/dl	160 mg/dl or greater	190 mg/dl or greater (160-189 mg/dl: LDL cholesterol lowering drug optional)

*CHD includes history of myocardial infarction, unstable angina, stable angina, coronary artery procedures (angioplasty or bypass surgery), or evidence of clinically significant myocardial ischemia.

†CHD risk equivalents include clinical manifestations of noncoronary forms of atherosclerotic disease, abdominal aortic aneurysm, and carotid artery disease (transient ischemic attacks, stroke of carotid origin, or greater than 50% obstruction of a carotid artery), diabetes, and 2+ risk factors with 10-year risk for CHD greater than 20%.

‡Consider the optional LDL cholesterol goal of less than 70 mg/dl in very high-risk patients. This includes patients with established cardiovascular disease plus multiple major risk factors (especially diabetes); severe and poorly controlled risk factors (especially continued cigarette smoking); multiple risk factors of the metabolic syndrome, especially high triglycerides greater than or equal to 200 mg/dl plus non-HDL cholesterol greater than or equal to 130 mg/dl with low high density lipoprotein (HDL) cholesterol; or patients with acute coronary syndromes.

§Risk factors include cigarette smoking, hypertension (blood pressure greater than or equal to 140/90 mmHg or on antihypertensive medication), low HDL cholesterol (less than 40 mg/dl), family history of premature CHD (CHD in male first-degree relative younger than 55 years of age; CHD in female first-degree relative younger than 65 years of age), and age (men older than or equal to 45 years; women older than or equal to 55 years).

From Grundy SM, Cleeman JI, Merz NB et al: Implications of recent clinical trials for the National Cholesterol Education Program Adult Treatment Panel III Guidelines, *Circulation* 110:227-239, 2004.

CHD, Coronary heart disease; *LDL,* low-density lipoprotein; *TLC,* therapeutic lifestyle changes.

control groups did not have a substantial difference in LDL cholesterol and CHD risk reduction. See Chapter 34 for further discussion of these trials.

HPS[9] and PROVE IT[13] demonstrated that additional CHD risk reduction occurred when LDL cholesterol was reduced well below the ATP III target level of less than 100 mg/dl in high-risk patients. The Treating to New Targets (TNT) Trial[15] reduced LDL cholesterol to a mean of 77 and 101 mg/dl with high- and low-dose statin therapy, respectively, in stable CHD patients. A 22 percent relative risk reduction for major cardiovascular events was seen in the high-dose statin group compared to the low-dose statin group. Therefore, it is reasonable to conclude that a lower LDL cholesterol goal may be necessary for high-risk patients. An update[14] to the ATP III guidelines, published in 2004, recommended that clinicians consider an LDL goal of less than 70 mg/dl in the highest risk patients: e.g., those with established cardiovascular disease plus multiple major risk factors (especially diabetes); those with severe and poorly controlled risk factors (especially continued cigarette smoking); those with multiple risk factors of the metabolic syndrome, especially high triglycerides of 200 mg/dl or higher plus non-HDL cholesterol of 130 mg/dl or higher with low HDL cholesterol; or those with acute coronary syndromes. Table 77-2 contains the risk stratification and recommended LDL cholesterol goals according to the ATP III update.

Risk assessment also includes the evaluation of life-habit risk factors and emerging risk factors. These are not included on the list of major risk factors (see Box 77-2) that modify LDL cholesterol goals. Life-habit risk factors include obesity, physical inactivity, and atherogenic diet. These factors are direct targets for clinical intervention. Emerging risk factors, discussed in detail in Chapter 43, include lipoprotein (a), homocysteine, prothrombotic and proinflammatory factors; impaired fasting glucose; and evidence of subclinical atherosclerotic disease. These risk factors signal the need to intensify risk-reduction therapies in select patients.

MODELS OF CARE FOR MANAGING DYSLIPIDEMIA

Over the past few decades, we have gained a much greater understanding of the process of atherosclerosis, the contribution of biological and lifestyle-risk factors, and the efficacy and cost-effectiveness of specific interventions in reducing CHD events.[16] Clinical trials have demonstrated that intensive programs of multifactor risk reduction in patients with CHD were more effective than usual care, slowed the rate of coronary artery luminal narrowing, and reduced hospitalizations for clinical cardiac events.[17,18]

These studies and others[19,20] show that nurse case managers, in collaboration with physicians, provide safe, efficacious care for patients with dyslipidemia. They oversee and coordinate patient care, while maximizing the use of available resources within the health care organization and community. They are well-prepared to address physiological, lifestyle, and emotional issues, while meeting the educational needs of patients. They provide a vehicle for ongoing communication with patients through more frequent office visits and telephone and mail follow-up.[16]

The ATP III guidelines[6] address the need for multidisciplinary methods to help patients and clinicians adhere to recommendations for primary and secondary prevention of CHD. Numerous studies have shown improved outcomes with a collaborative approach to CHD prevention. Murchie and colleagues[21] randomized 1343 CHD patients from general practices to either a nurse-led secondary prevention clinic or usual care. The secondary prevention clinic promoted medical and lifestyle components of secondary prevention, such as aspirin, blood pressure management, lipid management, healthy diet, exercise, and nonsmoking. Significant improvements were shown in the intervention group in all secondary prevention components except for smoking (after 1 year) and were sustained for 4 years (except for exercise). After 4.7 years, death rates were 14.5 percent in the intervention group and 18.9 percent in the control group ($p = 0.038$).

A study by Allen and associates[22] evaluated the effect of a nurse practitioner and physician partnership in the management of lipids in 228 patients with hypercholesterolemia and CHD. Patients were recruited during hospitalization after coronary revascularization and randomized to receive either case management by a nurse practitioner for 1 year after discharge in addition to their usual care, or to usual care enhanced with feedback on lipids to their primary care provider and/or cardiologist. Significantly more patients in the nurse case management group (65 percent) reached the LDL cholesterol target level of less than 100 mg/dl compared with 35 percent of patients in the usual care group. Similar differences between groups were observed in dietary and exercise patterns.

Kinn and Brow[23] described a nurse-managed lipid clinic in the Midwest Heart Specialists practice. Patients received an initial physician evaluation followed by lifestyle counseling by nurses. Risk assessment was performed and treatment goals determined. Nurses continued to provide follow-up care and work with patients on strategies to achieve treatment goals. Lipid clinic patients had extraordinary results: 97 percent had an LDL level noted on the chart (versus 47 percent in the Midwest Heart Specialists general practice and 44 percent in the National Quality Assurance Program), 71 percent were at goal (versus 22 percent and 11 percent, respectively), and 97 percent were taking a lipid-lowering drug (versus 51 percent and 39 percent, respectively).

Similarly, Ryan and colleagues[24] reported on a collaborative care clinic model established to improve the management of high-risk patients with dyslipidemia. Retrospective analysis of 417 patients showed that 56 percent of patients participating in the collaborative care clinic received combination therapy, 41 percent received monotherapy, and only 2 percent were not taking drug therapy. All lipoproteins improved from baseline ($p = <0.001$); 62 percent to 74 percent of patients reached a single lipid goal, while 35 percent achieved combined lipid goals. Of particular importance, the proportion of patients with a Framingham 10-year CHD risk of more than 20 percent was reduced from 6 percent to less than 1 percent.

In summary, collaborative approaches to clinical practice that facilitate aggressive drug and lifestyle treatment strategies are highly effective in assisting patients achieve lipid target levels, initiate and sustain healthy dietary and exercise habits, reduce CHD risk, and reduce mortality.

OVERVIEW OF DYSLIPIDEMIA MANAGEMENT

Although lipid abnormalities encompass more than elevation of LDL cholesterol, ATP III[6] and the updated guidelines[14] identify LDL cholesterol as the primary target of therapy. Other dyslipidemias, e.g., elevated triglycerides and low HDL cholesterol, are secondary targets of therapy. The two methods for lowering LDL cholesterol are therapeutic lifestyle changes (TLC) and drug therapy. TLC—a diet low in saturated fat and cholesterol and increased physical activity—is discussed in detail below. Table 77-2 shows ATP III LDL cholesterol goals and cut-points for TLC and drug therapy according to risk categories.

For high-risk patients (patients with CHD or CHD risk equivalents), the LDL cholesterol goal is less than 100 mg/dl, with an optional goal of less than 70 mg/dl for the highest risk patients. TLC should be started when the LDL is 100 mg/dl or higher; however, whenever a high-risk patient has contributing lifestyle risk factors (e.g., obesity, physical inactivity, elevated triglycerides, low HDL cholesterol, metabolic syndrome), TLC is necessary to modify these risk factors regardless of LDL cholesterol level. Drug therapy should be initiated simultaneously with TLC in high-risk patients who have an LDL cholesterol of 100 mg/dl or higher. However, on the basis of clinical trial evidence, an LDL cholesterol lower than 100 mg/dl can be treated with drug therapy to achieve an LDL cholesterol lower than 70 mg/dl.[14]

For moderately high-risk patients (patients with two or more risk factors and a 10-year CHD risk of 10 percent to 20 percent), the LDL cholesterol goal is lower than 130 mg/dl with a therapeutic optional goal of lower than 100 mg/dl. TLC is necessary when the LDL cholesterol level is 130 mg/dl or higher or for any moderately high-risk patient who has lifestyle risk factors. Drug therapy should be considered in any patient with a LDL cholesterol of 130 mg/dl or higher. However, if the LDL cholesterol is 100 to 129 mg/dl at baseline or on TLC, drug therapy may also be considered to achieve an LDL cholesterol level lower than 100 mg/dl.[14]

Patients at moderate risk (two or more risk factors and a 10-year CHD risk of less than 10 percent) have an LDL cholesterol goal of lower than 130 mg/dl. TLC should be started when LDL cholesterol is 130 mg/dl or higher, and drug therapy is considered when LDL cholesterol is 160 mg/dl or higher. Patients at lower risk (patients with one risk factor or no risk factors) have an LDL cholesterol goal lower than 160 mg/dl. TLC should be started when LDL cholesterol is 160 mg/dl or higher, and drug therapy is considered when LDL cholesterol is 190 mg/dl or higher.[6,14]

NONPHARMACOLOGIC APPROACHES: THERAPEUTIC LIFESTYLE CHANGES

The key features of TLC are (1) reduced intake of saturated fat and cholesterol, (2) the option of adding plant stanols/sterols (2 g/day) and viscous (soluble) fiber (10 to 25 g/day) to enhance LDL cholesterol lowering, (3) weight reduction, and (4) increased physical activity. ATP III[6] guidelines recommend that dietary therapy be initiated for 6 weeks for patients with elevated LDL cholesterol; however for high-risk patients (CHD or CHD risk equivalents), drug therapy is started concurrently. After 6 weeks of diet alone in intermediate or low-risk patients, other therapeutic options for LDL lowering can be added, such as plant stanols/sterols and viscous fiber. All sedentary patients who can engage in physical activity should be counseled on a physical activity program. Patients with metabolic syndrome should receive weight reduction and physical activity counseling.

Nutritional Management

Whether or not lipid-altering drug therapy is necessary for a given patient, a heart-healthy diet is an essential facet of CHD risk reduction. The nutrient components of the TLC diet are listed in Table 77-3. The total fat intake may range from 25 percent to 35 percent of total calories, predominantly in the form of unsaturated fatty acids, which will help reduce triglycerides and increase HDL cholesterol. Less than 7 percent of total calories should come from saturated fat (found in meat, dairy products, and tropical oils) and a very low intake of trans-fatty acids (found in commercially prepared fried foods, baked goods, snack foods, and hard margarine) is advised.

■ ■ ■

TABLE 77-3   NUTRIENT COMPONENTS OF THE THERAPEUTIC LIFESTYLE CHANGES (TLC) DIET

NUTRIENT	RECOMMENDED INTAKE
Saturated fat*	Less than 7% of total calories
Polyunsaturated fat	Up to 10% of total calories
Monounsaturated fat	Up to 20% of total calories
Total fat	25-35% of total calories
Carbohydrate†	50-60% of total calories
Fiber	20-30 grams/day
Protein	Approximately 15% of total calories
Cholesterol	Less than 200 mg/day
Total calories (energy)‡	Balance energy intake and expenditure to maintain desirable body weight/prevent weight gain

*Trans fatty acids are another low-density lipoprotein (LDL)-raising fat that should be minimized.
†Carbohydrates should be derived predominantly from foods rich in complex carbohydrates including grains (especially whole grains) fruits, and vegetables.
‡Daily energy expenditure should include at least moderate physical activity (contributing approximately 200 kcal per day).
From Expert Panel on Detection, Evaluation, and Treatment of High Blood Cholesterol in Adults: Executive Summary of the Third Report of the National Cholesterol Education Program (NCEP) Expert Panel on the Detection, Evaluation, and Treatment of High Blood Cholesterol in Adults (Adult Treatment Panel III), *JAMA* 285:2486-2497, 2001.

The major saturated fatty acids that raise cholesterol levels are lauric acid, myristic acid, and palmitic acid. When vegetable oils are partially hydrogenated to make them more solid, trans-fatty acids are produced. The process of hydrogenation has become common in the United States because it produces products low in cost, long in shelf life, and appropriate for commercial frying.[25] Saturated fats and trans-fatty acids elevate LDL cholesterol levels, with the strongest association between trans-fatty acids and CHD risk.[26] Fortunately, oils and margarines low in trans-fatty acids, as well as prepared snacks and other food items, are now readily available.

The two major types of polyunsaturated fat are omega-6 and omega-3 fatty acids. Linoleic acid is the predominant omega-6 fatty acid in the diet and is found in certain vegetable oils (e.g., soybean oil, corn oil, and high-linoleic forms of sunflower and safflower seed oils). Linoleic acid can reduce LDL cholesterol when substituted for saturated fat in the diet; however, increased intake is not recommended because of a lack of safety data.[25] ATP III[6] recommends that up to 10 percent of total calories come from polyunsaturated fatty acids. Most omega-3 fatty acids in the American diet are found in fish (e.g., herring, mackerel, salmon, tuna, rainbow trout). The omega-3 fatty acids are eicosapentaenoic acid **(EPA)** and docosahexaenoic acid **(DHA)**. Two decades ago, Greenland Eskimos, who consume a diet high in omega-3 fatty acids, were observed to have a low incidence of CHD. Recent studies have shown that weekly fish consumption is associated with a lower CHD death rate and a reduction in cardiac arrest.[27,28] The American Heart Association recommends at least two servings of fish per week.[29] Fish oil capsules in doses of 3 to 12 g daily are sometimes used in treatment of severe hypertriglyceridemia.

Up to 20 percent of total calories should be in the form of monounsaturated fatty acids **(MUFAs)**. The primary MUFA found in the diet is oleic acid, which is present in canola and olive oil and high in oleic forms of sunflower and safflower seed oils. Other good sources of MUFAs are avocados and nuts (almonds, pecans, walnuts, hazelnuts, peanuts, macadamia nuts). The diet of Mediterranean countries (Spain, Italy, and Greece) is high in MUFAs, mostly from high olive oil consumption, which has been shown to be protective against CHD. Similar to polyunsaturated fatty acids, MUFAs have a beneficial effect on the lipoprotein profile.[30]

Dietary cholesterol intake should be maintained at less than 200 mg/day[6] because a higher intake raises plasma cholesterol levels in some individuals. Individual differences are thought to arise from the percentage of dietary cholesterol absorbed in the intestine and the efficiency of converting cholesterol to bile acids in the liver. Key sources of dietary cholesterol are egg yolks, animal fat, and meat. If the ingestion of egg yolks and animal fat is kept at a minimum, the cholesterol in lean meat and low-fat and fat-free dairy products should not be a huge concern.[25]

The ATP III[6] guidelines recommend a carbohydrate intake of 50 percent to 60 percent of total calories. Carbohydrates are dietary sugars and starches. Although they do not influence LDL cholesterol level, a high intake of carbohydrates may elevate triglycerides and lower HDL cholesterol, which are the two lipid-related features of the metabolic syndrome. Refined sugar intake should be minimized; instead, intake of complex carbohydrates is advised (e.g., fruits, vegetables, whole-grain breads and cereals, legumes), which will also increase dietary fiber content.

Glycemic index **(GI)** is a useful way to evaluate the quality of carbohydrates. The GI ranks carbohydrates based on their rate of glycemic response. The GI scale is from 0 to 100, with higher values given to foods that cause a rapid rise in blood glucose. Carbohydrates with a low GI break down more slowly and release glucose gradually into the blood stream. Glycemic load **(GL)** is a measure of the density and digestion speed of carbohydrates (GL = GI/100 × Net Carbs—net carbs are equal to the total carbohydrates minus dietary fiber).[31] Foods with a low GI and a low GL include items such as apples, kidney beans, peanuts, and all-bran cereal. A recent study[32] showed that a high dietary GL predicts CHD risk. To lower the GL, which will reduce triglycerides and raise HDL cholesterol, the diet should be increased in the percent of calories from complex carbohydrates, protein, fat, or a combination of all three.[33]

The TLC diet includes 20 to 30 g of fiber each day, predominantly consisting of soluble (viscous) fiber. Soluble fiber found in oat beta-glucan and psyllium seed husk carry a Food and Drug Administration–approved health claim for reducing CHD risk. Studies have determined that 3 g per day of beta-glucan or 7 g per day of psyllium lowers LDL cholesterol by 4 percent to 5 percent. Other viscous fibers, such as pectin and guar gum, are available as dietary supplements; however, less data are available on viscous fibers regarding cholesterol-lowering ability.[33] Good food sources of soluble fiber are oat bran, dried beans and peas, barley, oranges, apples, and carrots.

Plant Sterols and Stanols

Plant (phyto) sterols and stanols lower cholesterol by reducing cholesterol absorption in the intestines. When incorporated into a fat medium, such as margarine, they have been shown to lower LDL cholesterol by 7 percent to 15 percent.[33] Two spreads are commercially available—Benecol (containing plant stanols) and Take Control (containing plant sterols)—along with Benecol chews. ATP III[6] recommends 2 g per day of plant stanols/sterols to enhance LDL cholesterol lowering, which corresponds to a daily intake of 2 tablespoons of spread or 4 chews. It is important to teach patients that these products must be used in the recommended amounts in order to achieve LDL cholesterol reduction.

Increased Physical Activity

Forty percent of American adults report engaging in no leisure-time physical activity, and only 15 percent achieve the public health recommendation of moderate physical activity for 30 minutes 5 or more days per week.[34] However, regular physical activity is important in both primary and secondary prevention of cardiovascular disease. Regular aerobic exercise has a beneficial effect on the lipoprotein profile and improves all of the other modifiable CHD risk factors. The predominant effects on the lipoprotein profile are a decrease in triglycerides and a dose-dependent increase in HDL cholesterol. Although most studies do not show a significant exercise effect on total or LDL cholesterol, LDL particle size increases.[35] The amount of weekly exercise (versus intensity) seems to be the most important variable for influencing lipoprotein changes, indicating that exercise should be at moderate intensity for 30 to 60 minutes, 5 to 7 days per week. Counseling patients on moderate-intensity exercise is a safe practice for patients with risk factors who do not have known CHD or symptoms of CHD. Patients with CHD or symptoms of CHD should have a stress test prior to initiating a regular exercise program.[36]

Weight Reduction

Over the past two decades, the prevalence of obesity has significantly increased in the United States, as discussed in detail in Chapter 36. Thirty percent of U.S. adults are obese. However, this health problem is not limited to adults. The percentage of overweight children and teens has more than tripled since 1980. Among children and teens ages 6 to 19, 16 percent are considered overweight. Overweight and obesity are associated with numerous health problems, such as hypertension, dyslipidemia, type 2 diabetes, CHD, stroke, gallbladder disease, osteoarthritis, sleep apnea, and certain cancers.[37]

In adults, overweight is defined as a body mass index (**BMI**) of 25 kg/m^2 or above; obesity is defined as a BMI of 30 kg/m^2 or above. Abdominal obesity tends to impart the greatest health risk, which is identified by an increased waist circumference (men more than 40 inches; women more than 35 inches). Both BMI and waist circumference should be measured in clinical practice at baseline and during follow-up to evaluate the effectiveness of weight loss interventions.

Weight loss in overweight/obese patients benefits the lipoprotein profile in patients with dyslipidemia, specifically by reducing triglycerides and increasing HDL cholesterol. However, low-fat diets decrease HDL cholesterol.[33] The most successful strategies for weight loss are calorie reduction, increased physical activity, and behavior therapy to facilitate adherence to healthy eating and physical activity habits. The initial goal should be a 10 percent weight reduction in 6 months, with a weight loss of 1 to 2 pounds per week. This corresponds to a calorie deficit of 500 to 1000 kcal/day.[38] Many nurses feel comfortable teaching patients about a heart-healthy diet and the importance of portion control for weight loss. ATP III[6] guidelines suggest that patients be referred to registered dietitians for precise dietary counseling. While patients are awaiting this appointment, it is helpful to ask them to keep a diet diary by writing down all foods consumed, as well as the amounts, during a given day over a 2-week period. A diet diary provides an excellent vehicle for discussion.

DRUG THERAPY FOR DYSLIPIDEMIA

Based on the magnitude of LDL cholesterol level and risk status, patients may require LDL-lowering drug therapy in addition to TLC to reach the appropriate LDL cholesterol goal. Several clinical trials in primary and secondary prevention of CHD have demonstrated that LDL cholesterol lowering reduces CHD events and mortality. In addition to a current lipoprotein panel, other baseline laboratory tests should be obtained prior to the initiation of drug therapy, specifically a metabolic panel, liver enzymes, and a thyroid-stimulating hormone (**TSH**) level. These assessments are important to detect baseline abnormalities in kidney and liver function that may worsen with medication and to rule out secondary causes of dyslipidemia, such as hypothyroidism, type 2 diabetes, cholestatic liver disease, nephrotic syndrome, and chronic renal failure.

After 12 weeks of drug therapy, the response to therapy should be assessed by repeating the lipid panel and any necessary safety tests (e.g., liver enzymes with statin therapy). Patients should be questioned about symptoms of adverse effects. If the LDL cholesterol goal is not achieved, drug therapy should be intensified, and frequent follow-up should continue. After the LDL cholesterol goal is attained, the focus may switch to other lipid (elevated triglycerides, low HDL cholesterol) and nonlipid risk factors (obesity, physical inactivity). When medication use is stabilized, patients should be assessed every 4 to 6 months for response to therapy (lipid panel, safety laboratory tests). More frequent clinic visits may be necessary for reinforcement and monitoring of TLC. Although age is not a reason to withhold dyslipidemia drug therapy, older patients require careful monitoring due to diminished renal function and may require lower doses.

Statins

The 3-hydroxy-3-methylglutaryl-coenzyme A (**HMG-CoA**) reductase inhibitors (statins) are the primary drugs used to lower LDL cholesterol because of their effectiveness, safety profile, and tolerance (Table 77-4). Statins inhibit the rate-limiting enzyme (HMG-CoA reductase) for cholesterol biosynthesis in the liver and thus decrease cholesterol synthesis. The six available statins differ in the magnitude of their LDL cholesterol lowering (17 percent to 63 percent) and their effect on triglycerides and HDL cholesterol[39] (Table 77-5). In addition to having a potent LDL cholesterol-lowering effect, statins have been shown to reduce CHD events and mortality in primary and secondary prevention trials.[9,10,12,40-45] The HPS[9] showed that older patients, men and women alike, and patients with diabetes receive the same risk-reducing benefits of statin therapy. More recently, pleiotropic (unanticipated) effects of statins have been recognized, namely the antiinflammatory, antioxidant, and plaque-stabilizing effects and the increased bioavailability of nitric oxide, a potent vasodilator.[46]

■■ ■

TABLE 77-4   SUMMARY OF HMG-CoA REDUCTASE INHIBITORS

AVAILABLE DRUGS*	LOVASTATIN, PRAVASTATIN, SIMVASTATIN, FLUVASTATIN, ATORVASTATIN, ROSUVASTATIN†
Lipid/lipoprotein effects	LDL cholesterol - ↓ 18-55% HDL cholesterol - ↓ 5-15% Triglycerides - ↓ 7-30%
Major use	To lower LDL cholesterol
Contraindications	
Absolute	Active or chronic liver disease
Relative	Concomitant use of cyclosporine, macrolide antibiotics, various antifungal agents, and cytochrome P-450 inhibitors (fibrates and nicotinic acid should be used with appropriate caution)
Efficacy	Reduce risk for CHD and stroke
Safety	Side effects minimal in clinical trials
Major side/adverse effects	Myopathy, increased liver transaminases
Usual starting dose	Lovastatin - 20 mg Pravastatin - 20 mg Simvastatin - 20 mg Fluvastatin - 20 mg Atorvastatin - 10 mg Rosuvastatin - 10 mg
Maximum FDA-approved dose	Lovastatin - 80 mg Pravastatin - 80 mg Simvastatin - 80 mg Fluvastatin - 80 mg Atorvastatin - 80 mg Rosuvastatin - 40 mg
Available preparations	Lovastatin - 10, 20, 40 mg tablets Pravastatin - 10, 20, 40 mg tablets Simvastatin - 5, 10, 20, 40, 80 mg tablets Fluvastatin - 20, 40 mg capsules, 80 mg XL tablets Atorvastatin - 10, 20, 40, 80 mg tablets Rosuvastatin - 10, 20, 40 mg tablets

*Cerivastatin was withdrawn from the market by the manufacturer in August, 2001.
†Rosuvastatin released after publication of ATP III.
From Expert Panel on Detection, Evaluation, and Treatment of High Blood Cholesterol in Adults: Executive Summary of the Third Report of the National Cholesterol Education Program (NCEP) Expert Panel on the Detection, Evaluation, and Treatment of High Blood Cholesterol in Adults (Adult Treatment Panel III), *JAMA* 285:2486-2497, 2001.
FDA, Food and Drug Administration; *CHD,* coronary heart disease; *LDL,* low-density lipoprotein; *HDL,* high-density lipoprotein; *HMG-CoA,* 3-hydroxy-3-methylglutaryl coenzyme A

Statins as a class of drugs have an excellent safety profile. However, they exhibit differences in metabolism through the cytochrome P-450 (CYP) system, as shown in Table 77-5. They have the potential for interacting with other drugs that use the same enzyme system for metabolism; e.g., both simvastatin and erythromycin use the CYP3A4 system. Other drugs metabolized by the CYP3A4 isoenzyme include cyclosporine, fibrates, antifungal drugs, certain antidepressants, and protease inhibitors. Providers should discuss the use of other medications with patients on statin therapy, and often a safer statin or an alternative medication can be chosen. Grapefruit juice inhibits intestinal CYP3A4 and can increase serum concentrations of CYP3A4 medications. Therefore, grapefruit juice consumption should be separated from the dose of CYP3A4 statin (atorvastatin, simvastatin, lovastatin) by 2 hours.[33] The well-publicized adverse effects of statin therapy are an increase in liver enzymes, myopathy, and the extremely rare condition of rhabdomyolysis. Patients must be alerted to all potential adverse effects. If they complain of muscle aches, it is prudent to check a creatine kinase level.

Cholesterol Absorption Inhibitors

Ezetimibe is in the newest class of LDL cholesterol-lowering agents (Table 77-6). It selectively inhibits the absorption of cholesterol at the brush border of the small intestine. Ezetimibe is extremely well tolerated as a single 10 mg tablet and may be used either alone or in combination with a statin to achieve additional LDL cholesterol lowering. In fact, a combination tablet of simvastatin and ezetimibe is available. Ezetimibe reduces LDL cholesterol an average of 18 percent, and, when used in combination with a statin, an additional 12 percent to 15 percent LDL cholesterol reduction may be expected. Adverse effects reported with ezetimibe are gastrointestinal problems, arthralgia, and back pain; however, these occur rarely.

Bile Acid Sequestrants

Bile acid sequestrants reduce LDL cholesterol by interrupting the enterohepatic circulation of bile acids (Table 77-7). They bind with bile acids in the intestine and cause excretion into the feces; therefore, more choles-

■■ ■

TABLE 77-5   CHARACTERISTICS OF HMG-CoA REDUCTASE INHIBITORS (STATINS)

STATIN	DOSE RANGE (mg)	LDL CHOLESTEROL REDUCTION (%)	ELIMINATION HALF-LIFE (HOURS)	SOLUBILITY	CYTOCHROME P450 METABOLISM AND ISOENZYME	OPTIMAL TIME OF ADMINISTRATION
Atorvastatin	10-80	38-54	15-30	Lipophilic	3A4	Evening
Fluvastatin	20-80	17-33	0.5-2.3	Lipophilic	2C9	Bedtime
Lovastatin	20-80	29-48	2.9	Lipophilic	3A4	With meals (AM and PM)
Pravastatin	10-80	19-40	1.3-2.8	Hydrophilic	—	Bedtime
Rosuvastatin	5-40	52-63	19	Hydrophilic	Limited 2C9	Anytime
Simvastatin	10-80	28-48	2-3	Lipophilic	3A4, 3A5	Evening

From Rosenson RS: Lipid lowering with statins, *UpToDate©,* 2005, *www.uptodate.com,* accessed April 30, 2005.
HMG-CoA, 3-hydroxy-3-methylglutaryl coenzyme A; *LDL,* low-density lipoprotein.

■ ■ ■

TABLE 77-6 SUMMARY OF INTESTINAL ABSORPTION BLOCKERS*

AVAILABLE DRUG	EZETIMIBE (ZETIA)
Lipid/lipoprotein effects	LDL cholesterol - ↓ 13% HDL cholesterol - ↑ 1 % Triglycerides - ↓ 8 %
Major uses	Primary hypercholesterolemia
Contraindications	Hypersensitivity to any component of the medication
Efficacy	
Safety	When used as monotherapy, the incidence of elevations of serum transaminases was similar to placebo. Avoid combining with fibrates.
Major side/adverse effects	Generally well tolerated
Usual daily dose	Zetia 10 mg every day
Maximum daily dose	Zetia 10 mg every day
Available preparations	10 mg tablets
Monitoring parameters and follow-up	Lipid effects

*Released after the NCEP Guidelines
HDL, High density lipoprotein; *LDL*, low density lipoprotein.

■ ■ ■

TABLE 77-7 SUMMARY OF BILE ACID SEQUESTRANTS

AVAILABLE DRUGS	CHOLESTYRAMINE, COLESTIPOL, COLESEVELAM
Lipid/lipoprotein effects	LDL cholesterol - ↓ 15-30% HDL cholesterol - ↓ 3-5% Triglycerides - no effect or increase
Major use	To lower LDL cholesterol
Contraindications	Familial dysbetalipoproteinemia
Absolute	Triglycerides greater than 400 mg/dl
Relative	Triglycerides greater than 200 mg/dl
Efficacy	Clinical trial evidence of CHD risk reduction Clinical trial evidence of lack of systemic toxicity
Safety	Gastrointestinal side effects common
Major side/adverse effects	Upper and lower gastrointestinal complaints common Decrease absorption of other drugs
Usual daily dose	Cholestyramine — 4-16 g Colestipol — 5-20 g Colesevelam — 2.6-3.8 g
Maximum daily dose	Cholestyramine — 24 g Colestipol — 30 g Colesevelam — 4.4 g
Available preparations	Cholestyramine — 9 g packets (4 g drug), 378 g bulk Cholestyramine — 5 g packets (4g drug) "light"—210 g bulk Colestipol — 5 g packets (5g drug), 450 g bulk, 1 g tablets Colesevelam — 625 mg tablets

From Expert Panel on Detection, Evaluation, and Treatment of High Blood Cholesterol in Adults: Executive Summary of the Third Report of the National Cholesterol Education Program (NCEP) Expert Panel on the Detection, Evaluation, and Treatment of High Blood Cholesterol in Adults (Adult Treatment Panel III), *JAMA* 285:2486-2497, 2001.
HDL, High-density lipoprotein; *LDL*, low-density lipoprotein.

terol from the liver is required to produce bile acids. Bile acid sequestrants are cumbersome to take because of frequency and large quantities and often difficult to tolerate because of gastrointestinal side effects (e.g., bloating, constipation). Colesevelam, the newest agent in this class, is more potent and better tolerated than the older agents (cholestyramine and colestipol). Bile acid sequestrants can also be added to statin therapy for additional LDL cholesterol lowering.

Niacin

Nicotinic acid (niacin) is a soluble B vitamin that beneficially impacts the entire lipid profile (Table 77-8). Niacin reduces secretion of Apo B, an apolipoprotein associated with very-low-density lipoprotein (**VLDL**) and LDL, thereby lowering these lipoproteins. It decreases the hepatic uptake of Apo A-I, the apolipoprotein associated with HDL, and therefore increases HDL cholesterol. Niacin is the most potent drug for raising HDL cholesterol and is commonly given to lower triglycerides. Niacin also

■ ■ ■

TABLE 77-8 SUMMARY OF NICOTINIC ACID

AVAILABLE DRUGS	CRYSTALLINE NICOTINIC ACID, SUSTAINED-RELEASE (OR TIMED-RELEASE) NICOTINIC ACID, EXTENDED-RELEASE NICOTINIC ACID (NIASPAN)
Lipid/lipoprotein effects	LDL cholesterol - ↓ 5-25% HDL cholesterol - ↑ 15-35% Triglycerides - ↓ 20-50%
Major use	Useful in most lipid and lipoprotein abnormalities
Contraindications	
Absolute	Chronic liver disease, severe gout
Relative	Hyperuricemia; high doses in type 2 diabetes
Efficacy	Clinical trial evidence of CHD risk reduction
Safety	Serious long-term side effects rare for crystalline form; serious hepatotoxicity may be more common with sustained-release form
Major side/adverse effects	Flushing, hyperglycemia, hyperuricemia or gout, upper gastrointestinal distress, hepatotoxicity, especially for sustained-release form
Usual daily dose	Crystalline nicotinic acid — 1.5-3 g Sustained-release nicotinic acid — 1-2 g Extended-release nicotinic acid (Niaspan®) — 1-2 g
Maximum daily dose	Crystalline nicotinic acid — 4.5 g Sustained-release nicotinic acid — 2 g Extended-release nicotinic acid (Niaspan) — 2 g
Available preparations	Many over-the-counter preparations by various manufacturers for both crystalline and sustained-release nicotinic acid. The extended-release preparation (Niaspan) is a prescription drug.

The American Heart Association recently recommended the dietary niacin should not be not be used as a substitute for prescription niacin and should not be used for lowering cholesterol because of potential very serious side effects.
From Expert Panel on Detection, Evaluation, and Treatment of High Blood Cholesterol in Adults. Executive Summary of the Third Report of the National Cholesterol Education Program (NCEP) Expert Panel on the Detection, Evaluation, and Treatment of High Blood Cholesterol in Adults (Adult Treatment Panel III), *JAMA* 285:2486-2497, 2001.
CHD, Coronary heart disease; *HDL*, high-density lipoprotein; *LDL*, low-density lipoprotein.

reduces lipoprotein (a) [Lp(a)], an LDL particle with an Apo(a) attached, which when elevated, increases CHD risk through enhanced atherogenesis and thrombosis.

The use of niacin in clinical practice requires extensive patient education due to tolerance issues. The prescription form, Niaspan™, is better tolerated, albeit more expensive, than over-the-counter preparations. The most common side effect is a prostaglandin-mediated subcutaneous vasodilatation that causes flushing and pruritus. Flushing usually diminishes after the first couple of weeks and can be reduced by taking niacin with a low-fat snack and taking an aspirin or ibuprofen 30 minutes before taking niacin. Patients should avoid concomitant intake of alcohol, spicy food, and hot liquids. Niacin is started at a low dose and titrated slowly. Niacin can cause hepatotoxicity; therefore, liver enzymes should be monitored. This is a particular issue for patients who use over-the-counter niacin, especially sustained–release preparations. Other adverse effects include gastrointestinal distress and an elevation in uric acid and blood glucose level. Niacin should not be used in patients with hyperuricemia and should be cautiously used in diabetic patients with careful monitoring of glucose control.

Niacin may be added to a statin in patients with combined hyperlipidemia (elevated LDL cholesterol and elevated triglycerides), especially if the HDL cholesterol is low or Lp(a) is high. A combination tablet containing both lovastatin and Niaspan™ is available. Monitoring for myopathy and hepatotoxicity is needed although these adverse effects are rare.

New agents for raising HDL cholesterol are currently in development and testing. Among these are the cholesteryl ester transfer protein **(CETP)** inhibiting drugs. CETP facilitates the transport of cholesteryl ester from HDL to apolipoprotein B containing particles (VLDL and LDL). CETP inhibition results in an increased level of HDL cholesterol and reduced levels of VLDL and LDL cholesterol. A vaccine has been shown to inhibit CETP by inducing the production of autoantibodies against the protein. Torcetrapib was a CETP inhibitor that showed great promise, because HDL increased by 61 percent when combined with atorvastatin in patients with low HDL cholesterol. However, a Phase 3 trial was recently stopped due to an increased mortality rate in patients receiving the combination compared to atorvastatin alone. Other CETP inhibitors currently are being studied in clinical trials.[47] The PPAR drugs (peroxisome proliferation activated receptor agonists) are medications that raise HDL cholesterol levels by stimulating a pro-HDL gene. However, the research on these drugs is not as developed as that for the CETP inhibitors. Human infusion studies with apoA-I Milano/ phospholipids complexes elevate HDL cholesterol and show a regression in total atheroma volume by intravascular ultrasound. Unfortunately, apoA-I must currently be given intravenously; therefore, it cannot be used for chronic therapy.[48]

Fibric Acid Derivatives

Two fibric acid derivatives (fibrates) are available in the United States, gemfibrozil and fenofibrate (Table 77-9). These medications increase activity of the enzyme, lipo-

■ ■ ■

TABLE 77-9   SUMMARY OF FIBRIC-ACID DERIVATIVES

AVAILABLE DRUGS	GEMFIBROZIL, FENOFIBRATE, FENOFIBRATE (MICRONIZED)
Lipid/lipoprotein effects	LDL cholesterol - ↓ 5-20% (in nonhypertriglyceridemic persons); may be increased in hypertriglyceridemic persons HDL cholesterol - ↑ 10-35% (more in severe hypertriglyceridemia) Triglycerides - ↓ 20-50%
Major uses	Hypertriglyceridemia, atherogenic dyslipidemia
Contraindications	Severe hepatic or renal insufficiency
Efficacy	Clinical trials indicate a moderate reduction in CHD risk
Safety	Serious side effects seemingly do not occur in the long term, although early studies suggested an increase in non-CHD mortality
Major side/adverse effects	Dyspepsia, various upper gastrointestinal complaints, cholesterol gallstones, myopathy
Usual daily dose	Gemfibrozil - 600 mg bid Fenofibrate - 160 mg daily Fenofibrate (micronized) 200 mg daily
Maximum daily dose	Gemfibrozil - 1200 mg Fenofibrate - 160 mg Fenofibrate(micronized) 200 mg
Available preparations	Gemfibrozil - 600 mg tablets Fenofibrate - 54 and 160 mg tablets Fenofibrate (micronized) 67, 134, and 200 mg capsules

Clofibrate is no longer available, dosages of fenofibrate have changed, micronized fenofibrate has been added.
From Expert Panel on Detection, Evaluation, and Treatment of High Blood Cholesterol in Adults. Executive Summary of the Third Report of the National Cholesterol Education Program (NCEP) Expert Panel on the Detection, Evaluation, and Treatment of High Blood Cholesterol in Adults (Adult Treatment Panel III), *JAMA* 285:2486-2497, 2001.
CHD, Coronary heart disease; *HDL*, high-density lipoprotein; *LDL*, low-density lipoprotein.

protein lipase, which causes greater catabolism of the triglyceride-rich lipoproteins (VLDLs). They also increase expression of Apo A-I. Therefore, fibrates reduce triglycerides and increase HDL cholesterol.[33] Fibrates compare favorably with statins in outcome trials. In the Veterans Affairs High-Density Lipoprotein Cholesterol Intervention Trial **(VA-HIT)**,[49] gemfibrozil reduced CHD events 22 percent in men with CHD and low HDL cholesterol.

The fibrates are usually well-tolerated. Adverse effects include upper gastrointestinal distress, headache, and myalgia. They are contraindicated in hepatic and renal dysfunction and preexisting gallbladder disease. Drug interactions may occur with other drugs that are highly protein bound or are metabolized through the CYP3A4 pathway. Statin-fibrate combinations should be used with caution. Statin doses should be low, and patients should be asked about muscle aches. Fenofibrate is the better choice for statin-fibrate combination therapy because fenofibrate can be taken as a single dose in the morning and the statin taken in the evening. This helps to avoid drug levels peaking at about the same time.[33] Gemfibrozil is usually dosed at 600 mg twice a day 30 minutes before the morning and evening meals. The new formulation of fenofibrate is 145 mg (48 mg for patients with renal insufficiency) once a day and can be taken with or without food. (See accompanying feature on alternative approaches to dyslipidemia management.)

Oral Hypoglycemics

Several of the medications used for the management of type 2 diabetes may have beneficial effects on lipid levels. The thiazolidinediones (TZDs) reduce hyperglycemia via their insulin- sensitizing effect. Studies on the two available TZDs, rosiglitazone and pioglitazone, demonstrate a tendency to raise total cholesterol and LDL, while decreasing triglyceride levels and raising HDL. Pioglitazone appears to have a more favorable effect on HDL and triglycerides than rosiglitazone.[50-52]

LIPID LOWERING IN ACUTE CORONARY SYNDROME, CEREBROVASCULAR DISEASE, AND PERIPHERAL ARTERIAL DISEASE

Extensive clinical trial evidence shows favorable outcomes with aggressive lipid-lowering therapy in patients with acute coronary syndrome, cerebrovascular disease, and peripheral arterial disease. The Myocardial Ischemia Reduction with Aggressive Cholesterol Lowering (MIRACL) study[53] evaluated treatment with atorvastatin 80 mg or placebo soon after hospital admission in 3086 patients with unstable angina or non–Q-wave acute myocardial infarction with respect to recurrent ischemic events and death. Patients were followed for 16 weeks. Atorvastatin treatment lowered recurrent ischemic events by 26 percent in the first 16 weeks compared with placebo; however, there were no differences in mortality or the composite end point of death or myocardial infarction.

PROVE IT—TIMI 22 trial[54] compared standard LDL cholesterol lowering to 100 mg/dl with pravastatin 40 mg with more intensive LDL cholesterol lowering to 70 mg/dl with atorvastatin 80 mg in 4162 patients hospitalized for acute coronary syndrome. After an average of 24 months of follow-up, there was a 16 percent reduction in death or major cardiovascular events with high-dose atorvastatin therapy. In an effort to understand the beneficial mechanism of early statin therapy, Okazaki and associates[55] assessed if early aggressive lipid lowering with atorvastatin reduced plaque volume by stabilizing vulnerable plaques in nonculprit lesions in 70 patients with acute coronary syndrome. Volumetric intravascular ultrasound analyses at baseline and 6 months showed a significant reduction in plaque volume in the atorvastatin group versus an increase in the placebo group. Change in plaque volume was significantly correlated with LDL cholesterol reduction.

Some of the statin trials in patients with CHD have shown a reduction in stroke events with treatment as well as a reduction in cardiovascular events.[43,44,56] A metaanalysis of 38 randomized trials of primary and secondary CHD prevention with lipid-lowering therapies showed a 17 percent relative risk reduction of strokes, with statin trials reducing stroke incidence by 26 percent.[57] Limited data are available on the secondary stroke prevention; however, a trial that is near completion is evaluating the effect of statin treatment in patients who previously had a stroke or transient ischemic attack but who have no history of CHD.

Recent studies show that statin use improves leg functioning in patients with peripheral arterial disease (PAD). In patients with low ankle brachial indices, statin therapy was associated with better 6-minute walk performance, faster walking velocity, and a higher summary performance score. These results were independent of cholesterol levels.[58] In a randomized, placebo-controlled, double-blind study, 86 hypercholesterolemic patients with PAD and intermittent claudication received either simvastatin 40 mg daily or placebo for 6 months. Simvastatin patients experienced a significant increase in pain-free walking distance, total walking distance, ankle brachial indices at rest and after exercise, and an improvement in claudication symptoms compared with patients in the placebo group.[59] A 12-month study with atorvastatin showed similar improvements in pain-free walking distance and community-based physical activity; however, maximal walking time was unchanged.[60]

Statin therapy has proven to be beneficial in patients with all forms of atherosclerosis not just coronary atherosclerosis. Therefore, ATP III recognizes all patients with atherosclerosis as CHD risk equivalents, considers them high-risk, and recommends aggressive LDL-lowering. According to the updated guidelines, many of

---

ALTERNATIVE THERAPIES ■ ■ ■

APPROACHES TO DYSLIPIDEMIA MANAGEMENT

Many supplements are touted to improve cholesterol levels in a safer and more "natural" way than prescription medications. However, supplements are not regulated by the Food and Drug Administration; therefore, the active ingredients lack standardization. There is also less clinical trial data pertaining to a supplement's efficacy and long-term safety than prescription medications. Nonetheless, some patients are intolerant to conventional medical therapy or insist upon supplement use. Nurses should be familiar with the following supplements and their effects.

Supplement	Effects
Omega-3 fatty acids (fish oil capsules) (2-4 g/day of EPA plus DHA)	↓ triglycerides
Soy protein (at least 25 g/day)	↓ LDL cholesterol, ↓ triglycerides ↑ HDL cholesterol
Garlic	Conflicting data for cholesterol
Psyllium (7 g/day)	↓ LDL cholesterol
Plant stanols/sterols (2 g/day)	↓ LDL cholesterol
Polycosinol	↓ LDL cholesterol, ↑ HDL cholesterol
Red yeast rice	↓ LDL cholesterol
Guggulipid	↓ LDL cholesterol, ↓ triglycerides ↑ HDL cholesterol
Pantothenic acid	↓ LDL cholesterol, ↓ triglycerides ↑ HDL cholesterol
Inositol hexanicotinate (flush-free niacin)	↓ LDL cholesterol, ↓ triglycerides ↑ HDL cholesterol

DHA, Docosahexaenoic acid; EPA, eicosapentaenoic acid.

these patients qualify for an LDL target of less than 70 mg/dl (see Table 77-2).

Pharmacotherapy may not be sufficient for those with marked hypercholesterolemia, particularly those with familial hyperlipidemia. In such cases, LDL apheresis may be used, which is an extracorporeal removal method available in specialized centers. LDL apheresis uses filtration, adsorption, or precipitation of LDL at weekly or biweekly intervals.[61] This treatment may relieve ischemic symptoms and be lifesaving.[62]

MANAGEMENT OF SPECIFIC DYSLIPIDEMIAS

The Metabolic Syndrome as a Secondary Target of Therapy

The metabolic syndrome is a constellation of risk factors that, when occurring together, significantly increase risk for CHD.[63] See Chapter 37 for a detailed discussion of metabolic syndrome. The underlying factors that promote the development of the metabolic syndrome are overweight/obesity, sedentary lifestyle, and an atherogenic diet (high saturated fat, high carbohydrate). Therefore, first-line therapies for lipid and nonlipid risk factors of the metabolic syndrome are weight reduction, increased physical activity, and the TLC diet (often with some carbohydrate restriction, especially simple sugars).[6,64] This approach should occur in concert with appropriate control of LDL cholesterol, if necessary. Weight reduction will contribute to LDL cholesterol lowering and treat all of the risk factors of the metabolic syndrome. Increasing physical activity facilitates weight loss and also benefits the other risk factors. If triglycerides remain high and HDL is low, nicotinic acid (niacin) and/or a fibric acid derivative (fibrate) may be necessary either alone or in combination with a statin.

Elevated Triglycerides

Elevated triglycerides increase risk of CHD, especially in women. VLDLs are the most triglyceride-rich lipoproteins, and, when partially degraded, these remnant lipoproteins are considered to be atherogenic. Certain factors play a role in elevated triglycerides, such as overweight/obesity, sedentary lifestyle, cigarette smoking, excess alcohol intake, high carbohydrate diets (more than 60 percent of calories), several diseases (type 2 diabetes, chronic renal failure, nephrotic syndrome), medications (corticosteroids, estrogens, retinoids, higher doses of beta-adrenergic blockers, certain agents used in treating human immunodeficiency virus [HIV] infection),[65] and genetic disorders (familial combined hyperlipidemia, familial hypertriglyceridemia, and familial dysbetalipoproteinemia).[6] Elevated triglycerides are also a risk factor indicating the metabolic syndrome. The ATP III classification of serum triglycerides is presented in Table 77-10.

VLDL is a clinical measurement of atherogenic remnant lipoproteins and, like LDL, can be a target for therapy. ATP III[6] distinguishes the sum of LDL and VLDL (all atherogenic lipoproteins) as a secondary target of therapy for persons with elevated triglycerides (200 mg/dl or higher). This is termed *non-HDL cholesterol* and is calculated by subtracting HDL cholesterol from total cholesterol. The goal for non-HDL cholesterol is 30 mg/dl higher than the LDL cholesterol goal (Table 77-11).

The treatment of elevated triglycerides depends on severity and cause. First, the LDL cholesterol goal should be achieved. When triglycerides are borderline high (150 to 199 mg/dl), the patient is counseled on weight reduction (if overweight) and increased physical activity. When triglyceride level is high (200 to 499 mg/dl), non-HDL cholesterol is a secondary target of therapy. Weight reduction and physical activity should always be part of the intervention plan; however, drug therapy can be considered as well. Either the LDL-lowering drug regimen can be intensified or a second drug (nicotinic acid or a fibrate) can be added. Whenever combination therapy is used, patients must be thor-

■ ■ ■

TABLE 77-10 ADULT TREATMENT PANEL (ATP) III CLASSIFICATION OF TRIGLYCERIDES

Normal triglycerides	Less than 150 mg/dl
Borderline-high triglycerides	150-199 mg/dl
High triglycerides	200-499 mg/dl
Very high triglycerides	Greater than or equal to 500 mg/dl

From Expert Panel on Detection, Evaluation, and Treatment of High Blood Cholesterol in Adults: Executive Summary of the Third Report of the National Cholesterol Education Program (NCEP) Expert Panel on the Detection, Evaluation, and Treatment of High Blood Cholesterol in Adults (Adult Treatment Panel III), *JAMA* 285:2486-2497, 2001.

■ ■ ■

TABLE 77-11 LDL CHOLESTEROL AND NON-HDL CHOLESTEROL GOALS ACCORDING TO RISK CATEGORIES

RISK CATEGORY	LDL GOAL (MG/DL)	NON-HDL GOAL (MG/DL)
CHD and CHD risk equivalent	Less than 100	Less than 130 (10-year risk for CHD greater than 20%)
Multiple (greater than or equal to 2) risk factors and 10-year risk less than or equal to 20%	Less than 130	Less than 160
0-1 risk factor	Less than 160	Less than 190

From Expert Panel on Detection, Evaluation, and Treatment of High Blood Cholesterol in Adults: Executive Summary of the Third Report of the National Cholesterol Education Program (NCEP) Expert Panel on the Detection, Evaluation, and Treatment of High Blood Cholesterol in Adults (Adult Treatment Panel III), *JAMA* 285:2486-2497, 2001.
CHD, Coronary heart disease; *HDL,* high-density lipoprotein; *LDL,* low-density lipoprotein.

oughly evaluated for side effects. For patients who have very high triglycerides (500 mg/dl or higher), triglycerides must be lowered to prevent pancreatitis. Patients should be counseled on a diet extremely low in fat (15 percent or less of calories) as well as weight reduction, physical activity, and cessation of alcohol. Either a fibrate or nicotinic acid is prescribed. When triglycerides are reduced below 500 mg/dl, LDL cholesterol lowering is also addressed to reduce CHD risk.[6] If another condition is present with hypertriglyceridemia, such as type 2 diabetes, this condition must be treated and controlled, which will help normalize the triglyceride level.

Low HDL Cholesterol

A low level of HDL cholesterol (less than 40 mg/dl) is also considered a risk factor for CHD since HDL is cardioprotective. Low HDL cholesterol is associated with other facets of insulin resistance, such as elevated triglycerides, overweight/obesity, sedentary lifestyle, and type 2 diabetes. Cigarette smoking, a very high carbohydrate diet (greater than 60 percent of calories), and certain drugs (beta blockers, anabolic steroids, progestational agents) lower HDL cholesterol.[6]

The management of low HDL cholesterol should be addressed after achieving the LDL cholesterol goal. If the metabolic syndrome is present, treatment should then focus on weight reduction and physical activity counseling. When low HDL cholesterol is associated with a triglyceride level of 200 to 499 mg/dl, the secondary target of therapy is the non-HDL goal, which is achieved through diet, exercise, and possibly drug therapy. If low HDL cholesterol is associated with triglycerides less than 200 mg/dl (isolated low HDL cholesterol), drug therapy with nicotinic acid or a fibrate can be considered.[6]

CONCLUSION

Dyslipidemia management often includes a complex regimen of one or more medications, a special diet, an exercise program, possibly smoking cessation, regular blood tests, and follow-up appointments. Although this type of plan is consistent with clinical practice guidelines, it is a challenge to implement for most patients and to incorporate these changes into their daily lives. It is no surprise that adherence rates for medications are approximately 50 percent and much lower for lifestyle behavior changes such as exercise and diet therapy.[66]

A comprehensive plan for cholesterol and lifestyle goal attainment requires a coordinated effort involving actions by patients, providers, and health care organizations.[67] Nurses with a keen interest in cardiovascular disease prevention are vital to this coordinated plan (Table 77-12). Nurse case-managed systems have shown excellent outcomes in cardiovascular risk reduction, specifically dyslipidemia treatment. Nurses may require additional education and training in behavior change techniques in order to impact motivation and goal attainment with their patients.[67,68] But nurses bring important skills and opportunities that make them ideal for these roles. For example, nurses are often afforded more time with patients than physicians are. Nurses are excellent at active listening to patients' concerns and helping to simplify treatment regimens. They are expert educators and often initiate telephone follow-up as well as interim office appointments to reinforce education, provide support, and reward patients for their adherence efforts. They incorporate successful adherence strategies, such as written instructions, reminders, and self-monitoring. A comprehensive approach to dyslipidemia management, with nurses at the forefront, is vital for reducing the morbidity and mortality of cardiovascular disease.

■ ■ ■

TABLE 77-12 MONITORING PARAMETERS AND FOLLOW-UP SCHEDULE

DRUG	MONITORING PARAMETERS	FOLLOW-UP SCHEDULE
Bile acid sequestrants	Indigestion, bloating, constipation, abdominal pain, flatulence, nausea	Evaluate symptoms initially, and at each follow-up visit. Also check time of administration with other drugs.
Nicotinic acid	Flushing, itching, tingling, headache, nausea, gas, heartburn, fatigue, rash	Evaluate symptoms initially, and at each follow-up visit.
	Peptic ulcer	Evaluate symptoms initially, then as needed.
	Fasting blood sugar (FBS) Uric acid	Obtain an FBS and uric acid initially, 6-8 weeks after starting therapy, then annually or more frequently if indicated.
	Alanine transaminase (ALT), Aspartate aminotransferase (AST)	Obtain an ALT/AST initially, 6-8 weeks after reaching a daily dose of 1500 mg, 6-8 weeks after reaching the maximum daily dose, then annually or more frequently if indicated
Statins	Muscle soreness, tenderness, or pain	Evaluate muscle symptoms and creatine kinase (CK) initially. Evaluate muscle symptoms at each follow-up visit. Obtain a CK when persons have muscle soreness, tenderness, or pain.
	ALT, AST	Evaluate ALT/AST initially, approximately 12 weeks after starting, then annually or more frequently if indicated.
Fibrates	Abdominal pain, dyspepsia, headache, drowsiness	Evaluate symptoms initially and at each follow-up visit.
	Cholelithiasis	Evaluate history and symptoms initially and then as needed.

From Expert Panel on Detection, Evaluation, and Treatment of High Blood Cholesterol in Adults: Executive Summary of the Third Report of the National Cholesterol Education Program (NCEP) Expert Panel on the Detection, Evaluation, and Treatment of High Blood Cholesterol in Adults (Adult Treatment Panel III), *JAMA* 285:2486-2497, 2001.

REFERENCES

1. Stamler J, Wentworth D, Neaton J: Is relationship between serum cholesterol and risk of premature death from coronary heart disease continuous and graded? Findings in 356,222 primary screenees of the Multiple Risk Factor Intervention Trial (MRFIT), *JAMA* 256:2823-2828, 1986.

2. Report of the National Cholesterol Education Program Expert Panel on Detection, Evaluation, and Treatment of High Blood Cholesterol in Adults, *Arch Intern Med* 148:36-69, 1988.

3. Tolonen H, Keil U, Ferrario M and et al for the WHO MONICA Project: Prevalence, awareness and treatment of hypercholesterolaemia in 32 populations: results from the WHO MONICA Project, *Int J Epidemiol* 34:181-192, 2005.

4. Jacobson TA, Griffiths GG, Varas C et al: Impact of evidence-based "clinical judgment" on the number of American adults requiring lipid-lowering therapy based on updated NHANES III data, *Arch Intern Med* 160:1361-1369, 2000.

5. Pearson TA, Laurora I, Chu H et al: The lipid treatment assessment project (L-TAP): a multicenter survey to evaluate the percentages of dyslipidemic patients receiving lipid-lowering therapy and achieving low-density lipoprotein cholesterol goals, *Arch Intern Med* 160:459-467, 2000.

6. Expert Panel on Detection, Evaluation, and Treatment of High Blood Cholesterol in Adults: Executive Summary of the Third Report of the National Cholesterol Education Program (NCEP) Expert Panel on the Detection, Evaluation, and Treatment of High Blood Cholesterol in Adults (Adult Treatment Panel III), *JAMA* 285:2486-2497, 2001.

7. Grundy SM, Cleeman JI, Daniels SR et al: Diagnosis and management of the metabolic syndrome: An American Heart Association/National Heart, Lung, and Blood Institute Scientific Statement: Executive Summary, *Circulation* 25;112:e285-290, 2005. Epub Sep 12, 2005.

8. American Heart Association: *Heart disease and stroke statistics—2007 update*, Dallas, TX, 2007, American Heart Association.

9. Heart Protection Study Collaborative Group: MRC/BHF Heart Protection Study of cholesterol lowering with simvastatin in 20,536 high-risk individuals: a randomized placebo-controlled trial, *Lancet* 360:7-22, 2002.

10. Shepherd J, Blauw GJ, Murphy MB et al: Pravastatin in elderly individuals at risk of vascular disease (PROSPER): a randomized controlled trial. PROspective Study of Pravastatin in the Elderly at Risk. *Lancet* 360:1623-1630, 2002.

11. ALLHAT Officers and Coordinators for the ALLHAT Collaborative Research Group: The Antihypertensive and Lipid-Lowering Treatment to Prevent Heart Attack Trial. Major outcomes in moderately hypercholesterolemic, hypertensive patients randomized to pravastatin vs usual care: the Antihypertensive and Lipid-Lowering Treatment to Prevent Heart Attack Trial (ALLHAT-LLT), *JAMA* 288:2998-3007, 2002.

12. Sever PS, Dahlof B, Poulter NR et al: Prevention of coronary and stroke events with atorvastatin in hypertensive patients who have average or lower-than-average cholesterol concentrations, in the Anglo-Scandinavian Cardiac Outcomes Trial—Lipid Lowering Arm (ASCOT—LLA): a multicentre randomized controlled trial, *Lancet* 361:1149-1158, 2003.

13. Cannon CP, Braunwald E, McCabe CH et al: Intensive versus moderate lipid lowering with statins after acute coronary syndromes, *N Engl J Med* 350:1495-1504, 2004.

14. Grundy SM, Cleeman JI, Merz NB et al: Implications of recent clinical trials for the National Cholesterol Education Program Adult Treatment Panel III Guidelines, *Circulation* 110:227-239, 2004.

15. LaRosa JC: TNT: *Treating to New Targets*. Presented at the American College of Cardiology 2005 Annual Scientific Sessions, March, 2005.

16. Allen JK: Cholesterol management: an opportunity for nurse case managers, *J Cardiovasc Nurs* 14:50-58, 2000.

17. DeBusk RF, Miller NH, Superko HR et al: A case-management system for coronary risk factor modification after acute myocardial infarction, *Ann Intern Med* 120:721-729, 1994.

18. Haskell WL, Alderman EL, Fair JM et al: Effects of intensive multiple risk factor reduction on coronary atherosclerosis and clinical cardiac events in men and women with coronary artery disease. The Stanford Coronary Risk Intervention Project (SCRIP), *Circulation* 89:975-990, 1994.

19. Shaffer J, Wexler LF: Reducing low-density lipoprotein cholesterol levels in an ambulatory care system, *Arch Intern Med* 155:2330-2335, 1995.

20. Becker DM, Raqueno JV, Yook RM et al: Nurse-medicated cholesterol management compared with enhanced primary care in siblings of individuals with premature coronary disease, *Arch Intern Med* 58:1533-1539, 1998.

21. Murchie P, Campbell NC, Lewis DR et al: Secondary prevention clinics for coronary heart disease: four year follow up of a randomized controlled trial in primary care, *BMJ* 326:1-6, 2003.

22. Allen JK, Blumenthal RS, Margolis S et al: Nurse case management of hypercholesterolemia in patients with coronary heart disease: results of a randomized clinical trial, *Am Heart J* 144:678-686, 2003.

23. Kinn JW, Brown AS: Cardiovascular risk management in clinical practice: the Midwest Heart Specialists experience, *Am J Cardiol* 89:23C-29C, 2002.

24. Ryan MJ, Gibson J, Simmons P et al: Effectiveness of aggressive management of dyslipidemia in a collaborative-care practice model, *Am J Cardiol* 91:1427-1431, 2003.

25. Gotto A, Pownall H: *Manual of lipid disorders. Reducing the risk for coronary heart disease*, ed 3, Philadelphia, 2003, Lippincott Williams & Wilkins.

26. Hu FB, Manson JE, Willett WC: Types of dietary fat and risk of coronary heart disease: a critical review, *J Am Coll Nutr* 20:5-19, 2001.

27. Daviglus ML, Stamler J, Orencia AJ et al: Fish consumption and the 30-year risk of fatal myocardial infarction, *N Engl J Med* 336:1046-1053, 1997.

28. Albert CM, Hennekens CH, O'Donnell CJ et al: Fish consumption and risk of sudden cardiac death, *JAMA* 279:23-28, 1998.

29. Krauss RM, Eckel RH, Howard B et al: AHA dietary guidelines. Revision 2000. a statement for healthcare professionals from the Nutrition Committee of the American Heart Association, *Circulation* 102:2284-2299, 2000.

30. Kris-Etherton PM, for the Nutrition Committee: Monounsaturated fatty acids and risk of cardiovascular disease, *Circulation* 100:1253-1258, 1999.

31. *Http://www.nutritiondata.com/glycemic-index.html*, accessed 9/22/2005.

32. Liu S, Willett WC, Stampfer MJ et al: A prospective study of dietary glycemic load, carbohydrate intake, and risk of coronary heart disease in US women, *Am J Clin Nutr* 71:1455-1461, 2000.

33. Davidson MH: *The mobile lipid clinic. A companion handbook*, Philadelphia, 2002, Lippincott Williams & Wilkins.

34. U.S. Department of Health and Human Services: *Healthy people 2010. understanding and improving health*, ed 2, Washington, DC, November, 2000, Government Printing Office.

35. Kraus WE, Houmard JA, Duscha BD et al: Effects of the amount and intensity of exercise on plasma lipoproteins, *N Engl J Med* 347:1483-1492, 2002.

36. American College of Sports Medicine: *ACSM's guidelines for exercise testing and prescription*, sixth ed, Philadelphia, Lippincott Williams & Wilkins, 2000.

37. *Http://www.cdc.gov/nccdphp/dnpa/obesity*, accessed April 28, 2005.

38. National Institutes of Health: *Clinical guidelines on the identification, evaluation, and treatment of overweight and obesity in adults*, Bethesda, MD, 1998, National Institutes of Health.

39. Rosenson RS: Lipid lowering with statins, *UpToDate©*, 2005, *www.uptodate.com*, accessed April 30, 2005.

40. Shepherd J, Cobbe SM, Ford I et al: Prevention of coronary heart disease with pravastatin in men with hypercholesterolemia. West of Scotland Coronary Prevention Study Group, *N Engl J Med* 333:1301-1307, 1995.

41. Downs JR, Clearfield M, Weis S et al: Primary prevention of acute coronary events with lovastatin in men and women with average cholesterol levels: results of AFCAPS/TexCAPS. Air Force/Texas Coronary Atherosclerosis Prevention Study, *JAMA* 279:1615-1622, 1998.

42. Simes J, Furberg CD, Braunwald E et al: Effects of pravastatin on mortality in patients with and without coronary heart disease across a broad range of cholesterol levels. The Prospective Pravastatin Pooling Project, *Eur Heart J* 23:207-215, 2002.

43. Randomised trial of cholesterol lowering in 4444 patients with coronary heart disease: the Scandinavian Simvastatin Survival Study (4S), *Lancet* 344:1383-1389, 1994.

44. Prevention of cardiovascular events and death with pravastatin in patients with coronary heart disease and a broad range of initial cholesterol levels. The Long-Term Intervention with Pravastatin in Ischaemic Disease (LIPID) Study Group, *N Engl J Med* 339:1349-1357, 1998.

45. Sacks FM, Pfeffer MA, Moye LA et al : The effect of pravastatin on coronary events after myocardial infarction in patients with average cholesterol levels. Cholesterol and Recurrent Events Trial Investigators, *N Engl J Med* 335:1001-1009, 1996.

46. Davignon J: Beneficial cardiovascular pleiotropic effects of statins, *Circulation* 109 (23 Suppl 1):III39-43, 2004.

47. Anonymous. Cholesterol: the good, the bad, and the stopped trials. *The Lancet* 368:2034, 2006.

48. Brewer HB, Remaley AT, Newfeld EB et al: Regulation of plasma high-density lipoprotein levels by the ABCA1 transporter and the emerging role of high-density lipoprotein in the treatment of cardiovascular disease, *Arterioscler Thromb Vasc Biol* 24:1755-1760, 2004.

49. Rubins HB, Robins SJ, Collins D et al : Gemfibrozil for the secondary prevention of coronary heart disease in men with low levels of high-density lipoprotein cholesterol. Veterans Affairs High-Density Lipoprotein Cholesterol Intervention Trial Study Group, *N Engl J Med* 341:410-418, 1999.

50. van Wijk JP, de Koning EJ, Martens EP et al: Thiazolidinediones and blood lipids in type 2 diabetes, *Arterioscler Thromb Vasc Biol* 23:1744-1749, 2003.

51. Yki-Jarvinen H: Thiazolidinediones, *N Engl J Med* 351:1106-1118, 2004.

52. Krauss RM: Lipids and lipoproteins in patients with type 2 diabetes, *Diabetes Care* 27:1496-1504, 2004.

53. Schwartz GG, Olsson AG, Ezekowitz MD et al: Effects of atorvastatin on early recurrent ischemic events in acute coronary syndromes. The MIRACL Study: a randomized controlled trial, *JAMA* 285:1711-1718, 2001.

54. Cannon CP, Braunwald E, McCabe CH et al: Intensive versus moderate lipid lowering with statins after acute coronary syndromes, *N Engl J Med* 350:1495-1504, 2004.

55. Okazaki S, Yokoyama T, Miyauchi K et al: Early statin treatment in patients with acute coronary syndrome. Demonstration of the beneficial effect on atherosclerotic lesions by serial volumetric intravascular ultrasound analysis during half a year after coronary event: The ESTABLISH Study, *Circulation* 110:1061-1068, 2004.

56. Plehn JF, Davis BR, Sacks FM et al: Reduction of stroke incidence after myocardial infarction with pravastatin: the Cholesterol and Recurrent Events (CARE) Study, *Circulation* 99:216-223, 1999.

57. Corvol JJ-C, Bouzamondo A, Sirol M et al: Differential effects of lipid-lowering therapies on stroke prevention. A meta-analysis of randomized trials, *Arch Intern Med* 163:669-676, 2003.

58. McDermott MM, Guralnik JM, Greenland P et al: Statin use and leg functioning in patients with and without lower-extremity peripheral arterial disease, *Circulation* 107:757-761, 2003.

59. Mondillo S, Ballo P, Barbati R et al: Effects of simvastatin on walking performance and symptoms of intermittent claudication in hypercholesterolemic patients with peripheral vascular disease, *Am J Med* 114:359-364, 2003.

60. Mohler III ER, Hiatt WR, Creager MA: Cholesterol reduction with atorvastatin improves walking distance in patients with peripheral arterial disease, *Circulation* 108:1481-1486, 2003.

61. Thompson GR: LDL apheresis, *Atherosclerosis* 167:1-13, 2003.

62. Bambauer R, Schiel R, Latza R: Low density lipoprotein apheresis in treatment of hyperlipidemia: experience with four different technologies, *Ther Apheresis* 4:213-217, 2000.

63. Grundy SM, Brewer HB, Cleeman JI et al: Definition of metabolic syndrome. Report of the National Heart, Lung, and Blood Institute/American Heart Association Conference on Scientific Issues Related to Definition, *Circulation* 109:433-438, 2004.

64. Grundy SM, Hansen B, Smith SC et al: Clinical management of metabolic syndrome. Report of the American Heart Association/National Heart, Lung, and Blood Institute/American Diabetes Association Conference on Scientific Issues Related to Management, *Circulation* 109:551-556, 2004.

65. Armstrong W, Calabrese L, Taege AJ: HIV update 2005. origins, issues, prospects, complications, *Cleveland Clinic J Med* 72:73-78, 2005.

66. Haynes RB, McDonald HP, Garg AX: Helping patients follow prescribed treatment. Clinical applications, *JAMA* 288:2880-2883, 2002.

67. Miller NH, Hill M, Kottke T et al for the Expert Panel on Compliance: The multilevel compliance challenge: recommendations for a call to action, *Circulation* 95:1085–1090, 1997.

68. Burke LE, Fair J: Promoting prevention. Skill sets and attributes of health care providers who deliver behavioral interventions, *J Cardiovasc Nurs* 18:256-266, 2003.

Management of Hypertension

Nancy T. Artinian
Carolyn B. Yucha
Jennifer Dungan

CHAPTER ABBREVIATIONS

AAMI American Association for the Advancement of Medical Instrumentation

ABP ambulatory blood pressure

ACE angiotensin-converting enzyme

ARB angiotensin receptor blocker

BB beta blocker

BHS British Hypertension Society

BMI body mass index

BP blood pressure

CCB calcium channel blocker

CMS Centers for Medicare and Medicaid Services

DASH Dietary Approaches to Stop Hypertension

HF heart failure

HTN hypertension

JNC VII Seventh Report of the Joint National Committee on Prevention, Detection, Evaluation, and Treatment of High Blood Pressure

MI myocardial infarction

Cardiovascular nurses in clinical practice, especially those in advanced practice, must be able to provide comprehensive health assessments and demonstrate a high level of autonomy and skill in the diagnosis and treatment of patients with hypertension **(HTN).** As described in Chapter 35, a large percentage of Americans with HTN is either unaware they have HTN, or, if they are aware of their HTN, it is untreated or uncontrolled. Unless those who are untreated or without adequate treatment receive evidence-based care, as outlined in the Seventh Report of the Joint National Committee on Prevention, Detection, Evaluation, and Treatment of High Blood Pressure **(JNC VII)** guidelines,[1] they will be at higher risk for stroke, myocardial infarction **(MI),** heart failure, and end-stage renal disease.[1] This chapter reviews the classification, assessment, and diagnosis of HTN; nonpharmacologic and pharmacologic therapy for HTN; and models of care for HTN.

DEFINITION AND CLASSIFICATION OF HYPERTENSION

Hypertension is defined as a systolic blood pressure **(SBP)** of at least 140 mm Hg and/or diastolic BP of at least 90 mm Hg, or taking antihypertensive medication.[2,3] The JNC VII has introduced a new classification for HTN[1] that specifically counters the previously held notion that mildly elevated BP is normal (Table 78-1). In earlier JNC guidelines, patients with significantly elevated BP could be classified as having stage 3 HTN. These individuals are now categorized under stage 2 HTN. The JNC-VII classification includes the new category of pre-HTN for those with BP ranging from 120 to 139 mm Hg systolic and/or 80 to 89 mm Hg diastolic BP.[1] This category of pre-HTN is intended to identify those at risk for developing HTN and those who could benefit from preventive interventions.

ASSESSMENT OF PATIENTS WITH HYPERTENSION

Assessment of patients with HTN includes a medical history (Box 78-1), including over-the-counter medications and herbal supplements (see the accompanying Alternative Therapy box) physical examination (Box 78-2), and laboratory assessment (Table 78-2) in order to (1) assess lifestyle and identify other cardiovascular risk factors or other comorbidities that may affect prognosis and/or guide treatment, (2) reveal identifiable causes of high BP, and (3) assess the presence or absence of target organ damage.[1] Currently genetic profiling is not part of a routine diagnostic workup. (See the accompanying Genetics feature.)

Measurement of Blood Pressure

Accurate BP measurement is an important component of the physical examination. Blood pressure classification is based on the average of two or more properly measured, seated BP readings on each of two or more office visits.[1] Before classifying BP as high, great care must be taken to measure it accurately (Box 78-3).

Conventional clinic BP measurements often give a poor representation of average or true BP. Even when the recommended procedure is used, there are innumerable sources of error related to the patient, the operator, and the environment. BP changes throughout the day and is influenced by various stimuli. It is altered by activity (e.g., waking, sleeping, talking, defecation), posture, location (work or home), food and fluid intake (e.g., tobacco, alcohol, caffeine, sodium intake, etc.), psychological state, and concomitant medication.

Errors related to the operator include use of improper technique or incorrect cuff size, leaky bulb, experience, and hearing acuity.[4] Office BP measurements vary depending on the health care provider assessing the BP. In a sample of 1062 patients seen by 10 physicians and one nurse, the mean systolic BP for the physi-

■ ■ ■

TABLE 78-1 CHANGES IN BLOOD PRESSURE CLASSIFICATION

JNC VI CATEGORY	SBP/DBP (mm Hg)	JNC VII CATEGORY
Optimal	<120/80	Normal
Normal	120-129/80-84	Pre-hypertension
Borderline	130-139/85-89	
Hypertension	>140/90	Hypertension
Stage 1	140-159/90-99	Stage 1
Stage 2	160-179/100-109	Stage 2
Stage 3	>180/110	

DBP, Diastolic blood pressure; *JNC VI,* Joint National Committee on Prevention, Detection, Evaluation, and Treatment of High-Blood Pressure, Sixth Report; *JNC VII,* Joint National Committee, Seventh Report; *SBP,* systolic blood pressure. Data from Chobanian AV, Bakris GL, Black HR et al: Seventh Report of the Joint National Committee on Prevention, Detection, Evaluation, and Treatment of High Blood Pressure, *Hypertension* 42:1206-1252, 2003.

BOX 78-1
ELEMENTS OF A MEDICAL HISTORY   ■ ■ ■

- Duration and previous blood pressure levels of BP—last known blood pressure, prior treatment of hypertension (HTN)
- History or current symptoms of target organ damage
- Concurrent cardiovascular risk factors
- Secondary causes of HTN (e.g., pheochromocytoma, primary aldosteronism, thyroid or parathyroid disease, sleep apnea, drug-induced HTN, coarctation of the aorta, chronic kidney disease, renovascular disease, chronic steroid therapy, and Cushing's syndrome)
- Family history of HTN and heart disease
- Assessment of lifestyle (e.g., diet, activity level, smoking, alcohol consumption)
- Assessment of foods or drugs that may be associated with HTN (e.g., illicit drug use, oral contraceptives, adrenal steroids, nonsteroidal anti-inflammatory drugs, greater than two drinks of alcohol/day, excessive sodium intake, herbal remedies)
- Cultural background, values, and beliefs
- Literacy level
- Family structure, availability of social support, level of education, employment status, socioeconomic status, and availability of health care resources

---

BOX 78-2
ELEMENTS OF PHYSICAL EXAMINATION
FOR PATIENTS WITH HYPERTENSION   ■ ■ ■

- Accurate measurement of blood pressure with verification in the contralateral arm
- Examination of optic fundi
- Calculation of body mass index (BMI)
- Auscultation of carotid, abdominal, and femoral bruits
- Palpation of the thyroid gland
- Thorough examination of the heart and lungs
- Examination of abdomen for enlarged kidneys, masses, distended urinary bladder, and abnormal aortic pulsation
- Palpation of the lower extremities for edema and pulses
- Neurological assessment

ALTERNATIVE THERAPY

EFFECTS ON BLOOD PRESSURE

Up to 90 percent of the U.S. population takes either over-the-counter medications or herbal supplements. Thus it is reasonable to assume that your patient with hypertension might be taking supplements. Specifically ask about alternative medicines and then consider their effects on treatment goals and drug-herb interactions. Herbal supplements such as ephedra or Ma Huang, St. John's wort, yohimbine, garlic, and licorice all may affect blood pressure (BP).[2]

Ephedra-containing substances have been associated with rises in BP, tachycardia, palpitations, cardiac arrest, strokes, and seizures.[2] St. John's wort may interact with cardiovascular drugs.[2] Although individuals use garlic to lower their BP, its BP-lowering effects have not been supported by any large randomized controlled trials.[2] Although yohimbine is known to increase BP, it is readily available in herbal and supplement stores and is advertised as treatment for erectile dysfunction.[2] Licorice also has been associated with rises in BP.[3]

[1] Winslow L, Kroll D: Herbs as medicines, *Arch Intern Med.* 1998;158:2192-2199.
[2] Mansoor G. Herbs and alternative therapies in the hypertension clinic: *Am J Hypertens.* 2001;14:971-975.
[3] Chobanian A, Bakris G, Black H, et al. Seventh Report of the Joint National Committee on Prevention, Detection, Evaluation, and Treatment of High Blood Pressure. *Hypertension.* 2003;42:1206-1252.

■ ■ ■

TABLE 78-2 LABORATORY TESTS AND OTHER DIAGNOSTIC PROCEDURES

TEST/PROCEDURE	RATIONALE
12-lead electrocardiogram	To determine the presence or absence of dysrhythmias, myocardial ischemia, left ventricular hypertrophy.
Urinalysis	To assess renal function. White and red blood cells with proteinuria or casts suggest the presence of accelerated or malignant hypertension (HTN) or chronic renal parenchymal disease.
Blood glucose and hematocrit	Obtain blood glucose to screen for diabetes mellitus. Higher hematocrit concentrations increase blood viscosity, thus higher hematocrits are found in hypertensives subsequent to the effort needed to circulate more viscous blood.
Serum potassium	Hypokalemia is a clue to secondary HTN (i.e., primary aldosteronism). Hyperkalemia is common in acute and chronic renal insufficiency.
Creatinine (or the corresponding estimated glomerular filtration rate)	To assess kidney function.
Calcium	To screen for hyperparathyroidism.
Lipoprotein profile	To screen for other cardiovascular risk factors (i.e., dyslipidemia).

From Chobanian A, Bakris G, Black H et al: Seventh Report of the Joint National Committee on Prevention, Detection, Evaluation, and Treatment of High Blood Pressure, *Hypertension* 42:1206-1252, 2003.
Gifford RW, Moser M: Initial workup of the hypertensive patient. In Izzo J, Black H, editors: *Hypertension primer,* Dallas, TX, 2003, American Heart Association, pp. 325-328.
Kaplan, NM: Primary hypertension: pathogenesis. In Kaplan NM, editor: *Kaplan's clinical hypertension*, Philadelphia, 2002, Lippincott Williams & Wilkins, pp. 56-135.

■■■ GENETICS

THE DIAGNOSTIC WORK-UP

Several positive outcomes may emerge from the identification of genes underlying blood pressure (BP) variation: (a) definition of primary physiological mechanisms underlying BP, thus clarifying pathogenesis; (b) provision of the opportunity for preclinical diagnosis; (c) identification of pathways and targets for therapeutic intervention; and (d) determination of treatment strategies tailored to underlying abnormalities in individual patients.[1] Unfortunately, studies of BP variation in the general population are complicated by multifactorial determination, with a variety of demographic, environmental, and genetic factors contributing to the trait of BP in any one person.[1] To date no genetic variants have been identified that account for a substantial BP effect.[1] Genetic profiling is not yet part of a diagnostic workup unless rare cases of secondary hypertension are suspected.[2] Ongoing research may lead to the future ability to conduct genotyping that can provide unique diagnostic and prognostic information as well as direct pharmacogenetic applications.[2]

[1]Lifton R, Gharavi A, Geller D: Molecular mechanisms of human hypertension. *Cell.* 2001;104:545-556.

[2]Gavras H: Genetic profiling in hypertension. In: Izzo J, Black H, eds: *Hypertension primer,* Dallas, TX, American Heart Association; 2003.

BOX 78-3   ■■■
PROTOCOL FOR ACCURATE BLOOD PRESSURE MEASUREMENT IN AN OFFICE OR CLINIC

- Measure blood pressure (BP) using equipment that has been regularly inspected and validated; measurement of BP should be performed by care providers who have been trained and retrained in standardized technique.
- Position individuals seated in a chair (rather than on an exam table) with their backs supported, feet flat on floor, and their arms bared and supported at heart level. Suggest they sit next to a table and rest their arm on the table during measurement. The lack of back and foot support can cause a transient rise in BP, averaging 5 mm Hg diastolic.
- Measurement of BP in a standing position is recommended for those at risk for postural hypotension. Standing is accompanied by a small increase in diastolic BP and a small decrease in systolic BP.
- Begin BP measurement after at least 5 minutes of rest. Resting helps eliminate activity- related factors that may cause elevation in BP.
- Refrain from smoking, ingesting caffeine (e.g., coffee or tea), and exercise for 30 minutes prior to measurement. Smoking and caffeine ingestion can cause a transient rise in BP.
- Use the appropriate size cuff—the cuff bladder should encircle at least 80 percent of the arm. Wrong cuff sizes cause inaccurate BP readings.
- Wrap the cuff smoothly and snugly around the upper arm with its bladder center directly over the antecubital fossa and the lower edge of the cuff 2.5 cm (approximately 2 fingerbreadths) above the antecubital fossa. Inappropriate cuff placement causes inaccurate readings.
- Take two or more readings and record the average.
- For manual BP, palpated radial pulse obliteration pressure should be used to estimate systolic BP. Inflate the cuff 20-30 mm Hg above the estimated SBP. Deflate the cuff at a rate of 2 mm Hg per second.
- The point at which the first of two or more Korotkoff sounds is heard defines systolic BP; the disappearance of the Korotkoff sound defines diastolic BP.
- Provide both verbal and written specific BP numbers and the BP goal of treatment.

From Chobanian A, Bakris G, Black H et al: Seventh Report of the Joint National Committee on Prevention, Detection, Evaluation, and Treatment of High Blood Pressure, *Hypertension* 42:1206-1252, 2003.
Grim CM, Grim CE: Blood pressure measurement. In Izzo J, Black H, editors: *Hypertension primer, ed 3,* Dallas, TX, 2003, American Heart Association, pp. 321-324.

---

cians was 162 ± 27/97 ± 15 and that for the nurse was 155 ± 24/88 ± 14 mm Hg.[5] Major differences were also observed among individual physicians.

More importantly, office BP measurements are associated with "white coat HTN," which refers to people who are hypertensive according to their in-office BP but normotensive according to their out-of-office readings[6] (Figure 78-1). For these individuals, there is a risk of false positive diagnoses of HTN and needless prescription of medications. Home monitoring is free of the white coat effect and thus may contribute to better diagnostic and prognostic accuracy than can be achieved by conventional syphgmomanometry.[7] For patients hypertensive in the office, high BP at home can confirm the diagnosis, while low home BP indicates the need for further assessment with ambulatory BP measurement.[8]

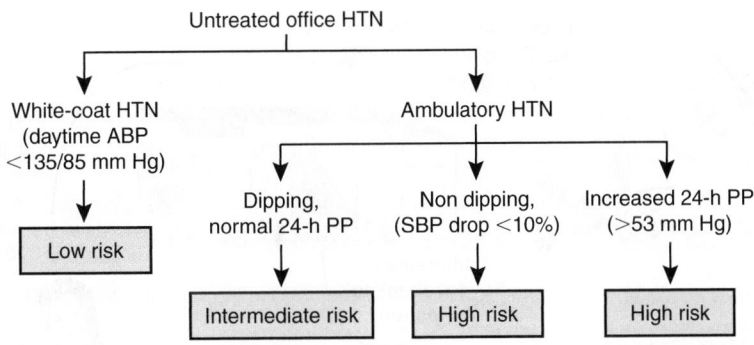

FIGURE 78-1 ■ The risk associated with various levels of blood pressure in untreated persons with hypertension. (Adapted from Verdecchia P: Prognostic value of ambulatory blood pressure: current evidence and clinical implications, *Hypertension* 35:844-851, 2000.) *ABP,* Ambulatory blood pressure; *HTN,* hypertension; *PP,* pulse pressure; *SBP,* systolic blood pressure.

■ ■ ■

TABLE 78-3 JNC VII CLASSIFICATION OF BLOOD PRESSURE AND RECOMMENDED FOLLOW-UP

BP CLASSIFICATION	SYSTOLIC BP (mm Hg)	DIASTOLIC BP (mm Hg)	RECOMMENDATIONS FOR FOLLOW-UP
Normal	<120	and <80	Recheck in 2 years
Pre-hypertension	120-139	or 80-89	Recheck in 1 year
Stage 1 hypertension	140-159	or 90-99	Confirm within 2 months
Stage 2 hypertension	≤160	or ≥100	Evaluate or refer to source of care within 1 month
			For blood pressure >180/110 mm Hg, evaluate and treat immediately or within 1 week, depending on clinical situation and complications

BP, Blood pressure.
From Chobanian A, Bakris G, Black H et al: Seventh Report of the Joint National Committee on Prevention, Detection, Evaluation, and Treatment of High Blood Pressure, *Hypertension* 42:1206-1252, 2003.

Individuals with HTN may not realize they have HTN based on how they are feeling, because the most common symptoms of HTN (i.e., headache and fatigue) can easily be attributed to some other cause. Encouragement is often needed to convince people to have their BP measured on a regular basis. Recommendations for follow-up based on initial BP measurements without end organ damage are described in Table 78-3.

Children and adolescents also should be assessed for BP elevation, especially those who are overweight. Because BP rises steadily from infancy until about age 18, there is no single cutoff point denoting HTN in children and adolescents. Using the appropriate cuff size is critically important in children, and the bladder width should be at least 40 percent of the arm circumference at a point midway between the olecranon and the acromion. The cuff bladder length should cover 80 percent to 100 percent of the circumference of the arm. BP measurements are overestimated to a greater degree with a cuff that is too small than they are underestimated by a cuff that is too large. Therefore, if a cuff is too small, the next larger cuff should be used.[9]

Blood Pressure Self-Measurement

Relatively inexpensive and automated devices are now available for self or home BP monitoring. BP self-monitoring has four advantages[10]:

1. Distinguishing sustained HTN from white coat HTN
2. Assessing response to antihypertensive medication
3. Improving individual adherence to treatment
4. Potentially reducing costs by reducing the number of clinic visits or the amount of medication needed to control BP

BP self-monitoring cannot be used for all patients. Those with cognitive and physical disabilities will not be able to master these devices although someone in the home might be able to assist. The automated devices all use the oscillometric technique,[4] which uses the small oscillations in the cuff pressure to identify the systolic, mean, and diastolic pressures. These devices cannot measure BP accurately in patients with dysrhythmias, such as rapid atrial fibrillation.[4]

A challenge to BP self-monitoring is observer error in reporting of self-measured BP values. Diaries of BP readings over time completed by patients lack reliability. In a sample of patients who were unaware that their home BP monitor had a memory device for all readings taken, Myers[11] found only 7 of 39 patients who performed BP self-monitoring twice daily for 1 week reported all their readings correctly. Fortunately, there are strategies for overcoming observer error, such as memory-equipped devices and/or telemonitoring (Figure 78-2). (See the accompanying Technology feature.)

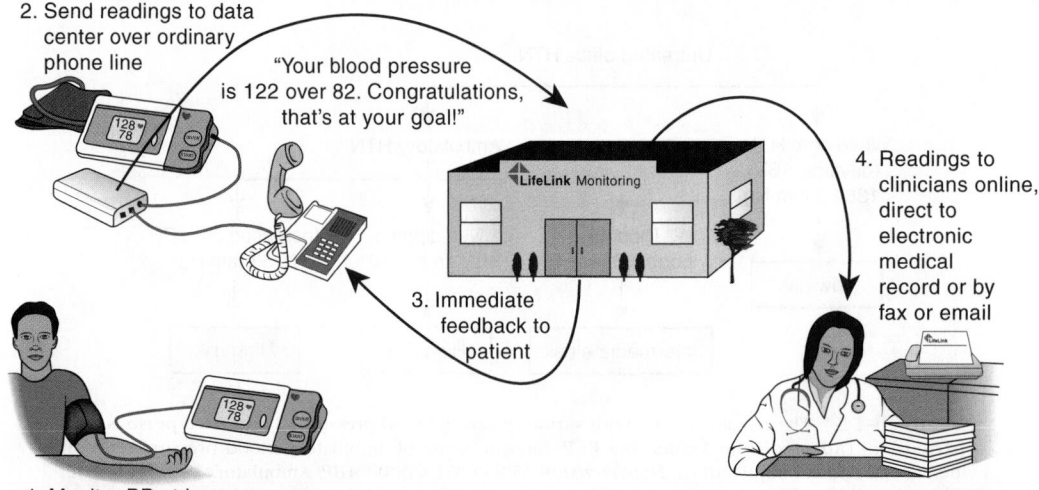

2. Send readings to data center over ordinary phone line

"Your blood pressure is 122 over 82. Congratulations, that's at your goal!"

LifeLink Monitoring

4. Readings to clinicians online, direct to electronic medical record or by fax or email

3. Immediate feedback to patient

1. Monitor BP at home

FIGURE 78-2 ■ The telemonitoring process. (Courtesy LifeLink Monitoring, Lake Katrine, New York.)

■■■ TECHNOLOGY

BLOOD PRESSURE TELEMONITORING

Telemonitoring refers to individuals self-monitoring their blood pressure (BP) at home and then transmitting their BP readings over existing telephone lines to a network server that is provided by a telemonitoring service.[1] The network server generates BP reports that are sent to care providers to facilitate telecounseling and treatment planning. Reports usually contain information about the mean systolic pressure, mean diastolic pressure, and mean heart rate. BP may also be displayed on a graph by date.

Telemonitoring improves on the use of BP self-monitoring alone. Investigators have found a substantial observer error in reporting of self-measured BP values.[2] Erroneous reporting has been found significantly more often in cases of uncontrolled BP and heart rate.[3] Under-reporting is a common bias that can be reduced by memory-equipped BP devices. Recent technological developments, such as BP telemonitoring that entails the use of low-cost monitors with memory and systems for sending stored readings over the telephone, overcome these barriers.[4] The new devices do not allow hypertensive individuals to edit their readings, enabling health care providers to confidently make clinical decisions based on home data.

Although more research is needed, BP telemonitoring appears to improve BP control. When compared to a group of individuals with hypertension who were receiving usual care, Artinian and colleagues[5] found that those using home BP telemonitoring had clinically and statistically significant drops in systolic and diastolic BP at 3-months follow-up, but little change in the usual care only group. Similar results have been found by others.[6-7]

[1]Artinian NT, Washington OGM, Klymko KW, Marburry CM, Miller WM, & Powell JL (2004). What you need to know about home blood pressure telemonitoring but may not know to ask. *Home Healthcare Nurse, 22*(10), 680-686.

[2]Mengden T, Medina RMH, Beltran B, Alvarez E, Kraft K, H. V. Reliability of reporting self-measured blood pressure values by hypertensive patients. *Am J Hypertens.* 1998;11:1413-1417.

[3]Johnson K, Partsch D, Rippole L, & McVey D. (1999). Reliability of self-reported blood pressure measurement. Archives of Internal Medicine, 159(22) 2689-2693.

[4]Pickering T, Gerin W, Holland J: Home blood pressure teletransmission for better diagnosis and treatment. Curr Hypertens Rep. 1999; 1, 1-5.

[5]Artinian NT, Washington OGM, Templin TN (2001). Effects of home telemonitoring and community-based monitoring on BP Control in urban African Americans: A pilot study. *Heart & Lung, 30*, 191-199.

[6]Gerin W, Pickering TG, Holland JK, Alter R. Telephone-linked home blood pressure monitoring in the management of hypertension. *Circulation.* 1998;98 (Suppl. 1):I-324.

[7]Bondmass M, Bolger N, Castro GM, Orgain J, B. A. Rapid control of hypertension in African Americans achieved utilizing home monitoring. *Circulation.* 1998;98 (Suppl.):I-517.

Selecting an Accurate Home Blood Pressure Monitor

There are numerous BP devices on the market (Table 78-4). Advise patients to purchase only those monitors that have passed evaluation by the American Association for the Advancement of Medical Instrumentation **(AAMI)** or the British Hypertension Society **(BHS)** criteria.[12] These criteria mean the monitors have undergone testing, were found to have the greatest agreement with the mercury standard, and to have a high degree of accuracy. The dabl Educational Trust website, *www. dableducational.com*, is an excellent source of information about BP measurement and about BP measurement devices. The link to "Device Tables" provides tables describing AAMI/BHS recommendations for various models of home BP devices.

■■■
TABLE 78-4 BLOOD PRESSURE SELF-MEASUREMENT DEVICES

TYPE OF DEVICE	DESCRIPTION
Upper arm	Recommended instead of wrist and finger devices due to greater accuracy of measurement.
Wrist	Wrist devices are more accurate than finger devices but also subject to inaccuracies due to the more distal site recording and the effect of arm placement on blood pressure (BP). A major disadvantage of wrist devices is that the wrist must be held at heart level during a BP measurement, and it must be kept at that level at the time of each subsequent measurement. If wrist placement is not correct, substantial systematic error may occur due to the influence of arm-heart hydrostatic pressure difference.
Finger	Inaccurate, not recommended Inaccuracies are due to measurement distortion caused by peripheral vasoconstriction, alteration in BP due to the more distal site recording, and the effect of hand position or placement on BP.

From Chobanian A, Bakris G, Black H et al: Seventh Report of the Joint National Committee on Prevention, Detection, Evaluation, and Treatment of High Blood Pressure, *Hypertension* 42:1206-1252, 2003.
Parati G, Asmar R, Stergiou G: Self blood pressure monitoring at home by wrist devices: a reliable approach? *J Hypertens* 20:573-578, 2002.
Wonka F, Thummler M, Schoppe A: Clinical test of a blood pressure measurement device with a wrist cuff, *Blood Press Monit* 1:361-366, 1996.
Zwieker R, Schumacher M, Fruhwald F et al: Comparison of wrist pressure measurement with conventional sphygmomanometry at a cardiology outpatient clinic, *J Hypertens* 18:1013-1018, 2000.

Ambulatory Blood Pressure Measurement

Ambulatory BP **(ABP)** measurement provides a means of monitoring BP at regular intervals throughout a 24-hour period. The noninvasive 24-hour ABP measurement systems use a standard arm cuff that is inflated by a small pump at predetermined intervals, for example, every 15 to 30 minutes during the day and every 30 to 60 minutes during the night.[13] Individual BP measurements are stored in the unit and later read by a computer that prints information such as day and night systolic and diastolic readings, pulse pressures, heart rate, mean plus or minus standard deviations for whatever intervals are desired, and BP load. Blood pressure load is the percentage of readings above a fixed threshold level, typically 140/90 mm Hg during the day and 120/80 mm Hg at night.

Ambulatory BP measurement is endorsed by experts.[10,14] Although it is used most commonly in persons with white coat HTN, it is also helpful in those with apparent drug resistance, hypotensive symptoms with antihypertensive medications, episodic HTN, and autonomic dysfunction.

Normal BP values taken by ambulatory BP monitors are lower than clinic readings when the individual is awake (below 135/85 mm Hg) and are even lower while sleeping (below 120/75 mm Hg).[10] In many persons whose clinic BP suggests a diagnosis of HTN, there is a large discrepancy between the two measurements, with the clinic readings being as much as 50 mm Hg higher.

Given that ABP values are lower than clinic readings, the standard cutoff level for defining HTN of 140/90 is inappropriate when considering ABP. Currently, there is no consensus about what constitutes the upper limit of normal ABP. Two general strategies have been used. First, the cutoff can be selected as the systolic BP or diastolic BP level that is exceeded by 95 percent of the normal population. This is problematic since approximately 20 percent of any population is likely to be hypertensive, and studies of normal populations exclude those with known HTN. Therefore, the upper limit of "normal" will depend to some extent on the criteria used to define HTN in the study population.

Second, ambulatory and clinic BP levels can be correlated and the level of ABP that corresponds to a clinic BP of 140/90 can be used as the cutoff. While acknowledging that there is no general agreement about cutoff levels for HTN, the American Society of Hypertension Ad Hoc panel has suggested limits for probably normal, borderline, and probably abnormal BP to be used when evaluating ABP measures. These have been widely accepted and are shown in Table 78-5. One of the benefits of using ABP monitors is that a number of BP measures may be measured or calculated as shown in Table 78-6. The automated systems are blind to bias, such as that introduced when assessing a patient expected to have high BP (e.g., an overweight or African American individual).

Lowered BP while sleeping is referred to as "dipping;" a "non-dipping" pattern is defined as a reduction in systolic or diastolic BP from day to night of less than 10 percent and an average 24-hour pulse pressure greater than 53 mm Hg.[15] Cardiovascular disease risk shows a direct and independent association with the observed ABP and an inverse association with the degree of dipping in untreated persons. The use of ABP has increased markedly in the last few years.[16] ABP can be used to identify a low-risk group with normal mean

■ ■ ■

TABLE 78-5 RECOMMENDED CUTOFF VALUES FOR MEASUREMENTS OBTAINED USING AMBULATORY BLOOD PRESSURE MONITORING

BLOOD PRESSURE (BP) MEASURE	PROBABLY NORMAL	BORDERLINE	PROBABLY ABNORMAL
SBP (mm Hg)			
Awake	<135	135-145	>140
Asleep	<120	120-125	>125
24 hour average	<130	130-135	>135
DBP (mm Hg)			
Awake	<85	85-90	>90
Asleep	<75	75-80	>80
24 hr average	<80	80-85	>85
Systolic Load (%)			
Awake	<15	15-30	>30
Asleep	<15	15-30	>30
Diastolic Load (%)			
Awake	<15	15-30	>30
Asleep	<15	15-30	>30

DBP, Diastolic blood pressure; *SBP*, systolic blood pressure.
Adapted from Pickering T: Recommendations for the use of home (self) and ambulatory blood pressure monitoring. American Society of Hypertension Ad Hoc Panel, *Am J Hypertens* 9:1-11, 1996.

■ ■ ■

TABLE 78-6 BLOOD PRESSURE PARAMETERS OBTAINED USING AMBULATORY BLOOD PRESSURE MONITORING

MEASURE	CALCULATION/UTILITY
SBP, DBP, MAP, and heart rate	Average values calculated for 24 hours, awake and asleep.
Peak and nadir BP	The range of BP reached over 24 hours.
BP load	Percentage of BP readings ≥140/90 while awake and ≥120/80 while asleep. An SBP or DBP load ≥40-50% is predictive of cardiovascular target organ damage.
BP variability	The standard deviation of the BP. It can be linked to activity if the patient diary is sufficiently explicit. High SBP variability is associated with more target organ damage
Diurnal changes— dippers vs. non-dippers	Dippers are those whose SBP or DBP drops 10 mm Hg between mean daytime and 5 mm Hg for nighttime BP. Others define dippers as those whose SBP or DBP drops 10% or more at night. Nondippers are those with an absent or diminished nocturnal decline in BP. Approximately 78.3% of hypertensives are dippers and 21.7 % are nondippers. Diminished or absent dipping has been associated with increased target organ damage

BP, Blood pressure; *DBP*, diastolic blood pressure; *MAP*, mean arterial pressure; *SBP*, systolic blood pressure.
From Prisant LM, Bottini PB, Carr AA: Ambulatory blood pressure monitoring: methodologic issues, *Am J Nephol* 16:190-201. 1996.
Schillaci G, Verdecchia P, Borgioni C et al: Predictors of diurnal blood pressure changes in 2042 subjects with essential hypertension, *J Hypertens* 14:1167-1173, 1996.

levels of ABP. Those with higher ABP and those with a non-dipping pattern are in a high-risk group. The remaining subjects belong to an intermediate-risk group.

Researchers have used ABP monitors to study normal BP patterns, complications of HTN, effects of antihypertensive drugs, and the prognosis of cardiovascular events.[17] ABP measurements that indicate high BP correlate much more strongly with target organ damage than do those acquired with static BP measurement techniques.[16] In their classic study, Perloff, Sokolow, and Cowan[18] showed that ABP measurements can discriminate between patients at high risk for HTN complications and those at low risk. Patients with lower-than-predicted ABP had a significantly lower cumulative mortality and cardiovascular morbidity than patients with higher-than-predicted ABP. Among those with HTN, ABP correlates more closely than clinic BP with a variety of measures of target organ damage, such as left ventricular hypertrophy. Higher values of 24-hour systolic BP variability (i.e., standard deviation of 24-hour BP) is related to the presence of silent cerebral white matter lesions, seen as silent manifestations of target organ damage; in persons with HTN, however, this relationship is partially dependent on absolute BP elevation.[19]

Currently, ABP monitoring is one of the best tools to confirm the diagnosis of white coat HTN. The Centers for Medicare and Medicaid Services (CMS) recently approved ABP monitoring for reimbursement in patients with suspected white coat HTN.

Circadian BP patterns

Ambulatory BP monitoring has provided a way to study circadian BP patterns. Blood pressure in both normotensive and hypertensive adults is characterized by a clear circadian pattern. In the early morning hours, BP rises and, within a relatively short period of time, reaches a plateau that extends from 0600 hours to 1800 hours. BP tends to be highest at work, lower at home, and lowest during sleep in both normotensive and hypertensive subjects. The typical BP pattern is characterized by two peaks, a prominent one in the morning, coincident with the commencement of daytime activity, and a second one in the early evening. Generally, there is a slight drop in BP in the afternoon and a profound dip nocturnally. Over 24 hours, BP can vary by more than 50 mm Hg.[20] In the majority of individuals, BP falls by 10 percent to 20 percent during the night.[21] This difference is more closely related to the pattern of sleep and wakefulness than to the time of day because BP rhythm follows the cycle of activity in nightshift workers.

The average day-night SBP difference is 11.6 mm Hg in men and 11.4 mm Hg in women; the average day-night DBP difference is 15.4 mmHg in men and 16.2 mm Hg in women.[22] A nocturnal decline equal to at least 10 percent of the daytime mean level constitutes a prominent characteristic of the profile of essential HTN.

Much of the day-night variability is thought to be due to behavioral factors that influence central modulation of autonomic drive to the heart and systemic blood vessels. The principal determinant of the circadian pattern appears to be the sympathetic nervous system because serial measurements of plasma catecholamines throughout a 24-hour period indicate that levels of both norepinephrine and epinephrine have patterns similar to that of BP. It is interesting that dipping is reduced or abolished after both ischemic and hemorrhagic stroke, regardless of the site of stroke.[23] This finding may provide further insight into the mechanisms responsible for the circadian pattern. Further, in centenarians, nocturnal dipping is abolished, presumably because of a derangement in the central sleep influences on the cardiovascular system.[24]

Those with HTN display significantly greater 24-hour variations in mean arterial pressure than do normotensives.[20] This difference may be due to greater pressor responses to emotional and other behavioral stimuli due to an increased central emotional reactivity.

Seasonal variations in 24-hour ABP have also been noted in patients with essential HTN. The winter-summer differences in daytime ambulatory systolic and diastolic BP were 3.5 mm Hg and 2.5 mm Hg, respectively, while the nighttime and average 24-hour BP showed no seasonal differences.[25] These authors suggest that this difference is due to the sympathetic nervous system as winter increases plasma and urinary noradrenaline.

Use of ABP monitors has also revealed racial differences in circadian BP patterns. A metaanalysis involving 2852 participants showed that Blacks had higher levels of systolic and diastolic BP during both the day and night. Subset analysis revealed that American Blacks experienced significantly less of a nocturnal dip in both systolic and diastolic BP in comparison to White subjects; nonAmerican Blacks did not differ in nocturnal dip when compared to White subjects.[26]

HYPERTENSION TREATMENT GOALS

The target BP goal of treatment is lower than 140/90 mm Hg or, in individuals with diabetes or renal disease, lower than 130/80 mm Hg; given the increased risks associated with the coexistence of HTN and diabetes, lower blood pressure goals are recommended.[1] The target goal for patients with HF is lower than 130/85 mm Hg, although effective treatment of HF frequently lowers BP values even lower, as afterload is reduced to improve myocardial performance.[27] Lowering BP protects target organs (e.g., heart, brain, kidney, eyes) from hypertension-related damage and reduces cardiovascular morbidity and mortality.

NONPHARMACOLOGIC AND PHARMACOLOGIC TREATMENT OF HYPERTENSION

Treatment of pre-HTN includes lifestyle modification; however, treatment of stage 1 and stage 2 HTN includes both lifestyle modification as well as drug therapy (Figure 78-3). Persons with pre-HTN who also have diabetes or kidney disease should be treated with antihypertensive medications if a trial of lifestyle modification does not reduce BP to 130/80 mm Hg or less (Table 78-7).

Lifestyle Modifications

Lifestyle modification is an essential component of prevention and treatment of HTN. Table 78-8 summarizes recommendations for lifestyle changes and associated expectations for BP reductions.

Weight Loss

Overweight individuals with HTN benefit from an individualized weight reduction program of reduced calorie intake and exercise.[28] An evidenced-based algorithm representing an overall approach to the treatment of obesity is shown in Figure 78-4.

Dietary Approaches

The Dietary Approaches to Stop Hypertension (**DASH**) diet has been shown to reduce BP and should be recommended to all individuals with HTN; it is especially beneficial in African Americans with HTN.[29] Several DASH diet trials have been conducted. In the first trial, 459 adults consumed one of the following three diets for 8 weeks: (a) a control diet, similar to the typical American diet; (b) a diet rich in fruits and vegetables, or (c) a combination diet rich in fruits and vegetables, low-fat dairy products, with reduced saturated and total fat, and thus rich in potassium and calcium content. All three diets were equal in sodium (3 g/day) and all participants maintained body weight. The largest reductions in BP occurred in those consuming the combination diet. The combination diet reduced systolic BP and diastolic BP by 5.5 and 3.0 mm Hg more, respectively,

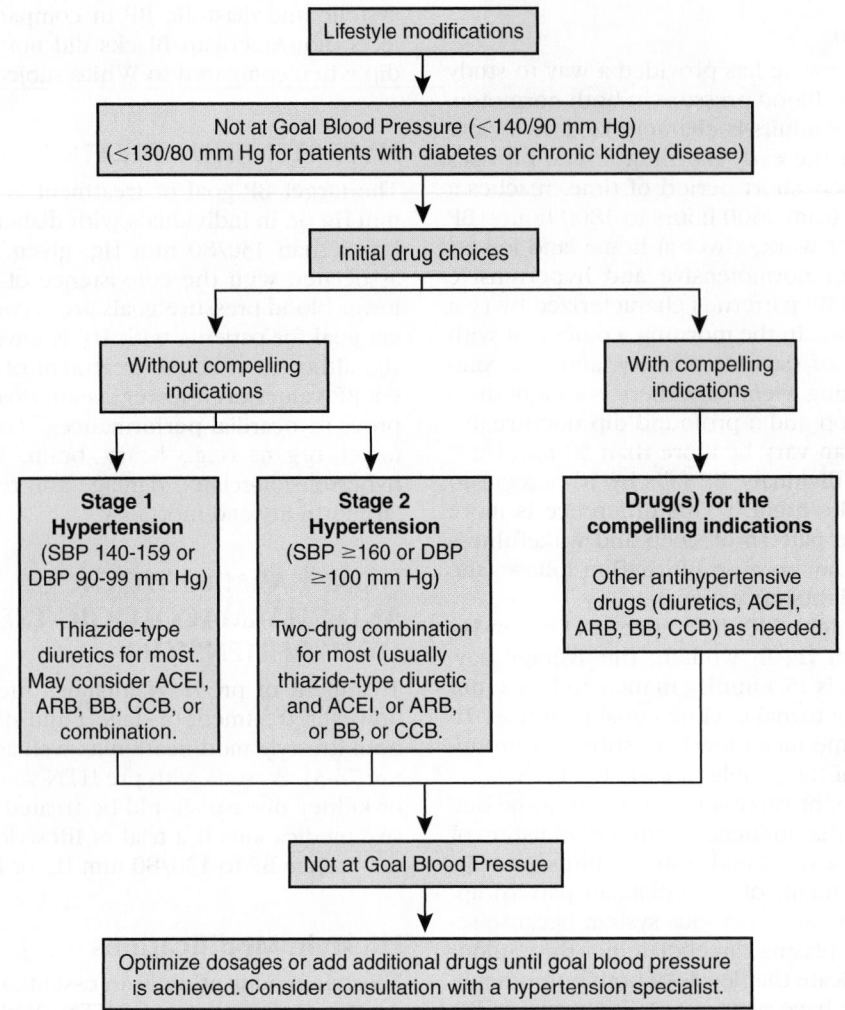

FIGURE 78-3 ■ Treatment of hypertension. *ACEI,* Angiotensin-converting enzyme inhibitor; *ARB,* angiotensin receptor blocker; *BB,* beta blocker; *CCB,* calcium channel blocker; *DBP,* diastolic blood pressure; *SBP,* systolic blood pressure.

■ ■ ■

TABLE 78-7   GUIDELINES FOR THE MANAGEMENT OF HYPERTENSION IN SPECIAL POPULATIONS

SPECIAL POPULATION	GUIDELINE
Individuals with ischemic heart disease, heart failure, diabetes, chronic kidney disease, minorities, older people, women, children, and adolescents	The Seventh Report of the Joint National Committee on Prevention, Detection, Evaluation, and Treatment of High Blood Pressure: the JNC 7 Report, *JAMA* 289:2560-2572, 2003 [pdf of document available at *www.dableducational.com/pdfs/index_page/jnc_vii_jama_may03.pdf*]
Individuals with diabetes, chronic renal disease, and established cardiovascular disease	British Hypertension Society Guidelines for Hypertension Management 2004 (BHS-IV): Summary, *BMJ* 328:643-640, 2004 [pdf available at *www.dableducational.com/pdfs/index_page/guidelines_bhs_bmj_2004.pdf*]
African Americans	Management of High Blood Pressure in African Americans: Consensus Statement of the Hypertension in African Americans Working Group of the International Society on Hypertension in Blacks, *Arch Intern Med* 163(5):525-541, 2003 [pdf available through the ISHIB website, link to ISHIB guidelines *ishib.org/supportfiles/Mgt_of_Hypertension_in_African_Americans.pdf*]
Elderly	Treatment of High Blood Pressure in the Elderly: A Position Paper from the Society of Geriatric Cardiology, *www.sgcard.org/position%20papers/new_treatment.htm*

than the control diet (p = <.001); the fruits and vegetables diet reduced systolic BP by 2.8 mm Hg more (p = <.001) and diastolic BP by 1.1 mm Hg more (p = .07) than the control diet. Among the 133 subjects with HTN, the combination diet reduced systolic and diastolic BP by 11.4 and 5.5 mm Hg more, respectively, than the control diet (p = <.001). Table 78-9 provides an overview of the DASH diet. Detailed information about the DASH eating plan may be found at this website: *www.nhlbi.nih.gov/health/public/heart/hbp/dash/*

Hypertensive individuals should limit their dietary sodium intake to no more than 2400 mg per day.[1] Those who are more sensitive to changes in dietary sodium intake, (e.g., African Americans, elderly, obese patients)

■ ■ ■

TABLE 78-8 LIFESTYLE MODIFICATIONS TO PREVENT AND MANAGE HYPERTENSION*

MODIFICATION	RECOMMENDATION	APPROXIMATE SBP REDUCTION (RANGE)‡
Weight reduction	Maintain normal body weight (body mass index 18.5-24.9 kg/m²)	5-20 mm Hg/10 kg
Adopt DASH† eating plan	Consume a diet rich in fruits, vegetables, and low-fat dairy products with a reduced content of saturated and total fat	8-14 mm Hg
Dietary sodium reduction	Reduce dietary sodium intake to no more than 100 mmol per day (2.4 g sodium or 6 g sodium chloride)	2-8 mm Hg
Physical activity	Engage in regular aerobic physical activity such as brisk walking (at least 30 minutes/day, most days of the week)	4-9 mm Hg
Moderation of alcohol consumption	Limit consumption to no more than 2 drinks (e.g., 24 oz beer, 10 oz wine, or 3 oz 80-proof whiskey) per day in most men and to no more than 1 drink per day in women and lighter weight persons.	2-4 mm Hg

*For overall cardiovascular risk reduction, stop smoking.
†Dietary Approaches to Stop Hypertension.
‡The effects of implementing these modifications are dose- and time-dependent and could be greater for some individuals.
From Chobanian AV, Bakris GL, Black HR et al: Seventh Report of the Joint National Committee on Prevention, Detection, Evaluation, and Treatment of High Blood Pressure, *Hypertension* 42(6):1206-1252, 2003.
Chobanian A, Hill M. National Heart, Lung, and Blood Institute Workshop on Sodium and Blood Pressure: a critical review of current scientific evidence, *Hypertension* 35:858-863, 2000.
He J, Whelton P, Appel L et al: Long-term effects of weight loss and dietary sodium reduction on incidence of hypertension, *Hypertension* 35:544-549, 2000.
Kelley G, Kelley K: Progressive resistance exercise and resting blood pressure: meta-analysis of randomized, controlled trials, *Hypertension* 35:838-843, 2000.
Sacks F, Svetkey LP, Vollmer WM et al: Effects on blood pressure of reduced dietary sodium and the Dietary Approaches to Stop Hypertension (DASH) diet. DASH-Sodium Collaborative Research Group, *N Engl J Med* 344:3-10, 2001.
Vollmer W, Sacks F, Ard J et al: Effects of diet and sodium intake on blood pressure: subgroup analysis of the DASH-sodium trial, *Ann Intern Med* 135:1019-1028, 2001.
Xin X, He J, Frontini M et al: Effects of alcohol reduction on blood pressure: a meta-analysis of randomized controlled trials, *Hypertension* 38:1112-1117, 2001.

should limit their sodium intake even further. Combining the DASH diet with reductions in sodium intake lowers BP more effectively than either intervention alone.[30]

Physical Activity

Aerobic physical activity for at least 30 minutes most days of the week is effective in controlling BP, independent of the change in body weight associated with exercise. Brisk walking, bicycling, swimming, stair walking, yard work, fast dancing are examples of physical activities than can lower BP.

Reduction of Alcohol Intake

The incidence and severity of HTN is linked to excessive alcohol intake. The effect on BP increases with age, independent of the type of beverage consumed, and is even more pronounced in those who are overweight, using contraceptives, and eating a high-salt diet.[28] Lowering alcohol intake can help to control BP.

Smoking Cessation

Smoking cessation is recommended for patients with HTN to reduce their risk of morbidity and mortality.[31] Additionally, smoking may reduce the effectiveness of antihypertensive medications. In one study, the antihypertensive efficacy of propranolol in the treatment of mild HTN was significantly impaired in cigarette smokers.[32]

Helping Patients Make Lifestyle Changes

While it is easy to recommend lifestyle modifications to lower BP, it is not easy to incorporate these changes into one's daily routine. As discussed in Chapters 83 and 84, certain capabilities such as knowledge, skills, and motivation, are needed to successfully carry out lifestyle modifications. Nurses play an important role in helping patients acquire knowledge, skills, and motivation. Information about HTN and the associated risks must be provided in a clear and understandable manner. Literacy level, cultural background, and age of the individual are some of the factors to be considered. An assessment of readiness to change, cognitive abilities that influence decision-making, and current skill levels such as goal setting and self-monitoring will suggest the manner in which to proceed. It is crucial to consider these factors in order to tailor a plan for lifestyle change with a pre-HTN or HTN individual. Assisting individuals to make comprehensive lifestyle changes requires time, attention, and consistent follow-up.

Pharmacological Treatment

Numerous drugs are available for the treatment and control of HTN (Table 78-10). The JNC VII guidelines recommend that thiazide diuretics be used as initial therapy, either alone or in combination with angiotensin-converting enzyme **(ACE)** inhibitors, angiotensin receptor blockers **(ARBs),** beta blockers **(BBs),** or calcium channel blockers **(CCBs).** Those with HF, MI, high risk of coronary disease, diabetes, chronic kidney disease, and risk of recurrent stroke require different antihypertensive drug classes (Table 78-11).[3]

Usually, two or more antihypertensive medications are needed to achieve BP control. JNC VII recommends the addition of a second drug from a different class when the use of a single drug in adequate doses fails to control BP to target goal. When the systolic BP is greater than 20 mm Hg and the diastolic BP is greater than 10 mm Hg above target, consider initiating therapy with two drugs, either as separate prescriptions or in fixed dose combinations.[3] Caution must be exercised when prescribing two drugs for elders or for those with diabetes or autonomic dysfunction due to the risk of ortho-

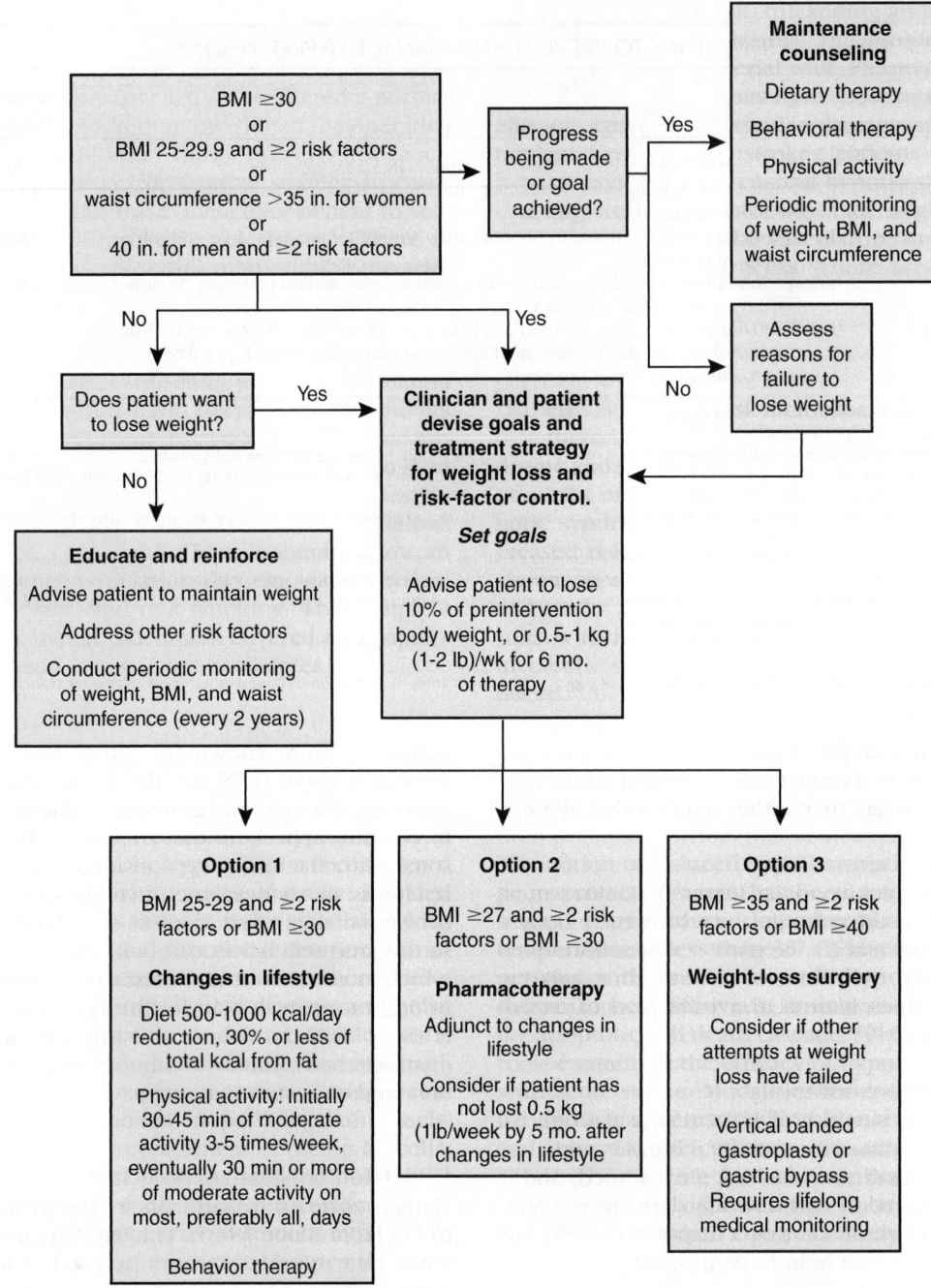

FIGURE 78-4 ■ Evidence-based algorithm for treatment of obesity. *BMI,* Body mass index.

static hypotension. (See the accompanying Conundrum feature on older hypertensive patients.) Once drug therapy is initiated, regular monthly follow-up visits are necessary until the target BP goal has been reached. Follow-up may need to be more frequent for those with stage 2 HTN or complicating comorbid conditions.

Although limited data are available about pharmacological treatment for HTN in African Americans and other minority groups, in terms of efficacy, there is no rationale to avoid certain classes of agents in African Americans with HTN; all drug classes are associated with BP-lowering efficacy in African Americans. Thiazide diuretics and calcium channel blockers may have

greater BP-lowering efficacy than other classes in African Americans, and, as monotherapy, beta blockers and ACE inhibitors may produce less BP lowering in African Americans than in Whites.[33] Clinical trial data suggest that pharmacological therapy effective in white populations is also effective in East Asian populations, but drug side effects such as cough or flushing may be greater among certain Asian ethnic subgroups.[34] African Americans also appear to be at increased risk for side effects associated with ACE inhibitors such as angioedema, cough, or both.[33]

Once medications are prescribed to control BP, adherence to therapy becomes important. Numerous fac-

■ ■ ■

TABLE 78-9   DIETARY APPROACHES TO STOP HYPERTENSION DIETARY PATTERN BASED ON 2000 KCAL DIET

FOOD GROUP	SERVINGS*	SERVING SIZES	IMPORTANCE TO DIET
Grains and grain products	7-8	1 slice bread ½ c dry cereal ½ c cooked rice, pasta, or cereal	Major sources of energy and fiber
Vegetables	4-5	1 c raw leafy vegetables ½ c cooked vegetables 6 oz vegetable juice	Rich sources of potassium, magnesium and fiber
Fruits	4-5	6 oz fruit juice 1 medium fruit ¼ c dried fruit ½ c fresh, frozen, or canned fruit	Important sources of potassium, magnesium, and fiber
Low-fat or fat-free dairy foods	2-3	8 oz milk 1 c yogurt 1.5 oz cheese	Major sources of calcium and protein
Meats, poultry, and fish	≤2	3 oz cooked meats, poultry or fish	Rich sources of protein and magnesium
Nuts, seeds, and dry beans and peas	4-5/wk	1½ oz or ⅓ c nuts ½ oz or 2 tbsp seeds ½ cup cooked dry beans and peas	Rich sources of energy, magnesium, potassium, protein and fiber
Fats and oils	2-3	1 tsp of margarine 1 tbsp low-fat mayonnaise 2 tbsp light salad dressing 1 tsp vegetable oil	Adds satiety, but remember that DASH diet has only 27% of energy as fat
Sweets	5/wk	1 tbsp sugar 1 tbsp jelly or jam ½ oz jelly beans 8 oz sugared lemonade	Sweets should be low in fat

*Daily servings, except as noted otherwise.
From Windhauser MM, Ernst DB, Karanja NM et al: Translating the Dietary Approaches to Stop Hypertension diet from research to practice: dietary and behavior change techniques. DASH Collaborative Research Group, *J Am Diet Assoc* 99(8 Suppl):S90-95, 1999.

tors influence the ability to adhere to a medication regimen: knowledge and understanding of the medication regimen, cognitive functioning, depression, frequent daily dosing regimens, complex dosing regimens, lower household income, individuals with multiple diseases and polypharmacy, impaired functional capacity such as finger dexterity to open pill containers, impaired sensory capacity such as visual or hearing impairments, low literacy levels, trouble swallowing large pills or taking medications, and side effects of medications.[35] The high cost of prescription drugs is another important barrier to medication adherence. Investigators report that two thirds of chronically ill adults who cut back on their medications because of cost do not tell their health care provider in advance.[36]

After identifying individuals at risk for poor medication adherence, interventions need to be designed; first and foremost is simplifying a complex drug regimen. Tailoring the medication to the individual's lifestyle or daily rituals and providing reminder strategies (e.g., reminder cards in strategic places) is important. Continuity of health care providers and professional follow-up by telephone or mail with those at-risk for poor adherence is recommended. If you are not responsible for writing prescriptions, advocate on behalf of patients for less expensive generic alternatives and once-a-day dosing. Suggest to patients that they ask for free samples, or help them complete pharmacy assistance forms if they cannot afford their medications. Box 78-4 provides an overview of some pharmacy assistance programs. Advise seniors to go to *www.Medicare.gov* for information about Medicare-approved drug discount cards.

RESISTANT HYPERTENSION

True refractory or resistant HTN is unusual in the general hypertensive population and may be more commonly encountered in HTN specialty clinics.[37] Resistant HTN refers to the persistence of out-of-the office BP above the appropriate goal of therapy, (i.e., above 140/90 mm Hg for most with HTN, above 130/80 mm Hg for those with diabetes or renal insufficiency, or above 140 mm Hg for those with isolated systolic HTN). True resistant HTN assumes that uncontrolled HTN persists even when the patient has been adherent to a regimen of three or more drugs from different classes, one of which is a diuretic, and that adequate drug doses have been prescribed.

When true resistance occurs, it may be due to factors that interfere with the efficacy of antihypertensive drugs, such as smoking, weight gain, or excessive alcohol intake.[38] Nonsteroidal antiinflammatory drugs also interfere with antihypertensive medications. Other drug-related causes of resistant HTN are sympathomimetics, nasal decongestants, appetite suppressants, cocaine and other illicit drugs, caffeine, oral contraceptives, adrenal steroids, licorice (as may be found in chewing tobacco), cyclosporine, tacrolimus, erythropoietin, and antidepressants.[37] Coexisting conditions that may interfere with BP control include obesity, anxiety disorders, sleep apnea, acute and chronic pain, hyperinsulinism with insulin resistance, and delirium that is associated with agitation and autonomic excess.[39] Physiological resistance also may be a cause of resistant HTN. Physiological resistance occurs when vasodilator

■ ■ ■

TABLE 78-10   ORAL ANTIHYPERTENSIVE DRUGS

CLASS	DRUG (TRADE NAME)	USUAL DOSE RANGE (mg/day)	USUAL DAILY FREQUENCY
Thiazide diuretics	Chlorothiazide (Diuril)	125-500	1-2
	Chlorthalidone (generic)	12.5-25	1
	Hydrochlorothiazide (Microzide, HydroDIURIL)	12.5-50	1
	Polythiazide (Renese)	2-4	1
	Indapamide (Lozol)	1.25-2.5	1
	Metolazone (Mykrox)	0.5-1.0	1
	Metolazone (Zaroxolyn)	2.5-5	
Loop diuretics	Bumetanide (Bumex)	0.5-2	2
	Furosemide (Lasix)	20-80	2
	Torsemide (Demadex)	2.5-10	1
Potassium-sparing diuretics	Amiloride (Midamor)	5-10	1-2
	Triamterene (Dyrenium)	50-100	1-2
Aldosterone receptor blockers	Eplerenone (Inspra)	50-100	1
	Spironolactone (Aldactone)	25-50	1
Beta blockers (BBs)	Atenolol (Tenormin)	25-100	1
	Betaxolol (Kerlone)	5-20	1
	Bisoprolol (Zebeta)	2.5-10	1
	Metoprolol (Lopressor)	50-100	1-2
	Metoprolol extended release (Toprol XL)	50-100	1
	Nadolol (Corgard)	40-120	1
	Propranolol (Inderal)	40-160	2
	Propranolol long-acting (Inderal LA)	60-180	1
	Timolol (Blocadren)	20-40	2
BB with intrinsic sympathomimetic activity	Acebutolol (Sectral)	200-800	2
	Penbutolol (Levatol)	10-40	1
	Pindolol (generic)	10-40	2
Combined alpha blockers and BBs	Carvedilol (Coreg)	12.5-50	2
	Labetalol (Normodyne, Trandate)	200-800	2
Angiotensin-converting enzyme (ACE) inhibitors	Benazepril (Lotensin)	10-40	1
	Captopril (Capoten)	25-100	2
	Enalapril (Vasotec)	5-40	1-2
	Fosinopril (Monopril)	10-40	1
	Lisinopril (Prinivil, Zestril)	10-40	1
	Moexipril (Univasc)	7.5-30	1
	Perindopril (Aceon)	4-8	1
	Quinapril (Accupril)	10-80	1
	Ramipril (Altace)	2.5-20	1
	Trandolapril (Mavik)	1-4	1
Angiotensin II antagonists	Candesartan (Atacand)	8-32	1
	Eprosartan (Teveten)	400-800	1-2
	Irbesartan (Avapro)	150-300	1
	Losartan (Cozaar)	25-100	1
	Olmesartan (Benicar)	20-40	1
	Telmisartan (Micardis)	20-80	1-2
	Valsartan (Diovan)	80-320	1-2
Calcium channel blockers (CCBs)— nondihydropyridine	Diltiazem extended release (Cardizem CD, Dilacor XR, Tiazac)	180-420	1
	Diltiazem extended release (Cardizem LA)	120-540	1
	Verapamil immediate release (Calan, Isoptin)	80-320	2
	Verapamil long acting (Calan SR, Isoptin SR)	120-480	1-2
	Verapamil (Coer, Covera HS, Verelan PM)	120-360	1
CCBs—dihydropyridine	Amlodipine (Norvasc)	2.5-10	1
	Felodipine (Plendil)	2.5-20	1
	Isradipine (Dynacirc CR)	2.5-10	2
	Nicardipine sustained release (Cardene SR)	60-120	2
	Nifedipine long-acting (Adalat CC, Procardia XL)	30-60	1
	Nisoldipine (Sular)	10-40	1
Alpha$_1$ blockers	Doxazosin (Cardura)	1-16	1
	Prazosin (Minipress)	2-20	1-2
	Terazosin (Hytrin)	1-20	2-3
Central alpha$_2$ agonists and other centrally acting drugs	Clonidine (Catapres)	0.1-0.8	2
	Clonidine patch (Catapres-TTS)	0.1-0.3	1 weekly
	Methyldopa (Aldomet)	250-1000	2
	Reserpine (generic)	0.1-0.25	1
	Guanfacine (Tenex)	0.5-2	1
Direct vasodilators	Hydralazine (Apresoline)	25-100	2
	Minoxidil (Loniten)	2.5-80	1-2

From Chobanian AV, Bakris GL, Black HR et al: Seventh Report of the Joint National Committee on Prevention, Detection, Evaluation, and Treatment of High Blood Pressure, *Hypertension* 42:1206-1252, 2003, with permission.

■■■

TABLE 78-11   CLINICAL TRIAL AND GUIDELINE BASIS FOR COMPELLING INDICATION FOR INDIVIDUAL DRUG CLASSES

	RECOMMENDED DRUGS						
COMPELLING INDICATION*	DIURETIC	BB	ACEI	ARB	CCB	ALDO ANT	CLINICAL TRIAL BASIS‡
Heart failure							ACC/AHA Heart Failure Guideline, MERIT-HF, COPERNICUS, CIBIS, SOLVD AIRE, TRACE ValHEFT, RALES, CHARM
Postmyocardial infarction							ACC/AHA Post-MI Guideline, BHAT, SAVE, Capricorn, EPHESUS
High coronary disease risk							ALLHAT, HOPE, ANBP$_2$, LIFE, CONVINCE, EUROPA, INVEST
Diabetes							NKF-ADA Guideline, UKPDS, ALLHAT
Chronic kidney disease							NKF Guideline, Captopril Trial, RENAAL, IDNT, REIN, AASK
Recurrent stroke prevention							PROGRESS

*Compelling indications for antihypertensive drugs are based on benefits from outcome studies or existing clinical guidelines; the compelling indication is managed in parallel with the BP.
ACC, American College of Cardiology; *ACEI,* angiotensin-converting enzyme inhibitor; *AHA,* American Hospital Association; *ARB,* angiotensin receptor blocker; *ALDO ANT,* aldosterone antagonist; *BB,* beta blocker; *CCB,* calcium channel blocker.
‡Conditions for which clinical trials demonstrate the benefit of specific classes of antihypertensive drugs.
From Chobanian AV, Bakris GL, Black HR et al: Seventh Report of the Joint National Committee on Prevention, Detection, Evaluation, and Treatment of High Blood Pressure, Hypertension 42:1206-1252, 2003.

■■■ CONUNDRUM

TREATING OLDER HYPERTENSIVE PATIENTS

Unfortunately, blood pressure (BPs) control rates are only about 20 percent in older hypertensives compared to 34 percent in all U.S. adults; estimates are that fewer than 25 percent of hypertensive individuals older than age 65 are being treated.[1,2] Many elders experience symptoms as their BP is lowered (fatigue, impaired cognition, dizziness, postural hypotension). Can patients older than age 75 or 80 have their BP lowered without it affecting their quality of life?

In general, treatment recommendations for elder hypertensive individuals, including those with idiopathic systolic hypertension, should follow the usual principles of hypertension management.[1] BP level and associated cardiovascular risk factors rather than age should determine treatment.[3] Investigators have found that elders respond similarly to antihypertensive treatment compared with younger persons. In a study comparing the safety and efficacy of fixed combinations of valsartan and hydrochlorothiazide versus valsartan monotherapy, both elderly and nonelderly persons responded similarly to combination therapy.[4]

In the frail elderly and those older than age 75 or 80, treatment may need to move a little bit more slowly, especially if symptoms occur as BP is lowered.[5] Blood pressure should be monitored in the upright position since a decrease in standing systolic BP of more than 10 mm Hg, when associated with dizziness or fainting, indicates postural hypotension. So as not to interfere with quality of life, medication doses should be titrated slowly, usually every 4 to 6 weeks, until the maximum reduction occurs; other agents may then be added until the BP goal is achieved.[6]

Nurses play a major role in helping elders achieve BP control and a good quality of life by helping them adapt to their antihypertensive regimens. Asking patients about the symptoms they experience and encouraging them to report those symptoms is important.

Lifestyle modification has been shown to be effective in lowering BP in elders and may reduce the need for antihypertensive medication. Restricting sodium to 1800 mg or less per day favorably reduced systolic and diastolic BP, and the combination of weight loss with sodium restriction reduced BP more than either strategy alone.[7,8] Institute dietary restrictions cautiously in elders, however, as they may have a lack of appetite or a diet poor in nutrition.

[1] Chobanian A, Bakris G, Black H, et al. Seventh Report of the Joint National Committee on Prevention, Detection, Evaluation, and Treatment of High Blood Pressure. *Hypertension.* 2003;42:1206-1252.
[2] Moser M, Cheitlin M, Gifford R: Treatment of high blood pressure in the elderly. A position paper from the Society of Geriatric Cardiology. Available at: *www.sgcard.org/position%20papers/new_treatment.htm;* accessed September 18, 2004.
[3] Baruch L. Hypertension and the elderly: More than just blood pressure control, *J Clin Hypertens* 6:249-255, 2004.
[4] Mallion J, Carretta R, Trenkwalder P, et al. Valsartan/hydrochlorothiazide is effective in hypertensive patients inadaquately controlled by valsartan monotherapy. *Blood Press Suppl.* 2003;Suppl. 1:36-43.
[5] Moser M, Alderman M, Wright J: Clinical problems in the management of hypertension: (1) Prehypertension: should we treat? (2) The very elderly: how should we treat? *J Clin Hypertens* 6:262-266, 2004.
[6] Basile J. Treatment of the elderly hypertensive: Systolic hypertension. In: Izzo J, Black H, eds. *Hypertension primer.* Dallas, TX: American Heart Association; 2003:446-448.
[7] Whelton P, Appel L, Espeland M, et al. Sodium reduction and weight loss in the treatment of hypertension in older persons: A randomized controlled trial of nonpharmacologic interventions in the elderly (TONE). TONE Collaborative Research Group. *JAMA.* 1998;279(11):839-846.
[8] Appel L, Espeland M, Easter L, Wilson A, Folmar S, Lacy C. Effects of reduced sodium intake on hypertension control in older individuals: Results from the Trial of Nonpharmacologic Interventions in the Elderly (TONE). *Arch Intern Med.* 2001;161(5):685-693.

therapy causes an initial fall in BP, which activates the sympathetic nervous and renin-angiotensin systems, which in turn cause sodium and water retention and volume overload.

Treatment of resistant HTN varies, depending on the cause. Inappropriate medication regimens, nonadherence to medication regimens, and secondary causes of HTN must be ruled out. If these issues have been addressed and BP control remains unattainable, consider referral to a HTN specialist.

BOX 78-4   ■ ■ ■
PHARMACY ASSISTANCE PROGRAMS

Most pharmaceutical manufacturers have special programs to assist people who cannot afford to buy the medications they need. Each company has its own pharmacy assistance program with its special requirements, forms, and procedures. Forms must be completed by the patient or for the patient, signed by the individual prescribing the medication, then submitted to the pharmaceutical company. These programs are intended to serve as a "last resort" for patients who are unable to use other programs and who otherwise would not be able to afford needed medications. The following websites can be used to find pharmacy assistance for persons with hypertension.

- **RxAssist** (*www.rxassist.org*). Nurses can search for assistance information by drug company, generic or brand name, or therapeutic class.
- **Needy Meds** (*www.needymeds.com*). Nurses can search lists of generic or trade names for the medication needed.

MODELS OF CARE FOR MANAGING HYPERTENSION
Community-Based Care

Public health nurses and community outreach workers in high-risk communities, such as the African American community, are an essential link in the effort to control HTN. They conduct BP screenings, identify cases of HTN, provide education about HTN, refer individuals for treatment, and track follow-up appointments.[1] BP control rates have a good chance of improving if interventions are provided in accessible community-based sites that reflect cultural characteristics and preferences.

Nurse-Managed Hypertension Clinics

Assisting individuals to make lifestyle changes and adhere to drug regimens requires time, attention, and consistent follow-up. Nurse-managed HTN clinics may be relatively more successful than other primary care settings in controlling BP because nursing care emphasizes the factors affecting patients' abilities to make lifestyle changes. Nurses are taught to facilitate lifestyle change and drug regimen adherence.

Evidence suggests nurse management effectively improves BP control. In a recent randomized controlled trial, patients received either usual care alone ($n = 76$) or usual care plus nurse management for HTN ($n = 74$). In nurse management, patients received baseline counseling about correct use of an automated home BP measurement device, information about how to enhance medication adherence and recognize potential drug side effects, printed educational information, and follow-up phone contacts (10-minute) at 1 week and 1-, 2-, and 4-months. Blood pressure reports were reviewed to determine if BP target goals were achieved and mailed to patients every 2 weeks. Nurses changed BP medication according to protocol as needed; physicians were contacted to initiate any new BP drug. Patients receiving nurse management achieved greater reductions in office BP values at 6 months than those receiving usual care.[40] Additionally, average daily adherence to medication, measured by electronic drug event monitors, was superior among nurse-managed subjects. Technological advancements such as BP telemonitoring in combination with additional supportive evidence for nurse-managed HTN may lead to virtual HTN clinics in the future. Virtual clinics would permit individuals to have their BP managed through telephone or internet-based interventions rather than through frequent clinic visits.

SUMMARY

Hypertension affects approximately 65 million U.S. adults and is associated with direct and indirect care costs totaling $59.7 billion.[41] Nurses are integral to providing information about HTN that is appropriate to individuals' literacy levels, cultural backgrounds, ages, and cognitive skills; helping them acquire the necessary skills and resources to be successful in making lifestyle changes; and assisting them to overcome barriers that may influence their abilities to adhere to an antihypertensive drug regimen.

REFERENCES

1. JNC-VII-Joint National Committee on Prevention Detection, Evaluation, and Treatment of High Blood Pressure: JNC 7: The Seventh Report of the Joint National Committee on Prevention, Detection, Evaluation, and Treatment of High Blood Pressure (NIH Publication No. 03-5233), Bethesda, MD, 2003, U.S. Department of Health and Human Services, National Institutes of Health, National Heart, Lung, and Blood Institute, National High Blood Pressure Education Program.
2. American Heart Association: *Heart disease and stroke statistics—2007 update*, Dallas, TX, 2007, American Heart Association.
3. Ong KL, Cheung BM, Man YB, et al: Prevalence, awareness, treatment, and control of hypertension among United States adults 1999-2004. *Hypertension.* Jan 2007;49(1):69-75.
4. O'Brien E: ABC of hypertension. Blood pressure measurement. Part IV—Automated sphygmomanometry: self blood pressure measurement, *BMJ* 322:1167-1170, 2001.
5. La Batide-Alanore A, Chatellier G et al: Comparison of nurse- and physician-determined clinic blood pressure levels in patients referred to a hypertension clinic: implications for subsequent management, *J Hypertens* 18:391-398, 2000.
6. Pickering T, Gerin W, Schwartz, AR: What is the white-coat effect and how should it be measured? *Blood Press Monit* 7:293-300, 2002.
7. Bobrie G, Chatellier G, Genes N et al: Cardiovascular prognosis of "masked hypertension" detected by blood pressure self-measurement in elderly treated hypertensive patients, *JAMA* 291:1342-1349, 2004.
8. Herpin D, Pickering T, Stergiou G et al: Clinical applications and diagnosis, *Blood Press Monit* 5:131-135, 2000.
9. National High Blood Pressure Education Program Working Group on High Blood Pressure in Children and Adolescents (NHBPEP): The Fourth Report on the Diagnosis, Evaluation, and Treatment of High Blood Pressure in Children and Adolescents. *Pediatrics* 114:555-576, 2004. (Also available at *www.pediatrics.org/cgi/content/full/114/2/S2/555*).
10. Shimizu M, Shibasaki S, Kario K: The value of home blood pressure monitoring. *Curr Hypertens Rep.* Oct 2006, 8(5):363-367.
11. Myers M: Reporting bias in self-measurement of blood pressure, *Blood Press Monit* 6:181-183, 2001.
12. O'Brien E, Waeber B, Parati G et al: Blood pressure measuring devices: recommendations of the European Society of Hypertension, *BMJ* 322:531-536, 2001.
13. Kaplan N: Measurement of blood pressure. In Kaplan N, editor: *Kaplan's clinical hypertension*, Philadelphia, 2002, Lippincott Williams & Wilkins, pp. 25-55.

14. Chalmers J, MacMahon S, Mancia G et al: 1999 World Health Organization—International Society of Hypertension Guidelines for Management of Hypertension. Guidelines Sub-Committee of the World Health Organization, *Clin Exp Hypertens* 21:1009-1060, 1999.

15. Stolarz K, Staessen JA, O'Brien ET: Night-time blood pressure: dipping into the future? *J Hyperten* 20:2131-2133, 2002.

16. Verdecchia P: Prognostic value of ambulatory blood pressure: current evidence and clinical implications, *Hypertension* 35:844-851, 2000.

17. Yucha CB: Ambulatory blood pressure monitoring: measurement implications for research, *J Nurs Meas* 9:49-59, 2001.

18. Perloff D, Sokolow M, Cowan R: The prognostic value of ambulatory blood pressures, *JAMA* 249:2792-2798, 1983.

19. Gomez-Angelats E, de La Sierra A, Sierra C et al: Blood pressure variability and silent cerebral damage in essential hypertension, *Am J Hypertens* 17:696-700, 2004.

20. Mancia G, Gamba PL, Omboni S et al: Ambulatory blood pressure monitoring, *Hypertens Suppl* 14:S61-66; discussion S66-68, 1996.

21. Pickering T: Recommendations for the use of home (self) and ambulatory blood pressure monitoring. American Society of Hypertension Ad Hoc Panel, *Am J Hypertens* 9:1-11, 1996.

22. Schillaci G, Verdecchia P, Borgioni C et al: Predictors of diurnal blood pressure changes in 2042 subjects with essential hypertension, *J Hypertens* 14:1167-1173, 1996.

23. Jain S, Namboodri KKN, Kumari S et al: Loss of circadian rhythm of blood pressure following acute stroke, *BMC Neurol* 4:1-6, 2004.

24. Bertinieri G, Grassi G, Rossi P et al: 24-hour blood pressure profile in centenarians, *J Hypertens* 20:1765-1769, 2002.

25. Minami J, Kawano Y, Ishimitsu T et al: Seasonal variations in office, home and 24 h ambulatory blood pressure in patients with essential hypertension, *J Hypertens* 14:1421-1425, 1996.

26. Profant J, Dimsdale JE: Race and diurnal blood pressure patterns: a review and meta-analysis, *Hypertens* 3:1099-1104, 1999.

27. Kostis J: Treatment of hypertensive patients with left ventricular systolic dysfunction. In Izzo J, Black H, editors: *Hypertension primer*, Dallas, TX, 2003, American Heart Association.

28. Joss J, Phillips B: Initiation of therapy. In Mutnick A, Hisel T, Joss J, Phillips B, editors: *Hypertension management for the primary care clinician*, Bethesda, MD, 2004, American Society of Health-System Pharmacists, pp. 61-89.

29. Appel L, Moore T, Obarzanek E et al: A clinical trial of the effects of dietary patterns on blood pressure. DASH Collaborative Research Group. *N Engl J Med* 336:1117-1124, 1997.

30. Svetkey L, Simons-Morton D, Proschan M et al: Effect of dietary approaches to stop hypertension diet and reduced sodium intake on BP control, *J Clin Hypertens* 6:373-381, 2004.

31. Critchley J, Capewell S: Mortality risk reduction associated with smoking cessation in patients with coronary heart disease: a systematic review, *JAMA* 290:86-97, 2003.

32. Greenberg G, Thompson S, Brennan P: The relationship between smoking and the response to anti-hypertensive treatment in mild hypertensives in the Medical Research Council's trial of treatment, *Int J Epidemiol* 16:25-30, 1987.

33. Douglas J, Bakris G, Epstein M et al: Management of high blood pressure in African Americans, *Arch Intern Med* 163:525-541, 2003.

34. Wong ND: Hypertension in East Asians and Native Hawaiians. In Izzo J, Black H, editors: *Hypertension primer*, Dallas, TX, 2003, American Heart Association, pp. 272-273.

35. Dunbar-Jacob J, Bohachick P, Mortimer M et al: Medication adherence in persons with cardiovascular disease, *J Cardiovasc Nurs* 18:209-218, 2003.

36. Piette J, Heisler M, Wagner T: Cost-related medication underuse, *Arch Intern Med* 164:1749-1755, 2004.

37. Venkata C, Ram S: Refractory hypertension. In Weber M, editor: *Hypertension medicine*, Totowa, NJ, 2001, Humana Press, pp. 419-427.

38. Kaplan N, Izzo J: Refractory hypertension. In Izzo J, Black H, editors: *Hypertension primer*, Dallas, TX, 2003, American Heart Association, pp. 382-384.

39. O'Rorke J, Richardson W: What do we do if our patient's blood pressure is "difficult-to-control"? In Mulrow C, editor: *Evidence-based hypertension*, London, 2001, BMJ Books, pp. 193-205.

40. Rudd P, Miller N, Kaufman J et al: Nurse management for hypertension. A systems approach, *Am J Hypertens* 17:921-927, 2004.

41. Fields L, Burt V, Cutler J et al: The burden of adult hypertension in the United States 1999 to 2000. a rising tide, *Hypertension* 44:1-7, 2004.

chapter 79

Heart Failure Disease Management

Anna Strömberg

CHAPTER ABBREVIATIONS

ACE angiotensin-converting enzyme
COACH Coordinating Study Evaluating Outcomes of Advising and Counseling in Heart Failure

The economic and societal impact of heart failure and the burden of disease to patients and their caregivers continue to increase despite modern advances in pharmacotherapy. Persons diagnosed with moderate to severe systolic dysfunction are disproportionately impacted by this chronic condition. Approximately two thirds of these severely ill individuals are hospitalized yearly, and one out of three dies within 1 year after hospitalization.[1,2] The heart failure population consumes a large proportion of health care resources—more than 2 percent of the total health care costs. The main cost is for hospitalizations.[3]

WHY "USUAL CARE" DOES NOT WORK

Usual care for heart failure means, in most countries, that patients only receive acute care when they request it because of escalating symptoms. That is, usual care for heart failure does not include any structured, health care system-initiated follow-up after the initial diagnosis or after hospitalization. It is not surprising that this approach causes problems if treatment is not optimal and education is not provided to newly diagnosed patients or those discharged home after a few days of intensive care. Without structured follow-up, these patients are at high risk for deterioration that will require a hospital admission since they are not completely stable. They need additional teaching and follow-up to maximize treatment adherence and self-care, and both the patient and his or her family need psychosocial support to cope with the illness and its effects on the family. Failure to provide structured follow-up with optimization of the medical treatment, patient education, psychosocial support, and easy access to care leads to anxiety and insecurity in patients and caregivers, poor self-care including low adherence to treatments, and unnecessary hospitalizations.[4,5]

There are several reasons why usual care typically means absence of structured follow-up in settings across the world. First, there are economic reasons. It is sometimes very difficult to implement new management strategies that need economic resources initially with the promise that they will save money in the long run. It is also often the case that the costs are taken on by one unit, and the savings will be in another. For example, follow-up is done in primary care, outpatient clinics, or home care, but the savings are accumulated in the hospitals. So despite evidence of cost-effectiveness, the decision becomes a political and financial issue.[6] Second, there are organizational factors that impair the development of structured care approaches. Organizing structured follow-up for the large heart failure population requires resources and structural changes. Third, explicit and clear recommendations in guidelines and other statements from influential organizations, such as the American Heart Association and the European Society of Cardiology, are needed to influence national guidelines, performance measures from major organizations, and local decision makers. Without such clear direction, disease management may not be made a priority.

Usual care, of course, differs within and between countries. Primary care and family physicians work differently across the world; nurses and other health care professionals have different levels of education and responsibilities as well. There are variations in the length of stay in the hospital, and other health care resources vary. However, an increasing body of research evidence illustrates the beneficial effects of heart failure disease management programs. Therefore, disease management initiatives are starting in many hospitals, primary care centers, and home care settings all over the world.[2,7-9]

ALTERNATIVE MODELS OF CARE
Heart Failure Disease Management

Until the last two decades, heart failure was a condition that did not receive special attention since it had very few treatment options. Over the last 20 years, new diagnostic tools and medical treatments have been developed. A large number of clinical trials have demonstrated significant reduction in mortality and morbidity among patients with heart failure who are treated with angiotensin-converting enzyme **(ACE)** inhibitors, beta blockers, angiotensin- and aldosterone-receptor blockers. Therefore, it is important to ensure that patients are prescribed optimal pharmacological treatment as summarized in clinical guidelines.[10,11] The number of patients suffering from heart failure also has increased as a consequence of decreased mortality from acute myocardial infarction and improved pharmacological treatment of heart failure. With longer life expectancy, this large heart failure population consumes a huge amount of health care resources.

Today, there are several issues in the management of patients with heart failure that need to be taken into account to improve outcomes. Many patients are not adequately diagnosed with echocardiography[12,13] and do not receive evidence-based care.[10,11] Patients hospitalized for heart failure often have a very short length of hospital stay, and discharge planning and follow-up after hospitalization are often not provided. Education aimed at improving heart failure self-care is often insufficient.[14] Patients' satisfaction with care is sometimes low, and patients ask for more support and education.[15,16] Studies from a wide variety of settings have shown that noncompliance with medication, diet, or symptom monitoring causes up to 50 percent of the hospital readmissions.[17] Heart failure disease management programs are designed to address these problems.

DEFINITION OF DISEASE MANAGEMENT

Disease management can be defined as a multidisciplinary care approach for patients with chronic illness, an approach that coordinates care along the continuum of illness and throughout the chain of care delivered by various heath care systems.[18] Multidisciplinary teams in heart failure disease management can include nurses, physicians, physical therapists, dieticians, social workers, psychologists, pharmacists, and others. In some settings, a full team with all the different health care professionals provides care to heart failure patients. However, most teams are nurse led with medical back up from a cardiologist and scarce collaboration with other physicians and health care professionals. The reason behind this structure is probably simply tradition. The roles of other heart failure team members need to be further developed and disseminated. These additional members have much to contribute to the care of these complex patients with a continuum of illness that proceeds toward the end of life with stable and unstable phases (Figure 79-1).[2,7-9]

Inclusion of a full range of disciplines can significantly improve the care provided for persons with heart failure. Physical therapists can evaluate physical capacity (e.g., 6-minute walk test), advise about training methods, and give practical advice on energy conservation. Their role is important since physical exercise has become an established part of heart failure rehabilitation. Dieticians can help to evaluate dietary intake, prescribe individualized diets, and help patients to improve adherence with diet recommendations. Being either overweight or underweight is serious in patients with heart failure. Weight reduction in obese heart failure patients and prevention and/or treatment of cachexia often need specialized guidance by a dietitian. Pharmacists can assist the patient in improving knowledge on heart failure treatment and to cope with medication side effects. They can also contribute in implementing guidelines and in preventing polypharmacy. Their knowledge on interactions and drug effects are useful in the heart failure team. Depression and cognitive dysfunction are common in heart failure, so there is room for extending the role of psychologists. Social workers also deal with psychosocial issues and support family and spouses[19] (see the accompanying Conundrum feature).

Development of Nurse-Managed Models

Nurses are increasingly involved in heart failure care, especially in patient education, follow-up, and drug titration. A nurse-led heart failure clinic was described in the literature for the first time in 1983 when Cintron and coworkers published the outcomes associated with their clinic in Puerto Rico.[20] During the latter part of the 1980s, the management of heart failure began to change in the United States, and heart failure clinics were initiated.[21] In 1995, Rich and coworkers[22] in the United States published a landmark study of a nurse-led, multidisciplinary intervention that combined telephone follow-up, outpatient, and home-based visits. They

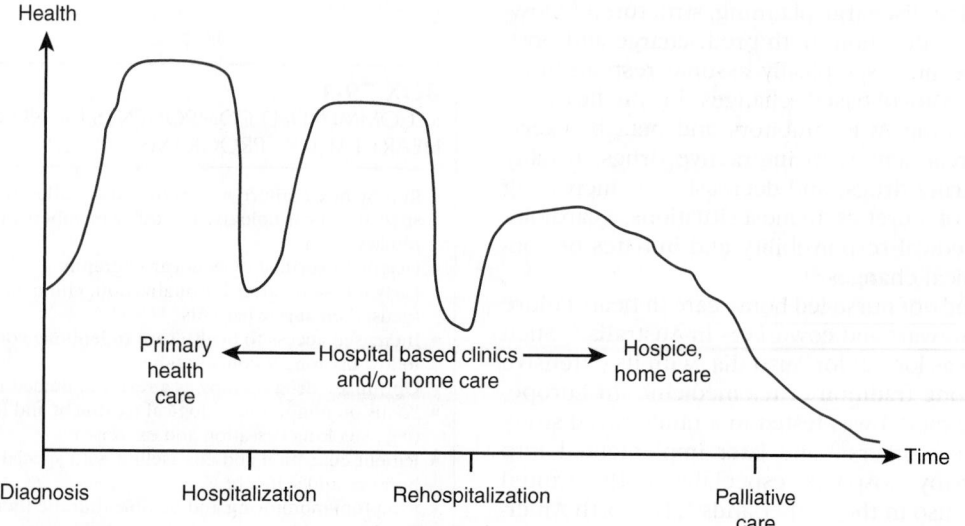

FIGURE 79-1 ▪ The continuum of heart failure with stable and unstable phases progressing toward the end of life. Also shown are the various health care systems involved in the different stages of heart failure.

■■■ CONUNDRUM

ELEMENTS OF DISEASE MANAGEMENT

Disease management, by definition, is a multifactorial intervention. What components of disease management are essential? Are some elements more effective than others? A recent meta-analysis attempted to answer this question by classifying the disease management interventions studied in 112 randomized and nonrandomized trials according to the chronic care model (CCM). Four elements of the six CCM elements—delivery system design, self-management support, decision support, and clinical information systems—were associated with better processes and outcomes. Too few investigators focused on community resources and health care organization to allow a full analysis of these CCM elements.

No single aspect of the CCM was essential to improve outcomes. Others have found that interventions with multiple components do better than single interventions, but in this meta-analysis, the number of CCM elements incorporated into the study intervention was not associated with better outcomes. Maybe delivery system design and self-management support had better outcomes than the other interventions. However, we remain uncertain at this point what components of disease management are essential to provide.

From Tsai AC, Morton SC, Mangione CM et al: A meta-analysis of interventions to improve care for chronic illnesses, *Am J Manag Care* 11:478-488, 2005.

---

demonstrated that a nurse-led intervention could decrease hospital admission and improve quality of life. These results echoed out over the Western world and resulted in many new nurse-led heart failure programs and randomized trials evaluating this initiative.[2,7-9]

Sweden was the first country in Europe to establish nurse-led heart failure clinics for patient education and follow-up, and there are currently heart failure clinics in more than 80 percent of Swedish hospitals.[23] There are also heart failure clinics in more that one third of the hospitals in Norway, Denmark, Iceland, the Netherlands, the United Kingdom, and Slovenia. Several other European countries are rapidly developing heart failure programs. Specially educated nurses staff these programs, providing discharge planning, structured follow-up, and patient education, both predischarge and postdischarge. The nurses typically assume responsibility for making protocol-based changes in medications, such as uptitrating ACE inhibitors and beta blockers; terminating treatment with interactive drugs; usually potassium-sparing drugs; and decreasing or increasing the daily dose of diuretics. In most situations, a cardiologist retains medical responsibility and initiates or confirms the medical changes.[24]

The first study of nurse-led home care in heart failure was done by Stewart and coworkers in Australia.[25] Such an approach was logical for Australia, with its extensive outback and long tradition of telemedicine. In Europe, the home-care model was tested in a randomized study by Blue and coworkers[26] and later implemented into practice in many hospitals, especially in the United Kingdom, but also in the Netherlands.[27] In North America, several different models (clinic and home-based in addition to telephone and telemonitoring programs) have been evaluated and are now used in routine clinical practice. Heart failure clinics in New Zealand use an integrated care model with collaboration between primary and secondary care.[28,29] So far there are no published scientific reports describing or evaluating nurse-led initiatives in heart failure care from Asia or Africa, but there are ongoing initiatives in clinical practice.

THE CLINIC MODEL
Components of Care

The clinic model of disease management focuses on early follow-up after hospitalization with symptom monitoring, optimized therapy, patient education, and psychosocial support. The care is often nurse led, with medical support by cardiologists with specialty training in heart failure. The patients come for an outpatient visit to a clinic often located close to or within a hospital. These clinics also provide telephone consultations, which are essential in the process of dealing with early symptom exacerbations. Box 79-1 summarizes the different components of the clinic and the home-based models. There is debate about which of these components of follow-up is most important and effective. But apart from education, which has been shown to have positive effects independent of the others,[30,31] none of the studies has attempted to answer this specific question. Therefore, it might be more relevant to consider disease management follow-up as a concept of care composed of several components with synergism instead of believing that just one single component could be enough to improve outcomes.

The advantages of the clinic model are first, its proximity to the hospital with all the medical facilities and equipment available. Secondly the physician, who retains medical responsibility, can be reached easily if the nurse needs a second opinion or advice, changes in medications, or tests. Thirdly, clinics are time and resource efficient because they negate the need to travel to patients' homes, and portable equipment is not needed.

BOX 79-1   ■■■
RECOMMENDED COMPONENTS OF NURSE-LED HEART FAILURE PROGRAMS

- Run by heart failure nurses in collaboration with heart failure specialized cardiologist and other members in a multidisciplinary team
- Diagnosis verified by echocardiography
- Early follow-up after hospitalization, clinic, or home based; focused on at-risk patients
- Increased access to health care (telephone consultation and follow-up, longer consultations)
- Optimized drug therapy as a result of guidelines
- Focus on nonpharmacological treatment and lifestyle changes (e.g., smoking cessation and exercise)
- Patient education and counseling with special emphasis on adherence and self-care
- Symptom monitoring and flexible diuretic therapy
- Psychosocial support to patients and family and/or caregiver
- Holistic, individualized care
- Evidence-based medicine and care

Evidence of Effectiveness

During the last years, several meta-analyses[2,7-9] have been performed evaluating the effects of heart failure disease management programs. Meta-analysis can be criticized for how the data are pooled since the original studies might be quite heterogeneous in design, intervention, outcome measures, and follow-up. However, since several of the studies evaluating disease management programs in heart failure have had small sample sizes, meta-analysis can be useful in guideline discussions and policymaking.

One of the recent meta-analyses included 30 randomized trials of almost 5000 patients cared for in disease management programs between 1993 and 2003.[2,7-9] This meta-analysis evaluated the effect of multidisciplinary, often nurse led, interventions with follow-up and patient education, often combined with optimization of treatment. The authors found that multidisciplinary care in a clinic or home-based setting significantly reduced mortality by 25 percent. Another meta-analysis by Philips and coworkers[7] found a trend toward decreased mortality, but a third by Gwadry-Sridhar and coworkers[9] did not find any effect on mortality. All meta-analyses showed that readmissions were also significantly reduced by multidisciplinary care in a clinic or home-based setting. The differences in the results regarding mortality in the meta-analyses may reflect the different aims and focus of the analyses or the fact that they categorized and analyzed the trials included differently. The reasons why some interventions were effective in improving survival in their study populations and others did not probably reflects both the components included in the intervention (e.g., if treatment was optimized and adherence and self-care improved) and the patients themselves (e.g., patients may have been severely ill and at high risk for a new event).

Currently available meta-analyses have analyzed different models of disease management and not included the same studies. McAlister and coworkers[2,7-9] found that, for the clinic model alone, the relative reduction in mortality was 34 percent in comparison with usual care; the absolute reduction in risk suggests that one life was saved for every 17 patients treated with this model of care. Readmissions also decreased by 21 percent, and clinics were shown to be cost-effective.[2,7-9] Gonseth and coworkers[8] stated that clinic models did not significantly reduce readmission or death alone, but the combined end point of mortality and hospitalization was significantly reduced (see the accompanying Evidence-Based Practice feature).

■ EVIDENCE-BASED PRACTICE

OUTCOMES IN DISEASE MANAGEMENT

Disease management is now the standard of care of persons with heart failure and other chronically ill patient groups (e.g., depression, diabetes, and asthma). Recent meta-analyses, reviews, and research syntheses have illustrated, without a doubt, that disease management is effective in improving outcomes. The question now is not *if* disease management should be used, but how it should be designed to fit within your setting.

HOME INTERVENTIONS
Components of Care

Home-based heart failure disease management programs contain components of care that are similar to that of the clinic model (see Box 79-1), but they are delivered in the patient's home. The home-based model of heart failure disease management has several distinct advantages over clinic-based models. First, patients do not need to be mobile or able to travel to a clinic. Second, it is much easier to assess the patients' needs, capabilities, and adherence to treatment in their own environment. Third, when palliative care is needed, the nurses, patients, and caregivers are already used to meeting in the familiar environment of the patient's home. Finally, it is easier to do a follow-up visit very shortly after hospitalization. In some cases, this means that patients can go home earlier from the hospital and receive some additional care in the home, which saves money for hospitals and improves the comfort of patients. In the future, with increasing average length of life and numbers of elderly, the use of home-based care is anticipated to increase.

Evidence of Effectiveness

Home-based care has been shown to significantly reduce morbidity. Stewart and coworkers have shown that the effects on mortality may persist as long as 18 months.[32] In the meta-analyses, the number of heart failure readmissions was reduced by home care by 28 percent to 39 percent as was the total number of hospitalizations reduced by 19 percent to 25 percent.[2,8] Because home-based interventions reduce readmissions, they are also cost-effective.[6] Interestingly, intervention with home-based education and support, but without optimization of treatment, also reduces the number of readmissions, showing the potent effect of these intervention components.[2]

TELEPHONE INTERVENTION
Components of Care

Telephone interventions can be provided through scheduled calls from a heart failure nurse or through a telephone service where the patients can call a heart failure nurse if questions arise or when deterioration occurs. The obvious limitation to this second approach is that patients must monitor their symptoms and be able to identify when deterioration has occurred. Another limitation is that these services are often regionally centralized and removed from the community in which the care is provided. McAlister and coworkers[2] showed that readmissions caused by heart failure were reduced by 25 percent, but all-cause morbidity and mortality was not reduced by telephone follow-up. One problem with the studies reviewed, however, was that many of these interventions included face-to-face counseling and education either before hospital discharge or during a clinic or home visit, in combination with the telephone intervention. This makes it difficult to determine exactly what the intervention was that was tested and found to be effective.

Evidence of Effectiveness

The previously cited meta-analysis by McAlister and co-workers[2,7-9] showed that telephone approaches were less effective in reducing morbidity than clinic- or home-based approaches. In addition, they did not affect mortality. In contrast to this result, a recently published study by Cleland and coworkers[33] showed that telephone follow-up by a specialist nurse improved 1-year survival significantly.

The advantages with telephone follow-up is that it can be provided at a low cost and is time saving and convenient both for the nurse and the patient since there is no need to travel to communicate. The disadvantages are that it can be difficult to assess, support, and educate a patient over the phone. Significant clinical expertise is needed to assess a patient when physical assessment is not an option and no tests can be performed.

SPECIAL TECHNOLOGICAL INTERVENTIONS

Components of Care

Telemonitoring allows daily monitoring of physiological variables and symptoms measured by patients or caregivers at home while allowing patients to remain under close supervision (Figure 79-2). Telemonitoring uses the

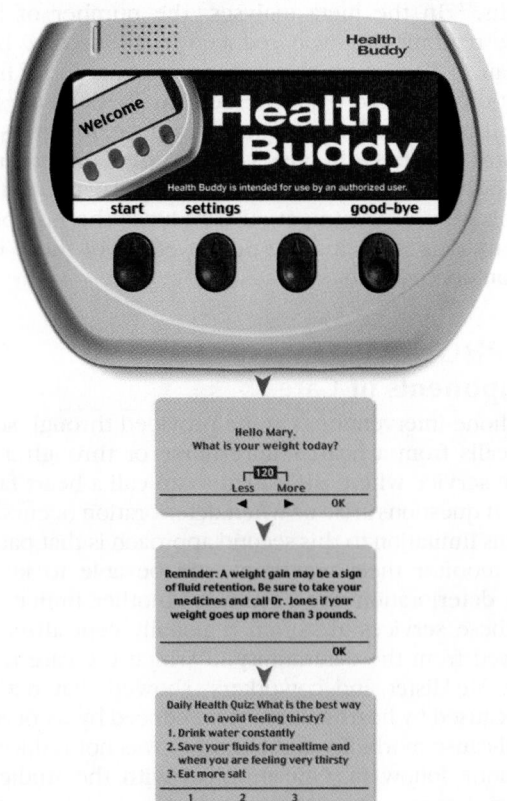

FIGURE 79-2 ■ Health care providers use the Health Hero Platform to send patients reminders, provide them with feedback on their progress, and provide tips for managing their disease more effectively. Shown here are samples of physician-to-patient dialogue using the *Health Buddy* messaging system. (Courtesy Health Hero Network, Inc.)

technology of special telecare devices and a telecommunication system standard telephone lines, cable-network, or broadband technology. The use of telemonitoring has increased in recent years but mainly in research settings. Before it spreads broadly to clinical practice, two things are needed: low-cost, user-friendly telemonitoring equipment and further evaluations of its effects.

Telemonitoring equipment may include blood pressure, pulse, electrocardiogram, oxygen saturation, electronic scales, symptom response systems, and video consultation equipment—all of which can be installed in the patient's home. Once collected, data are sent to a server, which is often housed in a hospital setting. A nurse monitors vital signs daily to detect early evidence of deterioration. He or she contacts the patient if signs of deterioration are detected or if no data are sent. Reports to date suggest that compliance with monitoring is good, and technical failures occur infrequently, so telemonitoring seems to be a feasible model of care.[34]

Evidence of Effectiveness

There are limited data evaluating the effectiveness of telemonitoring, and the few randomized trials conducted have had inconclusive results. Some trials have suggested that telemonitoring is ineffective, but the majority have shown reduced mortality and morbidity.[33,34] In a trans-European, multicenter study with 426 patients, telemonitoring was compared with usual care and nurse telephone support. The number of admissions and mortality were similar among the patients in the group receiving telemonitoring and the group getting telephone support from nurses, but significantly higher in the usual care group.[33] A randomized, multi-center study evaluating the effects of daily weight monitoring in almost 300 American patients with severe heart failure did not find any effect on readmissions, but mortality was reduced by more than 50 percent. In this study, experienced nurses evaluated symptoms and weight according to individualized protocols. Compliance with the monitoring system was almost 100 percent.[35] Another smaller study from the United Kingdom found similar results with very high compliance (*greater than* 75 percent) with measuring weight, pulse, and blood pressure.[36]

One problem may be that telemonitoring requires a steep learning curve for the patient and/or caregiver and the health care providers. There is still debate regarding which variables are most helpful to monitor, and new equipment with additional monitoring parameters is continuously under development. In the future, we can probably expect more advanced care moving into patients' homes. Telemonitoring is here to stay, and we will soon have more data on its overall efficacy as a distinct model of care and its overall cost-effectiveness.

WHICH MODEL IS BEST?

It is difficult to determine which of these models of care is optimal or best, at present. Both clinic- and home-based nurse-managed models effectively reduce mortality and all-cause morbidity in addition to costs. At present it appears that the home-based model may be the most effective model based on the results from the meta-analyses, especially for the population of fragile, older elderly patients and those who are not mobile. For the younger, fit elderly patients, the clinic model is probably more effective, from the perspective of the health care provider, since more patients can be seen in a day and hospital facilities are available. Telephone follow-up is probably an important aspect of care, but probably cannot replace face-to-face contact. Even a few visits with a heart failure nurse have been shown to have large effects on outcomes.

Local and national resources, patient needs, and setting infrastructure have to influence the decision regarding which model to use. In the United States, Australia, and Europe, all three models (clinic, home-based, and telecare) are used, either separately or combined. Regardless of the model chosen, though, the most important aspect of care is the inclusion of follow-up for previously hospitalized patients. Despite evidence-based recommendations in guidelines, most patients hospitalized for heart failure still do not receive an optimal follow-up. The effectiveness of heart failure disease management programs may be due to the inclusion of this one essential element.

IMPROVING CARE MODELS IN THE FUTURE

Perhaps care in the future will combine new technology with personal contact to allow patients to be assessed (e.g., using telemonitoring equipment in combination with a web camera) (Figure 79-3). Quality assurance using such an approach will need to be developed further and evaluated,[32] but every program should build in quality indicators, such as those shown in Box 79-2, to ensure continuous evaluation of programs.

Another ethical and equality issue is the need to make heart failure management programs suitable for as many heart failure patients as possible. Further evaluation is needed to determine which patients benefit the most from heart failure disease management and therefore are most cost-effective to enroll in such programs. To be most successful in reducing mortality and morbidity through heart failure disease management, populations most at risk need to be targeted. Further, there is a big need to find new ways of dealing with vulnerable populations, such as African-Americans and Hispanics living in the United States, aboriginals in Australia, and Maoris in New Zealand,[33,34] various immigrant groups in Europe, and persons with poor social support, depression, and/or low self-esteem. Hospitalized patients with moderate to severe heart failure appear to benefit more from disease management than those with mild heart failure, so research is needed to identify the best treatment approach for patients with mild or early heart failure. Mortality and morbidity from heart failure is much higher in vulnerable populations, and a paradox is that, despite this reality, these patients are seldom reached by effective, evidence-based interventions especially designed for their needs.

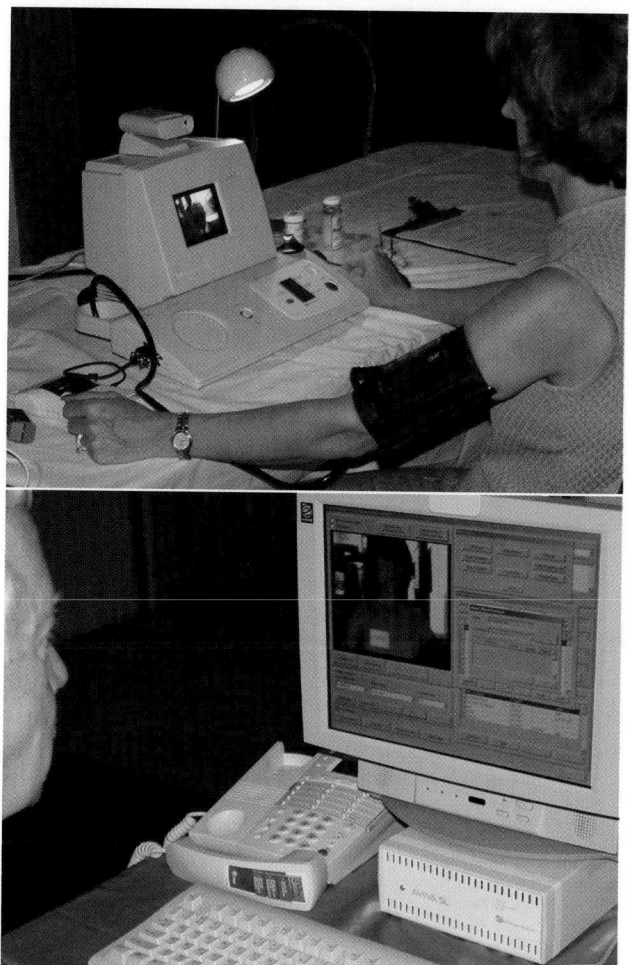

FIGURE 79-3 ▪ Telehealth with video monitoring is anticipated to be more widely used in the future. **A,** Patient's station. **B,** Nurse's station. (Courtesy Kathryn Bowles.)

Nurses' Contribution to Disease Management

Disease management programs are mainly coordinated and run by nurses with medical backup from a cardiologist and sometimes a multidisciplinary team. Heart failure nurses have long experience in cardiac care and a personal interest, in and additional education, in heart failure care and treatment. Many nurses have extended responsibilities, interpreting lab tests and echocardiography results, and initiating and titrating drugs based on changes in physiological status. For legal reasons, written delegation for tasks that represented extended practice may be needed. In the United States, many heart failure nurses have master's degrees and are clinical nurse specialists or nurse practitioners. In Europe, nurses working in heart failure clinics often have numerous years of clinical experience and additional heart failure education, but they are not necessarily master's prepared. In Sweden and Scotland, there are university courses that offer a degree in heart failure care. In several other European countries, there are shorter courses on how to set up and run a heart failure program.[23,37]

BOX 79-2
INDICATORS OF QUALITY CARE IN HEART FAILURE
MANAGEMENT PROGRAMS

Patient-Focused Indicators
- Documentation of cause
- Documentation of functional class (NYHA or equivalent)
- Documentation of physical findings
- Documentation of risk factors and reached target values
- Documentation of relevant laboratory reports
- Documentation of weight, body mass index, and nutritional status
- Documentation of cognitive dysfunction, learning needs, and barriers
- Proportion of patients with an objective diagnosis of cardiac dysfunction
- Proportion of patients receiving target doses of ACE inhibitors and beta blockers
- Proportion of patients receiving aldosterone-receptor blockers
- Proportion of patients receiving patient education
- Patient satisfaction scores
- Self-care behavior scores
- Quality-of-life scores
- Number of readmissions
- Mortality

Program-Focused Indicators
- Time from referral to first clinic visit
- Availability of telephone counseling
- Staff competencies
- Documentation of study visits and other educational activities
- Documentation of collaboration of other caregivers
- Costs

ACE, Angiotensin-converting enzyme; *NYHA*, New York Heart Association.
Adapted from Gustafsson F, Arnold J: Heart failure clinic and outpatient management: review of evidence and call for quality assurance, *Eur Heart J* 25:1596-1604, 2004.

It is important to delineate the core competencies and clinical responsibilities of the specialist heart failure nurse in contrast to nursing staff with limited training or experience in heart failure disease management. There are huge differences within and between countries in the education and competencies of registered nurses. There are also legal differences regarding what nurses are allowed to do with their license. The job description needs to be clear and in agreement with formal and real competence, and the whole heart failure team needs to agree on the roles and responsibilities assumed.

Nurses have a unique competence to bring to heart failure disease management programs. It is not by coincidence that nurses with their combined knowledge and skills within cardiology, nursing, teaching, and behavior science have been so successful in improving outcomes through delivering follow-up, education, and support to patients. It is important to provide holistic care of patients with heart failure that spans biomedical, psychological, social, emotional, and existential perspectives. The holistic nursing perspective involves a combination of all aspects of care.

Networks of heart failure nurses can be useful in the development of the individual heart failure nurse. Nurses who have already acquired specialized heart failure skills have an important role as teachers of future heart failure disease management nursing trainees. With the increasing number of patients with heart failure and the proven effectiveness of nurse-led heart failure man-

agement programs, there will be an increasing need for specialized nurses. Networks also improve our abilities to influence policymakers and stakeholders in the health care systems. Such networks now exist both in Europe through the Heart Failure Association within the European Society of Cardiology and in the United States through the American Association of Heart Failure Nurses and the Heart Failure Society of America.

Factors to Consider When Setting Up a Disease Management Program

There are several aspects in the organization of these nurse-led models of disease management that need further evaluation and comparison. It is still not clear which organizational model of care (e.g., home-based and/or clinic-based) or which educational model is most effective and optimal following a hospitalization. The timing of the first visit is still under debate. Early follow-up after discharge is, without doubt, essential, but does it matter whether it is done within the first days or weeks after discharge? There are differences in how quickly this first visit is done in different programs.[2,7-9] Other issues, such as how many visit are needed, how often, and for how long, are still being debated. That is, how long should a heart failure patient be maintained in a disease management program? Some programs continue to follow stable patients every 6 or 12 months. However, recent data show that the first 3 months of follow-up seem to make the most difference in terms of reducing hospital readmission.[38] There is also evidence that the number of visits can be few and individualized as a result of patients' needs and that stable, optimally treated, and well-informed patients can be referred back to their family physician, often a general practitioner or a cardiologist.[5,32]

Further follow-up is often performed in an outpatient clinic, through home visits or telephone consultations, or some combination is common as well. The place chosen for follow-up depends on resources, patient needs, and hospital or practice policy. Further research is needed to evaluate and compare various models of care. In the near future, a large scale Dutch trial called Coordinating Study Evaluating Outcomes of Advising and Counseling in Heart Failure (COACH) with more than 1000 patients will be presented and hopefully give us some answers regarding whether a more intense follow-up is more effective than a less intense regimen with fever visits to the heart failure nurse.[39] The key to designing a disease management program is to set up one that is adapted to the resources and organization of the local hospital.

Defining Goals and Key Components

Overall goals should be defined to include both the patient-centered and societal health care perspectives. On the patient level, goals can be to provide individualized patient education, increase self-care, and adaptation to life with chronic heart failure. A decision regarding whether the focus should be on both patients and spouses or other caregivers is needed. Caregivers often experience burden, and spouses might need special attention to prevent anxiety and depression.

Examples of goals on the health care level are to improve follow-up after hospitalization; improve quality of life and survival in patients with heart failure; reduce the number of hospital readmissions; provide evidence-based medicine and care regarding diagnostics, treatment, education, and support; and to perform quality assurance and audits of the program regularly. The key components should be discussed and decided on by the key participants. Usual key elements of nurse-managed programs are shown in Box 79-1.[40] These key elements aim at improving both societal and patient-centered goals. Quality indicators, as exemplified in Box 79-2, also should be set to ensure a continuous evaluation of quality of care and fulfillment of goals.

Defining Economic and Organizational Frames

The economic resources available for running a program influence how the service can be organized (e.g., the number of nurses, physicians, and other health care professionals that can be hired; what facilities can be afforded; and the extent of follow-up). In some cases, new resources are provided for starting up the program. In other cases, the program is financed by shrinking other departments. Often there are expectations that the program will be cost saving, but the savings are sometimes found in other parts of the organization (emergency department, cardiac care unit, other hospital units), making savings difficult to track.[6] Another important issue is whether it is most convenient for patients and the staff to have hospital-based clinic visits or home visits. If the visits are to be hospital based, a setting with close parking, little incline, few steps, etc. is crucial.

Optimizing Communication Between Providers

Establishing good collaboration throughout the whole chain of care providers, especially between primary and secondary care, is an important task for the staff in a nurse-led heart failure program. These good relations ensure that the competence and potential of the nurse-led program are used in the best way. It is essential to elucidate how and who can refer patients to the heart failure program and what service can be provided. It is also important to decide who has the responsibility for the total care and follow-up of stable heart failure patients to use resources and competence most effectively. For example, the protocol must address the issue of when patients are discharged from the program and to whom and when and how to admit or readmit them. The care and treatment of heart failure is often complex, with physicians and other health care professionals from different specializations involved. Good collaboration and communication can give additive effects that improve the care and safety. Poor communication can lead to duplication of work, misunderstandings, and mistakes.

The patients need to be optimally diagnosed, treated, and educated according to guidelines irrespective of the caregiver. Therefore, ongoing joint discussion and educational initiatives are needed for all caregivers in the chain of care.

Choosing the Patient Population

Before setting up a program, it is important to delineate the possible extent of the program. Patients with heart failure are a heterogeneous group that covers a large age span, different causes, and varied severity of heart failure and social situation. Most patients are older than age 70 and have several other comorbidities, such as diabetes, arthritis, cancer, chronic obstructive lung disease, and renal failure.[41]

The number of patients hospitalized each year as a result of heart failure and the percentage that is suitable for follow-up need to be estimated in addition to the number of patients that will be referred from other caregivers (e.g., primary care providers). It is crucial to discuss which patients would benefit the most from participating in the program. Most studies evaluating heart failure programs include hospitalized patients without severe cognitive dysfunction, and it is evident that these patients benefit from this type of follow-up. However, in some studies, patients have been younger than the average heart failure patient, and few studies have included socially deprived patients (e.g., immigrants, psychiatrically ill, and homeless).

DEFINING PROGRAM CONTENT

The content of heart failure disease management programs vary widely in different countries and health care settings. Some programs use a multidisciplinary approach; others are centered on heart failure specialist nurses. The programs can be initiated during hospitalization, at discharge, or during the first weeks after discharge. Follow-up can last between a week and a year, sometimes even longer. The intervention can be one single planned visit and then individualized depending on the condition of the patient up to a great number of planned follow-up visits at a clinic, at home, and/or through telephone calls.

The content of follow-up visits or telephone calls depends on how far along the patient is in the course of the disease. Figure 79-1 illustrates that the course of heart failure is not linear. It varies significantly and repeatedly with deteriorations and improvement, from the time of diagnosis to the time of death. It is important that optimal, guideline-based treatment and patient education be given immediately after the patient is first diagnosed rather than waiting until the patient experiences repeated hospitalizations. A heart failure management program can have an important role in the uptitration of drugs, such as ACE inhibitors, beta blockers, angiotensin- and aldosterone-receptor blockers. Since many nurses do not prescribe drugs autonomously, titration protocols and treatment algorithms need to be created and protocols developed that describe routines for prescriptions and consultations.[37]

The first educational session should include a definition of heart failure, the rationale for and importance of following the prescribed pharmacological and nonpharmacological treatment regimen, and a description of necessary self-care behaviors. Patients need to become proficient in symptom monitoring, and they need to understand the need for physical exercise, routine immunizations, and lifestyle changes, such as a restricted-sodium diet.[10,11]

The information about the diagnosis can trigger a crisis for both patients and their families as a result of the perception that life is threatened.[42] Support might be needed to facilitate their adaptation to the new situation of living with chronic illness. It is important to emphasize that the goal of treatment and self-care is to live with as little limitation as possible in daily life. However, it is important to also communicate that heart failure is not cured since many patients during periods of clinical stability feel that they do not suffer from heart failure anymore and might, for example, stop taking their medications or monitoring their symptoms.

Patients with heart failure who have been hospitalized are considered to be at high risk with a poorer prognosis and risk for readmissions.[3] An early outpatient visit is done to assess the physiological status to detect signs of deterioration, optimize treatment, and discuss side effects. Further, educational needs should be assessed, and additional education provided. Patients should learn to monitor symptoms and adjust their diuretics when signs and symptoms of fluid retention occur. After a period of deterioration, patients and their families often experience insecurity and anxiety and need support. Consultations in nurse-led programs are often longer (30 to 60 minutes) than visits to the physician and enable an extended, holistic assessment, with more time for education and psychosocial support.

To prevent readmission, the cause of a previous admission should be determined if possible, and eliminated. Increased access to care through daily telephone hours allows patients more opportunity to discuss symptoms, treatment, and self-care behavior with a specialized nurse.

The time when a high-risk patient goes into palliative care varies. Defining the prognosis of an individual patient is very difficult since heart failure is a fluctuating condition, and sudden death can occur during a stable phase. The medical treatment is seldom terminated in patients with heart failure since the treatment often is the best way to decrease symptoms.[43] This issue is discussed further in Chapter 64.

Each program must decide on the system of documentation to be used, but the physiological status, signs of heart failure, general health and life situation, treatment changes, education and psychosocial support provided, and the plan for further follow-up are important components of care that should be well documented.

REFERENCES

1. Jong P, Vowinckel E, Liu P et al: Prognosis and determinants of survival in patients newly hospitalized for heart failure: a population-based study, *Arch Intern Med* 162:1689-1694, 2002.
2. McAlister F, Stewart S, Ferrua S et al: Multidisciplinary strategies for the management of heart failure patients at high risk for admission. A systematic review of randomised trials. *J Am Coll Cardiol* 44:810-819, 2004.
3. McMurray JJ, Stewart S: Epidemiology, aetiology and prognosis of heart failure, *Heart* 83:596-602, 2000.
4. Vinson JM, Rich MW, Sperry JC et al: Early readmission of elderly patients with congestive heart failure, *J Am Geriatr Soc* 38:1290-1295, 1990.
5. Strömberg A, Mårtensson J, Fridlund B et al: Nurse-led heart failure clinics improve survival and self-care behaviour in patients with heart failure. Results from a prospective, randomised study, *Eur Heart J* 24:1014-1023, 2003.
6. Stewart S, Blue L, Walker A et al: An economic analysis of specialist heart failure nurse management in the UK; can we afford not to implement it? *Eur Heart J* 23:1369-1378, 2002.
7. Phillips C, Wright S, Kern D et al: Comprehensive discharge planning with postdischarge support for older patients with congestive heart failure: a meta-analysis, *JAMA* 291:1358-1367, 2004.
8. Gonseth J, Guallar-Castillon P, Banegas J et al: The effectiveness of disease management programmes in reducing hospital re-admission in older patients with heart failure: a systematic review and meta-analysis of published reports, *Eur Heart J* 25:1570-1595, 2004.
9. Gwadry-Sridhar F, Flintoft V, Lee D et al: A systematic review and meta-analysis of studies comparing readmission rates and mortality rates in patients with heart failure, *Arch Intern Med* 164:2315-2320, 2004.
10. ACC/AHA task force report: ACC/AHA guidelines for the evaluation and management of chronic heart failure in the adult: executive summary: a Report of the American College of Cardiology/American Heart Association Task Force on Practice Guidelines, *Circulation* 104:2996-3007, 2001.
11. The Task Force for the Diagnosis and Treatment of Chronic Heart Failure of the European Society of Cardiology: Guidelines for the diagnosis and treatment of chronic heart failure, *Eur Heart J* 26:1115-1140, 2005.
12. Philbin EF, DiSalvo TG: Influence of race and gender on care process, resource use and outcomes in congestive heart failure, *Am J Cardiol* 82:76-81, 1998.
13. Mejhert M, Holmgren J, Wändell P et al: Diagnostic tests, treatment and follow-up in heart failure patients—is there a gender bias in the coherence to guidelines? *Eur J Heart Fail* 1:407-410, 1990.
14. Carlson B, Riegel B, Moser D: Self-care abilities of patients with heart failure, *Heart Lung* 30:351-359, 2001.
15. Broström A, Strömberg A, Dahlström U et al: Patients with congestive heart failure and their conceptions of their sleep situation, *J Adv Nurs* 34:520-529, 2001.
16. Ekman I, Norberg A, Lundman B: An intervention aimed at reducing uncertainty in elderly patients with chronic heart failure, *International J Human Caring* 4:7-13, 2000.
17. Evangelista LS, Dracup K: A closer look at compliance research in heart failure patients in the last decade, *Prog Cardiovasc Nurs* 15:97-103, 2000.
18. Ellrodt G, Cook D, Lee J et al: Evidence-based disease management, *JAMA* 278:1687-1692, 1997.
19. Jaarsma T: Inter-professional team approach to patients with heart failure, *Heart* 91:832-838, 2005.
20. Cintron G, Bigas C, Linares E et al: Nurse practitioner's role in chronic heart failure clinic: in hospital time, costs, and patient satisfaction, *Heart Lung* 12:237-240, 1983.
21. Martens KH: The increasing role of nurses in the management of heart failure in the USA. In Stewart S, Blue L, editors: *Improving outcomes in chronic heart failure,* London, 2001, BMJ.
22. Rich MW, Beckham V, Wittenberg C et al: A multidisciplinary intervention to prevent the readmission of elderly patients with congestive heart failure, *N Engl J Med* 333:1190-1195, 1995.
23. Strömberg A, Mårtensson J, Fridlund B et al: Nurse-led heart failure clinics in Sweden, *Eur J Heart Fail* 3:139-144, 2001.
24. Jaarsma T, Strömberg A, DeGeest S et al: Heart failure management programmes in Europe, *Eur J Cardiovasc Nurs* 5:197-205, 2006.
25. Stewart S, Pearson S, Horowitz J: Effects of a home-based intervention among patients with congestive heart failure discharged from acute hospital care, *Arch Intern Med* 158:1067-1072, 1998.

26. Blue L, Strong E, McMurray JJV et al: Randomised controlled trial of specialist nurse intervention in heart failure, *BMJ* 323:715-718, 2001.

27. Jaarsma T, Haaijer-Ruskamp F, Sturm H et al: Management of heart failure in the Netherlands, *Eur J Heart Fail* 7:371-376, 2005.

28. Doughty RN, Wright SP, Walsh HJ et al: Integrated care for patients with chronic heart failure: the New Zealand experience. In Stewart S, Blue L, editors: *Improving outcomes in chronic heart failure,* London, 2001, BMJ.

29. Doughty RN, Wright SP, Pearl A et al: Randomized, controlled trial of integrated heart failure management: the Auckland Heart Failure Management Study, *Eur Heart J* 23:139-146, 2002.

30. Krumholz HM, Amatruda J, Smith GL et al: Randomized trial of an education and support intervention to prevent readmission of patients with heart failure, *J Am Coll Cardiol* 39:83-89, 2002.

31. Koelling T, Johnson M, Cody R et al: Discharge education improves clinical outcomes in patients with chronic heart failure, *Circulation* 111:179-185, 2005.

32. Stewart S, Marley JE, Horowitz JD: Effects of a multidisciplinary, home-based intervention on unplanned readmissions and survival among patients with chronic congestive heart failure, *Lancet* 354:1077-1083, 1999.

33. Cleland J, Louis A, Rigby A et al: Noninvasive home telemonitoring for patients with heart failure at high risk of recurrent admission and death: the Trans-European Network-Home-Care Management System (TEN-HMS) study, *J Am Coll Cardiol* 45:1654-1664, 2005.

34. Louis A, Turner T, Gretton M et al: A systematic review of telemonitoring for the management of heart failure, *Eur J Heart Fail* 5:583-590, 2003.

35. Goldberg L, Piette J, Walsh M et al: Randomized trial of a daily electronic home monitoring system in patients with advanced heart failure (WHARF) trial, *Am Heart J* 146:705-712, 2003.

36. de Lusignan S, Wells S, Johnson P et al: Compliance and effectiveness of 1 year's home telemonitoring. The report of a pilot study of patients with chronic heart failure, *Eur J Heart Fail* 3:723-730, 2001.

37. Blue L, McMurray J: How much responsibility should nurses take? *Eur J Heart Fail* 7:351-361, 2005.

38. Ledwidge M, Ryan E, O'Loughlin C et al: Heart failure care in a hospital unit: a comparison of standard 3-month and extended 6-month programs, *Eur J Heart Fail* 7:385-391, 2005.

39. Jaarsma T, Van Der Wal M, Hogenhuis J et al: Design and methodology of the COACH study: a multicenter randomised coordinating study evaluating outcomes of advising and counseling in heart failure, *Eur J Heart Fail* 6:227-233, 2004.

40. Grady KL, Dracup K, Kennedy G et al: Team management of patients with heart failure: a statement for healthcare professionals from the cardiovascular nursing council of the American Heart Association, *Circulation* 102:2443-2456, 2000.

41. Braunstein JB, Anderson GF, Gerstenblith G et al: Noncardiac comorbidity increases preventable hospitalizations and mortality among Medicare beneficiaries with chronic heart failure, *J Am Coll Cardiol* 42:1226-1233, 2003.

42. Stull DE, Starling R, Haas G et al: Becoming a patient with heart failure, *Heart Lung* 28:284-292, 1999.

43. Jaarsma T: End-of-life issues in cardiac patients and their families, *Eur J Cardiovasc Nurs* 1:223-225, 2002.

chapter 80

Cardiac Rehabilitation

Meg Gulanick
Kathy Berra

CHAPTER ABBREVIATIONS

AHCPR Agency for Health Care Policy and Research (now called the Agency for Healthcare Research and Quality)

AICD Automatic implantable cardioverter-defibrillator

ATP III Adult Treatment Panel III (Third Report of the Expert Panel on Detection, Evaluation, and Treatment of High Blood Cholesterol in Adults)

BMI body mass index

CABG coronary artery bypass graft

CHD coronary heart disease

CHESS Comprehensive Health Enhancement Support System

CR cardiac rehabilitation

CVD cardiovascular disease

ECG electrocardiogram

ETICA Exercise Training Intervention after Coronary Angioplasty Trial

ExTraMATCH Exercise training Meta-Analysis of Trials in Patients with Chronic Heart Failure

ENRICHD Enhancing Recovery in Coronary Heart Disease

HCFA Health Care Financing Agency (now called the Centers for Medicare and Medicaid Services)

MI myocardial infarction

NHLBI National Heart, Lung, and Blood Institute

SCRIP Stanford Coronary Risk Intervention Program

SHN Stanford Heart Network

HISTORICAL PERSPECTIVE

Lifestyle, medical, pharmacological, surgical, and technological advances greatly influenced the evolution of cardiac rehabilitation **(CR)**. Cardiovascular care from the 1920s to the 1940s offered limited choices. Coronary artery disease was felt to be an irreversible process. Home care for acute myocardial infarction **(MI)** was standard medical practice. The risk of thromboembolism was high as a result of a minimum of 6 weeks of strict bed rest and a lack of medical and surgical therapies. Significant morbidity and mortality was expected and accepted. Studies began to demonstrate the deleterious effects of strict bed rest and suggested that early mobilization following acute MI may be beneficial. These studies demonstrated a decrease in morbidity and mortality and improved psychological recovery with earlier ambulation.[1,2] Exercise-based CR played an important role in optimal recovery.

The 1960s brought the advent of coronary care units. Early and progressive ambulation resulted in earlier discharge and greatly improved outcomes. Dr. Nanette Wenger developed the "14 Steps of Cardiac Rehabilitation," providing physicians with a way to evaluate the safety of returning patients to activities of daily living and to work.[3] With earlier ambulation, patients with signs and symptoms of cardiovascular ischemia requiring further evaluation and therapy were identified and treated.[4,5] Programs in CR continued to meet the needs of patients with disabilities following acute MI resulting from myocardial injury and hospitalization.

In 1960, the Surgeon General's report on the health risk of cigarette smoking highlighted the importance of "prevention." Reducing coronary risk factors became an increasingly important role for CR professionals.

Sophisticated electrocardiogram **(ECG)** analysis, routine use of exercise testing, coronary arteriography, and bypass surgery were significant hallmarks of this time. Community-based interventions, such as CR and the widespread use of paramedics, flourished and became the standard of care.

The next 40 years brought major advances in our understanding of the pathophysiology of atherosclerosis. The importance of medications, such as aspirin, diuretics, beta blockers, calcium channel blockers, angiotensin-converting enzyme inhibitors, angiotensin-receptor uptake blockers, statins and other lipid-lowering drugs, and thrombolytics was identified. Angioplasty and coronary artery stenting became alternative therapies to bypass surgery. The Stanford Coronary Risk Intervention Program **(SCRIP)** demonstrated that systematic case management for risk reduction in persons with coronary artery disease stabilized disease; reduced lesion formation was documented angiographically.[6] In addition, a 45 percent reduction in clinical coronary events was found in the intervention group. This landmark clinical trial supported the importance of the CR multifactor risk reduction model.

Dramatic changes also were seen in the care of patients with heart failure. Cardiac transplantation became widely available. Pacemaker therapies were found to aid in resynchronization and improve myocardial function. The importance of early and intensive treatment for acute MI was the key to limiting damage and protecting myocardial tissue at risk. Atherosclerosis regression trials demonstrated safe and effective ways to prevent the growing epidemic of heart disease.[6,7] The development of the automatic implantable cardioverter-defibrillator **(AICD)** added greatly to the management of patients at high risk of sudden cardiac death.

At this same time, exercise-based CR programs continued to show their benefit in facilitating recovery and protection of patients with vascular diseases. Evidence accumulated showing that atherosclerotic plaque stabilized—progressing less and regressing more—in response to multifactor risk reduction.[6,7] Treatment for acute MI emphasized secondary prevention. Clinical practice guidelines suggested that participation in CR could decrease mortality up to 25 percent.[8]

CARDIAC REHABILITATION AND OUTCOMES

Consumers and health care providers alike require evidence-based information to guide informed decision making regarding the costs and benefits of the various CR services. Beneficial outcomes from CR can be classified as functional, psychosocial, and behavioral and/or lifestyle changes.

Functional Outcomes

Exercise provides important protection for patients with coronary artery disease and other cardiovascular related illnesses. Two meta-analyses by Oldridge[9] and O'Connor[10] were the first to demonstrate that exercise-based CR was associated with a 20 percent to 25 percent reduction in all-cause and cardiac mortality compared with usual care. Neither study found a significant reduction in nonfatal reinfarction.

In 1992 the Agency for Health Care Policy and Research (**AHCPR**, now known as the Agency for Healthcare Research and Quality) and the National Heart, Lung, and Blood Institute (**NHLBI**) of the National Institutes of Health commissioned the American Association of Cardiovascular and Pulmonary Rehabilitation to review the scientific literature on CR. From a total of 900 scientific reports, 334 studies were included in the final list of references that formed the basis for that early clinical practice guideline.[8] The guideline summarized the evidence on outcomes achieved with exercise training, cardiovascular risk reduction, and education. Exercise training was shown to:

- Improve exercise tolerance, regardless of gender or age, without significant cardiovascular complications. The authors concluded that "appropriately prescribed and conducted exercise training should be an integral component of CR services" (p.4).
- Improve symptoms of angina pectoris and heart failure.
- Reduce cardiovascular mortality by approximately 25 percent from multifactorial CR and 15 percent from exercise-only programs.
- Not be associated with increased mortality or morbidity.

Limitations of these early studies included preferential referral of middle-aged men recovering from uncomplicated MI. Many of these studies were not randomized controlled trials, and most were done with small samples. Further, most of the studies were done before the advent of major life-saving therapies and treatments for acute MI (i.e., coronary thrombolysis and angioplasty) and newer pharmacological therapies that significantly reduce cardiovascular risk.

In 2004, Taylor and coworkers conducted an extensive systematic review and meta-analysis of randomized controlled trials of CR services that incorporated newer models of delivery with a broader range of services in the setting of contemporary medicine.[11] This review included 8940 patients from 48 trials. Compared with usual care, CR exercise therapy reduced total mortality 20 percent and cardiac mortality 26 percent,[11,12] supporting the earlier AHCPR synthesis. The authors were unable to discern whether exercise-only or exercise combined with risk reduction therapies had the greatest benefit. There were no significant differences in the rate of nonfatal MI or revascularization.

The evidence is compelling that comprehensive, exercise-based CR reduces mortality.[11,13] Proposed cardioprotective benefits of exercise include improved endothelial function, reduced C-reactive protein levels, antiischemic effects, increased parasympathetic tone, reduced risk of sudden cardiac death, improved coagulation and clotting factors, and an improved risk factor profile.[14]

In particular, exercise has been shown to confer benefit in certain populations. For example, moderate intensity exercise training after percutaneous transluminal coronary angioplasty or stenting (as shown in the Exercise Training Intervention After Coronary Angioplasty [ETICA] Trial) improved functional capacity and lowered cardiac event rates and hospital readmission rates in treatment compared with control.[15] No differences were found in restenosis rates, however.

Persons with heart failure also benefit from aerobic exercise training.[16,17] Much of this benefit is from improvements in exercise tolerance and quality of life. There continues to be concern as to the cost-benefit ratio in the heart failure population, however. In a recent systematic review of 81 studies,[18] a broad range of exercise training programs for heart failure was shown to be safe and effective. Considered individually, adverse events and deaths were not significantly lower in the exercise group. However, when these end points were combined, the analysis neared statistical significance. Another review of 29 studies of patients with mild to moderate heart failure from the Cochrane collection supports the finding of improved exercise capacity and quality of life.[19] The short time period for most of these studies made it difficult to identify the effect of exercise on clinical outcomes. In contrast, the European Exercise Training Meta-Analysis of Trials in Patients with Chronic Heart Failure (ExTraMATCH) project reviewed nine prospective randomized controlled trials evaluating survival in patients with left ventricular systolic dysfunction. Supervised exercise programs were safe and significantly reduced mortality and time to hospital admission.[20]

The definitive study designed to answer the remaining questions about exercise training in heart failure is currently underway. HF-ACTION will randomize 3000 patients to a supervised exercise program followed by home exercise versus usual care for 3 years. The primary outcomes will include both all-cause mortality and readmissions.

It is important to remember that the trials included in these reviews continue to underrepresent women, elderly patients, ethnic groups, postrevascularization and angina patients, patients with heart failure, and those following heart transplantation or heart valve surgery.[13] More research is needed to evaluate the effects of alternative models for delivery of exercise-based therapies, such as home- and community-based approaches or virtual interventions delivered by the Internet. A recent community-based study demonstrated that the CR patients had a 3-year survival advantage of 95 percent compared with nonparticipants, 64 percent of whom survived, and this benefit was evident in all age groups and both genders.[21] Moreover, the CR participants had a 28 percent reduction in recurrent MI. This study highlighted the continued lower CR participation rates for women (38 percent versus 67 percent for men) and the elderly (see the accompanying Conundrum feature on special populations).

Although the benefits of physical activity are well established,[22,23] physical activity remains poorly prescribed for older patients with coronary artery disease. Older patients can participate safely in properly designed programs consisting of aerobic and strength training and flexibility and range of motion activities. However, there are no definitive studies demonstrating that CR exercise therapy for elders confers the same reduction in coronary and total mortality as that seen in the younger population. Only one study demonstrated that men (mean age 63 years) with coronary artery disease had significantly lower all-cause mortality over a 5-year follow-up period after participating in light-to-

moderate levels of physical activity compared with a sedentary cohort.[24] More studies of this type are greatly needed.

The Enhancing Recovery in Coronary Heart Disease (ENRICHD) trial provided an opportunity to examine the effects of exercise on morbidity and mortality in patients who were depressed or reporting low levels of social support following an MI.[25] Those who reported exercising ("In the past 6 months have you engaged in regular exercise?") had half the cardiac events (5.7 percent) than their sedentary counterparts (12 percent). Similarly, the exercisers had a lower rate of nonfatal acute MI (6.5 percent) compared with the nonexercisers (10.5 percent).

Psychosocial Outcomes

Reduced morbidity and mortality are important outcomes of CR.[26] Psychosocial variables, such as anxiety, depression, hostility, social isolation, and lack of social support, affect the prognosis of patients with coronary heart disease **(CHD)** and those undergoing revascularization procedures and device implants. Research demonstrating the effectiveness of CR in improving these outcomes is limited. Studies conducted were often poorly designed with limited follow-up. Participants often began the interventions with vastly different degrees of emotional disturbance. In spite of this, a few randomized controlled trials have documented beneficial effects of exercise training and comprehensive CR on quality of life, with increases in functional capacity, enhanced independence, reduced symptoms, and better overall psychological well-being.[27,28]

The 1995 AHCPR clinical practice guideline on CR reported beneficial effects of exercise training alone or with other CR services on psychological well-being.[8] Education, counseling, and behavioral CR interventions reduced stress and improved psychological functioning, but exercise alone did not positively affect anxiety or depression. Authors of that early guideline recommended exercise training in conjunction with education, counseling, and psychosocial intervention as part of a multifactorial CR program.

CR has been shown to enhance quality of life. A systematic review of 12 randomized clinical trials testing comprehensive CR approaches reported a significant positive effect.[29] Similarly the Women's Lifestyle Heart Trial found a significant improvement in quality of life among women participating in a comprehensive lifestyle change program.[30]

Interventions for depression have not been very effective in the CHD patient population. When cognitive behavioral therapy, supplemented with a selective serotonin uptake inhibitor antidepressant as needed, was tested in recovering depressed or socially isolated acute MI patients in the ENRICHD trial, the effect was minimal.[31] In the ENRICHD trial, 2481 patients were followed for a mean of 2 years. Although the treatment provided modest but significant improvement in depression and social isolation, there was no significant improvement in primary or secondary cardiac end points. A similar conclusion was reached by authors of a Co-

---

■■■ CONUNDRUM

SPECIAL POPULATIONS: WHY DO WOMEN, ELDERS, AND MINORITY POPULATIONS PARTICIPATE IN CARDIAC REHABILITATION LESS THAN WHITE MEN?

Research has convincingly demonstrated that women, older adults, and minority populations participate less in cardiac rehabilitation (CR) than white men. The reasons for this conundrum include failure to offer CR to these populations, insufficient financial resources, and family responsibilities, among others. Strategies for encouraging these populations to participate in CR are greatly needed. Here are some recommended strategies:

- Effective therapies, including CR, should be offered to women, elders, and minority populations whenever appropriate; consider ways to overcome barriers to participation.
- Clinical researchers must continue to recruit women, elders, and minority populations. Racial differences among women need to be studied. Gender specific differences in risk and treatments remain unknown in many situations.
- Clinical trials should be required to report results by gender and race.
- Evidence-based guidelines should be followed in all populations, including women, elders, and racial/ethnic minorities at risk for and with coronary heart disease.
- Efforts to increase awareness, access, and appropriate use of effective therapies in women, elders, and minority groups must continue.
- A specific focus on "successful aging" should be the focus of new agendas for research and clinical practice.

CHD, Coronary heart disease.

chrane review of psychological interventions for CHD patients.[32] They examined 36 trials with 12,841 acute MI, after cardiac surgery, and stable angina patients. Recognizing the limitations of poor quality trials, ill-defined interventions, and short follow-up periods, they concluded that psychological interventions for this population had small effects on reducing anxiety and depression, but no effect on total or cardiac mortality.

Patients with heart failure are also burdened by depression. Intervention studies aimed at treating this problem in a CR environment are severely lacking. In fact, the reviewers for the Cochrane database were unable to locate any valid randomized controlled studies to document outcomes.[32] A few observational studies suggest improvement in depressive symptoms following CR, but study methodological weaknesses preclude any definitive conclusions. Clearly, further study is indicated.

Behavioral and Lifestyle Changes

Education, counseling, and behavioral interventions provided in CR are effective in modifying risk factors, especially smoking cessation and blood lipid levels (Box 80-1).[8] Many studies report improved risk profiles following CR, but two will be highlighted here. One of the first randomized controlled trials to demonstrate the benefits of intensive Lifestyle changes (without lipid-lowering drugs) was the Lifestyle Heart Trial.[33] Though limited to only 48 patients, those receiving the treatment demonstrated comprehensive lifestyle changes that resulted in angiographically confirmed regression in coronary artery disease, which was maintained at 5 years. SCRIP also provided evidence of the positive effects of a physician-directed, nurse case managed multifactor risk reduction program.[6] This 4-year program focused on both lifestyle and medical therapies demonstrated marked reductions in all cardiac risk factors,

---

BOX 80-1 ■ ■ ■
COMPONENTS OF SUCCESSFUL BEHAVIOR CHANGE PROGRAMS

- Patient-centered approach
- Active partnership
- Empathic communication
- Assessing readiness to change
- Goal negotiation
- Individualized treatment plan
- Behavioral skill training and education
- Enhancing self-efficacy
- Guided problem solving
- Opportunities for self-monitoring
- Using reminder systems/cues
- Evaluation and personalized feedback
- Positive reinforcement/rewards
- Relapse prevention
- Ongoing counseling and support
- Empowerment

From Burke L, Fair J: Promoting prevention. Skill sets and attributes of health care providers who deliver behavioral interventions, *J Cardiovasc Nurs* 18:256-266, 2003.
Okene I, Hayman L, Pasternak R et al: Task Force #4—Adherence issues and behavior change: achieving a long-term solution, *J Am Coll Cardiol* 40:630-640, 2002.

---

which resulted in both clinical and angiographic benefits.

Based on the accumulated scientific evidence, the American Heart Association, the American Association of Cardiovascular and Pulmonary Rehabilitation, and the American College of Cardiology have developed national recommendations for CR and secondary prevention programs aimed at modifying global risk factors.[34-36] Existing CR programs are now challenged to modify their format from exercise only to a multifactorial program emphasizing comprehensive risk reduction.

ELIGIBILITY FOR CARDIAC REHABILITATION AND SECONDARY PREVENTION SERVICES

With the benefits, efficacy, and cost-effectiveness of CR and secondary prevention programs firmly established, it remains a puzzle why these services continue to be underused. Only 10 percent to 20 percent of eligible patients participate in traditional CR programs.[37] Barriers to participation include older age, female sex, lack of physician referral, lack of access to programs, inadequate reimbursement and limited financial resources, and patient attitudes.

Most persons with coronary artery disease can benefit greatly from the services provided by CR. Important services provided by CR, but not typically offered by health care providers, include help with behavioral change, medically supervised exercise and promotion of lifestyle physical activity, and psychosocial interventions.[38]

Initially, uncomplicated patients after an MI were the target population receiving CR services. Later, patients with other cardiac conditions, such as coronary artery bypass graft (**CABG**) surgery, percutaneous transluminal coronary angioplasty and/or stenting, valvular heart disease, chronic stable angina, severe heart disease including heart failure, cardiac transplantation, dysrhythmias, and AICDs, received CR. Patients with cerebrovascular and peripheral vascular disease also benefit from CR although these patients participate less frequently. With an increasing focus on secondary prevention and behavioral counseling, modern CR programs are well positioned to provide comprehensive disease management for all persons with atherosclerotic vascular disease.[14,16,36,39,40]

COMPONENTS OF SUCCESSFUL CARDIAC REHABILITATION AND SECONDARY PREVENTION PROGRAMS

CR has undergone a significant evolution, moving from a focused exercise intervention to a comprehensive disease management program. This change is evident from the variety of names used to describe the current CR programs: cardiovascular disease (**CVD**) risk reduction, preventive cardiology, center for the performing hearts, and cardiac therapy. The core components of these new programs have been defined as baseline and follow-up patient assessment; aggressive strategies for reducing modifiable risk factors (e.g., lipids, hypertension, diabetes, and obesity); counseling on heart-healthy nutrition, smoking cessation, and stress management; assistance in adhering to prescribed medications; promotion of lifestyle physical activity; exercise training; and psychosocial and vocational counseling.[14] As discussed in Chapter 25, these integrated services are best provided by an interdisciplinary team composed of physicians, nurses, health educators, exercise physiologists, dieticians, and behavioral medicine specialists. Recently, the nurse in CR has become the case manager.

Behavior Modification

Secondary prevention guidelines provide extensive lists of behavioral changes recommended for patients with CHD.[14,34] Even though lifestyle change is advocated for decreasing health risks, long-term adherence to healthy lifestyle behavior is difficult to maintain. During the acute episode of illness, patients often are motivated to make short-term changes when presented with their personal risk factors. However, with time many healthy behaviors are abandoned for a multitude of reasons. Although education has been a cornerstone of nursing practice for fostering these initial changes, its impact is limited in helping patients attain and maintain successful lifestyle change. Practical strategies are often missing from traditional patient education encounters. These practical strategies can help patients maintain recommended behavior change over time.

Several theories from psychological literature provide the basis for successful long-term behavior change. These theories include the following:

- Transtheoretical model of behavior change
- Health belief model
- Social cognitive theory
- Theory of reasoned action
- Relapse prevention model

Each theory provides information about variables that have been shown to affect long-term outcomes. The most critical assumptions about behavior change, drawn from these theories, are shown in Box 80-2. Each of these assumptions is discussed briefly below. See Chapters 83 and 84 for further detail.

Change as a Process

It is unrealistic to expect people to change if they are not prepared to do so, so assessing readiness to change is essential. Prochaska and Velicer reported that at any given time, only about 20 percent of people are in the "preparation" stage for change.[41] The remainder are either resistant to change or are contemplating the possibilities. Thus, we must assess *which* behaviors (such as taking medications) patients are ready to engage in and use this as a starting point to encourage healthy behaviors. Over time, attention can be directed to moving patients further along the change continuum for the other recommended lifestyle behaviors (such as smoking cessation).

Health Beliefs and Prior Experiences

Often we fall into paternalistic patterns of interaction, advocating for specific changes "because it is good for you." Even if patients are successful in achieving the mandated behavior change, change may be short-lived. That is, change that occurs to please the provider does not appear to hold up long term. Health may not be a prime motivator for everyone. We must be ready to understand patients' beliefs and culture, their unique lifestyle, and the meaning of the health experience. Some patients view illness as punishment or fate—something they cannot change. Others may not perceive excess body weight as a health problem. Rest may be valued over physical activity. Significant negative side effects from cardiac medications may be an unspoken deterrent to adherence. Some people prefer to focus on the present rather than the future. Prior attempts at smoking cessation may have led to feelings of hopelessness about quitting. Advocating change needs to begin with an exploration of what health means to the patient so that we can establish a common ground on which to begin the change process.

Reasoned Decision Making

Many people are capable of and want to make informed choices about their health behaviors. The reasons for wanting or not wanting to make changes in one's life are profoundly personal. Research has shown that patients carry out their own "cost-risk" analysis.[42] They weigh the costs and risks of each treatment (e.g., personal time required for exercise program, potential loss of smoking buddies, and financial cost) against the benefits as they perceive them (e.g., achievement of ideal weight, reduced risk of a future cardiac event). Moreover, they use this information to guide which behaviors they will initiate first and which can be deferred. These thoughtful evaluations are pivotal to such decision making.

Importance of Individualized Treatment Plans

Any new behavior needs to be compatible with the patient's lifestyle. The challenge is to help patients find a compatible treatment. The "one size fits all" approach simply does not work. The patient is the expert on what will work in his or her life. Thus, tailor-made interventions that take into account each person's uniqueness are most successful, for they recognize the importance of patient preferences and beliefs. The goal is to guide them in selecting the behavior to change, in setting realistic goals, and in designing the strategies for meeting their specific goals.

BOX 80-2   ■ ■ ■
CHALLENGES UNDERLYING BEHAVIORAL CHANGE

A large body of knowledge demonstrates that there are multiple challenges to behavior change. Some of the key points to consider include:

- Change is a process that occurs in stages.
- Health beliefs and prior experiences are central to change.
- Patients carry out a reasoned "cost-benefit" analysis.
- Treatment plans must be individualized.
- Patients must have sufficient self-efficacy to begin and continue with the change process.
- Helping relationships foster success.

Enhancing Self-Efficacy

Visualizing one's self being successful at a new behavior is paramount to successful change. Patients with low self-efficacy (a rating of *less than* 7 on a scale of 1 to 10) about the ability to perform a specific activity, such as quitting smoking, or taking daily hypertension medication, typically will not even try the new behavior.[43] The role of the nurse is to review past efforts with each suggested behavior, determine reasons for past successes or failures, and provide opportunities for ongoing skill building. Strategies found to be most useful for instilling confidence include starting with small steps to build mastery, providing ways to practice new behaviors, and using verbal persuasion and role modeling to instill confidence.

Promoting Helping Relationships

One of the cornerstones of CR is its supportive environment. Staff members are essential for providing the support needed for behavioral change. Recently, the concept of coaching has gained acceptance as a strategy for promoting change and adherence. Coaching is a patient-centered approach that empowers the patient to take an active role in the change process—but within a nurse-patient partnership. As a coach, the nurse assists the patient in making informed choices and taking ownership for health. Key components of successful coaching include mutual respect, supportive and persuasive communication, recognizing the importance of individual decision making, personalizing the experience for the patient, enthusiasm, and "being there for the long haul."

Social Support

Recovery from a cardiac event does not happen in isolation. During the acute episode, one's functional support systems are usually called into action. However, this support tends to wane over time. Several lines of evidence underscore the importance of a strong social support network. Patients with limited social ties have a significantly poorer prognosis compared with those with larger support systems. After an MI, patients who live alone have a 50 percent increased risk for recurrent events.[44] Low levels of social support also negatively affect outcomes from behavior change efforts. More isolated patients are less interested in smoking cessation, weight management, exercise, and the like. Women and elderly patients tend to be at even higher risk for recovery problems. Therefore, the CR team needs to be proactive in evaluating the quantity and quality of support available to each patient.

Enhancing social support is one of the hallmarks of the CR environment. Staff are creative in finding support opportunities for patients. One successful method of developing social support in CR is the "buddy system" for educational programs, physical activity, or weight loss. Family and friends also can be encouraged to join in selected activities. Some risk reduction CR centers offer "couples" programs to help foster positive support and attendance. Berkman[45] believes that interventions focused on restructuring and improving naturally occurring networks and support resources (i.e.,

family, friends, and coworkers) may be more effective than "newly constructed" support groups.

Patients may also benefit from the efforts of hospital- or community-based support groups, such as the Mended Hearts Program. The Internet can also provide opportunities for ongoing support through focused chat rooms. For example, the American Heart Association website: *www.mendedhearts.org* advertises a caring community for preventing heart attack and stroke, offering individually tailored health information along with chat rooms, and www.womenheart.org—the National Coalition for Women with Heart Disease—offers excellent opportunities for support.

EXPANDING CARDIAC REHABILITATION AND SECONDARY PREVENTION SERVICES

CR and secondary prevention are the standard of care for patients with CVD.[14] A paradigm shift is occurring in CR as care moves from an exercise model to multidimensional, global risk reduction programs with an array of individualized therapies that can be obtained in a variety of settings. This paradigm shift includes a focus on a broader audience of persons eligible for these services. These include women, elders, persons living in rural settings, the indigent, and minorities who represent a growing population of cardiac survivors who need comprehensive services.

Women

Women carry a great burden from CVD; almost half of women younger than age 65 who have a heart attack die within 8 years. At older ages, more women than men die from a first MI as a result of age and comorbid conditions. Women have more recurrent and severe angina, heart failure, and reinfarction rates than men. Women experience more depression, anxiety, slower return to work, and less symptom improvement after CABG than men. Further, CVD is a major issue for older women who are more likely to be disabled from the disease and living alone or in a nursing home on limited finances. The recent "Go Red For Women" (*www.americanheart.org*), "Heart Truth" (*www.nhlbi.nih.gov*), and "Tell A Friend" (*www.pcna.net*) campaigns have raised the awareness in women that heart disease is the number one killer and that they need to recognize and control their heart risk factors. Comprehensive secondary prevention services for women can dramatically reduce future CVD risk.[46]

Older Persons

The aging of the population poses additional challenges. As people live longer with CVD, their participation in CR becomes more important. Few older adults engage in regular physical activity despite the known benefits.[22,47] Physical activity has multiple health benefits in older adults, including significant improvements in aerobic fitness, decreased risks of CVD, lower risk of colon cancer and diabetes, greater muscular strength and bone health, reduced obesity, improved psychological well-being, and protection from falls and disability.[48] Elders also experiences challenges with medication adherence and monitoring of blood pressure, lipids, glucose, and nutrition. Secondary prevention programs must be integrated into the long-term care of older persons.

Racial and Ethnic Diversity

It is well established that women and older persons are less likely to be referred for CR compared with white men.[49] Low socioeconomic status is also a predictor of low CR referral rates. Yet CVD disproportionately affects racial and ethnic minorities, many of whom are of lower socioeconomic status. Issues of culture, cost, transportation, education, literacy, and language are a few of the reasons for this disparity. Lack of reimbursement for those who are uninsured or underinsured also creates a barrier for CR referral and participation. CR programs must examine their ability to create an environment that is welcoming to minorities, that seeks and supports their participation, and that can make their program affordable. Ideas to consider are:

- Developing scholarship opportunities
- Working with physicians who care for minority patients to develop a referral base
- Providing educational materials that are literacy appropriate
- Having bilingual staff available or supporting family members who are bilingual to attend for patients with language barriers
- Finding ways to overcome transportation barriers
- Making a commitment to greater inclusiveness of the medically underserved

New Models of Care

Another paradigm shift that must occur is expansion of the venue in which CR and secondary prevention services are offered. Traditionally, CR programs were hospital based, with a primary focus on supervised, monitored exercise sessions. Monitored exercise required expensive ECG-monitoring equipment, entry exercise stress tests, and high patient-staff ratios that escalated overall costs. However, not all patients require this high level of supervision during exercise. Compelling evidence supports the safety and effectiveness of exercise in the community and home environments.[21] Published guidelines are available to help clinicians determine the level of risk for individual patients.[34] Based on this assessment, the optimal level of supervision can be determined.

A number of programs have evolved for CVD risk reduction and facilitation of a heart-healthy lifestyle including risk reduction centers or clinics; nurse case management programs;[50-52] web-based programs that provide education, monitoring, and interactions with health professionals;[53] and community-based programs using nurses and allied health professionals to facilitate secondary prevention goals and long-term adherence to lifestyle change.[54] Some will join a community-based Mended Hearts club or other group support systems, such as WomenHeart (www.womenheart.org) to meet their psychosocial needs. No single model of care can meet the needs of all patients.

Using the "menu of services" approach discussed in Chapter 25, some patients may require a significant amount of one-on-one information and assistance for modifying multiple risk factors. Others may require assistance with nutrition and lipid management. For most, an important component of all services is ongoing monitoring and follow-up, beyond the traditional 3-month disease management program. Programs of the future will require several models and approaches to multifactor risk reduction that addresses a wide range of individual and community needs and capabilities.

Virtual Cardiac Rehabilitation Programs

"Virtual CVD risk reduction clinics" have been reported in the literature. Kinn and colleagues compared the use of an electronic medical record with paper and pencil charting for the management dyslipidemia in patients with CHD.[55] They followed 1109 patients with lipid disorders who were randomly assigned for 1 year to electronic medical records or usual care. The electronic medical record identified patients who were not at Adult Treatment Panel III (ATP III) goal, alerted physicians, and prompted modification of treatment as indicated. Physicians received positive reinforcement for behavioral changes including patient education, medication adjustment, and ordering laboratory tests. Monthly feedback of performance and comparison with peers was provided. After 1 year, 92 percent of patients in the virtual lipid clinic and 45 percent of patients in usual care had LDL documented in their medical record. The percent of patients at goal was 64 percent in the virtual lipid clinic compared with 22 percent in usual care.

Weight loss assistance has also been delivered by the Internet. Tate and colleagues randomized volunteers to Internet education or Internet education plus behavioral therapy and followed them for 6 months.[56] The Internet plus behavioral therapy showed significantly more weight loss (4 kg versus 2 kg) compared with Internet education alone for those volunteers who had measures at baseline, 3, and 6 months. The use of log in and frequent contact was significantly correlated with weight loss. This virtual approach has great potential because it can reach a large audience, be cost-effective, and convenient.

The Comprehensive Health Enhancement Support System (CHESS), a virtual approach developed in 1989 for use with a broad array of populations, provides access to a health library, communication services including live chat rooms, support groups, and access to expert advice. CHESS also provides health tracking that allows participants to self-monitor their health status. Results from the CHESS system show improved quality of life and reduced both hospital admissions and length of stay, even in minority populations.[57]

Other virtual programs have addressed multiple risk factors. An Internet-based case management system for secondary prevention of CVD included telephone, mail, and on-line discussion groups and communication with a nurse and registered dietitian.[53] In a 6-month trial of 104 patients with CHD randomized to usual care or intervention, weight loss, body mass index (BMI), and patient satisfaction improved significantly more in the intervention group than usual care. Lipids, blood pressure, and smoking did not change. Significantly fewer major cardiovascular events occurred in the usual care group compared with intervention (two versus eight). Another test of a computer generated behaviorally oriented risk reduction program (INTERxVENT) with counseling (face-to-face or over the Internet) was effective in helping 2390 ethnically diverse adults improve their CVD risk factors.[58] Similar benefits have been seen in a heart failure population.[59]

Based on the results of these promising trials, integrated health systems are moving toward the use of virtual programs to assess and triage persons at risk for CHD. The Stanford Heart Network (**SHN**) provides an Internet-based risk reduction program that uses a web-based CVD risk assessment.[60] Risk is calculated based on traditional risk factors, personal history of medical therapies for cardiovascular risk factors, and personal and family history of atherosclerotic vascular disease. Immediate feedback and health education is provided to participants. Comprehensive individual and group data are collected for the health care provider or health care system. By risk stratifying participants, providers can emphasize risk reduction for those at the highest risk of a CVD event. Participant confidentiality is ensured through unique passwords and additional Internet security systems.

Based on a review of five published studies evaluating Internet-based risk-reduction interventions for persons with CHD, Nguyen argued that Internet-based patient education and support has an emerging role in clinical practice (Box 80-3).[61] She noted barriers to innovation including adoption, literacy, and access. These problems currently limit the wide spread use of web-based technology.

FUTURE CHALLENGES

The Health Care Financing Administration (**HCFA,** now the Centers for Medicare and Medicaid Services), and other third party payers must recognize the overwhelming evidence supporting the beneficial effects of exercise training, global risk reduction, and promotion of healthy lifestyles. Secondary prevention is now recognized as an

---

■■■ CONUNDRUM

POLITICS OF HEALTH CARE

Idaho Senator Mike Crapo introduced legislation in July 2005 to include pulmonary and cardiac rehabilitation as a covered Medicare benefit. Senator Blanche Lincoln (D-Arkansas) joined Senator Crapo as an original co-sponsor (Senate Bill 1440). In January 2007, the same sponsors introduced the Pulmonary and Cardiac Rehabilitation Act (5.329) to include pulmonary and cardiac rehabilitation services as specific services covered by Medicare. If passed, this legislation would end the decade-long debate between providers, the Centers for Medicare and Medicaid Services (CMS), and the various fiscal intermediaries for reimbursing for these services.

Currently, there is no specific reference to pulmonary or cardiac rehabilitation services in the Medicare statute. While pulmonary and cardiac rehabilitation programs generally are often considered a covered service by Medicare under the "incident to physician services" clause, the absence of a national coverage policy decision has limited access to necessary care and lack of reimbursement in many instances.

Supporters of this legislation include the American Association for Cardiovascular and Pulmonary Rehabilitation, American Association for Respiratory Care, American College of Chest Physicians, American Hospital Association, American Thoracic Society, and the National Association for Medical Direction of Respiratory Care, National Home Oxygen Patients Association.

---

essential component of care for persons with CHD and heart failure.[46] Secondary prevention has become a standard of care, but reimbursement has not followed the scientific evidence. Professionals must continue to work within legislative and political arenas to advocate for reimbursement for secondary prevention services.

Patients need to be empowered to take responsibility for reducing their own risk of heart disease and stroke. By limiting the need for expensive equipment, CR programs can offer services at reduced cost over longer periods of time to larger numbers of patients. Patients can pay on a sliding scale for those services that they require. This model has been successfully used for many years by many CR programs around the United States. Average monthly rates range from $150 to $200. For patients without financial resources, community and hospital support for CR programs can help cover their costs. Many hospitals benefit from the "good will" and patient satisfaction generated by participation in CR as a method to market their services (see the accompanying Conundrum feature on politics in health care).

CONCLUSION

CR has undergone significant evolution and has changed from primarily an exercise-focused intervention into a comprehensive disease management program. Beneficial outcomes from participation in CR are functional, psychosocial, and behavioral and/or lifestyle. Convincing scientific evidence shows that multifactorial CVD risk reduction slows disease progression, stabilizes the atherosclerotic plaque, and promotes plaque regression. National recommendations aimed at modifying global risk factors consider participation in CR the standard of care. Our challenge is to find ways to expand these services to all eligible patients and families, using the model of care most appropriate for each.

BOX 80-3   ■■■
INNOVATIVE APPROACHES TO CARDIAC REHABILITATION

- Integrate services to include multiple risk reduction across disease entities.
- Use new delivery models including the Internet, e-mail, chat groups, and other electronic media tools (wireless, hand-held, digital television, etc.) to provide risk reduction, evaluation, and education.
- Use electronic media and technology to allow enhanced self-monitoring skills for participants in cardiac rehabilitation programs.
- Prevent geography from interfering with access to services.
- Work with governmental and health policy agencies to improve reimbursement for electronically facilitated cardiac rehabilitation programs.

REFERENCES

1. Winslow EH: Cardiovascular consequences of bedrest, *Heart Lung* 14:236-246, 1985.
2. Cassem NH, Hackett TP: Psychological rehabilitation of myocardial infarction patients in the acute phase, *Heart Lung* 2:382-388, 1973.
3. Wenger NK: Early ambulation after myocardial infarction. The in-patient exercise program, *Clin Sports Med* 3:333-348, 1984.
4. Wenger NK: Early ambulation physical activity: myocardial infarction and coronary bypass surgery, *Heart Lung* 13:14-18, 1984.
5. Wenger NK, Hellerstein HK, Blackburn H et al: Physician practice in the management of patients with uncomplicated myocardial infarction. Changes in the past decade, *Circulation* 65:421-427, 1982.
6. Haskell WL, Alderman EL, Fair JM et al: Effects of intensive multiple risk factor reduction on coronary atherosclerosis and clinical cardiac events in men and women with coronary artery disease. The Stanford Coronary Risk Intervention Project (SCRIP), *Circulation* 89:975-990, 1994.
7. Franklin BA, Kahn JK: Delayed progression or regression of coronary atherosclerosis with intensive risk factor modification. Effects of diet, drugs, and exercise, *Sports Med* 22:306-320, 1996.
8. Wenger NK, Froelicher ES, Smith LK et al: *Cardiac rehabilitation as secondary prevention*, Clinical practice guideline #17, Rockville, Md, 1995, US Department of Health and Human Services, Public Health Service, Agency for Health Care Policy and Research, and the National Heart, Lung, and Blood Institute, AHCPR Publication No 96-0672.
9. Oldridge NB, Guyatt GH, Fischer ME et al: Cardiac rehabilitation after myocardial infarction. Combined experience of randomized clinical trials, *JAMA* 260:945-950, 1988.
10. O'Connor GT, Buring JE, Yusuf S et al: An overview of randomized trials of rehabilitation with exercise after myocardial infarction, *Circulation* 80:234-244, 1989.
11. Taylor RS, Brown A, Ebrahim S et al: Exercise-based rehabilitation for patients with coronary heart disease: systematic review and meta-analysis of randomized controlled trials, *Am J Med* 116:682-692, 2004.
12. Thompson PD, Franklin BA: From case report to meta-analysis—additional evidence for the benefits of exercise training in cardiac patients, *Am J Med* 116:714-716, 2004.
13. Jolliffe JA, Rees K, Taylor RS et al: Exercise-based rehabilitation for coronary heart disease, *Cochrane Database Syst Rev* 1, CD001800, 2001.
14. Leon AS, Franklin BA, Costa F et al: AHA scientific statement. Cardiac rehabilitation and secondary prevention of coronary heart disease, *Circulation* 111:369-376, 2005.
15. Belardinelli R, Paolini I, Cianci G et al: Exercise training intervention after coronary angioplasty: the ETICA trial, *J Am Coll Cardiol* 37:1891-1900, 2001.
16. Pina IL, Apstein CS, Balady GJ et al: Exercise and heart failure. A statement from the American Heart Association Committee on Exercise, Rehabilitation and Prevention, *Circulation* 107:1210-1225, 2003.
17. Rees K, Taylor RS, Singh S et al: Exercise based rehabilitation for heart failure, *Cochrane Database Syst Rev* 1, 2005.
18. Smart N, Marwick TH: Exercise training for patients with heart failure: a systematic review of factors that improve mortality and morbidity, *Am J Med* 116:693-706, 2004.
19. Lane DA, Chong AY, Lip GYH: Psychological interventions for depression in heart failure, *Cochrane Database Syst Rev* 1, 2005.
20. Piepoli M, Daves C, Francis D et al: Exercise training meta-analysis of trials in patients with chronic heart failure (ExTraMATCH), *BMJ* 328:189-192, 2004.
21. Witt BJ, Jacobson SJ, Weston SA et al: Cardiac rehabilitation after myocardial infarction in the community, *J Am Coll Cardiol* 44:988-996, 2004.
22. Williams MA, Fleg, JL, Ades PA et al: Secondary prevention of coronary disease in the elderly (with emphasis on patients > 75 years of age), *Circulation* 105:1735-1743, 2002.
23. Thompson PD, Buchner D, Pina IL et al: Exercise and physical activity in the prevention and treatment of atherosclerotic cardiovascular disease, *Circulation* 107:3109-3116, 2003.
24. Wannamethee SG, Shaper AG, Walker M: Physical activity and mortality in older men with diagnosed coronary heart disease, *Circulation* 102:1358-1363, 2000.
25. Blumental JA, Babyak MA, Carney RM et al: Exercise, depression and mortality after myocardial infarction in the ENRICHD trial, *Med Sci Sports Exerc* 746-755, 2004.
26. Shephard RJ, Franklin B: Changes in the quality of life: a major goal of cardiac rehabilitation, *J Cardiopulm Rehabil* 21:189-200, 2001.
27. Ades PA, Green NM, Coello CF: Effects of exercise and cardiac rehabilitation on cardiovascular outcomes, *Cardiol Clin* 21:435-448, 2003.
28. Dugmore LD, Tipson RJ, Phillips MH et al: Changes in cardiorespiratory fitness, psychological wellbeing, quality of life, and vocational status following a12 month cardiac exercise rehabilitation programme, *Heart* 81:359-366, 1999.
29. McAlister FA, Lawson FM, Teo KK et al: Randomised trials of secondary prevention programmes in coronary heart disease: a systematic review, *BHJ* 323:957-962, 2001.
30. Toobert DJ, Glasgow RE, Radcliffe JL: Physiologic and related behavioral outcomes from the Women's Lifestyle Heart Trial, *Ann Behav Med* 22:1-9, 2000.
31. Berkman LF, Blumenthal J, Burg M et al: Effects of treating depression and low perceived social support on clinical events after myocardial infarction. The Enhancing Recovery in Coronary Heart Disease patients (ENRICHD) randomized trial, *JAMA* 289:3106-3116, 2003.
32. Rees K, Bennett P, West R et al: Psychological interventions for coronary heart disease (review), *Cochrane Database Syst Rev* 1, 2005.
33. Ornish D, Scherwitz LW, Billings JH et al: Intensive lifestyle changes for reversal of coronary heart disease, *JAMA* 280:2001-2007, 1998.
34. Balady GJ, Ades PA, Comoss P et al: Core components of cardiac rehabilitation/secondary prevention programs. A statement for healthcare professionals from the American Heart Association and the American Association of Cardiovascular and Pulmonary Rehabilitation, *Circulation* 102:1069-1073, 2000.
35. Smith SC, Allen J, Bonow RO et al: AHA/ACC guidelines for secondary prevention patients with atherosclerotic and other disease: 2006 update, *Circulation* 113:2363-2372, 2006.
36. Williams MA, Balady GJ, Carlson, JJ et al: *AACVPR guidelines for cardiac rehabilitation and secondary prevention programs*, ed 4, Champaign, Ill, 2004, Human Kinetics.
37. Ades P: Cardiac rehabilitation and secondary prevention of coronary heart disease, *N Engl J Med* 345:892-902, 2001.
38. Ades P, Balady GJ, Berra K: Transforming exercise based cardiac rehabilitation programs into secondary prevention centers: a national imperative, *J Cardiopulm Rehabil* 21:263-271, 2001.
39. Gordon N, Gulanick M, Costa F et al: AHA scientific statement. Physical activity and exercise recommendations for stroke survivors, *Circulation* 109:2031-2041, 2004.
40. Stewart KJ, Badenhop D, Brubaker PH et al: Cardiac rehabilitation following percutaneous revascularization, heart transplant, heart valve surgery, and for chronic heart failure, *Chest* 123:2104-2111, 2003.
41. Prochaska JO, Velicer WF: The transtheoretical model of health behavior change, *Am J Health Promot* 12:38-48, 1997.
42. Donovan JL, Blake DR: Patient non-compliance: deviation or reasoned decision-making? *Soc Sci Med* 34:507-513, 1992.
43. Bandura A: The assessment and predictive generality of self-percepts of efficacy, *J Behav Ther Exp Psychiatry* 13:195-199, 1982.
44. Berkman LF, Leo-Summers L, Horwitz RI: Emotional support and survival after myocardial infarction. *Ann Intern Med* 117:1003-1009, 1992.
45. Berkman LF: The role of social relations in health promotion, *Psychosomatic Med* 57:245-54, 1995.
46. Mosca L, Banka C, Benjamin EJ et al: Evidence-based guidelines for cardiovascular disease prevention in women:2007 Update, *Circulation* 115:1481-1501, 2007.
47. Fletcher GF, Balady GJ, Amsterdam EA et al: Exercise standards for testing and training: a statement for healthcare professionals from the American Heart Association, *Circulation* 104:1694-1740, 2001.
48. Agency for Healthcare Research and Quality and the Centers for Disease Control: *Physical activity and older Americans: bene-*

fits and strategies, Retrieved February 25, 2007 from www.ahrq. gov/ppip/actvity.htm.

49. Thomas RJ, Miller NH, Lamendola C et al: National survey on gender differences in cardiac rehabilitation programs. Patient characteristics and enrollment, *J Cardiopulm* 16:402-412, 1996.

50. Haskell WL: Cardiovascular disease prevention and lifestyle interventions. Effectiveness and efficacy, *J Cardiovasc Nurs* 18:245-255, 2003.

51. Berra K, Houston Miller N, Fair JM: Cardiovascular disease prevention program and disease management, *J Cardiopulm Rehabil* 26:197-206, 2006.

52. Petrilla AA, Benner JS, Battleman DS et al: Evidence-based interventions to improve patient compliance with antihypertensive and lipid-lowering medications, *Int J Clin Pract* 59(12):1441-1451, 2005.

53. Southard BH, Southard DR, Nuckolls J: Clinical trial of an internet case management system for secondary prevention of heart disease, *J Card Rehabil* 23:341-348, 2003.

54. Harris DE, Record NB: Cardiac rehabilitation in community settings, *J Cardiopulm Rehabil* 23:250-259, 2003.

55. Kinn JW, O'Toole MF, Rowley SM et al: Effectiveness of electronic medical record in cholesterol management in patient with coronary artery disease (virtual lipid clinic), *Am J Cardiol* 88:163-165, A5, 2001.

56. Tate D, Wing R, Winnett RA: Using the Internet technology to deliver a behavioral weight loss program, *JAMA* 285:1172-1177, 2001.

57. Gustafson DH, Hawkins RP, Boberg EW et al: CHESS: 10 years of research and development in consumer health informatics for broad populations, including the underserved, *Int J Med Inform* 65:169-177, 2002.

58. Gordon N, Salmon RD, Franklin BA et al: Effectiveness of therapeutic lifestyle changes in patients with hypertension, hyperlipidemia and/or hyperglycemia, *Am J Cardiol* 94:1558-1561, 2004.

59. Artinian N, Harden JK, Kronenberg MW et al: Pilot study of a web-based compliance monitoring device for patients with congestive heart failure, *Heart Lung* 32:226-233, 2003.

60. Berra K, Haskell W, Clark A et al: *Multifactor risk reduction in low income patients: opportunities and challenges in implementing a case management model*, April 11-13, National Cardiovascular Health Conference, 2002, National Heart, Lung, and Blood Institute.

61. Nguyen HQ, Carrieri-Kohlman V, Rankin A et al: Supporting cardiac recovery through eHealth technology, *J Cardiovasc Nurs* 19:200-208, 2004.

■■ ■■ chapter 81

Home Care and Heart Disease

Patricia S.A. Sparacino
Marianne Roncoli

Of the 31.7 million people discharged from nonfederal short-stay hospitals in 2000, almost 4.4 million (13.8 percent) had a primary diagnosis of heart disease, and about 999,000 (22.8 percent) of these had heart failure. Heart failure has the highest prevalence for any diagnosis-related group,[1] and thus is disproportionately represented in the home care population. In 2001, almost 7 percent of Medicare patients referred from the hospital[2] and about 5 percent of the patients referred from the community[3] to home care had a primary diagnosis of heart failure. Therefore, most of the clinical examples in this chapter address the heart failure population.

Clinical and demographic characteristics can be used to identify patients with heart disease who are at high risk for hospital readmission: previous diagnosis of heart failure, hospital admission within the previous year, diabetes, kidney failure, hypertension, a history of cardiac revascularization, and being older than age 65.[4-6] The greater the number of risk predictors, the higher the rate of rehospitalization.[4] There is also a significant association between readiness for discharge from and early readmission to a hospital.[4,7,8] We know, however, that there is a reduced risk of hospital readmission, improved functional status and survival, and an improvement in quality of life—without increasing the cost of medical care—for older patients with cardiac disease who receive coordinated care in the home, such as that provided by home health care nurses.[2,9,10] Patients who can benefit the most from referral to home care are those who have poor outcomes when discharged from a hospital.[7,11,12]

One of the standard outcome variables used to measure the effectiveness of home care is a decrease in the incidence of hospital readmissions. The goal of home care is to deliver care that integrates best evidence with clinician expertise and patient choices and decreases the rate of hospital readmission.

HOME CARE FOR PATIENTS WITH HEART DISEASE

Varying levels of providers care for home care patients with acute and chronic health care needs (see Chapter 26). Some home care agency nurses are specialists who provide expert care to a select subset of patients, focusing on a particular aspect of nursing, such as wound care, ostomy care, or care of the cardiac or diabetic patient. Home care agency nurses are usually generalists, though, who care for patients with wide-ranging ages, diagnoses, and socioeconomic circumstances.[13] A generalist nurse who is experienced in delivering care at home is able to address the care needs of patients with multiple chronic health problems. The structure of reimbursement for home care services does not necessarily support advanced practice nurses **(APNs),** despite evidence that APNs are more knowledgeable about effective interventions and are able to improve patient outcomes and reduce the risk of rehospitalization.[14]

There are unique challenges to home care. Most importantly the patient must be homebound. The skilled care that is provided is intermittent (services are only needed and provided a few hours a day or week). Other providers in the health care system may not communicate in a timely way to ensure coordinated care,[8,13] causing a breakdown in care or lack of care continuity. The patient's or family caregiver's goals for care may differ from those of the health providers and that difference may influence compliance with a treatment plan. The nurse or rehabilitation therapist is a guest in a patient's home, and treatment visits may be refused, cancelled, or limited by the patient or family. A patient or family caregiver manages the medications; financial status may influence the ability to purchase medicines or the decision to reduce the frequency or dosage of prescribed medicines.[15] Cognitive impairment may hamper symptom recognition or decrease compliance with a complex therapeutic or pharmacological regimen.

Health care continuity is especially critical for older people with multiple chronic diseases who experience repeated hospital admissions; therefore, discharge planning for a hospitalized patient, especially an older patient with a cardiac diagnosis, requires deliberate consideration. Deliberative care planning may include a variety of nursing interventions, such as those discussed below. There are special considerations for the home care patient after cardiac surgery or with heart failure.

After Cardiac Surgery

In 2000, 515,000 revascularization procedures were performed on 306,000 people in the United States, and 93,000 valve procedures were performed.[16] Patients who have had cardiac surgery are good candidates, and usually meet the admission criteria, for home care. There is little published about home care-specific interventions and outcomes of patients after cardiac surgery.[2]

The length of hospital stay for cardiac surgery patients has declined over the past decade. Many hospitals have early discharge programs for patients who have had an uncomplicated hospital stay and who meet specific discharge criteria. The short hospital stay allots little time for anticipatory guidance about recovery, diet education, activity and exercise guidelines, symptom recognition and monitoring, and pain management. Home care interventions and criteria for discharge from home care are focused on the most commonly encountered problems during recovery from cardiac surgery, such as pulmonary function; symptom recognition and monitoring; incision and wound care; medication management, especially anticoagulant therapy; pain management; activity progression and cardiac rehabilitation; nutrition education; risk factor modification; and education about mental health (Table 81-1).

■ ■ ■

TABLE 81-1   AFTER CARDIAC SURGERY: HOME CARE INTERVENTIONS AND PATIENT OUTCOMES

INTERVENTIONS: HOME CARE	OPTIMAL PATIENT OUTCOMES: READINESS FOR DISCHARGE
Assessment	
Blood pressure	Within parameters per PCP or cardiologist; no postural hypotension or hypertension
Pulse	Within parameters per PCP/cardiologist; without β blockade: *less than* 20 beats/min increase after ambulation
Respiratory rate	Within parameters per PCP or cardiologist; 10-20/min
Lung sounds	Clear or at baseline
Peripheral perfusion	Capillary refill: 2-3 sec, or at baseline
Ankle or dependent edema	Stable or decreasing edema and/or girth
Abdominal girth	At best weight or within acceptable range; recording daily weights
Weight	
Anticipatory guidance about recovery	Describes recovery trajectory: 4-6 wk to resume normal activity; ~ 3 mo to regain energy
Trajectory	Compares progress made with remaining recovery time
Nutrition education and counseling	
Low sodium	Describes relationship between sodium and intake and fluid retention
Low cholesterol diet	Describes effect of cholesterol on heart disease
Label reading	Describe label reading and need for compliance
Dietary limitations	Adaptation and adherence to prescribed diet; avoids restricted foods
Fluid limitations	Adaptation and adherence to prescribed fluid limits
Activity and exercise guidelines	
Activity progression	Demonstrates gradual increase in frequency and duration of walks
Cardiac rehabilitation	Has discussed cardiac rehabilitation with surgeon or cardiologist
Pulmonary function	Uses spirometer as needed; has increased volume from baseline
	Takes deep breaths and coughs regularly
	Splints sternum during coughing
Incision and wound care	Incisions are dry and intact, or wounds are healing
	Patient and/or caregiver able to perform wound care independently
Symptom Recognition and Monitoring	
Awareness	Recognizes and responds to cardiac and surgical wound signs and symptoms
Weight	Is knowledgeable about timely notification of PCP or cardiologist with symptom exacerbation
Edema	Control of fluid retention
Fatigue	Balances activity and rest and is increasing activity tolerance
Appetite	Appetite increasing; balanced diet within recommended dietary guidelines
Medication management (supervision of adjustment and titration)	
Compliance	Lists medication doses, purpose, frequency, action to take if dose missed, side effects
Interactions; untoward effects	Describes appropriate action if side effect
Response	Maintains medication schedule
Anticoagulation or antiplatelet therapy	Demonstrates how to reorder medications
Pain management	Takes pain medication before activities or exercises
	Need for pain medication is decreasing
	Recognizes the side effects of narcotic pain medications
Risk factor modification	
Stop smoking	Identifies personal risk factors
Alcohol and illicit drug limitations	Demonstrates strategies to control risk factors
Weight management	
Blood pressure control	
Diabetes management	
Mental health	Recognizes signs and symptoms of depression
	Uses family, social, and spiritual support systems as needed
	Reestablishing usual sleep cycles

PCP, Primary care physician.

Heart Failure

Heart failure is the most common hospital discharge diagnosis for those aged 65 years and older.[17] Older people with heart failure are more likely to incur higher health care costs than other elderly patients.[4,9,16] Issues that complicate self-care and thus have important implications for home care of persons with heart failure are multiple comorbidities, cognitive and functional impairments, inadequate financial resources, and poor social support.[8]

Cognitive impairment complicates the care of all elders, but especially those with heart failure.[18-20] The incidence of cognitive dysfunction and dementia is estimated to be 8 percent in people older than age 65[21] and about 30 percent at age 85.[22] The incidence of cognitive impairment, however, in people older than age 65 without a diagnosis of dementia is 17 percent—twice that of those diagnosed with dementia.[23] Cognitive impairment is almost two times greater in people with heart failure, independent of other variables.[24] Fifty-five percent of potentially preventable hospital admissions are due to heart failure exacerbations,[25] which appear to be related directly to the attention and memory deficits seen in people with heart failure.[26]

The association between heart failure and cognitive impairment is strongly supported by data, but the physiological mechanisms, neurological focus, specific cognitive deficits, and reversibility of heart failure-related cognitive impairment are poorly understood. These issues are assuredly complicated by the high rate of multiple medical comorbidities, associated polypharmacy, and neurological and cardiovascular aging. It is not fully understood if there are global, hemispheric, or regional neurological consequences of heart failure.

Cognitive impairment may be particularly difficult to detect in persons living in a familiar environment. Cognitive impairment is insidious, diminishing the ability to recognize symptoms, judge when to act, and comply with a complex health management regimen. Symptoms may not be reported by a patient or family because of vagueness about symptoms, misattribution of a symptom to a comorbid condition, or because cognitive dysfunction is impairing symptom recollection or appreciation of significance.

Home care interventions and criteria for discharge from home care are focused on the symptom recognition and monitoring; medication management, especially anticoagulant therapy; activity progression and cardiac rehabilitation; nutrition education; risk factor modification; cognitive assessment; and education about mental health (Table 81-2).

HOME CARE AND PRACTICE GUIDELINES

Evidence-based practice guidelines facilitate standardization of patient care, education, and documentation and permit tailoring of care to the individual patient. Guidelines also may include specific reference information for the home care nurse, especially when access to parameters is needed while in the patient's home. Two key components in the care of the cardiac patient at home are firsthand involvement of home care nurses in the design, implementation, and evaluation of practice guidelines to standardize care[27] and guidelines that are tailored to the patient population being served. Numerous national guidelines are available and easily accessed through the Internet. Although they are rarely specific to home care, they can be used as a resource for local efforts.

A performance improvement framework is useful in designing and implementing an evidence-based practice guideline for the home nursing care of a patient with a cardiac disorder and in measuring the effect on documentation and patient outcomes. A description of the cardiac disorder in general and the cardiac patient in particular (e.g., age, social resources) defines the pertinent associated prevalence, cost, and risks associated with the home care setting. Preliminary assessment of nursing practice and patient outcomes provides baseline reference data before the change process begins and identifies core areas for improvement.

Practice guidelines that are tailored to a specific patient population guide best nursing practice and ensure that care is individualized but consistent in quality. National practice guidelines are not available specifically for home care, but the National Guideline Clearinghouse (www.guideline.gov) offers resources that can be adapted for home care. Other practice guidelines specific to cardiac disease are available from the American Heart Association and American College of Cardiology websites.

Guidelines may address a general patient group (e.g., elders with multiple comorbid illnesses) or patients in a specific diagnostic category, such as heart failure (Table 81-3) or cardiac surgery. Home care goals include education of the patient and family caregiver, promotion of self-care, and prevention of functional and cognitive decline. The basic elements of a practice guideline may include a recommended frequency of home visits, physical and psychosocial assessment parameters, medication management, clinical interventions or procedures, patient education strategies and outcomes, desired outcomes, and criteria for discharge from home care. Because most home care nurses are generalists, useful additions to a practice guideline include classifications (e.g., New York Heart Association classification for heart failure); definitions (e.g., ejection fraction, ventricular systolic dysfunction, and ventricular diastolic dysfunction); normal and abnormal clinical parameters (e.g., blood pressure, pulse rate, respiratory rate, and weight); references (e.g., edema scale, capillary refill time, and dyspnea scale); common cardiac drugs, their side effects, and monitoring directives; and criteria for possible hospitalization (e.g., new onset altered mental status, symptomatic hypotension or syncope).

Clinical practice guidelines are developed using research findings and the consensus of experts. Guidelines should be printed or incorporated into an electronic patient record. Documentation mechanisms should be developed or refined, with decisions about whether to make them computer based or paper based. Patient education materials will need to be developed or refined with a record that tracks what, when, and how

■ ■ ■

TABLE 81-2   HEART FAILURE: HOME CARE INTERVENTIONS AND PATIENT OUTCOMES

INTERVENTIONS: HOME CARE	OPTIMAL PATIENT OUTCOMES: READINESS FOR DISCHARGE
Assessment	
Blood pressure	Within parameters per PCP or cardiologist; no postural hypotension or hypertension
Pulse	Within parameters per PCP or cardiologist; without β blockade: less than 20 beats/min increase after ambulation
Respiratory rate	Within parameters per PCP or cardiologist; 10-20/min
Lung sounds	Clear or at baseline
Peripheral perfusion	Capillary refill: 2-3 sec, or at baseline
Ankle or dependent edema	Stable or decreasing edema and/or girth
Abdominal girth	At best weight or within acceptable range; recording daily weights
Weight	
Nutrition education and counseling	
Sodium	Describes relationship between sodium intake and heart failure exacerbation
Label reading	Adaptation and adherence to prescribed diet; avoids restricted foods
Dietary limitations	Adaptation and adherence to prescribed fluid limits
Fluid limitations	
Activity and exercise guidelines	
Activity tolerance	If stable: demonstrates ability to perform daily activities (ADLs and IADLs) without heart failure symptoms
Activity pacing	Demonstrates gradual activity increase
Energy conservation	Demonstrates activity pacing to manage dyspnea
Activity endurance	Demonstrates self-monitoring: pulse and respiratory rate
Goal: regular low-level exercise to improve skeletal muscle efficiency	Functional capacity increased
	Balances activity and rest and is increasing activity tolerance
Symptom recognition and monitoring	
Awareness	Recognizes and responds to heart failure signs and symptoms
Weight	Timely notification of PCP or cardiologist with symptom exacerbation
Edema	Meticulous control of fluid retention
Fatigue	Lists causes of exacerbations and how to prevent
Appetite	
Chest pain	
Respiratory pattern and effort	
Timely notification of care provider	
Medication review and management (supervision of adjustment and titration)	
Compliance	Lists medication doses, purpose, frequency, action to take if dose missed, side effects
Interactions; untoward effects	Describes appropriate action if side effect
Response	Maintains medication schedule
Anticoagulation or antiplatelet therapy	Demonstrates how to reorder medications
Risk factor modification:	
Stop smoking	Identifies personal risk factors
Alcohol and illicit drug limitations	Demonstrates strategies to control risk factors
Weight management	
Blood pressure control	
Diabetes management	
Cognition	
Screen (e.g., MMSE) for baseline	MMSE greater than 24 or at baseline
Retest for changes	Improved cognition or at baseline
Living with heart failure: how to manage	
Causes of and responses to exacerbations	Complies with care regimen
Coping	Recognizes anxiety; identifies strategies to cope with anxiety; is aware of counseling resources
End of life	Uses social and psychological supports; accepts hospice referral if appropriate

ADL, Activities of daily living; *IADL,* independent activities of daily living. *MMSE,* Mini-Mental State Examination; *PCP,* primary care provider.

a patient was taught. Curriculum content for nurse education includes the cardiac disease process, physical assessment, nursing interventions, teaching content, and support skills.[28]

The new or updated material will need regular review and reinforcement in meetings, skills labs, and newsletters. Meetings at which home care nurses can discuss specific case studies and the usefulness of practice guideline is another strategy to augment didactic education and to reinforce best practices.[13] Measurement of change in practice and documentation is done after implementation of the practice guideline. Docu-

mentation of the outcomes helps to reinforce positive change and to refocus on areas that need further improvement.

The successful design, implementation, and evaluation of a practice guideline require the active involvement of home care nurses. A peer expert, or a small group of peer experts, provides the foundation and structure. The home care nurse who is, or becomes, a content expert assists in every step of the change process including collection of baseline data, training of peers, implementation, complex problem resolution, and follow-up.

■ ■ ■

TABLE 81-3 HEART FAILURE: PRACTICE, TEACHING, AND DOCUMENTATION GUIDELINES

GOALS, ASSESSMENT PARAMETERS, TEACHING GUIDELINES

Goals

Improve symptoms	Optimize physical and cognitive functioning
Promote self-care	Prevent hospital readmissions

Assessment

ADMISSION ASSESSMENTS	EVERY VISIT

1. Vital signs:
   a. BP: left and right arms, at least two positions
   b. P: apical and radial
   c. R
2. Weight and height
3. Edema: right and left, ankle thigh
4. Heart sounds
5. Lung sounds, dyspnea, orthopnea
6. Medications
   a. Prescriptions, OTC, herbal
   b. Possible interactions, side effects
   c. Compliance
7. Activity: endurance, tolerance; ADLs
8. Cognitive screen
9. Need for consults: nutritionist, pharmacist, SW
10. Barriers to care
	1. Vital signs:
	   a. BP: use same arm each visit; position
	   b. P: apical
	   c. R
	2. Weight
	3. Edema
	4. Heart sounds
	5. Lung sounds, dyspnea, orthopnea
	6. Medications
	   a. Compliance
	   b. Interactions or side effects
	   c. Response to therapy
	7. Activity: endurance, tolerance; ADLs
	8. Cognitive status
	9. Diet and fluid intake: compliance
	10. Recall of instruction from previous visit

Teaching: (See examples of education resources below)
1. Symptom recognition (e.g., weight gain, ankle edema, fatigue, appetite change, breathlessness, cough, change in mental status)
2. Daily weights: importance; same time in the morning (after void) with similar clothing; keep log
3. Reportable signs and symptoms; timely reporting to RN and/or MD
4. Medications: doses, scheduling, compliance
5. Diet and consequences of noncompliance
   a. Low sodium
   b. Low fat, low cholesterol
   c. Reading food labels
6. Fluid restriction
7. Activity
   a. Activity pacing and energy conservation techniques
   b. Regular, low-level exercise
8. How to manage heart failure

HEART FAILURE SPECIFIC INFORMATION

PARAMETERS	NORMAL	ABNORMAL (MD PARAMETERS PREVAIL)
Blood pressure	Systolic: 100-140 mm Hg Diastolic: 60-85 mm Hg	Hypotension: *less than* 95/60 Hypertension: *greater than* 160/95
Pulse	60-100/min	*greater than* 20/min increase with ambulation
Respirations	10-20/min	Dyspnea at rest and/or with exertion
Weight	Best or acceptable weight	Gain of *greater than or equal to* 2 lb/1 day or 5 lb in 7 or fewer days

Signs and Symptoms

Jugular venous distension (JVD)	Fatigue
Crackles (usually bibasilar), wheezes, diminished breath sounds	Exercise intolerance
Cough	Lightheadedness or syncope
DOE, PND; orthopnea; tachypnea	Decreased peripheral pulses
Tachycardia	Abdominal pain, anorexia
Lower extremity or sacral edema	Decreased urinary output

From the University of California, San Francisco, UCSF Home Health Care, Author. *ACE,* Angiotensin-converting enzyme; *ADL,* activities of daily living; *BP,* blood pressure; *CHF: practice, teaching, and documentation guidelines; DOE,* dyspnea on exertion; *LV,* left ventricular; *MD,* doctor; *OTC,* over-the-counter; *P,* pulse; *PND,* paroxysmal nocturnal dyspnea; *R,* respirations; *RN,* registered nurse.

■ ■ ■

TABLE 81-3 HEART FAILURE: PRACTICE, TEACHING, AND DOCUMENTATION GUIDELINES—cont'd

Definitions
Heart failure definition:
a. LV systolic dysfunction: reduced myocardial contractility, ejection fraction (EF) less than 55%
b. LV diastolic dysfunction: decreased LV filling, symptomatic but with normal EF

New York Heart Association Functional Classifications
Class 1   Asymptomatic with ordinary physical exertion
Class 2   Symptomatic with ordinary physical exertion
Class 3   Symptomatic with less than ordinary physical exertion
Class 4   Symptomatic at rest

Edema: depress your thumb over pretibial area for 5 sec
1+   2 mm depression
2+   4 mm depression
3+   6 mm depression
4+   8 mm depression

Patient Education Materials (Examples)
Congestive heart failure
Diet and congestive heart failure
How to choose foods low in cholesterol and saturated fat
Living with heart disease: is it heart failure?
Low-salt eating
Reading food labels to limit salt
Taking medicine to control heart failure
Taking your ACE inhibitor
Watching the salt when you are not cooking
Weighing yourself each day

NURSING CARE OF CARDIAC PATIENTS IN THE HOME

Medicare defines which interventions qualify in a Medicare-certified home care program. The determination of skilled nursing care is based on the knowledge and skills that are needed to intervene, taking into account the complexity of the intervention, a patient's condition, and nursing and medical standards of care. The principles of skilled nursing care include: (a) observing and assessing a patient's condition to identify problems or changes, to evaluate the need to modify medication or treatment, and monitor a patient's status until stabilized; (b) patient and family caregiver education and training about how to manage the treatment regimen; and (c) other interventions, including administration of necessary medications, wound care, and ostomy care.[29]

Assessment

A comprehensive history and physical assessment is essential to treating a patient receiving home care. Essential elements of a patient's history include medical and surgical histories, including cardiac and noncardiac events and procedures (see Chapter 45). Essential information from the referral source is often minimal or lacking. Baseline data, such as ejection fraction, New York Heart Association functional classification, best weight or acceptable weight range, and vital sign parameters, provide a useful reference for the home care nurse. In addition to a thorough general and cardiovascular physical assessment,[28,30] additional essential information includes a patient's or family caregiver's ability and willingness to provide care, the adequacy of social support or home support services, the patient's physical and cognitive functional capacity, and a risk factor inventory.

Screening of cognitive functional capacity can be easily performed in the home environment using the Mini-Mental State Examination **(MMSE).** This commonly used "bedside" or screening test is brief, psychometrically sound, and simple to use. The MMSE is an 11-question, 30-point test used to assess orientation to time and place, ability to recall, short-term memory, and arithmetic ability[31]; it does not assess abstraction, judgment, and appearance. The maximum MMSE score is 30 points, which is the total number of correct answers. A score of 23/24 is the most commonly used cut point at or below which cognitive impairment is defined. The MMSE is limited in its lack of sensitivity for mild cognitive impairment. Scores may need to be adjusted for people with a low educational level, different ethnic groups, and low socioeconomic status.

Medication Management

A complicated medication regimen and self-medication practices are two particularly important and sometimes overlooked aspects of medication management. Obtaining a comprehensive list of prescribed and over-the-counter medications, which also identifies drug allergies, is one of the essential first tasks for a home care nurse. The process of cataloging a patient's medications includes an assessment of understanding and management of the medication regimen. A complicated regimen, compounded by medications that are not in the formulary or are expensive, may influence compliance with the regimen. An older person with even mild cognitive impairment is particularly at risk for being unable to adhere to a complicated regimen. Self-medication practices include using over-the-counter medications and dietary and herbal supplements. Important aspects of a medication assessment include, but are not limited to, interactions between cardiovascular drugs and alternative therapies (see the accompanying Pharmacology feature), use of nonsteroidal antiinflammatory drugs (NSAIDs), presence of diabetes, and issues with sleep (see Chapter 17). Other drugs may cause fluid retention, and alternative therapies should be considered (see the accompanying Pharmacology feature on drugs that may exacerbate heart failure).

Interactions between cardiovascular drugs and alternative therapies are assessed by asking about self-medication practices, including all over-the-counter medications and dietary and herbal supplements. Such practices may cause drug interactions or inhibition of bioavailability.[32] Falls are common in older patients with heart failure,[33] which may be associated with drug interactions. Potential drug interactions should be evaluated by a pharmacologist.

Older people commonly seek treatment for pain related to inflammation, and NSAID use is common. The use of NSAIDs has been associated with the onset and exacerbation of heart failure.[34,35] Although some NSAIDs may be safer than others, in general, NSAIDS should be avoided in persons with heart failure because they cause fluid retention. Alternative pain management and antiinflammatory therapies should be tried.[36]

Patients with heart failure and comorbid diabetes must be taught that diuretics, such as furosemide, beta blockers,[37] and many psychotropic drugs can raise blood glucose levels, despite careful diet control. Chondroitin, a dietary supplement, also can raise blood glucose levels.[38]

■■■ PHARMACOLOGY

INTERACTIONS BETWEEN CARDIOVASCULAR DRUGS AND ALTERNATIVE THERAPIES

Commonly used supplements:	Supplements used more often by women:	Supplements used more often by men:
Megadose vitamins*	Black cohosh	Alpha lipoic acid
Multivitamins	Borage	Gingko biloba
Dietary supplements	Evening primrose	Grape seed extract
Iron†	Flaxseed oil	
Used most often:	Dehydroepiandrosterone	
Glucosamine‡	Grape seed extract	
Gingko biloba‡	Hawthorn	
Chondroitin‡	St. John's wort§	
Garlic‡		
Fish oil‡		

*Multivitamins with vitamin K can interact with warfarin if a patient is deficient in vitamin K.
†Correction of anemia improves resting energy expenditure; iron may decrease cough from ACE inhibitors.
‡Potential for increasing anticoagulation effect of warfarin and aspirin.
§There is evidence that St. John's wort may interact with many medications.

From Wold RS, Lopez ST, Yau CL et al: Increasing trends in elderly persons' use of nonvitamin, nonmineral dietary supplements and concurrent use of medications, *J Am Diet Assoc* 105:54-63, 2005.
Kurnik D, Lubetsky A, Loebstein R et al: Multivitamin supplements may affect warfarin anticoagulation in susceptible patients, *Ann Pharmacother* 37:1603-1606, 2003.
Buckley MS, Goff AD, Knapp WE: Fish oil interaction with warfarin, *Ann Pharmacother* 38:50-52, 2004.
Fugh-Berman A, Ernst E: Herb-drug interactions: review and assessment of report reliability, *Br J Clin Pharmacol* 52:587-595, 2001.

■■■ PHARMACOLOGY

DRUGS THAT MAY EXACERBATE HEART FAILURE

CLASS I DYSRHYTHMICS	PRODYSRHYTHMIC
Corticosteroids	Increased cardiac output
	Increased peripheral vascular tone
	Direct renal effect on sodium and water retention
Itraconazole	Negative inotropic effect
Nonsteroidal anti-inflammatory drugs	Fluid and sodium retention
	Decrease in renal blood flow and glomerular filtration
Thiazolidinediones (rosiglitazone and pioglitazone)	Fluid retention and increased plasma volume
Tricyclic antidepressants	Increased heart rate
	Orthostatic hypotension
	Conduction abnormalities; prodysrhythmic

From Bleumink GS, Feenstra J, Sturkenboom MC et al: Nonsteroidal anti-inflammatory drugs and heart failure, *Drugs* 63:525-534, 2003.
Aron DC, Findling JW, Tyrrell JB: Glucocorticoids and adrenal androgens. In Greenspan FS, Gardner DG, editors, *Basic and clinicaleEndocrinology*, ed 7, New York, 2004, Lange Medical Books/McGraw-Hill, pp. 334-376.
Sholter DE, Armstrong PW: Adverse effects of corticosteroids on the cardiovascular system, *Can J Cardiol* 16:505-511, 2000.
Nesto, RW, Bell D, Bonow RO et al: Thiazolidinedione use, fluid retention, and congestive heart failure, *Circulation* 108:2941-2948, 2003.
Ahmad SR, Singer SJ, Leissa BG: Congestive heart failure associated with itraconazole, *Lancet* 357:1766-1767, 2001.
Roose SP, Glassman AH, Attia E et al: Cardiovascular effects of fluoxetine in depressed patients with heart disease, *Am J Psychiatry* 155:660-665, 1998.

Two thirds of people with heart failure perceive that they either sleep too much or sleep too little. Although cardiovascular drugs, such as beta blockers, beta agonists, and antidysrhythmic drugs, are reported to interfere with sleep,[39] these data are primarily anecdotal and from case reports. More research is needed on the effects of cardiac medications on sleep.

Patient Education

Both general content and information specific to the diagnosis are taught by home care nurses. General content includes symptom recognition and management, instruction on when to seek medical care and the importance of consistently receiving care from the same provider, medication management and knowledge of interactions and side effects, nutrition and fluid intake guidelines and restrictions, daily weights and weight records, activity or exercise guidelines, and risk factor modification. Education specific to a patient with heart failure, the primary cardiac population seen in home care, includes reinforcement of the importance of recording daily weights, weight and diuretic parameters, energy conservation strategies, symptom recognition and management specific to heart failure, and the relationship between a change in mental status and heart failure. Education for patients after cardiac surgery includes pulmonary hygiene, incisional care, and pain management.

INNOVATIVE HOME-BASED INTERVENTIONS
Transitional Care

Is transitional care, such as APN-directed discharge planning and home care follow-up, contingent on an APN directing or providing care? A randomized clinical trial by Naylor and coworkers[8] that used an APN-directed intervention produced results similar to those of two previous trials.[9,40] Patients with heart failure in the intervention group received up to 3 months of home care directed and delivered by APNs with special training in heart failure and complications associated with comorbid conditions. The care began before patients were discharged from the hospital, where the APNs coordinated and planned the care in partnership with the patients' physicians and as guided by an evidence-based protocol. They consulted with multidisciplinary team members, patients, and family caregivers. During hospitalization medication regimens were simplified and improved. Efforts were made to prevent functional decline. Identifying the patients' goals for treatment adherence and behavioral change and teaching patients and caregivers early symptom recognition and effective intervention strategies were the major foci for home care.

After discharge an APN visited patients at home within 24 hours of discharge from the hospital and saw them at least eight times in 3 months. In addition to doing physical assessments and evaluating patients' responses to therapy, the APNs were the primary intermediaries who ensured continuity of care. They were the

conduits for the accurate and timely transfer of information critical for error prevention. They were able to detect problems early and adjust therapeutic regimens accordingly, communicating directly with the patient" physician or relying on physician-specific guidelines.

Heart failure patients in the control group received usual care, including management of heart failure and discharge planning; 58 percent of these were referred to a home care agency for skilled nursing or physical therapy. Outcomes were significantly better in the intervention group whose transition from hospital to home and home care were provided by an APN. Significantly fewer patients in the intervention group were hospitalized or died at 52 weeks than patients in the control group (47.5 percent versus 61.2 percent, $p = .01$). Time to first rehospitalization for patients in the intervention group was increased, controlling for self-rating of health status, living situation, hospitalizations within the previous 6 months, and number of daily medications. The median time of event-free survival was 241 days for patients in the intervention group compared with 131 days for those in the control group. There was a mean cost savings of \$4,845 per patient in the intervention group ($p = .002$).

It should be emphasized that the patients in the intervention group benefited from what is an ideal care model. The APNs provided expert clinical care that focused on symptom recognition and rapid management, holistic care that incorporated the complex needs and individualized goals of older patients with an average of 6.4 other health conditions, continuity of care from hospital to home, and coordination of care in a complex health care system that is often bewildering for older patients, especially when they have functional or cognitive impairments. APN care is costly and rarely used by home care agencies, although perhaps it should be.

Coordinated Discharge Planning

Recent meta-analyses have examined the impact of comprehensive discharge planning and support after hospitalization in older patients with heart failure and found that, despite inconsistent and variable reporting of data and elements of analysis, readmission rates were significantly reduced and health outcomes were improved without increasing the cost of care.[9,41] There are many forms of comprehensive discharge planning, but key components include medication review and counseling, monitoring daily weights and reporting heart failure symptoms, dietary counseling, telephone or telehealth monitoring, home care nurse visits, and increased communication between providers. The efficacy of each model or its variant continues to be analyzed and discussed; the most common outcomes under examination are the rate of readmission to a hospital, heart failure and all-cause mortality, quality of life, and cost of care.

Home Telehealth

Several investigators[42-47] have studied the use of different telecare interventions (e.g., telephone calls, video-based telecare, and telephonic communication devices) on outcomes and cost of care for older cardiac patients. The research designs usually included a study nurse who made home visits to collect data, but none of the telehealth studies used home care nurses. In heart failure samples, readmission rates and the costs of care were lower,[42-44] emergency room visits were fewer,[42,43] and symptoms improved,[45] but intervention costs were higher for patients receiving video-based telecare,[43,44] and there was little improvement in optimizing the medication regimen[42] or patient adherence to the treatment regimen.[44] At this point, it is not clear which patients would benefit most from telemedicine or if telemedicine could be a useful adjunct to home care.[46]

A feasibility study[47] used a home care team, including a nurse with advanced cardiovascular training and a teledisease management nurse, to improve medication adherence and reduce hospital readmissions. The home care nurse visited patients in their homes, physically assessed them, and taught them and their caregivers. Standardized (i.e., scripted) telephone calls were made by the teledisease nurse. Data were entered into a database that was used to update physicians and coordinate services. The intervention reduced rehospitalization rates, which was attributed to the consistency of skilled cardiac nurses providing the home visits, the increased number of scheduled home visits in the first 60 days after hospital discharge, enhanced patient education and self-care, and telehealth communication. Cost of the intervention was not reported.

One of the challenges in recruiting patients for a home care telemedicine intervention is the high cost of installing equipment and training patients who are expected to receive home care for a limited time. Likewise, telemedicine is less likely to provide a symptom monitoring and reporting benefit for patients whose needs require three or more skilled nurse visits a week.[46]

FREQUENCY OF HOME VISITS

After the initial home visit, subsequent visits are guided by home care agency standards or clinical guidelines, and are influenced by physical and self-care progress toward goals established by the patient, home care nurse, and physician. Changes in functional status, treatments, or the medication regimen and responses to medication modifications or adjustments will influence an increased or decreased visit frequency. Discharge from the agency occurs when a patient no longer meets home care eligibility requirements (e.g., he or she has met the plan of care goals, no longer requires medically necessary intermittent skilled care, or has met the goals mutually established by the patient and family caregiver, the home care nurse, and the patient's physician).

CONCLUSION

Home care is an indispensable link in the health care system that can promote, maintain, or restore a patient's health, maximize his or her level of independence, and minimize the effects of illness and disability. Few home care agencies are large enough to support disease-specific programs or APNs, but all home care nurses are obligated to implement evidence-based, best-practice guidelines. Though APN care is more expensive than that of a generalist home care nurse, the APN impact on patient outcomes and associated decrease in the cost of care, especially in a large agency, makes a compelling argument for an APN intervention that is continuous from hospital to home.

REFERENCES

1. Kozak LJ, Hall MJ, Owings MF: National hospital discharge survey: 2000, Series 13, *Vital Health Statistics* p 13, 2002.
2. *Basic statistics about home care*, National Association for Home Care, 2001.
3. *Home Health Community Beneficiaries 2001,* Department of Health and Human Services, Office of Inspector General, 2001.
4. Krumholz HM, Chen YT, Wang Y et al: Predictors of readmission among elderly survivors of admission with heart failure, *Am Heart J* 139:72-77, 2000.
5. Kossovsky MP, Sarasin FP, Perneger TV et al: Unplanned readmissions of patients with congestive heart failure: do they reflect in-hospital quality of care or patient characteristics? *Am J Med* 109:386-390, 2000.
6. Wexler DJ, Chen J, Smith GL et al: Predictors of cost of caring for elderly patients discharged with heart failure, *Am Heart J* 142:350-357, 2001.
7. Bowles KH, Naylor MD, Foust JB: Patient characteristics at hospital discharge and a comparison of home care referral decisions, *J Am Geriatr Soc* 50:336-342, 2002.
8. Naylor MD, Brooten DA, Campbell RL et al: Transitional care of older adults hospitalized with heart failure: a randomized, controlled trial, *J Am Geriatr Soc* 52:675-684, 2004.
9. Phillips CO, Wright SM, Kern DE et al: Comprehensive discharge planning with postdischarge support for older patients with heart failure: a meta-analysis, *JAMA* 291:1358-1367, 2004.
10. Naylor MD, Brooten D, Campbell R et al: Comprehensive discharge planning and home follow-up of hospitalized elders, *JAMA* 281:613-620, 1999.
11. Fortinsky RH, Fenster JR, Judge JO: Medicare and Medicaid home health and Medicaid waiver services for dually eligible older adults: risk factors for use and correlates of expenditures, *Gerontologist* 44:739-749, 2004.
12. Marcantonio ER, McKean S, Goldfinger M et al: Factors associated with unplanned hospital readmission among patients 65 years of age and older in a Medicare managed care plan, *Am J Med* 107:13-17, 1999.
13. Feldman PH, Peng TR, Murtaugh CM at al: A randomized intervention to improve heart failure outcomes in community-based home health care, *Home Health Care Serv Q* 23:1-23, 2004.
14. Stewart S, Horowitz JD: Home-based intervention in congestive heart failure: long-term implications on readmission and survival, *Circulation* 105:2861-2866, 2002.
15. Klein D, Turvey C, Wallace R: Elders who delay medication because of cost: health insurance, demographic, health, and financial correlates, *Gerontologist* 44:779-787, 2004.
16. *Heart disease and stroke statistics—2005 update*, Dallas, 2004, American Heart Association.
17. California HealthCare Foundation: *Improving quality of care for Californians with heart failure*, Oakland, Calif, 2002.
18. Almeida OP, Tamai S: Congestive heart failure and cognitive functioning amongst older adults, *Arqu Neuropsiquiatr* 59:324-329, 2001.
19. Antonelli Incalzi R, Trojano L, Acanfora D et al: Verbal memory impairment in congestive heart failure, *J Clin Exp Neuropsychol* 25:14-23, 2003.
20. Zuccalà G, Onder G, Pedone C et al: Cognitive dysfunction as a major determinant of disability in patients with heart failure: results from a multicentre survey. On behalf of the GIFA (SIGG-ONLUS) investigators, *J Neuro, Neurosurg Psychiatry* 70:109-112, 2001.

21. Erkinjuntti T, Ostbye T, Steenhuis R et al: The effect of different diagnostic criteria on the prevalence of dementia, *N Engl J Med* 337:1667-1674, 1997.

22. Lopez OL, Jagust WJ, DeKosky ST et al: Prevalence and classification of mild cognitive impairment in the cardiovascular health study cognition study, *Arch Neurol* 60:1385-1389, 2003.

23. Graham JE, Rockwood K, Beattie BL et al: Prevalence and severity of cognitive impairment with and without dementia in an elderly population, *Lancet* 349:1793-1796, 1997.

24. Almeida OP, Tamai S: Clinical treatment reverses attentional deficits in congestive heart failure, *BMC Geriatrics* 1:2, 2001.

25. Braunstein JB, Anderson GF, Gerstenblith G et al: Noncardiac comorbidity increases preventable hospitalizations and mortality among Medicare beneficiaries with chronic heart failure, *J Am Coll Cardiol* 42:1226-1233, 2003.

26. Bennett SJ, Sauve MJ: Cognitive deficits in patients with heart failure: a review of the literature, *J Cardiovasc Nurs* 18:219-242, 2003.

27. Sochalski J: Building a home healthcare workforce to meet the quality imperative, *J Healthc Qual* 26:19-23, 2004.

28. Whittier S: Cardiac assessment and disease management for home health nurses, *Geriatr Nurs* 25:248-249, 2004.

29. Centers for Medicare and Medicaid Services (CMS): *The Home Health Agency Manual— HCFA Publication 11,* Available at www.cms.hhs.gov/manuals/.

30. Coviello JS: Cardiac assessment 101: a new look at the guidelines for cardiac homecare patients, *Home Healthc Nurse* 22:116-123, 2004.

31. McDowell I, Newell C: *Measuring health: a guide to rating scales and questionnaires,* ed 2, New York, 1996, Oxford University Press.

32. Neafsey PJ: Self-medication practices that alter the efficacy of selected cardiac medications, *Home Healthc Nurse* 22:88-98, 2004.

33. Potocka-Plazak K, Plazak W: Orthostatic hypotension in elderly women with congestive heart failure, *Aging (Milano)* 13:378-384, 2001.

34. Feenstra J, Heerdink ER, Grobbee DE et al: Association of nonsteroidal anti-inflammatory drugs with first occurrence of heart failure and with relapsing heart failure: the Rotterdam study, *Arch Intern Med* 162:265-270, 2002.

35. Garcia Rodriguez LA, Hernandez-Diaz S: Nonsteroidal anti-inflammatory drugs as a trigger of clinical heart failure, *Epidemiology* 14:240-246, 2003.

36. Hudson M, Richard H, Pilote L: Differences in outcomes of patients with congestive heart failure prescribed celecoxib, rofecoxib, or non-steroidal anti-inflammatory drugs: population based study, *BMJ* 330:1370-1376, 2005.

37. Bell DS: Treatment of heart failure in patients with diabetes: clinical update, *Ethn Dis* 12:S1-12-18, 2002.

38. Wold RS, Lopez ST, Yau CL et al: Increasing trends in elderly persons' use of nonvitamin, nonmineral dietary supplements and concurrent use of medications, *J Am Diet Assoc* 105:54-63, 2005.

39. Parker KP, Dunbar SB: Sleep and heart failure, *J Cardiovasc Nurs* 17:30-41, 2002.

40. Rich MW, Beckham V, Wittenberg C et al: A multidisciplinary intervention to prevent the readmission of elderly patients with congestive heart failure, *N Engl J Med* 333:1190-1195, 1995.

41. McAlister FA, Lawson FM, Teo KK et al: A systematic review of randomized trials of disease management programs in heart failure, *Am J Med* 110:378-384, 2001.

42. Berg GD, Wadhwa S, Johnson AE: A matched-cohort study of health services utilization and financial outcomes for a heart failure disease-management program in elderly patients, *J Am Geriatr Soc* 52:1655-1661, 2004.

43. Jerant AF, Azari R, Nesbitt TS: Reducing the cost of frequent hospital admissions for congestive heart failure, *Med Care* 39:1234-1245, 2001.

44. Jerant AF, Azari R, Martinez C et al: A randomized trial of telenursing to reduce hospitalization for heart failure: patient-centered outcomes and nursing indicators, *Home Health Care Serv Q* 22:1-20, 2003.

45. Todero CM, LaFramboise LM, Zimmerman LM: Symptom status and quality-of-life outcomes of home-based disease management program for heart failure patients, *Outcomes Manag* 6:161-168, 2002.

46. Subramanian U, Hopp F, Lowery J et al: Research in home-care telemedicine: challenges in patient recruitment, *Telemed J E Health* 10:155-161, 2004.

47. Ohldin A: Observations from a home-based congestive heart failure intervention, *Home Care Provid* 6:213-217, 2001.

■■■ chapter 82
Hospice and Palliative Care

Cheryl Hoyt Zambroski

CHAPTER ABBREVIATIONS

ACE   angiotensin-converting enzyme

AHRQ   Agency for Healthcare Research and Quality

ANA   American Nurses Association

HIV   human immunodeficiency virus

ICD   implantable cardioverter-defibrillator

NHPCO   National Hospice and Palliative Care Organization

NSAID   nonsteroidal antiinflammatory drug

NYHA   New York Heart Association

SUPPORT   Study to Understand Prognosis and Preferences for Outcomes and Risks of Treatment

About 30 percent of all deaths worldwide are attributed to cardiovascular disease.[1] By the year 2020, cardiovascular disease will become the leading cause of death and disability worldwide, with the number of fatalities increasing to more than 20,000,000 annually.[2] In the United States alone, nearly 40 percent of all deaths are due to cardiovascular disease.[3] Additionally, cardiovascular diseases are responsible for 10 percent of the overall disease burden globally, evidenced by premature death and the years of productive life lost as a result of disability.[4]

Researchers and clinicians have emphasized the importance of cardiovascular disease prevention, early detection, and treatment in this text and elsewhere. Public awareness of the importance of diet and exercise, tobacco cessation, and symptom recognition continues to grow. What is missing from the public discourse and from our focus is the care of the patients who are dying from cardiovascular disease. According to the World Health Organization, palliative care is primarily associated with cancer or human immunodeficiency virus (HIV) rather than with cardiovascular disease, a major cause of disability and death worldwide.[2,4]

ADVANCED HEART FAILURE AS A FRAMEWORK TO DISCUSS PALLIATIVE CARE

Heart failure is the final common pathway for a wide variety of cardiovascular diseases that ultimately result in left ventricular dysfunction. Heart failure researchers and clinicians have recently embraced the need to improve palliative care for patients with advanced heart failure.[5-7] Thus, advanced heart failure will be used to frame this chapter on palliative care for patients with cardiovascular disease.

Tremendous advances have been made in pharmacological and technological interventions that reduce mortality and improve quality of life in patients with heart failure. Cytokine and endothelial antagonists, biventricular pacing, and left ventricular assist devices are only a few of the strategies being investigated for use in advanced heart failure.[8] Unfortunately, despite this dramatic progress in medical care, the mortality rate for patients with heart failure remains exceedingly high. Nearly 20 percent of patients with heart failure die within 1 year of diagnosis.[3] At 5 years, the mortality rate climbs to approximately 50 percent.[9] Once the patient has progressed to the stages of advanced heart failure, 1 year mortality is nearly 40 percent.[10] For heart failure patients, sudden death is six to nine times more likely than in the general population.[3]

Over and above the issue of high mortality, the end of life for many advanced heart failure patients is characterized by a progressive decline in physical functioning and a wide range of poorly managed physical and psychological symptoms that may remain unrelieved until the time of death.[11,12] To complicate matters, patients with heart failure typically experience a relatively unpredictable course of illness characterized by acute exacerbations of symptoms rather than by the progressive decline typical of conditions, such as cancer.[13] Like chronic illnesses, such as dementia and chronic lung disease, the dying process for heart failure patients can be long and protracted, requiring intermittent and often times progressive social and health care support until death.

The Institute of Medicine argued that improving end-of-life care for patients with advanced heart failure is a national imperative.[14] As a result, researchers and clinicians have joined forces to examine and improve the care of patients with heart failure.[5,6] Provision of expert palliative care is essential for nurses to respond to the needs of this growing population.

The purpose of this chapter is to define palliative care, identify major challenges affecting palliative care for patients with advanced heart failure, and recommend strategies to improve end of life for patients with advanced heart failure. For the purposes of this chapter, advanced heart failure is defined using the consensus statement for palliative and supportive care in advanced heart failure as "a state in which patients have significant cardiac dysfunction with marked symptoms of dyspnea, fatigue, or symptoms relating to end-organ hypoperfusion at rest or with minimal exertion despite maximal medical therapy".[5]

DEFINING PALLIATIVE CARE

The National Hospice and Palliative Care Organization (**NHPCO**) described palliative care as "treatment that enhances comfort and improves quality of an individual's life during the last phase of life.[15]" Using a broader definition, the National Consensus Project for Quality Palliative Care promotes the goal of palliative care as preventing and relieving suffering and supporting the best quality of life for patients and families regardless of the specific stages of a disease (Figure 82-1).[16]

Palliative care moves beyond traditional disease management models of care to include goals of enhancing the life of patients and their families, improving decision making, and optimizing function.[16] Palliative care is characterized by a multidimensional and interdisciplinary approach required to meet the physical, psychological, social, and spiritual needs of patients and their families. Patient's and families' values and decisions are vital in the philosophy of palliative care.

Ideally, palliative care is initiated at diagnosis of any life-threatening or debilitating illness and follows the patient and their family through the death and during the bereavement period. Palliative care should not be limited to patients with cancer or to those near death.[17] Although the time line for dying in patients with heart failure is often unclear, clinicians do recognize that heart failure does in fact reduce life expectancy.

Critical to the concept of palliative care is that no specific therapy is excluded from consideration. The test of palliative care versus curative care is that the expected outcome of palliative care is relief of distressing symptoms, the easing of pain, and/or enhancing quality of life. Palliative care can be delivered concurrently with life-prolonging care to meet the goals of comfort at the end of life. Therefore, mechanical ventilation, dialysis, blood transfusion, intravenous vasoactive therapies, and even balloon counter pulsation are not necessarily inappropriate care at the end of life for the heart failure patient if these therapies provide comfort, reduce symptoms, and improve quality of life at the end of life. Nevertheless, caution must be noted; interventions should be based on meeting the goals of palliative care rather than curing the underlying disease.

Integration of palliative care concepts into heart failure care ensures that patients and their families will receive holistic care designed to meet multiple needs across a variety of settings and the full continuum of health[16] (Box 82-1). Even following death, palliative care concepts warrant that the family is not abandoned but rather ensures the availability of bereavement support.

Hospice as a Model of Palliative Care Delivery

Hospice has provided the earliest example of expert palliative care delivery. Introduced to the United States in the early 1970s, hospices primarily targeted their interventions to improve pain and symptom management and spiritual support for patients with advanced cancer.[18] As the success of hospice has grown, more and more patients are referred to hospice for palliative care with a variety of noncancer diagnoses, including advanced heart failure.[19]

In 1998, nearly 66 percent of patients discharged from hospice had cancer diagnoses compared with 58 percent in 2000 and 49 percent in 2004.[20] Unfortunately, the numbers of patients with heart disease referred to hospice has not trended upward. In 1998, 8.6 percent of patients discharged from hospice had heart disease compared with only 6.8 percent in 2000.[20] Recent data indicate that between 7.9 percent and 11 percent had heart disease in 2003.[21] This is low considering that heart disease is the number one cause of death in the United States.

Confusion exists regarding the potential value of referring patients with heart failure to hospice, illustrating the need to better understand the role of hospice at the end of life. The philosophy of hospice is congruent with that of palliative care, with provisions that address physical, psychological, social, and spiritual needs of patients and families often missing from traditional models of care.[22] Guided by a holistic approach to care, hospice interdisciplinary teams of physicians, nurses,

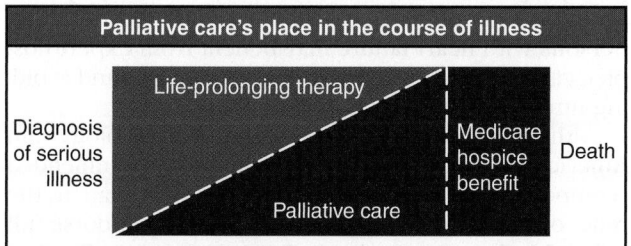

FIGURE 82-1 ■ Relationship between palliative care and life-prolonging therapy in life-threatening or debilitating illness, including heart failure. (From National Consensus Project for Palliative Care: *Clinical practice guidelines for quality palliative care,* Brooklyn, NY, 2004, National Consensus Project for Quality Palliative Care.)

BOX 82-1   ■ ■ ■
RESULT OF INTEGRATING PALLIATIVE CARE INTO ALL CARE FOR PATIENTS WITH HEART FAILURE

1. Patient and family needs will be addressed throughout the continuum of care.
   a. Pain and symptoms are managed.
   b. Psychosocial distress is diminished.
   c. Spiritual issues are addressed.
   d. Practical needs are met.
2. Patients and families will receive information in an ongoing and understandable manner so that:
   a. Condition and treatment options are discussed.
   b. Benefits and burdens of treatment are understood.
   c. Sensitivity to changes in the patient's condition will be ongoing.
3. Coordination of care across settings will be:
   a. Regular and of high quality to ensure communication among providers and family.
   b. Guided by effective case management incorporated into care.
4. Patient and family will be prepared for the dying process and death:
   a. Hospice options will explored.
   b. Opportunities for personal growth will be enhanced.
   c. Bereavement support will be available.

From National Consensus Project for Palliative Care: *Clinical practice guidelines for quality palliative care,* 2004, Brooklyn, NY, National Consensus Project for Quality Palliative Care.

social workers, chaplains, nutritionists, volunteers, and even music therapists effectively manage care. Hospice care can be delivered to patients and families in homes, long-term care or assisted living agencies, and in dedicated palliative care units.[22] Hospice supports patients and families through the process of dying and the family through the dying and bereavement periods.

The vast majority of hospices are certified by Medicare.[23] To be eligible for Medicare hospice benefits, patients must meet three specific criteria: (1) the patient's physician and hospice physician must certify that the patient is terminally ill with a life expectancy of 6 months or less; (2) the patient must choose to receive hospice care rather than curative treatment; and (3) the patient must enroll in a Medicare-approved hospice agency.[24] Consent to enroll in hospice does not preclude treatment for other illnesses (e.g., acute appendicitis) or injuries (e.g., hip fracture) not related to the terminal illness.

Formal guidelines were developed by the National Hospice Association in 1996 to assist physicians to determine 6-month life expectancy in patients with heart disease, including advanced heart failure.[25] The guidelines were designed to ease the process of referral while preventing the need for complex prognostic systems that use detailed clinical data. The guidelines have been updated to reflect current standards of practice (Box 82-2). General criteria include factors, such as diminished functional status, multiple emergency visits or inpatient hospitalizations within a 6-month period, and progressive unintentional weight loss. More specific criteria include factors, such as symptomatic heart failure despite optimal pharmacological management, history of cardiac arrest, or syncope.

Vital to understanding the hospice referral process as it relates to persons with heart failure is recognizing that the Medicare hospice benefit does not preclude expert nursing care, optimization of medication, education, and early attention to signs and symptoms of fluid overload. Components of heart failure disease management programs and hospice care are not mutually exclusive. Patients and families may need reassurance that enrollment in hospice is directed toward improving, not abandoning, care. They can benefit from the additional palliative care expertise of hospice clinicians. Furthermore, once the patient enrolls in hospice, they may choose to withdraw at anytime without penalty.

Cost-effectiveness data regarding hospice for patients with advanced heart failure is inconclusive. Recent evidence indicates that hospice enrollment may reduce cost in the last month of life, but not necessarily in the last year of life.[26] In a recent retrospective cohort study ($n = 245,326$) done to determine the financial impact of hospice care on Medicare payments during the last year of life, expenditures for patients with heart failure who received hospice care were as much as 16 percent higher than those who did not use hospice care during the last year of life.[26] Additional outcomes, such as quality of life and symptom management, were not studied. On the other hand, it has been reported that Medicare costs before enrollment in hospice are tremendous in patients with heart failure compared with other chronic illnesses.[27] For example, when compared with patients with advanced cancer, those with advanced heart fail-

---

BOX 82-2 ■ ■ ■

NATIONAL HOSPICE AND PALLIATIVE CARE ORGANIZATION GENERAL MEDICAL GUIDELINES FOR DETERMINING PROGNOSIS IN NONCANCER DISEASES AND HEART DISEASES

The Patient Should Meet All of the Following Criteria
I. The patient's condition is life limiting, and the patient and/or family knows this.
II. The patient and/or family have elected treatment goals directed toward relief of symptoms rather than the underlying disease.
III. The patient has either of the following:
  A. Documented clinical progression of the disease, which may include:
    1. Progression of the primary disease process as listed in the disease-specific criteria, as documented by serial physician assessment and laboratory, radiological, or other studies
    2. Multiple emergency department visits or inpatient hospitalizations over the prior 6 months
    3. For homebound patients receiving home health services, nursing assessment may be documented.
    4. For patients who do not qualify under 1, 2, or 3 above, a recent decline in functional status should be documented. Clinical judgment is required.
  B. Documented recent impaired nutritional status related to the terminal process:
    1. Unintentional, progressive weight loss of more than 10% over the prior 6 months
    2. Serum albumin of less than 2.5 g/dl may be a helpful prognostic indicator, but should not be used in isolation from other factors above.

Patients with Heart Disease Should Also Meet the Following Criteria
I. Intractable or frequently recurrent symptomatic heart failure or intractable angina pectoris with heart failure
II. Already optimally treated with diuretics, vasodilators, beta blockers, and spironolactone as indicated and tolerated*
III. Other factors contributing to a poor prognosis: symptomatic dysrhythmias, history of cardiac arrest and resuscitation or syncope, cardiogenic brain embolism, or concomitant HIV disease

HIV, Human immunodeficiency virus.
*This criterion is modified from the published guideline to reflect current, optimal medical management of heart failure.
From Pantilat SZ, Steimle AE: Palliative care for patients with heart failure, *JAMA* 291:2476-2482, 2004. (Adapted by *JAMA* with permission from National Hospice Organization.)

---

ure received more life-sustaining treatments and experienced longer hospital stays at the end of life.[28] Patients with heart failure may actually be discharged from hospice programs and then readmitted when symptoms again become unmanageable. These data illustrate that persons with heart failure may benefit from expert hospice care geared toward managing symptoms and avoiding unnecessary aggressive treatments.

Although the American College of Cardiology and American Heart Association guidelines recommended "components of hospice care that are appropriate to the relief of suffering"[8] they did not specifically endorse full referral to hospice. Lack of adequate data on effectiveness of the hospice model of care for patients with heart failure has contributed to a reluctance to endorse hospice, which must be overcome.

Efforts are being made to improve heart failure palliative care provided outside formal hospice agencies.[16,29]

Caution is noted, however; bypassing currently available hospice services in favor of developing an entirely new model of care could be an ineffective use of already strained health care resources.[30,31] Models of care that provide the best outcomes should guide practice.

CHALLENGES TO IMPROVING CARE AT THE END OF LIFE

According to the national consensus project, palliative care should be provided regardless of the stage of the illness.[16] In reality, the emphasis of palliative care is primarily directed toward improving the care at the end of life.[15] Before palliative care can be provided for earlier stages of heart failure, challenges must be overcome in providing end-of-life care for patients with advanced heart failure.

Defining End of Life

There are a variety of definitions associated with the phrase "end of life."[6,32] " End of life has been defined according to the timing of death. The phrase "actively dying" describes a patient's rapid clinical deterioration when they are reliably expected to die within hours to days.[32] End of life has been defined by the patient's readiness to die: when is the patient ready to address end-of-life discussions? Readiness to die can be contingent on understanding of age, social situation, depression, or even weariness with life.[32] End of life can also be defined by the patient's prognosis. Prognostication represents a likelihood of survival at a particular time rather than an actual prediction of how long a specific patient will live.[32]

Defining end of life according to prognosis is a major challenge for patients with heart failure. One of the most elusive definitions for end of life in patients with advanced heart failure is the Medicare definition of a prognosis of 6 months or less to live that determines hospice eligibility. In the landmark Study to Understand Prognosis and Preferences for Outcomes and Risks of Treatment (SUPPORT), investigators found that for patients with advanced heart failure, 54 percent had a median 6-month survival prediction even 3 days before death.[33]

Researchers have used a variety of methods to determine prognosis for patients with heart failure.[33-36] Although these studies are useful for improving outcomes in the heart failure population, they are far less useful in determining prognosis for individual patients.

Ellershaw and Ward proposed criteria for determining the dying phase of heart failure that may be useful for individual patients.[37] They reported that the dying phase of heart failure is characterized by a history of previous admissions to the hospital with worsening heart failure, having no clearly identifiable precipitant to a heart failure exacerbation, receiving optimal medications, exhibiting deteriorating renal function, and failure to respond to diuretics or vasodilators within 2 to 3 days of administration.

The essence of the heart failure illness trajectory is a course of long decline in functional status with intermittent life-threatening exacerbation and often ending with sudden death.[38] Goodlin and colleagues[5] proposed a schematic representation of the illness trajectory of Stage C and Stage D heart failure (Figure 82-2), which captures the phases of the trajectory through onset of

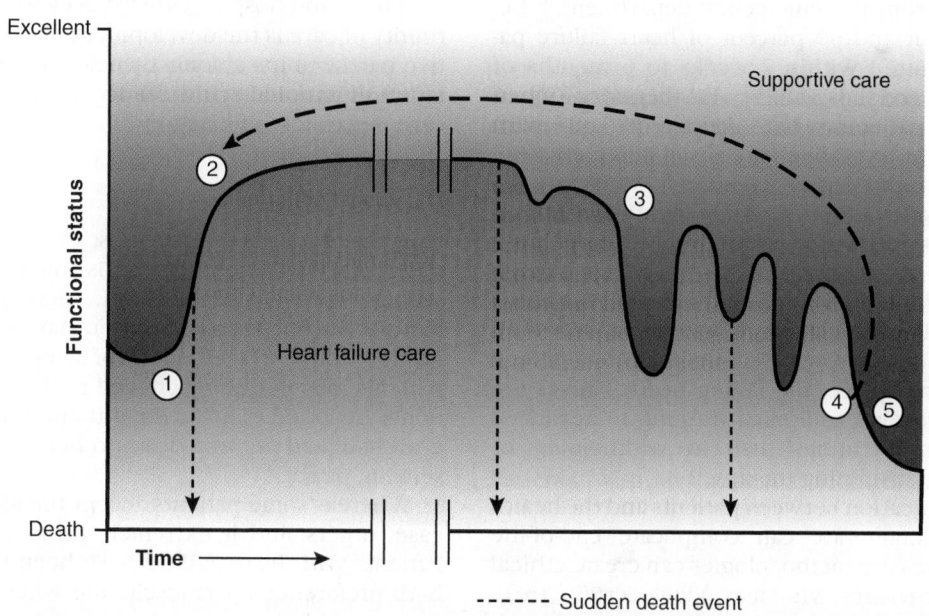

FIGURE 82-2 ▪ Schematic course of Stage C and D heart failure. Sudden death may occur at any point along the course of illness. (1) Initial symptoms of heart failure develop, and heart failure treatment begins. (2) Plateaus of variable length may be reached with initial medical management or after mechanical support or heart transplant. (3) Functional status declines with the variable slope, with intermittent exacerbations of heart failure that respond to rescue efforts. (4) Stage D heart failure, with refractory symptoms and limited function. (5) Patient reaches end of life. (From Goodlin SJ, Hauptman PJ, Arnold R et al: Consensus statement: palliative and supportive care in advanced heart failure, *J Card Fail* 10:203, 2004.)

symptoms to death. Importantly, even though there is a specific "end-of-life" phase, the illness trajectory for heart failure can be interrupted at any time by sudden death. Heart failure patients are six to nine times more likely to die of sudden death than the general population.[3]

Fox and colleagues[39] remind us that "the sickest patients are not necessarily the ones who die first." We know that the prognosis for heart failure patients is poor overall, but accurate estimation of the time of death may be an unrealistic expectation. Complexity of predicting death is not an adequate rationale for failure to use palliative interventions.

Recently, the National Institutes of Health identified two key components that can guide researchers and clinicians in determining the end of life.[6] First, there is the presence of chronic disease(s) or symptoms or functional impairment that persist, but may also fluctuate. Second, symptoms or impairments resulting from the underlying irreversible disease require formal or informal care and can lead to death. They agreed that there is no clear threshold that identifies the end of life. Use of the broad definition of end of life supports the concept of palliative care for those patients regardless of when they die.

Focus on Cure as Success in Acute Care Settings

End of life for patients with advanced heart failure has been characterized by chronic outpatient care punctuated by aggressive rescue efforts, preponderantly occurring in acute care settings.[5] Heart failure is second only to pneumonia as the most frequent reason for admission to the hospital from the emergency department.[40] Between 20 percent and 50 percent of heart failure patients are readmitted within 2 weeks to 6 months of discharge from the hospital.[41,42] Furthermore, when compared with patients with dementia, patients with heart failure were more likely to die in acute care (45 percent versus 18 percent, $p = 0.06$).

Once patients are admitted to the acute care setting, cure rather than death is often the implied outcome.[43] Live-saving devices or new treatments receive much greater publicity than palliation of symptoms using low-tech strategies. This is particularly true in patients with heart failure with the growing emphasis on technology to care for, even replace, the failing heart. Nurses are more likely to receive additional training in advanced technological interventions than in withholding or withdrawing life-sustaining therapy.[43]

Poor communication between patients and the health care team in acute care can complicate end-of-life care.[44] Aggressive care methodologies can create ethical dilemmas in providers who may view certain treatments as futile.[43-45] Poor communication can also result in failure to develop a clear treatment plan for chronically ill patients and ultimately an inability to discuss end-of-life issues with patients and families.[46]

Efforts have been made to address the conflict between aggressive care and caring interventions for dying patients.[43,46] Nurses recognize their lack of knowledge and clinical expertise in caring for dying patients.[44,46] Palliative care teams in acute care settings have been used to guide staff as they help patients and families at the end of life.

Inadequate Transition to End-of-Life Care

Patients with advanced heart failure are likely to receive care by many providers in a variety of settings. They potentially face multiple hospital readmissions, outpatient care, frequent physician visits, and even admission to long-term care. With lack of communication between settings, there is always a possibility of duplication and (particularly with end-of-life care) omission of services.

A descriptive study of advanced heart failure patients who died in hospice illustrates an inadequate transition to end-of-life care.[12] Even though the mean length of stay was close to national hospice statistics, median length of stay for patients with advanced heart failure was only 10 days. Functional status was significantly impaired with the majority of patients mostly bed bound. Over one third of the patients were admitted during the last week of life, diminishing the opportunities for effective palliative care delivery. In fact, 9 percent of the patients were actively dying on admission to hospice.[12] Although bereavement care is an important part of palliative care in general, this clearly indicates a bumpy transition to care with insufficient time to achieve critical outcomes of palliative care.

According to the national consensus project, continuity of care across settings is one of the key elements of palliative care.[16] A clear continuum of care should be available for advanced heart failure patients that includes home, emergency departments, outpatient care, long-term and hospice care.[16,47] Key to establishing continuity of care is the development of ongoing, collaborative partnerships among agencies to ensure implementation of national standards to ensure expert palliative care, regardless of location.

Patient Beliefs

Finucane[48] asserts that the most vital factor to providing good care at the end of life is maintaining sympathy with the person facing death: "perhaps what is most painful is to be dying" (p. 551). Having potentially survived multiple exacerbations of symptoms, heart failure patients may not be reconciled to their own deaths. Patients are asked to make the difficult transition between gravely ill and fighting death to being terminally ill and seeking peace.[49]

Whereas some patients accept the idea of dying with ease, others find it extremely difficult to surrender.[49] Patients with heart failure have been shown to have a high preference for resuscitation when compared with patients with cancer or dementia.[50] Examination of data following the death of 118 heart failure patients revealed that only about one third had do not resuscitate orders even though the deaths occurred a mean of 13 days following admission.[50]

Device therapies, new medications, and new surgical techniques offer continued hope to prolong life for patients with heart failure. Often these strategies are reported by the media without the information that they are not easily available, financially prohibitive, and not curative in nature.

Discussion of end-of-life issues with patients must be based on an awareness of the influence of culture on beliefs and values about dying and death. Ethnocentrism can block effective communication, decreasing the potential to relieve suffering in patients and their families (see Chapter 27).[51] Cultural assessment must include ethnicity, beliefs and values about religion and spirituality, and health practices. Specifically related to dying and death, it is important to assess meaning of dying and death, belief in afterlife, belief in fatalism, rituals surrounding death, and mourning and bereavement practices.

Pain and Symptom Management at the End of Life

Attention to relief of suffering is a central element of palliative care. Researchers and clinicians are challenged to prevent and relieve symptoms and symptom burden secondary to disease processes and their treatments. The end of life for patients with heart failure has been characterized by significant pain, shortness of breath, and diminished quality of life.[52-54] When researchers examined the meaning of a "good death," pain and symptom management emerged as a priority need.[55] As a result, the relief of pain and distressing symptoms is a priority outcome to assist patients with advanced heart failure to achieve a good death.

Before discussion of symptom management strategies, it is essential to more fully recognize symptoms that cause the greatest difficulties for heart failure patients at the end of life. In reports from the SUPPORT trial, researchers described physical and psychological symptoms experienced by patients with heart failure during the last 6 months of life.[53,54] As death approached, there were statistically significant increases in severe physical symptoms including severe pain and dyspnea.[53] Additionally, anxiety increased among hospitalized patients, and depression increased in both hospitalized and nonhospitalized heart failure patients. Although not describing specific symptoms, families reported that 64 percent of heart failure patients were either "extremely ill" or "very ill" during their last days of life.[54]

Nordgren and Sörenson reported 21 symptoms experienced by elderly persons with heart failure during the last 6 months of life.[11] Using a descriptive, retrospective chart review, they examined 80 medical records to determine the most prevalent symptoms recorded or inferred from treatments received. For example, when the patients received antidepressants, they documented depression or low mood. The most frequent symptom was breathlessness (88 percent), the least frequent was nocturia (4 percent). Other common symptoms were pain (75 percent), fatigue (69 percent), and anxiety (49 percent). Nausea was documented in nearly half of the patients. Patients had a mean of 6.7 symptoms documented. Symptom management strategies were rarely documented in the records.

Horne and Payne[56] conducted qualitative interviews to determine the palliative care needs of patients with heart failure. Of the 20 patients who consented to participate, 11 were New York Heart Association (NYHA) Class IV, seven were Class III, and two were Class II. Patients reported primarily physical symptoms related to decreased functional status, such as difficulty walking, fatigue, and inability to even do small tasks including personal care. Other physical symptoms included shortness of breath, sleeplessness, and loss of appetite. Psychological symptoms included feelings of frustration, anxiety, loss of self-esteem, loss of confidence, and fear.

To gain evidence of symptoms and symptom management strategies for patients with advanced heart failure in hospice, Zambroski and colleagues[12] examined medical records of 90 patients who died while receiving hospice care. The majority were admitted with markedly diminished functional status. As Nordgren and Sörenson[11] found, dyspnea was the most common symptom, present in 60 percent of the sample. Other symptoms commonly recorded were confusion at least some of the time (48 percent), edema (43 percent), and incontinence of the bowel and/or bladder (37 percent). Nine percent of the patients were "actively dying" on admission to hospice, with labored breathing, pulmonary congestion, mottling of the hands and feet, decreased consciousness, and little or no urinary output. Pain was documented far less often than others have found.[11,53] Chest pain was documented in only 3 percent of patients and other types of pain in only 20 percent. This discrepancy may have been related to expert palliative symptom management strategies provided in hospice, but this level of care was not clearly documented.

Evidence of the impact of specific interventions in improving pain and symptom management is essential.[57] To that end, the consensus statement for palliative and supportive care includes recommendations for symptom management in patients with advanced heart failure (Table 82-1).[5] The authors recognized that use of medications, device therapy, surgical therapy, and combination therapy may be effective for symptom management in this population.

Fundamental to all symptom management strategies is optimization of medications according to current heart failure guidelines.[8] Diuretics, angiotensin-converting enzyme **(ACE)** inhibitors or angiotensin-receptor blockers, and beta blockers or combined alpha-beta blockers are all potentially effect strategies for symptom management. However, specific pharmacological agents for palliation of dyspnea and fatigue require further study.[5]

There is a small but growing body of evidence on symptom management strategies used to improve end of life for patients with advanced heart failure. In one study describing heart failure symptom management strategies in hospice, there was clear evidence that multiple disciplines were involved.[12] Whereas most care was provided by nurses, patients also received care from physicians, chaplains, social workers, home health aids, volunteers, and in rare cases, music and massages therapists.

■ ■ ■

TABLE 82-1 CLINICAL RECOMMENDATIONS: CARE OF PATIENTS WITH ADVANCED HEART FAILURE

SUBJECT	RECOMMENDATION	LEVEL OF EVIDENCE RATED IN ACC/AHA GUIDELINES	SPECIAL CONSIDERATIONS	LIMITATIONS
Medical management	Diuretics to optimize volume status	Yes	Weight and estimated jugular venous pressure are clinical measures	
	ACE inhibitor or ARB	Yes	Dosage should be titrated to maximal doses in trials	Discontinuation indicated if patient develops a >30% rise in serum creatinine, or hypotension. Hydralazine and nitrates may then be an option
	B-blocker or α,β-blocker	Yes	Patient should be euvolemic before starting medication	Symptoms and quality of life were not reported in trials. Hypotension and negative inotropy may limit use
	Continuous outpatient support with inotropes	Yes	May allow outpatient care for otherwise seriously ill patients	Increased ventricular ectopy reported for all inotropes; increased mortality
	Oral inotropes	No	Study underway—no FDA-approved drugs	Combination with β-blockers may improve mortality seen in older studies
	CPAP for sleep-disordered breathing	No	Improve LV function and reduce norepinephrine levels with apnea or Cheynes-Stokes respiration	Equipment not well-tolerated by all patients; may also palliate fatigue
	Oxygen supplementation for sleep-disordered breathing	No		Recommended when CPAP not tolerated; no published data of effectiveness
Palliation of dyspnea	Oxygen	No	No clear evidence in HF	No physiological benefit in 1 study
	Opioids	No	Unstudied in HF	Physiological effects not known in HF
Palliation of fatigue	Psychostimulants	No	Unstudied in HF: benefit in cancer and HIV	
Treatment of depression	Antidepressants	No	Unstudied in HF	
Advanced technologies	VAD	No	Patients must manage the technology	Few VAD recipients in RE-MATCH survived beyond 2 years
	Implantable cardioverter defibrillator	No	Tested in patients with prior MI	Quality of life not assessed; uncertainty in patients with intolerable symptoms
	Cardiac resynchronization	No	Uncertain benefit for patients with advanced HF	
Communication	Advance care planning	No	Not tested in HF	Advance directives have no impact on care, symptoms or quality of life
	Honest communication about the course of HF	No	Not tested in HF	
	Understand patient needs for information and address their concerns	No	Not tested in HF, reduces anxiety in cancer patients	
Interdisciplinary supportive care	Concurrent supportive care and HF disease management	No	Not tested in HF	
Structure of care	Seamless transitions between sites of care	No	Not tested in HF or other diseases	
Hospice care		No	Not tested in HF or other diseases	Variable approaches to care by different agencies

ACE, Angiotensin-converting enzyme; *ARB*, angiotensin receptor blocker; *CPAP*, continuous positive airway pressure; *FDA*, Food and Drug Administration; *HF*, heart failure; *HIV*, human immunodeficiency virus; *LV*, left ventricular; *MI*, myocardial infarction; *REMATCH*, Randomized Evaluation of Mechanical Assistance for the Treatment of Congestive Heart Failure; *VAD*, ventricular assist device. From Goodlin SJ, Hauptman PJ, Arnold R et al: Consensus statement: palliative and supportive care in advanced heart failure, *J Card Fail* 10:203, 2004.

Nonpharmacological interventions used in hospice include teaching of patients and families, giving skin care, and providing family reassurance.[12] More specific interventions, such as positioning or monitoring fluid status, have not been documented and need to be stud-

ied. The care of patients with Stage D heart failure (see Chapter 64) must include the therapies provided in Stages A through C. It is not acceptable to abandon treatments, such as encouraging tobacco cessation, discouraging alcohol, and maintaining dietary sodium restrictions, at the end of life. Nurses must continue to educate patients and families about the importance of daily weighing as a strategy for monitoring fluid status; daily weighing should be continued as long as feasible. Effective fluid management decreases the risk of distressing respiratory symptoms.

In one study, oxygen therapy was the most common pharmacological intervention in hospice; 92 percent of heart failure patients used oxygen.[12] Recent consensus reports discourage the use of oxygen for breathlessness, as discussed in Chapter 27.[5,57] Additional pharmacological interventions included anxiolytic agents (79 percent) and antidepressants (30 percent).[12] In this sample, mainstays of heart failure medications were not consistently documented and not to the level of the current national standards.[8] Only 68 percent received diuretics, 24 percent received an ACE inhibitor, 20 percent a beta-blocker, and 32 percent digoxin. Caution is noted, however; this was a retrospective chart review rather than a prospective study, and the number may be artificially low.

Morphine is effective as a palliative agent for dyspnea. Nearly 75 percent of the heart failure patients in hospice received morphine or a morphine derivative.[12] Nevertheless, dyspnea rates were similar to previous reports, but pain was much less frequently reported than in prior studies.[11,53] In a randomized, double-blind placebo-controlled, crossover pilot study of 10 patients with advanced heart failure in an outpatient setting, Johnson and colleagues[58] assessed the effectiveness of oral morphine in managing breathlessness. Morphine improved breathlessness by the second day in 60 percent of patients. Side effects included sedation, which resolved by the fourth day, and constipation. Placebo had no effect on breathlessness or sedation. Further prospective studies of morphine derivatives would assist clinicians to determine the most effective symptom management strategies for patients with advanced heart failure. Concern about drug abuse should not preclude the appropriate medical use of opioid agents to manage symptoms whether in hospice or outside of hospice. (See the accompanying Conundrum feature.)

For patients with intractable symptoms, intravenous dobutamine or milrinone may provide symptomatic relief.[5,59] Dobutamine is a sympathomimetic agent that increases cardiac output by increasing heart rate and myocardial contractility as a result of stimulation of beta$_1$ receptors in the heart. It also decreases systemic vascular resistance and pulmonary wedge pressure, ultimately improving organ perfusion, decreasing dyspnea, and increasing exercise tolerance.[59] Milrinone is a phosphodiesterase inhibitor that can improve myocardial contractility and improve cardiac output as a result of arterial vasodilatation.[60] Beyond treatment of symptoms, home inotropic therapy reduces hospital admission, length of stay, and cost of care for patients with advanced heart failure.[61]

Another intravenous arterial and venous vasodilator, nesiritide, a form of brain natriuretic peptide, improves stroke volume, decreases aldosterone, and improves natriuresis and diuresis.[60,62] Nesiritide improves orthopnea, dyspnea, and sleeplessness in patients with advanced heart failure.[60] It has the advantage of not im-

■■■ CONUNDRUM

ETHICAL ISSUES AT THE END OF LIFE— THE DOUBLE EFFECT

Nurses provide a critical role in symptom management at the end of life. According to the Hospice and Palliative Nurses Association and the American Nurses Association, fear of sedation or of respiratory depression should not override adequate symptom management as long as it is consistent with the patient's wishes. Increasing titration of medication to achieve adequate symptom control, even at the expense of life and hastening death secondarily, is ethically justified. This is called the "rule of double effect." This rule says that if two or more possible effects are possible, at least one is good and the others are bad, the action is morally permissible if: (1) the action is good or morally neutral; (2) the action is undertaken with the intention of achieving only a good effect, and bad effects are not intended; (3) the action must not achieve a good effect by means of a bad effect; and (4) the benefits of the good outweigh the risk of the bad.

Honoring patient wishes to withdraw or withhold treatments that are not desired, are disproportionately burdensome, or will not benefit the patient can be ethically permissible. Even when this may risk hastening death, it does not constitute assisted suicide. Assisted suicide must not be confused with ethical end-of-life decisions. Assisted suicide includes activities that provide means for patients to end their own lives with the knowledge that suicide is the patient's intention. Active euthanasia means that someone other than the patient commits an action to end the patient's life. Nurses are ethically bound to not participate in assisted suicide or active euthanasia.

American Nurses Association: ANA position statement: active euthanasia. Dec 8. Available at: *www.nursingworld.org/readroom/position/ethics*. Accessed March 10, 2005.
American Nurses Associa tion: ANA position statement: assisted suicide. Dec 8. Available at: *www.nursingworld.org/readroom/position/ethics*. Accessed March 10, 2005.
Ersek M, Wagner B, Ferrell BR et al: HPNA position statement: providing opioids at the end of life, Oct 2003, Hospice and Palliative Nurses Association. Available at: *www.hpna.org/pdf/Providing_Opioid_at_the_End_of_Life_Position_Statement_PDF.pdf*. Accessed February 25, 2005.
Krakauer EL, Penson RT, Truog RD et al: Center rounds. Sedation for intractable distress of a dying patient: acute palliative care and the principle of double effect, *Oncologist* 5:53-62, 2000.

pacting heart rate as dobutamine does. Improved treatment of symptoms using nesiritide can decrease the need for hospitalization for symptom management.[60]

Before starting any infusion therapy for symptom palliation, it is essential for patients and families to understand that infusions do not cure heart failure.[63] Additionally, the decision to use these therapies in the home must be considerate of the caregivers. When unprepared for the caregiving role for patients receiving infusions, caregivers may become overwhelmed with the responsibility, even to the point of being unable to maintain their own health.[63]

A thorough evaluation of each patient's cardiac and noncardiac medications should be routine in caring for patients with advanced heart failure. Medications, such as nonsteroidal antiinflammatory agents (**NSAIDS**), most antidysrhythmic agents, and calcium channel blockers, may contribute to clinical deterioration and should be discontinued.[8] Nutritional supplements, such as coenzyme Q10, carnitine, ginseng, gingko, and taurine have not been demonstrated to be effective or may be harmful and are not recommended.[8,64]

Although clinicians agree on the use of diuretics, beta blockers, and ACE inhibitors for patients with advanced heart failure, actual clinical practice decisions are more difficult.[65] Palliation for symptoms may appear similar to standard medical therapy.[25] The American Nurses Association (ANA) position statement on pain management and control of distressing symptoms in dying patients states that patients should have "appropriate and sufficient medication by appropriate routes to control symptoms in whatever dosage, and by whatever route is needed to control symptoms as perceived by the patient."[66] Best evidence and clinical judgment are imperative in managing these complex patients.

Device Therapies

Patients with advanced heart failure may be treated with pacemakers, automatic implantable cardioverter-defibrillators (ICD), biventricular pacers, and/or ventricular assist devices (see Chapters 61 and 66). These devices are not curative, but rather supportive in nature as symptom management strategies at the end of life. Nevertheless, technology can also adversely affect end-of-life care.[67]

Goldstein and colleagues surveyed 100 family members of mostly men with an ICD that had been in place for a median of 2.3 years.[68] Of the 100 family members, only 27 reported having discussions about deactivation of the ICD before the patient's death. The discussions frequently occurred within the last few days of life; in 4 percent it was in the last few minutes. Even in those patients who had a written do not resuscitate order, nearly half of the family members did not recall discussions about device deactivation. The vast majority of patients died of nonsudden cardiac or noncardiac death rather than sudden cardiac death. As the family members recalled, 27 patients received a shock during the last month of life. Of those 27, 30 percent received a shock in the last few minutes of life. One patient reportedly experienced 12 shocks in one night.[68]

Patients and their families should have the opportunity to discuss their preferences regarding device deactivation at the end of life. To make an informed decision, patients and families should understand the potential outcomes of the deactivation.[69] Deactivation of a pacemaker could result in a more rapid death if the pacemaker is constantly functioning, but this is extremely unlikely.[70] More likely, deactivation of the pacemaker may cause a slow and more symptomatic end of life, particularly if it causes bradycardia resulting in further decreased cardiac output and progressive organ failure. Cardiac pacemakers generally do not keep dying patients alive, and removal does not necessarily hasten death in the terminally ill.[70]

It is essential to consider the benefit-to-burden ratio of an active ICD in dying patients. Deactivation of an ICD would be unlikely to hasten death or cause a decreased quality of life. Deactivation of the ICD will preclude treatment of life-threatening dysrhythmias, thereby allowing a natural death. The patient may have sudden death or may die from causes other than dysrhythmia. Patients and families may choose to deactivate the device rather than to experience the discomfort of receiving ongoing shocks. Newer ICD devices can be programmed to overdrive pace symptomatic tachydysrhythmias and subsequently reduce pain and discomfort rather than deliver shocks, which may be very effective in controlling anxiety in these patients.

Mechanical circulatory assist devices are being used with increasing frequency as a bridge to transplant and now as destination therapy for those ineligible for transplant.[71] Improvements are being made to increase patient mobility, improve safety, and decrease complications that may lead to death. At this time, deactivation of devices is not discussed in the literature. Ethical principles must guide decision making for this unique and growing subset of patients with advanced heart failure.

Communication

Effective communication is a central component of palliative care. Good communication allows providers to uncover and explore needs as the end of life approaches.[72] One example of inadequate communication was reported in a qualitative study of patients living with heart failure.[73] Shortly after the death of her husband, a chronically ill and homebound heart failure patient, a woman wrote: "*I didn't get to say goodbye! Or hold him, say I love you. He was just gone.*" He had been diagnosed with and treated for heart failure for more than 10 years. Before his death, he had experienced multiple 911 calls for his heart failure symptoms, even requiring defibrillation by paramedics to treat dysrhythmias. Despite that, his wife felt surprised when he died. It appeared that multiple opportunities to discuss end-of-life issues had been missed, and a wife was unable to tell her husband she loved him before he died.

The current medical system can deter good communication with short-term relationships between patients and clinicians, rapid movement through the health care system, and lack of opportunity for psychosocial care, including end-of-life discussion.[74] Patients and families may be reluctant to engage in end-of-life discussions because of fear of dying and death, inability to accept the advanced nature of the illness, regret, or even the influence of popular media continually hyping new treatments.[74]

In general, patients and families do value discussion about end-of-life concerns with providers. Unfortunately, providers often do not or are unable to attend to these needs.[45,72] Communication can be stifled by physicians and nurses who underestimate patient concerns and even block discussion of important issues for dying patients.[72] For example, inadequate communication about spiritual needs can contribute to feelings of hopelessness in patients with heart failure.

Murray and colleagues[75] compared the spiritual needs of people dying of lung cancer with those dying of heart failure. With a more clearly defined illness trajectory, lung cancer patients and their families were more able to plan for death. They experienced intermittent periods of despair and hope through disease progression and death. On the other hand, heart failure patients faced an unpredictable illness trajectory with gradual physical decline and periods of acute symptom exacerbation. Death was often sudden with no distinct terminal phase. Heart failure patients often felt abandoned by health and social services. They felt more dependent on others and hopeless. Both groups believed spiritual needs often were not addressed by clinicians.

Each block to effective communication diminishes the chance for nurses to decrease patient and family suffering. Using focus groups, Kirchoff and colleagues[76] found that family members experienced uncertainty surrounding prognoses and a conflict between technology and honoring patients' wishes. Even when a patient's wishes had been discussed, family members found it difficult to accept and carry out those wishes. This uncertainty did not necessarily disappear following the death, but lingered on even for months following. Good communication with providers assisted the families in dealing with decisions and relieving uncertainty. Effective communication is essential to decrease the turmoil experienced by family members during the hospitalization and death of a loved one.

Other Challenges

Barriers can diminish access to palliative care for patients with advanced heart failure. Physicians may fear financial consequences for inappropriate referral of heart failure patients to hospice.[77] Citing a lack of evidence of the effectiveness of hospice to manage outcomes for patients with heart failure, physicians also may be reluctant to yield care to another agency. Variable approaches to care provided by different hospice agencies may increase this reluctance.[5] Smaller hospices may be financially unable to provide more costly heart failure therapies.[78] Hospice staff may be unfamiliar with the complexities of heart failure symptom management when compared with cancer.[78] An additional barrier may be ambivalence of providers to introduce palliative care early in the disease course for fear that such discussions may bias patients toward choosing comfort care rather than more aggressive care directed at increasing survival.[79]

Hospice and palliative care as a strategy for patients with advanced heart failure may not even be on the radar screen for physicians who care for this population. When physicians were asked to articulate clinical questions arising in care of advanced heart failure patients for which there were no clear answers, of 318 questions, end of life was only addressed twice, and hospice was not mentioned.[65]

IMPROVING CARE FOR PATIENTS AT THE END OF LIFE

The Hospice and Palliative Care Nurses Association adopted Sackett and colleagues' 2001 definition of evidence-based practice to guide their clinical practice: best evidence must be integrated with clinical experience and patient values to determine the best care for patients.[80] Nurses who provide palliative care for patients with advanced heart failure have little evidence to guide their practice. Nevertheless, more and more researchers and

clinicians are recognizing this deficit and making commitments to gain this vital information.

The Agency for Healthcare Research and Quality (**AHRQ**) identified eight major domains for addressing end-of-life experiences (Box 82-3).[32] Assessment of each domain can guide researchers to identify interventions that may improve care not only of patients with advanced heart failure but of patients with a variety of cardiovascular diseases. Furthermore, the consensus panel for palliative and supportive care in advanced heart failure[5] proposed target areas of research that must be addressed as we develop the science of palliative care in heart failure (Table 82-2).

Researchers who are committed to improving palliative care are faced with a variety of methodological issues including recruitment, attrition, missing data, subject burden, and informed consent in an often increasingly debilitated patient population.[81] As palliative care researchers join forces with clinicians to clarify and improve these issues, they will improve the care in each of the AHRQ target domains.[32]

CONCLUSION

Within the next two decades, heart disease will become the number one cause of death across the globe. As a result, providers will be faced with a growing number of challenges in caring for patients with heart disease. Challenges, such as dealing with an unpredictable illness trajectory; smoothing transitions between care settings; educating providers regarding the wide range of pharmacological, nonpharmacological, and technological symptom management strategies available; and gaining critical expertise in communication about end-of-life issues. To meet these challenges, we must recognize that palliative care is as critically important if not more important than curative care.

Improving end of life for patients with advanced heart failure has gained national attention. Researchers have made significant headway in improving end of life and palliative care for patients with advanced cancer. Now we must eliminate the disparity between palliative care for patients with cancer and that provided to patients with advanced heart failure. A commitment to

---

> **BOX 82-3** ■ ■ ■
> CORE DOMAINS FOR EVALUATING
> THE END-OF-LIFE EXPERIENCE
>
> 1. Pain and other symptom management
> 2. Adequate support for families and caregivers, including bereavement
> 3. Continuity of health care
> 4. Treatment consistent with patient and family preferences and medical knowledge
> 5. Effective, empathetic communication about diagnosis, prognosis, and care plans
> 6. Well-being, including existential and spiritual concerns
> 7. Function and self-determination
> 8. Length of survival
>
> From Lorenz et al: End-of-life care and outcomes. Evidence report/ technology assessment No. 110. AHRQ Publication No.5-E004-2, Rockville, Md, Dec 2004, Agency for Healthcare Research and Quality.

■ ■ ■

TABLE 82-1 CLINICAL RECOMMENDATIONS: CARE OF PATIENTS WITH ADVANCED HEART FAILURE

TOPIC	RECOMMENDATION	SPECIFIC AREAS FOR RESEARCH
Prognosis and trajectory of illness in advanced HF	Descriptive, longitudinal study that includes a broad population of patients with advanced HF	1) Nature, severity, and pattern of symptoms in advanced HF 2) Identification of critical turning points in the course of the disease that require reexamination of goals, treatments, and patient preferences 3) Clinical features and psychosocial dynamics that distinguish a patient's course and outcomes with advanced technologies versus medical management or palliative care 4) Issues and needs are most important to patients and family members, and how these can be assessed in the course of care
Symptom treatment, optimizing quality of life for patients and family members	Studies to identify which interventions are effective in managing specific symptoms and optimizing quality of life. Addition to measurement of symptoms and quality of life to all trials in advanced HF	1) Outcome measures to best address patients' quality of life and patient/family needs in advanced HF 2) Use of opioids for dyspnea acutely or long-term in persons with advanced HF 3) Interventions to improve fatigue in HF 4) Impact of antidepressants on symptoms of anxiety, depression, and fatigue in HF and on the physiology of HF 5) Aspects of interdisciplinary care that benefit symptoms, quality of life, and patient/family needs in advanced HF
Communication with patients and family members about advanced HF	Studies to identify how best to communicate with patients and family members about the expected course of their illness, their concerns and fears and dying from HF	1) Patient and family member understanding about disease and its course 2) Information desired by patient and their family about their disease and effective formats for providing this information 3) Communication by primary care physicians, cardiologists, and HF specialists with patient and family members about dying from HF 4) Impact of specific training on communication between practicing physicians and their advanced HF patients
System of care	Studies to identify components of care and systems that positively impact patient and family outcomes; associated cost and cost-effectiveness	1) Treatments, staff skills, and knowledge essential to the provision of care for patients with advanced HF, and integration into hospice care 2) Models of care and payment structures to best meet patient/family needs most cost-effectively

HF, Heart failure.
From Goodlin SJ, Hauptman PJ, Arnold R et al: Consensus statement: palliative and supportive care in advanced heart failure, *J Card Fail* 10:203, 2004.

improving palliative care, strong interpersonal skills, advanced training in end-of-life care, and an understanding of the appropriate management of patients with cardiovascular disease, including advanced heart failure, are essential to meet the needs of this growing population.

REFERENCES

1. World Health Organization: The World Health Report 2004. Annex Table 2 Deaths by cause, sex and mortality stratum in WHO regions, estimates for 2002, 2004. World Health Organization. Available at: www.who.int/whr/2004/annex/topic/en/annex_2_en.pdf. Accessed April 5, 2005.
2. Mackay J, Mensah G: *Atlas of heart disease and stroke,* World Health Organization and US Centers for Disease Control and Prevention. Available at: www.who.int/cardiovascular_diseases/resources/atlas/en/print.html. Accessed April 4, 2005.
3. American Heart Association: Heart disease and stroke statistics-2005 update, Dallas, 2004, American Heart Association.
4. World Health Organization: The World Health Report 2004. Annex Table 3 Burden of disease by DALYs by cause, sex, and mortality stratum in WHO regions, estimates for 2002, 2004. World Health Organization. Available at: www.who.int/whr/2004/annex/topic/en/annex_3_en.pdf. Accessed April 5, 2005.
5. Goodlin SJ, Hauptman PJ, Arnold R et al: Consensus statement: palliative and supportive care in advanced heart failure, *J Card Fail* 10:200-209, 2004.
6. National Institutes of Health: State-of-the-science conference statement: improving end of life care, 2005, National Institutes

of Health. Available at: http://consensus.nih.gov/ta/024/EoL final011805pdf.pdf Accessed. March 1, 2005.
7. Addington-Hall JM, Gibbs JS: Heart failure now on the palliative care agenda, *Palliat Med* 14:361-362, 2000.
8. Hunt SA, Baker DW, Chin MH et al: ACC/AHA guidelines for the evaluation and management of chronic heart failure in the adult: executive summary a report of the American College of Cardiology/American Heart Association task force on practice guidelines (committee to revise the 1995 guidelines for the evaluation and management of heart failure): developed in collaboration with the International Society for Heart and Lung Transplantation; endorsed by the Heart Failure Society of America, *Circulation* 104:2996-3007, 2001.
9. Levy D, Kenchaiah S, Larson MG et al: Long-term trends in the incidence of and survival with heart failure, *New Engl J Med* 347:1397-1402, 2002.
10. Jaagolsild P, Dawson NV, Thomas C et al: Outcomes of acute exacerbation of severe congestive heart failure: quality of life, resource use, and survival, *Arch Intern Med* 158:1081-1089, 1998.
11. Nordgren L, Sorensen S: Symptoms experienced in the last six months of life in patients with end-stage heart failure, *Europ J Cardiovasc Nurs* 2:213-217, 2003.
12. Zambroski CH, Moser DK, Rosen LP et al: Patients with heart failure who die while in hospice, *Amer Heart J* 49:558-564, 2005.
13. Lynn J: Perspectives on care at the close of life. Serving patients who may die soon and their families: the role of hospice and other services, *JAMA* 285:925-932, 2001.
14. Institute of Medicine: *Priority areas for national action: transforming health care quality,* Washington, DC, 2003, The National Academies Press.

15. National Association of Hospice and Palliative Care: An explanation of palliative care. Available at: www.nhcpo.org/i4a/pages/index.cfm?pageid=3657. Accessed February 8, 2005.

16. National Consensus Project for Quality Palliative Care: Clinical practice guidelines for quality palliative care: executive summary, May 2004. Available at: www.nationalconsensusproject.org/summary.pdf. Accessed February 17, 2005.

17. Ward C: The need for palliative care in the management of heart failure, *Heart* 87:294-298, 2002.

18. Craven J, Wald FS: Hospice care for dying patients, *Amer J Nurs* 75:1816-1822, 1975.

19. Miller GW, Williams JR, Keyserling J: Delivering quality care and cost-effectiveness at the end of life: building on the 20-year success of the hospice benefit, Feb 2, 2002, National Hospice and Palliative Care Organization. Available at www.nhcpo.org. Accessed March 17, 2004.

20. National Center for Health Statistics: National home and hospice care data updated December, 2004. Available at: www.cdc.gov/nchs/about/major/nhhcsd/nhhcshomecare3.htm. Accessed August 9, 2005.

21. National Hospice and Palliative Care Organization: NHPCO facts and figures: updated November 2004. Available at: www.nhpco.org. Accessed August 9, 2005.

22. Egan KAL" MJ Hospice care: a model for quality end-of-life care. In Ferrell BR and Coyle N, editors: *Textbook of palliative nursing*, New York, 2001, Oxford University Press.

23. National Association of Hospice and Palliative Care: Medicare hospice benefit. Available at: www.nhcpo.org/i4a/pages/index.cfm?pageid=3283. Accessed February 23, 2005

24. Gage B, Miller S, Coppola K et al: US Department of Health and Human Services: important questions for hospice in the next century, 2002, US Department of Health and Human Services. Available at: http://aspe.hhs.gov/daltcp/reports/impques.htm#section2a. Accessed December 10, 2002.

25. Stuart B, Alexander C, Arnella C et al: Standards and accreditation committee medical guidelines task force, medical guidelines for determining prognosis in selected non-cancer diseases, 1999, National Hospice Organization. Available at: http://aspe.hhs.gov/daltcp/reports/impquesa.htm. Accessed February 23, 2005.

26. Campbell DE, Lynn J, Louis TA et al: Medicare program expenditures associated with hospice use, *Ann Intern Med* 40:269-277, 2004.

27. Gage B, Dao T: US Department of Health and Human Services: Medicare's hospice benefit: use and expenditures 1996 cohort, US Department of Health and Human Services. Available at: www.aspc.hhs.gov/daltcp/reports/96useexp.htm. Accessed December 10, 2002.

28. Tanvetyanon T, Leighton JC: Life-sustaining treatments in patients who died of chronic congestive heart failure compared with metastatic cancer, *Crit Care Med* 31:60-64, 2003.

29. Davidson PM, Paull G, Introna K et al: Integrated, collaborative palliative care in heart failure: the St George heart failure service experience 1999-2002, *J Cardiovasc Nurs* 19:68-75, 2004.

30. Zambroski CH: Hospice as an alternative model of care for older patients with end-stage heart failure, *J Cardiovasc Nurs* 19:76-83, 2004.

31. Gibbs JS, McCoy AS, Gibbs LM: Living with and dying from heart failure: the role of palliative care, *Heart (British Cardiac Society)* 88(suppl 2):ii36-39, 2002.

32. Lorenz K, Lynn J, Dy S et al: End-of-life care and outcomes. Evidence report/ technology assessment N. 110., (Prepared by the Southern California evidence-based practice center under Contract No. 290-02-0003), Vol AHRQ Publication No. 05-E004-2, Rockville, Md, 2004, Agency for Healthcare Research and Quality.

33. Fox E, Landrum-McNiff K, Zhong Z et al: Evaluation of prognostic criteria for determining hospice eligibility in patients with advanced lung, heart, or liver disease. SUPPORT investigators. Study to Understand Prognoses and Preferences for Outcomes and Risks of Treatments, *JAMA* 282:1638-45, 1999.

34. Poole-Wilson PA, Uretsky BF, Thygesen K et al: Mode of death in heart failure: findings from the ATLAS trial, *Heart* 89:42-48, 2003.

35. Anker SD, Ponikowski P, Varney S et al: Wasting as independent risk factor for mortality in chronic heart failure, *Lancet* 349:1050-1053, 1997.

36. Bittner V, Weiner DH, Yusuf S et al: Prediction of mortality and morbidity with a 6-minute walk test in patients with left ventricular dysfunction. SOLVD investigators. *JAMA* 270:1702-1707, 1993.

37. Ellershaw J, Ward C: Care of the dying patient: the last hours or days of life, *Brit Med J* 326:30-34, 2003.

38. Lunney JR, Lynn J, Foley DJ et al: Patterns of functional decline at the end of life, *JAMA* 289:2387-2392, 2003.

39. Fox E, Landrum-McNiff K, Zhong Z et al: Evaluation of prognostic criteria for determining hospice eligibility in patients with advanced lung, heart, or liver disease. SUPPORT investigators. Study to understand prognoses and Preferences for Outcomes and Risks of Treatments, *JAMA* 282:1638-1645, 1999.

40. Elixhauser A, Yu K, Steiner C et al: Hospitalization in the United States, 1997. HCUP fact book 1 AHRQ publication No. 00-0031, Agency for Healthcare Research and Quality. www.ahrq.gov/data/hcup/factbk1/hcupfbk1.pdf. Accessed January 13, 2003.

41. Krumholz HM, Parent EM, Tu N et al: Readmission after hospitalization for congestive heart failure among Medicare beneficiaries, *Arch Intern Med* 157:99-104, 1997.

42. Chin MH, Goldman L: Correlates of early hospital readmission or death in patients with congestive heart failure, *Amer J Cardiol* 79:1640-1644, 1997.

43. Campbell ML: End of life care in the ICU: current practice and future hopes, *Crit Care Nurs Clinic N Amer* 14:197-200, ix, 2002.

44. Kirchhoff KT, Spuhler V, Walker L et al: Intensive care nurses' experiences with end-of-life care, *Amer J Crit Care* 9:36-42, 2000.

45. Davidson P, Introna K, Daly J et al: Cardiorespiratory nurses' perceptions of palliative care in nonmalignant disease: data for the development of clinical practice, *Amer J Crit Care* 12:47-53, 2003.

46. Davidson P, Introna K, Daly J et al: Cardiorespiratory nurses' perceptions of palliative care in nonmalignant disease: data for the development of clinical practice, *Amer J Crit Care* 12:47-53, 2003.

47. Quaglietti S, Lovett S, Hawthorne C et al: Management of the patient with congestive heart failure using outpatient, home and palliative care, *Prog Cardiovasc Dis* 2;43: 259-274, 2002.

48. Finucane TE: Care of patients nearing death: another view, *J Amer Geriat Soc* 50:551-553, 2002.

49. Finucane TE: How gravely ill becomes dying: a key to end-of-life care, *JAMA* 282:1670-1672, 1999.

50. Haydar ZR, Lowe AJ, Kahveci KL et al: Differences in end-of-life preferences between congestive heart failure and dementia in a medical house calls program, *J Amer Geriat Soc* 52:736-740, 2004.

51. Mazanec P, Tyler MK: Cultural considerations in end-of-life care: how ethnicity, age, and spirituality affect decisions when death is imminent, *Amer J Nurs* 103:50-59, 2003.

52. Freeborne N, Lynn J, Desbiens NA: Insights about dying from the SUPPORT project. The Study to Understand Prognoses and Preferences for Outcomes and Risks of Treatments, *J Amer Geriat Soc* 48(suppl 5):S199-205, 2000.

53. Levenson JW, McCarthy EP, Lynn J et al: The last six months of life for patients with congestive heart failure *J Amer Geriat Soc* 48(suppl 5):S101-109, 2000.

54. Lynn J, Teno JM, Phillips RS et al: Perceptions by family members of the dying experience of older and seriously ill patients. SUPPORT investigators. Study to Understand Prognoses and Preferences for Outcomes and Risks of Treatments[comment], *Ann Intern Med* 126:97-106, 1997.

55. Steinhauser KE, Clipp EC, McNeilly M et al: In search of a good death: observations of patients, families, and providers, *Ann Intern Med* 132:825-832, 2000.

56. Horne G, Payne S: Removing the boundaries: palliative care for patients with heart failure, *Palliat Med* 18:291-296, 2004.

57. Booth S, Wade R, Johnson M et al: The use of oxygen in the palliation of breathlessness. A report of the expert working group of the scientific committee of the Association of Palliative Medicine [erratum appears in *Respir Med* 98:476, 2004.], *Resp Med* 98:66-77, 2004.

58. Johnson MJ, McDonagh TA, Harkness A et al: Morphine for the relief of breathlessness in patients with chronic heart failure-a pilot study, *Eur J Heart Fail* 4:753-756, 2002.

59. Rich MW, Shore BL: Dobutamine for patients with end-stage heart failure in a hospice program?, *J Palliat Med* 6:93-97, 2003.

60. Josephson S, Barnett PP: At the bedside. Nesiritide: practical approach and benefits in the outpatient setting, *J Cardiovasc Nurs* 19:358-363, 2004.

61. Harjai KJ, Mehra MR, Ventura HO et al: Home inotropic therapy in advanced heart failure: cost analysis and clinical outcomes *Chest* 112:1298-1303, 1997.

62. de Denus S, Pharand C, Williamson DR: Brain natriuretic peptide in the management of heart failure: the versatile neurohormone, *Chest* 125:652-668, 2004.

63. Scott LD: Caregiving and care receiving among a technologically dependent heart failure population, *Adv Nurs Sci* 23:82-97, 2000.

64. Albert NM, Davis M, Young J: Improving the care of patients dying of heart failure, *Cleveland Clinic J Med* 69:321-328, 2002.

65. Shah MR, Stevenson LW: Searching for evidence: refractory questions in advanced heart failure, *J Card Fail* 10:210-218, 2004.

66. American Nurses Association: Position statement on pain management and control of distressing symptoms in dying patients, Dec 5, 2003, American Nurses Association. Available at: www.nursingworld.org/readroom/position/ethics/etpain.pdf. Accessed February 28, 2005.

67. Enck RE: Management of cardiac devices as the end nears, *Amer J Hospice Palliat Med* 22:7-8, 2005.

68. Goldstein NE, Lampert R, Bradley E et al: Management of implantable cardioverter defibrillators in end-of-life care, *Ann Intern Med* 141:835-838, 2004.

69. Ballentine JM: Pacemaker and defibrillator deactivation in competent hospice patients: an ethical consideration, *Am J Hospice & Palliative Med* 22:14-19, 2005.

70. Braun TC, Hagan NA, Hatfield RE et al: Cardiac pacemakers and implantable defibrillators in terminal care, *J Pain Symp Manag* 18:126-131, 1999.

71. Cianci P, Lonergan-Thomas H, Slaughter M et al: Current and potential applications of left ventricular assist devices, *J Cardiovasc Nurs* 18:17-22, 2003.

72. Tulsky JA: Interventions to enhance communication among patients, providers, and families, Bethesda: National Institute of Nursing Research and the Office of Medical Application of Research at the National Institutes of Health, December 6-8 2004. Available at: http://consensus.nih.gov/. Accessed March 17, 2005.

73. Hoyt CA: Navigating to safe harbor: problems and processes of living with heart failure [dissertation], 1999, University of Kentucky.

74. Larson DG, Tobin DT: End-of-life conversations: evolving practice and theory, *JAMA* 1573-1578, 2000.

75. Murray SA, Boyd K, Kendall M et al: Dying of lung cancer or cardiac failure: prospective qualitative interview study of patients and their caregivers in the community, *Brit Med J* 325:929, 2002.

76. Kirchhoff KT, Walker L, Hutton A et al: The vortex: families' experiences with death in the intensive care unit, *Amer J Crit Care* 11:200-209, 2002.

77. Swiger H: Hospice care and the institutional barriers to success: an issues paper developed for NHPCO's public policy committee, March, 2002. Available at: www.nhpco.org. Accessed March 17, 2004.

78. Goodlin SJ, Kutner JS, Connor SR et al: Hospice care for heart failure patients, *J Pain Symptom Manag* 29:525-528, 2005.

79. Rosenfeld K, Rasmussen J: Palliative care management: a Veteran's Administration demonstration project, *J Palliat Med* 6:831-839, 2003.

80. Cliff B, Harte N, Kirschling J et al: HPNA position statement: evidenced based practice, April 2004, Hospice and Palliative Care Nurses Association. Available at: www.hpna.org/pdf/Evidenced_Based_Practice_Position_Statement_PDF.pdf. Accessed February 23, 2005.

81. McMillan SC, Weitzner MA: Methodological issues in collecting data from debilitated patients with cancer near the end of life, *Oncol Nurs Forum* 30:123-129, 2003.

chapter 83

Optimal Patient Education and Counseling

Victoria V. Dickson
Janet P. McMahon

CHAPTER ABBREVIATIONS

DVT deep vein thrombosis
JCAHO Joint Commission on the Accreditation of Healthcare Organizations (The Joint Commission)

Despite advances in pharmacological, surgical, and medical management, cardiovascular disease remains a leading cause of death and disability in the United States. Primary and secondary prevention efforts target modifiable risk factors, such as high blood pressure, high cholesterol, tobacco use, obesity, and lack of exercise. Education and counseling that help patients engage in self-care and change their lifestyle risk factors supports efforts to decrease the morbidity and mortality associated with cardiovascular disease. As discussed in Chapter 84, cardiovascular treatments will not improve outcomes if patients do not adhere to the regimen. These treatment regimens frequently involve the need to change lifelong behaviors and thus pose an extraordinary challenge to patients. Thirty-nine percent of patients with one or more cardiovascular disease are over age 65.[1] Many of these elders have some evidence of cognitive impairment,[2-5] and 75 percent suffer from comorbid conditions, such as diabetes, chronic obstructive pulmonary disease, and chronic renal disease,[6] that further complicate the management of their disease. Patient education aimed at increasing knowledge and improving self-care behaviors is a critical component of inpatient and outpatient care.

Nurses play a key role as patient educators. Understanding the components of optimal patient teaching and counseling strategies is essential, and the purpose of this chapter is to describe key elements. Principles that may be used to assess learning needs, develop a plan, and evaluate outcomes of the education strategy will be covered.

THEORETICAL FRAMEWORK

The importance of patient self-care has shifted the patient education paradigm from a traditional model characterized by authoritarian, prescriptive, and generalized information to a new emphasis on empowerment. This patient-centered, collaborative approach involves clarification of beliefs about himself or herself, about health, and about behavior.[7] With this paradigm shift, the importance of behavioral change has emerged as a key strategy to improving patient self-care and health outcomes. Therefore, the social learning theory and the transtheoretical model of change are used as the framework in this chapter to describe the development of patient education and counseling strategies (Table 83-1).

Social learning theory[8] emphasizes that human behavior can be understood as a reciprocal and dynamic interaction between personal (including cognitive, affective, and biological properties), behavioral, and environmental influences (Figure 83-1). According to this interactive model, human behavior can be viewed as self-organizing, proactive, self-reflecting, and self-regulating rather than controlled by the environment or inner impulses.[9] As such, humans are able to interpret the results of their behavior, understand the influences of personal factors and their environment, which in turn, allows them to alter these factors.

A basic premise of the social learning theory is that learning occurs within a social context. People learn from their own experiences and by observing the actions of others and the results of their actions. The six key concepts of social learning theory, illustrated in Table 83-1, can be used to assess learning needs, develop a teaching plan, and evaluate the success of the teaching strategy.

The transtheoretical model of change, discussed further in Chapter 84,[10] can be used to guide clinicians in counseling patients when behavioral change is the primary goal. The authors of this model suggest that we cycle through five stages of change (precontemplation, contemplation, preparation, action, and maintenance) before successfully achieving a preferred behavior. Specific strategies related to the patient's readiness to learn and processes of change can be used to motivate change and adopt the desired behavior. Maintenance of behavior can be supported using strategies to reinforce positive experiences associated with the behavior and to minimize relapse. The use of this model, which is augmented with concepts from the self-regulatory model of illness,[11] is discussed in more detail later in this chapter.

OVERVIEW OF PATIENT EDUCATION AND COUNSELING

Patient education is defined as "the process of influencing patient behavior through the provision of information and counseling that is designed to produce changes in knowledge, attitudes, and skills necessary to main-

■ ■ ■

TABLE 83-1   PRINCIPLES OF SOCIAL LEARNING THEORY

CONCEPT	DEFINITION	APPLICATION
Reciprocal determinism	Behavioral changes result from an interaction between person and environment; change is bidirectional.	Involve individual, social supports (significant others). Assess changes to environment (i.e., barriers to behavior).
Behavioral capability	Knowledge and skills influence behavior.	Provide information and training about action.
Expectations	Beliefs about results of actions	Incorporate information about likely results or outcomes related to the action.
Self-Efficacy	Confidence in ability to take action and persist in action	Identify strengths, use persuasion and encouragement. Approach behavior change in small steps.
Observational learning	Beliefs based on observing others take action and the results of those actions	Point out others' experience and results. Identify role models.
Reinforcement	Responses to a person's behavior that increases or decreases the chances of recurrence of the behavior	Provide incentives, rewards, praise; encourage self-reward. Decrease possibility of negative responses that deter positive changes.

National Cancer Institute: *Theory at a glance: a guide for health promotion practice,* Bethesda, Md, 2003, National Institutes of Health.

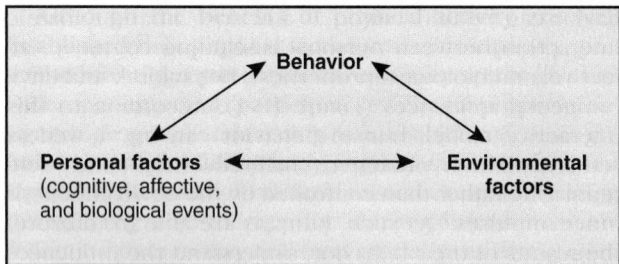

FIGURE 83-1 ■ Social learning theory which emphasizes that human behavior is the result of an interaction between personal, behavior, and environmental influences and therefore can be viewed as self-organizing, proactive, self-reflecting, and self-regulating rather than controlled by the external forces or inner impulses. (From Bandura A: A social cognitive approach to the exercise of control over AIDS infection. In DiClemente C, editor: *Adolescents and AIDS: a generation in jeopardy,* Beverly Hills, California 1991, Sage.)

tain or improve health.[12]" Patient education, as part of the total plan of patient care, can be incorporated into all interactions with patients—at the bedside, in clinic encounters, and home visits. The components of patient education include assessment of the patient's need to learn, assessment of motivation, setting of objectives, teaching-learning interaction and evaluation and re-teaching if needed (Table 83-2).

Patient teaching is often structured, but patient counseling techniques assume that the patient is not ready to change when the topic of learning or behavior change is first discussed. Since patients may underestimate their risk, believe they can control their situation without change, or express ambivalence, effective counseling allows the patient to lead the discussion with the nurse as facilitator. This collaborative approach results in a mutually acceptable plan of action, in which the patient is more likely to engage.

Principles of Learning

Patient teaching is a process, not a singular task. It is structured and sequenced to produce learning. Developing an effective teaching plan should consider the principles of adult learning[13] (Box 83-1), and the three general tenets of social learning theory: (1) individuals learn by observing the behaviors of others and the outcomes of those behaviors, (2) learning can occur without a change in behavior, and (3) expectations of future reinforcements or punishments affect the learner's behavior.

Observational learning includes techniques of vicarious learning and modeling. In this process, people gain an understanding of a behavior or action based on ob-

■ ■ ■

TABLE 83-2   PATIENT TEACHING AND COUNSELING

	TEACHING	COUNSELING
Assumptions	Patient may perceive a need to know or change.	Patient does not see a problem or wish to change.
Process	Provision of information and counseling Structured and sequential	Allow patient to lead the discussion. Present direct feedback. Provide menu of options for patient. Negotiate a plan of action.
Goals	To produce changes in knowledge, skills and attitudes necessary to maintain and improve health	To motivate behavioral change
Strategies	Often didactic instruction—lecture, written, audiovisual, discussion, may be incorporated into routine patient care sessions Skill exercises—demonstration, practice, feedback, role playing	Stages of change Motivational interviewing

BOX 83-1
KNOWLES ADULT LEARNING PRINCIPLES   ■ ■ ■

In 1978, Malcolm Knowles developed what he called the "adult learning principles," which are complementary to Bloom's taxonomy and are essential knowledge as well for effective patient education. According to Knowles, adults are autonomous and self-directed, and if a need is not perceived, then learning will not occur despite behavioral cues from the patient that would normally indicate interest and understanding.

Adults learn best when teaching progresses from the known to the unknown. Reteaching material that is well understood but on the clinical pathway chart for that day is condescending at best and may result in a patient's firm commitment to not participate in or seek further instruction. Always assess what a patient knows before a teaching session and if a patient is conversant on a topic, use the time wisely to teach more about the topic or what the patient deems as most important.

Active participation with dialogue between patient and nurse facilitates learning. A traditional didactic teaching relationship where the patient is supposed to learn simply because someone has spoken to them shows a lack of respect and denies the wealth of experiences that an adult brings to learning.

Adults need opportunities to practice and reinforce new skills. The majority of time teaching new manual skills should be spent on having the patient perform the skill until relative comfort and proficiency are demonstrated and verbalized by the patient.

Adults need reinforcement. Teaching about health needs frequent reinforcement and reevaluation. When a patient feels comfortable dialoguing with the nurse, misconceptions, fears, mistakes made, and new knowledge that a patient may have gained, especially from an Internet source, can be discussed.

Immediate feedback on the topic and any misconceptions increases learning. Family and significant others provide the patient with information, which may be inaccurate or even potentially fatal. If teaching has been done without acknowledgement of the role of the patient's social network, which often extends far beyond family and friends, misinformation may take greater authority and will be regarded as true, extinguishing teaching within days or less.

Knowles M: The modern practice of adult education: from pedagogy to andragogy, New York, 1980, Cambridge.

BOX 83-2
FEATURES OF AN EFFECTIVE PATIENT TEACHING PLAN   ■ ■ ■

Relevance
- Program is tailored to individual's knowledge, beliefs, situation, and prior experience of the learner.
- Content is appropriate for the patient.

Individualization
- The learner is given opportunities to have personal questions answered. Instruction is paced on individual progress.
- Specific goals and objectives are negotiated.

Feedback
- Information is given to the learner on progress and accomplishments.

Reinforcement
- Patient is given encouragement or rewards for progress.
- Social support is essential.
- Rewards may be tangible, such as incentives or recognition.

Facilitation
- Barriers or constraints to the behavior are eliminated or minimized so that learner is able to take action and perform behavior.
- Materials are provided to aid the patient in achieving behavioral change (e.g., equipment, transportation arrangements, and written instructions).

Kok G, van den Borne B, Mullen P: Effectiveness of health education and health promotion: meta-analysis of effect studies and determinants of effectiveness, *Patient Educ Couns* 30:19-27, 1997.

Learning, according to the social learning theory, is a cognitive and behavioral function. Therefore, understanding how domains of learning and learning styles affect patient education will increase the effectiveness of the assessment, planning, and teaching processes.

Domains of Learning

There are multiple systems or hierarchies that have been developed in education and training, but Bloom's taxonomy (classification system) is widely used and is easily understood. Bloom in 1956 identified the three domains of learning as knowledge, attitude, and skills.[15] Later revised to cognitive, attitude, and psychomotor, this taxonomy is applicable for learners of all age groups. Each of the three domains identifies ways of learning acquisition. Within each of the domains, learning is demonstrated on a continuum from simple to complex. This allows the measurement of learning by the level of complexity used by the learner as a result of teaching. The domains are also useful as classes of learning objectives, each of which requires a different set of conditions to achieve.

Cognitive Domain

The cognitive domain is evidenced by intellectual abilities. Cognitive learning behaviors are characterized by skills, such as comprehending information, organizing ideas, and evaluating information and actions. These skills are arranged in order of complexity, meaning that a learner who is able to perform at the higher levels of the taxonomy is demonstrating a more complex level of cognitive thinking.

serving others and the consequences of their actions. Vicarious learning—listening to others without demonstrating the behavior[8]—is beneficial in influencing expectations. In modeling, behavior is observed, learned, and ultimately repeated or performed. Modeling is effective in teaching new behaviors, influencing the frequency of previously learned behaviors, and increasing similar behaviors. For modeling to occur, four conditions must be met[14]: (1) attention, (2) retention or ability to remember the behavior, (3) motor reproduction or ability to replicate the action, and (4) motivation or desire to demonstrate what they have learned. In the absence of motivation, learning can occur without a change in behavior. Consistent with this theory, individuals are more likely to adopt a behavior if it results in an outcome they value (expectation), if they believe they are capable (self-efficacy), and if the model or behavior can fit with their environment. Based upon these principles of social learning theory, a patient education plan will be relevant, individualized, include feedback and reinforcement, and facilitate patient action (Box 83-2).

Affective Domain

The affective domain addresses a learner's emotions toward learning. Affective behaviors are demonstrated by attitude, interest, attention, awareness, and values. These emotional behaviors, which are grouped in a hierarchical order, can be thought of as a ladder that must be climbed to move onto the next category.

Psychomotor Domain

The psychomotor domain addresses the use of basic motor skills, coordination, and physical movement. Psychomotor skills are learned through repetitive practice. A learner's ability to perform these skills is measured by precision, speed, distance, and technique.[16]

Learning Styles

Learning styles refer to the manner in which an individual preferentially assimilates, organizes, and synthesizes information. It is common to characterize learning styles as being bipolar—visual or not, auditory or not, kinesthetic or not. In reality, learning styles exist on a continuum and people usually learn in multiple modes. There is also a stigma in classifying learning styles because, ultimately, classification is used to discuss differential performances of individuals and diverse cultural groups.

The Kolb model of learning styles[17] (Figure 83-2) identifies two separate learning activities: perception and processing. Perception can be further divided into opposites, concrete (touching, seeing, and hearing), and abstract (mental or visual conceptualization). Once information has been perceived, it must be processed. Like perception, processing can also be divided into op-

posites. Some people process information best by active experimentation (doing something while learning) or by reflective observation (cogitating before making a judgment, thinking about the meaning of what has been learned).

Based on Kolb learning styles, there are four types of learners[17]:

- Type I learners are primarily hands-on, more intuitive than logical. They are comfortable to depend on other's analyses and to apply learning in real-life situations.
- Type II learners are most comfortable watching rather than taking action. They tend to be highly imaginative, categorize information in detail, and are highly aware of feelings during learning.
- Type III learners are problem solvers who find practical answers and uses for new learning. They tend to shy away from social and interpersonal issues and enjoy technical tasks. Practicality is of greater importance than logic.
- Type IV learners are concise and logical. To this type of learner, abstract ideas and concepts are most important, not psychosocial issues.

There are numerous models of learning styles; this is just one. It is beyond the scope of this text to detail the many that exist, but familiarity and fluency with any single model allows assessment and refinement of one's patient education techniques.

Characteristics of an Effective Patient Educator

Recognition that patients have different domains and styles of learning leads to examining the qualities that enhance learning. To answer the question "what characteristics make an effective teacher, patient educator or counselor," reflect on personal experience as a student and recall effective instructors, mentors, and patient educators. Health education and clinical education studies report four general attributes of effective teachers and counselors as shown in Box 83-3.[18]

Many studies have shown that teaching by nurses increases patients' knowledge.[19] Delivering accurate and complete information that improves patient knowledge and corrects misconceptions reflects clinical expertise and experience. Demonstrating clinical acumen also increases patient confidence and trust and decreases patients' anxiety. One team of investigators[20] studied 300 nurses who worked in critical-care, telemetry, medical-surgical, and heart failure units to determine their knowledge of heart failure and how they went about patient teaching. The nurses who dealt with heart failure as a primary population were more likely to perform patient teaching as a part of their daily role. Familiarity with disease process and therapies increased self-confidence and allowed teaching to be a normal part of daily care rather than an event. In addition, the nurses' confidence in their clinical expertise and the content allowed them to focus on teaching strategies, answer patient questions, and facilitate behavioral change.

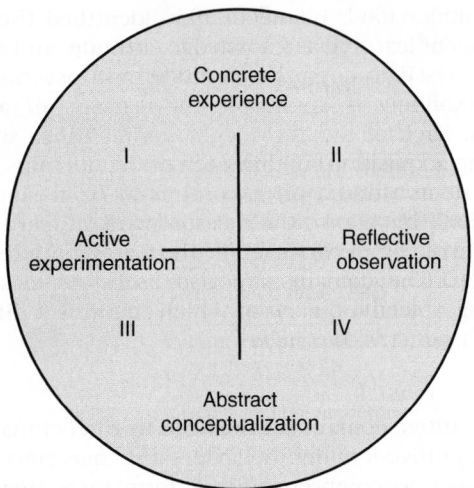

FIGURE 83-2 ■ Kolb theory of learning styles. According to the Kolb model of learning styles, once information has been perceived, it must be processed. Some people process information best by active experimentation or by reflective observation. (From Kolb D: Experiential learning: experiences as the source of learning and development, Englewood Cliffs, NJ, 1984, Prentice-Hall.)

Patient-provider communication is strongly linked to improved self-care and adherence behaviors,[21] important objectives of cardiovascular patient education. Good communication skills include listening and asking questions to gain clarity on the patient's point of view or concern. Effective teachers are also able to translate complex information into terms that are understandable to the patient. Providing the appropriate amount of information so that learning is enhanced and the patient is not overwhelmed is another important strength of an effective educator.

Clinicians and patients agree that positive and respectful interactions are important in patient interactions, such as teaching and counseling. Many patients believe that for the clinician to provide good care, the health care provider must "know" the patient.[22] This relationship between provider and patient is built on trust much like the trust established with a family member or friend. When viewed as a business arrangement, patients may feel like a commodity or subject; the lack of commitment by the provider is perceived as poor care and results in a lack of trust

Empathy, defined as identification with and understanding of another's situation, feelings, and motives, is important in behavioral change strategies and motivational approaches. Based on clinical education, practice, and professional guidelines, nurses know what patients should know about their disease. However, the illness is uniquely the patient's experience and is influenced by their significant others and environment. Displaying empathy includes understanding that unique experience or situation, feelings—which may include fear, helplessness, or hopelessness—and motivations that may be intrinsic or extrinsic. Empathy facilitates the open exploration of the patient's information needs *at the teaching moment* and leads to more efficient and focused teaching interventions.[23]

The Advanced Practice Nurse as Patient Educator

The advanced practice nurse plays several important roles in patient education: (1) providing direct patient education, (2) developing and coordinating patient education programs, and (3) mentoring other nurses through staff development programs and consultation[24] (Table 83-3). As an experienced clinician grounded in theoretical perspectives of patient education and counseling, advanced practice nurses may use more complex tactics to provide individualized patient teaching. Regardless of the setting—at the bedside, in specialty clinics, or primary care—the advanced practice nurse coordinates education among various providers. Many cardiovascular patients are cared for by an interdisciplinary team of providers. The advanced practice nurse supports the patient education process by coordinating available resources and ensuring communication among providers. Then through direct patient contact, the advanced practice nurse is often the provider to reinforce the information and answer questions from patients and families.

Development of staff educational programs is another role of advanced practice nursing. As experts in patient education, these professionals serve as mentors to new nurses both formally through professional training and informally through nurse consultations. By virtue of experience and advanced knowledge, advanced

---

BOX 83-3 ■ ■ ■
CHARACTERISTICS OF AN EFFECTIVE TEACHER

Demonstrates Clinical and Professional Competence
- Possesses clinical credibility (may include certification in specialty area)
- Experienced
- Provides teaching that is complete
- Able to answer questions
- Multilingual (especially essential for diverse patient populations)

Uses Good Communication and Listening Skills
- Communicates professionally
- Able to translate complex information into understandable terms
- Provides appropriate amount of information
- Listens and asks questions to gain clarity

Values Positive Human Relationships
- Compassionate
- Patient
- Attentive
- Respectful
- Honest
- Genuine

Displays Empathy
- Acknowledges the uniqueness of the patient's situation, feelings, and motivations

Langlais O, Shohet L: Part 2: Report on the needs assessment at the Montreal General Hospital. In Health literacy project, phase 1: needs assessment of the health education and information needs of hard-to-reach patients, Quebec, 2001, The Centre for Literacy.

■ ■ ■

TABLE 83-3 ROLE OF THE ADVANCED PRACTICE NURSE IN PATIENT EDUCATION

INTERVENTION	ROLE
Patient education and counseling	Provides direct patient education and counseling
	Uses a theoretical approach to assess learning needs, literacy, barriers to learning, cultural influences
	Develops patient educational materials
	Evaluates outcomes of teaching and counseling
Program development and coordination	Coordinates educational resources among multidisciplinary team
	Facilitates communication ensuring patient understanding
	Ensures consistent educational process
	Identifies additional resources for patient and family
Staff development and mentoring	Develops staff educational programs
	Assesses staff and provider knowledge and provides educational programs to meet needs of patient population
	Provides nurse consultation for difficult patient teaching situations

practice nurses can assist colleagues in tackling difficult patient education situations.

DEVELOPING AN EFFECTIVE PATIENT EDUCATION PLAN

Using these principles, a teaching plan can be developed that builds on what is known and progresses from simple concepts to more complex topics. Since adults learn best when there is a perceived need, assessment of the patients' understanding of their cardiovascular disease and perceived importance of self-care is the first step in formulating an effective teaching plan. For example, as Clark and Lan[16] reported, almost 25 percent of patients screened for a heart failure study did not know that they had been diagnosed with heart failure. Therefore, the first step in developing a patient teaching plan is assessment of the patient's baseline understanding of their diagnosis ("What did the doctor tell you about your heart condition?") and the meaning of the condition ("What does that mean to you?"). As discussed later in this chapter, cultural beliefs may influence the meaning of heart disease, the interpretation of their symptoms, and their choice of treatments. Culture is just one of the many important influences on a patient's understanding and behavior that should be assessed as part of developing an effective teaching plan.

Once baseline information knowledge and needs are assessed, patient teaching can proceed from general to specific, pertinent topics. Each topic should start with an assessment of a patient's current knowledge, which prevents unnecessary repetition and identifies knowledge gaps. For example, an explanation of the importance of taking prophylactic antibiotics with deep dental cleaning for patients with an artificial heart valve may start with an assessment question: "What did your doctor tell you about having your teeth cleaned?" Some patients may believe that they should only take antibiotics when they feel ill, a misconception that can guide their actions. Assessing the patient's current knowledge leads to an explanation of the purpose of prophylactic antibiotics in preventing endocarditis. Linking the association of an exposure to bacteria in the bloodstream with the need to protect seeding of the artificial valve reinforces the appropriate self-care behavior and illustrates the complications that may result if action is not taken.

Active participation in the teaching process increases learning and maintains interest and attentiveness. Self-care practices may be complex, so reinforcement through practice, observation, and immediate feedback will clarify misconceptions and support the new behavior. In teaching the patient with newly diagnosed coronary heart disease about a low-fat diet, the nurse may plan to observe a patient choosing foods from a menu to assess learning and to ensure accurate performance of the behavior. Role-playing how to ask a server for low-fat options helps the nurse assess the patient's comfort level with this behavior. In this manner, the behavior can either be reinforced through positive feedback

or misconceptions related to the behavior clarified and practice corrected.

Although provision of information likely increases patient knowledge about a topic, knowledge is not synonymous with behavior. For example, in a study of adherence to heart failure self-care, 40 percent of patients reported knowing little or nothing about heart failure despite evidence of instruction. Seventy-two percent of those patients who reported knowledge recalled instruction in a sodium-restricted diet, and 11 percent recalled being told to weigh themselves daily. However, only 67 percent followed a sodium-restricted diet, and 9 percent weighed themselves daily.[25] Motivation was identified as an important driver of patient behavior in this study.

The importance of motivation in the patient education process has implications for the approach taken in patient education. According to the social learning theory, patients may learn but not necessarily adopt the desired behavior. When the patient lacks motivation, patient counseling may be used to facilitate behavioral change.

PATIENT COUNSELING

Patient counseling allows the patient to lead the discussion and the nurse to follow as facilitator. Specific counseling tactics include presenting direct feedback, such as self-reports or lab results, offering advice only when solicited by the patient, exploring the importance of the behavior, and providing a menu of options or alternatives to support the patient's decisions about self-care. Ultimately, the goal of patient counseling as a teaching strategy is to negotiate a plan of action. For example, the nurse might start a counseling session by asking the patient what she or he would like to discuss. Using the patient's own self-report as feedback: "You said you noticed your ankles are swelling" or "You mentioned you were having difficulty with your breathing," can lead to a discussion of fluid accumulation as a mechanism of heart failure. Perhaps the patient voices concern over "keeping up" with grandchildren. Direct feedback on the implications of the cardiac-related symptom to quality of life often builds interest in learning. Let the patient choose the most important topic. Although exercise may be on the top of the list of important self-care behaviors for most patients with cardiovascular disease, patients may perceive that exercise is a low priority, but believe that daily blood pressure monitoring is a reasonable practice. Through collaboration a plan of action, often one behavior at a time, can be negotiated. At subsequent counseling sessions, positive behaviors can be reinforced through encouragement.

Specific Goals

According to the social learning theory, an effective program of patient education or includes four major components designed to alter the interacting behavioral, personal, and environmental factors that influence behavior change.[26] The first component is informational, designed to increase the patient's knowledge of a condition and awareness of health risks. Secondly, development of self-regulative skills results in effective preventive and coping behaviors, another important goal of patient education. The third component uses guided practice and feedback to build self-efficacy and skills. Finally, activating social supports is a critical component of an education or behavioral change program. Considering these four components, specific goals of patient education strategies may be categorized as increasing knowledge, self-efficacy, skill, and coping. The effectiveness of the education plan may be evaluated by measuring these outcomes linked to the specific goals of the educational strategy.

Knowledge

The 2001 Joint Commission on the Accreditation of Healthcare Organizations (**JCAHO,** now known as The Joint Commission) standards provide clear guidance on the goals of patient education (Box 83-4). A primary goal is to improve the patient's understanding of his or her health condition and treatment options including risks and benefits of the plan of care. For patients with cardiovascular disease, this means providing information on the pathophysiology or mechanisms of their disease and treatment plan (i.e., medication purpose, side effects, and testing procedures) so that they can recognize the relationship between the plan of care and their health. Lack of knowledge often complicates the patient's ability to perform self-care. Behavioral capability requires adequate knowledge and skills to perform a behavior. Therefore, patient teaching should include specific information that improves knowledge and leads to skill mastery.

Integrating information poses an additional challenge to the nurse and the patient. For example, a study of barriers to heart failure self-care found that although patient teaching sessions routinely include information on low-sodium diet, patients fail to integrate the facts learned with the behavioral outcome. That is, patients learned that certain foods had a high sodium content, but failed to link the intake of that food with physiological processes and their signs and symptoms (i.e., weight gain, shortness of breath).[27] Patient teaching plans that facilitate the patient's understanding of these important

links will contribute to the likelihood that patients will adhere to the plan of care.

Self-Efficacy

Self-efficacy is the confidence that an individual has in his or her ability to perform a specific action and to persist in performing that action or behavior. Self-efficacy affects behavior, motivation, thought patterns, and emotional response to situations.[28] Those with low self-efficacy may avoid difficult tasks, whereas those with high self-efficacy approach them as challenges.[9] Motivation will be stronger for individuals who believe that the goal behavior or task can be attained, and consequently, those with high self-efficacy are more persistent in overcoming obstacles than those with low self-efficacy.[29]

Since self-efficacy influences the choices that people make and the actions that they take, efforts to improve self-efficacy related to self-care, treatment adherence, and behavior change are critical. Specific strategies that have proven effective include the use of persuasion and encouragement; setting small, incremental goals to deter negative consequences; and providing feedback. It is also necessary to remember that self-efficacy is situation specific, so self-confidence in one context does not generalize to all situations.[28]

Skills

Maximizing self-care skills is another essential goal of patient education. Teaching skills includes an explanation of the entire procedure or task so that the patient understands (gains knowledge) the importance and integration of the task given the specific heart condition. Depending upon the learner's primary domain of learning, the nurse can adapt the teaching plan. However, skill mastery benefits from allowing the learner to practice the skill (e.g., during a return demonstration).

There are a number of skills associated with cardiovascular disease self-care. Adherence to dietary regimens is facilitated as the patient develops skills related to reading nutrition labels, selecting appropriate foods, and substituting low-sodium and low-fat foods for those high in salt or fat content. Many patients with cardiovascular disease need to learn to monitor their blood pressure at home. A patient teaching plan for this skill includes information about the meaning of blood pressure, the relation of the numbers (systolic to diastolic), factors that influence blood pressure, and symptom management so that the patient integrates the skill with a behavioral outcome. Demonstration of skill in monitoring blood pressure entails preparation, proper placement of the cuff, and use of the device. A return demonstration assesses skill development and allows the nurse to provide feedback to correct inaccurate technique and optimally reinforce skill acquisition.

Coping

Another important goal of patient education and counseling is improved patient and family coping. Coping is defined as "the constantly changing cognitive and be-

---

BOX 83-4 ■ ■ ■
JOINT COMMISSION GOALS FOR PATIENT AND FAMILY TEACHING

- Patient participation and decision making about health care options
- Increased potential to follow the health care plan
- Development of self-care skills
- Improved patient and family coping
- Increased participation in continuing care
- Adopting a healthy lifestyle

Rankin S, Stallings K, London F: *Patient education: principles and practice,* ed 4, Philadelphia, 2005, Lippincott.

havioral efforts to manage specific external and/or internal demands that are appraised as taxing or exceeding the resources of the person.[30]" Living with cardiovascular disease involves external and internal stresses that require the patient to tap into coping mechanisms. Patients use lifelong coping skills in response to the new and dynamic demands placed on them by their heart disease.

Blunters and Monitors

Two coping styles, "blunter" and "monitors" have been studied in a number of health care situations and found to be of clinical relevance in understanding patient decision making, adherence, anxiousness, and satisfaction.[31] Individuals who use a blunting coping style or "cognitive avoidance,[32]" tend to evade situations and information that are stressful. These individuals tend to be less anxious or apprehensive about their health status, procedures, or treatments. Those who use a monitoring coping style, also called "cognitive scanning,[32]" tend to be more vigilant and open to information, often attending more to preventive health care measures or instructions. The implication for patient teaching is to assess the coping style of the patient before teaching, especially in a potentially emotional situation, such as preceding an invasive procedure. Giving the wrong amount of information can increase stress for both "blunters" and "monitors." Providing the patient with a choice of the amount of information creates less stress and a more therapeutic patient teaching session.

Sensory Information

Patients also use specific sensory information to cope with health care events, such as procedures, treatment side effects, and even symptoms of their disease. As self-regulators, individuals use their perceptions and interpretations of their experiences to regulate their responses and behaviors to specific events (i.e., to cope).[33] Knowledge about expected sensations can influence a patient's expectations about what is likely to happen, his or her emotional responses, and actions to be taken. This information is represented in cognitive structures called "schemata," which are organized hierarchically from very specific to very abstract (e.g., from physical sensation to fear reaction).[33] When there is a discrepancy between the expected outcome and what exists, the normal response is to take action to minimize that discrepancy.

Because patients respond in a manner consistent with their understanding or expectation of the situation (i.e., procedure, treatment. or symptom), patient education can influence those interpretations and consequently, help patients cope. Patient teaching should include information about the physical sensations (see, hear, and feel) one might expect, such as the amount and duration of pain. For example, patients who are preparing for a cardiac catheterization will experience less distress if they understand that the room will be cold, they will remain awake, several people will be in the room, how long the procedure is expected to last, etc. An accurate explanation of pain, including its

cause, and a description of the sensation of catheter insertion or dye injection is likely to diminish apprehension. Studies have found that subjects who are accurately forewarned are less distressed and even require less sedation.[34] Similarly, patients undergoing surgery will benefit from patient teaching that explains what they might expect in the various stages of their preoperative and postoperative period.

Understandably, the patients' experience may differ from that described by the nurse. A surgical patient who develops a deep vein thrombosis (**DVT**) postoperatively may experience increased distress. An appropriate nursing response to facilitate coping with this unanticipated complication is to explain that blood clots postoperatively occur rarely and that the nurse did not want to prepare the patient to cope with something that was very unlikely to happen. The nurse can then help the patient to understand why the DVT occurred and the objective features of the plan of care and healing process (i.e., temporal characteristics—how long, use of a support stocking, how it will feel, etc.). The patient can then use that information to adjust the representation of the DVT and to cope with the event based on the revised representation.[33] Patient education aimed at improved coping also may be directed at important teaching topics, such as medication side effects and symptom management.

BEHAVIORAL CHANGE

Changing unhealthy behaviors is an important goal of education and counseling. Since the social learning theory acknowledges that learning may occur without a corresponding change in behavior, the advanced techniques of stages of change counseling and motivation interviewing are useful. The transtheoretical model of change has been studied in many health promotion and disease management programs. Evidence from these studies suggests that the model is effective in promoting positive lifestyle behavioral changes that lower risks in healthy and high risk populations. Therefore, readiness to learn and stages of change are useful in counseling cardiovascular patients on behavioral changes, such as smoking cessation, dietary restrictions, weight loss, and exercise programs.

Overview of the Transtheoretical Model of Behavioral Change

The transtheoretical model of change is an integrative model of behavior change developed from the principle theories used in psychotherapy—psychoanalytical, humanistic, gestalt, cognitive, and behavioral theories. The central construct of the transtheoretical model is the stages of change.[10] There are five temporal phases that individuals progress through in changing behavior: precontemplation, contemplation, preparation, action, and maintenance. Prochaska and colleagues[10] describe the stages of change as a sequential process; however, individuals frequently cycle through the stages before successfully achieving the preferred behavior. In the precontemplation stage, action is not intended in the foreseeable future, whereas those in contemplation stage intend to change in the next 6 months. In the preparation stage, action is intended in the immediate future and often has occurred in the past year. Action is the stage in which people make specific modifications to their behaviors, and maintenance signals the stage where individuals guard against relapses, but are increasingly confident that they can sustain the changed behavior.[35]

A second construct of the transtheoretical model of change is the processes of change that explain how shifts in behavior occur. Nine processes are identified and categorized into experiential or cognitive and behavioral processes (Table 83-4). Experiential processes increase the person's awareness that a problem exists, and action or change in behavior is needed. Behavioral processes focus directly on behavior change and support movement from preparation to the action stage.[10]

The decision-balance construct of the transtheoretical model, or the perceptions of pros and cons of a specific behavior, is influenced by the stage of change.[36] According to this model, individuals consider consequences to self and others of making change and reactions of self and others as a result of the change. For example, progression from the precontemplation or contemplation stage to the action stage is likely when the benefits of making the health behavior change or the cons of not making the change increase.[10]

Similar to the social learning theory, self-efficacy is used in the transtheoretical model of change as a representation of the situation-specific confidence an individual has that she or he can accomplish a behavior without relapsing. The opposite of self-efficacy is temptation, which represents the urges to engage in the unwanted behavior.[35]

The transtheoretical model of change is an appropriate model for patient education when behavioral change is a desired outcome. Specific tactics can be used to guide patients through the stages of behavioral change. First, an assessment of stage of change for each behavior is completed using specific definitions of the behavior. For example, assessment of a sodium-restricted diet should ask specifically about high-sodium foods, such as canned vegetables, processed foods, "fast food," and snacks, and the use of salt in cooking or at the table. A five-choice response format that includes the operational definition for each behavior is recommended to match the patient's stage of change to an appropriate intervention.[37] Response options include: "Yes, I have been doing X for more than 6 months" (maintenance stage), "Yes, I have been doing X for less than 6 months" (action stage), "No, but I am planning to start in the next 30 days" (preparation stage), "No, but I am planning to start in the next 6 months" (contemplation stage), and "No, and I don't have any plans to do X" (precontemplation stage). Table 83-5 describes an example of a patient education plan based upon the transtheoretical model of change.

■ ■ ■

TABLE 83-4 DEFINITIONS OF THE PROCESSES OF CHANGE

PROCESS	EXPLANATION
Experiential	
Consciousness raising	Increased awareness of causes, consequences, and cures for a problem; increasing information about self and the unhealthy behavior
Dramatic relief	Experiencing and releasing feelings about the possible consequences of the behavior; using feelings to help motivate change
Self-reevaluation	Cognitive and affective assessments of one's self-image with and without the behavior to change how one thinks about oneself in relation to the behavior
Environmental reevaluation	Cognitive and affective assessment of how the presence or absence of the behavior affects one's social environment; becoming aware that one can serve as a positive or negative role model to others
Social liberation	Recognizing changes in the environment or social changes that influence personal change
Behavioral	
Self-liberation	Recognizing choices related to available actions and making a commitment to change a behavior
Helping relationship	Seeking and accepting support from others in the form of caring, trust, acceptance, and openness
Reinforcement management	Applying consequences in the form of rewards to oneself for making change
Counterconditioning	Learning new and healthier alternative behavior substitute for the unhealthy behavior
Stimulus control	Avoiding or removing environmental cues for unhealthy behavior and adding cues for healthier alternatives

Prochaska J, Velicer W: The transtheoretical model of health behavior change, *Am J Health Promot* 12:38-48, 1997.

Self-Regulation

Maintenance of behavioral change is essential to improving cardiovascular health outcomes. Work from Leventhal and colleagues describes the individuals' decision to maintain behavior as a function of the behavioral, psychological, and physiological experiences associated with the new behaviors.[11] This self-regulatory model of illness extends our understanding of behavioral change by focusing on what would be described as maintenance in the transtheoretical model of change discussed above.

Generally, people who are satisfied with their new pattern of behavior are likely to maintain the change. Satisfaction indicates the decision to take action was justified and that the effort to perform the behavior is worthwhile. This assessment of satisfaction clearly shifts the decisional balance in favor of behavioral change.

According to the self-regulatory model of illness, behavior change occurs in four phases: initial response,

■■■

TABLE 83-5 EDUCATIONAL PLAN BASED ON TRANSTHEORETICAL MODEL OF CHANGE

PROCESS OF CHANGE	ACTIVITY

Stage: Precontemplation
Patient response: *"No, and I don't have plans to do X."*

Consciousness Raising
Encourage patients to increase level of awareness, seek information, and gain understanding and feedback.

- Provide educational pamphlets and Internet sites with information.
- Encourage questions.
- Invite patients to attend a (specific condition) support group.
- Have patients describe their condition in their own words.
- Share study results, especially findings about quality of life.

Dramatic Relief
Ask patients to consider ways in which heart disease affects the way they feel.

- Have patients recall how they felt before they had (condition) versus how they feel now.
- Share testimonials about how behavioral changes improved how they feel.

Environmental Reevaluation
Encourage patients to consider how their heart disease affects the physical and social environment.

- Have family members share experiences, thoughts, and emotions related to illness.
- Solicit physical and social changes since developing condition.

Stage: Contemplation
Patient Response: *"No, but I plan to start in the next 6 months."*

Consciousness Raising
Encourage patients to increase level of awareness, seek information, and gain understanding and feedback.

- Provide educational pamphlets and Internet sites with information.
- Encourage questions.
- Invite patients to attend a (specific condition) support group.
- Have patients describe their condition in their own words.
- Share study results, especially findings about quality of life.

Dramatic Relief
Ask patients to consider ways in which heart disease affects the way they feel.

- Have patients recall how they felt before they had (condition) versus how they feel now.
- Share testimonials about how behavioral changes improved how they feel.
- Role-play situations involving choices between healthy and unhealthy lifestyle changes.
- Have patients describe how body parts feel (e.g., swollen feet, chest pain).

Environmental Reevaluation
Encourage patients to consider how their heart disease affects the physical and social environment.

- Have patients and family members reverse role-play an episode of exacerbation of the condition.
- Have patients describe changes they have made in their physical environment.
- Discuss personal cost of illness.

Self-Reevaluation
Encourage patients to assess how they feel and think about themselves with respect to heart disease and the need to change behavior (i.e., exercise, restrict sodium in diet).

- Have patients describe changes in their lives associated with the condition.
- Assess quality of life.
- Have patient visualize what life would be like without signs and symptoms of condition.
- Review patients' behavior (i.e., diet record) and point out inconsistencies between values and behaviors.

Stage: Preparation
Patient Response: *"No, but I plan to start in the next 30 days."*

Self-Reevaluation
Encourage patients to assess how they feel and think about themselves with respect to heart disease and the need to change behavior (i.e., exercise, restrict sodium in diet).

- Assess beliefs about the condition; identify items that are incorrect and review corrected information.
- Help plan activities involving the lifestyle change (e.g., exercise plan, use of low-sodium recipes).

Self-Liberation
Encourage patients to believe in their ability to change and make the choice and commitment to act on that belief.

- Contract with patients about new behaviors.
- Explain importance of self-care in managing condition.
- Teach patients to read "nutrition facts" labels.
- Have patient speak with another patient in the maintenance stage about the effects of changes on quality of life.
- Encourage patients to obtain equipment needed for lifestyle change (e.g., comfortable walking shoes, scale).

Stimulus Control
Encourage patients to identify cues to remind them to increase positive behavior.

- Encourage removal of items from their home that are temptations (i.e., soup, cigarettes, alcohol).
- Encourage purchase of a low-salt cookbook, healthy snacks, pillbox.
- Place blood pressure home monitoring device and bathroom scale in convenient location.
- Post medication schedule in visible location.

Paul S, Sneed N: Strategies for behavior change in patients with heart failure, *Am J Crit Care* 13(4):305-313, 2004.

∎ ∎ ∎

TABLE 83-5   EDUCATIONAL PLAN BASED ON TRANSTHEORETICAL MODEL OF CHANGE—cont'd

PROCESS OF CHANGE	ACTIVITY

Stage: Action
Patient Response: *"Yes, I have been doing X for less than 6 months."*

Self-Liberation Encourage patients to believe in their ability to change and make the choice and commitment to act on that belief.	• Have patients keep daily weight, blood pressure, heart rate, diet and activity journal.
Counterconditioning Encourage patients to substitute healthier alternatives in situations and conditions that normally elicit signs or symptoms of heart disease.	• Identify situations that increase noncompliance and suggest ways to avoid those situations. • Review information on diet; provide low-sodium recipes, cookbooks, etc. • Develop an exercise plan or enroll patients in cardiac rehabilitation or fitness center.
Stimulus Control Encourage patients to identify cues to remind them to increase positive behavior.	• Remove temptations from the home. • Encourage purchase of supportive items, such as a low-fat cookbook. • Post daily reminder, such as an exercise plan. • Avoid restaurants that serve high-sodium foods.
Reinforcement Management Encourage patients to acknowledge and reward positive behavior changes.	• Help patients identify rewards for new behaviors.
Helping Relationships Encourage patients to use support system of family, friends, and health care team.	• Identify at least one person who is committed to helping them change. • Involve patients in a support group.

Stage: Maintenance
Patient Response: *"Yes, I have been doing X for more than 6 months."*

Counterconditioning Encourage patients to substitute healthier alternatives in situations and conditions that normally elicit signs or symptoms of heart failure or chest pain.	• Identify situations that increase noncompliance, and discuss ways to avoid those situations. • Provide additional information as needed, low-sodium recipes, cookbooks, etc.
Stimulus Control Encourage patients to identify cues to remind them to increase positive behavior.	• Remove temptations from the home. • Encourage purchase of supportive items, such as a low-fat cookbook. • Post daily reminders, such as an exercise plan. • Avoid restaurants that serve high-sodium foods. • Have patients complete quality of life survey and compare with previous results.
Reinforcement Management Encourage patients to acknowledge and reward positive behavior changes.	• Help patients identify rewards for new behaviors.
Helping Relationships Encourage patients to use support system of family, friends, and health care team.	• Ask patients to speak with other heart disease patients who are at an earlier stage of change.

continued response, maintenance, and habit. An individual may first initiate a change in behavior by intermittently exercising and move to the continued response phase by consistent performance of the desired behavior. In this phase, individuals shift their focus from expectations about the behavior to their experiences with it. Perhaps a patient who modifies his diet to eat less salt experiences less peripheral edema and a decrease in shortness of breath. Sustained effort and satisfaction with the new behavior and confidence in his ability to perform the behavior indicates movement to the maintenance phase where the perceived value of the behavior emerges and solidifies the behavior change. The habit phase is the self-perpetuating pattern of be-

havior where relapse is unlikely. The synthesis of the transtheoretical model of change and the self-regulatory model of illness provides a comprehensive model that can be used to guide behavior change strategies (Figure 83-3).

Building a patient education plan using the self-regulatory model of illness is also consistent with the social learning theory. According to the self-regulatory model, patients will continue to engage in behaviors, if they perceive that the behavior will prevent disruption of usual life activities (reinforcement) and will help them prevent discomfort or stress (prevent punishment). Therefore, patient teaching strategies should stress the psychological aspects of the desired behavior, which

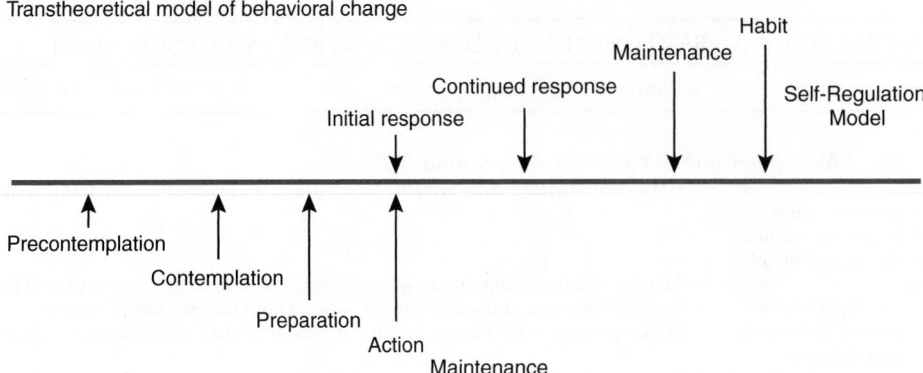

FIGURE 83-3 ■ Synthesis of transtheoretical model of change and self-regulation model. Together these two models illustrate that before behavioral change can be solidified, there is a pattern of ongoing behavior that is satisfying to the individual. Successful behavioral change results in self-perpetuating habit phase where relapse is unlikely.

may include increased comfort and improved quality of life. An example of a patient education plan using the self-regulatory model of illness is shown in Table 83-6.

Motivational Interviewing

Motivation, as a core construct of the social learning theory, is essential to behavioral change. For an individual to perform a behavior, she or he needs to be motivated to do so. A counseling strategy called motivational interviewing, developed by Miller and colleagues[38] as a way to encourage behavioral change in chronic alcohol abusers, has been studied extensively and found to be effective in myriad clinical populations and behaviors.[39] To promote behavioral change, motivational interviewing—and the adapted motivational approaches commonly used in health care—uses four basic tactics: empathic listening, encouraging patients to state their own reasons for change, rolling with resistance, and supporting self-efficacy.[40]

According to this approach, motivation is the likelihood that a person will do something to feel or get better and the product of the patient-provider interaction. Motivational interviewing assumes that people are ambivalent about changing their behavior. One of the goals of this approach is to help patients explore and resolve that ambivalence by placing the patient directly in the expert role. The patient must decide how to interpret and integrate information and determine if that information is relevant to his or her own situation.

Another underlying assumption of motivational interviewing is that the patient will change if and when they are committed to change. Motivational interviewing includes an assessment of the patient's readiness for change (see Transtheoretical Model of Change) and then selection of an appropriate strategy to use

■ ■ ■

TABLE 83-6   EDUCATIONAL PLAN BASED ON SELF-REGULATION MODEL

STAGE	ACTIVITY THEMES
Initiation Patients determine that the potential changes afforded by the new behavior compare favorably with their current situation.	* Have patients state expectations about the behavior and future outcomes. * Balance optimism with realistic expectations. * Support patient's confidence in performing behavior through reinforcement of positive practices. * Identify barriers to successful initiation and discuss ways to remove barriers and increase supports.
Continued Response Patients strive to gain a sense of mastery of the new behavior.	* Have patient explain how the experience with the behavior compares with their expectations. * Support patients' confidence in performing behavior through reinforcement of practices. * Provide additional informational resources, such as recipes, exercise options, to alleviate negative experiences. * Identify supports to new behaviors (family members, community resources, health care team) that can assist in sustaining efforts.
Maintenance Patients have successfully demonstrated their ability to perform behaviors and desire to sustain the new behaviors.	* Have patients identify the value of the new behavior. * Have patients recall changes in how they feel since adopting the behavior change. * Identify who will support the patient's new behavior.
Habit Patients engage in the behavior in the absence of any evaluation of costs or benefits.	* Involve the patient as support to other heart disease patients.

(Box 83-5 lists the essential principles of motivational interviewing).

The quality of the patient-provider interaction is the "spirit" of motivational interviewing.[41] This interaction should be empathic and nonjudgmental. The individualized, "nonrecipe" approach to each patient encounter is the key component. Patient interactions are gently guided to focus on ambivalence and its resolution (Box 83-6).

The four pillars of motivational interviewing technique are open-ended questions, affirmation, reflective listening, and summaries. Embedded in reflective listening is the idea that the feeling of being truly understood is empowering. Similarly, the technique of affirmation (i.e., affirming the patient's worth) promotes self-efficacy, which is essential to learning and behavioral change. Effectiveness of motivational interviewing is evidenced by the patient's "change talk." Change talk is defined as utterances of dissatisfaction with the status quo (current behavior), advantages of the change, optimism about change rather than resistance or difficulties of the new behavior, and intention to change. Ultimately, the patient will demonstrate motivation through performance of the new, desired behavior.[38]

Brief Motivational Counseling

Though the most effective applications of motivational interviewing are more time consuming than the standard short advice-giving sessions typically used in health care encounters, brief motivational counseling can be done rapidly. This brief approach is facilitated using a 10-point rating scale. For change to potentially occur, both importance and confidence must be rated highly by the patient (Figures 83-4 and 83-5).

Miller and Rollnick (2002) have developed a general strategy called FRAMES[38] to summarize the elements of brief motivational counseling:

- **F**eedback is given to patients, such as lab reports, physical findings.
- **R**esponsibility for change is the patient's. Expect resistance, denial, and ambivalence and do not be seduced into arguing.
- **A**dvice must be exquisitely timed based on the patient's request, not the provider's agenda.
- **M**enu of options, resources, and alternative choices are offered. Patients often need and want to discuss what is going on in their lives before addressing health issues.
- **E**mpathy must be truly present. Patients have emotional radar that accurately assesses our true interest in their lives. If empathy is absent, change will be too.
- **S**elf-Efficacy is supported and promoted. If a patient is not confident in their ability to change, they will probably not attempt it.

(See Table 83-7 for an example of a brief motivational interviewing plan.) Also see the accompanying Conundrum feature on the expert patient.

BOX 83-5 ■ ■ ■
ESSENTIAL PRINCIPLES OF MOTIVATIONAL INTERVIEWING

- The use of reflective listening
- Developing discrepancy between client goals and current problems by reflective listening and objective feedback
- Not arguing
- Not confronting or opposing resistance
- Supporting self-efficacy
- Optimism for change

Miller W, Rollnick S: *Motivational interviewing: preparing people for change,* ed 2, New York, 2002, Guilford.

BOX 83-6 ■ ■ ■
THE SPIRIT OF MOTIVATIONAL INTERVIEWING

- Readiness to change is not a client trait, but a fluctuating product of interpersonal interaction.
- The therapeutic relationship functions best as a partnership rather than an expert-recipient relationship.
- Motivation to change should be elicited from the client, not imposed by the counselor.
- It is the client's task, not the counselor's, to articulate and resolve his or her ambivalence.
- The counselor is directive in helping the client examine and resolve ambivalence.
- Rational arguments for change are presented to the client by the expert in what is known as direct persuasion.
- The counseling style is generally a quiet and eliciting one.

Miller W, Rollnick S: *Motivational interviewing: preparing people for change,* ed 2, New York, 2002, Guilford.

"On a scale of 1–10, how **important** is it for you to make a change in your...?"

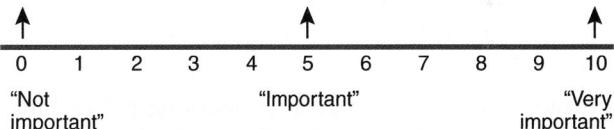

FIGURE 83-4 ■ Brief motivational evaluation—importance. This scale allows the individual to rate the importance of the behavioral change to provide immediate feedback during a brief motivational counseling interview.

"On a scale of 1–10, how **confident** are you that you could make a change if you wanted to?"

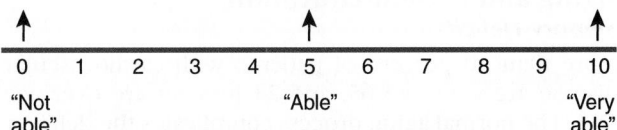

FIGURE 83-5 ■ Brief motivational evaluation—confidence. This scale allows individuals to rate their confidence in their ability to change behavior and provides immediate feedback during a brief motivational counseling interview. Confidence and importance of the desired change are valuable indicators of likelihood of behavioral change.

■ ■ ■

TABLE 83-7 EXAMPLE OF BRIEF MOTIVATIONAL INTERVIEW

GOAL	INTERVENTION COMPONENT BASED ON FRAMES	STRATEGY AND SAMPLE QUESTIONS
Understand patient's concerns and situation.	**Empathy** must be present and is essential to establishing rapport.	Use open-ended questions that demonstrate concern for patient as a person. • "How are you feeling today? Are you comfortable?" • "If I could see the situation through your eyes, what would I see?"
Get patient's agreement to talk about topic.	**Menu** of options, resources, and alternative choices are offered.	Request permission to discuss topic. • "Would you mind spending a few minutes talking about topic (e.g., diet, exercise) and how you see it affecting your health?"
Understand readiness to change behavior.	**Responsibility** for change is the patient's. **Advice** must be based on the patient's request, not the provider's agenda. Assess readiness to change.	Use an assessment tool to assess readiness and discuss results with patient. • "How do you feel about (topic)?" • "How ready are you to change your use of (topic)?"
Raise patient awareness of consequences of the behavior and share provider's concerns.	**Feedback** is given to patients, such as lab reports, physical findings.	Use objective data from individual's medical evaluation if possible and then elicit reactions from patient. • "What do you make of these results?"
Assure client that ongoing support is available.	**Self-efficacy** is supported and promoted. Offer continued support, targeted to patient's level of readiness to change.	For patients who are "not ready" to change: • "Is there anything else you want to know about (topic)?" • "What would it take to get you to consider thinking about a change?" For patients who are "unsure" about change: • "What are the good things you like about (topic)? What does it do for you?" • "What are the things you don't like about (topic)? What concerns do you have about it?" For patients who are "ready" to change: • "Here are some options for change. What do you think would work best for you?" Provide support and referral.

FRAMES, Feedback, responsibility, advice, empathy, self-efficiency.
D'Onofrio G, Bernstein E, Rollnick S: Motivating patients for change: a brief strategy for negotiation. In Bernstein E, Bernstein J, editors: *Case studies in emergency medicine and the health of the public,* Boston, 1996, Jones and Bartlett.

PATIENT EDUCATION IN SPECIAL SITUATIONS

As stated earlier in this chapter, learning is facilitated when four conditions are met: the patient is able to pay attention, retain or remember the information provided, perform the action, and is motivated to perform the behavior. In the cardiac patient population, nurses need to consider how age and sensory deficits will affect the learning process, cultural and literacy barriers to patient education, and the inherent cognitive deficits associated with the pathophysiology of many of the cardiovascular diseases (Table 83-8).

Aging and Patient Education
Sensory Deficits

More than 40 percent of patients with cardiovascular disease are over age 65, and 24 percent are over age 75.[42] The normal aging process complicates the delivery of patient education in many ways. Sensory changes include decreased vision acuity, diminished hearing, and alteration to the sense of smell, taste, and touch. Changes in visual acuity, such as cataracts, loss of peripheral

■ ■ ■ **CONUNDRUM**

THE EXPERT PATIENT: ALLY OR ENEMY

Patients today come armed with journal articles, research findings, studies, which you may not have seen or even be aware of. Though it is fashionable to term patients as "consumers," the worldview of health care professionals does not support this role. With the plethora of support groups and Internet resources, motivated patients can easily obtain information, and the conundrum is that by increasing their knowledge, they may be punished for stepping out of the traditional good patient role—the one who simply follows our instructions and thanks us effusively. These patients are often dismissed, ridiculed, labeled as difficult, humiliated, shortchanged, and all because tradition has taught that patients may not challenge us experts of knowledge.

In England in 1935, the director of the Peckham Health Centre in London, Dr. Scott Williamson, said that he only used his authority to stop anyone exercising control over another person.[68] In 2002 the UK Department of Health published *The Expert Patient,*[69] and England became the first country ever to undertake and fund a national initiative to fund self-management programs to create expert patients to improve the health care environment for both patients and providers and improve effectiveness of health care. When patients present new information or questions to us, they may actually be extending the tremendous honor of an invitation to work in greater partnership with them.

■■■

TABLE 83-8 TIPS FOR TEACHING IN SPECIAL SITUATIONS

Blind	• Identify self when approaching.
	• Use normal voice tone.
	• Audiotape teaching sessions.
	• Guide patient's hand with nurse's.
	• Warn when touching patients.
Hearing impaired	• Approach where patient can see you.
	• Use pamphlets, pictures, and videos.
	• Face person when speaking.
	• Use ASL interpreter.
Mute	• Watch nonverbal clues for frustration.
	• Provide slate or communication board, paper, and pencil.
Illiterate	• Use discussion and demonstration.
	• Use color-coded system and pictures to emphasize signs and symptoms.
	• Keep messages short, direct, and specific.
	• Present most important information first.
Patient from another culture	• Assess language ability, experience with health care system.
	• Use interpreter as necessary.
	• Use written materials in native language if literate.
	• Ask about client's values and beliefs.
	• If patient understands only a little English:
	• Speak slowly and clearly
	• Use simple words

vision, intolerance to glare, and inability to adjust from light to dark, affect the patient's ability to interact with the environment that includes reading material, medication dosing instruction, and even reading the bathroom scale.

Approach a hearing-impaired patient from an angle where you can be seen and face the person when speaking. Hearing aids for hard of hearing patients will help facilitate the learning process. Low-pitched voices are better heard, whereas shouting distorts the sounds making it more difficult for the hearing-impaired person. In addition, some high-frequency consonants (f, g, s, and t) and two-syllable words are more difficult to distinguish, so careful selection of words will decrease confusion and frustration. Use of pamphlets, videos, and pictures is recommended for delivery of information and allows for review and reinforcement after the session. An American sign language interpreter may be indicated for some patients.

Elders also frequently experience changes in the musculoskeletal system, such as arthritis, so the patient teaching setting should be easily accessible, have plenty of space in which to maneuver wheel chairs and walkers, and have comfortable chairs that are easy to get in and out of for patients with limited mobility. For example, many patients with cardiovascular disease take diuretics as part of their medication regimen, so including breaks in the patient teaching session conveys sensitivity to the patient's situation and will avert intentional noncompliance (i.e., patients deliberately not taking their medication so they do not have to use the restroom frequently).

Health Literacy

In all patient education scenarios, it is essential to assess the patient's functional literacy level (Table 83-9). About 20 percent of all Americans are functionally illiterate, and 25 percent are marginally illiterate (i.e., read at only a fifth to eighth grade level).[43] Illiterate patients generally speak and understand information, but have limited reading and writing capabilities. Functional illiteracy is higher in elders (71 percent of adults over age 60)[44] and highest in adults with chronic illness (75 percent).[45] Studies have shown a correlation between limited health literacy and worse health outcomes including poorer knowledge about health condition, lower use of prevention services, higher rates of nonadherence, higher hospitalization rates, and poorer self-reported health status.[46]

Illiteracy in the cardiovascular disease population poses a huge patient education challenge. These patients are often not able to read and understand the health care instructions, traditionally a printed set of materials, details on their medication prescriptions, or even the date and time on physician appointment slips. Further, patients with poor reading skills frequently have limited attention spans and poor memory. Therefore messages should be short, direct, and specific. Teaching should focus on essential information. Rather than inundate the low-literacy patient with complex explanations of cardiac pathophysiology, stress important information by presenting it first or last and providing frequent reinforcement. Sequential information needs to be presented logically (e.g., step-by-step) to minimize confusion. The patient should restate and demonstrate the instruction to ensure understanding. It is essential that information be very specific. For example, when instructing on medication regimens, list the exact times the medication is to be taken, not "twice a day" and reason for the medicine using the patient's

■■■

TABLE 83-9 ASSESSING INADEQUATE HEALTH LITERACY

SCREENING QUESTIONS	RESPONSES
1. How often do you have problems learning about your medical condition because of difficulty understanding written information?	Always Often Sometimes Occasionally Never
2. How confident are you filling out medical forms by yourself?	Extremely Quite a bit Somewhat A little bit Not at all
3. How often do you have someone (such as a family member, friend, hospital or clinic worker or caregiver) help you read hospital materials?	Always Often Sometimes Occasionally Never

Responses of "often or quite a bit" or "always or extremely" to any of the three questions may indicate inadequate health literacy.
Chew L, Bradley K, Boyko E: Brief questions to identify patients with inadequate health literacy, *Fam Med* 36:588-594, 2004.

terms. Use of pictures to supplement the demonstrations and discussion is helpful, but video or multimedia has not been shown to improve knowledge, memory, or adherence.[47] Even though the patient may not be able to read, printed instructions and materials should still be provided since family members or friends may use the instructions as a resource.

A pilot study for low-literacy patients with heart failure evaluated the efficacy of specially developed educational materials and questionnaires.[48] Teaching goals focused on building the key self-care skills of symptom and weight assessment and diuretic dose adjustment. Educational materials were developed to ensure readability at below the third grade level. A color-coded system of red, yellow, and green was developed to emphasize the signs and symptoms of worsening heart failure (weight gain and peripheral edema) and associated need for a change in the diuretic dosing. For low-literacy patients, this system eliminated the need for calculations or reading medication instructions. The color-coded system was used to guide patients' self-management decisions about other symptoms, such as shortness of breath while lying down, difficulty walking, and lower extremity edema, use the color-coded system to guide patients' self-management decisions. When the symptoms are in the red zone, or if they remain in the yellow zone for 3 days; the patient is instructed to contact the disease management team. Results of the pilot study were encouraging, with significant positive changes in self-care behavior and heart failure–related symptoms. Although the mean knowledge score did not improve after the intervention; the proportion of patients who reported weighing themselves daily increased from 32 percent to 100 percent at 12 weeks.[48] In addition, there was a meaningful increase in the Minnesota Living with Heart Failure Questionnaire (9.9 points) that indicated an improvement in heart failure–related quality of life. A complete version of the educational materials can be viewed at http://medicine.med.unc.edu/patient/dewalt.htm.[48]

Cultural Beliefs

Cardiovascular disease is a problem worldwide and affects people in varied ethnic groups with disproportionately higher morbidity and mortality. Research has uncovered differences in risk factors, pathophysiology of the disease, and health disparities that account for a portion of the discrepancy in health outcomes. This information can be used to frame interventions. Cultural factors that influence perceptions and beliefs about health and illness need to be incorporated into the patient teaching plan.

Explanatory models speak to the "notions about an episode of sickness and its treatment.[49]" According to the Kleinman explanatory model, people interpret the meaning of illness within the context of their culture. This representation influences their choices and behaviors, starting with the acceptance of patient teaching materials. Since clinicians and patients may hold divergent explanatory models of disease, assessment of the cultural perspectives is an important first step in teaching any patient, especially those from a different cultural background. Kleinman suggests that clinicians assess the explanatory model of illness by eliciting the patient's interpretation of their illness causality, symptoms, effects on body and mind, treatment, prognosis, and coping.[50] Eight questions (Box 83-7) are suggested to guide the interview. It is imperative that the nurse educator is nonjudgmental and shows genuine interest in the patient's beliefs and perceptions. Communicate that the information provided by the patient is important in planning an effective treatment and teaching plan.

A qualitative study that explored knowledge and communication difficulties[51] found that patients often had concerns about their medications and wondered about possible alternatives, but were reluctant to raise these issues. Other patients attributed their symptoms to advancing age and believed nothing could be done about their symptoms. These barriers to communication can be removed through respectful exploration of the patients' meaning of their illness, treatment, and prognosis.

The importance of cultural beliefs is seen in food choices, medicinal use of supplements, and choice of alternative therapies. The meaning of food as more than a source of nutrition may vary by cultures. Determination of foods for ingestion, medicinal purposes, or as sacred or profane drives dietary selection for many people.[50] Ask specifically about the medicinal use of foods and herbs and cultural food preferences to incorporate beliefs into the teaching plan. For example, in the black culture, foods with a high salt content (i.e., pork) bring luck to the household at certain times of the year. Traditional foods, such as collard greens, that are rich in potassium can affect blood clotting levels in heart patients taking anticoagulants (i.e., warfarin). Special attention in the teaching plan to these cultural beliefs is needed to negotiate a dietary plan that the patient can adhere to. Similarly, use of herbal supplements should be assessed to identify any contraindications to the medical regimen. Table 83-10 lists common characteristics associated with diverse populations and teaching strategies that should be considered as a patient teaching plan is developed.

BOX 83-7   ■ ■ ■

EIGHT QUESTIONS FOR ELICITING THE PATIENT'S EXPLANATORY MODEL OF AN ILLNESS

- What do you call the problem?
- What do you think has caused the problem?
- Why do you think it started when it did?
- What do you think the sickness does? How does it work?
- How severe is the sickness? Will it have a short or long course?
- What kind of treatment do you think you (the patient) should receive? What are the most important results you hope he or she receives from this treatment?
- What are the chief problems the sickness has caused?
- What do you fear most about the sickness?

Kleinman A: *Patients and healers in the context of culture,* Berkley, Calif, 1980, University of California Press.

■ ■ ■

TABLE 83-10   CULTURAL FACTORS AND TEACHING STRATEGIES

CULTURAL GROUP	CHARACTERISTICS	TEACHING STRATEGIES
Hispanic American	• Strong family ties • Obtain information from mass media • Either Spanish or English may be primary language • Categorize disease into "hot and cold," magical origin, emotional origin, folk defined • Often economically disadvantaged	• Encourage family's involvement in teaching sessions. • Provide adequate space for extended family. • Determine primary language. • Use an interpreter if needed. • Provide written materials in Spanish. • Incorporate religious beliefs into plan. • Respect cultural values and take time to learn beliefs. • Be considerate of feelings of modesty.
Asian/Pacific Islander	• Blend of four philosophies (Buddhism, Confucianism, Taoism, Phi) • Strong male authority • Strong family ties • "Saving face" or sense of pride • Respect for parents, elders, teachers, and authority figures	• Use friendly, nonthreatening approach. • Give permission to ask questions. Do not assume understanding with silence. • Ask questions in different ways to ensure understanding. • Consider language barrier and use an interpreter if needed. • Learning style is passive. • Learning is by repetition and rote memorization. • Give reassurance.
Native American	• Spiritual attachment to land • Strong association of religion and medicine • Strong ties to family and tribe • Children are important asset • Lack materialism • Believe witchcraft or supernatural cause of illness • Not future oriented—do not have control over destiny • Believe that looking into another's eyes reveals and may steal someone's soul	• Focus on giving information about diseases and risk factors. • Emphasize teaching of skills related to changes in diet and exercise. • Consider each tribe's unique customs and languages.
African American	• Often have economic or educational disadvantages • Extended family is very important. • Elders in family hold highest respect • Strong religious values • Some believe in voodoo or witchcraft, • May use folk remedies	• Assess folk practices and religious beliefs. • Incorporate folk practices into treatment plan if not harmful. • Assess dietary practices and beliefs. • Incorporate family members into teaching session.

Bastable S: Gender, Socioeconomic, and cultural attributes of the learner. In Bastable S, editor: *Nurse as educator: principles of teaching and learning,* Sudbury, Mass, 1997, Jones and Bartlett Publishers.

Cognition Deficits

Cognitive decline is considered a normal part of aging, with a prevalence of 25 percent in those over age 65 and 65 percent in those over age 85. Healthy older patients may show a decline in cognitive skills, such as abstract thinking, calculation, verbal comprehension, and decreased memory and recall. In heart failure patients, cognitive impairment occurs in more than 30 percent of patients[2] and may exceed 50 percent in older patients.[52] Carotid artery disease is associated with cognitive decline in individuals over age 65.[3] Midlife hypertension is also linked to cognitive impairment in later life. In fact, in a longitudinal study of hypertensive patients, psychomotor skills were 10 percent lower when compared with normotensive peers.[4]

Memory and attention are common deficits in the heart failure population.[53-55] Executive function deficits include difficulties in memory, attention, decision making, planning, cognitive flexibility, and abstract reasoning.[56] The underlying pathophysiological mechanisms of heart disease that lead to cognitive impairment is the subject of extensive research, clinical trials, and ongoing debate among experts. Although a consensus on what causes cognitive impairment has not yet been reached, clinicians and researchers do agree that deficits in memory, attention, and executive function affect self-care practices of medication taking, dietary modifications, and symptom management that are critical to managing disease and optimizing outcomes. In fact, several studies investigating predictors of hospital readmissions have identified cognitive impairment as a likely culprit. For example, in a study of medication compliance, that more than 50 percent of patients were unable to name their medication or dosage, and 75 percent failed to remember to take their medications despite extensive verbal and written information about their treatment regimen.[57] Since memory and attention are markedly impaired in older patients with cognitive dysfunction, they may be unable to be attentive during patient education sessions or to remember the verbal instructions later. Additionally, simply remembering to take medication on a daily basis may be difficult for a population with significant memory deficits.

As discussed in Chapter 64, self-care management requires that patients with cardiovascular disease learn to discern symptoms, such as shortness of breath, peripheral edema, fatigue, exercise or activity intolerance, and act on those changes. Patients are taught to self-adjust medication to manage symptoms or access health care resources to prevent emergency and life-threatening exacerbations. Daily self-care management requires that the patient has decision-making capabilities—monitoring and accurately identifying those subtle changes in symptoms, integrating that cue with action needed, and taking appropriate action.

Cognitive impairments contribute to the difficulty patients have in learning and practicing self-care behaviors. Frontal and temporal lobe dysfunction manifested in learning and memory loss likely influences knowledge attainment and retention, evidenced by difficulty in day-to-day adherence behaviors. Impairment in executive function attributed to subcortical damage may contribute to problems with complex decision-making processes through loss of memory, attention, and problem-solving skills needed to integrate self-care behaviors with symptom meaning.

According to Artinian,[58] "self-care is based on the acquisition of appropriate knowledge." Yet for the many patients with cognitive deficits, the gap between patient education, knowledge attainment, and adherence demonstrates the need for alternative and creative patient teaching strategies. Bridging this gap may include variation in messages, using audiotapes, pictures, etc. to enhance learning[59] or extending the patient education process into the home by including the family and other supporters in the learning process.

A great deal of success has been reported in self-care interventions that extend the patient education process beyond discharge. Interventions with multiple patient encounters, either home-based or specialized clinic programs, have been shown to improve self-care behaviors.[60] This success may be attributed in part to reinforcement of patient teaching and self-care instructions, clarification of misconceptions, and correction of behaviors. For example, hypertensive patients are often instructed to restrict the salt in their diet. These instructions may include an example to avoid canned soup or lunch meats in addition to choosing low-salt alternatives. For patients with a deficit in learning and memory, they may recall the specific instruction to avoid canned soup and sandwiches and therefore believe that a meal that includes fried chicken or pizza is within their dietary guidelines. An in-home visit by a nurse can reinforce the dietary restrictions after hospital discharge by reviewing the patient's specific food choices and correcting any misconceptions. Individualized patient teaching is more likely to be effective in patients with cognitive impairment since they are often unable to extrapolate specifics from generalities, such as "restrict your salt" or "eat only low-salt foods."

Remote interventions using mail and telephonic-based nurse encounters or telephonic weight and symptom monitoring have also resulted in significant improvement in self-care behaviors, knowledge, and hospital readmissions. Reminding the patient of important behaviors, such as blood pressure monitoring, medication taking, or dietary guidelines, by an outreach phone call or mailing is a prompt to the cognitively impaired patient. A telephone call may also provide an opportunity for them to ask questions. For patients with cognitive deficits that affect executive functions (such as flexibility in thinking), remote interventions also can assist in complex decision making by reinforcing symptoms and actions. The importance of patient education delivered as a component of disease management programs has emerged in successful home-based interventions that extend over a period of time because it allows information to be individualized and reinforced to patients with memory or attention deficits (see the accompanying Technology feature on Heart Messages).

CONCLUSION

Lack of knowledge about cardiovascular disease and how to perform self-care is widely recognized as a significant barrier to patient self-care.[27] Numerous patient education studies have demonstrated that education and support from a nurse in the hospital or at home can significantly increase self-care behaviors, especially when the patient teaching is individualized. However, cardiovascular patients pose a unique challenge to nurse educators. Teaching plans need to be developed that consider their special learning needs related to sensory impairments, cognitive deficits, and literacy level,

---

■ ■ ■ TECHNOLOGY

INNOVATION IN PATIENT EDUCATION: HEART MESSAGES

Heart messages is an innovative patient education tool designed as a computerized tailored message intervention that is delivered via the Internet. Heart messages is based on the health belief model which specifies that the likelihood that an individual will perform a specific health behavior depends on the individual's desire to prevent illness (or to get well) and the belief that a particular action will prevent illness or improve health. The program first asks patients to complete three surveys on diet beliefs, medication beliefs, self-monitoring beliefs, and a demographic survey. Then based on the patient's responses to those surveys, the program tailors the messages, pictures, and audio bytes that are delivered to the patient. Branching allows each patient's perceptions of the benefits of and barriers to dietary restriction, medication compliance, and self-monitoring behaviors to guide the presentation of tailored information. For example, if a black woman perceived foods on a low-sodium diet to lack flavor, information will be presented describing alternatives to salt that enhance the flavor of food, accompanied by a photograph of a black woman eating a healthy selection of foods. The program design allows the patient to progress at his or her own pace. Copies of the messages can be printed for patients to keep.

Advantages of the heart messages web-based program extend beyond the tailored messaging that is likely to increase the saliency of the information and enhance compliance behaviors. Presentation of information in alternative formats, such as pictures and audio bytes, and the repetition of information will accommodate visual impairments and cognitive deficits, such as poor attention, concentration, and memory. The program is written at a fifth grade reading level that will help low-literacy patients. In addition to the use of pictures and audio bytes, individuals can learn at their own pace and return to previous material that further facilitates learning.

Bennett S, Hays L, Embree J: Heart messages: a tailored message intervention for improving heart failure outcomes, *J Cardiovasc Nurs* 4:94-105, 2000.

in addition to the cultural factors that influence their individual beliefs and perceptions of illness.

Self-care practices of adherence with complex medication regimens, dietary modifications, and symptom management are critical to managing cardiovascular disease and optimizing outcomes. However, these self-care measures, which frequently involve the need to change lifelong behaviors, pose an extraordinary challenge. Therefore, effective patient teaching will incorporate the patient's readiness to change behavior and processes of change. For those patients who are not ready to learn or change behavior, counseling techniques, such as motivational interviewing, are most effective. Patient education aimed at improving knowledge about cardiovascular disease and self-care and motivating behavior change provides patients with the tools they need to successfully practice self-care that ultimately can improve cardiovascular outcomes.

REFERENCES

1. American Heart Association: Heart Disease and Stroke Statistics - 2005 Update, Dallas, 2004, American Heart Association.
2. Bennett S, Sauve M: Cognitive deficits in patients with heart failure: a review of the literature, *J Cardiovasc Nurs* 8:146-169, 2003.
3. Johnston S, O'Meara E, Manolia T et al: Cognitive impairment and decline are associated with carotid artery disease in patients without clinically evident cerebrovascular disease, *Ann Intern Med* 140:237-247, 2004.
4. Harrington F, Saxby B, McKeith I et al: Cognitive performance in hypertensive and normotensive older subjects, *Hypertension* 36:1079-1082, 2000.
5. Murray M, Lane K, Gao S et al: Preservation of cognitive function with antihypertensive medications: a longitudinal analysis of a community-based sample of African-Americans, *Ann Intern Med* 162:2090-2096, 2002.
6. Agency for Research and Quality: Medical expenditure panel survey, 1996.
7. Benson A, Latter S: Implementing health promoting nursing: the integration of interpersonal skills and health promotion, *J Adv Nurs* 27:100-107, 1998.
8. Knox D: Learning theories. In McEwen M, Wills E, editors: *Theoretical basis for nursing*, Philadelphia, 2002, Lippincott Williams & Wilkins.
9. Bandura A: *Social foundations of thought and action: a social cognitive theory*, Englewood Cliffs, NJ, 1986, Prentice Hall.
10. Prochaska J, Norcross J, DiClemente C: *Changing for good: a revolutionary six-stage program for overcoming bad habits and moving your life positively forward*, New York, 1994, Avon Books, Inc.
11. Jayne R, Rankin S: Application of Leventhals self-regulation model to Chinese immigrants with type 2 diabetes, *J Nurs Scholarsh* 33:53-59, 2001.
12. American Academy of Family Physicians. AAFP core educational guidelines: patient education, *Am Fam Physician* 62:1712, 2000.
13. Knowles M: *The modern practice of adult education: from pedagogy to andragogy*, New York, 1980, Cambridge.
14. Miller N, Dollard J: *Social learning and imitation*, New Haven, Conn, 1941, Yale University Press.
15. Bloom B: *All our children learning*, New York, 1980, McGraw-Hill.
16. Clark J, Lan V: Heart failure patient learning needs after hospital discharge, *Appl Nurs Res* 17:150-157, 2004.
17. Kolb D: *Experiential learning: experiences as the source of learning and development*, Englewood Cliffs, NJ, 1984, Prentice-Hall.
18. Langlais O, Shohet L: Part 2: Report on the needs assessment at the Montreal General Hospital. In Health literacy project, phase 1: needs assessment of the health education and information needs of hard-to-reach patients, Quebec, 2001, The Centre for Literacy.
19. Thesis S, Johnson J: Strategies for teaching patients: a meta-analysis, *Clin Nurse Spec* 9:100-5, 1995.
20. Coller A, Sumodi V, Wilkinson S et al: Nurse's knowledge of heart failure education principles, *Heart Lung* 31:102-112, 2002.
21. van Dam H, van der Horst F, van den Borne B et al: Provider-patient interaction in diabetes care: effects on patient self-care and outcomes: a systematic review, *Patient Educ Couns* 51:17-28, 2003.
22. Collins T, Clark J, Petersen L et al: Racial differences in how patients perceive physician communication regarding cardiac testing, *Med Care* 40:127-134, 2002.
23. Scott J, Thompson D: Assessing the information needs of post-myocardial infarction patients: a systematic review, *Patient Educ Couns* 50:167-177, 2003.
24. Dunbar S, Jacobson L, Deaton C: Heart failure: strategies to enhance patient self-management, *AACN Clin Issues* 9:244-56, 1998.
25. Ni H, Nauman D, Burgess D et al: Factors influencing knowledge of and adherence to self-care among patients with heart failure, *Arch Intern Med* 159:1613-1619, 1999.
26. Bandura A: A social cognitive approach to the exercise of control over AIDS infection. In DiClemente C, editor: *Adolescents and AIDS: a generation in jeopardy*, Beverly Hills, California, 1991, Sage.
27. Riegel B, Carlson B: Facilitators and barriers to heart failure self-care, *Patient Educ Couns* 46:287-295, 2002.
28. van der Bijl J, Shortridge-Baggett L: The theory and measurement of the self-efficacy construct, *Sch Inq Nurs Pract* 15:189-207, 2001.
29. Bandura A, Cervone D: Self-evaluative and self-efficacy mechanisms governing the motivational effects of goal systems, *J Pers Soc Psychol* 45:1017-1028, 1983.
30. Lazarus R, Folkman S: *Stress, appraisal and coping*, New York, 1984, Springer.
31. Johnson J, Roberts C, Cox C et al: Breast cancer patients' personality style, age, and treatment decision making, *J Surg Onc* 63, 1996.
32. Peterson L, Nordin K, Glimelius B et al: Differential effects of cancer rehabilitation depending on diagnosis and patients' cognitive coping style, *Psychosom Med* 64:971-980, 2002.
33. Johnson J: Self-regulation theory and coping with physical illness, *Res Nurs Health* 22:435-448, 1999.
34. Johnson J, Morrissey J, Leventhal H: Psychological preparation for an endoscopic examination, *Gastrointest End* 19:180-182, 1973.
35. Velicer W, Prochaska J, Fava J et al: Smoking cessation and stress management: applications of the transtheoretical model of behavior change, *Homeost Health Dis* 38:216-233, 1998.
36. Duran LS: Motivating health: strategies for the nurse practitioner, *J Am Acad Nurse Pract* 15:200-5, 2003.
37. Paul S, Sneed N: Strategies for behavior change in patients with heart failure, *Amer J Crit Care* 13:305-313, 2004.
38. Miller W, Rollnick S: *Motivational interviewing: preparing people for change*, ed 2, New York, 2002, Guilford.
39. Shinitzky H, Kub J: The art of motivating behavior change: the use of motivational interviewing to promote health, *Public Health Nurs* 18:178-185, 2001.
40. Kushner PR, Levinson W, Miller WR: Motivational interviewing: what, when and why, *Patient Care* 32:55-72, 1998.
41. Emmons K, Rollnick S: Motivational interviewing in health care settings: opportunities and limitations, *Am J Prev Med* 20:68-74, 2001.
42. Lethbridge-Cejku M, Schiller J, Bernadel L: Summary health statistics for US adults: national health interview survey, 2002. National Center for Health Statistics *Vital Health Statistics* 10, 2004.
43. Kirsch I, Jungeblut A, Jenkins L et al: Adult literacy in America: a first look at the findings of the national adult literacy survey. National Center for Education Statistics, 1993. 2002.
44. Brown B, Prisuta R, Jacobs B et al: Literacy of older adults in America: results from the national adult literacy survey. National Center for Education Statistics, 1996.

45. Schillinger D, Grumbach K, Piette J et al: Association of health literacy with diabetes outcomes, *JAMA* 288, 2002.

46. Chew L, Bradley K, Boyko E: Brief questions to identify patients with inadequate health literacy, *Fam Med* 36:588-594, 2004.

47. Rankin S, Stallings K, London F: *Patient education in health and illness,* ed 5, Philadelphia, 2005, Lippincott Williams & Wilkins.

48. DeWalt D, Pignone M, Malone R et al: Development and pilot testing of a disease management program for low literacy patients with heart failure, *Patient Educ Couns* 55:78-86, 2004.

49. Kleinman A: *Patients and healers in the context of culture,* Berkley, Calif, 1980, University of California Press.

50. George M: The challenge of culturally competent health care: applications for asthma, *Heart Lung* 30:392-400, 2001.

51. Rogers A, Addington-Hill J, Abery A et al: Knowledge and communication difficulties for patients with chronic heart failure: qualitative study, *Br Med J* 321:605-7, 2000.

52. Zuccala G, Onder G, Pedone C et al: Cognitive dysfunction as a major determinant of disability in patients with heart failure: results from a multicentre survey, *J Neurol Neurosurg Psychiatry* 70:109-112, 2001.

53. Trojano L, Incalzi R, Picone C et al: Cognitive impairment: a key feature of congestive heart failure in the elderly, *J Neurol* 250:1456-1463, 2003.

54. Almeida O, Tamai S: Congestive heart failure and cognitive functioning amongst older adults, *Arq Neuropsiquiartr* 59:324-329, 2001.

55. Zuccala G, Onder G, Pedone C et al: Hypotension and cognitive impairment: selective association in patients with heart failure, *Neurology* 57:1986-1992, 2001.

56. Ekman I, Fagerberg B, Skoog I: The clinical implications of cognitive impairment in elderly patients with chronic heart failure, *J Cardiovasc Nurs* 16:47-55, 2001.

57. Cline C, Mjorck-Linne A, Israelsson B et al: Non-compliance and knowledge of prescribed medication in elderly patients with heart failure. *Eur J Heart Fail* 1:145-149, 1999.

58. Artinian N, Magnan M, Sloan M et al: Self-care behaviors among patients with heart failure, *Heart Lung* 31:161-172, 2002.

59. Bennett S, Hays L, Embree J et al: Heart messages: a tailored message intervention for improving heart failure outcomes, *J Cardiovasc Nurs* 14:94-105, 2000.

60. Hershberger R, Hanyu N, Nauman D et al: Prospective evaluation of an outpatient heart failure management program, *J Card Fail* 7:64-74, 2001.

61. National Cancer Institute: Theory at a glance: a guide for health promotion practice. In title?} Bethesda, Md, 2003, National Institutes of Health.

62. Prochaska J, Velicer W: The transtheoretical model of health behavior change, *Am J Health Promot* 12:38-48, 1997.

63. D'Onofrio G, Bernstein E, Rollnick S: Motivating patients for change: a brief strategy for negotiation. In Bernstein E, Bernstein J, editors: *Case studies in emergency medicine and the health of the public,* Boston, 1996, Jones and Bartlett.

64. Bastable S: Gender, socioeconomic, and cultural attributes of the learner. In Bastable S, editor: *Nurse as educator: principles of teaching and learning,* Sudbury, Mass, 1997, Jones and Bartlett Publishers.

65. Kok G, van den Borne B, Mullen P: Effectiveness of health education and health promotion: meta-analysis of effect studies and determinants of effectiveness, *Patient Educ Couns* 30:19-27, 1997.

66. Dracup K, Baker D, Dunbar S et al: Management of heart failure: II counseling, education, and lifestyle modifications (review), *JAMA* 272:1442-1446, 1994.

67. Rankin S, Stallings K, London F: *Patient education: principles and practice,* ed 4, Philadelphia, 2005, Lippincott.

68. Illman J: Patient power, *Nurs Times* 96:28-30, 2000.

69. Department of Health: *The expert patient: a new approach to chronic disease management for the 21st century,* London, 2001, Department of Health.

chapter 84

Promoting Adherence to Treatment

Lorraine S. Evangelista
Nancy A. Pike

CHAPTER ABBREVIATIONS

HBM   Health Belief Model
TPB   Theory of Planned Behavior
TRA   Theory of Reasoned Action
TTM   Transtheoretical Model

Considerable time, effort, and expense have been spent in studying the causes of and treatments for various cardiovascular disorders. Despite advances in health care, people continue to succumb to conditions and complications that could have been prevented or treated. This occurs because the only way that a therapeutic or preventive regimen can be effective, assuming that the patient's condition has been accurately diagnosed and the appropriate treatment prescribed, is if the patient correctly follows the advice given.[1] However, it is widely accepted that this does not occur in many or even most instances.

Patient adherence is a multifactorial phenomenon that has become the topic of intense investigation in recent years. An enormous amount of research on the topic has been produced in the last few decades, illustrating its recognition as an increasingly important aspect of health care.[2] Areas of adherence studied include the full range of behaviors we ask of patients—appointment keeping, medication taking, and other lifestyle, treatment, and preventative health practices. The different types of nonadherence are summarized in Box 84-1. Nonadherence in any of these areas can affect the health of the individual and the health care system itself, depending on the seriousness of the condition and the degree of nonadherence.[3]

Recent research calls for a better understanding of factors that lead to nonadherence and identification of evidenced-based approaches to enhancing patient adherence. A patient-centered approach is needed that focuses on the patient's own ideas about the illness and treatment and the degree of concordance between the perceptions of the patient and the clinician.

The purpose of this chapter is to address the extent and relevance of nonadherence as it affects cardiovascular patients, to review the various patient, treatment, and provider factors associated with adherence to cardiovascular therapeutic regimens, to describe selected evidence-based models of behavioral change, and to summarize evidenced-based strategies that promote adherence in cardiovascular patients.

CONCEPTS AND ISSUES IN ADHERENCE
Defining Key Terms

Two terms often are used to describe performance of medically or psychologically prescribed behaviors: compliance and adherence. The classic, and most frequently cited, description is from Haynes who defined compliance as "the extent to which a person's behavior (in terms of taking medications, following diets, or executing lifestyle changes) coincides with medical advice.[2]" The term compliance has traditionally meant that the patient has to do as she or he is told by the clinician without taking into account the patient's concerns. In contrast, adherence implies a more active and collaborative involvement of the patient, working together with the clinician in planning and implementing the treatment regimen. Adherence implies awareness of and agreement to adopt a behavior (Figure 84-1). Whereas compliance seems to connote conformity and acquiescence to the demands of a health care professional, adherence suggests a more self-motivated perseverance with a treatment regimen. The term compliance also attributes more power to the provider in the provider-patient relationship, whereas adherence levels the relationship, to some extent. Table 84-1 compares these two common terms.

Adherence and nonadherence are far more nuanced than the terms would lead us to believe. Nonadherence may be the intentional result of a rational decision based on personal beliefs about the illness and treatment, or nonadherence may be the unintentional consequences of lack of ability to manage the treatment regimen. For example, it is not uncommon for some patients (e.g., elders) to have comorbid illnesses that cause functional and cognitive limitations. Significant declines in memory, attention, and executive function over time affect awareness of and ability to adopt or maintain a behavior. These specific cognitive issues will influence how patients make decisions to adhere to therapy and therefore need to be addressed.

BOX 84-1 ■■■
TYPES OF NONADHERENCE

- Delay in seeking care (population at risk)
- Nonparticipation in health programs (screening)
- Breaking of appointments (follow-up)
- Failure to follow physician's instructions (treatment)

Vermeire E, Hearnshaw H, Van Royen P et al: Patient adherence to treatment: three decades of research. A comprehensive review, *J Clin Pharm Therapeutics* 26:331-42, 2001.

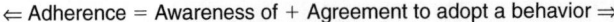

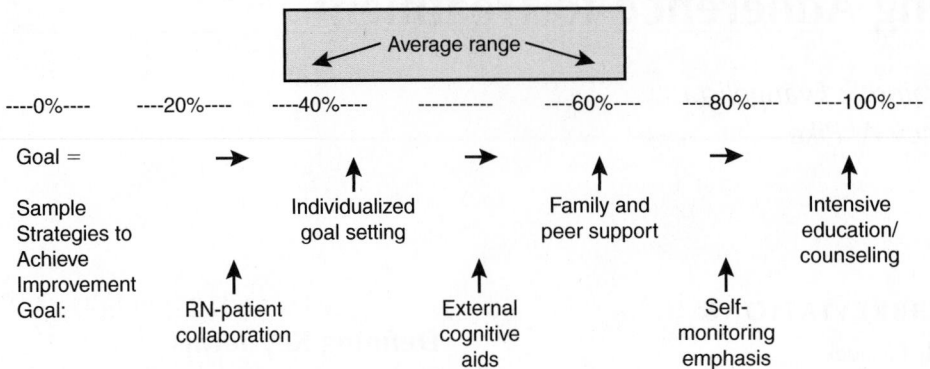

FIGURE 84-1 ▪ The sliding scale of adherence.

On the other hand, if a patient is aware of, but does not agree to adopt or maintain a recommended behavior, this can be described as noncompliance. That is a collaborative decision has not been reach about the behavior in question. True adherence depends on an interaction between the patient and the provider to ensure that the patient is fully informed regarding choices. This interaction should not reflect a value judgment regarding the patient's choice, but a validation of whether or not that choice was a fully informed choice.

Finally, when patient awareness of and agreement to adopt a behavior are both present, then this scenario appropriately may be labeled adherence. Periodic problem solving may occur as the patient and provider collaborate to meet the patient's self-care goals. Patients may not be satisfied with their ability to adhere to their own choices and may seek support from the provider and the team. In this chapter, consistent with recent literature that emphasizes collaboration, active participation, and self-control, we will use the less authoritarian term, adherence rather than compliance, whenever possible.

Extent and Significance of Nonadherence

Despite the plethora of highly effective and relatively safe therapies for various cardiovascular diseases, patients continue to be incapacitated or debilitated by conditions for which effective treatments are available. The process of seeking, receiving, and following treatments and advice has many stages and many opportunities for nonadherence. Highly advanced medical procedures and treatments are of limited use in improving health care status if the patient neglects to follow the recommendations provided. Likewise, although the risky behaviors associated with cardiovascular disease are known, millions of people continue to smoke, drink excessive amounts of alcohol, eschew exercise, and eat a high-fat, high-cholesterol, and high-salt diet. Several large-scale reviews of adherence in relation to cardiovascular disease have been published.[3-9]

Although the level of patient nonadherence in the general population varies depending on the definition of adherence, the medical condition, the treatment regimen, setting, and population, the available data suggest that the rates of nonadherence are alarmingly high. Poor adherence is estimated to involve 30 percent to 50 percent of all patients, irrespective of disease, prognosis, or setting.[10] In a comprehensive review of 256 articles reporting on studies of patient adherence, Sackett and Haynes suggested nonadherence rates between 20 percent and 60 percent,[11] whereas Dunbar-Jacob and colleagues report that between 20 percent and 80 percent of patients do not adhere to the basic requirements of their medical treatment regimen.[12] In a similar report, Burke and colleagues found nonadherence rates ranging from 15 percent to 90 percent in cardiovascular patients.[4] Haynes indicated that patients not only fail to seek medical attention, they also most likely will not stay in care or adhere with follow-up appointments more than 50 percent of the time.[13]

High rates of nonadherence have been consistently documented across all ages, ethnic groups, and socioeconomic strata. Patients of both genders are nonadherent, as are those with minor and severe medical problems. Nonadherence is costly; it wastes medical expertise and health care resources and is hazardous to patients. Nonadherence is an important impediment to the effectiveness of an intervention. The gap between efficacy (an effect under ideal conditions) and effectiveness (the effect in the general population) widens as nonadherence increases.

Nonadherence can have a profound effect not only on the individual patient's health status, but also on the health care system. The medical and economic implications of adherence go hand in hand. Although nonadherence-associated costs for specific issues vary widely, they are nearly universally high.[14] Nonadherence with a medi-

TABLE 84-1 COMPARING COMMON TERMS

	ADHERENCE	COMPLIANCE
Emphasis	Collaboration	Authoritarian
Focus	Patient-centered	Clinician-driven
Goal	Informed choice	Unquestioned performance
Outcome	Self-management	Clinician control

cation that is crucial to the maintenance of vital physiological functions is more likely to have serious consequences than a medicine intended for symptomatic relief and whose use can be optional.[6] Nonadherence results in tangible and intangible costs, such as patient suffering and death, provider and patient frustration and anger, and hopelessness. Nonadherence in patients enrolled in clinical trials can result in incorrect scientific research and clinical conclusions, which can undermine conclusions about the efficacy of treatments for future patients.[1] As such, nonadherence is truly a public health problem of serious proportion.

The effect of nonadherence on quality of life has been explored, but it remains poorly understood. Investigators have varying views of whether good or bad quality of life is a trigger for nonadherence or a consequence. Does the relationship work in two directions? Nonadherence may decrease quality of life, through negative health effects, or improve quality of life, by adapting the treatment schedule to fit a person's personal lifestyle. The relationship between nonadherence and quality of life needs further examination.

Variations in reports of nonadherence are related to difficulties in measuring adherence. Although it is beyond the scope of this chapter to review the various assessment tools used in adherence research, the more common approaches used in clinical practice and research are summarized in Box 84-2.[15] Interestingly, the rates of adherence to specific behaviors has been found to vary depending on cardiovascular disease characteristics. A brief summary of adherence rates for patients with coronary heart disease, heart failure, and hypertension is presented in the subsequent sections to further emphasize the point that wide variations exist in the levels and degrees of adherence among different patient populations.

BOX 84-2
METHODS OF MEASURING ADHERENCE

Subjective Reports
- Patient self-report
- Family member reports
- Health care provider reports

Biological Indicators
- Blood levels of medications
- Blood serum levels of targeted substances
- Medication tracers

Indirect Measurements
- Pill counts
- Prescription refill records
- Electronic medication monitoring

Direct Measurements
- Appointment keeping
- Physical activity monitors

Clinical Outcomes
- Hospitalization
- Disease severity
- Treatment response

Christiansen AJ: *Patient adherence to medical treatment regimens*, New Haven, Conn, 2004, Yale University Press.

Coronary Heart Disease

The extent of behavior and lifestyle modification required of patients with coronary heart disease depends upon their baseline risk factors. Nonadherence is common in general risk-reduction strategies. Nonadherence to the low-fat, low-cholesterol, low-sodium cardiac diet frequently recommended to coronary heart disease patients ranges from 15 percent to 88 percent.[12] Adherence to instructions to lose weight is *less than* 50 percent with long-term success of only 10 percent.[2] Drop-out rates for cardiac rehabilitation and preventative exercise programs averages 50 percent.[4,12] The risk for coronary heart disease is reduced by more than 50 percent after 1 year of smoking cessation,[16] but despite this benefit, adherence to smoking cessation is *less than* 50 percent, and long-term success is only 10 percent.[17]

Nonadherence rates for follow-up medical appointments in coronary heart disease patients range from 8.5 percent to 63.4 percent.[12] Even patients with cardiac symptoms often delay for hours before seeking treatment. In a review of the research related to delays in treatment-seeking behavior of patients with symptoms of acute myocardial infarction conducted over the past 2 decades, 26 percent to 44 percent of patients delayed longer than 4 hours.[18] See Chapter 51 for further discussion of delay in seeking care.

Heart Failure

For patients with heart failure, nonadherence with medications and diet restrictions exposes the patients to clinical destabilization, which can exacerbate symptoms and lead to acute hospitalization. As discussed in Chapter 64, 21 percent to 64 percent of patients who experienced heart failure exacerbation and hospitalization reported nonadherence with medication and diet.[19,20] Medication nonadherence rates between 10 percent and 96 percent have been reported in this population.[21,22] Adherence with a sodium-restricted diet varies from 50 percent to 88 percent; adherence with prescribed fluid restriction may be as low as 23 percent.[23] Adherence with daily weighing ranged from 12 percent to 75 percent in the various studies. In one study, although 87 percent of the patients had weighing scales, only 40 percent or less weighed themselves regularly.[24]

Long delays in care seeking have also been reported in patients with heart failure. Patients experiencing worsening symptoms delayed between one half day to 7 days, on average, before coming to the hospital.[25] In a similar study, Evangelista and colleagues reported that the mean time from the onset of worsening symptoms to the arrival at the hospital was $2.93 \pm .68$ days (70.5 hours).[26]

Hypertension

Although blood pressure control can significantly reduce the risk of stroke and myocardial infarction, hypertension is commonly associated with nonadherence, probably because it is often asymptomatic. Studies have shown that hypertensive patients have a six times higher rate of nonadherence than patients with angina.[27] The lack of adherence to prescribed antihypertensive medication has contributed to uncontrolled hypertension worldwide.[9]

Medication nonadherence for patients with treated hypertension is estimated to be between 30 percent and 50 percent.[4] Only half of patients with hypertension adhere to their prescribed dietary regimen and follow-up appointments.[27] Nonadherence in the form of delays in seeking treatment for care also has been documented in patients with elevated blood pressure. Following community screening for high blood pressure, 35 percent to 49 percent of those whose blood pressures were elevated failed to follow through with a referral for follow-up assessment. Once assessed and prescribed therapy, more than one third of patients drop out of care entirely, especially in the early months following their initial diagnosis.[13]

Section Summary

Nonadherence is rampant in cardiovascular patients, although the extent of nonadherence remains unclear because of wide variability in estimates. It is difficult to compare adherence rates between studies because of differences in measured outcomes, adherence measures, and patient characteristics. However, most studies support the statement that poor adherence is a widespread phenomenon in cardiovascular patients. On average, one third to one half of all patients is nonadherent,[15] leading to failure to achieve the goals of prevention and cure. As medical care becomes more sophisticated and efficacious in treating and preventing cardiovascular disease, patient adherence becomes more crucial.

Determinants of Adherence and Nonadherence

Many social and psychological factors are thought to influence adherence, with varying degrees of agreement among researchers. These factors will be discussed under three categories (patient, treatment, and provider), although some factors overlap, and it is difficult to isolate them. Examples of specific variables in each category are summarized in Box 84-3.[28]

Patient Factors

Most studies fail to find a clear association between adherence and patients' sociodemographic characteristics. For example, there is no consistent pattern of an association between adherence, gender, and age.[22] In some conditions, higher education and higher social class have been shown to contribute to greater levels of adherence. Further, even when associations are found, the direction of these associations has been inconsistent among studies.[22] Inconsistent findings may be attributed in part to different research designs, different study populations, and different forms of adherence measures.

The fact that many researchers have not been able to identify potentially nonadherent patients suggests that

---

> ### BOX 84-3
> #### DETERMINANTS OF NONADHERENCE
>
> **Personal Factors**
> - Knowledge and understanding of treatment regimen
> - Perceptions related to their illness and self-control over their condition
> - Beliefs and attitude toward the regimen
> - Doubts about expected benefit and efficacy of treatment
> - Support from spouse, family, and peers
> - Depression
>
> **Treatment-Related Factors**
> - Severity and duration of treatment
> - Complexity of treatment regimens
> - Number and costs of medications
> - Frequency of medication dosing
>
> **Provider-Related Factors**
> - Provider-patient communication
> - Patient empowerment
> - Inadequate follow-up and support from provider
> - Poor adherence of providers to adhere to evidenced-based clinical guidelines

Oldridge NB: Future directions: what paths do researchers need to take? What needs to be done to improve multi-level compliance? In Burke LE, Ockene JK, editors: *Compliance in healthcare and research,* Armonk, NY, 2001, Futura Publishing Company, Inc, pp 331-47.

sociodemographic characteristics are a poor explanation for adherence behaviors. However, authors of previous literature reviews have concluded that a wide assortment of patient-related factors, beyond sociodemographic characteristics, affect adherence in treatment of patients with heart disease. These factors include knowledge and understanding, perceptions related to their illness and self-control over their condition, beliefs and attitude toward the treatment regimen, and availability of support.

Knowledge of the medical condition does not increase adherence, but knowledge of the regimen does. Patients cannot be expected to fully and accurately follow through on treatment recommendations unless they understand and remember instructions about the regimen. Several studies have examined the degree to which patients understand and remember the clinician's instructions.

In a substudy of the medical outcomes study, conducted to determine recall of and adherence to physicians' recommendations among patients with chronic medical conditions, most patients failed to recall potentially important elements of medical advice.[29] Most of the patients (1291 of 1751) included in the study had heart disease. Among those who could recall the medical advice, they did not always adhere with that advice.[29] In a similar study, the extent of medication information recall and nonadherence to prescribed medication were examined in elderly patients with heart failure.[30] All patients received standardized verbal and written information regarding their medication, but only 12 (55 percent) could correctly name what medication had been prescribed, 11 (50 percent) were unable to state the prescribed doses, and 14 (64 percent) could not describe when the medication was to be taken.[30] This more recent, albeit smaller, study confirms that nonadherence is common in elders with heart failure and that failure to recall instructions adequately may influence adherence.

Another set of factors that influence patients' ability and willingness to carry out recommendations are psychosocial factors. Beliefs and attitudes, reactions to and perceptions of the illness, perceived control over the condition, support from family and others, and financial circumstances all have a profound impact on treatment adherence. Doubts about the expected benefits and efficacy of treatment, real or perceived barriers including side effects and financial constraints, unique demands of the regimen itself, and lack of help and support from family members and peers can all influence adherence.[31]

An important factor contributing to nonadherence is patients' unresolved concerns. These concerns may be related to the diagnosis, the absence of symptoms, failure to perceive a benefit in the interval between taking the drug and its effect, and the fear of adverse effects. Patients' beliefs about medications and about medicine in general are extremely influential. Their own knowledge, ideas, and experiences, in addition to those of family members and friends, correlate strongly with adherence. Patients' perceptions of increased disease severity is significantly related to the likelihood of adherence in some studies.[32] Clinical depression also accounts for an appreciable amount of nonadherence, probably because of the hopelessness, social isolation, fatigue, and cognitive impairment that accompany depression.[33] In one study, depressed elders with coronary artery disease were adherent on 45 percent of days compared with 69 percent of days for nondepressed patients.[34]

Treatment Factors

Other possible reasons for nonadherence include features of the disease itself, its diagnosis and severity, and its symptoms and chronicity. Although it seems logical that when failure to follow medical advice would be most harmful, patient adherence would be greatest; in many instances, this does not seem to be the case. A classic review by Haynes failed to find that features of the disease were important determinants of adherence, except for two important findings. First, increasing symptoms may be accompanied by decreasing adherence, but increased disability may be associated with increased adherence.[2]

Other factors related to low adherence include the duration of treatment, the number of medications prescribed, the cost of the regimen, and the frequency of dosing. Generally, the higher the duration, number, cost, and frequency of drug dosing, the lower the adherence.[3] Higher levels of adherence are achieved with more circumscribed regimens (medication taking as opposed to dietary changes). On the other hand, patients with more complex treatment regimens were less likely to adhere to their recommended care.[1] Most of the treatment-related factors examined are inconsistently correlated with adherence and thus cannot be used to adequately predict adherent behavior.

Provider Factors

Until recently, adherence had been viewed as purely a patient-related phenomenon. When considering the various patient characteristics that had been thought to be associated with nonadherence, however, clearly other factors must be taken into consideration. There is growing consensus that the behavior of the health care provider influences patient adherence.[3]

Recent efforts to understand the problem of nonadherence have focused on the interaction between the clinician and the patient. Although the patient and clinician share responsibility for the exchange of information, greater responsibility in this interchange lies with the clinician. It is the responsibility of the clinician to learn the necessary communication skills to adequately convey information to the patient. Communication skill involves more than simply conveying verbal information to the patient. Rather, attention must also be given to nonverbal aspects of communication and an understanding of the psychological, social, cultural, and situational variables that will either facilitate or impede the communication process.

Clinicians who provide consistent care within a truly caring relationship have higher adherence rates in their patients. This suggests that nonadherence is a problem in patient care and the treatment regimen. The provider's attitude towards the patient and his or her ability to elicit and respect the patient's concerns, to provide appropriate information, and to demonstrate empathy influence adherence.[3] Providers need to shift the emphasis away from attempting to persuade patients to follow their advice and toward a collaborative, problem-solving approach in which they contribute to patients' decisions about treatment adherence (see the accompanying Conundrum feature). Likewise, we need to understand that nonadherence may represent a rational choice made by patients to maintain their personal identity, achieve their goals, and preserve their quality of life.[1]

Section Summary

Although considerable time and effort have been and continue to be spent studying patient adherence and the variables that affect it, we remain unable to predict which patients will adhere and which will not. A variety

---

■■■ CONUNDRUM

PROMOTING ADHERENCE

Many clinicians believe that they have done their job in promoting adherence when they have instructed the patient on the need for, and details of, the regimen. However, simple instruction alone has little lasting effect on long-term adherence. Clinicians often believe that patients who have *sought* care from us must follow our advice. We need to understand, however, that patients have the right to refuse treatment and that this right must be respected. Coercing or intimidating patients to adhere does not work as well as positive reinforcement and supportive reminders. In fact, the paternalistic approach causes some patients with high anxiety levels to withdraw from care.

of factors determine an individual's reaction to illness and consequently, their reactions to the recommendations and advice given. Each patient has a personal, unique perspective on health, illness, and medical care. An understanding of how patient, treatment, and provider factors affect patient adherence is crucial to adequately addressing adherence behaviors.

EVIDENCED-BASED MODELS OF BEHAVIOR CHANGE

Behavioral change is required at nearly every stage of the medical process and for virtually every type of health-related intervention. Whether a medical intervention requires a patient to follow a prescribed medication regimen, make a dietary or other lifestyle change, or simply attend a clinic appointment, patient behavioral adherence is a necessary condition for safe, effective, and cost-efficient health care delivery.

Clearly, behavior can be changed, and those changes can influence health. Interventions designed to teach health-promoting behaviors and attenuate risky behaviors are often successful. However, maintaining behavioral change over time and across settings remains a problem. Health professionals have turned to models of behavioral change to guide the development of strategies that foster self-protective action, reduce risky behaviors, and facilitate effective adaptation to and coping with illness.

The role of patient beliefs or cognitions in influencing health-related behavior has held a prominent place in health behavior theory and research over three decades. Many theoretical models (e.g., health belief model, theory of reasoned action and theory of planned behavior, and transtheoretical model) focus on understanding, predicting, and improving adherence. As a group, these models suggest that programs that effectively change individual health behavior require a multifaceted approach to helping people adopt, change, and maintain behavior.[33] This section of the chapter provides a brief outline of selected behavior change models and provides examples of where they have been applied to adherence research. A summary of each model is provided in Box 84-4.

Health Belief Model

One of the earliest theoretical models developed for understanding health behavior is the health belief model.[35] This model was developed in the 1950s to explain why people failed to take up disease prevention measures or screening tests before the onset of symptoms to prevent or detect disease early. The original model proposed that the likelihood of someone carrying out a specific health behavior was a function of personal beliefs about the perceived threat of the disease (which is derived from beliefs about perceived seriousness of the threat and the individual's perceived susceptibility to it) and an assessment of the risk and benefits of the recommended course of action.

The health belief model has been modified several times to include additional variables, such as cues to ac-

---

> ### BOX 84-4
> ### SUMMARY OF MODELS OF BEHAVIOR CHANGE ■ ■ ■
>
> **Health Belief Model**
> The fundamental presupposition of the model is that individuals are rational decision makers who select a course of action after systematically evaluating and comparing the values and probabilities associated with each possible alternative.[35]
>
> **Theory of Reasoned Action**
> This theory examines the relationships between attitudes and behavior and takes account of social influences on behavior then explains how perceived threat and cost-benefit analysis are translated to action.[37]
>
> **Theory of Planned Behavior**
> This theory is a slightly reformulated version of the TRA in which the individual's perceived degree of control over a behavior is considered in addition to the social norm and attitudinal components of the theory of reasoned action.[38]
>
> **Transtheoretical Model**
> This behavioral model of change focuses on the concept of "readiness" and characterizes the continuum of steps that people take toward change and include the activities or processes to move people from one stage to another.[41]

tion and general health motivation. An important contribution of the model, which has been used in studies investigating adherence across a range of cardiovascular illnesses, is the recognition that prevention requires people to take action in the absence of illness. A fundamental assumption of the health belief model is that individuals are rational decision makers who select a course of action after systematically evaluating and comparing the values and probabilities associated with each possible alternative.[35]

The health belief model was originally intended as a predictive model for preventive behaviors and as such supported the premise that the likelihood of behavior change is increased if the perceived threat is high, if the benefits of behavior are thought to outweigh the barriers, and if certain cues are in place. Tests of the model and preventive health practices suggest a modest but fairly consistent association between these health beliefs and behavior. However, evidence regarding the utility of the model in the prediction of medical regimen adherence among patients with existing disease is more limited than is the case for preventive behaviors.[36] Nevertheless, the available evidence implies that our understanding of adherence may be enhanced by examining patients' own ideas about their illness and treatment and suggests that the cognitive variables specified in the health belief model may be prerequisites of adherence in some situations.

Theory of Reasoned Action and Theory of Planned Behavior

Ajzen and Fishbein[37] first proposed the theory of reasoned action to predict an individual's intention to engage in a behavior at a specific time and place. The theory examines the relationships between attitudes and behavior and takes account of social influences on behavior; it then explains how perceived threat and cost-benefit analysis are translated to action. The theory of reasoned action was intended to explain virtually all behaviors over which people have the ability to exert self-control. Factors that influence behavioral choices are mediated through the variable of behavioral intent. Behavioral intentions are influenced by the attitude about the likelihood that the behavior will have the expected outcome and the subjective evaluation of the risks and benefits of that outcome. The value or importance the individual places on how others will react to a behavioral decision is also deemed important. It is the social norm component that most distinguished the theory of reasoned action from the health belief model and other attitudinal or expectancy-based models of health-related behavior.[38]

Perceived behavioral control and perceived barriers have been added to the theory of reasoned action to form the theory of planned behavior.[38] This theory extends the theory of reasoned action to encompass behaviors, which may not be totally under the person's control. In the theory of planned behavior, attitudes and subjective norms exert their influence on behavior indirectly via their effect on intention. As is the case for the health belief model, the theories of reasoned action and planned behavior presume that the individuals engage in a rationalistic weighing of the evidence before coming to a decision.

The combined theory of reasoned action and planned behavior has predictive value in studies of various health behaviors, such as diet, smoking, weight loss, and dental care. More specifically, in the cardiovascular arena, the theory of reasoned action and planned behavior has been useful in predicting adherence to medication prescribed for myocardial infarction[39] and hypertension.[40] However, the two models have been found, almost universally, to be better predictors of behavioral intentions than of the actual target behavior.

Transtheoretical Model

The transtheoretical model (also known as the *stages of change* model) focuses on the concept of "readiness" and characterizes the continuum of steps that people take toward change. This model includes the activities or processes that move people from one stage to another.[41] In this model, the degree of intention to perform a behavior is combined with acquired habits vis-à-vis the behavior. When we consider two individuals who intend to perform a behavior, the one who has experience with the behaviors will be at a more advanced stage than the one who has never performed it.[42]

The earliest stage of behavior change starts with moving from being uninterested, unaware, or unwilling to change (precontemplation) to considering a change (contemplation). This is followed by the decision to take action (preparation) and the first steps toward behavioral change (action). With determined action, the requirement for maintenance and relapses are recognized as part of the process. In addition to these temporal stages, the transtheoretical model includes the concepts of decision criteria, self-efficacy, and change processes (consciousness-raising, relief from negative emotions

associated with unhealthy behavior, self-reevaluation, environmental reevaluation, committing to change, seeking support, substituting healthier alternative behaviors, contingency management, stimulus control, and recognizing supportive social norms).[42] Progress through stages may not be linear; it is more likely to take a cyclical route characterized by many brief or partially successful attempts before behavior change is established. It has been suggested that cognitions may be more important in particular stages than others and that interventions to promote behavior are likely to be more effective if they are targeted at the particular cognitions that characterize the stage that the individual has reached in their thinking about or implementation of the behavior.

The transtheoretical model has been applied to a broad range of behaviors and a wide variety of populations. Sneed and Paul (2003) used it to assess behavior change in patients with heart failure.[43] They suggested that once the patient's stage of readiness has been determined, appropriate strategies be instituted to assist patients to move through the stages. They argue that patients must successfully pass through three stages in which the pros and cons of making the change are considered, thus signifying that the person is prepared for action.[43] If true, perhaps interventions should focus twice as much emphasis on the benefits of change over those that address reducing the costs or barriers to change.[7]

Section Summary

Strong conceptual models are available to guide the development, implementation, and evaluation of health-related behavioral change interventions. Few models provide complete explanations of specific adherence behaviors, and no single model seems to be universally valid. Although the methods are useful constructs for thinking about behavioral change, they each have limitations, and each addresses different behavioral attributes. We have much to learn about how and when to intervene to facilitate adherence to treatment. The capacity of these theoretical models to generate effective interventions has yet to be fully evaluated; this remains a key challenge for future adherence research.

EVIDENCE-BASED STRATEGIES TO INCREASE ADHERENCE

With gradual recognition of the magnitude of the problem of nonadherence and the growing realization that the health professional is in a position to influence that problem, numerous strategies to enhance the likelihood of adherence have been recommended. In this section, a summary of general recommendations for promoting adherence specific to three selected cardiovascular conditions—coronary heart disease, heart failure, and hypertension—is presented. Instead of an exhaustive review of the published literature, an attempt has been made to include those articles that the authors believe have particular lessons for cardiovascular researchers and clinicians.

Coronary Heart Disease

There are multiple risk factors for coronary heart disease with myriad interventions that can be tailored to meet patient specific needs. Most common behavioral and lifestyle modifications in coronary heart disease focus on diet, exercise, smoking cessation, weight loss, and lifestyle and stress management.

Adherence to dietary regimens in cardiovascular disease can be challenging, particularly in culturally diverse populations. Various single and multiple intervention strategies have been employed; common intervention components are educational and behavioral counseling, written information, food diaries, reminder letters, physician prompting, urine monitoring, and spouse participation. A literature review by Newell and colleagues summarized the results of 15 studies addressing dietary adherence;[7] only five reported significant adherence to dietary regimens. These five studies all used patient education with the addition of behavioral counseling in one, the involvement of spouses in two studies, and the addition of self-monitoring of urine in four studies.

Exercise programs for coronary heart disease patients can be preventative or rehabilitative based. Interventions to increase exercise adherence are usually designed around supervised or independent exercise programs. In a review of exercise adherence, interventions included educational and behavior counseling, written educational material, reminder letters, behavioral contracts, audiovisual material, cardiovascular risk assessments, training of patients and spouses, self-monitoring of pulse rates, relaxation techniques, and monitoring feedback.[7] Adherence rates were higher in home verses group programs and in those that used self-monitoring, contractual agreements, and verbal persuasion.[7,8] Adherence declined over time.

Although the cardiovascular effects of cigarette smoking are well established, few clinical trials have focused on smoking cessation in cardiovascular populations. In a review of 12 studies examining smoking cessation interventions, the investigators reported little evidence to support nicotine replacement therapy or other adjuvant therapy and the use of self-help material or various counseling strategies (group, individual, or telephone).[16] Likewise, physician advice and nurse-delivered interventions demonstrated limited effectiveness in smoking cessation. The reasons why smoking cessation interventions are ineffective in cardiovascular patients remain unclear. Some authors have speculated that symptomatic cardiovascular patients (angina, after myocardial infarction, or heart surgery) may be more motivated to quit. The diagnosis of coronary heart disease alone does not appear to be a sufficient motivator for behavioral change.

Lifestyle and stress-management regimens are not frequently studied as part of interventional strategies to increase adherence. Most lifestyle-management interventions focus on providing written or audiovisual material and reminders. Stress-management interventions are usually a combination of educational and behavioral counseling. These interventions have very little or no significant effect on adherence.[7]

The risk-reduction interventions described above use a combination of cognitive, educational, and behavioral strategies. The most successful strategies for improving adherence include behavioral skill training, self-monitoring, telephone and/or mail contact, self-efficacy enhancement, and external cognitive aids.[4] Further randomized controlled clinical trials are necessary to clarify the effectiveness of these strategies in reducing risky behaviors in coronary heart disease patients.

Heart Failure

Several randomized studies designed to improve adherence in persons with heart failure were found in the literature. Hershberger and colleagues described the effect of education and counseling by a nurse in a heart failure clinic on treatment adherence.[44] Their intervention increased knowledge about sodium restriction, but only 35 percent of patients always avoided salty foods, and 52 percent reported reading labels when buying food. In a similar study, patients were educated about heart failure in a clinic visit and during telephone follow-up calls over a 6-month period. This structured diet education from a nurse decreased self-reported sodium intake.[19]

Intensive education and counseling by other members of the health care team also have been studied. Goodyer and Milligan measured the effect of intensive medication counseling by a pharmacist on medication adherence in 100 community-dwelling elders (older than age 70) in a randomized controlled trial.[45] The intervention consisted of three home visits at intervals of 2 to 4 weeks. Patients were given verbal counseling on the correct use of their medications using a standard written protocol, medication calendars, and information leaflets. Improvements in medication adherence ($p < 0.001$) were observed in the experimental group. Mean adherence scores by pill count were 49 percent for the control group and 61 percent for the experimental group. In another study examining the effect of education on diet and sodium restriction by a dietician, a significant decrease in fluid and sodium intake was found in a sample of heart failure patients.[46]

In a study of a nonpharmacological multidisciplinary intervention for heart failure, medication adherence was higher for elderly patients who received comprehensive education about prescribed medications compared with those randomized to a control group (87.9 percent versus 81.1 percent, $p = 0.003$).[47] In another study, medication and dietary adherence were predictive of recurrent symptoms and rehospitalization; those receiving a transitional care intervention were less likely to be rehospitalized.[48]

Hypertension

Hypertensive patients may fail to take their medications for a variety of reasons. Many different strategies have been used to improve medication adherence, but these methods can be complex, labor-intensive, and demonstrate minimal effectiveness.[49] McDonald and colleagues categorized interventions into common themes: patient instruction, increased communication and counseling, increased convenience of care, and involving patients more with self-monitoring, reminders, and rewards for adherence and treatment response.[49] The most common single intervention strategy effective in improving medication adherence was reducing dose frequency.[7,49] Complex multiple intervention strategies found to be effective combined home or work site visits, education information, reminders, written medication planner, drug packaging, support group referrals, and reinforcement.[49]

In a systematic review of adherence to antihypertensive medications, Schroeder and colleagues recommended reducing the number of daily doses as a first-line strategy to improve medication adherence.[9] This once daily dosing intervention, advocated in the medication adherence literature,[7,9,49] has increased adherence in seven of nine studies with a relative increase of 8 percent to 19.6 percent adherence. Patient education alone was unsuccessful with no reported effect on blood pressure. Motivational strategies were partly successful with small increases in adherence. Successful motivational interventions included daily drug reminder charts, training on self-determination, reminders and packaging, social support, nurse telephone calls, family member support, electronic medication aid cap, and telephone-linked computer counseling. Complex interventions increased adherence from 5 percent to 41 percent, but more evidence is needed on their effect through randomized controlled clinical trials.[7,9,49]

The ultimate outcome of medication adherence interventions is improved self-administration of medicines with secondary effects of reduced blood pressure and improved prognosis. Future studies are needed of a tailored approach to individual patients, using a combination of strategies of simplifying dosage regimens, patient motivation, and involvement of clinicians in a patient-centered approach.[9]

Section Summary

Although a large body of literature continues to develop around treatment adherence and methods to improve it, results continue to be contradictory, and few interventions have consistently been shown through rigorous research to improve adherence. Box 84-5 lists strategies shown in research to increase adherence.

Better patient education, aimed at improving patients' understanding of their treatment and their clinician's instructions is suggested as an adherence-enhancing strategy.[5] Patients cannot be expected to ad-

here to a treatment plan that they do not understand. However, patient education alone is dubious as a sole method of promoting adherence. A stronger predictor of improved adherence is the improvement of the clinician-patient relationship. Aspects of this relationship that are conducive to better adherence are clinician friendliness and approachability, clinician-patient cooperation, enhancement of patient centeredness, improved clinician teaching skills, accurate recognition of patients' problems, and taking into account the spiritual and psychological dimensions that may be of primary importance to patients.

Research addressing the way in which clinicians present information suggests that clarifying the link between the treatment and the illness could enhance treatment adherence. Other possibilities lie in the types of medication prescribed and techniques that encourage patients to take the correct dosages. Simplifying prescriptions and prescribing fewer concurrent medications can simplify the therapeutic regimen, but may not necessarily improve adherence unless the complexity of the regimen is one of the patient's concerns.

Some studies of behavioral techniques—differential reinforcement, extinction, shaping, modeling, and desensitization—suggest that these approaches have varying degrees of success in modifying patients' adherence behaviors. Additional factors to consider in helping patients improve adherence to medical regimens include reducing the barriers to adherence by tailoring the treatment and by identifying and helping to resolve difficulties the patient may have that are interfering with adherence. Clinicians are encouraged to increase the level of attention paid to patients who are having adherence difficulties by mobilizing professional and social support. The goal of this strategy is to develop a patient ally who can help ease behavioral change, reduce obstacles to adherence, and be supportive during failures and successes.

Combinations of educational and behavioral strategies have a better effect than either approach used alone. Good verbal communication and one-to-one counseling have a positive effect; written information increases knowledge and decreases medication utilization errors, but has no effect on adherence. On the other hand, written information with verbal reinforcement enhances adherence more than written information alone. Eliciting patients' beliefs is important before providing information. Patients' perceptions may thus be corrected or reinforced. Recall can be aided by presenting treatment instructions in a clear and simple manner, the use of concrete and specific advice, by repeating and stressing the importance of the critical components of the advice, and by checking understanding and by providing feedback.[3]

Although selected programs and interventions have been used with varying degrees of success in increasing adherence, most investigators also conclude that adherence drops when the specific intervention or special program designed to increase it is discontinued. Therefore it seems that any intervention designed to increase adherence, if it is to be effective on a long-term basis, must be ongoing rather than short-term.

BOX 84-5 ■ ■ ■
STRATEGIES TO INCREASE ADHERENCE

- Educational material with verbal reinforcement
- Tailor education to meet individual learning needs
- Simplify medication regimen (number of pills, frequency in dosing, dispensing)
- Identify behavioral barriers
- Elicit individual beliefs about treatment
- Identify lifestyle barriers
- Use of reminder techniques (memory issues)
- Support services (long-term)

Compared with the relatively straightforward research that has established the efficacy of many treatments, research into methods of improving adherence is often difficult and complex. Despite these limitations, there appears to be general consensus that multiple-strategy techniques are more effective than single-strategy techniques, especially with long-term treatments. Strategies could include: involvement of the patient in the negotiation of treatment goals, reduction of the complexity of the treatment regimen, tailoring the treatment to the patient's lifestyle, use of reminders, encouragement of family support, informing patients about side effects, monitoring of adherence, and provision of feedback to the patient.

CHAPTER SUMMARY

Patient adherence is a complex process. Patients' willingness and ability to carry out a regimen are influenced by the regimen's complexity and their knowledge of what to do, but multiple other influences, such as patient attitude and beliefs, values and perceptions, social support systems, and financial barriers, also have a considerable impact. Clearly, many treatment regimens require multiple behaviors, and complex regimens may lead to differential adherence rates for different behaviors. Therefore multidimensional approaches to dealing with the issue of adherence must be considered. Different individuals may be adherent to some behaviors and not others. Moreover, different approaches to increasing adherence may be necessary for different behaviors and for different individuals.

Our knowledge of the link between a specific intervention and subsequent behavior change, in addition to outcomes, is clearly limited. Many more practical and effective behavioral interventions in cardiovascular care are needed to significantly improve health and quality of life in this population. Nevertheless, clinicians need to recognize that each nonadherent patient's unique situation must be examined without resorting to categorization within only one underlying theoretical orientation. Rather, the clinician must appreciate the many interpersonal, familial, cultural, and situational factors that affect each individual. Only when such influences are understood can appropriate clinical interventions be designed and prescribed.

REFERENCES

1. DiMatteo MR: Variations in patients' adherence to medical recommendations: a quantitative review of 50 years of research, *Med Care* 42:200-9, 2004.
2. Haynes RB: Determinants of compliance: the disease and the mechanics of treatment. In Haynes RB, Taylor DW, Sackett DL, editors: *Compliance in health care*, Baltimore, 1979, The Johns Hopkins University Press, pp 49-62.
3. Vermeire E, Hearnshaw H, Van Royen P et al: Patient adherence to treatment: three decades of research. A comprehensive review, *J Clin Pharm Therapeutics* 26:331-42, 2001.
4. Burke LE, Dunbar-Jacobs JM, Hill MN: Compliance with cardiovascular disease prevention strategies: a review of the literature, *Ann Behav Med* 19:239-263, 1997.
5. DiMatteo MR: Variations in patients' adherence to medical recommendations: a quantitative review of 50 years of research, *Med Care* 42:200-209, 2004.
6. McDonald HP, Garg AX, Haynes RB: Interventions to enhance patient adherence to medication prescription: scientific review, *JAMA* 288:2868-2879, 2002.
7. Newell SA, Bowman JA, Cockburn JD: Can compliance with nonpharmacologic treatment for cardiovascular disease be improved? *Am J Prev Med* 18:253-261, 2000.
8. Newell SA, Bowman JA, Cockburn JD: A critical review of interventions to increase compliance with medication taking, obtaining medication refills, and appointment-keeping in the treatment of cardiovascular disease, *Preventative Medicine* 29:535-548, 1999.
9. Schroeder K., Fahey T, Ebrahim S: How can we improve adherence to blood pressure-lowering medication in ambulatory care: systematic review of randomized controlled trials, *Arch Intern Med* 164:722-732, 2004.
10. Sackett DL: The magnitude of compliance and noncompliance. In Haynes RB, Taylor DW, Sackett DL, editors: *Compliance in health care*, Baltimore, 1979, The Johns Hopkins University Press, pp 11-23.
11. Sackett DL, Haynes RB: *Compliance with therapeutic regimens*, Baltimore, 1976, John Hopkins University Press.
12. Dunbar-Jacob J, Erlen J, Schlenk E et al: Adherence in chronic disease, *Annu Rev Nurs Res* 18:48-90, 2000.
13. Haynes RB: Improving adherence: state of the art, with a special focus on medication taking for cardiovascular disorders. In Burke LE, Ockene JK, editors: *Compliance in healthcare and research*, Armonk, NY, 2001, Futura Publishing Co, Inc, pp 3-21.
14. Cleemput I, Kesteloot K, De Geest S: A review of the literature on the economics of noncompliance. Room for methodological improvement, *Health Policy* 59:65-94, 2002.
15. Christiansen AJ: *Patient adherence to medical treatment regimens*, New Haven, Conn, 2004, Yale University Press.
16. Wiggers LC, Smets EMA, de Haes JC et al: Smoking cessation interventions in cardiovascular patients, *Eur J Endovasc Surg* 26:467-75, 2003.
17. Haynes RB, McKibbon KA, Kanani R: Systematic review of randomised trials of interventions to assist patients to follow prescriptions for medications, *Lancet* 348:383-6, 1996.
18. McKinley S, Moser D, Dracup K: Treatment-seeking behavior for acute myocardial infarction symptoms in North America and Australia, *Heart Lung* 29:237-47, 2000.
19. Hamner JB, Ellison KJ: Predictors of hospital readmission after discharge in patients with congestive heart failure, *Heart Lung* 34:231-9, 2005.
20. Gwadry-Sridhar FH, Flintoft V, Lee DS et al: A systematic review and meta-analysis of studies comparing readmission rates and mortality rates in patients with heart failure, *Arch Intern Med* 164:2315-2320, 2004.
21. Cline CM, Bjorck-Linne AK, Israelsson BYA et al: Noncompliance and knowledge of prescribed medication in elderly patients with heart failure, *Eur J Heart Fail* 1:145-9, 1999.
22. Evangelista L, Berg J, Dracup K: Relationship between psychosocial variables and compliance in heart failure patients, *Heart Lung* 30:294-301, 2001.
23. van der Wal M, Jaarsma T, van Veldhuisen D: Non-compliance in patients with heart failure: how can we manage it?, *Eur J Heart Fail* 7:5-17, 2005.
24. de Lusignan S, Wells S, Johnson P et al: Compliance and effectiveness of 1 year's home telemonitoring. The report of a pilot study of patients with chronic heart failure, *Eur J Heart Fail* 3:723-30, 2001.
25. Friedman M: Older adults symptoms and their duration before hospitalization for heart failure, *Heart Lung* 26:169-76, 1997.
26. Evangelista L, Dracup K, Doering L: Treatment-seeking delays in heart failure patients, *J Heart Lung Transplant* 19:932-8, 2000.
27. Hamilton GA: Measuring adherence in a hypertension clinical trial, *Eur J Cardiovasc Nurs* 2:219-28, 2003.
28. Oldridge NB: Future directions: what paths do researchers need to take? What needs to be done to improve multi-level compliance? In Burke LE, Ockene JK, editors: *Compliance in healthcare and research*, Armonk, NY, 2001, Futura Publishing Co Inc, pp 331-47.

29. Kravitz R, Hays R, Sherbourne D et al: Recall of recommendations and adherence to advice among patients with chronic medical conditions, *Arch Intern Med* 153:1869-78, 1993.
30. Cline CM, Israelsson BYA, Willenheimer RB et al: Cost effective management programme for heart failure reduces hospitalisation, *Heart* 80:442-6, 1998.
31. DiMatteo MR, Giordani PJ, Lepper HS et al: Patient adherence and medical treatment outcomes, *Med Care* 40:794-811, 2002.
32. Scotto CJ: The lived experiences of adherence for patients with heart failure, *J Cardiopulm Rehab* 25:158-163, 2005.
33. DiMatteo MR, Martin LR: *Health psychology,* Boston, 2002, Allyn and Bacon.
34. Carney R, Freedland K, Eisen S et al: Major depression and medication adherence in elderly patients with coronary artery disease, *Health Psychology* 14:88-90, 1995.
35. Rosenstock I: The health belief model and preventative behavior, *Health Educ Mongraphs* 2:354-86, 1974.
36. Becker M, Green L: A family approach to medical treatment - a review of literature, *Intern J Health Educ* 18:1-11, 1975.
37. Ajzen I, Fishbein DP: *Understanding attitudes and predicting social behavior,* Englewood Cliffs, NJ, 1980, Prentice Hall.
38. Ajzen I: From intentions to actions: a theory of planned behavior. In Kuhl J, Beckmann J, editors: *Action-control: from cognition to behavior,* Heidelberg, 1985, Springer-Verlag.
39. Miller SP, Johnson NL, Garrett MJ et al: Health beliefs of and adherence to the medical regimen by patients with ischemic heart disease, *Heart Lung* 11:332-9, 1989.
40. Miller NH: Compliance with treatment regimens in chronic asymptomatic diseases, *Am J Med* 102:43-9, 1997.
41. Prochaska JJ, DiClemente CC: Stages and processes of self-change of smoking: toward an integrative model of change, *J Consulting Clinical Psychology* 51:390-5, 1983.
42. Prochaska JJ, Sallis JF, Rupp J: Screening measure for assessing dietary fat intake among adolescents, *Preventative Medicine* 33:699-706, 2001.
43. Sneed G, Paul SC: Readiness for behavior change in heart failure, *Am J Crit Care* 12:444-53, 2003.
44. Hershberger RE, Ni H, Nauman D et al: Prospective evaluation of an outpatient heart failure management program, *J Card Fail* 7:64-74, 2001.
45. Goodyer L, Miskelly F, Milligan P: Does encouraging good compliance improve patients' clinical condition in heart failure? *BJCP* 49:173-6, 1996.
46. Kuehneman T, Saulsbury D, Splett P et al: Demonstrating the impact of nutrition intervention in a heart failure program, *J Am Diet Asso* 102:1790-4, 2002.
47. Vinson J, Rich MW, Shah AS et al: Early readmission of elderly patients with congestive heart failure, *J Am Geriatr Soc* 38:1290-5, 1990.
48. Happ MB, Naylor MD, Roe-Prior P: Factors contributing to rehospitalization of elderly patients with heart failure, *J Cardiovasc Nurs* 11:75-84, 1997.
49. McDonald HP, Garg AX, Haynes RB: Interventions to enhance patient adherence to medication prescriptions, *JAMA* 22:2868-79, 2002.

SECTION VI

Interactions Between the Heart and Other Systems

Debra K. Moser and Barbara Riegel

Cardiovascular disease is rarely an isolated condition, and promotion of optimal patient outcomes demands that we not treat patients with only their cardiac condition in mind. A number of comorbid illnesses are extremely common in the setting of cardiovascular disease, and they have a profound impact on patient management, morbidity, prognosis, and the progression of cardiovascular disease.[1] These comorbidities, detailed in this section of the text, must be managed properly along with the cardiovascular condition, while attention is paid to potential disease-disease interactions, drug-drug interactions, disease-drug interactions, diet-drug-disease interactions, device-drug-disease interactions, and surgery-drug-diet-disease interactions.

Comorbidities produce their own sets of symptoms and pathophysiological manifestations that are superimposed on any underlying cardiovascular condition.[2] For example, in the case of heart failure, common noncardiac comorbidities include depression, hypertension, diabetes, chronic obstructive pulmonary disease, arthritis, cognitive dysfunction, anemia, and renal disease. Many patients have a combination of several or all of these.[2-5] Each of these comorbidities has the potential to make diagnostic and management decision-making extremely difficult. Thus it is essential that we are vigilant in detecting the presence of comorbidities and fully informed about current best practices for managing comorbidities.

It should be noted, however, that both practitioners and cardiovascular patients find it extremely challenging to manage comorbid illnesses. Few clinical practice guidelines consider the possibility of comorbidities, and strictly following the recommendations in guidelines could result in adverse drug and disease interactions.[6]

Further, patients commonly are confused by the different medication, dietary, and lifestyle change requirements imposed by different comorbidities.[7] They have difficulty differentiating their symptoms, which may contribute to delayed response to illness exacerbation. Moreover, patients with comorbid illnesses may believe that their health care needs are not being met and that health care providers are not adequately addressing their problems.[8]

The chapters in this section are designed to address these issues by providing vital information about common comorbid conditions in patients with cardiovascular disease so you can provide the best evidence-based care. Empirical research on the interactions of comorbid illnesses is scant, so the authors of the chapters in this section have been asked to include clinical pearls and in-depth information about the cardiovascular effects of disorders of other systems. More research is greatly needed on the interaction of cardiovascular disease and other illnesses that commonly afflict this population.

1. Gijsen R, Hoeymans N, Schellevis FG et al: Causes and consequences of comorbidity: a review, *J Clin Epidemiol* 54:661-674, 2001.
2. Dahlstrom U: Frequent non-cardiac comorbidities in patients with chronic heart failure, *Eur J Heart Fail* 7:309-316, 2005.
3. Junger J, Schellberg D, Muller-Tasch T et al: Depression increasingly predicts mortality in the course of congestive heart failure *Eur J Heart Fail* 7:261-267, 2005.
4. Konstam V, Moser DK, De Jong MJ: Depression and anxiety in heart failure, *J Card Fail* 11:455-463, 2005.
5. Lang CC, Mancini DM: Noncardiac comorbidities in heart failure, *Heart* Feb 17, 2006 [epub].

6. Boyd CM, Darer J, Boult C et al: Clinical practice guidelines and quality of care for older patients with multiple comorbid diseases: implications for pay for performance, *JAMA* 294:716-724, 2005.

7. Riegel B, Carlson B: Facilitators and barriers to heart failure self-care, *Patient Educ Couns* 46:287-295, 2002.

8. Kralik D: Patients with comorbidities perceived that acute care services did not fully acknowledge or accommodate the comprehensive care that they required, *Evidence Based Nurs* 8:30, 2005.

Diabetes and the Cardiovascular System

Deborah A. Chyun
Lawrence H. Young

CHAPTER ABBREVIATIONS

AHA   American Heart Association

ACE   angiotensin-converting enzyme

ARB   angiotensin-receptor blocker

BARI   Bypass Angioplasty Revascularization Investigation trial

CAN   cardiovascular autonomic neuropathy

CHD   coronary heart disease

CVD   cardiovascular disease

DIGAMI   Diabetes Insulin Glucose in Acute MI trial

ECG   electrocardiogram

GIK   glucose-insulin-potassium

HbA_1c glycosylated hemoglobin

HRV   heart rate variability

LDL   low-density lipoprotein

MI   myocardial infarction

NSTEMI   non–ST-segment elevation MI

PCI   percutaneous coronary intervention

STEMI   ST-segment elevation MI

TZD   thiazolidinedione

UKPDS   United Kingdom Prospective Diabetes Study

Individuals with type 1 or type 2 diabetes are at increased risk for cardiovascular disease **(CVD),** including hypertension, coronary heart disease **(CHD),** acute myocardial infarction (MI), heart failure, and sudden death.[1] Large, epidemiological trials have consistently shown a risk of CVD two to three times higher in those with diabetes than in those without diabetes.[2] In addition, data from the nurses' health study, demonstrated a 3.4 times greater mortality risk in women with diabetes and a 6.8 times greater risk in women with both diabetes and CHD.[3] This finding underscores the importance of diabetes as a risk factor in women. In the United Kingdom Prospective Diabetes Study **(UKPDS),** the overall incidence of CVD was 20 percent during a 10-year follow-up period after the new diagnosis of type 2 diabetes.[4]

Pathophysiological mechanisms responsible for CHD in patients with diabetes are complex, with traditional CHD risk factors not fully accounting for the increased risk. These risk factors are also associated with metabolic syndrome (see Chapter 37) and often precede the onset of type 2 diabetes. Lipid abnormalities in whites with diabetes include reduced high-density lipoprotein and increased triglyceride levels. Diabetes, although not associated with elevations in low-density lipoprotein **(LDL)** cholesterol, is associated with the presence of oxidized and small, dense LDL, which is relatively more atherogenic. Recent evidence regarding lipoprotein subfractions also suggests that these abnormalities may contribute to CVD in individuals with diabetes.[5]

Most people with type 2 diabetes also have hypertension, which has an important role in the development of left ventricular dysfunction, heart failure, and atrial fibrillation, in addition to being a risk factor for CHD and stroke. The importance of blood pressure control in the prevention of CVD in individuals with diabetes was clearly demonstrated in the UKPDS.[6] In addition to traditional risk factors, microalbuminuria and elevation of blood homocysteine levels[7] also appear to be significant risk factors for CVD in persons with diabetes. Hemostatic abnormalities (factor VIII, von Willebrand factor, plasminogen activator inhibitor, and platelet function), are more prevalent in diabetes, contribute to the atherogenic process, and promote thrombosis once CHD is established. Vascular inflammation, identified through a number of inflammatory markers (C-reactive protein, fibrinogen, and soluble cell adhesion molecules) is also increased in patients with diabetes and is thought to be an important contributor to the development of atherosclerosis.

There is some evidence that CHD risk factors vary among ethnic minority populations, and importantly, control of blood glucose and CHD risk factors are often suboptimal in minority populations.[8] The development of CHD in individuals with diabetes is multifactorial, and ongoing research in the area is likely to identify other important contributors. What is clear is that hyperglycemia alone is not responsible for the increased risk and that multifactorial risk-reduction efforts are needed to decrease the risk of CVD.[9]

Coronary atherosclerosis is more widespread in persons with diabetes, with stenoses in a greater number of vessels and more obstructive lesions in each vessel. Left main coronary artery disease is common, and individuals with diabetes tend to have less collateral blood flow. Although atherosclerosis primarily affects the epicardial or large surface arteries of the heart, diffuse disease involving long segments and/or distal aspects of the artery may also be present. Importantly, distal disease adversely affects the suitability of the vessels for either percutaneous or surgical revascularization, limiting treatment to medical intervention. In addition, small vessel or microvascular disease is common in those with diabetes, as is endothelial dysfunction, both of which may have important roles in limiting the augmentation of coronary blood flow.[10]

The atherosclerotic process results in plaque buildup that may culminate in plaque rupture, leading to acute coronary syndromes: unstable angina and acute MI, as discussed below. More advanced atherosclerosis significantly narrows the vessel lumen and restricts blood flow, leading to myocardial ischemia during exercise or emotional stress. CHD and hypertension contribute to the development of heart failure, reviewed in detail below. Although myocardial ischemia is often associated with symptoms, such as angina and dyspnea, many individuals with diabetes are asymptomatic. Asymptomatic myocardial ischemia is often associated with cardiovascular autonomic neuropathy (CAN), discussed at the conclusion of the chapter.

MEDICAL THERAPY FOR ACUTE CORONARY SYNDROMES

Acute coronary syndromes are common in individuals with diabetes. The incidence of MI in patients with type 2 diabetes was approximately 15 per 1000 patient years in the UKPDS, whereas the incidence of fatal MI was 7 per 1000 patient years.[4] Overall there is a consistent twofold higher mortality and increased morbidity associated with MI patients with diabetes.[11-13] In addition, acute coronary syndrome may occur without the warning of angina in patients with diabetes, who may also have atypical symptoms that delay their pursuing medical attention. Ischemic dysrhythmias leading to sudden death may prevent them from ever reaching the hospital.

Increased oxidative stress and vascular inflammation in persons with diabetes may render underlying plaque more vulnerable to rupture, which is problematic given their increased tendency toward thrombosis. In combination with accentuated platelet aggregation, which promotes thrombosis, and elevated plasminogen activator inhibitor-1, which impairs endogenous fibrinolysis and blood clot dissolution, those with diabetes are more prone to acute coronary syndrome and sudden death. In the setting of acute coronary syndrome, early and appropriate management is critical to limit myocardial damage and prevent complications.

Although early coronary reperfusion, aggressive CVD medication management, and coronary revascularization have dramatically improved the survival of patients with diabetes and acute coronary syndrome, patients with CVD and diabetes-related microvascular complications still have a higher risk of complications than patients without diabetes, both during and after hospitalization. The management and outcomes of patients with diabetes and acute coronary syndrome are also complicated by the higher number of comorbidities. The presence of hypertension, peripheral and cerebral vascular disease, left ventricular hypertrophy, and heart failure increase their overall risk. Cardiovascular autonomic dysfunction also complicates management by increasing heart rate as the result of a predominant parasympathetic neuropathy, and decreasing awareness of ischemic symptoms.

Pharmacological Therapy and Percutaneous Coronary Intervention

Patients with ST-segment elevation MI (STEMI), who typically have acute thrombotic occlusion of a coronary artery, benefit from prompt treatment to reestablish myocardial reperfusion. In many centers, this is achieved with thrombolytic therapy. Although thrombolytic therapy improves survival in patients with diabetes, both in-hospital and late mortality is 1.5- to 2-fold higher in those with diabetes compared with those without, with women and individuals treated with insulin being at particularly high risk. In addition, risk is elevated even in individuals with newly diagnosed diabetes.[14]

Although persons with diabetes tend to have non–ST-elevation MI (NSTEMI) more frequently than STEMI, making them less eligible for thrombolytics, overall acute coronary syndrome management appears to be less aggressive in individuals with diabetes.[15] Thrombolysis may take longer to achieve in this population and is more likely to fail.[16-18] Following thrombolytic therapy or percutaneous coronary intervention (PCI), underlying hemostatic abnormalities remain problematic and require subsequent antithrombotic treatment to prevent reocclusion. This is usually accomplished with aspirin, clopidogrel and glycoprotein IIb/IIIa inhibitors, which have been shown to have beneficial effects in this population.[19]

Individuals with diabetes, unstable angina, and NSTEMI are also at an increased risk for adverse outcomes, including death, progression to acute STEMI, and subsequent readmission for unstable angina within the next year.[20] Unstable angina is associated with coronary vascular instability and more extensive CHD, involving a greater number and longer segments of vessels and more often involving the left main coronary artery. Some of these patients have had a prior PCI or coronary artery bypass surgery. Imminent closure of a heavily diseased saphenous vein graft presents a particular challenge because symptoms often persist despite medical therapy, and revascularization strategies sometimes have limited efficacy.

As in patients without diabetes, the initial therapy of acute coronary syndrome includes the administration of beta blockers and nitrates to prevent ischemia,[21,22] recognizing the need for special consideration in patients with diabetes (Box 85-1). The approach to antithrombotic therapy depends on whether coronary intervention is under consideration. Aspirin should be administered to all patients; most should also receive clopidogrel, which has a synergistic effect to inhibit platelets. Heparin should be administered either intravenously in the unfractionated form or as subcutaneous low-molecular-weight heparin. When patients are unstable and coronary intervention is planned, clopidogrel and glycoprotein IIb/IIIa inhibitors should be given before PCI because they improve interventional outcomes in this setting. Recent investigations have suggested that high-dose clopidogrel (600 mg) results in better outcomes following PCI[23,24]; however, further research is needed to define the optimal treatment regimen, particularly in patients with diabetes.[25]

In the presence of ST-segment elevation, indicative of MI, patients with diabetes who are within 12 hours of the onset of symptoms should be considered for primary PCI with stent placement, particularly if they have evidence of heart failure or hemodynamic instability. Outcomes for patients with diabetes have been evalu-

---

BOX 85-1

SPECIAL CONSIDERATIONS FOR CARDIAC AND OVER-THE-COUNTER MEDICATIONS IN PATIENTS WITH DIABETES

■ ■ ■

ACE Inhibitors and ARBs
- Carefully monitor renal function and potassium levels (hyperkalemia), especially in the presence of renal insufficiency.

Beta Blockers
- Assess for worsening of glycemic and lipid control.
- Assess for hypoglycemic awareness and masking of hypoglycemia in patients treated with sulfonylureas or insulin.
- Assess for cardiovascular autonomic neuropathy and orthostatic hypotension.

Calcium Channel Blockers
- Non-dihydropyridines are contraindicated in heart failure with systolic dysfunction.
- Dihydropyridines may be used to treat hypertension or angina in patients with heart failure.

Digoxin
- Closely monitor renal function and electrolytes (hypokalemia and hypomagnesemia).

Diuretics
- Monitor serum potassium and renal function carefully.

Insulin
- Monitor patient carefully to prevent the development of hypoglycemia.
- Assess for autonomic neuropathy and/or hypoglycemic unawareness to identify high risk.

Lipid-Lowering Therapy
- Monitor liver function tests and closely monitor patients with renal dysfunction.
- Because fibrates and statins may be used together to treat lipid abnormalities in patients with diabetes, monitor carefully because of increased risk of rhabdomyolysis.
- Niacin may produce minor hyperglycemic effect.

Metformin
- Not intended for use in acute care setting.
- Monitor for development of lactic acidosis.
- Use cautiously with renal insufficiency.
- Avoid in heart failure.

Nitrates
- Contraindicated with use of phosphodiesterase inhibitors within previous 24 to 48 hours.
- Use cautiously in presence of cardiac autonomic neuropathy because hypotension may result.

Platelet Inhibitors and Anticoagulants
- Closely monitor renal function with use of low-molecular-weight heparin; serum creatinine should be below 2.5 mg/dl in men or 2.0 mg/dl in women or those older than age 75.

Thiazolidinediones
- Monitor patient for development of excessive weight gain, edema, or heart failure.
- Edema may be managed by increasing diuretic therapy or decreasing the thiazolidinedione dose.
- New or worsening heart failure may require discontinuation.
- Increase dose slowly in patients with structural heart disease or mild heart failure.
- Not intended for treatment of acute hyperglycemia in hospital because it has delayed onset of effect.

Over-the-Counter Medications
- Caution patient about cold and flu remedies; decongestants can raise blood pressure and interfere with antihypertensive medications.
- Weight-loss remedies may increase heart rate and blood pressure and interfere with cardiac medications and glucose control.
- Patients with diabetes should discuss all over-the-counter medications with their provider.

ACE, Angiotensin-converting enzyme; *ARB,* angiotensin receptor blocker.

---

ated in several primary angioplasty and stent trials, and those randomized to primary PCI showed improved short-term outcomes.[26] Long-term risks of restenosis, subsequent revascularization, and mortality remain elevated, however, with older individuals, women, and insulin-using patients being at higher risk.[19,27-30] In-stent restenosis is potentially a problem in those with diabetes for several reasons. First, smaller intraluminal diameter is achieved during the balloon dilatation. Second, accelerated neointimal hyperplasia occurs as a result of greater impairment in endothelial function and increased smooth muscle cell proliferation. Third, increased thrombus formation at the site of balloon dilatation triggers the smooth muscle cell response, which may be enhanced by hyperinsulinemia and insulin-like growth factor-1.[31] Long-term outcomes after acute coronary syndrome treated with primary PCI are also adversely influenced by the presence of multivessel disease, left ventricular dysfunction, and the development of restenosis, which are all more common in patients with diabetes.

The use of biologically coated coronary stents has reduced the initial incidence of restenosis from 40 percent to 50 percent to *less than* 10 percent to 20 percent in patients with diabetes.[32,33] Coronary stents achieve a greater luminal diameter than PCI alone. They also prevent or can be used to treat coronary artery dissection that can lead to complete vessel occlusion and MI. The development of smaller stents has permitted their more widespread use in patients with diabetes. Intermediate-term results are encouraging; however, long-term outcomes and the use of stents in patients with multivessel coronary artery disease remains to be determined. Use of other glycoprotein IIb/IIIa inhibitors (tirofiban, eptifibatide), clopidogrel and aspirin, and newer PCI techniques, along with aggressive control of diabetes and CHD risk factors on stent outcomes in diabetes need to be evaluated.

In patients with diabetes and acute coronary syndrome who respond to initial medical therapy, the decision whether to pursue angiography and revascularization needs to be individualized because some may remain at significant risk for subsequent cardiac events. This has led to the widespread use of an invasive strategy with early coronary angiography and revascularization in the management of acute coronary syndrome as discussed below. An invasive strategy may be preferable in high risk patients, including those with marked or widespread resting ST-segment depression, prior MI, decreased left ventricular function, heart failure, or ongoing evidence of ischemia. A noninvasive approach with further risk stratification based on stress echocardiography or myocardial perfusion imaging may be preferable in lower-risk patients and those with major comorbidity. Patients with renal insufficiency or severe peripheral vascular disease, frequently seen in individuals with diabetes, are at increased risk for an invasive approach.

Treating Diabetes and Acute Coronary Syndrome

Hyperglycemia in the setting of acute coronary syndrome is associated with poorer outcomes in patients with and without diabetes.[34-36] The Diabetes Insulin Glucose in Acute MI (DIGAMI) trial demonstrated that intravenous insulin infusion during the initial 24 hours after MI, followed by intensive insulin treatment for 3 months, significantly reduced mortality at 1 and 3 years.[37,38] In critically ill patients without diabetes, aggressive management of blood glucose level has also led to improvements in mortality.[39-41] Because many people previously not diagnosed with diabetes are found to have diabetes following the acute event, control of blood glucose level is critical. Current American College of Cardiology/American Heart Association guidelines call for the use of an insulin infusion to normalize blood glucose level in all patients with STEMI with complicated courses; this strategy is being considered in all patients, even in the absence of complications.[22]

It has long been known that the infusion of glucose-insulin-potassium (GIK) during acute coronary syndrome lowers free fatty acid concentrations, improves myocardial metabolism, and may prevent myocardial necrosis.[42] In addition to these early beneficial effects, intensive treatment of diabetes may stabilize the coronary vasculature and prevent recurrent events after acute coronary syndrome, in addition to exerting favorable effects on platelets, lipoproteins, plasminogen activator-1 activity, vascular reactivity, and ventricular remodeling. In the acute setting, the recommendation is that intravenous insulin be used, transitioning to subcutaneous insulin and/or other oral agents after the acute phase.[43] Oral agents should not be used to control blood glucose level in critically ill patients. Metformin should be stopped because of the risk of lactic acidosis (see Box 85-1).

The goal after discharge is to maintain glycosylated hemoglobin (HbA1c) levels below 7 percent. This may be accomplished with a variety of agents. However, in the UKPDS, obese patients with no known CVD who were treated with metformin had a lower risk of CVD.[44] In addition, recent evidence suggests that use of insulin-sensitizing thiazolidinediones (TZDs), such as rosiglitazone and pioglitazone, may contribute to lower restenosis rates following PCI[45] and improved outcomes following acute coronary syndrome in patients treated with glycoprotein IIb/IIIa inhibitors.[46] These agents not only have beneficial effects on blood pressure and lipids, but directly affect vascular inflammation and other mechanisms responsible for atherosclerosis. They may prove important for slowing the atherosclerotic process in individuals with diabetes. The role of these insulin sensitizers, compared with insulin, is currently being compared in patients randomized to either PCI or coronary bypass surgery in the Bypass Angioplasty Revascularization Investigation (BARI) 2D trial.[47]

There is some concern that intensive diabetes treatment may cause hypoglycemia and trigger myocardial ischemia in patients with diabetes. Hypoglycemia does trigger sympathetic activation and catecholamine release, leading to increases in heart rate and blood pressure that can increase myocardial oxygen demand or potentially trigger dysrhythmias. However, these potential negative effects need to be considered within the overall context of the benefits of improved glucose control. Although there was an increased risk of hypoglycemia in intensively treated patients in the DIGAMI study, this risk was outweighed by the benefits of intensive treatment. In critically ill patients, blood glucose levels should be kept as close to 110 mg/dl as possible and *less than* 180 mg/dl.[48] Although subcutaneous insulin may be used in patients who are not critically ill, this method of administration is more likely to lead to both hyperglycemia and hypoglycemia. Many institutions have successfully implemented insulin infusion protocols, which reduce these risks.[49]

Special Issues in Nursing Care

Beyond standard nursing care delivered to all patients with acute coronary syndrome, including those undergoing thrombolytic therapy and PCI, several issues are especially pertinent to patients with diabetes (Box 85-2). In relation to the initial patient assessment, because of the presence of atypical symptoms or the complete absence of pain, a high index of suspicion for ischemia should always be maintained for individuals with diabetes. In evaluating risks associated with thrombolysis, careful assessment of neurological status is needed because individuals with diabetes often have a previous history of hypertension and stroke. This evaluation should be documented both at baseline and during treatment. Changes in neurological status should be conveyed immediately so that fibrinolytic, antiplatelet, and anticoagulant therapy can be discontinued.

A baseline medication history including use of antihypertensive agents, agents to manage diabetes and other comorbidities, all over-the-counter medication and herbal preparation use, existing aspirin and/or antiplatelet therapy, and use of phosphodiesterase inhibitors for erectile dysfunction, should be obtained (see Box 85-1). The presence of erectile dysfunction or other evidence of autonomic neuropathy may place the patient at higher risk for adverse outcomes following acute coronary syndrome. Screening for alcohol, tobacco, and recreational drug use should be documented.

Because patients with diabetes have several factors that may lead to *less than* optimal thrombolysis and predispose to reocclusion, a careful ongoing assessment is needed to assess for adequacy of reperfusion and ongoing ischemia. The need for facilitated or "rescue" PCI should be anticipated in the event of ongoing ischemia. Importantly, patient teaching should stress the impor-

BOX 85-2   ▪ ▪ ▪
ACUTE CORONARY SYNDROME: NURSING CARE AND GOALS SPECIFIC TO PATIENTS WITH DIABETES

BASELINE: Early Identification of High-Risk Patients
- *Assess risk status:* History of peripheral vascular disease, stroke, MI, PCI, coronary artery bypass grafting, heart failure, autonomic neuropathy, renal insufficiency, and left ventricular dysfunction
- *History and physical exam:* Signs and symptoms of myocardial ischemia; cardiac, lung, neurological, and peripheral vascular exam; current medications; renal function, including urine microalbumin:creatinine ratio; blood glucose; full interpretation of 12-lead ECG

ONGOING: Prevention, Early Recognition, and Treatment of Complications
- Assess for evidence of ongoing or new ischemia, heart failure, or renal insufficiency and promptly treat: ECG changes, serum biomarkers, ST-segment evaluation, symptoms of ischemia, weight gain, intake and output, changes in chest x-ray, rales, S_3, S_4, murmur, serum BUN, creatinine, potassium.
- Assess for side effects of medications and be alert to specific considerations (see Box 85-1).
- In acute setting, keep blood glucose level as close to 110 mg/dl as possible and *less than* 180 mg/dl (see Box 85-1).
- Assess for specific complications during acute coronary syndrome or associated coronary revascularization.
  - *Acute coronary syndrome:* Heart failure, cardiogenic shock, postinfarct angina, heart block, atrial dysrhythmias, renal insufficiency, ongoing ischemia, reperfusion or reocclusion
  - *PCI:* MI, renal failure, stroke, restenosis, need for repeat revascularization, stroke, atheroembolic showering to the kidneys, mesenteric circulation, and periphery; retroperitoneal bleeding, femoral hematoma, femoral or iliac artery occlusion, or pseudoaneurysm formation
  - *Coronary artery bypass grafting:* MI, oliguria and renal failure, stroke, sternal wound infection, mediastinitis, sepsis, recurrent angina, and heart failure

DISCHARGE PLANNING: Prevent Recurrent Ischemia, MI, Heart Failure, and Death
- Emphasize need for combined management of anticoagulation, beta blockers, and ACE inhibitors, along with lifestyle management and glucose control (ensure adequate transition to long-term therapy).
- Make sure patient is aware of signs and symptoms of recurrent ischemia and HF and for need to alert provider.
- Identify patients at high risk of adverse events after discharge so that follow-up can be intensified.

ACE, Angiotensin-converting enzyme; *BUN,* blood-urea-nitrogen; *ECG,* electrocardiogram; *HF,* heart failure; *MI,* myocardial infarction; *PCI,* percutaneous coronary intervention.

tance of recognizing ischemic symptoms, both in the hospital and following discharge, and the need for CHD risk reduction efforts, discussed below.

The primary risk of PCI is coronary occlusion leading to MI; this risk is higher in the presence of multivessel angioplasty. The recent use of intensive antiplatelet treatment, including the glycoprotein IIb/IIIa inhibitors, has substantially lowered the risk of thrombosis formation, MI, and death during PCI in patients with diabetes so that immediate outcomes are similar to those in individuals without diabetes. However, monitoring for ongoing ischemia is especially important in these patients. When PCI fails, urgent coronary bypass surgery is sometimes required. However, this is an infrequent occurrence, occurring overall in more than 1 percent of patients with diabetes. In addition to the

cardiac risks, PCI may cause vascular complications or renal failure, particularly in older patients with diabetes who have underlying diffuse vascular disease and renal insufficiency. Stroke as a result of embolization of atheromatous material or thrombus from the aorta is the most serious vascular complication, occurring in *less than* 1 percent of patients with diabetes undergoing PCI. Patients with diabetes are also at increased risk for contrast nephropathy, which may be prevented in part by forced diuresis,[50] administration of the antioxidant acetylcysteine,[51] and use of nonionic contrast agents.

The long-term outcomes of PCI in individuals with diabetes, however, are less favorable than in patients without diabetes. This includes a higher risk of mortality, MI, need for coronary bypass surgery, and repeat PCI as a result of recurrent ischemia. Patients with diabetes, older patients, and those with decreased left ventricular function, heart failure, multivessel disease, and proteinuria have decreased survival after PCI.[52] With the advent of drug-eluting stents, restenosis rates have dropped dramatically to *less than* 8 percent.[14] Restenosis often leads to the recurrence of symptoms. However, even in the absence of symptoms, restenosis may contribute to long-term mortality in patients with diabetes following PCI.

Recent studies have demonstrated that patients with diabetes benefit from vigorous initial antiplatelet therapy after stent placement. Intensive early platelet inhibition also may prevent platelet vessel wall interaction that is important in initiating the restenosis process. Standard therapy during stent placement includes aspirin, clopidogrel, and heparin, followed by aspirin and clopidogrel for 6 months and then indefinite aspirin therapy. With the additional use of glycoprotein IIb/IIIa inhibitors before device delivery and for 12 hours afterward, the risks of stent thrombosis and resulting MI have decreased considerably, as has the need for repeat coronary revascularization.

Patients with diabetes have an increased incidence of complications associated with acute coronary syndrome, and these should be closely assessed for during hospitalization. Heart failure develops more commonly, even though the index infarctions are no larger than in those patients without diabetes. Heart failure may result from more extensive CHD causing ischemia in regions outside the infarct area or from prior scarring in remote regions. Underlying diabetes-related diastolic dysfunction and impaired systolic reserve may compromise the ability of the heart to cope with the stress of additional ischemia. Coexistent hypertension and renal disease, commonly found in individuals with diabetes, may further promote the development of symptomatic heart failure.

Patients with cardiac autonomic neuropathy or heart failure may have an increased heart rate contributing to increased myocardial oxygen demands, underscoring the importance of ongoing monitoring for continued ischemia. There is also evidence that individuals with diabetes and acute MI may have an increase risk of heart block (atrioventricular, fascicular, and bundle branch blocks), atrial dysrhythmias, renal insufficiency, and cardiogenic shock. These complications should be closely monitored for during hospitalization.

Following the acute management of the acute coronary syndrome, whether pharmacological or with PCI, an intensive effort is required to modify CHD risk factors. Since CVD is the result of numerous factors in patients with diabetes, secondary and tertiary prevention require a multifaceted approach. Although this requires intensive and often expensive treatments, recent evidence emphasizes that comprehensive reduction of multiple CHD risk factors along with glucose control prevents cardiac events in individuals with type 2 diabetes.[9] Aggressive treatment of dyslipidemia and hypertension, prevention of thrombosis with aspirin, and medications to reduce the occurrence of myocardial ischemia should be instituted. Careful, ongoing assessment should be made for restenosis and progression of CHD and for the development of heart failure.

The goals of this intensive therapy are to decrease the likelihood of subsequent cardiac events and death, to slow the progression of coronary atherosclerosis, and to prevent ischemic symptoms. Specific therapy for angina in patients with diabetes should include beta blockers, which prevent ischemia and improve exercise tolerance, in addition to reducing the risk of recurrent events. Angiotensin-converting enzyme (ACE) inhibitors have an important role in the treatment of CHD in patients with diabetes, particularly in the presence of heart failure, decreased left ventricular function, and hypertension. In addition, they may also have a more generalized benefit, stabilizing coronary plaques, and preventing acute coronary syndrome, thereby preventing cardiac events in patients with diabetes and with CHD.[53,54]

Despite the increased platelet reactivity that occurs in patients with diabetes, cardiac events are generally reduced by relatively low doses of aspirin. Aspirin inhibits platelet thromboxane synthesis and aggregation, preventing coronary thrombus formation in patients with diabetes. A second mechanism involved in thrombosis is adenosine diphosphate–mediated activation of platelets. Thienopyridine agents, such as clopidogrel, block this pathway and are effective in inhibiting platelet aggregation. Clopidogrel is used routinely following coronary stent placement and chronic CHD in patients allergic to or unable to take aspirin. All patients with diabetes, however, following acute coronary syndrome, should be taking daily aspirin unless there is a contraindication, in which case clopidogrel or warfarin should be used.

Treatment of lipid abnormalities and adequate control of blood pressure are critically important in patients with diabetes and CHD.[48] The beneficial effects of lipid lowering, both to stabilize existing plaque, thereby preventing acute coronary syndrome, and to slow the progression of atherosclerosis have been demonstrated. Both the American Diabetes Association and American Heart Association (AHA) recommend that diabetes be treated aggressively to reduce and maintain HbA1c concentrations below 7 percent and that lipids and blood pressure be brought under control. Blood pressure should be lowered to below 130/80 mm Hg. Lifestyle recommendations should include intensive dietary management, weight control, regular physical activity, mod-

eration in alcohol and sodium, and smoking cessation when indicated. Heavy drinking is classified as five or more drinks a day in men or four or more in women.[55] Individualized exercise recommendations are required in patients with peripheral CAN (discussed below), or severe retinopathy, or known CHD.

SURGICAL THERAPY FOR ACUTE CORONARY SYNDROMES

Although primary PCI or intracoronary stent placement is the preferred treatment for acute STEMI, patients with multivessel disease and left ventricular dysfunction remain at high risk following reperfusion. Multivessel disease is often identified in patients with diabetes at the time of primary angioplasty and presents a challenge in terms of management. Stent placement in the occluded vessel responsible for the infarction is preferable for initial treatment in most cases.[26] Only a small number of patients with diabetes require urgent surgical revascularization as a result of inaccessibility of the lesion or the presence of left main coronary artery disease.[26] In addition, when stent placement leaves the patient with significant residual obstructive CHD, evaluation of the need for additional revascularization should be weighed carefully.

The clinical presentation, coronary anatomy, and overall medical condition are considered when deciding whether and by what means a patient with diabetes should undergo PCI or revascularization. The decision depends upon a number of factors including the suitability of the target vessels and the number, location, morphology, and extent of residual coronary stenoses, in addition to the overall risk status of the patient. Patients with acute coronary syndrome and ischemic pulmonary edema are among those with the highest risk. PCI is usually performed for single vessel disease, whereas multivessel, long complex proximal lesions, or the presence of left main disease, frequently seen in patients with diabetes, often requires surgical revascularization.

Revascularization

The presence of far-advanced CHD, sometimes found during angiography in patients with diabetes, requires the use of coronary bypass surgery. This assumes that the distal vessels are suitable targets with good distal runoff, and that the patient does not have an excessive number of comorbid conditions because the surgical risk is increased by additional noncardiac morbidities, including renal insufficiency, cerebral or peripheral vascular disease, lung disease, and generalized immobility. In a small number of patients with diabetes, coronary angiography reveals multivessel disease, which is technically suitable for either PCI or coronary bypass surgery. In this case the lower initial morbidity of PCI is weighed against the greater prevalence of recurrent ischemia and need for future revascularization. In stable CHD, PCI has an important role in the treatment of single vessel disease in patients with diabetes, resulting in excellent symptomatic improvement. PCI is also attractive in that it avoids the initial complications of bypass surgery in patients at high risk for surgery because of significant comorbidity.

Concerns about the use of multivessel PCI were raised by the initial BARI trial, which randomized patients to either PCI with balloon angioplasty or coronary bypass surgery in the late 1980s and found a survival advantage associated with surgery in patients with diabetes, despite a higher risk of Q-wave MI and in-hospital mortality at the time of the initial procedure. More recently, the arterial revascularization therapy study trial[56] demonstrated a lower mortality risk with multivessel PCI at 1 year, although this was still higher in patients with diabetes (6.3 percent) compared with those without diabetes (3.1 percent). However, these patients were not aggressively treated with glycoprotein IIb/IIIa inhibitors, clopidogrel, drug-eluting stents, or more recent innovations during PCI.

Coronary artery bypass surgery has an important role in the management of CHD patients with diabetes, who generally derive excellent symptomatic improvement from this procedure. In the current era, mortality risks are *less than* 5 percent in patients with diabetes. The use of an internal mammary artery graft, whose long-term patency is superior to that of saphenous vein grafts, is important for survival in the overall population, but appears to be even more critical in patients with diabetes. However, many studies have noted that patients with diabetes are at risk for a number of postoperative complications. Less complete revascularization as a result of the presence of diffuse disease, more rapid progression of native disease, and increased risk for saphenous vein occlusion may contribute to a higher incidence of angina and heart failure following coronary bypass surgery in patients with diabetes.

Nursing Care to Prevent Complications

Postoperative nursing care is based on the recognition that patients with diabetes are at increased risk of a number of cardiac and noncardiac complications, thus requiring careful assessment so that complications can be promptly treated. The most concerning complications are postoperative MI, stroke, renal failure, mediastinitis, sternal wound infection, and sepsis.[57,58] The use of off-pump coronary bypass surgery in patients with diabetes has not consistently lowered the risk of early postoperative complications, with MI, reintubation, and balloon counterpulsation still needed in those undergoing off-pump procedures.[59]

The development of a new Q-wave MI is a serious complication of coronary bypass surgery, which occurs slightly more often in patients with diabetes compared with those without diabetes.[60] Potential causes of MI are ongoing ischemia before cardiopulmonary bypass, an inability to graft diseased vessels, and air or atherosclerotic coronary embolization. In-hospital mortality is higher in older patients and when surgery is performed on a nonelective basis following acute coronary syndrome.[56] Gender also has an impact on risk of bypass surgery in patients with diabetes, with women having a twofold higher operative mortality than men.

Patients with diabetes also have at least twice the risk for stroke during coronary bypass surgery.[58] Older patients with diabetes with a history of prior stroke and those with calcification of the ascending aorta or renal failure[61] are at particularly high risk. Postoperative renal failure occurs more commonly in patients with diabetes, with preoperative renal insufficiency being a strong risk factor. The use of ACE inhibitors immediately following surgery may precipitate oliguria in these patients. Preoperative renal insufficiency is also a marker of general, overall risk during coronary bypass surgery since it often occurs in older patients with diabetes and those with peripheral vascular disease, hypertension, or left ventricular dysfunction. Patients with diabetes who are on dialysis are at an increased risk of operative mortality that is as high as 10 percent to 15 percent.[62] These patients often require more prolonged mechanical ventilation and more frequently develop atrial fibrillation and gastrointestinal complications following surgery.

Sternal wound infections occur in 8 percent to 10 percent of patients with diabetes undergoing coronary artery bypass surgery, which is threefold to fivefold more often than in those without diabetes.[63] The majority of these are successfully treated with antibiotics, but occasionally operative debridement is needed. The risk of sternal wound infection may be increased when preoperative blood glucose levels are greater than 200 mg/dl.[64] Additionally, poor glycemic control has been linked to MI and stroke.[57] Intensive control of blood glucose with intravenous insulin during and following surgery is advocated because it has been shown to improve metabolic parameters and cardiac index and decrease the risk of immediate postoperative complications (need for pacing, atrial fibrillation, and infection), shorten the length of stay, and over 5 years, reduces the risk of death.[65]

After coronary artery bypass surgery, patients with diabetes should still be considered to have ongoing cardiovascular risk, with less favorable long-term outcomes, including lower survival than those individuals without diabetes. As with acute coronary syndrome outcomes, much of this risk is associated with the presence of diabetes-related comorbidities, particularly peripheral vascular disease and renal insufficiency. This reflects in part both their more advanced cardiac disease and comorbidity at the time of surgery. Predictors of worse outcomes following bypass surgery include preoperative stroke, hypertension, heart failure, high glucose levels, proteinuria, multivessel disease, male sex, left ventricular dysfunction, and surgery with *less than* three grafts.[66]

MEDICAL THERAPY FOR HEART FAILURE

Heart failure causes substantial morbidity in patients with diabetes, including both exertional limitation and recurrent hospitalizations. Early data from the Framingham Study indicating an increased risk in individuals with diabetes continues to be substantiated in more recent investigations. In the UKPDS the incidence of heart failure was 4 per 1000 patient years in conventionally treated subjects.[4] Whereas the risk of heart failure in men with diabetes appears to be doubled, it is four to five times greater in women, as is the risk in those patients treated with insulin. In middle-aged individuals with type 2 diabetes, prevalence of heart failure is approximately 12 percent, as compared with 5 percent in those without diabetes.[67] In elderly Medicare patients with diabetes, 22 percent had a diagnosis of heart failure with the prevalence increasing with increasing age.[68] Thus heart failure remains extremely common in patients with diabetes, and this risk is highest in the very elderly and in women.

Reducing Risk of Heart Failure

The prevention and treatment of heart failure in patients with diabetes requires optimal management of coexistent hypertension, CHD, and left ventricular dysfunction. Atherosclerotic CHD is the most common cause of heart failure in the United States and specifically in patients with diabetes. Myocardial ischemia resulting from CHD may contribute to heart failure through impairment in systolic and diastolic contractile function. In some cases, the patient with diabetes has a typical dilated ischemic cardiomyopathy and has clear evidence of underlying CHD, whereas frequently more diffuse CHD has caused patchy fibrosis, without a history or clear electrocardiogram (**ECG**) evidence of MI. Critical CHD may also impair systolic function as a result of recurrent ischemia in the absence of frank myocardial necrosis, a process referred to as stunned or hibernating myocardium. In assessing patients with diabetes and heart failure it is important to determine if underlying CHD is present because there may be a component of the left ventricular dysfunction that is reversible with revascularization and antiischemic medications (e.g., nitrates and beta blockers). Unexplained heart failure in a patient with diabetes should prompt evaluation for CHD, often including cardiac catheterization. Evaluation should also be made for secondary causes of heart failure, such as thyroid dysfunction and alcohol excess.

In the absence of CHD, hypertension, which is present in approximately 40 percent to 60 percent of patients with type 2 diabetes, is the most common cause of heart failure. The presence of hypertension almost doubles the risk of heart failure in men and nearly fourfold in women. Patients with hypertension and diabetes often develop heart failure despite normal systolic function, sometimes referred to as diastolic heart failure.[69] Although clinical heart failure is attributed in large part to coexistent CHD and/or hypertension, physiological abnormalities in left ventricular systolic and diastolic function related to diabetes may predispose the patient to heart failure.[70] Impaired left ventricular relaxation and compliance may result from myocardial fibrosis or ischemia and increases left ventricular diastolic pressures.

As discussed earlier, heart failure is frequently seen with acute MI and during long-term follow-up after acute coronary syndrome. Lower socioeconomic status,[68] older age,[67,68] female sex,[67] longer diabetes duration,[67] insulin use,[67] higher serum creatinine level,[67] and the presence of diabetes-related comorbidities, particularly nephropathy,[68] have been linked with an increased risk of heart failure in individuals with diabetes. Poorer glycemic control has also been shown to increase the risk of heart failure.[71-73] This association is not only strong, but shows that the level of risk increases as the

level of HbA1c rises above 7 percent. In women with diabetes, who are at such high risk of developing heart failure, risk factors for developing heart failure include a higher body mass index and decreased creatinine clearance.[73]

Special Issues in Nursing Care

In patients with diabetes, the prevention and management of heart failure follows standard recommendations (see Chapter 64), including intensive treatment of coexistent hypertension, CHD, renal disease, and hyperglycemia.[74] Because heart failure is extremely common in the elderly with diabetes,[69] comorbidities, such as chronic renal insufficiency, may complicate treatment.[75] Underlying pulmonary dysfunction,[76] susceptibility to fluid retention, and volume overload, not only cause exertional intolerance, but can also precipitate pulmonary edema. As discussed elsewhere, strategies supporting adherence to complex medical regimens (see Chapter 84) and discussion of advanced directives (Chapter 82) are important nursing considerations.

Optimal treatment of hypertension is critical to both the prevention and treatment of heart failure in patients with diabetes. The UKPDS of patients with newly diagnosed type 2 diabetes demonstrated that more intensive blood pressure control decreased the incidence of heart failure by 40 percent.[6] According to the Seventh Report of the Joint National Committee on Prevention, Detection, Evaluation, and Treatment of High Blood Pressure (commonly known as the JNC VII), optimal blood pressure is achieved with readings below 130/80 mm Hg.[77] ACE inhibitors are the cornerstone of prevention and treatment of heart failure in patients with diabetes.[78] Angiotensin-receptor blockers (**ARBs**) are also used widely for the prevention and treatment of heart failure, particularly when patients are unable to use ACE inhibitors because of the development of cough.[79,80] Special considerations for these and other medications used in the management of heart failure in patients with diabetes is provided in Box 85-1.

Historically, there is sometimes reluctance to use beta blockers in treating patients with diabetes with symptomatic heart failure because of concerns for worsening insulin resistance, masking hypoglycemia, or aggravating orthostatic hypotension. However, these agents have been shown to contribute to improved outcomes.[54,81,82] Careful monitoring and treatment for these effects, rather than avoidance, should be the goal. Loop diuretics have an important role in the treatment of symptomatic heart failure, particularly in patients with diabetes who are volume sensitive because of diastolic dysfunction and who have a tendency to retain fluid because of renal impairment. In addition, aldosterone antagonists may slow the progression of myocardial fibrosis and have the added benefit that they prevent hypokalemia resulting from loop diuretics.[83] However, serum potassium levels should be monitored because of an increased risk of hyperkalemia with their use, as with ACE inhibitors.

The treatment of patients with diabetes and heart failure caused by diastolic dysfunction requires specific attention. Poorly controlled hypertension, tachycardia, atrial fibrillation, active myocardial ischemia, and volume overload can all potentially exacerbate heart failure in these patients.[69,84] Aggressive blood pressure control, sodium restriction, and diuretics are important in symptomatic patients.[69] Although effectiveness of ACE inhibitors for diastolic dysfunction has not been demonstrated, they inhibit the renin-angiotensin-aldosterone system, thereby preventing adverse neurohormonal activation and reducing left ventricular mass.[85] Although calcium channel blockers theoretically may decrease intracellular calcium and improve diastolic relaxation in patients with heart failure caused by diastolic dysfunction, there is currently little support to use these agents in this setting. Although useful in treating hypertension, nondihydropyridine class drugs, such as diltiazem and verapamil, are contraindicated in patients with significant systolic dysfunction. The primary approaches to treat heart failure caused by diastolic dysfunction therefore include intensive treatment of hypertension to reduce afterload and left ventricular mass and diuretics to prevent volume overload.

In younger patients with diabetes who are unresponsive to medical therapy, their candidacy for cardiac transplantation is carefully considered. Although earlier studies have reported an increased risk following transplantation, recent data show similar survival experiences in selected patients with and without diabetes.[86] After transplant renal insufficiency is relatively common. Diabetes management may be complicated by the use of corticosteroids for immunosuppression, requiring high doses of insulin or oral agents. Infection is another concern, particularly in patients who need support from a left ventricular assist device while awaiting transplantation. Although all patients with diabetes require careful surveillance for the development of vasculopathy following heart transplant, insulin resistance and dyslipidemia increase that risk. Aggressive control of blood glucose and lipid lowering with statins are important to reduce the development of transplant vasculopathy.

Heart failure also affects the choice of medications used to treat type 2 diabetes. Metformin and TZDs are not recommended in patients with moderate-to-severe heart failure. Decreased clearance of metformin in patients with heart failure as a result of hypoperfusion or insufficiency can lead to potentially dangerous lactic acidosis. TZDs are sometimes associated with fluid retention, pedal edema, and weight gain, particularly when used in conjunction with insulin, and may contribute to heart failure.[87,88] However, recent observational data suggest that although there was a slightly higher risk of readmission for heart failure in patients treated with TZDs, use of both TZDs and metformin was associated with a lower risk of death.[89] Careful clinical assessment before initiation of TZDs, lower doses with slow dose escalation, and careful ongoing monitoring should be implemented when these drugs are used in the presence of known structural heart disease or a prior history of heart failure.

Although insulin treatment has been associated with poor outcomes in patients with heart failure, this largely reflects patient selection and the presence of more advanced microvascular and macrovascular disease. Duration of diabetes and the need to use any medication to control blood glucose, not a specific agent, contribute to heart failure.[90] Therefore insulin and insulin secretagogues are considered safe for use in patients with heart failure. Importantly the findings of the DIGAMI study support tighter control of blood glucose during MI and after discharge to reduce the subsequent rate of heart failure.[91]

CARDIOVASCULAR AUTONOMIC NEUROPATHY

CAN develops over time in at least 25 percent of individuals with diabetes.[92] Patients with diabetes and CAN have a high CVD risk, with CVD mortality approaching 25 percent to 40 percent over 5 years.[92] In addition, CAN is found in high risk patients who have established severe CHD, renal disease, poor glycemic control, and dyslipidemia. CAN is also a marker of CVD risk in patients with known cardiac disease without diabetes and in those with impaired fasting glucose and in relatives of individuals with diabetes.[93-98] The fact that many individuals with impaired autonomic function have been shown to be at risk of developing diabetes,[99] combined with the finding that even individuals newly diagnosed with diabetes may have significant CAN,[100] suggests that CAN and diabetes may develop in parallel, rather than CAN being solely a consequence of diabetes. Thus identification of CAN is likely to assume increasing importance in relation to CVD outcomes, beyond its role in diabetes.

Cardiovascular autonomic neuropathy may involve the parasympathetic and sympathetic innervation of the heart and peripheral vasculature, leading to a spectrum of manifestations. In its mildest form, cardiac neuropathy involves the parasympathetic innervation of the heart and may lead to a slightly increased resting heart rate. In more advanced cases, autonomic neuropathy causes severe orthostatic hypotension with recurrent lightheadedness, unsteadiness, or even frank syncope. CAN may contribute to abnormalities in left ventricular function, compromising exercise capacity and left ventricular contractile reserve.[10] Peak heart rate and blood pressure responses to exercise may be blunted even in the absence of detectable CHD and hypertension.

Studies have correlated autonomic neuropathy with prolongation of the QT interval and increased QT dispersion reflecting variability in ventricular repolarization. These measures have also been shown to predict adverse cardiac outcomes.[101] CAN-related repolarization abnormalities potentially predispose individuals with diabetes to sudden death. It has theorized that CAN creates an autonomic imbalance, predisposing to dysrhythmic events, or interferes with the perception of angina, predisposing to severe ischemic events. However, these concepts remain unproven, and CAN may simply be associated with other factors predisposing to cardiac events, such as severe CHD, prior MI, glycemic control, or poorly controlled lipid levels. Thus the exact mechanism by which CAN contributes to

CVD mortality remains uncertain. However, a high level of attention is warranted in patients with diabetes and CAN, and the presence of significant CHD should always be considered.

Cardiovascular Autonomic Neuropathy and Silent Heart Disease

Importantly, CAN may also have a role in the pathogenesis of silent ischemia in patients with diabetes.[92,102] Asymptomatic or "silent" ischemia often occurs in patients who also have symptomatic ischemia with angina, but some patients with diabetes only experience asymptomatic episodes. Abnormalities in cardiac autonomic function are associated with inducible myocardial ischemia in asymptomatic patients, with as many as 22 percent of patients with type 2 diabetes having evidence of ischemia without symptoms.[103]

Based on a growing body of evidence, the presence of CAN should alert providers to the possibility of asymptomatic CHD. At the very least, the ECG should be examined for abnormalities suggestive of prior MI or ischemia. Further testing is indicated when patients want to engage in high-intensity exercise or in those with long-standing diabetes, multiple CHD risk factors, or known diabetes-related complications (Box 85-3).[48,104] Although treadmill exercise ECG is perhaps the least expensive and most widely used approach, standard exercise electrocardiography has limitations, including a relatively low sensitivity and a significant incidence of false-positive test results, especially in patients with hypertension and in women. In addition, many older patients are unable to exercise adequately, decreasing the accuracy of the test.

Cardiac assessment with either myocardial perfusion imaging or echocardiography has a greater sensitivity and specificity than exercise testing with ECG monitoring alone.[105] These techniques can also be used along with pharmacological stress using adenosine or dobutamine infusions in patients unable to exercise well. Myocardial perfusion imaging not only improves the detection of CHD, but is also a well-recognized predictor of

---

BOX 85-3
NURSING CONSIDERATIONS IN THE ASSESSMENT OF CARDIAC AUTONOMIC NEUROPATHY AND ASYMPTOMATIC MYOCARDIAL ISCHEMIA

Identify Patients at High Risk of Cardiovascular Autonomic Neuropathy

- Older age
- Female sex
- Low level of education
- Higher body mass index
- Poor glucose control, insulin resistance
- Hypertension
- High resting heart rate
- Renal insufficiency
- High total cholesterol and triglyceride levels
- Beta blocker and diuretic use
- Increased QT interval corrected for heart rate and QT dispersion

Assess for Signs and Symptoms of Autonomic Neuropathy

- *Cardiac:* Resting tachycardia, exercise intolerance, orthostatic hypotension, syncope
- *Gastrointestinal:* Esophageal dysmotility, gastroparesis, constipation, diarrhea, fecal incontinence, gastric bloating after eating, upper GI symptoms
- *Genitourinary:* Neurogenic bladder, erectile dysfunction, retrograde ejaculation, female sexual dysfunction
- *Other:* Hypoglycemic unawareness, anhidrosis, heat intolerance, gustatory sweating, dry skin, sleep dysfunction

Identify Patients at High Risk of Asymptomatic Myocardial Ischemia

- Older age
- Male sex
- High total cholesterol level
- Proteinuria
- ST-T–wave abnormalities on resting ECG
- Decreased HRV on testing for CAN
- Electrocardiographic evidence of previous MI: significant Q waves, deep T-wave inversions, or left bundle branch block
- Ischemic ST-segment changes during monitoring without symptoms

Provide CHD Screening and Management: Annual Assessment of CHD Risk Factors and Appropriate Treatment

- Consider ACE inhibitor if patient is older than age 55 and has another CHD risk factor.
- Consider beta blocker if patient has prior MI or is undergoing major surgery.
- Exercise stress test in presence of typical or atypical symptoms; abnormal resting ECG; history of peripheral vascular disease or occlusive carotid disease; sedentary lifestyle, older than age 35, and plans to start a vigorous exercise program; and two or more CHD risk factors, including microalbuminuria or macroalbuminuria
- Cardiology referral for patients with signs and symptoms of CHD or abnormal ECG, echocardiogram, or exercise stress test

ACE, Angiotensin-converting enzyme; *CAN,* cardiovascular autonomic neuropathy; *CHD,* coronary heart disease; *ECG,* electrocardiogram; *GI,* gastrointestinal; *MI,* myocardial infarction.

American Diabetes Association: Consensus development conference on the diagnosis of coronary heart disease in people with diabetes, *Diabetes Care* 21:1551-1559, 1998.

American Diabetes Association: Standards of medical care in diabetes, *Diabetes Care* 28:S4-S36, 2005.

Gazzaruso C, De Amici E, Garzaniti A et al: Assessment of asymptomatic coronary artery disease in apparently uncomplicated type 2 diabetic patients, *Diabetes Care* 25:1418-24, 2002.

Janand-Delenne B, Savin B, Habib G et al: Silent myocardial ischemia in patients with diabetes. *Diabetes Care* 22:1396-1400, 1999.

Liao D, Carnethon M, Evans G et al: Lower heart rate variability is associated with the development of coronary heart disease in individuals with diabetes: the atherosclerosis risk in communities (ARIC) study, *Diabetes* 51:3524-31, 2002.

Low PA, Benrud-Larson LM, Sletten DM et al: Autonomic symptoms and diabetic neuropathy. *Diabetes Care* 27:2942-2947, 2004.

Stella P, Ellis D, Maser RE et al: Cardiovascular autonomic neuropathy (expiration and inspiration ratio) in type 1 diabetes. Incidence and predictors, *J Diabetes Complication* 14:1-6, 2000.

Vinik AI, Mitchell BD, Maser RE et al: Diabetic autonomic neuropathy, *Diabetes Care* 26:1553-79, 2003.

Wackers FJTH, Young LH, Inzucchi SE et al: Detection of silent myocardial ischemia in asymptomatic diabetic subjects: the DIAD study, *Diabetes Care* 27:1954-1961, 2004.

adverse cardiac outcomes in the overall population with either known or suspected CHD. The significance of asymptomatic ischemia depends on the extent of myocardium that is compromised, with some patients having only minor regions of ischemia and others having major ischemia. Large, reversible myocardial perfusion defects are sometimes found in patients with diabetes and indicate significant areas of potentially jeopardized myocardium. These patients should be referred for coronary angiography. Of particular concern is asymptomatic ischemia that has caused prior MI, decreased left ventricular function, heart failure, or ventricular dysrhythmias. These patients are at high risk for subsequent cardiac events and therefore require coronary angiography.

Diagnosis of Cardiovascular Autonomic Neuropathy

Symptoms of CAN may appear late in the disease course.[106] However, CAN should be considered in patients with diabetes who have peripheral neuropathy or other forms of autonomic neuropathy. Recent recommendations are that all patients with type 2 diabetes be screened at the time of diagnosis and those with type 1 diabetes be screened 5 years after diagnosis.[107] If screening is negative, it should be repeated yearly. The ECG can be used to determine heart rate–based changes, and the patient may easily be evaluated for orthostatic blood pressure changes.

An ECG rhythm strip that shows obvious sinus arrhythmia generally indicates that cardiac autonomic function is healthy in a patient with diabetes, whereas rapid, fixed heart rates may indicate CAN. A drop in the orthostatic systolic pressure *greater than* 15 mm Hg in the absence of acute hypovolemia is suggestive and *greater than* 20 mm Hg is fairly diagnostic of advanced autonomic dysfunction.

The diagnosis of CAN can be made using specific testing procedures. The standard approach involves analysis of changes in heart rate during deep breathing (the expiratory/inspiratory ratio), standing, and Valsalva maneuvers, along with blood pressure responses to hand grip and standing. Standard cut points for diagnosing abnormal tests are available; however, it is imperative that patients perform the tests correctly.[108,109] In regard to deep breathing, it is often difficult to ascertain that the patient is breathing deeply and slowly (six breaths per minute) enough. Failure to do this will result in inaccurate results, with the results possibly being falsely interpreted as abnormal. Similarly, it is necessary to hold the Valsalva maneuver for a full 15 seconds while maintaining a pressure of 40 mm Hg. Patients with proliferative retinopathy should not perform this test because of a small risk of intraocular hemorrhage. Even the relatively simple maneuver of rising from a lying to standing position is difficult for many patients with diabetes because of older age, functional limitations, and obesity. Recent meals, insulin administration, caffeine, alcohol, smoking, and medications may also influence results, so patients should be tested in a fasting state in the morning before they take their medica-

tion. A standard ECG machine or ambulatory Holter recorders may be used. In addition, newer, automated systems are available and facilitate analysis.

Analysis of heart rate variability **(HRV)** provides an important approach to the assessment of cardiac autonomic function in the patient with diabetes.[108,110] As the instantaneous heart rate (R-R) interval varies as a result of the influence of both parasympathetic and sympathetic modulation, R-R variability can be assessed by using either statistical analysis of R-R interval changes (time-domain) or power spectral analysis of successive R-R intervals (frequency-domain). The latter approach has the advantage of more readily differentiating between sympathetic and parasympathetic influences based on the frequency of the HRV and is able to distinguish between patients with different types of neuropathy (parasympathetic versus sympathetic) symptoms.[110] Variations in the high frequency range (0.15 to 0.40 Hz) are modulated more by parasympathetic activity, whereas low frequency (0.04 to 0.15 Hz) variability is modulated primarily by sympathetic activity. Because CHD can lead to diminished HRV, it is necessary to determine that individuals with diabetes do not have underlying CHD when attributing their abnormalities to diabetes. Newer monitoring systems measure low and high frequency power and calculate a ratio. In addition, they generally indicate whether a test result is considered normal or abnormal. Unlike earlier heart rate–based tests, cut points for defining an abnormal test based on HRV have not been standardized; however, lower values are indicative of CAN. Cardiac imaging with radiolabeled ^{123}I-meta-iodobenzyl-guanidine or ^{11}C-ephedrine have also been used to assess the integrity of cardiac sympathetic innervation. These approaches are largely investigative, although I-meta-iodobenzyl-guanidine is commercially available.

Special Issues in Nursing Care

Successful prevention and management of CAN involves multifactorial risk reduction, including intensive control of glucose, body mass index, blood pressure, and lipid levels, which may reduce both CAN progression and CHD risk.[9] Nursing has an important role in the identification of patients with CAN and asymptomatic myocardial ischemia and in facilitating appropriate follow-up and management (see Box 85-3). The presence of CAN complicates intensive glucose control because CAN may contribute to hypoglycemia unawareness, requiring increased vigilance on the part of the provider and patient. Special precautions for exercising are necessary in the presence of CAN and in the presence of peripheral neuropathy. Sedentary individuals should always initiate exercise programs at a low level and gradually increase the intensity of exercise. Because of the possibility of unrecognized CHD, patients with CAN should generally engage in moderate intensity exercise regimens. All patients should be educated about the symptoms of myocardial ischemia and instructed how to respond. Improving nutritional intake, decreasing alcohol intake, and cessation of smoking are also likely to benefit CAN. Other modalities, such as use of antioxidants, ACE inhibitors, and beta blockers, are being explored, as is the use of aldose-reductase inhibitors.[111]

In addition, the identification of asymptomatic CHD has clear implications for the care of the patient with diabetes. It strongly reinforces the need to aggressively reduce modifiable CVD risk factors, perhaps more fully motivating the patient to take multiple medications and engage in lifestyle modification. In some patients, it may lead to the initiation or intensification of lipid-lowering or blood pressure–lowering therapy. A heightened concern for CHD can motivate efforts at smoking cessation and weight reduction, which otherwise may be difficult to accomplish. Once CHD is identified, providers are more apt to ensure the patient's compliance with daily aspirin treatment and to consider the use of beta blockers to prevent ischemia. Recommendations for regular exercise are reinforced with limitations placed on strenuous activity that might place the patient at risk for a cardiac event.

SUMMARY

Short- and long-term outcomes following acute coronary syndrome, PCI, and coronary bypass surgery have improved in patients with diabetes over the past decade. However, these individuals still remain at high risk for ongoing ischemia, restenosis, heart failure, and cardiac-related mortality. The importance of identifying CAN in the clinical setting is receiving increased recognition because of its link to asymptomatic CHD and CVD mortality. The prevention of CHD, in addition to the prevention of complications once CHD is established, however, requires multifactorial CHD risk factor reduction, along with aggressive glucose control, in all patients with diabetes.

REFERENCES

1. Kannel WB, McGee DL: Diabetes and cardiovascular risk factors: the Framingham Study, *Circulation* 59:8-13, 1979.
2. Fox S, Coady S, Sorlie PD et al: Trends in cardiovascular complications of diabetes, *JAMA* 292:2495-2499, 2004.
3. Hu FB, Stampfer MJ, Solomon CG et al: The impact of diabetes mellitus on mortality from all causes and coronary heart disease in women, *Arch Intern Med* 161:1721-1723, 2001.
4. United Kingdom Prospective Diabetes (UKPDS) Group: Intensive blood-glucose control with sulfonylureas or insulin compared with conventional treatment and risk of complications in patients with type 2 diabetes (UKPDS 33), *Lancet* 352:837-853, 1998.
5. Jenkins AJ, Lyons TJ, Zheng D et al: Serum lipoproteins in the diabetes control and complications trial/epidemiology of diabetes intervention and complications cohort, *Diabetes Care* 26:810-818, 2003.
6. The UKPDS Group: Tight blood pressure control and risk of macrovascular and microvascular complications in type 2 diabetes: UKPDS 38, *Br Med J* 317:703-13, 1998.
7. Hoogeveen EK, Kostense PJ, Jakobs C et al: Hyperhomocysteinemia increases risk of death, especially in type 2 diabetes: 5-year follow-up of the Hoorn study, *Circulation* 101:1506-11, 2000.
8. Harris MI: Racial and ethnic differences in health care access and health outcomes for adults with type 2 diabetes, *Diabetes Care* 24:454-459, 2001.
9. Gaede P, Vedel P, Larsen N et al: Multifactorial intervention and cardiovascular disease in patients with type 2 diabetes, *N Engl J Med* 348:383-93, 2003.
10. Young LH, Chyun DA: Heart disease in patients with diabetes. In Porte D, Baron JA, Sherwin RS, editors: *Ellenberg and Rifkin's diabetes mellitus: theory and practice,* ed 6, New York, 2002, McGraw-Hill, pp 823-844.
11. Chyun DA, Vaccarino V, Murillo J: Acute myocardial infarction mortality in the elderly with diabetes, *Heart Lung* 327-39, 2002.
12. Chyun D, Vaccarino V, Murillo J et al: Cardiac outcome after myocardial infarction in elderly patients with diabetes mellitus, *Am J Crit Care* 11:504-519, 2002.
13. Murcia AM, Hennekens CH, Lamas GA et al: Impact of diabetes on mortality in patients with myocardial infarction and left ventricular dysfunction, *Arch Intern Med* 164:2273-2279, 2004.
14. Aguilar D, Solomon SD, Kober L et al: Newly diagnosed and previously known diabetes mellitus and 1-year outcomes of acute myocardial infarction, *Circulation* 110:1572-1578, 2004.
15. Franklin K, Goldberg RJ, Spencer F et al: Implications of diabetes in patients with acute coronary syndromes, *Arch Intern Med* 164:1457-1463, 2004.
16. Zairis MN, Lyras AG, Makrygianis SS et al: Type 2 diabetes and intravenous thrombolysis outcome in the setting of ST elevation myocardial infarction, *Diabetes Care* 27:967-971, 2004.
17. Roffi M, Chew DP, Mukherjee D et al: Platelet glycoprotein IIb/IIIa inhibitors reduce mortality in diabetic patients with non-ST-segment-elevation acute coronary syndromes. *Circulation* 204:2767-2771, 2001.
18. Tang WH, Lincoff AM: Diabetes, coronary intervention, and platelet glycoprotein IIb/IIIa blockade, *Circulation* 110:3618-3620, 2004.
19. Roffi M, Topol EJ: Percutaneous coronary intervention in diabetes patients with non–ST-segment elevation acute coronary syndromes, *Euro Heart J* 25:190-198, 2004.
20. Malmberg K, Yusuf S, Gerstein HC et al: Impact of diabetes on long-term prognosis in patients with unstable angina and non–Q-wave myocardial infarction: results of the OASIS (Organization to Assess Strategies for Ischemic Syndromes) registry, *Circulation* 102:1014-9, 2000.
21. Braunwald E, Antman EM, Beasley JW et al: ACC/AHA guidelines for the management of patients with unstable angina and non–ST-segment elevation myocardial infarction: executive summary and recommendations. A report of the American College of Cardiology/American Heart Association task force on practice guidelines (committee on the management of patients with unstable angina), *Circulation* 102:1193-209, 2000.
22. Antman EM, Anbe DT, Armstrong PW et al: ACC/AHA guidelines for the management of patients with ST-elevation myocardial infarction: executive summary, *Circulation* 110, 2004.
23. Patti G, Colonna G, Pasceri V et al: Randomized trial of high loading dose of clopidogrel for reduction of periprocedural myocardial infarction in patients undergoing coronary intervention, *Circulation* 111:2099-2106, 2005.
24. Gurbel PA, Bliden KP, Zaman KA et al: Clopidogrel loading with eptifibatide to arrest the reactivity of platelets, *Circulation* 111:1153-1159, 2005.
25. Leopold JA, Antman EM: Dual antiplatelet therapy for coronary stenting: a clear path for a research agenda, *Circulation* 111:1097-1099, 2005.
26. Hasdai D, Granger CB, Srivatsa SS et al: Diabetes mellitus and outcome after primary coronary angioplasty for acute myocardial infarction: lessons from the GUSTO-IIb angioplasty substudy. Global use of strategies to open occluded arteries in acute coronary syndromes (see comments), *J Am Coll Cardiol* 35:1502-12, 2000.
27. Laskey WK, Selzer F, Vlachos HA et al: Comparison of in-hospital and one-year outcomes in patients with and without diabetes undergoing percutaneous intervention (from the National Heart, Lung, and Blood Institute dynamic registry), *Am J Cardiol* 90:1062-1067, 2002.
28. Gilbert J, Raboud J, Zinman B: Meta-analysis of the effect of diabetes on restenosis rates among patients receiving coronary angioplasty stenting, *Diabetes Care* 27:990-994, 2004.
29. Matthew V, Gersh BJ, Willimas BA et al: Outcomes in patients with diabetes mellitus undergoing percutaneous coronary intervention in the current era, *Circulation* 109:476-480, 2004.
30. Wilson SR, Vakili BA, Sherman W et al: Effect of diabetes on long-term mortality following contemporary percutaneous coronary intervention, *Diabetes Care* 27:1137-1142, 2004.
31. Kornowski R, Lansky AJ: Current perspectives on interventional treatment strategies in diabetic patients with coronary artery disease, *Catheter Cardiovasc Interv* 50:245-54, 2000.

32. Morice MC, Serruys PW, Sousa JE et al: A randomized comparison of a sirolimus-eluting stent with a standard stent for coronary revascularization, *N Engl J Med* 346:1773-1780, 2002.

33. Moses JW, Leon MB, Popma JJ et al: Sirolimus eluting stents versus standard stents in patients with stenosis in native coronary artery, *N Engl J Med* 349:1315-1323, 2003.

34. Capes SE, Hunt D, Malmberg K et al: Stress hyperglycaemia and increased risk of death after myocardial infarction in patients with and without diabetes: a systematic overview (see comments), *Lancet* 355:773-8, 2000.

35. Stranders I, Diamant M, van Gelder RE et al: Admission blood glucose level as risk indicator of death after myocardial infarction in patients with and without diabetes, *Arch Intern Med* 164:982-988, 2004.

36. Suleiman M, Hammerman H, Boulos M et al: Fasting glucose is an important independent risk factor for 30-day mortality in patients with acute myocardial infarction, *Circulation* 111, 2005.

37. Malmberg K, Ryden L, Suad E et al: Randomized trial of insulin-glucose infusion followed by subcutaneous insulin treatment in diabetic patients with acute myocardial infarction (DIGAMI study): effects on mortality at 1 year, *J Am Coll Cardiol* 26:57-65, 1995.

38. Malmberg K, Norhammar A, Wedel H et al: Glycometabolic state at admission: important risk marker of mortality in conventionally treated patients with diabetes mellitus and acute myocardial infarction, *Circulation* 138:2626-2632, 1999.

39. Finney SJ, Zekveld C, Elia A et al: Glucose control and mortality in critically ill patients. *JAMA* 290:2041-2047, 2003.

40. Van den Berghe G, Wouters P, Weekers F et al: Intensive insulin therapy in critically ill patients, *N Engl J Med* 345:1359-1367, 2001.

41. Dandona P, Aljada A, Bandyopadhyay A: The potential therapeutic role of insulin in acute myocardial infarction in patients admitted to intensive care and those with unspecified hyperglycemia, *Diabetes Care* 26:516-519, 2003.

42. Clark R, English M, McNeil G et al: Effect of intravenous infusion of insulin in diabetics with acute myocardial infarction, *Br Med J* 291:303-305, 1985.

43. Clement S, Braithwaite SS, Magee MF et al: Management of diabetes and hyperglycemia in hospitals, *Diabetes Care* 27:553-591, 2004.

44. United Kingdom Prospective Diabetes Study Group: Effect of blood-glucose control with metformin on complications in overweight patients with type 2 diabetes (UKPDS-34), *Lancet* 352:854-865, 1998.

45. Choi D, Kim SK, Choi SH et al: Preventive effects of rosiglitazone on restenosis after coronary stent implantation in patients with type 2 diabetes, *Diabetes Care* 27:2654-2660, 2004.

46. McGuire DK, Newby LK, Bhapkar MV et al: Association of diabetes mellitus and glycemic control strategies with clinical outcomes after acute coronary syndromes, *Am Heart J* 147:246-252, 2004.

47. Sobel BE, Frye R, Detre KM: Burgeoning dilemmas in the management of diabetes and cardiovascular disease: rationale for the bypass revascularization investigation 2 diabetes (BARI 2D) trial, *Circulation* 107:636-642, 2003.

48. American Diabetes Association: Standards of medical care in diabetes, *Diabetes Care* 28:S4-S36, 2005.

49. Goldberg PA, Siegel MD, Sherwin RS et al: Implementation of a safe and effective insulin infusion protocol in a medical intensive care unit, *Diabetes Care* 27:461-467, 2004.

50. Stevens MA, McCullough PA, Tobin KJ et al: A prospective randomized trial of prevention measures in patients at high risk for contrast nephropathy: results of the P.R.I.N.C.E. Study: prevention of radiocontrast induced nephropathy clinical evaluation, *J Am Coll Cardiol* 33:403-11, 1999.

51. Tepel M, van der Giet M, Schwarzfeld C et al: Prevention of radiographic-contrast-agent-induced reductions in renal function by acetylcysteine (see comments), *N Engl J Med* 343:180-4, 2000.

52. Halon DA, Merdler A, Flugelman MY et al: Late-onset heart failure as a mechanism for adverse long-term outcome in diabetic patients undergoing revascularization (a 13-year report from the Lady Davis Carmel Medical Center registry), *Am J Cardiol* 85:1420-6, 2000.

53. Heart Outcomes Prevention Evaluation (HOPE) Study Investigators: Effects of ramipril on cardiovascular and microvascular outcomes in people with diabetes mellitus: results of the HOPE study and MICRO-HOPE substudy, *Lancet* 355:253-9, 2000.

54. Shekelle PG, Rich MW, Morton SC et al: Efficacy of angiotensin-converting enzyme inhibitors and beta-blockers in the management of left ventricular systolic dysfunction according to race, gender, and diabetic status: a meta-analysis of major clinical trials, *J Am Coll Cardiol* 41:1529-38, 2003.

55. National Institute of Alcohol Abuse and Alcoholism: *Helping patients who drink too much: a clinician's guide,* Rockville, Md, 2005, USDHHS (www.niaaa.nih.gov).

56. Abizaid A, Costa MA, Centemero M et al: Clinical and economic impact of diabetes mellitus on percutaneous and surgical treatment of multivessel coronary disease patients: insights for the Arterial Revascularization Therapy Study (ARTS) trial, *Circulation* 104:533-540, 2001.

57. McAlister FA, Man J, Bistritz L et al: Diabetes and coronary artery bypass surgery, *Diabetes Care* 26:1518-1524, 2003.

58. Leavitt BJ, Sheppard L, Maloney C et al: Effect of diabetes and associated conditions on long-term survival after coronary artery bypass graft surgery, *Circulation* 110:II-41-II-44, 2004.

59. Vermes E, Demaria RG, Martineau R et al: Increased early postoperative morbidity with off-pump coronary artery bypass grafting surgery in patients with diabetes, *Can J Cardiol* 20:1461-1465, 2004.

60. BARI Investigators: Seven-year outcome in the bypass angioplasty revascularization investigation (BARI) by treatment and diabetic status, *J Am Coll Cardiol* 35:1122-1129, 2000.

61. John R, Choudhri AF, Weinberg AD et al: Multicenter review of preoperative risk factors for stroke after coronary artery bypass grafting, *Ann Thoracic Surgery* 69:30-36, 2000.

62. Khaitan L, Sutter FP, Goldman SM: Coronary artery bypass grafting in patients who require long-term dialysis, *Ann Thoracic Surgery* 69:1135-1139, 2000.

63. Hirotani T, Kameda T, Kumamoto T et al: Effects of coronary artery bypass grafting using internal mammary arteries for diabetic patients, *J Am Coll Cardiol* 34:532-538, 1999.

64. Trick WE, Scheckler WE, Tokars JI et al: Modifiable risk factors associated with deep sternal site infection after coronary artery bypass grafting, *J Thor Cardiovasc Surgery* 119:108-114, 2000.

65. Lazar HL, Chipkins, SR, Fitzgerald CA et al: Tight glycemic control in diabetic coronary artery bypass graft patients improves perioperative outcomes and decreases recurrent ischemic events, *Circulation* 109:1497-1502, 2004.

66. Marso SP, Ellis SG, Gurm HS et al: Proteinuria is a key determinant of death in patients with diabetes after isolated coronary artery bypass grafting (see comments), *Am Heart J* 139:939-44, 2000.

67. Nichols GA, Erbey JR, Hillier TA et al: Congestive heart failure in type 2 diabetes, *Diabetes Care* 24:1614-19, 2001.

68. Bertoni AG, Bonds DE, Hundley WG et al: Heart failure prevalence, incidence, and mortality in the elderly with diabetes, *Diabetes Care* 27:699-703, 2004.

69. Piccini JP, Klein L, Gheorghiade M et al: New insights into diastolic heart failure: role of diabetes mellitus, *Am J Med* 116(suppl 5A):64S-75S, 2004.

70. Young LH, Russell RR, Chyun D: *Heart failure and cardiac dysfunction in diabetes,* Totowa, NJ, 2005, Humana Press.

71. Iribarren C, Karter AJ, Go AS et al: Glycemic control and heart failure among adult patients with diabetes, *Circulation* 103:2668-2673, 2001.

72. Stratton IM, Adler AI, Neil HA et al: Association of glycaemia with macrovascular and microvascular complications of type 2 diabetes (UKPDS 35): a prospective observational study, *BMJ* 321:405-412, 2000.

73. Bibbins-Domingo K, Lin F, Vittinghoff E et al: Predictors of heart failure among women with coronary disease, *Circulation* 110:1424-1430, 2004.

74. American College of Cardiology/American Heart Association Task Force on Practice Guidelines: ACC/AHA guidelines for the evaluation and management of chronic heart failure in the adult: executive summary, *Circulation* 104, 2001.

75. Havranek EP, Masoudi FA, Westfall KA et al: Spectrum of heart failure in older patients: results from the national heart failure project, *Am Heart J* 143:412-7, 2002.

76. Guazzi M, Brambilla R, Pontone G et al: Effect of non-insulin-dependent diabetes mellitus on pulmonary function and exercise

tolerance in chronic congestive heart failure, *Am J Cardiol* 89:191-7, 2002.

77. Chobanian AV, Bakris GL, Black HR et al: The Seventh Report of the Joint National Committee on Prevention, Detection, Evaluation, and Treatment of High Blood Pressure: the JNC 7 Report, *JAMA* 289:2560-2572.

78. The HOPE Study Investigators: Effects of an angiotensin-converting enzyme inhibitor, ramipril, on cardiovascular events in high-risk patients, *N Engl J Med* 342:145-153, 2000.

79. Pfeffer MA, McMurry JJV, Velazquez EJ et al: Valsartan, captopril, or both in myocardial infarction complicated by heart failure, left ventricular dysfunction, or both, *N Engl J Med* 349:1893-1906, 2003.

80. Barnett A, Bain S, Bouter P et al: Angiotensin-receptor blockade versus converting-enzyme inhibition in type 2 diabetes and nephropathy, *N Engl J Med* 351:1952-1961, 2004.

81. Haas SJ, Vos T, Gilbert RE et al: Are beta-blockers as efficacious in patients with diabetes mellitus as in patients without diabetes mellitus who have chronic heart failure? A meta-analysis of large-scale clinical trials, *Am Heart J* 146:848-53, 2003.

82. Domanski M, Krause-Steinrauf H, Deedwania P et al: The effect of diabetes on outcomes of patients with advanced heart failure in the BEST trial, *J Am Coll Cardiol* 42:914-22, 2003.

83. Pitt B, Perez A: Spironolactone in patients with heart failure, *N Engl J Med* 342:132, 2000.

84. Zile MR, Brutsaert DL: New concepts in diastolic dysfunction and diastolic heart failure: part II: causal mechanisms and treatment, *Circulation* 105:1503-8, 2002.

85. Wachtell K, Bella JN, Rokkedal J et al: Change in diastolic left ventricular filling after one year of antihypertensive treatment: the Losartan intervention for endpoint reduction in hypertension (LIFE) study, *Circulation* 105:1071-6, 2002.

86. Morgan JA, John R, Weinberg AD et al: Heart transplantation in diabetic recipients: a decade review of 161 patients at Columbia Presbyterian, *J Thorac Cardiovasc Surg* 127:1486-92, 2004.

87. Nesto RW, LeWinter M, Bell D et al: Thiazolidinedione use, fluid retention, and congestive heart failure, *Diabetes Care* 27:256-63, 2004.

88. Tang WH, Francis GS, Hoogwerf BJ et al: Fluid retention after initiation of thiazolidinedione therapy in diabetic patients with established chronic heart failure, *J Am Coll Cardiol* 41:1394-8, 2003.

89. Masoudi FA, Inzucchi SE, Wang Y et al: Thiazolidinediones, metformin, and outcomes in older patients with diabetes and heart failure, *Circulation* 111, 2005.

90. Maru S, Koch GG, Stender M et al: Antidiabetic drugs and heart failure risk in patients with type 2 diabetes in the UK primary care setting, *Diabetes Care* 28:20-26, 2005.

91. Malmberg K: Prospective randomised study of intensive insulin treatment on long term survival after acute myocardial infarction in patients with diabetes mellitus. DIGAMI (diabetes mellitus, insulin glucose infusion in acute myocardial infarction) study group (see comments). *BMJ* 314:1512-5, 1997.

92. Maser RE, Vinik AI, Mitchell BD et al: The association between cardiovascular autonomic neuropathy and mortality in individuals with diabetes, *Diabetes Care* 26:1895-1901, 2003.

93. Gerritsen J, Heine RJ, Dekker JM et al: Impaired autonomic function is associated with increased mortality, especially in subjects with diabetes, hypertension, or a history of cardiovascular disease, *Diabetes Care* 24:1793-8, 2001.

94. Wheeler SG, Ahroni JH, Boyko EJ: Prospective study of autonomic neuropathy as a predictor of mortality in patients with diabetes, *Diabetes Res Clin Practice* 58:131-8, 2002.

95. Liao D, Carnethon M, Evans G et al: Lower heart rate variability is associated with the development of coronary heart disease in individuals with diabetes: the atherosclerosis risk in communities (ARIC) study, *Diabetes* 51:3524-31, 2002.

96. Singh JP, Larson MG, O'Donnell CJ et al: Association of hyperglycemia with reduced heart rate variability (The Framingham Heart Study), *Am J Cardiol* 86:309-12, 2000.

97. Bigger JT, Fleiss JL, Steinman RC et al: RR variability in healthy, middle-aged persons compared with patients with chronic coronary heart disease or recent acute myocardial infarction, *Circulation* 91:1936-43, 1995.

98. Valensi P, Sachs RN, Harfouche B et al: Predictive value of cardiac autonomic neuropathy in diabetic patients with or without silent myocardial ischemia, *Diabetes Care* 24:339-43, 2001.

99. Carnethon MR, Golden SH, Folsom AR et al: Prospective investigation of autonomic nervous system function and the development of type 2 diabetes. The atherosclerosis risk in communities study, 1987-1998, *Circulation* 107:2190-5, 2003.

100. Valensi P, Paries J, Attali JR et al: Cardiac autonomic neuropathy in diabetic patients: influence of diabetes duration, obesity, and the microangiopathic complications. The French multicenter study, *Metabolism* 52:815-20, 2003.

101. Rana BS, Lim PO, Naas AAO et al: QT abnormalities are often present at diagnosis in diabetes and are better predictors of cardiac death than ankle brachial pressure index and autonomic function tests, *Heart* 91:44-50, 2005.

102. Vinik AI, Mitchell BD, Maser RE et al: Diabetic autonomic neuropathy, *Diabetes Care* 26:1553-79, 2003.

103. Wackers FJTH, Young LH, Inzucchi SE et al: Detection of silent myocardial ischemia in asymptomatic diabetic subjects: the DIAD study, *Diabetes Care* 27:1954-61, 2004.

104. American Diabetes Association: Consensus development conference on the diagnosis of coronary heart disease in people with diabetes, *Diabetes Care* 21:1551-1559, 1998.

105. Iskandrian AE: Risk assessment of stable patients (panel III): proceedings of the 4th invitational wintergreen conference wintergreen panel summaries, *J Nucl Cardiol* 6:93-155, 1999.

106. Low PA, Benrud-Larson LM, Sletten DM et al: Autonomic symptoms and diabetic neuropathy, *Diabetes Care* 27:2942-2947, 2004.

107. Boulton AJM, Vinik AI, Arezzo JC et al: Diabetic neuropathies: a statement by the American Diabetes Association, *Diabetes Care* 28:956-962, 2005.

108. Ewing DJ, Borsey DQ, Bellavere F et al: Cardiac autonomic neuropathy in diabetes: comparison of measures of R-R interval variation, *Diabetologia* 21:18-24, 1981.

109. O'Brien IA, O'Hare P, Corrall RJM: Heart rate variability in healthy subjects: effects of age and the derivation of normal ranges for tests of autonomic function. *Br Heart J* 55:348-54, 1986.

110. Task Force of the European Society of Cardiology and the North American Society of Pacing and Electrophysiology: Heart rate variability: standards of measurement, physiological interpretation, and clinical use, *Circulation* 93:1043-65, 1996.

111. Johnson B, Nesto RW, Pfeifer M et al: Cardiac abnormalities in diabetic patients with neuropathy, *Diabetes Care* 27:448-54, 2004.

112. Stella P, Ellis D, Maser RE et al: Cardiovascular autonomic neuropathy (expiration and inspiration ratio) in type 1 diabetes. Incidence and predictors, *J Diabetes Complication* 14:1-6, 2000.

113. Young LH, Jose P, Chyun D: Diagnosis of CAD in patients—who to evaluate, *Current Diabetes Reports* 3:19-27, 2002.

114. Janand-Delenne B, Savin B, Habib G et al: Silent myocardial ischemia in patients with diabetes, *Diabetes Care* 22:1396-1400, 1999.

115. Gazzaruso C, De Amici E, Garzaniti A et al: Assessment of asymptomatic coronary artery disease in apparently uncomplicated type 2 diabetic patients, *Diabetes Care* 25:1418-24, 2002.

■ ■ ■ ■ c h a p t e r **86**

Cardiorenal Syndromes

Robin J. Trupp
Mary C. Langford

CHAPTER ABBREVIATIONS

ACE angiotensin-converting enzyme

ACTIV Acute and Chronic Therapeutic Impact of Vasopressin Antagonist

ADH antidiuretic hormone

ADHERE Acute Decompensated Heart Failure National Registry

ARB angiotensin receptor blocker

AT angiotensin

AVP arginine vasopressin

BUN blood urea nitrogen

CHARM Candesartan in Heart Failure Assessment of Reduction in Mentality and Morbidity

COBRA Consolidated Omnibus Budget Reconciliation Act

CRIC Chronic Renal Insufficiency Cohort Study

DASH Dietary Approaches to Stop Hypertension

ESRD end stage renal disease

EVEREST Efficacy of Vasopressin Antagonist in Heart Failure: Outcome Study with Tolvaptan

FE$_{na}$ fractional urinary excretion of sodium

GFR glomerular filtration rate

IDNT Irbesartan Diabetic Nephropathy Trial

IL Interleukin

JGA juxtaglomerular apparatus

LIFE Losartan Intervention for Endpoint Reduction in Hypertension Trial

MDRD Modification of Diet in Renal Disease

NKF National Kidney Foundation

NSAIDs nonsteroidal anti-inflammatory drugs

OTC over the counter

PD peritoneal dialysis

PREVEND Prevention of Renal and Vascular End Stage Disease Trial

RAAS renin-angiotensin-aldosterone system

RENAAL Reduction of Endpoints in Non-Insulin Dependent Diabetes Mellitus with Angiotensin II Antagonist Losartan Trial

SOLVD Studies of Left Ventricular Dysfunction

The heart and the kidneys share an intimate relationship, jointly maintaining extracellular fluid balance, biochemical homeostasis, and intravascular function. Renal and myocardial function are integrated hemodynamically, metabolically, and neurohormonally.[1] It has been well-documented that cardiac impairment has profound effects on renal function. Conversely, intrinsic renal disease induces multiple cardiotoxic effects. Endothelial injury and dysfunction occurs in a parallel fashion within renal as well as myocardial tissue due to similar vasoconstrictive, inflammatory, and atherogenic processes.[2] Mortality and morbidity are markedly increased in persons who have both renal and cardiac dysfunction.[2] This chapter focuses on the complex interrelationships of renal and myocardial function.

INTIMATE RELATIONSHIP BETWEEN THE HEART AND THE KIDNEY

The kidneys receive approximately 20 percent of cardiac output, or approximately 1000 to 1200 ml/min total blood flow. Kidneys provide endocrine, metabolic, hemodynamic, and excretory functions within the body. The nephron performs multiple processes, including filtration, secretion, reabsorption, and excretion, with substantial impact on intravascular volume, intravascular biochemical content, extracellular homeostasis, and cardiovascular function.[3]

NEPHRON: A SPECIALIZED CAPILLARY

The nephron is the functional unit of the kidney (Figure 86-1). At birth an individual normally has approximately 2 million nephrons. The number of functional units naturally declines with age. Renal performance depends on the number of functioning nephrons as well as nephron responsiveness to the biochemical milieu of the body. The nephron can be visualized as a sequential capillary. Blood enters the kidney through renal arteries branching off the abdominal aorta. The initial renal capillary is the glomerulus, which is followed by a peritubular capillary system. These capillaries participate in a biochemical exchange along the nephron tubules and join to form renal veins emptying into the vena cava. The renal cortex includes the glomerulus and the afferent and efferent arterioles. The renal medulla encompasses the renal tubules and the peritubular capillaries (vasa recta). The distal convoluted tubule re-enters the renal cortex.

The glomerular basement membrane is delicate, highly oxygen-dependent, semipermeable, and preserves intravascular proteins and blood cells. It also filters out large molecules, such as glucose. Average plasma volume entering the glomerulus is 600 to 700 ml/min—of which approximately 125 ml/min is filtered into Bowman's capsule—and travels into the tubules as protein-free ultra-filtrate. Total plasma volume is filtered approximately 60 times daily. Ultra-filtrate flows across the glomerular basement membrane into Bowman's

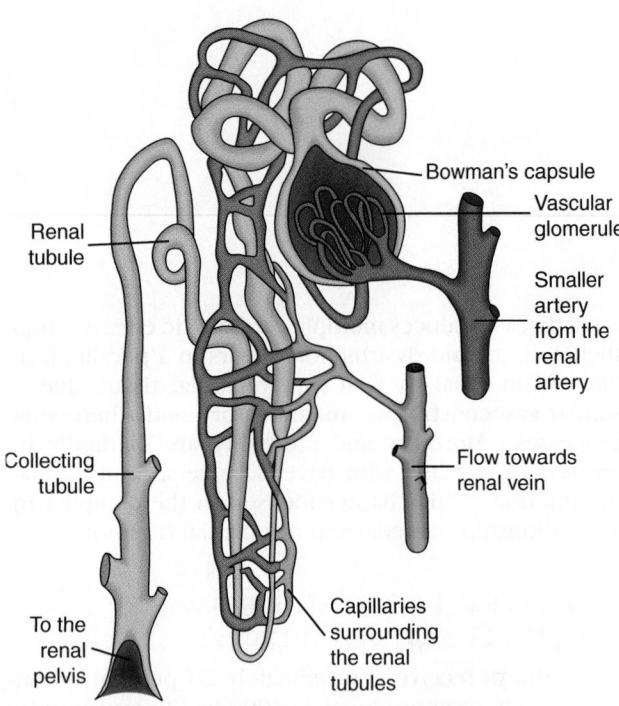

Renal tubule

Bowman's capsule

Vascular glomerule

Smaller artery from the renal artery

Collecting tubule

Flow towards renal vein

To the renal pelvis

Capillaries surrounding the renal tubules

FIGURE 86-1 ■ Anatomy of a nephron.

capsule and into the proximal convoluted tubules, the descending and ascending loop of Henle, and into the distal convoluted tubules throughout which active and passive biochemical and fluid exchange occurs. Because of the active biochemical work occurring throughout the tubular system, the renal medulla is exquisitely oxygen-dependent and vulnerable to ischemic injury. In general, renal excretion is equivalent to the rate of glomerular filtration plus the rate of tubular secretion, minus the rate of chemical reabsorption along tubule system. Fluid that remains within the tubule system enters the collecting ducts, draining into the renal pelvis as urine, and is excreted via ureters into the bladder. Pressures within the drainage system may exert backward influence within the tubular system, reducing efficiency of glomerular filtration.[3,4]

Specialized cells in the distal tubule, called *macula densa*, sense biochemical content, pressure, and osmolarity of tubular fluid. These cells communicate with the juxtaglomerular apparatus **(JGA),** a specialized tissue located adjacent to the afferent arteriole and distal collecting ducts. The JGA secretes a hormone renin that precipitates secretion of the vasopressor angiotensin II, integrating intrarenal biochemistry and intrarenal hemodynamics with systemic hemodynamic and biochemical regulation.[3,4] The hormonal cascade elicited by the secretion of renin is termed the *renin-angiotensin-aldosterone system* (RAAS).

Intrarenal Autoregulation

The filtration system of the nephron is pressure driven. Renal hemodynamic function is highly sensitive to intravascular volume, intravascular pressures, solute load (primarily sodium), acid-base balance, and to oxygen delivery. To maintain stable filtration, the glomerulus is flanked by

a unique dual arteriole system. The afferent arteriole leads into the glomerulus and the efferent arteriole exits from the glomerulus into peritubular capillaries. When renal perfusion pressure decreases, the afferent arteriole dilates and the efferent arteriole constricts, maintaining stable perfusion pressures within the glomerulus and preserving a consistent filtration rate. Excess perfusion pressure results in afferent arteriole constriction and efferent arteriole dilatation, reducing glomerular pressure and protecting the glomerular basement from hydrostatic damage. The afferent arteriole is exceptionally sensitive to effects of angiotensin (AT), while the efferent arteriole is more sensitive to effects of norepinephrine. Efferent arteriole function preferentially preserves glomerular function at the expense of peritubular capillary function. Prolonged or excess efferent constriction may precipitate tubular ischemia. In addition, endogenous or pharmaceutical vasopressors may induce peritubular artery constriction independently of glomerular filtration, altering biochemical exchange within nephron tubules.[1,3,4]

Intrarenal Neurohormonal Autoregulation

Intrarenal vasoconstriction is mediated by neurohormones, including epinephrine, norepinephrine, angiotensin II, aldosterone, and arginine vasopressin **(AVP),** also called *antidiuretic hormone* **(ADH).** Counterregulatory vasodilatation is mediated by nitric oxide, prostaglandins, and natriuretic peptides.[1,3,4] There are numerous complex interrelationships between various vasoactive peptides within the kidney that remain under active investigation. Overall neurohormonal processes maintain consistent renal perfusion pressure and glomerular filtration across wide variations of dietary intake and systemic hemodynamics. Intrarenal baroreceptors are acutely sensitive to changes in cardiac output. Chemoreceptors respond to extracellular biochemical changes. Vascular and biochemical processes within the nephron are also directly affected by sympathetic forces. The JGA responds to prompting of macular densa tissue as well as to sympathetic stimulation and secretes renin, which modulates intrarenal as well as systemic hemodynamics.[3,4]

RENAL EFFECT ON SYSTEMIC HEMODYNAMICS

The kidney participates in systemic hemodynamics via four primary processes: (1) sympathetic activation, (2) renin and AT secretion, (3) adrenal activation and extracellular expansion and contraction via water, and (4) sodium regulation.[5] Macula densa cells in renal distal and collecting tubules respond to changes in hydrostatic pressure, osmolarity (primarily determined by sodium content), hydrogen ion concentration, and oxygen content of tubular fluid. Decrease in distal tubular pressure, decreased sodium or oxygen content, or increased hydrogen ion stimulates macula densa cells, which activate the juxtaglomerular apparatus, and renin is secreted. Renin catalyzes the conversion of angiotensinogen to AT-I, which is subsequently converted to AT-II within pulmonary capillaries (Figure 86-2). AT-II

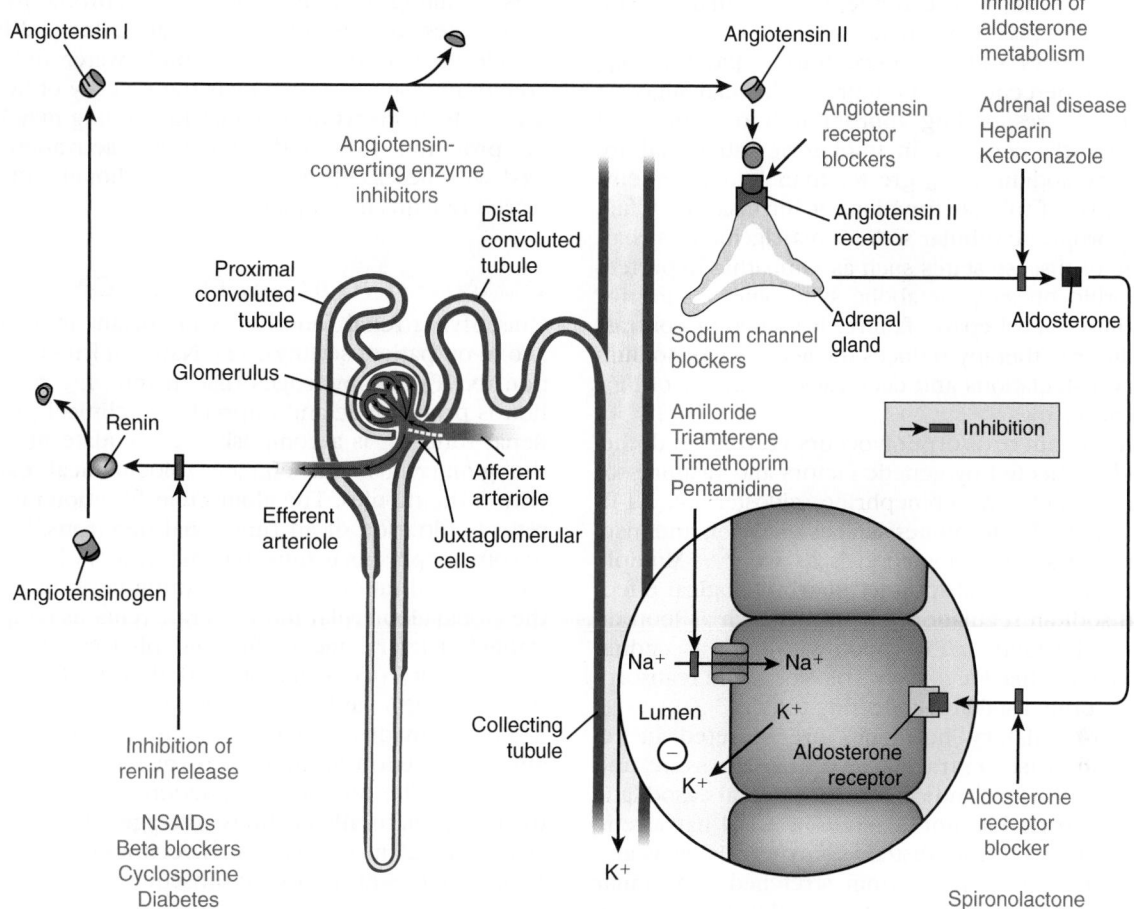

FIGURE 86-2 ■ Renin-angiotensin-aldosterone system. *NSAIDs,* Nonsteroidal anti-inflammatory drugs. *K⁺,* Potassium; *Na⁺,* sodium.

has profound systemic vasoconstrictive effects. AT-II directly stimulates norepinephrine release via the sympathetic nervous system, further augmenting its vasopressor effect. AT-II stimulates vasopressin release from the posterior pituitary gland. Vasopressin is a systemic vasoconstrictor and augments water reabsorption from the distal renal tubules.[1] AT-II also induces aldosterone release from the adrenal cortex. Aldosterone enhances systemic vasoconstriction. More importantly, aldosterone stimulates active tubular reabsorption of sodium at the expense of potassium in distal tubules. Sodium retention induces passive water retention, increasing intravascular volume and subsequently increasing blood pressure.[6]

Renal Sodium Management

The kidney dynamically maintains extracellular volume homeostasis by regulation of sodium and water. Sodium is the most abundant extracellular cation, while potassium is the most abundant intracellular cation. Ninety percent of extracellular fluid osmolarity is determined by sodium content (in combination with chloride and bicarbonate). Body cells actively extrude sodium from within the cell via sodium/potassium pump mechanisms to maintain a biochemical gradient across the cell membrane. The healthy kidney aggressively maintains

extracellular sodium concentration within the narrow range of 135 to 145 mEq/L in spite of widely variable dietary intake. The process of renal sodium excretion is termed *natriuresis.* Water follows sodium passively along an osmotic gradient. Renal water excretion is termed *diuresis.* Sodium is filtered at the glomerulus and reabsorbed throughout the tubular system. The majority of active sodium transport occurs in the proximal tubule, where 60 percent of filtered sodium is reabsorbed. Sodium that "escapes" into the distal tubule may be actively reabsorbed at that location as well. Distal tubule processes act as a "back-up" system for proximal tubular function.[1,5]

The kidney responds to changes in extracellular fluid milieu by adjusting sodium excretion. The baseline fractional urinary excretion of sodium (FE_{na}) of 1 percent will normally vary with dietary intake, such that increased sodium ingestion increases FE_{na}. Conversely when renal blood flow diminishes acutely, FE_{na} decreases as the kidney preserves serum sodium and subsequently intravascular volume. Inability to appropriately preserve extracellular sodium typifies acute renal failure. The FE_{na} is used in acute care settings to differentiate between prerenal and intrinsic renal failure. Calculation of fractional urine sodium excretion uses plasma and urine sodium and creatinine levels: $FE_{na} = (U_{na} \times P_{cr} \times 100) / (U_{cr} \times P_{na})$, where U_{na} = urinary sodium, P_{cr} = plasma creatinine, U_{cr} = urinary creatinine and P_{na} = plasma sodium.

A low urinary sodium concentration and low FE_{na} (less than 1 percent) in an oliguric individual suggests the kidney is responding appropriately to a prerenal stressor. On the contrary, in an oliguric patient, failure to conserve sodium (FE_{na} greater than 1 to 2 percent) suggests loss of tubular function, or intrinsic renal failure. Inappropriate tubular sodium management is characteristic of disease states such as idiopathic hypertension, morbid obesity, metabolic syndrome, congestive heart failure, and hepatic failure. Presence of contrast dye or diuretic therapy reduces the accuracy of sodium excretion calculations and decreases the utility of FE_{na} in clinical settings.[1,3,5]

Active sodium reabsorption occurs via renal endothelium and is affected by genetic factors and vasopressor substances, including epinephrine, aldosterone, AT-II, and endothelin-I.[7] Hormones such as glucagon and insulin influence sodium homeostasis as well.[1,3,5] Multiple drugs exert direct and indirect pharmacological effect on renal sodium regulation. Chemicals such as loop diuretics block sodium reabsorption within the ascending loop of Henle. Thiazide diuretics block sodium reabsorption within the distal and collecting tubules.[4]

Counter-regulatory hormones are secreted in response to increased extracellular volume, pressure, and biochemical content and promote intrarenal vasodilatation and increased sodium excretion. Atrial natriuretic peptide is released from distended myocardial atria and b-type natriuretic peptide from stretched ventricular myocardium, inducing intrarenal vasodilatation by way of nitric oxide pathways and stimulation of active sodium excretion in proximal tubules. Intrarenal prostaglandin secretion opposes the vasoconstrictive effects of renin, norepinephrine, and endothelin, enhancing sodium excretion and restoring normal hemodynamic balance within the nephron.[3-5]

Renal Water Management

AVP preserves intravascular water and augments blood pressure.[1,3] AVP is produced in the hypothalamus and stored in the posterior pituitary gland. Chemo- and baroreceptors within the hypothalamus are sensitive to intravascular pressure, volume, and tonicity. The hypothalamus communicates via nerve tissue with the posterior pituitary. Decreased systemic pressure, blood volume, or increased blood osmolarity results in posterior pituitary release of vasopressin that directly enhances water reabsorption in the distal renal tubules. AVP is also a potent systemic vasoconstrictor that intensifies sympathetic effects, including redistribution of blood flow from surface and splanchnic vessels into the great vessels.[3,4] This decreases renal blood flow, decreasing urine output and preserving extracellular volume. Intraarterial and intracardiac baroreceptors and osmoreceptors that are sensitive to diminished hydrostatic pressure and increased hemoconcentration activate adrenergic systems, with secondary activation of the renin-angiotensin aldosterone cascade. Catecholamine and vasopressin effects include activation of the thirst center in the hypothala-

mus, resulting in water craving.[3,4] In chronic hypervolemic states such as congestive heart failure, AVP levels are elevated regardless of total body water and the degree of AVP secretion parallels the severity of heart failure.[8,9] Mechanisms underlying this finding may include the profound RAAS and sympathetic activation associated with heart failure syndromes, although current research remains incomplete.[8,9]

QUANTIFYING RENAL FUNCTION

Quantifying renal function is important in acute care and in outpatient settings. The National Kidney Foundation **(NKF)** acknowledges that quantifying renal function is problematic and imprecise in clinical practice.[10] Renal function is a composite of adequate filtration at the glomerulus and efficient biochemical exchange within the tubules. The glomerular filtration rate **(GFR)** reflects filtration of all functional nephrons.[11] Damage to some nephrons results in compensatory hypertrophy and hyperfiltration of the remaining nephron units, so the global glomerular filtration rate remains temporarily stable.[14] Dietary, metabolic, and pharmacologic influences result in considerable variation in blood urea nitrogen (BUN) and serum creatinine. In addition, a healthy individual may demonstrate fluctuations in creatinine secretion up to 10 percent within a short time interval.[12] The number of functional nephrons within the kidney naturally declines with age. The normal GFR at age 30 (125 ml/min/1.73 m^2) declines by an estimated 1 ml/min/1.73 m^2 for every subsequent year.[10,12]

Measures of Renal Function

Urine output measurement, while helpful in assessing fluid balance, does not measure the ability of the kidney to process biochemically.[11] The most commonly used criteria of renal biochemical function in clinical practice are measurement of BUN and serum creatinine (Table 86-1). Rapidly rising serum BUN and Scr prompts aggressive reno-protective intervention in acute care settings. Examination of urine sediment for casts, erythrocytes, and leukocytes also provides information regarding tubular function and viability.[10] Comparing urine sodium content with serum sodium provides clues regarding prerenal versus intrarenal pathology. Serum creatinine alone should not be used to assess the

■ ■ ■

TABLE 86-1 COMMONLY MEASURED NORMAL RENAL PARAMETERS

NAME	ABBREVIATION	VALUE
Blood urea nitrogen	BUN	7-18 mg/dl
Serum creatinine	Scr	0.6-1.1 mg/dl (women)
		0.7-1.3 mg/dl (men)
Glomerular filtration rate	GFR	90 to 125 ml/min

Adapted from Kidney Disease Outcomes Quality Initiative (NKF K/DOQI): *Clinical practice guidelines for chronic kidney disease: evaluation, classification and stratification*, New York, 2002, National Kidney Foundation. *mg*, milligram; *dl*, deciliter; *ml*, milliliter; *min*, minute. *BUN*, blood urea nitrogen; *GFR*, glomerular filtration rate; *Scr*, serum creatinine.

level of renal function.[10] Using serum creatinine alone to monitor ongoing renal function can lead to serious over-estimation of renal function.[11] Serum creatinine is a product of steady-state creatinine metabolism from muscle and depends on an individual's muscle mass and muscle catabolism. Since muscle mass varies in individuals and is affected by age and gender, serum creatinine frequently underestimates decline in GFR. Substances such as cephalosporin antibiotics, inflammatory cytokines, glucose, uric acid, and catabolic states may directly alter serum creatinine levels independently of actual renal function.[10,11]

Renal Function Measured by Glomerular Filtration Rate

GFR, defined as the volume of plasma filtered across the glomerulus per unit time, is a more accurate reflection of nephron integrity than serum BUN and serum creatinine levels.[10,11] The best test available in clinical practice to measure GFR is a 24-hour measurement of urine creatinine clearance; however, errors in urine collection are common and measurement is cumbersome. Clearance of other molecules such as para-aminohippuric acid, inulin, or iothalamate or evaluation of GFR by means of radioisotope techniques are used to quantify renal function for research purposes. The utility of these techniques is limited in clinical settings due to substrate availability and cost considerations.[10,11]

Indirect estimations of GFR have been formulated by equations that consider serum creatinine and sodium, urine creatinine and sodium, gender, and body mass. GFR calculation is useful for bedside estimation of renal function.[11] Using GFR estimation allows for more accurate monitoring of renal efficiency than measuring BUN and serum creatinine. The most common GFR calculation for adults is the Cockcroft-Gault equation, which is gender adjusted by multiplying by 0.85 for female gender. In acute care settings weight used in calculation should be the ideal body weight or "dry weight." Newer equations such as developed by the Modification of Diet in Renal Disease Study Group incorporate ethnic variations. GFR calculators are readily available via internet access (search: "GFR calculator"), facilitating use in clinical settings[10,11] (Table 86-2).

All estimations of renal function have limitations in accuracy.[11] Earliest indicators of renal endothelial dys-

function such as von Willebrand factor levels, soluble P-selectin, or serum cystatin-C levels have been proposed as potential targets for initiating protective therapy but are not in common use at this time.[13] Urinary albumin levels increase with glomerular injury and spot microalbumin assessment (typically urine microalbumin/creatinine ratio) may add valuable information to other assessments of renal function. Current best clinical practice uses multiple indicators of renal function and maintains vigilant surveillance for early biochemical markers of renal stress.[10,11,13]

ACUTE RENAL IMPAIRMENT

Acute renal impairment is categorized by the likely site of pathology although combined pathologies are common. Prerenal dysfunction occurs when effective blood flow or pressure is diminished, decreasing glomerular filtration. Prerenal azotemia (build up of serum nitrogenous wastes due to impaired kidney perfusion) is distinguished from intrarenal and postrenal dysfunction to identify therapeutic strategies. Intrarenal dysfunction refers to glomerular or tubular injury. Postrenal impairment occurs when obstruction occurs in urine flow distal to the nephron. This results in increased hydrostatic intratubular pressure, causing backward impedance to glomerular filtration.[10]

Proteinuria: Early Marker of Glomerular Injury

Proteinuria is an early marker of glomerular endothelial injury and of generalized endovascular "leakiness."[14] Proteinuria occurs when renal perfusion pressure increases, leading to hyperfiltration of serum or other causes of damage to the delicate glomerular basement membrane. Proteinuria increases with age, hyperglycemia, and hypertension, particularly a hypertensive pattern of "nondipping" during the night.[15] Persistent proteinuria predicts progressive renal decline and failure.[14] Protein within the proximal tubule is a potent trigger of inflammatory cytokines and activates interstitial fibroblasts, leading to leukocyte adhesion, expression of growth factors, collagen deposits, fibrosis, and pathologic vascular remodeling, not only locally within the kidney but systemically as well[16,17] (Table 86-3).

■ ■ ■

TABLE 86-2 EQUATIONS TO PREDICT GLOMERULAR FILTRATION RATE IN STABLE CHRONIC KIDNEY DISEASE

Abbreviated MDRD Study equation	GFR (ml/min/1.73 m^2) = 186 × Scr$^{-1.154}$ × age$^{-0.203}$ × (0.742 if female) × (1.210 if African American)
Cockcroft-Gault equation	Ccr (ml/min) = ((140 x age) × weight (kg)) divided by (72 x Scr) × (0.85 if female)

Adapted from Kidney Disease Outcomes Quality Initiative (NKF K/DOQI): *Clinical practice guidelines for chronic kidney disease: evaluation, classification and stratification*, New York, 2002, National Kidney Foundation. *GFR*, Glomerular filtration rate; *MDRD*, Modification of Diet in Renal Disease; *Scr*, serum creatinine concentration (in mg/dl); *Ccr*, creatinine clearance.

■ ■ ■

TABLE 86-3 MEASURES OF URINE PROTEIN (SPOT MICROALBUMIN/CREATININE RATIO)

Normal urine protein	Less than 25 mg/g (women)
	Less than 17 mg/g (men)
Microalbuminuria	25-355 mg/g (women)
	17-250 mg/g (men)
Macro proteinuria (may be seen on urinalysis)	Greater than 355 mg/g (women)
	Greater than 250 mg/g (men)
Nephrotic syndrome	Greater than 2500 mg urine protein in 24 hr

Adapted from Kidney Disease Outcomes Quality Initiative (NKF K/DOQI): *Clinical practice guidelines for chronic kidney disease: evaluation, classification and stratification*, New York, 2002, National Kidney Foundation.

An early morning spot urine sample is used to measure urinary protein. When a small amount of urine protein, called microalbumin, is identified on a spot urine sample, findings should be confirmed using a 24-hour urine collection.[10] Serial samples are also useful to avoid diet- and activity-related bias. There are situations when the standard dipstick readings may not be accurate. Samples are noted in Table 86-4.

Presence of microalbuminuria defines stage I kidney damage even when GFR is normal (above 90 mg/ml/1.73 m²).[10] Increased protein excretion identifies elevated risk for progressive renal impairment. The rate of increase in proteinuria parallels progressive kidney decline. There exists an additional population, primarily individuals with hyperglycemia, where progressive renal dysfunction occurs without significant proteinuria. It is thought that this may occur due to widening and fibrosis of the mesangial space and collagen infiltration of the glomerular basement membrane.[14,15]

Microalbumin and Cardiovascular Disease

Excess renal endothelial permeability is reflective of systemic vascular endothelial dysfunction.[18,19] Microalbuminuria is considered a marker of generalized endothelial dysfunction and is consequently termed "an integrated risk factor" in evaluating cardiovascular disease.[19] Microalbumin has been documented in persons with impaired vasodilatory response to acetylcholine,[20] increased carotid intima-media thickness,[15] and increased risk of stroke.[19] Microalbuminuria is associated with left ventricular hypertrophy[21]; autonomic dysfunction[22]; and increased C-reactive protein, von Willebrand, and fibrinogen levels.[23] Microalbuminuria is an independent predictor of cardiovascular disease and heart failure in general populations.[19,23]

Even low levels of micoalbuminuria correlate with increased risk of cardiovascular events and death.[24] A sub-study of a general population cohort, the Third Co-penhagen City Heart Study, found that urinary microalbumin greater than 4.8 mcg/min (or approximately 6 mg/L) was associated with significantly increased coronary heart disease and death in men and women independent of age, hypertension, diabetes, and total cholesterol.[18] Measured urine albumin greater than 15 mcg/min corresponded with a three-fold increase in cardiovascular mortality in a general population independently of the serum creatinine level.[18] A cohort from the Heart Outcomes Prevention Evaluation Study demonstrated that presence of microalbuminuria in persons with known cardiovascular disease or diabetes increased the relative risk of major cardiovascular events by 1.83 and relative risk for congestive heart failure by 3.23.[25]

The degree of cardiovascular risk corresponds with increased urinary protein, and rapidly progressive proteinuria predicts worsened cardiovascular outcomes.[26] A general population study in Groningen demonstrated that progression of urinary protein over 1 year was associated with 29 percent increase in cardiovascular mortality.[24] Therapy targeted to decrease microalbuminuria has demonstrated positive impact on cardiac and vascular events.[19,26] The Reduction of Endpoints in Non-Insulin Dependent Diabetes Mellitus with the Angiotensin II Antagonist Losartan (RENAAL) data confirmed significant reduction in cardiovascular morbidity and mortality with AT blockade.[26] The Prevention of Renal and Vascular End Stage Disease (PREVEND) study included 864 persons from a general population cohort with documented microalbuminuria, randomized to fosinopril 20 mg or placebo and followed for 46 months. Fosinopril reduced urinary albumin by 26 percent and was associated with a 40 percent decrease in the relative risk of combined endpoint of cardiovascular mortality and hospitalization for CVD events (*p* = 0.098).[19] Reducing urine protein excretion with an AT blocker was found to significantly decrease the composite endpoint of cardiovascular disease death, myocardial infarction, and stroke in the Losartan Intervention for Endpoint Reduction in Hypertension (LIFE) Study.[19,27]

Microalbumin and All-cause Mortality

Microalbumin has been associated with increased risk for all-cause mortality in diabetic and in nondiabetic populations as well.[18,19,24,25,27] Microalbumin is associated with subclinical vascular inflammation, macrophage and platelet activation, and systemic hypercoagulability.[14,19] The Epic-Norfolk Study, a 6-year trial involving 22,368 individuals aged 40 to 79 years, demonstrated a significant increase in all-cause mortality when microalbuminuria was present in a general population, independent of all other risk factors.[19] The Nord-Trondelag Health Study (HUNT) of 2089 apparently healthy subjects over 4½ years demonstrated two times all-cause mortality with documented urinary microalbumin in the absence of diabetes or hypertension.[19] The Third Copenhagen City Heart Study using a general population cohort of 2762 men and women, aged 30 to 70, who were followed from 1992 to 2001, revealed a positive correlation between urine albumin and increased coronary heart disease (relative risk 2.0,

■ ■ ■

TABLE 86-4   CAUSES OF FALSE RESULTS IN URINE PROTEIN MEASUREMENTS

	FALSE POSITIVE	FALSE NEGATIVE
Fluid balance	Dehydration/urinary concentration	Overhydration/polyuria
Exercise	Exercise increases proteinuria	
Hematuria	Blood cells measured as protein	
Infection	Bacterial proteins	
Nonalbumin proteins		Do not interact with reagent as strongly as albumin
Pharmaceutical effects	Severely alkaline urine (pH greater than 8) reacts with dipstick reagent to give false positive	

Adapted from Kidney Disease Outcomes Quality Initiative (NKF K/DOQI): *Clinical practice guidelines for chronic kidney disease: evaluation, classification and stratification,* New York, 2002, National Kidney Foundation.

99 percent confidence interval) and death (relative risk 1.9, 95 percent CI), independent of age, sex, renal creatinine clearance, diabetes mellitus, hypertension, and plasma lipids.[18] The PREVEND Study Group used a population of 40,548 persons from Groningen, the Netherlands, aged 28 to 75 followed for a 3-year period. There was a significant positive dose-related correlation between urinary albumin and mortality. Increased urine albumin (defined as 20 and 200 mg/L) was positively associated with incidence of cardiac and noncardiac death after adjustment for tobacco use, age, diabetes, lipid levels, and hypertension. Noncardiac deaths were primarily due to malignant neoplasm. A two-fold increase in urinary albumin was associated with a relative risk of 1.29 for cardiovascular disease mortality (95 percent CI) and 1.2 relative risk for noncardiovascular disease mortality (95 percent CI).[24]

STAGES OF CHRONIC KIDNEY DISEASE

Chronic kidney disease is characterized by progressive nephron loss and inability to maintain extracellular fluid and biochemical balance. Chronic kidney disease is common, is associated with increased morbidity and mortality both in hospital and outpatient settings, and has important implications for clinical nursing practice[12] (Table 86-5).

Chronic Kidney Disease: Prevalence and Significance

Long-term health registries demonstrate that chronic kidney disease is a major and increasing health problem in the United States. Approximately 11 percent of U.S. citizens in 1994 had chronic kidney disease as defined by the NKF.[12,28] Incidence of chronic kidney disease has increased dramatically in the past decade. National longitudinal registries such as NHANES III estimate that currently 19.2 million persons in the United States have stage 1, 2, 3, or 4 chronic kidney disease and 300,000 have end-stage renal failure (stage 5 chronic kidney disease). Ongoing longitudinal trials, such as the Chronic Renal Insufficiency Cohort Study of 2001 (CRIC) supported by the National Institutes of Health, continue to provide insight into prevalence and progression of chronic kidney disease in the American population. Ad-

ditional data suggest an alarming growth in prevalence globally as well.[12] Causes of chronic kidney disease include diabetes; hypertension; infection; obstruction; toxic chemicals; and genetic, autoimmune, and infiltrative diseases. Prevalence of end stage renal disease (ESRD) varies with ethnic origin and increases with age.[29] Diabetes is the most common cause of end stage renal disease and uncontrolled hypertension contributes substantially to increased prevalence.[30] Diabetes accounted for 36 percent of persons on renal support therapies in one study.[30] The U.S. Renal Data System Fifteenth Annual Report anticipates that the incidence of end-stage renal disease incidence will approximate 460,000 per year by the year 2030 with a population of 2.24 million persons on renal replacement therapies. Two thirds of this population is anticipated to have diabetes as the primary cause of their renal failure.[30]

Economic Implications of Chronic Kidney Disease

Economic implications of the rise in chronic kidney disease and ESRD are substantial.[28,31,32] Persons with stage 1 to 4 chronic kidney disease make up approximately 3.3 percent of current Medicare populations; however, they account for 5.5 percent to 8 percent of the Medicare budget. Persons with any stage of chronic kidney disease had greater health-related costs across all categories of care over a 5.5 year observation study in a large northwestern health maintenance organization.[28] Categories of care included inpatient care, outpatient care, and pharmaceuticals. Total medical costs over the span of the study were double for persons with any stage chronic kidney disease without comorbidities than for age- and sex-matched persons with no chronic kidney disease and no comorbidities.[28] Ninety percent of ESRD patients in the United States are eligible for government Medicare support regardless of age and account for 1 percent of the Medicare population.[31] The per-person cost of care for the individual with ESRD is greater than six times the cost of care for a non-ESRD Medicare beneficiary. Non-accounted for economic costs of ESRD include chronic disability, premature death, and poor quality of life.[32] Costs for care of diabetic persons with ESRD are significantly higher than nondiabetic populations.[31] One recent study demon-

■ ■ ■

TABLE 86-5 STAGES AND PREVALENCE OF CHRONIC KIDNEY DISEASE

STAGE	DESCRIPTION	GFR ML/MIN/1.73 M²	PREVALENCE N × 1000	PERCENT OF POPULATION
1	Kidney damage with normal or increased GFR*	Greater than 90	5900	3.3
2	Kidney damage with mild decrease in GFR*	60-89	5300	3.0
3	Moderate decrease in GFR	30-59	7600	4.3
4	Severe decrease in GFR	15-29	400	0.2
5.	End stage renal disease	Less than 15 or renal support	300	0.1
Total			19,500	10.9

Adapted from Kidney Disease Outcomes Quality Initiative (NKF K/DOQI): *Clinical practice guidelines for chronic kidney disease: evaluation, classification and stratification,* New York, 2002, National Kidney Foundation.
*Kidney damage for stages 1 and 2 is estimated by two sequential spot urine samples with albumin-to-creatinine ratio greater than 17 mg/g for men or greater than 25 mg/g for women.
GFR, Glomerular filtration rate.

strated 69 percent increase in predialysis cost and 79 percent increase in postdialysis cost when diabetes coexisted with ESRD. On average, cost varied from $26,507 to $27,789 for the first month of renal replacement therapy, leveling off to an average of $5295 per month for individuals with diabetes.[31]

Chronic Kidney Disease and Cardiovascular Disease

Chronic kidney disease is an independent risk factor for cardiovascular disease morbidity and mortality.[12] The Hoorn Study evaluated a population-based cohort of persons aged 50 to 75 years with mild-to-moderate renal insufficiency, demonstrating a relative mortality risk of 1.17 and 1.15 for all-cause and cardiovascular mortality, respectively, with each 5 ml/min/1.73 m^2 decrease in creatinine clearance after adjustment for age, sex, glucose tolerance, and hypertension.[33] Moderate chronic kidney disease (GFR 60 ml/min/1.73 m^2, corresponding to serum creatinine 1.0 to 1.7 mg/dl) predicted cardiovascular disease in a sub-study of the Valsartan in Acute Myocardial Infarction Trial (VALIANT) in a community-based health maintenance organization population.[34] Renal dysfunction predicted reoccurrence of major cardiovascular events in a cohort of the Survival and Ventricular Enlargement (SAVE) Trial subjects.[35]

Cardiovascular disease mortality rates are ten to twenty times higher in persons with chronic kidney failure than the general population.[12,33] Although the number of individuals requiring dialysis is increasing, most persons with chronic kidney disease die of cardiovascular disease prior to the development of ESRD.[33] The American Heart Association's Council on Kidney and Cardiovascular Disease has designated chronic renal disease as "highest-risk status" for cardiovascular events.[12,34] In a 5.5-year longitudinal study of a large health maintenance organization, cardiovascular death was a more likely outcome than progression to end-stage renal failure for persons with chronic kidney disease, with 3.1 percent progressing to renal replacement therapy but with 24.9 percent mortality due to cardiovascular disease.[36] The burden of this increased risk begins with very low levels of proteinuria, the earliest stage of renal dysfunction.[18,28] Elevated serum Cystatin C level, another early marker of renal endothelial dysfunction, has also been associated with substantial cardiovascular mortality risk and increased all-cause mortality.[13]

Chronic Kidney Disease and Cardiomyopathy

Chronic kidney disease is also strongly associated with structural heart disease (cardiomyopathy) and heart failure.[15,19,37,38] Heart failure precipitates renal dysfunction by reducing renal perfusion and by activation of vasoactive inflammatory cytokines. A prospective cohort study confirmed that renal insufficiency is more prevalent in heart failure populations than the general population and, when present, is associated with wors-

ened outcomes whether the cause of heart failure is systolic or diastolic.[37] The Acute Decompensated Heart Failure National Registry (**ADHERE**) data reveals 31 percent of persons hospitalized with heart failure have chronic renal insufficiency on admission.[39] Twenty percent of persons hospitalized with heart failure had preexisting significant renal dysfunction, demonstrating a baseline serum creatinine greater than 2 mg/dl. ADHERE data demonstrate that persons with heart failure, regardless of cause, who have any degree of renal insufficiency suffer increased lengths of stay and increased mortality compared with age-matched control subjects.[39]

Conversely, persons with primary renal insufficiency are more likely to develop heart failure, and a combined diagnosis substantially increases mortality.[37] Eighty-five percent of persons starting renal replacement therapies are estimated to have myocardial abnormalities in structure and function by echocardiographic criteria.[12] Data from the Irbesartan Diabetic Nephropathy Trial (**IDNT**)[40] demonstrate a strong correlation between diabetic individuals with moderate renal insufficiency and subsequent development of heart failure. Twenty percent of one cohort study of 1715 participants with renal insufficiency developed heart failure over 2½ years.[19] The Medical Evidence Report of persons on renal replacement therapy describes incidence of coexisting cardiac pathology (i.e., heart failure, coronary artery disease, cardiac arrest, dysrhythmias, and pericarditis). The findings demonstrate that ESRD associated with hypertension alone results in a relative risk of heart failure of 2.8. When diabetes was included in the data, the relative risk of one cardiac condition was 5.9 and of three or more cardiac conditions was 4.8.[41] Proteinuria demonstrated a near linear predictive morbidity value using the RENAAL study population. Individuals with proteinuria greater than 3 g/g creatinine/24 hr demonstrated a 8.1-fold increased risk of developing ESRD compared with persons with under 1.5 g/g but also a 2.7-fold increased risk of congestive heart failure compared with those with less than 1.5 g/g creatinine/24 hr.[26] The change in proteinuria at 6 months was also predictive of adverse outcomes, with 30 percent increase in proteinuria demonstrating 141 percent increase in ESRD and 17 percent increase incidence of heart failure. Reductions in proteinuria using the AT receptor blocker losartan decreased ESRD by 52 percent and heart failure by 44 percent.[26]

Combined renal insufficiency and heart failure predicts worsened outcomes. Renal dysfunction is prevalent in persons with heart failure and is an independent negative prognostic factor during hospitalization for heart failure in both systolic and diastolic populations.[37,39] Evaluation of large database populations hospitalized for heart failure (73 percent with depressed ejection fraction) demonstrated that any detectable decrease in renal function is associated with increased mortality and prolonged hospital length of stay.[2,42] Evaluation of persons with ischemic cardiomyopathy following uncomplicated coronary bypass grafting demonstrated only 33 percent 5-year survival in persons with ejection fraction less than 35 percent who also had renal insufficiency (serum

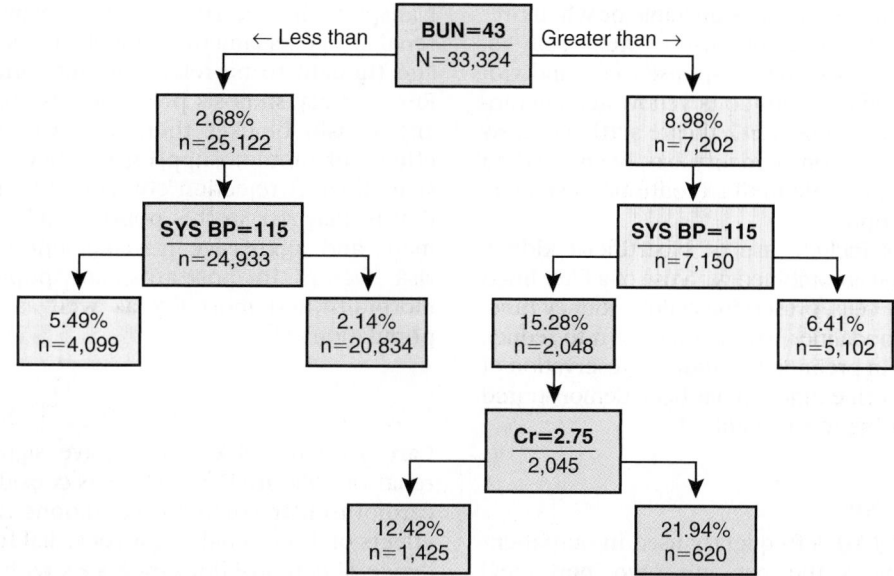

FIGURE 86-3 ■ Renal insufficiency predicts percent in-hospital mortality for persons with acutely decompensated heart failure. The patient populations presented are divided at three critical data points: when blood urea nitrogen (BUN) = 43, systolic blood pressure (BP) = 115, and creatinine (Cr) = 2.75. Patients with values less than the data point value are to the left, and those whose values exceed the data point are to the right at each level. *SYS BP*, Systolic blood pressure. (From the ADHERE data, Fonarow, GC et al. Risk stratification for in-hospital mortality in heart failure using classification and regression tree [CART] methodology. *JAMA*. 2005, 293:572-580.)

creatinine greater than 1.5 mg/dl), compared with 66 percent survival if they had normal renal function. The subjects with ejection fraction greater than 35 percent and normal renal function averaged a 5-year survival of 86 percent [43] (Figure 86-3).

Predialysis populations with serum creatinine greater than 3.0 mg/dl averaged 9.4 percent mortality when hospitalized with heart failure. A combination of blood urea nitrogen greater than 43 mg/dl, serum creatinine greater than 2.75 mg/dl, and systolic blood pressure less than 115 mm Hg conferred 19.5 percent mortality risk for any hospitalization for heart failure.[39] Morbidity and mortality are related to the degree of neurohormonal activation evident in cardiorenal syndromes. SAVE trial data revealed greatest absolute benefit for the angiotensin-converting enzyme inhibitor **(ACE)**, captopril, in persons with left ventricular dysfunction who had kidney disease following an acute coronary event. Captopril prevented 12.4 versus 5.5 events per 100 subjects with left ventricular dysfunction and chronic kidney disease versus left ventricular dysfunction and normal renal function, respectively.[35]

END-STAGE RENAL DISEASE: UREMIA

Uremia characterizes end stage renal disease and is an absolute indication for initiation of renal support therapies or transplantation.[12,29] Symptoms of uremia include anorexia, nausea, malaise, asterixis, muscular weakness, and mental status changes. Uremia has been associated with vascular inflammation, coagulopathy, pericarditis, and seizures. Cardiovascular symptoms of uremia are associated with accumulation of multiple toxic substances and do not directly correlate with serum BUN and creati-

nine levels.[12,29] Development of uremic symptoms confers very high mortality risk.[29,44]

Renal Replacement Therapies

Classic indications for renal replacement therapy include intractable extracellular volume overload, toxic electrolyte abnormalities (such as hyperkalemia), and signs and symptoms of uremic toxicity, especially uremic pericarditis or encephalopathy.[12] In recent years there has been increased incidence of acute renal failure as part of multi-organ system disease following high-risk cardiovascular surgery, subsequent to sepsis, and as drug-induced acute tubular necrosis.[44] Hemodynamic stability is used to determine onset and appropriate modality of renal replacement therapy. Hemodialysis is highly efficient and removes blood toxins and excess fluid by means of an extracorporeal semipermeable membrane and dialysate fluid. Anticoagulation is required to prevent thrombotic occlusion within the extracorporeal circuit. Complications associated with hemodialysis include accentuating hemodyamic instability and bio-incompatibility between blood and dialysis membranes. Complement activation, increased secretion of inflammatory cytokines, and coagulopathies may ensue with serious consequences. Synthetic dialysis membranes may decrease activation of inflammatory mediators and offer a survival advantage; however, increased research is indicated.[44]

Continuous renal replacement therapies are increasingly used in critical care settings due to decreased impact on hemodynamic stability. Toxins are removed via convection rather than diffusion of blood across a membrane. The slower rate of fluid and solute removal offers advantages when the individual is unstable or when preexisting coagulopathy precludes use of hemodialysis. Fluid and solute are replaced in response to the individual's electrolyte profile. Continuous venovenous hemofiltration is effective in most critical care settings. However, addition of diffusion modality has been used to increase removal of uremic toxins (continuous venovenous hemodiafiltration).[44]

Newer therapies include use of bioartificial kidney where hemofiltration is combined with use of a filter lined with human tubular cells, preserving cellular kidney functions. Bioartificial modalities have been shown to reduce cytokine activation in preliminary studies. Preservation of metabolic and endocrine function has been demonstrated in animal models using this modality.[44]

Peritoneal Dialysis

Peritoneal dialysis (PD) is frequently used in outpatient settings and employs the person's own peritoneal membrane to clear solutes and toxins. Fluid removal is accomplished by varying the tonicity of dialysate solution. PD requires an intact peritoneum, precluding use in most postoperative patients. PD is attractive in home settings where an individual can utilize a cycling device during sleep hours and disconnect during the day. PD is considered an optimal early replacement therapy for persons with end stage renal disease, reserving hemodialysis for PD failures.[45]

PD is associated with less anemia, better maintenance of nutrition status, and improved calcium and phosphorus homeostasis than is available with hemodialysis. Incidence of left ventricular hypertrophy and hypertension are decreased in PD populations, and some evidence points to improved success following transplantation in PD versus hemodialysis populations.[45] Disadvantages of PD include relatively high rate of infection. The need for hypertonic glucose solutions adversely affects metabolic control, especially in diabetic populations.[44] Hypertonic glucose triggers neoangiogenesis within the peritoneal cavity, associated with increased fibrosis of structures, occlusion of dialysis catheter, and loss of diffusion capacity.[44] Current research is focused on newer types of dialysate solutions such as icodextrin which are less likely to stimulate collagen deposits. Cardiovascular risk remains elevated in persons on renal replacement therapy. Tobacco cessation offers significant survival benefits and aggressive management of hyperglycemia, hypertension, and dyslipidemia are strongly advocated. ACE inhibitors and statins are considered the standard of care for chronic kidney disease populations.[45]

Cardiovascular Risk in the Postrenal Transplant Population

Heightened cardiovascular risk extends into the transplanted population as well, although to a lesser extent than dialysis patients.[15,28] Cardiovascular disease is implicated in up to 50 percent of deaths in the postrenal transplant populations.[15] Proteinuria, a marker of impaired glomerular function, has been demonstrated to herald increased cardiovascular mortality in the post-transplant individual.[15] Posttransplant stenosis of the renal artery serving the transplanted kidney is common and thought to be related to autoimmune processes.[4] Renal artery stenosis precludes use of reno-protective angiotensin blocker therapies. Adverse endovascular effects of immunosuppressant therapies and progressive allograft rejection contribute to an increased cardiovascular risk in this population.[15,28] Serial measurement and aggressive management of cardiovascular risk factors in posttransplant populations reduces morbidity and mortality as well as in pretransplant populations.[4,15]

CARDIORENAL RISK FACTORS

Cardiovascular risk factors have significant effect on renal vasculature.[15,28,32] There is considerable overlap in cardiovascular comorbid conditions that have adverse effects on both renal and myocardial function, and incidence of comorbidities increases with age.[2,28] Observational data continues to document under-utilization of cardiovascular and reno-protective therapies in individuals with vascular and metabolic disease. Recent review of NHANES III database reveals inadequate cardiovascular risk factor control in diabetic populations.[46] A large health maintenance organization database also reports significant under-treatment of diabetic populations with barely 32 percent of patients achieving HbA1c goal of under 7 percent. Only 22.5 percent achieved a target low density lipoprotein under 100 mg/dl, and 28.6 percent achieved blood pressure below 130/80.[47] Traditional cardiovascular risk factors are identified by the Framingham longitudinal database and tend to cluster in families.[32] Some risk factors can be altered to improve outcomes and some are nonmodifiable (e.g., age, gender). More recently, "nontraditional" risk factors have been recognized as having significant adverse impact on cardiovascular and renal outcomes[28,32] (Table 86-6).

Cardiorenal Comorbidities

Hypertension, dyslipidemia, anemia, calcium disturbance, vascular inflammation, and neuropathy are strongly associated with morbidity and mortality in both cardiac and kidney populations. The pathologic effect of these coexisting conditions is intensified when myocardial, metabolic, and renal diseases are all present together.[15,28]

Hypertension

Hypertension is independently associated with increased risk of endstage renal disease, cardiovascular, and cerebrovascular morbidity and mortality.[48,49] Incidence of hypertension varies with ethnicity and increases with age and body mass index. Proposed mechanisms of renal injury in hypertension include direct damage to small vessels from shear injury, disruption of renal autoregulation mechanisms, glomerular hyperfiltration, tubular injury from vasoactive and inflammatory substances, and volume overload. Nephron apoptosis is accelerated in inflammatory states. When hypertension coexists with organ dysfunction, such as left ventricular hypertrophy, cardiomyopathy, or renal

■■■

TABLE 86-6 TRADITIONAL AND "NONTRADITIONAL" CARDIOVASCULAR AND KIDNEY RISK FACTORS

TRADITIONAL RISK FACTORS	"NONTRADITIONAL" RISK FACTORS
Older age	Albuminuria/microalbuminuria
Male sex	Homocysteine
Hypertension	Lipoprotein (a) and isoforms
Higher LDL cholesterol	Lipoprotein remnants
Lower HDL cholesterol	Anemia
Diabetes	Abnormal calcium/phosphate balance
Tobacco	Extracellular fluid overload
Physical inactivity	Oxidative stress
Menopause	Inflammation
Family history of cardio- vascular disease	Malnutrition
Left ventricular hypertrophy	Thrombotic factors
Obesity	Sleep disturbances
	Altered nitric oxide/endothelin disturbance
	Hyperuricemia
	Depressed socioeconomic status/ poverty

HDL, High-density lipoprotein; *LDL,* low-density lipoprotein.
Adapted from Menon V, Sarnak MJ. The epidemiology of chronic kidney disease stages 1 to 4 and cardiovascular disease: a high risk combination, *Am J Kidney Dis* 45(1), 2005.

impairment morbidity, mortality risk is markedly increased as demonstrated by Framingham database population.[48] Elevated urinary microalbumin suggests need for intensified blood pressure management and intensified metabolic management as well.[19,40] Analysis of the RENAAL Study revealed that for every 50 percent reduction in albuminuria after initiation of antihypertensive therapy the risk of ESRD was decreased by 45 percent.[26]

Neurohormone-Induced Endothelial Dysfunction

Hypertension, hyperlipidemia, cardiac, and kidney disease each induce neurohormone activation systemically. This is also seen in obesity, metabolic syndrome, and diabetes. Regardless of the precipitating mechanism, neurohormonal activation results in systemic vasoconstriction leading to endothelial dysfunction and injury. Endothelial dysfunction subsequently augments renin, AT, aldosterone, and sympathetic cascades, setting up a vicious cycle of inflammation, injury, and neurohormonal activation.[6,30,40] Reactive oxygen species produced by stressed vascular endothelium directly stimulate AT-II secretion and stimulate platelet and macrophage activation, resulting in heightened intravascular coagulability.[14,17,30, 35,50]. Dysfunctional endothelium becomes increasingly permeable, allowing sorbitol and lipid infiltration into vascular media, producing endothelial cell edema and accelerating dysfunction. Cytokine activation stimulates smooth muscle cell proliferation with collagen infiltrating endothelial and surrounding tissues. This process results in intimal thickening, expansion of extracellular matrix, vascular fibrosis, and atherosclerotic plaque.[51] Capillary dysfunction is typified by loss of responsiveness to vasodilatation effects of nitric oxide and prostaglandins.[17,20]

When the vascular endothelium is impaired, oxygen delivery to microvasculature is inhibited and microvascular ischemia ensues. Vascular ischemia activates coagulation cascades within capillary beds as well as conduit vessels, and counter-regulatory fibrinolytic processes are disrupted.[51-53] Ischemic endothelium triggers inflammatory cytokines such as tumor necrosis factor and interleukin (IL)-6[52,53]. Inflammatory cytokines disrupt myocardial, renal, and pancreatic extracellular matrix, resulting in tissue necrosis, apoptosis, and fibrosis of organ parenchyma. Persistent and progressive subclinical vascular inflammation results in progressive end-organ functional decline.[53-55]

Neurohormone Blockade

Neurohormonal blockade interferes with multiple cascades involved in systemic vasoconstriction. In addition to reducing peripheral vasoconstriction and restoring normal systemic blood pressure, these interventions reduce vascular shear stress and protect heart, kidney, and brain tissue from inflammatory and ischemic injury. Neurohormone blockade includes blunting effects of the renin-angiotensin system, aldosterone, and the sympathetic nervous system. Additional vasoactive hormones such as endothelin-1 may exert significant pathologic effects when unmasked by blockade of other neurohormonal systems.[7,16]

Angiotensin Blockade

AT-II is one of the most potent vasoconstrictors within the body. AT-II causes constriction of preglomerular arterioles within the renal vasculature, provoking additional renin secretion before systemic effects on blood pressure are apparent.[5,14] AT-II increases glomerular pressures and induces proteinuria.[14] ACE inhibitors are established therapy for persons with cardiovascular, renal, or metabolic disease with numerous clinical trials demonstrating decreased morbidity and mortality with use in these populations.[5,12,14] ACE inhibitors reduce oxidative stress, lower glomerular capillary pressure, decrease proteinuria, and retard fibrosis independent of their effect on systemic blood pressure.[40,55] The African American Study of Kidney Disease and Hypertension (AASK) demonstrated a 46 percent reduction in renal impairment with the ACE inhibitor, ramipril, compared with amlodipine, a calcium blocker.[48] Blockade of AT-1 receptors inhibits release of oxygen-free radicals, increases nitric oxide expression, and reduces endovascular inflammation.[14] AT-II also has significant effects on lipid metabolism and plays a direct role in lipolysis. Lipolytic functions of AT-II are strongly associated with weight loss and cachexia in end-stage cardiac and renal disease. The release of free fatty acids from lipid degeneration promotes insulin resistance and has a direct toxic effect on end-organ function of the heart, kidney, and pancreas.[55] The lipid toxicity of AT-II is also modulated with ACE inhibitor therapy.

Angiotensin Receptor Blockers

ACE inhibitors blockers inhibit production of AT-II. However, serum AT-II levels have been noted to increase in spite of ACE inhibitor therapy. Blockade of angiotensin at the receptor level reduces this "escape" angiotensin effect.[40] Angiotensin receptor blockade has been demonstrated to decrease incidence of left ventricular hypertrophy and induce left ventricular hypertrophy regression in the LIFE study. A total of 9193 persons with hypertension and left ventricular hypertension were randomized to atenolol (a beta blocker) versus losartan (an ARB). Losartan reduced the incidence of stroke by 25 percent compared with atenolol. Losartan also reduced onset of diabetes in the treated population with 25 percent fewer persons on losartan developing diabetes than those on atenolol.[56] Benefits have been also demonstrated in persons with advanced renal disease. Using an Asian cohort from the RENAAL trial, losartan was found to decrease adverse renal outcomes by 36 percent and incidence of microalbuminuria by 47 percent.[57] The IDNT trial demonstrated a 23 percent decrease in development of end stage renal disease with irbesartan in a population with pre-terminal renal failure.[40]

More research is indicated before combined ACE inhibitor and angiotensin blockade therapy is recommended.[58,59] Preliminary data are promising. Addition of angiotensin receptor blocker, candesartan, to an ACE inhibitor decreased risk of cardiovascular death and decreased hospital heart failure admissions in the prospective Candesartan in Heart Failure Assessment of Reduction in Mortality and Morbidity (CHARM-added) trial.[58] Combination therapy with ACE inhibitors and ARB has been demonstrated to reduce urine microalbumin expression.[59] Myocardial remodeling following myocardial infarction was significantly decreased with combination therapy in an animal model compared with effects of either ACE inhibitors or angiotensin receptor blockade alone, and angiotensin receptor blockade conferred additional benefits in reducing interstitial collagen.[59]

Vasopressin Blockade

AVP potentiates catecholamine hemodynamic effects, systemically and within renal and myocardial vasculature.[11] Normally AVP release is triggered by baroreceptor and chemoreceptor stimulation responding to hypotension and increased serum osmolarity. However, vasopressin blood levels are inappropriately elevated in persons with reduced systolic function.[8,11] Vasopressin response to osmolarity remains intact, but overall serum levels are increased. Data from the Studies of Left Ventricular Dysfunction (SOLVD) substudy demonstrated that this occurs before the occurrence of symptomatic congestion.[11] Pure water retention contributes to hyponatremia common in heart failure. Increased preload and afterload increase wall stress and end-diastolic filling pressures. The degree of increased serum levels parallels the severity of heart failure. Vasopressin has additional metabolic effects, including platelet and cytokine activation. The role of AVP in endothelial inflammation remains under investigation.

Vasopressin antagonism therapy is currently undergoing clinical trials. Potential benefits include reduction in congestion, modulation of sympathetic and RAAS cascades, maintenance of electrolyte balance and normalization of serum sodium, and improved intrarenal hemodynamics.[11] Early studies, including the Acute and Chronic Therapeutic Impact of a Vasopressin Antagonist in Congestive Heart Failure (ACTIV in CHF) Trial ($n = 320$) revealed significant reduction in body water, symptoms of congestion, and normalization of serum sodium with administration of the AVP antagonist tolvaptan. This early study was underpowered to demonstrate mortality benefits.[8] The Efficacy of Vasopressin Antagonism in Heart Failure: Outcome Study with Tolvaptan (EVEREST) is ongoing with primary endpoint all-cause mortality. Secondary endpoints include perception of dyspnea and quality of life.

Endothelin Blockade

Similarly to AT-II, endothelin-I is a potent systemic vasoconstrictor and is implicated in congestive symptoms in left ventricular dysfunction. Endothelin-I directly activates sympathetic forces and increases norepinephrine release at postsynaptic sites.[53] Endothelin-1 acts on two receptors (A and B) within the nephron. Receptor A induces intrarenal vasoconstriction. Receptor B activation causes vasodilatation in renal vasculature.[7,16] ARB affect endothelin-I activity in certain populations. The ARB losartan was demonstrated to have a marked effect in lowering endothelin-I levels independent of hypertensive effects in a study of individuals with essential hypertension.[40] Blockade of endothelin A receptors was found to have reno-protective effects in persons with chronic kidney disease by lowering intrarenal vasoconstriction and decreasing proteinuria.[16] More research is indicated and clinical trials ongoing.

Aldosterone Blockade

The renin-angiotensin system also includes activation of aldosterone. Aldosterone, a mineralocorticoid hormone secreted from the adrenal cortex, promotes sodium retention in exchange for potassium and magnesium in renal tubules.[6] There may be significant aldosterone synthesis outside of the adrenal gland as well.[60] Aldosterone secretion is stimulated by renin, augmented by AT-II, and is directly affected by intravascular electrochemical balance. Serum catecholamines, nitric oxide, corticotropic hormone, and endothelin-1 also stimulate aldosterone release.[34] Aldosterone effects are accelerated by high sodium intake.[5] Aldosterone activates sympathetic forces; diminishes parasympathetic forces; promotes vascular, renal, and myocardial inflammation fibrosis; and contributes to baroreceptor dysfunction.[60,61] Aldosterone decreases bioavailability of endothelial nitric oxide and increases expression of reactive oxygen species, contributing to vascular inflammation and decreased arterial compliance.[60] Aldosterone antagonism reduced platelet activator-1 levels and decreased levels of tissue growth factor.[34]

Proteinuria is decreased with aldosterone receptor antagonism, suggesting an expanded role in preventing progressive renal failure with these agents.[6,60,62] Initially ACE inhibition and/or angiotensin receptor blockade effectively decreases serum aldosterone levels. However, aldosterone escape occurs eventually in approximately 20 percent of heart failure populations and in up to 40 percent of persons with diabetic renal disease.[62]

Persons with increased serum aldosterone levels exhibit progressive proteinuria and accelerated renal impairment.[62]

Renal nephrosclerosis, necrosis, and fibrosis were markedly decreased in animal models using aldosterone receptor blockers.[6] Clinical studies using eplerenone in persons with renal insufficiency demonstrated a 62 percent reduction in renal albumin excretion compared with 45 percent reduction using ACE inhibitors.[34] These findings were confirmed in the 4E study (Eplerenone, Enalapril, and Eplerenone/Enalapril Combination Therapy in Patients with Left Ventricular Hypertrophy), where eplerenone significantly decreased urinary microalbumin as solo therapy as well as in combination with the ACE inhibitor enalapril. Other studies have demonstrated these benefits were independent of blood pressure lowering.[60] One study of diabetic patients with renal insufficiency found significant decrease in proteinuria in persons who were given aldosterone receptor blocker in addition to either ACE inhibitor therapy or ARB (33 percent) as well as when combination renin-angiotensin blockade was used (22 percent).[62] Benefits were also seen in individuals with proteinuria at a nephrotic level (greater than 2500 mg urine albumin/24 hr), where a 35 percent reduction in proteinuria was seen.[62]

Aldosterone also plays a major role in hypertension. Hyperaldosteronism is found in many subjects with resistant hypertension.[61] Inflammatory cytokine expression is decreased with aldosterone receptor blockade independent of blood pressure effects.[60] In the Eplerenone Post-Acute Myocardial Infarction Heart Failure Efficacy and Survival Study (EPHESUS), the aldosterone blocker eplerenone was found to significantly decrease blood pressure and reduce vascular damage, endovascular inflammation, and necrosis.[63,64] Left ventricular wall stress was significantly reduced, associated with reduction in left ventricular end diastolic pressure with aldosterone antagonism.[63]

Unfortunately there is increased risk of hyperkalemia in persons with chronic kidney disease receiving aldosterone blockade therapy. This effect is dose dependent and a serious limiting factor in administration. Avoidance of vitamin preparations containing potassium and of nonsteroidal antiinflammatory pain medications is strongly recommended. Close monitoring of serum potassium is warranted. Antiandrogen effects including gynecomastia have also been observed in persons taking spironolactone, but this is not seen with eplerenone therapy.[62]

Dyslipidemia

Dyslipidemia is common in chronic kidney disease and has serious clinical implications.[54] Statin therapy reduces serum cholesterol and increases the stability of and decreases the size of vascular atherosclerotic lesions. Statins also have "pleiotropic" effects independent of serum cholesterol levels: decreasing endovascular inflammation and improving endovascular function.[64,65] An aggressive target of low density lipoprotein less than 70 mg/dl is recommended in high-risk subgroups such as those with diabetes, left ventricular dysfunction, and

■ ■ ■

TABLE 86-7 NATIONAL KIDNEY FOUNDATION K/DOQI GUIDELINES AND NCEP-ATP III GUIDELINES

NKF/K/DOQI GUIDELINES	NCEP-ATP III GUIDELINES
CKD confers highest risk category	No management differences from general population
Evaluate dyslipidemia at presentation, change in status, and annually	Evaluate dyslipidemia every 5 years
Drug therapy for LDL-C 100-129 mg/dl after 3 months TLC	Drug therapy is optional for LDL-C 100-129 mg/dl
Recommend initial drug therapy with statin	Drug therapy may be started with statin, bile acid sequestrant, or nicotinic acid
Fibrates may be used in Stage 5 CKD if triglycerides greater than 500 mg/dl or non- HDL-C greater than 130 mg/dl if statin not tolerated	Fibrates contraindicated in CKD
Gemfibrozil may be fibrate of choice to treat hypertriglyceridemia in CKD	No fibrate preference in hypertriglyceridemia

CKD, chronic kidney disease; *HDL*, high density lipoprotein cholesterol; *LDL-C*, low density lipoprotein cholesterol; *NCEP ATP III*, National Cholesterol Education Program: Adult Treatment Panel III; *TLC*, therapeutic lifestyle changes.

renal dysfunction when associated with cardiovascular disease[64,66] (Table 86-7).

Dyslipidemia and Endothelial Inflammation

Vascular inflammation is associated with progressive renal impairment. The Chronic Renal Impairment in Birmingham (CRIB) Study[54] compared inflammatory markers with renal function as quantified by serum Cystatin C levels and calculated creatinine clearance. Individuals with predialysis chronic kidney disease were found to have significantly elevated inflammatory markers compared to healthy subjects.[54] Hypercholesterolemia significantly activates systemic renin-angiotensin cascades.[67] Two-month administration of prevastatin significantly reduced expression of C reactive protein and thrombogenic substances, including prothrombin activator and von Willebrand factor in a diabetic cohort.[65] A subgroup analysis involving 1600 individuals from the GREek Atorvastatin and Coronary Heart Disease Evaluation (GREASE) Study revealed 8.2 percent reduction of the inflammatory marker serum uric acid with atorvastatin 24 mg per day, compared with 3.3 percent increase in serum uric acid in the untreated group. Serum uric acid was positively correlated with increased serum creatinine levels and inversely correlated with calculated GFR.[68]

Dyslipidemia and Chronic Kidney Disease

NKF guidelines recommend those with chronic kidney disease be designated a "highest risk" group for cardiovascular disease.[12] A recent meta-analysis of subgroups of large clinical trials found significant improvements with statin use in renal populations, reducing the progression of kidney disease.[69] The First United Kingdom Heart and Renal Protection (UK-HARP-1) study demonstrated safety and efficacy of statin therapy in persons with chronic kidney disease.[70] Mortality benefit of statin therapy in more advanced chronic kidney disease remains under investigation. Cholesterol profiles commonly seen in chronic kidney disease include decreased high density lipoprotein cholesterol and hypertriglyceridemia. Elevations in low density lipoprotein cholesterol are common as well with estimated 70 percent of persons using PD having low density lipoprotein cholesterol greater than 100 mg/dl and 45 percent low density lipoprotein cholesterol greater than 130 mg/dl.[66]

Treatment decisions for dyslipidemia in renal populations are confounded by different recommendations by national organizations. Data suggests low levels of low density lipoprotein cholesterol are associated with significant increased mortality in hemodialysis populations.[66] Chronic activation of inflammatory cytokines associated with protein energy malnutrition and cachexia associated with end-stage renal and cardiovascular disease may contribute to this finding and should not preclude dyslipidemia therapy in persons with chronic kidney disease.[12] When drug therapy is used for dyslipidemia in persons with chronic kidney disease, dose adjustments need to be considered and dose effects closely monitored[66] (Table 86-8).

Antiplatelet Therapy in Chronic Kidney Disease

Current recommendation by the American Heart Association is for low-dose aspirin in all adults with a 10-year cardiovascular risk of 10 percent or greater as defined by Framingham criteria. Persons with chronic kidney disease are considered in the highest risk category for cardiovascular disease.[71] However, they are also at higher risk for bleeding events due to associated anemia, platelet dysfunction, and fibrinolytic abnormalities associated with renal insufficiency.[71] The First United Kingdom Heart and Renal Protection (UK-HARP-1) Pilot Study evaluated the impact of low-dose (100 mg/day) aspirin in a population of 448 persons with chronic kidney disease. A three-fold increase in minor bleeding events was observed; however, there was no demonstrated increase in major bleeding. There was no significant change in hemoglobin levels with aspirin use from placebo. Low-dose aspirin effect on renal prostaglandin activity was assessed: there was no demonstrated difference in renal function from placebo. All-cause mortality was significantly reduced from 12 percent to 1 percent in the study group; however, the study was underpowered to make population general-

izations to all persons with chronic kidney disease.[70] The NKF recommends a prospective randomized trial to determine the role of antithrombotic therapy in chronic renal disease. Higher doses of aspirin have been demonstrated to act similarly to nonsteroidal antiinflammatory medications, antagonizing effects of renal prostaglandins, interfering with ACE inhibitor action, and precipitating renal dysfunction.[66,71,72]

Anemia and Chronic Kidney Disease

Anemia is common in renal disease, cardiomyopathy, and diabetes and adversely impacts outcomes in acute as well as chronic illness.[2,73-75] Degree of anemia is positively correlated with the extent and duration of renal impairment.[12] Anemia has metabolic and hemodynamic consequences and is associated with increased mortality in cardiorenal syndromes.[12,74,75] Anemia is defined by World Health Organization criteria as hemoglobin less than 13 mg/dl in men and under 12 mg/dl in women.[12] Anemia of chronic disease is normocytic and normochromic.[29] Anemia results in extracellular volume expansion, increased myocardial demand, left ventricular hypertrophy, cardiac failure, ischemic syndromes, progressive renal dysfunction, cognitive impairment, and decreased quality of life.[12,74,75] Conversely, an increase in cardiovascular mortality has been observed in persons with excess hemoglobin. This was thought to be related to excess blood viscosity and a tendency for thrombosis.[73] Correction of anemia is associated with improved outcomes in cardiorenal syndromes; however, recent observational studies suggest anemia remains under-recognized and under-treated in the chronically ill[75] (Table 86-9).

Anemia of chronic disease is a marker of excess expression of inflammatory cytokines.[74,75] Mortality increases with every decrease in hemoglobin below 12 mg/dl in chronic kidney as well as in cardiovascular disease.[75] The elderly are particularly susceptible to the adverse effects of anemia when exposed to acute illness, and mortality increases when underlying cardiac or renal disease are present.[2,75] In one Medicare-aged database of persons with end stage renal disease, hemoglobin less than 9 mg/dl was associated with a relative risk of death of 1.81 in men and 1.93 in women. Milder forms of anemia were associated with worsened outcome as well: for hemoglobin 9 to 10 mg/dl the relative risk was 1.66 for men and 1.60 for women when compared to elderly with normal blood counts. Compared

---

■ ■ ■

TABLE 86-8   DOSE ADJUSTMENTS FOR ANTI-LIPID THERAPIES IN CHRONIC KIDNEY DISEASE

	GFR 60-90 ML/MIN/1.73 M²	GFR 15-59 ML/MIN/1.73 M²	GFR <15 ML/MIN/1.73 M²	NOTES
Statin				
Lovastatin	None	Decrease by 50%	Decrease by 50%	Decrease by 50% for GFR less than 30
Pravastatin	None	None	None	Start 10 mg/day if GFR less than 60
Simvastatin	Unknown effect	Unknown effect	Unknown effect	Start 5 mg/day if GFR less than 10
Fibrate				
Gemfibrozil	None	None	None	No likely effect on serum creatinine

Weiner DE, Sarnak MJ: Managing dyslipidemia in chronic kidney disease, *J Gen Intern Med* 19(10):1045-1052, 2004.
GFR, glomerular filtration rate.

■ ■ ■

TABLE 86-9   PERCENT ANEMIA FOUND IN COMMON CHRONIC KIDNEY DISEASE COMORBIDITIES IN A MEDICARE POPULATION (n = 1,136,201)

COMORBIDITY	PERCENT WITH ANEMIA
CVA/TIA	23.1%
Diabetes	23.7%
Peripheral vascular disease	28.0%
Atherosclerotic heart disease	43.0%
Nonischemic cardiac disease	48.8%
Hypertension	66.7%

CVA, cerebrovascular disease; *TIA*, transient ischemic attack.
Herzog CA, Muster HA, Shuling L et al: Impact of congestive heart failure, chronic kidney disease, and anemia on survival in the Medicare population, *J Card Fail* 10:467-472, 2004.

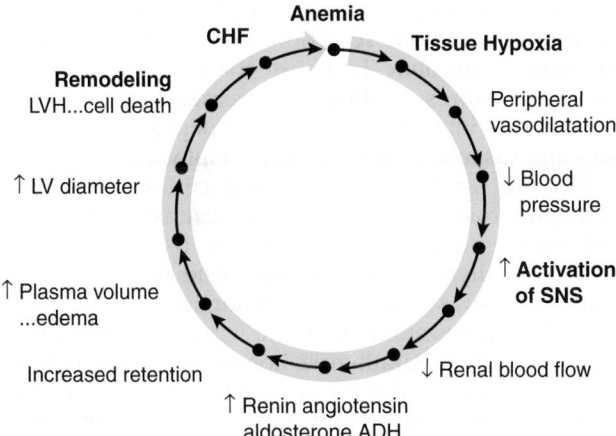

FIGURE 86-4 ■ Cycle of anemia and vascular inflammation. *ADH*, Antidiuretic hormone; *CHF*, congestive heart failure; *LDH, LV,* left ventricle; *LVH,* left ventricular hypertrophy; *SNS,* sympathetic nervous system.

with a healthy elderly population, anemia increased risk of death by 60 percent, chronic kidney disease by 64 percent, and congestive heart failure by 125 percent.[2] When all three conditions were present, mortality increased by four times that of age-matched healthy subjects[2].

Chronic Kidney Disease and Metabolic Effects of Anemia

The renal cortex is highly oxygen dependent. Erythrocyte lifespan is reduced in inflammatory states, including chronic kidney disease, heart failure, and diabetes.[73,74] Anemia decreases blood oxygen–carrying capacity to both the heart and kidney. Anemic states intensify renal oxygen extraction and decrease renal reserves.[75,76] Decreases in oxygen tension in proximal tubules stimulate sodium reabsorption at this location and activate renin secretion.[76] Sodium reabsorption expands extracellular volume and increases myocardial preload. Decreased oxygen-carrying capacity induces tissue hypoxia and reflex peripheral vasodilatation. Vasodilatation decreases effective renal blood flow, activating sympathetic forces. RAAS activation precipitates a vicious cycle of increased renal and myocardial demand in the setting of reduced oxygen delivery.[76] Cardiorenal stress is intensified by activation of inflam-

matory cytokines from ischemic tissue and vascular endothelium (Figure 86-4).

Bone Marrow Suppression and Chronic Kidney Disease

Activation of inflammatory cytokines contributes to hematopoietic tissue resistance to erythropoietin.[75] RAAS activation is associated with suppression of erythropoietin production in chronic heart failure.[76] Ischemic tissues and ischemic vascular endothelium release inflammatory cytokines, particularly IL-1, IL-6, and tumor necrosis factor-alpha.[76] Inflammatory cytokines cause osteocyte ischemia, bone marrow suppression, and destruction of boney pro-erythroblasts.[73] Red blood cell proliferation in response to recombinant human erythropoietin is blunted. Additional inflammatory markers such as tumor necrosis factor, C-reactive protein, and fibrinogen have been associated with anemia as well.[76]

Role of Blood Tranfusion. Anemia is a modifiable risk factor in cardiorenal syndromes.[73,74] Allogeneic blood transfusion has not been demonstrated to improve anemic states in chronic illness or tissue oxygen utilization in the short term.[74,77] Stored blood is deficient in 2,3 DPG reducing bioavailability of oxygen at the tissue level. Older blood cells (stored more than 28 days) may worsen splanchnic ischemia in spite of elevated hemoglobin levels. Transfused blood may activate inflammatory cascades and has been associated with metabolic acidosis, calcium depletion, bacterial and viral infection, and multiple organ failure.[77]

Iron Deficiency In Chronic Kidney Disease

Iron deficiency is common in cardiac and kidney disease and is associated with iron shift from serum to storage as ferritin.[73] Renal processing of iron is disrupted in chronic kidney disease, and iron conservation is impaired.[12] Iron deficiency is aggravated by intestinal malabsorption and malnutrition associated with chronic illness. Activated macrophages accumulate iron, reducing bioavailability to erythropoietic tissue.[73] Chronic malnutrition is also associated with B$_{12}$ and folate deficiency. Serum iron is inversely correlated with the degree of endovascular inflammation present in chronic kidney disease.[12] Proteinuria associated with endothelial dysfunction depletes iron stores.[75,76] Iron deficiency is seen in 21 percent of anemic persons with new onset heart failure and is prevalent in chronic kidney disease.[11,75] Transferrin saturation in combination with measurement of ferritin and serum iron levels is helpful in diagnosing functional iron deficiency.[12]

Iron is required for osteocyte production of hemoglobin. In the absence of adequate serum iron levels, erythropoietin efficacy is impaired.[73] Iron deficiency is corrected with oral iron preparations or intravenous preparations such as iron sucrose or ferric gluconate.

Role of Erythropoietin. Functional or absolute erythropoietin deficiency is the primary cause of anemia in chronic kidney disease.[10] GFR less than 60 ml/min/1.73 m^2 is associated with progressive loss of renal erythropoietin secretion.[12] Postrenal transplant patients have diminished erythropoietin secretion due to effects of immunosuppressive therapies or to subclinical inflammation from chronic organ rejection.[12] Stimulation of erythropoietin receptors inhibits cellular apoptosis and is thought to protect vulnerable hematopoietic tissue.[76] Recombinant human erythropoietin was demonstrated to improve reticulocyte count and serum transferrin receptor concentrations in a critically ill population.[78] Normalization of anemic states with recombinant human erythropoietin results in regression of left ventricular hypertrophy in persons with chronic kidney disease. Cardiocyte protection has been observed when erythropoietin was administered during ischemic events.[74,78] Recombinant human erythropoietin administration was found to decrease left ventricular end diastolic volume and improve myocardial stroke volume.[73] Recombinant human erythropoietin has beneficial effects on left ventricular remodeling, improved functional class and left ventricular ejection fraction.[37] Compensatory extracellular volume expansion resolved with less diuretic administration in persons with heart failure treated with recombinant human erythropoietin.[78] Improvement in exercise capacity was found when iron infusions were coupled with recombinant human erythropoietin administration.[73,75] Erythropoietin administration decreased need for diuretic therapy in hypervolemic states and reduced pulmonary capillary wedge pressure.[73,76]

Therapeutic targets for administration of recombinant human erythropoietin are not clearly defined in kidney or heart failure populations. However, the American Diabetes Association recommendations include administration of recombinant human erythropoietin when hemoglobin levels are under 11 mg/dl to achieve hemoglobin 12 to 13 g/dl.[79] The Anemia Correction in Diabetes (ACCORD) Study is ongoing to clarify outcomes associated with recombinant human erythropoietin therapy.[79] Intravenous recombinant human erythropoietin has been used in dialysis populations; however, more frequently subcutaneous administration is used, resulting in more sustained plasma concentrations. Darbepoietin (Aranesp, Amgen) has a longer half life than standard recombinant human erythropoietin preparations (48 hrs) and is successfully used with once or twice monthly subcutaneous administration.[78]

Adverse effects of recombinant human erythropoietin have been observed. Over-administration of hematopoietic therapy can increase blood viscosity and predispose to thrombosis. Hypertension is a relative contradiction to erythropoietin administration. Seizures have been reported in persons on renal replacement therapies receiving recombinant human erythropoietin therapy. Some preparations of erythropoietin have been found to induce autoimmune antibodies, suppressing existing bone marrow function.[73] Cost of care is increased with administration of hematopoietic therapy, which may preclude its use in uninsured populations.[73,78]

Calcium, Phosphorus, and Magnesium Homeostasis

Renal involvement in bone metabolism has serious implications for quality of life of the person with chronic kidney disease and for cardiovascular health.[12] Normally, the kidney participates in a delicate homeostasis of calcium and phosphorus within the extracellular milieu and within bone tissue, maintaining serum levels in a narrow therapeutic range.[80] Calcium has three primary physiological roles: maintenance of the structural integrity of the bony skeleton, as a critical serum electrolyte in intracellular dynamics, and as a key component of hemostasis.[80] Ninety-nine percent of total body calcium is stored within the bony matrix. Calcium is transported in bound form (primarily attached to serum albumin) and in a free (ionized form). Parathyroid hormone is released from the parathyroid gland in response to low serum (ionized) calcium or elevation in serum phosphorus.

Bone abnormalities associated with chronic renal disease are primarily due to inability of the kidney to produce activated Vitamin D (calcitrol) and to impairment of renal phosphorous excretion. Vitamin D (calcitrol) is required for dietary calcium absorption. Inadequate calcitrol impairs dietary calcium absorption via the small intestine, resulting in decreased availability of calcium. Phosphorus excretion is reduced in renal insufficiency. Elevated serum phosphorus levels stimulate parathyroid hormone secretion. Under the influence of parathyroid hormone, bone osteoblasts release calcium from bony stores, leading to increased ionized serum calcium and inappropriate calcium deposits in soft tissues and vascular endothelium (calciphylaxis).[80]

Chronic renal insufficiency induces secondary hyperparathyroidism: the parathyroid gland hypertrophies and secretes abnormal amounts of parathyroid hormone. Parathyroid hormone secretion results in high bone turnover, subsequently causing increased cortical bone demineralization and bone weakening (osteitis fibrosa cystica).[80] Parathyroid hormone elevations have also been associated with myocardial fibrosis, left ventricular hypertrophy, and valvular and vascular calcification.[80] Mineral wasting (osteodystrophy) is common in chronic kidney disease and intensifies with renal decline and uremia.[12,29] Bone disease has been documented between 40 percent to 100 percent of persons with chronic renal insufficiency and increases with severity of renal impairment.[12] Bone wasting is associated with chronic pain and with heightened risk of fracture. Bone fractures are common in persons on renal replacement therapies and are associated with significant mortality. One-year mortality is 2.5 times greater for persons on dialysis therapy following hip fracture than in the general population.[80] Intracardiac calcium abnormalities are associated with arrhythmia, predisposing to left ventricular dysfunction, ischemia, and cardiac death.[12] Soft tissue calcium deposits precipitate skin lesions that are easily infected, adding to morbidity and mortality of end stage renal disease[12] (Table 86-10).

Elevated parathyroid hormone levels occur in early stages of renal dysfunction and secretion accelerates when creatinine clearance decreases below 60 ml/minute/1.73 m².[12,29] Chronic renal insufficiency may lead to depletion of parathyroid hormone. Decreased parathyroid secretion impairs bone formation (osteomalacia). Adynamic bone disease (near complete loss of bone formation) has been observed in end-stage renal disease.[29] Decreased bone responsiveness to parathyroid hormone is also observed in chronic kidney disease and contributes to progressive loss of bone matrix.[80] Inadequate parathyroid hormone secretion is associated with hyperphosphatemia and hypomagnesemia and is augmented in metabolic acidosis.[12] Osteoblast resistance to parathyroid hormone may occur in inflammatory states.[80]

■ ■ ■

TABLE 86-10   TARGET RANGES OF PARATHYROID HORMONE, CALCIUM, PHOSPHORUS, AND MAGNESIUM FOR STAGES OF CHRONIC KIDNEY DISEASE

CKD STAGE	GFR ML/MIN/1.73M²	PARATHYROID HORMONE TARGET RANGE	PHOSPHORUS TARGET RANGE	IONIZED CALCIUM TARGET RANGE	MAGNESIUM TARGET RANGE
2	60-89	35-65 pg/ml	2.7-4.6 mg/dl	4.65-5.28 mg/dl	1.3-2.1 mEq/L
3	30-59	Less than 70 pg/ml	2.7-4.6 mg/dl	4.65-5.28 mg/dl	1.3-2.1 mEq/L
4	15-29	70-110 pg/ml	2.7-4.6 mg/dl	4.65-5.28 mg/dl	1.3-2.1 mEq/L
5	Less than 15 or renal support	150-300 pg/ml	3.5-5.5 mg/dl	4.65-5.28 mg/dl	1.3-2.1 mEq/L

Legg V: Complications of chronic kidney disease: a close look at osteodystrophy, nutritional disturbances and inflammation, *Am J Nurs* 105(6):40-49, 2005.
CKD, Chronic kidney disease; *GFR,* glomerular filtration rate; *pg,* picogram; *ml,* milliliter; *mEq,* millequivalent; *L,* liter.

Parathyroid hormone elevations are modulated by restricting dietary phosphorous (beans, nuts, dairy products) and administration of calcium and vitamin D supplements (rocaltrol).[29] Calcium, phosphorus, and parathyroid hormone levels are closely monitored in persons with chronic renal insufficiency. Calcium levels are adjusted for accuracy when serum albumin is low: corrected total serum calcium = measured serum calcium mg/dl + 0.8 × (4 − measured serum albumin (g/dl)). Direct measure of ionized (free, unbound) calcium levels are more commonly used in renal populations.[12]

Neuropathy

Neuropathy is common in chronic kidney disease and diabetes. Neuropathic abnormalities include cognitive dysfunction, autonomic dysfunction, and peripheral sensorimotor dysfunction. Neuropathic cognitive dysfunction consists of loss of short-term memory, delayed speed of decision making, and decreased attention span.[12] Cognitive dysfunction improves with renal replacement therapy. Sleep disturbances are common in the chronically ill with chronic kidney disease, cardiomyopathy, or diabetes. Autonomic neuropathy affects response to sympathetic and parasympathetic forces and is associated with increased incidence of sudden death.[81,82]

Autonomic Neuropathy

Autonomic neuropathy is defined as decreased parasympathetic activity. It is seen in up to 80 percent of persons with kidney disease and diabetes and in up to 66 percent of nondiabetic persons with stage 4 or 5 renal disease or who are on renal replacement therapies.[12] Autonomic neuropathy is a common cause of positional orthostasis. Autonomic dysfunction is responsible for common complaints, including impaired gastric emptying (gastroparesis), bowel dysfunction (diabetic diarrhea), and loss of bladder control (neurogenic bladder).[81] Autonomic dysfunction is a common source of arrhythmia and has been associated with significantly increased morbidity and mortality in cardiovascular syndromes, including sudden death.[81,83] A dyslipidemia profile typical of insulin resistance also was found to have significant correlation with abnormal heart rate recovery in a population-based study of 4963 men. This abnormality in heart rate recovery following exercise was also associated with significant increase in all-cause mortality.[82]

Cardiac autonomic neuropathy was significantly associated with excretion of urinary protein in a small population of elderly diabetics.[22] Lower heart rate variability was correlated with higher urine microalbumin-to-creatinine ratio. This was thought to reflect a pattern of endothelial dysfunction within the kidney as well as in nerve tissue. Another small observational study found significant correlation between resting electrocardiogram ST abnormalities, QT interval lengthening, decreased heart rate variability, and end stage renal disease in a cohort of 565 diabetics in Wisconsin.[84] Interestingly, serum fibrinogen was also elevated in persons with evidence of autonomic dysfunction, suggesting heightened tendency for coagulopathy. In addition, decreased peak expiratory flow rates were similarly correlated with autonomic dysfunction, suggesting associated decreased pulmonary function in this population.[84] Findings of association between QT lengthening, left ventricular hypertrophy, and increased ventricular arrhythmia were also found in a study of 296 nondiabetic persons with end stage kidney disease. Interestingly, a similar pattern of autonomic and functional cardiac abnormality was seen in a postrenal transplant population.[85]

Autonomic dysfunction was found to predict development of diabetes in a cohort of 8185 subjects from the Atherosclerosis Risk in Communities (ARIC) Study.[81] After controlling for age, race, body mass index, tobacco, and cardiovascular disease, the relative risk for developing diabetes was 60 percent in the highest, compared with the lowest, quartile of heart rate variability indices. Cardiac autonomic neuropathy was associated with 3.5-fold increase in all-cause mortality in a diabetic population and was especially predictive in the setting of silent ischemia.[22] Inability to achieve 85 percent of predicted heart rate response on exercise testing was found associated with increase incidence of coronary disease and was predictive of all-cause mortality in a cohort of 1575 asymptomatic healthy men from the Framingham database.[85]

Peripheral Neuropathy

Peripheral neuropathy is common in chronic kidney disease with sensory impairment occurring in up to 90 percent of affected persons and motor impairment in 40 percent.[12] Painful sensorimotor neuropathies are also common in diabetic patients and are a consequence of endothelial dysfunction and microvascular disease.[81]

Sensory impairment in diabetic populations is associated with peripheral vascular disease, lower limb amputations, and worsened outcomes.[86] Renal transplantation is thought to significantly improve peripheral neuropathy. Pain associated with peripheral neuropathy is particularly difficult to treat. Some newer anticonvulsants have shown promise in reducing discomfort. Although tricyclic antidepressants have demonstrated some benefit, higher doses are arrhythmogenic.[12] Aldose reductase inhibitors reduce influx of sorbitol into nerve endings and decrease endothelial dysfunction but are less effective in long-term neuropathy when more permanent nerve damage has occurred.[12]

NURSING IMPLICATIONS FOR CARE OF PERSONS WITH CARDIAC AND KIDNEY DISEASE

Elderly populations bear the burden of increased incidence of chronic illness, such as renal and cardiovascular disease. Anemia is common in the chronically ill. Incidence of kidney disease, cardiovascular disease, and diabetes each significantly increase with age. There is wide individual variation in the degree of functional and physiological decline corresponding to chronological age.[87] Aging is associated with loss of structural, physiological, and functional reserve and inadequate response to physiological stress.[2,87] Age affects all body systems even when the individual has no documented chronic disease.[2]

A study evaluating a Medicare database of elderly individuals ($n = 1,136,201$) demonstrated substantial cardiorenal morbidity and mortality in this age group.[2] For all patients in the database 3.2 percent had chronic kidney disease, 13.2 percent had heart failure, and 14.8 percent were anemic. Of persons with chronic kidney disease, 51.9 percent had at least one inpatient claim per year. 46.9 percent of persons with heart failure had one or more inpatient hospitalizations; 46.3 percent of persons with anemia had one or more inpatient hospitalizations. Annual mortality rate was also striking in persons over 65 years of age with cardiac or kidney disease. For persons with no anemia, heart failure, or chronic kidney disease, annual mortality was 3.8 percent. For persons with chronic kidney disease only, mortality per year was 8.2 percent. Persons with chronic kidney dis-

ease and anemia demonstrated 13.7 percent mortality. One-year mortality for individuals with chronic kidney disease, heart failure, and anemia was 22.9 percent.[2]

Aging is associated with multiple chronic conditions including obesity, anemia, degenerative joint disease, and depression each of which increases the potential for disability.[87] Maladaptive lifestyle patterns, including physical inactivity, alcohol consumption and tobacco use, add to risk of physical disability as the individual ages (Table 86-11).

Renal Alterations of Aging

After the age of 40, renal function is noted to decline on average of 1 percent per year of life. In one study a healthy 70-year-old had 60 percent the renal function of a 25-year-old.[88] Age-related nephron loss is accompanied by decreased nephron function and diminished kidney size. Muscle mass reduction in elderly affects accuracy of creatinine clearance as an indicator of renal function.[88] Persons at age 80 commonly have a creatinine clearance less than 50 ml/min in the absence of intrinsic renal disease.[87,88]

Aging is associated with impaired renal sodium and water processing that may contribute to hypervolemic states and heart failure.[87] Diuretic-induced electrolyte disorders are more common in elderly populations due to impaired renal electrolyte processing.[88] Chronic urinary incontinence is common in the elderly and incidence increases with diuretic and ACE inhibitor therapy. Importance of urinary incontinence as a cause of medication nonadherence is likely under-appreciated in clinical practice.[87]

Nursing Implications Related to Polypharmacy

Persons with kidney disease, cardiovascular disease, or diabetes require multiple medications for optimal outcomes.[87] One study found an average of seven prescriptions medications in a population of older diabetics and this increased with the number of comorbidities.[89,90]

Recent national surveys indicate that more than 40 percent of populations 65 years or older used five or more medications per week, and 12 percent used more than ten different medications. Adherence to prescribed

■ ■ ■

TABLE 86-11   INCIDENCE OF CHRONIC ILLNESS IN NON-INSTITUTIONALIZED POPULATION (PER 100,000 PERSONS)

CONDITION	MEN (AGE) 45-64 YRS	65-74 YRS	GREATER THAN OR EQUAL TO 75 YRS	WOMEN (AGE) 45-64 YRS	65-74 YRS	GREATER THAN OR EQUAL TO 75 YRS
Hypertension	242.4	319.4	281.0	254.4	422.8	415.6
Heart disease	152.7	290.4	324.2	116.9	229.1	372.2
Diabetes	57.9	97.3	95.1	57.0	109.0	91.1
Kidney disease	16.7	18.0	23.7	17.9	27.9	29.9
Cerebrovascular disease	12.9	63.4	77.0	19.0	54.1	66.3

Nagle BA, Erwin WG: Geriatrics. In Dipiro JT et al, editors: *Pharmacotherapy: a pathophysiologic approach*, Stamford, Conn, 1997, Appleton-Lange, pp. 87-100.

regimens decreases with the number of medications and complexity of the treatment plan.[90] Dosing schedules need to be adapted to individual lifestyles and work schedules. Visual deficits are common in elderly and chronically ill populations and vision assessment is critical to determine if instructions can be read. One study found the incidence of diabetic retinopathy was 35.6 percent in a population of diabetics with renal disease.[17]

Cognitive impairments and memory loss interfere with comprehension and interpretation of instructions.[87] Cognitive dysfunction is one component of neuropathy common in diabetic and renal populations. Confusion between generic and brand names of medications is common in chronically ill populations, and error risk increases with number of medications prescribed.[91] Written medication lists that the individual is able to read back to you are useful. Black marker may be helpful to improve visualization. Family support is invaluable in accurate medication administration. Prohibitive cost of medications remains a substantial factor in nonadherence.[89] Consideration should be given to enlisting pharmaceutical medical assist programs for persons with chronic illness who are financially indigent.

Prescription errors, patient confusion, nonadherence, and inadequate monitoring and surveillance were the most frequent causes of adverse drug-related events in a large Medicare cohort.[90] Adverse events are common, particularly when the individual has multiple comorbidities. Adverse drug reactions result in 5.5 percent to 27 percent of hospitalizations for Medicare enrollees with cardiovascular disease, and this may underestimate incidence for elderly overall.[90,92] Medication adverse events occurred in up to 50.1 per 1000 person years in one observational study with up to 27.6 percent events deemed preventable.[90] The highest incidence of adverse events occurred with cardiovascular drugs (up to 60 percent of adverse events). Adverse events occurred in up to a fourth of individuals on renal regimens as well.[90]

Drug Marketing Targeted to the Elderly and Disabled

The elderly and chronically ill are increasingly subject to targeted marketing in written, televised, and web-based media who offer magical cures and multiple herbal, homeopathic, and supplemental products of dubious value.[92] These marketers provide testimonies and other enticements to encourage purchase of products with little regulation from government agencies. Over-the-counter (OTC) supplements add substantially to the cost of medical care in vulnerable populations and may interfere with medications whose efficacy is supported by large clinical trials. One United Kingdom study found 64 percent of hospitalized patients used OTC nonprescription medications, with little knowledge of potential adverse effects or drug interactions,[92] and many of these were continued during acute hospitalization. Well-meaning but uninformed family members may contribute to this practice.

Patients may take the marketed product preferentially over prescribed medication unless the importance of each prescribed medication is clearly explained.[92] Patient use of OTC medications needs to be addressed and family assistance enlisted. Successful care of the chronically ill includes maintaining a trusting relationship, encouraging disclosure of OTC medication use, and supporting use of approved therapies. Increased public advocacy is needed to discourage direct marketing to the chronically ill and elderly.[92]

Nursing Implications Related to Chronic Noncardiac Pain

Chronic noncardiac pain is common in chronic kidney disease, cardiovascular disease, and diabetes.[16,93] Chronic pain is prevalent in elderly populations with multiple comorbidities, has an adverse impact on quality of life and medical adherence, and is a major cause of disability in this population.[87] Uncontrolled pain is associated with increased hospitalization, poor sleep, decreased functional status, and adversely affects self-management.[93,94] Sources of chronic pain in cardiorenal populations include hyper-uricemia, gout, osteodystrophy, degenerative joint disease, inflammatory arthritis, and neuropathy.[93] Pain may be augmented by chronic subclinical vascular inflammation associated with cardiorenal syndromes.[53]

Pain management appropriately begins with careful assessment. Pain is subjective. It is a multidimensional sensation with physical, psychological, and spiritual aspects.[93,94] Pain assessment tools such as the McGill Pain Questionnaire have been successfully used in clinical practice. Assessment may also be structured using a mnemonic approach (Table 86-12).

Current medical practice recommends nonsteroidal antiinflammatory drugs (NSAIDs) as first-line therapy for chronic pain. However, adverse effects of NSAIDs preclude their use in cardiorenal populations.[72] These cyclooxygenase inhibitors reduce blood flow within the renal medulla by blocking prostaglandin release. This leads to unopposed vasoconstriction within the nephron. NSAIDs have been found to precipitate acute renal failure by a factor of three in previously healthy populations compared with non–NSAID users, and this effect may be more common in the elderly.[72] NSAIDs promote renal water and sodium retention and antagonize beneficial effects of ACE inhibitors and ARBs within the renal tubule. NSAIDs are implicated in increased heart failure admission rates in elderly populations.[72,87] NSAIDs are more likely to precipitate renal failure and hyperkalemia when taken with diuretic therapy.[72] NSAIDs have also been implicated in impaired ligament repair after injury and delayed bone healing following fracture.[95] Tylenol is not as effective in inflammatory pain as NSAIDs, and

■ ■ ■

TABLE 86-12 PAIN ASSESSMENT MNEMONIC

P	**Place of pain:** Location (s) of discomfort
A	**Amount of pain:** Use pain scale, patient descriptors, colors of intensity, faces of pain
I	**Intensifies:** Rate pain at the worst, describe triggers that increase pain
N	**Negates:** Rate pain at the best, relief measures currently used to reduce pain (nonpharmacological and pharmacological)

Wheeler M, Wingate S: Managing noncardiac pain in heart failure patients, *J Cardiovas Nurs* 19(s6):s75-s83, 2004.

clearance may be decreased in hepatic insufficiency. In addition, chronic renal and hepatic insufficiency decreases drug clearance of narcotic pain medications. Interventions to relieve pain include nonpharmacological as well as pharmacological. Treatment strategies must be tempered by comorbidities and adapted to the needs of the individual. Best clinical practice will use a variety of strategies to reduce pain in chronically ill populations[93] (Table 86-13).

Nursing Implications Related to Financial Limitations

Financial concerns are paramount in the lives of the chronically ill and their families, and worries about finances may lead to therapy nonadherence and worsening outcomes.[91,92] Increased use of biotechnology has had dramatic impact on cost for the chronically ill. In the United States, insurance coverage is employer dependent. As health costs have risen exponentially, strategies have increasingly shifted costs to the employee and reimbursement schedules have been reduced. Loss of employment-based insurance coverage can be catastrophic, resulting in rapid impoverishment not only for the individual but the family as well. Health care crises are the most common cause of bankruptcy in the United States today. Although there are laws to provide increased insurance portability, the cost of insurance coverage under Consolidated Omnibus Budget Reconciliation Act (commonly known as COBRA) provisions is not restricted. The costs of chronic illness are increasingly shifted to government-based programs, such as Medicare, yet it is clear that these programs are underfunded and acceptable solutions have been elusive. Persons with chronic kidney disease make up 3.3 percent of Medicare populations but account for up to 8 percent of the Medicare budget.[23]

Dialysis modalities significantly increase cost of care for persons with chronic kidney disease.[17] There are

■ ■ ■

TABLE 86-13   CHRONIC PAIN MANAGEMENT OPTIONS IN CARDIORENAL POPULATIONS

INTERVENTION	EXAMPLES FOR CARDIORENAL PATIENTS
Exercise	Low impact (senior) aerobics, water aerobics, walking, stationary bike, recumbent bike
Rehabilitation	Cardiac rehabilitation programs, individual rehabilitation
Meditation, relaxation	Yoga, Tai Chi
Cognitive and behavioral therapy	Specialty pain management programs
Over-the-counter medications	Acetaminophen
Adjuvant medications	Anticonvulsants, antidepressants, anesthetics, medications such as colchicine or allopurinol for gout
Opioid medications	Methadone, long-acting morphine (MS contin), Tramadol, combination therapy such as codeine with acetaminophen

Wheeler M, Wingate S: Managing noncardiac pain in heart failure patients, *J Cardiovas Nurs* 19(s6):s75-s83, 2004.

minimal financial incentives for early proactive preventive care or for patient educational programs to correct maladaptive lifestyle patterns. New paradigms are urgently needed to provide financial support for the chronically ill.

Nursing Implications Related to Family Dynamics

Lack of social support is consistently associated with worse outcomes in chronic illness, including cardiorenal syndromes and diabetes.[87] Social isolation, particularly after the death of a spouse, is common in elderly populations. Nursing considerations need to include family members in care planning, both for strategies to manage illness but also in end-of-life strategies. End-of-life medical care has been estimated to represent 10 percent to 12 percent of the U.S. total health care costs.[96] While less than 5 percent of Medicare recipients die each year, the last year of life accounts for nearly 25 percent of annual Medicare costs. Costs for the last year of life averaged $31,000 in 1997 and have continued to rise exponentially since.[96]

Data from the SUPPORT Trial demonstrate the tremendous financial burden borne by patients and families in the last 6 months of life. By the time the patient was within 3 days of death, 16 percent of family members had lost a major source of income, 13 percent had a family member quit work to provide care, and 23 percent reported the family had depleted most of their savings in the care of the individual.[96] When the family is supportive, the individual is better able to maintain restrictive lifestyle regimens and follow complex pharmacy directions. Family financial support is often crucial to maintaining quality of life in the chronically ill. Transportation needs for health maintenance and testing and basic home care needs are often borne by family members.

Nursing Implications Related to Dietary Sodium

High sodium diets typical of Western societies have significant adverse effects on morbidity and mortality of persons with cardiorenal syndromes.[5,97] Diet modifications that include increased fruit, vegetables, legumes, and whole grains have demonstrated significant reduction in cardiovascular complications.[98] Increased intake of fish, nuts, and low fat dairy products are also beneficial as long as energy intake does not exceed expenditure. Evidence associates diets such as the Mediterranean diet with reduction in cardiovascular disease risk and all-cause mortality.[98] The Dietary Approaches to Stop Hypertension **(DASH)** diet developed by the National Institutes of Health was demonstrated to lower blood pressure in adults with stage 1 hypertension.[99] When sodium restriction was added, additional antihypertensive benefits were obtained.[99]

High sodium intake is implicated in development and perpetuation of hypertension and has been listed as a primary cause of resistant hypertension.[100] High sodium proximal tubules stimulates the renin-angiotensin-aldosterone cascade and promotes inflammatory cytokine production.[52] Animal models have demonstrated significant impairment in sodium/potassium pump mechanisms with high salt intake.[97] Intratubular renal dysfunction may attenuate diuretic natriuretic effectiveness and ability to reduce extracellular volume. High sodium intake has also been associated with sympathetic activation.[98] In one Finnish study an increase of urine sodium excretion of 100 mmol/day was associated with a 45 percent increase in cardiovascular disease and 25 percent increase in all cause mortality.[99] Proteinuria and left ventricular hypertrophy have also been associated with high dietary sodium independently of blood pressure effects.[99]

Typical guidelines recommend reducing sodium intake to less than 2000 mg per day for persons with cardiorenal impairment.[100] However, calculating sodium intake per day is cumbersome and difficult for patients to follow in real world settings, and this strategy may be ineffective if sodium intake occurs in bulk fashion during a given meal. The kidney responds immediately to sodium ingestion, so isolated sodium loading can lead to persistent fluid retention. One heart failure treatment program found that restricting sodium intake to foods containing less than 200-mg sodium per serving based on food labels was more practical and facilitated improved diet adherence.[101]

Nursing Implications Related to Protein Intake

Protein restriction is recommended in persons with end-stage renal disease to reduce glomerular stress and injury. Excess protein consumption is associated with alterations in renal hemodynamics, glomerular hyperfiltration, and urinary protein secretion.[102] Presence of protein within the proximal renal tubule induces inflammatory cytokine activation.[52] It is also true that protein-calorie malnutrition develops during the course of chronic kidney disease and accelerates as GRF declines.[12] Causes of malnutrition in chronic kidney disease include appetite loss, anorexia, and uremic toxicity. Cachexia associated with protein energy malnutrition is intensified by protein catabolism associated with subclinical inflammation of chronic kidney disease.[51,53] Hormonal influences also participate in progressive malnutrition, including effects of metabolic acidosis associated with chronic kidney disease. Protein energy malnutrition is a major predictor of adverse outcome in renal populations.[12] The Modification of Diet in Renal Disease **(MDRD)** Study found inadequate evidence that protein retards progression of kidney disease. Recent research continues to define optimal medical nutrition therapy. Current guidelines for protein and calorie intake are related to GFR (Table 86-14).

NEW HORIZONS: FUTURE RESEARCH

The complexity and intricate dynamics of cardiorenal syndromes have generated intense interest across medical disciplines and subspecialties. Neurohormonal similarities between cardiac, renal, and endocrine patholo-

■ ■ ■

TABLE 86-14   RECOMMENDATIONS FOR PROTEIN AND ENERGY RESTRICTION IN CHRONIC KIDNEY DISEASE

CKD STAGE	MONITORING INTERVAL	GOAL PROTEIN INTAKE	GOAL ENERGY INTAKE
CKD Stage 1-3 (GFR 30-60 ml/min/1.73 m²)	6-12 month	0.75 g/kg/day	35 kcal/kg/day
CKD Stage 4-5 (GFR less than 30 ml/min/1.73 m²)	1-3 month	0.60 g/kg/day	35 kcal/kg/day

Adapted from Kidney Disease Outcomes Quality Initiative (NKF K/DOQI): *Clinical practice guidelines for chronic kidney disease: evaluation, classification and stratification,* New York, 2002, National Kidney Foundation. Body mass index of 23.6-24 kg/m2 is ideal. Nutritional monitoring includes serum albumin, body weight, global assessment, assessment of protein intake, prealbumin, transferrin, total cholesterol.
CKD, Chronic kidney disease; *GFR,* glomerular filtration rate.

gies continue to be evaluated. In general, important areas of research include diagnostic strategies and prognostic indicators, therapeutic interventions, and outcome research. Research will continue to expand, evaluating the genetic basis leading to predisposition for cardiovascular disease, renal disease, obesity, and diabetes. The regenerative role of multipotent stem cells is another area of rapidly growing research in cardiorenal syndromes.[103]

Clinical research continues to focus on therapies to prevent and modulate multiple comorbidities associated with end stage renal disease. Role of vascular endothelium and nitric oxide dysregulation leading to cytokine activation and inflammation remain areas of intense investigation.[104] Reno-protection strategies and prevention of renal failure continues to be emphasized in clinical trials.[105] Early detection and aggressive intervention for proteinuria, anemia, parathyroid abnormalities, hypertension, and dyslipidemia are increasingly becoming standards of care in chronic kidney disease.[45,105] Optimal medical nutritional therapy is a critical area of future research.[12] Research continues to seek optimal treatment strategies in high-risk patients.

Improved renal support therapies reduce burden of care for persons with chronic kidney disease.[44] Improved organ salvage techniques and advances in immuno-modulation therapy following transplantation have led to increased organ availability and viability for many. Recognition of the prevalence of cardiovascular disease in persons with predialysis renal impairment, persons on renal support therapies, and in the postrenal transplant population has intensified management of cardiovascular risk factor modification.[45] There has also been increased interest in evaluation of outcomes associated with intensified sympathetic and neurohormonal blockade therapy in renal populations. Future research will evaluate outcome benefits using these agents in kidney populations. The value of cytokine blockade is also being investigated in chronic kidney disease.[106,107]

CONCLUSION

Nurses in critical care settings have long operated under the axiom, "the kidney is the window to the heart." Chronic kidney disease, cardiovascular disease, and diabetes are intimately related and share multiple layers of pathology. Morbidity and mortality increase when both the kidneys and the heart are impaired and are accelerated when metabolic disease is also present. Quality of life is increasingly important as chronic illness progresses. Nurses' ability to think holistically and appreciate patient and family perspectives provides an immense advantage when caring for the chronically ill with multiple comorbidities. Understanding complex interrelationships between renal, cardiac, and vascular function is critical to caring for the chronically critically ill. Nurses who recognize early signs and symptoms of cardiovascular and kidney impairment are better prepared to proactively intervene, minimizing complications. Nurses have substantial roles within multidisciplinary teams to optimize management of persons with chronic illness, improving patient outcomes.

REFERENCES

1. Costello-Boerrigter LC, Boerrigter G, Burnett JC: Revisiting salt and water retention: new diuretics, acquaretics, and natriuretics, *Med Clin N Am* 87:475-492, 2003.
2. Herzog CA, Muster HA, Shuling L et al: Impact of congestive heart failure, chronic kidney disease, and anemia on survival in the Medicare population, *J Card Fail* 10:467-472, 2004.
3. Abraham WT, Schrier RW: Renal salt and water handling in congestive heart failure. In Hosenpud JD, Greenberg, BH, editors: *Congestive heart failure, pathophysiology, diagnosis and comprehensive approach to management*, New York, 1994, Springer-Verlag.
4. Pastan SO, Braunwald E: Renal disorders and heart disease. In Braunwald E, editor: *Heart disease: a textbook of cardiovascular medicine*, ed 6, Philadelphia, 2001, WB Saunders.
5. Strazzullo P, Galletti F, Barba G: Altered renal handling of sodium in human hypertension, *Hypertension* 41:1000-1005, 2003.
6. Rocha R, Funder JW: The pathophysiology of aldosterone in the cardiovascular system, *Ann NY Acad Sci* 970:89-100, 2002..
7. Montanari A, Carra N, Perinotto P et al: Renal hemodynamic control by endothelin and nitric oxide under angiotensin II blockade in man, *Hypertension* 31:715-720, 2002..
8. Goldsmith SR: Vasopressin: a therapeutic target in congestive heart failure? *J Card Failure* 5:347-356, 1999.
9. Gheorghiade M, Orlandi C, Burnett JC et al: Rationale and design of the multicenter randomized double-blind, placebo-controlled study to evaluate the efficacy of vasopressin antagonism in heart failure: outcome study with Tolvaptan (EVEREST), *J Card Failure* 11:260-269, 2005.
10. Kidney Disease Outcomes Quality Initiative (NKF K/DOQI): *Clinical practice guidelines for chronic kidney disease: evaluation, classification and stratification*, New York, 2002, National Kidney Foundation.
11. Verhave JC, Gansevoort RT, Hillege HL et al: Drawbacks in the use of indirect estimates of renal function to evaluate the effect of risk factors on renal function, *J Am Soc Nephrol* 15:1316-1322, 2004.
12. Podrazik PM, Schwartz JB: Cardiovascular pharmacology of aging. In Friesinger, G, editor: *Cardiology clinics*, Philadelphia, 1999, WB Saunders, pp. 17-34.
13. Shiplak MG, Sarnak MJ, Katz R et al: Cystatin C and risk of death and cardiovascular events among elderly persons, *N Engl J Med* 352:2049-2060, 2005.
14. Trevisan R, Viberti G: The renin-angiotensin system, nephropathy and hypertension. In Marso SP, Stern DM, editors: *Diabetes and cardiovascular disease*, Philadelphia, 2004, Lippincott & Williams, pp. 315-336.
15. Sarnak MJ, Levey AS, Schoolwerth AC: Kidney disease as a risk factor for development of cardiovascular disease, *Circulation* 108:2154-2185, 2003.
16. Goddard J, Johnston NR, Hand MF et al: Endothelin A receptor antagonism reduces blood pressure and increases renal blood flow in hypertensive patients with chronic renal failure: a comparison of selective and combined endothelin receptor blockade, *Circulation* 109:1186-1193, 2004.
17. Ritz E: Albuminuria and vascular damage: the vicious twins, *N Engl J Med* 348:2349-2352, 2003.
18. Klausen K, Borch-Johnsen K, Feldt-Rasmussen B et al: Very low levels of microalbuminuria are associated with increased risk of coronary heart disease and death independently of renal function, hypertension and diabetes, *Circulation* 110:32-35, 2004.
19. Yunyun MF, Adler AI, Wareham NJ: What is the evidence that microalbuminuria is a predictor of cardiovascular disease events? *Curr Opin Nephrol Hypertension* 14:271-276, 2005.
20. Perticone F, Maio R, Tripepi G et al: Endothelial dysfunction and mild renal insufficiency in essential hypertension, *Circulation* 110:821-825, 2004.
21. Wachtell K, Palmieri V, Olsen MH et al: Urine albumin/creatinine ratio and echocardiographic left ventricular structure and function in hypertensive patients with electrocardiographic left ventricular hypertrophy: the LIFE study, *Am Heart J* 143:319-326, 2002.
22. Moran A, Palmas V, Field L et al: Cardiovascular autonomic neuropathy is associated with microalbuminuria in older patients with type 2 diabetes, *Diabetes Care* 27:972-977, 2004.
23. Barzilay JI et al: The relationship of cardiovascular risk factors to microalbuminuria in older adults with or without diabetes mellitus or hypertension: the Cardiovascular Health Study, *Am J Kidney Dis* 44:25-34, 2004.
24. Hillege HL et al: Urinary albumin excretion predicts cardiovascular and noncardiovascular mortality in general population, *Circulation* 106:1777-1782, 2002.
25. Gerstein HC et al: Albuminuria and risk of cardiovascular events, death and heart failure in diabetic and nondiabetic individuals, *JAMA* 286:421-426, 2001.
26. Mitch WE et al: Detecting and managing patients with type 2 diabetic kidney disease, proteinuria and cardiovascular disease, *Kidney Internat* 66(s 92): 97-98. 2004.
27. Ibsen H et al: Reduction in albuminuria translates to reduction in cardiovascular events in hypertensive patients, *Hypertension* 45:198-209, 2005.
28. Menon V, Sarnak MJ: The epidemiology of chronic kidney disease stages 1 to 4 and cardiovascular disease: a high risk combination. *Am J Kidney Dis* 45:223-232, 2005.
29. Snively CS, Gutierrez C: Chronic kidney disease: prevention and treatment of common complications, *Am Fam Physician* 70:1921-1930, 2004.
30. El-Atat FA, Stas SN, McFarlane SL et al: The relationship between hyperinsulinemia, hypertension and progressive renal disease, *J Am Soc Nephrol* 15: 2816-282, 2004.
31. Joyce AT et al: End stage renal disease–associated managed care costs among patients with and without diabetes, *Diabetes Care* 27:2829-2835, 2004.
32. McClellan WM et al: Epidemiology and risk factors for chronic kidney disease. *Medical clinics of North America, 89 (3)*.
33. Henry RM et al: Mild renal insufficiency is associated with increased cardiovascular mortality: the Hoorn Study, *Kidney Internat* 62:1402-1407, 2002.
34. Hostetter TH: Chronic renal disease predicts cardiovascular disease, *N Engl J Med* 351:1344-1346, 2004.
35. Tokmakova MP et al: Chronic kidney disease, cardiovascular risk, and response to angiotensin-converting enzyme inhibition after myocardial infarction: survival and ventricular enlargement (SAVE) Study, *Circulation* 110:3617, 2004.

36. Go AS et al: Chronic kidney disease and the risks of death, cardiovascular events and hospitalization, *New Engl J Med* 351(13):1296-1305, 2004.

37. McAlister, FA, Ezekowitz J, Tonelli M: Renal insufficiency and heart failure: prognostic and therapeutic implications from and prospective cohort study, *Circulation* 109:1004-1009, 2004.

38. de Zeeuw D et al: Albuminuria, a therapeutic target for cardiovascular protection in type 2 diabetic patients with nephropathy, *Circulation* 110(8):921-927, 2004.

39. Heywood TJ: The cardiorenal syndrome: lessons from the ADHERE database and treatment options, *Heart Failure Rev* 9:195-201, 2004.

40. Lewis EJ et al: Renoprotective effect of the angiotensin-receptor antagonist irbesartan in patients with nephropathy due to type 2 diabetes, *New Engl J Med* 345(12):851-860, 2001.

41. Xue JL, Frazier ET, Herzog CA, Collins AJ: Association of heart disease with diabetes and hypertension in patients with ESRD, *Am J Hypertension* 45(2):316-323, 2005.

42. Gottlieb SS, Abraham W, Butler J: The prognostic importance of different definitions of worsening renal function in congestive heart failure, *J Card Failure* 8(3):136-148, 2002.

43. Soltero ER et al: Long-term results of coronary artery bypass grafting in patients with ischemic cardiomyopathy: the impact of renal insufficiency and noncardiovascular disease, *J Card Failure* 11(3):206-212, 2005.

44. Quan A, Quigley R: Renal replacement therapy and acute renal failure, *Curr Opin Pediatr* 17(2):205-209, 2005.

45. Bloomgarden ZT: The European Association for the Study of Diabetes: perspectives in the news, *Diabetes Care* 28(5):1250-1257, 2005.

46. Saydah SH, Fradkin J, Cowie CC: Poor control of risk factors for vascular disease among adults with previously diagnosed diabetes, *JAMA* 291(3):335-342, 2004.

47. Beaton SJ, Nag SS, Gunter MJ: Adequacy of glycemic, lipid, and blood pressure management for patients with diabetes in a managed care setting, *Diabetes Care* 27(3):694-698, 2004.

48. Douglas JG et al: Management of high blood pressure in African Americans, *Arch Internal Med* S2S:55-541, 2003.

49. Freitag MH, Vasan RS: What is normal blood pressure? *Curr Opin Nephrol Hypertension* 12:285-292, 2003.

50. Derweesh IH, Novick AC: Mechanisms of renal ischemic injury and their clinical impact, *Brit J Urol* 95(7):948-950, 2005.

51. Mann DL: Inflammatory mediators and the failing heart: past, present and the foreseeable future, *Circulation Res* 91(11):988-998, 2002.

52. Creager MA, Luscher TA: Diabetes and vascular disease, clinical consequences and medical therapy, part I, *Circulation* 108:1527-1542, 2003.

53. Virdis A, Schifrin L: Vascular inflammation: a role in vascular disease and hypertension? *Curr Opin Nephrology Hypertension* 12:181-187, 2003.

54. Landray MJ, Wheeler DC, Lip GY: Inflammation, endothelial dysfunction, and platelet activation in patients with chronic kidney disease: the chronic renal impairment in Birmingham (CRIB) study, *Am J Kidney Dis* 43:244-253, 2004.

55. Cabassi A et al: Sympathetic modulation by carvedilol and losartan reduces angiotensin II mediated lipolysis in subcutaneous and visceral fat, *J Clin Endocrinol Metabol* 90(5):2888-2897, 2005.

56. Lindholm LH et al: Cardiovascular morbidity mortality in patients with diabetes in the Losartan Intervention for Endpoint Reduction in Hypertension Study (LIFE): a randomized trial against atenolol, *Lancet* 359(9311):1004-1010, 2002.

57. Chan JC, Wat NM, So WY: Renin, angiotensin, aldosterone system blockade and renal disease in patients with type 2 diabetes, *Diabetes Care* 27(4):874-879, 2004.

58. McMurray JJ et al: Effects of candesartan in patients with chronic heart failure and reduced left ventricular systolic function taking angiotensin converting enzyme inhibitors: the CHARM-added Trial, *Lancet* 362:767-771, 2003.

59. Kim YK et al: Adding angiotensin II type receptor blockade to angiotensin converting enzyme inhibition limits myocyte remodeling after myocardial infarction, *J Card Failure* 9(3):238-245, 2003.

60. Brown NJ: Aldosterone and end-organ damage, *Curr Opin Nephrol Hypertension* 14(3):235-241, 2005.

61. Nishizaka MK, Calhoun DA: Use of aldosterone antagonists in resistant hypertension, *J Clin Hypertension* VI(VIII):458-460, 2004.

62. Rossing K et al: Beneficial effects of adding spironolactone to recommended antihypertensive treatment in diabetic nephropathy, *Diabetes Care* 28(9):2106-2112, 2005.

63. Manrique C et al: Hypertension and the cardiometabolic syndrome, *J Clin Hypertension* 7(8):471-476, 2005.

64. Grundy S et al: Implications of recent clinical trials for the National Cholesterol Education Program Adult Treatment Panel III Guidelines, *Circulation* 110:227-239, 2004.

65. Sommeijer DW et al: Anti-inflammatory and anticoagulant effects of pravastatin in patients with type 2 diabetes, *Diabetes Care* 27(2):468-473, 2004.

66. Weiner DE, Sarnak MJ: Managing dyslipidemia in chronic kidney disease, *J Gen Intern Med* 19(10):1045-1052, 2004.

67. Daugherty A et al: Hypercholesterolemia stimulates angiotensin peptide synthesis and contributes to atherosclerosis through the AT-1 receptor, *Circulation* 110(25):3849-3857, 2004.

68. Athyros VG et al: Effect of statins versus untreated dyslipidemia on serum uric acid levels in patients with coronary heart disease: a subgroup analysis of the GREek Atorvastatin and Coronary Heart Disease Evaluation (GREASE) Study, *Am J Kidney Dis* 43(4):589-599, 2004.

69. Shah S, Paparello J, Danesh FR: Effects of statin therapy on the progression of chronic kidney disease, *Advance Chronic Kidney Dis* 12(2):187-195, 2005.

70. Baigent C, Landray M, Warren M: Statin therapy in kidney disease populations: potential benefits beyond lipid lowering and need for clinical trials, *Curr Opin Nephrol Hypertension* 13(6):601-605, 2004.

71. Antithrombotic Trialists' Collaboration Group: Collaborative metaanalysis of randomized clinical trials of anti-platelet therapy for prevention of death, myocardial infarction and stroke in high risk patients, *Brit Med J* 324:71-82, 2002.

72. Huerta C et al: Nonsteroid anti-inflammatory drugs and risk of ARF in the general population, *Am J Kidney Dis* 45(3):531-539, 2005.

73. Paul S: Anemia in heart failure: implications, management and outcomes, *J Cardiovas Nurs* 19(6 suppl):s57-s66, 2004.

74. Pearl RG, Pohlman A: Understanding and managing anemia in critically ill patients, *Crit Care Nurs Supplement* s1-s12, 2002.

75. Ezekowitz JA, McAlister FA, Armstrong PW: Anemia is common in heart failure populations and is associated with poor outcomes, *Circulation* 107:223-225, 2003.

76. Okono DO, Anker SD: Anemia in chronic heart failure: pathogenetic mechanisms, *J Card Failure* 10(suppl):s5- s9, 2004.

77. Surgenor SD, Hampers MJ, Corwin HL: Is blood transfusion good for the heart? *Crit Care Med* 29(9s):s189-s90, 2001.

78. Van Iperen CE et al: Response of erythropoiesis and iron metabolism to recombinant human erythropoietin in intensive care patients, *Crit Care Med* 29(9s):s193-s197, 2001.

79. American Diabetes Association: Clinical practice recommendations, *Diabetes Care* 22(suppl 1):s1-s150, 2004.

80. Legg V: Complications of chronic kidney disease: a close look at osteodystrophy, nutritional disturbances and inflammation, *Am J Nurs* 105(6):40-49, 2005.

81. Carnethon MR et al: Prospective investigation of autonomic system function in the development of type 2 diabetes, *Circulation* 107:2190-2208, 2003.

82. Shishehbor MH, Hoogwerf BJ, Lauer MS: Association of triglyceride to HDL cholesterol ratio with heart rate recovery, *Diabetes Care* 27(4):936-941, 2004.

83. Bloomgarden ZT: Consequences of diabetes, *Diabetes Care* 27(7):1825-1831, 2004.

84. Klein BE et al: Electrocardiographic abnormalities in individuals with long duration type 1 diabetes, *Diabetes Care* 28(1):145-147, 2005.

85. Stewart GA et al: Electrocardiographic abnormalities and uremic cardiomyopathy, *Kidney International* 67(1):217-226, 2005.

86. Zimny S, Schatz H, Pfohl M: The role of limited joint mobility in diabetics with an at risk foot, *Diabetes Care* 27(4):94-96, 2004.

87. Rich MW: Heart failure in the oldest patients: the impact of comorbid conditions, *Am J Geriatr Cardiol* 14(3):134-141, 2005.

88. Nagle BA, Erwin WG: Geriatrics. In Dipiro JT et al, editors: *Pharmacotherapy: a pathophysiologic approach*, Stamford, Conn, 1997, Appleton-Lange, pp. 87-100.

89. Piette JD, Heisler M, Wagner TH: Problems paying out-of-pocket medication costs among older adults with diabetes, *Diabetes Care* 27(2):384-391, 2004.

90. Gurwitz JH et al: Incidence and preventability of adverse drug events among older persons in the ambulatory setting, *J Am Med Assoc* 289(9):1107-1116, 2003.

91. Tang WH, Francis GS: Polypharmacy of heart failure, *Cardiol Clin* 19(4):583-596, 2001.

92. Osborne CA, Luzac ML: Over-the-counter medicine use prior to and during hospitalization, *Am J Nurs Pract* 9(4):25-30, 2005.

93. Wheeler M, Wingate S: Managing noncardiac pain in heart failure patients, *J Cardiovas Nurs* 19(s6):s75-s83, 2004.

94. Krein SL et al: The effect of chronic pain on diabetes patients' self management, *Diabetes Care* 28(1):65-70, 2005.

95. Dahners LE, Mullis BH: Effects of nonsteroidal anti-inflammatory drugs on bone formation and soft tissue healing, *J Am Acad Orthoped Surg* 12(3):139-143, 2004.

96. Brumley RD, Enguidanos S, Cherin DA: Effectiveness of a home based palliative care program for end of life, *J Palliative Med* 6:715-724, 2003.

97. Periyasamy SM, Lin J, Tanta F et al: Salt-loading induces redistribution of the plasmalemma 1 Na/K-ATPase in proximal tubule cells. Kidney International 2005; 67 (5): 1868-1877.

98. Kokkinos P, Panagiotakos DB, Polychronopoulos E: Dietary influences on blood pressure: the effect of the Mediterranean diet on the prevalence of hypertension, *J Clin Hypertension* 7:165-170, 2005.

99. Kaplan NM: Lifestyle modifications for prevention and treatment of hypertension, *J Clin Hypertension* VI(XII):716-719, 2004.

100. Chobanian AV et al: Seventh Report of the Joint National Committee on Prevention, Detection, Evaluation and Treatment of High Blood Pressure, *Hypertension* 42(6):1206-1252, 2003.

101. Josephson S, Morikawa S: *Personal communication*, Kaiser Permanente Mid-Atlantic Heart Failure Treatment Program, April 1, 2000.

102. Tuttle KR: Renal manifestations of the metabolic syndrome, *Nephrol Dialysis Transplant* 20(5):861-868, 2005.

103. Bates CM, Lin F: Future strategies in the treatment of acute renal failure: growth factors, stem cells and other novel therapies, *Curr Opin Pediatr* 17(2):215-220, 2005.

104. Herrera M, Garvin JL: Recent advances in the regulation of nitric oxide in the kidney, *Hypertension* 45(6):1062-1067, 2005.

105. Perico N et al: Scientific care for prevention: global perspectives in renal failure, *Kidney International* 67(suppl 94):s8-s13, 2005.

106. Bakris GL: Hypertension and nephropathy, *Am J Med* 115(8A):s49-s54, 2003.

107. Mallamaci F et Al: Prognostic value of combined use of biomarkers of inflammation, endothelial dysfunction and myocardiopathy in patients with ESRD, *Kidney International* 67:2330-2337, 2005.

Pulmonary Hypertension and the Cardiovascular System

Dorothy Lee

Pulmonary arterial hypertension **(PAH)** represents one of the most serious, progressive, and potentially life-threatening conditions of the pulmonary vasculature.[1] Because there is no single agreed-upon definition, PAH can be viewed as a constellation of diseases whereby a progressive increase in pulmonary resistance results in right ventricular failure and untimely death.[5-7] It was thought that PAH was a rare phenomenon, seldom encountered in the clinical setting. Current research and evidence-based guidelines along with numerous clinical trials for novel treatment modalities have increased awareness, screening efforts, and identification of PAH.

Because the cause and pathological conditions of PAH are diverse and the onset of the disease is insidious with vague symptomology that can be related to a multiplicity of medical conditions, many patients are misdiagnosed. Patients can have a cause of PAH that is idiopathic, familial, or associated with several preexisting diseases and conditions. Some of the conditions or diseases include but are not limited to congenital heart defect, connective tissue disease, human immunodeficiency virus, portopulmonary liver disease, thromboembolic disease, and exposure to drugs or toxins.[1-3] Although the specific molecular mechanisms for the diverse causes of PAH remain unclear, a common feature among the conditions is the involvement of progressive vasculopathic changes in the vessels of the pulmonary microcirculation causing hemodynamic abnormality.[4]

Since the 1990s, PAH research has focused on the vascular abnormalities that lead to the development and progression of endothelial dysfunction. Critical to the list of abnormalities are (a) decrease in nitric oxide **(NO)** and prostacyclin synthesis, (b) increase in the production of thromboxane A_2 and endothelin, (c) potassium channel dysfunction, and (d) proliferation of the matrix of the adventitia. During the past decade, many life-extending pharmaceutical treatment options have been marketed, and several more are awaiting approval from the U.S. Food and Drug Administration **(FDA)**.[5,7-15] Although there is no cure, these treatment advances have greatly added to the armamentarium of modalities to attenuate disease progression and prolong survival in certain groups of patients with PAH.

CAUSES

PAH is just one dimension of the grouping of diseases and conditions termed pulmonary hypertension **(PH).** PH can be subdivided into the following five classifications:

- PAH
- PH associated with left heart disease
- PH associated with respiratory disease or from hypoxemia
- PH from thromboembolic disease
- PH caused by other causes, such as sarcoidosis.[2,16-18]

All of these forms of PH share a common characteristic clinical description expressed in the form of hemodynamic criteria. These clinical criteria are used by the National Institutes of Health patient registry for the characterization of primary pulmonary hypertension: mean pulmonary artery pressure **(MPAP)** greater than 25 mm Hg at rest and greater than 30 mm Hg with exercise, along with a pulmonary capillary wedge or left atrial pressure less than 15 mm Hg.[13,19,20] This definition is most often used in clinical trials regarding inclusion criteria for PH.

In 2003, the Third World Conference on Pulmonary Hypertension was held in Venice, Italy, resulting in a revised classification system for PH (Box 87-1). The purpose of the new nomenclature was to extend the scope of the term PH to describe the aforementioned hemodynamic state that is shared in varying manifestations by the conditions listed under the five main categories.[6,18] The previous classification system (referred to as the Evian classification, 1998) was modified to provide a more comprehensive tool with greater utility for use by clinicians and scientists.[2,16,21] Central to the current classification nomenclature is the elimination of the terms primary and secondary PH and the division of the spectrum of PH into five categories. The terms primary and secondary PH were eliminated because each category now denotes a common pathogenesis for the disease states listed under that heading.

In the 2003 organizational reclassification, the five classification groups are arranged such that mechanisms for detection and more specifically modalities for treatment are unique to each group.

BOX 87-1 ■ ■ ■
CLINICAL CLASSIFICATION OF PULMONARY HYPERTENSION

1. Pulmonary arterial hypertension (PAH)
   1.1. Idiopathic (IPAH)
   1.2. Familial (FPAH)
   1.3. Associated with (APAH)
      1.3.1. Connective tissue disease
      1.3.2. Congenital systemic to pulmonary shunts
      1.3.3. Portal hypertension
      1.3.4. HIV infection
      1.3.5. Drugs and toxins
      1.3.6. Other (thyroid disorders, glycogen storage disease, Gaucher disease, hereditary hemorrhagic telangiectasia, hemoglobinopathies, myeloproliferative disorders, splenectomy)
   1.4. Associated with significant venous or capillary involvement
      1.4.1. Pulmonary venoocclusive disease (PVOD)
      1.4.2. Pulmonary capillary hemangiomatosis (PCH)
   1.5. Persistent pulmonary hypertension of the newborn (PPHN)
2. PH associated with left heart diseases
   2.1. Left-sided atrial or ventricular heart disease
   2.2. Left-sided valvular heart disease
3. PH associated with lung respiratory diseases and/or hypoxia
   3.1. Chronic obstructive pulmonary disease
   3.2. Interstitial lung disease
   3.3. Sleep disordered breathing
   3.4. Alveolar hypoventilation disorders
   3.5. Chronic exposure to high altitude
   3.6. Developmental abnormalities
4. PH caused by chronic thrombotic and/or embolic disease
   4.1. Thromboembolic obstruction of proximal pulmonary arteries
   4.2. Thromboembolic obstruction of distal pulmonary arteries
   4.3. Nonthrombotic pulmonary embolism (tumor, parasites, foreign material)
5. Miscellaneous
   Sarcoidosis, histiocytosis X, lymphangiomatosis, compression of pulmonary vessels (adenopathy, tumor, fibrosing mediastinitis)

ESC Guidelines on diagnosis and treatment of pulmonary arterial hypertension, *European Heart Journal* 25:2243-2278, 2004.

Pulmonary Artery Hypertension

PAH includes idiopathic PAH **(IPAH)**, familial PAH **(FPAH)**, and associated PAH **(APAH)**. IPAH is diagnosed when the cause of PAH is determined to be unknown and all other causative conditions have been excluded.

FPAH is associated with mutations in the bone morphogenetic protein receptor II gene **(BMPR2)**. The gene is located on chromosome 2q33 and although the BMPR2 gene is autosomal dominant, it is thought to have incomplete penetrance.[6] This means FPAH is not manifest in each person with the mutated gene, whereby disease expression can skip generations further obscuring the presence in family history.[17,18] BMPR2 plays a pivotal role in regulation of cell growth and proliferation, and the mutation is present in approximately 50 percent of patients with FPAH and 10 percent to 20 percent of patients with IPAH.[2,27] It has been suggested that the absence of the BMPR2 gene mutation in the remaining FPAH and the majority of IPAH patients is cause to believe that there are more genes present in the BMP-transforming growth factor beta **(TGF-beta)** molecular pathway that have yet to be identified.[27]

APAH is a subcategory of PAH that generally occurs somewhat later in life and generates from several diverse causes including connective tissue disease, congenital systemic to pulmonary shunts, portal hypertension, human immunodeficiency virus infection, drugs (e.g., Fen-Phen, illicit drugs, such as cocaine), toxins (e.g., rapeseed oil), and other disorders that occur in the spectrum of PAH.[2,16,21] Patients with PAH benefit from oral, inhaled, or intravenous medications targeted to inhibit vascular growth and proliferation.

Pulmonary Hypertension with Left Heart Disease

PH associated with left heart disease involves left heart dysfunction, which can be systolic, diastolic, or valvular in cause. Patients in this category receive appropriate surgical and/or medical treatment for valvular or left heart disease to alleviate the primary pathological condition.

Pulmonary Hypertension with Respiratory Disease or Hypoxemia

For patients with PH associated with lung respiratory diseases and/or hypoxia, treatment revolves around the primary pathological condition as in chronic obstructive pulmonary disease, interstitial lung disease, or obstructive sleep apnea, whereby medication, supplemental oxygen, and bilevel positive airway pressure **(BiPAP)** would be prescribed, along with further evaluation of the contributing causes.

Pulmonary Hypertension from Thromboembolic Disease

For patients with PH as a result of chronic thrombotic and/or embolic disease, surgical intervention (pulmonary thromboendarterectomy) can result in a "cure" for some patients or at least provide substantial improvement in hemodynamic profile, functional status, and length of survival.[22] Lifelong warfarin therapy and a superior vena cava filter are also indicated.

Pulmonary Hypertension from Other Causes

The miscellaneous category of PH necessitates pharmacological treatment and medical intervention specific to the primary disorder. Disease conditions in this category include sarcoidosis, histiocytosis X, lymphangiomatosis, and compression of pulmonary vessels.

In tandem with clinical classification, patients with PAH are classified according to functional status via the New York Heart Association **(NYHA)** classification of dyspnea. The NYHA classification was modified and streamlined by the World Health Organization to categorize PH according to severity of symptoms. NYHA classification is an important metric because it yields a strong correlation with mortality.[2,13,21,23] Clinicians use the NYHA classification (Table 87-1) at the baseline evaluation, during treatment to monitor disease progression, response to therapy, and to aid in prediction of survival.[16] It is also used as part of inclusion and exclusion criteria and to monitor therapeutic progress in many clinical trials.[1]

INCIDENCE AND PREVALENCE
Idiopathic Pulmonary Artery Hypertension

IPAH is mostly a disease of younger women, with a female-to-male ratio of 2 to 3 to 1.[2,17,21] IPAH typically appears in the 30s and 40s, with a mean age of 36.[2,21,26] IPAH is sporadic in nature and diagnosis is based on exclusion of associated disease conditions. IPAH has an estimated annual occurrence of 1 to 2 cases per million.[17,19,21,26]

■ ■ ■

TABLE 87-1 NEW YORK HEART ASSOCIATION/WORLD HEALTH ORGANIZATION CLASSIFICATION OF FUNCTIONAL STATUS OF PATIENTS WITH PULMONARY HYPERTENSION

CLASS	DESCRIPTION
I	Patients with PH in whom there is no limitation of usual activity; ordinary physical activity does not cause increased dyspnea, fatigue, chest pain, or presyncope.
II	Patients with PH who have mild limitation of physical activity. There is no discomfort at rest, but normal physical activity causes increased dyspnea, fatigue, chest pain, or presyncope.
III	Patients with PH who have a marked limitation of physical activity. There is no discomfort at rest, but less than ordinary activity causes increased dyspnea, fatigue, chest pain, or presyncope.
IV	Patients with PH who are unable to perform any physical activity and who may have signs of right ventricular failure at rest. Dyspnea and/or fatigue may be present at rest and symptoms are increased by almost any physical activity.

PH, Pulmonary hypertension.
ESC guidelines on diagnosis and treatment of pulmonary arterial hypertension, *European Heart Journal* 25:2243-2278, 2004.

Familial Pulmonary Artery Hypertension

The incidence and prevalence of FPAH in the general population is unknown because genetic investigation is not considered routine in the diagnosis and treatment of PAH. Therefore an unidentified percentage of IPAH patients may carry a BMPR2 gene mutation or other mutation in the TGF-beta pathway associated with PAH.

Associated Pulmonary Artery Hypertension

This heterogenous group of diseases and exposures are associated with or facilitate the development of PAH in certain susceptible individuals. In the connective tissue disease category, specific diseases have varying percentages of PAH prevalence. In scleroderma PAH affects between 6 percent and 60 percent of all cases, and when associated with lupus, PAH affects between 4 percent to 14 percent of the cases.[21] The incidence of APAH is somewhat higher when related to amphetamine or appetite suppressant use and has been estimated between 25 to 50 cases per million annually.[26] In human immunodeficiency virus infection, the incidence of PAH is 0.5 percent and develops irrespective of viral load.[17,21]

PROGRESSIVE NATURE (NATURAL HISTORY)

In 1987 data from the patient registry for the characterization of primary pulmonary hypertension was used to investigate factors associated with survival in PAH patients. A strong correlation between right-sided heart function and survival was revealed.[28] The estimated median of survival for untreated IPAH patients from diagnosis was 2.8 years, with group survival rates of 68 percent at 1 year, 48 percent at 3 years, and 34 percent at 5 years.[1,23] APAH median survival statistics from disease-related causes include congenital heart disease (5 years), Eisenmenger (3 years), portopulmonary hypertension (2 years), human immunodeficiency virus (1 to 2 years), sickle cell disease (1 to 2 years), and appetite suppressants or amphetamines (2 to 3 years).[21] Variables most associated with mortality were mean MPAP, right atrial **(RA)** pressure, cardiac index **(CI),** and NYHA functional class. Using these values, a regression equation was formulated to describe the correlation between the variables and thus predict survival.[12,13,28] Because there was no effective treatment at the time of publication of registry findings, it is reasonable to conclude that these survival estimates predict the natural history of untreated PAH.

Pulmonary Artery Hypertension and Right Heart Failure

PAH has an insidious nature most often having a gradual onset of symptoms common to a multiplicity of illnesses. When symptoms become prevalent, the disease has usually progressed to a moderate or severe stage with diffuse and extensive arterial damage.[16] This damage causes an increase in pulmonary vascular resistance

(PVR), such that the right ventricle **(RV)** hypertrophies to adapt to the pressure overload.[16] There is progressive deterioration of RV function in advanced disease demonstrated by an increase in MPAP, PVR, and RV afterload.[16,19,26] The presence of enlarged RA, RV, and tricuspid valve regurgitation are morphological manifestations of progressive right heart decompensation.[16] In later stages of the disease, some patients show a progressive decline in MPAP and CI because the heart is no longer able to compensate for the excessive workload.[12,16,23] The patient is symptomatic at rest, and ultimately the afterload-intolerant RV fails and death is inevitable.

PATHOPHYSIOLOGY

In contrast to the systemic circulation, the pulmonary circulation is viewed as high-flow, low-pressure, and low-resistance circulation, with the capacity to enlist unperfused vessels of the pulmonary vasculature when needed (Figure 87-1).[20,27,29] This is most evident when a comparison is made between the pressures in the systemic and pulmonary circuits. Pulmonary artery pressure **(PAP)** in a young adult residing at sea level is normally 25/10 mm Hg with a mean MPAP of 15 mm Hg.[3] PVR is described as resistance to blood flowing through the pulmonary circulation and is primarily dictated by the radius of the pulmonary arteries, according to Poiseuille law.

Poiseuille law:

$$R = 8?L/pr^4$$
(? = viscosity, L = length, r = radius, p = pi (3.1415 . . .)

This means that even very small changes in the radius of the pulmonary vessels have a profound effect on resistance. Also, increases in viscosity of air (e.g., moisture in a sauna) can add to the work of breathing.

In the aforementioned normal young adult, PVR is likely to be reported at 1.5 mm Hg/liter/min, not exceeding 3.0 mm Hg/liter/min. PVR can be calculated by the following equation:

$$PVR = \frac{(MPAP - PCWP)}{CO}$$

(where PCWP = the pulmonary capillary wedge pressure and CO = cardiac output). PVR can also be expressed in dynes/sec/cm[5].

The conducting arteries of the pulmonary circulation are classified as elastic and are exceedingly distensible in nature (Table 87-2). However, as the arteries progress toward the capillary bed, they decrease in radius, intimal and elastic laminal thickness, and are classified as terminal arterioles. These precapillary terminal arterioles measure *less than* 100 μm and are composed of a single layer of intima and a narrow elastic lamina.[29] The capillaries are composed of a continuous layer of endothelium that rests on a thin continuous basement membrane, with central connections to intermittent pericytes found inferior to the basement membrane. This arrangement of vascular structures allows the pulmonary circulation to have the qualities of high flow, low pressure, and low resistance to facilitate gas exchange.[29]

Histopathology

The vascular pathological changes that occur in the pulmonary arteries are neither disease specific nor diagnostic (Figure 87-2). The changes begin with medial thickening and lead to intimal hyperplasia and fibrosis, smooth muscle hypertrophy, and in situ thrombosis.[26,30] The most advanced lesion is called the plexiform lesion, which is characterized by an aneurismal dilatation revealing endothelial hyperplasia, extracellular matrix, suspected evidence of angiogenesis, and organizing thrombi.[2,26,30] It is the presence of these structural alterations in the pulmonary vasculature that result in the increase in resistance reflected by the increase in MPAP. Further, the increase in PVR causes a profound effect on cardiac structure and morphology.

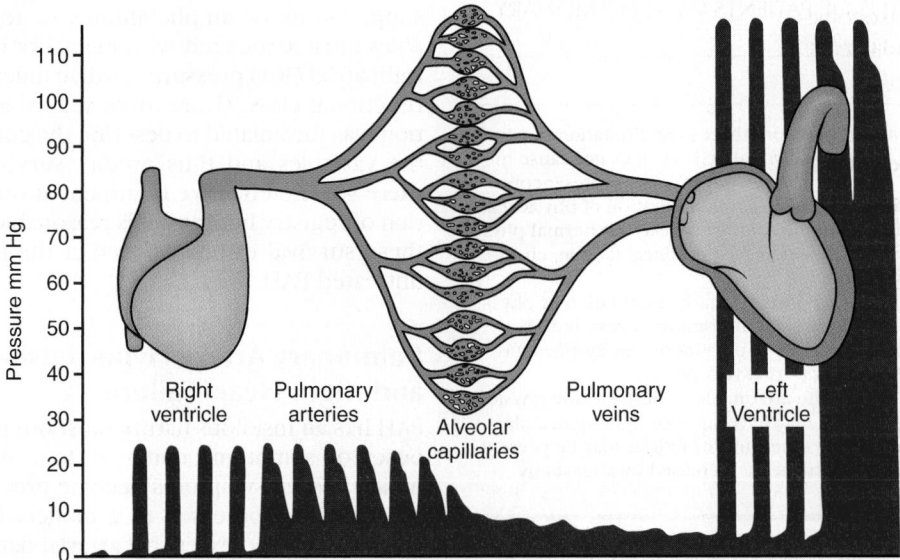

FIGURE 87-1 ■ Pulmonary circulation pressures. (From Rushmer, RF: *Organ physiology: structure and function of the cardiovascular system*, ed 2, Philadelphia, 1976, WB Saunders, p 31.)

■■■

TABLE 87-2 COMPARISON OF PULMONARY AND SYSTEMIC CIRCULATIONS

	SYSTEMIC	PULMONARY
Vascular Physical Characteristics	Thick walled Heavily muscled Nondistensible Narrow lumina	Thin walled Scant smooth muscle Distensible Wide lumina
Physiological Characteristics	Dilate in response to acidemia and hypoxemia	Constrict in response to acidemia and hypoxemia
Pressures and Blood Flow		
Arterial (mm Hg)	120/80	25/8
Mean	90	15
Pressure gradient driving flow (mm Hg)	90	9
Mean capillary (mm Hg)	18	8
Mean venous (mm Hg)	0-8	4-12
Blood flow (liter/min)	5	5
Vascular resistance	High	Low

From Rushmer, RF: *Organ physiology: structure and function of the cardiovascular system*, ed 2, Philadelphia, 1976, WB Saunders, p 31.

Pathogenesis

In IPAH the cause of the disease is unknown, but in all three categories of PAH, three components appear to be central: a preexisting condition of individual susceptibility, a risk factor, and a triggering factor (Figure 87-3).[2,26] Risk factors include but are not limited to female gender, familial predisposition, and associated diseases.[6] Trigger factors include but are not limited to appetite suppressants, amphetamine or cocaine use, hypoxemia from high altitude, interstitial lung disease or sleep apnea, hormones as in pregnancy or oral contraceptives, and viruses (e.g., human herpes virus 8). The trigger factor is pivotal in providing the initial insult to the pulmonary artery endothelium causing a cascade of mediators to provoke changes in the vessel. The normal order of homeostasis is shifted to a progressive pathological process that promotes vasoconstriction, cell proliferation, and progressive vascular remodeling.

Mediators

The proposed mediators are as follows:

- Prostacyclin I2
- Thromboxane A_2
- Nitric oxide (NO)
- Endothelin 1
- Serotonin
- Estrogen
- Arginine deficiency
- Dysfunctional Ca^{2+}-sensitive K^+ channels
- Vascular endothelial growth factor (**VEGF**)
- TGF-beta superfamily (related to the BMPR2 gene)

These mediators affect every component of the arterial wall (intima, media, and adventitia).[26,27] The extensive list of proposed mediators suggests that the pulmonary vascular damage wrought by the endothelial dysfunction, smooth muscle cell hyperplasia, and matrix changes result from a complex multifactorial pathobiology involving a variety of biochemical pathways and cell types.*

Vasoconstriction

Vasoconstriction and medial hypertrophy occur early in the vascular remodeling process and may be the result of the initial endothelial cell injury. The injury causes an increase in the release of potent vasoconstrictive agents endothelin 1, thromboxane A_2, and a suppression of potent vasodilators, such as prostacyclin and NO.[17,26,27] Endothelial cell dysfunction has been linked with chronic impairment in NO synthase and prostacyclin synthase production and excessive expression of endothelin 1 (**ET1**).[27] ET1 is associated with both acute and chronic detrimental effects on the pulmonary vasculature. Acute effects include vasoconstriction and inflammation, whereas chronic effects include fibrosis, neurohormonal secretion, and cellular proliferation. Acute (leading to chronic) vasoconstriction has been associated with dysfunctional Ca^{2+}-sensitive K^+ channels and endothelial dysfunction.[31] It appears that chronic hypoxia in PAH down-regulates the K^+ channels in smooth muscle cells causing a release of Ca^{2+} leading to vasoconstriction.[18,27,31] The presence of VEGF immunolocalization in the plexiform lesions suggests the lesion, in part, represents a vasoproliferative process associated with disordered angiogenesis.[27] Serotonin transporter overexpression has been associated with medial layer smooth muscle hypertrophy in the arterial walls of PAH patients.[27]

---

*References 8, 18, 26, 27, 30, 31.

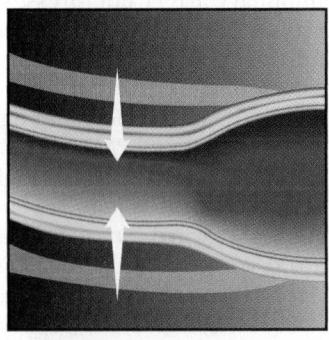
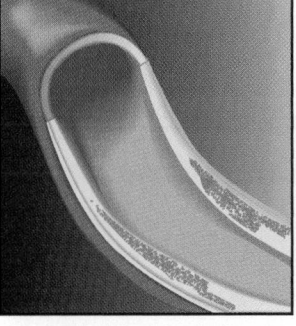
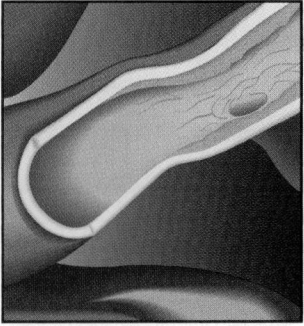

Pulmonary vasconstriction   Hypertrophy   Fibrosis

FIGURE 87-2 ■ Vascular changes in pulmonary artery hypertension.

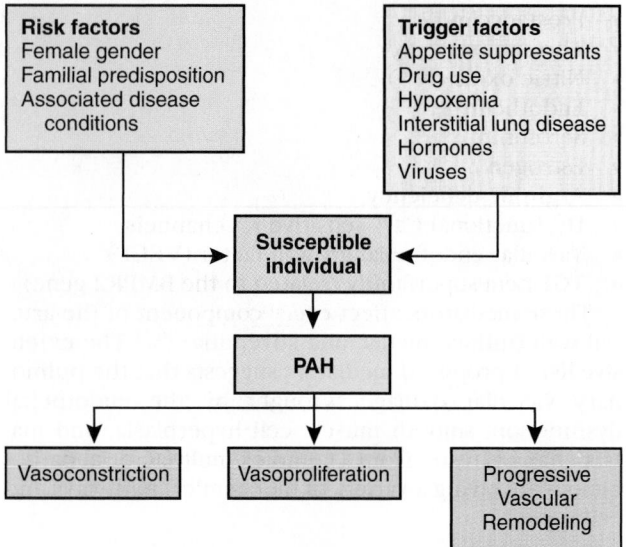

FIGURE 87-3 ■ Central components of pulmonary artery hypertension. *PAH,* Pulmonary artery hypertension.

Vasoproliferation

Of all the mediators, ET1 plays a preponderant and significant multifactorial role in the pathogenesis of PAH. ET1 is an endogenous 21 amino acid peptide released from the endothelium that exerts potent vasoconstrictor, mitogenic, and profibrotic effects.[32] ET1 is formed when endothelin-converting enzyme **(ECE)** cleaves big ET1 (Figure 87-4).[9] There are two ET1 receptor isoforms pertinent to cell proliferation in PAH; they are ETa and ETb. ETa receptors are located and mediate sustained vasoconstriction and cellular proliferation on vascular smooth muscle and fibroblasts.[8] Similar to ETa receptors, ETb receptors are found on vascular smooth muscle cells and fibroblasts, but are also located on endothelial cells, macrophages, and in the sympathetic nervous system. In a nondisease environment, ETb receptors mediate endothelial-dependent vasodilatation, but in disease states, ETb is down-regulated on endothelium to favor vasoconstriction, and it is up-regulated on vascular smooth muscle to maintain a proliferative state. The down-regulated Ca^{2+}-dependent K^+ channels also play a role in cell proliferation.[27] Additionally, ETb receptors are responsible for the clearance of approximately 50 percent of the circulating ET1 during pulmonary perfusion.[9] Evidence of this ET1-driven process is found in the plasma of PAH patients, where increased levels of ET1 are linearly correlated with disease severity and prognosis.[18,27]

Progressive Pulmonary Vascular Remodeling

ET1 is associated with hyperplasia and vascular remodeling as seen in the plexiform lesions of PAH. Specific structural remodeling of the vasculature is manifest by cellular intimal thickening, intimal fibrosis, in situ thrombosis, and ultimately, the plexiform lesion.[30] Characteristics of intimal thickening include oval-shaped nuclei and copious cytoplasm with scarce traces of elastin. Other characteristics of vascular remodeling include the presence of macrophages, intimal fibrosis, endothelial cell proliferation, and immature smooth muscle cells.[30] Prostacyclin is a potent endogenous vasodilator that is activated via the cyclic adenosine monophosphate (cAMP)–dependent pathways.[17,27] Prostacyclin also has an inhibitory effect on platelet aggregation, smooth muscle proliferation, and inflammation.[21] Prostacyclin synthase is decreased in endothelial cells of PAH patients. Further, endothelium vasodilatory support is suppressed by the reduction of NO synthase. NO likewise has potent smooth muscle vasodilatory and antiproliferative properties through activation of the cyclic guanosine monophosphate phosphodiesterase-type 5 **(cGMP)** pathway.[27] Thus progressive proliferative pulmonary vascular remodeling continues unopposed in the absence of prostacyclin and NO vasodilatory effects.

MANIFESTATIONS

Dyspnea upon exertion is present in 60 percent of the patients in early stages of PAH and is common among all patients with disease progression.[19] Limited exercise capacity, fatigue, and weakness can be easily and mistakenly attributed to deconditioning. Other symptoms include angina or chest discomfort, palpitations, presyncope or syncope, Raynaud phenomenon, and (less commonly) hoarseness or voice changes.[2,16,21,26] The presence of a hoarse voice is related to a phenomenon known as Ortner syndrome. Hoarseness results when the dilated pulmonary artery compresses the recurrent laryngeal nerve as it courses around the ligamentum arteriosum and travels up toward the larynx alongside the trachea and esophagus.[21,26]

Common physical examination findings may be subtle, dependent on severity of PAH, and are likely to reflect right ventricular hypertrophy and right-sided valvular insufficiency. They include jugular-venous distention with a prominent "a" wave, an accentuated pulmonic component of the second heart sound, right ventricular heave palpable at the left sternal border, pansystolic murmur of tricuspid regurgitation, soft blowing diastolic murmur of pulmonary insufficiency, and a right ventricular S_3 gallop best detected at the left sternal bor-

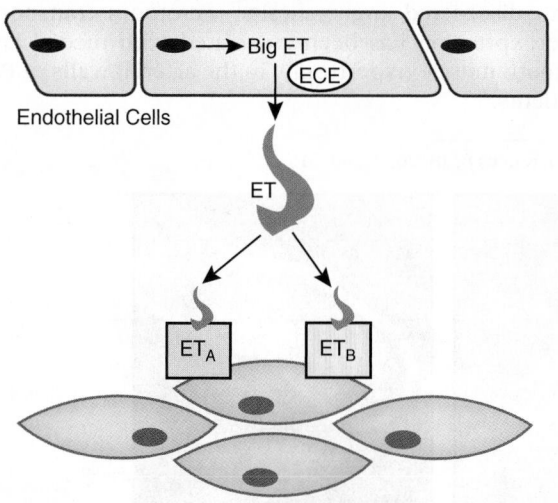

FIGURE 87-4 ■ Production of endothelin. *ECE,* Endothelin converting enzyme; *ET,* endothelin.

der.[2,16,21,26] Pedal edema, ascites, central or peripheral cyanosis, tricuspid valve regurgitation, and RV failure are manifestations of more advanced disease.[2,16]

Signs and Symptoms of Related Conditions

The history and physical exam can provide evidence of APAH. Specific components of the history should include anorexigen use, reports of loud nightly snoring with breath holding, smoking history, alcohol and illicit drug abuse, and lifestyle risks related to possible human immunodeficiency virus infection. The physical exam should note the presence of crowded oropharynx as in obstructive sleep apnea, joint swelling, sclerodactyly, tight skin, cutaneous telangiectasia and other signs of connective tissue disease, and hepatomegaly or pulsatile liver as in portopulmonary hypertension.[2,16] These findings are useful to raise clinical suspicion to begin screening for PAH.

SCREENING

Patients may come in for screening for one of three reasons: gradually worsening unexplained dyspnea; incidental findings that appear on a chest x-ray **(CXR)**, echocardiogram, or ECG; and having a first-degree family member with IPAH. Screening should proceed within a logical framework with the goal of identifying and then categorizing the cause of PH because this will dictate the treatment approach. Assessing the level of functional impairment, and delineating the specific hemodynamic profile, with subsequent response to vasodilator challenge are key to diagnosis and treatment.[2,16]

Electrocardiogram

Although the ECG is nonspecific, it is likely to show evidence of RV hypertrophy and right-heart dilatation. RV hypertrophy is seen in 87 percent, and right-axis deviation is present in 79 percent of patients with IPAH (Box 87-2).[16] The right precordial leads may show ST-T segment wave depression and inversion and RA enlargement as demonstrated by a tall P wave greater than 2.5 mm in leads II, III, and aV_F. However, this evidence should be considered suggestive or supportive only because the ECG lacks sensitivity (55 percent) and specificity (70 percent) for use as a screening tool in PAH.[16,26]

Chest X-ray

Subtle abnormal findings can be revealed in the CXR of PAH patients, but sensitivity and specificity are lacking such that a normal CXR is not used to exclude the diagnosis.[2,16,26] Prominent main and hilar pulmonary arterial shadows with "pruning" (a decrease in pulmonary vascular markings in the lung fields) are classic for PAH; however, absence of pruning is not cause for exclusion.[2,16] Although not considered a screening tool, the CXR can prove valuable in assessment of PAH as a result of interstitial lung disease.[26]

6-Minute Walk Test

Although not officially part of the screening algorithm, the 6-minute walk test is an objective measure that yields valuable information regarding functional status and exercise capacity.[2,55] It is used as a primary end point in a great majority of PAH clinical trials and is well established, has worldwide acceptance, is noninvasive and inexpensive, and has prognostic importance.[1,8,11,13] The test is accepted by researchers and clinicians as a means for evaluating treatment efficacy, monitoring treatment response, and is a predictor of survival with poor prognosis for distances of *less than* 250 meters.[16]

Transthoracic Doppler Echocardiogram

Transthoracic echocardiography **(TTE)** is often the first screening test for diagnosis of PAH.[22] It is noninvasive and useful in determining an estimation of the pulmonary artery systolic pressure, which is deemed equivalent to the right ventricular systolic pressure, given there is no pulmonic valve disease. Tricuspid regurgitant jets can be determined in approximately 74 percent of PH patients.[2] Other measurements of diagnostic value and confirmation include RA and RV dimension and function; tricuspid, pulmonic, and mitral valve abnormalities; characteristics of RV ejection and left ventricular filling; inferior vena cava diameter; left displacement of the ventricular septum; and presence of pericardial effusion.[2,22]

Ventilation Perfusion Scan

A ventilation perfusion scan should be performed to rule out the presence of chronic thromboembolic PH. Abnormal scans reveal multiple segmental mismatched defects; however, the magnitude of the defect is usually an underestimation of the actual degree of thromboembolic obstruction.[22] Therefore positive scan results are followed by pulmonary angiography to help determine if the obstruction is surgically accessible.[2,16,22] Scanning to differentiate between IPAH and chronic thromboembolic PH has a sensitivity of 90 percent to 100 percent and a specificity of 94 percent to 100 percent.[2] The value in substituting computed tomography instead of a ventilation perfusion scan is equivocal and not clearly defined.[2,16,22]

BOX 87-2   ■ ■ ■
ELECTROCARDIOGRAPHIC FINDINGS IN PULMONARY HYPERTENSION

- Right axis deviation
- Tall R wave and small S wave with R/S ratio greater than 1 in lead V_1
- QR complex in lead V1
- rSR pattern in lead V1
- Large S wave and small R wave with R/R ratio less than 1 in lead V_5 or V_6
- S_1, S_2, S_3 pattern

McGoon M, Gutterman D, Steen V et al: Screening, early detection, and diagnosis of pulmonary arterial hypertension: ACCP evidence-based clinical practice guidelines, *Chest* 126:14S-34S, 2004.

Computed Tomography Scan

High resolution computed tomography can be used to provide detailed images of the lung parenchyma useful for the diagnosis of emphysema or interstitial lung disease. Advanced left ventricular failure can be manifest as ground-glass opacification, whereas pulmonary veno-occlusive disease is suggested by the presence of a thickened interlobular septum.[2] Other findings indicative of concomitant lung disease include lymphadenopathy, pleural effusions, and the presence of pulmonary nodules.

Pulmonary Function Testing

A complete pulmonary function test should be ordered to exclude or characterize the contribution of underlying obstructive or restrictive lung disease as the cause of dyspnea. The diffusion of carbon monoxide yields information regarding the presence of interstitial lung disease.[2] However, in the absence of interstitial lung disease, the diffusion of carbon monoxide in PAH patients can be reduced to 60 percent to 80 percent of predicted.[16] Arterial blood gases provide an index of arterial oxygenation, where hypoxemia can be due to a ventilation-perfusion mismatch and/or secondary to a reduction in mixed venous oxygen saturation as a consequence of decreased cardiac output.

Laboratory Tests

Serological assessment should be performed to measure levels of antinuclear antibody, sedimentation rate, and certain specific autoantibodies for suspicion of APAH and connective tissue disease. Human immunodeficiency virus infection testing should be done. Liver function tests and hepatitis profile are necessary to rule out portopulmonary hypertension. Serum b-type natriuretic peptide level, protein C and S, and thyroid studies (TSH and Free T_4) can be of diagnostic value.[21,33]

Right-Heart Catheterization

The right-heart catheterization is the most important test in the assessment of PH because it confirms the presence of PH and establishes the diagnosis by providing a precise hemodynamic profile, which defines the severity.[16,17,26,33] It is also required to test the vasoreactive response in the pulmonary circulation. Parameters of significance are RA pressure; PAP, including pulmonary artery occlusion pressure; CI; PVR; and arterial and mixed venous oxygen saturation.[2,16] Right heart catheterization is also useful in the diagnosis of PAH by excluding intracardiac or extracardiac shunts and left-heart disease.[16] Lastly the hemodynamic parameters attained through right heart catheterization aid in the determination of pharmacological management and have prognostic value.[2,16,18,26]

Vasoreactivity of the pulmonary circulation is challenged through the selection of any of these three short-acting vasodilators: intravenous adenosine or prostacyclin, or inhaled NO.[12] In the past, intravenous calcium channel blockers were used; however, because of the deleterious systemic effects of hypotension, shock, and death in some patients, they are no longer recommended.[34,35] NO is very commonly used because it is specific for the pulmonary vascular bed and does not affect the systemic circulation.[18] The purpose of a vasodilator test is to assess the safety and likelihood of a favorable response to oral calcium channel blocker therapy. Calcium channel blocker responders make up a disproportionately small group of IPAH patients, and long-term response to treatment with oral calcium channel blocker therapy is not always sustained; approximately half of patients require a different therapeutic option.[2] Varying parameters for defining vasoreactive response have been used in the past; however, current recommendations define a positive acute response to be a decrease in mean PAP *greater than* 10 mm Hg to reach an absolute value of MPAP of 40 mm Hg or less *with* an increase or unchanged cardiac output.[2,16]

MANAGEMENT

See Figure 87-5 for an overview of the management of PAH. The aim of therapy for PAH patients from a clinical standpoint is to reverse or inhibit the three primary abnormalities of vasoconstriction, smooth muscle proliferation, and vascular remodeling with the goals of decreasing PAP and PVR, improving RV function, and increasing CI. From a more holistic standpoint, improvement of functional status and quality of life are patient-focused expectations from therapy. Recently, many therapeutic developments have occurred broadening the once limited number of pharmacological options. This is especially fortuitous because some medication regimens involve a somewhat sophisticated level of complexity. Conventional therapy is considered to be oxygen, warfarin, diuretics, digoxin, and calcium channel blockers. No randomized clinical trials have been conducted using these agents for treatment of PAH because they do not affect any of the biomolecular pathways pertinent to disease pathogenesis.[36] These therapies basically treat potential complications of PAH.

Oxygen should be used in patients with hypoxemia with a saturation of peripheral oxygen (**SpO₂**) maintained at greater than 90 percent at rest and with exercise.[2,21,26,36] Consistent data with regard to the efficacy of long-term oxygen use in PAH is lacking.[2]

Warfarin has been tested in uncontrolled trials retrospectively.[2] Recommendations for use support maintaining the international normalized ratio (**INR**) between 1.5 and 2.5 for IPAH; however, the INR range differs from1.5 to 4.0 between PAH centers in the United States and Europe.[21,36] Use of warfarin in patients with APAH is controversial, and guidelines encourage providers to carefully consider the benefit-risk ratio in each case.[2,36]

Diuretics are used when decompensated right heart failure results in fluid retention.[2,21,26,36] Loop diuretics, thiazides, and spironolactone are commonly used. Long-term diuretic use involves careful maintenance of near-normal intravascular volume and attention to electrolyte levels and renal function.[17,36]

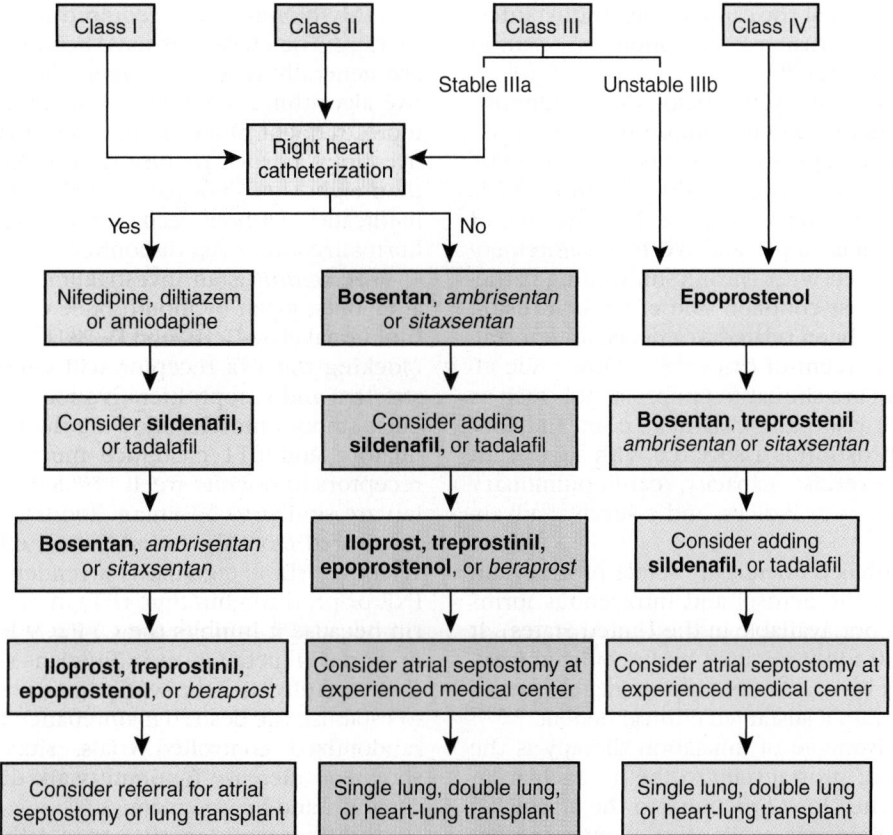

FIGURE 87-5 ■ Management of pulmonary artery hypertension is facilitated by using right-heart catheterization to determine vasoreactivity in the pulmonary circulation by challenge with any of the three short-acting vasodilators mentioned in the text. A patient is considered vasoreactive (YES) if the vasodilator provocation yields a decrease in MPAP of more than 10 mm Hg to reach an absolute mean value for MPAP of 40 mm Hg or less with increased or unchanged cardiac output.[2,16] Patients who do not meet these criteria for vasoreactivity (NO) start with more aggressive initial therapy as seen in the middle arm of the figure. Patients in classes IIIb and IV start with an even more potent therapy regimen, as seen to the right. (Treatment algorithm courtesy of Kamal Mubarak, MD.)

Digoxin is used to address the decreased contractility in the progression of right heart failure to improve cardiac output.[2,36] Overall the use of digitalis in PAH is controversial.[21,26] Drug levels and renal function must be monitored.

Calcium channel blockers are only used for a select group of PAH patients who respond to the calcium channel blocker challenge, reflecting a near normalization of PAPs and cardiac output.[2,36] An acute vasoreactive response is estimated to be present in approximately 10 percent of IPAH patients. Sustained long-term response is estimated to be maintained in about 50 percent of this total group, representing an exceedingly small number (6 percent) of IPAH patients.[2,36] It is thought that patients exhibiting an acute vasoreactive response are in the early stages of PAH where fibrosis and increased vascular proliferation have not advanced to the point of vasodilatory impairment. The most common calcium channel blockers used in PAH treatment are diltiazem and nifedipine. Diltiazem is the likely choice for patients with relative tachycardia, and nifedipine is selected for those with bradycardia.[2]

Prostacyclin is a metabolite of arachidonic acid, produced by endothelial cells and yields a potent vasodilatory response.[2,21,36] Synthetic prostacyclin and its analogs (prostanoids) are indicated in PAH for the inhibition of platelet aggregation, cytoprotective effects, antiproliferative influence on vascular growth, antiinflammatory effects, and enhancing cardiac output.[18,21,26,36] Synthesis of prostacyclin is impaired in PAH as evidenced by a reduction of the enzyme prostacyclin synthase; therefore use of prostanoids aids in replacement of impaired and suppressed prostacyclin production.

Epoprostenol (synthetic prostacyclin) has been tested in clinical trials in IPAH and in scleroderma patients with APAH. Epoprostenol significantly improved exercise capacity, functional capacity, hemodynamics, and survival in IPAH patients.[7,13,19,25,36] Epoprostenol is available in a freeze-dried preparation and must be reconstituted by the patient before use for continuous intravenous administration. An indwelling central venous catheter is required for drug delivery through the use of an infusion pump. Epoprostenol has a half-life of 3 to 5 minutes, and because the drug is not stable at room temperature, it must be kept cold with ice packs.[13,21,36] Side effects include jaw pain, anorexia, nausea, headache, flushing, diarrhea, skin rash, and musculoskeletal aches in the feet and legs, with most of the side effects being dose related.[36] Adverse effects and morbidity are associated with chronic indwelling catheter use and include local infections at the catheter site, tunnel infections, and sepsis.[13,36] Infusion interruption can result in death from rebound PAH.[36]

Treprostinil is a prostacyclin analog that is administered subcutaneously via a continuous infusion pump.[24] Dose preparation of treprostinil must be performed by the patient before each drug infusion. Treprostinil is chemically stable at room temperature, has a half-life of 3 to 4 hours, has a neutral pH, and averts the aforementioned risks associated with chronic indwelling catheter use.[2,24,26] The most common side effect is infusion site pain, which has been related to a decision to terminate therapy in 8 percent of cases.[21,24,37] Other side effects of treprostinil are similar to epoprostenol, such as nausea, headache, jaw pain, diarrhea, rash, and foot and leg pain. Treprostinil is associated with significant improvement in exercise capacity, cardiopulmonary hemodynamics, dyspnea indices, and a survival advantage.[2,21]

Iloprost is an inhaled chemically stable prostacyclin analog available in the aerosol and intravenous forms (intravenous form not available in the United States). It has a half-life of 60 to 90 minutes, and nebulized treatments are taken every 2 hours, approximately six to nine times daily attain a sustained clinical benefit.[21,24,37] The theoretical advantage of inhalation therapy is the direct application of prostacyclin to the intraacinar arteries because of the close proximity to the alveoli.[6,36] The vasodilatory response to iloprost is more potent than NO.[36] Side effects include headache, mild coughing, jaw pain, syncope, and flushing. Overall iloprost is a well-tolerated, safe, and effective therapy for severe PAH.

Endothelin Receptor Antagonists

The pulmonary vascular bed is an important and abundant site for ET1 production and clearance.[9] In PAH ET1 production is enhanced, and production of prostacyclin and NO is diminished. ET1 interacts with the ETa and ETb receptors to promote an environment that facilitates vasoconstriction, vasoproliferation, and vascular remodeling in the pulmonary circulation. Endothelin receptor antagonists are prescribed to antagonize the receptor perturbations of PAH and restore normal functioning of the endothelial and vascular smooth muscle cells. Endothelin receptor antagonists are highly teratogenic and are also noted to cause irreversible testicular injury and sterility in laboratory animals.

Bosentan is the first orally active nonselective (ETa and ETb) endothelial receptor-antagonist to improve symptoms, increase 6-minute walk distance, and improve hemodynamics in PAH patients.[5,37] It is indicated for and has shown improvement in NYHA functional class III and IV patients; however, class II patients also have benefited from this therapy.[2,5,21,37] Bosentan has demonstrated improvement in echocardiographic variables (left ventricle to RV areas ratio) and time to clinical worsening.[2,5,37] Bosentan is taken by mouth twice daily, with minor side effects of headache, nausea, dizziness, and fluid retention. The major side effect of bosentan is elevation in hepatic transaminases, and

monthly monitoring is required for all patients on this therapy. The elevations have been dose dependent and are generally reversible when the suggested prescriptive algorithm is followed. Mild elevations are cause for more frequent monitoring. Liver enzymes greater than five times normal require dose reduction, and greater than eight times normal require discontinuation of the medication without rechallenge. Liver enzymes should normalize after drug discontinuation.

Sitaxsentan is an investigational, oral, selective ETa antagonist given by mouth once daily for use in NYHA functional class II, III, and IV PAH.[5,8,36] It is believed that blocking the ETa receptor will decrease the vasoconstrictive and vasoproliferative focus of ET1 on the vascular smooth muscle, allowing the benefits of the vasodilatory and ET1 clearance mechanisms of the ETb receptors to operate freely.[5,8,36] Side effects of sitaxsentan are similar to bosentan, and liver function must be monitored monthly. An additional effect of this potent selective ETa antagonist is a tendency to increase the INR or prothrombin time (PT) in patients taking warfarin because it inhibits the CYP2C9 P-450 enzyme used in warfarin metabolism.[2] Clinicians should monitor the INR carefully, and the warfarin dose should be reduced to establish the desired maintenance INR range. In early randomized controlled trials, sitaxsentan has been shown to increase 6-minute walk distance, functional capacity, and hemodynamics.[2,8]

Ambrisentan is another once daily oral selective ETa antagonist currently being tested. Preliminary reports show benefits similar to the bosentan and sitaxsentan with respect to improved exercise capacity and hemodynamics.[2,21,36] The side effect profile is also expected to be similar except that ambrisentan is not metabolized in the same molecular pathway as sitaxsentan and is not expected to affect the PT and INR values. Efficacy and long-term safety trials are still underway.

Phosphodiesterase-5 (PDE-5) inhibitors achieve clinical efficacy in PAH patients by modulating the cGMP content in vascular smooth muscle cells to reduce tone, proliferation, and remodeling.[2,21,36,37] Drugs that selectively inhibit breakdown of cGMP in the pulmonary circulation augment the pulmonary vascular response to NO, which is diminished in PAH.[36]

Sildenafil is the first PDE-5 inhibitor to be approved by the FDA for treatment of functional class II and III PAH because of its potent selective pulmonary vasodilatory and antiproliferative effects.[2,21,36] Sildenafil is available as an oral preparation with the dose ranging from 25 to 75 mg that must be taken three times daily because of its short half-life of 4 to 6 hours. Sildenafil has been shown to increase exercise capacity, decrease echocardiographic estimates of systolic PAP, and improve hemodynamics.[2,36] Side effects are relatively few including headache, nasal congestion, and visual disturbances; however, the development of nonarteritic anterior ischemic optic neuropathy at high doses remains a cause for concern.[36]

Tadalafil is an oral PDE-5 inhibitor currently being tested for use in PAH through randomized controlled trials. It has the compliance advantage of once daily dosing, with a half-life of 17.5 hours.

Combination therapy is being used with more frequency for treatment of PAH. Because there are multiple therapeutic targets in the pathophysiology of PAH, it makes sense to use a combination of mechanistic pathways in lieu of treatment failure with monotherapy. A few studies have investigated combination therapy.[11,25] In one study, a PDE-5 inhibitor was added to an endothelin receptor antagonist for patients with insufficient response to monotherapy.[11] Improvement in 6-minute walk distance and maximum oxygen uptake in cardiopulmonary exercise were reported. In another study, investigators examined adding PDE-5 inhibitor to an inhaled prostacyclin, showing synergistic improvement by reduction in PVR through vasodilatory effects.[25] Questions remain as to whether switching to the second agent would have shown the same improvement or whether the combination of the two medicines augmented the effects. Long-term data regarding safety, efficacy, and sustained effect of combination therapy is an important area for future study.

Lung transplantation (either single or double) is an option for the patient with functional Class III or IV who shows disease progression in spite of aggressive medical therapy.[2,18,26] Most U.S. lung transplant centers prefer to perform double lung transplants because it affords the patient extra reserve in the case of infection or rejection.[2] In lung transplantation, improvement of RV dysfunction is significant with normalization of PVR.[18] Median survival for lung transplantation is approximately 2½ years, and 5-year survival of patients on epoprostenol therapy has been shown to surpass that of lung-transplanted patients, thus reducing the need for this surgical option.[21] However, patients refractory to medical treatment face an operative mortality range between 16 percent and 29 percent, with a 5-year survival rate of 40 percent to 45 percent.

Atrial septostomy is a procedure conducted to decrease RV strain and improve cardiac output in patients refractory to diuretic therapy.[26] An atrial right-to-left shunt is constructed to decompress the right heart, subsequently increasing filling pressures in the left heart.[2] The resulting decrease in oxygen saturation is thought to be mitigated by the global improvement in cardiac output and systemic oxygen transport.[2,26] Although this procedure has been used in an extremely small sample of patients, it is either performed as a palliative bridge to lung transplantation or as a single palliative intervention. Atrial septostomy has a mortality rate between 5 percent and 15 percent and is indicated in NYHA class III to IV patients experiencing recurrent syncope and treatment refractory right heart failure.[2] Atrial septostomy should only be performed at medical centers with experience in this procedure.[21]

TREATMENT SUCCESS

Treatment success can be judged by subjective and objective measures. Subjective methods include:

- Questionnaires that measure health-related quality of life, such as the SF-36

- Scales that measure intensity of symptoms, such as the Borg dyspnea scale, which rates shortness of breath
- Qualitative interviews exploring the impact of living with PAH

Objective measures include the following:

- 6-minute walk distance
- NYHA functional class level
- Hemodynamic improvements in diagnostic tests, such as right heart catheterization and echocardiogram
- Overall survival and mortality

The NYHA functional class assessment has been shown to correlate well with survival in PAH patients.[2,16,21,28] Hemodynamic variables, such as RA pressure and CI also correlate with survival. Distance walked in the 6-minute walk test correlates with survival and correlates inversely with NYHA functional status.[2] In many clinical trials, the 6-minute walk test is linked with a subjective measure, most commonly the Borg scale, to gain a more holistic view of treatment success.

PAH can afflict some patients in the prime of their lives and other patients as they are approaching their golden years, with the devastation associated with a progressively debilitating disease. Depending on the type of pharmacological therapy, there can be a complex and labor-intensive medication regimen along with changes in body image and role functioning, which may contrast greatly with a clinician's or researcher's definition of treatment success. In a qualitative study exploring patient experiences in living with PAH, two overarching themes were identified: coping with uncertainty and living with treatment.[38] The advances in pharmacological therapeutic options do not translate into a cure for PAH. A patient can be compliant with oral therapy for 6 months only to find that they now require central line catheter placement and intravenous prostacyclin therapy. Intravenous epoprostenol or treprostinil requires in-depth teaching and reinforcement by health care providers to enable the patient and family to feel comfortable with the intricacies of medicine preparation, titration schedules, side effects, backup batteries and pumps, and maintenance of an infection-free infusion site.[2,36,38]

Patient and family education can facilitate coping with this disorder. Many resources are available and should be used for patient support. A reliable online source of information is the Pulmonary Hypertension Association website *(http://phassociation.org)* where patients and family can acquire useful and vital information and links regarding: (a) newest pharmacological advances; (b) chat rooms (special for PH children); (c) caregiver information; (d) information and rationale regarding common procedures, such as central line placement; and (e) investigational drugs and clinical trials. Patients and families empowered with education communicate more effectively with health care providers, develop pertinent questions, and better participate in informed decision making. For patients and family without Internet access, many PH centers have support groups that encourage sharing of personal experiences and hardship challenges. Patients and families can experience improved quality of life through relationship development and the exchange of comfort and support.

REFERENCES

1. McLaughlin VV, Presberg KW, Doyle RL et al: Prognosis of pulmonary arterial hypertension: ACCP evidence-based clinical practice guidelines, *Chest* 126:78S-92S, 2004.
2. Galie N, Torbicki A, Barst R et al: Guidelines on diagnosis and treatment of pulmonary arterial hypertension. The task force on diagnosis and treatment of pulmonary arterial hypertension of the European Society of Cardiology, *Eur Heart J* 25:2243-78, 2004.
3. Koerner SK: Pulmonary hypertension: etiology and clinical evaluation, *J Thorac Imaging* 3:25-31, 1988.
4. Pietra GG, Capron F, Stewart S et al: Pathologic assessment of vasculopathies in pulmonary hypertension, *J Am Coll Cardiol* 43:25S-32S, 2004.
5. Galie N, Hinderliter AL, Torbicki et al: Effects of the oral endothelin-receptor antagonist bosentan on echocardiographic and Doppler measures in patients with pulmonary arterial hypertension, *J Am Coll Cardiol* 41:1380-6, 2003.
6. Simonneau G, Galie N, Rubin LJ et al: Clinical classification of pulmonary hypertension, *J Am Coll Cardiol* 43:5S-12S, 2004.
7. Galie N, Humbert M, Vachiery JL et al: Effects of beraprost sodium, an oral prostacyclin analogue, in patients with pulmonary arterial hypertension: a randomized, double-blind, placebo-controlled trial, *J Am Coll Cardiol* 39:1496-502, 2002.
8. Barst R, Langleben D, Frost A et al: Sitaxsentan therapy for pulmonary arterial hypertension, *Am J Respir Crit Care Med* 169:441-447, 2004.
9. Bauer M, Wilkens H, Langer F et al: Selective upregulation of endothelin B receptor gene expression in severe pulmonary hypertension, *Circulation* 105:1034-6, 2002.
10. Feinstein JA, Goldhaber SZ, Lock JE et al: Balloon pulmonary angioplasty for treatment of chronic thromboembolic pulmonary hypertension, *Circulation* 103:10-13, 2001.
11. Hoeper MM, Faulenbach C, Golpon H et al: Combination therapy with bosentan and sildenafil in idiopathic pulmonary hypertension, *Eur Respir J* 24:1007-1010, 2004.
12. Kawut SM, Horn EM, Berekashvili KK et al: New predictors of outcome in idiopathic pulmonary arterial hypertension, *Am J Cardiol* 95:199-203, 2005.
13. McLaughlin VV, Shillington A, Rich S: Survival in primary pulmonary hypertension: the impact of epoprostenol therapy, *Circulation* 106:1477-82, 2002.
14. Preston IR, Tang G, Tilan JU et al: Retinoids and pulmonary hypertension, *Circulation* 111:782-790, 2005.
15. Ribas J, Angrill J, Barbera JA et al: Isosorbide-5-mononitrate in the treatment of pulmonary hypertension associated with portal hypertension, *Eur Respir J* 13:210-212, 1999.
16. McGoon M, Gutterman D, Steen V et al: Screening, early detection, and diagnosis of pulmonary arterial hypertension: ACCP evidence-based clinical practice guidelines, *Chest* 126:14S-34S, 2004.
17. Cheever KH: An overview of pulmonary arterial hypertension: risks, pathogenesis, clinical manifestations, and management, *J Cardiovasc Nurs* 20:108-116, 2005.
18. Gaine S: Pulmonary hypertension, *JAMA* 284:3160-8, 2000.
19. Rich S, Dantzker DR, Ayres SM et al: Primary pulmonary hypertension. A national prospective study, *Ann Intern Med* 107:216-23, 1987.
20. Rubin LJ: Diagnosis and management of pulmonary arterial hypertension: ACCP evidence-based clinical practice guidelines, *Chest* 126:7S-10S, 2004.
21. Sirithanakul K, Mubarak KK: Pulmonary arterial hypertension: new treatments are improving outcomes, *J Fam Pract* 53:959-69, 2004.
22. Fedullo PF, Auger WR, Channick RN et al: Chronic thromboembolic pulmonary hypertension, *Clin Chest Med* 16:353-74, 1995.
23. D'Alonzo GE, Barst RJ, Ayres SM et al: Survival in patients with primary pulmonary hypertension. Results from a national prospective registry, *Ann Intern Med* 115:343-9, 1991.
24. Simonneau G, Barst R, Gaile N et al: Continuous subcutaneous infusion of treprostinil, a prostacyclin analogue, in patients with pulmonary arterial hypertension, *Am J Respir Crit Care Med* 165:800-804, 2002.
25. Ghofrani HA, Wiedemann R, Rose F et al: Combination therapy with oral sildenafil and inhaled iloprost for severe pulmonary hypertension, *Ann Intern Med* 136:515-522, 2002.
26. Gaine SP, Rubin LJ: Primary pulmonary hypertension, *Lancet* 352:719-25, 1998.
27. Humbert M, Morrell NW, Archer SL et al: Cellular and molecular pathobiology of pulmonary arterial hypertension, *J Am Coll Cardiol* 43:13S-24S, 2004.
28. Humbert M: Improving survival in pulmonary arterial hypertension, *Eur Respir J* 25:218-20, 2005.
29. Berne RM, Levy MN: *Cardiovascular physiology,* ed 8, St Louis, 2001. Mosby.
30. Mitani Y, Ueda M, Komatsu R et al: Vascular smooth muscle cell phenotypes in primary pulmonary hypertension, *Eur Respir J* 17:316-20, 2001.
31. Bonnet S, Savineau JP, Barillot W et al: Role of Ca^{2+} - sensitive K= channels in the remission phase of pulmonary hypertension in chronic obstructive pulmonary diseases, *Cardiovasc Res* 60:326-336, 2003.
32. Barst RJ, McGoon M, Torbicki A et al: Diagnosis and differential assessment of pulmonary arterial hypertension, *J Am Coll Cardiol* 43:40S-47S, 2004.
33. Widmar B: When cure is care: diagnosis and management of pulmonary arterial hypertension, *J Am Acad Nurse Pract* 17:104-112, 2005.
34. Ricciardi MJ, Knight BP, Martinez FJ et al: Inhaled nitric oxide in primary pulmonary hypertension, *J Am Coll Cardiol* 32:1068-1073, 1998.
35. Sitbon O, Humbert M, Jagot JL et al: Inhaled nitric oxide as a screening agent for safely identifying responders to oral calcium-channel blockers in primary pulmonary hypertension, *Eur Respir J* 12:265-70, 1998.
36. Badesch DB, Abman SH, Ahearn G et al: Medical therapy for pulmonary arterial hypertension: ACCP evidence-based clinical practice guidelines, *Chest* 126:35S-62S, 2004.
37. Galie N, Seeger W, Naeije R et al: Comparative analysis of clinical trials and evidence-based treatment algorithm in pulmonary arterial hypertension, *J Am Coll Cardiol* 43:81S-88S, 2004.
38. Flattery MP, Pinson JM, Savage L et al: Living with pulmonary artery hypertension: patients' experiences, *Heart Lung* 34:99-107, 2003.

chapter 88

Neurological Disorders and the Cardiovascular System

Mary Jo Kocan

CHAPTER ABBREVIATIONS

ACE angiotensin-converting enzyme

ATP adenosine triphosphate

AV atrioventricular

ECG electrocardiogram

GBS Guillain-Barré Syndrome

SAH subarachnoid hemorrhage

SF-36 Short Form 36

The relationship between neurological disorders and cardiovascular abnormalities has been observed since the late 19th century, when myocardial abnormalities were identified in patients with muscular dystrophy.[1] In 1903, Cushing noted the occurrence of bradycardia, increased systolic blood pressure, and widening pulse pressure in response to a rise in intracranial pressure.[2] The advent of the electrocardiogram (**ECG**) resulted in the identification of abnormal patterns that developed with the onset of acute cerebrovascular events. Several genetic disorders have been identified that are characterized by structural defects in both the nervous system and the cardiovascular system. The interactions between the nervous and cardiovascular systems in these disorders have been well-described and therapeutic interventions identified. In contrast, the pathophysiological basis for abnormalities occurring in response to acquired neuropathological processes, such as immune-mediated neuromuscular disease and cerebrovascular disease, is less clear. Despite advances in diagnostic testing, cardiac and neurological imaging, and sophisticated physiological monitoring, many questions remain as to the mechanisms responsible for neurocardiac interactions, the physiologic basis for dysfunction, and effective interventions to treat them. The purpose of this chapter is to describe the interactions between the cardiovascular system and the genetic and immune-mediated neuromuscular disorders. Also briefly covered in this chapter is the interaction between cerebrovascular disease and the cardiovascular system. A complete discussion of stroke and its impact on the cardiovascular system can be found in Chapter 76.

GENETIC NEUROMUSCULAR DISORDERS
Muscular Dystrophies

The muscular dystrophies are comprised of a variety of disorders characterized by progressive weakness of skeletal muscles. The inheritance patterns and specific genetic defects of each disorder are summarized in Table 88-1.

Duchenne Muscular Dystrophy

Duchenne muscular dystrophy is due to the absence of the protein dystrophin, which is normally found in the muscle cell membrane. Dystrophin is responsible for maintaining the structural and functional integrity of the muscle cell membrane; its absence leaves the muscle cell membrane susceptible to damage from contraction[3] and results in disruption of the cell membrane and necrosis of the muscle fiber.[4] Dystrophin is normally found in skeletal muscle, cardiac muscle, smooth muscle and the brain. Patients with Duchenne muscular dystrophy develop progressive muscle weakness, especially of the proximal muscles. Lower extremities are usually more affected than the upper extremities. Muscle hypertrophy, especially of the calf muscles, is a prominent feature. The weakness is usually noted in early childhood and progresses rapidly; most are wheelchair-bound by the teen years. Muscles of respiration are also weak, often leading to respiratory failure. Many have decreased intellectual functioning. Serum creatine kinase levels are elevated at birth and may be used as a diagnostic marker of the disease.[5]

In the heart, as myocardial fibers are destroyed, they are replaced by connective tissue and fat.[4,6] This leads to hypokinesis and may serve as an arrhythmogenic focus. On echocardiogram, patients demonstrate regional wall motion abnormalities, systolic dysfunction, and left ventricular dilatation. Common ECG abnormalities consist of sinus tachycardia, atrial arrhythmias including premature atrial contractions, atrial fibrillation or flutter, shortened PR interval, tall R waves in the first precordial lead, deep Q waves, and increased QT dispersion.[6] Cardiac involvement may be asymptomatic initially in Duchenne muscular dystrophy patients, with reduced demands on the heart due to severe motor deficits and resultant impaired physical activity.[6,7] However, given the progressive nature of cardiac dysfunction, early diagnosis and treatment can prolong life. Consensus recommendations for management include ECG and echocardiogram at diagnosis, every 2 years until age 10, and yearly thereafter.[8] In a study of 84 patients with Duchenne muscular dystrophy followed for a median of 76 months, left ventricular systolic dysfunction on echocardiogram was a better predictor of mortality than ECG alterations or the presence of ventricular arrhythmia.[9] Due to the lack of controlled clinical trials on the management of cardiomyopathy in muscular dystrophy, treatment recommendations are based on accepted methods of treatment for heart failure and cardiomyopathy from other etiologies and include the use of angiotensin-converting enzyme (**ACE**) inhibitors for afterload reduction and the use of beta blockers.[8,10]

■ ■ ■

TABLE 2-6   GENETIC DEFECTS IN NEUROMUSCULAR DISEASES

DISEASE	GENETIC TRANSMISSION	GENETIC DEFECT, IF IDENTIFIED
Muscular Dystrophies		
Duchenne muscular dystrophy	X-linked	Xp21[5]
Becker muscular dystrophy	X-linked	Xp21[5]
Emery-Dreifuss muscular dystrophy	X-linked	Xq28[5,16]
	Autosomal dominant	1q[5]
Limb-girdle muscular dystrophy	Variety of autosomal recessive and autosomal dominant	Map to a variety of genetic defects, many of which result in sarcoglycan protein deficiencies[19]
Myotonic muscular dystrophy type 1	Autosomal dominant	Cytosine-thymine-guanine (CTG) triplet repeat on chromosome 19[21,23]
Friedreich's Ataxia	Autosomal recessive	Guanine-adenine-adenine (GAA) triplet repeat on the X25 gene on chromosome 9q13[36]

Although Duchenne muscular dystrophy is a disease of males, approximately 10% of female carriers will display cardiac involvement with or without signs of clinical skeletal muscle weakness.[4,8] (See the accompanying Genetics feature.) While often asymptomatic, carriers

■ ■ ■ **GENETICS**

COUNSELING PATIENTS WITH NEUROMUSCULAR DISORDERS

- Prenatal diagnosis is possible in Duchenne and Becker muscular dystrophy; carriers should be referred to a center specializing in the laboratory diagnosis of the disorders.
- Prenatal diagnosis of myotonic dystrophy type 1 is available, and pre-implantation diagnosis is available at a few centers.
- Female carriers of Duchenne and Becker muscular dystrophy may develop some degree of muscle weakness and/or cardiac involvement[5]; they should be advised to have a formal cardiac evaluation.
- Female carriers of X-linked Emery-Dreifuss muscular dystrophy may exhibit cardiac involvement requiring pacemakers.
- Since cardiac involvement is often the first evidence of lamin A/C gene mutation and the clinical course and prognosis is so severe, some recommend familial screening for patients with autosomal dominant Emery-Dreifuss muscular dystrophy (8% prevalence in one study).
- In limb-girdle muscular dystrophies, it is important to make the genetic diagnosis (especially to distinguish from dystrophin deficiency diseases) since many of the limb-girdle diseases have autosomal recessive inheritance.
- Genetic testing can identify carrier status for Friedreich's ataxia in individuals with a family history or for spouses of carriers or individuals with the disease.

Bushby K, Muntoni F, Bourke JP: 107th ENMC International Workshop: The Management of Cardiac Involvement in Muscular Dystrophy and Myotonic Dystrophy, June 7-9, 2002, Naarden, The Netherlands, *Neuromuscul Disord* 13:166-172, 2003.
Die-Smulders CEM, Jennekens FGI, Howeler CJ: Myotonic dystrophy type 1. In Cassidy SB, Allanson JE, editors: *Management of genetic syndromes*, ed 2, Hoboken, NY, 2005, Wiley-Liss, pp. 351-367.
Emery AEH: The muscular dystrophies, *Lancet* 359:687-695, 2002.
Grain L, Cortina-Borja M, Forfar C et al: Cardiac abnormalities and skeletal muscle weakness in carriers of Duchenne and Becker muscular dystrophies and controls, *Neuromuscul Disord* 11:186-191, 2001.
Lynch DR, Farmer JM, Balcer IJ et al: Friedreich's ataxia: effects of genetic understanding on clinical evaluation and therapy, *Arch Neurol* 59:743-747, 2002.
Taylor MRG, Fain PR, Sinagra G et al: Natural history of dilated cardiomyopathy due to main A/C gene mutations, *J Am Coll Cardiol* 41:771-780, 2003.
Bushby K: Genetics and the muscular dystrophies, *Dev Med Child Neurol* 42:780-784, 2000.

can develop progressive cardiomyopathy, which can become so severe as to require transplant.[6] ECG alone may not be adequate in screening for cardiac involvement in these patients, as studies have shown echocardiographic abnormalities in carriers with normal ECGs.[11] Recommendations for management include an echocardiogram and ECG at the time of diagnosis or at age 16 and every 5 years afterward if there are no abnormalities. If significant abnormalities develop, ACE inhibitors should be used.[8]

The outlook for patients with Duchenne muscular dystrophy has been bleak; the disease is always fatal, usually by the early 20s. Treatment with corticosteroids has been shown to preserve strength and functional ability[5,12]; however, research is needed to develop a universally accepted treatment regimen. Patients often have compromised pulmonary function, related to weakness of the respiratory muscles and skeletal deformities of the thorax, making them prone to pneumonia and respiratory insufficiency.[5] Improvements in supportive therapy, such as pulmonary hygiene, noninvasive nocturnal ventilation, and even elective tracheostomy, have improved survival.[5,13] New treatment approaches using gene and stem cell therapy are being explored as a way to replace the dystrophin-deficient cells in the heart and skeletal muscles.[5,10]

Becker Muscular Dystrophy

Becker muscular dystrophy has a similar clinical presentation to Duchenne muscular dystrophy, with later onset and slower progression of muscular weakness. Dystrophin protein is deficient rather than absent, as in Duchenne muscular dystrophy, which explains the reduced severity of symptoms. Patients usually become symptomatic in their teenage years and are wheelchair-bound by mid-life. Intellectual impairment occurs in about 25 percent of cases.[5] Serum creatine kinase levels are also elevated and may be the only sign of the disease in the first decade of life.[6]

Cardiac involvement is more prominent in Becker muscular dystrophy than Duchenne muscular dystrophy, perhaps due to the milder course of muscular weakness. Patients frequently have ECG abnormalities, most typically decreased R or large Q waves in leads I, AV_L, and V_6.[6] Echocardiograms are also frequently abnormal, showing myocardial thickening, left and right ventricular dilatation, and wall motion abnormalities.[6,7] Cardiomyopathy may be a more prominent symptom than skeletal muscle weakness in these patients, and recognition, prevention, and treatment of cardiac failure is important. Recommendations for management and treatment of cardiac involvement in patients with Becker muscular dystrophy are identical to that of patients with Duchenne muscular dystrophy (see discussion above). Whereas heart transplant is usually not indicated in patients with Duchenne muscular dystrophy due to complications from respiratory failure,[8] transplant has been successful in patients with Becker muscular dystrophy and should be considered for patients who fail medical therapy.[14,15]

As in Duchenne muscular dystrophy, Becker muscular dystrophy carriers may also be at risk for developing cardiac involvement. Recommendations for diagnosis, follow-up, and treatment are identical to those for carriers of Duchenne muscular dystrophy.

Emery-Dreifuss Muscular Dystrophy

Emery-Dreifuss muscular dystrophy has several different modes of genetic transmission, two of which result in cardiac involvement. The X-linked variant causes a deficiency of the protein emerin, which is normally found in the muscle cell nuclear membrane. The autosomal dominant variant causes a deficiency in lamins A and C, proteins which make up the inner membrane of the nucleus. The disease is characterized by contractures of the Achilles tendons, elbows, and neck, followed by progressive weakness and atrophy in the proximal muscles of the upper extremities and the distal muscles of the lower extremities.[5] Treatment is generally supportive and consists of muscle strengthening exercises, prevention of contractures, and preservation of respiratory function.[16]

Cardiac effects are usually more pronounced than muscle weakness. Conduction system defects are prominent, characterized by a prolonged PR interval that progresses to complete heart block.[4] Atrial arrhythmias are common, including small P waves, atrial fibrillation, and atrial flutter. Atrial involvement can evolve to complete atrial standstill.[4,17] Although cardiomyopathy may develop, the conduction system defects are often life-threatening and patients may require a pacemaker. Recommended follow-up includes an ECG at the time of diagnosis and annually, with a 24-hour Holter monitor to assess for tachyarrhythmias or bradyarrhythmias and an echocardiogram.[8] Pacemakers are recommended even for asymptomatic patients when the ECG shows sinus or atrioventricular nodal disease.[17] Patients with atrial fibrillation should receive antiembolic prophylaxis to prevent stroke.[4,8,17]

The autosomal dominant variant of Emery-Dreifuss muscular dystrophy tends to have a higher degree of cardiac involvement and more severe progression of disease.[4,17,18] Dilated cardiomyopathy may develop along with conduction defects.[4,8] In autosomal dominant disease, implantable defibrillators may be more appropriate than pacemakers, based on cases of sudden death in patients with implanted pacemakers.[8] End-stage heart failure may be an indication for cardiac transplant.[17,18]

Limb-Girdle Muscular Dystrophy

Limb-girdle muscular dystrophy is due to a variety of genetic abnormalities, which result in deficiencies of various muscle cell membrane proteins. It occurs in both males and females and leads to variable progression of weakness, primarily in the shoulder and pelvic muscles; the facial muscles are usually spared. Some genetic types result in mutations of the sarcoglycan complex, which leads to cardiac involvement.[8] ECG abnormalities include abnormal P waves and inverted T waves.[19,20] Left ventricular dysfunction with dilated cardiomyopathy has also been identified. Those patients with sarcoglycanopathy should be followed using the same criteria to diagnose and treat cardiac involvement as patients with Duchenne muscular dystrophy.

Myotonic Muscular Dystrophy

Myotonic dystrophy Type I is a multisystem disorder that affects skeletal, cardiac, and smooth muscle.[21] Muscle weakness initially involves the face and distal extremities and then progresses proximally. The respiratory muscles are also involved and may progress to respiratory failure with the need for assisted ventilation. Smooth muscle is also affected, leading to difficulty swallowing, gastroesophageal reflux, and decreased peristalsis. Patients may develop cataracts. Testicular atrophy also occurs. The disease is characterized by myotonia, a delay in the ability to relax a muscle after forceful contraction. Apathy and an increase in daytime sleepiness are prominent features in some patients, which can hinder effective treatment. Age at onset of symptoms varies from infancy to late adulthood.

Most patients have cardiac abnormalities, primarily arrhythmias and conduction defects, which may be presenting signs of the disease[21] and tend to progress over time.[22] Myocardial fibrosis occurs, which often affects the conduction system.[23] Atrioventricular conduction delays occur more frequently than intraventricular delays. In addition to **(AV)** block, atrial tachyarrhythmias and ventricular tachyarrhythmias also occur, possibly due to re-entry mechanisms.[21] Progression of conduction and rhythm disturbances are correlated with age and length of the abnormal nucleotide repeat.[23] The PR interval and QRS duration on ECG have been found to be markers of cardiac involvement. Recommendations for cardiac evaluation and follow-up include ECG at the time of diagnosis and annually with Holter monitoring if the PR interval is increased or if there is an increased risk of bradycardia.[8] This recommendation is supported by a study of asymptomatic patients with infranodal conduction delays, with implanted pacemakers that found a high incidence of transient AV block.[24] Because the PR interval and QRS duration tend to become progressively longer with aging, medications that prolong the PR interval or QRS duration or cause bradycardia should be used with caution.[25] Electrophysiological studies may be warranted if conduction delays or tachyarrhythmias are noted. Pacemaker insertion is recommended in patients with third-degree block (American Heart Association Class I recommendation) and in patients with any degree of AV or fascicular block (Class

II indication), whether or not the patient is symptomatic, because the rate of disease progression is unpredictable.[26] The utility of electrophysiological studies and the use of implanted defibrillators is still under debate.[8,22]

Friedreich's Ataxia

Friedreich's ataxia occurs as the result of a deficiency of the mitochondrial protein frataxin. The exact function of frataxin is unknown, but it appears to be involved in oxidative phosphorylation and mitochondrial iron homeostasis; its absence leads to mitochondrial iron accumulation, generation of free radicals, and oxidative damage.[27-29] The disease is characterized by progressive gait and limb ataxia, loss of deep tendon reflexes and proprioception in the lower extremities, and dysarthria, with onset usually before age 25.[30] Many patients display impaired glucose tolerance and most patients develop hypertrophic cardiomyopathy.[27,31,32] One theory on the development of cardiac hypertrophy links the condition to decreased mitochondrial adenosine triphosphate (ATP) production.[33,34] Nonspecific ECG abnormalities often occur as well as T-wave inversion in the left precordial leads. Echocardiography provides the best assessment of cardiac involvement, the most common feature being left ventricular wall thickening. Echocardiographic abnormalities may be used to differentiate Friedreich's ataxia from other neurological disorders.[35]

Treatment has primarily consisted of supportive care: however, recent research has focused on the role of antioxidants in slowing the progression or improving the clinical course of the disease, particularly of cardiac function. The aim is to enhance mitochondrial function and to decrease free radical production.[36] Idebenone, an analog of coenzyme Q and a free-radical scavenger, resulted in a decrease in myocardial hypertrophy when used from 6 to 12 months in small groups of patients.[28,37] In a longer term study, Hart and associates used a combination of vitamin E and coenzyme Q for a total of 47 months, which resulted in improved mitochondrial energy synthesis, associated with improved cardiac functioning.[29]

IMMUNE-MEDIATED NEUROMUSCULAR DISEASES
Guillain-Barré Syndrome

Guillain-Barré Syndrome (GBS), or acute inflammatory demyelinating polyradiculoneuropathy, refers to a group of disorders caused by an autoimmune response that destroys the myelin sheath or axon of peripheral nerves. It results in weakness and areflexia. Although not always clinically significant, autonomic dysfunction occurs in about 65 percent of patients and warrants cardiac monitoring to detect life-threatening arrhythmias. Treatment of GBS is aimed at reversing the immune process and supportive care. The primary immunotherapies are plasma exchange and intravenous immunoglobulin, both of which are supported by Class I or II evidence and are considered equivalent in effectiveness.[38] The choice of treatment may be based upon patient-specific clinical factors. Limitations to the use of plasma exchange include difficulty with venous access and lack of equipment and trained personnel. Side effects of immunoglobulin therapy include renal failure and anaphylaxis.[39]

Most patients recover; the majority with little or no disability.[40] Supportive nursing care is essential to recovery. Cardiac monitoring is recommended for patients who display symptoms of autonomic involvement.

Dysautonomia occurs most often in patients with severe weakness and respiratory failure. The clinical presentation of autonomic dysfunction in GBS is highly variable and can consist of over-activity or impaired functioning of either the sympathetic or parasympathetic nervous system. In patients who display sympathetic hyperactivity, tachyarrhythmias and hypertension may be persistent or paroxysmal.[41] Inverted T waves on the ECG have been reported and linked with over-activity of the sympathetic nervous system. Sympathetic hyperactivity has been identified as the cause of reversible left ventricular dysfunction in some patients.[41,42] Lack of sympathetic activity can result in hypotension, which may be exacerbated by fluid shifts during plasma exchange. Hypotension is usually responsive to fluid administration or positioning with head of bed flat, but vasopressors may be required. Persistent hypotension may be a limiting factor in the use of plasma exchange to treat the underlying disease.[39]

The dramatic variations in blood pressure demonstrated by some patients are one of the major patient management challenges, since attempts to treat blood pressure at one extreme can complicate treatment when blood pressure suddenly shifts to the other extreme. This extreme lability of blood pressure was commonly associated with bradycardic episodes in a group of artificially ventilated GBS patients.[43] The author describes one patient with episodes of bradycardia that eventually required a pacemaker, whose systolic blood pressure could vary between 100 and 250 mm Hg in minutes.[43] Autonomic dysfunction is reversible and tends to parallel the course of motor recovery.

Myasthenia Gravis

Myasthenia gravis is an autoimmune disease that results in impaired neuromuscular impulse transmission due to destruction of acetylcholine receptors in the neuromuscular junction. The lack of acetylcholine receptors at the neuromuscular junction results in weakness, which typically presents in the ocular or bulbar muscles, resulting in ptosis, diplopia, or difficulty swallowing. Symptoms may remain localized or may become generalized and tend to become worse with exertion.[44] Patients may require intensive care management if the bulbar or respiratory muscles are involved. Treatment consists of maintenance therapy with acetylcholinesterase inhibitors, such as pyridostigmine, which prevent the conversion of acetylcholine and allow it to remain active in the neuromuscular junction. Immunomodulators, such as steroids or plasma exchange, aimed at reversing the autoimmune process, may be required to prevent or treat acute exacerbations.

BOX 88-1
DRUGS TO AVOID OR USE WITH CAUTION IN PATIENTS WITH MYASTHENIA GRAVIS

Neuromuscular Blocking Agents
- *Nondepolarizing agents.* Effects are prolonged. Use greatly reduced dose.
- *Depolarizing agents.* Require higher doses, probably from loss of receptor sites. Patients receiving cholinesterase inhibitors may have prolonged neuromuscular blockade from decreased metabolism of the blocking agent.
- *Local anesthetics.* Decrease sensitivity to acetylcholine and may potentiate neuromuscular blockade. Ester forms are metabolized by cholinesterase, so use of anticholinesterase drugs to treat myasthenia can prolong their effect.

Antibiotics
- *Aminoglycosides.* Impair neuromuscular transmission through a variety of mechanisms and should be avoided.
- Practically all antibiotics have been shown to exacerbate symptoms in select patients with myasthenia gravis; if use is clinically indicated, observe the patient closely for signs of increased weakness when starting antibiotics.

Cardiovascular Drugs
- *Procainamide.* Alters binding of acetylcholine to receptors.
- *Beta-adrenergic blockers.* May cause increased weakness; use with caution. Systemic absorption of ocular preparations used to treat glaucoma may cause symptoms.
- *Quinidine and quinine-containing agents.* Impair acetylcholine release and should not be used.
- *Calcium channel blockers.* May alter potassium outflow at the motor endplate.

Miscellaneous
- *Phenytoin.* Conflicting reports of increased weakness in some patients and safe use in others.
- *Magnesium supplements and magnesium-containing drugs.* Inhibit release of acetylcholine.

Abel M, Eisenkraft JB: Anesthetic implications of myasthenia gravis, *Mount Sinai J Med* 69:31-37, 2002.
Pascuzzi RM: *Medications and myasthenia gravis,* Myasthenia Gravis Foundation of America, 2000. Retrieved May 31, 2005 from *www.myasthenia.org/drug/reference.htm*
Rubino FA: Perioperative management of patients with neurologic disease, *Neurol Clin N Am* 22:261-276, 2004.
Wittbrodt ET: Drugs and myasthenia gravis: an update, *Arch Intern Med* 157:399-408, 1997.

Thymic hyperplasia or thymoma has been implicated in the pathogenesis of the disease; about 10 percent of patients are found to have a tumor of the thymus gland.[44,45] Thymectomy may result in improvement in symptoms, even in patients with no evidence of abnormalities in the thymus gland.[46] In rare instances, myocarditis has been associated with myasthenia gravis with the presence of thymoma. ECG abnormalities that have been observed include ST- and T-wave changes, premature atrial and ventricular beats, and sinus bradycardia.[47]

One important aspect in the care of these patients is avoidance of drugs that can interfere with neuromuscular transmission (Box 88-1). Use of neuromuscular blocking agents, for example, during intubation or operative procedures, can result in prolonged muscle weakness as can use of aminoglycoside antibiotics.[48] Myasthenia gravis often occurs in elderly patients who may also have cardiovascular disease. Many cardiovascular drugs have been associated with increased weakness in individual cases, even unmasking previously

undetected cases of the disease. Patients should be observed closely for increased symptoms, in particular diplopia, ptosis, difficulty swallowing, or generalized weakness, when any new medication is initiated.

CEREBROVASCULAR DISEASE

Acute stroke, both ischemic and hemorrhagic, has been associated with the development of cardiovascular abnormalities, often manifested by changes in the ECG. These ECG changes are most prominent and most widely researched in subarachnoid hemorrhage **(SAH)** although they occur in all types of stroke. See Chapter 76 for information on management of acute stroke.

Virtually every known type of arrhythmia, conduction defect, and morphological change in the ECG pattern has been found to occur in patients following SAH. In a recent review by Sakr and associates, morphological changes were the abnormality reported most frequently, with T-wave changes, ST-segment changes, and presence of U waves cited most frequently.[49] Prolongation of the QT interval was also frequently reported. Rhythm disturbances, especially sinus bradycardia, sinus tachycardia, and premature ventricular contractions, were also common. Potentially lethal ventricular arrhythmias have also been identified, including torsades de pointes (Figure 88-1).

In addition to ECG abnormalities, evidence of cardiac injury has been identified in SAH patients, consisting of elevated cardiac enzymes (creatine kinase, troponin) and echocardiographic abnormalities. There seems to be a relationship between cardiac troponin I levels and left ventricular dysfunction on echocardiogram.[50] Troponin I levels may be a useful tool to screen for patients with reversible cardiac injury versus those with acute myocardial infarction.[51] Patients with more severe neurological events appear to be at greater risk for cardiac involvement. A study that used the level of cardiac troponin I as a measure of cardiac injury found that patients with more severe neurological injury had a greater degree of cardiac injury.[52]

The direct cause of cardiac involvement, including ECG changes, enzyme elevations, and ventricular dysfunction, is thought to be a massive sympathetic activation triggered by neurological injury. Focal cardiac damage may be related to direct local release of catecholamines from sympathetic nerve terminals in the myocardium.[52,53] The end result is termed *myocardial stunning*, reflecting the reversible nature of the injury in many patients.

The etiology and consequences of ECG changes in SAH have been debated, but there is now general agreement that the changes are transient, that underlying cardiac damage is reversible, and that monitoring and supportive care are key to the management of these patients.[50,53,54] Early intervention to secure the aneurysm, either through surgical or endovascular procedures, is important to reduce the risk of rebleeding. Evidence of cardiac involvement has sometimes led to delay in definitive treatment of the aneurysm. Further research is needed to identify markers that would indicate which patients are most at risk for deterioration

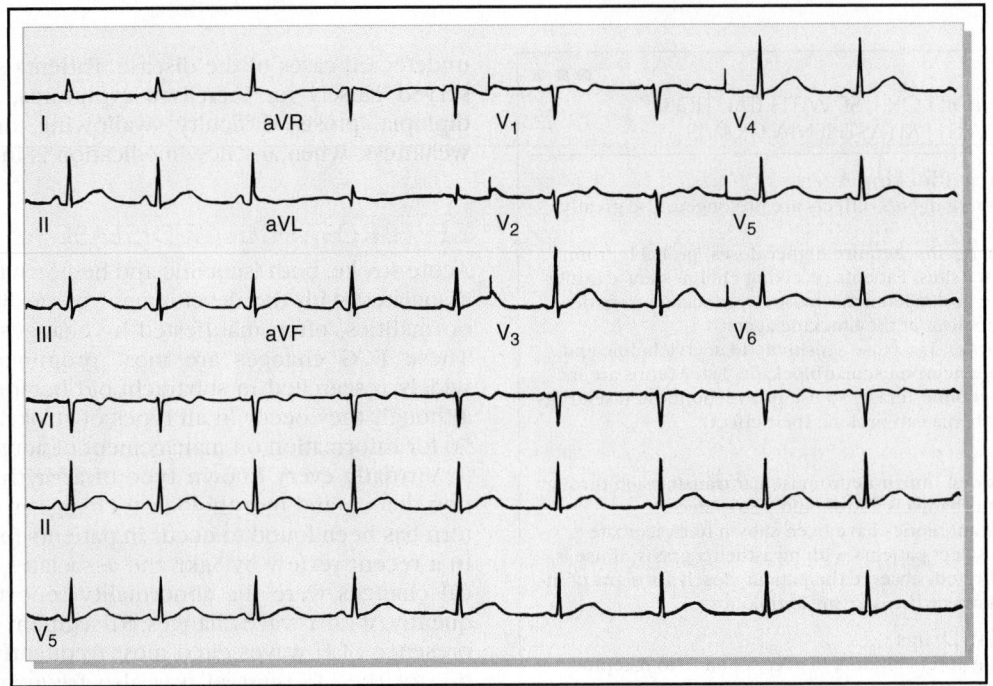

A

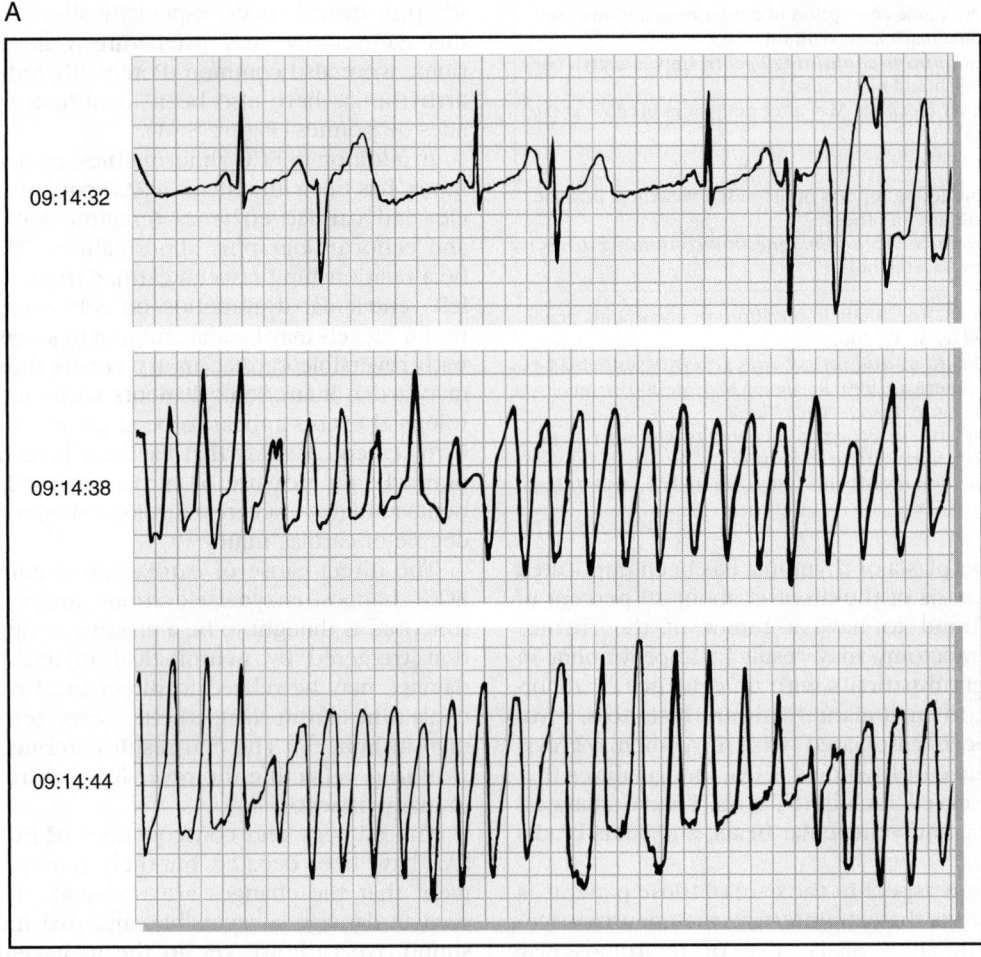

B

FIGURE 88-1 ■ A 49-year-old patient with cerebral hemorrhage. **A,** Electrocardiogram recorded within 3 hours of admission and 4 hours after onset of symptoms. The QT interval is prolonged. **B,** Electrocardiographic monitoring 6 hours after admission. Ventricular bigeminy precedes the onset of polymorphic ventricular tachycardia. Cardioversion was required. The patient was treated with a beta-adrenergic blocker without further ventricular tachycardia.

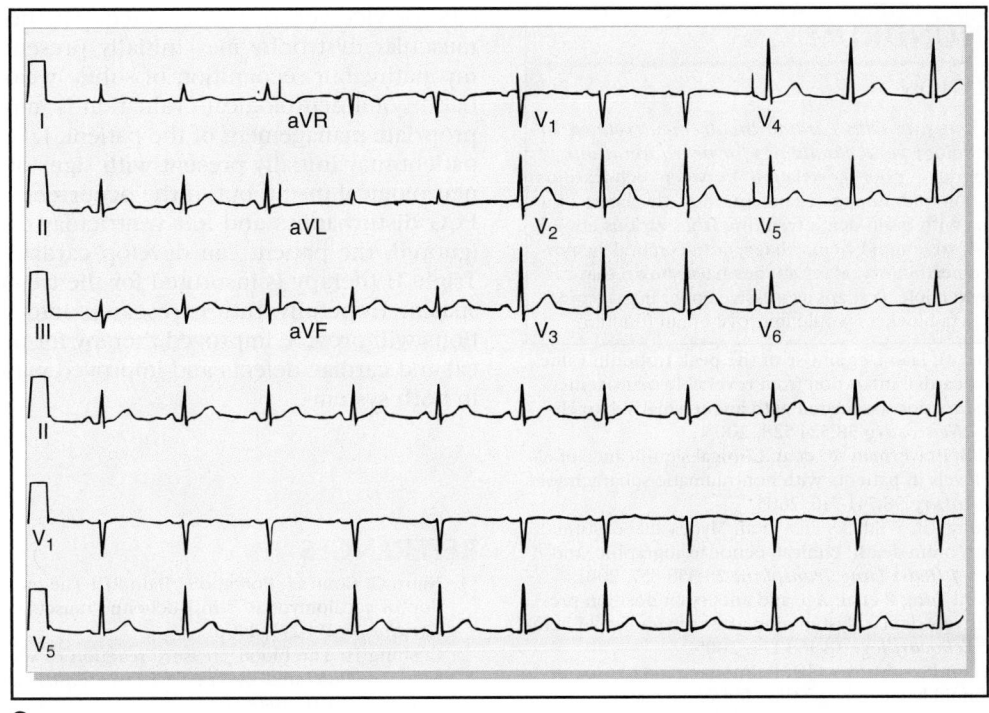

C

FIGURE 88-1, cont'd ■ **C**, Electrocardiogram done 2 weeks after admission. The QT interval has normalized. (From Zipes DP, Libby P, Bonow R, Braunwald E, editors: *Braunwald's heart disease: a textbook of cardiovascular medicine*, ed 7, Philadelphia, 2005, Elsevier Saunders, pp. 2158-2159.)

due to cardiac involvement so patients can be managed optimally.

After SAH, patients are at risk for vasospasm, a sustained constriction of the cerebral vessels triggered by the breakdown of red blood cells in the subarachnoid space. Treatment for vasospasm consists of improving cerebral blood flow through hypertension, hypervolemia, and hemodilution (Triple H therapy). Depressed cardiac function as a result of myocardial stunning can complicate the treatment of vasospasm, putting the patient at risk for further cerebral ischemia. Nimodipine, a calcium channel blocker, has been found to be effective in preventing adverse neurological outcomes due to delayed cerebral ischemia from vasospasm,[55] but its side effect of decreased blood pressure may limit its use in patients who are hypotensive from cardiac involvement. Decreased blood pressure puts those patients at further risk of developing neurological deficits from cerebral ischemia. Magnesium sulfate infusion has been found to reduce the incidence of delayed cerebral ischemia from vasospasm[56] perhaps due to its vasodilating effect. Hypomagnesemia has been noted in SAH patients and was related to prolonged PR interval.[57] Although this research is still ongoing, monitoring serum magnesium levels is recommended.

The relationship between the occurrence of cardiac complications after SAH and eventual neurological outcome for the patient has also been studied. In a retrospective review, an association was found between the occurrence of ST-segment depression and poor outcome as measured by the Glasgow outcome scale at 1 to 3 months following hospitalization.[58] In patients who develop cardiac complications after SAH, any resultant hypotension can contribute to neurological injury and add to long-term physical and cognitive deficits.[54] In a prospective study, which followed patients by telephone interview at 3, 6, and 12 months, Crago and associates found a negative effect on recovery in patients who displayed cardiac complications.[59] In this study, outcomes were measured by Glasgow outcome scale, Modified Rankin scale, Barthel index, and the Physical Function Subscale of the Medical Outcomes Survey Short Form 36 **(SF-36).** The authors found that, although there was no difference in mortality, those who developed cardiac complications had a significantly worse outcome as measured by Barthel index and SF-36 than the group without cardiac complications at 3 months after hemorrhage. The negative effect on physical functioning as measured by the SF-36 continued at the 6-month interview. One interesting aspect of this study was the inclusion of patients with prior known cardiac disease, such as hypertension and coronary artery disease, a group frequently excluded from studies of cardiac complications after SAH. Curiously, the authors noted fewer cardiac complications in this group than in patients with no prior history of cardiovascular disease and speculated that pharmacological therapy for cardiovascular disorders prior to the neurological event may have had a protective effect.[59] (See the accompanying Conundrum feature.)

Ischemic stroke has also been linked to the development of ECG abnormalities, including QT-interval prolongation, T-wave changes, ST-segment changes, and U waves. Strokes involving the insula, the area of cortex

■■■ CONUNDRUM

HEART DONATION

Are brain-dead patients with cardiac involvement related to intracranial pathology good candidates for heart donation?

One study found a poor correlation between echocardiographic dysfunction and autopsy examination of the heart in a subset of patients with brain death resulting from various etiologies, including subarachnoid hemorrhage, intracerebral hemorrhage, and closed-head injury. Many studies have shown that cardiac effects are reversible. Perhaps aggressive donor management using alpha and beta blockers would improve organ function.

Bulsara KR, McGirt MJ, Liao L et al: Use of the peak troponin value to differentiate myocardial infarction from reversible neurogenic left ventricular dysfunction associated with aneurysmal subarachnoid hemorrhage, *J Neurosurg* 98:524-528, 2003.

Deibert E, Barzilai B, Braverman AC et al: Clinical significance of elevated troponin I levels in patients with nontraumatic subarachnoid hemorrhage, *J Neurosurg* 98:741-746, 2003.

Dujardin KS, McCully RB, Wijdicks EFM et al: Myocardial dysfunction associated with brain death: clinical, echocardiographic, and pathologic features, *J Heart Lung Transplant* 20:350-357, 2001.

Khush I, Kopelnik A, Tung P et al: Age and aneurysm position predict patterns of left ventricular dysfunction after subarachnoid hemorrhage, *J Am Soc Echocardiogr* 18:168-174, 2005.

Macmillan CSA, Grant IS, Andrews PJD: Pulmonary and cardiac sequelae of subarachnoid haemorrhage: time for active management? *Intensive Care Med* 28:1012-1023, 2002.

Sakr YL, Ghosn I, Vincent JL: Cardiac manifestations after subarachnoid hemorrhage: a systematic review of the literature, *Prog Cardiovasc Dis* 45:67-80, 2002.

beneath the Sylvian fissure that separates the temporal, parietal, and frontal lobes,[60] may result in ECG abnormalities and even in an increased incidence of sudden death.[61] Lesions of the right insula in particular have been associated with more complex arrhythmias[62] and with an increased risk of death within 3 months of stroke,[60] possibly related to a disruption in autonomic balance.

While research continues to try to identify targeted therapies to prevent adverse outcomes related to cardiac involvement in acute stroke, the benefits of cardiac monitoring have been validated. Providing care in dedicated stroke units as opposed to care delivered on a general ward has been shown to improve patients' functional outcomes.[63] Caring for patients in a dedicated stroke unit, which provides continuous monitoring of ECG, blood pressure, and oxygen saturation (among other parameters), resulted a greater degree of independence related to self-care and a shorter length of hospital stay, despite identification of a greater number of complications in the stroke unit patients. The authors postulated that the results were due to earlier identification of complications, such as adverse cardiac events, hypotension and hypertension, and prompt intervention, many times before patients became clinically symptomatic.[64,65]

SUMMARY

There are intricate linkages between the neurological and the cardiovascular systems. Patients may present primarily with cardiac symptoms, and health care practitioners must be alert for evidence of neurological deficits (or vice versa). For instance, patients with Becker muscular dystrophy may initially present with cardiomyopathy, but recognition of subtle weakness and initiation of a neurological evaluation is important for appropriate management of the patient. Likewise the SAH patient may initially present with signs of a devastating neurological insult, but, if the occurrence of associated ECG disturbances and left ventricular dysfunction are ignored, the patient can develop cardiac failure when Triple H therapy is instituted for the treatment of vasospasm. Hopefully future research into these interactions will provide improved therapy for both neurological and cardiac defects and improved patient outcomes in both systems.

REFERENCES

1. Nigro G, Comi LI, Politano L, Bain RJI: The incidence and evolution of cardiomyopathy in Duchenne muscular dystrophy, *Int J Cardiol* 26:271-277, 1990.
2. Cushing H: The blood pressure reaction of acute cerebral compression illustrated by cases of intracranial hemorrhage, *Am J Med Sc* 125:1017-1044, 1903.
3. Lapidos KA, Kakkar R, McNally EM: The dystrophin glycoprotein complex: signaling strength and integrity for the sarcolemma, *Circ Res* 94:1023-1031, 2004.
4. Muntoni F: Cardiomyopathy in muscular dystrophies, *Curr Opin Neurol* 16:577-583, 2003.
5. Emery AEH: The muscular dystrophies, *Lancet* 359:687-695, 2002.
6. Finsterer J, Stollberger C: The heart in human dystrophinopathies, *Cardiology* 99:1-19, 2003.
7. Kirchman C, Kececioglu D, Korinthenberg R, Dittrich S: Echocardiographic and electrocardiographic findings of cardiomyopathy in Duchenne and Becker-Kiener muscular dystrophies, *Pediatr Cardiol* 26:66-72, 2005.
8. Bushby K, Muntoni F, Bourke JP: 107th ENMC International Workshop: The Management of Cardiac Involvement in Muscular Dystrophy and Myotonic Dystrophy, June 7-9, 2002, Naarden, The Netherlands, *Neuromuscul Disord* 13:166-172, 2003.
9. Corrado G, Lissoni A, Beretta S et al: Prognostic value of electrocardiograms, ventricular late potentials, ventricular arrhythmias, and left ventricular systolic dysfunction in patients with Duchenne muscular dystrophy, *Am J Cardiol* 89:838-841, 2002.
10. McNally EM, Towbin JA: Cardiomyopathy in muscular dystrophy workshop, September 28-30, 2003, Tucson, Arizona, *Neuromuscul Disord* 14:442-448, 2004.
11. Grain L, Cortina-Borja M, Forfar C et al: Cardiac abnormalities and skeletal muscle weakness in carriers of Duchenne and Becker muscular dystrophies and controls, *Neuromuscul Disord* 11:186-191, 2001.
12. Bushby K, Muntoni F, Urtizberea A et al: Report on the 124th ENMC International Workshop. Treatment of Duchenne Muscular Dystrophy; Defining the Gold Standards of Management in the Use of Corticosteroids, April 2-4, 2004, Naarden, The Netherlands, *Neuromuscul Disord* 14:526-534, 2004.
13. Eagle M, Baudouin SV, Chandler C et al. Survival in Duchenne muscular dystrophy: improvements in life expectancy since 1967 and the impact of home nocturnal ventilation, *Neuromuscul Disord* 12:926-929, 2002.
14. Melacini P, Gambino A, Caforio A et al: Heart transplantation in patients with inherited myopathies associated with end-stage cardiomyopathy: molecular and biochemical defects on cardiac and skeletal muscle, *Transplant Proc* 33:1596-1599, 2001.
15. Ruiz-Cano MJ, Delgado JF, Jimenez C et al. Successful heart transplantation in patients with inherited myopathies associated with end-stage cardiomyopathy, *Transplant Proc* 35:1513-1515, 2003.
16. Emery AEH. Emery-Dreifuss muscular dystrophy—a 40 year retrospective, *Neuromuscul Disord* 10:228-232, 2000.

17. Boriani G, Gallina M, Merlini L et al: Clinical relevance of atrial fibrillation/flutter, stroke, pacemaker implant, and heart failure in Emery-Dreifuss muscular dystrophy: a long-term longitudinal study, *Stroke* 34:901-908, 2003.

18. Kichuk Chrisant MR, Drummond-Webb J, Hallowell S, Friedman NR: Cardiac transplantation in twins with autosomal dominant Emery-Dreifuss muscular dystrophy, *J Heart Lung Transplant* 23:496-498, 2004.

19. Politano L, Nigro V, Passamano L et al: Evaluation of cardiac and respiratory involvement in sarcoglycanopathies, *Neuromuscul Disord* 11:178-185, 2001.

20. Poppe M, Bourke J, Eagle M et al: Cardiac and respiratory failure in limb-girdle muscular dystrophy 2I, *Ann Neurol* 56:738-741, 2004.

21. Die-Smulders CEM, Jennekens, FGI, Howeler CJ: Myotonic dystrophy type 1. In Cassidy SB, Allanson JE, editors: *Management of genetic syndromes*, ed 2, Hoboken, NJ, 2005, Wiley-Liss, pp. 351-367.

22. Duboc D, Eymard B, Damian MS: Cardiac management of myotonic dystrophy. In Harper PS, van Engelen B, Eymard B, Wilcox DE, editors; *Myotonic dystrophy: present management, future therapy,* Oxford, 2004, Oxford University Press, pp. 85-97.

23. Groh WJ, Lowe MR, Zipes DP: Severity of cardiac conduction involvement and arrhythmias in myotonic dystrophy type 1 correlates with age and CTG repeat length, *J Cardiovasc Electrophysiol* 13:444-448, 2002.

24. Lazarus A, Varin J, Babuty D et al: Long-term follow-up of arrhythmias in patients with myotonic dystrophy treated by pacing, *J Am Coll Cardiol* 40:1645-1652, 2002.

25. Merlevede K, Vermander D, Theys P et al: Cardiac involvement and CTG expansion in myotonic dystrophy, *J Neurol* 249:693-698, 2002.

26. Gregoratos G, Abrams J, Epstein AE et al: ACC/AHA/NASPE 2002 Guideline Update for Implantation of Cardiac Pacemakers and Antiarrhythmia Devices, summary article, *J Am Coll Cardiol* 40:1703-1719, 2002.

27. Hart PE, Lodi R, Rajagopalan B et al: Antioxidant treatment of patients with Friedreich ataxia, *Arch Neurol* 62:621-626, 2005.

28. Lynch DR, Farmer JM, Balcer LJ et al: Friedreich ataxia: effects of genetic understanding on clinical evaluation and therapy, *Arch Neurol* 59:743747, 2002.

29. Buyse G, Mertens L, Di Salvo G et al: Idebenone treatment in Friedreich's ataxia: neurological, cardiac, and biochemical monitoring, *Neurology* 60:1679-1681, 2003.

30. McDaniel DO, Keats B, Vedanarayanan VV, Subramony SH: Sequence variation in GAA repeat expansions may cause differential phenotype display in Friedreich's ataxia, *Movement Disord* 16:1153-1158, 2001.

31. Durr A: Friedreich's ataxia: treatment within reach, *Lancet Neurol* 1:370-374, 2002.

32. Cooper JM, Schapira AHV: Friedreich's ataxia: disease mechanisms, antioxidant and coenzyme Q10 therapy, *BioFactors* 18:163-171, 2003.

33. Lodi R, Rajagopalan B, Blamire AM et al: Cardiac energetics are abnormal in Friedreich ataxia patients in the absence of cardiac dysfunction and hypertrophy: an in vivo 31P magnetic resonance spectroscopy study, *Cardiovasc Res* 52:111-119, 2001.

34. Bunse M, Bit-Avragim N, Riefflin A et al: Cardiac energetics correlates to myocardial hypertrophy in Friedreich's ataxia, *Ann Neurol* 53:121-123, 2003.

35. Alizad A, Seward JB: Echocardiographic features of genetic diseases: part 1. Cardiomyopathy, *J Am Soc Echocardiogr* 13:73-86, 2000.

36. Puccio H, Koenig M: Recent advances in the molecular pathogenesis of Friedreich ataxia, *Hum Mol Genet* 9:887-982, 2000.

37. Hausse AO, Aggoun Y, Bonnet D et al: Idebenone and reduced cardiac hypertrophy in Friedreich's ataxia, *Heart* 87:346-349, 2002.

38. Hughes RAC, Wijdicks EFM, Barohn R et al: Practice parameter: immunotherapy for Guillain-Barré syndrome, *Neurology* 61:736-740, 2003.

39. Lindenbaum Y, Kissel JT, Mendell JR: Treatment approaches for Gullain-Barré syndrome and chronic inflammatory demyelinating polyradiculoneuropathy, *Neurol Clin* 19:187-204, 2001.

40. Chalela JA: Pearls and pitfalls in the intensive care management of Guillian-Barré syndrome, *Semin Neurol* 21:399-405, 2001.

41. Bernstein R, Mayer SA, Magnano A: Neurogenic stunned myocardium in Guillian-Barré syndrome, *Neurology* 54:759-762, 2000.

42. Yoshii F, Kozuma R, Haida M et al: Giant negative T waves in Guillain-Barré syndrome, *Acta Neurol Scand* 101:212-215, 2000.

43. Pfeiffer G, Schiller B, Kruse J, Netzer J: Indicators of dysautonomia in severe Guillain-Barré syndrome, *J Neurol* 246:1015-1022, 1999.

44. Vincent A, Palace J, Hilton-Jones D: Myasthenia gravis, *Lancet* 357:2112-2128, 2001.

45. Sanders DB: Myasthenia gravis and Lambert-Eaton myasthenic syndrome. In Pourmand R, editor: *Neuromuscular diseases: expert clinicians' views.* Boston, 2001, Butterworth-Heinemann, pp. 439-457.

46. Saperstein DS, Barohn RJ: Management of myasthenia gravis, *Semin Neurol* 24:41-48, 2004.

47. Gibson TC: The heart in myasthenia gravis, *Am Heart J* 90:389-396, 1975.

48. Rubino FA: Perioperative management of patients with neurologic disease, *Neurol Clin N Am* 22:261-276, 2004.

49. Sakr YL, Ghosn I, Vincent JL: Cardiac manifestations after subarachnoid hemorrhage: a systematic review of the literature, *Prog Cardiovasc Dis* 45:67-80, 2002.

50. Deibert E, Barzilai B, Braverman AC et al: Clinical significance of elevated troponin I levels in patients with nontraumatic subarachnoid hemorrhage, *J Neurosurg* 98:741-746, 2003.

51. Bulsara KR, McGirt MJ, Liao L et al: Use of the peak troponin value to differentiate myocardial infarction from reversible neurogenic left ventricular dysfunction associated with aneurysmal subarachnoid hemorrhage, *J Neurosurg* 98:524-528, 2003.

52. Tung P, Kopelnik A, Banki N et al: Predictors of neurocardiogenic injury after subarachnoid hemorrhage, *Stroke* 35:548-553, 2004.

53. Khush I, Kopelnik A, Tung P et al: Age and aneurysm position predict patterns of left ventricular dysfunction after subarachnoid hemorrhage, *J Am Soc Echocardiogr* 18:168-174, 2005.

54. Macmillan CSA, Grant IS, Andrews PJD: Pulmonary and cardiac sequelae of subarachnoid haemorrhage: time for active management? *Intensive Care Med* 28:1012-1023, 2002.

55. Rinkel GJE, Feigin VL, Algra A et al: Calcium antagonists for aneurismal subarachnoid haemorrhage, *Cochrane Database Syst Rev* CD000277, 2005.

56. van den Bergh WM: Magnesium sulfate in aneurysmal subarachnoid hemorrhage: a randomized controlled trial, *Stroke* 36:1011-1015, 2005.

57. van den Bergh WM, Algra A, Rinkel GJE: Electrocardiographic abnormalities and serum magnesium in patients with subarachnoid hemorrhage, *Stroke* 35:644-648, 2004.

58. Sakr YL, Lim N, Amaral ACKB et al: Relation of ECG changes to neurological outcome in patients with aneurysmal subarachnoid hemorrhage, *Int J Cardiol* 96:369-373, 2004.

59. Crago EA, Kerr ME, Kong Y et al: The impact of cardiac complications on outcome in the SAH population, *Acta Neurol Scand* 110:248-253, 2004.

60. Christensen H, Boysen G, Christensen AF, Johannesen HH: Insular lesions, ECG abnormalities, and outcome in acute stroke, *J Neurol Neurosurg Psychiatry* 76:269-271, 2005.

61. Cheung RTF, Hachinski V: The insula and cerebrogenic sudden death, *Arch Neurol* 57:1685-1688, 2000.

62. Colivicchi F, Bassi A, Santini M, Caltagirone C: Cardiac autonomic derangement and arrhythmias in right-sided stroke with insular involvement, *Stroke* 35:2094-2098, 2004.

63. Rudd AG, Hoffman A, Irwin P et al: Stroke unit care and outcome: results from the 2001 National Sentinel Audit of Stroke, *Stroke* 36:103-106, 2005.

64. Cavallini A, Micieli G, Marcheselli S, Quaglini S: Role of monitoring in management of acute ischemic stroke patients, *Stroke* 34:2599-2603, 2003.

65. Sulter G, Elting JW, Langedijk M et al: Admitting acute ischemic stroke patients to a stroke care monitoring unit versus a conventional stroke unit: a randomized pilot study, *Stroke* 34:101-104, 2003.

■ ■ ■ c h a p t e r **89**

Rheumatic Diseases and the Cardiovascular System

Suzette Sewell

CHAPTER ABBREVIATIONS

ANA antinuclear antibodies

APLS antiphospholipid syndrome

CBC complete blood count

CHD coronary heart disease

CK creatinine kinase

COX-2 cyclooxygenase-2

CREST Calcinosis, Raynaud's phenomenon, esophageal involvement, sclerodactyly, telangiectasia

CRP C-reactive protein

CTD connective tissue diseases

DMARD disease-modifying antirheumatic drug

dsDNA double-stranded deoxyribonucleic acid

ESR erythrocyte sedimentation rate

GCS glucocorticosteroids

HDL high-density lipoprotein

IL interleukin

LDL low-density lipoprotein

MCTD mixed connective tissue disorders

MRI magnetic resonance imaging

MTX methotrexate

NSAID nonsteroidal antiinflammatory drug

OA osteoarthritis

PSS progressive systemic sclerosis

PTT partial thromboplastin time

RA rheumatoid arthritis

RHUPUS RHU-rheumatic; PUS-lupus

RNP ribonucleoprotein

SLE systemic lupus erythematosus

TNF tumor necrosis factor

UCTD undifferentiated connective tissue disorders

Increasing evidence indicates that rheumatoid arthritis (RA) and other connective tissue diseases (CTD) are associated with increased cardiovascular morbidity and mortality.[1] Cardiovascular manifestations associated with rheumatic diseases are noted in Box 89-1. These manifestations are related to the proinflammatory activity of rheumatic diseases in conjunction with atherogenic factors previously linked to the development of cardiovascular disease.[2] Possible explanations include endothelial dysfunction; altered lipid metabolism; proatherogenic factors, such as platelet activation; and proinflammatory cytokines.[1]

PATHOPHYSIOLOGICAL CARDIOVASCULAR-RHEUMATOLOGICAL INTERACTIONS

Vasculitis and endothelial dysfunction are common in patients with RA and systemic lupus erythematosus **(SLE)**.[3] Inflammation plays a key role in their development.[4] Alteration of the endothelial wall is initiated by increased leukocyte and low-density lipoprotein **(LDL)** production, with platelet adhesion to the endothelium. LDL can damage the endothelium when it becomes oxidized by free radicals. Endothelial dysfunction is caused by subsequent attraction and adhesion of LDL and macrophages.[5] Inflammation-induced endothelial dysfunction and chronic vascular changes contribute to the premature development of atherosclerosis and coronary artery disease in patients with CTD.[6]

Patients with untreated RA have altered patterns of lipid metabolism.[7] This altered pattern of lipid metabolism and other proatherogenic factors associated with the immune inflammatory response in RA may contribute to atherosclerosis. These patterns include increased triglycerides, decreased high-density lipoprotein **(HDL)** cholesterol, and increased LDL cholesterol. Treatment with disease-modifying antirheumatic drugs **(DMARDs)**, such as infliximab, can change lipid levels. Administration of infliximab, used in clinical trials to treat RA, resulted in changes in lipid levels after 2 weeks of treatment that included an increase in total cholesterol and HDL with no changes noted in triglycerides or LDL.[7] It is unknown whether DMARDs reduce cardiovascular morbidity and mortality. See the accompanying Evidence-Based Practice feature. Further study of this relationship is necessary to explore the link between RA, its treatments, and cardiovascular disease outcomes.

Rheumatic diseases, such as RA and SLE, contribute to platelet activation through a variety of stimuli including those leading to tissue inflammation. Under normal conditions, activation of platelets enhances the inflammatory response for the purposes of hemostasis, wound healing, and tissue repair. However, in the rheumatic diseases, the process is associated with the secretion of adhesion molecules and activation of platelets caused by the influence of excessive stimulatory signals, not tissue repair. This proatherogenic influence on platelets in conjunction with other proinflammatory factors contributes to the development of vascular changes and thrombosis resulting in peripheral vascular disease and premature coronary and cerebral artery disease.

A number of proinflammatory signals are released from various cells during activation of the immune response (Box 89-2). Acute phase reactants and cytokines, such as C-reactive protein **(CRP)**, interleukin (IL)-6, and

■ EVIDENCE-BASED PRACTICE

EFFECTS OF INFLIXIMAB

Infliximab (anti–tumor necrosis-alpha), used in clinical trials to treat RA, has resulted in changes in lipid and cholesterol levels that included an increase in total cholesterol.[7] This occurred because of statistically significant increases in HDL, although there were no changes in triglycerides or LDL after 2 weeks of treatment.

HDL cholesterol before and after treatment with infliximab versus placebo

LDL cholesterol before and after treatment with infliximab compared to placebo

C-Reactive Protein in RA before and after infliximab compared to placebo

HDL, High-density lipoprotein; *RA,* rheumatoid arthritis; *TNF,* tumor necrosis factor.
Adapted from Popa C et al: Influence of anti-tumor necrosis factor therapy on cardiovascular risk factors in patients with active rheumatoid arthritis, *Ann Rheum Dis* 64:303-305, 2005.

tumor necrosis factor **(TNF alpha)** are increased in patients with RA and are independently associated with increased risk of cardiovascular disease. Increased homocysteine levels resulting from antifolate therapies, such as the RA treatment, methotrexate **(MTX),** are also

associated with an increased risk for cardiovascular disease.[8] From a rheumatological standpoint, elevations of these markers in conjunction with expression of clinical features signal uncontrolled inflammation in the patient with rheumatic diseases. A number of inflammatory markers and lipids are associated with an increased risk of cardiovascular events[7] as noted in Figure 89-1.

The increased mortality associated with cardiovascular and cerebrovascular disease among patients with RA (especially prominent in women) provides evidence of the impact of chronic inflammation.[9,10] Patients with RA have an increased risk of developing cardiovascular events, such as myocardial infarction and congestive heart failure, compared with normal controls and those with osteoarthritis **(OA)** who do not have chronic inflammation.[2] Other research has shown that RA patients are more likely to die from a cardiac event compared with patients with OA or the general population.[3] Risk of cardiovascular death is increased even after controlling for traditional cardiovascular risk factors and comorbidities.[11] The relationship between rheumatic diseases and cardiovascular disease deserves further investigation to reveal the link between the two diseases.

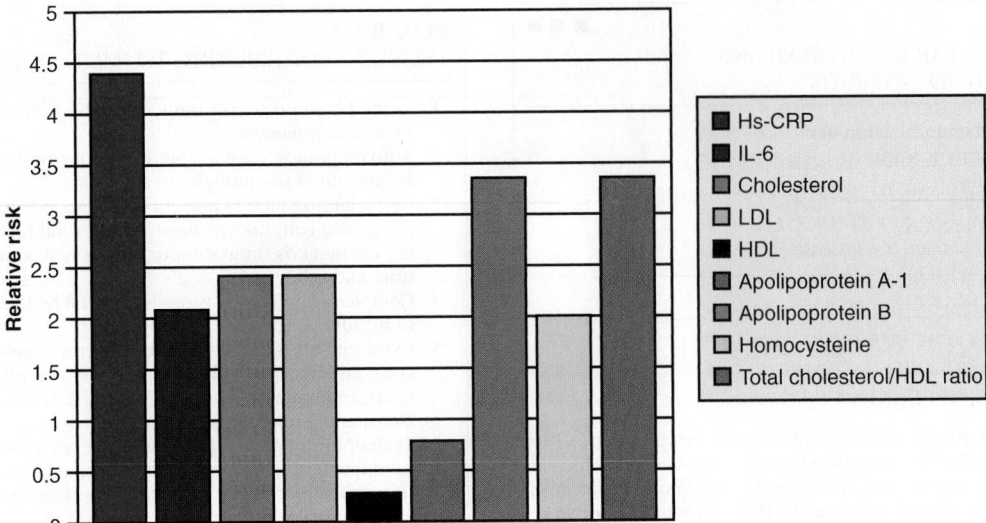

FIGURE 89-1 ■ Relative risks of cardiovascular disease associated with inflammatory markers and lipids. (Data from Ridker P, Hennekens C, Buring J: C-reactive protein and other markers of inflammation in the prediction of cardiovascular disease in women, *N Engl J Med* 342:836-843, 2000.) *HDL,* High-density lipoprotein; *HS-CRP,* highly sensitive C-reactive protein; *IL-6,* interleukin 6; *LDL,* low-density lipoprotein.

RHEUMATIC DISEASES
Rheumatoid Arthritis

Proinflammatory responses that occur as a result of systemic immune stimulation usually protect the host from infection. In some instances, these retaliatory responses to infection or injury may damage normal tissue in their response. In RA the joints and synovial tissue are targets of inflammatory responses. On occasion the blood vessels, the pericardium, and the pleura are also affected. Researchers have examined these structures histologically for pathological features, including the influence of lymphocytic and nonlymphocytic cells, enzymes, cytokines, antibodies, complement, and many others. Every inflammatory mediator may be present serologically in patients with RA. Cytokines, such as IL-1beta, and TNF-alpha have been the focus of much research in the treatment of RA. Other research has focused on suppression of B-cell lymphocyte activity and the autoantibodies produced by them. Despite substantial research, the cause of RA and associated CTD remains unknown.

Synovial Damage and Apoptosis

In RA the articular tissues appear to be affected by two complex mechanisms: chronic inflammation and failure of the immune modulatory system (apoptosis) to restore the integrity of damaged tissue. Chronic inflammation is attributed to the effects of TNF-alpha (Table 89-1). Macrophages or activated T cells produce TNF-alpha and other proinflammatory cytokines, such as IL-1 and IL-12, which cause increased inflammation. This process mediates the acute phase response and leads to increased CRP in the serum.

Apoptosis is the process of tissue modulation that creates a balance between new cell growth and death. In RA the body fails to repair the articular damage and cannot keep up with the degree of damage resulting in destruction of the joint's surface (Figure 89-2). The se-

■ ■ ■

TABLE 89-1 ACTIONS OF TUMOR NECROSIS FACTOR-ALPHA

TARGET	MECHANISM	ACTION
Macrophages	Increases production of cytokines	Increased Inflammation
Endothelium	Increased production of adhesion molecules and vascular endothelial growth factor	Increased infiltration of cells Increased angiogenesis
Synoviocytes	Increases acute phase response	Increased C-reactive protein
	Increased synthesis of metalloproteinase	Increases degradation of collagen

verity and duration of the inflammatory process influences the destruction of the joint and if untreated, irreversible deformity will result. Severity of RA is directly related to the level of functional impairment and disability.

The incidence of RA is variable depending on age and gender. It increases with age, is most likely diagnosed between ages 30 and 50, and is observed in twice as many women as men. RA is seen in all races and in all parts of the world. RA is a chronic, disabling disease that may shorten the life span by as much as 18 years.[12] Symptoms of RA in women sometimes improve during pregnancy and with the use of oral contraceptives. RA affects about 1 percent of the U.S. population[12] (see the accompanying Genetics feature).

Rheumatoid Arthritis and Cardiovascular Morbidity

Cardiovascular disease accounts for 35 percent to 50 percent of all RA deaths.[13] Traditional risk factors and manifestations of RA inflammation contribute to carotid atherosclerosis in RA.[14,15] In one clinical trial, cardiovascular risk (diabetes mellitus, hypercholesteremia, ciga-

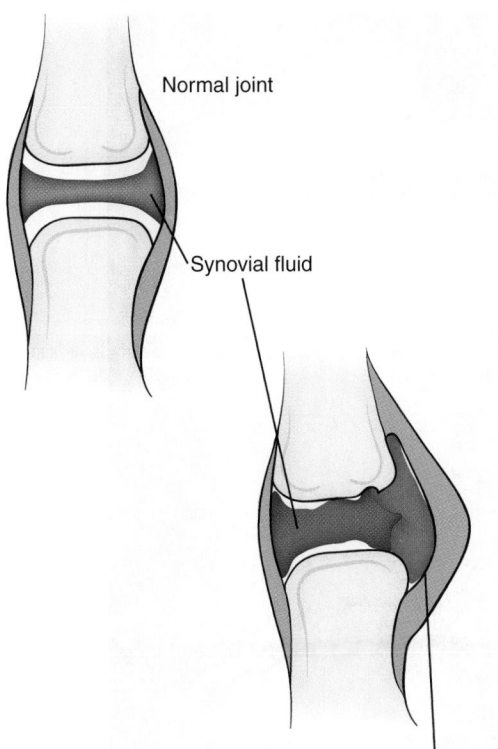

FIGURE 89-2 ■ Normal joint versus joint in an individual with rheumatoid arthritis.

Labels on figure:
- Normal joint
- Synovial fluid
- Inflamed synovial membrane

■ ■ ■ GENETICS

LINK TO RHEUMATOID ARTHRITIS

Family studies of rheumatoid arthritis (RA) patients suggest a four times higher risk of disease in blood relatives than in unrelated family members. Other research notes a genetic disposition to RA with a concordance rate for monozygotic twins of 25 percent. Of particular interest to science, is the association of RA with particular alleles of the class II major histocompatibility complex genes. Certain human leukocyte antigen molecules are associated with the development and severity of RA and represent a genetic disposition.

Data from Alarcon G: Epidemiology of rheumatoid arthritis, *Rheum Dis Clin North Am* 21:589-604, 1995.

rette smoking, hypertension, and body mass index) contributed to the development of atherosclerosis[14]; however, these did not fully explain all the risk.[16] Among RA patients with no history of coronary heart disease **(CHD)**, use of glucocorticosteroids **(GCS)** was associated with a 78 percent increased risk of cardiovascular death compared with those that did not receive steroids. However, among those with RA and CHD, the risk of cardiovascular death among those who received GCS was *less than* the risk of those who did not.[17] GCS are used in patients with more severe disease and they can promote hypertension, dyslipidemia, and diabetes. It has been suggested that these agents may be risk factors for increased cardiovascular mortality in RA.[17,18] Yet patients treated with biologicals to reduce disease activity have a lower incidence of an initial cardiovascular event than those not treated.[19]

Several mechanisms have been proposed to explain the increased cardiovascular mortality in RA patients.

First, decreased emphasis on reduction of risk factors, such as smoking and obesity, may contribute to increased mortality overall. Undertreatment of cardiovascular comorbidities, such as hyperlipidemia or dyslipidemia, may result in the increased risk. Yet another mechanism may be that patients with chronic RA share a higher prevalence for traditional risk factors compared with those without RA. Alternatively, inflammation may act independently of traditional risk factors to increase the risk. Possibly all of the mechanisms mentioned may contribute to the overall risk. Additional studies are needed to address whether aggressive treatment of RA to control systemic inflammation would reduce the risk of cardiovascular mortality.[20]

Traditional risk factors increase the risk of cardiovascular death in RA patients, but increased erythrocyte sedimentation rate **(ESR),** presence of RA vasculitis, and RA-related lung disease were strong predictors of cardiovascular mortality. Markers of systemic inflammation (e.g., TNF-alpha, CRP) present a statistically significant risk for cardiovascular death among patients with RA, even after controlling for traditional cardiovascular risk factors and comorbidities.[17] Heart failure is twice as likely to occur in patients with RA compared with those of the same age and sex without RA.[21] The increased risk is not explained by traditional risk factors or the presence of ischemic heart disease.[22]

Diagnosis and Clinical Presentation

In the absence of unique clinical features, diagnosis has been made easier using classification criteria like those developed for epidemiological studies of RA patients.[23] However, the clinical presentation of the patient with rheumatic disease may be subtle and insidious; so patients with true disease may or may not meet all research criteria for diagnosis to occur. RA is a systemic disease characterized by variable inflammation of the connective tissue, particularly the diarthrodial joints (hands and feet). Chronic, symmetrical polyarthritis affecting the hands and feet is the classic presentation of a patient with RA. The clinical features of RA are listed in Box 89-3.

RA is characterized by joint swelling that obscures the margins of the joint and extensive synovial-based articular inflammation or synovitis (Figure 89-3) that causes erythema with heat and pain noted on palpation. The "squeeze test" has been validated as a diagnostic test for synovitis in early RA. It is performed by compressing a group of small, adjacent joints between your thumb and forefinger like one would when approaching a handshake (Figure 89-4). A positive finding is noted when pain is elicited by mild compression of the metatarsal or

BOX 89-3   ■ ■ ■
CARDINAL FEATURES OF RHEUMATOID ARTHRITIS

- Early morning stiffness longer than 45 min
- Symmetric articular pain with insidious onset
- Articular tenderness
- Pain on motion
- Joint swelling "red and warm"
- Limitation of motion
- Joint deformity and rheumatoid nodules

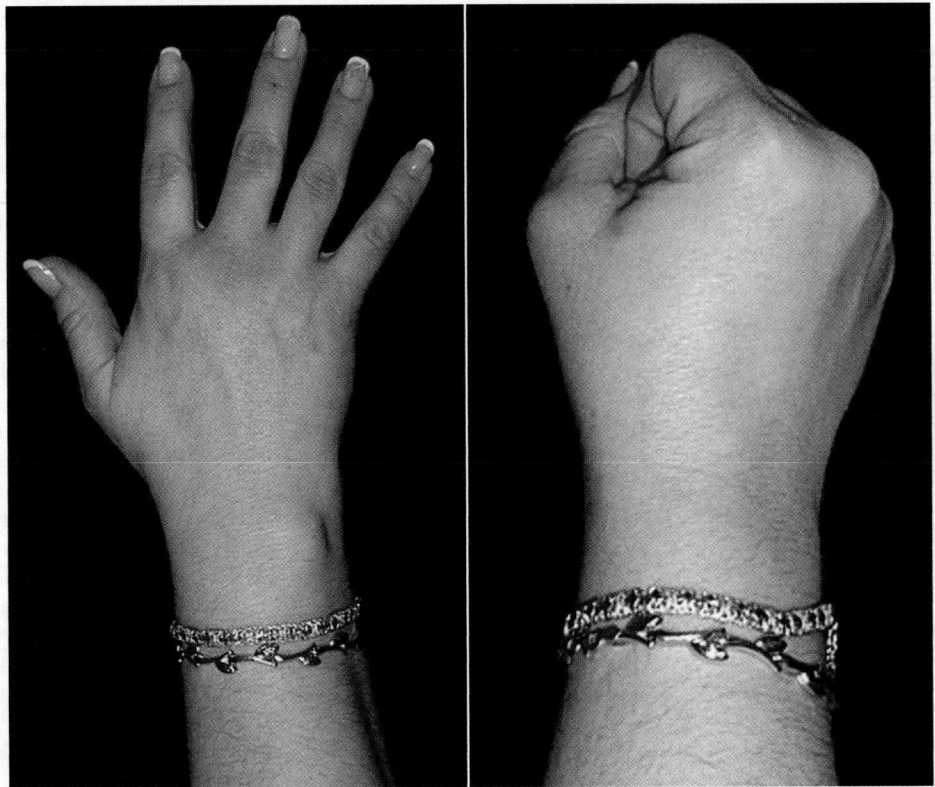

FIGURE 89-3 ■ Two views of characteristic early inflammatory changes seen in a 33-year-old patient with rheumatoid arthritis (RA). Note the mild joint swelling that obscures the margins of the first and second metacarpal joints and swelling and erythema of the wrist joint. Suspect early RA in a patient with any of the following: three or more swollen joints, metacarpophalangeal and/or metatarsophalangeal joint involvement (squeeze test positive), or morning stiffness for 30 minutes or longer.

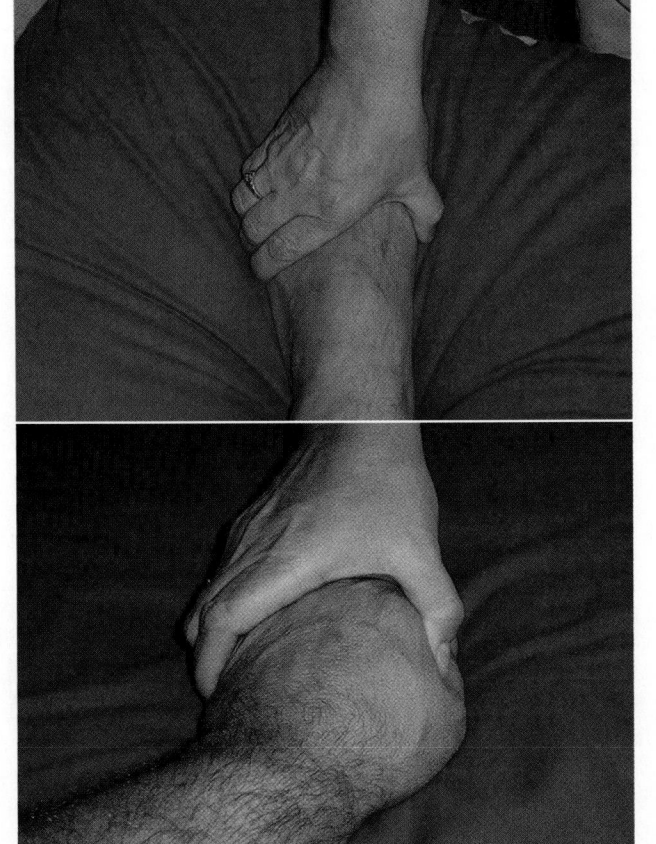

A

B

FIGURE 89-4 ■ Squeeze test on foot (**A**) and hand (**B**).

metacarpal joints as a group. Individual joints are also assessed this way to isolate single joint involvement.[24] Extent of involvement is categorized as monoarticular (one joint), oligoarticular (two to four joints), or polyarticular (more than four joints). Morning stiffness in excess of an hour is also commonly present in RA patients and patients with other inflammatory diseases. Other extraarticular manifestations associated with RA are noted in Box 89-4. Weight loss and persistent inflamma-

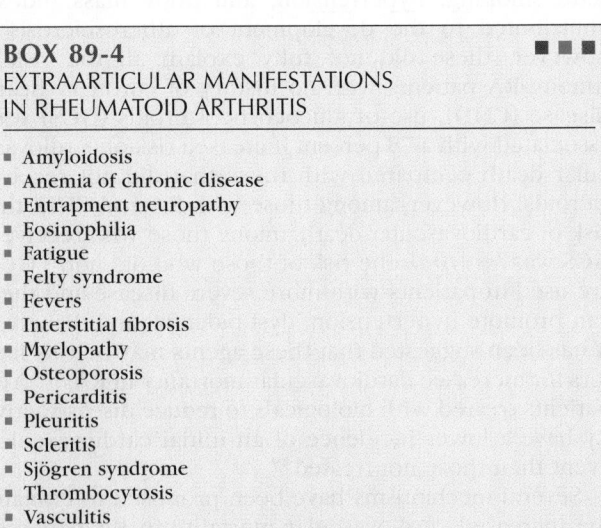

BOX 89-4 ■ ■ ■
EXTRAARTICULAR MANIFESTATIONS
IN RHEUMATOID ARTHRITIS

- Amyloidosis
- Anemia of chronic disease
- Entrapment neuropathy
- Eosinophilia
- Fatigue
- Felty syndrome
- Fevers
- Interstitial fibrosis
- Myelopathy
- Osteoporosis
- Pericarditis
- Pleuritis
- Scleritis
- Sjögren syndrome
- Thrombocytosis
- Vasculitis
- Weakness

tion resulting in joint destruction can cause significant declines in functional status and premature mortality.

With increased recognition, early diagnosis, and effective treatment with available therapeutic agents that suppress the immune proinflammatory response, deformities that are known to occur in RA (Figure 89-5) are less severe and may be prevented. Categories of medications commonly used are noted in Box 89-5. Treatments for RA are effective in slowing the progression of the disease (see the accompanying Technology feature).

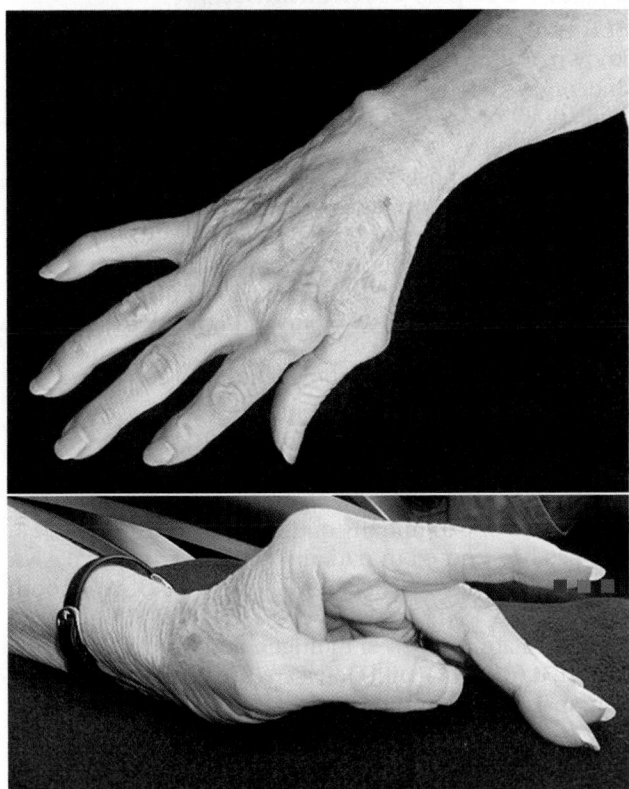

FIGURE 89-5 ■ Two views of severe deformity in rheumatoid arthritis.

BOX 89-5
CATEGORIES OF DRUGS USED FOR RHEUMATOID ARTHRITIS ■ ■ ■

- NSAIDs and COX-2 inhibitors
- DMARDs and cytotoxic drugs
- Glucocorticoids

COX-2, Cyclooxygenase-2; *DMARDS*, disease-modifying antiinflammatory drugs; *NSAIDs*, nonsteroidal antiinflammatory drugs.

■ ■ ■ **TECHNOLOGY**

EFFECTS OF A BIOLOGICAL AGENT

Abatacept, the new biological agent for RA, appeared to improve RA symptoms in about half the patients treated in clinical trials. Results from clinical trials indicated that 48.3 percent of patients receiving Abatacept achieved a 50 percent improvement in disease activity compared with 18.2 percent receiving placebo.

1. Update on clinical aspects of rheumatology at the 2004 American College of Rheumatology meeting, San Antonio, TX, University of Alabama School of Medicine.

RA, Rheumatoid arthritis.

These medications are used to modify the severity of the disease, suppress the activity of the immune system, and manage pain. Side effects of the treatments themselves may contribute to the disease process and should be monitored by a knowledgeable physician or nurse practitioner (see the accompanying Conundrum feature). Whether DMARD therapy will reduce all-cause and cardiovascular disease mortality in rheumatic diseases requires further study.

Diagnostic Testing

Although there is no gold standard test for RA, serological tests for RA includes measurement of rheumatoid factor. Rheumatoid factor is present in 75 percent to 85 percent of patients with RA,[25] but is not exclusive to RA. It may be increased in SLE, OA, Sjögren syndrome, hepatitis, bacterial endocarditis, and other serious conditions. Rheumatoid factor is an IgM reacting anti-IgG autoantibody. It is normally detected in *less than* 5 percent of people and is not used as a screening test for RA.

Useful tests to the diagnosis of RA include a complete blood count (CBC) and measurement of acute phase reactants, such as ESR or CRP. The CBC of a patient with active RA may show anemia (normocytic, normochromic) and thrombocytosis. Both findings are manifestations of chronic inflammation involved in the disease process. Thrombocytosis often occurs in patients with active RA and correlates with the extent of joint inflammation and acute phase proteins, such as ESR and

■ ■ ■ **CONUNDRUM**

Should prescription of antiinflammatories, such as cyclooxygenase-2 (COX-2) inhibitors, be based on collateral cardioprotective benefits, cardiovascular risk, gastrointestinal protection, or antiinflammatory benefits for arthritis pain?

Aspirin and nonsteroidal antiinflammatory drugs (NSAIDs) are used for treating rheumatoid arthritis pain. Aspirin has been used to prevent myocardial infarction. Most experts considered NSAIDs, such as nonselective NSAIDs and COX-2 inhibitors, to have the same cardioprotective, antithrombotic effect as aspirin. However, a meta-analysis of at least 23 studies using Vioxx (rofecoxib) failed to support this assumption.[2] Recent investigations into the increased risk of cardiovascular events associated with COX-2 inhibitors, such as Vioxx and Bextra (valdecoxib), compared with placebo has resulted in these two medications being removed from the market by Food and Drug Administration[3] recommendation.[45] Vioxx returned to the market with a strong recommendation to monitor patients for the development of cardiovascular disease. Bextra remains off the market. Many experts in rheumatology have debated the use of these agents. Trials are currently looking at the clinical implications of these findings and the risk factors that are associated with their use.[4]

1. Ray W et al: Non-steroidal antiinflammatory drugs and risk of serious coronary heart disease: an observational cohort study, *Lancet* 359:118-123, 2002.
2. Konstam M, Weir M, Reicin A: Cardiovascular thrombotic events in controlled trials of rofecoxib, *Circulation* 104:280-288, 2001.
3. Vioxx: arthritis advisory committee meeting. Feb 8, 2001, Gaithersburg, Md, Food and Drug Administration.
4. Johnsen S et al: Risk of hospitalization for myocardial infarction among users of rofecoxib, celecoxib, and other NSAIDs: a population-based case-control study, *Arch Intern Med* 165:978-984, 2005.

CRP. The underlying cause of this phenomenon is unknown.

The erythrocyte sedimentation rate **(ESR)** and CRP have been used as indicators for progression of rheumatic diseases and outcomes in RA patients. Several disease activity scales use these measures to quantify the severity and progression of RA for research purposes; however, these acute phase reactants may not always be increased in patients with active symptoms. Elevations of CRP have been noted as an independent, noncausal risk factor for cardiovascular disease and an indicator of inflammation in rheumatic disease in both men and women.[26] Further study is necessary to explore the causal link between rheumatic and cardiovascular diseases and the relationship between the tests used to diagnosis and treat them.

■ **EVIDENCE-BASED PRACTICE**

CALCULATING MODIFIED SHARP SCORE

The modified Sharp score is a quantitative measure of radiographic progression that assigns a score for the number of erosions present on hand and foot x-rays and the number of joint spaces with narrowing present. Erosions and joint-space narrowing contribute equally to structural damage in early and late rheumatoid arthritis (RA). An *erosion score* is obtained by counting the number of surfaces that contain erosions in 40 joints. If erosions are confluent, estimate the extent of erosion. If damage is noted in all four surface quadrants and the joint is destroyed, the score is 5.

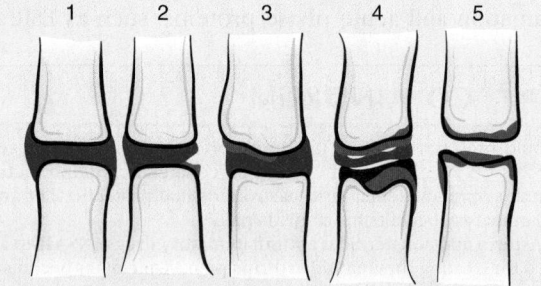

Joint-space narrowing is assessed in 44 joints using the following scale:

   0 = No narrowing
   1 = Asymmetrical or minimal narrowing, *less than* 25 percent
   2 = Narrowing 25 percent to 49 percent
   3 = Narrowing 50 percent to 99 percent, or subluxation
   4 = No visible joint space, presumed ankylosis, or dislocation

The total Sharp score = erosion score + joint-space narrowing.

Imaging Techniques

Almost 70 percent of patients will develop bony erosions within 2 years of disease onset.[25] Radiological images, such as x-rays of the hands, are not as helpful to the early diagnosis of RA because they cannot show images of the soft tissue. However, ongoing progression of joint destruction and erosion may be evaluated using x-rays of the hands. For research purposes, this evaluation may be quantified by calculating the Sharp score. This score is a significant predictor of progressive joint destruction used frequently in clinical trials to judge progression of disease. See the accompanying Evidence-Based Practice feature on using a modified Sharp score. Erosions of the joint are most likely seen in the wrist, metacarpal, and metatarsal joints, but may be seen in any joint.[24]

According to most experts, the most effective imaging method for assessment of articular inflammation and erosion is magnetic resonance imaging **(MRI).** MRI images demonstrate erosions and soft tissue involvement much earlier than conventional x-rays and have superior detail. Unfortunately, the cost of such procedures is prohibitive in many cases because of insurance or out-of-pocket costs to the patient.

Systemic Lupus Erythematosus

SLE is a group of inflammatory disorders, with an unknown cause, that collectively affects multiple tissues and organs. It is not a common disease, although the availability of serological testing (anticardiolipin, antinuclear antibodies **[ANA],** and anti-DNA antibodies) has increased its diagnosis. The conditions for SLE are created by a dysregulated immune system that produces autoantibodies against the nucleus of the host cells. These autoantibodies work in concert with proinflammatory mediators resulting in widespread damage to the skin, joints, kidneys, lungs, nervous system, and other organs.

Autoantibodies and Antiphospholipid Syndrome

Ninety-eight percent of patients with SLE have positive test results for ANA; however, only 10 percent of persons with ANA actually have lupus. Therefore a patient suspected of having SLE with a negative ANA test result would lead one to initially question the diagnosis of SLE. SLE has been noted in patients who have negative ANA test results. The presence of ANA to native DNA, smooth muscle, and RNP are seen exclusively in SLE patients and correlate to different antigen activity. Anti–double-stranded **(dsDNA)** antibodies are the most useful to the diagnosis of SLE and occur in more than 50 percent of SLE patients. Almost 10 percent of patients with SLE develop antiphospholipid antibodies that interfere with coagulation. This is also referred to as lupus anticoagulant, which will result in a prolonged partial thromboplastin time **(PTT)** in vitro. This appearance of anticoagulation is misleading, however, if it results in antiphospholipid syndrome **(APLS).** This syndrome is manifested by enhanced thrombosis, not anticoagulation. APLS is linked to cardiovascular complications, such as myocardial infarction and stroke, resulting from vascular thrombosis and infarction. APLS increases morbidity during pregnancy and can result in premature delivery or spontaneous abortion.

Cardiovascular manifestations reported in SLE patients are listed in Box 89-6. Inflammation of the heart

---

BOX 89-6   ■ ■ ■
CARDIOVASCULAR MANIFESTATIONS ASSOCIATED WITH SYSTEMIC LUPUS ERYTHEMATOSUS

- Pericarditis
- Myocarditis
- Endocarditis
- Coronary artery disease
- Unexplained tachycardia
- Cardiomegaly
- Congestive heart failure
- Sterile, vegetative lesions on valves

resulting in exudative pericarditis is the most commonly reported cardiovascular manifestation of SLE, but is still an uncommon development. Congestive heart failure, although less common than pericarditis, is associated with the use of corticosteroids and concomitant hypertension in SLE. Early death in SLE is associated with renal disease, infection, acute thromboembolic events, and central nervous system vasculitis; although cardiovascular disease is a major cause of death in patients with long term SLE.[27,28]

There are five types of lupus listed in Box 89-7. Each type has unique clinical subsets that may be confused with other overlapping clinical features associated with other diseases, including fibromyalgia, RA, and polymyositis. SLE is the most common type (70 percent) of lupus. The disease course varies from mild to severe and is marked by periods of exacerbation and remission. SLE is 10 times more common in women, with their diagnosis most likely occurring during the childbearing years, ages 15 to 40. The incidence of SLE is four times higher in blacks than in whites.

Systemic Lupus Erythematosus and Cardiovascular Morbidity

Cardiovascular morbidity and mortality is increased in patients with SLE, particularly in females ages 35 to 44, in whom the risk of myocardial infarction is raised 50-fold.[22] Myocarditis is a major cause of sudden death in young adults with SLE.[13] Heart valve abnormalities and thromboses are the most commonly reported cardiac manifestations in APLS associated with SLE. The reasons for these pathological conditions are not fully understood.

Traditional risk factors, such as hypertension and diabetes mellitus, do not completely account for the increased cardiovascular risk in SLE. It is theorized that increased cardiovascular risk factors encourage vascular damage resulting in impairment of normal endothelial function. In SLE oxidized lipoproteins, along with inflammatory cytokines, and suppression of fibrinolytic parameters enhance atherogenesis.

Despite the high risk of cardiovascular disease in SLE, assessment of cardiovascular risk factors is surprisingly lacking among health care professionals. Greater attention needs to be paid to cardiovascular disease risk factor screening in patients with SLE.[29] Consideration should be given to those factors specific to lupus that may influence the development of CHD, including chronic inflammation, antiphospholipid antibodies and therapy, especially GCS use. Treatment with GCS may accelerate atherosclerosis in these patients. As health care providers, we need to be proactive in our approach to risk-factor management in SLE patients. It is proposed that like diabetes mellitus, SLE should be considered a CHD equivalent condition for baseline risk and that assessment of cardiovascular risk should be done routinely.[30] In addition to lifestyle changes or modifications, blood pressure and cholesterol levels should be stringently controlled, and administration of aspirin should be considered in selected patients. The increased use of certain interventions, such as statins, also needs to be more widely investigated in this population.

Diagnosis and Clinical Presentation

SLE is commonly referred to as lupus. The term "lupus" is a derivative of Latin for the word "wolf."[31] Historically, this term was used to describe the facial lesions that resembled animal bites and ulcers about the face. This is now described as the malar or butterfly rash, the most recognizable feature of SLE. The most common complaints associated with SLE are joint pain, skin rashes, and fatigue.[31] A list of the clinical signs and symptoms of SLE patients and their frequency of occurrence are noted in Table 89-2.

Arthralgias and arthritis are the most common complaints of patients with SLE. The arthritis seen in SLE is a symmetrical polyarthritis, typically affecting the hands, wrists, and knees. The arthritis associated with SLE is usually not erosive or deforming. If deforming arthritis occurs, also known as Jaccoud arthropathy, it results from recurrent inflammation of the tendons and supporting structures of the joints.

A facial rash may be an early sign of SLE. Skin rashes include malar, discoid, and subacute lesions. Lupus rashes are photosensitive. Chronic scarring rashes called discoid can involve the face, scalp, ears, and upper extremities. Subacute lesions are generally widespread and symmetric. Other common dermatological manifestations of SLE include alopecia, ulcerations of the mouth and nose, and periungual erythema.

Cutaneous vasculitis of the hands and feet can occur resulting in breakdown of the skin and splinter hemorrhages of the nail beds. Infarctions of the fingers or toes can be a complication of cutaneous vasculitis, Raynaud phenomenon or disease, APLS, or thrombotic events. Treatment of lupus includes nonsteroidal antiinflammatory drugs (**NSAIDs**) and antimalarials, particularly hydrochloroquine. GCS are routinely used for SLE manifestations despite the adverse side effects associated with them. High doses of oral steroids (1 mg/kg/d) or

■ ■ ■

TABLE 89-2 CLINICAL FEATURES OF ACTIVE SYSTEMIC LUPUS ERYTHEMATOSUS

	CLINICAL FEATURE	PATIENTS REPORTING
Constitutional symptoms	Fatigue	80%
	Fever	40%
	Anorexia	20%
	Weight loss	25%
Cutaneous manifestations	Increased photosensitivity	65%
	Alopecia	30%
	Malar rash	35%
	Discoid rash	20%
	Oral ulcerations	20%
	Pigment changes to the skin	10%
	Urticaria	10%
Vasculocutaneous manifestations	Raynaud phenomenon	30%
Musculoskeletal system	Arthralgia	90%
	Polyarthritis	50%
	Morning stiffness	50%
	Inflammatory arthritis	50%
	Tendon involvement	10%
	Subcutaneous nodules	10%
	Myalgia	50%
	Inflammatory myositis	11%
	Secondary fibromyalgia	15%
	Osteoporosis	25%
Cardiopulmonary system	Chest pain	60%
	Pericarditis	25%
	Myocarditis	Rare
	Hypertension	25%
	Coronary artery disease	15-50%
	Pleurisy	60%
	Interstitial lung disease	20%
	Pulmonary embolism	10%
Neuro/Psychiatric	Cerebral vasculitis	10%
	Lupus headache	15%
	Cognitive dysfunction	50%
	Fibromyalgia	20%
	Depression	40%
Eye symptoms	Discoid lesions of eye	10%
	Dry eyes	20%
Esophageal symptoms	Dysphagia	25%
	Hepatomegaly	10%
	Heartburn with reflux*	25%
Hematological	Lymphadenopathy	50%
	Anemia	80%
	Hemolytic anemia	10%
	Leukopenia	20%
Renal system	Nephritis (increased urinary sediment)	25-50%
	Nephropathy (proteinuria)	25-50%

*Most likely related to drugs.
Data from Wallace D, Metzer A: Systemic lupus erythematosus: clinical aspects and treatment. In Koopman W, editor: *Arthritis and allied conditions: a textbook of rheumatology,* Philadelphia, 1997, Williams and Wilkins, pp 3-34.

boluses of methylprednisolone (120 to 1080 mg) may be required to gain control of the disease, but should be tapered as rapidly as disease activity permits[25] (see the accompanying Pharmacology feature).

Other immunosuppressive agents, such as azathioprine and cyclophosphamide, may be used to spare steroid use. Other priorities include management of hypertension and clotting diatheses. Patients with APLS should be treated with anticoagulants as needed to prevent endothelial dysfunction and thrombosis.

Diagnostic Testing

Typically, when SLE is suggested by clinical presentation, autoantibody testing is performed in addition to routine medical tests. Increased ANA with a pattern associated with dsDNA is the characteristic finding in SLE (sensitivity), although ANA may be found in other diseases (specificity). The ANA test defines specific antibodies that react with certain cells and may correlate with particular organ involvement. It is frequently used in the clinical area in determining prognosis of these diseases. Autoantibodies most commonly seen with SLE are ANA, anti-dsDNA, anti–Sm, and anti-ribonucleoprotein (**RNP**). Other laboratory findings in patients with SLE are seen in Box 89-8.

Antiphospholipid antibodies, such as anticardiolipin, interfere with lipid metabolism and coagulation. The anticardiolipin antibody is associated with the lupus anticoagulant that paradoxically is associated with intravascular thrombosis. Tests for APLS are noted in Box 89-9.

BOX 89-8 ■ ■ ■
LABORATORY FINDINGS IN SYSTEMIC LUPUS ERYTHEMATOSUS

- Decreased blood counts including anemia, leukopenia, and thrombocytopenia
- Decreased serum complement levels
- Hematuria
- Hemolytic anemia
- Increased anti-DNA and anti–smooth muscle antibodies
- Increased antiphospholipid antibodies
- Increased antinuclear antibodies
- Increased urinary sediment (casts)
- Presence of lupus anticoagulant
- Prolonged partial thromboplastin time
- Proteinuria

DNA, Deoxyribonucleic acid.

BOX 89-9 ■ ■ ■
TESTS FOR ANTIPHOSPHOLIPID SYNDROME

- VDRL—(venereal disease research laboratories) antiphospholipid yields a false-positive result in this test for syphilis
- RPR—(rapid plasma reagin) antiphospholipid yields a false-positive result in this test for syphilis
- PTT—(partial thromboplastin time) prolongs in response to lupus anticoagulant
- Anticardiolipin antibodies—isolated using enzyme-linked immunosorbent assay (**ELISA**)

■ ■ ■ **PHARMACOLOGY**

TAPERING CORTICOSTEROIDS

If dose is *greater than* 40 mg	Taper by 5-mg increments per day.
If dose is 20 to 40 mg	Taper by 5-mg increments.
If does is 10 to 20 mg	Taper by 2.5-mg increments.
If does is *less than* 10 mg	Taper by 1-mg increments.

Progressive Systemic Sclerosis (PSS) or Scleroderma

Progressive systemic sclerosis **(PSS)** (also called scleroderma) is characterized by thickening of the skin and degenerative changes to the blood vessels, skeletal muscle, gastrointestinal tract, lungs, heart, and kidneys. PSS is an uncommon disease reported more in women than men and usually diagnosed between ages 30 and 55. Like other inflammatory diseases, activation of the immune system causes pathological endothelial changes in the arteries and capillaries. This autoimmune response results in the widespread vasculopathy and fibrosis that sets PSS apart from other CTD. Although the cause of of PSS is unknown, several potential factors have been investigated. Examples of agents causing scleroderma-like illnesses include: silica dust, urea formaldehyde, vinyl chloride, bleomycin, and L-tryptophan. Other studies noting increased risk of PSS included lifestyle factors, such as smoking, alcohol consumption, pet ownership, and silicone breast implants.[32] Retrospective studies in women with silicon implants have not revealed an increased incidence of PSS; however, this remains a highly litigated area. A potential role between PSS and several known viruses has been suggested including feline sarcoma virus, cytomegaly virus, human immunodeficiency virus, herpes simplex virus I, and Epstein-Barr virus.

Progressive Systemic Sclerosis and Cardiovascular Morbidity

PSS is associated with an increased prevalence of atherosclerosis[33]; however, published research reporting on the relationship between PSS and cardiovascular disease is limited. In one investigation, PSS was characterized by vascular lesions and fibrosis of the pulmonary organs resulting in impaired right ventricular filling. Myocardial fibrosis and coronary vessel involvement are known to affect both left and right ventricles in these patients.[34]

Diagnosis and Clinical Presentation

The hallmark of PSS is scleroderma or skin thickening caused by abnormal accumulation of connective tissue, most commonly noted in the fingers, hands, and face. The disease ranges from the classic presentation of scleroderma only to more severe manifestations involving the organs. The initial symptoms are generally nonspecific and include Raynaud phenomenon, fatigue, and polyarthritis. These symptoms may persist for months. Nearly all patients with PSS have Raynaud phenomenon and sclerodactyly. Raynaud phenomenon is associated with arterial vasospasm of the hands in response to temperature changes or stress.[25] The hands undergo color changes from pale to bluish color and become cold to touch. Raynaud is noted in as many as 15 percent of normal persons; however, it is usually mild and not associated with vascular changes or tissue damage. Skin changes in the fingers or sclerodactyly are the first clue to scleroderma because the skin experiences changes in which it is swollen, shiny, taut, and progressively hardened.

PSS is classified into subsets of disease defined by the degree of involvement, noted as limited, diffuse, and mixed. Limited scleroderma is cutaneous thickening

---

BOX 89-10
OTHER CLINICAL MANIFESTATIONS NOTED IN PROGRESSIVE SYSTEMIC SCLEROSIS

- Carpal tunnel syndrome
- Diverticula and atrophy of large intestine and rectum
- Dry mucous membranes
- Dysphagia
- Generalized edema
- Gastroesophageal reflux disease (GERD)
- Hypomotility of the small intestine
- Hypothyroidism
- Impotence
- Joint stiffness
- Left ventricular or biventricular failure
- Nonmalignant hypertension
- Pericarditis with or without effusion
- Periodontal disease
- Primary myopathy
- Sausaging of the fingers
- Sjögren syndrome
- Small oral aperture (mouth opening)
- Supraventricular tachycardia
- Symmetric polyarthralgias
- Tendon friction rub
- Vaginal dryness and constricted introitus
- Weakness and atrophy of skeletal muscle

---

without involvement of the trunk. CREST syndrome is considered a limited form of scleroderma. CREST syndrome is a mnemonic term used to describe the clinical findings of PSS that includes **c**alcinosis, or hard calcium deposits under the skin; **R**aynaud phenomenon; **E**sophageal involvement; **S**clerodactyly, or skin thickening of the hands only; and **T**elangiectasia, or dilated vessels on the skin of the fingers, face, or inside of the mouth.

Patients with diffuse disease have thickening over the limbs and trunk with severe visceral disease. Diffuse disease is also called systemic sclerosis. Inflammatory signs include edematous skin, arthralgia, tendon friction rubs, and others listed in Box 89-10. This type is associated with a poor prognosis and survival. Almost 80 percent of these patients develop some form of esophageal dysfunction, resulting in complaints from the patient that something is "stuck" in their esophagus. Three out of four patients have lung involvement as a result of fibrosis. Pulmonary arterial hypertension may occur in 25 percent to 50 percent of persons with PSS, and interstitial lung disease may occur in 10 percent of this population.[34] The most common symptom is exertional dyspnea.

Diffuse PSS is manifested by accelerated hypertension and progressive renal failure. Twenty five percent of patients with PSS develop renal crisis (hematuria and proteinuria) followed by oliguric renal failure. Laboratory data will reveal normal to high creatinine levels, anemia, proteinuria, and hematuria (microscopic).

Patchy fibrosis throughout the myocardium is characteristic of PSS. Thallium scintigraphy performed in PSS patients revealed perfusion defects and necrotic bands occurring as a result of vasospasm of distal coronary arteries.[25] Overt signs of any cardiovascular, pulmonary, or renal disease in the patient with PSS are a poor prognostic sign. As a result of damage caused by diffuse systemic sclerosis, lung involvement and renal disease are common comorbidities in this disease; however, cardiovascular disease remains the number one cause of death in PSS

BOX 89-11 ■ ■ ■
LABORATORY FINDINGS IN PROGRESSIVE
SYSTEMIC SCLEROSIS

- Anemia
- Proteinuria
- Hematuria
- Reduced creatinine clearance
- Normal to high serum creatinine level
- Antinuclear antibodies (both limited and diffuse)
- Anticentromere antibody (limited)

BOX 89-12 ■ ■ ■
DERMATOLOGICAL FINDINGS IN DERMATOMYOSITIS

- Gottron papules—scaly, raised, erythematous, nontender lesions, commonly seen on the hands and knees
- Heliotope rash—purplish rash over the eyelids, usually associated with periorbital edema
- Rashes noted in sun-exposed area
- Periungual edema of the nail beds
- Hyperkeratosis and calcinosis of the hands resulting in scaling of the fingers

---

patients.[25] Patients with PSS are usually managed symptomatically. They should be encouraged to stop smoking and take precautions to prevent gastroesophageal reflux. Vasodilating agents including calcium channel blockers and angiotensin-converting enzyme inhibitors are used to prevent Raynaud phenomenon. Corticosteroids are used in limited and diffuse forms of the disease; however, there is evidence that high-dose steroids in PSS also lead to renal failure; thus careful monitoring of patients requiring GCS is a necessity. Penicillamine has also demonstrated clinical improvements in the course of this disease.

Diagnostic Testing

The patient with PSS or scleroderma will most likely show no abnormalities on their hemogram, blood chemistries, or urinalysis. If abnormalities are noted, they will include those listed in Box 89-11. If PSS is being considered based on clinical presentation, the vast majority of PSS patients have ANA positive test results. Anticentromere antibodies are noted in up to 50 percent of limited scleroderma patients, and a small number of patients have anti-RNP antibodies. Pulmonary function tests will be abnormal in 30 percent of diffuse PSS patients.

Polymyositis and Dermatomyositis

Polymyositis and dermatomyositis are idiopathic inflammatory myopathies, characterized by proximal muscle weakness, skeletal muscle damage on biopsy, and elevated concentrations of muscle-derived proteins (e.g., creatine kinase [**CK**]). The cause of these autoimmune diseases remains unknown. Like SLE the incidence is four times greater in blacks than whites, for both sexes. For all ethnicities, it is twice as common in females. Polymyositis is more common in adults, whereas dermatomyositis is more likely to occur in a child or young adult.

Inflammatory Myopathies and Cardiovascular Morbidity

Very little research has been published on patients with myopathy and its influence on cardiovascular morbidity and mortality. Research is needed to evaluate the effects of inflammatory myopathy on the cardiovascular system including interventions to decrease morbidity and autoimmune activity.

Diagnosis and Clinical Presentation

Patients with polymyositis or dermatomyositis usually have fatigue, fever, and myalgia. Complaints of weakness involving the large muscles of the legs and arms causing difficulties with activities of daily living are commonly reported. In moderate cases, skeletal muscle involvement of the head and neck causes neck weakness, pharyngeal dysphagia, and aspiration, whereas more extreme disease involving the respiratory muscles may cause dyspnea, respiratory failure, or even death. More than half of the patients diagnosed with polymyositis will have cardiac involvement manifested as dysrhythmias, electrocardiogram changes, and congestive heart failure.[25] Persistent chronic disease may result in irreversible weakness and muscle loss that causes substantial adverse effects on the person's functional capacities. Young patients with inflammatory myositis and dermatological manifestations are more characteristic of dermatomyositis. More than 70 percent of patients with dermatomyositis will have Gottron papules. These scaly, erythematous lesions are commonly seen over the metacarpals and the knees. Other dermatological manifestations are listed in Box 89-12.

Corticosteroids are the main treatment of polymyositis and dermatomyositis. Patients not responding satisfactorily or requiring high doses of steroids are commonly prescribed methotrexate or azathioprine. Infusions of immunoglobin have also been used successfully to treat polymyositis and dermatomyositis.

Diagnostic Testing

A variety of investigations may be performed to yield useful information including markers for skeletal muscle injury, electromyography, muscle biopsy, autoantibody testing, and acute phase reactants. Increased markers of muscle damage, such as CK, are observed in almost 90 percent of patients with polymyositis and dermatomyositis, making it the most commonly used diagnostic test. Increases in CK within polymyositis and dermatomyositis patients are usually 25 to 50 times normal.[25] Diagnostic findings associated with polymyositis and dermatomyositis are noted in Box 89-13. Recognition and careful management of polymyositis and dermatomyositis is crucial to prevent irreversible muscle damage and disability from chronic inflammation and myositis.

Undifferentiated or Mixed Connective Tissue Disorders

Often patients with undifferentiated connective tissue disorders (**UCTD**) or mixed connective tissue disorders (**MCTD**) have one or more clinical or serological features, but do not fit the clinical criteria for just one of the rheumatic diseases. These conditions are often referred to as overlap syndromes that have clinical and

> **BOX 89-13** ■ ■ ■
> DIAGNOSTIC FINDINGS IN POLYMYOSITIS AND DERMATOMYOSITIS
>
> **Markers of Muscle Damage**
> - Increased creatine kinase
> - Increased aldolase
> - Increased lactate dehydrogenase
> - Increased aspartate aminotransferase
> - Increased alanine transaminase
>
> **Electromyography**
> - Abnormal, low amplitude motor potential
>
> **Muscle Biopsy**
> - Inflammatory cellular infiltrate
> - Perivascular, myofibril necrosis
>
> **Autoantibodies**
> - Positive antinuclear antibodies
> - Positive antisynthetase
>
> **Other**
> - Increased C-reactive protein
> - Increased erythrocyte sedimentation rate

> **BOX 89-15** ■ ■ ■
> TREATING SICCA SYMPTOMS
>
> - Treat dry eyes with lubricating agents, such as eyedrops.
> - Use sugar-free hard candies to treat dry mouth symptoms.
> - Wear eyeglasses to reduce the drying effects of the environment.
> - Referral to ophthalmology is recommended.
> - Dental care is extremely important to prevent dental caries.
> - Use humidifiers to increase moisture.

serological features from a variety of the connective tissue disorders reviewed. Examples include symptoms of a systemic rheumatic disease, such as RA with Sjögren syndrome, RA with SLE symptoms (RHUPUS, in which RHU refers to rheumatoid and PUS refers to lupus), PSS with SLE and polymyositis, primary biliary cirrhosis, or Sjögren syndrome and scleroderma (CREST). These UCTD and MCTD share clinical features as noted in Box 89-14, including Raynaud phenomenon or disease, anemia, interstitial lung disease, polyarthritis, pleuritis, pericarditis, and vasculitis. Patients with UCTD or MCTD should be treated accordingly with NSAIDs, GCS, and other therapies to prevent serious end-organ involvement.

Sjögren Syndrome

Sjögren syndrome is an immune-mediated disorder of the salivary, lacrimal, and other exocrine glands. Sjögren syndrome is classified as primary if symptoms are not associated with any other autoimmune disease and secondary Sjögren if RA, SLE, or PSS are present.

Diagnosis and Clinical Presentation

The most common complaints are keratoconjunctivitis sicca (dry eyes) and xerostomia (dry mouth). Physical exam reveals tenderness and swelling of parotid gland and extremely dry mucous membranes, notably the mouth, throat, vagina, and skin. Extraglandular symptoms include rashes, dysphagia, Raynaud phenomenon,

> **BOX 89-14** ■ ■ ■
> SHARED CLINICAL FEATURES OF CONNECTIVE TISSUE DISEASES
>
> - Raynaud phenomenon
> - Anemia
> - Interstitial lung disease
> - Polyarthritis
> - Pleuritis
> - Pericarditis
> - Vasculitis

arthralgia, and myalgia. Systemic involvement is rare, but can include interstitial pneumonitis, glomerulonephritis, vasculitis, thyroid disease, and neuropathy. Autoantibodies test results are commonly positive in Sjögren syndrome patients. ANA titers positive for anti-SS-A and anti-SS-B antibodies provides evidence of a systemic autoimmune response. Although sicca symptoms are found in patients with depression or fibromyalgia, these patients usually lack autoantibodies and do not progress to an autoimmune process.[35] Sicca symptoms are managed using the guidelines in Box 89-15. Corticosteroids should be avoided unless vasculitis, pleuropericarditis, or hemolytic anemia occurs.

TREATMENT OF CONNECTIVE TISSUE DISEASES

Treatment of rheumatic diseases first requires a thorough history and physical examination including joint assessment, medication history, pain assessment, morning stiffness assessment, assessment of functional capacity, and clinically indicated laboratory tests.[32] Serious evaluation of patient complaints by the primary care provider coupled with collaboration and referral to a rheumatological specialist may assist with early identification and treatment of rheumatic diseases. It is imperative that connective tissue disorders be identified and treated with an aggressive approach to prevent joint damage, deformities, vascular complications, and functional limitations.

Treatment of various rheumatic conditions depends on the diagnosis, the severity of the disease, and the response to therapy by the patient. The steps after establishing the diagnosis include (1) evaluating and initiating treatment; (2) monitoring clinical status and response to therapy including complications and toxicity; (3) modifying therapy for inadequate efficacy, toxicity, or acceptable response; and (4) rehabilitation. In some diseases, beneficial effects of drugs may be modest; therefore nondrug therapies also play an important role in the treatment of rheumatic diseases. Nondrug modalities frequently used in the treatment of arthralgia and/or myalgia and functional impairments are noted in Box 89-16 and Box 89-17.

Pharmaceutical treatments frequently employed in rheumatic diseases are noted in the accompanying Pharmacology feature. These agents are usually employed to relieve pain and stiffness, prevent progression of the disease, maintain or restore function, and improve the quality of life. Medications that relieve pain and inflammation include NSAIDs and cyclooxygenase-2 (COX-2) inhibitors. COX-2 inhibitors are a selective NSAID that

PHARMACOLOGICAL AND BIOLOGICAL AGENTS USED IN TREATING RHEUMATIC DISEASES

DRUG/DRUG CLASS	MECHANISM OF ACTION	POTENTIAL ADVERSE EFFECTS	CLINICAL IMPLICATIONS
NSAIDs Aspirin, diclofenac, fenoprofen, ibuprofen, indomethacin, ketoprofen, meclofenamate, meloxicam, nabumetone, naproxen, piroxicam, sulindac	Inhibit prostaglandin by blocking cyclooxygenase produced in the setting of inflammation.	Increased GI symptoms Monitor for fluid retention/HTN. Decreased creatinine clearance Monitor for liver inflammation. Increased liver enzymes Monitor for hematological toxicity including agranulocytosis, anemia, leukopenia, and thrombocytopenia. Interacts with anticoagulants, other NSAIDs, MTX, diuretics, lithium	Suppresses inflammation, pain, and fever. Monitor CBC and LFTs during therapy. Use with caution in patients with heart and renal failure. May cause NSAID-associated gastric ulcer.
COX-2 inhibitors Celecoxib, rofecoxib, valdecoxib	Block COX-2 produced in the setting of inflammation.	Less gastric irritation than NSAIDs Monitor for fluid retention/HTN. Decreased creatinine clearance Monitor for liver inflammation. Increased liver enzymes Monitor for hematological toxicity, including agranulocytosis, anemia, leukopenia, and thrombocytopenia. Interacts with anticoagulants, other NSAIDs, MTX, diuretics, lithium	Suppresses inflammation, pain, and fever. Monitor CBC and LFTs while on therapy. Use cautiously in patients with heart or renal failure. Less GI toxicity than NSAIDs
Glucocorticosteroids Dexamethasone, methylprednisolone, prednisone, solu-Cortef, soluMedrol	Glucocorticoid with wide range of effects on inflammatory cells, their migration, and the production of inflammatory mediators Used in RA, SLE, PM, DM, and PsA.	Toxic side effects include worsening diabetes, HTN, infections, peptic ulcer, fractures, and cirrhosis. Monitor for adrenal insufficiency with prolonged therapy and abrupt withdraw. Leukocytosis and neutrophilia occur with administration. Other common side effects include hypokalemia, bruising, moodiness, insomnia, and skin fragility. Drug interactions include hepatic enzyme inducers, such as rifampin, phenytoin, and diuretics.	Powerful antiinflammatory that improves function and controls acute inflammation Short courses of 20 mg/d recommended with tapering off over several days. Adverse events are usually related to dose/length of therapy. Monitor potassium, glucose, and BMD with chronic use.
DMARDs Azathioprine	Antimetabolite, immunosuppressive agent that acts as a purine antagonist. The active metabolite is 6-mercaptopurine that interferes with DNA synthesis. Used in refractory RA, SLE, DM, PM as a steroid sparing agent to decrease prolonged high doses in a variety of autoimmune diseases.	Suppresses bone marrow and increases infections. Monitor CBC, especially platelets and LFTs. Increases risk of malignancy. Common side effects; GI symptoms, fever, chills, thrombocytopenia, leukopenia Less common side effects include stomatitis, rashes, hepatotoxicity, pneumonitis, and herpes zoster. Avoid in pregnancy. Drug interactions with allopurinol, other immunosuppressants, and live vaccines	Used in refractory RA. Is safe and effective. Mostly replaced by MTX. Use with caution in renal disease or liver impairment. Avoid live vaccines. Patient should report persistent sore throat, unusual bleeding, bruising, and fatigue.
Cyclophosphamide	Antineoplastic, alkylating agent interferes with DNA synthesis by alkylating and cross-linking DNA strands. Used in vasculitis, PSS, RA, vasculitis, PM/DM, SLE, and RA. Frequent monitoring of CBC, especially platelets and WBCs	Side effects include myelosuppression, infections, gastrointestinal symptoms, rashes, and fluid retention. Pretreat for nausea and hypersensitivity. Consider using Mesna to reduce hemorrhagic cystitis. Toxic side effects include thrombocytopenia, leukopenia, stomatitis, pulmonary fibrosis. May cause permanent sterility. Increases potential for malignancies.	Causes depletion of B cells and T cells in lymphoid tissue. Alkylating agents appear to be overall immunosuppressive and anti-inflammatory. May boost immune system by inhibiting suppressor cells. Reduction of dose and use of intermittent dosing may decrease side effects. Monitor for opportunistic infections. Hydration during/after administration extremely important to prevent cystitis.

AS, Ankylosing spondylitis; ASA, acetylsalicylic acid; BP, blood pressure; CBC, complete blood count; CDC, Centers for Disease Control and Prevention; COX-2, cyclooxygenase-2; CXR, chest x-ray; DM, dermatomyositis; DMARD, disease-modifying antirheumatic drug; DNA, deoxyribonucleic acid; GCS, glucocorticosteroids; GI, gastrointestinal; HA, headache; HIV, human immunodeficiency virus; HTN, hypertension; HX, history; IBD, inflammatory bowel disease; IL, interleukin; JRA, juvenile rheumatoid arthritis isoniazid; LFTs, liver function tests; MS, multiple sclerosis; MTX, methotrexate; NSAID, nonsteroidal antiinflammatory drug; PM, polymyositis; PsA, psoritic arthritis; PSS, progressive systemic sclerosis; RA, rheumatoid arthritis; SLE, systemic lupus erythematosus; TB, tuberculosis; TNF, tumor necrosis factor; WBCs, white blood cells.

■■■ PHARMACOLOGY

PHARMACOLOGICAL AND BIOLOGICAL AGENTS USED IN TREATING RHEUMATIC DISEASES—cont'd

DRUG/DRUG CLASS	MECHANISM OF ACTION	POTENTIAL ADVERSE EFFECTS	CLINICAL IMPLICATIONS
Cyclosporine	An immunosuppressant that inhibits production of IL-2, an immunomodulator Used in RA, psoriasis, PsA, SLE, and PM.	Avoid use in immunosuppression, past or present malignancy, renal or hepatic dysfunction, or uncontrolled hypertension. Common side effects include hypertension, nausea, cramps, hyperkalemia, hypomagnesemia, hyperuricemia, HA. Drug interactions with grapefruit juice, antibiotics, antivirals, rifampin, phenytoin, INH, potassium-sparing diuretics, lovastatin, and nephrotoxic drugs.	Indicated for refractory RA Monitor BP & chemistries including creatinine at start. Use with caution in renal failure. Decrease or stop with elevations of creatinine.
Hydroxychloroquine	Antimalarial that interacts with the macrophage, antigen, and T cell to modify inflammation in RA, SLE, and PsA	May lead to retinal problems. Annual eye exam recommended. Side effects include GI irritation, HA, rashes, blurred vision. Less common side effects are irreversible retinal toxicity, ototoxicity, blood dyscrasias, and hypersensitivity. Drug interactions with penicillamine	Single agent used for mild or early disease or combined with other agents for more severe disease. Use with caution in hepatic disease, and psoriasis. May worsen psoriasis, but is used to treat PsA.
Leflunomide	Inhibits pyrimidine and tyrosine kinase using dihydroorotate dehydrogenase causing inhibition of activated T cells. Used in RA.	Monitor CBC and LFTs. Avoid in pregnancy and liver disease. Most common side effects include diarrhea, nausea, rash, and alopecia.	Efficacy is similar to MTX. Is a suitable replacement for those intolerant to MTX or who have failed it. Use with caution in liver failure.
MTX	Antimetabolite, cytotoxic, antiinflammatory DMARD that inhibits dihydrofolate reductase resulting in inhibition of folic acid metabolism Used in RA, JRA, PsA, SLE, PM and vasculitis.	Avoid in liver disease, alcoholism, pregnancy, renal impairment, HIV, severe hepatitis, and marked leukopenia. Monitor CBC, platelets, LFTs, chemistries, and CXR. May cause pneumonitis. May cause mouth sores and folate deficiency. Other side effects include nausea, diarrhea, fatigue, hair loss, impotence, osteoporosis, increased risk of infection, leucopenia, and increased uric acid level. Drug interactions with other immunosuppressants, NSAIDs, probenecid, trimethoprim-sulfamethoxazole.	Slows radiographic progression and damage in RA. Used alone or in combination. Dose reduction is necessary for increases in LFTs and pneumonitis. Review HX for other hepatotoxic agents. Supplement folate 1mg/d. MTX is used as a steroid-sparing therapy. MTX may be given orally, or parenterally. Injectable form may be used orally if cost is an issue. May cause photosensitivity; encourage use of sunscreen. Most studied DMARD
Penicillamine	Chelating agent with unknown DMARD action, but thought to inhibit T-cell function Used in RA, scleroderma, and primary biliary cirrhosis.	Monitor CBC and urinalysis for protein. Common side effects include rashes, pruritis, metallic taste, proteinuria. Rare side effects include hematologic toxicity including agranulocytosis, thrombocytopenia, aplastic anemia, leukopenia. Avoid in pregnancy. Drug interactions include antacids, iron supplements, and food.	Has largely been replaced by MTX, but still used by those not able to tolerate MTX. Take on an empty stomach. Penicillamine is associated with a high frequency of side effects.
Sulfasalazine	Sulfa and aspirin combination known as a sulfonamide with an unknown mechanism of action Used with RA, JRA, AS, PsA, and IBD.	Avoid in patients with sulfa or ASA allergy. Monitor CBC and LFTs initially. May cause hemolysis with G6PD deficiency. Side effects include GI effects (nausea, vomiting, diarrhea, cramps) rashes, pruritis, dizziness, HA. Toxic side effects include anemia, Stevens-Johnson syndrome, SLE-like syndrome, nephrotic syndrome, neutropenia, agranulocytosis. May cause folate deficiency. Drug interactions with warfarin and MTX.	Efficacy appears similar to MTX with more minor side effects and less serious ones. Use with caution in renal dysfunction. GI symptoms are usually prominent at the start and with high doses. Used as a single DMARD or in combination with MTX and hydroxychloroquine. Supplement folate 1 mg/day.

Continued

▪▪▪ PHARMACOLOGY

PHARMACOLOGICAL AND BIOLOGICAL AGENTS USED IN TREATING RHEUMATIC DISEASES—cont'd

DRUG/DRUG CLASS	MECHANISM OF ACTION	POTENTIAL ADVERSE EFFECTS	CLINICAL IMPLICATIONS
Biological Modifying DMARDS			
Etanercept	Biological response modifier A fusion protein that forms immunoglobin that decoys TNF-alpha from binding to cellular receptors Used in RA, PsA, psoriasis, JRA, AS, and IBD.	Increased risk of infection Monitor CBC and TB test Common side effects include chills, cough, fever, sneezing. Less common include chest congestion, depression, tachycardia, swelling. Most common complaint is site reactions.	Clinical improvement over that of MTX alone. Usually employed in MTX failure. Patient gives self subcutaneous injection. Avoid live vaccines. Hold treatment with antibiotics.
Adalimumab	First human anti-TNF-alpha monoclonal antibody (IgG) Used in RA, PsA, AS.	Monitor for infections including TB, fungal infections, and invasive opportunistic infections. May be associated with an increased risk for demyelinating diseases and malignancies. Common side effects include chills, cough, fever, sneezing.	Clinical response similar to that of etanercept. Reduces symptoms of RA and progression of structural damage for those who have had an insufficient response to one or more DMARDS. Monitor CBC and TB test.
Infliximab	Chimeric, monoclonal molecule It is an antibody to TNF-alpha. It binds TNF in the blood or as it attaches to its cellular receptor. Used in RA, IBD, PsA, AS.	Increased incidence of *Mycobacterium tuberculosis* in patients receiving infliximab. Monitor CBC, chemistries routinely. May be associated with an increased risk for demyelinating diseases (MS) and malignancies (lymphoma). Monitor for hives, back pain, and flushing during infusions. Anaphylaxis occurs rarely.	Infliximab results in clinical improvement and halts erosions and joint space improvement. Drug given as an IV infusion. Evaluate patient for exposure to TB. If positive TB, perform CXR and treat prophylactically for TB according to CDC guidelines. Pretreatment may be necessary with GCS and antihistamine before infusions. Hold treatment with antibiotics.
Anakinra	A recombinant form of human IL-1 receptor antagonist used to inhibit inflammation Used in RA.	Monitor CBC for toxicity. Most common side effects was injection site reactions and increased infections.	Used for moderate to severe RA who have failed one or more DMARDs or biologics. Given by patient as a daily subcutaneous injection. Hold treatment with antibiotics.

ABX, Antibiotics; *CBC,* complete blood count; *CDC,* Centers for Disease Control and Prevention; *CXR,* chest X-ray; *DM,* dermatomyositis; *DMARD,* disease-modifying antirheumatic drug; *GCS,* glucocorticosteroids; *GI,* gastrointestinal; *HA,* headache; *HTN,* hypertension; *LFTs,* liver function tests; *NSAID,* nonsteroidal antiinflammatory drug; *PM,* polymyositis; *RA,* rheumatoid arthritis; *SQ,* subcutaneously; *TB,* tuberculosis.

BOX 89-16 ▪▪▪
MODALITIES USED IN THE TREATMENT OF PAIN AND MUSCLE SPASM

- Heat
- Hydrotherapy
- Electrotherapy using transcutaneous nerve stimulation (TENS)
- Cryotherapy
- Traction
- Manipulation of contractures
- Acupuncture

BOX 89-17 ▪▪▪
TREATMENT OF PHYSICAL IMPAIRMENTS

- Rest can reduce inflammation and pain and should be used in the acute phase of inflammation causing pain.
- Exercise with short periods of rest has demonstrated preserved joint motion, strength, endurance, and promotion of a sense of well-being.
- Stretching improves range of motion and prevents contractures.
- Splinting and positioning may be necessary to restore function, reduce pain, and rest the joint.

---

blocks only COX-2 while preserving the protective COX-1 enzyme. These agents were developed to decrease pain and inflammation while also decreasing the gastrointestinal toxicity associated with the nonselective NSAIDs. They are beneficial in the rheumatic diseases because they reduce pain; however, they do not alter disease progression and are therefore a symptomatic

treatment only. Patients may also be prescribed narcotic and nonnarcotic analgesics for severe pain.

An acute inflammatory response will likely be treated with a steroid preparation. Corticosteroids have broad spectrum antiinflammatory effects that reduce symptoms associated with RA, SLE, polymyositis or dermatomyositis, PSS, and MCTD. A higher dose is used for acute inflammation or "flares" and then tapered off. However, some patients may require daily oral low-dose prednisone (*less than* 10 mg/d) or an intraarticular injection for more local inflammatory processes. When these fail or higher doses are required, more aggressive therapies, including investigational ones, are necessary to prevent damage in these chronic, progressive diseases.

DMARDs are used early in the patient with aggressive disease. Most of these medications are given for their ability to alter the progression of the disease and thus decrease the symptoms. When a single agent fails, combinations of DMARDs are useful in the patient's treatment to enhance efficacy and reduce toxicity. Eventually, all patients experience difficulty with sustained efficacy even when the various agents are used in combination to treat their disease. Several experimental therapies involving inflammatory cytokines have shown promise in clinical trials. Marketed biological DMARDs, such as adalimumab, etanercept, and infliximab, have consistently improved disease outcomes and reduced progression of diseases, such as RA, in clinical trials and report relatively good safety profiles in these patients. The recent encouraging results from these clinical trials using TNF-alpha inhibitors in RA have prompted the study of other cellular targets and cytokines including B cells, T cells, metaproteinase inhibitors, adhesion molecules, interleukins, anti-campath-1H, anti-CD7 mab, and anti-CD4 in other autoimmune diseases. Gene therapy may be another approach to treating autoimmune disorders and requires further study.

Treatment of RA has significantly improved with new therapies for patients who have either not responded to conventional therapies (e.g., MTX) or who do not continue to achieve a beneficial effect. These same therapies are being investigated in other CTD with hopes of altering the progression of structural damage and impaired quality of life that typically evolves from these diseases. Although most experts have not agreed on how patients will advance from simple therapies to aggressive treatments in the management of their disease, the ultimate goal of treatment is clinical remission. Progressive diseases like these warrant the use of aggressive therapies that produce the greatest clinical impact.[36] All practitioners providing treatment of rheumatic diseases, such as RA, should consider the goals noted in Box 89-18.

Ongoing treatment consists of rehabilitation, monitoring drug therapy, and responding to adverse events. Rehabilitation is the process that spans from the prevention of disability to the integration of the disabled person into society.[37] Known risk factors for increased disability are listed in Table 89-3. Assessment of physical impairment includes joint and musculoskeletal examination and evaluation of functional limitations. General guidelines for reducing functional impairments are listed in Box 89-19.

Disease modification rather than symptom control is desired as a final treatment outcome. Just as important is treatment that decreases disease progression, but that is also tolerable to the patient. In fact, suppression of disease activity with single agents has been challenging and difficult to sustain.[20] Patients should be periodically reassessed for evidence of disease progression and for any toxic effects of treatment.[36] A common list of ICD-9 codes for rheumatic diseases is noted in Box 89-20.

■ ■ ■

TABLE 89-3   RISK FACTORS FOR DISABILITY

RISK FACTOR	EFFECT
Socioeconomic	Morbidity and mortality are increased among the poor and uneducated.
Marital status	Unmarried are at higher risk for disability.
Social support	Morbidity and morality are increased among those with poor social support.
Lifestyle factors	Increased age, low education, and lower socioeconomic status are risk factors for disability.
	Increased body mass index is associated with increased disability.
Health care factors	Availability of health care, presence, and type of insurance has an effect on disability.
Functional factors	The level of functional capacity is highly predictive of disability.

BOX 89-19   ■ ■ ■
WAYS OF REDUCING FUNCTIONAL LIMITATIONS

- Improve ambulation and gait training
- Improving awareness of and prevention of falls
- Use of adaptive aids and self-care devices
- Increasing exercise and recreational activities
- Referral to pain management centers
- Appropriate counseling for sexual problems

BOX 89-18   ■ ■ ■
GOALS FOR MANAGING AUTOIMMUNE DISEASES, SUCH AS RHEUMATOID ARTHRITIS

- Arrest disease progression with a treatment goal of complete remission.
- Eliminate pain and swelling.
- Maximize the quality of life for your patient.
- Prevent loss of function and disability.
- Prevent or control joint damage.

American College of Rheumatology subcommittee on rheumatoid arthritis guidelines. Guidelines for the management of rheumatoid arthritis, *Arthritis Rheum* 46:328-346, 2002.

BOX 89-20   ■ ■ ■
ICD9 CODES

DISEASE	CODES
Dermatomyositis	710.3
Discoid lupus	695.4
Drug-induced SLE	695.4
Lupus coagulant	286.5
MCTD	710.8
Polymyositis	710.4
PSS or scleroderma	710.1
RA nodules	729.89
RA vasculitis	447.6
RA	714.0
Raynaud disease	443.0
Sjögren syndrome	710.2
SLE nephritis	583.81
SLE	710.0

MCTD, Mixed connective tissue disorders; *PSS*, progressive systemic sclerosis; *RA*, rheumatoid arthritis; *SLE*, systemic lupus erythematosus.

SUMMARY: AUTOIMMUNE DISEASES AND CARDIOVASCULAR MORBIDITY

Cardiovascular disease is the leading cause of death in the United States and the most common cause of death in persons with RA and SLE. There are many similarities between the pathological conditions of autoimmune diseases and the cardiovascular system, and yet traditional cardiovascular risk factors do not predict all the risk of cardiovascular morbidity and mortality in patients with autoimmune diseases, such as RA and SLE, compared with those without these diseases. It is likely that the pathological conditions of these diseases contribute to the development of early atherosclerosis and enhance the morbidity of those with a history of CHD. Atherosclerosis is an inflammatory process with abnormalities similar to other inflammatory conditions. Atherosclerosis and RA have shared immunological features involving inflammatory cytokines, T cells, and macrophages.[38] The inflammatory response associated with autoimmune diseases is likely to predispose the heart, in particular to increased damage. Cytokines associated with increased heart disease include TNF-alpha, IL-1ß, IL-18, and IL-4. These have been known to contribute to heart failure.[13] Cytokines may influence or mediate cardiac remodeling. Cytokines produced endogenously that reduce inflammatory disease include interferon alpha and IL-12. Research is ongoing to determine how these factors affect disease activity in these patients.

Epidemiological studies on cardiovascular disease have highlighted several novel cardiovascular risk factors including homocysteine, thrombotic markers, insulin resistance, and markers of inflammation.[39] Similarly, RA patients have abnormal homocysteine metabolism including that resulting from methotrexate use,[39] although supplementing folic acid is a preventative measure for hyperhomocysteinemia. Thrombotic markers and proatherosclerotic factors are present in RA and SLE. These factors promote changes in the endothelium including atherosclerotic changes from the systemic effects of inflammation and influences from increased markers present in the blood during enhanced disease activity.

Increased markers of inflammation are associated with dyslipidemia and hypercholesteremia. Some experts have proposed that statin therapy including inhibitors of 3-hydroxy-3-methylglutaryl coenzyme A (HMG-CoA) reductase might be of benefit to patients with autoimmune diseases, such as A or SLE. Statins have been used to lower serum lipid levels, specifically LDL cholesterol. Statins are proposed to modulate the inflammatory component of autoimmune diseases; clearly, more clinical trials are needed to evaluate this therapy in RA and SLE.[40] Ongoing research is needed to evaluate the benefits of these agents in reducing cardiovascular morbidity and autoimmune activity.

REFERENCES

1. Wolfe F, Michaud K: Heart failure in rheumatoid arthritis: rates, predictors, and the effect of anti-tumor necrosis factor therapy, *Am J Med* 116:305-311, 2004.
2. DeMaria A: Relative risk of cardiovascular events in patients with rheumatoid arthritis, *Am J Cardiol* 89(suppl):33D-38D, 2002.
3. Wang L, Feng G: Rheumatoid arthritis increases the risk of coronary heart disease via vascular endothelial injury, *Medical Hypotheses* 63:442-445, 2004.
4. Bijil M: Endothelial activation, endothelial dysfunction and premature atherosclerosis in systemic autoimmune diseases, *Netherland J Med* 61(9):273-277, 2003.
5. Patrick L, Uzick M: Cardiovascular disease: C reactive protein and the inflammatory disease paradigm: HMG-CoA reductase inhibitors, alpha-tocopherol, red yeast rice, and olive oil polyphenols. A review of the literature, *Alternat Med Rev* 6:248-271, 2001.
6. Park Y et al: Effects of antirheumatic therapy on serum lipid levels in patients with rheumatoid arthritis: a prospective study, *Am J Med* 113:188-193, 2002.
7. Popa C et al: Influence of anti-tumor necrosis factor therapy on cardiovascular risk factors in patients with active rheumatoid arthritis, *Ann Rheum Dis* 64:303-305, 2005.
8. van Ede A et al: Homocysteine and folate status in methotrexate treated patients with rheumatoid arthritis, *Rheumatology* 41:658-665, 2002.
9. Wolfe F, Freundlich B, Rimm E: Increase in cardiovascular and cerebrovascular disease prevalence in rheumatoid arthritis, *J Rheumatol* 30:36-40, 2003.
10. Soloman D et al: Cardiovascular morbidity and mortality in women diagnosed with rheumatoid arthritis, *Circulation* 107:1303-1307, 2003.
11. Maradit-Hremers H et al: Cardiovascular death in rheumatoid arthritis: a population based study, *Arthrit Rheumat* 52:722-732, 2005.
12. Felson D: Epidemiology of the rheumatic diseases. In Koopman W, editor: *Arthritis and allied conditions: a textbook of rheumatology*, Philadelphia, 1997, Williams and Wilkins, pp 3-34.
13. Fairweather D, Rose N: Inflammatory disease; a role for cytokines, *Lupus* 14:646-651, 2005.
14. del Rincon I et al: Relative contribution of cardiovascular risk factors and rheumatoid arthritis clinical manifestations to atherosclerosis, *Arthritis and Rheumatism* 52:3413-3423, 2005.
15. Hurlimann D, Enseleit F, Ruschitzka F: Rheumatoid arthritis, inflammation and atherosclerosis, *Herz* 29:760-768, 2004.
16. Warrington K et al: Rheumatoid arthritis is an independent risk factor for multi-vessel coronary artery disease: a case control study, *Arthritis Research and Therapy* 7:R984-991, 2005.
17. Maradit-Hremers H et al: Cardiovascular death in rheumatoid arthritis: a population based study, *Arthrit Rheumat* 52:722-732, 2005.
18. del Rincon I et al: Effect of glucocorticoids on the arteries in rheumatoid arthritis, *Arthritis and Rheumatism* 50:3813-3822, 2004.
19. Jacobsen S et al: Treatment with tumor necrosis factor blockers is associated with a lower incidence of first cardiovascular events in patients with rheumatoid arthritis, *J Rheumatol* 32:1213-1218, 2005.
20. Madhok R, Capell H: Outstanding issues in use of disease modifying agents in RA, *Lancet* 353:257-259, 1999.
21. Crowson C et al: How much of the increased incidence of heart failure in rheumatoid arthritis is attributable to traditional cardiovascular risk factors and ischemic heart disease? *Arthritis and Rheumatism* 52:3039-3044, 2005.
22. Haque S, Bruce I: Therapy insight: systemic lupus erythematosus as a risk factor for cardiovascular disease, *Nat Clin Pract Cardiovasc Med* 2:423-430, 2005.
23. Arnett F et al: The American Rheumatism Association 1987 revised criteria for the classification of rheumatoid arthritis, *Arthritis and Rheumatism* 31:315-324, 1988.
24. Emery P, Breedveld F, Dougados M: Early referral recommendation for newly diagnosed rheumatoid arthritis; evidence based development of a clinical guide, *Ann Rheum Dis* 61:290-297, 2002.
25. Cush J et al: *Rheumatology: diagnosis and therapeutics*, Philadelphia, 2000, Lippincott Williams & Wilkins.
26. Dessein P, Joffe B, Singh S: Biomarkers of endothelial dysfunction, cardiovascular risk factors and atherosclerosis in rheumatoid arthritis, *Arthritis Research and Therapy* 7:R634-643, 2005.

27. Bessant R et al: Risk of coronary heart disease and stroke in large British cohort of patients with systemic lupus erythematosus, *Rheumatology* 43:924-929, 2004.

28. Doherty N, Siegel R: Cardiovascular manifestations of systemic lupus erythematosus, *Am Heart J* 110:1257-1265, 1985.

29. Al-Herz A et al: Cardiovascular risk factor screening in systemic lupus erythematosus, *J Rheumatol* 30:493-496, 2003.

30. Thomas G et al: Accelerated atherosclerosis in patients with systemic lupus erythematosus: a review of the causes and possible prevention, *Hong Kong Med J* 8(1):26-32, 2002.

31. Wallace D, Metzer A: Systemic lupus erythematosus: clinical aspects and treatment. In Koopman W, editor: *Arthritis and allied conditions: a textbook of rheumatology,* Philadelphia, 1997, Williams and Wilkins, pp 3-34.

32. Anderson R: Clinical and laboratory features. In Klippel J, editor: *Primer on rheumatic diseases,* Atlanta, 1997, Official publication of the Arthritis Foundation.

33. Palmer C et al: Association of common variation in glutathione S transferase genes with premature development of cardiovascular disease in patients with systemic sclerosis, *Arthritis and Rheumatism* 48(3):854-855, 2003.

34. Guinta A et al: Right ventricular diastolic abnormalities in systemic sclerosis. Relation to left ventricular involvement and pulmonary hypertension, *Ann Rheum Dis* 59:94-98, 2000.

35. Fox R: Clinical features, pathogenesis and treatment of Sjögren's syndrome, *Curr Opin Rheumatol* 8:438-445, 1996.

36. American College of Rheumatology Subcommittee on rheumatoid arthritis guidelines. Guidelines for the management of rheumatoid arthritis, *Arthritis Rheum* 46:328-346, 2002.

37. Straaton K, Sandoval D: Rehabilitation in the rheumatic diseases. In Koopman W, editor: *Arthritis and allied conditions: a textbook of rheumatology,* Philadelphia, 1997, Williams and Wilkins, pp 3-34.

38. Wasko MC: Comorbid conditions in patients with rheumatoid diseases: an update, *Curr Opin Rheumatol* 16:109-113, 2004.

39. Gerli R, Goodson J: Cardiovascular involvement in rheumatoid arthritis, *Lupus* 14:679-682, 2005.

40. Jury E, Ehrenstein M: Statins: immunomodulators for autoimmune rheumatic disease, *Lupus* 14:192-196, 2005.

chapter 90

The Cardiovascular System and Pregnancy

Jerome Yankowitz
Kristi Borowski

CHAPTER ABBREVIATIONS

ACC American College of Cardiology

AHA American Heart Association

AMI acute myocardial infarction

BP blood pressure

CO cardiac output

CPR cardiopulmonary resuscitation

HR heart rate

IUGR intrauterine growth retardation

SV stroke volume

The cardiovascular system adapts to pregnancy via multiple mechanisms. Cardiovascular changes are seen in all pregnancies. These changes alter physical exam findings, cardiovascular testing, and pharmacotherapy for cardiovascular disease in pregnancy. Pregnancy is a unique situation in that there are two patients to consider with all treatments and testing.

CARDIOVASCULAR ADAPTATION TO PREGNANCY
Hematological Changes

Maternal blood volume undergoes marked expansion throughout pregnancy. These increases are first appreciated in the first trimester, at approximately 6 weeks of gestation, increase significantly in the second trimester and less dramatically in the third trimester.[1] The average expansion of the blood volume during pregnancy is 40 percent to 50 percent.[1] The increase in blood volume results from increases in both the plasma volume and the red blood cell volume. The plasma volume increase is *greater than* the red cell volume, leading to a reduction in hematocrit and physiological hemodilution noted especially in the early third trimester (Figure 90-1).[2] Hemoglobin concentrations at term average 12.5 g/dl and throughout pregnancy remain above 11 g/dl in normal iron-supplemented pregnant women.[3] The World Health Organization defines anemia in pregnancy as *less than* 11 g/dl, and the Centers for Disease Control defines it as *less than* 11 g/dl in the first and third trimesters and *less than* 10.5 g/dl in the second trimester.[3,4] Approximately 50 percent of pregnant women could be described as anemic at some point in their pregnancy.[3] By approximately 6 weeks postpartum, the hemoglobin and hematocrit return to normal unless excessive bleeding has occurred during delivery or in the puerperium.

The average blood loss from a vaginal delivery of a term infant is 500 ml and from an uncomplicated cesarean section is 1000 ml.[1] The increase in blood volume throughout pregnancy and the physiological anemia of pregnancy play a role in protecting the parturient from hemorrhage associated with delivery and the puerperium. The decreased viscosity of the blood caused by the exaggerated plasma volume expansion may facilitate uteroplacental perfusion as a result of reduced vascular resistance as well.

Cardiovascular Changes

Pregnancy produces profound changes in the cardiovascular system. Cardiac output **(CO)** is noted to rise during pregnancy an average of 30 percent to 50 percent.[5] In a longitudinal study, 21 percent of the total increase in CO of pregnancy was noted by 5 weeks of gestation.[6] In a review of 33 cross-sectional and 19 longitudinal studies on CO in pregnancy, CO was noted to be highest in the second trimester.[5] CO is the product of stroke volume **(SV)** and heart rate **(HR).** It appears that in early pregnancy the increase in CO is due to increased SV, whereas late pregnancy is more dependent on increased HR.[6,7] HR is not noted to significantly increase until after 16 weeks of gestation.[7] The average increase in HR during pregnancy is 15 beats/min (Table 90-1).

Position also appears to play a role in CO, especially in late pregnancy. CO decreases by as much as 30 percent with maternal change from the left lateral recumbent position to the supine position.[2] This can be explained by compression or near occlusion of the inferior vena cava by the gravid uterus in the supine position in late pregnancy. Compression of the inferior vena cava can significantly decrease preload and in some women lead to supine hypotensive syndrome manifested by maternal hypotension, tachycardia, syncope, nausea, visual disturbances, paresthesias, pallor, and cyanosis.[8]

Blood pressure **(BP)** is the product of CO and systemic vascular resistance. BP decreases during pregnancy. The decline in systemic BP mimics the simultaneous decline in systemic vascular resistance, despite the increased CO. The cause of the decrease in systemic vascular resistance is not known, but proposed mechanisms include vasodilatory effects of progesterone and decreased responsiveness to pressors.

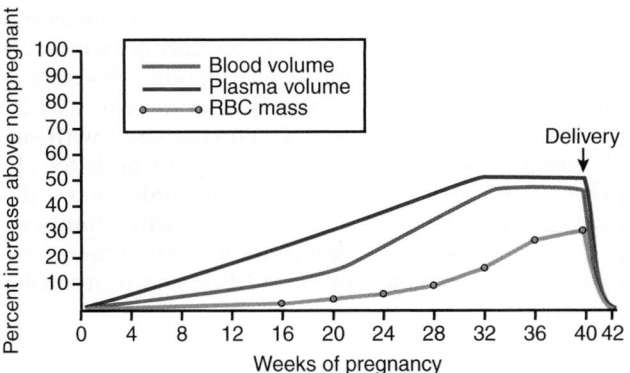

FIGURE 90-1 ■ Changes in blood volume in pregnancy. (From Scott DE: Anemia in pregnancy, *Obstet Gynecol Annu* 1:219-244, 1972.) *RBC,* Red blood cell.

■ ■ ■

TABLE 90-1   CARDIOVASCULAR CHANGES
AND PREGNANCY

	FIRST TRIMESTER	SECOND TRIMESTER	THIRD TRIMESTER	POSTPARTUM
BP	Unchanged	Decreased	Minimally increased	Unchanged
CO	Moderately increased	Unchanged	Unchanged	Decreased
HR	Minimally increased	Unchanged	Minimally increased	Decreased

Coagulation Changes

Pregnancy is a hypercoagulable state as a result of both venous stasis and alterations in the coagulation cascade proteins.[9] Compression from a gravid uterus leads to venous stasis. Changes in coagulation proteins during pregnancy produce a procoagulant state. Increases in factors II, VII, VIII, X, and XII are seen in normal pregnancy in conjunction with a decrease in protein S, an anticoagulant.[10]

In addition to the venous stasis and changes in coagulation proteins, pregnancy is occasionally associated with prolonged bed rest, surgery, and infection. These factors may play a role in clot formation as well. Venous thromboembolism has been reported in 1 in 1000 to 2000 pregnancies.[11] The risk of venous thromboembolism was eightfold greater in pregnant women with an established deficiency of antithrombin, protein C, or protein S.[12] In a study of pregnant women with venous thromboembolism, the controls were tested and 7.7 percent were found to have factor V Leiden, whereas 1.3 percent had prothrombin G20210A, both common inherited thrombophilias.[13]

Screening for inherited and acquired (antiphospholipid antibodies) thrombophilia has been recommended for all patients with a history of venous thromboembolism, fetal loss *greater than* 10 weeks, placental abruption, severe preeclampsia, and severe intrauterine growth retardation **(IUGR)**.[14] Anticoagulation in pregnancy is recommended for women with venous thromboembolism history and known inherited thrombophilia. The benefit of anticoagulation in women with

prior venous thromboembolism and a nonrecurring risk factor without inherited thrombophilia, in addition to in asymptomatic patients with known inherited thrombophilia, has been questioned. Recent evidence suggests that maternal heterozygous carriage of factor V Leiden mutation is associated with a low risk of venous thromboembolism, and thus universal screening or treatment in pregnancy is not warranted for women with no other adverse history.[15]

LABOR AND DELIVERY HEMODYNAMICS

There is a superimposed increase in CO in labor over that of pregnancy. Uterine contractions lead to increases in CO because of the autotransfusion of 300 to 500 ml of blood into maternal circulation with each contraction. Position changes from the supine to the left lateral recumbent also lead to increased CO in labor. Pain associated with labor and the exertion of labor can both lead to increased CO as well. With epidural anesthetic, the pain and anxiety of labor are reduced, and the CO is noted to decrease. Epidural anesthetic is beneficial in most cardiac patients because it minimizes fluctuations in CO associated with pain and labor. The concern with epidural and spinal anesthetics is that of decreased systemic vascular resistance and hypotension. If general anesthetic is needed, care to maintain normal to low HR and prevention of large swings in BP with hypertension at induction followed by hypotension with drug administration is crucial. Prelabor consultation with obstetrical anesthesia is critical for optimal patient management in the pregnant patient with severe cardiovascular disease.

Postpartum there is an increase in preload caused by significant decreases in blood flow through the uteroplacental unit. During the postpartum period, marked fluctuations in CO, SV, and HR occur and can make care complicated. Accurate monitoring of blood loss, fluid balance, and maternal hemodynamics is crucial because the increased preload, positive fluid balance from labor and delivery, and the antidiuretic properties of oxytocin (contractile agent used in many labors and after delivery) may predispose to fluid overload.

CARDIOVASCULAR EVALUATION IN PREGNANCY

Both altered physical exam findings and maternal symptoms during pregnancy can be similar to cardiovascular disease and require special attention. Common findings in pregnant women include dyspnea, fatigue, decreased tolerance to exercise, and peripheral edema. Pregnant women are also often noted to have an elevated HR with bounding pulses. Because of an enlarging uterus, the diaphragm gets progressively elevated and leads to displacement of the heart to the left and anterior and rotated slightly transverse. Pregnancy can also alter the normal heart sounds. It is typical to note a third heart sound caused by rapid diastolic filling and a systolic ejection murmur along the left sternal border as a result of increased blood flow across both the aortic and pulmonic valves. Splitting of the first and second heart sounds is also common in pregnancy. Auscultation of a fourth heart sound or a diastolic murmur, although possible in pregnancy, requires further evaluation to rule out a pathological cause.

Abnormal findings during pregnancy on chest radiographs, electrocardiograms, and echocardiograms may suggest cardiac disease. The altered positioning of the heart as a result of pregnancy may give the impression of cardiomegaly and ventricular hypertrophy on chest radiograph. The rotation of the heart may also be noted on electrocardiogram with evidence of left axis deviation. Echocardiograms performed on pregnant women also frequently find mild regurgitation at the pulmonic and tricuspid valves.[16]

Although assessment of cardiac symptoms can be difficult in the pregnant patient, frequent monitoring for subtle clinical signs is paramount. Frequent physical exams of the cardiopulmonary system combined with vital sign assessment and weight may alert the clinician to early changes in the clinical condition that may require further work-up or cardiac consultation. In addition to patients with diastolic murmurs and fourth heart sounds, patients with multiple cardiovascular symptoms or acute onset symptoms should be evaluated. Complaints such as chest pain, orthopnea, and nocturnal symptoms cannot be explained by pregnancy alone and require further evaluation. The decision to evaluate a pregnant patient for cardiac disease is based on symptoms, patient history, physical exam, and the timeline of the concerns. (See the accompanying Evidence-Based Practice feature.)

CARDIOVASCULAR ADAPTATION TO PREGNANCY COMPLICATIONS
Multifetal Gestation

Pregnancies complicated by multifetal gestation place further demands on the maternal cardiovascular system. This results from the increase in blood volume re-

quired to support the multifetal gestation. Kametas and colleagues studied cardiac function during twin pregnancy using two-dimensional and M-mode echocardiography. They found that CO was further increased by 20 percent in twin pregnancies when compared with single gestations, caused by an increase in both SV (15 percent) and HR (3.5 percent).[17] In addition to the marked hyperdynamic state, women with multifetal gestation are also at increased risk for hypertensive disease during pregnancy, preterm labor, and postpartum hemorrhage.

Preeclampsia

In pregnancies complicated by preeclampsia, a marked plasma volume reduction is noted with a concomitant hemoconcentration in proportion to the severity of the disease.[18] Multiple studies using pulmonary artery catheterizations in pregnant women with and without preeclampsia have demonstrated hyperdynamic left ventricular function in those women with preeclampsia.[19,20,21] Other studies have shown variable CO in preeclamptic patients, and the current thought is that initially increased CO decreases owing to an increase in systemic vascular resistance.[22]

Postpartum Hemorrhage

Traditionally, postpartum hemorrhage has been defined as blood loss following vaginal delivery of *greater than* 500 ml or blood loss of *greater than* 1000 ml following cesarean section. A better definition of postpartum hemorrhage may be excessive bleeding postpartum in conjunction with symptoms of hemodynamic compromise. Signs and symptoms that can be seen even with normal blood loss include palpitations, dizziness, and tachycardia. As blood loss increases, patients may experience weakness, pallor, sweating, oliguria, increased respiratory rate, and syncope.

Postpartum hemorrhage occurs in approximately 3 percent of all deliveries and is one of the leading causes of maternal mortality worldwide. Postpartum hemorrhage can be due to uterine atony, retained placenta, or lacerations either from vaginal delivery or cesarean section. Factors predisposing to uterine atony include multifetal pregnancy, fetal macrosomia, polyhydramnios, induced or prolonged labor, general anesthetic, and infection. To prevent postpartum hemorrhage from uterine atony, easy availability of uterotonic medications (oxytocin, Methergine, and misoprostol) should be secured.

Cardiopulmonary Resuscitation and Pregnancy

Modifications to cardiopulmonary resuscitation (**CPR**) in the pregnant woman are required. The gravid uterus may compress the inferior vena cava and lead to hypotension and shock. Modifications recommended for advanced challenges in resuscitation are as follows:

■ Place in left lateral tilt position, with right-sided wedge or manual uterine manipulation.

- Perform chest compressions higher on the sternum to adjust for gravid uterus.
- If resuscitation fails and the fetus is viable, consider immediate perimortem cesarean section, with the goal of delivery within 4 to 5 minutes of arrest.
- Delivery will increase blood return to the mother and allow resuscitation of the neonate.[23]

CARDIAC DISEASE AND PREGNANCY

Maternal risk associated with pregnancy in women with known cardiovascular disease depends on the type of cardiovascular disease and the severity of the disease. Counseling a pregnant woman with cardiovascular disease regarding her risks of mortality can be difficult because death is rare, but women with pulmonary hypertension, Marfan syndrome, cardiomyopathy, coronary artery disease, endocarditis, and sudden cardiac arrhythmia seem to be at the highest risk (Table 90-2). In women at high risk of maternal mortality based on their cardiac disease, recommendations against pregnancy and consideration of termination of any ongoing pregnancy should be discussed in detail. Maternal life expectancy and ability to care for a child in women with limited functional status should also be addressed in preconception planning. Associated risk factors that may complicate these pregnancies include dysrhythmia, heart failure, teratogenic medications, anticoagulation, and cardiovascular surgery.[24]

In a prospective study on pregnancy outcomes in women with heart disease, there was evidence that women with cardiac disease are at increased risk for both neonatal complications and maternal cardiovascular complications.[25] Predictors of maternal primary cardiac events are: prior cardiac event or dysrhythmia, baseline New York Heart Association Class III or IV, left heart obstruction, and ventricular systolic function.[26] The risk for neonatal complications in this group of women is increased by the presence of obstetrical risks, such as age *less than* 20 or *greater than* 35, multiple gestation, smoking, and need for anticoagulant medication.[25] Known neonatal risks in women with cardiovascular disease include preterm birth, intrauterine growth restriction, and increased risk of fetal congenital heart disease. The background risk for fetal congenital heart disease is 0.5 percent to 1 percent. When a first-degree relative is affected, the fetal risk increases 8- to 10-fold.[27,28] Maternal congenital heart disease appears to have a greater risk than paternal or sibling disease.

In addressing cardiac disease in pregnancy, it is often useful to look at the cardiac diseases in groups because the risks, treatment, and recommendations may be more similar within similar groups of cardiac disease.

Valvular Heart Disease

Mitral stenosis occurs most commonly as a result of rheumatic heart disease. This valvular lesion can lead to pulmonary edema and atrial dysrhythmias as a result of the expanded blood volume of pregnancy and physiological tachycardia that decreases left ventricular filling time. Recommendations for management of patients with mild to moderate mitral stenosis is to treat with diuretics to relieve pulmonary congestion and beta blockers to prevent tachycardia and optimize diastolic filling.[29] The severity of mitral stenosis is classified by mitral valve area with normal being 4 to 5 cm^2, mild mitral stenosis being *greater than* 1.5 cm^2, moderate mitral stenosis being 1.1 to 1.5 cm^2, and severe mitral stenosis being 1 cm^2 or less.[30] In patients with severe mitral stenosis who are symptomatic before pregnancy, the American College of Cardiology/American Heart Association **(ACC/AHA)** recommends percutaneous balloon valvotomy before conception.[29] Balloon mitral valvotomy has been performed during pregnancy for patients with persistent heart failure with success. Close monitoring of HR during labor is important because increased HR leads to decreased time for filling and decreased CO. Beta blockers may be required during labor to control HR. Control of pain with epidural anesthetic may help to prevent tachycardia and can be safely administered with monitoring for hypotension.

In general, regurgitant valvular lesions cause fewer problems in pregnancy as a result of the increase in CO and decrease in systemic vascular resistance that corresponds with pregnancy. Mitral regurgitation is most commonly caused by mitral valve prolapse. Because of the physiological changes of pregnancy, there are rarely cases of mitral regurgitation that cannot be managed medically. Patients are often managed on diuretics if pulmonary congestion is encountered. The risk of atrial fibrillation may be increased in pregnant women with mitral regurgitation.[31] Mitral valve prolapse has a reported prevalence of up to 12 percent to 17 percent in reproductive-aged women.[32]

■ ■ ■

TABLE 90-2   MATERNAL MORTALITY IN SPECIFIC CARDIAC DISEASE

RISK	CONDITION
Group I: Minimal risk of complications (mortality *less than* 1%)	Atrial septal defect*
	Ventricular septal defect*
	Patent ductus arteriosus*
	Pulmonic and/or tricuspid disease
	Corrected Tetralogy of Fallot
	Bioprosthetic valve
	Mitral stenosis, New York Heart Association Class I or II
	Marfan syndrome with normal aorta
Group II: Moderate risk of complications (mortality 5%-15%)	Mitral stenosis with atrial fibrillation†
	Artificial valve*†
	Aortic stenosis
	Uncorrected Tetralogy of Fallot
	Mitral stenosis, New York Heart Association Class III or IV
	Uncomplicated coarctation of the aorta
	Previous myocardial infarction
Group III: Major risk of complications or death (mortality *greater than* 25%)	Pulmonary hypertension
	Complicated coarctation of aorta
	Marfan syndrome with aortic involvement

*If unassociated with pulmonary hypertension.
†If anticoagulation with heparin, rather than Coumadin, is elected.
From Dildy GA, Belfort M, Saade G et al: *Critical care obstetrics,* ed 4, Malden, Mass, 2004, Blackwell Publishing.

The most common cause of aortic stenosis in women of reproductive age is a congenital bicuspid aortic valve.[22] Most patients with mild or moderate aortic stenosis can be managed medically throughout their pregnancy. For women with severe aortic stenosis, with a pressure gradient across the valve of *greater than* 50 mm Hg or persistent symptoms, the ACC/AHA recommends delaying pregnancy until aortic stenosis is surgically treated.[29] Forceps or vacuum-assisted vaginal delivery is often recommended for pregnant women with aortic stenosis and mitral stenosis to shorten the second stage of labor because it places high cardiac demand on patients with a fixed CO.[30] Cesarean section is typically reserved for obstetrical indications because it is associated with increased blood loss, infection, and thrombosis when compared with vaginal delivery. The decision for mode of delivery is individualized and based on both obstetrical history and cardiac disease history, but in general cesarean section is recommended for obstetrical indications, aortic dissection, Marfan syndrome with aortic root dilatation, and warfarin therapy within 2 weeks.[24]

Aortic regurgitation can generally be managed medically during pregnancy. Aortic regurgitation can be associated with a congenital bicuspid valve that does not close completely and with rheumatic valve disease. This valvular lesion is generally well tolerated in pregnancy because of the increase in HR, which decreases diastole.

Mechanical Heart Valves

Women of reproductive age requiring valve replacement surgery must contemplate the risks and benefits of both mechanical and bioprosthetic valves. The bioprosthetic valves degenerate more quickly and require reoperation, but do not require anticoagulation, which during pregnancy can be problematic. Mechanical valves have a longer lifespan, but do require anticoagulation. Pregnancy in women with mechanical heart valves is associated with a 1 percent to 4 percent mortality rate, usually caused by prosthetic valve thrombosis.[33] Women with mechanical heart valves who become pregnant must be informed of the risks and benefits of both warfarin and heparin therapy in pregnancy. Treatment recommendations for pregnant women with mechanical heart valves are shown in Table 90-3. Also see the accompanying Conundrum feature, Anticoagulation with Mechanical Heart Valves in Pregnancy.

Congenital Heart Disease

Congenital heart disease in pregnancy is now becoming more common than rheumatic heart disease because women are surviving to reproductive age. The risk to the fetus of acquiring a congenital heart defect depends on the defect.[30] Atrial septal defects and ventricular septal defects are generally well tolerated during pregnancy. Atrial septal defects can be associated with atrial dysrhythmias, most commonly atrial fibrillation, and heart failure. Paradoxical embolization, causing neurological symptoms, is also a potential complication in any patient with a left to right shunt.

Eisenmenger syndrome occurs when a congenital left to right shunt produces pulmonary hypertension, and then either bidirectional or reversed shunting occurs. This most commonly results from a large ventricular septal defect, but can be caused by patent ductus arteriosus or an atrial septal defect. A recent review of patients with Eisenmenger syndrome showed a maternal mortality rate of 36 percent, which is not significantly improved from earlier studies.[34] General care recommendations for pregnant patients with Eisenmenger syndrome include continuous oxygen therapy, bed rest, and anticoagulation. Older studies showed an increase in maternal mortality with cesarean delivery compared with vaginal delivery, but that was not shown in the more recent review by Weiss and colleagues.[35] Monitoring patients in the third trimester for fetal growth is also important because fetal growth restriction is common in patients with Eisenmenger syndrome.

There is now a generation of reproductive-aged women who have had cyanotic congenital heart disease repaired surgically as a child. Although most of these women are no longer cyanotic, they may experience

■ ■ ■

TABLE 90-3 ANTICOAGULATION DURING PREGNANCY IN WOMEN WITH MECHANICAL HEART VALVES

	RISKS	RECOMMENDATIONS
Warfarin	Warfarin embryopathy at 6 to 12 weeks of gestation, risk of 4% to 10%. Possible increased risks of spontaneous abortion, prematurity, stillbirth, and fetal cerebral hemorrhage	Rarely used in the first trimester because of known teratogenicity. Fetal cerebral hemorrhage can complicate labor and delivery, and some advocate cesarean section if on warfarin when labor begins.
Heparins	Increased maternal risk for fatal valve thrombosis and known risks of osteoporosis, thrombocytopenia, and bleeding	Therapy throughout pregnancy has been used with goal midinterval aPTT two to three times normal. The patient must understand increased risk of maternal valve thrombosis that can be fatal and that maternal complications jeopardize pregnancies.
Combination therapy: First and third trimester heparin with interim warfarin	The risk of warfarin embryopathy is eliminated by early heparin therapy, and the risk of fetal cerebral hemorrhage should be decreased with resumption of heparin at 35 to 36 weeks of gestation.	Generally recommended to patients following extensive counseling regarding fetal and maternal risks

aPTT, Activated partial thromboplastin time.

■■■ **CONUNDRUM**

ANTICOAGULATION WITH MECHANICAL HEART VALVES IN PREGNANCY

Pregnant women with mechanical heart valves require anticoagulation. Outside of pregnancy, these women are treated with warfarin to keep the INR at 2.5 to 3.5. During pregnancy warfarin is associated with fetal risks that must be discussed with the patient. The alternative anticoagulant is heparin, which has been associated with an increased risk of valve thrombosis and maternal mortality. Both unfractionated heparin **(UFH)** and low-molecular-weight heparin **(LMWH)** have been used in pregnancy, but there is controversy regarding the use of LMWH for anticoagulation in pregnant women with mechanical heart valves because of a warning placed by Aventis Pharmaceuticals, the maker of enoxaparin.[1]

Warfarin crosses the placenta, and its use in pregnancy has been associated with warfarin embryopathy, which consists of nasal hypoplasia and epiphyseal stippling when administered between 6 and 9 weeks of gestation.[2] Review of the literature shows the risk of warfarin embryopathy to be *less than* 5 percent when administered between 6 and 12 weeks of gestation, *less than* some case series or reports stating up to 30 percent.[3] Maternal hemorrhage and fetal intracranial hemorrhage have also been reported with warfarin use throughout gestation.

UFH does not cross the placenta and thus is not teratogenic to the fetus. Maternal concerns have been raised because of reports of thrombosed valves, leading to increased maternal morbidity and mortality.[1] This has been attributed to inadequate dosing during pregnancy, but not confirmed. Risks involved with UFH use also include immune, immunoglobulin G **(IgG)**-mediated thrombocytopenia.[4] Long-term use of UFH has been associated with osteoporosis with vertebral fractures and sterile abscesses at the injection site.[5] LMWH has also been associated with valve thrombosis and maternal mortality, although the exact risk is unknown. LMWH has the advantage over UFH of once daily dosing and decreased risks of thrombocytopenia and osteoporosis. Adjunctive aspirin has been recommended for both women using warfarin to decrease the necessary dose and with patients receiving UFH, especially if they are considered to be high risk. Women considered to be high risk according to American College of Cardiology and American Heart Association are those with a history of thromboembolism and older generation mechanical prosthesis in the mitral position or atrial fibrillation.[5]

1. Ginsberg JS et al: Anticoagulation of pregnant women with mechanical heart valves, *Arch Intern Med* 163:694-698, 2003.
2. Jones KL: *Smith's recognizable patterns of human malformation*, ed 5, Philadelphia, 1997, WB Saunders.
3. Chan WS, Anand S, Ginsberg JS: Anticoagulation of pregnant women with mechanical heart valves, *Arch Intern Med* 160:191-196, 2000.
4. Warkentin TE et al: Heparin-induced thrombocytopenia in patients treated with low-molecular-weight heparin or unfractionated heparin, *N Engl J Med* 332:1330-1335, 1995.
5. Bonow RO et al: ACC/AHA guidelines for the management of patients with valvular heart disease, *J Am Coll Cardiol* 32:1486-1588, 1998.

problems during pregnancy including dysrhythmias, thromboembolism, ventricular failure, and recurrence of cyanosis.[30] Maternal prepregnancy arterial oxygen saturation and hemoglobin concentration may be the best predictors of pregnancy outcome in women with cyanotic heart disease.

Marfan syndrome is an autosomal dominant disorder of connective tissue that can lead to aortic root dilatation, aneurysm, and aortic dissection. Historically, maternal mortality has been estimated at 50 percent for women with an abnormal aortic valve or aortic dilatation.[36] Because of this high rate of maternal mortality,

pregnancy is contraindicated in women with Marfan syndrome and aortopathy. A more recent prospective study found that women with Marfan syndrome with an aortic root diameter of *less than* 4 cm have a small risk of aneurysm and have favorable maternal and neonatal outcomes.[37] Routine use of beta blockers is recommended and monitoring of the aortic root for evidence of dilatation in women who do become pregnant because rapidity of aortic root dilatation also plays a role in aortic dissection.[38]

Peripartum Cardiomyopathy

Peripartum cardiomyopathy was first defined in 1971 as cardiomyopathy developing in the last month of pregnancy or the first 5 months postpartum in a woman without preexisting heart disease and exclusion of other causes of heart failure.[39] Echocardiographic criteria were more recently added to the definition, including ejection fraction *less than* 45 percent, M-mode fractional shortening *less than* 30 percent, and a left ventricular end-diastolic dimension of more than 2.72 cm/m^2.[40] The incidence of the disease is 1:3000 to 4000 with associated risk factors of multiparity, advanced maternal age, multifetal gestation, preeclampsia, and black race.[41] Therapy generally includes sodium restriction, diuretics, positive inotropes, and afterload reduction. Anticoagulation for patients with an ejection fraction of *less than* 35 percent may be of benefit because of the increased risk of thrombotic emboli.[41] Angiotensin-converting enzyme inhibitors, which are commonly used outside of pregnancy, are contraindicated in pregnancy (Table 90-4).

The risk of death associated with peripartum cardiomyopathy in women with persistent left ventricular dysfunction 6 months postpartum has been reported as high as 85 percent over 5 years.[41] Risks in subsequent pregnancies have not been fully elucidated. A recent retrospective study of heart failure and death in women with peripartum cardiomyopathy in their subsequent pregnancies found that in women with normal left ventricular function at the start of pregnancy there was 21 percent risk of heart failure and 0 percent maternal mortality compared with 44 percent and 19 percent, respectively, in the group with abnormal left ventricular function at the start of pregnancy.[42]

Ischemic Heart Disease

Acute myocardial infarction **(AMI)** is a rare event in reproductive-aged women, so is rarely encountered in pregnant women. A population-based study estimated the incidence to be 1:35,700 deliveries.[43] A recent retrospective review of AMI revealed it is more common in the third trimester and in multigravidas older than age 33.[44] The overall maternal mortality associated with AMI in this study was 21 percent, with a fetal mortality of 13 percent correlating with maternal mortality.[44] Delivery within 2 weeks of AMI is associated with increased mortality, therefore allowing time for myocardial healing is recommended if possible. Considerations for labor in a woman with a history of AMI include oxygen therapy, epidural anesthetic, and vaginal delivery

■ ■ ■

TABLE 90-4 CARDIOVASCULAR MEDICATIONS IN PREGNANCY

MEDICATION	FIRST TRIMESTER RISKS	SECOND AND/OR THIRD TRIMESTER RISKS	MATERNAL PREGNANCY RELATED RISKS	BREAST-FEEDING
Angiotensin-converting enzyme inhibitors	None documented	Fetal hypocalvaria Fetal renal defects Oligohydramnios		AAP compatible
Amiodarone	Congenital goiter	Congenital goiter and/or hypothyroidism Hyperthyroidism Prolonged QT interval and/or transient bradycardia Questionable IUGR		Breast-feeding not recommended
Aspirin	No evidence of increased congenital defects	Increased risk of neonatal hemorrhage At high doses an increase in perinatal mortality, IUGR, and premature closure of the ductus arteriosus	Increased risk of maternal hemorrhage	AAP recommends caution with use of aspirin in breast-feeding women
Beta blockers	No evidence of increased congenital defects	IUGR Neonatal beta blockade Nonreactive nonstress tests		AAP compatible—infants should be monitored for signs of beta blockade
Coumadin	Fetal warfarin syndrome Increased spontaneous abortions	CNS defects Increased stillbirths and neonatal deaths Increased neonatal hemorrhage	Increased risk of maternal hemorrhage	AAP compatible
Digoxin	None documented	Possible accelerated labor		AAP compatible
Heparin	None documented	None documented	Increased risk of maternal hemorrhage Osteopenia Thrombocytopenia	Heparin is not excreted in breast milk
Nifedipine	Digital anomalies in rats and rabbits, no teratogenic effect noted in humans	None documented	Severe reactions can occur if administered with magnesium sulfate.	AAP compatible

AAP, American Academy of Pediatrics; *IUGR*, intrauterine growth retardation.

with forceps or vacuum-assisted second stage, all with the goal to decrease myocardial oxygen demand.

Maternal and fetal outcome data of pregnancy in patients with a history of AMI are extremely limited, so counseling these patients is difficult. The risks to subsequent pregnancy may be determined by factors, such as interval from infarction to pregnancy, amount of myocardial damage, left ventricular function, underlying coronary anatomy, ongoing myocardial ischemia, and medication requirements.[44] Pharmacological stress tests should be performed in these patients and close clinical follow-up is recommended. Troponins are useful markers for myocardial damage in pregnancy. Medications typically used in secondary prevention either have not been studied in pregnant women (clopidogrel) or have been shown to be teratogenic in animal or human studies (statins and angiotensin-converting enzyme inhibitors). Management of labor and delivery should be comparable with management of other patients with a history of AMI undergoing a major surgical procedure.

Dysrhythmias

An increase in HR is a normal cardiovascular adaptation to pregnancy. Sinus tachycardia defined as HR *greater than* 100 beats/min is therefore common in the pregnant patient. Benign dysrhythmias, such as ventricular

and atrial ectopic beats, are also common and do not require treatment in pregnancy, unless associated with symptoms. Significant dysrhythmias not associated with congenital heart disease or valvular disease are rare. Treatment of dysrhythmias is the same in the pregnant patient as in the nonpregnant patient with the exception that amiodarone is usually avoided. Please see the chapter on dysrhythmias for further management. Also see the accompanying Technology feature.

Bacterial Endocarditis Prophylaxis

Bacteremia is a rare event with obstetrical deliveries, occurring in 1 percent to 5 percent of patients.[45] Patients who require antibiotics for dental procedures may not require them for delivery. According to the AHA and ACC, prophylaxis for bacterial endocarditis is only recommended for patients with suspected bacteremia or active infection.[29,46] See Table 90-5 for complete recommendations and endocarditis prophylaxis regimens. Controversy exists regarding these recommendations because in obstetrics it is difficult to both predict who is at risk for infection intrapartum or laceration into the gastrointestinal or genitourinary tract. Many obstetricians are very conservative and treat patients with any structural heart defect with endocarditis prophylaxis intrapartum.

■ ■ ■

TABLE 90-5 RECOMMENDED PROPHYLAXIS FOR PREGNANT PATIENTS WITH BACTERIAL ENDOCARDITIS

PATIENT	PROPHYLAXIS RECOMMENDED	DRUG TREATMENT	REGIMEN
High risk	Optional for routine delivery. Recommended for delivery complicated by suspected bacteremia.	Ampicillin and gentamycin Or	2 g ampicillin IV or IM and 1.5 mg/kg gentamycin (maximum dose 120 mg) IV or IM; with 1 g ampicillin IV or IM or 1 g amoxicillin 6 hr later
		Vancomycin and gentamycin for penicillin-allergic patient	1 g vancomycin IV and 1.5 mg/kg gentamycin IV or IM (maximum dose 120 mg)
Moderate risk	Not recommended for routine delivery Recommended for delivery complicated by suggested bacteremia	Amoxicillin or ampicillin Or Vancomycin for penicillin-allergic patient	Amoxicillin 2 g PO or ampicillin 2 g IV or IM Vancomycin 1 g IV

Adapted and modified from Dajani AS et al: Prevention of bacterial endocarditis: recommendations by the American Heart Association. *JAMA* 277:1794-1801, 1997, and Durack DT: Prevention of infective endocarditis, *N Engl J Med* 332:38-44, 1995.

■ ■ ■ TECHNOLOGY

TECHNOLOGY IN PREGNANCY

Treatment of dysrhythmias in pregnancy is complicated by concerns of safety for the fetus and the mother. Cardioversion and implantable cardioverter-defibrillators (**ICDs**) are methods of treatment that have been questioned in pregnancy. Electrical (DC) cardioversion is safe in all trimesters of pregnancy.[1] The concern about using cardioversion in pregnancy is induction of fetal dysrhythmia, which is unlikely because of the small amount of current reaching the fetus and the high fibrillation threshold in the fetus.[1] A retrospective review of 44 pregnant women with ICDs in place during pregnancy found negligible risks to the pregnant woman or her fetus.[2] Eleven of the 44 women received shocks during their pregnancy with no adverse fetal outcomes reported. Given this information it seems reasonable to counsel women with ICDs in place that pregnancy should not be discouraged just because an ICD is in place.

1. Tan HL, Lie KI: Treatment of tachyarrhythmias during pregnancy and lactation, *Euro Heart J* 22:458-464, 2001.
2. Natale A et al: Implantable cardioverter-defibrillators and pregnancy: a safe combination? *Circulation* 96:2808-2812, 1997.

THE PREGNANT PATIENT

Many pregnant patients are admitted to the hospital for medical complications and require nonobstetrical care. If the patient is previable (*less than* 23 to 24 weeks of gestation), heart tones should be obtained at admission and both before and after surgical procedures. Obstetrical consult should be obtained at admission to determine frequency of obstetrical assessment. Patients with viable pregnancies need to be monitored much more closely because delivery would be recommended for fetal distress. Generally twice weekly nonstress tests are recommended, but if the maternal status is critical, continuous monitoring may be recommended. Labor can have symptoms of abdominal or back pain, contractions, vaginal bleeding or spotting, and rupture of membranes. These symptoms warrant an obstetrical consult. Lack of fetal movement and signs or symptoms of preeclampsia (elevated BP, proteinuria, persistent headache, visual changes, and right upper quadrant pain) also warrant immediate obstetrical consult. Accurate fluid balance, weight, and vital sign assessment are critical to the care of the pregnant patient.

SUMMARY

Although the evidence is limited compared with management of other cardiac conditions, use of a systematic, evidence-based approach whenever possible in the care of pregnant patients with cardiovascular conditions can improve both maternal and fetal outcomes. Recommendations for pregnancy in women with cardiac conditions include the following:

- Preconception counseling regarding maternal and fetal risks associated with pregnancy, maternal life expectancy with cardiac disease and recurrence of congenital heart disease in the offspring
- Antenatal monitoring by a team of cardiology, obstetrics, anesthesia, and neonatology
- Activity limitation may be helpful for patients with New York Heart Association Class III or IV.[24]
- Continuous fetal monitoring during labor and continuous maternal monitoring
- Vaginal delivery with the exception of aortic dissection, Marfan syndrome with dilated aortic root, and warfarin therapy within 2 weeks of delivery **or** obstetrical indications for a cesarean section[24]
- Preterm induction is not warranted routinely, once fetal lung maturity has been determined, planned induction may be beneficial to allow for ideal multidisciplinary care at delivery and postpartum.
- Discontinuation of heparin 12 hours before delivery and resumption of heparin 6 to 12 hours after delivery
- Postpartum monitoring for 72 hours in intermediate- and high risk patients and possibly for up to 7 days in patients with Eisenmenger syndrome because of increased risk of death postpartum as a result of hemodynamic fluid shifts and changing cardiac demand.

REFERENCES

1. Pritchard JA: Changes in the blood volume during pregnancy and delivery, *Anesthesiology* 26:393-399, 1965.
2. Metcalfe J, Ueland K: Maternal cardiovascular adjustments to pregnancy, *Prog Cardiovasc Dis* 16:363-374, 1974.
3. CDC criteria for anemia in children and child-bearing aged women, *MMWR* 38:400-404, 1989.

4. World Health Organization: Nutritional anemias, *Tech Rep Ser* 503: 1972.

5. van Oppen AC, Stigter RH, Bruinse HW: Cardiac output in normal pregnancy: a critical review, *Obstet Gynecol* 87:310-318, 1996.

6. Robson SC et al: Serial study of factors influencing changes in cardiac output during human pregnancy, *Am J Physiol* 256: H1060-65, 1989.

7. Capeless EL, Clapp JF: Cardiovascular changes in early phase of pregnancy, *Am J Obstet Gynecol* 161:1449-1453, 1989.

8. Kinsella SM, Lohmann G: Supine hypotensive syndrome, *Obstet Gynecol* 83:774-779, 1994.

9. Toglia MR, Weg JG: Venous thromboembolism during pregnancy, *N Engl J Med* 335:108-114, 1996.

10. Delorme MA et al: Thrombin regulation in mother and fetus during pregnancy, *Semin Thromb Hemost* 18:81-90, 1992.

11. Rutherford S et al: Thromboembolic disease associated with pregnancy: an 11 year review. *Am J Obstet Gynecol* 164 (suppl):286, 1991 (abstract).

12. Friederich PM et al: Frequency of pregnancy-related venous thromboembolism in anticoagulant factor deficient women, implications for prophylaxis, *Ann Intern Med* 125:955-960, 1996.

13. Gerhardt A et al: Prothrombin and factor V mutations in women with a history of thrombosis during pregnancy and puerperium, *N Engl J Med* 342(6):374-380, 2000.

14. Lockwood CJ: Inherited thrombophilias in pregnant patients: detection and treatment paradigm, *Obstet Gynecol* 99:333-341, 2002.

15. Dizon-Townsend D et al: The relationship of the factor V Leiden mutation and pregnancy outcomes for mother and fetus, *Obstet Gynecol* 106:517-524, 2005.

16. Campos O et al: Physiologic multivalvular regurgitation during pregnancy: a longitudinal Doppler echocardiographic study, *Int J Cardiol* 40:265-268, 1993.

17. Kametas NA et al: Maternal cardiac function in twin pregnancy, *Obstet Gynecol* 102:806-15, 2003.

18. Chesley LC: Plasma and red cell volumes during pregnancy, *Am J Obstet Gynecol* 112:440-450, 1972.

19. Clark SL et al: Central hemodynamic observations in normal third trimester pregnancy, *Am J Obstet Gynecol* 161:1439-1442, 1989.

20. Cotton DB et al: Hemodynamic profile of severe pregnancy induced hypertension, *Am J Obstet Gynecol* 158:523-529, 1988.

21. Mabie WC, Ratts TE, Sibai BM: The central hemodynamics of severe preeclampsia, *Am J Obstet Gynecol* 161:1443-1448, 1989.

22. Bosio PM et al: Maternal central hemodynamics in hypertensive disorders of pregnancy, *Obstet Gynecol* 94:978-984, 1999.

23. ECC Guidelines, part 8: Advanced challenges in resuscitation, *Circulation* 102I:229-252, 2000.

24. Siu SC, Colman JC: Congenital heart disease: heart disease and pregnancy, *Heart* 85:710-715, 2001.

25. Siu SC et al: Adverse neonatal and cardiac outcomes are more common in pregnant women with cardiac disease. *Circulation* 105:2179-2184, 2002.

26. Siu S et al: Prospective multicenter study of pregnancy outcomes in women with heart disease, *Circulation* 104:515-521, 2001.

27. Burn J et al: Recurrence risks in offspring of adults with major heart defects: results from first cohort of British collaborative study, *Lancet* 351:311-316, 1998.

28. Siu S et al: Pregnancy in women with congenital heart defects: what are the risks?, *Heart* 81:225-226, 1999.

29. Bonow RO et al: ACC/AHA guidelines for the management of patients with valvular heart disease, *J Am Coll Cardiol* 32:1486-1588, 1998.

30. Klein LL, Galan HL: Cardiac disease in pregnancy, *Obstet Gynecol Clin N Am* 31:429-459, 2004.

31. Szekely P, Turner R, Snaith L: Pregnancy and the changing pattern of rheumatic heart disease, *Br Heart J* 35:1293-1303, 1973.

32. Savage DD et al: Mitral valve prolapse in the general population. I. epidemiologic features: The Framington study, *Am Heart J* 106:571-576, 1983.

33. Reimold SC, Rutherford JD: Valvular heart disease in pregnancy, *N Engl J Med* 349:52-59, 2003.

34. Weiss BM et al: Outcome of pulmonary vascular disease in pregnancy: a systematic overview from 1978 through 1996, *J Am Coll Cardiol* 31:1650-1657, 1998.

35. Gleicher N et al: Eisenmenger syndrome and pregnancy, *Obstet Gynecol Surv* 34:721-741, 1979.

36. Pyeritz RE: Maternal and fetal complications of pregnancy in the Marfan syndrome, *Am J Med* 71:784-90, 1984.

37. Rossiter JP et al: A prospective longitudinal evaluation of pregnancy in Marfan syndrome, *Am J Obstet Gynecol* 173:1599-1606, 1995.

38. Shores J et al: Progression of aortic dilatation and benefit of long-term β-adrenergic blockade in Marfan syndrome, *N Engl J Med* 330:1335-1341, 1994.

39. Demakis JG et al: Natural course of peripartum cardiomyopathy, *Circulation* 44:1053-1061, 1971.

40. Hibbard JU, Lindheimer M, Lang RM: A modified definition for peripartum cardiomyopathy and prognosis based on echocardiography, *Obstet Gynecol* 94:311-316, 1999.

41. Pearson GD et al: Peripartum cardiomyopathy, *JAMA* 283:1183-8, 2000.

42. Elkayam U et al: Maternal and fetal outcomes of subsequent pregnancy in women with peripartum cardiomyopathy, *N Engl J Med* 344:157-171, 2001.

43. Ladner HE et al: Acute myocardial infarction in pregnancy and the puerperium: a population-based study, *Obstet Gynecol* 105:480-484, 2005.

44. Roth A, Elkayam U: Acute myocardial infarction associated with pregnancy, *Ann Intern Med* 125:751-762, 1996.

45. Sugrue D et al: Antibiotic prophylaxis against infective endocarditis after normal delivery—is it necessary?, *Br Heart J* 44:499-502, 1980.

46. Dajani AS et al: Prevention of bacterial endocarditis: recommendations by the American Heart Association, *JAMA* 277:1794-1801, 1997.

Index

Note: Page numbers ending in f indicate figures; t, tables; b, boxes.

1383

John L. Atlee, MD

Professor of Anesthesiology
Department of Anesthesiology
Medical College of Wisconsin
Milwaukee, Wisconsin

Complications in Anesthesia

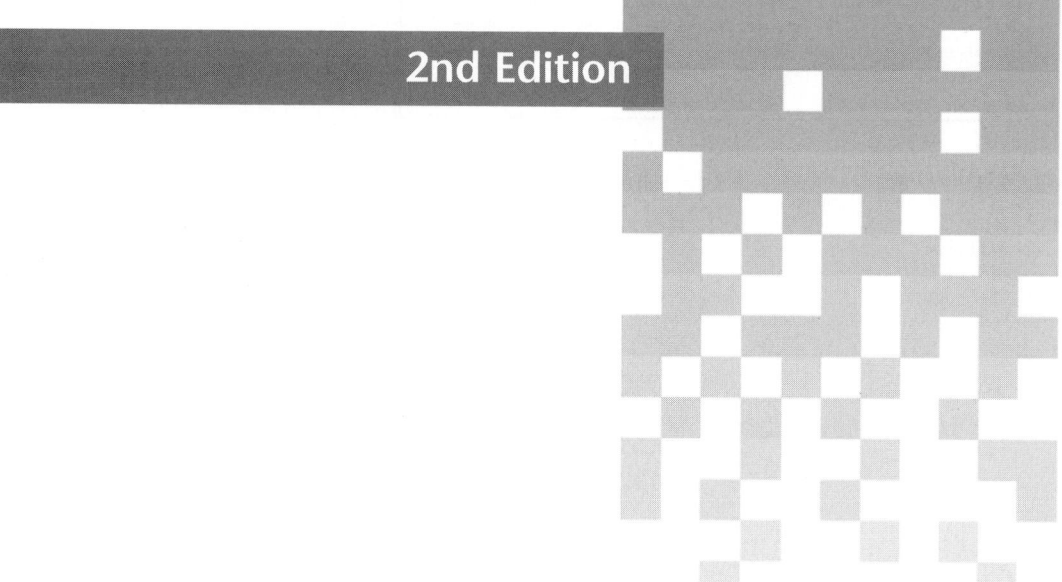

2nd Edition

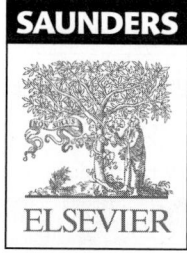

SAUNDERS

ELSEVIER

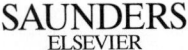

SAUNDERS
ELSEVIER

1600 John F. Kennedy Blvd.
Ste 1800
Philadelphia, PA 19103-2899

COMPLICATIONS IN ANESTHESIA, 2nd edition
ISBN-13: 978-1-4160-2215-2
ISBN-10: 1-4160-2215-5

Notice

Library of Congress Cataloging-in-Publication Data
Complications in anesthesia / [edited by] John L. Atlee. -- 2nd ed.
    p. ; cm.
    Includes bibliographical references and index.
    ISBN-13: 978-1-4160-2215-2   ISBN-10: 1-4160-2215-5
  1. Anesthesia--Complications.   I. Atlee, John L.
    [DNLM: 1. Anesthesia--adverse effects. 2. Anesthetics--adverse effects.   WO 245 C7369 2007]
    RD82.5.C63 2007
    617.9'6041--dc22   2006040549

ISBN-13: 978-1-4160-2215-2
ISBN-10: 1-4160-2215-5

Executive Publisher: Natasha Andjelkovic
Developmental Editor: Jean Nevius
Publishing Services Manager: Tina Rebane
Project Manager: Amy Norwitz
Marketing Manager: Dana Butler

Printed in the United States of America

Last digit is the print number: 9   8   7   6   5   4   3

To all who have contributed to this work, and to the patients we serve.

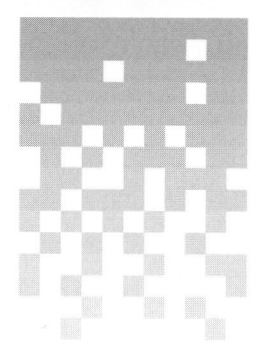

Preface

An ounce of prevention is worth a pound of cure.
— ANONYMOUS

The second edition of *Complications in Anesthesia*, like its first edition, is intended to provide all practitioners of anesthesia and critical care medicine with a comprehensive source of information for most complications that might be faced in clinical practice. Topics are addressed in ten sections: Pharmacology; General Anesthesia; Regional Anesthesia and Pain Management; Cardiothoracic and Vascular Surgery; Physiologic Imbalance and Coexisting Disease; Equipment and Monitoring; Pediatrics and Neonatology; Neurosurgery, Ophthalmology, and ENT; Other Surgical Subspecialties (subdivided into Obstetrics and Gynecology, General Surgery, Urologic Surgery, and Orthopedic Surgery); and Special Topics (subdivided into Postanesthesia Care Unit, Diagnostic or Therapeutic Intervention, and Medicolegal Aspects). Section Editors were selected based on their special expertise and knowledge of the topics addressed in each section.

Each chapter is presented in a highly structured format (in accordance with problem-based learning) under the following headings and subheadings: Case Synopsis, Problem Analysis (divided into Definition, Recognition, Risk Assessment, Implications), Management, and Prevention; in chapters with more than one topic, each topic is addressed using the same headings. Schematics, figures, and tables are used liberally to illustrate key points or to summarize important information. Key references are listed at the end of each chapter under "Further Reading," avoiding in-text citations that might distract the reader. Some chapters contain footnotes that provide further explanations. In this way, the reader can gain useful insight into a topic of interest in the minimal amount of time and with maximal retention. Also, thumb indexing and liberal cross-referencing are intended to reduce the need for time-consuming index searches. Finally, under Further Reading, in text, or in footnotes, there are references to Web sites for more or updated information. In that way, the reader can keep abreast of new developments.

I hope this unconventional treatment of complications in anesthesia and critical care will serve several purposes: first, to permit quick location and researching of topics of interest to busy practitioners in the least amount of time; second, to organize the thought processes involved in medical decision-making in an attractive format—i.e., akin to Sherlock Holmes' "who done it?"; and third and most importantly, to reduce the risk to our patients for unexpected and untoward events.

John L. Atlee, MD

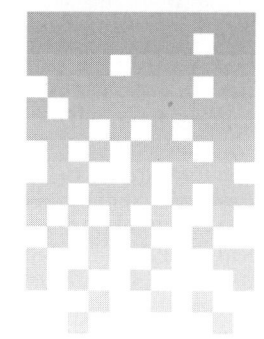

Contributors

Mark Abel, MD
Clinical Assistant Professor, Department of Anesthesiology, Mount Sinai Medical Center, New York, New York
Vaporizers

Gaury S. Adhikary, MD, FRCA
Assistant Professor, Department of Anesthesiology, University of Michigan Hospitals, Ann Arbor, Michigan
Carbon Dioxide Absorbers

Maurice S. Albin, MD, MSc (Anes)
Professor of Anesthesiology, Department of Anesthesiology, University of Alabama School of Medicine, Birmingham, Alabama
Venous Air Embolism

Stacey L. Allen, MD
Assistant Professor of Anesthesiology, Department of Anesthesiology, University of Texas Health Science Center at San Antonio, San Antonio, Texas
Corneal Injury; Open Globe Injury

Steven J. Allen, MD
Professor of Anesthesiology, Ohio State University College of Medicine; Chief Executive Officer, Columbus Children's Hospital, Columbus, Ohio
Autonomic Hyperreflexia

Jonathan M. Anagnostou, MD
Associate Professor of Clinical Anesthesia, Department of Anesthesia, Indiana University School of Medicine; Staff Anesthesiologist, Medical Director of Respiratory Care, Department of Anesthesia, Respiratory Care, Indiana University Hospital, Indianapolis, Indiana
Blood and Blood Products: Hepatitis and HIV

Maged Argalious, MD
Staff Anesthesiologist, Departments of General Anesthesiology and Critical Care Medicine, Cleveland Clinic Foundation, Cleveland, Ohio
Complications of Trauma Surgery

George A. Arndt, MD
Professor (CHS), Department of Anesthesiology, University of Wisconsin Medical School, Madison, Wisconsin
Difficult Airway: Cannot Ventilate, Cannot Intubate

Lori A. Aronson, MD, FAAP
Assistant Professor of Clinical Anesthesia and Pediatrics, Department of Anesthesia, University of Cincinnati College of Medicine; Assistant Professor, Clinical Anesthesia and Pediatrics, Department of Anesthesia, Cincinnati Children's Hospital Medical Center, Cincinnati, Ohio
Hypoxemia

John L. Atlee, MD
Professor of Anesthesiology, Department of Anesthesiology, Medical College of Wisconsin, Milwaukee, Wisconsin
Adenosine; Disorders of Potassium Balance; Nonbarbiturate Anesthetics; Chemotherapeutic Agents; Cardiac Risk Assessment; Postobstruction Pulmonary Edema; Perioperative Tachyarrhythmias; Tachyarrhythmias with Ventricular Preexcitation; Long QT Syndromes and Ventricular Arrhythmias; Patients with Cardiac Rhythm Management Devices; Disorders of Water Homeostasis: Hyponatremia and Hypernatremia

Michael S. Avidan, MD
Associate Professor of Anesthesiology and Surgery; Division Chief, CT Anesthesiology and CT Intensive Care, Washington University School of Medicine, St. Louis, Missouri
HIV Infection and AIDS

Isaac Azar, MD
Professor of Anesthesiology, Albert Einstein College of Medicine; Consultant, Department of Anesthesiology, Beth Israel Medical Center, New York, New York
Scavenging Systems

James E. Baker, MD, FRCPC
Assistant Professor and Anesthesiologist, Department of Anesthesia and Perioperative Care, University of California, San Francisco, San Francisco, California
Postoperative Pulmonary Hypertension

Narayan Baliga, MD
Staff Anesthesiologist, Kenosha Hospital and Medical Center, Kenosha, Wisconsin
Difficult Airway: Opiate-Induced Muscle Rigidity

Shahar Bar-Yosef, MD
Assistant Professor, Department of Anesthesiology and Critical Care, Duke University School of Medicine, Durham, North Carolina
Complications of Laparoscopic Surgery

Juliana Barr, MD
Associate Professor, Department of Anesthesiology,
Stanford University School of Medicine, Stanford,
California; Staff Intensivist and Anesthesiologist, Veterans
Affairs Palo Alto Health Care System, Anesthesiology
Service, Palo Alto, California
Reversal Agents: Naloxone and Flumazenil

Curtis L. Baysinger, MD
Associate Professor, Department of Anesthesiology,
Vanderbilt University School of Medicine, Nashville,
Tennessee
Hypertensive Disorders of Pregnancy

Eric Bedell, MD
Associate Professor, Department of Anesthesiology,
University of Texas Medical Branch, Galveston,
Texas
Posterior Fossa Surgery

Joan Benca, MD
Associate Professor, Department of Anesthesiology,
University of Wisconsin Hospital and Clinics, Madison,
Wisconsin
Bronchospasm

Patrick E. Benedict, MD
Assistant Professor of Anesthesiology, University of
Michigan Medical School, Ann Arbor, Michigan
Transesophageal Echocardiography

David G. Bjoraker, MD
Associate Professor, Department of Anesthesiology,
University of Florida College of Medicine, Gainesville,
Florida
Anaphylaxis and Anaphylactoid Reactions

Susan Black, MD
Professor, Department of Anesthesiology,
University of Alabama School of Medicine,
Birmingham, Alabama
Antidepressants

William S. Blau, MD, PhD
Associate Professor of Anesthesiology, University of
North Carolina School of Medicine, Chapel Hill,
North Carolina
Opioid Tolerance

Steffan Blumenthal, MD
Assistant Professor, Department of Anesthesiology and
Reanimation, Orthopedic University Clinic Balgrist/Zurich,
Zurich, Switzerland
Interscalene Nerve Block: Potential Severe Complications

John C. Boncyk, MD
Assistant Professor, Department of Anesthesiology,
University of Wisconsin Hospital and Clinics, Madison,
Wisconsin
Perioperative Hypoxia

Alain Borgeat, MD
Professor and Chief of Staff, Department of Anesthesiology
and Reanimation, Orthopedic University Clinic
Balgrist/Zurich, Zurich, Switzerland
Interscalene Nerve Block: Potential Severe Complications

Lois L. Bready, MD
Professor and Vice Chair, Department of Anesthesiology,
University of Texas Health Science Center at San Antonio,
San Antonio, Texas
Corneal Injury

Thomas P. Broderick, MD
Assistant Professor, Department of Anesthesiology,
University of Wisconsin Hospital and Clinics, Madison,
Wisconsin
Preanesthetic Evaluation: Inadequate or Missing Test Result

David L. Brown, MD
Edward Rotan Distinguished Professor and Chairman,
Department of Anesthesiology and Pain Medicine, M.D.
Anderson Cancer Center, Houston, Texas
Celiac Plexus Block: Side Effects and Complications

Adrie Bruijnzeel, MD
Assistant Professor, Department of Psychiatry, Evelyn and
William McKnight Brain Institute, University of Florida
College of Medicine, Gainesville, Florida
Chemical Dependency: Opioids

Brenda A. Bucklin, MD
Associate Professor of Anesthesiology, Department of
Anesthesiology, University of Colorado Health Sciences
Center, Denver, Colorado
Fetal Distress

Matthew D. Caldwell, MD
Assistant Professor, Department of Anesthesiology,
University of Michigan Medical School, Ann Arbor,
Michigan
Pulmonary Artery Pressure Monitoring

William R. Camann, MD
Associate Professor, Department of Anesthesia, Harvard
Medical School; Director of Obstetric Anesthesia, Brigham
and Women's Hospital, Boston, Massachusetts
Pulmonary Aspiration in the Parturient

Maria I. Castro, PhD
Assistant Professor, Department of Anesthesiology,
University of Arkansas for Medical Sciences, Little Rock,
Arkansas
*Class II Antiarrhythmic Drugs: β-Blockers—Heart Block or
Bradycardia*

Kevin P. Chan, MD
Fellow in Cardiovascular Anesthesia, Stanford University
School of Medicine, Stanford, California
Nonbarbiturate Anesthetics

Mark A. Chaney, MD
Associate Professor of Anesthesiology, Department of
Anesthesia and Critical Care, University of Chicago Pritzker
School of Medicine, Chicago, Illinois
*Perioperative Myocardial Ischemia and Infarction; Adverse
Neurologic Sequelae: Central Neurologic Impairment;
Hypercoagulable States: Thrombosis and Embolism*

Amit V. Chawla, MD
Consultant, Department of Anesthesia, Guy's Hospital,
London, United Kingdom
Inspiratory and Expiratory Gas Monitoring

David C. H. Cheng, MD, MSc, FRCPC
Professor and Chair, Department of Anesthesia and
Perioperative Medicine, University of Western Ontario;
Anesthesiologist in Chief, London Health Sciences Center
and St. Joseph's Health Care, London, Ontario,
Canada
Fast-Track Cardiac Surgery

S. Devi Chiravuri, MD
Assistant Professor, Department of Anesthesiology,
University of Michigan Medical School, Ann Arbor,
Michigan
Rapid Fluid and Blood Delivery Systems

Gordon Lee Collins, MD
Clinical Fellow, Department of Anesthesiology, Washington
University School of Medicine, St. Louis, Missouri
Complications after Pneumonectomy

Lois A. Connolly, MD
Associate Professor, Department of Anesthesiology,
Medical College of Wisconsin, Froedtert Memorial Lutheran
Hospital, Milwaukee, Wisconsin
Unstable Cervical Spine, Atlantoaxial Subluxation

D. Ryan Cook, MD
Professor of Anesthesiology, Department of Anesthesiology,
Children's Hospital of Pittsburgh, Pittsburgh,
Pennsylvania
Hypoglycemia and Hyperglycemia

Scott D. Cook-Sather, MD
Assistant Professor of Anesthesia, Department of
Anesthesiology and Critical Care Medicine, University of
Pennsylvania School of Medicine; Associate
Anesthesiologist, Children's Hospital of Philadelphia,
Philadelphia, Pennsylvania
Ophthalmic Problems and Complications

Victoria Coon, CRNA, MS
Perioperative Director and Anesthesiology Department
Administrator, Kaiser Permanente, West Los Angeles,
Los Angeles, California
Quality Assurance; Cost Containment

John R. Cooper, Jr., MD
Clinical Associate Professor of Anesthesiology, University of
Texas Health Science Center; Associate Chief,
Cardiovascular Anesthesia; Co-Director, Cullen
Cardiovascular Research Laboratories, Texas Heart Institute,
Houston, Texas
*Troubleshooting Common Problems during
Cardiopulmonary Bypass*

Charles J. Coté, MD
Director of Clinical Research in Pediatric Anesthesia,
Department of Anesthesiology, Massachusetts General
Hospital, Boston, Massachusetts
Sedation of Pediatric Patients

Douglas B. Coursin, MD
Professor of Anesthesiology and Internal Medicine,
Department of Anesthesiology, University of Wisconsin
School of Medicine and Public Health, Madison,
Wisconsin
Adrenal Insufficiency

James C. Crews, MD
Associate Professor of Anesthesiology, Section of Regional
Anesthesia and Acute Pain Management, Department of
Anesthesiology, Wake Forest University School of Medicine,
Winston-Salem, North Carolina
Infectious Complications of Central Neuraxial Block

Deborah A. Davis, MD
Clinical Professor of Anesthesiology, Department of
Anesthesiology, Thomas Jefferson University – Jefferson
Medical College, Philadelphia, Pennsylvania; Pediatric
Anesthesiologist/Intensivist, Nemours Cardiac Center,
A.I. duPont Hospital for Children, Wilmington,
Delaware
Pulmonary Hypertension

Martin L. De Ruyter, MD
Associate Professor of Anesthesiology, Department of
Anesthesiology, Kansas University School of Medicine,
Kansas City, Kansas
Hyperglycemia and Diabetic Ketoacidosis; Sarcoidosis

Hernando De Soto, MD
Associate Professor, Department of Pediatric Anesthesia,
University of Florida Health Science Center; Staff
Anesthesiologist/Medical Director of the OR, Department
of Anesthesiology, SHANDS Jacksonville, Jacksonville,
Florida
Difficult Pediatric Airway

Donn M. Dennis, MD, FAHA
Joachim S. Gravenstein, MD, Professor of Anesthesiology,
Department of Anesthesiology, University of Florida College
of Medicine, Gainesville, Florida; Vice President-
Pharmacology, ARYx Therapeutics, Inc., Santa Clara,
California
*Class III Antiarrhythmic Drugs: Potassium Channel Blockers;
Class IV Antiarrhythmic Drugs: Calcium Channel Blockers*

Ronak Desai, DO
Resident, CA-2, Department of Anesthesia and Critical
Care, University of Chicago Pritzker School of Medicine,
Chicago, Illinois
Peripheral Vascular Surgery

Cheryl DeSimone, MD
Associate Professor of Anesthesiology, Obstetrics and
Gynecology, Department of Anesthesiology, Albany Medical
College; Director of Obstetric Anesthesia, Albany Medical
Center, Albany, New York
Embolic Events of Pregnancy

Cyrus DeSouza, MB,BS, FANZCA
Acting Assistant Professor, Cardiothoracic Anesthesiologist,
Department of Anesthesiology, University of Washington
Medical Center, Seattle, Washington; Staff Specialist
Anaesthetist, Department of Anaesthetics, St. Georges
Hospital, Sydney, NSW, Australia
Chronotropic Drugs

Clifford S. Deutschman, MD
Professor, Department of Anesthesia and Surgery,
Hospital of the University of Pennsylvania, Philadelphia,
Pennsylvania
*Sepsis, Systemic Inflammatory Response Syndrome, and Multiple
Organ Dysfunction Syndrome*

Pema Dorje, MD
Clinical Assistant Professor, Department of Anesthesiology,
University of Michigan Medical School, Ann Arbor,
Michigan
Arterial Blood Pressure Monitoring

Anthony R. Doyle, BSc, MB,BS, FRCA
Formerly, Visiting Instructor in Anesthesiology, University of
Michigan Medical School, Ann Arbor, Michigan;
Consultant Anaesthetist, Dorset County Hospital,
Dorchester, United Kingdom
Fires in the Operating Room

Kenneth Drasner, MD
Professor, Department of Anesthesiology and Perioperative
Care, University of California, San Francisco, San Francisco,
California
*Local Anesthetic Neurotoxicity: Cauda Equina
Syndrome*

Catherine Drexler, MD
Vice Chair, Department of Anesthesiology, Columbia-
St. Mary's-Milwaukee Campus, Milwaukee,
Wisconsin
Angioedema and Urticaria

Ellen Duncan, MD
Tejas Anesthesia, San Antonio, Texas
Open Globe Injury

Martin W. Dünser, MD
Resident in Anesthesiology and Critical Care Medicine,
Department of Anesthesiology and Critical Care
Medicine, Medical University Innsbruck, Innsbruck,
Austria
Vasopressors: Vasoconstrictor Drugs

Jörg Dziersk, MD, FRCA
Assistant Professor of Anesthesiology, Department of
Anesthesiology, University of Washington School of
Medicine, Seattle, Washington
Vasodilator Drugs

Michael P. Eaton, MD
Associate Professor, Department of Anesthesiology,
University of Rochester School of Medicine and Dentistry,
Rochester, New York
Proportioning Systems; Patient Warming Systems

Charles E. Edmiston, Jr., MS, PhD
Associate Professor, Department of Surgery; Director,
Surgical Microbiology Research Laboratory, Medical College
of Wisconsin, Milwaukee, Wisconsin
Nosocomial Infections: Bacterial Pneumonia

James B. Eisenkraft, MD
Professor of Anesthesiology, Mount Sinai School of
Medicine, New York, New York
Vaporizers

John Ellis, MD
Professor of Anesthesiology, Department of Anesthesia
and Critical Care, University of Chicago Pritzker School of
Medicine, Chicago, Illinois
Carotid Endarterectomy; Thoracic Aortic Aneurysm

Brenda G. Fahy, MD, FCCP, FCCM
Professor, Department of Anesthesiology, University of
Kentucky; Director of Critical Care, Department of
Anesthesiology, AB Chandler Medical Center,
Lexington, Kentucky
*Disorders of Water Homeostasis: Hyponatremia and
Hypernatremia*

Zhuang T. Fang, MD, MSPH
Assistant Clinical Professor, Department of Anesthesiology,
David Geffen School of Medicine at University of California,
Los Angeles, Los Angeles, California
Unanticipated Hospital Admission and Readmission

Doron Feldman, MD
Associate Professor of Clinical Anesthesiology, State
University of New York at Buffalo School of Medicine;
Attending in Anesthesiology, Children's Hospital of Buffalo,
Buffalo, New York
The Hostile-Combative Patient

Lynne R. Ferrari, MD
Associate Professor, Department of Anesthesia, Harvard
Medical School; Medical Director, Perioperative Services,
Children's Hospital, Boston, Massachusetts
Adenotonsillectomy

Matthew P. Feuer, MD
Staff Anesthesiologist, Department of Anesthesiology,
Virginia Mason Medical Center, Seattle,
Washington
Spinal Anesthesia: Post–Dural Puncture Headache

Stephanie S. F. Fischer, MD
Visiting Associate in Cardiothoracic and Critical Care,
Division of Pediatric Anesthesiology, Duke University School
of Medicine, Durham, North Carolina
Cardiomyopathies

M. Pamela Fish, MB,ChB
Associate Professor, Department of Anesthesiology, Stanford
University School of Medicine, Stanford, California; Staff
Physician, Veterans Affairs Palo Alto Health Care System,
Palo Alto, California
Antiemetic Drugs

Randall Flick, MD, MPH
Assistant Professor of Anesthesiology and Pediatrics,
Department of Anesthesiology and Pediatrics,
Mayo Clinic College of Medicine; Chair, Section
of Pediatric Anesthesiology, Mayo Clinic, Rochester,
Minnesota
Anterior Mediastinal Mass

Michael P. Ford, MD
Assistant Professor of Anesthesiology, Department of
Anesthesiology, University of Wisconsin Medical School,
Madison, Wisconsin
*Preanesthetic Evaluation: False-Positive Tests; Difficult Airway:
Cannot Ventilate, Cannot Intubate*

Jennifer T. Fortney, MD
Assistant Clinical Professor, Department of Anesthesiology,
Duke University School of Medicine, Durham, North
Carolina
Fat Embolism Syndrome

James M. T. Foster, MD
Clinical Assistant Professor of Anesthesiology, Department of Anesthesiology, State University of New York at Buffalo School of Medicine; Director of Anesthesiology Services, Kaleida Health, Buffalo, New York
The Hostile-Combative Patient

Melissa Franckowiak, MD
Resident, Department of Anesthesiology, State University of New York at Buffalo School of Medicine, Buffalo, New York
Cardioversion

Eugene B. Freid, MD
Associate Professor, Departments of Anesthesiology and Pediatrics, University of North Carolina Hospitals, Chapel Hill, North Carolina
Succinylcholine

Kimberly Frost-Pineda, MD
Assistant in Psychiatry, Department of Psychiatry, Director of Public Health Research, University of Florida College of Medicine, Gainesville, Florida
Chemical Dependency: Opioids; Chemical Dependency: Nonopioids

Jeffrey L. Galinkin, MD
Associate Professor, Department of Anesthesia, Children's Hospital, Denver, Colorado
Fetal Intrauterine Surgery

Arjunan Ganesh, MD
Assistant Professor of Anesthesia, Department of Anesthesia, University of Pennsylvania School of Medicine; Assistant Anesthesiologist, Department of Anesthesiology and Critical Care Medicine, Children's Hospital of Philadelphia, Philadelphia, Pennsylvania
Upper Respiratory Tract Infection

Hind M. Gautam, MD
Clinical Assistant Professor, Department of Anesthesiology, Veterans Affairs Medical Center, Buffalo, New York
Magnetic Resonance Imaging

Rodolfo Gebhardt, MD
Assistant Professor of Clinical Anesthesiology, Department of Anesthesiology, Department of Clinical Anesthesiology, Veterans Affairs Medical Center, Buffalo New York
Uncontrolled Pain

Jeremy M. Geiduschek, MD
Clinical Professor, Department of Anesthesiology, University of Washington School of Medicine; Director, Clinical Anesthesia Services, Department of Anesthesiology, Children's Hospital and Regional Medical Center, Seattle, Washington
Intraoperative Cardiac Arrest

J. C. Gerancher, MD
Associate Professor and Section Head, Regional Anesthesia and Acute Pain Management, Department of Anesthesiology, Wake Forest University School of Medicine, Winston-Salem, North Carolina
Epidural Anesthesia: Unintended Intrathecal Injection; Epidural Anesthesia: Unintended Subdural Injection

Mark S. Gold, MD
Distinguished Professor and Chief, Departments of Psychiatry, Neuroscience, Anesthesiology, Community Health and Family Medicine, Evelyn and William McKnight Brain Institute, University of Florida College of Medicine, Gainesville, Florida
Chemical Dependency: Opioids; Chemical Dependency: Nonopioids

Stuart Grant, MD
Assistant Professor, Department of Anesthesiology, Duke University School of Medicine, Durham, North Carolina
Continuous Nerve Blocks: Perineural Local Anesthetic Infusion

Glenn P. Gravlee, MD
Professor, Department of Anesthesiology, Ohio State University Hospitals, Columbus, Ohio
Hemodilution and Blood Conservation

Ivar Gunnarsson, MD
Staff Anesthesiologist, Department of Anesthesia and Intensive Care, Landspitalinn, University Hospital, Reykjavik, Iceland
Oxygen Flush Valve

Mary Ann Gurkowski, MD
Professor of Anesthesiology, University of Texas Health Science Center at San Antonio; Clinical Staff/Director of Medical Students, Department of Anesthesiology/Cross-appointed to Otorhinolaryngology, University Hospital; Attending Staff, Department of Anesthesiology, Audie Murphy Veterans Affairs Hospital, San Antonio, Texas
Foreign Body Aspiration

Jacob Gutsche, MD
Physician, Department of Anesthesia, Hospital of the University of Pennsylvania, Philadelphia, Pennsylvania
Sepsis, Systemic Inflammatory Response Syndrome, and Multiple Organ Dysfunction Syndrome

Thomas S. Guyton, MD
Staff Anesthesiologist, Methodist Healthcare of Memphis, Memphis, Tennessee
Magnesium; Antibiotics

Ali Habibi, MD
Adjunct Clinical Faculty, Anesthesiology, Stanford University School of Medicine, Stanford, California
Antihistamines: H_1- and H_2-Blockers

Saeed Habibi, MD
Chair, Department of Anesthesiology, Columbia–St. Mary's–Milwaukee Campus, Milwaukee, Wisconsin
Angioedema and Urticaria

Charles B. Hantler, MD
Professor, Department of Anesthesiology, Washington University School of Medicine, St. Louis, Missouri
Bradyarrhythmias

H. David Hardman, MD, MBA
Assistant Clinical Professor, Department of Anesthesiology, Duke University School of Medicine, Durham, North Carolina
Extremity Tourniquets

Barry A. Harrison, MB,BS
Assistant Professor of Anesthesiology, Department of Anesthesiology, Mayo Clinic College of Medicine, Jacksonville, Florida
Hyperglycemia and Diabetic Ketoacidosis; Sarcoidosis

Joy L. Hawkins, MD
Professor of Anesthesiology and Director of Obstetric Anesthesia, University of Colorado School of Medicine, Denver, Colorado
Nonobstetric Surgery during Pregnancy

Christopher M. B. Heard, MB,ChB, FRCA
Research Assistant Professor, Department of Anesthesiology and Division of Pediatric Critical Care, State University of New York at Buffalo School of Medicine; Assistant Attending, Children's Hospital of Buffalo, Buffalo, New York
Magnetic Resonance Imaging; Alleged Malpractice; The Hostile-Combative Patient

Stephen O. Heard, MD
Interim Chair, Professor of Anesthesiology and Surgery, University of Massachusetts Medical School, Worcester, Massachusetts
Perioperative Care of Immunocompromised Patients

James R. Hebl, MD
Assistant Professor, Department of Anesthesiology, Mayo Clinic College of Medicine, Rochester, Minnesota
Anticoagulants and Peripheral Nerve Block

Robert F. Helfand, MD
Associate Professor, Cleveland Clinic Lerner College of Medicine; Staff Anesthesiologist; Vice Chairman, Department of General Anesthesiology; Section Head of Orthopedic Anesthesia, Glickman Urological Center, Cleveland Clinic Foundation, Cleveland, Ohio
Thromboembolic Complications

Rosemary Hickey, MD
Professor and Program Director, Department of Anesthesiology, University of Texas Health Science Center at San Antonio, San Antonio, Texas
Intracranial Hypertension

George A. Higgins, BSN, MS, CRNA
Adjunct Faculty, Department of Nursing, University of Southern California; Senior Nurse Anesthetist, Department of Anesthesiology, Department of Veterans Affairs Medical Center, Los Angeles, California
Embolization Procedures

Scott Holliday, MD
Resident, Department of Anesthesiology, University of Texas Health Science Center at San Antonio, San Antonio, Texas
Foreign Body Aspiration

William Hope, MD, PhD
Assistant Professor, Department of Anesthesiology, Medical College of Wisconsin, Froedtert Memorial Lutheran Hospital East, Milwaukee, Wisconsin
Laryngeal and Tracheal Injury

Terese T. Horlocker, MD
Professor, Department of Anesthesiology, Mayo Clinic College of Medicine, Rochester, Minnesota
Spinal Hematoma; Persistent Paresthesia

Liana Hosu, MD
Assistant Professor of Anesthesia and Pediatrics, Department of Anesthesiology, University of Cincinnati College of Medicine; Staff Anesthesiologist, Department of Anesthesiology, Cincinnati Children's Hospital Medical Center, Cincinnati, Ohio
Postoperative Apnea in Infants

Kate Huncke, MD
Clinical Associate Professor, Department of Anesthesiology, New York University School of Medicine, New York, New York
Radiation Oncology

Samuel A. Irefin, MD
Associate Professor of Anesthesiology, Cleveland Clinic Lerner College of Medicine; Staff Anesthesiologist, Department of Anesthesiology and Critical Care Medicine, Cleveland Clinic Foundation, Cleveland, Ohio
Complications of Thyroid Surgery

William Jacobs, MD
Associate Professor, Departments of Psychiatry and Anesthesiology, University of Florida College of Medicine, Gainesville, Florida
Chemical Dependency: Opioids; Chemical Dependency: Nonopioids

Eric Jacobsohn, MB,ChB, MHPE, FRCPC
Associate Professor of Anesthesiology, Department of Anesthesiology, Washington University School of Medicine, St. Louis, Missouri
Complications after Pneumonectomy

J. Michael Jaeger, MD, PhD
Associate Professor of Anesthesiology and Neurological Surgery; Director, Thoracic Anesthesia, Department of Anesthesiology, University of Virginia Health Sciences Center, Charlottesville, Virginia
Class IV Antiarrhythmic Drugs: Calcium Channel Blockers

Michael F. M. James, MB,ChB, PhD, FRCA, FCA(SA)
Professor and Head, Department of Anesthesia, University of Cape Town; Professor and Chief Anaesthetist, Department of Anaesthesia, Groote Schuur Hospital, Cape Town, Western Cape, South Africa
Complications of Adrenal Surgery

Gregory M. Janelle, MD
Assistant Professor, Chief of Cardiovascular Anesthesia, Department of Anesthesiology, University of Florida College of Medicine, Gainesville, Florida
Phosphodiesterase Inhibitors

David R. Jobes, MD
Professor of Anesthesia, Department of Anesthesia and Critical Care Medicine, Children's Hospital of Philadelphia, Philadelphia, Pennsylvania
Complications of Massive Transfusion

Nicola Jones, MA, MB,BS, DTM&H, MRCP, MRCPath, PhD
Consultant in Microbiology and Infectious Diseases, Departments of Microbiology and Infectious Diseases, Nuffield Department of Clinical Laboratory Sciences, John Radcliffe Hospital, University of Oxford, Oxford, United Kingdom
HIV Infection and AIDS

Shailendra Joshi, MD
Assistant Professor of Anesthesiology, Department of Anesthesiology, College of Physicians and Surgeons of Columbia University, New York, New York
Arteriovenous Malformation: Normal Perfusion Pressure Breakthrough

Zeev N. Kain, MD
Professor of Anesthesiology, Department of Anesthesiology, Yale University School of Medicine, New Haven, Connecticut
Perioperative Psychological Trauma

Wendy B. Kang, MD
Associate Professor and Chair, Residency Education Committee, Department of Anesthesiology, University of Texas Health Science Center at San Antonio, San Antonio, Texas
Retrobulbar Block

Shubjeet Kaur, MD
Clinical Vice Chair, Department of Anesthesiology, University of Massachussets Memorial Medical Center, Worcester, Massachusetts
Perioperative Care of Immunocompromised Patients

Robert D. Kaye, MD
Assistant Professor of Clinical Anesthesiology and Pediatrics, State University of New York at Buffalo School of Medicine; Attending Anesthesiologist, Children's Hospital of Buffalo, Buffalo, New York
Alleged Malpractice

Paul E. Kazanjian, MD
Clinical Assistant Professor, Department of Anesthesiology, University of Michigan Medical School, Ann Arbor, Michigan
Fires in the Operating Room; Pulmonary Artery Pressure Monitoring

Jeffrey S. Kelly, MD
Associate Professor of Anesthesiology, Section of Critical Care, Wake Forest University School of Medicine, Winston-Salem, North Carolina
Complications from Toxic Ingestion

Kevin J. Kelly, MD
Professor and Chair, Department of Pediatrics; Associate Dean, School of Medicine, Children's Mercy Hospital and Clinics, University of Missouri, Kansas City, Missouri
Latex Reactions in Health Care Personnel

Robert E. Kettler, MD
Associate Professor, Department of Anesthesiology, Medical College of Wisconsin, Froedtert Memorial Lutheran Hospital East, Milwaukee, Wisconsin
Patients with Seizure Disorders; Latex Reactions in Health Care Personnel

Jonathan T. Ketzler, MD
Associate Professor of Anesthesiology; Associate Director, Trauma and Life Support Center, Department of Anesthesiology, University of Wisconsin School of Medicine and Public Health, Madison, Wisconsin
Adrenal Insufficiency

Evan D. Kharasch, MD, PhD
Assistant Dean for Clinical Research; Professor and Research Director, Department of Anesthesiology, University of Washington School of Medicine, Seattle, Washington
Volatile Anesthetics: Organ Toxicity

M. Sean Kincaid, MD
Resident, Department of Anesthesiology, University of Washington Medical Center, Seattle, Washington
Head Injury

Kathryn P. King, MD
Associate Clinical Professor, Department of Anesthesiology, Duke University School of Medicine, Durham, North Carolina
Methylmethacrylate

Kai T. Kiviluoma, MD, PhD
Associate Professor, Department of Anaesthesiology, University of Oulu Faculty of Medicine; Head of the Department, Paediatric Anaesthesia, Oulu University Hospital, Oulu, Finland
Disorders of Potassium Balance

Jerome M. Klafta, MD
Associate Professor and Associate Chair for Education, Department of Anesthesia and Critical Care, University of Chicago Pritzker School of Medicine, Chicago, Illinois
Mediastinal Masses

Pattricia S. Klarr, MD
Clinical Assistant Professor, Department of Anesthesiology, University of Michigan Medical School; Associate Clinical Director, Department of Anesthesiology, University of Michigan Medical Center, Ann Arbor, Michigan
Laser Complications

Sandra L. Kopp, MD
Instructor, Department of Anesthesiology, Mayo Clinic College of Medicine, Rochester, Minnesota
Supraclavicular and Infraclavicular Block: Pneumothorax

Donald A. Kroll, MD, PhD
Staff Anesthesiologist, Department of Surgery, Veterans Affairs Medical Center, Biloxi, Mississippi
Quality Assurance; Cost Containment; Adverse Outcomes: Withheld Information or Misinformation

Kenneth Kuchta, MD
Assistant Clinical Professor, Department of Anesthesiology, David Geffen School of Medicine at University of California, Los Angeles, Los Angeles, California
Misidentification of a Patient

C. Dean Kurth, MD
Professor of Anesthesia and Pediatrics, University of
Cincinnati College of Medicine; Anesthesiologist-in-Chief;
Chair, Institute for Pediatric Research; Cincinnati Children's
Hospital Medical Center, Cincinnati, Ohio
Postoperative Apnea in Infants

Arthur M. Lam, MD, FRCPC
Professor of Anesthesiology, Department of Anesthesiology,
University of Washington School of Medicine; Head of
Neuroanesthesia, Harborview Medical Center, Seattle,
Washington
Head Injury

Jeffrey L. Lane, MD
Assistant Professor of Clinical Anesthesia and Director,
Human Simulation Laboratory, Department of Anesthesia,
Indiana University School of Medicine; Staff Anesthesiologist,
Clarian Health Partners, Indianapolis, Indiana
Postoperative Respiratory Insufficiency

Paul B. Langevin, MD
Associate Professor, Department of Anesthesiology, Veterans
Affairs–West Haven, West Haven, Connecticut
Chemotherapeutic Agents

Melissa A. Laxton, MD
Assistant Professor of Anesthesiology, Wake Forest
University School of Medicine, Winston-Salem,
North Carolina
Pituitary Tumors: Diabetes Insipidus

Marcia M. Lee, MD, MBA
Assistant Chief, Department of Anesthesiology,
Kaiser Permanente–South Bay, Harbor City, California
Awareness under Anesthesia

Mijin Lee, MD
Assistant Clinical Professor, Department of Anesthesiology,
David Geffen School of Medicine at University of California,
Los Angeles, Los Angeles, California
Anesthesia for Electroconvulsive Therapy

Peter J. Lee, MD, MPH
Formerly, Assistant Professor, Department of
Anesthesiology, University of Michigan Medical School,
Ann Arbor, Michigan
Central Venous Pressure Monitoring

Philip Levin, MD
Associate Professor, Department of Anesthesiology, David
Geffen School of Medicine at University of California,
Los Angeles, Los Angeles, California
Postoperative Delirium

Jerrold H. Levy, MD
Professor and Department Chair/Research, Department of
Anesthesiology, Emory University School of Medicine,
Atlanta, Georgia
Perioperative Hypertension

Ian Lewis, MB,BS, MRCP, FRCA
Associate Professor, Department of Anesthesiology, University
of Michigan Medical School, Ann Arbor, Michigan
Surgical Diathermy and Electrocautery

Ray P. Liao, MD
Acting Assistant Professor, Department of Anesthesiology,
University of Washington School of Medicine, Seattle,
Washington
Inotropic Drugs

Spencer S. Liu, MD
Clinical Professor of Anesthesiology, Department of
Anesthesiology, Virginia Mason Medical Center, Seattle,
Washington
Spinal Anesthesia: Post–Dural Puncture Headache

Emilio B. Lobato, MD
Professor of Anesthesiology, Department of Anesthesiology,
University of Florida College of Medicine; Chief,
Cardiovascular Anesthesia, Department of Anesthesia
Service, Malcom Randall Veterans Affairs Hospital,
Gainesville, Florida
Digitalis

Robert G. Loeb, MD
Associate Professor of Anesthesiology, University of Arizona
College of Medicine, Tucson, Arizona
Flowmeters

Celeste M. Lombardi, MD
Fellow in Interventional Pain Medicine, Department of
Anesthesiology, University of Florida College of Medicine,
Gainesville, Florida
Chronic Nonsteroidal Anti-inflammatory Drug Use

Prashant Lotlikar, MD
Clinical Assistant Professor, Department of Anesthesiology,
University of Texas Health Science Center, Texas Heart
Institute, Houston, Texas
*Troubleshooting Common Problems during
Cardiopulmonary Bypass*

Michelle L. Lotto, MD
Assistant Professor of Anesthesiology, Department of
General Anesthesiology and Critical Care Medicine,
Cleveland Clinic Lerner College of Medicine; Associate
Staff Anesthesiologist, Cleveland Clinic Foundation,
Cleveland, Ohio
Complications of Spinal Surgery

Katarzyna Luba, MD
Assistant Professor of Clinical Anesthesiology, Department
of Anesthesia and Critical Care, University of Chicago
Pritzker School of Medicine, Chicago, Illinois
*Perioperative Management of Patients with Muscular
Dystrophy*

Stewart J. Lustik, MD
Associate Professor of Anesthesiology, University of
Rochester School of Medicine and Dentistry, Rochester,
New York
Proportioning Systems; Patient Warming Systems

Vinod Malhotra, MD
Professor and Vice Chair for Clinical Affairs,
Department of Anesthesiology, Weill Medical College of
Cornell University, New York–Presbyterian Hospital,
New York, New York
Complications of Transurethral Surgery

Christina M. Matadial, MD
Assistant Professor, Department of Anesthesiology, Leonard M. Miller School of Medicine at the University of Miami; Staff Physician, Department of Anesthesiology, Jackson Memorial Hospital, Miami, Florida
Surgery in the Morbidly Obese

Viktoria D. Mayr, MD
Resident in Anesthesiology and Critical Care Medicine, Department of Anesthesiology and Critical Care Medicine, Medical University Innsbruck, Innsbruck, Austria
Vasopressors: Vasoconstrictor Drugs

Deborah A. McClain, MD
Chief, Anesthesiology Section, Veterans Affairs Medical Center, Biloxi, Mississippi
Delayed Emergence

Thomas McCutchen, MD
Assistant Professor, Department of Anesthesiology, Wake Forest University School of Medicine, Winston-Salem, North Carolina
Epidural Anesthesia: Unintended Intrathecal Injection; Epidural Anesthesia: Unintended Subdural Injection

David L. McDonagh, MD
Resident, Department of Anesthesiology, Duke University School of Medicine, Durham, North Carolina
Autonomic Dysreflexia

Susan B. McDonald, MD
Staff Anesthesiologist, Department of Anesthesiology, Virginia Mason Medical Center, Seattle, Washington
Side Effects of Neuraxial Opioids

Lynda J. Means, MD
Professor of Anesthesia and Surgery, Department of Anesthesia, Indiana University School of Medicine, Indianapolis, Indiana
Postobstruction Pulmonary Edema in Pediatric Patients

Mark Meyer, MD
Assistant Professor of Clinical Anesthesia, Department of Anesthesia, University of Cincinnati College of Medicine; Assistant Professor, Clinical Pediatrics, Cincinnati Children's Hospital Medical Center, Cincinnati, Ohio
Perioperative Aspiration Pneumonitis

Mohammed Minhaj, MD
Assistant Professor, Department of Anesthesia and Critical Care, University of Chicago Pritzker School of Medicine, Chicago, Illinois
Adverse Neurologic Sequelae: Peripheral Nerve Injury

Vivek Moitra, MD
Assistant Professor of Anesthesiology, Department of Anesthesiology, College of Physicians and Surgeons of Columbia University, New York, New York
Carotid Endarterectomy

Constance L. Monitto, MD
Assistant Professor of Anesthesiology, Department of Anesthesiology and Critical Care Medicine, Johns Hopkins Medical Institute, Baltimore, Maryland
Muscle Relaxants

Terri G. Monk, MD
Professor, Department of Anesthesiology, Duke University Medical Center, Durham, North Carolina
Intraoperative Penile Erection; Complications of Radical Urologic Surgery

Lisa M. Montenegro, MD
Assistant Professor of Anesthesiology, University of Pennsylvania School of Medicine and Children's Hospital of Philadelphia; Attending Anesthesiologist, Department of Anesthesiology, Children's Hospital of Philadelphia, Philadelphia, Pennsylvania
Complications of Massive Transfusion

Timothy E. Morey, MD
Associate Professor of Anesthesiology, Department of Anesthesiology, University of Florida College of Medicine, Gainesville, Florida
Magnesium; Antibiotics

Lucille A. Mostello, MD
Assistant Professor of Anesthesiology and Pediatrics, Department of Anesthesiology, George Washington University School of Medicine; Staff Anesthesiologist, Department of Anesthesiology, Children's National Medical Center, Washington, DC
Latex Allergy

Isobel Muhiudeen-Russell, MD
Professor, Department of Anesthesia, University of California, San Francisco, San Francisco, California
Postoperative Pulmonary Hypertension

J. Thomas Murphy, MD, FRCPC
Associate Professor, Department of Anesthesiology, University of Kentucky College of Medicine, Lexington, Kentucky
Disorders of Water Homeostasis: Hyponatremia and Hypernatremia

Catherine Friederich Murray
Research Associate, Department of Anesthesiology, Mayo Clinic College of Medicine, Jacksonville, Florida
Parkinson's Disease; Alzheimer's Disease

Michael J. Murray, MD, PhD
Professor of Anesthesiology and Chair, Department of Anesthesiology, Mayo Clinic College of Medicine, Jacksonville, Florida
Parkinson's Disease; Alzheimer's Disease

David Muzic, MD
Fellow in Cardiac Anesthesia, Department of Anesthesia and Critical Care, University of Chicago Pritzker School of Medicine, Chicago, Illinois
Adverse Neurologic Sequelae: Central Neurologic Impairment

Nader D. Nader, MD
Associate Professor of Anesthesiology, Surgery and Pathology, State University of New York at Buffalo School of Medicine, Buffalo, New York
Uncontrolled Pain; Hemodynamic Instability; Cardioversion

Carsten Nadjat-Haiem, MD
Assistant Professor, Department of Anesthesiology,
David Geffen School of Medicine at University of California,
Los Angeles, Los Angeles, California
Syringe Swaps

Mohamed Naguib, MB,Bch, MSc, FFARCSI, MD
Professor, Department of Anesthesia, Roy J. and Lucille A.
Carver College of Medicine, University of Iowa,
Iowa City, Iowa
Myasthenic Disorders

Bhiken Naik, MD
Fellow, Department of Anesthesiology, University of Florida
College of Medicine, Gainesville, Florida
Intrathecal Opiates; Ketamine; Steroids

David A. Nakata, MD
Associate Clinical Professor and Vice Chair, Residency
Development, Department of Anesthesia, Indiana University
School of Medicine, Indianapolis, Indiana
*Postoperative Peripheral Neuropathy; Intractable Nausea and
Vomiting*

Charles A. Napolitano, MD, PhD
Associate Professor; Director, Division of Cardiothoracic
Anesthesia; Co-Director, Residency Program, Department of
Anesthesiology, University of Arkansas for Medical Sciences,
Little Rock, Arkansas
*Class II Antiarrhythmic Drugs: β-Blockers—Heart Block or
Bradycardia*

Bradly J. Narr, MD
Associate Professor and Chair, Department of
Anesthesiology, Mayo Clinic College of Medicine,
Rochester, Minnesota
Porphyrias

Krishna M. Natrajan, MB,BS, FRCA
Assistant Professor of Adult and Pediatric Cardiothoracic
Anesthesiology, Department of Anesthesiology,
University of Washington School of Medicine; Attending
Anesthesiologist, Department of Anesthesiology,
University of Washington Medical Center, Seattle,
Washington
Inotropic Drugs

Norah Naughton, MD
Associate Professor of Anesthesiology and Associate
Professor of Obstetrics and Gynecology, University of
Michigan Medical School, Ann Arbor, Michigan
Intracranial Pressure Monitoring

Patrick Neligan, MD
Assistant Professor, Department of Anesthesia, University
of Pennsylvania School of Medicine, Philadelphia,
Pennsylvania
Metabolic Acidosis and Alkalosis

Philippa Newfield, MD
Assistant Clinical Professor of Anesthesia and Neurosurgery,
University of California, San Francisco, School of Medicine;
Attending Anesthesiologist, Department of Anesthesiology,
California Pacific Medical Center, San Francisco,
California
*Intracranial Aneurysms: Rebleeding; Intracranial Aneurysms:
Vasospasm and Other Issues*

Hector F. Nicodemus, MD
Pediatric Anesthesiologist, Department of Anesthesiology,
Holy Cross Hospital, Silver Spring, Maryland
Delayed Emergence in Pediatric Patients

Susan C. Nicolson, MD
Professor of Anesthesia, Department of Anesthesia,
University of Pennsylvania School of Medicine; Division
Director, Cardiothoracic Anesthesia, Department of
Anesthesiology and Critical Care Medicine, Children's
Hospital of Philadelphia, Philadelphia, Pennsylvania
Upper Respiratory Tract Infection

Susan H. Noorily, MD
Clinical Professor, Department of Anesthesiology,
University of Texas Health Science Center at San Antonio,
San Antonio, Texas
Laryngoscopy and Microlaryngoscopy

Mark Nunnally, MD
Assistant Professor, Department of Anesthesia and Critical
Care, University of Chicago Pritzker School of Medicine,
Chicago, Illinois
*Postoperative Acute Renal Failure; Metabolic Acidosis and
Alkalosis*

Christopher J. O'Connor, MD
Associate Professor, Department of Anesthesiology, Rush
University Medical Center, Chicago, Illinois
Abdominal Aortic Aneurysm Repair

Michael F. O'Connor, MD
Associate Professor, Department of Anesthesia and Critical
Care, University of Chicago Pritzker School of Medicine,
Chicago, Illinois
Thermally Injured Patients

Jerome F. O'Hara, Jr., MD
Associate Professor, College of Medicine, Case Western
Reserve University; Vice Chairman, Department of General
Anesthesiology; Section Head of Anesthesia, Glickman
Urological Center, Urology Department, Cleveland Clinic
Foundation, Cleveland, Ohio
Complications of Lithotripsy

Maria A. K. Öhrn, MD
Anesthesiology Associates of North Florida, PA, North
Florida Regional Medical Center, Gainesville, Florida
Nondepolarizing Neuromuscular Relaxants

Nollag O'Rourke, MD
Fellow in Obstetric Anesthesia, Department of Anesthesia,
Brigham and Women's Hospital, Boston, Massachusetts
Pulmonary Aspiration in the Parturient

Sheela S. Pai, MD
Assistant Professor, Department of Anesthesiology, Baylor
College of Medicine; Staff Anesthesiologist, Department of
Anesthesiology and Critical Care, Michael E. DeBakey
Veterans Affairs Medical Center, Houston, Texas
Mechanical Assist Devices

Craig M. Palmer, MD
Professor of Clinical Anesthesiology; Director, Obstetric
Anesthesia, University of Arizona College of Medicine,
Tucson, Arizona
Preterm Labor

C. Lee Parmley, MD, JD
Professor of Anesthesiology, Department of Anesthesiology, Vanderbilt University Medical Center, Nashville, Tennessee
Autonomic Hyperreflexia

Komal Patel, MD
Fellow in Cardiac Anesthesia, Department of Anesthesia and Critical Care, University of Chicago Pritzker School of Medicine, Chicago, Illinois
Hypercoagulable States: Thrombosis and Embolism

D. Janet Pavlin, MD
Professor, Department of Anesthesiology, University of Washington School of Medicine; Head of Teaching and Research in Ambulatory Anesthesia, Department of Anesthesia, University of Washington Medical Center, Seattle, Washington
Postoperative Urinary Retention

Padmavathi Perala, MD
Anesthesiologist, Department of Anesthesiology, Veterans Affairs Medical Center, Buffalo, New York
Hemodynamic Instability

Patricia H. Petrozza, MD
Professor of Anesthesiology, Associate Dean for Graduate Medical Education, Wake Forest University School of Medicine, Winston-Salem, North Carolina
Pituitary Tumors: Diabetes Insipidus

Linda S. Polley, MD
Associate Professor, Department of Anesthesiology, University of Michigan Medical School, Ann Arbor, Michigan
Postpartum Hemorrhage

David Porembka, FCCM
Professor of Anesthesia, Surgery and Internal Medicine (Cardiology), Department of Anesthesiology; Associate Director of Surgical Intensive Care; Director of Perioperative Echocardiography, University of Cincinnati College of Medicine, Cincinnati, Ohio
Postoperative Respiratory Failure

Claudia Praetel, MD
Research Fellow, Department of Anesthesiology, College of Physicians and Surgeons of Columbia University, New York, New York
Nitrous Oxide: Neurotoxicity

Joseph Previte, MD
Associate Professor of Pediatrics and Anesthesiology, Project Leader of Anesthesia Centricity IS, Cincinnati Children's Hospital Medical Center, Cincinnati, Ohio
Anesthetic Complications of Fetal Surgery: EXIT Procedures; Perioperative Aspiration Pneumonitis

Richard C. Prielipp, MD, FCCM
JJ Buckley Professor and Chair, Department of Anesthesiology, University of Minnesota Medical School, Minneapolis, Minnesota
Hypothyroidism: Myxedema Coma; Hyperthyroidism: Thyroid Storm

William Prince, MD
Department of Anesthesiology, Kaiser Permanente Oakland Medical Center, Oakland, California
Central Venous Pressure Monitoring

Lester T. Proctor, MD
Professor, Departments of Anesthesiology and Pediatrics, University of Wisconsin Medical School, Madison, Wisconsin
Blood and Blood Products: Transfusion Reaction

Donald S. Prough, MD
Professor and Chair, Department of Anesthesiology, University of Texas Medical Branch, Galveston, Texas
Perioperative Fluid Management; Posterior Fossa Surgery

M. J. Pekka Raatikainen, MD
Division of Cardiology, Oulu University Central Hospital, Oulu, Finland
Adenosine; Class III Antiarrhythmic Drugs: Potassium Channel Blockers

Lee M. Radke, DDS
Assistant Professor, Oral and Maxillofacial Surgery, Medical College of Wisconsin, Froedtert Memorial Lutheran Hospital, Milwaukee, Wisconsin
Dental Injuries

Sivam Ramanathan, MD
Professor of Anesthesiology, University of Pittsburgh School of Medicine, Magee-Womens Hospital, Pittsburgh, Pennsylvania
Humidifiers; Peripartum Neurologic Complications

James G. Ramsay, MD
Professor of Anesthesiology, Program Director, Anesthesiology Critical Care Medicine, Department of Anesthesia, Emory University School of Medicine; Anesthesiology Service Chief, Department of Anesthesiology, Emory University Hospital, Atlanta, Georgia
Central Venous Pressure Monitoring

Monica N. Riesner, MD
Lecturer, Obstetric Anesthesia, Department of Anesthesiology, University of Michigan Medical School, Ann Arbor, Michigan
Postpartum Hemorrhage

Edward T. Riley, MD
Associate Professor, Department of Anesthesia, Stanford University School of Medicine, Stanford, California
Antihistamines: H_1- and H_2-Blockers

Pamela R. Roberts, MD, FCCM, FCCP
Professor and Division Chief, Critical Care Medicine, John A. Moffitt Endowed Chair, Department of Anesthesiology, University of Oklahoma Health Science Center, Oklahoma City, Oklahoma
Hypothyroidism: Myxedema Coma; Hyperthyroidism: Thyroid Storm

Kerri M. Robertson, MD
Associate Clinical Professor of Anesthesiology; Chief, General, Vascular, High-Risk Transplant and Surgical Critical Care Medicine Division; Chief, Transplant Services, Duke University School of Medicine, Department of Anesthesiology, Durham, North Carolina
Postoperative Hepatic Dysfunction; Complications of Carcinoid Tumors; Complications of Deliberate Hypotension: Visual Loss

Marnie Robinson, MD
Assistant Professor of Anesthesiology and Pediatrics, Department of Anesthesiology, University of Cincinnati College of Medicine, Cincinnati Children's Hospital Medical Center, Cincinnati, Ohio
Anesthetic Complications of Fetal Surgery: EXIT Procedures

John B. Rose, MD
Director, Pain Management Service, Department of Anesthesiology and Critical Care Medicine, Children's Hospital of Philadelphia, Philadelphia, Pennsylvania
Delayed Emergence in Pediatric Patients

Mark I. Rossberg, MD
Assistant Professor of Anesthesiology, Department of Anesthesia and Critical Care Medicine, Johns Hopkins Medical Institute, Baltimore, Maryland
Postintubation Croup

David M. Rothenberg, MD
Professor of Anesthesiology; Associate Dean, Academic Affiliations; Co-Medical Director, Surgical Intensive Care Unit, Rush University Medical Center, Chicago, Illinois
Acute Pancreatitis

Daniel D. Rubens, MB,BS, FANZCA
Assistant Professor, Department of Anesthesia, University of Washington School of Medicine, Children's Hospital and Regional Medical Center, Seattle, Washington
Intraoperative Cardiac Arrest

Senthilkumar Sadhasivam, MD
Assistant Professor in Anesthesia and Pediatrics, Department of Anesthesia, University of Cincinnati College of Medicine, Cincinnati Children's Hospital Medical Center, Cincinnati, Ohio
Postoperative Nausea and Vomiting

Tetsuro Sakai, MD, PhD
Resident, Department of Anesthesiology, University of Pittsburgh School of Medicine, Pittsburgh, Pennsylvania
Complications in Orthopedic Outpatients Not Receiving Peripheral Nerve Blocks

Francis V. Salinas, MD
Clinical Assistant Professor, Department of Anesthesiology, University of Washington School of Medicine; Staff Anesthesiologist, Department of Anesthesiology, Virginia Mason Medical Center, Seattle, Washington
Local Anesthetic Systemic Toxicity

Theodore J. Sanford, Jr., MD
Clinical Professor of Anesthesiology, Department of Anesthesiology, University of Michigan Medical School, Ann Arbor, Michigan
Difficult Airway: Opiate-Induced Muscle Rigidity

Ramachandran Satya-Krishna, MD, FRCA
Lecturer, Department of Anesthesiology, University of Michigan Medical School, Ann Arbor, Michigan; Consultant, Department of Anaesthesia, John Radcliffe Hospital, Oxford, United Kingdom
Anesthesia Circuit

Scott R. Schulman, MD
Associate Professor of Anesthesiology and Pediatrics, Division of Pediatric Anesthesia and Critical Care Medicine, Duke University Medical Center, Durham, North Carolina
Malignant Hyperthermia

Annette Schure, MD
Anesthesiologist and Pediatric Anesthesiologist, Department of Anesthesia, Tufts-New England Medical Center, Boston, Massachusetts
Thoracic Aortic Aneurysm

Jeffrey J. Schwartz, MD
Associate Professor, Department of Anesthesiology, Yale University School of Medicine; Attending Physician, Department of Anesthesiology, Yale-New Haven Hospital, New Haven, Connecticut
Electrical Safety

Christian Seefelder, MD
Assistant in Anaesthesia, Harvard Medical School; Instructor in Anaesthesia, Department of Anaesthesiology, Perioperative and Pain Medicine, Children's Hospital, Boston, Massachusetts
Air Emboli

Rajamani Sethuraman, MD, FRCA
Consultant Anaesthetist, Department of Anaesthesia, Princess Alexandra Hospital, Essex, United Kingdom
Intravenous Drug Delivery Systems

Christoph N. Seubert, MD
Assistant Professor, Department of Anesthesiology, University of Florida College of Medicine, Gainesville, Florida
Barbiturates: Porphyrias

Jack S. Shanewise, MD
Chief, Division of Cardiothoracic Anesthesiology, Department of Anesthesiology, College of Physicians and Surgeons of Columbia University, New York, New York
Transesophageal Echocardiography

Kelly T. Shannon, MD
Associate Professor of Anesthesiology, University of Pittsburgh School of Medicine; Associate Chief, Department of Anesthesiology, Magee-Womens Hospital, Pittsburgh, Pennsylvania
Humidifiers

Gauhar Sharih, MD, FRCA
Formerly, Visiting Instructor, Department of Anesthesiology, University of Michigan Medical School, Ann Arbor, Michigan; Specialist Registrar, Department of Anaesthetics, City Hospital, Birmingham, West Midlands, United Kingdom
Inspiratory and Expiratory Gas Monitoring

Aarti Sharma, MD, DA(UK)
Assistant Professor of Anesthesiology, Department of Anesthesiology, Weill Medical College of Cornell University; Attending Anesthesiologist, Department of Anesthesiology, New York–Presbyterian Hospital, New York, New York
Complications of Deliberate Hypotension: Visual Loss

Robert N. Sladen, MD
Professor and Vice Chair, Department of Anesthesiology; Chief, Division of Critical Care, College of Physicians and Surgeons of Columbia University, New York, New York
Postoperative Acute Renal Failure; Hypothermia

Peter D. Slinger, MD
Professor of Anesthesia, Department of Anesthesiology, Toronto General Hospital, Toronto, Ontario, Canada
One-Lung Ventilation

Tod B. Sloan, MD
Professor of Anesthesiology, University of Colorado Health Sciences Center, Denver, Colorado
Spinal Cord Injury

Jonathan H. Slonin, MD
Chief Resident, Department of Anesthesiology, Leonard M. Miller School of Medicine at the University of Miami, Miami, Florida
Surgery in the Morbidly Obese

Paul Smythe, MD
Assistant Professor of Anesthesiology, University of Michigan Medical School; Adjunct Clinical Lecturer in Dentistry, Department of Oral and Maxillofacial Surgery/Hospital Dentistry, University of Michigan School of Dentistry, Ann Arbor, Michigan
Intracranial Pressure Monitoring

Jennifer E. Souders, MD
Clinical Associate Professor, Department of Anesthesiology, University of Washington School of Medicine, Seattle, Washington
Venous Air Embolism

Scott R. Springman, MD
Professor, Departments of Anesthesiology and Surgery, University of Wisconsin Medical School, Madison, Wisconsin
Preanesthetic Evaluation: False-Positive Tests; Preanesthetic Evaluation: Inadequate or Missing Test Result

James M. Steven, MD
Associate Professor of Anesthesia and Pediatrics, Department of Anesthesia, University of Pennsylvania School of Medicine; Chief Medical Officer, Children's Hospital of Philadelphia, Philadelphia, Pennsylvania
Upper Respiratory Tract Infection

Robert K. Stoelting, MD
Emeritus Professor and Chair, Department of Anesthesia, Indiana University School of Medicine, Indianapolis, Indiana
Postoperative Peripheral Neuropathy; Intractable Nausea and Vomiting

Mark D. Stoneham, MD, FRCA
Honorary Senior Clinical Lecturer, Nuffield Department of Anaesthesia, John Radcliffe Hospital, Oxford, United Kingdom
Pulse Oximetry

E. Price Stover, MD*
Clinical Assistant Professor, Department of Anesthesia, Stanford University Medical Center, Stanford, California
Nonbarbiturate Anesthetics

Laura Stover, MD, MASc, FRCP(C)
Acting Instructor, Department of Anesthesiology, University of Washington School of Medicine; Acting Instructor, Department of Cardiothoracic Anesthesiology, University of Washington Medical Center, Seattle, Washington; Assistant Professor of Anesthesiology, Hamilton Health Sciences, Hamilton, Ontario, Canada
Drugs Affecting the Renin-Angiotensin System

Vijayendra Sudheendra, MD
Clinical Instructor, Department of Surgery and Anesthesiology, Brown University School of Medicine; Staff Anesthesiologist, Miriam Hospital, Providence, Rhode Island; Chief of Anesthesia, East Bay Surgery Center, Swansea, Massachusetts
Complications of Transurethral Surgery

Kevin J. Sullivan, MD
Assistant Professor of Anesthesiology, Mayo Clinic College of Medicine; Clinical Assistant Professor of Pediatrics, University of Florida College of Medicine, Jacksonville; Staff Member, Department of Anesthesiology, Nemours Children's Clinic; Staff Pediatric Anesthesiologist and Intensivist, Department of Anesthesia and Critical Care Medicine, Wolfson Children's Hospital, Jacksonville, Florida
Anticholinergics; Hypothermia in Pediatric Patients

Christer H. Svensén, MD
Associate Professor, Department of Anesthesiology, University of Texas Medical Branch, Galveston, Texas
Perioperative Fluid Management

James F. Szocik, MD
Associate Professor, Department of Anesthesiology, University of Michigan Medical School; Chair, Technical Support Committee, Department of Anesthesiology, University of Michigan Medical Center, Ann Arbor, Michigan
Pipeline Source Failure

Kenichi A. Tanaka, MD
Assistant Professor, Department of Anesthesiology, Emory University School of Medicine, Atlanta, Georgia
Perioperative Hypertension

Mark D. Tasch, MD
Associate Professor of Clinical Anesthesia, Department of Anesthesia, Indiana University School of Medicine, Indianapolis, Indiana
Pulmonary Aspiration

*Deceased

Peter Tassani-Prell, MD
Professor of Cardiac Anesthesia, Department of Anesthesia,
German Heart Center Munich, München, Germany
  *Anticoagulation Initiation and Reversal for Cardiac Surgery;
  Bleeding after Cardiac Surgery*

Lisa Thannikary, MD
Adjunct Assistant Professor, Department of Anesthesiology,
University of Florida College of Medicine, Gainesville,
Florida
  Intrathecal Opiates; Ketamine; Steroids

Klaus D. Torp, MD
Assistant Professor of Anesthesiology, Department of
Anesthesiology, Mayo Clinic College of Medicine,
Jacksonville, Florida
  Perioperative Management of Dialysis-Dependent Patients

Laurence C. Torsher, MD
Assistant Professor of Anesthesiology, Department of
Anesthesiology, Mayo Clinic College of Medicine,
Rochester, Minnesota
  *Perioperative Care for Patients with Hepatic Insufficiency
  (Cirrhosis)*

Mark F. Trankina, MD
Staff Anesthesiologist, Carraway Methodist Medical Center
and University of Alabama Hospital at Birmingham,
Birmingham, Alabama
  Class I Antiarrhythmic Drugs: Ventricular Proarrhythmia

Kenneth W. Travis, MD
Associate Professor Emeritus, Department of
Anesthesiology, Dartmouth-Hitchcock Medical Center,
Lebanon, New Hampshire
  Postobstruction Pulmonary Edema

Lawrence C. Tsen, MD
Associate Professor of Anesthesia, Department of
Anesthesia, Harvard Medical School; Director of Anesthesia,
Center for Reproductive Medicine, Department of
Anesthesiology, Perioperative and Pain Medicine, Brigham
and Women's Hospital, Boston, Massachusetts
  Antepartum Hemorrhage

Avery Tung, MD
Associate Professor, Department of Anesthesia and Critical
Care, University of Chicago Pritzker School of Medicine,
Chicago, Illinois
  *Major Organ System Dysfunction after Cardiopulmonary
  Bypass; Mechanical Assist Devices; Thermally Injured Patients*

Manuel C. Vallejo, MD, DMD
Associate Professor, Department of Anesthesiology,
University of Pittsburgh School of Medicine, Pittsburgh,
Pennsylvania
  Peripartum Neurologic Complications

Gail A. Van Norman, MD
Clinical Associate Professor of Anesthesiology, Affiliate
Associate Professor of Medical History and Ethics,
University of Washington School of Medicine, Seattle,
Washington; Physician, Department of Anesthesiology,
St. Joseph Medical Center, Tacoma, Washington
  *Patient Confidentiality; Do-Not-Resuscitate Orders in the
  Operating Room; The Jehovah's Witness Patient*

Karen M. Van Tassel, MD
Chief Resident, Department of Anesthesiology,
Duke University Medical Center, Durham,
North Carolina
  Malignant Hyperthermia

Gurinder M. S. Vasdev, MB,BS
Assistant Professor of Anesthesiology, Department
of Anesthesiology, Mayo Clinic College of Medicine,
Rochester, Minnesota
  Cardiopulmonary Bypass in Pregnancy

Melissa M. Vu, MD
Instructor of Anesthesiology, Department
of Anesthesiology, Mayo Clinic College of Medicine,
Jacksonville, Florida
  Hyperthermia

Mehernoor F. Watcha, MD
Associate Professor of Anesthesia, Department of
Anesthesiology and Critical Care Medicine,
University of Pennsylvania School of Medicine,
Children's Hospital of Philadelphia, Philadelphia,
Pennsylvania
  Postoperative Nausea and Vomiting

Eileen Watson, MD
Clinical Assistant Professor, Department of Anesthesiology,
State University of New York at Buffalo; Attending
Anesthesiologist, Children's Hospital of Buffalo,
Buffalo, New York
  Hemodynamic Instability

B. Craig Weldon, MD
Associate Professor, Department of Anesthesiology
and Pediatrics, Duke University School of Medicine,
Durham, North Carolina
  Cardiomyopathies; Emergence Agitation

Robert S. Weller, MD
Associate Professor of Anesthesiology, Department of
Anesthesiology, Wake Forest University School of Medicine;
Staff Anesthesiologist, Department of Anesthesiology,
North Carolina Baptist Hospitals, Inc., Winston-Salem,
North Carolina
  Psoas Compartment Block: Potential Complications

Lynda Wells, MD
Associate Professor of Anesthesiology, University of Virginia
Health System, Charlottesville, Virginia
  Pediatric Neurosurgery

Volker Wenzel, MD, MSc
Associate Professor of Anesthesiology and Critical Care
Medicine, Department of Anesthesiology and Critical Care
Medicine, Medical University of Innsbruck, Innsbruck,
Austria
  Vasopressors: Vasoconstrictor Drugs

Harshdeep Wilkhu, MD
Clinical Assistant Professor, Department of Anesthesiology,
University of Florida College of Medicine, Gainesville,
Florida
  Nonbarbiturate Anesthetics

Brian A. Williams, MD
Associate Professor, Department of Anesthesiology, University of Pittsburgh School of Medicine; Director of Outpatient Regional Anesthesia Service, Department of Anesthesiology, University of Pittsburgh Medical Center, Pittsburgh, Pennsylvania

Complications in Orthopedic Outpatients Not Receiving Peripheral Nerve Blocks

Glyn D. Williams, MB,ChB, FFA
Associate Professor, Department of Anesthesia, Stanford University School of Medicine, Lucile Packard Children's Hospital, Palo Alto, California

Catheter Ablation for Arrhythmias

Lisa Wise-Faberowski, MD
Assistant Professor, Departments of Anesthesiology and Pediatrics, University of Colorado School of Medicine, Denver, Colorado

Antidepressants; Air Emboli

Eric P. Wittkugel, MD
Associate Professor of Clinical Anesthesia and Critical Care; Staff Anesthesiologist; Director, Preoperative Services, Cincinnati Children's Hospital Medical Center, Cincinnati, Ohio

Pediatric Laryngospasm

David J. Wlody, MD
Clinical Associate Professor of Anesthesiology and Vice Chair for Clinical Affairs, Department of Anesthesiology, State University of New York-Downstate Medical Center; Interim Chair, Department of Anesthesiology, Long Island College Hospital, Brooklyn, New York

Postpartum Headache Other Than Post–Dural Puncture Headache

Gilbert Y. Wong, MD
Assistant Professor of Anesthesiology and Consultant Physician, Division of Pain Medicine, Department of Anesthesiology, Mayo Clinic College of Medicine, Rochester, Minnesota

Celiac Plexus Block: Side Effects and Complications

Brian J. Woodcock, MD
Assistant Professor of Anesthesiology, Department of Anesthesiology, University of Michigan Medical School, Ann Arbor, Michigan

Mechanical Ventilators

Christopher C. Young, MD, FCCM
Assistant Clinical Professor of Surgery, Associate Clinical Professor of Anesthesiology, Chief of Critical Care Medicine Division, Department of Anesthesiology, Duke University School of Medicine, Durham, North Carolina

Hypothermia

William L. Young, MD
James P. Livingston Professor and Vice Chair, Department of Anesthesia and Perioperative Care, University of California, San Francisco, San Francisco General Hospital, San Francisco, California

Arteriovenous Malformation: Normal Perfusion Pressure Breakthrough

Christine M. Zainer, MD
Assistant Professor of Anethesiology, Department of Anesthesiology, Medical College of Wisconsin, Froedtert Memorial Lutheran Hospital East, Milwaukee, Wisconsin

Herbals and Alternative Medicine

Mark A. Zakowski, MD
Chief, Section of Obstetric Anesthesia, Department of Anesthesiology, Cedars-Sinai Medical Center, Los Angeles, California

Peripartum Neurologic Complications

Paul B. Zanaboni, MD, PhD
Anesthesiologist, St. John's Mercy Health Care, St. Louis, Missouri

Bradyarrhythmias

R. Victor Zhang, MD, PhD
Assistant Professor, Department of Anesthesiology, University of Florida College of Medicine, Gainesville, Florida

α_2-Adrenoreceptor Agonists

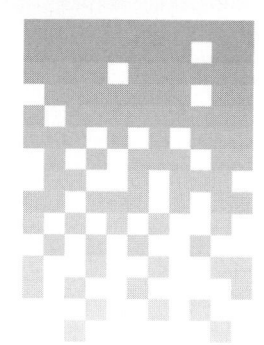

Acknowledgments

First, I wish to acknowledge the contributions to this work of my wife Barbara, my in-house administrative and editorial assistant. Thank you, Barbara! Your literary skills (you did major in English and minor in Philosophy) were much needed and greatly appreciated! I am deeply indebted to the Section Editors for this edition of *Complications in Anesthesia*, some of whom were Section Editors for the first edition as well. Organizing the topics for their sections or subsections, recruiting contributors, and seeing to it that the chapter manuscripts were submitted and pre-edited in a timely fashion were some of their tasks. Special appreciation goes to Natasha Andjelkovic (Executive Publisher), Jean Nevius (Senior Developmental Editor), and Amy Norwitz (Senior Project Manager). Once again, I salute Lewis Reines (former President of WB Saunders) and Leslie Day (former Medical Editor at WB Saunders), who in 1996-1997 convinced me of the need for this conceptually new work as a resource for busy practitioners in anesthesia and critical care. Finally, I express my sincere appreciation to John P. Kampine, MD, PhD, former Professor and Chair of the Department of Anesthesiology at the Medical College of Wisconsin, and to my colleagues in that department (some of whom have contributed to this work) for providing me the time and encouragement for yet again undertaking this work.

John L. Atlee, MD

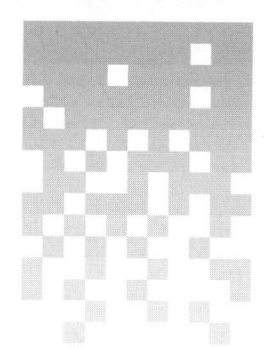

Contents

Section 2
GENERAL ANESTHESIA
Scott R. Springman • John L. Atlee

Preanesthetic Assessment,   141

Anesthetic Management Issues,   159

*Deceased

Section 6
EQUIPMENT AND MONITORING
Kevin K. Tremper

Anesthetic Equipment, 515

Ancillary Systems, 546

Monitoring Devices, 570

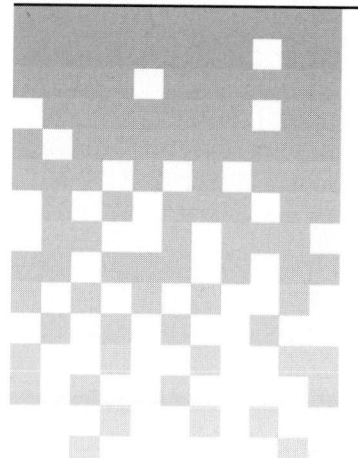

Pharmacology

Donn M. Dennis

Timothy E. Morey

pathways are the primary pathways for the metabolism of sildenafil. Thus, potent inhibitors of the these cytochromes (e.g., cimetidine, erythromycin, digoxin, some statins) may increase sildenafil's plasma concentration. In such patients, and in those with severely compromised renal or hepatic function, reduced starting doses of sildenafil have been advocated to reduce the incidence of significant untoward effects.

Further Reading

Cheitlin MD, Hutter AM Jr, Brindis RG, et al: Use of sildenafil (Viagra) in patients with cardiovascular disease: ACC/AHA expert consensus document. Circulation 99:168-177, 1999.

Hermann HC, Chang G, Klugherz BD, et al: Hemodynamic effects of sildenafil in men with severe coronary artery disease. N Engl J Med 342:1622-1626, 2000.

Hetman JM, Robas N, Baxendale R, et al: Cloning and characterization of two splice variants of human phosphodiesterase 11A. Proc Natl Acad Sci U S A 97:12891-12895, 2000.

Jaski BE, Fifer MA, Wright RF, et al: Positive inotropic and vasodilator actions of milrinone in patients with severe congestive heart failure: Dose-response relationships and comparison to nitroprusside. J Clin Invest 75:643-649, 1985.

Kulkarni SK, Patil CS: Phosphodiesterase 5 enzyme and its inhibitors: Update on pharmacological and therapeutical aspects. Methods Find Exp Clin Pharmacol 26:789-799, 2004.

Landesberg G, Mosseri M, Wolf Y, et al: Perioperative myocardial ischemia and infarction: Identification by continuous 12-lead electrocardiogram with online ST-segment monitoring. Anesthesiology 96:264-270, 2002.

Viagra (sildenafil citrate): US prescribing information. In Physicians' Desk Reference, 57th ed. Montvale, NJ, Medical Economics, 2003, pp 2653-2656.

Zusman RM, Morales A, Glasser DB, et al: Overall cardiovascular profile of sildenafil citrate. Am J Cardiol 83(Suppl):35C-44C, 1999.

Digitalis

Emilio B. Lobato

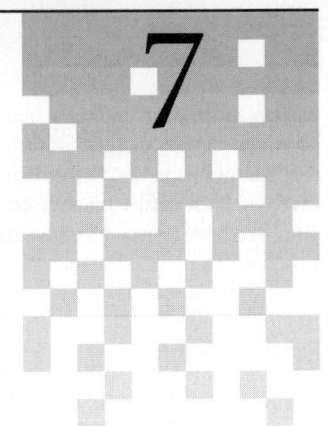

7

Case Synopsis

A 70-year-old man is scheduled for a subtotal colectomy under general anesthesia. He has a history of anterior myocardial infarction and intermittent atrial fibrillation and is receiving digoxin. His preoperative serum digoxin and potassium concentrations are 1.5 ng/dL and 3.9 mEq/L, respectively. Preparation for surgery includes colonic enemas (given until clear). His digoxin is withheld. Soon after the patient is placed on mechanical ventilation, he develops atrioventricular junctional tachycardia (AVJT) at 95 to 100 beats per minute (Fig. 7-1). Pulse oximetry reveals an arterial blood oxygen saturation of 100%. The end-tidal carbon dioxide partial pressure is 22 mm Hg, and the serum potassium concentration is 3.0 mEq/L. Digitalis toxicity is the suspected cause of the AVJT. Intravenous potassium chloride is given, and ventilation is reduced. Eventually, AVJT gives way to sinus rhythm, and the surgical procedure continues uneventfully.

PROBLEM ANALYSIS

Definition

The use of digitalis to treat congestive heart failure (CHF) has been eclipsed by the current widespread use of angiotensin-converting enzyme (ACE) inhibitors and β-blockers to treat this condition. Prospective, randomized clinical trials have shown conclusively that both ACE inhibitors and β-blockers reduce mortality, whereas digoxin does not. However, one meta-analysis of available clinical trials (2001) showed that digoxin had beneficial effects, even in patients treated with ACE inhibitors; these findings may extend to β-blockers, but specific data were lacking. The results of this meta-analysis strengthen the concept that digoxin still has beneficial clinical effects in symptomatic patients with CHF, including the ability to reduce hospitalizations. Further, most patients in these reviewed trials were also receiving diuretics. Thus, clinicians still offer digoxin to symptomatic patients or those at appreciable risk for hospitalization for CHF, with a reasonable expectation of some benefit.

Digitalis increases myocardial contractility in patients with heart failure and reduces the ventricular rate in those with atrial fibrillation. Cardiac complications can result from therapeutic or toxic effects of digitalis, primarily due to inhibition of membrane Na⁺,K⁺-ATPase. Extracardiac complications usually involve the central nervous system and gastrointestinal tract. Monitoring serum concentrations of digoxin (normally, 0.9 to 2.0 ng/dL) may help prevent toxic effects; however, there is considerable overlap between digoxin's toxic and therapeutic effects, especially with hypokalemia or increased sensitivity to its effects (e.g., patients with severe cardiac disease or hypothyroidism). To avoid sampling errors due to slow digoxin equilibration, blood must be drawn at least 4 hours after intravenous dosing or 12 hours after oral dosing. Elevated serum digoxin concentrations may be due to the following:

- Overdose or increased bioavailability (e.g., digitalis gel caps)
- Reduced volume of distribution (especially in elderly patients)

- Reduced excretion (e.g., renal failure, patients receiving quinidine)
- Displacement from binding sites (e.g., with calcium channel blockers)

Recognition

Digitalis toxicity may be immediately apparent or difficult to recognize, especially if cardiac manifestations are due to underlying heart disease. The presenting signs and symptoms depend on whether the digitalis toxicity is acute or chronic. If acute, gastrointestinal symptoms may be prominent. If chronic, patients may present with nonspecific symptoms (e.g., weakness and malaise). However, the sole evidence of chronic toxicity may be new arrhythmias.

CARDIAC MANIFESTATIONS

Cardiac manifestations of digitalis toxicity (primarily arrhythmias) include the following:

- Sinus bradycardia
- Ventricular premature beats
- Nonparoxysmal AVJT
- Wenckebach atrioventricular (AV) block
- Atrial tachycardia with varying AV block
- Bidirectional ventricular tachycardia
- Ventricular fibrillation

When interpreting electrocardiogram (ECG) findings in patients receiving digitalis, one must distinguish between

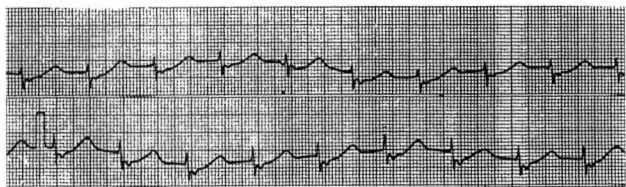

Figure 7–1 ■ Nonparoxysmal atrioventricular junctional tachycardia at 100 beats per minute. Negative P waves after each QRS complex indicate retrograde atrial capture.

normal and toxic effects. Normal ECG changes with therapeutic levels of digitalis include the following:

- T-wave changes (often the earliest sign), ranging from flattening to inversion or peaking of the terminal portion of the T wave
- Shortening of the Q-T interval
- ST-T segment flattening or depression, resulting in the classic concave ("scooped") appearance (often more pronounced in ECG leads with tall R waves)
- Increased U-wave amplitude

Also, a slowed but irregular ventricular rate in atrial fibrillation implies a therapeutic digitalis effect. Regularization of the ventricular rate suggests toxicity and is usually due to the development of AV junctional rhythm (rate ≤70 beats per minute) or AVJT (rate >70 beats per minute).

Cardiac complications can also result from the *therapeutic* effects of digitalis and include the following:

- Increased risk for ventricular tachycardia and ventricular fibrillation in patients with Wolff-Parkinson-White syndrome and atrial fibrillation. Digitalis shortens refractoriness and speeds conduction in accessory AV conducting pathways. This may lead to preferential accessory pathway conduction and a greatly increased ventricular rate with atrial fibrillation (see Chapter 80). The latter can exceed 300 beats per minute and is limited solely by accessory pathway refractoriness. If this rate is sustained, there is a strong potential for early degeneration into ventricular tachycardia or ventricular fibrillation.
- Increased ventricular outflow tract obstruction in patients with asymmetrical ventricular septal hypertrophy, due to the positive inotropic effects of digitalis.
- Aggravation of myocardial ischemia in patients with coronary artery disease; this is "demand" ischemia due to digitalis-increased myocardial oxygen consumption.

Digitalis is ill-advised in any of these circumstances. The associated risks outweigh any potential benefits.

ECG signs of toxicity occur in 5% to 20% of patients receiving digitalis. Almost any arrhythmia can result from the direct toxic or neurally mediated electrophysiologic effects of digitalis on cardiac muscle or the specialized conducting tissues (Table 7-1). The most common arrhythmia

in patients with sinus rhythm is the appearance of ventricular extrasystoles. With atrial fibrillation, regularization of the ventricular rate occurs due to the development of AV junctional rhythm or AVJT; this may be the first manifestation of digitalis toxicity. In fact, the development of accelerated AV junctional rhythm or idioventricular rhythm in patients with AV heart block is highly suggestive of digitalis toxicity.

Two other arrhythmias are characteristically identified with digitalis toxicity:

1. Paroxysmal atrial tachycardia with AV heart block. This is due to increased atrial conduction time and reduced refractoriness, along with AV node conduction block.
2. Bidirectional ventricular tachycardia. In this case, QRS complexes alternate between two distinctly different morphologies. In some leads, distinct R and S waves alternate between each other.

Table 7-2 lists arrhythmias associated with digitalis toxicity in decreasing order of frequency. Worsening of preexisting CHF is often the first symptom of digitalis-induced arrhythmias and should alert the clinician to possible toxicity.

EXTRACARDIAC MANIFESTATIONS

Extracardiac manifestations of digitalis toxicity include the following:

- Gastrointestinal symptoms, including nausea, vomiting, diarrhea, and increased salivation, from stimulation of central vagal nuclei
- Central nervous system manifestations (more common in the elderly), including blurred vision, abnormal color perception (e.g., green halos), hallucinations, and frank delirium
- Acute life-threatening hyperkalemia, occurring with severe digitalis overdose and caused by paralysis of the Na^+-K^+ pump and outward intracellular K^+ leak

Risk Assessment

Knowledge of factors that may alter digitalis pharmacokinetics or myocardial sensitivity and thus predispose patients to digitalis toxicity is of paramount importance (Table 7-3). Elderly patients are at greater risk than younger ones, and

Table 7–1 ■ Electrophysiologic Effects of Therapeutic and Toxic Digitalis

Tissue	Therapeutic Effects	Clinical Manifestations	Toxic Effects	Clinical Manifestations
Sinus node	Slows sinus rate	Sinus bradycardia	Sinus pause or arrest; SA conduction block	Sinus pause; SA conduction block
Atrium	None	None	↑ Conduction; ↓ refractoriness	↑ Atrial rate (atrial flutter/fibrillation)
AV node/AVJ	↓ Conduction time	↓ Ventricular rate; ↑ P-R interval	AV heart block; ↑ AVJ automaticity	Mobitz type I-II second or third degree heart block; AVJR or AVJT
Purkinje fibers	↓ Refractoriness; ↑ repolarization	None; ST-T segment depression	↑ Automaticity; DAD-triggered activity	VPB; VT
Ventricle	↓ Refractoriness	↓ Q-T interval	↑ Automaticity; DAD-triggered activity	VPB; VT

AV, atrioventricular; AVJ, atrioventricular junction; AVJR, atrioventricular junctional rhythm; AVJT, atrioventricular junctional tachycardia; DAD, delayed after depolarization; SA, sinoatrial; VPB, ventricular premature beats; VT, ventricular tachycardia.

Table 7–2 ▪ Digitalis-Caused Arrhythmias in Decreasing Order of Frequency

Premature ventricular beats
Accelerated AV junctional rhythm or tachycardia
Wenckebach (Mobitz type I) AV block
Sinus bradycardia or arrest
Atrial tachycardia with variable AV block*
Bidirectional ventricular tachycardia*
Atrial flutter
Ventricular fibrillation

*Almost always due to the toxic effects of digitalis.
AV, atrioventricular.

reduced body mass lowers the volume of distribution for digitalis. Other drugs administered concomitantly may interact with digoxin and affect serum concentrations. Also, a progressive decline in renal function and reduced serum albumin may elevate serum digoxin concentrations, as does reduced creatinine clearance if no adjustment in dosage is made. Importantly, dialysis is not effective for clearing digoxin.

In hypothyroidism, the activity of membrane Na^+,K^+-ATPase is reduced, which means that lower digoxin doses are needed to achieve a therapeutic effect, and toxicity can occur with usual doses. Hypoxemia enhances digitalis's acceleration of lower pacemaker activity and may trigger arrhythmias from delayed afterpotentials. In patients receiving digitalis, ectopic beats or tachycardia can be exacerbated by the concomitant use of β-adrenergic agonists and diuretics.

Hypokalemia potentiates the effects of digitalis owing to impaired Na^+-K^+ pump function. Low serum K^+ concentrations increase the binding of digitalis to myocardium. Hypomagnesemia reduces the activity of membrane Na^+,K^+-ATPase and may increase kaliuresis and cause hypokalemia. Hypercalcemia increases digitalis activity by increasing intracellular Ca^{2+}. In addition, many drugs and other factors interact with digoxin to alter its pharmacokinetics, displace it from tissue binding sites, or reduce its clearance to increase serum drug concentrations (see Table 7-3).

Table 7–3 ▪ Factors that Predispose to Digitalis Toxicity

Older age
Electrolyte imbalance (hypokalemia, hypomagnesemia, hypercalcemia)
Renal insufficiency
Severity of heart disease
Hypoxemia
Hypothyroidism
Drug interactions
  Angiotensin-converting enzyme inhibitors
  Benzodiazepines
  Quinidine or quinine
  Calcium channel blockers
  Erythromycin
  Cyclosporine
  Amiodarone

Implications

Digitalis toxicity constitutes a serious condition that merits hospitalization. Hemodynamic deterioration with associated arrhythmias in patients with significantly impaired cardiac function may cause acute hemodynamic decompensation. In addition to hemodynamic compromise, some arrhythmias themselves are life threatening. Therefore, early recognition of the toxic effects of digitalis is imperative. Some extracardiac manifestations may be debilitating and may, in fact, precipitate arrhythmias. In surgical candidates, all but the most urgent procedures should be postponed until the digitalis toxicity has been resolved.

MANAGEMENT

The treatment of digitalis toxicity depends on the severity of the clinical manifestations (Table 7-4). However, all patients suspected of digitalis intoxication should have an assessment of serum electrolytes, potassium, magnesium, and calcium, as well as a determination of serum digoxin concentration.

For patients with mild symptoms, temporary discontinuation of the drug, cardiac monitoring, and supportive measures are sufficient. For patients with severe or life-threatening arrhythmias (complete heart block, ventricular tachyarrhythmias), in addition to discontinuing digitalis, the administration of potassium chloride (in the absence of hyperkalemia) and magnesium sulfate should be considered. For heart block, 1 mg of atropine is usually effective in counteracting the vagal effects of digoxin. For ventricular arrhythmias, in addition to monitoring serum levels, lidocaine is the drug of choice, with a loading dose of 1 to 2 mg/kg, followed by an infusion of 1 to 2 mg/minute. Phenytoin was used in the past but, owing to its myocardial depressant properties and its tendency to produce hypotension when given intravenously, has largely been replaced by digoxin-specific antibodies (Digibind).

There is no evidence to support the use of amiodarone to treat ventricular tachycardia or to prevent recurrences of ventricular fibrillation in patients with digitalis toxicity. At least in theory, the complementary electrophysiologic actions of amiodarone and digitalis to promote sinus bradycardia and increase sinoatrial and AV node conduction times and refractoriness might promote or precipitate asystole. More important is that amiodarone is known to

Table 7–4 ▪ Management of Digitalis Toxicity

Withhold further digitalis
Assess electrolytes (K^+, Ca^{2+}, Mg^{2+})
Administer potassium chloride in the absence of hyperkalemia
Administer magnesium sulfate
Treat bradyarrhythmias
  Atropine
  Temporary or (possibly) permanent artificial pacing
Treat ventricular arrhythmias
  Lidocaine
  Phenytoin (diphenylhydantoin)
  Digoxin-specific antibodies (Digibind)

increase serum digoxin levels. Systemic clearance of digoxin is significantly prolonged owing to reduced renal and non-renal clearance, which lengthens its half-life of elimination by approximately 20%. However, amiodarone does not appear to affect the volume of distribution for digoxin.

Electrical countershock (direct-current cardioversion) is contraindicated because it can exacerbate the severity of arrhythmias. Administration of digoxin-specific antibodies (Digibind) is the treatment of choice for life-threatening arrhythmias and for digoxin-induced refractory hyperkalemia. The use of an antibody rapidly reduces the percentage of unbound digoxin in the serum from 75% to less than 5%. The antibody-digoxin complex then undergoes renal excretion. Side effects are infrequent but include allergic reactions and rebound toxic digoxin effects in patients treated with inadequate doses of Digibind. Importantly, conventional serum assays for digoxin cannot distinguish between free and bound digoxin; thus, serum digoxin concentrations appear markedly elevated following Digibind treatment. The results of treatment are monitored by manifestations of clinical improvement; however, free digoxin determinations can be obtained in patients who show a poor response to treatment.

PREVENTION

Knowledge of the multiple factors that affect digoxin pharmacokinetics and pharmacodynamics is important to avoid its toxic effects. Regular determination of serum digoxin concentrations and dose adjustments in patients with conditions that increase the risk of digitalis toxicity are important measures, especially in the elderly.

Further Reading

Antman EM, Wenger TL, Butler VP Jr, et al: Treatment of 150 cases of life-threatening digitalis intoxication with specific Fab antibody fragments: Final report of a multicenter study. Circulation 81:1744-1750, 1990.

Fenster PE, White NW Jr, Hanson CD: Pharmacokinetic evaluation of the digoxin-amiodarone interaction. J Am Coll Cardiol 5:108-112, 1985.

Hauptman PJ, Kelly RA: Digitalis. Circulation 99:1265-1270, 1999.

Hood WB Jr, Dans AL, Guyatt GH, et al: Digitalis for treatment of congestive heart failure in patients in sinus rhythm. Update of Cochrane Database Syst Rev 3:CD002901, 2001; PMID: 11687032.

Kelly RA, Smith TW: Recognition and management of digitalis toxicity. Am J Cardiol 69:108G-119G, 1992.

Ma G, Brady WJ, Pollack M, et al: Electrocardiographic manifestations: Digitalis toxicity. J Emerg Med 20:145-152, 2000.

Ooi H, Colucci WS: Pharmacological treatment of heart failure. In Hardman JG, Limbird LE (eds): Goodman and Gilman's The Pharmacological Basis of Therapeutics, 10th ed. New York, McGraw-Hill, 2001, pp 901-932.

Spratt KA, Doherty JE: Principles and practice of digitalis. In Messerli FH (ed): Cardiovascular Drug Therapy, 2nd ed. Philadelphia, WB Saunders, 1996, pp 1136-1146.

Anticholinergics

Kevin J. Sullivan

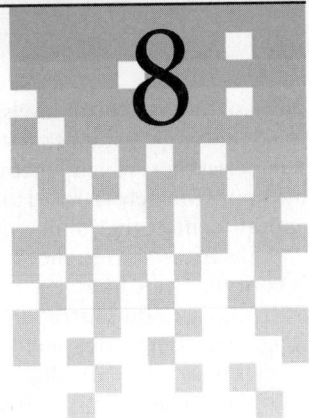

8

Case Synopsis

A 1-year-old child weighing 10 kg is in the pediatric intensive care unit with respiratory failure and a difficult airway. Prior attempts at laryngoscopy and endotracheal intubation have been unsuccessful, and mask ventilation is difficult. The infant, who becomes hypoxic and bradycardic during resuscitation efforts, is unintentionally given 4 mg of intravenous atropine, instead of the 0.2 mg that was ordered. Endotracheal intubation is performed to reverse the respiratory failure and hypoxia. Shortly thereafter, the patient is noted to be tachycardic (225 beats per minute), with warm, red, dry skin and fever (39°C). He appears disoriented, agitated, and inconsolable.

PROBLEM ANALYSIS

Definition

Because infants and young children have a relatively enhanced vagal tone compared with adults, vagotonic physiologic perturbations, such as airway instrumentation, can result in bradycardia. Thus, in pediatric anesthesia and critical care settings, bradycardia can be seen during laryngoscopy and induction of anesthesia with volatile inhalational agents (most commonly halothane), as well as with hypoxemia and elevated intracranial pressure. Bradycardia and the consequent reduced cardiac output can be prevented by premedication with oral, intravenous, or intramuscular anticholinergic drugs. In the case synopsis, an inadvertently high dose of atropine (about 20-fold too high) was given to increase the patient's heart rate during bradycardia.

Anticholinergic (antimuscarinic) toxicity is commonly seen in infants and young children after the accidental ingestion of belladonna alkaloids and their synthetic congeners, antiparkinson medications, histamine receptor antagonists, tricyclic antidepressants, and phenothiazines. For persons of all ages, the ingestion of plants that contain large quantities of belladonna alkaloids can cause anticholinergic toxicity. Such plants include deadly nightshade (*Atropa belladonna*), jimsonweed (*Datura stramonium*), and angel's trumpet (*Brugmansia candida*).

Anticholinergics used in anesthesia include atropine, glycopyrrolate, and scopolamine. They compete with neurally released acetylcholine to attach to muscarinic cholinergic receptors and block the effects of acetylcholine, and they antagonize muscarinic agonist actions at noninnervated muscarinic cholinergic receptors. Further, presynaptic muscarinic receptors on adrenergic nerve terminals inhibit norepinephrine release. Thus, muscarinic antagonists (anticholinergics) can enhance sympathetic activity. Except for the fact that quaternary ammonium compounds (glycopyrrolate) do not readily cross the blood-brain barrier to exert central nervous system (CNS) actions, there is little difference in the qualitative actions of atropine, glycopyrrolate, and scopolamine. However, some quantitative differences in effect may be seen. For example, both atropine and scopolamine have a shorter duration of action than glycopyrrolate. Further, the antisialagogue effects of glycopyrrolate and scopolamine are greater than those of atropine. In addition, heart rate is most increased by atropine, then by glycopyrrolate, and least by scopolamine. Finally, although both atropine and scopolamine are tertiary amines that readily cross the blood-brain barrier, they differ in CNS effects: atropine causes CNS stimulation, whereas scopolamine produces sedation and amnesia.

Human tissues vary with respect to both the density and the type of muscarinic receptors present. Five subtypes of muscarinic receptors have been identified (M_1, M_2, M_3, M_4, M_5), each with a different location and function. For example, M_1 receptors are found in the cerebral cortex, sympathetic ganglia and postganglionic neurons, and some presynaptic sites. M_2 receptors are present in myocardium, smooth muscle cells, and some presynaptic sites. M_3 receptors are found in exocrine glands, and M_4 receptors in heart. M_5 receptors are found mostly in brain.

All muscarinic receptor subtypes interact with heterotrimeric, guanine nucleotide-binding regulatory proteins (G proteins) linked to cellular effectors. Although selectivity is not absolute, stimulation of M_1 or M_3 receptors causes hydrolysis of polyphosphoinositides and mobilization of intracellular Ca^{2+}, which is due to interaction with a G protein (Gq) that activates phospholipase C. The latter causes a variety of Ca^{2+}-mediated events, either directly or via phosphorylation of target proteins. In contrast, M_2 and M_4 muscarinic receptors inhibit adenylyl cyclase and regulate specific ion channels (e.g., enhancement of K^+ conductance in cardiac atrial tissue) through subunits released from pertussis toxin-sensitive G proteins (G_1 and G_0). These are distinct from the G proteins used by the M_1 and M_3 receptors. Finally, M_5 receptors may inhibit M-type (KCNQ2/KCNQ3) K^+ channels via the activation of a common G protein.

Recognition

Table 8-1 lists the effects of anticholinergics in various organ systems. Appreciation of the range of organ systems affected by anticholinergic drugs is required to maximize their benefits while minimizing side effects. Drugs in common use (atropine, scopolamine, glycopyrrolate) are nonselective muscarinic receptor antagonists. They have similar side effects, but to a varying extent. As stated earlier, atropine and

Table 8–1 ■ Clinical Effects of Anticholinergic Drugs

Cardiovascular effects (observed at moderate doses)
  Increased rate of sinoatrial (SA) node discharge
  Decreased rate of SA node discharge (low doses of atropine)
  Enhanced atrioventricular node conduction
  Little or no effect on ventricular function
  Little effect on peripheral vasculature
  Cutaneous vasodilatation in high doses
Respiratory effects (observed at low doses)
  Drying of respiratory secretions
  Relaxation of bronchial smooth muscle
  Increased anatomic dead space
Central nervous system effects (observed at larger doses)
  Wide range of symptoms, from sedation and depression to
    agitation and delirium
Gastrointestinal effects (observed at larger doses)
  Decreased salivation
  Reduced gastric secretions and motility
  Decreased lower esophageal sphincter tone
Ophthalmic effects (observed at moderate doses)
  Mydriasis
  Cycloplegia
Genitourinary effects (observed at larger doses)
  Decreased ureter and bladder tone
  Urinary retention
Thermoregulation effects (observed at small doses)
  Inhibition of sweat gland secretions (function most sensitive
    to anticholinergics)
  Elevated temperature

in the 1980s and reestablished anticholinergics as a therapy for bronchospastic disorders. Although ipratropium is structurally similar to atropine and has similar actions if given parenterally, it is a quaternary ammonium compound. Ipratropium is poorly absorbed when inhaled and has few extrapulmonary effects, even with very large inhaled doses. When inhaled, 90% of ipratropium is swallowed, and only 1% of the total dose is absorbed systemically. When given to normal volunteers, the drug provides almost complete protection against bronchospasm induced by a variety of provocative agents. However, in asthmatics, the results can vary. Whereas the bronchospastic effects of some agents (e.g., methacholine, sulfur dioxide) are completely blocked, there is little blocking of leukotriene-induced bronchoconstriction. Also, unlike atropine, ipratropium has no negative effect on ciliary clearance. In general, this drug and other anticholinergics are more effective in chronic obstructive pulmonary disease, especially when cholinergic tone is high. The development of new drugs that affect specific muscarinic receptor subtypes will provide more effective therapy with fewer adverse or troublesome side effects than the drugs used today.

The child in the case synopsis displayed many of the signs and symptoms of anticholinergic toxicity, which can be divided into two types: CNS and peripheral antimuscarinic. CNS toxicity can manifest as agitation, delirium, seizures, or coma. Systemic anticholinergic effects are most prominent in tissues or organs with dense parasympathetic innervation and include tachycardia; dry mucous membranes; urinary retention; dry, flushed skin; dilated pupils with cycloplegia; fever; and ileus. The child in the case illustrated the typical findings accompanying anticholinergic overdose in pediatric patients. Although the cause of his condition was known, the differential diagnosis includes other potentially life-threatening conditions (Table 8-3). Physical examination and the natural history of the disease process should allow the clinician to differentiate among these conditions. Physical and laboratory findings of anticholinergic toxicity that help exclude other conditions are summarized in Table 8-4. Although the conditions in the differential diagnosis share overlapping features with anticholinergic toxicity, the combination of abolition of pupillary responses and sweating is very specific for anticholinergic toxicity.

Many clinicians confuse anticholinergic toxicity with the diametrically opposed toxidrome associated with anticholinesterase poisoning, which results in excessive cholinergic tone. Physician familiarity with toxic syndromes due to anticholinesterase poisoning has increased dramatically with the proliferation of chemical weapons of mass destruction. In contrast to the symptoms and signs of anticholinergic

scopolamine cross the blood-brain barrier, whereas glycopyrrolate does not. Scopolamine is more sedating than atropine but causes less of a heart rate increase; similar to atropine, it is a moderately potent antisialagogue. Glycopyrrolate is the most potent antisialagogue, causes moderate tachycardia, and is nonsedating. The pharmacologic effects of anticholinergics used in anesthesia are summarized in Table 8-2.

Another anticholinergic agent, ipratropium (Atrovent), is used primarily in pulmonary care. This drug was introduced

Table 8–2 ■ Pharmacologic Effects of Anticholinergics Used in Anesthesia

Atropine
  Causes greater vagolysis than glycopyrrolate
  Increases heart rate and enhances atrioventricular node
    conduction
  Paradoxical slowing of heart rate at low doses
  Little sedation
  Moderately potent antisialagogue
Glycopyrrolate
  Moderate vagolytic effect on heart, but less than that
    of atropine
  No sedation (charged quaternary amine; does not cross
    blood-brain barrier)
  Highly potent antisialagogue
Scopolamine
  Marked sedation-amnesia (tertiary amine structure; lipid
    soluble; crosses blood-brain barrier)
  Most likely to cause central anticholinergic syndrome (easily
    reversed with physostigmine)
  Moderately potent antisialagogue

Table 8–3 ■ Differential Diagnosis of Anticholinergic Toxicity

Hypoxemia and/or hypercarbia
Sepsis
Malignant hyperthermia
Thyroid storm (crisis)
Pheochromocytoma
Carcinoid syndrome

Table 8–4 ■ Distinguishing Features of Anticholinergic Toxicity*

Relatively normal arterial O_2 and CO_2 tensions (rules out hypoxemia and hypercarbia)
Cycloplegia (pupillary light reflexes remain intact for most other conditions)
Mydriasis (pupils may also be dilated in MH due to elevated circulating catecholamines)
Anhidrosis; warm, red skin (sweating is preserved in other disorders within the differential diagnosis; see Table 8-3)
Lack of muscle rigidity (commonly seen with MH)
No ventricular arrhythmias (not characteristic of carcinoid syndrome, but common with MH, pheochromocytoma, and thyrotoxicosis)
Minimal to modest increase in end-tidal CO_2 due to hyperthermia (usually far greater with MH or thyrotoxicosis)
Mild (or no) hypertension (as in MH), or paroxysmal, severe hypertension (thyroid storm, pheochromocytoma, or carcinoid tumor[†]), especially with gland or tumor manipulation
Mild to no metabolic acidosis (far more severe in MH)

*In anesthetized patients, the modulatory effects of anesthesia must be considered.
[†]Serotonin released by carcinoid tumors has little if any direct effect on the heart. However, positive chronotropic and inotropic effects, and possibly arrhythmias, may occur with the release of norepinephrine. Effects of serotonin on the peripheral vasculature include both vasoconstriction and vasodilatation.
MH, malignant hyperthermia.

overdose, poisoning with carbamate insecticides or organophosphates leads to CNS excitation and excessive nicotinic and muscarinic receptor activation. CNS signs include ataxia, restlessness, agitation, convulsions, and coma. Muscarinic signs include excessive salivation, perspiration, vomiting, diarrhea, abdominal cramps, tenesmus, bradycardia or heart block, pupillary constriction, lacrimation, wheezing, hypotension, blurred vision, and urinary and fecal incontinence. Nicotinic signs include muscle twitching, fasciculations, cramping, paralysis, respiratory compromise, and subsequent cardiac arrest.

Risk Assessment

Patients with heart disease are at far greater risk for anticholinergic complications. In this respect, atropine and glycopyrrolate produce more vagolysis than scopolamine does, causing a much greater increase in the sinus rate and speed of atrioventricular (AV) node conduction. An increased heart rate is more dangerous in patients with coronary artery disease and valvular or subvalvular restrictive cardiac lesions (e.g., aortic and mitral valve stenosis, idiopathic hypertrophic subaortic stenosis). Further, in patients with functional accessory AV pathways and a history of AV reciprocating tachycardia or atrial flutter or fibrillation (e.g., Wolff-Parkinson-White syndrome), atropine or glycopyrrolate (especially in a relative overdose) may precipitate dangerously fast tachyarrhythmias (see Chapter 80). Also, because both drugs facilitate AV node conduction, they are contraindicated in patients with supraventricular tachyarrhythmias, especially atrial flutter or fibrillation.

Implications

Anticholinergics exert their effects in many organ systems (see Table 8-1). Therapeutic effects in one organ system may be accompanied by undesirable side effects in others. Careful selection of the anticholinergic agent and its dose allows the clinician to target the appropriate organ system and simultaneously minimize undesirable side effects in other organ systems (see Table 8-2).

Although atropine is considered relatively safe and benign in adults, an atropine overdose is very dangerous in pediatric patients, especially infants. Deaths due to anticholinergic poisoning have been reported with doses as low as 2 mg of atropine in infants.

Anticholinergics have complex gastrointestinal actions. Salivary gland secretions are reduced and are the most sensitive to cholinergic block. Gastric secretions are also reduced, but this requires larger doses. Both gastrointestinal motility and lower esophageal sphincter tone are reduced. However, it is important to remember that anticholinergic premedication does not confer protection against aspiration of gastric contents and chemical or bacterial pneumonitis.

Also, the function of a number of other organs can be impaired by anticholinergic therapy. In the eye, anticholinergic drugs can precipitate narrow-angle glaucoma. Individuals with a shallow anterior chamber can suffer acute increased intraocular pressure due to impaired drainage via the canal of Schlemm. Postsurgical patients, especially elderly men with prostatic hypertrophy, are at risk for severe urinary retention after taking anticholinergics. Further, confusion, agitation, and delirium are CNS side effects of anticholinergics that cross the blood-brain barrier (scopolamine, atropine). Patients at greatest risk for mental status changes are those at the extremes of age, those with preexisting abnormalities of mental status, and those taking drugs with significant anticholinergic properties (e.g., antiparkinson drugs, phenothiazines, tricyclic antidepressants, butyrophenones, antihistamines, cycloplegics, antispasmodics).

Impaired thermoregulation due to the inability to sweat can result in hyperpyrexia. Children and infants are especially vulnerable owing to their high metabolic rate and immature thermoregulatory mechanisms. It is clear that hyperpyrexia involves an impaired ability to dissipate heat through sweating. Whether there is a central effect on thermal regulation remains unclear.

Finally, atropine and glycopyrrolate are commonly given with or prior to anticholinesterase drugs to reverse nondepolarizing neuromuscular blockade. Because of similarities in onset of drug action, atropine is commonly administered with edrophonium, which has a very rapid onset. Similarly, glycopyrrolate is often administered with neostigmine because both have a slower onset and a longer duration of action. By selecting an anticholinergic that matches the anticholinesterase drug's onset and duration of action, heart rates that are too fast or too slow can be avoided. It also appears that lower doses of anticholinergics are required to antagonize the weaker and shorter-lived muscarinic effects of edrophonium compared with those of neostigmine.

MANAGEMENT

Most complications related to anticholinergic drugs are self-limited and can be effectively treated with supportive care. For example, urinary retention in elderly men may require short-term or intermittent bladder catheterization. However, some complications, such as fast sinus or non-paroxysmal atrial tachycardias in patients with myocardial ischemia or infarction, aortic or mitral valve stenosis, or idiopathic hypertrophic subaortic stenosis, require prompt treatment. Therapeutic options include β-blockers and calcium channel antagonists. If paroxysmal supraventricular tachycardia is likely, adenosine is useful. However, the current advanced cardiovascular life support guidelines advise early cardioversion for most hemodynamically disadvantageous tachyarrhythmias, rather than a trial of drugs (see Chapter 79). Likewise, severe hyperthermia should be treated aggressively with cooling blankets and, if needed, immersion in ice water and irrigation of body cavities with cold saline. With careful consideration of the underlying medical history and the pharmacodynamics of the various anticholinergics, it is possible to maximize the benefits of this class of medications while minimizing undesirable side effects of therapy.

PREVENTION

Prevention of the side effects of anticholinergic drugs begins with an appreciation of the fact that they affect different organ systems with different intensities (see Tables 8-1 and 8-2) but do so in a predictable, dose-related fashion. To avoid complications, it is most important to recognize that certain subsets of patients are at greater risk for morbidity related to the use of anticholinergic drugs. Therefore, it is crucial to evaluate the specific vulnerabilities of the patient, delineate the goals of anticholinergic therapy, and select a drug with a pharmacodynamic profile that most closely suits the goals of therapy.

Further Reading

Brown JH, Taylor P: Muscarinic receptor agonists and antagonists. In Hardman JG, Limbird LE (eds): Goodman and Gilman's The Pharmacological Basis of Therapeutics, 10th ed. New York, McGraw-Hill, 2001, pp 155-173.

Das G: Therapeutic review: Cardiac effects of atropine in man: An update. Int J Clin Pharmacol 27:473-477, 1989.

Feldman MD: The syndrome of anticholinergic intoxication. Am Fam Physician 34:113-116, 1986.

Friesen RH, Lichtor JL: Cardiovascular depression during halothane anesthesia in infants: A study of three induction techniques. Anesth Analg 61:42-45, 1982.

Goyal RK: Muscarinic receptor subtypes: Physiology and clinical implications. N Engl J Med 321:1022, 1989.

Gross NJ: Ipratropium bromide. N Engl J Med 319:486-494, 1988.

Guo J, Schofield GG: Activation of muscarinic M5 receptors inhibits recombinant KCNQ2/KCNQ3 K$^+$ channels expressed in HEK293T cells. Eur J Pharmacol 462:25-32, 2003.

Mirakhur RK: Antagonism of the muscarinic effects of edrophonium with atropine or glycopyrrolate. Br J Anaesth 57:1213-1216, 1985.

Moss J, Glick D: The autonomic nervous system. In Miller RD (ed): Miller's Anesthesia, 6th ed. Philadelphia, Churchill Livingstone, 2005, pp 617-677.

Patton WDM: The principles of drug action. Proc R Soc Med 53:815-820, 1965.

Polak RL: Effects of hyoscine on the output of acetylcholine into preferred cerebral ventricles on cats. J Physiol 181:317-323, 1965.

Adenosine

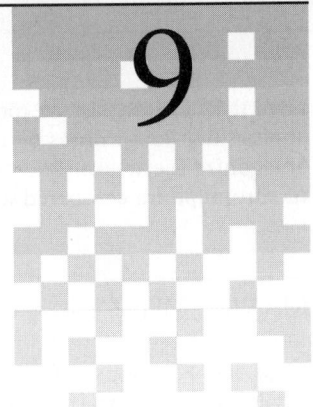

M. J. Pekka Raatikainen and John L. Atlee

9

Case Synopsis

A 63-year-old man with a history of transient ischemic attacks is admitted to the hospital for elective surgery. His medications include aspirin 250 mg/day orally and dipyridamole 75 mg orally three times a day. During the operation under regional anesthesia, a regular supraventricular tachycardia (SVT) is observed. The tachycardia terminates after intravenous bolus adenosine (12 mg) and is followed by a long sinus pause and angina-like pain (Fig. 9-1).

PROBLEM ANALYSIS

Definition

The first step is to determine whether the signs or symptoms are due to tachycardia. If they are, the existing advanced cardiovascular life support guidelines advise immediate cardioversion rather than a trial of antiarrhythmic drugs. If cardioversion is not indicated (e.g., ectopic atrial tachycardia), the guidelines stress making a specific diagnosis and identifying patients with impaired cardiac function (ejection fraction <40%). Importantly, the 2000 guidelines downplay the use of adenosine to differentiate wide QRS tachycardia due to ventricular aberration versus ectopy. This unnecessarily exposes patients to adenosine's unpleasant side effects, possibly worsens arrhythmias, and may destabilize heart rate and pressure.

However, given the history of the patient described in the case synopsis, the circumstances, and the apparent suddenness of onset, it was reasonable to administer adenosine to terminate this regular, narrow QRS complex tachycardia, especially because it was associated with apparent ST segment depression in the lead depicted. The advantage of adenosine (versus intravenous calcium channel antagonists, such as verapamil or diltiazem, or β-blockers) for the chemical conversion of sudden-onset, narrow QRS tachycardia is related to its rapid action and ultrashort half-life. Although adenosine rarely causes severe side effects, minor adverse effects such as facial flushing and chest discomfort are frequently observed. In the majority of patients, these are well tolerated and resolve rapidly without intervention. However, the concomitant administration of drugs that inhibit the elimination of adenosine from blood, and the presence of some clinical conditions (e.g., asthma), may render some patients more susceptible to the development of severe adverse effects with adenosine.

Recognition

Endogenous adenosine is involved in numerous physiologic and pathophysiologic processes in mammalian organs and tissues. Most, if not all, of these actions are mediated by specific cell surface receptors (A_1-, A_{2A}-, A_{2B}-, and A_3-adenosine receptors). Because of the ubiquitous nature and distribution of these receptors, administration of adenosine to terminate SVT may cause adverse effects unrelated to the heart.

Following are the most common patient complaints after the administration of adenosine:

- Facial flushing
- Dyspnea
- Chest discomfort

Less common side effects are nausea, lightheadedness, headache, dizziness, and palpitations. These adverse side effects often occur concomitantly with tachycardia termination and persist for 2 to 3 minutes. Many, but not all, of these effects are attributable to vasodilatation with activation of the A_2-adenosine receptors. For example, facial flushing is caused by cutaneous vasodilatation. Direct stimulation of carotid chemoreceptors and cardiac pain receptors may explain respiratory stimulation and the sensation of dyspnea and chest discomfort (angina-like pain), respectively. Adenosine may also cause bronchoconstriction, especially in asthmatics.

Like all antiarrhythmics, adenosine may be proarrhythmic, provoking new or worse arrhythmias. Given the potent depressant effects of adenosine in the sinoatrial (SA) and atrioventricular (AV) nodes, it is not surprising that adenosine

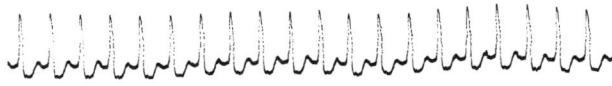

A Rhythm strip during the tachycardia

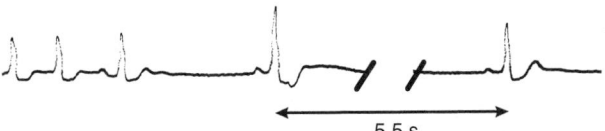

5.5 s

B 20 sec after 12 mg adenosine bolus

Figure 9–1 ■ *A,* Intraoperative rhythm strip from the patient described in the case synopsis (paper speed, 25 mm/second). It shows a regular, narrow QRS tachycardia (180 beats per minute). *B,* Rhythm strip 20 seconds after the administration of intravenous bolus adenosine (12 mg). Sinus arrest lasting 5.5 seconds occurs after termination of the tachycardia. The patient was receiving dipyridamole, which is a potent nucleoside transport blocker and likely potentiated adenosine's effects. In later ambulatory electrocardiographic recordings and electrophysiologic testing, there was no evidence of sinoatrial node dysfunction.

often causes transient sinus bradycardia and AV block. In fact, adenosine's efficacy in terminating AV nodal reentrant tachycardia and AV reciprocating tachycardia depends on the production of transient AV block. In addition to commonly associated bradyarrhythmias, clinicians report that adenosine occasionally induces atrial fibrillation, ventricular premature beats, brief episodes of nonsustained ventricular tachycardia (VT), and torsades de pointes VT (a polymorphic VT in association with Q-T interval prolongation; see Chapter 81).

The following proarrhythmias have been observed after the intravenous administration of adenosine:

- Sinus bradycardia; transient sinus arrest
- Transient AV block
- Supraventricular premature beats
- Atrial flutter
- Atrial fibrillation
- Ventricular premature beats
- Nonsustained VT
- Torsades de pointes–type polymorphic VT

The potent negative chronotropic (slowed sinus rate) and dromotropic (slowed AV node conduction) effects of adenosine explain its ability to cause pronounced bradycardia or sinus arrest or AV heart block. The induction of atrial flutter or fibrillation by adenosine appears to be due to shortening of atrial repolarization and refractoriness. Although the drug effectively terminates most paroxysmal SVT, some reports have demonstrated its proarrhythmic potential, including the induction of VT. However, the mechanisms of adenosine-induced ventricular premature beats and nonsustained or even sustained VT are less clear. Adenosine has no known direct effect on ventricular myocytes. Thus, it seems unlikely that adenosine exerts a direct proarrhythmic effect, at least in normal ventricles. Further, ventricular premature beats are not specific for adenosine but may also be seen after termination of SVT by calcium channel blockers (e.g., verapamil, diltiazem) or AV node ablation. Some reports suggest that termination of SVT by adenosine may occasionally lead to the development of torsades de pointes polymorphic VT. Adenosine markedly slows the sinus and ventricular rates and, when given intravenously, leads to increased sympathetic discharge. In fact, adenosine has been used to reproduce clinical torsades de pointes in patients with congenital long Q-T interval syndrome during electrophysiologic testing. Thus, one might speculate that an adenosine-slowed ventricular rate and an increased sympathetic discharge interact adversely to facilitate early afterdepolarizations, the proximate cause of ventricular tachyarrhythmias in experimental models.

One group attempted to define the proarrhythmic effects of adenosine used to terminate 187 episodes of SVT in 127 patients admitted to the emergency room over a 5-year period. In two thirds of cases, adenosine induced ventricular ectopy after successful termination of SVT, including premature ventricular beats and nonsustained VT, both of which were transient and self-terminating. Based on morphologic criteria, more than half the arrhythmias appeared to originate in the inferior left ventricular septum, which may be more susceptible to adenosine's proarrhythmic effects. Although this high incidence of ventricular arrhythmias was surprising, no further intervention was required. These proarrhythmic effects may be due to abnormal electrophysiologic mechanisms facilitated by adenosine-increased sympathetic discharge. To recognize transient or sustained ventricular proarrhythmias after the administration of adenosine for the treatment of paroxysmal SVT, one should monitor the electrocardiogram (ECG) continuously for at least 2 minutes following each intravenous adenosine bolus.

Risk Assessment

The reported incidence of adverse extracardiac symptoms after an intravenous bolus injection of adenosine ranges from less than 30% to more than 70%. Proarrhythmic effects are less common; for example, the incidence of atrial fibrillation is 1% to 5%, and the incidence of ventricular premature beats is approximately 10% to 30%. Only occasionally do case reports describe more severe proarrhythmic actions. However, it is known that interactions with drugs inhibiting adenosine metabolism and some clinical conditions may sensitize patients to the effects of adenosine and thus render them susceptible to more severe adverse effects. For example, in patients receiving dipyridamole, the cellular uptake of adenosine is blocked, and the half-life of the nucleoside is markedly prolonged. Consequently, these patients are much more vulnerable to the development of prolonged bradycardia, AV node conduction disturbances, and extracardiac adverse effects. Likewise, patients with preexisting AV node conduction disturbances, sick sinus syndrome, myocardial ischemia, and cardiac allografts are more sensitized to the cardiac effects of adenosine, and asthmatic patients are more susceptible to adenosine-induced bronchoconstriction. In view of the finding that abrupt slowing of the heart rate may cause torsades de pointes VT, adenosine, like any other agent that promotes the development of sudden bradycardia, may be arrhythmogenic in patients with long QT syndrome.

Factors and clinical conditions that predispose patients to the adverse effects of adenosine include the following:

- Medications that inhibit the elimination of adenosine from blood (e.g., dipyridamole)
- Myocardial ischemia (especially inferior myocardial infarction or ischemia)
- Heart transplantation
- Preexisting AV node conduction disturbances
- Preexisting SA node disease
- Acquired or congenital long QT syndrome

Nevertheless, compared with calcium channel antagonists, β-blockers, and other antiarrhythmic agents, adenosine has many important advantages related to its rapid onset of action and less severe and shorter-lived adverse effects. Initial experience also indicates that adenosine can be relatively safely administered to patients in whom the use of calcium channel antagonists may be hazardous (e.g., those with heart failure, ischemic heart disease, Wolff-Parkinson-White syndrome, or wide-complex tachycardia or those taking β-blockers). In addition, adenosine may still have utility for differentiating wide QRS complex SVT from VT and for identifying the arrhythmogenic mechanism of a variety of tachycardias, especially in the cardiac catheterization laboratory during electrophysiologic testing (Fig. 9-2). However, as stated earlier, for arrhythmias involving

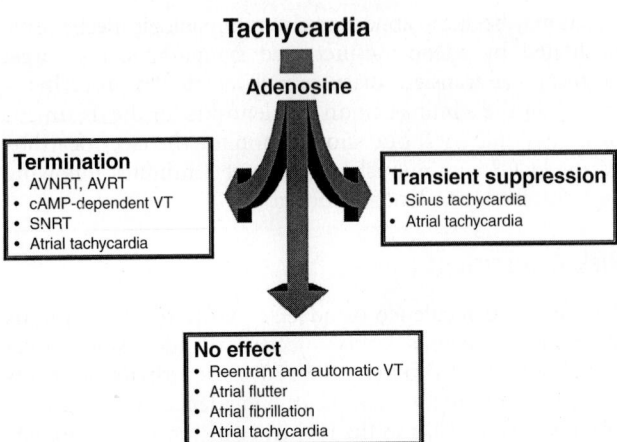

Figure 9–2 ■ Possible effects of adenosine on cardiac arrhythmias. Because important diagnostic information can be obtained during the drug's peak effect, the cardiac rhythm should be monitored by electrocardiogram for at least 2 minutes after each adenosine bolus. Rapid intravenous bolus adenosine (6 mg, followed by 12 mg if necessary) terminates more than 90% of supraventricular tachycardias that involve the atrioventricular (AV) node, including AV nodal reentrant tachycardia (AVNRT) and AV reentrant tachycardia (AVRT) involving the AV node and accessory AV conduction pathways. Some catecholamine-dependent (e.g., cyclic adenosine monophosphate [cAMP]) ventricular tachycardia (VT) and sinoatrial node reentrant tachycardia (SNRT) are also terminated by adenosine. Depending on the tachycardia mechanism and the location of the arrhythmogenic focus, the effect of adenosine on atrial tachycardias can vary considerably. Although adenosine may terminate some atrial tachyarrhythmias, it can also precipitate atrial fibrillation or flutter.

severe hemodynamic compromise, immediate cardioversion is recommended rather than a trial of antiarrhythmic drugs.

Implications

Among the drugs used for the acute treatment of paroxysmal SVT, adenosine appears to be the least likely to cause significant adverse hemodynamic effects. It can also be used safely throughout the perioperative period. However, caution is necessary when administrating adenosine to patients receiving dipyridamole or other agents that inhibit the elimination of adenosine. Likewise, patients with myocardial ischemia, SA or AV node dysfunction, and cardiac allografts seem to be sensitized to both the therapeutic and the adverse effects of adenosine.

MANAGEMENT

Because of adenosine's extremely short half-life, any adverse effects caused by its intravenous bolus injection are usually transient and require observation only. Again, to recognize transient or sustained ventricular proarrhythmias after the administration of adenosine for paroxysmal SVT, the ECG must be monitored continuously for at least 2 minutes after each injection.

The nonselective A_1- and A_2-adenosine receptor antagonists aminophylline and theophylline are highly effective in reversing any unfavorable side effects of adenosine injection or infusion. In addition, these agents have been used to

restore sinus rhythm in patients with ischemia-induced AV node block during the early phase of inferior myocardial infarction. They can also relieve angina-like pain in patients treated with adenosine.

The principles for the management of proarrhythmias associated with adenosine administration are outlined in Figure 9–3. With hemodynamically unstable AV heart block or bradyarrhythmias, cardiopulmonary resuscitation must be started without delay. Likewise, patients with adenosine-induced tachyarrhythmias and hemodynamic compromise require emergency direct-current cardioversion. Otherwise, an adenosine receptor antagonist (e.g., theophylline, aminophylline) is the initial drug of choice. The recommended dose of theophylline is 150 to 250 mg as a slow intravenous bolus injection (approximately 100 mg/minute). If bradycardia or AV block does not respond to theophylline, adrenergic drugs, atropine, or cardiac pacing may be effective. If antiarrhythmic drugs are used to treat adenosine-induced tachyarrhythmias, they should be selected according to the type or mechanism of tachycardia. However, cardioversion is generally preferred to drugs.

PREVENTION

There are only a few absolute contraindications for the use of adenosine. Adenosine should not be administered to patients with second or third degree AV block or sick sinus syndrome unless the patient has a pacemaker. In addition, patients with asthma or severe obstructive pulmonary disease probably should not be given adenosine.

When administering adenosine therapeutically, physicians should be aware of important drug interactions. Drugs that inhibit the metabolism of adenosine, either by blocking the nucleoside transporter or by directly inhibiting adenosine-metabolizing enzymes (adenosine kinase and adenosine deaminase), significantly prolong the half-life of the adenosine and dramatically potentiate its effects. For example, the concurrent use of dipyridamole potentiates the effects of adenosine by a factor of four. Accordingly, clinicians

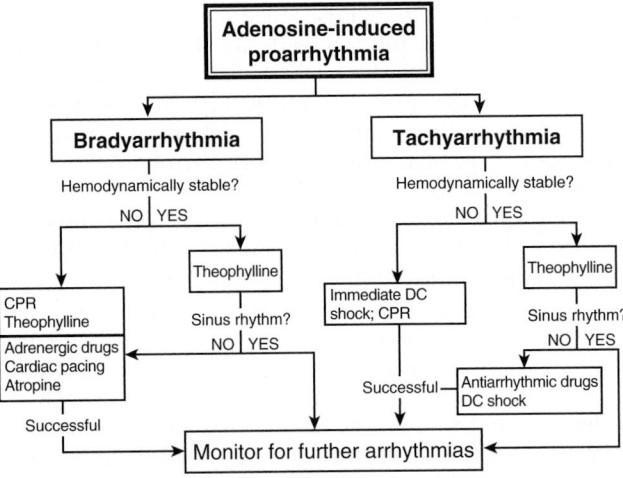

Figure 9–3 ■ Algorithm for the management of proarrhythmias associated with the administration of adenosine. CPR, cardiopulmonary resuscitation; DC, direct current.

recommend that the initial dose of adenosine in patients receiving dipyridamole should not exceed 1 mg, compared with the typical initial dose of 6 mg rapidly administered via a peripheral vein. It is also advisable to use lower-than-usual doses if adenosine is given via a central vein or to patients with myocardial ischemia or to cardiac transplant recipients. In contrast, larger doses (≥12 mg) may be needed to terminate SVT in patients receiving adenosine receptor antagonists such as aminophylline or theophylline.

The response to adenosine may be attenuated in patients who consume food or drink containing methylxanthines (e.g., coffee, cola, chocolate). Although no severe interactions with anesthetic drugs have been reported, it may be important to recognize that benzodiazepines block nucleoside transport in the brain, albeit to a lesser extent than dipyridamole. Adenosine may also lower anesthetic requirements (reduced minimum alveolar concentration) and potentiate nondepolarizing neuromuscular blockade.

The following actions may help prevent adverse effects associated with the use of adenosine:

- Identify and correct factors that may predispose patients to proarrhythmia and other adverse effects.
- Reduce the dosage in patients receiving dipyridamole or other agents that inhibit the elimination of adenosine.
- Reduce the dose when using central vascular access.
- Always use incremental adenosine dosing, starting with a low initial dose. An unnecessarily large initial dose will not improve adenosine's efficacy in terminating SVT but will certainly increase the risk for adverse effects.
- Warn patients about adenosine's common side effects and reassure them that these effects will resolve within 2 minutes.
- Monitor the ECG continuously for several minutes after each intravenous bolus of adenosine. This facilitates early diagnosis and treatment of proarrhythmia and may provide valuable diagnostic information.

In summary, an understanding of the pharmacologic basis of adenosine's actions (pharmacokinetics and drug interactions), combined with meticulous attention to minimizing the factors predisposing to adverse effects, is crucial to this drug's safe and effective use.

Further Reading

Bertolet BD, McMurtrie EB, Hill JA: Theophylline for the treatment of atrioventricular block after myocardial infarction. Ann Intern Med 123:509-511, 1995.

Blomström-Lundqvist C, Scheinman MM, Aliot EM, et al: ACC/AHA/ESC guidelines for the management of patients with supraventricular arrhythmias—executive summary. J Am Coll Cardiol 42:1493-1531, 2003.

Camm AJ, Garratt CJ: Adenosine and supraventricular tachycardia. N Engl J Med 325:1621-1629, 1991.

Celiker A, Tokel K, Cil E, et al: Adenosine induced torsades de pointes in a child with congenital long QT syndrome. Pacing Clin Electrophysiol 17:1814-1817, 1994.

Guidelines 2000 for cardiopulmonary resuscitation and emergency cardiovascular care. Part 6: Advanced cardiovascular life support. Section 5: Pharmacology. I: Agents for arrhythmias. The American Heart Association in collaboration with the International Liaison Committee on Resuscitation. Circulation 102(8 Suppl):I112-I128, 2000.

Guidelines 2000 for cardiopulmonary resuscitation and emergency cardiovascular care. Part 6: Advanced cardiovascular life support. 7D: The tachycardia algorithms. The American Heart Association in collaboration with the International Liaison Committee on Resuscitation. Circulation 102(8 Suppl):I158-I165, 2000.

Harrington GR, Froelich EG: Adenosine-induced torsades de pointes. Chest 103:1299-1301, 1993.

Pelleg A, Pennock RS, Kutalek SP: Proarrhythmic effects of adenosine: One decade of clinical data. Am J Ther 9:141-147, 2002.

Raatikainen MJP, Dennis DM, Belardinelli L: Cardiac electrophysiology of adenosine: Cellular basis and clinical implications. In Pelleg A, Belardinelli L (eds): Effects of Extracellular Adenosine and ATP on Cardiomyocytes. Austin, Tex, RG Landes, 1998, pp 87-132.

Sylven C: Mechanisms of pain in angina pectoris: Critical review of the adenosine hypothesis. Cardiovasc Drug Ther 7:745-759, 1993.

Tan HL, Spekhorst HH, Peters RJ, et al: Adenosine induced ventricular arrhythmias in the emergency room. Pacing Clin Electrophysiol 24:450-455, 2001.

Wesley RC Jr, Turnquest P: Torsades de pointe after intravenous adenosine in the presence of prolonged QT syndrome. Am Heart J 123:794-796, 1992.

Class I Antiarrhythmic Drugs: Ventricular Proarrhythmia

10

Mark F. Trankina

Case Synopsis

A 56-year-old man with stable angina and paroxysmal atrial fibrillation is scheduled for ambulatory inguinal hernia repair. He takes sublingual nitroglycerin as needed, quinidine (400 mg four times a day), and metoprolol (50 mg/day). His preoperative electrocardiogram (ECG) shows normal sinus rhythm at 60 beats per minute, with a corrected Q-T interval of 490 msec and possible left atrial enlargement. He refuses regional anesthesia. He is induced with fentanyl (150 μg), thiopental (350 mg), and succinylcholine (100 mg). His airway is secured without difficulty. However, the pulse oximeter malfunctions within minutes of induction. A sporadic carotid pulse is felt, and the ECG shows twisting of QRS complexes around the isoelectric baseline (Fig. 10-1).

PROBLEM ANALYSIS

Definition

The Cardiac Arrhythmia Suppression Trial (CAST) in 1989 and CAST II in 1992 tested the idea that chronic suppression of lesser ventricular arrhythmias (e.g., ventricular premature beats and nonsustained ventricular tachycardia) by class I antiarrhythmics would reduce mortality in survivors of myocardial infarction. Such arrhythmias were believed to be the inciting events for lethal (malignant) ventricular arrhythmias such as sustained ventricular tachycardia (VT) or ventricular fibrillation. Although encainide and flecainide reduced the incidence of lesser ventricular arrhythmias, they also conferred excess mortality (7.7% in the treatment group versus 3.0% in placebo groups). This excess mortality was attributed to proarrhythmia. Further, deaths in the treatment group were equally distributed throughout the treatment period, suggesting that the proarrhythmic response could occur any time after the start of drug therapy.

Proarrhythmia is defined as the provocation of new or worse arrhythmias by antiarrhythmic drugs. The incidence can be as high as 9% to 10% with some class IA, IB, IC, or III drugs and is lowest (2% to 3%) with amiodarone (a class III antiarrhythmic that also has class I, II, and IV actions). Ventricular proarrhythmia manifests as (1) incessant monomorphic VT or polymorphic VT *without* Q-T interval prolongation or (2) polymorphic VT *with* Q-T interval prolongation, or torsades de pointes (TDP). Because the patient in the case synopsis had Q-T prolongation, his arrhythmia was TDP (see Fig. 10-1). Early afterdepolarizations (EADs) are believed to be the inciting mechanism for TDP. EADs are oscillations in the transmembrane potential of ventricular myocytes that occur during the repolarization phase. EADs are caused by the blockage of outward potassium (K$^+$) repolarization currents; however, this blockage also leads to Q-T interval prolongation and increased ventricular refractoriness. This is conducive to reentry of excitation, the likely sustaining mechanism for TDP. However, because the increase in refractoriness is uneven (greater in some ventricular fibers than in others), VT induced by EADs has a multiform rather than a uniform morphology.

Ischemia-related regional differences in cardiac conduction delay and refractoriness promote ventricular reentry. Ischemia also leads to heterogeneity in antiarrhythmic drug concentrations in myocardium, which augments ischemic cellular electrophysiologic changes. However, the reentry circuits are larger (i.e., macroreentry versus microreentry), and the associated VT is often monomorphic as opposed to polymorphic. When polymorphic VT occurs in patients without Q-T interval prolongation, it is simply polymorphic VT; in association with Q-T interval prolongation, it is TDP. Both have the same ECG appearance (see Fig. 10-1).

Mechanisms for the development of clinical arrhythmias include automaticity, which refers to spontaneous cardiac impulse formation without the need for prior stimulation; it can be normal or abnormal. Normal automaticity occurs in the sinoatrial node (the primary pacemaker) or in latent pacemakers (e.g., subsidiary atrial or Purkinje fibers). Abnormal automaticity can occur in any myocardial fiber type, although it usually occurs in fibers that do not normally exhibit automaticity, such as atrial and working ventricular muscle fibers. Such fibers manifest automaticity only if their cell membrane potentials become depressed by the effects of disease, drugs, or imbalance (i.e., the loss of cell membrane potential). At these low cell membrane potentials, ionic currents responsible for automaticity become activated. Arrhythmias ascribed to enhanced normal automaticity are atrioventricular (AV) junctional and ventricular escape rhythms with advanced second degree or complete (third degree) AV heart block or increased AV node refractoriness.

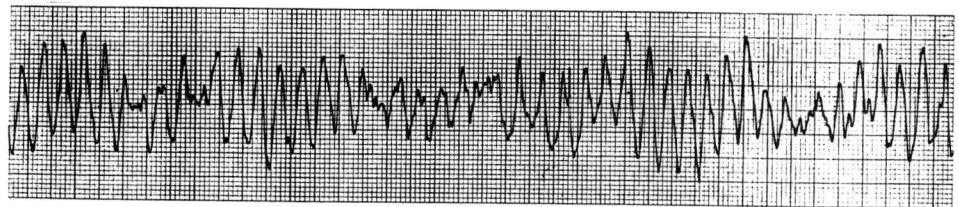

Figure 10–1 ■ Torsades de pointes after induction of general anesthesia. Note "twisting" of the QRS complexes around the isoelectric baseline.

Those ascribed to abnormal automaticity include automatic atrial and AV junctional tachycardia, as well as accelerated idioventricular rhythm or tachycardia following cardiopulmonary bypass or in patients with acute coronary syndromes.

Triggered activity is initiated by depolarizing oscillations in the cell transmembrane potential (afterdepolarizations) that occur before EADs or after full cell repolarization (delayed afterdepolarizations). Thus, triggered activity is the result of a preceding impulse or series of impulses, without which electrical quiescence occurs. Not all afterdepolarizations reach the threshold potential for a regenerative action potential. However, if they do, they can trigger further afterdepolarizations and thus become self-perpetuating. Arrhythmias caused by digitalis toxicity are triggered by delayed afterdepolarizations. Some ectopic atrial tachycardia may also be triggered.

As already noted, there is strong evidence that EADs and EAD-triggered activity are the cause of polymorphic VT associated with congenital or acquired long QT syndromes (e.g., TDP). Some causes of EADs are listed in Table 10-1. In addition, there has been a great deal of controversy over the Food and Drug Administration's "black box" warning about the clinical significance of Q-T prolongation due to droperidol, a drug that has been used safely for decades by anesthesiologists and other health care providers. A more comprehensive listing of drugs associated with TDP (and thus likely causes of EADs) can be found in Chapter 81 or on the Web site http.//www.torsades.org.

Table 10–1 ■ Causes of Early Afterdepolarizations and Triggered Activity

α-Adrenergic stimulation
Imbalance
  Hypoxia
  Hypercarbia
  Acidosis
Hypokalemia
Anitarrhythmic drugs
  Quinidine
  Ibutilide
  Sotalol
Local anesthetics
  Bupivacaine
  Etidocaine
Miscellaneous
  Cesium

Recognition

The Vaughan-Williams antiarrhythmic drug classification divides drugs into four classes based on their principal mode of action: class I, sodium channel blockers; class II, β-adrenergic blockers; class III, potassium channel blockers; and class IV, calcium channel blockers. Class I antiarrhythmic drugs are further subdivided into classes IA, IB, and IC.

Signs of toxicity caused by class I antiarrhythmics include the following:

- Lengthened Q-T interval (class IA) or widened QRS complexes (class IC) manifesting as proarrhythmia
- Long Q-T interval (corrected Q-T interval of 440 to 450 msec)
- History of dizziness or syncope preoperatively
- Change in dosing or the recent initiation of antiarrhythmic therapy
- Occurrence of TDP (see Fig. 10-1)

Class IA Antiarrhythmic Drugs. All class I antiarrhythmics are sodium channel blockers, and some also affect the currents involved in action potential repolarization. Class IA drugs (e.g., quinidine, procainamide, disopyramide) reduce action potential upstroke velocity and prolong its duration. The kinetics of these drugs' onset and offset of effect are of intermediate rapidity (<5 seconds).

Class IB Antiarrhythmic Drugs. Class IB drugs (e.g., mexiletine, phenytoin, lidocaine) do not reduce upstroke velocity, but they do shorten action potential duration. They have fast onset and offset kinetics (<500 msec).

Class IC Antiarrhythmic Drugs. Class IC drugs (e.g., flecainide, propafenone, moricizine) reduce upstroke velocity (primarily by slowing conduction) and also prolong refractoriness somewhat. They have slow onset and offset kinetics (10 to 20 seconds).

The Vaughan-Williams classification is still widely used, but it has many limitations because of the complexity of drug actions. The "Sicilian gambit" (see Further Reading) provides a more realistic view. Some drugs exert greater effects at slow rates than at fast rates (reverse use dependence); this is particularly true of drugs that lengthen repolarization (class IA). Thus, the Q-T interval becomes prolonged at slow rates rather than at fast rates, which is exactly the opposite of what an ideal antiarrhythmic drug should do. Prolongation of refractoriness should be increased at fast rates to interrupt or prevent a reentrant tachycardia and minimal at slow rates to avoid precipitating TDP.

Finally, it is important to remember that anesthesiologists must evaluate the *patient* with a rhythm disturbance, not the rhythm disturbance itself. Some arrhythmias are hazardous to the patient *regardless of* the clinical setting, whereas others are hazardous *because of* the clinical setting (e.g., anesthesia and surgery, acute coronary syndromes, post cardiopulmonary bypass).

Risk Assessment

Conditions associated with Q-T interval prolongation and thus predisposition to TDP are listed in Table 10-2. A variety of commonly prescribed drugs belonging to many different therapeutic classes, including antiarrhythmics, antibiotics, antihistamines, and prokinetic drugs, can adversely prolong cardiac repolarization. However, arrhythmias related to drug-induced Q-T prolongation do not occur in every patient treated with such drugs; they occur only in susceptible patients. It has been postulated that these individuals may be silent carriers of genes responsible for congenital long QT syndromes. Up to 70% of these patients have normal Q-Tc intervals until exposed to a Q-T interval–prolonging drug.

The primary objective of pharmacologic therapy for a patient with a cardiac arrhythmia is to achieve an effective and well-tolerated plasma drug concentration as quickly as possible and to maintain that concentration for as long as required without producing adverse effects. In many circumstances (but not with all drugs), the plasma concentration after equilibration correlates with the pharmacodynamic and adverse effects of the drug. However, the therapeutic concentration for any given patient is the amount of drug required to suppress or terminate the specific cardiac arrhythmia without producing adverse side effects.

Table 10–2 ■ Factors that Predispose to Q-T Interval Prolongation
Congenital or acquired long QT syndromes
Coexisting disease
Hypothyroidism
Cardiomyopathies
Bradycardia
Physiologic imbalance
Hypokalemia
Hypomagnesemia
Hypocalcemia
Antiarrhythmics
Class IA, IC, and III drugs
Combined class IA and III drugs
Other drugs
Potassium-wasting diuretics
Tricyclic antidepressants
Phenothiazines
Erythromycin
Terfenadine
Astemizole
Liquid protein diets

For a more complete listing, see Chapter 81 or go to http.//www.torsades.org.

Given the fact that automaticity, triggered activity, or reentry can cause cardiac arrhythmias, the mechanisms by which antiarrhythmic agents suppress cardiac arrhythmias can be postulated. Antiarrhythmic agents can slow the spontaneous discharge frequency of an automatic pacemaker by depressing the slope of diastolic depolarization, shifting the threshold voltage toward zero, or hyperpolarizing the resting membrane potential. Mechanisms by which different drugs suppress normal or abnormal automaticity may not be the same. In general, most antiarrhythmic drugs in therapeutic doses depress automaticity at ectopic sites while minimally affecting automaticity of the sinus node. However, calcium channel blockers (e.g., verapamil) and β-blockers (e.g., propranolol) can depress the sinus rate, and drugs that exert vagolytic effects (e.g., disopyramide, quinidine) can increase the sinus rate. Drugs can also suppress early or delayed afterdepolarizations to eliminate triggered arrhythmias.

Proarrhythmia with antiarrhythmic drugs is an important clinical problem. Electrophysiologic mechanisms include prolongation of repolarization, development of delayed after depolarizations (e.g., arrhythmias with digitalis toxicity) or EADs (to initiate TDP), or alterations in conduction and refractoriness that are conducive to reentry and the initiation or maintenance of VT or ventricular fibrillation.

The acquired form of Q-T interval prolongation (see Table 10-2) is caused by various agents and conditions that reduce the magnitude of outward repolarizing K^+ currents, enhance inward depolarizing Na^+ or Ca^{2+} currents, or both, which leads to the development of EADs that initiate TDP. Proarrhythmic events can occur in as many as 5% to 10% of patients. Congestive heart failure increases proarrhythmic risk. In one recent study, patients with atrial fibrillation receiving antiarrhythmic drugs had a 4.7 relative risk of cardiac death if they had a history of heart failure, compared with a 3.7 relative risk among those not receiving antiarrhythmic drugs. Patients without a history of congestive heart failure had no increased risk of cardiac mortality during antiarrhythmic drug therapy. Reduced left ventricular function, treatment with digitalis and diuretics, and longer pretreatment Q-T interval are often seen in patients who develop drug-induced ventricular fibrillation. Usually the proarrhythmic events occur within several days of beginning drug therapy or after a change in dosage and are manifest by the development of VT, Q-T interval prolongation, or TDP (long QT syndrome).

Doses for class I antiarrhythmic drugs are listed in Table 10-3. Proarrhythmic effects are likely additive when multiple drugs are used. Mortality with TDP is approximately 30%. With acquired long QT syndromes, the therapeutic challenge is to maintain prolonged repolarization but interrupt the arrhythmogenic cascade.

MANAGEMENT

It is possible that multiple drugs have a cumulative effect in provoking EADs and TDP. Antiarrhythmics may paradoxically produce malignant ventricular tachyarrhythmias via proarrhythmia, and preoperative antiarrhythmic treatment does not preclude the generation of more ominous perioperative arrhythmias. The ECG should be carefully scrutinized

Table 10–3 ■ Dosing for Class I Antiarrhythmic Agents

Drug	IV Loading	IV Maintenance	PO Loading	PO Maintenance
Quinidine	6-10 mg/kg at 0.3-0.5 mg/kg/min	600-1000 mg	300-600 mg q6h	300-600 mg q6h
Procainamide	6-13 mg/kg at 0.2-0.5 mg/kg/min	2-6 mg/min	500-1000 mg	350-1000 mg q3-6h
Disopyramide	1-2 mg/kg over 15-45 min	1 mg/kg/hr		100-400 mg q6-8h
Lidocaine	1-3 mg/kg at 20-50 mg/min	1-4 mg/min	NA	NA
Mexiletine	500 mg	0.5-1.0 g/24 hr	400-600 mg	150-300 mg q6-8h
Tocainide	750 mg		400-600 mg	400-600 mg q8-12h
Phenytoin	100 mg q5min to <1000 mg		1000 mg	100-400 mg q12-24h
Flecainide	2 mg/kg	100-200 mg q12h		
Propafenone	1-2 mg/kg		600-900 mg	150-300 mg q8-12h
Moricizine			300 mg	100-400 q8h

NA, not applicable.

preoperatively for signs of toxic effects caused by drugs (e.g., prolonged Q-Tc interval or widened QRS complex). Specific management for TDP includes the following:

- Atrial or ventricular pacing to increase the K⁺ current and shorten refractoriness at faster heart rates
- Intravenous bolus magnesium sulfate
- Lidocaine by intravenous bolus (does not prolong the Q-T interval)
- Calcium channel blocker by intravenous bolus (if other interventions fail)
- Cautious use of isoproterenol to increase the heart rate if pacing is not available

PREVENTION

Prevention includes providing a stress-free perioperative period (to the extent possible) to reduce myocardial ischemia and related increased dispersion of myocardial refractoriness. In addition, the following points should be noted:

- Regional anesthesia is advised.
- Consider cardiology reevaluation for drug dosing and appropriateness.
- Consider stopping quinidine before anesthesia administration.
- Avoid conditions that prolong the Q-T interval (see Table 10-2).

Booker and colleagues have provided a comprehensive review of anesthetic management for patients with congenital and acquired long QT syndromes, including specific recommendations for the perioperative management of such patients.

Further Reading

Atlee JL: Drug treatment for arrhythmias. In Atlee JL (ed): Arrhythmias and Pacemakers: Practical Management for Anesthesia and Critical Care Medicine. Philadelphia, WB Saunders, 1996, pp 154-204.

Atlee JL: Overview of mechanisms for arrhythmias. In Atlee JL (ed): Arrhythmias and Pacemakers: Practical Management for Anesthesia and Critical Care Medicine. Philadelphia, WB Saunders, 1996, pp 25-58.

Booker PD, Whyte SD, Ladusans EJ: Long QT syndrome and anaesthesia. Br J Anaesth 90:349-366, 2003.

Charbit B, Albaladejo P, Funck-Brentano C, et al: Prolongation of QTc interval after postoperative nausea and vomiting treatment by droperidol or ondansetron. Anesthesiology 102:1094-1100, 2005.

Effect of the antiarrhythmic agent moricizine on survival after myocardial infarction. The Cardiac Arrhythmia Suppression Trial II investigators. N Engl J Med 327:227-233, 1992.

Preliminary report: Effect of encainide and flecainide on mortality in a randomized trial of arrhythmia suppression after myocardial infarction. The Cardiac Arrhythmia Suppression Trial (CAST) investigators. N Engl J Med 321:406-412, 1989.

Soroker D, Ezri T, Szmuki P, et al: Perioperative torsades de pointes ventricular tachycardia induced by hypocalcemia and hypokalemia. Anesth Analg 80:630-633, 1995.

Tan HL, Hou CJ, Laver MR, et al: Electrophysiologic mechanisms of the long QT interval syndromes and torsades de pointes. Ann Intern Med 122:701-714, 1995.

Task Force of the Working Group on Arrhythmias of the European Society of Cardiology: The Sicilian gambit: A new approach to the classification of antiarrhythmic drugs based on their actions on arrhythmogenic mechanisms. Circulation 84:1831-1851, 1991.

Class II Antiarrhythmic Drugs: β-Blockers—Heart Block or Bradycardia

11

Charles A. Napolitano and Maria I. Castro

Case Synopsis

A 60-year-old woman with a history of mitral valve stenosis and atrial fibrillation is scheduled for abdominal hysterectomy. Her current medications include verapamil and digoxin. Following induction of anesthesia with etomidate and maintenance with sevoflurane, oxygen, fentanyl, and vecuronium, her ventricular rate increases acutely to 140 beats per minute. Esmolol therapy results in acute bradycardia (30 beats per minute). Electrocardiogram (ECG) monitoring reveals third degree atrioventricular (AV) heart block with regular, wide QRS complexes.

PROBLEM ANALYSIS

Definition

β-Blockers are commonly used in the management of arrhythmias, hypertension, and heart failure. However, by producing β-adrenergic block, they have the potential to cause sinus bradycardia or sinoatrial (SA) or AV heart block at the AV node. These effects can be aggravated by drugs used during anesthesia (e.g., potent volatile anesthetics, high-dose opiates, local anesthetic toxicity, succinylcholine). Some β-blockers also have vasodilator activity (e.g., carvedilol, labetalol) and may be better tolerated in patients with heart failure.

Sinus bradycardia in adults is a heart rate less than 60 beats per minute with a rhythm that originates in the SA node. Third degree AV heart block is the complete absence of impulses conducted from the atria to the ventricles, with the ventricles controlled by impulses originating in subsidiary (latent) cardiac pacemakers located distal to the site of block. If the site of conduction block is perinodal (SA exit block or AV node block), the heart rate typically ranges from 45 to 55 beats per minute, and the QRS interval is of normal duration (≈120 msec). Infranodal block (below the AV node) is characterized by a ventricular rate of 30 to 40 beats per minute and wide QRS complexes. The conduction defect depicted in the case synopsis represents infranodal third degree block with slow secondary pacemaker activity; this can lead to cardiac arrest.

Although the third degree AV heart block in this case likely resulted from synergistic depression of AV node function by esmolol (a class II antiarrhythmic) and verapamil (a class IV antiarrhythmic), the other drugs, including digoxin, sevoflurane, and fentanyl, likely contributed. Esmolol, a short-acting β₁-selective adrenergic antagonist (β-blocker), is indicated when immediate control of the heart rate or blood pressure is needed and prolonged β-blockade is undesirable. The peak onset of action (6 to 10 minutes) and short half-life (8 minutes) make esmolol appropriate for the management of perioperative tachyarrhythmias. Like all β-blockers, esmolol reduces the sinus rate and AV node conduction time while increasing AV node functional refractoriness.

Owing to its inhibitory effects on AV node conduction, verapamil, a calcium channel antagonist, is also useful for reducing the ventricular rate in patients with atrial flutter or fibrillation. However, the effects of verapamil can be potentiated by the concomitant use of β-blockers.

As mentioned, the use of sevoflurane, digoxin, and fentanyl, and possibly the surgical procedure itself, likely contributed to the development of heart block in this case. To maintain cardiac output and prevent left ventricular failure or pulmonary edema, tight control of left ventricular preload, heart rate, and systemic vascular resistance is critical for patients with mitral or aortic stenosis and restrictive cardiomyopathies. Thus, the selection of etomidate as an anesthetic induction agent was, at least in theory, a good choice, because etomidate minimizes reflex increases in heart rate and generally maintains systemic vascular resistance and blood pressure within normal limits. However, like other potent inhalational agents, sevoflurane reduces systemic vascular resistance and preload (by dilating the venous capacitance bed to decrease venous return) and may have contributed to the intraoperative increase in ventricular rate via a reflex increase in adrenergic tone. Further, it may have contributed to the third degree AV block and bradycardia by direct effects on AV node conduction and refractoriness. Other potent volatile anesthetics, with the possible exception of desflurane, may also decrease the rate of AV node conduction and SA node discharge. Digoxin's central actions stimulate vagal tone to reduce heart rate and increase AV node conduction time and refractoriness. Fentanyl, especially at high doses, may inhibit AV node function by causing centrally increased parasympathomimetic and reduced sympathomimetic tone. Finally, peritoneal retraction slows the heart rate and AV node conduction by increasing vagal tone. Thus, any of these factors could have exacerbated the effects of verapamil and esmolol on SA and AV node function.

Although this patient had third degree AV heart block and severe bradycardia, any condition within the spectrum of bradycardia (including asystole) could have occurred. Anesthesiologists must be prepared for this possibility with the appearance of severe bradycardia.

Recognition

ECG monitoring is the definitive means of detecting bradycardia or AV conduction block. Sinus bradycardia (<60 beats per minute) or asystole is easily recognized on ECG. AV node or infranodal third degree conduction block requires closer ECG inspection (Fig. 11-1). With AV node or perinodal heart block, P waves are dissociated from the QRS complex, but with an AV junctional pacemaker and normal conduction through the ventricles. The QRS complex is of normal width (≈120 msec duration). In contrast, with infranodal block, conduction from latent pacemakers below the AV node or His bundle leads to wide QRS complexes.

Other, less reliable methods of detecting bradycardia or heart block include the following:

- Pulse oximetry plethysmographs reveal a reduced heart rate and possibly reduced arterial oxygen saturation.
- Capnography may show low end-tidal carbon dioxide values due to reduced pulmonary flow.
- Noninvasive blood pressure monitoring may reveal hypotension and a reduced heart rate or may simply provide a default "error" message.

- Invasive blood pressure monitoring reveals reduced frequency and possibly amplitude of the arterial waveform.
- Palpation of peripheral pulses indicates decreased frequency and intensity of the pulses.

Although these modalities can assist in assessing the hemodynamic impact of bradycardia, only ECG allows definitive diagnosis of its cause.

Risk Assessment

Although the incidence of new intraoperative heart block is unknown, its incidence in animal and prospective clinical studies appears to be greater when antagonists and β-blockers are used in combination. The potential risk of developing bradyarrhythmias and AV node conduction disturbances in patients receiving β-blockers varies. It is greatest with verapamil, somewhat less with diltiazem, and least with dihydropyridine (DHP) calcium channel antagonists such as nicardipine, amlodipine, and nifedipine. DHP calcium channel antagonists have a much higher affinity for L-type Ca^{2+} channels in vascular smooth muscle as opposed to cardiac myocytes.

Animal studies show synergism between the cardiac electrophysiologic effects of β-blockers and calcium channel antagonists (e.g., verapamil, diltiazem). When the latter are given at low doses, propranolol enhances their effect on heart rate and AV node conduction. When given at high doses

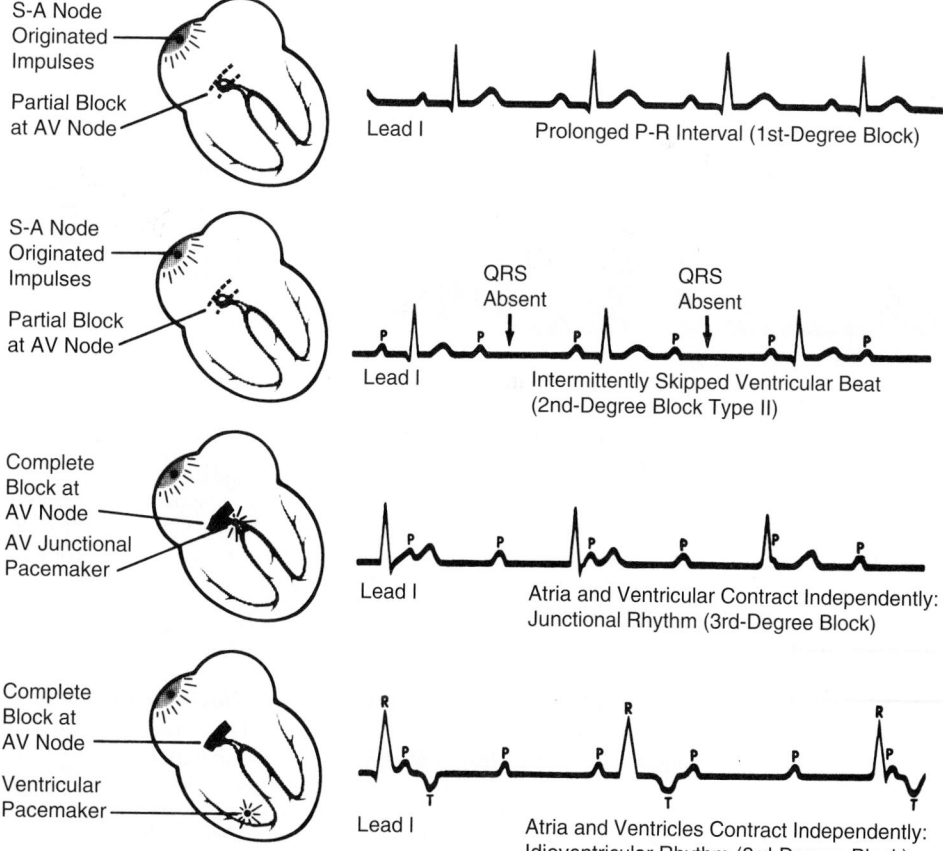

Figure 11–1 ■ Atrioventricular (AV) block. Diagrammatic representation of the conduction pathology and resultant electrocardiogram. S-A, sinoatrial. (Adapted with permission from the American Heart Association: Textbook of Advanced Cardiac Life Support, 2nd ed. New York, AHA, 1990; and Netter FH: CIBA Collection of Medical Illustrations. West Caldwell, New Jersey, CIBA Medical Education Division, 1987.)

S-A Node Originated Impulses
Partial Block at AV Node
Lead I   Prolonged P-R Interval (1st-Degree Block)

S-A Node Originated Impulses
Partial Block at AV Node
QRS Absent   QRS Absent
Lead I   Intermittently Skipped Ventricular Beat (2nd-Degree Block Type II)

Complete Block at AV Node
AV Junctional Pacemaker
Lead I   Atria and Ventricular Contract Independently: Junctional Rhythm (3rd-Degree Block)

Complete Block at AV Node
Ventricular Pacemaker
Lead I   Atria and Ventricles Contract Independently: Idioventricular Rhythm (3rd-Degree Block)

with verapamil or diltiazem, propranolol causes significant heart block, hypotension, or left ventricular dysfunction.

Clinical studies support the findings in animal models. In patients with chronic stable angina, therapy with a β-blocker and verapamil (versus diltiazem or nifedipine) causes a significant (10% to 15%) increase in the incidence of adverse cardiac or hemodynamic effects (bradycardia, heart block, hypotension, syncope, or congestive heart failure). However, diltiazem in combination with various β-blockers does not cause significant AV heart block, although it does increase the risk for P-R interval prolongation and bradycardia. Also, intraoperative bradycardia, first degree AV block, and AV junctional rhythms occurred more often in patients having coronary artery bypass graft surgery who took non-DHP calcium channel antagonists and β-blockers before surgery. Finally, transient AV block after aortic cross-clamp release during coronary artery bypass surgery was significantly increased in patients receiving preoperative propranolol (5% higher) or propranolol-nifedipine (15% higher).

Patients whose medical treatment may include a β-blocker, calcium channel antagonist, or both are listed in Table 11-1. Other preoperative and intraoperative factors that place patients at increased risk for heart block during anesthesia and surgery are listed in Tables 11-2 and 11-3.

Implications

Bradycardia with AV heart block can lead to severe hemodynamic compromise. In the absence of SA node activity, cardiac arrest is possible if perinodal or ventricular escape rhythms do not occur promptly. Severe hypotension due to reduced heart rate and lack of AV synchrony may cause myocardial ischemia. Heart failure may follow if cardiac output is not maintained by a compensatory increase in stroke volume. Hypotension, increased pulmonary artery pressure, and increased left ventricular end-diastolic pressure

have been observed in both animal and clinical studies of combined β-blocker and non-DHP calcium channel antagonist therapy.

MANAGEMENT

After verification of third degree AV heart block and hemodynamic assessment, optimal oxygenation, ventilation, and perfusion are ensured by increasing the fraction of inspired

---

Table 11–2 ■ Preoperative Risk Factors for the Development of Intraoperative Heart Block

Age older than 60 years
Chronic administration of β-blockers, calcium channel antagonists, amiodarone, or other drugs that prolong AV node or AV conduction (e.g., class IC antiarrhythmics, long-acting local anesthetics)
Underlying conduction system disease (e.g., congenital heart disease, repair of atrial secundum defects, repair of transposition of the great vessels)
Electrolyte or metabolic imbalance (e.g., hyperkalemia, hypothermia)
Systemic disease (e.g., hypothyroidism-myxedema, intracardiac rheumatoid nodules, rheumatic heart disease)
Preexisting heart disease (e.g., coronary artery disease, idiopathic degeneration or fibrosis, aortic or mitral valve surgery, Lyme disease, bacterial endocarditis, chagasic myocarditis,* calcific aortic stenosis)
Preoperative bradycardia (<60 beats per minute)
Myocardial infiltrative processes (e.g., sarcoidosis, amyloidosis, scleroderma)

*Common in Central and South America.
AV, atrioventricular.

Table 11–1 ■ Patient Populations Managed with β-Blockers or Calcium Channel Blockers

Coronary Artery Disease
Chronic stable angina or previous myocardial infarction
Native coronary arteries or autografts prone to spasm
Perioperative management of myocardial ischemia in selected patients

Arrhythmias
Prevention or treatment of supraventricular tachyarrhythmias (especially paroxysmal supraventricular tachycardia)
Prevention or treatment of focal ventricular tachycardia in patients without structural heart disease (e.g., right ventricular outflow tract tachycardia, idiopathic left ventricular tachycardia*)

Cardiovascular Disease
Hypertension
Heart failure (β-blockers along with other drugs, such as angiotensin-converting enzyme inhibitors or angiotensin II receptor blockers)
Symptomatic patients treated with β-blockers for mitral valve prolapse

*Focal ventricular tachycardias that originate in the left ventricular outflow tract, epicardium, or midseptum.

Table 11–3 ■ Intraoperative Risk Factors Associated with the Development of Atrioventricular Heart Block

Drugs
β-blockers
Calcium channel antagonists
High-dose volatile anesthetics or opiates
IV anesthetic drugs (e.g., propofol, high-dose opiates, succinylcholine)
Anticholinesterase therapy
Digitalis glycosides
IV amiodarone or sotalol
Class IA or IB antiarrhythmic drugs, especially high IV doses

Increased Vagal Tone or Stimulation
Peritoneal retraction or retraction of ocular muscles
Direct laryngoscopy and endotracheal intubation
Urinary bladder catheterization
Esophageal instrumentation
Baroreceptor reflex activation with acute hypertensive episodes (e.g., aortic cross-clamp application)
Rectal or cervical dilatation

Imbalance
Hypoxia
Hypothermia
Hyperkalemia

oxygen to 1.0 and discontinuing the use of volatile anesthetics. If the blood pressure and cardiac output are not adequate, cardiopulmonary resuscitation should be started immediately. The surgeon should discontinue any maneuvers that could increase vagal tone (e.g., peritoneal retraction) until the condition has been resolved. The treatment of mild (sinus bradycardia) to severe (asystole) complications includes the following:

- Ephedrine 5 to 10 mg intravenously (IV); repeat if necessary
- Atropine 0.4 mg IV or glycopyrrolate 0.2 mg IV (up to a total of 2 or 1 mg IV, respectively, if necessary)
- Calcium 250 mg IV; repeat up to a total of 1 g if necessary
- Epinephrine 10 μg IV; repeat with increased doses as needed
- Isoproterenol 1 to 10 μg/minute IV
- Perform noninvasive (transcutaneous) pacing before instituting invasive transvenous pacing; noninvasive esophageal atrial pacing is ineffective in third degree AV block.
- Perform cardiopulmonary resuscitation if systolic blood pressure is 40 to 50 mm Hg (while attempting or repeating the above measures).
- Anticipate adverse drug interactions.
- Maintain hemodynamic stability.
- Perform intraoperative hemodynamic monitoring.
- Select drugs to treat tachycardia.
- Consider cardioversion in place of drugs for symptomatic supraventricular tachycardia.

PREVENTION

The patient in the case synopsis developed third degree AV heart block after esmolol was given to control a rapid ventricular rate with atrial fibrillation. Her preexisting heart disease required the avoidance of extreme increases or decreases in heart rate to maintain hemodynamic stability and vital organ perfusion. Prevention of hemodynamic instability in such patients requires careful preoperative assessment, anticipation of adverse drug interactions, and attention to surgical or procedure-related interventions that might lead to wide fluctuations in heart rate or blood pressure. In addition to a thorough history and physical examination and the necessary laboratory tests, the preoperative assessment should include knowledge of the patient's baseline heart rate, blood pressure, and intravascular volume status. Anesthesiologists should be able to anticipate adverse events and must be prepared to manage them early to minimize complications.

Intraoperatively, care should be taken to ensure an adequate depth of anesthesia and analgesia and to maintain appropriate hydration. The placement of a Swan-Ganz catheter or intraoperative transesophageal echocardiography to monitor cardiac hemodynamic parameters should be considered for high-risk patients. If significant tachycardia develops in a patient receiving a non-DHP calcium channel antagonist, a reduced dose of esmolol (0.1 to 0.25 mg/kg) can be given to minimize any synergistic effect. To terminate

reentrant supraventricular tachycardia involving the AV node, adenosine (6 to 12 mg IV) can be used; it is an ultra-short-acting nucleoside with an efficacy equal to or better than that of the DHP calcium channel antagonists. Other alternatives are diltiazem (0.25 to 0.35 mg/kg IV), neostigmine (1 mg IV), edrophonium (10 mg IV), or phenylephrine (50 to 100 μg IV); vagal maneuvers (e.g., carotid sinus massage, Valsalva's maneuver, ocular massage); or medications the patient is already receiving (e.g., verapamil 1.25 to 2.5 mg or digoxin 0.125 to 0.5 mg IV).

Although synergistic effects with β-blockers are most often reported with verapamil, heart block is a theoretical possibility with any of the previously mentioned drugs, particularly when they depress AV node function by different cellular mechanisms. Finally, early direct-current cardioversion is the treatment of choice for atrial fibrillation or flutter causing hemodynamic compromise due to a rapid ventricular response.

Further Reading

Atlee JL: Perioperative cardiac dysrhythmias: Diagnosis and management. Anesthesiology 86:1397-1424, 1997.

Auerbach AD, Goldman L: Beta-blockers and reduction of cardiac events in noncardiac surgery: Scientific review. JAMA 287:1435-1444, 2002.

Baraka AS, Taha SK, Yasbeck VK, et al: Transient atrioventricular block after release of aortic cross-clamp. Anesth Analg 80:54-57, 1995.

Devereaux PJ, Beattie WS, Choi PT, et al: How strong is the evidence for the use of perioperative beta-blockers in non-cardiac surgery? Systematic review and meta-analysis of randomised controlled trials. BMJ 331:313-321, 2005.

Henling CE, Slogoff S, Kodal SV, et al: Heart block after coronary artery bypass: Effects of chronic administration of calcium-entry blockers and β-blockers. Anesth Analg 63:515-520, 1984.

Hoffman BB: Catecholamines, sympathomimetic drugs, and adrenergic receptor antagonists. In Hardman JG, Limbird LE (eds): Goodman and Gilman's The Pharmacological Basis of Therapeutics, 10th ed. New York, McGraw-Hill, 2001, pp 215-268.

Kapur PA, Matarazzo DA, Fung OM, et al: The cardiovascular and adrenergic actions of verapamil or diltiazem in combination with propranolol during halothane anesthesia in the dog. Anesthesiology 66:122-129, 1987.

Kerins DM, Robertson RM, Robertson D: Drugs used for the treatment of myocardial ischemia. In Hardman JG, Limbird LE (eds): Goodman and Gilman's The Pharmacological Basis of Therapeutics, 10th ed. New York, McGraw-Hill, 2001, pp 843-870.

Krum H: Tolerability of carvedilol in heart failure: Clinical trials experience. Am J Cardiol 93:58B-63B, 2004.

Lopez-Sendon J, Swedberg K, McMurray J, et al: Task Force on Beta-Blockers of the European Society of Cardiology. Expert consensus document on beta-adrenergic receptor blockers. Eur Heart J 25:1341-1362, 2004.

McMurray JJ, Pfeffer MA: Heart failure. Lancet 365:1877-1889, 2005.

Messerli FH, Grossman E: Beta-blockers in hypertension: Is carvedilol different? Am J Cardiol 93:7B-12B, 2004.

Oates JA, Brown NJ: Antihypertensive agents and the drug therapy of hypertension. In Hardman JG, Limbird LE (eds): Goodman and Gilman's The Pharmacological Basis of Therapeutics, 10th ed. New York, McGraw-Hill, 2001, pp 871-900.

Priebe HJ: Perioperative myocardial infarction—aetiology and prevention. Br J Anaesth 95:3-19, 2005.

Schwartz AB, Moskowitz RM, Klausner SC: The electrophysiological effects of nicardipine hydrochloride in man. Can J Cardiol 3:14-17, 1987.

Strauss WE, Parisi AF: Combined use of calcium-channel and beta-adrenergic blockers for the treatment of chronic stable angina: Rationale, efficacy, and adverse effects. Ann Intern Med 109:570-581, 1988.

Class III Antiarrhythmic Drugs: Potassium Channel Blockers

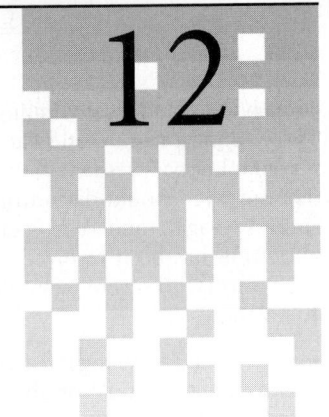

M. J. Pekka Raatikainen and Donn M. Dennis

Case Synopsis

A 76-year-old woman with a history of paroxysmal atrial fibrillation is admitted to the hospital for elective surgery. Her antiarrhythmic medication is 80 mg of sotalol twice daily. Before the operation, she has a sudden syncopal attack, and an electrocardiogram (ECG) shows a wide QRS self-terminating tachycardia.

PROBLEM ANALYSIS

Definition

The patient's medical history and ECG (Fig. 12-1) are consistent with drug-induced Q-T prolongation and proarrhythmia. It is well known that prolongation of ventricular repolarization (i.e., long Q-T interval), the electrophysiologic basis for class III antiarrhythmic drug action, can paradoxically cause polymorphic torsades de pointes (TDP). TDP is a polymorphic ventricular tachycardia (VT) that occurs in the setting of Q-T interval prolongation; in the absence of Q-T prolongation, it is known as simply polymorphic VT. With TDP or polymorphic VT, the distinctive ECG pattern is characterized by a continuous twisting of the QRS axis around the isoelectric ECG baseline.

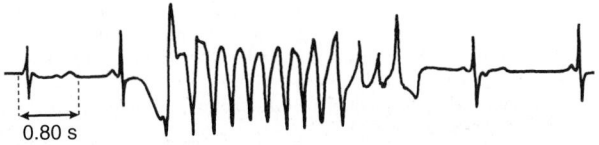

A Rhythm strip during the tachycardia

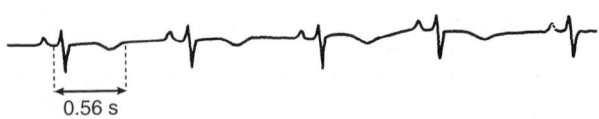

B ECG (lead II) before the syncope

Figure 12–1 ■ *A,* Electrocardiogram (ECG) rhythm strip obtained from a 76-year-old woman immediately after syncope. Note the extremely long Q-T interval (0.80 second) immediately before the onset of the arrhythmia and twisting of the QRS axis around the isoelectric baseline during the tachycardia (220 beats per minute) (paper speed 25 mm/second). *B,* ECG (lead II) from the same patient showing a significant prolongation of the Q-T interval (Q-Tc = 0.56 second) during normal sinus rhythm (62 beats per minute) (paper speed 25 mm/second). After cessation of class III antiarrhythmic drugs (sotalol 80 mg twice daily), the Q-Tc interval returned to a value of 0.40 second.

Although the precise mechanisms underlying TDP are unclear, most experimental and clinical evidence suggests that triggered activity initiated by early afterdepolarizations, along with delayed ventricular repolarization, provokes the onset of TDP. In general, TDP manifests as brief, repetitive episodes of self-terminating VT. Unabated, it can deteriorate into ventricular fibrillation.

Recognition

The diagnosis of drug-induced long QT syndrome and TDP (see also Chapter 81) is based on the characteristic ECG findings and the patient's medical history. In particular, special attention should be focused on concurrent use of other Q-T–prolonging drugs, including class IA antiarrhythmics (e.g., quinidine), macrolide antibiotics (e.g., erythromycin), nonsedating antihistamines (e.g., terfenadine), and psychotropic drugs (e.g., antipsychotics, tricyclic antidepressants). A more complete listing can be found at http://www.torsades.org.

ECG features of long QT syndrome include the following:

- Prolonged ventricular repolarization (Q-Tc >0.44 second)
- Alternating T waves or prominent U waves
- Increased dispersion of ventricular repolarization (Q-T dispersion)

ECG features of drug-induced TDP include the following:

- Polymorphic tachycardia (160 to 250 beats per minute), with characteristic twisting of the QRS axis around the isoelectric ECG baseline
- Characteristic "short-long-short" initiation sequence (i.e., R-R intervals)
- Initiation frequently caused by extra systoles with a long coupling interval

In patients with acquired long QT syndrome, TDP typically follows long pauses, whereas in patients with congenital (idiopathic) long QT syndrome, the initiation of TDP is commonly associated with an increase in catecholamines and heart rate (e.g., stress, fright, physical exercise).

Although TDP may present as a monomorphic VT in a *single* monitored ECG lead, confusion with monomorphic ventricular arrhythmias is rare when a 12-lead ECG is obtained. The characteristic "short-long-short" initiation sequence and the patient's medical history help distinguish TDP from other forms of polymorphic VT. Importantly, these other forms of polymorphic VT occur without ECG evidence of Q-T interval prolongation, and often in the setting of an acute coronary syndrome (e.g., myocardial ischemia or infarction, reperfusion injury).

Risk Assessment

Experience with the perioperative use of class III antiarrhythmic agents is limited, and there is little information on interactions between these drugs and anesthetic agents. The major perioperative complications related to long-term therapy with class III antiarrhythmics include proarrhythmia (e.g., TDP) and noncardiac amiodarone interactions and toxicity. The latter is discussed in more detail later in this chapter.

Proarrhythmic Risk

The following factors predispose to the development of class III antiarrhythmic drug-induced TDP during anesthesia:

- Female gender
- Electrolyte disturbances (e.g., hypokalemia, hypomagnesemia, severe hypocalcemia)
- Structural heart disease and myocardial ischemia
- Excessive dosing
- Genetic defects behind the enzymes metabolizing the drug or defective cardiac ion channels responsible for congenital long QT syndrome (see Chapter 81)
- Drug interactions or simultaneous use of drugs that prolong ventricular repolarization

Critical values for Q-T prolongation are lacking. Available data indicate that Q-T dispersion (i.e., difference between the longest and shortest Q-T intervals assessed by 12-lead ECG) may predict the proarrhythmia more accurately than absolute Q-T interval prolongation or the latter corrected for heart rate (Q-Tc interval). For example, amiodarone—which, unlike the other class III agents, prolongs the Q-T interval uniformly (i.e., does not increase Q-T interval dispersion)—has a significantly lower proarrhythmic risk (2% to 3%) than the other class III antiarrhythmics (5% to 10%). Other factors that may explain amiodarone's lower proarrhythmic risk compared with "pure" class III antiarrhythmics (which selectively inhibit cardiac potassium channels) include a heart rate–independent action on ventricular repolarization, and β-adrenergic blocking, α-adrenergic blocking, and calcium channel blocking properties.

The incidence of TDP with amiodarone is only 0.7%, whereas sotalol and quinidine induce TDP in about 5% and 8% of cases, respectively. Further, in contrast to sotalol and ibutilide (a class III antiarrhythmic), acute intravenous amiodarone seldom if ever prolongs the Q-T interval. However, in the setting of electrolyte abnormalities, bradycardia, or abrupt changes in the heart rate, the proarrhythmic risk increases significantly. Thus, although definitive clinical studies have yet to be conducted, one could speculate that anesthetics that reduce heart rate, depress atrioventricular (AV) node conduction, and lengthen ventricular repolarization might increase the proarrhythmic effects of class III antiarrhythmic drugs during surgery. Given the data indicating that patients with acquired long QT syndrome may suffer from variant forms of the congenital syndrome (e.g., electrically silent gene defects that manifest only with Q-T interval–prolonging drugs), genetic analyses of genes encoding the cardiac sodium and potassium channels may provide valuable information about the risk of drug-induced proarrhythmias.

The following ECG findings before anesthesia indicate an increased risk for perioperative proarrhythmia:

- Excessive prolongation of the Q-T interval
- Increased Q-T interval dispersion
- T-wave alternans or prominent U waves
- Polymorphic premature ventricular complexes
- Sinus bradycardia and AV conduction disturbances
- Abrupt slowing of the heart rate (e.g., conversion of atrial fibrillation to normal sinus rhythm)

Amiodarone Interactions and Toxicity

Several groups have noted a greater incidence of cardiac rhythm and conduction disturbances (e.g., atropine-resistant bradycardia, slow AV junctional rhythms, complete AV heart block, pacemaker dependency), an increased need for perioperative circulatory support (including inotropes or intra-aortic balloon counterpulsation), and more noncardiac complications in patients receiving amiodarone. However, perioperative hemodynamic instability with amiodarone and a poor response to inotropic drugs may be explained, in part, by the drug's antiarrhythmic actions. In addition to class III activity, these include sodium channel blockade (class I), noncompetitive blockade of β- and α-adrenergic receptors (class II), and inhibition of calcium channels (class IV). The reader is referred to Chapters 10, 11, and 13, respectively, for complications related to these antiarrhythmic classes of drugs.

The role of general anesthetic agents in the development of amiodarone's pulmonary toxicity remains controversial. Although some groups have found a higher incidence of postoperative acute respiratory distress syndrome and other pulmonary disorders in patients receiving amiodarone, others have been unable to show this relationship. Nonetheless, pulmonary toxicity is the most feared long-term complication of amiodarone therapy and should not be forgotten in the risk assessment of patients receiving this drug.

Implications

Owing to their potent cardiac electrophysiologic properties, class III drugs not only exhibit important antiarrhythmic actions but also have the potential to induce life-threatening proarrhythmias, typically TDP. Therefore, anesthesiologists should be familiar with the adverse effects of these drugs and their interactions with other Q-T interval–prolonging drugs and anesthetics. Also, amiodarone has special implications in terms of pulmonary complications.

MANAGEMENT

Actions to take when treating drug-induced TDP include the following:

- Immediate electrical cardioversion in hemodynamically unstable patients
- Infusion of magnesium sulfate (MgSO$_4$)
- Interventions that shorten the Q-T interval and prevent pause-dependent bradycardia (preferably atrial or ventricular overdrive pacing, or atropine or isoproterenol)
- Alleviation of electrolyte disturbances and bradycardia (preferably with temporary pacing) and other permissive factors
- Withdrawal of any offending drugs, along with correction of imbalance

Therapy of drug-induced TDP must focus on immediate TDP termination and the prevention of early recurrence. If TDP causes early hemodynamic collapse, it must be treated with prompt direct-current cardioversion or defibrillation, depending on whether the ECG R or S waves are distinct (cardioversion) or not (defibrillation). Other therapy includes intravenous MgSO$_4$, which is effective against TDP even in patients with normal serum magnesium levels.

MgSO$_4$ is given as a 1- to 2-g intravenous bolus. If necessary, it is repeated after 10 to 15 minutes, followed by continuous intravenous infusion at 3 to 20 mg/minute for 24 to 48 hours. If this is ineffective, atropine, isoproterenol, or overdrive pacing is used to prevent long sinus pauses to shorten the Q-T interval. Isoproterenol infused at a dose that maintains the ventricular rate at about 90 beats per minute (1 to 8 µg/minute) may suppress TDP within minutes. However, given this drug's proarrhythmic actions and other adverse effects, isoproterenol should be used only while pacing is instituted, especially in patients with ischemic heart disease. Preferably, temporary atrial or ventricular overdrive pacing is initiated at a rate of 120 to 130 beats per minute and adjusted to the lowest effective rate. Temporary pacing should be continued until the offending drug is completely eliminated.

The role of antiarrhythmic drugs in the treatment of TDP is controversial. In experimental preparations and in some patients, calcium channel blockers, lidocaine, mexiletine, and recently developed potassium channel openers (e.g., nicorandil, pinacidil) have been effective. However, the clinical evidence is marginal and has yet to be verified in large prospective clinical studies. Drugs that prolong ventricular repolarization should be avoided in the therapy of acquired long QT syndrome.

Once acute TDP episodes have been controlled, attention should focus on identifying and correcting predisposing metabolic and electrolyte factors and eliminating causative drugs. In patients with congenital long QT syndrome, β-blockers are the drugs of choice, and catecholamines must be avoided.

Patients receiving class III antiarrhythmics, especially amiodarone, may be more vulnerable to the development of perioperative bradycardia, AV node conduction disturbances, and circulatory failure. If these conditions do not respond to atropine, adrenergics, or other positive chronotropes, cardiac pacing or intra-aortic counterpulsation should be instituted.

PREVENTION

Prevention includes the following measures:

- Identify and correct any factors that predispose patients to proarrhythmia (e.g., electrolyte imbalance, bradycardia, myocardial ischemia).
- Stop any drugs that prolong the Q-T interval (e.g., macrolide antibiotics, nonsedating antihistamines, tricyclic antidepressants).
- Consider reassessing the dosage or withdrawing class III antiarrhythmics and postponing elective operations, especially if the Q-Tc is greater than 0.60 second.
- Consider regional anesthesia in patients receiving amiodarone.
- Monitor hemodynamic and respiratory functions throughout the perioperative period.

Q-T prolongation with class III antiarrhythmic drugs is a therapeutic end point. Mechanisms by which this effect becomes proarrhythmic are not easily separated from antiarrhythmic actions. Thus, the cornerstone of preoperative risk reduction in patients receiving class III antiarrhythmics is identification and elimination of predisposing risk factors. Of special importance is correction of electrolyte imbalance and withdrawal of drugs that cause additional Q-T interval prolongation (e.g., macrolide antibiotics, nonsedating antihistamines, tricyclic antidepressants). Likewise, patient reassurance and adequate sedation and analgesia can eliminate preoperative catecholamine increases and help prevent abrupt changes in heart rate during the induction of anesthesia.

Amiodarone is the most effective intravenous antiarrhythmic for life-threatening arrhythmias. However, its extremely long elimination half-life and serious adverse extracardiac effects (especially with chronic therapy) make it the most complicated of the class III agents. Importantly, amiodarone significantly augments the cardiac depressant effects of general anesthesia. In addition, amiodarone-associated pulmonary toxicity may become apparent during emergence and recovery from general anesthesia. Attention to these shortcomings and careful intraoperative monitoring of respiratory and hemodynamic parameters should help anesthesiologists avoid these severe complications.

Some case reports suggest that regional anesthesia is preferable in patients receiving amiodarone, but this remains to be confirmed in controlled clinical studies. Likewise, although some experimental data suggest that intravenous anesthetics have different effects on ventricular repolarization in acquired (drug-induced) long QT syndrome, until clinical trials are completed, no specific advice can be given on the selection of general anesthetics for patients receiving class III antiarrhythmics. Finally, because most patients receiving class III agents have severe arrhythmias and other cardiac disease, it is prudent to consult a cardiologist before anesthesia and surgery.

Further Reading

Atlee JL: Perioperative cardiac dysrhythmias: Diagnosis and management. Anesthesiology 86:1397-1424, 1997.

Balser JR: The rational use of intravenous amiodarone in the perioperative period. Anesthesiology 84:974-987, 1997.

Belardinelli L, Antzelevitch C, Vos MA: Assessing predictors of drug-induced torsades de pointes. Trends Pharmacol Sci 24:619-625, 2003.

Haverkamp W, Breithardt G, Camm AJ, et al: The potential for QT prolongation and proarrhythmia by non-antiarrhythmic drugs: Clinical and regulatory implications. Report on a policy conference of the European Society of Cardiology. Eur Heart J 21:1216-1231, 2000.

Priori SG, Napolitano C: Genetic defects of cardiac ion channels: The hidden substrate for torsades de pointes. Cardiovasc Drugs Ther 16:89-92, 2002.

Roden DM: Drug-induced prolongation of the QT interval. N Engl J Med 350:1013-1022, 2004.

Shah RR: Pharmacogenetic aspects of drug-induced torsades de pointes: Potential tool for improving clinical drug development and prescribing. Drug Saf 27:145-172, 2004.

Viskin S, Justo D, Halkin A, et al: Long QT syndrome caused by noncardiac drugs. Prog Cardiovasc Dis 45:415-427, 2003.

Wolbrette DL: Risk of proarrhythmia with class III antiarrhythmic agents: Sex-based differences and other issues. Am J Cardiol 91:39D-44D, 2003.

Class IV Antiarrhythmic Drugs: Calcium Channel Blockers

13

J. Michael Jaeger and Donn M. Dennis

Case Synopsis

An obese 48-year-old woman with a history of hypertension treated with diltiazem undergoes a laparoscopic cholecystectomy. Following insufflation of the abdomen with carbon dioxide, she becomes hypertensive and develops sinus tachycardia at a rate of 110 beats per minute; the tachycardia is unresponsive to deepening the level of anesthesia with isoflurane and fentanyl. Propranolol 1 mg is administered intravenously. The patient develops a marked sinus bradycardia, with a P-R interval of 0.24 second on the electrocardiogram (ECG), and becomes hypotensive.

PROBLEM ANALYSIS

Definition

This case illustrates many of the common toxic effects of L-type (long-lasting) calcium channel antagonists (specifically the class IV antiarrhythmic drugs verapamil and diltiazem) or of interactions between calcium channel antagonists and other cardiodepressant drugs. The marked bradycardia, first degree atrioventricular (AV) node block, and hypotension are manifestations of the pharmacologic interaction of several drugs, most notably diltiazem and propranolol. Each drug has a depressive effect on conduction in both the sinoatrial (SA) node and the AV node, although by different cellular mechanisms. However, both diltiazem and propranolol have little effect on ventricular conduction (Fig. 13-1).

Although therapeutic doses of diltiazem and propranolol by themselves generally do not produce this magnitude of response, the concurrent use of a calcium channel antagonist and a β-receptor antagonist can lead to cardiovascular collapse, particularly when other cardiac depressants (e.g., volatile inhalational anesthetics) are involved. Such patients require heightened vigilance by anesthesiologists because AV node conduction blockade can reduce the compensatory reflex increase in cardiac output observed with pathophysiologic conditions (e.g., hypercarbia, hypoxemia, hypovolemia, anemia). In addition to SA and AV node conduction block, this drug combination can precipitate acute heart failure in patients with cardiac disease and limited functional reserve.

Both L-type (e.g., verapamil, diltiazem, nifedipine) and T-type (transient) calcium channel antagonists (e.g., mibefradil) have been implicated as the cause of adverse drug interactions. They alter the pharmacokinetics and pharmacodynamics of a wide variety of drugs, including carbamazepine, neuromuscular blockers, digoxin, quinidine, statins, theophylline, and volatile inhalational anesthetics (Table 13-1).

Recognition

The toxic effects of class IV antiarrhythmic drugs, or their interactions with other depressants of cardiac conduction, can be recognized by the following ECG features:

- Sinus bradycardia (<60 beats per minute)
- P-R intervals greater than 0.2 second (first degree block) or P waves not always followed by QRS complexes (second degree block)
- Normal QRS complex duration (≤0.1 second)
- Normal Q-T interval relationships and ST segment configurations unless myocardial ischemia is present

Note that the QRS complex and ST segment remain normal in duration and configuration. This distinguishes direct toxicity by class IV antiarrhythmics or indirect toxicity through their interaction with other depressants of myocardial conduction (e.g., β-blockers) from other disturbances of conduction (e.g., bundle branch or fascicular block, myocardial ischemia). In addition, the interaction of calcium channel antagonists with other drugs should not be confused with preexisting conditions that can have a similar clinical presentation. For example, sick sinus syndrome, preexisting AV node block of varying degrees, amyloidosis, myotonic dystrophy, or cardiomyopathy may confound the ECG diagnosis, although the clinical history and presentation should allow clarification.

Risk Assessment

The following factors influence the risk of toxicity:

- Therapeutic spectrum
- Clinical pharmacology
- Mechanism of action

Verapamil and diltiazem are widely used to treat and prevent supraventricular tachycardias, to limit ventricular rates with atrial flutter or fibrillation, and as adjuncts for the

Figure 13–1 ▪ Cardiac conduction system, with examples of "slow-response" action potentials recorded from the sinoatrial (SA) and atrioventricular (AV) nodes and a "fast-response" action potential recorded from a Purkinje fiber in a bundle branch. Note the smaller action potential upstrokes characteristic of slow-conducting SA and AV node (i.e., slow-response) cells versus the much faster and larger action potential upstroke typical of fast-conducting (i.e., fast-response) Purkinje fibers. Atrial and ventricular muscle fibers also have fast-response action potentials (not shown), similar to those of Purkinje fibers. Verapamil and diltiazem have a greater impact on the conduction of slow-response action potentials in the heart. Contractility is also reduced because of the reduced influx of calcium ions during the cardiac action potential plateau.

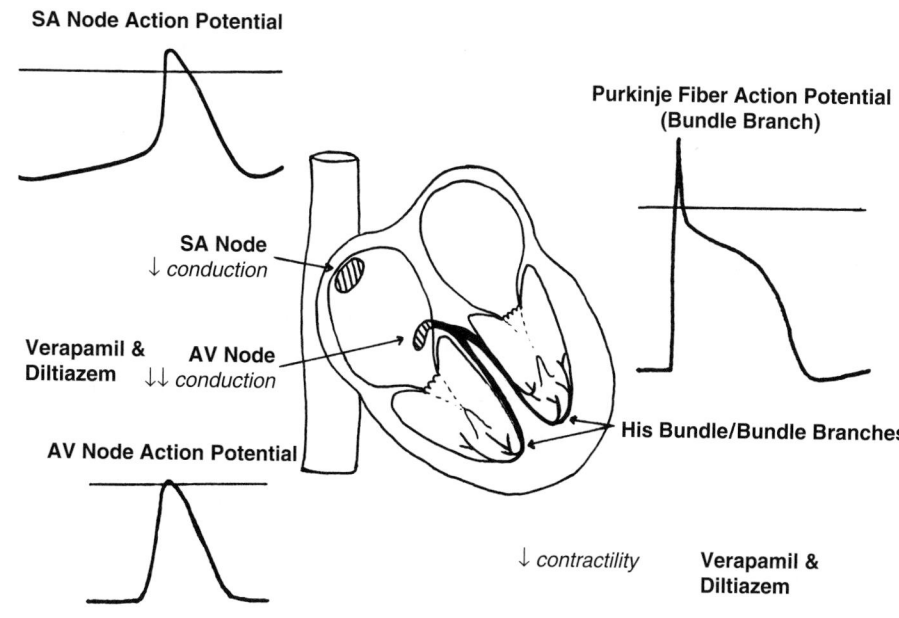

SA Node Action Potential

Purkinje Fiber Action Potential (Bundle Branch)

SA Node
↓ *conduction*

Verapamil & Diltiazem   **AV Node**
↓↓ *conduction*

His Bundle/Bundle Branches

AV Node Action Potential

↓ *contractility*   **Verapamil & Diltiazem**

Table 13–1 ▪ Selected Drug Interactions with Calcium Channel Antagonists

Drug	Nature of Interaction	Effect of Interaction
Antiarrhythmics		
Amiodarone (AM)	Possible potentiation of AM class IV activity at SA and AV nodes*	AV node block and hypotension; possible bradycardia
	Possible increase in L-type Ca^{2+} channel block by AM in vascular smooth muscle*	
Adenosine	Additive effect	Prolonged bradycardia
Quinidine	↓ Clearance	AV node block
β-Blockers		
Atenolol	Noncompetitive	Hypotension; AV node block
Metoprolol	Potentiation	Hypotension; AV node block
Propranolol	Potentiation	Hypotension; AV node block
Carbamazepine	↓ Clearance	Neurotoxicity;
Clonidine	Additive effect	Hypotension; AV node block
Cyclosporine	↑ Serum concentration	Nephrotoxicity
Digoxin	Modest ↑ serum concentration	AV node block
Lithium	Synergism	Muscle weakness, ataxia
Magnesium sulfate	Potentiation	Muscle weakness, hypotension
Midazolam	↓ Clearance	Profound and prolonged sedation
Phenytoin	↑ Serum concentration	Neurotoxicity
Quinidine	↑ Serum concentration	Potentiate hypotensive effects
Rifampin	↑ Clearance of verapamil	Supraventricular tachycardia
Statin drugs	↑ Serum concentration	Rhabdomyolysis
Succinylcholine	Potentiation	Possible prolonged effect
Theophylline	↓ Clearance	Theophylline toxic effects
Vecuronium	Potentiation	Prolonged neuromuscular block
Volatile anesthetics		
Desflurane	Unknown† (possible ↓ heart rate?)	No reported interactions in humans†
Enflurane	Potentiation	Rare AV node block
Halothane	Potentiation	↓ Cardiac output, AV node block
Isoflurane	Potentiation	No significant interactions in humans
Sevoflurane	Unknown	No reported interactions in humans†

*Speculation.
†MEDLINE database search Sept 27, 2005: no reports of adverse interactions in animal models or humans.
AV, atrioventricular; SA, sinoatrial.

treatment of vasospastic angina and essential hypertension. Although the probability of having to administer an anesthetic to a patient taking either of these calcium channel antagonists is high, actual clinical experience reveals that doing so is generally not a significant problem for anesthesiologists. Nonetheless, the potential for problems exists, and vigilance is important. In large clinical trials, verapamil and diltiazem caused the following cardiovascular abnormalities, in decreasing order of frequency: first degree AV block (2.4%), bradycardia (1.7%), second or third degree AV block (0.8%), and congestive heart failure (<1% to 1.8%).

Understanding the clinical problem and identifying patients at risk for complications require an appreciation of the relevant cardiac electrophysiology and pharmacology of all classes of calcium channel antagonists. Six types (T, L, N, P/Q, and R) of mammalian voltage-dependent calcium channels (VDCCs) have been identified. They are distinguishable by location and electrophysiologic characteristics (voltage thresholds for activation; kinetics of channel opening and closing). VDCCs have been classified into two general groups: (1) high-voltage-activated (HVA) calcium channels (threshold activation = −40 to −10 mV), and (2) low-voltage-activated (LVA) calcium channels (threshold activation = −60 to −70 mV). HVA channels include calcium channels of the L, N, P/Q, and R types, whereas LVA channels include only the T type. At times, the R-type channel is classified as an intermediate voltage activated (IVA) calcium channel with threshold activation voltages being intermediate between those of HVA and LVA.

Key characteristics of the different types of calcium channels include the following:

- T-type calcium channels include a heterogeneous group of **T**ransient (or low voltage) activated–type calcium channels, which are primarily located in the SA and AV nodes, cardiac Purkinje cells, and central nervous system.
- L-type calcium channels are **L**ong-lasting voltage-gated channels located in both excitable and nonexcitable tissue, which are responsible for normal myocardial and vascular smooth muscle contractility. The alpha-1 subunit of L-type calcium channel is the binding site for calcium channel blockers (e.g., dihydropyridine [DHP]-based calcium channel antagonists.
- N-type calcium channels are widely distributed in **N**eural tissue. Omega toxins inhibit the function of these types of calcium channels by changing their voltage dependence.
- P-type calcium channels were first identified within the **P**urkinje cells of the cerebellum. They play a role in regulating neuronal stimulation-secretion coupling.
- Q-type calcium channels are located in neurons. Because Q- (letter derived from the following letter of P) type current is rapidly inactivated, it requires prior blockade of P- and N-type calcium current components to isolate this current for study.
- R-type calcium channels are located in neurons. They are inhibited by the marine snail toxin, omega conotoxin MVIIC. A notable feature of the R-type channels is their resistance to all known calcium channel blockers. The R-type current (which was named after the following letter of Q, or **R**emaining channel) is defined as the residual HVA calcium current observed after the application of toxins that selectively block N, L, P, and Q-type currents.

Calcium channels in cardiac muscle and vascular smooth muscle cells are generally of the T and L types, which impart distinct characteristics to the cardiac action potential and influx of calcium into the cell. The T-type channel contributes significantly to the slow upstroke of the action potential found in the SA and AV nodes and, therefore, controls one of the pacemaker currents responsible for the initiation of the heartbeat. This channel exists in ventricular muscle but plays a less significant role in initiating the action potential. The L-type calcium channel produces the plateau of the cardiac action potential and is responsible for the influx of extracellular Ca^{2+} into the cell. This influx of extracellular Ca^{2+} is thought to serve as the trigger for the release of internally stored (sarcolemmal) Ca^{2+}. The latter leads to cardiac contraction. The entire process is known as excitation-contraction coupling.

Verapamil and diltiazem alter the function of L-type but not T-type calcium channels. Hence, they have a greater impact on the conduction and repolarization of cardiac action potentials (especially within the SA and AV nodes) and on the influx of extracellular Ca^{2+} than they do on the initiation of cardiac (or smooth) muscle action potentials (see Fig. 13-1). At first, this might seem counterintuitive, given that sinus bradycardia is occasionally observed with verapamil (less often with diltiazem). However, for heartbeats to occur, the SA node must first generate an action potential. In turn, it must be propagated to surrounding atrial muscle and the rest of the heart in a properly synchronized fashion. As more and more L-type calcium channels become blocked, SA node impulse formation slows, and SA conduction and refractoriness increase. Together, these lead to failure of SA node impulse formation and propagation. Reduction of the magnitude of extracellular Ca^{2+} influx—through fewer functional L-type calcium channels or a shorter duration of their open state—also reduces the strength of cardiac contraction. Because L-type calcium channels are also found in vascular smooth muscle, inhibition of excitation-contraction coupling here leads to vasodilatation. Whereas verapamil affects primarily cardiac L-type calcium channels, diltiazem affects L-type calcium channels in both cardiac and vascular smooth muscle. Finally, the dihydropyridine (DHP) calcium channel blockers (e.g., nifedipine, nicardipine, nimodipine) are highly selective for L-type calcium channels in vascular smooth muscle.

Among the L-type calcium channel blockers, verapamil (a diphenylalkylamine) and diltiazem (a benzothiazepine) markedly depress AV node conduction and increase refractoriness, whereas the DHP calcium channel blockers mentioned earlier are primarily vasodilators and have minimal to no effect on SA or AV node tissue or cardiac contractility. Verapamil and diltiazem are useful for treating reentrant supraventricular tachycardias involving the AV node and for achieving ventricular rate control in most patients with atrial flutter or fibrillation. They are also used as therapy for essential hypertension and chronic stable angina, especially vasospastic angina. However, DHP calcium channel blockers are increasingly used in these conditions, especially for patients who are also receiving β-blockers.

Implications

Increased AV node refractoriness with non-DHP calcium channel blockers increases the risk for high-degree AV block when combined with other drugs that also slow AV node conduction. Although this list is lengthy, it includes any drugs that are vagomimetic (e.g., opioids, anticholinesterases, digoxin) or sympatholytic (β-receptor antagonists, clonidine), as well as other drugs (e.g., adenosine, amiodarone, volatile inhalational anesthetics).

Accentuation of high-degree AV heart block can lead to cardiovascular collapse. Also, because non-DHP calcium channel blockers have the potential to increase the ventricular rate with atrial flutter or fibrillation and precipitate fatal ventricular tachyarrhythmias, diltiazem or verapamil should not be used in patients with Wolff-Parkinson-White syndrome or its variants, especially when the state of accessory pathway refractoriness is unknown. Essentially, accessory pathways are extensions of atrial muscle and have similar electrophysiologic properties (i.e., they are "fast-response" fibers). Thus, accessory pathway conduction is not blocked, nor is its refractoriness increased. However, both conduction and refractoriness at the AV node are impaired by diltiazem or verapamil. Because low-dose non-DHP calcium channel blockers (diltiazem more so than verapamil) cause vascular relaxation and hypotension before significant AV node block, reflex tachycardia can occur and cause angina in susceptible patients with nonvasospastic (fixed) coronary artery disease. Also, patients with limited cardiovascular reserve (i.e., cardiomyopathy) are at risk for acute worsening of heart failure when subjected to the additional negative inotropic effect of non-DHP calcium channel blockers.

Last, aside from their cardiac effects, calcium channel blockers may significantly inhibit hepatic cytochrome enzymes and alter hepatic or renal blood flow and drug binding. Thus, the pharmacologic properties of a wide variety of drugs may be affected (see Table 13-1). This problem was most pronounced with mibefradil, a T-type calcium channel blocker that was developed for the treatment of hypertension and chronic stable angina. Because mibefradil was a very potent inhibitor of CYP3A4, the single most important P-450 enzyme for metabolizing therapeutic agents, it caused many severe adverse drug reactions and was removed from the market. One interesting drug-drug interaction with mibefradil was increased blood levels of HMG-CoA reductase inhibitors (statin cholesterol-lowering agents) that depended on CYP3A4 for metabolic clearance (e.g., lovastatin, simvastatin, atorvastatin), leading to severe rhabdomyolysis.

MANAGEMENT

Because bradycardia, AV block, and hypotension can occur in patients receiving regional or general anesthesia, the first step is to determine the level of consciousness and then the adequacy of the airway and ventilation. Administer 100% oxygen and, if bradycardia is hemodynamically significant, immediately send for a transcutaneous or transvenous pacing device. Transesophageal atrial pacing is ineffective with high-degree (second or third degree) AV node block. Secure the airway if necessary. In the interim, attempt to reduce as many negative chronotropic, dromotropic, and inotropic influences as possible by decreasing (or turning off) the inspired concentration of volatile inhalational agents and ceasing the manipulation of any organs (e.g., bowel, reproductive organs, eyes) known to elicit vagal responses. Atropine can be given as a first-line drug to reduce vagal tone and enhance SA and AV node conduction. If the patient remains hypotensive and does not respond to atropine, β-sympathomimetic drugs, such as epinephrine or isoproterenol, are used to enhance SA and AV node conduction if pacing is not yet available, especially if reduced myocardial contractility is evident. Intravenous calcium chloride has been used successfully in cases of deliberate verapamil overdose. In some cases, high-degree AV heart block resistant to pharmacologic intervention may require cardiac pacing. Once stabilized, the patient requires prolonged monitoring because the α-elimination half-life of calcium channel blockers ranges from 10 to 35 minutes (depending on age), and the β-elimination half-life is 5 to 12 hours. Depending on the duration of calcium channel blocker therapy, the latter parameter is variable and may increase to 16 hours or more with hepatic insufficiency.

PREVENTION

Prevention relies on a full understanding of the patient's underlying pathophysiology and the effects of all concurrent drugs, including antiarrhythmics, calcium channel blockers, β-adrenergic blockers, opiates, and digitalis; automaticity of the sinus node; subsidiary atrial, AV junctional, or ventricular escape pacemakers; electrophysiologic properties of specialized atrial, AV, and ventricular conducting tissues (i.e., conduction times and refractoriness); and potential interactions with any drugs used during anesthesia or in perioperative settings.

Take the following specific precautions:

- Assess the patient's history (duration of drug use, dose, side effects, response).
- Determine the presence of heart failure or arrhythmias by a focused cardiac and pulmonary examination, and assess a 12-lead ECG for arrhythmias and AV conduction abnormalities.
- Use caution if block of the cardioaccelerator nerves is anticipated (e.g., activation of vagal, cardioinhibitory reflexes), and evaluate whether regional anesthesia might be preferable to intravenous or inhalation general anesthesia.
- If inhalation anesthesia is chosen, isoflurane, sevoflurane, or desflurane is preferable to enflurane or halothane in patients receiving calcium channel blockers (or β-adrenergic blockers).
- Use careful opiate dosing. Use of muscle relaxants must be guided by neuromuscular function monitoring.

Many patients receiving calcium channel blockers have successfully undergone a variety of surgical procedures under both regional and general anesthesia. Although the safety of these drugs in perioperative settings is supported by the paucity of reports of adverse outcomes, calcium channel blockers have a recognized potential to cause significant adverse events in perioperative settings. Given recent clinical trials showing the safety and efficacy of calcium channel blockers for the treatment of cardiovascular disease, anesthesiologists can expect to see a substantial increase in the number of patients receiving these drugs. Large prospective, controlled clinical trials (e.g., the INVEST trial) have shown that (1) for patients with hypertension, therapy with calcium channel blockers, angiotensin-converting enzyme inhibitors, or angiotensin receptor blockers reduces the risk for diabetes more effectively than does therapy with β-blockers and diuretics; and (2) for patients with hypertension and coronary artery disease, therapy with sustained-release verapamil or trandolapril was as clinically effective as atenolol-hydrochlorothiazide.

Further Reading

Altier C, Zamponi GW: Targeting Ca^{2+} channels to treat pain: T-type versus N-type. Trends Pharmacol Sci 25:465-470, 2004.

Atlee JL: Perioperative cardiac dysrhythmias: Diagnosis and management. Anesthesiology 86:1397-1424, 1997.

Atlee JL, Hamann SR, Brownlee SW, et al: Conscious state comparisons of the effects of the inhalation anesthetics and diltiazem, nifedipine, or verapamil on specialized atrioventricular conduction times in spontaneously beating dog hearts. Anesthesiology 68:519-528, 1988.

Bakris GL, Gaxiola E, Messerli FH, et al: Clinical outcomes in the diabetes cohort of the International Verapamil SR-Trandolapril [INVEST] study. Hypertension 44:637-642, 2004.

Durant NN, Nguyen N, Katz R, et al: Potentiation of neuromuscular blockade by verapamil. Anesthesiology 60:298-303, 1984.

Elmslie KS: Neurotransmitter modulation of neuronal calcium channels. J Bioenerg Biomembr 35:477-489, 2003.

Opie L: Calcium channel antagonists in the treatment of coronary artery disease: Fundamental pharmacological properties relevant to clinical use. Prog Cardiovasc Dis 38:273-290, 1996.

Packer M, Meller J, Medina N, et al: Hemodynamic consequences of combined beta-adrenergic and slow calcium channel blockade in man. Circulation 65:660-668, 1982.

Pepine CJ, Cooper-Dehoff RM: Cardiovascular therapies and risk for development of diabetes. J Am Coll Cardiol. 44:509-512, 2004.

Reves JG, Kissin I, Lell W, et al: Calcium entry blockers: Uses and implications for anesthesiologists. Anesthesiology 57:504-518, 1985.

Rosenthal T, Ezra D: Calcium antagonists: Drug interactions of clinical significance. Drug Saf 13:157-187, 1995.

ADJUNCT THERAPY

Disorders of Potassium Balance

John L. Atlee and Kai T. Kiviluoma

14

Case Synopses

Hypokalemia

A 56-year-old man with chronic renal failure underwent cardiopulmonary bypass (CPB) for coronary artery revascularization. His pre-CPB serum potassium (K^+) concentrations ranged between 5.5 and 6.6 mEq/L. After separation from CPB, the patient had frequent premature atrial beats and nonsustained ectopic atrial tachycardia ($\leq$15 seconds). Lead II of the monitored electrocardiogram (ECG) revealed prominent U waves (Fig. 14-1). Repeated post-CPB serum K^+ concentrations were 4.5 and 4.7 mEq/L.

Hyperkalemia

A 74-year-old man with severe coronary artery disease had coronary artery bypass grafting with five distal anastomoses. Because of impaired myocardial function (ejection fraction 22%), a high-dose glucose-insulin-potassium infusion was started intraoperatively. Postoperatively the patient was hemodynamically stable, and he was extubated 12 hours after surgery. However, 2 days later, ventricular arrhythmias, peaked T waves, and transient second degree atrioventricular (AV) block developed.

PROBLEM ANALYSIS

Definition

HYPOKALEMIA

There is a lack of consensus over what constitutes hypokalemia. Although a number of studies have addressed this issue, many fall short because (1) a single K^+ value is not confirmed, (2) there is no information regarding the patient's usual range of K^+ values (i.e., is the hypokalemia acute or chronic?), and (3) possible confounding effects of concurrent diseases and other metabolic imbalances are not considered.

As the case synopsis illustrates, the reported "normal" serum K^+ values may be misleading unless interpreted within the context of the patient's history and clinical status. Notably, the patient has ECG changes and arrhythmias consistent with hypokalemia, despite seemingly "normal" serum K^+ concentrations of 4.5 and 4.7 mEq/L.

HYPERKALEMIA

With regard to the patient described in the case synopsis, it is probable that after stopping glucose-insulin treatment, a new balance between intracellular and extracellular K^+ concentrations was established. Because up to 98% of the total body potassium pool is located intracellularly, dramatic changes in serum K^+ may be observed. Normal values for serum K^+ range from 3.5 to 5.3 mEq/L. Hyperkalemia increases myocardial membrane permeability to K^+ to increase the

speed of repolarization and reduce action potential duration. In moderate hyperkalemia, these actions may even reduce the likelihood for arrhythmias. The increase in K^+ permeability with hyperkalemia decreases the rate of spontaneous diastolic (phase 4) depolarization in the sinus node and subsidiary pacemakers to cause bradycardia and even asystole at very high extracellular K^+ concentrations. AV and intraventricular conduction abnormalities are also observed with severe hyperkalemia. This latter group of patients has

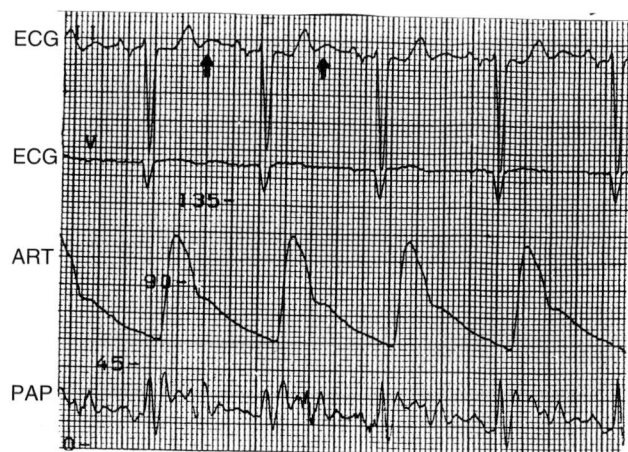

Figure 14–1 ■ Electrocardiogram changes after separation from cardiopulmonary bypass. Note the prominent U waves *(arrows).* (From Atlee JL: Arrhythmias and Pacemakers. Philadelphia, WB Saunders, 1996, p 90.)

a very high risk of developing fatal arrhythmias, including persistent ventricular fibrillation or asystole. Excessive serum K+ concentrations not only profoundly affect the electrical properties of the heart but also cause severely depressed myocardial contractility. These myocardial effects of hyperkalemia are potentiated in patients with concomitant hypocalcemia or hyponatremia.

Recognition

HYPOKALEMIA

Low serum K+ concentrations can exist without significant associated ECG changes. The following are common ECG changes with acute hypokalemia (serum K+ ≤ 3.0 mEq/L) in normokalemic patients (serum K+ 3.5 to 4.5 mEq/L):

- The appearance of U waves (see Fig. 14-1, lead II), which may fuse with T waves to cause *apparent* Q-T interval prolongation
- "Bowl-shaped" (concave or scooped) ST segment depression (see the last four QRS complexes in Fig. 14-1, lead II)
- Increased amplitude of QRS complexes (see Fig. 14-1, lead II)
- Flattened or inverted T waves
- Arrhythmias: atrial or ventricular extrasystoles or ectopic atrial tachycardia

Aside from arrhythmias and ECG changes, hypokalemia can affect cardiovascular, central nervous system, neuromuscular, renal, or metabolic function (Table 14-1).

HYPERKALEMIA

To recognize hyperkalemia, one must be aware of the possibility. It is confirmed by measuring serial serum K+ concentrations. Also, the ECG is analyzed for the following features:

- Peaking and narrowing of the T wave
- Progressive widening of the QRS complex as hyperkalemia worsens
- Prolongation of the P-Q and disappearance of P waves

The earliest manifestation of hyperkalemia is peaking and narrowing of the T wave. This is usually observed when plasma K+ concentrations exceed 5.5 mEq/L (Fig. 14-2). These T-wave changes are seen most clearly in the precordial leads of the ECG. With more severe hyperkalemia, the P-Q interval is prolonged, the QRS amplitude is decreased, and the QRS interval widens (usually seen at potassium concentrations >6.5 mEq/L). Ultimately, the P wave disappears. With preterminal hyperkalemia, the markedly widened QRS complex merges with the T wave, giving the ECG a "sine-wave" appearance (see Fig. 14-2). Ventricular flutter, fibrillation, or asystole usually ensues shortly thereafter.

The correlation between the degree of hyperkalemia and tissue effects is better at higher K+ concentrations than at lower ones. Thus, widening of the QRS complex more reliably predicts serum K+ levels than does peaking of the T wave. Although ECG changes can be detected during the early phase of hyperkalemia, a high index of clinical suspicion and serial measurement of serum K+ concentrations are essential for the definitive diagnosis of hyperkalemia and to avoid the morbidity and mortality associated with it.

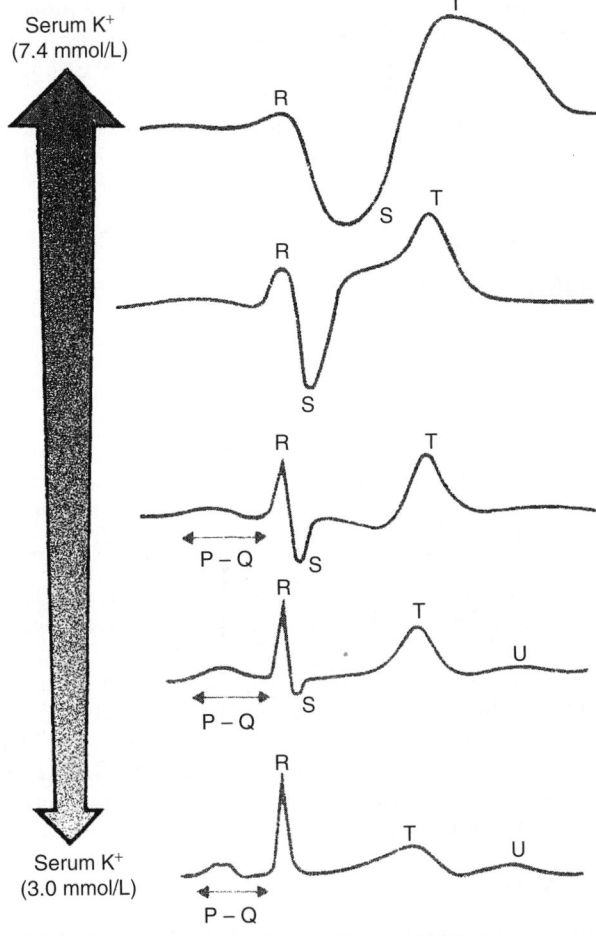

Serum K+ (7.4 mmol/L)

Serum K+ (3.0 mmol/L)

Figure 14–2 ▪ Schematized electrocardiogram (ECG) changes accompanying acute changes in serum potassium (K+) concentration. Note flattening of the T wave and prominent U waves with hypokalemia. As the serum K+ increases toward hyperkalemia, there is a small reduction in the QRS amplitude, QRS complex widening, P-R interval prolongation, reduced P-wave amplitude, and increased T-wave amplitude. Finally, the QRS and T waves merge, giving the ECG a sine-wave appearance. (From Sandøe E, Sigurd B: Arrhythmia. St. Galen, Belgium, Fachmed AG, 1984, p 403.)

Table 14–1 ▪ Effects of Hypokalemia
Cardiovascular
Autonomic neuropathy with postural hypotension
Impaired contractility and vasopressor responses
Potentiation of toxic effects of digitalis
Neuromuscular and Central Nervous System
Potentiation of neuromuscular blockade
Weakness and lethargy
Peripheral neuropathy and hyporeflexia
Respiratory depression
Confusion and depression
Renal and Gastrointestinal
Polyuria; reduced urine concentrating ability
Hypoperistalsis
Metabolic
Glucose intolerance
Potentiation of hypomagnesemia and hypocalcemia

Risk Assessment

HYPOKALEMIA

Hypokalemia is more likely than hyperkalemia to cause clinically important arrhythmias. It often results from excessive dialysis, thiazide or loop diuretics, mechanical hyperventilation, or therapy with insulin or β-adrenergic agonists. Cellular repolarization abnormalities and loss of transmembrane potential with hypokalemia alter cardiac conduction and refractoriness to facilitate reentry. They are also conducive to disturbed automaticity or triggered activity. Arrhythmias caused by severe hypokalemia resemble those accompanying digitalis toxicity (see Chapter 7) and likely have similar mechanisms. Arrhythmias include atrial and ventricular extrasystoles, ectopic atrial tachycardia, reentrant (paroxysmal) supraventricular tachycardia, and AV heart block. These are not caused by changes in serum K$^+$ concentration per se, but rather by changes in the ratio between intra- and extracellular K$^+$. This is the most important determinant of resting cell membrane potential and cellular electrophysiologic properties. Only extreme extracellular K$^+$ changes (<2.7 or >10 mEq/L) significantly depolarize cell transmembrane potential in atrial, Purkinje, or ventricular muscle fibers. However, loss of transmembrane potential is conducive to automatic, triggered, or reentrant arrhythmias. Between these values, transmembrane potential increases toward more normal values. Further, electrophysiologic changes due to K$^+$ imbalance are likely heterogeneous, with some cells or tissues affected more than others.

Thus, the patient described in the first case synopsis was likely *relatively* hypokalemic, because his pre-CPB serum K$^+$ concentrations ranged from 5.5 to 6.5 mEq/L. Indeed, treatment with intravenous potassium chloride (KCl) restored this patient's serum K$^+$ concentration to his normal range and abolished the U waves, ectopic atrial beats, and nonsustained ectopic atrial tachycardia.

HYPERKALEMIA

Causes of hyperkalemia are listed in Table 14-2. Surgery or underlying pathophysiology can cause large changes in potassium excretion and balance. Patients receiving potassium therapy or potassium-sparing diuretics preoperatively are at risk for the development of intra- and postoperative hyperkalemia. Renal failure also renders patients extremely susceptible to hyperkalemia. Patients with advanced renal failure do not respond normally to aldosterone. Thus, their ability to excrete potassium is impaired.

Cell disruption of any kind causes intracellular potassium leak and is often associated with hyperkalemia. Hyperkalemia is commonly associated with major trauma, large surface area third-degree burns, and rhabdomyolysis. During hemolytic processes, massive amounts of potassium are liberated over a short period. Reperfusion of ischemic areas can mobilize potassium, and hyperkalemia is worsened by ischemic acidosis. Anesthesiologists commonly encounter these problems in patients having vascular surgery that requires the application of an aortic cross-clamp.

Succinylcholine muscle depolarization causes transient increases in serum K$^+$ that are especially dangerous in the setting of chronic hyperkalemia. Owing to a proliferation in

Table 14–2 ■ Causes of Hyperkalemia

Potassium supplementation and potassium-sparing diuretics
Acute or chronic renal insufficiency
Trauma and large burns
Succinylcholine
Neuromuscular disorders, myopathies, muscle denervation, massive muscle injury, tetanus
Hemiplegia or paraplegia
Diffuse head injury and encephalitis
Rhabdomyolysis, hemolysis, or massive blood transfusions
Primary or secondary hypoaldosteronism
Addison's disease (chronic adrenocortical insufficiency)
Angiotensin-converting enzyme inhibitors
Prostaglandin synthetase inhibitors
Heparin therapy or digitalis poisoning
Respiratory or metabolic acidosis

the number of nicotinic receptors or alterations in the kinetics of potassium channel opening (i.e., the channels remain open longer), succinylcholine may cause life-threatening increases in serum K$^+$ concentrations in a variety of disorders, especially large surface area third-degree burns, spinal cord injury leading to hemi- or quadriplegia, and neuromuscular diseases.

Potassium distribution between the intra- and extracellular spaces is strongly pH dependent. A 0.1 decrease in pH causes about a 1.0 mEq/L increase in serum K$^+$. Thus, acidemia of metabolic or respiratory origin can cause severe hyperkalemia by moving intracellular K$^+$ out of the cell. Hypoventilation and respiratory acidosis are important causes of hyperkalemia during anesthesia. Likewise, diabetic ketoacidosis due to insulin-dependent diabetes, especially when compounded by acidosis due to circulatory or hemorrhagic shock, is a common cause of hyperkalemia in emergency rooms. However, despite seeming hyperkalemia, these patients actually have total body K$^+$ depletion.

A number of other conditions can cause clinically significant hyperkalemia, albeit more rarely. Massive blood transfusion can cause hyperkalemia by liberating potassium accumulated during blood preservation. Massive amounts of citrate can also bind calcium and worsen the cardiac effects of hyperkalemia. In addition, digitalis preparations have the potential to cause clinically significant hyperkalemia by inhibiting the Na$^+$,K$^+$-ATPase pump.

Implications

HYPOKALEMIA

There is no unequivocal serum K$^+$ concentration below which the risk for arrhythmias is certain. The development of clinically significant hypokalemia is context sensitive and depends on the following factors:

- Concurrent disease and associated pathophysiology
- Nature of the planned surgery or other therapeutic intervention
- Acute imbalance imposed by the circumstances of anesthesia and surgery

The last can include stress-induced catecholamine surges, exaggerated temperature changes, impaired ventilation and oxygenation, and the effects of drugs and other interventions.

Therefore, the decision to proceed with elective surgery in the face of *chemical evidence* of hypokalemia depends on many factors: whether the condition is acute or chronic, its effect on perioperative risk, the urgency of the planned surgery or intervention, and the implications of the associated imbalance and the patient's current medications.

HYPERKALEMIA

Concerns about anesthesia and surgery in a patient with hyperkalemia (especially if acute) involve the risk of cardiac electrical and mechanical dysfunction:

- First, second, and third degree AV heart block
- Potential for bradycardia and asystole
- Ventricular and AV junctional escape rhythms
- Ventricular fibrillation
- Decreased contractility

Hyperkalemia can impair cardiac function by causing disturbances of cardiac rhythm or mechanical dysfunction. Although cardiac electrophysiologic abnormalities related to hyperkalemia can cause many different types of arrhythmias, heart block and bradycardia are most common. However, ventricular extrasystolic beats, ventricular fibrillation, and asystole are also possible. Importantly, far more adverse events occur with rapid changes in serum K^+ concentration than with chronic hyperkalemia.

MANAGEMENT

The decision to proceed with surgery or other major therapeutic interventions requiring anesthesia in patients with hypo- or hyperkalemia remains controversial. However, it is now clear that the duration of hypo- or hyperkalemia is more important than some arbitrary serum K^+ value. Chronic imbalances are much better tolerated than their acute counterparts. Other considerations before proceeding with surgery in patients with hypokalemia or hyperkalemia include the following:

- Severity and urgency of the planned surgery or therapeutic intervention
- Presence of associated physiologic or metabolic imbalances
- Presence of concurrent systemic disease that may be aggravated by acute hypokalemia or hyperkalemia, especially cardiovascular and central nervous system afflictions
- Presence of uncontrolled hypertension
- Presence of renal insufficiency, heart failure, or coronary heart disease

Hypokalemia

Roizen and Fleisher addressed some unresolved issues concerning the perioperative management of patients with hypokalemia:

- In patients with modest hypokalemia, should surgery be delayed to subject them to the risks of intravenous or even oral K^+ supplementation therapy?
- What is the definition of modest hypokalemia: less than 3.4 mEq/L? less than 3.0 mEq/L?

- Is modest hypokalemia context sensitive? That is, is modest hypokalemia (however defined) safe for some surgeries but not for others (e.g., coronary artery bypass grafting)?
- Are some individuals more sensitive than others to even minor K^+ depletion?
- Are risk measures for modest hypokalemia (e.g., ventricular premature beats per hour) appropriate and context sensitive? (Such frequency might be more meaningful for patients with evolving myocardial infarction or following cardiopulmonary bypass.)

Based on the available evidence and the realization that context-sensitive and adequately powered outcome studies are lacking, we suggest the following guidelines for patients with hypokalemia.

WHETHER TO PROCEED WITH ANESTHESIA AND SURGERY

- Serum K^+ below 2.5 mEq/L: Confirmed serum K^+ values less than 2.5 mEq/L, especially if associated with ECG changes or arrhythmias, justify the delay of all but truly emergency interventions requiring anesthesia, owing to the increased risk of periprocedural complications. This delay provides the time needed to determine the cause and chronicity of the imbalance and to correct it.
- Serum K^+ between 2.5 and 3.0 mEq/L: Confirmed values in this range, especially when associated with ECG changes consistent with hypokalemia or the anticipated presence of other factors that increase the risk for perioperative arrhythmias (Table 14-3), justify the postponement of elective surgery in order to identify the cause of hypokalemia and correct the imbalance. Emergent and urgent procedures can proceed as the imbalance is being corrected.
- Serum K^+ between 3.1 and 3.5 mEq/L: With serum K^+ values in this range, provided there has not been an acute decrease of 1.5 mEq/L or more, there is little risk of significant arrhythmias without overt digitalis toxicity, catecholamine excess, acute myocardial infarction, heart

Table 14–3 ■ **Risk Factors for Perioperative Arrhythmias**
Unstable coronary artery disease
Chronic pulmonary disease
Hypertensive urgencies* or emergencies†
NYHA class III or IV or ACC/AHA stage C or D heart failure‡
Acute or chronic renal failure
Morbid obesity
Malnutrition or cachexia
Excess catecholamines
Autonomic dysfunction
Sick sinus syndrome
Increased intracranial pressure

*Subacute or chronic stage 2 blood pressure increase to ≥160/100 mm Hg; no end-organ damage.

†Acute stage 2 blood pressure increase with evidence of end-organ damage.

‡New York Heart Association (NYHA): class I—no symptoms of heart failure (HF) at rest; class II—HF symptoms with ordinary exertion; class III—HF symptoms with less than ordinary exertion; class IV—HF symptoms at rest. The American College of Cardiology/American Heart Association (ACC/AHA) staging emphasizes the evolution and progression of HF: stage A—high risk for developing HF, but no structural heart disease; stage B—structural heart disease (SHD), but no HF symptoms; stage C—SHD and past or current HF symptoms; stage D—end-stage heart disease and need for advanced HF treatment (continuous inotropes, mechanical circulatory support, cardiac transplantation, hospice care).

failure, or other significant comorbidities. In other words, there is no compelling reason to delay elective surgery or other therapeutic interventions to correct the imbalance.

POTASSIUM REPLACEMENT

Treatment for hypokalemia, especially with arrhythmias, consists of K^+ repletion, correction of alkalosis, and removal of drugs that are likely to exaggerate its effects (e.g., insulin, potassium-wasting diuretics, β_2-adrenergic agonists, catecholamines). If total body K^+ is depleted, as with chronic hypokalemia, oral repletion is prudent. For intravenous repletion, KCl is used because coexisting chloride depletion may limit the ability of the kidney to conserve K^+. KCl is administered cautiously (no more than 10 to 20 mEq/hour), especially if the absolute deficit and its acuteness are not known. However, if the deficit is known to be acute and large (e.g., the result of massive diuresis or overly aggressive dialysis), intravenous KCl can be administered more rapidly; however, this should be done with simultaneous ECG monitoring. Special care should be exercised during K^+ repletion in patients with diabetes, acidemia, and renal tubular acidosis and in those receiving angiotensin-converting enzyme inhibitors, β-adrenergic blockers, or nonsteroidal anti-inflammatory agents. All these conditions and drugs delay the movement of K^+ into cells and could lead to significant hyperkalemia.

Finally, keep in mind that hypomagnesemia is commonly associated with hypokalemia; it aggravates the effects of the latter by impairing K^+ conservation. Hypomagnesemia is common in critically ill patients with chronic ethanolism, acute myocardial infarction, diarrhea, cachexia, malnutrition, and starvation. It is also common following CPB and dialysis and in patients receiving digitalis or chronic diuretic therapy.

Hyperkalemia

It is unknown what a safe concentration of K^+ is in patients with hyperkalemia. In *experimental* hyperkalemia, there is good correlation between the magnitude of serum K^+ increases and ECG changes (see Fig. 14-2). In *clinical* hyperkalemia, however, abnormalities of impulse formation and propagation may occur at lower K^+ concentrations than in experimental hyperkalemia; in addition, the correlation between serum K^+ concentration and ECG changes is not as reliable. However, if hyperkalemia is associated with conduction disturbances, arrhythmias, or reduced contractility, acute therapy is warranted, as follows:

- Antagonize the cardiac effects of K^+ with intravenous calcium gluconate or chloride.
- Redistribute K^+ into the cells with β-adrenergic agonists, sodium bicarbonate, hyperventilation, or glucose-insulin.
- Remove K^+ from the body with furosemide or potassium-binding resin (Kayexalate).
- Use hemo- or peritoneal dialysis.

In emergencies, one must rapidly reduce the extracellular concentration of K^+ to counteract its effects on myocardial function. Although normalizing total body K^+ is the long-term goal of therapy, calcium gluconate or chloride is used acutely to antagonize the effects of increased K^+ on cardiac cell membranes. Insulin and β-adrenergic agents redistribute K^+ intracellularly and produce a positive inotropic effect.

Correction of acid-base imbalance and moderate alkalosis have the same effect. Sodium bicarbonate (1 to 2 mEq/kg) and moderate hyperventilation (pH 7.45 to 7.50) are also effective for acutely lowering serum K^+. Infusion of glucose (1.5 g/kg) and insulin (1 unit/3 g glucose) are relatively rapid means of moving K^+ intracellularly. One must measure serum K^+ repeatedly, because marked hypokalemia can result from overly rapid intracellular K^+ shifts.

Total body K^+ content is reduced with loop diuretics (e.g., furosemide) or cation exchange resins (e.g., Kayexalate). The latter bind K^+ in the gut. Although both therapies are effective, their actions develop more slowly. Thus, they are used after initial treatment in emergencies. Dialysis (hemodialysis or peritoneal dialysis) or hemofiltration (our preference) is indicated in patients with severe renal insufficiency or when physiologic stability cannot be achieved by other means.

PREVENTION

In the critically ill patient, sequential perioperative measurement of serum K^+ and arterial blood gases for acid-base status is important. Although hypokalemia can be easily treated by giving potassium, the principles of potassium homeostasis must be kept in mind. Before and during anesthesia, it is often wise not to treat mild hypokalemia ($K^+ \leq 3.0$ to 3.4 mEq/L), or to do so very slowly (≤ 10 mEq KCl/hour). Circulatory insufficiency can cause tissue hypoperfusion and severe metabolic acidosis, which in turn moves intracellular K^+ to the extracellular space. Respiratory acidosis acts similarly. In hyperkalemic patients, succinylcholine should be avoided because it causes a transient rise in serum K^+. This rise can be dramatic and potentially lethal if succinylcholine is given to patients with large surface area burns, certain neuromuscular disorders (see Chapters 23 and 153), or a large mass of denervated muscle (i.e., spinal hemiplegia or paraplegia).

Hypokalemia

One must be knowledgeable about the causes of hypokalemia and its associated conditions. Also, one must have a high index of suspicion for this condition in critically ill patients or those receiving chronic therapy with potassium-wasting diuretics (e.g., patients with hypertension or heart failure). Finally, one must be able to recognize the ECG signs of hypokalemia and monitor the ECG for evidence of its development.

Hyperkalemia

Clinical awareness of the possibility of hyperkalemia is the most important factor in preventing it and its complications. To this end, take the following steps:

- Identify patients at risk.
- Monitor the ECG for signs of hyperkalemia.
- Measure serial serum K^+ concentrations.
- Monitor acid-base status.
- Avoid unnecessary potassium supplementation.
- Avoid respiratory or metabolic acidosis and succinylcholine.

Preoperative use of potassium supplementation or the use of potassium-sparing diuretics must be kept in mind. During anesthesia, continuous ECG monitoring and end-tidal carbon dioxide monitoring are essential; with the latter, respiratory acidosis can be avoided. With suspected hyperkalemia, T-wave changes usually manifest well before heart block, bradycardia, escape rhythms, or deterioration in myocardial contractile function. Widening of the QRS complex indicates more severe changes. Asystole or ventricular fibrillation occurs with extreme hyperkalemia or after inadvertent intracardiac administration of potassium.

Further Reading

Atlee JL: Perioperative cardiac arrhythmias. Anesthesiology 86:1397-1425, 1997.

Atlee JL: Perioperative Cardiac Dysrhythmias, 2nd ed. Chicago, Year Book Medical Publishers, 1990, pp 128-129.

Cox M: The renal system and metabolic function. In Carlson RW, Geheb MA (eds): Principles and Practice of Medical Intensive Care, 3rd ed. Philadelphia, WB Saunders, 1993, pp 1155-1334.

Davis RF: Etiology and treatment of perioperative cardiac arrhythmias. In Kaplan JA, Reich DL, Konstadt SN (eds): Cardiac Anesthesia, 4th ed. Philadelphia, WB Saunders, 1999, pp 177-213.

Juurlink DN, Mamdani MM, Lee DS, et al: Rates of hyperkalemia after publication of the randomized aldactone evaluation study. N Engl J Med 351:543-551, 2004.

Roizen MF, Fleisher LA: Anesthetic implications of concurrent diseases. In Miller RD (ed): Miller's Anesthesia, 6th ed. Philadelphia, Churchill Livingstone, 2005, pp 1017-1149.

Winkler AW, Hoff HE, Smith PK: Electrocardiographic changes and concentration of potassium in serum following intravenous injection of potassium chloride. Am J Physiol 124:478-483, 1948.

Magnesium

Thomas S. Guyton and Timothy E. Morey

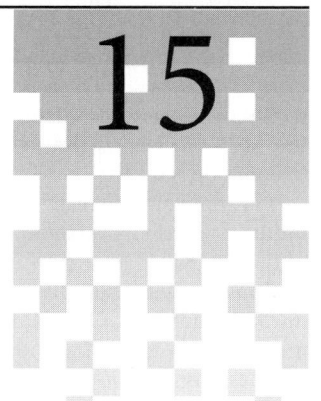

Case Synopsis

While recovering from hip surgery, a 54-year-old man suffering from alcoholism experiences recurrent episodes of ventricular tachycardia that are resistant to therapy with lidocaine. His serum magnesium level is 1.1 mEq/L. While receiving intravenous magnesium sulfate replacement, the patient complains of feeling hot and has difficulty breathing. Within 15 minutes of initiating replacement therapy, the patient has a respiratory arrest.

PROBLEM ANALYSIS

Definition

MAGNESIUM HOMEOSTASIS

Magnesium is the fourth most abundant cation in the body, with total body stores of about 2000 mEq. Normal serum magnesium (Mg^{2+}) concentrations are between 1.4 and 2.1 mEq/L, equivalent to 1.7 and 2.5 mg/dL, respectively (see Table 15-1 for unit conversions). Serum Mg^{2+} concentrations correlate poorly with total body stores, reflecting less than 1% of the amount stored. Gastrointestinal absorption in the duodenum and jejunum represents the principal source of Mg^{2+} (8 to 9 mEq/day). The amount of Mg^{2+} lost from the body via gastrointestinal secretions is relatively constant (2 mEq/day). In contrast, the kidney can dramatically affect losses in response to lowered serum Mg^{2+} concentrations due to reabsorption of Mg^{2+} in the proximal renal tubules and the loop of Henle.

ROLE IN CELLULAR FUNCTION

Magnesium serves as an essential cofactor for many important cellular enzymes (e.g., adenylyl cyclase, Na^+,K^+-ATPase). In addition, the magnesium complex with adenosine triphosphate serves as a substrate for the enzymatic reaction mediating muscle contraction and relaxation. Magnesium also regulates cellular function by antagonizing the cellular effects of calcium and modulating several potassium currents (Table 15-2).

Increased serum Mg^{2+} concentrations cause vascular smooth muscle relaxation by directly competing with Ca^{2+} to inhibit muscle contraction. Alterations in serum Mg^{2+} concentrations affect multiple organ systems. For example, hypermagnesemia produces relaxation of vascular smooth muscle by directly competing with Ca^{2+} to inhibit smooth muscle contraction, increasing the release of prostacyclin and decreasing catecholamine release after sympathetic stimulation. At the motor neuromuscular junction, increased Mg^{2+} causes presynaptic inhibition of Ca^{2+} release; this facilitates acetylcholine release, which depresses sarcolemmic excitability. In the heart, reduced Mg^{2+} slows the heart rate owing to suppressed automaticity and depressed atrioventricular conduction. Hypermagnesemia also reduces the amplitude of early afterdepolarizations to oppose triggered arrhythmias (see later). In the brain, increased Mg^{2+} serves as an anticonvulsant by blocking neuronal Ca^{2+} channels associated with the *N*-methyl-D-aspartate receptor.

ROLE IN THERAPEUTICS

Magnesium infusions may be therapeutic in the case of triggered ventricular arrhythmias. They are also used as adjunct therapy for atrial fibrillation in cardiac surgery, as tocolytic agents in preterm labor, and to prevent seizures with preeclampsia. The frequency of automatic or triggered ventricular arrhythmias with hypomagnesemia (e.g., torsades de pointes, digitalis ventricular arrhythmias) is reduced by intravenous magnesium infusions that double the serum Mg^{2+} concentration. Thus, such infusions may increase inwardly

---

Table 15–1 ■ Unit Conversions for Magnesium Compounds and Serum Concentrations

Compound	Unit Conversions
Magnesium sulfate ($MgSO_4$)	1 g = 8.13 mEq of Mg^{2+}
Magnesium oxide (MgO)	1 g = 46 mEq of Mg^{2+}
Magnesium acetate ($MgC_4H_6O_4$)	1 g = 9.35 mEq of Mg^{2+}
Magnesium chloride ($MgCl_2$)	1 g = 9.75 mEq of Mg^{2+}
Serum concentrations (all compounds)	1 mg/dL = 0.83 mEq/L = 0.415 mmol/L

Table 15–2 ■ Mechanisms for Magnesium's Effect on Cellular Function

Ca^{2+} Antagonism
Modulates handling of Ca^{2+} by sarcoplasmic reticulum
Inhibits Ca^{2+} influx into myocyte through sarcolemmal channels
Modulates second messenger system (i.e., adenyl cyclase–adenosine monophosphate)
Competes with Ca^{2+} for high affinity site on actin

K^+ Current
Enhances function of Na^+,K^+-ATPase
Blocks outward K^+ current to result in an increase in inward rectifying K^+ current
Mediates inwardly rectifying properties

rectifying potassium currents to reduce the amplitude of the early afterdepolarizations that serve as the triggers for torsades de pointes.

Proposed mechanisms for magnesium's effect on digitalis-induced ventricular arrhythmias include improved function of the Na^+,K^+-ATPase pump and reduction in the amplitude of delayed afterdepolarizations owing to a reduction in the intracellular rise of Ca^{2+}. However, most ventricular arrhythmias are due to reentry and do not respond to intravenous magnesium. In contrast, preoperative β-blockers and calcium channel antagonists with adjunct Mg^{2+} therapy can reduce the occurrence of atrial fibrillation in postoperative cardiac surgery patients. Hypomagnesemia can result from hemodilution with cardiopulmonary bypass and diuretic therapy. Finally, increasing the serum Mg^{2+} concentration by 4 to 6 mEq/L has been used to decrease uterine activity in preterm labor and to prevent seizure activity in women diagnosed with preeclampsia.

Recognition

HYPOMAGNESEMIA

Alterations in serum Mg^{2+} concentrations are often occult and occur along with alterations in other serum electrolytes, such as calcium and potassium. Hypomagnesemia is best diagnosed by recognizing those conditions associated with it (e.g., chronic ethanol abuse, diuretic or digitalis therapy). Hypomagnesemia alone does not result in electrocardiogram changes; however, the associated disturbances in calcium and potassium may do so.

HYPERMAGNESEMIA

Hypermagnesemia is most often diagnosed by associating the timing of adverse effects with the administration of magnesium. In patients with gastrointestinal diseases leading to increased absorption or renal failure leading to decreased excretion, large doses of cathartics, antacids, or analgesics containing magnesium salts may result in significant hypermagnesemia. Under these conditions, the temporal association with magnesium administration is often not apparent.

Hypermagnesemia is also diagnosed by recognizing the progressive pattern of its adverse effects and then confirming that suspicion with serum Mg^{2+} measurements. Hypermagnesemia can produce the following adverse effects:

- Generalized vasodilatation
- Lethargy
- Muscle weakness
- Respiratory depression
- Sinus bradycardia
- Atrioventricular block
- Asystole

Table 15-3 lists common adverse effects of hypermagnesemia and the associated serum Mg^{2+} concentration at which these effects first appear. It is noteworthy that the serum concentration at which a particular adverse reaction occurs in a given individual varies considerably, depending on the associated metabolic disturbances.

Table 15–3 ▪ Correlation between Serum Magnesium Concentration and Systemic Effects	
Concentration (mEq/L)	Systemic Effects
<0.8	Arrhythmias may be resistant to therapy When associated with hypocalcemia: disorientation, muscle twitching, choreiform movements, seizures
1.4-2.1	Normal range
3-4	Flushing 7%-13% increase in PR interval 0%-11% increase in QRS interval No change in Q-T interval
5-6	Slight reduction in blood pressure Slight increase in heart rate 10% reduction in FEV_1 and FVC Blurred vision from diminished accommodation and convergence Lethargy
10	Loss of deep tendon reflexes
20	Respiratory arrest Atrioventricular conduction block Progressive QRS widening and bradycardia
>25	Cardiac arrest

FEV_1, forced expiratory volume in 1 second; FVC, forced vital capacity.

Risk Assessment

HYPOMAGNESEMIA

Hypomagnesemia has an incidence of 470 per 1000 individuals suspected of having serum electrolyte abnormalities. Persons with congestive heart failure who are treated with diuretics and digitalis have a 7% to 37% incidence of hypomagnesemia. Alcoholics have a 30% to 40% incidence of hypomagnesemia.

HYPERMAGNESEMIA

Hypermagnesemia has an incidence of 57 per 1000 individuals suspected of having serum electrolyte abnormalities. Because of the kidney's remarkable ability to reduce the reabsorption of magnesium, respiratory and cardiac arrests are extremely rare during continuous magnesium infusions for arrhythmias, tocolysis, or seizure prevention in preeclampsia. To prevent the adverse effects of hypermagnesemia, it is best to avoid administering magnesium to individuals with renal failure. In individuals with congestive heart failure, a therapeutic regimen consisting of 0.3 mEq/kg of magnesium given as an intravenous bolus over 10 minutes, followed by a continuous infusion of 0.08 mEq/kg per hour, resulted in serum Mg^{2+} concentrations of 3.5 mEq/L. In women with preeclampsia, an intravenous bolus of 32 mEq of magnesium sulfate over 20 minutes, followed by 16 mEq/hour, resulted in average serum Mg^{2+} levels of 4 to 6 mEq/L.

Implications

Ventricular arrhythmias resulting from increased automaticity or triggered activity due to magnesium deficits clearly warrant the replacement of those deficits. The use of magnesium infusions to reduce the risk of acute myocardial infarction is controversial and is still under investigation. The use of magnesium for preterm labor tocolysis seems to be a safe alternative to β-sympathomimetics. In comparison to phenytoin, magnesium appears to be more efficacious in preventing seizures in women with preeclampsia.

MANAGEMENT

The key to the management of both hypomagnesemia and hypermagnesemia is recognition. Hypomagnesemia can be treated either orally or parenterally. Table 15-1 gives the elemental content of the various magnesium-containing formulations used to treat hypomagnesemia. In patients with normal renal function, 16 to 32 mEq of magnesium sulfate can be infused intravenously over 30 minutes to 1 hour for rapid correction or over 8 to 24 hours for slower correction.

As stated earlier, serum Mg^{2+} represents less than 1% of the total body stores of magnesium. Thus, achieving sustained elevations in serum Mg^{2+} concentrations with hypomagnesemia involves multiple doses to replete total body stores. In contrast, the treatment of hypermagnesemia includes any or all of the following:

- Removal of all potential ex vivo sources of magnesium
- In cases of respiratory arrest, intubation and support of ventilation
- Administration of furosemide and magnesium-free salt solutions to increase the renal excretion of magnesium
- Calcium chloride (5 to 10 mEq every 5 to 10 minutes) to antagonize hypermagnesemia
- Dialysis with magnesium-poor dialysate

PREVENTION

The best prevention for hypermagnesemia is to not give magnesium-containing salts or compounds to patients with renal failure. Magnesium-containing compounds include the following:

- Cathartics (e.g., magnesium citrate)
- Antacids (e.g., magnesium oxide)
- Analgesics (e.g., buffered aspirin)
- Magnesium supplements

During the administration of cathartics to individuals with gastrointestinal disturbances (e.g., paralytic ileus, ulcerative colitis, perforated duodenal ulcer), massive amounts of magnesium absorption can occur.

Further Reading

Dube L, Granry JC: The therapeutic use of magnesium in anesthesiology, intensive care and emergency medicine: A review. Can J Anaesth 50: 732-746, 2003.

Ducceschi V, Di Micco G, Sarubbi B, et al: Ionic mechanisms of ischemia-related ventricular arrhythmias. Clin Cardiol 19:325-331, 1996.

Hazelrigg SR, Boley TM, Cetindag IB, et al: The efficacy of supplemental magnesium in reducing atrial fibrillation after coronary artery bypass grafting. Ann Thorac Surg 77:824-830, 2004.

Kelepouris E, Agus ZS: Hypomagnesemia: Renal magnesium handling. Semin Nephrol 18:58-73, 1998.

Sibai BM: Magnesium sulfate prophylaxis in preeclampsia: Lessons learned from recent trials. Am J Obstet Gynecol 190:1520-1526, 2004.

Surawicz B: The interrelationship of electrolyte abnormalities and arrhythmias. In Mandel WJ (ed): Cardiac Arrhythmias: Their Mechanisms, Diagnosis, and Management. Philadelphia, JB Lippincott, 1995, pp 89-109.

Perioperative Fluid Management

Donald S. Prough and Christer H. Svensén

Case Synopses

Case 1

A 72-year-old man is scheduled to undergo transverse colectomy and primary reanastomosis for a nonobstructing carcinoma. He has a history of hypertension that is well controlled by a diuretic and is otherwise healthy.

Case 2

A 35-year-old woman is scheduled to undergo laparoscopic cholecystectomy for cholelithiasis. Other than mild obesity (preoperative weight, 88 kg), she is healthy.

PROBLEM ANALYSIS

Definition

Complications are related to either insufficient or excessive fluid therapy, and in both instances, complications can range from relatively minor to life threatening. Recent studies strongly suggest that both the frequency and the importance of complications of perioperative fluid therapy have been underestimated in the past.

Life-threatening complications of insufficient fluid therapy are hypoperfusion and related vital organ system complications. Acute renal failure and multisystem organ failure are associated with the worst outcomes. Less serious complications are postoperative thirst, dizziness, nausea, vomiting, fatigue, and drowsiness. Postoperative exercise capacity and pulmonary function may be transiently impaired by insufficient fluid therapy.

The most feared complication of excessive fluid therapy is primary or secondary pulmonary edema. With primary pulmonary edema, there is increased venous return and right ventricular preload. This leads to increased right ventricular outflow and pulmonary artery flow and, ultimately, increased pulmonary capillary hydrostatic pressure. If this increase is sufficient and sustained, it can cause pulmonary alveolar capillary leak and alveolar flooding. This mechanism is similar to that associated with naloxone overreversal of opiates (see Chapter 33). Secondary pulmonary edema is due to left ventricular overload and "forward" (cardiogenic) failure. This is more likely in patients with at least some left ventricular functional impairment. Less threatening but still bothersome late complications related to excessive fluid therapy include peripheral edema, periorbital edema, and impaired gastrointestinal function or wound healing. These occur after discharge from the postanesthesia care unit or in the intensive care unit and are thus less readily apparent to anesthesia personnel.

Historical Perspective

Because fluid restriction was the predominant strategy of perioperative fluid management until the mid-1960s, the complications of insufficient fluid administration have been emphasized for the past 40 years. In the 1960s, Shires and colleagues emphasized the concept that extracellular fluid volume was decreased during hemorrhage or major surgery and required replacement with crystalloid fluids. As a consequence of their studies, infusion of large amounts of crystalloids became the standard of care for combat casualties during the Vietnam conflict. This new treatment method was associated with an apparent reduction in the rate of renal failure and was subsequently adopted for the perioperative management of civilian surgical patients. Morris and associates reported in 1991 that of 72,757 admissions to nine regional trauma centers, only 78 patients (0.11%) required dialysis for acute renal failure, perhaps as a result of more liberal fluid therapy. Yet as the perioperative administration of larger crystalloid volumes became more prevalent, "shock lung" or the "Da Nang lung syndrome," now termed acute respiratory distress syndrome (ARDS), was clinically recognized.

Although a strict cause-and-effect relationship between increased fluid resuscitation and ARDS has never been established, the possible association has troubled clinicians. In 1999, Arieff reported 13 patients who developed postoperative pulmonary edema. Of these, 10 were generally healthy, and 3 had serious medical comorbidities. However, collectively, the group had a net fluid retention of 67 mL/kg within the first 24 intraoperative and postoperative hours. An accompanying retrospective review of the surgical experience during 1 year at a major teaching hospital found that among 8195 patients having major inpatient surgery, 7.6% developed postoperative pulmonary edema. One third of these patients had no preexisting comorbidity. The overall mortality rate was 11.9%, and the mortality rate among those without comorbidities was 3.9%. Based on this single-institution experience, Arieff projected that between 8300 and 74,000 patients die from perioperative pulmonary edema in the United States each year.

Recognition

Clinicians can easily recognize the extremes of insufficient or excessive fluid therapy. Hypotension, tachycardia, and oliguria are obvious, though not specific, signs of hypovolemia; pulmonary edema is an obvious but not specific sign of hypervolemia. Recognition of subtle hypovolemia or hypervolemia is often more difficult.

The clinical assessment of blood and extracellular volume begins with the recognition of deficit-generating situations, such as bowel obstruction, preoperative bowel preparation, chronic diuretic use, sepsis, burns, and trauma. Physical signs suggesting hypovolemia include oliguria, supine hypotension, and a positive tilt test. Although oliguria implies hypovolemia, hypovolemic patients may be nonoliguric, and normovolemic patients may be oliguric because of renal failure or stress-induced endocrine responses. Supine hypotension implies a blood volume deficit of more than 30%, although a normal arterial blood pressure could represent relative hypotension in an elderly or chronically hypertensive patient. A positive tilt test is defined as an increase in heart rate of at least 20 beats per minute and a decrease in systolic blood pressure of 20 mm Hg or more when a patient assumes the upright position. However, young, healthy subjects can withstand acute loss of 20% of blood volume while exhibiting only postural tachycardia. In contrast, orthostasis may occur in 20% to 30% of elderly patients, despite normal blood volume.

Laboratory evidence that suggests hypovolemia or extracellular volume depletion includes azotemia, low urinary sodium, metabolic alkalosis (if hypovolemia is mild), and lactic acidosis (if hypovolemia is severe). Hematocrit is virtually unchanged by acute hemorrhage until fluids are administered or fluid shifts from the interstitial to the intravascular space occur. Blood urea nitrogen (BUN), normally 8 to 20 mg/dL, is increased by hypovolemia, high protein intake, gastrointestinal bleeding, or accelerated catabolism; it is reduced by severe hepatic dysfunction. Serum creatinine (SCr), a product of muscle catabolism, may be misleadingly low in elderly adults, females, and debilitated or malnourished patients; however, in muscular or acutely catabolic patients, it may exceed the normal range (0.5 to 1.5 mg/dL). A BUN/SCr ratio exceeding the normal range (10 to 20) suggests dehydration. In prerenal oliguria, enhanced sodium reabsorption should reduce urinary $[Na^+]$ to 20 mEq/L or less. Enhanced water reabsorption should increase the urine concentration (urine osmolality >400; urine-plasma creatinine ratio >40:1). However, sensitivity and specificity of these urinary variables may be misleading.

Assessment of the adequacy of intraoperative fluid resuscitation integrates multiple clinical variables, including sodium concentrations, estimates of intraoperative blood loss and monitoring of heart rate, blood pressure, urine output, arterial oxygenation, and pH. Visual estimation of intraoperative blood loss is notoriously inaccurate. Moreover, tachycardia is an insensitive, nonspecific indicator of hypovolemia. In patients receiving potent inhalational anesthetics, maintenance of a satisfactory blood pressure implies adequate intravascular volume, as does a central venous or pulmonary artery occlusion pressure within the normal range (6 to 12 mm Hg). However, during profound hypovolemia, indirect blood pressure measurements may underestimate direct arterial pressure. Another advantage of direct arterial pressure monitoring may be the recognition of increased systolic blood pressure variation accompanying positive-pressure ventilation with hypovolemia.

Urine output often declines precipitously during moderate to severe hypovolemia. Therefore, in the absence of glycosuria or diuretic administration, a urine output of 0.5 to 1.0 mL · kg⁻¹ · hr⁻¹ during anesthesia suggests adequate renal perfusion. Arterial pH may decrease only when tissue hypoperfusion becomes severe. Cardiac output may remain normal, despite severely reduced regional blood flow. Mixed venous oxygen saturation is a specific indicator of poor systemic tissue and vital perfusion; however, it reflects average perfusion in multiple organs and cannot supplant regional monitors such as urine output.

Risk Assessment

Anesthesia personnel have considerable experience and expertise in recognizing patients at high risk for the extremes of perioperative hypovolemia and hypervolemia. Preoperative determination of the patient's American Society of Anesthesiologists (ASA) physical status and assessment of the likely duration and magnitude of physiologic stress imposed by the planned surgery can be accomplished quickly. However, to date, anesthesia training has not adequately emphasized the relationship between intraoperative fluid therapy and (1) mild symptomatic outcomes (e.g., nausea, vomiting, drowsiness) or (2) less immediate but more important outcomes (e.g., integrity of bowel anastomosis, likelihood of satisfactory wound healing or postoperative wound infection). As further evidence accumulates, anesthesia personnel should approach fluid management for all patients with the expectation that careful attention to the rate and volume of fluid administration will improve the postoperative course.

Implications

The potential complications of improper perioperative fluid management suggest that additional studies in certain patient populations are needed to develop specific and comprehensive fluid management algorithms. The input needed to develop such algorithms is now available for patients undergoing colon surgery or laparoscopic cholecystectomy.

Brandstrup and colleagues randomized 172 elective colon surgery patients to restrictive or standard perioperative fluid management. In the fluid-restricted group, the primary measure was maintenance of preoperative body weight. All patients underwent combined epidural and general anesthesia. Important details of the standard (liberal) and restrictive protocols are detailed in Table 16-1. By design, the fluid-restricted group received less perioperative fluid and acutely gained less than 1 kg, in contrast to more than 3 kg in the standard fluid therapy group. More important, total postoperative complications were 33% in the fluid-restricted group and 51% in the standard fluid therapy group. Cardiopulmonary complications were also significantly reduced in association with fluid restriction (7% in the restricted group versus 24% in the liberal group), as were tissue healing complications (16% in the restricted group versus 31% in the liberal group).

Holte and coworkers randomized 48 ASA I to II patients having laparoscopic cholecystectomy to receive either 15 or 40 mL/kg of lactated Ringer's solution intraoperatively. They found that the higher dose was associated with improved

Table 16–1 ■ Restricted versus Liberal Perioperative Fluids

Group	Restricted Fluids	Liberal Fluids
Preload	None	Hydroxyethyl starch
Maintenance	5% dextrose in water	0.9% normal saline
Third-space fluid replacement	None	0.9% normal saline
Blood replacement	Hydroxyethyl starch 1:1 for blood loss ≤1500 mL; components for blood loss >1500 mL	0.9% normal saline or hydroxyethyl starch for blood loss ≤1500 mL; components for blood loss >1500 mL

From Brandstrup B, Tonnesen H, Beier-Holgersen R, et al: Effects of intravenous fluid restriction on postoperative complications: Comparison of two perioperative fluid regimens—a randomized assessor-blinded multicenter trial. Ann Surg 238:641-648, 2003.

postoperative pulmonary function and exercise capacity, reduced neurohormonal stress response, and improvements in nausea, general sense of well-being, thirst, dizziness, drowsiness, fatigue, and balance function.

MANAGEMENT

For the patients described in the case synopses, there is enough class I evidence from randomized clinical trials to propose appropriate approaches to perioperative fluid therapy (although one clinical trial for each condition would be insufficient to support formal standards or guidelines). For the 72-year-old man having transverse colectomy, a reasonable option is to manage fluids as in the trial conducted by Brandstrup and colleagues. Using that approach, the patient would receive no preload and minimal crystalloid during induction. Postinduction hypotension, if it developed, would be treated with a pressor while awaiting the onset of surgical stimulation. Maintenance fluids would consist of 5% dextrose in water, and no additional fluid would be given to cover third-space losses. All blood loss would be replaced with 6% hydroxyethyl starch in a ratio of 1:1 unless blood loss exceeded 1500 mL, in which case blood components would be given as appropriate. (For details on the management of changes in blood pressure unrelated to blood loss and other perturbations, such as oliguria, the original publication by Brandstrup's group should be consulted.) In addition, it is essential to note that in patients undergoing colon surgery, laparoscopic cholecystectomy, or other surgery, it may be necessary to modify the preoperative fluid management plan.

For the 35-year-old woman undergoing laparoscopic cholecystectomy, the fluid strategy would be diametrically opposite. Infusing 40 mL/kg of crystalloid over the course of the case would likely exceed what such patients typically receive, but the available evidence suggests that this approach is associated with improved postoperative symptoms. Also, there are important differences between laparoscopic cholecystectomy and colon surgery:

- Postoperative cardiovascular, pulmonary, infectious, and wound complications occur much less commonly with laparoscopic cholecystectomy than with colon surgery. Thus, the goals of fluid therapy may be quite different for the two types of surgery.

- In contrast to colon surgery, in which fluid sequestration and blood loss are common, laparoscopic cholecystectomy is associated with minimal fluid sequestration and usually minimal blood loss. Also, based on Brandstrup's study, it is likely that replacement of blood loss with colloid limits postoperative hypovolemia.

So far, clinical trials have examined the influence of relative extremes of fluid therapy in only two types of surgery. It is likely that subsequent trials will examine more intermediate fluid restriction in colon surgery and less liberal fluid administration in laparoscopic cholecystectomy.

PREVENTION

Prevention of the complications of insufficient or excessive perioperative fluid administration requires a multifaceted, flexible approach. A reasonable starting point for the fluid management of individual patients is to plan to replicate a strategy that has been effective in a prospective, randomized clinical trial in a similar population of patients undergoing the same procedure. In addition, each perioperative fluid plan must take into account the physiologic status of the individual patient. If no trials are available for identical surgical procedures, fluid management is based on trials in similar patients and adjusted for the invasiveness of the planned surgery (e.g., amount of tissue manipulation and trauma leading to increased third-space losses, amount of associated bleeding). Also, ambulatory patients without cardiovascular, pulmonary, or renal disease could reasonably be managed with a strategy similar to that used by Holte and coworkers in patients undergoing laparoscopic cholecystectomy. Data reported by Yogendran and associates suggest that such a strategy is advantageous, although improved outcomes in their trial were attained with less isotonic crystalloid preload (20 mL/kg). In patients undergoing major surgical procedures other than bowel surgery, the fluid strategy used by Brandstrup's group might be used; bowel surgery may impose some procedure-specific constraints.

One possible refinement of fluid management in major surgical procedures is better monitoring of fluid requirements. In that regard, studies in which esophageal Doppler monitoring (EDM) was used to measure descending aortic flow are provocative. EDM also quantifies the percentage of time that the descending aortic flow is systolic (i.e., corrected flow time). For example, Gan and colleagues randomized 100 patients undergoing surgery in which the predicted blood loss was greater than 500 mL to fluid management based on conventional criteria versus EDM (the treatment group). In the latter, 6% hydroxyethyl starch was given in 200-mL increments to increase corrected flow time if it was less than 0.35 second. The treatment group had a shorter hospital length of stay and resumed eating solid food more quickly. Venn and associates randomized 90 patients having repair of proximal femoral fractures to one control and two treatment groups: (1) conventional fluid management (control), (2) repeated challenges with colloid guided by central venous pressure monitoring, or (3) the same colloid challenges guided by EDM. Both treatment groups had significantly fewer episodes of intraoperative hypotension and were discharged from the hospital sooner than the controls. Importantly, noninvasive EDM was equivalent to more invasive central venous pressure monitoring for assessing intraoperative fluid requirements.

Further Reading

Arieff AI: Fatal postoperative pulmonary edema: Pathogenesis and literature review. Chest 115:1371-1377, 1999.

Brandstrup B, Tonnesen H, Beier-Holgersen R, et al: Effects of intravenous fluid restriction on postoperative complications: Comparison of two perioperative fluid regimens—a randomized assessor-blinded multicenter trial. Ann Surg 238:641-648, 2003.

Gan TJ, Soppitt A, Maroof M, et al: Goal-directed intraoperative fluid administration reduces length of hospital stay after major surgery. Anesthesiology 97:820-826, 2002.

Hirsch EF: United States Navy surgical research Republic of Vietnam 1966-1970: A retrospective review. Mil Med 152:236-240, 1987.

Holte K, Klarskov B, Christensen DS, et al: Liberal versus restrictive fluid administration to improve recovery after laparoscopic cholecystectomy: A randomized, double-blind study. Ann Surg 240:892-899, 2004.

Knight RJ: Resuscitation of battle casualties in South Vietnam: Experiences at the First Australian Field Hospital. Resuscitation 2:17-31, 1973.

Lipsitz LA: Orthostatic hypotension in the elderly. N Engl J Med 321:952-957, 1989.

Morris JA Jr, Mucha P Jr, Ross SE, et al: Acute posttraumatic renal failure: A multicenter perspective. J Trauma 31:1584-1590, 1991.

Perel A: Assessing fluid responsiveness by the systolic pressure variation in mechanically ventilated patients. Anesthesiology 89:1309-1310, 1998.

Rooke GA, Schwid HA, Shapira Y: The effect of graded hemorrhage and intravascular volume replacement on systolic pressure variation in humans during mechanical and spontaneous ventilation. Anesth Analg 80:925-932, 1995.

Shires GT, Brown FT, Canizaro PC: Distributional changes in extracellular fluid during acute hemorrhagic shock. Surg Forum 11:115, 1960.

Shires GT, Coln D, Carrico J, et al: Fluid therapy in hemorrhagic shock. Arch Surg 88:688-693, 1964.

Shires GT, Williams J, Brown F: Acute changes in extracellular fluid associated with major surgical procedures. Ann Surg 154:803-810, 1961.

Stoneham MD: Less is more . . . using systolic pressure variation to assess hypovolaemia. Br J Anaesth 83:550-551, 1999.

Tavernier B, Makhotine O, Lebuffe G, et al: Systolic pressure variation as a guide to fluid therapy in patients with sepsis-induced hypotension. Anesthesiology 89:1313-1321, 1998.

Venn R, Steele A, Richardson P, et al: Randomized controlled trial to investigate influence of the fluid challenge on duration of hospital stay and perioperative morbidity in patients with hip fractures. Br J Anaesth 88:65-71, 2002.

Yogendran S, Asokumar B, Cheng DC, et al: A prospective randomized double-blinded study of the effect of intravenous fluid therapy on adverse outcomes on outpatient surgery. Anesth Analg 80:682-686, 1995.

Zaloga GP, Hughes SS: Oliguria in patients with normal renal function. Anesthesiology 72:598-602, 1990.

ANESTHETIC DRUGS

Volatile Anesthetics: Organ Toxicity

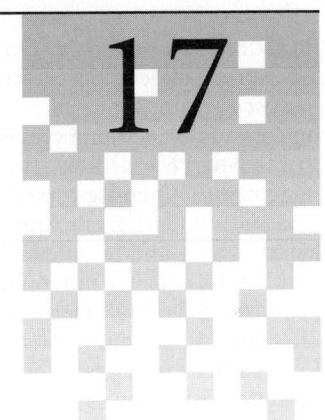

Evan D. Kharasch

Case Synopsis

A 53-year-old woman has laser excision of vocal cord papillomas under anesthesia with halothane and spontaneous ventilation. She has had several prior excisions, including one a month earlier, all with halothane; all were uneventful. However, 1 week after this surgery, she develops fever, nausea, and malaise, along with severe jaundice and markedly elevated serum transaminase concentrations.

PROBLEM ANALYSIS

Definition

Organ toxicity caused by volatile anesthetics is the result of alterations in cellular structure or function that persist beyond the period of anesthetic administration and elimination. Of greatest concern with volatile anesthetics are hepatic toxicity and renal toxicity.

Not discussed here, but worthy of mention, is the potential for volatile inhalational anesthetics to interact with desiccated carbon dioxide absorbents to form potentially toxic compounds, such as carbon monoxide and compound A. Pulmonary and renal toxicity can occur, and fires and explosions have also been reported. (For more details, see the works by Baum and Woehlck listed under "Further Reading.")

HEPATIC TOXICITY

Hepatic toxicity occurs most commonly after halothane administration, but it has also been observed with less frequency after enflurane, isoflurane, sevoflurane, and desflurane. Halothane causes two types of liver damage:

- Fulminant hepatic necrosis ("halothane hepatitis")
- Mild subclinical hepatotoxicity

Fulminant hepatic necrosis is clinically characterized by fever and jaundice, with grossly elevated serum transaminase levels. Liver biopsies show massive centrilobular necrosis. Today, fulminant hepatic necrosis is considered an immune phenomenon that is initiated by oxidative metabolism of halothane to an intermediate. This subsequently binds to liver proteins and induces trifluoroacetylation, which renders the proteins antigenic. These antigens stimulate the formation of antibodies that, on re-exposure to halothane (or enflurane, isoflurane, or desflurane), initiate immune-mediated hepatic necrosis. Such necrosis is rare, occurring in 1 in 6000 to 35,000 persons after halothane administration and in 2 in 1 million persons after enflurane; there have been a few reports of cases after isoflurane and one confirmed case after desflurane. Hepatic dysfunction after sevoflurane administration has also been reported, but it is not thought to represent immune-mediated necrosis, and the relationship to anesthesia is unknown.

Mild hepatotoxicity occurs commonly after halothane administration (approximately 25% of cases) but not after the administration of other volatile anesthetics. It is characterized by mild, transient elevations in serum transaminase and glutathione-S-transferase concentrations and altered postoperative drug metabolism. However, clinically evident hepatocellular disease is not a characteristic of mild hepatic toxicity. Rather, it is attributed to reductive (anaerobic) halothane metabolism, with reactive metabolites causing lipid peroxidation and binding to cytochrome P-450. The two forms of hepatic anesthetic toxicity are thought to be unrelated.

ACUTE RENAL FAILURE

Acute renal failure is a common perioperative problem, but it is now rarely the direct result of volatile anesthetics. Several terms require definition:

- *Renal failure* is a reduction in renal function sufficient to cause alterations in serum biochemistry; it may be oliguric, nonoliguric, or polyuric.
- *Renal insufficiency* is a lesser reduction in renal function with normal serum biochemistry.
- *Oliguria* is urine output less than 20 mL/hour (in a 70-kg adult) and implies renal failure.
- *Nonoliguric renal failure* is more common than oliguric failure, and it is thought to represent a milder renal insult.
- *Polyuria* is urine output greater than 100 mL/hour (in a 70-kg adult).

Both oliguric and nonoliguric renal failure may be postrenal (obstructive), prerenal (renal hypoperfusion due to hypovolemia, hypotension, decreased renal blood flow, or cardiovascular surgery), or intrinsic (caused by nephrotoxins such as aminoglycosides, myoglobin, hemoglobin, radiocontrast media, or nonsteroidal anti-inflammatory agents). Polyuric renal failure with reduced concentrating ability is due to either central diabetes insipidus (insufficient antidiuretic hormone secretion, usually due to pituitary dysfunction) or nephrogenic diabetes insipidus (renal unresponsiveness to antidiuretic hormone).

Anesthesia-related renal insufficiency is often prerenal and is caused by hypotension or altered renal perfusion. It is limited to the duration of the anesthetic and is reversible. Renal failure specifically attributable to anesthetic agents has been observed only with methoxyflurane, which can cause vasopressin-resistant polyuria, hypernatremia, hyperosmolality, and dehydration; it also increases blood urea nitrogen (BUN) and creatinine levels. Methoxyflurane nephrotoxicity is due to dose-related methoxyflurane metabolism. Associated plasma fluoride concentrations range from greater than 50 to 80 μM. A mild but reversible concentrating defect following prolonged enflurane use has been noted. Direct nephrotoxicity has not been observed with enflurane, isoflurane, desflurane, or sevoflurane, even with systemic fluoride concentrations far exceeding 50 μM. The role of systemic fluoride concentrations as a factor in nephrotoxicity has been discounted.

Recognition

Fulminant hepatic necrosis manifests clinically as fever, nausea, anorexia, chills, malaise, and rash that appear 3 to 6 days postoperatively, followed by severe jaundice that occurs 6 to 10 days postoperatively. Laboratory manifestations include grossly elevated serum transaminase levels, hyperbilirubinemia, and prolonged prothrombin time, but these are not specific for the disease. Pathologic findings include centrilobular and midzonal necrosis, but again, these findings are not specific. Mild hepatotoxicity after halothane is usually clinically silent, consisting of only mild, reversible increases in liver enzymes (aspartate aminotransferase, alanine aminotransferase, γ-glutamyl transferase, and glutathione-S-transferase) on laboratory studies. These elevations appear 1 to 2 days postoperatively and usually resolve within days. However, levels may remain elevated for up to 2 weeks.

A specific diagnosis of anesthetic-related hepatitis is difficult at best. Both the clinical presentation and the morphologic features strongly resemble those of viral hepatitis. Indeed, the incidence of occult perioperative hepatitis (viral, infectious, alcoholic) is 1 in 700, and in 30% of these cases, postoperative jaundice develops; this is far greater than the incidence of anesthetic-related fulminant hepatitis. Positive serologic markers for hepatitis A, B, C, or D or other infectious agents (e.g., cytomegalovirus, Epstein-Barr virus) may help exclude anesthesia as the cause of postoperative hepatitis, but negative serologic findings are inconclusive, especially if infection is recent. A few laboratories can detect antitrifluoroacetylated protein antibodies in serum, which favors a diagnosis of anesthetic-related hepatitis. However, the assay lacks sufficient specificity and is not routinely available. Hepatitis C is the most common cause of postoperative hepatitis, but hepatic ischemia, other drugs, transfusion, and cholestasis should also be excluded.

The clinical characteristics of renal insufficiency and acute renal failure were listed earlier. Differentiation of central and nephrogenic diabetes insipidus is based on response to water deprivation and vasopressin. The cause of oliguric renal failure is determined by the BUN-creatinine ratio, urine sodium and osmolality, urine-plasma osmolality, urine-plasma creatinine, fractional excretion of sodium, and response to volume challenge. The diagnosis of renal failure specific to a volatile anesthetic is extremely rare in the postmethoxyflurane era.

Risk Assessment

Clinical risk factors for fulminant hepatic necrosis include the following:

- Repeated halothane exposure
- Prior history of postanesthetic fever or jaundice
- Obesity
- Female sex
- Middle age

Halothane is oxidatively metabolized by cytochrome P-450 2E1. Thus, enzyme induction (alcohol, isoniazid, obesity) increases antigen formation and increases risk, whereas enzyme inhibition (disulfiram) reduces metabolism. Multiple, repeated exposures at short intervals (<6 weeks) is the greatest risk factor for halothane hepatitis.

Children are at greatly diminished risk, for unknown reasons, even after repeated halothane exposure. Liver disease itself is not a risk factor for halothane hepatitis. Clinical risk factors for mild hepatotoxicity are those that increase reductive halothane metabolism. Halothane is reduced anaerobically by P-450 3A4 and 2A6; thus, enzyme induction (e.g., by barbiturates, phenytoin, valproic acid) increases metabolism, as does reduced hepatic blood flow. The latter is further reduced by halothane. Although enflurane, isoflurane, and desflurane also cause neoantigen formation, the degree of such formation is far less than with halothane, so the risk of hepatitis with these agents in halothane-sensitized patients is far less.

The only clearly identified clinical risk factors for postoperative renal failure are the following:

- Poor preoperative renal function (increased BUN or creatinine levels)
- Advanced age
- Cardiac failure

Treatment and prevention of hypovolemia and preoperative hydration are primary goals in ameliorating the cardiovascular and renal blood flow effects of volatile anesthetics in general. Mechanical ventilation and positive endexpiratory pressure are other factors peripherally related to volatile anesthetics that diminish renal function. Although not pertinent to contemporary anesthesia, certain inducers of drug metabolism (barbiturates, isoniazid, ethanol) potentiate methoxyflurane metabolism and toxicity.

Implications

Fulminant hepatic necrosis after halothane is fatal in nearly half of all cases. There are no known clinical implications of mild hepatotoxicity. Perioperative acute renal failure accounts for half of all patients who require acute dialysis and is associated with a 50% mortality rate. This has remained unchanged for decades.

MANAGEMENT

There is no specific management for either fulminant hepatic necrosis or mild hepatotoxicity. No therapy is needed for mild hepatotoxicity, whereas only supportive therapy and orthotopic liver transplantation are available for hepatic necrosis. Treatment for acute renal dysfunction includes restoration of normovolemia and renal blood flow; administration of mannitol, loop diuretics (controversial), dopamine, and fenoldopam (experimental); and dialysis.

PREVENTION

No measures for the prevention of mild hepatotoxicity are necessary. The only fail-safe method of preventing fulminant hepatic necrosis is total avoidance of halothane, enflurane, isoflurane, and desflurane in patients previously exposed to halothane. Hepatitis is rare in children and in adults with only a single exposure to halothane. A conservative approach is to avoid halothane in patients with known risk factors for fulminant necrosis, especially recent halothane anesthesia. The ultraconservative approach is to avoid halothane altogether.

The single most effective measure to prevent postoperative renal failure is to minimize renal ischemia by maintaining renal perfusion. Maintenance of adequate hydration is essential. Mannitol may be an effective prophylactic.

Further Reading

Baden JM, Mazze RI: Polyuria. In Gravenstein N, Kirby RR (eds): Complications in Anesthesiology, 2nd ed. Philadelphia, Lippincott-Raven, 1996, pp 493-498.

Baum JA, Woehlck HJ: Interaction of inhalational anaesthetics with CO_2 absorbents. Best Pract Res Clin Anaesthesiol 17:63-76, 2003.

Brown BR: Inhalation anesthesia and hepatic injury. In Gravenstein N, Kirby RR (eds): Complications in Anesthesiology, 2nd ed. Philadelphia, Lippincott-Raven, 1996, pp 701-710.

Dooley JR, Mazze RI: Oliguria. In Gravenstein N, Kirby RR (eds): Complications in Anesthesiology, 2nd ed. Philadelphia, Lippincott-Raven, 1996, pp 479-491.

Gut J, Christen V, Frey N, et al: Molecular mimicry in halothane hepatitis: Biochemical and structural characterization of lipoylated autoantigens. Toxicology 97:199-224, 1995.

Novis BK, Roizen MF, Aronson S, et al: Association of preoperative risk factors with postoperative acute renal failure. Anesth Analg 78: 143-149, 1994.

Pearson JD, Gelman S: Liver complications after anesthesia. In Benumof JL, Saidman LJ (eds): Anesthesia and Perioperative Complications. St. Louis, Mosby–Year Book, 1992, pp 413-433.

Prough DS, Zaloga G: Hypovolemia and renal dysfunction. In Benumof JL, Saidman LJ (eds): Anesthesia and Perioperative Complications. St. Louis, Mosby–Year Book, 1992, pp 434-465.

Ray DC, Drummond GB: Halothane hepatitis. Br J Anaesth 67:84-99, 1991.

Woehlck HJ: Sleeping with uncertainty: Anesthetics and desiccated absorbent. Anesthesiology 101:276-278, 2004.

Nitrous Oxide: Neurotoxicity

18

Claudia Praetel

Case Synopsis

Two weeks after surgery for prostate adenoma, a 69-year-old man developed ascending paresthesia of the limbs, severe ataxia, tactile sensory loss in the limbs and trunk, and absent tendon reflexes. After a second surgical intervention, the patient became confused. Four months after onset, the patient demonstrated paraplegia, severe weakness of the upper limbs, cutaneous anesthesia sparing the head, and confusion.

PROBLEM ANALYSIS

Definition

Nitrous oxide (N_2O) has been safely used for anesthesia for almost 140 years, since it first became available in compressed gas cylinders in 1868. However, there are increasing reports of the neurotoxic potential of N_2O associated with recreational use, with chronic occupational exposure in unscavenged environments, and after exposure during general anesthesia. A small subset of patients routinely seen during preoperative anesthetic assessment may indeed be at high risk for postoperative neurologic deterioration if exposed to N_2O. Schilling postulated that N_2O may precipitate neurologic disease in patients with unrecognized vitamin B_{12} deficiency.

The patient described in the case synopsis was diagnosed with previously unrecognized pernicious anemia with subacute combined degeneration of the spinal cord after exposure to N_2O anesthesia. Marié and coworkers published this case report in 2000. During the past 20 years, numerous well-documented case reports have substantiated this potentially devastating complication. Table 18-1 highlights recent reports of neurologic complications after N_2O in both children and adults.

Recognition

N_2O is a potent oxidant. It irreversibly oxidizes methylcobalamin through inhibition of the methionine synthesis pathway, thereby inactivating the active form of vitamin B_{12}. The latter is essential for methionine synthase, the key enzyme for converting homocysteine to methionine (an essential amino acid) using tetrahydrofolate (the bioactive form of folate) as the methyl source. Therefore, insufficient availability of either cobalamin[1] or folate results in a decrease of methionine, with the accumulation of homocysteine. N_2O also directly

inactivates methionine synthase, possibly due to the production of free radicals. Inhibition of methionine synthase activity has deleterious consequences for DNA synthesis, leading to megaloblastic changes in all rapidly dividing cells, macrocytosis in erythroid precursors, and ineffective erythropoiesis.

Lack of methionine can also result in defective myelination and demyelination. Neurologic sequelae include paresthesias, peripheral neuropathy, and subacute combined degeneration of both the posterior and lateral columns of the spinal cord. Subacute combined degeneration is reversible if diagnosed and treated early with cobalamin. Psychological symptoms such as memory loss, disorientation, and depression have been described. These conditions may be observed with or without macrocytic changes in erythrocytes.

Risk Assessment

Inhibition of methionine synthase by N_2O anesthesia does not cause a problem in healthy individuals with sufficient vitamin B_{12} stores. However, any patient with even subclinical deficits of vitamin B_{12} is at increased risk for the development of myeloneuropathy because occult cobalamin deficiency, combined with subsequent N_2O exposure, compounds inhibition of the methionine synthesis pathway. Insufficient availability of cobalamin may have the following causes:

- Inadequate intake (e.g., alcoholics, long-term strict vegetarians, breast-fed infants of vitamin B_{12}-deficient mothers)
- Impaired absorption (e.g., gastric atrophy, long-term use of drugs that interfere with acid production, Crohn's disease, lack of intrinsic factor due to autoimmune destruction of parietal cells or after surgery such as gastrectomy and gastric bypass)
- Rare congenital disorders (e.g., deficiencies of transcobalamin II, familial selective vitamin B_{12} malabsorption)

Folate deficiency is very rare due to the dietary fortification of wheat and corn grains with folic acid. Inherited defects in folate metabolism (5,10-methylenetetrahydrofolate reductase deficiency) are a contraindication to N_2O exposure.

---

[1]The terms *cobalamin* and *vitamin B_{12}* are used interchangeably as generic terms for all the cobalamides active in human beings. Preparations of vitamin B_{12} for therapeutic use contain either cyanocobalamin or hydroxocobalamin, because only these derivatives remain active following storage.

Table 18–1 ■ Selected Case Reports of Neurologic Complications after Nitrous Oxide (N₂O) Anesthesia

Reference	Demographics	Onset Time and Symptoms	Findings
Selzer et al	3 mo old; excisional biopsy (45 min); 4 days later, tumor resection (270 min), for a total N₂O exposure time of 315 min	25 days: hypotonia, ataxic ventilation, absent reflexes	Methylenetetrahydrofolate reductase deficiency; died 46 days postoperatively
Felmet et al	8 mo old; laparoscopic orchiopexy; N₂O exposure of 180 min	6 days: hypotonia, fine motor tremor, athetoid movements	Profound dietary cobalamin deficiency (<20 pg/mL); hyperhomocysteinemia; normal folate levels; megaloblastic abnormalities in bone marrow
McNeely et al	4 mo old; repair of cranisynostosis; N₂O exposure of 80 min	3 wk: hypotonia, lethargy, feeding difficulty, severe acidosis, dehydration	Severe dietary cobalamin deficiency (<45 pg/mL); normal folate levels; MRI revealed diffuse cerebral atrophy
Ilnicziky et al (case 1)	57-yr-old man; cranial artery bypass; duration of N₂O exposure unspecified	2 mo: gait imbalance, lower extremity paresthesias	Cobalamin deficiency (135 pmol/L); borderline anemia; abnormal Schilling test; MRI revealed signal changes of posterior spinal columns; SSEP showed severe spinal cord conduction disturbance; EMG and NCS showed mixed polyneuropathy
Ilnicziky et al (case 2)	52-yr-old man; gallbladder removal; duration of N₂O exposure unknown	1 wk: paresthesias in both feet, ascending to trunk and upper extremities; weakness and clumsiness in all limbs	Normal cobalamin level (<166 pmol/L); low folate; macrocytic, hyperchromic anemia; bone marrow exam revealed megaloblastic hematopoiesis; MRI showed signal changes in posterior columns along cervical cord segments: EMG and NCS showed mild demyelinative polyneuropathy
Sesso et al	63-yr-old woman; gallbladder removal; N₂O exposure of 80 min	1 day: rapidly ascending paresthesias in hands/feet; 2 mo: moderate tabetic-spastic gait, with impaired proprioception and sensation	Macrocytic anemia; MRI revealed signal changes in posterior and lateral spinal columns

EMG, electromyography; MRI, magnetic resonance imaging; NCS, nerve conduction velocity study; SSEP, somatosensory evoked potentials.

Implications

A recently published multicenter study in Great Britain examined blood samples of 1562 patients aged 65 to 74 years and 75 years or older. Among men, 11% and 24%, respectively, were at high risk of vitamin B_{12} deficiency; the corresponding numbers were slightly lower for women (9% and 17%, respectively). Similar results were reported for the United States. This high prevalence of borderline or low vitamin B_{12} concentrations in the elderly (due to the decline in digestive efficiency, atrophic gastritis, and the ubiquitous use of acid-reducing drugs) is particularly worrisome because the clinical presentation varies considerably and rarely includes all the classic features. Hematologic signs of macrocytosis and anemia are often missing. Apparently, a dissociation of neurologic and hematologic findings is common.

Cobalamin deficiency in young adults is uncommon, except among strict long-term vegetarians. The potential risks of N₂O are increased in children with enzyme disorders and noncompliance with vitamin supplements, as described in a patient with phenylketonuria. There is growing evidence that markers such as holotranscobalamin II, methylmalonic acid, and total serum homocysteine constitute a better index of early cobalamin deficiency and allow the differentiation between storage depletion and functional deficiency.

Presently, these tests are very expensive and are not used as routine assays to investigate functional vitamin B_{12} status. Low cobalamin status is significantly correlated to increased plasma homocysteine, which is recognized as an independent atherothrombotic risk factor. The latency in onset of neurologic symptoms following exposure to N₂O may confound the true incidence of this anesthesia-related complication.

MANAGEMENT

The preoperative risk assessment should include careful attention to the following:

- Hematologic abnormalities (e.g., anemia, macrocytosis)
- Increased prevalence of subclinical vitamin B_{12} deficiency in the elderly
- Rare genetic enzyme disorders
- Diet (strict vegetarian or vegan)

- History of gastric or small bowel surgery (e.g., gastric bypass in the morbidly obese, resection of the terminal ileum in Crohn's disease)
- Inflammatory bowel disease
- Long-term use of antacids, histamine (H_2) receptor antagonists, or proton pump inhibitors (e.g., aluminum and magnesium hydroxide, ranitidine, omeprazole)
- Severe depression in the elderly
- Unexplained neurologic symptoms
- Previous exposure to inhaled anesthesia (including N_2O) that was associated with postoperative neurologic complications
- Increased prevalence of folate deficiency in patients with chronic liver disease or malabsorption syndromes, long-term use of anticonvulsants (e.g., valproic acid, phenytoin), and antimetabolite therapy (e.g., methotrexate)

PREVENTION

Avoidance of N_2O anesthesia in patients with an elevated risk of cobalamin deficiency appears prudent in view of the possibly serious neurologic sequelae. The fact that subclinical or clinical deficits are not always accompanied by hematologic changes deserves special emphasis. Routine N_2O use may be detrimental to patients with marginal cobalamin status. Vitamin pretreatment of at-risk patients is an option, but an impractical one, because anesthesiologists generally see patients immediately before surgery. Optimal management of patients with confirmed or suspected cobalamin deficiency includes an anesthetic regime devoid of N_2O. N_2O-induced postoperative neurologic complications are preventable with

a proper focus on the recognition of preexisting vitamin B_{12} deficiency as outlined here.

Further Reading

Badner NH, Freeman D, Spence JD: Preoperative oral B vitamins prevent nitrous oxide-induced postoperative plasma homocysteine increase. Anesth Analg 95:787, 2002.

Clarke R, Refsum H, Birks J, et al: Screening for vitamin B_{12} and folate deficiency in older persons. Am J Clin Nutr 77:1241-1247, 2003.

Deleu D, Hanssens Y, Louon A: Nitrous oxide-induced cobalamin deficiency. Arch Neurol 58:134-135, 2001.

Felmet K, Robins B, Tilford D, Haflick SJ: Acute neurologic decompensation in an infant with cobalamin deficiency exposed to nitrous oxide. J Pediatr 137:427-428, 2000.

Hadzic A, Glab K, Sanborn KV, Thys DM: Severe neurologic deficit after nitrous oxide anesthesia. Anesthesiology 83:863-866, 1995.

Herrmann W, Geisel J: Vegetarian lifestyle and monitoring of vitamin B_{12} status. Clin Chim Acta 326:47-59, 2002.

Ilniczky S, Jelencsik, Kenéz J, Szirmai I: MR findings in subacute combined degeneration of the spinal cord caused by nitrous oxide anaesthesia—two cases. Eur J Neurol 9:101-104, 2002.

Marié RM, Le Biez E, Busson P, et al: Nitrous oxide anesthesia-associated myelopathy. Arch Neurol 57:380-382, 2000.

McNeely JK, Buczulinski B, Rosner DR: Severe neurological impairment in an infant after nitrous oxide anesthesia. Anesthesiology 93:1549-1550, 2000.

Nunn JF: Clinical aspects of the interaction between nitrous oxide and vitamin B_{12}. Br J Anaesth 59:3-13, 1987.

Royston BD, Nunn JF, Weinbren HK, et al: Rate of inactivation of human and rodent methionine synthase by nitrous oxide. Anesthesiology 68:213-216, 1988.

Schilling RF: Is nitrous oxide a dangerous anesthetic for vitamin B_{12}-deficient subjects? JAMA 255:1605-1606, 1986.

Selzer RR, Rosenblatt DS, Laxova R, Hogan K: Adverse effect of nitrous oxide in a child with 5,10-methylenetetrahydrofolate reductase deficiency. N Engl J Med 349:45-50, 2003.

Sesso RM, Iunes Y, Melo AC: Neuropathy following nitrous oxide anesthesia in a patient with macrocytic anaemia. Neuroradiology 41:588-590, 1999.

Intrathecal Opiates

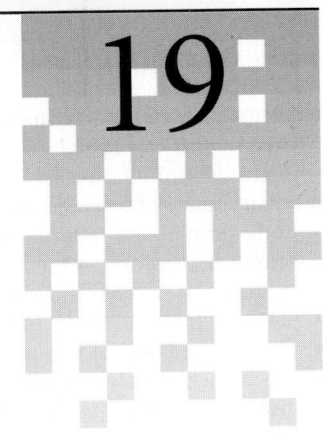

Lisa Thannikary and Bhiken Naik

Case Synopsis

An otherwise healthy 26-year-old woman undergoes cesarean section for delivery of a breech infant. Spinal anesthesia is used, consisting of hyperbaric bupivacaine (12 mg) with preservative-free morphine (0.3 mg). The surgery is uneventful, and the infant has Apgar scores of 9 and 9 at 5 and 10 minutes, respectively. The patient remains in the recovery room for 2 hours and is then transferred to the floor. She is treated with diphenhydramine 50 mg intravenously (IV) for generalized pruritus 4 hours after surgery and promethazine 25 mg IV for vomiting 7 hours after surgery. Ten hours after surgery, she is found to be somnolent, with a respiratory rate of 6 breaths per minute, and is minimally responsive to deep tactile stimulation.

PROBLEM ANALYSIS

Definition

Intrathecal administration of opioids is an effective means of providing analgesia. A combination of opioids and local anesthetics is often administered intrathecally in an effort to reduce drug dosages while limiting the side effects of both classes of drugs. Morphine is commonly chosen for intrathecal administration, because a single dose may provide analgesia for up to 24 hours. Side effects of intrathecal opioids include early and late respiratory depression, nausea and vomiting, pruritus, sedation, and urinary retention (Table 19-1).

Early respiratory depression occurs in the first 2 hours after intrathecal administration and is believed to be due to vascular uptake and redistribution. This occurs more often with lipophilic opioids such as fentanyl and sufentanil than with less lipophilic opioids such as morphine. Delayed respiratory depression occurs 6 to 12 hours after intrathecal administration and is believed to be the result of rostral spread of the opioid in the cerebrospinal fluid. The target receptors are likely located in the respiratory center of the brainstem. However, the occurrence of clinically significant respiratory depression is very low, typically less than 0.5%.

Pruritus, either generalized or localized, occurs frequently in patients receiving intrathecal opioids. Although the mechanism is not fully understood, histamine release is not postulated to be a causative factor. Nausea and vomiting are believed to be due to rostral spread of the opioid in the cerebrospinal fluid. The opioid stimulates the vomiting center and the chemoreceptor trigger zone in the fourth ventricle. Sedation is believed to result from opioid spread through the cerebrospinal fluid to the thalamus, limbic system, or cerebral cortex. Sedation may be exacerbated by hypercarbia with carbon dioxide narcosis. Urinary retention is believed to be due to inhibition of sacral parasympathetic outflow. This results in relaxation of the bladder detrusor muscle and the concomitant inability to relax the sphincter.

Recognition

The most serious complication of intrathecal opioid administration is delayed respiratory depression because it usually occurs when the patient is no longer under an anesthesiologist's or intensivist's care. In the operating room, labor suite, recovery room, or critical care unit, patients are more closely monitored than they are on the floor. It is also important to recognize that respiratory depression is often a late finding. Increasing somnolence, bradypnea, and smaller tidal volumes are early signs of respiratory compromise. Late signs are hypoxia, unresponsiveness, and cardiopulmonary arrest.

Table 19–1 ■ Cause and Treatment of Complications of Intrathecal Medications

Complication	Cause	Treatment
Early respiratory depression	Rapid vascular uptake and redistribution	Ventilatory support, naloxone
Late respiratory depression	Rostral CSF spread to brainstem respiratory center	Ventilatory support, naloxone
Pruritus	Unknown (unlikely due to histamine release)	Naloxone, antihistamines, propofol
Nausea, vomiting	Rostral CSF spread to vomiting center or chemoreceptor trigger zone in fourth ventricle	Naloxone, antiemetics, droperidol, transdermal scopolamine
Urinary retention	Inhibited sacral parasympathetic outflow	Naloxone (large doses), urinary catheterization
Sedation	Rostral spread in CSF to thalamus, limbic system, or cortex; hypercarbia	Naloxone

CSF, cerebrospinal fluid.

Further, intrathecal opioids can impair the ventilatory response to carbon dioxide, which can exacerbate respiratory depression. A high index of suspicion and early recognition of delayed respiratory depression are paramount to timely and effective management. Otherwise, there may be fatal or permanent injuries.

Risk Assessment

Careful selection of patients for the administration of intrathecal opioids is important. Patients at increased risk for respiratory depression include those who are debilitated or elderly, suffer from coexisting respiratory disease, and are placed in Trendelenburg's position following intrathecal opioid injection. Also, patients receiving hydrophilic opioids, large or frequent doses of opioids, large-volume injections, and concomitant parenteral or oral sedatives are at increased risk for respiratory depression.

Implications

Anesthesiologists commonly administer intrathecal opioids to provide postoperative analgesia. It is important to remember that side effects of intrathecal opioids can occur after the patient has left the anesthesiologist's care. Good communication with the nursing staff caring for the patient is crucial for the prevention of many complications.

MANAGEMENT

The immediate treatment for neuraxial opiate-induced respiratory depression is ventilatory support until the opiate is metabolized or pharmacologically antagonized. The patient must be ventilated with positive-pressure mask ventilation and 100% oxygen. Tracheal intubation and mechanical ventilation may be necessary in some patients. Opiate reversal is accomplished with small doses (40 to 80 µg) of parenteral naloxone. Repeated naloxone doses or infusions may be necessary because its half-life is shorter than that of intrathecal morphine. Also, advanced cardiovascular life support is required for patients with cardiac arrest due to narcotic-caused respiratory depression. Arterial blood gas measurements for carbon dioxide concentrations are helpful to ascertain the degree of inhibition of respiration or the adequacy of ventilation. Finally, narcotics administered by other routes (intravenous, oral, epidural, intramuscular) must be discontinued.

PREVENTION

The best way to prevent delayed respiratory depression in patients receiving spinal opioids is to not give parenteral opioids or other sedating medications until at least 24 hours after intrathecal administration. Pruritus and nausea are common side effects of intrathecal opioids and can be treated effectively with naloxone. If other drugs are used for the treatment of pain or side effects, it is important to use nonsedating ones, such as nonsteroidal anti-inflammatory drugs for patients with pain.

Good communication between anesthesia and nursing personnel is essential to prevent and treat adverse sequelae of intrathecal opioid administration. Nursing staff must be educated about intrathecal opioid side effects and their appropriate management. One effective measure is to use a preprinted order signed by the anesthesiologist stating that the patient received intrathecal opioids and should not receive further sedating drugs for at least 24 hours without clearance from the anesthesia staff. Signs posted above the head of the patient's bed indicating that intrathecal opioids have been used may also be helpful.

Monitoring the patient at frequent intervals is critical to prevent significant respiratory depression. The patient must be assessed for rate and quality of respirations and level of sedation. For very high-risk patients, the usual floor-monitoring interval may not be adequate. If so, the patient may have to be admitted to a unit where more staff are available to monitor the patient more closely. Pulse oximetry monitoring with data telemetry to a centralized nursing station is also helpful but may not be available to all patients or in all hospitals.

Further Reading

Ballantyne JC, Loach AB, Carr DB: Itching after epidural and spinal opiates. Pain 33:149-160, 1988.

Brill S, Gurman GM, Fisher A: A history of neuraxial administration of local analgesics and opioids. Eur J Anaesthesiol 20:682-689, 2003.

Gustafsson LL, Schildt B, Jacobsen K: Adverse effects of extradural and intrathecal opiates: Report of a nationwide survey in Sweden. Br J Anaesth 54:479-485, 1982.

Ready LB: Acute perioperative pain. In Miller RD (ed): Anesthesia, 5th ed. Philadelphia, Churchill Livingstone, 2000, pp 2323-2350.

Reiz S, Westberg M: Side effects of epidural morphine. Lancet 2:203-204, 1980.

Sinatra RS: Acute pain management and acute pain services. In Cousins MJ, Bridenbaugh PO (eds): Neural Blockade in Clinical Anesthesia and Management of Pain, 3rd ed. Philadelphia, Lippincott-Raven, 1998, pp 793-835.

Barbiturates: Porphyrias

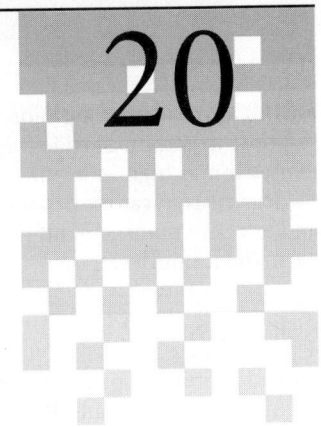

20

Christoph N. Seubert

Case Synopsis

An anxious 24-year-old woman presents with nausea, vomiting, and abdominal pain and is scheduled for an exploratory laparotomy. The past medical history indicates a negative exploratory laparotomy 2 years ago. The patient's blood pressure is 150/90 mm Hg and pulse is 105 beats per minute. The physical examination reveals abdominal tenderness. Electrolyte levels and white blood cell count are normal. With direct questioning about family history, the patient declares that her mother may have had porphyria.

PROBLEM ANALYSIS

Definition

Although barbiturates are widely used in anesthetic practice, they may cause an acute attack in susceptible patients with inducible porphyria. Porphyrias are a heterogeneous group of genetic disorders wherein genetic, physiologic, and environmental factors interact to cause disease. Although porphyrias can be classified on the basis of the underlying genetic defects involved in hemoglobin synthesis, the simple clinical division into inducible-acute and noninducible-chronic forms remains useful. An example of the latter is porphyria cutanea tarda (PCT), the most common form of porphyria. Apart from the friability of the patient's skin and the association with hepatitis C, human immunodeficiency virus (HIV), and alcohol abuse, PCT presents no anesthetic concerns and does not restrict the choice of drugs. In contrast, all patients with acute porphyrias are at risk for porphyric crisis, particularly in the perioperative period. Drugs administered in the perioperative period for the condition requiring surgery, stress, or fasting may precipitate acute attacks of porphyria. If the attack goes untreated or unrecognized, it may be fatal. Conversely, control of precipitating factors or prompt treatment can avert or mitigate the attack and allow the safe conduct of surgery. Acute porphyrias, therefore, present important anesthetic concerns.

Porphyrin synthesis occurs in all cells and is of particular importance in the bone marrow and liver. Porphyrins are essential components of proteins involved in the utilization, transport, and storage of oxygen. These proteins include the ubiquitous cytochrome oxidases of the respiratory chain, the hepatic cytochrome P-450 enzymes, and transport proteins such as hemoglobin. Synthesis of porphyrins involves a series of enzymes (Fig. 20-1). Genes for key enzymes of porphyrin synthesis are duplicated in the genome, allowing for separate regulation of heme synthesis in the bone marrow and the liver. In the liver, most heme is used for the production of cytochrome P-450 enzymes. Heme synthesis and P-450 production are regulated in a coordinated fashion.

The four acute porphyrias are acute intermittent porphyria (AIP), variegate porphyria (VP), hereditary coproporphyria (HCP), and δ-aminolevulinic acid dehydratase-deficient porphyria (ADP) (Table 20-1). The gene defects that underlie the acute porphyrias are loss-of-function mutations and typically reduce enzyme activity by half. This reduction results in a pattern of inheritance that is either recessive for the rare ADP or dominant with variable penetrance for the three more frequent acute porphyrias. Although the location of the defective hepatic enzyme in the synthetic pathway for heme varies among the acute porphyrias (see Fig. 20-1), all four may present with acute attacks that are similar in terms of symptoms and treatment. It is not known why enzymatic defects in chronic or erythropoietic porphyrias do not lead to acute attacks. HCP and VP may cause accumulation of excess porphyrins in the skin, where excitation by ultraviolet light causes blistering and scarring skin lesions.

Recognition

Acute attacks of inducible porphyria are difficult to recognize in the perioperative setting because symptoms may be nonspecific and varied. Typical symptoms are summarized in Table 20-2. Attacks rarely occur before puberty and seldom recur throughout adult life. They last for several days and are characterized by intense abdominal pain that is steady and poorly localized. The pain intensity contrasts sharply with the paucity of physical findings, sometimes resulting in emergent exploratory laparotomy. Nausea, vomiting, and decreased bowel sounds are common but do not dominate

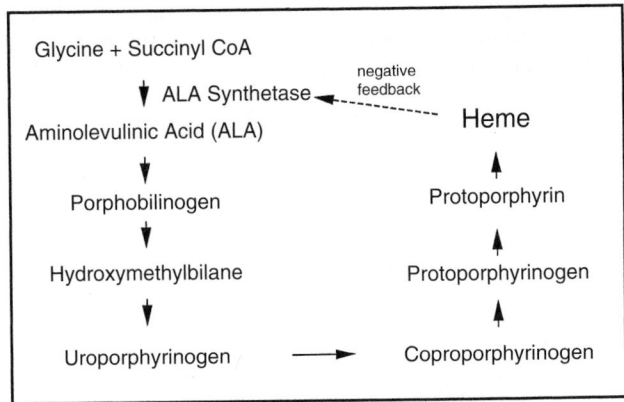

Figure 20–1 ■ Heme synthesis.

Table 20–1 ■ Acute-Inducible Porphyrias

Type	Incidence	Inheritance	Neurovisceral Symptoms	Photosensitivity
δ-Aminolevulinic acid dehydratase-deficient porphyria (ADP)	Exceedingly rare (only 7 cases reported)	Autosomal recessive	++	−
Acute intermittent porphyria (AIP)	1:10,000 (higher in Scandinavia)	Autosomal dominant	+++	−
Hereditary coproporphyria (HCP)	Rare (1:1 million)	Autosomal dominant	++	+
Variegate porphyria (VP)	1:300,000 (higher in South Africa)	Autosomal dominant	++	+

the clinical picture; fever, leukocytosis, and abdominal tenderness are usually absent. Acute attacks of inducible porphyria may involve the peripheral nervous system in the form of a proximally accentuated motor weakness. This weakness occasionally occurs after resolution of the abdominal pain and may resemble Guillain-Barré syndrome, without the characteristic albumin increase in cerebrospinal fluid. Cranial nerves and sensory nerves may be affected, and progression of neurologic involvement to respiratory and bulbar paralysis and death is possible. In a quarter of patients the central nervous system may be involved, resulting in psychiatric symptoms such as anxiety, hallucinations, and paranoia. Generalized seizures may occur as a neurologic manifestation of central nervous system involvement or as a manifestation of severe hyponatremia caused by inappropriate secretion of antidiuretic hormone or vomiting. If acute porphyria is suspected, the diagnosis can be confirmed by screening for and quantifying the porphyrin precursors δ-aminolevulinic acid and porphobilinogen in urine. Daylight can convert the colorless porphobilinogen to porphyrins, causing a darkening and red to purple discoloration of the urine. Resolution of symptoms is usually rapid, but weakness may persist for days or months.

In asymptomatic patients, the perioperative diagnosis of acute porphyria relies on a detailed family history. Because the more frequent forms are all inherited as autosomal dominant diseases, many susceptible patients know of blood relatives with a diagnosis of acute porphyria. In contrast, laboratory investigations may be negative because the patient's metabolic situation is compensated. Positive diagnosis of porphyria therefore belongs in the hands of a specialist.[1]

Risk Assessment

The prevalence of acute porphyrias (see Table 20-1) is difficult to estimate because as many as 80% of affected patients may never experience an acute attack in their lifetimes. The prevalence of AIP is estimated to be about 1 in 10,000 in North America but may be as high as 1 in 1000 in Scandinavia or in people of Scandinavian descent. Clinically, AIP accounts for three quarters of acute attacks. VP is less prevalent, except in South Africans of Dutch descent; more than 20,000 cases have been traced to a single immigrant couple. HCP is rare, with an estimated prevalence of 1 in 1 million. Only seven cases of ADP have been reported.

More important to risk assessment than prevalence data is the fact that acute attacks are always multifactorial. Even prior uneventful exposure to porphyrinogenic drugs does not rule out a diagnosis of acute porphyria. A high index of suspicion is therefore justified if the constellation of symptoms (see Table 20-2) fits that of an acute attack of porphyria.

Implications

Failure to diagnose and treat an acute attack of porphyria confers up to a 10% risk of mortality. Such failure not only prolongs the attack but also puts the patient at risk of further morbidity from the following:

- Further up-regulation of hepatic heme synthesis, because of decreased glucose intake
- Progression of motor involvement to include respiratory muscles and cranial nerves
- Residual paresis that persists even after resolution of the attack
- Seizures, which may be treated with porphyrinogenic drugs
- Exposure to porphyrinogenic drugs for other supportive treatment
- Unwarranted surgery

Table 20–2 ■ Symptoms of a Porphyric Crisis

Parameter	Symptom
Peripheral nervous system	
Sensory	Abdominal pain
Motor	Proximally accentuated weakness; may involve cranial nerves and respiratory muscles
Autonomic	Tachycardia; hypertension
Central nervous system	
Psychiatric	Anxiety; hallucinations; paranoia
Endocrine	SIADH
Neurologic	Seizures
Miscellaneous	Nausea, vomiting
Laboratory	Increased ALA and PBG in urine; light-exposed urine turns dark red or pink

ALA, δ-aminolevulinic acid; PBG, porphobilinogen; SIADH, syndrome of inappropriate secretion of antidiuretic hormone.

[1]Information can be found on the American Porphyria Foundation Web site: www.porphyriafoundation.com.

MANAGEMENT

Perioperative care of patients with porphyria involves more than the avoidance of barbiturates. Preoperative assessment should identify whether symptoms of an acute attack are present. In the absence of an acute attack, the anesthetic prescription should consist of nonporphyrinogenic drugs. Details, as well as additional measures to minimize the risk of an acute attack, are discussed later. If the preoperative assessment suggests an acute attack of porphyria, both symptomatic and specific therapies should be instituted in an appropriate inpatient setting.

Acute Attack of Porphyria in the Perioperative Period

Therapy for acute attacks of porphyria consists of three interventions: (1) administration of hematin and (2) administration of glucose, both of which inhibit δ-aminolevulinic acid synthase and thus correct the metabolic abnormality; and (3) identification and removal of the precipitating factor to decrease enzyme induction. Hematin (Panhematin, Ovation Pharmaceuticals, Deerfield, Ill) contains alkaline heme from processed human red blood cells. It is a lyophilized powder that is best reconstituted in albumin to form a stable solution and minimize thrombophlebitis and anticoagulation. Depending on the severity of an attack, hematin is given at a dose of 3 to 4 mg/kg for up to 4 days. Hematin replenishes the hepatic heme pool and normalizes the activity of the heme synthesis pathway by providing negative feedback (see Fig. 20-1). Given the mortality risk and the potential for severe or protracted neurologic symptoms with acute attacks of porphyria, hematin therapy should be initiated as early as possible.

Glucose, at a dose of 300 to 400 g/day, is less effective than hematin but has been shown to decrease the excretion of porphyrin precursors. Furthermore, fasting and low-carbohydrate diets can precipitate acute attacks. Although glucose is effective when administered enterally, the nausea and decreased intestinal motility accompanying an acute attack make parenteral administration more feasible.

Finally, identification and removal of precipitating factors should include a careful assessment of the patient's drug therapy to determine the safety implications of such drugs in a patient with suspected acute porphyria (Table 20-3). Given that the causes of an acute attack may be multifactorial, complete removal of all precipitating factors may not be possible.

Supportive therapy focuses on the symptoms associated with the attack. Pain is treated with opiates, and electrolyte imbalances are corrected. Cranial nerve involvement may require aspiration prophylaxis, whereas involvement of respiratory muscles may require mechanical ventilation or close monitoring in an intensive care unit. Seizures present a particular challenge because barbiturates, phenytoin, and some other antiseizure drugs are potent triggers for an acute attack. Hyponatremia should be excluded as a cause of seizures, and midazolam or clonazepam can be used safely to stop seizure activity.

Table 20–3 ▪ Safety of Drugs in Patients with Acute Porphyria

Unsafe/Avoid	Use with Caution/ Avoid	Probably Safe
Barbiturates	Ketorolac	Opiates
Etomidate	Macrolides	Neuromuscular blockers
Phenytoin	Tetracyclines	Glycopyrrolate
Valproic acid	Quinolones	Atropine
Succinimides	Hydralazine	Neostigmine
Pyrazolones	Calcium channel	Naloxone
Clindamycin	blockers	Midazolam
Erythromycin		Flumazenil
Doxycycline		Nitrous oxide
Sulfonamides		Halothane
Amiodarone		Local anesthetics
		Procainamide
		β-Blockers
		Scopolamine
		Diphenhydramine
		Chlorpromazine

This list is incomplete, and unlisted drugs cannot be assumed to be safe. These categories are intended to provide guidance and not to replace the clinical judgment of the prescribing physician. Some drugs are categorized based on clinical experience, irrespective of the presence or absence of warnings in the package insert. Porphyrics should be treated with the minimum number of drugs necessary.

Anesthetic Management of Patients with Acute Porphyria

Assessment of the safety profile of drugs in porphyria is difficult. On the one hand, drugs are the most frequent precipitating factor of acute attacks. On the other hand, not every exposure of susceptible patients to porphyrinogenic drugs results in an acute attack. Information about drug safety in porphyria is derived from three sources, listed in order of decreasing clinical applicability: (1) actual human cases that suggest a temporal or causal relationship, (2) animal models of induced porphyria, and (3) cell culture. The last two sources tend to overstate the risks to patients and frequently provide conflicting information.[2] Volatile anesthetics, for example, are porphyrinogenic in animal models, but clinical experience with halothane and isoflurane suggests that they are safe to use. Many drugs can be used with caution, provided they are indicated and the potential benefits outweigh the risks.

The anesthetic plan for patients with porphyria should avoid agents that are known to precipitate acute attacks (see Table 20-3). For general anesthesia, propofol is considered the induction agent of choice, whereas barbiturates and etomidate should be avoided. Muscle relaxants and opioids are safe. As stated earlier, volatile agents appear safe, although data on sevoflurane and desflurane are limited. Local and regional anesthesia can be used safely in patients with porphyria, but during an acute attack, autonomic instability, psychiatric symptoms, weakness, and hypovolemia

---

[2]More detailed drug information and lists of safe and potentially unsafe drugs can be found on the following Web sites: http://web.uct.ac.za/depts/porphyria/professional/prof%20index.htm and http://www.porphyries.com.fr.

may present relative contraindications. Clinical experience suggests that both amide- and ester-type local anesthetics are safe, even though lidocaine increases δ-aminolevulinic acid synthase activity in tissue culture.

PREVENTION

Perioperative prevention of acute attacks in patients with acute porphyria requires careful planning and good communication among all caregivers. Admission on the night before surgery allows prophylactic administration of glucose, thus minimizing the impact of the preoperative fast. Reassurance and premedication can relieve anxiety and stress. Drug administration should be minimized, and each drug should be assessed for its risk of precipitating an acute attack. Because a delayed porphyric crisis may develop 3 to 5 days after the precipitating event, discharge instructions should stress the symptoms of a porphyric crisis as reportable postoperative complaints. The workup for symptoms should include screening for and quantification of the urinary porphyrin precursors δ-aminolevulinic acid and porphobilinogen. Such an integrated approach allows for the safe conduct of surgery in patients with acute porphyria.

Further Reading

Dover SB, Plenderleith L, Moore MR, et al: Safety of general anesthesia and surgery in acute hepatic porphyria. Gut 35:1112-1115, 1994.

Elder GH, Hift RJ, Meissner PN: The acute porphyrias. Lancet 349:1613-1617, 1997.

Harrison GG, Meissner PN, Hift RJ: Anesthesia for the porphyric patient. Anaesthesia 48:417-421, 1993.

James MFM, Hift RJ: Porphyrias. Br J Anaesth 85:143-153, 2000.

Palmieri C, Vigushin DM, Peters TJ: Managing malignant disease in patients with porphyria. Q J Med 97:115-126, 2004.

Ketamine

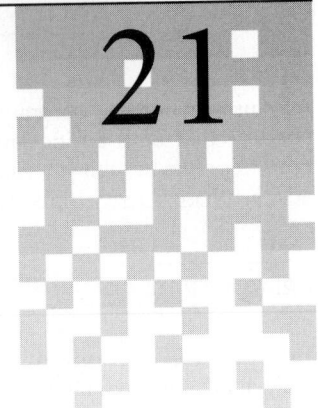

Lisa Thannikary and Bhiken Naik

Case Synopsis

A 68-year-old man is brought to the operating room emergently for exploratory laparotomy after suffering a gunshot wound to the abdomen. He is tachycardiac with a heart rate of 114 beats per minute and hypotensive with a blood pressure of 86/47 mm Hg. He was resuscitated with 2 L of crystalloid in the emergency room. Although he was not intubated, he was unable to give any history owing to acute ethanol intoxication. A rapid-sequence induction with cricoid pressure is performed with intravenous ketamine (3 mg/kg) and succinylcholine (1.5 mg/kg). Intubation occurs without difficulty. Following intubation, the patient's blood pressure decreases precipitously to 65/33, and an ST segment depression of 2 mm is noted in lead V_5. The patient is treated with intravenous fluids and ephedrine, with minimal improvement in blood pressure. A transesophageal echocardiogram shows decreased myocardial contractility.

PROBLEM ANALYSIS

Definition

Ketamine is a phencyclidine derivative used for the induction of anesthesia; it provides anterograde amnesia as well as intense analgesia. It is the only induction agent that stimulates the sympathetic nervous system centrally, which can lead to an increase in blood pressure and heart rate of approximately 30% from baseline values. These hemodynamic effects are seen after 3 to 5 minutes of intravenous injection and slowly decrease to predrug levels after about 20 minutes. The cardiovascular stimulating effects can be blunted by the prior administration of benzodiazepines or concomitant use of inhalation agents.

The mechanisms for the increase in hemodynamic variables are complex. Ketamine is believed to stimulate the central nervous system directly, leading to increased sympathetic outflow. Increased plasma levels of epinephrine and norepinephrine that occur after injection of the drug are also believed to play a role in increasing the heart rate and blood pressure. Ketamine has direct negative inotropic effects, however, that are usually overshadowed by the sympathetic stimulation. These negative inotropic effects are usually seen with depletion of endogenous catecholamine stores or with exhaustion of the sympathetic nervous system compensatory mechanisms in patients who are critically ill or in shock.

Recognition

If a patient has an attenuated or blunted response to an induction dose of ketamine, the possibility of depleted catecholamine stores or exhausted sympathetic nervous system compensatory mechanisms, with unmasking of the direct myocardial depressant effects of ketamine, must be considered.

Risk Assessment

Clinical scenarios in which the negative inotropic effects of ketamine can be unmasked include the following:

- Prolonged critical illness
- Uncompensated shock
- Inadequate volume resuscitation
- Underlying ischemic heart disease
- Chronic β-blocker therapy
- Cocaine use

Implications

Ketamine antagonizes *N*-methyl-D-aspartate receptors. It also interacts with μ, δ, and κ opioid receptors, as well as with monoaminergic receptors, muscarinic receptors, and voltage-sensitive calcium channels. It produces dissociative anesthesia resembling a cataleptic state in which the patient is noncommunicative but appears awake. Because ketamine is a phencyclidine derivative, emergence delirium is possible, but this can be reduced with concomitant use of benzodiazepines.

Ketamine has a rapid onset of action, a relatively short duration of action, and high lipid solubility. It does not bind significantly to plasma proteins and is initially distributed to highly perfused tissues, such as the brain. Ketamine rapidly crosses the blood-brain barrier owing to its high lipid solubility. Ketamine's pharmacokinetic characteristics (Table 21-1), coupled with its sympathomimetic effects, make it an ideal induction agent for patients who are hemodynamically unstable.

Table 21–1 ■ Pharmacokinetic Properties of Intravenous Ketamine	
Parameter	**Value**
pK$_a$	7.5
Protein binding (%)	12
Distribution half-life (min)	11-16
Distribution volume at steady state (L/kg)	2.5-3.5
Clearance (mL/kg/min)	12-17
Elimination half-life (hr)	2-4
Breakdown product	Norketamine (20%-30% potency of ketamine)
Elimination	Renal

Caution should be exercised, however, when using ketamine in the aforementioned high-risk patients.

MANAGEMENT

Before induction of anesthesia, anesthesiologists should attempt to identify patients who might be at risk for developing a hypotensive response to ketamine. Patients with hypovolemic or hemorrhagic shock should be volume-resuscitated before induction, if possible. Invasive monitoring, including central venous pressure, pulmonary artery catheter, or transesophageal echocardiography, can be used in the perioperative period to optimize filling pressures and contractility. If the patient remains hypotensive after induction—despite adequate fluid resuscitation—an inotropic agent or pressor (or both) may be needed to ensure adequate perfusion pressure to the vital organs. The optimal inotropic agent in these patients is a direct-acting sympathomimetic, such as epinephrine or norepinephrine.

PREVENTION

It is important to recognize risk factors that may lead to hypotension with the use of ketamine. In these patients, an alternative induction agent should be used.

Further Reading

Reich DL, Silvay G: Ketamine: An update on the first 25 years of clinical experience. Can J Anaesth 36:186-197, 1989.

Rogers RJ: Intravenous anesthetic agents. In Kirby RR, Gravenstein N, Lobato EB, et al (eds): Clinical Anesthesia Practice. Philadelphia, WB Saunders, 2002, pp 636-637.

Stoelting RK: Nonbarbiturate induction drugs. In Stoelting RK (ed): Pharmacology and Physiology in Anesthetic Practice. Philadelphia, Lippincott-Raven, 1999, pp 148-155.

Tweed WA, Minuck MS, Mymin D: Circulatory response to ketamine anesthesia. Anesthesiology 37:613-619, 1972.

Nonbarbiturate Anesthetics

22

Harshdeep Wilkhu, Kevin P. Chan, E. Price Stover, and John L. Atlee

Case Synopsis

A 53-year-old, 75-kg man with no significant past medical history or allergies is scheduled for a screening colonoscopy. During anesthetic induction he receives a bolus of propofol (80 mg) with additional propofol (170 mg) titrated in divided doses over the course of the procedure. The patient maintains spontaneous ventilation throughout the procedure. Upon completion of the procedure, the patient is responsive to verbal commands and is transferred to the recovery room. Ten minutes after arrival, the patient develops gross arrhythmic jerking of all limbs that appears to be a grand mal seizure.

PROBLEM ANALYSIS

Definition

In addition to ketamine (see Chapter 21), nonbarbiturate anesthetics include midazolam, etomidate, and propofol. Midazolam is more commonly used as a sedative-anxiolytic than as an intravenous (IV) anesthetic induction agent. Both etomidate and propofol are used as IV induction agents; the former is often preferred for patients with or at risk for hemodynamic instability.

Recognition

MECHANISM OF ACTION

Midazolam is a benzodiazepine that increases the frequency of chloride channel opening by facilitating γ-aminobutyric acid (GABA) receptor binding, and it has an inhibitory effect on neural function. GABA is the principal central nervous system neuroinhibitory transmitter.

Etomidate is an imidazole derivative. It inactivates the reticular activating system and may also increase GABA receptor availability.

Propofol is an alkylphenol. It is presumed to act on GABA receptors in the central nervous system to increase the frequency of chloride channel opening. Thus, propofol too has a neuroinhibitory action.

PHARMACOKINETICS

Midazolam is water soluble in a buffered acid medium (pH = 3.5) and highly lipophilic at physiologic pH. Other pharmacokinetic data for propofol, etomidate, and midazolam are listed in Table 22-1.

Etomidate is water soluble and is dissolved in 35% propylene glycol. Its short duration of action is the result of redistribution after an initial distribution time of 3 minutes. It is metabolized by the liver into inactive metabolites that are excreted by the kidneys (85%) and in the bile (13%). Age decreases its clearance, whereas in cirrhosis, clearance is normal but the volume of distribution and elimination half-time are doubled.

Parameter	Drug		
	Propofol	*Etomidate*	*Midazolam*
Distribution half-life (min)	2-8	Initial: 3 Late: 29	3-10
Elimination half-life (hr)	0.5-1.5	2-5	1-4
Biotransformation	Hepatic; extrahepatic (lungs)	Hepatic	Hepatic
Metabolites	Inactive	Very weakly active	Inactive
Excretion	Renal	Renal (85%); bile (13%)	Renal
IV induction dose	1-2.5 mg/kg	0.2-0.5 mg/kg	0.1-0.2 mg/kg
IV sedation dose	10-75 μg/kg/min	5-8 μg/kg/min	0.5-1 mg incremental dosing
IV maintenance dose	50-150 μg/kg/min	10 μg/kg/min (with N_2O-opiate)	0.05-0.1 μg/kg/min

Table 22–1 ■ Pharmacokinetic Data for Propofol, Etomidate, and Midazolam

Propofol is highly lipophilic and is formulated in a soybean oil–egg yolk–lecithin emulsion. Pharmacodynamic properties of propofol are dependent on the plasma concentration of the drug. The induction dose of propofol in adults is 1 to 2.5 mg/kg, producing blood concentrations of 2 to 6 μg/mL. Awakening is rapid even after prolonged infusions and typically occurs at plasma concentrations of 1.0 to 1.5 μg/mL. Steady-state propofol blood concentrations are generally proportional to infusion rates. The context-sensitive half-time of propofol is minimally influenced by infusion duration, owing to rapid metabolic clearance. Biotransformation occurs in the liver. Clearance exceeds hepatic blood flow, suggesting the existence of extrahepatic metabolism. Metabolites are secreted in the urine. Hepatic or renal dysfunction does not reduce the clearance of the parent drug.

Hemodynamic and Other Effects

Midazolam has little effect on hemodynamic parameters (Table 22-2). At a dose of 0.2 mg/kg, midazolam appears to be safe in patients with cardiovascular disease. Any increase in heart rate is likely a reflex-caused response to modestly decreased stroke volume and blood pressure, with reduced sympathetic tone secondary to anxiolysis. Hypovolemia accentuates these effects. In contrast, midazolam can cause apnea and decrease the ventilatory response to carbon dioxide (CO_2), especially after bolus dosing. Also, midazolam is commonly given with an opiate (e.g., fentanyl, alfentanil) for sedation in the preoperative or ambulatory surgery holding area. Such opiates potentiate midazolam's effect on respiration, so patients receiving this combination of drugs must be closely monitored for signs of respiratory insufficiency.

Etomidate does not affect sympathetic activity or baroreflex function. It confers reliable hemodynamic stability in patients with or without cardiac disease. The myocardial oxygen (O_2) supply-demand ratio is maintained. A slightly negative inotropic effect occurs with its solvent (propylene glycol), which likely explains any observed hemodynamic changes (see Table 22-2). In hemorrhagic shock models, etomidate is associated with increased survival compared with thiopental. However, some studies suggest that the cardiovascular depression with etomidate is similar to that with propofol. Finally, etomidate is less likely to cause apnea or decrease the ventilatory response to CO_2 than is midazolam.

Propofol has potent cardiovascular depressant effects. It decreases mean arterial pressure by as much as 40% due to myocardial depression and vasodilatation. Preload and afterload are reduced secondary to decreased venous return and systemic vascular resistance, respectively. This is brought about by propofol's action to reduce sympathetic tone and directly relax vascular smooth muscle. However, the myocardial O_2 supply-demand balance is maintained. Propofol also impairs the vasoconstrictor reflex in acute hemorrhage. Propofol has neuroexcitatory side effects that range from mild, involuntary myoclonic limb movements to grand mal seizures; their timing is quite variable and may occur with induction, in the recovery room, or even many days afterward. However, most neuroexcitatory events related to propofol occur during induction or emergence from anesthesia, when both plasma and cerebral concentrations of the drug are in a dynamic state of flux. They also occur in a variety of scenarios: lengthy or short, major or minor surgical procedures; with or without a prior history of neurologic events.

Risk Assessment

When choosing a nonbarbiturate anesthetic for short outpatient procedures, there are several options, including midazolam, etomidate, propofol, and ketamine (see Chapter 21). The most commonly used drug is propofol, owing to its rapid onset of action and recovery and lack of serious side effects. However, when choosing among these nonbarbiturates as IV induction agents, one must consider whether any of the following is present or possible:

- Hypovolemia or circulatory shock
- Cardiovascular disease

Table 22–2 ■ Hemodynamic, Respiratory, and Other Effects of Propofol, Etomidate, and Midazolam

Parameter	Drug		
	Propofol	*Etomidate*	*Midazolam*
Heart rate	↓	0/↑	0/↑
Mean arterial pressure	↓↓	0/↓	0/↓
Systemic vascular resistance	↓↓	0/↓	0/↓
Mean pulmonary artery pressure	0	0/↑	0
Cardiac index	↓↓	0/↑	0/↓
Stroke volume	↓↓	0/↓	0/↓
Myocardial contractility	0/↓	0/↓	0/↓
Apnea	↑↑↑	↑	↑↑
Ventilatory response to CO_2	↓↓↓	↓	↓↓
Bronchodilatation	+ in COPD	0	0
Nausea and vomiting	Decrease	Increase	Minimal
Analgesia	Minimal	Minimal	Minimal
Pain on injection	Severe	Possible	Minimal

COPD, chronic obstructive pulmonary disease.

- Respiratory insufficiency
- Central nervous system injury or impairment
- Hepatic or renal impairment and any related pharmacokinetic implications
- Drug interactions
- Full stomach or history of acid reflux

MIDAZOLAM

As earlier noted, midazolam has minimal adverse cardiovascular effects and appears to be safe in patients with coronary or heart disease (at doses of 0.2 mg/kg); however, it has the potential to aggravate respiratory insufficiency (see Table 22-2). Other considerations include the following:

- Hepatic biotransformation with inactive metabolites; renal excretion
- Slight reduction in cerebral O_2 consumption, with little or no decrease in cerebral blood flow
- Small decrease in intracranial pressure (ICP); small increase in seizure threshold
- Maintains cerebral autoregulation; large decrease in intraocular pressure (IOP)
- Slower loss of consciousness and longer recovery period for return of cognitive functions
- Potential for coughing, hiccups, or involuntary skeletal muscle movements when used for induction of anesthesia

ETOMIDATE

Etomidate has generally supportive and beneficial effects on both cardiovascular and cerebral function. However, as noted earlier, there is a slightly negative inotropic effect with its solvent (propylene glycol). Etomidate has minimal effects on ventilation and does not trigger histamine release. It is not an analgesic. Similar to the effects of midazolam, coughing, hiccups, or involuntary skeletal muscle movements (nonepileptogenic) may occur if etomidate is used for anesthetic induction. Although grand mal seizures have occurred with etomidate, it induces electroencephalographic burst suppression at high doses. Other considerations are the following:

- Increased incidence of nausea and vomiting
- Irritation at peripheral vein injection site
- Clinically significant adrenocortical inhibition with prolonged infusions
- May reduce IOP, but this is counteracted by myoclonus, mydriasis, or coughing
- Unlikely to cause apnea or impair the ventilatory response to CO_2
- Hepatic metabolism; inactive metabolites; renal elimination
- Initial distribution half-life of 3 minutes and redistribution half-life of about 30 minutes
- Elimination half-life of 3 to 5 hours

PROPOFOL

Propofol reduces systemic blood pressure by vasodilatation and negative inotropic effects. The inhibition of efferent sympathetic activity results in vascular smooth muscle relaxation and blood pressure reduction. Propofol's negative inotropic effects are due to reduced myocardial intracellular calcium availability, caused by Ca^{2+} influx inhibition. Overall, propofol decreases sympathetic more than parasympathetic activity, leading to parasympathetic dominance.

Propofol produces dose-dependent respiratory depression that acts in synergy with opioids and benzodiazepines. Further, it has a high potential to impair the ventilatory response to CO_2 and cause apnea (see Table 22-2). Continuous infusions reduce both the tidal volume and the frequency of breathing; opiates potentiate this effect. Propofol has a bronchodilating effect, and it decreases the intraoperative incidence of bronchospasm with reactive airways disease. In February 2001 the Food and Drug Administration noted that abrupt discontinuation of propofol after prolonged infusion may result in agitation, tremulousness, and hyperirritability in pediatric patients. This led to a pediatric exclusivity labeling change: propofol is not indicated for prolonged use in the pediatric intensive care unit. Other effects to consider are the following:

- Coughing, hiccups, and involuntary skeletal muscle movements with induction
- Vein irritation and pain on injection (lidocaine helps reduce this, but slow, incremental, "desensitizing" injections are more reliable)[1]
- Antiemetic, antipruritic, and anxiolytic properties
- Reports of delayed seizures, hallucinations, and opisthotonos
- Formerly, anaphylactic reactions and bacterial growth were possible with the lipid solvent (less of a problem with the current formulation)
- Hepatic and possible extrahepatic biotransformation, with inactive metabolites and renal (85%) and bile (13%) excretion
- Reduction in cerebral O_2 consumption, blood flow, and ICP and IOP
- No effect on seizure threshold, and not an analgesic

Implications

The delayed onset of neurologic excitatory events (especially with etomidate or propofol) has serious implications for ambulatory surgery (outpatient) anesthesia practice. When patients are discharged home 1 to 2 hours after surgery or other procedures, they are at serious risk of harm to themselves or others. The patient or family can be traumatized during a seizure, and loss of the airway during this event can have dire consequences. Adverse neurologic sequelae also increase health care costs because many of these patients must be admitted to an intensive care unit to rule out serious pathology and undergo costly diagnostic studies (e.g., magnetic resonance imaging, computed tomography, electroencephalography). In addition, consultant care may be requested for these events.

---

[1]We have found that 1-, 2-, and 3-mL "desensitizing" increments of propofol spaced 30 to 45 seconds apart, followed by an IV "push" of the remaining induction dose, are effective at reducing the discomfort associated with propofol induction. Lidocaine (50 mg) can be either mixed with or given before propofol.

Patients with cardiovascular disease or hypovolemia are at increased risk for cardiovascular collapse and myocardial ischemia or infarction after IV anesthesia induction (greatest risk with propofol, followed by midazolam and then etomidate). Hemorrhagic shock results in lactic acidosis, and hepatorenal lactate clearance must be maintained. End-organ perfusion in general must be preserved. Also, the risk of irreversible brain or ocular injury must be carefully evaluated during the selection of a rapid IV induction agent.

MANAGEMENT

Selection of an appropriate nonbarbiturate IV induction agent must take the following issues into consideration:

- Hypovolemia or hypotension due to hemorrhage
  - Restore intravascular volume (preload) and use blood or blood products as needed.
  - Optimize ventilation and oxygenation.
  - Restore acid-base balance.
  - Consider the use of vasoactive drugs.
  - Initiate invasive monitoring, transesophageal echocardiography, or both, if needed.
  - Choose a nonbarbiturate anesthetic and method of delivery according to the aforementioned considerations.
- Airway management
  - Use awake intubation followed by an IV induction agent or inhalational anesthetic.
  - Assess the need for rapid or modified rapid-sequence intubation.
- Increased ICP
  - Choose an IV induction agent accordingly (propofol or etomidate decreases ICP).
  - Consider hypocapnia, mannitol, and corticosteroids (see also Chapters 174 and 182).

Hypovolemia and Airway Management

Resuscitation begins with securing a compromised airway, optimizing O₂ delivery, restoring intravascular volume, and correcting acidosis. A rapid-sequence induction is usually necessary to minimize the risk of aspiration. In the case of a difficult airway or an unstable cervical spine, awake intubation is indicated in a cooperative patient. The choice of an IV anesthetic is dictated by its cardiovascular, cerebrovascular, and pharmacokinetic effects (see Tables 22-1 and 22-2). Of the agents discussed here, etomidate is probably the safest agent for patients with significant hypovolemia or blood loss. However, regardless of which agent is selected, its dose must be reduced in the presence of significant hemorrhage or reduced intravascular volume, because either of these conditions will increase the amount of drug delivered to the heart or brain due to redistribution of blood flow to vital organs.

Increased Intracranial or Intraocular Pressure

Midazolam, etomidate, and propofol exert a beneficial decrease in ICP, in contrast to ketamine, which increases ICP and can produce emergence delirium. However, slower emergence with midazolam can hinder early postoperative neurologic assessment.

Both midazolam and propofol decrease IOP. Etomidate has the same effect, but it can be counteracted by myoclonic activity, mydriasis, and cough caused by etomidate. Ketamine increases IOP.

Neuroexcitatory Events

Initially, no treatment may be necessary because the majority of neuroexcitatory events resolve spontaneously. Benzodiazepines are the drugs of choice for events that do not resolve spontaneously. They depress spinal reflexes and reduce the spontaneous electrical activity in all regions of the brain and spinal cord. All benzodiazepines elevate the seizure threshold and thus are considered anticonvulsants. These drugs are quite safe and are rarely fatal, unless taken concomitantly with other sedatives. Second-line therapy for neuroexcitatory events is a barbiturate. This family of drugs depresses the activity of all excitable central nervous system tissue. In general, barbiturates possess a low therapeutic index, along with low selectivity. Hence, they must be dosed cautiously.

PREVENTION

Avoidance of complications with nonbarbiturate IV induction agents requires attention to the following issues:

- Volume repletion and administration of blood or blood products, if indicated
- Appropriate selection of the IV anesthetic induction agent. Consider time of onset and emergence, amnesia, analgesia, coronary and cerebral perfusion, systemic blood pressure, myocardial and cerebral O₂ consumption, onset of apnea, and effects on ICP and IOP.
- Slow titration and adjustment of induction doses. Careful titration to effect generally prevents abrupt, deleterious changes in blood pressure, unless a rapid-sequence induction is indicated. If so, a vasopressor may be needed for the patient to tolerate the induction. Doses of IV induction agents should be adjusted based on the patient's age, ideal weight, and hepatic and renal function.
- Side effects of and relative contraindications to the various IV anesthetic induction agents

For the patient described in the case synopsis, prevention of future neuroexcitatory events suggests that propofol (or etomidate) should not be administered to him in the future. This advice might also apply to patients with a history of neuroexcitatory events. However, no single diagnosis or combination of diagnoses has been implicated as the cause of such events. The seeming rarity of major neuroexcitatory events with administration of propofol or etomidate, along with the lack of reported long-term adverse sequelae, has resulted in their continued use in ambulatory and inpatient settings, especially propofol. The overall risk-benefit ratio for propofol is extremely low, and the decision whether to use the drug should not be based on reports of rare associated neurologic phenomena.

Further Reading

Dearlove JC, Dearlove OR: Cortical reflex myoclonus after propofol anaesthesia. Anaesthesia 57:834-835, 2002.

Reves JG, Glass PSA, Lubarsky DA, et al: Intravenous nonopioid anesthetics. In Miller RD (ed): Miller's Anesthesia, 6th ed. Philadelphia, Churchill Livingstone, 2005, pp 317-378.

Strachan AN, Raithatha HH: Propofol myoclonus. Can J Anaesth 43:536-537, 1996.

Sutherland MJ, Burt P: Propofol and seizures. Anaesth Intensive Care 22:733-737, 1994.

Walder B, Tramer MR, Seeck M: Seizure-like phenomena and propofol: A systematic review. Neurology 58:1327-1332, 2002.

ANESTHETIC ADJUNCTS

Succinylcholine

Eugene B. Freid

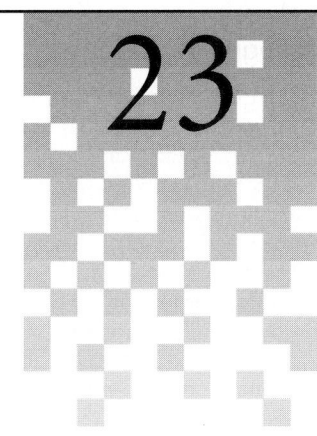

23

Case Synopsis

A 32-year-old woman undergoes emergent open reduction of bilateral femoral fractures sustained in a fall. Past history is pertinent only for mild, hemiparetic, static encephalopathy as a result of meningitis in infancy. Rapid-sequence induction of anesthesia with 20 mg of etomidate and 80 mg of succinylcholine is uneventful. At the end of the 2-hour procedure, she is clinically weak, with four diminished twitches and moderate fade on a train-of-four. She is extubated 1 hour after completion of surgery. Evaluation reveals a pseudocholinesterase activity of 95% and a dibucaine number of 25, which is consistent with an abnormal genetic variant of pseudocholinesterase.

PROBLEM ANALYSIS

Definition

The onset and offset characteristics of succinylcholine provide distinct advantages over other neuromuscular blocking drugs. Unfortunately, succinylcholine also has a number of well-described complications related to its mechanism of action or pharmacokinetics or that occur as an idiosyncratic effect (Table 23-1). Observations show that hyperkalemia and cardiac arrest develop soon after succinylcholine administration to patients with thermal injury, trauma, upper and lower motor neuron injuries, and various myopathies (Table 23-2).

Prolonged relaxation may occur after succinylcholine administration because of the development of a phase II blockade or decreased metabolism. After a single large dose, repeated doses, or a prolonged continuous infusion of succinylcholine, the postjunctional receptor may not respond normally to acetylcholine, even after the receptor-nicotinic channel has repolarized. This is termed a *phase II block* and is preferred to the terms *dual block* and *nondepolarization block* because *phase II block* does not imply a specific mechanism.

Under normal circumstances, the short duration of the effect of succinylcholine is the result of rapid hydrolysis by pseudocholinesterase. Ninety percent of an intravenous dose of succinylcholine is rapidly hydrolyzed to a nearly inactive metabolite in the plasma and liver by pseudocholinesterase. Neuromuscular blockade terminates by the diffusion of succinylcholine from the end plate into the extracellular fluid because there is no pseudocholinesterase at the motor end plate. Pseudocholinesterase influences the onset and duration of action by controlling the rate of hydrolysis in plasma. A prolonged duration of succinylcholine neuromuscular block may occur when quantities of normal pseudocholinesterase are decreased or when an atypical or abnormal variant of pseudocholinesterase is present.

Table 23–1 ■ Complications of Succinylcholine Administration

Cardiovascular
  Tachycardia (ganglionic stimulation)
  Bradycardia, sinus arrest, junctional rhythm
Hyperkalemia
Fasciculations; myalgia*
Myoglobinuria, elevated plasma creatine phosphokinase
Sustained muscle contraction (myotonic dystrophy, congenital myotonia)
Malignant hyperpyrexia
Masseter muscle rigidity
Prolonged relaxation
  Phase II block
  Inadequate pseudocholinesterase activity
Increased intraocular pressure*
Increased intracranial pressure
Increased intragastric pressure*
Histamine release

*May be reduced with succinylcholine pretreatment (defasciculation).

Table 23–2 ■ Conditions Predisposing to Exaggerated Potassium Release with Succinylcholine

Thermal injury
Traumatic injury
Neurologic disease
  Spinal cord trauma
  Hemiparesis, lower motor neuron lesions
  Multiple sclerosis
  Stroke
  Guillain-Barré disease
  Encephalitis
  Central nervous system trauma
Myopathy, muscular dystrophy
Disuse atrophy
Tetanus

Recognition

T-wave elevation, QRS complex prolongation and a sinusoidal QRS waveform (see Chapter 14, Fig. 14-2), and arrhythmias (ventricular tachycardia or fibrillation) occurring shortly after succinylcholine administration are the characteristic alterations seen on the electrocardiogram (ECG) in patients with hyperkalemia and exaggerated potassium (K^+) release. Measurement of serum K^+ concentrations confirms hyperkalemia. However, if the ECG is abnormal, treatment should precede confirmation of serum K^+ concentrations.

Prolonged relaxation after succinylcholine is indicated by apnea and neuromuscular weakness or paresis. The diagnosis is confirmed by characteristic findings on peripheral nerve stimulation, including a train-of-four (T_4/T_1) of less than 0.3 and the presence of fade and post-tetanic facilitation.

The presence of low levels of normal pseudocholinesterase, or atypical or abnormal forms of pseudocholinesterase, leads to variable prolongation of neuromuscular blockade (Table 23-3). The presence of abnormal pseudocholinesterase is frequently recognized only after moderately or very prolonged blockade occurs in an otherwise healthy patient who received a normal dose of succinylcholine. Nerve monitoring characteristics typical of a phase II block should be expected when abnormal pseudocholinesterase is present due to the large concentration of unmetabolized succinylcholine at the neuromuscular junction.

Risk Assessment

POTASSIUM RELEASE

Under normal conditions, depolarization of skeletal muscle occurs at acetylcholine receptors at the motor end plate. Fluxes in sodium (Na^+) and K^+ after succinylcholine typically lead to an increase in serum K^+ concentrations of up to 0.5 mEq/dL. In a number of pathologic conditions, however, exaggerated K^+ release following succinycholine causes plasma K^+ concentrations to rise excessively (see Table 23-2). In patients with denervation states, up-regulation of acetylcholine receptors leads to muscle supersensitivity. In effect, the entire muscle membrane acts as a motor end plate.

The increased zone of permeability to Na^+ and K^+ leads to exaggerated movement of these ions after the administration of succinylcholine and consequent increased efflux of K^+ from the myocytes into the extracellular fluid.

The timing of the development of exaggerated K^+ release with succinylcholine administration depends on the nature of the injury and follows the timing of the development of acetylcholine receptor supersensitivity. Typically, it begins 5 to 15 days after thermal injury or trauma, peaks at 20 to 60 days, and persists for up to 3 months. In patients with upper and lower motor neuron disease, it begins at 7 days and persists for about 6 months. *Pretreatment with a nondepolarizing relaxant does not reliably abolish the hyperkalemic response.* In infants and children, myopathy may be clinically unapparent and may be diagnosed only after succinylcholine-hyperkalemic cardiac arrest. In contrast, patients with static encephalopathies (e.g., cerebral palsy) typically do not have exaggerated K^+ release after succinylcholine, because their nervous system damage is remote and stable.

PHASE II BLOCK

Clinically relevant phase II block can occur with total succinylcholine doses as low as 4 mg/kg in some patients, with either repeat dosing or continuous infusions. Such block may be evident with tetanic stimulation in highly sensitive ("fine") muscle groups (e.g., extraocular muscles) before it occurs in the larger muscles involved in respiration. Development of tachyphylaxis, which manifests as an increase in the amount of infused succinylcholine, often occurs concurrently with the development of clinically relevant phase II block.

PSEUDOCHOLINESTERASE

Low pseudocholinesterase activity occurs in the newborn and the elderly; with pregnancy, liver disease, malignancy, or thermal injury; and with the use of certain medications (glucocorticoids, estrogens, echothiophate, bambuterol, phenelzine, and cyclophosphamide) and organophosphate pesticides. Pseudocholinesterase levels may drop precipitously

---

Table 23–3 ■ Characteristics of Normal, Atypical, and Abnormal Pseudocholinesterase

Pseudocholinesterase Type	Genotype	Duration of Clinical Block	Dibucaine No.	Fluoride No.
Homozygous normal	Eu Eu	Normal	80	60
Heterozygous dibucaine	Eu Ea	Slightly prolonged	60	50
Heterozygous fluoride	Eu Ef	Slightly prolonged	75	50
Heterozygous silent	Eu Es	Slightly prolonged	80	60
Dibucaine fluoride	Ea Ef	Moderately prolonged	50	50
Dibucaine silent	Ea Es	Very prolonged	20	20
Fluoride silent	Ef Es	Moderately prolonged	65	35
Homozygous dibucaine (atypical)	Ea Ea	Very prolonged	20	20
Homozygous fluoride	Ef Ef	Slightly prolonged	65	35
Homozygous silent	Es Es	Very prolonged	—	—

Adapted from Pantuck EJ, Pantuck CB: Prolonged apnea following succinylcholine administration. In Azar I (ed): Muscle Relaxants. New York, Marcel Dekker, 1987, pp 206-229.

after plasmapheresis. Low levels of normal pseudocholinesterase generally do not prolong succinylcholine block to a clinically significant degree; this occurs only when normal pseudocholinesterase activity is reduced by at least 75% (normal, 4.9 to 12 IU/mL). In contrast, in patients with genetically atypical or abnormal pseudocholinesterase, the delay in return of normal neuromuscular function can range from mild (10 to 15 minutes) to severe (2 to 4 hours), depending on the variant. The difference among normal, atypical, and abnormal pseudocholinesterase variants is shown in the laboratory with compounds (e.g., dibucaine, fluoride) that inhibit benzoylcholine hydrolysis by pseudocholinesterase.

The most common forms of abnormal pseudocholinesterase are the dibucaine-resistant and atypical variants (Eu Ea and Ea Ea, respectively). The homozygous atypical form (Ea Ea) occurs in 1 in 3200 patients, and the heterozygous form (Eu Ea) occurs in 1 in 480 patients. Dibucaine inhibits benzoylcholine hydrolysis by normal pseudocholinesterase by more than 70%; it inhibits benzoylcholine hydrolysis by the atypical (Ea Ea) form by less than 30%. Other forms of pseudocholinesterase include fluoride-resistant variants and a "silent" variant that shows neither dibucaine- nor fluoride-induced inhibition. Table 23-3 summarizes the characteristics of normal, atypical, and abnormal pseudocholinesterase variants.

Implications

The consequences of succinylcholine-induced hyperkalemia include arrhythmias and cardiac arrest. Prolonged relaxation after succinylcholine requires airway management and mechanical ventilation (with sedation) until the neuromuscular weakness subsides. Patients with atypical or abnormal pseudocholinesterase also demonstrate prolonged metabolism of mivacurium and ester local anesthetics. Because red blood cell esterase hydrolyzes esmolol, its metabolism is unaffected in patients with atypical or abnormal pseudocholinesterase.

MANAGEMENT

Hyperkalemia

Ventricular tachyarrhythmias and fibrillation are treated with standard advanced cardiovascular life support protocols. In addition, hyperkalemia must be aggressively treated with hyperventilation, calcium salts (chloride or gluconate), sodium bicarbonate, and epinephrine. Hyperventilation, bicarbonate, and β-adrenergic receptor agonists help drive K^+ intracellularly, and calcium reduces the cellular effects of high K^+ concentrations in the heart. Milder degrees of hyperkalemia are treated with hyperventilation, calcium salts, sodium bicarbonate, and parenteral or inhaled β-adrenergic receptor agonist therapy (albuterol or terbutaline). Glucose and insulin can also be used, but because their effects are more delayed, they are not considered first-line therapy. For children with hyperkalemic cardiac arrest, a postoperative evaluation by a neurologist or physical and rehabilitation medicine specialist for an occult myopathy should be performed.

Prolonged Block

Treatment for prolonged relaxation includes ensuring an adequate airway and gas exchange until phase II block is no longer evident (neuromuscular function monitoring) and adequate muscle strength is present. Pure phase II block is reversible with anticholinesterase. However, the block caused by succinylcholine overdose or with atypical or abnormal pseudocholinesterase is mixed (phase I and phase II block). In this case, anticholinesterase therapy may lengthen the duration of phase I block. Most practitioners simply continue ventilatory support until the block wanes and muscle strength has returned to its baseline level. With prolonged block due to atypical or abnormal pseudocholinesterase, ventilatory support must be continued until muscle strength returns. Although banked blood and plasma contain active pseudocholinesterase, the risk associated with their transfusion outweighs the possible benefit of reversing prolonged block. Patients suspected of having atypical or abnormal pseudocholinesterase should be tested for pseudocholinesterase activity and type and made aware of their condition. There should be a note in the patient's chart indicating an "allergy" to succinylcholine, and the patient should wear a MedicAlert bracelet.

PREVENTION

One way to prevent complications with succinylcholine is to avoid it altogether, unless there is a compelling indication for or advantage to its use. This is especially true in young children, who might have clinically unapparent myopathies. Rarely, an unexpected hyperkalemic response may occur, but with the avoidance of succinylcholine in at-risk patients, this should be quite unusual.

With the availability of short- and intermediate-acting nondepolarizing agents, the need for large doses or infusions of succinylcholine should be uncommon. If repeated doses or infusions of succinylcholine are used, keeping the total dose under 5 to 6 mg/kg will help. During the preoperative evaluation, a family history of prolonged weakness or delay in awakening from anesthesia should be elicited. There are some geographic regions in which pseudocholinesterase exists because of its hereditary nature. In these regions, preoperative laboratory screening for pseudocholinesterase activity may be useful.

Further Reading

Goldhill DR, Martyn JA Jr: Succinylcholine-induced hyperkalemia. In Azar I (ed): Muscle Relaxants. New York, Marcel Dekker, 1987, pp 93-113.

Jensen FS, Viby-Mogensen J: Plasma cholinesterase and abnormal reaction to succinylcholine: Twenty years' experience with the Danish Cholinesterase Research Unit. Acta Anaesth Scand 39:150-156, 1995.

Larach MG, Rosenberg H, Gronert GA, et al: Hyperkalemic cardiac arrest during anesthesia in infants and children with occult myopathies. Am J Anesth 24:241-247, 1997.

Levano S, Ginz H, Siegemund M, et al: Genotyping the butyryl-cholinesterase in patients with prolonged neuromuscular block after succinylcholine. Anesthesiology 102:531-535, 2005.

Martyn JA Jr, White DA, Gronert GA, et al: Up-and-down regulation of skeletal muscle acetylcholine receptors. Anesthesiology 76:822-843, 1992.

Pantuck EJ: Plasma cholinesterase: Gene and variations. Anesth Analg 77:380-386, 1993.

Pantuck EJ, Pantuck CB: Prolonged apnea following succinylcholine administration. In Azar I (ed): Muscle Relaxants. New York, Marcel Dekker, 1987, pp 206-229.

Viby-Mogensen J: Correlation of succinylcholine duration of action with plasma cholinesterase activity in subjects with the genotypically normal enzyme. Anesthesiology 53:517-520, 1980.

Nondepolarizing Neuromuscular Relaxants

24

Maria A. K. Öhrn

Case Synopsis

Following emergence and extubation after general anesthesia, a 52-year-old woman with a history of chronic renal insufficiency has a labored breathing pattern, including paradoxical movement of the chest wall and abdomen and intermittent upper airway obstruction.

PROBLEM ANALYSIS

Definition

Prolonged (residual) neuromuscular relaxant blockade is due to the presence of a nondepolarizing muscle relaxant (NDMR) at the neuromuscular junction beyond its expected duration of action. Residual neuromuscular relaxant block must be sufficient to cause motor weakness in response to peripheral nerve stimulation or to cause clinical signs of impaired muscle function. Unrecognized, residual neuromuscular relaxant block may cause respiratory insufficiency or arrest.

Under controlled circumstances, each NDMR is metabolized, excreted, or both at a rate that can be predicted based on its pharmacokinetic profile. Clinically, however, it is important to recognize that coexisting disease processes, intraoperative events, and some concurrent drug therapy may prolong the duration of action of all NDMRs.

Recognition

After anesthesia, if the patient is unable to sustain a head lift for at least 5 seconds or has fade with 50-Hz tetanic peripheral nerve stimulation for 5 seconds or more, evidence exists of significant block at the neuromuscular junction. To prevent the overaccumulation of NDMR at the neuromuscular junction, one must consider the following:

- Coexisting diseases or conditions that may affect any particular NDMR's route of elimination or metabolism
- Expected recovery times with low or high doses of NDMRs (Table 24-1)
- Routine monitoring of neuromuscular function with a peripheral nerve stimulator

With train-of-four (T_1/T_4) stimulation, titration of twitch responses, and knowledge of the usual recovery time for specific NDMRs, clinicians can detect early evidence of impaired drug metabolism or excretion.

Risk Assessment

Whether by known, unknown, or postulated mechanisms, all the following agents can potentiate the actions of NDMRs:

- Antibiotics (especially aminoglycosides)
- Loop diuretics (e.g., furosemide)
- Magnesium sulfate

Table 24-1 ■ Approximate Recovery Time to Baseline Twitch Height with Nondepolarizing Muscle Relaxants (NDMRs)

	Dose Range (mg/kg)	Recovery Time from Low Dose* (min)	Recovery Time from High Dose* (min)
Long-acting NDMRs			
Pancuronium[†]	0.1		40-60
Doxacurium	0.05-0.08	50-130 (mean 91)	74-268 (mean 177)
Intermediate-acting NDMRs			
Vecuronium	0.10		25-45
Rocuronium	0.6-1.2	15-85 (mean 31)	38-160 (mean 67)
Atracurium[†]	0.5		20-45
Cisatracurium[‡]	0.15-0.20	28-65 (mean 46)	31-103 (mean 59)
Short-acting NDMRs			
Mivacurium[†]	0.25	11-29 (mean 19)	

*Approximate duration of recovery based on package inserts and variability in manufacturers' definitions of recovery. Unless otherwise specified, the value given is for recovery to 25% of twitch height.
[†]Range for recovery time from high dose is that until a first maintenance dose is needed.
[‡]Value for recovery to 5% of twitch height.

- Lithium salts
- Calcium channel blockers
- Quinidine or procainamide

Along with drugs that may potentiate NDMR actions, there are patient factors that impair the metabolism or excretion of NDMRs. Renal or hepatic insufficiency can alter the duration of action of some NDMRs (Table 24-2). Intraoperative temperature fluctuations and acid-base imbalance also affect the pharmacokinetic and pharmacodynamic properties of NDMRs, which can make their duration of action and effects unpredictable.

Implications

It is known that some NDMRs (e.g., D-tubocurarine, atracurium, cisatracurium, doxacurium, metocurine, mivacurium) may cause nonimmunologic histamine release. The magnitude of this response is species dependent (e.g., greater in cats than in rats or dogs) and varies with the dose, the rapidity of injection, and, in clinical situations, the individual patient. Although the response may at first appear anaphylactic, any histamine release is more direct (anaphylactoid), often self-limited, and easily managed with judicious use of short-lived vasoconstrictors to counter the associated vasodilatation.

Recent studies indicate that NDMRs account for more than half of all anaphylactoid reactions during general anesthesia. NDMRs, collectively, cause more such reactions than any other class of drugs commonly given during general anesthesia. However, the incidence of true anaphylaxis during anesthesia is quite low (estimated at 1 in 5000 to 1 in 25,000 cases).

Concerning other NDMR complications, if these are recognized early enough, prolonged block can be managed without incident. If not (e.g., those that occur at the end of anesthesia), the need for patient care and the health care costs increase. Prolonged block can also increase operating room times, especially if patients must be extubated before admission to the postanesthetic care unit, as required in some ambulatory surgery centers. With severe NDMR overdose, postoperative mechanical ventilatory support may be needed for some time. If so, the patient must be sedated to avoid subsequent recall of unpleasant events due to partial or complete paralysis.

Unrecognized residual neuromuscular blockade can cause further complications. With partial block, patients may have insufficient motor strength to protect the airway, increasing the risk for pulmonary aspiration. This can also cause respiratory insufficiency, hypercarbia, and hypoxemia. Collectively, these conditions may cause hemodynamic instability, arrhythmias, or respiratory arrest.

MANAGEMENT

Use of smaller NDMR doses titrated to twitch, train-of-four, and tetanic responses and early recognition of prolonged NDMR block are important for expectant management. If prolonged recovery from the initial intubating NDMR dose is detected, the cause of the drug's reduced elimination or potentiation must be sought and corrected, if possible.

Alternatively, in longer cases, subsequent use of shorter-acting NDMRs with a different route of elimination may help address the problem, assuming that the cause of reduced metabolism or elimination of the first drug is known. Even so, at least initially, the kinetics of the second NDMR will be more like those of a longer-acting agent. For example, changing from pancuronium (a long-acting drug) to mivacurium (a short-acting drug) will not immediately alter the pharmacokinetics to those of mivacurium. Instead, mivacurium's duration of action will be more similar to that of pancuronium. Not until several pancuronium half-lives have passed will the pharmacokinetics resemble those of mivacurium. Also, combining steroid-derivative NDMRs (identified by the suffix "curonium") with benzylisoquinolone-derivative NDMRs (identified by the suffix "curium") may have an initial supra-additive effect on the duration of action.

If prolonged neuromuscular block is not detected until the case's conclusion, the patient is kept sedated with nitrous oxide or low-dose volatile inhalation anesthesia. If the patient continues to show weakness, even with evidence for adequate neuromuscular relaxant reversal by head lift or peripheral nerve stimulation, an amnestic is given while arrangements are made for postoperative ventilatory support

Table 24–2 ▪ **Routes of Metabolism or Elimination for Neuromuscular Blocking Agents**				
	Route			
Drug	*Renal*	*Hepatic*	*Ester Hydrolysis**	*Hoffman Elimination†*
Pancuronium	Major	Intermediate	Negligible	Negligible
Doxacurium	Major	Major	Negligible	Negligible
Vecuronium	Minor	Major	Negligible	Negligible
Rocuronium	Minor	Major	Negligible	Negligible
Atracurium	Negligible	Negligible	Major	Major
Cisatracurium	Minor	Minor	Negligible	Major
Mivacurium	Minor	Minor	Major	Negligible

All categories were derived from data on elimination and metabolism from package inserts.
*Plasma (pseudo) cholinesterase.
†Butyrylcholinesterase and spontaneous (nonenzymatic) degradation.

in the postanesthesia care unit. Evidence that a problem exists includes the following:

- Inability to sustain a head lift for at least 5 seconds
- Fade with 50-Hz tetanic stimulation lasting 5 seconds (the patient must be sedated, because this is extremely painful)
- Detectable difference in two responses elicited by double-burst stimulation

While in the postanesthesia care unit, the patient should remain sedated until head lift or results of peripheral nerve stimulation indicate adequate recovery of motor strength.

An unfortunate occurrence is the one described in the case synopsis. Apparently, the patient was not adequately assessed before extubation, so the clinician was confronted with a patient struggling to breathe. Prompt action was needed to ensure adequate oxygenation and ventilation, which could be achieved with a face or laryngeal mask, while preparing for reintubation. The patient did not need additional muscle relaxation for reintubation, but she did require an amnestic agent.

PREVENTION

Preventing prolonged neuromuscular blockade begins with the selection of an appropriate NDMR. An understanding of the comorbidities affecting hepatic or renal elimination of various NDMRs will help clinicians choose one that is not overly dependent on the liver or kidneys for its metabolism or elimination.

Continual intraoperative surveillance of the magnitude of neuromuscular block requires a peripheral nerve stimulator and documentation of the time course for recovery of twitch, double-burst, train-of-four, and tetanic responses. This allows early detection of block prolongation. Ideally, the train-of-four response is measured after induction of anesthesia, but before giving a neuromuscular relaxant, whether succinylcholine or an NDMR. The peripheral nerve stimulator must be tested for adequate battery voltage, and it should display the current (amperes) delivered to the patient. Ball-electrode, hand-held peripheral nerve stimulators are not as reliable as those secured at one site with electrode gel adhesive pads. Any monitoring site that avoids misleading effects

of direct muscle stimulation is acceptable, bearing in mind that there are slight differences in recovery times among the various muscle groups. For example, the diaphragm and pharyngeal muscles recover relatively more quickly than the other muscle groups.

The train-of-four response, which is preferred for intraoperative monitoring, poorly predicts adequate recovery from blockade. For clinical recovery of respiratory muscle function to occur, the T_4/T_1 ratio should be at least 0.7. Experienced clinicians, however, are unable to detect any fade with T_4/T_1 ratios as low as 0.3. Therefore, many patients are still significantly weak, based solely on train-of-four responses. Selecting double-burst stimulation or 5-second, 50-Hz tetanus, combined with clinical signs, provides far greater sensitivity for the detection of residual block. Even with anticholinesterase therapy, the time to full recovery is dependent on full metabolism *and* elimination of the NDMR. Further, there may be active metabolites. If these or the parent drug have slow metabolism or elimination, the recovery time can be even more delayed.

Further Reading

Bevan DR, Donati F: Muscle relaxants. In Barash PG (ed): Clinical Anesthesia, 2nd ed. Philadelphia, Lippincott-Raven, 1996, pp 481-508.

Erkola O, Rautoma P, Meretoja OA, et al: Mivacurium when preceded by pancuronium becomes a long-acting muscle relaxant. Anesthesiology 84:562-565, 1996.

Goudsouzian NG: Muscle relaxants in children. In Coté CJ, Todres ID, Goudsouzian N, Ryan J (eds): A Practice of Anesthesia for Infants and Children, 3rd ed. Philadelphia, WB Saunders, 2001, pp 196-215.

Mertes PM, Laxenaire MC, Alia F: Groupe d'Etudes des Reactions Anaphylactoides Peranesthesiques. Anaphylactic and anaphylactoid reactions occurring during anesthesia in France in 1999-2000. Anesthesiology 99:536-545, 2003.

Naguib M, Lien CA: Pharmacology of muscle relaxants and their antagonists. In Miller RD (ed): Miller's Anesthesia, 6th ed. New York, Churchill Livingstone, 2005, pp 481-572.

Nejman AM: Muscle relaxants. In Kirby R, Gravenstein N, Lobato E, Gravenstein J (eds): Clinical Anesthesia Practice, 2nd ed. Philadelphia, WB Saunders, 2002, pp 707-714.

Plaud B, Debaene B, Lequeau F, et al: Mivacurium neuromuscular block at the adductor muscles of the larynx and adductor pollicis in humans. Anesthesiology 85:77-81, 1996.

Viby-Mogensen J: Neuromuscular monitoring. In Miller RD (ed): Anesthesia, 4th ed. New York, Churchill Livingstone, 1994, pp 1345-1361.

Antihistamines: H$_1$- and H$_2$-Blockers

Ali Habibi and Edward T. Riley

25

Case Synopsis

A 75-year-old man presents with acute urinary retention, tremors, blurred vision, and confusion. His past medical history is significant for allergic rhinitis, chronic renal failure, and hypertension. He is currently taking diphenhydramine and diltiazem.

PROBLEM ANALYSIS

Definition

Antihistamines (H$_1$-blockers) are a family of drugs used for hypersensitivity reactions of various types. Antihistamines are easily obtained, even without a prescription, but are not free of adverse side effects. Also, most first-generation H$_1$-antagonists, such as diphenhydramine, inhibit muscarinic receptors to cause anticholinergic effects; the elderly are especially prone to these side effects of H$_1$-blockers. Common side effects of first-generation antihistamines are sedation, confusion, tremors, blurred vision, diplopia, nervousness, insomnia, tinnitus, dry mouth, and dilated pupils. Second-generation H$_1$-blockers (e.g., terfenadine, astemizole) can cause Q-T interval prolongation and torsades de pointes (see Chapter 81). H$_2$-blockers can have significant effects on the hepatic metabolism of drugs and alcohol absorption.

Recognition

An overview of the side effects associated with antihistamines is provided in Table 25-1. A more detailed description of the physiology behind these effects follows.

H$_1$-BLOCKERS

H$_1$-receptor antagonists competitively inhibit the interaction of histamine with the H$_1$-receptor, thereby inhibiting the vasodilator effects of histamine and preventing the occurrence of edema, flare, and wheal. H$_1$-antagonists are taken primarily for acute allergies that present as rhinitis, urticaria, congestion, or conjunctivitis. However, H$_1$-receptor antagonists may not oppose histamine-induced allergic bronchoconstriction, anaphylaxis, laryngeal edema, or angioedema. This is probably due to the involvement of other mediators (e.g., leukotriene, platelet-activating factor). H$_1$-antagonists are well absorbed from the gastrointestinal tract, and they are metabolized by the hepatic microsomal

Table 25–1 ■ Adverse Reactions to Antihistamines

Reaction Type	First-Generation H$_1$-Blockers	Second-Generation H$_1$-Blockers	H$_2$-Blockers
Cardiovascular	Tachycardia; no vasodilatation or vasoconstriction	Long Q-T interval; torsades de pointes	With rapid IV administration: decreased blood pressure, bradycardia, potential asystole
Nervous system	Adults: sedation, dry mouth, seizures, tremors, confusion Children: fixed, dilated pupils; flushed face; fever; possible coma	Minimal	Coma, headaches (famotidine), dizziness, drowsiness, confusion, seizures, agitation
Genitourinary, gastrointestinal, endocrine, skin, miscellaneous	Urinary retention; diarrhea, nausea, vomiting, constipation; no endocrine effects; allergic dermatitis (topical application)	Minimal genitourinary or endocrine effects; diarrhea or constipation	Transient ↑ serum creatinine; constipation or diarrhea; ↓ hepatic blood flow, gastric acidity; rare hepatotoxicity (ranitidine); gynecomastia; impotence (cimetidine); can facilitate bacterial infection
Interactions	Potentiated by alcohol	Potentiated by cytochrome P-450 inhibitors	Cimetidine inhibits cytochrome P-450; ↑ alcohol absorption

92

P-450 system. Most H_1-antagonists induce hepatic microsomal enzymes to facilitate their metabolism. The metabolites, whether active or inactive, are renally excreted.

The newer types of H_1-receptor antagonists (second-generation or specific H_1-blockers) were designed to eliminate the unwanted central nervous system and anticholinergic side effects of older H_1-blockers.

H_2-BLOCKERS

Histamine binds to the H_2-receptors located on the acid-secreting gastric parietal cells. This initiates a cascade that eventually increases the intracellular cyclic adenosine monophosphate (cAMP). Cyclic AMP activates the hydrogen-potassium pump, causing secretion of hydrogen ions. H_2-receptor antagonists are competitive inhibitors of histamine at H_2-receptors, thereby reducing acid secretion. Currently there are several H_2-blockers approved in the United States for the treatment of duodenal and gastric ulcer disease. They are all orally absorbed but have different degrees of bioavailability. Cimetidine and ranitidine are eliminated primarily by hepatic metabolism through cytochrome P-450 enzymes. Famotidine and nizatidine are primarily renally excreted.

Risk Assessment and Implications

H_1-BLOCKERS

As noted earlier, the elderly are especially prone to the anticholinergic side effects of older H_1-blockers. Urinary retention, confusion, hallucinations, tremors, dry mouth, and tachycardia may occur in older patients, even with moderate amounts of first-generation antihistamines. At higher doses, the central excitatory effects may cause convulsions. Concurrent ingestion of alcohol can potentiate the sedative effects of older H_1-blockers.

In contrast, second-generation H_1-blockers have a minimal effect on muscarinic receptors. They do not cross the blood-brain barrier and thus have a less sedating effect. However, the second-generation H_1-blockers (terfenadine, astemizole) can prolong the Q-Tc interval, which on rare occasion can cause polymorphic ventricular tachycardia. The latter in association with Q-Tc interval prolongation is known as torsades de pointes (see Chapter 81). Hepatic dysfunction or the coadministration of drugs that inhibit cytochrome P-450 (e.g., erythromycin, clarithromycin, ketoconazole, itraconazole) can also prolong the Q-Tc interval and trigger torsades de pointes.

H_2-BLOCKERS

H_2-blockers are relatively safe when the manufacturer's prescribing guidelines are followed. Cimetidine inhibits cytochrome P-450. This can impair the metabolism and potentiate the actions of certain drugs (e.g., phenytoin,

carbamazepine, quinidine, nifedipine, theophylline, warfarin, tricyclic antidepressants). Cimetidine and ranitidine inhibit the renal excretion of procainamide and its metabolite N-acylprocainamide to increase their plasma concentrations. Further, cimetidine, ranitidine, and nizatidine may potentiate the absorption of alcohol by inhibiting gastric alcohol dehydrogenase. Renal dysfunction can potentially increase the plasma levels of H_2-blockers, which may contribute to a lower threshold for adverse effects.

MANAGEMENT

Therapy for anticholinergic side effects of first-generation H_1-blocking antihistamines is supportive. Each adverse effect must be addressed and treated separately. The drug causing the adverse side effects must be stopped immediately. With urinary retention, a Foley catheter should be inserted. If the patient has coronary artery disease or cardiovascular instability, tachycardia is treated with β-blockers or calcium channel blockers. The patient should be reassured about the transient central nervous system effects of diphenhydramine and closely monitored. Management for torsades de pointes with second-generation H_1-blockers is discussed in Chapter 81.

PREVENTION

Avoid giving antihistamines to patients at increased risk for their adverse side effects. First-generation H_1-blockers should be avoided in the elderly. Patients receiving first-generation H_1-blockers and H_2-blockers should avoid alcohol. Second-generation H_1-blockers should not be given to persons with Q-Tc interval prolongation; this advice may apply to those susceptible to ventricular tachyarrhythmias (or with a history thereof) as well, although there is no concrete evidence to back this recommendation. One must consider potential drug interactions (see Table 25-1), and doses should be adjusted on the basis of underlying renal or hepatic diseases.

Further Reading

Feldman M: Pros and cons of over-the-counter availability of histamine-2 receptor antagonists. Arch Intern Med 153:2415-2418, 1993.

Kosoglou T, Vlasses PH: Drug interactions involving renal transport mechanisms: An overview. Ann Pharmacother 23:116-122, 1989.

Sax MJ: Clinically important adverse effects and drug interactions with H-2 antagonists: An update. Pharmacotherapy 7:110S-115S, 1987.

Simons FER, Simons KJ: H₁-receptor antagonist treatment of chronic rhinitis. J Allergy Clin Immunol 81:975-980, 1988.

Simons FER, Simons KJ: The pharmacology and use of H₁ receptor-antagonist drugs. N Engl J Med 330:1663-1670, 1994.

Woosley RL, Chen Y, Freiman JP: Mechanism of the cardiotoxic actions of terfenadine. JAMA 269:1532-1536, 1993.

α₂-Adrenoreceptor Agonists

26

R. Victor Zhang

Case Synopsis

A 44-year-old woman presents for an abdominal incisional hernia repair. She is on several medications for hypertension, including oral clonidine (0.3 mg twice daily), which she did not take on the day of surgery. On preoperative examination, her blood pressure is 195/95 mm Hg, and her heart rate is 86 beats per minute. Surgery under general anesthesia proceeds uneventfully. On awakening, the patient has excellent pain control with narcotics, but her blood pressure has increased to 230/120 mm Hg, with a heart rate of 110 to 120 beats per minute. She is treated with intravenous (IV) boluses of labetalol and hydralazine and an IV infusion of esmolol. An IV bolus of clonidine 100 µg is also given but does not provide immediate hemodynamic improvement.

PROBLEM ANALYSIS

Definition

The case synopsis typifies rebound hypertension after the abrupt withdrawal of clonidine in a patient with hypertension. The stress response associated with surgery under general anesthesia makes clonidine withdrawal more pronounced and difficult to control.

Clonidine is a centrally acting α₂-adrenoreceptor agonist (α₂-agonist). It is commonly used by anesthesiologists and critical care physicians to treat patients with hypertension. In addition, it is used as a preanesthesia medication owing to its sedative, anxiolytic, hemodynamic, analgesic, antisialagogic, and anesthetic-sparing properties. A newer, more selective, and shorter acting α₂-agonist, dexmedetomidine, has a similar pharmacologic profile to clonidine and is increasingly used in general anesthesia and intensive care settings. α₂-Agonists reduce sympathetic tone, as well as plasma aldosterone and catecholamine concentrations and plasma renin activity. Perioperatively, these agents reduce heart rate, cardiac output, hypertension, and myocardial ischemia. They also improve survival in high-risk patients undergoing noncardiac surgery. Also, clonidine is used in conjunction with local anesthetics in neuraxial and peripheral nerve blocks to enhance and prolong analgesia. α₂-Agonists are becoming more important as anesthetic adjuncts and analgesics. Clonidine is also used in therapy for withdrawal from alcohol, nicotine, and benzodiazepines, as well as in narcotic detoxification. Further, it has been used successfully in the treatment of migraine headaches, Tourette's syndrome, attention-deficit disorder, premenstrual tension, and diabetic diarrhea.

Perioperative use of α₂-agonists is associated with adverse effects, including the following:

- Increased incidence of hypotension and bradycardia during anesthesia
- Transient hypertension following rapid IV administration
- Mild respiratory depression
- Rebound hypertension on abrupt withdrawal

Hypotension and bradycardia during anesthesia are caused by the sympatholytic and anesthetic-sparing properties of α₂-agonists. They often occur when dosages of other anesthetic agents and adjuncts are not properly adjusted in patients receiving α₂-agonists. Transient hypertension after rapid IV injection of α₂-agonists is due to direct binding with postsynaptic, vascular smooth muscle α₂-adrenergic receptors. This causes vasoconstriction in peripheral resistance vessels via an endothelium-independent process. α₂-Agonist-mediated respiratory depression is often mild, except at high doses or in association with other sedatives or narcotics. Rebound hypertension after abrupt cessation of α₂-agonists is due to sympathetic hyperactivity. It occurs most often with clonidine, especially after prolonged use. It may produce a hypertensive crisis that is accompanied by other signs of sympathetic hyperactivity, such as nervousness, tachycardia, headache, and sweating.

Recognition

Adverse effects of α₂-agonists are related primarily to the extension of their pharmacologic activities, especially when compounded by the effects of anesthetics and anesthetic adjuncts. Thus, knowledge of potentially untoward perioperative physiologic effects is necessary for the recognition, management, and prevention of adverse effects of α₂-agonists. These drugs exert their effects mainly via activation of presynaptic α₂-adrenoreceptors in various locations in the central nervous system, especially within the brainstem. This results in a decreased efferent sympathetic outflow, with reduced blood pressure and heart rate, along with sedative, anxiolytic, and anesthetic-sparing effects that are often desirable during the perioperative period.

Most adverse effects from α₂-agonists are hemodynamic. In this case, early detection relies on close monitoring of blood pressure, heart rate, and electrocardiogram (ECG).

Sinus bradycardia is the most common form of bradycardia caused by α₂-agonists. However, atrioventricular (AV) junctional and ventricular escape rhythms (bradycardia) and high-degree AV heart block can also occur. Therefore, the ECG is important for its ability to detect cardiac rhythm changes.

Blood pressure and heart rate should be closely monitored in patients receiving α₂-agonists, especially during induction and maintenance of anesthesia. For patients with poorly controlled hypertension, especially those on clonidine, an arterial line should be considered for perioperative blood pressure monitoring.

The preoperative interview should focus on the patient's history of hypertension and medications to control it, to identify those at high risk for clonidine withdrawal. Close monitoring of blood pressure and heart rate should continue for several hours postoperatively in such patients. In awake patients, other signs of clonidine withdrawal, such as nervousness, headache, and sweating, can aid in the diagnosis.

Respiratory depression from α₂-agonists is normally mild. Nevertheless, for patients sedated with an α₂-agonist, respiratory rate and pulse oximetry must be monitored.

Risk Assessment

All α₂-agonists cause sympatholysis, which results in decreased sympathetic outflow. Patients whose hemodynamic stability depends on increased sympathetic tone are at increased risk for severe hypotension with α₂-agonists, especially those with anemia, hypovolemia, or heart failure. Patients with sinus node dysfunction or AV conduction delay or block are also at increased risk for severe bradycardia or complete AV block when treated with α₂-agonists. Anesthetic adjuncts with sympatholytic properties, such as high doses of a potent narcotic, also increase the risk of bradycardia in patients receiving α₂-agonists, especially during anesthesia induction.

The risk of hypotension and bradycardia is also significantly increased if the anesthesiologist fails to take into account the anesthetic-sparing effect of α₂-agonists and properly reduce the dose of IV or volatile anesthetic agents. Another risk factor for hypotension and bradycardia is renal insufficiency, which reduces the renal clearance of α₂-agonists. Patients older than 65 years are also at increased risk for hypotension and bradycardia due to age-related renal insufficiency and reduced cardiovascular compensation. Transient hypertension after rapid IV injection of α₂-agonists is enhanced in patients with hypertension, who are more sensitive to vasoconstrictors. Avoiding such rapid IV injections can reduce transient hypertension.

Sudden cessation of clonidine can cause worrisome and sometimes severe rebound hypertension. The risk of this withdrawal response is higher in patients who have been chronically treated with clonidine, especially at high doses. It can occur from 8 to 36 hours after the last dose. Rebound hypertension is also possible after stopping guanfacine, another α₂-agonist, but it occurs later (2 to 4 days) and with less frequency, presumably owing to its longer half-life.

Respiratory depression from α₂-agonists is often mild. However, at high doses or with other sedative-narcotics, deep sedation and respiratory depression can occur, especially in the elderly.

Implications

Bradycardia or hypotension from α₂-agonists is usually mild. These conditions can be treated effectively with anticholinergics or positive chronotropes and therefore do not present serious problems. In contrast, severe bradycardia and hypotension are associated with a significant reduction in cardiac output and compromised perfusion to vital organs. Owing to the prevalence of hypertension and coronary artery disease in the elderly, these patients are at increased risk for myocardial and cerebral ischemia.

Clonidine withdrawal is especially worrisome in the elderly. Rebound hypertension increases the risk of cerebral hemorrhage. Hypertension and tachycardia increase myocardial oxygen consumption, possibly leading to myocardial ischemia or infarction. Hypertension after rapid IV boluses of α₂-agonists can be more pronounced in patients with hypertension. Although transient, this too increases the risk for adverse cardiovascular events.

Mild sedation and respiratory depression can be well tolerated in healthy patients. However, those with hypertension or coronary artery disease are at increased risk for myocardial and cerebral ischemia.

MANAGEMENT

Bradycardia is treated effectively with IV anticholinergics (e.g., atropine, glycopyrrolate). IV ephedrine is also useful, especially with associated hypotension. However, ephedrine's action is brief, so it may not be effective for bradycardia of long duration. Vasoconstrictors and IV fluids are used for α₂-agonist-mediated hypotension. Because this is due to sympatholysis, α₁-adrenergic agonists, especially phenylephrine, can reverse hypotension. Ephedrine has both α₁- and β-agonist effects and is sometimes used to reverse α₂-agonist-mediated hypotension.

The anesthetic-sparing effect of α₂-agonists likely contributes to hypotension and bradycardia during induction or maintenance of general anesthesia. Hemodynamics are stabilized with IV fluids and vasoconstrictors, along with readjustment of anesthetic dosing.

Transient hypertension from overly rapid IV injection of α₂-agonists is often mild and followed by hypotension from central α₂-adrenoreceptor activation. Treatment with long-acting antihypertensive agents can result in undesired hypotension.

For rebound hypertension, labetalol is a good choice owing to its ability to block α- and β-adrenergic receptors. Labetalol alone might be inadequate to control hypertension and tachycardia; more selective β-blockers (e.g., metoprolol, esmolol, atenolol) are often needed to control tachycardia. β-Blockers should not be used alone, however, because they can worsen hypertension due to unopposed vasoconstriction from peripheral α-adrenergic activity. β-Blockers may even increase the risk of rebound hypertension with abrupt clonidine withdrawal. Vasodilators (e.g., hydralazine, dihydropyridine calcium channel blockers) are often required to control hypertension. Also, IV infusions of nitroglycerine or sodium nitroprusside are options for uncontrolled severe hypertension. IV clonidine is another option, but it does not offer immediate relief for rebound hypertension and has the potential to aggravate hypertension transiently; subsequently, it may cause hypotension and bradycardia.

PREVENTION

Awareness of the potential adverse effects of α_2-agonists and their proper management is the key to preventing complications associated with their use. Dosages for IV anesthetic induction agents and volatile anesthetics must be adjusted downward. For patients at increased risk for bradycardia and hypotension, α_2-agonists should not be used at all or should be given in smaller doses. Avoiding the rapid IV injection of clonidine or high doses of dexmedetomidine helps prevent transient hypertension with α_2-agonists.

To prevent adrenergic hyperactivity with withdrawal, patients receiving α_2-agonists should continue therapy throughout the perioperative period. If the α_2-agonist must be discontinued, this should be done over 1 week. For patients at risk for rebound hypertension, a transdermal clonidine patch may be applied preoperatively to abate perioperative sympathetic hyperactivity. Parenteral agents are also used to prevent rebound hypertension (e.g., labetalol, esmolol, propranolol, hydralazine, diltiazem, dihydropyridine calcium channel blockers, nitrates).

Finally, severe respiratory depression is rare with therapeutic α_2-agonist doses. For patients receiving other sedatives or narcotics, these must be used with caution to avoid overly deep sedation or severe respiratory depression.

Further Reading

Ghignone M, Calvillo O, Quintin L: Anesthesia and hypertension: The effect of clonidine on perioperative hemodynamics and isoflurane requirements. Anesthesiology 67:3-10, 1987.

Ghignone M, Quintin L, Duke PC, et al: Effects of clonidine on narcotic requirements and hemodynamic response during induction of fentanyl anesthesia. Anesthesiology 64:36-42, 1986.

Husserl FE, Messerli FH: Adverse effects of antihypertensive drugs. Drugs 22:188-210, 1981.

Kamibayashi T, Maze M: Clinical uses of α_2-adrenergic agonists. Anesthesiology 93:1345-1349, 2000.

Levitan D, Massry SG, Romoff M, et al: Plasma catecholamines and autonomic nervous system function in patients with early renal insufficiency and hypertension: Effect of clonidine. Nephron 36:24-29,1984.

Manhem P, Paalzow L, Hökfelt B: Plasma clonidine in relation to blood pressure, catecholamines, and renin activity during long-term treatment of hypertension. Clin Pharmacol Ther 31:445-451, 1982.

Mercado DL, Petty BG: Perioperative medication management. Med Clin North Am 87:41-57, 2003.

Talke P, Lobo E, Brown R: Systemically administered α_2-agonist-induced peripheral vasoconstriction in humans. Anesthesiology 99:65-70, 2003.

Talke PO, Lobo EP, Brown R, et al: Clonidine-induced vasoconstriction in awake volunteers. Anesth Analg 93:271-276, 2001.

Weber MA: Discontinuation syndrome following cessation of treatment with clonidine and other antihypertensive agents. J Cardiovasc Pharmacol 2(Suppl 1):S73-S89, 1980.

Weitz HH: Perioperative cardiac complications. Med Clin North Am 85:1151-1169, 2001.

Wijeysundera DN, Naik JS, Beattie WS: Alpha-2 adrenergic agonists to prevent perioperative cardiovascular complications: A meta-analysis. Am J Med 114:742-752, 2003.

MISCELLANEOUS DRUGS AND RELATED TOPICS

Anaphylaxis and Anaphylactoid Reactions

27

David G. Bjoraker

Case Synopsis

A 40-year-old man has brachial plexus block with a lidocaine-tetracaine mixture containing a 1:200,000 concentration of epinephrine. Initially he complains of dizziness, difficulty breathing, and retrosternal chest discomfort. He rapidly develops acute respiratory distress and pulmonary edema, urticaria over the blocked extremity and shoulder, and marked hypotension.

PROBLEM ANALYSIS

Definition

Parenteral medications may cause anaphylaxis. Although it varies in severity, anaphylaxis is the most severe of the immediate hypersensitivity reactions. Anaphylactic shock refers to the complete cardiovascular collapse that may result. The classic anaphylactic reaction is mediated by immunoglobulin E (IgE) antibodies formed in response to prior exposure to a foreign antigen. In many cases, low-molecular-weight drugs are too small to be antigenic alone, but they may combine as haptens with endogenous protein carriers to form an antigenic complex.

In the early 20th century, Richet and Portier administered large doses of sea anemone toxin to dogs. The animals survived the initial dose but died within minutes when given a minute dose weeks later. They termed this phenomenon *anaphylaxis,* indicating that attempted immunization failed to provide prophylaxis against sea anemone toxin.

Anaphylactoid reactions may be clinically indistinguishable from anaphylactic reactions. The same chemical mediators released via the IgE-antigen pathway in anaphylaxis are also released by nonimmunologic mechanisms in anaphylactoid reactions.

Recognition

DRUG REACTIONS: ALLERGIC AND NONALLERGIC

Drug reactions are common during anesthesia, but less than 10% are true allergic reactions. Nonallergic drug reactions are generally predictable, dose dependent, and related to the known properties of the drug. Often the reactions are either enhanced desired effects or side effects of the drug resulting from overdosage, inadvertent route of administration, impaired elimination, low individual tolerance, or interaction with another drug. Allergic drug reactions are generally not predictable, not dose dependent, and not related to the pharmacology of the drug.

CLINICAL MANIFESTATIONS OF ANAPHYLAXIS

The clinical manifestations of anaphylaxis depend on the route of administration of the antigen or hapten, as well as the exact type, quantity, and anatomic site of the various physiologic mediators released (Table 27-1) and the end-organ responses to them. These mediators result from the initial degranulation of mast cells and basophils and the ensuing biochemical events. Symptoms of anaphylaxis occur within 2 to 20 minutes of exposure to the antigen or hapten and may persist for up to 36 hours. Before induction and during regional anesthesia and monitored anesthesia care, both symptoms (Table 27-2) and signs (Table 27-3) of an allergic reaction can facilitate an early diagnosis. After the induction of general anesthesia, however, the patient cannot express symptoms and is hidden from view by the surgical drapes; in this case, serious respiratory and cardiovascular signs are often the first indicators of anaphylaxis. In addition, many signs, such as tachypnea, laryngeal edema, small increases in

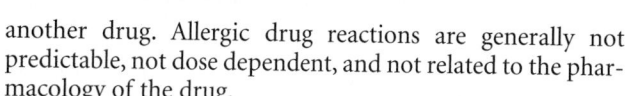

Table 27–1 ▪ Mediators Released during Anaphylaxis

Complement (C3a, C5a anaphylatoxins)
Heparin
Histamine
Kinins
Leukoagglutinins
Leukotrienes
Lysosomal enzymes
Platelet-activating factor
Prostaglandins and other arachidonic acid metabolites
Serotonin

Table 27–2 ■ Symptoms of Anaphylaxis

Cutaneous
   Pruritus
   Burning
   Tingling
Respiratory
   Nasal stuffiness
   Breathing difficulty
   Chest tightness, discomfort
Cardiovascular
   Dizziness
   Malaise; confusion
   Retrosternal oppression
Other Organ Systems
   Aura
   Nausea
   Abdominal pain

bronchial tone, and early decreases in systemic vascular resistance, may be obscured by anesthetic drugs and management.

DIFFERENTIAL AND LABORATORY DIAGNOSES

Generally, the differential diagnosis of anaphylaxis is not difficult owing to the immediacy of the response after exposure to a foreign antigen or hapten. Because anaphylaxis is a systemic condition, signs in multiple organ systems differentiate it from a primary cardiac event or sudden exacerbation of bronchospasm in patients with asthma. Differentiation of anaphylactic and anaphylactoid reactions is academic, because the immediate medical management is identical.

Table 27–3 ■ Signs of Anaphylaxis

Cutaneous
   Urticaria (hives); angioedema
   Erythema (flushing)
   Periorbital, facial edema
Respiratory
   Coughing; sneezing
   Hoarseness
   Perioral and intraoral edema
   Laryngeal edema; stridor
   Intercostal and substernal retractions
   Cyanosis
   Tachypnea
   Wheezing
   Reduced pulmonary compliance
   Pulmonary edema
   Acute respiratory distress
Cardiovascular
   Diaphoresis
   Hypotension
   Tachycardia
   Arrhythmias
   Reduced systemic vascular resistance
   Pulmonary hypertension
Other Organ Systems
   Vomiting
   Diarrhea
   Acute intravascular coagulation

Laboratory diagnosis of anaphylaxis is retrospective, owing to the rapidity of its onset; after a reaction, however, several uncommon tests may substantiate its diagnosis. Circulating complement C3 and C5 activation products (C3a, C3d, and C5a) may be increased. IgE blood concentrations may be reduced, and plasma histamine concentrations may be briefly elevated. In addition, the concentration of tryptase, a protease released from mast cells, may be increased. If multiple drug exposures occur in close temporal proximity to an anaphylactic reaction, these tests will not assist in differentiating the causative agent.

Risk Assessment

All patients receiving parenteral drugs are at risk for anaphylaxis, but those with a notable allergic history or atopy have a greater risk. The risk of an allergic reaction to a drug is approximately 1% to 3%. Anaphylaxis occurs in about 1 of 4000 to 25,000 anesthetic administrations.

Table 27-4 lists drugs and other agents frequently used in the perioperative period that may cause anaphylactic or anaphylactoid reactions. For induction agents used in the United States, severe allergic reactions are uncommon. Neuromuscular relaxants are the most common cause of allergic reactions (about two thirds) during anesthesia. Neuromuscular relaxants such as atracurium, cisatracurium, tubocurarine, doxacurium, metocurine, and mivacurium occasionally cause signs of an allergic response due to non-immunologic histamine release. Morphine, meperidine, and codeine also may release sufficient amounts of histamine to be confused with an allergic reaction. Other materials that come into contact with the patient, such as vascular graft material, methylmethacrylate bone cement, chlorhexidine, and latex rubber, have been implicated in anaphylactoid reactions. Latex allergy is the second most common cause of anaphylaxis during anesthesia (approximately one eighth of cases), and antibiotics are the third most common cause.

Implications

An allergic reaction during anesthesia is usually unexpected and may range from a mild urticarial reaction to anaphylactic shock with cardiorespiratory arrest. Although a patient's preexisting medical conditions may affect or otherwise complicate therapy, a fatal outcome can also occur in patients classified as status I or II by the American Society of Anesthesiologists (ASA) system.

MANAGEMENT

Management of anaphylaxis and anaphylactoid reactions includes the following:

- Removal or reduction of the offending agent
- Aggressive airway management
- Circulatory management: volume, epinephrine
- Adjunct pharmacologic management

If an anaphylactic or anaphylactoid reaction is suspected, the administration of any possible causative agents should

Table 27–4 ■ Perioperative Drugs and Other Factors Associated with Anaphylactic or Anaphylactoid Reactions

Anesthetic Agents

Induction agents used in the United States
- Barbiturates
- Benzodiazepines
- Etomidate
- Ketamine
- Propofol

Induction agents not approved in the United States but used elsewhere
- Althesin
- Propanidid

Neuromuscular relaxants
- Succinylcholine (see Chapter 23)
- Nondepolarizing neuromuscular relaxants (see Chapter 24)

Opioids
- True allergic reactions and systemic anaphylactoid reactions to opioids are rare
- Anaphylactoid reactions have been reported after IV morphine or codeine (rare)

Local anesthetics
- Para-aminobenzoic ester local anesthetics
- Amide local anesthetics (rare)
- Methylparaben or propylparaben preservatives
- Sulfite, bisulfite, or metabisulfite antioxidants

Other Drugs and Miscellaneous Products

Antibiotics
- Aminoglycosides
- Amphotericin B
- Cephalosporins
- Nitrofurantoin
- Penicillin
- Tetracycline
- Vancomycin

Intravenous fluids, blood products, volume expanders, hemostatics
- Albumin, dextran, hetastarch, purified protein fraction
- Aprotinin, protamine, vitamin K (phytonadione)
- Blood and blood products (all)
- Hypertonic solutions*: mannitol, sodium bicarbonate

Dyes
- Isosulfan blue, methylene blue, iodinated radiopaque contrast dyes*

Hormones
- Corticosteroids
- Insulin
- Vasopressin

Immunosuppressive agents
- Cyclosporin
- FK-506
- Antithymocyte globulin

Latex

Nonsteroidal anti-inflammatory drugs*
- Acetylsalicylic acid
- Aminopyrine
- Indomethacin

Other drugs
- Chlorhexidine
- Chymopapain
- Streptokinase
- Tetanus antitoxin

*Usually anaphylactoid reactions.

be stopped immediately. Although a reaction is not strictly dose dependent, the less antigen or triggering agent administered, the better the situation. Also, use of a venous extremity tourniquet can prevent subcutaneously and intramuscularly administered antigenic or triggering material from reaching the central circulation.

Oxygenation is monitored by pulse oximetry, and supplemental oxygen is used if necessary. Airway edema can progress rapidly, so the airway must be carefully and continuously monitored. Anesthesiologists should be predisposed to early endotracheal intubation.

Discontinuation of general anesthesia is advised to help stabilize the circulatory dynamics, and rapid intravascular volume expansion should be started. Epinephrine is the drug of choice for hypotension because it attenuates associated mediator release and counters bronchospasm. In selecting a dose, the patient's current hemodynamic state must be considered; doses range from an initial intravenous bolus of 0.2 to 1 μg/kg for moderate hypotension to 3 to 15 μg/kg intravenously for circulatory collapse. Repeated administration or an infusion is appropriate and often necessary.

Other adjunct therapy may help after initial stability is achieved. If further antigen will likely be introduced into the central circulation, antihistamines (e.g., diphenhydramine 0.5 to 0.7 mg/kg or cimetidine 4 to 6 mg/kg) and corticosteroids (e.g., methylprednisolone 15 to 25 mg/kg or hydrocortisone 4 to 15 mg/kg) should be considered. For bronchospasm, along with β-adrenergic aerosols (e.g., albuterol), aminophylline 5 to 6 mg/kg over 20 minutes, followed by an infusion at 0.5 to 1 mg/kg per hour, may be useful. Sodium bicarbonate is used to correct measured acidosis.

The Joint Task Force on Practice Parameters has published diagnostic and management guidelines for anaphylaxis (see "Further Reading"). Although not limited to intraoperative anaphylaxis, these guidelines recognize that anaphylaxis is a significant perioperative problem, and they provide a broader context for patient care both before and after anesthesia.

PREVENTION

Prevention includes avoiding risky practice patterns, as well as the following measures:

- Intradermal skin testing
- Radioallergosorbent test (RAST)

- Leukocyte histamine release test
- Pharmacologic prophylaxis

The ultimate prevention of anaphylaxis and anaphylactoid reactions would be the elimination of exposure to all foreign materials, substances, and drugs, which of course is absurd. The practical approach is to prevent re-exposure to known allergens and to avoid risky patterns of practice, such as the repeated use of aprotinin or dextran infusions without the prior use of dextran 1 (Promit) or the use of a nonsteroidal anti-inflammatory drug when another such drug has caused a serious reaction. A careful history of prior incidents should be obtained, including review of the medical records and discussion with medical personnel who treated a previous reaction. If avoidance of a reactive drug compromises medical treatment, pretesting should be performed before actual use. Fortunately, an acceptable anesthetic regimen can almost always be formulated that excludes any questionable agents.

Skin testing is the least expensive and most widely used method for pretesting anesthetic drugs. Fisher and Doig described intradermal skin testing for anesthetic agents and recommended dilution—usually a 1:1000 to 1:10,000 dilution of the commercial concentration. However, the irritant effect of the injection or direct histamine release by opioids or muscle relaxants may result in false-positive findings. False-negative findings are also possible, especially if the patient uses antihistamines or sympathomimetic preparations. Because anaphylaxis can occur in response to even small quantities (0.02 mL) of an agent, even when diluted 1000-fold, resuscitation agents and skilled personnel must be readily available.

In vitro testing is much more convenient and completely safe for the patient. RAST is the most useful test and involves exposure of the patient's serum to the questionable allergen. The latter is bound to an insoluble, drug allergen-matrix complex, and if the patient is capable of reacting to the allergen, his or her serum IgE will bind to the drug allergen-matrix complex as well. To measure the quantity of the patient's serum IgE bound to the drug allergen-matrix complex, they are combined with radiolabeled antihuman IgE, and the radioactivity is measured. A low level of radioactivity indicates high occupation of the drug allergen-matrix complex by the patient's serum IgE, or true allergy. Conversely, a high level of radioactivity indicates unlikely allergy. However, a deficiency of RAST is that many drug allergen-matrix complexes are not available commercially.

Another in vitro test, the leukocyte histamine release test, does not require commercial allergen-matrix complexes. This test is conducted through direct exposure of a suspension of the patient's leukocytes to the allergen. Histamine release is measured fluorometrically or with a radioenzymatic assay.

For patients requiring treatment with a drug that has previously caused an allergic or anaphylactoid response, or

for atopic patients with multiple drug allergies, pharmacologic prophylaxis may be required. For anaphylactoid reactions to iodinated radiopaque contrast material, Greenberger and colleagues recommended the following protocol:

- Ephedrine 25 mg and H_1-receptor blockade (diphenhydramine 50 mg orally or intramuscularly) 1 hour before exposure
- Prednisone 50 mg 13 hours, 7 hours, and 1 hour before exposure
- Another 25 mg of oral ephedrine just before exposure, unless contraindicated

H_2-blockade with cimetidine also was examined but was not found to be helpful.

Recommendations for drug pretreatment in other situations are anecdotal and similar to those for radiocontrast material. H_2-blockade in other circumstances can be achieved with 4 to 6 mg/kg of cimetidine or 1 to 2 mg/kg of ranitidine, preferably started 24 hours before exposure. Terbutaline, a β_2-adrenergic agonist, and cromolyn sodium (which blocks the release of histamine and other autacoids from basophils and mast cells) have been proposed as prophylactic treatment, but their role in preventing anaphylactic or anaphylactoid reactions is unproved.

Further Reading

Ebo DG, Hagendorens MM, Bridts CH, et al: Allergic reactions occurring during anaesthesia: Diagnostic approach. Acta Clin Belg 59:34-43, 2004.
Fisher MM, Doig GS: Prevention of anaphylactic reactions to anaesthetic drugs. Drug Saf 27:393-410, 2004.
Fukuda K: Intravenous opioid anesthetics. In Miller RD (ed): Miller's Anesthesia, 6th ed. Philadelphia, Churchill Livingstone, 2005, pp 379-437.
Greenberger PA, Patterson R, Tapio CM: Prophylaxis against repeated radiocontrast media reactions in 857 cases: Adverse experience with cimetidine and safety of β-adrenergic antagonists. Arch Intern Med 145:2197-2200, 1985.
Gutstein HB, Akil H: Opioid analgesics. In Hardman JG, Limbird LE (eds): Goodman and Gilman's The Pharmacological Basis of Therapeutics, 10th ed. New York, McGraw-Hill, 2001, pp 569-619.
Joint Task Force on Practice Parameters, American Academy of Allergy, Asthma and Immunology; American College of Allergy, Asthma and Immunology; Joint Council of Allergy, Asthma and Immunology: The diagnosis and management of anaphylaxis: An updated practice parameter. J Allergy Clin Immunol 115:S483-S523, 2005.
Levy JH: Anaphylactic Reactions in Anesthesia and Intensive Care, 2nd ed. Stoneham, Mass, Butterworth-Heinemann, 1992.
Mertes PM, Laxenaire MC: Allergic reactions occurring during anaesthesia. Eur J Anaesthesiol 19:240-262, 2002.
Moneret-Vautrin DA, Kanny G: Anaphylaxis to muscle relaxants: Rationale for skin tests. Allerg Immunol (Paris) 34:233-240, 2002.
Pepys J, Whitwam JG, Baldo BA, et al: Anaphylactic/anaphylactoid reactions to anaesthetic and associated agents: Skin prick tests in aetiological diagnosis. Anaesthesia 49:470-475, 1994.
Soetens FM: Anaphylaxis during anaesthesia: Diagnosis and treatment. Acta Anaesthesiol Belg 55:229-237, 2004.
Terr AI: In vitro tests for immediate hypersensitivity. Annu Rev Med 39:135-145, 1988.

Antibiotics

Timothy E. Morey and Thomas S. Guyton

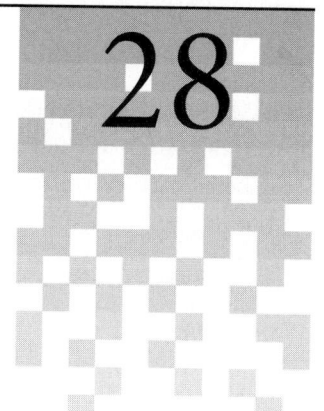

Case Synopsis

A 23-year-old man presents for reduction and fixation of an open tibial fracture after falling off a horse. Following thiopental and succinylcholine administration and successful endotracheal intubation, anesthesia is maintained with isoflurane, nitrous oxide 50% and oxygen 50%, and fentanyl 2 μg/kg per hour. The surgeon requests that the patient be given vancomycin 1 g before incision. Three minutes after vancomycin is given, the patient suffers cardiovascular collapse.

PROBLEM ANALYSIS

Definition

Anesthesiologists frequently administer antibiotic prophylaxis to surgical patients and should be knowledgeable about the indications, dosages, complications, and interactions between antibiotics and anesthetics and other medications used in the perioperative period. Antibiotics possess a diverse spectrum of side effects (Table 28-1) and interact with a number of anesthetic adjuvants. For these reasons, anesthesiologists must understand and anticipate possible complications associated with antibiotic administration.

Vancomycin is a glycopeptide antibiotic commonly used for bacterial prophylaxis in orthopedic, neurologic, and vascular surgery and as an alternative antibiotic for patients who are allergic to penicillins and cephalosporins. An unusual feature of vancomycin is its ability to nearly double histamine release from basophils and cutaneous mast cells through a poorly understood dose-dependent mechanism that is neither immunologic nor cytotoxic. The liberated histamine causes dilatation of peripheral blood vessels and simultaneously increases cardiac output, stroke volume, and pulmonary artery pressure. However, peripheral vascular dilatation is the most prominent physiologic feature and may induce severe hypotension and cardiovascular collapse. There have been several reports of hypotension and cardiac arrest during concurrent vancomycin and anesthesia administration, but cardiovascular collapse can also occur in unanesthetized patients receiving vancomycin.

Recognition

Recognition of vancomycin as the cause of hypotension relies primarily on the exclusion of other intraoperative events as the cause, the temporal relationship between cardiovascular instability and vancomycin infusion, and the observation of other manifestations of histamine release. Signs of elevated plasma levels of histamine include the following:

- "Red neck" or "red man" syndrome, consisting of cutaneous flushing, erythema, urticaria, pruritus, and maculopapular rash primarily on the face, neck, arms, and chest
- Perioral, periocular, and facial edema

- Bronchospasm due to stimulation of bronchial histamine receptors
- Hypoxia caused by histamine-induced inhibition of pulmonary vasoconstriction and subsequent formation of pulmonary shunts
- Systemic hypotension
- Pulseless electrical activity cardiac arrest (electromechanical dissociation)

In addition, a "pain and spasm" syndrome has been described following vancomycin infusion, but it is unknown whether this is a histamine-mediated complication or whether another mechanism is responsible. Anesthesiologists must be cognizant that contaminants in the vancomycin solution may cause a true anaphylactic reaction, although hypotension is much more likely to result from vancomycin-induced histamine release.

Risk Assessment

Because vancomycin-induced histamine release results from nonspecific degranulation of basophils or mast cells, it is classified as an anaphylactoid reaction, not anaphylaxis. That is, histamine liberation is mediated not by an immune system response but by an unclear mechanism. Consequently, a patient's risk for hypotension and cardiovascular collapse is independent of previous exposure to vancomycin, may occur with the first dose, and does not increase with multiple administrations of the antibiotic. Hence, a patient with a history of "red man" syndrome or vancomycin-induced hypotension can safely receive this antibiotic if it is administered appropriately.

Anesthesiologists may be concerned about a greater risk of hypotension when vancomycin and a volatile anesthetic are administered concurrently (i.e., vancomycin infusion after anesthetic induction), because both agents can potentially depress blood pressure. Although hypotension during vancomycin administration is more common in anesthetized than in nonanesthetized patients, this difference is probably due to more intensive monitoring and observer vigilance during anesthesia rather than an actual interaction between vancomycin and anesthetics.

In one study investigating hypotension during concurrent vancomycin and anesthetic administration in adult patients undergoing orthopedic surgery (see Von Kaenel under "Further Reading"), no difference was noted (either before

Table 28–1 ■ Complications of Antibiotics Used for Prophylaxis

Antibiotic	Common	Occasional	Rare
Aminoglycosides	Nephrotoxicity Ototoxicity	Rash Nausea, vomiting Potentiation of neuromuscular blockade	Peripheral neuritis Anaphylaxis Electrolyte disturbances
Cephalosporins	Painful when given IM	Nausea Drug fever Diarrhea Phlebitis	Anaphylaxis Hypotension Bronchospasm Angioedema Urticaria
Clindamycin		Diarrhea Pseudomembranous colitis Rash Metallic taste Inhibition of neuromuscular transmission Potentiation of neuromuscular blockade	Anaphylaxis Cardiac arrest Erythema Granulocytopenia Thrombocytopenia
Erythromycin	Phlebitis when given IV Painful when given IM	Nausea, vomiting Diarrhea Pseudomembranous colitis	Long QT syndrome Fever Rash Eosinophilia
Metronidazole	Nausea, vomiting Metallic taste Disulfiram-like reaction if alcohol consumed	Burning tongue Urethral/vaginal burning Dark urine Rash	Convulsions Ataxia Peripheral neuropathy Encephalopathy Cerebellar dysfunction
Penicillin G, ampicillin		Rash Drug fever Diarrhea Leukopenia	Anaphylaxis Bronchospasm Angioedema Electrolyte disturbances Interstitial nephritis
Trimethoprim-sulfamethoxazole		Rash	Erythema multiforme Diarrhea Aplastic anemia Neutropenia Thrombocytopenia Neutropenia
Vancomycin	Phlebitis Severe pain when given IM	"Red man" syndrome "Pain and spasm" syndrome Hypotension Anaphylaxis Nephrotoxicity Ototoxicity	

Adapted from Cheng EY, Nimphius N, Hennen CR: Antibiotic therapy and the anesthesiologist. J Clin Anesth 7:425-439, 1995.

or after anesthetic induction) in hemodynamic parameters, anesthetic depth, ephedrine use, or volume of intravenous fluid administration following an infusion of either vancomycin or a saline carrier solution over 30 to 60 minutes (Table 28-2). In contrast, children and patients undergoing cardiopulmonary bypass and coronary bypass grafting are apparently more sensitive to the vasodilating effects of vancomycin. Anesthetized pediatric patients demonstrated a 35% incidence of hypotension following vancomycin infusion. Likewise, 30% of adults undergoing cardiopulmonary bypass required a postbypass infusion of norepinephrine following the addition of vancomycin 500 mg to the cardiopulmonary bypass pump prime solution, compared with 7% in a control group given saline. However, vancomycin administration via aortic cannula using flow rates necessary for cardiopulmonary bypass (60 to 70 mL/kg per minute) is probably too rapid

to maintain hemodynamic stability even in some healthy patients.

Critically ill patients have a diminished risk of vancomycin-induced reactions compared with healthy patients presenting for elective procedures. Vancomycin 1 g infused over 30 minutes did not affect cardiac index, heart rate, blood pressure, pulmonary venous pressure, central venous pressure, systemic vascular resistance, or pulmonary vascular resistance in 16 hemodynamically stable patients who were given the antibiotic within 24 hours of coronary artery bypass grafting or cardiac valve replacement. Remarkably, little rise in histamine concentrations occurred, despite substantially elevated vancomycin concentrations. Failure to develop cardiovascular side effects may be explained in part by the depletion of histamine from its previous liberation in response to illness, perioperative stress, and protamine administration.

Table 28–2 ■ Complications of Vancomycin Administration before or after Induction of Anesthesia in Studies Noting Adverse Events

Study (Year)	Subjects	No. Preinduction	No. Postinduction	End Points (No. of Patients)
Blomstedt et al (1988)	Adults	—	169	"Red man" syndrome (6), hypotension (5), bronchospasm (1), hypoxia (1)
Von Kaenel et al (1993)	Adults	17	19	No differences in HR, BP, end-tidal enflurane concentration, ephedrine use, IV fluid administration compared with placebo
Odio et al (1984)	Children	—	20	"Red man" syndrome (7), hypotension (1)
Romanelli et al (1993)	Adults	30*	30*	No differences in HR, SBP, CVP, CO, SVR, or intraoperative fluid balance after anesthetic induction and before cardiopulmonary bypass, but higher HR and CO combined with lower BP, CVP, and SVR after cardiopulmonary bypass and surgery in patients receiving vancomycin compared with placebo; also, 9 of 30 patients receiving vancomycin required norepinephrine infusion, compared with 2 of 28 patients in the control group

*Patients received vancomycin both before anesthetic induction and at the initiation of cardiopulmonary bypass for coronary artery bypass grafting.
BP, blood pressure; CO, cardiac output; CVP, central venous pressure; HR, heart rate; SBP, systemic blood pressure; SVR, systemic vascular resistance.

Consistent with this hypothesis is an investigation that demonstrated significantly elevated histamine concentrations in 28 patients who were studied immediately after multiple traumatic injuries and compared with a control group. Alternatively, critically or chronically ill patients may possess a diminished response to histamine stimulation when compared with the response of healthy volunteers or patients presenting for ambulatory surgery. For example, patients with cancer exhibit less pruritus and diminished wheal and flare responses following an intradermal histamine challenge. Regardless, anesthesiologists would be prudent to carefully monitor such patients during vancomycin administration, because even mild or moderate hypotension may be poorly tolerated in critically ill patients.

Implications

Vancomycin can be safely administered to patients in the perioperative period either before or after induction of anesthesia. Prudent anesthesiologists follow the manufacturer's recommendations regarding the duration of vancomycin infusion, especially in patients at greater risk (e.g., children) or who poorly tolerate even mild hypotension (e.g., patients with aortic stenosis). Hemodynamic depression requires prompt detection and treatment to avoid potentially life-threatening cardiovascular collapse.

MANAGEMENT

Managing vancomycin-induced hypotension grows progressively more difficult the longer it takes to detect the drug's toxic effects, and detecting the toxic effects grows progressively more difficult the longer the drug is administered.

That is, treatment options should become more aggressive with later detection, greater histamine release, and more severe hypotension. Management options include the following:

- Discontinue or slow the vancomycin infusion.
- Administer an intravenous fluid bolus.
- Discontinue or decrease concentrations of other agents that are capable of inducing hypotension (e.g., anesthetics, sodium nitroprusside).
- Administer H_1-antihistamines (e.g., diphenhydramine).
- Consider inhaled β-agonists if bronchospasm is present.
- Administer vasopressors (e.g., ephedrine, phenylephrine, epinephrine) for severe hypotension.
- Initiate advanced cardiovascular life support maneuvers in the event of cardiac arrest.

PREVENTION

Histamine release and the severity of reactions during vancomycin administration are directly dependent on the rate of infusion. Consequently, vancomycin should be infused over 60 minutes to minimize adverse reactions, as recommended by the manufacturer. In a study of nonanesthetized patients, rapid vancomycin infusion (1 g over 10 minutes) caused a 25% to 50% decrease in systolic blood pressure lasting 2 to 3 minutes in 11 of 56 patients, whereas no hypotension was observed in patients receiving a slow vancomycin infusion (1 g over 30 minutes). The key element is slow administration over 30 to 60 minutes, which may be impractical when attempting to complete a dose before surgical incision or tourniquet inflation. In this situation, preoperative infusion may be warranted if there is insufficient time to safely infuse vancomycin. Regardless, frequent monitoring of blood pressure; observation of skin color of the head, neck, and trunk; and auscultation of breath sounds are necessary for prompt detection and treatment of vancomycin's toxic effects.

Finally, some patients with extreme sensitivity to vancomycin may require this antibiotic to treat infections with multidrug-resistant organisms. In this situation, protocols for vancomycin desensitization have been developed to allow this patient population to safely receive intravenous vancomycin. This treatment revolves around gradual desensitization of mast cells by gradually increasing the serum concentration of vancomycin. This can be accomplished in as little as 24 hours for acutely ill patients. This preventive protocol is, of course, reserved for patients in duress and requires planning before the day of surgery if operative prophylactic vancomycin administration is envisioned.

Further Reading

Cheng EY, Nimphius N, Hennen CR: Antibiotic therapy and the anesthesiologist. J Clin Anesth 7:425-439, 1995.

Levy JH, Kettlekamp N, Goertz P, et al: Histamine release by vancomycin: A mechanism for hypotension in man. Anesthesiology 67:122-125, 1987.

Polk RE: Anaphylactoid reactions to glycopeptide antibiotics. J Antimicrob Chemother 27B:17-29, 1991.

Romanelli VA, Howie MB, Myerowitz PD, et al: Intraoperative and postoperative effects of vancomycin administration in cardiac surgery patients: A prospective, double-blind, randomized trial. Crit Care Med 21:1124-1131, 1993.

Sokoll MD, Gergis SD: Antibiotics and neuromuscular function. Anesthesiology 55:148, 1981.

Stier GR, McGory RW, Spotnitz WD, Schwenzer KJ: Hemodynamic effects of rapid vancomycin infusion in critically ill patients. Anesth Analg 71:394-399, 1990.

Von Kaenel WE, Bloomfield EL, Amaranath L, Wilde AA: Vancomycin does not enhance hypotension under anesthesia. Anesth Analg 76:809-811, 1993.

Wazny LD, Daghigh B: Desensitization protocols for vancomycin hypersensitivity. Ann Pharmacother 35:1458-1464, 2001.

Antidepressants

Lisa Wise-Faberowski and Susan Black

29

MONOAMINE OXIDASE INHIBITORS

Case Synopsis

A 32-year-old woman with a 38-week intrauterine pregnancy presents for cesarean section due to failure to progress. The patient has a 2-year history of depression and is currently taking 15 mg of phenelzine orally, twice daily. The patient refuses general anesthesia. A lumbar epidural block is placed without complication, and a T6 level of anesthesia is achieved. The surgical procedure proceeds and is uneventful. In the recovery room, the nurse requests intravenous meperidine for postoperative shivering. Later, the anesthesiologist is informed that the patient is tachycardic, hypertensive, and hyperpyrexic.

PROBLEM ANALYSIS

Definition

Monoamine oxidase inhibitors (MAOIs) block oxidative deamination to cause the accumulation of endogenous catecholamines (serotonin, norepinephrine, and dopamine) at adrenergically active tissue sites (e.g., brain). This is the proposed mechanism for the antidepressant actions of MAOIs. Meperidine increases serotonin (5-hydroxytryptamine) and catecholamine concentrations in synaptic clefts by inhibiting their uptake. In combination, meperidine and MAOIs can lead to increased serotonin and catecholamine levels in brain and peripheral tissue sites, causing signs of sympathetic nervous system overactivity (e.g., hypertension, tachycardia, hyperpyrexia) and potentially coma.

Recognition

Use of narcotics in patients receiving MAOIs can lead to one of three clinical presentations:

1. No adverse effects
2. Hypertension, hyperpyrexia, and tachycardia—a more common clinical presentation, especially with meperidine
3. Hypotension and loss of consciousness—reported with morphine sulfate

Risk Assessment

Inhibition of approximately 80% of monoamine oxidase (MAO) activity is necessary to achieve a therapeutic antidepressant effect with MAOIs. There are two MAO enzymes (A and B), which differ in their tissue distribution (active sites) and preference for substrates.

Because the brain contains predominantly MAO A (approximately 60% of the total), selective inhibitors could potentially minimize (or eliminate) the side effects associated with MAOIs. Two types of MAOI derivatives (hydrazine and nonhydrazine analogues) exist.

Implications

The use of narcotics in the setting of MAOI treatment remains controversial. Morphine has been reported to cause adverse outcomes in patients taking MAOIs, presumably via histamine-mediated release of catecholamines. In addition, MAOIs reduce intrahepatic enzyme function and thus can prolong the effects of other drugs. The most well-known adverse interactions, however, are those between MAOIs and meperidine; such adverse outcomes have been reported from at least 12 independent sources. Even the use of synthetic narcotics (e.g., fentanyl) that do not release histamine has been questioned. The synthetic opioids increase norepinephrine release and inhibit its reuptake in sympathetic nerve terminals. Fentanyl may also increase the release of serotonin. Despite three reports of adverse outcomes with fentanyl-based anesthesia in patients receiving MAOIs and having cardiac surgery, many other reports have described the safety of high-dose fentanyl in that setting.

The newer selective MAOI moclobemide has not been associated with adverse outcomes in patients receiving morphine or synthetic opioids. Volatile anesthetics and intravenous agents, including ketamine, have also been used safely in patients receiving moclobemide. Although there is some concern about the use of local anesthetic solutions containing epinephrine in patients receiving moclobemide, data to support or refute this concern are unavailable.

Hyperdynamic circulatory responses have been reported in patients receiving MAOIs who are given indirect-acting vasopressors such as ephedrine. Indirect-acting adrenergic agonists can cause an unpredictable release of catecholamines from presynaptic stores into the nerve terminal and lead to a grossly exaggerated sympathetic response. Therefore, these drugs are best avoided in patients receiving MAOIs. In contrast, MAOIs do not significantly alter the hemodynamic effects of exogenously administered direct-acting vasopressors such as phenylephrine.

MANAGEMENT

The hyperdynamic circulatory responses elicited with the use of meperidine and indirect-acting sympathomimetic agents in patients receiving MAOIs can be controlled with the use of arterial vasodilators such as nitroprusside and nicardipine. In comatose patients, supportive care, including airway management, is imperative. Hypotensive episodes during surgery are best treated with reduced intravenous doses of phenylephrine or other direct-acting sympathomimetic agents.

PREVENTION

The preceding considerations suggest the discontinuance of MAOIs 2 weeks before elective surgery to permit the synthesis of new MAO enzyme. However, the pharmacologic effects of nonhydrazine MAOIs are absent after the drug has been discontinued for 24 hours. The nonhydrazine MAOIs are reversible inhibitors of MAO and are not associated with

adverse outcomes during anesthesia and surgery. Thus, discontinuing such therapy is generally not warranted and must be carefully weighed against exacerbations of the underlying psychiatric illness.

Neither general nor regional anesthesia is contraindicated in patients receiving nonhydrazine MAOIs. If central neuraxial regional anesthesia is chosen, however, volume loading before the introduction of sympathectomy is advised. Further, with hypotension, the use of direct-acting vasopressors is recommended. MAOIs have a minor role in terminating the release and action of norepinephrine at nerve terminals. For cardiac surgical patients, some authors recommend the use of benzodiazepines and β-adrenergic blockers with high-dose narcotic anesthesia, whereas others recommend the use of etomidate or thiopental in doses appropriate to the patient's hemodynamic status.

TRICYCLIC ANTIDEPRESSANTS

Case Synopsis

A 24-year-old man presents emergently to the operating room for surgical exploration of the abdomen after a motor vehicle accident. In the emergency room, the patient is very difficult to arouse and is intubated. Vital signs are stable except for mild tachycardia. The head computed tomography scan is normal, and no other injuries are noted. During induction of anesthesia with low-dose thiopental and pancuronium, the patient becomes extremely hypotensive and bradycardic, with wide QRS complexes on the electrocardiogram (ECG). Epinephrine (100 μg) is given, and profound sustained hypertension and tachycardia ensue. An attempt at arterial line placement reveals severe scarring on both wrists. Intravenous fluid resuscitation is initiated, and sodium nitroprusside 1 μg/kg per minute is administered. Later, the family reveals that the patient has had suicidal depression for at least 3 months and is taking imipramine.

PROBLEM ANALYSIS

Definition

Reduced concentrations of norepinephrine and serotonin in the central nervous system (CNS) are thought to underlie depression. Thus, the condition is effectively treated by agents that block catecholamine reuptake in the CNS. Although tricyclic antidepressants (TCAs) do this, they also bind to other CNS receptors (γ-aminobutyric acid [GABA], muscarinic, α-adrenergic, and histamine). In addition to CNS actions, TCAs have important cardiac implications. Depending on serum TCA concentrations, these drugs may exert proarrhythmic or antiarrhythmic properties. However, TCAs have not been implicated as a direct cause of left ventricular dysfunction.

Recognition

The width of the QRS complex represents the relatively brief duration of phase 0 and phase I of the cardiac action potential (AP) relative to phases II, III, and IV (plateau, repolarization, and isoelectric phases, respectively). Phase 0 is the rapid depolarization phase that results from the influx of sodium

ions into the cardiac muscle and conducting fibers. Phase I is early, rapid depolarization that precedes the AP plateau phase (phase II). Phase I is believed to be due to several potassium repolarizing currents and to sodium "window" and calcium currents.

Blockage of voltage-gated sodium channels that generate fast inward current required for AP phase 0 depends on the heart rate. Profound block, especially with toxic TCA concentrations, occurs at fast heart rates. However, such block accumulates over time and eventually leads to bradycardia with widened QRS complexes. Early signs of TCA toxicity are PR interval prolongation and T-wave flattening. Also, most patients display anticholinergic effects with TCAs, leading to an early increase in heart rate. However, bradycardia with wide QRS complexes may follow.

Risk Assessment

QRS complex widening is the harbinger of seizures and cardiac arrhythmias with acute TCA intoxication. With therapeutic TCA concentrations, most patients show a 10% to 20% increase above their baseline heart rate due to TCAs' anticholinergic effects. Further, PR and Q-Tc interval prolongation is not infrequent with therapeutic concentrations of TCAs.

Implications

With TCAs, hypotension can occur due to bradycardia, volume depletion, or vasodilatation secondary to α-adrenergic receptor blockade. One's first impulse might be to administer a direct-acting vasoconstrictor, such as phenylephrine or even epinephrine. However, the use of epinephrine can lead to profound hypertension and tachycardia (as illustrated in the case synopsis) in the presence of increased circulating concentrations of catecholamines with TCAs. Use of epinephrine in local anesthetic solutions should also be avoided. Increased circulating catecholamines may lead to ventricular tachycardia and arrest in the presence of halothane and pancuronium. Ketamine should also be avoided owing to its potential sympathomimetic effects. ECG evidence of Q-T interval prolongation precludes the use of stellate ganglion blocks for treating reflex sympathetic dystrophy. In fact, TCAs are an alternative but often overlooked therapy for these patients.

MANAGEMENT

In the presence of ventricular arrhythmias, class IA antiarrhythmic agents (e.g., quinidine, procainamide, disopyramide) are of no benefit and in fact should not be used. TCAs and class IA antiarrhythmics have similar effects on the myocardium that are compounded by combined use, especially the risk for Q-T interval prolongation and proarrhythmia (i.e., torsades de pointes). In cardiac arrest, resuscitation should proceed as usual with intravenous lidocaine (a class IB agent) or amiodarone (the class III agent with the lowest proarrhythmia risk) and direct-current cardioversion for ventricular tachycardia or defibrillation for ventricular fibrillation. If cardiac arrest is due to ventricular tachycardia or fibrillation, epinephrine should be avoided. Assurance of ventilation and oxygenation, mechanical chest compressions, and early cardioversion or defibrillation are mandatory. If a vasopressor is needed, the best alternative may be vasopressin in reduced dosages. Then, attention should be directed toward the correction of acidosis and hypokalemia and the replacement of intravascular volume. Bradycardia or asystole may respond to atropine, but if not, temporary transcutaneous pacing is used. In a comatose patient, airway management is the primary concern, not only to ensure adequate ventilation and oxygenation but also to protect against pulmonary aspiration.

PREVENTION

In the case of elective surgery, a preoperative ECG should be obtained in all patients receiving TCAs. Unless the history or physical examination reveals significant heart disease or heart failure, a preoperative echocardiogram is generally not necessary, because left ventricular function is usually well preserved in patients taking TCAs. Further, the preoperative discontinuation of TCAs is not warranted. However, close observation of the intraoperative ECG and knowledge and awareness of the drug's cardiac implications are of utmost importance in the care of these patients. Drugs to avoid include direct-acting catecholamines, sensitizing inhalation agents (e.g., halothane more than enflurane; but sensitization unlikely with desflurane or sevofurane), induction agents that facilitate this interaction (e.g., thiopental), and intravenous agents such as ketamine (owing to its sympathomimetic actions).

SELECTIVE SEROTONIN REUPTAKE INHIBITORS

Case Synopsis

After an orthopedic procedure performed with an axillary block and sedation, a 28-year-old woman develops hyperthermia, hyperreflexia, and agitation in the recovery room. She is currently being treated with sertraline because of postpartum depression.

PROBLEM ANALYSIS

Definition

Selective serotonin reuptake inhibitors (SSRIs) inhibit the presynaptic 5-hydroxytryptamine reuptake transport system. This leads to an acute increase in serotonin concentrations at the synaptic cleft. The therapeutic effects, which take approximately 2 weeks to develop, are the result of neuro-adaptive changes that result in increased serotonin release and transmission. Because SSRIs are highly specific for serotonin and have less effect on other neurotransmitter systems (e.g., adrenergic, muscarinic, histamine, and dopaminergic pathways) and channels (e.g., sodium, potassium), they have a significantly better safety profile than TCAs.

Recognition

In patients receiving SSRIs, concurrent nonanesthetic drugs and some anesthetic drugs may cause adverse reactions, including the serotonin syndrome, which is identified by any three of the following symptoms: mental status changes, including agitation; hyperreflexia; diaphoresis; shivering; tremor; hypertension; oculogyric crisis (i.e., extreme eyeball rotation); diarrhea; and hyperthermia. Drugs that can cause adverse reactions or the serotonin syndrome in concert with SSRIs include the following:

- Nonanesthetic drugs: L-dopa, lithium, bromocriptine, fenfluramine, dextromethorphan, pethidine, and pentazocine can increase serotonin activity by blocking the reuptake or increasing the presynaptic release of serotonin.
- Anesthetic drugs: highly protein-bound anesthetic drugs (e.g., fentanyl, midazolam, local anesthetics) may increase the free (unbound) fraction of sertraline (Zoloft).

Risk Assessment

SSRIs are the most frequently used antidepressants in the United States. Fluoxetine (Prozac) is the least specific of the SSRIs, especially at higher doses, and may be associated with greater CNS effects. Paroxetine (Paxil) is more specific but also has mild antimuscarinic effects. Sertraline (Zoloft) is the most specific SSRI.

Implications

SSRIs inhibit cytochrome P-450 enzymes. Their use with drugs that have narrow therapeutic windows, including phenytoin, TCAs, tolbutamide, carbamazepine, clozapine, haloperidol, class IC antiarrhythmics (see Chapter 10), and warfarin, can cause clinically significant adverse drug interactions. Thus, for some surgeries, preoperative evaluation of coagulation status may be warranted. The syndrome of inappropriate antidiuretic hormone secretion (SIADH) may occur in geriatric patients and warrants preoperative evaluation for hyponatremia. Postoperative delirium can be confused with neuroleptic malignant syndrome, SIADH, and withdrawal of SSRIs.

MANAGEMENT

Most adverse events associated with SSRIs are due to drug interactions. If this is the case, the preferred initial therapy is to discontinue the inciting drug. Supportive measures include cooling for hyperthermia, artificial ventilation for inadequate ventilation, clonazepam for myoclonus, anticonvulsants for seizures, and chlorpromazine for its antipyretic and sedative properties.

PREVENTION

SSRIs should be continued perioperatively to prevent a withdrawal syndrome. Neither general nor regional anesthesia is contraindicated. SSRIs are metabolized by hepatic transformation involving the cytochrome P-450 enzyme and can potentially inhibit the metabolism of other drugs similarly metabolized. For example, prolonged sedation with midazolam has been observed in patients receiving SSRIs. Decreased analgesic effects of μ opioids, such as morphine, have also been noted with fluoxetine.

ST. JOHN'S WORT

Case Synopsis

A 19-year-old, otherwise healthy man undergoes general anesthesia with midazolam, propofol, fentanyl, rocuronium, and nitrous oxide for an appendectomy. The intraoperative course is uncomplicated, with a total anesthesia time of 1 hour. Later, in the recovery room, the patient is difficult to arouse. His pupils are equal and reactive but constricted. Despite the administration of naloxone and flumazenil, and normal electrolytes and arterial blood gas measures, he remains difficult to arouse. An hour and a half later, he is arousable and purposeful. Upon subsequent interview, he states that he uses St. John's wort for depression.

PROBLEM ANALYSIS

Definition

Increasing numbers of surgical patients are taking herbal remedies that can complicate the perioperative period (see also Chapter 39). A survey of the general U.S. population reported a 380% increase in the use of herbal preparations over the past decade. Up to 22% of all surgical patients use homeopathic medications.

St. John's wort is an extract from the flowers and leaves of the plant *Hypericum perforatum*. It is used for the short-term treatment of mild to moderate depression but is not effective for major depression. Although St. John's wort is used for other psychiatric conditions (e.g., anxiety), there is little evidence to support its use outside of depression, and even then, its efficacy for clinical depression is controversial. Meta-analyses of some studies have reported response rates similar to those for placebo; others have shown efficacy comparable to that of conventional antidepressants. St. John's wort appears to have fewer side effects than conventional antidepressants.

Recognition

Six classes of compounds in St. John's wort extracts are believed to be its active components:

1. Naphthodianthones (i.e., hypericin, pseudohypericin)
2. Acylphloroglucinols (i.e., hyperforin, adhyperforin)
3. Proanthocyanidins
4. Flavanol glycosides

5. Phenylpropanes
6. Biflavones

Although hypericin was formerly believed to be the principal active compound in St. John's wort, more recent evidence suggests that hyperforin is more important for its antidepressant effects. Hyperforin has the following actions:

- Inhibition of serotonin reuptake
- Weak in vitro inhibition of MAO A and B (demonstrated in one report but not confirmed in several others)
- Inhibition of norepinephrine and dopamine reuptake
- High affinity for $GABA_A$ and $GABA_B$ receptors, as well as adenosine, dopamine, and benzodiazepine receptors
- Significant increase in the metabolism of many concurrently used drugs by induction of cytochrome P-450 microsomal enzymes to nearly double their metabolic activity

The most affected enzyme appears to be CYP3A4, which is responsible for the metabolism of more than half of clinical drugs subject to cytochrome P-450 oxidative metabolism. Interactions with the CYP3A4 substrates indinavir, ethinyl estradiol, and cyclosporin have been reported. This interaction led to a 50% reduction in cyclosporin concentrations in one series of organ transplant recipients. There have also been reports of acute heart transplant rejection. Other CYP3A4 substrates in perioperative use are alfentanil, midazolam, lidocaine, calcium channel blockers, and SSRIs. It is likely that metabolism of these drugs is also increased. Further, St. John's wort induces CYP2C9. Its clinical substrates include nonsteroidal anti-inflammatory drugs, diphenylhydantoin (phenytoin), and, importantly, warfarin. Finally, St. John's wort lowers digoxin serum concentrations by induction of the P-glycoprotein transporter.

St. John's wort can be associated with adverse drug reactions in patients undergoing anesthesia and surgery, including the development of serotonin syndrome. Because it increases serotonin levels, serotonin syndrome is most commonly seen in patients also taking TCAs and is even more problematic with MAOIs.

Delayed emergence from anesthesia is a relatively common occurrence with St. John's wort and is often due to potentiation of the effects of other drugs used in anesthesia. Less common is thromboembolic stroke in patients on warfarin. Metabolic imbalance is rare.

Risk Assessment

Because the most active ingredient in St. John's wort was formerly believed to be hypericin, most preparations are still standardized to hypericin content. However, extracts contain other active constituents, especially hyperforin. Because herbals such as St. John's wort are not subject to stringent licensing regulations, the hypericin percentage does not guarantee the amounts or pharmacologic biopotential of any other components.

Implications

The antidepressant effects of St. John's wort are believed to be a synergistic combination of MAO inhibition, decreased serotonin reuptake, and GABA activity. The anesthetic implications are mostly theoretical, with rare case reports. Of greatest concern is the potential for a decreased response to inotropic agents, because long-term use of St. John's wort alters G-protein coupling mechanisms and down-regulates adrenergic receptors.

MANAGEMENT

Because of its effect on anesthetics and other drugs used in perioperative settings, the preoperative discontinuation of St. John's wort is important. This is critical in certain organ transplant patients owing to the increased risk of rejection. Also included are patients receiving warfarin for prophylaxis of thromboembolic events. Further, delayed emergence from anesthesia has been associated with St. John's wort. In particular, the sedative effects of agents acting at GABA receptors are potentiated by the preoperative use of St. John's wort. Also, it inhibits norepinephrine reuptake and down-regulates adrenergic receptors, thus increasing the risk of cardiovascular collapse.

PREVENTION

The use of herbal medications cannot be discounted and must be addressed in the preoperative assessment. Because of the long median elimination half-lives of hyperphorin (9 hours), hypericin (43 hours), and pseudohypericin (25 hours), patients should be advised to discontinue the use of St. John's wort 5 to 7 days before anesthesia and surgery, if possible.

Further Reading

Ang-Lee M, Yuan C-S, Moss J: Complementary and alternative therapies. In Miller RD (ed): Miller's Anesthesia, 6th ed. Philadelphia, Churchill Livingstone, 2005, pp 605-615.

Atlee JL: Management of perioperative dysrhythmias. Anesthesiology 86:1397-1424, 1997.

Atlee JL, Bosnjak ZJ: Mechanisms for cardiac dysrhythmias during anesthesia. Anesthesiology 72:347-374, 1990.

Boehnert MT, Lovejoy FH: Value of the QRS duration versus the serum drug level in predicting seizures and ventricular arrhythmias after an acute overdose of tricyclic antidepressants. N Engl J Med 313:474-479, 1985.

El-Ganzouri AR, Ivankovich AD, Braverman B, et al: Monoamine oxidase inhibitors: Should they be discontinued preoperatively? Anesth Analg 64:592-596, 1985.

Glassman AH, Bigger JT: Cardiovascular effects of therapeutic doses of tricyclic antidepressants: A review. Arch Gen Psychiatry 38:815-820, 1981.

Hodges PJ, Kam PC: The perioperative implications of herbal medicines. Anaesthesia 57:889-899, 2002.

Kam PC, Chang GW: Selective serotonin reuptake inhibitors: Pharmacology and implications in anaesthesia and critical care medicine. Anaesthesia 52:982-988, 1997.

Kudoh A, Katagai H, Takazawa T: Antidepressant treatment for chronic depressed patients should not be discontinued prior to anesthesia. Can J Anaesth 49:132-136, 2002.

Mcfarlane HJ: Anesthesia and the new generation monoamine oxidase inhibitors. Anaesthesia 49:597-599, 1994.

Scher CS, Anwar M: The self-reporting of psychiatric medications in patients scheduled for elective surgery. J Clin Anesth 11:619-621, 1999.

Stack CG, Rogers P, Linter SPK: Monoamine oxidase inhibitors and anesthesia. Br J Anaesth 60:222-227, 1988.

Chemotherapeutic Agents

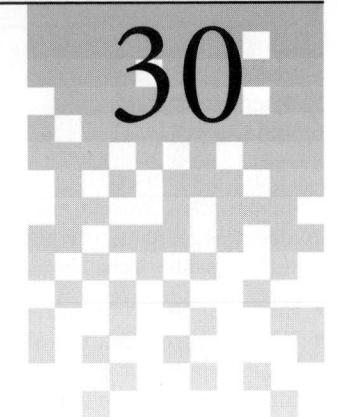

30

Paul B. Langevin and John L. Atlee

Case Synopsis

A 45-year-old woman presents for elective cholecystectomy. During the preoperative consultation, she states that she had a lump removed from her breast 10 years earlier after "they found cancer under my arm." She underwent six cycles of chemotherapy with radiation therapy, and the cancer has not recurred. She feels fine and denies any cardiac history.

PROBLEM ANALYSIS

Definition

CLASSIFICATION AND USE

There are numerous chemotherapeutic agents in use today. The major classes, along with their subclasses and some specific agents, are as follows:

- Alkylating agents: nitrogen mustards (mechlorethamine, cyclophosphamide, ifosfamide, melphalan, chlorambucil); ethylenimines and methylmelamines (triethylenemelamine [TEM], thiotepa [triethylene thiophosphoramide], altretamine [hexamethylmelamine]); alkyl sulfonates (busulfan); nitrosoureas (carmustine [BCNU], streptozocin); triazenes (dacarbazine)
- Antimetabolites: folic acid analogues (methotrexate); pyrimidine analogues (fluorouracil, floxuridine, cytarabine, gemcitabine); purine analogues (mercaptopurine, azathioprine, thioguanine, fludarabine phosphate, pentostatin, cladribine)
- Natural products and synthetic congeners: antimitotics (vinca alkaloids, paclitaxel and its more potent analogue docetaxel); epipodophyllotoxins (etoposide, teniposide); camptothecin analogues (the parent compound [camptothecin] had significant antitumor activity but was subsequently discarded in favor of analogues with less severe and more predictable toxicity, such as irinotrecan and topotecan); antibiotics (dactinomycin [actinomycin D], daunorubicin, doxorubicin, idarubicin), newer synthetic analogues of doxorubicin (valrubicin, epirubicin, mitoxantrone), bleomycins (bleomycin sulfate, mitomycin)
- Enzymes (L-asparaginase)
- Miscellaneous agents: platinum coordination complexes (cisplatin, carboplatin, oxaliplatin); hydroxyurea; procarbazine; mitotane
- Hormones: adrenocorticosteroids
- Aminoglutethimide and two newer classes of aromatase inhibitors (the enzyme that converts androgens to estrogens): analogues that block this conversion (formestane, exemestane) and the imidazole inhibitors (anastrozole, vorozole, letrozole); steroidals (progestins, estrogens and androgens, antiestrogens [tamoxifen, raloxifene], antiandrogens [flutamide, nilutamide, bicalutamide]); gonadotropin-releasing hormone analogues (leuprolide, goserelin, triptorelin, buserelin); biologic response

modifiers (interleukin-2, granulocyte colony-stimulating factor [filgrastin], granulocyte-macrophage colony-stimulating factor [sargramostim]); monoclonal antibodies (trastuzumab, rituximab, tositumomab)

The potential perioperative complications associated with all chemotherapeutics cannot be addressed here. This chapter focuses on two commonly used anthracycline antibiotics and a synthetic analogue. Information about other important, representative chemotherapeutic agents is provided in Table 30-1.

Anthracycline antibiotics and their derivatives are among the principal chemotherapeutics in use today. Daunorubicin (Cerubidine, daunomycin, rubidomycin) and doxorubicin (Rubex, Adriamycin) were first isolated from the fungus *Streptomyces peucetius*. Synthetic derivatives are available (e.g., idarubicin [Idamycin]). Although they differ slightly in chemical structure, daunorubicin and idarubicin are used, along with cytarabine (see Table 30-1), against acute myelogenous and lymphocytic leukemias. In fact, daunorubicin is among the most active drugs against acute myelogenous leukemia in adults. A daunorubicin citrate liposomal drug preparation (DaunoXome) is used to treat Kaposi's sarcoma related to acquired immunodeficiency syndrome (AIDS). Doxorubicin has activity against acute leukemias, malignant lymphomas, and other human neoplasms. A doxorubicin liposomal product (Doxil) is used against AIDS-related Kaposi's sarcoma. In contrast to daunorubicin, doxorubicin has activity against solid tumors. Along with cyclophosphamide, procarbazine, and vincristine (or others), it is critical for the successful treatment of Hodgkin's and non-Hodgkin's lymphomas. Doxorubicin is also used in regimens against breast and small cell lung carcinomas; adult and pediatric sarcomas (osteogenic, Ewing's, soft tissue); cancer of the cervix or endometrium, prostate, testes, and head and neck; and plasma cell myeloma.

However, the clinical value of these "parent" anthracycline antibiotics (daunorubicin, doxorubicin) is limited by an unusual and often irreversible cardiomyopathy that is directly related to the total amount of agent received. Thus, in the search for agents with higher antineoplastic activity but less cardiotoxicity, numerous derivatives have been prepared, some of which have shown promise in clinical studies:

- Idarubicin (leukemia)
- Epirubicin (solid tumor chemotherapy)
- Mitoxantrone (prostate cancer, leukemia, high-dose chemotherapy)

Table 30–1 ■ Mechanisms, Uses, and Toxicities of Selected Chemotherapeutic Agents Other than Anthracycline Antibiotics

Drug	Mechanism of Antineoplastic Effect	Important Indications	Clinical Toxicities	Clinical Considerations
Dactinomycin or actinomycin D (Cosmegen)	Antibiotic; binds to DNA to form highly stable drug-DNA complexes that block DNA transcription by RNA polymerase; this inhibits any rapidly proliferating cells	Pediatric tumors: Wilms' and Ewing's tumors Additional activities: Kaposi's sarcoma, choriocarcinoma, metastatic testicular sarcoma	Myelosuppression (pancytopenia), N/V, anorexia, diarrhea, proctitis, cheilitis, ulcerations (oral and GI mucosa, skin), alopecia	With SC extravasation, marked local inflammation; very potent immunosuppressant
Anastrozole (Arimidex)	Nonsteroidal; inhibits imidazole aromatase; effectively blocks the biosynthesis of estrogen	Primary therapy: estrogen or unknown receptor Postmenopausal, advanced, or metastatic breast cancer; recurrence of disease after tamoxifen	Reduced toxicity: acne ("androgenic skin"), alopecia, N/V	No androgenic effects; metabolized in liver; dosing unaffected by renal dysfunction; long half-life (50 hr); can be given orally once daily; suppresses estrogen to below detectable concentrations; has a favorable toxicity profile
L-Asparaginase (Oncaspar, Elspar)	Catalyzes the hydrolysis of L-asparagine (required by some neoplastic cells—e.g., acute lymphoblastic leukemia—for protein synthesis) to aspartic acid and ammonia, which deprives neoplastic cells of an essential amino acid, leading to cell death	Useful component of therapy for acute lymphoblastic leukemia and other lymphoid malignancies	Few effects on bone marrow or GI mucosa; severe toxicity due to antigenicity and protein synthesis inhibition; hypersensitivity reactions in 5%-20% of patients (may be fatal); deficient insulin or clotting factors	Hypoalbuminemia; hyperglycemia; thrombosis; less often, hemorrhagic events Most thromboses are in patients with gene defects: factor V Leiden; protein S, C, or AT III; low or ↑ homocysteine
Bleomycin (Blenoxane)	Antibiotic; cleaves DNA The drug in clinical use is a mixture of two copper-chelating peptides (bleomycin A_2 and B_2); interactions with O_2 and Fe^{2+} lead to scission of DNA	Highly effective for ovarian or testicular germ cell tumors With cisplatin and vinblastine or etoposide, curative for testicular cancer With cisplatin and other agents, highly active for GU tract squamous cell, esophageal, and head and neck carcinomas Sometimes used as a component of therapy for Hodgkin's and non-Hodgkin's lymphomas	Pulmonary toxicity (dry cough, fine rales, diffuse infiltrates leading to possibly fatal pulmonary fibrosis), worsened by ↑ Fio_2 Skin toxicity: erythema, hyperkeratoses, hyperpigmentation, ulcerations, N/V Unusual toxicity in patients with lymphomas: severe hyperthermia and hypotension; then sustained cardiorespiratory arrest Nonimmune? Endogenous pyrogen?	Little myelosuppression; avoid high Fio_2; judicious IV fluids in patients with pulmonary toxicity, especially with fibrosis
Busulfan (Myleran, Busulfex)	Alkylating agent; few actions other than myelosuppression at conventional doses; at low doses, selective depression of granulocytopoiesis	For chronic granulocytic leukemia, expect remission in 85%-90% of patients after initial therapy; however, the drug has largely been replaced by interferon-α and hydroxyurea	Low doses: cytotoxic action does not appear to extend to lymphoid or GI tissues High-dose regimens: pulmonary fibrosis and hepatic veno-occlusive disease	Allopurinol reduces renal damage from urate deposits Expect lower leukocyte counts by 3 wk, then a reduction in spleen size in CML

Continued

111

Table 30–1 ■ Mechanisms, Uses, and Toxicities of Selected Chemotherapeutic Agents Other than Anthracycline Antibiotics—cont'd

Drug	Mechanism of Antineoplastic Effect	Important Indications	Clinical Toxicities	Clinical Considerations
		In AML, busulfan (high doses) + cyclophosphamide is given for bone marrow transplants Also used in polycythemia vera and myeloid fibrosis-metaplasia	Thrombocytopenia (prolonged) is possible Initially, rapid cell destruction leads to extensive purine catabolism and renal damage from precipitation of urates	Prevent N/V with ondansetron and high-dose corticosteroids For electrolyte imbalance, use K^+, Mg^{2+} repletion therapy Anaphylactic-like reactions may occur minutes after administration (facial edema, bronchospasm, tachycardia, hypotension) and are treated with IV epinephrine + corticosteroids or antihistamines.
Cisplatin (Platinol-AQ)	Enters cells by diffusion Replacement of Cl^- by water yields a positively charged molecule that may be responsible for drug activity; this can react with nucleic acids and proteins Acquation is favored at low [Cl^-]; high [Cl^-] stabilizes cisplatin Platinum complexes react with DNA, forming intra- and interstrand cross-links; DNA adducts inhibit replication and transcription of DNA breaks and miscoding; ability to form these adducts predicts efficacy	Combined chemotherapy with cisplatin, bleomycin, etoposide, and vinblastine is 85% curative for advanced testicular carcinoma If combined with paclitaxel, doxorubicin, or cyclophosphamide, it is beneficial in ovarian carcinoma Also produces responses in cancers of the head and neck, endometrium, small cell lung carcinoma, and some childhood neoplasms Sensitizes cells to cytotoxic effects of radiation therapy	N/V in almost all patients Nephroxicity can be mostly prevented with hydration and diuresis Tinnitus and high-frequency hearing loss more frequent or severe with repeat dosing in children Peripheral neuropathy may worsen after repeated cycles of therapy Electrolyte imbalance ($\downarrow Ca^{2+}$, Mg^{2+}, K^+, PO_4) common and can cause tetany or promote arrhythmias Hemolytic anemia, hyeruricemia, and seizures Cardiac abnormalities have been reported	
Cyclophosphamide (Cytoxan, Neosar)	Most widely used alkylating drug; converted by liver P-450 enzymes to acyclic aldophosphamide and 4-hydroxycyclophosphamide (tautomers that are in steady-state equilibration with each other); the latter is metabolized to inactive metabolites that may limit liver damage; aldophosphamide is converted in malignant cells to phosphoramide mustard and acrolein; the former, an alkylating agent, is antineoplastic Pretreatment with phenobarbital (which induces liver P-450 enzymes) enhances drug activation but does not affect its toxicity or therapeutic efficacy	Alone, for susceptible lymphomas and chronic leukemia Higher doses with other drugs: breast cancer, lymphomas Key drug in non-Hodgkin's or Burkitt's lymphoma Used with methotrexate (or doxorubicin) + fluorouracil after breast cancer surgery Other uses: multiple myeloma; lung cancers; cancer of the breast, ovaries, or cervix; childhood neuroblastoma or retinoblastoma As immunosuppressant: organ transplants, Wegener's granulomatosis, rheumatoid arthritis, pediatric nephrotic syndrome	Myelosuppression (platelet sparing), N/V, alopecia, SIADH, GI mucosal ulcerations and (less common) interstitial pulmonary fibrosis With high-dose IV therapy, renal, hepatic, and cardiac toxicities may occur; sterile hemorrhagic cystitis occurs in 5%-10% of patients secondary to acrolein	No SC extravasation reactions or thrombophlebitis Reduce cystitis incidence with mesna + diuresis Stop drug if dysuria or hematuria occurs Hepatic P-450 required for activation; may be less effective with liver dysfunction Caution: renal dysfunction is possible; ample fluids advised, but water intoxication is possible Cyclophosphamide and others (mechlorethamine) prolong block with some muscle relaxants (i.e., act as anticholinesterases)

Drug	Mechanism	Clinical Applications	Toxicity	Notes
Cytarabine or ara-C (Cytosar-U, Tarabine PFS)	Antimetabolite, pyrimidine analogue; penetrates cells by a carrier-mediated process; activated by conversion to ara-CMP (a 5′-monophosphate nucleotide), which reacts with nucleotide kinases to form diphosphate-triphosphate nucleotide residues (ara-CDP, ara-CTP), potent inhibitors of DNA polymerase; effects extend not only to DNA synthesis but also to repair Precise mechanism of cellular death is not understood; fragmentation of DNA is observed in ara-C–treated cells, and there is evidence of apoptosis in tumor and normal cells Kinetic properties also affect results of therapy Intracellular concentrations of ara-CTP must be at inhibitory levels for ≥1 cell cycle Response to ara-C is strongly affected by proportion of drug converted to ara-CTP	Best agent for inducing remissions in AML in children and adults; as single therapy, remission rates of 20%-40% reported, but more effective with anthracyclines or mitoxantrone Given as a single IV injection or by continuous infusion (varying dosage); children may tolerate higher doses than adults Intrathecal ara-C has been used against meningeal leukemia Liposomal ara-C (DepoCyt) appears to be as effective as IV ara-C Especially useful for adult, acute nonlymphocytic leukemia Used in aggressive non-Hodgkin's lymphomas and for acute lymphocytic leukemia relapses in patients of all ages	As a potent myelosuppressant, toxicity includes thrombocytopenia, severe leukopenia, and anemia with striking megaloblastic changes Causes fever, GI disturbances, stomatitis, mild reversible hepatic dysfunction, pneumonitis, and dermatitis After intrathecal administration, seizures and other neurotoxic manifestations can occur; also possible when high IV doses (>3 g/m²) are given to patients ≥40 yr and/or with renal dysfunction or abnormal alkaline phosphatase	Response to therapy affected by proportion of drug converted to ara-CTP, which depends on relative activities of a number of anabolic or catabolic enzymes (see Chabner under "Further Reading") Relationships exist between ara-CTP synthesis and its retention in leukemic cells, and remission duration in AML; cells' ability to transport ara-CTP is another important factor in determining clinical response Owing to a rapid fall in plasma drug concentrations to levels less than those needed to saturate drug transport or activation processes, many clinicians use high-dose regimens to attain 20- to 50-fold higher serum levels; this has improved the induction of remissions
Imatinib mesylate (Gleevec)	FMS-like TK 3 (FLT3) receptor exists in myeloid and some lymphoid leukemias The bcr-abl translocation in CML encodes for abnormal TK, needed for cell proliferation and survival; it causes the Philadelphia chromosome abnormality in CML GISTs may harbor oncogenic TK mutations and are targets for TK receptor inhibitors such as imatinib	CML (with bcr-abl translocation); some GISTs (mostly stomach) and lymphoid CML; possibly some activity against other solid tumors As a single agent, imatinib has remarkable remission-inducing activity Some GIST subsets have mutations that confer in vitro resistance to imatinib	Periorbital and leg edema, muscle cramping, GI hemorrhage	Metabolism by cytochrome P-450 system (primarily by CYP3A4) mandates careful surveillance for possible drug-drug interactions
Methotrexate (Folex, Mexate, Rheumatrex, others)	Folic acid is an essential dietary factor; from it are derived tetrahydrofolate (TH₄) cofactors that provide single carbon groups for the synthesis of precursors of DNA (thymidylate and purines) and RNA (purines) The enzyme DHFR is the primary site of action for MTX and most other folate analogues; MTX's inhibition of DHFR leads to toxic effects via (1) partial depletion of TH₄ cofactors needed for synthesis of purines and	Acute lymphoblastic leukemia in high doses in children Valuable for remission induction or consolidation and for maintaining remissions in leukemia; less valuable for adult leukemia, except for treatment or prevention of leukemic meningitis Intrathecal MTX: therapy or prophylaxis of meningeal leukemia, lymphoma, or carcinoma Proven value in choriocarcinoma and related trophoblastic tumors in women	Major toxicity: GI epithelium, bone marrow Patients possibly at risk for spontaneous hemorrhage or severe infections Side effects often last for weeks Chronic bone marrow suppression with renal dysfunction due to slow MTX excretion Other toxicities: alopecia, dermatitis, lung (interstitial pneumonitis), kidneys, defective oogenesis or spermatogenesis, teratogenesis or abortion	Potent immune suppressant that reduces platelets, hemoglobin, and leukocytes Eliminated renally via glomerular filtration and tubular secretion; ensure adequate hydration to avoid MTX precipitation in renal tubules; also, avoid drugs that decrease renal flow or are weak acids or direct nephrotoxins (NSAIDs, piperacillin, aspirin, cisplatin) Half of MTX is bound to plasma proteins and is displaced from plasma albumin by salicylates, chloramphenicol, sulfonamides, tetracyclines, and phenytoin

Continued

Table 30–1 ■ Mechanisms, Uses, and Toxicities of Selected Chemotherapeutic Agents Other than Anthracycline Antibiotics—cont'd

Drug	Mechanism of Antineoplastic Effect	Important Indications	Clinical Toxicities	Clinical Considerations
	thymidylate, (2) inhibition of folate-dependent enzymes required in thymidylate-purine metabolism, and (3) accumulation of a toxic DHFR inhibitory substrate—FH$_2$ polyglutamate	Also used in osteosarcoma and mycosis fungoides Part of combined therapy in Burkitt's and non-Hodgkin's lymphomas and in carcinomas of the breast, lung, head and neck, ovary, and bladder Also used in therapy of severe and disabling psoriasis	Liver dysfunction is often reversible but may lead to cirrhosis (e.g., chronic continuous therapy, as in psoriasis) Intrathecal use often causes inflammatory response in CSF or meningismus Seizures, coma, and death (rare occurrences)	Folinic acid (Leukovorin) does not reverse neurotoxicity
Streptozocin (Zanosar)	Natural antibiotic derived from *Streptomyces acromogenes*; also a nitrosourea alkylating agent that affects all stages of the mammalian cell cycle MNU has high affinity for insulin-producing β cells of pancreatic islets of Langerhans and causes diabetes in animal models	Advanced and metastatic pancreatic islet cell tumors; beneficial response results in significant increase in 1-yr survival rate and doubling of median survival time Also shows promise as therapy with fluorouracil or dacarbazine for advanced carcinoid tumors	Nausea (common) Renal or hepatic toxicity in about two thirds of patients; renal toxicity is usually reversible, dose related, and cumulative, but may be fatal; proximal tubular damage is the most important effect; urinary protein assays are used to detect early toxicity; not given with nephrotoxic drugs	Unmodified MNU (active moiety) causes delayed myelosuppression; streptozocin does not Also, MNU carbamoylates lysine residues of proteins; it is attached to these to alter specificity, distribution, and toxicity (e.g., carmustine and lomustine are lipophilic and cross the blood-brain barrier and are used for brain tumors; unlike streptozocin, they cause profound, cumulative myelosuppression)
Vincristine (Oncovin, Vincasar PFS, others) and vinblastine (Velban)	Important vinca alkaloids; cell cycle–specific agents that block cells in mitosis—specifically, binding to tubulin to block its ability to polymerize into microtubules; this disrupts microtubules of the mitotic apparatus to arrest cell	Vincristine and corticosteroids are first-line therapy for inducing remission of leukemia in children Adults with lymphomas (Hodgkin's or non-Hodgkin's) usually receive vincristine as part of a combined protocol	Hematologic toxicity occurs in 20% of patients and includes anemia, leukopenia, and thrombocytopenia Vincristine: toxicity is predictable, cumulative, and mostly neurologic—extremity numbness or tingling and loss of deep tendon reflexes (early, common), followed by motor weakness; the former usually do not warrant an	Neurologic toxicity is avoided or reversed by stopping therapy or reducing the dosage when motor dysfunction first occurs Severe constipation or obstipation is prevented with laxatives or hydrophilic agents

division in metaphase (microtubules are important for other cell functions as well: movement, axonal transport, phagocytosis)

Without an intact mitotic spindle, chromosomes disperse throughout the cytoplasm ("exploded mitosis") or cluster oddly

Incorrect chromosomal segregation during mitosis causes cell death

Normal and malignant cells exposed to these agents undergo changes characteristic of apoptosis

Vinblastine was once used with bleomycin and cisplatin to cure metastatic testicular tumors, but etoposide has largely replaced it

Other indications for vinblastine are breast cancer, Hodgkin's disease, Kaposi's sarcoma, histiocytosis, neuroblastoma, and choriocarcinoma

immediate dose reduction, but motor loss dictates re-evaluation of therapy; vocal cord paralysis or extraocular muscle function loss is rare

In high doses, vincristine can cause severe constipation or obstipation; intrathecal injection causes fatal CNS toxicity; SIADH occurs rarely

Vinblastine: nadir of leukopenia occurs by 7-10 days, with recovery by 7 days; other toxicities include neurotoxicity (as for vincristine), GI disturbances, and SIADH; alopecia, oral mucositis, and dermatitis are rare; extravasation during injection may lead to cellulitis and phlebitis

Alopecia occurs in about 20% of patients but is always reversible (often without stopping therapy)

Myelodepression (leukopenia, anemia, thrombocytopenia) is more common with vincristine than vinblastine

Hyponatremia, high urinary Na^+, and SIADH are occasionally seen

In view of the rapid action of vinca alkaloids, one must prevent hyperuricemia with allopurinol

Vinca alkaloids are extensively metabolized by the liver, so caution is advised in patients with decreased hepatic function

Vinca alkaloids are very irritating to tissues

AML, acute myelogenous leukemia; AT, antithrombin; CML, chronic myelogenous leukemia; CSF, cerebrospinal fluid; DHFR, dihydrofolate reductase; FiO₂, fractional inspired oxygen; GI, gastrointestinal; GIST, gastrointestinal stromal tumor; GU, genitourinary; IV, intravenous; MNU, methylated nitrosourea; MTX, methotrexate; N/V, nausea or vomiting; NSAIDs, nonsteroidal anti-inflammatory drugs; SC, subcutaneous; SIADH, syndrome of inappropriate antidiuretic hormone secretion; TK, tyrosine kinase.

From Chabner BA, Ryan DP, Paz-Ares L, et al: Antineoplastic agents. In Hardman JG, Limbird LE (eds): Goodman and Gilman's The Pharmacological Basis of Therapeutics, 10th ed. New York, McGraw-Hill, 2001, pp 1389-1459; and www.pdr.net.

Mitoxantrone (an anthracenedione) has significantly less cardiotoxicity than the anthracyclines.

MECHANISM OF ACTION

The anthracycline antibiotics have three major biochemical effects that may explain their antineoplastic efficacy (if not their toxicity). First, they function as electron-accepting and electron-donating agents. They intercalate with the DNA helix to affect many of its functions. Single- and double-strand breaks and sister chromatid exchanges interfere with the transcription of RNA and the replication of DNA. As a result, toxicity occurs in the S phase of the cell cycle, but the cell dies on entering the G_2 phase. Genetic material is exchanged between chromatids, which, in addition to causing breaks in the DNA strand, renders this material mutagenic and carcinogenic. Breaks in the helix occur because intercalation disturbs the action of topoisomerase II. Second, the anthracycline antibiotics produce free radicals, giving rise to potent alkylating agents. For example, with reduced NADPH, they react with cytochrome P-450 reductase to generate semiquinone radical intermediates. In the presence of oxygen, superoxide anion radicals form to generate reactive species (e.g., H_2O_2, NO, and OH^-) that attack DNA. At least with doxorubicin, iron catalyzes free radical production. Insertion of these free radicals into the DNA helix may also cause breaks in the DNA sequence. Third, anthracycline antibiotics interact with cell membranes to form lipid peroxides. Peroxides alter cell membrane function and, therefore, cell function. Which of these three diverse actions is primarily responsible for the efficacy or toxicity of the anthracyclines is still a matter of speculation.

Recognition

Patients almost invariably know their primary tumor type but may not know or recall exactly what drugs they received or their dosages. This is especially true when patients received complex chemotherapeutic regimens or were treated in the distant past. In addition, many patients now receive their chemotherapy as outpatients, and the specific protocol used may not be included in the medical record. As a result, anesthesiologists should at least be aware of the agents used to treat the more common malignancies and the side effects of some typically used antineoplastics.

The goal of chemotherapy is to administer a dose of drug that maximizes the cytotoxic effect on neoplastic cells or tissues without impairing the patient's lifestyle when the course of therapy is completed. However, these drugs may significantly reduce the patient's functional reserve, which becomes apparent only in the perioperative period when the patient is physiologically stressed. Anesthesiologists should maintain a high index of suspicion that such a patient's physiologic reserve may be significantly impaired (in spite of a healthy appearance) and be prepared to evaluate this condition appropriately and initiate the indicated remedial therapy.

Risk Assessment

CLINICAL CONSIDERATIONS

Daunorubicin, doxorubicin, epirubicin, and idarubicin are usually administered intravenously and are cleared by hepatic metabolism and biliary excretion. Doxorubicin has biphasic clearance, with 3- and 30-hour half-lives of elimination. Idarubicin has monophasic clearance and a half-life of elimination of 15 hours. The clearance of all anthracyclines is delayed in patients with hepatic dysfunction, and at least a 50% reduction in dose should be considered in patients with abnormal serum bilirubin concentrations.

Daunorubicin and doxorubicin are converted to a variety of less active or inactive products. Idarubicin is metabolized primarily to idarubicinol, which accumulates in plasma and resembles the parent compound in activity. Daunorubicin and doxorubicin are converted to their alcohols, aglycons, and other derivatives.

Rapid uptake of these anthracyclines occurs in the heart, kidneys, lungs, liver, and spleen. The anthracyclines do not cross the blood-brain barrier. Superoxide dismutase and catalase help protect against anthracycline toxicity, an effect increased by exogenous antioxidants. Both daunorubicin and doxorubicin may impart a red color to urine. Appropriate care is exercised to prevent inadvertent extravasation during intravenous administration of anthracyclines because a severe local vesicant action and tissue necrosis may result.

TOXICITY

The anthracycline antibiotics cause myelosuppression. This results in leukopenia and, to a lesser degree, anemia and thrombocytopenia, reaching a nadir around 10 to 14 days after beginning therapy. Stomatitis, alopecia, and gastrointestinal symptoms are also common.

The anthracycline antibiotics produce a dose-dependent cardiotoxicity that is unique to this class of drugs. This cardiotoxicity may be acute or chronic and is resistant to digitalis. Acute myocardial damage is often revealed by electrocardiogram (ECG), showing flattened T waves, ST segment depression, or cardiac rhythm disturbances (notably, sinus tachycardia and extrasystoles). Often, these are self-limited and rarely cause serious complications. However, life-threatening arrhythmias have occurred within hours of doxorubicin administration in some patients. Further, the cardiac ejection fraction may be depressed within 24 hours of a single dose of these agents, but even this is often transient and rarely problematic.

The pericarditis-myocarditis syndrome is a potentially life-threatening manifestation of acute cardiotoxicity with anthracycline antibiotics. Features include severe conduction disturbances or arrhythmias and frank congestive heart failure (CHF), often associated with pericardial effusion. Although this usually occurs outside of perioperative settings, it may first manifest after anesthetic induction, with surgical stress, or in the postanesthetic or intensive care unit after anesthesia and surgery. Fortunately, pericarditis-myocarditis syndrome is an uncommon occurrence.

CHF that is unresponsive to cardiac glycosides is the hallmark of chronic cardiac toxicity with anthracycline antibiotics. It may develop years after the completion of chemotherapy but often develops within 6 months. Electron microscopy reveals cardiac mitochondrial changes, a reduction in myocardial fibrils, and cellular cardiac degeneration after the administration of these agents. On ECG, the QRS voltage is reduced, and the systolic time interval is prolonged. The extent of myocardial damage is directly proportional to the cumulative dose of the anthracycline antibiotic or synthetic congeners. Although practical and completely reliable tests are unavailable, serious cardiomyopathy with doxorubicin occurs in 1% to 10% of patients with total doses less than 450 mg/m^2 of body surface area (BSA). This risk increases to more than 20% of patients with total doses greater than 550 mg/m^2 BSA. Such total dosage should rarely be exceeded, and then only with the concomitant administration of dexrazoxane (Zinecard), a cardioprotective, intracellular chelating agent (see "Confounding Issues and Variables").

The mortality rate with significant anthracycline-related cardiomyopathy can exceed 50%. Total doses as low as 250 mg/m^2 can cause myocardial toxicity, as revealed by subendocardial biopsies. Children appear to be at even greater risk, because anthracyclines impair myocardial growth. Among pediatric patients, 5% to 10% will have overt CHF by the time they become adults, and subclinical cardiac dysfunction will develop in 40%. Finally, cardiac irradiation or the coadministration of high doses of cyclophosphamide or other anthracyclines may increase the risk of cardiotoxicity.

EVALUATION AND WORKUP

The first and most important element when assessing risk in patients who are receiving (or have received) anthracycline antibiotic chemotherapeutics is a high index of suspicion for associated cardiotoxicity. This cannot be overemphasized. Often, these patients do not appear physically handicapped based on their history, physical examination, and routine laboratory test results. Only when their cardiac functional reserve is tested (e.g., during exercise stress testing) does it become apparent that further (i.e., perioperative) cardiac stress will be poorly tolerated.

Once the anesthesiologist suspects that a patient has received a chemotherapeutic agent that could compromise cardiopulmonary function, every effort must be made to determine the regimen used, including the dose and pathway of concurrent or subsequent irradiation therapy. The drugs, their associated toxicities, and therapeutic implications (see Table 30-1) must be carefully assessed. This includes defining the patient's baseline physiologic functional status and the anticipated insult from any surgical or other intervention requiring anesthesia.

Radionuclide-gated blood pool studies may be the most sensitive test for detecting CHF, but an echocardiogram is a reasonable alternative. The patient should have an ECG and evaluation of the cardiac ejection fraction before the initiation of anthracycline chemotherapy and before each cycle of such therapy after cumulative doses of 400 mg/m^2. No test can predict which patients will develop CHF with therapy. Acute or chronic toxicity is unpredictable. Common sense suggests reducing the cumulative dose in patients with preexisting heart disease.

The preoperative evaluation should include the following:

- Cumulative dose of drugs administered
- Date of final administration
- Associated therapy (e.g., irradiation? if so, how directed?)
- Results of cardiac functional evaluation (ECG, echocardiogram, multiple gated image analysis, exercise stress testing, or a combination) before therapy was initiated and 6 months after the last cycle of chemotherapy

Because myocardial injury may progress for years after therapy, ideally, cardiac function should be evaluated within 1 month of interventions requiring anesthesia. However, given current cost concerns, this may not be justified unless the patient's history suggests a deteriorating functional status.

CONFOUNDING ISSUES AND VARIABLES

Irradiation of the mediastinum; exposure to cyclophosphamide, vincristine, or fluorouracil; or the addition of another drug can exacerbate the toxicity associated with these drugs. Indeed, in one study, all cases of CHF in patients who had received radiation therapy to the mediastinum occurred after anthracycline antibiotic doses of less than 315 mg/m^2. Calcium channel blockers also may increase the risk for cardiotoxicity. As noted earlier, when CHF does develop, the mortality rate can exceed 50%.

Dexrazoxane appears to reduce cardiotoxicity with the anthracycline antibiotics. Its addition to the regimen may allow higher cumulative doses of these agents. Newer anthracycline analogues (e.g., epirubicin, mitoxantrone, idarubicin) may have less cardiotoxicity but retain near full cytotoxic potential against some malignant cells. Thus, although they may have a narrower spectrum of action, they may be inherently safer.

Finally, doxorubicin can cause red streaks near the infusion site (i.e., Adriamycin flare), even without extravasation of the vesicant. Also, doxorubicin can cause severe local toxic effects in irradiated tissues, even when chemotherapy and irradiation therapy are not concurrent.

Implications

Cancer has now surpassed heart disease as the leading cause of death in the United States. Patients with cancer live longer and, increasingly, present to hospitals or ambulatory care facilities for treatment requiring an anesthesiologist's services—anesthesia for surgical or other painful interventions, pain management, critical care, or treatment for disease progression, a new malignancy, or another problem. Regardless, patients who have received anthracycline antibiotics tolerate anesthetics or other myocardial depressants poorly, even without evidence of loss of myocardial function (e.g., reduced ejection fraction). Invariably, these patients have reduced inotropy that is difficult to assess with echocardiography or cardiac catheterization. If anesthesia is required for such patients, the anesthesiologist must give serious consideration to a regional anesthetic technique, if suitable. Perioperative care should include the following:

- Limiting intravenous fluids
- Improving the inotropic state
- Reducing afterload to optimize cardiac output
- Careful selection of the intravenous induction agent
- Judicious use of invasive cardiovascular monitoring
- Availability of mechanical circulatory assistance, if needed (however, this intervention often proves minimally beneficial)

Although this chapter focuses on anthracycline-induced cardiotoxicity, anesthesiologists should be aware of the mechanisms of action, important indications, and clinical toxicities and indications of other important and widely used chemotherapeutic agents (see Table 30-1).

MANAGEMENT

Therapy for anthracycline-induced CHF includes the following:

- Diuretics
- Afterload reduction
- Low-sodium diet
- Bed rest

Therapy should also include cardiac glycosides, despite their limited benefit (anthracycline-induced cardiotoxicity is resistant to digitalis). Although these interventions may provide some symptomatic and functional improvement, the direct effects of cardiotoxicity are irreversible. Finally, because of the loss of contractile elements, mitochondrial damage, and unsatisfactory geometry of a dilated ventricle, the response to nondigitalis inotropes may be quite limited. An intensive care unit should be available postoperatively to receive the patient if needed.

PREVENTION

There is no acceptable therapeutic alternative to chemotherapeutic drugs in many patients. Even after a successful course of chemotherapy, a patient may continue to require the services of an anesthesiologist for related or nonrelated surgery or other painful interventions or for chronic pain management. With the anthracycline antibiotics, prevention focuses on how best to minimize the risk for further depression of myocardial function. Thus, awareness that some myocardial injury has occurred and evaluation of its severity are critical to anesthetic or pain management. With such knowledge, the anesthesiologist will be able to tailor any anesthetics or drugs used for pain management to the needs of the patient.

Further Reading

Capizzi RL: Principles of treatment of cancer. In Stein JH (ed): Internal Medicine, 4th ed. New York, Mosby–Year Book, 1994, pp 707-729.

Chabner BA, Ryan DP, Paz-Ares L, et al: Antineoplastic agents. In Hardman JG, Limbird LE (eds): Goodman and Gilman's The Pharmacological Basis of Therapeutics, 10th ed. New York, McGraw-Hill, 2001, pp 1389-1459.

Corless CL, Schroeder A, Griffith D, et al: PDGFRA mutations in gastrointestinal stromal tumors: Frequency, spectrum and in vitro sensitivity to imatinib. J Clin Oncol 23:5357-5364, 2005.

de Mestier P, des Guetz G: Treatment of gastrointestinal stromal tumors with imatinib mesylate: A major breakthrough in the understanding of tumor-specific molecular characteristics. World J Surg 29:357-361, 2005.

Di Cosimo S, Ferretti G, Fazio N, et al: Docetaxel in advanced gastric cancer—review of the main clinical trials. Acta Oncol 42:693-700, 2003.

Kouvaraki MA, Ajani JA, Hoff P, et al: Fluorouracil, doxorubicin, and streptozocin in the treatment of patients with locally advanced and metastatic pancreatic endocrine carcinomas. J Clin Oncol 22: 4762-4771, 2004.

Kvolik S, Glavas-Obrovac L, Sakic K, et al: Anaesthetic implications of anticancer chemotherapy. Eur J Anaesthesiol 20:859-871, 2003.

McCollum AD, Kulke MH, Ryan DP, et al: Lack of efficacy of streptozocin and doxorubicin in patients with advanced pancreatic endocrine tumors. Am J Clin Oncol 27:485-488, 2004.

Roizen MF, Fleisher LA: Anesthetic implications of concurrent disease. In Miller RD (ed): Miller's Anesthesia, 6th ed. New York, Churchill Livingstone, 2005, pp 1017-1149.

Selvin BL: Cancer chemotherapy: Implications for the anesthesiologist. Anesth Analg 60:425-434, 1981.

Sternberg DW, Licht JD: Therapeutic intervention in leukemias that express the activated FMS-like tyrosine kinase 3 (FLT3): Opportunities and challenges. Curr Opin Hematol 12:7-13, 2005.

Sun W, Lipsitz S, Catalano P, et al: Phase II/III study of doxorubicin with fluorouracil compared with streptozocin with fluorouracil or dacarbazine in the treatment of advanced carcinoid tumors: Eastern Cooperative Oncology Group Study E1281. J Clin Oncol 23: 4897-4904, 2005.

Chemical Dependency: Opioids

31

Mark S. Gold, Adrie Bruijnzeel, Kimberly Frost-Pineda, and William Jacobs

Case Synopsis

A 38-year-old anesthesiologist is found unresponsive and cyanotic in the call room after failing to return from a break in the case of a patient undergoing a craniotomy for tumor. Both fresh and recent venipuncture sites are found on his left forearm, along with a 1-mL insulin syringe and a rubber tourniquet.

PROBLEM ANALYSIS

Definitions

The American Medical Association defines an impaired physician as "one unable to fulfill professional or personal responsibilities due to psychiatric illness, alcoholism or drug dependency." This definition is in stark contrast to that for a professional athlete or a pilot, who is defined as impaired if "he or she is unfit for duty, shows up at work under-the-influence, or with residual effects." As defined in the *Diagnostic and Statistical Manual of Mental Disorders*, drug dependence is a maladaptive pattern of substance use leading to clinically significant distress or impairment. Individuals are considered to be drug dependent when three or more of the following behaviors exist within the same 12-month period:

- Tolerance, which is the need for more of the drug to achieve intoxication or the desired effect, or a decreased effect with continued use of the same amount of the drug.
- Withdrawal, in which a characteristic withdrawal syndrome appears without the substance, or the same or similar substance is taken to relieve or avoid withdrawal.
- The drug is taken in larger quantities or over a longer period than was intended.
- There is a persistent desire or unsuccessful efforts to cut down or control use.
- A significant amount of time is spent in obtaining, using, or recovering from use.
- Important social, occupational, or recreational activities are reduced or stopped because of use.
- Use continues despite adverse consequences.

Recognition

Although drug testing is used in emergencies because clinical diagnosis is so unreliable, a medical history and physical examination coupled with confirmatory laboratory testing are useful for diagnosing drug dependence. Direct observation of a health professional using drugs, inappropriately carrying or procuring drugs, or having withdrawal symptoms makes the diagnosis possible. This is so because lying and denial are part of the disease of addiction. Naturally, the intensity of withdrawal depends on whether a tolerant and dependent person is given an antagonist (e.g., naloxone, naltrexone) to provoke withdrawal or whether opiates are slowly discontinued. Abrupt withdrawal from opiates often results in nausea, vomiting, diarrhea, goose flesh, dilated pupils, perspiration, increased vital signs (pulse rate, respiratory rate, blood pressure), bone and muscle aches, and a delusional fear that death will occur without opiates. These symptoms are associated with a very strong drive for the drug. Track marks and other physical evidence of parenteral use may be found during examination of a chemically dependent anesthesiologist. Most anesthesiologists, however, are quite adept at using needles and finding discreet intravenous injection sites. Patients, physician colleagues, and loved ones often recognize the drug seeking, acquisition, and consumption after it becomes clear that addiction is the cause of observed problems. Clinicians and experienced addicts recognize that a protracted syndrome, which may last for months and include episodes of sweats, night terrors, dysphoria, drug craving, and malaise, generally follows the acute withdrawal phase with its dramatic symptoms.

Laboratory diagnosis is the gold standard. Drug testing is available and reliable when the correct methodology is used and the correct body fluid for the particular opioid being abused is tested. Thin-layer chromatography is the most inexpensive and commonly used comprehensive test. Enzyme-linked immunoassays can detect opiates, methadone, and propoxyphene even in the microgram or picogram per milliliter range. Gas chromatography with mass spectroscopy is a gold standard for testing. Blood testing using this method or radioimmunoassay is necessary for some very potent opioids (e.g., fentanyl).

Risk Assessment

Opiates have been important analgesics and drugs of abuse for centuries. With the availability of parenterally administered opiates and the invention of the hypodermic syringe, opiate addiction and withdrawal distress are now major, worldwide public health problems. Drug dependence is a disorder characterized by compulsive drug use, tolerance, and withdrawal symptoms with cessation of drug use.

The concept of drug tolerance was originally based on the observation that opioids lose their physiologic effects with repeated use. As tolerance develops, drug-dependent subjects progressively increase the dose of the drug to achieve the originally experienced euphoric effects.

In the psychopharmacologic context, tolerance is an organism's adaptive response to supraphysiologic levels of an exogenous substance. A major drawback of this adaptation is that on cessation of drug use, the physiologic adaptations remain unopposed and induce a physiologic withdrawal syndrome. After chronic opioid use, cessation can induce a severe physical withdrawal syndrome including diarrhea, hypertension, vomiting, and muscle cramps. Depression, dysphoria, or negative affective symptoms (e.g., anhedonia) are associated with the cessation of almost all drugs of abuse. Depression and suicide are common comorbidities with drug abuse and dependence. In contrast to drug use, drug dependence is characterized by loss of control over drug intake and the development of tolerance and withdrawal.

Addiction among health professionals is a significant public health problem. Without treatment, impaired professionals harm themselves, their families, and their patients. Although treatment outcomes for physician addicts are remarkably positive, there is a dearth of research on the primary prevention of substance abuse and dependence in this population. Researchers have studied opioid-addicted physicians for decades, reported on the use of clonidine and naltrexone in this population, and followed them for many years after detoxification. Although physicians are overrepresented among prescription drug addicts, their rates of alcohol abuse and dependence are similar to those of appropriately matched controls.

All medical schools and hospitals encounter cases of physician opioid abuse, dependence, and overdose. However, they attribute these events to poor self-regulation or ease of drug access. Substance abuse appears to be an occupational hazard among physicians, but why is this so? To become a physician, one must be a high achiever throughout high school and college to obtain the required grades and test scores for medical school admission. Additionally, potential physicians must continue to excel throughout medical school to gain internships and residencies.

Physicians seem unlikely candidates for opioid injection and self-administration. However, they are 30 to 100 times more likely to become addicted to narcotics than the general population. One study estimated that 12.5% of male physicians are drug dependent, compared with 0.1% of men in the general population. Although alcohol-related disorders and cigarette smoking rates were comparable between physicians and other Harvard University graduates, physicians had higher rates of drug use and prescription drug abuse, depression, depression with substance abuse, and suicide than other age- and sex-matched professionals. At least 15% of all physicians will become markedly impaired during their careers. Stress and access have dominated the theories for physician use and dependence, but basic scientists who conduct research with cocaine or narcotics do not usually use these drugs themselves. Further, not all medical subspecialties are equally represented among physicians with substance use disorders (Fig. 31-1). Perhaps anesthesiologists suffer a high rate of drug abuse because they administer

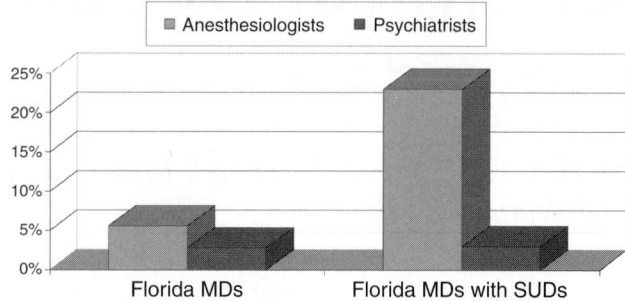

Figure 31–1 ▪ Substance use disorders (SUDs) among anesthesiologists and psychiatrists in Florida.

highly potent anesthetics or other drugs to patients; they also work in a confined space around the patient's head and are exposed in the workplace to discarded drugs (e.g., narcotics, benzodiazepines) that can affect the brain, emotions, and behavior. This intriguing hypothesis merits further consideration in future investigations.

Fentanyl and its analogues deserve special mention as a risk to anesthesiologists. Fentanyl abuse, overdose deaths, and dependence have been limited to health care professionals for many years. Fentanyl is a narcotic analgesic developed in the early 1960s by Janssen Pharmaceutica in Belgium. Like morphine, fentanyl is an opioid receptor agonist that preferentially binds μ-opioid receptors. Fentanyl's chemical structure, however, is distinct from that of morphine analogues. Also, new and more potent fentanyl analogues have been developed. The most potent is 3-methylfentanyl, which is about 6000 times as potent as morphine and 600 times as potent as heroin. Unfortunately, these potent analgesics also have an extremely high abuse potential and have been associated with a large number of drug overdose deaths. Between 1979 and 1988, 108 drug overdose deaths were related to fentanyl analogues in California alone. The respiratory depressant effects of fentanyl, combined with its extreme potency, may account for the high number of overdose deaths. It has been reported that fentanyl concentrations vary between 1 and 10 ng/mL in the body fluids of those dying of fentanyl overdose, which is very low compared with the concentrations of other abused opioids. For example, free morphine concentrations in heroin overdose deaths vary between 462 and 1350 ng/mL. In 2004, prescription methadone, OxyContin-like analgesics, and fentanyl were more likely to cause an overdose death in Florida than was heroin.

Implications

At the onset of therapy, a full medical and psychiatric evaluation helps predict the outcome of therapy. Intravenous drug abuse is associated with a number of medical conditions, including bacterial or viral endocarditis, hepatitis, acquired immunodeficiency syndrome, tuberculosis, cellulitis, cerebritis, wound abscess, sepsis, arterial thrombosis, renal infarction, and thrombophlebitis. The most common severe complications from intravenous drug use, however, are accidents, head injuries, memory failure, sexually transmitted diseases, seizures, depression, suicidal thinking, and suicide attempts. Opioid dependence is associated with a very high death rate, with an annual incidence of about 10 per 1000 persons among those who are untreated. Death is most often due to overdose, accidents, injuries, or general medical complications. In some places, violence accounts for more opioid-related deaths than does overdose or human immunodeficiency virus infection. Beyond these medical issues, physician addicts are exposed to significant professional risk in medical credentialing and licensure, as well as marital and other personal problems.

MANAGEMENT

Detoxification and abstinence are the treatment of choice for physician addicts; replacement or maintenance treatments (e.g., methadone) are not used for this class of addicts. In the detoxification phase, clonidine not only provides an effective nonopiate treatment for opiate withdrawal but also allows a rapid progression from opiate dependence to maintenance, especially when coupled with naltrexone. Together, clonidine and naltrexone reduce the detoxification process from 14 days to 8 to 24 hours. This combination has rapidly become a new standard of treatment, along with opiate maintenance, detoxification and abstinence, 12-step fellowships, and therapeutic communities. Clonidine and naltrexone, however, also reveal the limitations of pharmacologic advances in the prevention and treatment of opiate addiction, for none of these treatments has greatly impacted the long-term natural history of the disease.

Nevertheless, the treatment of physicians in specialized physician programs has been remarkably efficacious. Whereas most treatment programs for addicts have been shortened, physician and health care provider treatment programs have been extended to include inpatient, residential, and rehabilitation phases. Using these techniques, long-term treatment outcomes for physicians are far better than those reported for similarly diagnosed addicts in the general population. In the most recent study of randomly selected Physician Recovery Network physician addicts at 5 years, 91.4% had returned to work. This rate is comparable to the results of other studies of physician addicts. In summary, good management options exist to care for physicians addicted to narcotics and allow them to obtain meaningful recovery and return to their professional duties.

PREVENTION

Our research confirms other studies' findings that anesthesiologists have an increased rate of opiate abuse and dependence. Left untreated, addiction has numerous adverse health consequences for anesthesiologists, as well as their patients and families. Early detection is critical and makes outpatient treatment more successful. For prevention and early detection,

consideration should be given to random testing until the cause is identified and remedied.

Further Reading

Aach RD, Girard DE, Humphrey H, et al: Alcohol and other substance abuse and impairment among physicians in residency training. Ann Intern Med 116:245-254, 1992.

American Psychiatric Association Diagnostic and Statistical Manual of Mental Disorders. Washington, DC, American Psychiatric Press, 1994.

Bohigian GM, Croughan JL, Sanders K: Substance abuse and dependence in physicians: An overview of the effects of alcohol and drug abuse. Mo Med 91:233-238, 1994.

Gold MS: Opiate addiction and the locus coeruleus. Psychiatr Clin North Am 16:61-73, 1993.

Gold MS, Frost-Pineda K, Pomm R: Is addiction an occupational hazard for anesthesiologists? College on Problems of Drug Dependence, 2004. Available online at http://biopsych.com:81/CPDD04_Web/MeetProgAbSearch_04.html

Gold MS, Miller NS: Intoxication and withdrawal from opiates and inhalants. In Miller NS, Gold MS, Smith DE (eds): Manual of Therapeutics for Addictions. New York, Wiley-Liss, 1992, pp 72-86.

Gold MS, Redmond DE Jr, Kleber HD: Clonidine may relieve opiate withdrawal symptoms. JAMA 240:25-27, 1978.

Goldberger BA, Merves ML, Frost-Pineda K, et al: Use, misuse and diversion of methadone and hydrocodone: The deaths continue to increase J Clin Pharmacol 43:83, 2003.

Henderson GL: Blood concentrations of fentanyl and its analogs in overdose victims. Proc West Pharmacol Soc 26:287-290, 1983.

Henderson GL: Designer drugs: Past history and future prospects. J Forensic Sci 33:569-575, 1988.

Herridge P, Gold MS: Pharmacological adjuncts in the treatment of opioid and cocaine addicts. J Psychoactive Drugs 20:233-242, 1988.

Jacobs WS, Hall JD, Pomm R: Prognostic factors for physician addiction outcomes at five years. J Addict Dis 22:140, 2003.

Janssen PAJ: 1-Aralkyl-4-(n-aryl-carbonyl-amino)-piperidines and related compounds. US Patent Office No. 3,164,600, 1965.

Koob GF: Neuroadaptive mechanisms of addiction: Studies on the extended amygdala. Eur Neuropsychopharmacol 13:442-452, 2003.

Maguire P, Tsai N, Kamal J, et al: Pharmacological profiles of fentanyl analogs at mu, delta and kappa opiate receptors. Eur J Pharmacol 213:219-225, 1992.

Miller NS, Mahler JC, Gold MS: Suicide risk associated with drug and alcohol dependence. J Addict Dis 10:49-61, 1991.

Moriya F, Hashimoto Y: Distribution of free and conjugated morphine in body fluids and tissues in a fatal heroin overdose: Is conjugated morphine stable in postmortem specimens? J Forensic Sci 42:736-740, 1997.

Repetto M, Frost-Pineda K, Gold MS: Pharmacological therapeutics for alcohol, cocaine and opioid intoxication and detoxification. In Miller NS, Wadland WC (eds): Addictions in Medicine: Principles and Practice. Hoboken, NJ, John Wiley & Sons, 2004.

Shook JE, Watkins WD, Camporesi EM: Differential roles of opioid receptors in respiration, respiratory disease, and opiate-induced respiratory depression. Am Rev Respir Dis 142:895-909, 1990.

Talbott GD, Richardson AC Jr, Mashburn JS, et al: The Medical Association of Georgia's Disabled Doctors Program—a 5-year review. J Med Assoc Ga 70:545-549, 1981.

Vaillant GE, Brighton JR, McArthur C: Physicians' use of mood-altering drugs: A 20-year follow-up report. N Engl J Med 282:365-370, 1970.

Van Bever WF, Niemegeers CJ, Janssen PA: Synthetic analgesics: Synthesis and pharmacology of the diastereoisomers of N-(3-methyl-1-(2-phenylethyl)-4-piperidyl)-N-phenylpropanamide and N-(3-methyl-1-(1-methyl-2-phenylethyl)-4-piperidyl)-N-phenylpropanamide. J Med Chem 17:1047-1051, 1974.

Chemical Dependency: Nonopioids

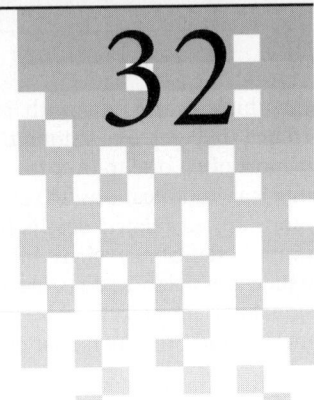

Mark S. Gold, Kimberly Frost-Pineda, and William Jacobs

Case Synopses

Alcohol

Dr. P is a 60-year-old white male anesthesiologist with a 40-year history of alcohol abuse. Five years ago, he was questioned about alcohol on his breath before starting an 8:00 AM case. He immediately took a blood alcohol concentration (BAC) test, which was below detectable limits, and proceeded with the case. Two years later, the operating room staff thought they detected the smell of alcohol on his breath; that time, his BAC was 0.12. Dr. P denied having had anything to drink since midnight but admitted to drinking vodka tonics the night before. He was referred to the state physician's health program (PHP), where he was evaluated by an addictionologist certified by the American Society for Addictive Medicine. Dr. P successfully completed an intensive outpatient program and then entered into a monitoring agreement with the PHP. He actively participated in the facilitated group meetings and attended 12-step meetings but did not get a sponsor or work the steps. Random urine testing was negative until 1 month ago. Dr. P had had three drinks after his wife retired for the night and was selected for a random urine drug screen the following morning. He notified the PHP facilitator of his relapse before the positive result was reported.

Tobacco

Dr. K is a 62-year-old white male anesthesiologist with a 100 pack-year history of cigarette smoking. He has smoked two packs a day since age 12 and has suffered from chronic bronchitis and chronic obstructive pulmonary disease for at least the past 12 years. He has made numerous attempts to stop smoking—including cold turkey, hypnosis, and nicotine patch—without success. He now believes that he is "too old" to quit. He slipped on a wet floor in the operating room last week and fell against the anesthesia machine. Since then, he has had left-sided chest pain at the site of the impact and had a lateral chest film taken today. He reads the film himself and sees a cavitating lesion in the right upper lobe.

Cannabis

Dr. B is a 28-year-old black male anesthesiologist who joined a prestigious private practice after finishing his chief residency at a major university anesthesiology program. He immediately became a favorite of many surgeons and operating room staff. He was seen smoking cigars on his way home on a number of occasions. After 6 months in private practice, he purchased a new car that was valued at over $100,000. The following Friday, after finishing his cases and leaving the hospital, he was arrested for misdemeanor possession of marijuana and drug paraphernalia after a police officer saw his car pulled to the side of the road. Dr. B was caught with six rolled "joints." The incident was discovered by his partners within 24 hours, and he was given no option but to self-report to the state PHP. He was evaluated and found to have a long history of polysubstance dependence that had evolved into cannabis dependence and alcohol abuse. He was treated in a long-term residential treatment program and entered into a 5-year monitoring agreement with the PHP. His license was placed on probation for 2 years after treatment and then restored to unencumbered active status. He returned to private practice after completing residential treatment.

Cocaine

Dr. W is a 44-year-old white male anesthetist who was reported to his state PHP after being seen snorting a white powder, presumed to be cocaine, in the men's room during the hospital Christmas party. He was contacted 2 days after the party and denied any drug abuse. A urine drug screen was requested immediately, and Dr. W reluctantly complied. It was positive for benzyleconine, a cocaine metabolite. Dr. W was not allowed to continue working and, after an evaluation by an addiction psychiatrist, was admitted to a residential substance abuse treatment program.

PROBLEM ANALYSIS

Definition

Nonopiate abuse and dependence are common among health care professionals. Alcohol and tobacco are the most commonly abused chemical substances, but marijuana is the most commonly abused *illicit* chemical substance in the general population.

It is widely believed that tobacco, alcohol, and marijuana are the most commonly abused substances among physicians. Alcohol dependence appears to be as common among physicians as among their age-, sex-, socioeconomic-matched controls. Cannabis abuse is quite common among medical students and younger physicians, and alcohol dependency is more common among older physicians. Although the abuse of other illicit or licit substances, such as cocaine, is not as prevalent, it may cause significant impairment and have detrimental effects on the lives of health care providers, their patients, and their families. Although the diversion and abuse of prescription drugs by physicians and other health care personnel are also a concern, this problem is not discussed here.

Definitions for impairment and chemical (substance) dependence are found in Chapter 31. Substance dependence can have a number of negative impacts, including severe medical and legal implications. Chemical dependence can impair function in relation to acute intoxication, drug-seeking behavior, chronic dependence, and substance withdrawal. In this chapter, we focus on the recognition of nonopiate dependence—specifically, alcohol, tobacco, marijuana, and cocaine. Also, we consider behaviors associated with such substance use, the diagnosis of dependence, its implications, and the management and prevention of substance dependency.

Recognition and Risk Assessment

DIAGNOSIS

Several screening tests are available for the diagnosis of substance abuse, such as the CAGE and AUDIT programs for alcohol; these have now been modified for marijuana abuse. Clinical diagnosis of substance abuse is often difficult, because denial and lying are part of the disease of addiction. Denial is the hallmark of many initial clinical interviews. Physicians may admit to use, but only on occasion. They may quote the *New York Times* or *High Times* to defend their use, as opposed to a respected medical, addiction, or psychiatric text or journal. They may actually say that marijuana smoke is not dangerous to one's health and deny any similarities to tobacco smoking or secondhand smoke. Among health care professionals, direct observation of drug use, possession, inappropriate procurement of drugs, or signs and symptoms of intoxication or withdrawal can help make the diagnosis. The diagnosis of abuse or dependence is based on *Diagnostic and Statistical Manual of Mental Disorders (DSM-IV)* criteria (see Chapter 31). The medical history and physical examination, along with confirmatory laboratory testing, are useful for diagnosis. Although there could be other reasons for changes in personality, family problems, infertility (males), withdrawal from social activities, and impaired ability to perform professional duties, a positive drug test moves a substance use disorder to the top of the differential diagnosis.

Physicians rarely refer themselves to addiction specialists for drug abuse or dependence problems. Laboratory testing is the gold standard for confirming substance use and is also helpful during treatment. Drug testing cannot detect all marijuana, cocaine, or other illicit drug users, however. Random testing does not detect all substances of abuse and may not detect infrequent use. For example, even daily users have only a 50-50 probability of testing positive in any given month when urine testing is done eight times per year. Urine testing is standard for the evaluation and treatment of substance abuse; detection times for some common drugs of abuse are given in Table 32-1. There have also been advances in the testing of other biologic substrates, including hair, sweat, and oral fluid. Thin-layer chromatography and enzyme-linked antibody testing are the most comprehensive, inexpensive, and widely used drug screening tests, but combined gas chromatography with mass spectroscopy is the gold standard for drug testing. Marijuana impairment must be diagnosed with blood tetrahydrocannabinol (THC) concentrations. Random drug testing should be a mandatory part of all health care provider health programs.

Laboratory tests may also help in the diagnosis of a chronic substance abuse problem, but they are usually performed late in the course of the disease. Heavy consumption of alcohol (e.g., one bottle of wine a day) for a few months almost always results in macrocytosis (mean corpuscular volume between 100 and 110 fL), even before anemia occurs. Alcohol-related liver disease may be reflected in abnormal serum γ-glutamyltransferase, aspartate transaminase, and alanine transaminase levels. In fact, unlike in other liver diseases, aspartate transaminase may be more than two times greater than alanine transaminase when alcoholic hepatitis is present. The Food and Drug Administration has also approved a new test that measures serum carbohydrate-deficient transferrin to identify long-term excessive alcohol use.

ALCOHOL AND TOBACCO

Symptoms of alcohol or tobacco dependence include the following:

- Impaired control over use
- Preoccupation with obtaining the substance
- Continued use, despite adverse consequences
- Distorted thinking, especially denial of substance dependency
- Development of tolerance to the effects
- Withdrawal symptoms when use is discontinued

Table 32–1 ■ Substance Detection Time in Urine	
Substance	**Detection Times**
Amphetamines	Up to 24 hr
Barbiturates	5-10 days
Benzodiazepines	5-7 days
Cannabinoids	1-3 days; greater with chronic use
Cocaine	1-3 days
Opiates	1-3 days
Phencyclidine	Up to 3 days

Although no specific constellation of symptoms is specific for the diagnosis of alcohol abuse or dependence, physical examination findings consistent with alcohol abuse are elevated blood pressure, evidence of physical harm, tremors, obstructive lung disease (due to concurrent tobacco use), and unexplained tachycardia, hepatosplenomegaly, or peripheral neuropathy. In contrast to alcohol, the health consequences of tobacco dependence generally take years to develop and are related primarily to lung cancer or chronic pulmonary disease. Just quitting smoking has immediate positive health effects, reduces the risk for adverse consequences over time, and increases the smoker's life expectancy. (see www.cancer.org for more details).

COCAINE

A number of clinical and behavioral signs and symptoms of cocaine use are usually evident. Some are related to acute intoxication, and others appear after chronic use or during withdrawal (Table 32-2). Although cocaine is more commonly abused as a "street drug" (snorted as powder or smoked as crack), it is also used medicinally as a topical anesthetic and vasoconstrictor (e.g., in awake oral or nasal intubation). If so, health care professionals may have access to unadulterated cocaine, similar to fentanyl and other highly potent narcotics (see Chapter 31). Street cocaine is often adulterated or "cut" with other substances that have the potential to cause additional harm.

MARIJUANA

In the 1960s and 1970s, marijuana was perceived as a safe and natural drug that produced a "high" (euphoria) without the risk of negative side effects or addiction. Some young physicians still do not believe that marijuana dependence is possible and may smoke marijuana more frequently than cigarettes. Dependence on marijuana is related to the THC concentration in its smoke and the duration of use; signs of marijuana withdrawal can be provoked by the administration of a THC antagonist. Today, the THC concentration in "street" marijuana has been increased to encourage repeat use. Researchers at Harvard and Columbia have shown that with this increased potency, chronic marijuana use can lead to tolerance, dependence (even subhuman animal species will self-administer THC), and a distinct withdrawal syndrome. Marijuana is now one of the leading substances of abuse in persons institutionalized for the treatment of substance abuse.

As defined in *DSM-IV*, marijuana intoxication begins with a feeling of being "high." Symptoms vary but generally include grandiosity, euphoria, and inappropriate laughter. Acute use also causes difficulty with concentration and complex thought processes; distorted sensory and time perception; lethargy and sedation; and impaired judgment, memory (especially short-term memory), and motor performance. Marijuana use sometimes provokes anxiety and panic, which may require treatment. During and after intoxication, there is generally increased appetite, red eyes, dry mouth, and increased heart rate. As these effects subside, there is often depressed mood, anger, irritability, or social withdrawal. Experimental cannabinoid antagonists, which are now in clinical trials, appear to be the most effective treatment for the overeating and memory problems related to chronic marijuana dependence. The long-term health effects of marijuana smoke are difficult to determine because persons who use marijuana often use tobacco products as well. Recent studies have shown, however, that there are many carcinogens in marijuana smoke, which actually has 50% higher levels of tar and carcinogens than tobacco smoke does. Also, case-control studies have linked marijuana smoke to head and neck cancers.

Table 32–2 ■ Signs and Symptoms of Acute Cocaine Intoxication and Chronic Cocaine Abuse or Dependence

Acute Cocaine Intoxication		Chronic Cocaine Abuse or Dependence	
Signs	**Clinical Symptoms**	**Physical and Mental Symptoms**	**Behavioral and Social Signs**
Sociability—most users become overly "chatty" at low doses Hypervigilance Impaired judgment Grandiose thinking and plans Increased anxiety and tension Quick mood changes Increased libido	Blood pressure changes Breathing difficulties Dilated pupils Mental confusion Muscle weakness Tachycardia, chest pain Nausea or vomiting Psychomotor agitation or retardation, seizures Sweating or chills	Anxiety, delirium, depression, hallucinations, insomnia, memory loss, confusion, slurred speech, reflex changes, blackouts, acute vision changes, incoordination, dizziness, tremors, impotence Hypertension, irregular heartbeat, bradycardia Bronchitis, lingering colds and flu symptoms, frequent respiratory tract infections Bumps and bruises due to falls Craving for sweets or avoidance, loss of appetite, poor nutrition, liver enlargement Increased or reduced alcohol or drug tolerance Red, puffy face; red, swollen nasal mucosa	Car and boat accidents Problems with family or job (e.g., tardiness, absenteeism) Legal or financial problems Increased reliance on drugs Passive-aggressive behavior, suicidal thoughts or gestures, violent or aggressive behavior, suspiciousness

People who become dependent on marijuana usually use it daily, often for months or years. When they try to stop using it, they often cannot do so for longer than 30 days. They are also easily angered by questions about their marijuana use, because they are psychopathologically attached to the substance. Often, this has a negative impact on their health, families, and careers. Moreover, they may choose parties, social contacts, or friends on the basis of whether marijuana is going to be available, and they may spend many hours each day thinking about using marijuana and later recovering from the effects. Further, they may smoke cigarettes or take psychostimulants in an attempt to reverse the effects of marijuana on their memory or performance. Dependence interferes with family life and work, but use continues despite the development of chronic problems, such as a smoker's cough or psychological problems (e.g., excessive sedation resulting from repeated use of high doses), or social consequences.

Implications

Maladaptive behavior problems are usually the first sign of chemical dependency. However, these often are not attributed to drug abuse until after an addiction is recognized. Health care professionals are generally better equipped than others to hide and deny substance abuse. Most often, family and social problems related to use occur far in advance of problems on the job. Health care professionals who are using drugs may experience changes in mood, energy level, and the ability to concentrate. They also miss work or arrive late. They may use the drug more often and at inappropriate times, taking more frequent breaks than their colleagues. In addition, they may have alcohol on their breath or smell of tobacco or marijuana smoke. Often family and friends become aware of the drug-seeking, -acquiring, and -consuming behaviors before patients and other physicians recognize the problems.

Chemical-dependent health care professionals often have problems in their interpersonal relationships, and they are exposed to significant professional risk in terms of medical credentialing and licensure, as well as criminal investigations. A physician might come to attention by propositioning a prostitute or experiencing money problems related to gambling or purchasing drugs. However, these are late-stage behaviors. Early detection requires a high degree of suspicion both at the workplace and at home. Common severe complications from drug abuse include accidents, head injuries, memory failure, financial collapse, sexually transmitted diseases, seizures, depression, impulsivity, suicidal thinking, and suicide attempts.

Negative affective symptoms (e.g., anhedonia), depression, and dysphoria are symptoms associated with the cessation of almost all drugs of abuse (see also Chapter 31). The chemical withdrawal syndrome specific to the drug of choice may be another sign of chronic use and dependence. The desire for the drug is probably greatest during withdrawal, because the addicted person wishes to alleviate unpleasant withdrawal symptoms. Health care professionals who abuse or become dependent on drugs have higher rates of depression, which may lead to suicide without intervention and treatment.

ALCOHOL AND TOBACCO

Alcohol and tobacco are the most widely used drugs. Alcohol is generally considered safe and may even have a beneficial effect when used in moderation. However, there are no established moderate or safe levels of tobacco use. People who smoke often drink, and those who abuse alcohol usually use tobacco; thus, dependence on both alcohol and tobacco is common. Tobacco smoking is the leading cause of death among alcoholics. Alcohol can also be potent and dangerous, causing more death and personal destruction than any other drug except for tobacco. Each year, alcohol misuse causes more than 100,000 deaths and injury to more than 2 million people; tobacco is reportedly responsible for more than 400,000 deaths annually.

COCAINE

The pathologic attraction to cocaine can be intense, with many experts agreeing that it is the most intense among the substances of abuse. Although detoxification is usually unnecessary, discontinuation is clinically significant and difficult to manage outside of a hospital or highly controlled environment. Craving for cocaine, anhedonia, feelings of helplessness, and drive for the drug make relapse likely. Animal self-administration models suggest that the amount of work or punishment an animal will expend or endure for a dose of cocaine is greater than for most other drugs.

Once the physician addict discontinues the drug, treatment begins. We have reported on cocaine sniffing, cocaine injecting, and even crack addiction among physicians. Cocaine addiction is so profound and relapse so common that the *DSM* had to change the diagnostic criteria to allow addiction to be diagnosed in the absence of significant signs and symptoms of withdrawal. Addicted physicians often sign contingency contracts, agree to random and at least biweekly urine testing, and are sent to inpatient and residential treatment facilities.

MARIJUANA

Possessing, smoking, growing, and purchasing marijuana are all illegal. Physicians who do so are a phone call or two away from losing their licenses. This usually does not occur, however. Their spouses, children, or angry patients may call an anonymous tip line to report their behavior. Marijuana use may bring doctors into contact with other illicit drugs, leading to further experimentation. Sometimes, marijuana smoking or the use of other illicit substances brings physicians into contact with drug dealers and other criminals. Physicians are usually undertrained for this social network and may be easily blackmailed or robbed by their dealers or new "friends."

MANAGEMENT

Changes in thinking and behavior, along with a positive drug test, are usually taken as definitive evidence of substance abuse by hospital staffs, physician employment groups, and state physician health monitoring programs. Detoxification and abstinence, followed by involvement in 12-step fellowships and therapeutic communities, remain the treatment of choice for professional health care addicts. It is important to note that detoxification is not sufficient treatment. Numerous treatment programs are designed to meet the special needs of addicted health care professionals. There are also a number of pharmacologic therapies that may be useful in the treatment of alcohol, tobacco, marijuana, and cocaine dependence (Table 32-3). Physicians have the best outcomes when there is long-term follow-up, random routine drug testing, 12-step group attendance, and individual follow-up with a psychiatrist and treatment facilitator.

Alcohol and Tobacco

Both psychosocial and pharmacologic therapies can help in overcoming alcohol and tobacco addiction. Some of these can be purchased over the counter (e.g., nicotine replacements), but others require a prescription. For alcohol, a number of pharmacologic therapies have been approved for use in the United States, including disulfiram (Antabuse), naltrexone, and acamprosate.

Cocaine

Treatment for cocaine dependence includes both residential and outpatient approaches. One primary approach is behavioral intervention. After stabilization, recovery begins with a learning process of breaking old habits, breaking ties with cocaine-using friends, and identifying "triggers" that increase the desire to use cocaine; once these triggers are identified, patients are encouraged to restructure their lifestyles to avoid them. Cognitive-behavioral coping skills provide another alternative that, in the short term, focuses on helping cocaine-addicted individuals become abstinent through a learning process. This therapy is compatible with a range of other treatments, such as pharmacotherapy. Active membership in 12-step programs, such as Narcotics Anonymous and Cocaine Anonymous, is one of the most beneficial tools for continued abstinence from cocaine and other drugs of abuse. For addicted health care professionals, regular random drug testing, a contract, and chronic follow-up care improve the long-term success of treatment. It is imperative that any positive drug tests be promptly identified and that any necessary changes in treatment plans be made quickly. Waiting can be associated with a rapid and complete relapse. Finally, cocaine abstinence and long-term use are associated with depression,

suicidal ideation, and suicide attempts; thus, cocaine-dependent physicians must be closely monitored.

Marijuana

Treatments under study include use of the synthetic marijuana dronabinol (Marinol). This is similar to the use of methadone for heroin addicts. Relapse prevention is an important factor in the successful treatment of marijuana dependence. Recovering addicts must change their behaviors and be able to resist social and environmental cues for continued drug use. Psychosocial treatments, such as cognitive-behavioral therapy, can be successful. Pharmacologic therapies under study may be useful as maintenance therapy.

PREVENTION

Prevention of substance abuse and dependence starts with abstinence—that is, no experimentation. Physicians are well educated and are therefore used as examples of the limitations of knowledge as a protective factor against addiction. Drug use, abuse, and dependence are now observed in medical students and house staff, not just in older practicing physicians. Physicians who have learned to balance their lives and manage their stress, anxiety, and workplace problems without drugs should mentor medical students to help them learn to do the same. Addiction among health care professionals is a significant public health problem that requires intervention. Without treatment, addiction leads to harm to self, family, and patients. At least 15% of all physicians will become markedly impaired sometime during their careers; however, there continues to be a dearth of research on the primary prevention of substance abuse and dependence among health care providers.

Generally, the best way to prevent drug dependence is to prevent drug use in the first place. For example, there is a strong genetic risk for alcohol dependence among those who have a positive family history, especially among first-degree relatives. Such persons should refrain from using alcohol. Prevention of exposure to drugs and drug use during early childhood and adolescence is key to reducing later dependence. Prevention efforts and appropriate training should also be a focus in medical schools and other

Table 32–3 ▪ Pharmacologic Treatment for Nonopioid Dependency

Substance	Pharmacologic Treatment
Alcohol	Antabuse—deters drinking by causing painful symptoms when alcohol is used
	Naltrexone—likely reduces craving and may reduce pleasurable effects of alcohol
	Acamprosate—reduces craving for alcohol and prevents relapse
Tobacco	Nicotine replacement: gum, patch, inhaler, spray
	Detoxification: bupropion (Zyban, Wellbutrin)—originally prescribed as an antidepressant but now used primarily for smoking cessation
Marijuana	Maintenance: Marinol—in clinical trials
	Antagonist: Rimonblat—in clinical trials
Cocaine	Definitive: none at present
	Supportive: antidepressants, mood stabilizers (e.g., lithium)

health care professional educational programs to minimize the risk of future chemical dependency problems. If primary prevention has failed, there is still the opportunity for early intervention.

Even if dependence has developed, we know that treatment works, especially for physician addicts, who have remarkably positive 5-year outcomes. Treatment can prevent or reduce the incidence of a number of adverse health outcomes. Another method to detect and prevent drug use that is increasingly being used in training, workplace, and treatment settings is random drug testing. Some leading institutions, such as Massachusetts General Hospital, have incorporated random testing into their substance abuse policy and now routinely test residents and house staff.

Further Reading

Aach RD, Girard DE, Humphrey H, et al: Alcohol and other substance abuse and impairment among physicians in residency training. Ann Intern Med 116:245-254, 1992.

American Psychiatric Association: Diagnostic and Statistical Manual of Mental Disorders, 4th ed [DSM-IV]. Washington, DC, American Psychiatric Press, 1994.

Bohigian GM, Croughan JL, Sanders K: Substance abuse and dependence in physicians: An overview of the effects of alcohol and drug abuse. Mo Med 91:233-238, 1994.

Gold MS, Aronson MD: Screening and diagnosis of patients with alcohol problems, and treatment of alcohol abuse and dependence. Harvard University's UpToDate Web site and CD-ROM Educational Program, 2005.

Gold MS, Frost-Pineda K: Substance abuse and psychiatric dual disorders: Focus on tobacco. J Dual Diagnosis 1:15-36, 2005.

Gold MS, Frost-Pineda K, Jacobs WS: In Galanter M, Klever HD (eds): Textbook of Substance Abuse Treatment, 3rd ed. New York, American Psychiatric Press, 2004, pp 167-188.

Gold MS, Jacobs W: Cocaine (and crack): Clinical aspects. In Lowinson JH, Ruiz P, Millman RB (eds): Substance Abuse: A Clinical Textbook, 2nd ed. Baltimore, Williams & Wilkins, 2004, pp 218-251.

Herridge P, Gold MS: Pharmacological adjuncts in the treatment of opioid and cocaine addicts. J Psychoactive Drugs 20:233-242, 1988.

Jacobs WS, Hall JD, Pomm R, et al: Prognostic factors for physician addiction: Outcomes at five years. J Addict Dis 22:140, 2003.

Jacobs WS, Repetto M, Vinson S: Random urine testing as an intervention for drug addiction. Psych Ann 34:781-785, 2004.

Koob GF: Neuroadaptive mechanisms of addiction: Studies on the extended amygdala. Eur Neuropsychopharmacol 13:442-452, 2003.

Miller NS, Mahler JC, Gold MS: Suicide risk associated with drug and alcohol dependence. J Addict Dis 10:49-61, 1991.

Repetto M, Frost-Pineda K, Gold MS: Pharmacological therapeutics for alcohol, cocaine and opioid intoxication and detoxification. In Miller NS, Wadland WC (eds): Addictions in Medicine: Principles and Practice. Hoboken, NJ, John Wiley & Sons, 2004.

Repetto M, Gold MS: Cocaine (and crack): Neurobiology In Lowinson JH, Ruiz P, Millman RB (eds): Substance Abuse: A Clinical Textbook, 2nd ed. Baltimore, Williams & Wilkins, 2004, pp 195-218.

Robinson TE: Addicted rats. Science 305:951-953, 2004.

Talbott GD, Richardson AC Jr, Mashburn JS, et al: The Medical Association of Georgia's Disabled Doctors Program—a 5-year review. J Med Assoc Ga 70:545-549, 1981.

Vaillant GE, Brighton JR, McArthur C: Physicians' use of mood-altering drugs: A 20-year follow-up report. N Engl J Med 282:365-370, 1970.

Reversal Agents: Naloxone and Flumazenil

33

Juliana Barr

Case Synopsis

An otherwise healthy 65-year-old, 80-kg man with coronary artery disease is given fentanyl (2 mg), midazolam (20 mg), and vecuronium (15 mg) intravenously during a 3-hour coronary artery bypass grafting procedure. He remains intubated and mechanically ventilated after surgery and is transferred to the intensive care unit (ICU) in stable condition. The surgeons elect for early extubation, but the patient remains deeply sedated, does not respond to painful stimuli, and is not "fighting" the ventilator. He is given intravenous (IV) naloxone (2 mg) and flumazenil (1 mg) over 5 minutes. He becomes acutely hypoxemic, with increasing rales and frothy pulmonary secretions. A chest radiograph reveals acute pulmonary edema, and the electrocardiogram shows ventricular ectopy.

PROBLEM ANALYSIS

Definition

Naloxone. Naloxone (Narcan) is an opioid antagonist that competitively inhibits the sedative, analgesic, and cardiopulmonary depressant effects of opioids at various opioid receptors. Typically, it is used to reverse the sedative and respiratory depressant effects of opioids. Following a single IV bolus injection, the onset of naloxone is rapid, with a short duration of effect (Table 33-1). It is metabolized hepatically, with renal excretion of its inactive metabolites. Small IV doses of naloxone (e.g., 20 to 40 μg) may reverse the respiratory depressant and sedative effects of opioids, but with incomplete reversal of the analgesic effects (Table 33-2). Larger doses may cause acute cardiopulmonary instability, especially in critically ill patients. Hypertension, tachycardia, arrhythmias, or acute fulminant pulmonary edema may occur following the administration of naloxone, even with incomplete reversal of the opioid's analgesic and sedative effects.

Flumazenil. Flumazenil (Romazicon) is a benzodiazepine antagonist with weak agonist activity at the γ-aminobutyric acid (GABA) receptor. It is given intravenously to reverse benzodiazepine-induced sedation, amnesia, disorientation, hypoventilation, or cardiovascular instability. After a single IV bolus dose, flumazenil's onset of action and peak effect occur within minutes (see Table 33-1). Because of its rapid hepatic clearance, flumazenil is short acting. It has no active or toxic metabolites. Flumazenil's duration of effect may be prolonged in patients with severe liver disease owing to reduced hepatic clearance. Unlike naloxone, flumazenil does not precipitate the acute onset of cardiopulmonary instability in critically ill patients, although it can cause signs of withdrawal or seizures in some patients.

Recognition

Naloxone. The onset of naloxone's cardiopulmonary side effects is rapid. Acute pulmonary edema results from increased hydrostatic pressure across the pulmonary capillary bed and increased pulmonary capillary permeability. This causes rapid extravasation of protein-rich fluid into the lung parenchyma. Hypertension is due to increased cardiac output, as well as increased systemic and pulmonary vascular resistance. The cardiovascular side effects of naloxone may resolve more quickly than the pulmonary edema and pulmonary hypertension.

Flumazenil. Like naloxone, the onset of flumazenil action is rapid. Because of its short duration of action, flumazenil does not precipitate cardiopulmonary instability; however, resedation and respiratory depression may recur after its administration. The total dose of flumazenil needed to achieve a full and sustained reversal of the side effects of benzodiazepines may vary with the potency and residual plasma concentration of the benzodiazepine used. Respiratory depression may not be fully reversed, however, even with maximal doses of flumazenil. In patients with a history of chronic benzodiazepine use, those undergoing benzodiazepine withdrawal, or those with tricyclic antidepressant overdose, flumazenil can cause seizures or other

Table 33–1 ■ Clinical Parameters of Intravenous Reversal Agents

Drug	Onset (min)	Peak Effect (min)	Duration of Effect (min)	Elimination Half-life (min)
Naloxone*	1-2	5-15	60-240	40-60†
Flumazenil	1-2	2-10	45-90	50‡

*Can also be given intramuscularly, subcutaneously, or endotracheally, although time to onset, peak effect, and duration and magnitude of effect may vary considerably among patients.

†Doubled in neonates.

‡Halved in neonates and prolonged in patients with liver disease.

Table 33–2 ■ Dosing Reversal Agents for Postoperative Sedation and Respiratory Depression

Drug	Intermittent IV Bolus Dosing*	Continuous IV Infusion*
Naloxone	20-40 µg q1-2 min (5-20 µg q1-2 min)	4-8 µg/kg/hr (4-8 µg/kg/hr)
Flumazenil	0.2 mg q2-5 min to ≤1 mg; may repeat q20 min; maximum dose 3 mg/hr (4-20 µg/kg)	0.5-1 µg/kg/min to ≤3 mg/hr (0.5-1 µg/kg/min)

*Pediatric doses are in parentheses.

signs of drug withdrawal. There are no reports of seizures following flumazenil administration to ICU patients who received benzodiazepines for chronic sedation.

Risk Assessment

Naloxone. The incidence of cardiopulmonary instability after naloxone administration is not known. Although it appears to occur more commonly in patients with preexisting cardiopulmonary disease, it has also been reported in patients without such disorders. Cardiopulmonary instability is more likely in critically ill patients and after cardiac surgery, because much larger doses of highly potent opioids (e.g., alfentanil, fentanyl, sufentanil) are used in these patients. Patients with a history of opioid use and physical dependency also appear to be at increased risk for cardiopulmonary instability, as well as seizures and other symptoms of opioid withdrawal (e.g., nausea, vomiting, diaphoresis, agitation), after naloxone. The risk for cardiopulmonary instability is increased with rapid administration of high IV doses of naloxone (400 µg).[1]

Flumazenil. Flumazenil is an effective means of reversing the residual sedative or respiratory depressant effects of benzodiazepines following the small doses typically used for anesthesia or conscious sedation. However, owing to flumazenil's short duration of action, ICU patients who receive chronic infusions or large doses of benzodiazepines may experience resedation and recurrent respiratory depression once flumazenil's antagonistic effects wear off. Therefore, flumazenil should not be used to hasten the termination of benzodiazepine sedation in these patients. However, a trial of flumazenil may be diagnostically useful in critically ill patients who fail to awaken within a reasonable time after discontinuing benzodiazepines. If the patient fails to awaken after receiving the maximal dose of IV flumazenil (3 mg over 1 hour), other causes of the persistent sedation or respiratory depression should be considered. Patients who do respond to flumazenil should be carefully monitored for up to 2 hours after the last dose of flumazenil for signs of resedation or recurrent respiratory depression.

Implications

Acute-onset hypertension, tachycardia, arrhythmias, or pulmonary edema after naloxone, or seizures after flumazenil, may not be well tolerated, especially in critically ill patients with preexisting cardiopulmonary disease. Cardiac surgical patients appear to be at even greater risk for hemodynamic instability after naloxone due to compromised myocardial performance and postoperative arrhythmias. Also, hemodynamic profiles can fluctuate rapidly with rewarming or increased circulating catecholamines. Moreover, the pulmonary capillary bed becomes more permeable owing to systemic inflammatory mediators released during cardiopulmonary bypass. If so, early postoperative naloxone may trigger acute, life-threatening cardiopulmonary changes in cardiac surgical patients. In contrast, flumazenil does not precipitate acute anxiety, hypertension, tachycardia, myocardial ischemia, or ventricular dysfunction in postoperative cardiac surgical patients who do not take benzodiazepines chronically.

MANAGEMENT

Avoid IV boluses and continuous naloxone infusions if cardiopulmonary instability occurs. Treat the patient symptomatically, as follows, until naloxone's effects resolve:

- Control blood pressure with short-acting IV antihypertensives (see Chapter 77).
- Treat myocardial ischemia with nitrates (see Chapter 76).
- Treat tachycardia with β-blockers (see Chapter 11).
- Treat arrhythmias with pacing, cardioversion, or defibrillation and antiarrhythmic drug therapy (see Chapters 10-13, 79-82, and 229).
- Minimize intravascular volume to minimize extravasation of fluid into lung tissues (see Chapter 16).
- Support oxygenation and ventilation.
- Provide treatment for exacerbating conditions or imbalances (e.g., acidosis, hypercarbia, hypoxia, hypokalemia, hypomagnesemia, agitation, pain).

Flumazenil can precipitate withdrawal symptoms (e.g., seizures, agitation, confusion) in patients with a physical dependence on benzodiazepines and can cause seizures in patients with tricyclic antidepressant overdose. Patients with any of these symptoms after flumazenil should be treated symptomatically, as follows:

- Seizures: antiepileptics, including benzodiazepines, phenytoin, or barbiturates

[1]Over a period of 2 months, shortly after naloxone became available for the reversal of high-dose opioid effects, the editor saw three cases of acute fulminant pulmonary edema that developed within 15 to 20 minutes after IV bolus naloxone (400 µg) was given in the postanesthesia care unit to patients who had had lengthy, major noncardiac surgeries. ICU admissions were not planned.

- Acute agitation and delirium: short-acting anxiolytics, including benzodiazepines
- Observation: careful monitoring for resedation or recurrent respiratory depression for up to 2 hours after benzodiazepine reversal with flumazenil

PREVENTION

Naloxone. Avoid high doses of naloxone, especially in critically ill patients. Small IV bolus doses (20 to 40 μg) or continuous infusions (4 to 8 μg/kg per hour) may reverse opioid-induced respiratory depression and sedation without reversing the analgesic effects of opioids or precipitating cardiopulmonary instability. The duration of naloxone's effect is brief and variable. Resedation and respiratory depression may occur following a single dose of naloxone.

Although naloxone can be given intramuscularly, subcutaneously, or endotracheally, IV dosing is preferred because of the variable uptake with other routes of administration. Further, the dose does not need to be adjusted in patients with hepatic or renal insufficiency, although the elimination half-life and duration of clinical effect may be prolonged in neonates. Naloxone readily crosses the placenta and may precipitate acute withdrawal symptoms or seizures in neonates or their opioid-dependent mothers.

Flumazenil. Flumazenil is safe and effective for reversing short-term sedation and respiratory depression with benzodiazepines, but not for chronically dependent patients.

It should be given in small divided doses, and patients must be carefully observed for signs of resedation and respiratory depression for at least 2 hours. Small repeat IV boluses (0.2 mg) or a low-dose continuous IV infusion (0.5 to 1 μg/kg per minute, up to 3 mg/hour) can be titrated to the desired level of sedation and ventilation. This more reliably prevents resedation of postoperative patients and also avoids abrupt or complete reversal of anxiolysis. Finally, avoid flumazenil in patients with chronic dependence on benzodiazepines or suspected tricyclic antidepressant overdose.

Further Reading

Bertaccini E, Geller E: Benzodiazepine antagonists and their role in anesthesia and critical care. Anaesth Pharmacol Rev 3:74-81, 1995.

Murray MJ, DeRuyter ML, Harrison BA: Opioids and benzodiazepines. In Cheng EY (ed): Sedation of the critically ill patient. Crit Care Clin 11:849-874, 1995.

Rudolph U, Crestani F, Möhler H, et al: Sedatives, anxiolytics, and amnestics. In Evers AS, Maze M (eds): Anesthetic Pharmacology: Physiologic Principles and Clinical Practice. Philadelphia, Churchill Livingstone, 2004, p 431.

Sasada M, Smith S: Flumazenil. In Drugs in Anaesthesia and Intensive Care, 3rd ed. New York, Oxford University Press, 2003, pp 162-163.

Sasada M, Smith S: Naloxone. In Drugs in Anaesthesia and Intensive Care, 3rd ed. New York, Oxford University Press, 2003, pp 266-267.

Stoelting RK: Benzodiazepines. In Pharmacology and Physiology in Anesthetic Practice, 3rd ed. Philadelphia, JB Lippincott–Williams & Wilkins, 1999, p 138.

Stoelting RK: Opioid agonists and antagonists. In Pharmacology and Physiology in Anesthetic Practice, 3rd ed. Philadelphia, JB Lippincott–Williams & Wilkins, 1999, pp 106-107.

White PF, Shafer A, Boyle WA, et al: Benzodiazepine antagonism does not provoke a stress response. Anesthesiology 70:636-639, 1989.

Steroids

Bhiken Naik and Lisa Thannikary

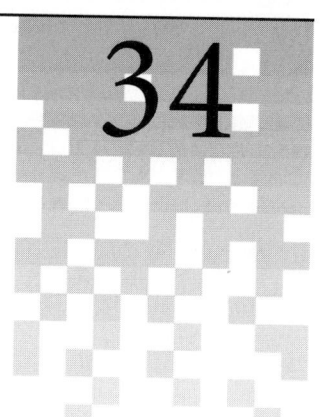

Case Synopsis

A 55-year-old man with severe chronic obstructive airway disease and steroid dependence is taken to the operating room emergently for an acute abdomen due to a perforated colonic diverticulum. The patient has been maintained on this dose of steroids for 1 year. Intraoperatively, he demonstrates hemodynamic instability requiring large-volume fluid resuscitation and the use of vasopressors. Postoperatively, he is transferred to the intensive care unit, where he is intubated and ventilated and remains hemodynamically unstable.

PROBLEM ANALYSIS

Definition

Steroids are the mainstay of therapy for a variety of disorders, including autoimmune diseases, and for immune suppression following solid organ transplantation. With chronic steroid therapy, there is a risk of triggering an addisonian crisis if cortisol levels are insufficient to meet the increased physiologic, perioperative demands. Following surgery, peak plasma cortisol concentrations are achieved after 4 to 5 hours and may remain elevated for 48 to 72 hours, especially following major surgery. Minor surgery induces less than 50 mg of cortisol production during the first 24 hours, but after major surgery, 75 to 100 mg of cortisol is produced in the same period. With maximal stress (e.g., septic shock), the adrenals may produce as much as 300 to 500 mg of cortisol per day.

Adrenal insufficiency is classified as primary, secondary, or tertiary, based on the anatomic level of impairment within the hypothalamic-pituitary-adrenal (HPA) axis. With primary adrenal insufficiency, the abnormality is in the adrenal gland. More than 90% of the adrenal gland must be destroyed before symptoms of glucocorticoid and mineralocorticoid deficiency are evident. The most common cause of primary adrenal insufficiency in the United States is autoimmune in nature. In secondary adrenal insufficiency, the abnormality is at the level of the pituitary gland. Such patients show symptoms of glucocorticoid deficiency but usually have intact mineralocorticoid function. Tertiary adrenal insufficiency is the most common type and is caused by suppression of the HPA axis by chronic exogenous steroids. However, there is a lack of prospective, randomized trials investigating perioperative steroid supplementation in patients receiving chronic steroids. Most available data are based on small case series and personal preference.

Recognition

The clinical presentation of an addisonian crisis varies from mild, nonspecific constitutional symptoms to the presence of profound shock unresponsive to vasopressor therapy. Clinicians should maintain a high index of suspicion when caring for patients receiving chronic steroids during the perioperative period. Mild symptoms or signs of adrenal insufficiency include nausea, vomiting, and abdominal pain. With associated hypoglycemia, there may be subtle neurologic symptoms (e.g., restlessness, lethargy). Mineralocorticoid deficiency occasionally accompanies an addisonian crisis and presents as hyponatremia and hyperkalemia with metabolic acidosis. With severe adrenal insufficiency, arterial hypotension with postural accentuation is common. Such hypotension may be refractory to fluid and vasopressor therapy.

Risk Assessment

The following are important predictors of risk for the development of adrenal insufficiency during the perioperative period:

- Total daily dose of steroids
- Duration of steroid therapy
- Type of surgery and degree of perioperative stress
- Response to short (rapid) adrenocorticotropic hormone (ACTH) stimulation test

It has been shown that the total daily dose of steroids determines the responsiveness of the HPA axis to stress. LaRochelle and colleagues demonstrated that when the total daily dose of prednisone was less than 5 mg, there was a normal response to the short ACTH test. With doses greater than 5 mg/day, however, responses to the short ACTH test varied widely. Although these authors reported that the duration of steroid therapy did not affect HPA axis recovery, there is evidence that HPA axis responsiveness may be impaired for up to 9 months after chronic steroid therapy. The nature of the surgery and the degree of perioperative stress are important determinants for steroid replacement therapy. Subjects undergoing major surgery have elevated glucocorticoid concentrations commensurate with the degree of stress and nature of the surgery. Finally, the response to the short ACTH test can help the clinician determine whether the HPA axis has returned to normal. It is sensitive for determining HPA axis impairment in subjects on chronic steroid therapy. Following measurement of baseline plasma cortisol concentrations, 250 µg of cosyntropin is administered intravenously (IV). Blood cortisol concentrations are then determined at 30 and 60 minutes. A normal response is a peak cortisol concentration greater than 18 µg/dL and a minimal increase of 7 µg/dL above baseline.

Table 34–1 ■ Steroid Supplementation Guidelines

Dose and Duration of Steroid Therapy*	Perioperative Management
<5 mg/day	Normal HPA axis; no supplemental steroids necessary
>5 mg/day—minor surgery	Hydrocortisone 25 mg at anesthetic induction; resume oral steroids
>5 mg/day—moderate surgery	Hydrocortisone 75-100 mg/day; taper over 1-2 days to usual dose
>5 mg/day—major surgery	Hydrocortisone 100-150 mg/day; taper over 1-2 days to usual dose
Steroids stopped <6 mo	Assume HPA axis impaired; dose steroids according to type of surgery
Steroids stopped >6 mo	Assume HPA axis intact; no supplemental steroids necessary
Septic shock with abnormal ACTH test	Hydrocortisone 100 mg q 8 h for 5-7 days
Late fibroproliferative ARDS	Methylprednisolone 2 mg/kg/day tapered to 0.125 mg/kg/day over 32 days

*Based on dose of cortisol (hydrocortisone). For relative potencies of synthetic corticosteroids, see Table 34-2.
ACTH, adrenocorticotropic hormone; ARDS, acute respiratory distress syndrome; HPA, hypothalamic-pituitary-adrenal.

Implications

Although addisonian crisis secondary to inadequate steroid supplementation is rare, vigilance by the anesthesiologist for subtle signs of adrenal insufficiency is important. The cumulative daily dose, the duration of chronic steroid therapy, and the nature of surgery are important factors for determining the integrity and responsiveness of the HPA axis. Further, there is increasing evidence of the importance of physiologic replacement doses of steroids in patients with sepsis and septic shock. Although supraphysiologic steroid doses have not been shown to improve outcomes, studies by both Annane and Bollaert and their coworkers have shown the benefits of physiologic replacement doses of steroids in septic shock. There also appears to be a beneficial role for steroid therapy in the late fibroproliferative phase of acute respiratory distress syndrome (ARDS). Although this conclusion is based on a small study by Meduri and associates, a larger multicenter trial is being conducted by the ARDS Network.

MANAGEMENT

As discussed earlier, the decision to supplement steroids in the perioperative period is based on the history of steroid intake and the severity of the planned surgery (Tables 34-1 and 34-2). *A standard dose for all patients should be avoided.* Supplemental doses should be individualized based on total daily dose, duration of therapy, and severity of perioperative stressors. Although the short ACTH test is useful for determining the integrity of the HPA axis, it may be impractical to perform the test in all patients. When steroids have been stopped for at least 6 months, it can be assumed that the HPA axis has returned to normal. Although some data suggest that a minimum of 2 months is sufficient time for the resumption of normal cortisol production, it is prudent to assume that HPA axis function will be impaired for up to 6 months. Patients taking less than 5 mg/day of prednisone or its equivalent can be assumed to have an intact HPA axis and do not require supplemental doses of steroids; however, it is important to continue the daily dose of the steroid.

With minor surgery, a supplemental dose of 25 mg of hydrocortisone should be given IV at induction of anesthesia; normal oral replacement therapy should be resumed postoperatively. With moderate surgical stress, the chronic daily steroid dose should be given IV preoperatively. Additional doses of hydrocortisone between 75 and 100 mg/day should be given IV. If there are no postoperative complications, the supplemental steroid should be weaned rapidly over 1 to 2 days, and the normal oral steroid dose should be restarted. With major surgery, the preoperative oral steroid dose should be followed by an additional 100 to 150 mg of intravenous hydrocortisone administered over 24 hours. In uncomplicated cases, this dose can be rapidly tapered within 24 to 48 hours. Patients with septic shock who are refractory to

Table 34–2 ■ Steroid Comparisons: Relative Glucocorticoid and Mineralocorticoid Potencies and Duration of Action

Steroid	Glucocorticoid Potency	Mineralocorticoid Potency	Duration of Action (hr)
Cortisol*	1	1	8-10
Prednisone	4	0.8	18-36
Prednisolone	4	0.8	12-36
Methylprednisolone	5	0.5	18-36
Dexamethasone	25-30	0	36-54
Fludrocortisone	10	120	18-36

*Identical to hydrocortisone.

fluid and vasopressor therapy can be treated with hydrocortisone 100 mg IV every 8 hours or with a continuous infusion of 10 mg/hour. Before initiating therapy, a short ACTH test should be performed to document adrenal insufficiency. When surgery is urgent or emergent and time constraints prevent the performance of a short ACTH test, dexamethasone can be given, because this will not interfere with future tests to determine normal blood cortisol concentrations in response to a short ACTH test.

PREVENTION

The following steps are useful for preventing a steroid-induced crisis:

- Identify patients who are at risk of developing adrenal insufficiency.
- Be vigilant for subtle signs of hypoadrenalism.
- Have a low threshold for treating patients with possible adrenal insufficiency.
- Use postoperative steroids in patients with septic shock, based on emerging evidence of their beneficial role in this patient subgroup.

- Consider the possible benefit of steroids for attenuating the late fibroproliferative phase of ARDS and reducing mortality.

Further Reading

Annane D, Sebille V, Charpentier C, et al: Effect of treatment with low doses of hydrocortisone and fludrocortisone on mortality in patients with septic shock. JAMA 288:862-871, 2002.

Bollaert PE, Charpentier C, Levy B, et al: Reversal of late septic shock with supraphysiologic doses of hydrocortisone. Crit Care Med 26:645-650, 1998.

Friedman RJ, Schiff CF, Bromberg JS: Use of supplemental steroids in patients having orthopaedic operations. J Bone Joint Surg Am 77:1801-1806, 1995.

LaRochelle GE Jr, LaRochelle AG, Ratner RE, et al: Recovery of the hypothalamic-pituitary-adrenal (HPA) axis in patients with rheumatic diseases receiving low-dose prednisone. Am J Med 95:258-264, 1993.

Meduri GU, Headley AS, Golden E, et al: Effect of prolonged methylprednisolone therapy in unresolving acute respiratory distress syndrome: A randomized controlled trial. JAMA 280:159-165, 1998.

Salem M, Tainsh RE Jr, Bromberg J, et al: Perioperative glucocorticoid coverage: A reassessment 42 years after emergence of a problem. Ann Surg 219:416-425, 1994.

Antiemetic Drugs

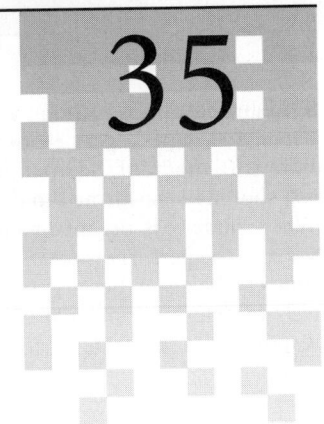

35

M. Pamela Fish

Case Synopsis

A 21-year-old woman (American Society of Anesthesiologists [ASA] status 1) presents with a suspected ectopic pregnancy for outpatient laparoscopy. She has no history of previous psychiatric illness or drug use. Metoclopramide 10 mg and glycopyrrolate 0.2 mg are administered intravenously as premedication. The patient becomes severely agitated and verbally abusive and refuses to proceed with surgery. She returns the following day and receives no premedication. Anesthesia and surgery proceed uneventfully.

PROBLEM ANALYSIS

Definition

Complications of antiemetic therapy are undesirable effects resulting from the administration of medications to prevent or treat nausea and vomiting. Untreated, up to 30% of surgical patients will suffer postoperative nausea and vomiting (PONV). For high-risk patients, the incidence can be as high as 80%. Thus, antiemetic drugs are commonly used in the perioperative period.

Recognition

Conditions such as hypotension, hypoxemia, hypoglycemia, raised intracranial pressure, and bowel obstruction should be considered in the differential diagnosis of PONV.

Currently available antiemetics produce their effect by antagonizing neurotransmitters in the brainstem. The major receptor sites at which these drugs act are listed in Table 35-1. Except for antiserotonin (5-HT$_3$) antagonists, most antiemetics antagonize more than one neurotransmitter. The antiemetic action of the corticosteroids is not well understood; some of the proposed mechanisms include prostaglandin antagonism, tryptophan depletion, and reduced 5-HT$_3$ concentrations. Common side effects with antiemetic therapy are provided in Table 35-2.

Risk Assessment

All patients who receive antiemetic therapy are at risk for related side effects. The following factors increase the likelihood that a patient will require treatment with antiemetic drugs:

PATIENT FACTORS

- Female sex and children under the age of puberty
- Nonsmoking history

Table 35–1 ■ Receptor Site Affinity of Antiemetic Drugs

Drug	Dopamine Receptor	Cholinergic (Muscarinic) Receptor	Histamine Receptor	Serotonin Receptor
Phenothiazine				
Chlorpromazine (Thorazine)	+++	++	+++	+
Prochlorperazine (Compazine)	+++	+	++	+
Antihistamine				
Diphenhydramine (Benadryl)	+	++	+++	−
Promethazine (Phenergan)	++	+++	++++	−
Butyrophenone				
Droperidol (Inapsine)	++++	−	+	+
Benzamide				
Metoclopramide (Reglan)	++	−	+	++
Antiserotonin				
Ondansetron (Zofran)	−	−	−	++++
Dolasetron (Anzemet)	−	−	−	++++
Granisetron (Kytril)	−	−	−	++++
Anticholinergic				
Scopolamine (Hyoscine)	+	++++	−	−

The number of plus signs indicates the relative degree of activity from least (+) to most (++++); a minus sign indicates no activity.
Adapted from Watcha MF, White PF: Postoperative nausea and vomiting. Anesthesiology 77:162-184, 1992.

Table 35–2 ■ Side Effects of Antiemetic Drugs

Drug	Sedation	Restlessness/Agitation	Extrapyramidal Movements	Dysphoria	Disturbed Coordination	Headache	Dizziness	Hypotension	Tachycardia	Dry Mouth	Visual Effects/Diplopia	Hallucinations	Neuroleptic Malignant Syndrome	Cutaneous Flushing/Perineal Itching	ECG Changes
Phenothiazine															
Chlorpromazine	+	+	+					+	+				+		
Prochlorperazine	+	+	+				+	+	+	+	+		+		
Antihistamine															
Diphenhydramine	+				+	+	+	+	+	+	+				
Promethazine	+	+	+		+		+	+	+	+	+		+		+
Anticholinergic															
Scopolamine	+	+		+			+			+	+	+			
Benzamide															
Metoclopramide	+	+	+			+	+	+	+			+	+		+
Butyrophenone															
Droperidol	+	+	+	+			+	+	+		+	+	+		+
Antiserotonin															
Ondansetron					+	+									+
Dolasetron					+	+									+
Granisetron					+	+									+
Corticosteroid															
Dexamethasone														+	+

ECG, electrocardiogram.

- Prior history of motion sickness or PONV
- Preoperative anxiety or pain
- Any disease process that delays gastric emptying

SURGICAL FACTORS

- Strabismus repair, head and neck surgery, or dental surgery
- Laparoscopic gynecologic procedures, shoulder surgery
- Plastic surgery (especially breast augmentation)
- Adenotonsillectomy, hernia repair, orchiopexy, and penile surgery in children

ANESTHESIA FACTORS

- Inadequate fluid replacement
- Duration of surgery (risk increases for length up to 3 hours)
- General anesthesia with volatile anesthetic agents
- Nitrous oxide use, due to gastrointestinal distention or increased middle ear (labyrinthine, vestibular apparatus) pressure
- Use of narcotic analgesics
- Use of certain hypnotic agents (etomidate, ketamine)
- Use of neostigmine (>2.5 mg)

POSTOPERATIVE FACTORS

- Pain
- Sudden motion

- Overly early or aggressive fluid intake, or requirement of oral fluid intake before discharge home

Implications

The following list describes some considerations and potential complications with antiemetic therapy:

- Sedation
  - This is the most common side effect with all antiemetic drugs.
- Metoclopramide
  - Causes an increased risk of extrapyramidal reactions in children and the elderly
  - Avoid in patients with hypertension or those taking monoamine oxidase inhibitors
  - Painful stimulation may provoke supraventricular tachycardia after administration.
  - Use is contraindicated in patients with epilepsy
  - Because of its short half-life, not effective when administered at start of surgery
- Antihistamines
  - Often cause dizziness, sedation, and hypotension in elderly patients
- Serotonin receptor antagonists
  - Headache (dose dependent), dizziness, blurred vision, and abnormal liver enzymes have been reported.
  - Blockage of cardiac sodium and potassium channels can cause transient electrocardiogram (ECG) changes.

- Cross-reactive hypersensitivity (anaphylactic, anaphylactoid) reactions among different 5-HT₃ receptor antagonists have been reported.
- Droperidol
  - A Food and Drug Administration (FDA) advisory was issued concerning potential Q-T prolongation and fatal arrhythmias with droperidol use (see Chapter 81).
  - Contraindicated in patients with Parkinson's disease
- Phenothiazines
  - Drug ampules contain sodium bisulfite and sodium sulfite, which may cause an allergic-type reaction, especially in patients with a history of asthma.
  - Perphenazine, the most potent antiemetic among the phenothiazines, is reserved for intractable vomiting.
- Scopolamine
  - Use of the transdermal route is limited by long onset time and excessive drowsiness.
  - Psychosis may be seen in the elderly and has also occurred in pediatric patients.
- Dexamethasone
  - Wound infection and adrenal suppression have not been noted after a single bolus dose in otherwise healthy patients.
  - Phosphate (injectable solution) is linked to perineal itching and cutaneous flushing.

MANAGEMENT

Management of the complications of antiemetic drugs can range from simple observation after discontinuing the drug to treatment with specific agents. Sedation is a common side effect of antiemetc drug therapy, frequently resulting in delayed transfer from the recovery room or discharge home after ambulatory surgery. There is no specific therapy other than continued observation. Hypotension usually responds to increased intravenous fluids. However, parenteral phenothiazines may produce hypotension, requiring therapy with a vasoconstrictor such as phenylephrine.

As noted earlier, ECG changes with antiserotonin antagonists are usually temporary. Although there have been reports of Q-T interval prolongation and fatal arrhythmias (torsades de pointes) with larger doses of droperidol, there have been no reports in any peer-reviewed journal of Q-T prolongation, arrhythmias, or cardiac arrest associated with the much smaller intravenous doses (0.125 mg) used for the management of PONV. Extrapyramidal disorders can present as dystonic reactions (especially in children), motor restlessness (akathisia), or signs and symptoms of parkinsonism (especially in the elderly). Treatment of extrapyramidal effects involves the administration of benztropine (a centrally acting anticholinergic) or diphenhydramine. For akathisia, antiparkinsonian drugs, benzodiazepines, or propranolol may be useful.

Clinical manifestations of the neuroleptic malignant syndrome include hyperpyrexia, muscle rigidity, altered mental status, and evidence of autonomic instability. Management is discontinuation of nonessential drugs, intensive correction of fluid and electrolyte imbalance, and therapy with dopamine agonists such as bromocriptine or dantrolene.

PREVENTION

The following list describes measures to avoid complications with drugs used to treat or prevent PONV:

- Prophylaxis for PONV
  - In general, there is no rationale for routine prophylactic antiemetic therapy.
  - Prophylaxis in some high-risk patients may be appropriate, however (see "Risk Assessment").
  - Dexamethasone requires 4 to 5 hours for an optimal effect, so it is best administered before induction of anesthesia.
  - Low-dose dexamethasone or droperidol and a 5-HT₃ receptor antagonist have been shown to be effective prophylaxis for patients at high risk for PONV.
- Appropriate preoperative antiemetic management
  - Use premedication with oral clonidine or benzodiazepines.
  - In females, avoid elective laparoscopic surgery around the time of their menses.
  - Acupressure or acupuncture at the P-6 (Neiguan) point should be considered.
- Anesthetic technique
  - Use regional anesthesia when possible.
  - Choose appropriate anesthetic agents (e.g., total intravenous anesthesia with propofol).
  - Avoid gastric distention from high positive-pressure facemask ventilation.
  - Consider prophylactic gastric decompression (oro- or nasogastric tube) before endotracheal extubation (especially for patients having emergency surgery, with a history of PONV, or at high risk for PONV).
  - Avoid ingestion of blood with throat packs, or insert an oro- or nasogastric tube.
  - Ensure adequate fluid replacement.
  - Provide effective postoperative analgesia (consider epidural analgesia, peripheral nerve blocks, or local anesthetic wound infiltration). This will reduce opiate needs and the associated increased risk for PONV.
  - Use analgesics that are less likely to cause PONV (e.g., ketorolac, COX-2 inhibitors).
- Antiemetic therapy
  - Should PONV occur, select the antiemetic agent most appropriate for the patient.
  - Serotonin receptor antagonists are more effective against vomiting than nausea.
  - Repeated low doses of droperidol (0.125 mg) increase the drug's antinausea efficacy, with reduced side effects. However, current FDA guidelines require that ECG monitoring be performed before and continued for 2 to 3 hours after droperidol use, thus limiting its use in outpatient settings.
  - Antihistamines are the agents of choice following middle ear surgery.
  - Ephedrine, an indirect-acting sympathomimetic, is effective for treating emesis due to hypotension associated with spinal anesthesia.
  - A new class of drugs, the neurokinin-1 (NK₁) receptor antagonists, is currently under investigation for the prevention of PONV.

Further Reading

Apfel CC, Laara E, Koivuranta M, et al: A simplified risk score for predicting postoperative nausea and vomiting. Anesthesiology 91:693-700, 1999.

Caldwell C, Rains G, McKiterick K: An unusual reaction to preoperative metoclopramide. Anesthesiology 67:854-855, 1987.

Gan TJ, Meyer T, Apfel CC, et al: Consensus guidelines for managing postoperative nausea and vomiting. Anesth Analg 97:62-71, 2003.

Sinclair DR, Chung F, Mezei G: Can postoperative nausea and vomiting be predicted? Anesthesiology 91:109-118, 1999.

Watcha MF, White PF: Postoperative nausea and vomiting. Anesthesiology 77:162-184, 1992.

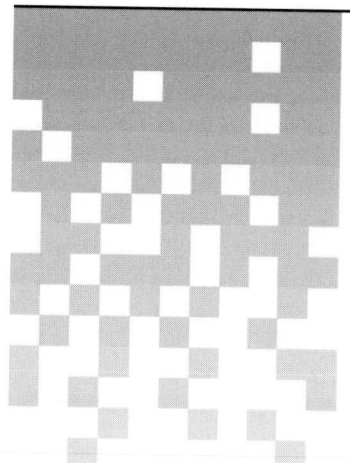

General Anesthesia

Scott R. Springman

John L. Atlee

Preanesthetic Evaluation: False-Positive Tests

36

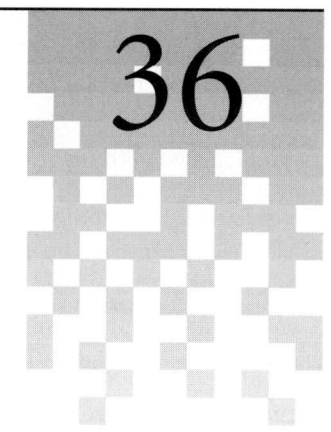

Michael P. Ford and Scott R. Springman

Case Synopsis

A 25-year-old male athlete presents for repair of the anterior cruciate ligament of his knee. He is taking no medications. He has a negative personal and family history of abnormal clotting or bleeding or easy bruising. Multiple tests, including prothrombin time and partial thromboplastin time (PTT), are ordered. The PTT results are reported as above normal. The surgery is postponed, and an extensive hematology workup is performed. The final report concludes, "normal variant, no coagulation defect."

PROBLEM ANALYSIS

Definition

A test is useful only to the extent that clinicians can understand the implications of a positive or negative result. Few, if any, tests always correctly identify the presence or absence of disease in all patients. Clinicians can decide what to do with a "positive" test result only when they have a clear knowledge of the test's characteristics and its statistical predictive value when applied to a specific patient population. Such "medical decision analysis" directly affects the clinical care of patients.

Some tests provide a qualitative positive or negative result. Many test results, however, are quantitative and define a range of "normal" values around a mean. Therefore, a few members of any population will have an "abnormal" test result but not actually have a disease. This means that a test result may be misleading owing to variability in the patient population.

The test itself can give an incorrect result due to (1) inaccuracy, (2) imprecision, or (3) incorrect performance. The *accuracy* of a test is the difference between the mean value of test results and the true result, as measured by a gold standard test. The *precision* of a test is the reproducibility of results between instruments or persons performing the test. An *incorrectly performed* test can invalidate any result.

Test accuracy can be described in several ways. The *sensitivity* of a test measures the proportion of individuals who have a disease and are correctly identified as being positive for that disease, based on the test. *Specificity* measures the proportion of individuals who do not have a disease and are identified as being disease free, based on the test. False-positive results are more likely with tests that have a high sensitivity, low specificity, or both. Sensitivity and specificity are characteristics of the test and do not change with the prevalence (frequency) of disease in the population. Said another way: a test's sensitivity and specificity do not affect the probability of a patient having a disease.

The *predictive value* of tests, in contrast, depends on the prevalence of a disease in a population of patients.

The predictive value of a positive test indicates the proportion of those with a positive test who actually have the disease. Often, the predictive value of tests is expressed as the probability, or odds, that a condition is present. *Likelihood ratios* express the amount that the odds change when the results of the test are available (Table 36-1). In this respect, an important concept is Bayes' theorem, which "relates the probability of an item (e.g., a patient) being a member of a particular group (e.g., clinical class), given the presence of an attribute (e.g., an abnormal test result), to the probability of known group members having the attribute and the probability of

Table 36–1 ■ Accuracy and Predictive Value of Tests

Diagnostic Test Results	Target Disorder, Based on Gold Standard Test		Number of Patients with This Test Result
	Present	*Absent*	
Positive	a	b	a + b
Negative	c	d	c + d
Total	a + c	b + d	

1. a/(a + c) = Sensitivity.
2. d/(b + d) = Specificity.
3. a/(a + b) = Positive predictive value, or post-test probability of having the target disorder among patients with positive test results.
4. d/(c + d) = Negative predictive value, or post-test probability of not having the target disorder among patients with negative test results.
5. c/(c + d) = Post-test probability of having the target disorder for patients with negative test results.
6. (a + c)/(a + b + c + d) = Prevalence or pretest probability of having the target disorder.
7. Sensitivity/(1 − Specificity) = Likelihood ratio (of having the target disorder) for a positive test result = [a/(a + c)]/[b/(b + d)].
8. (1 − Sensitivity)/Specificity = Likelihood ratio (of having the target disorder) for a negative test result = [c/(a + c)]/[d/(b + d)].
9. Post-test probability of the target disorder (expressed as odds) = Pretest probability of target disorder (expressed as odds) × Likelihood ratio for the test result.
10. Odds = Probability/[1 − Probability].

Adapted from Sackett DL: A primer on the precision and accuracy of the clinical examination. JAMA 267:2638-2644, 1992.

obtaining a group member when picking at random an item from the universe of items."[1] It allows the calculation of changes in the probability of disease as new information (e.g., test results) becomes available. The post-test probability is calculated with the Fagan nomogram, similar to that shown in Figure 36-1. A Web-based interactive nomogram can be accessed at http://www.cebm.net/nomogram.asp.

Recognition

A positive test result may turn out to be false if the test was performed incorrectly. Alternatively, a patient may not actually have a disease if the results of a gold standard test are normal. Other, non–gold standard tests may falsely indicate that a patient has a disease when he or she does not. Finally, because of population variability, a patient may truly test positive for a disease (be outside the "normal" range) yet be clinically normal.

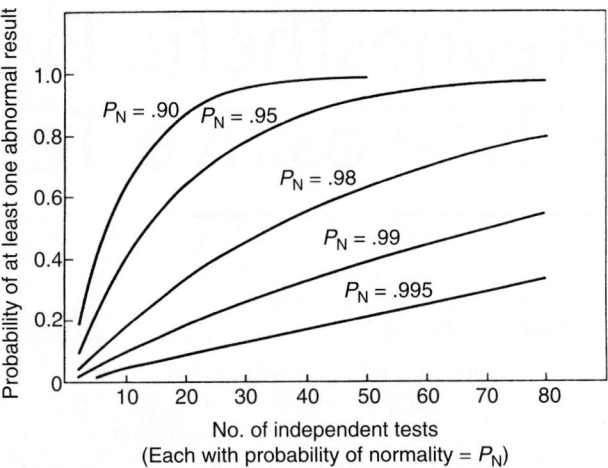

Figure 36–2 ▪ Probability of at least one falsely abnormal result for multiple tests, each with a probability of a normal result (P_N), for selected values of P_N. (From Berwick DM: Screening in health fairs. JAMA 254:1495, 1985.)

Risk Assessment

If we assume that tests are being performed correctly and that their precision is high, then the accuracy of the test and the prevalence of the disease are the main factors that determine whether a test result will be "correct." Patients who undergo multiple tests are likely to have at least one that is falsely positive. This is true especially if the tested patient population has a low prevalence of the condition. This scenario often occurs when asymptomatic patients undergo large numbers (a battery) of preoperative screening tests (Fig. 36-2).

Implications

In the preoperative setting, the most likely outcome of a false-positive test is the delay or cancellation of surgery. Physicians often repeat the test, hoping that the first result was due to an improperly performed test. Other tests to corroborate the diagnosis may be performed. However, both these options add to costs. Further, if the test is invasive, it adds to the risk of physical harm to the patient. Yet if elective surgery is not delayed and the test was not falsely positive, the providers run the risk of professional or medicolegal scrutiny. In addition, any unnecessary alteration in perioperative management may add cost and risk to the patient's care. Finally, a false-positive result, such as for human immunodeficiency virus (HIV), may cause unnecessary psychological stress for the patient, as well as for providers.

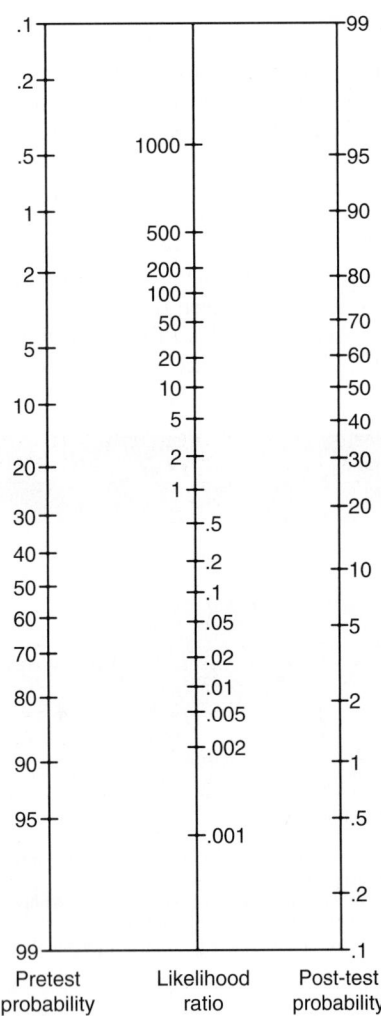

Figure 36–1 ▪ Draw a line from the pretest probability through the likelihood ratio to determine the post-test probability. (Adapted from Fagan TJ: Nomogram for Bayes's theorem. N Engl J Med 293:257, 1975.)

MANAGEMENT

The decision to accept a positive test result as "true" must depend on knowledge of the test's characteristics and its performance pitfalls. The decision also depends on knowledge of the incidence of the tested condition in the patient population in question. Every test result should be examined to determine whether it fits the overall picture of the patient's condition. If it does not, and if there are no corroborative

---

[1]This definition is found in the 25th edition of *Stedman's Medical Dictionary,* Baltimore, Williams & Wilkins, 1990.

findings, further investigation may be required before accepting the result as true. In many cases, a lone finding should be suspect unless it is known that the specificity of the test is high, the incidence of the condition is high, or both.

PREVENTION

Clearly, the best way to minimize the chances of a false-positive test result is to avoid any unnecessary testing. Appropriate guidelines may take into account available scientific studies and local and national expert medical opinion. Selection of tests with a high specificity can also reduce the number of false-positive results. However, both physicians and patients abhor adverse outcomes, and the consequences of missing a true-positive result may be serious; therefore, testing and the acceptance of a certain incidence of false-positive results are commonplace. The use of cost-benefit and risk-benefit analysis may help decide whether a test should be performed at all, in spite of the complexity of such evaluations and the need for subjective value judgments.

Further Reading

Pasternak LR: Preoperative laboratory testing: General issues and considerations. Anesthesiol Clin North Am 22:13-25, 2004.

Practice Advisory for Preanesthesia Evaluation: A Report by the American Society of Anesthesiologists Task Force on Preanesthesia Evaluation. Anesthesiology 96:485-496, 2002.

Roizen MF, Foss JF, Fischer SP: Preoperative evaluation. In Miller R (ed): Anesthesia. New York, Churchill Livingstone, 2000, pp 824-883.

Ross AF, Tinker JH: Preoperative evaluation of the healthy patient. In Longnecker DE, Tinker JH, Morgan GE (eds): Principles and Practice of Anesthesiology. St. Louis, Mosby–Year Book, 1998, pp 3-51.

Sackett DL: A primer on the precision and accuracy of the clinical examination. JAMA 267:2638-2644, 1992.

Vitez TS: Principles of cost analysis. J Clin Anesth 6:357-363, 1994.

Preanesthetic Evaluation: Inadequate or Missing Test Result

37

Thomas P. Broderick and Scott R. Springman

Case Synopsis

A 44-year-old man with a history of hypertension, obesity, and episodes of epigastric pain is scheduled for elective laparoscopic cholecystectomy. No preoperative electrocardiogram is obtained. The patient subsequently sustains perioperative myocardial infarction secondary to undiagnosed coronary artery disease.

PROBLEM ANALYSIS

Definition

Effective preoperative test selection is best achieved by knowing how outcome is affected by the performance or omission of a test. The following are three important outcomes:

1. Adverse medical events
2. Cost of care
3. Litigation

These may or may not be related. Simply knowing the result of a preoperative test cannot ensure a good outcome. Moreover, the accuracy and usefulness of a test depend greatly on its sensitivity and specificity, combined with the frequency of the condition in the patient population.

Recognition

It is easy to determine whether a test was not done, not reviewed, or not available. A more difficult issue is whether a specific test was actually indicated. Hindsight may not be adequate to determine actual preoperative need. Only well-structured clinical studies and logical analysis can provide direction for clinicians who wish to provide evidenced-based care.

Risk Assessment

Patients are at risk for adverse outcomes when tests are not done owing to an oversight, inadequate history and physical examination, inadequate guidelines, or inappropriate emphasis on cost reduction. Process failures also occur when tests are done but the results are unavailable or lost or when providers fail to review the results before an anesthetic is administered.

Implications

If a test is mandated by policy but is not done, the outcome may or may not be affected. For example, if a patient has a slightly elevated serum calcium level or is slightly anemic, for most operations, adverse perioperative outcomes are unlikely.

However, if a patient has severe, unrecognized coronary disease and sustains a perioperative myocardial infarction, there will definitely be more medical care required, greater time spent in the hospital, increased costs, and possible long-term disability or risk of death. Further, emotional, professional, economic, and medicolegal risks for the providers will be increased.

MANAGEMENT

If a test is found to be missing before an anesthetic is administered and the surgery is elective, the anesthesiologist and the surgeon must determine whether official internal or external policies absolutely mandate the test. If so, the test should be obtained, or the providers must justify in the medical record why they were willing to proceed with anesthesia or surgery without the test results. Of course, for emergent or urgent procedures, physicians should always weigh the expected benefits of a test against the risks of delay.

If the test is discovered to be missing after anesthesia or surgery has commenced, the providers must determine whether obtaining the test result will make a real difference and whether the procedure should be terminated (fortunately, rare). Tests may, of course, be obtained during the provision of an anesthetic and serve the same purpose as a preoperative test. This is not true, however, if a preoperative test would have changed the decision to proceed with the procedure or if the test would have substantially affected the initial anesthetic plan. An example of this would be the finding of an elevated prothrombin time before the administration of a neuraxial anesthetic.

If a test is discovered to be missing after surgery, is there a need to obtain the test? It may be wise to do so if postoperative or long-term medical management would be altered by the results.

PREVENTION

VALUE-BASED MEDICAL CARE

If the absence of a test leads to an adverse outcome, the system should be reexamined to prevent future problems.

Caution should be used, however, in ascribing causality. Bad outcomes do not necessarily mean that more defensive testing is indicated. Consider whether testing really would have made a difference in the outcome. In addition, short-term and long-term benefits versus the potential harmful effects of testing must be considered. This is consistent with the concept of value-based anesthesia care. Complex cost-benefit analysis may be needed; time has actual value in medicine, and a seemingly more costly process may turn out to be less expensive in the long run than a less costly but lengthier process. A thoughtfully managed continuous quality improvement program may provide process and systems benefits, minimizing the pitfalls of arbitrarily assigning value based purely on cost to clinical decision making.

EVIDENCE-BASED MEDICAL CARE

Ideally, all tests should be ordered using the principle of evidence-based medical care. Many articles have been written about preoperative assessment, but few cite sufficient rigorous evidence to be of significant use. Recently, an American Society of Anesthesiologists task force found that there were insufficient scientific outcome studies to support a specific scheme for preoperative testing, other than sound medical practice based on a careful history and physical examination. The National Institute for Clinical Excellence (NICE) in the United Kingdom published a lengthy set of preoperative testing guidelines based on both patient disease and severity of surgery (www.nice.org.uk). The American College of Cardiology–American Heart Association guideline update (see also Chapter 38) can help determine the need for cardiac testing based on criteria that rely heavily on the history and physical examination.

FOCUSED PREOPERATIVE TESTING

The proper use of the history and physical examination is to focus further preoperative testing. However, it is important to note that many symptoms are sensitive but not highly specific indicators of problems. Interobserver variability also may be high. In addition, the value of the history depends on the adequacy of the past medical record and the patient's reliability and communication skills.

NONSELECTIVE VERSUS SELECTIVE TESTING

Pathology can exist without significant symptoms or signs. With that in mind, most schemes for preoperative testing distinguish between nonselective and selective testing. The former requires that every patient be tested or screened, even if asymptomatic. Although this approach was commonly used in the past, few recommend it today. Selective testing requires that certain groups of criteria be used to determine the need for testing.

Patient Factors. The first group of criteria involves patient factors. These include, but are not limited to, symptoms, age, past medical history, gender, and physical findings. Other factors, such as the ability to obtain a reliable history or perform an adequate examination, should also be considered.

Type of Surgery. The second group of criteria involves the type of surgery. Baseline values may be required because the surgery itself will alter these values or because of possible physiologic derangements caused by the surgery.

Type of Anesthesia. The last group of criteria relates to the type of anesthesia. Although local or regional anesthesia may require a different testing scheme or perhaps fewer tests, there is always the possibility that local or regional anesthesia may be inadequate, and conversion to general anesthesia may be required.

TESTING GUIDELINES

Lacking rigorous outcome studies, criteria must be based on local and national experience. Policies or guidelines need to be constantly updated to be credible, and local consensus is an absolute necessity. Published guidelines may be simple (Table 37-1) or complex, such as the NICE guidelines. Others may simply recommend testing "as indicated by history and examination." Experience has shown, however, that such nonspecific guidelines often result in many more or fewer tests than needed, especially when nonanesthesia providers are responsible for ordering the tests.

Importantly, there are good reasons to omit nonindicated tests. Even if the tests cost nothing, they can do harm by leading to further testing, inappropriately altering case

Table 37–1 ■ Preanesthetic Testing and Type of Anesthesia

Age	General or Major Conduction Anesthesia (Asymptomatic Individuals)		Sedative-Hypnotics for IV Monitored Anesthesia	Peripheral Nerve Blocks
	Men	*Women*		
6 mo-<40 yr	None	HCT ± pregnancy test	None	None
40-<50 yr	ECG	HCT ± pregnancy test	None	None
50-<65 yr	ECG	HCT ± pregnancy test, ECG	HCT (≤6 mo)	None
65-74 yr	HGB or HCT, ECG, BUN, GLU	HGB or HCT, ECG, BUN, GLU	HCT (≤6 mo), ECG (≤1 yr)	HCT (≤6 mo)
≥75 yr	HGB or HCT, ECG, BUN, GLU, ± chest radiograph	HGB or HCT, ECG, BUN, GLU, ± chest radiograph	HCT (≤6 mo), ECG (≤1 yr), BUN (≤6 mo), GLU (≤6 mo)	HCT (≤6 mo), ECG (≤1 yr)

BUN, blood urea nitrogen; ECG, electrocardiogram; GLU, glucose; HCT, hematocrit; HGB, hemoglobin; IV, intravenous.
Adapted from Roizen MF, Fisher SP: Preoperative evaluation: Adults and children. In White PF (ed): Ambulatory Anesthesia and Surgery. Philadelphia, WB Saunders, 1997, p 164.

management, giving the anesthesiologist and surgeon a false sense of security, and even distracting them from more important issues. Performing tests when there is no plan to review them before surgery is medically useless and legally dangerous.

COMPUTERIZED PREOPERATIVE ASSESSMENT SYSTEMS AND PREANESTHETIC EVALUATION CLINICS

A preanesthetic evaluation clinic can provide a systematic, logical, cost-effective, and streamlined approach to preoperative testing. Also, a well-structured computerized preoperative assessment system (which must comply with the Health Insurance Portability and Accountability Act) can both enhance the collection of patient data and reduce the volume of unnecessary or missed preoperative visits. Further, an electronic medical record employing integrated "decision support" may substantially improve both the quality and the availability of preoperative evaluation and testing. The anesthesiologist's review of a patient's workup is then more convenient, complete, and useful.

Gaining consensus about the indications for testing, the timing of testing, who orders the tests, and who reviews the test results is the first step in optimizing a preoperative evaluation process.

Further Reading

American Society of Anesthesiologists: Practice advisory for preanesthesia evaluation: A report by the American Society of Anesthesiologists Task Force on Preanesthesia Evaluation. Anesthesiology 96:485-496, 2002.

Eagle KA, Berger PB, Calkins H, et al: ACC/AHA guideline update for perioperative cardiovascular evaluation for noncardiac surgery—executive summary: A report of the American College of Cardiology/American Heart Association Task Force on Practice Guidelines (Committee to Update the 1996 Guidelines on Perioperative Cardiovascular Evaluation for Noncardiac Surgery). Anesth Analg 94:1052-1064, 2002.

Ferrari LR: Preoperative evaluation of pediatric surgical patients with multisystem considerations. Anesth Analg 99:1058-1069, 2004.

Fischer S: Development and effectiveness of an anesthesia preoperative evaluation clinic in a teaching hospital. Anesthesiology 85:196-206, 1996.

Fisher S: Cost-effective preoperative evaluation and testing. Chest 115: 96S-100S, 1999.

Gibby G: How preoperative assessment programs can be justified financially to hospital administrators. Int Anesthesiol Clin 40:17-30, 2002.

Hildred W, Watkins L: The nearly good, the bad, and the ugly in cost effectiveness analysis of health care. J Econ Issues 30:755-775, 1996.

Orkin FK: Moving toward value-based anesthesia care. J Clin Anesth 5: 91-98, 1993.

Roizen MF, Fisher SP: Preoperative evaluation: Adults and children. In White PF (ed): Ambulatory Anesthesia and Surgery. Philadelphia, WB Saunders, 1997, pp 155-172.

Cardiac Risk Assessment

John L. Atlee

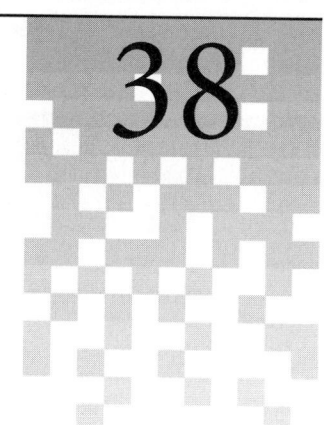

Case Synopsis

A 70-year-old man with intermittent claudication, hypertension, non-insulin-dependent diabetes mellitus, and hyperlipidemia is admitted for same-day right axillary–bifemoral and right femoral–popliteal bypass surgery for arterial occlusive disease. His past medical history is significant for myocardial infarction (MI) 5 years ago and 50 pack-years of smoking before that. His left ventricular ejection fraction is 45%, but his exercise capacity is limited by claudication. The 12-lead electrocardiogram (ECG) shows sinus bradycardia (56 beats per minute), old anterior wall infarction, and occasional ventricular extrasystoles (VES). In the preoperative holding area, his blood pressure is 168/95 mm Hg, and the monitored ECG shows 4 to 6 VES/minute. His current medications include metoprolol, glyburide, atorvastatin, and a long-acting nitrate. His primary physician has cleared him for surgery.

PROBLEM ANALYSIS

Definition

Cardiovascular disease and all types of surgeries are increasing globally, both in prevalence and in number. Cardiovascular conditions that may affect the postoperative outcomes of cardiac and noncardiac surgery alike include hypertensive crisis,[1] coronary artery disease, valvular heart disease, arrhythmias or conduction disturbances, and hypertrophic or dilated cardiomyopathy. Cardiomyopathies also increase the risk for perioperative congestive heart failure. Chronic pulmonary disease, hepatic or renal insufficiency, diabetes mellitus, and other severe systemic disease can also have an adverse impact on postoperative cardiovascular outcomes.

The cardiovascular complication of most concern is perioperative acute MI. Others are acute heart failure, thromboembolism (e.g., stroke, pulmonary embolism), arrhythmias and conduction disturbances, and hypertensive crisis.

Recognition

The initial history, physical examination, and ECG assessment should focus on identifying potentially serious cardiac disorders, including coronary artery disease (defined as previous MI or angina), heart failure, and symptomatic arrhythmias; the presence of an implanted cardiac rhythm management device, such as a pacemaker or internal cardioverter-defibrillator (see Chapter 97); or a history of orthostatic intolerance. The Framingham Heart Study identified major, predisposing, and conditional risk factors for coronary artery disease (Table 38-1). Although age per se is not a modifiable risk factor, it relates to the length of time a person is exposed to risk factors that increase the severity of atherosclerosis; it is also an important index in the Framingham risk equation. Because obesity, family history of early coronary artery disease, and physical inactivity contribute to other risk factors, they too are considered major risk factors.

Risk Assessment

Clinical predictors of increased risk for perioperative MI, heart failure, or death are listed in Table 38-2. Major predictors

Table 38–1 ■ Risk Factors for Coronary Artery Disease
Major
Cigarette smoking
Elevated blood pressure
Elevated serum total and LDL cholesterol
Low serum HDL cholesterol
Diabetes mellitus
Advanced age
Other (Predisposing) Risk Factors
Obesity
Abdominal obesity
Physical inactivity
Family history of premature coronary heart disease
Ethnic characteristics
Psychosocial factors
Conditional Risk Factors
Elevated serum triglycerides
Small LDL particles
Elevated serum homocysteine
Elevated serum lipoproteins
Prothrombogenic factors (e.g., fibrinogen)
Inflammatory markers (e.g., C-reactive proteins)

HDL, high-density lipoprotein; LDL, low-density lipoprotein.
Adapted from Eagle KA, Brundage BH, Chaitman BR, et al: Guidelines for perioperative cardiovascular evaluation for noncardiac surgery. Circulation 93: 1278-1317, 1996; and Eagle KA, Berger PB, Calkins H, et al: ACC/AHA update for perioperative cardiovascular evaluation for noncardiac surgery. Circulation 105: 1257-1267, 2002.

---

[1]Hypertensive crisis includes urgencies and emergencies. Both require severe (stage 2) blood pressure elevation above 160/100 mm Hg. For emergencies, end-organ damage is also evident.

Table 38–2 ■ Clinical Predictors of Increased Risk for Perioperative Myocardial Infarction, Heart Failure, or Death

Major

Unstable coronary syndromes
  Acute or recent MI*
  Unstable or severe angina† (Canadian class III or IV)‡
  Evidence of large ischemic burden by clinical symptoms or noninvasive testing
Decompensated heart failure
Significant arrhythmias
  High-grade atrioventricular block
  Symptomatic ventricular arrhythmias in the presence of underlying heart disease
  Supraventricular arrhythmias with uncontrolled ventricular rate
Severe valvular heart disease

Intermediate

Mild angina pectoris
Previous MI by history or pathologic Q waves
Compensated or prior heart failure
Diabetes (particularly insulin-dependent)
Renal insufficiency

Minor

Advanced age
Abnormal ECG (left ventricular hypertrophy, left bundle branch block, ST-T abnormalities)
Rhythm other than sinus (e.g., atrial fibrillation)
Low functional capacity (e.g., inability to climb one flight of stairs with a bag of groceries)
History of stroke
Uncontrolled systemic hypertension

*Acute MI is within 7 days; recent MI is >7 days but ≤30 days.
†May include "stable" angina in patients who are unusually sedentary.
‡See Campeau L: Grading of angina pectoris. Circulation 54:522-523, 1976.
ECG, electrocardiogram; MI, myocardial infarction.
Adapted from Eagle KA, Brundage BH, Chaitman BR, et al: Guidelines for perioperative cardiovascular evaluation for noncardiac surgery. Circulation 93: 1278-1317, 1996; and Eagle KA, Berger PB, Calkins H, et al: ACC/AHA update for perioperative cardiovascular evaluation for noncardiac surgery. Circulation 105: 1257-1267, 2002.

Table 38–3 ■ Factors that Increase the Risk for Perioperative Cardiac Events and Are Indications for β-Blocker Therapy

Risk Variables	Odds Ratio (95% CI)	β-Blocker Indicated
Clinical features		
Coronary artery disease (CAD)*	2.4 (1.3-4.2)	Yes
Heart failure (HF)	1.9 (1.1-3.5)	Yes
Diabetes mellitus†	3.0 (1.3-7.1)	Yes
Renal insufficiency	3.0 (1.4-6.8)	Probably yes, if secondary to CAD or HF
Poor functional status‡	1.8 (0.9-3.5)	Probably yes, if secondary to CAD or HF
High-risk surgery§	2.8 (1.6-4.9)	Yes

*Includes angina and prior myocardial infarction.
†Especially if insulin required.
‡Inability to walk four blocks or climb two flights of stairs.
§See Table 38-4.
CI, confidence interval.
Adapted from Fleisher LA, Eagle KA: Clinical practice: Lowering cardiac risk in noncardiac surgery. N Engl J Med 345:1677-1682, 2001.

increase the risk of perioperative cardiac complications, as well as indications for perioperative β-blocker therapy, are listed in Table 38-3. Cardiac risk for various types of surgery is stratified in Table 38-4.

Note that a remote history of MI or abnormal Q waves by ECG is an intermediate predictor of increased risk for perioperative cardiovascular events, whereas an acute MI (documented MI ≤7 days before preoperative evaluation) or recent MI (>7 but <30 days before preoperative evaluation),

Table 38–4 ■ Cardiac Risk Stratification for Various Types of Surgical Procedures

High risk (reported cardiac risk* ≥ 5%)
  Emergency major operations, especially in the elderly
  Aortic, major vascular, and peripheral vascular surgery
  Extensive operations with large volume shifts and/or blood loss
Intermediate risk (reported cardiac risk ≥ 1% but < 5%)
  Intraperitoneal surgery
  Intrathoracic surgery
  Carotid endarterectomy
  Head and neck surgery
  Orthopedic surgery
  Prostate surgery
Low risk (reported cardiac risk† < 1%)
  Endoscopic procedures
  Superficial biopsy
  Cataract surgery
  Breast surgery

*Combined incidence of cardiac death and nonfatal MI
†Does not generally require further preoperative cardiac testing
Adapted from Eagle KA, Brundage BH, Chaitman BR, et al: Guidelines for perioperative cardiovascular evaluation for noncardiac surgery. Circulation 93:1278-1317, 1996.

of increased risk are unstable coronary syndromes or evidence of large ischemic burden, decompensated heart failure, significant arrhythmias, or severe valvular heart disease. Evidence of such risk factors is found in clinical symptoms or results of noninvasive testing. Anemia also may increase the risk for perioperative cardiovascular events. Further, the patient's underlying cardiac condition, which might be stable at present (e.g., angina, heart failure, valvular disease), may become manifest with perioperative stress (e.g., pain, high circulating catecholamines, hypoxia, hypercarbia, acute electrolyte imbalance). Also, one should identify serious comorbid conditions (e.g., diabetes, peripheral vascular disease, renal insufficiency, stroke, pulmonary disease), because these too may affect perioperative outcome. Intermediate predictors of increased risk for perioperative cardiovascular events are mild angina, more remote previous MI, compensated heart failure, creatinine 2.0 mg/dL or greater, and diabetes mellitus. Minor predictors are advanced age, abnormal ECG, low functional capacity, history of stroke, and uncontrolled systemic hypertension. Odds ratios for variables that with evidence of important ischemic burden by symptoms or noninvasive study, is a major predictor. This definition of acute and recent MI was a consensus recommendation and avoids the traditional division of MI into 3-month and 6-month intervals.

Finally, current management of MI provides for risk stratification during convalescence. If a recent stress test does not indicate residual myocardium at risk (ischemic burden), the likelihood of perioperative reinfarction with noncardiac surgery is low. Although there are no adequate clinical trials on which to base firm recommendations, it appears reasonable to wait 4 to 6 weeks after acute MI to perform elective surgery.

Implications

Preoperative cardiac risk assessment is important for reducing perioperative morbidity and mortality, especially for patients having noncardiac surgery. Such risk is best evaluated by a multidisciplinary, integrated approach. This requires good communication among the patient, primary physician, consultant, anesthesiologist, and surgeon.

MANAGEMENT

The goal of cardiac risk assessment and any remedial therapy is to improve intra- and postoperative and long-term outcomes. Optimization of associated medical conditions may include control of hypertension, coronary revascularization, treatment for congestive heart failure and other important systemic conditions (e.g., hepatic or renal insufficiency, pulmonary insufficiency), and management for coagulation or anticoagulation disorders.

PREVENTION

Perioperative β-blockers are used to prevent postoperative atrial fibrillation and perioperative hypertension. Anticoagulation may be required to reduce the risk of thromboembolism and stroke in patients at increased risk (e.g., those with atrial fibrillation, hemoglobinopathies, coagulopathies, heart failure, prolonged bed rest). For patients with systemic anticoagulation or coagulopathies who are at increased risk for bleeding complications, special precautions must be taken if regional anesthesia will be used or is contemplated.

Further Reading

Boersma E, Poldermans D, Bax JJ, et al: Predictors of cardiac events after major vascular surgery. JAMA 285:1865-1873, 2001.

Dupuis J-Y, Wang F, Nathan H, et al: The cardiac anesthesia risk evaluation score. Anesthesiology 94:194-204, 2001.

Eagle KA, Berger PB, Calkins H, et al: ACC/AHA update for perioperative cardiovascular evaluation for noncardiac surgery. Circulation 105:1257-1267, 2002.

Eagle KA, Brundage BH, Chaitman BR, et al: Guidelines for perioperative cardiovascular evaluation for noncardiac surgery. Circulation 93:1278-1317, 1996.

Fleisher LA, Eagle KA: Clinical practice: Lowering cardiac risk in noncardiac surgery. N Engl J Med 345:1677-1682, 2001.

Grundy SM: Age as a risk factor: You are as old as your arteries. Am J Cardiol 83:1455-1457, 1999.

Grundy SM, Pasternak R, Greenland P, et al: Assessment of cardiovascular risk by use of multiple-risk-factor assessment equations: A statement for healthcare professionals from the American Heart Association and the American College of Cardiology. Circulation 100:1481-1492, 1999.

Lee TH, Marcantonio ER, Mangione CM, et al: Derivation and prospective validation of a simple index for prediction of cardiac risk of major noncardiac surgery. Circulation 100:1043-1049, 1999.

Mukherjee D, Eagle KA: Perioperative cardiac assessment for noncardiac surgery. Circulation 107:2771-2774, 2003.

Nashef SA, Roques F, Michel P, et al: European system for cardiac operative risk evaluation (EuroScore). Eur J Cardiothorac Surg 16:9-13, 1999.

Ouattara A, Niculescu M, Ghazouani S, et al: Predictive performance and variability of the cardiac anesthesia risk score. Anesthesiology 100:405-410, 2004.

Park KW: Preoperative cardiology consultation. Anesthesiology 98:754-762, 2003.

Tu JV, Jaglal SB, Naylor D: The Steering Committee of the Provincial Adult Cardiac Care Network of Ontario: Multicenter validation of a risk index for mortality, intensive care unit stay, and overall hospital length of stay after cardiac surgery. Circulation 91:677-684, 1995.

Wilson PWF, D'Agostino RB, Levy D: Prediction of coronary heart disease using risk factor categories. Circulation 97:1837-1847, 1998.

Herbals and Alternative Medicine

Christine M. Zainer

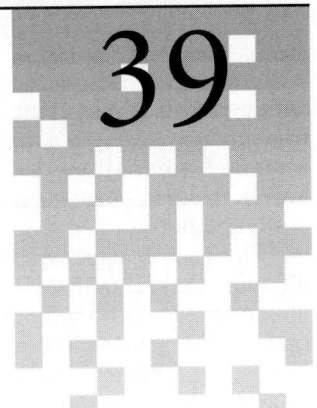

Case Synopsis

A 47-year-old female executive with breast cancer is scheduled to have a lumpectomy and sentinel node biopsy under general anesthesia. She has a history of mild depression and a 1-week history of an upper respiratory infection that is resolving. The patient denies allergies and medications. Upon further questioning, she admits to taking St. John's wort, *Ginkgo biloba*, dong quai, multivitamin and calcium supplements, and vitamin E. She also admits to taking ginseng and echinacea for the past week to treat her upper respiratory symptoms, because she did not want to postpone her surgery.

PROBLEM ANALYSIS

Definition

Many complementary and alternative medicine (CAM) systems rely on herbs or dietary supplements or modifications. These substances are also called nutraceuticals—anything that can be considered a food or part of a food and provides medical or health benefits, including the prevention and treatment of disease. Such CAM systems include Ayurveda (India), traditional Chinese medicine, homeopathy, and naturopathy. Other CAM systems do not necessarily include nutraceuticals but may involve manipulative, body-based, or energy therapies. These include the following:

- Chiropractic
- Acupuncture
- Bioelectromagnetic field therapies
- Qi gong
- Reiki
- Therapeutic touch

Under the 1994 Dietary Supplement Health and Education Act, herbals are considered dietary supplements, not drugs. According to the Food and Drug Administration (FDA), dietary supplements are nutrients (vitamins, minerals, amino acids), botanicals (herbs or extracts from plants, including flowers, trees, shrubs, algae, ferns, fungi, seaweeds, and grasses), and glandular extracts from animal or synthetic sources.

Manufacturers are allowed to state that their products affect the "structure or function" of the body, provided that there is a disclaimer that the product has not been evaluated by the FDA. Manufacturers are responsible for their products' quality and safety, but the FDA does not require proof of efficacy or purity or reporting of adverse effects. The FDA may withdraw products shown to be harmful (e.g., fen-phen, cholestin, contaminated L-tryptophan, ephedra). Also, since 1998, FDA regulations require that dietary supplements that claim to "diagnose, treat, prevent, or cure disease" are to be regarded as drugs and must meet safety and efficacy standards; hence the disclaimers on so many product labels. Homeopathic and parenteral nutritional products are registered by the FDA but are not approved as drugs.

Recognition

Herbal medicines have been used for many thousands of years and are still used by 80% of the world's population. Herbal medicines are prescribed in Europe, and the German Commission E monographs for over 400 herbs are a resource for physicians. One third of conventional drugs are plant derived; aspirin (willow bark), digoxin (foxglove), ephedrine (ma huang), and atropine (belladonna alkaloids) are some common examples.

More than 5000 suspected herb-related adverse effects were reported to the World Health Organization prior to 1996. Between 1993 and 1998, the FDA received 2621 reports of adverse events, with 101 deaths associated with dietary supplements. In contrast, in 1995 the FDA received reports of 7000 deaths related to adverse prescription drug effects. One meta-analysis estimated that 100,000 deaths per year are associated with adverse drug reactions in hospitalized patients.

Given the widespread use of herbals and other dietary supplements, reported adverse effects are relatively few. However, lack of recognition and underreporting are possible reasons for this disparity. Many reports of adverse effects lack documentation of temporal effects, concomitant drug use, and positive identification of the herb in question, and they exclude the possible effects of contaminants or adulterants. For any substance that may have pharmacologic effects, vigilance is prudent, especially during anesthesia and surgery.

Consumers consider nutraceuticals to be safe, effective, and natural; as a result, their use is often not reported to physicians. As many as 20% of adults in the United States may use nutraceuticals, including herbs, and these numbers are increasing. One survey of more than 1000 adults undergoing preanesthetic evaluation revealed that about 40% were using at least one supplement, and 32% of these patients took herbals. More than 70% of these patients failed to report this use during routine preanesthetic assessment. A survey of more than 1000 preoperative pediatric patients showed that 12% used herbal remedies.

Supplement use is more prevalent among the following groups: females, nonsmokers, those with higher incomes, those who exercise regularly, those educated beyond high school, those in generally good health (albeit with one or more health problems), presurgical patients, and patients with cancer, liver disease, human immunodeficiency virus (HIV), asthma, and rheumatologic disorders.

By sales, the 10 top-ranked herbs in 2001 were echinacea, garlic, *Ginkgo biloba,* saw palmetto, ginseng, grapeseed extract, green tea, St. John's wort, bilberry, and aloe. Studies have shown statistically significant efficacy in the case of garlic, *Ginkgo biloba,* saw palmetto, and St. John's wort.

Risk Assessment

Although mechanical and infectious complications have been reported after some CAM therapy, an extensive review is beyond the scope of this chapter. Given that there are more than 20,000 herbal products in the United States, this chapter focuses on those substances most commonly used or most likely to have adverse pharmacologic effects in the perioperative period.

Assessment of risk is difficult, given the relative paucity of reports, incomplete information, and multiple patient and product variables. Dietary supplements, including vitamins, may contain a variety of substances with herbal ingredients. Product labels may not accurately reflect the contents or amounts. Also, lot-to-lot potency may vary owing to many factors, such as growing conditions, part of the plant used, time of harvest, preparation and extraction methods, and storage techniques. Standardization of compounds extracted from herbs is sometimes attempted, but the pharmacologic effects may be due to the combined or synergistic effects of the many compounds present in the herb. Further, products may be misused or adulterated with contaminants, such as misidentified botanical species, pesticides, herbicides, heavy metals, and conventional drugs.

Asian products have a high rate of contamination (about 30%). For example, contaminants in L-tryptophan resulted in eosinophilia-myalgia syndrome. Also, substitution of *Aristolochia fangchi* (fang-ji, a known nephrotoxin) for *Stephania tetrandra* (huang-fang ji) in a Chinese weight-loss preparation sold in Belgium caused more than 100 cases of renal failure and urothelial carcinoma.

The safety of raw animal glandular products (e.g., melatonin) is not known, especially those originating from the brains of animal species capable of transmitting spongiform encephalopathies. Synthetic sources are available for some of these substances.

Possible adverse effects are often based on in vitro studies of isolated compounds in animal models, isolated case reports, or small observational clinical trials. Often, any observed adverse effects are assumed to be related to the active ingredients. Randomized, controlled trials of the effects of herbs in the perioperative period are lacking. Future risk assessment must distinguish a "no observed effect level" and a "no observed *adverse* effect level" similar to that adopted for food additives and contaminants. More study is definitely needed.

Dietary substances affect enzyme systems and have clinical effects. For example, foods in the nightshade family (e.g., tomato, potato, eggplant) decrease acetylcholinesterase and pseudocholinesterase activity. These foods may influence the levels of drugs metabolized by these routes, including the neuromuscular blocking agent succinycholine.

Dietary regimens that lead to subclinical vitamin deficiency states may predispose patients to complications. Neurologic complications after nitrous oxide anesthesia have been reported in patients with vitamin B_{12} deficiency, including one patient on a restricted vegan diet.

Implications

Common side effects include gastrointestinal upset, allergic reactions, and dermatitis. Direct, indirect, synergistic, antagonistic, and toxic pharmacologic effects are possible when herbs are taken alone or in combination with conventional drugs. Herbs and nutraceuticals associated with organ system toxicity or physiologic effects are listed in Table 39-1. Table 39-2 summarizes the common uses for these herbs, the perioperative concerns, and other pertinent information.

The risk of toxicity with conventional medications is increased for patients at the extremes of age, as well as those who are pregnant, have a chronic illness or metabolic dysfunction, or are receiving chronic drug treatment. These patients may also be at increased risk for adverse effects or drug interactions with some nutraceuticals.

MANAGEMENT

There are no formal guidelines for the perioperative management of patients who are taking herbals or nutraceuticals. It may be reasonable to postpone elective surgery in those who are using nutraceuticals that may affect coagulation or cardiovascular, central nervous system, or other major organ function.

The American Society of Anesthesiologists has made no formal statement about the known therapeutic properties of herbal medications, and it has no formal policy or standards of care that apply specifically to phytopharmaceuticals. It does advise, however, that patients inform their physicians if they are using phytopharmaceuticals, that physicians specifically ask their patients about such use, and that patients discontinue these products 2 to 3 weeks before anesthesia and surgery.

Just as discontinuing some conventional medications is associated with increased morbidity and mortality, the discontinuation of herbal preparations may have similar effects. Abruptly stopping the use of some herbs may produce withdrawal symptoms. Individual management based on available pharmacokinetic data is recommended by some authors and may be the most practical approach in some clinical scenarios (Table 39-3).

As for neuraxial blocks, herbal medicines alone are not thought to create a risk that would mandate the cancellation of surgery. Concurrent use of oral anticoagulants or heparin may increase the risk for bleeding. There are no wholly accepted tests for hemostasis in patients using

Table 39–1 ■ Organ System or Pharmacologic Effects of Herbals and Nutraceuticals

Effects	Herbal/Nutraceutical	Other Names	Specific Effects/Comments
Abortifacient effects	Devil's claw		Oxytocic
	Dong quai		
	Goldenseal		
Analgesic effects	Aromatherapy		
	Salicylate sources: willow bark, meadowsweet		
	Feverfew (↓ migraines)		Withdrawal possible
	Fish oils (ω-3 fatty acids)		Decreases pain associated with migraines, sickle cell, rheumatoid arthritis
	Ginseng (↓ opioid effects)		
Anti-inflammatory effects	Blueberry	*Vaccinium myrtillus*	
	Devil's claw	*Harpagophytum procumbens*	
	Ginkgo biloba	*Ginkgo biloba*	
	Ginger	*Zingiber officinale*	
	Green tea	*Camellia sinensis*	
	Milk thistle	*Silybum marianum*	
	Red grapes	*Vitus vinifera*	
	Stinging nettle	*Urtica dioica*	
	Turmeric	*Curcuma longa*	
	Willow bark	*Salix alba*	
	Yarrow	*Achillea millefolium*	
Blood pressure effects	Black cohosh (↓)		
	Celery (↓)		
	Fenugreek (↓)		
	Garlic (↓)		
	Hawthorn (↓)		
	Horseradish (↓)		
	Capsicum (↑)		
	Ephedra (↑)		
	Goldenseal (↑)		
	Licorice (↑)		
	Ginger (↓ or ↑)		
	Ginkgo (↑ or ↓)		
	Ginseng (↓ or ↑)		
	St. John's wort (↓ or ↑)		
Carcinogen	Calamus		
	Sassafras		
Cardiac effects	Aconite		Arrhythmias
	Black cohosh		↓ HR, vasodilator
	Ephedra		Arrhythmias
	Fenugreek		↑ HR
	Fish oils		↓ Sudden death, ↓ lipids
	GBL, BD, GHB		↓ HR, death
	Ginger		↓ HR, inotrope in vitro
	Ginkgo biloba		Vasodilator, but HTN noted
	Goldenseal		Cardiac stimulant, ↓ coronary blood flow
	Hawthorn		Arrhythmias; potentiation of digitalis; possible β-blocker, ACE inhibitor properties
	Jimsonweed		↑ HR, anticholinergic effects
	Licorice		HTN, hypokalemia
	Lobelia		↑ HR
Cardiac glycoside–like effects	Foxglove (yellow, purple)	*Digitalis lanata; purpurea*	
	Kyushin		
	Milkweed	*Apocynum androsaemifolium*	
	Lily of the valley		
	Plantain (adulterated with foxglove)		
	Siberian ginseng	*Eleutherococcus senticosus*	
	Hawthorn berries		
	Uzara root		
Cardiac effects— ischemic preconditioning	Antioxidants (free radicals are involved in ischemic preconditioning in animals)		Vitamin C–attenuated beneficial effect of ischemic preconditioning in pigs
CNS effects			
Cognitive function	Melatonin		Case report—used to treat/prevent postoperative delirium
Seizures	Ginkgo toxin in seed and leaf		Neurotoxin; decreased seizure threshold
Sedative effects	Celery		
	Chamomile		Unconsciousness, slow respirations

Table continued on following page

Table 39–1 ■ **Organ System or Pharmacologic Effects of Herbals and Nutraceuticals—cont'd**

Effects	Herbal/Nutraceutical	Other Names	Specific Effects/Comments
	GBL, BD, GHB		
	Ginseng		
	Goldenseal		
	Hops		
	Kava kava		
	Passionflower		
	St. John's wort		Serotonergic syndrome with SSRIs (tremor, headache, myalgias, restlessness, mental status changes)
	Valerian		Withdrawal syndrome
Coagulation effects	Chinese herbs (most P)		Coumarin-containing plants: alfalfa, capsicum, celery, chamomile, fenugreek, ginseng, horseradish, licorice, passsionflower, red clover
	Dan-shen (P)		
	Dong quai (P)		
	Vitamin E (P) (>800 mg = 1200 IU/day)		
	Feverfew (P)		
	Fish oils (P)		
	Garlic (P)		
	Ginger (P) (inhibits thromboxane synthetase)		
	Ginkgo biloba (P) (inhibits platelet-activating factor)		
	Ginseng—*Panax* (P, F) (prolongs PT, PTT; but ↓ INR on warfarin)		
	Ginseng—American (↓ INR)		
	Kava kava (P)		
Drug interactions			
Digoxin	Hawthorn		↑ Toxicity
	Licorice		
	St. John's wort		↓ Digoxin levels
Digoxin assay: interference/ without toxicity	Kyushin (false ↑)		Traditional Chinese medicine "to save the heart"
	Siberian ginseng (false ↑)		
Dilantin	Shankhapushpi (Ayurvedic)		↓ Plasma concentration
MAOIs	Ginseng (*Panax*)		
	Licorice		
	St. John's wort		
SSRIs	St. John's wort		Serotonergic syndrome with concomitant use
Warfarin			
↓ INR	St. John's wort		
	Coenzyme Q$_{10}$		
	Ginseng (*Panax,* American)		Vitamin K analogue
↑ INR	Dan-shen		
	Dong quai		
	Garlic		
Potentiation of effect	Ginger		
	Ginkgo		
Drug metabolism			
Hepatic enzyme inducers ↓ drug concentrations (subtherapeutic)	St. John's wort		
Hepatic enzyme inhibitors ↑drug levels (toxicity)	Echinacea		
	Grapefruit juice		
Esterase inhibitors (↓ metabolism of cocaine, heroin, esmolol, local ester anesthetics, cholinesterase inhibitors, neuromuscular blocking drugs)	Glycoalkyloids of *Solanaceae* (nightshades—potato, tomato, eggplant)		
Electrolyte abnormalities	Aloe		Cathartic, hypokalemia
	Artichoke		Diuretic
	Celery		Diuretic
	Dandelion		Diuretic

Table continued on following page

Table 39–1 ■ Organ System or Pharmacologic Effects of Herbals and Nutraceuticals—cont'd

Effects	Herbal/Nutraceutical	Other Names	Specific Effects/Comments
	Glossypol		Hypokalemia
	Goldenseal		Aquaretic (water, not Na+, excreted; ↑ HTN, edema)
	Licorice		Hypokalemia, pseudoaldosteronism
Glucose blood levels			
Increased	Devil's claw		
	Ephedra		
	Ginseng		
	Licorice		
Decreased	Chromium		
	Cinnamon		
	Fenugreek		
	Garlic		
	Ginseng		
	Karela	*Momordica charantia*	
	Sage		
Hepatic toxicity	Chaparral		
	Comfrey		
	Germander		
	Kava kava		Need for liver transplant or death
	Pennyroyal		
	Yohimbe		Multicomponent product
Immune function	Echinacea		Not recommended for patients with autoimmune diseases
Nausea and vomiting	Ginger (↓ motion sickness)		
Neuromuscular blockade	Potato glycoalkaloids		Inhibits pseudocholinesterase (in vitro, human; in vivo, rabbit)
	Solanaceae (nightshade—tomato, potato, eggplant)		Inhibits pseudocholinesterase and acetylcholinesterases
Renal toxicity	*Aristolochia fangchi*		Urothelial carcinoma, renal failure
Skin effects	Kava kava		Kava dermopathy (yellow, dry, flaky skin)
	Dong quai		Photosensitizer
	St. John's wort		Photosensitizer
Withdrawal syndromes	Valerian (GABAergic)		Consider tapering over 2 wk; give benzodiazepines for withdrawal

ACE, angiotensin-converting enzyme; BD, 1,4-butanediol; CNS, central nervous system; F, fibrin formation inhibitor; GABA, γ-aminobutyric acid; GBL, γ-butyrolactone; GHB, γ-hydroxybutyrate; HR, heart rate; HTN, hypertension; INR, international normalized ratio; MAOI, monoamine oxidase inhibitor; P, platelet aggregation inhibitor; PT, prothrombin time; PTT, partial thromboplastin time; SSRI, selective serotonin reuptake inhibitor.

herbal preparations, nor are there specific concerns or recommendations regarding the timing of neuraxial block placement or catheter removal.

Information and vigilance are key to recognizing potentially adverse reactions and responding to them appropriately. Also, the recognition of potentially advantageous effects may come with further research.

PREVENTION

Physicians should be informed about and familiar with the effects of commonly used herbals and nutraceuticals, whether positive and negative. They should ask patients about their use and be willing to act as resource for them.

Patients should consult with their physicians before using herbals or nutraceuticals and then report any beneficial or adverse side effects. Consumers who use these substances should be cautious about product quality, especially with foreign manufacturers or distributors. They may want to consider requesting independent laboratory test results for product content and the presence of contaminants.

Information about herbals and nutraceuticals is available from many public and private resources (Table 39-4). Suspected adverse effects should be reported to the FDA's Center for Food Safety and Applied Nutrition (http://vm.cfsan.fda.gov/~dms/supplmnt.html) or to the FDA MedWatch Program (www.fda.gov/medwatch; 1-800-FDA-1088).

Table 39–2 ■ Common Uses of and Potential Problems with Herbals and Nutraceuticals

Herbal/Nutraceutical	Common Uses	Potential Perioperative Concerns	Potential Bleeding	Other Concerns
Aloe	Digestion, cathartic	Hypokalemia		Cross-allergenicity with ragweed
Chamomile (*Matricaria chamomilla*)	Insomnia	Sedation		
Coenzyme Q₁₀ (ubiquinone, ubidecarenone)	Congestive heart failure, cardiovascular health; used with statins	↓ INR on warfarin		Structurally related to vitamin K
Dong quai (*Angelica sinensis*)	Menopausal symptoms	Possible inhibition of platelet aggregation and cyclooxygenase; ↑ INR on warfarin	Yes	Photosensitivity
Echinacea (*E. angustifolia, E. pallida, E. purpurea*)	Upper respiratory infections, flu	Immunostimulant; inhibits CYP3A4, so risk of toxicity for drugs metabolized by CYP3A4 (alprazolam, calcium channel blockers, protease inhibitors)		Tachyphylaxis; autoimmune disease exacerbation; potentially hepatotoxic, but lacks 1,2 unsaturated necrine ring associated with other hepatotoxic pyrrolizidine alkaloids
Ephedra, ma huang (*Ephedra sinica*)	Weight loss; antitussive; asthma	HTN, arrhythmias, sympathomimetic effects		Banned by FDA in 2004; interactions with cardiac glycosides
Vitamin E	Antioxidant; antiaging; cardiovascular health and cancer prophylaxis; fibrocystic breast syndrome		Yes	Possible bleeding with doses >800 mg = 1200 IU/day
Feverfew (*Tanacetum parthenium*)	Migraines; fever	Inhibits platelets	Yes	Abrupt withdrawal can cause headache, insomnia, nervousness, arthralgias, fatigue, stiffness; aphthous ulcers
Garlic (*Allium sativum*)	HTN; hyperlipidemia; respiratory, digestive, liver complaints	Inhibits platelet aggregation; ↑ INR with warfarin	Yes	Case of elderly man who developed spontaneous epidural hematoma while gardening—4 raw cloves/day
Ginger (*Zingiber officinale*)	Nausea, vomiting; vertigo; motion sickness; antispasmodic; digestive complaints	Inhibits thromboxane synthetase	Yes	Possible mutagenesis
Ginkgo (*Ginkgo biloba*)	Dementia; claudication; increased mental acuity; tinnitus; vertigo	Inhibits platelet-activating factor; seed and leaf contain a neurotoxin	Yes	Spontaneous hyphema, subdural hematoma; no known interaction with cardiac glycosides or hypoglycemics
Ginseng American (*Panax quinquefolius*) Asian (*Panax ginseng*) Sanchi (*Panax pseudoginseng var notoginseng*) Siberian (*Eleutherococcus senticosus*)	Adaptogen; immunomodulation; tonic for many conditions	HTN; tachycardia; bleeding; ↓ INR with warfarin; CNS stimulation; hypoglycemic effects in type 2 diabetes	Yes	Stevens-Johnson syndrome; epistaxis; vaginal bleeding; mastalgia Siberian ginseng interferes with digoxin assay—false elevation of digoxin levels without toxicity
GBL, BD, GHB	Illegally distributed (not approved by FDA) for bodybuilding, weight loss, sleep aid			Death; seizures; unconsciousness; bradycardia; slowed respirations requiring intubation

Continued

Table 39–2 ■ Common Uses of and Potential Problems with Herbals and Nutraceuticals—cont'd

Herbal/Nutraceutical	Common Uses	Potential Perioperative Concerns	Potential Bleeding	Other Concerns
Goldenseal (*Hydrastis canadensis*)—turmeric root	Diuretic; anti-inflammatory; laxative; hemostatic	HTN; edema; paralysis with overdosage		Oxytocic; aquaretic, not diuretic (no Na⁺ excreted, just free water)
Kava kava (*Piper methysticum*)	Insomnia; sedation; anxiety	Coma with alprazolam; GABA effects; potentiates barbiturates and benzodiazepines; hepatotoxicity		Kava dermopathy (red eyes; dry, flaky, yellow skin and nails); inhibits cyclooxygenase
Kyushin	Chinese medicine "to save the heart"	False elevations of digoxin levels without toxicity		Cross-reacts with digoxin assays
Licorice (*Glycyrrhiza glabra*)	Digestion; ulcers	HTN; K⁺ loss; edema; pseudoaldosteronism		Glycyrrhizic acid inhibits 11-β-hydroxysteroid dehydrogenase resulting in mineralocorticoid effects; transient myopathy (2 wk)
Saw palmetto (*Serenoa repens*)	Benign prostatic hypertrophy	None known		Inhibits dihydrotestosterone binding and 5α-reductase activity; possible interaction with other hormone therapies
St. John's wort (*Hypericum perforatum*)	Depression; anxiety; sleep disorders	Possible weak MAOI; possible SSRI (mechanism uncertain); use caution with β-sympathomimetic amines, SSRIs, MAOs		Photosensitivity; induction of hepatic cytochromes P-450, 3A4; decreased digoxin levels; decreased HIV protease inhibitors and NNRTIs
Valerian (*Valeriana officinalis*)	Insomnia; sedation; anxiety	Prolongs barbiturate-induced sleep		Withdrawal possible; treat with benzodiazepines

BD, 1,4-butanediol; CNS, central nervous system; FDA, Food and Drug Administration; GABA, γ-aminobutyric acid; GBL, γ-butyrolactone; GHB, γ-hydroxybutyrate; HIV, human immunodeficiency virus; HTN, hypertension; INR, international normalized ratio; MAOI, monoamine oxidase inhibitor; NNRTI, non-nucleoside reverse transcriptase inhibitor; SSRI, selective serotonin reuptake inhibitor.

Table 39–3 ■ Recommended Preoperative Discontinuation of Herbs

Herb	Preoperative Discontinuation
Aloe	No data
Echinacea	No data
Ephedra (banned)	At least 24 hr
Garlic	At least 7 days
Ginkgo	At least 36 hr
Ginseng	At least 7 days
Kava kava	At least 24 hr
St. John's wort	At least 5 days
Valerian	No data (benzodiazepine-like acute withdrawal possible)

Table 39–4 ■ Herbal and Dietary Supplement Resources

Organization	Web Address/Phone	Information/Comments
Alternative Medicine Foundation	http://www.herbmed.org	Research publication summaries; MEDLINE links
American Botanical Council	www.herbalgram.org	News, information; German Commission E Monographs
Certificates of analysis	Various sources; available on request from manufacturers or distributors	Amount of active ingredient in given lot; presence of contaminants
Epocrates Rx Pro	www.epocrates.com	Alternative medicine tables
FDA, Center for Food Safety and Applied Nutrition	http://vm.cfsan.fda.gov/~dms/supplmnt.html 1-888-723-3366	Report adverse events; safety, industry regulations
FDA Medwatch	www.fda.gov/medwatch 1-800-FDA-1088	Report adverse events
NCI, Division of Cancer Prevention and Control, Chemoprevention Program	www.cancer.gov	Search "alternative medicine"
NIH, National Center for Complementary and Alternative Medicine	http://nccam.nih.gov 1-888-644-6226	Fact sheets, consensus reports, databases
NIH, Office of Alternative Medicine and Office of Dietary Supplements	www.altmed.od.nih.gov	
NIH, Office of Dietary Supplements, International Bibliographic Information on Dietary Supplements (IBIDS)	www.ods.od.nih.gov	Abstracts of peer-reviewed literature
PDR for Herbal Medicines	ISBN 1-56363-292-6; Medical Economics Co., Montvale, NJ	
Quackwatch	http://www.quackwatch.com	General health care; CAM Search "alternative medicine"
US Department of Health and Human Services	www.healthfinder.gov	
US Pharmacopoeia	www.usp.org	Private organization; quality standards

CAM, complementary and alternative medicine; FDA, Food and Drug Administration; NCI, National Cancer Institute; NIH, National Institutes of Health; PDR, *Physicians' Desk Reference*.

Further Reading

Abebe W: Herbal medication: Potential for adverse interactions with analgesic drugs. J Clin Pharm Ther 27:391-401, 2002.

Adusumilli PS, Ben-Porat L, Pereira M, et al: The prevalence and predictors of herbal medicine use in surgical patients. J Am Coll Surg 198:583-590, 2004.

Anesthesiologists warn: If you're taking herbal products, tell your doctor before surgery. Information for patients: http://www.asahq.org/patientEducation/insiderherb.html. Information for doctors: http://www.asahq.org/patientEducation/herbal.html.

Ang-Lee MK, Moss J, Yuan C: Herbal medicines and perioperative care. JAMA 286:208-216, 2001.

Bent S, Ko R: Commonly used herbal medicines in the United States: A review. Am J Med 116:478-485, 2004.

Borins M: The dangers of using herbs—what your patient needs to know. Postgrad Med 104:91-100, 1998.

Chagan L, Ioselovich A, Asherova L, Cheng JWM: Use of alternative pharmacotherapy in management of cardiovascular diseases. Am J Manag Care 8:270-285, 2002.

Considerations for anesthesiologists—what you should know about your patients' use of herbal medicines and other dietary supplements. American Society of Anesthesiologists brochure, 2003. Available at www.ASAhq.org.

De Smet PAGM: Herbal remedies. N Engl J Med 347:2046-2056, 2002.

Ernst E: The risk-benefit profile of commonly used herbal therapies: Ginkgo, St John's wort, ginseng, echinacea, saw palmetto, and kava. Ann Intern Med 136:45-53, 2002.

Ezzo J, Berman BM, Vickers AJ, et al: Complementary medicine and the Cochrane collaboration. JAMA 280:1628-1630, 1998.

Fugh-Berman A: Herb-drug interactions. Lancet 355:134-138, 2000.

Get the facts—what is complementary and alternative medicine (CAM). National Institutes of Health Center for Complementary and Alternative Medicine. Available at http://nccam.nih.gov/health/whatiscam/index.htm.

Hanania M, Kitain E: Melatonin for treatment and prevention of postoperative delirium. Anesth Analg 94:338-339, 2002.

Horlocker TT, Wedel DJ, Benzon H, et al: Regional anesthesia in the anticoagulated patient: Defining the risks. Reg Anesth Pain Med 29:1-11, 2004.

Izzo AA, Ernst E: Interactions between herbal medicines and prescribed drugs. Drugs 61:2163-2175, 2001.

Kaye AD, Clarke RC, Sabar R, et al: Herbal medicines: Current trends in anesthesiology practice—a hospital survey. J Clin Anesth 12:468-471, 2000.

Kaye AD, Kucera I, Sabar R: Perioperative anesthesia clinical considerations of alternative medicines. Anesthesiol Clin North Am 22:125-139, 2004.

Kottke MK: Scientific and regulatory aspects of nutraceutical products in the United States. Drug Dev Indust Pharm 24:1177-1195, 1998.

Lazarou J, Pomeranz BH, Corey PN: Incidence of adverse drug reactions in hospitalized patients. JAMA 279:1200-1205, 1998.

Lee P, Smith I, Piesowicz A, Brenton D: Spastic paraparesis after anaesthesia. Lancet 353:554, 1999.

Lin Y, Bioteau AB, Ferrari LR, Berde CB: The use of herbs and complementary and alternative medicine in pediatric preoperative patients. J Clin Anesth 16:4-6, 2004.

McGehee DS, Krasowski MD, Fung DL, et al: Cholinesterase inhibition by potato glycoalkaloids slows mivacurium metabolism. Anesthesiology 93:510-519, 2000.

Miller LG: Herbal medicinals—selected clinical consideration focusing on known or potential drug-herb interactions. Arch Intern Med 158:2200-2211, 1998.

Murphy JM: Preoperative considerations with herbal medicines. AORN J 69:173-183, 1999.

Niggemann B, Gruber C: Side-effects of complementary and alternative medicine. Allergy 58:707-716, 2003.

Norred CL: A follow-up survey of the use of complementary and alternative medicines by surgical patients. AANA J 70:119-125, 2002.

Norred CL, Brinker F: Potential coagulation effects of preoperative complementary and alternative medicines. Altern Ther Health Med 7:58-67, 2001.

Norred CL, Zamudio S, Palmer SK: Use of complementary and alternative medicines by surgical patients. AANA J 68:13-18, 2000.

Pinn G: Adverse effects associated with herbal medicine. Aust Fam Physician 30:1070-1075, 2001.

Pribitkin E, Boger G: Herbal therapy—what every plastic surgeon must know. Arch Facial Plast Surg 3:127-132, 2001.

Rados C: Ephedra ban: No shortage of reasons. FDA Consumer Magazine, July 2004. Available at http//www.fda.gov/fdac/features/2004/204_ephedra.html.

Rose KD, Croissant PD, Parliament CF, Levin MB: Spontaneous spinal epidural hematoma with associated platelet dysfunction from excessive garlic ingestion: A case report. Neurosurgery 26:880-882, 1990.

Rosener M, Dichgans J: Severe combined degeneration of the spinal cord after nitrous oxide anaesthesia in a vegetarian. J Neurol Neurosurg Psychiatry 60:354, 1996.

Sabar R, Kaye AD, Frost EAM: Perioperative considerations for the patient on herbal medicines. Middle East J Anesthesiol 16:287-314, 2001.

Skyschally A, Schulz R, Gres P, et al: Attenuation of ischemic preconditioning in pigs by scavenging of free oxyradicals with ascorbic acid. Am J Physiol Heart Circ Physiol 284:698-708, 2003.

Walker R: Criteria for risk assessment of botanical food supplements. Toxicol Lett 149:187-195, 2004.

Yuan CS, Wei G, Dey L, et al: Brief communication: American ginseng reduces warfarin's effect in healthy patients: A randomized controlled trial. Ann Intern Med 141:23-27, 2004.

ANESTHETIC MANAGEMENT ISSUES

Difficult Airway: Cannot Ventilate, Cannot Intubate

Michael P. Ford and George A. Arndt

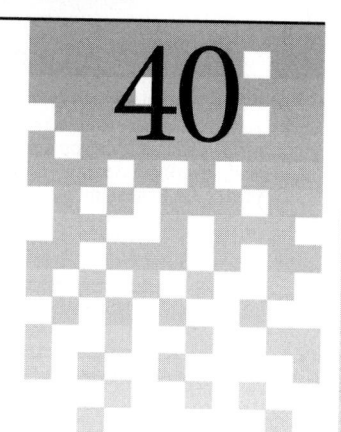

40

GENERAL ANESTHESIA

Case Synopsis

A moderately obese man with lung contusions and a closed head injury requires endotracheal intubation on admission to the hospital. Two days later, after neurologic and respiratory recovery, his trachea is extubated. The patient immediately develops respiratory difficulty. Attempts to ventilate the lungs via facemask are unsuccessful. As the patient loses consciousness, laryngoscopy is performed, but the laryngeal structures cannot be visualized. The patient's oxygen saturation decreases rapidly.

PROBLEM ANALYSIS

Definition

CANNOT VENTILATE, CANNOT INTUBATE

The cannot ventilate, cannot intubate (CVCI) situation is defined as the inability to ventilate the patient's lungs via facemask despite multiple attempts, and the inability to intubate the patient's trachea via conventional direct laryngoscopy. In 2003 the American Society of Anesthesiologists (ASA) Task Force on Management of the Difficult Airway updated the applicable practice guidelines. It is hoped that use of the ASA difficult airway algorithm (Fig. 40-1) will reduce the likelihood of adverse outcomes.

The CVCI situation can develop quickly but often occurs after repeated attempts at direct laryngoscopy or after a failed rapid-sequence induction or intubation. No more than two or three attempts should be made at direct laryngoscopy, because repeated attempts may worsen the patient's outcome. The CVCI portion of the ASA algorithm entails the use of rescue options with varying degrees of invasiveness. Before resorting to invasive airway rescue techniques, it is crucial that every effort be made to achieve oxygenation and ventilation through noninvasive techniques, such as optimal facemask ventilation (two-person mask technique, ensuring adequate jaw thrust and facemask seal, with an oral or nasal airway [or both]) or supraglottic ventilation using a laryngeal mask airway. Although potentially lethal, the CVCI situation is, fortunately, a rare occurrence. El-Ganzouri and colleagues evaluated the airways of 10,507 consecutive patients and found that 107 (1%) had a poor laryngoscopic view (grade 4—neither laryngeal structures nor epiglottis visualized), 535 (5.3%) patients had a grade 3 laryngeal view, and only 8 patients (0.07%) could not be adequately ventilated using a facemask.

DIFFICULT AIRWAY

A difficult airway is defined as a clinical situation in which a conventionally trained anesthesiologist experiences difficulty with facemask ventilation of the airway, difficulty with tracheal intubation, or both. Intubation is difficult when multiple attempts, maneuvers, blades, and endoscopies are required. Some patients with a difficult airway for mask ventilation may be relatively easy to intubate, and vice versa. Reasons for the majority of airway complications and management failures are listed in Table 40-1.

DIFFICULT FACEMASK VENTILATION

Difficult facemask ventilation occurs when positive-pressure ventilation, by an unassisted anesthesiologist, fails to maintain oxygen saturation above 90% (with an inspired oxygen concentration of 100%) or the ventilation effort fails to prevent or reverse signs of inadequate gas exchange. Inadequate facemask ventilation is secondary to inadequate facemask seal, excessive gas leak, or excessive resistance to the ingress or egress of gas. Signs of inadequate facemask ventilation are listed in Table 40-2. The incidence of difficult facemask ventilation is approximately 5%. The incidence of difficult ventilation, despite optimization of the mask airway using supraglottic adjuncts, is less than 0.5%.

All patients should be oxygenated before the induction of general anesthesia; doing so decreases the incidence of and prolongs the time interval to oxygen desaturation when facemask ventilation is inadequate or not attempted (rapid-sequence induction). In pediatric and uncooperative patients, however, the effectiveness of preoxygenation may be limited. In obese patients, preoxygenation using continuous positive airway pressure and the reverse Trendelenburg position lengthens the time to decreased oxygen saturation after the onset of apnea or inadequate ventilation. Patient factors associated with difficult facemask ventilation, as well as some suggestions for dealing with them, are listed in Table 40-3. Multiple factors indicate a high likelihood of difficult facemask ventilation. Placing a laryngeal mask airway permits adequate positive-pressure ventilation to occur in most patients and should be used early when difficulty with facemask ventilation (or difficult intubation) is encountered.

159

1. Assess the likelihood and clinical impact of basic management problems:
    A. Difficult ventilation
    B. Difficult intubation
    C. Difficulty with patient cooperation or consent
    D. Difficult tracheostomy
2. Actively pursue opportunities to deliver supplemental oxygen throughout the process of difficult airway management
3. Consider the relative merits and feasibility of basic management choices:

A.	Awake intubation	vs.	Intubation attempts after induction of general anesthesia
B.	Noninvasive technique for initial approach to intubation	vs.	Invasive technique for initial approach to intubation
C.	Preservation of spontaneous ventilation	vs.	Ablation of spontaneous ventilation

4. Develop primary and alternative strategies:

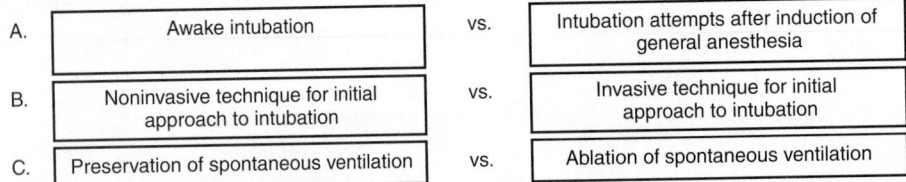

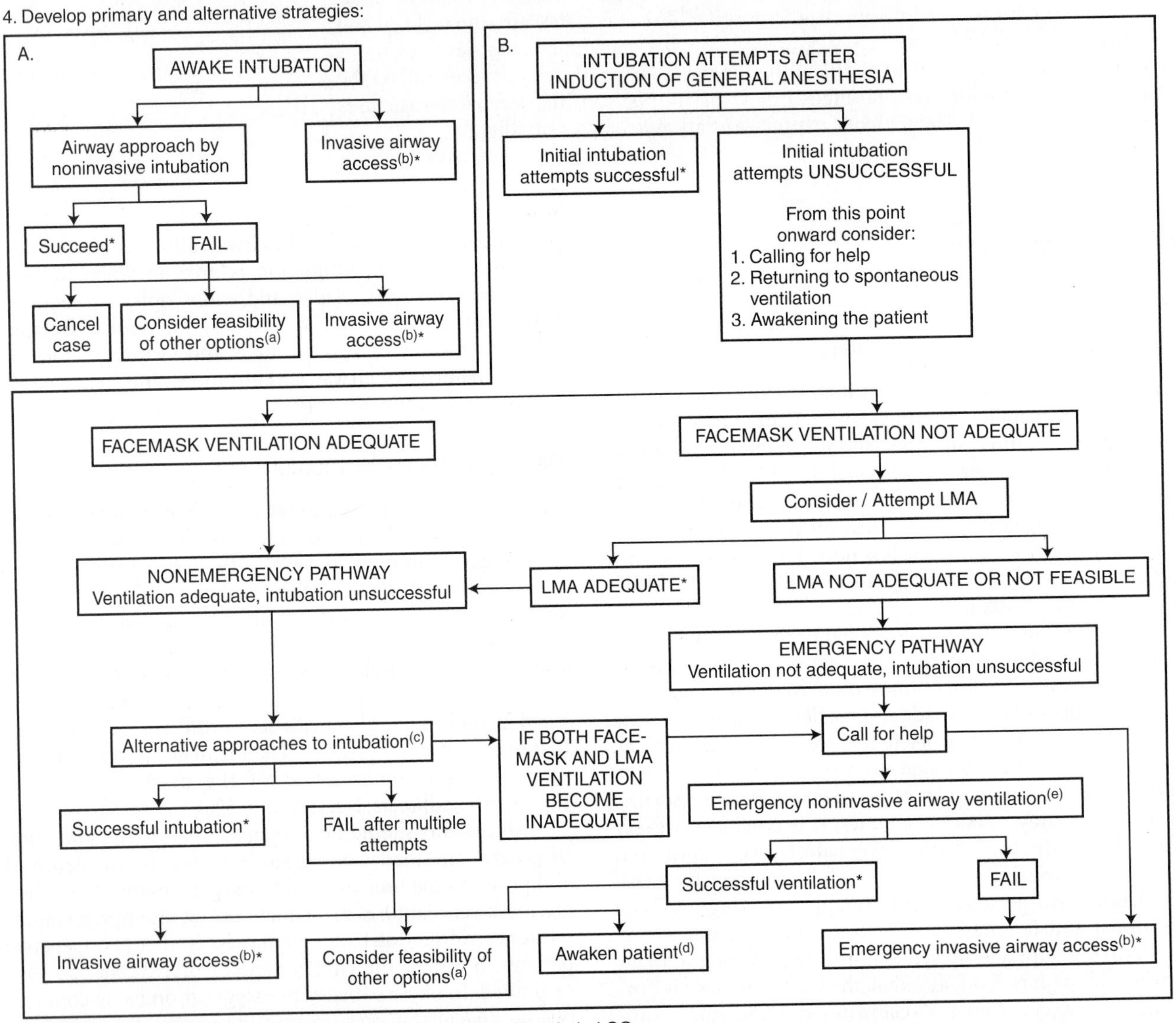

* Confirm ventilation, tracheal intubation, or LMA placement with exhaled CO_2.
a. Other options include (but are not limited to): surgery utilizing facemask or LMA anesthesia, local anesthesia infiltration or regional nerve blockade. Pursuit of these options usually implies that mask ventilation will not be problematic. Therefore, these options may be of limited value if this step in the algorithm has been reached via the Emergency Pathway.
b. Invasive airway access includes surgical or percutaneous tracheostomy or cricothyrotomy.
c. Alternative noninvasive approaches to difficult intubation include (but are not limited to) use of different laryngoscope blades, LMA as an intubation conduit (with or without fiberoptic guidance), fiberoptic intubation, intubating stylet or tube changer, light wand, retrograde intubation, and blind oral or nasal intubation.
d. Consider repreparation of the patient for awake intubation or canceling surgery.
e. Options for emergency noninvasive airway ventilation include (but are not limited to) rigid bronchoscope, esophageal-tracheal Combitube ventilation, or transtracheal jet ventilation.

Figure 40–1 ▪ American Society of Anesthesiologists difficult airway algorithm. LMA, laryngeal mask airway. (From Practice guidelines for management of the difficult airway—an updated report by the American Society of Anesthesiologists Task Force on Management of the Difficult Airway. Anesthesiology 98:1269-1277, 2003.)

Table 40–1 ■ Reasons for Airway Complications and Management Failures

Inaccurate or incomplete preoperative airway assessment
Incorrect prediction of:
  Easy mask airway
  Routine direct laryngoscopy-guided intubation
  Uncomplicated extubation
Unwillingness to abandon failed airway management plan
Failure to call for help early, when difficult airway is first apparent
Incomplete preparation of backup plan
Deterioration of performance under stress
Failure in judgment

Table 40–3 ■ Patient Factors Associated with Difficult Facemask Ventilation and Suggested Solutions

Facial Hair

Place adhesive plastic sheet, with mouth and naris openings, over facial hair to achieve better mask seal
Place oral, nasal, or laryngeal mask airway early

Edentulous

Consider leaving dentures in place until laryngoscopy to improve facemask seal
Place laryngeal mask airway early

Body Mass Index >26

Preoxygenate patient with continuous positive airway pressure and use 20- to 30-degree reverse Trendelenburg position
  Increases time interval to desaturation after onset of apnea or difficult mask ventilation
  Reverse Trendelenburg "unloads" diaphragm, improving pulmonary compliance
Use laryngeal mask airway early for positive-pressure mask ventilation

Snoring and Obstructive Sleep Apnea

Place oral, nasal, or laryngeal mask airway early

Age >55 yr
History of Smoking
Supraglottic, Glottic, and Subglottic Pathology or Stridor

Consider prospective placement of translaryngeal jet ventilation catheter
Strongly consider awake airway management
Avoid sedation if stridor is present

Bronchospasm (active or at risk for)

Nebulize with bronchodilator before induction

DIFFICULT INTUBATION

Difficult intubation occurs when endotracheal intubation requires multiple attempts. The ASA Task Force defines difficult intubation as more than three attempts at conventional direct laryngoscopy or more than 10 minutes to achieve intubation. Difficult laryngoscopy is the inability to visualize any portion of the vocal cords after multiple attempts using conventional rigid laryngoscopy. The incidence of difficult direct laryngoscopy (more than two attempts) is between 0.5% and 2%. The first attempt must be optimized, including adequate depth of anesthesia and muscle relaxation, proper positioning of the head and neck, use of a styletted tube, and application of laryngeal manipulation. External laryngeal pressure or manipulation by the laryngoscopist's right hand (or by an assistant) may convert a grade 3 visualization of the larynx to a grade 2 (Fig. 40-2). Straight laryngoscope blades can be efficacious with "anterior" anatomy. Alternative, specialized laryngoscopes should be employed only by those experienced with their use. No more than two or three attempts should be made at direct laryngoscopy, because repeated attempts may worsen the patient's outcome (e.g., conversion of a can-ventilate to a cannot-ventilate situation, or laryngeal edema causing glottic airway obstruction after tracheal extubation). Facemask ventilation must occur between attempts, and direct laryngoscopy must be stopped if oxygen saturation falls below 90% to 92% (maintenance of oxygenation takes precedence). The most experienced anesthesiologist available should perform the final attempt at direct laryngoscopy.

Table 40–2 ■ Signs of Inadequate Facemask Ventilation

Insufficient or absent chest movement
Absent or inadequate breath sounds
Audible signs of airway obstruction, gastric air insufflation, or gastric dilatation
Inadequate or decreasing oxygen saturation
Cyanosis
Absent, inadequate, or elevated end-tidal carbon dioxide
Absent or inadequate exhaled gas flow (spirometry)
Hemodynamic consequences of hypercarbia or hypoxemia (e.g., tachycardia, hypertension, dysrhythmias)

Recognition

The cause of the majority of difficult endotracheal intubations is limited oropharyngeal space, decreased atlanto-occipital extension, decreased pharyngeal space, or decreased submandibular compliance. Recognition of potentially difficult direct laryngoscopy and endotracheal intubation is facilitated by a systematic search for abnormalities during the preoperative airway examination (Table 40-4). Unfortunately, airway examination findings have low and variable sensitivity and marginal specificity; however, worrisome findings, particularly in combination, suggest a difficult intubation. A Mallampati class higher than II (Fig. 40-3) in association with other airway findings signifies potential difficulty during traditional direct laryngoscopy. Reviewing the patient's prior anesthetic history and previous records of airway management (if available) is extremely helpful when formulating the airway management plan. Anesthesiologists must accurately document the ease or difficulty of facemask ventilation, laryngoscopy attempts and blades used, the laryngoscopic view obtained (see Fig. 40-2), how intubation was ultimately achieved, and any special maneuvers or devices used. Assume high reliability if the patient self-reports a difficult airway. Consider any systemic diseases or congenital abnormalities that require special attention during airway management.

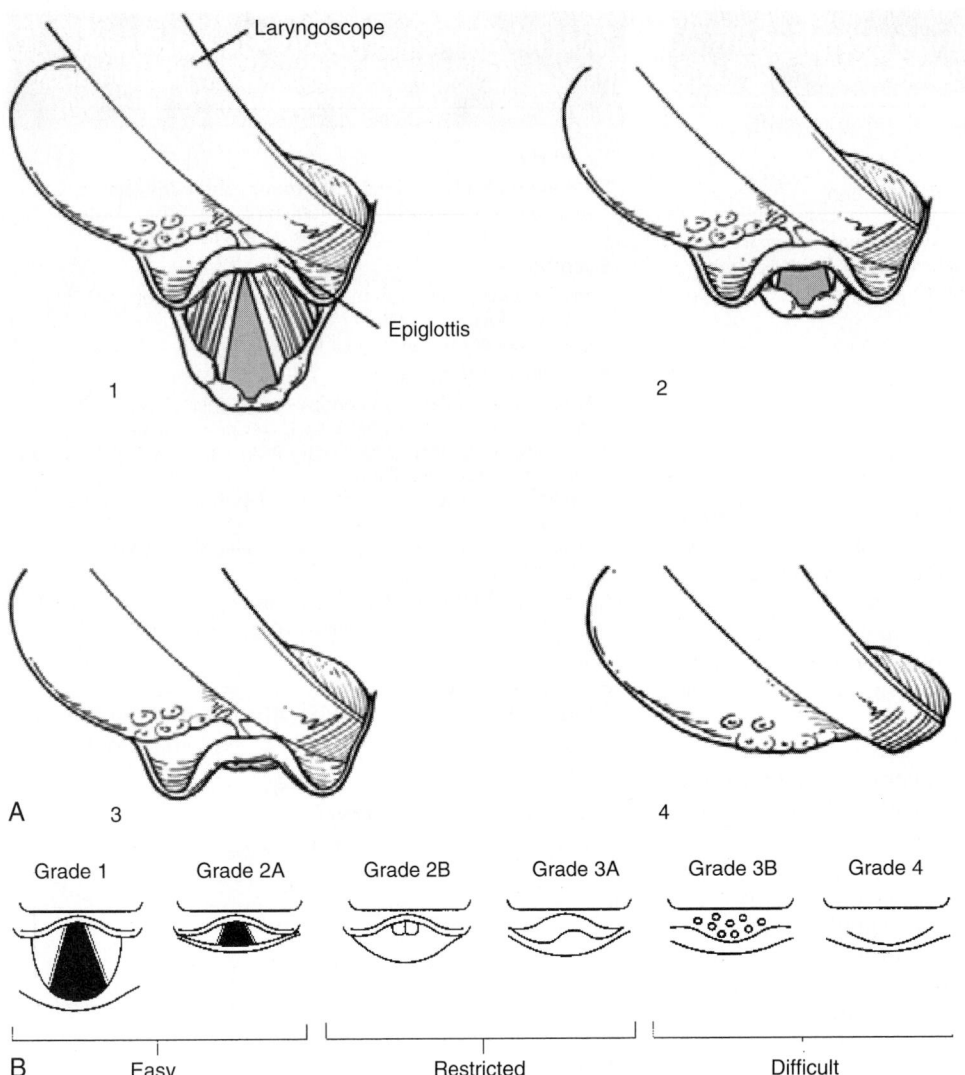

Figure 40–2 ■ Laryngoscopic view grading systems. *A,* Cormack-Lehane system: grade 1, visualization of the entire laryngeal aperture; grade 2, visualization of only the posterior portion of the laryngeal aperture; grade 3, visualization of only the epiglottis; grade 4, visualization of only the soft palate. *B,* Modified grading system of view at direct laryngoscopy: grade 1, most of cords visible (direct intubation); grade 2A, posterior cord visible (direct intubation); grade 2B, only arytenoids visible (indirect intubation); grade 3A, epiglottis visible and liftable (indirect intubation); grade 3B, epiglottis adherent to pharynx (specialist required for intubation); grade 4, no laryngeal structures seen (specialist required for intubation). (*A,* From Cormack RS, Lehane J: Difficult tracheal intubation in obstetrics. Anaesthesia 39:1105, 1984. *B,* From Cook TM: A new practical classification of laryngeal view. Anaesthesia 55:274-279, 2000.)

ENDOTRACHEAL INTUBATION INTRODUCERS AND INTUBATING CATHETERS

A malleable tracheal tube introducer (gum-elastic bougie [GEB], length 60 cm) or an intubating catheter can be placed blindly and gently under the epiglottis (or directed through partially visible, posterior vocal cords) into the trachea during one of the laryngoscopic attempts. The anesthesiologist will not see the GEB entering the larynx with a grade 3 or 4 laryngoscopic view. Tactile "clicking" may be felt as the angled (about 60 degrees), anteriorly directed tip of the GEB passes over (hits against) the tracheal rings. If clicks are not perceived, the GEB should be gently advanced to a maximum depth of 45 cm (in an adult patient). If distal hold-up is sensed, such as slight resistance to further advancement, the GEB is likely "caught up" in the bronchial tree, and the patient may cough if not completely paralyzed. If neither clicks, hold-up, nor coughing is evoked, the GEB is probably in the esophagus and should be removed. A second attempt at passing the GEB blindly into the trachea can be considered, unless there is a grade 4 laryngeal view or the epiglottis

cannot be elevated (the epiglottis is "adherent" to the pharynx). If the GEB is believed to be in the trachea, an internally lubricated endotracheal tube (ETT) is advanced ("railroaded") over the GEB. Leaving the laryngoscope blade in the mouth and rotating the ETT 90 degrees counterclockwise facilitates ETT advancement (orientation of the Murphy eye at the 12 o'clock position prevents the ETT tip from hanging up on the right vocal cord or arytenoids during passage). Tracheal location is confirmed by auscultation of equal bilateral breath sounds and sustained end-tidal carbon dioxide waveforms. The rule is, "if in doubt, take the ETT out," unless immediate flexible bronchoscopy via the ETT confirms a tracheal location. Optimal results achieving intubation with the GEB are dependent on experience and regular use.

DIFFICULT EXTUBATION

The risks for difficult facemask ventilation and difficult intubation, as well as other events, herald difficult extubation. Patients with a difficult airway should meet the usual criteria for extubation and be fully awake. They also should cough

Table 40–4 ▪ Airway Examination Predictors of Difficult Direct Laryngoscopy and Endotracheal Intubation

Interincisor Gap

If distance between upper and lower incisors is less than 3-4 cm, direct laryngoscopy may be difficult because of:
    Insufficient space for blade insertion and blade "traction" without dental injury
    Less room for endotracheal tube passage and direction
    Possible obscured line of sight to glottic opening

Length of Upper Incisors

Long incisors impede alignment of oral and pharyngeal axes during direct laryngoscopy
Relatively long, protruding upper incisors are worrisome

Mallampati Oropharyngeal Classification (see Fig. 40-3)

With Mallampati class I or II, tongue should be easily retracted from the line of site during direct laryngoscopy
Mallampati class >II is worrisome

Mandibular Space

With hyomental and thyromental distances (estimates of mandibular space) >6 and 7 cm, respectively, larynx should be sufficiently
    posterior for favorable line of sight with direct laryngoscopy
Distance <3 ordinary fingerbreadths (5 cm) is worrisome

Length and Thickness of Neck

Short, thick neck reduces ability to align upper airway axes during direct laryngoscopy
In obese patients, large neck circumference and Mallampati class >II are worrisome

Head and Neck Range of Motion

Atlanto-occipital (AO) extension or neck flexion on chest of <35 degrees predicts difficult direct laryngoscopy; this amount of AO
    extension and neck flexion is required for proper alignment of oral, pharyngeal, and laryngeal axes
Obese body habitus may preclude optimal alignment of oral, pharyngeal, and laryngeal axes
Direct laryngoscopy in obese patients is facilitated when head, neck, and shoulders are elevated ("stacked"), bringing chin level with
    sternum; fiberoptic bronchoscopy intubation is rarely necessary with proper positioning
Higher Mallampati class and large neck circumference are reliable predictors of difficult intubation in obese patients
Inability to touch chin to chest is worrisome

Maxillary-Mandibular Overbite (Buck Teeth)

Buck teeth reduce the ability to align oral and pharyngeal axes during direct laryngoscopy

Mandibular Translation

Ability to protrude lower jaw by more than 1 cm often predicts good direct laryngoscopic view
Ability to touch bottom incisors to the upper lip–skin border is reassuring

Mandibular Space Compliance

Worrisome findings include stiffness, induration, and presence of mass

Palate Configuration

Narrow or highly arched palate reduces oropharyngeal volume and ability to visualize glottis with both laryngoscope blade and
    endotracheal tube in mouth

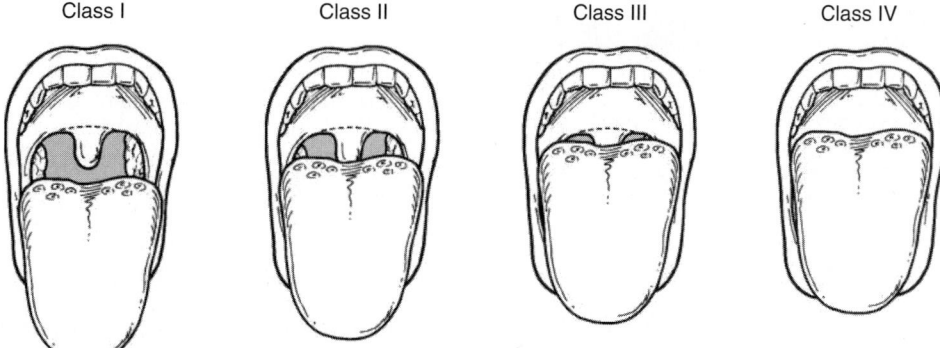

Class I   Class II   Class III   Class IV

Figure 40–3 ▪ Mallampati classification. With the patient seated and the head in the neutral position, the patient is asked to open the mouth as wide as possible and to protrude the tongue out as far as possible (the patient should not phonate during this evaluation). Class I, soft palate, fauces, uvula, and anterior and posterior tonsillar pillars are visible; class II, soft palate, fauces, and uvula are visible; class III, soft palate and base of uvula are visible; class IV, only hard palate is visible. (Modified from Mallampati S, Gatt S, Gugino L, et al: A clinical sign to predict difficult tracheal intubation: A prospective study. Can J Anaesth 32:429, 1985; and Samsoon GLT, Young JRB: Difficult tracheal intubation: A retrospective study. Anaesthesia 42:487, 1987.)

Table 40–5 ■ Factors to Consider When Formulating an Extubation Strategy

Relative advantages of awake extubation vs tracheal extubation before return of consciousness
    Was intubation difficult?
    Was facemask ventilation difficult?
    Is risk for aspiration high?
Upper airway edema or bleeding may have adverse impact on effective ventilation after extubation
    Bleeding, tissue edema, or nerve injury can cause airway obstruction after neck surgery
    Edema risk may be higher with recent neck infection or prior irradiation
Direct or indirect trauma to peritracheal, laryngeal, and supraglottic structures
    Manipulation during surgery increases potential for airway obstruction
    Edema may occur after difficult or multiple laryngoscopies but not be apparent until after extubation
Recurrent laryngeal nerve injury
Predetermined plan for airway management if patient is unable to maintain adequate ventilation after removal of endotracheal tube
Extubation over previously inserted endotracheal tube exchange catheter
    Functions as a guide for rapid reintubation
    Can facilitate ventilation if tube exchanger has a lumen
Extubation over flexible fiberoptic bronchoscope
    Endotracheal tube can be readvanced into trachea if necessary
    Trachea and glottic and supraglottic structures can be examined for abnormalities as bronchoscope is slowly removed
    Bronchoscope removal can be stopped if significant airway concerns are identified
    Bronchoscope may be readvanced into trachea, with subsequent passage of "loaded" endotracheal tube
    Wire can be inserted through fiberoptic bronchoscope suction channel before bronchoscope's gradual removal to serve as guide for reintroduction of bronchoscope or airway exchange catheter into trachea

and phonate during ETT cuff deflation. Patients at high risk should have the ETT removed over an intubating stylet (bougie or exchange catheter), guidewire, or fiberoptic bronchoscope, with an experienced surgeon (for cricothyrotomy and tracheostomy) at the bedside. Factors to consider in formulating an extubation strategy are listed in Table 40-5.

Risk Assessment

Risk assessment for a potentially difficult airway is multifactorial (Table 40-6). Reduction of risk with the CVCI situation begins with a thorough assessment of the patient's airway before induction, predicting which patients may be difficult or impossible to ventilate via facemask (see Table 40-2) or intubate (see Table 40-4).

Table 40–6 ■ Risk Assessment of the Difficult Airway

Physical examination predictors suggestive of difficult facemask or supraglottic ventilation
Physical examination predictors suggestive of difficult intubation
Preexisting medical conditions and congenital abnormalities
Actual difficulties with mask ventilation or laryngoscopy-guided intubation
    How was effective ventilation achieved?
    How was intubation achieved?
Preexisting or current airway pathology
    Airway infection
    Tumor; prior head or neck surgery or radiation treatment
    Supraglottic or subglottic edema
    Presenting injuries of the airway, facial bones, and cervical spine
Postoperative effects on airway
    From prior surgery
    From just-completed surgical procedure
    From multiple laryngoscopic attempts or traumatic intubation

Implications

The inability to provide adequate ventilation to a patient may rapidly result in disability or death. ASA closed claims analysis revealed that the most common mechanisms of adverse respiratory events were inadequate ventilation, difficult intubation, and esophageal intubation. The airway sites most frequently injured were the larynx (33%), pharynx (19%), and esophagus (18%). Injuries to the trachea and esophagus were more commonly associated with difficult endotracheal intubation. Injuries to temporomandibular joint and the larynx were more frequently associated with intubations that were classified as "nondifficult." Injuries to the esophagus were more devastating and resulted in larger payments to the plaintiffs than did claims for injuries to other locations. Although the CVCI situation is rare, the consequences can be devastating.

MANAGEMENT

Optimal airway management requires recognition of the causes of a difficult airway and familiarity with the methods to secure it. Goals include maintenance of adequate oxygenation, ventilation, and protection of the airway from aspiration. Many airway management devices and techniques are available. The ASA difficult airway algorithm (see Fig. 40-1) favors no single method. It is unlikely that an individual anesthesiologist will be adept at all techniques and devices; each anesthesiologist should use the airway techniques at which he or she is adept. All anesthesiologists must have clinical familiarity with a number of airway devices and techniques, however, including (but not limited to) fiberoptic intubation, a method for emergency nonsurgical ventilation that allows blind supraglottic placement (laryngeal mask airway or esophageal-tracheal Combitube), and a method for emergency nonsurgical ventilation that allows subglottic

Table 40-7 ■ Indications for Awake Airway Management

History of difficult intubation
Anticipated difficult airway
    Prominent protruding teeth
    Small mouth opening
    Narrow mandible
    Micrognathia
    Macroglossia
    Short, muscular neck
    Very long neck
    Limited neck extension
    Congenital airway anomalies
    Obesity
    Known airway pathology
    Known airway malignancy
    Upper airway obstruction
Trauma
    Facial
    Upper airway
    Cervical spine
Anticipated difficult mask ventilation
Severe risk of aspiration
Respiratory failure
Severe hemodynamic instability

From Sanchez A, Trivedi NS, Morrison DE: Preparation of the patient for awake intubation. In Benumof JL (ed): Airway Management: Principles and Practice. St. Louis, Mosby, 1996, pp 159-182.

placement (transtracheal jet ventilation or percutaneous dilatational cricothyrotomy). If there is any reason to believe that conventional facemask or supraglottic ventilation may be unsuccessful, awake management of the airway is indicated (Table 40-7).

Recently, Rosenblatt published a decision tree for organizing preoperative airway information (Fig. 40-4). This approach asks a series of questions regarding management of the airway. A positive answer leads the operator to the next question, and a negative answer directs the clinician to the appropriate location in the ASA algorithm (see Fig. 40-1). Predicting specific difficulties with airway management prospectively (preoperatively) and integrating this information into the airway approach strategy may avoid the need to use the emergency branches of the ASA algorithm (e.g., encourage the anesthesiologist to use awake intubation initially rather than intubation after induction of general anesthesia, apnea, and paralysis).

The CVCI situation, once recognized, must be managed quickly and decisively. "Rapid" options for management include the following:

- Laryngeal mask airway
- Esophageal-tracheal Combitube
- Laryngeal tube
- Transtracheal jet ventilation
- Cricothyrotomy

The first three methods of establishing ventilation are supraglottic ventilatory mechanisms, and the latter two are subglottic ventilatory mechanisms. Only the most invasive method, cricothyrotomy with insertion of a cuffed airway device, is capable of definitively securing the airway, allowing positive-pressure ventilation, and preventing aspiration

1) Must the airway be managed? (Is airway control necessary?)
  • If NO, is regional anesthesia or monitored anesthesia care an acceptable alternative for the patient, surgeon, and anesthesiologist? If NOT, continue on to question 2.
    – Regional anesthesia doesn't always preclude airway management.
2) Is there potential for a difficult laryngoscopy?
  • If NO, enter ASA-DAA @ Intubation Attempts After Induction of General Anesthesia.
3) Can supraglottic ventilation be utilized? (LMA or Combitube for rescuing the airway, if the cannot-ventilate, cannot-intubate scenario occurs).
  • If NO, enter ASA-DAA @ Awake Intubation.
4) Is the stomach empty? (Is there an aspiration risk?)
  • If NO, enter ASA-DAA @ Awake Intubation.
5) Will the patient tolerate an apneic period if unable to ventilate?
  • If NO, enter ASA-DAA @ Awake Intubation.
  • If YES, enter ASA-DAA @ Intubation Attempts After Induction of General Anesthesia with supraglottic airway/ventilation device present.

A "NO" answer to any of the AAA questions directs the anesthesiologist to a "root point" of the American Society of Anesthesiologists–Difficult Airway Algorithm (ASA-DAA). A "YES" answer leads the anesthesiologist to the subsequent question. The AAA does not suggest particular procedures or specific pathways, but rather is meant to organize the anesthesiologist's own beliefs and choices along the lines of the ASA-DAA.

Figure 40–4 ■ Airway approach algorithm (AAA). LMA, laryngeal mask airway. (Modified from Rosenblatt W: The airway approach algorithm: A decision tree for organizing preoperative airway information. J Clin Anesth 16:312-316, 2004.)

of gastric material. Regardless of the temporary measures taken to ventilate a patient in the CVCI situation, efforts should be made to definitively secure the airway as soon as possible. The following techniques are commonly employed in managing the difficult airway.

Fiberoptic Bronchoscopy and Endotracheal Intubation

Many anesthesiologists prefer to use fiberoptic bronchoscopy (FOB) to manage a known or suspected difficult airway and for an unrecognized difficult intubation when supraglottic ventilation is achieved and maintained. FOB can be performed in awake or anesthetized patients. Success requires careful patient selection and preparation, as well as sufficient operator skill and experience. The decision to perform the procedure in an awake or sedated patient versus after the induction of general anesthesia depends on the patient's ability to cooperate and the ability to maintain ventilation and oxygenation. Fiberoptic intubation under general anesthesia should be considered only if the anesthesiologist believes that adequate ventilation and oxygenation can be readily maintained. It is often better to maintain spontaneous ventilation and consciousness, especially in a patient with a difficult airway.

INDICATIONS AND CONTRAINDICATIONS

Tumors, abscesses, maxillofacial trauma, and suspected or actual cervical spine injuries are indications for FOB intubation, provided the airway can be safely navigated.

Other indications include the following situations: (1) neck extension for optimal alignment of the oral, pharyngeal, and laryngeal axes is difficult or ill advised; (2) difficult direct laryngoscopy is predicted on the basis of airway risk assessment; (3) risk of aspiration is high; (4) patient who cannot tolerate a period of apnea; and (5) patient with an injury to or near the airway.

Absolute contraindications to FOB intubation include (1) high risk of dislodging friable tissue or rupturing an abscess, (2) bleeding or swelling that prevents visualization of airway structures or passage of the bronchoscope, and (3) life-threatening airway obstruction or hemodynamic instability (lack of time). Relative contraindications include (1) copious secretions despite an anticholinergic drying agent, (2) friable tissues that cannot be navigated despite careful manipulation, (3) edema of the pharynx or tongue, (4) hematoma, (5) tracking infections, and (6) infiltrating masses.

PATIENT PREPARATION

Nasal FOB intubation is generally easier to perform than oral FOB intubation because the angle of curvature of the inserted ETT naturally approximates that of the patient's upper airway. The ETT serves as a channel for the bronchoscope, and the gag reflex is less pronounced with the nasal approach. The sitting position is preferred to the supine position because it facilitates passage of the bronchoscope and drainage of secretions. Extension of the cervical spine (if not contraindicated) provides the optimal position for the performance of fiberoptic laryngoscopy. For awake or sedated patients, nasal or oral oxygen is administered, monitors are applied, and an anticholinergic drying agent (to increase the effectiveness of topical anesthetics and decrease secretions) and sedation are administered, according to the anesthesiologist's preferences. Good topical anesthesia (with adequate time allowed) is essential for awake techniques. The naris and nasopharynx are anesthetized with cocaine or lidocaine-phenylephrine, if vasoconstrictors are not contraindicated. The superior laryngeal nerve (innervates the epiglottis, aryepiglottic folds, and laryngeal mucosa) is blocked by the advancement of cotton-tipped applicators into the pyriform fossa. The oropharynx, base of tongue, and larynx are sprayed with a topical anesthetic, or the patient can gargle with a topical anesthetic. A lidocaine and phenylephrine mixture can be nebulized via a facemask; lidocaine can also be sprayed onto the vocal cords and into the tracheal lumen via the bronchoscope as they are encountered or viewed. The use of transtracheal lidocaine, superior laryngeal nerve blocks, and glossopharyngeal blocks is optional. Insufflation of oxygen through the suction port of the bronchoscope serves as a defogging mechanism, blows secretions away from the tip of the bronchoscope, and provides supplemental oxygen during the procedure. When performing FOB in apneic patients, transnasal jet ventilation, via a nasal airway, often effectively oxygenates the patient for a short time.

TECHNIQUES

Nasal Intubation.   Care must be taken to minimize the risk of epistaxis. Nasal intubation is contraindicated in patients with coagulation disorders, who cannot tolerate vasoconstrictors, and with facial or basilar skull trauma. Often one side of the nose has a larger "passage," which can be determined with trials of nasal airways of progressively increasing diameters. "Softened" ETTs (warmed in warm water) usually pass more easily. The largest ETT possible should be used— 8 mm internal diameter in adults, if a 34 French soft nasal airway readily passes. The ETT is positioned proximally over the bronchoscope. The most patent naris is intubated first, preventing it from exiting the Murphy eye of the ETT during bronchoscope advancement. If the ETT is inserted through the naris first, the bronchoscope should be visualized following the stripe on the ETT to the beveled tip. This prevents passage of the bronchoscope through the Murphy eye. Lidocaine is sprayed via the bronchoscope on or in airway structures as they are identified. Inflating the cuff of the ETT can create more space in the pharynx and directs the FOB channel (ETT) anteriorly. The bronchoscope is advanced until the epiglottis or glottis is identified, maneuvered past the glottis into the trachea, and advanced to the carina. Subsequently, the ETT is advanced into the trachea. The ETT may hang up on supraglottic structures as it is advanced over the bronchoscope. Rotation of the ETT 90 degrees counterclockwise may facilitate passage. The appropriate depth of the ETT can be determined by visualizing the distance between the carina and the tip of the ETT as the bronchoscope is removed. If the ETT does not advance or the bronchoscope cannot easily be removed from the ETT, both must be removed together (to avoid bronchoscope damage), and FOB intubation should be reattempted, possibly with a smaller ETT. Factors affecting the success of FOB-guided intubation are summarized in Table 40-8.

Oral Intubation.   Oral FOB intubation is well suited for apneic or anesthetized patients, as well as for awake or sedated patients who are well anesthetized topically. Preparation of the nasal passageway is unnecessary, and the oral route can be used in patients when the nasal route is contraindicated. Neck extension, if not contraindicated, reduces the angle between the oropharynx and larynx, facilitating advancement of the bronchoscope into the trachea. The bronchoscope can be advanced through a fiberoptic-compatible oral airway (FCOA) or advanced above and around a "pulled-out" or protruded tongue. The FCOA serves as a channel for the bronchoscope, prevents "bite" damage to it, and facilitates midline positioning by mechanically guiding the bronchoscope (Fig. 40-5). An FCOA with an "anterior channel" may be better at directing the bronchoscope toward the glottic opening. Performing a jaw thrust or pulling the tongue forward can be helpful. Oral FOB intubation can readily be accomplished by using a laryngeal mask as the channel for the bronchoscope. Ventilation is continuous via the laryngeal mask airway (LMA), either spontaneously or by positive pressure, as the bronchoscope is passed through a bronchoscope port adapter, through the LMA ventilating tube, and into the trachea.

Blind Nasal Intubation

Blind nasal intubation is much less stimulating than direct laryngoscopy. The patient must breathe spontaneously and be adequately sedated and cooperative. Topical anesthesia and nasal vasoconstriction precede the insertion of a

Table 40–8 ▪ Factors Affecting Successful Fiberoptic Bronchoscopy and Intubation

Factor	Comments and Possible Solutions
Patient Selection	
Oropharyngeal bleeding	Frequent suctioning and topical vasoconstrictor will help reduce small amounts of bleeding
Uncooperative patient	Rarely a problem with elective FOB but may be in trauma or emergency situations
	Titrate sedation as indicated
	Amount of sedation inversely proportional to degree of airway difficulty
Unstable patient	Inadequate time to safely anesthetize patient and intubate trachea
	Skill and experience can decrease FOB intubation time
Patient Preparation	
Topical anesthesia	Reduce and remove secretions so topical agents are in contact with mucosa
	Allow sufficient contact time
	Spray lidocaine (via suction port of bronchoscope) onto structures as they are identified
	Nerve blocks are often unnecessary
Secretions, blood	Administer anticholinergic drying agent and vasoconstrictor
	Suction oral pharynx with tonsil tip suction before starting
	Connect O_2 source to suction port of bronchoscope to blow away secretions
Decreased O_2 saturation	Use nasal prongs or mask O_2 during FOB
	Maintain spontaneous ventilation
	Attach O_2 source to suction port of bronchoscope
	Instruct patient to breathe during procedure
	Avoid excessive sedation
	Ventilate with LMA
	Use LMA as channel or conduit for bronchoscope
	Jet-ventilate via nasal airway
Endoscopist Experience	
Abnormal anatomy	Full knowledge of normal anatomy necessary to negotiate abnormal anatomy with difficult airway
	Maintain spontaneous ventilation
	Use nasal route; allow sufficient laryngeal space
	Use channel for bronchoscope (ETT, FCOA)
Large, floppy epiglottis	Awake patient: instruct patient to pant, say "ahh," or stick out tongue
	Unconscious or anesthetized patient: jaw thrust, pull out tongue, use FCOA, use nasal route
Fogging of objective	Warm and wipe bronchoscope lens with dilute detergent before use
	Insufflation of O_2 via suction port decreases fogging
Inability to advance ETT	Lubricate bronchoscope
	If tube becomes hung up, try rotating it counterclockwise 90 degrees
Inability to remove bronchoscope	May exit Murphy eye of ETT
	Remove tube and bronchoscope as unit and try again

ETT, endotracheal tube; FCOA, fiberoptic-compatible oral airway; FOB, fiberoptic bronchoscopy; LMA, laryngeal mask airway; O_2, oxygen.

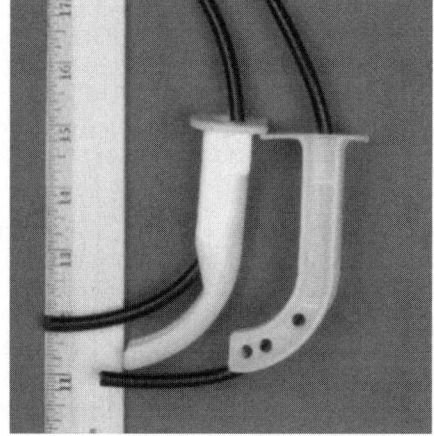
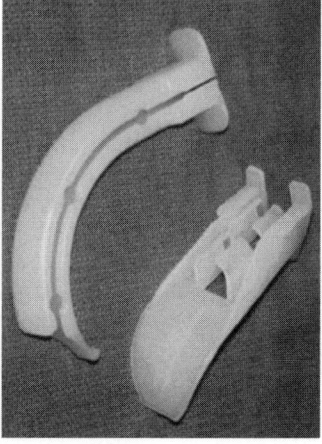

A   **B**

Figure 40–5 ▪ Fiberoptic-compatible oral airways (FCOAs). *A,* Two FCOAs, with anterior versus posterior channels compared. On the left is the Williams airway intubator, with an anterior channel; on the right is a Luomanen FCOA, with a posterior channel. Note that an anterior channel may offer more immediate entry into an anteriorly oriented glottis. *B,* Berman and Ovassapian oral intubating airways. (*A,* From Atlas GM: A comparison of fiberoptic-compatible oral airways. J Clin Anesth 16:66-73, 2004. *B,* From Stackhouse R: Fiberoptic airway management. Anesthesiol Clin North Am 20:933-951, 2002.)

Table 40–9 ■ Endotracheal Tube Malpositioning and Corrective Measures during Blind Nasal Intubation
Vocal cords outside larynx
Obstructed tube passage despite good detection of breath sounds
Can often be corrected by gentle rotation
Vallecula
Often causes midline supralaryngeal bulge in neck
Retract tube a few centimeters, followed by gentle pressure just above larynx or slight flexion of head
Left or right pyriform fossa
Often results in corresponding lateral bulge in neck
Gently use tongue depressor or laryngoscope blade to see if endotracheal tube is in midline
Correct this problem by:
Displacing patient's larynx slightly in direction of bulge
Rotating tube
Moving head toward side of displacement
Using lighted stylet to transilluminate endotracheal tube tip location
Esophagus
Pull back endotracheal tube and try again

Table 40–10 ■ Lighted Stylet–Assisted Oral Intubation
Indications
Elective, asleep, oral intubation
Patients with the following:
Restricted movement of cervical spine (e.g., cervical spine instability)
Limited mouth opening
Capped teeth
Severe overbite
Poor dentition
Facial trauma
Direct "blind" passage of endotracheal tube through intubating laryngeal mask airway
To facilitate intubation using direct laryngoscopy
Difficult airway alternative in experienced hands
Situations in which a fiberoptic bronchoscope is unavailable
Situations in which fiberoptic bronchoscopy is difficult to perform (e.g., secretions, blood)
Contraindications
Airway pathology
Foreign body
Laryngeal fracture
Pharyngeal mass
Retropharyngeal abscess

"warmed" ETT. The ETT is gently passed and advanced. Breath sounds (or air movement) heard through the ETT become louder as the tube tip nears the glottis. Tracheal passage is facilitated during patient inspiration. Palpation bilaterally under the patient's mandible may detect passage of the ETT off the midline and guide redirection by rotation of the ETT. Other ETT tip locations outside the trachea and corrective measures that may enable successful blind nasal intubation are listed in Table 40-9. Multiple blind passages must be avoided. Bleeding can compromise subsequent attempts at FOB intubation or direct laryngoscopy. Switch to FOB-guided intubation if blind passage is not successful.

Lighted Stylet Oral Intubation

The lighted stylet (LS) or light wand is sometimes used for routine elective and difficult endotracheal intubations. The LS is inserted into the lumen of the ETT until its tip is within 5 mm from the end of the ETT. The LS and distal ETT tip are bent or curved about 90 degrees and advanced during tongue retraction (the LS tip must point anteriorly). Light transilluminates through the anterior neck tissue (darken the room if necessary), facilitating redirection of the ETT-LS tip toward and into the trachea. Once past the glottis, the LS transilluminates brightly through the trachea, producing a distinct jack-o'-lantern effect (well-circumscribed glow through the anterior neck if in the trachea; diffuse glow if in the esophagus). The ETT is stabilized while the LS is removed. Transillumination may be inadequate in obese patients. Indications for LS intubation and contraindications to blind passage of the LS are listed in Table 40-10.

SUPRAGLOTTIC AIRWAY DEVICES

Many supraglottic airway devices are available, and they have changed our approach to airway management. Most, if not all anesthesiologists commonly use the laryngeal mask. Both the LMA and the esophageal-tracheal Combitube are useful for emergency airway management unless the cause of airway obstruction is glottic or subglottic in nature. The recently introduced laryngeal tube has also been used to manage the difficult airway.

LARYNGEAL MASK AIRWAY

The LMA plays an important role in the management of the difficult airway, serving as an airway ventilating device, a conduit for achieving endotracheal intubation, or both. The incidence of the cannot-ventilate situation decreased dramatically after the adoption and widespread use of the LMA, which is now an integral part of the ASA difficult airway algorithm (see Fig. 40-1). The LMA is blindly inserted into the hypopharynx until the leading edge of the mask is behind the arytenoids and cricoid cartilage and lies just above the upper esophageal sphincter. The LMA "mask" is inflated to form a low-pressure seal (20 cm H_2O or less; about 30 cm H_2O with a ProSeal LMA) around the laryngeal inlet. Spontaneous or controlled positive-pressure ventilation can be used. Disadvantages of the LMA include the following:

- It is a supraglottic device and may be ineffective in the presence of glottic or subglottic pathology.
- It does not protect the trachea against pulmonary aspiration of gastric contents.
- It may be placed over the esophageal inlet, resulting in gastric distention, especially when positive-pressure ventilation is employed.
- It may not be able to achieve adequate airway sealing pressures in patients with poor pulmonary compliance who require positive-pressure ventilation.

The aperture of a properly positioned classic LMA aligns itself anatomically with the glottis and can serve as a conduit to endotracheal intubation. An FOB wire-guided exchange technique for achieving endotracheal intubation via a classic laryngeal mask is as follows:

- Place a classic LMA while adequate ventilation is occurring.
- Pass a fiberoptic bronchoscope through a bronchoscope port adapter attached to the classic LMA ventilating tube.
- Guide the bronchoscope visually through the LMA aperture into the trachea, without interrupting ventilation.
- Pass a wire through the working channel of the bronchoscope into the trachea.
- Remove the bronchoscope.
- Place an airway exchange catheter over the wire into the trachea.
- Subsequently, remove the LMA over the airway exchange catheter.
- Pass an ETT over the airway exchange catheter into the trachea.

The intubating LMA (ILMA) was specially designed to facilitate endotracheal intubation, either blindly or by fiberoptic guidance. In a recent study by Combs and associates using a treatment algorithm (the gum-elastic bougie [GEB] and ILMA were proposed as the first and second steps in the case of impossible laryngoscope-assisted tracheal intubation, respectively), 100 cases of unexpected difficult airway were recorded among 11,257 intubations (0.9%), with no cases of impossible ventilation. Deviation from the algorithm was recorded in three cases, and two patients were wakened before any alternative intubation technique was attempted. All remaining patients were successfully ventilated with either the facemask (89 of 95) or the ILMA (6 of 95). Six difficult-to-ventilate patients required the ILMA before completion of the first intubation step. Eighty patients were intubated using the GEB, and 13 required a blind intubation through the ILMA. Two patients ventilated with the ILMA were never intubated.

In emergency situations, the ProSeal LMA may prove especially useful when positive-pressure ventilation is required and gastric distention or regurgitation is a major concern (e.g., cannot intubate in the obstetric patient). The ProSeal is not useful as a channel for FOB (smaller lumen for the bronchoscope; channel off the midline).

Esophageal-Tracheal Combitube

The esophageal-tracheal Combitube (ETC, Sheridan Catheter, Argyle, NY) was developed for emergency airway management. The ETC is a double-lumen airway containing a "tracheoesophageal" lumen with an open distal end. The second "pharyngeal" lumen, resembling an esophageal obturator-type airway, contains a distally blocked end and perforations in the lumen through which ventilation occurs. Dual standard airway connectors allow ventilation in either the esophageal or the tracheal position. The ETC comes in 37 and 41 French sizes for patients 4 to 6 feet tall and greater than 6 feet tall, respectively.

With the neck in a neutral position (the sniffing position may hinder insertion), the ETC is inserted through the mouth. It is advanced over and beyond the tongue using a gentle, downward-curved, dorsocaudal movement and then advanced parallel to the patient's horizontal plane until the proximal marker rings are at the upper incisors (or the

alveolar ridge in edentulous patients). When inflated, the proximal, 100-mL, latex oropharyngeal balloon essentially seals the patient's mouth and nose (some titrate the oropharyngeal balloon volume to air leak). The distal tracheoesophageal 15-mL balloon (use 10 to 15 mL air) seals either the esophagus or the trachea after insertion and inflation. Insertion results in esophageal intubation more than 96% of the time. Ventilation is initiated via tube 1 (the longer blue tube), with ventilation occurring via perforations in the "pharyngeal lumen" between the two balloons. Air is forced past the epiglottis into the trachea because the two balloons seal off all other "escape routes" (nose, mouth, esophagus). If there are no breath sounds or expired carbon dioxide (<4% of the time), tube 2 (the shorter clear tube) is ventilated (via the tracheoesophageal lumen), because the ETC has presumably entered the trachea.

The ETC is an important method of out-of-hospital emergency airway management and can be used as a rescue ventilation device in the management of the difficult airway. When properly positioned, the ETC allows higher airway sealing pressures than a classic LMA. The distal balloon may prevent gastric distention and protect from gastric regurgitation and pulmonary aspiration. The risk of aspiration should theoretically be less than that with an LMA because the esophagus is sealed by the distal cuff. The ETC is a useful device to facilitate airway control in trauma patients with possible cervical spine injury because it is placed with the neck in the neutral position. In addition, the ETC is useful in patients with massive airway bleeding or regurgitation or limited access to the airway. Laryngoscopy can also be performed to ease placement of the ETC and may decrease soft tissue trauma compared with blind passage. The ETC has a good safety record, with only rare reports of esophageal injury.

Laryngeal Tube

The laryngeal tube (LT) is a new supraglottic ventilatory device consisting of an airway tube and two low-pressure balloons (cuffs). When inserted, the LT lies along the length of the tongue with the distal tip (blind end; no gastric access) positioned in the upper esophagus. The distal (esophageal) balloon seals the airway distally, protecting from regurgitation. The proximal (pharyngeal) balloon seals both the oral and nasal cavities. The two balloons are inflated sequentially. Openings in the airway tube are situated between the two balloons and allow ventilation to occur. Fiberoptic tracheal intubation through the LT using an "exchange technique" is also possible. Recently, the LT was fitted with a second lumen for suctioning and free gastric drainage, but not for ventilation, as with the Combitube.

Invasive Airway Techniques

Retrograde Tracheal Intubation

Retrograde tracheal intubation has been used with good success to manage difficult airways and is a useful alternative in difficult (or anticipated to be difficult) intubations. The entry site for transtracheal puncture is made midline through the cricothyroid membrane. The risk of significant bleeding is low because the cricothyroid membrane is relatively avascular. The patient is placed supine—ideally, in the sniffing position, if it is not contraindicated. Under sterile technique, an epidural needle or intravenous needle-catheter (18 gauge), with a saline (or lidocaine) half-filled syringe attached, is advanced in a 30- to 40-degree cephalad direction through the cricothyroid membrane. Upon air aspiration, lidocaine can be injected into the trachea. The patient's tongue is pulled or protruded anteriorly. An epidural catheter, or spring guidewire, is passed "retrograde" back through the glottis into the mouth or naris. The guidewire needs to be long enough to pass out of the mouth or naris (a 100-cm wire is recommended to allow the use of adjunct equipment or manipulation of the ETT). An ETT is advanced over the epidural catheter or guidewire past the glottis into the trachea. The guidewire or epidural catheter is removed via the mouth (or naris) in the retrograde direction to prevent contamination of the cervical soft tissues at the puncture site. Unfortunately, the ETT may fall back into the hypopharynx upon release of the guide. Tracheal location of the ETT is confirmed using standard techniques. A guidewire technique using a commercially available retrograde intubation kit (Cook Critical Care, Bloomington, Ind) is shown in Figure 40-6. Indications, contraindications, and alternative methods for retrograde tracheal intubation are summarized in Table 40-11.

SURGICAL AIRWAY

The rapid development of severe hypoxemia, especially if associated with bradycardia, is an indication for immediate intervention with an invasive technique, because rapid reoxygenation is essential. Surgical methods to secure the airway include cricothyrotomy and surgical tracheostomy. The cricothyroid membrane is the most accessible portion of the trachea below the level of the glottis. Cricothyrotomy is easier and preferred for transtracheal jet ventilation (TTJV). Contraindications to cricothyrotomy are listed in Table 40-12.

Tracheostomy. The classic emergency surgical tracheostomy involves incision through the skin and platysma, division of the isthmus of the thyroid gland, hemostasis, incision of the tracheal cartilage, and insertion of a cuffed tracheostomy tube. Emergency tracheostomy can be very difficult to perform and may result in serious complications. Although a few surgeons may be able to perform a tracheostomy in 3 minutes or less, most take longer. Delay in completing a tracheostomy during the CVCI scenario may result in serious morbidity or death of the patient. Some patients require awake tracheostomy as the initial airway management method.

Cannula Cricothyrotomy with Percutaneous Transtracheal Jet Ventilation. Compared with emergency surgical cricothyrotomy or tracheostomy, establishment of percutaneous TTJV via needle-cannula cricothyrotomy is quicker and simpler. TTJV permits continuous, uninterrupted ventilation and oxygenation in patients without an anatomic impediment to passive exhalation through the upper airway. This allows time to secure the patient's airway by alternative techniques. Some anesthesiologists place a "prophylactic" TTJV catheter before intubation attempts in patients with suspected difficult airways so that a ready conduit is available in the event of difficulty with ventilation.

The cricothyroid membrane is identified, and a 12- to 16-gauge over-the-needle catheter, attached to a partially

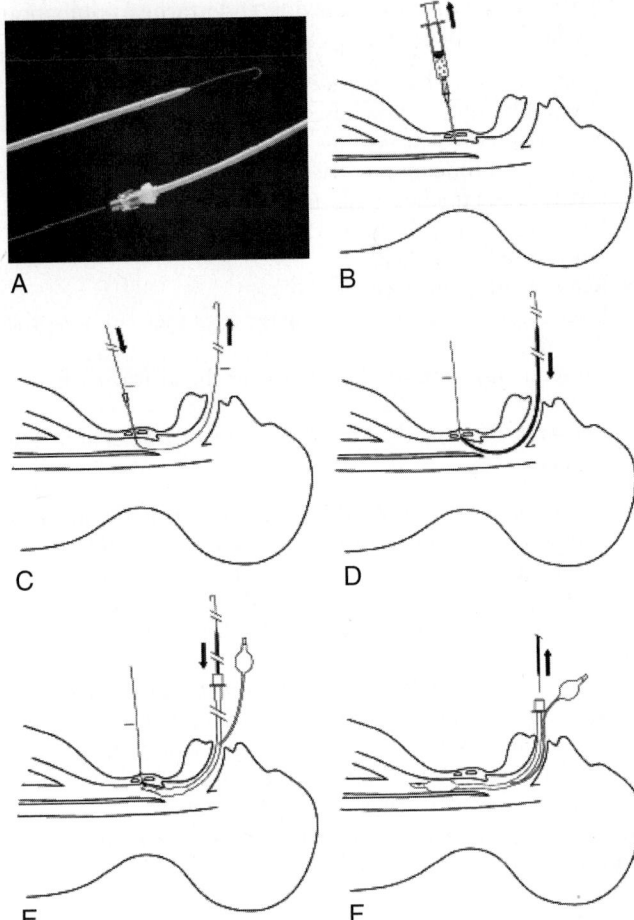

Figure 40-6 ▪ Retrograde intubation using the guidewire technique. *A,* The J-tip of the guidewire and the guiding catheter. *B,* After standard preparation of the access site, advance the 18-gauge sheath needle (attached to a 6-mL disposable syringe) in a cephalad direction through the cricothyroid membrane and into the trachea. Free flow of air aspirated into the syringe confirms correct positioning. Remove the needle and syringe, leaving the sheath in place. *C,* Advance the J end of the guidewire through the sheath and up the trachea in a cephalad direction, until the tip of the guidewire can be retrieved through the mouth or nose. Note: The black proximal positioning mark of the guidewire should be visible at the access site, ensuring that enough guidewire is exposed orally or nasally for control of subsequent catheter introduction. Remove the sheath, leaving the guidewire in place. *D,* Advance the catheter antegrade over the guidewire by way of the mouth or nose and into the trachea until tenting is noted at the cricothyroid access site. *E,* With the catheter is position, advance the endotracheal tube over the catheter and into position below the level of the vocal cords. Note: Always maintain control and position of the guidewire during advancement of the endotracheal tube. *F,* Remove the guidewire and catheter from the endotracheal tube and inflate the balloon cuff of the endotracheal tube. Verify the position, and secure in a standard fashion. (From Behringer ED: Approaches to managing the upper airway. Anesthesiol Clin North Am 20:813-832, 2004; courtesy of Cook Critical Care, Bloomington, Ind.)

saline-filled syringe, is inserted at a 30- to 45-degree angle caudally into the "air vessel." Easy aspiration of air into the syringe confirms placement (Fig. 40-7). Kink-resistant catheters are recommended because standard intravenous catheters are readily bent. The catheter hub is connected (preferably by a Luer-Lok connector) to a TTJV system. An alternative technique is to use a Seldinger catheter introducer set (8.5 French introducer kit commonly used for

Table 40–11 ▪ Retrograde Tracheal Intubation

Indications

Multiple intubation attempts have caused bleeding or edema
Patients with limited mouth opening or neck movement
Facial trauma
Failed endotracheal intubation
Elective management of difficult airway

Contraindications

Unfavorable anatomy in area of cricoid cartilage and cricothyroid membranes
Nonpalpable landmarks
Pretracheal mass
Severe flexion deformity of neck
Laryngotracheal pathologic condition
Malignancy
Tracheal stenosis
Severe trauma to larynx or laryngotracheal separation
Infection
Significant coagulopathy
Patients requiring immediate intubation and ventilation (can take up to 5 min to complete)
Complete upper airway obstruction

Alternative Techniques

Needle placement through infracricoid membrane instead of cricothyroid membrane (may increase success rate because it facilitates passage of ETT through larynx)
Introduction of guidewire or epidural catheter (previously passed retrograde into mouth or naris) through hollow airway exchange catheter; passage of tube exchanger down over guidewire into trachea; subsequent advancement of ETT down over tube exchanger into trachea; guide lessens chance of dislodgment or hang-up of ETT tip in vocal cords, arytenoid cartilage, vallecula, or pyriform sinus
Insertion of guide (previously passed retrograde into mouth or naris) through distal lateral eye of ETT before passing ETT over guide into trachea; can prevent entrapment of ETT tip in arytenoids or epiglottis
Use of pulling techniques, either by creating loop around side eye or simply knotting epidural catheter with Murphy's eye; can increase success rate of retrograde tracheal intubation
Insertion of bronchoscope with preloaded ETT over guidewire via bronchoscope's suction channel; allows visualization of airway structures as bronchoscope is advanced; wire is removed while observing bronchoscope remaining in trachea, with subsequent advancement of ETT into trachea

ETT, endotracheal tube.

---

pulmonary artery catheters). The needle is used to make the initial puncture, air is aspirated, the guidewire is inserted into the distal trachea, and the catheter is threaded over the guidewire using the dilator. These 8.5 French catheters may allow some exhalation to take place via the catheter if the system can be vented. The TTJV system should provide 50 pounds per square inch of pressure (using an adjustable high-pressure device, driven by gas pipeline pressure) for adequate inspiratory gas flow. The oxygen flush systems of most modern anesthesia machines do not provide

Table 40–12 ▪ Contraindications to Cricothyrotomy

Preexisting laryngeal disease
   Acute inflammation
   Chronic inflammation
   Malignancy
Translaryngeal intubation >3 days
   Increased incidence of subglottic stenosis
Coagulopathy
Distortion of normal airway anatomy
Infants and children <6 yr
Inexperience in cricothyrotomy procedure (experience decreases complications)

sufficient pressure. Jaw thrust facilitates exhalation. The catheter must be stabilized during ventilation, or else the jet pressure may force it out of the trachea.

TTJV should be considered a temporary measure because it can maintain adequate oxygenation for only about 30 to 60 minutes. Progressive hypercapnia is likely to occur because overall minute ventilation is usually inadequate. When air entry exceeds air exit during TTJV, lung hyperinflation, tension pneumothorax, pneumomediastinum, and subcutaneous emphysema will inevitably occur. Strategies to minimize barotrauma are listed in Table 40-13. Major changes in cardiovascular parameters should be assumed to be related to TTJV and possible barotrauma. TTJV can sometimes facilitate endotracheal intubation using standard methods because the high intratracheal pressure from TTJV can lift up and open the glottis. The escape of gas under high pressure causes the edges of the glottis to flutter, which may facilitate the identification of the glottic opening. If TTJV fails or surgical emphysema or another complication occurs, convert immediately to surgical cricothyrotomy.

Surgical Cricothyrotomy. Surgical cricothyrotomy may allow the rapid restoration of oxygenation and ventilation in the CVCI scenario. Surgical cricothyrotomy is also indicated in the setting of severe maxillofacial trauma preventing oral intubation, known unstable cervical spine fracture,

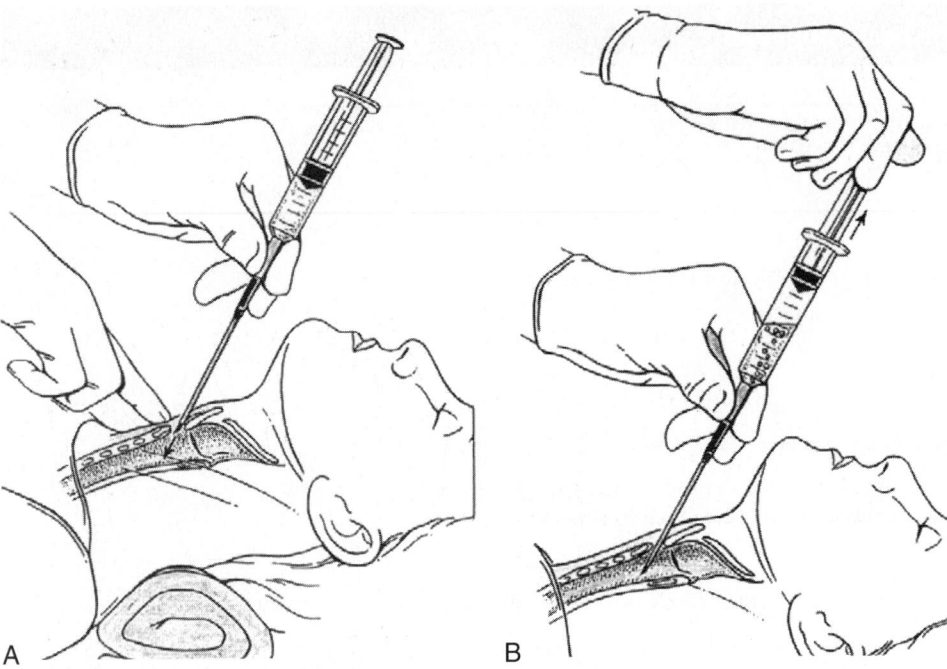

Figure 40–7 ■ Needle insertion for cricothyrotomy and transtracheal jet ventilation (TTJV). *A*, A 14-gauge (or larger) angiocatheter is directed caudad, using an angle of approximately 30 degrees to the skin, and passed through the cricothyroid membrane. *B*, The free return of air on aspiration through the syringe confirms the position of the tip of the needle in the tracheal lumen. The catheter is advanced over the needle into the tracheal lumen, the needle is removed, and the hub of the catheter is connected to the TTJV tubing (Luer-Lok connector recommended). (From Patel RG, Norman JR: The technique of transtracheal ventilation. J Crit Illness 11:803-808, 1996.)

A   B

laryngotracheal trauma (except for tracheal transection), complete upper airway obstruction, oropharyngeal obstruction, or inability to secure the airway by other intubation techniques. It is contraindicated in patients younger than 12 years and in the case of laryngotracheal separation or tracheal transection (the transected airway may be tenuously held together by cervical fascia), tracheal foreign body, or penetrating trauma to the neck (in either high zone 2 or zone 3) associated with an expanding hematoma. The surgical cricothyrotomy technique uses low-pressure ventilation through a cuffed tube placed in the trachea. A simplified cricothyrotomy technique (consisting of palpation, incision, insertion, and intubation) can be performed in approximately 30 seconds in experienced hands (Table 40-14). Invasive airway access is a temporary measure to restore oxygenation. Definitive airway management follows, such as surgical tracheostomy; alternatively, because oxygenation and ventilation have been established, there may be time to achieve tracheal intubation. Guidewire techniques of cricothyrotomy have been developed, and some claim that these techniques can restore the airway as quickly as the

standard surgical technique. Percutaneous dilatational cricothyrotomy (PDC) kits are commercially available. PDC is a rapid, relatively straightforward procedure that is touted as having a decreased operative time and lower late complication rate compared with surgical cricothyrotomy.

PREVENTION

Prevention of complications related to difficult airway management requires the following:

- Ability to recognize a potentially difficult airway
- Well-thought-out plan with suitable alternatives for all patients
- Willingness to call for help at the first sign of difficulty
- Availability of all necessary equipment (i.e., difficult airway cart)

Table 40–13 ■ Minimizing Barotrauma during Transtracheal Jet Ventilation

Preset jet ventilator to 25-50 psi by using additional in-line regulator
Use lowest effective psi
Limit inspiratory time to <1 sec
Keep natural airway maximally patent with bilateral jaw thrust and oropharyngeal or nasopharyngeal airway (or both)
If laryngeal mask airway was used, leave in place to facilitate exhalation
Confirm ventilation of lungs and exhalation through upper airway

psi, pounds per square inch.

Table 40–14 ■ Technique of Rapid Cricothyrotomy

Identify cricothyroid membrane (CTM)
  Palpate and stabilize larynx by bracing laryngeal cartilage with thumb and middle finger
  Maintain position of CTM with index finger
Make horizontal stab incision through skin and CTM, just above cricoid cartilage
Immediately insert tracheal hook (preferred), hemostat, or blade handle into opening
  Do not lose control of opening
  Apply caudal traction on CTM (if tracheal hook used)
Intubate trachea with appropriately sized, preferably cuffed, endotracheal tube
  Tube insertion can be facilitated by passage of introducer (bougie) through incision or use of tracheal retractor
  Avoid excessive insertion depth (endobronchial tube placement)
Confirm breath sounds and expired carbon dioxide

- Adequate technical assistance (i.e., knowledgeable staff, dedicated to the task)
- Immediate availability of another anesthesiologist experienced with difficult airway management

It is also incumbent on any clinician who is confronted with a difficult airway to enroll the patient in the MedicAlert system (1-800-344-3226) to apprise other clinicians of the patient's history.

Further Reading

Agro F, Frass M, Benumof JL, Krafft P: Current status of the Combitube: A review of the literature. J Clin Anesth 14:307-314, 2002.

Atlas GM: A comparison of fiberoptic-compatible oral airways. J Clin Anesth 16:66-73, 2004.

Behringer EC: Approaches to managing the upper airway. Anesthesiol Clin North Am 20:813-832, 2002.

Blanda M, Gallo UE: Emergency airway management. Emerg Med Clin North Am 21:1-26, 2003.

Bogetz M: Using the laryngeal mask to manage the difficult airway. Anesthesiol Clin North Am 20:863-870, 2002.

Cheney FW, Posner KL, Caplan RA: Adverse respiratory events infrequently leading to malpractice suits: A closed claims analysis. Anesthesiology 75:932-939, 1991.

Combes X, Le Roux B, Suen P, et al: Unanticipated difficult airway in anesthetized patients: Prospective validation of a management algorithm. Anesthesiology 100:1146-1150, 2004.

Cook TM: A new practical classification of laryngeal view. Anaesthesia 55:274-279, 2000.

Davis L, Cook-Sather SD, Schreiner MS: Lighted stylet tracheal intubation: A review. Anesth Analg 90:745-756, 2000.

Domino KB, Posner KL, Caplan RA, Cheney FW: Airway injury during anesthesia: A closed claims analysis. Anesthesiology 91:1703-1711, 1999.

Dorges V, Ocker H, Wenzel V, et al: The Laryngeal Tube S: A modified simple airway device. Anesth Analg 96:618-622, 2003.

el-Ganzouri AR, McCarthy RJ, Tuman KJ, , et al: Preoperative airway assessment: Predictive value of a multivariate risk. Anesth Analg 82:1197-1204, 1996.

Ezri T, Szmuk P, Warters RD, et al: Difficult airway management practice patterns among anesthesiologists practicing in the United States: Have we made any progress? J Clin Anesth 15:418-422, 2003.

Gaitini LA: The esophageal-tracheal Combitube. Anesthesiol Clin North Am 20:893-906, 2002.

Genzwuerker H, Vollmer T, Ellinger K: Fibreoptic tracheal intubation after placement of the laryngeal tube. Br J Anaesth 89:733-738, 2002.

Hagberg CA: Special devices and techniques. Anesthesiol Clin North Am 20:907-932, 2002.

Hagberg CA: Current concepts in the management of the difficult airway. ASA Refresher Course, 2004.

Henderson JJ, Popat MT, Latto IP, et al: Difficult Airway Society guidelines for management of the unanticipated difficult intubation. Anaesthesia 59:675-694, 2004.

Langeron O, Masso E, Huraux C, et al: Prediction of difficult mask ventilation. Anesthesiology 92:1229-1236, 2000.

Levitan RM: Patient safety in emergency airway management and rapid sequence intubation: Metaphorical lessons from skydiving. Ann Emerg Med. 42:81-87, 2003.

Melker RJ, Florete OG: Cricothyrotomy: Review and debate. Anesthesiol Clin North Am 13:565, 1995.

Mort TC: Emergency tracheal intubation: Complications associated with repeated laryngoscopic attempts. Anesth Analg 99:607-613, 2004.

Patel RG, Norman JR: The technique of transtracheal ventilation. J Crit Illness 11:803-808, 1996.

Practice guidelines for management of the difficult airway—an updated report by the American Society of Anesthesiologists Task Force on Management of the Difficult Airway. Anesthesiology 98:1269-1277, 2003.

Rosenblatt W: The airway approach algorithm: A decision tree for organizing preoperative airway information. J Clin Anesth 16:312-316, 2004.

Stackhouse R: Fiberoptic airway management. Anesthesiol Clin North Am 20:933-951, 2002.

Weksler N, Klein M, Weksler D, et al: Retrograde tracheal intubation: Beyond fiberoptic endotracheal intubation. Acta Anaesthesiol Scand 48:412-416, 2004.

Wilson WC: Emergency airway management. In Brown D (ed): Cardiac Intensive Care. Philadelphia, WB Saunders, 1998, pp 705-734.

Wong EK, Bradrick JP: Surgical approaches to airway management for anesthesia practitioners. In Hagberg CA (ed): Handbook of Difficult Airway Management. Philadelphia, Churchill Livingstone, 2000, pp 209-210.

Difficult Airway: Opiate-Induced Muscle Rigidity

Narayan Baliga and Theodore J. Sanford, Jr.

Case Synopsis

Anesthetic induction is being performed in a 70-kg, 65-year-old man undergoing elective coronary artery bypass graft surgery. Following 3 minutes of preoxygenation, fentanyl (3000 µg) is administered intravenously over 5 minutes. The chest and abdominal wall become rigid, and it becomes very difficult to ventilate the patient's lungs with a mask and bag. The oxygen saturation drops rapidly, and the anesthesiologist cannot maintain the airway. It is difficult to open the patient's mouth to insert an oropharyngeal airway.

PROBLEM ANALYSIS

Definition

Opioid-induced muscle rigidity usually occurs with large doses of potent opioids given intravenously. These include drugs such as fentanyl, alfentanil, sufentanil, and remifentanil. Morphine and meperidine can also cause such reactions, but this is not common with the doses used during balanced anesthesia. There have been published reports of muscle rigidity occurring with relatively small doses of highly potent opiates such as sufentanil and alfentanil. The phenomenon of muscle rigidity is usually seen during induction of anesthesia when opioids are the sole or primary anesthetic agent. All the skeletal muscles are involved. The rigidity starts within 1 or 2 minutes of opioid administration and typically lasts 10 to 20 minutes. The mechanism is thought to originate in the central nervous system. Rigidity of the torso muscles leads to a fall in chest wall compliance, hypoventilation, respiratory acidosis, and systemic arterial hypotension.

Recognition

MUSCLE RIGIDITY

The rigidity is immediate and occurs in all skeletal muscles. Sometimes the rigidity is accompanied by explosive myoclonus and vertical nystagmus, resembling seizures. There is an increase in electromyographic activity, but the electroencephalogram does not indicate seizure activity. It has been shown that this increase in muscle tone is most likely central in origin.

CARDIORESPIRATORY EFFECTS

The sudden onset of muscle rigidity immediately following the intravenous (IV) administration of opioids, accompanied by apnea and rapid oxygen desaturation, suggests that the opioid is the causative agent. Chest wall rigidity makes it difficult to ventilate the patient with a mask and bag. Inability to open the mouth may make it impossible to insert an oropharyngeal or laryngeal mask airway. Although a nasopharyngeal airway can be inserted, airway obstruction caused by glottic closure may make it difficult to ventilate the patient manually.

Chest wall rigidity leads to a rise in intrathoracic pressure, which causes an immediate rise in right atrial pressure. If sustained, this leads to a reduction in venous return and cardiac output and, ultimately, systemic arterial blood pressure.

Risk Assessment

The differential diagnosis for inability to maintain the airway and oxygen desaturation includes the following:

- Muscle rigidity from rapid narcotic administration
- Laryngospasm from a noxious stimulus during light anesthesia
- Seizures, if there is a history of epilepsy or an intracranial lesion

The incidence of muscular rigidity is between 50% and 100% in unpremedicated patients given large doses of the contemporary synthetic opioids (e.g., fentanyl, alfentanil, sufentanil, remifentanil). The doses noted to cause rigidity from various studies are as follows: fentanyl, 12 to 15 µg/kg; alfentanil, 175 µg/kg; sufentanil, 2.6 µg/kg. Much smaller doses may cause rigidity when given rapidly as an IV bolus.

Little time is available for making a diagnosis. Rapid muscular paralysis and control of the airway are imperative and must be done immediately to prevent cerebral hypoxia.

Implications

Chest wall rigidity and respiratory insufficiency can lead to cardiovascular collapse and cerebral hypoxia. Unlike thiopental, opioids do not sufficiently reduce cerebral oxygen consumption to protect the brain during a global hypoxic event. Prompt intervention is required to prevent cerebral hypoxia. Patient awareness does not seem to be a problem; patients have no recall of the event when questioned postoperatively.

MANAGEMENT

Attempts to manually ventilate the patient's lungs without muscle relaxants are usually inadequate. Management consists of IV administration of either a depolarizing or a rapidly acting nondepolarizing neuromuscular blocking agent in the usual intubating doses (succinylcholine 1 mg/kg, vecuronium 150 μg/kg, or rocuronium 100 μg/kg). Manual ventilation is performed easily within 60 seconds after the administration of succinylcholine, and the airway can then be secured with an endotracheal tube. Once the airway has been secured, IV or inhaled anesthetics are administered to continue the anesthesia.

A 7.6% incidence of delayed postoperative muscle rigidity has been reported when large doses (100 μg/kg) of fentanyl are used for induction of anesthesia. If this is severe enough to cause failure of ventilation, either a muscle relaxant or naloxone can be administered to reverse muscle rigidity.

PREVENTION

Opioid-induced rigidity is difficult to prevent. The incidence can be reduced by slow injection of the opioid agent and pretreatment with midazolam (0.1 mg/kg) or α_2-agonists, such as clonidine and dexmedetomidine. Rigidity cannot be prevented or significantly reduced by pretreatment with small doses of nondepolarizing muscle relaxants. Careful attention to the time frame over which the newer synthetic opioids are administered and pretreatment with midazolam are the most important measures for prevention.

Further Reading

Bailey PL, Wilbrink J, Zwanikken P, et al: Anesthetic induction with fentanyl. Anesth Analg 64:48-53, 1985.

Benthuysen JL, Smith NT, Sanford TJ, et al: Physiology of alfentanil-induced rigidity. Anesthesiology 64:440-446, 1986.

Janis KM: Acute rigidity with small intravenous dose of Innovar: A case report. Anesth Analg 51:375-376, 1972.

Lui PW, Tsen LY, Fu MJ, et al: Involvement of locus coeruleus and noradrenergic neurotransmission in fentanyl-induced muscular rigidity in the rat. Neurosci Lett 96:114-119, 1989.

Muller P, Vogtmann C: Three cases with different presentation of fentanyl-induced muscle rigidity—a rare problem in intensive care of neonates. Am J Perinatol 17:23-26, 2000.

Sanford TJ, Weinger MB, Smith NT, et al: Pretreatment with sedative-hypnotics, but not with nondepolarizing muscle relaxants, attenuates alfentanil-induced muscle rigidity. J Clin Anesth 6:473-480, 1994.

Streisand JB, Bailey PL, LeMaire L, et al: Fentanyl-induced rigidity and unconsciousness in human volunteers: Incidence, duration, and plasma concentrations. Anesthesiology 78:629-634, 1993.

Weinger MB, Segal IS, Maze M: Dexmedetomidine, acting through central alpha$_2$-adrenoceptors, prevents opiate-induced muscle rigidity in the rat. Anesthesiology 71:242-249, 1989.

Weinger MB, Smith NT, Blasco TA, et al: Brain sites mediating opiate-induced muscle rigidity in the rat: Methylnaloxonium mapping study. Brain Res 544:181-190, 1991.

GENERAL ANESTHESIA

Unstable Cervical Spine, Atlantoaxial Subluxation

42

Lois A. Connolly

Case Synopsis

A 79-year-old man presents with C1 and odontoid fractures sustained in a fall down stairs while he was intoxicated. He was found at the bottom of the stairs 2 days after the injury. In addition to alcoholism, the patient has a history of hypertension and smokes 1 to 2 packs of cigarettes per day. The patient is not oriented to time, place, or person and has inappropriate verbal responses, but there is no apparent neurologic deficit.

PROBLEM ANALYSIS

Definition

Cervical spine stability is defined as the ability of the spine to maintain relationships between vertebrae during physiologic loading, so as not to damage contained neural structures. Cervical spine instability occurs when physiologic loading causes patterns of vertebral displacement that jeopardize the cervical spinal cord. The muscles of the neck, along with ligamentous structures, intervertebral disks, and osseous articulations, all play a role in cervical spine stability.

Upper cervical spine stability may be affected by trauma, congenital disorders, and inflammatory diseases, all of which may result in atlantoaxial instability (Table 42-1).

TRAUMATIC ATLANTOAXIAL INSTABILITY

The transverse ligament normally allows no more than 3 mm of anteroposterior translation between the odontoid and the anterior arch of the atlas. If disruption of this ligament occurs, displacement of the odontoid reduces the space available for the spinal cord (Fig. 42-1). In the normal spine, the space available for the spinal cord is about 20 mm. Cord compression does not occur when the space is greater than 18 mm, but it does occur if it is less than 14 mm.

CONGENITAL ATLANTOAXIAL INSTABILITY

Congenital or chromosomal anomalies may contribute to atlantoaxial instability by means of either odontoid hypoplasia or laxity of the transverse ligaments. The stabilizing action of the odontoid during extension is lost with odontoid hypoplasia, and subluxation of the atlas occurs on the axis anteriorly, reducing the space available for the spinal cord. Laxity of the transverse ligament is present in 14% to 22% of patients with trisomy 21. Excessive laxity of other joints correlates with the presence of atlantoaxial instability.

INFLAMMATORY ATLANTOAXIAL INSTABILITY

Cervical spine involvement is common in inflammatory arthropathies such as rheumatoid arthritis (RA). The pathophysiology involves pannus formation, with subsequent destruction of cartilage and subchondral bone, along with

Table 42–1 ■ Conditions Associated with Atlantoaxial Subluxation

Congenital
Down's syndrome
Odontoid anomalies
Mucopolysaccharidoses
Acquired
Rheumatoid arthritis
Juvenile rheumatoid arthritis
Ankylosing spondylitis
Psoriatic arthritis
Enteropathic arthritis
   Crohn's disease
   Ulcerative colitis
Reiter's syndrome
Trauma
   Odontoid fracture
   Ligamentous disruption

From Crosby ET: The adult cervical spine: Implications for airway management. Can J Anaesth 37:77-93, 1990.

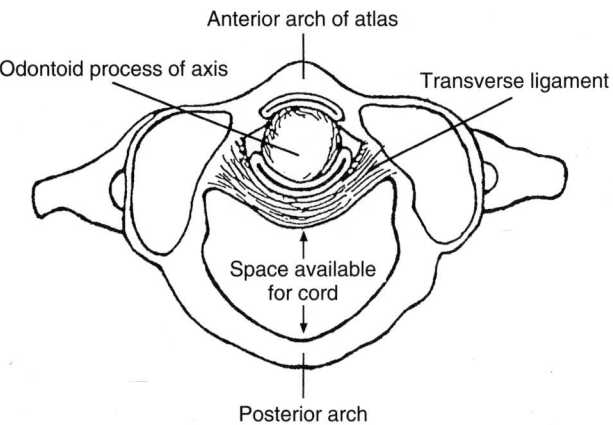

Figure 42–1 ■ Atlantoaxial articulation—view from above. (From Crosby ET: The adult cervical spine: Implications for airway management. Can J Anaesth 37:77-93, 1990.)

ligamentous laxity and instability. Atlantoaxial subluxation occurs in about 25% of patients with RA. It occurs more frequently in men, in those with disease of long duration, in patients with subcutaneous nodules or seropositive disease, and in those receiving steroid therapy. Vertical subluxation of the odontoid process through the foramen magnum may also occur in patients with RA.

EPIDEMIOLOGY

- Cervical spine injuries occur in 1.5% to 7.7% of all major trauma cases.
- The peak distribution of injury is at the C2 and C5-C6 levels.
- The highest prevalence is in 15- to 24-year-old males, with a smaller peak occurring in persons older than 55 years.
- Most cervical spine injuries result from motor vehicle accidents (42% to 56%), falls (19% to 30%), or gunshots and sports-related activities (6% to 7%).
- Motor vehicle accidents and sports-related activities account for the majority of cervical spine injuries in younger patients, whereas falls account for most cervical spine injuries in older patients.
- Young children are less susceptible to cervical spine injury because they weigh less and have more cartilage than adults do; vulnerability increases with age.
- Cervical spine injuries in children younger than 2 years are exclusively C1-C2 injuries, because facet joints at this level are more horizontal and the ligaments more lax.

The cervical spinal cord is particularly prone to injury because of spinal flexibility and the mass of the head. The spinal cord is injured when the ligaments, muscles, and osseous structures fail to dissipate the energy of impact. Transmission of this energy results in microhemorrhage in the spinal cord central gray matter and loss of neurotransmission in the surrounding white matter. A biochemical cascade that destabilizes the neurologic axon membrane and promotes vasospasm creates a secondary injury pattern after the initial insult. Also, primary cervical spinal cord injury leads to altered autonomic tone, loss of autoregulation, depressed cardiovascular function, and hypotension. Current pharmacologic treatment is concerned with minimizing the deleterious effects of secondary injury.

Recognition

HISTORY AND PHYSICAL EXAMINATION

Recognition of a cervical spine injury begins with the history. High-risk causes (e.g., motor vehicle accident, fall, long-standing RA) or known chromosomal abnormalities may alert the clinician to the presence of an unstable cervical spine. For example, a patient with RA may complain of clicking on neck flexion and pain and stiffness of the neck. An alert trauma patient may complain of neck pain or tenderness. An alert patient without neck pain or neurologic deficit does not require further cervical spine evaluation, immobilization, or special precautions during airway manipulation. If the patient is not fully alert, complains of neck pain, has neurologic deficits, or has other painful injuries, cervical spine precautions should be maintained.

Vertebral injury can occur without cord damage because the spinal canal is widest in the cervical region. Neurologic deficits are present in 46% of patients and are more frequent with injuries involving C5-C7. A thorough neurologic examination should enable classification and identification of the level of the spinal cord lesion.

Autonomic instability may occur acutely and is termed *spinal shock*. With spinal shock, loss of sympathetic tone leads to generalized hemodynamic instability characterized by bradycardia, peripheral arterial and venous vasodilatation, hypotension, and arrhythmia.

Respiratory compromise may occur acutely due to loss of intercostal muscle innervation or, with high cervical lesions, due to phrenic nerve loss. In normal individuals, expansion of the rib cage accounts for 60% of resting tidal volume. Therefore, alveolar ventilation and the ability to cough are decreased with loss of intercostal muscle innervation, even if phrenic nerve function remains intact. Thus, acute cervical cord injury may cause hypoxia, atelectasis, and respiratory failure. The possibility of aspiration pneumonitis may compound the situation. In addition, neurogenic pulmonary edema may be associated with spinal cord injury due to massive sympathetic discharge associated with trauma.

RADIOGRAPHIC EVALUATION

Radiographic evaluation of the cervical spine is indicated for all of the following patients:

- Alert, sober patients who complain of neck pain or tenderness
- Patients who have neurologic deficits or multiple traumatic injuries, including craniofacial injuries
- Inebriated or unconscious patients

A missed cervical spine injury can have devastating long-term consequences. Therefore, coexistent cervical spine injury should be assumed until the diagnosis is excluded. Patients with no significant mechanism of injury and who are fully alert and oriented, with no evidence of head trauma or a distracting injury, may be cleared clinically if they have no neck pain or tenderness and have a normal neurologic examination.

The most appropriate method for clearing the cervical spine in patients with mental status changes is controversial. There is no national or international consensus for the optimal approach to this patient population. The Eastern Association for the Surgery of Trauma's 1998 practice management guidelines state that "trauma patients with altered levels of consciousness who are unable to complain of neck pain or neurological deficits for 24 hours or more may be considered to have a stable cervical spine if adequate three-view radiography and thin-cut CT images through C1 and C2 are read as normal." Others recommend a passive extension-flexion examination under fluoroscopy to assess ligamentous stability. Ligamentous injury is the type most often missed on other radiographic studies, even though unstable cervical spine ligamentous injury without fracture is rare (<0.5%). Others suggest indefinite cervical immobilization. However, collar complications such as rash, skin breakdown, and pressure-related injuries; difficult central venous access; and delay in tracheostomy are possible when collars are left on for more than 72 hours.

A lateral cervical spine radiograph is assessed first. All seven cervical vertebrae should be evaluated, because 20% of cervical spine injuries are at C7. A swimmer's view may be used if necessary to view C7. Alignment of the vertebral bodies, transverse processes, and spinous processes is best assessed on the lateral view (Fig. 42-2). Each vertebra should be examined for bony integrity, intervertebral disk spaces, facet joints, and interspinous distance. Sensitivity of the cross-table lateral view alone is 80%; that is, 20% of patients with cervical spine injury have a normal lateral view. The sensitivity increases to 93% by adding the anteroposterior and odontoid views. The cervical spine cannot be considered cleared on the basis of the lateral view alone. A diagnostic algorithm for the evaluation of cervical spine fractures is shown in Figure 42-3.

Computed tomography (CT) is considered the gold standard for diagnosis. It is superior to plain films in evaluating injuries to C1-C2. Fractures in the axial plane may be difficult to identify by CT scan, and ligamentous injury may not be appreciated. Magnetic resonance imaging (MRI) provides excellent visualization of spinal soft tissue structures and clear definition of canal compromise. In an emergent situation, however, MRI may be impractical.

In conditions associated with the possibility of atlantoaxial subluxation (e.g., RA, Down's syndrome), lateral cervical spine films are obtained in neutral, flexed, and extended positions. Evidence of both anterior and vertical subluxation should be sought, and the space available for the spinal cord

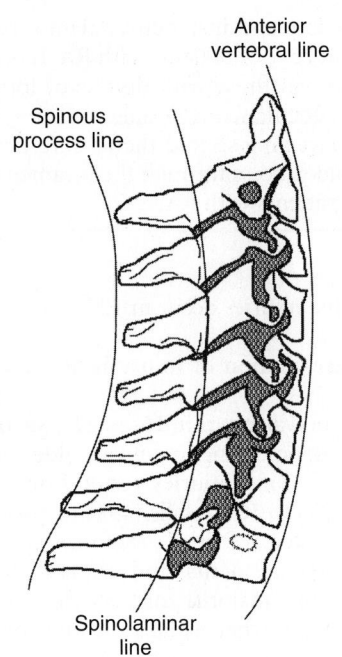

Figure 42–2 ■ Lateral cervical spine.

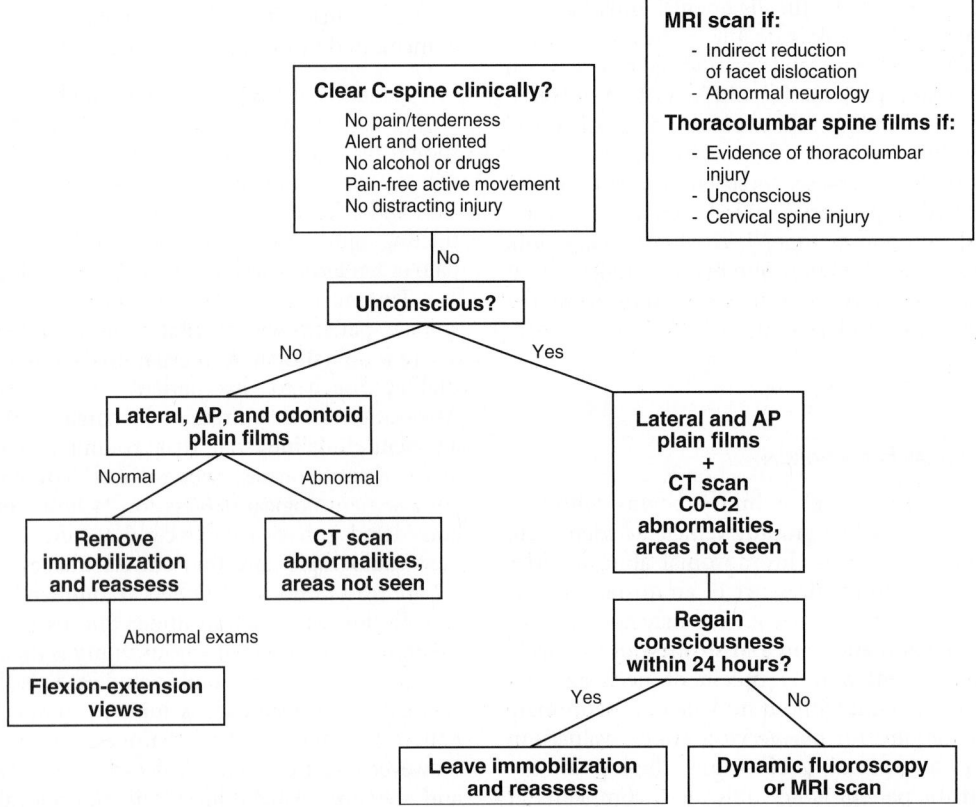

Figure 42–3 ■ Algorithm for evaluation of cervical spine injury. AP, anteroposterior; CT, computed tomography; MRI, magnetic resonance imaging. (From Brohi K, Wilson-Macdonald J: Evaluation of unstable cervical spine injury: A 6-year experience. J Trauma 49:76-80, 2000.)

should be measured. In patients with RA, the anteroposterior view may be examined for the presence of laryngeal deviation.

Risk Assessment

Preoperative assessment in a patient with a known unstable cervical spine should include the following:

- Evaluation of the cervical spine radiographically
- Determination of the adequacy of respiration (blood gas analysis or spirometry)
- Examination for evidence of spinal shock (blood pressure, heart rate, arrhythmia, electrocardiographic changes, need for vasopressors)
- Evaluation of the injury's effect on the central nervous system (neurologic evaluation, evidence of closed cranial trauma)
- Examination of associated injuries (chest radiograph or CT and electrocardiogram to rule out chest injuries)
- Determination of hemoglobin, electrolyte levels, coagulation status, and creatinine level
- Assessment of temperature balance

Implications

As discussed, multiple organs are affected by acute spinal cord trauma. Spinal shock requires invasive arterial monitoring, central venous pressure monitoring, and titration of vasopressors to ensure adequate perfusion pressure. If neurogenic pulmonary edema exists, further monitoring with a pulmonary artery catheter may be warranted. Acute spinal cord injuries are treated with high-dose methylprednisolone. This is believed to reduce edema, have anti-inflammatory effects, and protect neuronal membranes by scavenging free radicals. However, complications of such therapy include an increased rate of wound infection and a greater risk of gastrointestinal hemorrhage. Initial immobilization, with supervised reduction and realignment, is achieved with skeletal traction. Cervical immobilization is paramount and must be maintained during airway manipulation.

MANAGEMENT

Intraoperative Concerns

The primary intraoperative concerns are as follows:

- Monitoring
- Airway management
- Positioning
- Administration of anesthetic drugs (succinylcholine)
- Fluid management, glucose administration

Intraoperative management requires tracheal intubation. The urgency of airway intervention is probably the most important factor in planning for airway management. Other factors include patient cooperation, assessment of the airway, and risk to the cord with neck movement. Direct laryngoscopy requires atlanto-occipitoaxial extension and mild inferior rotation of C3-C5, although there is minimal movement below C3. Accordingly, unstable C1-C2 injuries

are most likely to cause neurologic damage. Manual in-line traction reduces atlanto-occipital extension during intubation, and several published series detail the use of direct laryngoscopy with in-line traction without evidence of neurologic deterioration.

The use of a Miller-type blade results in less movement (i.e., axial distraction) than the use of curved (e.g., Macintosh) blades. Preintubation techniques, such as jaw-thrust and chin-lift maneuvers, cause the most motion and narrowing of the space available for the cord; therefore, great care must be taken when performing these maneuvers. Failed intubation is a danger, however, and the laryngoscopist's view may be hindered by the stabilization. Direct laryngoscopy with in-line stabilization is most useful when it is vital to gain rapid control of the airway (e.g., patients with respiratory failure, hemodynamic instability, increased intracranial pressure). Use of a laryngeal mask airway is not advised because it can exert a great deal of pressure against the cervical vertebrae. Indeed, it may produce posterior displacement of the cervical spine (C2-C6) and possible rupture of the posterior longitudinal ligament.

Awake tracheal intubation is probably the ideal way to secure the airway in a patient with an unstable cervical spine, although it may be inappropriate if rapid intubation is necessary. Use of the fiberoptic scope allows intubation under direct vision, but it may be difficult if the patient has pharyngeal bleeding or is uncooperative. Other awake techniques include blind nasal intubation or retrograde intubation over a wire.

Cricothyrotomy or tracheotomy may be considered if attempts at placing an endotracheal tube by other means are unsuccessful.

Once tracheal intubation is achieved in a conscious patient, positioning for surgery requires that continuous cervical spine stability be maintained. Often, the patient is positioned awake, so that any neurologic deterioration can be identified immediately.

In addition to securing the airway and correct patient positioning, choice of anesthetic agents is paramount. Beyond the first 24 hours after injury, succinylcholine may cause hyperkalemia. In denervated muscle, motor end plates proliferate, and succinylcholine produces an exaggerated depolarizing response with a large release of potassium. This acute increase in potassium may lead to arrhythmia, cardiac arrest, and death.

Anesthetic drugs are chosen based on preserved spinal cord perfusion and autoregulation and neuroprotective effects. If somatosensory evoked potential monitoring is done intraoperatively, anesthetic drugs may affect the latency or amplitude of evoked potentials. Hypotension and hypothermia may also affect somatosensory evoked potential monitoring. A drug regimen based on nitrous oxide, opiates, and nondepolarizing muscle relaxants, with minimal use of potent inhalational agents, appears most advantageous.

Fluid management should balance the need to maintain intravascular volume to ensure adequate perfusion with the avoidance of interstitial edema. Avoidance of glucose-containing solutions is important. Worsening neurologic outcomes have been demonstrated with transient spinal cord ischemia and exposure to modest elevations in plasma glucose concentrations.

Postoperative Concerns

Extubation relies on the level of the neurologic lesion and the absence of associated injuries to the head and chest. Weaning criteria used for other patients, which include a maximum inspiratory force of -20 cm H_2O, a vital capacity of 1000 mL, and a PaO_2/FiO_2 ratio greater than 250, may not be appropriate for a quadriplegic patient. If the surgical approach includes the anterior neck, a leak test around the endotracheal tube is helpful to rule out edema or airway compression from a neck hematoma. Both the recurrent laryngeal nerve and branches of the vagus may be damaged during neck dissection (more common on the right side than the left), leading to vocal cord paralysis and stridor on extubation, as well as dysphagia.

PREVENTION

Prevention of neurologic deterioration with an unstable cervical spine requires the following:

- Recognition of cervical spine injury and stabilization of the cervical spine during airway maneuvers and positioning
- Preservation of spinal cord perfusion by optimizing mean arterial pressure
- Minimization of spinal cord edema by careful attention to fluid management
- Use of high-dose steroids
- Prompt treatment of respiratory compromise to prevent hypoxia and further neurologic deterioration

In summary, the unstable cervical spine requires prompt recognition, evaluation of neurologic deficits, and evaluation and treatment of systemic effects, as well as meticulous airway management to ensure optimal outcome from the cervical spine injury.

Further Reading

Ajani AE, Cooper DJ, Scheinkestel CD, et al: Optimal assessment of cervical spine trauma in critically ill patients: A prospective evaluation. Anaesth Intensive Care 26:487-491, 1998.

Brohi K, Wilson-Macdonald J: Evaluation of unstable cervical spine injury: A 6-year experience. J Trauma 49:76-80, 2000.

Chin WC, Haan JM, Cushing BM, et al: Ligamentous injuries of the cervical spine in unreliable blunt trauma patients: Incidence, evaluation, and outcome. J Trauma 50:457-464, 2001.

Cornelius RS, Leach JL: Imaging evaluation of the cervical spine trauma. Neuroimaging Clin N Am 5:451-463, 1995.

Crosby ET, Lui A: The adult cervical spine: Implications for airway management. Can J Anaesth 37:77-93, 1990.

Davis JW, Kaups KL, Cunningham MA, et al: Routine evaluation of the cervical spine in head-injured patients with dynamic fluoroscopy: A reappraisal. J Trauma 50:1044-1047, 2001.

Donaldson WF, Heil BV, Donaldson VP, et al: The effect of airway maneuvers on the unstable C1-C2 segment: A cadaver study. Spine 22:1215-1218, 1997.

Edge CJ, Hyman N, Addy V, et al: Posterior spinal ligament rupture associated with laryngeal mask insertion in a patient with undisclosed unstable cervical spine. Br J Anaesth 89:514-517, 2002.

Gerling MC, Davis DP, Hamilton RS, et al: Effects of cervical spine immobilization technique and laryngoscope blade selection on an unstable cervical spine in a cadaver model of intubation. Ann Emerg Med 36:293-300, 2000.

Hastings RH, Marks JD: Airway management for trauma patients with potential cervical spine injuries. Anesth Analg 73:471-482, 1991.

http://www.dhfs.state.wi.us/Disabilities/Physical/SCI.htm

Keller C, Brimacombe J, Keller K: Pressures exerted against the cervical vertebrae by the standard and intubating laryngeal mask airways: A randomized, controlled, cross-over study in fresh cadavers. Anesth Analg 89:1296-1300, 1999.

Laine FJ, Smoker WRK: Neuroradiology. In Cottrell JE, Smith DS (eds): Anesthesia and Neurosurgery, 4th ed. St. Louis, Mosby–Year Book, 2001, pp 151-156.

Mackenzie CF, Geisler FH: Management of acute cervical spinal cord injury. In Albin MS (ed): Textbook of Neuroanesthesia. New York, McGraw-Hill, 1997, pp 1083-1136.

Marshall WK, Mostrom JL: Neurosurgical diseases of the spine and spinal cord: Anesthetic considerations. In Cottrell JE, Smith DS (eds): Anesthesia and Neurosurgery, 4th ed. St. Louis, Mosby–Year Book, 2001, pp 557-590.

Netterville JL, Koriwchak MJ, Winkle M, et al: Vocal fold paralysis following the anterior approach to the cervical spine. Ann Otol Rhinol Laryngol 105:85-91, 1996.

Pasquale M, Fabian T: Practice management guidelines for trauma from the Eastern Association for the Surgery of Trauma. J Trauma 44:941-957, 1998.

Short DJ, El Masry WS: High dose methylprednisolone in the management of acute spinal cord injury—a systematic review from a clinical perspective. Spinal Cord 38:273-286, 2000.

Slucky AV, Eismont FJ: Treatment of acute injury of the cervical spine. Instr Course Lect 44:67-80, 1995.

Stewart M, Johnston RA, Stewart I, et al: Swallowing performance following anterior cervical spine surgery. Br J Neurosurg 9:605-609, 1995.

Walker DAJ: Management of the patient with spinal cord injury. In Fleisher LA, Prough DS (eds): Problems in Anesthesia: Traumacare, vol 13. Philadelphia, JB Lippincott–Williams & Wilkins, 2001, pp 340-347.

Dental Injuries

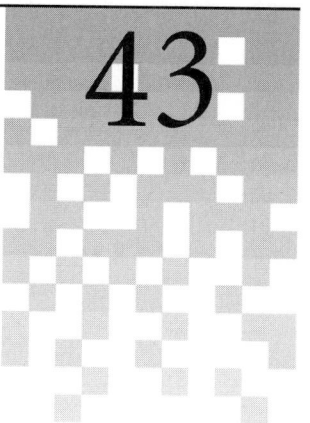

Lee M. Radke

Case Synopsis

A 55-year-old man is taken to the operating room for hernia repair. He has cervical ankylosis, and intubation proves to be difficult. Two maxillary incisors are fractured. Hernia repair is completed, and the dental service is contacted for consultation.

PROBLEM ANALYSIS

Definition

Most anesthesia references identify damage to teeth and dental prostheses as the most common complication of endotracheal intubation. In fact, dental complications are the most common reason for complaints against anesthesiologists. The incidence of dental trauma during general anesthesia has been reported to be as high as 12% and as low as 0.04%. A large survey in which more than 1 million endotracheal intubations were examined reported an incidence of approximately 1 dental injury per 1000 intubations.

Recognition

Modern dental materials and techniques make dental injury difficult to recognize and diagnose. Restorations are often quite natural appearing, and to the untrained eye, it may be difficult to differentiate whether damage has occurred to a natural tooth or a restored tooth.

Intubation-related dental injuries include fractured teeth, displaced restorations, subluxation, and avulsion. Individual teeth are numbered according to a system (Fig. 43-1), and damage to a tooth is classified in the following manner:

- Class I: fracture confined to enamel
- Class II: fracture involving dentin layer
- Class III: fracture resulting in exposure of dental pulp
- Class IV: fracture of tooth root
- Class V: subluxation of tooth
- Class VI: tooth avulsion

Risk Assessment

The greatest risk of dental injury occurs during laryngoscopy and tracheal intubation. The anterior maxillary teeth are most commonly damaged, with the left incisors affected most often. Damage to oral hard and soft tissues can usually be attributed to use of the maxillary anterior teeth as a fulcrum or resting place for the proximal laryngoscope blade during tracheal intubation. However, dental injuries occur in other ways as well. During airway maintenance, a poorly positioned airway or bite block can damage the dentition. During recovery, especially when volatile anesthetic agents have been used, powerful masseter muscle spasms can occur. If an oropharyngeal airway device has been left in place, the spastic biting and grinding forces against the airway can be sufficient to cause dental injury.

Patients with preexisting dental problems are at greater risk for dental injury during general anesthesia. During the preanesthetic evaluation, the anesthesiologist should note the patient's risk for dental injury, especially the condition of the number 9 and 10 incisors (see Fig. 43-1), which are the teeth at highest risk for injury. Any potential dental problems should be noted in the patient's chart:

- Teeth that are decayed and not restored are susceptible to chipping or fracture.
- Teeth with dental restorations (e.g., large fillings or crowns), although strong and functional, can fracture when subjected to impact stresses.
- Endodontically treated teeth (e.g., root canal therapy) are weaker and more brittle than healthy, vital teeth.
- Periodontal disease results in decreased bony support. In this situation, laryngoscopy, tracheal intubation, or insertion of a laryngeal mask airway makes subluxation or avulsion of affected teeth more likely.
- Elderly patients may experience thinning of the tooth enamel due to aging and attrition. Such enamel is more easily damaged during instrumentation of the airway.
- Loose, exfoliating deciduous teeth are at risk for displacement in young patients.

Although deciduous teeth often are considered expendable, premature loss can result in problems. Deciduous teeth maintain space in the dental arch and help guide the permanent teeth into the proper position. If deciduous teeth are lost prematurely, the dental arch could collapse, with a resultant crowding of the permanent teeth. Further, any damage to a deciduous tooth may harm the underlying permanent tooth.

Difficulty of endotracheal intubation can be a contributing factor to dental injury. Emergent, hurried intubations are more likely to result in tooth damage. Unfavorable anatomic features, such as mandibulofacial abnormalities or a short neck, complicate intubation, as do conditions that cause decreased mobility of the mandible or the neck.

Although not well studied, another factor contributing to dental injury during general anesthesia is the experience level of the person performing the intubation.

Implications

As stated, patients with preexisting dental problems are at the greatest risk for dental injuries related to intubation. If the patient is aware of dental problems or is informed of such risk before general anesthesia, liability is greatly diminished, even if damage occurs. Affected teeth should be noted

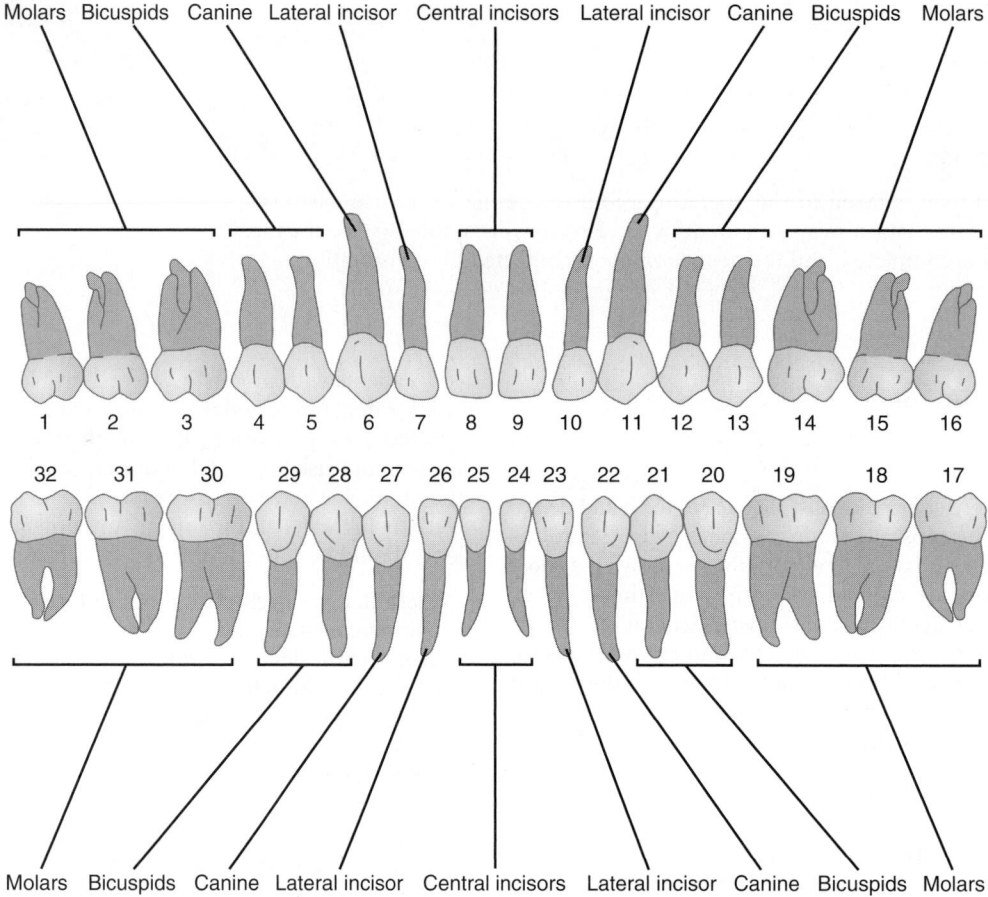

Molars Bicuspids Canine Lateral incisor Central incisors Lateral incisor Canine Bicuspids Molars

1 2 3 4 5 6 7 8 9 10 11 12 13 14 15 16

32 31 30 29 28 27 26 25 24 23 22 21 20 19 18 17

Molars Bicuspids Canine Lateral incisor Central incisors Lateral incisor Canine Bicuspids Molars

Figure 43–1 ▪ Nomenclature and universal numbering system for permanent (adult) dentition.

by number (see Fig. 43-1) during the preanesthetic airway evaluation.

The consequences of dental trauma during general anesthesia can range from minor to severe. Many dental injuries can be repaired easily with standard restorative dental procedures, such as replacement of a displaced filling or repair of chipped enamel. More severe damage, such as dentoalveolar injury, "healthy" tooth loss, or damaged crowns or bridgework, is costly to rectify, causes substantial patient dissatisfaction and upset, and may result in litigation. Endobronchial aspiration of a natural, restored, or prosthetic tooth is the most serious adverse outcome of dental injury.

MANAGEMENT

Ideally, management of an intubation-related dental injury is undertaken by a dental consultant shortly after the injury occurs. Because this service is not always immediately available, the anesthesia staff usually provides early management of such injuries.

If a fragment of a tooth or restoration is displaced, the pieces must be located and recovered. If it is apparent that not all pieces have been retrieved, radiographs should be obtained to ensure that the object has not passed through the glottic opening. Anteroposterior and lateral chest radiographs and lateral head and neck views should be taken.

If a tooth is loosened but not avulsed, it should be returned to its original position as soon as possible. The inner and outer alveolar bone should be compressed with digital pressure to realign bone fragments. Temporary splinting should be done with tape or suture, especially if the tooth is very loose and aspiration is a concern.

If a tooth is avulsed, it should be replanted immediately into its original position. Care must be taken not to wipe or dry the root surface. Tooth roots attach to the alveolar socket through a network of collagenous fibers, which form the periodontal ligament. Wiping or drying the root disrupts the attachment fibers, making successful replantation less likely. In addition, the less time a tooth is out of its socket, the more likely it is that replantation will be successful. Teeth replanted within 30 minutes can usually be retained. Temporary splinting with tape or suture is indicated.

Often, a tooth cannot be safely replanted until the patient awakens because of concern about aspiration. If this is the case, the tooth should be handled carefully by the crown and placed in a suitable medium. Saline is readily available and works well, but milk is better. Milk may be available from the lunch bag of an understanding employee or from a nearby cafeteria.

In the case of significant dental injury, arrangements should be made for immediate referral to a dentist for further evaluation. Loosened or avulsed teeth usually require splinting, and root canal therapy is often necessary if the teeth are to be retained.

The circumstances of a dental injury should be documented in the patient's chart and discussed with the patient as soon as he or she is able to understand the situation. Hospital policy usually requires that an incident report be filed. Administrative personnel from risk management or an equivalent department should become involved to help prevent public-relations, legal, or economic problems for the hospital and physicians involved. Responsibility for reimbursement of the patient for anesthesia-related dental injury could rest with the hospital, anesthesia department, or physician, depending on the hospital's policy.

PREVENTION

Preoperative Evaluation

Prevention of anesthesia-related dental injuries begins during the preoperative anesthetic evaluation. Clinicians should determine whether the patient has any difficulty opening his or her mouth and whether any fixed or removable prostheses are present. The patient should be asked whether he or she is aware of any carious teeth or teeth that have been loosened by periodontal disease, especially any anterior teeth (numbers 6 to 11 and 21 to 27; see Fig. 43-1). Many patients do not receive regular dental care and may be totally unaware of their dental and periodontal status.

If any teeth have periodontal disease (e.g., gingival recession, gingivitis, stain, calculus deposits, exudate), an evaluation for hypermobility should be done. This can be done using a tongue depressor blade or wooden cotton-tipped applicator to apply pressure to the facial aspect of the tooth while bracing the lingual aspect with the index finger of the other hand. Subtle, almost imperceptible movement is normal. Do not attempt to evaluate mobility by wiggling a tooth with the fingertips alone, because the sponginess of the fleshy part of the fingertip could be perceived as tooth movement.

Accurate documentation of preexisting conditions (e.g., loose teeth, decay, restorations) and honest discussion of the risk of dental injury with the patient and his or her family members or representatives will greatly reduce liability if damage to the teeth should occur during anesthesia. If time permits (i.e., elective surgery) and there are serious concerns related to poor dental health, a dental consultation may be requested to thoroughly evaluate and possibly treat dental problems before the planned surgery.

Tooth protection devices should always be considered for patients undergoing laryngoscopy or endoscopy, especially those who have known risk factors for dental injury. Prefabricated rubber or plastic protectors are available but are not universally used or accepted. Concerns that tooth protectors may hinder visualization during direct laryngoscopy may account for their limited use. Custom-made protectors can be fabricated by a dentist before surgery if the need exists and time permits. Custom-made protectors are somewhat expensive, but they offer a high degree of protection with minimal hindrance to visualization of the larynx. It has been reported that some degree of tooth protection may be provided by applying several layers of surgical adhesive tape to the teeth or the back of opposing surface of the laryngoscope blade. In an attempt to minimize contact between the teeth and the laryngoscope, many modifications to the shape of the blade have been proposed. It is suggested that an angulated straight blade with a low heel offers greater visualization between the posterior end of the blade and the upper teeth.

Regardless, it is apparent that most anesthesia-related dental injuries can be prevented with a knowledge of dental factors that predispose teeth to such injury and the use of devices or strategies to protect the teeth.

Further Reading

Burton JF, Baker AB: Dental damage during anaesthesia and surgery. Anaesth Intensive Care 15:262-268, 1987.

Chadwick RG, Lindsay SM: Dental injuries during general anesthesia. Br Dental J 180:255-258, 1996.

Givol N, Gershtansky Y, Halamish-Shani T, et al: Perianesthetic dental injuries: Analysis of incident reports. J Clin Anesth 16:173-176, 2004.

Lockhart PB, Feldbau EV, Gabel RA, et al: Dental complications during and after tracheal intubation. J Am Dent Assoc 112:483, 1986.

Skeie A, Schwartz O: Traumatic injuries of the teeth in connection with general anaesthesia and the effect of use of mouthguards. Endodont Dental Traumatol 15:33-36, 1999.

Warner ME, Benenfeld SM, Warner MA, et al: Perianesthetic dental injuries: Frequency, outcomes, and risk factors. Anesthesiology 90:1302-1325, 1999.

Watanabe S, Suga A, Asakura N, et al: Determination of the distance between the laryngoscope blade and the upper incisors during direct laryngscopy. Anesth Analg 79:638-641, 1994.

Laryngeal and Tracheal Injury

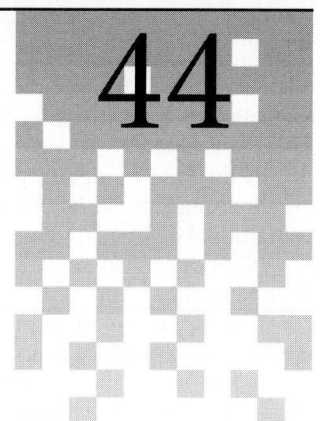

44

William Hope

Case Synopsis

A 65-year-old man describes persistent hoarseness and stridor after prolonged tracheal intubation and mechanical ventilation for treatment of respiratory insufficiency after emergent abdominal aortic aneurysm repair.

PROBLEM ANALYSIS

Definition

Acute and chronic injuries associated with laryngoscopy and tracheal intubation include but are not limited to the following:

- Tracheobronchial laceration and rupture
- Laryngeal and tracheal edema and scarring
- Tracheal ulceration and stricture
- Subglottic and posterior glottic stenosis
- Dislocation of the arytenoid cartilages
- Vocal cord paralysis
- Ductal retention cysts

These complications can result in vocal cord dysfunction and airway obstruction of variable severity. In addition, laryngoscopy and placement of a tracheal tube may cause acute problems related to excessive autonomic stimulation and device malposition or malfunction.

An endotracheal tube always lies in and exerts pressure on the posterior larynx, with potential damage to the arytenoid cartilages and cricoarytenoid joints, posterior glottis, and subglottis involving the inner surface of the cricoid cartilage. The degree of damage from intubation differs among patients. Damage has been shown to occur within a few hours and increases with the duration of intubation. Changes such as edema and hyperemia are seen initially. Progression to mucosal ulcerations and granuloma formation can lead to scar tissue formation and strictures, with chronic airway obstruction. Depending on the site of the injury and the presence of granulation or scar tissue, there can be stenosis and adhesions at, above, or below the level of the vocal cords, possibly with vocal cord dysfunction. Ductal retention cysts form due to irritation and obstruction of subglottic mucous gland ducts. Tracheal erosion caused by tracheal tube trauma may ultimately lead to tracheoesophageal fistula or tracheomalacia and potential tracheal collapse.

Recognition

Laryngeal and tracheal injuries can be divided into those occurring after short-term or prolonged intubation.

SHORT-TERM TRACHEAL INTUBATION

Acute injury, including mucosal and vocal cord edema, usually manifests within hours after extubation and may produce a barking, brassy cough and varying degrees of respiratory obstruction. Dyspnea, stridor, tachypnea, tachycardia, and suprasternal retraction are common presenting signs. Vocal cord dysfunction from recurrent laryngeal nerve injury or arytenoid dislocation presents as partial airway obstruction, dysphonia, and dysphagia. Although usually unilateral, bilateral vocal cord paralysis can present as complete airway obstruction necessitating emergency airway management. Tracheobronchial rupture is suspected with subcutaneous emphysema, respiratory distress, pneumomediastinum, and pneumothorax. Radiography and fiberoptic bronchoscopy confirm the diagnosis.

PROLONGED TRACHEAL INTUBATION

Chronic disorders often present weeks to months after prolonged intubation. Patients present with persistent voice dysfunction, dysphagia, and symptoms of airway obstruction. The lesion can be diagnosed endoscopically or radiographically. In the case of arytenoid dislocation, direct laryngoscopy with the patient under general anesthesia allows testing of the mobility of the cricoarytenoid joint. Flow-volume loops can be used to detect airway obstruction and provide valuable information about its location and functional importance. For example, in patients with airway obstruction, flows are reduced over the full range of lung volume from total lung capacity to residual volume (Fig. 44-1).

Risk Assessment

Because late complications of tracheal intubation present weeks to months after the injury, the acute care practitioner is often unaware of the true incidence of the problem. There is evidence that even with short-term intubation, laryngoscopy results in radiographic and endoscopic evidence of laryngeal damage in a high percentage of patients. As many as 4% of young children experience symptomatic tracheal or laryngeal edema after intubation. The incidence of granuloma formation in adults reportedly ranges from 1 in 800 to 1 in 20,000 tracheal intubations. Granuloma formation occurs more commonly in women than in men and is relatively rare in children.

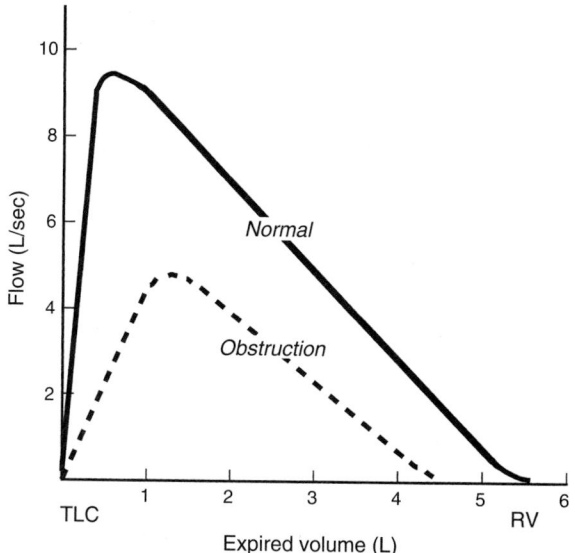

Figure 44–1 ■ Hypothetical expiratory flow-volume curve for a patient with severe airway obstruction due to tracheal stenosis compared with that for a normal person. Note that flows are reduced over the full range of lung volumes, from total lung capacity (TLC) to residual volume (RV).

The following factors have been identified as contributing to intubation trauma:

- Laryngeal abnormalities (external trauma, inflammatory conditions)
- Difficult, traumatic, or repeated attempts at tracheal intubation
- Endotracheal tube movement (during coughing, swallowing, mechanical ventilation)
- Impairment of mucociliary clearance mechanisms or stasis of secretions
- Bacterial superinfection (prolongs healing and increases scar formation)
- Gastroesophageal reflux with spillover of acid into the laryngeal and subglottic region
- Nasogastric tube (increases the likelihood of gastroesophageal reflux and can cause pressure necrosis in the posterior cricoid region)
- Acute or chronic disease states with altered consciousness, poor tissue perfusion, or hypoxemia
- Long duration of intubation (5 to 7 days in adults and 1 to 2 weeks in children)
- Endotracheal tube characteristics (larger size, high-pressure cuff)

Implications

Laryngeal and tracheal injuries after laryngoscopy and tracheal intubation can be a significant cause for perioperative morbidity and, possibly, mortality. Tracheal rupture can lead to mediastinitis and pneumothorax. Acute airway edema can result in significant obstruction; this is especially true in young children because of their small airway diameter. Sedatives, anesthetics, and muscle relaxants oppose the necessary compensatory increased activity of the accessory muscles of breathing in patients with severe airway obstruction to cause respiratory embarrassment. Bilateral recurrent laryngeal nerve palsy and flaps of granulation tissue can cause sudden and complete airway obstruction, necessitating the immediate establishment of an artificial airway.

MANAGEENT

For acute laryngeal edema, nebulized racemic epinephrine (0.5 mL of a 2% solution diluted in a volume of 2 to 4 mL, given every 4 hours) can improve the symptoms of stridor. This dose should not be repeated more frequently than every 2 hours, and the patient must be observed for at least 4 to 6 hours after the last dose for possible rebound effects. Although its efficacy has not been proved, dexamethasone (0.2 to 0.4 mg/kg; maximum dose, 10 mg) may be beneficial.

With prolonged intubation (adults, 5 to 7 days; children, 1 to 2 weeks), consultation for endoscopic laryngeal assessment is advised. Minor injuries usually resolve spontaneously after removal of the endotracheal tube. However, the finding of deep ulcerations calls for immediate extubation or tracheotomy, in addition to precautions to reduce the risk of infection (antibiotic therapy).

If extubation is attempted in a patient with laryngeal edema, steroids can be administered in addition to the interim placement of a smaller endotracheal tube for 24 to 48 hours. The removal of granulation tissue may be required for successful extubation.

Chronic injury secondary to intubation trauma may require laser ablation of scar tissue; tracheal dilatation, resection, reconstruction, or stents; or even anterior cricoid arch resection. Tracheal rupture usually requires emergent thoracotomy for repair.

PREVENTION

Attempt to treat modifiable risk factors as follows:

- Judicious use of intubating stylet
- Use of smallest endotracheal/tracheostomy tube diameter possible
- Aggressive gastroesophageal reflux treatment
- Antibiotic treatment for tracheostomy site infection

Further Reading

Benjamin B: Prolonged intubation injuries of the larynx: Endoscopic diagnosis, classification, and treatment. Ann Otol Rhinol Laryngol Suppl 160:1-15, 1993.
Flemming DC, Orkin FK, Kirby RR: Hazards of tracheal intubation. In Gravenstein N, Kirby RR (eds): Complications in Anesthesiology, 2nd ed. Philadelphia, Lippincott-Raven, 1996, pp 229-239.
Reidenbach MM, Schmidt HM: Membranous tracheal rupture after endotracheal intubation. Ann Thorac Surg 60:1367-1371, 1995.

Pulmonary Aspiration

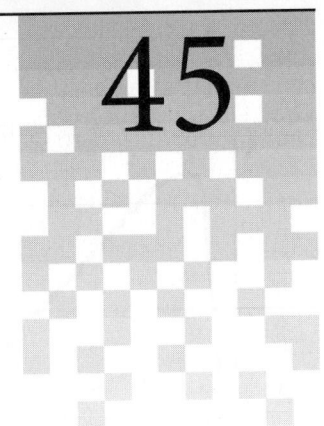

Mark D. Tasch

Case Synopsis

An obese, agitated, 43-year-old man presents for exploratory laparotomy following a gunshot wound to the abdomen. He is uncooperative for examination of the airway. Following rapid-sequence induction of anesthesia, laryngoscopy is unexpectedly difficult. As neuromuscular function returns, the patient vomits a massive quantity of semi-digested food.

PROBLEM ANALYSIS

Definition

The pulmonary aspiration of gastric contents can produce a variety of hazardous sequelae, depending on the nature of the aspirate. Aspirations may include the following:

- Large food fragments, which can obstruct the airway, rapidly causing asphyxia
- Small particles (e.g., particulate antacids), which can produce severe granulomatous inflammation
- Gastric acids, which can induce chemical pneumonitis
- Blood and digestive enzymes, which are relatively innocuous
- Feculent material, which can cause severe infectious pneumonia

Recognition

Unwanted materials can enter the lungs in either a subtle or a dramatic manner. Signs and symptoms (Table 45-1) can appear immediately or after several hours. Rales and rhonchi may be audible in affected lung regions, whereas wheezing may be prominent in only one third of patients with pulmonary aspiration. Dyspnea and tachypnea may develop in an awake patient. Both bronchial obstruction and pulmonary edema can induce profound hypoxemia. Pulmonary edema may also be associated with pink, frothy sputum. Tachycardia can result from respiratory distress as well as from intravascular hypovolemia. The latter can be due to a massive leakage of fluid through damaged pulmonary capillaries.

Radiographic infiltrates may appear promptly or after a variable delay, and they may continue to worsen even as the clinical picture begins to improve. No particular radiographic

Table 45–1 ■ Signs and Symptoms of Pulmonary Aspiration
Rales and rhonchi
Wheezing
Dyspnea and tachypnea
Hypoxemia
Tachycardia
Pulmonary infiltrates or edema

pattern is specific to pulmonary aspiration; it depends on the volume of material inhaled and the patient's position during aspiration. In supine adult patients, the bronchial anatomy most commonly directs foreign matter into the right lower lobe and, less frequently, into the left upper lobe.

Risk Assessment

Several large surveys have found that the incidence of clinically significant aspiration ranges from 0.5 to 4.7 per 10,000 cases. In some studies, the likelihood of pulmonary aspiration is three to four times greater for emergency surgery than for elective surgery. Children and the elderly are more likely to aspirate than are patients of intermediate ages. It may be troubling to note that whereas one third to one half of manifest pulmonary aspirations occur during anesthetic induction or laryngoscopy, one fifth to one third occur during emergence from anesthesia and extubation, when vigilance for this complication is lessened. The preoperative factor most often associated with aspiration is gastrointestinal obstruction. When aspiration occurs in the absence of known predisposing factors, two thirds of such episodes are complications of unanticipated difficulties in airway management.

Pulmonary aspiration has two basic components. First, gastric contents must either escape or be propelled from the stomach into the oropharynx. Second, they must enter the lungs. Active vomiting can be provoked by opioids, cricoid pressure, gastrointestinal obstruction, or hypotension (Table 45-2). Passive regurgitation is promoted by increased intragastric volume or pressure or reduced lower esophageal sphincter (LES) tone. Failure of protective laryngeal reflexes can result from neurologic or neuromuscular disorders, sedative or narcotic medications, or general medical debility.

Among the factors that influence the risk of pulmonary aspiration and its sequelae are the volume and character of gastric contents (Table 45-3). Increased volume alone may overcome any protection afforded by the strength of LES tone. Although the normal stomach apparently passes clear liquids within 2 to 3 hours, clearance of solids may require 6 hours or longer. Gastric acid secretion is thought to be stimulated by ethanol, hypoglycemia, and anxiety. In contrast, antegrade gastric emptying may be inhibited by diabetic gastroparesis, opioids, and pain. LES tone is weakened by nicotine, caffeine, fats, and gastric acid. Although a nasogastric tube permits gastric decompression, it also prevents LES closure. Finally, it is important to seek a history of gastroesophageal reflux

Table 45–2 ■ Risk Factors for Pulmonary Aspiration: Escape of Gastric Contents

Vomiting
Gastrointestinal obstruction
Opioids
Cricoid pressure
Hypotension

Regurgitation
Gastrointestinal obstruction
Diabetic gastroparesis
Gastroesophageal reflux
Increased intragastric pressure
Decreased lower esophageal sphincter tone

Other Factors
Impaired laryngeal protective reflexes
Difficult airway management

from all patients and to recognize that elderly individuals may have feeble gag or cough reflexes.

Some large clinical studies have failed to confirm conventional notions regarding the risk for aspiration. In these studies, patient factors that did not reliably predict gastric fluid acidity or volume were outpatient status, reflux history, anxiety, obesity, duration of fasting, and pregnancy. Similarly, the intake of alcohol, nicotine, or opioids had limited predictive value.

Implications

When pulmonary aspiration of gastric contents occurs, the possible consequences range from benign to lethal. In one series of more than 200,000 operations, nearly two thirds of obvious aspirations produced no signs or symptoms within 2 hours. In this fortunate majority, no related complications ensued. For those patients who developed coughing, wheezing, infiltrates, or hypoxemia within 2 hours of aspiration, more than half required mechanical ventilation for at least several hours. Half the patients who required mechanical ventilation for more than 24 hours never fully recovered. In this and other large series, overall mortality from pulmonary aspiration was less than 5%; however, others reported much higher mortality rates. In two major surveys, pulmonary aspiration was never fatal in healthy patients after elective surgery. Even in Mendelson's historic 1946 report of peripartum aspiration, the only fatalities resulted from rapid asphyxiation caused by food solids.

Table 45–3 ■ Risk Factors for Pulmonary Aspiration: Volume and Character of Gastric Contents

Increased volume of gastric contents
Increased acidity of gastric contents
Particulate matter in stomach
Feculent matter in aspirate

MANAGEMENT

When gastric contents enter the pharynx, the first priority is to clear the upper airway and prevent asphyxia. Tracheal intubation should follow promptly, even if difficult intubation precipitated the aspiration. Bronchoscopic suctioning of the lower airways may be indicated for pulmonary toilet. It is utterly useless, at best, to attempt to neutralize or dilute inhaled acids with an alkaline or saline chaser. Gastric acids experimentally instilled into the bronchi appear at the surface of the lung in less than 20 seconds. Thus, pulmonary parenchymal damage occurs almost immediately.

It had been hoped that corticosteroids might interrupt the pulmonary inflammatory response to acid aspiration and ameliorate the subsequent clinical course. Unfortunately, after 3 decades of investigation, no beneficial effect has been shown. Although corticosteroids may attenuate inflammatory pneumonitis, the immunosuppressant effect of glucocorticoids may exacerbate any secondary bacterial pneumonia or sepsis. Also, prophylactic antibiotics are now considered useless in cases of pulmonary aspiration and may promote rather than prevent secondary infection with resistant pathogens. However, when the aspirate is feculent, antibiotic coverage may be indicated.

The most important therapeutic measure after any pulmonary aspiration is maintenance of pulmonary gas exchange. Often, mechanical ventilation is instituted immediately after any major pulmonary aspiration. Although the prophylactic benefits of positive-pressure ventilation and positive end-expiratory pressure on the development of subsequent lung injury have been debated, such measures are often required merely to provide adequate arterial oxygenation.

PREVENTION

Prevention of pulmonary aspiration includes careful, skilled airway management, as well as pharmacologic alteration of gastric contents and emptying with the following agents:

- Nonparticulate antacids
- H_2-receptor antagonists (or other suppressants of gastric acid secretion)
- Gastroprokinetic drugs

Several classes of drugs are used as chemoprophylaxis to alter gastric fluid volume and pH and to reduce both the likelihood of pulmonary aspiration and any associated complications (Table 45-4). Nonparticulate citrate antacids can

Table 45–4 ■ Prophylaxis for Pulmonary Aspiration

Safe airway management
Cricoid pressure
Gastric tube decompression
Chemoprophylaxis
    Clear citrate antacids
    H_2-receptor histamine antagonists
    Proton pump inhibitors
    Gastroprokinetic agents

elevate gastric pH in most patients, although gastric acids do reaccumulate. Commonly, 15 or 30 mL of sodium citrate or Bicitra is given before cesarean section and has been shown to raise gastric fluid pH to a presumably safe level in the vast majority of parturients. When given before nonobstetric emergency surgery in nonfasting patients, citrates reportedly have less consistent effects. In nonobstetric patients, 30 mL of citrate appears to be more reliable than 15 mL. However, the effects of citrates can never be presumed to persist through emergence and extubation. Particulate antacids are hazardous to the lungs and are therefore contraindicated preoperatively.

Various H_2-receptor histamine antagonists (e.g., cimetidine, ranitidine, famotidine) have been evaluated in many oral and parenteral regimens. Such drugs effectively suppress gastric acid secretion in most patients for several hours. However, they exert no effect on secretions already present in the stomach. Thus, their clinical utility is limited in truly emergent surgical patients. Proton pump inhibitors (e.g., omeprazole) are similarly effective in reducing further gastric acid production, but they have no demonstrable advantage over the H_2-receptor histamine antagonists for aspiration prophylaxis.

Gastroprokinetics (e.g., metoclopramide) may both facilitate antegrade gastric emptying and strengthen LES barrier pressure. However, their efficacy is somewhat inconsistent. Diabetics and others with known or suspected gastroparesis are likely the best candidates for gastroprokinetic medications. When preparing a patient for emergency surgery, a 10- or 20-mg intravenous dose of metoclopramide can empty the stomach within 10 to 20 minutes, whereas an oral dose takes 30 to 60 minutes. Erythromycin is also known to accelerate gastric emptying. Of course, individual responses vary, and it is potentially dangerous (and contraindicated) to attempt to increase gastrointestinal motility in the presence of intestinal obstruction.

Prevention of pulmonary aspiration rests primarily on proper airway management. Chemoprophylaxis is useful, but it is only an adjunct. Although a variety of drugs can safely reduce the pulmonary threat imposed by gastric contents, their routine use is generally not advocated in otherwise healthy, nongravid surgical patients without apparent risk factors for aspiration. Owing to the infrequency of aspiration pneumonitis in such patients, it is unlikely that these drugs will ever be shown to have a statistically significant effect on clinical outcome.

Whenever possible, a difficult airway should be identified preoperatively. Gastrointestinal obstruction and airway morphology may warrant tracheal intubation before protective laryngeal reflexes are pharmacologically ablated. Although a gastric tube may not completely empty the stomach, it can provide a vent for increased intragastric pressure. Cricoid pressure (Sellick's maneuver), when properly applied, can help prevent the passage of gastric contents into the oropharynx. However, it may also provoke active vomiting in an unanesthetized patient. In recent years, more authors have questioned the primary benefits of this maneuver. It is physically difficult to maintain cricoid pressure at the recommended level or force for more than a few minutes. In addition, backward pressure on the cricoid cartilage facilitates laryngoscopy in some patients but interferes with it in others. In fact, in some patients, pushing the larynx posteriorly, cephalad, and to the right provides the best view of the vocal cords. Cricoid pressure can also impede mask or laryngeal mask airway ventilation. Although Sellick's maneuver remains a standard component of aspiration prophylaxis, oxygenation, ventilation, and securing the airway must always take precedence.

Further Reading

ASA Task Force: Practice guidelines for preoperative fasting and the use of pharmacologic agents to reduce the risk of pulmonary aspiration: Application to healthy patients undergoing elective procedures: A report by the American Society of Anesthesiologists Task Force on Preoperative Fasting. Anesthesiology 90:896-905, 1999.

Ljungqvist O, Soreide E: Preoperative fasting. Br J Surg 90:400-406, 2003.

LoCicero J: Bronchopulmonary aspiration. Surg Clin North Am 69:71-76, 1989.

Marik PE: Primary care: Aspiration pneumonitis and aspiration pneumonia. N Engl J Med 344:665-671, 2001.

Mendelson CL: The aspiration of stomach contents into the lungs during obstetric anesthesia. Am J Obstet Gynecol 52:191-205, 1946.

Ng A, Smith G: Gastroesophageal reflux and aspiration of gastric contents in anesthetic practice. Anesth Analg 93:494-513, 2001.

Sellick BA: Cricoid pressure to control regurgitation of stomach contents during induction of anaesthesia. Lancet 2:404-406, 1961.

Warner MA, Warner ME, Weber JG: Clinical significance of pulmonary aspiration during the perioperative period. Anesthesiology 78:56-62, 1993.

Bronchospasm

Joan Benca

Case Synopsis

A 4-year-old boy with cerebral palsy has general anesthesia for repair of an inguinal hernia. Following intubation, peak inspiratory pressure increases acutely from 18 to 35 cm H_2O. This is accompanied by a decrease in oxygen (O_2) saturation from 100% to 82%, a decrease in blood pressure from 98/64 to 68/34 mm Hg, and an increase in heart rate from 90 to 140 beats per minute. Chest auscultation reveals diffuse bilateral expiratory wheezes.

PROBLEM ANALYSIS

Definition

In asthmatics, bronchospasm is caused by the spasmodic contraction of the bronchial smooth muscle. However, it occurs rarely during general anesthesia. In one series, wheezing occurred in only 0.17% of nonasthmatic and 0.8% of asthmatic patients. However, following induction with thiopental, wheezing has been reported in 6.7% to 8.1% of normal patients and in up to 45% of asthmatics. One review of a large number of asthmatic patients who received general anesthesia concluded that bronchospasm was a rare event and that associated adverse outcomes were uncommon. Thus, the relationship between intraoperative wheezing due to bronchospasm and severe adverse outcomes is unclear. However, data from the American Society of Anesthesiologists (ASA) closed claims study indicate that severe bronchospasm can result in death or brain injury.

Patients who have bronchial asthma or chronic bronchitis may exhibit exaggerated responses to mechanical or chemical irritants or toxins, such as severe bronchoconstriction. Other factors can contribute to increased airway resistance with bronchospasm, such as mucosal edema, excessive mucus production and plugging, and desquamation of bronchial epithelium. Likely, all these in combination (bronchoconstriction, mucosal edema, mucus production, and inflammation) constitute bronchospasm, not just bronchial smooth muscle contraction.

Normal airways are slightly constricted in their baseline condition. Bronchial smooth muscle tone is controlled by the parasympathetic nervous system via efferent vagal activity. Histamine also directly stimulates afferent parasympathetic pathways and directly increases bronchial smooth muscle tone. Muscarinic receptors can be blocked with atropine or glycopyrrolate.

The parasympathetic nervous system is an important pathway in bronchoconstriction caused by inhaled irritants. Asthmatics have a smaller baseline airway caliber and hypertrophied bronchial smooth muscle, giving irritants greater access to receptors mediating bronchoconstriction. The smaller baseline airway caliber of asthmatic patients is significant; any further decrease in diameter will have a major effect on airway resistance, because laminar flow is proportional to the fourth power of the radius (Poiseuille's law).

Large airways account for 80% of airflow resistance. The remaining 20% is accounted for by small airways and peripheral bronchioles. These smaller airways are sometimes referred to as the silent zone because their resistance can increase before there is a significant change in total airway resistance.

Different factors trigger bronchospasm in pediatric patients versus adult patients with obstructive airway disease. In pediatric patients, environmental allergens and viral respiratory illnesses are the most common causes of acute bronchospasm, whereas in adults, mechanical and chemical irritants are probably the most common causes. Further, viral illnesses can exacerbate symptoms in patients with asthma and can cause normal patients to exhibit increased airway reactivity. Thus, it is important to consider these mechanisms when tailoring therapy for individual patients.

Recognition

Symptoms and signs of acute bronchospasm include wheezing, prolonged expiration, reduced breath sounds, and increased airway pressure during positive-pressure ventilation. O_2 saturation may decrease, and the patient may become hypotensive. Owing to ventilation-perfusion mismatch, end-tidal carbon dioxide (CO_2) concentration may decrease, even with an increased arterial CO_2 concentration. End-tidal CO_2 monitoring shows an upsloping curve, but this alone is not specific for bronchospasm; it indicates only obstruction to exhalation somewhere along the expiration pathway (i.e., from the patient's alveolus to where the end-tidal CO_2 sensor is positioned in the breathing circuit). Further, bronchospasm is not the only cause of wheezing. Table 46-1 lists other causes of wheezing in anesthetized, ventilated patients, and Table 46-2

Table 46-1 ■ Causes of Nonbronchospastic (Asthmatic) Wheezing in Anesthetized Patients

Mechanical obstruction of endotracheal tube
Negative-pressure expiration
Tension pneumothorax
Pulmonary edema
Pulmonary aspiration of gastric contents
Pulmonary embolism

Table 46-2 ■ Causes of Increased Peak Airway Pressure during Ventilation

Increased inspiratory flow rate
Excessive tidal volume: "alveolar overdistention"
Increased intrapleural pressure
    Coughing
    Pleural effusion, ascites
    Abdominal gas insufflation, abdominal packs
    Restraints, bandages
    Head-down position
    Tension pneumothorax
Increased resistance of endotracheal tube
    Small caliber, kinks, secretions
Increased resistance of patient's airway
    Secretions, bronchospasm*

*If confronted with wheezing and increased peak inspiratory pressure, other causes must be ruled out before making the diagnosis of acute bronchospasm.

Table 46-3 ■ Causes of Acute Bronchospasm in Anesthetized Patients

Nonspecific bronchial hyperresponsiveness
Allergic or anaphylactic reaction to drugs or blood transfusion
Allergic or anaphylactic reaction to other allergens (e.g., latex)
Exacerbation of asthma
Pharmacologic factors (e.g., β-blockers, prostaglandin inhibitors, anticholinesterases)
Stimulation of parasympathetic fibers and M2 and M3 muscarinic receptors
Tracheal irritation from intubation

lists causes of increased peak inspiratory pressure during ventilation. Table 46- 3 lists causes of acute bronchospasm in anesthetized patients.

Risk Assessment

Many patients with bronchospasm do not have a history of obstructive pulmonary disease. Also, most patients with obstructive pulmonary disease do not have bronchospasm under anesthesia. Factors that increase the risk for intraoperative bronchospasm are the following:

- Recent viral upper respiratory infection
- Recent exacerbation of pulmonary symptoms
- Recent hospital admission for treatment of asthma
- Exposure to tobacco smoke

Bronchospasm may be more common in patients with tracheal intubation. One study showed a reversible component of increased airway system resistance after placement of an endotracheal tube, but not after placement of a laryngeal mask airway.

Implications

Acute bronchospasm requires early diagnosis and treatment. Untreated, it causes hypoxemia, hypotension, and possibly brain damage or death. In the 1991 ASA closed claims study, 2% of the claims involved bronchospasm, and in 90% of these, the result was brain injury or death. The majority of these cases occurred during induction of general anesthesia and airway instrumentation. Airway instrumentation may precipitate acute bronchospasm, likely due to mechanical irritation and parasympathetic stimulation.

MANAGEMENT AND PREVENTION

Acute bronchospasm is not limited to patients with a history of bronchial hyperreactivity. It is helpful, however, to make sure that patients with such a history receive bronchodilators and possibly steroids before the induction of general anesthesia. Patients with a history of asthma or chronic bronchitis who are scheduled for elective surgery should continue all their medications, and the chest examination should be at their baseline. Preoperative physical examination on the day of surgery must include chest auscultation. Active wheezing, worsening cough, more than usual sputum production, shortness of breath, and fever are reasons to delay anesthesia and surgery. A review of any previous anesthesia records may help in planning anesthetic management. For severe asthmatics, preoperative investigation may include a chest radiograph, 1-second forced expiratory volume (FEV_1), and arterial blood gas analysis. For patients who are asymptomatic, no laboratory tests are necessary.

Guidelines for the treatment of asthmatic patients were described by the 1997 National Heart, Lung, and Blood Institute's Expert Panel on Asthma and include the use of steroids as anti-inflammatory agents (Table 46-4). It is unnecessary to treat all patients with a history of wheezing with steroids and bronchodilators, however. There is about an 8% incidence of asthma in the United States, so checking the FEV_1 and starting all patients with asthma on steroids before anesthesia would be excessively costly. Those at highest risk for postoperative pulmonary complications (e.g., those having cardiac surgery, thoracotomy or airway surgery, or abdominal surgery, and those with a history of significant pulmonary symptoms) should probably receive steroids and have a baseline pulmonary function assessment.

Interventions that may attenuate bronchial hyperreactivity during induction of anesthesia and airway manipulation include pretreatment with a nebulized β-agonist (e.g., albuterol, salbutamol, ipratroprium); intravenous (IV), nebulized, or intratracheal lidocaine; IV propofol induction; and preoperative oral or inhaled steroids. It is difficult to compare studies of interventions to attenuate bronchial hyperreactivity because some report airway resistance changes in response to tracheal intubation, others report responses to a histamine challenge, and still others report the incidence of perioperative clinical wheezing.

Clearly, patients with significant bronchial hyperreactivity will benefit from the administration of steroids before anesthesia and surgery. A combination of steroids and β-agonists is clearly superior to either agent alone. For patients requiring general anesthesia, potent inhalational agents (at least equal to or greater than one minimum alveolar concentration) are the mainstays of anesthetic technique. All potent inhalational agents effectively reduce airway resistance. Using propofol as an induction agent, instead of thiopental or etomidate, reduces the incidence of postintubation wheezing in both

Table 46–4 ■ Approach to Asthma Management in Adults and Children Older than Five Years

Step and Asthma Type	Daily Medications
Step 4 Severe, persistent Asthma	Anti-inflammatory: inhaled steroid (high dose) and long-acting inhaled β_2-agonist; possibly systemic steroids Short-acting bronchodilator: inhaled β_2-agonist as needed for symptoms
Step 3 Moderate, persistent Asthma	Anti-inflammatory: inhaled steroid (medium dose) or inhaled steroid (low to medium dose) and inhaled long-acting β_2-agonist Short-acting bronchodilator: inhaled β_2-agonist as needed for symptoms
Step 2 Mild, persistent Asthma	Anti-inflammatory: inhaled steroid (low dose) or cromolyn or nedrocromil Short-acting bronchodilator: inhaled β_2-agonist as needed for symptoms
Step 1 Mild, intermittent Asthma	Anti-inflammatory: no daily medication needed Short-acting bronchodilator: inhaled β_2-agonist as needed for symptoms

Adapted from National Heart, Lung, and Blood Institute National Asthma Education and Prevention Program EPR-2, 1997.

asthmatic and nonasthmatic patients. Both inhaled and IV lidocaine attenuate histamine-induced bronchospasm; however, the use of inhaled lidocaine attenuates histamine-induced bronchospasm at lower serum levels of local anesthetic than does IV lidocaine. This effect appears to be independent of topical airway anesthesia, because inhaled dyclonine provides excellent topical anesthesia but does not attenuate bronchial hyperreactivity to histamine.

Laryngeal mask airways do not provoke bronchospasm and should be used if endotracheal intubation is not necessary, especially for pediatric patients with upper respiratory infections. Regional anesthesia is another option that avoids the problems associated with tracheal intubation. However, a neuraxial block may adversely affect pulmonary function. For patients with primarily reactive airway disease but without increased mucus production, the reduced ability to cough with a high neuraxial block is not a problem. Further, there is some evidence that a high epidural block does not exacerbate symptoms of asthma, but it is unclear whether it is the lack of tracheal intubation, serum concentration of local anesthetic, or some other effect of epidural anesthesia that contributes to the lower incidence of bronchospasm.

Bronchospasm may still occur despite careful patient preparation and choice of an appropriate anesthetic technique. Treating bronchospasm under anesthesia can be difficult. One should administer 100% O_2 and use a potent inhalational anesthetic, but these steps are not always effective. With bronchospasm, it can be difficult to deepen anesthesia with an inhalational agent if ventilation is severely compromised.

Adjunctive measures to treat the bronchospasm include IV lidocaine, IV propofol, subcutaneous (SC) terbutaline, SC or IV epinephrine, and a nebulized β-agonist. With severely impaired ventilation due to bronchospsam, SC or IV epinephrine should be given, and anesthesia should be deepened with an IV agent until effective ventilation is possible. Table 46-5 lists therapeutic steps for acute bronchospasm.

β-Agonists given via a breathing circuit elbow adapter and a metered-dose inhaler are not as effective as those administered via a nebulizer or aerosol-enhancing chamber. Much of the delivered dose is contained in large (>5 μm) particles that do not reach the distal airways (a particle size of 1 to 5 μm is required for deposition in the distal airways). Therefore, only 10% to 20% of a dose delivered by a metered-dose inhaler reaches the small airways under optimal conditions in nonintubated patients. Delivery systems for intubated patients are even less effective, with as little as 1% to 2% of the delivered dose reaching the distal airways.

Corticosteroids do not have an immediate beneficial effect in acute bronchospasm. However, they should be given to patients with acute bronchospasm to help reduce ongoing inflammatory changes that contribute to the problem.

Finally, the most important factor in preventing bronchospasm during general anesthesia is to provide an adequate depth of anesthesia before and during airway manipulation and tracheal intubation, as well as during the surgical procedure itself. It is important to use anesthetic adjuncts, such as lidocaine and narcotics, in addition to potent inhalational agents to achieve this goal.

Table 46–5 ■ Therapy for Acute Bronchospasm

Deepen anesthesia with potent inhalational anesthetics or IV anesthetics
Administer β-agonist bronchodilators (albuterol, metoproterenol, salbutamol, ipratropium) using a metered-dose inhaler through an aerosolization chamber or by solution in a nebulizer placed in the anesthesia circuit
Epinephrine
    Adult dose: 0.1 to 0.5 mL of 0.1% epinephrine solution SC
    Pediatric dose: 0.01 mL/kg of 0.1% epinephrine solution SC (maximum, 0.3 mL); 0.10 to 0.01 μg/kg/min infusion
Isoproterenol
    Pediatric dose: 0.01 μg/kg SC up to a maximum of 0.3 mg; 0.01 to 0.1 μg/kg/min infusion
Corticosteroids
    Hydrocortisone
    Methylprednisolone
    Dexamethasone

Further Reading

Berry A, Brimacombe J, Keller C, Verghese C: Pulmonary airway resistance with the endotracheal tube versus laryngeal mask airway in paralyzed anesthetized adult patients. Anesthesiology 90:395-397, 1999.

Bishop MJ: Preoperative corticosteroids for reactive airway? Anesthesiology 100:1047-1049, 2004.

Bishop MJ, Cheney FW: Anesthesia for patients with asthma: Low risk but not no risk. Anesthesiology 85:455-456, 1996.

Cheney FW, Posner KL, Caplan RA: Adverse respiratory events infrequently leading to malpractice suits. Anesthesiology 75:932-939, 1991.

Eames WO, Rooke GA, Wu RS, Bishop MJ: Comparison of the effects of etomidate, propofol, and thiopental on respiratory resistance after tracheal intubation. Anesthesiology 84:1307-1310, 1996.

Gold MI, Helrich M: A study of the complications related to anesthesia in asthmatic patients. Anesth Analg 42:283-293, 1963.

Groeben H, Grosswendt T, Silvanus M-T, et al: Airway anesthesia alone does not explain attenuation of histamine-induced bronchospasm by local anesthetics: A comparison of lidocaine, ropivicaine, and cyclonine. Anesthesiology 94:423-426, 2001.

Groeben H, Silvanus M-T, Beste M, Peters J: Combined intravenous lidocaine and inhaled salbutamol protect against bronchial hyper-reactivity more effectively than lidocaine or salbutamol alone. Anesthesiology 89:862-865, 1998.

Kil H-K, Rooke GA, Ryan-Dykes MA, Bishop M: Effect of prophylactic bronchodilator treatment on lung resistance after tracheal intubation. Anesthesiology 81:43-46, 1994.

Kim ES, Bishop MJ: Endotracheal intubation, but not laryngeal mask airway insertion, produces reversible bronchoconstriction. Anesthesiology 90:391-393, 1999.

National Institutes of Health Guidelines for the Diagnosis and Management of Asthma: Clinical Practice Guidelines Expert Panel Report-2. Bethesda, Md, National Institutes of Health, 1997.

Olsson GL: Bronchospasm during anaesthesia: A computer aided incidence study of 136,929 patients. Acta Anaesthesiol Scand 31:244-252, 1987.

Pizov R, Brown RH, Weiss YS, et al: Wheezing during induction of general anesthesia in patients with and without asthma: A randomized, blinded trial. Anesthesiology 82:1111-1114, 1995.

Rooke GA, Choi J-H, Bishop M: The effect of isoflurane, halothane, sevoflurane, and thiopental/nitrous oxide on respiratory system resistance after tracheal intubation. Anesthesiology 86:1294-1297, 1997.

Scalfaro P, Sly PD, Sims C, et al: Salbutamol prevents the increase of respiratory resistance caused by tracheal intubation during sevoflurane anesthesia in asthmatic children. Anesth Analg 93:888-890, 2001.

Shnider SM, Papper EM: Anesthesia for the asthmatic patient. Anesthesiology 22:886-892, 1961.

Silvanus M-T, Groeben H, Peters J: Corticosteroids and inhaled salbutamol in patients with reversible airway obstruction markedly decrease the incidence of bronchospasm after tracheal intubation. Anesthesiology 100:1052-1057, 2004.

Tait AR, Pandit U, Voepel-Lewis T, et al: Use of the laryngeal mask airway in children with upper respiratory tract infections: A comparison with endotracheal intubation. Anesth Analg 86:706-709, 1998.

Warner DO, Warner MA, Barnes RD, et al: Perioperative respiratory complications in patients with asthma. Anesthesiology 85:460-464, 1996.

Perioperative Hypoxia

John C. Boncyk

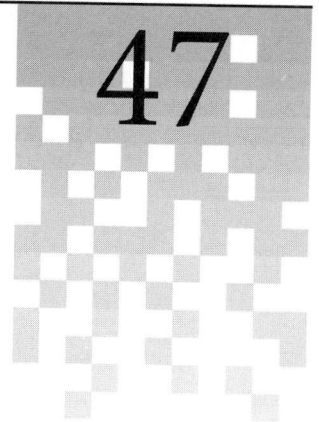

Case Synopsis

A 70-year-old, 63-inch, 110-kg woman has laparoscopic cholecystectomy. After satisfactory anesthesia (nitrous oxide-oxygen, isoflurane, and a muscle relaxant) and surgery, she is transported to the postanesthesia care unit (PACU). Upon arrival in the PACU, the oxygen saturation of her arterial blood by pulse oximetry (SpO_2) is 85% with 40% oxygen by facemask. She does not appear to be in any distress, and her other vital signs are stable. Over the next few minutes, her SpO_2 trends down to 70%, and she becomes dyspneic.

PROBLEM ANALYSIS

Definition

Hypoxia is reduced oxygen (O_2) tension within or outside the body; however, it is usually construed as reduced O_2 tension at the tissue level. The oxygen cascade (Fig. 47-1) depicts the movement of O_2 down its partial-pressure gradient from that of dry ambient air to the mitochondria. There are four categories of hypoxia: hypoxemia, anemic hypoxia, circulatory hypoxia, and histiocytic hypoxia.

HYPOXEMIA

Hypoxemia is decreased blood O_2 tension. The lungs play a central role in all causes of hypoxemia:

- Low fraction of inspired O_2 (FiO_2)
- Hypoventilation
- Alveolar ventilation-perfusion ($\dot{V}A/\dot{Q}$) mismatch
- Increased shunt
- Diffusion limitations

How these affect the alveolar-arterial O_2 partial-pressure difference [$P(A-a)O_2$], the response to breathing 100% O_2, and the arterial partial pressure of carbon dioxide (CO_2) is shown in Table 47-1.

Low Inspired Oxygen Concentration. In addition to altitude and incorrect flowmeter settings, low FiO_2 may be caused by faulty tank or hose connections, central gas distribution, or excessive inspired concentrations of nitrous oxide or nitrogen. The inspired partial pressure of O_2 (PiO_2) is directly related to atmospheric minus saturated water (H_2O) vapor pressure (47 mm Hg at 37°C, regardless of altitude) and FiO_2.

Hypoventilation. With hypoventilation, alveolar ventilation ($\dot{V}A$) cannot remove all produced CO_2, so arterial and alveolar CO_2 concentrations increase. With constant O_2 consumption, hypoxia inevitably results. However, even a small increase in FiO_2 will increase the arterial partial pressure of O_2 (PaO_2), as predicted by the alveolar gas equation:

$$PAO_2 = FiO_2 \cdot (PB - PiH_2O) - (PACO_2/RQ)$$

where PAO_2 and $PACO_2$ are alveolar partial pressures of O_2 and CO_2, respectively; FiO_2 is the fraction of inspired O_2;

PB is atmospheric (barometric) pressure; PiH_2O is saturated H_2O vapor pressure; and RQ is the respiratory quotient (0.8).

Assuming an FiO_2 of 0.21, sea-level PB (760 mm Hg) and PiH_2O (47 mm Hg), and variable $PACO_2$, PAO_2 decreases from 100 to 50 mm Hg as $PACO_2$ increases from 40 to 80 mm Hg. Simply increasing FiO_2 to 0.3 ($PACO_2$ 80 mm Hg) will increase PAO_2 to 114 mm Hg.

Ventilation-Perfusion Mismatch. Matching alveolar ventilation ($\dot{V}A$) and perfusion ($\dot{Q}$) involves many factors:

- Ventilation volume
- Alveolar pressure
- Lung compliance
- Chest wall compliance
- Airway resistance
- Gravity (posture)
- Pulmonary blood flow
- Mode of ventilation

When ventilation and perfusion are matched, $\dot{V}A/\dot{Q}$ is equal to 1.0. However, the lung does not have uniform $\dot{V}A/\dot{Q}$ (Fig. 47-2). *Dead space* refers to ventilation without perfusion, and perfusion without ventilation is called *shunt*. Note in Figure 47-2 that the top of the lung has more dead-space ventilation (and higher PAO_2) than the bottom, and the bottom of the lung has relatively more shunt (and lower PAO_2).

The reason PaO_2 is decreased with $\dot{V}A/\dot{Q}$ mismatch is that capillary blood leaving the high-$\dot{V}A/\dot{Q}$ regions has higher-than-normal PO_2 but only minimally enhanced O_2 content (owing to the shape of the oxyhemoglobin dissociation curve). Blood leaving the low-$\dot{V}A/\dot{Q}$ regions has both low PO_2 and low O_2 content; this situation reduces O_2 transfer to blood far more than high-$\dot{V}A/\dot{Q}$ regions can increase it, thereby increasing the $P(A-a)O_2$ gradient. $\dot{V}A/\dot{Q}$ mismatch also interferes with the uptake and elimination of anesthetic gases. Denitrogenation and the uptake and elimination of inhalational anesthetic agents are slowed in patients with significant $\dot{V}A/\dot{Q}$ mismatch.

Increased Shunt. Anatomic right-to-left shunt ($\dot{Q}s/\dot{Q}t$) is not considered here (see Chapter 157). Right-to-left transpulmonary shunt (i.e., mixed venous blood traverses the pulmonary capillary bed without being oxygenated) is the primary mechanism for hypoxia in anesthetized patients and in those with pneumonia and pulmonary edema. Right-to-left shunt (either anatomic or transpulmonary) is the only mechanism

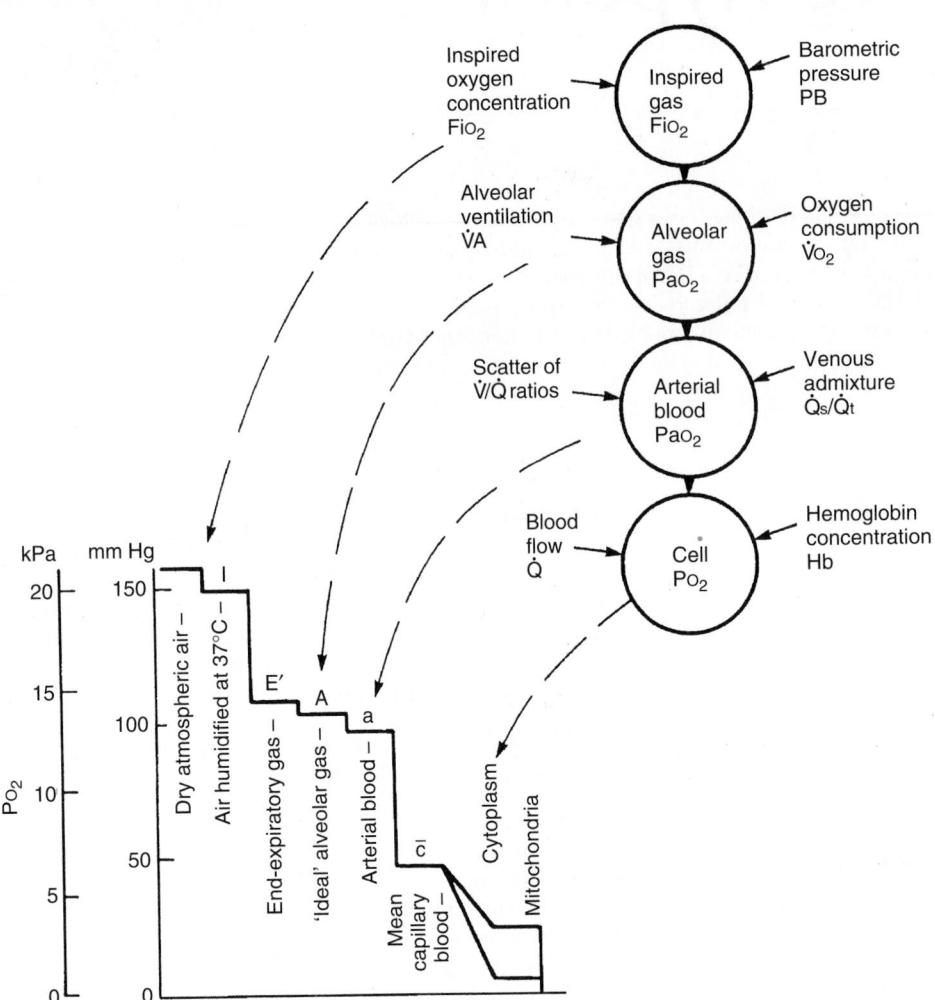

Figure 47–1 ■ Oxygen partial-pressure cascade from dry atmospheric air (160 mm Hg) to the mitochondria (3 to 20 mm Hg). (From Lumb AB: Nunn's Applied Respiratory Physiology, 5th ed. London, Butterworth-Heinemann, 2000, p 250.)

Table 47–1 ■ Causes of Hypoxemia and Their Effects on Alveolar-Arterial Oxygen Partial Pressure Difference, Response to 100% Oxygen, and Arterial Partial Pressure of Carbon Dioxide

Cause	$P(A-a)O_2$	100% O_2	$PaCO_2$
Low FiO_2	Normal	Increased PaO_2	Normal
Hypoventilation	Normal	Increased PaO_2	Increased
$\dot{V}A/\dot{Q}$ mismatch	Increased	Increased PaO_2	Normal
Shunt ($\dot{Q}s/\dot{Q}t$)	Increased	No change	Normal
Diffusion limitation	Increased	Increased PaO_2	Normal

FiO_2, fraction of inspired oxygen; PaO_2, arterial partial pressure of oxygen; $P(A-a)O_2$, alveolar-arterial oxygen partial pressure difference; $PaCO_2$, arterial partial pressure of carbon dioxide; $\dot{V}A/\dot{Q}$, alveolar ventilation-perfusion.

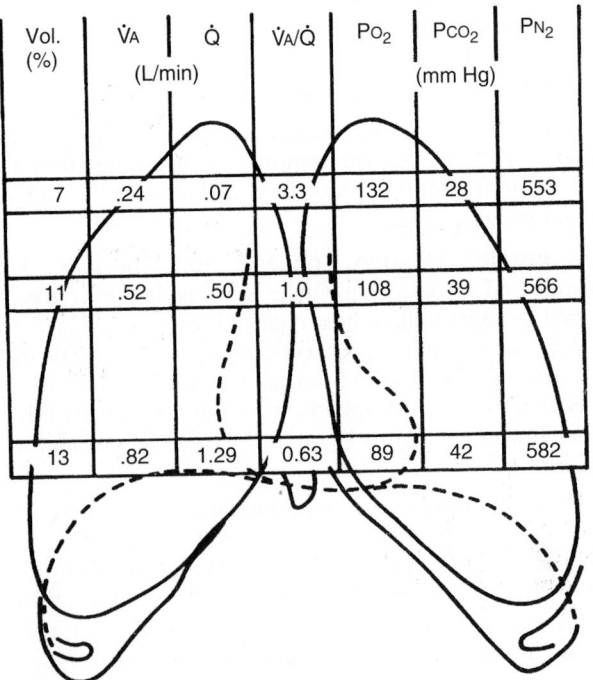

Vol. (%)	$\dot{V}A$ (L/min)	$\dot{Q}$	$\dot{V}A/\dot{Q}$	PO_2	PCO_2 (mm Hg)	PN_2
7	.24	.07	3.3	132	28	553
11	.52	.50	1.0	108	39	566
13	.82	1.29	0.63	89	42	582

Figure 47–2 ■ Regional lung alveolar ventilation-perfusion ($\dot{V}A/\dot{Q}$) ratios and gas composition for three zones of the upright lung. (From West JB: Pulmonary Pathophysiology: The Essentials. Baltimore, Williams & Wilkins, 1980.)

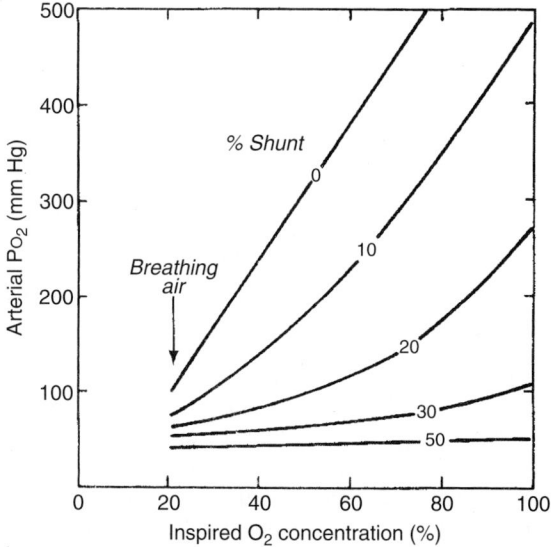

Figure 47–3 ■ Relationship between arterial partial pressure of oxygen (PaO$_2$) and fraction of inspired oxygen (FiO$_2$) for shunts of various percentages (isoshunt diagram). Isoshunt lines hold for hemoglobin of 10 to 14 g/dL and arterial partial pressure of carbon dioxide (PaCO$_2$) of 25 to 40 mm Hg. (Modified from Nunn JF: Applied Respiratory Physiology, 4th ed. London, Butterworth-Heinemann, 1993, p 184.)

for hypoxemia in which PaO$_2$ stays well below PAO$_2$, even with an FiO$_2$ of 1.0 (Fig. 47-3).

Diffusion Limitation.   Alveolar-capillary gas exchange is limited by the diffusing capacity of a particular gas across the alveolar-capillary membrane (D). The normal resting diffusing capacity for O$_2$ (DO$_2$) is 21 mL/minute per mm Hg P(A-a)O$_2$. During exercise, DO$_2$ can increase to 65 mL/minute per mm Hg P(A-a)O$_2$ owing to increased capillary exchange and improved V̇A/Q̇ matching. Diffusion limitation is an unusual cause of clinical hypoxemia.

GENERAL ANESTHESIA

ANEMIC HYPOXIA

Anemic hypoxia is caused by a low hemoglobin concentration or abnormal hemoglobin function. The following considerations are relevant to the discussion of anemic hypoxia:

- Hemoglobin structure-function relationship
- Oxygen-hemoglobin (O$_2$-Hb) dissociation curve
- Oxygen content
- Other hemoglobin species
- Minimum hemoglobin concentration

Hemoglobin Structure-Function Relationship.   Hemoglobin is composed of four subunits to form a tetrameric molecule. There are several different subunits (denoted α through ε), but only two are contained in a single hemoglobin molecule. Normal adult hemoglobin has two α and two β subunits. Heme, the iron-containing moiety, fits into each hemoglobin subunit, allowing it to bind one molecule of O$_2$ (oxygenation). Interactions between hemoglobin subunits (subunit cooperativity) are responsible for the increased O$_2$ affinity that occurs as each successive O$_2$ molecule is bound to hemoglobin. This property accounts for the sigmoid shape of the O$_2$-Hb dissociation curve (Fig. 47-4).

Oxygen-Hemoglobin Dissociation Curve.   The O$_2$-Hb dissociation curve is sigmoidal and describes the affinity of hemoglobin for O$_2$. P50 is the value for PO$_2$ when hemoglobin is 50% saturated with O$_2$. For normal hemoglobin in adults, this is 26.6 mm Hg (see Fig. 47-4). A shift to the right means that hemoglobin unloads its O$_2$ to tissues more easily, and a shift to the left means that hemoglobin unloads its O$_2$ with more difficulty. Four factors regulate the affinity of hemoglobin for O$_2$:

1. Hydrogen ion (Bohr effect)
2. 2,3-Diphosphoglycerate

Figure 47–4 ■ Oxyhemoglobin dissociation curve relates arterial oxygen saturation (SaO$_2$; left ordinate) and content (CaO$_2$ [mL/dL]; right ordinate) to tension (PaO$_2$; abscissa). This assumes hemoglobin = 15 g/dL, CaO$_2$ = 20 mL/dL, and arteriovenous CaO$_2$ difference = 5 mL/dL. (From Luce JM, Pierson DJ, Tyler ML: Intensive Respiratory Care, 2nd ed. Philadelphia, WB Saunders, 1993, p 27.)

3. CO_2 (Haldane effect)
4. Temperature

An increase in any of these factors decreases the affinity of hemoglobin for O_2 and shifts the O_2-Hb dissociation curve to the right (i.e., increases P50), with more O_2 unloaded to tissues for a given Po_2. A decrease shifts the O_2-Hb dissociation curve to the left, with less O_2 unloaded to tissues at any given Po_2.

Oxygen Content.   Four moles of O_2 bind with each mole of hemoglobin. The O_2 carrying capacity of hemoglobin is 1.39 mL O_2/g; however, this is typically lower in patients (about 1.34 mL/g), owing to the small amounts of methemoglobin and carboxyhemoglobin that are normally present. In addition, there is physically dissolved O_2 in plasma (0.003 mL/dL per mm Hg of Po_2), so arterial O_2 content (Cao_2) is expressed as follows:

$$Cao_2 = Sao_2 \cdot [Hb] \cdot 1.34 + Pao_2 \cdot 0.003$$

or 20 mL/dL (see Fig. 47-4). However, the amount of O_2 given off to the tissues is dependent on O_2 content and the P50 of the hemoglobin species.

Other Hemoglobin Species.   Myoglobin serves both as an O_2 buffer and to store O_2 in muscle. All known vertebrate myoglobins and β-hemoglobin subunits are similar in structure, but myoglobin binds O_2 more avidly at low Po_2 (Fig. 47-5) because it is a monomer (i.e., it does not undergo a significant conformational change with oxygenation). Thus, myoglobin remains fully saturated at O_2 tensions between 15 and 30 mm Hg and unloads its O_2 to the muscle mitochondria only at very low O_2 tensions. Note that fetal hemoglobin also functions at a lower Po_2 than adult hemoglobin (see Fig. 47-5).

Minimum Hemoglobin Concentration.   The American Society of Anesthesiologists (ASA) addressed optimal hemoglobin concentrations in its Practice Guidelines for Blood Component Therapy. The ASA task force reviewed the pertinent literature and made the following recommendations: Transfusion is rarely indicated when hemoglobin values are greater than 10 g/dL and is almost always indicated when values are less than 6 g/dL. Determining whether a transfusion is indicated when the hemoglobin is between 6 and 10 g/dL is based on the risk of tissue hypoxia in the individual patient, as judged by the patient's physician. The organ at highest risk during anemia is normally the heart, because it has a baseline O_2 extraction ratio greater than 50%. In a study evaluating outcomes for critically ill patients transfused to hemoglobins of 7 to 9 g/dL versus greater than 10 g/dL, patients had better outcomes when maintained at the lower range, unless they had clinically significant cardiac disease.

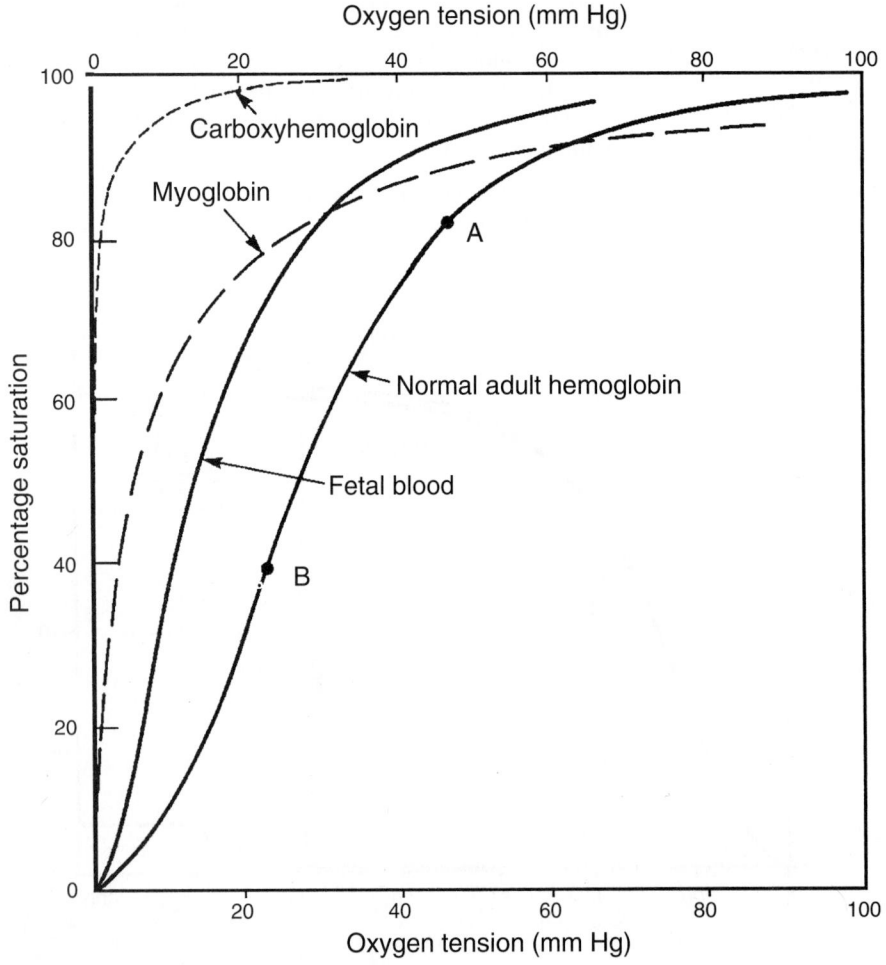

Figure 47–5 ▪ Oxyhemoglobin dissociation curves for adult and fetal hemoglobin and carboxyhemoglobin and myoglobin. Note that fetal hemoglobin and myoglobin function at much lower oxygen tension (Po_2) levels than adult hemoglobin, and carboxyhemoglobin has a very left-shifted curve. (From Lumb AB: Nunn's Applied Respiratory Physiology, 5th ed. London, Butterworth-Heinemann, 2000, p 266.)

CIRCULATORY HYPOXIA

Circulatory hypoxia results from insufficient cardiac output. All conditions that reduce heart rate or stroke volume also reduce cardiac output. However, cardiac output must increase with increased tissue O_2 utilization (O_2 demand). Basal O_2 delivery (DO_2) is about 200 mL O_2 per liter of cardiac output per minute (or 1000 mL O_2 for a cardiac output of 5 L/minute). But what is critical for survival? One study in conscious, resting volunteers reported a rate of 7.5 mL/kg per minute (525 mL/minute for a 70-kg adult). A case report of a Jehovah's Witness patient found critical DO_2 to be 184 mL/minute per square meter.

HISTIOCYTIC HYPOXIA

Histiocytic hypoxia occurs if the cell is unable to use delivered O_2. Cyanide (CN^-) toxicity is a classic example and may occur with the administration of large amounts of sodium nitroprusside. CN^- binds to mitochondrial cytochrome oxidase, disrupting aerobic metabolism and resulting in anaerobic metabolism. Early signs of CN^- toxicity are tachycardia, increased mixed venous O_2 saturation, bright red venous blood, and lactic acidosis. All are due to the inability of tissue to utilize O_2.

Carbon monoxide (CO), in addition to binding to hemoglobin and shifting the oxyhemoglobin curve to the left, binds to cytochrome c and interferes with oxidative metabolism at the mitochondrial level. The high affinity of CO for hemoglobin (200 times that of O_2) requires a high concentration of O_2 (100% at 1 to 3 atmospheres) to effectively treat CO poisoning. The subsequent regeneration of functional cytochrome c by the displacement of CO with O_2 may be the mechanism by which neuronal death is prevented.

Recognition

CYANOSIS

Before the widespread use of pulse oximetry, the early recognition of hypoxemia (PaO_2 <60 mm Hg) was difficult. The presence of cyanotic mucosal membranes or dark blood in the operative field often provided the earliest warning, because the anesthetic agents in use before the availability of SpO_2 measurement tended to attenuate the physiologic (tachycardia, hypertension, tachypnea) and mental status (restlessness, somnolence) changes caused by hypoxia.

Even so, cyanosis is an imprecise monitor of O_2 status, because hemoglobin saturation must be below 85% before cyanosis is clinically apparent. Anemia makes detection even more difficult. More than 50 years ago, Comroe and Botehlo used ear oximetry to assess whether hypoxia was invariably associated with clinical cyanosis. Of 1723 SpO_2 measurements with values between 71% and 80%, 12% were said to be associated with a normal skin color. It is possible that anemia skewed the results in some patients, because 5 g of reduced hemoglobin must be present to allow the detection of cyanosis.

ARTERIAL BLOOD GAS ANALYSIS

The gold standard for the diagnosis of hypoxemia is direct PaO_2 measurement with a Clark electrode; however, this is invasive and is rarely a continuous parameter.

PULSE OXIMETRY

Pulse oximetry provides an early warning of hypoxemia (for SpO_2 from 70% to 100%), *provided that* reduced or oxyhemoglobin is the only hemoglobin present. Carboxyhemoglobin and methemoglobin have similar absorption spectra to oxyhemoglobin and may provide misinformation; in fact, carboxyhemoglobin and oxyhemoglobin are indistinguishable. Pulse oximetry readings are falsely high in the presence of carboxyhemoglobin. As methemoglobin concentrations increase, pulse oximetry readings tend to approach 85%. Fluorescent lighting can also cause a falsely elevated SpO_2. Blue nail polish, tape adhesive, methylene blue, indigo carmine, and isosulfan blue may cause falsely low SpO_2 measurements. A co-oximeter measures the amounts of deoxyhemoglobin, oxyhemoglobin, carboxyhemoglobin, and methemoglobin in a blood sample. Such testing is indicated if SpO_2 readings are dubious (e.g., intravenous dyes have been injected or infiltrated for surgical mapping) or CO poisoning is suspected. One major manufacturer has developed a pulse co-oximeter using eight light wavelengths and capable of measuring deoxyhemoglobin, oxyhemoglobin, carboxyhemoglobin, and methemoglobin.

SPECIFIC ORGANS

Methods used to assess the adequacy of O_2 delivery to organs and tissues are summarized in Table 47-2.

Table 47-2 ■ Methods to Assess the Adequacy of Organ and Tissue Oxygen Delivery

Organ/Tissue	Method
Brain	Cerebral perfusion pressure (CPP = MAP − ICP), transcranial Doppler monitoring, electroencephalography, jugular venous O_2 saturation, near-infrared spectroscopy, SSEPs/MEPs
Heart	Electrocardiography, transesophageal echocardiography, coronary sinus O_2 saturation, pulmonary artery catheter
Lungs	PaO_2/FiO_2 ratio, lung injury score, pulmonary arterial pressures, airway pressures (lung compliance and resistance), bronchoalveolar lavage
Liver, kidneys, gut	Lactate production, hepatic enzymes, urine output and specific gravity, blood urea nitrogen and creatinine, gastric tonometry

CPP, cerebral perfusion pressure; FiO_2, fraction of inspired oxygen; ICP, intracranial pressure; MAP, mean arterial pressure; MEP, motor evoked potential; PaO_2, arterial partial pressure of oxygen; SSEP, somatosensory evoked potential.

Table 47–3 ■ Measures to Reduce the Risk of Perioperative Hypoxia Based on Cause

Cause	Measure
Hypoxemia	Verify O_2 supply (check anesthesia machine), confirm fail-safe function; use in-line O_2 analyzer; preoxygenate; increase FiO_2
Hypoventilation	Confirm breath sounds and end-tidal CO_2; increase FiO_2; assess lung compliance; use bronchodilators; maintain bronchopulmonary toilet
$\dot{V}A/\dot{Q}$ mismatch	Increase FiO_2; restrict volatile agents (inhibit hypoxic pulmonary vasoconstriction)
Shunt	Use larger tidal volumes (10-15 mL/kg), intermittent sighs, frequent suctioning; add PEEP in high-risk patients (low FRC, obesity, hypoalbuminemia)
Diffusion limitation*	Increase FiO_2
Anemia	Evaluate hematocrit frequently; give transfusions; increase FiO_2
Circulatory failure	Increase cardiac output (volume, inotropes, circulatory assist device); relieve surgical compression or traction; increase FiO_2
O_2 utilization	Limit SNP to ≤1 mg/kg over 1-3 hr and 0.5 mg/kg/hr over 24 hr, use another vasodilator[†], or combine another vasodilator or SNP with a β-blocker to reduce the need for SNP; increase FiO_2 (especially with CO poisoning)

*Uncommon cause in healthy patients; may contribute to hypoxia after lung resection in patients with a reduced alveolar capillary bed (emphysema) and high cardiac output (sepsis).

[†]Nicardipine IV may be preferred to SNP owing to the possibility of cyanide toxicity with large doses of the latter (see Chapters 1 and 77).

CO, carbon monoxide; CO_2, carbon dioxide; FiO_2, fraction of inspired oxygen; FRC, functional residual capacity; PEEP, positive end-expiratory pressure; SNP, sodium nitroprusside; $\dot{V}A/\dot{Q}$, alveolar ventilation-perfusion.

Risk Assessment

Inhalational anesthetics reduce the slope of the CO_2-ventilation response curve in direct proportion to dose. Intravenous anesthetics (except ketamine) have the same effect. Inhalational anesthetics and propofol have also been shown to depress the ventilatory response to hypoxia, even at low doses. Functional residual capacity decreases upon the induction of anesthesia and does not return to normal until hours after anesthesia has been terminated. This contributes to atelectasis in alveoli with low $\dot{V}A/\dot{Q}$ ratios. Volatile (but not intravenous) anesthetic agents oppose hypoxic pulmonary vasoconstriction and increase the risk of hypoxia due to $\dot{V}A/\dot{Q}$ mismatch. During recovery, elimination of nitrous oxide lowers PAO_2 for several minutes. Anesthetics also reduce the tone in muscles involved in maintaining pharyngeal patency, increasing the risk of partial or complete airway obstruction. For these reasons, any patient having an anesthetic is at risk for hypoxia.

Patients at increased risk for hypoxia include those with significant cardiopulmonary disease, morbid obesity, major trauma, thromboembolism, sepsis, head injury, pulmonary aspiration, and drug overdose. Risk also increases when diagnostic or therapeutic procedures are performed with the patient under intravenous sedation and inattentive, untrained, or preoccupied personnel are responsible for patient monitoring (e.g., interventional radiology or cardiology, magnetic resonance imaging). The risk for postoperative hypoxia is increased with long-acting anesthetic agents or neuromuscular blockers and with hypothermia or impaired drug metabolism and elimination.

Implications

Severe hypoxia leads to ischemia or death. The central nervous system is most vulnerable to hypoxia (tolerating ≤5 minutes of normothermic ischemia). With hypoxia, anaerobic metabolism replaces aerobic metabolism, with a consequent fall in intracellular high-energy compounds and acidosis.

Insufficient high-energy compounds leads to the failure of intracellular pumps and the release of calcium from intracellular stores, damaging the intracellular elements. Acidosis and consequent anaerobic metabolism of glucose (causing lactic acidosis) produce further cell damage. As noted, the brain is most vulnerable, followed by the heart, the liver, and the kidneys.

MANAGEMENT

- Identify and correct the primary cause.
- Supply supplemental oxygen; increase FiO_2.
- Increase O_2 delivery (transfusion, inotropes, or both).
- Treat $\dot{V}A/\dot{Q}$ mismatch (positive end-expiratory pressure, sighs, inhaled nitric oxide, patient posturing).
- Protect vital organs (hypothermia, drugs, spinal drainage, steroids).
- Administer amyl nitrate, sodium nitrite, or thiosulfate for CN^- toxicity.

PREVENTION

Measures to reduce the risk of perioperative hypoxia from the causes discussed herein are listed in Table 47-3.

Further Reading

Comroe JH, Botehlo S: The unreliability of cyanosis in the recognition of arterial hypoxemia. Am J Med Sci 214:1, 1947.

Comroe JH, Forster RE, Dubois AB, et al: Diffusion. In The Lung: Clinical Physiology and Pulmonary Function Tests, 2nd ed. Chicago, Year Book Medical Publishers, 1962, pp 111-139.

Hall AH: Systemic asphyxiants. In Irwin RS, Rippe JM (eds): Intensive Care Medicine, 5th ed. Philadelphia, JB Lippincott–Williams & Wilkins, 2003, pp 1608-1616.

Herbert PC, Wells G, Blajchman MA, et al: A multicenter, randomized, controlled clinical trial of transfusion requirements in critical care. N Engl J Med 340:409-417, 1999.

Kelly SD, Lieberman J, Feiner JR, et al: Critical oxygen delivery in resting conscious humans is less than 7.5 mL O_2 /kg/min [abstract]. Anesthesiology 87:58, 1997.

Lumb AB: Anaesthesia. In Nunn's Applied Respiratory Physiology, 5th ed. London, Butterworth Heinemann, 2000, pp 420-459.

Lundsgaard C, Van Slyke DD: Cyanosis. Medicine 2:1, 1923.

Martin RL, Lloyd HGE, Cowan AI: The early events of oxygen and glucose deprivation: Setting the scene for neuronal death? Trends Neurosci 17:251-256, 1994.

Moon RE, Camporesi EM: Clinical care at altered environmental pressure. In Miller RD (ed): Anesthesia, 5th ed. Philadelphia, Churchill Livingstone, 2000, pp 2271-2301.

Moon RE, Camporesi EM: Respiratory monitoring. In Miller RD (ed): Anesthesia, 5th ed. Philadelphia, Churchill Livingstone, 2000, pp 1255-1295.

Stehling LC, Doherty DO, Faust RJ, et al: Practice guidelines for blood component therapy. Anesthesiology 84:732-747, 1996.

van Woerkens ECSM, Trouwborst A, van Lanshot JJB: Profound hemodilution: What is the critical hemodilution at which oxygen delivery-dependent oxygen consumption starts in an anesthetized human? Anesth Analg 75:818-821, 1992.

Wilson WC, Shapiro B: Perioperative hypoxia: The clinical spectrum and current oxygen monitoring methodology. Anesth Clin North Am 19:769-812, 2001.

GENERAL ANESTHESIA

Patients with Seizure Disorders

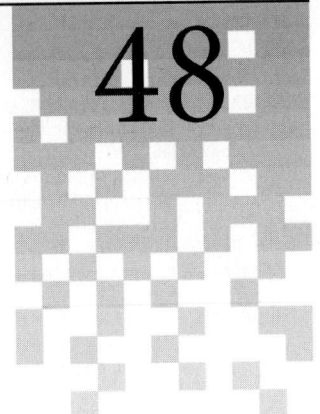

Robert E. Kettler

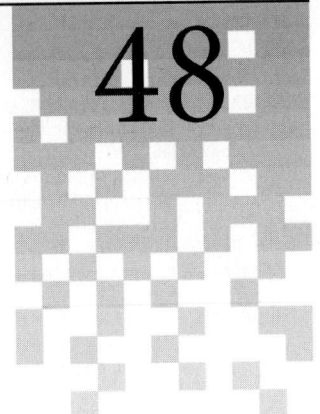

Case Synopsis

A 45-year-old man presents for repair of an inguinal hernia. Other than a history of epilepsy, his past medical history is unremarkable. Except for the inguinal hernia, his physical examination is also unremarkable.

PROBLEM ANALYSIS

Definition

Epilepsy presents clinically as sudden, usually spontaneous episodes of involuntary motor activity with an altered level of consciousness. Epilepsy is a chronic condition. It has an annual incidence of 30 to 55 per 100,000 persons and affects about 2 million people in the United States. In addition, many patients with chronic pain syndromes are treated with anticonvulsants. Thus, anesthesiologists have a high probability of managing patients receiving these drugs.

Epilepsy is classified according to seizure type, which also determines which drug will be used to manage the epileptic syndrome. Partial seizures originate in part of one cerebral hemisphere, whereas more generalized seizures originate throughout the hemispheres. Partial seizures are further classified as follows:

- Simple partial seizures (i.e., with no impairment of level of consciousness)
- Complex partial seizures (i.e., with impairment of level of consciousness)
- Partial seizures that progress to generalized seizures

Generalized seizures are associated with an altered level of consciousness and are further classified as follows:

- Absence seizures
- Myoclonic seizures
- Tonic-clonic seizures
- Atonic seizures

Complex partial seizures are the most common type of seizures in both adult and pediatric epileptic populations, constituting 23% and 39% of seizures in these groups, respectively. Generalized tonic-clonic seizures are second in frequency; this seizure type accounts for 25% of adults and 19% of children with epilepsy.

The pathologic mechanism of epilepsy is unknown; however, several mechanisms have been proposed. It is thought that absence seizures may result from disruption of normal thalamocortical activity. As a result, cortical activity typical of non–rapid eye movement sleep occurs during periods of wakefulness. Such activity may be due to the abnormal function of T-type calcium channel or γ-aminobutyric acid (GABA) receptors. Other more generalized seizures may be caused by an abnormality of the sodium channel, resulting in frequent depolarization. Additional evidence suggests that there is a reduction in potassium channel activity, which also increases the frequency of depolarization. Partial seizures may be due to structural alterations that result in hyperexcitability and altered GABA receptor functioning. The result of these neuronal changes is a pool of neurons that have the following characteristics:

- Increased excitability
- Increased excitatory input
- Increased effectiveness of excitatory input
- Decreased inhibition

Primary physicians caring for patients with epilepsy must evaluate such patients with the goals of (1) determining that the patient does indeed have a seizure disorder, (2) the cause of the disorder, and (3) the type of seizure disorder.

Goals of pharmacotherapy are reduction in seizure frequency, maximization of overall function, and minimal adverse effects. Typically, patients who present with one seizure but have no family history of epilepsy, no history of brain injury or mass lesion, and a normal electroencephalogram (EEG) are not treated. Such patients have only a 24% rate of seizure recurrence in the subsequent 2 years. However, patients who have a second seizure should be treated because the risk of recurrence then rises to 80%. Patients presenting with a new seizure, a history of brain injury or lesion, and an abnormal EEG have a 65% chance of recurrence in 2 years; therefore, these patients receive treatment.

Most patients can be adequately managed with one drug. The principles that guide therapy are (1) the slow titration of medications to attain satisfactory seizure control, or (2) increased doses of medication until, in the absence of any appreciable effect on seizures, unacceptable side effects occur. If one medication fails, the physician should try a drug with a different mechanism of action rather than one with the same mechanism. If several trials of monotherapy are ineffective, polydrug therapy is a reasonable option.

The risk of congenital anomalies is apparently increased in offspring of epileptic women, but extant studies contain a number of methodologic flaws. The presumption that antiepileptic drugs cause such anomalies is based on the observations that (1) a dose-response relationship seems to exist, and (2) multidrug therapy seems to increase the frequency of seizures owing to decreased serum levels of anticonvulsant drugs caused by the physiologic changes of pregnancy. Therefore, it is prudent to monitor serum drug concentrations in pregnant women. Also, pregnant women taking antiepileptic medications appear to be at 1.5- to 3-fold greater risk for hemorrhage, preterm labor, toxemia, placental abruption, and stillbirth than normal parturients.

Recognition

No data exist regarding the incidence of epilepsy that first presents in the perioperative period. It is likely that the vast majority of patients with seizure disorders (aside from those associated with local anesthetic systemic toxicity; see Chapter 56) have been diagnosed and placed on antiseizure medications before they present for elective surgery. The history should suffice for recognizing the presence of epilepsy and assessing the patient's compliance with the prescribed therapy. However, it is useful to query these patients about seizure frequency, known triggers, compliance with medications and dosing, and side effects of antiseizure medications.

Risk Assessment

Patients with epilepsy have a mortality rate about 20 times that of the general population. Causes of death include accidents, arrhythmias, pulmonary edema, and myocardial infarction. Perioperative risk of morbidity and mortality has not been quantified with rigorous methodology. Likely, the most important consideration is to maintain the best possible control of seizure activity by maintaining appropriate antiepileptic therapy during the perioperative period.

Antiepileptic medications typically have sedative effects, which could affect the speed of the patient's recovery from general anesthesia, opiates, or sedative-hypnotics. Many of the anticonvulsants interfere with the hepatic metabolism of other drugs, and anesthesiologists must be aware of this issue. The drugs gabapentin, levetiracetam, tiagabine, and topiramate are less likely to affect hepatic metabolism.

Finally, anesthesiologists may be called on to assist with the management of patients in status epilepticus (especially those with airway and cardiovascular issues). Patients in status epilepticus can have a very high mortality (10% to 30%) when not properly managed.

Implications

Because of the prevalence of epilepsy and the increased use of anticonvulsants to manage various pain syndromes, anesthesiologists are likely to care for patients receiving anticonvulsants. Though unquantified, the risk of adverse outcomes in these patients is likely low. Awareness of the potential problems and use of the measures outlined in the next section are probably sufficient. There are no data to support the notion that one anesthetic technique is preferable to another.

MANAGEMENT AND PREVENTION

Anesthesiologists should evaluate patients' compliance with antiepileptic therapy and its effectiveness with a careful history.

A patient's report of the success of therapy is more meaningful than serum concentrations of the drugs used; the latter are used to evaluate compliance with therapy. Patients should take their usual medications with a sip of water before surgery and resume their regimens as soon as possible after surgery. If patients are unable to take oral medications, tablets can be crushed and given via a gastric tube. Consultation with a pharmacist may be necessary. If the enteric route is inappropriate, consider administering a parenteral form or substituting a comparable parenteral agent. Consultation with a neurologist may be needed. Because pain and sleep deprivation may provoke seizures, adequate pain management, combined with sedatives and anxiolytics, may be beneficial during the perioperative period.

Anesthesiologists may be called on to assist with the management of status epilepticus. They have the necessary expertise in airway management, ventilation, intravascular line placement, cardiopulmonary monitoring, assessment and management of acid-base derangements, and use of neuromuscular blockade. It is important to keep in mind that untreated electrical brain activity can be associated with morbidity, even without seizure-related motor activity.

When standard anticonvulsants fail to control status epilepticus, the anesthesiologist may have to administer general anesthesia with either midazolam or propofol. Effective general anesthesia for status epilepticus is induced with intravenous midazolam in a dose of 0.2 mg/kg and an intravenous maintenance dose of 0.75 to 10 µg/kg per minute. If propofol is used, it is induced with 1 to 2 mg/kg intravenously and maintained at 10 mg/kg per hour intravenously. The EEG is used to monitor the therapeutic effectiveness of either drug. If midazolam and propofol are ineffective, continuous intravenous thiopental or pentobarbital may be necessary. Patients under general anesthesia may require aggressive intravenous fluid therapy and hemodynamic support with dopamine or dobutamine to maintain adequate vital organ perfusion.

Further Reading

Brodie MJ, Dichter MA: Antiepileptic drugs. N Engl J Med 334:168-175, 1996.

Broune TR, Holmes GR: Epilepsy. N Engl J Med 344:1145-1151, 2001.

Chang BS, Lowenstein DH: Epilepsy. N Engl J Med 349:1257-1266, 2003.

Dichter MA, Brodie MJ: New antiepileptic drugs. N Engl J Med 334: 1583-1590, 1996.

Lowenstein DH, Alldredge BK: Status epilepticus. N Engl J Med 338: 970-976, 1998.

McNamara JC: Drugs effective in the therapy of the epilepsies. In Hardman JG, Limbird LE (eds): Goodman and Gilman's The Pharmacological Basis of Therapeutics, 10th ed. New York, McGraw-Hill, 2001, pp 521-547.

Pedley TA: The epilepsies. In Goldman L, Bennett JC (eds): Cecil Textbook of Medicine, 21st ed. Philadelphia, WB Saunders, 2000, pp 2151-2163.

Rowbotham MC, Petersen KL: Anticonvulsants and local anesthetic drugs. In Loeser JD, Butler SH, Chapman CR, Turk DC (eds): Bonica's Management of Pain, 3rd ed. Philadelphia, JB Lippincott–Williams & Wilkins, 2001, pp 1727-1735.

Blood and Blood Products: Transfusion Reaction

49

Lester T. Proctor

Case Synopsis

A 40-year-old woman undergoing an abdominal hysterectomy receives a unit of blood for a hematocrit of 24. Shortly after the transfusion begins, the patient's blood pressure decreases by 20 mm Hg. The urine is noted to be bloody.

PROBLEM ANALYSIS

Definition

Transfusion reactions are broadly defined as any unfavorable consequence of blood transfusion. This chapter addresses primarily transfusion reactions that are immune mediated (Table 49-1).

Recognition

When the transfusion of blood or a blood product is associated with fever, chills, flank pain, hemodynamic instability, wheals, nausea, and symptoms of anaphylaxis, this suggests the occurrence of a transfusion reaction. Certain symptoms (fever, chills, dyspnea, urticaria) can be helpful in delineating the type of reaction involved (Table 49-2). The identification of a transfusion reaction may be more challenging in anesthetized patients, when the only obvious symptoms may be hypotension, hemoglobinuria, or a bleeding diathesis. The features of the major immune-mediated transfusion reactions are noted in Table 49-3 and discussed individually in the paragraphs that follow.

ACUTE HEMOLYTIC TRANSFUSION REACTION

Acute hemolytic transfusion reactions (AHTRs) result from the binding of donor red blood cell antigens with recipient antibodies to form immune complexes. Complexes trigger the fixing of complement to red cell membranes, resulting in hemolysis and the release of cellular debris, which may trigger the development of disseminated intravascular hemolysis. Immune complexes also induce the formation of cytokines, which results in hypotension, fever, and the mobilization and activation of leukocytes. The elaboration of sympathetic amines in response to hypotension contributes to renal failure by renal vasoconstriction.

AHTRs usually involve antibodies to antigens from the ABO blood group. Because these antibodies are readily identifiable, most AHTRs are the result of clerical errors. Symptoms of an AHTR, especially those occurring while a patient is anesthetized, are limited to hemoglobinuria, hemodynamic instability, bleeding diathesis, and failure to achieve the expected rise in hematocrit. A positive direct antiglobulin (Coombs') test confirms the diagnosis. In contrast, evidence of hemolysis (e.g., hemoglobinuria, high free serum hemoglobin, low serum haptoglobin) with a negative direct Coombs' test suggests hemolysis from a nonimmune cause (Table 49-4).

FEBRILE NONHEMOLYTIC TRANSFUSION REACTION

Febrile nonhemolytic transfusion reactions (FNTRs) present as a temperature increase of at least 1°C associated with

---

Table 49–1 ■ Immune-Mediated Transfusion Reactions

Acute
Hemolytic
Nonhemolytic
  Febrile
  Allergic: anaphylactoid (immediate generalized reaction) or anaphylactic
  Transfusion-related acute lung injury

Delayed
Hemolytic

Table 49–2 ■ Determination of Transfusion Reaction Type by Presenting Symptom

Fever or chills
  Hemolytic transfusion reaction: acute or delayed
  Bacterial contamination of blood product
  Febrile nonhemolytic reaction
Hemolysis (may present as hemoglobinuria)
  Acute hemolytic transfusion reaction
  Bacterial contamination of blood product
Dyspnea
  Anaphylactic reaction
  Transfusion-related acute lung injury
  Congestive heart failure or volume overload
Urticaria
  Urticarial transfusion reaction

Adapted from Welborn JL, Hersch J: Blood transfusion reactions: Which are life-threatening and which are not? Postgrad Med 90:125-138, 1991.

Table 49–3 ■ Nonimmune-Mediated Causes of Hemolysis

Type	Cause	Characteristics	Incidence per Unit	Mortality
Acute hemolytic transfusion reaction	Recipient Ab vs donor RBC Ag	Hemolysis, hypotension, DIC, hypoperfusion, renal failure, fever	1 in 25,000	10%
Febrile nonhemolytic transfusion reaction	Recipient Ab vs donor granulocyte Ag	Fever	1 in 200	None reported
Allergic reaction	Recipient Ab vs donor Ag	IGR: hives only Anaphylactic: potentially severe hypotension and bronchospasm	Urticaria: 1 in 200 Anaphylaxis: 1 in 150,000	Rare
Transfusion-related acute lung injury	Donor Ab vs recipient leukocyte Ag	Respiratory distress with noncardiogenic pulmonary edema	1 in 2400	5%
Delayed hemolytic transfusion reaction	Recipient Ab vs donor RBC Ag	Fever, jaundice, decreasing hemoglobin	1 in 2500	Rare

Ab, antibody; Ag, antigen; DIC, disseminated intravascular coagulation; IGR, immediate generalized reaction; RBC, red blood cell.

a transfusion and without any other explanation. FNTRs are usually caused by binding of the recipient's antibodies to antigens on donor granulocytes, lymphocytes, or platelets. An FNTR often presents with chills and rigor and is a diagnosis of exclusion once AHTR and bacterial contamination of transfused blood are ruled out.

ALLERGIC REACTION

Allergic reactions are either immunoglobulin E (IgE) mediated (anaphylactic) or not IgE mediated (anaphylactoid or immediate generalized reaction; see Chapter 27). Immediate generalized reactions are typically mild, involving reactions to transfused serum proteins, medications taken by the donor (e.g., penicillin), or additives from blood product preparation. Diagnosis is based on the presence of only mild allergic symptoms that respond to an antihistamine.

Anaphylactic reactions are typically more severe in presentation and usually manifest within minutes after the transfusion begins. Symptoms include shock, respiratory distress, dermatologic findings, and generalized enteritis, usually in the absence of fever. Although most such reactions commence immediately after the transfusion begins, the presentation may be delayed for up to an hour after the transfusion has been completed. Anaphylactic reactions are most commonly mounted by patients who lack immunoglobulin A (IgA) but have an anti-IgA antibody. IgA deficiency occurs in 1 in 700 patients in the general population, although only 20% of IgA-deficient patients develop antibodies to IgA. Of these, only 20% have clinically significant reactions. The diagnosis is usually based on the striking presentation and confirmed by finding anti-IgA antibody in the patient's serum.

Table 49–4 ■ Nonimmune-Mediated Causes of Hemolysis

Mechanical trauma to red blood cells
  Thermal injury
    Overheating (>40°C)
    Freezing or partial freezing
  Osmotic injury
    Sterile water for bladder irrigation during cystoscopy
    Reconstitution of red blood cells with nonisotonic solutions
  Shearing injury
    High-pressure infusion or small catheter size
    Mechanical valves, vascular grafts, hematomas
    Extracorporeal circulation
Bacterial contamination (gram-negative bacteremia)
Drug-induced hemolysis: penicillin, quinidine, methyldopa
Disease-mediated hemolysis
  Hemolytic anemias: glucose-6-phosphate dehydrogenase deficiency, autoimmune anemias
  Paroxysmal nocturnal hemoglobinuria; hemolytic uremic syndrome
  Thrombotic thrombocytopenic purpura; malaria; mononucleosis
  Sepsis with disseminated intravascular coagulation

Modified from Cooper CL: Complications of transfusion therapy. In Lake CL, Moore RA (eds): Blood: Hemostasis, Transfusion, and Alternatives in the Perioperative Period. New York, Raven Press, 1995, p 320.

TRANSFUSION-RELATED ACUTE LUNG INJURY

Transfusion-related acute lung injury (TRALI) presents as a syndrome of respiratory distress, fever, hypoxia, hypotension, and noncardiogenic pulmonary edema that occurs 1 to 6 hours after the transfusion of plasma containing blood products. The proposed mechanism involves the reaction between the donor's antibodies and the recipient's leukocytes. Cytokines present in the donated unit may also augment this response. An aggressive search for cardiogenic or other noncardiogenic sources of pulmonary edema must be undertaken, because TRALI is relatively rare. The diagnosis may be confirmed by identifying an antileukocyte antibody in the donor blood unit that corresponds to the patient's human leukocyte antigen type.

DELAYED HEMOLYTIC TRANSFUSION REACTION

Delayed hemolytic transfusion reactions (DHTRs) present with red blood cell hemolysis from 2 days to several months after a transfusion. Symptoms and signs include fever, mild jaundice, and an inexplicable decline in hemoglobin concentration. Other serious symptoms, more typical of an AHTR (e.g., renal failure, hemoglobinuria), are uncommon.

DHTRs commonly result in postoperative jaundice and may significantly lower the patient's hemoglobin level. The cause of DHTRs is the delayed generation of an antibody to a donor antigen to which the recipient has been previously exposed. The culprit antibody binds a non-ABO group such as the Rh, Kidd, Kell, or Duffy groups. The diagnosis of a DHTR may be difficult. A direct antiglobulin test is not positive until several days after the transfusion and then remains positive only while there are active symptoms.

Risk Assessment

The risk of developing a transfusion reaction varies, depending on the type of reaction.

An AHTR typically results from an antibody against an antigen of the ABO blood group. Because antibodies to the ABO group are readily identifiable, an AHTR is usually the result of a clerical error, typically involving the administration of a unit of blood to a patient without confirming the patient's identification. Careful attention to paperwork, especially during multiple-unit transfusions, should reduce the incidence of AHTRs.

FNTRs occur more frequently in multiparous women and in patients who have received multiple transfusions, because antibody production is induced by prior exposure to foreign antigens. It has been estimated that up to 55% of women develop leukoagglutinins after three pregnancies.

Allergic reactions can occur in any patient, although certain groups of patients are at higher risk than others. The most severe reactions are noted in IgA-deficient patients. Most of these persons are genetically deficient in IgA, although some with common variable immune deficiency who receive multiple gamma globulin injections may also develop anti-IgA antibodies. Less severe reactions are typical of non-IgA-deficient patients. Renal dialysis patients are particularly prone to allergic reactions because they may develop a sensitivity to sterilizers or plasticizers found in dialysis equipment and react to these substances in transfusion equipment. Atopic patients are more sensitive to vasoactive substances released during reactions, and they manifest more clinically significant reactions than do nonatopic individuals.

TRALI does not appear to be any more common in one patient population than another. Screening of donor serum is discussed under the section on prevention.

DHTRs occur almost exclusively in patients who have undergone multiple transfusions in the past or in multiparous women. In most cases, these individuals have become sensitized to non-ABO blood groups that are undetectable in the serum until after the patient has been re-exposed to the antigen via transfusion.

Implications

The risk of death associated with the major immune-mediated transfusion reactions is given in Table 49-3. The majority of transfusion-related deaths are related to AHTRs. It is estimated that 1 out of 33,000 transfused units of blood are incompatible. This estimate predicts a mortality of 20 deaths per year due to AHTRs in the United States. TRALI is a rare complication but results in an estimated 5% mortality. FNTRs and allergic reactions rarely result in death.

MANAGEMENT

Management of transfusion reactions varies with the type of reaction. Often the clinician must base therapy on only one or two symptoms. The management of any reaction begins by stopping the transfusion while maintaining intravenous access. Next, the type of reaction must be identified. This section outlines an appropriate diagnostic plan based on the presenting symptom. Once the type of transfusion reaction has been identified, more specific therapy can be applied. Therapies for immune-mediated transfusion reactions are given in Table 49-5.

Fever and Chills

Fever and chills, the most common presenting symptoms of a transfusion reaction, are usually due to an FNTR, AHTR, or sepsis from bacterial contamination. The primary goal is to rule out an AHTR by (1) confirming that the patient is receiving the intended unit of blood and (2) drawing a sample of the patient's blood for a free hemoglobin and direct antiglobulin (Coombs') test. Ruling out septic contamination requires (1) examination of the unit for discoloration or gas and (2) stain and culture for bacteria in the transfused blood and the patient's blood. In the absence of positive results, the diagnosis of exclusion is FNTR. The occurrence of hemoglobinuria, hypotension, or bleeding diathesis should prompt a second look for AHTR or septic contamination, because these findings are not characteristic of FNTR.

Hemoglobinuria

Hemoglobinuria may be the sole indicator of a transfusion reaction, and its presence should prompt a search for evidence of hemolysis, which may be caused by an AHTR, bacterial contamination, or a nonimmune-mediated source (see Table 49-4). Hemolysis in the absence of other symptoms is characteristic of a nonimmune-mediated hemolytic cause.

Dyspnea

Dyspnea may be caused by an anaphylactic reaction, cardiogenic pulmonary edema from fluid overload, or (more rarely) TRALI. The management of dyspnea relies less on making the diagnosis than on supportive care for the patient's condition, which may require mechanical ventilation. Invasive monitoring or transesophageal echocardiography to determine whether the cause of the pulmonary edema is cardiogenic or noncardiogenic is often helpful.

Urticaria

Urticaria in the absence of other symptoms is characteristic of an immediate generalized reaction, although the patient should be reevaluated periodically for progression to a full-blown anaphylactic reaction.

Table 49–5 ■ Treatment of Immune-Mediated Transfusion Reactions

Reaction Type	Treatment
Acute hemolytic transfusion reaction (AHTR) with positive direct antiglobulin test	1. Stop the transfusion 2. Maintain systolic blood pressure >100 mm Hg 3. Maintain urine output (diuretics; fluids ≥100 mL/hr) 4. Support blood pressure with pressors as needed 5. Maintain vigilance for DIC and treat as needed
Febrile reaction secondary to bacterial contamination	1. Treat as for AHTR (above) 2. After Gram stain and cultures, cover with broad-spectrum antibiotic for gram-positive and -negative organisms
Febrile nonhemolytic transfusion reaction	1. Stop the transfusion 2. Rule out AHTR and bacterial contamination 3. Administer an antipyretic 4. Consider a leukocyte filter (blood products) or antipyretics before the next transfusion
Allergic: urticarial reaction	1. Stop the transfusion 2. Administer diphenhydramine 20-50 mg IV 3. Restart blood slowly after 30 min 4. Consider giving an antihistamine before the next transfusion
Allergic: anaphylaxis	1. Stop the transfusion 2. Administer epinephrine 400 μg SC 3. Support ventilation; use bronchodilators or intubation if needed 4. Support circulation; administer vasopressors if needed
Transfusion-related acute lung injury	1. Stop the transfusion 2. Rule out cardiogenic pulmonary edema and other sources of noncardiogenic pulmonary edema 3. Support ventilation as needed
Delayed hemolytic transfusion reaction	1. Usually, no acute treatment required 2. Maintain urine output with evidence of renal failure 3. Maintain hemoglobin level with additional transfusions after identifying responsible antibody

DIC, disseminated intravascular coagulation.

Data from Jenner PW, Holland PV: Diagnosis and management of transfusion reactions. In Petz LD, Swisher SN, Kleinman S, et al (eds): Clinical Practice of Transfusion Medicine. New York, Churchill Livingstone, 1996, p 908; and Welborn JL, Hersch J: Blood transfusion reactions: Which are life-threatening and which are not? Postgrad Med 90:125-138, 1991.

PREVENTION

Vigilance and a high index of suspicion lead to early recognition of transfusion reactions and may limit their severity. In addition, specific measures can be taken to reduce the risk of certain immune-mediated transfusion reactions:

- AHTRs are usually the result of misidentification of the patient or the unit of blood. Because one third of all transfusion reactions occur in the operating room, the anesthesiologist should carefully match the patient with the blood unit to limit the risk of AHTR.
- FNTRs may be limited by the use of leukocyte filters to reduce the number of leukocytes in transfused blood. Prophylactic antipyretics may help limit the symptoms.
- Antihistamines can be used before transfusion to pretreat patients with a history of mild allergic reactions. The use of washed blood products is generally reserved for patients who do not benefit from antihistamines.
- Patients with known IgA deficiency should receive blood products from IgA-deficient donors. In an emergency situation, washing of red blood cells or platelets should limit the risk of a fatal reaction.
- TRALI can be prevented if the antibody responsible for the antileukocyte reaction can be determined. If so, the administration of blood products containing this antibody can be avoided.
- DHTRs usually cannot be prevented before the first episode, because the antibody responsible for the reaction is present in undetectable titers. Once a DHTR has occurred, however, and the culprit antibody has been identified, blood with the corresponding antigen should be avoided.

Further Reading

Brand A: Immunological aspects of blood transfusions. Transpl Immunol 10:183-190, 2002.

Cooper CL: Complications of transfusion therapy. In Lake CL, Moore RA (eds): Blood: Hemostasis, Transfusion, and Alternatives in the Perioperative Period. New York, Raven Press, 1995, pp 319-334.

Gilstad CW: Anaphylactic transfusion reactions. Curr Opin Hematol 10:419-423, 2003.

Heddle NM: Universal leukoreduction and acute transfusion reactions: Putting the puzzle together. Transfusion 44:1-4, 2004.

Janatpour K, Holland PV: Noninfectious serious hazards of transfusion. Curr Hematol Rpt 1:149-155, 2002.

Jenner PW, Holland PV: Diagnosis and management of transfusion reactions. In Petz LD, Swisher SN, Kleinman S, et al (eds): Clinical Practice of Transfusion Medicine. New York, Churchill Livingstone, 1996, pp 905-929.

Lozano M, Cid J: The clinical implications of platelet transfusions associated with ABO or Rh(D) incompatibility. Transfus Med Rev 17:57-68, 2003.

Noninfectious Complications of Blood Transfusion. *In* Technical Manual of the American Association of Blood Banks. Bethesda, Md., American Association of Blood Banks, 543-562, 1996.

Sharma AD, Grocott HP: Platelet transfusion reactions: febrile nonhemolytic reaction or bacterial contamination? Diagnosis, detection, and current preventive modalities. J Cardiothorac Vasc Anes 14:460-466, 2000.

Telen MJ: Principles and problems of transfusion in sickle cell disease. Sem Hematol 38:315-323, 2001.

Welborn JL, Hersch J: Blood transfusion reactions: Which are life-threatening and which are not? Postgrad Med 90:125-138, 1991.

Blood and Blood Products: Hepatitis and HIV

50

Jonathan M. Anagnostou

Case Synopsis

An otherwise healthy 40-year-old woman experiences 2000 mL blood loss while undergoing abdominal hysterectomy. She receives 2 units of packed red blood cells during the course of her resuscitation. Following surgery, the patient's husband is very upset that his wife "probably caught something from the blood she received."

PROBLEM ANALYSIS

Definition

Blood-borne infections are a concern of patients, family members, and health care providers alike. Individuals may be exposed to these infections through the transfusion of banked blood products or through blood-contaminated injuries (e.g., needle sticks). Although blood products (especially platelets) can transmit bacterial infections, viral infections are more common. Despite the modern screening of blood products, hepatitis C is a major cause of post-transfusion hepatitis, although hepatitis B remains a clinical concern. Hepatitis D is a blood-borne viral infection that affects only patients infected with hepatitis B, because it requires the hepatitis B virus for replication. Although the parenteral spread of hepatitis A has been reported, it is normally spread through the oral-fecal route. Human immunodeficiency virus (HIV) has become an increasing concern since its recognition in the early 1980s.

Recognition

Given the emotional impact associated with the risk of blood-borne infections, this issue must be put in its proper perspective during the patient's preoperative visit. In the case of any procedure that might involve significant blood loss, a discussion of the potential risks of transfusion should take place. Many hospitals include a separate consent form for blood products in their admission paperwork.

Blood-contaminated injuries to health care providers are another important issue. Each health care facility should have defined infection-control procedures to deal with such events. Although painful needle-stick or scalpel injuries are obvious, practitioners should also recognize that blood seepage under torn or defective gloves onto a preexisting hand wound also constitutes a blood-contaminated injury. Clearly, risks from patient blood contact are significant. In the United States, approximately 0.2% to 0.4% of the population are carriers of the hepatitis B virus, and 0.5% carry hepatitis C. The incidence of HIV infection varies widely from near zero in some areas to well over 5% in certain urban populations.

Following transfusion or other blood exposure, the diagnosis of hepatitis or HIV infection depends on an index of suspicion and the development of viral symptoms weeks to months after exposure. Initial HIV infection is often asymptomatic, although roughly half of infected patients develop a viral syndrome (e.g., fever, pharyngitis, myalgia, lymphadenopathy) within 6 weeks of exposure. Similarly, initial infection with hepatitis B or C may be asymptomatic or may involve a flulike syndrome weeks or even months after exposure. Clinical jaundice develops in less than one third of patients. A chronic infection may result in 10% of those infected with hepatitis B and in up to 80% to 90% of patients with hepatitis C. The development of symptoms consistent with hepatitis (e.g., malaise, jaundice) several weeks after exposure to blood should prompt referral for appropriate hematologic studies, such as hepatic enzyme levels and antigen-antibody testing. Antibody testing for hepatitis B has been available for many years, and similar testing for hepatitis C is now available. Serologic evidence of anti-HIV antibodies by enzyme-linked immunosorbent assay (ELISA) testing confirms HIV infection.

Risk Assessment

The risk of transfusion-related infection is estimated as follows (per unit of blood):

- Hepatitis: 1 in 180,000 to 220,000
- HIV: 1 in 900,000 to 1.4 million

The risk of needle-stick infection is estimated as follows (per incident):

- HIV-positive: 1 in 250 to 300
- Hepatitis C-positive: 1 in 20

Improved blood screening has reduced but not eliminated the risk of transfusion-associated infections. False-negative test results can occur, and in the case of antibody testing (e.g., for HIV), there is an interval between infection with the virus and the appearance of detectable antibodies in blood. It was estimated in 1996 that the risk of transfusion-related hepatitis in the United States was approximately 0.3 per 10,000 units transfused, and the risk of HIV infection from a single transfused blood unit was roughly 1 in 493,000 transfusions.

Blood-contaminated injuries are a significant occupational hazard for health care workers. The risk of infection via a hepatitis C–contaminated needle stick is estimated to be 0.5%, and that for anti-HIV antibody seroconversion after an HIV-contaminated needle stick is approximately 0.004%. The risk of infection may be greater under certain circumstances (e.g., hollow-core needles, large virus inoculum).

Implications

Infections from blood-borne viruses can be benign or lethal, and the emotional impact of blood transfusion can represent a distinct psychological complication. The manifestations of hepatitis range from an asymptomatic infection to fulminant hepatic dysfunction and death. Chronic infection with hepatitis B or C can result in cirrhosis, hepatic failure, or hepatocellular carcinoma. Although HIV infection commonly leads to acquired immunodeficiency syndrome (AIDS), many otherwise healthy individuals remain asymptomatic for years after documented HIV seroconversion.

MANAGEMENT

Management of transfusion-related hepatitis or AIDS is clearly beyond the typical anesthesia provider's scope of practice. Recognition and appropriate referral are of the utmost importance, although transmission of these illnesses is only retrospectively linked with a patient's history of blood product transfusion or a provider's history of occupational exposure.

PREVENTION

Avoiding contact with blood and blood products is the obvious key to prevention. Blood or banked blood products should not be administered as generic volume expanders but should be given only for specific indications, such as to increase oxygen carrying capacity or increase clotting factor levels. The predonation of autologous blood, the use of isovolumic hemodilution, or both may be useful in avoiding exposure to homologous blood products. For practitioners, strict adherence to universal precautions (Table 50-1) should minimize the risk of contact with potentially infectious blood and body fluids. Needle-stick injuries can be minimized by careful operating technique and by the use of alternative equipment when possible (e.g., needleless intravenous injection systems, "blunt" suture needles).

Vaccination is an important preventive measure for many infectious diseases. Although no vaccines are currently available for HIV or hepatitis C, hepatitis B vaccination is strongly advised for high-risk health care providers, including anesthesia personnel. For those who have received the vaccination, no set schedule for booster doses has been established. With the recent recommendation of the U.S. Public Health Service for childhood hepatitis B vaccination, the overall incidence of hepatitis in the United States (including hepatitis D) should continue to decline.

When a blood-contaminated injury occurs, the affected area should be washed immediately with soap and water. Involved mucous membranes are flushed with water or an appropriate salt solution. Injuries contaminated with blood should be reported to the institution's infection-control office for documentation, counseling, and management. There is no accepted postexposure prophylaxis available for hepatitis C, but if the source patient is infected with hepatitis B and the provider has not been immunized, passive immunization with hepatitis immune globulin (0.06 mL/kg intramuscularly), followed by hepatitis B vaccination, is advised.

If the source patient is HIV infected, the initiation of postexposure chemoprophylaxis within 24 to 36 hours may be appropriate to reduce the risk of HIV infection. Although data regarding efficacy are limited, chemoprophylaxis after percutaneous exposure normally includes the use of two or even three antiretroviral drugs (e.g., zidovudine, lamivudine, stavudine, didanosine). In practice, the timely institution of chemoprophylaxis may be complicated if the source patient's HIV status is unknown and by the legal difficulties involved in obtaining informed consent for HIV testing. The National HIV/AIDS Clinician's Consultation Center offers a 24-hour postexposure prophylaxis hotline (1-888-HIV-4911). The Centers for Disease Control and Prevention has current information on its Web site (http://www.cdc.gov/niosh/topics/bbp).

Table 50–1 ■ Highlights of Universal Precautions

Barrier precautions with *all* patients to prevent blood and body fluid contact
    Gloves when contacting blood or body fluids or nonintact skin (do not wash or disinfect gloves, because disinfectants can cause deterioration)
    Gown, mask, eyewear if splash or spray is likely
Avoid sharps injuries
    Prompt disposal in appropriate container
    Avoid recapping needles
Hand washing after glove removal or any blood or body fluid contact
Artificial mouthpieces and airways for cardiopulmonary resuscitation
Providers with exudative or weeping cutaneous lesions should refrain from direct patient contact until condition resolves

From Centers for Disease Control and Prevention: Recommendations for prevention of HIV transmission in the health-care setting. MMWR Morb Mortal Wkly Rep 36:3-18, 1987; updated MMWR Morb Mortal Wkly Rep 37:377-388, 1988.

Further Reading

Centers for Disease Control and Prevention: Updated US Public Health Service guidelines for the management of occupational exposures to HBV, HCV, and HIV and recommendations for postexposure prophylaxis. MMWR Morb Mortal Wkly Rep 50:1-54, 2001.

Goodnough LT: Risks of blood transfusion. Crit Care Med 31:S678-S686, 2003.

Murray DJ: Blood component therapy: Indications and risks. In Rogers MC, Tinker JH, Covino BG, et al (eds): Principles and Practice of Anesthesiology. St. Louis, Mosby–Year Book, 1993, pp 2482-2498.

Ockner RK: Acute viral hepatitis. In Wyngaarden JB, Smith LH Jr, Bennett JC (eds): Cecil Textbook of Medicine. Philadelphia, WB Saunders, 1992, pp 763-771.

Perillo RG, Regenstein FG: Viral and immune hepatitis. In Kelly WN (ed): Textbook of Internal Medicine. Philadelphia, Lippincott-Raven, 1997, pp 822-833.

Petrovitch CT: Hemostasis and hemotherapy. In Barash PG, Cullen BF, Stoelting RK (eds): Clinical Anesthesia, 3rd ed. Philadelphia, Lippincott-Raven, 1997, pp 189-217.

Rehm SJ: Approach to the patient with human immunodeficiency virus exposure. In Kelly WN (ed): Textbook of Internal Medicine. Philadelphia, Lippincott-Raven, 1997, pp 1867-1868.

Schreiber GB, Busch MP, Kleinman SH, et al: The risk of transfusion-transmitted viral infections. N Engl J Med 334:1685-1690, 1996.

GENERAL ANESTHESIA

Nosocomial Infections: Bacterial Pneumonia

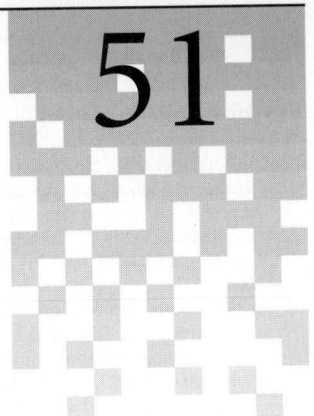

51

Charles E. Edmiston, Jr.

Case Synopsis

A 78-year-old man is diagnosed with pneumonia 4 days after exploratory abdominal laparotomy. While the patient was mechanically ventilated, a fever and purulent tracheal secretions developed. Radiographic evidence was consistent with pneumonia involving both lower lobes.

PROBLEM ANALYSIS

Definition

Nosocomial, or hospital-acquired, pneumonia is defined as pneumonia occurring more than 48 hours after hospital admission. However, this definition excludes any infection that is incubating at the time of hospital admission.

Pneumonia is the second most common nosocomial infection. The proportion of patients who acquire pneumonia in the intensive care unit (ICU) ranges from 10% to 65%. This is associated with significant morbidity and mortality. Data from the National Nosocomial Infection Surveillance program indicate that 75% of all cases of nosocomial bacterial pneumonia occur postoperatively. Patients having a thoracoabdominal procedure have a 38-fold higher risk than other patients do.

Those with mechanically assisted ventilation constitute the population at highest risk for the development of nosocomial pneumonia. Ventilator-associated pneumonia occurs in 8% to 28% of mechanically ventilated patients. Rates of ventilator-associated pneumonia are dependent on the duration of mechanical ventilation; the incremental risk is 1% to 3% per day (5% at 5 days, and >68% for patients ventilated for ≥30 days). Along with causing significant morbidity and mortality, ventilator-associated pneumonia is an important determinant of excessive hospital length of stay and inpatient resource utilization.

The most probable cause of nosocomial pneumonia is colonization of the aerodigestive tract by pathogenic microorganisms. Subsequently, these contaminated secretions are aspirated into the lower airways. Aerobic microorganisms are the predominant isolates recovered, including gram-negative bacilli such as *Escherichia coli*, *Klebsiella* species, *Enterobacter* species, and *Pseudomonas aeruginosa*. *Staphylococcus aureus* and *Streptococcus pneumoniae* are other important isolates and may express drug resistance (e.g., methicillin-resistant *S. aureus* [MRSA], penicillin-resistant pneumococci). Late-onset infections (occurring >72 hours after admission) are most often associated with multidrug-resistant microorganisms such as *Acinetobacter*, *Pseudomonas*, and MRSA. Yeasts such as *Candida albicans* or other *Candida* species are an infrequent cause of nosocomial pneumonia (<4%).

Pneumonia-associated morbidity prolongs hospitalizations by 4 to 9 days and is associated with significant institutional costs. Death from nosocomial pneumonia accounts for 60% of all nosocomial-associated fatalities.

Recognition

Nosocomial bacterial pneumonia is extremely difficult to diagnose, especially in intubated ICU patients with mechanically assisted ventilation. Generally accepted criteria include the following: fever, cough with productive or purulent sputum, and radiographic evidence of a pulmonary infiltrate. The diagnosis of pneumonia in these patients is especially difficult because traditional culture methods may be highly nonspecific or have low sensitivity. Endotracheal aspiration is the most common sampling technique used in mechanically ventilated patients. The accuracy of the method, however, is compromised by contamination with upper respiratory flora.

A consensus recommendation proposed a standardized method for diagnosing pneumonia in this patient population. It is based on direct—rather than clinical—evidence and includes one of the following:

- Bronchoscopically acquired protective specimen brush (PSB) with quantitative culture
- Bronchoalveolar lavage (BAL)
- Protected BAL

The sensitivity of these procedures is reported to vary from 70% to 100%, and their specificity varies from 60% to 100%. PSB is widely accepted as the reference method for pneumonia diagnosis in ventilator patients. False-positive findings have been reported, however, and may be related to prior antibiotic therapy.

Risk Assessment

Tracheal intubation and mechanical ventilation alter the patient's first-line barrier defenses and greatly enhance the risk of nosocomial pneumonia. This risk is 6 to 21 times greater than that for patients who do not receive ventilator support. In addition to a thoracoabdominal procedure or intubation, other risk factors include the following:

- Mean age older than 70 years
- Reintubation or self-extubation

- Depressed level of consciousness (e.g., closed head trauma)
- Underlying chronic lung disease
- Supine head position
- Conditions favoring aspiration or reflux
- 24-hour ventilator circuit changes
- Stress-bleeding prophylaxis with cimetidine (with or without antacid)
- Antimicrobial administration
- Exposure to contaminated respiratory equipment

In addition, manipulation of the ventilator circuit or endotracheal tube increases the potential for cross-contamination. Recent studies have shown that interdisciplinary educational initiatives coupled with appropriate infection-control practices can reduce the risk of cross-contamination.

Implications

The high morbidity and mortality associated with pneumonia in ventilator-dependent patients encourage a more aggressive approach to diagnosis and treatment. Yet invasive bronchoscopic techniques (e.g., PSB, protected BAL) may be associated with complications, including hypoxemia, bleeding, or arrhythmia.

MANAGEMENT

Once the diagnosis of nosocomial pneumonia has been made, the choice of therapeutic agent is based on which organisms are associated with hospital-acquired pneumonia in the specific ICU environment, as well as the sensitivity and resistance patterns of those organisms. Recent studies suggest that selecting an inappropriate antibiotic for the treatment of nosocomial pneumonia is an independent risk factor for mortality, especially with highly resistant gram-negative bacilli (e.g., *Pseudomonas, Acinetobacter*, MRSA). In addition, if the patient received prior antibiotic therapy, it is likely that an extended-spectrum agent will be needed.

Selected empirical antimicrobial agents for the treatment of nosocomial pneumonia include the following:

- Early-onset infections: third- or fourth-generation cephalosporin (ceftriaxone, ceftizoxime, cefepime), β-lactam inhibitor combination (ampicillin-sulbactam or piperacillin-tazobactam), new extended-spectrum fluoroquinolone (moxifloxacin), or aztreonam plus clindamycin
- Late-onset infections: aminoglycoside or fluoroquinolone (ciprofloxacin) plus one of the following: imipenem, antipseudomonal broad-spectrum β-lactam, or aztreonam

A glycopeptide (vancomycin) or oxazolidinone (linezolid) should be added for the treatment of MRSA infection. Recent studies suggest that linezolid for documented MRSA nosocomial pneumonia reduces patient mortality compared with traditional glycopeptide therapy.

Resistant gram-negative pathogens such as *Enterobacter* species have been successfully treated with either imipenem or ciprofloxacin. If *P. aeruginosa* is recovered or suspected, ceftazidime or ciprofloxacin is included. If anaerobic species involvement is suspected, especially in an aspiration-prone patient, the addition of clindamycin is appropriate.

However, the emerging resistance among some anaerobic gram-negative bacteria suggests that a β-lactam inhibitor combination or fourth-generation fluoroquinolone (e.g., moxifloxacin) should be considered.

The rate of MRSA infections in the ICU population continues to increase, and resistance among gram-negative microbial pathogens (e.g., *Klebsiella, E. coli*) to extended-spectrum third-generation cephalosporins is being reported with greater frequency. Therefore, prior knowledge of existing patterns of gram-positive and gram-negative resistance within the ICU is crucial for the development of an appropriate therapeutic strategy for nosocomial pneumonia. Once microbiologic results are available, broad-spectrum antimicrobial therapy should be de-escalated to a specific antimicrobial agent in an effort to minimize the emergence of resistance.

PREVENTION

Prevention of nosocomial pneumonia is complex and requires attention to patient-, device-, and personnel-related factors. The use of antimicrobial prophylaxis to prevent nosocomial pneumonia is highly questionable and may lead to superinfection.

An attempt should be made to prevent microbial colonization of the oropharynx, trachea, and stomach by gram-negative pathogens. For instance, the use of sucralfate rather than antacids or H_2-blockers to prevent stress bleeding in critically ill, postoperative, or mechanically ventilated patients may prevent gastric bacterial overgrowth by preserving gastric acidity.

Other interventions aimed at reducing the risk of postoperative pneumonia include earlier ambulation, deep-breathing exercises, chest physiotherapy, use of incentive spirometry, intermittent positive-pressure breathing, and continuous positive airway pressure by facemask. Simply placing a patient in a semirecumbent position may reduce the aspiration of oropharyngeal secretions with potential nosocomial pathogens. Studies have shown that the longer a patient remains supine, the greater the volume of secretions aspirated. Control of pain in the immediate postoperative period with intravenous or regional analgesia has also been shown to be beneficial in decreasing the incidence of pulmonary complications after surgery.

Bacteria rapidly adhere to biomaterial surfaces. Over time, they can produce a biofilm that is effective at protecting them from antibiotic and host defense mechanisms. These organisms can be dislodged by mechanical ventilatory flow, tube manipulations, or suctioning. Therefore, gentle suctioning and barrier precautions by the caregiver can decrease the incidence of cross-contamination to patients from either contaminated respiratory therapy devices or the hands of health care professionals. Appropriate hand hygiene should be emphasized among health care workers.

For intubated patients, chlorhexidine-based oral hygiene can reduce the risk of endotracheal tube colonization. It is difficult to prevent the pooling of secretions around the endotracheal cuff, but this situation can provide bacteria with direct access to the lower respiratory tract.

The internal machinery of mechanical ventilators is rarely associated with bacterial contamination of inhaled gases.

However, bacterial contamination from the patient's oropharynx or condensate in the inspiratory-limb tubing of the ventilator circuit may occur rapidly after the initiation of mechanical ventilation (33% at 2 hours, and 80% after 24 hours).

Tracheobronchial tree spillage may occur when the endotracheal tube is manipulated. Therefore, less frequent ventilator circuit tube changing (every 24 to 48 hours versus 6 to 8 hours) has been suggested as a way to reduce such contamination.

Further Reading

American Thoracic Society: Hospital-acquired pneumonia in adults: Diagnosis, assessment of severity, initial antimicrobial therapy, and preventive strategies: A consensus statement, American Thoracic Society, November 1995. Am J Respir Crit Care 153:1711-1725, 1996.

Babcock HM, Zack JE, Garrison T, et al: An educational intervention to reduce ventilator-associated pneumonia in an integrated health system. Chest 125:224-231, 2004.

Croce MA, Fabian TC, Stewart RM, et al: Empiric monotherapy versus combination therapy of nosocomial pneumonia in trauma patients. J Trauma 35:303-309, 1993.

Eggimann P, Hugonnet S, Sax H, et al: Ventilator-associated pneumonia: Caveats for benchmarking. Intensive Care Med 29:2086-2089, 2003.

Guidelines for prevention of nosocomial pneumonia. MMWR Morb Mortal Wkly Rep RR-I:1-79, 1997.

Hoffken G, Niedermann MS: Nosocomial pneumonia: The importance of a de-escalating strategy for antibiotic treatment of pneumonia in the ICU. Chest 122:2183-2196, 2002.

Leroy O, Soubrier S: Hospital-acquired pneumonia: Risk factors, clinical features, management and antibiotic resistance. Curr Opin Pulm Med 10:171-175, 2004.

Pringleton SK, Fagon J-Y, Leeper KV: Patient selection for the clinical investigation of ventilator-associated pneumonia: Criteria for evaluating diagnostic technique. Chest 102(Suppl 5):553S-556S, 1992.

Pugin J, Auckenthaler R, Lew DP, et al: Oropharyngeal decontamination decreases incidence of ventilator-associated pneumonia. JAMA 265:2704-2710, 2001.

Sanford JP, Gilbert DN, Sande M: The Sanford Guide to Antimicrobial Therapy, 25th ed. Dallas, Antimicrobial Therapy Inc, 1996, pp 26-28.

Postobstruction Pulmonary Edema

Kenneth W. Travis and John L. Atlee

52

Case Synopsis

Progressive Respiratory Distress

After 3 days of malaise and fever, a 5-year-old, 16-kg girl develops a barking cough, stridor, and progressive respiratory distress. Her respiratory rate is 32 breaths per minute. Lung auscultation reveals reduced breath sounds and coarse rales. Her room air oxygen (O_2) saturation is 82%, and the chest radiograph shows bilateral infiltrates.

Postextubation Stridor

A 22-year-old, 90-kg triathlete has marked inspiratory stridor lasting about 1 minute after tracheal extubation in the operating room, after an otherwise uneventful general anesthetic for septorhinoplasty. Within 15 minutes, he has tachycardia and tachypnea, with forced exhalations. His O_2 saturation is 88% while breathing O_2 via facemask at 6 L/minute.

PROBLEM ANALYSIS

Definition

Acute pulmonary edema that develops during or shortly after relief of severe upper airway obstruction is called postobstruction or negative-pressure pulmonary edema. The precipitating event is the generation of extreme negative intrapleural pressure, which increases the pulmonary transvascular hydrostatic pressure gradient (Table 52-1). In addition, associated hypoxia, catecholamine excess, exaggerated hemodynamic changes, and increased pulmonary vascular permeability disrupt the dynamic fluid equilibrium in the lung (Figs. 52-1 and 52-2). The accelerated movement of fluid from the pulmonary vasculature to the interstitium eventually exceeds the clearing capacity of the pulmonary lymphatic system, and the alveolar epithelial barrier becomes compromised; alveolar flooding is the end result. Owing to the rapidity and the severe pathophysiology associated with postobstruction pulmonary edema (POPE), prompt recognition and management of the condition are mandatory.

Recognition

PRESENTATION

POPE is suspected in the following situations:

- A child (see also Chapter 157) or adult has hypoxemia, prolonged expiration, wheezing, and rales, with or without signs of bilateral pulmonary infiltrates.
- Pink, frothy tracheal secretions accumulate suddenly after tracheal intubation for acute or chronic upper airway obstruction.
- Oxygenation deteriorates after resolution of acute laryngospasm or removal of a foreign body (see Table 52-1).

Usually, POPE develops immediately or within minutes after intubation or extubation of the trachea. Sometimes, however, symptoms and signs of POPE do not appear for several hours, prompting some physicians to advise up to 18 hours of close surveillance for patients who have had significant perioperative or out-of-hospital obstructive events.

NOTABLE FINDINGS

In the most severe cases, the voluminous pulmonary edema fluid is pink and frothy and high in protein content. The chest radiograph frequently reveals bilateral, perihilar, patchy infiltrates and edema around the major pulmonary arteries. These arteries are believed to have endothelial damage as a result of high intravascular volumes and pressures.

TIME COURSE

In general, the more rapid the onset of the obstruction, the more severe the associated acute pulmonary edema. It has been postulated that patients with fixed upper airway obstruction, in whom the negative inspiratory forces are largely compensated for by forced expiration (Valsalva's maneuver) or the development of air trapping (which causes increased positive end-expiratory pressure—auto-PEEP), are more likely to develop pulmonary edema following relief of the obstruction. Patients with variable upper airway obstruction that is more severe during inspiration are more prone to develop pulmonary edema during the obstruction.

DIFFERENTIAL DIAGNOSIS

With prompt treatment, POPE usually resolves within 12 to 24 hours, but recovery may take as long as 96 hours. Many mild cases probably go undetected. Common differential diagnoses include aspiration pneumonitis and other causes of increased capillary permeability edema (e.g., fat or amniotic

Table 52–1 ■ Mechanisms, Recognition, and Management of Postobstruction Pulmonary Edema

Mechanism	Recognition	Management

Severe upper airway obstruction:
    Partial or complete laryngospasm
    Upper airway tumor or foreign body
    Relaxed tongue or other
        oropharyngeal soft tissue structure
    Hypertrophy of tonsils or adenoids
    Croup or epiglottitis
	Airway-related causes:
	    Inspiratory stridor
	    Wheezing
	    Barking cough
	    Emesis (aspiration pneumonitis)
		Ensure and maintain patent airway:
		    Insert naso- or oropharyngeal airway
		    Insert laryngeal mask airway
		    Suction or remove upper airway secretions, blood,
		        vomit, particulate matter, foreign body
		    Perform endotracheal intubation or reintubation
		    Perform cricothyrotomy or tracheostomy

Extremely negative intrapleural
    pressures:
    Increased pulmonary transvascular
        hydrostatic pressure gradient
    Hypoxia, hypercarbia, acidosis:
        associated vasoconstriction of
        the pulmonary bed leads to
        myocardial depression and
        increased capillary permeability
    Hyperadrenergic state: peripheral
        arterial or venous constriction
        leads to increased preload or
        afterload, "forward heart failure,"
        increased capillary permeability
	Pulmonary edema with airway
	    obstruction:
	    Variable obstruction (most severe
	        with inspiration)
	    Hypoxia, rales, prolonged expiration,
	        wheezing
	    Chest radiograph—perihilar,
	        fluffy (patchy) infiltrates
		Respiratory management:
		    Ensure adequate oxygenation and ventilation
		    Increase Fio_2
		    Facial, endotracheal or tracheal CPAP
		    Mechanical ventilation with pressure support or PEEP

Associated hemodynamic changes:
    Marked increase in venous return
        to RV
    Ventricular interdependence
    Reduced LV compliance
    Increased RV and LV
        preload and afterload
    Reduced LV stroke volume
    Increased pulmonary vascular
        volume and pressure
    Increased alveolar interstitial fluid
	Pulmonary edema after relief of
	    upper airway obstruction:
	    Fixed obstruction compensated
	        by Valsalva's maneuver or
	        auto-PEEP
	    Florid, pink, frothy, proteinaceous
	        ("cotton candy") airway fluids
	    Onset can be immediate, within
	        minutes after relief of obstruction,
	        or delayed (hours)
	    Progressive respiratory distress
	    Chest radiograph—often shows
	        bilateral infiltrates
		Additional measures:
		    IV sedation and muscle relaxants
		    Diuretics; vasoactive medications
		    Invasive cardiovascular monitoring
		    Specific therapy directed at cause
		    Indicated therapy for complications
		    Admission to an appropriate facility for postevent
		        observation and treatment

Other pathophysiologic mechanisms:
    Pulmonary lymphatic system
        overwhelmed
    Alveolar epithelial barrier breached
    Alveolar flooding
	Common differential diagnoses:
	    Aspiration pneumonitis
	    Iatrogenic fluid overload
	    Cardiogenic fulminant heart failure	

CPAP, continuous positive airway pressure; Fio_2, fraction of inspired oxygen; LV, left ventricle; PEEP, positive end-expiratory pressure; RV, right ventricle.

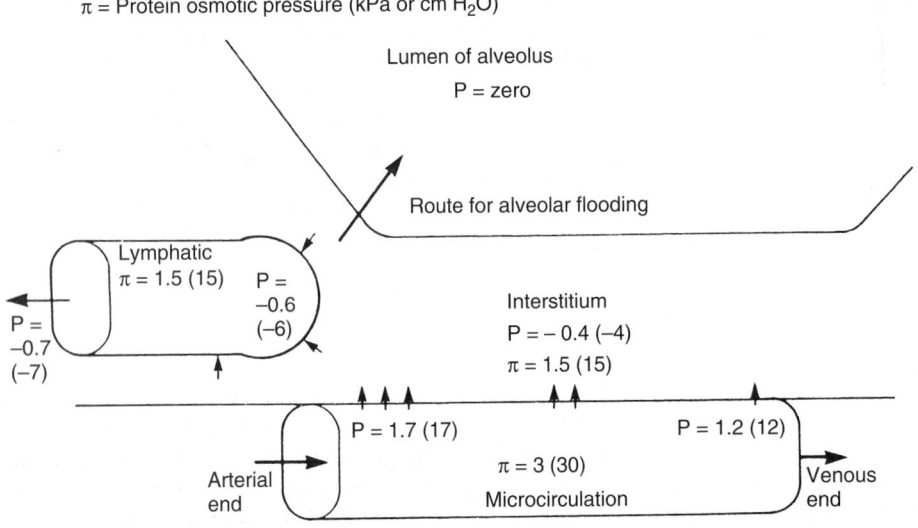

P = Hydrostatic pressure (kPa or cm H_2O) – relative to atmosphere

π = Protein osmotic pressure (kPa or cm H_2O)

Lumen of alveolus

P = zero

Route for alveolar flooding

Lymphatic
π = 1.5 (15)   P = –0.6 (–6)

P = –0.7 (–7)

Interstitium
P = – 0.4 (–4)
π = 1.5 (15)

P = 1.7 (17)

P = 1.2 (12)

Arterial end

π = 3 (30)
Microcirculation

Venous end

Figure 52–1 ■ The Starling equation describes fluid flux in pulmonary capillaries: $Q = K [(P_{mv} – P_{pmv}) – \Sigma(\pi mv – \pi pmv)]$, where K is the hydraulic conductance, P_{mv} is the hydrostatic pressure in the microvasculature, P_{pmv} is the hydrostatic pressure in perivascular tissue (interstitium), Σ is the reflection coefficient for albumin, πmv is the osmotic pressure within the microvasculature, and πpmv is the osmotic pressure in the perimicrovascular tissue. Extremely negative intrapleural pressure increases the pulmonary transvascular hydrostatic gradient. (Modified from Nunn JF: Nunn's Applied Respiratory Physiology, 4th ed. Oxford, Butterworth-Heinemann, 1993, p 487.)

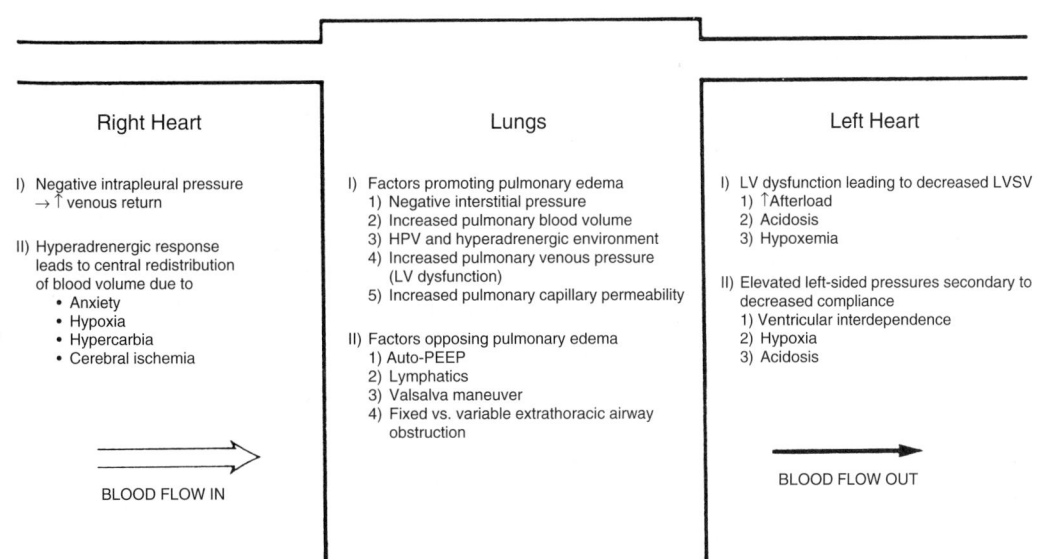

Figure 52–2 ▪ Hypoxia causes pulmonary vasoconstriction, increased capillary permeability, and myocardial depression. The hyperadrenergic state, which results from hypoxia, anxiety, hypercarbia, acidosis, and cerebral ischemia, favors a central redistribution of blood volume. This, combined with the markedly negative intrapleural pressure during inspiration, dramatically increases venous return to the right ventricle (RV) and afterload stress to both the RV and the left ventricle (LV). Increased right ventricular volumes and pressures also cause a leftward shift of the interventricular septum. This reduces left ventricular compliance (ventricular interdependence) and raises end-diastolic and pulmonary microvascular pressures. Hypoxia, hypercarbia, and acidosis contribute to left ventricular dysfunction. Reduced left ventricular stroke volume causes a further rise in pulmonary blood volume and vascular pressure, which mechanically increases the transudation of fluid into the alveolar interstitium. When the rate of interstitial fluid flux exceeds the capacity of lymphatic clearance mechanisms, discontinuities appear in the alveolar epithelial cells, accompanied by crescentic alveolar fluid filling, flooding, and atelectasis. (Modified from Lang SA, Duncan PG, Shephard DAE, et al: Pulmonary oedema associated with airway obstruction. Can J Anaesth 37:213, 1990.)

fluid embolism, sepsis, cardiogenic causes, iatrogenic fluid overload). Acute pulmonary edema has also been reported in patients with head injury, heroin or other narcotic overdose, overly abrupt reversal of intraoperative narcotics (e.g., using 400 μg of naloxone as opposed to 20- to 40-μg increments), venous air embolism, pulmonary embolectomy, and high-altitude exposure. Usually, careful review of the patient's past medical history and temporal events points to a cause. However, if it is still unclear, echocardiography, invasive hemodynamic monitoring, or both may be needed to rule out other causes. Patients with POPE have shown normal hemodynamic measurements after relief of upper airway obstruction. Other causes of extremely negative pulmonary interstitial pressures and pulmonary edema are rapid expansion of a collapsed lung and overly aggressive pleural suctioning during chest tube thoracentesis.

Risk Assessment

Anyone strong enough to generate significant sustained negative intrapleural pressure against a closed glottis (Müller's maneuver) or severely restricted upper airway is at risk for the development of POPE. This condition more commonly occurs in younger, healthy patients. Although the exact incidence is unknown, it is estimated that 11% to 12% of adult or pediatric patients who require urgent tracheal intubation or tracheostomy due to upper airway obstruction of various causes have associated POPE. Laryngospasm during emergence from general anesthesia accounts for 50% of reported cases in adults. In children younger than 10 years old,

croup and epiglottitis are associated with more than half the reported cases of POPE.

Implications

In most instances, establishment of a patent airway improves the clinical condition of patients with significant upper airway obstruction. The dramatic appearance of pulmonary edema before, during, or after the relief of upper airway obstruction in a previously healthy individual is, to say the least, disconcerting. Further, without prompt recognition and treatment, it can lead to severe morbidity. However, it is important to remember that when POPE occurs in such patients and is appropriately managed, it is usually self-limited. If so, staff, family, and friends can be reassured that there is likely to be a favorable outcome and that the problem is unlikely to recur.

MANAGEMENT

After recognition, management includes maintenance of a patent airway and the provision of adequate arterial oxygenation. Supplemental O_2 is required, with or without continuous positive airway pressure (CPAP) or mechanical ventilation with PEEP (see Table 52-1). Tracheal intubation or reintubation is necessary to sustain the airway in 85% of adults and children. Slightly more than 50% of adults and just under 50% of children require mechanical ventilation.

It therefore seems prudent, after ensuring upper airway patency, to first administer 100% O_2 and CPAP in some form (e.g., spontaneous breathing with CPAP, tracheal intubation and CPAP, mechanical ventilation with pressure support and PEEP) while assessing the severity of the POPE and ruling out other causes of acute pulmonary edema. Along with appropriate sedation, treatment includes titrating the fraction of inspired O_2 (FiO_2) into the range of 0.4 as the alveolar-arterial O_2 difference improves and the patient no longer demonstrates respiratory distress. The ventilatory and airway pressure supports can then be reduced. If fluid overload or coexisting cardiogenic dysfunction compounds the problem, diuretics or vasoactive agents may be indicated. Often, however, no additional medication is needed. Patients with a mild case may require only supplemental O_2.

The decision of where to manage patients with POPE depends on local capabilities and the availability of experienced caregivers. The most severely affected patients and those in whom the diagnosis is less certain benefit from admission to a designated critical care facility. Well-staffed freestanding ambulatory surgery centers might retain less severe cases of POPE in the postanesthesia care unit, but others might choose to transfer patients to an affiliated institution with critical care facilities. Office-based practitioners are best advised to transfer such patients to an acute care facility.

PREVENTION

Vaccination against invasive *Haemophilus influenzae* type B has effectively reduced the number of cases of severe epiglottitis and, by inference, the number of cases of severe POPE from that cause in children. Other measures to protect against POPE include the following:

- Use of bite blocks to prevent patients from biting and obstructing the endotracheal tube while attempting to inhale at the same time

- Avoidance of factors that cause laryngospsam: (1) repeated failed attempts at endotracheal intubation ("Woody Woodpecker" syndrome), (2) inadequate anesthetic depth or skeletal muscle relaxation for tracheal intubation, and (3) excessive oropharyngeal secretions
- Careful timing of tracheal extubation after general anesthesia to avoid stimulation during the excitement phase

The immediate, judicious use of CPAP after tracheal intubation or extubation in patients at high risk for POPE might mitigate the severity of the syndrome and minimize the need for reintubation and mechanical ventilation.

Further Reading

Benumof JL: Anesthesia for Thoracic Surgery, 2nd ed. Philadelphia, WB Saunders, 1995, pp 43-56.

Capatanio MK, Kirkpatrick JA: Obstruction of the upper airway in children as reflected by the chest radiograph. Pediatr Radiol 107:159-161, 1973.

Lang SA, Duncan PG, Shephard DAE, et al.: Pulmonary oedema associated with airway obstruction. Can J Anaesth 37:210-218, 1990.

Meissner HH, Robinson L, Dubinett SM, et al: Pulmonary edema as a result of chronic upper airway obstruction. Respir Med 92:1174-1176, 1998.

Nunn JF: Nunn's Applied Respiratory Physiology, 4th ed. Oxford, Butterworth-Heinemann, 1993, pp 484-493.

Oswalt CE, Gates GA, Holmstrom FMG: Pulmonary edema as a complication of upper airway obstruction. JAMA 238:1833-1835, 1977.

Ringold S, Klein EJ, Del Beccaro MA: Postobstructive pulmonary edema in children. Pediatr Emerg Care 20:391-395, 2004.

Staub NA: Pathophysiology of pulmonary edema. In Staub NA, Taylor AE (eds): Edema. New York, Raven Press, 1984, pp 719-741.

Travis KW, Todres ID, Shannon DC: Pulmonary edema associated with croup and epiglottitis. Pediatrics 59:695-698, 1977.

Van Kooy MA, Gargiulo RF. Postobstructive pulmonary edema. Am Fam Physician 62:401-404, 2000.

Wilson WC, Benumof JL: Respiratory physiology and respiratory function during anesthesia. In Miller RD (ed): Miller's Anesthesia, 6th ed. Philadelphia, Churchill Livingstone, 2005, pp 679-722.

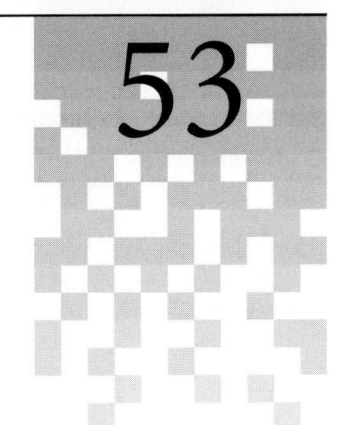

Latex Reactions in Health Care Personnel

53

Kevin J. Kelly and Robert E. Kettler

Case Synopsis

A 44-year-old anesthesiologist notes a rash on his right middle finger that has recently progressed to urticaria. He has been in good general health all his life; however, he is allergic to fish and ragweed pollen, and he was treated for eczema as a child. The rash has been intermittently present for several years and is exacerbated by wearing gloves to perform medical procedures. In the past 2 weeks, he has experienced chest tightness and rhinoconjunctivitis on entering the operating room. His only medication is an antihistamine taken during autumn for hay fever.

PROBLEM ANALYSIS

Definition

Natural rubber latex allergy (see also Chapter 161) is an issue of clinical importance for health care workers in terms of both patient management and occupational health. Use of rubber gloves dates to the late 1800s, when Halsted apparently produced them to protect the hands of his scrub nurse from the disinfectant solution she used to wash her hands. Skin lesions on the hands caused by the wearing of rubber gloves were first described in the medical literature in the 1930s. The increasing prevalence of latex-induced reactions is due to a confluence in the late 1980s of a number of factors: the increasing prevalence of hepatitis and acquired immunodeficiency syndrome (AIDS) led to the need for universal precautions; this led to increased demand for and use of barrier devices, including gloves made from natural rubber latex.

The rubber industry responded to meet this demand, but final product quality may have been compromised by new entrants into the field, new geographic locations for rubber production, political turmoil in rubber-producing countries, and changes in the manufacturing process to increase output while complying with environmental and occupational health concerns. This increase in demand was associated with a greater number of medical gloves imported into the United States.

As the use of latex gloves increased, allergic reactions in patients and health care providers were reported, leading to greater awareness of the problem, which in turn led to efforts to recognize and report it. This growing medical awareness was reflected by an increase in MEDLINE citations of journal articles published with *latex* as a key word, as shown in Table 53-1. There was an increase in both the absolute number of these citations and the number of these citations relative to the entire database. By mid-2004, the number of latex citations had increased to 0.1% of the MEDLINE database.

Natural latex contains several polypeptides that bind immunoglobulin E (IgE) and that may be altered during denaturation, polymerization, or breakdown during the manufacturing process. Most latex gloves have a cornstarch powder to facilitate donning. This powder binds various latex antigens and can be dispersed in the atmosphere, readily facilitating exposure through the respiratory system.

Recognition

Three types of untoward latex reactions are recognized (Table 53-2): irritant dermatitis, type I IgE-mediated reactions, and type IV delayed contact hypersensitivity reactions.

IRRITANT DERMATITIS

Irritant reactions occur because the glove creates a local environment that can cause physical or chemical irritation to the skin. Risk factors for irritant reactions include increased age, cold weather, and excessive sweating. The skin breaks down over several days, and erythema and fissures are noted on inspection of the affected area. These reactions are not immunologically mediated. However, by disrupting the cutaneous barrier to allergens, they may be risk factors for the development of immunologically mediated reactions.

Table 53–1 ■ Latex Citations in MEDLINE Database		
Year	Number (%) of Latex Citations	Total Literature Citations (Millions)*
1966-1974	445 (0.02)	2.0
1975-1979	241 (0.02)	1.3
1980-1984	286 (0.02)	1.4
1985-1989	348 (0.02)	1.7
1990-1993	472 (0.03)	1.5
1994-1997	679 (0.07)	1.0
1966-1997	2471 (0.03)	8.8

*All entries are rounded to nearest 100,000. In August 2004 the MEDLINE database contained 14 million citations, of which 14,372 (10%) were about latex.

Table 53–2 ■ Manifestations of Irritant, Immediate, and Delayed Reactions to Latex

Reaction Type	Time of Onset	Clinical Signs	Immune Mechanism
Irritant dermatitis	Often gradual (days)	Erythema; scalded or parched appearance; chapped, cracked, fissured, or scaling skin; possibly vesicles or blisters	None
IgE-mediated reaction (type I)	Within minutes; rarely >2 hr	Swelling, pruritus, urticaria, rhinoconjunctivitis, asthma, hypotension, anaphylaxis	IgE release of mast cell mediators; antigens are natural latex proteins
Delayed contact hypersensitivity reaction (type IV)	6-48 hr after contact	Acute: erythema, pruritus, vesicles, blisters, cracking, crusting, desquamation Chronic: dryness, scaling, fissures, thickening or darkening of skin	Delayed or cell-mediated immunity; T-cell response to small rubber chemicals acting as haptens

From Ownby DR: Manifestations of latex allergy. Immunol Allergy Clin North Am 15:34, 1995.

TYPE I IGE-MEDIATED REACTION

Type I reactions are mediated by IgE and usually occur within minutes of contact with latex proteins. The allergen binds to IgE, resulting in the release of vasoactive substances from mast cells (i.e., histamine, bradykinin, leukotrienes, prostanoids). There are several potential manifestations of IgE-mediated reactions, including urticaria, pruritus, bronchospasm, rhinoconjunctivitis, flushing, hypotension, angioedema, and anaphylaxis.

TYPE IV DELAYED HYPERSENSITIVITY REACTION

Type IV reactions to latex gloves are cell-mediated reactions to chemicals retained in the glove. The symptoms are apparent within several days and include erythema, pruritus, vesicles, fissuring, scaling, and thickening. The rash usually extends beyond the site of contact. Natural rubber latex is usually not the cause of type IV reactions; additives from the manufacturing process, such as thiuram and mercaptobenzathiazole, are more likely causes.

Risk Assessment

There are few studies on the natural history and clinical course of natural rubber latex reactions; in addition, owing to differences in their methodology, there is variation in the reported prevalence. Even so, the prevalence of latex allergy in the general population has been consistently reported as less than 1%. Although a study of blood donors revealed detectable antibody in 6.5% of subjects, this does not indicate the presence of clinical allergy. The pediatric spina bifida population has been estimated to have a prevalence of 28% to 67%. The prevalence of latex allergy in health care workers is 5% to 17%, but its prevalence in health care workers with a history of atopy is 24% to 36%.

Latex reaction risk factors include a history of environmental allergy, food allergy (especially to banana, kiwi, or avocado), hay fever, eczema, asthma, and chronic latex exposure (either occupational or as a result of repeated therapeutic procedures, with both frequency and exposure intensity being factors). The skin is relatively impermeable to latex proteins. However, disruption of the skin by irritant or contact reactions may predispose subjects to the development of IgE-mediated disease and subsequent systemic reactions. Cornstarch powder lubricant, which binds latex protein, and any activity that disperses these particles in the atmosphere can increase the quantity of respiratory exposure. If a patient's history indicates a risk of latex allergy, a serum level of IgE reactive to latex allergens or skin testing from an allergist may be obtained. Further workup can be performed as outlined in Table 53-3.

Table 53–3 ■ Manifestations of Irritant, Immediate, and Delayed Reactions to Latex

Negative	Positive
Patient at Risk of Latex Allergy*	
No symptoms; no latex allergy; no testing needed	Symptomatic; possible latex allergy; perform diagnostic tests
Serum Test	
Negative; do further testing	Positive; no further testing needed (latex allergy confirmed)
Latex Use Test	
Negative; do further testing	Positive; no further testing needed (latex allergy confirmed)
Skin Test	
Negative; no latex allergy	Positive; no further testing needed (latex allergy confirmed)

*Some investigators have advocated latex testing in all patients with spina bifida. This approach would identify asymptomatic patients who have positive serum test results. Until further studies are performed, this patient group should be considered to be allergic to latex.
From Kelly KJ, Kurup VP, Reijula KE, et al: The diagnosis of natural rubber latex allergy. J Allergy Clin Immunol 93:814, 1994.

Implications

The severity of a latex reaction can range from a minor annoyance to life-threatening anaphylaxis and can include disabling symptoms (e.g., asthma). In addition to these medical complications, there are social implications, such as the need to change responsibilities or careers and the cost of disability payments. Institutions and individuals may have to change aspects of their medical practice to reduce the risk of latex reactions in others.

MANAGEMENT

The mainstays of management are as follows:

- Avoidance of allergens
- Topical therapy
- Systemic therapy (see Chapter 27)

Antigen avoidance can be difficult because of the ubiquitous presence of natural rubber products, especially in the health care environment. However, steps can be taken, such as wearing nonlatex gloves or using some type of barrier between the latex gloves and the skin (e.g., vinyl gloves). Using gloves only when necessary can also reduce exposure. Individuals who suffer severe reactions and cannot avoid allergens may have to change their specialty or profession. Airborne exposure can be eliminated or reduced to levels that are clinically insignificant by the exclusive use of powder-free, low-allergen latex gloves or synthetic gloves. Topical therapy with steroids and moisturizers can relieve the symptoms of irritant and type IV reactions. Therapy for systemic IgE-mediated reactions includes airway management, ventilatory and circulatory support if necessary (including the use of epinephrine), antihistamines, and bronchodilators.

PREVENTION

Susceptible individuals should be advised to avoid latex products, but as already noted, this can be difficult. They should wear allergy-alert identification and carry an autoinjectable device for the emergency administration of epinephrine. Institutions should consider managing prevention through a multidisciplinary committee that develops guidelines for patients, health care workers, and other employees. This committee should provide guidelines for the identification of latex-containing medical products, the identification and purchase of latex-free substitutes, the establishment of latex-free treatment areas for susceptible individuals, and the use of powder-free gloves.

Further Reading

Garabrant DH, Schweitzer S: Epidemiology of latex sensitization and allergies in health care workers. J Allergy Clin Immunol 110:S82-S95, 2002.

Kelly KJ: Management of the latex-allergic patient. Immunol Allergy Clin North Am 15:139-157, 1995.

Kelly KJ, Kurup VP, Reijula KE, et al: The diagnosis of natural rubber latex allergy. J Allergy Clin Immunol 93:813-816, 1994.

Landwehr LP, Boguniewicz M: Current perspectives on latex allergy. J Pediatr 128:305-312, 1996.

Ownby DR: Manifestations of latex allergy. Immunol Allergy Clin North Am 15:31-43, 1995.

Ranta PM, Owenby DR: A review of natural-rubber latex allergy in health care workers. Clin Infect Dis 38:252-256, 2004.

Sussman GL, Beezhold DH: Allergy to latex rubber. Ann Intern Med 122:43-46, 1995.

Truscott W: The industry perspective on latex. Immunol Allergy Clin North Am 15:89-121, 1995.

SECTION 3

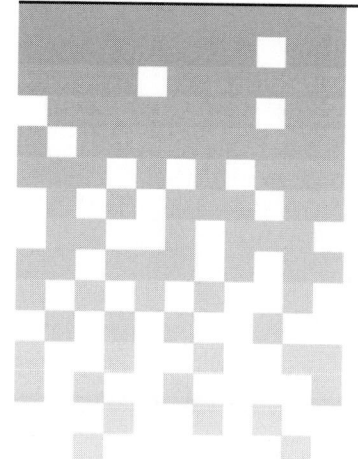

Regional Anesthesia and Pain Management

Brian M. Ilfeld

Spinal Anesthesia: Post–Dural Puncture Headache

54

Matthew P. Feuer and Spencer S. Liu

REGIONAL ANESTHESIA &
PAIN MANAGEMENT

Case Synopsis

A 25-year-old woman undergoes spinal anesthesia with a 25-gauge Quincke needle for outpatient knee arthroscopy. The following day, she complains of a severe frontal-occipital headache in the upright position that resolves when she is supine.

PROBLEM ANALYSIS

Definition

Post–dural puncture headache (PDPH) is a well-known complication of spinal anesthesia. It commonly occurs 24 to 48 hr after dural puncture (in 92% of affected patients), but the presentation can be delayed for as long as 5 days. Current evidence from laboratory and clinical imaging studies strongly supports the theory that loss of cerebrospinal fluid (CSF) from the puncture site is the key initiating factor (Fig. 54-1). Reduction in CSF fluid and pressure allows sagging of the brain and supporting structures when the patient assumes the upright position. Sagging of the brain places direct traction on pain-sensitive structures and can also cause painful reflex vasodilatation of cerebral blood vessels. This theory is also supported by PDPH's pathognomonic feature of occurrence or exacerbation in the upright position and resolution in the supine position. Typically, 70% of PDPHs resolve spontaneously by 1 week after dural puncture, and 95% resolve by 6 weeks.

Recognition

PDPH should be considered a diagnosis of exclusion. Medical conditions that have been misdiagnosed as PDPH include hypothalamic tumors, eclampsia, spinal meningitis, and superior sagittal sinus thrombosis.

Clinical features of PDPH include the following:

- History of dural puncture
- Delayed presentation of headache (usually 24 to 48 hours after dural puncture)
- Positional nature of headache (exacerbated when upright and resolved when supine)
- Headache that is typically frontal or occipital in nature
- Presence of common associated symptoms: neck ache (57%), backache (35%), nausea (22%)
- Presence of less common associated symptoms: shoulder pain, cranial nerve dysfunction, auditory complaints
- Spontaneous resolution between 1 and 6 weeks after dural puncture

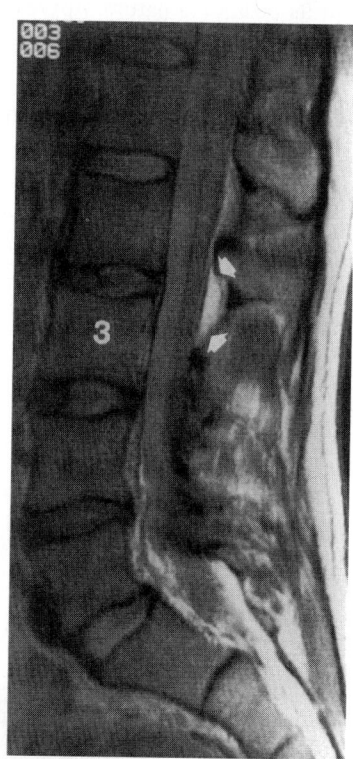

Figure 54–1 ■ Lumbar spine magnetic resonance image in a patient with post–dural puncture headache before the administration of an epidural blood patch. The static collection of fluid at L2-L3 *(arrows)* corresponds to leakage of cerebrospinal fluid from the dural puncture site. (From Vakharia SB, et al: Magnetic resonance imaging of cerebrospinal fluid leak and tamponade effect of blood patch in postdural puncture headache. Anesth Analg 84:585, 1997.)

Risk Assessment

With current anesthetic practice, the incidence of PDPH typically ranges from 1% to 7% after spinal anesthesia. Both patient characteristics and anesthetic technique have been implicated as risk factors for the subsequent development of PDPH.

Patient factors that increase the risk include the following:

- Younger age, probably owing to changes in the elastic properties of the dura with aging
- Female gender
- Previous history of PDPH

Anesthetic factors that reduce the risk of PDPH are the following:

- Smaller-diameter spinal needles, probably owing to smaller dural punctures (Figs. 54-2 and 54-3)
- Use of pencil-point rather than cutting-tip spinal needles—the former result in less CSF leakage in vitro (see Figs. 54-2 and 54-3)
- Orientation of the bevel of cutting-tip needles parallel to the long axis of the dura, which may produce a smaller rent in the dura because of the longitudinal splitting of fibers, as opposed to direct transection (cutting)

Implications

PDPH can result in significant discomfort and limitation of activity owing to its positional nature. Approximately 60% of affected patients can be treated with mild analgesics until spontaneous resolution occurs. Of these patients, approximately 18% will have slight restriction of physical activity, 31% will be partially bedridden with restricted physical activity, and 51% will be entirely bedridden.

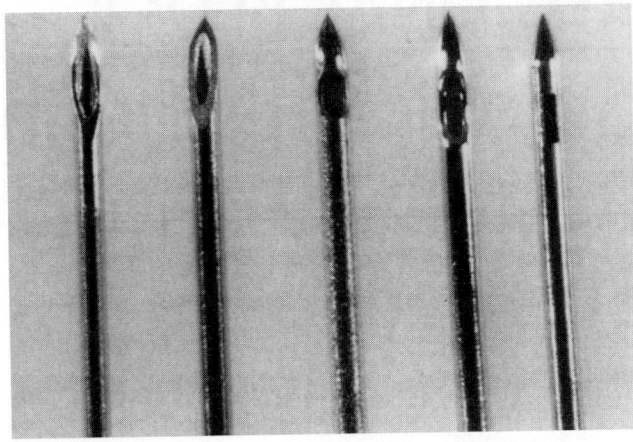

Figure 54–2 ■ From the left: Atraucan, Quincke, Gertie Marx, Sprotte, and Whitacre needles. Note the cutting points on the Atraucan and Quincke needles. Also, note the differences in the configuration of the lateral eyes of the pencil-point needles. The eye of the Gertie Marx needle is the smallest and situated closest to the needle tip. The left horizontal markings are in 2-mm increments. (From Vallejo MC, et al: Postdural puncture headache: A randomized comparison of five spinal needles in obstetric patients. Anesth Analg 91:916, 2000.)

MANAGEMENT

Both systemic and invasive therapies have been advocated for the treatment of PDPH. It is reasonable to try systemic treatments before instituting more invasive therapies (Fig. 54-4).

Systemic Therapy

Because the proposed pathophysiology of PDPH includes reflex vasodilatation of cerebral blood vessels, systemic

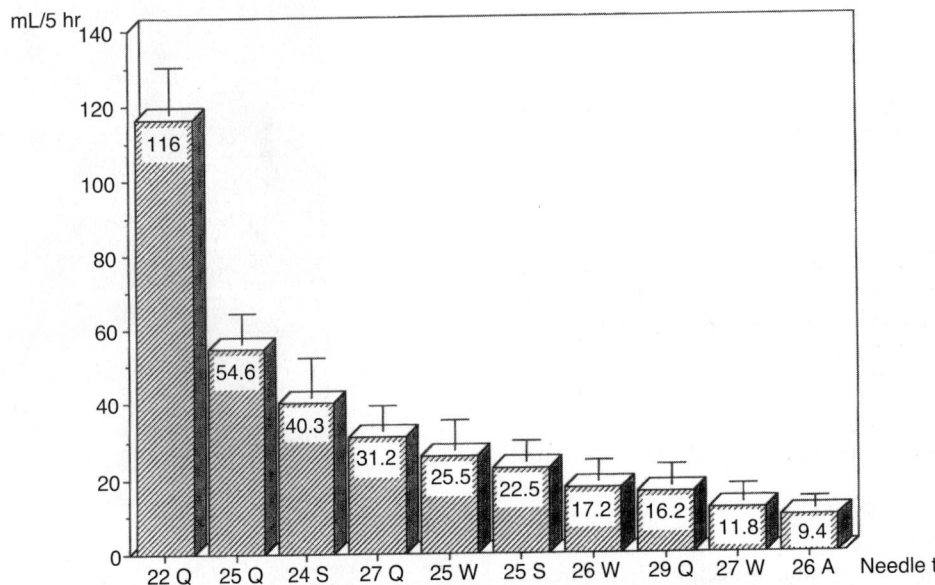

Figure 54–3 ■ Relationship between needle size and bevel type and leakage of cerebrospinal fluid after dural puncture in a laboratory model. (From Holst D, et al: In vitro investigation of cerebrospinal fluid leakage after dural puncture with various spinal needles. Anesth Analg 87:1331, 1998.)

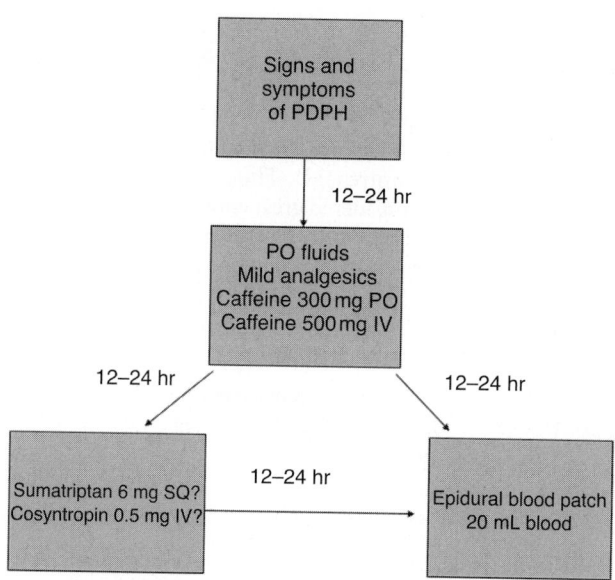

Figure 54–4 ▪ Suggested treatment algorithm for post–dural puncture headache.

therapies generally focus on the administration of vasoconstrictive agents or adrenocorticotropic hormone (ACTH).

Caffeine. The intravenous administration of caffeine (500 mg) has been observed to decrease cerebral blood flow by 22% in patients suffering from PDPH. Success rates with intravenous caffeine therapy range from 40% to 80%, with mild side effects (dizziness, flushing). Oral caffeine can also be an effective therapy, with an approximately 50% success rate after 300 mg of oral caffeine.

Sumatriptan. This serotonin type 1d receptor agonist is a potent cerebral vasoconstrictor that is an effective treatment for migraine and cluster headaches. Sumatriptan can be administered intranasally, orally, or by subcutaneous injection. Case reports on the use of sumatriptan to treat PDPH are conflicting, and the sole available small randomized trial showed no benefit.

Adrenocorticotropic Hormone. ACTH and its synthetic analogues have been administered intravenously for the treatment of PDPH. Proposed mechanisms of action include increased CSF production, dural edema secondary to aldosterone production, and increased β-endorphin production. Anecdotal evidence suggests a success rate of 70% to 95%, but the sole randomized controlled trial to date showed no benefit. There have been case reports of seizures in obstetric patients treated with ACTH analogues.

Invasive Therapy

Loss of CSF pressure due to leakage of CSF from the dural puncture site has prompted investigators to inject substances into the epidural space to try to return CSF pressure to normal:

Epidural Blood Patch. Epidural injection of autologous blood was first proposed as a treatment for PDPH in 1960, after anecdotal observations of a reduced incidence of PDPH

after "bloody" dural punctures. Epidural blood patch (EBP) is currently the gold standard for PDPH treatment, with a success rate ranging from 90% to 99%. Its mechanisms of action are thought to involve increased intracranial CSF pressure due to mass effect and sealing of the dural puncture site with fibrin clot (Fig. 54-5). Injection of blood into the epidural space results in an immediate mass effect persisting for at least 3 hours. Mature clot formation and sealing of the dural rent occurs by 7 hours after injection. Initial reports of EBP used small volumes of blood (2 to 3 mL), but recent recommendations are for larger volumes (15 to 20 mL). These larger volumes provide greater spread of clot (five to nine spinal segments), greater mass effect, and a higher incidence of successful treatment. Although safe and effective, the use of EBP is not risk free. Contraindications to EBP include systemic infection, localized infection of the back, and active neurologic disease. Reported complications of EBP include transient backache (35% to 100% incidence), mild temperature elevation (5%), sudden bradycardia, and radicular pain. Prolonged sequelae from EBP may also occur. Less successful epidural analgesia after prior EBP has been reported.

Epidural Injection of Other Solutions. Both saline and dextran have been injected into the epidural space for the treatment of PDPH. Highly variable success rates have been reported, ranging from no effect to 90% success. The variable and often temporary nature of relief from saline or dextran,

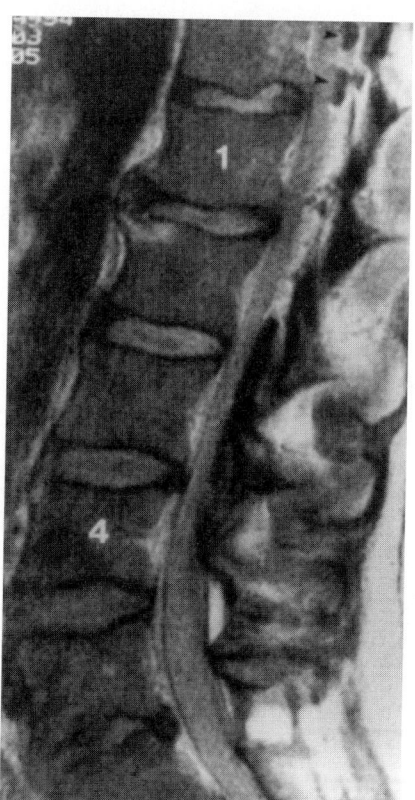

Figure 54–5 ▪ Magnetic resonance image of 20-mL epidural blood patch demonstrating sealing of the dural leak and spread from L4 to T12 *(arrowheads)*. (From Vakharia SB, et al: Magnetic resonance imaging of cerebrospinal fluid leak and tamponade effect of blood patch in postdural puncture headache. Anesth Analg 84:585, 1997.)

coupled with the inherent risk of an epidural injection, makes their use questionable. A recent case report documented the successful use of 3 mL of fibrin glue to treat a PDPH resistant to three EPBs.

PREVENTION

The cornerstone of preventing PDPH is the selection of small, non-cutting-tipped needles for dural puncture. The prophylactic administration of systemic therapies has not been well studied, and results are disappointing. The prophylactic administration of EBP is controversial. Because not all patients undergoing dural puncture will develop PDPH, many experts recommend EBP only after the development of symptoms. Another argument against the prophylactic use of EBP is its questionable efficacy when administered early (<24 hours after dural puncture). Several studies of the early administration of relatively small volumes of blood (7 to 10 mL) via an epidural catheter after dural puncture with a large-gauge Tuohy needle reported virtually no effects on the subsequent development of PDPH. However, these studies have been criticized for using small volumes of blood. A recent study administering a larger volume of blood (15 mL) via an epidural catheter after dural puncture with a large-gauge Tuohy needle reported

a marked reduction in the incidence of PDPH in obstetric patients (5% in treated versus 88% in untreated patients). Another recent controlled trial demonstrated the efficacy of the immediate injection of 10 mL of saline after inadvertent dural puncture (32% of treated patients developed PDPH, versus 62% of those untreated). Thus, if patient and anesthetic risk factors are considered great enough to warrant prophylactic therapy, a large-volume EBP or immediate saline injection may be a reasonable and effective therapy.

Further Reading

Canovas L, Barros C, Gomez A, et al: Use of intravenous tetracosactin in the treatment of postdural puncture headache: Our experience in forty cases. Anesth Analg 94:1369, 2002.

Connelly NR, Parker RK, Rahimi A, Gibson CS: Sumatriptan in patients with postdural puncture headache. Headache 40:316-319, 2000.

Halpern S, Preston R: Postdural puncture headache and spinal needle design: Metaanalyses. Anesthesiology 81:1376-1383, 1994.

Harrington BE: Postdural puncture headache and the development of the epidural blood patch. Reg Anesth Pain Med 29:136-163, 2004.

Kroin JS, Nagalla SK, Buvanendran A, et al: The mechanisms of intracranial pressure modulation by epidural blood and other injectates in a postdural puncture rat model. Anesth Analg 95:423-429, 2002.

Lybecker H, Djernes M, Schmidt J: Postdural puncture headache (PDPH): Onset, duration, severity, and associated symptoms. Acta Anaesthesiol Scand 39:605-612, 1995.

Local Anesthetic Neurotoxicity: Cauda Equina Syndrome

55

Kenneth Drasner

Case Synopsis

A 48-year-old man underwent right inguinal hernia repair under spinal anesthesia. With the patient in a sitting position, a 24-gauge pencil-point needle was inserted at the L4-L5 level, and 75 mg of 5% lidocaine hydrochloride with 7.5% glucose, 0.1 mg of epinephrine, and 25 μg of fentanyl was administered, resulting in an L3 block after 5 minutes. The patient was then placed in the right lateral decubitus position, and an additional 50 mg of 5% lidocaine with glucose was administered intrathecally. A T10 block was achieved, and surgery proceeded uneventfully. Twelve hours postoperatively, perineal numbness persisted, and the patient was unable to void. Anal sphincter tone was diminished, and anal reflexes were absent. Lumbosacral spine films and lumbosacral magnetic resonance imaging results were within normal limits. Six months postoperatively, the patient had to strain to urinate, was unable to have a spontaneous bowel movement, and continued to have diminished sensation in the S3-S5 region bilaterally.

PROBLEM ANALYSIS

Definition

As the term cauda equina syndrome (CES) implies, clinical manifestations are related to injury to the nerve roots below the conus medullaris. Consequently, CES results in varying degrees of bowel and bladder dysfunction, perineal sensory loss, and lower extremity motor weakness. Although there are multiple potential causes, two are of most concern to anesthesiologists: (1) compressive injuries (e.g., epidural hematoma or epidural abscess), and (2) direct toxicity of substances administered into the intrathecal space. Recent clinical experience and experimental data suggest that, under certain circumstances, local anesthetics in current clinical use have the potential to induce neurotoxic damage. That is the focus of this chapter.

Recognition

Throughout the last century of clinical use, sporadic reports of neurologic injury associated with spinal and epidural anesthesia raised the concern that local anesthetics might be neurotoxic. Clinical and experimental evidence accumulated over the last decade, beginning with reports of CES associated with continuous spinal anesthesia (CSA), has substantiated this concern. All the CSA-related cases shared certain common elements: there was evidence of a restricted sacral block that required repetitive doses of local anesthetic to achieve adequate surgical anesthesia, and the cumulative dose far exceeded that commonly used with single-injection spinal anesthesia. It was suggested that the combination of maldistribution and high dose of anesthetic led to neurotoxic concentrations in a restricted area of the subarachnoid space, a mechanism supported by subsequent in vitro and in vivo experimental data. Although most of the injuries involved the administration of 5% lidocaine through small-bore microcatheters, not all were associated with lidocaine, and some involved intrathecal delivery of anesthetic through an epidural catheter. Therefore, withdrawal of microcatheters from clinical practice has not eliminated the risk of injury, as practitioners remain at liberty to use epidural equipment for CSA. Further, some clinicians routinely convert to a continuous spinal technique if dural puncture accidentally occurs during attempted epidural placement.

Factors that lead to neurotoxic injury with CSA are not unique to this technique; they also apply to single-injection spinal anesthesia. Specifically, inadequate sensory block with single-injection spinal anesthesia is often the result of maldistribution. Under such circumstances, there is the potential for repeat injections to distribute in the same pattern, resulting in neurotoxic concentrations of local anesthetic within a restricted area of the subarachnoid space. Case reports and review of the closed claims database appear to support this concern.

There is a third mechanism by which high doses of anesthetic may be administered into the subarachnoid space. If a practitioner is administering an epidural anesthetic and fails to appreciate that the needle or catheter has traversed the dura or arachnoid, the doses administered may achieve neurotoxic concentrations in the subarachnoid space. Such doses may be sufficient to induce injury even in the absence of maldistribution, as evidenced by case reports.

Reports of neurologic injury with CSA, repetitive injection after failed spinal anesthesia, and inadvertent intrathecal injection of anesthetic intended for the epidural space established the potential toxicity of anesthetics administered at a dose exceeding the usual clinical range for spinal anesthesia. More surprising, two fairly recent reports raised the suspicion that neurologic deficits might occur with the administration of lidocaine at doses recommended for single-injection spinal anesthesia. One was a case report of CES following the intrathecal injection of 100 mg of lidocaine with epinephrine. The second was a prospective study of regional anesthesia from France. In both reports there were persistent deficits following single injections of lidocaine that could not be otherwise explained. In all cases, relatively high doses (≥75 mg) were used, and cases of permanent injury occurred only after injection of the maximum recommended clinical dose (100 mg).

Risk Assessment

In prospective studies, retrospective reviews, and epidemiologic studies, the incidence of CES resulting from neurotoxic reactions to local anesthetic varies. Such information is potentially misleading, however, because the incidence depends on practice patterns. For example, the very high incidence associated with the repetitive administration of high doses of anesthetic through continuous spinal catheters has little relevance to current anesthetic practice. Similarly, the roughly 1 in 5000 incidence of permanent deficits with single-injection lidocaine spinal anesthesia in the aforementioned report from France may overestimate the risk, because modifications have been made to reduce the risk of injury (see "Prevention"). Nonetheless, when assessing the likelihood that postoperative CES is the result of a neurotoxic reaction, one should consider the circumstances of the case relative to factors known to be associated with clinical toxicity (e.g., inadvertent intrathecal injection of an intended epidural dose of anesthetic).

In addition to the rare occurrence of CES following spinal or epidural anesthesia, transient neurologic symptoms—defined as pain or dysesthesia in the buttocks and lower extremities—may occur in up to a third of individuals receiving lidocaine for spinal anesthesia. Known risk factors include outpatient status and surgical positioning (e.g., patients undergoing knee arthroscopy or placed in the lithotomy position). However, transient neurologic symptoms can be readily distinguished from CES because the former is not associated with sensory or motor deficits or disturbance of bladder and bowel function. Although there has been considerable speculation that these transient symptoms and CES may represent opposite ends of a spectrum of toxicity, recent evidence suggests that these two entities are not mediated by the same mechanism.

Implications

CES is a rare but disastrous complication that may result from neurotoxic injury to the nerve roots below the conus medullaris. Because of its seriousness and lack of effective treatment, attention must be focused on the adoption of clinical strategies that minimize risk (see "Prevention").

MANAGEMENT

Although some advocate the use of high-dose steroids, these agents have no proven benefit for nerve root injuries resulting from local anesthetic toxicity. As mentioned earlier, there are many potential causes of CES. It is critical to consider the possibility that clinical manifestations may be due to a compressive lesion (e.g., hematoma, abscess). Unlike neurotoxic damage, injury from compression is readily reversible, and the extent of recovery is related to the degree of functional loss and the time from the onset of deficits to surgical decompression. The clinical circumstances, such as coagulation status, may provide guidance as to the likelihood of this alternative. Also, local anesthetic neurotoxicity presents with a block that does not recede, whereas a period of normal postoperative function followed by progressive loss in the absence of ongoing administration of local anesthetic is strongly suggestive of a compressive lesion. Because time is of the essence, any suspicion should be investigated by emergent magnetic resonance imaging.

PREVENTION

Analysis of the clinical reports of CES occurring with spinal and epidural anesthesia and data generated in experimental studies of neurotoxicity has led to the identification of factors that appear to potentiate risk. This information forms the basis of practice modifications.

Continuous Spinal Anesthesia

Injuries occurred with CSA because high doses of anesthetic were administered intrathecally to compensate for a restricted sensory block. Guidelines have been proposed that emphasize reliance on a test dose, adjustment of technique, and abandonment of the technique if adequate block is not achieved within the normal clinical dose range for single-injection spinal anesthesia (Table 55-1).

Repeat Injection after Failed Spinal Anesthesia

Similar to CSA, guidelines for the management of failed spinal anesthesia have been proposed. These include an assessment of the likelihood of technical error (e.g., failure to inject the drug intrathecally) and appropriate adjustment of the dosage for the repeat injection. However, a more efficient

---

Table 55–1 ■ Continuous Spinal Anesthesia: Guidelines for Administration

Insert the catheter just far enough to confirm and maintain placement.
Use the lowest effective anesthetic concentration.
Place a limit on the amount of anesthetic to be used.
Administer a test dose, and assess the extent of block.
If maldistribution is suspected, use maneuvers to increase the spread of local anesthetic (e.g., change the patient's position, alter the lumbosacral curvature, switch to a solution with a different baricity).
If well-distributed sensory anesthesia is not achieved before the dose limit is reached, abandon the technique.

Adapted from Rigler ML, Drasner K, Krejcie TC, et al: Cauda equina syndrome after continuous spinal anesthesia. Anesth Analg 72:275-281, 1991.

(and perhaps safer) strategy is to simply limit the combined anesthetic dosage to the maximum amount a clinician would consider reasonable to administer as a single intrathecal injection.

Epidural Anesthesia

The potential for toxicity with inadvertent intrathecal injection of an epidural dose of anesthetic underscores the importance of a test dose and the fractional administration of anesthetic. Additionally, should high doses of anesthetic be administered through a misplaced catheter, repetitive withdrawal of small volumes of cerebrospinal fluid and replacement with saline should be considered, regardless of the anesthetic agent.

Lidocaine Spinal Anesthesia

Most of the recent injuries associated with spinal and epidural anesthesia have been associated with the use of lidocaine. Experimental investigations have reinforced concerns about this anesthetic, suggesting that its inherent toxicity exceeds that of bupivacaine. Modified guidelines for the use of this agent are summarized in Table 55-2 and detailed in the following paragraphs (although lidocaine is the focus, most of these considerations apply to any intrathecal anesthetic agent).

Dose. Most studies indicate that the potency ratio of lidocaine to bupivacaine is approximately 1:4. Yet the maximum recommended doses of 100 mg and 20 mg, respectively, or the administration of whole ampules of these agents (100 mg and 15 mg), result in ratios of 5:1 or 6.7:1. The issue of relative toxicity aside, 100 mg exceeds the dose of lidocaine required for reliable spinal anesthesia. This, combined with case reports of probable neurotoxicity at the upper end of the dose range, leaves little justification for the continued use of a 100-mg ceiling. The data are inadequate to make a firm recommendation regarding the maximum safe dose, but it is my personal practice not to exceed 60 mg.

Concentration. Abundant data suggest that anesthetic neurotoxicity is, to some extent, concentration dependent. It is therefore hard to justify the continued use of concentrations that far exceed that required for adequate blockade.

Table 55–2 ■ Lidocaine Spinal Anesthesia: General Guidelines

Dosage should be limited to 60 mg.
Concentration should not exceed 2%.
Epinephrine should not be used to enhance anesthesia or prolong the duration of block.

Modified from Drasner K: Lidocaine spinal anesthesia: A vanishing therapeutic index? Anesthesiology 87:469-472, 1995.

With respect to lidocaine, the injected concentration should not exceed 2% lidocaine because it will produce sensory anesthesia that is clinically equivalent to a 5% solution.

Glucose. A feature common to most recent cases of clinical injury is the use of an anesthetic solution with a high concentration of glucose and a tonicity far exceeding the normal physiologic range. Despite this association, 7.5% glucose does not affect the compound action potential in vitro or potentiate anesthetic-induced conduction failure. Moreover, dose-dependent loss of sensory function produced by intrathecal lidocaine in vivo is unaffected by the presence of 7.5% glucose, and the administration of 10% glucose does not induce impairment or morphologic damage. These findings suggest that it is appropriate to continue to use glucose to increase baricity.

Vasoconstrictors. Vasoconstrictors might contribute to toxicity by promoting ischemia, decreasing anesthetic uptake, or directly affecting neural elements. Recent data indicate that epinephrine potentiates sensory impairment induced by intrathecal lidocaine. Combined with the clinical report of a deficit following the intrathecal injection of 100 mg lidocaine with epinephrine, these data argue against using a vasoconstrictor with lidocaine for spinal anesthesia. Moreover, if the goal is to provide a longer duration of surgical anesthesia, this can be readily achieved with bupivacaine. Thus, there is no cogent argument for the continued use of epinephrine with lidocaine.

Further Reading

Auroy Y, Narchi P, Messiah A, et al: Serious complications related to regional anesthesia: Results of a prospective survey in France. Anesthesiology 87:479-486, 1997.

Drasner K: Lidocaine spinal anesthesia: A vanishing therapeutic index? Anesthesiology 87:469-472, 1997.

Drasner K, Rigler M: Repeat injection after a "failed spinal"—at times, a potentially unsafe practice. Anesthesiology 75:713-714, 1991.

Drasner K, Rigler M, Sessler D, Stoller M: Cauda equina syndrome following intended epidural anesthesia. Anesthesiology 77:582-585, 1992.

Freedman J, Li D, Drasner K, et al: Transient neurologic symptoms after spinal anesthesia: An epidemiologic study of 1863 patients. Anesthesiology 89:633-694, 1998.

Hampl KF, Schneider MC, Ummenhofer W, Drewe J: Transient neurologic symptoms after spinal anesthesia. Anesth Analg 81:1148-1153, 1995.

Hashimoto K, Bollen A, Ciriales R, Drasner R: Comparative toxicity of glucose and lidocaine administered intrathecally in the rat. Reg Anesth Pain Med 23:444-450, 1998.

Hashimoto K, Hampl K, Nakamura Y, et al: Epinephrine increases the neurotoxic potential of intrathecally administered local anesthetic in the rat. Anesthesiology 94:876-883, 2001.

Lambert L, Lambert D, Strichartz G: Irreversible conduction block in isolated nerve by high concentrations of local anesthetics. Anesthesiology 80:1082-1093, 1994.

Pollock JE, Neal JM, Stephenson CA, Wiley CE: Prospective study of the incidence of transient radicular irritation in patients undergoing spinal anesthesia. Anesthesiology 84:1361-1367, 1996.

Rigler M, Drasner K: Distribution of catheter-injected local anesthetic in a model of the subarachnoid space. Anesthesiology 75:684-692, 1991.

Rigler M, Drasner K, Krejcie T, et al: Cauda equina syndrome after continuous spinal anesthesia. Anesth Analg 72:275-281, 1991.

Local Anesthetic Systemic Toxicity

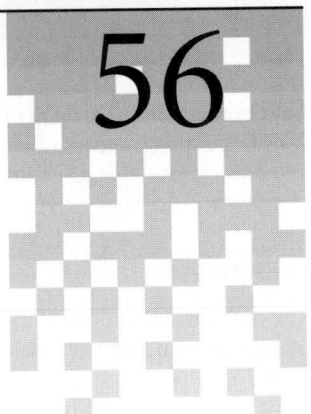

56

Francis V. Salinas

Case Synopsis

A 65-year-old man (183 cm, 87 kg, American Society of Anesthesiologists [ASA] status 1) was scheduled for a left total knee arthroplasty revision. His only medical problem was hypertension that was well controlled with atenolol 50 mg/day. After resolution of an uneventful 15-mg isobaric bupivacaine subarachnoid block, a continuous femoral nerve block was planned for postoperative analgesia. The patient was positioned supine for the femoral nerve block, and a brisk quadriceps response was obtained at a minimal current of 0.4 mA. A perineural catheter was advanced 10 cm beyond the needle tip, and the stimulating needle was removed. After a negative catheter aspiration test, ropivacaine 0.5% with epinephrine 2.5 μg/mL (30 mL) was injected slowly over 60 seconds. Near the end of the injection, the patient complained of unfocused vision and suddenly developed a generalized tonic-clonic seizure.

PROBLEM ANALYSIS

Definition

Local anesthetics are used to block the generation and propagation of electrical impulses (action potentials) in electrically excitable tissues. They bind to voltage-gated sodium channels and prevent conformational changes within those channels that allow the movement of ions for the propagation of action potentials. Clinically, local anesthetics are usually injected directly into perineural tissues (central neuraxis, major plexus, or peripheral nerves), joint spaces, and subcutaneous tissues. Additionally, they can be applied topically to mucosal surfaces to provide anesthesia of the airway or interpleural and intraperitoneal spaces. They may also be administered intravenously to provide regional anesthesia or treat arrhythmias.

Adverse reactions to local anesthetics are either systemic or localized (e.g., direct neurotoxicity; see Chapter 55). Systemic toxicity involves primarily the central nervous system (CNS) and the cardiovascular system (CVS). In practice, systemic toxicity occurs as a result of the inadvertent intravascular injection or systemic absorption of excessive doses of local anesthetics from the injection site. Less commonly, systemic toxic reactions are due to methemoglobinemia, allergic reactions, or direct myo- or neurotoxicity. For example, *ortho*-toluidine (a metabolite of benzocaine and prilocaine) may oxidize deoxyhemoglobin to methemoglobin; deoxyhemoglobin does not bind oxygen or carbon dioxide.

Recognition

CENTRAL NERVOUS SYSTEM TOXICITY

Based on studies of unsedated human volunteers receiving intravenous infusions of local anesthetics, the early symptoms of local anesthetic-induced CNS toxicity include perioral numbness, lightheadedness or dizziness, tinnitus, difficulty focusing visually, paresthesia, disorientation, and drowsiness. As the local anesthetic's plasma concentration increases, common signs include dysarthria, skeletal muscle twitching, and tremors; these can progress to generalized tonic-clonic seizures. With still higher plasma concentrations, CNS toxicity may cause unconsciousness, respiratory arrest, and coma. Symptoms of CNS excitation are thought to be related to an initial blockade of inhibitory neurons in the cerebral cortex, thereby allowing facilitative neurons to function in an unopposed manner. This may ultimately lead to generalized seizures. With further increases in plasma and CNS concentrations of local anesthetics, both inhibitory and facilitative neurons are blocked, leading to more global CNS depression.

This stereotypical pattern of initial CNS excitation relates primarily to slow intravenous injection or absorption of local anesthetics. Because the most common cause of clinical systemic toxicity is inadvertent intravenous injection of large amounts of local anesthetics, symptoms and signs of toxicity may progress much more rapidly, and generalized seizures may be the initial presentation of CNS toxicity. Also, the use of intravenous sedatives during the performance of an epidural or peripheral nerve block can attenuate early signs and symptoms of CNS toxicity. If so, skeletal muscle twitching and tremors or loss of consciousness may be the initial presentation.

CARDIOVASCULAR SYSTEM TOXICITY

Local anesthetics' inhibition of cardiac sodium channels reduces the action potential duration, the effective refractory period, and the maximal depolarization rate of Purkinje fibers and ventricular muscle. Electrophysiologic studies in animal models have shown that local anesthetics produce dose-dependent depression of cardiac conduction, leading to a prolonged P-R interval and QRS duration and depression of sinoatrial and atrioventricular activity. Local anesthetics also exert direct dose-dependent negative inotropic effects on the ventricular myocardium, which may be related to the blockage of calcium channels and mitochondrial energy metabolism. Further, local anesthetics are peripheral vasodilators and exert potent inhibitory effects on sympathetic smooth muscle vasoconstriction. CVS toxicity from local anesthetics' direct actions on both myocardium and the peripheral vasculature may present as arrhythmias (refractory ventricular arrhythmias, sinus bradycardia or arrest), profound hypotension (due to negative inotropic effects or vasodilatation), or cardiovascular collapse.

METHEMOGLOBINEMIA

Methemoglobinemia is characterized by central cyanosis that is refractory to supplemental oxygen. Central cyanosis usually develops with methemoglobin levels greater than 15%. Higher concentrations may result in anxiety, dyspnea, headache, weakness, nausea, and vomiting. Severe methemoglobinemia (>50% to 60% methemoglobin) may cause confusion, seizures, arrhythmias, hemodynamic instability, and death. The diagnosis is suggested by the presence of "chocolate-colored" blood that does not change color when exposed to air and an arterial percentage of oxygen saturation gap when analyzed by pulse oximetry and arterial blood gases. The diagnosis is confirmed by qualitative measures of methemoglobin concentrations by co-oximetry.

Risk Assessment

Multiple factors determine the risk of developing local anesthetic–induced systemic toxicity and its severity:

- Regional anesthetic technique
- Pharmacokinetic factors
- Physiochemical and stereoselective properties of individual local anesthetics
- Individual patient characteristics

Based on several large series from the mid-1980s to the late 1990s, the reported overall incidence of seizures and cardiac arrest is relatively low (Table 56-1). Because premonitory signs precede the vast majority of seizures, they are most likely the result of acutely increased plasma levels of local anesthetic secondary to inadvertent intravascular injection. Seizures are five times more frequent after peripheral nerve block than after epidural anesthesia; this difference may be explained by the fact that the former usually requires larger

doses of local anesthetics than the latter does. In contrast, the frequency of cardiac arrest is low with either technique.

Although the systemic toxic effects of local anesthetics are dose dependent, the rate of change in plasma levels is also an important factor. In the absence of intravascular injection, local anesthetics are absorbed into the systemic circulation by uptake and distribution from the surrounding perineural tissue. Subsequent plasma levels are governed by the following factors:

- Amount of administered drug
- Physiochemical properties (e.g., lipid solubility, protein binding) of the individual local anesthetic
- Regional blood flow
- Presence of perineural tissue and fat that can bind local anesthetics
- Concomitant use of vasoconstrictors with local anesthetics

In general, perineural tissue with greater regional blood flow has a more rapid and complete uptake of local anesthetic, regardless of its type. Based on technique, the rates of systemic absorption generally decrease, in the following order: interpleural, intercostal, epidural, brachial plexus, sciatic-femoral (Table 56-2). The greater the total dose administered, the greater the systemic absorption and peak plasma levels. Within clinically recommended doses, and with the exception of speed of injection, this relationship is nearly linear. The addition of epinephrine causes a 20% to 30% reduction in peak plasma levels during epidural anesthesia and peripheral nerve blocks.

After systemic absorption, local anesthetics are rapidly distributed throughout different tissues in the body, based on organ perfusion. Because the CNS and CVS are highly perfused, initial tissue levels of local anesthetics may not correlate with systemic blood levels. Thus, regional pharmacokinetics play an important role in the subsequent systemic pharmacodynamic effects of these anesthetics.

The severity of local anesthetic–induced toxicity can also be influenced by the patient's acid-base status. With increased arterial carbon dioxide tension or decreased pH, the seizure threshold is reduced. Increased hydrogen ion concentrations enhance cerebral blood flow, so that more local anesthetic is delivered to the CNS. Also, hypercapnia or acidosis reduces plasma protein binding of local anesthetics, which increases the amount of free drug available to diffuse across cell membranes. Patients with advanced liver disease may be particularly susceptible to local anesthetic–induced toxicity with the amide class of drugs, owing to the combination of reduced protein synthesis and hepatic degradation.

Implications

In general, more potent local anesthetics produce seizures at lower plasma concentrations and doses than do less potent local anesthetics. The relative CNS toxicity of bupivacaine and lidocaine is approximately 4:1, which mirrors their relative anesthetic potency. The cardiovascular manifestations during the excitatory phase of CNS toxicity can include increased heart rate, blood pressure, and cardiac output. The CVS is much more resistant to the toxic effects of local anesthetics than the CNS is. Severe CVS toxicity is rare with the less potent amide local anesthetics, and severe direct myocardial

Table 56–1 ■ Reported Incidence of Seizures and Cardiac Arrest after Regional Anesthesia

Technique	Seizures	Cardiac Arrest
Peripheral nerve block	36/72,746 (4.9/10,000)	4/72,746 (0.54/10,000)
Epidural	9/52,844 (1.3/10,000)	3/52,844 (0.57/10,00)
Intravenous regional	3/11,229 2.6/10,000	0/11,229 0

Table 56–2 ■ Typical Maximal Plasma Concentrations of Common Local Anesthetics, by Regional Technique

Local Anesthetic	Technique	Dose (mg)	C_{max} (µg/mL)	T_{max} (min)	Toxic Plasma Concentration (µg/mL)
Bupivacaine	Brachial plexus	150	1.00	20	3
	Epidural	50	1.50	1.7	3
	Intercostal	140	1.26	20	3
	Sciatic/femoral	400	1.89	15	3
Lidocaine	Brachial plexus	400	4.00	25	5
	Epidural	400	4.27	20	5
	Intercostal	400	6.80	15	5
	Sciatic/femoral*	650	2.39	30	5
Mepivacaine	Brachial plexus	500	3.68	24	5
	Epidural	500	4.95	16	5
	Intercostal	500	8.06	9	5
	Sciatic/femoral	500	3.59	31	5
Ropivacaine	Brachial plexus	190	1.30	53	4
	Epidural	150	1.07	40	4
	Intercostal	140	1.10	21	4
	Femoral†	150	0.65	30	4
	Psoas compartment†	150	1.19	15	4
Levobupivacaine	Brachial plexus‡	250	1.20	55	>4
	Epidural	150	1.02	2	>4

*Data from Elmas C, Atanassoff PG: Combined inguinal paravascular (3-in-1) and sciatic nerve blocks for lower limb surgery. Reg Anesth 18:88-92, 1993.

†Data from Kaloul I, Guay J, Cote C, et al: Ropivacaine plasma concentrations are similar during continuous lumbar plexus block using the anterior three-in-one and the posterior psoas compartment techniques. Can J Anaesth 51:52-56, 2004.

‡Data from Crews JC, Weller RS, Moss J, James RL: Levobupivacaine for axillary brachial plexus block: A pharmacokinetic and clinical comparison in patients with normal renal function or renal disease. Anesth Analg 95:219-223, 2002.

C_{max}, maximal plasma concentration; T_{max}, maximal time.

From Salinas FV: Ion channel ligands/sodium channel blockers/local anesthetics. In Evers AS, Maze M (eds): Anesthetic Pharmacology: Physiologic Principles and Clinical Practice, 1st edition. Philadelphia, Churchill Livingstone, 2004, pp 507-537.

depression and peripheral vasodilatation occur only with extremely high levels of either lidocaine or mepivacaine. Conversely, more potent amide local anesthetics, such as bupivacaine, have a significantly narrower margin of CVS safety, expressed as the ratio of the dosage or plasma concentration required to produce irreversible cardiovascular collapse (CC) to that required to produce CNS toxicity (generalized seizures). In contrast to lidocaine, the CC/CNS ratio for bupivacaine can result in nearly simultaneous progression from CNS toxicity to cardiovascular collapse, in large part owing to bupivacaine's ability to cause malignant ventricular arrhythmias.

Bupivacaine's enhanced ability to precipitate ventricular arrhythmias is thought to be related primarily to differences in the recovery of sodium channel block between bupivacaine and lidocaine. Both drugs rapidly block sodium channels during systole; however, bupivacaine dissociates from the sodium channel receptor much more slowly than lidocaine during diastole. Thus, within the physiologic range of heart rate, lidocaine dissociates rapidly (fast on–fast off) from the sodium channel, whereas bupivacaine remains avidly bound to it during diastole (fast on–slow off). The net electrophysiologic effect is slowed ventricular conduction and prolonged refractoriness, both of which are conducive to reentry ventricular arrhythmias.

Although bupivacaine has the advantage of prolonged duration of block, with enhanced sensory-motor dissociation, concerns about its potent cardiotoxicity led to the development of alternative long-acting amide local anesthetics with the same beneficial properties but an enhanced margin of safety.

Ropivacaine is the propyl homologue of mepivacaine and bupivacaine. In contrast to older amide local anesthetics, which exist as racemic mixtures, ropivacaine is an enantiomerically pure (levorotatory isomer) local anesthetic. In general, the levorotatory isomer has less potential for systemic toxicity than the dextrorotatory isomer of the same local anesthetic. Animal and human volunteer studies have confirmed that ropivacaine is approximately 30% to 40% less cardiotoxic than racemic bupivacaine. Ropivacaine causes less prolongation of cardiac conduction and less direct negative inotropic effects than equivalent doses of bupivacaine. During cardiac resuscitation after incremental overdosage in anesthetized dogs, free plasma concentrations of ropivacaine causing cardiac arrest were more than twice those of bupivacaine. Further, the inability to resuscitate dogs with bupivacaine was higher than with ropivacaine (50% versus 10%). Recent case reports attest to ropivacaine's lower cardiotoxicity, even after the injection of large doses sufficient to cause cardiac arrest.

Although the incidence of severe systemic toxicity from local anesthetics appears to be decreasing, the potential catastrophic outcomes from cardiotoxicity cannot be underestimated. In the most recent ASA closed claims analysis of injuries associated with regional anesthesia, unintentional intravascular injections were the second largest category of neuraxial anesthesia claims that were block related and resulted in high-severity outcome (death or brain damage). Of 12 such cases, 11 occurred in the 1980s and only 1 in the 1990s; 75% of these were associated with cardiac arrest.

Clinically significant methemoglobinemia can occur when large doses of prilocaine (>600 mg) are administered.

After several cases reports of methemoglobinemia after intravenous prilocaine was used for regional anesthesia, it was withdrawn for such use. However, it is still available as a eutectic mixture of prilocaine 2.5% and lidocaine 2.5% (EMLA cream), commonly used as a topical anesthetic. Neonatal patients have immature reductase enzyme pathways that may predispose them to methemoglobinemia with the application of EMLA cream.

Benzocaine is an ester-type local anesthetic commonly used for topical anesthesia before fiberoptic intubation, bronchoscopy, transesophageal echocardiography, and upper gastrointestinal endoscopy procedures. The Food and Drug Administration's adverse event reporting system described 132 cases of methemoglobinemia secondary to benzocaine between 1997 and 2002. These resulted in two deaths (1.5%) and 55 (42%) life-threatening complications. Potential risk factors include concomitant use of other oxidizing agents and excessive absorption from either breaks in the mucosal barrier or delivery of excessive dosages. Clinically significant toxicity is effectively treated with intravenous methylene blue (1 mg/kg).

Immunologic-mediated (allergic) reactions to preservative-free amide local anesthetics are extremely rare. However, ester local anesthetics may produce allergic reactions due to their metabolism to *para*-aminobenzoic acid (PABA), a known allergen. Amide local anesthetics are not metabolized to PABA unless preservatives (e.g., methylparaben) are used in their formulation; methylparaben is metabolized to PABA. Patients with true allergic reactions to ester local anesthetics should be treated with preservative-free local anesthetics.

MANAGEMENT

Management of systemic toxicity depends on the severity of the event. Because plasma levels of local anesthetics associated with minor reactions fall rapidly, as long as normal metabolic processes are functional, such events can be allowed to terminate spontaneously, provided attention is paid to maintaining airway patency and providing supplemental oxygen and hemodynamic support. Seizures can be terminated with small doses of intravenous midazolam (0.05 to 0.1 mg/kg), sodium thiopental (1 to 2 mg/kg), or propofol (0.5 to 1.5 mg/kg). If generalized tonic-clonic seizures are not aborted with these doses of intravenous anesthetics, administration of succinylcholine followed by endotracheal intubation is indicated. Prompt termination of seizure activity is important to prevent the rapid development of severe metabolic acidosis associated with tonic-clonic muscular contractions.

Cardiovascular depression should be treated by fluid resuscitation and vasopressors, if required. Because hypotension is usually due to a combination of direct myocardial depression and peripheral vasodilatation, agents with both β_1 and α_1 activity are recommended: ephedrine or phenylephrine or both (even epinephrine or norepinephrine) in incremental doses until the desired response is obtained. With cardiovascular collapse refractory to these drugs, vasopressin should be considered. Malignant ventricular arrhythmias should be managed with direct-current cardioversion and amiodarone if needed to prevent recurrences. If CVS toxicity is not responsive to any of these measures, intravenous lipid infusion or cardiopulmonary bypass should be considered. Recent animal models have demonstrated that intravenous lipid emulsion can facilitate resuscitation from acute bupivacaine overdose.

PREVENTION

Because the vast majority of systemic toxic reactions to local anesthetics are the result of either inadvertent intravascular injection or systemic absorption of excessive doses, efforts should be made to minimize that potential. The anesthesiologist must be aware of the risk factors associated with both the regional technique and physiologic status of the patient that predispose to clinically significant systemic toxic reactions. Proper patient preparation includes appropriate monitoring of heart rate, blood pressure, and oxygenation; recent data indicate the added value of continuous electrocardiography. Resuscitative drugs and equipment should be immediately available. Sedatives may increase the seizure threshold but also attenuate the patient's ability to report subjective symptoms of CNS toxicity, as well as reducing the heart rate's response to the traditional 15-μg epinephrine "test dose."

Techniques that reduce the likelihood of direct intravascular injection should be used. Although no single measure is 100% reliable in preventing severe systemic toxicity, the following measures are recommended:

- Inject local anesthetics in small, fractionated doses, with frequent aspiration of the syringe to assess for intravascular placement of either the needle or catheter.
- In the absence of contraindications, add epinephrine to local anesthetic solutions to aid in the identification of intravascular injections ("test dose") and to decrease systemic absorption from the injection site.
- Be aware of the different criteria for a positive epinephrine test dose during different clinical scenarios (Table 56-3).

Table 56–3 ■ Criteria for Positive Epinephrine (15 μg) Test Dose in Adults			
Clinical Scenario	**Heart Rate Increase (bpm)**	**Systolic Blood Pressure Increase (mm Hg)**	**T-Wave Amplitude**
Age <60 yr (not on β-blockers)	>20	>15	Decrease ≥25%
β-blockers	NA	>15	NA
Age >60 yr	>9	>15	Decrease ≥25%
General anesthesia	>8	>15	Decrease ≥25%

bpm, beats per minute; NA, not applicable.

REGIONAL ANESTHESIA & PAIN MANAGEMENT

- Although the scientific basis for maximum recommended doses is tenuous, and actual plasma levels vary with the site of injection, always administer the minimum effective dose.
- For blocks with a higher risk of intravascular injection or systemic absorption, consider using ropivacaine.
- During the administration of the local anesthetics, be vigilant for symptoms and signs of toxicity. Early intervention can reduce the complications of local anesthetic–induced toxicity.

Further Reading

Albright GA: Cardiac arrest following regional anesthesia with etidocaine or bupivacaine [editorial]. Anesthesiology 51:285-287, 1979.

Auroy Y, Benhamou D, Barguues L, et al: Major complications of regional anesthesia in France: The SOS regional anesthesia hotline service. Anesthesiology 97:1274-1280, 2002.

Auroy Y, Narchi P, Messiah A, et al: Serious complications related to regional anesthesia: Results of a prospective survey in France. Anesthesiology 87:479-486, 1997.

Berkum Y, Ben-Zvi A, Levy Y, et al: Evaluation of adverse reactions to local anesthetics: Experience with 236 patients. Ann Allergy Asthma Immunol 91:342-345, 2003.

Bernards CM, Carpenter RL, Rupp SM, et al: Effects of midazolam and diazepam premedication on the central nervous system and cardiovascular toxicity of bupivacaine in pigs. Anesthesiology 70:318-323, 1989.

Braid DP, Scott DB: The effect of adrenaline on the systemic absorption of local anaesthetic drugs. Acta Anaesthesiol Scand Suppl 23:334-346, 1996.

Brown DL, Ransom DM, Hall JA, et al: Regional anesthesia and local anesthetic-induced systemic toxicity: Seizure frequency and accompanying cardiovascular changes. Anesth Analg 81:321-328, 1995.

Butterworth JF, Brownlow RC, Leith JP, et al: Bupivacaine inhibits cyclic-3′, 5′-adenosine monophosphate production: A possible contributing factor to cardiovascular toxicity. Anesthesiology 79:88-95, 1993.

Butterworth JF, Strichartz GR: Molecular mechanisms of local anesthesia: A review. Anesthesiology 72:711-734, 1990.

Chazalon P, Tourtier JP, Villevielle T, et al: Ropivacaine-induced cardiac arrest after peripheral nerve block: Successful resuscitation. Anesthesiology 99:1449-1451, 2003.

Clarkson CW, Hondeghem LM: Mechanism for bupivacaine depression of cardiac conduction: Fast block sodium channels during the action potential with slow recovery during diastole. Anesthesiology 62:396-405, 1985.

Dernedde M, Furlan D, Verbesselt R, et al: Grand mal convulsions after accidental intravenous injection of ropivacaine. Anesth Analg 98:521-523, 2004.

Gall H, Kaufmann R, Kalveram CM: Adverse reactions to local anesthetics: Analysis of 197 cases. J Allergy Clin Immunol 97:933-937, 1996.

Groban L: Central nervous system and cardiac effects from long-acting amide local anesthetic toxicity in the intact animal model. Reg Anesth Pain Med 28:3-11, 2003.

Groban L, Butterworth J: Lipid reversal of bupivacaine toxicity: Has the silver bullet been identified? [editorial] Reg Anesth Pain Med 28:167-169, 2003.

Groban L, Deal DD, Vernon JC, et al: Cardiac resuscitation after incremental overdosage with lidocaine, bupivacaine, levobupivacaine, and ropivacaine in anesthetized dogs. Anesth Analg 92:37-43, 2001.

Heavner JE: Cardiac toxicity of local anesthetics in the intact isolated heart model: A review. Reg Anesth Pain Med 27:545-555, 2002.

Huet O, Eyrolle LJ, Mazoit JX, Ozier YM: Cardiac arrest after injection of ropivacaine for posterior lumbar plexus blockade. Anesthesiology 99:1451-1453, 2003.

Knudsen K, Suurkula MB, Blomberg S, et al: Central nervous and cardiovascular effects of IV infusions of ropivacaine, bupivacaine, and placebo in volunteers. Br J Anaesth 78:507-514, 1997.

Lee LA, Posner KL, Domino KB, et al: Injuries associated with regional anesthesia in the 1980s and 1990s: A closed claims analysis. Anesthesiology 101:143-152, 2004.

Liu PL, Feldman HS, Giasi R, et al: Comparative CNS toxicity of lidocaine, etidocaine, bupivacaine, and tetracaine in awake dogs following rapid intravenous administration. Anesth Analg 62:375-379, 1983.

Lofstrom JB: 1991 Labat lecture: The effects of local anesthetics on the peripheral vasculature. Reg Anesth 17:1-11, 1992.

Moore JM, Liu SS, Neal JM: Premedication with fentanyl and midazolam decreases the reliability of intravenous lidocaine test dose. Anesth Analg 86:1015-1017, 1998.

Moore TJ, Walsh CS, Cohen MR: Reported adverse event cases of methemoglobinemia associated with benzocaine products. Arch Intern Med 164:1192-1196, 2004.

Mulroy MF: Systemic toxicity and cardiotoxicity from local anesthetics: Incidence and preventative measures. Reg Anesth Pain Med 27:556-561, 2002.

Orringer CE, Eustace JC, Wunsch CD, Gardner LB: Natural history of lactic acidosis after grand-mal seizures. N Engl J Med 297:796-799, 1977.

Salinas FV: Ion channel ligands/sodium channel blockers/local anesthetics. In Evers AS, Maze M (eds): Anesthetic Pharmacology: Physiologic Principles and Clinical Practice, 1st ed. Philadelphia, Churchill Livingstone, 2004, pp 507-537.

Scott DB: Evaluation of the toxicity of local anesthetic agents in man. Br J Anaesth 47:56-59, 1975.

Soltesz EG, van Pelt F, Byrne JG: Emergent cardiopulmonary bypass for bupivacaine cardiotoxicity. J Cardiothorac Vasc Anesth 17:357-358, 2003.

Stewart J, Kellett N, Castro D: The central nervous system and cardiovascular effects of levobupivacaine and ropivacaine in healthy volunteers. Anesth Analg 97:412-416, 2003.

Szocik JF, Gardener CA, Webb RC: Inhibitory effects of bupivacaine and lidocaine on adrenergic neuroeffector junctions in rat-tail artery. Anesthesiology 78:911-917, 1993.

Tanaka M, Nishikawa T: T-wave amplitude as in indicator for detecting intravascular injection of epinephrine test dose in awake and anesthetized elderly patients. Anesth Analg 93:1332-1337, 2001.

Tanaka M, Sato M, Nishikawa T: The efficacy of simulated intravascular test dose in sedated patients. Anesth Analg 93:1612-1617, 2001.

Weinberg GL: Current concepts in resuscitation of patients with local anesthetic cardiac toxicity. Reg Anesth Pain Med 27:568-575, 2002.

Weinberg GL, Ripper R, Feinstein DL, Hoffman W: Lipid emulsion infusion rescues dogs from bupivacaine-induced cardiac toxicity. Reg Anesth Pain Med 28:198-202, 2003.

Xuecheng J, Xiaobin W, Bo G, et al: The plasma concentration of lidocaine after slow versus rapid administration of an initial dose of epidural anesthesia. Anesth Analg 84:570-573, 1997.

Spinal Hematoma

Terese T. Horlocker

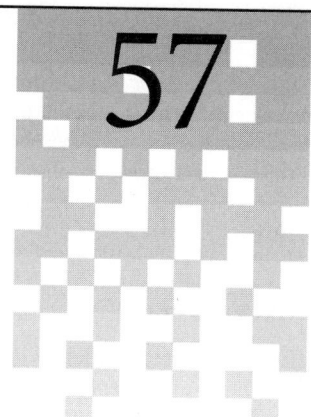

57

Case Synopsis

A 75-year-old man undergoes total knee replacement under continuous epidural anesthesia. The epidural catheter is left indwelling to provide postoperative analgesia with 0.125% bupivacaine. Thromboprophylaxis with low-molecular-weight heparin (LMWH), 30 mg twice daily, is initiated 24 hours after surgery. Forty-eight hours later, the epidural catheter is removed 1 hour after a dose of LMWH. The patient's sensory and motor block progresses, however, despite discontinuation of the local anesthetic infusion. A magnetic resonance image reveals an epidural hematoma at T12. Immediate surgical decompression results in complete neurologic recovery.

PROBLEM ANALYSIS

Definition

The actual incidence of neurologic dysfunction resulting from hemorrhagic complications associated with neuraxial blockade is unknown; however, estimates in the literature are less than 1 in 150,000 for epidural anesthesia and less than 1 in 220,000 for spinal anesthesia. In a review of the literature between 1906 and 1994, Vandermeulen and colleagues reported 61 cases of spinal hematoma associated with epidural or spinal anesthesia. In 42 of the 61 patients (69%) with spinal hematomas associated with central neural blockade, there was evidence of hemostatic abnormality. Twenty-five of the patients had received intravenous or subcutaneous (unfractionated or low-molecular-weight) heparin, and an additional five patients were presumably administered heparin during vascular surgical procedures. In addition, 12 patients had evidence of coagulopathy or thrombocytopenia or were treated with antiplatelet drugs (aspirin, indomethacin, ticlopidine), oral anticoagulants (phenprocoumon), thrombolytics (urokinase), or dextran 70 immediately before or after the spinal or epidural anesthetic. Needle and catheter placement was difficult in 15 patients (25%) and bloody in 15 patients (25%). Overall, in 53 of 61 cases (87%), either a clotting abnormality or difficult needle placement was noted. A spinal anesthetic was administered in 15 patients. The remaining 46 patients received an epidural anesthetic, including 32 patients with indwelling catheters. In 15 of the latter, spinal hematoma occurred immediately after removal of the epidural catheter. These results suggest that catheter removal is not entirely atraumatic and that the patient's coagulation status should be optimized at the time of both catheter placement and removal.

Recognition

In Vandermeulen's series, neurologic compromise presented as progression of sensory or motor block (68% of patients) or bowel or bladder dysfunction (8% of patients), rather than severe radicular back pain. Spinal hematoma should be ruled out in patients exhibiting early signs of cord compression in the postoperative period. The differential diagnosis includes cauda equina syndrome, epidural abscess, and anterior spinal artery syndrome (Table 57-1). If spinal hematoma is suspected, radiographic confirmation must be sought immediately,

Table 57–1 ■ Differential Diagnosis of Epidural Abscess, Epidural Hemorrhage, and Anterior Spinal Artery Syndrome

Finding	Epidural Abscess	Epidural Hemorrhage	Anterior Spinal Artery Syndrome
Age of patient	Any age	50% >50 yr	Elderly
Previous history	Infection*	Anticoagulants	Arteriosclerosis, hypotension
Onset	1-3 days	Sudden	Sudden
Generalized symptoms	Fever, malaise, back pain	Sharp, transient back and leg pain	None
Sensory involvement	None or paresthesias	Variable, late	Minor, patchy
Motor involvement	Flaccid paralysis, later spastic	Flaccid paralysis	Flaccid paralysis
Segmental reflexes	Exacerbated*; later obtunded	Abolished	Abolished
Myelogram/CT scan	Signs of extradural compression	Signs of extradural compression	Normal
Cerebrospinal fluid	Increased cell count	Normal	Normal
Blood data	Rise in sedimentation rate	Prolonged coagulation time*	Normal

*Infrequent findings.
CT, computed tomography.
From Wedel DJ, Horlocker TT: Risks of regional anesthesia—infectious, septic. Reg Anesth 21:57-61, 1996.

because delay can lead to irreversible cord ischemia. Although spontaneous recovery has been reported, the treatment of choice is decompressive laminectomy. Complete neurologic recovery is unlikely if surgery is postponed for more than 8 hours.

Risk Assessment

The risk of spinal hematoma depends on the timing of needle or catheter placement and removal and the degree of anticoagulation with the following drugs:

- Standard heparin (intravenous and subcutaneous)
- Low-molecular-weight heparin (LMWH)
- Oral anticoagulants
- Antiplatelet medications

STANDARD HEPARIN

Ruff and Dougherty reported spinal hematomas in 7 of 342 patients (2%) who underwent diagnostic lumbar puncture with subsequent heparinization. Three factors were associated with increased risk: less than 60 minutes between the administration of heparin and the lumbar puncture, traumatic needle placement, and concomitant use of other anticoagulants (aspirin). These findings have been used to define safe practice protocols for patients undergoing neuraxial blockade during systemic heparinization, particularly in the case of vascular surgery.

Intrathecal and epidural anesthesia and analgesia, along with complete heparinization and cardiopulmonary bypass, have been reported without neurologic sequelae. However, at this time, there are insufficient data and experience to quantify the risk of spinal hematoma among this patient population.

Low-dose subcutaneous, unfractionated heparin is administered for thromboprophylaxis in patients undergoing major thoracoabdominal surgery and in those at increased risk for hemorrhage with oral anticoagulant or LMWH therapy. A review by Schwander and Bachmann noted no spinal hematomas in more than 5000 patients who received subcutaneous heparin with spinal or epidural anesthesia. There were five cases of spinal hematoma associated with neuraxial blockade in patients receiving low-dose heparin. This confirms the limited risk associated with the use of epidural and spinal anesthesia in the presence of subcutaneous heparin treatment.

LOW-MOLECULAR-WEIGHT HEPARIN

Despite a notable safety record in Europe, in the first 5 years after the release of LMWH in North America, there were 40 cases of spinal hematoma associated with LMWH and neuraxial anesthesia. The risk of spinal hematoma, based on LMWH sales, prevalence of neuraxial techniques, and reported cases, was estimated to be approximately 1 in 3000 continuous epidural anesthetics, compared with 1 in 40,000 spinal anesthetics. However, this risk was later found to be much higher. Similar to the Vandermeulen series, severe radicular back pain was not the presenting symptom. Most patients complained of new-onset numbness, weakness, or bowel and bladder dysfunction. About half of patients undergoing a continuous technique reported neurologic deficits 12 hours or more after catheter removal. The median interval between initiation of LMWH therapy and neurologic dysfunction was 3 days, and the median time to onset of symptoms and laminectomy was more than 24 hours. Less than one third of patients reported fair or good neurologic recovery. Over the past 5 years, the number of reported cases of spinal hematoma associated with LMWH therapy has declined markedly. This may be a result of decreased reporting, improved management, or simple avoidance of all neuraxial techniques in patients receiving LMWH. Continued monitoring is necessary.

Indications and labeled uses for LMWH continue to evolve, including for thromboprophylaxis and the treatment of deep venous thrombosis. In addition, several off-label applications of LMWH are of special interest to the anesthesiologist and warrant discussion. LMWH has been shown to be efficacious as "bridge therapy" for patients chronically anticoagulated with warfarin, including parturients and patients with prosthetic cardiac valves, a history of atrial fibrillation, or preexisting hypercoagulable conditions. The patient is therapeutically anticoagulated with LMWH while the warfarin effect is allowed to resolve before surgery. Doses of LMWH are two- to threefold higher than those used for thromboprophylaxis. At least 24 hours is required for normal hemostais following this level of LMWH anticoagulation.

ORAL ANTICOAGULANTS

Few data exist regarding the risk of spinal hematoma in patients with indwelling epidural catheters who are anticoagulated with warfarin. The optimal duration of an indwelling catheter and the timing of its removal in an anticoagulated patient are also controversial. A combined series of 651 patients reported no spinal hematomas in those receiving neuraxial block in conjunction with low-dose warfarin therapy. The mean international normalized ratio (INR) at the time of catheter removal was 1.4. However, marked variability in patient response to warfarin was noted.

ANTIPLATELET MEDICATIONS

Several large studies have demonstrated the relative safety of neuraxial blockade in obstetric, surgical, and ambulatory pain clinic patients receiving antiplatelet medications. In a prospective study involving 1000 patients, Horlocker and colleagues reported that preoperative antiplatelet therapy did not increase the incidence of blood present at the time of needle or catheter placement or removal, suggesting that trauma during needle or catheter placement is neither increased nor sustained by these medications. The paucity of case reports among these patients is notable, given the prevalence of aspirin and other nonsteroidal anti-inflammatory drug (NSAID) use among patients with acute, chronic, or cancer pain who receive interventional therapy.

No series involving the performance of neuraxial blockade in the presence of thienopyridine derivatives (clopidogrel and ticlopidine) or platelet glycoprotein IIb/IIIa receptor antagonists has been reported. Although case reports are inconsistent, increased perioperative bleeding has been noted in patients undergoing cardiac and vascular surgery after receiving ticlopidine, clopidogrel, and glycoprotein IIb/IIIa antagonists. This suggests that these medications may increase the risk of regional anesthesia–related hemorrhagic complications.

Implications

Whether to perform spinal or epidural anesthesia or analgesia and the timing of catheter removal in a patient receiving thromboprophylaxis should be decided on an individual basis, weighing the small but definite risk of spinal hematoma against the benefits of regional anesthesia for the particular patient. Alternative anesthetic and analgesic techniques exist for patients considered to be at an unacceptably high risk.

MANAGEMENT

Before surgery, the patient's history should be reviewed for medical conditions associated with bleeding tendencies, and the patient should be questioned about previous episodes of sustained bleeding after trauma or surgery. Because patients respond to anticoagulants with varying sensitivities, it may be helpful to verify the reversal of heparin's or warfarin's effects before the performance of epidural or spinal blockade (Table 57-2).

The following guidelines will assist in the management of patients with altered hemostasis undergoing regional anesthetic techniques. Except in the most extraordinary circumstances, spinal and epidural blockade should be avoided in fully anticoagulated patients or those who have received thrombolytic therapy.

- Intravenous heparin
  - Administer heparin 60 minutes after needle placement.
  - Monitor the effect of the heparin.
  - Remove the catheter when heparin activity is low or completely reversed.

- Subcutaneous heparin
  - Consider delaying administration until after needle or catheter placement in patients with anticipated technical difficulties.
  - Monitor platelet count in patients receiving heparin for more than 4 days.

- Low-molecular-weight heparin
  - Proceed cautiously.
  - For preoperative LMWH, administer spinal anesthesia 12 to 24 hours after the administration of LMWH, depending on dose (i.e., treatment versus thromboprophylaxis).
  - Epidural catheters may remain indwelling with once-daily dosing of LMWH. Place or remove catheters in the morning; administer LMWH in the evening.
  - Epidural catheters should not remain indwelling with twice-daily dosing of LMWH. Remove the epidural catheter 2 hours before the initiation of twice-daily LMWH therapy.

- Oral anticoagulants
  - Preoperative administration does not preclude regional technique.
  - Monitor the prothrombin time postoperatively; there is marked variability in patient response.
  - Remove the catheter when the INR is less than 1.5.

- Antiplatelet agents
  - NSAIDs do not represent significant risk.
  - Allow the antiplatelet effects of clopidogrel, ticlopidine, and glycoprotein IIb/IIIa inhibitors to resolve before neuraxial block.

PREVENTION

The patient's coagulation status should be optimized at the time of spinal or epidural needle or catheter placement, and

---

Table 57–2 ▪ Pharmacologic Activities of Anticoagulants, Antiplatelet Agents, and Thrombolytics

Agent	Effect on Coagulation Variables		Time to Peak Effect	Time to Normal Hemostasis after Discontinuation
	PT	aPTT		
Intravenous heparin	↑	↑↑↑	Minutes	4-6 hr
Subcutaneous heparin	—	↑	40-50 min	4-6 hr
Low-molecular-weight heparin	—	—	3-5 hr	12-24 hr
Warfarin	↑↑↑	↑	4-6 days (less with loading dose)	4-6 days
Antiplatelet agents	—	—		
Aspirin			Hours	5-8 days
Other NSAIDs			Hours	1-3 days
Ticlopidine, clopidogrel			Hours	1-2 wk
Platelet glycoprotein IIb/IIIa receptor inhibitors			Minutes	8-48 hr
Fibrinolytics	↑	↑↑	Minutes	24-36 hr

aPTT, activated partial thromboplastin time; NSAID, nonsteroidal anti-inflammatory drug; PT, prothrombin time; —, no effect; ↑, clinically insignificant increase; ↑↑, possibly clinically significant increase; ↑↑↑, clinically significant increase.

the level of anticoagulation must be carefully monitored during the period of epidural catheterization. It is important to note that patients respond with variable sensitivities to anticoagulant medications. Indwelling catheters should not be removed in the presence of therapeutic anticoagulation, because this appears to significantly increase the risk of spinal hematoma. In addition, communication among clinicians involved in the perioperative management of patients receiving anticoagulants for thromboprophylaxis is essential to decrease the risk of serious hemorrhagic complications.

Further Reading

Bergqvist D, Lindblad B, Matzsch T: Low molecular weight heparin for thromboprophylaxis and epidural/spinal anaesthesia: Is there a risk? Acta Anaesthesiol Scand 36:605-609, 1992.

Chaney MA: Intrathecal and epidural anesthesia and analgesia for cardiac surgery. Anesth Analg 84:1211-1221, 1997.

CLASP (Collaborative Low-Dose Aspirin Study in Pregnancy): A randomized trial of low-dose aspirin for the prevention and treatment of preeclampsia among 9364 pregnant women. Lancet 343:619-629, 1994.

Ho AM, Chung DC, Joynt GM: Neuraxial blockade and hematoma in cardiac surgery: Estimating the risk of a rare adverse event that has not (yet) occurred. Chest 117:551-555, 2000.

Horlocker TT, Bajwa ZH, Ashraft Z, et al: Risk assessment of hemorrhagic complications associated with nonsteroidal antiiflammatory medications in ambulatory pain clinic patients undergoing epidural steroid injection. Anesth Analg 95:1691-1697, 2002.

Horlocker TT, Wedel DJ, Benzon H, et al: Regional anesthesia and anticoagulation—defining the risk. The Second ASRA consensus conference on neuraxial anesthesia and anticoagulation. Reg Anesth Pain Med 28:172-197, 2003.

Horlocker TT, Wedel DJ, Offord KP, et al: Preoperative antiplatelet therapy does not increase the risk of spinal hematoma associated with regional anesthesia. Anesth Analg 80:303-309, 1995.

Odoom JA, Sih IL: Epidural analgesia and anticoagulant therapy. Anaesthesia 38:254-259, 1983.

Rao TLK, El-Etr AA: Anticoagulation following placement of epidural and subarachnoid catheters: An evaluation of neurologic sequelae. Anesthesiology 55:618-620, 1981.

Ruff RL, Dougherty JH: Complications of lumbar puncture followed by anticoagulation. Stroke 12:879-881, 1981.

Schroeder DR: Statistics: Detecting a rare adverse drug reaction using spontaneous reports. Reg Anesth Pain Med 23:183-189, 1998.

Schwander D, Bachmann F: Heparin and spinal or epidural anesthesia: Decision analysis [review]. Ann Fr Anesth Reanim 10:284-296, 1991.

Tryba M: Epidural regional anesthesia and low molecular heparin: Pro [German]. Anasth Intensivmed Notfallmed Schmerzther 28:179-181, 1993.

Vandermeulen EP, Van Aken H, Vermylen J: Anticoagulants and spinal-epidural anesthesia. Anesth Analg 79:1165-1177, 1994.

Wu CL, Perkins FM: Oral anticoagulant prophylaxis and epidural catheter removal. Reg Anesth 21:517-524, 1996.

Infectious Complications of Central Neuraxial Block

58

James C. Crews

Case Synopsis

A 63-year-old woman with a history of diabetes mellitus, hypertension, and chronic low back pain underwent a small bowel resection for obstruction secondary to metastatic colon cancer. A thoracic epidural catheter was placed for perioperative analgesia, and the patient received an epidural infusion of bupivacaine and morphine for 3 days postoperatively. At the time of epidural catheter removal, the insertion site was surrounded by a small area of erythema, with a scant amount of serosanguineous drainage. The patient was followed by the Acute Pain Service for an additional 2 days, at which time she reported severe thoracolumbar back pain, low-grade fever, and heaviness in her legs. Examination of the back revealed a small erythematous area at the previous epidural catheter insertion site with a small amount of purulent drainage. The neurologic examination was unremarkable. Laboratory studies demonstrated leukocytosis. Owing to the patient's history and complaints, a magnetic resonance imaging (MRI) scan with and without gadolinium contrast was obtained of the thoracic, lumbar, and sacral spine. MRI demonstrated an extensive posterior spinal epidural abscess from T10 to L2. The patient underwent a laminotomy drainage procedure and culture-directed antibiotic therapy for *Staphylococcus aureus*. The remainder of her hospital recovery was uneventful, and she was discharged home without neurologic sequelae.

PROBLEM ANALYSIS

Definition

Infectious complications of central neuraxial anesthetic and analgesic procedures occur rarely but may be associated with significant patient morbidity, including sepsis, epidural or paravertebral abscess formation, meningitis, and paraplegia. A high index of suspicion, early diagnosis, and prompt intervention with appropriate therapy are important for achieving optimal outcomes.

Infectious complications of central neuraxial block techniques may range from superficial infection at the percutaneous puncture site to more consequential infections, such as epidural abscess or meningitis. Most consequential infectious complications are associated with percutaneous catheter techniques, although epidural abscess and meningitis have been reported after single-injection epidural anesthesia or corticosteroid injections. Potential mechanisms for infection associated with central neuraxial block include (1) direct inoculation during needle or catheter placement; (2) infection at the catheter exit site, with spread along the catheter track; (3) contamination of the injectate; and (4) hematogenous spread ("bacteremic seeding") from a distant site of infection.

Progressive neurologic impairment of bowel and bladder function or lower extremity sensory and motor function may result from epidural or paravertebral abscess with spinal cord or nerve root compression. The specific pathogenesis underlying spinal cord dysfunction with spinal epidural abscess is thought to be related to direct mechanical compression or vascular damage, with resultant spinal cord hypoxia.

Recognition

Superficial infectious complications usually present with localized erythema and drainage at the needle or catheter insertion site. Deep infections may present with local symptoms at the needle or catheter insertion site in addition to the following:

- Back pain
- Fever
- Localized tenderness
- Leukocytosis

Neurologic impairment due to deep tissue abscess and spinal cord or nerve root compression may present with the following:

- Radicular irritation
- Progressive sensory or motor neurologic deficit
- Bowel and bladder incontinence

The clinical features of meningitis include the following:

- Nuchal rigidity
- Headache
- Leukocytosis and fever
- Photophobia

Patients with evidence of superficial infection should be evaluated and monitored for the development of symptoms associated with deep infection. Culture of purulent drainage at the site of infection or epidural catheter tip may be important to direct appropriate antibiotic therapy. Before hospital discharge, patients must be instructed to notify appropriate health care personnel or to seek emergency medical evaluation in the event of any of the following:

- New onset of back pain
- Fever
- Redness or soreness at the needle or catheter insertion site
- Subtle signs or symptoms of neurologic impairment

Patients with signs or symptoms suggestive of spinal or epidural abscess should be urgently evaluated for fever and leukocytosis and have a thorough neurologic evaluation. Radiographic diagnosis of spinal epidural abscess is best made by gadolinium-enhanced MRI scan of the spine (Figs. 58-1 and 58-2). Diagnosis and treatment of epidural abscess should *not* be delayed until neurologic deficits become apparent.

Risk Assessment

In a meta-analysis of 915 patients with spinal epidural abscess reported in the world literature between 1954 and 1997, neuraxial anesthesia or analgesia had been performed in 5.5% of them; other invasive procedures as diverse as vascular access and spinal surgery accounted for 16.5%. Estimates of the incidence of spinal epidural abscess after central neuraxial block range from 1 in1930 for continuous epidural catheter techniques to 1 in 100,000 for single-injection and short-term techniques. For patients with chronically implanted epidural catheter systems, infectious risk has been reported as 1 per 1702 catheter-days. Although the specific incidence is unclear, the presence of any of the following factors suggests a higher risk for infection following central neuraxial block:

- Immunocompromised state (e.g., acquired immunodeficiency syndrome [AIDS], cancer chemotherapy, organ transplantation, chronic dialysis, intravenous drug abuse, chronic alcoholism)
- Diabetes mellitus
- Concomitant steroid treatment

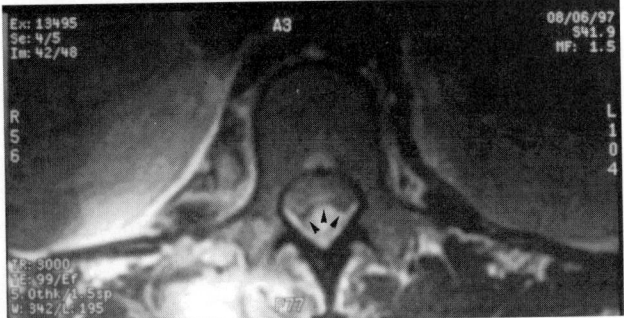

Figure 58–1 ▪ Axial T2-weighted magnetic resonance image of the spine at the level of L1. There is a large, high-signal fluid collection in the posterior epidural space. The abscess is causing anterior displacement of the dural sac *(arrowheads)*, producing approximately 30% reduction in the anteroposterior diameter of the spinal canal. (From Rathmell JP, Garahan MB, Alsofrom GF: Epidural abscess following epidural analgesia. Reg Anesth Pain Med 25:79-82, 2000.)

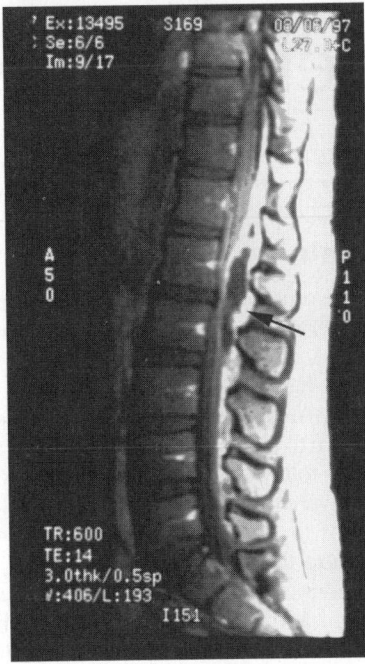

Figure 58–2 ▪ Sagittal T1-weighted magnetic resonance image of the spine following intravenous administration of gadolinium. There is a large gadolinium-enhanced mass (arrow) in the posterior epidural space extending from T9 to L3. The area of low signal density within the abscess represents a poorly perfused area of liquefaction. (From Rathmell JP, Garahan MB, Alsofrom GF: Epidural abscess following epidural analgesia. Reg Anesth Pain Med 25:79-82, 2000.)

- Localized infection at insertion site
- Sepsis
- Long-term catheter use
- Bacteremia

Implications

Both meningitis and epidural abscess can be life threatening or result in permanent neurologic sequelae if not treated immediately. A high index of clinical suspicion, early diagnosis, and prompt treatment before massive neurologic symptoms occur are key to optimizing patient outcomes.

MANAGEMENT

Patients with superficial infectious complications can be managed by local drainage and antibiotic therapy. However, even these patients, especially those at increased risk for more serious infectious complications, should be carefully instructed and monitored for the development of any signs or symptoms of epidural or spinal abscess or meningitis. They should also be advised to seek immediate medical attention for progressive back pain, fever, or the development of subtle neurologic changes. This will facilitate timely detection, diagnosis, and therapy. Patients with a history of central neuraxial block who present with back pain and fever should undergo a thorough evaluation for serious infectious complications as part of the differential diagnosis. Epidural abscess following central neuraxial block has been diagnosed days, weeks, and even months after the intervention.

Although more conservative treatment approaches have been reported, surgical drainage and antibiotic therapy for epidural abscess are still the definitive treatment of choice. Epidural abscess with neurologic signs or symptoms requires urgent surgical intervention to prevent progressive and possibly permanent neurologic injury.

Antibiotic therapy should be initiated promptly. The initial agent used should be effective against *Staphylococcus aureus* and able to penetrate bone. Ultimately, antibiotic therapy should be directed by specific culture and sensitivity determinations, as well as by clinical or institutional considerations. Depending on the nature and severity of the infection, antibiotic therapy may be required for 4 to 6 weeks or longer.

PREVENTION

As with any invasive procedure, the risks associated with a planned central neuraxial block must be weighed against its potential benefits. Although infectious complications are rare, patients who might benefit most from such blocks are often those with associated morbidities or other factors that increase the risk for serious infectious complications. If central neuraxial blocks are used in patients at increased risk for complications, especially if the extended use of indwelling catheters is anticipated for postoperative or post-traumatic injury pain relief, a higher index of suspicion is required when evaluating these patients for potential infectious complications.

Meticulous attention to sterile technique is vital for reducing infectious complications associated with central neuraxial blocks or catheters. Thorough hand washing, sterile gloves, surgical caps or hoods and masks, and sterile block techniques are all important considerations. A wide area of skin should be prepared with povidone-iodine, iodophor-in-isopropyl alcohol, or chlorhexidine. Adequate time must be given for the solution to dry before the central neuraxial block is performed. Also, use of a "no-touch" technique (i.e., landmarks identified and marked, if necessary, before skin preparation) helps reduce the risk of central neuraxial infectious complications. Chlorhexidine and iodophor-in-isopropyl alcohol reportedly provide better antimicrobial skin disinfection and prevention of bacterial regrowth compared with povidone-iodine. Use of clear plastic surgical drapes offers the advantage of being able to visualize landmarks during the block procedure. Further, covering epidural catheters with clear sterile dressings allows daily assessment of the insertion site.

Sterile technique should be maintained for dosing catheters and when changing infusion connections for continuous epidural infusions. Maintaining a tightly closed infusion system throughout therapy should help reduce catheter contamination during line or infusate changes. Infusion solutions should be prepared by pharmacy personnel with sterile technique and under a laminar flow hood.

Central neuraxial block in patients with bacteremia remains controversial. If such blocks are deemed necessary or appropriate in patients with bacteremia, one should consider performing the block only after appropriate antibiotic coverage has been provided. For patients with indwelling epidural catheters who become bacteremic, it is my practice to remove the catheter, provide indicated antibiotic therapy, and then replace the catheter at a different level if continuous epidural therapy is still desired. Both for cost considerations and because of its low predictive value in identifying contamination and infection, routine culture of epidural catheter tips is not advised. However, if the epidural catheter insertion site is surrounded by an area of localized inflammation or drainage, bacteriologic examination of the epidural catheter tip may suggest appropriate antibiotic therapy.

Although preventive measures are important, they cannot entirely eliminate the risk of infectious complications of central neuraxial block. A high index of suspicion for the development of infectious complications, prompt diagnosis, and immediate therapy are paramount for reducing patient morbidity and permanent neurologic injury.

Further Reading

Aota Y, Onari K, Suga Y: Iliopsoas abscess and persistent radiculopathy: A rare complication of continuous infusion techniques of epidural anesthesia. Anesthesiology 96:1023-1025, 2002.

Birnbach DJ, Meadows W, Stein DJ, et al: Comparison of povidone iodine and DuraPrep, an iodophor-in-isopropyl alcohol solution, for skin disinfection prior to epidural catheter insertion in parturients. Anesthesiology 98:164-169, 2003.

Dawson S: Epidural catheter infections. J Hosp Infect 47:3-8, 2001.

Du Pen SL, Peterson DG, Williams A, Bogosian AJ: Infection during chronic epidural catheterization: Diagnosis and treatment. Anesthesiology 73:905-909, 1990.

Hooten WM, Kinney MO, Huntoon MA: Epidural abscess and meningitis after epidural corticosteroid injection. Mayo Clin Proc 79:682-686, 2004.

Huang RC, Shapiro GS, Lim M, et al: Cervical epidural abscess after epidural steroid injection. Spine 29:E7-E9, 2004.

Kindler CH, Seeberger MD, Staender SE: Epidural abscess complicating epidural anesthesia and analgesia: An analysis of the literature. Acta Anaesthesiol Scand 42:614-620, 1998.

Kinirons B, Mimoz O, Lafendi L, et al: Chlorhexidine versus povidone iodine in preventing colonization of continuous epidural catheters in children: A randomized, controlled trial. Anesthesiology 94:239-244, 2001.

Koka VK, Potti A: Spinal epidural abscess after corticosteroid injections. South Med J 95:772-774, 2002.

Lee BB, Kee WD, Griffith JF: Vertebral osteomyelitis and psoas abscess occurring after obstetric epidural anesthesia. Reg Anesth Pain Med 27: 220-224, 2002.

Leys D, Lesoin F, Viaud C, et al: Decreased morbidity from acute bacterial spinal epidural abscesses using computed tomography and nonsurgical treatment in selected patients. Ann Neurol 17:350-355, 1985.

Rathmell JP, Garahan MB, Alsofrom GF: Epidural abscess following epidural analgesia. Reg Anesth Pain Med 25:79-82, 2000.

Reihsaus E, Waldbaur H, Seeling W: Spinal epidural abscess: A meta-analysis of 915 patients. Neurosurg Rev 23:175-204, 2000.

Sorensen P: Spinal epidural abscesses: Conservative treatment for selected subgroups of patients. Br J Neurosurg 17:513-518, 2003.

Steffen P, Seeling W, Essig A, et al: Bacterial contamination of epidural catheters: Microbiological examination of 502 epidural catheters used for postoperative analgesia. J Clin Anesth 16:92-97, 2004.

Trautmann M, Lepper PM, Schmitz FJ: Three cases of bacterial meningitis after spinal and epidural anesthesia. Eur J Clin Microbiol Infect Dis 21:43-45, 2002.

Wang LP, Hauerberg J, Schmidt JF: Incidence of spinal epidural abscess after epidural analgesia: A national 1-year survey. Anesthesiology 91: 1928-1936, 1999.

Wittum S, Hofer CK, Rolli U, et al: Sacral osteomyelitis after single-shot epidural anesthesia via the caudal approach in a child. Anesthesiology 99:503-505, 2003.

REGIONAL ANESTHESIA & PAIN MANAGEMENT

Epidural Anesthesia: Unintended Intrathecal Injection

59

Thomas McCutchen and J. C. Gerancher

Case Synopsis

A frail, 55-kg, 79-year-old woman is admitted for elective hip replacement as the first surgery of the day in a busy ambulatory surgery center. An epidural catheter is placed for surgical anesthesia and postoperative analgesia. With the patient sitting on the operating room table, catheter placement is uneventful. Fifteen milliliters of a slightly hypobaric solution (2% lidocaine with 5 μg/mL of both fentanyl and epinephrine) is administered via the catheter in three 5-mL doses over 3 minutes. Pain in the arthritic hip is immediately relieved, and the patient's lower extremities become insensate. Five minutes later, she complains of weakness and experiences difficulty breathing. She then becomes apneic and unconscious, with subsequent oxygen desaturation and hypotension. She is ventilated with a mask and then intubated. Blood pressure is maintained with ephedrine and intravenous fluid.

PROBLEM ANALYSIS

Definition

When local anesthetic in volumes typically used for epidural analgesia or anesthesia is unintentionally administered into the subarachnoid (intrathecal) space, morbidity and mortality may result due to high spinal anesthesia. Such injection may occur if local anesthetic is delivered through a needle or catheter that has fully or partially penetrated the dura and arachnoid membranes.

Recognition

The clinical consequences of unintended intrathecal injection depend on the amount of local anesthetic introduced into the cerebrospinal fluid (CSF). Small amounts result in numbness of the lower extremities; larger amounts result in extensive spread and possibly unconsciousness and respiratory arrest secondary to brainstem anesthesia.

Risk Assessment: Anatomic Considerations

The epidural space lies outside the dura mater. This tough outer layer of the meninges fuses with periosteum at the foramen magnum. The epidural space extends laterally to the spinal nerve roots, where it fuses with epineurium in the intervertebral foramina, caudad to the sacrococcygeal ligament and anterior to the posterior longitudinal ligament, ligamentum flavum, and laminae. It communicates with the paravertebral space via intervertebral foramina. The contents of the epidural space consist of fat, which is found predominantly posteriorly and laterally. Valveless veins are found predominantly in the lateral and anterior epidural space.

The arachnoid membrane is a delicate membrane that abuts the inner surface of the dura mater. It consists of layers of flattened cells with connective tissue fibers running between these layers. The cells are interconnected by tight junctions, which likely accounts for the fact that the arachnoid is the principal physiologic barrier for drugs diffusing from the epidural space to the intrathecal space. In the region of the foramina, where spinal nerve roots traverse both the arachnoid and the dura mater, the arachnoid membrane herniates through the dura to form granulations. Both spinal and intracranial arachnoid granulations serve as portals for CSF and its constituents to exit the central nervous system.

The pia mater is an even more delicate layer of the meninges that is adherent to the spinal cord. The intrathecal space lies between the arachnoid membrane and the pia mater and contains CSF. Spinal CSF directly communicates with intracranial CSF.

Implications

The epidural space is a potential space, as the majority of the dura is in contact with the walls of the vertebral canal. It is also a discontinuous series of compartments that become continuous only when liquid or air is injected. Thus, a larger dose of local anesthetic is required for epidural anesthesia or analgesia compared with spinal anesthesia. This anatomy also explains the bandlike block that develops in dermatomes just above and below the level of epidural local anesthetic injection, with further spread directly related to the volume of local anesthetic injected. In contrast, when local anesthetic is introduced into and diffuses throughout CSF within the intrathecal space to produce spinal anesthesia, it can produce block well above and below the level of injection. In addition to the volume of drug delivered and its concentration, spread of an intrathecally administered local anesthetic is related to the patient's position, depending on whether a hypotonic or hypertonic local anesthetic solution is injected. If the solution is isotonic, spread of the block is more dependent on the volume and concentration of the local anesthetic injected intrathecally, regardless of whether vasoconstrictors are used to prolong the block.

The C3-C5 spinal nerve roots, which contribute to the phrenic nerves, may be anesthetized with "high" epidural blocks. Thus, phrenic nerve paralysis may result from high epidural anesthesia. This can lead to respiratory paralysis with complete awareness. However, because intracranial and vertebral spinal fluid are continuous, spinal anesthetics can reach and anesthetize the brainstem. Finally, direct communication between the epidural and paravertebral spaces may result in a one-sided epidural block, especially if the epidural catheter is placed near, or the majority of local anesthetic is deposited into, a nerve root foramen laterally or the posterior longitudinal ligament anteriorly.

MANAGEMENT

Early recognition of unintentional spinal injection is paramount to prevent further injections and limit the potential for morbidity. If the patient is in pain as the epidural is being dosed (e.g., an obstetric patient in active labor), the first sign of an unintended intrathecal injection may be almost immediate, total cessation of all pain after injection of a small test dose. This may be followed by motor and sensory block that develops more rapidly and extensively than expected with epidural injection.

Treatment for unintended spinal injection is supportive and consists of ensuring a patent airway, oxygenating and ventilating the patient, and supporting blood pressure with fluids (volume) and vasopressors (if needed) until the high block resolves. In any setting where neuraxial anesthesia is used, basic airway equipment must be readily available, along with a well-thought-out plan for managing unconscious and apneic patients with possible complete cardiovascular collapse.

PREVENTION

Prevention requires a high index of suspicion during epidural needle and catheter placement, with careful aspiration and appropriate test dosing of the needle and catheter before the administration of the planned epidural volume of local anesthetic. With obvious free flow of CSF via the epidural needle or catheter during attempts to locate the epidural space, epidural-strength doses and volumes of local anesthetic should not be administered. Often, inadvertent intrathecal needle or catheter placement is not obvious. For example, a dural rent or small tear may be made by the tip of the needle intended for epidural placement. This rent or tear may be large enough to admit an epidural catheter, but there would be no CSF return from the needle because its tip resides mostly in the epidural space. In this case, slow, deliberate aspiration of the catheter before injection might identify CSF.

If saline is used for the loss-of-resistance technique or an epidural catheter is being replaced after recent dosing via a previously placed epidural catheter, it may be difficult to determine whether the clear fluid aspirated from the supposed epidural space is previously injected saline or local anesthetic or CSF. Several maneuvers have been suggested to distinguish CSF from other fluids, including measurement of pH, temperature, glucose, and turbidity when mixed with thiopental. Unfortunately, none of these methods has broad clinical utility. If bubbles are aspirated along with the clear fluid and the total amount of clear fluid that can be aspirated is less than 3 to 5 mL, the catheter is *not* likely to be in the intrathecal space. However, the catheter should not be used until it has been adequately tested.

Epidural test doses consist of a small amount of local anesthetic. The rationale is that such small amounts injected into the intrathecal space would produce an easily recognizable motor and sensory spinal block without producing unacceptably high spinal anesthesia; if the same test dose were injected epidurally, it should produce minimal or no obvious effects. A typical test dose might be 40 to 60 mg of lidocaine, which would quickly produce signs and symptoms of relatively low-level spinal block if injected intrathecally. One must also keep in mind that if combined spinal-epidural anesthesia is performed and the patient has received sufficient spinal local anesthetic for high- or low-level surgical anesthesia, any subsequent epidural test dose might result in an unacceptably high level of spinal anesthesia.

In all instances, repeat dosing of an in situ epidural catheter should be incremental. Case reports have noted catheter migration into the intrathecal space. Providing an appropriate time interval between incremental dosing to assess for intrathecal injection should allow for the detection of migrated catheters. Finally, intrathecal catheters left in place intentionally should be clearly labeled as such, to prevent accidental dosing with epidural volumes of local anesthetic.

Further Reading

Bernards CM: Epidural and spinal anesthesia. In Barash PG, Cullen BF, Stoelting RK (eds): Clinical Anesthesia, 4th ed. Philadelphia, Lippincott Williams & Wilkins, 2001, pp 689-713.

Bernards CM, Hill H: The spinal nerve root sleeve is not a preferred route for redistribution of drugs from the epidural space to the spinal cord. Anesthesiology 75:827, 1991.

Calimaran AL, Strauss-Hoder TP, Wang WY, et al: The effect of epidural test dose on motor function after a combined spinal-epidural technique for labor analgesia. Anesth Analg 96:167-172, 1996.

Hogan Q: Epidural catheter tip position and distribution of injectate evaluated by computed tomography. Anesthesiology 90:964-970, 1994.

Poblete B, Van Gessel EF, Gaggero G, Gamulin Z: Efficacy of three test doses to detect epidural catheter misplacement. Can J Anaesth 46:34-39, 1999.

Reisner LS: Epidural test solution or spinal fluid? Anesthesiology 44:451, 1976.

Tessler MJ, Wiesel S, Wahba RM, Quance DR: A comparison of simple identification tests to distinguish cerebrospinal fluid from local anaesthetic solution. Anaesthesia 49:821-822, 1994.

Visser WA: Delayed subarachnoid migration of an epidural catheter. Anesthesiology 88:1414-1415, 1998.

Waters JH, Rizzo VL, Ramanathan S: A re-evaluation of the ability of thiopental to identify cerebrospinal fluid in epidural catheter aspirate. J Clin Anesth 7:224-227, 1995.

Epidural Anesthesia: Unintended Subdural Injection

60

Thomas McCutchen and J. C. Gerancher

Case Synopsis

A healthy, 80-kg primigravida (38 weeks' gestation) is admitted in active labor, with a cesarean section (C-section) planned for breech presentation. Because of an anticipated 1-hour delay before the C-section can begin, a lumbar epidural block is requested for analgesia and anesthesia. This is placed without incident. The patient experiences a significant amount of pain with injection of the 3-mL test dose (1.5% lidocaine with 1:200,000 epinephrine). There are no signs of intrathecal or intravenous administration. The catheter is pulled back 1 cm, and 10 mL of 2% lidocaine is injected in 5-mL increments, with less pain. Her contraction pain resolves completely, and she develops a T6-level block to temperature. Fifteen minutes before the C-section, an additional 15 mL of 2% lidocaine is administered through the epidural catheter, with total loss of sensation below T6 5 minutes after arrival in the operating room. Fifteen minutes later, the patient complains of difficulty breathing; her hand grip and biceps strength are weak. The patient becomes lethargic, followed by a loss of consciousness and finally apnea. She is successfully intubated, and the case proceeds under general anesthesia. She is mechanically ventilated in the operating room and postanesthesia care unit for 3 hours after the initial epidural dosing. She then begins to awaken, gains strength, and is successfully extubated. Later that day, radiopaque contrast material is injected through the epidural catheter and reveals cephalad, parallel, "train-tracking" of the contrast medium.

PROBLEM ANALYSIS

Definition

If local anesthetic in volumes typically used for epidural analgesia or anesthesia are unintentionally administered into the subdural space, considerable morbidity and mortality may result. Also, such injections may result in inadequate blockade.

Recognition

Classically, subdural injection has been described as an unexpectedly high block 15 to 35 minutes after intended lumbar epidural injection. When investigated with radiographic contrast material, a stereotypical cephalad "railroad tracking" of contrast material (outlining the subdural space circumferentially around the thecal sac) has been seen (Figs. 60-1 to 60-3). Since 1975, there have been 30 reports of unusually extensive blocks with subdural injection that were confirmed by radiocontrast radiography. Because the subdural space extends above the foramen magnum, some cases presented as unconsciousness with centrally mediated apnea.

Recent work, mainly by Collier, suggests that cases with the latter presentation are merely one subset of the possible clinical manifestations of subdural injection. Other presentations, including low block, unilateral block, and dermatomal block, are usually not investigated with radiographic contrast material and thus are not recognized as attributable to local anesthetic subdural injection. The myriad possible presentations of subdural injection have not been identified owing to the dearth of investigation. Collier recently used radiography to investigate 35 cases of atypical or inadequate epidural blocks for cesarean delivery and found four instances (11.4%) of subdural radiocontrast injection. Each patient had severe pain with injection of less than 5 mL of "epidural" local anesthetic. Three had low blocks, and one had a one-sided block. With time (25 to 50 minutes), and after the injection of 10 to 20 mL of additional local anesthetic, all patients eventually achieved surgical anesthesia.

Depending on the volume injected and the force and direction of injection, local anesthetic may track cephalad, caudad, or laterally toward a nerve root or form a well-localized "pocket" of local anesthetic. Further, use of multiple orifice catheters may facilitate multicompartment (e.g., subdural-epidural or subdural-intrathecal) injections. Collier further speculates that several potential tissue planes exist within the arachnoid membrane and the arachnoid-dura interface, "with each plane having its own radiographic findings and clinical significance."

Risk Assessment

Subdural injections are not injections into a potential space, as epidural injections are. Rather, the injectate produces

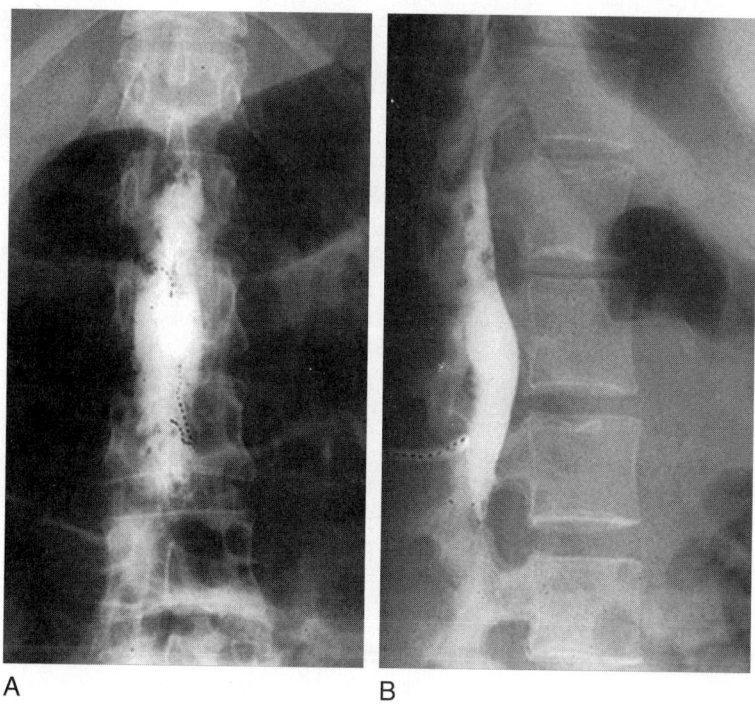

Figure 60–1 ■ Anteroposterior *(A)* and lateral *(B)* views of the lumbar spine after radiocontrast injection through a lumbar catheter *(dotted line)* reveal a focal collection of contrast material in the subdural space anterior to the thecal sac. (From Collier CB: Accidental subdural injection during attempted lumbar epidural block may present as failed or inadequate block: Radiographic evidence. Reg Anesth Pain Med 29:45-51, 2004.)

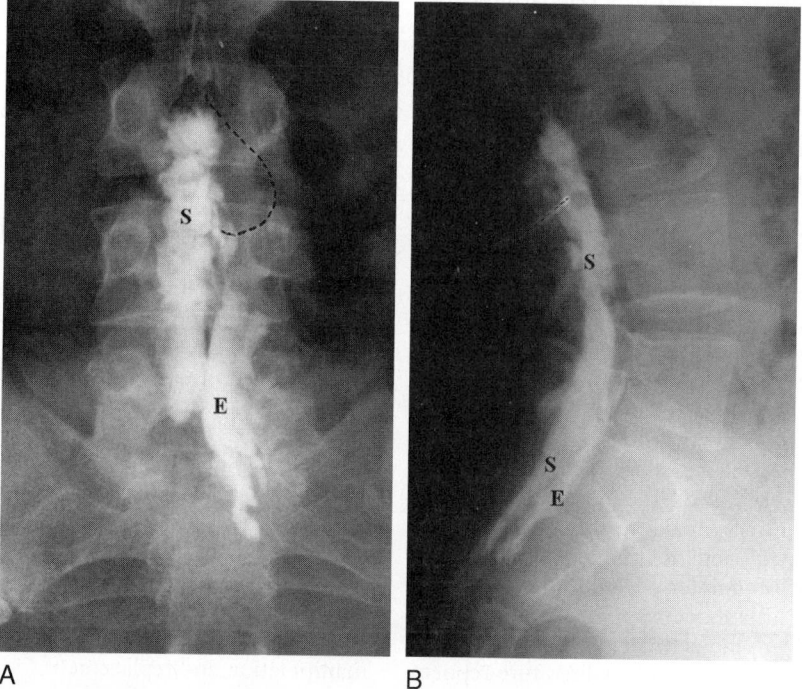

Figure 60–2 ■ Anteroposterior *(A)* and lateral *(B)* views of the lumbar spine after contrast injection through a lumbar catheter *(dotted line)* reveal multicompartment spread of radiocontrast around the thecal sac in the subdural space of L3-L5 (S), and anterior-caudad spread of radiocontrast into the sacral canal (E). (From Collier CB: Accidental subdural injection during attempted epidural block may present as failed or inadequate block: Radiographic evidence. Reg Anesth Pain Med 29:45-51, 2004.)

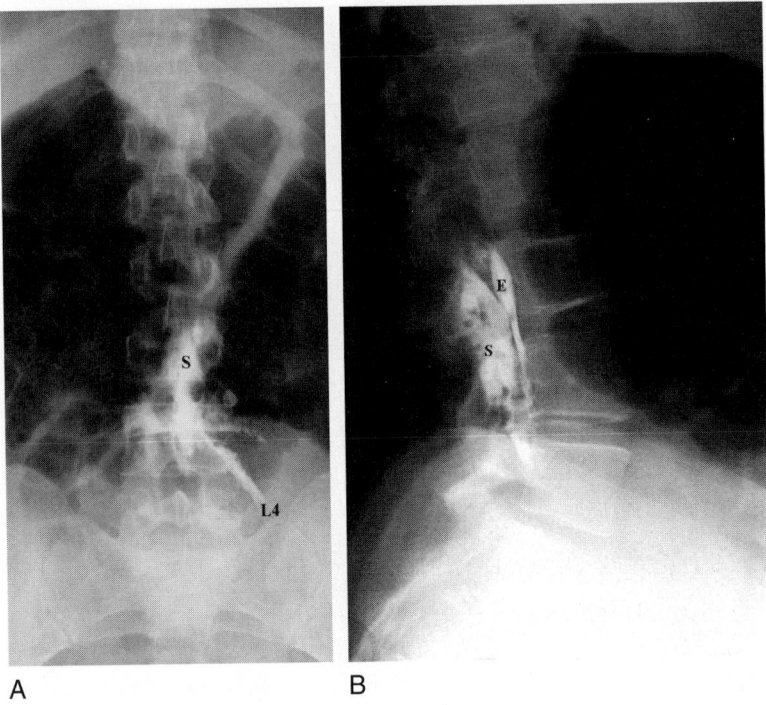

A   B

Figure 60–3 ■ Anteroposterior *(A)* and lateral *(B)* views of the lumbar spine after radiocontrast injection through a lumbar catheter reveal multicompartment subdural spread of radiocontrast (S), including localized extension along the L4 nerve root (visible in *A*) and into the epidural space (E) of L3. (From Collier CB: Accidental subdural injection during attempted lumbar epidural block may present as failed or inadequate block: Radiographic evidence. Reg Anesth Pain Med 29:45-51, 2004.)

a disruptive dissection between two tissue planes. Both Collier and Reina and colleagues describe the subdural space as the dura-arachnoid interface formed by a cellular junction between the two membranes. This junction is composed of neuroepithelial cells surrounded by an amorphous substance. There is no subdural space in nontraumatized tissues. Both groups hypothesize that a subdural space may appear if the neuroepithelial cells break up as a result of pressure exerted by mechanical shear forces, air, or injected fluids. Any of these have the potential to create fissures within the amorphous substance of the dura-arachnoid interface. Such fissures could readily expand toward weaker areas, especially laterally, where the amorphous substance is more prolific.

Unintended subdural injection occurs when local anesthetic is injected through a needle or catheter that has created a disruption in the subdural space large enough to accommodate local anesthetic. Subdural injections are unpredictable. Given the flimsy nature of the arachnoid and its intimate relationship with the dura, it is remarkable that subdural injections are even possible. Indeed, the most skilled neurosurgeons have difficulty incising the dura under direct vision without disrupting the arachnoid membrane.

The reported rate of unintended subdural injection during epidural anesthesia is about 0.8%. However, it is now believed that subdural injections are more common than previously thought. Indeed, the radiology literature reports a 10% rate of subdural injection during attempted spinal myelography. A likely explanation for this discrepancy is that radiologists have readily available radiocontrast materials for detecting subdural injections. Thus, unusual blocks following

epidural injection that are not investigated radiographically may be the result of subdural injection.

Implications

Patients may have transient pain with the injection of small volumes of local anesthetic. This is uncommon with epidural or intrathecal injection of similar volumes. This pain is thought to be caused by either cleaving of meningeal tissues or nerve root compression due to the mass effect of subdural injectates. Pain is short-lived and without sequelae. Additional doses cause little if any pain.

Subdural local anesthetic injection can present in multiple ways, depending on the spread and direction of the dissecting injectate and the amount that enters the epidural, subdural, or intrathecal compartment. Subdural and multicompartment injections may present as a high block, low block, radicular block, "patchy" block, or one-sided block. High blocks caused by subdural injections have a clinical presentation similar to that of high spinal blockade (unconsciousness, centrally mediated apnea, hypotension). High subdurals may be difficult to distinguish from high epidurals, because both blocks mature over a relatively long period (15 to 30 minutes). With additional local anesthetic and time, inadequate blocks may eventually resemble a normal epidural block, or they may require catheter manipulation and replacement.

Attempted intrathecal block after subdural injection may be difficult, because the needle and injectate tend to reenter the newly created subdural space. This may occur even several months after suspected subdural injection, suggesting that a permanent defect may be formed that predisposes the patient to subsequent subdural injections. Indeed, two of Collier's most recent cases involved one patient who experienced subdural injection during what appeared to be uncomplicated epidural catheter placements for two cesarean deliveries.

MANAGEMENT

Treatment of extensive blockade is supportive, as for unintended high intrathecal injection. Inadequate subdural blockade may be overcome with additional doses of local anesthetic, but there is the associated risk of more extensive block.

PREVENTION

Unlike the situation with intrathecal needle or catheter placement, aspiration and incremental dosing do not prevent subdural injection. However, removing a needle or catheter through which small injections of local anesthetic produced pain may prevent subdural blockade.

Further Reading

Bernards CM: Epidural and spinal anesthesia. In Barash PG, Cullen BF, Stoelting RK (eds):Clinical Anesthesia, 4th ed. Philadelphia, Lippincott Williams & Wilkins, 2001, pp 689-713.

Collier CB: Accidental subdural block: Four more cases and a radiographic review. Anesth Intensive Care 20:215-232, 1992.

Collier CB: Accidental subdural injection during attempted lumbar epidural block may present as a failed or inadequate block: Radiographic evidence. Reg Anesth Pain Med 29:45-51, 2004.

Jones M, Newton T: Inadvertent extra-arachnoid injections in myelography. Radiology 80:818, 1963.

Lubenow T, Keh-Wong E, Kristof K, et al: Inadvertent subdural injection: A complication of epidural block. Anesth Analg 67:175, 1988.

Reina MA, De Leon Casasola O, Lopez A, et al: The origin of the spinal subdural space: Ultrastructure findings. Anesth Analg 94:991-995, 2002.

Schultz GH, Brogden BG: The problem of subdural placement in myelography. Radiology 79:91-95, 1962.

REGIONAL ANESTHESIA &
PAIN MANAGEMENT

Interscalene Nerve Block: Potential Severe Complications

61

Alain Borgeat and Steffan Blumenthal

Case Synopsis

A 25-year-old man presents for rotator cuff repair and has an interscalene block and catheter placed. The block is performed using Winnie's landmarks and with the aid of a nerve stimulator. A triceps response is obtained at a depth of 2.5 cm. The catheter is threaded 6 cm past the tip of the stimulating needle. The procedure is uneventful, except for transient resistance encountered during catheter placement. After negative aspiration for blood and cerebrospinal fluid, 0.5% bupivacaine is slowly injected through the catheter. After 10 mL is injected, the patient becomes drowsy, then unresponsive and apneic, with loss of muscle tone in all extremities; his pupils are widely dilated. The patient is given oxygen with manual assisted ventilation, followed by tracheal intubation.

PROBLEM ANALYSIS

Definition

Total spinal anesthesia is one of the most severe complications that can occur during the performance of an interscalene block. Other severe complications include injection of the local anesthetic into the vertebral artery, high epidural anesthesia, subdural injection, pneumothorax, and neuropathy.

Recognition

The signs and symptoms of total spinal anesthesia result from blockade of the cervicothoracic segments of the central neuraxis. Symptoms of central nervous system involvement are virtually always present and range from the inability to phonate to unconsciousness and the rapid development of bilateral flaccid paralysis. Bilateral dilated, nonreactive pupils are frequently observed, consistent with a block of parasympathetic efferent activity from the Edinger-Westphal nucleus. The latter sign demonstrates that some amount of local anesthetic entered the cranium. Apnea is usually (but not always) present, due to the close proximity of the phrenic nerve roots (C3-C5) to the site of interscalene injection (C6-C7). The development of bradycardia and hypotension is explained by either cervicothoracic spinal block of the cardiac accelerator fiber (T1-T4) or penetration of local anesthetic into the medullary region of the central nervous system. The application of local anesthetic in this structure results in hypotension, bradycardia, and ventricular arrhythmias.

The differential diagnosis includes injection of local anesthetic into the vertebral artery. When this occurs, seizures and unconsciousness are almost immediate. Hypotension and bradycardia may also be due to the cardiotoxic effects of local anesthetics. After epidural injection, such signs and symptoms develop more slowly. Moreover, the epidural space does not extend intracranially. Therefore, signs and symptoms related to intracranial spread of local anesthetic are unlikely. Subdural injection is also part of the differential diagnosis. In this case, the development of clinical block is even slower and usually asymmetrical and incomplete. Intravascular injection or rapid reabsorption of the local anesthetic should always be considered with both central nervous system toxicity and hemodynamic instability. However, the presence of bilateral flaccid paralysis makes this diagnosis very unlikely.

Different mechanisms may be implicated in the occurrence of total spinal anesthesia following interscalene block (Table 61-1). Direct injection into the subdural or epidural space may be the consequence of incorrect needle placement through an intervertebral foramen. A perineural or intraneural injection may lead to secondary migration of the drug into the subdural space. Finally, long dural sleeves have been shown in autopsy studies, extending as far as 3 to 5 cm beyond the intervertebral foramen. Placement of a needle into an abnormally long dural root sleeve may explain the spread of local anesthetic into the intrathecal space.

Risk Assessment

Total spinal anesthesia following interscalene block, either with or without a perineural catheter, is a rare but serious complication. Such events are often documented as case

Table 61–1 ■ Proposed Mechanisms of Intrathecal Migration of Local Anesthetics

Injection through intervertebral foramen
Direct intraneural injection
Injection into dural root sleeve

Table 61–2 ■ **Interscalene Block Techniques: Relative Advantages and Disadvantages**

Advantages/ Disadvantages	Winnie	Posterior	Modified Lateral
Spinal injection	++	++	–
Epidural injection	++	++	–
Vertebral artery injection	+	+/–	–
Intravenous injection	+	+	+
Pneumothorax	+	+	+
Discomfort	+/–	++	+/–
Ease of catheter placement	–	+	++

++, most likely/easiest; +, less likely/easy; +/–, possible; – unlikely/difficult.

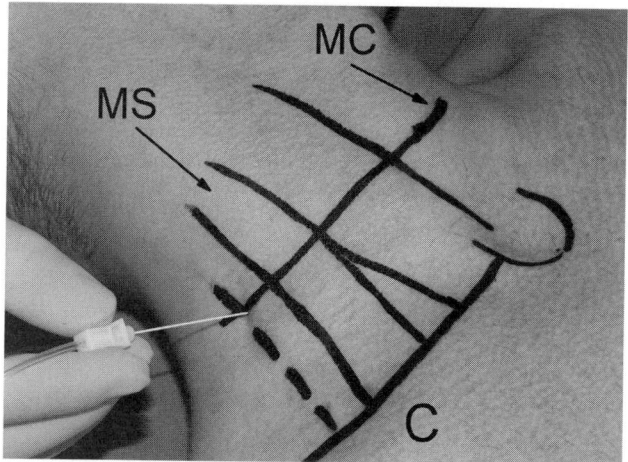

Figure 61–1 ■ Winnie's technique. The needle is directed medially, caudad, and slightly posteriorly toward the transverse process of C6. The needle is close to the spinal structures. C, clavicle; MC, cricothyroid membrane; MS, clavicular head of sternocleidomastoid muscle; dotted line, interscalene groove.

reports. Thus, there is no way to estimate the specific risk for this complication. The only identifiable factor that increases risk is the approach used to perform the block. Three main techniques are used: the Winnie approach, the posterior approach, and the modified lateral approach. The relative advantages and disadvantages of each technique are given in Table 61-2.

Implications

Total spinal anesthesia is a rare complication following interscalene block. However, its diagnosis should be prompt. The differential diagnoses of vertebral artery or intravenous injection should be rapidly ruled out so that the appropriate remedial measures can be instituted. Spontaneous breathing often ceases promptly, so assisted manual or mechanical ventilation will be necessary. Bradycardia and hypotension may occur as a result of vasodilatation and block of the cardiac accelerator fibers, which may lead to cardiac arrest if not treated urgently.

MANAGEMENT

The first step is to immediately cease the local anesthetic injection. Further management includes the following:

- Provide assisted manual or mechanical ventilation with 100% oxygen. Tracheal intubation is often necessary but not always mandatory.
- Consider the patient's mental status, drugs administered, and surgical procedure.
- Volume expansion may be required to treat or prevent hemodynamic instability.
- Vasopressors, positive chronotropic drugs, or temporary pacing may be required to treat bradycardia or hypotension.
- Monitor the patient in the intensive care unit or recovery room until the block wears off.

PREVENTION

The most important precaution is to administer the drug slowly, with repeated aspiration; however, intravenous,

intra-arterial, or intrathecal drug administration is still possible. The choice of approach for performing the interscalene block has implications in the occurrence of complications. Winnie's approach (Fig. 61-1) directs the needle more toward the spine and therefore increases the risk of injection through an intervertebral foramen, especially if the needle is directed too horizontally. The posterior approach is a paravertebral block. All paravertebral blocks carry at least some risk of puncturing the dural cuff (whether abnormally long or not) that accompanies spinal nerves distal to the intervertebral foramina. The modified lateral approach (Fig. 61-2) directs the needle away from spinal structures and is likely the safest technique for avoiding intervertebral or inadvertent dural puncture Advancing the catheter more than 2 to 3 cm past the tip of the stimulating needle carries no advantage. In fact, by threading it

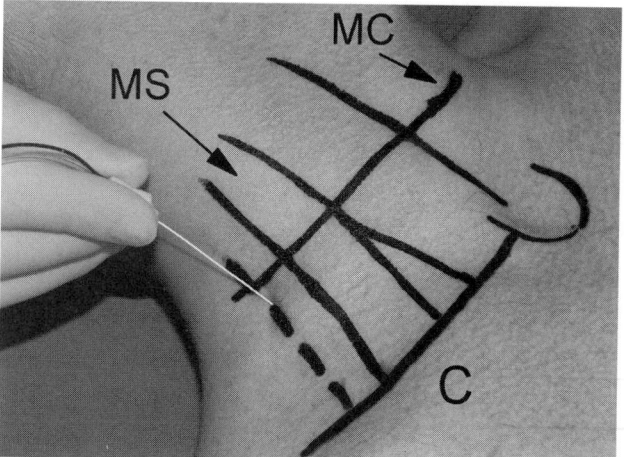

Figure 61–2 ■ Modified lateral approach. The needle is inserted toward the plane of the interscalene space at an angle of between 45 and 60 degrees. The needle avoids the spinal structures. C, clavicle; MC, cricothyroid membrane; MS, clavicular head of sternocleidomastoid muscle; dotted line, interscalene groove.

farther, the anesthesiologist loses control over its position (e.g., interscalene catheters have been placed within the pleura). Last, an important precaution is to perform the interscalene block only in awake or lightly sedated patients. This allows the patient to report paresthesia (needle encounters a nerve root) or pain due to intraneural injection, and it allows the operator to more promptly recognize early signs of central nervous system toxicity.

Further Reading

Borgeat A, Dullenkopf A, Ekatodramis G, Nagy L: Evaluation of the lateral modified approach for continuous interscalene block after shoulder surgery. Anesthesiology 99:436-442, 2003.

Borgeat A, Ekatodramis G, Kalberer F, Benz C: Acute and nonacute complications associated with interscalene block and shoulder surgery: A prospective study. Anesthesiology 95:875-880, 2001.

Brown AR: Regional anesthesia for shoulder surgery. Tech Reg Anesth Pain Manage 3:64-78, 1999.

Iocolano CF: Total spinal anesthesia after an interscalene block. J Perianesth Nurs 12:163-170, 1997.

Long TR, Wass CT, Burkle CM: Perioperative interscalene blockade: An overview of its history and current clinical use. J Clin Anesth 14:546-556, 2002.

Norris D, Klahsen A, Milne B: Delayed bilateral spinal anaesthesia following interscalene brachial plexus block. Can J Anaesth 43:303-305, 1996.

Supraclavicular and Infraclavicular Block: Pneumothorax

62

Sandra L. Kopp

Case Synopsis

A 42-year-old man complains of shortness of breath and mild right-sided chest pain in the outpatient recovery area, shortly after a right wrist fusion. A preoperative brachial plexus block was placed using the supraclavicular approach. Upon examination, the patient's respiratory rate is 20 breaths per minute, and his room-air saturation is 94%. His blood pressure and heart rate are normal. A chest radiograph is positive for a small, right-sided pneumothorax.

PROBLEM ANALYSIS

Definition

Pneumothorax is an accumulation of air or gas in the space between the lung and the chest wall (pleural space). With the supraclavicular approach, the brachial plexus is blocked at the level of its three trunks, where it is most compactly arranged (Fig. 62-1). There are several advantages to the supraclavicular brachial plexus technique, including neutral position of the arm, quick onset of blockade, and a very homogeneous block. Limitations of this approach include difficulty describing or teaching the technique and the risk of pneumothorax. This block is best avoided in uncooperative patients or those with unclear landmarks. Special consideration must be given to patients who could not tolerate the respiratory distress that may accompany a pneumothorax or phrenic nerve block, such as those with severe respiratory disease.

The infraclavicular approach to brachial plexus block allows local anesthetic injection above the level where the musculocutaneous and axillary nerves branch off the plexus. This approach is more proximal than the axillary technique and more distal than the supraclavicular approach, thus leading to blockade of all the nerves derived from the plexus, but with a lower incidence of pneumothorax (Fig. 62-2). As with the supraclavicular approach, the arm can remain in a neutral position. This approach has recently gained favor for use in patients requiring a continuous catheter technique, because maintaining an aseptic dressing at this site is much more practical than in the axilla.

Recognition

Recognition of a pneumothorax is based largely on the clinical presentation. A pneumothorax may occur immediately during block placement, or it may present hours later. The diagnosis of pneumothorax should be suspected if air is aspirated through the needle during performance of the block, or if a patient becomes acutely dyspneic after block placement.

Unilateral phrenic nerve paralysis and concomitant elevation of the hemidiaphragm must be ruled out, as this is very common after proximal brachial plexus blocks (e.g., interscalene blocks). Although the incidence of hemidiaphragmatic paresis is significantly lower in patients having supraclavicular block compared with interscalene block, it is still estimated to occur in approximately 50% of all patients. Infraclavicular block is rarely associated with changes in pulmonary function. If a patient's clinical condition suddenly deteriorates during mechanical ventilation, pneumothorax must be considered.

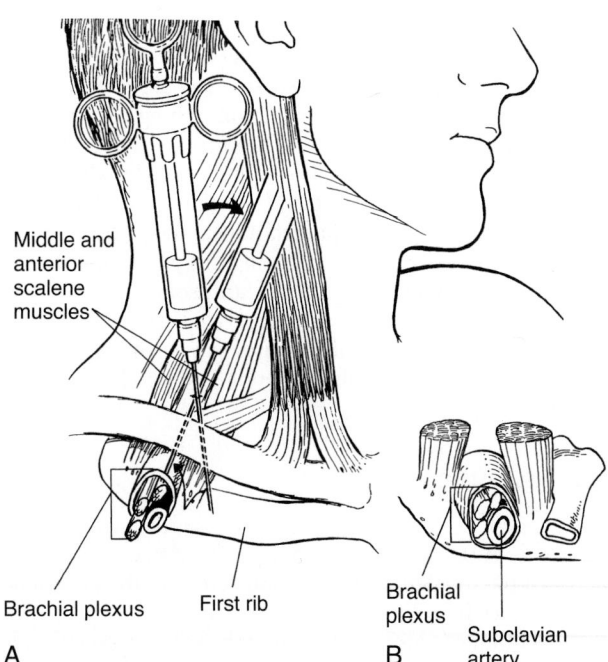

Middle and anterior scalene muscles

Brachial plexus

First rib

Brachial plexus

Subclavian artery

A

B

Figure 62–1 ■ *A,* Supraclavicular block. The needle is systematically walked anteriorly and posteriorly along the rib until the brachial plexus is located. *B,* Trunks of the brachial plexus are compactly arranged at the level of the first rib. (From Miller RD [ed]: Anesthesia, 5th ed. Philadelphia, Churchill Livingstone, 2000, p 1524.)

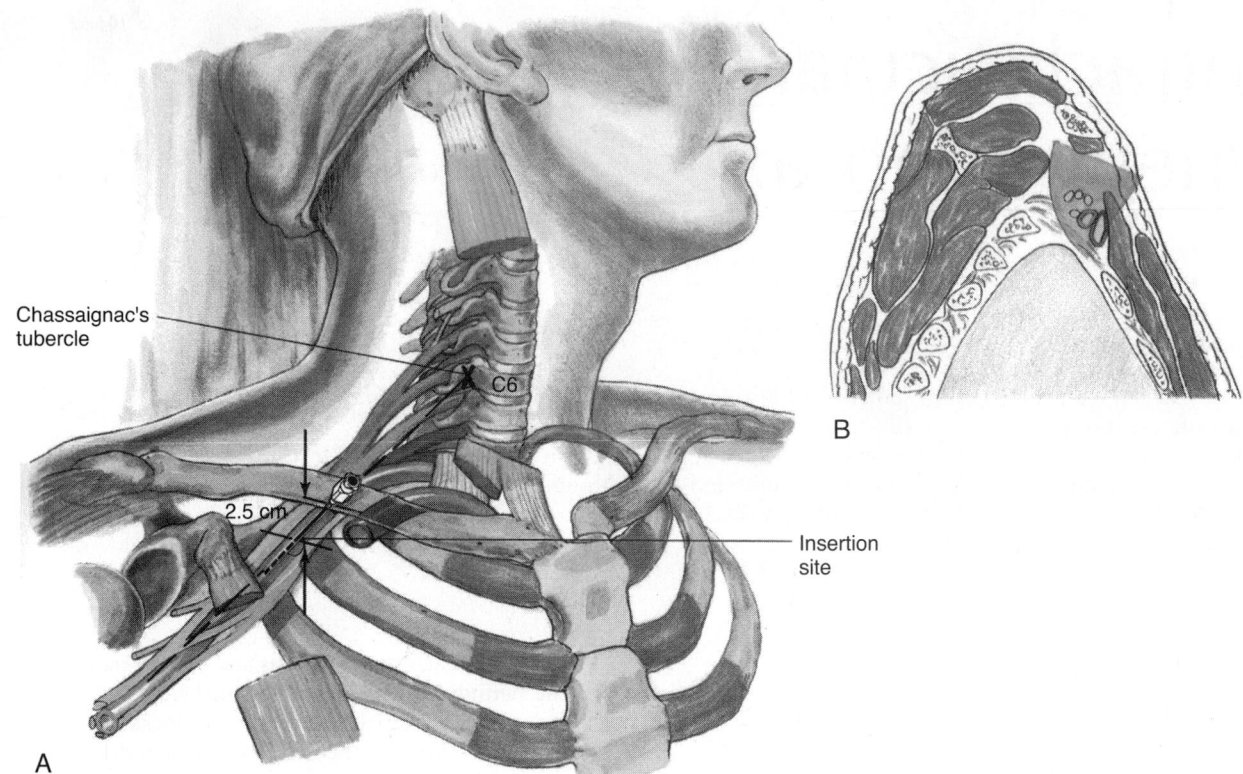

Chassaignac's tubercle

C6

2.5 cm

Insertion site

A

B

Figure 62–2 ■ *A*, Surface markings for the infraclavicular approach to brachial plexus block. *B*, Cephalocaudad arc of needle redirection. (From Brown DL: Atlas of Regional Anesthesia, 2nd ed. Philadelphia, WB Saunders, 1999, p 47.)

Patients who are being ventilated with volume-controlled ventilators present with increased peak and plateau pressures; those ventilated with pressure-controlled ventilators have reduced tidal volumes with a new pneumothorax.

The chest may have a hyperresonant or tympanitic sound during percussion. There may also be absent breath sounds on the affected side. These signs are most notable when there is at least a 25% reduction in lung volume.

Although a computed tomography (CT) scan is the most sensitive study, a chest radiograph is usually diagnostic. Radiographs obtained at the end of expiration allow easier visualization because the pneumothorax takes up a greater proportion of the hemithorax during this part of the respiratory cycle. The main radiographic feature of a pneumothorax is a white visceral pleural line, separated from the parietal pleura by an avascular collection of gas. In most cases, no pulmonary vessels are visible beyond the visceral pleural edge (Fig. 62-3).

Risk Assessment

The incidence of pneumothorax during supraclavicular block ranges from 0.5% to 6.1%. There is an inverse relationship between the incidence of pneumothorax and the experience of the anesthesiologist performing the block. Relatively new techniques, such as the "plumb-bob" approach, have been used to reduce the risk of pneumothorax. Routine chest radiography following a supraclavicular block is not justified because of the low incidence of pneumothorax and the fact that the onset of symptoms may take up to 24 hours.

Implications

Normally, the pressure in the pleural space is negative with respect to the alveolar pressure during the entire respiratory cycle. If the needle punctures the chest wall during block placement, it creates a communication between the atmosphere and the pleural space. Air begins to enter the pleural space until

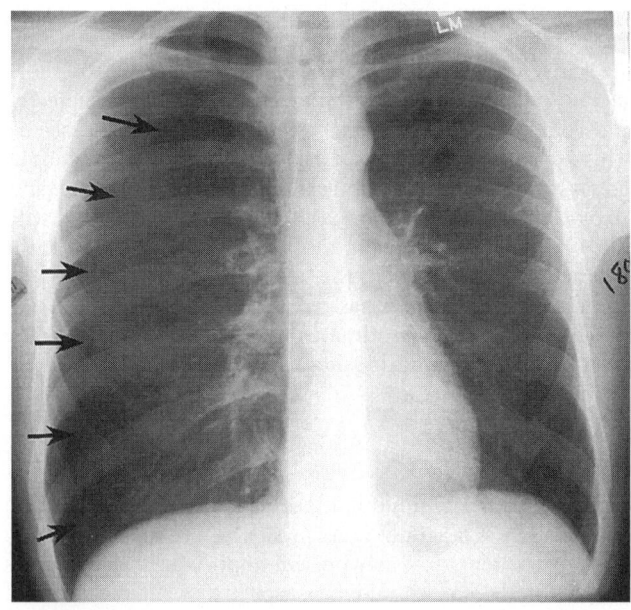

Figure 62–3 ■ Right-sided 40% pneumothorax. *Arrows* mark the visceral pleural line.

the pressure gradient is eliminated or the communication is repaired. The main physiologic changes associated with a pneumothorax are decreased arterial partial pressure of oxygen (PO_2) and decreased vital capacity. The consequences are much more pronounced in patients with poor lung function, because a decrease in vital capacity can lead to respiratory insufficiency, which manifests as hypoventilation and ultimately respiratory acidosis.

Although a tension pneumothorax is unlikely in a spontaneously breathing patient, those who have positive-pressure mechanical ventilation are at significantly increased risk. A tension pneumothorax occurs when the positive pressure of inspiration forces more air into the pleural space than exits during expiration. A sudden decline in the patient's cardiopulmonary status should raise suspicions of the presence of a tension pneumothorax. The deterioration in cardiopulmonary status is likely due to the combination of decreased cardiac output secondary to decreased venous return and extreme hypoxia due to ventilation-perfusion mismatching.

MANAGEMENT

If the patient has minimal symptoms and the pneumothorax is less than 15% of the lung volume, simple observation is advised. It is also necessary to provide the patient with supplemental oxygen, which will increase the rate of absorption of the pneumothorax. Because nitrogen is the primary gas in the pleural space, the gradient for nitrogen absorption into the blood is the main factor in determining the rate of reabsorption of a pneumothorax. Reabsorption can be accelerated by breathing 100% oxygen, which lowers the partial pressure of nitrogen in the blood, thereby increasing the gradient for nitrogen absorption from the pleural space.

If the patient has more than minimal symptoms or if the pneumothorax occupies more than 15% of the hemithorax, aspiration with a plastic catheter is the treatment of choice. If aspiration does not prevent expansion of the pneumothorax, tube thoracostomy should be performed.

Treatment of patients who are undergoing positive-pressure mechanical ventilation should include tube thoracostomy to prevent the development of a tension pneumothorax.

Most often, the chest tube is inserted via an incision at the fourth or fifth intercostal space in the anterior axillary or midaxillary line and directed apically.

A tension pneumothorax is a medical emergency. When it is suspected, the patient should immediately receive 100% oxygen to alleviate hypoxia. A large-bore angiocatheter should be inserted into the pleural space through the second intercostal space, along the midclavicular line. If the diagnosis is confirmed by the aspiration of air through the catheter, the patient should undergo immediate tube thoracostomy.

PREVENTION

Many modifications have been made to supraclavicular and infraclavicular blocks to decrease the complication rate. In 1949 Bonica and colleagues first recommended a careful, gentle technique; thorough familiarity with anatomic relationships; use of the first rib as a protective shield over the lung; and use of a short, fine needle to help prevent complications, including pneumothorax. Although many years have passed, and several reviews have been published since then, this careful approach is still the best advice for any anesthesiologist planning to perform these techniques.

Further Reading

Bonica JJ, Moore DC, Orlov M: Brachial plexus block anesthesia. Am J Surg 65, 1949.

Brown DL, Bridenbaugh LD: The upper extremity: Somatic block. In Cousins MJ, Bridenbaugh PO (eds): Neural Blockade in Clinical Anesthesia and Management of Pain, 3rd ed. Philadelphia, Lippincott-Raven, 1998, pp 345-371.

Brown DL, Cahill DR, Bridenbaugh LD: Supraclavicular nerve block: Anatomic analysis of a method to prevent pneumothorax. Anesth Analg 76:530-534, 1993.

Light RW, Broaddus VC: Pneumothorax, chylothorax, hemothorax, and fibrothorax. In Murray JF, Nadel JA (eds): Textbook of Respiratory Medicine, 3rd ed. Philadelphia, WB Saunders, 2000, pp 2043-2066.

Neal JM, Moore JM, Kopacz DJ, et al: Quantitative analysis of respiratory, motor, and sensory function after supraclavicular block. Anesth Analg 86:1239-1244, 1998.

Rodriquez J, Barcena M, Rodriguez V, et al: Infraclavicular brachial plexus block effects on respiratory function and extent of the block. Reg Anesth Pain Med 23:564-568, 1998.

REGIONAL ANESTHESIA & PAIN MANAGEMENT

Celiac Plexus Block: Side Effects and Complications

63

Gilbert Y. Wong and David L. Brown

Case Synopsis

A 55-year-old woman presents with epigastric abdominal pain of several months' duration and a recent diagnosis of pancreatic cancer. To manage her pain, a neurolytic celiac plexus block is performed using the classic posterior percutaneous approach. Soon after injection of the neurolytic solution, she notices sensory loss and impaired motor control of her lower extremities.

PROBLEM ANALYSIS

Definition

Neurolytic celiac plexus block (CPB) is an effective analgesic technique used primarily for pain management in patients with intra-abdominal malignancies, especially pancreatic cancer. Neurolytic solutions are injected in the area of the celiac plexus or splanchnic nerves, which are the neural structures transmitting the majority of visceral pain from the abdomen. Because the targeted area of neurolysis is in close proximity to vascular and other neurologic structures (Fig. 63-1), neurologic side effects and complications are the primary concerns associated with CPB.

Neurologic side effects such as orthostatic hypotension or bowel hypermotility often occur after an effective neurolytic CPB. The celiac plexus and splanchnic nerves are primarily sympathetic nervous system structures. Neurolysis of these structures results in sympatholysis and a relative increase in parasympathetic tone in the splanchnic region. As a result, vasodilatation of the splanchnic vasculature, especially the venous capacitance bed (which effectively reduces venous return and cardiac preload), can result in orthostatic hypotension. In addition, the relative increase in parasympathetic outflow to the viscera can result in increased peristalsis and bowel hypermotility.

Neurologic complications are the most serious concerns associated with neurolytic CPB. Although they are rare, these complications can include sensory and motor deficits of the lower trunk and lower extremities, loss of bladder or bowel control or both, and impotence in males. Neurolysis of sensory or motor nerves can occur from direct contact of the neurolytic solution, such as alcohol or phenol, spreading to the intrathecal or epidural space or thoracic or lumbar nerve roots (see Fig. 63-1). In a separate mechanism, alcohol has been shown to cause arterial spasm of feeding arteries to the spinal cord, which can result in ischemia and permanent neurologic deficits (Fig. 63-2).

Recognition

Neurologic side effects, such as orthostatic hypotension and bowel hypermotility, are not appreciated until after the neurolytic procedure is completed. Patients with intra-abdominal malignancies often have decreased oral intake owing to pain or nausea. Decreased intravascular volume can potentiate the hypotensive effects of neurolytic CPB. Symptoms associated with orthostatic hypotension include syncope or dizziness in the upright position, which may be exacerbated during a rapid shift from the supine position. These symptoms may occur immediately after the CPB. Orthostatic hypotension can be diagnosed based on blood pressure measurements performed before and after the neurolytic CPB with the patient in the supine and upright positions. Bowel hypermotility effects may not be noticed until hours after the neurolytic CPB. Because patients experiencing pain associated with intra-abdominal malignancies are frequently treated with opioid medications, and because constipation is a common side effect of opioid medications, such patients often consider increased bowel motility to be beneficial.

Neurologic complications, such as sensory and motor changes of the lower trunk and extremities, must be carefully evaluated both during and after the CPB procedure. Although not completely reliable, needle aspiration for cerebrospinal fluid or blood should occur both before and during the incremental injections of neurolytic solution. If cerebrospinal fluid or blood is aspirated, no additional injections should occur until the needle position is reevaluated. Before the injection of a neurolytic agent, a functional test consisting of local anesthetic injection is important to rule out incorrect needle placement. Neurologic deficits occurring as a result of local anesthetic injection into the intrathecal or epidural space or in contact with the thoracolumbar nerve roots confirm incorrect needle positioning. Radiographic guidance, such as fluoroscopy or CT, can also be used to recognize grossly inaccurate needle placement.

Risk Assessment

The risks of neurologic side effects and complications must be carefully considered and weighed against the benefits of neurolytic CPB in patients with intra-abdominal malignancies and limited life expectancy.

Meta-analysis of the literature regarding patients undergoing neurolytic CPB found that hypotension occurred in

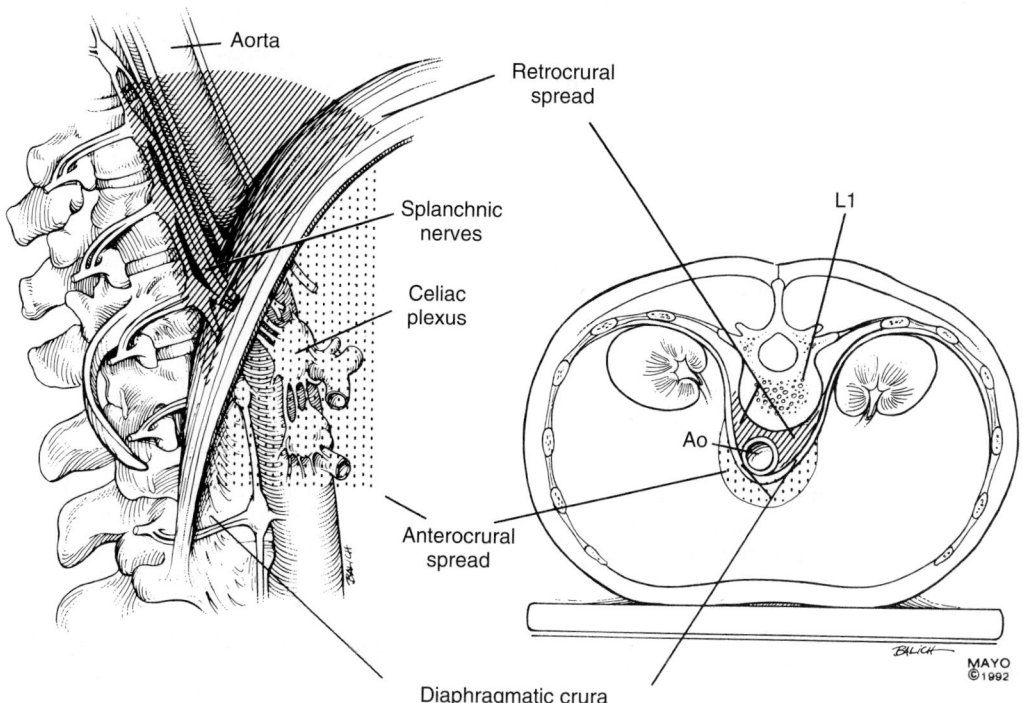

Figure 63–1 ■ The spread of neurolytic solution in a celiac plexus block occurs in anterocrural or retrocrural regions. The neurolytic solution is in close proximity to vital structures associated with the spine, including the intrathecal and epidural spaces, thoracic and lumbar nerve roots, and major feeding arteries of the spinal cord.

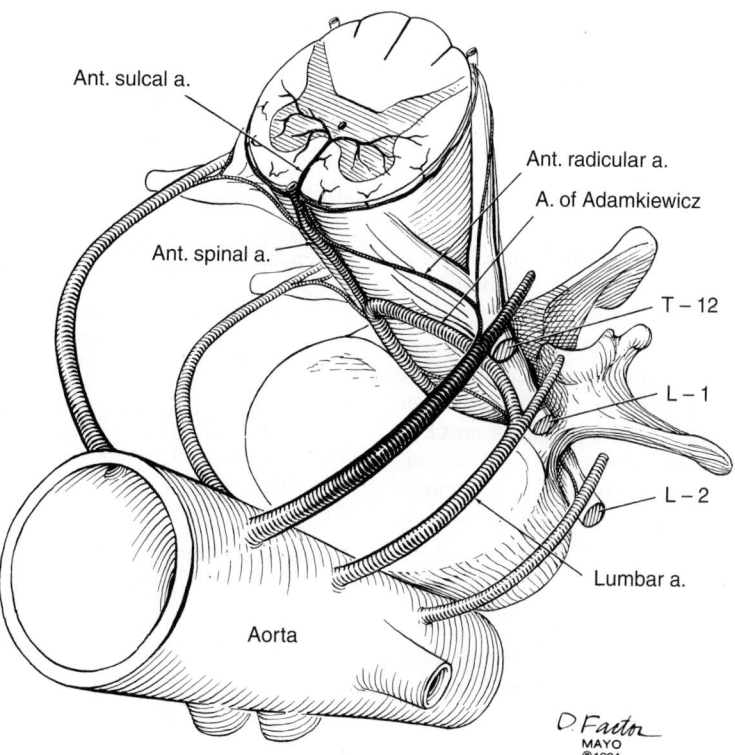

Figure 63–2 ■ Arterial supply of the spinal cord at low thoracic and high lumbar vertebral levels. The largest feeding artery to the spinal cord is the artery of Adamkiewicz (anterior radicular artery), which branches from the lumbar artery (in this case).

38% of cases and bowel hypermotility occurred in 31% to 44% of cases. A case series of 136 patients who had neurolytic CPB reported that 8 patients (6%) with symptomatic orthostatic hypotension required treatment. Another study (61 patients) that prospectively compared different CPB techniques reported a 38% incidence of transient decreases in systolic blood pressure greater than 33% compared with baseline measurements. Bowel hypermotility also occurred in 31% of these patients.

In the largest series (2730 patients) evaluating neurologic complications associated with neurolytic CPB, four cases (0.15%) of permanent paraplegia were identified. In three of these cases, there was also loss of anal and bladder sphincter function. Radiographic guidance with radiocontrast dye was used for CPB in all four cases. In a case series by Brown and coworkers, there were no cases of permanent paraplegia in 136 patients undergoing neurolytic CPB. Meta-analysis of the literature revealed a 1% incidence of neurologic complications, including lower extremity weakness, paresthesia, epidural anesthesia, and lumbar puncture, after neurolytic CPB.

Implications

Benign neurologic side effects can occur in patients receiving neurolytic CPB. These side effects can usually be treated in a symptomatic manner with no significant impact on the patient. Orthostatic hypotension typically improves shortly after equilibration of the intravascular volume. Bowel hypermotility is usually transient and may actually be desirable in many patients. The potential for neurologic side effects should be discussed with the patient and family before the procedure.

Neurologic complications are very uncommon but can have a significant impact. In patients with intra-abdominal malignancies, these neurologic deficits are likely to continue for the remainder of their lives.

MANAGEMENT

The management of neurologic side effects is directed toward symptomatic relief. Orthostatic hypotension, if symptomatic, can be treated by increasing oral fluid intake or intravenous fluids. Leg wrappings with elastic bandages or support stockings can also decrease venous capacitance and improve hypotension. Antihypertensive medications, if any, should be discontinued until equilibration of intravascular volume is reached. If symptoms are sustained and not responsive to conservative therapy, pharmacologic treatment with an α_1-agonist, such as midodrine, can be considered. Bowel hypermotility can be treated symptomatically with antihypermotility medications such as diphenoxylate with atropine.

The management of neurologic complications is more complicated. If neurologic deficits occur during neurolytic CPB, the procedure should be terminated immediately. Aspiration of the injectate can be attempted but is unlikely to be effective. Emergency consultation with a neurologist is recommended. If ischemia of the spinal cord is suspected as a result of spasm of a lumbar radicular artery, the immediate involvement of an interventional radiologist for arterial vasodilatation should be considered.

PREVENTION

The neurologic side effects of orthostatic hypotension and bowel hypermotility are not preventable; they are merely the result of a successful CPB.

The ability to prevent neurologic complications with the use of radiographic guidance is controversial. Traditionally, the CPB procedure relies on anatomic landmarks rather than radiographic guidance. Needle position is confirmed with a functional test of injected local anesthetic. If the patient notes an appropriate improvement in preexisting pain with no neurologic deficits, the needle position is considered to be correct. This approach requires that the patient not be oversedated, so that he or she can provide reliable responses.

The large case series of 2730 patients undergoing neurolytic CPB revealed four cases of permanent paraplegia, all of which involved the use of radiography and radiocontrast dye to confirm final needle placement. Thus, radiographic guidance cannot ensure the prevention of neurologic complications. Despite these observations, the use of radiographic guidance provides the advantage of confirming needle position and the spread of injectate, as traced by the radiocontrast dye, before the injection of neurolytic solution.

Further Reading

Brown DL, Bulley CK, Quiel EL: Neurolytic celiac plexus block for pancreatic cancer pain. Anesth Analg 66:869-873, 1987.

Davies DD: Incidence of major complications of neurolytic coeliac plexus block. J R Soc Med 86:264-266, 1993.

Eisenberg E, Carr DB, Chalmers TC: Neurolytic celiac plexus block for treatment of cancer pain: A meta-analysis. Anesth Analg 80:290-295, 1995.

Goudas L, Carr DB, Bloch R, et al: Management of Cancer Pain: Evidence Report/Technology Assessment No. 35 (AHCPR Publication No. 02-E002). Rockville, Md, Agency for Healthcare Research and Quality, 2001. (Prepared by the New England Medical Center Evidence-Based Practice Center under Contract No. 290-97-0019.)

Ischia S, Ischia A, Polati E, et al: Three posterior percutaneous celiac plexus block techniques. Anesthesiology 76:534-540, 1992.

Wong GY, Brown DL: Transient paraplegia following celiac plexus block. Reg Anesth 20:352-355, 1995.

Wong GY, Schroeder DR, Carns PE, et al: Effect of neurolytic celiac plexus block on pain relief, quality of life, and survival in patients with unresectable pancreatic cancer—a randomized controlled trial. JAMA 291:1092-1099, 2004.

Psoas Compartment Block: Potential Complications

64

Robert S. Weller

Case Synopsis

A 76-year-old man with a mechanical aortic valve was scheduled for left above-knee amputation. Chronic warfarin (Coumadin) was stopped, and a heparin infusion was begun on admission but stopped 4 hours before surgery. On arrival in the preoperative area, his prothrombin time, international normalized ratio, and activated partial thromboplastin time were normal; hemoglobin was 13 g/dL. A posterior approach to the lumbar plexus block (psoas compartment block) was performed, in combination with a subgluteal sciatic block. His vital signs remained stable, and the surgery and recovery room stay were uneventful. The estimated blood loss was 300 mL. The patient was returned to the floor, and heparin was restarted 8 hours postoperatively at 1200 units/hour. His blood pressure gradually declined overnight from his usual 140/90 to 95/55 mm Hg, and he became confused and oliguric. He received several 500-mL normal saline fluid challenges. The blood pressure improved, but urine output remained low. The next morning, his hemoglobin was 7.3 g/dL. Two units of packed red blood cells were given. Hemoglobin was 7.7 g/dL. He was moved to the intensive care unit, heparin was discontinued, and a computed tomography (CT) scan of the abdomen showed a large left retroperitoneal hematoma.

PROBLEM ANALYSIS

Definition

Retroperitoneal hemorrhage after psoas compartment block (PCB) results from arterial bleeding into the retroperitoneal space. Signs and symptoms of PCB depend on the rate and extent of bleeding and whether the hematoma compresses adjacent structures. The most rapid and dramatic bleeding occurs with aortic rupture, which is often fatal. However, bleeding from smaller arteries after PCB can also cause morbidity or mortality.

Numerous cases of retroperitoneal hemorrhage have been reported following interventional radiology procedures requiring femoral artery cannulation, especially if the artery is injured proximal to the inguinal ligament. The incidence following cardiac catheterization is reportedly 0.12%. Only a few cases of retroperitoneal hemorrhage have been reported after PCB or lumbar sympathetic block; anticoagulant therapy at the time of or after the block was involved in each of those cases. Spontaneous retroperitoneal hematoma may also occur in patients on chronic anticoagulant therapy. The risk of this complication increases as the degree of anticoagulation increases. Finally, spontaneous iliopsoas hemorrhage with femoral nerve palsy is the most common nerve palsy caused by spontaneous bleeding in hemophiliacs.

Recognition

Retroperitoneal bleeding is deep, concealed, and rarely obvious until significant blood loss has occurred. The most common signs of retroperitoneal hemorrhage are hypotension and tachycardia due to intravascular volume depletion, and anemia (Table 64-1). In one series, 64% of patients had hypotension (systolic blood pressure <90 mm Hg), and 73% showed progressive anemia. Ultimately, there is hemorrhagic shock, with oliguria and mental status changes. Oliguria can also result from ureteral obstruction, although retroperitoneal hematoma usually does not extend across the midline. Therefore, oliguria is more commonly due to hypovolemia.

Symptoms of retroperitoneal hematoma include abdominal, flank, groin, or leg pain, as well as lumbar plexus irritation or dysfunction. In the series noted earlier, 45% of patients complained of pain in the lower extremity, and 55% had femoral nerve palsy. Over time, patients may also develop flank ecchymoses (Grey Turner's sign; Fig. 64-1).

In addition to the complications of PCB itself, the differential diagnosis for hypotension and anemia hours after PCB includes inadequate surgical blood replacement or continued surgical bleeding, which is usually obvious after lower extremity surgery. Perioperative hypotension may also be due to sepsis, with anemia absent and fever usually present. Abdominal CT should be performed if retroperitoneal bleeding is suspected; it readily demonstrates retroperitoneal hematoma (Fig. 64-2).

Table 64-1 ■ Signs and Symptoms of Retroperitoneal Hemorrhage
Hypotension
Anemia
Shock
Abdominal, flank, groin, or leg pain
Femoral neuropathy
Flank ecchymoses (Grey Turner's sign)

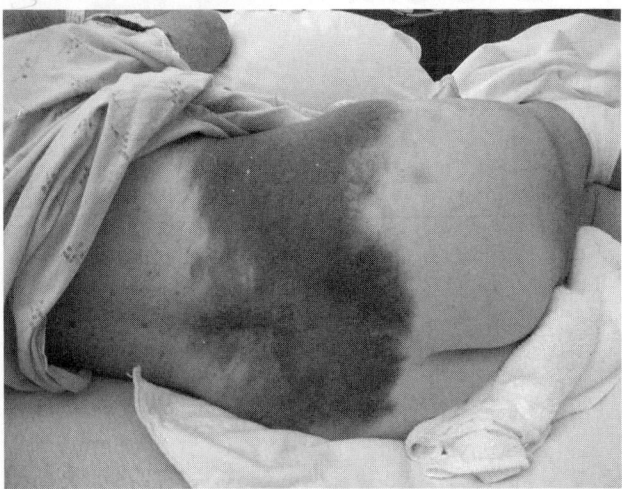

Figure 64–1 ■ Patient in the left lateral decubitus position showing widespread flank ecchymoses (Grey Turner's sign) due to retroperitoneal hematoma after psoas compartment block.

Risk Assessment

The translumbar, posterior approach to lumbar plexus block or PCB was described in 1974. The approach and landmarks have since been modified. The most popular contemporary approach for PCB requires the use of a nerve stimulator to identify the femoral nerve component of the lumbar plexus. Local anesthetic injection through a PCB needle or catheter has a much higher rate of success in blocking the femoral, lateral femoral cutaneous, and obturator branches (especially the last) of the lumbar plexus, compared with about a 25% success rate with the inguinal perivascular (three-in-one) block of these branches.

PCB has also been used to provide analgesia following hip replacement. Some have found that PCB provides equivalent analgesia to epidural local anesthetic, with fewer side effects; others have found it inferior to intrathecal morphine. Continuous PCB has been used for patients with femoral neck fracture, and although it is inadequate for surgical anesthesia, PCB produces analgesia that is superior to systemic

meperidine analgesia. When used alone for analgesia following knee replacement surgery, continuous PCB is equivalent to a continuous femoral block; both blocks are superior to intravenous patient-controlled morphine.

The incidence of epidural spread of local anesthetic after PCB ranges from 2% to 25% and must be considered a side effect of this approach. Epidural and even intrathecal catheter placement has occurred during attempted continuous PCB. This is not unexpected, given the anatomic proximity of the intervertebral foramen to the intended site of needle or catheter placement. Although PCB is usually safe and successful, a number of serious complications have been reported in addition to retroperitoneal hematoma (Table 64-2). In a survey of major complications associated with regional anesthesia, Auroy and colleagues cautioned that PCB may be associated with a higher rate of life-threatening complications (8:1000) than other peripheral nerve block procedures. However, this survey included only 394 PCBs, a small percentage of the total number of peripheral nerve blocks performed.

The retroperitoneal space contains a rich network of arteries and veins. Segmental lumbar arteries arise from the aorta, run along the vertebral bodies, and then course behind the psoas major and lumbar plexus between the lumbar transverse processes. The iliolumbar arteries ascend from their origin at the hypogastric arteries and anastomose with the fourth lumbar artery at the medial border of the psoas major. Segmental lumbar veins connect to each other by the ascending lumbar vein (Fig. 64-3), which feeds into the inferior vena cava. With this abundant vascular supply in the vicinity of the lumbar plexus, it is not surprising that needles or catheters may occasionally enter or injure these vessels during PCB, producing hemorrhage or systemic local anesthetic toxicity.

The potential for concealed, significant hemorrhage must be taken into account when calculating the risk-benefit ratio of PCB for each patient. Alternative techniques, the use of anticoagulant or antiplatelet drugs, and the degree of anticoagulation must be included in this analysis. The American Society of Regional Anesthesia and Pain Medicine (ASRAPM) has developed consensus guidelines for the performance of central neuraxial blocks in the setting of anticoagulant therapy (see Chapter 67), but no such guidelines exist for the performance of peripheral nerve and plexus blocks. The incidence of clinically significant retroperitoneal bleeding following single-injection or continuous PCB with the typical dose of drugs used for perioperative thromboprophylaxis or anticoagulation therapy is not known.

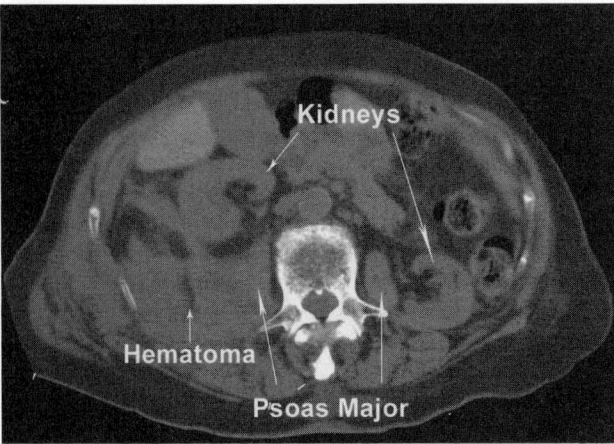

Figure 64–2 ■ Abdominal computed tomography scan showing a large retroperitoneal hematoma after psoas compartment block.

Table 64–2 ■ Complications following Psoas Block
Retroperitoneal hematoma
Renal injury and hematoma
Intrathecal, epidural, and intra-abdominal catheter placement
Development of severe phantom limb pain
Femoral neuropathy
Total spinal anesthesia with cardiac arrest
Systemic toxicity with cardiac arrest
Death

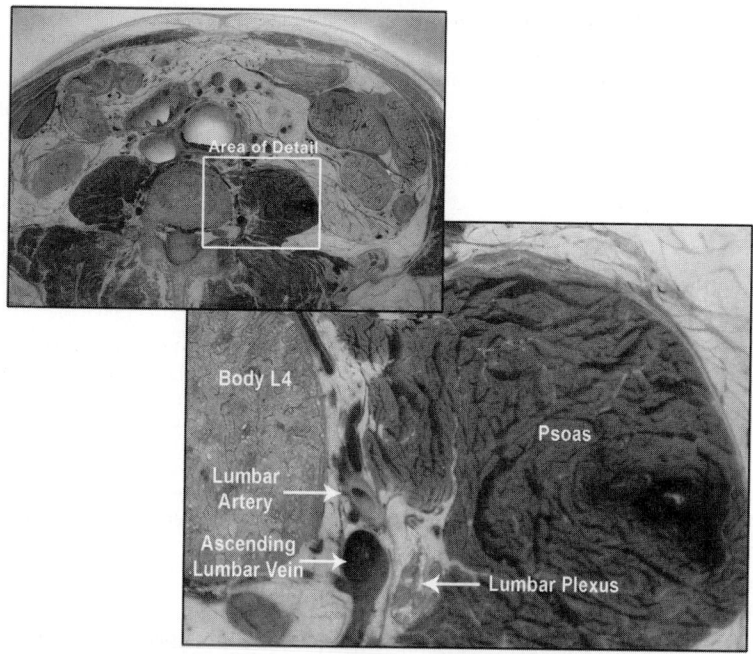

Figure 64–3 ■ Anatomic cross section through the L4 vertebral body. The enlarged image shows the lumbar artery and much larger ascending lumbar vein close to the lumbar plexus.

In contrast to retroperitoneal hematoma following PCB, epidural hematoma with spinal cord compression after epidural block requires urgent diagnosis and surgical decompression to reduce the risk of catastrophic injury to the patient (i.e., paraplegia). However, retroperitoneal bleeding after PCB, if diagnosed early and treated with transfusion and supportive care, typically results in complete recovery and usually does not require surgical intervention. For this reason, some believe that it is not necessary to apply the ASRAPM guidelines to PCB. Others argue that, at a minimum, significant retroperitoneal hemorrhage requires substantial transfusion, an extended hospital stay, and the reversal of anticoagulation, with its attendant risks. Even worse, retroperitoneal hemorrhage after PCB can cause persistent femoral neuropathy, life-threatening hemorrhagic complications, and even death. Therefore, the more conservative approach is to avoid PCB in patients with coagulation abnormalities that preclude epidural or spinal anesthesia.

Implications

Consideration of PCB as a component of surgical anesthesia or postoperative analgesia must take into account its success rate and benefits compared with those of alternative techniques, as well as the potential for severe complications, including life-threatening bleeding. This is especially true for patients with significant bleeding abnormalities, including those who are fully anticoagulated or on high-dose antithrombolytic therapy. The risk is less well established for those receiving antiplatelet drugs or perioperative thromboprophylaxis. Because the signs and symptoms of retroperitoneal hemorrhage are well known, one must maintain a strong index of suspicion for bleeding-related complications in any patient receiving PCB, especially those with seemingly less consequential acquired or intrinsic coagulation abnormalities (e.g., patients taking nonsteroidal anti-inflammatory drugs).

MANAGEMENT

The most common presentation of retroperitoneal hematoma is hypovolemia and anemia. In this case, intravascular volume repletion is the first priority (Table 64-3). Hemoglobin concentration, platelet count, and coagulation parameters should be measured to guide transfusion and other therapy. Discontinuation or reversal of anticoagulation may be necessary, although this must be weighed against the risk of venous thrombosis and embolism that such therapy was intended to prevent. It might be necessary to transfer the patient to a high-observation unit until cardiovascular stability has been achieved. Once the patient has stabilized, a CT scan can confirm the diagnosis and demonstrate the extent of bleeding. If active bleeding continues, technetium 99 scanning can help identify its source and guide embolization of the bleeding vessel.

Many authorities believe that patients with continued or progressive nerve dysfunction from compression of branches

---

Table 64–3 ■ Management of Retroperitoneal Hemorrhage following Psoas Block

Restore intravascular volume
Measure blood count and coagulation activity
Transfuse blood and coagulation factors as indicated
Reverse anticoagulation pharmacologically
Transfer to high-acuity unit until cardiovascular stability achieved
Perform abdominal computed tomography scan to confirm diagnosis when stable
Consider interventional radiology for continued hemorrhage
Consider surgical exploration for continued hemorrhage or femoral palsy

of the lumbar plexus should undergo urgent decompressive surgery. Others believe that surgical intervention is a last resort and recommend that evolving femoral neuropathies be managed more expectantly, especially in patients with congenital coagulopathies.

PREVENTION

The vascularity of the tissues through which the needle passes for PCB makes it impossible to completely avoid arterial or venous trauma. Because the larger needles and catheters used for continuous epidural anesthesia carry a higher risk for epidural hematoma than does single-injection spinal anesthesia, it seems logical that this would also be true for peripheral nerve blocks, including PCB.

If an insulated needle and nerve stimulator are used to locate the lumbar plexus for PCB, vascular puncture might go unrecognized. Even with hollow-core needles, vascular injury might not be obvious. Regardless of the type of needle used, retroperitoneal hematoma following PCB has been reported. Thus, the following precautions are prudent:

- Avoid PCB in fully anticoagulated patients or if thrombolytic therapy is likely.
- Maintain an index of suspicion for concealed bleeding in patients who have undergone PCB and are anticoagulated postoperatively.
- If known vascular puncture has occurred during PCB, communicate this to the surgical team and delay potent thromboprophylactic therapy postoperatively. Also, careful patient follow-up and monitoring of serial hematocrits are advised.
- Avoid PCB catheter removal during therapeutic anticoagulation, and maintain a high index of suspicion for bleeding after catheter removal in patients on more modest prophylactic anticoagulation postoperatively.
- Communicate the potential for concealed bleeding with members of the primary surgical service so that they too have the appropriate index of suspicion for bleeding complications after PCB, especially when unanticipated anemia or hypovolemia occurs in the postoperative period.

Further Reading

Auroy Y, Benhamou D, Bargues L, et al: Major complications of regional anesthesia in France: The SOS Regional Anesthesia Hotline Service. Anesthesiology 97:1274-1280, 2002.

Capdevila X, Biboulet P, Morau D, et al: Continuous three-in-one block for postoperative pain after lower limb orthopedic surgery: Where do the catheters go? Anesth Analg 94:1001-1006, 2002.

Capdevila X, Marcaire P, Dadure C, et al: Continuous psoas compartment block for postoperative analgesia after total hip arthroplasty: New landmarks, technical guidelines, and clinical evaluation. Anesth Analg 94:1606-1613, 2002.

Chudinov A, Berkenstadt H, Salai M, et al: Continuous psoas compartment block for anesthesia and perioperative analgesia in patients with hip fractures. Reg Anesth Pain Med 24:563-568, 1999.

Kaloul I, Guay J, Cote C, Fallaha M: The posterior lumbar plexus (psoas compartment) block and the three-in-one femoral nerve block provide similar postoperative analgesia after total knee replacement. Can J Anaesth 51:45-51, 2004.

Klein SM, D'Ercole F, Greengrass RA, Warner DS: Enoxaparin associated with psoas hematoma and lumbar plexopathy after lumbar plexus block. Anesthesiology 87:1576-1579, 1997.

Levine MN, Raskob G, Landefeld S, Kearon C: Hemorrhagic complications of anticoagulant treatment. Chest 119(1 Suppl):109S-121S, 2001.

Maier C, Gleim M, Weiss T, et al: Severe bleeding following lumbar sympathetic blockade in two patients under medication with irreversible platelet aggregation inhibitors. Anesthesiology 97:740-743, 2002.

Souron V, Delaunay L, Schifrine P: Intrathecal morphine provides better postoperative analgesia than psoas compartment block after primary hip arthroplasty. Can J Anaesth 50:574-579, 2003.

Sreeram S, Lumsden AB, Miller JS, et al: Retroperitoneal hematoma following femoral artery catheterization: A serious and often fatal complication. Am Surg 59:94-98, 1993.

Tokarz VA, McGrory JE, Stewart JD, Croslin AR: Femoral neuropathy and iliopsoas hematoma as a result of postpartum factor-VIII inhibitor syndrome. J Bone Joint Surg Am 85:1812-1815, 2003.

Turker G, Uckunkaya N, Yavascaoglu B: Comparison of the catheter-technique psoas compartment block and the epidural block for analgesia in partial hip replacement surgery. Acta Anaesthesiol Scand 47:30-36, 2003.

Weller R, Gerancher JC, Crews JC, Wade KL: Extensive retroperitoneal hematoma without neurologic deficit in two patients who underwent lumbar plexus block and were later anticoagulated. Anesthesiology 98:581-585, 2003.

Williams P: Gray's Anatomy: The Anatomical Basis of Medicine and Surgery, 38th ed. New York, Churchill Livingstone, 1995, pp 1562, 1558, 1600.

Wilson MW, Fidelman N, Lull RJ, et al: Evaluation of active bleeding into hematomas by technetium-99m red blood cell scintigraphy before angiography. Clin Nucl Med 27:763-766, 2002.

Winnie A, Ramamurthy S, Durrani Z, Radonjic R: Plexus blocks for lower extremity surgery: New answers to old problems. Anesthesiol Rev 1:11-16, 1974.

Witz M, Cohen Y, Lehmann JM: Retroperitoneal haematoma—a serious vascular complication of cardiac catheterisation. Eur J Vasc Endovasc Surg 18:364-365, 1999.

Side Effects of Neuraxial Opioids

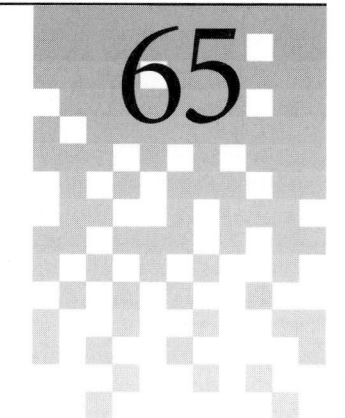

65

Susan B. McDonald

Case Synopsis

A 55-year-old obese woman undergoes a total vaginal hysterectomy under spinal anesthesia comprising local anesthetic and 100 μg of morphine. Later that evening, her oxygen saturation is normal with oxygen supplementation by nasal cannula, but she appears excessively somnolent.

PROBLEM ANALYSIS

Definition

Epidural and intrathecal administration of opioids in humans was first described in 1979. It was termed "selective spinal analgesia" because it offered profound segmental analgesia without the motor, sensory, and autonomic blockade of local anesthetics. Since then, neuraxial opioids have been widely accepted as a means of providing prolonged analgesia in acute postoperative, obstetric, and chronic pain scenarios. There is evidence that patients may have better postoperative outcomes with neuraxial opioid analgesia than with conventional opioid use. The addition of intrathecal fentanyl to spinal anesthesia prolongs the duration of sensory blockade without increasing the time to discharge, making it a popular choice in the ambulatory surgery setting. Intrathecal narcotics for labor analgesia, or "walking epidurals," are a desirable option for parturients.

Recognition

The most common side effects associated with neuraxial opioids are the following:

- Respiratory depression
- Sedation
- Pruritus
- Nausea and vomiting
- Urinary retention

In general, the adverse effects associated with neuraxial opioids are similar to those seen with intravenous, intramuscular, or oral opioids. However, the severity, incidence, and timing differ owing to the interaction of receptors in the spinal cord and the brain. The most serious complication is respiratory depression, which can be early or delayed.

Risk Assessment

Respiratory Depression

The degree and rate of the opioid's rostral spread in the cerebrospinal fluid (CSF) determine the side effect profile for respiratory depression. The natural circulation of CSF brings residual drug into direct contact with the brain's respiratory center, which lies on the floor of the fourth ventricle. Typically, lumbar CSF reaches the brain in about 4 to 6 hours. Thus, factors that determine the amount of drug reaching the rostral CSF include where the drug was placed (intrathecally versus epidurally; thoracic versus lumbar area), its dose, and its lipid solubility.

When a highly lipophilic drug such as fentanyl or sufentanil is placed intrathecally, it rapidly penetrates the spinal cord tissues to directly act on the dorsal horn neurons. Low residual concentrations of the drug remain in the CSF; therefore, such drugs have a more segmental analgesic effect.

In contrast, morphine is not highly lipophilic and has a slower uptake into the spinal cord and efflux from the CSF (via arachnoid granulations). Therefore, higher concentrations of drug remain in the CSF for longer periods. As a result, morphine is much more likely to reach the brain's respiratory center and cause delayed respiratory depression than is fentanyl or sufentanil.

If an opioid is placed epidurally, it can have spinal or supraspinal (systemic) effects, imparting a biphasic nature to respiratory depression. This may manifest early (<2 hours) due to vascular uptake and redistribution, similar to what occurs after intramuscular dosing, or late (6 to 12 hours) due to rostral migration of the drug in the CSF. The ratio of spinal to supraspinal effects depends on how much of the drug is absorbed into the epidural venous plexus, how much is deposited in epidural fat, and how much penetrates the meninges and passes into the CSF. The drug's lipid solubility and molecular weight and shape in large part determine dural penetration and the amount that remains in the CSF long enough to spread rostrally. This explains why hydrophilic morphine or hydromorphone has more dural penetration (and therefore spinal activity) than highly lipophilic drugs such as fentanyl or sufentanil. For the same reason, there is a much greater risk of respiratory depression when morphine or hydromorphone is placed in the high thoracic or cervical epidural space.

Patients considered at increased risk for respiratory depression include the elderly and debilitated, those with significant pulmonary disease (including sleep apnea), and those receiving concomitant opioids or central nervous system depressants. Patients receiving chronic opioid therapy are drug tolerant and thus much less likely to experience centrally mediated, neuraxial opioid respiratory depression. Postpartum patients also demonstrate less respiratory depression, possibly because of their younger age and increased ventilatory drive due to pregnancy. Finally, the overall reported incidence of significant respiratory depression (i.e., that requiring treatment) from neuraxial opioids is 0.2% to 2%, which is not much different from that associated with more conventional use (about 1%). Table 65-1 lists risk factors for respiratory depression.

SEDATION

Sedation correlates with respiratory depression for two reasons. First, the opioid may have a direct effect on the thalamus, limbic system, or cerebral cortex from rostral spread in the CSF. Second, if significant respiratory depression does occur, resultant hypercapnia may create carbon dioxide narcosis. Therefore, when a patient becomes increasingly somnolent after neuraxial opioids, episodic hypoventilation and respiratory depression should be carefully considered, even when respiratory rate and oxygenation are within acceptable limits.

PRURITUS

The incidence of pruritus with neuraxial opioids ranges from 30% to 100%, but it is severe in only about 1% of patients. Larger doses and intrathecal administration carry a higher risk for pruritus, as does pregnancy (possibly owing to high plasma estrogen).

Fentanyl and morphine are more likely to cause itching, but all opioids have been implicated. The exact mechanism is unclear. Neuraxial opioids appear to interact with medullary inhibitory pathways in the spinal cord. The time course for itching correlates with the analgesic effect. Opioids may also act on an "itch center" in the medulla, which is associated with the trigeminal nucleus; this may explain why facial itching is most common. Histamine release is not a cause of neuraxial opioid-induced pruritus.

NAUSEA AND VOMITING

Nausea is less likely with neuraxial administration than with more conventional dosing. The incidence is about 30%. The risk is higher in female patients and with morphine and intrathecal use, probably due to the drug's direct interaction with the vomiting center and chemoreceptor trigger zone located in the fourth ventricle.

URINARY RETENTION

The incidence of urinary retention with neuraxial opioids varies widely but is higher than that seen after parenteral or oral administration. The opioid's effect on the sacral spinal cord receptors likely interferes with parasympathetic outflow and causes detrusor muscle relaxation and decreased sensation of the urge to void. It occurs more often in males and is dose dependent in duration. Time to complete recovery can be more than 5 hours after intrathecal sufentanil and more than 15 hours after intrathecal morphine.

Implications

Proper patient selection and careful vigilance can reduce serious adverse effects from neuraxial opioid use, especially central respiratory depression. Appropriate postoperative care requires the recognition that hydrophilic drugs (morphine, hydromorphone) can lead to a delayed onset and longer duration of respiratory depression. Monitoring is necessary for at least 24 hours after the administration of neuraxial morphine or hydromorphone. Excessive somnolence may be the first sign, which is why mental status checks should be performed during postoperative observation. Most hospitals provide thorough nurse education and have precise written protocols for monitoring and treatment in the case of significant respiratory depression. An example is given in Table 65-2. Also, concomitant administration of other narcotics or central nervous system depressants should be avoided, especially in opioid-naïve patients.

Small doses of lipophilic drugs such as fentanyl can be safely used in ambulatory surgery settings. Studies have shown that the risk of respiratory depression is minimal with intrathecal doses of less than 25 μg of fentanyl, even in elderly patients. For patients receiving postoperative epidural analgesia, no special monitoring is necessary if fentanyl is used in reasonable doses, even with thoracic epidural catheters.

Side effects such as pruritus, nausea and vomiting, and urinary retention may be viewed as nuisance or minor complications, but even so, there can be undesirable consequences. If they are severe enough, there may be an unanticipated hospital admission or a delay in discharge, unpleasant side effects from the treatment medications, or unwanted procedures such as an indwelling bladder catheter for inability to void.

Use of intrathecal narcotics for labor and delivery has become increasingly popular. Complications such as prolonged early labor and severe fetal bradycardia have been reported,

---

Table 65–1 ■ Factors That Increase the Risk of Respiratory Depression

Opioid Characteristics
Larger doses
Intrathecal administration
Hydrophilic morphine or hydromorphone
Repeated boluses versus continuous infusion
Patient Characteristics
Elderly
Debilitated
Significant pulmonary disease
Sleep apnea
Opioid naïve
Concomitant opioids or central nervous system depressants

Table 65–2 ▪ **Example of Postoperative Orders for Patients Receiving Neuraxial Morphine**
Postoperative Orders for Intrathecal or Epidural Morphine
Pain Service beeper no: _____
Patient received morphine _____mg (dose)
Intrathecal Epidural (circle correct route) at _____(time)
Epidural morphine _____mg bolus every _____hours
DO NOT administer any narcotic until patient reports discomfort
No other opioids or sedative-hypnotics are to be given without notifying the Pain Service
☐ Vitals: check respiratory rate and level of sedation q1hr × 12 hr, q2hr × 12 hr, and q4hr thereafter
NOTIFY the Pain Service in case of the following:
• Respiratory depression: respiratory rate <8 and patient unarousable
• Inadequate analgesia
☐ Activity: assisted ambulation only
☐ IV fluids: maintain IV access for 12 hours following intrathecal or epidural morphine dose
Medications (medication management of side effects to be discontinued 12 hours after epidural discontinued):
Naloxone 0.1mg IV STAT (may repeat ×3) for respiratory rate <8 and patient unarousable
Droperidol 0.5 mg IV q4hr PRN for nausea or vomiting
Diphenhydramine 25 to 50 mg IV or PO q4hr PRN for itching
Nalbuphine 2.5 mg IV q4hr PRN for itching
Other: _____

Table 65–3 ▪ **Common Treatment Modalities for Neuraxial Opioid Side Effects**
Respiratory Depression
Naloxone
Close observation and frequent monitoring
Supplemental oxygen
Avoid concomitant opioids and central nervous system depressants
Pruritus
Nalbuphine
Diphenhydramine
Propofol
Ondansetron
Nausea or Vomiting
Droperidol
Ondansetron
Propofol
Nalbuphine
Urinary Retention
Naloxone
Bladder catheterization

REGIONAL ANESTHESIA & PAIN MANAGEMENT

but a causal relationship is still debated in the obstetric literature. The incidence of fetal heart rate abnormalities, especially bradycardia, may be dose dependent. The presumed cause is uterine hyperactivity due to an imbalance in circulating catecholamines after the rapid onset of analgesia. It should be emphasized that such heart rate abnormalities respond to conservative measures and are not associated with poor neonatal outcomes.

MANAGEMENT

For serious adverse effects, including respiratory depression, the best reversal agent is a pure opioid antagonist such as naloxone. Although intravenous naloxone has a rapid onset, the duration of a single bolus may be insufficient, and infusions are often warranted. For less critical side effects (e.g., pruritus), naloxone may be hard to titrate to effect without the reversal of at least some analgesia. If so, a mixed agonist-antagonist such as nalbuphine may be more suitable. Studies have shown that nalbuphine can effectively treat pruritus, nausea, or vomiting without altering the level of pain control.

Other agents have been used to treat the side effects of neuraxial opioids (Table 65-3). Serotonin 5-HT$_3$ antagonists (e.g., ondansetron) are effective for the treatment of both pruritus and nausea. Droperidol, with its weak serotonin antagonist activity, may help treat pruritus but is more useful against nausea and vomiting, whether administered intravenously or epidurally. Propofol inhibits dorsal horn signal transmission and can effectively treat nausea and pruritus; however, the management and cost of a propofol infusion

for this purpose probably outweigh the benefits. Although histamine release is not the mechanism for opioid-induced pruritus, the sedating effect of antihistamines such as diphenhydramine may be beneficial by breaking the itch-scratch cycle, but they do not directly reduce the itch.

Future directions include the development of peripheral opioid antagonists. These may reduce side effects such as pruritus and postoperative nausea and vomiting without affecting analgesia. Respiratory depression, however, is less likely to be treated with such agents, as it is a centrally mediated effect.

PREVENTION

Limiting the dose of a neuraxial opioid can reduce the incidence of side effects. Thus, a multimodal approach to postoperative analgesia may be the best prophylactic regimen. Nonsteroidal anti-inflammatory drugs, for example, reduce opioid requirements, provide analgesia, and perhaps even prevent pruritus by inhibiting prostaglandin synthesis. Dexamethasone is also an effective prophylaxis against nausea and vomiting and, in higher doses, may enhance analgesia. Droperidol may help reduce postoperative nausea and vomiting. Prophylactic ondansetron has been shown to reduce nausea, vomiting, and pruritus. Nalbuphine, however, may be a better drug for treatment than for prophylaxis. Intraoperative propofol infusions do not prevent either pruritus or nausea in the postoperative period. For continuous epidural analgesia, adding a low concentration of local anesthetic to the infusion reduces the opioid dose via a synergistic effect.

Further Reading

Bates JJ, Foss JF, Murphy DB: Are peripheral opioid antagonists the solution to opioid side effects? Anesth Analg 98:116-122, 2004.
Chaney MA: Side effects of intrathecal and epidural opioids. Can J Anaesth 42:891-903, 1995.

Cousins MJ, Mather LE: Intrathecal and epidural administration of opioids. Anesthesiology 61:276-310, 1984.

de Leon-Casasola OA, Lema MJ: Postoperative epidural opioid analgesia: What are the choices? Anesth Analg 83:867-875, 1996.

Etches RC, Sandler AN, Daley MD: Respiratory depression and spinal opioids. Can J Anaesth 36:165-185, 1989.

Kuipers PW, Kamphuis ET, van Venrooij GE, et al: Intrathecal opioids and lower urinary tract function: A urodynamic evaluation. Anesthesiology 100:1497-1503, 2004.

Szarvas S, Harmon D, Murphy D: Neuraxial opioid-induced pruritus: A review. J Clin Anesth 15:234-239, 2003.

Van de Velde M, Teunkens A, Hanssens M, et al: Intrathecal sufentanil and fetal heart rate abnormalities: A double-blind, double placebo-controlled trial comparing two forms of combined spinal epidural analgesia with epidural analgesia in labor. Anesth Analg 98:1153-1159, 2004.

Complications in Orthopedic Outpatients Not Receiving Peripheral Nerve Blocks

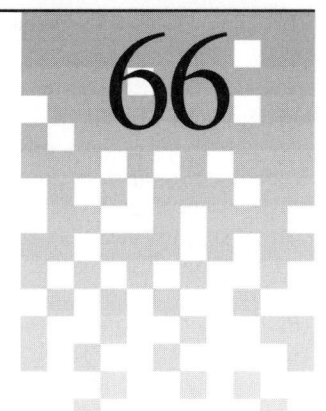

66

Brian A. Williams and Tetsuro Sakai

Case Synopsis

An otherwise healthy 30-year-old man underwent outpatient high tibial osteotomy. The uncomplicated procedure was performed with the patient under general anesthesia with endotracheal intubation. After emergence, the patient experienced severe, uncontrolled pain and then postoperative nausea and vomiting (PONV) after opioids were used in the postanesthesia care unit for pain control. He later required unplanned hospital admission for intractable pain, PONV, and somnolence. The patient was discharged after 2 days, when he was finally able to tolerate oral intake. However, he was readmitted to the emergency room 5 days later with constipation, episodic nausea, and wound dehiscence. The wound cultured positive for methicillin-resistant *Staphylococcus aureus* and vancomycin-resistant *Enterococcus faecalis*.

REGIONAL ANESTHESIA &
PAIN MANAGEMENT

PROBLEM ANALYSIS

Definition

The development of anesthesia techniques for outpatient surgery has led to great improvements in the management of PONV and postoperative pain. A growing demand for ambulatory surgery and anesthesia has resulted, because these adverse sequelae are the most common causes of unplanned hospital admissions. Multimodal analgesic techniques are especially recommended in ambulatory surgery patients to reduce many of the complications associated with high-dose opioid analgesia. Successful same-day discharge also protects patients from nosocomial and iatrogenic complications inherent to hospitalization.

Currently, many complex procedures are performed on an outpatient basis. This trend will continue in order to meet patients' desire for a more rapid return of cognitive and social function, as well as the public desire to reduce health care expenditures. The evolving subspecialties of outpatient orthopedic anesthesia and acute postoperative pain management are increasingly recognized for their positive effect on reducing hospital length of stay and improving functional recovery and patient satisfaction. Complications in the setting of outpatient orthopedic anesthesia and surgery require a multidisciplinary approach by anesthesiologists, nursing staff, surgeons, and hospital administrators.

The goals of ambulatory surgery are as follows:

- To maintain or improve quality and safety of care
- To schedule cases efficiently

- To minimize complications, such as poorly controlled pain and PONV
- To avoid unplanned postoperative hospital admissions
- To minimize readmissions after initial hospital discharge

The choice of anesthetic technique has paramount importance in achieving these goals, particularly in orthopedic surgery.

Recognition

Traditional belief in the safety and efficacy of general endotracheal anesthesia (GETA) in the inpatient setting should be reexamined in the context of outpatient surgery. In the setting of same-day surgery, a postoperative in-hospital care "buffer" is not necessarily available to manage such common problems as uncontrolled pain and PONV.

For orthopedic outpatients, problems associated with GETA include the following:

- Dental or oral mucosal injury from airway instrumentation
- Respiratory complications from mechanical ventilation
- Complications from volatile anesthetics (e.g., PONV, malignant hyperthermia)
- Prolonged or adverse effects from induction agents and systemic muscle relaxants
- Side effects from opioids (e.g., PONV, somnolence, delayed awakening, pruritus, respiratory depression, urinary retention, constipation)

Prolonged recovery from GETA often requires labor-intensive admission to a postanesthesia care unit for prolonged surveillance with physician-directed/interpreted monitoring and intervention. Significant cardiopulmonary changes caused by GETA are to be expected among elderly patients or those with predisposing medical risk factors. Unplanned admissions to an intensive care unit may also be necessary if prolonged mechanical ventilation or other patient support measures are required for cardiorespiratory or other complications.

Regional anesthesia, including peripheral nerve block (PNB), has traditionally been reserved for patients with contraindications to GETA. In outpatient orthopedic surgery, however, there is a shift toward the preferential use of PNB among progressive practitioners, whereas GETA (with volatile agents and no PNB) is reserved for outpatients in whom PNB is contraindicated.

PNB for orthopedic outpatients can help avoid the risks associated with GETA mentioned earlier. Williams and colleagues recently reviewed 1200 consecutive cases of outpatient knee surgery and reported that general anesthesia with a volatile agent was associated with a 200% increase in nursing interventions for pain control in the same-day recovery unit and a 300% increase in unplanned hospital admissions compared with anesthesia consisting of sedation and femoral-sciatic nerve block techniques. In addition, continuous PNB using indwelling catheters and portable infusion pumps can offer excellent postoperative pain control for 2 to 3 days at home.

Risk Assessment

Absolute contraindications to PNB for outpatient surgery include the following:

- Patient refusal (with appropriate patient education by the anesthesiologist, which may take 10 to 15 minutes, many patients who initially refuse PNB ultimately will accept it)
- Coagulopathies (systemic anticoagulants such as warfarin should be converted to intravenous heparin preoperatively, if PNB is indicated)
- Infection at the site of needle placement
- Systemic bacteremia or sepsis

In practice, these contraindications are highly unlikely in outpatients presenting for same-day orthopedic surgery.

Preexisting neurologic conditions are relative contraindications to PNB. Careful documentation of any preexisting neurologic deficit is mandatory if PNB will be performed in such patients.

To perform successful ambulatory surgery with PNB, the environment and resources must be coordinated. Good communication between the anesthesiologist and the surgical team is mandatory. To select the appropriate PNB modality, the anesthesiologist must be familiar with the surgical procedure, its invasiveness, and the dermatomes that must be covered. Also, the anesthesiologist must be comfortable performing the indicated PNB. All precautions for conversion to general anesthesia must be immediately available. This includes proper preoperative airway assessment and preparation of the required airway equipment before any regional procedure is performed. Ideally, an induction room or separate facility where PNB can be performed is preferable, to reduce time in the operating room.

Anesthesiologists and nursing staff need to be aware of PNB-associated risks. These include central nervous system and cardiovascular toxicity of local anesthetics and potential peripheral nerve damage with the PNB procedure; the incidence of the latter ranges from 4 in 1000 to 2 in 10,000.

The centerpiece of anesthesia care in outpatient orthopedic surgery is multimodal analgesia, including the use of PNB, the prevention of PONV with routine multimodal antiemetic prophylaxis, and the avoidance of general anesthesia with volatile agents whenever possible. A propofol-based intravenous anesthesia technique should be considered as an adjunct to PNB if sedation is required.

Implications

Preferential (but careful) use of PNB in orthopedic outpatients is beneficial in terms of reducing hospital costs and improving patient satisfaction. The use of PNB for anesthesia has been associated with earlier discharge (fewer nursing interventions for pain or PONV and fewer unplanned hospital admissions) when compared with GETA in patients undergoing ambulatory orthopedic surgery.

MANAGEMENT

There are two methods of PNB: single-injection PNB and continuous PNB with an indwelling catheter. Although single-injection techniques are effective, they offer postoperative analgesia for only a few hours—certainly no more than 12 to 24 hours—depending on the local anesthetic and adjuncts used. Consequently, the duration of the block may be too brief to provide adequate postoperative analgesia or sufficient analgesia to initiate physical therapy. Early physical therapy is essential to optimize functional recovery after orthopedic surgery. Continuous PNB catheter techniques have the following advantages over single-injection or neuraxial techniques:

- Longer duration of postoperative analgesia
- Titratable dosage
- Preferential sensory block, when active physical therapy is required
- Avoidance of the neuraxis and associated complications (especially in the context of systemic anticoagulation)

Once it is established that PNB is indicated, one must select the correct PNB modality according to the invasiveness of the planned orthopedic procedure. An example of a PNB algorithm for the care of outpatients undergoing knee surgery is given in Table 66-1. Use of a peripheral nerve stimulator facilitates PNB and catheter placement (Fig. 66-1). The patient can later be discharged with the PNB catheter in place and a portable infusion pump. Written instructions for catheter and pump management should be provided and explained to the patient at the time of discharge. Further, the anesthesia care team should make daily contact with the patient by telephone and be available by pager if the patient has questions.

PNB can be used safely in patients who require postoperative anticoagulation with intravenous unfractionated heparin or subcutaneous low-molecular-weight heparin to prevent deep venous thrombosis and pulmonary embolism. Systemic anticoagulation is seldom used in surgical outpatients.

Table 66–1 ■ Recommended Peripheral Nerve Blocks for Outpatient Knee Surgery

Category I (Mild)
No blocks unless unanticipated postoperative pain occurs

Category II (Moderate)
Single-injection femoral nerve block recommended: arthrotomy, deep hardware removal, microfracture, mosaicplasty or chondroplasty, ACL allograft
   Femoral bolus: 30 mL of preferred long-duration local anesthetic
   No sciatic block unless unanticipated pain refractory to femoral block
Continuous catheter recommended: ACL patellar tendon autograft, femoral osteotomy
   Femoral catheter initial bolus: 20 to 30 mL of preferred long-duration local anesthetic
   Femoral catheter infusion: 5 mL/hr of low-concentration, long-duration local anesthetic
   No sciatic block unless unanticipated pain refractory to femoral block

Category III (Severe)

Procedure	Femoral Nerve Block	Sciatic Nerve Block
Most Invasive Category III*		

Total knee replacement
High tibial osteotomy
Multiligament reconstruction
  (including PCL, LCL, MCL, POL)
    Posterolateral corner reconstruction
	Continuous femoral catheter–initial bolus: 20-30 mL of intermediate-concentration, long-duration local anesthetic
	Catheter dose: 5 mL/hr of low-concentration, long-duration local anesthetic
		Continuous sciatic catheter–initial bolus: 5-10 mL of low-concentration, long-duration local anesthetic
		Catheter dose (postoperatively): 5-20 mL bolus as needed, followed by 3 mL/hr of low-concentration, long-duration local anesthetic

Moderately Invasive Category III		
ACL hamstring autograft Meniscal reconstruction Unicompartmental knee arthroplasty	Continuous femoral catheter–initial bolus: 20 mL of low- concentration, long-duration local anesthetic Catheter dose: 5 mL/hr of low-concentration, long-duration local anesthetic	Single-injection sciatic: 20 mL of intermediate-concentration, long-duration local anesthetic
Less Invasive Category III		
Distal patella realignment	Single-injection femoral: 30 mL of intermediate-concentration, long-duration local anesthetic	Single-injection sciatic: 20 mL of low- to intermediate-concentration, long-duration local anesthetic

Algorithm for the use of nerve block additives:
–If a catheter is used, clonidine is not routinely added.
–If no catheter is used, clonidine is routinely recommended if ropivacaine is the local anesthetic used.
–Regardless of catheter status, buprenorphine may be a useful analgesic adjunct (as part of the catheter bolus dose or single-injection dose). The buprenorphine dose should be restricted to a total of 150 µg for an adult patient to prevent nausea, vomiting, and pruritus associated with higher doses.

*Test for dorsiflexion postoperatively before ablating sciatic nerve motor response.
ACL, anterior cruciate ligament; LCL, lateral collateral ligament; MCL, medial collateral ligament; PCL, posterior cruciate ligament; POL, posterior oblique ligament.

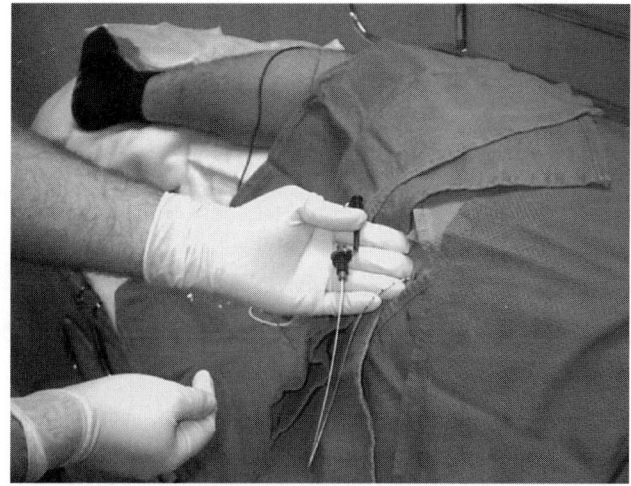

Figure 66–1 ■ Patient receiving a continuous sciatic nerve block catheter after already having received a femoral nerve block catheter (not shown). Note that the catheter is a stimulating catheter (StimCath, Arrow International, Reading, Pa) and that its proper placement can be confirmed with nerve stimulation before the nerve block catheter is dosed with local anesthetic. The operator's hand is highlighting the attachment of a nerve stimulator adapter clip to the catheter's Luer-Lok connection device. This catheter can later be attached to an infusion pump containing low-dose local anesthetic that can be infused for up to 72 hours after surgery.

Finally, use of a continuous propofol infusion as an adjunct to PNB is beneficial for ambulatory surgery patients to reduce the risk of PONV, especially if intraoperative sedation or total intravenous anesthesia is indicated.

PREVENTION

One should avoid the underutilization of PNB techniques in outpatient orthopedic surgery, assuming the availability of anesthesiologists who are skilled in such techniques. Anesthesiologists must be proactive and educate patients and surgeons about the benefits of PNB techniques. Using PNB, either as the main anesthetic or as an adjunct to total intravenous anesthesia with propofol, facilitates rapid emergence and perioperative analgesia.

Finally, to prevent nosocomial wound infections and unplanned hospital admissions, it is important to discharge patients home the same day. This requires a comprehensive plan for symptom management as part of the total anesthesia and analgesia care plan.

Further Reading

Chelly JE, Ben-David B, Williams BA, Kentor ML: Anesthesia and postoperative analgesia: Outcomes following orthopedic surgery. Orthopedics 26(8 Suppl):S865-S871, 2003.

Gupta A, Wu CL, Elkassabany N, et al: Does the routine prophylactic use of antiemetics affect the incidence of postdischarge nausea and vomiting following ambulatory surgery? A systematic review of randomized controlled trials. Anesthesiology 99:488-495, 2003.

Ilfeld BM, Morey TE, Enneking FK: Continuous infraclavicular brachial plexus block for postoperative pain control at home: A randomized, double-blinded, placebo-controlled study. Anesthesiology 96:1297-1304, 2002.

Ilfeld BM, Morey TE, Wright TW, et al: Continuous interscalene brachial plexus block for postoperative pain control at home: A randomized, double-blinded, placebo-controlled study. Anesth Analg 96:1089-1095, 2003.

Klein SM, Nielsen KC, Greengrass RA, et al: Ambulatory discharge after long-acting peripheral nerve blockade: 2382 blocks with ropivacaine. Anesth Analg 94:65-70, 2001.

Williams BA, Kentor ML, Vogt MT, et al: Femoral-sciatic nerve blocks for complex outpatient knee surgery are associated with less postoperative pain before same-day discharge: A review of 1200 consecutive cases from the period 1996-1999. Anesthesiology 98:1206-1213, 2003.

Williams BA, Kentor ML, Vogt MT, et al: The economics of nerve block pain management after anterior cruciate ligament reconstruction: Significant hospital cost savings via associated PACU bypass and same-day discharge. Anesthesiology 100:697-706, 2004.

Williams BA, Vogt MT, Kentor ML, et al: Nausea and vomiting after outpatient ACL reconstruction with regional anesthesia: Are lumbar plexus blocks a risk factor? J Clin Anesth 16:276-281, 2004.

Anticoagulants and Peripheral Nerve Block

67

James R. Hebl

REGIONAL ANESTHESIA &
PAIN MANAGMENT

Case Synopsis

A 73-year-old man with a history of ischemic heart disease and diabetes mellitus is scheduled to undergo an elective total hip arthroplasty. The patient has been receiving daily anticoagulation with warfarin since his aortic valve replacement 3 years ago. Five days before surgery, the patient's warfarin was discontinued by his primary care physician, at which time he began therapeutic anticoagulation bridging therapy with low-molecular-weight heparin (LMWH). The patient's last injection of LMWH was about 24 hours ago. The orthopedic surgeon intends to reinitiate anticoagulation with LMWH 12 hours after surgery. During the preanesthetic interview, the patient requests spinal anesthesia and a peripheral nerve catheter for extended postoperative analgesia.

PROBLEM ANALYSIS

Definition

The use of peripheral nerve blocks (PNBs) for perioperative anesthesia and analgesia has increased dramatically over the past several years. Importantly, this shift in practice does not appear to be a transient phenomenon. For example, more than 40% of clinicians surveyed in 1998 in the United States estimated that their use of PNB techniques would increase over the next several years. Further, use of PNB in France increased approximately 18-fold between 1980 and 1996. Reasons for the increased use of PNB include not only its potential benefits (Table 67-1) but also the avoidance of complications that may accompany central neuraxial techniques, including concerns about perioperative anticoagulation, hemodynamic instability due to sympathetic block, and delayed discharge after outpatient surgery.

However, the use of PNB is associated with its own unique set of concerns and complications. In particular, hemorrhagic complications have been reported with greater frequency as changes in clinical practice occur (e.g., more aggressive perioperative anticoagulation, new regional techniques, continuous perineural catheters) and the popularity of PNB continues to increase. Although hemorrhagic complications are quite rare, they can be among the most devastating complications

Table 67-1 ■ Potential Benefits of Peripheral Nerve Block

Superior postoperative analgesia
Improved rehabilitative efforts (owing to analgesia)
Decreased perioperative nausea and vomiting
Faster emergence and recovery
Earlier mobilization (unilateral blockade)
Faster outpatient discharge
Improved blood flow to affected extremity
Benefits extended with continuous catheter techniques

of PNB. Such injury has been reported with a variety of PNBs, including interscalene, axillary, intercostal, paravertebral, femoral, ilioinguinal, posterior lumbar plexus, and lumbar sympathetic blocks. Patients at greatest risk include those receiving unfractionated heparin, LMWH, warfarin, antiplatelet aggregation medications, or antithrombolytic therapy.

Recognition

In general, localized bruising and tenderness are very common following PNB, with reported frequencies ranging from 8% to 23%. True hemorrhagic complications appear to be much less common. For example, the reported frequency of hematoma formation after brachial plexus block ranges from 0.2% to 3%. Most hematomas are small, unrecognized, and clinically inconsequential. However, there have been reports of more severe hemorrhagic complications, as well as significant neurologic impairment after hematoma formation. Recognition of bleeding complications relies on astute clinical vigilance throughout the perioperative period; this is especially important in patients receiving perioperative anticoagulation with intravenous heparin, warfarin, LMWH, or antiplatelet drugs. Significant hypotension, localized pain or tenderness, severe ecchymosis, unexplained anemia, or the development of neurologic deficits may signal underlying hemorrhage or a compressive hematoma. Computed tomography (CT), magnetic resonance imaging, or ultrasonography may be required for confirmation and to determine the location and extent of injury.

Risk Assessment

There are no reports on the frequency or severity of hemorrhagic complications with PNB in patients receiving anticoagulants. However, there are reports of serious complications following neurovascular sheath cannulation for central vascular access. Although this intervention is not the same as PNB, it *may* predict what can occur after PNB

269

needle- or catheter-caused vascular injury in patients receiving anticoagulants or antiplatelet drugs.

Fransson and Nylander reported vascular complications in 0.26% of 4879 patients having cardiac catheterization, coronary angiography, or angioplasty at one university hospital. These included pseudoaneurysm (12 cases), thromboembolism (4 cases), and excessive bleeding (3 cases). There was no neurologic impairment in any patient. Among those with vascular complications, 58% were receiving anticoagulation, compared with 10% of those with no complications.

Reports of vascular injury after PNB are limited to case reports. Such complications have occurred in patients with normal hemostasis and in those receiving anticoagulation therapy. Complications include anemia with profound hypotension and the need for transfusion, myocardial ischemia, acute renal insufficiency, localized pain and tenderness, neurologic injury, and even death. Of note, all reported adverse neurologic sequelae were transient and self-limited, with full recovery by 12 months. Thus, in contrast to central neuraxial bleeding, bleeding into a more compliant peripheral nerve site seems unlikely to be associated with irreversible, permanent nerve injury.

The majority of severe hemorrhagic complications after PNB have been associated with either posterior lumbar plexus (i.e., psoas compartment; see Chapter 64) or lumbar sympathetic blocks. In all instances, patients received anticoagulants before, during, or after PNB. Klein and associates reported one case of psoas compartment hematoma with transient neuropathy after lumbar plexus block for below-knee amputation. That patient received 30 mg of enoxaparin 20 hours before the attempted PNB and also 4 hours afterward. After several attempts at posterior lumbar plexus block, an anterior three-in-one block (lumbar plexus and sciatic nerves) was performed. On postoperative day 1, the patient had right hip pain, which progressed to complete paralysis by day 9. A CT scan revealed a large retroperitoneal hematoma in the psoas compartment, displacing the kidney anteriorly. Her coagulation profile and platelet count were normal. She was treated conservatively, enoxaparin was stopped, and motor function gradually returned over the next 5 days, with complete return by 4 months. Also, Weller and coworkers reported extensive retroperitoneal hemorrhage in two patients, both of whom were anticoagulated after three-in-one blocks. Neither had new neurologic deficits, and both had normal coagulation profiles at the time of the block. One received enoxaparin (30 mg) 90 minutes after removal of a catheter within the neurovascular sheath (postoperative day 2) and later developed severe right paravertebral low back pain, hypotension (hemoglobin 7.1 g/dL), and transient renal insufficiency. A CT scan revealed a large retroperitoneal hematoma with renal displacement. The other patient had previously undergone aortic valve replacement and was taking warfarin (Coumadin); this drug was stopped, and the coagulation profile was normal before single-injection three-in-one block for knee arthroscopy. Heparin was started 8 hours after the block, and Coumadin was restarted the evening of postoperative day 1. On day 3, the patient had back pain at the block site, with a slow decline in hemoglobin from 12.8 to 8.5 g/dL. The CT scan revealed moderate retroperitoneal hematoma, which was treated conservatively, without residual neurologic impairment.

Irreversible platelet aggregation inhibitors (e.g., ticlopidine, clopidogrel) are implicated as contributing to hemorrhagic complications in patients with PNB. Maier and colleagues reported two cases of severe bleeding after lumbar sympathetic block (LSB). The first patient had peripheral vascular disease, and his medications included ticlopidine (500 mg/day) for stroke prevention. After his first LSB, hemoglobin decreased from 13.5 to 10.3 g/dL, and he complained of groin pain and medial thigh numbness. Inadvertent vascular puncture occurred during a second LSB performed 6 days later. The next night, the patient experienced severe groin pain, with a simultaneous drop in blood pressure and hemoglobin to 8.9 g/dL. A large retroperitoneal hematoma was diagnosed. He was transfused and discharged 5 days later, with no permanent neurologic deficits. The second patient was referred for diagnostic LSB and was receiving clopidogrel (75 mg/day). This drug was discontinued 3 days before the LSB, which was uneventful. Nine hours later, the patient complained of burning groin and medial thigh pain, which was treated with intravenous opioids. Twelve hours after LSB, she was found pulseless. Attempted resuscitation was unsuccessful. At autopsy, there was a massive, congealed retroperitoneal hematoma.

As these cases show, severe hemorrhage, but not permanent neurologic injury, may be the most serious complication of PNB in anticoagulated patients. It appears to be most likely if PNB is performed at concealed, noncompliant sites (e.g., psoas compartment). Further, such occult bleeding may go unrecognized for several hours to days.

Implications

Perioperative anticoagulation for the prevention of venous thromboembolism can result in significant morbidity, mortality, and resource allocation. Knowledge of specific clinical risk factors for thromboembolism (Table 67-2) is the basis for the proper use of perioperative anticoagulation treatment or prophylaxis. These risk factors are present alone or in combination

Table 67–2 ■ Clinical Risk Factors for Venous Thromboembolism
Increased age
Prolonged immobility
Prior stroke or paralysis
Previous venous thromboembolism
Cancer
Major surgery
Abdominal surgery
Pelvic surgery
Lower extremity surgery
Trauma
Obesity
Varicose veins
Cardiac dysfunction
Indwelling central venous catheter
Inflammatory bowel disease
Nephrotic syndrome
Pregnancy or estrogen use

From American College of Chest Physicians: Sixth ACCP Consensus Conference on Antithrombotic Therapy. Chest 119(Suppl), 2001.

in a high proportion of hospitalized patients. Consequently, many patients who present for elective or emergency surgery are, or will be, receiving medications that alter normal hemostasis. All clinicians should be aware of this, especially when performing regional anesthesia.

MANAGEMENT

Patients receiving anticoagulants may be at the greatest risk of hemorrhagic complications after PNB. Therefore, astute clinical vigilance is mandatory. If such a complication is suspected, immediate clinical evaluation should occur, including the following:

- Focused review of the patient's perioperative history
  - Past medical history
  - Preoperative coagulation status
  - Pre- and perioperative medications (e.g., hemostasis-altering drugs, herbals)
  - Surgical course, including intra- and postoperative blood loss
  - Immediate postoperative course
- Consideration of the patient's chief complaint
  - Pain (location, duration, nature)
  - Neurologic deficits (sensory or motor, onset, duration, fluctuation)
  - Orthostatic symptoms
  - Fatigue, syncope, lightheadedness, postural hypotension

- Physical examination (including a detailed neurologic assessment)
- Laboratory investigation (complete blood count, coagulation profile, electrolytes)
- Radiographic imaging for definitive diagnosis (CT, magnetic resonance imaging, ultrasonography)

Surgical decompression with hematoma evacuation may be necessary if (1) the hematoma continues to expand, (2) there is progressive neurologic deterioration, (3) neural dysfunction does not improve despite hematoma resolution, or (4) there is evidence of airway, vascular, or lymphatic obstruction. In select cases, when these criteria are not satisfied, observation and conservative management may be appropriate. However, prompt assessment and appropriate intervention are critical in *all* patients to prevent hemorrhagic catastrophes and irreversible neurologic impairment.

PREVENTION

Development of a central neuraxial hematoma due to bleeding into a fixed and noncompressible site is clearly the most significant and potentially devastating hemorrhagic complication of regional anesthesia. In an effort to reduce this risk, the American Society of Regional Anesthesia and Pain Medicine (ASRAPM) developed consensus guidelines for central neuraxial anesthesia and analgesia in anticoagulated patients (Table 67-3). Because the risk of such complications

---

Table 67–3 ▪ American Society of Regional Anesthesia and Pain Medicine Guidelines for Central Neuraxial Anesthesia in Patients Receiving Thromboprophylaxis

Anticoagulant	Recommendation
Antiplatelet medications	No contraindication with NSAIDs Discontinue ticlopidine for 14 days Discontinue clopidogrel for 7 days Discontinue glycoprotein IIb/IIIa inhibitors 8-48 hr in advance

Unfractionated heparin
  Subcutaneous
  Intravenous
	No contraindication; consider delaying heparin until after block if technical difficulty is anticipated
	Heparinize 1 hr after neuraxial technique
	Remove catheter(s) 2-4 hr after last heparin dose
	No mandatory delay if traumatic needle placement

Low-molecular-weight heparin (LMWH)	Preoperative dosing:
	    Needle placement should occur at least 10-12 hr after last LMWH dose (prophylactic dosages) or at least 24 hr after higher doses (treatment dosages)
	Postoperative twice-daily dosing:
	    LMWH 24 hr after surgery, regardless of technique
	    Remove neuraxial catheter(s) 2 hr before first LMWH dose
	Postoperative once-daily dosing:
	    LMWH 6-8 hr after surgery
	    Give second postoperative dose no sooner than 24 hr after first dose
	    Indwelling catheter(s) can be safely maintained
	    Remove catheter(s) 10-12 hr *after* last dose of LMWH and 2 hr *before* subsequent dosing

Warfarin	Document normal INR after discontinuation (before neuraxial technique) Remove catheter(s) when INR ≤1.5 (within initiation of therapy)
Thrombolytics	No data on safe performance of neuraxial techniques or catheter removal
Herbal therapy	No evidence of mandatory discontinuation before neuraxial techniques Be mindful of potential drug interactions (see Chapter 39)

INR, international normalized ratio; NSAID, nonsteroidal anti-inflammatory drug.
Adapted from Horlocker TT, Wedel DJ, Benzon H, et al: Regional anesthesia in the anticoagulated patient: Defining the risks (the Second ASRA Consensus Conference on Neuraxial Anesthesia and Anticoagulation). Reg Anesth Pain Med 28:172-197, 2003.

in anticoagulated patients undergoing PNB is not clearly defined, one approach might be to apply these guidelines to all patients receiving regional anesthesia, including PNB. However, this might be overly cautious. Instead, it might be more prudent to consider the compressibility of the PNB needle insertion site and the vascular structures at risk.

Also, it is strongly advised that, in patients with inherent or drug-induced coagulopathies, PNB be used only after a careful risk-benefit analysis, and that it be performed with extra caution. This is especially true if the PNB will be performed in a region where an expanding hematoma could compress the airway (e.g., deep cervical plexus, interscalene, or "plumb-bob" supraclavicular block) or might not become apparent for several hours to days in a noncompressible site (e.g., psoas compartment with a lumbar plexus block). Regardless, good communication among all clinicians involved in the perioperative care of any patient receiving drugs that affect hemostasis is critical to provide optimal patient care and to reduce the risk of serious hemorrhagic complications.

Further Reading

Aida S, Takahashi H, Shimoji K: Renal subcapsular hematoma after lumbar plexus block. Anesthesiology 84:452-455, 1996.

American College of Chest Physicians: Sixth ACCP Consensus Conference on Antithrombotic Therapy. Chest 119(Suppl), 2001.

Ben-David B, Stahl S: Axillary block complicated by hematoma and radial nerve injury. Reg Anesth Pain Med 24:264-266, 1999.

Bergman BD, Hebl JR, Kent J, Horlocker TT: Neurologic complications of 405 consecutive continuous axillary catheters. Anesth Analg 96:247-252, 2003.

Clergue F, Auroy Y, Perquignot F, et al: French survey of anesthesia in 1996. Anesthesiology 91:1509-1520, 1999.

Ekatodramis G, Macaire P, Borgeat A: Prolonged Horner syndrome due to neck hematoma after continuous interscalene block. Anesthesiology 95:801-803, 2001.

Fransson SG, Nylander E: Vascular injury following cardiac catheterization, coronary angiography, and coronary angioplasty. Eur Heart J 15:232-235, 1994.

Hadzic A, Vloka JD, Kuroda MM, et al: The practice of peripheral nerve blocks in the United States: A national survey. Reg Anesth Pain Med 23:241-246, 1998.

Horlocker TT: Peripheral nerve blocks: Regional anesthesia for the new millennium. Reg Anesth Pain Med 23:237-240, 1998.

Horlocker TT, Wedel DJ, Benzon H, et al: Regional anesthesia in the anticoagulated patient: Defining the risks (the Second ASRA Consensus Conference on Neuraxial Anesthesia and Anticoagulation). Reg Anesth Pain Med 28:172-197, 2003.

Johr M: A complication of continuous blockade of the femoral nerve [German]. Reg Anaesthesie 10:37-38, 1987.

Klein SM, D'Ercole F, Greengrass RA, Warner DS: Enoxaparin associated with psoas hematoma and lumbar plexopathy after lumbar plexus block. Anesthesiology 87:1576-1579, 1997.

Maier C, Gleim M, Weiss T, et al: Severe bleeding following lumbar sympathetic blockade in two patients under medication with irreversible platelet aggregation inhibitors. Anesthesiology 97:740-743, 2002.

Neal JM, Hebl JR, Gerancher JC, Hogan QH: Brachial plexus anesthesia: Essentials of our current understanding. Reg Anesth Pain Med 27:402-428, 2002.

Nielsen CH: Bleeding after intercostal nerve block in a patient anticoagulated with heparin. Anesthesiology 71:162-164, 1989.

Sada T, Kobayashi T, Murakami S: Continuous axillary brachial plexus block. Can Anaesth Soc J 30:201-205, 1983.

Thomas PW, Sanders DJ, Berrisford RG: Pulmonary haemorrhage after percutaneous paravertebral block. Br J Anaesth 83:668-669, 1999.

Vaisman J: Pelvic hematoma after an ilioinguinal nerve block for orchialgia. Anesth Analg 92:1048-1049, 2001.

Weller RS, Gerancher JC, Crews JC, Wade KL: Extensive retroperitoneal hematoma without neurologic deficit in two patients who underwent lumbar plexus block and were later anticoagulated. Anesthesiology 98:581-585, 2003.

Chronic Nonsteroidal Anti-inflammatory Drug Use

68

Celeste M. Lombardi

Case Synopsis

A 60-year-old man with a history of osteoarthritis has been taking naproxen for the past 3 years without complications or side effects. He experienced sudden severe nausea and vomited frank blood. He was taken to the emergency room and underwent an urgent upper gastrointestinal (GI) endoscopy, which revealed a bleeding gastric ulcer.

PROBLEM ANALYSIS

Definition

Nonsteroidal anti-inflammatory drugs (NSAIDs) are widely used drugs that act by inhibiting cyclooxygenase and the formation of prostaglandins. Prostaglandins are derived from arachidonic acid, formed by phospholipase A_2 acting on cell membrane phospholipids (Fig. 68-1). NSAIDs are among the most commonly used drugs worldwide and are usually well tolerated. However, like all medications, NSAIDs are not without side effects. They are known to cause the following:

- GI toxicity, leading to the formation of peptic ulcers
- Unwanted antiplatelet effects (nonselective inhibitors of cyclooxygenase)
- Potential for increased thrombogenicity (selective cyclo-oxygenase-2 [COX-2] inhibitors)
- Renal toxicity, with potential alterations of potassium and fluid balance, decreased renal function, nephrotic syndrome with interstitial nephritis, papillary necrosis, and rhabdomyolysis
- Anaphylactic and anaphylactoid reactions in select patients

Recognition

GASTROINTESTINAL EFFECTS

NSAID use is the second most important cause of peptic ulcers after *Helicobacter pylori* infection. The primary mechanism of ulcer formation is from suppression of gastric prostaglandins, although decreases in nitric oxide and calcitonin gene-related peptide may also be involved. This leads to decreases in epithelial mucus, bicarbonate secretion, and mucosal resistance to injury. NSAIDs also reduce gastric mucosal blood flow, with subsequent damage to the vascular endothelium (an early effect of NSAID administration) in conjunction with an enhanced adherence of neutrophils to the vascular endothelium. The neutrophil adherence causes endothelial injury by release of oxygen-derived free radicals.

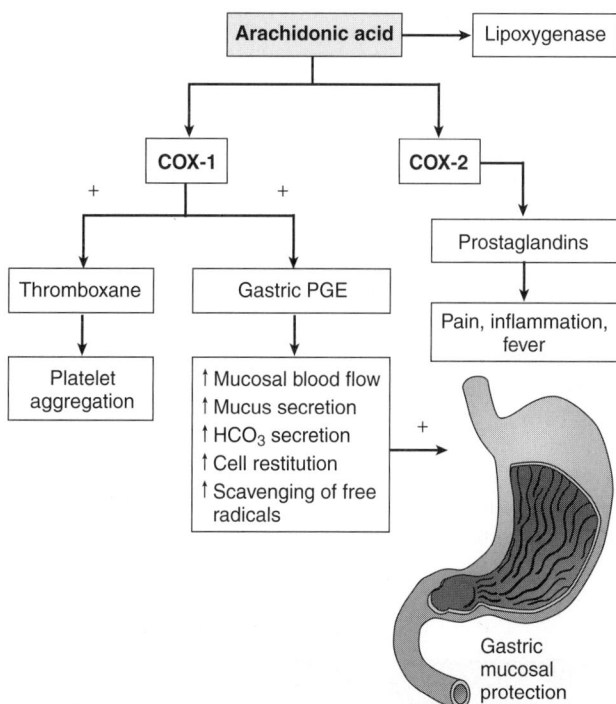

Figure 68–1 ■ Biosynthesis of prostaglandins from arachidonic acid via the cyclooxygenase (COX-1 and COX-2) pathways. Arachidonic acid, the immediate precursor of prostaglandins, is derived from membrane phospholipids in reactions catalyzed by the two COX isoenzymes. The gene for COX-1 (the "housekeeping" enzyme) is expressed constitutively and maintains organ homeostasis, including integrity of the gastric mucosa. The gene for COX-2 (the "inflammatory" enzyme) is inducible. Thromboxane derived via COX-1 causes platelet aggregation or the listed gastric mucosal protective effects. In contrast, prostaglandins such as prostacyclin (PGI_2) derived via COX-2 are mediators of pain, inflammation, and fever. PGE, prostaglandin E. (Adapted from Wolfe MM: Therapy and prevention of NSAID-related gastrointestinal disorders. In Wolfe MM [ed]: Therapy of Digestive Disorders: A Companion to Sleisenger and Fordtran Gastrointestinal Diseases. Philadelphia, WB Saunders, 2000, pp 96-112.)

273

THROMBOGENIC EFFECTS

Thromboxane A_2 is a major product of COX-1 metabolism in platelets (see Fig. 68-1). It causes platelet aggregation, vasoconstriction, and smooth muscle proliferation. In patients with peripheral vascular disease, increased thromboxane production is associated with increased risk of major vascular events. Aspirin is a potent inhibitor of platelet cyclooxygenase (COX-1), which blocks thromboxane production for the life of the platelet. With other NSAIDs, this process lasts 24 hours or less. This effect underlies aspirin's ability to reduce the incidence of cardiovascular death, myocardial infarction, and stroke in high-risk patients. However, high doses or toxic doses of aspirin can inhibit vitamin K–dependent coagulation factors, leading to an increase in prothrombin time and international normalized ratio.

In contrast, prostacyclin is a product of COX-2 metabolism in vascular endothelium. This is postulated from the finding that pharmacologic inhibition of COX-2 leads to the inhibition of prostacyclin formation. Prostacyclin inhibits platelet aggregation and smooth muscle proliferation and causes vasodilatation. Nabumetone, etodolac, and nonacetylated salicylates (relatively COX-2–selective NSAIDs) inhibit COX-2–mediated prostacyclin biosynthesis and seem to have little or no effect on platelet aggregation. Other NSAIDs block COX-1 thromboxane biosynthesis and COX-2 prostacyclin production with less selectivity (Table 68-1; Fig. 68-2).

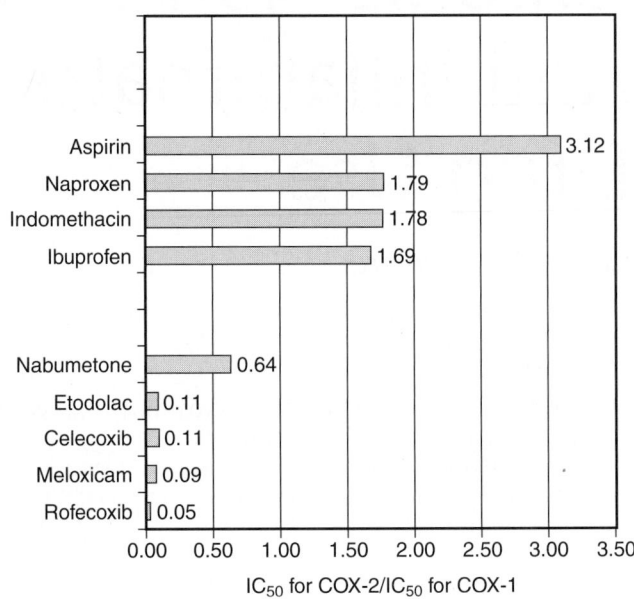

Figure 68–2 ▪ Selectivity of COX-2 inhibitors. Comparison of in vivo inhibitory concentration (IC_{50}) ratios (COX-2/COX-1) of selective and nonselective nonsteroidal anti-inflammatory drugs. A lower ratio indicates an increased degree of selectivity for COX-2. (Adapted from Feldman M, McMahon AT: Do cyclooxygenase-2 inhibitors provide benefits similar to those of traditional anti-inflammatory drugs, with less gastrointestinal toxicity? Ann Intern Med 132:134-143, 2000.)

RENAL EFFECTS

Up to 5% of patients on regular NSAID therapy develop one or more nephrotoxic side effects, including fluid and electrolyte abnormalities, acute renal failure, and nephrotic syndrome (Table 68-2). The mechanism of action of these side effects is inhibition of the production of prostaglandins I_2, E_2, and D_2 by blocking of the COX-1 isoenzyme. This reduces renal perfusion by causing acute renal artery vasoconstriction, medullary ischemia, and, in some cases, acute renal failure. NSAIDs also decrease the efficacy of antihypertensive medications because they require intact renal prostaglandin function. The exceptions are calcium channel blockers and angiotensin II receptor antagonists, which are not influenced by renal prostaglandins. Various NSAIDs have different effects on blood pressure, depending on their capacity to inhibit renal vasodilatory prostaglandins. Sulindac, for instance, may be a weaker inhibitor of renal prostaglandins and thus exert less effect on blood pressure in hypertensive individuals. Blood pressure needs to be closely monitored in patients who are started on NSAID therapy and take antihypertensive medication, especially those 55 years and older.

Fluid and electrolyte disturbances are common NSAID-associated renal side effects. They occur as a result of inhibition of prostaglandin formation in the thick ascending limb of the loop of Henle and the distal renal tubule, leading to hypotonic sodium and water retention. With the inhibition

Table 68–1 ▪ Inhibition of Prostacyclin and Thromboxane Biosynthesis and Risk of Thrombosis

Drug	Prostacyclin	Thromboxane	Thrombosis Risk
Low-dose aspirin	+/–	⇓⇓	⇓
Conventional	⇓	⇓	Unclear
COX-2 specific inhibitors	⇓	+/–	Unclear

COX, cyclooxygenase; NSAID, nonsteroidal anti-inflammatory drug.
From Catella-Lawson F, Crofford LJ: Cyclooxygenase inhibition and thrombogenicity. Am J Med 110:28-32, 2001.

Table 68–2 ▪ Renal Syndromes Related to Therapy with Conventional Nonsteroidal Anti-inflammatory Drugs

Fluid and electrolyte abnormalities
Acute renal failure
Hemodynamic compromise
Nephrotic syndrome (minimal-change glomerulopathy, interstitial nephritis)
Acute papillary necrosis (typically, single drug cause)
Other systemic interactions
Hypernatremia
Water retention
Hyperkalemia
Membranous glomerulopathy
Chronic papillary necrosis (typically, multidrug causes)
Chronic heart failure
Hypertension (treated)

of the cyclooxygenase pathway, there is a theoretical increase in leukotriene formation via the 5-lipoxygenase pathway, leading to increased capillary permeability and edema formation. This is often seen in patients who develop congestive heart failure.

Hyperkalemia is a rare but serious complication of chronic NSAID therapy. This can occur as a result of inhibition of prostaglandin-mediated renin release. This, in turn, leads to decreased aldosterone formation and decreased secretion of potassium in the distal renal tubules.

The development of nephrotic syndrome with interstitial nephritis is rare and is not clearly understood. It is theorized that the preferential formation of leukotrienes and inhibition of prostaglandins increase vascular permeability, leading to nephrotic-range proteinuria and interstitial nephritis.

Renal papillary necrosis is also rare and is thought to occur in cases of NSAID overdose in severely dehydrated patients. The combination of prostaglandin inhibition and high intrapapillary doses of NSAIDs, which may be cytotoxic themselves, leads to papillary necrosis. This is unlikely to occur with conventional doses of NSAIDs.

ANAPHYLACTIC AND ANAPHYLACTOID REACTIONS

A small number of patient experience allergic and pseudoallergic reactions to aspirin and NSAIDs. Some reactions are caused by the similar pharmacologic properties of traditional NSAIDs, which inhibit both COX-1 and COX-2. Prostaglandin E_2 formation is blocked by the inhibition of COX-1, leading to a relative increase in leukotriene formation and histamine release from mast cells. Such a pseudoallergic reaction occurs after the first exposure to the NSAID, which makes prior sensitization impossible. Aspirin and other NSAIDs that are more specific for COX-1 than COX-2 (see Fig. 68-2) can induce rhinorrhea, bronchospasm, and laryngospasm in patients with a prior history of sinusitis and asthma. Cross-sensitivity of aspirin and other relatively COX-1–specific NSAIDs with newer COX-2–selective antagonists does not occur. This is further evidence that COX-1 inhibition is the inciting event in aspirin-induced respiratory symptoms.

Some patients display a true allergy to a specific NSAID, with prior exposure leading to the formation of immunoglobulin E (IgE) antibodies. On subsequent exposure, they experience symptoms, including urticaria, angioedema, and anaphylaxis. Assays for specific drug haptens have not been developed, and IgE antibodies are rarely found in the blood of these patients. Therefore, the term *anaphylactoid* has been used to describe such reactions. These reactions are caused by a specific NSAID, and patients are able to take other NSAIDs without difficulty.

Risk Assessment and Implications

GASTROINTESTINAL INJURY

Dyspepsia is not a reliable means of assessing GI mucosal damage. Ten percent to 20% of patients on NSAID therapy complain of dyspepsia, yet 50% of endoscopic findings show normal GI mucosa. Most patients do not complain of GI symptoms until they develop a life-threatening upper GI bleed. Risk factors for the development of ulcers include advanced

age (older than 65 years), renal or hepatic impairment, prior history of ulcers, smoking, alcohol use, concomitant use of oral corticosteroids or anticoagulants, high doses of NSAIDs, and prolonged duration of therapy.

Since recognition of the two isoforms of cyclooxygenase, the COX-1 enzyme has been identified as the one responsible for the formation of gastric prostaglandin E_1, and nonselective NSAIDs have been implicated in a higher risk of GI complications. It is important to understand the relative selectivity of the NSAIDs for COX isoforms, because this may influence the decision of which drug to choose for a patient. For example, etodolac, meloxicam, and nabumetone have a relatively higher affinity for COX-2 than for COX-1 (see Fig. 68-2) and have a safer profile with respect to GI toxicity.

The Celecoxib Long-Term Arthritis Safety Study (CLASS) was a 6-month randomized, double-blind, controlled trial comparing the GI toxicity of celecoxib (400 mg twice a day) with that of more traditional NSAIDs (diclofenac 75 mg twice a day; ibuprofen 800 mg three times a day). The primary end point was ulcer-related complications (gastric perforation, gastric outlet syndrome, GI bleeding), and the secondary end point was symptomatic ulcers. Although there appeared to be a difference in symptomatic and complicated ulcers, this was not statistically significant. Two confounding factors in the study were the supratherapeutic doses of celecoxib used and the inclusion of 21% of patients on low-dose aspirin for cardiovascular prophylaxis. Aspirin is known to increase the risk of upper GI hemorrhage. The ulcer complication rate among the nonaspirin users who took celecoxib was similar to that of the general population, but because there was no placebo group, it was difficult to assess the risk of ulcers with celecoxib. However, we were able to ascertain that patients tolerate celecoxib better than diclofenac and ibuprofen, with less decline in hematocrit, a reduced incidence of dyspepsia, and fewer required endoscopies.

The Vioxx Gastrointestinal Outcomes Research (VIGOR) was a 12-month trial performed to compare the GI toxicity of rofecoxib (Vioxx)[1] 50 mg daily to the more traditional NSAID naproxen 500 mg twice a day. The primary end point was confirmed clinical upper GI events, including symptomatic gastroduodenal ulcers, perforation, or obstruction or upper GI bleeding. The secondary end point was complicated GI events causing severe patient compromise. Results showed a statistically significant reduction in GI events with rofecoxib compared with naproxen. The reduced incidence of GI toxicity with rofecoxib was even present in patients with risk factors for GI events, including advanced age, corticosteroid use, prior history of GI perforation or obstruction, and *H. pylori* infection. This was the first study to demonstrate a definitive benefit with the use of a selective COX-2 inhibitor.

THROMBOGENICITY

COX-2–selective antagonists preferentially block the formation of prostacyclin, with little effect on thromboxane production. Thus, there is a theoretical concern about an increased risk

---

[1]Rofecoxib (Vioxx) was voluntarily withdrawn from the market by its manufacturer (Merck) on September 30, 2004, owing to an increased risk of coronary events.

of thrombosis.[2] This may be especially true among elderly patients, who are at higher risk of atherosclerotic disease.

In the CLASS study, there was no notable difference in cardiovascular events among patients taking celecoxib compared with diclofenac or ibuprofen. In the VIGOR study, there was a statistically significant increase in major cardiovascular events among patients taking rofecoxib versus naproxen. However, in my view, this is not necessarily indicative of a higher cardiovascular risk for patients taking rofecoxib: 27% of patients from the celecoxib study group and 100% of patients from the rofecoxib study group had rheumatoid arthritis, which increases the risk of cardiovascular events. Further, 21% of patients in the celecoxib study were on low-dose aspirin for cardiovascular prophylaxis; low-dose aspirin was an exclusion criterion in the rofecoxib study.

RENAL INJURY

Patients with the greatest risk of developing renal insufficiency due to the inhibition of renal prostaglandins are the elderly and those with renal or liver disease, hypertension, some degree of cardiovascular compromise, congestive heart failure, or hypovolemia. It has been noted that COX-2 is also produced in the kidney, so both nonselective and selective inhibition of COX-2 can lead to edema formation.

Celecoxib has been evaluated for its ability to impair renal function—specifically, nephrotic syndrome, interstitial nephritis, increased serum creatinine levels, and papillary necrosis. Celecoxib seems to cause less renal impairment compared with nonselective COX inhibitors, but this has not been tested rigorously. Therefore, at least for now, selective COX-2 inhibitors must be used with caution in patients with preexisting renal disease, just as with traditional NSAIDs.

ALLERGIC REACTIONS

There have been rare reported cases of aseptic meningitis in patients with arthritis who were treated for months with specific NSAIDs. In these cases, the aseptic meningitis is thought to be an immune reaction to the NSAID. IgG and immune complexes have been found in the cerebrospinal fluid of patients with aseptic meningitis. This has not been reported with aspirin. There have also been rare reports of cough, fever, pulmonary infiltrates, and eosinophilia after exposure to multiple NSAIDs, except aspirin. Such allergic alveolitis or hypersensitivity pneumonitis is also thought to be mediated by an immune reaction, because interstitial lymphocytes and eosinophils were found in lung biopsies taken from these patients. This could be either an IgE-mediated reaction or delayed hypersensitivity.

MANAGEMENT

Gastrointestinal Toxicity

About 15,000 people die each year as a result of major GI complications from NSAIDs, including hemorrhage, perforation, and obstruction. NSAID-induced ulcers heal spontaneously, but slowly, once the NSAID is discontinued; antisecretory therapy accelerates ulcer healing. Althoughe H_2-antagonists are inexpensive, proton pump inhibitors are generally preferred. They cause more rapid ulcer healing and early symptomatic relief. If patients continue to take NSAIDs while on ulcer therapy with an H_2-antagonist (e.g., ranitidine 150 mg twice a day) or proton pump inhibitor (e.g., omeprazole 20 mg daily), there is a high rate of ulcer recurrence. Surgery is reserved for patients who present with severe GI hemorrhage or perforation.

Allergic Reactions

Aspirin desensitization has been successfully undertaken, with patients receiving aspirin 650 mg twice a day for up to 2 weeks. Urine leukotrienes have been followed, with a significant decrease noted after desensitization. Such desensitization may be especially beneficial for older patients with cardiovascular disease who need to be on long-term aspirin therapy.

PREVENTION

Peptic Ulcers

Misoprostol, a prostaglandin E_1 analogue, decreases the risk of gastric and duodenal ulcers. H_2-antagonists and proton pump inhibitors are used to reduce the incidence of duodenal ulcers and gastric ulcers, respectively. For patients at high risk of developing GI complications, a selective COX-2 antagonist is preferred.

Thrombogenicity

If patients are taking traditional NSAIDs and COX-2–selective antagonists, those at risk for cardiovascular events should be on low-dose aspirin. Because the traditional NSAIDs and aspirin inhibit COX-1, there may be competitive antagonism. There is also the added risk of upper GI bleeding. Thus, for patients taking aspirin, an H_2-antagonist may be the better choice for GI prophylaxis. Omeprazole increases aspirin's rate of absorption. It may rapidly increase salicylate levels, with potential toxic effects.

Renal Toxicity

In general, patients with a serum creatinine level of 2.5 mg/dL or higher should not be started on conventional NSAID therapy. Those on antihypertensive therapy need to have their blood pressure closely monitored during the initiation of NSAID therapy. Patients at risk of developing congestive heart failure should also be closely monitored while on NSAID therapy.

Further Reading

Boyce EG, Takiya L: Nonsteroidal anti-inflammatory drugs: Review of factors guiding formulary selection. Formulary 35:142-168, 2000.
Buttgereit F, Burmester GR, Lee LS: Gastrointestinal toxic side effects of nonsteroidal anti-inflammatory drugs and cyclooxygenase-2-specific inhibitors. Am J Med 110(Suppl 3A):13S-19S, 2001.

---

[2]See footnote 1 and Topol EJ: Failing the public health—rofecoxib, Merck, and the FDA. N Engl J Med 351:1707-1709, 2004; and Fitzgerald GA: Coxibs and cardiovascular disease. N Engl J Med 351:1709-1711, 2004.

Catella-Lawson F, Crofford LJ: Cyclooxgenase inhibition and thrombogenicity. Am J Med 110(Suppl 3A):28S-32S, 2001.

Frishman WH: Effects of nonsteroidal anti-inflammatory drug therapy on blood pressure and peripheral edema. Am J Card 89:18D-25D, 2002.

Oviedo JA, Wolfe MM: Gastroprotection by coxibs: What do the Celecoxib Long-Term Arthritis Safety Study and the Vioxx Gastrointestinal Outcomes Research Trial tell us? Rheum Dis Clin North Am 29:769-788, 2003.

Shiotani A, Graham DY: Pathogenesis and therapy of gastric and duodenal ulcer disease. Med Clin North Am 86:1447-1466, 2002.

Stevenson DD: Anaphylactic and anaphylactoid reactions to aspirin and other nonsteroidal anti-inflammatory drugs. Immunol Allergy Clin North Am 21:745-768, 2001.

Stevenson DD: Aspirin and NSAID sensitivity. Immunol Allergy Clin North Am 24:491-503, 2004.

Whelton A: Renal aspects of treatment with conventional nonsteroidal anti-inflammatory drugs versus cyclooxygenase-2-specific inhibitors. Am J Med 110(Suppl 3A):33S-42S, 2001.

REGIONAL ANESTHESIA & PAIN MANAGMENT

Opioid Tolerance

William S. Blau

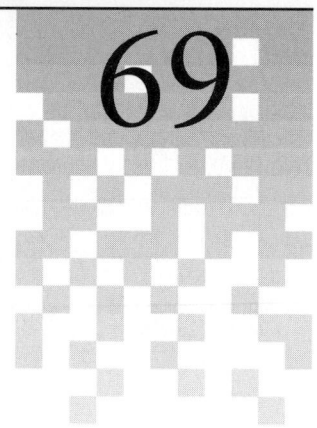

69

Case Synopsis

A 32-year-old woman with ovarian carcinoma, chronic cancer-related pain, and a previous history of intravenous drug abuse presents with small bowel obstruction and is posted for an emergency laparotomy. Her current medications include continuous-release morphine and an oxycodone-acetaminophen preparation that she takes for breakthrough pain (8 to 12 pills daily).

PROBLEM ANALYSIS

Definition

Tolerance occurs when increasing doses of a substance are required to sustain a given effect. It may develop within 1 to 2 weeks after initiating opioid therapy, although recent evidence suggests that its onset may be faster, especially with potent, ultra-short-acting opioids such as remifentanil. The degree of tolerance depends on the magnitude and duration of exposure. Variable degrees of cross-tolerance occur between different opioids and different routes of administration (e.g., systemic versus epidural). It is important to distinguish tolerance (a predictable, involuntary physiologic response to drug exposure) from the related phenomena of physical dependence, addiction, and pseudoaddiction (Table 69-1).

Recognition

Tolerance should be suspected when a patient requires greater than the usual dose of analgesic or fails to obtain appropriate relief at the usual dose. Any patient receiving opioid medications for 2 weeks or more can be presumed to have some degree of tolerance, related to the dose of opioid medication. Some patients who present for surgery may have developed opioid tolerance from prolonged therapy for chronic or cancer-related pain or from prior substance abuse. Tolerance is often not readily detectable from the preoperative history in drug abusers. Suspicion should be raised in patients who report multiple "allergies" to opioid medications, express a preference for specific medications, or are known to abuse alcohol or other substances. Prior medical records or history from family members may provide further evidence. In some cases, an unexpectedly high intraoperative or postoperative opioid requirement may be the first indication of prior exposure; however, it is important to recognize that there is a wide range of interindividual variability in opioid requirements, even among patients who are opioid naïve.

Risk Assessment

Any patient with prolonged hospitalization, multiple surgeries, or history of chronic or cancer pain is at risk and should be carefully assessed for the possibility of tolerance. The lifetime prevalence of nonalcohol drug addiction ranges from 5% to 6%. There is probably a higher prevalence of chemical dependency among hospitalized individuals with acute pain problems caused by medical illnesses, trauma, or surgical procedures than among the general population. As many as half of acute trauma victims use drugs or alcohol before injury and may be habitual users. Patients receiving daily methadone or buprenorphine for chemical dependency should be assumed to have significant tolerance and cross-tolerance to other opioids as well.

Implications

Patients with opioid tolerance are difficult to assess and are at risk for inadequate postoperative pain control. These patients require higher than customary doses of opioids,

Table 69–1 ■ Definition of Terms

Term	Definition
Tolerance	Phenomenon whereby exposure to a drug results in diminution of effect or the need for a higher dose to maintain that effect
Physical dependence	Physiologic phenomenon characterized by the development of an abstinence syndrome following abrupt discontinuation of therapy, substantial dose reduction, or administration of an antagonist drug
Addiction	Psychological and behavioral syndrome characterized by (1) intense desire for a drug and overwhelming concern about its continued availability; (2) evidence of compulsive drug use; or (3) evidence of one or more associated behaviors, including manipulation of the treating physician or medical system for the purpose of obtaining additional drugs, acquisition of drugs from other medical or nonmedical sources, drug hoarding or sale, or unapproved use of other drugs during opioid therapy
Pseudoaddiction	Iatrogenic syndrome of abnormal behavioral symptoms, mimicking those of addiction, that is a direct consequence of inadequate pain management

yet many physicians are inclined to undermedicate. As patients become more vocal about their needs, hospital staff may react negatively or even punitively, ultimately leading to the syndrome of pseudoaddiction. The risk of side effects from pain therapy, such as oversedation or respiratory depression, is also increased in patients with opioid tolerance.

Many opioid-tolerant patients also exhibit physical dependence and are at risk of experiencing withdrawal during the postoperative period, especially when surgery eliminates the source of chronic pain and opioids are rapidly tapered or discontinued. Symptoms generally begin 8 to 12 hours after the last dose of an intermediate-acting opioid and may be difficult to distinguish from those of undertreated pain (e.g., hypertension, tachycardia, abdominal pain).

MANAGEMENT

General Considerations

Effective management of a patient with opioid tolerance begins with the preoperative assessment. The possibility of tolerance should be identified and anticipated, based on the patient's history. Particular attention should be paid to preexisting sites and intensity of pain, baseline functional limitations, and the success of previous pain therapies. It is essential to establish a good therapeutic relationship with the patient as early as possible. Make the patient a partner in developing the analgesic plan, provide reassurance that every effort will be made to provide adequate pain control, but be direct and honest about the limitations of therapy. Patients can help establish realistic goals for pain and activity; for example, obtaining a score of 3 out of 10 after surgery may be unrealistic if the baseline score at home is 7 out of 10. Reassure the patient that his or her reporting of postoperative pain will be taken seriously but will also be corroborated by objective data whenever possible (e.g., quality of sleep; ability to cough, move, and participate in therapy). Involvement of family members may be helpful. Seek preoperative consultation from a pain specialist, as necessary. The patient's preferences and requests for particular analgesics should be honored to the extent allowable by institutional policy and principles of safe pharmacologic practice. Plans and goals should be clearly communicated to the anesthesia team, postanesthesia care unit staff, and postoperative ward.

The overriding principle of acute pain management for patients with opioid tolerance is to titrate analgesic therapy to effect, while anticipating the need for higher than usual doses. Frequent assessment, intervention, and reassessment are required. These patients are at increased risk for anxiety or sedation, and special arrangements may be necessary for postoperative monitoring of respiration and level of consciousness. Whenever possible, the cause or mechanism of pain should be identified and treated primarily. A multimodal approach should be taken, and the pain management plan should be initiated as early as possible. In some cases, preoperative intervention may have preemptive effects. Pharmacologic therapy for symptom control should be based on sound pharmacologic principles. Trials of alternative opioids or routes of delivery should be considered, owing to the possibility of incomplete cross-tolerance. Additional alternative therapies include nonopioid analgesics or adjuncts, regional analgesia, and nonpharmacologic interventions (e.g., transcutaneous electrical nerve stimulation, relaxation, heat or cold, massage, distraction). Every effort should be made to avoid the discontinuation of routine daily psychotropic medications that may promote psychological coping mechanisms.

Medications

For patients receiving chronic opioids preoperatively, the daily baseline medication dose or analgesic equivalent should be continued throughout the perioperative period. In many cases, this may need to be administered parenterally and can often be incorporated into a basal infusion as part of a patient-controlled analgesia (PCA) prescription. For patients in substance abuse maintenance programs, continuation of the baseline methadone or buprenorphine dose is equally important. Also, avoid substituting medications if at all possible. On the day of surgery, the usual oral dose can be administered in the morning, with the remainder of the daily requirement titrated intravenously intraoperatively and after surgery. Additional intraoperative dosing above baseline requirements should be expected; double doses or greater of morphine, methadone, hydromorphone, or fentanyl may be required. It may be helpful to allow muscle relaxation to wear off near the end of general anesthesia and titrate additional opioid to a mild slowing of the spontaneous respiratory rate.

Postoperatively, avoid administering analgesic medications solely on an as-needed basis. Intravenous PCA therapy is often appropriate and effective, even in a patient with a history of drug abuse. A loading dose should be provided and titrated to the level of pain so that the patient starts from a position of adequate pain control. If the patient is able to continue oral medications, PCA bolus dosing can be added, in combination with the baseline oral opioid dose. Otherwise, the total daily opioid dose can be converted to the intravenous morphine, hydromorphone, or fentanyl equivalent using standard conversion tables (Table 69-2) and provided as a basal infusion over 24 hours. Bolus dosing requirements

Table 69–2 ■ Equianalgesic Opioid Conversion*

Drug	Oral Equivalent (mg)	Parenteral Equivalent (mg)
Morphine	60 (acute)	10
	30 (chronic)	10
Methadone (Dolophine)	†	†
Fentanyl (Duragesic)	—	0.125
Hydromorphone (Dilaudid)	7.5	1.5
Codeine	180-200	130
Hydrocodone (Lorcet, Vicodin)	15	—
Oxycodone (Percocet, Tylox)	15	—

*Based on single-dose studies only.
†Conversions to and from methadone are unpredictable; they vary among patients and with the overall magnitude of opioid dose. However, acutely, the parenteral equivalent for methadone is the same as morphine (10 mg).

1.5 to 3 times greater than those of opioid-naïve patients should be anticipated, correlating with the magnitude of the preoperative dose, intraoperative opioid requirements, and titrated loading dose. It should also be anticipated that the duration of therapy for acute or postoperative pain will be longer than for opioid-naïve patients.

Most opioids have no specific toxicity, so there is no upper limit to dose titration. However, the agonist-antagonists and partial agonists, such as butorphanol and buprenorphine, exhibit an analgesic ceiling that limits dose titration and may precipitate withdrawal in patients with physical dependence. Meperidine and propoxyphene have active metabolites that may cause central nervous system toxicity, especially in the setting of impaired renal function. Combination drugs (e.g., oxycodone with acetaminophen) are relatively contraindicated because of the risk of acetaminophen or aspirin toxicity. Morphine alone and at extremely high doses, especially when delivered intrathecally, can rarely produce a state of paradoxical pain, which may be related to metabolite accumulation.

Morphine and other opioid agonists are more or less equivalent in terms of clinical efficacy. Nevertheless, converting to an alternative opioid can improve analgesia in some cases, owing to incomplete cross-tolerance. In particular, methadone sometimes provides effective analgesia even at modest doses in the setting of inadequate pain control with high and rapidly escalating doses of morphine. Methadone can be administered at a dose of 20 to 40 mg orally (or half as much parenterally) over 24 hours, with additional breakthrough doses of 1 to 2.5 mg intravenously as often as every 5 to 10 minutes. However, care must be taken to avoid rapid dose escalation with methadone because of its prolonged half-life and variable pharmacokinetics.

In addition to opioids, adjunctive medications should be used for pain. These include nonsteroidal anti-inflammatory drugs, tricyclic antidepressants and anticonvulsants for neuropathic sources of pain, muscle relaxants, and anxiolytics. There is accumulating evidence that some other medications, when administered perioperatively, may have novel analgesic applications that enhance the chance of successful pain modulation. These include gabapentin, clonidine, adenosine, lidocaine, and ketamine. Of these, ketamine has the most evidence supporting an analgesic benefit. It is my practice to infuse ketamine at 0.1 mg/kg per hour intraoperatively, along with the administration of 1 to 2 g magnesium intravenously, to suppress NMDA receptor activation in patients with opioid tolerance.

The pain management plan continues through the hospital discharge process. The 24-hour parenteral opioid dose should be converted to an oral equivalent, with two thirds as the standing dose and one third administered on an as-needed basis. Depending on the severity and persistence of postoperative pain, the patient may be discharged on his or her baseline preoperative analgesic with a provision for breakthrough pain; often, however, upward adjustment of the baseline dose is required, at least temporarily. It is essential to have a clear postdischarge plan, with a responsible physician willing to manage and taper pain medications on an outpatient basis.

Regional Anesthesia

Continuous regional anesthesia techniques can be invaluable in enhancing pain control and avoiding the escalation of opioid doses, but they do not eliminate the need for ongoing administration of baseline analgesic medications in tolerant or dependent patients. Epidural analgesia is an acceptable and useful adjunct. For drug abusers or patients at high risk for opioid withdrawal, it may be advantageous to infuse only local anesthetic through the epidural catheter (e.g., bupivacaine 0.1% to 0.25%) and give the patient systemic analgesics to cover baseline needs.

Drug Abusers

In patients with opioid tolerance due to active drug abuse or addiction, all the previously discussed principles of pain management apply; however, there are some special considerations. The first and foremost goal is satisfactory control of pain. This is not an appropriate time to attempt detoxification or assume a punitive role. It is essential to engage in a frank discussion with the patient preoperatively to (1) reassure him or her that all reasonable efforts will be made to provide satisfactory pain control and (2) set reasonable expectations and clear limits to avoid excessive negotiation about drug choices or doses. Avoid multiple pain managers, and aim for consistency of response rather than negotiation. Drug abuse–related behaviors should not be tolerated; ignore negative behaviors and reward cooperation with therapy. Consider the use of urine toxicologic screens, especially with the occurrence of oversedation or respiratory depression or the suspicion of unsanctioned drug use.

Intravenous PCA is an acceptable technique for pain management. Offering the patient some degree of control, within specified limits, helps reduce negotiation and confrontation with hospital staff. Care must be taken, however, to monitor closely for evidence of tampering with the PCA device. Tapering and discontinuation of pain therapy should proceed according to a predetermined schedule, usually over 3 to 4 weeks. At discharge, clear instructions should be provided, along with a limited supply of pain medication, and only one physician should be responsible for any refills. Aberrant drug-related behaviors should not be tolerated. Some patients may require transfer to a detoxification center rather than discharge to home.

Patients with a remote history of substance abuse do not necessarily require special treatment and can be managed with standard techniques. If the risk of relapse is deemed high, however, efforts should be made to rely minimally on systemic opioid analgesics in favor of other modalities, including single or continuous peripheral nerve blocks or epidural analgesia. Consultation with an addiction specialist should be obtained, and intensification of a formal relapse prevention program should be considered.

PREVENTION

Tolerance is a predictable neurophysiologic response to continued opioid exposure. The possibility of tolerance is not a reason to avoid analgesic therapy if it is indicated. Propensity toward addiction is more a characteristic of the person using the drug than of the drug itself. The risk of creating a drug addiction problem when opioids are part of an analgesia plan for acute pain control is extremely low and is no reason to withhold therapy or to underdose.

Care must be taken to prevent withdrawal after the transition to epidural therapy or during the tapering of therapy as pain resolves. A daily 10% to 50% dose reduction is usually well tolerated. Conversion to methadone before weaning can be helpful because of methadone's longer half-life. The addition of clonidine 6 µg/kg per day, divided in four to six doses, can help prevent many autonomic features of withdrawal; this dose can be increased to 17 µg/kg per day as necessary and tolerated. Once symptoms are suppressed, clonidine can be weaned over several days.

Further Reading

De Kock M, Lavand'homme P, Waterloos H: "Balanced analgesia" in the perioperative period: Is there a place for ketamine? Pain 92:373-380, 2001.

Dirks J, Fredensborg BB, Christensen D, et al: A randomized study of the effects of single-dose gabapentin versus placebo on postoperative pain and morphine consumption after mastectomy. Anesthesiology 97:560-564, 2002.

Doverty M, Somogyii AA, White JM, et al: Methadone maintenance patients are cross-tolerant to the antinociceptive effects of morphine. Pain 93:155-163, 2001.

Fukunaga AF, Alexander GE, Stark CW: Characterization of the analgesia actions of adenosine: Comparison of adenosine and remifentanil infusions in patients undergoing major surgical procedures. Pain 101:129-138, 2003.

Goyagi T, Tanaka M, Nishikawa T: Oral clonidine premedication enhances postoperative analgesia by epidural morphine. Anesth Analg 89: 1487-1497, 1999.

Groudine SB, Fisher HAG, Kaufman RP Jr, et al: Intravenous lidocaine speeds the return of bowel function, decreases postoperative pain, and shortens hospital stay in patients undergoing radical retropubic prostatectomy. Anesth Analg 86:235-259, 1998.

Guignard B, Bossard AE, Coste C, et al: Acute opioid tolerance: Intraoperative remifentanil increases postoperative pain and morphine requirement. Anesthesiology 93:409-417, 2000.

Mitra S, Sinatra RS: Perioperative management of acute pain in the opioid-dependent patient. Anesthesiology 101:212-227, 2004.

Rapp SE, Ready LB, Nessly ML: Acute pain management in patients with prior opioid consumption: A case-controlled retrospective review. Pain 61:195-201, 1995.

Steindler EM: ASAM addiction terminology. In Graham AW, Schultz TK (eds): Principles of Addiction Medicine, 2nd ed. Chevy Chase, Md, American Society of Addiction Medicine, 1998, pp 1301-1304.

Weissman DE, Haddox JD: Opioid pseudoaddiction: An iatrogenic syndrome. Pain 36:363-366, 1989.

REGIONAL ANESTHESIA & PAIN MANAGEMENT

Continuous Nerve Blocks: Perineural Local Anesthetic Infusion

70

Stuart Grant

Case Synopsis

A 62-year-old man undergoing unilateral total knee arthroplasty has lumbar plexus and sciatic nerve perineural catheters placed for surgical anesthesia and postoperative analgesia. He receives ropivacaine 0.2% by patient-controlled infusion through the lumbar plexus catheter and ropivacaine 0.2% as a continuous infusion via the sciatic nerve catheter. In the recovery room he is pain free, but during the first postoperative night he complains of pain. This is managed using bolus 0.5% ropivacaine, but the next day, the physical therapist and surgeon complain because of the profound motor block.

PROBLEM ANALYSIS

Definition

Numerous studies have shown that perineural local anesthetic infusions provide profound analgesia. These techniques have been used to provide both intraoperative anesthesia and postoperative analgesia. Certain complications are block specific, such as a pneumothorax with classic (non-"plumb-bob") supraclavicular or infraclavicular blocks or epidural spread with a lumbar plexus block. This chapter does not discuss block-specific complications; rather, the focus is on those complications that can occur using continuous perineural local anesthetic infusions at any insertion site. A variety of complications have been reported, including the following:

- Insertion difficulty or inability to insert a catheter, leading to block failure
- Local anesthetic toxicity
- Catheter migration into a vessel
- Retained catheter fragments
- Infectious complications
- Neurologic complications
- Prolonged motor block
- Pain during injection or infusion via the perineural catheter

Recognition

The clinical features of local anesthetic toxicity are discussed in Chapter 56. The clinical features of infectious complications include the following:

- Late onset of symptoms, 2 to 3 days after peripheral nerve catheter placement
- Tissue erythema and swelling at catheter insertion site
- Leukocytosis and fever
- Pain and tenderness at catheter insertion site

The clinical features of neurologic complications include the following:

- Prolonged motor block long after cessation of local anesthetic infusion
- Reduced touch or paresthesias that persist or worsen after cessation of infusion
- Pain that is neuropathic in nature

The clinical features of motor block and inadequate analgesia include the following:

- Numbness and perception of a heavy or weak extremity
- Loss of proprioception
- Increasing or high patient-reported pain score
- Increased opioid-related side effects

Risk Assessment

The incidence of complications following peripheral nerve block is low and must be balanced against the risks of general anesthesia and central neuraxial techniques. Auroy and coworkers reported the incidence of serious complications related to regional anesthesia in a prospective study using data from 103,730 cases. The incidence of cardiac arrest and neurologic injury related to regional anesthesia was low, but both complications were more than three standard deviations greater after spinal anesthesia than after other regional procedures. These data did not discriminate between single-injection and continuous peripheral nerve block techniques, but peripheral nerve blocks in general were associated with fewer neurologic injuries and cardiac arrests than were central neuraxial techniques.

Bergman and coworkers retrospectively examined the neurologic complications after 405 consecutive continuous axillary nerve block catheter procedures. They found no greater incidence of neurologic complications using continuous catheter techniques than using single injections for axillary nerve block. Borgeat and colleagues prospectively examined complications associated with interscalene block and shoulder surgery and found no differences between catheter techniques and single-injection blocks.

Leaving a catheter in situ entails the potential risk of infection and catheter migration into a vessel. This risk must be balanced against the improved analgesia. Although Cuvillon and coworkers were able to isolate bacterial colonization in 57% of 208 femoral nerve catheters, no clinically relevant infectious complications occurred. There was one case (0.1% incidence) of a serious infection (abscess), and superficial erythema was observed in 0.7% of the patients in Borgeat's series (cited earlier). Only superficial skin infections (5% incidence) were reported in the recent series by Boezaart and associates. Only one case report of migration into a vessel has been reported in the literature, so the incidence of that complication is unknown.

After resolution of the primary block with long-acting amide local anesthetics, inadvertent catheter dislodgment or incorrect initial catheter positioning is the most common cause of pain 12 hours or more after the initial block. This can occur in up to 10% to 20% of patients and is by far the most common complication of continuous perinural nerve blocks. Some patients with infusions of low concentrations of local anesthetics in a functional perineural catheter suffer breakthrough pain. Use of a patient-controlled bolus, in addition to the background basal infusion, can reduce the severity of breakthrough pain. As the case synopsis illustrates, the challenge for the clinician is to balance the risk of motor block or even local anesthetic toxicity against the patient's discomfort from inadequately controlled pain.

Implications

Infection can result in discomfort and limitation of activity. Neurologic complications can result in weakness and chronic pain, with reduced functional capacity after surgery. Careful technique and patient selection are important factors in reducing these complications. Prolonged motor block produced by high local anesthetic concentrations may delay early ambulation but has not been shown to affect long-term functional outcomes following arthroplasty. In fact, patients given either epidural or peripheral nerve catheters after knee arthroplasty have increased rates of recovery for the first 6 weeks after surgery compared with those on opioid analgesia regimens. Failed blocks result in pain and reduced patient satisfaction. This can lead to increased use of opioid analgesics and opioid-related side effects such as respiratory depression, pruritus, nausea, vomiting, and constipation.

MANAGEMENT

Infection

- Remove the infected catheter.
- Culture the catheter tip and obtain antibiotic sensitivities.
- Commence treatment with a broad-spectrum antibiotic.
- Convert to an appropriate multimodal analgesic regimen.

Neurologic Complications

- Obtain a careful history and complete neurologic examination.

- Refer the patient to a neurologist.
- Consider computed tomography to exclude hematoma (e.g., in the psoas compartment around the lumbar plexus; see Chapter 64).
- Perform early electromyography (EMG) to document any preexisting neurologic deficit, followed by late EMG to identify any perioperative nerve injury.
- Consider commencing gabapentin (Neurontin), especially in patients with symptoms of neuropathic pain.

Pain

Pain should be assessed using the patient-reported analog scale. Peripheral nerve catheter techniques should be part of any balanced analgesic regimen. Use of nonsteroidal anti-inflammatory agents and COX-2 enzyme inhibitors should be considered in all cases, unless contraindicated. The postoperative management of peripheral nerve catheters for pain control includes the following:
- Postoperative pain assessment
- Clinical examination for evidence of nerve block

PREVENTION

Infectious complications can be reduced by the use of appropriate skin preparations. Chlorhexidine is more effective than iodine-based preparations in this regard. Care must be taken to ensure that the chlorhexidine has dried before needle insertion, because of the potential for neurotoxicity. Additionally, the choice of catheter insertion site is important. For example, a femoral nerve catheter placed in an obese patient with a large pannus is more likely to become infected. Surgeons fully appreciate that best medical practice supports the use of prophylactic antibiotics whenever foreign material is being inserted. The perineural nerve catheter is a foreign material, and if the surgical team prescribes prophylactic antibiotics, it makes sense to start these before peripheral nerve catheter insertion. If the surgeon does not prescribe antibiotics for the patient, the anesthesiologist may want to consider prescribing them for prophylaxis of perineural catheter infection.

Evidence regarding the prevention of neurologic perineural catheter complications is scant, but by performing blocks in lightly sedated patients, minimizing pressure when injecting local anesthetics, and stopping injections immediately when pain is experienced, a practitioner may be able to reduce the likelihood of nerve injury. The use of blunt versus sharp needles is often debated in the literature, as is the technique of eliciting paresthesia versus the use of a nerve stimulator.

The likelihood of motor block can be reduced by using lower concentrations of drug in perineural local anesthetic infusions. There is also evidence of better sensory versus differential motor blockade with ropivacaine than bupivacaine. Careful attention to the details of catheter fixation at the time of insertion, use of bolus local anesthetic via the catheter for breakthrough pain, and use of a patient-controlled regional anesthesia catheter can help reduce the likelihood of postoperative pain.

Further Reading

Auroy Y, Narchi P, Messiah A, et al: Serious complications related to regional anesthesia: Results of a prospective survey in France. Anesthesiology 87:479-486, 1997.

Bergman BD, Hebl JR, Kent J, Horlocker TT: Neurologic complications of 405 consecutive continuous axillary catheters. Anesth Analg 96:247-252, 2003.

Boezaart AP, De Beer JF, Nell ML: Early experience with continuous cervical paravertebral block using a stimulating catheter. Reg Anesth Pain Med 28:406-413, 2003.

Borgeat A, Dullenkopf A, Ekatodramis G, Nagy L: Evaluation of the lateral modified approach for continuous interscalene block after shoulder surgery. Anesthesiology 99:436-442, 2003.

Borgeat A, Kalberer F, Jacob H, et al: Patient-controlled interscalene analgesia with ropivacaine 0.2% versus bupivacaine 0.15% after major open shoulder surgery: The effects on hand motor function. Anesth Analg 92:218-223, 2001.

Capdevila X, Barthelet Y, Biboulet P, et al: Effects of perioperative analgesic technique on the surgical outcome and duration of rehabilitation after major knee surgery. Anesthesiology 91:8-15, 1999.

Cuvillon P, Ripart J, Lalourcey L, et al: The continuous femoral nerve block catheter for postoperative analgesia: Bacterial colonization, infectious rate and adverse effects. Anesth Analg 93:1045-1049, 2001.

Gillespie WJ, Walenkamp G: Antibiotic prophylaxis for surgery for proximal femoral and other closed long bone fractures. Cochrane Database Syst Rev 2000(2):CD000244, 2000.

Grant SA, Nielsen KC, Greengrass RA, et al: Continuous peripheral nerve block for ambulatory surgery. Reg Anesth Pain Med 26:209-214, 2001.

Tuominen MK, Pere P, Rosenberg PH: Unintentional arterial catheterization and bupivacaine toxicity associated with continuous interscalene brachial plexus block. Anesthesiology 75:356-358, 1991.

Yentur EA, Luleci N, Topcu I, et al: Is skin disinfection with 10% povidone iodine sufficient to prevent epidural needle and catheter contamination? Reg Anesth Pain Med 28:389-393, 2003.

Persistent Paresthesia

71

Terese T. Horlocker

Case Synopsis

A 58-year-old woman with insulin-dependent diabetes mellitus is scheduled to undergo total wrist arthroplasty. An axillary block is performed with the transaxillary technique using 45 mL of 1.5% mepivacaine containing 5 µg/mL of epinephrine. Total tourniquet time is 130 minutes. After surgery, the patient has residual numbness in her fourth and fifth fingers. Electromyography performed at 8 weeks demonstrates a diffuse sensori-motor neuropathy and an ulnar neuropathy at the level of the axilla. The symptoms slowly and completely resolve over a period of 10 weeks.

PROBLEM ANALYSIS

Definition

Perioperative nerve injuries have long been recognized as a complication of regional anesthesia. Fortunately, severe or disabling neurologic complications rarely occur. Cheney and coworkers examined the American Society of Anesthesiologists' closed claims database to determine the role of nerve damage in malpractice claims filed against anesthesia care providers. Of the 4183 claims reviewed, 670 (16%) were for anesthesia-related nerve injury. The most frequent sites of injury were the ulnar nerve (190 claims), brachial plexus (137 claims), lumbosacral roots (105 claims), and spinal cord (84 claims). Upper extremity nerve injuries were more often associated with general anesthesia. However, spinal cord and lumbosacral nerve root injuries having identifiable causes were associated predominantly with regional anesthetic techniques and were related to paresthesias during needle or catheter placement or pain during injection of local anesthetic. It is also notable that despite intensive medicolegal investigation, a definite mechanism of injury is rarely determined. The lack of an apparent mechanism often leads the patient (and consulting specialists) to assume that something must have been done incorrectly during the perioperative period to cause the nerve injury.

This review demonstrates that although perioperative nerve injury is a significant source of anesthesia-related claims, the exact mechanism of injury is often unclear. The potential risk of nerve injury due to needle trauma, local anesthetic toxicity, or neural ischemia during regional anesthetic techniques increases the probability that neurologic deficits will be attributed to anesthetic agents. However, several series have demonstrated that neurologic deficits are more likely to be associated with a cause that is unrelated to regional anesthesia. For example, Horlocker and colleagues reported 61 nerve injuries after 1614 upper extremity surgical procedures performed under axillary block, for a 3.8% overall frequency of neural dysfunction. Only 7 of the 61 injuries (11%) were the result of the anesthetic; the remaining 54 (89%) were related to surgical factors. The anesthesiologist must therefore be aware of the surgical, medical, and anesthetic risk factors associated with perioperative nerve injuries to reduce the incidence of neurologic complications.

Recognition

Neurologic complications associated with regional anesthesia can be divided into two broad categories: those that are unrelated to the regional anesthetic but coincide temporally, and those that are the direct result of the regional anesthetic agent or technique.

Causes of nerve injury unrelated to the regional anesthetic agent or technique include the following:

- Surgical trauma
- Surgical retractor
- Patient positioning
- Tourniquet ischemia
- Improperly placed dressings or casts
- Preexisting neurologic diseases

Causes of nerve injury directly related to the regional anesthetic agent or technique include the following:

- Direct or indirect needle or catheter trauma
- Neural ischemia
- Local anesthetic neurotoxicity
- Infection

Risk Assessment

Trauma, ischemia, infection, and local anesthetic neurotoxicity contribute to the development of neurologic complications after peripheral neural block. Patient and anesthetic factors that may be associated with an increased risk of neurologic complications after regional anesthetic agents or techniques include the following:

- Preexisting neurologic disorder or diagnosis
- Needle bevel and configuration
- Local anesthetic (drug and concentration)
- Use of vasoconstrictors

The elicitation of a paresthesia while performing an axillary block may represent direct needle-induced trauma and increased risk of persistent paresthesia associated with regional anesthesia. Selander and coworkers reported a 2.8% incidence of postoperative nerve injury in patients in whom paresthesia was sought during axillary block, compared with a 0.8% incidence in those undergoing a perivascular technique (the difference was not statistically significant, however).

The neurologic deficits ranged from slight hypersensitivity to severe paresis and persisted from 2 weeks to more than 1 year. Theoretically, using a nerve stimulator to localize neural structures should allow a high success rate without increasing the risk of neurologic complications, but this hypothesis has not been formally tested. Fanelli and colleagues prospectively evaluated 3996 patients undergoing sciatic-femoral, axillary, and interscalene blocks using multiple-injection and nerve stimulator techniques. During the first month after surgery, 69 patients (1.7%) developed neurologic dysfunction; recovery was complete in all but 1 patient by 4 to 12 weeks. (This frequency and outcome are similar to those reported using a paresthesia technique.)

Direct needle trauma also may cause disturbances in nerve conduction without clinical evidence of a neuropathy. After sciatic nerve impalement with an axillary block needle in rats, histologic changes consistent with axonal injury persisted for 28 days. However, clinical evidence of hind leg hyposensitivity was present for only 2 weeks. Similar findings have been reported after sciatic nerve penetration with a microneurographic electrode in rats. These data suggest that a subclinical neuropathy may occur with greater frequency and longer duration than anticipated. Needle gauge, type (short versus long bevel), and bevel configuration may also influence the degree of nerve injury, although evidence from animal models is unclear, and there are no relevant human studies.

The passage into and presence of an indwelling catheter in a peripheral nerve sheath represent an additional source of direct trauma. Although difficulty during catheter insertion may lead to vessel puncture, tissue trauma, and bleeding, significant complications are uncommon, and permanent sequelae are rare. The largest series of continuous brachial plexus blocks with indwelling catheters included only 405 patients. Bergman and coworkers reported nine complications in eight patients, for an overall frequency of 2.2%, including one each of the following: localized infection (treated with catheter removal and antibiotics), axillary hematoma, and retained catheter fragment requiring surgical excision. Two patients reported signs and symptoms of systemic local anesthetic toxicity manifesting as preseizure activity. Four patients (1%) reported new neurologic deficits postoperatively, only two of which were anesthesia related.

Peripheral nerves have a dual blood supply consisting of intrinsic endoneural vessels and extrinsic epineural vessels. A reduction in or disruption of nerve blood flow may result in neural ischemia. Intraneuronal injection of volumes as small as 50 to 100 μL may generate intraneuronal pressures that exceed capillary perfusion pressure for as long as 10 minutes, thus causing neural ischemia. Endoneural hematomas have also been reported after intraneuronal injection. Epineural blood flow is responsive to adrenergic stimuli. Theoretically, the use of local anesthetic solutions containing epinephrine can produce local nerve ischemia, especially in patients with microvascular disease; however, the actual risk of significant neurologic ischemia in patients given local anesthetic solutions containing vasoconstrictors is unknown.

Neurologic complications after regional block may be a direct result of local anesthetic toxicity. There is both laboratory and clinical evidence that local anesthetic solutions are potentially neurotoxic. Differences in neurotoxicity are dependent on pKa, lipid solubility, protein binding, and potency.

In histopathologic, electrophysiologic, and neuronal cell models, lidocaine and tetracaine appear to have a greater potential for neurotoxicity than does bupivacaine at clinically relevant concentrations. Additives such as epinephrine and bicarbonate may also affect neurotoxicity.

Patients with microangiopathic processes, such as diabetes, demonstrate a reduction in neural blood flow and local anesthetic uptake. Concurrently, the presence of a peripheral neuropathy reduces the amount of local anesthetic required to produce neural block and toxicity. Therefore, these patients are more sensitive to the clinical effects of local anesthetic solutions. The concentration of local anesthetic selected, as well as the use of vasoconstrictors, must be carefully evaluated in patients with peripheral neuropathies, because prolonged exposure to or high concentrations of local anesthetic solutions within the neurovascular compartment may result in permanent neurologic deficits.

The presence of a preexisting neurologic condition may predispose a nerve to injury by the neurotoxic effects of local anesthetics. The presumed mechanism is a "double crush" of the nerve at two locations, resulting in a nerve injury of clinical significance. The double-crush concept suggests that nerve damage caused by traumatic needle placement, local anesthetic toxicity, or neural ischemia during the performance of regional anesthesia may worsen neurologic outcome in the presence of an additional patient factor or surgical injury.

Implications

Neurologic deficits that arise within the first 24 hours most likely represent extraneural or intraneural hematoma, intraneural edema, or a lesion involving a sufficient number of nerve fibers to permit immediate diagnosis. However, in many cases of persistent paresthesias after regional anesthesia, the symptoms of nerve injury do not develop until days to weeks later. The presentation of late disturbances in nerve function suggests an alternative cause, such as tissue reaction or scar formation, although it is unknown whether this reaction is due to mechanical trauma, chemical toxicity, or both.

MANAGEMENT

Major complications after regional anesthetic techniques are rare but can be devastating to the patient and the anesthesiologist. Prevention and management begin during the preoperative visit with a careful evaluation of the patient's medical history and a discussion of the risks and benefits of the available anesthetic techniques. Patients with preexisting neurologic disorders such as multiple sclerosis, poliomyelitis, or amyotrophic lateral sclerosis may develop new neurologic deficits perioperatively, and it is often difficult to differentiate between surgical and anesthetic causes. In these patients, if a regional anesthetic is indicated (or requested), the patient's preoperative neurologic examination should be formally documented, and the patient must be made aware of the possible progression of the underlying disease process. Stable preexisting neurologic conditions (e.g., documented peripheral neuropathy, inactive lumbosacral radiculopathy, hemiparesis due to an old cerebrovascular accident) are not contraindications to the use of regional anesthesia. However, the underlying cause of such neurologic deficits requires careful evaluation.

PREVENTION

Preventive measure include all of the following:

- Appropriate patient selection
- Meticulous regional anesthetic technique
- Avoidance of direct needle trauma and intraneuronal injection
- Weighing of the risks and benefits of vasoconstrictors
- Use of appropriate local anesthetic concentrations
- Prompt evaluation of perioperative neuropathies

Meticulous technique must be used during any central neuraxial or peripheral nerve block. Paresthesias elicited during needle or catheter placement or injection of local anesthetic should be documented. Painful paresthesias are associated with nerve injury and should be avoided. The total local anesthetic dose and concentration, as well as the addition of vasoconstrictors, must be carefully considered.

Hadzic and associates recently evaluated the use of peripheral nerve stimulators to identify the nerves to be blocked to achieve regional anesthesia. They found that the nerve stimulators in common use in the United States vary greatly in terms of accuracy of current output and manufacturer-selected electrical characteristics (e.g., current duration, stimulating frequency, maximum voltage output). They also noted that most authors recommend obtaining a motor response with a current of 0.5 mA or less before injecting a local anesthetic, and they suggested that stimulation at currents higher than 0.5 mA may result in failure of the block; this was attributed to the needle being too far from the nerve to be blocked. In contrast, injection after nerve stimulation thresholds of 0.1 mA or less may increase the risk of nerve injury because of the possibility of intra-neuronal local anesthetic injection.

Finally, although postoperative neurologic complications may present immediately after surgery, some require days to weeks to emerge. Should such neurologic dysfunction occur, timely evaluation with a multidisciplinary approach involving neurology, radiology, internal medicine, and surgery will allow appropriate treatment.

Further Reading

Auroy Y, Narchi P, Messiah A, et al: Serious complications related to regional anesthesia: Results of a prospective survey in France. Anesthesiology 87:479-486, 1997.

Bergman BD, Hebl JR, Kent J, Horlocker TT: Neurologic complications of 405 consecutive continuous axillary catheters. Anesth Analg 96: 247-252, 2003.

Cheney FW, Domino KB, Caplan RA, Posner K: Nerve injury associated with anesthesia: A closed claims analysis. Anesthesiology 90: 1062-1069, 1999.

Fanelli G, Casati A, Garancini P, et al: Nerve stimulator and multiple injection technique for upper and lower limb blockade: Failure rate, patient acceptance, and neurologic complications. Anesth Analg 88:847-852, 1999.

Hadzic A, Vloka J, Hadzic N, et al: Nerve stimulators used for peripheral nerve blocks vary in their electrical characteristics. Anesthesiology 98:969-974, 2003.

Horlocker TT, Kufner RP, Bishop AT, et al: The risk of persistent paresthesia is not increased with repeated axillary block. Anesth Analg 88:382-387, 1999.

Kalichman MW, Calcutt NA: Local anesthetic-induced conduction block and nerve fiber injury in streptozotocin-diabetic rats. Anesthesiology 77:941-947, 1992.

Neal JM: Effects of epinephrine in local anesthetics on the central and peripheral nervous systems: Neurotoxicity and neural blood flow. Reg Anesth Pain Med 28:124-134, 2003.

Neal JM, Hebl JR, Gerancher JC, Hogan QH: Brachial plexus anesthesia: Essentials of our current understanding. Reg Anesth Pain Med 27: 402-428, 2002.

Rice ASC, McMahon SB: Peripheral nerve injury caused by injection needles used in regional anaesthesia: Influence of bevel configuration, studied in a rat model. Br J Anaesth 69:433-438, 1992.

Selander D, Dhuner KG, Lundborg G: Peripheral nerve injury due to injection needles used for regional anesthesia. Acta Anaesthesiol Scand 21: 182-188, 1977.

Selander D, Edshage S, Wolff T: Paresthesiae or no paresthesiae? Acta Anaesthesiol Scand 23:27-33, 1979.

Selander D, Sjostrang J: Longitudinal spread of intraneurally injected local anesthetics. Acta Anaesthesiol Scand 22:622-634, 1978.

Stan TC, Krantz MA, Solomon DL, et al: The incidence of neurovascular complications following axillary brachial plexus block using a transarterial approach: A prospective study of 1000 consecutive patients. Reg Anesth 20:486-492, 1995.

REGIONAL ANESTHESIA & PAIN MANAGEMENT

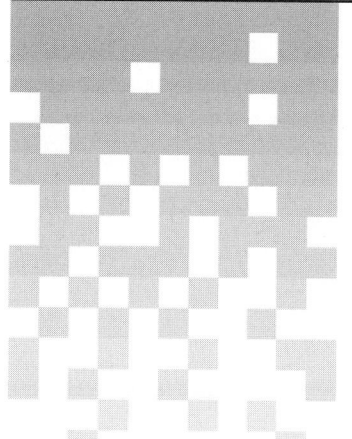

Cardiothoracic and Vascular Surgery

Mark A. Chaney

John Ellis

SECTION 4

Cardiothoracic and Vascular Surgery

Anticoagulation Initiation and Reversal for Cardiac Surgery

72

Peter Tassani-Prell

Case Synopsis

An 81-year-old woman with dyspnea at rest due to aortic stenosis (valve area 0.4 cm^2, mean gradient 50 mm Hg) presents for aortic valve replacement. Past medical history is significant for a recent pulmonary embolism, for which she received intravenous heparin therapy. At the time of operation, antithrombin III (AT-III) levels are low, and the activated partial thromboplastin time is elevated. After heparinization (375 units/kg), the activated clotting time (ACT) increases to 325 seconds. An additional 125 units/kg heparin and 2000 units of AT-III concentrate are given. Thereafter, the ACT increases to 866 seconds, and cardiopulmonary bypass (CPB) is commenced without further complications.

PROBLEM ANALYSIS

Definition

Unfractionated heparin is a heterogeneous mixture of sulfated oligosaccharides with molecular weights ranging from 5000 to 50,000 daltons. The anticoagulant activity of heparin is initiated via binding to AT-III, which results in a conformational change that increases its inactivation of thrombin and factors Xa and IXa. Thus, in the setting of low AT-III activity, the clinical effect of heparin is reduced.

Recognition, Risk Assessment, and Implications

There is wide individual variability in the clinical anticoagulant response to a single dose of heparin. This necessitates evaluation with on-site or laboratory coagulation testing. Owing to the extreme importance of ensuring sufficient anticoagulation before initiating CPB, on-site testing is preferred. A number of options are available to clinically assess heparin-induced anticoagulation.

The activated partial thromboplastin time is sensitive to low plasma heparin concentrations (0.1 to 1.0 units/mL). However, with the high doses of heparin required for the initiation of CPB, values exceed this method's detection limit.

The ACT assesses the clinical anticoagulation effect of the large doses of heparin (200 to 400 units/kg) required for the initiation of CPB. Though somewhat controversial, ACT values between 400 and 600 seconds are generally considered safe for anticoagulation during routine CPB, based on the observation of a lack of fibrin deposits on extracorporeal circuits. Even so, ACT values may be misleading because they can be prolonged by factors other than heparin, such as hypothermia, hemodilution, and thrombocytopenia. Further, clinical investigations have shown that ACT values correlate poorly with plasma heparin concentrations in patients during mild hypothermic CPB. Commercially available ACT measurement devices use two different activators. Celite-activated clotting time is prolonged by aprotinin, which may lead to inadequate heparinization during CPB. Kaolin-activated clotting time is unaffected by aprotinin. If aprotinin is used and only celite ACT testing is available, most clinicians prefer to maintain the ACT at greater than 800 seconds during CPB to ensure adequate heparinization.

Heparin-protamine titration has been proposed as an alternative and more specific method for ensuring adequate heparin levels or protamine reversal in patients during CPB. However, the advantages of heparin-protamine titration (if any) over traditional methods have yet to be proved.

Heparin resistance results in an unanticipated small increase in ACT values after initial and subsequent heparin dosing. Approximately 1 in 2000 patients has a heterozygotic deficiency (40% to 70% activity) of AT-III and is thus predisposed to developing deep vein thrombosis and pulmonary embolism. Significant reductions in AT-III levels may also occur secondary to AT-III consumption during heparin therapy. Other causes of heparin resistance include left ventricular clot, use of oral contraceptives, and thrombocytosis. These entities may be due to reduced plasma concentrations of heparin caused by its increased binding to plasma proteins and endothelium.

Heparin may cause thrombocytopenia via immune- and nonimmune-mediated mechanisms. There are two types of heparin-induced thrombocytopenia (HIT) that can result from heparin use. Type I is nonimmune mediated, and type II is immune mediated. For standardization, the term *non-heparin immune-associated thrombocytopenia* is recommended for type I HIT. This is a benign condition, with no heparin-dependent antibodies present. The term *heparin-induced thrombocytopenia* is recommended for type II HIT, in which heparin-dependent antibodies are detectable and produce thrombocytopenia.

MANAGEMENT

Three different aspects of anticoagulation during cardiac surgery with CPB are discussed: routine management using anticoagulation with heparin and neutralization with protamine, management of AT-III deficiency (as in the case synopsis), and HIT.

For the initiation of CPB, the heparin dose is based on body weight (300 to 400 units/kg, or 3 mg/kg). It is essential to obtain an ACT of about 480 seconds before initiating CPB. Determining the ACT before initiating CPB allows one to detect inadequate heparin dosing or AT-III deficiency. It is also recommended that the heparin injection be given via a central venous line after aspirating blood to ensure central vascular delivery. Patient-specific heparin dosing can be automatically extrapolated by several commercially available heparin monitoring systems.

Subsequent heparin can be dosed empirically during CPB (e.g., 5000 to 10,000 units/hour, one third the initial dose every hour) if the ACT is less than 400 to 480 seconds or if plasma heparin concentration values are appropriate. Some commercial systems also calculate a heparin concentration corresponding to an ACT greater than 480 seconds. Hypothermia and hemodilution prolong ACT values independent of heparin concentration. Thus, basing subsequent heparin doses on ACT values may lead to inadequate inhibition of thrombin activity and subclinical thrombosis, fibrinolysis, and depletion of coagulation factors and platelets. Maintenance of patient-specific heparin concentrations during CPB may result in more accurate heparin dosing, more complete thrombin inhibition, and reduced postoperative bleeding and blood product use.

With suspected heparin resistance, one must first confirm that the heparin was indeed given intravenously, followed by the administration of additional heparin from another vial or lot to exclude lot-specific reduced heparin activity. If the ACT values still remain below those expected, despite large doses of heparin, AT-III concentrates should be given, with an initial dose of at least 2000 units. Because of the danger of AT-III deficiency (thrombosis during CPB), the routine clinical practice in some centers is to confirm adequate AT-III levels in patients before any operation is performed requiring extracorporeal circulation.

Non-heparin immune-associated thrombocytopenia (type I HIT) implies absent heparin-dependent antibodies. This entity is probably caused by direct nonimmune platelet activation by heparin. Type I HIT is usually associated with larger doses of heparin. In contrast, type II HIT can occur with any heparin dose. Further, type I HIT occurs earlier in the clinical treatment course (usually within 4 days) in 30% of patients receiving intravenous heparin therapy. The induced platelet abnormality is usually mild and reversible, even with

continued heparin administration. Type I HIT is self-limited and usually causes no important complications (e.g., thrombosis). Heparin therapy is continued despite low platelet counts. The clinical importance of type I HIT lies in the necessity to differentiate it from the more serious type II HIT.

Type II HIT (or heparin-induced thrombocytopenia with thrombosis [HITT] syndrome) is an immune-mediated reaction to heparin that is often underdiagnosed and may lead to venous and arterial thrombosis. Type II HIT exists as three distinct entities: (1) latent (antibodies without thrombocytopenia), (2) HIT (antibodies with thrombocytopenia), and (3) HITT (antibodies with thrombocytopenia and thrombosis).

Type II HIT is potentially more dangerous than type I HIT because it can be associated with thromboembolic complications (absent in type I). About 0.5% to 3% of patients given heparin develop type II HIT and moderate thrombocytopenia. In some, this leads to venous or arterial thrombosis. Thrombosis frequently leads to disastrous clinical sequelae, including loss of limbs and even death. The basis for this severe adverse drug reaction is production of an immunoglobulin G antibody that reacts with heparin and platelet factor 4 antigenic complexes. The diagnosis of type II HIT is made with the heparin-induced platelet aggregation (HIPA) assay. Alternatively, an enzyme-linked immunosorbent assay (ELISA) can detect the binding of antibodies to immobilized heparin–platelet factor 4 antigenic complexes.

For patients with type II HIT who will be exposed to CPB, treatment generally includes either the use of alternative anticoagulants or combined treatment with platelet function inhibitors and heparin. Examples include the following:

- *Danaproid sodium.* This is a low-molecular-weight heparinoid (i.e., a mixture of dermatan, glycosaminoglycans, and chondroitin sulfates) that does not contain heparin.
- *Ancrod.* This is an inhibitor of fibrin derived from Malayan pit viper venom. It provides a treatment option for patients with type II HIT who require anticoagulation.
- *Hirudin and lepirudin.* This combination is also used for anticoagulation in type II HIT patients. Hirudin is a direct inhibitor of thrombin, acting independently of cofactors such as antithrombin. Lepirudin (a form of recombinant hirudin derived from yeast cells) is a highly specific, direct, irreversible inhibitor of thrombin (one molecule of lepirudin binds with one of thrombin). Typically, patients given hirudin have more perioperative bleeding, require multiple allogeneic blood product transfusions, and have higher rates of mediastinal re-exploration for bleeding after CPB.
- *Bivalirudin.* This is a direct thrombin inhibitor and an analogue of the peptide fragment hirugen derived from hirudin. Bivalirudin is approved by the U.S. Food and Drug Administration for patients with unstable angina undergoing coronary angioplasty who are also receiving aspirin. Randomized clinical trials in cardiac surgery are currently in progress.
- *Argatroban.* This is a synthetic, competitive thrombin inhibitor derived from L-arginine. It reversibly binds to thrombin's catalytic site. One recent case report described the successful use of argatroban as an alternative to heparin during CPB in a patient with type II HIT, end-stage renal failure, and ischemic cardiomyopathy with ventricular fibrillation.

The management of patients with HIT antibodies who require heart surgery is challenging, because heparin anticoagulation is an integral part of cardiac operations, with or without extracorporeal circulation. A standard approach to patients with HIT has not been established, although several options have been proposed for using the previously listed nonheparinoid anticoagulants. However, there is little experience with approved alternative anticoagulants, specific antidotes are not available, and special tests (which are not readily available) are needed to ascertain their effectiveness.

In patients with a history of HIT but no detectable antibodies, heparin is currently the safest approach to the high-dose anticoagulation required for CPB. However, before and after surgery, alternative anticoagulants should be used. The risk of clinical HIT after cardiac surgery may be reduced by substituting low-molecular-weight heparin for postoperative anticoagulation in patients with type II HIT antibodies found immediately before surgery. Alternatively, hirudin can be used as the anticoagulant for CPB in these patients. If hirudin is used, the ecarin clotting time (instead of ACT) can be used to guide anticoagulation therapy during CPB.

A more recent approach in patients with a history of HIT is to selectively block platelet aggregation using monoclonal antibodies directed toward glycoprotein IIb/IIIa (GP IIb/IIIa) or to use a specific GP IIb/IIIa inhibitor (e.g., tirofiban). An 80% block of GP IIb/IIIa receptors and suppressed platelet aggregation (<20%) permit the use of unfractionated heparin and CPB in the usual way. After CPB, as usual, unfractionated heparin is neutralized with protamine.

After approximately 2 to 12 months, most patients with a history of type II HIT no longer have laboratory evidence of heparin-induced platelet aggregation. If so, heparin use is likely acceptable. However, caution is advised with regard to further heparin exposure during the postoperative period (e.g., heparin flushes, cardiac catheterization). Use of aspirin or dipyridamole for anticoagulation in patients with type II HIT has been successful.

Heparin reversal after CPB is usually accomplished with protamine, a protein derived from salmon sperm. The appropriate dosage is controversial. Most cardiac anesthesiologists use 1.0 to 1.3 mg/100 units of previously administered heparin. Commercial systems for whole blood, circulating heparin assays may allow exact titration of the required amount of protamine; however, despite their theoretical advantage, a fixed dose based on the amount of heparin used is more conventional. Additional protamine may be given about 30 minutes after heparin reversal. Protamine has a high number of positively charged arginine residues that form stable complexes with negatively charged heparin and are eliminated via the reticuloendothelial system.

Protamine has been associated with significant clinical complications, consisting of three major types of adverse responses:

- Type I is the most common, consisting of hypotension from too rapid administration of protamine. It is likely related to the release of histamine, and hypotension can be associated with a marked decrease in systemic vascular resistance.
- Type II is anaphylaxis and can be mediated by immunoglobulins. It occurs more frequently in patients with a history

of fish allergy. Subsequent release of histamine and leukotrienes results in systemic and pulmonary capillary leakage.

- Type III is associated with the formation of heparin-protamine complexes. Pulmonary macrophages activate complement and leukocyte aggregation, causing the release of free radicals and activation of the arachidonic acid pathway, which leads to the formation of thromboxane. This causes intense pulmonary vasoconstriction, pulmonary hypertension, and reduced left atrial pressure. The net result is right heart chamber dilatation and heart failure. Fortunately, type III responses are very uncommon.

PREVENTION

The appearance of heparin resistance can delay surgery and disrupt the operating room schedule. Consequently, some clinicians advise preoperative AT-III level screening for all patients having cardiac surgery requiring CPB. Determination of the heparin dose-response curve can also alert clinicians to heparin resistance before CPB. This allows advance planning for subsequent heparin dosing. If possible, surgery is delayed in patients with type II HIT until antibody titers are absent. New drugs, such as bivalirudin, may be useful alternatives to heparin in such patients.

To eliminate protamine reactions, antihistamines can be used. Also, protamine should be given slowly, preferably via a peripheral vein after substantial dilution. Some surgeons inject it into the aortic root to bypass the lungs during its initial distribution. Although heparin-bonded CPB circuitry may allow lower doses of intravenous heparin, this technology remains unproved.

Further Reading

Anderson EF: Heparin resistance prior to cardiopulmonary bypass. Anesthesiology 64:504-507, 1986.

Bull BS, Huse WM, Brauer FS, et al: Heparin therapy during extracorporeal circulation. II. The use of a dose-response curve to individualize heparin and protamine dosage. J Thorac Cardiovasc Surg 69:685-689, 1975.

DeBois WJ, Liu J, Lee LY, Girardi LN: Diagnosis and treatment of heparin-induced thrombocytopenia. Perfusion 18:47-53, 2003.

Despotis GJ, Joist JH, Hogue CW Jr, et al: The impact of heparin concentration and activated clotting time monitoring on blood conservation. J Thorac Cardiovasc Surg 110:46-54, 1995.

Despotis GJ, Joist JH, Hogue CW Jr, et al: More effective suppression of hemostatic system activation in patients undergoing cardiac surgery by heparin dosing based on heparin blood concentrations rather than ACT. Thromb Haemost 76:902-908, 1996.

Despotis GJ, Levine V, Joist JH, et al: Antithrombin III during cardiac surgery: Effect on response of activated clotting time to heparin and relationship to markers of hemostatic activation. Anesth Analg 85:498-506, 1997.

Edwards JT, Hamby JK, Worrall NK: Successful use of argatroban as a heparin substitute during cardiopulmonary bypass: Heparin-induced thrombocytopenia in a high-risk cardiac surgical patient. Ann Thorac Surg 75:1622-1624, 2003.

Greinacher A: The use of direct thrombin inhibitors in cardiovascular surgery in patients with heparin-induced thrombocytopenia. Semin Thromb Hemost 30:315-327, 2004.

Koster A, Spiess B, Chew DP: Effectiveness of bivalirudin as a replacement for heparin during cardiopulmonary bypass in patients undergoing coronary artery bypass grafting. Am J Cardiol 93:356-359, 2004.

Levy JH: New concepts in anticoagulation and reversal. In Stanley TH, Bailey PL (eds): Anesthesiology and the Cardiovascular Patient. Norwell, Mass, Kluwer Academic Publishers, 1996.

Makhoul RG, McCann RL, Austin EH, et al: Management of patients with heparin-associated thrombocytopenia and thrombosis requiring cardiac surgery. Ann Thorac Surg 43:617-621, 1987.

Messerli FH (ed): Cardiovascular Drug Therapy, 2nd ed. Philadelphia, WB Saunders, 1996.

Nuttall GA, Oliver WC Jr, Santrach PJ: Patients with a history of type II heparin-induced thrombocytopenia with thrombosis requiring cardiac surgery with cardiopulmonary bypass: A prospective observational case series. Anesth Analg 96:344-350, 2003.

Pravinkumar E, Webster NR: HIT/HITT and alternative anticoagulation: Current concepts. Br J Anaesth 90:676-685, 2003.

Sabbagh AH, Chung GKT, Shuttleworth P, et al: Fresh frozen plasma: A solution to heparin resistance during cardiopulmonary bypass. Ann Thorac Surg 37:466-468, 1984.

Sane DC, Califf RM, Topol EJ, et al: Bleeding during thrombolytic therapy for acute myocardial infarction: Mechanisms and management. Ann Intern Med 111:1010-1022, 1989.

Visentin GP, Ford SE, Scott JP, et al: Antibodies from patients with heparin-induced thrombocytopenia/thrombosis are specific for platelet factor 4 complexed with heparin or bound to endothelial cells. J Clin Invest 93:81-88, 1994.

Walenga JM, Jeske WP, Prechel MM: Newer insights on the mechanism of heparin-induced thrombocytopenia. Semin Thromb Hemost 30(Suppl 1):57-67, 2004.

Hemodilution and Blood Conservation

73

Glenn P. Gravlee

Case Synopsis

A 61-year-old, 80-kg man is scheduled for removal and replacement of a total hip prosthesis. He is concerned about blood transfusion and the transmission of infectious diseases, particularly human immunodeficiency virus (HIV). He requests that transfusion of homologous blood be avoided, if possible. He predonated 2 units of autologous blood. During surgery, blood loss is more than 2000 mL, and the hemoglobin level is 7.5 g/dL after both units of autologous blood are given. Vital signs and urine output remain within normal limits. An additional 500 mL of intraoperative blood loss is expected.

PROBLEM ANALYSIS

Definition, Recognition, and Risk Assessment

Complications arising from the transfusion of homologous (also called allogeneic) blood products have been recognized since the beginning of modern transfusion therapy. Bacterial blood contamination was fairly common before the introduction of refrigerated storage and sterile plastic bags. Subsequently, contamination with viruses (e.g., cytomegalovirus, hepatitis B and C, HIV, and human T-cell lymphotropic virus) became a source of greater morbidity. Now, West Nile virus and possibly variant Creutzfeldt-Jakob disease have been added to the list of viral diseases transmissible by blood transfusion. Fortunately, improvements in donor screening and blood component testing have reduced the risk of both HIV and hepatitis C transmission to less than 1 per 1 million units, and that for hepatitis B to about 1 per 137,000 units. Cytomegalovirus remains prevalent in the blood pool, but its transmission is generally not a problem in the absence of clinical immunosuppression. Nevertheless, many blood banks now routinely apply leukoreduction techniques to all cellular blood components before dispensing them, which has greatly reduced the risk of cytomegalovirus transmission. Thus, viral transmission by blood transfusion is now so rare that bacterial contamination once again poses the highest risk for infectious complications, which is 1 in 30,000 red blood cell (RBC) units and 1 in 2000 to 3000 platelet units. Blood group incompatibility and anaphylactic reactions remain rare.

Implications

Considerable evidence supports immunosuppression as a significant consequence of blood transfusion. This increases the risk of cancer recurrence and of bacterial infection among transfusion recipients.

Large blood loss and hemodilution also raise the question of what constitutes a reasonable minimum hemoglobin level in an anesthetized patient with acceptable intravascular volume and vital signs. This is a surprisingly complex issue, but in general, healthy patients safely tolerate hemoglobin concentrations as low as 6 g/dL. Sicker patients may require hemoglobin concentrations as high as 10 g/dL.

Assuming that the hypothetical patient described in the case synopsis is otherwise healthy, the limiting factor may be the rate and predictability of blood loss, because some margin of safety is desirable if sudden additional blood loss should occur. Also, one must consider the possibility of significant postoperative bleeding. Consequently, the patient's hemoglobin concentration of 7.5 g/dL signals the possible need for homologous transfusion, unless shed blood is being effectively salvaged.

MANAGEMENT

This section focuses on available techniques (Table 73-1) and a cost-benefit analysis of autotransfusion techniques that may reduce or avoid the need for homologous RBC or blood component therapy.

Autologous Predonation

Patients can donate blood up to 42 days before operation, which constitutes the maximum storage period for modern

Table 73–1 ■ Autotransfusion Techniques

Technique	Cost	Risk	Advisability*
Autologous predonation	Moderate	Low	Yes
Acute normovolemic hemodilution	Low	Low	No
Intraoperative salvage	High	Low	Yes
Postoperative salvage, unwashed	Low	Moderate	No
Postoperative salvage, washed	Moderate	Low	Yes

*For the patient described in the case synopsis.

anticoagulant and storage solutions. The frequency and amount of donation depend on the patient's ability to tolerate serial phlebotomy while maintaining an adequate hemoglobin level. Typically, a patient donates 2 units of blood per week starting 2 to 4 weeks before surgery. The minimum recommended hemoglobin level for donation is 11 g/dL. To maintain this level, patients are routinely given iron supplementation. Erythropoietin can be used to increase hemoglobin levels during predonation, which enables patients to donate more units; this is quite expensive, however, costing approximately $800 per unit of erythropoietin "manufactured." Erythropoietin augmentation of autologous predonation may be justified if some combination of the following factors exists:

- The preoperative timeline is short (e.g., cancer resection).
- Homologous transfusion is not possible (e.g., Jehovah's Witness).
- The patient is anemic.
- The anticipated surgical blood loss is large (>2000 mL).

Autologous predonation is most effective at avoiding homologous transfusion when used in combination with other autotransfusion techniques, such as intraoperative blood salvage. The cost-effectiveness of autologous donation varies widely, but it often fails to meet the usual standards of efficacy. For this reason, its popularity has dropped substantially over the past several years. The donation itself carries a hospitalization risk of approximately 1 in 17,000, which is 12 times that for community donations by healthy individuals. Even though the blood is autologous, its use still incurs some of the usual homologous transfusion risks, including bacterial contamination or clerical errors leading to incompatible blood transfusions. Compared with allogeneic blood units, autologous units typically require the same testing procedures but more complex storage and identification procedures, so the cost for each unit is higher.

Acute Normovolemic Hemodilution

Acute normovolemic hemodilution involves the removal of blood just before or after the induction of anesthesia, combined with volume replacement using crystalloid or colloid. The technique requires standard anesthesia monitors (electrocardiogram, blood pressure, pulse oximetry, and temperature) and large-bore intravenous access with a 14- or 16-gauge peripheral or central venous catheter. Blood is collected into standard citrate-phosphate-dextrose bags. Removed blood is then stored in anticoagulated sterile bags and returned to the patient intraoperatively or postoperatively.

The rationale is that the patient will be losing fewer RBCs into the surgical field because shed blood has a lower hematocrit due to hemodilution. Assuming that the lowest hematocrit remains acceptable (>20%) and that intravascular volume also remains intact, tissue perfusion will be maintained (and perhaps enhanced). Also, oxygen delivery will be sufficient owing to reduced blood viscosity. Additional clinical advantages include low cost, simple storage, and ease of transportation and record keeping.

Acute normovolemic hemodilution risks hypovolemia if volume replacement is inadequate. Further, the obligatory drop in hemoglobin concentration could induce unanticipated end-organ ischemia if there is an undiagnosed condition such as critical stenosis of a coronary artery or carotid artery. Mathematical analyses strongly suggests that the blood loss savings are fairly minor unless this technique is used quite aggressively—for example, hemodilution from a starting hematocrit of 40% to one of 20% or lower. Typically, this would require withdrawing 6 to 10 500-mL bags of blood. One study found no difference in allogeneic transfusion exposure when 3 units of acute normovolemic hemodilution were compared with a similar volume of autologous predonation in patients undergoing total hip arthroplasty.

Postoperative Blood Salvage

This technique involves the collection and reinfusion of blood shed postoperatively. The blood is collected through a relatively large filter and reinfused through a small-pore filter. This blood can be reinfused unmodified ("unwashed"), or it can be washed and concentrated in the same way as for intraoperative blood salvage.

Reinfused blood typically contains very low concentrations of plasma coagulation factors and platelets. It also contains elevated levels of fibrin degradation products, free hemoglobin, and inflammatory products such as cytokines. With total hip arthroplasty, it might also contain fat and bone spicules. As a result, many clinicians elect to administer salvaged blood only after it has been washed. This somewhat controversial technique reduces the need for allogeneic blood only when postoperative blood losses are large (e.g., >1000 mL), because the hematocrit of blood shed postoperatively is typically in the 15% to 20% range.

Intraoperative Blood Salvage

This method involves using a suction apparatus to collect the patient's blood as it is shed intraoperatively into the surgical field. An anticoagulant solution is added to the shed blood, and it is then stored in a filtered reservoir. Once an adequate amount of blood has been collected (typically >700 mL), it is washed and concentrated so that the final product usually has a hematocrit between 55% and 70%.

Because intraoperative blood salvage conserves RBCs but not plasma or platelets, a dilutional coagulopathy should be anticipated if blood losses approach or exceed one blood volume. Otherwise, the risks of this technique are low if appropriate procedures and standards are followed and the blood is not contaminated with bacteria. The ability to conserve RBCs with this technique depends largely on the surgeon's ability to capture shed blood using suction. In this regard, total hip arthroplasty is in an intermediate category between laparotomy for aortic aneurysm repair, where blood pools in a body cavity and is easily captured, and a more superficial procedure such as reduction mammaplasty, where blood typically runs off the surgical field onto the drapes or is absorbed by sponges.

Table 73–2 ■ Other Potential Blood-Conservation Techniques			
Technique	**Cost**	**Risk**	**Advisability***
Induced hypotension	Varies	Varies	Questionable; patient's age is cause for some concern
Prophylactic aprotinin	Expensive	Low	Unclear; reduces blood loss, but expensive
Spinal or epidural anesthesia	Low	Low	Facilitates blood pressure control; reduces deep vein thrombosis

*For the patient described in the case synopsis.

PREVENTION

Often, clinicians fail to appreciate how much blood loss can be safely tolerated by patients before the need for transfusion. This can be estimated using the following formula:

$$ABL = V \times (H_i - H_d)/H_m,$$

where ABL is allowable blood loss; V is blood volume; H_i and H_d are the initial and lowest desired hematocrit values, respectively; and H_m is the hematocrit average of H_i and H_d. Assuming a blood volume of 5600 mL (80 kg × 70 mL/kg), an H_i of 40%, and an H_d of 25%, the patient in the case synopsis can tolerate a blood loss of almost 2600 mL without transfusion therapy. Intraoperative RBC salvage increases this figure in direct proportion to the efficacy of salvage.

Autologous Predonation

In retrospect, if one could have predicted the amount of blood loss experienced by the patient in the case synopsis based on the surgeon's track record with reoperative hip arthroplasties, the patient should have been given supplemental iron therapy and predonated 3 or 4 units of autologous blood over 3 to 4 weeks before surgery. If the patient's original hematocrit was less than 40%, supplementation with erythropoietin would have been reasonable, although health insurance policies often do not cover the cost of erythropoietin used for this purpose.

Acute Normovolemic Hemodilution

Arguably, the most common application of this procedure is to withdraw 2 units in smaller patients (e.g., those <70 kg) and 3 units in larger ones. This saves 1 to 2 units of allogeneic packed RBCs if the intraoperative blood loss is between 3000 and 6000 mL, which crudely approximates one half to one normal blood volume. As blood losses exceed 6000 mL, the number of units saved gradually diminishes (to 0.5 to 1 unit) with this technique.

Initially, one bag containing approximately 450 mL of blood is collected. As this is occurring, either 500 mL of colloid solution or about 1500 mL of crystalloid solution is infused into the patient to maintain intravascular volume. Hypotension or tachycardia suggests inadequate volume replacement. The exchange continues to the desired end point, as long as the patient tolerates the procedure. Checking the hematocrit or hemoglobin concentration periodically is advisable to reassess the appropriateness of the calculated end point. The blood is then stored at room temperature if it will be used within 8 hours; otherwise, refrigerated storage is required.

Intraoperative Blood Salvage

In the case presented here, intraoperative blood salvage may offer the best chance of respecting the patient's wish to avoid homologous blood. Further, effective use of this technique tends to override any theoretical benefits of acute normovolemic hemodilution. Alternatively, if the patient is otherwise completely healthy, one might "tough it out" to a hematocrit as low as 20%. Considering this patient's age, however, reducing the hematocrit below that level is probably ill advised.

Postoperative Blood Salvage

Because the cost of this technique is low and the likelihood of substantial postoperative bleeding is high in the patient described in the case synopsis, postoperative salvage is appropriate. Wound drainage contains various undesirable elements, however, so washing the product before reinfusion is advisable. Bacterial contamination can also occur, so this strategy should be avoided unless the drainage exceeds 500 mL over an 8-hour period. After this time, the collection device should be replaced if reinfusion is planned.

Alternative Blood Conservation Techniques

Other potential blood-conserving options are listed in Table 73-2. Moderate deliberate hypotension is reasonable if the patient is otherwise healthy; for a patient in his 60s, however, setting a relatively conservative lower mean arterial pressure limit, in the range of 70 mm Hg for 1 to 2 hours, might be prudent.[1] Another reasonable approach for deliberate hypotension might be to reduce the mean arterial pressure

---

[1] Because our hypothetical patient is male and older than 60 years, and assuming no coronary artery disease or risk factors for it (hyperlipidemia, hypertension, or smoking history; see Chapter 38), another way to estimate the minimal acceptable pressure for deliberate hypotension (i.e., that required to maintain coronary perfusion pressure) is diastolic blood pressure – left ventricular end-diastolic pressure = 50 mm Hg. The value for adequate coronary perfusion pressure may be higher in patients with advanced age, diastolic heart failure, or a strong family history of coronary artery disease, hypertension, or other heart disease (all associated with some amount of elevated left ventricular end-diastolic pressure).

by about 20% below the patient's preoperative baseline level, which could probably be safely sustained for several hours if necessary. Aprotinin and its lysine analogues (e.g., tranexamic acid) can also reduce blood loss in hip replacement surgery with a low risk of complications, but the high cost of aprotinin must be considered.

Further Reading

American Association of Blood Banks: All about blood (2004). Available at www.aabb.org/All_About_Blood.

American Society of Anesthesiologists Task Force on Blood Component Therapy: Practice guidelines for blood component therapy. Anesthesiology 84:732-747, 1996.

Birkmeyer JD, Goodnough LT, AuBuchon JP, et al: The cost effectiveness of preoperative autologous blood donation for total hip and knee replacement. Transfusion 33:544-551, 1993.

Goodnough LT: Red blood cell support in the perioperative setting. In Simon TL, Dzik WH, Snyder EL, et al (eds): Rossi's Principles of Transfusion Medicine, 3rd ed. Philadelphia, JB Lippincott–Williams & Wilkins, 2002, pp 590-601.

Goodnough LT, Despotis GJ, Merkel K, Monk TG: A randomized trial comparing acute normovolemic hemodilution and preoperative autologous blood donation in total hip arthroplasty. Transfusion 40:1054-1057, 2000.

Goodnough LT, Monk TG, Brecher ME: Autologous blood procurement in the surgical setting: Lessons learned in the last 10 years. Vox Sang 71:133-141, 1996.

Jacobs MR, Palavecino E, Yomtovian R: Don't bug me: The problem of bacterial contamination of blood components—challenges and solutions. Transfusion 41:1331-1334, 2001.

Wu W-C, Rathore SS, Wang Y, et al: Blood transfusion in elderly patients with acute myocardial infarction. N Engl J Med 345:1230-1236, 2001.

Troubleshooting Common Problems during Cardiopulmonary Bypass

Prashant Lotlikar and John R. Cooper, Jr.

COMPLICATIONS OF AORTIC ROOT CANNULATION: ACUTE AORTIC ROOT DISSECTION

Case Synopsis

A 75-year-old man with a history of calcific aortic stenosis was scheduled for valve replacement. Induction of anesthesia, sternotomy, and placement of cannulas were uneventful. The aortic tissue, however, appeared thin and calcified. The aortic purse strings and cannula appeared well placed, but on beginning cardiopulmonary bypass (CPB), the pump arterial line pressure increased, and systemic blood pressure (radial artery) decreased. The aorta appeared acutely dilated.

PROBLEM ANALYSIS

Definition

Acute aortic dissection following aortic cannulation is an infrequent but serious complication of cardiac surgery. The diagnosis must be made early and thus requires a high index of suspicion. Dissection may also occur during CPB or after decannulation.

In this case, the cannula orifice was situated within the media of the arterial wall rather than the true lumen, owing to a dissection created during cannulation. For aortic dissection to occur, blood under pressure must gain access to the media of the aortic wall. In this case, access was obtained via cannula insertion and initiation of perfusion. Additional manipulation of the ascending aorta (e.g., aortic cross-clamp, antegrade cardioplegia line, proximal bypass grafts) may increase the risk of dissection. Predisposing factors that increase the risk for acute aortic dissection include conditions that weaken the aortic wall, such as the following:

- Cystic medial necrosis
- Elastic or medial degeneration associated with aging
- Poststenotic dilatation (aortic stenosis)
- Atheromatous disease

Dissection may occur spontaneously in the operating room or during the postoperative period in the intensive care unit.

Recognition

A sudden, unexplained decrease in mean arterial pressure and venous return is usually seen, associated with an acute elevation in arterial line pressure and bluish discoloration and enlargement of the aortic root. Myocardial ischemia, aortic insufficiency, or both may develop, and signs of organ hypoperfusion (including oliguria and pupil asymmetry) may be present if the dissection extends to other major arterial vessels. If transesophageal echocardiography is used, dissection may be evident on examination of the thoracic aorta (Fig. 74-1).

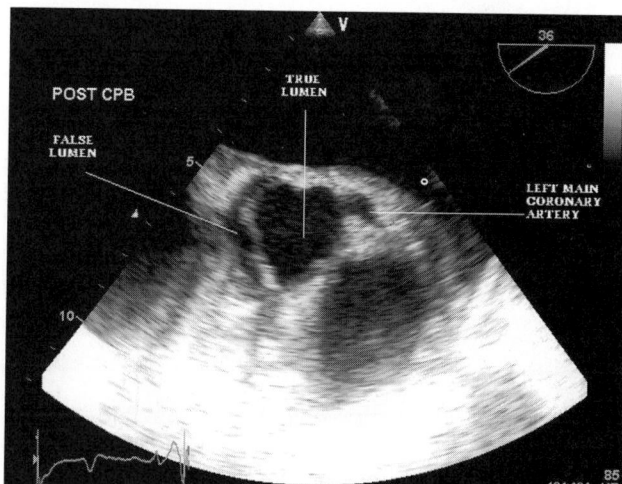

Figure 74–1 ■ Transesophageal echocardiography of the ascending aorta just distal to the aortic valve, with an intraoperative aortic dissection evident showing true and false lumens. This dissection propagated from the antegrade cardioplegia administration site.

MANAGEMENT

CPB must be discontinued immediately. The surgeon must then either reposition or replace the arterial cannula into the true lumen at a more distal site on the aortic arch or initiate femoral artery cannulation. Surgical repair of the aortic dissection is almost always necessary, including coronary artery reimplantation if patency of the coronary arteries is threatened.

PREVENTION

Measures that may be effective in reducing the incidence of aortic dissection during cannulation include the following:

- Blood pressure control (to avoid hypertension) at the time of cannulation
- Insertion of the cannula at a right angle to the aorta to prevent dissection into tissue planes
- Special care in locating the tip in the true lumen of the aorta
- Blood pressure reduction when the aortic cross-clamp is applied or removed
- Use of atraumatic clamps, with as few applications to the aorta as possible
- Continuous monitoring of arterial cannula pressure by the perfusionist

CAROTID OR INNOMINATE ARTERY HYPERPERFUSION

Case Synopsis

A 58-year-old woman underwent CPB for coronary artery bypass grafting. After successful aortic and venous cannulation by the surgeon, the anesthesiologist noted right-sided facial blanching. Further examination showed the presence of a right carotid thrill.

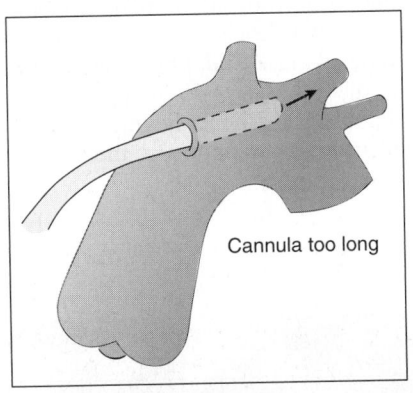

Cannula too long

A

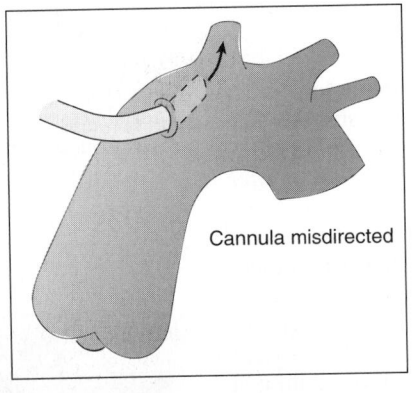

Cannula misdirected

B

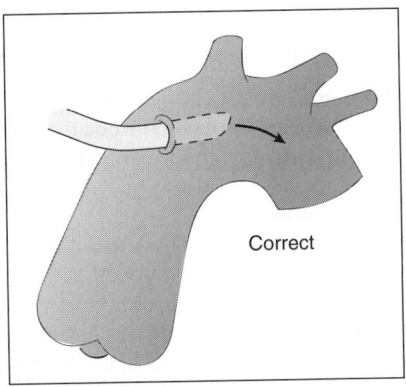

Correct

C

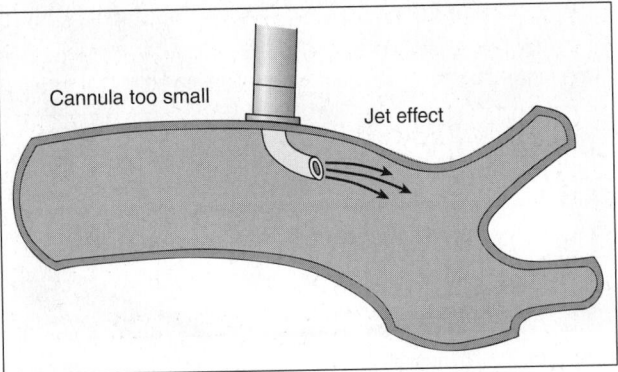

Cannula too small

Jet effect

D

Figure 74–2 ▪ Carotid or innominate artery hyperperfusion. *A,* The cannula is too long, causing it to enter the left carotid artery. *B,* The cannula angulation is incorrect, directing the majority of flow to the innominate artery. *C,* Correct position. *D,* The cannula is too small, resulting in a high-velocity jet. See Definition (next page) for further discussion. (From Moores WY: Cardiopulmonary bypass strategies in patients with severe aortic disease. In Utley JR [ed]: Pathophysiology and Techniques of Cardiopulmonary Bypass, vol 2. Baltimore, Williams & Wilkins, 1983, p 190.)

PROBLEM ANALYSIS

Definition

Pump flow can be directed primarily into the carotid or innominate artery instead of the aorta. This can result in cerebral edema or arterial rupture due to high perfusion pressure or the creation of an intimal flap that obstructs arterial flow (Fig. 74-2).

Recognition

Signs of innominate artery cannulation include ipsilateral facial blanching, pupillary dilatation, and conjunctival chemosis. Hypotension measured via a left radial or femoral artery catheter may be observed, but a right radial artery catheter may show hypertension.

MANAGEMENT

Repositioning of the cannula is necessary. Measures to reduce cerebral edema, including diuretics or head-up position, may be indicated.

PREVENTION

Use of a short aortic cannula with a flange to prevent insertion too far into the aorta is usually effective. The anesthesiologist can check for bilateral carotid pulses without thrills after cannulation and initiation of CPB, but this may not reliably detect problems caused by carotid or innominate artery hyperperfusion.

OBSTRUCTION TO VENOUS RETURN

Case Synopsis

A 60-year-old man was placed on CPB after uneventful aortic cannulation and use of a single venous cannula in the right atrium. There was an immediate decrease in both arterial pressure and pump-oxygenator venous reservoir volume. Obvious venous engorgement in the patient's face and neck was noted immediately.

PROBLEM ANALYSIS

Definition

Obstruction of venous return to the pump-oxygenator may have several causes:

- An "air lock" created by the presence of large air bubbles within the venous cannula or tubing
- Failure to remove a venous line clamp
- Lifting of the heart within the chest by the surgeon
- Use of venous cannulas too small for the patient
- Presence of thrombus or tumor
- Kinked or malpositioned cannula (most common)

When two cannulas are used, the superior vena cava cannula may be placed into the azygos vein or, if advanced too far cephalad, into the innominate vein. The inferior vena cava cannula may be placed into the hepatic vein. In this case synopsis, the single cannula was placed so far into the inferior vena cava that there could be no venous return from the superior vena cava.

Recognition

Decreasing venous reservoir volume in the pump-oxygenator is the first sign. Failure to reduce pump flow immediately can result in emptying of the venous reservoir, with a risk of massive arterial air embolism. Increased central venous pressure occurs, along with obvious venous engorgement in the face and neck and later conjunctival chemosis. Also, lack of drainage from the right side of the heart may result in compression of the left ventricle, detected by direct visualization or by an increase in pulmonary artery or left atrial pressure.

MANAGEMENT

Pump flow should be reduced until the cause of obstruction to venous return is found. The surgeon can propel an air lock through the venous tubing by progressively raising and tapping the tubing downstream from the bubble. Venous cannulas will probably have to be repositioned. Only after adequate venous return is established, with recovery of volume in the venous reservoir, should full-flow CPB be continued.

PREVENTION

The surgeon should inspect the venous cannula for large bubbles and ensure proper venous cannula position. The anesthesiologist should routinely check the patient's face, neck, and conjunctiva for signs of high venous pressures. Monitoring central venous pressures may not detect a superior vena cava obstruction because the catheter tip may be below the obstruction point.

MASSIVE GAS EMBOLISM

Case Synopsis

A 65-year-old woman undergoing mitral valve replacement was placed on CPB after uneventful insertion of aortic and venous cannulas. Before application of the aortic cross-clamp, the surgeon inserted a vent cannula into the left atrium via the left superior pulmonary vein. Blood initially began to drain normally toward the venous reservoir but then reversed direction, and a large quantity of air entered the heart and was ejected systemically.

PROBLEM ANALYSIS

Definition

Systemic gas embolism is the most common serious adverse event associated with CPB and is largely preventable. Principal causes include the following:

- Vortexing—air being pumped out of an empty or near empty oxygenator reservoir

- Reversed roller-pump tubing in the vent line or arterial cannula
- Disconnection, leak, oxygenator disruption, or line occlusion proximal to the arterial pump, with air entrainment or cavitation
- Development of positive pressure in the cardiotomy reservoir, producing retrograde airflow into the heart or aorta
- Injection of air into the aortic root from the cardioplegia delivery system
- Clotted oxygenator or runaway pump head

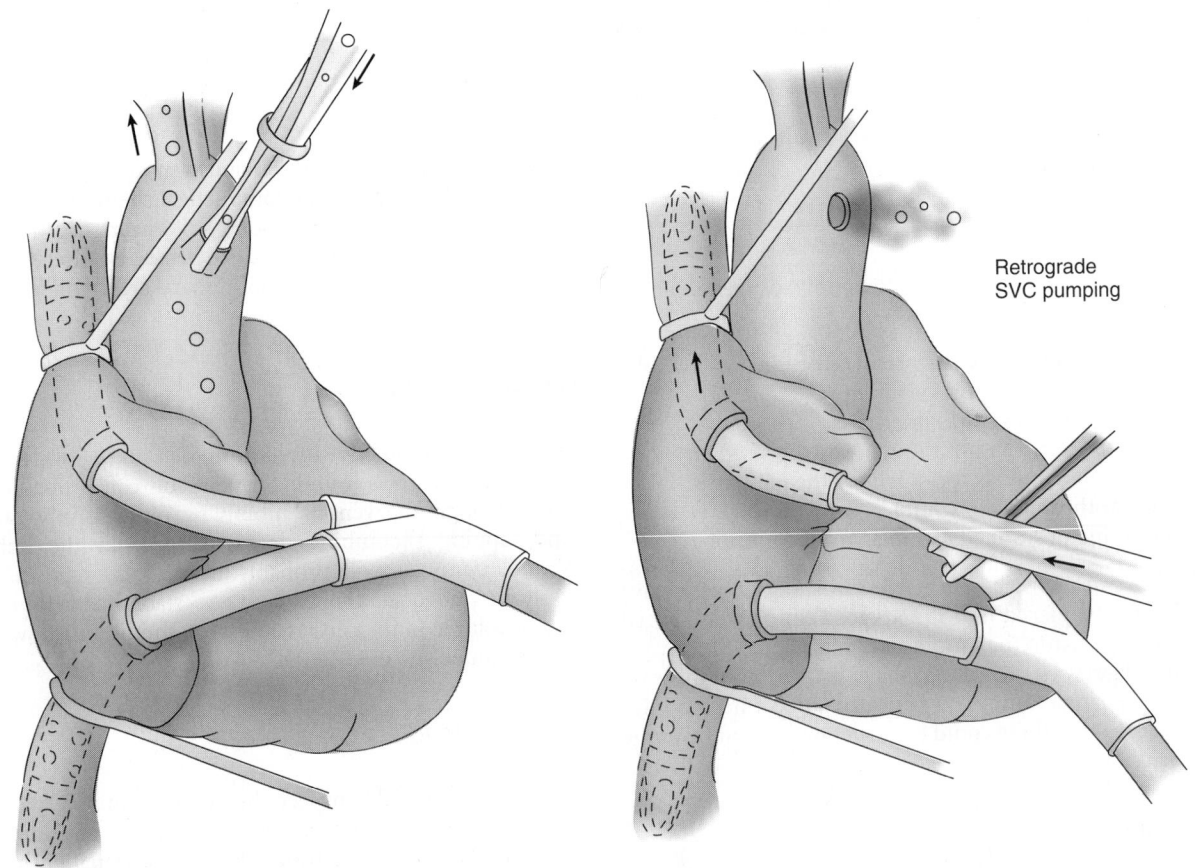

A   B

Figure 74–3 ▪ *A,* Massive air embolus through the aortic cannula. (*circles* represent the aortic root) *B,* The aortic cannula is removed, purged of air (*circles*), and inserted into the divided superior vena cava (SVC) cannula. Retrograde perfusion at 1200 mL/minute at 20°C is carried out for 1 to 2 minutes. Air exits the aortic cannulation site. (From Mills NL, Ochsner JL: Massive air embolism during CPB: Causes, prevention and management. J Thorac Cardiovasc Surg 80:713, 1980.)

- Ejection of blood before the removal of air from the heart, or opening a beating heart
- Disconnection or rupture of the oxygenator or lines during CPB
- Failure to clamp the aortic line at the end of CPB, resulting in air infusion if the pump head is accidentally restarted

Recognition

Air in the arterial cannula is usually visually apparent, but signs of myocardial or other organ ischemia may also occur. Rarely, withdrawal of air from an arterial pressure monitoring line indicates air embolism.

MANAGEMENT

After recognition, if the embolus is massive, CPB must be discontinued. The patient is then placed in a steep Trendelenburg position, the aortic cannula is removed, and the CPB circuit is reprimed. Retrograde perfusion of the superior vena cava is initiated (Fig. 74-3). CPB is then restarted with hypothermia, increasing perfusion pressure, and

100% oxygen. Consideration can then be given to pharmacologic interventions to reduce cerebral injury, including mannitol, steroids, and barbiturates. Postoperative interventions may include initiation of hyperbaric oxygen treatment, reverse Trendelenburg position, initiation of slight hyperventilation, and avoidance of hyperglycemia and hyponatremia.

PREVENTION

Special attention must be paid to maintaining a safe volume of blood in the oxygenator reservoir. Low-level alarms and bubble detectors should be used. The surgical team must protect the venous lines and communicate with the perfusionist when venous return is likely to be compromised. Other measures include the use of the following:

- Centrifugal pumps
- Arterial line filters
- Bubble traps with an open air purge line guarded by a one-way valve
- Collapsible reservoirs
- One-way valves placed in the left heart vent line

PUMP OR OXYGENATOR FAILURE

Case Synopsis

A 68-year-old man underwent CPB for combined mitral valve replacement and coronary bypass grafting. Five minutes after initiation of CPB, dark blood was observed by the anesthesiologist in the aortic cannula. An immediate blood gas sampling revealed a low arterial oxygen tension (PaO_2).

PROBLEM ANALYSIS

Definition

This situation can be caused by oxygenator failure, with three possible causes of arterial inflow desaturation: (1) the gas supply system, (2) the oxygenator itself, or (3) specific patient characteristics or pathophysiology.

Low PaO_2 can also be caused by pump failure. This can occur by means of electrical or mechanical failure, tubing rupture or disconnection, or automatic shutoff by the bubble or reservoir level detector. A runaway pump head may inappropriately raise the pump flow rate to maximum. If the occlusion of a roller pump is improperly set, excessive regurgitation can cause reduced forward blood flow, hypotension, and metabolic acidosis.

Recognition

Oxygenator failure results in dark blood in the arterial cannula and severe vasodilatation. Blood leaking into the heater-cooler water may also be seen with oxygenator rupture. With pump failure and low PaO_2, one observes hypotension, metabolic acidosis, and perhaps hemolysis.

MANAGEMENT

If oxygenator failure is suspected, a blood gas measurement from the arterial inflow line should be obtained, and the perfusionist should increase oxygen gas flows and determine the adequacy of mechanical pump flow. Additionally, the following actions should be taken:

- Careful inspection of the gas circuit, including gas sources, all connections, tubing, gas line filter, and vaporizer
- Inspection of the oxygenator for appropriate blood levels and adequacy of foaming (bubble oxygenator), and examination of the shell for leaks or cracks
- Inspection of the venous and arterial cannulas for appropriate patient connections
- Assurance of adequate muscle relaxation, appropriate patient temperature, and depth of anesthesia

If the heart is still beating, one should consider allowing it to eject blood into the pulmonary circulation for additional oxygenation and continue ventilation of the lungs until apparent arterialization of blood is observed in the aortic cannula.

If there is pump failure, a hand crank can be used until a replacement is obtained or tubing is replaced. In the case of a runaway pump head, the machine must be unplugged, and the tubing must be switched to a different roller head. If flow will be low or absent for more than a few minutes, and if the patient cannot be weaned immediately from CPB, hypothermia should be induced. One should then consider packing the head and heart in ice for additional protection.

PREVENTION

Vigilance is paramount. Use of a pump arterial line oxygen saturation monitor and/or a partial pressure of oxygen analyzer may be beneficial. Backup equipment should always be available.

CLOTTED OXYGENATOR OR CIRCUIT

Case Synopsis

A 60-year-old man underwent aortocoronary bypass and concurrent abdominal aortic aneurysm repair. After weaning from CPB, while the aneurysm was being repaired, the CPB circuit was used for blood salvage and reinfusion. After 1 hour, as blood was given through the aortic cannula, a large clot was discovered in the oxygenator. The activated clotting time was greater than 400 seconds.

PROBLEM ANALYSIS

Definition

This adverse event can prevent CPB flow, cause massive gas embolus, and interfere with gas exchange. Causes include inadequate heparinization, stagnation in the bypass circuit (no flow in the circuit during circulatory arrest), and, occasionally, addition of unheparinized blood products during CPB.

Recognition

Visual inspection of the circuit for clots is most reliable, but the observation of air exiting from a bubble oxygenator or high arterial cannula pressure may also indicate a large clot.

MANAGEMENT

Stop CPB and reheparinize the patient using a different lot of heparin, if possible. Hypothermia should be initiated, and open cardiac massage should be performed if the patient cannot be acutely weaned from CPB. The oxygenator may need to be replaced. The protocol for massive air embolism should be followed, if appropriate.

PREVENTION

The surgical team should ensure adequate heparin administration and monitoring in prolonged cases, plus visual inspection of the circuit and arterial line filter for clots. Heparinizing any blood products added to the circuit should be considered, and stagnant blood pooling in the CPB circuit should be avoided, even if heparinization is "adequate" by laboratory measurements.

Further Reading

Gravlee GP, Davis RF, Krusz M, Utley JR: Cardiopulmonary Bypass: Principles and Practice. Philadelphia, JB Lippincott–Williams & Wilkins, 2000, pp 69-97, 578-612.

Hensley FA Jr, Martin DE, Gravlee GP: A Practical Approach to Cardiac Anesthesia, 3rd ed. Philadelphia, JB Lippincott–Williams & Wilkins 2003, pp 513-556.

Mills NL, Ochsner JL: Massive air embolism during cardiopulmonary bypass: Causes, prevention, and management. J Thorac Cardiovasc Surg 80:708-717, 1980.

Mora CT: Cardiopulmonary Bypass: Principles and Techniques of Extracorporeal Circulation. New York, Springer-Verlag, 1995, pp 302-307.

Reed CC, Kurusz M, Lawrence AE Jr: Safety and Techniques in Perfusion. Stafford, Tex, Qualimed, 1988, pp 123-133.

Bleeding after Cardiac Surgery

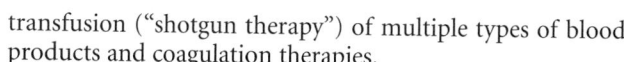

Peter Tassani-Prell

Case Synopsis

A 73-year-old man presents with a history of aortic stenosis, coronary artery disease, peripheral vascular disease, dyspnea at rest, and chronic renal failure (creatinine level 1.6 mg/dL). Myocardial function is reduced (left ventricular ejection fraction is 35%). Combined aortic valve replacement and coronary artery bypass graft surgery is performed. Total cardiopulmonary bypass (CPB) time is 142 minutes. Increased bleeding is noted via the mediastinal tubes after surgery. Blood loss via these tubes is 2200 mL in the first 24 hours postoperatively.

PROBLEM ANALYSIS

Definition

Excessive bleeding after cardiac surgery is broadly categorized as surgical or nonsurgical. Surgical bleeding can originate from multiple locations, including bypass graft anastomoses, cannulation sites, mammary beds, sternal wires, or wherever blood vessel integrity has been interrupted. Nonsurgical or microvascular bleeding can result from hemostatic abnormalities involving the endothelium, platelets, coagulation factors, or fibrinolysis. The combined effects of large heparin and protamine doses required for cardiac surgery, CPB circuitry, blood scavenging systems, hypothermia, and, occasionally, massive transfusion can contribute to postoperative bleeding.

Recognition

Surgical exploration for bleeding begins in the operating room (OR) following heparin neutralization with protamine after separation from CPB or completion of "off-pump" cardiac surgery. There are great individual differences in the amount of bleeding that can be detected by direct observation of the operative field. The multifactorial nature of coagulation disorders often makes the distinction between surgical and nonsurgical bleeding difficult. The typical delay in obtaining laboratory test results further complicates the decision as to what therapeutic treatment is needed (e.g., platelets, fresh frozen plasma, cryoprecipitate). Postoperatively, mediastinal chest tube drainage is monitored hourly. As a rule, drainage should not exceed 100 to 125 mL/hour for the first 4 postoperative hours, 250 mL for any hour during this period, or 50 to 75 mL/hour for the subsequent 24 hours.

Life-threatening hypotension from postoperative bleeding can result from cardiac tamponade or hypovolemia. It is essential to initiate diagnostic efforts long before the patient's arrival in the postoperative intensive care unit. Nonsurgical bleeding may be detected in the OR by the surgical team. Appropriate laboratory analysis should be initiated early to obtain results in the OR. Early detection of specific hemostatic deficiencies leads to specific therapy instead of nonspecific transfusion ("shotgun therapy") of multiple types of blood products and coagulation therapies.

Risk Assessment

Risk factors for postoperative bleeding include the following:

- Prolonged duration of CPB
- Repeat cardiac procedures
- Combined procedures (e.g., bypass grafting and valve surgery)
- Low body temperature after surgery
- Increased cell salvage usage
- Advanced age
- Chronic steroid use
- Intra-aortic balloon counterpulsation
- Internal mammary artery harvesting
- Female sex
- Preoperative use of anticoagulant drugs

Individual screening in the preoperative period is essential to identify patients at increased risk for postoperative bleeding. Clinical observation and the patient's medical history are extremely important. Drugs that alter the coagulation system or platelet function are commonly used in patients scheduled for cardiac surgery. Glycoprotein IIb/IIIa inhibitors, including abciximab, eptifibatide, and tirofiban, are used extensively as short-term adjuncts to heparin or aspirin therapy in patients with acute coronary syndromes or in those having preoperative percutaneous coronary interventions. It is also likely that many patients requiring emergency cardiac surgery will have received anticoagulation therapy before arriving in the OR. When in doubt, additional laboratory analysis for specific coagulation disorders may be indicated.

Implications

Use of CPB during cardiac surgery disrupts the normal hemostatic system in several ways. Combined effects of hypothermia, hemodilution, blood loss, and transient activation of platelets are often seen. Activated platelets following exposure to CPB are "exhausted" and have lost their function.

However, with normal CPB duration, detrimental quantitative and qualitative platelet defects are usually short-lived.

Hemodilution.
Crystalloid CPB priming and cardioplegia solutions dilute platelets and coagulation factors. The significance of this depends on their baseline concentrations, as well as the volume used relative to the patient's circulating blood volume. Recent efforts to reduce the volume of CPB priming solutions by using different CPB circuits for adults with lower body weight or using blood versus crystalloid cardioplegia may significantly reduce the amount of clinical hemodilution. Even so, hemodilution is rarely the sole cause of postoperative bleeding, because coagulation factor concentrations of 25% to 30% and platelet counts of 50,000 to 100,000/mm^3 can be tolerated without excessive bleeding if platelet function is normal.

Cardiopulmonary Bypass Circuitry.
The exposure of blood to nonendothelial surfaces of the CPB circuit activates platelets and the coagulation and fibrinolytic pathways. Platelet dysfunction is the single most important cause of bleeding after cardiac surgery. Use of pericardial suction devices during surgery traumatizes blood cells and returns activated coagulation factors to the circulation via the venous reservoir. The use of closed reservoirs, coated CPB circuits, and retransfusion of the suctioned blood after preparation in an autotransfusion device have all been proposed to reduce the detrimental effects of CPB on coagulation.

Hypothermia.
Hypothermia may result in impaired platelet function and reduced function of temperature-dependent coagulation factors. Also, laboratory coagulation system assessment is uniformly done at 37°C. Therefore, misleading results might be obtained when analyzing cold blood samples obtained during hypothermic CPB. Cooling to more tepid temperatures (mild hypothermia) has been proposed by some to reduce the activation of inflammatory cascades and lessen coagulation abnormalities.

Cell Salvage Systems.
Because coagulation factors and platelets are removed during routine red cell salvage, reinfused products from cell salvage devices are deficient in these components. Thus, red cell salvage may contribute to abnormalities of coagulation.

Heparin.
Despite initial neutralization with protamine, heparin rebound can occur 2 to 6 hours afterward, leading to inhibition of platelet function. Antibody-mediated, heparin-induced thrombocytopenia and thrombosis (type II HIT; see Chapter 72) is a distinct, severe, and rare entity that involves accelerated clearance or activation of platelets. The target antigen is generated in the presence of platelet factor 4 and heparin at a concentration that allows the formation of heparin–platelet factor 4 complexes. Such interaction then exposes neoepitopes, which bind to the heparin-dependent antibodies. These antibodies are generated in a minority of heparin-treated patients, and occasionally one subgroup develops thrombocytopenia associated with thrombosis.

MANAGEMENT

Treatment of postoperative bleeding can be challenging because of its complex and multifactorial causes. Excessive mediastinal tube drainage, especially when accompanied by hemodynamic instability, indicates a probable surgical source of bleeding and requires surgical re-exploration in the OR. However, the amount of mediastinal drainage does not allow one to differentiate between surgical and nonsurgical causes of bleeding—a distinction that is of the utmost importance. Therefore, a scientifically based algorithm (based on laboratory values) should be used for the precise diagnosis of specific hemostatic abnormalities.

When the activated clotting time (ACT) returns to baseline values, this is often interpreted as meaning that heparin neutralization is complete. However, the ACT is insensitive to low circulating heparin concentrations. Even when the ACT has returned to baseline, heparin plasma concentrations can be as high as 0.2 unit/mL, which corresponds to an activated partial thromboplastin time (aPTT) of 1.5 times control. More sensitive tests for residual heparin following surgery include whole blood or plasma aPTT, thrombin time, whole blood heparin concentration measurements, or heparinase ACT values.

Continued bleeding in the absence of detectable heparin concentrations warrants further evaluation of the coagulation system. Results of laboratory-based coagulation studies (e.g., prothrombin time, aPTT, platelet count) may take an hour or more to obtain. Commercially available on-site or point-of-care testing methods can provide clinically relevant coagulation test results in about 5 minutes. Such testing can provide a whole blood determination of prothrombin time and aPTT (i.e., plasma separation is not required). Because of the relative importance of quantitative and qualitative platelet defects following CPB, it is important to evaluate and correct such defects as soon as possible. It is difficult to obtain adequate surgical hemostasis without at least 50,000 to 100,000/mm^3 of fully functional platelets. Therefore, use of an OR-based hemocytometer can provide rapid information about platelet concentrations. Normal counts, however, do not guarantee adequate platelet function. Modified computerized thromboelastography provides more rapid results than conventional thromboelastography and may be useful. This system allows rapid whole blood coagulation testing with different activators and additives, typically reaching the maximal amplitude after about 15 minutes. It is also possible to see this process in the OR while the test is still running in the laboratory. It is important to initiate diagnostic evaluation early, when microvascular bleeding ("oozing") in the surgical field is first observed. Timely point-of-care, laboratory-assisted assessment of coagulation leads to reduced and more appropriate use of blood products in the OR.

Platelet Dysfunction

Once the determination of thrombocytopenia or qualitative platelet dysfunction has been made, treatment includes the administration of desmopressin acetate (DDAVP), platelet transfusions, or both. DDAVP, a synthetic analogue of antidiuretic hormone, is thought to augment platelet function by the release of factor VIII and von Willebrand's factor from endothelial cells. Other studies, however, indicate that DDAVP may have direct beneficial effects on platelets, such as increased expression of the adhesive receptor (glycoprotein Ib). The usual dose of DDAVP is 0.3 µg/kg, given intravenously over

Table 75–1 ■ Antifibrinolytic Drugs to Reduce Blood Loss and Requirements for Blood Transfusion after Cardiac Surgery

Drug	Mechanism of Action	Dose	Comments
Aprotinin (full-dose regimen)	Broad-spectrum serine protease inhibitor Interacts with trypsin, kallikrein, chymotrypsin Blood-sparing effects likely related to plasmin inhibition, with platelet function preserved Reduced activation of the hemostatic system via inhibition of contact (kallikrein inhibitor) and tissue factor (binding of VIIa-TF) pathways, with resultant reductions in thrombin and anti-inflammatory properties	Test dose: 1 mL (10,000 units) to test for anaphylaxis Loading dose: 200 mL (2 million units) over 30 min before starting CPB Maintenance dose: 50 mL/hr (0.5 million units/hr); 200 mL in CPB prime solution	Aprotinin prolongs the celite ACT, which may lead to inadequate heparinization during CPB; kaolin ACT is unaffected by aprotinin Whole blood heparin concentrations (>3 units/mL) can also be maintained with the heparin-protamine titration method If only celite ACT is available, ACT should be kept >800 sec during CPB, or fixed heparin dosing should be used
Aprotinin (half-dose regimen)	See above	Test dose: 1 mL (10,000 units) to test for anaphylaxis Loading dose: 100 mL (1 million units) over 30 min before starting CPB Maintenance dose: 25 mL/hr (0.25 million units/hr); 100 mL in CPB prime solution	Half-dose regimen is effective for reducing blood loss for complex or repeat CABG surgery Anti-inflammatory effects with the full-dose regimen may affect other outcomes
∈-aminocaproic acid (EACA)	Binds to plasmin, inhibiting fibrinolysis	Loading dose: 100-150 mg/kg or 5-10 g (adults) over 30 min Maintenance dose: 10-20 mg/kg/hr or 1 g/hr (adults)	Renal excretion; dose must be reduced in patients with renal failure Contraindicated with DIC or in presence of hematuria, because ureteral obstruction may result Risks include thrombotic complications Not approved by FDA for prophylaxis of cardiac surgical bleeding
Tranexamic acid	Binds to plasmin, inhibiting fibrinolysis	Loading dose: 10 mg/kg Maintenance dose: 1 mg/kg/hr	Renal excretion; dose must be reduced in patients with renal failure Contraindicated with DIC or in presence of hematuria, because ureteral obstruction may result Risks include thrombotic complications Not approved by FDA for prophylaxis of cardiac surgical bleeding

ACT, activated clotting time; CABG, coronary artery bypass graft; CPB, cardiopulmonary bypass; DIC, disseminated intravascular coagulation; FDA, Food and Drug Administration; TF, tissue factor.

30 minutes. The principal adverse side effect is hypotension. A similar beneficial effect, but without hypotension, can be achieved by giving 4 μg/kg of DDAVP intranasally.

Platelet transfusion should consist of an appropriate number of units, preferably obtained by apheresis from a single donor. During cardiac transplantation, blood from the organ donor can be acquired during cardiac explantation, from which platelet-rich plasma is derived by separation plasmapheresis. Such platelet-rich plasma is then transfused into the organ recipient. This can substantially reduce the need for perioperative blood transfusion in cardiac transplant recipients.

Coagulation Factor Deficiencies

When the prothrombin time is greater than 16 seconds or the aPTT is greater than 57 seconds, coagulation factor deficiencies are treated with fresh frozen plasma. Although the amount needed varies, depending on initial factor concentrations and circulating blood volume, 1 mL/kg of fresh frozen plasma usually increases coagulation factor concentrations by 1% to 2%. Cryoprecipitate provides a concentrated source of fibrinogen, which is beneficial when deficiencies of this coagulation factor are documented. A prothrombin complex concentrate may be useful when liver function is compromised or liver-generated coagulation factors have been chemically reduced by warfarin. Substitution or supplementation of native antithrombin III leads to higher ACT values and reduced concentrations of fibrin monomer and D-dimer. Substitution of antithrombin III is essential when its activity is less than 60%, because the heparin effect is dependent on it. Several case reports have described using recombinant activated factor VII in cases of life-threatening hemorrhage after cardiac surgery. Randomized, controlled trials to assess the efficacy and safety of such therapy are under way.

PREVENTION

Measures to prevent bleeding after cardiac surgery include the following:

- Minimal CPB duration
- Autologous blood procurement before CPB to provide a source of fresh whole blood with functioning platelets and coagulation factors for use after heparin neutralization
- Maintenance of normothermia
- Judicious postoperative blood pressure control

The fibrinolytic system is known to be up-regulated during CPB owing to the activation of multiple physiologic systems. This results in clot dissolution, coagulation factor consumption, and platelet dysfunction. Multiple clinical studies indicate that the prophylactic administration of antifibrinolytic drugs reduces blood loss and the number of transfusions in patients after cardiac surgery, particularly reoperations (Table 75-1).

Further Reading

Cammerer U, Dietrich W, Rampf T, et al: The predictive value of modified computerized thromboelastography and platelet function analysis for postoperative blood loss in routine cardiac surgery. Anesth Analg 96:51-57, 2003.

Caputo M, Bryan AJ, Calafiore AM, et al: Intermittent antegrade hyperkalaemic warm blood cardioplegia supplemented with magnesium prevents myocardial substrate derangement in patients undergoing coronary artery bypass surgery. Eur J Cardiothorac Surg 14:596-601, 1998.

Despotis GJ, Filos KS, Zoys TN, et al: Factors associated with excessive postoperative blood loss and hemostatic transfusion requirements: A multivariate analysis in cardiac surgical patients. Anesth Analg 82:13-21, 1996.

Hekmat K, Zimmermann T, Kampe S, et al: Impact of tranexamic acid vs aprotinin on blood loss and transfusion requirements after cardiopulmonary bypass: A prospective, randomized, double-blind trial. Curr Med Res Opin 20:121-126, 2004.

Herbertson M: Recombinant activated factor VII in cardiac surgery. Blood Coagul Fibrinolysis 15(Suppl 1):S31-S32. 2004.

Levi M, Cromheecke ME, de Jonge E: Pharmacological strategies to decrease excessive blood loss in cardiac surgery: A meta-analysis of clinically relevant endpoints. Lancet 354:1940-1947, 1999.

Levy JH, Despotis GJ, Szlam F, et al: Recombinant human transgenic antithrombin in cardiac surgery: A dose-finding study. Anesthesiology 96:1095-1102, 2002.

Mongan PD, Hosking MP: The role of desmopressin acetate in patients undergoing coronary artery bypass surgery: A controlled clinical trial with thromboelastographic risk stratification. Anesthesiology 77:38-46, 1992.

Nuttall GA, Fass DN, Oyen LJ, et al: A study of a weight-adjusted aprotinin schedule during cardiac surgery. Anesth Analg 94:283-289, 2002.

Nuttall GA, Oliver WC, Santrach PJ, et al: Efficacy of a simple intraoperative transfusion algorithm for nonerythrocyte component utilization after cardiopulmonary bypass. Anesthesiology 94:773-781, 2001.

Ohata T, Sawa Y, Kadoba K, et al: Effect of cardiopulmonary bypass under tepid temperature on inflammatory reactions. Ann Thorac Surg 64:124-128, 1997.

Remadi JP, Marticho P, Butoi I, et al: Clinical experience with the mini-extracorporeal circulation system: An evolution or a revolution? Ann Thorac Surg 77:2172-2175, 2004.

Richter JA, Meisner H, Tassani P, et al: Drew-Anderson technique attenuates systemic inflammatory response syndrome and improves respiratory function after coronary artery bypass grafting. Ann Thorac Surg 69:77-83, 2000.

Spiess BD, Gillies BS, Chandler W, et al: Changes in transfusion therapy and reexploration after institution of a blood management program in cardiac surgical patients. J Cardiothorac Vasc Anesth 9:168-173, 1995.

Tassani P, Otto D, Szekely A, et al: Transfusion of platelet-rich plasma from the organ donor during cardiac transplantation. J Clin Anesth 9:409-414, 1997.

Woodman RC, Harker LA: Bleeding complications associated with cardiopulmonary bypass. Blood 76:1680-1697, 1990.

Perioperative Myocardial Ischemia and Infarction

76

Mark A. Chaney

Case Synopsis

A 62-year-old man is scheduled for elective coronary artery bypass grafting. Immediately after uneventful induction of general anesthesia and tracheal intubation, new ST segment depression is observed on the electrocardiogram (ECG) tracing.

PROBLEM ANALYSIS

Definition

Myocardial ischemia results from an imbalance between myocardial oxygen supply and demand. If this persists, ischemia eventually leads to myocardial infarction (MI). Patients in whom perioperative ischemia develops are at increased risk for subsequent cardiac morbidity and mortality. Postoperative MI and major cardiac complications occur in more than 4% of patients who have either an established diagnosis of coronary artery disease or risk factors for it and who undergo major noncardiac surgery. In the United States alone, 1.5 to 2 million patients are at such risk for postoperative MI each year. There is marked variability in the reported short-term mortality (<10% to 70%), but few data exist for long-term prognosis after postoperative MI.

Well over 50,000 patients a year sustain perioperative MI, adding substantial cost to postoperative care. Unlike nonsurgical MI, the clinical diagnosis of perioperative MI is often difficult or impossible, especially if it is based on the classic triad of (1) cardiac symptoms, (2) typical ECG findings, and (3) biochemical markers. The silent nature of perioperative MI, the subtle and transient ST depression changes on ECG (resulting in non-Q-wave MI), and the low specificity of the creatine kinase (CK) MB isoenzyme all lead to inconsistencies in the diagnosis of MI and uncertainty about the long-term significance of perioperative markers of MI.

Recognition

Ischemia

Anginal symptoms and hemodynamic alterations are not necessarily reliable indicators of myocardial ischemia. Reliance on increased pulmonary artery wedge pressure for the detection of ischemia is controversial at best. In fact, acutely increased pulmonary artery wedge pressure probably signifies only global ischemia. Detection of regional wall motion abnormalities with transesophageal echocardiography is the most sensitive of the currently available, clinically useful techniques for detecting myocardial ischemia. In addition to wall motion abnormalities, decreased systolic wall thickening or abnormal diastolic filling patterns, detected by Doppler interrogation across the left ventricular inflow region at the tips of the mitral valve, may also contribute to the recognition of myocardial ischemia. However, transient systolic wall motion abnormalities without accompanying hemodynamic or ECG changes indicative of ischemia are not always related to ischemia. Nevertheless, patients who demonstrate new, persistent wall motion abnormalities perioperatively are more likely to experience a postoperative adverse cardiac outcome than are those with normal wall motion.

INFARCTION

The ECG is the most commonly used modality to detect myocardial ischemia and acute MI. Transmural MI presents initially with prominent T waves, hyperacute ST segment elevation, or both. This evolves over minutes, hours, or even days to a pattern of significant Q waves (i.e., >40 msec duration, >30% of QRS amplitude) or persistent ST-T wave changes. Subendocardial (non-Q-wave) MI is less clearly defined because it may present only as subtle ST-wave or T-wave changes. Detection of non-Q-wave MI often relies on other modalities (e.g., CK, cardiac-specific troponins, transesophageal echocardiographic radionuclide imaging) to confirm the diagnosis. Most perioperative MIs are subendocardial in nature.

Serum CK exceeds the normal range within 4 to 8 hours following acute MI and declines to normal by 2 to 3 days. Three isoenzymes of CK (BB, MM, MB) have been identified. Brain and kidney contain predominantly BB, skeletal muscle MM (with 1% to 3% MB), and myocardium both MM and MB (isoforms MB_1 and MB_2). One study found 59% and 92% sensitivity for the diagnosis of acute MI at 2 to 4 and 4 to 6 hours, respectively, for $CKMB_2$ greater than 1 unit/L or $CKMB_2/CKMB_1$ ratio greater than 1.5.

Cardiac troponins are highly sensitive and specific chemical markers for myocardial necrosis and predict increased risk of mortality and reinfarction in patients presenting with acute coronary syndrome. The troponin (Tn) complex consists of three subunits (TnC, TnI, TnT) that regulate calcium-mediated contraction in striated muscle. TnC binds to calcium, TnI binds to actin, and TnT binds to tropomyosin. Both TnI and TnT are present in skeletal and cardiac muscle, but they are encoded by different genes and have different amino acid sequences. This permits the production of specific antibodies for cardiac Tn (cTn) and the development of quantitative assays for cTnI and cTnT. In patients with acute MI, cTnT and cTnI levels first begin to rise above their normal reference limits by 3 hours after the onset of chest pain. Elevations of cTnI may persist for 7 to 10 days, and cTnT for 10 to 14 days, following acute MI. The kinetics of release are similar in those with Q-wave or non-Q-wave acute MI. The assay for cTnI is currently the most sensitive and specific marker of myocardial injury. In surgical patients, cardiac troponins have been shown to identify postoperative MI better than CKMB isoenzymes.

Finally, the cTnT assay is probably capable of detecting episodes of myocardial necrosis below the detection limit of current CKMB assays. Hence the terms *minor myocardial damage* and *microinfarction* have been coined to describe myocardial changes in patients with chest pain and elevated TnT but normal CKMB levels. Regardless, it is well established that such patients are at increased risk for an adverse clinical outcome (e.g., recurrent MI, need for revascularization, death).

Risk Assessment

Most studies have focused on historical predictors of cardiac risk discovered during preoperative assessment. Of these, only recent MI (<6 months) and congestive heart failure are significant predictors of perioperative cardiac morbidity. New data show that postoperative ischemia is also a significant predictor of subsequent cardiac morbidity.

All cardiac surgical patients are considered at risk for the development of perioperative ischemia, which may occur preoperatively (up to 20% of patients), intraoperatively (up to 50% of patients), and postoperatively (up to 30% of patients). A smaller proportion of noncardiac surgical patients are at risk for perioperative ischemia, depending on their underlying disease. In such patients, most ischemic episodes occur postoperatively.

Contributing factors to perioperative myocardial ischemia are listed in Table 76-1. Traditionally, increases in myocardial oxygen demand were thought to be the most important causes of perioperative ischemia; however, recent data reveal that decreases in supply may also be a significant cause.

Coronary artery vasoconstriction or vasospasm and thrombosis likely account for a large percentage of episodes of perioperative ischemia that occur without hemodynamic aberrations. Also, because oxygen extraction is near maximum in working myocardium, maintenance of normal blood oxygen content is critical in the presence of restrictions to coronary flow.

Implications

Myocardial ischemia may initiate both systolic and diastolic myocardial dysfunction, lead to arrhythmias, or progress to MI. There is a proven association between the occurrence of perioperative ischemia and increased cardiac morbidity and mortality. Moreover, studies suggest a causal relationship between perioperative ischemia and MI. In cardiac surgical patients, intraoperative ischemia exhibits the strongest correlation with perioperative MI. In noncardiac surgical patients, postoperative ischemia exhibits the strongest correlation with perioperative MI. Perioperative MI increases mortality in both cardiac and noncardiac surgical patients.

Development of acute MI is often preceded by a period of myocardial ischemia. Thus, early detection of perioperative myocardial ischemia should prompt therapeutic measures to relieve the ischemia, thereby reducing the incidence or size of any subsequent MI.

MANAGEMENT

Management of perioperative myocardial ischemia is based on interventions that decrease myocardial oxygen demand or increase its oxygen supply (Table 76-2).

Nitroglycerin. Nitroglycerin reduces myocardial oxygen demand by lowering left ventricular end-diastolic volume and afterload. It increases oxygen delivery by coronary artery vasodilatation and a reduction in left ventricular end-diastolic volume. Nitroglycerin is often the initial drug of choice for the management of perioperative myocardial ischemia. However, if such ischemia is associated with tachycardia, β-blockers are also indicated.

Table 76–1 ▪ Factors that Contribute to Myocardial Ischemia

Increased Myocardial Oxygen Demand
Increased heart rate
Increased contractility
Increased left ventricular end-diastolic volume
Increased wall tension (afterload)

Decreased Myocardial Oxygen Supply
Decreased coronary blood flow
 Vasoconstriction
 Thrombosis
 Decreased diastolic time
 Decreased aortic diastolic pressure
 Increased ventricular end-diastolic pressure
Decreased blood oxygen content
 Decreased hematocrit
 Decreased oxygen saturation

Table 76–2 ▪ Management of Myocardial Ischemia

Reduce Myocardial Oxygen Demand
Decrease heart rate
Decrease contractility
Decrease left ventricular end-diastolic volume
Reduce afterload

Increase Myocardial Oxygen Supply
Increase coronary blood flow
 Decrease vasoconstriction
 Decrease thrombosis
 Increase diastolic time
 Increase aortic diastolic pressure
 Reduce ventricular end-diastolic pressure
Increase blood oxygen content
 Optimize hematocrit
 Increase oxygen saturation

β-Blockers. β-Blockers decrease myocardial oxygen demand by reducing heart rate and contractility. They increase oxygen supply by increasing diastolic time and reducing ventricular wall stress, especially in patients with left ventricular hypertrophy. Recent data indicate that β-adrenergic antagonists may decrease morbidity and mortality associated with myocardial ischemia and MI.

Calcium Channel Blockers. The calcium channel blockers diltiazem and verapamil, but not the dihydropyridine calcium channel blockers (e.g., nicardipine), decrease myocardial oxygen demand by reducing heart rate and contractility and may increase oxygen supply via coronary artery vasodilatation,[1] an increase in diastolic time, or a reduction in wall stress. Although still somewhat controversial, dihydropyridines such as sublingual nifedipine or intravenous nicardipine may be specifically indicated when coronary artery vasospasm is suspected.

α-Adrenergic Agonists. α_1-Receptor agonists can increase myocardial oxygen supply by increasing aortic diastolic blood pressure, but they may also increase myocardial oxygen demand by increasing left ventricular end-diastolic volume and wall stress. α_1-Agonists also have the potential to cause coronary artery vasoconstriction or vasospasm. These drugs should be used cautiously, and only in patients who would clearly benefit from systemic vasoconstriction and increased aortic diastolic pressure.[2] α_2-Receptor agonists reduce central nervous system sympathetic efferent tone. This leads to decreased myocardial oxygen demand secondary to reduced heart rate, blood pressure, and left ventricular end-diastolic volume and wall stress (i.e., dilatation of splanchnic venous capacitance bed).

Sodium Nitroprusside. The physiologic benefits of sodium nitroprusside are similar to those of nitroglycerin, with the added benefit of afterload reduction. However, the precise role of sodium nitroprusside in the management of myocardial ischemia is controversial because of the possibility of coronary artery steal (from vasodilatation of coronary artery resistance vessels).[3]

β-Receptor Agonists. The physiologic effects of β-agonists may be beneficial (decreased left ventricular diastolic volume, increased aortic diastolic pressure) or detrimental (increased heart rate, reduced diastolic time, increased contractility). Their precise role, if any, in the management of myocardial ischemia is determined by the specific clinical hemodynamic aberration present.

Phosphodiesterase Inhibitors. The physiologic benefits are similar to those of β-adrenergic agonists. However, systemic and pulmonary vasodilatation, along with little effect on heart rate, makes these drugs more appealing than the traditional β-adrenergic agonists.

In summary, if myocardial ischemia occurs in association with tachycardia or hypertension, initially one must ensure adequate anesthesia, oxygenation, and ventilation. If all of these are present, nitroglycerin or β-blockers (or both) should be used. If myocardial ischemia is associated with tachycardia and hypotension, judicious volume expansion or careful use of α_1-receptor agonists is instituted. If ischemia is associated with a normal heart rate and hypotension, therapy should be directed toward the suspected cause of hypotension (e.g., left ventricular pump failure, hypovolemia, reduced systemic vascular resistance). Intra-aortic balloon counterpulsation, via afterload reduction and diastolic augmentation, may also be beneficial and should be considered. When ischemia is not associated with hemodynamic aberrations, coronary vasodilator drugs (e.g., nitroglycerin) or those that both dilate coronary arteries and relieve coronary vasospasm (e.g., nifedipine,[4] nicardipine) are used.

PREVENTION

Perioperative myocardial ischemia and infarction result from a complex interaction among hemodynamic parameters, vascular tone, neural influences, and the coagulation system. Most attempts to prevent perioperative ischemia and infarction (especially with a single drug) have failed. Patients receiving cardiac medications should continue taking them until the time of operation. Preoperative antiischemic therapy should be directed at optimizing the cause of ischemia (myocardial oxygen supply and demand imbalance) and treating its consequences (e.g., congestive heart failure, arrhythmias). Anesthesia should be administered to maintain stable perioperative hemodynamic parameters. No evidence exists that the type of anesthesia (general versus regional, inhalation versus intravenous) affects the incidence of perioperative ischemia or MI in patients at risk. However, prophylactic use of β-blockers may significantly decrease the incidence of perioperative ischemia and subsequent cardiac morbidity. Prophylactic perioperative nitroglycerin is controversial, and the role of drugs that reduce the risk of coronary thrombosis remains to be determined.

Aggressive control of postoperative pain with regional anesthesia and analgesia to attenuate associated stress may decrease cardiac morbidity and mortality in both cardiac and noncardiac surgical patients. Perioperative use of thoracic epidural anesthesia with local anesthetics may benefit all patients by blocking cardiac sympathetic efferent activity and improving the balance between myocardial oxygen demand and supply. Finally, studies have revealed that maintenance of normothermia may decrease perioperative myocardial ischemia and subsequent cardiac morbidity.

---

[1]It is likely that diltiazem and verapamil also relieve coronary vasospasm.

[2]Many believe that α_1-mediated venoconstriction of the splanchnic venous capacitance bed (increasing venous return and preload) is mechanistically more important for any noted blood pressure increase than increased systemic vascular resistance per se.

[3]Sodium nitroprusside also dilates the venous capacitance bed to reduce venous return and left ventricular preload. This enhances the effect of systemic arterial vasodilatation to reduce blood pressure.

[4]Caution: Nifedipine is not available in intravenous form. It is available in capsule form for oral or sublingual use. However, owing to variable absorption after sublingual dosing and potentially adverse hemodynamic actions due to the drug's polysorbate vehicle (direct depression of myocardial contractility, systemic venous and arterial dilatation), in 1985 the Food and Drug Administration advised against using nifedipine in hypertensive emergencies. Among the adverse effects reported with sublingual nifedipine in this setting were fatalities due to acute MI.

CARDIOTHORACIC & VASCULAR SURGERY

Further Reading

Antman EM, Braunwald E: Acute myocardial infarction. In Braunwald E (ed): Heart Disease, 5th ed. Philadelphia, WB Saunders, 1997, pp 1184-1188.

Apple FS, Wu AHB: Myocardial infarction redefined: Role of cardiac troponin testing. Clin Chem 47:337-339, 2001.

Badner NH, Knill RL, Brown JE, et al: Myocardial infarction after non-cardiac surgery. Anesthesiology 88:572-578, 1998.

Beattie C, Fleisher LA: Perioperative myocardial ischemia and infarction: Preface. Int Anesthesiol Clin 30:xix-xxii, 1992.

Brown CS, Bertolet BD: Cardiac troponin: See ya later, CK! Chest 111:2-4, 1997.

Carrier M, Pellerin M, Perrault LP, et al: Troponin levels in patients with myocardial infarction after coronary artery bypass grafting. Ann Thorac Surg 69:435-440, 2000.

Chaney MA: Intrathecal and epidural anesthesia and analgesia for cardiac surgery. Anesth Analg 84:1211-1221, 1997.

Duke PC (ed): Myocardial ischemia and performance. Anesthesiol Clin North Am 9:455-730, 1991.

Fleisher LA, Barash PG: Preoperative cardiac evaluation for noncardiac surgery: A functional approach. Anesth Analg 74:586-598, 1992.

Keats AS: Adventures in perioperative myocardial ischemia. Texas Heart Inst J 20:5-11, 1993.

Leslie JB: Prevention and treatment of intraoperative myocardial ischemia Anesth Analg 84(Suppl):79-89, 1997.

Mangano DT: Perioperative cardiac morbidity. Anesthesiology 72:153-184, 1990.

Mangano DT, Goldman L: Preoperative assessment of patients with known or suspected coronary disease. N Engl J Med 333:1750-1756, 1995.

Perez-Carceles MD, Osuna E, Vieira DN, et al: Biochemical assessment of acute myocardial ischaemia. J Clin Pathol 48:124-128, 1995.

Perioperative Hypertension

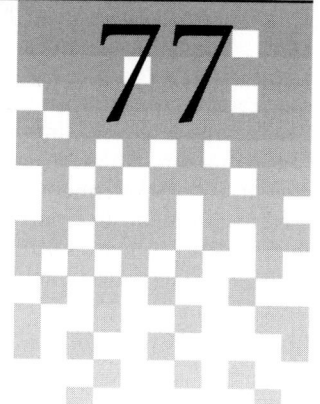

77

Jerrold H. Levy and Kenichi A. Tanaka

Case Synopsis

A 58-year-old man has just had abdominal aortic aneurysm repair. He is noted to be hypertensive, with a blood pressure of 160/110 mm Hg. His heart rate is 72 beats per minute in sinus rhythm, pulmonary artery pressure is 45/25 mm Hg, pulmonary artery occlusion pressure is 6 mm Hg, and central venous pressure is 5 mm Hg. The patient also has ST segment depression in the anterior precordial electrocardiogram (ECG) leads. Preoperative evaluation revealed no prior history of hypertension, but a history of peripheral vascular disease.

PROBLEM ANALYSIS

Definition

The definition of perioperative hypertension differs from that of chronic hypertension. Perioperatively, patients may have acute changes in blood pressure (BP) because of multiple factors, including rapid intravenous volume shifts and changes in sympathetic tone secondary to surgical stimulation, stress responses, or pain. Patients with otherwise normal BP may develop hypertension perioperatively because of these factors. Also, because oral antihypertensive therapy is not possible at this time, patients require parenteral treatment. Hypertension is a major problem after both cardiac and noncardiac surgery. The incidence of postoperative hypertension ranges from 6% to 20% in various noncardiac surgical studies, occurring more commonly in patients with preoperative hypertension, irrespective of anesthetic regimen.

Recognition

Because BP monitoring is an essential part of perioperative management, either invasive or noninvasive methods may be acceptable for diagnosis and institution of therapy. In cardiac surgical patients, BP is usually kept at lower levels to avoid graft or suture line disruption. Based on data collected from an international survey, hypertension following cardiac surgery is defined as a sustained BP greater than 140/90 mm Hg. When pressures exceed this, most anesthesiologists institute therapy. Recently, new BP guidelines in medical patients were formulated following the Seventh Report of the Joint National Committee on Prevention, Detection, Evaluation, and Treatment of High Blood Pressure.

Risk Assessment

Reported risk factors for hypertension in the postanesthesia care unit include increasing age, smoking, and renal disease. Patients with a preoperative history of angina and those with inadequate ventilation during the postoperative period are also at increased risk for hypertension. Hypertension and tachycardia are associated with increased long-term morbidity and mortality. Preexisting hypertension is also a risk factor.

Hypertension following surgery for coronary artery bypass grafting has been reported in 30% to 80% of patients. Augmentation of the stress response because of cardiopulmonary bypass has been suggested as the pathophysiologic basis of increased vascular resistance. Other factors to consider are rapid weaning from mechanical ventilation following cardiac surgery and coronary graft spasm. Ventricular dysfunction is common even in patients with normal preoperative function.

Implications

When to treat perioperative hypertension and how rapidly to decrease the BP are not well-resolved issues. Management goals to maintain hemodynamic stability depend on many factors, especially preoperative BP—that is, the patient's "normal" pressure. There are few data to guide management, and in selected patients (e.g., neurosurgical and cardiac surgical patients), BP may be kept at even lower values immediately following surgery to avoid complications such as hemorrhage, rupture of suture lines, cerebrovascular accidents, myocardial ischemia, and arrhythmias.

MANAGEMENT

Therapeutic approaches to perioperative hypertension include the following:

- Intravenous vasodilators, dihydropyridine (DHP) calcium channel blockers such as nicardipine,[1] dopamine receptor agonists (fenoldopam), hydralazine, or, potentially, angiotensin-converting enzyme (ACE) inhibitors (enalaprilat)
- Intravenous β-adrenergic blockers
- Deepening anesthesia

Vasodilators

Nitroprusside and nitroglycerin release nitric oxide to produce arterial vasodilatation and venodilatation, which

---

[1]Clevidepine, another rapid-acting DHP calcium channel blocker, is similar to nicardipine and has a similar hemodynamic profile. It, too, is suitable for intravenous administration and was set to enter phase III clinical trials in 2005.

contribute significantly to the labile hemodynamic state. In a hypertensive patient, intravenous volume administration is often used to allow nitroprusside to be infused when the patient is hypovolemic.[2] Although nitroprusside is often used to control postoperative hypertension in other surgical interventions, it may contribute to myocardial ischemia by producing nonspecific coronary vasodilatation and coronary steal. Hydralazine, a more arterioselective vasodilator, is also used in obstetric patients and in perioperative settings, often concomitantly with a β-blocker.

Calcium Channel Blockers

There are three types of calcium channel blockers: verapamil, diltiazem, and the DHPs (e.g., nicardipine). Vasodilatation can be produced by any of these drugs, which reduce calcium entry into vascular smooth muscle. DHP calcium channel blockers act by binding with high affinity to the L-type calcium channels, which modulates their voltage-dependent calcium conductivity. DHPs are mainly dilators of the peripheral resistance arteries. In doses that effectively reduce BP, the DHPs have little or no direct negative effect on cardiac contractility or conduction. Their lack of negative chronotropic effect allows an initial reflex increase in heart rate, which decreases during prolonged antihypertensive treatment. Calcium channel blockers do not affect venous smooth muscle; therefore, unlike nitrodilators, they are not venodilators and have little influence on filling pressure and preload. As a result, cardiac output is well maintained or increased when calcium channel blockers are given to reduce arterial pressure. Nicardipine also is a potent coronary and cerebral vasodilator, with important applications in neurosurgical and cardiac surgical patients.

Other Agents

Although ACE inhibitors are widely used to treat heart failure, the only intravenous form available is enalaprilat, an indirect-acting agent that is used on occasion to treat perioperative hypertension. ACE inhibitors are complex drugs that interfere with angiotensin II synthesis and may increase nitric oxide release from blood vessels by increasing bradykinin levels. Specific dopamine (DA) receptor agonists are a new class of agents that are under clinical investigation. Fenoldopam, a selective agonist to peripheral DA_1-receptors, produces vasodilatation, increases renal perfusion, and enhances natriuresis but may have variable effects on BP and heart rate.

β-Adrenergic Blockers

β-Adrenergic blockers reduce heart rate and myocardial contractility, decreasing cardiac output and thus reducing both diastolic and systolic BP. Therefore, β-blockers should be considered in treating perioperative hypertension in patients with tachycardia. Because heart rate is a major determinant of myocardial blood supply, tachycardia must be treated aggressively in patients with ischemic heart disease, and β-blockers should be used as first-line therapeutic agents. Several β-blockers can be administered intravenously and are used as antihypertensive agents in the perioperative period: propranolol, metoprolol, atenolol, esmolol, and labetalol. Distinct advantages of esmolol are its short elimination half-life (<10 minutes) and $β_1$-selectivity.

Deepening Anesthesia

Increasing anesthetic depth is always a potential means of treating increased BP during surgery, but it may not always be possible or effective. Regional anesthetic techniques may also be effective at preventing perioperative hypertension. Not to be overlooked is the effect of positive-pressure ventilation or continuous positive airway pressure to impede venous return, effectively reducing preload and systemic BP.

PREVENTION

Perioperative hypertension commonly occurs as part of the normal response to induction, surgery, emergence, and pain. Continuing treatment for chronic hypertension is important in the perioperative management of hemodynamic stability. Increasing use of regional anesthetic techniques to better control perioperative pain may also have important effects in preventing perioperative hypertension. Although increasing anesthetic depth can be effective in maintaining hemodynamic control, this technique may not always be feasible; thus, use of the specific antihypertensive agents reviewed here may be required.

Further Reading

Aronson S, Boisvert D, Lapp W: Isolated systolic hypertension is associated with adverse outcomes from coronary artery bypass grafting surgery. Anesth Analg 94:1079-1084, 2002.

Bailey JM, Tanaka KA, Levy JH: Cardiac surgical pharmacology. In Cohn LH, Edmunds H (eds): Adult Cardiac Surgery, 2nd ed. New York, McGraw-Hill, 2003, pp 85-118.

Rose DK, Cohen MM, DeBoer, et al: Cardiovascular events in the postanesthesia care unit: Contribution of risk factors. Anesthesiology 84: 772-781, 1996.

Seventh Report of the Joint National Committee on Prevention, Detection, Evaluation, and Treatment of High Blood Pressure (JNC 7). Available at www.nhlbi.nih.gov/guidelines/hypertension/.

Tanaka KA, Tsuda A, Yamaguchi K, et al: In vitro effects of antihypertensive drugs on thromboxane agonist (U46619)-induced vasoconstriction in human internal mammary artery. Br J Anaesth 93:257-262, 2004.

Vuylsteke A, Feneck RO, Jolin-Mellgard A, et al: Perioperative blood pressure control: A prospective survey of patient management in cardiac surgery. J Cardiothorac Vasc Anesth 14:269-273, 2000.

---

[2]Nitroprusside has prominent vasodilatory effects on the venous capacitance bed (i.e., is a potent venodilator) in addition to its arteriodilator effect. Venodilatation reduces venous return and cardiac preload. Because patients with chronic hypertension are often preload restricted—an adaptive response to chronic increased systemic vascular resistance and ventricular wall stress (i.e., afterload)—they may become relatively hypovolemic when given antihypertensive drugs with prominent venodilator effects.

Postoperative Pulmonary Hypertension

Isobel Muhiudeen-Russell and James E. Baker

Case Synopsis

A 46-year-old woman with primary pulmonary hypertension requires assessment in the postanesthesia care unit. She underwent laparoscopy for acute cholecystitis but required conversion to an open procedure (via a right subcostal incision) to remove the gallbladder. She was mechanically ventilated for 2 hours postoperatively but has since been extubated. Her blood pressure is 78/50 mm Hg, with a heart rate of 110 beats per minute (sinus rhythm). Oxygen saturation is 93% despite receiving oxygen via a facemask with a reservoir bag. A pulmonary artery catheter was placed in the operating room, and her pulmonary artery pressure is 75/45 mm Hg. Temperature is 35.5°C. The patient is dyspneic, complains of moderate abdominal pain, and appears to be splinting, with rapid, shallow tidal volumes. Her blood pressure has not improved despite a volume challenge with 250 mL of intravenous colloid solution.

PROBLEM ANALYSIS

Definition

Pulmonary artery pressure (PAP) is normally substantially lower than systemic arterial blood pressure. Mean PAP greater than 25 mm Hg, or peak pressure greater than 40 mm Hg, is usually interpreted as pulmonary hypertension. Degrees of pulmonary hypertension are inconsistently defined and may be classified as mild (systolic PAP 40 to 49 mm Hg), moderate (systolic PAP 50 to 59 mm Hg), or severe (systolic PAP 60 mm Hg or above). In keeping with its low-pressure workload, the right ventricle (RV) is a low-pressure, thin-walled structure, but it is able to transmit all its blood to the left atrium owing to the large cross-sectional area and high compliance of the pulmonary vascular bed. Indeed, whereas systemic vascular resistance (SVR) is normally 900 to 1500 dynes•sec•cm^{-5}, pulmonary vascular resistance (PVR) is usually 90 to 120 dynes•sec•cm^{-5} (1.1 to 1.5 Wood's units).

Thus, pulmonary hypertension is due to either increased PVR, which requires a commensurate increase in the pressure generated by the RV, or a hyperdynamic cardiac state that increases PAP despite a normal PVR.

Many disease entities that elevate PVR are chronic processes that, in addition to damaging pulmonary parenchyma, damage or destroy pulmonary blood vessels at both the arteriolar and capillary levels. Notable causes of pulmonary hypertension are listed in Table 78-1 and include chronic obstructive pulmonary disease and interstitial lung disease.

Less commonly, pulmonary hypertension due to increased PVR may be congenital (persistent pulmonary hypertension of the newborn) or acquired as an idiopathic entity (primary pulmonary hypertension), as exemplified by the case synopsis. Also, systemic or extrathoracic disease processes may act on previously normal lungs to increase PVR (see Table 78-1).

Abnormal cardiac physiology may cause secondary pulmonary hypertension in the absence of elevated PVR.

Table 78–1 ■ Causes of and Risk Factors for Pulmonary Hypertension

Idiopathic (primary pulmonary hypertension)
Congenital heart disease with increased pulmonary artery blood flow or pressure
Cardiac disease with elevated left atrial pressure (e.g., left-sided valvular disease or left ventricular failure)
Respiratory system disorders with pulmonary parenchymal or vascular damage
   Chronic obstructive pulmonary disease
   Interstitial lung disease (idiopathic or secondary to rheumatoid arthritis, systemic lupus erythematosus, sarcoidosis)
Alveolar hypoxemia (e.g., obstructive sleep apnea, chronic high-altitude exposure)
Chronic pulmonary thrombosis or thromboembolism (also, sickle cell disease)
Congenital (e.g., persistent pulmonary hypertension of the newborn)
Portal hypertension
Compression of pulmonary veins (e.g., by tumor, lymphadenopathy, anastomotic stricture after lung transplantation)
Miscellaneous causes
   Drugs or toxins
   Infections, including schistosomiasis and opportunistic infections with human immunodeficiency virus

Congenital heart disease with left-to-right intracardiac shunting may cause pulmonary hypertension by subjecting the lungs to increased blood flow (e.g., atrial septal defect) or backpressure from the left ventricle (LV; e.g., ventricular septal defect). Also, any cardiac disease that leads to increased left atrial pressure (e.g., dilated cardiomyopathy, ischemic heart disease, mitral stenosis) can also result in pulmonary hypertension, because mean PAP must be sufficiently higher than left atrial pressure to allow blood to flow through the pulmonary vasculature. Unfortunately, many sustained processes that begin as pulmonary hypertension with a normal PVR eventually lead to pulmonary arterial and arteriolar remodeling. This compounds the problem by causing a secondary increase in PVR. Such pulmonary remodeling includes increased muscularity of the medial layer, thickening of the connective tissue within the adventitial layer, and abnormal pulmonary endothelial regulatory function. These changes are usually at least partially irreversible and may perpetuate pulmonary hypertension, even when the underlying hemodynamic problem is corrected.

Recognition and Risk Assessment

The ability to recognize pulmonary hypertension has important perioperative implications. It begins with being able to recognize which patients are at risk. When reviewing the patient's preoperative history, special note should be made of congenital heart disease (whether corrected or not) and chronic pulmonary disease. Such patients constitute the majority of those at risk for significant perioperative pulmonary hypertension, but the other predisposing factors (see Table 78-1) should also be kept in mind. In some of these patients, pulmonary hypertension may have been diagnosed already, and they may have undergone an evaluation to define or quantify the problem. Cardiac catheterization is the gold standard for diagnosing pulmonary hypertension, although noninvasive echocardiography can also be used. In the absence of preoperative information that specifically confirms the diagnosis of pulmonary hypertension, a chest radiograph may show evidence of right-sided cardiac enlargement, and the electrocardiogram may show right axis deviation, right atrial enlargement, or an RV strain pattern.

In the case synopsis, a pulmonary artery catheter was inserted preoperatively, prompted by the prior diagnosis of primary pulmonary hypertension. In such instances, the pulmonary artery catheter can confirm any significant elevation in PAP. Generally, mean PAP greater than 40 mm Hg or greater than two thirds of systemic arterial pressure can be interpreted as severe pulmonary hypertension. Although no degree of pulmonary hypertension is necessarily associated with adverse consequences, no degree is necessarily safe either. Indeed, many patients with pulmonary hypertension may tolerate PAP levels that appear quite alarming. Others may suffer adverse consequences even with relatively minor elevations, especially when the increase is acute. The difference is probably related to the RV's ability to adapt to chronically elevated afterload by concentric hypertrophy, as does the LV in patients with systemic hypertension. Finally, many stresses related to surgery or the conduct of anesthesia influence the degree of perioperative pulmonary hypertension and patient tolerance.

Implications

It must be remembered that the real significance of perioperative pulmonary hypertension is not its presence or any particular degree of hypertension but rather the RV's ability to tolerate any increased afterload. Although pulmonary hypertension is an important cause of hemodynamic instability, the pattern depends on the RV's inability to eject against increased afterload and to provide adequate LV filling to maintain cardiac output. As the RV fails, both its diastolic and systolic dimensions increase, displacing the ventricular septum to the left. LV function is subsequently impaired due to inadequate diastolic filling and its inability to adequately contract during systole. RV coronary perfusion is also reduced due to RV wall stretching and intracavitary hypertension (recall that unlike the LV, the RV normally receives significant coronary perfusion during systole and is therefore vulnerable to increased systolic and diastolic intracavitary pressures). If systemic hypotension develops from reduced LV stroke volume, RV coronary perfusion pressure is further reduced, and the problem becomes self-propagating. Severe shock and cardiovascular collapse may be the ultimate expression of postoperative pulmonary hypertension.

MANAGEMENT

Although pulmonary hypertension can be difficult to manage, especially when it is chronic and associated with pulmonary vascular remodeling, treatment is based on evidence that elevated PVR may be at least partly reversible. In any event, some factors may actually aggravate PVR, and care must be taken to avoid them to the extent possible. Table 78-2 summarizes the current approach to management.

Ventilatory Management

Ventilation has an important impact on PVR and may worsen or improve pulmonary hypertension. Either a very high fraction of inspired oxygen (FiO_2 1.0) or severely reduced arterial carbon dioxide tension ($PaCO_2$ <30 mm Hg; significant respiratory alkalosis) may appreciably improve PVR. To reduce PVR, especially with respiratory acidosis, one can increase minute ventilation to lower $PaCO_2$ (keeping it >20 mm Hg) or increase pH (keeping it <7.6). It is likely that pH mediates changes in pulmonary arteriolar tone, not $PaCO_2$ itself. Therefore, if pulmonary parenchymal disease precludes this degree of hyperventilation, systemic alkalinization (sodium bicarbonate) might be considered.

Ventilatory management must be conducted to avoid significant increases in lung volume and airway pressure. As lung volumes increase above functional residual capacity, the alveolar capillaries are stretched. This can lead to progressive collapse and reduction in the total cross-sectional area of the pulmonary capillary bed. Conversely, low lung volumes may contribute to the collapse of extra-alveolar vessels and alveolar atelectasis. The former directly increases PVR, whereas the latter increases it through hypoxic pulmonary vasoconstriction.

Table 78–2 ▪ Management of Severe Pulmonary Hypertension with Right Ventricular Heart Failure

Type of Treatment	Features of Therapy
Conservative and remedial measures to lower PVR	High FiO$_2$; avoid hypercarbia and acidosis; correct respiratory alkalosis (pH <7.6); avoid hypothermia or shivering; prevent both alveolar collapse and overdistention; optimize pain control
Pharmacologic therapy to lower PVR	Nitrates; PGE$_1$; inhaled NO; prostacyclin
Inotropic support for right ventricle	Milrinone, dobutamine, or isoproterenol for adequate SAP; norepinephrine or epinephrine if SAP is marginal or inadequate
Maintenance of coronary perfusion	Add α-adrenergic agonist (e.g., phenylephrine) to a combined inotrope-vasodilator (e.g., milrinone); consider norepinephrine for combined inotropic support and elevation of SAP; avoid RV distention
Optimization of RV preload	Avoid RV distention and underfilling; consider invasive (RAP or PAP) monitoring or transesophageal echocardiography where appropriate
Mechanical support	RV assist device; intra-aortic balloon pump

FiO$_2$, fraction of inspired oxygen; NO, nitric oxide; PAP, pulmonary artery pressure; PGE$_1$, prostaglandin E$_1$; PVR, pulmonary vascular resistance; RAP, right atrial pressure; RV, right ventricular; SAP, systemic systolic arterial blood pressure.

Other Nonpharmacologic Management

Other factors that may promote acutely elevated PVR and PAP include hypothermia, excess circulating catecholamines due to light anesthesia or uncontrolled postoperative pain, and sepsis. Patients having cardiac surgery are vulnerable to increased PVR due to an increase in circulating inflammatory mediators associated with cardiopulmonary bypass. Although not all of these factors can be controlled, it is important to maintain or reestablish normothermia postoperatively and to treat or prevent postoperative pain as effectively as possible.

Pharmacologic Management

Pharmacologic management of pulmonary hypertension is undertaken to (1) lower PVR directly, (2) support RV inotropic function, and (3) maintain sufficient systemic arterial blood pressure for adequate RV coronary perfusion. Many drugs reduce PVR and have been used in patients with pulmonary hypertension. Nitroglycerin, nitroprusside, calcium channel antagonists, and especially prostaglandin E$_1$ may be effective in reducing PVR and PAP. However, all these drugs have the same limitation: lack of specificity for the pulmonary vasculature. To whatever extent PVR is lowered by these agents, SVR may be similarly decreased. Given the importance of maintaining adequate RV coronary perfusion pressure, any significant reduction in SVR may be poorly tolerated and precipitate acute RV failure. Similarly, some inotropes, such as dobutamine, isoproterenol, and milrinone, are well known for their ability to lower PVR while also increasing inotropy, but use of these drugs is limited by their potential to reduce SVR and cause systemic hypotension when coronary perfusion pressure must be maintained. Use of α-agonists (e.g., phenylephrine) to reduce systemic hypotension may negate any salutary effects of other drugs given to reduce PVR. Thus, inotropes or systemic vasodilators that are also pulmonary vasodilators may be used with caution in patients with preserved systemic blood pressure, but the possibility of an overall deleterious effect

and the need to support systemic blood pressure should be kept in mind.

Although intravenous drugs that selectively reduce PVR are lacking, inhaled nitric oxide (NO) directly dilates the pulmonary vasculature. By virtue of its rapid degradation by circulating hemoglobin, its vasodilating action is effectively confined to the pulmonary vasculature; SVR is not significantly altered. NO dosages range from 10 parts per million (ppm) to a maximum of 80 ppm. These doses reduce RV afterload without compromising systemic blood pressure or coronary perfusion. Beneficial effects are achieved with NO in many perioperative and critical care settings, including lung or heart transplantation and surgery for congenital heart disease. Improved ventilation-perfusion matching and arterial oxygen tension (PaO$_2$) may also be achieved because inhaled NO increases blood flow to those lung units that are best ventilated. Inhaled prostacyclin also selectively lowers PVR in patients with pulmonary hypertension.

Although norepinephrine has the potential to increase PVR, it has been used successfully in many patients with critical pulmonary hypertension. In fact, it is preferred when systemic blood pressure is low or marginal. Owing to well-balanced α- and β-adrenergic effects, coronary perfusion pressure is well maintained or improved, while RV contractility is enhanced. To the extent that high left-sided heart pressures contribute to pulmonary hypertension (e.g., severe mitral valve disease, ischemic LV failure), inotropic support for the LV may also reduce RV afterload by lowering left atrial pressure.

Judicious volume therapy is important in patients with impaired RV function. An excessively low RV preload reduces cardiac output. However, RV overload increases RV wall stress, reduces coronary perfusion (via increased RV intracavitary pressure), and worsens tricuspid insufficiency. Most patients with severely elevated PAP, especially with RV failure or tricuspid insufficiency, do not require more RV preload unless volume or blood loss is significant. If so, any volume loading should be done with caution. For example, patients without improved hemodynamics after a 250-mL colloid or blood product challenge are unlikely to benefit from more volume.

Also, invasive monitoring may be of some help. A central venous or right atrial pressure greater than 15 mm Hg suggests that more volume is unlikely to be beneficial. If available, transesophageal echocardiography provides the best assessment of left- or right-sided intracardiac volume status.

PREVENTION

Unfortunately, pulmonary hypertension severe enough to cause perioperative RV failure is likely the result of a chronic or preexisting condition. Although it cannot be prevented, it may be mitigated or optimized by careful anesthetic management. An exception is new-onset or aggravated pulmonary hypertension caused by intraoperative protamine. This can be prevented by giving the drug more slowly or not giving it at all in patients with a history of protamine-associated pulmonary hypertension.

Most other pulmonary hypertension cases, and any attendant cardiac dysfunction, should be diagnosed and quantified during preoperative assessment. Then perioperative management can be adjusted to prevent the development of further PAP increases in at-risk patients. This may require PAP monitoring, transesophageal echocardiography, or both to assess the effects of surgical stress and anesthetic drugs and techniques on PVR, cardiac output, and RV function.

Most nonpharmacologic strategies for treating pulmonary hypertension are also used in preventive intraoperative management for high-risk patients. Ventilator and overall blood gas management should aim to promote appropriate alveolar expansion, oxygenation, and respiratory alkalosis. If possible, agents that might increase PVR (e.g., histamine-releasing muscle relaxants, opioids) should be avoided. If necessary, systemic arterial blood pressure should be supported to maintain RV coronary perfusion. Also, as the case synopsis illustrates, the anesthetic plan must address the need for optimal postoperative pain control, especially when pain impairs ventilatory mechanics. Consider the use of regional analgesia when appropriate, use patient warming devices, and provide an appropriate duration of postoperative mechanical ventilation. Tracheal extubation should be attempted only when the patient is likely to have adequate respiratory mechanics and gas exchange without mechanical assistance.

Further Reading

Fischer LG, Van Aken H, Burkle H: Management of pulmonary hypertension: Physiological and pharmacological considerations for anesthesiologists. Anesth Analg 96:1603-1616, 2003.

Meyer KC, Love RB, Zimmerman JJ: The therapeutic potential of nitric oxide in lung transplantation. Chest 113:1360-1371, 1998.

Stobierska-Dzierzek B, Awad H, Michler RE: The evolving management of acute right-sided heart failure in cardiac transplant recipients. J Am Coll Cardiol 38:923-931, 2001.

Perioperative Tachyarrhythmias

79

John L. Atlee

Case Synopsis

A 62-year-old man sustains sudden-onset monomorphic ventricular tachycardia (Fig. 79-1) after separation from cardiopulmonary bypass (CPB) for aortic valve replacement and coronary artery bypass grafting. The tachycardia terminates with internal cardioversion. The patient is returned to CPB for revision of a vein graft. Subsequent separation from CPB and the early postoperative course are uneventful. However, 16 hours after arrival in the intensive care unit, the patient has atrial fibrillation (Fig. 79-2), which is terminated by cardioversion. Antiarrhythmic drug therapy with intravenous amiodarone is begun. However, atrial fibrillation recurs two times over the next 12 hours. On each occasion, it is terminated by cardioversion. After this, the patient stabilizes. He is continued on intravenous amiodarone, with transition to the oral form during his hospitalization and after discharge home. At 1-year follow-up, there has been no recurrence of atrial fibrillation.

PROBLEM ANALYSIS

Definition

Ventricular tachycardia, ventricular flutter or fibrillation, and atrial flutter or fibrillation commonly complicate cardiovascular and thoracic surgery in the early postoperative course. Indeed, without prophylaxis, the incidence of postoperative atrial flutter or fibrillation approaches 50%, especially after valve repair or replacement. Other tachyarrhythmias that may complicate the perioperative course of patients undergoing cardiothoracic or vascular surgery (or other high-risk surgery in high-risk patients) include paroxysmal supraventricular tachycardia, ectopic (uniform or multiform) atrial tachycardia, and junctional or idioventricular tachycardia. Tachyarrhythmias with ventricular preexcitation (i.e., Wolff-Parkinson-White syndrome) or long QT syndromes are discussed in Chapters 80 and 81, respectively.

Recognition

Electrocardiographic and other features of tachyarrhythmias are provided in Table 79-1. When confronted with a sustained tachyarrhythmia, it is useful (time permitting), for purposes of diagnosis and patient follow-up, to record an electrocardiogram (ECG) rhythm strip and place a copy in the patient's chart. Other attributes that aid in arrhythmia diagnosis are (1) the presence or absence of cannon a waves (indicative of atrioventricualr dissociation), (2) the suddenness of onset and termination (paroxysmal tachycardias), and (3) a gradual rate increase at onset ("warm-up") and slowing at termination ("fade"), which are characteristic of automatic or ectopic, in contrast to reentrant, tachycardias. The latter usually have a more abrupt onset (often following a supraventricular or ventricular extrasystole) and termination. Also, the onset of tachyarrhythmias can often be recognized by a sudden change in the patient's hemodynamic status, which should prompt a look at the ECG monitor.

Risk Assessment

Predisposing factors for perioperative tachyarrhythmias include (1) advanced age; (2) a history of tachyarrhythmias,

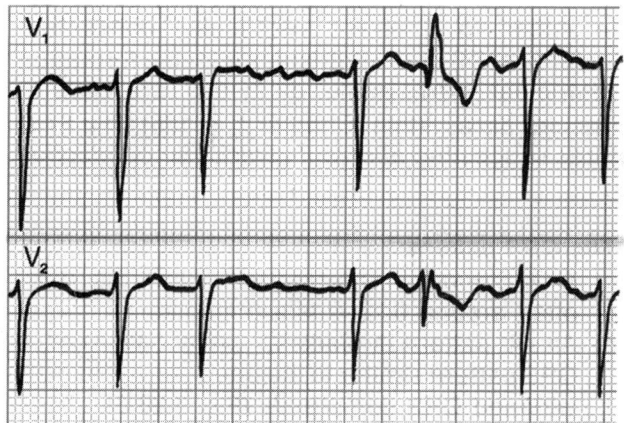

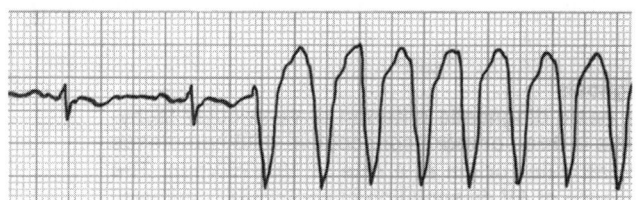

Figure 79–1 ■ Onset of monomorphic ventricular tachycardia.

Figure 79–2 ■ Atrial fibrillation.

Table 79–1 ■ **Characteristic Electrocardiographic Rates and Rhythms of Perioperative Tachyarrhythmias**

Arrhythmia	Rate (bpm)	Rhythm	Comments
Accelerated idioventricular rhythm	A: 50-100* V: 50-110	A: regular V: fairly regular; may be irregular	Hemodynamic insufficiency; intermittent cannon a waves; not amenable to cardioversion
Atrial fibrillation	A: 400-600 V: 100-160	A: highly irregular V: highly irregular	No a waves; ventricular rate slows with CSM but remains highly irregular
Atrial flutter	A: 250-360 V: 75-180	A: regular V: regular (with fixed AVHB) or "regularly" irregular (with varying AVHB)	Flutter waves; ventricular rate slows with CSM but remains "regularly" irregular; type 1 flutter (atrial rate ≤340 bpm) may be converted by rapid atrial pacing
AV junctional tachycardia†	A: 70-130* V: 70-130	A: regular or irregular (with AVHB) V: fairly regular	Hemodynamic insufficiency; intermittent cannon a waves; may slow slightly with vagal maneuvers or β-blocker; not amenable to cardioversion; can be overdriven by atrial pacing
Ectopic atrial tachycardia	A: 100-250 V: ≥100‡	A: abnormal P waves (uniform or multiform); may be irregular V: normal appearance; may be irregular with AVHB	More a waves than c or v waves; possible slowing with vagal maneuvers or CSM, followed by return to usual rate; not amenable to cardioversion
Paroxysmal supraventricular tachycardia	A: 150-250§ V: 150-250	A: very regular (if apparent), except at onset and termination V: very regular, except at onset and termination; normal QRS contour	Constant cannon a waves; CSM or vagal maneuvers may cause abrupt slowing and termination of tachycardia or have no effect
Sinus tachycardia	A: 100-180 V: 100-180	A: regular V: regular unless patient has ≥ second degree AVHB	Rate may gradually slow with CSM or vagal maneuvers, then gradually return to former rate
Ventricular fibrillation	A: 60-100 V: 400-600	A: normal, but difficult to see on surface leads V: grossly irregular and multiform appearance	Cannon a waves; imminently lethal unless early termination by DC defibrillation
Ventricular flutter	A: 60-100* V: 150-300	A: normal, but difficult to see on surface leads V: regular, sine waves	Cannon a waves; imminently lethal unless terminated by DC cardioversion
Ventricular tachycardia	A: 60-100* V: 110-250	A: normal, but often not seen on surface leads unless capture beats are present (confirming VT) V: regular (R-R interval may vary by ≥20 msec in 20% of patients, unless interrupted by capture beats from higher pacemakers	Intermittent cannon a waves; "slow" VT may be tolerated hemodynamically; prompt DC cardioversion recommended for most VT

*Constant and same as ventricular rate (AV junctional tachycardia, accelerated idioventricular rhythm, or ventricular flutter or tachycardia with retrograde atrial activation).
†Also known as accelerated AV junctional rhythm or nonparoxysmal AV junctional tachycardia.
‡Usually <250 bpm or limited by AV block.
§P waves often nonapparent or may be inverted, depending on mechanism for reentry, which could be the AV node or the AV node with retrograde atrial activation via an electrically silent accessory pathway (i.e., the accessory pathway does not conduct from atria to ventricles during sinus rhythm to produce a δ wave associated with ventricular preexcitation).
A, atrial; AV, atrioventricular; AVHB, AV heart block; bpm, beats per minute; CSM, carotid sinus massage; DC, direct current; V, ventricular; VT, ventricular tachycardia.

even if the patient is receiving adequate treatment and is now asymptomatic; (3) cardiovascular or chronic pulmonary disease; (4) the presence of an implanted cardiac rhythm management device (e.g., pacemaker, defibrillator, cardiac resynchronization device); (5) hepatic or renal insufficiency; (6) central nervous system disease or space-occupying lesion; (7) dysautonomias; and (8) metabolic or physiologic imbalance (e.g., circulatory or hemorrhagic shock, sepsis, hypercarbia, hypoxia, acid-base imbalance, adverse drug effects or interactions, stress, pain, anxiety, hyperthyroidism, other hyperadrenergic states). Also, some surgical procedures are more likely to be associated with tachyarrhythmias. Aside from cardiothoracic and vascular surgery, neurosurgery for

aneurysms and posterior fossa tumors is not uncommonly associated with bradycardia or tachyarrhythmias.

Among the causes of perioperative tachyarrhythmias are ischemia-reperfusion injury, CPB, high circulating catecholamines secondary to physiologic stress (pain, anxiety), and physiologic or metabolic imbalance. Generally, it is uncommon for a patient with a structurally normal heart to develop sustained ventricular tachyarrhythmias. The most common cardiac disorder associated with sustained ventricular tachycardia is coronary artery disease with an acute coronary syndrome (e.g., myocardial ischemia or infarction) or healed myocardial infarction with scar (the substrate) and a superimposed trigger (e.g., ischemia, proarrhythmia, stress).

Table 79–2 ■ Causes, Prevention, and Treatment of Tachyarrhythmias

Arrhythmia	Cause	Prevention	Treatment
Accelerated idioventricular rhythm	Ischemia; myocardial reperfusion injury; acute MI; digitalis toxicity	Measures to correct cause; usually transient (seconds to minutes), so little or no effect on outcome	Often transient (after establishing coronary reperfusion); overdrive atrial pacing preferred to drugs (atropine or other positive chronotropes) to increase atrial rate; easily overdriven by atrial pacing
Atrial fibrillation (AFB)	Clinical or subclinical cardiovascular disease; cardiac surgery, especially valve surgery; history of treated hypertension, left atrial enlargement, stroke, valvular heart disease, or CHF, COPD; occult or manifest thyrotoxicosis	Amiodarone; left or biatrial pacing or β-blockers for primary prevention in cardiac surgery; sotolol (class II and III activity) may also be effective; in thoracic surgery, primary prophylaxis with a β-blocker; indicated therapy for predisposing disease or conditions to facilitate more specific measures	If hemodynamically destabilizing and acute, DC cardioversion; drugs for chemical conversion of acute AFB include class IA, IC, and III antiarrhythmics, but consider proarrhythmia risk (up to 8%-10% with ibutilide and dofetilide)
Atrial flutter (AFT)	See AFB; also, may occur after congenital heart disease surgery	See AFB	DC cardioversion is preferred initial therapy (promptly restores sinus rhythm in most cases); IV ibutilide converts 60%-90% of episodes (but 8%-10% risk of proarrhythmia); rapid atrial pacing (AFT ≤340 bpm) converts some AFT (also, see AFB)
AV junctional tachycardia (AVJT)	Inferior wall MI; open heart surgery; acute rheumatic fever; myocarditis; digitalis toxicity*	Possibly β-blockers; indicated treatment for predisposing factors; possibly magnesium supplementation in pediatric congenital heart surgery	If digitalis is the cause, stop it; potassium, β- blockers, lidocaine, or phenytoin may also be used; atrial or AV overdrive pacing (slowly reduce rate to wean from pacing); DC cardioversion should *not be used* if digitalis could be the cause; otherwise, it might be effective if AVJT is not caused by enhanced automaticity (e.g., if AVJT occurs with myocardial reperfusion injury)
Ectopic atrial tachycardia: uniform (EAT) or multiform (MAT)	EAT: possibly digitalis toxicity; more likely, significant structural heart disease	Optimize treatment for COPD or CHF; stop digitalis and give potassium if not elevated; consider magnesium if hypomagnesemia is present	EAT: digitalis; consider β-blocker or CCB to slow ventricular rate; possibly add class IA, IC, or III antiarrhythmic; does not respond to DC cardioversion
	MAT: commonly COPD or CHF; digitalis is an unlikely cause; theophylline has been implicated		MAT: possibly a β-blocker (nonasthmatics); give potassium or magnesium if low; antiarrhythmics include verapamil, diltiazem, or amiodarone; does not respond to DC cardioversion

Table continued on following page

Table 79–2 ■ Causes, Prevention, and Treatment of Tachyarrhythmias—cont'd

Arrhythmia	Cause	Prevention	Treatment
Paroxysmal supraventricular tachycardia	Anxiety; panic attacks; caffeine; theophylline; catecholamines; WPW	Rest, reassurance, or sedation may abort attacks; provide adequate pain control and avoid triggers; RF ablation of APs or AVN pathways is definitive for prevention	After vagal maneuvers, adenosine, edrophonium, or CCB; if patient is unstable, immediate DC cardioversion; class IA antiarrhythmics increase AP conduction time and refractory periods; class II antiarrhythmics, adenosine, and digitalis increase AVN conduction time and refractory periods; class IC and III antiarrhythmics increase conduction time and refractory periods in both APs and AVN
Sinus tachycardia	Stress, anxiety, or pain; sepsis; hypovolemia, hypercarbia, or hypoxia; light anesthesia; MH; sympathomimetic, anticholinergic, and some illicit drugs	Treat, remove, or avoid the underlying cause	None unless symptomatic or causes myocardial ischemia; β-blockers
Ventricular flutter or fibrillation	Myocardial ischemia, MI, reperfusion injury; cardiomyopathy (end stage) due to any cause; idiopathic	Indicated treatment for primary heart disease	Immediate DF followed by IV amiodarone or procainamide to prevent recurrences; search for and correct causative conditions
Ventricular tachycardia	Myocardial ischemia, MI, reperfusion injury; cardiomyopathy (end stage) due to any cause; specific types of VT†; severe imbalance due to physiologic or metabolic imbalance or drug related (e.g., proarrhythmia)	Indicated treatment for primary heart disease; removal of offending drug(s); correction of physiologic or metabolic imbalance	If destabilizing (some slow VT is not), immediate DC followed by IV amiodarone or procainamide to prevent recurrences; search for and correct identifiable causative or contributing conditions

*Recognized by regularization of rate in patients with AFB receiving digitalis, and signs of digitalis toxicity.
†Idiopathic VT or that associated with arrhythmogenic right ventricular dysplasia, a surgical scar involving the right ventricular outflow tract (e.g., after correction of tetralogy of Fallot), bundle branch reentry, or mitral valve prolapse.
AP, accessory pathway; AV, atrioventricular; AVN, AV node; bpm, beats per minute; CCB, calcium channel blocker; CHF, congestive heart failure; COPD, chronic obstructive pulmonary disease; DC, direct current; DF, defibrillation; IV, intravenous; MH, malignant hyperthermia; MI, myocardial infarction; RF, radiofrequency; WPW, Wolff-Parkinson–White syndrome.

Idiopathic left ventricular tachycardia and right ventricular outflow tract tachycardia are two uncommon but specific types of ventricular tachycardia that occur in patients without demonstrable heart disease. In addition, idiopathic ventricular fibrillation is a potentially lethal tachyarrhythmia that occurs in otherwise healthy individuals and requires aggressive management.

Implications

Hemodynamic tolerance of tachycardia depends on the inherent stability of the rhythm, its rate and duration, and the status of atrial transport function, ventricular compliance, and ventricular function. Ventricular fibrillation, polymorphic ventricular tachycardia, and fast ventricular tachycardia are inherently unstable and pose an immediate threat to life. Tachyarrhythmias with sustained high ventricular rates impair ventricular filling, reduce diastolic time and coronary perfusion, and increase myocardial oxygen demand. Atrial transport function loss (which occurs with atrial fibrillation, junctional tachycardia, and all ventricular tachyarrhythmias) reduces ventricular filling and is especially disadvantageous for patients with reduced ventricular compliance. Finally, patients with marginally compensated heart failure may rely on sinus rhythm or a paced equivalent to meet their basic metabolic needs. Otherwise, they may develop overt heart failure.

MANAGEMENT

Prompt direct-current cardioversion or defibrillation is the preferred initial treatment for all hemodynamically disadvantageous tachyarrhythmias that can be terminated by such shocks. Those that cannot be terminated by these methods are ectopic atrial tachycardias (uniform or multiform), accelerated atrioventricular junctional rhythm or idioventricular tachycardia, and tachyarrhythmias due to digitalis toxicity. For all tachyarrhythmias with distinct QRS complexes, synchronized shocks (direct current) are used. This applies to most non-sinus-origin supraventricular tachycardia and ventricular tachycardia. Defibrillation is used for ventricular fibrillation and polymorphic ventricular tachycardia if QRS complexes and T waves are indistinguishable. Antiarrhythmic drugs can be used for cardioversion if the arrhythmia does not pose an imminent threat to life. Examples are intravenous ibutilide or amiodarone for "chemical" conversion of atrial flutter or fibrillation. However, the use of drugs for cardioversion carries the risk of inducing a proarrhythmic event (ventricular tachycardia or fibrillation); this risk is greatest for patients with structural heart disease. Among the antiarrhythmic drugs approved for intravenous use, amiodarone carries the least risk of proarrhythmia (1% to 2%). The risk of proarrhythmia can be as high as 8% to 10% with some class IA or IC drugs and with ibutilide or dofetilide, especially in patients with structural heart disease.

PREVENTION

The old adage "an ounce of prevention is worth a pound of cure" is especially applicable to perioperative tachyarrhythmias. Meticulous attention to the preservation of optimal physiologic and metabolic balance is fundamental to the prevention of adverse arrhythmic events. Also, multiple antiarrhythmic drug therapy may have an adverse impact on cardiac arrhythmia "substrates" (any diseased myocardium). Further, one must be mindful of drug interactions that might promote arrhythmias or have other untoward circulatory or neuroregulatory consequences. Causes, prevention, and treatment of specific tachyarrhythmias (aside from those associated with ventricular preexcitation or long QT syndromes) are outlined in Table 79-2.

Further Reading

Atlee J: Perioperative cardiac dysrhythmias. Anesthesiology 86:1397-1424, 1997.

Crystal E, Connolly SJ, Sleik K, et al: Interventions on prevention of postoperative atrial fibrillation in patients undergoing heart surgery. Circulation 106:75-80, 2002.

Dorman BH, Sade RM, Burnette JS, et al: Magnesium supplementation in the prevention of arrhythmias in pediatric patients undergoing surgery for congenital heart defects. Am Heart J 139:522-528, 2000.

Ho RT, Cullans DJ: Malignant ventricular arrhythmias. In Antman EM (ed): Cardiovascular Therapeutics. Philadelphia, WB Saunders, 2002, pp 477-501.

Hollenberg SM, Dellinger RP: Noncardiac surgery: Postoperative arrhythmias. Crit Care Med 28:145-150, 2000.

Mangrum JM, DiMarco JP: Acute and chronic pharmacologic management of supraventricular tachyarrhythmias. In Antman EM (ed): Cardiovascular Therapeutics. Philadelphia, WB Saunders, 2002, pp 423-444.

Olgin JE, Zipes DP: Specific arrhythmias: Diagnosis and management. In Braunwald E, Zipes DP, Libby P (eds): Heart Disease, 6th ed. Philadelphia, WB Saunders, 2001, pp 815-889.

Thomas RG: Supraventricular tachycardia: Implications for the intensivist. Crit Care Med 28:129-135, 2000.

Waktare JEP, Camm AJ: Atrial fibrillation: A comprehensive approach. In Antman EM (ed): Cardiovascular Therapeutics. Philadelphia, WB Saunders, 2002, pp 458-476.

CARDIOTHORACIC & VASCULAR SURGERY

Tachyarrhythmias with Ventricular Preexcitation

80

John L. Atlee

Case Synopsis

A 61-year-old woman has paroxysmal, irregular, wide QRS tachycardia in the recovery room following general anesthesia for left thoracotomy and upper lobe lung resection (Fig. 80-1). The ventricular rate exceeds 220 beats per minute for some beats, and the rhythm disturbance is poorly tolerated. Her preoperative electrocardiogram (ECG) during sinus rhythm revealed δ waves consistent with ventricular preexcitation.

PROBLEM ANALYSIS

Definition

The association of paroxysmal tachycardia with ECG evidence of ventricular preexcitation during sinus rhythm (δ waves) is known as Wolff-Parkinson-White (WPW) syndrome. Ventricular preexcitation requires functional accessory atrioventricular (AV) pathways that bypass normal AV conduction via the AV node during sinus rhythm to cause ventricular preexcitation. The fast conduction and refractory periods of accessory pathways (APs) are similar to those of atrial muscle. APs may also conduct from the ventricles to the atria (retrograde or ventriculoatrial conduction) to participate in AV reciprocating tachycardia (AVRT) (Fig. 80-2). Further, they may conduct atrial impulses more rapidly during atrial flutter or fibrillation than would otherwise be the case with conduction via the AV node. Usually, the ventricular rate during atrial flutter or fibrillation is limited by the AV node refractory period (300 msec) to less than 200 beats per minute. In contrast, the AP refractory period is shorter (240 msec), which allows ventricular rates greater than 250 beats per minute. If such rates are sustained, rapid deterioration to ventricular fibrillation is possible.

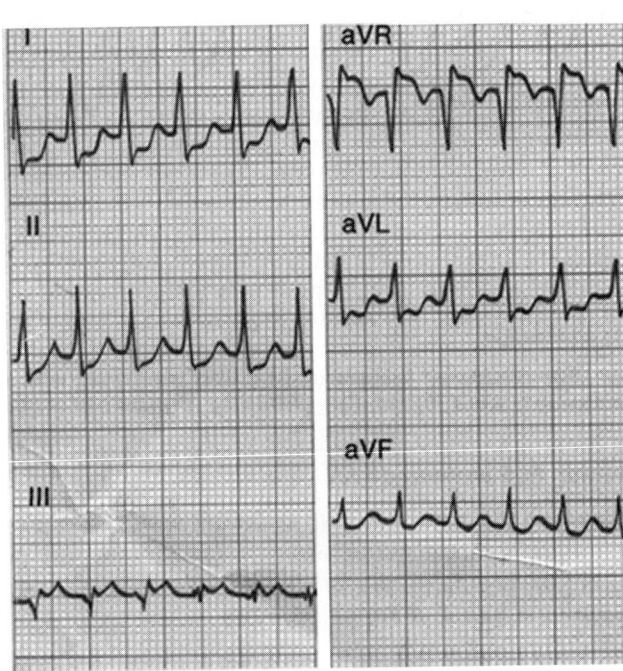

Figure 80–2 ■ Atrioventricular reciprocating tachycardia (AVRT) in a patient with ventricular preexcitation (δ waves) during sinus rhythm. During AVRT, conduction to the ventricles (i.e., orthodromic conduction) is via the AV node, giving rise to a narrow QRS complex tachycardia. The propagating impulse returns to the atria via the accessory pathway (i.e., antidromic conduction) to complete the reentry circuit. The rate of tachycardia is about 210 beats per minute and is associated with evidence of myocardial ischemia (elevated or depressed ST segments, depending on which lead is viewed). Although retrograde P waves often accompany antidromic AVRT, in this example, the P waves are not apparent, possibly due to the ST segment changes related to ischemia.

Figure 80–1 ■ Electrocardiogram from the recovery room (leads V₁-V₃). Note the highly irregular, wide QRS tachycardia, with ventricular rates ranging from 150 to 300 beats per minute.

Recognition

Features of WPW syndrome and ventricular preexcitation include the following:

- Short P-R interval (<0.12 second)
- Wide QRS complex (>0.12 second) with slurred initial QRS (δ wave) in some leads
- Usually, normal terminal QRS
- ST-T changes commonly directed opposite to the major δ wave and QRS vectors

The QRS appearance with ventricular preexcitation may be confused with bundle branch block, ventricular hypertrophy, or even myocardial infarction. It varies, depending on the location of APs (left or right anterior, posterior septal, or free walls) and coexisting ECG abnormalities. APs may conduct antegradely (atria to ventricles) to cause δ waves or preexcited tachycardia, or retrogradely (ventricles to atria) to cause orthodromic AVRT, the mechanism for more than 40% of paroxysmal supraventricular tachycardias (PSVTs) in all patients, with or without WPW syndrome. Preexcited tachycardias include wide QRS antidromic AVRT and preexcited atrial flutter or fibrillation (see Fig. 80-1). Finally, APs may "manifest" (cause δ waves or preexcited tachycardia) at any time during one's lifetime, but not at others.

The ECG appearance with supraventricular tachyarrhythmias in WPW syndrome is as follows:

- During orthodromic AVRT, inverted P waves (leads II, III, aVF) usually follow a narrow QRS complex. This contrasts with AV nodal reentry PSVT (the other >40% of all PSVTs), where P waves are usually nonapparent.
- With antidromic AVRT (<5% of PSVTs), retrograde P waves (if apparent) are upright in the inferior leads, and the QRS complex is widened (i.e., maximal preexcitation). Antidromic AVRT may be difficult to distinguish from monomorphic or polymorphic ventricular tachycardia. The appearance depends on whether single or multiple APs participate in ventricular activation during tachycardia.
- During atrial flutter or fibrillation in patients with WPW syndrome, antegrade conduction may occur via the AV node or APs. In this case, there might be no, incomplete, or maximal preexcitation. With maximal preexcitation, atrial flutter or fibrillation may be difficult to distinguish from polymorphic ventricular tachycardia; however, it may be better tolerated, and the R-R intervals are more irregular. Irregular R-R intervals with wide QRS tachycardia, with minimally or maximally preexcited beats (see Fig. 80-1), suggest atrial flutter or fibrillation as the mechanism for tachycardia.

Risk Assessment

- Preexcitation can be highly variable (present or absent) over one's lifetime.
- The most common paroxysmal tachycardia in WPW syndrome is orthodromic AVRT (70% to 80%); this is a narrow QRS tachycardia.
- Atrial flutter or fibrillation accounts for most other (20% to 25%) tachycardias in WPW syndrome.
- Ninety percent to 95% of AVRT in WPW syndrome is orthodromic tachycardia (narrow QRS), and 5% to 10% is antidromic tachycardia (wide QRS, preexcited tachycardia).

- Primary ventricular tachycardia or fibrillation is rare in WPW syndrome (<1% of tachycardias).

The incidence of WPW syndrome is 1 to 3 per 1000 persons (60% to 70% male preponderance). However, the incidence is difficult to estimate, because the presence of ventricular preexcitation can be highly variable on the same day in the same individual. Indeed, APs may manifest (i.e., antegrade conduction over the AP during sinus rhythm) only at certain times in one's lifetime. For example, the incidence of orthodromic AVRT in patients with WPW syndrome increases from 10% in adults younger than 40 years to 35% or more in those older than 60 years. The most common paroxysmal tachycardia with WPW syndrome is AVRT (70% to 80%), with orthodromic AVRT accounting for 90% to 95% of AVRT. Atrial fibrillation accounts for 15% to 30%, and atrial flutter for 5% of paroxysmal tachycardias in WPW syndrome. In the absence of coronary artery disease, heart failure, or other causes for arrhythmias, primary ventricular tachycardia is uncommon (<1% of tachyarrhythmias in patients with WPW syndrome). This is important to remember when confronted with a paroxysmal wide QRS tachycardia in a patient with WPW syndrome. For example, lidocaine to treat "presumed" ventricular tachycardia (see Fig. 80-1) might further reduce AP refractoriness and accelerate AP conduction, thereby increasing the rate of preexited tachycardia and possibly causing ventricular fibrillation.

Any event that temporarily dissociates conduction via the AV node and APs can initiate paroxysmal AVRT. This could be an atrial, junctional, or ventricular extrasystole, asynchronous atrial or ventricular pacing, sinus tachycardia with rate-dependent AV block, or the use of certain drugs (e.g., theophylline, catecholamines, caffeine, illicit stimulants). Also, the risk of tachyarrhythmia is increased by stress, anxiety, fatigue, exercise, and alcohol abuse. No studies have shown that anesthetic drugs (except ketamine) facilitate the induction of tachyarrhythmias in patients with WPW syndrome. Indeed, many anesthetic drugs act directly or indirectly to increase AV node and AP refractoriness, so that AVRT is uncommon during anesthesia and surgery. However, orthodromic AVRT or preexcited tachyarrhythmias may occur in preoperative holding areas or postanesthesia care units in patients with WPW syndrome in response to stress, pain, anxiety, or some imbalance. Except for patients at increased risk for postoperative atrial tachyarrhythmias (e.g., cardiac surgery), anesthesia and surgery should have little effect on the incidence of perioperative atrial flutter or fibrillation in patients with WPW syndrome.

Implications

Due to the fast rates with orthodromic or antidromic AVRT (180 to 250 beats per minute—faster than AV node reentry PSVT) and the fact that the rate of atrial flutter or fibrillation may exceed 300 beats per minute, ischemia with early hemodynamic collapse and rapid deterioration to ventricular fibrillation is possible. Prompt intervention is thus required for most paroxysmal tachycardias in patients with WPW syndrome.

Patients with WPW syndrome require a different approach to management, because AV conduction may occur exclusively or preferentially over the APs rather than over the AV node. A paradoxical acceleration of rate after the administration of cardiac glycosides, calcium channel blockers, or adenosine is due to both direct and indirect effects of these drugs, and they should generally be avoided in patients known to have WPW syndrome.

MANAGEMENT

- Narrow QRS AVRT
  - Vagal maneuvers
  - Drugs that increase AV node or AP refractoriness, such as β-blockers, amiodarone, class IA or IC antiarrhythmics, or sotalol (a β-blocker possessing class III activity)
  - Cardioversion, if hemodynamically unstable
- Wide QRS tachycardias: antidromic AVRT and preexcited atrial flutter or fibrillation
  - Cardioversion with hemodynamic instability (equipment should be available at bedside when treating any wide QRS tachycardia with drugs in a patient with WPW syndrome)
  - Intravenous amiodarone to terminate and prevent recurrences if not hemodynamically unstable
  - A drug that increases AV node refractoriness (β-blocker) along with one that increases AP refractoriness (class IA or IC antiarrhythmic, amiodarone, sotalol)

For narrow QRS (orthodromic) AVRT, vagal maneuvers (e.g., carotid sinus massage) are attempted first, followed by drugs that increase AV node refractoriness (e.g., β-blockers, adenosine, and possibly verapamil if adenosine is ineffective). Verapamil will compound any hypotension that may ensue if AVRT fails to terminate, mandating immediate cardioversion. Early cardioversion is required for any AVRT that causes hemodynamic compromise (angina, heart failure, or hypotension). β-Blockers, diltiazem, or verapamil may help prevent recurrences. As a rule, however, patients with recurrent AVRT are best treated with catheter or surgical AP ablation. Although digitalis prolongs conduction time and refractoriness in the AV node, it has been reported to shorten refractoriness in the APs and speed the ventricular response in some patients with WPW syndrome and atrial fibrillation. Therefore, digitalis should not be used as a single drug in patients with WPW syndrome who are prone to or have atrial flutter or fibrillation. Further, because atrial fibrillation can develop during AVRT in many patients with WPW syndrome, this caveat probably applies to all patients with tachycardia and WPW syndrome. Instead, drugs that prolong refractoriness in the APs should be used, such as class IA and IC drugs.

For preexcited (wide QRS) tachycardia with hemodynamic compromise, early cardioversion is required. Procainamide or flecainide (both increase AP refractoriness and reduce conduction over the APs) can be used if supine systolic blood pressure is >90 mm Hg. Either may reduce the ventricular rate and terminate preexcited tachycardia. Amiodarone increases AP and AV node refractoriness and may be effective. After direct-current cardioversion for hemodynamically unstable preexcited tachycardia, the previously mentioned drugs that increase AP refractoriness are used to prevent recurrences. Amiodarone increases AV node, atrial, and AP refractoriness and can be used when other drugs fail to prevent recurrences. However, AP ablation is definitive therapy.

With atrial flutter or fibrillation in a WPW patient, dangerous ventricular rates and rapid deterioration into ventricular fibrillation are of paramount concern. If cardioversion is not readily available, the immediate goal is to slow the ventricular rate. Drugs that increase refractoriness and conduction time in the AV node (β-blockers, verapamil, diltiazem), along with those that increase AP refractoriness (sotalol, procainamide, amiodarone), may temporarily reduce the ventricular rate while awaiting direct-current cardioversion.

PREVENTION

- Provide stress-free circumstances (e.g., reassurance, sedation).
- Regional or general anesthesia (except ketamine) is safe.
- Risk of paroxysmal tachycardia is greatest during emergence from anesthesia and during the first few days following major or stressful surgery.
- Continue any antiarrhythmic drugs the patient may be taking.

For WPW patients with a history of tachyarrhythmias and facing surgery with a high risk of postoperative atrial fibrillation or flutter (e.g., cardiac surgery), consideration should be given to AP ablation before elective surgery. For all other surgery, the circumstances should be as stress free as possible. Reassurance, adequate preoperative sedation and analgesia, and local anesthesia for vascular access will help prevent attacks of paroxysmal tachycardia before surgery. Except for ketamine, it makes little difference which anesthetic agents or techniques are chosen, provided that the patient is adequately anesthetized for periods of maximal stress (e.g., airway or surgical manipulation). There is no literature suggesting that regional or general anesthesia is preferable for procedures that can be performed with either. The risk of paroxysmal tachyarrhythmias is likely highest during emergence and recovery from anesthesia due to sudden awareness and pain, and possibly during the first few postoperative days due to physiologic imbalance and increased stress (e.g., uncontrolled pain). Attention to minimizing these factors should help reduce the risk of paroxysmal tachycardias. Finally, as for any systemic condition requiring chronic medication, it is important that patients receiving antiarrhythmic drugs to prevent recurrences be given these medications up to and throughout the perioperative period. When there is any doubt, a cardiologist should be consulted.

Further Reading

Atlee J: Perioperative cardiac dysrhythmias. Anesthesiology 86:1397-1424, 1997.

Kastor J: Arrhythmias. Philadelphia, WB Saunders, 2000.

Mangrum JM, DiMarco JP: Acute and chronic pharmacologic management of supraventricular tachyarrhythmias. In, Antman EM (ed): Cardiovascular Therapeutics. Philadelphia, WB Saunders, 2002, pp 423-444.

Olgin JE, Zipes D: Specific arrhythmias: Diagnosis and treatment. In Braunwald E, Zipes DP, Libby P (eds): Heart Disease, 7th ed. Philadelphia, WB Saunders, 2005, pp 803-863.

Thomas RG: Supraventricular tachycardia: Implications for the intensivist. Crit Care Med 28:129-135, 2000.

Long QT Syndromes and Ventricular Arrhythmias

81

John L. Atlee

Case Synopsis

A 48-year-old woman takes amitriptyline for depression and combined hydrochlorothiazide and triamterene for hypertension. In the recovery room following general anesthesia for abdominal hysterectomy, she has sudden-onset polymorphic ventricular tachycardia. This is poorly tolerated, does not respond to intravenous bolus lidocaine, and recurs following direct-current cardioversion. The corrected Q-T interval on her preoperative electrocardiogram (ECG) was 0.48 second, and her serum potassium concentration was 3.2 mEq/L.

PROBLEM ANALYSIS

Definition and Causes

The long QT syndrome (LQTS) is the association of polymorphic ventricular tachycardia (PMVT) with Q-T interval prolongation on the ECG (Fig. 81-1). Such PMVT is known as torsades de pointes (TdP). Without Q-T interval prolongation, often in association with an acute coronary syndrome, it is just termed PMVT. This distinction is important, because causes, management, and prevention differ. PMVT is discussed in Chapter 79, along with other perioperative tachyarrhythmias.

LQTS has two forms: congenital and acquired. Although congenital LQTS was once thought to be caused by left-sided sympathetic imbalance, it is now known that LQTS is due to intrinsic (congenital) or acquired abnormalities of ionic currents that underlie cardiac repolarization. Prolongation of cardiac repolarization is critical to the generation of early afterdepolarizations (EADs), which in turn can generate spontaneous or triggered action potential upstrokes. If these propagate throughout the heart, ventricular extrasystoles preceded by normal sinus beats with long Q-T intervals are recorded on the surface ECG (see Fig. 81-1). Available evidence implicates EADs and triggered activity in the genesis of TdP. Notably, conditions that elicit EADs experimentally (e.g., slow heart rate, hypokalemia, drugs that prolong the Q-T interval) are known to be associated with clinical TdP. Also, certain populations of cells within the ventricles (Purkinje fibers, midmyocardium or M cells) are more likely to develop EADs on drug challenge. EADs with heterogeneity in the development of prolonged cardiac action potentials result in a myocardial substrate vulnerable to reentry of excitation, the probable proximate cause for TdP.

Genetic studies have now identified at least six separate genes that, if mutated, may cause congenital LQTS. Study of one of these genes (*HERG*), which encodes a potassium channel protein that regulates a major repolarizing current in cardiac fibers (I_{Kr}), has been especially informative with regard to drug-associated TdP. Mutations in *HERG* reduce I_{Kr} and thus prolong action potentials in individual cells, causing congenital LQTS. Further, virtually all drugs that prolong the Q-T interval and cause TdP also block I_{Kr}. Unfortunately, this finding is nonspecific, because many drugs that do not cause TdP also block I_{Kr}.

It is also known that congenital LQTS can show incomplete penetrance; that is, family members with near-normal Q-T intervals may carry the same genetic mutations associated with LQTS that increase the risk of sudden death in their relatives. Available evidence also suggests that 5% to 10% of persons in whom TdP develops on exposure to drugs or other factors that prolong the Q-T interval harbor mutations associated with congenital LQTS and therefore can be viewed as having a subclinical form of the syndrome. This observation is consistent with the clinical concept of reduced repolarization reserve arising from an ion channel gene mutation that predisposes the carrier to drug or other forms of stress-induced TdP.

Recognition

The upper limit of normal for the Q-Tc interval (Q-T interval corrected for heart rate using Bazett's formula: Q-Tc = $Q\text{-}T/[R - R^{1/2}]$) is 0.46 second for men and 0.47 second for women. In patients with either form of LQTS, there may be U-wave or T-wave abnormalities, such as notched or biphasic T waves or T-wave alternans. These reflect the heterogeneity

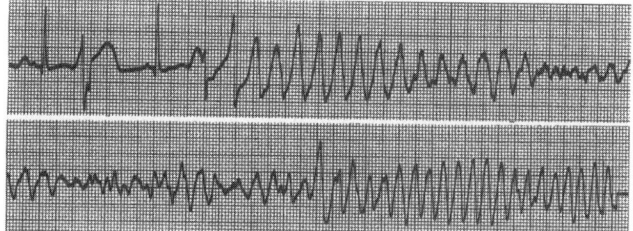

Figure 81–1 ■ Wide QRS, polymorphic tachycardia (PMVT) in lead II (contiguous tracings). The rate of tachycardia is about 250 beats per minute. Note that normal sinus beats preceding tachycardia in the upper tracing are associated with prolonged Q-T intervals. Therefore, this PMVT qualifies as torsades de pointes, which begins with an extrasystole during inscription of the T wave.

of ventricular repolarization. ECG features of TdP with either form of LQTS are as follows (see Fig. 81-1):

- QRS complexes that vary in amplitude and appear to twist around the isoelectric baseline
- Rate of tachycardia usually between 200 and 250 beats per minute
- Often associated with bradycardia or heart block (especially acquired LQTS)

Risk Assessment

There are two forms of congenital LQTS. One (Jervell and Lange-Nielsen syndrome) is accompanied by deafness, and the other (Romano-Ward syndrome) is not. With either, there may be a history of syncope or sudden death due to TdP. With congenital LQTS, TdP is often precipitated by stress, sudden noise, or adrenergic stimulation. Adrenergic dependence may be explained as follows: (1) Mutant cardiac ion channels respond abnormally to adrenergic stimulation in a manner conducive to prolongation of repolarization; and (2) prolonged repolarization increases intracellular Ca^{2+} accumulation and the likelihood of EAD-triggered activity and TdP. In contrast, TdP with acquired LQTS is facilitated by bradycardia or sinus pauses (i.e., bradycardia- or pause-dependent TdP).

Syncope with congenital LQTS may initially be misdiagnosed as a seizure disorder, and ECGs may not be obtained. About 30% of patients are diagnosed during clinical evaluation for unexplained syncope or aborted sudden death. Another 60% are identified when family members of an individual with syncope or cardiac arrest (the proband) undergo ECG screening. The remaining 10% are identified by Q-T prolongation on routine ECG testing.

What is the risk for syncope or cardiac arrest in individuals with congenital LQTS? Among 328 families with at least one affected family member, 50% of probands, 8% of affected family members, and 2% of unaffected family members experienced one or more cardiac events by 12 years of age. During 10 years of follow-up, 37% of probands, 5% of affected family members, and less than 1% of unaffected family members experienced a cardiac event. Among probands, event rates for syncope and sudden death were 5% and 0.9% per year, respectively. Risk factors for these included length of Q-T interval, history of cardiac event, and heart rate.

Implications

Factors that predispose to Q-T interval prolongation and increase risk for TdP include baseline Q-T interval prolongation, high concentrations or rapid infusions of Q-T interval-prolonging drugs, older age, female sex, low left ventricular ejection fraction, congestive heart failure, left ventricular hypertrophy, digitalis, ischemia, bradycardia, hypokalemia or hypomagnesemia, and recent conversion from atrial flutter or fibrillation, especially with drugs that prolong the Q-T interval (e.g., dofetilide, ibutilide). Drugs that may prolong the Q-T interval and cause TdP are listed in Table 81-1. A more extensive list of such drugs can be found at http.//www.torsades.org.

Table 81-1 ■ Drugs that May Prolong the Q-T Interval and Cause Torsades de Pointes*

Antiarrhythmics	Anti-infectives
Amiodarone[†]	Azithromycin
Bepridil	Ciprofloxacin
Disopyramide	Clarithromycin
Dofetilide	Clindamycin
Ibutilide	Erythromycin
Procainamide	Fluconazole
Quinidine	Gatifloxacin
Sotalol	Halofantrine
Antidepressants	Levofloxacin
Amitriptyline	Pentamidine
Desipramine	Sparfloxacin
Fluoxetine	Trimethoprim-sulfamethoxazole
Imipramine	**Antiemetics**
Paroxetine	Domperidone
Sertraline	Droperidol
Venlafaxine	**Migraine Drugs**
Antipsychotics	Sumatriptan
Chlorpromazine	Zolmitriptan
Haloperidol	**Miscellaneous**
Mesoridazine	Arsenic trioxide
Olanzapine	Cisapride
Pimozide	Isradipine
Risperidone	Lidoflazine[‡]
Thioridazine	Methadone
Ziprasidone	Nicardipine

*For relative risk, consult http://www.torsades.org.
[†]Least likely of listed antiarrhythmic drugs to cause acquired long QT syndrome and torsades de pointes (<2%).
[‡]Calcium channel blocker not marketed in the United States.

When an antiarrhythmic drug promotes arrhythmias, these are termed proarrhythmic events. For example, in patients with structural heart disease (especially ischemic cardiomyopathy), the class IC drugs flecainide or propafenone may cause proarrhythmia but not TdP; the proarrhythmia in this setting is incessant monomorphic ventricular tachycardia. Potent inhalational anesthetics also prolong the Q-T interval, but this prolongation is small and is not known to be associated with TdP. Bupivacaine and etidocaine, both of which avidly bind to cardiac sodium channels and have very slow offset kinetics, may be associated with malignant ventricular arrhythmias and severe myocardial depression (cardiotoxicity), but they are not listed as associated with Q-T interval prolongation or TdP (see http.//www.torsades.org). However, in an older study in pentobarbital-anesthetized dogs, both bupivacaine and etidocaine were associated with PMVT resembling TdP following ventricular burst pacing.[1] In my view, it is prudent to avoid either local anesthetic in patients with congenital LQTS.

---

[1]Burst pacing is a series of rapidly paced beats (often 10 to 15) intended to initiate or reproduce clinical atrial or ventricular tachyarrhythmias.

MANAGEMENT

Torsades de Pointes with Congenital Long QT Syndrome

- Patients with congenital LQTS and a history of syncope or aborted sudden death will likely have an implanted cardiac rhythm management device (CRMD[2]; see Chapter 97). The CRMD provides rate support (pacing) for bradycardia and internal cardioversion or defibrillation for TdP or ventricular fibrillation.
- For patients without CRMDs, institute maximally tolerated doses of β-blockers in those with a history of syncope, aborted sudden death, or complex ventricular tachyarrhythmias.
- If, despite maximally tolerated doses of β-blockers, the patient continues to experience complex ventricular arrhythmias or syncope and does not have a CRMD, consider left stellate ganglion block for patients requiring urgent or emergent surgery. If surgery is elective or can be postponed until after CRMD implantation, consider doing so.
- Treat TdP with class IB antiarrhythmics (e.g., lidocaine, mexiletine, diphenylhydantoin) and magnesium sulfate. Temporary pacing is advised for patients with bradycardia or pause-dependent TdP to reduce heterogeneity of repolarization with slow rates. Even in patients without profound bradycardia, temporary pacing at 75 to 100 beats per minute may provide rhythm stabilization.
- If temporary pacing is not feasible or practical, cautious use of isoproterenol to increase heart rate to 75 to 100 beats per minute may prevent recurrences of TdP.

Torsades de Pointes with Acquired Long QT Syndrome

- If known, correct or remove the cause of Q-T interval prolongation.
- Intravenous magnesium sulfate is the initial drug of choice for TdP from an acquired cause. Also, consider administering intravenous potassium if the serum potassium concentration is low.
- Institute prophylactic atrial, dual-chamber, or ventricular pacing at 75 to 100 beats per minute for bradycardia or pause-dependent TdP. If pacing is not feasible or practical, cautious use of isoproterenol can achieve the same rates.
- If antiarrhythmic drugs are used to suppress TdP, they must be ones that do not prolong the Q-T interval (see Table 81-1).

Polymorphic Ventricular Tachycardia Resembling Torsades de Pointes

With PMVT resembling TdP and a normal Q-T interval, antiarrhythmic drugs used for ventricular tachycardia in the absence of Q-T interval prolongation (see Chapter 79) are used for treatment and to prevent recurrences. These include antiarrhythmic drugs that prolong the Q-T interval. With instability or tachycardia intolerance, immediate direct-current cardioversion is advised.

PREVENTION

- With any Q-T interval prolongation, avoid drugs that might further prolong it.
- Provide stress-free perioperative circumstances, to the extent possible.
- Continue effective antiarrhythmic drugs (i.e., ones that do not cause Q-T interval prolongation).
- Consider prophylactic temporary pacing for bradycardia or pause-dependent tachycardia.
- If the patient is not receiving β-blockers (congenital LQTS), perioperative β-blockade is advised.

For patients with congenital LQTS facing anesthesia and surgery, it is important to provide circumstances that are as stress free as possible. Reassurance, adequate preoperative sedation and analgesia, and local anesthesia for vascular access can help prevent attacks of paroxysmal tachycardia before surgery. Except for ketamine and "sensitizing" inhalational anesthetics (halothane or enflurane, especially if preceded by thiopental induction), it makes little difference which anesthetic agents or techniques are used, provided the patient is adequately anesthetized during periods of maximal stress. There is no literature suggesting that either regional or general anesthesia is preferable for procedures that can be performed with either type. Risk for TdP may be increased during emergence and recovery from anesthesia and possibly for the first few days after major or stressful surgery. If a patient with congenital LQTS is receiving β-blockers, these should be continued throughout the perioperative period. Finally, consideration should be given to temporary perioperative pacing if the patient does not already have a functioning CRMD, and an external cardioverter-defibrillator should be available on site.

For patients having elective surgery with ECG evidence of acquired LQTS (i.e., receiving drugs known to cause Q-T interval prolongation) and with a history of syncope, it is prudent to postpone surgery until the cause of syncope is explored thoroughly, and TdP should be high on the list of suspects. If TdP is identified as the cause of syncope, elective surgery should be delayed until the Q-T interval is normalized by withdrawal of the offending drugs. It is almost always possible to substitute another drug (or drugs) less likely to cause Q-T interval prolongation and TdP. Similar precautions apply when physiologic or nutritional imbalance causes acquired LQTS and TdP.

---

[2]A task force was commissioned by the American Society of Anesthesiologists (ASA) in 2003 to prepare a practice advisory for the management of patients with CRMD. This was approved by the ASA House of Delegates during the 2004 annual ASA meeting. See Further Reading.

Further Reading

Al-Khatib SM, LaPointe NMA, Califf RM: What clinicians should know about the QT interval. JAMA 289:2120-2127, 2003.

American Society of Anesthesiologists Task Force on Perioperative Management of Patients with Cardiac Rhythm Management Devices: Practice advisory for the perioperative management of patients with cardiac rhythm management devices: pacemakers and implantable cardioverter-defibrillators: A report by the American Society of Anesthesiologists Task Force on Perioperative Management of Patients with Cardiac Rhythm Management Devices. Anesthesiology 103:186-198, 2005.

Atlee JL: Management of perioperative dysrhythmias. Anesthesiology 86:1397-1424, 1997.

Chaudhry G, Muqtada G, Haffagee CI: Antiarrhythmic agents and proarrhythmia. Crit Care Med 28:158-164, 2000.

El-Sherif N, Turitto G: The long QT syndrome and torsade de pointes. Pacing Clin Electrophysiol 22:91-110, 1999.

Ho RT, Cullans DJ: Malignant ventricular arrhythmias. In Antman EM (ed): Cardiovascular Therapeutics. Philadelphia, WB Saunders, 2002, pp 477-501.

Kasten GW: Amide local anesthetic alterations of effective refractory period temporal dispersion: Relationship to ventricular arrhythmias. Anesthesiology 65:61-66, 1986.

Keating MT, Sanguinetti MC: Molecular and cellular mechanisms of cardiac arrhythmias. Cell 104:569-580, 2001.

Olgin JE, Zipes DP: Specific arrhythmias: Diagnosis and treatment. In Braunwald E, Zipes DP, Libby P (eds): Heart Disease, 7th ed. Philadelphia, WB Saunders, 2001, pp 815-889.

Roden DM: Drug-induced prolongation of the QT interval. N Engl J Med 350:1013-1022, 2004.

Bradyarrhythmias

Paul B. Zanaboni and Charles B. Hantler

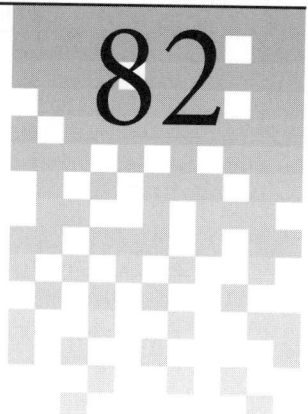

Case Synopsis

During an open abdominal aortic aneurysm repair, a 71-year-old man suddenly becomes profoundly hypotensive following acute blood loss. The mean arterial blood pressure is 40 mm Hg, and the electrocardiogram (ECG) shows a wide complex rhythm of 35 beats per minute. The patient's preoperative ECG showed a first degree heart block with a bifascicular bundle branch block pattern.

PROBLEM ANALYSIS

Definition

Bradyarrhythmias include cardiac rhythm abnormalities associated with a slow ventricular depolarization rate (<60 beats per minute). Such rhythm disturbances are clinically significant when associated with abnormalities of vital organ function, such as central nervous system impairment (syncope, altered mental status), postural hypotension, heart failure, or other major organ system dysfunction (especially renal, hepatic, or gastrointestinal).

Bradyarrhythmias are caused by failure of impulse formation, failure of impulse conduction, or both (Table 82-1). Anatomic structures involved in the generation and propagation of electrical impulses within the heart (i.e., its specialized conduction system) are depicted in Figure 82-1.

The maximum diastolic potential of the sinoatrial (SA) node is between −50 and −60 mV. When maximum diastolic potential is reached, SA node cells immediately begin to depolarize. Spontaneous phase 4 depolarization is due to an imbalance between slowly decaying delayed rectifier (an outward potassium current) and slowly recovering inward calcium currents. The latter cause the cell interior to become progressively less negative with respect to the exterior. A pacemaker current is involved only when the cell interior is less negative than −50 mV. In SA node cells, this current is probably subserved by L-type calcium channels. However, T-type current may be activated during the latter half of spontaneous

phase 4 depolarization (i.e., normal automaticity). Cells of the SA node depolarize to +10 mV, their maximum action potential overshoot. Thus, maximum amplitudes are 60 to 70 mV. Once these are reached, SA node cells repolarize. During early repolarization, especially in atrial or ventricular muscle or Purkinje fibers (i.e., "fast-response" fibers),[1] sodium "window" and calcium currents contribute, along with several different potassium repolarizing (outward) currents. Regardless, in all fiber types, net ionic movements during repolarization favor net outward movement of positive charges (mainly potassium), in addition to a variable contribution of reduced inward calcium and sodium current. During the action potential upstroke (depolarization), net ionic movements favor the net inward movement of positive charges. These are carried mainly by sodium and calcium, but there is also reduced outward movement of potassium.

The normal SA firing rate is 60 to 100 beats per minute. Drugs, neural input (both sympathetic and parasympathetic), temperature, and hormones influence the rate of sinus node depolarization by affecting either the rate of spontaneous (phase 4) depolarization or the threshold for a regenerative (self-sufficient) action potential upstroke.

In addition to sinus bradycardia (sinus rhythm with a rate <60 beats per minute; Fig. 82-2), there may be bradycardic (slow) escape rhythms arising in lower pacemakers. Such escape pacemaker rhythms (i.e., originating below the atrioventricular [AV] junction) are often associated with advanced second and third degree AV heart block.[2]

Subsidiary Atrial Pacemakers. These pacemakers are found along the sulcus (crista) terminalis and around the coronary sinus orifice. Subsidiary atrial pacemaker rhythms are identified by flattened, biphasic, or negative P waves (e.g., wandering atrial pacemaker) in leads with normally upright P waves (leads II, III, and aVF). Both lower and upper rate cutoffs for subsidiary atrial pacemakers appear to be similar to those for the SA node. The P-R interval may be the same or slightly less than that of the SA node (<0.10 second).

Table 82–1 ■ Causes of Bradyarrhythmias

Failure of Impulse Formation
Sinus bradycardia
    Slow sinus node automatic rate
    Sinoatrial conduction block
Carotid sinus hypersensitivity
    Neurocardiogenic syncope (with decrease in sympathetic outflow)

Failure of Impulse Conduction
Atrioventricular node heart block
    First degree
    Second degree
        Type I
        Type II
    Third degree

---

[1]Fast-response fibers have higher action potential maximum amplitudes and overshoots and faster rates of conduction than do SA or AV node cells. They also have more prominent early rapid (phase 1) repolarization.

[2]Advanced second degree AV heart block is defined as two or more successive, blocked P waves, but with some that are conducted. With third degree (complete) AV heart block, no P waves are conducted to the ventricles.

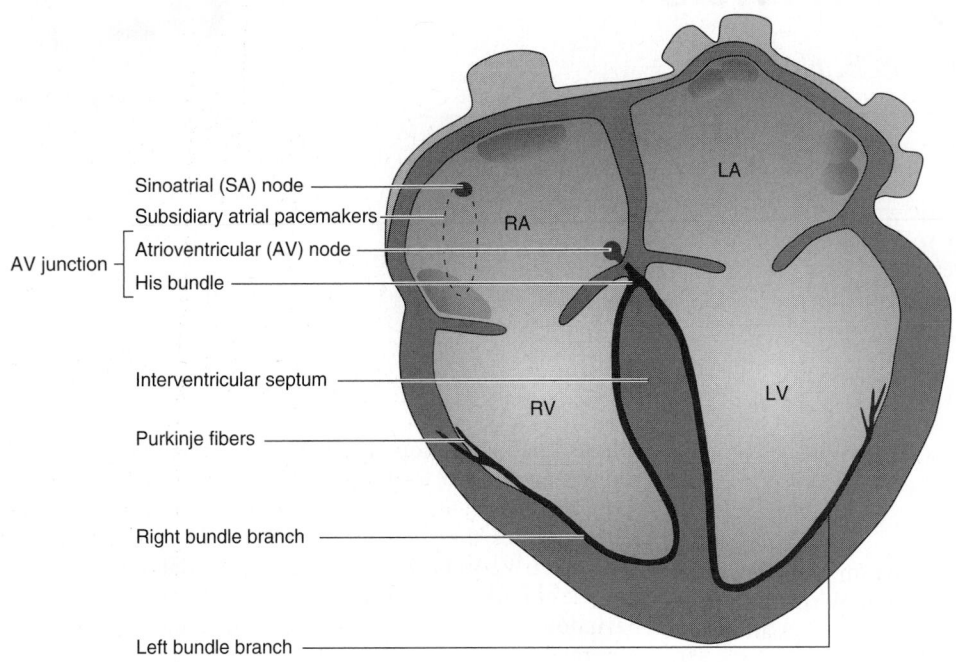

Figure 82–1 ■ Anatomic structures involved in the generation and propagation of electrical impulses within the heart (i.e., its specialized conduction system). LA, left atrium; LV, left ventricle; RA, right atrium; RV, right ventricle.

Atrioventricular Junctional Pacemakers.   With AV junctional bradycardia, there may be no apparent P waves, or they may be inverted in ECG leads with normally upright P waves during sinus rhythm. Associated, inverted P (retrograde) waves may occur just before the QRS complex (P-R interval <0.10 second) or, less commonly, after the QRS complex.

Purkinje Fibers.   Typically (e.g., during escape rhythms associated with advanced second degree or complete [third degree] AV heart block), escape rates are less than 50 beats per minute (may be lower in adults). Commonly, there are no associated P waves; however, there may be dissociated, upright P waves. These originate in the SA node or subsidiary atrial pacemakers but are blocked and bear no relationship to QRS complexes. However, even with advanced second or third degree AV heart block, retrograde (ventriculoatrial) conduction may be intact, so that associated P waves may be possible. If so, these will be inverted in leads with normally positive P waves.[3]

Ventricular Muscle Fibers.   Rarely, ventricular fibers exhibit automaticity. When this occurs, it is due to loss of resting membrane potential. The partial depolarization of these fibers may be the result of disease, usually in association with myocardial ischemia or infarction. Ventricular rates are generally less than 40 beats per minute, and retrograde

P waves are uncommon. Not uncommonly, the atria beat independently of the ventricles (AV dissociation).

Following SA node depolarization, the impulse is conducted via specialized atrial conducting tissue. SA conduction block is failure of conduction within the atrial tissue; it is characterized by the absence of P waves on the ECG. When this occurs (or the SA node fails to depolarize), lower pacemaker fibers must assume control of the ventricles. Finally, as alluded to earlier, the SA node is most influenced by altered parasympathetic or sympathetic (autonomic) control. Often, this is mediated by baroreceptors and cardiac mechanoreceptors.

Recognition

ECG features of sinus bradycardia and lower pacemaker escape rhythms were already discussed. In addition, bradycardia may also be due to AV conduction delay or block. First degree AV block is simply delayed AV impulse transmission (P-R interval >0.12 second), with no dropped ventricular beats (QRS complexes). Second degree AV block is block of

---

[3]During advanced second or third degree AV heart block, the sinus node beats independently of the ventricles, and its rate is faster than that of the pacemaker controlling the ventricles. This is because sinus nodes are under autonomic control, blood pressure is lower with ventricular escape rhythm, and there is a baroreflex-mediated increase in sympathetic efferent activity.

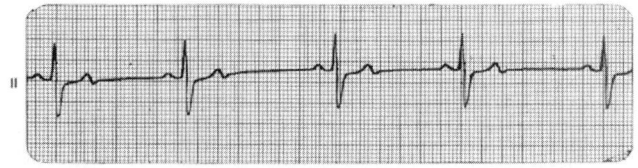

Figure 82–2 ■ In sinus bradycardia, there is a regular relationship between the P waves and QRS complexes. The rate is less than 60 beats per minute.

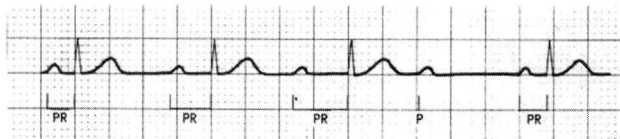

Figure 82–3 ■ With Mobitz type I (Wenckebach) second degree atrioventricular (AV) block, there is progressive P-R interval prolongation before blocked P waves (i.e., the fourth P wave). As with first degree AV block, the P-R interval is greater than 0.12 second, but there are no dropped ventricular beats. In this example, block would be variable (not shown) if the ratio of conducted to nonconducted atrial beats varied (e.g., 3:2, 4:3), as commonly occurs with Mobitz type I second degree AV block. Block usually occurs within the AV node or at its margins.

some impulses between the atria and ventricles. It is further subdivided into Mobitz type I, Mobitz type II, and advanced second degree AV block. With Mobitz type I (Wenckebach) AV block (Fig. 82-3), some but not all atrial beats are blocked in a recurring pattern, with progressively prolonged P-R intervals before dropped beats. The ratio of conducted to dropped beats may be fixed (e.g., 3:2, 4:3) or variable (e.g., 4:3 and 3:2). With Mobitz type II block, there are no progressively prolonged P-R intervals before dropped beats, but the block may also be variable (Fig. 82-4). With advanced second degree AV block, there are two or more dropped beats between conducted beats; again, the ratio between the two can vary. Finally, with third degree (complete) AV block, there are no conducted atrial beats (Fig. 82-5). The atria and ventricles are controlled by different pacemakers, and the QRS complexes may be narrow (if the pacemaker that controls the ventricles is above the bifurcation of the bundle of His) or widened (if below the bifurcation). Thus, in third degree AV heart block, there is complete AV dissociation (independent beating of the atria and ventricles).

Risk Assessment

Bradyarrhythmias can arise from either intrinsic myocardial causes or external influences, such as increased vagal tone or electrolyte imbalance. Implanted artificial pacemakers (see Chapter 97) are indicated for patients with symptomatic bradyarrhythmias (e.g., easy fatigability, near or true syncope) without reversible causes.

GENERAL ANESTHESIA AND SURGERY

Bradyarrhythmias that occur during general anesthesia can have many causes. Deep inhalation anesthesia (especially with older volatile agents) and opiates are well-known

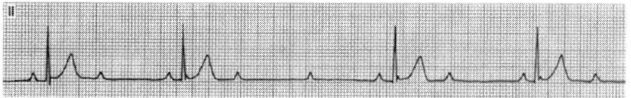

Figure 82–4 ■ With Mobitz type II second degree atrioventricular (AV) block, there may be no P-R interval variability (fixed block), or block may be variable (as shown) or intermittent. If fixed, block is constant at some fixed ratio of atrial to conducted beats (e.g., 2:1, 3:1, 4:1). If variable, block varies on a recurring basis (e.g., 2:1 and 3:1). If block is intermittent, periods of normal AV conduction are interrupted by occasional dropped beats, but not on a recurring basis. Type II second degree AV block most commonly occurs at or below the bundle of His.

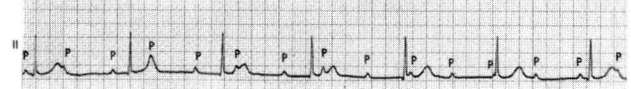

Figure 82–5 ■ With third degree atrioventricular (AV) heart block (almost always at or below the bundle of His), P waves are independent of the QRS complexes (i.e., complete AV dissociation, as with ventricular-origin brady- or tachyarrhythmias). With third degree AV heart block, the QRS complexes can be narrow (as shown) if the pacemaker that controls the ventricles is within or above the bifurcation of the bundle of His, or widened if the pacemaker controlling the ventricles is more distal.

causes of significant bradycardia during anesthesia. Surgical stimulation may be associated with a relative increase in vagal tone, leading to slowing of SA node automaticity, AV node conduction, or both. Well-known examples are the oculocardiac reflex, peritoneal stimulation, and stimulation of the carotid body; such responses terminate when the stimulation is discontinued. Although both drug- and surgery-induced bradyarrhythmias usually respond to drugs—either anticholinergics (atropine, glycopyrrolate) or sympathomimetics (epinephrine, isoproterenol)—if temporary transvenous or pacing wires are available (e.g., during cardiac surgery), pacing is always preferable to drugs. Drugs have the potential to cause excessive tachycardia, are not easily reversed, and may cause arrhythmias. If AV conduction is intact and transesophageal pacing is available, it is preferred over drugs as treatment for sinus bradycardia and AV junctional rhythms. Drug-resistant, clinically significant bradyarrhythmias should always be treated with external (transesophageal or transcutaneous) or internal (transvenous or epicardial) pacing to improve hemodynamics.

NEURAXIAL BLOCKADE

Neuraxial blockade, involving the high thoracic level, may lead to vagal dominance (bradycardia) by blocking sympathetic outflow from the cardiac accelerator fibers that originate in the upper thoracic spinal cord. This bradycardia usually responds well to treatment with anticholinergic agents.

DRUG-INDUCED BRADYCARDIA

Many patients undergoing surgery are taking medications that slow the sinus heart rate or AV node conduction (e.g., β-blockers, nondihydropyridine calcium channel blockers). The combination of these medications, anesthesia, and surgery may result in significant bradyarrhythmias. Again, bradycardia is usually reversed with either anticholinergic or sympathomimetic agents. However, caution is advised, because excess tachycardia can put patients with ischemic heart disease or arrhythmias at further risk. In the case of elective surgery, one should consider a preoperative dose reduction of any drugs that may cause untoward bradycardia due to reduced heart rate or AV conduction block.

METABOLIC CAUSES

Metabolic conditions may cause significant preoperative or intraoperative bradyarrhythmias. These include hypothermia (now rare with the widespread use of forced air warming blankets), endocrine disorders, and electrolyte abnormalities.

With severe hypothermia, there may be sinus bradycardia or escape rhythms, with or without associated Osborne or J waves.[4] Patients with hypothyroidism and Addison's disease often have preoperative bradycardia that may become more clinically significant during surgery and anesthesia due to effects of anesthetic drugs. Hyperkalemia (which hyperpolarizes cells of the SA and AV nodes) can also cause significant sinus bradycardia or slow AV node conduction. The ECG may show a slow, wide-complex rhythm. Severe hyperkalemia can result in AV heart block or asystole. Hypermagnesemia may also cause sinus bradycardia by reducing the slow, inward, depolarizing calcium current. Both hyperkalemia and hypermagnesemia should be corrected before elective surgery to prevent bradyarrhythmias.

Implications

Because cardiac output is often reduced with bradyarrhythmias, especially with impaired or loss of atrial transport function (e.g., slow atrial fibrillation or escape rhythms), bradyarrhythmias may be poorly tolerated during anesthesia. Moreover, any vasodilatation, hypovolemia, or myocardial depression is even more poorly tolerated with significant bradycardia. For example, the normal physiologic response to acute hypotension is impaired if there can be no increase in heart rate or cardiac output to maintain tissue perfusion. It is important to remember that cardiac output is the product of both heart rate and stroke volume. Whereas stroke volume is altered by contractility and preload, in addition to the effects of increased heart rate,[5] cardiac output is reduced by bradycardia and bradyarrhythmias, especially if the latter are associated with loss of atrial transport function. Properly timed atrial contractions are critical for left ventricular filling in patients with impaired ventricular relaxation (diastolic dysfunction). These include aged patients and those with chronic hypertension, aortic stenosis, or hypertrophic cardiomyopathy. Patients with impaired ventricular systolic function may also tolerate slow heart rates poorly. In this case, stroke volume is reduced by increased end-systolic volume; forward flow must be increased by higher heart rates. Valvular regurgitation, such as mitral regurgitation, is more severe at slower heart rates, possibly due to an increase in mitral annular size.

MANAGEMENT

Failure of Impulse Formation

SINUS BRADYCARDIA

Clinically significant sinus bradycardia is treated according to the severity of any physiologic impairment. Conservative management includes removing or reducing the dose of drugs known to inhibit the SA node or removing the surgical stimulus (e.g., oculocardiac reflex). If this is not effective or possible, use of anticholinergics (e.g., atropine) or sympathomimetics (e.g., ephedrine, epinephrine, isoproterenol) is considered. If this is ineffective, or if sinus bradycardia results in severe hemodynamic compromise or collapse, artificial pacing (transcutaneous, transvenous, or transesophageal) should be instituted.

ATRIOVENTRICULAR JUNCTIONAL ESCAPE RHYTHM

AV junctional rhythms, whether bradycardia or tachycardia (rate >100 beats per minute), abolish any atrial transport function and may also be associated with tricuspid or mitral regurgitation. In patients dependent on atrial transport function (those with severe diastolic dysfunction), restoration of sinus rhythm is highly desirable. Anticholinergic or sympathomimetics are often ineffective or only increase the rate of AV junctional rhythm. Use of a β-adrenergic blocker (e.g., esmolol) may restore dominance of the SA node during general anesthesia. However, use of a drug that may exacerbate bradycardia is risky and should be attempted only when the AV junctional rhythm is greater than 60 beats per minute. Other measures include changing to an intravenous anesthetic that may have less impact on the SA node compared with volatile anesthetics. Transesophageal atrial pacing restores atrial transport function and improve preload.

SICK SINUS SYNDROME

Sick sinus syndrome includes sinus bradycardia, sinus arrest, and chronotropic incompetence; it also may be associated with supraventricular tachyarrhythmias (bradycardia-tachycardia, or "brady-tachy" syndrome), the most common of which is atrial flutter or fibrillation. Regardless, treatment for bradycardia is as described earlier for sinus bradycardia. Management of associated tachycardia is discussed in Chapter 79. Always keep in mind, especially in patients with sick sinus syndrome and a history of tachyarrhythmias, that excessive tachycardia or tachyarrhythmias are a distinct possibility with any positive chronotropic treatment. Often, patients with symptomatic sick sinus syndrome have had dual-chamber pacemakers implanted, as well as drug treatment to prevent tachyarrhythmias and to slow AV node conduction.

Failure of Impulse Propagation

FIRST DEGREE ATRIOVENTRICULAR BLOCK

No treatment is indicated for first degree AV block, unless it is associated with symptomatic or hemodynamically significant bradycardia or escape rhythms. There are, however, rare exceptions. For example, after cardiac surgery, shorter P-R intervals may improve diastolic filling (preload), especially after hypertrophic cardiomyopathy repair. Thus, dual-chamber sequential (AV) pacing with surgically placed temporary pacing wires to shorten the P-R interval may result in improved ventricular filling. Also, if hemodynamic insufficiency is due to P-R interval prolongation, both perioperative and long-term (if symptomatic) dual-chamber pacing should be considered.

SECOND DEGREE ATRIOVENTRICULAR BLOCK

Mobitz type I AV block is usually due to impaired AV node conduction. It rarely progresses to complete heart block.

---

[4]Osborne or J waves consist of prominent notching of the terminal QRS complex with ST segment elevation.

[5]Except for the treppe or Bowditch effect, whereby an increase in heart rate increases cardiac contractile force.

Pacing (temporary or permanent) is indicated only when any associated bradycardia is hemodynamically significant or severely symptomatic. Mobitz type II AV block can be treated conservatively in the absence of preoperative symptoms. It is likely due to intra- or infra-Hisian disease and frequently progresses to advanced second or third degree heart block. Symptomatic, hemodynamically disadvantageous bradycardia is an indication for temporary pacing (surgery) and, if persistent, permanent pacing.

THIRD DEGREE ATRIOVENTRICULAR BLOCK

Some children with congenital complete AV heart block are asymptomatic, and permanent pacemaker implantation can be postponed until adolescence. However, pacing is indicated for all adult patients with third degree block unless it has a reversible cause (e.g., digoxin intoxication, β-blocker overdose).

PREVENTION

Patients undergoing surgery have similar indications for permanent pacemaker placement as the general population. The American Heart Association, American College of Cardiology, and North American Society for Pacing and Cardiac Electrophysiology (now the Heart Rhythm Society)

have published guidelines for the implantation of permanent pacemakers (see "Further Reading"). Indications for temporary perioperative pacing are less well established. However, temporary pacing should be strongly considered for patients without an implanted cardiac rhythm management device and with debilitating symptoms or documented disadvantageous bradycardia, escape rhythms, or AV heart block and facing intermediate- or high-risk surgery.

Further Reading

Atlee JL: Perioperative cardiac arrhythmias: Diagnosis and management. Anesthesiology 86:1397-1423, 1997.

Atlee JL, Pattison CZ, Mathews EL, et al: Transesophageal atrial pacing for intraoperative sinus bradycardia or AV junctional rhythm: Feasibility as prophylaxis in 200 anesthetized adults and hemodynamic effects of treatment. J Cardiothorac Vasc Anesth 7:436-441, 1993.

De Costa D, Brady WJ, Edhouse J: Bradycardias and atrioventricular conduction block. BMJ 324:535-538, 2002.

Goodacre S, McLeod K: ABC of clinical electrocardiography. BMJ 324: 1382-1385, 2002.

Gregoratos G, Abrams J, Epstein AE, et al: ACC/AHA/NASPE 2002 guideline update for implantation of cardiac pacemakers and antiarrhythmia devices: A report of the American College of Cardiology/American Heart Association Task Force on Practice Guidelines (ACC/AHA/NASPE Committee on Pacemaker Implantation). Circulation 106:2145-2161, 2002.

Zimetbaum PJ, Josephson ME: Use of the electrocardiogram in acute myocardial infarction. N Engl J Med 348:933-940, 2003.

Adverse Neurologic Sequelae: Peripheral Nerve Injury

83

Mohammed Minhaj

Case Synopsis

A 62-year-old man underwent coronary artery bypass graft surgery via a median sternotomy, with harvesting of the internal mammary artery. During a routine postoperative visit, the patient complains of a "tingling" sensation in the fourth and fifth fingers of his left hand. On physical examination, he has decreased sensation over those fingers, with minimally reduced muscular function in the ulnar distribution. A neurologic consultation is obtained, and the patient is diagnosed with a brachial plexus injury.

PROBLEM ANALYSIS

Definition

Nerve injuries are a well-recognized complication of anesthesia, causing substantial morbidity for patients and liability for anesthesiologists. Despite their prominence in closed claims analyses (16% of injuries in the most recent American Society of Anesthesiologists [ASA] Closed Claims Project database), no single cause has been clearly delineated. Although the proportion of nerve injuries has remained relatively constant over the last two closed claims surveys, there has been a relative decrease in the proportion of ulnar nerve-related injuries. The reason for this decrease is probably more stringent attention to proper positioning, but given the multifactorial nature of this complication, it is unlikely that simple improvements in positioning can entirely eradicate this problem in the future. The ASA closed claims study found that anesthesia care was appropriate in 66% of all nerve injury claims, reinforcing the notion that multiple factors likely contribute to such complications. These factors include the following:

- Ischemia to the brachial plexus
- Direct trauma (e.g., during central venous cannulation of the internal jugular vein via the needle or postprocedural hematoma)
- Needle injury, metabolic insults, and idiopathic injuries

The clinical syndrome of idiopathic brachial neuritis has been reported in a wide range of patient populations, including obstetric, arthritic, and noncardiac surgical patients. However, injuries to the ulnar nerve and brachial plexus occur more frequently during cardiac than noncardiac surgery. For example, the incidence of nerve injury in noncardiac surgery ranged from 0.02% to 0.06%, whereas that in cardiac surgery ranged from 2% to 38%.

Recognition

Most often, nerve injuries that occur during cardiac surgery are identified postoperatively. Intraoperative identification of injury is limited, given that most patients are under general anesthesia (85% of all ulnar nerve injuries in ASA closed claims analyses were associated with general anesthesia). Further, there is no intraoperative monitoring that reliably detects nerve injury.

Although some investigators have attempted to identify intraoperative signs that may predict postoperative dysfunction, these have not proved very reliable. Somatosensory evoked potentials (SEPs) reportedly allow the early identification of nerve injury, especially when harvesting of the internal mammary artery is involved. Such harvesting is typically associated with greater chest retraction, potentially producing excessive stretch on the brachial plexus. Transient intraoperative changes in SEPs obtained during venous cannulation have not reliably predicted postoperative sequelae, although SEPs obtained at the conclusion of surgery may do so.

In general, nerve injury in cardiac surgical patients differs from that in noncardiac patients. As mentioned earlier, such injuries are more common in the former. Cardiac patients also typically demonstrate sensory deficits in the lower roots of the brachial plexus (C8-T1), compared with more upper and middle nerve root distributions in noncardiac surgical patients. Further, sensory deficits are typically more prominent than motor deficits in cardiac surgical patients; the opposite is true in noncardiac patients. Finally, symptoms are usually present in the early postoperative period in both groups of patients.

Risk Assessment

Most peripheral nerve injuries are attributed to ischemia of the intraneural vasculature. The interruption of adequate oxygen and nutrient delivery leads to injury and postoperative deficits. Such ischemia is generally thought to be a result of stretching or compression of the plexus caused by patient malpositioning.

There is, however, some debate regarding "appropriate" positioning during cardiac surgery. One study reported a higher rate of nerve injury in patients whose arms were at their sides compared with those whose arms were abducted (23.5% versus 14.5%), although this difference was not statistically significant. Some authorities advocate a "hands-up" position, with the arms abducted 90 degrees but flexed at the shoulder by 15 to 20 degrees, and the forearm flexed at the elbow by 90 to 110 degrees to reduce stretch on the brachial plexus and the associated risk of nerve injury. However, no data exist to show that this significantly reduces brachial plexus injuries when compared with the more traditional practice of tucking patients' arms at their sides and padding the elbows.

Because patient positioning is a concern in all surgeries, there has been considerable debate about ideal positioning. Also, because the incidence of postoperative nerve injury is higher with cardiac surgery than noncardiac surgery, investigators have searched for mechanisms (other than ischemia) specific to cardiac surgery. Multiple mechanisms have been postulated by various authors (Table 83-1); however, excessive sternal retraction is the most commonly accepted risk factor for brachial plexus injury.

Understanding the anatomy of the brachial plexus and the effects of sternal retraction on it may help determine causative factors for perioperative injury. The nerve roots of the brachial plexus are fixed at their points of exit from the vertebral canal and are distally anchored to the axillary fascia. Moreover, the plexus lies close to many bony structures, such as the head of the humerus, first rib, clavicle, and coracoid process, making it vulnerable to compression at these sites. Autopsy studies have shown that excessive spread of the sternal retractor pushes the clavicles into the retroclavicular space and rotates the first rib upward. These movements may result in stretch of the brachial plexus. Finally, some investigators have postulated that fracture of the first rib during sternal retraction may cause direct penetration injury to the plexus.

In addition, preexisting anatomic and pathophysiologic disease processes have been reported as risk factors not only for brachial plexus injury but also for delayed postoperative recovery (Table 83-2).

Table 83–1 ■ Risk Factors for Perioperative Nerve Injury during Cardiac Surgery

Sternal retraction
    Positioning of sternal retractors
    Asymmetrical sternal retraction
Internal mammary artery harvesting
Duration of surgery
Duration of cardiopulmonary bypass
Hypothermia
Penetration injury due to first rib fracture during sternotomy
Injury during cannulation of internal jugular vein
    Direct, needle-related injury
    Hematoma formation resulting in compression of brachial plexus

Table 83–2 ■ Preexisting Anatomic and Pathophysiologic Risk Factors for Perioperative Nerve Injury

Diabetes
Neuropathy
Alcoholism
Herpes zoster
Polyarteritis nodosa
Peripheral vascular disease
Coagulopathies
Hypertension
Hypothyroidism
Cervical rib
Deformities in shoulder or derivation of brachial plexus

Implications

Most cardiac patients with postoperative brachial plexus injury recover quickly. It has been estimated that more than 90% of such patients recover substantially within 1 month of surgery. In one study, 94% of patients were asymptomatic by the time of hospital discharge.

Subsequent referral to a hand clinic for continued symptoms has been reported in only 0.2% of all cardiac surgical patients. Even when recovery is prolonged, most patients recover fully within a year, and it is rare to have a patient with incomplete recovery. Coexisting diseases such as diabetes have been implicated in more prolonged or incomplete recoveries.

MANAGEMENT

Because most cases resolve quickly and spontaneously, supportive management is often sufficient. Splints and physical therapy have been reported to be beneficial, even immediately postoperatively. These measures help prevent muscle atrophy and provide support until symptoms resolve. Only if symptoms are prolonged (>3 months) should more comprehensive interventions be considered.

Electrophysiologic studies are usually performed only if symptoms persist and spontaneous recovery is prolonged. Electromyography may be performed to evaluate signs and symptoms of denervation during rest, reinnervation of motor units during weak effort, and loss of motor units during maximal effort. In one clinical study in which bilateral nerve conduction studies were performed in patients who experienced perioperative ulnar neuropathy, 12 of 14 patients with unilateral symptoms had abnormal nerve conduction studies on the contralateral side. These findings suggest that preexisting neuropathies may manifest during the perioperative period.

Surgical intervention is usually limited to conditions that involve anatomic abnormalities, such as thoracic outlet syndrome, fracture of the first rib resulting in penetration of the brachial plexus, or compression by bony prominences.

PREVENTION

Prevention of perioperative nerve injuries is difficult, given that the mechanisms of injury are incompletely understood.

Although proper patient positioning, along with adequate padding of pressure points and avoidance of brachial plexus stretch, may not prevent all nerve injuries, the importance of such measures cannot be overemphasized. A thorough understanding of the anatomy involved and the potential mechanisms of injury enables anesthesiologists to reduce such postoperative complications.

In addition to awareness of the specific risk factors postulated to contribute to postoperative nerve injury in cardiac surgery, most clinicians advocate the following:

- Proper vigilance with regard to patient positioning and position changes
- Minimal sternal retraction, especially during harvesting of the internal mammary artery, and placement of sternal retractors as caudally as possible
- Maintenance of a neutral (midline) head position to minimize tension on the brachial plexus produced by head rotation
- Avoidance of asymmetrical retraction when possible (perform true median sternotomy)

Further Reading

Alvine FG, Schurrer ME: Postoperative ulnar-nerve palsy: Are there predisposing factors? J Bone Joint Surg Am 69:255-259, 1987.

Ben-David B, Stahl S: Prognosis of intraoperative brachial plexus injury: A review of 22 cases. Br J Anaesth 79:440-445, 1997.

Cheney FW, Domino KB, Caplan RA, Posner KL: Nerve injury associated with anesthesia: A closed claims analysis. Anesthesiology 90:1062-1069, 1999.

Dumitru D, Liles RA: Postpartum idiopathic brachial neuritis. Obstet Gynecol 73:473-475, 1989.

Eggers KA, Asai T: Postoperative brachial plexus neuropathy after total knee replacement under spinal anaesthesia. Br J Anaesth 75:642-644, 1995.

Hanson MR, Breuer AC, Furlan AJ, et al: Mechanism and frequency of brachial plexus injury in open-heart surgery: A prospective analysis. Ann Thorac Surg 36:675-679, 1983.

Hickey C, Gugino LD, Aglio LS, et al: Intraoperative somatosensory evoked potential monitoring predicts peripheral nerve injury during cardiac surgery. Anesthesiology 78:29-35, 1993.

Jellish WS, Martucci J, Blakeman B, Hudson E: Somatosensory evoked potential monitoring of the brachial plexus to predict nerve injury during internal mammary artery harvest: Intraoperative comparisons of the Rultract and Pittman sternal retractors. J Cardiothorac Vasc Anesth 8:398-403, 1994.

Kroll DA, Caplan RA, Posner K, et al: Nerve injury associated with anesthesia. Anesthesiology 73:202-207, 1990.

Lederman RJ, Breuer AC, Hanson MR, et al: Peripheral nervous system complications of coronary artery bypass graft surgery. Ann Neurol 12:297-301, 1982.

Tomlinson DL, Hirsch IA, Kodali SV, Slogoff S: Protecting the brachial plexus during median sternotomy. J Thorac Cardiovasc Surg 94:297-301, 1987.

Vahl CF, Carl I, Muller-Vahl H, Struck E: Brachial plexus injury after cardiac surgery: The role of internal mammary artery preparation: A prospective study on 1000 consecutive patients. J Thorac Cardiovasc Surg 102:724-729, 1991.

Vander Salm TJ, Cereda JM, Cutler BS: Brachial plexus injury following median sternotomy. J Thorac Cardiovasc Surg 80:447-452, 1980.

Vander Salm TJ, Cutler BS, Okike ON: Brachial plexus injury following median sternotomy. Part II. J Thorac Cardiovasc Surg 83:914-917, 1982.

Adverse Neurologic Sequelae: Central Neurologic Impairment

84

David Muzic and Mark A. Chaney

Case Synopsis

A 68-year-old man with a history of non-insulin-dependent diabetes mellitus, hypertension, alcohol abuse, and heavy smoking is scheduled for four-vessel off-pump coronary artery bypass grafting (CABG). After uneventful induction of anesthesia, severe aortic atheromatous disease is observed via transesophageal echocardiography (TEE) in the descending aorta, and the aortic root is not well visualized. Epiaortic ultrasound scanning is performed to ascertain the best location for a planned radial artery graft anastomosis. The patient's biventricular function is adequate, and the CABG is performed successfully. The postoperative course is complicated, however, by significant short-term memory loss, and the patient is discharged first to a skilled nursing facility and eventually to an assisted-living home.

PROBLEM ANALYSIS

Definition

Central neurologic injury following CABG is much more common than was previously recognized. Such impairment was formerly observed primarily as stroke, which currently has a perioperative incidence of 1% to 5% for CABG surgery. However, studies of postoperative neuropsychological function using rigorous testing strategies have shown neurocognitive dysfunction in 50% to 90% of patients at discharge and in 20% to 40% throughout the first year after CABG. Accordingly, postoperative central nervous system (CNS) impairment is often divided into two types of adverse outcomes, along these same lines:

- Type I outcomes due to macroembolic focal injury, associated with stupor and coma
- Type II outcomes due to macroembolic global injury, associated with deterioration of intellectual function or memory

The focal neurologic deficits representing overt stroke (type I outcomes) are caused mainly by macroemboli of atheroma debris, thrombus, and air. Current data suggest that microemboli of similar materials and debris such as bone wax, marrow, and lipid particles from retransfused cardiotomy suction blood are major contributors to the more diffuse (and much more common) injuries associated with type II outcomes. The systemic inflammatory response of surgical stress and blood contact with the cardiopulmonary bypass (CPB) circuit are believed to contribute importantly to type II injury. Other causes of both type I and type II CNS injury include cerebral hyperthermia during rewarming, arterial hypotension, and neurohormonal derangements.

A recent randomized, controlled trial comparing type II neurocognitive outcomes in patients undergoing conventional CABG with and without CPB showed a nonsignificant trend toward a benefit of off-pump CABG at 3 and 12 months postoperatively. The incidence of type II outcomes was 29% versus 21% at 3 months ($P = 0.15$) and 33% versus 31% at 12 months ($P = 0.69$) for conventional CABG versus off-pump CABG, respectively. Importantly, these findings suggest that type II neurologic outcomes are more common than previously thought and that rigorous neurocognitive testing is necessary for detection. For example, an earlier multicenter study demonstrated only a 3% incidence of type II outcomes at discharge for patients undergoing conventional CABG, whereas a more recent study with more thorough neurocognitive testing revealed incidences of 53%, 36%, 24%, and 42% at discharge, 6 weeks, 6 months, and 5 years after discharge following CABG, respectively.

Recognition

The presence of type I CNS injury is often apparent in the immediate postoperative recovery period. This type of injury commonly presents with failure to awaken from anesthesia, obtundation, generalized or localized hypertonicity, aphasia, visual field deficits, hemineglect, or seizures and is thought to be caused by intraoperative embolic phenomena or global or regional cerebral hypoperfusion. Progressive deficits or signs of elevated intracranial pressure, especially in the presence of anticoagulation, suggest intracranial hemorrhage and require immediate evaluation. Computed tomography (CT) is often used in the first 24 hours to evaluate for hemorrhage and then again after 48 hours to detect evidence of infarction (infarcted brain tissue often appears normal on CT imaging before 48 hours). Magnetic resonance imaging is sometimes used in the first 24 hours owing to its higher

339

sensitivity for diagnosing hemorrhage and brain ischemia; however, it cannot be used in the presence of implanted cardiac rhythm management devices. Worsened or new deficits postoperatively also warrant echocardiography for detection of a cardiac embolic source.

Recognition of type II CNS injury is much more difficult. The first sign is often the patient's report of "not feeling right" or the patient's family members noting that their loved one has "slowed down" or become more forgetful. Studies to measure intellectual deterioration and memory deficits related to type II injury rely on changes in neurocognitive test scores compared with a preoperative baseline; in practice, however, such a baseline test is almost never performed. Therefore, any neurocognitive decline noted after CABG is rarely quantifiable.

Risk Assessment

Perioperative neurologic risk can be divided into patient-related preoperative risk factors and intraoperative procedure-related factors. Recognized independent patient-related risk factors for type I injury include the following:

- Advanced age
- Proximal aortic atherosclerosis
- Previous CABG
- Peripheral vascular disease
- Preexisting neurologic disease
- Diabetes mellitus
- Hypertension
- Pulmonary disease
- Unstable angina

Patient-related risk factors for type II injury include the following:

- Advanced age
- Systolic hypertension greater than 180 mm Hg on admission
- Excessive alcohol consumption
- Previous CABG
- Arrhythmia on day of surgery
- Antihypertensive therapy

Whether the presence of the apoE ε-4 allele, which is associated with late-onset Alzheimer's disease and poorer outcome after stroke or subarachnoid hemorrhage, is a risk factor for type I or type II injury remains controversial.

Intraoperative procedure-related factors also play a major role in type I and type II injury after cardiac surgery, perhaps owing to increased microembolic and macroembolic load to the brain, cerebral hypoperfusion, or normal or increased cerebral metabolic rate. Manipulation of the aorta by CPB cannulation, cross-clamping, side-clamping, unclamping, or lifting of the heart and the use of an intra-aortic balloon pump are also believed to increase the risk of CNS injury. Microembolic load to the brain, as measured by transcranial Doppler, has been shown to correlate with the severity of neurocognitive decline, and an association between microembolization and such aortic manipulations has been demonstrated. Similarly, manipulation of the CPB circuit itself and prolonged CPB time have been implicated as risk factors for CNS injury by increasing the embolic load of air and microthrombi. Open-heart procedures, such as valve surgery or septal defect repair, also appear to be associated with a greater risk of CNS injury.

Possibly the most important intraoperative risk factor is the surgeon's choice of aortic cannulation site for CPB. Approximately 20% of patients undergoing CABG have moderate to severe ascending aortic atherosclerotic disease. If so, it is critical that the anesthesiologist be involved in the decision making to determine the optimal cannulation site. It has been shown that TEE is more accurate than direct palpation for locating aortic plaques. Therefore, TEE-guided aortic cannulation has become standard in most centers. More recent data show that detecting these plaques is best accomplished with direct epiaortic scanning using a sterile-sheathed surface ultrasound probe applied directly to the aorta. Additionally, TEE is helpful in diagnosing other procedure-related risk factors for type I and II adverse neurologic outcomes, including intracardiac thrombi and air, septal defects, and iatrogenic aortic dissection.

Maintaining a somewhat depressed cerebral metabolic rate intraoperatively is thought to help prevent CNS injury. Procedures performed under normothermic conditions, or those allowing rapid rewarming after CPB, increase the risk of type I and II injury. Rapid rewarming has been shown to cause a desaturation of jugular venous hemoglobin and is believed to correlate with poorer CNS outcomes. Similarly, avoiding glucose-containing CPB priming fluids and maintaining normoglycemia are believed to reduce risk.

One might think that avoiding CPB altogether, by performing off-pump CABG whenever possible, would greatly reduce the risk of CNS injury. However, as mentioned earlier, a recent randomized, controlled trial failed to show any significant difference in type I or II CNS injuries for off-pump versus conventional CABG. Whether off-pump CABG involving bilateral internal mammary artery grafting and the avoidance of aortic manipulation could reduce CNS injury has yet to be shown.

Implications

Perioperative CNS injury, whether overt type I or more subtle type II, can be devastating in terms of quality of life and resource utilization. In-hospital mortality is about 10-fold and 5-fold higher for type I and type II injuries, respectively. The need for skilled nursing facilities on hospital discharge also increases approximately 6-fold for type I and 4-fold for type II injury. The economic burden for CNS injury after cardiac surgery reaches well above the billion dollar mark annually.

MANAGEMENT AND PREVENTION

Preventing or reducing the risk of neurologic injury during cardiac surgery is of the utmost importance. Even more subtle and common type II injuries have a great impact on postoperative autonomy and patient lifestyle and undermine the primary goal of surgery, which is to improve longevity and quality of life. Therefore, all patients should be considered at risk, and certain steps should be taken to identify and reduce specific risks for neurologic injury.

Aortic Imaging. Intraoperative TEE or direct epiaortic scanning allows informed aortic cannulation. Without such imaging, an unacceptably large fraction of patients is unnecessarily exposed to large cerebral embolic loads from cannulation and clamping through or near aortic atheromas.

Moderate Hypothermia.
Cooling during CPB to approximately 32°C reduces the cerebral metabolic rate and provides cerebral protection. Careful rewarming is equally important in preventing unnecessary increases in cerebral metabolism.

Avoidance of Arterial Hypotension.
Some data suggest that higher mean arterial pressure during CPB is associated with better neurologic outcomes in higher-risk patients as identified by TEE evaluation or direct epiaortic scanning, but this is controversial. It is hypothesized that in these patients, optimizing collateral cerebral flow minimizes the risk of embolic neurologic injury. However, there is little evidence that maintaining a specific mean or cerebral perfusion pressure range improves outcome.

Alpha-Stat pH Management.
During cooling, targeting a pH of 7.4 corrected to 37°C (i.e., alpha-stat pH management) and maintaining cerebral autoregulation may provide improved neurologic outcomes when compared with pH-stat management. The latter requires the addition of carbon dioxide to the CPB circuit in order to maintain the pH at 7.4 measured at the hypothermic patient's actual body temperature. However, pH-stat may be beneficial during procedures requiring deep hypothermia, because it may provide better cerebral protection by decoupling cerebral autoregulation and enhancing cerebral blood flow. Even so, the relative importance of these techniques remains unclear.

Avoidance of Retransfusion of Unprocessed Blood.
Retransfusion of unprocessed cardiotomy suction blood delivers particulate microemboli consisting of cell aggregates, bone wax, lipids, and surgical debris to the circulation. This has been implicated in neurologic injury.

Antifibrinolytic Therapy.
Aprotinin, a serine protease inhibitor, reduces the inflammatory response to CPB and has the potential to reduce the incidence of stroke in CABG patients.

Pharmacotherapy.
Many drugs have been evaluated for their ability to reduce neurologic injury after cardiac surgery, but with conflicting results. Thiopental, propofol, etomidate, glucocorticoids, nimodipine, inhalational anesthetics, and others have been studied for their ability to reduce cerebral metabolic rate, inhibit inflammation and brain edema, and limit the embolic load through cerebral vasoconstriction. However, none has yet been shown to improve neurologic outcome.

Devices.
Newly developed sutureless and clampless grafting devices allow surgeons to perform aortic proximal anastomoses without the need for aortic side-clamping. This may reduce the embolic load and improve neurologic outcome.

Other Surgical Techniques.
Minimizing CPB time or performing off-pump CABG may improve neurologic outcomes, but so far, the data have been inconsistent. Also, left and right internal mammary artery grafts (which avoid aortic manipulation), nontraditional aortic cannulation sites, and deep hypothermia have been advocated. However, further study is required to determine whether any of these techniques is truly effective.

Further Reading

Arrowsmith JE, Grocott HP, Newman MF: Neurologic risk assessment, monitoring, and outcome in cardiac surgery. J Cardiothorac Vasc Anesth 13:736-743, 1999.

Gringore AM, Grocott HP, Mathew JP, et al: The rewarming rate and increased peak temperature alter neurocognitive outcome after cardiac surgery. Anesth Analg 94:4-10, 2002.

Mackensen GB, Ti LK, Phillips-Bute BG, et al: Cerebral embolization during cardiac surgery: Impact of aortic atheroma burden. Br J Anaesth 91:656-661, 2003.

Mark DB, Newman MF: Protecting the brain in coronary artery bypass graft surgery. JAMA 287:1448-1450, 2002.

Mora CT, Henson MB, Weintraub WS, et al: The effect of temperature management during cardiopulmonary bypass on neurologic and neuropsychologic outcomes in patients undergoing coronary revascularization. J Thorac Cardiovasc Surg 112:514-522, 1996.

Murkin JM: Attenuation of neurologic injury during cardiac surgery. Ann Thorac Surg 72:S1838-S1844, 2001.

Newman MF, Wolman R, Kanchuger M, et al: Multicenter preoperative stroke risk index for patients undergoing coronary artery bypass graft surgery. Circulation 94:II74-II80, 1996.

Roach GW, Kanchuger M, Mangano CM, et al: Adverse central nervous system outcomes following coronary artery bypass graft surgery in a multicenter study: Incidence, predictors and resource utilization. N Engl J Med 335:1857-1863, 1996.

Scarborough JE, White W, Derilus FE, et al: Combined use of off-pump techniques and a sutureless proximal aortic anastomotic device reduces cerebral microemboli generation during coronary artery bypass grafting. J Thorac Cardiovasc Surg 126:1561-1567, 2003.

Van Dijk D, Jansen EW, Hijman R, et al: Cognitive outcome after off-pump and on-pump coronary artery bypass graft surgery: A randomized trial. JAMA 287:1405-1412, 2002.

CARDIOTHORACIC & VASCULAR SURGERY

Postoperative Acute Renal Failure

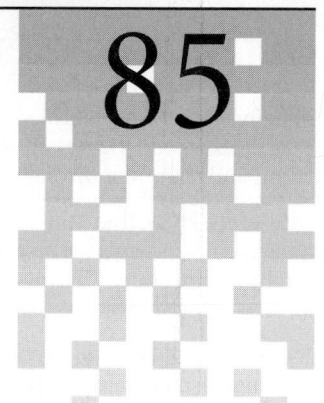

Mark Nunnally and Robert N. Sladen

Case Synopsis

A 75-year-old man with long-standing hypertension and type 2 diabetes mellitus underwent open repair of an infrarenal aortic aneurysm. His baseline creatinine was 1.6 mg/dL and rose to 2.0 mg/dL on the second postoperative day. On the fifth postoperative day, he developed progressive hypoxemia, fever, and hypotension. A contrast-enhanced scan of the pulmonary vessels was not suggestive of pulmonary embolism. He was started on a β-lactam and an aminoglycoside for probable pneumonia. Over the next 12 hours, he became hypotensive and anuric. Renal replacement therapy was started, and antibiotic therapy was shifted to a quinolone. The patient's renal function returned after several weeks, and he was eventually discharged.

PROBLEM ANALYSIS

Definition

Postoperative acute renal failure (ARF) describes a spectrum of renal dysfunction that occurs after surgery. Unfortunately, multiple definitions of this complication exist, including those based on intervention (dialysis required or not), relative or absolute decline in glomerular filtration rate (GFR), or relative or absolute increase in serum creatinine (S_{Cr}) level. It can include new-onset renal failure as well as acute worsening of chronic renal failure. The fractional change in S_{Cr} has emerged as a practical and consistent index of the severity of perioperative renal injury; however, the need for dialysis is a potent predictor of outcome. In one study of patients undergoing coronary artery bypass grafting (CABG), mortality associated with ARF was 14%, but this doubled to 28% when dialysis was required.

The cause of ARF has traditionally been classified as prerenal (decreased perfusion), renal (parenchymal injury), or postrenal (urinary obstruction). Although these distinctions remain useful for directing diagnostic strategy, they frequently overlap. In about 90% of cases, postoperative ARF is a consequence of sustained prerenal injury that culminates in ischemic acute tubular necrosis (ATN). ATN can also be caused by nephrotoxic insults, which may themselves exacerbate ischemic injury.

In animal models, transient low perfusion creates a prerenal state characterized by oliguria and low urine sodium, with salt and water retention. This is the normal renal tubular response to hypovolemia. With increased perfusion, urine flow returns to normal. This is a hemodynamically mediated event with preserved tubular function; it is reversed by restoration of normal hemodynamic function. More prolonged perfusion deficits result in oliguria (with high urine sodium) that does not reverse when perfusion increases. In this scenario, ATN occurs, characterized by tubular obstruction and "backleak." The latter is a hemodynamically mediated event with loss of tubular function; it is not reversed by restoration of normal hemodynamic function. Even so, intrinsic renal architecture is preserved, and the kidney may ultimately recover.

The pathogenesis of ARF reflects the kidney's unique sensitivity to insult. Figure 85-1 demonstrates several sensitive areas of the nephron. The medulla and inner cortex have marginal blood flow and are therefore at risk for ischemic ATN from alterations in renal oxygen delivery. This could result from intravascular volume depletion, hypotension, diminished cardiac output, or anemia. In nephrotoxic ATN, damage to the tubules is the result of inflammatory signaling, free radical damage, disturbances in cellular metabolism, and disruption of intrinsic renal vasodilators such as prostaglandins and nitric oxide. Tubular cell necrosis and apoptosis lead to loss of function, disruption of architecture, and nephron obstruction by cellular debris. Once this has occurred, restoration of renal blood flow can no longer reestablish GFR.

Recognition

Perioperative oliguria is an unreliable index of renal function because it is almost inevitably prerenal in nature. It reflects absolute or relative hypovolemia, with vasoconstriction and sodium retention as a consequence of activation of the sympathoadrenal, renin-angiotensin-aldosterone, and antidiuretic hormone systems. With two very important exceptions (sepsis and liver failure), it is reversed by restoration of normal renal hemodynamics. In contrast, when postoperative ATN occurs, it is often a culmination of multiple lesser insults in a protected milieu, resulting in nonoliguric renal failure, defined as ARF with urine flow 15 to 80 mL/hour. In summary, oliguria is common but seldom implies ARF, but the presence of a normal urine flow rate does not exclude it.

When ARF does ensue, loss of renal solute clearance begins to result in the buildup of serum concentrations of electrolytes, urea, water, and other osmotic elements (azotemia). Blood urea nitrogen and S_{Cr} are the most commonly used indicators of renal function. Urea depends on

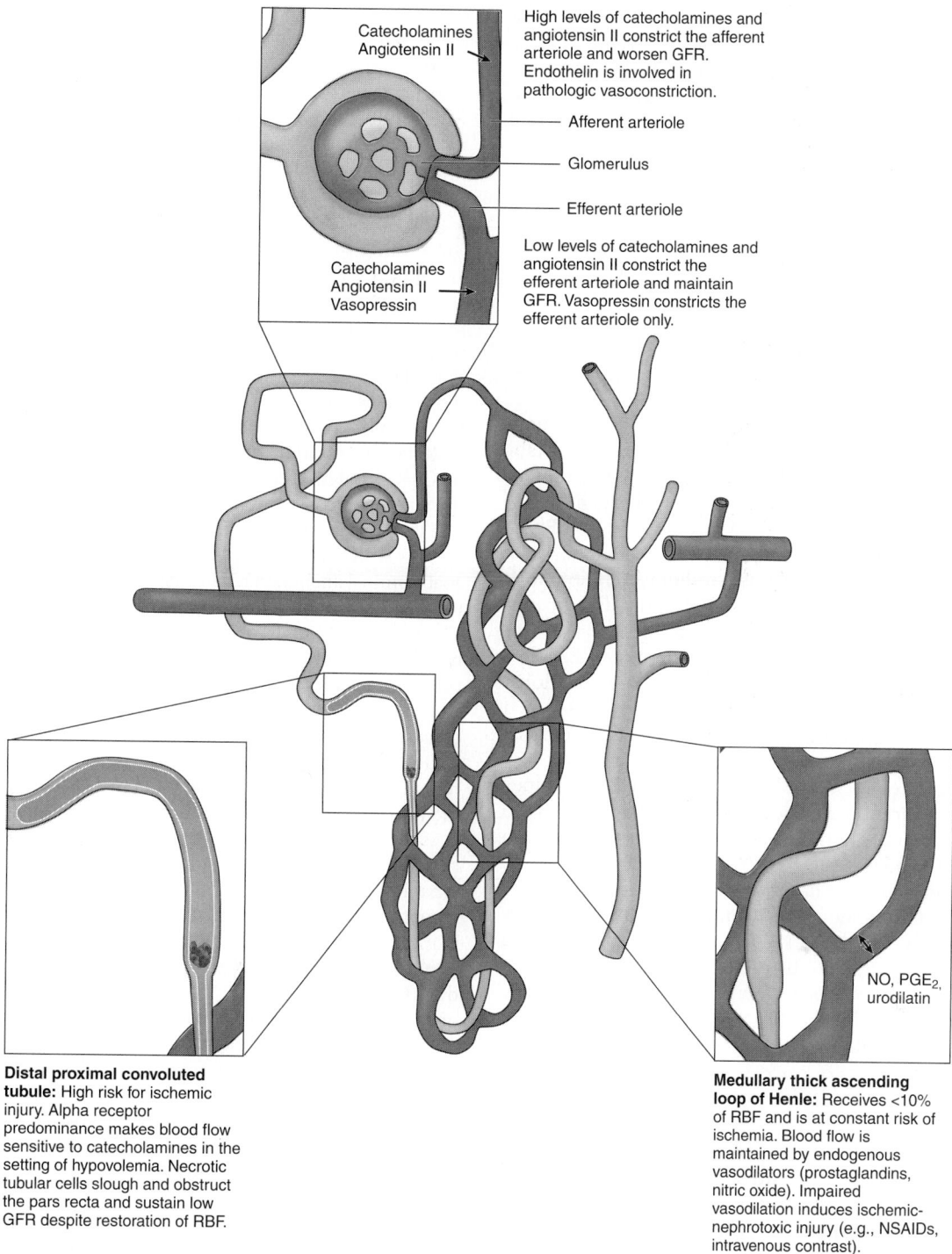

Catecholamines
Angiotensin II

High levels of catecholamines and angiotensin II constrict the afferent arteriole and worsen GFR. Endothelin is involved in pathologic vasoconstriction.

— Afferent arteriole

— Glomerulus

— Efferent arteriole

Low levels of catecholamines and angiotensin II constrict the efferent arteriole and maintain GFR. Vasopressin constricts the efferent arteriole only.

Catecholamines
Angiotensin II
Vasopressin

Distal proximal convoluted tubule: High risk for ischemic injury. Alpha receptor predominance makes blood flow sensitive to catecholamines in the setting of hypovolemia. Necrotic tubular cells slough and obstruct the pars recta and sustain low GFR despite restoration of RBF.

NO, PGE$_2$, urodilatin

Medullary thick ascending loop of Henle: Receives <10% of RBF and is at constant risk of ischemia. Blood flow is maintained by endogenous vasodilators (prostaglandins, nitric oxide). Impaired vasodilation induces ischemic-nephrotoxic injury (e.g., NSAIDs, intravenous contrast).

Figure 85–1 ■ The proximal tubule and medullary thick ascending loop of Henle are potential sites of ischemic and nephrotoxic tubular injury. Both segments have high oxygen consumption and are at risk owing to supply-demand imbalance. GFR, glomerular filtration rate; NO, nitric oxide; NSAIDs, nonsteroidal anti-inflammatory drugs; PGE$_2$, prostaglandin E$_2$; RBF, renal blood flow.

tubular excretion but may be a misleading surrogate for tubular function because its blood level is affected by nonrenal pathology, such as gastrointestinal hemorrhage and protein catabolism (abnormally increased) or malnutrition and end-stage liver disease (abnormally decreased). S_{Cr} reflects the balance between creatinine production and excretion. These come into equilibrium when renal function is in a steady state. Therefore, S_{Cr} is a reliable surrogate for GFR.

However, the relationship between S_{Cr} and GFR is not direct; it is exponentially inverse. That is, a doubling of S_{Cr} implies a halving of GFR. Thus, a "trivial" increase in S_{Cr} from 0.6 to 1.2 mg/dL implies a 50% decrease in GFR. Moreover, S_{Cr} does not increase above normal limits until GFR has decreased below 50 mL/minute. In cachectic patients with low creatinine production, S_{Cr} may be "normal" with a GFR as low as 30 mL/minute.

CARDIOTHORACIC &
VASCULAR SURGERY

Creatinine clearance provides a real-time estimate of GFR because its calculation (UV/S_{Cr}, where U is urine creatinine and V is urine flow rate) incorporates the creatinine excretion rate (UV), which is directly proportional to GFR. If a patient has a urinary catheter and the urine flow rate is carefully measured, reliable estimates of GFR can be obtained with urine collection times of 2 hours or less. A shortcut that is often used in perioperative studies of renal function is to forgo the necessity of urine collection by calculating creatinine clearance from a nomogram—the Cockroft-Gault formula:

Creatinine clearance =

$$\frac{[(140 - \text{Age [years]}) \times \text{Weight [kg]} \times 1.73 \text{ m}^2 \times 0.85^*]}{72 \times S_{Cr} \text{ [mg/dL]} \times \text{Body surface area [m}^2]}$$

In the presence of oliguria, evaluation of tubular function may help distinguish a prerenal syndrome from established ARF. The prerenal state is characterized by avid tubular sodium and water retention, leading to small quantities of concentrated urine with low urinary sodium (<10 mEq/L) and a fractional excretion of sodium (FE_{Na}) less than 1%. Prerenal states leading to elevated sodium excretion with intact tubular function (e.g., metabolic alkalosis, diuretic use) may spuriously elevate the FE_{Na} to greater than 3%. In this setting, a high FE_{Na} is unreliable, but persistence of FE_{Na} less than 1% is highly suggestive of a prerenal state. Fractional excretion of urea nitrogen has recently been proposed as a more sensitive and specific method to differentiate prerenal azotemia from ATN, especially when diuretics are used.

In established ARF, tubular function is lost. The kidney is unable to concentrate urine and retain sodium, leading to small quantities of dilute urine with high urinary sodium (>80 mEq/L) and high FE_{Na} (>3%).

Additional objective data may be derived from electrolyte disturbances and hemodynamic monitoring. Ultrasonography of the renal vasculature, kidneys, and urinary drainage system can help rule out obstructive uropathy and confirm the diagnosis of ATN (normal renal blood flow) or ischemic injury (regional or global deficits). Risk assessment serves to clarify suspicion and evaluate for treatable risk factors.

Risk Assessment

Identification of patients at risk permits more accurate prediction of postoperative ARF and offers the opportunity for intervention. Risk assessment is achieved by integrating patient factors, the surgical procedure, and the perioperative milieu. The potential for acute renal injury increases exponentially as risk factors accumulate. For example, exposure to a single nephrotoxin (e.g., ketorolac) seldom causes a problem, but if combined with other nephrotoxins (e.g., gentamicin) and decreased perfusion (hypovolemia), the risk for ARF becomes extremely high.

Of all preoperative risk factors, the most predictive is preexisting renal dysfunction. Renal risk increases exponentially when the preoperative S_{Cr} exceeds 2.0 mg/dL. Other important risk factors include advancing age and markers for vascular disease and end-organ damage, such as diabetes, abnormal cholesterol metabolism, and hypertension. Severe obstructive jaundice and the hepatorenal syndrome are associated with abnormal portal absorption of endotoxin, which induces renal vasoconstriction and a refractory prerenal state characterized by low urine sodium. Sepsis induces a similar milieu, along with the insults of hypotension and sympathetic renal vasoconstriction. Finally, there may be a genetic predisposition to renal injury, as suggested by the finding of a decreased risk associated with a specific apolipoprotein genotype.

Intraoperative risk factors are related to the type of surgery (potential for complications such as bleeding, hypotension, or low cardiac output states) and specific interventions that may cause renal injury (e.g., aortic cross-clamping, cardiopulmonary bypass). Suprarenal aortic cross-clamping leads to a complete cessation of GFR, and full recovery may take 24 to 48 hours. Infrarenal cross-clamping also induces a decrease in GFR through reflex vasoconstriction. In either event, the duration of cross-clamping correlates with the risk for ARF. The risk of postoperative renal dysfunction and ARF requiring dialysis is 12% to 25% and 3% to 8%, respectively, for thoracoabdominal aneurysm repair; the risk is 2% to 30% and 0.6% to 1%, respectively, for abdominal aortic aneurysm repair.

Cardiopulmonary bypass also increases the risk of ARF, but this is remarkably well tolerated by patients with normal preexisting renal function who have an uncomplicated course. Despite early optimism, off-pump CABG does not consistently decrease the incidence of perioperative renal injury. The most important risk factors in cardiac surgery remain preoperative renal insufficiency, the complexity of the procedure, and postoperative cardiac dysfunction.

For all types of surgery, the most important postoperative risk factor is circulatory instability. Sepsis alone may induce renal injury through local vasoconstriction and nephrotoxicity without substantial hemodynamic perturbations. The risk is markedly exacerbated by the concomitant occurrence of nephrotoxic insults. These include pigment nephropathy due to rhabdomyolysis, intravascular hemolysis, severe obstructive jaundice, contrast nephropathy, and drugs. In the case synopsis, the patient had preoperative renal dysfunction (i.e., high S_{Cr}), underwent a high-risk procedure (aortic aneurysm repair, even though infrarenal), and was later exposed to several other renal insults (sepsis, contrast exposure, and an aminoglycoside antibiotic).

Implications

Overall outcome is substantially determined by the severity of renal injury, but it is adversely affected even when renal dysfunction is moderate. For example, ARF requiring dialysis is uncommon after CABG but is associated with high mortality. Renal dysfunction (S_{Cr} increased >1 mg/dL above baseline) is considerably more common and is associated with significantly greater mortality compared with patients with no renal dysfunction. This may be explained by concomitant cardiac dysfunction, or it may be related to an independent adverse effect of renal failure on global organ function. For high-risk surgeries, in-hospital mortality can exceed 60% with ARF; this also leads to a substantial increase in resource utilization.

---

*0.85 conversion factor is used for females only.

This forbidding mortality rate has been little altered despite the development of improved renal replacement therapies (RRTs), including continuous venovenous hemodialysis. Although RRT consistently controls electrolyte and acid-base abnormalities, circulatory overload, and acute uremia, it does not eliminate the risk of sepsis, multiorgan system dysfunction, or impaired wound healing, which also contribute substantially to postoperative morbidity and mortality.

Isolated ATN is inherently reversible, but additional ischemic or nephrotoxic insults may convert it into protracted ARF or even established chronic renal failure. In particular, there is compelling evidence that autoregulation is lost in ARF, so when dialysis causes hypotension, it injures the tubular cells and paradoxically delays renal recovery.

MANAGEMENT

A coherent strategic approach is predicated on vigilance for worsening renal function and its associated complications, judicious diuresis, and timely institution of RRT. Hyponatremia, acidosis, azotemia, and elevations in serum potassium, magnesium, and phosphate should be anticipated and treated promptly. Above all, maintenance of adequate renal blood flow and perfusion pressure helps avoid further damage.

Diuretics may be helpful for the management of pulmonary congestion and electrolyte disorders, thereby delaying or even avoiding the need for RRT. With aggressive hydration, diuretics form an essential component of "tubular washout" therapy for pigment nephropathy (intravascular hemolysis, rhabdomyolysis). However, tubular delivery of loop diuretics is impaired because of the accumulation of organic acids that compete for active transport in the proximal tubule. Double or triple the normal doses may be required. Continuous infusion of furosemide (1 to 10 mg/hour) is a pharmacokinetically rational means of enhancing the drug's tubular concentration at lower doses and is effective even in states of low GFR. Another effective strategy is dual segment blockade of sodium reabsorption, at the medullary thick ascending loop of Henle and the distal tubule, by combined administration of a loop diuretic (furosemide, ethacrynic acid, torsemide) and a thiazide diuretic (metolazone, hydrochlorothiazide).

Initiation of RRT is required when pulmonary edema, acidosis, or hyperkalemia threaten life or when manifestations of acute uremia (encephalopathy, enteropathy, serositis, thrombocytopathy) are profound. There is limited evidence that early elective RRT may be favorable in ARF, but there is no established threshold for intervention on the basis of blood urea nitrogen or S_{Cr} values. Continuous venovenous hemodialysis provides both hemodialysis and ultrafiltration with minimal hemodynamic perturbation, allowing its use in much sicker patients. Nonetheless, because autoregulation is impaired, it is imperative to avoid episodic hypotension. Animal data suggest that intrarenal vascular responsiveness to norepinephrine is markedly decreased in ARF. If this applies to human patients, the use of this drug for the treatment of hypotension is unlikely to compromise renal blood flow.

PREVENTION

The simplest approach to preventing ARF is the maintenance of hemodynamic stability. This is predicated on the fact that 25% of the cardiac output normally goes to the kidneys. Ultimately, it is wiser to err on the side of hypervolemia rather than to restrict fluids and precipitate ARF.

Hemodynamic stability implies the maintenance of both renal blood flow and renal perfusion pressure, especially in states in which autoregulation is lost (ARF) or impaired (vasodilatory shock). Nephrotoxic insults should be minimized or avoided, keeping in mind that the risk of nephrotoxic ATN is exponentially related to the number of insults, which are far more damaging in the presence of shock or sepsis.

There are no pharmacologic "magic bullets" for the prevention of ARF. Osmotic diuresis with mannitol can prevent or even reverse tubular obstruction by cellular debris. This is of particular benefit in pigment nephropathy and is routinely used for renal protection during suprarenal aortic cross-clamping. However, although mannitol increases urine flow in infrarenal cross-clamping, it is no better than saline hydration in preserving GFR.

Furosemide may decrease oxygen consumption in the thick ascending loop of Henle by diminished ion transport. To obtain its protective effects, however, furosemide must be administered before the insult occurs, and adequate intravascular volume must be maintained.

"Renal dose" dopamine has become an increasingly controversial intervention because a number of studies have shown either no effect or possibly harm associated with prophylactic low-dose dopamine. In part, this may be due to the almost 30-fold variability in intersubject plasma dopamine levels, such that patients on low-dose dopamine may have plasma dopamine levels akin to high-level infusions, and vice versa. Nevertheless, we should not discount dopamine's potential therapeutic role as an inotropic agent to restore normal renal perfusion in patients who are putatively normovolemic but have impaired cardiac function.

Fenoldopam is a selective DA-1 receptor agonist and pure vasodilator that increases renal blood flow and blocks tubular sodium reabsorption. Unlike dopamine, it has predictable dose-related effects and is not arrhythmogenic. However, it may cause reflex tachycardia. It may prove to be useful for the prevention of ARF, but human outcome data are lacking, and a recent prospective study failed to show any benefit for reducing radiocontrast nephropathy.

Human recombinant B-type natriuretic peptide (nesiritide) is approved by the Food and Drug Administration for the management of decompensated cardiac failure. It is a balanced venous and arterial vasodilator with natriuretic properties that can relieve pulmonary congestion and promote diuresis. Its role in perioperative renal protection is currently being investigated.

Early results showing a decrease in radiocontrast renal injury with the prophylactic administration of oral *N*-acetylcysteine, a free radical scavenger, prompted considerable interest. However, subsequent studies were more equivocal and suggested that the benefit is no greater than that offered by hydration with saline. Most recently, sodium bicarbonate appeared to prevent contrast nephropathy in a small randomized, controlled trial, but corroboration by larger clinical trials is needed. The low acquisition costs of these interventions make them particularly appealing.

Other novel agents being investigated are prostaglandin analogues, human growth factors, and selective adenosine agonists and antagonists. All have theoretical advantages in ARF, but outcome data are preliminary.

Further Reading

Bellomo R, Champman M, Finfer S, et al: Low-dose dopamine in patients with early renal dysfunction: A placebo-controlled randomised trial. Australian and New Zealand Intensive Care Society (ANZICS) Clinical Trials Group. Lancet 356:2139-2143, 2000.

Birck R, Krzossok S, Markowetz F, et al: Acetylcysteine for prevention of contrast nephropathy: Meta-analysis. Lancet 362:598-603, 2003.

Braams R, Vossen V, Lisman BAM, et al: Outcome in patients requiring renal replacement therapy after surgery for ruptured and non-ruptured aneurysm of the abdominal aorta. Eur J Vasc Endovasc Surg 18:323-327, 1999.

Brezis M, Rosen S: Hypoxia of the renal medulla—its implications for disease. N Engl J Med 332:647-655, 1995.

Carvounis CP, Nisar S, Guro-Razuman S: Significance of the fractional excretion of urea in the differential diagnosis of acute renal failure. Kidney Int 62:2223-2229, 2002.

Chen G, Paka L, Kako Y, et al: A protective role for kidney apolipoprotein E: Regulation of mesangial cell proliferation and matrix expansion. J Biol Chem 276:49142-49147, 2001.

Chertow GM, Lazarus JM, Christiansen CL, et al: Preoperative renal risk stratification. Circulation 95:878-884, 1997.

Cockcroft DW, Gault MH: Prediction of creatinine clearance from serum creatinine. Nephron 16:31-41, 1976.

Conlon PJ, Stafford-Smith M, White WD, et al: Acute renal failure following cardiac surgery. Nephrol Dial Transplant 14:1158-1162, 1999.

Forni LG, Hilton PJ: Continuous hemofiltration in the treatment of acute renal failure. N Engl J Med 336:1303-1309, 1997.

Gines P, Guevara M, Arroyo V, et al: Hepatorenal syndrome. Lancet 362:1819-1827, 2003.

Huynh TTT, Miller CC III, Estrera AL, et al: Determinants of hospital length of stay after thoracoabdominal aortic aneurysm repair. J Vasc Surg 35:648-653, 2002.

Kelleher S, Robinette J, Miller F, et al: Effect of hemorrhagic reduction in blood pressure on recovery from acute renal failure. Kidney Int 31:725-730, 1987.

MacGregor DA, Smith TE, Prielipp RC, et al: Pharmacokinetics of dopamine in healthy male subjects. Anesthesiology 92:338-346, 2000.

Marik PE: Low-dose dopamine: A systematic review. Intensive Care Med 28:877-883, 2002.

Merten GJ, Burgess WP, Gray LV, et al: Prevention of contrast-induced nephropathy with sodium bicarbonate. JAMA 291:2328-2334, 2004.

Modi KS, Rao VK: Atheroembolic renal disease. J Am Soc Nephrol 12:1781-1787, 2001.

Novis BK, Roizen MF, Aronson S, et al: Association of preoperative risk factors with postoperative acute renal failure. Anesth Analg 78:143-149, 1994.

Ryckwaert F, Boccara G, Frappier J-M, et al: Incidence, risk factors, and prognosis of a moderate increase in plasma creatinine early after cardiac surgery. Crit Care Med 30:1495-1498, 2002.

Singri N, Ahya SN, Levin ML: Acute renal failure. JAMA 289:747-751, 2003.

Stone GW, McCullough PA, Tumlin JA, et al: Fenoldopam mesylate for the prevention of contrast-induced nephropathy. JAMA 290:2284-2291, 2003.

Tang ATM, El-Gamel A, Keevil B, et al: The effect of "renal-dose" dopamine on renal tubular function following cardiac surgery: Assessed by measuring retinol binding protein (RBP). Eur J Cardiothorac Surg 15:717-722, 1999.

Wahlberg E, DiMuzio PJ, Stoney RJ: Aortic clamping during elective operations for infrarenal disease: The influence of clamping time on renal function. J Vasc Surg 36:13-18, 2002.

Postoperative Respiratory Failure

David Porembka

Case Synopsis

A 25-year-old person involved in a high-speed motor vehicle accident required prolonged extrication and underwent an emergency laparotomy for a positive diagnostic abdominal ultrasonogram. Injuries included a ruptured spleen, a grade III liver laceration, multiple right-sided rib fractures with an ipsilateral pulmonary contusion, and a vertical shear pelvic fracture. The initial vital signs were heart rate 120 beats per minute, respiratory rate 35, and systolic arterial blood pressure 80 mm Hg. Resuscitation required multiple transfusions (approximately 5 L). Following corrective surgery, the patient underwent embolization for the pelvic fracture. In the surgical intensive care unit, a continuous right ventricular ejection catheter with mixed venous saturation capabilities was placed. Also, transesophageal echocardiography (TEE) was used for initial diagnostic interrogation (ventricular function and volume, ventricular interaction, aortic interrogation) and for continuous postoperative hemodynamic assessment. During subsequent aggressive hemodynamic resuscitation, the patient's hemodynamic instability improved, but oxygenation saturation status deteriorated (arterial oxygen tension [PaO_2] 60 mm Hg with fraction of inspired oxygen [FiO_2] of 1.0). After sedation and an appropriate level of analgesia (with continuous infusions of lorazepam and fentanyl) to a modified Ramsey score of 3 to 4, initial ventilator adjustments to improve static compliance did not improve PaO_2.

PROBLEM ANALYSIS

Definition

Numerous issues are involved in the trauma situation described in the case synopsis. The patient arrived at the hospital in hypovolemic shock with end-organ ischemia due to several life-threatening injuries (splenic rupture, liver injury, severe pelvic injury). Significant occult blood loss can occur with pelvic fractures alone, especially those involving vertical shear injury. Often, severe lactic acidosis accompanies such traumatic injuries and the associated hypovolemia and hypotension. Because the patient also sustained chest wall trauma with multiple rib fractures and pulmonary contusion, hypoxemia is inevitable. Indeed, with multiple trauma and associated lung injury, the potential for significant acute respiratory failure is high.

In this case, aggressive blood and fluid resuscitation and immediate corrective surgery are required. However, these may compound the risk for acute respiratory failure. Fortunately, after surgery, the need for blood products and fluid replacement will be reduced. In the case described, however, the patient's oxygenation worsened, suggesting associated severe lung injury or early acute respiratory distress syndrome (ARDS) and associated cellular, humoral, and oxidative pathophysiologic processes (Table 86-1).

Recognition

Diagnostic criteria for ARDS are listed in Table 86-2. Early diagnosis and corrective measures are key to a successful outcome. Initially, the work of breathing is greatly increased. Therefore, patients become tachypneic, tachycardic, and agitated. Typically, arterial blood gas measurement reveals respiratory alkalosis with hypoxemia or relative hypoxemia with supplemental oxygen. Subsequently, this progresses to an increase in the alveolar-arterial oxygen gradient. Without intervention (i.e., airway control and mechanical ventilatory support with positive end-expiratory pressure [PEEP]), the

Table 86–1 ▪ Pathophysiologic Aspects of Acute Respiratory Distress Syndrome

Cellular	Oxidative
Endothelial cells	Antioxidant depletion
Eosinophils	Hypoxia-reoxygenation phenomena
Epithelial cells	
Fibroblasts	Oxygen toxicity
Neutrophils	Reactive oxygen species
Monocytes and macrophages	Superoxide radical
Humoral	Hydrogen peroxide
Arachidonic acid metabolites	Singlet oxygen
Thromboxane A₂	Hypochlorous acid
Leukotrienes	Reactive nitrogen species
Complement	Nitric oxide
C5a, C3a	Peroxynitrite
Cytokines	Transition metal ion catalysts
TNF-α, IL-1β, IL-6, IL-8	Xanthine oxidase
Endotoxin	
Platelet-activating factor	
Prostaglandins	

IL, interleukin, TNF, tumor necrosis factor.

347

Table 86–2 ■ Diagnostic Criteria for Acute Respiratory Distress Syndrome

Clinical Criteria

Appropriate risk factors or precipitating causes
Respiratory distress with severe hypoxemia
Radiographic evidence of noncardiac pulmonary edema
Loss of lung compliance
No obvious cardiac failure

NHLBI Criteria

Widespread, bilateral infiltrates on chest radiograph <7 days
  duration
Hypoxemia with PaO_2/FiO_2 <150 off PEEP or <200 on PEEP
Pulmonary artery occlusion pressure <18 mm Hg

*0, no lung injury; 0.1 to 2.5, mild to moderate lung injury; >2.5, severe lung injury (acute respiratory distress syndrome).

FiO_2, fraction of inspired oxygen; NHLBI, National Heart, Lung, and Blood Institute; PaO_2, arterial oxygen tension; PEEP, positive end-expiratory pressure.

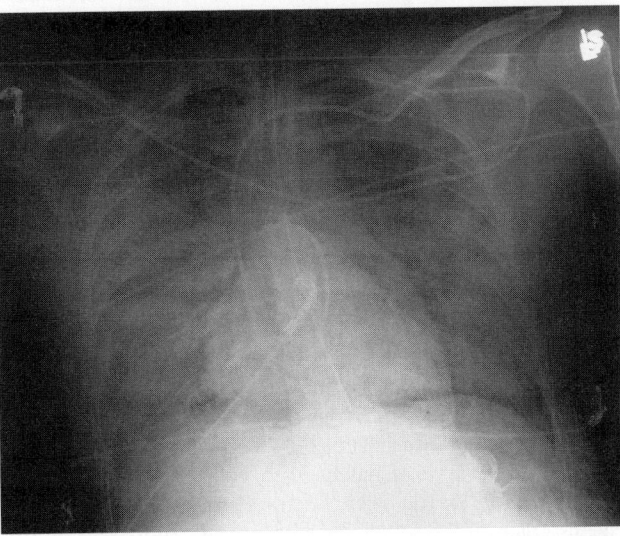

Figure 86–2 ■ Chest radiograph with bilateral fluffy infiltrates (panacinar pattern), consistent with severe acute respiratory distress syndrome.

work of breathing is so great that severe hypoxemia occurs. This is compounded by increased alveolar fluid, a significant decrease in the functional residual capacity, atelectasis, and loss of lung compliance. Metabolic acidosis may ensue if the hypoxemia is not reversed or becomes refractory, leading to end-organ and cellular damage. In addition to hypoxemia, the chest radiograph may reveal a pattern consistent with early ARDS, including bilateral patchy interstitial infiltrates (Fig. 86-1). Later, with severe ARDS, this pattern progresses to bilateral, fluffy infiltrates with a panacinar pattern (Fig. 86-2). These findings may worsen or even appear to dissipate with positive-pressure ventilation, especially if plateau pressures and PEEP are significantly elevated.

Although patients were once considered to have ARDS if the pulmonary artery occlusion (wedge) pressure was less than 18 mm Hg, today, with the greater use of echocardiography, this criterion may not apply to acidotic, underresuscitated patients. Because the left ventricle may be noncompliant, even if relatively empty, the pulmonary artery occlusion pressure may be falsely elevated. Even in the static phase of resuscitation, ongoing cellular injury occurs, and the phenomena of reperfusion injury proceed and continue to impair left ventricular function, which is inadequately measured by information derived from a pulmonary artery catheter. Even with correction of the medical or surgical pathology associated with ARDS, the pathophysiologic processes initiated by severe acute lung injury are unabated, leading to pulmonary microcirculation compromise.

Risk Assessment

Conceptually, there are several categories of pulmonary edema, depending on cause and associated factors. *Hydrostatic pulmonary edema* results from volume overload, left ventricular failure, valvular heart disease, and lymphatic insufficiency. *Permeability pulmonary edema* (alveolar capillary leak) is associated with the systemic inflammatory response syndrome (SIRS; see Chapter 119) due to shock (e.g., traumatic, septic, cardiogenic, anaphylactic), pulmonary contusion, thermal injury, fat embolism, closed head injury, infectious agents, near-drowning, inhaled toxins, pancreatitis, drug ingestion, multiple transfusions, and so forth. *Mixed pulmonary edema* combines elements of both and often occurs in patients with subtle heart failure (due to systolic or diastolic dysfunction) with superimposed SIRS.

The presence of mixed pulmonary edema in the intensive care unit is not well documented. However, it is a definite entity in gravely ill surgical and trauma patients, and it perplexes physicians with regard to the modulation of intravascular volume. Again, echocardiography (especially TEE) can help clinicians diagnose pathologic entities that might be involved and assess the patient's hemodynamic

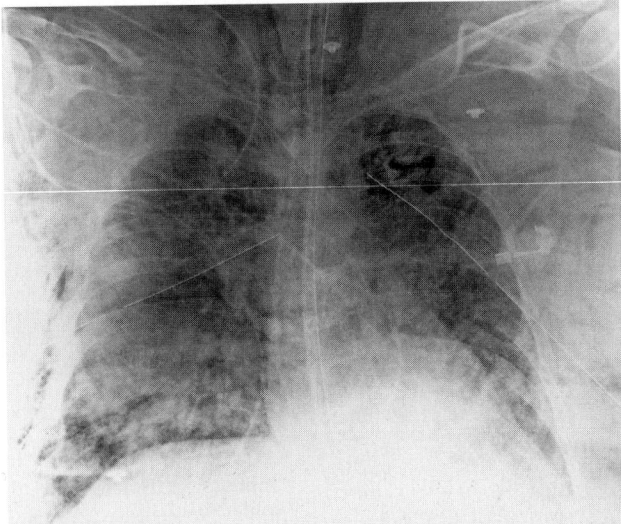

Figure 86–1 ■ Chest radiograph consistent with the pattern of early acute respiratory distress syndrome following right-sided pulmonary contusion with multiple rib fractures. In addition to diffuse patchy infiltrates, note diffuse subcutaneous emphysema from either the traumatic insult or pulmonary barotrauma.

status, particularly biventricular performance and interactions. Until clinicians have the capability to construct right-left heart pressure-volume loops, clinical interventions are optimized with the appropriate use of pulmonary artery catheters and TEE.

The pathogenesis of ARDS is complex. Our understanding of initiating factors in ARDS, as well as disease progression, resolution, and healing, is ever-changing. Recent strides in both basic and clinical research have increased our understanding of ARDS. Also, since the establishment of the ARDS Network, we have finally reduced earlier stagnant mortality rates (40% to 60%) by such simple interventions as reducing mechanical ventilatory tidal volumes and plateau pressures.

The incidence of ARDS in the United States approaches 150,000 patients per year (75 per 100,000 population per year). The incidence depends on the primary cause of ARDS and associated pathophysiology: SIRS (41%), multiple transfusions (36%), near-drowning (33%), pulmonary aspiration (21%), multiple fractures (11%), drug overdose (8.5%). In patients with two risk factors, the incidence increases to 42%; in those with three risk factors, it is 85%. The 1-year outcome for ARDS survivors is not necessarily benign. Rapid resolution of lung injury, even without associated multiorgan system dysfunction, is more often observed in previously healthy patients. Even so, muscle wasting and weakness may occur, possibly related to critical myopathic illness that may accompany prolonged stays in the intensive care unit. By 6 months, pulmonary function generally improves in ARDS patients. However, most have a persistent reduction in carbon monoxide diffusing capacity. Only about half of ARDS survivors return to work in their prior capacity.

There are many pathogenic processes involved in ARDS. However, because ARDS is a continuum, these are not easily subdivided. Nonetheless, in the *acute phase* of lung injury, there is an influx of protein-enriched fluid into the alveolar spaces. Transmigration of gases across the alveolar membrane is impaired owing to a breakdown of the alveolar-capillary barrier. This sets the stage for problematic management of ARDS patients. The alveolar epithelium (90% type I cells; 10% type II [cuboidal] cells) is also injured in early ARDS, and the extent of such injury is a predictor of ARDS mortality. Type I cells produce surfactant and are involved in ion transport. They also proliferate and differentiate into type II cells following lung injury. The loss of vital type I cell functions reduces the integrity of the barrier, leading to (1) pneumonia, sepsis, and septic shock and (2) cellular disorganization that interferes with epithelial repair and fibrosis. Neutrophil transmigration and consequent injury are well known in ARDS and contribute to continued injury and interference with healing.

Extrapulmonary and pulmonary proinflammatory substances and cytokines are also implicated in the aggressive pathophysiology of ARDS involving alveolar epithelial cells, neutrophils, and fibroblasts. With such overwhelming inflammation and the production of interleukin-8 (IL-8) and tumor necrosis factor-α, any glucocorticoid-mediated inhibition is ineffective. Thus, the balance between pro- and anti-inflammatory cytokines and mediators is altered, but this is not yet well understood.

ARDS also increases alveolar epithelial cell apoptosis and dysfunction. This process is enhanced by a kinase-1 signaling pathway that regulates hydrogen peroxide-induced apoptosis in pulmonary vascular endothelial cells. Also, the impaired coagulation observed in patients with septic shock may improve with activated protein C. It is unknown whether the use of such pharmacotherapy may benefit ARDS patients with impaired fibrinolysis and enhance platelet-fibrin thrombus formation.

Although intensive glucose control is considered standard in critically ill patients, there are no prospective randomized trials of this practice in patients with severe ARDS. However, conventional wisdom dictates that such a course may be prudent.

Ventilation-induced lung injury is a well-known entity, but it has only recently gained attention because of the unexpected results from the ARDS Network multicenter study. Patient enrollment was halted in that study because patients who received standard ventilatory support (12 mL/kg tidal volume) with a maximal plateau pressure of 50 cm H_2O had a mortality rate of 39.8%, compared with 31.0% for those with 6 mL/kg and a maximal plateau pressure of 30 cm H_2O ($P = .007$). However, in clinical practice, there is varying compliance with the lowered ventilatory settings promulgated by the ARDS Network. This is disconcerting, and clinicians must be encouraged to use more protective ventilatory strategies.

What is also clear from the ARDS Network study is that ARDS is not a homogeneous process. Some alveoli will be overdistended by high pressure and volumes; others will never be opened, even with higher pressures and volumes. The latter include dependent regions of the lung.

More recent studies show that simple alterations in mechanical ventilation can have deleterious effects. It is now known that systemic cytokine up-regulation is possible with high-pressure, high-volume ventilation. Another benefit of protective lung strategies is that systemic cytokine levels are significantly lower with lower-pressure, lower-volume ventilation. These levels decrease significantly over time owing to reduced lung injury (overdistention), while lung recruitment is maintained throughout the ventilatory cycle by more modest maximal plateau pressure.

Other investigators have examined plasma chemokines (MCP-1, IL-8, and GRO) in patients with conventional (high volume, high plateau pressure) and protective (lower volume, lower plateau pressure) ventilation strategies. Plasma cytokines were increased in patients with conventional ventilation. Thus, there may be an associated risk of end-organ damage and the development of multiple organ failure. Circulating pro-apoptotic soluble factors (e.g., soluble Fas ligand) may contribute. Finally, studies in a rat model of ischemic gut suggest that patients with acute lung injury and ischemic gut may be at even higher risk for ARDS. This might be due to more pronounced release of inflammatory cytokines from ischemic gut.

Implications

In the past, mortality from ARDS was significant, ranging from 53% to 69%. Recently, mortality from isolated ARDS has declined to 26% to 47%. This has been attributed to the following factors:

- Better ventilator management: pressure-controlled ventilation, reduced tidal volumes, permissive hypercapnia, and measures to recruit alveoli and avoid derecruitment

- Altering the patient's position to improve ventilation-perfusion mismatch, such as the use of special beds that can be tilted horizontally or vertically ("posturing") to improve ventilation-perfusion matching by increasing hydrostatic pressure in the dependent lung[1]
- Better control of circulatory dynamics, early and more aggressive management of nosocomial pneumonia, therapy with corticosteroids in late-phase ARDS, and anti-inflammatory modalities
- More timely, aggressive hemodynamic assessment and therapy; increased understanding of underlying pathophysiology; use of echocardiography, computed tomography, and electrical impedance tomography

Despite the apparent decline in mortality associated with isolated ARDS, mortality for multiorgan system failure has not declined. No matter what severity scoring system is used, mortality for ARDS with the failure of one, two, three, or four additional organs is 54%, 72%, 84%, and 99%, respectively. Reducing mortality from multiorgan system failure involves early intervention and aggressive treatment of the underlying causes, with meticulous attention to ventilatory management.

MANAGEMENT

Understanding the pathogenesis of ARDS is critical to minimizing the numerous potential adverse consequences. If possible, underlying causes that may have precipitated ARDS must be identified and treated, and associated pathophysiology must be ameliorated or reversed (see Table 86-1).

Maintaining adequate (not necessarily optimal) oxygenation and delivery can be challenging. Aggressive interventional strategies should be used to inhibit the activation of inflammatory responses. Especially in patients with sepsis, early treatment may prevent or minimize associated ARDS. An important caveat is that ARDS is a heterogeneous disease in terms of both cause and pathophysiology. Not all alveolar lung units are equally affected, and this can change during acute and resolving ARDS. Early identification of the extent and distribution of the disease process (collapsed lung areas) by computed tomography can guide clinicians in use of PEEP and posturing to improve regional distribution of gas flow and ventilatory pressures.

With hypoxia due to ARDS, supplemental oxygenation is required, usually with an artificial airway. With mild acute lung injury, high-flow continuous positive airway pressure (CPAP) mask ventilation may be sufficient. With more severe injury, tracheal intubation and ventilator support may be required to deliver adequate oxygen and reduce the work of breathing. Assisted modes include proportional assist ventilation and synchronized intermittent mandatory ventilation with pressure support. Proportional assist ventilation proportionally amplifies instantaneous patient ventilatory efforts. With very severe injury, PEEP with increased mean airway pressure and lower tidal volumes (matched to the patient's

ideal body weight) is used to recruit alveoli and improve ventilation-perfusion matching. Mean airway pressure depends on the degree of lung injury and hemodynamic tolerance, with caution required to avoid barotrauma or volume trauma.

"Best" PEEP is difficult to define. Generally, pressure between 5 and 15 cm H_2O is sufficient, with mean airway pressures initially maintained at less than 35 cm H_2O. PEEP greater than 15 cm H_2O may open collapsed alveoli but could expose normal alveoli to injury. PEEP greater than 20 cm H_2O may be required on occasion, but this should be critically evaluated on a case-by-case basis. Recruitment of collapsed airways is crucial, especially during mechanical or assisted ventilation, so that derecruitment does not occur. The latter has been observed in dynamic studies in both animal models and humans. Thus, there is still uncertainty about the best level of PEEP for a given patient—one that will avoid untoward pulmonary volume trauma or barotrauma.

Prone and, in some centers, postural positioning is used to manage patients with severe acute lung injury. This method is more prevalent in Europe and Canada than in the United States and may be more efficacious early in ARDS. In my opinion, once the clinician has identified the extent of injury to all pulmonary segments, increased PEEP and prone positioning may benefit some patients. However, with a predominant parenchymal component of ARDS (e.g., pulmonary contusion), increasing PEEP may actually worsen oxygenation, even in the prone position or with posturing.

Surfactant instillation is used to replenish endogenous surfactant lost due to injury to type I alveolar epithelium. Although surfactant is useful in infants, only anecdotal reports show any benefit in adults. A multicenter study in progress, with direct administration of surfactant into 15 distal lung segments, has shown no encouraging results to date.

Although inhaled nitric oxide initially showed some promise in severely ill patients, it has not withstood the test of time or well-designed prospective clinical trials. However, in an animal model of the effects of L-NAME (a nitric oxide synthetase inhibitor) and inhaled nitric oxide on ventilator-induced lung injury (perfused rabbit lung), L-NAME attenuated the resultant microvascular leak, while nitric oxide appeared to further the induced lung injury. Of note in this study, measuring nitric oxide metabolites in bronchoalveolar lavage fluid may provide a method of measuring lung injury induced by mechanical stress.

Prolonged exposure to high inspired oxygen concentrations can produce lung injury similar to ARDS. Thus, FiO_2 should be adjusted to the lowest level possible to ensure adequate oxygenation (arterial blood oxygen saturation >90%).

Today, lower tidal volumes (6 mL/kg of ideal body weight) are used in patients with ARDS. The idea is to avoid barotrauma while providing satisfactory oxygenation and alveolar ventilation. However, because alveolar ventilation may be decreased by up to 50% with these lower tidal volumes, arterial carbon dioxide tension ($PaCO_2$) invariably rises ("permissive hypercapnia") to greater than 80 mm Hg. Such high $PaCO_2$ levels are not always benign and may have detrimental hemodynamic effects. Although increasing ventilator rates may reduce such high $PaCO_2$ levels, ventilator rates greater than 30 are often ineffective. Judicious sedation

---

[1]The editor (JLA) benefited from such posturing therapy when he was treated in 2003 for ARDS secondary to pneumonia and empyema (due to *Streptococcus pneumoniae*). His condition was compounded by septic shock and multiorgan system failure.

and neuromuscular relaxation (rarely) may help reduce agitation, carbon dioxide production, and high spontaneous respiratory rates with permissive hypercapnia. Also, coordinating spontaneous respiratory efforts with any mechanical ventilation is key to avoiding lack of synchrony, diaphragmatic wasting, or the triggering of mechanical ventilator responses to spontaneous respirations.

The strategy for selecting the best inspiration/expiration (I/E) ratio is based on a consideration of internal or external PEEP. Internal PEEP may be increased with higher tidal volumes, shorter expiratory time, or higher ventilatory constants (e.g., inverse I/E ratio). External PEEP is applied from the ventilator. It must be remembered that respiration is dynamic, and distended alveoli can collapse during expiration if the pressure applied is too low. Fast alveolar compartments expire easily and may collapse prematurely; external PEEP may be helpful in this situation. Conversely, increased internal PEEP may be required to match slower alveolar compartments and to make ventilation and perfusion more homogeneous. This can be accomplished by shortening expiratory time (inverse I/E ratio ventilation). In general, patients with ARDS have more fast compartments, so PEEP is ideal to prevent alveolar collapse. Yet with inverse I/E ratio ventilation, both external and internal PEEP should be monitored to limit internal PEEP.

In summary, management of postoperative ARDS should be problem oriented and aggressive. Causes and contributing factors should be identified and corrected or treated. Aggressive monitoring (pulmonary artery catheter, TEE) is indicated to assess volume status, pulmonary and peripheral hemodynamics, oxygen supply and demand, and right and left heart function. For optimal ventilatory management, a strategy should be implemented to ensure adequate arterial oxygen saturation (>90%) with the lowest possible FiO_2. Protective lung strategies, including a tidal volume of 6 mL/kg of predicted body weight, a plateau pressure of 30 to 35 cm H_2O, optimal PEEP to avoid derecruitment and overdistention of a significant proportion of compliant alveoli, permissive hypercapnia (in patients without increased intracranial pressure), sedation, and neuromuscular blockers, are required. However, treatment must always be individualized in an effort to optimize outcome. The approach to these patients may be quite diverse, considering the pathologic differences between pulmonary ARDS and extrapulmonary ARDS.

PREVENTION

At present, there are no clinically proven interventions to prevent ARDS in patients at risk. However, prompt recognition and treatment or removal of mitigating factors (e.g., heart failure, source of sepsis), along with the institution of supportive therapy, may favorably modify the course of ARDS and reduce associated morbidity and mortality. New measures and criteria for ventilatory management, as promulgated by the ARDS Network (www.ardsnet.org) have changed the standards of practice. The goal of maintaining optimal recruitment of alveoli without triggering airway collapse is critical. Thus, it may be necessary for clinicians to obtain dynamic computed tomography scans early in ARDS to characterize lung involvement and then use such scans to determine the appropriate management strategy (e.g., higher PEEP levels, prone or postural positioning). There is no proven method (evidence-based practice standard) of preventing all lung injury during ARDS treatment. However, the use of newer protective management strategies discussed in this chapter may help minimize such injury.

Further Reading

Acute Respiratory Distress Syndrome Network: Ventilation with lower tidal volumes as compared with traditional tidal volumes for acute lung injury and the acute respiratory distress syndrome. N Engl J Med 342:1301-1308, 2000.

Bouadma L, Schortgen F, Ricard J-D, et al: Ventilation strategy affects cytokine release after mesenteric ischemia-reperfusion in rats. Crit Care Med 32:1563-1569, 2004.

Brower RG, Lanken PN, MacIntyre N, et al: Higher versus lower positive end-expiratory pressures in patients with the acute respiratory distress syndrome. N Engl J Med 351:327-336, 2004.

Gainnier M, Michelet P, Thirion X, et al: Prone position and positive end-expiratory pressure in acute respiratory distress syndrome. Crit Care Med 31:2719-2726, 2003.

Galic O, Dara SI, Mendez JL, et al: Ventilator-associated lung injury in patients without acute lung injury at the onset of mechanical ventilation. Crit Care Med 32:1817-1824, 2004.

Goss CH, Brower RG, Hudson LD, et al: ARDS Network: Incidence of acute lung injury in the United States. Crit Care Med 31:1607-1611, 2003.

Gunther A, Mosavi P, Heinemann S, et al: Alveolar fibrin formation caused by enhanced procoagulant and depressed fibrinolytic capacities in severe pneumonia: Comparison with the acute respiratory distress syndrome. Am J Respir Crit Care 161:454-462, 2000.

Herridge MS, Cheung AM, Tansey CM, et al: One-year outcomes in survivors of the acute respiratory distress syndromes. N Engl J Med 348:683-693, 2003.

Hickling KG: Low tidal volume ventilation: A PEEP at the mechanism of derecruitment. Crit Care Med 31:318-320, 2003.

Hotchkiss RS: The pathophysiology and treatment of sepsis. N Engl J Med 348:138-150, 2005.

Ince C: Microcirculation in distress: A new resuscitation end point? Crit Care Med 32:1963-1964, 2004.

Lew TWK, Kwek TK, Tai D, et al: Acute respiratory distress syndrome in critically ill patients with severe acute respiratory syndrome. JAMA 290:374-380, 2003.

Lim C-M, Jung H, Koh Y, et al: Effect of alveolar recruitment maneuver in early acute respiratory distress syndrome according to antirecruitment strategy, etiological category of diffuse lung injury, and body position of the patient. Crit Care Med 31:411-418, 2003.

Machino T, Hashimoto S, Maruoka S, et al: Apoptosis signal-regulating kinase 1-mediated signaling pathway regulates hydrogen peroxide-induced apoptosis in human pulmonary vascular endothelial cells. Crit Care Med 31:2776-2781, 2003.

Oczenski W, Hormann C, Keller C, et al: Recruitment maneuvers after a positive end-expiratory pressure trial do not induce sustained effects in early adult respiratory distress syndrome. Anesthesiology 101: 620-625, 2004.

van Genderingen HR, van Vught AJ, Jansen JRC: Regional lung volume during high-frequency oscillatory ventilation by electrical impedance tomography. Crit Care Med 32:787-794, 2004.

van Kaam AH, Haitsma JJ, Dik WA, et al: Response to exogenous surfactant is different during open lung and conventional ventilation. Crit Care Med 32:774-780, 2004.

Victorino JA, Borges JB, Okamoto VN, et al: Imbalances in regional lung ventilation: A validation study on electrical impedance tomography. Am J Respir Crit Care Med 169:791-800, 2004.

Young MP, Manning HL, Wilson DL, et al: Ventilation of patients with acute lung injury and acute respiratory distress syndrome: Has new evidence changed clinical practice? Crit Care Med 32:1260-1265, 2004.

CARDIOTHORACIC & VASCULAR SURGERY

Major Organ System Dysfunction after Cardiopulmonary Bypass

87

Avery Tung

Case Synopsis

A 78-year-old man with chronic ischemic cardiomyopathy and renal insufficiency underwent redo coronary artery bypass grafting and mitral valve repair. Cardiopulmonary bypass time was 200 minutes. Upon weaning from bypass, persistent hypoxemia (PaO_2/FiO_2 ratio <100) and a low systemic vascular resistance (500 dyne·sec·cm^{-5}) were noted. Intravenous norepinephrine was begun, an intra-aortic balloon pump was placed, and the patient was transferred to the intensive care unit. Over the next 48 hours, the patient continued to require intravenous norepinephrine for reduced systemic vascular resistance. His creatinine levels increased, and there were radiographic changes consistent with acute respiratory deficiency syndrome, with continued hypoxemia despite 15 cm H_2O positive end-expiratory airway pressure. He was intermittently agitated and had nonfocal neurologic changes. On the morning of the third postoperative day, he developed atrial fibrillation.

PROBLEM ANALYSIS

Definition

Complications specific to cardiopulmonary bypass (CPB) range from minor to severe and include mechanical issues, introduction of air and other debris, damage to blood elements, metabolic and electrolyte derangements, and alterations in vital organ perfusion. Mechanical complications of CPB involve abnormalities of blood flow between the CPB machine and the patient and include obstruction, embolization, and damage to the native vasculature. In addition, CPB triggers a systemic inflammatory response that can have significant effects on end-organ function during the immediate postbypass period. Organs commonly affected by the inflammatory response to CPB include the lungs, heart, gastrointestinal tract, brain, and kidneys.

Although surgical trauma, blood loss, and hypothermia can all induce an inflammatory response, the physiologic response to CPB is unusual in its complexity. Three distinct mechanisms likely participate in the post-CPB inflammatory state:

1. Direct activation of the cellular and humoral immune system by artificial surfaces of the CPB circuit. This process involves complement and cytokines, leading to activation of both leukocytes and the vascular endothelium.
2. Aortic cross-clamping leads to ischemia-reperfusion injury and the resultant activation of the inflammatory mediator cascade.
3. Damage to mucosal barriers due to hypoperfusion induces endotoxin translocation and immune system activation. This leads to a systemic inflammatory response that alters microvascular perfusion, systemic pressure, endothelial integrity, and end-organ perfusion postoperatively. Figure 87-1 depicts pathways of inflammatory activation during CPB.

Recognition

A number of mechanical complications of CPB have been described. Obstruction to either arterial flow or venous drainage, embolization of air or debris, aortic dissection, dislodgment of aortic debris, and malposition of inflow and outflow cannulas can all cause catastrophic injury. Table 87-1 lists mechanical complications of bypass and their detection.

Clinical signs and symptoms of the inflammatory response mediated by CPB are more subtle and involve primarily end-organ dysfunction and systemic hypotension. Renal function may decline slowly after CPB and progress to acute renal failure of sufficient severity to require temporary dialysis. Increased capillary endothelial leak may lead to pulmonary edema, with altered lung compliance and worsened gas exchange. Microvascular occlusion from leukocyte aggregates may produce an altered mental status, commonly without focal neurologic findings. Depressed myocardial contractility and arrhythmias can result, leading to increased fluid or vasopressor requirements and worsened perfusion. Finally, systemic activation of complement and cytokines can induce vasodilatation and consequent hypotension.

Because of the protean manifestations of the CPB-mediated inflammatory response, related signs and symptoms are similar to those resulting from any inflammatory insult and may not be universally present. For example, white blood cell counts may not be elevated, and fever may or may not be present. Urine volumes are typically low,

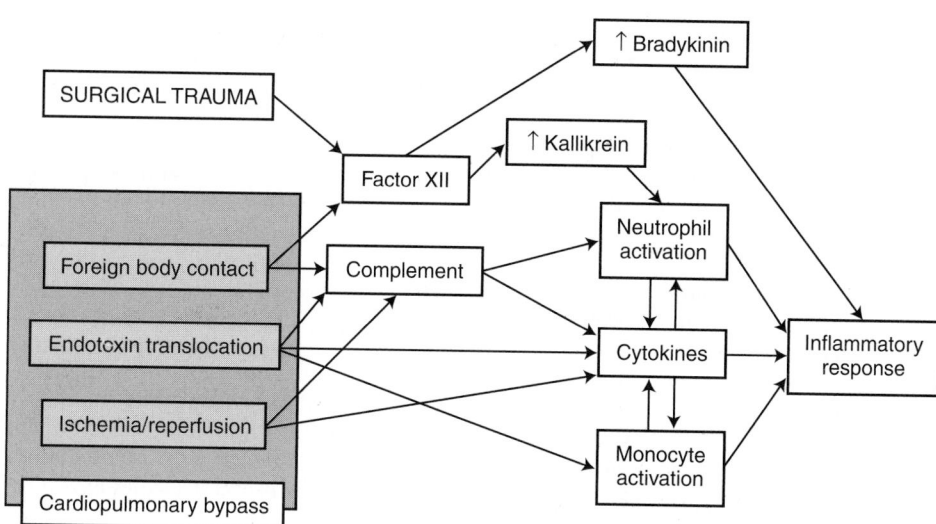

Figure 87–1 ■ Pathways of inflammatory activation during cardiopulmonary bypass.

and urine sediment frequently demonstrates only acute tubular necrosis. Altered pulmonary mechanics and gas exchange are nonspecific, resemble those of acute respiratory distress syndrome, and can be severe. Neurologic dysfunction may not be focal, manifesting instead as agitation, delirium, or delayed emergence from anesthesia. Hypotension may result from decreased cardiac output or vascular resistance. Systemic vasodilatation responds to α-adrenergic agonists such as norepinephrine, phenylephrine, or vasopressin.

Risk Assessment

Almost any exposure to CPB induces some degree of systemic inflammation. Nonetheless, several pre-, intra-, and post-CPB factors are known to predispose patients to a clinically relevant, increased inflammatory response.

Preoperative Factors.   Although the amount and degree of cytokine release does not vary with age, both ischemic heart disease and perioperative left ventricular dysfunction appear to increase the intensity of the cytokine response to CPB. This increased response has been correlated with impaired postoperative hemodynamics and an increase in perioperative complications. Diabetes, particularly when poorly controlled, also appears to increase the inflammatory response. Renal failure, perhaps by impairing the kidneys' ability to clear pro- and anti-inflammatory mediators, intensifies the inflammatory response as well. In general, a greater perioperative severity of illness predicts a greater inflammatory response.

Intraoperative Factors.   Both splanchnic hypoperfusion and increased gastrointestinal mucosal permeability occur during CPB. Consequent ischemia-reperfusion injury leads to free radical production, sequestration of pulmonary neutrophils, and possible bacterial translocation and endotoxin formation. Cytokine levels appear to be higher in heart or heart-lung transplant patients, possibly owing to their more severe illness. However, the cytokine levels in patients undergoing valve surgery are similar to the levels in those having coronary artery bypass grafting.

Anesthetic Agents.   Although most anesthetic agents have some immunomodulatory activity, the clinical impact of their use in patients undergoing CPB is unknown. Both propofol and thiopental (Pentothal) inhibit neutrophil activation, and propofol may enhance anti-inflammatory cytokine production. Morphine down-regulates immune cell function and suppresses the antibody response. Sevoflurane and isoflurane reduce inflammatory cytokine activity.

Table 87–1 ■ **Detection of Mechanical Complications of Cardiopulmonary Bypass**	
Complication	**Detection**
Aortic dissection	Visual inspection of cannula or aorta
	Abnormal inflow pressure
	Alterations in peripheral arterial waveform
Dislodgment of aortic debris	Chest radiography
	Aortography
	Transesophageal or epivascular echocardiography
	Direct palpation
Obstruction to venous drainage	Inspection of head and jugular veins
	Sudden or unexpected changes in CVP while on CPB
Embolization	Transesophageal echocardiography
	Transcranial Doppler
	Bubble detectors in CPB circuit
	Arterial line filters
Cerebral hypoperfusion	Arterial pressure and flow monitoring during CPB
	Hypothermia
	Mixed venous oxygen saturation monitoring
	Electroencephalography

CPB, cardiopulmonary bypass; CVP, central venous pressure.

Although thoracic epidural anesthesia decreases the perioperative stress response, it does not significantly alter the cytokine response due to CPB.

Cardiopulmonary Bypass Factors.
The data are unclear regarding what effect the type of oxygenator, pump, or extracorporeal circuit and the temperature during CPB have on the duration and extent of the inflammatory response. The duration of CPB has been correlated with interleukin (IL)-8 concentrations and measures of neutrophil adhesion and may alter clinical outcomes for several reasons. Although warm CPB increases the inflammatory response when compared with cold CPB, warm cardioplegia appears to reduce consequent inflammation. Membrane oxygenators produce less inflammation than bubble oxygenators do, but the effects are not sustained and do not alter clinical pulmonary function. No clear effect on outcome has been observed based on CPB prime, type of pump, or pulsatility, although pulsatile flow is associated with less endotoxin release and lower cytokine levels.

Transfusion Factors.
Allogeneic blood transfusion clearly increases the intensity of the CPB inflammatory response. Autotransfusion of mediastinal blood may not be any better, because such blood contains high levels of tumor necrosis factor-α and IL-6. CPB reservoir blood processed through washing devices typically has higher neutrophil counts than blood in the circulation but significantly lower levels of inflammatory mediators (e.g., IL-1, IL-6, tumor necrosis factor-α). However, cell-saver or similar techniques have no significant effects on bleeding or other CPB-related morbidity and mortality.

Implications

The effects of CPB-mediated systemic inflammation can be severe. Global immunosuppression can predispose to sepsis, potentially altering outcomes in susceptible individuals. CPB results in neutrophil sequestration into the lung, with damage to pulmonary epithelial and endothelial surfaces. The consequent increase in pulmonary vascular permeability produces interstitial and alveolar edema, reducing oxygenation and lung compliance. Detectable changes in lung function are present in up to 12% of CPB patients, with severe acute lung injury in as many as 3%. Increased duration of CPB increases both the likelihood and the severity of lung injury.

Postoperative neurologic dysfunction is also linked to the CPB inflammatory response. Mechanisms include neutrophil-mediated vascular endothelial damage and loss of vasomotor control from inappropriate production of nitric oxide. Mild cognitive dysfunction has been documented in up to 69% of patients, seizures in 5% to 10%, and focal cerebral deficits in 1% to 3%.

Perioperative renal dysfunction occurs in 7% to 13% of patients and may increase mortality 20- to 30-fold. The need for dialysis is associated with even greater mortality. Although specific mechanisms linking progression of the CPB inflammatory response to renal dysfunction are incompletely understood, ischemia-reperfusion injury has been shown in animal models. Impaired vascular regulation may play a role in altering glomerular perfusion along with elevated cytokine levels.

Coagulation disorders are an especially relevant sign of the CPB inflammatory response. CPB-induced platelet dysfunction, complement and fibrinolytic cascade activation, and elevated cytokine levels have all been implicated in the hemostatic defects following CPB. Evidence that a reduction in cytokine levels during bypass correlates with less postoperative blood loss supports an inflammatory cause for some of the coagulation deficits that occur after CPB.

MANAGEMENT

Management of the inflammatory state following CPB centers primarily on prevention and secondarily on supportive care for end-organ dysfunction. Although no specific agent has been identified that directly modulates the inflammatory response, a number of potentially useful strategies have been studied.

Avoidance of Cardiopulmonary Bypass and Aortic Cross-clamping.
Current evidence suggests that although off-pump cardiac surgery does not prevent CPB-induced inflammation, it does diminish the intensity of the response. It is unclear whether this actually improves clinical outcomes.

Heparin-Coated Bypass Circuits.
The goal of using heparin-coated bypass circuits is to reduce contact-mediated complement activation by decreasing factor XII activation. Use of such circuits does reduce neutrophil and complement activation. When combined with leukocyte filtration, there is a synergistic effect. Trials have shown a benefit only in high-risk groups, with no improvement in outcome in low-risk patients. It may be that the benefits of heparin-coated circuits are maximal only with prolonged bypass and cross-clamp times.

Selective Digestive Decontamination.
By reducing the endotoxin burden contained in the gut, adverse consequences of gut translocation due to poor perfusion during CPB may be reduced. Early trials of preoperative administration of oral nonabsorbable antibiotics showed decreased endotoxin and cytokine levels after CPB and fewer postoperative infections. However, no decrease in mortality has been observed to date.

Hemofiltration and Leukocyte Depletion.
By removing inflammatory mediators from the circulation, the CPB inflammatory response may be reduced in scope. In high-risk patients, hemofiltration improves post-CPB renal function and reduces the magnitude of pulmonary complications but has no significant effect on overall outcome.

Aprotinin and Other Modulators of the Immune Response.
Aprotinin is the best known of the class of agents known as serine protease inhibitors. These drugs reduce systemic inflammation by blocking hydrolysis and activation of inflammatory cascade mediators. Aprotinin is known to reduce blood loss during cardiac surgery, but it also has several anti-inflammatory actions, including limiting platelet activation and decreasing complement and leukocyte activation as well as cytokine levels. Clinical studies have not shown a definite improvement in mortality but have demonstrated reduced blood loss, decreased reoperation rates, fewer perioperative strokes, and less lung reperfusion injury.

Steroids. Although steroids would seem to have utility in blunting the consequences of uncontrolled inflammation, little outcome benefit has been demonstrated with peri-CPB steroid use. In small studies, steroids have been shown to decrease endotoxin and proinflammatory cytokine levels after CPB. Animal studies have shown that steroids reduce the indicators of pulmonary inflammation and may reduce inflammatory effects on pulmonary, cardiac, renal, and hematologic function. However, no outcome studies clearly show a benefit from perioperative steroid use.

PREVENTION

All the previously described measures are mainly preventive. Once the inflammatory reaction is initiated, treatment is primarily supportive. Maintenance of hemodynamic stability can reduce the extent of subsequent ischemia-reperfusion injury and is obviously mandatory. Mechanical ventilation should be adjusted to avoid overdistention of alveoli and consequent lung injury. Postoperative renal failure may require dialysis; in hemodynamically unstable patients, continuous venovenous hemodialysis may be better tolerated. Hyperglycemia worsens outcomes in cardiac surgery patients, and postoperative blood glucose levels should be kept below 150 mg/dL. Although no truly effective prophylaxis exists for postoperative atrial fibrillation, maintenance of normal electrolytes, perioperative β-blockade, and possibly temporary left or biatrial pacing may reduce its incidence and should be considered in high-risk patients.

Finally, it should be remembered that systemic infection can mimic the clinical presentation of CPB-related systemic inflammation. The postoperative presence of vasodilatation, pulmonary capillary leak, renal dysfunction, and cardiac dysfunction should thus prompt not only supportive care but also a careful search for infection as a potential treatable cause. Catheter sepsis, mediastinitis, endocarditis, and preexisting pulmonary or urinary tract infections all represent possible sources of systemic infection in postoperative cardiac surgery patients. These causes must be excluded in the presence of systemic inflammation.

Further Reading

Anselmi A, Abbate A, Girola F, et al: Myocardial ischemia, stunning, inflammation, and apoptosis during cardiac surgery: A review of evidence. Eur J Cardiothorac Surg 25:304-311, 2004.

Asimakopoulos G, Gourlay T: A review of anti-inflammatory strategies in cardiac surgery. Perfusion 18:7-12, 2003.

Chaney MA: Corticosteroids and cardiopulmonary bypass: A review of clinical investigations. Chest 121:921-931, 2002.

Laffey JG, Boylan JF, Cheng DCH: The systemic inflammatory response to cardiac surgery: Implications for the anesthesiologist. Anesthesiology 97:215-252, 2002.

Mojcik CF, Levy JH: Aprotinin and the systemic inflammatory response after cardiopulmonary bypass. Ann Thorac Surg 71:745-754, 2001.

Paparella D, Yau TM, Young E: Cardiopulmonary bypass induced inflammation: Pathophysiology and treatment. An update. Eur J Cardiothorac Surg 21:232-244, 2002.

Rady MY, Ryan T, Starr NJ: Early onset of acute pulmonary dysfunction after cardiovascular surgery: Risk factors and clinical outcome. Crit Care Med 25:1831-1839, 1997.

CARDIOTHORACIC & VASCULAR SURGERY

Fast-Track Cardiac Surgery

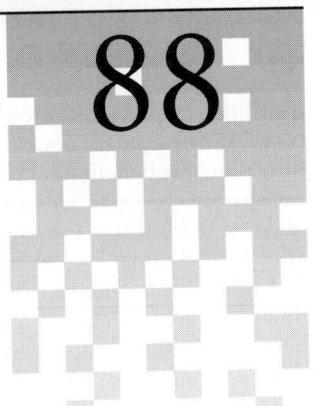

88

David C. H. Cheng

Case Synopsis

An 80-year-old man presents with crescendo angina and is scheduled for urgent coronary bypass surgery. Significant medical history includes prior tobacco use, non-insulin-dependent diabetes mellitus, and prior transient ischemic attacks with occasional slurred speech. Heart catheterization reveals significant coronary artery disease with subtotal occlusion of the left anterior descending coronary artery, complete occlusion of the right coronary artery, and 90% stenosis of the circumflex and acute obtuse marginal branch. Left ventricular ejection fraction is 45%, and the electrocardiogram shows right bundle branch block and an old inferior myocardial infarction. Off-pump coronary artery bypass grafting (CABG) is attempted but is electively converted to on-pump CABG during revascularization, owing to an intramural left anterior descending coronary artery. The aortic cross-clamp is positioned after epiaortic scanning, and all four coronary vessels are revascularized under cardiopulmonary bypass (CPB). A low-dose narcotic and inhalation anesthesia are used for the operation. The patient is separated from CPB with low-dose epinephrine for heart rate control and is transferred to the intensive care unit (ICU) with a sedative dose of propofol. His recovery is uneventful. He is extubated after about 6 hours in the ICU and discharged from the hospital 5.5 days after surgery.

PROBLEM ANALYSIS

Definition and Recognition

The costs related to the morbidity and mortality associated with cardiac surgery are increasing by about $1.2 billion per year owing to more severe disease, older patients, more extensive medical therapy, and often prior angioplasty or revascularization. Moreover, the number of CABG surgeries doubles every 5 years in the elderly population. With the escalating number of patients requiring cardiac surgery, more efficient use of limited facilities and resources is vital for cost containment in health care delivery.

Fast-track cardiac anesthesia (FTCA) is a perioperative anesthetic management regimen designed to facilitate the early tracheal extubation of patients, within 8 hours after cardiac surgery. Although it is feasible to extubate some post-CPB patients in the operating room, the risks (e.g., cardiorespiratory instability, bleeding) outweigh the potential cost-saving benefits, and it is not recommended at most centers. However, it has been demonstrated that early extubation anesthesia is safe and cost-effective and can improve resource use in some cardiac patients. It is important to realize, however, that early tracheal extubation does not necessarily mean early discharge from the ICU or hospital. To achieve maximal cost benefit, a team approach to a FTCA and surgery program must be implemented. This process includes preoperative patient education, same-day admission surgery, an anesthetic protocol conducive to early extubation, expeditious and meticulous surgery, flexibility in ICU nursing shifts, early postoperative extubation, avoidance of complications, horizontal integration between the step-down unit and the ICU, and good communication among cardiac patient management team members.

Risk Assessment

Key considerations for the patient described in the case synopsis are the following: (1) elderly patient with high comorbidity risks (prior myocardial infarction, diabetes, transient ischemic attacks) and critical coronary artery disease; (2) planned off-pump CABG surgery, with unanticipated need for conversion to CPB; and (3) perioperative anesthetic agents and techniques, monitoring, and preventive measures for perioperative anesthetic complications.

Implications

MEDICAL

Early extubation anesthetic management provides more stable perioperative hemodynamics and adequately suppresses the perioperative stress response without increasing the requirement for vasoactive medications. There is no significant laboratory evidence of greater myocardial injury during the first 48 hours with early versus conventional late extubation (Fig. 88-1). Respiratory mechanics after extubation are comparable between early- and late-extubation patients. The first hour after extubation is most crucial for respiratory care (Table 88-1). Tidal volume and central respiratory drive progressively improve over the first hour after extubation. There is no increased risk for respiratory acidosis, hypoxemia, or atelectasis with early extubation.

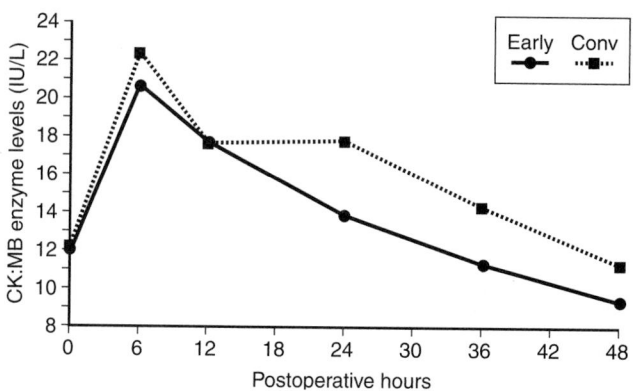

Figure 88–1 ■ Comparison of postoperative creatine kinase MB (CK-MB) enzyme levels between early and conventional (Conv) extubation groups over 48 hours. (From Cheng DCH, Karski J, Peniston C, et al: Morbidity outcome in early versus conventional tracheal extubation after coronary artery bypass grafting: A prospective randomized controlled trial. J Thorac Cardiovasc Surg 112:755-764, 1996.)

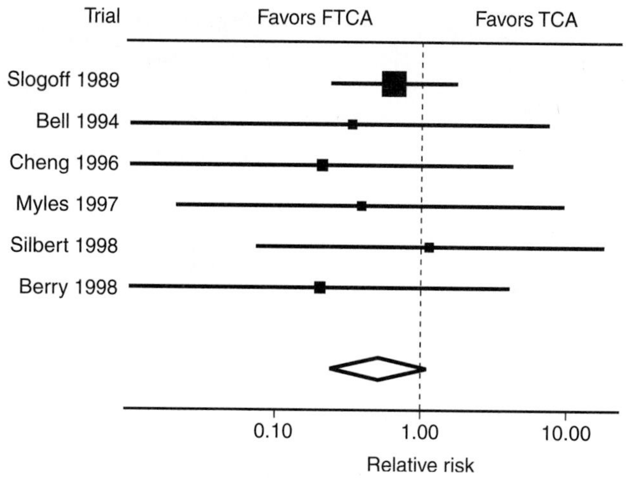

Figure 88–2 ■ Relative risk of mortality with a low-dose opioid regimen (fast-track cardiac anesthesia [FTCA]) and the more traditional high-dose opioid regimen (traditional cardiac anesthesia [TCA]). (From Myles PS, Daly DJ, Djaiani G, et al: A systematic review of the safety and effectiveness of fast track cardiac anesthesia. Anesthesiology 99:982-987, 2003.)

Also, early extubation improves the intrapulmonary shunt fraction by 30% to 40% after CABG. Cognitive function has also been shown to return to baseline earlier in patients given early extubation versus conventional anesthetic management. This allows earlier mobilization and oral intake of food in the early postoperative period, resulting in shorter ICU and hospital length of stay. Importantly, early extubation does not increase ICU readmission or mortality rates.

A systematic review and meta-analysis of 10 randomized trials in adult cardiac surgical patients undergoing CABG or valve surgery with CPB showed a nonsignificant reduction in mortality in patients undergoing FTCA versus traditional care based on high-dose opioids, as well as no significant difference between groups with respect to major morbidity (Fig. 88-2).

Currently, approximately 25% of all CABG surgery in the United States is off-pump CABG. A meta-analysis of 37 randomized trials revealed that off-pump bypass does not significantly reduce mortality, stroke, myocardial infarction, or renal dysfunction compared with conventional CABG with CPB. Further, off-pump CABG may improve selected 30-day clinical outcomes (e.g., reduced postoperative atrial fibrillation, respiratory infections, and need for inotropic support or blood transfusions) without measurable increased risk to the patient. At the same time, off-pump CABG reduces resource utilization, including ventilation time and ICU and total hospital length of stay, leading to potential reductions in hospitalization costs. However, there is an increased risk for significant mortality and morbidity in patients emergently converted from off-pump to conventional CABG with CPB.

Economic

The strongest predictors of cost for cardiac surgical patients are patient age, operating room time, ICU and hospital length of stay, and postoperative complications. Differences in CABG costs are primarily a reflection of accounting methods (e.g., charges, actual patient costs, reimbursed costs). Additional important factors are the following:

- Are costs reimbursed by a health maintenance organization or managed care provider?
- Is CABG performed in a teaching hospital or a community cardiac center?
- Are physician fees or cardiac catheterization costs included?
- What is the impact of patient-specific factors (e.g., number of coronary vessels grafted, extent and severity of postoperative complications)?

Early extubation protocols significantly lower CABG costs compared with more traditional management methods. They also reduce the intensity of nursing care by reducing ICU and hospital length of stay and by allowing more timely patient mobilization and hospital discharge. Early extubation

Table 88–1 ■ Apnea* in Early- and Late-Extubated Patients after Coronary Artery Bypass Grafting		
	Early	**Late**
Incidence of apnea episodes	27.5% (14/51)	33.3% (17/51)
Duration of apnea (sec)	17.7 ± 23.0	15.7 ± 28.6
Index (apnea episodes/hr)		
1 hr	13	15
2 hr	4	8
3 hr	2	9
4 hr	2	8

*Apnea is defined as expiratory pause of more than 10 seconds or tidal volume of less than 100 mL as measured with inductive plethysmography.

From Cheng DCH, Karski J, Peniston C, et al: Morbidity outcome in early versus conventional tracheal extubation after coronary artery bypass grafting: A prospective randomized controlled trial. J Thorac Cardiovasc Surg 112:755-764, 1996.

CARDIOTHORACIC & VASCULAR SURGERY

Table 88–2 ▪ Total Costs for Early- and Late-Extubation Anesthesia, Including Complications			
	Costs (Canadian $)		
	Early (n = 50)	Late (n = 50)	P
Preoperative	1347 ± 104	1353 ± 92	.76
Operating room	7619 ± 499	7755 ± 653	.24
Cardiovascular ICU	6463 ± 4943	12,046 ± 16,573	.026
Postoperative ward	4169 ± 1426	4963 ± 3068	.25
CABG: mean	19,596 ± 5766	26,116 ± 18,175	.019
CABG: median	17,269	19,372	.019

CABG, coronary artery bypass grafting; ICU, intensive care unit.
From Cheng DCH, Karski J, Peniston C, et al: Early tracheal extubation after coronary artery bypass graft surgery reduces costs and improves resource use: A prospective randomized controlled trial. Anesthesiology 85:1300-1310, 1996.

also improves ICU use and allows for increased caseloads with significantly fewer surgery cancellations (0.3% versus 2.0%). Finally, it results in up to a 28% lower rate of ICU readmission.

Importantly, to reduce perioperative costs, in addition to improving efficiency, perioperative morbidity rates must be minimized. This is because postoperative complications are far more costly than uncomplicated recoveries. Postoperative myocardial infarction or stroke can increase the cost of CABG three- to fivefold, infection two- to fourfold, and repeat surgery for postoperative bleeding or atrial arrhythmia control by 30% to 40%.

Early extubation anesthesia can be performed without increasing CABG complication rates while reducing ICU costs by 53% and overall costs by 25% (Table 88-2). In a 1-year follow-up study of FTCA patients after surgery, there was also evidence of reduced resource utilization after their index hospital discharge. Fifteen patients (25%) from both groups were readmitted to acute care hospitals during the follow-up period. The mean length of stay for acute care readmission was 0.3 day in the FTCA group and 1.6 days in the conventional group at 3 months (95% confidence interval [CI], 0.1 to 5.7; P = .01); it was 0.8 and 2.9 days, respectively, at 12 months (95% CI, 0.2 to 7.5; P = .01). The cost reduction associated with FTCA was 68% at 3 months and 50% at 1 year.

MANAGEMENT

An effective FTCA program requires appropriate patient selection, a balanced anesthetic technique (i.e., low-dose opioids and inhalational agents), early tracheal extubation, a short stay in a postoperative unit, and coordinated perioperative care. It is also necessary to avoid postoperative complications such as excessive bleeding, myocardial ischemia, low cardiac output states, stroke, arrhythmias, and renal failure. Finally, it is important for anesthesiologists to participate in the development and implementation of an FTCA and surgery program, based on their knowledge of perioperative medicine and skills with perioperative management.

Preoperative Care

Preoperative patient education is important to reduce anxiety and to establish realistic patient expectations. A preadmission clinic and same-day surgery program can reduce hospital length of stay by 1 to 2 days. Further, it reduces surgery cancellation or delays due to abnormal test results or patients' suboptimal clinical condition.

Intraoperative Care

The anesthetic regimen consists of balanced anesthesia with a low-dose narcotic, propofol, and inhalational agents:

- Sedation: intravenous midazolam (1 to 3 mg) for line instrumentation
- Prophylactic antifibrinolytic treatment: intravenous tranexamic acid (50 to 100 mg/kg over 15 minutes) or aprotinin (6 million units total for induction, CPB, and post-CPB)
- Induction: propofol (0.5 mg/kg) or thiopental (1 mg/kg), low-dose narcotic (up to 10 μg/kg fentanyl, or 1 to 2 μg/kg sufentanil, or 1 μg/kg per minute remifentanil), rocuronium (0.10 mg/kg), and midazolam (1 to 3 mg)
- Before CPB: inhalational agent (isoflurane, sevoflurane, or desflurane)
- During CPB: inhalational agents
- After CPB: postoperative analgesia (indomethacin 50 to 100 mg as needed, if not contraindicated) is essential, and sedation (propofol) is titrated to allow tracheal extubation within 1 to 6 hours
- Fluids and arrhythmia: tight fluid balance and aggressive arrhythmia control

Trials of remifentanil in cardiac surgery suggest that it provides excellent hemodynamic stability, minimal elevation of catecholamines, and reliable awakening, with most patients being eligible for early extubation. A remifentanil infusion and a low-dose fentanyl-based anesthetic regimen appear to be equivalent in the following respects: time to tracheal extubation, need for less intense monitoring, ICU and hospital length of stay, and resource utilization after CABG surgery. However, remifentanil's short duration of action necessitates the use of one or more supplementary methods for postoperative analgesia. These must be started before cessation of the remifentanil infusion.

Inhalational anesthetic agents have been recommended to provide cardioprotective effects via preconditioning and the reduction of reperfusion injury. The cardioprotective effects of sevoflurane appear to be most efficacious when the agent is administrated throughout the operation.

Shorter-acting neuromuscular blocking drugs should be used in FTCA; at a minimum, reversal of pancuronium neuromuscular blockade should be done before commencing weaning from mechanical ventilation. Hemofiltration, but not steroids, results in earlier tracheal extubation following CPB.

Intrathecal morphine doses as low as 250 μg are effective for reducing pain scores and postoperative parenteral opiate requirements, but their effect on time to tracheal extubation is not clear. Also, numerous well-conducted clinical trials have demonstrated a reduced time to tracheal extubation with thoracic epidural anesthesia in patients undergoing cardiac surgery. However, when compared with general anesthesia designed to facilitate early tracheal extubation, the differences are arguably of little clinical significance, because the majority of patients receiving thoracic epidural anesthesia still require ICU admission for a brief period of ventilation. Also, the majority of patients having general anesthesia can be extubated within 8 hours, so either technique appears to be consistent with FTCA.

Transesophageal echocardiography (TEE) during CABG surgery remains a class II indication and is valuable or informative in 15% to 50% of cases and essential in 5% to 20%. Epiaortic echocardiography is the current gold standard for diagnosing and evaluating patients for ascending aortic atherosclerosis during heart surgery. Results of urgent TEE in hemodynamically unstable patients or those with thromboembolic phenomena in the post-cardiac surgery ICU are unpredictable in more than half of cases. Clinical management is often modified based on TEE findings, and TEE is essential for the management of hemodynamically unstable patients after cardiac surgery.

Postoperative Care

Although high-risk patients are more likely to incur postoperative complications, both intraoperative and postoperative complications ultimately determine whether early extubation and reduced ICU length of stay are possible (Table 88-3). All patients should be assessed for the feasibility of tracheal extubation once certain criteria are met (Table 88-4).

Nonsteroidal anti-inflammatory drugs have been used widely in cardiac surgery patients who lack contraindications such as peptic ulcer, renal impairment, or coagulopathies. Diclofenac appears to be more effective than indomethacin and ketoprofen. Enteric-coated aspirin is routinely given postoperatively and is associated with a reduced risk of death and major complications after CABG surgery.

Nursing support is needed to achieve 1-day ICU stays and transfer to the floor or a step-down unit. There must be appropriate changes in analgesia and sedation practices and adherence to accelerated weaning and tracheal

Table 88–4 ■ Tracheal Extubation Guidelines

Central nervous system: Responsive and cooperative
Cardiovascular system: CI >2.0; absence of uncontrolled arrhythmia
Respiratory system: VC >10 mL/kg, NIF >–20 mm Hg; pH >7.30, PaO_2 >80 on FiO_2 <0.5
Bleeding: Chest tube drainage <100 mL/hr
Renal: Urine output >0.5 mL/kg/hr
Temperature: >36.5°C

CI, cardiac index; FiO_2, fraction of inspired oxygen; NIF, negative inspiratory force; PaO_2, arterial oxygen tension; VC, vital capacity.

extubation protocols. Early extubation may allow for chest tube removal, mobilization, and food intake on postoperative day 1, facilitating early ICU discharge and hospital discharge by days 4 to 5. Finally, health care providers should be cognizant of the need for continuous improvement in quality of care and for cost savings, which can be facilitated by following appropriate weaning and extubation guidelines, arrhythmia management regimens, post-valvular anticoagulation protocols, and ICU and hospital discharge guidelines (Table 88-5).

PREVENTION

Bleeding and Chest Re-exploration. The incidence of postoperative bleeding necessitating chest re-exploration ranges from 1% to 5%. The common use of the potent antiplatelet medications (glycoprotein IIb/IIIa receptor antagonists) abciximab, eptifibatide, and tirofiban necessitates the delay of elective cardiac surgery for 1 to 2 days, 2 to 4 hours, or 3 to 4 hours, respectively, after discontinuing these medications. Aprotinin is more effective in preventing postoperative bleeding than either tranexamic acid or ε-aminocaproic acid, and it may provide additional anti-inflammatory protection. Because of its high cost, aprotinin is usually reserved for cases with a high likelihood of allogeneic blood transfusion (e.g., reoperations, combined CABG-valve procedures, aortic surgery).

Atrial Arrhythmia. Atrial fibrillation is common after cardiac surgery, occurring in up to 35% of patients. Drugs with β-blocking properties are effective at reducing the frequency of postoperative atrial fibrillation. The added benefit versus

Table 88–3 ■ Independent Predictors of Delayed Extubation by Multiple Logistic Regression Analysis

Independent Predictors	No. of Patients (%)	Odds Ratio	P
Age (versus <60 yr)			
60-69 yr	338 (38.1)	1.67	.0004
70-79 yr	193 (21.8)	2.22	.0004
≥80 yr	18 (2.0)	1.86	.0004
Intraoperative inotropes	61 (6.9)	1.86	.004
Intraoperative IABP	57 (6.4)	3.58	.0001
Postoperative atrial arrhythmias	109 (12.3)	1.85	.003

IABP, intra-aortic balloon pump.
From Wong DT, Cheng DCH, Kustra R, et al: Risk factors of delayed extubation, prolonged length of stay in the intensive care unit, and mortality in patients undergoing CABG with fast track cardiac anesthesia: A new cardiac risk score. Anesthesiology 91:936-944, 1999.

Table 88–5 ■ Intensive Care Unit Discharge Guidelines

Central nervous system: Alert and cooperative
Cardiovascular system: No uncontrolled arrhythmia; stable hemodynamics
Respiratory system: PaO_2 >80, $PaCO_2$ <60, SaO_2 >90% at ≤60% facemask
Bleeding: Chest tube drainage <50 mL/hr × 2 hr
Renal: Urine output >0.5 mL/kg/hr

$PaCO_2$, arterial carbon dioxide tension; PaO_2, arterial oxygen tension; SaO_2, arterial oxygen saturation.

the safety of combining class III antiarrhythmic activity (e.g., amiodarone) with β-blocking activity is not clearly defined. Therefore, the use of amiodarone to prevent or manage postoperative atrial fibrillation should be considered on a case-by-case basis (assessing risk versus benefit). The role of magnesium for the prevention of atrial fibrillation is not clearly defined, but it is usually well tolerated. Biatrial pacing is likely to reduce the incidence of postoperative atrial fibrillation, but the ideal pacing strategy (i.e., left, right, or biatrial pacing) remains to be defined.

Stroke.   Stroke occurs in 2% to 4% of patients after cardiac surgery and carries a high 1-year mortality of 15% to 30%. Steps to reduce the perioperative stroke rate have been suggested and include routine epiaortic scanning for cannulation and cross-clamping, higher CPB perfusion pressure, avoidance of unprocessed cardiotomy blood, and preservation of cerebral oximetry.

Renal Failure.   Approximately 8% to 15% of cardiac surgery patients sustain moderate renal injury (>1.0 mg/dL peak creatinine rise), with 1% to 5% requiring dialysis. Patients with preexisting renal dysfunction are at greater risk for needing dialysis. However, patients with preexisting renal dysfunction are not at greater risk for additional renal injury relative to baseline. Steps to minimize postoperative acute renal injury include higher CPB flow rates and avoidance of excessive hemodilution during CPB (e.g., hematocrit <20%).

Further Reading

Chaney MA: Intrathecal and epidural anesthesia and analgesia for cardiac surgery. Anesth Analg 84:1211-1221, 1997.

Cheng DCH: Fast track cardiac surgery pathways: Early extubation, process of care, and cost containment. Anesthesiology 88:1429-1433, 1998.

Cheng DC, Bainbridge D, Martin JE, et al: Does off-pump coronary artery bypass reduce mortality, morbidity and resource utilization when compared to conventional coronary artery bypass? A meta-analysis of randomized trials. Anesthesiology 102:188-203, 2005.

Cheng DCH, Byrick RJ, Knobel E: Structural models for intermediate care areas. Crit Care Med 27:2266-2271, 1999.

Cheng DCH, Karski J, Peniston C, et al: Early tracheal extubation after coronary artery bypass graft surgery reduces costs and improves resource use: A prospective randomized controlled trial. Anesthesiology 85:1300-1310, 1996.

Cheng DCH, Karski J, Peniston C, et al: Morbidity outcome in early versus conventional tracheal extubation after coronary artery bypass grafting: A prospective randomized controlled trial. J Thorac Cardiovasc Surg 112:755-764, 1996.

Cheng DCH, Newman M, Duke P, et al: Efficacy and resource utilization of remifentanil and fentanyl in fast track CABG surgery: A prospective randomized double blind controlled multicenter trial. Anesth Analg 92:1094-1102, 2001.

Cheng DCH, Wall C, Djaiani G, et al: A randomized assessment of resource utilization in fast-track cardiac surgery one-year after hospital discharge. Anesthesiology 98:651-657, 2003.

Cohen DJ, Breall JA, Ho KKL, et al: Economics of elective coronary revascularization: Comparison of costs and charges for conventional angioplasty, directional arthrectomy, stenting and bypass surgery. J Am Coll Cardiol 22:1052-1059, 1993.

De Hert SG, Van der Linden PJ, Cromheecke S, et al: Cardioprotective properties of sevoflurane in patients undergoing coronary surgery with cardiopulmonary bypass are related to the modalities of its administration. Anesthesiology 101:299-310, 2004.

Dowd N, Cheng DCH, Karski J, et al: Intraoperative awareness in fast track cardiac anesthesia. Anesthesiology 89:1068-1073, 1998.

Dowd NP, Karski JM, Cheng DCH, et al: Cognitive recovery and resource utilization following fast track cardiac anesthesia for CABG surgery in the elderly: Propofol versus benzodiazepines. Br J Anaesth 86:68-76, 2001.

Edgerton JR, Dewey TM, Magee MJ, et al: Conversion in off-pump coronary artery bypass grafting: An analysis of predictors and outcomes. Ann Thorac Surg 76:1138-1143, 2003.

Engelman RM, Rousou JA, Flack JE, et al: Fast-track recovery of the coronary bypass patient. Ann Thorac Surg 58:1742-1746, 1994.

Hynninen MS, Cheng DC, Hossain I, et al: Non-steroidal anti-inflammatory drugs in treatment of postoperative pain after cardiac surgery. Can J Anaesth 47:1182-1187, 2000.

Kogan A, Cohen J, Raanani E, et al: Readmission to the intensive care unit after "fast-track" cardiac surgery: Risk factors and outcomes. Ann Thorac Surg 76:503-507, 2003.

Mangano D: Aspirin and mortality from coronary bypass surgery. N Engl J Med 347:1309-1317, 2002.

Myles PS, Daly DJ, Djaiani G, et al: A systematic review of the safety and effectiveness of fast track cardiac anesthesia. Anesthesiology 99:982-987, 2003.

Wake PJ, Ali M, Carroll J, et al: Clinical and echocardiographic diagnoses disagree in patients with unexplained hemodynamic instability after cardiac surgery. Can J Anaesth 48:778-783, 2001.

Westaby S, Pillai R, Parry A, et al: Does modern cardiac surgery require conventional intensive care? Eur J Cardiothorac Surg 7:313-318, 1993.

Wong DT, Cheng DCH, Kustra R, et al: Risk factors of delayed extubation, prolonged length of stay in the intensive care unit, and mortality in patients undergoing CABG with fast track cardiac anesthesia: A new cardiac risk score. Anesthesiology 91:936-944, 1999.

Hypercoagulable States: Thrombosis and Embolism

89

Komal Patel and Mark A. Chaney

Case Synopsis

An obese 53-year-old woman with right-sided heart failure and ovarian cancer has an exploratory laparotomy under general anesthesia for tumor debulking. On postoperative day 1, she experiences sudden-onset shortness of breath.

CARDIOTHORACIC &
VASCULAR SURGERY

PROBLEM ANALYSIS

Definition and Recognition

More than 150 years ago, Virchow suggested a triad that leads to intravascular coagulation: injury to blood vessels, venous stasis, and hypercoagulability. Injury to blood vessels, as might occur with direct trauma, major burns, surgical manipulation, or central venous access, causes endothelial damage, leading to the formation of local clot (thrombus) and subsequent propagation (thromboembolism). Venous stasis, as might occur in anesthetized surgical or immobilized patients, results in sluggish venous flow and a propensity for thrombus formation. An understanding of hypercoagulability requires a basic knowledge of the coagulation process.

Thrombus formation is triggered by endothelial injury, exposing subendothelial collagen to circulating platelets. These adhere and form a platelet plug. As this is forming, the clotting cascade is activated via one of two pathways. In the *intrinsic pathway*, subendothelial collagen is activated through activation of factor XII (which requires factors VIII, IX, and XI). In the *extrinsic pathway*, tissue thromboplastin (tissue factor) is released by injured tissue to activate factor VII. The final (common) pathway begins with activated factor X (Xa). Once factor X is activated, it binds with its cofactor, factor V, and platelet phospholipid, and this complex activates prothrombin (factor II) to form thrombin (factor IIa). Thrombin, bound to platelet phospholipid, cleaves fibrinogen to fibrin monomers. These aggregate to form a fibrin polymer that is loosely held together by hydrogen bonds (soluble fibrin, or fibrin S). Subsequently, factor XIII (fibrin stabilizing factor), which is activated by thrombin and calcium ions, mediates the formation of covalent peptide bonds between the fibrin monomers to yield a stable fibrin clot (insoluble fibrin, or fibrin I).

Normally, the clotting process is balanced by an endogenous anticoagulant and thrombolytic system that limits clot formation and eventually dissolves the clot. Thrombolysis is initiated by tissue-type plasminogen activator (t-PA) from injured cells near the fibrin clot. As t-PA cleaves circulating plasminogen to plasmin, this dissolves fibrin within the clot matrix.

Several physiologic mechanisms regulate the coagulation process, thus limiting clot formation to the injured area and preventing excessive clotting (i.e., disseminated intravascular coagulation [DIC]):

- Coagulation factors circulate in inactive form.
- Normal blood flow dilutes the concentration of activated factors and removes them from the site of injury. These are subsequently removed from the circulation by the liver and reticuloendothelial system.
- Some coagulation factors (e.g., factor Xa) require a phospholipid surface (tissue factor, platelet phospholipid) for proper interaction.
- Antithrombin (AT; formerly known as antithrombin III) complexes with and inactivates thrombin as well as other circulating coagulation factors (with the exception of factor VII). AT molecules have two critical domains: one binds to thrombin and other activated clotting factors, and the other binds heparin. In the presence of heparin, the rate of AT binding to thrombin and other activated clotting factors is markedly accelerated.
- Thrombin binds to thrombomodulin (a protein located on the vascular endothelial surface), which activates protein C, thereby inactivating factors Va and VIIIa.
- Protein S is a cofactor (along with protein C) in the inactivation of factors Va and VIIIa.
- Tissue factor pathway inhibitor is synthesized by vascular endothelium and inhibits factor X in two ways: it directly inhibits factor Xa, and it complexes with factor Xa to inhibit tissue factor VIIIa, thereby inhibiting the extrinsic pathway.

Hypercoagulable states represent a spectrum of processes that increase the activation of coagulation, decrease endogenous anticoagulation, or decrease the activity of thrombolytic systems. These disorders may be qualitative or quantitative, and their clinical manifestations depend on the severity of the disorder. Hypercoagulable disorders are classified as inherited disorders (conditions for which specific defects of the endogenous anticoagulation system have been identified; Table 89-1) or acquired disorders (disease or states associated with increased risk of thrombotic complications compared with that in general population; Table 89-2).

Table 89–1 ■ Inherited Disorders Causing Hypercoagulable States

Affected Component	Expression
Factor V gene mutation	Resistance to activated protein C by factor V
Prothrombin gene mutation	Increased prothrombin production
Antithrombin	Deficiency and dysfunction
Protein C	Deficiency and dysfunction
Protein S	Deficiency
Fibrinogenemia	Dysfunctional protein
Heparin cofactor II	Deficiency
Procoagulant factor	Deficiency
Plasminogen	Deficiency or dysfunctional protein
Plasminogen activator	Deficiency
Plasminogen activator inhibitor-1	Elevation

INHERITED HYPERCOAGULABLE DISORDERS

Factor V Leiden Mutation and Resistance to Activated Protein C.   Activated factor V serves as a cofactor in the conversion of prothrombin to thrombin. Factor Va is inactivated by activated protein C. A single point mutation in the factor V gene (R506Q [factor V Leiden]) makes the molecule resistant to degradation by activated protein C and thus leads to a hypercoagulable state by increasing the generation of thrombin. About 3% of the general population is heterozygous for this mutation. It accounts for 21% to 25% of patients with recurrent deep venous thrombosis (DVT).

Prothrombin Gene Mutation.   A specific point mutation in the prothrombin gene (G20210A) results in a 30% increase in the plasma prothrombin levels. Heterozygotes account for about 6% to 18% of patients with recurrent DVT.

Table 89–2 ■ Acquired Disorders Predisposing to Thrombosis

Venous Stasis	Diabetes
Immobilization	Homocysteinemia
Pregnancy	Cigarette smoking
Congestive heart failure	Estrogen therapy
Varicosities	Prosthetic cardiovascular
Obesity	device
Coagulation Activation	Indwelling vascular catheters
	Vascular Occlusive
Trauma	**Disorders**
Surgery	
Malignancies	Hyperviscosity, polycythemia
Factor IX concentrates	Sickle cell disease
Lupus inhibitor	Plasma cell dyscrasias
Myocardial infarction	**Increased Platelet**
Myeloproliferative disorders	**Reactivity**
Nephrotic syndrome	Thrombocytosis
Oral contraceptives	Surgery
Abnormal Vascular Surface	
Atherosclerosis, hyperlipidemia	

Antithrombin Deficiency.   AT is an α_2-globulin synthesized in the liver that inactivates thrombin; factors XIIa, XIa, Xa, and IXa; and kallikrein. AT deficiency was the first identified cause of hereditary hypercoagulable disorders. It is inherited in an autosomal dominant fashion and accounts for approximately 0.5% to 1% of patients with recurrent DVT.

Protein C and Protein S Deficiency.   Proteins C and S are vitamin K–dependent plasma proteins that inactivate factors Va and VIIIa. Their deficiency is transmitted in an autosomal dominant fashion and accounts for 5% to 10% of patients with recurrent DVT.

ACQUIRED HYPERCOAGULABLE DISORDERS

Acquired Protein C Deficiency.   Acquired protein C deficiency has been observed in patients with DIC, acute leukemia, hepatic disease, and nephrotic syndrome; renal transplant patients; and patients taking warfarin or oral contraceptives.

Malignancy.   The incidence of clinical thromboembolic disease in patients with cancer has been estimated to be as high as 11%. Thrombotic episodes may precede the diagnosis of malignancy by months to years. It may present as migratory superficial thrombophlebitis (Trousseau's syndrome), DVT, DIC, nonbacterial thrombotic endocarditis, or, rarely, arterial thrombosis. Tumors may secrete procoagulants (cysteine protease, tissue factor–like procoagulant). Tumors can also lead to venous thrombosis by external compression, vascular invasion (renal tumor), or hepatic involvement and dysfunction.

Pregnancy.   Pregnancy and the postpartum period are associated with the presence of all three components of Virchow's triad: venous stasis within the lower extremity veins (the gravid uterus impedes venous return), endothelial injury to the pelvic veins produced during delivery, and hypercoagulability. Pregnancy is also associated with increases in factors I, II, VII, VIII, IX, and X, along with decreases in protein S and AT activity. In addition, the activity of fibrinolytic inhibitors PAI-1 and PAI-2 is increased during pregnancy.

Surgery.   DVT and pulmonary emboli may occur postoperatively. Thrombosis in surgical patients appears to be related to surgical tissue trauma and the liberation of tissue factor, leading to thrombin formation. In addition, inflammation (leukocyte reactivity) and surgery-induced hemostatic changes may contribute to thromboembolism (Table 89–3). Hemostatic changes appear to correlate with the type of surgery and magnitude of surgical intervention and are maximal during the first 48 hours after surgery.

Immobilization.   It is postulated that venous stasis contributes to thrombosis by causing local hypoxia (with resulting endothelial injury) and inadequate clearance of activated procoagulant proteins.

Myeloproliferative Disease.   Patients with myeloproliferative disorders (e.g., polycythemia rubra vera, essential thrombocythemia, myelofibrosis with myeloid metaplasia, agnogenic myeloid metaplasia, megakaryocytic myelosis, chronic myelocytic leukemia) have an increased incidence of

Table 89-3 ■ Surgery-Induced Hemostatic Changes

Increased Platelet Reactivity ↑ Aggregation ↑ Dense granule release	↑ Von Willebrand's factor ↑ Thrombin formation
Increased Leukocyte Reactivity ↑ Free radical release ↑ Surface adhesion molecules	**Decreased Endogenous Anticoagulants** ↓ Antithrombin III ↓ Heparin cofactor II ↓ Tissue factor pathway inhibitor ↓ Protein C, protein S
Increased Coagulation Cascade Activation ↑ Fibrinogen ↑ Factor VIII	**Decreased Fibrinolysis** ↑ Plasminogen activator inhibitor-1

thrombotic events. Both arterial and venous thrombosis may occur at unusual anatomic sites, including the mesenteric, renal, splenic, portal, and hepatic (Budd-Chiari syndrome) circulations.

Hyperviscosity Syndrome. Blood viscosity is increased when there is an elevated red cell mass (polycythemia), increased immature adherent leukocytes (aplastic anemia), deformed red cell membrane (sickle cell anemia), and increased globulin concentrations (plasma cell disorders). Sluggish flow associated with these conditions can result in vascular occlusion in any vascular bed. It is believed that immature white cells cause leukostasis; this in turn releases proteases, which promote thrombus formation.

Lupus Anticoagulant. Lupus anticoagulants are antiphospholipid antibodies (usually immunoglobulin [Ig] G and, rarely, IgM) directed against plasma proteins (e.g., β_2-glycoprotein I, prothrombin, annexin V) bound to anionic phospholipids. Lupus anticoagulants occur in about 5% to 10% of patients with systemic lupus erythematosus. They block the in vitro assembly of the prothrombinase complex, resulting in a prolongation of protein assays such as activated partial thromboplastin time, dilute Russell viper venom time, kaolin plasma clotting time, and, rarely, prothrombin time. Although these changes suggest impaired coagulation, patients with lupus anticoagulants have a paradoxical increase in the frequency of arterial and venous thrombotic events. The mechanism for thrombosis is incompletely understood but may involve IgG binding to phospholipids that are essential for the normal activating and degrading effects of protein C and protein S, thus shifting the balance in favor of thrombus formation.

Hyperhomocysteinemia. High levels of homocysteine are associated with both venous and arterial thrombosis. The mechanism by which hyperhomocysteinemia predisposes to thrombosis is unclear; however, potential mechanisms include endothelial activation, proliferation of smooth muscle cells, changes in endothelial nitric oxide production, or changes in endothelial sterol metabolism. The disorder can be congenital or acquired. Acquired forms are found in patients with dietary deficiencies of folate, vitamin B_{12}, or vitamin B_6. Congenital hyperhomocysteinemia is most commonly due to

mutations affecting the cystathion β-synthase *(CBS)* gene or the methylenetetrahydrofolate reductase *(MTHFR)* gene.

Other Factors. Other factors that may be associated with hypercoagulable states are nephrotic syndrome, oral contraceptive use, hormone replacement therapy, prolonged travel, heavy smoking, hypertension, paroxysmal nocturnal hemoglobinuria, heparin-induced thrombocytopenia, thrombocytosis, and inflammatory bowel disease.

THROMBOEMBOLISM

Arterial thromboembolism may lead to cerebral or other vital end-organ infarction. For all intents and purposes, venous thromboembolism is pulmonary embolism, which has the following pathophysiologic effects:

- Increased pulmonary vascular resistance secondary to vascular obstruction, neurohumoral mediators, cytokines, and reflex vasoconstriction
- Impaired gas exchange secondary to increased alveolar dead space, ventilation-perfusion mismatch, and right-to-left shunt
- Compensatory alveolar hyperventilation
- Right heart dysfunction and dilatation secondary to increased pulmonary artery pressure, wall tension, oxygen consumption, and ischemia
- Bronchoconstriction and increased airway resistance
- Reduced lung compliance secondary to edema, hemorrhage, and surfactant loss

Risk Assessment

INHERITED HYPERCOAGULABLE STATES

The prevalence of factor V Leiden mutation and prothrombin gene mutation in patients with DVT is about 21% to 25% and 6% to 18%, respectively. However, patients with these mutations have a relatively low risk for thrombosis. By age 65 years, only about 6% of carriers of these mutations have experienced venous thrombosis, with most thrombotic events occurring during high-risk periods such as surgery. The frequency of factor V Leiden varies by ethnicity; it is common in people of European descent but rare in those of African or Asian descent.

AT deficiency accounts for only 0.5% to 1% of patients with DVT, but more than 50% of affected patients experience venous thrombotic events by age 60 years. Protein C and protein S deficiency accounts for 0.5% to 4% and 1% to 7% of patients with DVT, respectively.

ACQUIRED HYPERCOAGULABLE STATES

Malignancy. Intravascular thrombus formation can occur with any malignancy but is more common with neoplasms of the mucin-secreting organs (gastrointestinal and pulmonary). Migratory superficial thrombophlebitis occurs in up to 10% of patients with pancreatic carcinoma. Patients with malignancy also have other predisposing factors for venous thrombosis (e.g., surgery, immobilization).

Pregnancy. Pregnancy is associated with an approximate sixfold increased risk of venous thromboembolism compared

CARDIOTHORACIC & VASCULAR SURGERY

with nonpregnant patients (see also Chapter 196). Risk is greatest in the third trimester and first month post partum. The incidence of DVT and pulmonary embolism has been estimated to be as high as 0.05% to 0.1%. Pulmonary embolism is estimated to account for 12% of fatalities during pregnancy. Risk factors for thrombosis in pregnancy include increasing age, cesarean delivery, prolonged immobilization, obesity, prior thromboembolism, and coexistent thrombophilia.

Surgery.   Orthopedic procedures on the hip and lower extremities are among the most thrombogenic surgical procedures. In the absence of prophylaxis, the risk of DVT after total knee replacement ranges from 45% to 70%, and fatal pulmonary embolism has been reported to occur in 1% to 3% of patients undergoing hip surgery. Coronary artery bypass grafting surgery is associated with up to a 20% risk of DVT and a 4% risk of pulmonary embolism. Although the risk of thromboembolism is greatest during the first 2 postoperative days, embolic events may occur weeks to months after knee or hip surgery.

Immobilization.   Conditions leading to prolonged immobility (e.g., heart failure, stroke, spinal cord injury, old age, obesity, major trauma, surgery) increase the risk for hypercoagulability. DVT incidence rates of 58% in patients after major trauma and 33% in immobilized patients requiring medical intensive care have been reported.

Myeloproliferative Disease.   There is a correlation between elevated hematocrit, blood viscosity, and occlusive vascular events.

Indwelling Vascular Catheters.   Thrombotic complications are common with central venous catheters and are often associated with catheter sepsis. Thrombosis can be due to fibrin deposition or vascular occlusion.

Implications

Because the heparin effect (anticoagulation) depends on adequate AT levels, patients with AT deficiency may not respond appropriately to heparin. The use of warfarin may produce a deficiency in protein C and protein S before anticoagulation, which is responsible for warfarin-induced skin necrosis. For patients with hypercoagulable states, heparin therapy may be indicated for conditions that significantly increase the risk of venous thrombosis and pulmonary embolism (e.g., surgery, major trauma, immobilization).

MANAGEMENT

Except for AT deficiency (see Prevention), there is no specific therapy for hypercoagulable states other than anticoagulation with heparin (standard unfractionated or low molecular weight) or warfarin to prevent pulmonary embolism and thrombolysis (streptokinase, urokinase, recombinant t-PA) to dissolve clots. Nonspecific measures include hemodilution and avoidance of factors that might increase blood viscosity or facilitate coagulation (e.g., packed red blood cells, plasma, calcium).

Treatment of pulmonary embolism may be primary or secondary. Primary treatment to remove clot includes thrombolysis, catheter embolectomy, clot fragmentation, or surgical embolectomy. Secondary treatment for the prevention of recurrences includes systemic anticoagulation (heparin, warfarin) and inferior vena cava filters (e.g., bird's nest or Greenfield filters).

PREVENTION

Preventive measures for venous thrombosis and pulmonary embolism in high-risk patients include subcutaneous low-molecular-weight or unfractionated heparin, graduated compression stockings, and pneumatic compression devices. Fondaparinux (a synthetic heparin pentasaccharide) has been approved by the Food and Drug Administration for the prophylaxis of DVT in patients undergoing surgery for hip fracture or hip or knee replacement. Recombinant hirudin preparations have been used as prophylactic agents for DVT in European countries. In the United States, they are currently approved only for the treatment of heparin-induced thrombocytopenia. The following preventive measures should be considered for patients with acquired or inherited hypercoagulable states.

Antithrombin Deficiency.   AT concentrations routinely decrease after surgery but can be increased with the administration of plasma. Recombinant human AT is also available, and its use should be considered perioperatively in patients with AT deficiency, keeping in mind that heparin can decrease AT concentrations.

Protein C and Protein S Deficiency.   Concentrations of protein C and protein S can be increased by the administration of plasma. Specific protein C concentrate is also available.

Myeloproliferative Disease.   Because there is a correlation between occlusive vascular events and elevated hematocrit, blood viscosity, and leukocytosis, these three parameters should be returned to a more normal range with the appropriate use of phlebotomy, chemotherapy, or crystalloid solutions.

Further Reading

Bucur SZ, Levy JH, Despotis GJ, et al: Uses of antithrombin III concentrate in congenital and acquired deficiency states. Transfusion 38:481-498, 1998.

Loscalzo J, Schafer A: Thrombosis and Hemorrhage, 3rd ed. Philadelphia, JB Lippincott–Williams & Wilkins, 2003.

Martinelli I, Mannucci PM, De Stefano VD, et al: Different risk of thrombosis in four coagulation defects associated with inherited thrombophilia: A study of 150 families. Blood 92:2353-2358, 1998.

Mateo J, Oliver A, Borrell M, et al: Laboratory evaluation and clinical characteristics of 2132 consecutive unselected patients with venous thromboembolism: Results of the Spanish Multicentric Study on Thromboembophilia (EMET-Study). Thromb Haemost 77:444-451, 1997.

Santoro SA: Antiphospholipid antibodies and thrombotic predisposition: Underlying pathologic mechanisms. Blood 83:2389-2391, 1994.

Sixth ACCP guidelines for antithrombotic therapy for prevention and treatment of thrombosis. American College of Chest Physicians. Chest 119(1 Suppl):1S-370S, 2001.

Van Guldener C, Stehouwer CD: Hyperhomocysteinemia, vascular pathology and endothelial dysfunction. Semin Thromb Hemost 26:281-289, 2000.

THORACIC SURGERY

One-Lung Ventilation

Peter D. Slinger

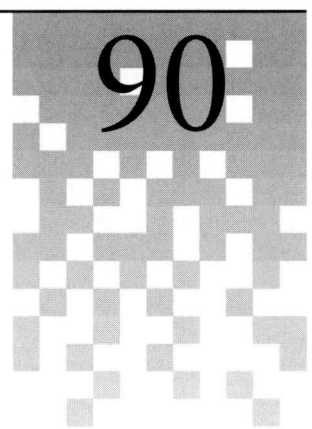

90

Case Synopsis

A 70-year-old woman with recurrent carcinoma of the right lung is scheduled for a right thoracotomy and possible pneumonectomy (Fig. 90-1). After induction of general anesthesia, a 37 French left-sided double-lumen endotracheal tube is placed, and satisfactory positioning is confirmed through auscultation (Figs. 90-2 and 90-3). After the patient is turned to the left lateral decubitus position, the tracheal (right) lumen of the double-lumen tube is clamped, and the bronchial cuff is inflated with 3 cm³ of air. On thoracotomy, the right lung remains inflated, and the patient's pulse oximetric saturation falls below 85%.

PROBLEM ANALYSIS

Definition

This case synopsis demonstrates two of the major complications of one-lung ventilation: inadequate lung isolation and hypoxemia (Table 90-1). Persistent inflation of the operative lung results from one of three potential causes: (1) double-lumen tube or bronchial blocker malposition or migration due to surgical manipulation or patient positioning;

(2) delayed lung deflation in a patient with obstructive airway disease, bullae or both; or (3) iatrogenic tracheal or bronchial rupture, or both, from the tube.

Although there are many potential causes of intraoperative hypoxemia during one-lung ventilation, it usually results from pulmonary shunting through the nonventilated lung. Hypoxemia due to shunting usually becomes clinically evident 10 to 20 minutes after the start of one-lung ventilation. Arterial desaturation very early in the course of one-lung ventilation is often due to inadequate gas exchange in the dependent lung due to malposition of the double-lumen tube. The concurrence of inadequate lung isolation and early desaturation in the patient described in the case synopsis suggests intraoperative migration of the double-lumen tube as the most likely cause.

Recognition

Management of arterial desaturation takes precedence over the diagnosis of tube malposition. Once adequate oxygenation has been ensured, fiberoptic bronchoscopy is performed to confirm double-lumen tube position or assist with repositioning of the bronchial blocker. If a bronchoscope is not immediately available, palpation of the lung hilum and carina by the surgeon may be useful to determine the position of the double-lumen tube. Surgical exploration also helps rule out pneumomediastinum, the most common presenting sign of tracheal or bronchial laceration by the double-lumen tube.

There are many other methods that can aid in the intraoperative diagnosis of double-lumen tube malposition, including the following:

- *Chest auscultation.* This is difficult to perform after the patient has been prepped and draped for surgery, and it may fail to diagnose lobar obstruction from distal migration of a double-lumen tube.
- *Changes in lung mechanics.* These may be revealed by airway pressure changes or changes in flow-volume or pressure-volume loops. Although any of these is a fairly sensitive indicator of changes in lung mechanics, they are

Figure 90–1 ■ Preoperative chest radiograph of a 70-year-old woman with recurrent carcinoma of the right lung who is scheduled for right thoracotomy and possible completion pneumonectomy. Tracheal deviation is a warning that double-lumen tube placement may be difficult.

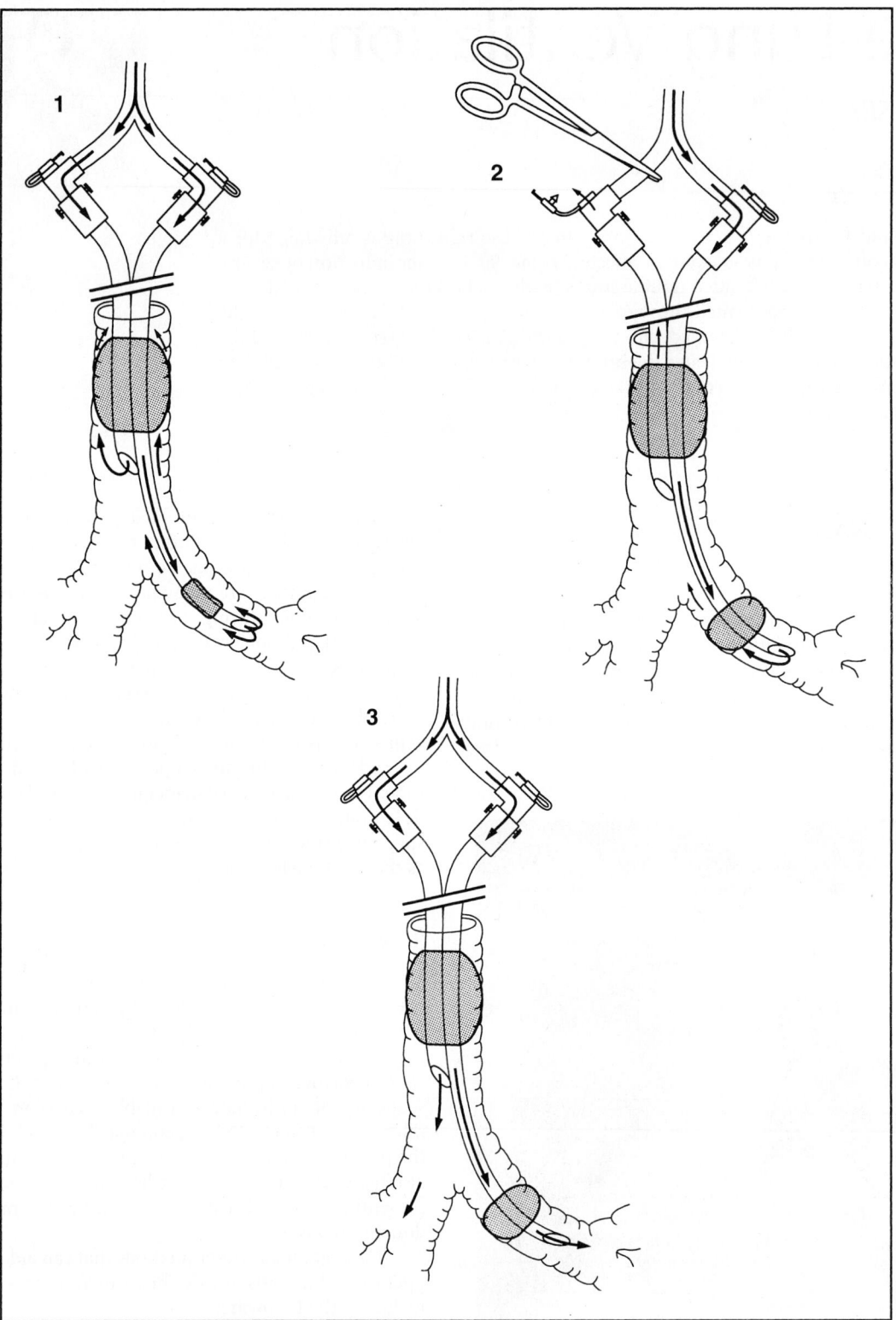

Figure 90–2 ■ Three-step method of auscultation to confirm double-lumen endobronchial tube positioning. Step 1: Inflate the tracheal cuff. Auscultate to confirm bilateral ventilation. Step 2: Clamp the tracheal lumen proximally (clamp the short side short) and inflate the bronchial cuff. Open the tracheal port and ventilate. Auscultate to confirm correct unilateral ventilation. Step 3: Release the tracheal lumen clamp, and close the tracheal port. Auscultate to confirm resumption of bilateral ventilation.

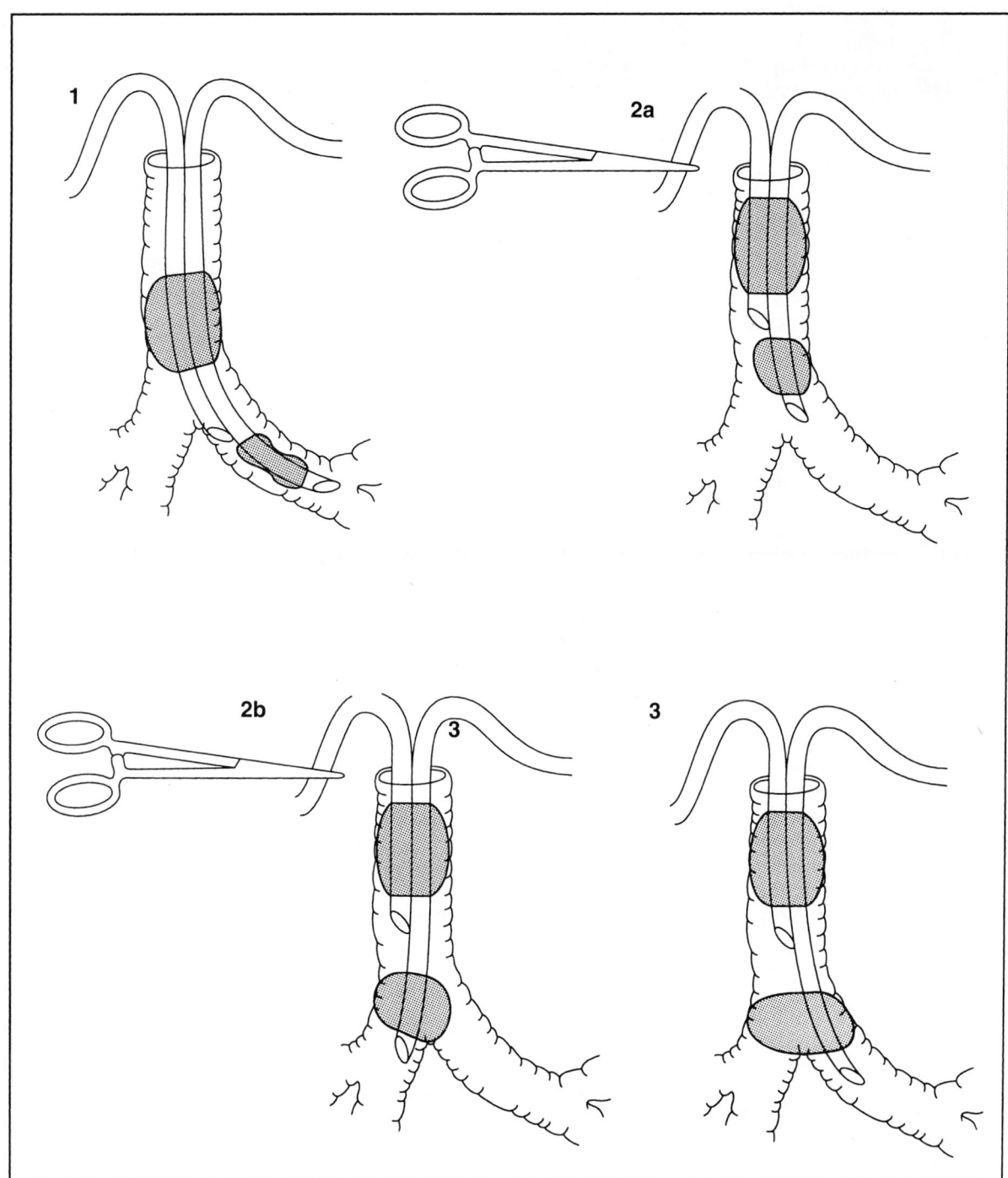

Figure 90–3 ▪ Common initial malpositions of double-lumen endobronchial tubes can be detected sequentially during the three-step method of auscultation. Step 1: Overly distal placement in either main bronchus is revealed by unequal breath sounds. Step 2a: Overly proximal placement results in inability to achieve unilateral ventilation during ventilation by the bronchial lumen. Step 2b: Incorrect side of bronchial intubation is revealed by unilateral breath sounds in the incorrect hemithorax. Step 3: Slightly too proximal placement results in appropriate isolation but unequal auscultation with resumption of bilateral ventilation.

all relatively nonspecific and can be due to surgical manipulation, pulmonary air leaks, airway blockage due to secretions or tube malposition, inadequate muscle relaxation, and many other causes.

- *Changes in end-tidal carbon dioxide (CO_2) tension.* The onset of one-lung ventilation is usually associated with a small ($\leq$5 mm Hg) and transient ($\leq$5 minutes) drop in end-tidal CO_2. Sudden, severe, or prolonged declines in end-tidal CO_2 suggest inadequate gas exchange in the dependent lung. Because similar changes in end-tidal CO_2 can be caused by alterations in cardiac output, this is also a fairly nonspecific indicator.

Table 90–1 ▪ Complications of One-Lung Ventilation and Double-Lumen Endobronchial Tubes
Hypoxemia
Malpositioning (primary or delayed)
Soiling of healthy lung regions
Inadequate ventilation
Interference with surgery
Airway trauma
Laryngeal
Tracheal
Bronchial
Difficulty managing secretions
Surgical damage to distal bronchial lumen

Risk Assessment

Difficult Lung Isolation. Although techniques to predict difficult *endotracheal* intubation are well described, the methods of assessment for difficult *endobronchial* intubation are not widely appreciated. Problems with double-lumen tube or bronchial blocker placement can occasionally be anticipated on the basis of the preoperative history, the physical examination, or a bronchoscopy report that suggests abnormal tracheobronchial anatomy. The majority of potentially difficult endobronchial intubations can be anticipated by examining the preoperative chest radiograph and computed tomography (CT) scan.

Hypoxemia during One-Lung Ventilation. Factors associated with increased risk of oxygen desaturation during one-lung ventilation include (1) a larger proportion of preoperative ventilation or blood perfusion to the operative lung, (2) an increased alveolar-arterial oxygen gradient during two-lung ventilation, (3) right-sided thoracotomy, and (4) predictive preoperative spirometry.

Implications

Although lung isolation is usually performed to facilitate surgery, in certain circumstances (e.g., bronchopleural fistula, pulmonary hemorrhage, lung abscess), the inability to adequately isolate the lungs can be life-threatening. Iatrogenic tracheal or bronchial rupture due to double-lumen tubes or bronchial blockers is estimated to occur in 0.5 to 2 in 1000 cases.

MANAGEMENT

Inadequate Lung Isolation

Immediate treatment for inadequate lung isolation is deflation of the bronchial cuff (or blocker, if one is used) and manual ventilation of both lungs to assess compliance. Ventilation of the dependent lung can be confirmed by observing mediastinal movement with lung inflation in the open chest. Ventilation of the nondependent lung can be observed directly. If ventilation of both lungs is not quickly confirmed, the double-lumen tube should be withdrawn

until the distal end of the bronchial lumen is above the carina (<25 cm by the tube markings from the inferior alveolar ridge for most adults) and ventilation is resumed. Once ventilation of both lungs is ensured by the return of satisfactory pulse oximetric oxygen saturations and end-tidal CO_2 concentrations, definitive repositioning of the double-lumen tube can be undertaken.

The fiberoptic bronchoscope should be passed via the bronchial lumen, and the carina should be identified. During repositioning, if the tube persistently tends to enter the right main-stem bronchus, tube rotation or right flexion or rotation of the patient's head often facilitates left main-stem bronchial intubation. If this fails, the bronchoscope should be advanced into the left main-stem bronchus and used as a guide to advance the bronchial lumen. This is easier to perform with fiberoptic bronchoscopes, which are specifically designed for anesthesia (e.g., Olympus LF-1 or LF-2) and are more rigid than pediatric bronchoscopes of similar diameter (<4 mm).

If bronchoscopy does not help achieve tube repositioning, an attempt can be made to advance a partially withdrawn tube into the left main-stem bronchus while the surgeon compresses the right main-stem bronchus. If this fails, an attempt can be made to ventilate the left lung via the tracheal (incorrect) lumen of the left double-lumen tube with the bronchial lumen malpositioned in the right main-stem bronchus.

If it is not possible to position the left-sided double-lumen tube satisfactorily, there are two major options (Fig. 90-4):

1. Continue the surgery with the double-lumen tube positioned above the carina and two-lung ventilation.
2. Replace the airway catheter or choose another technique for lung isolation (e.g., right-sided double-lumen tube, single-lumen endotracheal tube plus a bronchial blocker or single-lumen left endobronchial tube). The left double-lumen tube can be changed to a single-lumen tube or a right-sided tube without repositioning the patient with the use of a specifically designed, commercially available tube exchanger or with the fiberoptic bronchoscope. The problem of obstruction of the right upper lobe, which is seen commonly with right double-lumen tubes, is not a concern during left lung ventilation.

If a single-lumen tube is used, a bronchial blocker (e.g., Arndt Blocker, Cook Critical Care, Bloomington, Ind.) can be passed intraluminally and positioned in the right main-stem bronchus under direct fiberoptic bronchoscopic vision. Alternatively, some bronchial blockers can be passed through the vocal cords extraluminally to a single-lumen tube. Another method for bronchial blockade is the use of a Univent tube (Fugi Corp., Tokyo), which is a single-lumen tube with an enclosed bronchial blocker. However, all forms of bronchial blockers are more likely than double-lumen tubes to migrate intraoperatively, causing loss of lung isolation, particularly when placed in the shorter right main-stem bronchus. A final option is to advance a small (<7 mm internal diameter) single-lumen tube as an endobronchial tube under fiberoptic guidance. However, this may be difficult in a patient with distorted carinal anatomy.

Figure 90–4 ■ Management options for failure to achieve lung isolation with a left-sided double-lumen tube.

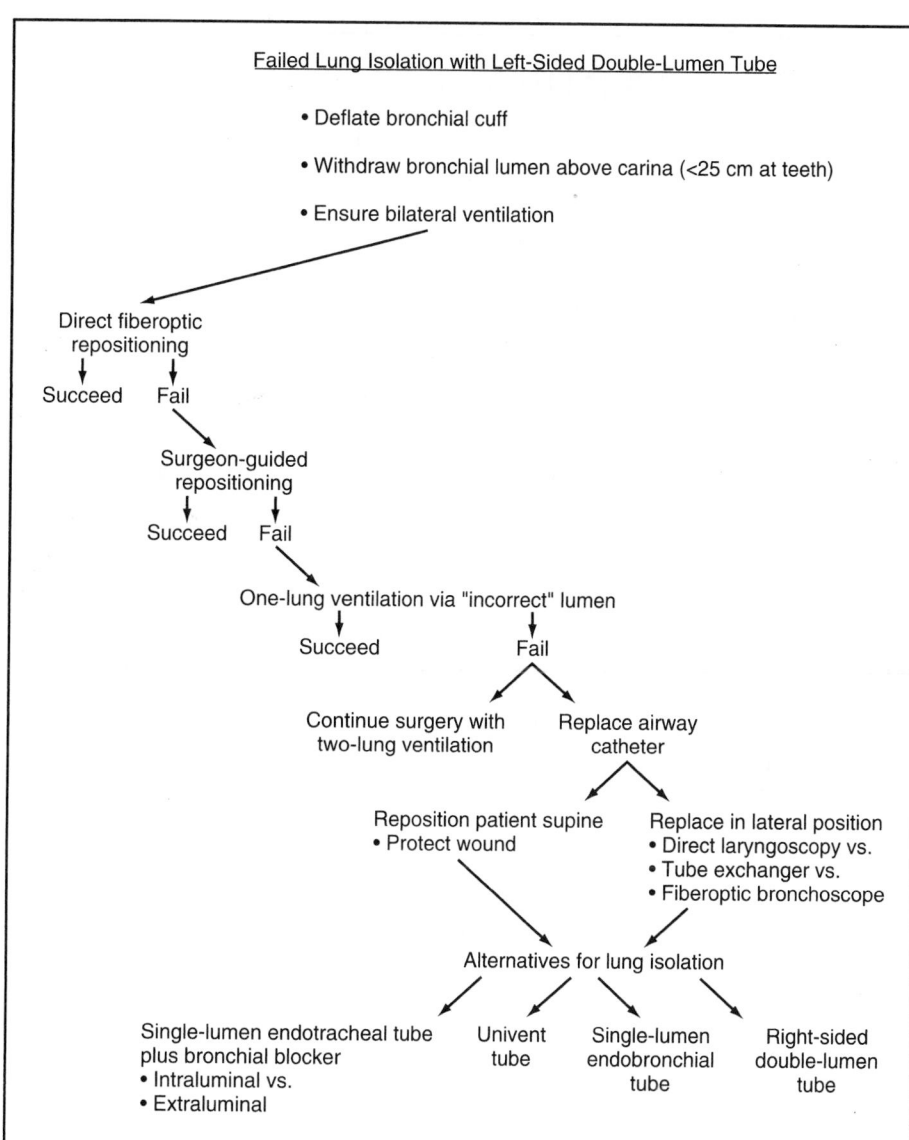

Failed Lung Isolation with Left-Sided Double-Lumen Tube

- Deflate bronchial cuff
- Withdraw bronchial lumen above carina (<25 cm at teeth)
- Ensure bilateral ventilation

Direct fiberoptic repositioning
Succeed   Fail

Surgeon-guided repositioning
Succeed   Fail

One-lung ventilation via "incorrect" lumen
Succeed   Fail

Continue surgery with two-lung ventilation   Replace airway catheter

Reposition patient supine
• Protect wound

Replace in lateral position
• Direct laryngoscopy vs.
• Tube exchanger vs.
• Fiberoptic bronchoscope

Alternatives for lung isolation

Single-lumen endotracheal tube plus bronchial blocker
• Intraluminal vs.
• Extraluminal

Univent tube

Single-lumen endobronchial tube

Right-sided double-lumen tube

Hypoxemia

Hypoxemia should resolve with reinstitution of two-lung ventilation. During one-lung ventilation with an appropriately placed double-lumen tube or blocker and a fraction of inspired oxygen (FiO$_2$) of 1.0, hypoxemia occurs in less than 5% of cases. Airway suctioning should be performed to ensure that thick bronchial secretions are not obstructing ventilation. When hypoxemia occurs during one-lung ventilation despite correct double-lumen tube positioning, continuous positive airway pressure (CPAP) with 2 to 5 cm H$_2$O to the reinflated, nonventilated lung is the only therapy required in most cases. Positive end-expiratory pressure (PEEP) to the ventilated lung is not useful in patients with obstructive lung disease who develop auto-PEEP during one-lung ventilation. However, low levels of PEEP (<5 cm H$_2$O) are useful in children or patients with normal lungs.

PREVENTION

Inadequate lung isolation can be prevented by following the "ABCs":

- *Anatomy:* A thorough knowledge of the lobar bronchial anatomy is necessary to achieve successful lung isolation (Fig. 90-5). Understanding the lengths and diameters of the bronchi and their variations with age and sex enables the anesthesiologist to plan the appropriate technique for lung isolation.
- *Bronchoscope:* The anesthesiologist should always use a fiberoptic bronchoscope to assess double-lumen tube or bronchial blocker position and to gain familiarity with bronchial anatomy. This familiarity will be useful when there is distorted anatomy or blood or pus in the airway. Because double-lumen tubes or bronchial blockers commonly

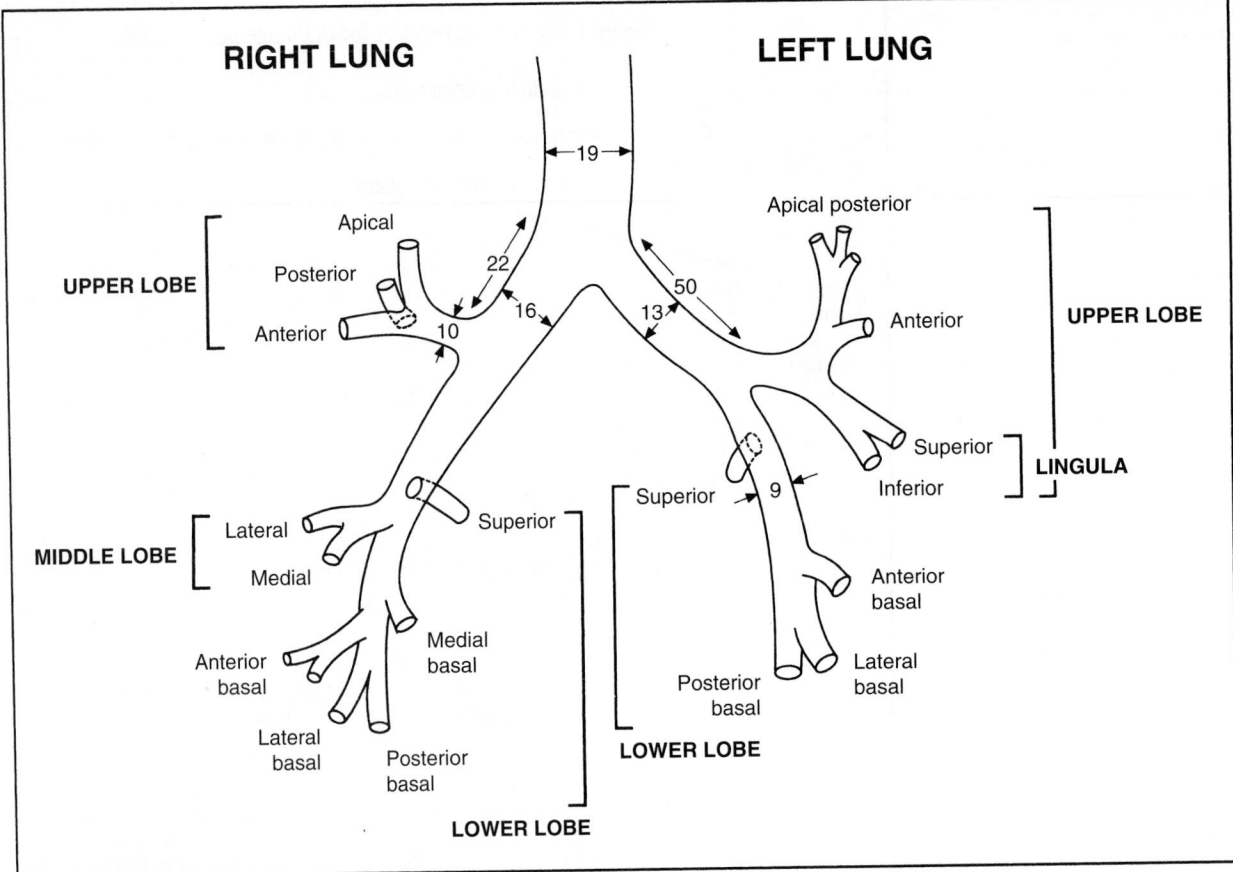

Figure 90–5 ■ Diagram of the tracheobronchial tree. Mean lengths and diameters are given in millimeters. Note that the right middle lobe bronchus exits directly anteriorly, whereas the superior (also called apical) segments of both lower lobes exit posteriorly. If the superior segment of the right lower lobe is called the apical, the segments from top to bottom on the right spell the mnemonic APALM.

migrate during patient positioning, the most important time to perform bronchoscopy is after final positioning of the patient for surgery and just before the start of one-lung ventilation.

• *Chest radiography and CT scanning:* Examining the preoperative chest radiographs and CT scans can provide information about anatomic problems and airway size (see Fig. 90-1). This information is useful when selecting lung isolation methods and tube sizes.

Prevention of hypoxemia is most reliably performed with the use of an FiO$_2$ of 100% and prophylactic application of CPAP to the nonventilated lung in selected high-risk patients (e.g., those with large alveolar-arterial oxygen gradients during two-lung ventilation, right-sided thoracotomies, and good preoperative spirometry). CPAP must be applied to a reinflated lung for optimal effect.

To reduce the risk of tracheobronchial trauma during endobronchial tube or blocker insertion, use the appropriate size tube; avoid nitrous oxide, which can cause bronchial cuff overinflation; always manipulate the tube or blocker gently; and position the double-lumen tube under direct bronchoscopic guidance when problems are anticipated

or encountered. The suggested double-lumen tube sizes based on gender and height are as follows: females less than 160 cm tall, 35 French; females greater than 160 cm tall, 37 French; males less than 170 cm tall, 39 French; and males greater than 170 cm tall, 41 French. Smaller double-lumen tubes (26 to 28 French) are available for children and small adults.

The bronchial cuff volume required to seal the airway is usually less than 3 mL. The bronchial cuff should be slowly inflated to the minimal volume required to achieve isolation. It is important to be aware that airway trauma is always a risk whenever a double-lumen tube or blocker is used.

Further Reading

Arndt GA, Kranner PW, Rusy DA, Love R: Single-lung ventilation in a critically ill patient using a fiberoptically directed wire-guided endobronchial blocker. Anesthesiology 90:184-186, 1999.

Bardoczky G, Szegedi L, d'Hollander A: Two-lung and one-lung ventilation in COPD patients: The effects of position and FiO$_2$. Anesth Analg 90:35-41, 2000.

Bauer C, Winter C, Hentz JG, et al: Bronchial blocker compared to double-lumen tube for one-lung ventilation during thoracoscopy. Acta Anaesth Scand 45:250-254, 2001.

Fujiwara M, Abe K, Mashimo T: The effect of positive end-expiratory pressure and continuous positive airway pressure on the oxygenation and shunt fraction during one-lung ventilation with propofol anesthesia. J Clin Anesth 13:473-477, 2001.

Licker M, de Perrot M, Spiliopoulos A: Risk factors for acute lung injury after thoracic surgery for lung cancer. Anesth Analg 97:1558-1565, 2003.

Russell WJ, James MF: The effects of increasing cardiac output with adrenalin or isopenaline on arterial haemoglobin oxygen saturation and shunt during one-lung ventilation. Anaesth Intensive Care 28:636-641, 2000.

Slinger P, Kruger M, McRae K, Winton T: The relation of the static compliance curve and positive end-expiratory pressure to oxygenation during one-lung ventilation. Anesthesiology 95:1096-1102, 2002.

Mediastinal Masses

Jerome M. Klafta

91

Case Synopsis

A 23-year-old previously healthy man presents with a 3-month history of cough (worse when he is lying flat). He says he has "head fullness." His chest radiograph demonstrates mediastinal lymphadenopathy with no other abnormalities. He is scheduled for parasternal mediastinotomy. After induction with propofol and succinylcholine, the patient is easily intubated, but manual ventilation is extremely difficult.

PROBLEM ANALYSIS

Definition

Patients with anterior mediastinal masses are prone to develop certain potentially life-threatening complications because of the influence of these masses on neighboring structures (superior vena cava, tracheal bifurcation or main-stem bronchi, main pulmonary artery, aortic arch, and heart). Principal anesthetic considerations for patients with anterior mediastinal masses involve the following three potential complications:

- Tracheobronchial tree compression or obstruction
- Superior vena cava syndrome
- Compression of the heart and pulmonary vessels

Also, patients may present for anesthesia or monitored anesthesia care for a variety of reasons, including:

- Excision of intrathoracic tumor (primary or metastatic)
- Lymph node biopsy (for tissue diagnosis)
- Central line placement (for chemotherapy)
- Biopsy of intrathoracic mass (open or thoracoscopic)
- Any other procedure, either related to the disease (e.g., open reduction and internal fixation of pathologic fracture) or not (cesarean section)
- Imaging studies (children)

Although these masses are referred to as "anterior," they are often at the confluence of the anterior, superior, and middle mediastinum (Fig. 91-1).

Recognition

TRACHEOBRONCHIAL TREE COMPRESSION OR OBSTRUCTION

Tracheobronchial tree compression or obstruction is the most common of the three potential complications arising from anterior mediastinal masses. There can be both static and dynamic components to such compression or obstruction. The dynamic components may not be unmasked until

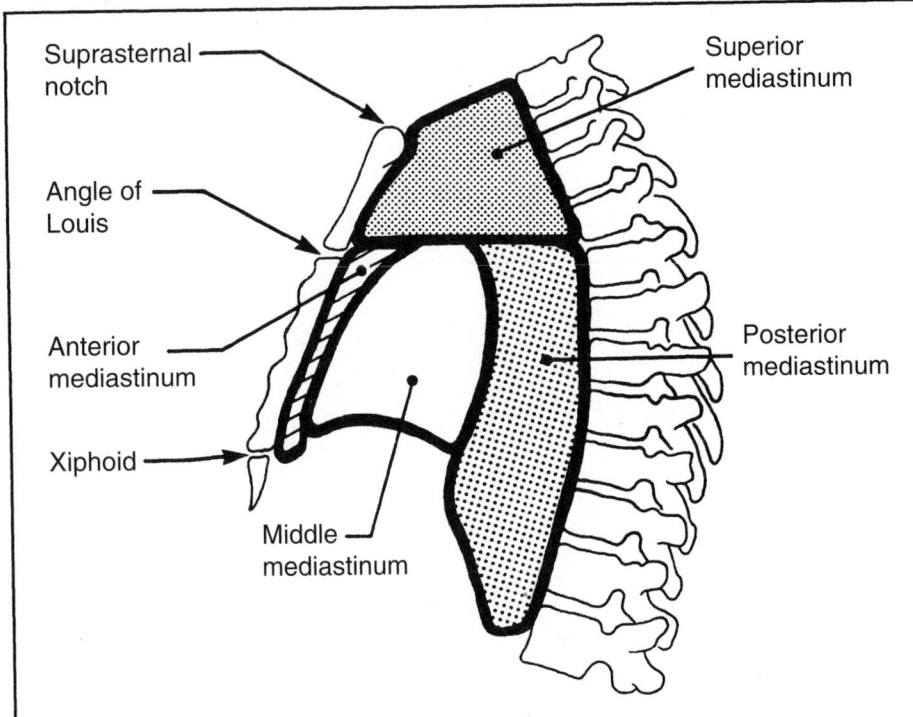

Figure 91–1 ■ The mediastinum is divided into superior and inferior portions. The inferior mediastinum is divided into anterior, middle, and posterior portions. (From Benumof JL: Anesthesia for Thoracic Surgery, 2nd ed. Philadelphia, WB Saunders, 1995, p 39.)

Suprasternal notch

Superior mediastinum

Angle of Louis

Anterior mediastinum

Posterior mediastinum

Xiphoid

Middle mediastinum

Figure 91–2 ■ Fiberoptic bronchoscopic appearance of the lower trachea in an anesthetized patient in the supine position *(A)* with a large anterior mediastinal mass that almost totally obstructs the trachea in the anteroposterior plane. With the patient in the sitting position *(B)*, the lumen appears normal. (From Prakash UBS, Abel MD, Hubmayr RD: Mediastinal mass and tracheal obstruction during general anesthesia. Mayo Clin Proc 63:1004-1011, 1988.)

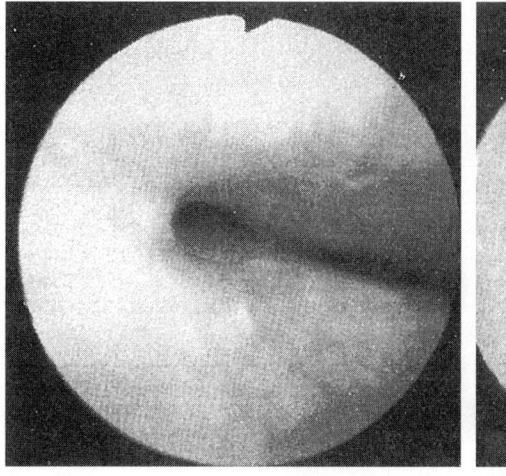

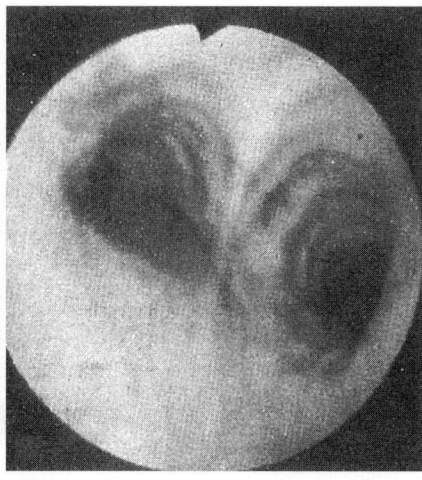

A

B

after supine positioning (Fig. 91-2), induction of general anesthesia, or administration of paralytic agents (Table 91-1). Difficulty in mask ventilation or difficulty ventilating despite successful endotracheal intubation is a classic scenario.

Preoperative features include the following:

- History of orthopnea, positional dyspnea
- Chest radiograph showing large mass, airway compression
- Chest computed tomography (CT) scan showing compression of airway or other structures (Fig. 91-3)
- Flow-volume loops with truncation of expiratory and possibly inspiratory limbs (Fig. 91-4)

SUPERIOR VENA CAVA SYNDROME

Superior vena cava syndrome occurs as a result of tumor compression or direct invasion of the superior vena cava and has the following features:

- Facial or upper extremity edema
- Dilated facial or upper extremity veins with collateralization
- Respiratory symptoms (nasal congestion, cough, orthopnea)
- Central nervous system effects (mental status changes, headache)
- Collateralization evident on chest CT with contrast enhancement

Table 91–1 ■ Possible Contributory Causes of Tracheobronchial Tree Compression or Cardiovascular Obstruction after the Induction of General Anesthesia and Tracheal Intubation in Patients with Mediastinal Masses

Cause	Result
Loss of lung volume	The mass remains constant in size, but pressure on the lung increases with applied positive airway pressure
Increase in central blood volume	The mass remains constant in size, but an increased transmural pressure gradient* created by the mass interferes with cardiac filling, thereby increasing central blood volume
Reduction in cardiac output	The mass remains constant in size, but pressure on more compliant superior, middle, or posterior mediastinal cardiovascular structures (superior or inferior vena cava, left or right atria, or even right ventricle) impairs venous filling and cardiac preload, effectively reducing cardiac output
Loss of negative pleural pressure	The mass increases the transmural pressure gradient and increases intrapleural pressure and (potentially) vital organ perfusion
Tracheobronchial obstruction at the endotracheal tube tip	The mass compresses the wall of the tracheobronchial tree, resulting in tracheobronchial distortion (e.g., bending, unusual curves), and can produce mechanical obstruction at the endotracheal tube tip
Associated tracheobronchial tree malacia	Airway collapse, atelectasis, increased intrapulmonary shunt, and arterial O_2 desaturation can occur
Intraoperative increase in tumor size	Tumor size can increase intraoperatively as a result of surgical manipulation, leading to edema or bleeding into the tumor mass (hematoma)
Creation of turbulent airway flow	Turbulence created by extrinsic airway compression by the tumor mass may be aggravated by overly vigorous positive-pressure ventilation
Injury to the recurrent laryngeal nerve (RLN)	Especially when the tumor mass involves the RLN, surgical dissection to remove the tumor may damage the nerve, leading to partial or complete vocal cord paralysis

*Transmural pressure gradient is the difference between a cardiac chamber pressure and the juxtacardiac or pericardial pressure.
Modified from Benumof JL: Anesthesia for Thoracic Surgery, 2nd ed. Philadelphia, WB Saunders, 1995, p 569.

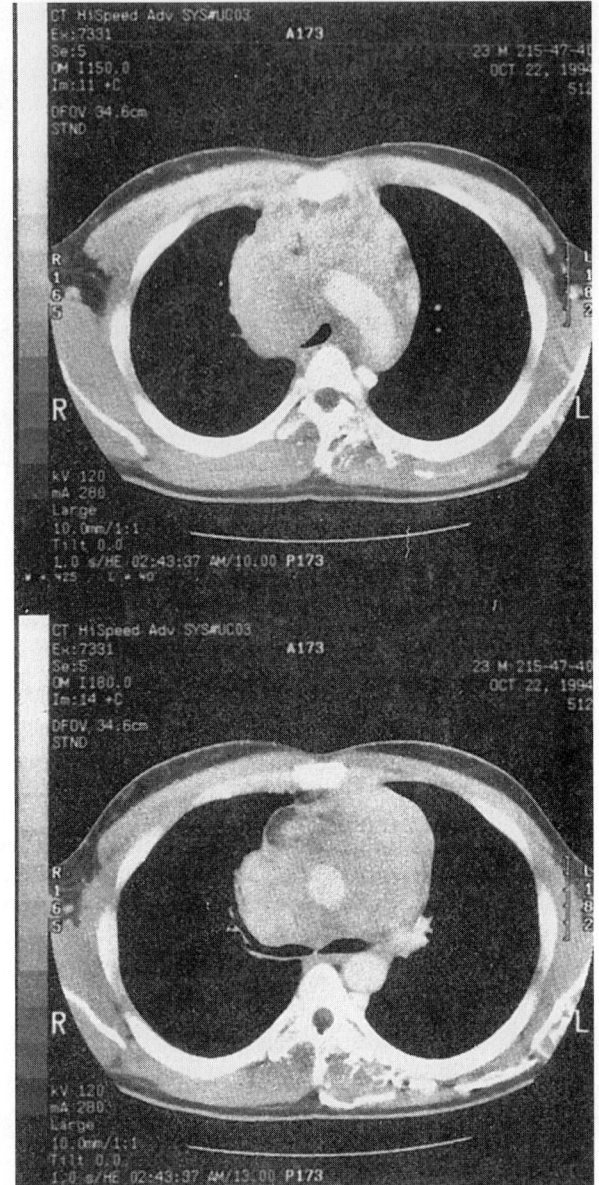

Figure 91–3 ■ Chest computed tomography scan showing extrinsic compression at the level of the trachea (*top*) and main-stem bronchi (*bottom*).

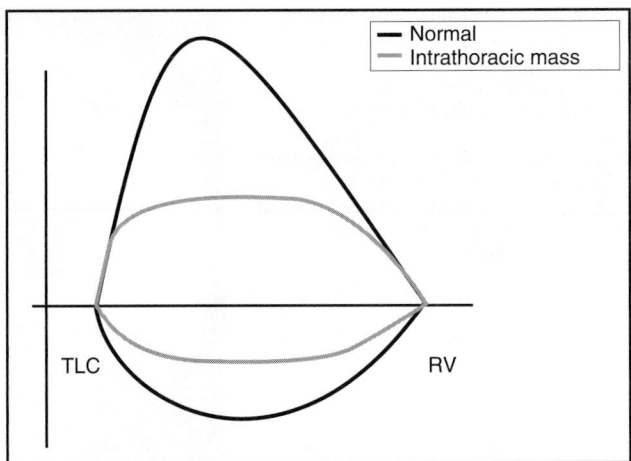

Figure 91–4 ■ Flow-volume loop for a patient with a normal airway and for a patient with an intrathoracic mass. TLC, total lung capacity; RV, residual volume. (From Pullerits J, Holzman R: Anaesthesia for patients with mediastinal masses. Can J Anaesth 36:681-688, 1989.)

COMPRESSION OF HEART AND PULMONARY ARTERY

Compression of the heart or pulmonary artery is a rare but life-threatening complication. A history of syncope or with Valsalva's maneuver is suggestive and merits at least a focused preoperative two-dimensional echocardiographic examination (look for extrinsic compression of cardiac chambers or of the pulmonary artery).

Risk Assessment

Generally, the larger the mass, the greater physiologic embarrassment it is likely to cause. However, the ability to prospectively identify which patients with mediastinal masses are at high risk for perioperative cardiorespiratory complications with general anesthesia is limited. The incidence of these complications may be significantly higher in pediatric patients. This can be explained by the fact that infants and small children are more susceptible than adults to extrinsic airway obstruction because their airways are more compressible and because small decreases in airway diameter result in proportionally greater effects on airway cross-sectional area and resistance.

In children, tracheal cross-sectional area (as measured by CT) less than 50% to 66% of predicted has been suggested as a cutoff below which general anesthesia should be avoided if possible. The only symptom that has been shown to strongly correlate with the degree of tracheal narrowing is orthopnea; however, its value in predicting intraoperative airway collapse is questionable.

In another report, pulmonary function testing performed in both sitting and supine positions revealed peak expiratory flow rates below 50% of predicted in 5 of 31 children in whom the tracheal cross-sectional area was more than 50% of predicted. Therefore, peak expiratory flow rate may be more sensitive than cross-sectional area alone in detecting airflow compromise due to the compressive effects of a mediastinal mass.

In adults, the presence of a pericardial effusion or mixed pattern of obstructive and restrictive pulmonary disease is associated with a high rate of postoperative respiratory complications. However, in all these studies (both children and adults), patients in the highest risk groups were anesthetized with a local anesthetic and sedation, thus limiting any conclusions regarding the safety of a general anesthetic technique.

Implications

- Tracheobronchial tree compression
  - Inability to ventilate or oxygenate, with hypercarbia or hypoxia
  - Possible cardiorespiratory arrest
- Superior vena cava syndrome
  - Excessive bleeding if the surgical site involves the head, neck, or upper extremities
  - Unreliable drug or fluid delivery via upper extremity intravenous (IV) lines

- Relative contraindication for jugular or subclavian central IV access
- Potential for airway edema
- Compression of heart and pulmonary vessels
- Hypotension; cardiovascular collapse

MANAGEMENT

Tracheobronchial Tree Compression

The best approach is prevention. However, if tracheobronchial tree compression does occur, the following maneuvers should be attempted:

- Change the patient's position to a lateral or semi-Fowler's position.
- Resume spontaneous ventilation.
- Attempt to advance the endotracheal tube past the obstruction (however, this could cause severe hemorrhage).
  - Consider using fiberoptic bronchoscopic guidance or an endotracheal tube changer.
  - Consider a smaller endotracheal tube.
- Attempt to bypass the obstruction and ventilate with a rigid bronchoscope.
- Oxygenate via femorofemoral cardiopulmonary bypass.

Superior Vena Cava Syndrome

- Recognize the effect of associated airway edema on intubation.
- Elevate the head of the bed to reduce venous pressure.
- Use lower extremity IV access as a more reliable route to the central circulation.
- Consider the use of diuretics and steroids.

Compression of Heart and Pulmonary Artery

- Perform intraoperative echocardiography to assess the degree of impairment.
- Position the patient to minimize compression (lateral or even prone).
- Maintain venous return, pulmonary artery pressure, and cardiac output as needed with fluids, pressors, and inotropic agents.
- Spontaneous ventilation may help.
- Have cardiopulmonary bypass available on a standby basis (have the groins prepped and draped).

PREVENTION

In patients with significant vascular, cardiac, or airway compromise, preoperative radiation therapy to shrink the tumor or local anesthesia for the procedure (if feasible) should be strongly considered. A potential disadvantage of preoperative radiation therapy is that it may obscure the histologic diagnosis and jeopardize treatment. CT-guided transsternal core biopsy is an alternative diagnostic technique at some centers. A multidisciplinary approach (oncology, radiation oncology, surgery, and anesthesiology) is required to make an intelligent decision regarding the risk-benefit ratio for proceeding with therapy.

The anesthetic plan and required setup vary, depending on the proposed operation (and surgical approach), the severity of the patient's symptoms, and other coexisting conditions and diseases. However, the following guidelines can be used:

- Have a low threshold for placing a preinduction arterial line in patients undergoing general anesthesia who have any symptoms or other evidence (e.g., CT scans) of airway compression. This will provide beat-to-beat blood pressure monitoring in the event of respiratory or hemodynamic compromise.
- A rigid bronchoscope should be available with the attending surgeon in the operating room for induction if there is particular concern about airway collapse.
- In the absence of contraindications (e.g., aspiration risk, difficult mask airway), slow induction of general anesthesia is preferred (IV or inhalation). Maintain spontaneous ventilation until effective positive-pressure ventilation is confirmed. If needed, perform tracheal intubation with succinylcholine (unless contraindicated); its short duration of action is advantageous in the event that muscle relaxation has a deleterious effect on the ability to ventilate the patient. Also, use the smallest dose of succinylcholine possible (≤1.0 mg/kg ideal or lean body weight).
- If feasible, perform fiberoptic intubation in an awake, spontaneously breathing patient. The fiberoptic bronchoscope can also be used to assess positional or dynamic airway collapse.
- Aim for a very smooth emergence and extubation sequence, because excessive coughing and straining can exacerbate both airway obstruction and the symptoms of superior vena cava syndrome.
- If central venous access or monitoring is required (indications are related to coexisting disease), access should be obtained via the femoral route.

Further Reading

Bechard P, Letourneau L, Lacasse Y, et al: Perioperative cardiorespiratory complications in adults with mediastinal mass. Anesthesiology 100:826-834, 2004.

Hnatiuk OW, Corcoran PC, Sierra A: Spirometry in surgery for anterior mediastinal masses. Chest 120:1152-1156, 2001.

Hoerbelt R, Keunecke L, Grimm H, et al: The value of a noninvasive diagnostic approach to mediastinal masses. Ann Thorac Surg 75: 1086-1090, 2003.

Johnson D, Hurst T, Cujec B, et al: Cardiopulmonary effects of an anterior mediastinal mass in dogs anesthetized with halothane. Anesthesiology 74:725-736, 1991.

Neuman GG, Weingarten AE, Abramowitz RM, et al: The anesthetic management of the patient with an anterior mediastinal mass. Anesthesiology 60:144-147, 1984.

Pullerits J, Holzman R: Anaesthesia for patients with mediastinal masses. Can J Anaesth 36:681-688, 1989.

Shamberger RC, Holzman RS, Griscome NT, et al: CT quantitation of tracheal cross-sectional area as a guide to the surgical and anesthetic management of children with anterior mediastinal masses. J Pediatr Surg 26:138-142, 1991.

Shamberger RC, Holzman RS, Griscome NT, et al: Prospective evaluation by computed tomography and pulmonary function tests of children with mediastinal masses. Surgery 118:468-471, 1995.

Tempe DK, Arya R, Dubey S, et al: Mediastinal mass resection: Femorofemoral cardiopulmonary bypass before induction of anesthesia in the management of airway obstruction. J Cardiothorac Vasc Anesth 15:233-236, 2001.

Complications after Pneumonectomy

92

Gordon Lee Collins and Eric Jacobsohn

Case Synopsis

A 74-year-old man is scheduled for a right-sided pneumonectomy for lung cancer. He has a past medical history of hypertension and coronary artery disease, with a coronary artery stent placed in his left anterior descending artery. He has mild chronic obstructive pulmonary disease, with no reversible airway obstruction. He does moderate (>4 METS) daily physical activity without any difficulty. A nuclear medicine stress test performed 1 year previously was negative for myocardial ischemia. Medications include aspirin, simvastatin, and atenolol. Aspirin therapy was discontinued 7 days before surgery.

His anesthetic and surgical course is uncomplicated and includes a combined general anesthetic-thoracic epidural technique. There is minimal blood loss, and he receives limited intra- and postoperative fluid. The chest tube is removed on postoperative day 1. Aspirin therapy is restarted on postoperative day 2. On postoperative day 3, the patient has increasing dyspnea, and a chest radiograph shows that the left lung has diffuse bilateral pulmonary infiltrates, in keeping with pulmonary edema. Because of progressive respiratory distress, he is intubated, and mechanical ventilation is commenced. The patient's oxygen saturation remains between 90% and 94% on 100% oxygen, 10 cm H_2O positive end-expiratory pressure, and optimal ventilator settings. A pulmonary artery catheter is judiciously inserted, and appropriate placement is confirmed by chest radiograph. The cardiac output and wedge pressure are low, there is moderate pulmonary artery hypertension and a transpulmonary gradient, and the right atrial pressure is elevated. A transesophageal echocardiogram shows mild right ventricular and right atrial dilation, with no demonstrable intracardiac shunt. A diagnostic bronchoalveolar lavage is performed and is negative for inflammatory cells or organisms (subsequent cultures are negative). A diagnosis of postpneumonectomy pulmonary edema, complicated by right ventricular dysfunction, is made. Supportive therapy includes diuresis, lung-protective ventilatory support, low-dose dobutamine, and inhaled prostacyclin (for increased pulmonary artery pressure and refractory hypoxemia). On postoperative day 5, hemodynamically unstable atrial fibrillation develops, and the patient is cardioverted. An amiodarone infusion is commenced. The patient's troponin level increases to 1.1 ng/mL. He is fully heparinized, and β-blockade is intensified. After 14 days of supportive therapy, including an early tracheostomy, he is successfully weaned from mechanical ventilation. After discharge from the intensive care unit, an angiogram shows stable coronary artery disease.

PROBLEM ANALYSIS

Definition and Recognition

Pneumonectomy is most frequently performed for bronchogenic carcinoma involving the hilum. Occasionally it is performed for inflammatory lung disease, traumatic lung injury, congenital lung disease, and irreversible atelectatic conditions. It is a major operation that results in changes in anatomy and cardiopulmonary physiology. Potentially serious and sometimes life-threatening postpneumonectomy pulmonary, cardiovascular, or other complications are relatively frequent. These are summarized in Table 92-1.

Risk Assessment

Many postoperative complications can be minimized by appropriate patient selection. This involves an assessment of pulmonary function, as well as the evaluation of and optimal therapy for any coexisting diseases or conditions, including obesity, cigarette smoking, reversible lung disease, coronary artery disease, and physical nonconditioning. Although baseline pulmonary function testing may have limited predictive value, the results of lung spirometry, lung diffusing capacity, maximal oxygen uptake, and arterial blood gas analysis are the cornerstones of most clinical decisions (Fig. 92-1). There may be less adverse physiologic impact from lung resection in some situations (e.g., resection of an obstructed, nonperfused lobe; concomitant resection of emphysematous bullae).

Implications

Right-sided pneumonectomy is associated with greater mortality compared with left-sided pneumonectomy (10% to 12% versus 1% to 3.5%). The indication for pneumonectomy

Table 92–1 ■ Complications after Pneumonectomy

Pulmonary
Hypoxemia
Postoperative respiratory failure
Chronic pulmonary debility or deficiency
Postpneumonectomy pulmonary edema
Postpneumonectomy syndrome
Bronchopleural fistula
Pulmonary embolism
Empyema
Esophagopleural fistula
Hemothorax
Chylothorax
Contralateral pneumothorax
Pneumomediastinum
Mediastinal infection (mediastinitis)
Vocal cord paralysis

Cardiovascular
Arrhythmias
Myocardial infarction
Intracardiac shunt
Cardiac tamponade or herniation
Pneumopericardium

Miscellaneous
Postpneumonectomy paralysis
Postpneumonectomy scoliosis
Difficulty interpreting pulmonary artery catheter data

may affect outcome; for example, pneumonectomy for lung cancer has a mortality of 3% to 4%, whereas that performed for benign disease may be as high as 26%. Emergent pneumonectomy in cases of trauma or massive hemoptysis is associated with mortality rates greater than 30%. Also, pneumonectomy performed by thoracic surgeons has a lower mortality than that performed by general surgeons. Associated lung disease, history of coronary artery disease, history of congestive heart failure, hypertension, atrial fibrillation, cerebrovascular accident, cigarette smoking, and a 10% or greater weight loss over the 6-month period before surgery all contribute to higher mortality.

MANAGEMENT AND PREVENTION

Complications occurring after pneumonectomy may be pulmonary, cardiac, or unrelated to either of these systems.

Pulmonary Complications

Intraoperative Hypoxemia. The differential diagnosis and approach to the prevention and management of hypoxemia during one-lung ventilation are discussed in Chapter 90.

Postoperative Respiratory Failure. Proper patient selection and the identification and treatment of reversible disorders involving the heart and lungs have greatly reduced postoperative respiratory failure. The following factors may also reduce the incidence of perioperative respiratory complications associated with pneumonectomy:

- Surgery performed by a certified thoracic surgeon in a medical center that does a large volume of pulmonary surgeries
- Appropriate perioperative use of pulmonary rehabilitation, bronchodilators, steroids, and antibiotics
- Smoking cessation before surgery
- Effective postoperative physical therapy and incentive spirometry
- Good postoperative pain control (e.g., thoracic epidural analgesia)

Chronic Pulmonary Insufficiency. This condition is largely preventable by appropriate patient selection and preoperative assessment of lung function.

Postpneumonectomy Pulmonary Edema. This syndrome develops in up to 5% of patients undergoing pneumonectomy. Mortality exceeds 50%. Postpneumonectomy pulmonary edema results in hypoxemic respiratory failure, with chest radiograph findings of diffuse infiltrates resembling those of acute respiratory distress syndrome. It usually occurs on about the third postoperative day. Its pathogenesis is multifactorial, including the following:

- Excessive fluid administration or use of fresh frozen plasma
- Hyperinflation injury during one-lung ventilation
- Coexisting pulmonary hypertension
- Impaired lymphatic drainage due to surgical dissection of hilar lymph nodes
- Occult pulmonary aspiration

There are no specific methods for managing or preventing postpneumonectomy pulmonary edema. Likely beneficial measures include avoidance of hypervolemia and excessive diuresis, lung-protective ventilatory support, and

CARDIOTHORACIC & VASCULAR SURGERY

Figure 92–1 ■ Algorithm for the preoperative pulmonary assessment of pneumonectomy patients. DLCO, diffusing capacity of the lung for carbon monoxide; FEV_1, forced expiratory volume over 1 second; PFT, pulmonary function test; PPO, predicted postoperative; VO_2 max, maximum oxygen uptake.

Routine PFTs $\Rightarrow$ FEV_1 >60% and DLCO >60% $\Rightarrow$ Proceed to surgery
$\Downarrow$
FEV_1 <60% and DLCO <60% $\Rightarrow$ Proceed to lung scan
$\Downarrow$
PPO FEV_1 >40% and PPO DLCO >40% $\Rightarrow$ Proceed to surgery
$\Downarrow$
PPO FEV_1 <40% and PPO DLCO <40%
$\Downarrow$
Exercise testing with VO_2 max >15 mL/kg/min $\Rightarrow$ Proceed to surgery
$\Downarrow$
VO_2 max <15 mL/kg/min $\Rightarrow$ Consider other options before surgery

inhaled pulmonary artery vasodilators if pneumonectomy is associated with refractory hypoxemia or elevated pulmonary artery pressures. Patients with this condition may also benefit from early tracheostomy.

Postpneumonectomy Syndrome.   This syndrome is the result of extrinsic compression of the distal trachea and mainstem bronchus, caused by a mediastinal shift toward the side of pneumonectomy and hyperinflation of the remaining lung. It occurs about 6 months after surgery, is more common in patients having pneumonectomy during childhood, and is usually a complication of right pneumonectomy. Treatment involves repositioning the mediastinum and filling the empty thorax with a nonabsorbable material.

Bronchopleural Fistula.   The incidence of bronchopleural fistula ranges from 1.5% to 4.5%; it is associated with 30% to 80% mortality and is more common after right pneumonectomy. It often presents 1 to 2 weeks after pneumonectomy as fever, productive cough, hemoptysis, and subcutaneous emphysema. Other associations include large bronchial stump size, incomplete tumor resection, concurrent radiation or chemotherapy, and poor wound healing (e.g., debilitated patients, steroid therapy). Treatment includes antibiotics, longer-term drainage of the pleural space, and repair of any air leaks with muscle flap procedures when appropriate.

Pulmonary Embolism.   Most pulmonary emboli arise from the deep veins of the legs. Rarely, they can arise from the pulmonary artery stump or the tumor itself. This complication can be devastating for patients with an already reduced pulmonary vascular reserve. Proper prophylaxis for perioperative deep venous thrombosis is critical. Management includes anticoagulation, but emergent embolectomy may be required immediately postoperatively. In patients further removed from surgery, intravenous thrombolytics should be considered. In those presenting with significant deep venous thrombosis and no pulmonary embolism, retrievable inferior vena cava filter placement may be indicated.

Other Pulmonary Complications.   Other complications include empyema, chylothorax and acute hemithorax, esophagopleural fistula, contralateral pneumothorax, and vocal cord paralysis. Management may require surgery (incision and drainage, fistula closure, mediastinal repositioning and filling of the empty thorax with nonabsorbable material). For partial or complete vocal cord paralysis, consultation with an otolaryngologist is recommended.

Cardiac Complications

Arrhythmia.   Atrial tachyarrhythmias (see Chapter 79), especially atrial flutter or fibrillation, are common after thoracic surgical procedures and occur in about 20% of cases. Eighty percent occur within the first 72 hours after surgery. Risk factors for such arrhythmias include age older than 60 years, right pneumonectomy, intrapericardial pneumonectomy, preexisting coronary artery disease, and chronic hypertension. Primary prophylaxis for atrial tachyarrhythmias after pneumonectomy is a β-blocker—either a primary β-blocker or sotalol, which is a β-blocker but also has class III antiarrhythmic activity (see Chapters 11, 12, and 79).

Amiodarone[1] may also be effective, but its role in the prophylaxis of postpneumonectomy or thoracotomy atrial tachyarrhythmias has not been established. In addition, pulmonary toxicity with *chronic* amiodarone administration is known to occur. It is possible that intravenous amiodarone for the prophylaxis or treatment of postpneumonectomy or thoracotomy atrial tachyarrhythmias might aggravate acute lung injury. Hemodynamically unstable atrial flutter or fibrillation requires immediate direct-current cardioversion, with further management and prevention according to established (advanced cardiovascular life support) guidelines (see Chapter 79).

Myocardial Infarction.   Perioperative myocardial infarction (MI) occurs in 1% to 5% of patients after thoracic surgery. Prophylactic perioperative β-blockers should reduce the incidence of acute MI and other cardiac events after thoracic surgery. Preoperative risk stratification for patients having pneumonectomy should follow existing American Heart Association–American College of Cardiology guidelines, which classify pneumonectomy as an intermediate-risk surgical procedure (see Chapter 38). The patient described in the case synopsis had only one intermediate-risk predictor (remote history of non-Q-wave MI), but he had been revascularized and was physically active. He also had a negative stress test a year before the planned pneumonectomy, making further preoperative testing unnecessary. All patients receiving chronic β-blocker therapy should continue these drugs. Patients with known coronary artery disease or peripheral vascular disease, and those with two or more risk factors for coronary disease (age older than 65 years, treated or untreated hypertension, diabetes mellitus, hypercholesterolemia, current or recent mI [≤6 months]), should receive perioperative β-blockers.

Routine withdrawal of aspirin therapy before major surgery in patients with coronary artery disease or peripheral vascular disease is probably contraindicated. However, the decision whether to cease such therapy must be individualized. Patients with coronary artery disease on chronic aspirin therapy may develop an aspirin withdrawal syndrome leading to acute MI. Factors such as the severity of cardiovascular and cerebrovascular disease and the presence and age of any stents must also be considered. The risk of withdrawing aspirin must be weighed against the risk of possible increased bleeding.

There is accumulating evidence that statin therapy may be protective in the perioperative period in patients with cardiovascular disease. This is likely related to the drugs' pleiotropic effects. Patients taking statins should not have their therapy interrupted in the perioperative period.

Intracardiac Shunting.   A patent foramen ovale may be present in 30% of the population. This can cause significant right-to-left shunting and severe hypoxemia if right heart pressure becomes elevated. This could occur due to poor patient selection, increased preoperative pulmonary artery pressures, pulmonary embolism, pneumonia, pneumothorax, postpneumonectomy pulmonary edema, or pulmonary aspiration.

---

[1]Amiodarone is listed as a class III drug, but it has all four Vaughan-Williams antiarrhythmic class actions.

Treatment for the underlying cause of increased right atrial pressure is critical. This includes optimizing right ventricular function and reducing pulmonary artery pressures, if elevated. Measures include inhaled pulmonary artery vasodilators, such as prostacyclin or nitric oxide. Percutaneous closure of the shunt may have to be done in some patients.

Cardiac Herniation.

Herniation of the heart through a defect in the pericardium can occur at any time after the surgical procedure. In addition to herniation through a pericardial defect, the heart or mediastinal contents may herniate into the pleural space if a chest tube is inadvertently placed on suction. Hence, many surgeons believe that routine chest tubes, even for short periods, are contraindicated after pneumonectomy. Cardiac herniation presents as sudden-onset hypotension and shock, cyanosis, chest pain, and symptoms of the superior vena cava syndrome. Emergent reopening of the thoracotomy is required to immediately reposition the heart. Suturing the edges of the pericardium to the myocardium or placing a prosthetic patch over the pericardial defect during surgery can prevent this complication. If it is caused by inadvertent chest tube suctioning, this must be stopped immediately. Repositioning the patient with the pneumonectomy side up may also be helpful.

Complications Unrelated to the Cardiopulmonary System

Only a few of the more common and difficult to manage complications unrelated to the heart and lungs are discussed here.

Postpneumonectomy Spinal Cord Ischemia and Paralysis.

This is a rare complication caused by intraoperative injury of the intercostal arteries to the thoracolumbar region of the spinal cord, leading to an anterior spinal artery syndrome. Treatment options are limited and largely unproved. They include maintaining a high spinal cord perfusion pressure and use of cerebrospinal fluid drainage.

Postpneumonectomy Scoliosis.

Scoliosis is estimated to affect 90% of patients undergoing pneumonectomy. This complication is due to shrinkage of the thoracic cage after surgery. Associated symptoms are usually mild and mostly inconsequential.

Difficulty Interpreting Pulmonary Artery Catheter Data.

A pulmonary artery catheter or central venous access is not routinely required for pneumonectomy. However, if a pulmonary artery catheter is used during thoracic surgery, it is important to note that data derived from the catheter may vary, depending on which lung or segment it floats to (e.g., dependent or nondependent zone), whether one-lung ventilation is used, and when the readings are made. Depending on the clinical circumstances, a pulmonary artery catheter has the potential to provide misleading data. If placed in the postoperative period, caution must be exercised when floating and inflating the balloon in the newly sutured or stapled pulmonary artery. Further, one should consider floating the pulmonary artery catheter under fluoroscopy or echocardiographic guidance.

Other Complications.

Other complications after pneumonectomy involve primarily the gastrointestinal system and include motility disorders and gastric volvulus. Optimal management may be medical or surgical; if necessary, appropriate consultation should be sought as soon as these complications become apparent.

Further Reading

Attar S, Hankins JR, Turney SZ, et al: Paraplegia after thoracotomy: Report of five cases and review of the literature. Ann Thorac Surg 59:1410-1415, 1995.

Bachamn DS: Discontinuing chronic aspirin therapy: Another risk factor for stroke? Ann Neurol 51:137-138, 2002.

Cerfolio RJ, Bryant AS, Thurber JS, et al: Intraoperative Solu-Medrol helps prevent postpneumonectomy pulmonary edema. Ann Thorac Surg 76:1029-1033, 2003.

Datta D, Lahiri B: Preoperative evaluation of patients undergoing lung resection surgery. Chest 123:2096-2103. 2003.

De Wet CJ, Affleck DJ, Jacobsohn E, et al: Inhaled prostacyclin is safe, effective, and affordable in patients with pulmonary hypertension, right heart dysfunction, and refractory hypoxemia after cardiothoracic surgery. J Thorac Cardiovasc Surg 127:1058-1067, 2004.

De Wet CJ, McConnell K, Jacobsohn E: Progress in postoperative ICU management. Thorac Surg Clin 15:159-180, 2005.

Eagle KA, Berger PB, Calkins H, et al: ACC/AHA update for perioperative cardiovascular evaluation for noncardiac surgery. Circulation 105:1257-1267, 2002.

Guggino G, Doddoli C, Barlesi F, et al: Completion pneumonectomy in cancer patients: Experience with 55 cases. Eur J Cardiothorac Surg 25:449-455, 2004.

Handschin AE, Lardinois D, Schneiter D, et al: Acute amiodarone-induced pulmonary toxicity following lung resection. Respiration 70:310-312, 2003.

Hoff WS, Hoey BA, Wainwright GA, et al: Early experience with retrievable inferior vena cava filters in high-risk trauma patients. J Am Coll Surg 199:869-874, 2004.

Kertai MD, Boersma E, Westerhout CM, et al: A combination of statins and beta-blockers is independently associated with a reduction in the incidence of perioperative mortality and nonfatal myocardial infarction in patients undergoing abdominal aortic aneurysm surgery. Eur J Vasc Endovasc Surg 28:343-352, 2004.

Khan SN, Stansby G: Cerebrospinal fluid drainage for thoracic and thoracoabdominal aortic aneurysm surgery. *The Cochrane Database of Systematic Reviews* 2003, Issue 4. Art. No.: CD003635. DOI: 10.1002/14651858. CD003635.pub2.

Miller DL, Deschamps C, Jenkins GD, et al: Completion pneumonectomy: Factors affecting operative mortality and cardiopulmonary morbidity. Ann Thorac Surg 74:876-883, 2002.

Poldermans D, Boersma E, Bax JJ, et al: The effect of bisoprolol on perioperative mortality and myocardial infarction in high-risk patients undergoing vascular surgery. Dutch Echocardiographic Cardiac Risk Evaluation Applying Stress Echocardiography Study Group. N Engl J Med 341:1789-1794, 1999.

Rahimtoola A, Bergin JD: Acute pulmonary embolism: An update on diagnosis and management. Curr Probl Cardiol 30:61-114, 2005.

Senior K: Aspirin withdrawal increases risk of heart problems. Lancet 362:1558, 2003.

Sugarbaker DJ, Jaklitsch MT, Bueno R, et al: Prevention, early detection, and management of complications after 328 consecutive extrapleural pneumonectomies. J Thorac Cardiovasc Surg 128:138-146, 2004.

Van Mieghem W, Coolen L, Malysse I, et al: Amiodarone and the development of ARDS after lung surgery. Chest 105:1642-1645, 1994.

Vaporciyan AA, Correa AM, Rice DC, et al: Risk factors associated with atrial fibrillation after noncardiac thoracic surgery: Analysis of 2588 patients. J Thorac Cardiovasc Surg 127:779-786, 2004.

CARDIOTHORACIC & VASCULAR SURGERY

VASCULAR SURGERY

Carotid Endarterectomy

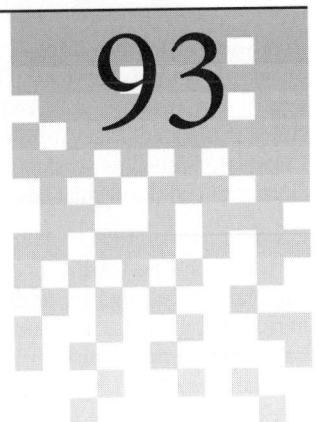

93

Vivek Moitra and John Ellis

Case Synopsis

A 72-year-old woman with a significant past medical history of hypertension and coronary artery disease undergoes carotid endarterectomy under general anesthesia. Electroencephalogram (EEG) monitoring is used. Her intraoperative course includes placement of a carotid artery shunt. On the following day, the patient experiences right upper extremity weakness.

PROBLEM ANALYSIS

Definition

Stroke is the third leading cause of death in the United States. Little can be done after a cerebrovascular accident (stroke) to reverse any permanent vascular brain injury. Stroke may result from aneurysm rupture with intracerebral bleeding, occlusion of intracerebral arteries, or carotid artery occlusion or thromboembolism. For the last, the focus is on prevention. Carotid endarterectomy and stenting are the most commonly performed procedures to minimize the risk of further stroke in patients with carotid atherosclerosis, a systemic and progressive disease.

Both symptomatic and asymptomatic patients with carotid lesions (i.e., atheromatous plaques) may benefit from carotid endarterectomy. Frequently, such plaques involve the proximal internal carotid artery and the carotid bifurcation. This may result in luminal narrowing and compromised blood supply to the brain, especially with contralateral atheromatous disease or disease involving the circle of Willis. In addition to luminal narrowing, atheromatous plaques may rupture, leading to thrombus formation and thromboembolism. Transient ischemic attacks and reversible ischemic neurologic deficits are believed to be the result of embolism or hypoperfusion. In many patients, however, carotid disease may manifest only as an asymptomatic carotid bruit.

The anesthetic management of candidates for carotid endarterectomy or stenting requires a clear understanding of cerebral circulation and physiology, appropriate monitoring techniques, and the potential for cardiovascular compromise.

Recognition

During carotid endarterectomy, the carotid artery is surgically occluded. Early recognition of cerebral ischemia is essential to guide subsequent surgical and anesthetic management. Many surgeons elect to place a shunt to maintain ipsilateral carotid flow, and the use of intraoperative monitors of cerebral perfusion and ischemia can aid the surgeon in making that decision. Placement of a surgical shunt may be routine, or the need for one may be determined by various methods (discussed later). Surgical shunting is not without risk; vessel wall disruption, dislodgment of atheromatous plaque with thromboembolism, shunt kinking, or air embolism may occur.

Methods used to assess the need for a shunt include neurologic assessment of awake patients (if carotid endarterectomy is performed under local or regional anesthesia, such as deep and superficial cervical plexus block), transcranial Doppler, EEG, somatosensory evoked potentials (SEPs), measurement of distal cerebral artery stump pressures (i.e., pressure created by backflow from the contralateral carotid artery across the circle of Willis), or direct measurement of cerebral blood flow with xenon (Table 93-1). The purpose of these measures is to avoid routine shunting, which can cause air embolism or thromboembolism. Different techniques or combinations of these methods may be preferred by different centers. However, the sensitivity of any technique for detecting perioperative ischemia or strokes is limited, because most strokes occur after surgery and are likely caused by thromboembolic phenomena.

The gold standard for cerebral monitoring is neurologic assessment of an awake patient. Awake patients having carotid endarterectomy have fewer EEG changes, and many practitioners advocate the use of regional anesthesia to allow the detection of cerebral ischemia, which manifests as acute changes in mental status or motor response to verbal commands. A successful regional anesthetic requires that the patient be comfortable and cooperative throughout the surgery. If combined with general anesthesia, regional blocks may reduce general anesthetic requirements, hasten awakening, and reduce the need for opiate analgesia after surgery.

Table 93–1 ■ Monitors of Cerebral Ischemia during Carotid Endarterectomy

Regional Anesthesia
Repeated neurologic examination of the awake patient

General Anesthesia
Electroencephalogram
Somatosensory evoked potentials
Internal carotid artery stump pressure
Xenon 133 washout
Transcranial Doppler ultrasonography
Jugular venous oxygen saturation
Transconjunctival oxygen saturation

Use of superficial or deep cervical plexus block may also minimize the hemodynamic changes associated with general anesthesia. Even so, the vast majority of patients undergo carotid surgery under general anesthesia, and several monitors are available to evaluate the adequacy of collateral circulation and cerebral perfusion.

Carotid stump pressure can be measured manually or invasively. The presence of a palpable pulse or a mean stump pressure greater than 60 mm Hg suggests sufficient backflow to prevent ischemia. However, ischemia may occur despite adequate carotid stump pressures if there is middle cerebral artery stenosis on the operative side and distal to the circle of Willis.

The EEG represents cortical electrical activity, which decreases with cerebral ischemia. Disadvantages of EEG monitoring include the inability to monitor deep brain structures, the presence of false-negative findings due to pre-existing or fluctuating neurologic deficits, and the influence of general anesthesia on EEG patterns.

Unlike EEG monitoring, SEPs can monitor deeper brain structures. SEPs are a result of electrical impulses that originate peripherally and travel through first- and second-order neurons to synapse in the brainstem. Subsequently, these impulses are transmitted to the somatosensory cortex. As with EEG monitoring, false-negatives may result if anesthetics produce SEP changes that mimic cerebral hypoxia.

Transcranial Doppler measures the velocity of blood flow in the middle cerebral artery. It can be used to detect acute thrombotic occlusion or embolization during or after carotid surgery, or to identify patients at risk for developing a postoperative hyperperfusion syndrome. However, the need for temporal ultrasound probe placement limits surgical and anesthetic access to the head.

Cerebral blood flow can also be measured by the intravenous or intracarotid administration of radioactive xenon or krypton. This method requires considerable expertise for the interpretation of data, and it is highly specialized and expensive.

Risk Assessment

Important risk factors for carotid disease include advanced age, hypertension, tobacco abuse, and a history of diabetes mellitus. Patients with left main coronary artery disease or other peripheral vascular disease are also more likely to have carotid disease. Conversely, patients with carotid disease often have concomitant coronary artery disease. Because these patients are at high risk for stroke but are more likely to die from myocardial infarction, the preoperative risk assessment, workup, and timing of surgery can be challenging and controversial.

Cardiac risk assessment may include exercise or dobutamine stress testing to determine the need for preoperative coronary revascularization (e.g., coronary artery bypass grafting or percutaneous coronary transluminal angioplasty, with or without stenting). The appropriate amount of preoperative risk assessment and subsequent preventive intervention is debatable for several reasons. Both the surgeon and the anesthesiologist must consider the risk of neurologic insult if carotid surgery is delayed in favor of a coronary intervention that may prevent the cardiac morbidity associated with

carotid endarterectomy. Also, both the anesthesiologist and the surgeon must assess the possibility of stroke in patients with carotid stenosis who undergo coronary artery bypass grafting.

There are no clear guidelines for anesthesiologists who are managing patients with both carotid and coronary artery disease, and the decision to pursue an invasive intervention is often based on the patient's clinical history, stability of symptoms, and institutional preference.

Implications

A number of trials have demonstrated the benefit of carotid endarterectomy for the prevention of stroke in both symptomatic and asymptomatic patients. This procedure is not without risk, however. In the postoperative period, patients may develop a second neurologic insult, respiratory insufficiency, hemodynamic instability, carotid body damage, hyperperfusion syndrome, or wound hematoma (Table 93-2).

Because most perioperative strokes are a result of postoperative thrombus, many vascular surgeons are asking their patients to continue taking antiplatelet agents (e.g., clopidogrel) up until the time of surgery. The use of aggressive antiplatelet therapy in patients with postoperative hypertension may predispose to wound hematoma, which may compromise the airway through laryngeal edema or extrinsic compression.

A number of randomized trials have compared carotid endarterectomy to carotid angioplasty and stenting. The challenge during angioplasty is to limit stroke from distal embolization of plaque. Transcranial Doppler has demonstrated that embolic events are far more common with carotid angioplasty than with endarterectomy. Even so, such events are not necessarily associated with increased rates of cognitive dysfunction. "Umbrella" devices that capture embolic particles may improve the results of angioplasty. The ischemic time for angioplasty and stenting is much shorter than for carotid endarterectomy, which may have benefits. Large randomized trials are currently under way, but it will be several years before definitive results are available.

Several studies have sought to elucidate predictors of outcome after carotid endarterectomy. Risk factors such as age older than 70 years, history of angina, coronary artery disease, congestive heart failure, severity of preoperative neurologic symptoms, occlusion of the contralateral internal

Table 93–2 ■ **Common Postoperative Problems**
Hemodynamic instability
Hypertension
Hypotension
Myocardial infarction
Wound hematoma
Glossopharyngeal edema with loss of airway
Cranial nerve damage
Respiratory insufficiency through loss of carotid body function
Neurologic dysfunction
Acute graft thrombosis (may require re-exploration)
Minor focal deficits
Hyperperfusion syndrome

carotid artery, and so-called siphon stenosis[1] have been both supported and refuted, leading many to question their prognostic significance. Perioperative risk may also be affected by the surgeon's experience.

MANAGEMENT AND PREVENTION

The two main goals of intraoperative management are protecting the brain and protecting the heart, but these two goals are often in conflict. For example, increasing blood pressure to augment cerebral blood flow can increase afterload or myocardial contractility, thereby increasing the oxygen demand of the heart. Also, although hypothermia may provide effective cerebral protection, it poses a severe challenge to cardiac homeostasis if the patient is awake and shivering. Thus, the anesthetic plan involves trade-offs if both organs are to be protected.

Cerebral Protection

Several strategies have been proposed to protect the brain during carotid endarterectomy. A stable high-normal blood pressure is maintained throughout surgery on the assumption that because blood vessels in ischemic or hypoperfused areas of the brain have lost their normal autoregulation, flow is directly proportional to pressure.

Manipulation of arterial carbon dioxide tension ($PaCO_2$) also affects cerebral blood flow. Although permissive hypercapnia dilates cerebral vessels in nonischemic areas of the brain, it may be detrimental if blood flow is diverted from already maximally dilated cerebral arteries perfusing ischemic areas. Conversely, hypocapnia may constrict vessels in adequately perfused, nonischemic areas of the brain to reroute blood to ischemic areas, thereby causing inverse steal. Because neither of these responses is predictable, most experts recommend normocarbia.

Hyperglycemia may worsen ischemic brain injury. Elevated blood sugar is associated with elevated glucose levels in the brain and cerebral lactic acidosis from anaerobic glycolysis. Many candidates for carotid endarterectomy are diabetic, and the administration of dextrose-containing intravenous solutions may adversely affect cerebral injury. Although the exact mechanism of hyperglycemia's adverse effect on ischemic brain injury is unknown, maintaining normoglycemia may be protective. However, isovolemic hemodilution with dextran or hetastarch may be beneficial in cases of cerebral ischemia. Blood viscosity may be reduced, with attendant microcirculatory disturbances thereby ameliorated.

Some volatile anesthetic agents (e.g., isoflurane) may offer cerebral protection by reducing cerebral metabolism and decreasing the brain's requirement for oxygen. Under these circumstances, the brain's tolerance for temporary ischemia may be enhanced. Barbiturates also offer a degree of brain protection during periods of regional ischemia by

decreasing cerebral metabolic oxygen requirements to about 50% of baseline. Maximal reductions in oxygen requirements correspond to an electrically silent or isoelectric EEG.

Hypothermia can depress neuronal activity and reduce reperfusion injury sufficiently to put cellular oxygen requirements below the minimal levels normally required for viability. In theory, hypothermia represents the most effective method of cerebral protection. Even a mild decrease in temperature by about 2°C to 3°C during cerebral arterial hypoxemia has the potential to reduce ischemic damage to the brain.

Cardiac Protection

Adequate preoperative preparation and intraoperative monitoring to protect the myocardium can prevent perioperative myocardial infarction. Maintaining the patient's hemodynamic stability begins before surgery. Patient reassurance during the preoperative evaluation may prevent anxiety-induced myocardial ischemia. If sedatives are necessary, a short-acting premedication facilitates early preoperative neurologic assessment. Blood pressure and heart rate values obtained from the preoperative visit or previous hospital admissions determine the acceptable hemodynamic range for the patient. Chronic antianginal, antihypertensive, and aspirin therapy is generally continued on the day of surgery. β-Blockade has been shown to be cardioprotective in vascular patients with a positive stress test. The American Heart Association and American College of Cardiology 2002 guidelines recommend β-blockers in vascular patients with evidence of stress test–induced ischemia or symptomatic angina, arrhythmias, or hypertension (class I), as well as for patients with untreated hypertension, coronary artery disease, or risk factors for coronary artery disease (class IIa). However, β-blockade may make efforts to increase blood pressure during carotid clamping more difficult, and it may be associated with exaggerated bradycardia if the carotid sinus is stimulated during surgery.

Monitoring during carotid endarterectomy includes the usual measures for general or regional anesthesia: temperature probe, blood pressure cuff, pulse oximeter, and end-tidal carbon dioxide. Often, an intra-arterial catheter is placed for beat-to-beat blood pressure monitoring for earlier detection and treatment of changes in blood pressure.

Leads II and V_4 or V_5 of the electrocardiogram should be monitored for ST-T segment changes due to the high incidence of myocardial ischemia after carotid reperfusion. In high-risk patients, monitoring with transesophageal echocardiography may be added.

Further Reading

Crawley F, Stygall J, Lunn S, et al: Comparison of microembolism detected by transcranial Doppler and neuropsychological sequelae of carotid surgery and percutaneous transluminal angioplasty. Stroke 31:1329-1334, 2000.

Endarterectomy for asymptomatic carotid artery stenosis. Executive Committee for the Asymptomatic Carotid Atherosclerosis Study. JAMA 273:1421-1428, 1995.

Jordan WD Jr, Voellinger DC, Doblar DD, et al: Microemboli detected by transcranial Doppler monitoring in patients during carotid angioplasty versus carotid endarterectomy. Cardiovasc Surg 7:33-38, 1999.

---

[1]Flow to the brain at risk for ischemia or stroke is siphoned from the ipsilateral diseased internal carotid artery by the more normal contralateral internal carotid artery to increase ischemia or stroke risk.

Munro FJ, Makin AP, Reid J: Airway problems after carotid endarterectomy. Br J Anaesth 76:156-159, 1996.

Naylor AR, Rothwell PM, Bell PR: Overview of the principal results and secondary analyses from the European and North American randomised trials of endarterectomy for symptomatic carotid stenosis. Eur J Vasc Endovasc Surg 26:115-129, 2003.

Riles TS, Imparato AM, Jacobowitz GR, et al: The cause of perioperative stroke after carotid endarterectomy. J Vasc Surg 19:206-214, 1994.

Tangkanakul C, Counsell CE, Warlow CP: Local versus general anaesthesia in carotid endarterectomy: A systematic review of the evidence. Eur J Vasc Endovasc Surg 13:491-499, 1997.

Wilke HJ II, Ellis JE, McKinsey JF: Carotid endarterectomy: Perioperative and anesthetic considerations. J Cardiothorac Vasc Anesth 10:928-949, 1996.

Zvara DA: Pro: Regional anesthesia is the best technique for carotid endarterectomy. J Cardiothorac Vasc Anesth 12:111-114, 1998.

CARDIOTHORACIC & VASCULAR SURGERY

Thoracic Aortic Aneurysm

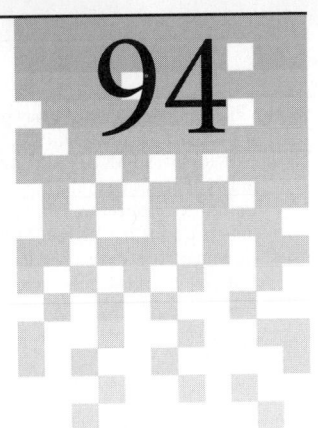

94

Annette Schure and John Ellis

Case Synopsis

A 67-year-old man underwent repair of a thoracoabdominal aortic aneurysm. The aortic occlusion time was 37 minutes, and left atriofemoral bypass was used during cross-clamping for distal perfusion. Blood pressure and heart rate were maintained within 20% of the patient's preoperative values. Urine output exceeded 0.5 mL/kg per hour in the postrepair period. On emergence from anesthesia, the patient was paraplegic.

PROBLEM ANALYSIS

Definition

Diseases of the thoracic aorta fall into four categories:

1. Aortic aneurysm: an atheromatous dilatation of the entire vessel wall
2. Aortic dissection (often incorrectly referred to as "dissecting aneurysm"): an expanding hematoma within the aortic wall, caused by either an intimal tear or degeneration of the media
3. Aortic rupture: secondary to trauma involving major shear forces
4. Coarctation: congenital stenosis of the aorta.

Exact information about type, location, and extent of the lesion is extremely important, both for surgical approach and for anesthetic management.

Aortic dissections are commonly described according to the Stanford classification (types A and B) or the DeBakey classification (types I, II, IIIA, and IIIB) (Fig. 94-1); for aortic aneurysms, the Crawford classification (types I to IV) is used (Fig. 94-2).

Both aneurysms and dissections involving the ascending aorta and the aortic arch are usually approached via a median sternotomy and require cardiopulmonary bypass, often with deep hypothermic circulatory arrest or retrograde or antegrade cerebral perfusion. The perioperative complications and anesthetic management of these aneurysms and dissections are beyond the scope of this chapter. The following discussion focuses on the management of patients with descending thoracic aneurysms.

Recognition

Patients with lesions of the descending thoracic aorta may be completely asymptomatic, and the aneurysm may be

DeBakey Classification			Stanford Classification	
Type I	Type II	Type III	Type A	Type B
		A B		

Figure 94–1 ■ DeBakey (types I, II, IIIA, and IIIB) and Stanford (types A and B) classifications of aortic dissection. (From Kouchoukos NT, Dougenis D: Surgery of the thoracic aorta. N Engl J Med 336:1876-1888, 1997.)

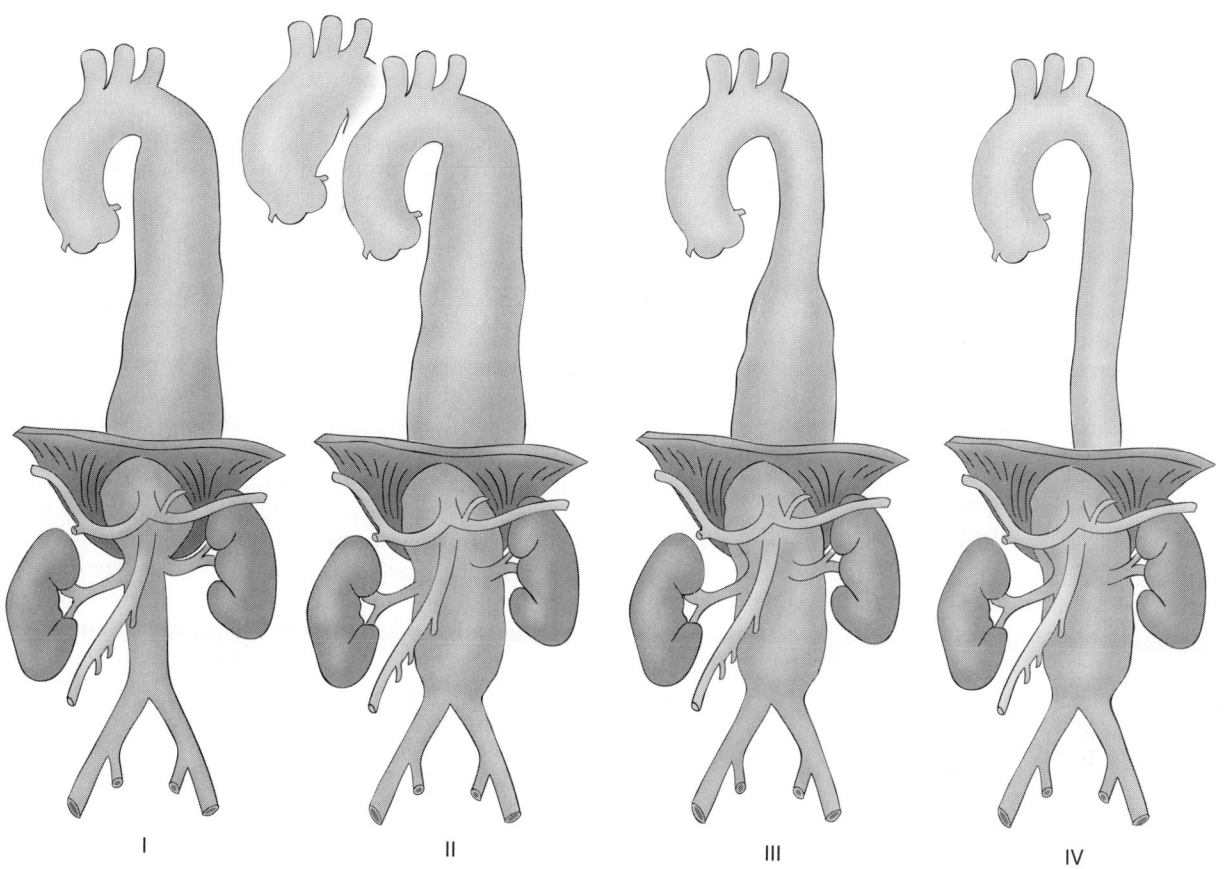

Figure 94–2 ■ Crawford classification of aortic aneurysms. (From Norris EJ, Frank SF: Anesthesia for vascular surgery. In Miller RD [ed]: Anesthesia, 5th ed. Philadelphia, Churchill Livingstone, 2000, p 1870.)

discovered incidentally on a chest radiograph or computed tomography (CT) scan. Alternatively, these aneurysms can present with a wide range of symptoms, depending on type, location, and extent of the lesion (Table 94-1).

Imaging studies include a chest radiograph (revealing the classic widened mediastinum and aortic knob), spiral CT, and magnetic resonance imaging to assess the exact location and size of the aneurysm or dissection. Transesophageal echocardiography is useful for the diagnosis of dissections, especially in unstable patients. Angiography is still considered the gold standard; however, it is invasive, is associated with a high rate of complications (e.g., hemorrhage, nephropathy), and should be reserved for selected cases. Electrocardiogram and laboratory tests provide useful but nonspecific information.

Risk Assessment

Patients with aortic disease have a high incidence of comorbidities: coronary artery disease (66%), hypertension (42%), chronic obstructive pulmonary disease (23%), peripheral

Table 94–1 ■ Presenting Clinical Signs and Symptoms of Thoracic Aortic Aneurysm and Dissection

	Aneurysm	Dissection
General presentation	Chronic or acute with leak or rupture	Dramatic onset and fulminant course
Location of pain	Chronic back pain	Acute-onset back or midscapular pain
Cardiovascular	Normal or elevated blood pressure	Elevated blood pressure due to pain; hypotension (possibly shock) if ruptured
Respiratory	Dyspnea if associated with left main-stem bronchial obstruction; hoarseness with laryngeal nerve compression; hemoptysis due to erosion	Dyspnea if associated with left main-stem bronchial obstruction; hemorrhagic pleural effusion
Gastrointestinal (GI)	Usually normal	Acute abdomen or GI bleeding
Renal	Possible renal insufficiency with aortic occlusive disease	Renal insufficiency with involvement of renal arteries
Neurologic	Commonly no associated neurologic symptoms or signs	Paraplegia if blood supply to spinal cord is impaired

Modified from Skeehan TM, Cooper R Jr: Anesthetic management for thoracic aneurysms and dissections. In Hensley FA, Martin DE, Gravlee GP (eds): A Practical Approach to Cardiac Anesthesia, 3rd ed. Philadelphia, Lippincott Williams & Wilkins, 2003, pp 624-625.

vascular disease (22%), cerebrovascular disease (14%), diabetes mellitus (8%), and chronic renal disease (3%). The preoperative evaluation should assess the extent, severity, and therapy for any of these comorbidities. Further assessment should focus on the following:

- Risk of aspiration (i.e., recent oral intake)
- Airway evaluation and evidence of tracheal or left mainstem compression on chest radiograph or CT
- Cardiac evaluation (left ventricular function, regional wall motion abnormalities)
- Vascular access
- Preexisting renal insufficiency (diabetic nephropathy, contrast dye load)
- Preexisting neurologic impairment (possibly associated with dissection or diabetes)

A wide variety of severe perioperative complications can be associated with the surgical repair:

- Difficult airway management
- Acute heart failure, myocardial infarction or disadvantageous tachy- or bradyarrhythmias
- Pulmonary hemorrhage and postoperative respiratory failure
- Hemorrhage and coagulopathy
- Hepatic and intestinal ischemia
- Renal failure
- Paraplegia

Implications

SURGICAL APPROACH

The thoracic aorta is usually approached via a left-sided thoracotomy, with the patient in the right lateral decubitus position. Single-lung ventilation and, depending on the surgeon's preference and experience, either a simple cross-clamping technique ("clamp and sew") or various forms of distal circulatory support are used. These include heparin-bonded shunts (Gott shunts, 7 or 9 mm) that connect the proximal aorta with the femoral artery and provide adequate proximal decompression and maintenance of distal perfusion. Unfortunately, they can be difficult to place and tend to kink. Extracorporeal circulation via an atriofemoral or axillofemoral bypass (partial bypass without oxygenator) and full femorofemoral bypass are alternatives, but they require some degree of heparinization, with the associated risk of increased bleeding.

AIRWAY MANAGEMENT

Single-lung ventilation is critical for optimal surgical exposure and prevention of tissue trauma. Preoperative evaluation of the chest radiograph, CT scan, or magnetic resonance image is important, because large thoracic aneurysms can distort or compress the left main-stem bronchus, impairing proper positioning of a left-sided double-lumen tube. If in doubt, the double-lumen tube should be advanced only after fiberoptic examination of the left main bronchus. Right-sided double-lumen tubes, in contrast, easily dislodge and tend to obstruct the right upper lobe. Appropriate alternatives,

especially in the case of difficult airways, are Univent tubes and Arndt endobronchial blockers. Additionally, extensive postoperative airway edema and facial swelling can complicate extubation or the change of a double-lumen tube to a single-lumen tube, even with a tube exchanger. Sometimes, it is safer to refrain from any such attempt, pull the double-lumen tube tip back into the trachea, and reassess the patient in 24 to 36 hours.

HEMODYNAMIC CHANGES WITH CLAMPING AND UNCLAMPING

Cross-clamping of the thoracic aorta is often associated with severe hemodynamic and neuroendocrine responses. In contrast to infrarenal clamping, exclusion of the splanchnic circulation significantly reduces the available venous capacitance vasculature, so the sudden increase in impedance to aortic outflow, as well as the proximal shift of blood volume, results in drastic increases in afterload and preload, with the potential for cardiac decompensation or cerebral hemorrhage. Injudicious use of vasodilators (nitroprusside, nitroglycerine, milrinone, inhalational agents) can interfere with hypoxic pulmonary vasoconstriction, which is essential for adequate gas exchange; it can also decrease distal blood flow via the collateral circulation. The goal is careful titration of vasodilators to balance "permissive hypertension" for the maintenance of distal perfusion against the risk of cardiac decompensation. Finally, unclamping of the thoracic aorta can result in severe hypotension. Causes include reactive hyperemia, acidosis, hypercarbia, release of humoral factors such as cytokines and thromboxane, cardiac depression, and blood loss from the anastomosis.

HEMORRHAGE

Patients undergoing thoracic aneurysm or dissection repair are at increased risk for intra- and postoperative bleeding. Along with renal and cardiac dysfunction, intraoperative blood loss correlates directly with perioperative mortality. In addition to bleeding from the aorta, intrapulmonary hemorrhage may occur due to adhesions and lung manipulations. Heparin use and hypothermia and coagulopathy associated with massive transfusions and liver ischemia are other contributing factors. Liver and bowel ischemia can lead to severe hypocalcemia and endotoxin-induced disseminated intravascular coagulation.

RENAL PROTECTION

The incidence of perioperative acute renal failure ranges from 3% to 14%. Aortic cross-clamping decreases renal blood flow from 80% to 90%, resulting in an ischemic insult. The risk is higher in older patients with coronary artery disease, diabetes, or preexisting renal dysfunction. Acute renal failure is a major predictor of increased morbidity and mortality.

Intraoperative urine output is not predictive of postoperative renal function. Acute renal failure may occur despite apparently adequate perfusion (using distal circulatory support) or infrarenal clamping. Various methods of renal protection have been tried, including mannitol, furosemide, fenoldopam, dopexamine, and cold perfusion, all without good scientific evidence. It seems that maintenance of intravascular volume and myocardial function are the most important determinants.

SPINAL CORD PROTECTION

Paraplegia occurs in about 1% to 11% of surgeries involving the thoracic aorta and is probably the most devastating complication. It usually presents as an anterior spinal artery syndrome with loss of motor function (anterior horn) and partially intact sensation (posterior columns), either immediately on emergence or within the first 24 hours. Interruption of spinal cord blood flow or prolonged hypoperfusion (>30 minutes) results in spinal cord ischemia. The blood supply for the spinal cord is provided by a single anterior spinal artery (75%) and two posterior spinal arteries (25%). In the upper cervical area, the anterior spinal artery is formed by branches of the vertebral arteries, with multiple collaterals from deep cervical and costovertebral arteries. In the middle portion, only a few intercostal arteries provide additional blood supply; the lower part of the spinal cord is almost entirely supplied by one intercostal artery branch (artery of Adamkiewicz). This artery is quite variable in origin, arising somewhere between T5 and T8 in 15%, T9 and T12 in 75%, and L1 and L2 in 10% of patients (Fig. 94-3). In addition to an unpredictable blood supply for vulnerable areas, increased cerebrospinal fluid (CSF) pressure can contribute to spinal cord ischemia. Spinal cord perfusion pressure is the mean arterial pressure minus CSF pressure. During aortic cross-clamping, hypertension and increased preload lead to increased intracranial pressure, followed by redistribution of CSF toward the spine and increased CSF pressure. Spinal cord edema after prolonged clamping or with reperfusion can further decrease spinal cord perfusion and contribute to neurologic dysfunction.

Somatosensory evoked potentials (SEPs) and motor evoked potentials (MEPs) are used to monitor spinal cord ischemia. However, SEPs monitor only posterior column function, not the more vulnerable anterior part of the spinal cord, which likely explains the number of case reports of patients with paraplegia despite normal SEPs during clamping. MEPs appear to be more promising in this respect. Also, there can be a substantial delay between the onset of ischemia

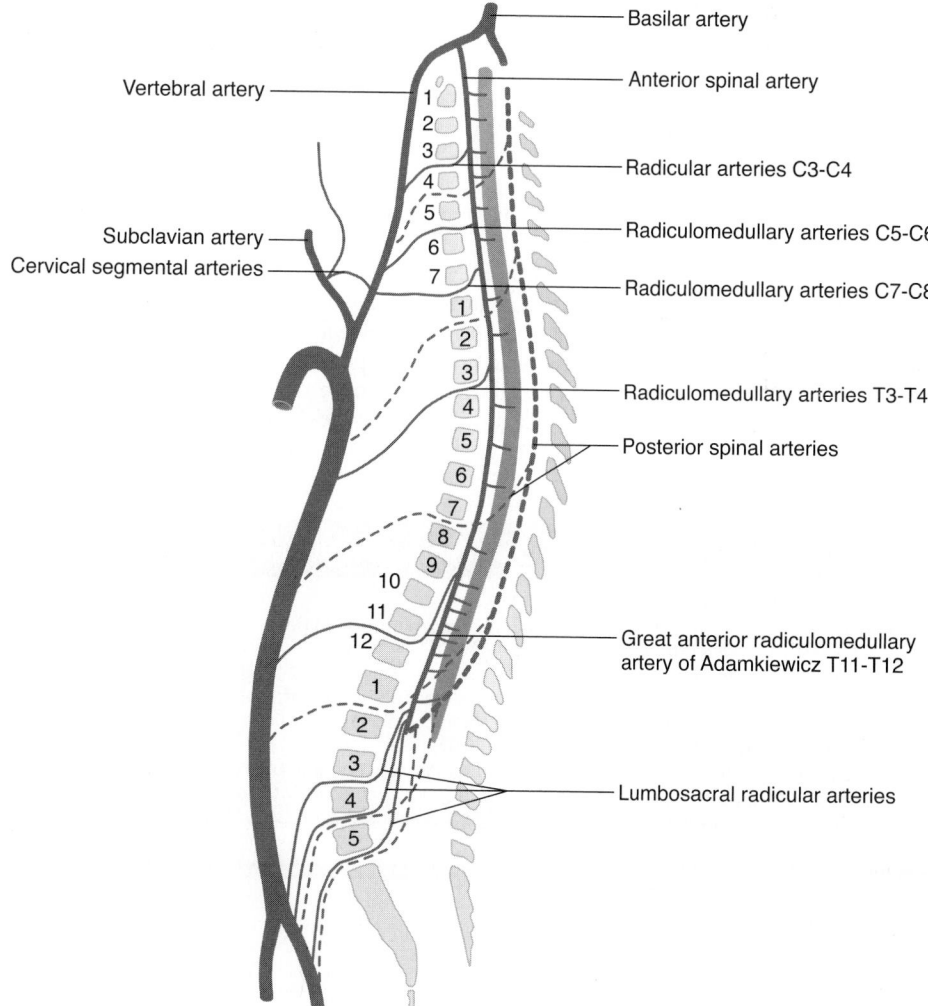

Figure 94-3 Blood supply of the spinal cord. (From Marijic J, El-Magharbel I, Weiss L, Mahajan A: Anesthesia for patients with thoracic aortic disease. In Leung J [ed]: Cardiac and Vascular Anesthesia: The Requisites in Anesthesiology. Philadelphia, Mosby, 2004, p 180.)

Basilar artery
Anterior spinal artery
Vertebral artery
Radicular arteries C3-C4
Radiculomedullary arteries C5-C6
Subclavian artery
Cervical segmental arteries
Radiculomedullary arteries C7-C8
Radiculomedullary arteries T3-T4
Posterior spinal arteries
Great anterior radiculomedullary artery of Adamkiewicz T11-T12
Lumbosacral radicular arteries

and the appearance of SEP changes. Finally, SEP and MEP monitoring in the operating room is technically cumbersome and influenced by many factors, including anesthetic agents, hypercarbia, temperature, and electrical interference.

MANAGEMENT

Monitoring and Intravascular Access

Blood pressure should be monitored proximal and distal to the aortic cross-clamp, usually via a right radial artery line (because blood flow to the left subclavian artery might be compromised by the cross-clamp) and a right femoral line. A pulmonary artery catheter and transesophageal echocardiography are useful monitors to assess ventricular function and volume status during clamping and unclamping. In preparation for massive blood loss, one or two 9 French introducers, possibly a dialysis-type catheter in a femoral vein, and one or two large-bore peripheral intravenous lines are advised. Blood warmer and rapid infusion devices should be set up and ready, and an adequate number of blood products should be typed and crossmatched. Also, one or two lumbar CSF drains can be placed and monitored for CSF pressure.

Clamping and Unclamping

Anesthetic management depends on the surgical technique and the use of distal circulatory support or electrophysiologic monitoring. An important goal is the prevention of hemodynamic instability (hypertension or hypotension) and myocardial ischemia. Usually, "balanced anesthesia" is used: a combination of potent opioids, benzodiazepines, and low-dose inhalational agents, with or without muscle relaxants. Inotropes or vasodilators are used as required. Some centers advocate the use of combined general-epidural or general-spinal anesthesia, despite the risk of hematoma and medicolegal concerns. In preparation for simple aortic cross-clamping (without bypass), the patient should be allowed to become slightly hypovolemic (pulmonary capillary wedge pressure

5 to 15 mm Hg). Mannitol is often given as a free radical scavenger for renal and spinal cord protection. During clamping, as discussed earlier, vasodilators and inhalational agents should be carefully titrated to balance distal perfusion via permissive hypertension with cardiac function. Before aortic cross-clamp removal, vasodilators and anesthetics are reduced, preload is optimized, and blood products, bicarbonate, and calcium are prepared. A temporary low-dose norepinephrine drip, epinephrine, and occasionally sequential release of the clamp by the surgeon are other useful measures of providing hemodynamic support after aortic cross-clamp release.

Adverse hemodynamic changes are usually much less of a concern when extracorporeal circulation systems are used. Flow rates and volume status can be adjusted according to pre- and postclamp pressures, trying to achieve distal aortic pressures greater than 50 to 60 mm Hg.

PREVENTION

Many techniques and methods have been described to reduce the risk of spinal cord ischemia (Table 94-2). Unfortunately, the scientific evidence supporting these modalities is inadequate or controversial.

Some recent studies support the use of CSF drainage, but only as a component of a multimodal approach to spinal cord protection. Others suggest preoperative identification and selective or serial reimplantation of critical intercostal arteries under SEP or MEP guidance.

At present, a combined strategy involving short cross-clamp time, some form of distal circulatory support, CSF drainage, adjunctive pharmacotherapy, hypothermia, and avoidance of hyperglycemia is recommended.

Finally, the current trend toward endovascular repair has provided a new perspective. So far, the results are promising, but paraplegia can still occur. Further experience and larger case series are necessary before a final recommendation can be made. For the time being, this minimally invasive technique presents anesthesiologists with new challenges.

Table 94–2 ■ **Methods of Spinal Cord Protection during Descending Thoracic Aortic Surgery**

Limitation of cross-clamp duration (<30 min)
Distal circulatory support: shunt, atriofemoral or femorofemoral bypass
Reattachment of critical intercostal arteries
Cerebrospinal fluid drainage
Moderate systemic hypothermia (32°C-34°C), epidural cooling, or circulatory arrest
Maintenance of proximal blood pressure to improve collateral blood flow
Neuroprotective pharmacotherapy
    Systemic: corticosteroids, barbiturates, naloxone, calcium channel blockers, free radical scavengers, NMDA receptor antagonists,
        mannitol, magnesium, vasodilators (adenosine, papaverine, prostacyclin), perfluorocarbons, colchicine
    Intrathecal: papaverine, magnesium, tetracaine, perfluorocarbons
Avoidance of postoperative hypotension
Sequential aortic clamping
Neurologic monitoring for spinal cord ischemia
    Somatosensory evoked potentials
    Motor evoked potentials
Avoidance of hyperglycemia

From Ellis JE, Roizen MF, Mantha S, et al: Anesthesia for vascular surgery. In Barash PG, Cullen BF, Stoelting RK (eds): Clinical Anesthesia, 4th ed. Philadelphia, JB Lippincott–Williams & Wilkins, 2001, p 952.

Further Reading

Coselli JS, LeMaire SA, Köksey C, et al: Cerebrospinal fluid drainage reduces paraplegia after thoracoabdominal aortic aneurysm repair: Results of a randomized clinical trial. J Vasc Surg 35:631-639, 2002.

Ellis JE, Roizen MF, Mantha S, et al: Anesthesia for vascular surgery. In Barash PG, Cullen BF, Stoelting RK (eds): Clinical Anesthesia, 4th ed. Philadelphia, JB Lippincott–Williams & Wilkins, 2001, pp 929-967.

Gelman S: The pathophysiology of aortic cross-clamping. Anesthesiology 82:1026-1060, 1995.

Greenberg R, Resch T, Nyman U, et al: Endovascular repair of descending thoracic aortic aneurysms: An early experience with intermediate-term follow up. J Vasc Surg 31:147, 2000.

Khan RA, Moskowitz DM, Marin M, Hollier L: Anesthetic considerations for endovascular aortic repair. Mt Sinai J Med 69:57-67, 2002.

Khan SN, Stansby G: Cerebrospinal fluid drainage for thoracic and thoraco-abdominal aortic aneurysm surgery. Cochrane Library, vol 2, 2004.

Ling E, Arellano R: Systematic overview of the evidence supporting the use of cerebrospinal fluid drainage in thoracoabdominal aneurysm surgery for prevention of paraplegia. Anesthesiology 93:1115-1122, 2000.

Lippman M, Lingham K, Rubin S, et al: Anesthesia for endovascular repair of abdominal and thoracic aortic aneurysms: A review article. J Cardiovasc Surg 44:443-451, 2003.

Marijic J, El-Magharbel I, Weiss L, Mahajan A: Anesthesia for patients with thoracic aortic disease. In Leung J (ed): Cardiac and Vascular Anesthesia: The Requisites in Anesthesiology. Philadelphia, Mosby, 2004, pp 169-185.

O'Connor CJ, Rothenberg DM: Anesthetic considerations for descending thoracic aortic surgery: Part I. J Cardiothorac Vasc Anesth 9:581-588, 1995.

O'Connor CJ, Rothenberg DM: Anesthetic considerations for descending thoracic aortic surgery: Part II. J Cardiothorac Vasc Anesth 9:734-747, 1995.

Oliver WC Jr, Nuttall G, Murray MJ: Thoracic aortic disease. In Kaplan JA (ed): Cardiac Anesthesia, 4th ed. Philadelphia, WB Saunders, 1999, pp 821-859.

Skeehan TM, Cooper R Jr: Anesthetic management for thoracic aneurysms and dissections. In Hensley FA, Martin DE, Gravlee GP (eds): A Practical Approach to Cardiac Anesthesia, 3rd ed. Philadelphia, JB Lippincott–Williams & Wilkins, 2003, pp 617-647.

Svensson LG, Patel V, Robinson MF, et al: Influence of preservation or perfusion of intraoperatively identified spinal cord blood supply on spinal motor evoked potentials and paraplegia after aortic surgery. J Vasc Surg 13:355-365, 1991.

CARDIOTHORACIC &
VASCULAR SURGERY

Abdominal Aortic Aneurysm Repair

95

Christopher J. O'Connor

Case Synopsis

A 74-year-old man with chronic stable angina, hypertension, and a previous myocardial infarction undergoes repair of an infrarenal abdominal aortic aneurysm (AAA) with the use of combined epidural and general anesthesia. Preoperative dipyridamole thallium testing revealed a large, fixed myocardial defect with no evidence of reversible disease. Transient hypotension during aneurysm exposure responds promptly to phenylephrine. After placement of the aortic cross-clamp, there is 1-mm ST segment depression and an increase in the pulmonary capillary wedge pressure. Both resolve with intravenous nitroglycerin therapy. However, moderate hypotension occurs after release of the aortic cross-clamp. Aggressive fluid and cell-saver blood replacement and the administration of phenylephrine restore blood pressure to normal. The patient is successfully extubated at the completion of the procedure and transported to the intensive care unit with an epidural infusion of bupivacaine-fentanyl for perioperative analgesia.

PROBLEM ANALYSIS

Definition

Hypotension is relatively common during infrarenal AAA repair, although it is usually transient and well tolerated. The cause is multifactorial, and treatment depends on the specific cause. Myocardial ischemia, although less frequent, is often encountered in patients with known or previously undiagnosed coronary artery disease (CAD) and may be accompanied by increased pulmonary capillary wedge pressure, reduced cardiac output (Fig. 95-1), and transesophageal echocardiogram (TEE) evidence of regional wall motion abnormalities.

In addition to hypotension and myocardial ischemia, other important intraoperative complications include hypertension and left ventricular (LV) dysfunction after aortic occlusion; hypothermia; hypoxemia due to abdominal retraction and underlying obstructive pulmonary disease; severe hemorrhage; and coagulopathy as a result of dilutional changes, hypocalcemia, and acidosis. Mild hypertension is typically encountered after placement of the aortic cross-clamp, although the magnitude of the blood pressure rise is substantially less than that with occlusion at the level of the thoracic aorta. Hypertension during aortic clamping may be absent, however, if blood and third-space fluid losses have not been adequately replaced. Table 95-1 compares the hemodynamic changes with supraceliac and suprarenal versus infrarenal aortic occlusion.

Recognition

Recognition of these hemodynamic events is facilitated by the use of direct arterial and central venous pressure monitoring. A pulmonary artery catheter and TEE are monitors for the assessment of preload and LV function and are also used to detect myocardial ischemia. Pulmonary artery catheter and TEE are likely indicated in patients with severe CAD or LV dysfunction. Hypovolemia is diagnosed on the basis of a significant decline in pulmonary capillary wedge pressure, pulmonary artery end-diastolic pressure, or central venous pressure and diminished LV end-diastolic area on TEE. Myocardial ischemia typically manifests as ST segment changes and new regional wall motion abnormalities on TEE. Alterations in pulmonary artery pressure, which also may be observed, are less sensitive indicators of myocardial ischemia.

The cause of intraoperative hypotension depends, in part, on the stage of the procedure in relation to the application of

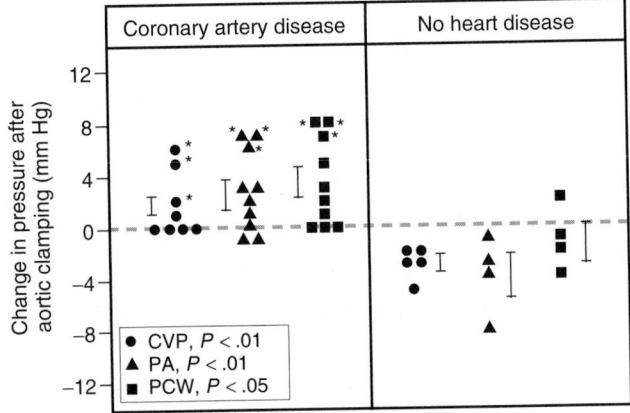

Figure 95–1 ■ Comparison of changes in central venous pressure (CVP), pulmonary artery (PA) pressure, and pulmonary capillary wedge (PCW) pressure in patients with and without coronary artery disease (CAD). Values with asterisks refer to patients developing myocardial ischemia during infrarenal aortic occlusion. Significance values refer to the comparison between patients with and without heart disease. (From Attia RR, Murphy JD, Snider M, et al: Myocardial ischemia due to infrarenal aortic cross-clamping during aortic surgery in patients with severe coronary artery disease. Circulation 53:961-965, 1976.)

Table 95–1 ■ Percentage Change in Cardiovascular Variables on Initiation of Aortic Occlusion during Supraceliac versus Infrarenal Aortic Aneurysm Surgery			
	Level of Aortic Occlusion		
Variable	*Supraceliac*	*Suprarenal-Infraceliac*	*Infrarenal*
Mean arterial blood pressure	+54	+5*	+2*
Pulmonary capillary wedge pressure	+38	+10*	0*
End-diastolic area	+28	+2*	+9*
End-systolic area	+69	+10*	+11*
Ejection fraction	−38	−10*	−8*
Patients with wall motion abnormalities	+92	+33	0
New myocardial infarction	+8	0	0

*Statistically different (*P* <.05) from group undergoing supraceliac aortic occlusion.
From Roizen MF, Beaupre PN, Alpert RA, et al: Monitoring with two-dimensional transesophageal echocardiography: Comparison of myocardial function in patients undergoing supraceliac, suprarenal-infraceliac, or infrarenal aortic occlusion. J Vasc Surg 1:300-305, 1984.

the aortic cross-clamp. Hypotension before placement of the cross-clamp may be secondary to prostacyclin release from bowel eventration and mesenteric traction, causing profound vasodilatation, tachycardia, and facial flushing–the so-called mesenteric traction syndrome. Although this is a transient event, it usually requires treatment with a vasopressor such as phenylephrine. Further, the concomitant use of regional anesthesia may contribute to arterial hypotension by means of reduced vascular resistance and venous return (preload).

Hypotension during the period of aortic occlusion is typically due to hypovolemia from ongoing blood loss, evaporative fluid loss from exposure of the abdominal cavity and its contents, and third-space loss. These operative fluid losses, when superimposed on the potential effects of preoperative diuretics, contrast dye administration, and bowel

preparation, may substantially reduce preload, cardiac output, and blood pressure. Also, if myocardial ischemia develops, LV dysfunction may further diminish cardiac output, thereby augmenting the effects of hypovolemia and vasodilatation. It is critical to recognize that hypotension during this stage of the procedure suggests profound hypovolemia, because aortic occlusion usually results in mild hypertension. A thorough assessment of cardiac filling pressures, surgical blood loss, and current fluid replacement is indicated in this situation.

Hypotension after release of the aortic cross-clamp is a common and expected event. It is attributed to a decrease in vascular resistance and central hypovolemia. Ischemic vasodilatation develops in the lower extremities during the period of occlusion. With reperfusion of these vascular beds, ischemic metabolites and humoral factors released into the systemic circulation cause a fall in systemic vascular resistance. In addition, pooling of blood in these dilated venous and arterial vessels contributes to reduced venous return. The degree of hypotension encountered depends on the level and duration of occlusion, speed of clamp removal, intravascular volume status before aortic clamp release, and persistent effects of anesthetics and pharmacologic vasodilators. Severe hypotension can be largely avoided with appropriate fluid loading and replacement of blood losses before unclamping the aorta, as well as gradual release of the occlusion. The pathophysiology of hypotension resulting from cross-clamp release is depicted in Figure 95-2.

Risk Assessment

Patients with underlying CAD are at the highest risk for myocardial ischemia and ventricular dysfunction during abdominal aortic surgery. Up to two thirds of patients with AAAs have angiographic evidence of significant CAD, and 30% of these will sustain a perioperative cardiac complication, such as myocardial infarction with or without associated heart failure. Although there is ongoing controversy regarding the appropriate preoperative cardiac evaluation of vascular surgical patients, a careful clinical and functional assessment is essential, along with noninvasive tests of

Figure 95–2 ■ Cause of hypotension after aortic unclamping.

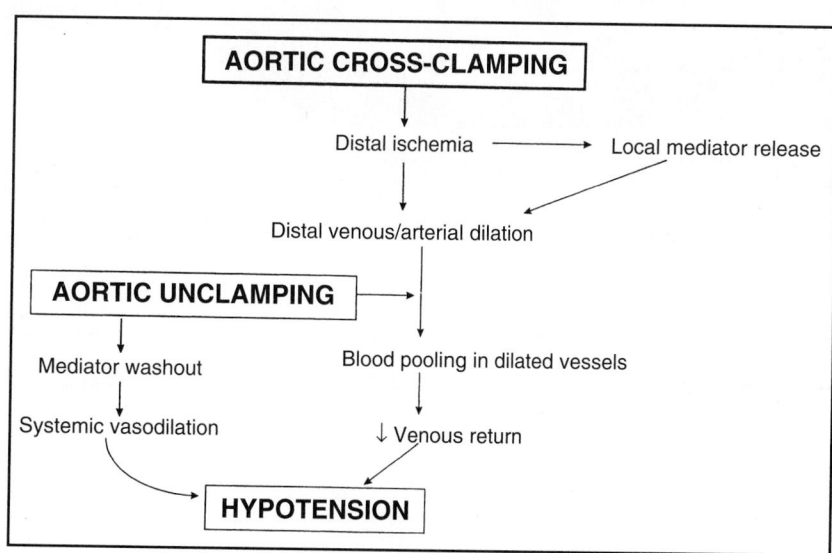

coronary vascular reserve, when appropriate. Individuals with LV dysfunction may be more susceptible to intraoperative hemodynamic instability. In addition, blood pressure changes are less pronounced in patients with aorto-occlusive disease compared with those undergoing simple aneurysm repair. Chronic occlusive disease results in the formation of extensive periaortic collateral vessels that continue to perfuse the lower extremities during the period of aortic occlusion; thus, changes in vascular resistance with both aortic clamping and release are considerably attenuated.

In addition to these preoperative factors, the degree of preexisting volume depletion and the rate of intraoperative blood loss determine the response to aortic cross-clamping and release. Although blood loss typically ranges from 800 to 1500 mL, hemorrhage may be severe enough to require fresh frozen plasma or platelet transfusions if a dilutional coagulopathy develops.

Implications

Hypotension and myocardial ischemia are poorly tolerated in patients with CAD. Mortality rates for elective AAA repair are 2% to 7%. The majority of deaths are due to myocardial infarction and other fatal cardiac events (e.g., acute heart failure, ventricular tachyarrhythmias). Mortality rates may be as much as fivefold higher in patients with clinically evident CAD. In addition, owing to coexisting renal disease, sustained and prolonged intraoperative hypotension and renal artery embolization may contribute to postoperative renal failure. The incidence rates of postoperative complications and a comparison of the causes of early mortality after elective and ruptured AAA repair are given in Tables 95-2 and 95-3, respectively.

Endovascular stent-graft repair has become an important alternative to the open treatment of AAA, and it is associated with less morbidity. Even though endovascular repair is typically recommended for high-risk patients, it is still associated with lower complication rates. These devices are typically placed in the operating room by a team of vascular surgeons and interventional radiologists. Anesthesia is easily provided with either spinal or combined spinal-epidural anesthesia, although some institutions prefer general anesthesia. Comparisons of open versus endovascular repair have demonstrated reduced 30-day mortality rates, bleeding, duration of time in the intensive care unit, and incidence of cardiac and pulmonary complications in patients treated with endovascular devices (Table 95-4). The long-term durability and rupture-free periods following placement of these devices are not yet well established, and large-scale, prospective, randomized comparisons of these two approaches are still under way.

MANAGEMENT

When hypotension develops, aggressive evaluation of the intravascular volume and degree of blood loss is the first diagnostic maneuver, because hypovolemia is the most

Table 95-3 ■ Causes of Early Mortality after Elective and Ruptured Abdominal Aortic Aneurysm Repair

Cause	Mortality Rate (%)	
	Elective	Ruptured
Cardiac	58	20
Pulmonary	6	3
Renal	4	9
Colon infarction	1	9
Hemorrhage	0	18
Multisystem organ failure	1	35
Other	24	6

From Cronenwett JL, Sampson LN: Aneurysms of the abdominal aorta and iliac arteries. In Dean RH, Yao JS, Brewster D (eds): Diagnosis and Treatment in Vascular Surgery. Norwalk, Conn., Appleton & Lange, 1995, pp 230-233.

Table 95-2 ■ Incidence of Immediate Postoperative Complications after Elective Abdominal Aortic Aneurysm Repair

Complication	Incidence (%)
Cardiac	15
Myocardial infarction	2-8
Pulmonary	8-12
Pneumonia	5
Renal insufficiency	5-12
Renal failure requiring dialysis	1-6
Hemorrhage	2-5
Lower extremity ischemia	1-4
Ischemic colitis	1
Stroke	1
Ureteral injury	<1

From Cronenwett JL, Sampson LN: Aneurysms of the abdominal aorta and iliac arteries. In Dean RH, Yao JS, Brewster D (eds): Diagnosis and Treatment in Vascular Surgery. Norwalk, Conn., Appleton & Lange, 1995, pp 230-233.

Table 95-4 ■ Perioperative Complications: Open versus Endovascular Repair of Abdominal Aortic Aneurysms

Complication	Open Repair	Endovascular Repair
30-day mortality (%)	1-4	0-3*
Cardiac complications (%)	4-22	3-11*
Pulmonary complications (%)	13-16	3-4*
Neurologic complications (%)	3	1*
Renal complications (%)	4-8	4.3-5†
ICU stay (days)	2	0.5-1*
Transfusion (% transfused)	51	26*
Blood loss (mL)	1200	450*
Graft-related complications	3.8	13.8*

*P <.05; endovascular versus open repair.
†Not significant; endovascular versus open repair.
ICU, intensive care unit.
From Miraude A, Bosch JL, Halpern EF, et al: Elective endovascular versus open surgical repair of abdominal aortic aneurysms: Systematic review of short-term results. Radiology 224:739-747, 2002; Elkouri S, Gloviezki P, McKusick MA, et al: Perioperative complications and early outcome after endovascular and open surgical repair of abdominal aortic aneurysms. J Vasc Surg 39:497-505, 2004.

likely cause. Evidence of myocardial ischemia should be assessed with ST segment analysis, TEE, or both. It is treated by providing adequate coronary perfusion pressure, possibly intravenous nitroglycerin, and β-blockers when there is associated tachycardia. Maintenance of β-blockade throughout the perioperative period is *essential* for patients at risk for postoperative cardiac morbidity due to CAD.

Management of hypotension depends on its relation to aortic occlusion:

- Hypotension before aortic occlusion: Consider the effects of epidural anesthesia, mesenteric traction, or preoperative hypovolemia.
- Hypotension during occlusion: Consider severe hypovolemia. Aggressive volume resuscitation with blood and crystalloid solutions is indicated before release of the aortic cross-clamp, to increase central venous pressure or pulmonary capillary wedge pressure by 10% to 20% above baseline levels.
- Hypotension after release of the aortic cross-clamp: Administration of all anesthetic agents and vasodilators should be temporarily discontinued. Vasopressors such as dopamine or phenylephrine should be available to counteract the accompanying vasodilatation and preload reduction. Blood must be available in case hemorrhage is severe, and cell-saver systems for intraoperative blood salvage are strongly recommended.

PREVENTION

Prevention of intraoperative hypotension requires an understanding and anticipation of the specific surgical events that precipitate vasodilatation and blood loss. A fastidious approach to monitoring cardiac filling pressures, along with frequent assessment of ongoing blood and fluid losses, is essential to maintaining a stable blood pressure. Discontinuation of anesthetics and vasodilators, along with appropriate volume loading before the release of aortic occlusion, attenuates accompanying vasodilatation. The incidence of myocardial ischemia may be reduced by recognizing and controlling the determinants of myocardial oxygen supply and demand in high-risk patients. Prophylactic intravenous nitroglycerin is not consistently effective for preventing myocardial ischemia or myocardial infarction in high-risk patients. Although it may be reasonable therapy in patients receiving preoperative nitrates, careful monitoring of preload is essential to avoid possibly deleterious reduced coronary

perfusion pressure. Finally, substantial data suggest that prophylactic perioperative oral β-blockers and α_2-agonists can reduce the incidence of postoperative cardiac events in patients undergoing major noncardiac surgery.

Further Reading

ACC/AHA guidelines for perioperative cardiovascular evaluation for noncardiac surgery. Circulation 93:1280-1317, 1996.

Attia RR, Murphy JD, Snider M: Myocardial ischemia due to infrarenal aortic cross-clamping during aortic surgery in patients with severe coronary artery disease. Circulation 53:961-965, 1976.

Cronenwett JL, Sampson LN: Aneurysms of the abdominal aorta and iliac arteries. In Dean RH, Yao JS, Brewster D (eds): Diagnosis and Treatment in Vascular Surgery. Norwalk, Conn., Appleton & Lange, 1995, pp 230-233.

Elkouri S, Gloviezki P, McKusick MA, et al: Perioperative complications and early outcome after endovascular and open surgical repair of abdominal aortic aneurysms. J Vasc Surg 39:497-505, 2004.

Ellis JE, Roizen M, Mantha S, et al: Anesthesia for vascular surgery. In Barash PG, et al (eds): Clinical Anesthesia. Philadelphia, Lippincott-Raven, 1997, pp 871-910.

Gelman S: The pathophysiology of aortic cross-clamping and unclamping. Anesthesiology 82:1026-1060, 1995.

Gewertz BL, Kremser PC, Zarins CK, et al: Transesophageal echocardiographic monitoring of myocardial ischemia during vascular surgery. J Vasc Surg 5:607-613, 1987.

Johnston WE, Balestrieri FJ, Plonk G, et al: The influence of periaortic collateral vessels on the intraoperative hemodynamic effects of acute aortic occlusion in patients with aorto-occlusive disease or abdominal aortic aneurysm. Anesthesiology 66:386-389, 1987.

Mangano DT, Layug E, Wallace A, et al: Effect of atenolol on mortality and cardiovascular morbidity after noncardiac surgery. Multicenter Study of Perioperative Ischemia Research Group. N Engl J Med 335:1713-1720, 1996.

Miraude A, Bosch JL, Halpern EF, et al: Elective endovascular versus open surgical repair of abdominal aortic aneurysms: Systematic review of short-term results. Radiology 224:739-747, 2002.

Pevec WC: Morbidity associated with vascular surgery. In Callow A, Ernst C (eds): Vascular Surgery. Stamford, Conn., Appleton & Lange, 1995, pp 1373-1395.

Poldermans D, Boersma E, Bax JJ, et al: The effect of bisoprolol on perioperative morbidity and myocardial infarction in high-risk patients undergoing vascular surgery. Dutch Echocardiographic Cardiac Risk Evaluation Applying Stress Echocardiography Study Group. N Engl J Med 341:1789-1794, 1999.

Roizen MF, Beaupre PN, Alpert RA, et al: Monitoring two-dimensional transesophageal echocardiography: Comparison of myocardial function in patients undergoing supraceliac, suprarenal-infraceliac, or infrarenal aortic occlusion. J Vasc Surg 1:300-305, 1984.

Wallace A, Galindez D, Salahieh A, et al: Effect of clonidine on cardiovascular morbidity and mortality after noncardiac surgery. Anesthesiology 101:284-293, 2004.

Wallace A, Layug E, Tateo I, et al: Prophylactic atenolol reduces postoperative myocardial ischemia. McSPI Research Group. Anesthesiology 88:7-17, 1998.

Peripheral Vascular Surgery

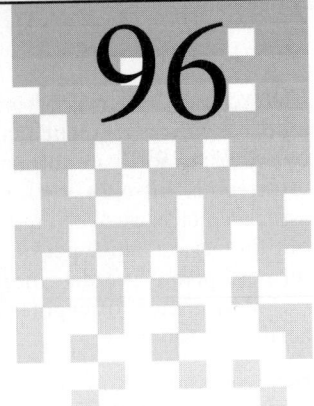

96

Ronak Desai

Case Synopsis

A 74-year-old woman with insulin-dependent diabetes, hypertension, and a long-standing history of smoking requires a redo right lower limb revascularization on a semiurgent basis. There is a possibility of using upper extremity vessels as graft material. A general orotracheal anesthetic is planned. An hour after uneventful surgery, while the patient is in the recovery unit, the surgeon recognizes impending graft thrombosis after the loss of Doppler signals. The graft must be re-explored in the operating room. The surgeon also mentions the possible intraoperative use of urokinase, a thrombolytic agent.

PROBLEM ANALYSIS

Definition

Lower limb atherosclerotic peripheral vascular disease (PVD) is common in the elderly but is asymptomatic in more than 90% of cases. When it is symptomatic, intermittent claudication is by far the most common complaint. Indications for elective peripheral vascular surgery (PVS) include claudication, ischemic pain at rest, ulceration, and gangrene. Goals of revascularization are to improve the natural course of PVD and ultimately to avoid amputation. However, bypass grafts may fail acutely or long term, with 25% to 60% of grafts occluded after 5 years.

Critical leg ischemia occurs in less than 10% of patients and is defined as pain at rest or the presence of gangrene or ulcers. Because such patients are at risk for imminent limb loss, surgery is semiurgent or urgent. During revascularization, aortoiliac (inflow) or distal (outflow) obstructions are bypassed with axillofemoral or femoropopliteal distal bypass grafts, respectively.

Recognition

The prevalence of cardiac risk factors is usually greater in patients undergoing PVS than in those having nonvascular surgery. Therefore, careful attention to metabolic and cardiac status is critical. Also, successful surgery and long-term survival of the graft depend on blood flow through the graft, blood coagulability, and the future development of atherosclerotic changes in the graft. Anesthesia care can have an important impact on immediate and longer-term outcomes.

Risk Assessment

Primary concerns are the impact of the planned anesthetic technique on the surgical revascularization procedure, the patient's tolerance of the anesthetic and surgery (which often takes many hours), and preoperative cardiopulmonary risk factors. Another important concern is the effect of anesthetic technique—regional anesthesia (RA) versus general anesthesia (GA)—on the success of revascularization and perioperative outcomes. The following factors should be considered:

- *Sympathectomy.* This procedure dilates the venous capacitance bed to reduce cardiac preload, thus increasing fluid requirements to maintain cardiac output. It also reduces systemic vascular resistance. If this decreases cardiac afterload and work, it may improve global and regional left ventricular function for the duration of the sympathetic block.
- *Analgesia.* Successful RA provides analgesia and reduces or eliminates the need for systemic narcotics. This benefit is extended with continuous RA techniques.
- *Surgical stress.* RA attenuates the surgical stress response, including renin-angiotensin-aldosterone system activation and the associated increased release of vasopressin and catecholamines.
- *Postoperative hypercoagulability.* Sympathetic block may reduce stress-related hypercoagulability.

Although it is difficult to compare studies of anesthetic techniques, medications, and surgical factors related to PVD, recent prospective randomized trials have found no difference in mortality between spinal or epidural RA and GA (Table 96-1). The lack of reported differences in outcome may be attributed to improved cardiovascular management in these trials compared with earlier ones.

RA continued as postoperative analgesia may improve graft patency, as indicated by a reduced need for regrafting, thrombectomy, or amputation. Two studies in Table 96-1 (Tuman and Christopherson) showed marked differences in graft failure rates between GA alone and RA with or without GA; the other studies found no such difference. Conflicting outcomes may be ascribed to differences in methodology, type of graft material, extent of distal vessel disease, and adjunct anesthetic drugs. Thus, RA for PVD surgery may benefit patients at highest risk for early graft failure or those who require reoperation for whatever reason. For limb salvage surgery, hypercoagulable states and prosthetic conduits are independent risk factors for graft failure.

RA may have beneficial effects on some procoagulant parameters (e.g., platelet function, fibrinogen and plasminogen

Table 96–1 ■ Summary of Studies Comparing Regional Anesthesia and General Anesthesia for Peripheral Vascular Surgery

Study	Number of Patients		Perioperative Mortality (%)		Cardiovascular Complications (%)		PVS Graft Thrombosis (%)		Remarks
	GA	RA	GA	RA	GA	RA	GA	RA	
Cook et al 1986	51	50	5.9	2.0	7.8	4.0	—	—	Spinal anesthesia; higher incidence of hypotension (RA) and HTN (GA); blood loss less with spinal anesthesia; risk of postoperative MI similar
Tuman et al 1991	40	40	0	0	27	10	—	—	GA with postoperative epidural analgesia vs GA with postoperative PCA Controls (N = 40) were randomly selected GA patients (non-CV surgery), but no PVD
Christopherson et al 1993	51	49	3.9	4.1	7.8	8.2	21*	4*	EA for surgery followed by epidural analgesia, or GA for surgery and IV PCA 11 (GA) vs 2 (RA) patients had regrafting or embolectomy
Bode et al 1996	138	285	2.9	3.1	19	23	—	—	EA (N = 149); spinal anesthesia (N = 136); GA (N = 138) Overall, the patient population included 86% with DM, 69% with HTN, 36% with prior MI, and 41% with a history of smoking
Pierce et al 1997	96	86/82	—	—	—	—	2.1	2.3/2.4	Of 423 patients randomized to GA, spinal anesthesia, or EA, 76 did not meet protocol standards, 32 had inadequate anesthesia, 51 were lost to follow-up There were no differences among groups for 30-day graft patency, reoperation rates, 30-day graft occlusion, death, amputation, or length of hospital stay
Schunn et al 1998	158	145	5.0	3.4	—	—	9.4	14	EA vs GA; retrospective analysis of femoral-popliteal-tibial bypass graft patients with similar demographic profiles Conclusion was that EA vs GA choice should be based on preanesthesia findings

*P ≤.05.

CV, cardiovascular; DM, diabetes mellitus; EA, epidural anesthesia; GA, general anesthesia; HTN, hypertension; IV, intravenous; MI, myocardial infarction; PCA, patient-controlled analgesia; PVD, peripheral vascular disease; PVS, peripheral vascular surgery; RA, regional anesthesia.

CARDIOTHORACIC & VASCULAR SURGERY

activator inhibitor levels). Furthermore, serologically proven hypercoagulability is known to be associated with inferior long-term graft patency and lower rates of limb salvage and survival after infrainguinal bypass grafts. However, whether RA protects against graft thrombosis remains controversial.

As for preoperative cardiopulmonary risk assessment, 20% to 60% of patients with PVD have manifest or silent coronary artery disease. The preoperative history and physical examination should focus on identifying cardiac functional status and associated risk factors (see Chapter 38). In a post hoc review of 10 studies on outcomes after femoropopliteal bypass graft surgery, combined perioperative mortality was 0.8% for patients at low risk versus 4.7% for those at high risk. The cause of death was similar for both groups (multi-organ failure, stroke, or cardiac complications). Cardiac risk factors for those having PVS are similar to those for patients having other major noncardiac surgery (see Chapter 38). They include the following:

- History of ischemic heart disease
- History of congestive heart failure
- Uncontrolled stage 2 hypertension, especially if associated with evidence of end-organ damage[1]
- Associated cerebrovascular disease
- Preoperative treatment with insulin
- Preoperative serum creatinine greater than 2 mg/dL
- High-risk surgery

Implications

Although multiple anesthetic techniques have been evaluated to date, the ideal technique for lower limb revascularization surgery, especially femoral-popliteal-tibial (distal) bypass grafting, remains unclear. Nonetheless, a number of medical and surgical factors may help determine the best technique for a particular patient. The duration of surgery is one important consideration. Surgeons may expend considerable time harvesting the patient's own veins because acute and chronic patency is significantly enhanced with these grafts compared with frozen veins or prosthetic materials. Repeat revascularization procedures are typically longer and more complex. Certainly RA may still be possible, because continuous epidural infusions and spinal catheters are available and routinely employed. However, patients may have difficulty tolerating intravenous sedation for long periods. Another consideration is whether arm veins will be harvested, particularly for reoperations. Reconstructions of this type may preclude the use of RA alone, but combined RA and GA may be appropriate.

Patients with severe pulmonary disease may also benefit from RA, but lengthy surgeries that require them to lie flat for prolonged periods may be difficult to tolerate. Further, sudden patient movement due to spasmodic coughing secondary to bronchitis, chronic pulmonary disease, smoking, or reactive airway disease may make creating delicate vascular anastomoses nearly impossible. Similarly, patients with cardiovascular disease may experience orthopnea, especially those with low cardiac ejection fractions (≤ 0.35) or a past history of congestive heart failure, and they may be unable to remain supine for long periods. Use of modified semi-Fowler positioning[2] and back supports may help reduce discomfort or reduce or eliminate orthopnea.

If it is determined that RA is optimal for a patient, the use of perioperative anticoagulation must be given consideration. Guidelines of the American Society of Regional Anesthesia address the implications of anticoagulation and offer advice for the prevention and management of bleeding complications with RA (see Chapter 67).

MANAGEMENT

In general, all prescribed cardiac medications should be given preoperatively to optimize the cardiovascular dynamics (see Chapter 38). If RA is used, perioperative anticoagulation status must be determined, and appropriate precautions exercised (see Chapter 67).

Monitoring

Indicated monitoring includes at least a two-lead electrocardiogram with precise placement of V_4 or V_5 leads, surface pulse oximetry, end-tidal carbon dioxide and inhalational anesthetic monitoring, and noninvasive blood pressure monitoring. Invasive monitoring is indicated for some patients, especially those with symptomatic or severe cardiovascular disease (e.g., stage III or IV heart failure, chronic atrial fibrillation, symptomatic arrhythmias, stage 2 hypertension). Such monitoring includes an arterial line, central venous pressure, and possibly a pulmonary artery catheter. These are placed before or after anesthesia induction. With severe hypertension,[3] poor left ventricular function (ejection fraction ≤ 0.35), or symptomatic coronary artery disease, preinduction invasive monitoring allows tighter control of hemodynamic changes during induction and tracheal intubation and during periods of increased cardiovascular stress. The anesthetic technique (RA versus GA) should not affect the decision to institute central venous pressure or pulmonary artery catheter monitoring. Central lines may be required for patients with poor peripheral access or when arm veins will be used. Transesophageal echocardiography is useful for monitoring cardiac function and volume status when GA is used, especially for hemodynamically unstable patients or if a cardiac (atrial fibrillation) or aortic (unstable plaque) source for thromboembolism is present.

---

[1]Stage 2 hypertension is systemic blood pressure of 160/100 mm Hg or higher (sequential measurements on separate days). If stage 2 hypertension is associated with evidence of end-organ damage (e.g., aortic dissection, renal failure, cerebral symptoms, heart failure, retinopathy), this constitutes a true hypertensive emergency; if not, it is a hypertensive crisis. The former requires more urgent therapy (intravenous drugs) than the latter (oral drugs). See Chapter 77.

[2]Namely, 15- to 30-degree versus 30- to 45-degree head-up tilt, without compromising surgical groin access.

[3]Stage 1 (blood pressure >140/90 but <160/100 mm Hg) or stage 2 hypertension (see footnote 1).

Hemodynamic Changes

Careful assessment of hemodynamic parameters and myocardial ischemia during a stress test is invaluable. The purpose of serially recording the patient's blood pressure during stress (e.g., admission to hospital, invasive procedures) is to gain knowledge of its range and lability. Notation of the range of blood pressure at night provides an idea of how well low blood pressure values will be tolerated. Also, during RA, vasopressor support (e.g., phenylephrine) for hypotension may be better (safer) than increased fluid infusion.

Sustained tachycardia is one of the least tolerated hemodynamic alterations. It is important to determine and correct the cause, such as surgical stimulation or excessive or rapid blood loss; the latter often occurs during thrombectomy. Changing anesthetic depth or administering β-blockers is first-line therapy. Patients at high risk for cardiovascular complications (see Chapter 38) benefit from perioperative β-blockade, especially when GA is used. However, it is unclear whether this advice applies to similar patients having the same surgical procedures performed under RA. In large part, this will depend on whether RA produces cardiac sympathetic blockade (which, in itself, blocks against heart rate increases).

Emergence from GA is a common time for perioperative myocardial ischemia to occur. It may be associated with hypertension and tachycardia due to subconscious or conscious pain awareness. Labetalol or esmolol can attenuate elevated heart rate responses. These drugs as well as nitroglycerin, hydralazine, or nicardipine can be used to reduce blood pressure or treat ischemia if it persists after a favorable heart rate has been restored.

Fluid Management

Most patients having PVS require careful attention to fluid status, because there is a fine line between fluid overload with pulmonary edema and hypovolemia with impaired flow to the graft and vital organs. Maintenance crystalloid is used to replace preoperative insensible deficits (e.g., caused by lack or oral intake or by bowel preparation). Inpatients are often dehydrated or may have received dye loads during preoperative angiograms and require volume repletion. Third-space fluid loss is moderate for typical lower extremity PVS. The starting point is often 5 mL/kg per hour.

Blood replacement is accomplished with colloids or red blood cells as needed. However, vascular surgeons are especially cognizant of the fact that reduced blood viscosity increases blood flow through the bypass graft.[4] Thus, some degree of anemia may be beneficial for high-risk grafts; however, it is also associated with reduced vital organ and tissue oxygen delivery. A reasonable trade-off for intraoperative hemoglobin concentration is maintaining a hematocrit of 28 in high-risk patients.

Temperature

Temperature homeostasis is important owing to the detrimental cardiovascular effects associated with hypothermia.

Hypothermia increases the risk for myocardial ischemia, promotes instability in heart rate and blood pressure, and may cause postoperative confusion. Thus, forced air warming blankets, a warm operating room, warmed intravenous fluids, a humidifier on the ventilator circuit, or low fresh gas flows are appropriate for maintaining normothermia.

PREVENTION

Any patient having lower extremity PVS is presumed to have generalized atherosclerotic disease and coronary artery disease. Therefore, preoperative considerations are similar to those for patients with known cardiac disease having major noncardiac surgery (see Chapter 38). Aggressive preventive strategies such as risk factor modification and drug therapy (e.g., β-blockers, lipid-lowering agents, antiplatelet drugs) are needed. Antiplatelet drugs and RA may reduce the rate of postoperative graft thrombosis. β-Blockers reduce the risk for myocardial ischemia and myocardial infarction, which are responsible for most of the morbidity associated with PVS.

The superiority of RA or GA for preventing adverse cardiovascular outcomes, graft thrombosis, or mortality has not been established. As discussed earlier, a number of proposed mechanisms may explain the trend toward improved outcomes with RA, but these have not been firmly established. Thus, the choice of anesthetic management should be made on a case-by-case basis after discussions with both the surgeon and the patient. Medical and surgical factors, as well as patient preferences, can help determine the best strategy for each patient.

Further Reading

Bode RH, Lewis KP, Zarich SW, et al: Cardiac outcome after peripheral vascular surgery: Comparison of general and regional anesthesia. Anesthesiology 84:3-13, 1996.

Breslow MJ, Parker SD, Frank SM, et al: Determinants of catecholamine and cortisol responses to lower extremity revascularization. The PIRAT study group. Anesthesiology 79:1202-1209, 1993.

Caldicott L, Lumb A, McCoy D: Lower limb revascularization. In Caldicott L, Lumb A, McCoy D (eds): Vascular Anaesthesia: A Practical Handbook. Oxford, Butterworth-Heinemann, 1999, pp 198-224.

Christopherson R, Beattie C, Frank SM, et al: Perioperative morbidity in patients randomized to epidural or general anesthesia for lower extremity vascular surgery. Anesthesiology 79:422-434, 1993.

Collins CC, Peterson NJ, Suarez-Almazor M, et al: The prevalence of peripheral arterial disease in a racially diverse population. Arch Intern Med 163:1469-1474, 2003.

Cook PT, Davies MJ, Cronin KD, et al: A prospective randomized trial comparing spinal anaesthesia using hyperbaric cinchocaine with general anaesthesia for lower limb vascular surgery. Anaesth Intensive Care 14:373-380, 1986.

Criqui MH, Denenberg JO: The generalized nature of atherosclerosis: How peripheral arterial disease may predict adverse events from coronary artery disease. Vasc Med 3:241-245, 1998.

Curi MA, Skelly CL, Baldwin ZK, et al: Long-term outcome of infrainguinal bypass grafting in patients with serologically proven hypercoagulability. J Vasc Surg 37:301-306, 2003.

Dormandy J, Heeck L, Vig S: The fate of patients with critical leg ischemia. Semin Vasc Surg 12:142-147, 1999.

Frank SM, Beattie C, Christopherson R, et al: Unintentional hypothermia is associated with postoperative myocardial ischemia. Anesthesiology 78:468-476, 1993.

Hertzer NR, Beven EG, Young JR, et al: Coronary artery disease in peripheral vascular patients: A classification of 1000 coronary angiograms and results of surgical management. Ann Surg 199:223-233, 1984.

---

[4]From Poiseuille's formula.

Hickey NC, Wilkes MP, Howes D, et al: The effect of epidural anaesthesia on peripheral resistance and graft flow following femoro-distal reconstruction. Eur J Endovasc Surg 9:93-96, 1995.

Horlocker TT, Wedel DJ, Benzon H, et al: Regional anesthesia in the anticoagulated patient: Defining the risks (the Second ASRA Consensus Conference on Neuraxial Anesthesia and Anticoagulation). Reg Anesth Pain Med 28:172-197, 2003.

Hunink MGM, Wong JB, Donaldson MC, et al: Revascularization for femoropopliteal disease: A decision and cost-effectiveness analysis. JAMA 274:165-171, 1995.

Johnson WC, Lee KK: A comparative evaluation of polytetrafluoroethylene, umbilical vein, and saphenous vein bypass grafts for femoral-popliteal above-knee revascularization: A prospective randomized Department of Veterans Affairs cooperative study. J Vasc Surg 32:268-277, 2000.

Lee TH, Marcantonio ER, Mangione CM, et al: Derivation and prospective validation of a simple index for prediction of cardiac risk of major noncardiac surgery. Circulation 100:1043-1049, 1999.

Mangano DT, Layug EL, Wallace A, et al: Effect of atenolol on mortality and cardiovascular morbidity after non-cardiac surgery. N Engl J Med 335:1713-1720, 1996.

Modig J, Borg T, Bagge L, et al: Role of extradural and of general anesthesia in fibrinolysis and coagulation after total hip replacement. Br J Anaesth 55:625-629, 1983.

Nelson AH, Fleisher LA, Rosenbaum SH: Relationship between postoperative anemia and cardiac morbidity in high-risk vascular patients in the intensive care unit. Crit Care Med 21:860-866, 1993.

Pierce ET, Pomposelli FB, Stanley GD, et al: Anesthesia type does not influence early graft patency or limb salvage rates of lower extremity bypass. J Vasc Surg 25:226-233, 1997.

Poldermans D, Boersma E, Bax JJ, et al: The effect of bisoprolol on perioperative mortality and myocardial infarction in high-risk patients undergoing vascular surgery. Dutch Echocardiographic Cardiac Risk Evaluation Applying Stress Echocardiography Study Group. N Engl J Med 341:1789-1794, 1999.

Raby KE, Brull SJ, Timimi F, et al: The effect of heart rate control on myocardial ischemia among high-risk patients after vascular surgery. Anesth Analg 88:477-482, 1999.

Roizen MF: Anesthesia for vascular surgery. In Barash PG, Cullen BF, Stoelting RK (eds): Clinical Anesthesia. Philadelphia, JB Lippincott, 1989, pp 1041-1043.

Rosenfeld BA, Beattie C, Christopherson R, et al: The effects of different anesthetic regimens on fibrinolysis and the development of postoperative arterial thrombosis. Anesthesiology 79:435-443, 1993.

Schunn CD, Hertzer NR, O'Hara PJ, et al: Epidural versus general anesthesia: Does anesthetic management influence early infrainguinal graft thrombosis? Ann Vasc Surg 12:65-69, 1998.

Sixth report of the Joint National Committee on Prevention, Detection, Evaluation, and Treatment of High Blood Pressure. Arch Intern Med 157:2413-2446, 1997; erratum, Arch Intern Med 158:573, 1998.

Stone JG, Foex P, Sear JW, et al: Myocardial ischemia in untreated hypertensive patients: Effect of a single small oral dose of a beta-adrenergic blocking agent. Anesthesiology 68:495-500, 1988.

Summary of the second report of the National Cholesterol Education Program (NCEP) Expert Panel on Detection, Evaluation, and Treatment of High Blood Cholesterol in Adults (Adult Treatment Panel II). JAMA 269:3015-3023, 1993.

Tuman KJ, McCarthy RJ, March RJ, et al: Effects of epidural anesthesia and analgesia on coagulation and outcome after major vascular surgery. Anesth Analg 73:696-704, 1991.

Vandermeulen EP, Van Aken H, Vermylen J: Anticoagulants and spinal-epidural anesthesia. Can J Anaesth 43:R129-R141, 1996.

Wildsmith JA, McClure JH: Anticoagulant drugs and central nerve blockade [editorial]. Anaesthesia 46:613-614, 1991.

Wulf H: Epidural anaesthesia and spinal haematoma. Can J Anaesth 43:1260-1271, 1996.

CARDIOVASCULAR DEVICE THERAPY

Patients with Cardiac Rhythm Management Devices

97

John L. Atlee

CARDIOTHORACIC & VASCULAR SURGERY

Case Synopsis

A 32-year-old man with congenital complete heart block has been pacemaker dependent since early childhood. He has an adaptive-rate atrioventricular (AV) universal pacemaker (DDDR) and presents for elective orthognathic surgery. His preoperative electrocardiogram (ECG) reveals sinus rhythm with AV synchronous (atrial-triggered) pacing artifacts. The electrocautery grounding pad is placed on the patient's left thigh before surgery. Intermittently, with electrocautery, the anesthesiologist notices no pulse pressure in the radial artery pressure tracings. Several hours into the procedure, the patient suffers cardiac arrest. Despite aggressive attempts at resuscitation, including external pacing, the resuscitation is unsuccessful and the patient dies.

PROBLEM ANALYSIS

Definition

Pacemakers (PMs) and internal cardioverter-defibrillators (ICDs) have evolved rapidly since the first asynchronous single-chamber PM and ICD implantations in 1958 and 1980, respectively. Today, more than 500,000 persons in the United States have PMs, and more than 115,000 new devices are implanted each year. Also, more than 50,000 ICDs are implanted worldwide each year.

Contemporary single- and dual-chamber PMs and ICDs are sophisticated devices. Both types of cardiac rhythm management devices (CRMDs) incorporate some or all of the following features or capabilities:

- *AV universal pacing:* single- or dual-chamber sequential sensing and pacing.
- Adaptive-rate pacing: activity or metabolic sensors[1] increase pacing rates in response to exercise-related increases in metabolic demand.
- *Multisite pacing:* two or more pacing electrodes are used to synchronize left ventricular (LV) or right ventricular (RV) contractions (or both) in patients with ventricular conduction delay.
- *Cardiac resynchronization therapy (CRT):* biventricular or LV pacing to synchronize RV and LV contractions (Fig. 97-1). With LV pacing alone, LV contraction must be timed with

respect to atrial and RV contractions (i.e., RV conduction cannot be delayed).
- *Programmable lead configuration:* this can be unipolar or bipolar.
- *Tachycardia sensing and discrimination:* detects and diagnoses tachyarrhythmias as atrial or ventricular in origin and decides on the sequence of therapy (pacing or shocks).
- *Antitachycardia pacing (ATP):* ATP terminates reentry atrial or ventricular arrhythmias.
- *Biphasic shock waveforms:* such shocks are delivered when ATP fails to terminate a tachyarrhythmia or the disturbance is not amenable to termination by a programmed pacing sequence (e.g., atrial or ventricular fibrillation). Such shocks are more efficient (require less energy) than their monophasic counterparts used in earlier ICDs.

Recognition

Pacing may be temporary or permanent. If temporary, an external pulse generator (PG) transmits pulses either indirectly to the heart via leads on the body's surface or within the esophagus or directly to the heart via endocardial or epicardial electrodes within or on the heart's surface. For permanent pacing, an implantable PG (or "can") transmits pulses directly to the heart via endocardial or epicardial leads to electrodes within the heart or on its surface, respectively.

Pacing leads can have a unipolar or bipolar configuration. With the former, the PG serves as an anode (+) and the cardiac electrode as a cathode (−). With the latter, both electrodes are within the heart (endocardial), on its surface (epicardial), immediately behind the heart (transesophageal), or on the body's surface (transcutaneous).

With implanted CRMDs, the PG is often located in the left or right pectoral region. However, it may be subcostal,

---

[1]Piezoelectric crystals or accelerometers that detect changes in motion, acceleration, vibration, or pressure with exercise. However, minute ventilation or stimulus or Q-T interval sensors may provide a rate response that is more proportional to increased metabolic demand with exercise.

DCM baseline

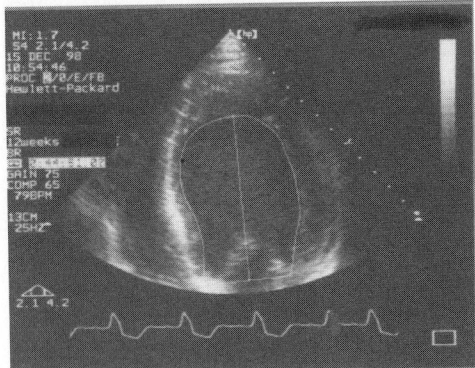

A   DCM—abnormal LV contraction
pattern; early septal movement

DCM-CRT

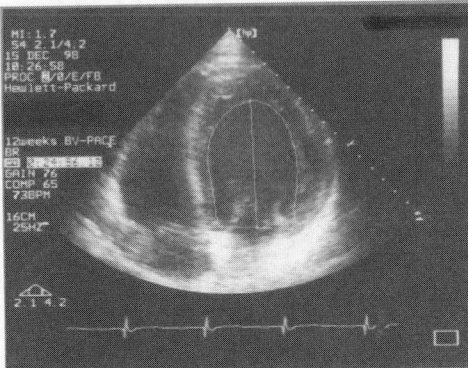

B   CRT—better LV contraction pattern
with decreased systolic dimension

Figure 97–1 ■ Cardiac resynchronization therapy (CRT) in a patient with dilated cardiomyopathy (DCM) and left ventricular (LV) conduction delay. *A,* Before CRT, the echocardiogram (EC) shows early septal movement, with the lower interventricular septum moving toward the LV cavity. Note that the lateral wall of the left ventricle has not yet begun to contract (due to conduction delay), and on the electrocardiogram (ECG), the QRS complex beneath the EC is widened. *B,* After CRT (biventricular pacing to synchronize contraction of both ventricles), the LV septum and lateral wall contract nearly simultaneously, and the ECG QRS complexes beneath the EC are now narrowed.

especially in infants or small children. Knowledge of the PG's location and leads is important for predicting the CRMD's susceptibility to malfunction in the hospital or other environments where electromagnetic interference (EMI), or "noise," is present (see "Implications").

Aside from pacing in cases of acute myocardial infarction, there are no consensus indications for temporary pacing (see later). Temporary pacing is often used for rate support with transient, hemodynamically disadvantageous bradycardia or escape rhythms or for slow atrial fibrillation, bradyasystole, or high-degree AV heart block in acute myocardial infarction. It is widely used in cardiac surgery; in fact, epicardial pacing wires are routinely placed as a precautionary measure in many centers. In other settings, atrial or ventricular transvenous pacing leads (or both) are widely used (especially in cardiac intensive care units and in high-risk patients before cardiac surgery). Noninvasive pacing includes transcutaneous pacing (causes global myocardial depolarization) and transesophageal pacing (primarily for atrial pacing, but feasibility for ventricular pacing has been shown). Indications for temporary pacing are summarized in Table 97-1.

Indications for permanent PMs and ICDs are summarized in Tables 97-2 and 97-3. These indications are based on the 1998 American College of Cardiology (ACC)–American Heart Association (AHA) guidelines and the most recent (2002) update by a task force comprising ACC and AHA members and a committee appointed by the North American Society of Pacing and Electrophysiology (NASPE; now the Heart Rhythm Society). Only class I and III indications are listed. Class I indications are conditions for which there is evidence or general agreement that a procedure or treatment is useful and effective. Class III indications are those for which there is evidence or general agreement that the procedure or treatment is not useful or effective and in some cases may be harmful. Class II indications are conditions for which there is conflicting evidence or a divergence of opinion about the usefulness or efficacy of a procedure or treatment. Class II indications are subdivided into IIa if the weight of evidence favors usefulness or efficacy and IIb if usefulness or efficacy is less well established by evidence or opinion (hereafter, class IIa and IIb indications are collectively considered as "possible" indications).

Table 97–1 ■ Indications for Temporary Pacing in Children or Adults

Common Indications	Less Common Indications
Sinus bradycardia or escape rhythms due to reversible causes, with symptoms or signs of disadvantageous hemodynamics As a bridge to insertion of an implanted CRMD for any class I or IIa indication (see text and Tables 97-2 and 97-3) With acute MI: asystole; new bifascicular block with first degree AVHB; alternating BBB; bradycardia with symptoms of hemodynamic compromise not responsive to drugs*; type II second degree† or advanced second degree AVHB‡ Bradycardia-dependent tachyarrhythmias (e.g., torsades de pointes with long QT syndromes)	During acute MI: new or age-indeterminate right BBB with LAFB, LPFB, or first degree AVHB, or with left BBB; recurring sinus pauses refractory to atropine; overdrive pacing for incessant VT; new or age-indeterminate bifascicular block or isolated right BBB During heart surgery: during overdrive disadvantageous lower pacemaker escape rhythms; to pace or terminate reentry SVT or VT; to prevent pause- or bradycardia-dependent tachyarrhythmias; during PAC insertion with left BBB

*Especially in cardiac surgery or if atrioventricular conduction is intact and transesophageal atrial pacing is available, pacing is preferable to drugs because they may have unpredictable and deleterious effects on cardiac rate and rhythm.
†No progressive P-R prolongation before nonconducted atrial beats, as with type I second degree AVHB.
‡Two or more nonconducted atrial beats before conducted atrial beats.
AVHB, atrioventricular heart block; BBB, bundle branch block; CRMD, cardiac rhythm management device; LAFB, left anterior fascicular block; LPFB, left posterior fascicular block; MI, myocardial infarction; PAC, pulmonary artery catheter; SVT, supraventricular tachycardia; VT, ventricular tachycardia.

Table 97–2 ■ Class I and III indications for Permanent Pacing in Adults

Class I (Useful and Effective)	Class III (Not Useful or Effective)
Acquired Atrioventricular Heart Block	**Acquired Atrioventricular Heart Block**
Third degree and advanced second degree AVHB at any anatomic level, with any of the following: AVHB and bradycardia with symptoms Arrhythmias or conditions that require drugs leading to bradycardia with symptoms Proven asystole ≥3.0 sec or escape rate <40 bpm (awake patient without symptoms) After catheter ablation or modification of AV junction Postoperative AVHB not expected to resolve after cardiac surgery Neuromuscular diseases with AVHB (with or without symptoms owing to unpredictable disease progression) Second degree AVHB, regardless of type or site, with bradycardia and symptoms	Asymptomatic first degree AVHB Type I* second degree AVHB above the His bundle without symptoms AVHB expected to resolve or unlikely to recur (e.g., drug toxicity, Lyme disease, sleep apnea without symptoms)
Atrioventricular Heart Block after Acute Myocardial Infarction	**Atrioventricular Heart Block after Acute Myocardial Infarction**
Persistent second degree AVHB in His-Purkinje system with bilateral BBB or third degree AVHB within or below the His-Purkinje after acute MI Transient advanced (second or third degree) infranodal AVHB with BBB; if site is uncertain, EPS may be necessary Persistent second or third degree AVHB with symptoms	Transient AVHB in absence of intraventricular conduction defects Transient AVHB with isolated LAFB without AVHB Acquired LAFB in absence of AVHB Persistent first degree AVHB with old or age-indeterminate BBB
Sinus Node Dysfunction	**Sinus Node Dysfunction**
SND with documented bradycardia and symptoms, including frequent sinus pauses (possibly the result of essential long-term drug therapy for which there are no acceptable alternatives) Symptomatic chronotropic incompetence	SND in asymptomatic patients, including those with substantial sinus bradycardia (heart rate <40 bpm) caused by long-term drug treatment SND in patients with symptoms suggesting bradycardia that is clearly documented as not being associated with slow heart rate SND with bradycardia and symptoms due to nonessential drug therapy
Hypersensitive Carotid Sinus and Neurally Mediated Syndromes	**Hypersensitive Carotid Sinus and Neurally Mediated Syndromes**
Recurrent syncope with CSS; minimal carotid sinus pressure induces ventricular asystole >3 sec in absence of drug that depresses sinus node or AV conduction	Hyperactive cardioinhibitory response to CSS with no symptoms or vague ones (e.g., dizziness, lightheadedness) Recurrent syncope, lightheadedness, or dizziness in absence of hyperactive cardioinhibitory response Situational vasovagal syncope in which avoidance behavior is effective

AV, atrioventricular; AVHB, AV heart block; BBB, bundle branch block; bpm, beats per minute; CSS, carotid sinus stimulation; EPS, electrophysiologic study (cardiac); LAFB, left anterior fascicular block; MI, myocardial infarction; SND, sinus node dysfunction.

Table 97–3 ■ Class I and III Indications for an Internal Cardioverter-Defibrillator for Primary* or Secondary Prevention†

Class I (Always Indicated)	Class III (Never Indicated)
Cardiac arrest due to VT or VF not due to transient or reversible cause Spontaneous sustained VT (lasting >30 sec) in patients with SHD Syncope of undetermined origin with clinically relevant, hemodynamically significant sustained VT or VF induced at EPS when AD therapy is ineffective, not tolerated, or not preferred NSVT in patients with CAD, prior MI, LV dysfunction, and inducible VF or sustained VT at EPS not suppressed by class I AD Spontaneous sustained VT in patients without SHD amenable to other treatments	Syncope of undetermined cause in patients without inducible tachyarrhythmias or SHD Incessant VT or VF VT or VF due to arrhythmias amenable to surgical or catheter ablation (e.g., atrial tachyarrhythmias in WPW, RV outflow tract VT, idiopathic LV VT, fascicular VT) VT or VF due to transient or reversible cause (e.g., acute MI, electrolyte imbalance, drugs, trauma) when correction is feasible and will likely reduce risk for further VT or VF Significant psychiatric illness that may be aggravated by ICD implantation or may preclude systematic follow-up Terminal illness and life expectancy <6 mo CAD patients with LV dysfunction and QRS >130 msec, and without spontaneous or inducible sustained or NSVT having CABG NYHA class IV drug-refractory congestive heart failure in patients not candidates for cardiac transplantation

*ICDs are used for primary prevention in patients with class I or II indications but without a history of cardiac arrest due to VT or VF or without inducible sustained VT or VF at EPS.

†ICDs are used for secondary prevention in patients with a history of sudden cardiac death or who have documented or inducible (at EPS) sustained VT or VF.

AD, antiarrhythmic drug; CABG, coronary artery bypass grafting; CAD, coronary artery disease; EPS, electrophysiologic study (cardiac); ICD, internal cardioverter-defibrillator; LV, left ventricular; MI, myocardial infarction; NSVT, nonsustained VT; NYHA, New York Heart Association; RV, right ventricular; SHD, structural heart disease; VF, ventricular fibrillation; VT, ventricular tachycardia; WPW, Wolff-Parkinson-White syndrome.

Permanent pacing is indicated for any patient with symptomatic bradycardia or slow escape rhythms due to sinus node dysfunction or AV heart block. Also, pacing is indicated for syncope due to neurally mediated syndromes (e.g., hypersensitive carotid sinus syndrome) with a more prominent cardioinhibitory component in response to carotid sinus stimulation (i.e., bradycardia or escape rhythm) than a vasodepressor response (i.e., vasodilatation with hypotension). Further, the syncope must not be due to a reversible condition or a medication for which there is no suitable alternative therapy.

In the 1998 and 2002 guidelines, the indications for pacing in infants, children, or adolescents with congenital heart disease are similar to those in adults, except that they are based on the correlation of symptoms with bradycardia rather than on arbitrary rate criteria per se. Also, pacing is indicated for bradycardia only after the exclusion of other causes (e.g., seizures, breath holding, apnea, neurally mediated mechanisms). Revisions in the 2002 guidelines include the following: (1) substituting "ventricular dysfunction" for "congestive heart failure" in pacing for advanced second or third degree AV heart block, (2) specifying greater than 7 days for advanced second or third degree AV heart block after cardiac surgery, and (3) adding the qualifier "with complex ventricular ectopy" to class I indications for congenital third degree AV heart block. New qualifiers for class IIa indications in children with congenital heart disease are the following: (1) congenital third degree AV heart block "associated with symptoms," (2) increasing the resting heart rate from 35 to 40 beats per minute in children with complex congenital heart disease, and (3) adding the phrases "and impaired hemodynamics due to sinus bradycardia" or "loss of AV synchrony" to the indication for pacing in children with complex congenital heart disease. For updates to Class IIb indications for pacing in patients with congenital heart disease, see the 2002 ACC-AHA-NASPE guidelines.

The indications for pacing in other conditions (e.g., chronic bifascicular and trifascicular block, hypertrophic or obstructive cardiomyopathy, idiopathic dilated cardiomyopathy, cardiac transplantation, detection and pacing to terminate tachycardias) are beyond the scope of this chapter (see the 1998 and 2002 ACC-AHA-NASPE guidelines).

Class II indications are constantly evolving. For example, what constitutes a class II indication in AV heart block revolves around whether second or third degree block at any anatomic site is expected to persist, and certainly not any arbitrary rate if the block is associated with cardiomegaly or LV dysfunction. Even asymptomatic first degree AV heart block is a class IIa indication if associated symptoms are similar to those of the pacemaker syndrome.[2] However, the patient must have LV dysfunction and symptoms of heart failure, especially when first degree AV heart block is associated with neuromuscular disease. This is due to the unpredictable progression of associated AV conduction system disease.

For sinus node dysfunction, the important element is whether there is a clear association between bradycardia (<40 beats per minute) and symptoms. A clear association constitutes a class I indication, and the 2002 guidelines specify that even in the absence of a clear, documented association between significant symptoms and the actual presence of bradycardia, this constitutes a class IIa indication. The 1998 guidelines specified chronic heart rates less than 30 beats per minute with minimal symptoms as class IIb. For hypersensitive carotid sinus syncope, there must be recurrent syncope, no clear provocative events, and a hypersensitive cardioinhibitory response. For neurocardiogenic syncope, the patient must be significantly symptomatic. Also, syncope must be associated with bradycardia documented spontaneously or during tilt-table testing (class IIa). Finally, biventricular pacing (simultaneous LV and RV pacing) in medically refractory and symptomatic New York Heart Association class III or IV heart failure or dilated ischemic cardiomyopathy, with a QRS duration of ≥130 msec, LV end-diastolic diameter of ≥55 mm, or ejection fraction of 0.35, is listed as a class IIa indication for CRT in the 2002 ACC-AHA-NASPE Guidelines. However, given recent additional evidence (e.g., COMPANION trial, CARE-HF study) and similar findings from other large trials of biventricular pacing in comparable patients, it is possible that it might soon become a class I indication.

Finally, ICDs are prescribed for the primary or secondary prevention of destabilizing atrial or ventricular tachyarrhythmias (see Table 97-3). For primary prevention, ICDs have been used in patients with asymptomatic coronary artery disease and nonsustained ventricular tachyarrhythmias. Other settings include after coronary artery bypass surgery or percutaneous coronary intervention in patients with ejection fractions less than 35%. Also, they have been used in patients with abnormal signal-averaged ECGs or those awaiting heart transplantation. For secondary prevention, the patient must have survived an incident of sudden death, usually due to coronary artery disease, but possibly due to other causes, such as the following:

- Congenital or acquired long QT syndromes
- Brugada syndrome
- Idiopathic ventricular fibrillation
- Ventricular tachycardia with infiltrative, dilated, or hypertrophic cardiomyopathy
- Bundle branch reentry ventricular tachycardia
- Idiopathic monomorphic ventricular tachycardia (subdivided into RV outflow tract obstruction or arrhythmogenic RV dysplasia)
- Idiopathic LV tachycardia

Tachycardia discrimination algorithms used with ICDs have evolved and can now distinguish between atrial fibrillation with ventricular aberration and polymorphic ventricular tachycardia or fibrillation. Thus, ICDs are prescribed that provide lower-energy atrial shocks for atrial fibrillation (i.e., indicated for "atrioversion").

Risk Assessment

Both PMs and ICDs are subject to primary or secondary malfunction. The former is due to device failure. The latter

---

[2]This syndrome was originally reported with ventricular-inhibited pacing but can occur with any pacing mode if there is associated AV dissociation. The most common symptoms are shortness of breath, dizziness, fatigue, pulsations in the back or abdomen, apprehension, and cough.

may be caused by electromagnetic or mechanical interference. Because all ICDs incorporate at least single- or dual-chamber and adaptive-rate pacing, they are also subject to any PM malfunction. Malfunctions unique to devices for CRT have not yet been adequately defined.[3]

PACEMAKER MALFUNCTION

Primary PM malfunction is rare (<2% of all device-related problems in one large center over a 6-year period). Some devices have programmed functions (e.g., rate hysteresis), whereby the pacing cycle duration lengthens after sensed versus paced events. Although this simulates true CRMD malfunction, it is actually a pseudomalfunction. True PM malfunction includes the following:

- *Failure to pace:* no pacing artifacts in one or both chambers (atrium and ventricle).
- *Failure to capture:* visible (12-lead ECG) pacing artifacts are present for one or both chambers, but there are no or only intermittent atrial or ventricular depolarizations.
- *Pacing at an abnormal rate:* this can occur in a single- or dual-chamber device and may be normal (elective battery replacement indicator or response to an adaptive-rate sensor) or abnormal behavior (e.g., pacemaker runaway due to more than two system component failures, with the upper rate limited by contemporary devices to 200 beats per minute). Dual-chamber PMs may show such behavior as PM reentrant tachycardia[4] or 1:1 tracking of supraventricular tachycardia by the ventricular chamber.
- *Undersensing (failure to sense):* the intracardiac electrogram must have a sufficient amplitude and frequency to be sensed properly, and there are many potential causes of failure (e.g., progression of cardiac disease, effect of drugs; component malfunction).
- *Oversensing:* any electrical signal of sufficient amplitude occurring during the PM alert period (i.e., sensing in one or both chambers) can reset the device's timing. For example, if the atrial chamber senses ventricular depolarization, this may inhibit atrial stimulus delivery.

INTERNAL CARDIOVERTER-DEFIBRILLATOR MALFUNCTION

Specific ICD malfunctions include inappropriate delivery of ATP therapy, failure to deliver or ineffective pacing or shock therapies, and interactions with drugs or other devices that affect the efficacy of such therapies. Because any unsuccessful ATP is sequenced to shock delivery, such ATP "malfunction" is not really a true ICD malfunction. In fact, in studies cited by Atlee and Bernstein, ATP effectively converted 89% to 96% of episodes of ventricular tachycardia,

thereby significantly reducing the need for painful shocks. Actual ICD malfunctions include the following:

- *Inappropriate delivery of shocks:* electrical artifact due to lead malfunction or caused by surgical electrocautery artifact may be misinterpreted as tachycardia, leading to shocks.
- *Failure to deliver or ineffective pacing or shock therapies:* magnet application may disable sensing and therefore the ability to deliver therapy for tachyarrhythmias. Lead-related problems may also cause such failure. Acute myocardial infarction, drugs, and other imbalances may also affect sensing or increase shock thresholds, influencing the efficacy of ICD therapies. Imbalances may also affect the rate or morphology of ventricular tachycardia, leading to misdiagnosis or unnecessary pacing or shock therapies.
- *Interactions with drugs or other implanted devices:* antiarrhythmic drugs are prescribed with ICDs to suppress the need for frequent shocks and for other reasons (e.g., to suppress atrial fibrillation). Possible adverse effects of such interactions are (1) proarrhythmia (see Chapters 12 and 81); (2) slowing of the heart rate below the detection threshold (e.g., with the use of amiodarone); (3) increased defibrillation thresholds; (4) altered P or T waves or QRS intervals, leading to overcounting and spurious shocks; or (5) morphologic alterations, leading to failure to detect or discriminate ventricular tachycardia or fibrillation.
- *Device-device interactions:* in the past, it was not uncommon for patients to have both a PM and an ICD, with the potential for adverse interactions between the two. This is rare today.

Implications

PMs and ICDs are subject to EMI from nonphysiologic sources. Most devices implanted today are effectively shielded or protected from EMI. The use of bipolar lead configurations (electrodes on PM or ICD leads) reduces the sensing "antenna" and has greatly reduced EMI-related CRMD malfunction (Fig. 97-2). With unipolar leads, the PG is the anode, and electrodes on the lead are the cathode, greatly increasing the antenna and the susceptibility to EMI (Fig. 97-3). Importantly, EMI signal frequencies between 5 and 100 Hz are not filtered by CRMDs because they overlap the frequency range of intracardiac signals. Therefore, EMI entering the CRMD in this frequency range has the potential to cause abnormal behavior, including the following:

- Inhibition or triggering of pacing stimulation.
- Asynchronous pacing (asynchronous interference mode) when continuous EMI is sensed throughout the lower rate interval (e.g., surgical electrocautery). The device appears to have reverted to asynchronous pacing (VOO), but in fact, it senses EMI as noise after the ventricular refractory period and restarts the ventricular refractory period. This continues until the programmed lower rate interval times out with the delivery of stimulation—in effect, VOO pacing.
- EMI may cause a change to another mode that persists after the noise stops (backup or reset mode). The rate may be similar to the battery end-of-life indicator. Random or "phantom" reprogramming, reported in the early 1980s,

---

[3]A MEDLINE OVID database search (April 6, 2005) failed to identify any case reports or other literature pertaining to primary or secondary malfunction unique to CRT devices.

[4]The PM must be programmed to an atrial tracking mode (VAT, VDD, DDD; see ASA practice advisory for code designations), and the patient must have intact retrograde (ventriculoatrial) conduction; PM reentrant tachycardia is often initiated by a premature ventricular beat.

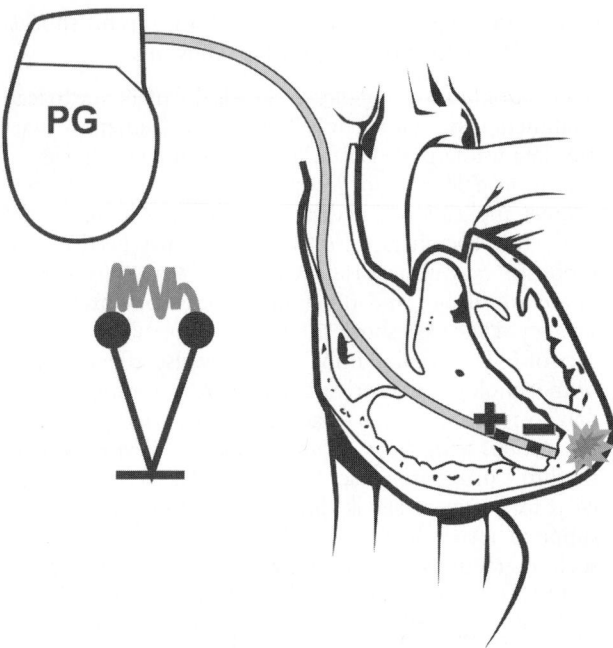

Figure 97–2 ■ Illustration of a cardiac rhythm management device with a bipolar lead configuration. With bipolar leads, both the anode (+) and the cathode (−) are on the lead and near the site of stimulation (apex of the right ventricle [RV]). Such proximity reduces interelectrode distance and the "antenna" (as shown by the TV antenna). PG, pulse generator.

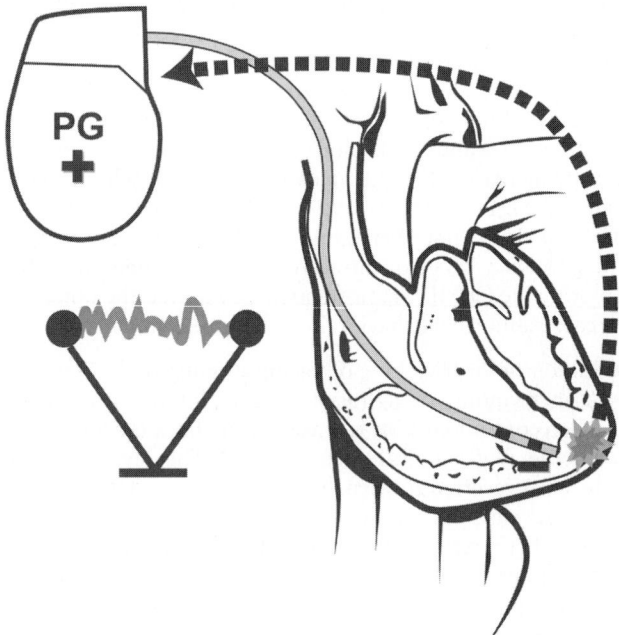

Figure 97–3 ■ With unipolar leads, the cardiac rhythm management device's pulse generator serves as the anode (+), and the most distal electrode on the pacing lead serves as the cathode (−). Compared with the bipolar configuration (see Fig. 97-2), this greatly increases the "antenna" and susceptibility to electromagnetic interference.

is considered virtually impossible with today's CRMDs, because unique radiofrequency sequences (code) are required to reprogram a CRMD.

- Damage to the CRMD's PG or circuitry, causing output failure, PM runaway (see earlier), or other malfunction that necessitates PG replacement.
- Triggering of unnecessary (spurious) ICD shocks and ATP therapies.

Although unipolar surgical electrocautery (bovie)[5] is the most widely recognized source of EMI in hospitals, other sources also exist: external defibrillator-cardioverter shocks, magnetic resonance imaging (MRI), radiation therapy (but not diagnostic radiographs or computed tomography scans), electroconvulsive therapy, extracorporeal shock wave lithotripsy, radiofrequency catheter ablation, and transcutaneous nerve stimulation units. (For a more complete discussion of the risks associated with specific EMI, see part II of the review by Atlee and Bernstein and the American Society of Anesthesiologists [ASA] practice advisory under "Further Reading.")

Less risky alternatives to surgical electrocautery include bipolar cautery and the harmonic scalpel, neither of which appears to pose a risk of EMI-related malfunction of implanted CRMDs. With bipolar cautery, the current pathway is between the two tips (electrodes) of the cautery tool, which are usually less than 1 cm apart during the application of bipolar cautery. Unless the CRMD leads are actually between these electrodes (in the current pathway) or in the immediate vicinity (within 1 cm of the PG or leads) when bipolar cautery is used, there is virtually no risk of CRMD malfunction, because the "antenna" (i.e., the ability to sense EMI) is very small.

MANAGEMENT

Patients with CRMDs have significant heart disease and often significant coexisting medical conditions as well. They may be taking medications with implications for perioperative CRMD management. Preoperative and preprocedural evaluation is indicated before any planned intervention, regardless of where it will be performed (e.g., operating room, radiology suite, critical care unit, ambulatory facility), that might put a CRMD patient at risk for adverse events related to EMI or other device malfunction.

It is important to determine what risk the planned intervention poses to the patient or the CRMD. This may require consultation with the hospital's CRMD follow-up service or a cardiologist. Most patients with implanted CRMDs carry cards that identify the device and manufacturer, the date of implantation, serial numbers of the CRMD and lead systems, and a 24-hour toll-free hotline; thus, relevant information can be obtained, even in emergencies, from the manufacturer. Based on the advice given, it may be

---

[5]With unipolar cautery, the cautery tool (cathode) is variably removed from the grounding plate (anode), which creates a small or large current pathway between the two, depending on the distance between them.

necessary to have the device reprogrammed to an asynchronous mode (i.e., if the patient is PM dependent) or to have ATP or shock therapies programmed off. This can be done by a manufacturer's representative, a cardiologist, or the hospital CRMD service.

For any elective intervention, all the necessary information for optimal CRMD perioperative or peri-interventional management must be obtained. If the risk to the patient is high (e.g., MRI scans, therapeutic radiation, unipolar cautery in the vicinity of the PG, leads in the current pathway) or even moderate, the PM is programmed to sense (e.g., AAI, VVI, VAT, VDD, DDI, DDD; see ASA practice advisory for code designations), and the patient is mostly PM dependent, then it may be necessary to interrogate and reprogram the CRMD to an asynchronous mode (AOO, VOO, DOO).

Generally, it is ill advised to place a magnet over the PG of a CRMD without knowing what the magnet response is. Again, this information can be obtained from the manufacturer or CRMD service. In some devices, the magnet response may be programmed off; in others, it may not confer immunity to sensing and potential malfunction during the planned intervention or after the patient has been discharged. However, for emergent intervention or surgery, when one cannot take the previously mentioned precautions (or have someone else obtain the needed information), it is reasonable to place a magnet over the PG if unusual pacing behavior is observed or spurious shocks or ATP therapies are initiated in response to sensed EMI.

Finally, the CRMD should be interrogated after the procedure for any alteration in programmed settings. For patients with CRMDs who are receiving sequential radiation therapy for the treatment of cancer, the CRMD should be checked after each session.

PREVENTION

Precautions for some specific EMI are listed here. However, these cannot guarantee that there will be no CRMD-related malfunction due to EMI during surgical or other interventions.

- Evaluate the patient before the procedure to determine whether a CRMD is present, the type of device, and whether the patient is PM dependent and the device is functioning.
- For a patient undergoing a procedural or surgical intervention:
  - Determine whether EMI is likely to occur.
  - Program the PM adaptive-rate therapy off.
  - Program the PM to an asynchronous mode, especially if the patient is PM dependent.
  - Program all antitachycardia therapies off.
  - Use bipolar electrocautery or a harmonic scalpel if possible.
  - Ensure the availability of external temporary pacing and a cardioverter-defibrillator.
  - Consider possible untoward effects of any drugs or interventions on CRMD function.
- Use appropriate monitoring:
  - Continuous ECG and arterial oxygen saturation monitoring by pulse oximetry.

- End-tidal carbon dioxide monitoring when general anesthesia is used.
- For procedures that require surgical electrocautery:
  - Use bipolar cautery or harmonic scalpel if possible.
  - Position the electrocautery grounding (receiving) plate so that the current pathway does not pass through or near the PG or leads.
  - Avoid proximity or contact of the cautery tool with the PG or leads.
  - Use short, intermittent, irregular bursts of cautery and the lowest possible energy.
- For radiofrequency ablation (e.g., for arrhythmogenic foci or reentry pathways):
  - Avoid direct contact between the radiofrequency catheter and CRMD or leads.
  - Keep the current path (electrode to return plate) as far away from the PG or leads as possible.
- For MRI and radiation therapy:
  - MRI is generally contraindicated for CRMD patients, but exceptions have been reported (consult the device manufacturer before proceeding with MRI).
  - CRMD malfunction or damage to PG circuitry or components is related to the cumulative dose of radiation; thus, device function should be checked after each session. Alternatively, the device may have to be explanted and reimplanted away from the ionizing beam of radiation; shielding can also be used.

Further Reading

American Society of Anesthesiologists Task Force on Perioperative Management of Patients with Cardiac Rhythm Management Devices: Practice advisory for the perioperative management of patients with cardiac rhythm management devices: Pacemakers and implantable cardioverter-defibrillators. Anesthesiology 103:186-198, 2005 (additional material available at http://www.anesthesiology.org).

Atlee JL, Bernstein AD: Cardiac rhythm management devices (part I). Anesthesiology 95:1265-1280, 2001.

Atlee JL, Bernstein AD: Cardiac rhythm management devices (part II). Anesthesiology 95:1492-1506, 2001.

Baller MR, Kirsner KM: Anesthetic implications of implanted pacemakers: A case study. AANA J 63:209-216, 1995.

Bristow M, Saxon LA, Boehmer J, et al: Comparison of medical therapy, pacing, and defibrillation in heart failure (COMPANION) investigators: Cardiac-resynchronization therapy with or without an implantable defibrillator in advanced chronic heart failure. N Engl J Med 350:2140-2150, 2004.

Cleland JGF, Daubert J-C, Erdmann E, et al: The effect of cardiac resynchronization therapy on morbidity and mortality in heart failure. N Engl J Med 352:1539-1549, 2005.

Epstein MR, Mayer JE Jr, Duncan BW: Use of an ultrasonic scalpel as an alternative to electrocautery in patients with pacemakers. Ann Thorac Surg 65:1802-1804, 1998.

Furman S, Robinson G: The use of an intracardiac pacemaker in the correction of total heart block. Surg Forum 9:245-248, 1958.

Gregoratos G, Abrams J, Epstein AAE, et al: ACC/AHA/NASPE 2002 guideline update for implantation of cardiac pacemakers and antiarrhythmia devices. Summary article: A report of the American College of Cardiology/American Heart Association Task Force on Practice Guidelines (ACC/AHA/NASPE Committee to Update the 1998 Pacemaker Guidelines). Circulation 106:2145-2161, 2002.

Gregoratos G, Cheitlin M, Conill A, et al: ACC/AHA guidelines for implantation of cardiac pacemakers and antiarrhythmia devices: A report of the ACC/AHA Task Force on Practice Guidelines (Committee on Pacemaker Implantation). Circulation 97:1325-1335, 1998.

CARDIOTHORACIC & VASCULAR SURGERY

Kleinman B, Hamilton J, Heriman R, et al: Apparent failure of a precordial magnet and pacemaker programmer to convert a DDD pacemaker to VOO mode during use of the electrosurgical unit. Anesthesiology 86:247-250, 1997.

Mirowski M, Reid PR, Mower MM, et al: Termination of malignant ventricular arrhythmias with an implanted automatic defibrillator in human beings. N Engl J Med 303:322-324, 1980.

Nichol G, Kaul P, Huszti E, et al: Cost-effectiveness of cardiac resynchronization therapy in patients with symptomatic heart failure. Ann Intern Med 141:343-351, 2004.

Ozeren M, Dogan OV, Duzgun C, et al: Use of an ultrasonic scalpel in the open-heart reoperation of a patient with a pacemaker. Eur Cardiothorac Surg 21:761-762, 2002.

Smith CL, Frawley G, Hamar A: Diathermy and the telectronics "META" pacemaker. Anaesth Intensive Care 21:452-454, 1993.

Mechanical Assist Devices

98

Sheela S. Pai and Avery Tung

Case Synopsis

A 78-year-old man with New York Heart Association class III heart failure, hypertension, type 2 diabetes mellitus, and chronic renal insufficiency had coronary artery bypass grafting with mitral valve repair. A prebypass transesophageal echocardiogram (TEE) revealed an ejection fraction of 20%, septal akinesis, severe mitral regurgitation with annular dilatation, and a patent foramen ovale. Owing to the low prebypass ejection fraction, an intra-aortic balloon pump (IABP) was placed before initiation of cardiopulmonary bypass (CPB). Total CPB time was 210 minutes. Despite the use of IABP support and dobutamine and epinephrine infusions, repeated attempts to separate the patient from CPB failed. Therefore, a left ventricular assist device (LVAD) was placed. On postoperative day 2, the patient developed acute right-sided weakness and facial palsy. A computed tomography scan revealed a large translucent defect in the territory supplied by the left middle cerebral artery.

PROBLEM ANALYSIS

Definition

Mechanical circulatory assist devices are artificial devices that perform some or all of the functions of the heart. They vary significantly in design and indication but are typically used to provide either partial or full support for a heart that is unable to function adequately. Those used for temporary support include the IABP, extracorporeal membrane oxygenation (ECMO), LVAD, and right ventricular assist device (RVAD). Those used for full support include biventricular assist device (BiVAD) and total artificial heart (TAH). Indications for mechanical assist devices are evolving but fall into three broad categories:

1. Temporary support for a heart that is expected to recover
2. Bridge therapy to cardiac transplantation
3. Destination therapy for a patient whose heart is unlikely to regain adequate function

Also, as shown in Table 98-1, devices are classified according to (1) the indication for the device (emergent versus urgent), (2) the expected duration of therapy (short versus long term), or (3) the degree of support provided (augmentation of intrinsic cardiac function versus full cardiac support).

The modern era of mechanical cardiac assist devices began in 1957, with the first successful use of CPB. Although it was first intended to provide intraoperative circulatory support, CPB's success led physicians to consider mechanical circulatory support for other indications as well. In 1966 DeBakey first used a pneumatic ventricular assist device (VAD) for a patient with left ventricular failure. In 1967 the IABP was first used to treat patients with acute heart failure, but it subsequently became a mainstay of therapy for severe, decompensated heart failure and unstable angina. In 1994 pneumatically driven VADs for partial (LVAD or RVAD) or complete (BiVAD) support of the heart were approved by the Food and Drug Administration. Today, single-chamber assist devices (e.g., IABP, LVAD, RVAD) are used to treat failure due to a wide variety of causes; dual-chamber assist devices (BiVAD, TAH) allow patients without any native heart function to survive.

Unlike an IABP or VAD, ECMO is similar to CPB because it provides both oxygenation and circulatory support, bypassing the heart and lungs altogether. Although experience with ECMO in adults is limited, venoarterial ECMO is a therapeutic option if intractable cardiovascular instability and inadequate pulmonary gas exchange are encountered after cardiac surgery. ECMO drains blood from either the arterial or venous circulation and delivers it to the arterial circulation.

Table 98–1 ■ Classification of Mechanical Assist Devices

By Indication

Urgent (unstable angina or uncontrolled congestive heart failure with worsening symptoms)
   IABP
   VAD

Emergent (hypotension incompatible with life or inability to separate from cardiopulmonary bypass)
   IABP
   VAD
   ECMO

By Duration of Therapy

Short term
   IABP
   Abiomed VAD
   ECMO

Long term
   Thoratec VAD
   Implantable VAD

By Degree of Support Provided

Augmentation (IABP)
LVAD or RVAD alone
Total support (BiVAD, ECMO)

BiVAD, biventricular assist device; ECMO, extracorporeal membrane oxygenation; IABP, intra-aortic balloon pump; LVAD, left ventricular assist device; RVAD, right ventricular assist device; VAD, ventricular assist device.

Institution of ECMO can be quick (i.e., CPB tubing can be used), but an experienced CPB perfusionist must be present to monitor and adjust anticoagulation and to troubleshoot. Although ECMO has been used successfully in children, good outcomes in adults are mostly anecdotal. Because the management of patients on ECMO is by CPB perfusionists under the supervision of cardiovascular surgeons and is confined to intensive care settings, ECMO is not discussed further here.

Recognition

INTRA-AORTIC BALLOON PUMP

The IABP is the most commonly used assist device in cardiac surgery. IABPs are inserted percutaneously or via surgical cutdown from the femoral artery. A Seldinger introducer is used for placement of the large-diameter IABP introducer sheath. The IABP catheter is passed via the introducer and positioned with its tip at the junction of the descending aorta and the aortic arch, just distal to the subclavian artery. This position minimizes the risk of subclavian or renal artery injury or occlusion. If the IABP is placed intraoperatively, TEE can determine proper balloon tip location before pump initiation. Patients with femoral atherosclerotic vascular disease may require IABP insertion into a subclavian artery or directly into the aorta with transthoracic access.

Patient suitability for IABP depends on the presence of appropriate access, the stability of the proximal descending aorta, the absence of aortic dissection, and the absence of aortic insufficiency. Perioperative indications for IABP include the following:

- Preoperative placement for patients undergoing emergent coronary artery bypass grafting or with low ejection fractions
- Intraoperative placement for left ventricular failure despite maximal inotropic support or unabated regional myocardial ischemia not amenable to surgical revascularization

The definitions used for low ejection fraction, left ventricular failure, maximal inotropic support, and ongoing regional myocardial ischemia can vary widely among institutions performing coronary artery bypass graft surgery.

Contraindications to placement of an IABP are aortic insufficiency, sepsis, and severe vascular disease. Because the IABP inflates in the descending thoracic aorta during diastole to promote retrograde flow into the ascending aorta, this has the potential to increase aortic regurgitation and further distend the left ventricle at the expense of coronary perfusion. As with any prosthetic intravascular device, infectious bacteremia is difficult to treat if surfaces of the prosthesis become seeded with bacteria. In addition to technical difficulties with placing an IABP in patients with severe vascular disease, such patients are prone to aortic rupture and thromboembolic complications (see "Risk Assessment" and "Implications").

Although use of an IABP was once considered primarily after one or more failed attempts at separation from CPB in the operating room, today the number of IABPs placed in the cardiac catheterization laboratory approaches or exceeds the number placed in the operating room in some centers.

VENTRICULAR ASSIST DEVICE

VADs are designed to completely replace the function of the native heart. They can be left-sided (LVAD), right-sided (RVAD), or biventricular (BiVAD). VADs bypass the left or right ventricle by withdrawing blood from the circulation as it enters the failing ventricle and pumping it back into the circulation immediately downstream from the failing ventricle. Flow from the patient into the VAD is from systemic (RVAD inflow) or pulmonary (LVAD inflow) venous drainage. Venous cannulas are placed in the ventricle (series cannulation) or the atria (parallel cannulation). Outflow is via pulmonary (RVAD) or systemic (LVAD) arterial cannulas. Arterial cannulas are usually placed in the aorta (LVAD), pulmonary artery (RVAD), or both (BiVAD or TAH).

The two primary types of VADs are displacement and rotary pumps. The former are used mostly in adults, and the latter are used in both children and adults. Displacement pumps can be intracorporeal or extracorporeal, designating the pumping chamber's location within or outside the body, respectively. Displacement pumps provide pulsatile flow, and rotary pumps do not. Rotary pumps are smaller in size and weight, operate more quietly, and have relatively low power consumption. However, they are more prone than displacement pumps to thrombus formation and bearing failure, which limits their longevity to several weeks.

Indications for VADs are as follows:

- *Post-CPB:* Patients with post-CPB ventricular failure that persists despite maximal pharmacologic support (often in combination with IABP support) require placement of a pneumatic VAD if they are to survive the immediate postoperative period.
- *Post–myocardial infarction:* Formerly, mortality rates associated with early VAD placement for severe left ventricular failure after acute myocardial infarction were dismal (>75%). However, more recent rates are closer to 15%. This is encouraging, given the high mortality rate reported for this patient population without such therapy.
- *Bridge to cardiac transplantation:* Technologic advances have allowed VADs to become mostly intracorporeal, with increasingly smaller extracorporeal components. Also, as the incidence of adverse side effects has declined, the acceptable duration of VAD circulatory support has increased to longer than 3 months.
- *Destination therapy:* Improved VAD portability and reduced associated morbidity have enabled more patients to survive many months with intracorporeal VADs. As a result, and because of the limited availability of human hearts, VADs are now being given serious consideration as "destination therapy" (i.e., TAH as an alternative to cardiac transplantation).

Accepted hemodynamic criteria for long-term VAD placement include the following:

- Cardiac index less than 2 L/minute per square meter
- Pulmonary capillary wedge pressure greater than 20 mm Hg
- Systolic blood pressure less than 80 mm Hg

Other considerations can also affect the decision to implant a VAD. For example, for LVADs, the status of right ventricular function is an important concern. Associated right ventricular disease (e.g., high preoperative central venous pressure, TEE evidence of right ventricular free wall hypokinesis) may be aggravated by the sudden increase in cardiac output and right ventricular preload following LVAD placement.

Risk Assessment

INTRA-AORTIC BALLOON PUMP

The incidence of IABP complications has decreased significantly since its first use, but significant associated morbidity still exists. The most frequent complications are vascular in nature, with a reported morbidity of 6% to 33%:

- Limb ischemia
- Compartment syndrome
- Mesenteric infarction
- Aortic perforation
- Aortic dissection

Risk factors for these complications include a history of peripheral vascular disease, female gender, tobacco smoking, diabetes mellitus, and postoperative IABP placement.

Other complications of IABP include infection (primarily at the groin site of the IABP introducer sheath), coagulopathies, and balloon rupture with gas embolism. The last may be related to aortic arteriosclerotic severity and associated aortic calcifications, which become increasingly severe in elderly patients.

VENTRICULAR ASSIST DEVICE

Patients who require a VAD are severely ill, and the necessary surgery is extensive. Thus, the decision to place a VAD should involve a careful, individualized evaluation of benefit, risk, and likelihood of an acceptable outcome. In addition, careful attention should be paid to patient status at the time of device placement. Although VADs are typically reserved for acute, lifesaving indications, placement during a more stable period may be better tolerated.

Ideal candidates for VAD placement are patients with preserved end-organ function. Further, post-VAD survival appears to be better in patients who are hemodynamically stable and have lower APACHE scores than in those in shock or with higher APACHE scores.

Although altered mental status and pulmonary or hepatic dysfunction do not predict outcome after VAD placement, preplacement confirmation of adequate renal function plays a critical role. For example, preplacement dependence on dialysis has been associated with 50% or more mortality after VAD placement. Additional predictors of adverse outcomes after VAD placement include age older than 65 years and the presence of multiple medical comorbidities.

Technical aspects of placement should also play a significant role in the decision to implant a VAD. Increased bleeding and poor myocardial function often accompany repeat sternotomy and CPB. Further, there may be injury to myocardial structures that adhere to the sternum or to previously placed bypass grafts. Finally, VAD cannulas have the potential to limit intrathoracic volume, prevent complete ventricular filling, and possibly decrease coronary blood flow by compressing bypass grafts.

Implications

INTRA-AORTIC BALLOON PUMP

IABP inflation exerts mechanical stress forces on the aortic wall. Therefore, known aortic dissection or a proximal aortic graft is a contraindication to IABP placement. Also, in patients with aortic insufficiency, the IABP will exacerbate regurgitant blood flow into the left ventricle during diastole, leading to ventricular dilatation and compromised coronary perfusion.

There are few restrictions to IABP use. However, it is important to remember that the IABP provides support to the left ventricle only and is unlikely to improve primary right ventricular systolic dysfunction.

Further, the IABP's ability to augment cardiac output and unload the left ventricle is limited because it does not directly alter left ventricular function. With severe left ventricular failure, an IABP will not provide enough flow to sustain the circulation, and a VAD will have to be considered.

The risk of air embolism to the brain from the IABP pressure monitoring line is greater than that from a radial or femoral arterial line. This is because the IABP monitoring port is at the tip of the balloon catheter, which resides close to the origin of the carotid arteries. Samples for blood gas determinations should be drawn from the IABP monitoring line only if there is no other suitable site. Also, one must be sure that no air bubbles or other debris is flushed through the IABP line.

Inappropriate timing of IABP inflation and deflation can worsen myocardial oxygen supply and increase myocardial oxygen balance. Early inflation (before closure of the aortic valve) can be detected by an arterial waveform demonstrating IABP inflation before the dicrotic notch and results in dramatically increased afterload, end-diastolic wall stress, and myocardial oxygen consumption. Delayed IABP inflation (after aortic valve closure) is detected by balloon inflation after the dicrotic notch and results in suboptimal coronary perfusion. Similarly, early deflation during diastole results in suboptimal coronary perfusion and afterload reduction, as well as increased myocardial oxygen consumption. Also, late deflation may lead to ineffective afterload reduction and excessive impedance of left ventricular ejection.

IABPs are foreign bodies and may promote clot formation. Although anticoagulation is not routine with IABP placement, a low degree of anticoagulation may be required to prevent thromboembolic phenomena. As with any large-bore femoral arterial access catheter, the IABP introducer sheath poses a significant infectious risk. It must be placed under strictly sterile conditions and removed as soon as possible.

VENTRICULAR ASSIST DEVICE

The venous cannula may be placed in either the ventricle (series cannulation) or the atria (parallel cannulation). Often, series cannulation allows more effective ventricular emptying, but it requires that the cannula be placed through ventricular myocardium. Although the associated myocardial trauma is less important to a transplant candidate, even a small amount of direct myocardial injury in a post-CPB patient with cardiogenic shock may significantly impede myocardial recovery.

CARDIOTHORACIC & VASCULAR SURGERY

MANAGEMENT AND PREVENTION

Intra-aortic Balloon Pump

In the United States, IABP balloon catheters are available in four lengths: 25, 34, 40, and 50 inches. The patient's height determines the appropriate length; 34 inches (for patients 64 inches tall or less) and 40 inches (for taller patients) are the most commonly used sizes. Placement of an IABP may be technically difficult in patients with extensive atherosclerosis, and these patients are more prone to arterial thrombosis during use of an IABP. Therefore, for patients with severe aortoiliac or femoral artery disease, another option is to place the balloon directly into the descending thoracic aorta. Proper balloon tip placement is 2 inches below the origin of the left subclavian artery. This is necessary to prevent occlusion of the artery during balloon inflation. Correct placement can be confirmed radiographically or by TEE.

The balloon is timed to inflate immediately after aortic valve closure (dicrotic notch, which signals aortic valve closure and the start of diastole). Inflation too early will impede left ventricular ejection. If inflation is too late, its effectiveness for increasing coronary perfusion pressure and reducing afterload will be less than optimal. Also, balloon deflation must be timed so that arterial pressure has reached its minimal level at the onset of the next ventricular systole. If it deflates too soon, the aorta will not be maximally evacuated before the next ventricular systole, and coronary perfusion will be suboptimal. If the balloon deflates too late, it will impede left ventricular ejection systole. Appropriate timing of balloon inflation and deflation is depicted in Figure 98-1.

Two methods are used to synchronize the IABP inflations with the cardiac rhythm: (1) the largest detectable ventricular electrocardiographic (ECG) signal (e.g., QRS complex) or (2) the arterial pressure waveform. If intrinsic arterial pulse pressure is greater than 40 mm Hg, the arterial waveform is preferred in the operating room because electrocautery artifact can inhibit some ECG-triggered IABP consoles. However, this has become less of a problem with the incorporation of electronic artifact suppression circuitry that makes IABPs less susceptible to electrocautery inference. Further, contemporary IABP consoles can differentiate pacing artifacts, thereby allowing proper balloon inflation timing, even if atrial or ventricular pacing is used.

Balloon inflation is often initiated at a ratio of 1:2 (one IABP beat for every two cardiac beats). Thus, natural and augmented ventricular beats can be compared to determine IABP timing and efficacy. Depending on the patient's condition, the ratio may be increased to 1:1 to produce maximal augmentation, or it may be decreased to 1:3, 1:4, or less during weaning. Typically, the volume of balloon inflation is set at 50% to 60% of the patient's ideal stroke volume. Overinflation risks balloon rupture and arterial gas embolization.

During extended use of IABP, anticoagulation is generally indicated. However, in the early postoperative period, anticoagulation may not be instituted until the chest tube drainage is acceptable (<100 to 150 mL/hour). Some surgeons prefer low-molecular-weight dextran to heparin because its antithrombogenic effects are fairly mild, even though no specific reversal agent exists.

Ventricular Assist Device

Patients with valvular dysfunction or artificial heart valves are challenges to VAD placement. The cannulas should be

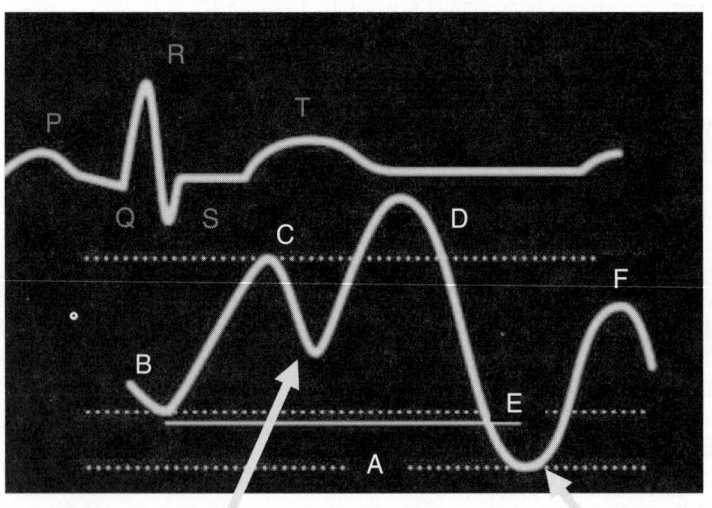

A = cardiac cycle

B = unassisted aortic end-diastolic pressure (EDP)

C = unassisted systole

D = diastolic augmentation

E = reduced aortic EDP

F = reduced systolic pressure

Figure 98–1 ■ Appropriate timing of IABP balloon inflation and deflation. (Adapted from Rao V, Slater JP, Edwards NM, et al: Surgical management of valvular heart disease in patients requiring left ventricular assist device support. Ann Thorac Surg 71:1448-1453, 2001.)

Inflation occurs at the onset of diastole (aortic valve closure—i.e., dicrotic notch), giving rise to the sharp V wave on the arterial waveform. This leads to increased coronary perfusion.

Deflation occurs at the end of diastole prior to systole, resulting in reduced aortic end-diastolic and systolic pressures. This leads to decreased afterload, myocardial oxygen consumption (MVO_2), and increased cardiac output.

aligned such that there is maximal flow across the mechanical valve. There is also some evidence that maximizing flow across the valves (valve washing) by adjusting VAD flow rates (depending on myocardial recovery) may decrease the incidence of thrombus formation. If aortic valve insufficiency is present, regurgitant flow may prevent a VAD from effectively decompressing the left ventricle to reduce myocardial oxygen consumption. Inadequate decompression is particularly problematic when aortic insufficiency is severe and with apical versus left atrial LVAD placement. Because VAD placement can (and is expected to) reduce left atrial and left ventricular pressures, atrial and ventricular septal defects should be identified and repaired before VAD placement to prevent potentially dangerous right-to-left shunting.

The presence of native or prosthetic valvular heart disease can complicate VAD placement. Severe mitral stenosis limits VAD filling during serial cannulation and may result in restricted VAD flow. In contrast, VAD placement in patients with mitral regurgitation results in complete unloading of the left ventricle and improved valve function. Aortic stenosis alone is not a contraindication to placement of an LVAD. However, aortic insufficiency will allow regurgitant blood flow from the VAD outflow cannula across the incompetent aortic valve to distend the left ventricle and compromise end-organ perfusion. Even mild to moderate aortic insufficiency may become more severe with institution of LVAD support.

Because inflow and outflow VAD cannulas must be placed in the thoracic cavity, they may compromise cardiac filling in the early postoperative period. Therefore, most VADs are approved for use in patients with a body surface area greater than 1.5 m² or weighing more than 42 kg. Often, left ventricular preload improves over 12 to 24 hours as intrathoracic contents shift to accommodate the VAD cannulas.

Anticoagulation is usually required with most VAD devices except the HeartMate LVAS (for left ventricular assist system; Thoratec Laboratories, Pleasanton, Calif.). The goal for anticoagulation is the same as for patients with prosthetic valves. The usual practice is to start heparin after postoperative bleeding from the chest tubes is less than 50 mL/hour and then to switch to warfarin after adequate anticoagulation has been obtained. With the HeartMate LVAS, only aspirin (80 mg/day) is required after the initial postoperative bleeding has subsided.

Infectious complications of VAD placement are classified into two types: device related and non–device related. Non-device-related infections include pneumonia, urinary tract infection and sepsis. Device-related infections tend to involve the blood-contacting surface of the VAD, the outer surface of an implanted VAD, or the VAD inflow or outflow cannulas. Because the VAD cannot be removed, all infections with the potential for VAD colonization are potentially life threatening. Usually, *Staphylococcus*, *Pseudomonas*, *Enterococcus*, or *Candida* species are the offending agents, but other infectious causes have been described.

Patient risk factors for infectious complications include preoperative infection, malnutrition, immunosuppressive medications (steroids), mechanical ventilation, and intravascular catheters. It is imperative to correct as many of these factors as possible before device implantation. Further, all vascular access lines and drains should be removed as soon as possible, drive-line sites should be inspected routinely, and aseptic conditions should be aggressively maintained during dressing changes. Treatment depends on the type of infection. Pocket infections may require surgical drainage. VAD-related endocarditis is extremely challenging. Often, the VAD must be explanted and replaced, with all the attendant complications of reoperation.

Many patients requiring VAD implantation for left ventricular failure have coexistent pulmonary disease and pulmonary hypertension. For such patients, placement of an LVAD may result in inadequate VAD flow rates due to right ventricular failure and reduced blood flow to the left ventricle, where the inflow cannula is located. In these patients, careful attention to factors influencing pulmonary vascular resistance (e.g., hypoxemia, hypercarbia, acidosis, bronchospasm, vasopressors) is important to reduce the likelihood of right ventricular failure. In extreme cases, an RVAD may be necessary to ensure adequate blood return to the LVAD.

Further Reading

Baskett RJF, Ghali WA, Maitland A, et al: The intraaortic balloon pump in cardiac surgery. Ann Thorac Surg 74:1276-1287, 2002.

Datascope Cardiac Assist CS100. Datascope Corporation, Cardiac Assist Division, Fairfield, NJ. Available at http://www.datascope.com/ca/caeducmaterials.html.

Frazier OH, Delgado RM: Mechanical circulatory support for advanced heart failure: Where does it stand in 2003? Circulation 108:3064-3068, 2003.

Harter RL, Michler RE: Circulatory assist devices. In Hensley FA Jr, Martin DE, Gravlee GP (eds): Practical Approach to Cardiac Anesthesia, 3rd ed. Philadelphia, JB Lippincott–Williams & Wilkins, 2003, pp 557-573.

Holman WL, Rayburn BK, McGiffin DC, et al: Infection in ventricular assist devices: Prevention and treatment. Ann Thorac Surg 75:S48-S57, 2003.

Ko W, Jin C, Chen RJ, et al: Extracorporeal membrane oxygenation support for adult postcardiotomy shock. Ann Thorac Surg 73:538-545, 2002.

Loebe M, Koerner MM, Lafuente JA, et al: Patient selection for assist devices: Bridge to transplant. Curr Opin Cardiol 18:141-146, 2003.

Melhorn U, Kroner A, deVivie ER: 30 Years of clinical intra-aortic balloon pumping: Facts and figures. Thorac Cardiovasc Surg 47(Suppl 2): 298-303, 1999.

Rao V, Slater JP, Edwards NM, et al: Surgical management of valvular heart disease in patients requiring left ventricular assist device support. Ann Thorac Surg 71:1448-1453, 2001.

Rose EA, Gelijns AC, Moskowitz AJ, et al: Randomized Evaluation of Mechanical Assistance for the Treatment of Congestive Heart Failure (REMATCH) study group: Long-term mechanical left ventricular assistance for end-stage heart failure. N Engl J Med 345:1435-1443, 2001.

Smedira NG, Blackstone EH: Postcardiotomy mechanical support: Risk factors and outcomes. Ann Thorac Surg 71:S60-S66, 2001.

Smith C, Bellomo R, Raman JS, et al: An extracorporeal membrane oxygenation-based approach to cardiogenic shock in an older population. Ann Thorac Surg 71:1421-1427, 2001.

Thoratec TLC-II VAD Portable Driver and System Operator's Manual, rev ed. Pleasanton, Calif, Thoratec Corporation, 2004. Available at www.thoratec.com.

Tisol WB, Mueller DK, Hoy FB, et al: Ventricular assist device use with mechanical heart valves: An outcome series and literature review. Ann Thorac Surg 72:2051-2055, 2001.

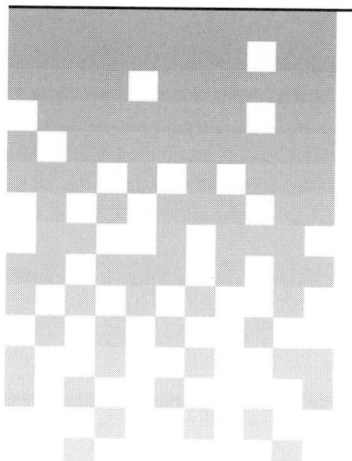

Physiologic Imbalance and Coexisting Disease

Michael J. Murray

Michael F. O'Connor

PHYSIOLOGIC AND METABOLIC IMBALANCE

Hyperglycemia and Diabetic Ketoacidosis

99

Martin L. De Ruyter and Barry A. Harrison

Case Synopsis

A 75-year-old woman with type 2 diabetes mellitus, controlled by glyburide 5 mg twice a day, presents for scheduled coronary artery bypass grafting. She has diabetic nephropathy with a serum creatinine of 1.8 mg/dL. The patient did not take her oral antidiabetic medication before surgery, and her fasting plasma glucose was 130 mg/dL. After cardiopulmonary bypass, the intraoperative plasma glucose was 236 mg/dL. There was a brisk diuresis. The serum potassium was 5.8 mEq/L with a base deficit of −4.0 mEq/dL. The patient received furosemide and mannitol while on cardiopulmonary bypass and repeated doses of cardioplegia. Cardiopulmonary bypass took 130 minutes.

PROBLEM ANALYSIS

Definition

Hyperglycemia in adults is defined as a random plasma glucose level greater than 200 mg/dL, but this definition does not reflect today's target for glucose control. Perioperative plasma glucose levels are determined by many factors, including preoperative glucose and nutritional status, metabolic activity, catecholamines, cortisol, glucagon, and insulin levels.

At times of illness or acute severe stress, hyperglycemia may be present; this is referred to as hyperglycemic stress syndrome. In some patients this may reflect the unmasking of an abnormality of glucose tolerance, which should be treated to reduce the risk of increased morbidity and mortality. The patient should subsequently be reevaluated and reclassified after recovering from surgery or acute illness. A similar approach is used in the management of gestational diabetes.

Diabetes mellitus (DM) is a chronic, multisystem disease heralded by signs and symptoms of persistent hyperglycemia and confirmed by a random plasma glucose level greater than 200 mg/dL, a fasting plasma glucose level greater than 126 mg/dL, or a plasma glucose level of 200 mg/dL or greater based on 2-hour postprandial testing or 2 hours following an oral glucose tolerance test. In the absence of acute metabolic decompensation or severe hyperglycemia, these criteria should be reconfirmed at least 24 hours apart. Type 1 DM is due to a failure to produce endogenous insulin. Type 2 DM is a metabolic syndrome characterized by relative degrees of reduced insulin secretion, increased insulin receptor resistance, and increased glucose availability. Impaired glucose tolerance is defined as a 2-hour postprandial or glucose tolerance test plasma glucose level between 140 and 200 mg/dL. Normal values for plasma glucose are given in Table 99-1.

Diabetic ketoacidosis is usually associated with type 1 DM. It generally occurs in the setting of absent insulin, poor glucose utilization, and often some pathologic stressor (e.g., illness, infection, trauma). The body attempts to preserve energy stores via gluconeogenesis, which is the mobilization of fats and amino acids into glucose-producing pathways, resulting in hyperglycemia and ketosis (Fig. 99-1).

Nonketotic hyperosmolar syndrome occurs in type 2 diabetics with insufficient production of insulin or altered receptor sensitivity to insulin. Endogenous insulin is present in sufficient quantities to prevent these patients from developing ketoacidosis; however, they present with an anion gap metabolic acidosis secondary to lactic acidosis. This acid-base derangement occurs as a result of cellular hypoxia, likely due to hypovolemia, inadequate organ perfusion, or a shock state. Nonketotic hyperosmolar syndrome is characterized by severe hyperosmolarity (>320 mOsm/L), hyperglycemia (>600 mg/dL), and marked dehydration.

Recognition

Preoperatively, clinical symptoms and signs of hyperglycemia may be absent or vary widely. One third of patients with DM are unaware that they have the condition. Symptoms and signs include the following:

- Polyphagia
- Polydipsia

Table 99–1 ■ Normal Values for Plasma Glucose

Fasting plasma glucose: <100 mg/dL
Peak plasma glucose*: <200 mg/dL
2-hr postprandial glucose: <140 mg/dL

*After glucose tolerance testing.

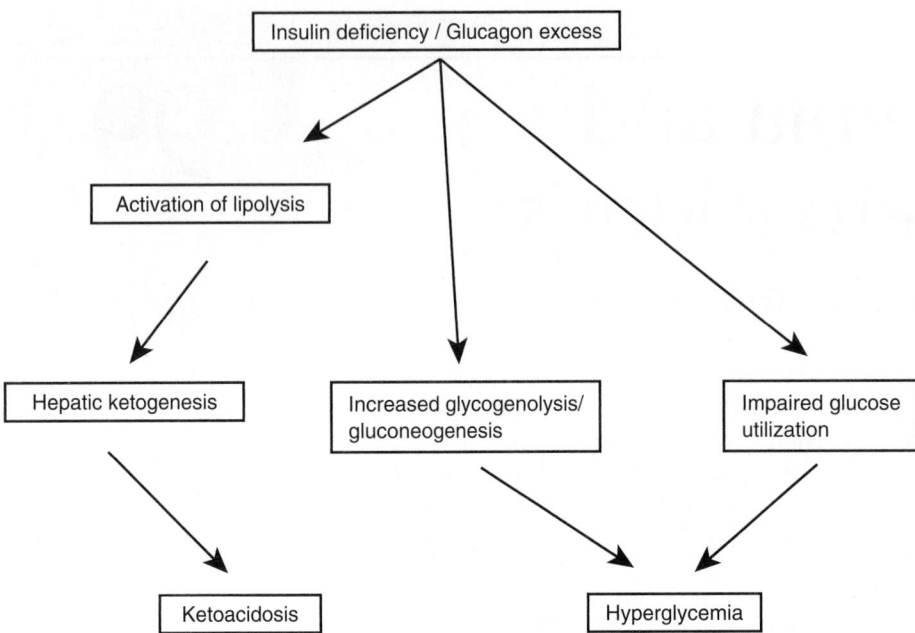

Figure 99–1 ▪ Pathogenesis of diabetic ketoacidosis.

- Polyuria
- Confusion
- Coma

Intraoperative signs are as follows:

- Unexplained diuresis
- Tachycardia and hypotension
- Anion gap metabolic acidosis
- Hyponatremia and hyperkalemia

Frequently hyperglycemia is first recognized by an increased plasma blood glucose level.

Risk Assessment

Causes of perioperative hyperglycemia are listed in Table 99-2. Emergency surgery increases the risk of type 1 diabetics developing diabetic ketoacidosis and type 2 diabetics developing nonketotic hyperosmolar syndrome. In emergency situations (e.g., trauma), patients may miss their usual insulin dose, interrupt their usual caloric intake, or encounter excessive pathologic stresses, which alter the normal counterregulatory hormone balance. The patient's inability to increase insulin production results in hyperglycemia.

DM is associated with significant complications, including retinopathy, neuropathy, gastropathy, and nephropathy. DM also accelerates atherosclerosis, leading to increased coronary artery disease, cerebrovascular disease, and peripheral vascular disease.

Implications

The effects of hyperglycemia are related to the severity and duration of increased plasma glucose levels.

Cellular. Hyperglycemia leads to nonenzymatic glycosylation of immunoglobulins, granulocyte dysfunction, and reduction

of both CD4 and CD8 lymphocyte populations. It also exaggerates ischemia-reperfusion cellular injury, induces cardiac cell death, and reduces coronary collateral blood flow. Hyperglycemia induces platelet hyperreactivity, which increases thrombosis, and it increases levels of interleukin-6, interleukin-8, and tumor necrosis factor-α, reflecting

Table 99–2 ▪ **Causes of Perioperative Hyperglycemia**
Diabetes mellitus (types 1 and 2)
Dextrose-containing intravenous fluids
Maintenance solutions or parenteral nutrition
Medications
Catecholamine-induced stress response
Burns
Trauma
Surgery
Sepsis
Stroke
Pain
Cardiopulmonary bypass
Excess counterregulatory hormones
Cushing's disease or syndrome
Pheochromocytoma
Acromegaly
Glucagonoma
Drugs
Thiazide diuretics
Glucocorticosteroids
Phenytoin
Pentamidine
β-Adrenergic receptor blockers
Oral contraceptives
Pancreatic disease
Pancreatitis or pancreatic trauma
Hemochromatosis
Pregnancy

a proinflammatory action. Hyperglycemia and insulin resistance lead to endothelial cell dysfunction, inactivation of nitric oxide, decreased synthesis of prostacyclin, and increased synthesis of endothelin-1, which all lead to decreased local blood flow.

Renal. Blood glucose levels in excess of 250 mg/dL overwhelm renal tubular absorption capabilities, which leads to hypovolemia secondary to an osmotic diuresis. A profound diuresis may result in prerenal azotemia, altered organ perfusion, cellular hypoxia, and lactic acidosis.

Cerebral. Patients with DM or newly recognized hyperglycemia are at increased risk for severe strokes and increased mortality. A meta-analysis of studies of stroke patients found increased mortality in patients with blood glucose levels of 110 to 126 mg/dL. Serum osmolarity greater than 330 mOsm/L is associated with central neurologic dysfunction and coma.

Cardiovascular. A meta-analysis of patients admitted for acute myocardial infarction, with or without a prior diagnosis of DM, found that hyperglycemia (>110 mg/dL) was associated with increased hospital mortality and congestive heart failure.

Inpatients. Newly noted hyperglycemia in medical and surgical inpatients resulted in an 18-fold increase in hospital mortality and longer hospital stays.

Major Surgery. Thirty percent to 40% of cardiac surgical patients have DM. Hyperglycemia is associated with increased mortality and deep-seated infections in cardiac surgical patients.

Critical Illness. In 1826 critically ill patients, there was a direct and proportional correlation between increasing blood glucose levels and mortality.

MANAGEMENT

Intraoperative Hyperglycemia

In December 2003 the American Association of Clinical Endocrinologists published a position statement on inpatient diabetes and metabolic control. For intensive care unit patients (including cardiac, vascular, thoracic, and major surgical patients), the consensus as to the tolerable upper limit for glucose is 110 mg/dL. For non–critically ill patients, the consensus is 110 mg/dL for preprandial plasma glucose levels and 180 mg/dL for maximal glucose levels. During the perioperative period, intravenous (IV) infusion of insulin is advocated. In hospitalized patients, high IV doses of insulin may be necessary to achieve acceptable plasma glucose levels. Studies have demonstrated that the use of standardized protocols, developed by multidisciplinary teams, can successfully control hyperglycemia, decrease hypoglycemia, decrease length of stay, and improve outcome in diabetic patients. A continuous IV insulin infusion algorithm is presented in Table 99-3. Subcutaneous regular insulin is not advocated in the critically ill and those undergoing major surgery but may find applications in less severe cases. Table 99-4 illustrates a regimen of regular insulin dosing via the subcutaneous route.

Table 99–3 ■ Algorithm for Continuous Intravenous Infusion of Insulin*

Blood Glucose (mg/dL)	Insulin Infusion Rate (U/hr)
>400	8
351-400	6
301-350	4
250-300	3
200-249	2.5
150-199	2
120-149	1.5
100-119	1
70-99	0
<70	0

*Algorithm is designed for the average 70-kg patient. Adjustments should be based on hourly glucose determinations.

Diabetic Ketoacidosis

Diabetic ketoacidosis is a medical emergency. Initial assessment includes the following:

- Identification of the precipitating event—infection, ischemia, missed insulin administration
- Volume status
  - Tachycardia, hypotension
  - Increased urea and creatinine
- Mental status—cerebral edema
- Hyperglycemia—increased plasma glucose and urine glucose
- Ketosis—increased serum ketones and β-hydroxybutyrate
- Increased anion gap acidosis
  - Increased respiratory rate (Kussmaul's respiration)
  - Serum bicarbonate <15 mEq/dL; pH <7.3
- Potassium—initially increased secondary to metabolic acidosis, but decreased total potassium stores
- Sodium—laboratory measurement secondary to hyperglycemia

Fluid resuscitation, IV insulin administration, and correction of electrolytes are crucial.

Fluid Resuscitation. The fluid deficit is often between 4 and 8 L of sodium and free water. Initial resuscitation includes infusion of normal saline (0.9% NaCl). Within the first 2 hours, patients should receive enough fluid to stabilize their hemodynamic parameters (usually 2 to 3 L of non-glucose-containing crystalloid solution). After initial rehydration with isotonic saline, subsequent administration of

Table 99–4 ■ Subcutaneous Supplementation of Regular Insulin

Blood Glucose (mg/dL)	Regular Insulin Dose (U)*
200-250	2
251-300	4
301-350	6
>350	8

*Subcutaneous insulin dosing is approximately every 4 to 6 hr.

0.45% normal saline should be started, because free water loss typically exceeds the natriuresis. Once blood glucose levels have declined to less than 250 mg/dL, 5% dextrose is added to the IV fluids to maintain acceptable glucose levels and reduce the risk of cerebral edema. Infusions with hypotonic fluid may cause cerebral edema secondary to reverse osmotic shifts. Hypertonic solutions have no role because they may worsen the acidosis, dehydration, and hyperosmolar state.

Insulin Therapy. Regular insulin is administered as a bolus (0.1 to 0.2 unit/kg), followed by a continuous IV insulin infusion (0.1 unit/kg per hour) and hourly determinations of blood glucose levels. Additional glucose supplementation may be necessary, but care must be taken to avoid hypoglycemia. Blood glucose levels of 200 to 250 mg/dL are a reasonable initial goal. As the patient improves, titration to 150 to 200 mg/dL should be the goal. A continuous IV infusion algorithm is presented in Table 99-3.

Metabolic Acidosis. The administration of bicarbonate is controversial. A paradoxical rebound central nervous system acidosis can be observed with excessive bicarbonate therapy. IV bicarbonate replacement should be reserved for patients with an arterial pH less than 7.0 after initial rehydration, and it should be discontinued once the pH rises above this value.

Electrolytes. Serum potassium may be elevated despite a depletion in total body stores. Hyperglycemic osmotic diuresis causes systemic potassium wasting (up to 10 mEq/kg), whereas an extracellular shift in potassium secondary to metabolic acidosis results in an elevated serum concentration. Provided the patient's urine output is adequate, acute renal failure is not evident, and a normal serum potassium level is documented, potassium should be repleted promptly. In general, replacement with potassium chloride at a rate of 20 to 30 mEq/hour should be sufficient. Electrocardiographic monitoring is recommended during repletion of potassium. Measured hyponatremia is a laboratory phenomenon secondary to the dilutional effect of hyperglycemia. In general, for each 100 mg/dL increase in glucose above normal levels, serum sodium levels decrease by 1.6 to 2.0 mEq/L. No specific therapy is required other than correction of the hyperosmolar state. Phosphate levels may be depleted because this anion is excreted with osmotic diuresis. Routine replacement is controversial because rapid replacement can cause hypocalcemia. Phosphate replacement should be guided by periodic surveillance of magnesium, calcium, and phosphate levels.

PREVENTION

Diabetes affects 18.2 million Americans and is the seventh leading cause of death in the United States. Preoperatively, random plasma glucose testing is advised for patients older than 60 years and those with symptoms or with DM. Diabetic patients need a complete medical evaluation to detect diabetic complications and comorbidities. Oral agents need to be stopped before surgery. Long-acting sulfonylureas or chlorpropamide are stopped for at least 72 hours, whereas shorter-acting sulfonylureas and metformin are stopped the night before surgery.

For type 1 DM patients and patients with uncontrolled type 2 DM, it is essential to administer insulin. The aim of any regimen is to maintain good control without hypoglycemia. It also must be practical and easy to use as the patient is transferred from the ward to the operating room, to the recovery room, and back to the ward. It is important to monitor plasma glucose at frequent intervals. One regimen that fulfills all these criteria is the continuous IV administration of regular insulin. With an increasing number of type 1 DM patients on continuous subcutaneous insulin maintenance, the use of a continuous IV infusion perioperatively is advised. For stable type 2 DM patients having minor or moderately stressful surgery, oral therapy can resume postoperatively. Unless insulin is part of a type 2 diabetic patient's usual regimen, it can be reserved for glucose levels exceeding 180 mg/dL.

Further Reading

American College of Endocrinology position statement on inpatient diabetes and metabolic control. Endocr Pract 10:77-82, 2004.

Clement S, Braithwaite SS, Mangee MF, et al: Management of diabetes and hyperglycemia in hospitals. Diabetes Care 27:553-591, 2004.

Coursin DB, Connery LE, Ketzler JT: Perioperative diabetic and hyperglycemic management issues. Crit Care Med 32:S116-S125, 2004.

Expert Committee on the Diagnosis and Classification of Diabetes Mellitus: Report of the Expert Committee on the Diagnosis and Classification of Diabetes Mellitus. Diabetes Care 20:1183-1197, 1997.

Furnary AP, Gao G, Grunkemeier GL, et al: Continuous insulin infusion reduces mortality in patients with diabetes undergoing coronary artery bypass grafting. J Thorac Cardiovasc Surg 125:1007-1021, 2003.

Malmberg K, Norhammar A, Wedel H, Rydén L: Glycometabolic state at admission: Important risk marker of mortality in conventionally treated patients with diabetes mellitus and acute myocardial infarction: Long-term results from the Diabetes and Insulin-Glucose Infusion in Acute Myocardial Infarction (DIGAMI) study. Circulation 99:2626-2632, 1999.

Pittas AG, Siegel RD, Lau J: Insulin therapy for critically ill hospitalized patients: A meta-analysis of randomized controlled trials. Arch Intern Med 164:2005-2011, 2004.

Savage MW, Mah PM, Weetman AP, Newell-Price J: Endocrine emergencies Postgrad Med J 80:506-515, 2004.

Van den Berghe G, Wouters P, Weekers F, et al: Intensive insulin therapy in critically ill patients. N Engl J Med 345:1359-1367, 2001.

Wass T, Lanier W: Glucose modulation of ischemic brain injury: Review and clinical recommendations. Mayo Clin Proc 71:801-812, 1996.

Hypothermia

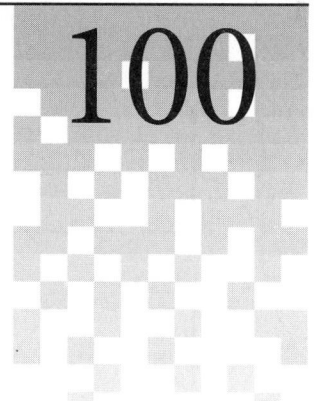

Christopher C. Young and Robert N. Sladen

Case Synopsis

A 74-year-old woman with insulin-dependent diabetes mellitus is found several hours after a fall. She is admitted for emergency surgery with epidural and general anesthesia for repair of a fractured hip. She receives 4 units of packed red blood cells. In the postanesthesia care unit, she is confused and disoriented after tracheal extubation. Her heart rate is 110 beats per minute; blood pressure, 160/90 mm Hg; temperature, 33.8°C (oral); arterial oxygen tension (PaO_2), 63 mm Hg; and arterial carbon dioxide tension ($PaCO_2$), 54 mm Hg (on nasal oxygen at a rate of 6 L/minute).

PROBLEM ANALYSIS

Definition

Normal body temperature is 37°C (98.6°F). Hypothermia is classified as mild to moderate (33°C to 36°C), severe (23°C to 33°C), or profound (<23°C). Accidental (Table 100-1) or iatrogenic (Table 100-2) causes may contribute to hypothermia.

The patient in the case synopsis is at increased risk for hypothermia owing to the following factors:

- Age-impaired thermoregulatory responses
- Anesthesia-impaired thermoregulatory responses
- Ambient factors (e.g., cold environment, air conditioning)

Age-related impairment involves decreased perception of cold, decreased ability to prevent heat loss (blunted vasoconstrictor response), and diminished ability to increase heat production (reduced muscle mass). Microvascular atheroma and diabetic autonomic neuropathy also impair thermoregulatory vasoconstriction in response to cold.

General and regional anesthesia disrupts physiologic thermoregulatory responses (Fig. 100-1). For example, the hypothermic vasoconstriction threshold (about 37°C) is suppressed 2°C to 4°C in a dose-dependent manner by volatile or opioid anesthesia, with significantly greater suppression occurring in the elderly. Regional anesthesia induces a sympathetic blockade that prevents vasoconstriction in the affected dermatomes, and heat generation from muscle activity is reduced in proportion to the extent of segmental motor blockade. Spinal thermoregulatory centers may be depressed by central neuraxial anesthesia or analgesia. Shivering is abolished by anesthetic agents and neuromuscular blocking agents. Conversely, physiologic thermoregulatory responses to warmth (i.e., vasodilatation and sweating) are also suppressed by anesthetic agents, such that their thresholds are elevated about 1°C above normal.

The *interthreshold range* is the range of core temperatures within which no physiologic responses are evoked. Normally, this is very narrow (about 0.5°C). However, from Figure 100-1, it is apparent that anesthesia widens the interthreshold range to as much as 4°C. This implies, for example, that the central temperature could vary from 34°C to 38°C without any physiologic responses to conserve or eliminate heat. Within this range, the patient is poikilothermic (i.e., the central temperature varies directly with ambient temperature).

This and the widespread use of air conditioning in operating rooms put anesthetized patients at high risk for inadvertent hypothermia.[1] Also, heat balance is the sum of heat production and loss, with heat production (via exercise or metabolism) negligible during anesthesia. In fact, heat loss dominates due to the following physical factors, in decreasing order of importance:

- Radiation (heat exchange from one surface to another), such as from the skin or mucosa to the colder environment of the operating room

---

[1]Before air conditioning was introduced, inadvertent hyperthermia was not uncommon.

Table 100-1 ▪ Accidental Causes of Hypothermia

Environmental
Wind chill
Cold water immersion

Impaired Thermoregulation
Extremes of age (neonates, elderly)
Prolonged immobilization
Drugs
   Alcohol
   Central nervous system depressants
   Drug overdose

Medical Conditions
Hypothyroidism
Large body surface area burns
Infection or sepsis
Malnutrition
Hypoglycemia
Hypothalamic stroke or tumor
Unconsciousness

Table 100-2 ▪ Iatrogenic Causes of Hypothermia

Prolonged anesthesia and surgery
Prolonged cardiopulmonary resuscitation
Blood or blood product transfusions*
Large-volume fluid resuscitation*

*Without adequate warming.

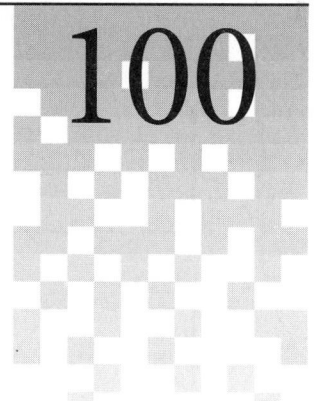

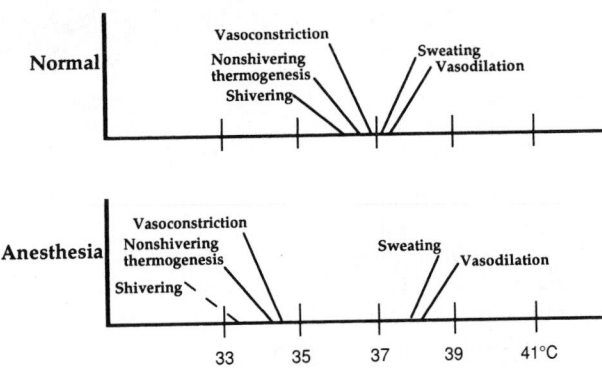

Figure 100–1 ■ Schematic illustration of thermoregulatory thresholds in nonanesthetized (normal) and anesthetized humans. The intersection of each regulatory response (e.g., shivering, sweating) with the temperature scale (core body temperature) is the threshold. The interthreshold range is shown as the distance between the first cold response (vasoconstriction) and the first warm response (sweating); temperatures within this range do not elicit autonomic thermoregulatory compensation. Because each thermoregulatory response has its own threshold and gain, there is an orderly progression of responses, and response intensities, in proportion to need. During general anesthesia *(bottom)*, the thresholds for vasoconstriction and nonshivering thermogenesis are shifted down to 34.5°C (depending on anesthetic type and dose). Similarly, thresholds for active precapillary vasodilatation and sweating are increased about 1°C. Interthreshold range thus increases from 0.2°C to about 4°C. (From Sessler DI: Temperature monitoring. In Miller RD [ed]: Anesthesia, 4th ed. New York, Churchill Livingstone, 1994, pp 1363-1382.)

- Evaporation (heat lost by the movement of molecules from liquid to gas phase), such as from cold skin preparation and irrigation solutions, and evaporative loss from exposed body serosal surfaces
- Convection (heat lost by eddy currents), such as from drafts and the infusion of cold blood and fluids
- Conduction (heat exchanged by direct molecular contact), such as from the skin to the cold operating table

Recognition

During general and regional anesthesia, intraoperative hypothermia has three distinct stages:

1. Internal redistribution: abrupt decline of about 0.5°C to 1.0°C in central temperature caused by redistribution of heat from the warm central core to the cold periphery due to anesthetic-induced peripheral vasodilatation. The colder the skin at anesthetic induction, the greater the central temperature decline.
2. Environmental heat loss: passive heat loss by radiation, evaporation, convection, and conduction continues to the extent that physiologic responses are depressed, usually to about a central temperature of 34°C to 35°C. Advanced age and diabetes can contribute to depression of the vasoconstrictor threshold to less than 34°C, as in the patient described in the case synopsis.
3. Plateau phase: once thermoregulatory vasoconstriction is evoked, heat loss becomes constrained, and the central temperature reaches a plateau. However, further declines can be caused by massive blood loss and transfusion, for example.

Risk Assessment and Implications

Hypothermia may benefit the patient by providing organ protection against ischemia. Oxygen utilization is halved for each 10°C decrease in normal body temperature. Mild hypothermia (33°C to 36°C) provides important central nervous system protection. There is increasing evidence that it may play a protective role after stroke and cardiac arrest due to ventricular fibrillation.

Even mild hypothermia induces platelet dysfunction and may increase intraoperative bleeding. Platelet thromboxane generation, required for platelet aggregation and local hemostatic vasoconstriction, is impaired by cold. Quantitative laboratory assessment is misleading because blood samples are warmed to 37°C. Massive transfusion of cold blood can induce severe hypothermic coagulopathy with irreversible bleeding. There is now evidence that even mild intraoperative hypothermia may increase the risk for postoperative wound infection, possibly due to vasoconstriction with low tissue oxygen tension. This impairs chemotaxis and facilitates bacterial growth.

Severe hypothermia (<33°C) has adverse effects on almost every organ system (Table 100-3; Fig. 100-2).

Emergence from anesthesia may be delayed by a number of cold-induced factors, including impairment of central nervous system function (e.g., obtundation, confusion, somnolence), slowed hepatic or renal clearance of anesthetic drugs and neuromuscular blocking agents, and impaired ventilatory response to hypoxemia and hypercarbia.

Cold-induced vasoconstriction and increased systemic vascular resistance may exacerbate postoperative hypertension (blood pressure of 160/90 mm Hg in the patient in the case synopsis is characteristic). Together with high norepinephrine concentrations, both may produce myocardial ischemia in susceptible patients.

The consequences of rewarming from hypothermia may outweigh the implications of hypothermia itself. Postoperative shivering greatly increases oxygen demand and carbon dioxide production, leading to increased minute ventilation, work of breathing, and oxygen consumption. If minute ventilation is fixed (mechanical ventilation) or suppressed (by anesthetic agents or opioids), hypercarbia and acute respiratory acidosis may result. When oxygen consumption is increased but cardiac output cannot compensate, oxygen extraction increases, setting the stage for hypoxemia and its sequelae. Shivering can also cause patient discomfort and other adverse sequelae, such as wound disruption and increased bleeding or intracranial and intraocular pressures.

Subsequently, rewarming vasodilatation may unmask hypovolemia, resulting in even more dangerous hypotension and tachycardia.

MANAGEMENT AND PREVENTION

The management and prevention of hypothermia are inseparable and include the following.

- Preoperative skin warming
- Adjusted ambient temperature in the operating room
- Intraoperative temperature monitoring

Table 100–3 ■ Adverse Effects of Hypothermia on Organ System Function

Cardiovascular

Early: tachycardia, hypertension, increased cardiac output, vasoconstriction (catecholamine release)
Late: bradycardia, decreased cardiac output, hypotension
ECG: Generalized slow conduction, sinus bradycardia, T-wave inversion, Q-T prolongation, ventricular ectopy (32°C, Osborne waves; 30°C, ventricular fibrillation; see Fig. 100–2)

Respiratory

Early: increased respiratory rate
Late: reduced respiratory rate and tidal volume, diminished hypoxic pulmonary vasoconstriction and responsiveness to hypoxemia and hypercarbia, diminished mucociliary activity

Renal

Early: initial "cold" diuresis (increased central blood volume with peripheral vasoconstriction); diuresis continues due to impaired renal tubular sodium reabsorption
Late: oliguria and azotemia

Hematologic

Early: hemoconcentration, increased viscosity (sludging, poor tissue perfusion, ischemia), decreased oxygen availability (left shift of oxyhemoglobin dissociation curve)
Late: disseminated intravascular coagulation, thrombocytopenia

Metabolic

Early: hyponatremia, hyperkalemia, hyperglycemia (inhibition of insulin release and block of its cellular uptake)
Late: metabolic acidosis

Neurologic

Cerebral blood flow decreases 6% to 7% per 1°C decrease in temperature:
   34°C: amnesia
   30°C: obtundation
   26°C: loss of pupillary and deep tendon reflexes
   18°C: loss of brain activity (isoelectric electroencephalogram)

Gastrointestinal

Early: decreased intestinal motility (full stomach), diminished hepatic clearance
Late: ulceration of stomach, ileum, and colon; hemorrhagic pancreatitis

ECG, electrocardiogram.

- Heated and humidified anesthesia circuits
- Forced-air warming blankets and other devices
- Warmed intravenous fluids and blood products
- Postoperative mechanical ventilation
- Prevention and treatment of postoperative shivering
- Anticipation and treatment of rewarming vasodilatation

A simple way to prevent redistribution hypothermia is to warm the patient's skin before anesthetic induction. In many cases, warming with a forced-air blanket can be initiated in the preoperative holding area or preinduction room. Before anesthetic induction, the ambient temperature in the operating room should be increased to 23°C to 26°C to maintain normothermia. Once the patient is fully draped and protected, the temperature can be decreased so that it does not impair the performance of the surgeon or assistants. Ambient room temperature should be increased again at the end of the operation.

Temperature monitoring is mandatory for all procedures lasting 30 minutes or longer. However, "normal" temperature (like blood pressure) depends on where it is measured. Monitors for core body temperature include the tympanic membrane (susceptible to injury), nasopharynx (influenced by anesthetic gas temperature), esophagus

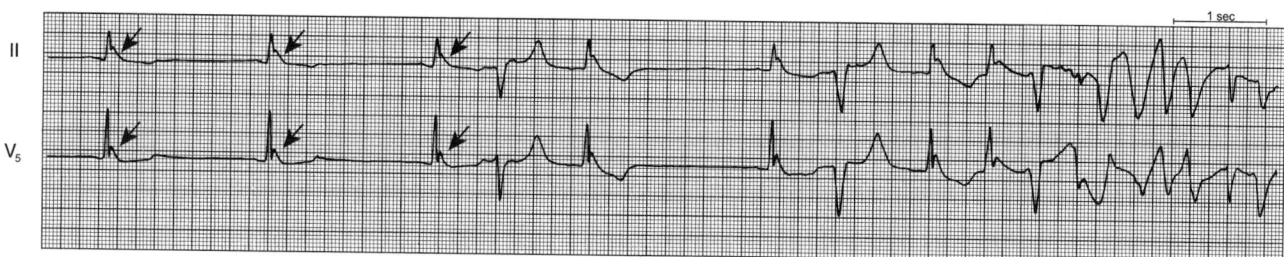

Figure 100–2 ■ Two electrocardiographic leads obtained during cooling with cardiopulmonary bypass. Sinus bradycardia (about 30 beats per minute) and prominent J (Osborne) waves *(arrows)* distinguish the first three complexes. Ventricular ectopy increases in frequency and progresses to fibrillation as the patient rapidly becomes hypothermic. Bladder and nasopharyngeal temperatures were 35.8°C and 31.4°C, respectively. (From Mark JB: Atlas of Cardiovascular Monitoring. New York, Churchill Livingstone, 1997, p 331.)

(dependent on depth of insertion),[2] and pulmonary artery (if a thermistor-equipped pulmonary artery catheter is used). The rectum and bladder may reflect central core body temperature if the patient is warm and vasodilated, or peripheral body temperature if the patient is cold and vasoconstricted. Skin temperature may be useful to evaluate gradients but may have little or no relationship to core temperature changes.

Routine use of heated and humidified anesthesia circuits is not warranted in adult patients except to reduce further heat loss in an already hypothermic patient or for extended, major surgical procedures. Such circuits do little to increase core temperature. After the induction of anesthesia, reduction of the total fresh gas flow to less than 2 L/minute will help reduce heat and moisture loss from the airway, as will an "artificial nose" (i.e., a heat- and moisture-exchanging filter or hygroscopic condenser humidifier).

A forced-air warming blanket should be placed to prevent intraoperative hypothermia and even induce rewarming. Full-body or half-body blankets are available, and this convection-based device is by far the most effective system for perioperative warming. One caveat is that it should not be placed over the lower body[3] during aortic cross-clamping, because this will exacerbate the tissue oxygen demand-supply imbalance. Passive insulation (blankets, drapes) and circulating water mattresses are not nearly as effective, and there is a risk of thermal injury with the latter if water temperature exceeds 40°C. Although an overhead radiant heater is frequently used for infants and small children, the patient's skin must be left exposed for heat transfer to occur. Heat transfer is blocked by interposed surgical or nursing personnel. Also, overhead heaters restrict access to the patient.

Whenever large volumes of crystalloid, colloid, or blood products are infused, a fluid warming device should be used. Four units of refrigerated blood at 4°C or 1 L of room-temperature crystalloid can decrease mean body temperature by about 1°C. During massive blood transfusion, the use of a rapid infusion device (which can deliver up to 1000 mL/minute at 37°C) is essential to prevent potentially life-threatening hypothermia and irreversible hypothermic coagulopathy.

When patients are hypothermic to less than 35°C following anesthesia and surgery, it is prudent to consider deferring tracheal extubation and providing mechanical ventilation until the core temperature has normalized. Capnometry is useful to detect early increases in carbon dioxide production and facilitate appropriate adjustments in minute ventilation.

The most effective means of preventing postoperative shivering is to warm the skin (e.g., with a forced-air warming blanket). Impulses from skin thermoreceptors govern the hypothalamic response to cold; the warmer the skin, the lower the central temperature threshold for the onset of shivering. There is considerable evidence that premedication with α_2-adrenergic receptor agonists (clonidine, dexmedetomidine) suppress postoperative shivering. Active shivering can be treated with intravenous meperidine (12.5 to 25 mg), which likely has a specific hypothalamic effect. However, it is effective only about 50% to 60% of the time. Intravenous dexmedetomidine is also an effective treatment for postoperative shivering and has an additive effect when used with meperidine.

Rewarming vasodilatation begins variably after the patient's arrival in the postanesthesia care unit and depends on hypothermia severity. Increased muscle tone (i.e., subclinical shivering) initially generates heat during persistent peripheral vasoconstriction. As a result, core temperature climbs and may even "overshoot" to 38°C to 40°C, especially after hypothermic cardiopulmonary bypass. When peripheral vasodilatation finally occurs, heat generation is balanced by heat loss, so that the central temperature reaches a plateau before returning to normal. If patients are hypovolemic, rewarming vasodilatation can produce acute hypotension, reflex tachycardia, and myocardial ischemia. Thus, in the early postoperative period, patients who are hypothermic, vasoconstricted, and hypertensive may benefit from vigorous fluid replacement, along with judicious use of vasodilator therapy (e.g., nitroprusside, nitroglycerin). Once rewarming vasodilatation occurs, fluid replacement is essential, together with a vasopressor if needed.

Further Reading

Doufas AG, Lin CM, Suleman MI, et al: Dexmedetomidine and meperidine additively reduce the shivering threshold in humans. Stroke 34: 1218-1223, 2003.

Frank SM, Higgins MS, Breslow MJ, et al: The catecholamine, cortisol, and hemodynamic responses to mild perioperative hypothermia: A randomized clinical trial. Anesthesiology 82:83-93, 1995.

Giesbrecht GG, Ducharme MB, McGuire JP: Comparison of forced-air patient warming systems for perioperative use. Anesthesiology 80:806-810, 1994.

Kurz A, Sessler DI, Lenhardt R: Perioperative normothermia to reduce the incidence of surgical-wound infection and shorten hospitalization. N Engl J Med 334:1209-1215, 1996.

Nesher N, Zisman E, Wolf T, et al: Strict thermoregulation attenuates myocardial injury during coronary artery bypass graft surgery as reflected by reduced levels of cardiac-specific troponin I. Anesth Analg 96:328-335, 2003.

Sessler DI: Temperature monitoring. In: Miller RD (ed): Miller's Anesthesia, 6th ed. Philadelphia, Churchill Livingstone, 2005, pp 1571-1598.

Young CC, Sladen RN: Temperature monitoring. Int Anesth Clin 34: 149-174, 1996.

---

[2] If the thermistor is behind the trachea, core temperature will be <0.2°C below its true value.

[3] Or, if a lower body warming blanket is in place, it must not be used at this time.

Hyperthermia

Melissa M. Vu

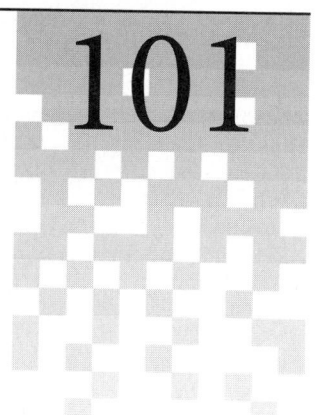

101

Case Synopsis

A 24-year-old, 62-kg, gravida I para 0 woman presents at 39 + 5 weeks for elective induction of labor under combined spinal-epidural analgesia. After approximately 5 hours of labor, the patient's oral temperature is noted to be 38°C (100.4°F). The fetal heart rate is 120 to 130 beats per minute, with normal variability.

PROBLEM ANALYSIS

Definition

Normal core body temperature is 36.7°C to 37.0°C ± 0.2°C to 0.4°C and is maintained via a complex system of neuroregulatory sensors and responses. A person's age and level of activity, the time of day, medications, the hormonal milieu, and other factors determine the hypothalamic "setpoint" to which core body temperature is compared. Consequently, whether the core temperature is below or above this setpoint determines whether the body will generate, conserve, or lose heat. Hyperthermia exists if body temperature during homeostatic conditions rises above the normal range. This may be due either to heat production exceeding heat loss or to heat storage. The opposite is true for hypothermia.

During general and regional anesthesia, thermoregulation is impaired via pharmacologic and central mechanisms. Mild hypothermia commonly occurs in a characteristic pattern during anesthesia and surgery due to this impairment, as well as exposure to the cooler operating room environment. Thus, a less common but more functional definition of hyperthermia is a rise in core temperature more than 2°C per hour or more than 0.5°C over 15 minutes. Such a rise typically warrants further investigation.

Recognition

Optimal detection of temperature disturbances during anesthesia is achieved by monitoring core body temperature. Core temperature can be assessed from a variety of locations, including the pulmonary artery (the gold standard, but even this may be misleading in some surgeries), nasopharynx, tympanic membrane (a reflection of brain temperature), and distal esophagus.[1] Sites outside the core compartment include the bladder, rectum, axilla, and skin, with the last being the least reliable. These sites can be used when clinical circumstances preclude the use of core temperature monitoring, such as surgery under regional anesthesia.

Peripheral temperature (skin, extremity) may show a large discrepancy with core temperature as a result of the physiologic thermal gradient between the two sites. A reasonable alternative is axillary temperature, which may be closer to core temperature values. Transitional zone temperatures (rectal, bladder) fall between core and peripheral temperatures.

Risk Assessment

Hyperthermia itself has a variety of physiologic implications. Of greatest significance is that hyperthermia or fever may be a sign of a more serious underlying pathologic process (Table 101-1). As previously mentioned, hyperthermia occurs far less often than hypothermia during general anesthesia. The incidence of hyperthermia depends largely on its cause.

Malignant hyperthermia is reported to occur in 1 in 5000 to 65,000 cases of general anesthesia in which triggering agents such as inhalational agents or succinycholine are used. Approximately 50% of patients in whom malignant hyperthermia is triggered (see also Chapter 162) have undergone prior uneventful general anesthesia.

Ninety percent of all transfusion reactions are associated with increased temperature. Temperature elevation occurs in about 1% to 2% of all transfusions.

The incidence of other causes of hyperthermia (e.g., infection, thyrotoxicosis, neuroleptic malignant syndrome, other hypermetabolic conditions) is variable. Passive hyperthermia is common in pediatric patients brought to a heated operating room and placed on the operating table under warming lights. Nonetheless, hyperthermia should alert the anesthesiologist to search for a cause rather than to simply treat the elevated temperature elevation itself.

Implications

Hyperthermia has physiologic effects on multiple organ systems. First, elevated temperature results in increased metabolic rates, with consequent increased oxygen consumption. To meet this increase in oxygen demand, cardiac output and heart rate are increased. Acidosis may develop if cellular metabolic demand exceeds oxygen delivery. Myocardial ischemia will occur if the oxygen supply is insufficient. Also, compensatory thermoregulation (perspiration, vasodilatation) may lead to decreased intravascular volume and preload, with possible worsening of oxygen delivery. Perspiration may also cause electrolyte abnormalities due to loss of electrolytes or free water.

Hypothermia is known to provide some measure of cerebral protection during periods of ischemia, whereas

---

[1]The thermistor element should be 2 to 3 cm beyond the tracheal bifurcation or point of best breath sounds. Exposure to cooler inspired gases will reduce core temperature by about 0.3°C, depending on inspired gas flow, respiratory rate, and tidal volume.

Table 101–1 ■ Causes of Hyperthermia during General Anesthesia

Iatrogenic
Increased room temperature
Warming devices
Airway humidifiers or warmers
Excessive rewarming after cardiopulmonary bypass

Infectious
Preoperative fever associated with upper respiratory tract
    infection or condition related to surgical indication
Sepsis
Bacteremia or sepsis associated with surgical manipulation
    (e.g., oral surgery)

Pulmonary
Aspiration pneumonia
Atelectasis
Deep venous thrombosis or pulmonary embolus

Metabolic
Pheochromocytoma
Thyrotoxicosis or thyroid storm
Adrenal insufficiency

Central Nervous System
Status epilepticus
Hypothalamic pathology
Parkinson's disease

Drug Induced
Malignant hyperthermia
Neuroleptic malignant syndrome
Anticholinergic effect
Cocaine, tricyclic antidepressants
Antibiotic-induced drug fever
Monoamine oxidase inhibitors interacting with opioids,
    especially meperidine

Miscellaneous
Monitoring error
Connective tissue diseases
Hematoma
Transfusion reactions
Infusion of blood components with infectious contamination

hyperthermia has been shown to worsen neurologic injury following ischemic events or status epilepticus. Numerous central nervous system effects may occur, including the following:

- Cerebral blood flow increases 5% to 7% for each degree change in temperature.
- Release of excitatory neurotransmitters, such as glutamate, is increased with temperatures greater than 39°C during ischemia.
- Hyperthermia can result in seizure activity in children.
- Permanent central nervous system damage can occur with temperatures above 42°C.
- Increased temperature affects somatosensory evoked potentials by reducing latency.

Hyperthermia causes a rightward shift of the oxygen-hemoglobin dissociation curve. This rightward shift means that hemoglobin has a lower affinity for oxygen and is less saturated at a given arterial oxygen tension.

Further, the cause of hyperthermia may have a variety of untoward effects. Malignant hyperthermia may lead to acidosis, renal dysfunction, hematologic disturbances, or even death. Transfusion reactions may be fatal. Pheochromocytoma and thyrotoxicosis are associated with severe hemodynamic disturbances as well as endocrine complications. Neuroleptic malignant syndrome may behave very similarly to malignant hyperthermia. Although elevated temperature is typically not the only sign of these conditions, it may serve as an early indicator of underlying pathology and assist in the diagnosis.

MANAGEMENT

Management for hyperthermia is directed primarily at the underlying cause (i.e., fever from infection versus other conditions). One should review the patient's history and examine the patient for clues to possible causes of hyperthermia. The perioperative course, including drugs administered, the nature of the surgical procedure, and any other perioperative complications, should also be examined. Patients with sepsis require antibiotics and possibly hemodynamic support as well. Patients with malignant hyperthermia should be treated with dantrolene and supportive therapy. Those in whom fever develops during a transfusion need to be evaluated to rule out a possibly severe transfusion reaction.

Active patient cooling should be considered when the temperature exceeds 39°C. Treatment of hyperthermia itself may be as simple as lowering the room temperature, removing drapes or coverings, turning off warming devices, and blowing cool air over the patient. In more severe cases, one may consider the following:

- Apply ice to the groin, axilla, or neck.
- Use cooled intravenous solutions.
- Undertake ice-water lavage into the surgical wound, bladder, stomach, or rectum (ice-water peritoneal lavage has also been used in extreme cases).
- In desperate situations, use cardiopulmonary bypass to provide rapid cooling.

PREVENTION

Prevention of intraoperative hyperthermia begins with a preoperative history and physical examination. Does the patient have a history of malignant hyperthermia? Does the patient have known sepsis, pheochromocytoma, thyroid dysfunction, or other possible preoperative causes of hyperthermia? What was the patient's temperature preoperatively?

Iatrogenic hyperthermia or hypothermia is prevented by monitoring the patient's core body temperature after the establishment of a baseline temperature and using a blanket cooling or warming device as necessary. If hyperthermia occurs, one should review recent intraoperative events:

- Has a transfusion just begun?
- Were malignant hyperthermia–triggering agents used?
- Where is the site of surgery?
- What drugs have been given recently?

Although some mild hyperthermia or fever may be beneficial with infection, the potential physiologic effects on the heart and brain can be detrimental, especially in the elderly. If so, the condition must be treated aggressively.

Further Reading

Baughman V: Brain protection during neurosurgery. Anesthesiol Clin North Am 20:315-327, 2002.

Cereda M, Maccioli GA: Intraoperative temperature monitoring. Int Anesthesiol Clin 42:41-54, 2004.

Chiharu N, Lenhardt R: Fever during anaesthesia. Best Pract Res Clin Anesthesiol 17:499-517, 2003.

Oku G, Rosenberg H: Thermoregulation in the postoperative patient. In Brown M, Brown EM (eds): Comprehensive Postanesthesia Care. Baltimore, Williams & Wilkins, 1997, pp 283-301.

Rosenberg H, Frank S: Causes and consequences of hypothermia and hyperthermia. In Benumof JL, Saidman U (eds): Anesthesia and Perioperative Complications. St. Louis, Mosby–Year Book, 1999, pp 338-356.

Sessler DI: Temperature monitoring. In Miller RD (ed): Anesthesia, 6th ed. Philadelphia, Churchill Livingstone, 2004, pp 1571-1597.

PHYSIOLOGIC IMBALANCE & COEXISTING DISEASE

Angioedema and Urticaria

102

Saeed Habibi and Catherine Drexler

Case Synopsis

A 24-year-old woman with a vague history of swelling of the lips and tongue and wheezing associated with exercise, anxiety, and cold temperature receives general anesthesia for shoulder arthroscopy. After induction of general anesthesia and tracheal intubation, severe bronchospasm develops, followed by generalized angioedema and cardiovascular collapse.

PROBLEM ANALYSIS

Definition

Angioedema and urticaria are clinical signs that may result from a vast array of causes, including immune-mediated and non-immune-mediated mechanisms. They often occur together and represent a clinical spectrum ranging from a minor irritating reaction to life-threatening laryngeal edema or anaphylaxis.

Urticaria is characterized by erythematous, pruritic wheals of cutaneous edema. These blanch with pressure but remain surrounded by a "flare" of erythema. Although angioedema is a similar process, it occurs in the deeper subcutaneous tissues and produces more diffuse swelling.

Sites of involvement may include the face, tongue, larynx, and gastrointestinal tract, as well as the extremities. Involvement of the upper respiratory tract has potential to cause life-threatening airway obstruction.

Most episodes of urticaria and angioedema are acute but may recur during a period of 6 weeks or less. Periodic episodes lasting longer than 6 weeks are viewed as chronic, and most are idiopathic in origin.

Hereditary angioneurotic edema (HAE), or complement 1 esterase inhibitor (C1-INH) deficiency, is a rare form of angioedema. HAE is an autosomal dominant inherited disease characterized by absolute (type 1) or relative (type 2) deficiency of C1-INH activity. The deficiency of C1-INH allows C1 esterase to cleave C1 and subsequently to activate the complement cascade, resulting in vasodilatation and angioedema. The diagnosis of HAE is crucial, because the treatment for an acute episode of C1-INH deficiency differs dramatically from that for other types of angioedema. Further, HAE has a significant mortality rate due to associated laryngeal edema.

Acquired C1-INH deficiency is associated with systemic diseases such as autoimmune disorders, B-cell lymphomas (type I), and carcinomas. It can also be secondary to immunoglobulin (Ig) G anti–C1-INH autoantibodies (type II).

Acute urticaria or angioedema results from activation and degranulation or degradation of mast cells and basophils due to IgE-mediated or non-IgE-mediated mechanisms (e.g., complement-mediated or direct mast cell–releasing agents). These cells release or generate several mediators that cause vasodilatation and increased vascular permeability. These include histamine, histamine-releasing factors, prostaglandin D_2, leukotrienes C_4 and D_4, platelet-activating factor, anaphylatoxins (C3a, C4a, C5a), bradykinin, kallikrein, cytokines such as interleukin (IL)-4 and IL-5, and interferon γ. The clinical features of mast cell degradation are similar, regardless of the classification and underlying cause (Table 102-1).

Recognition

Perioperative urticaria or angioedema warrants immediate recognition and careful evaluation for laryngeal edema, which may be life threatening, particularly in pediatric patients with small airways.

Intraoperative diagnosis of urticaria or angioedema may be difficult for several reasons. Surgical drapes, warming blankets, and surgical preparation solutions may obscure and limit patient exposure, thereby delaying recognition of

Table 102–1 ■ Classification of Angioedema

Idiopathic
Immune-mediated angioedema
   Immunoglobulin E mediated
   Physical urticaria
   Contact reactions

Complement Mediated
C1 esterase inhibitor (C1-INH) deficiency
   Hereditary angioneurotic edema
   Acquired C1-INH deficiency
Serum sickness
Urticarial vasculitis
Systemic lupus erythematosus
Transfusion reactions

Non–Immune Mediated
Direct mast cell or histamine release
Angiotensin-converting enzyme inhibitor related

Other Rare Syndromes
Systemic mastocytosis
C3b inactivator deficiency
Infection
   Helminthic
   Fungal
   Viral
Systemic diseases
   Hyperthyroidism
   Collagen vascular diseases
Malignancies

any cutaneous manifestations. Further, bronchospasm secondary to histamine release may be incorrectly attributed to airway manipulation or asthma. Also, hypotension consequent to vasodilatation from more generalized reactions may wrongly be assumed to be secondary to myocardial depression, anesthetic effects, or blood loss. Finally, multiple drugs capable of immunologic or nonimmunologic mast cell activation and degranulation may be administered over a brief period; these include antibiotics, induction and neuromuscular blocking agents, and opioids. Therefore, even when a reaction is recognized, it is often difficult to identify the cause or to determine whether a true "allergic" reaction has occurred.

Once urticaria or angioedema is recognized, it is crucial to document the temporal relation between the administration of drugs and the onset of the reaction. The reaction may be significantly delayed from the presumed time of contact with the causal agent.

Risk Assessment

Approximately 15% to 20% of the population will experience an episode of angioedema or urticaria during their lifetime, and it is more prevalent in middle-aged women. However, it is extremely difficult to identify patients at risk for angioedema or urticaria because of the multitude of potential initiators. Patients with a history of past reactions, HAE, collagen vascular diseases, B-cell lymphoma or other malignancies, occult infections, or thyroid disorders may be at increased risk.

The mainstays of the evaluation of acute or chronic urticaria and angioedema are a thorough history, physical examination, and identification of all medication administered. The appropriate initial laboratory evaluation of chronic urticaria is controversial. In general, it may include a complete blood cell count with (manual) differential cell count, erythrocyte sedimentation rate, and thyroid gland studies (thyroid-stimulating hormone, antithyroglobulin, and antithyroid peroxisomal antibody titers). In atypical cases, or if urticarial vasculitis is suspected, complement studies, hepatocellular enzyme tests, and skin biopsies are advised. Further testing depends on the individual circumstances. It may include blood chemistries, serologic studies, skin testing for IgE-mediated reactions, and radioallergosorbent testing (RAST) for specific IgE antibodies.

In the evaluation of patients with suspected intraoperative urticaria or angioedema reactions, meticulous documentation of the time course of events in relation to drug administration is of paramount importance. Unfortunately, even when a specific drug is suspected, proving a causal relationship is often difficult.

Specific IgE antibodies may be demonstrated in immunologically mediated reactions (e.g., to thiopental, latex, succinylcholine, blood products, protamine, plasma expanders, antibiotics). A positive skin test or RAST indicates sensitization and a potential risk of generalized reaction with re-exposure to the agent. Although rechallenge with the drug may confirm the diagnosis, it is potentially dangerous and not usually recommended.

Although a past history of anaphylaxis to a specific drug contraindicates its future use, a nonimmunologic reaction is more difficult to interpret and may not be a contraindication to such use (e.g., for drugs causing histamine release,

the magnitude of reaction is related to both the dose and the rate of administration).

Implications

Acute intraoperative urticaria or angioedema can progress to laryngeal edema or anaphylaxis with respiratory failure or hemodynamic collapse. In an immune-mediated reaction, repeated exposure may increase the risk of a reaction. In a patient with a past history of intraoperative urticaria or angioedema reactions, the options for anesthetic drugs are limited, depending on the mechanism and cause of such reactions. Preoperative prophylaxis with anabolic steroids (danazol, stanozolol) or glucocorticoids may be useful in certain patients with a history of perioperative angioedema.

MANAGEMENT AND PREVENTION

It is essential to avoid known causative agents and those with the potential for cross-reactivity. Although prophylactic use of antihistamines or corticosteroids is common, and although leukotriene antagonists have been used with some success, their efficacy in preventing and modulating perioperative allergic or nonimmunologic reactions is unknown.

With suspected acute urticaria or angioedema, the causative agent should be removed when possible. Because laryngeal edema may develop rapidly, the adequacy of ventilation must be assessed immediately. If indicated, the airway should be secured by tracheal intubation. Difficult intubation should be anticipated, and the airway must be evaluated for residual edema before extubation.

Urticaria or angioedema may be associated with significant intravascular volume depletion. Consequently, fluid resuscitation is mandatory. Epinephrine is used if cardiovascular collapse, anaphylaxis, or severe respiratory compromise occurs. Other β-agonists (e.g., terbutaline, albuterol) may replace epinephrine for the treatment of isolated bronchospasm.

Antihistamines may be used alone or in conjunction with epinephrine when clinical features do not warrant the sole use of epinephrine. Although H_2-blockers alone have minimal effects, they may be effective when used in combination with H_1-blockers.

Corticosteroids are used for the management of acute, recurrent, or persistent angioedema or urticaria. However, long-term use of these drugs is associated with frequent complications.

In HAE, the goal is to increase C1-INH activity to at least 50% of its normal level. This can be achieved by transfusion of fresh frozen plasma, which contains C1-INH, antifibrinolytics, attenuated androgens, and C1-INH concentrate. ε-Aminocaproic acid and tranexamic acid have been used for perioperative prophylaxis. Anabolic steroids (danazol, stanozolol) can induce hepatic synthesis of C1-INH and provide effective preoperative prophylaxis for HAE. For short-term prophylaxis, these agents are administered for several days before and after the scheduled surgery (e.g., danazol 10 mg/kg per day, to a maximum of 600 mg/day; stanozolol 6 mg/day). C1-INH concentrate has been used as preoperative prophylaxis in a dose of 500 or 1000 units;

however, C1-INH is expensive and is currently not available in the United States. It has been used mainly in Europe. Antihistamines, corticosteroids, and epinephrine are usually ineffective in treating acute episodes of HAE, but they are often administered when the specific mechanism of the reaction is unclear.

Further Reading

Abraham D, Grammer L: Idiopathic anaphylaxis. Immunol Allergy Clin North Am 21:783-794, 2001.

Agostoni A, Aygoren-Pursun E, Binkley KE, et al: Hereditary and acquired angioedema: Problems and progress. Proceeding of the third C1 esterase inhibitor deficiency workshop and beyond. J Allergy Clin Immunol 114(Suppl):S51-S131, 2004.

Dibbern DA Jr, Dreskin SC: Urticaria and angioedema: An overview. Immunol Allergy Clin North Am 24:141-162, 2004.

Hepner DL, Castells MC: Anaphylaxis during the peioperative period. Anesth Analg 97:1381-1395, 2003.

Ledford DK: Allergy, anaphylaxis, and general anesthesia. Immunol Allergy Clin North Am 21:795-812, 2001.

Lieberman P: Anaphylactic reactions during surgical and medical procedures. J Allergy Clin Immunol 110(Suppl):S64-S69, 2002.

Mertes PM, Laxenaire MC, Alla F: Anaphylactic and anaphylactoid reactions occurring during anesthesia in France in 1999-2000. Anesthesiology 99:536-545, 2003.

Muller BA: Urticaria and angioedema: A practical approach. Am Fam Physician 69:1123-1128, 2004.

Disorders of Water Homeostasis: Hyponatremia and Hypernatremia

103

Brenda G. Fahy, J. Thomas Murphy, and John L. Atlee

HYPONATREMIA

Case Synopsis

A 55-year-old man with small cell lung carcinoma presents for preanesthetic evaluation for right upper lobectomy. His past medical history includes emphysema, hypertension, and insulin-dependent diabetes mellitus. On physical examination, his blood pressure is 140/80 mm Hg, and his pulse is 86 beats per minute, with good skin turgor. His laboratory values are as follows: serum sodium, 126 mEq/L; serum osmolality, 390 mOsm/kg; serum uric acid, 3.7 mg/dL; urine sodium, 30 mEq/L; and normal glucose, blood urea nitrogen (BUN), and thyroid and adrenal function tests. The patient denies nausea, lethargy, or weakness.

PROBLEM ANALYSIS

Definition

Serum sodium concentration and osmolality are closely regulated by water homeostasis. This is mediated by thirst, arginine vasopressin, and the kidneys. A disruption in water homeostasis is manifested by an abnormal serum sodium concentration—either hyponatremia or hypernatremia. The former is defined as a serum sodium concentration less than 135 mEq/L, with severe hyponatremia occurring at values less than 120 mEq/L. The patient described in the case synopsis had hypo-osmotic hyponatremia and was euvolemic with normal thyroid and adrenal function. Causes of true hyponatremia are listed in Table 103-1; causes of pseudo-hyponatremia are listed in Table 103-2. The case presented is due to the syndrome of inappropriate secretion of antidiuretic hormone (SIADH) related to small cell lung carcinoma (Table 103-3).

Recognition

Symptoms of hyponatremia are related to the serum sodium concentration and how rapidly it decreases. The blood-brain barrier is virtually impermeable to sodium. Thus, rapid decreases in serum sodium cause water entry into the cells of the brain and other tissues. This can lead to cerebral edema, with progression to intracranial hypertension.

Both the magnitude and the rapidity of water entry into brain cells explain the central nervous system (CNS) symptoms associated with hyponatremia. These also correlate with symptom severity (Fig. 103-1). Early symptoms of hyponatremia-related CNS water entry are lethargy, weakness, and somnolence. Unabated, there may be progression to seizures, coma, and death. Therefore, hyponatremia must always be considered in the differential diagnosis of any mental status deterioration.

The diagnosis of hyponatremia is based on laboratory testing, specifically, serum sodium concentration (Fig. 103-2). The next step is to measure plasma osmolality. This may help establish the diagnosis of pseudohyponatremia (see Table 103-2). Pseudohyponatremia occurs when the extracellular fluid compartment contains an impermeable solute (e.g., lipids) or there has been translocation or extravasation of large volumes of non-salt-containing fluids (e.g., transurethral resection of prostate or bladder tumor, hysteroscopy). This causes a shift of water from the intracellular to extracellular fluid compartment, causing dilutional hyponatremia. With more laboratories using ion-selective electrodes to measure serum sodium concentrations, dilutional hyponatremia has become less of a problem. Normal values for plasma osmolality range from 274 to 290 mOsm/kg. Calculated plasma osmolality (P_{osm}) is determined by the following formula:

$$P_{osm} = (2.0 \times [Na^+]) + Glucose\ (mg/dL)/18 + BUN\ (mg/dL)/2.8$$

Patients with disorders such as hyperproteinemia or hyperlipidemia, which cause increased osmolality and pseudohyponatremia, have an abnormal osmolality gap (measured P_{osm} − calculated P_{osm} >10 mOsm/L). These disorders highlight

Table 103–1 ■ Causes of True Hypo-osmotic Hyponatremia

Hypovolemia

Renal losses (urinary sodium >20 mEq/L)
  Diuretic therapy
  Mineralocorticoid deficiency
  Cerebral salt wasting syndrome (e.g., subarachnoid hemorrhage)
  Renal disease
    Renal tubular acidosis (bicarbonaturia with renal tubular acidosis and metabolic alkalosis)
    Renal tubular defect (salt wasting nephropathy)
Extrarenal losses (urinary sodium <20 mEq/L)
Gastrointestinal diseases—vomiting, diarrhea, and gastric suctioning
Skin—burns, sweating, cystic fibrosis
Pancreatitis
Trauma

Hypervolemia

Renal causes (urinary sodium >20 mEq/L)
  Renal failure
Other causes (urinary sodium <20 mEq/L)
  Congestive heart failure
  Hepatic cirrhosis
  Nephrotic syndrome
  Pregnancy

Euvolemia (Urinary Sodium >20 mEq/L)

Glucocorticoid deficiency
Hypothyroidism
Syndrome of inappropriate antidiuretic hormone (SIADH)
Reset osmostat—psychosis, malnutrition

Table 103–3 ■ Causes of Syndrome of Inappropriate Secretion of Antidiuretic Hormone

Malignancy
Lung (especially small cell carcinoma)
Central nervous system
Pancreas

Pulmonary
Pneumonia
Tuberculosis
Fungal
Abscess

Neurologic
Infection
Trauma
Cerebrovascular accident

Drugs (Most Common)
Amitriptyline
Chlorpropamide
Cyclophosphamide
Desmopressin
Morphine
Nicotine
Nonsteroidal anti-inflammatory drugs
Oxytocin
Selective serotonin reuptake inhibitors
Vincristine

the importance of measuring plasma osmolality in hyponatremic patents. Other important laboratory tests are urine osmolality and sodium and a complete chemistry panel, including uric acid concentrations. Other electrolyte abnormalities (e.g., hypokalemia, hypomagnesemia) are often associated with hyponatremia.

Once pseudohyponatremia has been excluded, the next diagnostic step is to determine the volume status, because true hypo-osmotic hyponatremia may be hypovolemic, hypervolemic, or euvolemic (see Table 103-1). This is assessed by clinical signs and symptoms in conjunction with hemodynamic and laboratory data. The serum uric acid level may be helpful in determining the patient's volume status. A low serum uric acid level (<4 mg/dL) likely indicates euvolemia, whereas an elevated uric acid level may be present with hypovolemia or hypervolemia.

Table 103–2 ■ Causes of Pseudohyponatremia

Normal Plasma Osmolarity

Hyperlipidemia
Hyperproteinemia
Transurethral resection of prostate or bladder tumor; hysteroscopy

Increased Plasma Osmolarity

Hyperglycemia
Mannitol administration

From Rose BD: Hypoosmolal states: Hyponatremia. In Jeffers JD, Navrozov M (eds): Clinical Physiology of Acid-Base and Electrolyte Disorders. New York, McGraw-Hill, 1994, pp 651-694.

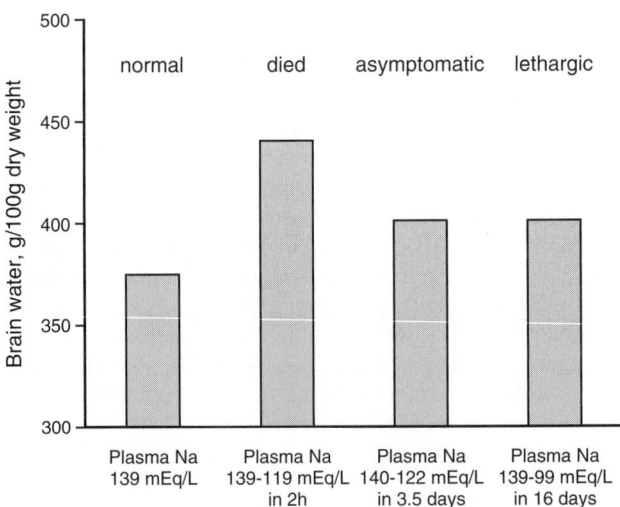

Figure 103–1 ■ Brain water content in control and hyponatremic rabbits. When plasma sodium was acutely lowered to 119 mEq/L over 2 hours, brain water content increased to 17% above normal. This was associated with severe symptoms and death. In contrast, slowly lowering plasma sodium to the same level over 3.5 days resulted in a smaller increase in brain water (7%) and no symptoms. Finally, gradually reducing plasma sodium to extremely low levels (99 mEq/L) produced a small increase in brain water and only mild neurologic symptoms. (From Arieff AI, Llach F, Massry SG: Neurological manifestations and morbidity of hyponatremia: Correlation with brain water and electrolytes. Medicine 55:121-129, 1976.)

Figure 103–2 ■ Major steps in the initial evaluation of hyponatremia and the syndrome of inappropriate antidiuretic hormone secretion (SIADH).

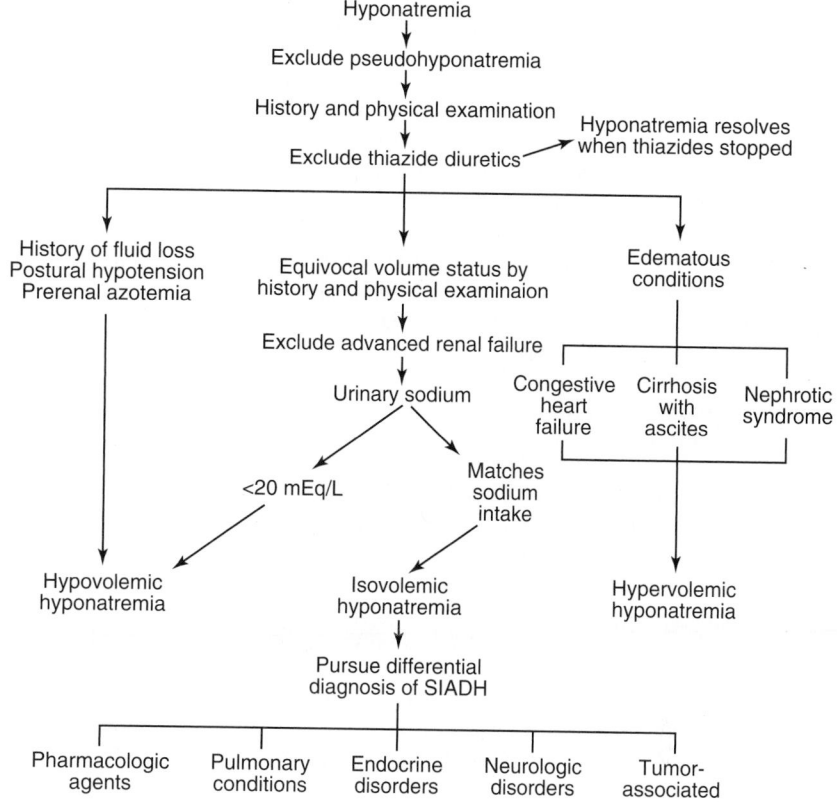

Risk Assessment

Hyponatremia is a common clinical electrolyte disorder. Fifteen percent to 22% of hospitalized patients have serum sodium values less than 135 mEq/L, and 1% to 4% have values less than 130 mEq/L. Hyponatremia can occur preoperatively, intraoperatively, or postoperatively. It can be diagnosed during the preoperative assessment as being caused by SIADH (as was the case in the patient presented earlier) or as a known side effect of medical management (e.g., thiazide diuretics, carbamazepine).

Hyponatremia often presents perioperatively as hypovolemic hyponatremia. Intraoperative hypervolemic hyponatremia occurs with transurethral resection of prostate (TURP), transurethral resection of bladder tumor (TURBT), or hysteroscopy with intravascular translocation of irrigating solutions (e.g., glycine, sorbitol). The manifestations of such absorption are due to combined hyponatremia and hypoosmolality. Severe hyponatremia can cause problems in the absence of hypo-osmolality, however. Most other causes of hyponatremia also result in hypo-osmolality, and the manifestations attributed to low serum sodium concentrations cannot be separated from those occurring as a consequence of concomitant hypo-osmolality. During procedures utilizing irrigating solutions, hyponatremia can develop quickly, presenting with CNS manifestations. Prompt recognition and therapy are key.

One cause of postoperative hyponatremia is the increased effect of antidiuretic hormone (ADH). This occurs if the sodium in perioperative intravenous fluids is excreted while some of the infused water is retained. If extreme, postoperative hyponatremia may cause death.

Hyponatremia is often accompanied by other electrolyte abnormalities (see also Chapters 14 to 16). For example, hypokalemia may be associated with hypovolemic hyponatremia due to gastrointestinal losses (vomiting, diarrhea), use of loop diuretics, or renal tubular acidosis. Metabolic alkalosis may accompany vomiting or diuretic use, and metabolic acidosis may accompany diarrhea or mineralocorticoid deficiency. With euvolemic hyponatremia, there may be associated hypokalemia due to SIADH and polydipsia (psychogenic water drinking). In contrast, hyperkalemia accompanies glucocorticoid deficiency. Azotemia is common with hypervolemic hyponatremia. Serum sodium serves as a marker for disease severity with hypervolemic hyponatremia.

Implications

The risk for hyponatremia is related to the absolute level of serum sodium. However, more critical is how rapidly the serum sodium falls due to accompanying fluid shifts. Upon exclusion of pseudohyponatremia, it is necessary to determine the type of hyponatremia, because therapy differs.

Whether correction of hyponatremia is required and how fast it should be accomplished depend on the severity of symptoms. With acute CNS symptoms, the risk of cerebral edema outweighs the risk of rapid correction; thus, correction is undertaken quickly, while realizing that too rapid correction may cause excess morbidity or even mortality.

MANAGEMENT

Major steps in the initial evaluation of hyponatremia are outlined in Figure 103-2. Treatment involves two basic principles: identifying and treating the underlying cause, and increasing serum sodium safely when indicated. With serious CNS symptoms or serum sodium less than 110 mEq/L, rapid sodium replacement with hypertonic saline (3%) may be required to prevent death. Under these circumstances, the goal of hypertonic saline replacement should be to increase serum sodium 1 to 2 mEq/L per hour over a maximum of 3 hours. Careful monitoring is required throughout this process. Sodium replacement should not exceed 12 mEq/L over 24 hours, or 25 mEq/L over 48 hours. Despite the risks associated with acute, severe hyponatremia, too rapid correction may cause demyelinating lesions in the pons, which can develop over several days. This disorder, termed central pontine myelinolysis or the osmotic demyelination syndrome, can lead to quadriparesis, coma, and death. Diagnostic confirmation is by computed tomography or magnetic resonance imaging; however, changes may not be detectable for up to 4 weeks. Risk factors for central pontine myelinolysis include (1) sodium correction rate greater than 12 mEq/L in 24 hours or 25 mEq/L in 48 hours, (2) overcorrection of serum sodium greater than 140 mEq/L within 2 days, (3) hypoxic or anoxic episodes before therapy, (4) hypercatabolic states (e.g., burns) or malnutrition (e.g., chronic alcoholism), and (5) chronic rather than acute hyponatremia. Unfortunately, determining the duration of hyponatremia may be difficult. Chronic hyponatremia is less likely to be accompanied by CNS manifestations because it develops more slowly.

If rapid correction of serum sodium is not required, a hypovolemic hyponatremic patient may receive isotonic saline with any required electrolyte supplementation to correct the fluid deficit and hyponatremia. If diuretics are the cause, these should be stopped, and appropriate fluids and electrolytes administered. Mineralocorticoids should be replaced if indicated.

Euvolemic hyponatremia therapy requires free water restriction. Steroid or thyroid hormone replacement may be required. If SIADH is determined to be the cause, treatment includes strict fluid restriction, especially free water. Isotonic saline should not be used to treat SIADH hyponatremia because it can result in urinary sodium excretion, exacerbate water retention, and worsen hyponatremia. Reversible causes of SIADH should be sought and treated (see Table 103-3). If SIADH is caused by medications that inhibit ADH (e.g., demeclocycline, phenytoin, loop diuretics, lithium), these may need to be discontinued.

Hypervolemic hyponatremia is due to excessive secretion of ADH. This occurs when a disease process (e.g., cirrhosis, nephritic syndrome, congestive heart failure) results in increased total body fluids (i.e., hypervolemia), but there is an associated decrease in effective circulating intravascular volume and glomerular filtration rate. This triggers ADH secretion. Therapy focuses on the underlying disease process and fluid restriction, especially free water.

The patient in the case synopsis had SIADH from small cell carcinoma of the lung, with euvolemic hypo-osmotic hyponatremia. His hyponatremia was likely chronic, based on absent CNS symptoms. Free water should be restricted, with serial serum sodium monitoring. Aggressive intraoperative hydration with isotonic saline could potentially worsen this patient's hyponatremia.

PREVENTION

Identifying high-risk patients and having a high index of suspicion for hyponatremia can help prevent hyponatremic complications. Because of the high frequency of hyponatremia in hospitalized patients, serum sodium should be monitored. Hyponatremia can occur throughout the perioperative period, and vigilance for its development during procedures that use irrigating solutions (TURP, TURBT, hysteroscopy) is required. Once hyponatremia is diagnosed, and pseudohyponatremia has been excluded, it is important to evaluate the patient's volume status to seek treatable causes of hypo-osmotic hyponatremia. Careful monitoring of serum sodium can help prevent the development of hyponatremia during high-risk procedures, as well as in high-risk patients.

If slower correction of serum sodium is indicated for hypo-osmotic hyponatremia, the volume status determines treatment. With euvolemia, free water is restricted; with hypervolemia, free water and salt are restricted; with hypovolemia, isotonic saline is administered.

HYPERNATREMIA

Case Synopses

Case 1

A 62-year-old woman with postoperative ileus had a nasogastric suctioning tube placed. Within 3 days, she had reduced skin turgor and mild orthostatic hypotension. Her serum sodium was 155 mEq/L, serum potassium was 3.8 mEq/L, and body weight was 62 kg.

Case 2

A 7-year-old boy with severe colitis had a diverting colostomy placed. Subsequently, he received intravenous and nasogastric nutrition for several years. Over that period, he presented two times with confusion, hypernatremia, and weight gain. However, on both occasions, there was no fever, diarrhea, or vomiting. Plasma and urine samples collected on the second visit revealed plasma and urine sodium concentrations of 155 and 172 mEq/L, respectively.

PROBLEM ANALYSIS

Definition

Hypernatremia is defined as a serum sodium concentration greater than 145 mEq/L. In both children and adults, hypernatremia is seen primarily in persons with restricted access to water for a variety of reasons (e.g., patients in hospitals, convalescence facilities, or homes for the elderly; those who are debilitated or mentally impaired). Hypernatremia can also be iatrogenic, resulting from inappropriate fluid therapy or excessive administration of sodium bicarbonate during cardiopulmonary resuscitation.

The body has two defense mechanisms to protect against hypernatremia: the ability to produce concentrated urine, and a powerful thirst mechanism. Release of ADH occurs when plasma osmolality exceeds 275 to 280 mOsm/kg, and the urine becomes maximally concentrated when plasma osmolality exceeds 290 to 295 mOsm/kg. Thirst provides the ultimate protection against hypernatremia, however. If the thirst mechanism is intact and there is unrestricted access to free water, it is rare for an individual to develop sustained hypernatremia from either excess sodium ingestion or a renal concentrating effect.

Recognition

The signs and symptoms of hypernatremia mostly reflect CNS dysfunction. They are more prominent when the increase in serum sodium concentration is large or occurs rapidly (i.e., over a few hours). Most outpatients with hypernatremia are either very young or very old.

Common presenting symptoms in the young include hyperpnea, agitation, irritability, insomnia, and a typical high-pitched cry. These can progress to muscle weakness, confusion, listlessness, lethargy, and coma. Neurologic examination often reveals increased tone, nuchal rigidity, and brisk reflexes. Myoclonus, asterixis, and chorea can be present. Tonic-clonic and absence seizures have been described. Hyperglycemia is an especially common consequence of hypernatremia in children. Severe hypernatremia also can result in rhabdomyolysis. Finally, although hypocalcemia was once believed to be associated with hypernatremia, this has not been a common finding in more recent reports.

Unlike infants, elderly patients generally have few symptoms until the serum sodium concentration exceeds 160 mEq/L. Intense thirst may be present early, but it dissipates as the disorder progresses, and it is absent in those with hypodipsia. Convulsions in either age group are typically absent, except with inadvertent sodium loading or overly aggressive rehydration. The level of consciousness correlates with the severity of hypernatremia. Muscle weakness, confusion, and coma may be manifestations of coexisting disorders rather than of hypernatremia itself. Finally, unlike outpatient hypernatremia, that acquired in hospital settings affects patients of all ages. In addition, the clinical symptoms are even more elusive, because these patients often have pre-existing neurologic dysfunction. As in children, rapid sodium loading can result in convulsions and coma. In patients of all ages, orthostatic hypotension and tachycardia reflect marked hypovolemia.

Risk Assessment

Hypernatremia represents a deficit of water relative to whole body sodium stores. This can result from a net water loss or a gain in hypertonic sodium Table 103-4. Net water loss accounts for the majority of cases. Because sustained hypernatremia can occur only when the thirst sensation is impaired or access to water is limited, persons at highest risk are those with impaired mental status, those on mechanical ventilators, infants, and the elderly. Hypernatremia in infants usually results from gastroenteritis (vomiting and diarrhea); in the elderly it is usually associated with thirst impairment, febrile illness, or infirmity. Also, frail nursing home residents and hospitalized patients are prone to hypernatremia because they depend on others for their water requirements.

Implications

Hypernatremia results in the efflux of fluid from the intracellular space to the extracellular space to maintain osmotic equilibrium. This leads to transient cerebral dehydration and brain shrinkage. Brain cell volume can decrease by as much as 10% to 15% acutely, but it adapts quickly. Within 1 hour, the brain significantly increases its intracellular content of sodium and potassium, amino acids, and unmeasured organic substances or idiogenic osmoles (i.e., rapid adaptation). Normalization of brain volume is completed by 1 week (slow adaptation), as the brain regains approximately 98% of its water content. When severe hypernatremia develops acutely, the brain may not be able to increase its intracellular solute sufficiently to preserve its volume. If so, resulting cellular shrinkage can lead to structural changes. Cerebral dehydration from hypernatremia can result in physical separation of the brain from the meninges, leading to rupture of delicate bridging veins and subarachnoid or intracerebral hemorrhage, with permanent neurologic damage or death. Venous sinus thrombosis progressing to cerebral infarction can also develop. Acute hypernatremia has also been shown to cause cerebral demyelinating lesions in both animal models and humans. Patients with hepatic encephalopathy appear to be at higher risk for developing such lesions.

Table 103–4 ■ Causes of Water Deficit Relative to Whole Body Sodium Stores

Net Free Water Deficit

Pure Water

Unreplaced insensible loss
Hypodipsia
Neurogenic diabetes insipidus
   Post-traumatic
   Due to brain tumor, cyst, histiocytosis, tuberculosis, sarcoidosis
   Idiopathic
   Due to aneurysm, meningitis, Guillain-Barré syndrome
   Due to ethanol ingestion (transient)
Congenital or acquired nephrogenic diabetes insipidus
   Renal disease (e.g., medullary cystic disease)
   Hypercalemia or hypokalemia
   Drugs (lithium, demeclocycline, foscarnet, methoxyflurane, amphotericin B, vasopressin V2-receptor antagonists)

Hypertonic Fluids

Renal causes
   Loop diuretics
   Osmotic diuresis (glucose, mannitol, urea)
   Postobstructive diuresis
   Polyuric phase of acute tubular necrosis
   Intrinsic renal disease
Gastrointestinal causes
   Vomiting
   Nasogastric drainage
   Enterocutaneous fistula
   Diarrhea
   Osmotic cathartics (e.g., lactulose)
Cutaneous causes
   Burns
   Excessive sweating

Hypertonic Sodium Gain

Hypertonic sodium bicarbonate
Hypertonic feeding preparations
Ingestion of sodium chloride
Ingestion of sea water
Sodium chloride–rich emetics
Hypertonic saline enemas
Intrauterine injection of hypertonic saline
Hypertonic sodium chloride infusion
Hypertonic dialysis
Primary hyperaldosteronism
Cushing's syndrome

From Adrogué HJ, Madias NE: Hypernatremia. N Engl J Med 342:1493-1499, 2000.

MANAGEMENT AND PREVENTION

Treatment for hypernatremia must correct the underlying cause, normalize the serum sodium concentration, and restore the normal circulatory volume. The therapeutic cornerstone is the provision of adequate free water to correct the serum sodium concentration. The free water deficit cannot be easily assessed by physical examination in patients with hypernatremic dehydration, because most of the free water losses are intracellular. Accordingly, the signs of volume depletion are less apparent owing to better preservation of extracellular volume. A simple method for estimating the minimum amount of fluid necessary to correct the serum sodium concentration is the following equation:

$$\text{Free water deficit (mL)} = 4 \text{ mL} \times \text{Lean body weight (kg)} \times [\text{Desired } \Delta \text{serum Na}^+ \text{ (mEq/L)}]$$

The amount of fluid required depends on the fluid composition. For example, to correct a 3-L free water deficit, approximately 4 L of 0.2% saline or 6 L of 0.45% saline would be needed, because these solutions contain approximately 75% and 50% free water, respectively.

The calculated deficit does not account for insensible or ongoing urinary or gastrointestinal losses. Maintenance fluids, which include replacement of urine volume with hypotonic fluids, are given in addition to the deficit. If there are signs of severe hypovolemia or circulatory collapse, fluid resuscitation with normal saline, lactated Ringer's solution, or colloid should be instituted before correcting the free water deficit. The type of therapy depends largely on the cause of hypernatremia and should be tailored to the pathophysiologic events involved in each patient (Table 103-5). Oral hydration should be started as soon as it can be safely tolerated. Plasma electrolytes should be measured every 2 to 3 hours until the patient is neurologically stable.

In patients with hypernatremia that has developed over hours (e.g., accidental sodium overloading), rapid correction improves the prognosis without increasing the risk of cerebral edema. This is because accumulated electrolytes are rapidly extruded from brain cells. In such patients, reducing the serum sodium concentration by 1 mEq/L per hour is appropriate. A slower pace of correction is advised for patients with hypernatremia of longer or unknown duration, because full dissipation of brain solutes occurs over a period of days. In such patients, reducing the serum sodium concentration at a maximal rate of 0.5 mEq/L per hour prevents cerebral edema and convulsions. Consequently, some authorities (e.g., Adrogué and Madias) advise a target reduction in serum sodium concentration of 10 mEq/L per day for all patients with hypernatremia, except those in whom the disorder has developed over a period of hours. The goal of treatment is to reduce serum sodium concentration to 145 mEq/L.

The preferred route for administering fluids is orally or via a feeding tube. If neither is feasible, fluids are given intravenously. The more hypotonic the fluid is (see Table 103-5), the lower the infusion rate should be. This reduces the risk for cerebral edema formation. Finally, except in cases of

Table 103–5 ■ Management of Hypernatremia

Cause	Treatment
Sodium and water loss* Gastroenteritis	0.45% NaCl in 5% dextrose and water
Primary water loss* Ineffective breast feeding Hypodipsia	0.2% NaCl in 5% dextrose and water
Nephrogenic diabetes insipidus*	0.1% NaCl in 2.5% dextrose and water†
Central diabetes insipidus*	Desmopressin acetate
Sodium overload*	5% dextrose and water‡

*See also Table 103-4.
†Acute management.
‡Diuretics may be needed.

Adapted from Moritz ML, Ayus JC: Disorders of water metabolism in children. Pediatr Rev 23:371-380, 2002; and Adrogué HJ, Madias NE: Hypernatremia. N Engl J Med 342:1493-1499, 2000.

frank circulatory compromise, 0.9% normal saline or lactated Ringer's solution is *unsuitable* therapy for hypernatremia.

Further Reading

Adrogué HJ, Madias NE: Hypernatremia. N Engl J Med 342:1493-1499, 2000.

Adrogué HJ, Madias NE: Hyponatremia. N Engl J Med 342:1581-1589, 2000.

Arieff AI, Llach F, Massry SG: Neurological manifestations and morbidity of hyponatremia: Correlation with brain water and electrolytes. Medicine 55:121-129, 1976.

Berl T: Treating hyponatremia: Damned if we do and damned if we don't. Kidney Int 37:1006-1018, 1990.

Brunner JE, Redmond JM, Haggar AM, et al: Central pontine myelinolysis and pontine lesions after rapid correction of hyponatremia: A prospective magnetic resonance imaging study. Ann Neurol 27:61-66, 1990.

Coulthard MG, Haycock GB: Distinguishing between salt poisoning and hypernatraemic dehydration in children. BMJ 326:157-160, 2003.

Estes CM, Maye JP: Severe intraoperative hyponatremia in a patient scheduled for elective hysteroscopy: A case report. AANA J 71:203-205, 2003.

Issa MM, Young MR, Bullock AR, et al: Dilutional hyponatremia of TURP syndrome: A historical event in the 21st century. Urology 64:298-301, 2004.

Janicic N: Evaluation and management of hypo-osmolality in hospitalized patients. Endocrinol Metab Clin North Am 32:459-481, 2003.

Moritz ML, Ayus JC: Disorders of water metabolism in children. Pediatr Rev 23:371-380, 2002.

Nguyen MK, Kurtz I: New insights into the pathophysiology of the dysnatremias: A quantitative analysis. Am J Physiol Renal Physiol 287: F172-F180, 2004.

Norenberg MD, Papendick RE: Chronicity of hyponatremia as a factor in experimental myelinolysis. Ann Neurol 15:544-547, 1984.

Ofran Y, Lavi D, Opher T, et al: Fatal voluntary salt intake resulting in the highest ever documented sodium plasma level in adults (255 mmol L⁻¹): A disorder linked to female gender and psychiatric disorders. J Intern Med 256:525-528, 2004.

Oster JR, Singer I: Hyponatremia, hypoosmolalilty and hypotonicity: Tables and fables. Arch Intern Med 159:333-336, 1999.

Rose BD: Hypoosmolal states: Hyponatremia. In Jeffers JD, Navrozov M (eds): Clinical Physiology of Acid-Base and Electrolyte Disorders. New York, McGraw-Hill, 1994, pp 651-694.

Steele A, Gowrishankar M, Abrahamson S, et al: Postoperative hyponatremia despite near-isotonic saline infusion: A phenomenon of desalination. Ann Intern Med 126:20-25, 1997.

Weisberg LS: Pseudohyponatremia: A reappraisal. Am J Med 86:315-318, 1989.

Metabolic Acidosis and Alkalosis

104

Mark Nunnally and Patrick Neligan

Case Synopsis

A 56-year-old man is chronically critically ill. Serum chemistries and blood gas analysis are performed. The data are as follows: sodium (Na^+) 130 mEq/L, potassium (K^+) 4 mEq/L, chloride (Cl^-) 100 mEq/L, total carbon dioxide (CO_2) 24 mEq/L, urea 10 mg/dL, creatinine 1.0 mg/dL, albumin 1.0 g/dL, lactate 6.0 mEq/dL, pH 7.42, CO_2 tension (Pco_2) 40 mm Hg, bicarbonate (HCO_3) 24 mEq/L, and base excess (BE)+1 mEq/L.

PROBLEM ANALYSIS

Definition

Acid-base analysis is a method of identifying abnormalities of ventilation or electrolyte balance that relies on the chemical properties of water. Water is a highly ionizing solvent and exists in high concentration (55 M), but there is little dissociation into its components: hydrogen and hydroxyl ions. The potential for such dissociation is determined by electrical charge and temperature. Electrical neutrality is always constant.

Clinical quantification of water dissociation relies on measurement of the hydrogen ion concentration in arterial blood, which averages 0.00004 mEq/L. For convenience, this is expressed in negative logarithmic form as pH. The physiologic pH of serum is meticulously maintained by the body and is 7.4 at 37°C. If serum pH is less than 7.35, a state of acidemia exists. If it is greater than 7.45, a state of alkalemia exists.

The extracellular fluid is a cellular and ionic mix of chemicals and organic proteins whose charges influence the dissociation of water. An acid substance may increase the hydrogen ion concentration of extracellular fluid (lower the pH), whereas a base substance may decrease the hydrogen ion concentration of extracellular fluid (raise the pH). Acids either dissociate in solution to yield an anion or associate with a hydroxyl ion to form water. Bases either dissociate to form a cation plus a hydroxyl ion or associate with a hydrogen ion to form water. Thus, anions are acids, and cations bases. This process is governed by three principles:

1. *Electrical neutrality:* The number of positive charges must equal the number of negative charges.
2. *Mass conservation:* The quantity of a substance remains constant unless added, generated, or destroyed.
3. *Dissociation equilibria:* The dissociation equilibria for all partially dissociated substances must be satisfied. In all cases, the water dissociation equilibrium readjusts to the ionic milieu.

Although a variety of complicated approaches have been used to explain acid-base chemistry, the approach proposed by Stewart is most applicable to perioperative medicine.

Using a complex mathematical model, Stewart determined that only three independent variables govern water dissociation and thus acid-base balance (Table 104-1):

1. *Arterial partial pressure of carbon dioxide ($Paco_2$):* CO_2 hydrates to form carbonic acid, which is transported in blood bound to hemoglobin and as bicarbonate.
2. *Strong ion difference (SID):* Strong ions are fully dissociated in solution. One example is lactate, whose pKa is 3.4. The SID is the electrical difference between the positively charged strong cations (sodium, potassium, magnesium, calcium) and the negatively charged strong anions (chloride, lactate, ketones, sulfate, formate). The SID is always positive and is determined mainly by the relative concentrations of sodium and chloride. Removal of strong cations or anions, or a change in their volume of distribution (e.g., the extracellular fluid volume of free water), alters the SID. Normally, the SID is 44 mEq/L. If it increases, the net effect is alkalinizing; if it decreases, the net effect is acidifying.
3. *Total concentration of partially dissociated weak anions (A_{TOT}):* The major weak acids are albumin and phosphate. Both quantity and dissociation equilibria determine the effect of A_{TOT} on water dissociation.

There are two reasons why acid-base disorders are important. First, tissue dysfunction occurs at extremes of acidosis and alkalosis. Second, and perhaps more important, acidosis and alkalosis may be indicators of serious underlying pathology, such as tissue hypoperfusion, dehydration, and renal failure. As such, acid-base abnormalities are critical manifestations of underlying pathologies.

Recognition

Four primary disturbances of acid-base balance exist: respiratory acidosis, respiratory alkalosis, metabolic acidosis, and metabolic alkalosis. Mixed respiratory acidosis and metabolic acidosis is common in severely injured or infected patients, while mixed respiratory acidosis and metabolic alkalosis is seen in chronic respiratory failure.

Respiratory acid-base disorders arise from the partial pressure of CO_2 in the blood and are related to ventilation. Respiratory acidosis results from hypoventilation due to loss

Table 104–1 ■ Classification of Primary Acid-Base Abnormalities

	Acidosis	Alkalosis	At-a-Glance Pearls
Respiratory	Increased P_{CO_2}	Decreased P_{CO_2}	$\downarrow$pH 0.08 for each 10 mm Hg in P_{CO_2}
Metabolic			
Abnormal SID			
Due to water	Water excess, dilutional $\downarrow$ SID, $\downarrow$ [Na$^+$]	Water deficit, contraction $\uparrow$ SID, $\uparrow$ [Na+]	Dilutional acidosis is usually present when NaCl <136 mEq/L, contraction alkalosis when >148 mEq/L
Due to electrolytes Chloride	Chloride excess $\downarrow$ SID, $\uparrow$ [Cl$^-$]	Chloride deficit $\uparrow$ SID, $\downarrow$ [Cl$^-$]	Hyperchloremic acidosis is usually present if corrected serum Cl$^-$ >112 mEq/L, hypochloremic alkalosis if <100 mEq/L [Cl$^-$ CORRECTED] = [Cl$^-$ MEASURED] × ([Na$^+$ NORMAL] / [Na$^+$ MEASURED])
Unmeasured anions [A$^-$], e.g., lactate, keto acids	$\downarrow$ SID, $\uparrow$ [A$^-$]		Most, but not all, [A$^-$] behave as strong anions; in renal failure, [A$^-$] consist of formate and sulfate (hyperphosphatemia is also a common acidosis)
Abnormal A$_{TOT}$			
Albumin [Alb]	$\uparrow$ [Alb] (rare)	$\downarrow$ [Alb]	Hypoalbuminemic alkalosis is usually present when the serum albumin is >35 g/dL
Phosphate [Pi]	$\uparrow$ [Pi]	$\downarrow$ [Pi]	Hyperphosphatemic acidosis is usually present when the serum phosphate is >2.0 mmol/L

A$_{TOT}$, total concentration of partially dissociated weak anions; SID, strong ion difference.
From Fencl V, Jabor A, Kazda A, et al: Diagnosis of metabolic acid-base disturbances in critically ill patients. Am J Respir Crit Care Med 162:2246-2251, 2000.

of respiratory drive, neuromuscular or chest wall disorders, rapid or shallow breathing, ventilation-perfusion mismatching, or an increase in the fraction of dead space ventilation. Respiratory alkalosis arises from increased alveolar minute ventilation (e.g., with pain, anxiety, sepsis, or hepatic insufficiency). Acute respiratory alkalosis usually accompanies acute metabolic acidosis.

Metabolic acidosis is caused by a decrease in SID or an increase in A$_{TOT}$. A change in SID can be caused by anion gain (as occurs with lactic, renal, keto-, and hyperchloremic acidosis) or cation loss (severe diarrhea, renal tubular acidosis). Acidosis can also be caused by strong ion dilution in a larger extracellular volume (dilutional acidosis), excessive hypotonic fluid intake, certain poisons (methanol, ethylene glycol, isopropyl alcohol), hyperglycemia, mannitol administration, or reduced ability to excrete free water. In acute metabolic acidosis, three possible diagnoses should be investigated immediately:

1. *Lactic acidosis:* This is caused by increased glycolysis and lactate production. It may be due to hypoxemia, hypoperfusion, congenital errors of metabolism, or exposure to biguanide or toxins.
2. *Ketoacidosis:* Ketones include acetate, acetoacetate, and β-hydroxybutyrate. All act as strong anions. Ketoacidosis results from starvation or insulin deficiency. Diabetic ketoacidosis is characterized by ketosis and hyperglycemia.
3. *Acute renal failure:* Renal acidosis is caused by the accumulation of ions excreted exclusively by the kidney—sulfate, formate, and the weak acid phosphate.

A variety of other processes can also cause metabolic acidosis. Low serum sodium (<135 mEq/L) should alert the clinician to the possibility of a dilutional acidosis.

Alcohol toxicity is suspected with an osmolar gap. A difference between measured and calculated serum osmolality greater than 12 mOsm indicates the presence of unmeasured osmoles. Following infusion of large volumes of 0.9% saline, 5% albumin, or 6% hetastarch, hyperchloremic acidosis is common. All of these contain 154 mEq of both Na$^+$ and Cl$^-$ (SID = 0) and thus reduce serum SID.

Metabolic alkalosis can be caused by chloride loss, an increase in sodium relative to chloride, or loss of weak acid. Renal chloride loss is a compensatory response to chronic respiratory acidosis. Chloride may also be lost via the gastrointestinal tract with vomiting or nasogastric suctioning. The sodium concentration increases due to a loss of free water (contraction alkalosis) or after administration of sodium with a weak anion (e.g., bicarbonate, citrate, acetate). Finally, albumin is the most contributory weak acid, and hypoalbuminemia is a common cause of metabolic alkalosis in critically ill or malnourished patients.

Risk Assessment

Historically, the gradual introduction of serum assays directly influenced the evaluation of acid-base abnormalities. Early assays for pH resulted in quantification of serum or blood by titration to a pH of 7.4. The base deficit-excess (BDE) is the amount (in mEq/L) of strong cation or anion required to return pH to 7.4, with PaCO$_2$ adjusted to 40 mm Hg. Current algorithms for computing BDE are derived from the Van Slyke equation. Modern analyzers sample PCO$_2$, electrolytes, and lactate and make more comprehensive analysis possible. However, BDE is still a useful tool for quantitative comparison. Figure 104-1 demonstrates a stepwise approach to acid-base disorders that includes BDE.

PHYSIOLOGIC IMBALANCE & COEXISTING DISEASE

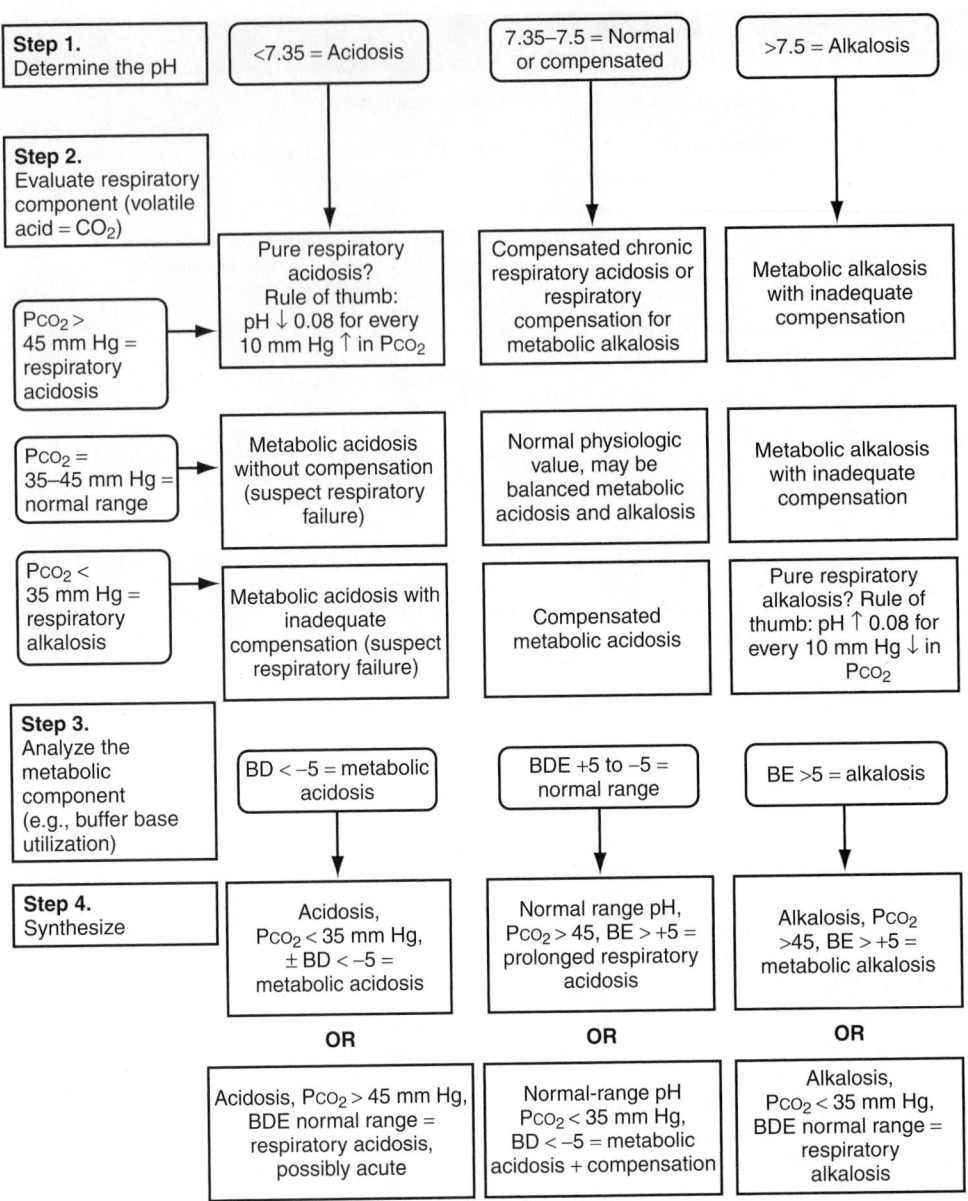

Figure 104–1 ■ Stepwise approach to blood gas analysis. Analysis of measured variables and base deficit-excess (BDE). If the acid-base picture does not conform to any of these, a mixed picture is present, and the Stewart-Fencl-Gilfix method should be used to tease out coexisting acidifying and alkalinizing processes. BD, base deficit; BE, base excess.

Implications

The anion gap theory was developed by Emmett and Narins in 1977 as a method to evaluate simple metabolic acidosis. The system is based on the contribution of weak acids (i.e., phosphate and albumin) and unmeasured anions to electrical neutrality. The sum of the difference in charge of common extracellular ions reveals an unaccounted for "gap" of 10 to 12 mEq/L—the anion gap: $Na^+ + K^+ - (Cl^- + HCO_3^-)$.

If a patient develops a metabolic acidosis and the gap widens to, for example, 16 mEq/L, the acidosis is caused by unmeasured anions, such as lactate or ketones. If the gap does not widen, then the anions are measured and the acidosis is hyperchloremic. Figure 104-2 depicts an approach to the diagnosis of metabolic acidosis using the anion gap. Although this is a useful tool, it is weakened by the assumption of what is or is not a "normal" gap and should be corrected in critically ill patients for hypoalbuminemia using the following formula: Anion gap = Calculated anion gap + 2.5 × (4.5 g/dL – Observed albumin [g/dL]).

The most comprehensive approach to acid-base physiology is Stewart's quantitative approach. This technique permits quantitative comparison of the relative contributions of the different components of acid-base balance. It is the most complete assessment of the variables influencing acid-base chemistry, but it is too cumbersome for rapid application.

A simpler, more workable approach is to use a modification of this approach, the BDE gap. This allows recalculation of BDE using strong ions, free water, and albumin. The resulting BDE gap should mirror the SID and reveal the true anion gap:

$$BDE = Standard\ base\ deficit\text{-}excess$$

Modern blood gas analyzers calculate the BDE by the following equation:

$$BDE = 0.9287 \times [HCO_3^- - 24.4 + 14.83 \times (pH - 7.4)]$$

$$BEfw = Changes\ in\ free\ water = 0.3 \times (Na - 140)$$

$$BECl = Changes\ in\ chloride = 102 - ([Cl] \times 140\ [Na])$$

Figure 104–2 ■ Evaluation of metabolic acidosis using the anion gap. BUN, blood urea nitrogen.

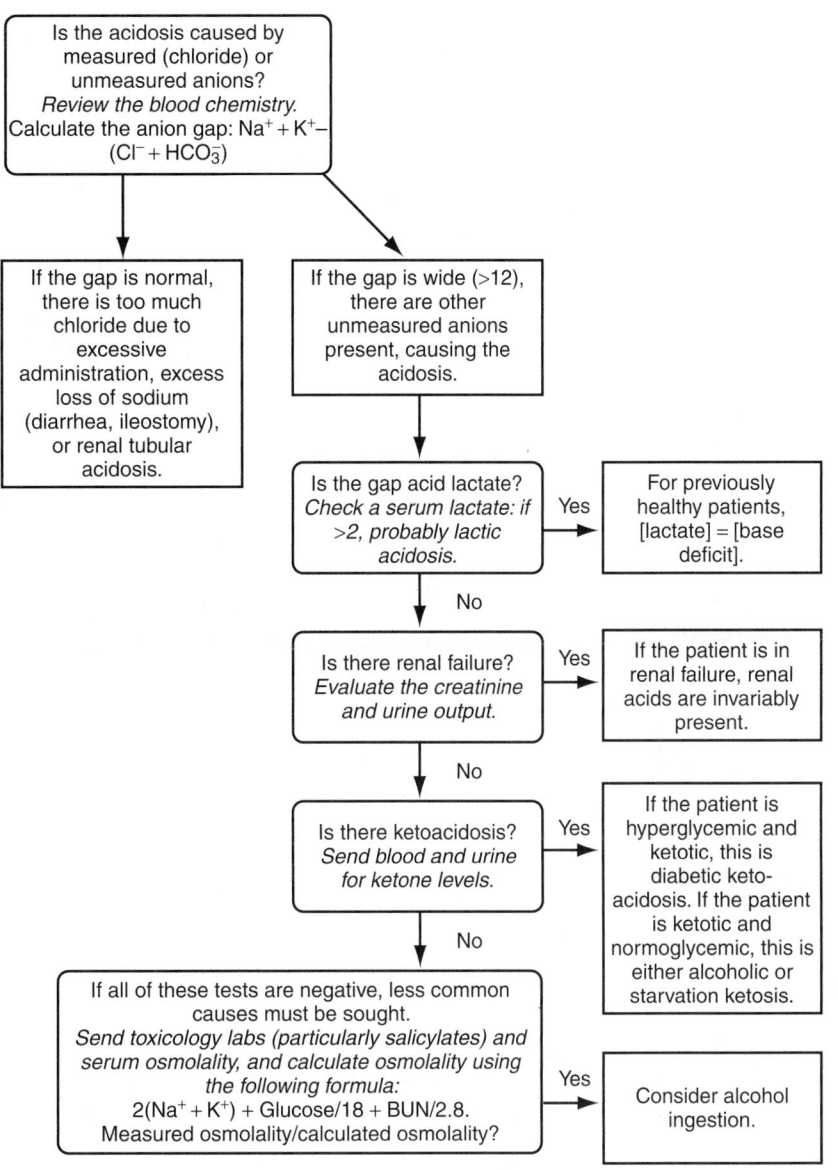

BEalb = Changes in albumin = $3.4 \times (4.5 - \text{Albumin [g/dL]})$

CBE = Calculated BDE = BEfw + BECl + BEalb

BEG = Base excess caused by unmeasured anions = BDE − CBE

This useful approach separates multiple simultaneous acid-base disturbances, such as those that occur in critically ill patients. A further simplification of this approach has been proposed and validated by Story and colleagues:

Sodium-chloride effect (mEq/L) = $[\text{Na}^+] - [\text{Cl}^-] - 38$

Albumin effect (mEq/L) = $0.25 \times (42 - [\text{Albumin (g/L)}])$

Thus, the sodium-chloride effect on the BDE plus the albumin effect minus the calculated BDE equals the BDE gap.

MANAGEMENT

Therapy is directed at the cause of the acid-base abnormality. Respiratory alkalosis is corrected by reducing iatrogenic hyperventilation or removing the causes of an increased respiratory drive (e.g., hypoxemia, pain, anxiety). Respiratory acidosis may require reversal of hypnotics or opioids or an increase in minute ventilation, but in isolation it is probably a minor abnormality. Hypercapnia is often well tolerated (e.g., patients with acute respiratory distress syndrome and multiorgan system dysfunction). Lactic acidosis due to circulatory failure is treated with resuscitation and hemodynamic optimization. Electrolyte abnormalities are corrected by replacement of specific deficiencies, correction of free water disturbances, and hemodialysis, if necessary. Toxic ingestions may require specific therapies (e.g., ethanol infusion in methanol poisoning, methemoglobin induction in cyanide toxicity), purging, adsorption, or hemodialysis. Ketoacidosis compels a search for a cause (starvation, diabetes, excessive alcohol consumption) and appropriate therapy. Figure 104-2 outlines an approach to the management of metabolic acidosis. Metabolic alkalosis (Fig. 104-3) is generally well tolerated but may be treated with chloride replacement if it is the result of hypochloremia. This is accomplished by the administration of 0.9% saline solution.

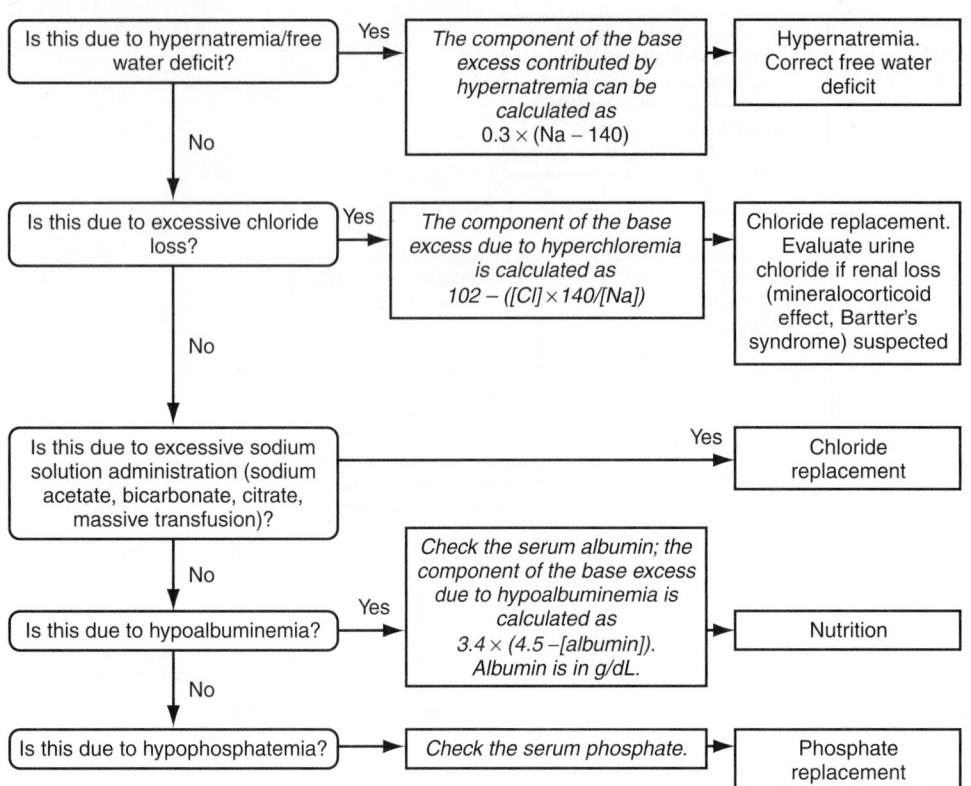

Figure 104–3 ■ Evaluation of metabolic alkalosis.

Hypoalbuminemia is a marker of severe illness and resolves with treatment of the underlying cause.

PREVENTION

Significant perioperative acid-base derangements are better avoided rather than managed after the fact. Adequate prevention requires vigilance for common sources of acid-base abnormalities. Serum lactate is used to follow the quality of resuscitation for patients in shock, particularly hemorrhagic shock. The magnitude of the base deficit and speed of resolution have prognostic implications. Type 1 diabetics should be treated with insulin perioperatively, and patients with acute or chronic renal failure may have to undergo dialysis. Care should be taken to avoid hyperventilation, especially in the setting of chronic respiratory acidosis. Hyperventilation reduces the central respiratory drive, making it more difficult to subsequently wean the patient from the ventilator. Appropriate fluid selection avoids SID disturbances due to dilution or excess chloride administration. Hypotonic and dextrose-containing fluids are best avoided. Fluid choice makes little difference in patients having small-volume resuscitation. If larger-volume resuscitation is expected, then solutions that more closely match the electrolyte content of extracellular fluid (lactated Ringer's, Normosol, Plasma-Lyte) are advised. Many commercially available colloids also contain high concentrations of chloride. Human albumin solution, some hetastarches, and gelatins are formulated in sodium chloride; large volumes of these can cause hyperchloremic acidosis. In the setting of chloride loss from nasogastric suctioning, normal saline can be administered until the base excess returns to zero. Normal saline is also therapeutic with excess sodium citrate administration (e.g., large-volume blood or fresh frozen plasma transfusions). Proactive management strategies minimize the risk of patients developing multiple complex acid-base disturbances in the postoperative setting.

Using the approach advocated by Fencl and colleagues and Gilfix and associates, correcting the BDE for acidifying and alkalinizing processes for the patient presented in the

Table 104–2 ■ Correction of Base Deficit-Excess

Acidifying Process	Magnitude	BDC	Alkalinizing Process	Magnitude	BEC
Hyponatremia	130 mEq/L	−3	Hypoalbuminemia	1.0 g/dL	+11.9
Hyperchloremia	100 mEq/L	−3			
Lactate	6 mEq/L	−6			
Total		−12	Total		+11.9

BDC, base deficit corrected; BEC, base excess corrected.
BDC − BEC = 0.9

case synopsis is complex (Table 104-2). In this example, the patient has three significant acidifying processes. The presence of lactic acidosis is ominous. However, by using traditional approaches to acid-base analysis (bicarbonate or BDE), the presence of this abnormality would not be apparent.

Further Reading

Alfaro V, Torras R, Ibanez J, et al: A physical-chemical analysis of the acid-base response to chronic obstructive pulmonary disease. Can J Physiol Pharmacol 11:1229-1235, 1996.

Balasubramanyan N, Havens PL, Hoffman GM: Unmeasured anions identified by the Fencl-Stewart method predict mortality better than base excess, anion gap, and lactate in patients in the pediatric intensive care unit. Crit Care Med 27:1577-1581, 1999.

Emmett M, Narins RG: Clinical use of the anion gap. Medicine 56:38-54, 1977.

Fencl V, Jabor A, Kazda A, et al: Diagnosis of metabolic acid-base disturbances in critically ill patients. Am J Respir Crit Care Med 162:2246-2251, 2000.

Figge J, Jabor A, Kazda A, et al: Anion gap and hypoalbuminemia. Crit Care Med 26:1807-1810, 1998.

Figge J, Rossing TH, Fencl V: The role of serum proteins in acid-base equilibria. J Lab Clin Med 117: 453-467, 1991.

Gilfix BM, Bique M, Magder S: A physical chemical approach to the analysis of acid-base balance in the clinical setting. J Crit Care 8:187-197, 1993.

Hickling KG: Permissive hypercapnia. Respir Care Clin N Am 8:155-169, 2002.

Morgan TJ, Clark C, Endre ZH: Accuracy of base excess—an in vitro evaluation of the Van Slyke equation. Crit Care Med 28:2932-2936, 2003.

Morgan TJ, Venkatesh B, Hall J: Crystalloid strong ion difference determines metabolic acid-base change during in vitro hemodilution. Crit Care Med 30:157-160, 2002.

Rutherford EJ, Morris JA Jr, Reed GW, et al: Base deficit stratifies mortality and determines therapy. J Trauma 33:417-423, 1992.

Salem MM, Mujais SK: Gaps in the anion gap. Arch Intern Med 152:1625-1629, 1992.

Schlichtig R, Grogono AW, Severinghaus JW: Human $PaCO_2$ and standard base excess compensation for acid-base imbalance. Crit Care Med 26:1173-1179, 1998.

Siggaard-Andersen O: The Van Slyke equation. Scand J Clin Lab Invest 37:S15-S20, 1977.

Stewart PA: Modern quantitative acid-base chemistry. Can J Physiol Pharmacol 61:1444-1461, 1983.

Story DA, Morimatsu H, Bellomo R: Strong ions, weak acids and base excess: A simplified Fencl-Stewart approach to clinical acid-base disorders. Br J Anaesth 92:54-60, 2004.

Adrenal Insufficiency

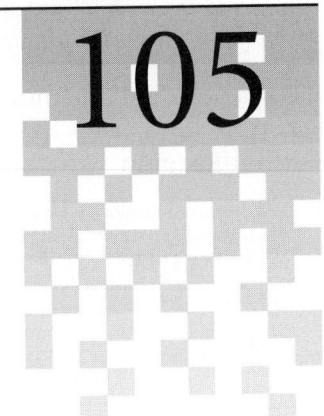

105

Jonathan T. Ketzler and Douglas B. Coursin

Case Synopsis

A 68-year-old, 5-foot 10-inch tall, 100-kg man develops refractory hypotension toward the end of a laparotomy to remove the left colon because of recurrent diverticulitis and suspected peridiverticular abscess. The patient remains intubated at the end of the procedure and is taken to the intensive care unit (ICU), where a pulmonary artery catheter is placed. The pulmonary artery occlusion pressure is 6 mm Hg, the systemic vascular resistance is 475 dynes/cm^5, cardiac output is 10 L/minute and cardiac index is 6 L/minute/m^2. The patient is being mechanically ventilated; he has a heart rate of 128 beats per minute in sinus rhythm and blood pressure of 88/42 mm Hg on norepinephrine at 0.1 µg/kg per minute and dobutamine at 5 µg/kg per minute. The patient's medical history is remarkable for hypertension and type 2 diabetes chronically treated with lisinopril and metformin (Glucophage), respectively. Both were withheld on the day of surgery. Shortly after his admission to the ICU, a diagnostic test is performed and a new medication is added to the therapeutic regimen. After several hours, the patient is hemodynamically stable, and vasopressors have been discontinued.

PROBLEM ANALYSIS

Definition

Adrenal insufficiency (AI) is a relatively rare but potentially life-threatening condition that can be quiescent until unmasked by medical stressors such as sepsis, traumatic insults, or surgical procedures.

Sir Thomas Addison described primary AI in 1855. Approximately a century later Harvey Cushing developed the concept of secondary AI. Causes for primary and secondary AI are listed in Table 105-1.

The hypothalamic-pituitary-adrenocortical (HPA) axis (Fig. 105-1) regulates the amount of cortisol released by the adrenals. The cycle begins with the release of corticotropin-releasing factor from the hypothalamus, which stimulates the release of adrenocorticotropic hormone (ACTH) from the anterior pituitary. ACTH then stimulates the release of cortisol from the adrenal cortex at a rate of about 20 mg/day. Cortisol (or a synthetic analogue) acts on the hypothalamus to inhibit the release of corticotropin-releasing factor and on the anterior pituitary to inhibit the release of ACTH. The associated diurnal variation in cortisol release peaks in the morning and midafternoon and then tapers off to a nadir in the evening. Although normal adults secrete about 5 to 10 mg/m^2 of cortisol (or hydrocortisone) each day, during periods of acute stress the adrenal cortex can secrete as much as 100 mg/m^2 per 24 hours.

Primary adrenal failure is rare and may be caused by trauma, hemorrhage, infection, or infiltrative disease. Secondary adrenal failure may be brought about by adrenal atrophy due to acute or chronic glucocorticoid therapy. Patients with adrenal atrophy may show no symptoms of AI.

However, when subjected to the stress of even modest surgery or acute illness, these patients may develop life-threatening symptoms of AI.

Along with the classification of AI as a primary or secondary process, there is now recognition of absolute or relative AI. Classic Addison's disease due to autoimmune destruction of the adrenals is an example of primary, absolute AI. In contrast, the normal stress-induced increase in cortisol production may be blunted during life-threatening illnesses (e.g., sepsis) in some patients owing to relative AI. Alternatively, there may be down-regulation of cortisol binding and adrenergic receptors despite the normal stress-induced increase in steroid genesis, another explanation for relative AI. It is still uncertain whether etomidate blunts normal adrenal steroid genesis (see Table 105-1) to cause relative AI in critically ill patients. Finally, as illustrated in the case synopsis, relative AI may underlie life-threatening hemodynamic instability. However, if it is recognized as such and treated with stress doses of glucocorticoids, this process may be reversed.

Recognition

The presentation of acute AI varies from a gradual onset over many days in a patient who is not stressed to a sudden fall in blood pressure associated with major stress such as an operation, trauma, or infection. Hypotension associated with AI can be severe and refractory to treatment. Chronic AI can be insidious and nonspecific in onset and remain undiagnosed for months. The prevalence of signs and symptoms associated with AI are detailed in Table 105-2. The most specific sign of primary AI is hyperpigmentation of the skin and mucosal surfaces caused by the high levels of corticotropin resulting from decreased cortisol feedback.

Table 105–1 ■ Causes of Adrenal Insufficiency

Primary Adrenal Insufficiency
Autoimmune
  Polyglandular autoimmune syndrome types I and II
Infectious
  Tuberculosis
  Histoplasmosis
  Blastomycosis
  Coccidiomycosis
  Cryptococcosis
  Human immunodeficiency virus
  Cytomegalovirus
  Mycobacterium avium-intracellulare
  Cryptococcus
  Toxoplasmosis
  Kaposi's sarcoma
Fibrosis
Infarction
Adrenal hemorrhage
  Waterhouse-Friderichsen syndrome
  Lupus anticoagulant
  Antiphospholipid antibodies
  Immune thrombocytopenic purpura
  Heparin-induced
  Thrombocytopenia
  Anticoagulants
Metastatic disease
  Lung
  Gastric
  Breast
  Malignant melanoma
  Lymphoma
Drugs
  Decreased steroid synthesis
    Metyrapone
    Aminoglutethimide
    Mitotane
    Etomidate*
    Ketoconazole
  Increased steroid catabolism
    Rifampin
    Dilantin
    Phenobarbital
Familial
  Familial glucocorticoid deficiency
  Adrenoleukodystrophy
  Adrenomyeloneuropathy

Secondary Adrenal Insufficiency
Exogenous steroid administration
Pituitary or hypothalamic diseases
  Infiltrative tumor (adenoma)
  Sarcoid
  Hemorrhage
  Autoimmune
Isolated ACTH deficiency
Surgical
  Pituitary surgery
  Removal of a functioning adrenal adenoma

*Still unproven and therefore speculative.
ACTH, adrenocorticotropic hormone.

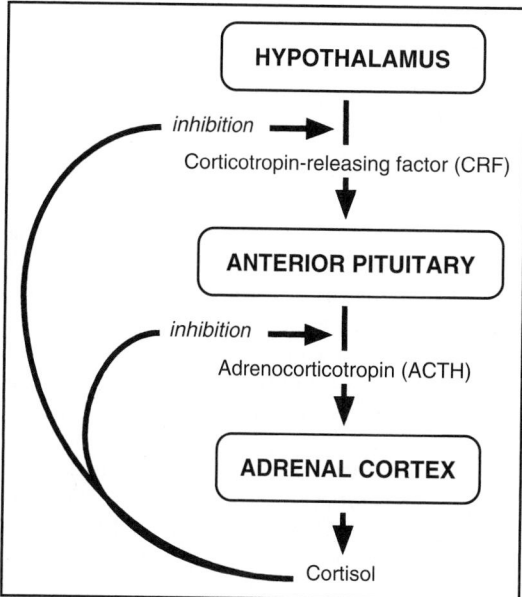

Figure 105–1 ■ Hypothalamic-pituitary-adrenocortical axis.

this is not related to sodium excretion but rather to water intoxication secondary to an elevated level of antidiuretic hormone (ADH), as well as a primary defect in free water excretion related to glucocorticoid deficiency.

Hypotension can be a common finding in both chronic and acute AI. Hypotension associated with acute AI has been reported as high-output circulatory failure with hallmarks of elevated cardiac output and index, normal pulmonary artery occlusion pressure, and decreased systemic vascular resistance. The pathogenesis of such hypotension is unknown but may include a combination of three possible mechanisms: (1) impairment of the direct effect of glucocorticoids on vascular smooth muscle, (2) loss of the "permissive" glucocorticoid effect on catecholamine synthesis and action, and (3) a decrease in the effects of glucocorticoids on vasoactive peptides. Dehydration can also be a factor in the hypotension associated with acute and chronic AI.

Table 105–2 ■ Prevalence of Signs and Symptoms of Chronic Adrenal Insufficiency

Signs and Symptoms	Prevalence (%)
Weakness and fatigue	74–100
Weight loss	56–100
Hyperpigmentation	92–96
Hypertension	59–88
Hyponatremia	88–96
Hyperkalemia	52–64
Gastrointestinal symptoms	56
Postural dizziness	12
Adrenal calcification	9–33
Hypercalcemia	6–41
Muscle and joint pain	6
Vitiligo	4

Data from De Rosa G, Corsello SM, Cecchin L, et al: Clinical study of Addison's disease. Exp Clin Endocrinol 90:232-242, 1987.

Because primary AI (Addison's disease) develops from failure of the adrenal gland itself, there is evidence of both glucocorticoid and mineralocorticoid deficiencies. Because secondary AI is an interruption of the pituitary-hypophysial axis that stimulates the adrenal glands to secrete cortisol, but spares the gland itself, it presents as pure glucocorticoid deficiency. In this case, the patient may also have hyponatremia;

Risk Assessment

Using clinical indicators, there is no way to predict consistently which patients are at risk for developing AI during the stress of a surgical procedure or severe illness. Patients with certain comorbid diseases such as asthma, inflammatory bowel disease, collagen vascular disease, and rheumatoid arthritis may have received corticosteroids within 1 year, and the HPA axis can be suppressed by a relatively modest dose of exogenous steroids administered for as short a period as 7 to 10 days. Except for low-dose (prednisone ≤5 to 7.5 mg/day) and alternate-day regimens, chronic administration of corticosteroids suppresses the HPA axis, and recovery of its function can take up to 12 months. Normalization of pituitary function comes first; adrenocortical function returns more gradually.

The reported incidence of perioperative AI is between 0.01% and 0.7%. A report by Rivers and colleagues suggested that older patients may have a greater risk of relative AI. The incidence during septic shock also appears to be significant, and steroid replacement therapy has been reported to significantly improve outcome in a selected subpopulation of such patients.

Even though there are ample case reports of hypotension and even death secondary to AI, there are also many reports of glucocorticoid-treated patients undergoing major surgery without any perioperative glucocorticoid coverage. Most of these patients had uneventful perioperative courses, probably because they had normal perioperative biochemical indices of HPA function. This suggests that a historical assessment of glucocorticoid administration alone is unreliable.

Endocrine evaluation is necessary in patients with suspected adrenal failure. A random screening cortisol level less than 25 µg/dL is abnormal when measured during the stress of an acute illness. A higher level does not preclude a subsequent abnormal cosyntropin stimulation test. A low cortisol level (<25 µg/dL) during a stressful illness or following stressful surgery mandates further evaluation. Major trauma and surgical stress usually result in a two- to threefold increase in plasma cortisol levels, with levels returning to normal 4 to 5 days after the stress. Levels may remain increased if there are complications.

The cosyntropin stimulation test is still the best test for evaluating adrenal function in critically ill patients. After injection of 250 µg of cosyntropin, cortisol levels are compared with baseline levels at 30 and 60 minutes. The exact interpretation of test results remains controversial, but the best outcomes in septic patients occur in those with baseline values greater than 36 µg/dL and with at least a 9 µg/dL difference between baseline and peak values.

Finally, if life-threatening AI is strongly suspected, treatment need not be delayed for diagnostic testing. Dexamethasone provides glucocorticoid coverage without interfering with cosyntropin studies.

Implications

An acute adrenal crisis can occur spontaneously or in response to significant emotional or physiologic stress. Stressors may include extreme psychological stress, trauma, withdrawal from alcohol or opioids, infection, general anesthesia, or surgery. During such times of stress, the patient is unable to secrete adequate amounts of cortisol to maintain hemodynamic stability.

MANAGEMENT

Because AI can progress rapidly, early recognition and intervention are essential to improve outcome. Adrenal crisis is a medical emergency, and treatment cannot be delayed for extensive diagnostic studies. Therapy is directed toward rapidly increasing the circulating levels of cortisol. Without such treatment, even symptomatic treatment for volume depletion and electrolyte imbalance is inadequate.

If AI is suspected, baseline plasma cortisol levels can be obtained just before treatment. Serum electrolytes, complete blood count, glucose, blood urea nitrogen, and creatinine are analyzed to assess for sodium depletion, potassium retention, and hypoglycemia.

During adrenal crisis, patients can lose up to 20% of their circulating intravascular blood volume. This can result in hypovolemic shock and tissue hypoperfussion, both of which can lead to lactic acidemia. Therefore, rapid infusion of intravenous fluid is started to correct dehydration and hypovolemia. Normal saline is the initial fluid of choice. Subsequent treatment of electrolyte abnormalities, volume deficits, and hypoglycemia can be guided by laboratory measurements and the patient's response to treatment.

If a patient is known to have AI, replacement therapy should be individualized, depending on the degree of surgical or medical stress. For patients at high risk who undergo major procedures or have life-threatening injuries or illnesses, hydrocortisone 100 mg can be given, with additional intravenous doses of 50 to 100 mg every 6 to 8 hours (see also Chapter 34). Such doses can usually be rapidly tapered as the patient's clinical condition improves. If the patient has no known history of AI, dexamethasone 4 to 10 mg can be given as an intravenous bolus. Dexamethasone does not interfere with the measurement of serum cortisol levels, so diagnostic tests can still be performed. However, because dexamethasone has no aldosterone activity, fludrocortisone, a mineralocorticoid, may also be needed.

Patients usually respond quickly to initial therapies, and improvement is usually seen within several hours. Adrenal dysfunction has been shown to be present in as many as 70% of patients with septic shock, and the outcome can be significantly improved with replacement therapy in 20% of such patients. Finally, because 40% to 65% of critically ill patients have high plasma renin activity, previous recommendations did not include the administration of a mineralocorticoid. Based on more recent data, some experts now advise the addition of fludrocortisone 50 µg/day or greater by mouth in patients with sepsis-induced relative AI.

PREVENTION

There are many ways to approach the administration of steroids in stressed patients with likely adrenal suppression. Some studies suggest tailoring the dose of hydrocortisone to the magnitude of the stress. Others advocate testing the HPA axis in patients at risk for AI. This is done using the cosyntropin stimulation test, which is easy and safe. However, there is controversy over how to interpret the test and even over what dose of cosyntropin to use. Some advocate the use of a more physiologic dose (e.g., 1 µg) instead of the currently recommended 250 µg for stimulation. Because the risk of steroids is so small in most stressed patients, most authorities suggest the use of stress doses in any patient at risk for AI. Because cortisol production under extreme stress is as much as 300 mg/day, hydrocortisone can be administered in 100-mg intravenous doses every 8 hours for 2 days or as a continuous infusion of 300 mg/day for 2 days (see also Chapter 34). In the absence of continued stress, these doses can be tapered to 50 mg every 8 hours for 1 to 2 days and then stopped, or continued at 25 mg every 8 hours for 1 to 2 days and then stopped. How steroids are tapered must be determined on a case-by-case basis, depending on the amount and duration of stress in patients with likely adrenal suppression. Finally, some have reported better outcomes with weight-related dosing for the treatment of chronic AI.

Further Reading

Connery LE, Coursin DB: Assessment and therapy of selected endocrine disorders. Anesthesiol Clin North Am 22:93-123, 2004.

Cook DM: Safe use of glucocorticoids: How to monitor patients taking these potent agents. Postgrad Med 93:145-154, 1992.

Coursin DB, Wood KE: Corticosteroid supplementation in adrenal insufficiency. JAMA 287:236-240, 2002.

Eichacker PQ, Parent C, Kalil A, et al: Risk and the efficacy of anti-inflammatory agents: Retrospective and confirmatory studies of sepsis. Am J Respir Crit Care Med 9:1197-1205, 2002.

Goldberg PA, Inzucchi SE: Critical issues in endocrinology. Clin Chest Med 24:583-606, 2003.

Holmes CL, Walley KK: The evaluation and management of shock. Clin Chest Med 24:775-789, 2003.

Mah PM, Jenkins RC, Rostami-Hodjegan A: Weight-related dosing, timing and monitoring hydrocortisone replacement therapy in patients with adrenal insufficiency. Clin Endocrinol 61:367-375, 2004.

Marik PE, Zaloga GP: Adrenal insufficiency in the critically ill: A new look at an old problem. Chest 122:1784-1796, 2002.

Minneci PC, Deans KJ, Banks SM, et al: Meta-analysis: The effect of steroids on survival and shock during sepsis depends on the dose. Ann Intern Med 1:47-56, 2004.

O'Brien JM Jr, Abraham E: New approaches to the treatment of sepsis. Clin Chest Med 24:521-548, 2003.

Oelkers W: Adrenal insufficiency. N Engl J Med 335:1206-1211, 1996.

Rivers EP, Gaspari M, Saad GA, et al: Adrenal insufficiency in high-risk surgical ICU patients. Chest 119:889-896, 2001.

Salem M, Tainsh RE, Bromberg J, et al: Perioperative glucocorticoid coverage: A reassessment 42 years after emergence of a problem. Ann Surg 219:416-425, 1994.

HIV Infection and AIDS

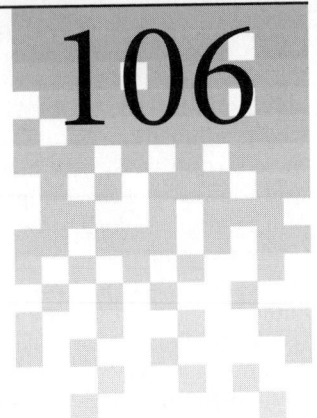

106

Michael S. Avidan and Nicola Jones

Case Synopsis

A 34-year-old woman with known human immunodeficiency virus (HIV) infection and a recent diagnosis of acquired immunodeficiency syndrome (AIDS) with *Pneumocystis jirovecii* (previously *carinii*) pneumonia presents for elective cesarean section at 38 weeks' gestation. She has been taking antiretroviral therapy throughout her pregnancy. She is very short of breath and has a dry cough, and her peripheral arterial oxygen saturation is 84% on room air. She weighs 62 kg, and her height is 164 cm. Her tympanic temperature is 37.2°C. She is alert and oriented, with no localizing neurologic signs. Her blood pressure is 90/50 mm Hg; her heart rate is 115 beats per minute, with no respiratory variation; and her respiratory rate is 26 breaths per minute. Recent laboratory tests show a CD4 T-cell count of 186 cells/mL and an HIV viral load of 240,000 copies/mL.

PROBLEM ANALYSIS

Definition

AIDS was first described in 1981 in the United States. HIV and the AIDS pandemic pose a major threat to global health. It is estimated that more than 40 million people worldwide are infected with HIV, which is thought to have caused more than 20 million deaths to date. The infection continues to spread apace, with the most rapid increases observed in southern and central Africa and in South Asia. The predominant mode of HIV transmission is heterosexual sex, and women represent a high proportion of new infections, including in developed countries.

Increasing numbers of patients presenting for surgery are HIV-seropositive or have AIDS. Anesthesiologists should be familiar with this disease and be aware of the impact of HIV on anesthesia. An understanding of the pathogenesis of HIV and an awareness of the possible drug interactions occurring with HIV therapy may help guide the choice of anesthetic technique. The possibility of nosocomial transmission of HIV highlights the need for anesthesiologists to enforce rigorous infection control policies to protect themselves, other health care workers, and their patients. Antiretroviral therapy decreases the rate of disease progression, but there is no cure available, nor is a vaccine likely in the foreseeable future.

Recognition

HIV belongs to the family Retroviridae and the genus *Lentivirus*. Members of this genus are cytopathic (cell damaging), have long latent periods, and run a chronic course. When cases of AIDS first appeared, its pathogenesis was frustratingly elusive because the disease does not appear immediately on infection with HIV. There is a variable period during which the patient remains healthy but is viremic.

Acute seroconversion illness occurs with a high viral load soon after infection. After several months, there is a gradual decrease in the viremia as the immune response occurs. The viral load is often at a steady state as the rate of viral production equals the rate of destruction. Up to 98% of T-helper lymphocytes (CD4 T cells) are located in lymph nodes, which are the major site of viral replication and T-cell destruction. There is a gradual involution of the lymph nodes, with a concomitant decrease in CD4 T cells and an increase in viral load as the inexorable onset of AIDS occurs (Fig. 106-1).

Before 1995, prospects for the treatment of HIV were gloomy. Subsequently, the situation changed dramatically as a result of four factors:

1. Improved understanding of the pathogenesis of HIV infection
2. Availability of surrogate markers of immune function and plasma viral burden
3. Development of new and more powerful drugs, such as the protease inhibitors and non-nucleoside reverse transcriptase inhibitors
4. Completion of several large clinical end-point trials that conclusively demonstrated that antiretroviral combinations significantly delayed the progression of HIV disease to AIDS and improved survival

Risk Assessment

HIV is a virus found mainly in CD4 T cells, macrophages, and monocytes, and it requires a large infecting dose for transmission. HIV has been isolated from blood, cerebrospinal fluid, tears, saliva, semen, synovial fluid, pleural fluid, peritoneal fluid, pericardial fluid, amniotic fluid, vaginal secretions, and breast milk. Modes of transmission are through oral, rectal, and vaginal sexual intercourse, blood product transfusion, shared intravenous needles, occupational acquisition, and vertical transmission from mother to child. The screening of blood products for HIV antibodies has reduced the risk of transfusion-associated infection (<1 per 750,000 donor units); the exact risk is difficult to quantify, however, and it may increase as the HIV infection rate increases in the general population. Antibody screening fails to detect the virus in the so-called window period before antibody formation, which lasts about 3 months. Nuclear amplification is an alternative technique that may allow for early virus detection.

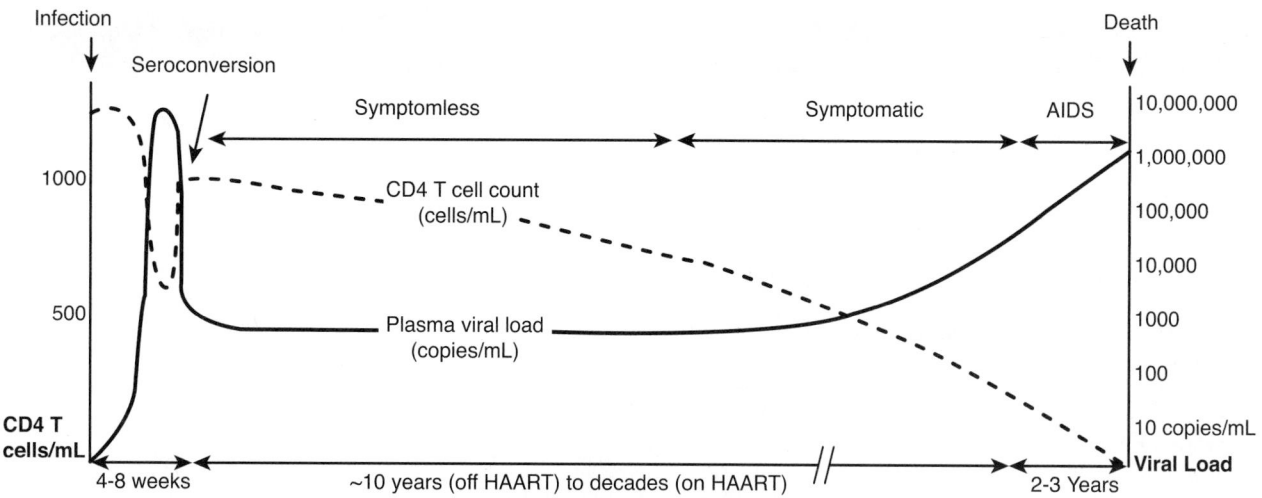

Figure 106–1 ■ Progression to acquired immunodeficiency syndrome (AIDS) of those infected with human immunodeficiency virus (HIV). Note that highly active antiretroviral therapy (HAART) greatly delays development of clinical AIDS.

Implications

UNIVERSAL PRECAUTIONS

Universal precautions for the prevention of transmission of blood-borne viruses were recommended in 1987 by the Centers for Disease Control. These precautions advise that every patient be regarded as potentially infected with a blood-borne virus.

POSTEXPOSURE PROPHYLAXIS

Following accidental exposure to a high-risk body fluid, such as a (hollow) needle-stick injury, postexposure prophylaxis is recommended for health care workers. This should commence as soon as possible after the injury, ideally within 1 to 2 hours, but it can be considered up to 1 to 2 weeks after the injury. Very-high-risk exposures may be treated beyond this time with a view to modifying rather than preventing infection. A recommended postexposure prophylaxis regimen of 4 weeks' duration is the following:

- Zidovudine 300 mg every 12 hours
- Lamivudine 150 mg every 12 hours
- Indinavir 800 mg every 8 hours

However, the high rate of toxicity and noncompliance may necessitate other regimens.

MANAGEMENT

Antiretroviral Drug Therapy

Three major classes of antiretroviral agents are currently in use (Table 106-1):

1. Nucleoside analogue reverse transcriptase inhibitors (NRTIs) bind to the evolving viral DNA and prevent the completion of reverse transcription.
2. Non-nucleoside reverse transcriptase inhibitors (NNRTIs) interfere with the transcriptional activity of reverse transcriptase by binding to it directly, downstream of the active catalytic site.
3. Protease inhibitors (PIs) inhibit the HIV protease, which cleaves the polyprotein precursors that ultimately make up the core proteins of the mature virions. PIs bind specifically to the active cleavage site.

Table 106-1 lists examples of these major classes of antiretroviral agents currently in use, as well as routes of administration and common side effects. A typical antiretroviral regimen consists of three agents: a PI or NNRTI combined with two NRTIs. Such combined therapy has been termed highly active antiretroviral therapy (HAART). In some circumstances, combinations of four or more drugs are used. The aim of therapy in treatment-naïve patients is to achieve an undetectable viral load by 24 weeks of therapy and to improve and extend the length and quality of life.

However, there is a downside to HAART. The AIDS pandemic, one of the most devastating to ever affect humankind, has now entered its third decade, and there is still no cure in sight. The initial enthusiasm that greeted HAART has been tempered by the recent discovery of multidrug-resistant viral strains. Also, there is the issue of important adverse side effects.

SIDE EFFECTS OF HAART REGIMENS

Numerous side effects and drug interactions complicate HAART regimens and decrease compliance. Patients may experience drug hypersensitivity reactions, causing fever, hypotension, and acute interstitial pneumonitis with respiratory failure. Concurrent use of zidovudine and corticosteroids may result in severe myopathy and respiratory muscle dysfunction. In addition, reports have documented several cases of respiratory failure related to HAART initiation and immune reconstitution resulting in a paradoxical worsening of *Pneumocystis* pneumonia; distinguishing this event from a superimposed respiratory infection is often clinically challenging. Of particular importance to anesthesiologists is that patients receiving HAART are subject to

Table 106–1 ■ **Major Classes of Antiretroviral Agents Currently in Use**

Drug Name	Dosing	Common Side Effects
Nucleoside Analogue Reverse Transcriptase Inhibitors		
Zidovudine (AZT/ZDV)	Oral/IV	Bone marrow suppression (neutropenia), GI upset, headache
Didanosine (DDI)	Oral	Peripheral neuropathy, pancreatitis, diarrhea
Zalcitabine (DDC)	Oral	Peripheral neuropathy, pancreatitis, oral ulcers
Stavudine (D4T)	Oral	Peripheral neuropathy
Lamivudine (3TC)	Oral	Anemia, GI upset
Abacavir	Oral	GI upset, potentially fatal acute hypersensitivity
Non-nucleoside Analogue Reverse Transcriptase Inhibitors		
Nevirapine	Oral	Rash, hepatitis, increased liver enzymes
Delavirdine	Oral	Rash, increased liver enzymes
Efavirenz	Oral	Dizziness, rash, dysphoria, increased liver enzymes
Protease Inhibitors		
Saquinavir	Oral	Diarrhea, raised transaminases, hyperlipidemia, cytochrome P-450 inhibition
Indinavir	Oral + ≥1.5 L H_2O/24 hr	Nephrolithiasis, hyperbilirubinemia, hyperlipidemia, lipodystrophy, cytochrome P-450 inhibition
Ritonavir	Oral	GI upset, circumoral paresthesia, hyperlipidemia, lipodystrophy, cytochrome P-450 inhibition
Nelfinavir	Oral	Diarrhea, hyperlipidemia, lipodystrophy, cytochrome P-450 inhibition

GI, gastrointestinal.

long-term metabolic complications, including lipid abnormalities and glucose intolerance, which may result in the development of diabetes, coronary artery disease, and cerebrovascular disease.

A syndrome resembling acute gram-negative sepsis has been reported in patients taking NRTIs. Lactic acidosis and hepatic steatosis are usually found. Patients develop high fever and can rapidly become confused and comatose. Nucleoside analogue drugs may cause inhibition of DNA polymerase gamma, the sole DNA polymerase required for the replication of mitochondrial DNA. This in turn causes mitochondrial dysfunction and impaired aerobic cellular respiration. Inhibition of oxidative phosphorylation and derangement of respiratory chain enzymes have been implicated. Riboflavin has been suggested as a potential treatment. Unfortunately, most patients die despite intensive care unit (ICU) support.

HAART Drug Interactions

PIs, particularly ritonavir, are inhibitors of cytochrome P-450 (see Table 106-1). In contrast, drugs such as nevirapine are inducers of hepatic microsomal enzymes. These variable effects on liver enzymes complicate the dosing of drugs, including anesthetic and analgesic agents, many of which undergo hepatic metabolism.

Respiratory Complications

Pneumocystis jirovecii pneumonia (PJP) does not usually occur until the CD4 T-cell count is less than 200 cells/mL. Breathlessness, night sweats, and weight loss are frequent complaints. The chest examination of may be unremarkable, and the chest radiograph is normal in many instances. Complications include respiratory failure, pneumothorax. and chronic pulmonary disease.

The chest radiograph typically shows bilateral "ground-glass" shadowing. Pneumothoraces may be evident, and there may be multiple pneumatoceles. High-resolution computed tomography scanning reveals a ground-glass appearance even when the radiograph is normal. Lung function tests show reduced lung volumes with decreased compliance and diminished diffusing capacity for carbon monoxide. Oxygen saturation measurements during exercise may be more helpful than lung function tests. If PJP is suspected, fiberoptic bronchoscopy and bronchoalveolar lavage should be performed. The advantage of an early diagnosis compensates for the high frequency of negative examinations.

Combined high-dose sulfamethoxazole (100 mg/kg per day) with trimethoprim (20 mg/kg per day) remains the treatment of choice. Systemic steroid therapy, such as prednisolone 1 mg/kg per day, is advised for patients with low oxygen saturation values. Respiratory support and supplementary oxygen are invariably required. Use of continuous positive airway pressure can, in some instances, obviate the need for positive-pressure mechanical ventilation. The prognosis for patients who require mechanical ventilation despite adjunct corticosteroid therapy is poor. Further, the use of positive end-expiratory pressure may cause pneumothorax.

Cavitary lung disease can be due to a pyogenic bacterial lung abscess, pulmonary tuberculosis (TB), fungal infection, and *Nocardia* species. Kaposi's sarcoma (KS) and lymphoma can also affect the lung. Adenopathy can lead to tracheobronchial obstruction or compression of the great vessels. Endobronchial KS may cause massive hemoptysis. HIV also directly affects the lungs, causing a destructive pulmonary syndrome similar to emphysema.

Disseminated TB is a potential cause of severe respiratory failure, and respiratory secretions should be examined routinely for acid-fast bacilli in AIDS patients with pulmonary infiltrates. Bacterial pneumonia *(Streptococcus pneumoniae, Moraxella catarrhalis, Haemophilus influenzae, Staphylococcus aureus, Pseudomonas aeruginosa)* can also cause severe acute respiratory failure. Empirical antibacterial treatment to cover these microorganisms should be given when a bacterial agent is suspected. Outbreaks of multidrug-resistant TB have occurred in patients with HIV infection and in health care workers. Airborne transmission by inhalation of infective aerosols justifies appropriate isolation measures to protect medical staff and other patients from TB transmission.

Central Nervous System Complications

Neurologic disease ranging from AIDS dementia to infectious or neoplastic involvement may complicate AIDS. Three entities constitute mostly focal cerebral processes: cerebral toxoplasmosis, primary central nervous system (CNS) lymphoma, and progressive multifocal leukoencephalopathy. Focal lesions may increase intracerebral pressure, thereby precluding neuraxial anesthesia. Spinal cord involvement, peripheral neuropathy, and myopathy may occur with cytomegalovirus or HIV infection itself. Giving succinylcholine may be hazardous in this setting. *Cryptococcus neoformans*, HIV, and TB can cause meningitis. HIV infection is associated with autonomic neuropathy, and this can manifest as hemodynamic instability during anesthesia or in the ICU.

Cardiovascular Disease

Cardiac involvement in the course of HIV is common but is often clinically silent. Up to 50% of patients with HIV have abnormal echocardiographic findings at some point in their disease. Approximately 25% have pericardial effusions. Myocarditis is more common in advanced HIV and may be caused by toxoplasmosis, disseminated cryptococci, coxsackievirus B, cytomegalovirus, lymphoma, *Aspergillus* species, and HIV itself. Ventricular dilatation and cardiac dysfunction may result. With PIs, glucose intolerance and disorders of lipid metabolism are common. Aggressive generalized vascular disease, including cardiac and cerebral, may occur as a complication of antiretroviral therapy. If patients exhibit unexplained hypotension, adrenal insufficiency should be considered, because this may occur with advanced HIV infection.

Surgery and Anesthesia

HIV infection does not increase the risk for postprocedural complications, including death, up to 30 days after the procedure. Thus, surgical intervention should not be limited because of HIV status and concern for subsequent complications. However, during anesthesia, tachycardia is more frequently seen in HIV-seropositive patients. Also, high fever, anemia, and tachycardia are more frequent postoperatively.

Several studies indicate that general anesthesia and opiates may impair immune function. Although this is likely of little clinical importance in healthy individuals, the implications for HIV-infected patients are not known. Immunosuppression due to general anesthesia occurs within 15 minutes of induction and may persist for as long as 3 to 11 days. Postoperative immunosuppression may last longer in inherently immunosuppressed patients and may predispose to the development of postoperative infections or facilitate tumor growth or metastasis.

Obstetric Patients

HIV and AIDS are increasing in women of childbearing age. In one study, zidovudine monotherapy was shown to dramatically reduce the incidence of vertical transmission of HIV from 25.5% to 8.3%. However, zidovudine monotherapy has limited long-term benefits because HIV resistance develops rapidly. Therefore, in pregnancy, combination therapy is now believed to be preferable.

There are limited data on the use of PIs in pregnancy. A recent meta-analysis strongly suggested that cesarean section independently reduces the incidence of vertical transmission. Combined antiretroviral therapy and elective cesarean section reduce the rate of vertical transmission to 2%. However, cesarean section is a major surgical intervention with well-known complications (see Section 9). There is a higher incidence of morbidity following cesarean compared with vaginal delivery, even in healthy women, including more prolonged and intense pain, longer duration of bed rest, increased blood loss, and more frequent venous thrombosis and wound infection. Many practitioners today do not recommend elective cesarean section to HIV-infected women who are compliant with antiretroviral therapy and have undetectable HIV viral loads. Unfortunately, HIV-positive women with low CD4 lymphocyte counts, whose infants would theoretically benefit most from cesarean delivery, are also those who are most likely to experience significant postoperative complications.

In a study of HIV-seropositive parturients receiving regional anesthesia, there were no infectious or neurologic complications related to the anesthetic or obstetric courses. In the immediate postpartum period, immune function measurements remained essentially unchanged, as did the severity of the disease. There have been concerns that epidural and lumbar puncture in HIV-seropositive patients may allow entry of the virus into the CNS. However, the natural history of HIV includes CNS involvement early in the clinical course, and expression of CNS infection varies widely.

Finally, epidural blood patches for the treatment of post–dural puncture headache have been reported as safe and effective in HIV-seropositive patients. Nevertheless, given the very small theoretical risk of introducing virus to the CNS, other analgesic strategies should be tried first.

Intensive Care Unit Complications

APACHE II scoring significantly underestimates mortality risk for HIV-seropositive patients admitted to a medical ICU with a total lymphocyte count less than 200 cells/mL. This is particularly true for those admitted with pneumonia or sepsis. There is a diverse range of indications for critical care in patients with HIV infection. Historically, respiratory failure due to PCP has been the most common reason for admission to an ICU, accounting for 34% of cases. Mechanical ventilation for PCP and other pulmonary disorders is associated with a mortality rate greater than 50%. In contrast, ICU admission and mechanical ventilation for nonpulmonary disorders are associated with a mortality rate less than 25%. In patients with septic shock, HIV infection is an independent predictor of poor outcome. In the era of HAART, fewer patients with HIV infection are admitted to ICUs with AIDS-defining illnesses such as PJP. In fact, many patients are now admitted with unrelated critical illnesses and are coincidentally found to be infected with HIV. Nonetheless, initiation of HAART in patients with PCP is known to improve outcome. However, this benefit must be weighed against problems associated with immune reconstitution, which may occur in septic patients when HAART is initiated.

PREVENTION

There is little specific information concerning the overall risk of anesthesia and surgery in HIV-seropositive patients. The American Society of Anesthesiologists' physical status assessment and the inherent surgical risk probably provide a measure of global risk. This information, when combined with the Centers for Disease Control and Prevention stage of HIV infection, the degree of immunosuppression, and the presence and severity of opportunistic infection or neoplasm, may offer the best predictor of global preoperative risk for HIV-seropositive patients. With regard to choice of anesthetic technique to minimize complications, regional anesthesia is the technique of choice, except in certain cases of neuropathies.

Finally, anesthesiologists and intensivists have contact with a broad range of patients, many of whom may be HIV-seropositive. Therefore, rigorous adherence to infection control practices is imperative. Further, all clinicians should keep abreast of current knowledge about HIV therapy to ensure that their patients are receiving optimal treatment.

Further Reading

Afessa B, Green B: Bacterial pneumonia in hospitalized patients with HIV infection: The Pulmonary Complications, ICU Support, and Prognostic Factors of Hospitalized Patients with HIV (PIP) Study. Chest 117:1017-1022, 2000.

Avidan MS, Groves P, Blott M, et al: Low complication rate associated with cesarean section under spinal anesthesia for HIV-1-infected women on antiretroviral therapy. Anesthesiology 97:320-324, 2002.

Avidan MS, Jones N, Pozniak AL: The implications of HIV for the anaesthetist and the intensivist. Anaesthesia. 55:344-354, 2000.

Casalino E, Mendoza-Sassi G, Wolff M, et al: Predictors of short- and long-term survival in HIV-infected patients admitted to the ICU. Chest 113:421-429, 1998.

Casalino E, Wolff M, Ravaud P, et al: Impact of HAART advent on admission patterns and survival in HIV-infected patients admitted to an intensive care unit. AIDS 18:1429-1433, 2004.

Evron S, Glezerman M, Harow E, et al: Human immunodeficiency virus: Anesthetic and obstetric considerations. Anesth Analg 98:503-511, 2004.

Hughes SC, Dailey PA, Landers D, et al: Parturients infected with human immunodeficiency virus and regional anesthesia: Clinical and immunologic response. Anesthesiology 82:32-37, 1995.

Morris A, Wachter RM, Luce J, et al: Improved survival with highly active antiretroviral therapy in HIV-infected patients with severe *Pneumocystis carinii* pneumonia. AIDS 17:73-80, 2003.

Vincent B, Timsit JF, Auburtin M, et al: Characteristics and outcomes of HIV-infected patients in the ICU: impact of the highly active antiretroviral treatment era. Intensive Care Med 2004;30:859-866.

Hypothyroidism: Myxedema Coma

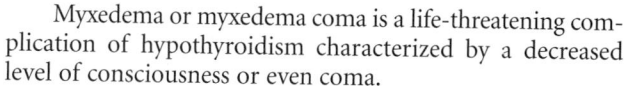

Pamela R. Roberts and Richard C. Prielipp

107

Case Synopsis

A 59-year-old man with history of a previous myocardial infarction with preserved left ventricular function underwent three-vessel coronary artery bypass grafting. He remained intubated and was taken to the intensive care unit (ICU) for postoperative care. On arrival in the ICU, he was receiving continuous infusions of propofol, phenylephrine, and fenoldopam. After several hours, he was awake and following commands and showed evidence of good perfusion and cardiac function, but he had a mild respiratory acidosis ($PaCO_2$ 49 mm Hg). Subsequently he was extubated and had persistent respiratory acidosis over the next few hours. His vital signs were remarkable overnight for a temperature that remained below 36°C (measured via a pulmonary artery catheter), heart rate paced at 90 beats per minute, blood pressure 95/62 to 105/68 mm Hg, respiratory rate 10 to 18 breaths per minute, and cardiac index greater than 2.4 L/minute/m². About 8 hours after extubation, his oxygenation, ventilation, cardiac index, and mental status deteriorated, and he was reintubated. A chest radiograph showed mild pulmonary edema. Thyroid function studies revealed very elevated thyrotropin and very low thyroxine levels; the cortisol level was appropriate for a stress response. Therapy with thyroid hormone was initiated, after which the patient improved; he was extubated the following day. Later discussions with the patient revealed a previous diagnosis of hypothyroidism and noncompliance with medical therapy.

PROBLEM ANALYSIS

Definition

Hypothyroidism is thyroid gland hypoactivity with decreased synthesis and secretion of thyroxine (T_4). Normal regulation and activity of thyroid hormone can be summarized as follows:

- Thyrotropin-releasing hormone (TRH) is released from the hypothalamus.
- TRH stimulates the synthesis and release of thyrotropin (also called thyroid-stimulating hormone [TSH]) from the pituitary gland.
- Circulating TSH stimulates the thyroid gland to produce and secrete thyroid hormone (about 80% as T_4 and about 20% as triiodothyronine [T_3]).
- The remainder of T_3 (the physiologically active form of thyroid hormone) is produced in extrathyroidal tissues (mainly the liver and kidneys) by monodeiodination of circulating T_4.
- T_3 and T_4 circulate bound to serum proteins, but free T_3 and T_4 are metabolically active.
- T_3 feeds back on the pituitary gland to inhibit the production of TSH.
- Some of the circulating T_4 is metabolized to the inactive product "reverse T_3."
- Both T_3 and reverse T_3 are rapidly cleared from the serum.
- Thyroid hormone activity begins with the binding of T_3 to receptors on cell nuclei, which is needed for normal cellular function.

Myxedema or myxedema coma is a life-threatening complication of hypothyroidism characterized by a decreased level of consciousness or even coma.

Recognition

HISTORY

Patients may present with previously undiagnosed hypothyroidism or may have been noncompliant with thyroid hormone replacement therapy. They may manifest decreased mental acuity, hoarseness, somnolence, cold intolerance, dry skin, brittle hair, and weight gain. Myxedema is usually precipitated by a stressful event such as an acute infection, trauma, myocardial infarction, or surgery or following anesthesia.

PHYSICAL EXAMINATION

The following findings may be evident on physical examination:

- Hypothermia (core temperature typically <35°C)
- Dry skin, with a thickened and doughy appearance
- Facial and generalized puffiness (periorbital edema, large tongue)
- Depressed mental status (lethargy, coma)
- Hypoventilation (slow respiratory rate, shallow breaths)
- Sinus bradycardia
- Hypotension
- Low-output cardiac failure and cardiomyopathy (possibly pericardial effusion with muffled heart sounds)

- Disorders of muscle function (paralytic ileus, urinary retention, atonic bowel)

Thyroid hormone is essential for the normal metabolism of all cells, and deficiency presents with widespread symptoms. For example, thyroid hormone is required for the synthesis of many proteins (e.g., β-receptors), and deficiency contributes to a lack of responsiveness to vasoactive drugs.

In myxedema, decreased circulating levels of thyroid hormones contribute to decreased mental responsiveness, bradycardia, and reduced stroke volume. This leads to low cardiac output and decreased cerebral perfusion. Hypothermia results from a decreased metabolic rate and an inability to shiver. Decreased plasma volume and intense peripheral vasoconstriction are common. Alveolar hypoventilation is secondary to (1) respiratory center depression (exacerbated by use of analgesics, sedatives, and anesthesia); (2) defective respiratory muscle function; and (3) occasionally, airway obstruction due to tongue enlargement.

The actual mechanism whereby hypothyroidism deteriorates into severe illness and coma is poorly understood, but it most often occurs after a stressful event, as illustrated in the case synopsis. Regardless of the cause, the resulting syndrome consists of a severe hypometabolic state. The reported mortality rate for untreated myxedema coma is over 80%. However, with treatment, the mortality rate is decreased to less than 10%.

Hypothyroidism occurs secondary to autoimmune thyroid disease (Hashimoto's thyroiditis), previous chronic treatment with lithium or amiodarone, iodine excess or deficiency (extremely rare in the United States, but an important cause of goitrous hypothyroidism in many countries), radioactive thyroid ablation, surgical resection, and pituitary or hypothalamic disease. The last two can be secondary or tertiary causes of hypothyroidism. Occasionally a patient may have thyroid hormone resistance or congenital thyroid agenesis. The incidence of hypothyroidism is three times higher in females than in males, and elderly women seem to be most susceptible to myxedema coma.

Risk Assessment and Implications

The diagnosis of myxedema is based on clinical suspicion, and confirmation relies on thyroid studies with the following results (Table 107-1):

- Decreased T_4
- Decreased T_3
- Elevated TSH (but not in secondary or tertiary hypothyroidism)

Other routine studies include complete blood count, electrolytes, urinalysis, arterial blood gases, chest radiograph, electrocardiogram, and blood and urine cultures. Serum cortisol levels should be drawn initially to evaluate for concomitant adrenal insufficiency. Additional studies should evaluate for infection as indicated by the history and physical examination.

Associated laboratory abnormalities that may be present include hyponatremia, hypoglycemia, hypercholesterolemia, and normochromic normocytic anemia. The chest radiograph may reveal signs of pleural or pericardial effusion or infection. The electrocardiogram may reveal many associated or potential abnormalities, including sinus bradycardia, small-voltage

Table 107–1 ▪ Thyroid Function Studies in Thyroid Disorders

	Disorder		
Test	Hyperthyroid	Hypothyroid	Euthyroid Sick Syndrome
TSH	Low	High	Low to slightly high
Total T_4	High	Low	Low to normal
Total T_3	High	Low	Low
Reverse T_3	High	Low to normal	High
Free T_4	High	Low	Normal
T_3 resin uptake*	High	Low	Normal to high

*Approximates serum hormone binding by thyroxine-binding globulin (normal range is 33–48%).

T_3, triiodothyronine; T_4, thyroxine; TSH, thyroid-stimulating hormone.

QRS complexes, prolonged Q-T intervals, isoelectric T-wave changes, or supraventricular tachycardia. Arterial blood gases may reveal hypoxemia, hypercarbia, and respiratory acidosis.

Sepsis should be considered in the differential diagnosis. Other causes for depressed mental status, such as stroke, electrolyte disturbances (e.g., hyponatremia), hypoglycemia, or renal failure with uremia, should also be considered. Hypopituitarism causing both hypothyroidism and adrenal insufficiency should be ruled out. Finally, the differential diagnosis should include hypothermia and drug overdose with β-receptor or calcium channel antagonists, encephalitis, and hypothalamic strokes.

MANAGEMENT AND PREVENTION

Do *not* wait for laboratory values to begin treatment if there is sufficient clinical suspicion of myxedema. Appropriate treatment includes the following:

- Thyroid hormone replacement
  - Intravenous (IV) administration is necessary owing to unreliable gastrointestinal absorption.
  - The best therapeutic regimen remains controversial, and clinical trials are unlikely because the disease is so rare. We prefer a combination of T_3 and T_4: T_3 20 μg IV bolus followed by 10 μg every 8 hours and T_4 200 μg IV followed by 100 μg IV every 24 hours for 1 to 2 days, followed by T_4 alone.
  - If IV T_3 is not immediately available, IV T_4 (in the preceding dosage) can be given with oral T_3 (25 μg every 12 hours) until the patient can be treated with oral T_4 alone.
  - Previously, T_4 alone was frequently used (200 to 500 μg IV bolus followed by 50 to 100 μg IV every 24 hours).
  - Peripheral conversion of T_4 to T_3 requires the presence of some T_3 for enzyme activity.
  - An advantage of IV T_3 includes a more rapid onset of action than T_4; also, peripheral conversion of T_4 is not required for activity.
  - T_3 is more arrhythmogenic than T_4, so careful monitoring is essential.

- Monitor T_3 and T_4 levels after 5 days, and adjust doses accordingly if the patient remains unconscious.
- General supportive measures
  - Give IV fluids to restore intravascular volume.
  - Use passive warming (active warming can cause peripheral vasodilatation and worsen shock).
  - Mechanical ventilation may be required.
  - Seizures can be treated with standard anticonvulsant drugs.
  - Use sedatives judiciously.
  - Hydrocortisone (100 mg IV every 8 hours) should be given until initial evaluation of hypothalamic-pituitary-adrenal axis function is performed; this therapy may be lifesaving in patients with secondary or tertiary hypothyroidism.
- Cardiovascular supportive measures
  - After restoring intravascular volume, inotropic or vasopressor therapy may be required for cardiovascular support.
  - Hypotension is poorly responsive to vasopressors until thyroid hormone replacement is initiated.
  - Monitor for the presence of arrhythmias (the dosage of thyroid hormone replacement may have to be decreased).
  - Hypothyroidism is associated with a high incidence of coronary artery disease, and patients should be monitored for evidence of myocardial ischemia, which is exacerbated by increased myocardial oxygen consumption during T_3 and T_4 treatment.
- Special considerations
  - Euthyroid patients tolerate short-term administration of thyroid hormone well.
  - Delay of treatment in a myxedematous patient can make the difference between survival and death.
  - This treatment regimen should *not* be routinely instituted in hypothyroid patients without clinical evidence of myxedema coma because of potential cardiac complications.

In addition, definitive treatment may require diagnosis and treatment of the underlying cause (e.g., infection, stroke, myocardial infarction, narcotics, gastrointestinal bleeding). Mortality in myxedema coma may approach 80%, and improved survival depends on early, aggressive therapy.

One retrospective study suggested that delaying surgery did not improve the outcome in patients with severe hypothyroidism. However, optimizing a patient's chance for the best outcome may be achieved by preoperative therapy when the need for surgery is not urgent.

Further Reading

Cone AM: Anaesthesia in a patient with untreated myxoedema coma. Anaesth Intensive Care 22:295-298, 1994.

Hellman DE: The thyroid gland. Contemp Anesth Pract 3:109-145, 1980.

James ML: Endocrine disease and anaesthesia: A review of anaesthetic management in pituitary, adrenal, and thyroid diseases. Anaesthesia 25:232-252, 1970.

Marcaine JM: Anesthesia and hypothyroidism: A review of thyroxine physiology, pharmacology, and anesthetic implications. Anesth Analg 61:371-383, 1982.

Myers L, Hays J: Myxedema coma. In Zaloga GP (ed): Critical Care Clinics—Endocrine Crises. Philadelphia, WB Saunders, 1991, pp 43-56.

O'Connor CJ, March R, Tuman K: Severe myxedema after cardiopulmonary bypass. Anesth Analg 96:62-64, 2003.

Rodriguez I, Fluiters E, Perez-Mendez LF, et al: Factors associated with mortality of patients with myxoedema coma: Prospective study in 11 cases treated in a single institution. J Endocrinol 180:347-350, 2004.

Smallridge RC: Metabolic and anatomic thyroid emergencies: A review. Crit Care Med 20:276-291, 1992.

Weinberg AD, Brennan MD, Gorman CA, et al: Outcome of anesthesia and surgery in hypothyroid patients. Arch Intern Med 143:893-897, 1983.

PHYSIOLOGIC IMBALANCE & COEXISTING DISEASE

Hyperthyroidism: Thyroid Storm

108

Richard C. Prielipp and Pamela R. Roberts

Case Synopsis

A 32-year-old woman undergoes general anesthesia with 1% isoflurane in a mixture of 60-40 nitrous oxide and oxygen for open fixation of a humeral fracture. Preoperative history is significant for anxiety and intolerance to heat. Physical examination is noteworthy for periorbital swelling; warm, moist skin with sweaty palms; and a midline lower neck mass consistent with an enlarged thyroid. Thirty minutes after induction, sinus tachycardia (128 beats per minute), arterial hypertension (190/100 mm Hg), and hyperpyrexia (core temperature 38.1°C despite a cool operating room environment) are noted. Increasing the depth of anesthesia with 2% isoflurane results in occasional ventricular premature beats. Muscle rigidity is absent.

PROBLEM ANALYSIS

Definition

Normal regulation and activity of thyroid hormone are summarized in Chapter 107. The following definitions apply to the discussion of hyperthyroidism:

- *True hyperthyroidism* is thyroid gland hyperactivity with increased synthesis and secretion of thyroid hormone.
- *Thyrotoxicosis* refers to the clinical and biochemical manifestations of excess thyroid hormone. It affects 2% of women and 0.2% of men in the general population.
- *Thyrotoxic crisis* or *thyroid storm* is a life-threatening complication of hyperthyroidism characterized by a severe, sudden exacerbation of thyrotoxicosis. Patients with uncontrolled hyperthyroidism presenting for surgical or trauma care are at considerable risk of developing thyrotoxicosis. Therefore, anesthesiologists should ensure that patients are euthyroid before proceeding with elective surgery.
- *Thyrotoxicosis factitia* refers to thyrotoxicosis without true hyperthyroidism (e.g., ingestion of thyroid hormone, ectopic thyroid hormone production) and is associated with *decreased* synthesis of thyroid hormone.

Recognition, Risk Assessment, and Implications

History

Patients with undiagnosed hyperthyroidism often have a history of anxiety (occasionally progressing to psychosis or even coma), significant recent weight loss, heat intolerance, gastrointestinal disturbances (diarrhea, nausea, vomiting, abdominal pain), unexplained fever, muscle weakness, and tremor. Thyroid storm is usually precipitated by a stressful event such as surgery, childbirth, infection, myocardial infarction, diabetic ketoacidosis, or trauma.

PHYSICAL EXAMINATION FINDINGS

Findings on physical examination that support the diagnosis of hyperthyroidism include the following symptoms (in decreasing order of frequency):

- Altered mental status (nervousness, agitation, anxiety, confusion, possible psychosis or even coma)
- Sweating, heat intolerance
- Weight loss, fatigue, muscle weakness
- Increased appetite, diarrhea, other gastrointestinal symptoms
- Prominent, dry eyes
- Leg swelling

Signs of hyperthyroidism include the following (in decreasing order of frequency):

- Sinus tachycardia (virtually 100% incidence) and tachyarrhythmias
- Goiter—neck mass with potential airway compromise (Fig. 108-1)
- Warm, moist skin
- Muscle tremor
- Systolic hypertension; widened pulse pressure
- Enlarged thyroid with thyroid bruit
- Ophthalmic signs, including exophthalmos, lid lag, lid retraction, periorbital swelling, and conjunctival injection
- Pretibial edema
- Atrial fibrillation, classically in the elderly (about 10% incidence)

PATHOPHYSIOLOGY

The actual mechanism whereby thyrotoxicosis decompensates into thyroid crisis is poorly understood, but it most often develops after a stressful precipitating event. Whatever the cause, the resulting syndrome resembles prolonged, severe β-adrenergic agonist overdose. Catecholamine concentrations appear to be normal, despite the apparent hypermetabolic state.

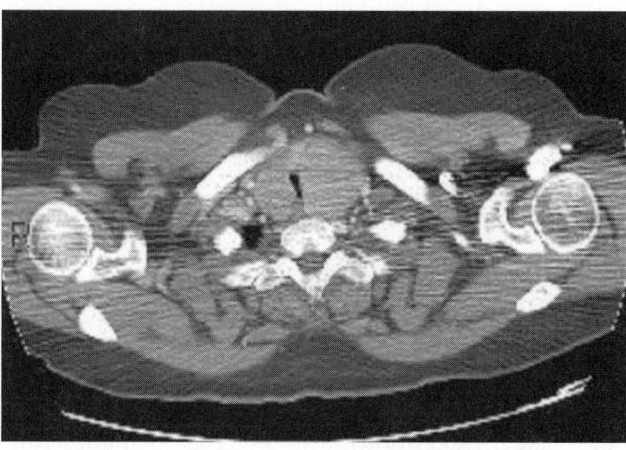

Figure 108–1 ■ Computed tomography scan (with intravenous contrast) of lower neck–upper thorax region reveals an enlarged thyroid gland (goiter) compressing the trachea and esophagus. Anesthetists must recognize the potential for significant airway compromise during induction of anesthesia in patients with large goiters in the neck and anticipate possible extension of the goiter to the retrosternal space. Up to 6% of tracheal intubations in patients anesthetized for thyroid surgery are difficult.

CAUSE

Undiagnosed hyperthyroidism (usually Graves' disease or toxic multinodular goiter) in a patient with major stress is the most common cause of thyroid storm. Another cause may be inadequate treatment in a known hyperthyroid patient. Disorders associated with thyrotoxicosis are listed in Table 108-1. The many causes of thyrotoxicosis can be distinguished by a 24-hour radioactive iodine uptake study performed when the patient's condition is stable.

DIAGNOSIS

The diagnosis of thyroid storm is clinical. Corroboration and confirmation rely on thyroid studies with the following findings (Table 108-2):

- Elevated thyroxine (T_4)
- Elevated triiodothyronine (T_3)
- Decreased thyroid-stimulating hormone (TSH)

Table 108–1 ■ Disorders Associated with Thyrotoxicosis

Graves' disease (may account for 85% of cases)
Toxic multinodular goiter
Toxic adenoma
Subacute thyroiditis
Neonatal thyrotoxicosis (consequent to maternal Graves' disease)
TSH-secreting pituitary tumor
Labor and childbirth
Hydatidiform mole
Metastatic (hyperfunctioning) thyroid carcinoma
Thyrotoxicosis factitia

TSH, thyroid-stimulating hormone.

Table 108–2 ■ Results of Thyroid Function Studies in Patients with Thyroid Disorders

Test	Disorder	
	Hyperthyroid	*Hypothyroid*
TSH	Low	High
Total T_4	High	Low
Total T_3	High	Low
Reverse T_3	High	Low to normal
Free T_4	High	Low
T_3 resin uptake*	High	Low

*Approximates serum hormone binding by thyroxine-binding globulin (normal range is 33-48%).

T_3, triiodothyronine; T_4, thyroxine; TSH, thyroid-stimulating hormone.

However, T_4 and T_3 concentrations may correlate poorly with the severity of clinical signs. Other routine studies include complete blood cell count, electrolyte levels, urinalysis, chest radiograph, and electrocardiogram. Additional studies looking for infectious processes should be performed.

Associated laboratory abnormalities (present 5% to 20% of the time) include hypercalcemia, hypokalemia, hyperglycemia, hypocholesterolemia, microcytic anemia, lymphocytosis, granulocytopenia, hyperbilirubinemia, and increased alkaline phosphatase level.

DIFFERENTIAL DIAGNOSIS

Malignant hyperthermia must be investigated simultaneously and treatment initiated if triggering anesthetic agents are used. This is especially true in children or when severe hypercarbia, acidosis, hyperkalemia, and increased creatine phosphokinase are present. Other hypermetabolic states such as sepsis, pheochromocytoma, or thyrotoxicosis without crisis should be considered. Last, the differential diagnosis should include severe drug intoxication with either cocaine or amphetamines.

MANAGEMENT

Do not wait for laboratory results to begin treatment if there is sufficient clinical suspicion. Appropriate treatment includes general supportive measures; inhibition of thyroid hormone synthesis, thyroid hormone release, peripheral β-adrenergic activity, and peripheral conversion of T_4 to T_3; and regulation of intracellular calcium.

General Supportive Measures

- Intravenous (IV) fluids to restore intravascular volume
- Acetaminophen for hyperthermia (avoid aspirin, because it displaces T_4 from thyroid-binding globulin, thereby increasing free T_4)
- Cooling blankets
- Magnesium salts to reduce the severity and incidence of cardiac arrhythmias

Inhibition of Thyroid Hormone Synthesis

- Propylthiouracil (PTU)—up to 1000 mg initially as a loading dose, then 200 to 300 mg orally or via nasogastric tube every 4 to 6 hours. It may take 6 to 8 weeks to achieve a full euthyroid state; PTU also inhibits peripheral conversion of T_4 to T_3.
- Methimazole—20 to 30 mg orally or via nasogastric tube every 4 to 6 hours. Achieves a euthyroid state more quickly than PTU and has a lower incidence of agranulocytosis, hepatitis, and vasculitis.

Iodide Therapy

Iodide inhibits thyroid hormone synthesis (Wolff-Chaikoff effect). Delay iodide therapy at least 4 hours after beginning PTU therapy.

- Sodium iodide—1 g intravenously every 8 hours
- Potassium iodide (SSKI, a saturated solution of potassium iodide), such as Lugol solution—10 drops orally every 6 hours. Lugol solution was once widely administered for 7 to 10 days before elective thyroidectomy in an effort to reduce vascularity of the gland.
- Iopanoic acid—0.5 to 1.0 g/day (also blocks peripheral conversion of T_4 to T_3)

Inhibition of Peripheral β-Adrenergic Activity

- β-blockers, which also block peripheral conversion of T_4 to T_3
  - Propranolol—0.5 to 1.0 mg/minute intravenously, up to a total dose of 2 to 10 mg; repeat every 3 to 4 hours. After initial control with IV drug, treat with 20 to 40 mg orally every 6 hours; occasionally, a patient may require up to 2 g/day orally owing to the variability of hepatic metabolism in thyrotoxic individuals.
  - Esmolol—IV bolus with 0.5 to 0.75 mg/kg, followed by IV infusion with 50 µg/kg per minute. If effect is inadequate after 5 minutes, repeat IV bolus and increase IV infusion to 100 µg/kg per minute; it may even be necessary to increase the infusion to 300 µg/kg per minute.
  - Titrate β-blockade to achieve a heart rate of 80 to 90 beats per minute.
  - If the patient has a history of reactive airway disease, use caution and a short-acting cardioselective agent such as esmolol, atenolol, or metoprolol.
  - If β-blockers are contraindicated, other sympatholytic drugs (e.g., reserpine, a depleter of catecholamines, or guanethidine, an inhibitor of catecholamine release) may be useful as second-line agents.

Inhibition of Peripheral Conversion of T_4 to T_3

- PTU (see dosages given earlier)
- β-blockade (see dosages given earlier)

- Dexamethasone 2 mg intravenously or orally every 6 hours, or hydrocortisone 50 mg intravenously every 6 hours

Intracellular Calcium Regulation

Dantrolene in doses of 1 mg/kg (equivalent to that used for malignant hyperthermia) has been reported in anecdotal cases; however, its utility and efficacy in the setting of thyroid storm are not well defined.

PREVENTION

Prevention of complications in patients with hyperthyroidism (especially thyroid storm) relies on recognition of the stigmata of undiagnosed hyperthyroidism during the preoperative evaluation. In addition, anesthesiologists must anticipate potential airway difficulties during tracheal intubation, which occurs in 6% of patients anesthetized for thyroid surgery (see Fig. 108-1). Mortality with thyroid storm may be as high as 20%. Improved survival relies on early, aggressive therapy. In addition, definitive therapy requires treatment of any associated disorders, such as infection or diabetic ketoacidosis.

Further Reading

Ambus T, Evans S, Smith NT: Thyrotoxicosis factitia in the anesthetized patient. Anesthesiology 81:254-256, 1994.

Bennett MH, Wainwright AP: Acute thyroid crisis on induction of anaesthesia. Anaesthesia 44:28-30, 1989.

Benua RS, Becker DV: Thyroid storm. In Bardin CW (ed): Current Therapy in Endocrinology and Metabolism, 4th ed. Philadelphia, BC Decker, 1991, pp 68-70.

Burch HB, Wartofsky L: Life-threatening thyrotoxicosis. Endocrinol Metab Clin North Am 22:263-277, 1993.

Connery LE, Coursin DB: Assessment and therapy of selected endocrine disorders. Anesthesiol Clin North Am 22:93-123, 2004.

Farling PA: Thyroid disease. Br J Anaesth 85:15-28, 2000.

Gavin LA: Thyroid crises. Med Clin North Am 75:179-193, 1991.

Knighton JD, Crosse MM: Anaesthetic management of childhood thyrotoxicosis and the use of esmolol. Anaesthesia 52:62-76, 1997.

Lacoste L, Gineste D, Karayan J, et al: Airway complications in thyroid surgery. Ann Otol Rhinol Laryngol 102:441-446, 1993.

Nishiyama K, Kitahara A, Natsume H, et al: Malignant hyperthermia in a patient with Graves' disease during subtotal thyroidectomy. Endocr J 48:227-232, 2001.

Pandey CK, Raza M, Dhiraaj S, et al: Rapid preparation of severe uncontrolled thyrotoxicosis due to Graves' disease with iopanoic acid. Can J Anaesth 51:38-40, 2004.

Peters KR, Nance P, Wingard DW: Malignant hyperthyroidism or malignant hyperthermia? Anesth Analg 60:613-615, 1991.

Pugh S, Lalwani K, Awal A: Thyroid storm as a cause of loss of consciousness following anaesthesia for emergency caesarean section. Anaesthesia 49:35-37, 1994.

Sarcoidosis

109

Barry A. Harrison and Martin L. De Ruyter

Case Synopsis

A 50-year-old African American woman with stage III pulmonary sarcoidosis is scheduled to undergo a thoracotomy for resection of a right upper lobe aspergilloma. Chronically, she has a hoarse voice, dyspnea at rest, and swollen ankles. She is receiving corticosteroids and ambulatory oxygen therapy at a rate of 2 L/minute. She complains of palpitations and fainting spells.

PROBLEM ANALYSIS

Definition

Sarcoidosis is a systemic granulomatous disease of unknown cause. A complex interaction of genetic, environmental, and infectious agents triggers a type 1 T-lymphocyte response that is characterized by chronic inflammation, monocyte recruitment, and granuloma formation. Characteristic pathohistologic findings include noncaseating granulomas that are both discrete and compact. These granulomas are composed of mononuclear phagocytes, including epithelioid cells, multinucleated central giant cells, and lymphocytes. The multinucleated central giant cells are surrounded by fibroblasts and mast cells (Fig. 109-1).

Recognition

CLINICAL FEATURES

Sarcoidosis occurs mainly in individuals between the ages of 20 and 40 years, with a prevalence in the United States of approximately 20 in 100,000. It is slightly more common in females than in males and has a black-white ratio of 15:1.

Sarcoidosis may present acutely, subacutely, or insidiously. Between 30% and 60% of cases are asymptomatic, detected incidentally by an abnormal chest radiograph. Constitutional symptoms may occur and consist of fever, fatigue, anorexia, cough, dyspnea, and vague retrosternal discomfort. Syndromes such as erythema nodosum, anterior uveitis, arthritis, parotid enlargement, and facial nerve palsy occur in acute sarcoidosis. In patients with an insidious presentation, respiratory symptoms usually predominate.

Diagnosis requires relevant clinical features and a tissue biopsy showing characteristic noncaseating granulomas. The degree and variability of disease activity together with the organ involved determine the clinical presentation. These factors contribute to the delay in diagnosis observed in sarcoid patients.

Death from sarcoidosis usually results from progressive pulmonary, cardiac, or neurologic involvement.

PULMONARY PRESENTATION

Upper Airway. Although laryngeal sarcoid involvement may be an isolated finding, it is usually associated with systemic manifestations. It occurs in <5% of patients with sarcoidosis. Symptoms and signs of laryngeal sarcoidosis include dysphagia, hoarseness, throat pain, dyspnea, and stridor. Granulomas or nodules involving the supraglottic larynx or the entire larynx are often found (Fig. 109-2). Airway obstruction can occur, and a tracheostomy may be necessary in some cases. Recurrent laryngeal nerve involvement can result in unilateral vocal cord paralysis.

Lower Airway. Enlarged intrathoracic lymph nodes can compress large airways, potentially causing tracheal and bronchial stenosis, airflow obstruction, and pulmonary atelectasis.

Pulmonary Parenchyma. The lung and intrathoracic lymph nodes are involved in >90% of cases. Approximately 50% of patients develop permanent pulmonary abnormalities, with 5% to 15% developing pulmonary fibrosis. Chronic hypoxemic respiratory failure and cor pulmonale may result from pulmonary sarcoidosis.

Chest Radiographic and Laboratory Findings. Ninety percent of patients with sarcoidosis have an abnormal chest radiograph at some time. Three classic chest radiographic patterns have been described, with higher stages correlating with an increased frequency of dyspnea (Table 109-1). An increase in the serum concentration of angiotensin-converting enzyme (ACE), which is secreted by sarcoid granulomas, can assist in making the diagnosis. Unfortunately, other chronic inflammatory conditions are also associated with increased

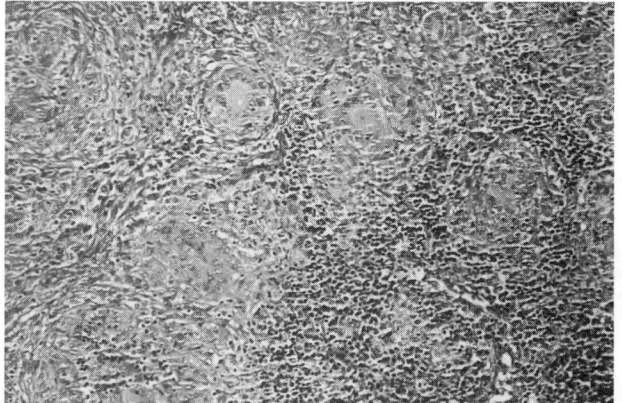

Figure 109–1 ■ Sarcoid granulomas in lung tissue. (Photomicrograph courtesy of Dr. Thomas A. Gaffey, Department of Pathology, Mayo Clinic and Foundation, Rochester, Minn.)

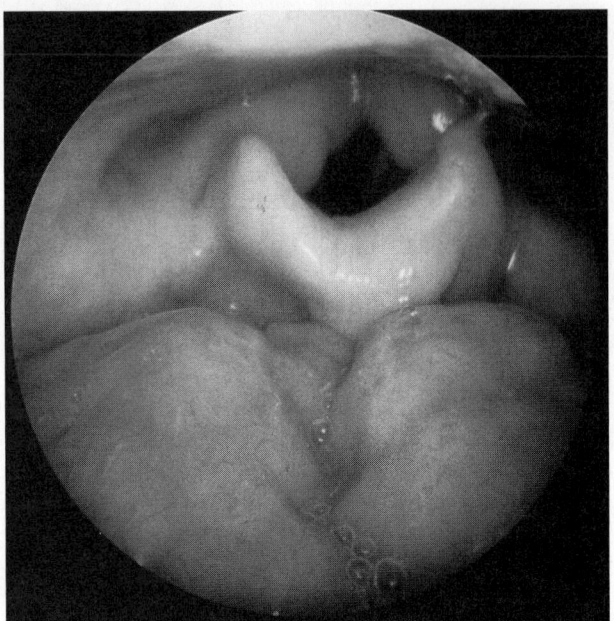

Figure 109–2 ■ Granulomas involving the supraglottic region. (From Neel HB, McDonald TJ: Laryngeal sarcoidosis. Ann Otol Rhinol Laryngol 91:361, 1982.)

serum ACE. Recent findings demonstrate that serum ACE is not consistently correlated with disease activity or treatment response.

Computed Tomography. High-resolution computed tomography (CT) is helpful if the chest radiograph is equivocal; a diagnosis can be made in up to 75% of cases. High-resolution CT can be used to diagnose small, well-defined nodes and peribronchial interstitial thickening, whereas conventional CT is better for the evaluation of diffuse parenchymal sarcoidosis (Fig. 109-3).

Transbronchial Biopsy. Transbronchial biopsy is diagnostic in 90% of cases. The yield is excellent even if interstitial infiltrates are not detectable on chest radiography.

Bronchoalveolar Lavage. Lavage may be helpful, especially if the lymphocyte population is analyzed. A CD4/CD8 ratio greater than 3.5 is 94% specific for sarcoidosis.

CARDIAC PRESENTATION

Clinically overt cardiac involvement occurs in about 5% of patients with sarcoidosis, usually without evidence of disease elsewhere. Cardiac involvement may manifest as cardiac arrhythmias (ventricular more often than supraventricular), conduction disorders, cardiomyopathy, pericarditis, wall motion abnormalities, or cardiac arrest. Electrocardiography, echocardiography, and, in select patients, cardiac catheterization with myocardial biopsy may be helpful in evaluating patients with cardiac findings. Myocardial sarcoidosis may be difficult to diagnose in the absence of systemic manifestations. Myocardial biopsy may be falsely negative owing to sampling bias. Cor pulmonale may result from pulmonary parenchymal disease. Sudden death is associated with cardiac sarcoidosis; however, with progress in the development of antiarrhythmic drugs, cardiac pacemakers, and implantable defibrillators, congestive heart failure associated with myocardial sarcoidosis is now a more frequent cause of death.

MULTISYSTEM PRESENTATION

Sarcoidosis is a systemic disease; multiple organ systems can be involved and have implications for the anesthesiologist (Table 109-2).

Risk Assessment

Risk assessment is dependent on the extent and severity of sarcoidosis and the organ system affected.

PULMONARY ASSESSMENT

As elastic resistance of the lungs is increased, patients with sarcoidosis adapt to reduce the work of breathing by taking rapid, shallow breaths. Most commonly there are reductions in lung volume and the diffusing capacity for carbon monoxide (Fig. 109-4). Expiratory flow rates may also be decreased, suggesting airflow obstruction. Arterial hypoxemia with exercise occurs frequently; arterial hypoxemia at rest indicates severe disease. Although sarcoid lung pathology is caused by granuloma and fibrosis, pulmonary function testing may reflect disease extent but not necessarily disease activity. However, such testing may provide objective data when following a patient's response to therapy.

CARDIAC ASSESSMENT

Electrocardiography and 24-hour electrocardiographic monitoring, echocardiography, and cardiac catheterization with myocardial biopsy may be helpful in the evaluation of cardiac sarcoidosis. Thallium 201 myocardial imaging may demonstrate segmental defects consistent with sarcoid granulomas or fibrous scars. Magnetic resonance imaging has

Table 109–1 ■ **Three Classic Chest Radiograph Patterns in Sarcoidosis**		
Chest Radiograph Pattern	**Radiographic Findings**	**Incidence of ACE Elevation (%)**
Stage I	Hilar and mediastinal abnormality without pulmonary parenchymal abnormality	67
Stage II	Hilar and mediastinal abnormality associated with pulmonary parenchymal abnormality	88
Stage III	Diffuse pulmonary disease without node enlargement	95

ACE, angiotensin-converting enzyme.

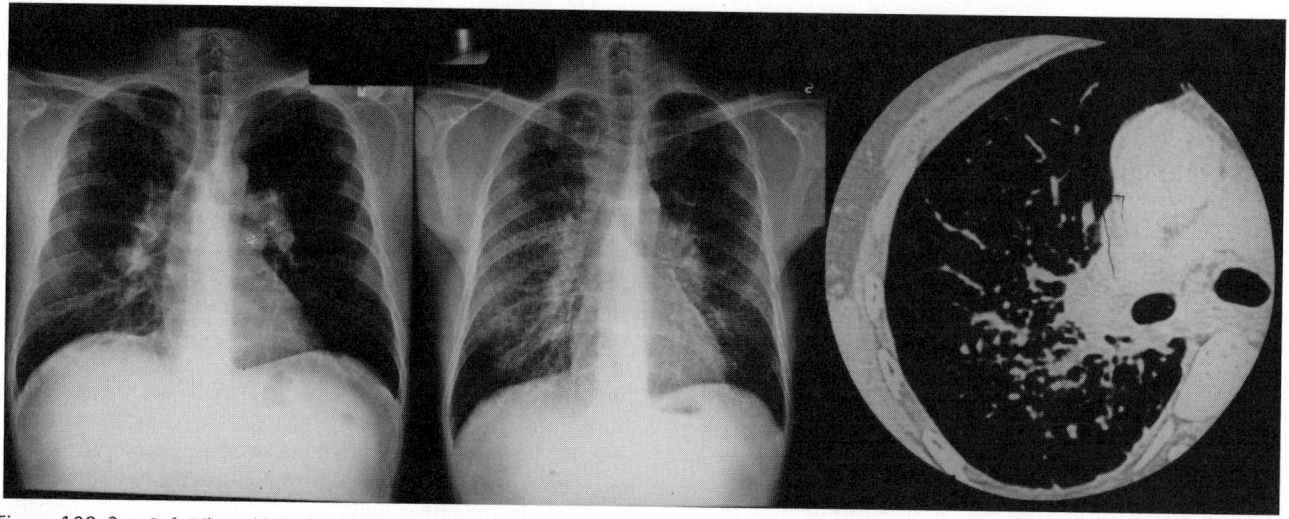

Figure 109–3 ■ *Left*, Bilateral hilar lymphadenopathy (stage I). *Middle*, Bilateral hilar lymphadenopathy and interstitial infiltrates (stage II). *Right*, High-resolution chest computed tomography scan showing extensive nodular interstitial process. (Radiographs courtesy of Department of Radiology, Mayo Clinic and Foundation, Rochester, Minn.)

also been used to identify areas of myocardium affected by sarcoidosis and to guide myocardial biopsy.

Implications

Patients with sarcoidosis undergo procedures for biopsy and diagnosis that may require anesthesia. These include fiberoptic bronchoscopy with transbronchial biopsy, scalene node biopsy, and mediastinoscopy for hilar lymph node biopsy and lung biopsy, either by video-assisted thoracoscopy or thoracotomy. Many patients with sarcoidosis require anesthesia owing to a complication of therapy (e.g., perforated duodenal ulcer secondary to corticosteroid therapy). Sarcoid patients routinely require anesthesia for comorbid conditions. In the case synopsis, the patient had developed an aspergilloma fungus ball in a lung cavity due to cystic destruction of lung tissue by sarcoidosis. Progressive pulmonary sarcoidosis with chronic hypoxemic respiratory failure and right heart failure or progressive cardiac sarcoidosis can cause problems with anesthesia and increase risk.

MANAGEMENT

Self-Limited Disease

Over a 3-year period following diagnosis, approximately 30% to 50% of cases remit spontaneously. Of the remaining approximately 50% of cases that do not show remission, over the next 5 to 10 years, 30% of those patients show disease progression, while the remaining 20% remain stable. Thus, not all patients with sarcoidosis require specific therapy, especially those with a stage I radiographic pattern.

Corticosteroids, Cytotoxics, and Immunosuppressive Therapy

Treatment for sarcoidosis is indicated for progressive symptomatic disease. Clear-cut examples include cardiac and neurologic sarcoidosis and hypocalcemia secondary to sarcoidosis. Pulmonary sarcoidosis with respiratory symptoms

PHYSIOLOGIC IMBALANCE & COEXISTING DISEASE

Table 109–2 ■ Multisystem Involvement in Sarcoidosis

Organ System (Incidence of Involvement)	Manifestations	Anesthetic Implications
Nervous (5%)	Peripheral neuropathies, central nervous system symptoms: meningitis, encephalitis, epilepsy, cranial nerve disturbances	Use caution with muscle relaxants
Musculoskeletal (1%)	Arthritis of peripheral joints: ankles, knees, wrists, hands; ankylosis of temporomandibular joints	Examine the airway
Renal (1%)	Hypercalciuria with or without hypercalcemia, nephrocalcinosis, nephrolithiasis	Altered drug excretion
Hepatic (12%)	Hepatomegaly, abnormal liver function tests	Altered drug metabolism
Hematopoietic (26%)	Anemia, thrombocytopenia, neutropenia, eosinophilia, splenomegaly	Check complete blood count
Eye (12%)	Uveitis, conjunctival nodules, keratoconjunctivitis sicca	Standard eye precautions
Skin (15%)	Erythema nodosum, plaques, subcutaneous nodules	Lesions may be tender and painful
Endocrine (4%)	Posterior pituitary: diabetes insipidus, hypercalcemia	Monitor serum Ca^{2+}, Na^+, and urine output

From Baughman RP, Teirstein AS, Judson MA, et al: Clinical characteristics of patients in a case control study of sarcoidosis. Am J Respir Crit Care Med 164:1885–1889, 2001.

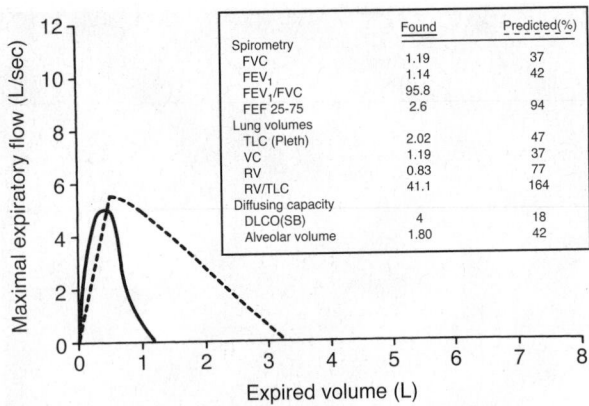

Figure 109–4 ■ Expiratory flow volume loop. *Solid line* is the patient with sarcoid; *dashed line* is the normal predicted loop. The *insert* contains the values of spirometry, lung volumes, and diffusing capacity of a patient with pulmonary sarcoidosis. DLCO(SB), diffusing capacity of carbon monoxide, single breath; FEF$_{25-75}$, forced expiratory flow rate between 25% and 75% of a forced vital capacity; FEV$_1$, forced expiratory volume in 1 second; FVC, forced vital capacity; RV, residual volume; TLC, total lung capacity; VC, vital capacity. (Data from Pulmonary Function Laboratory, Mayo Clinic and Foundation, Rochester, Minn.)

associated with progressive loss of lung function also requires treatment.

A systemic evidence-based review of corticosteroids in sarcoidosis found that they improved radiographic assessment (stage II and III radiographic patterns) and pulmonary function. However, no data exist demonstrating that corticosteroids have a significant effect on long-term disease progression. A 3-month trial of corticosteroids is required before reevaluating the patient. Although inhaled corticosteroids have been tried, insufficient clinical trials have been conducted to determine their efficacy.

Cytotoxics and antimalarials are used in sarcoidosis to control disease progression, especially if cortocosteroids have failed or in an effort to decrease the corticosteroid dosage. Methotrexate, azathioprine, and chloroquine have all been used. However, such use has usually been reported anecdotally or in small case series. There have been only four studies evaluating these drugs in a prospective, controlled manner. Results were inconclusive, and all the drugs were associated with severe side effects.

Activated T lymphocytes secreting interleukin-2 may play a role in sarcoidosis, which has led to trials of cyclosporine for the treatment of sarcoidosis. Unfortunately, these trials have also failed to show any benefit. Thalidomide and antagonists to tumor necrosis factor-α are currently undergoing therapeutic trials.

Lung Transplantation

Single or bilateral lung transplantation has been tried in patients with end-stage lung disease who are refractory to aggressive medical therapy. Recurrence of sarcoid granulomas within the lung allografts occurs in a majority of patients but rarely causes clinical symptoms. The survival rate for single- or double-lung transplantation is 70% at 2 years.

Chronic Hypoxemic Respiratory Failure and Cor Pulmonale

Long-standing progressive pulmonary sarcoidosis may give rise to chronic hypoxemic respiratory failure and cor pulmonale. The latter is pulmonary arterial hypertension resulting from diseases affecting lung structure or function. Pulmonary arterial hypertension results in right ventricular enlargement (hypertrophy or dilatation) and may progress over time to right heart failure. The treatment of both conditions is first and foremost the titration of continuous oxygen to increase arterial oxygen saturation to above 90%. If right-sided heart failure is present, diuresis, initially with bed rest and then, if necessary, with diuretics (often furosemide), should be initiated. Excessive fluid loss is dangerous, however, because it may decrease right ventricular preload. Digitalis use is controversial because the potential for digitalis toxicity is high, even with low serum concentrations, when hypoxemia, alkalosis-induced hypokalemia, and cor pulmonale are present. The use of pulmonary vasodilators is undergoing investigation.

PREVENTION

Preoperative

Because sarcoidosis is a multisystem disease, all systems must be evaluated for possible sarcoid involvement during the preoperative assessment. Symptoms and signs of upper airway involvement with sarcoidosis must be specifically addressed before tracheal intubation. Chronic corticosteroid use and the associated potential for adrenal insufficiency must be evaluated, and preoperative corticosteroids should be administered if necessary.

Operative

If chronic hypoxemic respiratory failure and right-sided heart failure are present, hypoxia, hypercapnia, and acidosis must all be avoided because they act to increase pulmonary artery pressure, further exacerbating right heart failure. Central venous pressure monitoring to guide intravascular fluid administration and the use of a pulmonary artery catheter to determine pulmonary artery pressure and cardiac output may also be necessary. Regional anesthesia may be advantageous if the surgical site is below the level of the umbilicus. In patients with ventilatory compromise, the usual accessory function of the intercostal muscles may make a larger contribution to overall ventilation. If so, high central neuraxial blockade may interfere with intercostal muscle function and exacerbate the tenuous oxygen supply-demand balance. Large-volume intravenous fluid administration to treat hypotension associated with sympathetic blockade may exacerbate right-sided heart failure. Therefore, blood pressure is maintained with intravenous vasopressors (e.g., phenylephrine) to ensure adequate venous return to the right heart. During general anesthesia, mechanical ventilation may be necessary. If so, titration of positive end-expiratory pressure and oxygen to maintain an oxygen saturation of at least 90% is necessary. Limit the plateau airway pressure to less than 35 cm H_2O by adjusting the tidal volume and inspiratory flow rates. Careful titration of all these parameters may help prevent further lung injury.

Postoperative

With sarcoidosis-induced chronic hypoxemic respiratory failure and right-sided heart failure, careful consideration must be given to postoperative analgesia. Systemic opioid administration may depress ventilation and precipitate hypoxia. Thus, a central neuraxial technique may be preferable, with the use of local anesthetic agents, opioids, or both. Also, use of local anesthetics via continuous peripheral nerve blockade optimizes analgesia and limits respiratory side effects. Titration of inspired oxygen is advised to maintain oxygen saturation greater than 92%.

Further Reading

Baughman RP, Lower EE, Du Bois R: Sarcoidosis. Lancet 361:1111-1118, 2003.

Clark D, Mitchell AW, Dick R, et al: The radiology of sarcoidosis [review]. Sarcoidosis 11:90-99, 1994.

Karl TK: Sarcoidosis. JAMA 289:3300-3303, 2003.

Paramothayan S, Jones PW: Corticosteroid therapy in pulmonary sarcoidosis: A systematic review. JAMA 287:1301-1307, 2002.

Paramothayan S, Lasserson T, Walters EH: Immunosuppressive and cytotoxic therapy for pulmonary sarcoidosis. Cochrane Database of Syst Rev 2:2004.

Weitzenblum E: Chronic cor pulmonale. Heart 89:225-230, 2003.

Wills MH, Harris MM: An unusual airway complication with sarcoidosis. Anesthesiology 66:554-555, 1987.

PHYSIOLOGIC IMBALANCE & COEXISTING DISEASE

Perioperative Management of Dialysis-Dependent Patients

110

Klaus D. Torp

Case Synopsis

A 43-year-old gas station attendant is scheduled for emergency exploratory laparotomy after sustaining an abdominal stab wound during an attempted robbery. He is dialysis dependent and awaiting renal transplantation. His last hemodialysis was 52 hours earlier. He is awake and alert. His blood pressure is 102/90 mm Hg; heart rate, 114 beats per minute; and respiratory rate, 24 breaths per minute. His hemoglobin level is 8.2 g/dL after receiving 3 units of packed red blood cells; the serum potassium level before the transfusion was 6.0 mEq/L. While cricoid pressure is applied, anesthesia is induced with etomidate, fentanyl, and rocuronium. Soon after the operation begins, the surgeon complains of difficulty achieving hemostasis. T waves on the electrocardiogram are tall and peaked.

PROBLEM ANALYSIS

Definition

Approximately 500,000 patients are affected by end-stage renal disease (ESRD) in the United States, with an estimated incidence of about 333 per 1 million persons (quadrupled from 1980) and a prevalence of 1435 per 1 million (quintupled from 1980). Prevalence rates are 1.4 times higher for males than for females and 4 times higher for African Americans than for whites. Those aged 45 to 64 years account for the largest number of patients. About 45% of all ESRD patients have a primary diagnosis of diabetes, another 30% are hypertensive, and less than 20% have glomerulonephritis; the remainder have rarer diseases, such as the following:

- Polycystic kidney disease
- Immunoglobulin (Ig) A and IgM nephropathies
- Systemic lupus erythematosus
- Wegener's granulomatosis
- Multiple myeloma
- Amyloidosis
- Acquired immunodeficiency syndrome (AIDS) nephropathy
- Miscellaneous causes or conditions

Patients with these rarer causes tend to be younger and are less likely to present with the typical comorbidities of dialysis patients.

In 2002 about 100,000 patients began treatment for ESRD with hemodialysis, peritoneal dialysis, or renal transplantation. Dialysis is usually required when the glomerular filtration rate falls below 20 mL/minute. Dialysis may also be indicated for hospitalized patients with volume overload refractory to diuretics, severe metabolic acidosis, hyperkalemia, seizures or other neurologic symptoms, or pericarditis. It is usually started when the blood urea nitrogen is greater than 100 mg/mL or the creatinine level approaches 10 mg/dL. Regardless of cause, ESRD affects virtually all organ systems (Table 110-1) and has implications for anesthesiologists, intensivists, and surgeons. These abnormalities result from the failure to excrete urea and other waste products of metabolism or the loss of metabolic and endocrine functions normally performed by the kidney.

Recognition

Perioperative complications of ESRD are listed in Table 110-2. The most frequent life-threatening perioperative complication is hyperkalemia. It is frequently associated with acidosis and with trauma due to the release of potassium from damaged tissue and hematomas. Hyperkalemia can cause progressive cardiac conduction defects, ending in ventricular fibrillation or, less commonly, asystole (Table 110-3). Electrocardiographic changes are critically dependent on the rate of rise in serum potassium levels (i.e., acute versus chronic hyperkalemia).

An increased propensity for bleeding often occurs in the presence of uremia because of an acquired defect in primary hemostasis. Tests of coagulation are typically normal, although a slight reduction in platelet counts may be seen. The pathogenesis is multifactorial, and the major defects involve decreased platelet–vessel wall adhesion and platelet-platelet interactions manifesting as impaired aggregation in response to epinephrine, adenosine diphosphate, collagen, and fibrinogen. Platelets from uremic patients release less adenosine triphosphate and serotonin and also display reduced cyclooxygenase activity. The activation-dependent receptor function of the glycoprotein IIb/IIIa complex is defective in uremia, as shown by decreased binding of both von Willebrand's factor (vWF) and fibrinogen to stimulated platelets. Cutaneous bleeding time remains the most readily

462

Table 110–1 ■ Clinical Abnormalities in End-Stage Renal Disease

Nervous System

Sleep disorders
Motor weakness
Polyneuritis
Asterixis
Seizures
Coma

Hematologic System

Anemia
Increased fragility of red blood cells
Platelet dysfunction with bleeding
Thrombosis

Metabolic and Endocrine Systems

Glucose intolerance
Hyperparathyroidism
Hypogonadism

Immunologic System

Increased susceptibility to infection

Integumentary System

Pruritus

Cardiovascular System

Hypertension
Hypotension
Cardiomyopathy
Diastolic dysfunction
Left ventricular hypertrophy
Congestive cardiac failure
Pericarditis

Gastrointestinal System

Gastrointestinal bleeding
Pancreatitis

Acid-Base and Electrolytes

Anion gap metabolic acidosis
Hyperkalemia
Hyponatremia
Hypermagnesemia or hypomagnesemia
Hyperphosphatemia

Musculoskeletal System

Renal osteoporosis or osteomalcia

Table 110–3 ■ Electrocardiographic Changes with Progressive Hyperkalemia

K^+ (mEq/L)	Electrocardiographic Abnormality
5.0	Usually none or tenting of T waves
6.0	Tall and peaked T waves
7.0	Prolonged P-R interval with depressed ST segments
8.0	Sinoatrial arrest with "sine wave" QRS complex
9.0	Ventricular fibrillation

frequently noted. In fact, some patients receive antiplatelet agents to prevent thrombosis of arteriovenous grafts, as well as for cardiovascular disease, which in turn may contribute to the bleeding tendency.

Cardiovascular dysfunction is common in patients with ESRD. This is not surprising, given the high prevalence of hypertension, left ventricular hypertrophy, and coronary artery disease in patients on chronic dialysis. Further, diminished responsiveness of cardiac α- and β-adrenergic receptors due to dysautonomia results in poor compensatory responses to acute hemodynamic changes.

Hypoxemia and dysequilibrium syndrome are two complications of which anesthesiologists should be aware. They can occur either during or soon after dialysis. Hypoxemia is more common when acetate rather than bicarbonate is used in the dialysate, and it is due to both alveolar hypercapnia and complement-induced pulmonary inflammation. Any associated hypoxemia is usually transient. Dysequilibrium is caused by rapid removal of urea and other osmotically active agents while the blood-brain barrier prevents their rapid removal from brain cells. These become relatively hypertonic. Fluid diffuses into brain cells along an osmotic gradient. Therefore, cerebral edema may result.

Risk Assessment

Patients who are dialysis dependent and undergo major surgical procedures have a higher perioperative mortality rate than patients with normal renal function. It is particularly high for patients undergoing open-heart surgery (approximately 12%, versus 2.9% in nondialysis patients). The risk of major surgery is related to abnormalities directly attributable to ESRD, as well as to the underlying disease process (e.g., hypertension). In dialysis patients, diastolic dysfunction is as common a cause of congestive heart failure as dilated cardiomyopathy is. Therefore, in patients with ESRD, a relatively small excess of ingested sodium chloride and water can lead to a large increase in left ventricular end-diastolic pressure, resulting in pulmonary edema. The probability of having angina or a myocardial infarction requiring hospitalization is 10% per year, and cardiac disease accounts for 45% of deaths in patients on dialysis. Anemia and hypertension are independent predictors of mortality. The 5-year survival rate after the initiation of dialysis is around 33%, and the life expectancy is only about one fourth that of the general population.

Anesthetic drugs such as succinylcholine (which causes an increase in serum potassium levels after intubating doses)

available test of platelet function, although its accuracy is often questioned. A markedly prolonged bleeding time with a relatively normal platelet count should trigger efforts to correct this abnormality. Despite the bleeding tendency in patients with ESRD, hypercoagulability markers (e.g., elevated vWF activity and thromboelastographic amplitudes) are

Table 110–2 ■ Perioperative Complications of End-Stage Renal Disease

Hyperkalemia
Bleeding
Cardiovascular dysfunction
Hypertension or hypotension
Congestive heart failure
Ischemia
Sepsis
Graft thrombosis

can contribute to the risk of death. The need for multiple blood transfusions also increases serum potassium levels, as does acidosis resulting from long periods of hypoperfusion or the failure to adequately compensate for increasing metabolic acidosis with an increase in minute ventilation. Drug overdoses can occur owing to reduced renal clearance of the drug itself or its active metabolites, which is more of a concern with repeat dosing. However, increased unbound fractions of a drug caused by decreased plasma proteins may lead to relative overdose with initial intravenous dosing of some drugs (e.g., thiopental, methohexital, diazepam).

All anesthetic techniques have the potential to reduce renal perfusion and adversely affect any residual renal function, with important implications for the patient's health.

Implications

The potential for serious life-threatening problems relating to electrolyte, coagulation, and acid-base problems is always present. This is compounded by any underlying or coexistent diseases, especially serious cardiovascular abnormalities.

MANAGEMENT

General principles for the management of all ESRD patients undergoing surgery, regardless of the cause of ESRD, are listed in Table 110-4.

Hyperkalemia

The management of acute hyperkalemia can be divided into three steps (Table 110-5). First, treatment is directed toward antagonizing the adverse effects of increased potassium by administering intravenous calcium. Second, potassium is shifted intracellularly by stimulating Na^+,K^+-ATPase or using its electrochemical gradient. Third, potassium is removed from the body with dialysis or exchange resins.

Bleeding in Uremic Patients

Treatment with erythropoietin or infusion of washed red blood cells has been shown to significantly reduce bleeding times in uremic patients with a hematocrit above 30%. Erythrocytes enhance platelet function by releasing adenosine

Table 110–4 ■ **General Management Principles for Patients with End-Stage Renal Disease Undergoing Surgery**

Dialysis within 24 hr of surgical procedure
Serum potassium in normal range
Serum bicarbonate ≥20 mEq/L desirable
Euvolemic or minimally hypovolemic before surgical procedure
Hematocrit around 30%
Use potassium-free fluid; wash red blood cells to minimize transfused potassium load
Use caution with succinylcholine
Choose drugs that do not depend on renal elimination; adjust (decrease) dosages of drugs that depend on renal metabolism or that are highly protein bound
Use strict aseptic techniques when placing intravascular devices
Identify and adequately protect functioning shunts during surgical procedures
Pay attention to padding of pressure points

diphosphate, inactivating prostacyclin, and increasing platelet–vessel wall contact (i.e., directing platelets toward the vessel wall instead of the usual axial flow). Infusion of desmopressin (DDAVP), which has less pressor effect than vasopressin, stimulates the release of vWF from endothelial cells. This may explain its therapeutic effect in uremia. DDAVP is given intravenously at a dose of 0.3 μg/kg in 50 mL of normal saline over 15 to 30 minutes. It shortens bleeding times in 50% to 75% of uremic patients. This correction occurs in 30 to 60 minutes and lasts for about 4 hours, correlating with increased plasma concentrations of vWF, as well as an increase in the proportion of high-molecular-weight multimers of vWF. Tachyphylaxis typically occurs after the second DDAVP dose, possibly owing to depletion of endothelial multimer stores. Cryoprecipitate, which is rich in factor VIII and vWF, can also be used at an initial dose of 10 to 20 units. Its onset of action is similar to that of desmopressin, but the beneficial effects persist for 24 to 36 hours.

Conjugated estrogen (Premarin 0.6 mg/kg per day intravenously for 5 days) is effective before elective major operations, and its beneficial effects persist for 3 to 4 weeks.

Hemodialysis significantly ameliorates platelet dysfunction and should be used, if required, within 24 hours of the planned operation.

Table 110–5 ■ **Treatment Modalities for Acute Hyperkalemia**

Mechanism	Intervention
Antagonism of K+ effects	Calcium chloride or calcium gluconate 1-2 g (*slow* IV push)
Shift K+ intracellularly (effective within 30 min)	Moderate hyperventilation
	Insulin 20 units/dextrose 50 g IV infusion over 20-30 min
	Sodium bicarbonate 50-100 mEq IV
	Albuterol 10 mg (nebulized)
	Epinephrine 0.01 μg/kg/min IV
Remove K+ from the body	Sodium polystyrene sulfonate (Kayexalate: 30 g sodium polystyrene sulfonate in 100 mL 20% sorbitol) administered via nasogastric tube (100 mL = 30 g) or rectally (100-200 mL = 30-60 g) *Caution: This exchanges potassium for sodium and may lead to pulmonary edema*
	Emergency hemodialysis (even intraoperatively, if required) *Caution: Increases risk for hypotension and bleeding*

PREVENTION

Complications of ESRD in the perioperative period are best prevented by consulting a nephrologist to perform dialysis the day before surgery and to arrange for dialysis in the immediate postoperative period or intraoperatively if necessary. There is accumulating evidence that more aggressive treatment of predialysis hypertension is a potent intervention for reducing subsequent perioperative cardiovascular mortality. Also, early treatment of anemia is recommended because it may delay or prevent left ventricular hypertrophy and reduce bleeding problems. Prevention and treatment of acidosis (serum bicarbonate >20 mEq/L) to establish an acid buffer can help reduce the risk of hyperkalemia. After major surgery, any of these methods has the potential to reduce the high morbidity and mortality rates formerly associated with ESRD and improve patient outcomes.

Further Reading

Boccardo P: Platelet dysfunction in renal failure. Semin Thromb Hemost 30:579-589, 2004.

Foley RN, Parfrey PS, Harnett JD, et al: Clinical and echocardiographic cardiovascular disease in patients starting end stage renal disease therapy: Prevalence, association and progress. Kidney Int 47:186-192, 1995.

Janson PA, Jubelirer SJ, Weinstein MJ, et al: Treatment of bleeding tendency in uremia with cryoprecipitate. N Engl J Med 303:1318-1322, 1980.

Kasiske BL: Dialysis in special clinical situations: Anesthesia. In Jacobs C, et al (eds): Replacement of Renal Function by Dialysis. Dordrecht, The Netherlands, Kluwer Academic Publishers, 1996, pp 954-957.

Kentro TB, Lottenberg R, Kitchens CS: Clinical efficacy of desmopressin acetate for hematocrit control in patients with primary platelet disorder undergoing surgery. Am J Hematol 24:215-219, 1987.

Morbidity and mortality of renal dialysis: An NIH consensus conference statement. Ann Intern Med 121:62-70, 1994.

Remuzzi G, et al: Effect of renal failure on hemostasis. In Brenner & Rector's The Kidney, 7th ed. Philadelphia, WB Saunders, 2004, pp 2173-2178.

Sladen R: Anesthetic considerations for the patient with renal failure. Anesthesiol Clin North Am 18:863-882, 2000.

United States Renal Data System 2004 Annual Data Report. Bethesda, Md, National Institute of Diabetes and Digestive and Kidney Diseases, 2004. Available at www.usrds.org.

Perioperative Care for Patients with Hepatic Insufficiency (Cirrhosis)

111

Laurence C. Torsher

Case Synopsis

A 67-year-old man is scheduled for a right total hip arthroplasty. He has consumed more than 80 g/day of alcohol for the past 15 years. The physical examination is remarkable for numerous spider angiomas, hepatosplenomegaly, and moderate ascites. Laboratory results (with range of normal values) are as follows: hemoglobin, 11.2 g/dL (13.6 to 17.2 g/dL); platelet count, 87×10^9/L (150 to 300×10^9/L); total bilirubin, 2.4 mg/dL (0.3 to 1.0 mg/dL); aspartate aminotransferase, 117 units/L (0 to 35 units/L); alanine aminotransferase, 52 units/L (0 to 35 units/L); and prothrombin time, prolonged by 5 to 15 seconds, with an international normalized ratio (INR) of 1.5.

PROBLEM ANALYSIS

Definition

As the prevalence of liver disease, as well as the survival of those affected, increases, patients with hepatic insufficiency presenting for elective surgery will become more common.

Cirrhosis is a disease characterized by irreversible fibrous scarring of the liver in response to hepatocyte injury and death, with regenerative parenchymal nodule formation that disrupts the normal hepatic architecture. Cirrhosis results in loss of functioning hepatocyte mass, and associated scarring and hepatocellular regeneration disorganize the usual hepatic vasculature, leading to portal hypertension.

Cirrhosis impairs the liver's normal function, which includes filtration of portal blood; metabolism of protein, carbohydrates, fat, hormones, and exogenous chemicals, including drugs; synthesis and excretion of bile; and synthesis of coagulation factors.

The most common cause of cirrhosis in the United States is excessive and prolonged consumption of alcohol, but it can result from other chronic diseases as well (Table 111-1). Complications of cirrhosis are listed in Table 111-2.

Recognition

As many as 10% of men and 5% of women are alcoholic at some time in their lives; however, only 10% to 15% of alcoholics develop cirrhosis. Up to 50% of all hospitalized patients have abused alcohol at one time or another. Ten percent of patients with liver disease undergo operative procedures during the final 2 years of their lives.

Cirrhosis has numerous signs and symptoms that may involve many organ systems.

Cardiovascular. Cirrhosis is usually associated with a hyperdynamic circulatory state and an increased cardiac output.

The increase in cardiac output may be secondary to arteriovenous malformations, especially in the lungs; hypoviscosity secondary to anemia; and increased intravascular volume. Chronic alcohol ingestion can also lead to an alcohol-induced cardiomyopathy that manifests with arrhythmias, low cardiac output, and congestive heart failure.

Table 111–1 ■ Causes of Cirrhosis

Alcohol
Biliary cirrhosis
    Primary
    Secondary
        Sclerosing cholangitis
        Biliary atresia
        Bile duct stricture or tumor
Infection
    Viral (hepatitis A, B, C; cytomegalovirus; Epstein-Barr; herpes)
    Bacterial (brucellosis)
    Parasitic (capillariasis, echinococcosis, schistosomiasis, toxoplasmosis)
Autoimmune chronic active hepatitis
Drugs and toxins
    Methotrexate
    Methyldopa
    Amiodarone
    Isoniazid
    Steroids
    Oral contraceptives
    Arsenic
Inherited and metabolic disorders
    Hemochromatosis
    Wilson's disease
    α_1-Antitrypsin deficiency
    Galactosemia
    Cystic fibrosis
Cryptogenic
Graft-versus-host disease
Nonalcoholic steatohepatitis

Table 111–2 ▪ Complications of Cirrhosis

Portal hypertension
  Varix formation and variceal bleeding
  Splenomegaly with hypersplenism and platelet sequestration
  Ascites formation
    Spontaneous bacterial peritonitis
    Decreased gastric emptying
    Decreased appetite
    Hydrothorax
Hepatorenal syndrome
Hepatic encephalopathy
Portopulmonary hypertension
Coagulopathy
  Thrombocytopenia
  Decreased coagulation factor production
  Low-grade disseminated intravascular coagulation
Anemia
Hepatocellular carcinoma
Malnutrition
Osteoporosis
Altered immune defenses

Pulmonary. Hepatopulmonary syndrome, which results in an increased alveolar-arterial gradient due to the reduced transit time of blood through the lungs (caused by the hyperdynamic circulatory state and the presence of right-to-left intrapulmonary and intrahepatic shunts), occurs to some degree in 47% of patients. Resultant hypoxia may be worsened by ventilation-perfusion mismatching from altered respiratory mechanics, impairment of diaphragmatic function by ascites, presence of hydrothorax, or generalized weakness from malnutrition. Hyperventilation with primary respiratory alkalosis is common. Two percent of patients may exhibit portopulmonary hypertension—the presence of pulmonary hypertension in conjunction with portal hypertension.

Hematologic. Patients with liver disease have multiple hemostatic defects due to reduced synthesis of clotting and fibrinolytic factors. Vitamin K–dependent factors (II, VII, IX, and X) are decreased, as are plasminogen and fibrinogen levels. Owing to splenomegaly caused by portal hypertension, thrombocytopenia and leukopenia are common. Abnormal platelet function has also been observed in patients with cirrhosis. Anemia is due to acute and chronic gastrointestinal blood loss, nutritional deficiency, and bone marrow depression.

Gastrointestinal. Portal hypertension may lead to collateral circulation, causing large varices of the stomach, esophagus, anus (hemorrhoids), and umbilicus. These are susceptible to bleeding. Portal venous blood flow is reduced. Ascites and splanchnic congestion can lead to decreased bowel motility and gastric emptying.

Renal. Fluid and electrolyte disorders can present as ascites, edema, hyponatremia, hypokalemia, or the hepatorenal syndrome. There is also the potential for hypoalbuminemia and hypoglycemia. Patients with cirrhosis have decreased glomerular filtration rate, avid sodium and water retention, and impaired free water clearance. Secondary hyperaldosteronism and diuretic-induced hypovolemia may lead to increased water retention, hyponatremia, and other electrolyte abnormalities. Multiple factors may lead to abnormalities in functional circulating fluid volume. Thus, prerenal renal failure is common. Measurement of creatinine levels may underestimate the degree of renal impairment.

Central Nervous System. The symptoms of hepatic encephalopathy can range from apathy and restlessness to coma. It is believed to be secondary to inadequate removal of toxins or nitrogenous compounds. Asterixis is a common finding in hepatic encephalopathy. Also, patients who are still actively consuming alcohol are at risk for alcohol withdrawal during hospitalization.

Risk Assessment

The history should focus on (1) risk factors for liver disease (e.g., alcohol, drug, or chemical exposure), (2) family history, and (3) symptoms suggestive of liver disease (e.g., jaundice, easy bleeding, expanding abdominal girth). The physical examination focuses on identifying findings compatible with liver disease (e.g., hepatosplenomegaly, right upper quadrant tenderness, ascites, encephalopathy, asterixis, palmar erythema, gynecomastia in men). If the history and physical examination suggest liver disease, blood should be tested for prothrombin time, aspartate aminotransferase and alanine aminotransferase concentrations, total and direct bilirubin, alkaline phosphatase, albumin, complete blood count, creatinine, electrolytes, glucose, and hepatitis viral serology. Other laboratory tests based on comorbid conditions should be carried out as indicated. Table 111-3 lists other perioperative risk factors.

Implications

The modified Child-Pugh score (Table 111-4) identifies patients as class A, B, or C, based on prothrombin time, albumin and bilirubin concentrations, and the presence of ascites or encephalopathy. Although originally developed for the risk stratification of patients undergoing esophageal surgery, the Child-Pugh score has also been validated for patients undergoing other abdominal surgeries. Mortality rates for abdominal surgery in one study were 10%, 30%, and 80% for Child-Pugh class A, B, and C patients, respectively. Although patients with mild chronic liver disease tolerate surgery well, for those with higher Child-Pugh scores, an honest discussion of nonsurgical options is warranted.

Table 111–3 ▪ Factors Associated with Poor Perioperative Outcomes in Patients with Cirrhosis

Elevated creatinine
American Society of Anesthesiologists risk classification ≥3
History of gastrointestinal bleeding
Perioperative infection
Need for intraoperative blood transfusion
Intraoperative hypotension
Hepatic encephalopathy
Emergency operation

Table 111–4 ■ Modified Child-Pugh Score

Presentation	Points*		
	1	2	3
Albumin (g/dL)	>3.5	2.8-3.5	<2.8
Prothrombin time			
Prolonged (sec)	<4.0	4-6	6.0
INR	<1.7	1.7-2.3	>2.3
Bilirubin (mg/dL)†	<2	2.0-3.0	>3.0
Ascites	Absent	Slight-moderate	Tense
Encephalopathy	None	Grade I-II	Grade III-IV

*Class A, 5-6 points; class B, 7-9 points; class C, 10-15 points.
†For cholestatic diseases (e.g., primary biliary cirrhosis), the bilirubin level is disproportionate to the impairment of hepatic function. For these conditions, assign 1 point for bilirubin level <4 mg/dL, 2 points for bilirubin 4-10 mg/dL, and 3 points for bilirubin >10 mg/dL.
INR, international normalized ratio.

Usual causes of perioperative mortality include hemorrhage, sepsis, and acute hepatic function decompensation with or without associated hepatorenal syndrome. Abnormalities in protein concentration, drug clearance, and volume of distribution may have unexpected effects on the onset and duration of medications. Reduced platelet numbers and function and coagulation factor deficiencies associated with low-grade disseminated intravascular coagulation can lead to significant hemorrhage. Moreover, reduced intravascular volume, surgical traction, poor patient positioning, hypocapnia, and impairment of autoregulatory mechanisms may lead to decreased hepatic blood flow, with possible further liver damage. Finally, untreated alcohol withdrawal in the perioperative period with delirium tremens has a mortality rate of 20%. However, with appropriate treatment, mortality rates from withdrawal can be reduced to 1%.

MANAGEMENT AND PREVENTION

Preoperatively, if diaphragmatic movement is impaired by tense ascites, respiratory function may be improved by paracentesis. Coagulopathy should be corrected with platelet transfusion (for severe thrombocytopenia), administration of vitamin K, and transfusion of fresh frozen plasma (for prolonged prothrombin time). Cryoprecipitate and desmopressin (DDAVP) may also be helpful. If hemoglobin is less than 10 g/dL, transfusion of red blood cells should be considered to maintain oxygen carrying capability, particularly to the liver. Careful assessment of volume status (with normalization, if necessary) is important, especially for patients receiving diuretics to control ascites or who have undergone recent paracentesis. Evaluation of the patient's preoperative mental status and function is helpful if there are concerns about worsening encephalopathy perioperatively. Preoperative nutrition consultation may be helpful. Premedication with sedative drugs is usually unnecessary and may have unpredictable effects.

In addition to routine intraoperative monitors, an arterial cannula is useful for beat-to-beat monitoring of blood pressure and frequent blood sampling. Use of a peripheral nerve stimulator to monitor the response to neuromuscular blocking agents is necessary. A pulmonary artery catheter may help with fluid management for patients with significant ascites or for procedures in which large fluid shifts are anticipated. Transesophageal echocardiography may also be helpful for assessing volume status and cardiac function. However, one must be cautious when placing the probe in patients at risk for or with known esophageal varices. Rapid volume administration may be necessary. If so, one should consider at least two large-bore cannulas for venous access.

Medication doses may need to be individually tailored owing to altered drug metabolism and volume of distribution in cirrhotic patients. The influence of cirrhosis on a specific drug's pharmacokinetics depends on its first-pass hepatic extraction. Most sedatives and opioids have prolonged effects and may exacerbate encephalopathy. Neuromuscular blocking agents that depend on hepatic elimination may have prolonged effects. Because atracurium and cisatracurium are eliminated by Hoffman degradation, they offer the advantage of increased predictability of duration of action. The effects of succinylcholine may be prolonged owing to reduced pseudocholinesterase concentrations, but this is rarely clinically significant. Titration to effect, rather than using precalculated doses, is the safest approach for various anesthetic drugs. One must be cautious of medications with potential hepato- and nephrotoxicity (e.g., halothane, nonsteroidal anti-inflammatory drugs, aminoglycoside antibiotics).

Patients with cirrhosis may undergo a regional anesthetic technique if no coagulopathy exists and blood pressure is well maintained. With a general anesthetic, rapid-sequence induction is necessary. Decreased arterial blood pressure or cardiac output, positive-pressure ventilation, and elevated central venous pressure impair hepatic blood flow, as does surgical trauma to the liver or splanchnic bed. Isoflurane and desflurane appear to increase hepatic blood flow, and sevoflurane maintains it, provided that blood pressure and cardiac output are maintained.

Fluid management to correct hypovolemia due to bleeding or reaccumulation of ascites is required to maintain cardiac output and hepatic blood flow. Colloid-containing solutions have theoretical benefits as replacement fluids, especially for patients with hypoalbuminemia. However, this has not been conclusively shown in clinical trials.

Postoperatively, observation in a closely monitored setting facilitates the management of fluids, electrolytes, coagulation, respiratory function, and alcohol withdrawal.

Finally, if the patient is cirrhotic because of viral hepatitis, the risk of transmission to caregivers is an important concern. All health care workers should be vaccinated against hepatitis B. Universal precautions are recommended for all patients, not just those with a diagnosis of viral hepatitis. In the event of high-risk exposure of a health care worker to contaminated body fluids or tissues from a patient with viral hepatitis, the hospital employee health service should be notified immediately.

Further Reading

Gatecel C, Losser M, Payen D: The postoperative effects of halothane versus isoflurane on hepatic artery and portal vein blood flow in humans. Anesth Analg 96:740-745, 2003.

Ginès R, Càrdenas A, Arroyo V, et al: Management of cirrhosis and ascites. N Engl J Med 350:1646-1654, 2004.

Mansour A, Watson W, Shayani V, et al: Abdominal operations in patients with cirrhosis: Still a major surgical challenge. Surgery 122:730-735, 1997.

O'Riordan J, O'Beirne HA, et al: Effects of desflurane and isoflurane on splanchnic microcirculation during major surgery. Br J Anaesth 78:95-96, 1997.

Patel T: Surgery in the patient with liver disease. Mayo Clin Proc 74: 593-599, 1999.

Schuckit MA: Alcohol and alcoholism. In Braunwald E, Fauci AS, Kaper DL, et al (eds): Harrison's Principles of Internal Medicine. New York, McGraw-Hill, 2001, p 2561.

Ziser A, Plevak DJ, Wiesner RH, et al: Morbidity and mortality in cirrhotic patients undergoing anesthesia and surgery. Anesthesiology 90:42-53, 1999.

PHYSIOLOGIC IMBALANCE & COEXISTING DISEASE

Porphyrias

Bradly J. Narr

112

Case Synopsis

A 56-year-old woman with a 23-year history of intermittent abdominal pain was admitted to the hospital. For 24 hours before admission, she had nausea, vomiting, and palpitations, and on admission, she was "out of her head." She retched during the evaluation, so rapid-sequence induction was performed with thiopental (350 mg) and succinylcholine (100 mg); maintenance was with nitrous oxide and fentanyl (700 μg). Following abdominal computed tomography (the scan was normal), she was lethargic and had increased pulse (125 beats per minute) and blood pressure (196/110 mm Hg). Because the bladder appeared distended, catheterization was performed, which produced 400 mL of dark red urine.

PROBLEM ANALYSIS

Definition

The porphyrias are rare, inherited disorders of one of the steps in the biosynthesis of heme (Fig. 112-1). Each porphyria has a characteristic set of symptoms and a specific pattern of heme precursor (porphyrin) overproduction that distinguish it from the others. Carriers of abnormal genes encoding porphyrias often do not have clinical symptoms.

Porphyrins that accumulate as a result of individual enzyme defects may be deposited into a variety of tissues, based on the lipid solubility and size of the porphyrin molecule. The porphyrins that occur in the first half of the heme synthetic pathway (see Fig. 112-1) are water soluble and are excreted in urine. Those that accumulate in the nervous system cause neuroporphyrias, and those that accumulate in skin cause cutaneous porphyrias. Those that accumulate in both cause neurocutaneous porphyrias.

The disorders of most interest to anesthesiologists fall into the class called acute porphyrias (Table 112-1). Enzyme-inducing drugs are the most important triggering factor during anesthesia.

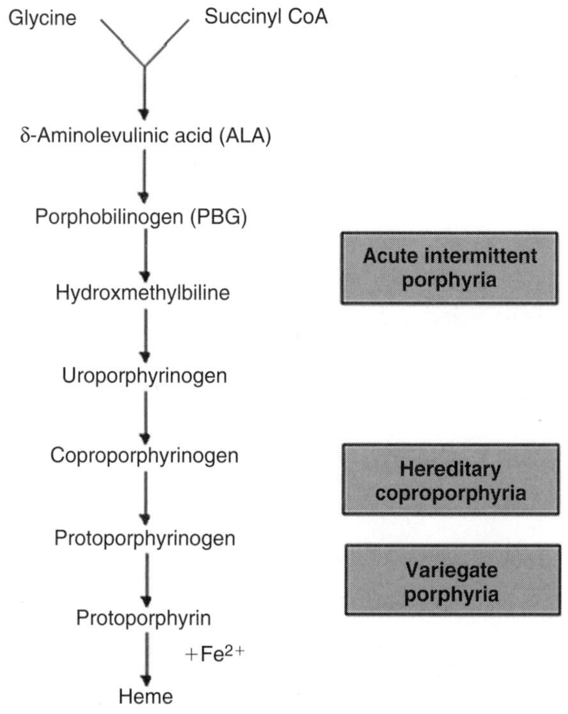

Recognition

The neuroporphyrias and neurocutaneous porphyrias are characterized by acute attacks that can be precipitated by infection, fasting, alcohol intoxication, or administration of some drugs (Tables 112-2 and 112-3). These events stimulate heme synthesis, but because of the enzyme defects, heme is not produced. Therefore, negative feedback to the rate-limiting step (glycine + succinyl coenzyme A → δ-aminolevulinic acid catalyzed by the enzyme δ-aminolevulinic acid synthetase) does not occur. The resulting buildup of porphyrins is believed to cause acute symptoms and signs.

The disease is hereditary and is transmitted most often by an autosomal dominant path. Everyone inherits two copies of each of the heme synthetic enzyme genes. Mutation of one allelle, which results in a 50% reduction in enzyme activity, may be completely asymptomatic until the stresses on the heme synthetic system noted earlier provoke an acute problem. More than 90 mutations that cause acute intermittent porphyria have been identified. There is no evidence that any specific genotype determines the severity of an acute attack.

Figure 112–1 ■ Simplified diagram of the metabolic pathways for heme synthesis. As shown, the porphyrias are inherited disorders of one of the steps in the biosynthesis of heme.

Table 112–1 ■ Disorders of Heme Biosynthesis of Most Importance to Anesthesiologists
Acute intermittent porphyria
Variegate porphyria
Hereditary coproporphyria
δ-Aminolevulinic acid dehydratase deficiency

Table 112–2 ▪ Conditions That May Precipitate Acute Porphyrias
Fasting
Hormones
Alcohol (excessive use)
Drugs (barbiturates and sulfonamides)

The clinical presentation includes recurrent unexplained abdominal pain, sensory or motor neuropathy, autonomic dysfunction (e.g., hypertension, tachycardia), nausea, vomiting, and a history of red or dark urine. Acute porphyria attacks are always associated with elevated levels of δ-aminolevulinic acid, porphobilinogen, or both. Diagnosis is based on biochemical investigation. Only a doubling of the upper normal limits for δ-aminolevulinic acid and porphobilinogen justifies further workup. Also, symptoms should not be attributed to porphyria without a marked increase (several times normal) in urinary porphyrin excretion.

Risk Assessment

In the past, anesthesia posed a real risk for patients with unrecognized porphyria. In South Africa, which had the highest world incidence of variegate porphyria, a study was conducted at Groote Schur Hospital in Cape Town between 1950 and 1971. It showed that 31 of 145 hospital admissions for acute attacks of porphyria were likely precipitated by thiopental induction of anesthesia. Since that time, this incidence has been markedly reduced by better clinical and historical assessment, improved biochemical testing, and an awareness of the potential for drug interactions in patients with porphyria.

Historically, acute porphyria was always considered in the differential diagnosis of patients presenting with an acute abdomen. However, the proliferation of modern imaging techniques has made exploratory surgery a thing of the past in most medical centers. This evolution in patient care, in concert with modern, balanced anesthetic techniques—including the use of drugs with no or low risk (see Table 112-3)—has made the risk of inducing acute porphyria during administration of anesthesia a remote possibility.

Implications

Data comparing drugs of different classes are incomplete in that there are no prospective, randomized studies. Lists have been published categorizing drugs as safe, probably safe, and unsafe (see Table 112-3), based on personal experience, case reports, and the screening of different drugs in animal (chemically primed rats) or tissue (chick embryo) models.

Recent reviews have recommended a more permissive attitude toward precipitating factors, especially during the quiescent phase of the disease, which accounts for a great majority of patients with porphyria. Triggering events vary among patients. Those who are very sensitive may require strict avoidance of all potentially porphyrinogenic events.

MANAGEMENT

Appropriate therapy is difficult without an accurate diagnosis, which is hindered by other variables. These include lack of specific symptoms, latent disease that may recur in only 10% of susceptible individuals, and the high response rate of acute porphyria to supportive therapy. Supportive therapy includes dextrose-containing intravenous fluids because fasting, dehydration, or alcohol intoxication[1] may induce acute porphyria. Additional measures include analgesics and anxiety relief (anxiolytics)[2] and treatment of any associated hypertension and tachycardia. The use of intravenous heme preparations (hematin and its analogues) to provide exogenous negative feedback to the rate-limiting steps in heme synthesis may be lifesaving when employed early in severe attacks.

[1]Alcohol (ethanol) inhibits the release of antidiuretic hormone, resulting in enhanced diuresis.

[2]Droperidol and phenothiazines, but possibly not all benzodiazepines, appear to be safe (see Lambrecht, Gildemeister, Pepe, et al under "Further Reading").

Table 112–3 ▪ Drugs Relevant to Anesthesia that May Produce Acute Porphyrias

Use/Safety*	Induction	Maintenance	Other
Do not use (unsafe)	Barbiturates	Enflurane	Pentazocine, hydralazine, calcium channel blockers†, chlordiazepoxide, ketorolac, sulfonamides
Use carefully (probably safe)	Ketamine Etomidate	Isoflurane Sevoflurane Desflurane	Atracurium, mivacurium, vecuronium, rocuronium, mepivacaine, benzodiazepines, cimetidine, ranitidine, ondansetron, sodium nitroprusside, metoclopramide, clonidine, ACE inhibitors, β-blockers‡
Use (safe)	Propofol	Nitrous oxide Halothane	Analgesics or antagonists: narcotics, aspirin, acetaminophen, naloxone Muscle relaxants or reversal agents: pancuronium, succinylcholine, glycopyrrolate, neostigmine Local anesthetics: procaine, bupivacaine, tetracaine, prilocaine Supportive: droperidol, phenothiazines, atropine, corticosteroids, α-agonists

*The evidence against the use of drugs in the "do not use" category is robust. There is much less evidence, conflicting evidence, or only educated guesses based on chemical structure–activity relationships (CSAR) in the "use carefully" category. For drugs in the "use" category, there is no hard or CSAR evidence against their use.
†Based on animal studies, dihydropyridine calcium channel blockers are more likely than diltiazem or verapamil to cause acute porphyria.
‡Based on a single report (Moore et al; see "Further Reading"), β-blockers appear to be safe for treating tachycardia associated with acute porphyria.
ACE, angiotensin-converting enzyme.

PREVENTION

Many drugs considered unsafe for patients who have been diagnosed with porphyria have been implicated on theoretical grounds. Such drugs either induce heme synthesis or stimulate the cytochrome P-450 system. *There is sufficient evidence to recommend complete avoidance of barbiturates, sulfonamides, and excessive alcohol use.* Enzyme-inducing drugs remain the most important triggering factor related to porphyria and anesthesia. Use of drugs based on the recommendations in Table 112-3 should provide a good outcome for patients with documented porphyria. Blood loss with a resultant increase in heme demand does not stimulate the heme synthetic pathway enough to result in acute porphyria.

Further Reading

Elder GH, Hift RJ, Meissner PN: The acute porphyrias. Lancet 349: 1613-1617, 1997.

Harper P, Hybinette T, Thunell S: Large phlebotomy in variegate porphyria. J Intern Med 242:255-259, 1997.

Harrison GG, Meissner PN, Hift RJ: Anaesthesia for the porphyric patient. Anaesthesia 48:417-421, 1993.

James MFM, Hift RJ: Porphyrias. Br J Anaesth 85:143-153, 2000.

Kauppinen R, Mustajoki P: Prognosis of acute porphyria: Occurrence of acute attacks, precipitating factors, and associated disease. Medicine 71:1-13, 1992.

Lambrecht RW, Gildemeister OS, Pepe JA, et al. Effects of antidepressants and benzodiazepine-type anxiolytic agents on hepatic porphyrin accumulation in primary cultures of chick embryo liver cells. J Pharmacol Exp Ther 291:1150-1155, 1999.

Lambrecht RW, Gildemeister OS, Williams A, et al: Effects of selected antihypertensives and analgesics on hepatic porphyrin accumulation: Implications for clinical porphyria. Biochem Pharmacol 58:887-896, 1999.

Marks GS, Goldman DR, McCluskey SA, et al: The effects of dihydropyridine calcium antagonists on heme biosynthesis in chick embryo liver cell culture. Can J Physiol Pharmacol 64:438-443, 1986.

Meissner PN, Meissner DM, Sturrock ED, et al: Porphyria: The University of Cape Town experience. S Afr Med J 72:755-761, 1987.

Moore MR, McColl KE, Goldberg A: The porphyrias. Diabete Metab 5: 323-336, 1979.

Mustajoki P, Nordmann Y: Early administration of heme arginate for acute porphyric attacks. Arch Intern Med 153:2004-2008, 1993.

Pierach CA: Did Ulysses have porphyria? J Lab Clin Med 144:7-10, 2004.

Tefferi A, Colgan JP, Solberg LA Jr: Acute porphyrias: Diagnosis and management. Mayo Clin Proc 69:991-995, 1994.

Tefferi A, Solberg LA Jr, Ellefson RD: Porphyrias: Clinical evaluation and interpretation of laboratory tests. Mayo Clin Proc 69:289-290, 1994.

Acute Pancreatitis

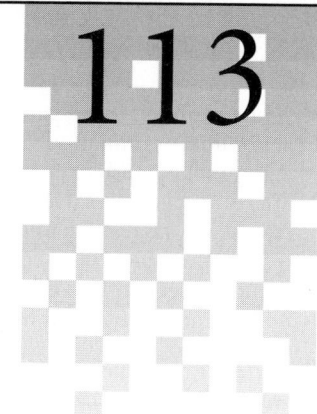

David M. Rothenberg

Case Synopsis

A 56-year-old woman is admitted to the intensive care unit (ICU) following 5 days of increasing abdominal pain, nausea, and vomiting. The patient describes repeated episodes of right upper quadrant pain after certain meals for the past 2 years, but she has not sought medical attention. On physical examination she is noted to have tachypnea, tachycardia, and hypotension. Her sclerae are mildly icteric. Breath sounds are diminished in the lower left lung field, and abdominal palpation reveals diffuse rebound tenderness. Arterial blood gas analysis reveals a mixed respiratory and metabolic alkalosis with an arterial oxygen tension (PaO_2) of 70 mm Hg (fraction of inspired oxygen [FiO_2], 0.5). The white blood cell count is 8000/mm³. The serum amylase level is normal, although lipase, bilirubin, and alanine aminotransferase levels are elevated. Computed tomography (CT) of the abdomen shows an enlarged pancreas with two peripancreatic fluid collections.

PROBLEM ANALYSIS

Definition

Acute pancreatitis commonly presents as a mild, self-limited disorder, but severe systemic manifestations may develop in 20% to 25% of patients, resulting in sepsis, shock, and multiorgan dysfunction syndrome. The majority of cases of acute pancreatitis are associated with gallstones and alcohol abuse, but the link between cause and pathogenesis remains poorly understood.

It appears that dysfunction of the acinar cell, the most active protein-synthesizing cell in the body, is responsible for initiating a host response that may lead to local edema, hemorrhage, or necrosis, with subsequent release of inflammatory mediators into the peritoneal space and circulation. The acinar cell normally secretes and packages digestive and lysosomal enzymes into vacuoles; these enzymes eventually mature into zymogen granules and lysosomes, respectively. Fusion occurs at the luminal surface, allowing the release of enzyme precursors in a process known as exocytosis. Experimental studies have noted that luminal enzyme secretion is decreased in acute pancreatitis, whereas synthesis remains normal. It is speculated that the clinical process is the result of reflux of bile into or septal compression of the pancreatic ductal tree.

Intra-acinar activation of the proteolytic enzyme trypsin, from its precursor trypsinogen, is instrumental in precipitating acute pancreatitis. Intracellular activation of trypsin leads to the conversion of other proteolytic enzymes, such as elastase and phospholipase A_2, to their active forms, causing autodigestive damage of the pancreas. In mild cases of acute pancreatitis it is presumed that trypsin combines with intracellular α_1-antitrypsin to inactive trypsin. The complex is transferred to α_2-macroglobulin for eventual consumption by circulating monocytes and macrophages. In severe forms of acute pancreatitis this process is overwhelmed, resulting in a more systemic inflammatory response. The release of elastase into the peripancreatic space may cause degradation of blood vessels and produce local hemorrhage; the release of phospholipase A_2 may degrade surfactant and be the factor by which acute lung injury occurs. Mediators such as kallikreins, complement, thrombin, and chymotrypsin are also released and modulate the degree of local or systemic injury, most likely through a complex interplay of cytokines and reactive oxygen metabolites.

The more common causes of acute pancreatitis are listed in Table 113-1.

Recognition

Signs and symptoms of acute pancreatitis include the following:

- Diffuse, constant abdominal pain, typically radiating to the back and flank areas, in association with nausea and vomiting
- Tachycardia and tachypnea (common findings)
- Hypotension relative to the degree of hypovolemia, hemorrhage, or systemic vasodilatation

Table 113–1 ■ Causes of Acute Pancreatitis

Biliary tract disease (e.g., choledocholithiasis, ampullary tumor, pancreas divisum)
Ethanol abuse
Hypertriglyceridemia
Hypercalcemia
Trauma
Postsurgical (e.g., cardiopulmonary bypass, endoscopic retrograde cholangiopancreatography)
Vascular insufficiency (e.g., hypoperfusion, shock, vasculitis)
Drugs (e.g., azathioprine, furosemide, pentamidine)
Infection (e.g., mumps, ascariasis, *Mycobacterium tuberculosis*, AIDS)
Other toxins (e.g., methanol, scorpion bites)
Idiopathic

AIDS, acquired immunodeficiency syndrome.

- Tenderness, guarding, and diminished bowel sounds on abdominal examination
- Periumbilical and flank ecchymosis (Cullen's and Grey Turner's signs, respectively; these occur less commonly and represent pancreatic hemorrhage and dissection of blood into the retroperitoneal space)
- Jaundice (seen in 15% of cases, usually in association with biliary tract obstruction from gallstones)

Elevation of the serum amylase level is a characteristic, albeit somewhat nonsensitive, marker of acute pancreatitis. Amylase is released early in the course of the disease and tends to peak within 5 days of the onset of symptoms, yet it may be undetectable in 20% to 30% of cases. Hyperamylasemia is also nonspecific, as it may exist in other disease states (e.g., perforated peptic ulcer, small bowel obstruction, mesenteric infarction, pelvic inflammatory disease, diabetic ketoacidosis, all of which are characterized by acute abdominal pain). Fractionated serum amylase levels, urine amylase levels, and amylase-creatinine clearance ratios do not appear to contribute to diagnostic accuracy in acute pancreatitis. The serum lipase level is a more accurate test for acute pancreatitis (90% sensitive and specific), and it tends to remain elevated long after the onset of symptoms. Elevation in alanine aminotransferase, alkaline phosphatase, and bilirubin levels points toward a diagnosis of gallstone-induced pancreatitis. Additional serum markers that may be useful in predicting the severity of acute pancreatitis include C-reactive protein (a nonspecific acute-phase reactant), polymorphonuclear elastase, and trypsinogen-activating peptide. Elevated trypsinogen-activating peptide levels in either urine or peritoneal fluid have been shown to be highly indicative of pancreatic necrosis.

Imaging techniques are invaluable in diagnosing acute pancreatitis. Chest radiographs may show basilar atelectasis or pleural effusions (these effusions are exudative in nature and characterized by high levels of amylase and lipase). Plain abdominal films may be useful if only to rule out a perforation or to reveal a "sentinel loop," signifying a localized ileus due to acute pancreatitis. Ultrasonography, though important in detecting gallstones or complications of acute pancreatitis (e.g., pseudocysts, abscesses), has a limited role in the detection of acute pancreatitis, because findings may be obscured by obesity or the presence of overlying bowel gas. Contrast-enhanced CT of the abdomen is the most accurate method of diagnosing acute pancreatitis and its local complications. Pancreatic abnormalities are discovered in more than 90% of patients with acute pancreatitis, the severity of which can be graded by CT to correlate with pancreatic abscess or necrosis. Table 113-2 presents a useful grading system for acute pancreatitis. Patients with grades A through D have a less than 2% incidence of abscess formation, whereas those classified as grade E have a 57% incidence of abscess formation. In addition to contrast-enhanced CT, dynamic CT pancreatography offers the possibility of detecting pancreatic perfusion abnormalities that correlate with the location and extent of pancreatic and retroperitoneal fat necrosis. Finally, magnetic resonance imaging may be beneficial in distinguishing between uncomplicated pseudocysts and those associated with necrosis. Identifying these patients early in the course of the disease is critical for the prevention of subsequent infection and in the timing of surgical debridement.

Table 113–2 ▪ Grading System for Pancreatitis

Grade A: Normal pancreas
Grade B: Pancreatic enlargement, focal or diffuse
Grade C: Pancreatic enlargement with mild peripancreatic inflammation
Grade D: Enlarged pancreas associated with fluid in anterior pararenal space
Grade E: Enlarged pancreas with fluid collections in at least two areas

Risk Assessment

A number of prognostic grading systems have been used to gauge the severity of acute pancreatitis and determine optimal treatment. Despite their inability to predict late morbidity or mortality, Ranson's criteria (Table 113-3) are the most frequently used method of predicting early complications of acute pancreatitis. Mortality rates are 1% for patients with fewer than three signs, 15% for those with three to four signs, 40% for those with five to six signs, and up to 100% for patients with seven or more signs. The addition of CT data may improve the accuracy of this scoring system.

The acute physiologic assessment and chronic health evaluation (APACHE) II scoring system (Table 113-4) is a specific and sensitive method of assessing the severity of acute pancreatitis. Unlike Ranson's criteria, it is applicable throughout the course of the illness. One study in young patients with gallstone pancreatitis identified heart rate greater than 110 beats per minute, white blood cell count greater than $14.5/mm^3$, blood urea nitrogen greater than 12 mmol/L, serum glucose greater than 150 mg/dL, and APACHE II score greater than 5 as predictive of the development of serious complications, such as necrotizing pancreatitis. Finally, obesity is thought to be a major risk factor for increased mortality from acute pancreatitis (36% in obese patients versus 6.9% in nonobese patients). The higher mortality is thought to be due to increased peripancreatic fat and greater necrosis.

Table 113–3 ▪ Causes of Acute Pancreatitis

At Admission

Age >55 yr
White blood cell count >16,000/mm³
Blood glucose level >200 mg/dL
Serum lactate dehydrogenase level >350 IU/L
Serum glutamic-oxaloacetic transaminase level >250 units/dL

During Initial 48 Hours

Hematocrit decline >10%
Blood urea nitrogen level rise >5 mg/dL
Serum calcium level <8 mg/dL
Arterial Po₂ <60 mm Hg
Base deficit >4 mEq/L
Estimated fluid sequestration >6 L

From Ranson JHC: Etiological and prognostic factors in human acute pancreatitis: A review. Am J Gastroenterol 77:633-638, 1982.

Table 113–4 ■ APACHE II Severity of Disease Classification System

Physiologic Variable	High Abnormal Range			Low Abnormal Range					
	+4	+3	+2	+1	0	+1	+2	+3	+4
Temperature, rectal (°C)	≥41	39-40.9		38.5-38.9	36-38.4	34-35.9	32-33.9	30-31.9	≤29.9
Mean arterial pressure (mm Hg)	≥180	130-179	110-129		70-109		50-69		≤49
Heart rate (ventricular response)	≥180	140-179	110-139		70-109		55-69	40-54	≤39
Respiratory rate (nonventilated or ventilated)	≥50	35-49		25-34	12-24	10-11	6-9		≤5
Oxygenation: P_{AO_2} – Pa_{O_2}, or Pa_{O_2} (mm Hg)									
a. Fi_{O_2} ≥0.5: record P_{AO_2} – Pa_{O_2}	500	350-499	200-349		<200				
b. Fi_{O_2} <0.5: record only Pa_{O_2}					Po_2 >70	Po_2 61-70		Po_2 55-60	Po_2 <55
Arterial pH	≥7.7	7.6-7.69		7.5-7.59	7.33-7.49		7.25-7.32	7.15-7.24	<7.15
Serum sodium (mmol/L)	≥180	160-179	155-159	150-154	130-149		120-129	111-119	<110
Serum potassium (mmol/L)	≥7	6-6.9		5.5-5.9	3.5-5.4	3-3.4	2.5-2.9		<2.5
Serum creatinine (mg/100 mL) (double point score for acute renal failure)	≥3.5	2-3.4	1.5-1.9		0.6-1.4		<0.6		
Hematocrit (%)	≥60		50-59.9	46-49.9	30-45.9		20-29.9		<20
White blood cell count (total/mm³, in 1000s)	≥40		20-39.9	15-19.9	3-14.9		1-2.9		<1
Glasgow coma score (GCS): Score = 15 minus actual GCS									
A Total APS: Sum of the 12 individual variable points									
Serum HCO_3 (venous, mmol/L) (not preferred; use if no arterial blood gases)	≥52	41-51.9		32-40.9	22-31.9		18-21.9	15-17.9	<15

B Age points:
Assign points as follows:

Age (yr)	Points
≥44	0
45-54	2
55-64	3
65-74	5
≥75	6

C Chronic health points:
If the patiet has a history of severe organ system insufficiency or is immunocompromised, assign points as follows:
a. For nonoperative or emergency postoperative patients— 5 points
or
b. For elective postoperative patients—2 points

APACHE II Score
Sum of A + B + C
A APS points _____
B Age points _____

C Chronic health points _____

Total APACHE II _____

APS, APACHE score.
From Knaus WA, Draper EA, Wagner DP, et al: APACHE II: A severity of disease classification system. Crit Care Med 13:818-829, 1985.

Implications

Although the majority of patients with acute pancreatitis have an uncomplicated course, 20% to 25% develop sequelae that may be life threatening, requiring either ICU support or surgical intervention. Local complications include sterile or infected tissue necrosis, pseudocysts, abscesses, colonic fistulas, gastrointestinal hemorrhage, and splenic rupture. Systemic complications include shock, acute renal failure, acute lung injury, coagulopathy, hyperglycemia, hypocalcemia, retinopathy, and psychosis.

MANAGEMENT

The treatment of uncomplicated acute pancreatitis is primarily supportive, with the judicious use of intravenous fluids and parenteral analgesia. Nasogastric suctioning is beneficial only in patients with documented ileus. Recent randomized, controlled trials have confirmed the benefits of early enteral feedings in patients with severe acute pancreatitis, noting less end-organ failure, a diminished systemic inflammatory response, and shorter length of hospital stay compared with parenteral feedings. The use of prophylactic antibiotics for severe acute pancreatitis remains controversial. A 1998 meta-analysis of eight prospective, randomized, controlled trials found that reduced mortality was limited to patients who were administered broad-spectrum antibiotics that could penetrate pancreatic tissue. However, a more recent study cited an increase in the incidence of fungal infections and higher perioperative mortality. Also, controlled trials investigating the use of H_2-antagonists, protease inhibitors, and peritoneal lavage were unable to document improved outcomes.

Early use of endoscopic retrograde cholangiopancreatography (ERCP) and papillotomy for biliary pancreatitis is also controversial. One prospective multicenter study in the late 1990s failed to show a benefit from ERCP. In more severe forms of acute pancreatitis, ICU support with mechanical ventilation for respiratory failure, dialysis for acute renal failure, and infusions of vasoactive drugs may be required. Urgent surgery is indicated only in cases of deteriorating condition or evidence of pancreatic sepsis. The diagnosis of

PHYSIOLOGIC IMBALANCE & COEXISTING DISEASE

infected necrotizing pancreatitis is often made by CT-guided fine-needle aspiration and signals the need for urgent surgical debridement.

The role of surgical intervention for sterile necrotizing pancreatitis remains controversial. Intraoperative management relies on the maintenance of intravascular volume, monitoring of serum electrolytes and glucose levels, and recognition of sepsis and acute lung injury. In this regard, pulmonary artery catheterization may be useful in directing vasopressor or other supportive therapies.

PREVENTION

Episodes of acute pancreatitis are prevented by avoiding exposure to precipitating factors such as alcohol and by early surgical therapy for choledocholithiasis. Use of biochemical and radiographic markers to facilitate the early recognition of necrotizing pancreatitis may further reduce the morbidity and mortality from acute pancreatitis.

Further Reading

Arnell TD, de Virgilio C, Chang L, et al: Admission factors can predict the need for ICU monitoring in gallstone pancreatitis. Am Surg 62: 815-819, 1996.

Balthazar EJ: Acute pancreatitis: Assessment of severity with clinical and CT evaluation. Radiology 223:603-613, 2002.

Folsch UR, Nitsche R, Ludtke R, et al: Early ERCP and papillotomy compared with conservative treatment for acute biliary pancreatitis: The German Study Group on Acute Biliary Pancreatitis. N Engl J Med 336:237-242, 1997.

Funnell IC, Bornman PC, Weakley SP, et al: Obesity: An important prognostic factor in acute pancreatitis. Br J Surg 80:484-486, 1993.

Golub R, Siddiqi F, Pohl D: Role of antibiotics in acute pancreatitis. J Gastrointest Surg 2:496-503, 1998

Gudgeon AM, Heath DI, Hurley P, et al: Trypsinogen activation peptides assay in the early prediction of severity of acute pancreatitis. Lancet 335:4-8, 1990.

Gumaste V, Dave P, Sereny G: Serum lipase: A better test to diagnose acute alcoholic pancreatitis. Am J Med 92:239-242, 1992.

Isenmann R, Runzi M, Kron M, et al: Prophylactic antibiotic treatment in patients with predicted severe acute pancreatitis: A placebo-controlled, double-blind trial. Gastroenterology 126:997-1004, 2004.

Ranson JHC: Etiological and prognostic factors in human acute pancreatitis: A review. Am J Gastroenterol 77:633-638, 1982.

Swaroop VS, Chari ST, Clain JE: Severe acute pancreatitis. JAMA 291: 2865-2868, 2004.

Wilson C, Heath DI, Imrie CW: Prediction of outcome in acute pancreatitis: A comparative study of APACHE II, clinical assessment and multiple factor scoring systems. Br J Surg 77:1260-1264, 1990.

Yousaf M, McCallion K, Diamond T: Management of severe acute pancreatitis. Br J Surg 90:402-420, 2003.

Autonomic Hyperreflexia

114

C. Lee Parmley and Steven J. Allen

Case Synopsis

A 25-year-old woman develops headache and severe hypertension following a urologic procedure performed with topical anesthesia. She has C6 quadriplegia resulting from a motor vehicle accident 5 years ago. Examination reveals blood pressure 240/130 mm Hg, pulse 45 beats per minute, facial flushing, and cool lower extremities.

PROBLEM ANALYSIS

Definition

Autonomic hyperreflexia is a disturbance arising in patients with chronic spinal cord injury. It is also termed autonomic dysreflexia, hypertensive autonomic crisis, and mass reflex. Autonomic hyperreflexia is characterized by massive sympathetic activity set off by reflex stimulation from a variety of triggers (Table 114-1). It has been reported in 85% of patients within 2 to 3 weeks of spinal cord injury. Because it requires viable spinal cord below the level of injury or transaction, the disturbance does not occur in patients with paraplegia due to spinal cord infarction.

Autonomic hyperreflexia occurs when the hypothalamus and brainstem can no longer modulate segmental spinal sympathetic nerves and thereby inhibit their output. In the acute phase following spinal cord injury, there is low sympathetic activity. However, sympathetic activity returning to viable cord below the lesion is isolated from upper inhibitory control. This can result in an uncontrolled sympathetic response to a stimulus. The sympathetic activity causes vasoconstriction in the vasculature below the spinal cord lesion, leading to systemic hypertension. The hypertension stimulates the baroreceptors in the aortic arch and carotid sinus, inducing bradycardia and vasodilatation above the spinal cord defect. The vasodilatation is thought to be the cause of headaches and flushing. The severity of autonomic hyperreflexia is dependent on the amount of cord below the lesion that is involved with sympathetic outflow. Thus, higher cord lesions have a more profound response than do lower lesions.

Table 114–1 ▪ Autonomic Hyperreflexia Triggers

Bladder or large or small bowel distention
Cutaneous stimulation
Uterine contractions
Lower or upper extremity surgery
Sexual pathology
Urogenital pathology
Cystoscopy and other genitourinary instrumentation
Extracorporeal lithotripsy

Recognition

Autonomic hyperreflexia should be suspected when headache or hypertension develops in any patient with paraparesis of greater than 2 weeks' duration. Autonomic hyperreflexia's onset is variable among patients, and some may exhibit signs as early as the fourth postinjury day. Clinical findings are related to the level of intact innervation. Evidence of sympathetic stimulation below the level of the lesion may include skin pallor, pilomotor erection, spastic muscle contraction, and increased muscle tone. Above the lesion, one may find flushing of the face and neck, diaphoresis, mydriasis, and lid retraction. Awake patients frequently complain of headache, dyspnea, blurred vision, chest pain, nausea, and a sense of ill ease.

Risk Assessment

The severity of autonomic hyperreflexia is dependent on the amount of cord below the lesion that is involved with sympathetic outflow. Thus, lesions below T10 generally are not associated with autonomic hyperreflexia, because there are few sympathetic spinal synapses to disinhibit. Conversely, lesions above T5 tend to be associated with the worst autonomic hyperreflexia–related problems, because the majority of spinal sympathetic efferents arise below this level.

The site and nature of the planned procedure may also play a role. The majority of patients come to the operating room for urologic procedures, all of which are likely to produce autonomic hyperreflexia. One group of at-risk patients that has been the subject of increased interest in recent years is spinal cord–injured parturients. Because uterine contractions may result in strong sympathetic outflow, these patients pose a unique challenge during labor. The literature suggests that the incidence of autonomic hyperreflexia is as high as 75% in this population. In addition, it may be difficult to distinguish autonomic hyperreflexia from preeclampsia. Accordingly, some clinicians advise epidural anesthesia for all spinal cord–injured women in labor to prevent autonomic hyperreflexia.

Implications

If untreated, autonomic hyperreflexia can lead to serious complications and even death. Cardiovascular complications include left ventricular failure, myocardial ischemia, and possibly arrhythmias, all related to increased demands related to severe hypertension or central nervous system complications.

Central nervous system complications are typically those associated with hypertensive encephalopathy, such as confusion, seizures, and stroke. Autonomic hyperreflexia may also increase surgical blood loss.

MANAGEMENT

The onset of hypertension requires immediate intervention, because systemic blood pressure can quickly escalate to dangerous levels. The first maneuver should be to remove the offending stimulus (e.g., relieving a distended bladder). If hypertension develops during a general anesthetic, the concentration of volatile agent should be increased. If an epidural catheter is being used, raising the level of the block may help.

Pharmacologic intervention can consist of any agent that interrupts the sympathetic reflex and has the characteristics of rapid onset, short duration, and low toxicity. The most frequently recommended drugs are sodium nitroprusside and nifedipine. Sodium nitroprusside has the advantages of reliability, rapid onset, and titratability. However, continuous use may require monitoring for cyanide toxicity. Also, nitroprusside may be harder to titrate to the desired effect (requiring more dosing changes), and it may be associated with untoward hypotension.[1] Nifedipine has an acceptable degree of effectiveness in treating autonomic hyperreflexia. Its advantages are oral (sublingual) administration, relatively short duration, and minimal toxicity in this patient population. Disadvantages are unreliable or delayed absorption, possibly leading to excessive dosing and hypotension. Nicardipine's actions are similar to those of nifedipine; it has a short half-life of elimination (minutes) after intravenous bolus administration and no specific organ toxicity during prolonged infusion.[2] For these reasons, nicardipine might be preferred over nifedipine or sodium nitroprusside for hypertensive emergencies in patients with autonomic hyperreflexia, but there is little precedent for such use. There are also anecdotal reports of excellent results with magnesium sulfate.

PREVENTION

The main goal in patients at risk for autonomic hyperreflexia is to prevent hypertension. The purpose of anesthetic management is not to prevent pain in an insensate area but rather to prevent enhanced sympathetic activity due to visceral organ stimulation. Although topical and general anesthesia may be used, regional anesthesia is associated with the lowest incidence of perioperative hypertension.

This is because regional techniques most directly block conduction of the afferent nerves in the spinal cord. For urologic procedures, most of the stimulation is via the sacral nerves, suggesting that a subarachnoid block is an appropriate technique. Lumbar epidural anesthesia is less reliable, because the sacral nerve roots may not be completely blocked. Regional anesthesia also has the advantage of providing muscle relaxation and preventing sudden leg flexion during visceral organ manipulation. Some clinicians are reluctant to perform a regional technique in the presence of a neurologic deficit. One reason is that the level of the block is difficult to determine owing to the lack of sensation. As an alternative, some clinicians employ nifedipine or nicardipine for hypertension prophylaxis.

General anesthesia can be problematic in patients with autonomic hyperreflexia. Inadequate anesthesia (especially for tracheal intubation, electroconvulsive therapy, aortic cross-clamping, and the like) may trigger dangerous hypertension, whereas anesthetic overdose may result in profound hypotension. Typically, anesthesia must be deep to prevent autonomic hyperreflexia. For that reason, a technique based solely on nitrous oxide and opioids may not be satisfactory. Isoflurane and sevoflurane have been used successfully, likely owing to their salutary vasodilatory effects (i.e., reducing both preload and afterload). Emergence must be carefully managed, because patients with high spinal cord injury have some degree of respiratory compromise. The adequacy of ventilation must be ensured before and after extubation.

Further Reading

Amzallag M: Autonomic hyperreflexia. Int Anesthesiol Clin 31:87-102, 1993.
Baker ER, Cardenas DD, Benedetti TJ: Risks associated with pregnancy in spinal cord-injured women. Obstet Gynecol 80:425-428, 1992.
Bernstein A, Richlin D, Sotolongo JR Jr: Nifedipine pretreatment for prevention of autonomic hyperreflexia during anesthesia-free extracorporeal shock wave lithotripsy. J Urol 147:676-677, 1992.
Jones NA, Jones SD: Management of life-threatening autonomic hyperreflexia using magnesium sulphate in a patient with a high spinal cord injury in the intensive care unit. Br J Anaesth 88:434-438, 2002.
Kobayashi A, Mizobe T, Tojo H, et al: Autonomic hyperreflexia during labour. Can J Anaesth 42:1134-1136, 1995.
Krassioukov AV, Furlan JC, Fehlings MG: Autonomic dysreflexia in acute spinal cord injury: An underrecognized clinical entity. J Neurotrauma 20:707-716, 2003.
Lambert DH, Deane RS, Mazuzan JE Jr: Anesthesia and the control of blood pressure in patients with spinal cord injury. Anesth Analg 61:344-348, 1982.
Maehama T, Izena H, Kanazawa K: Management of autonomic hyperreflexia with magnesium sulfate during labor in a woman with spinal cord injury. Am J Obstet Gynecol. 813:492-493, 2000.
Pereiara L: Obstetric management of the patient with spinal cord injury. Obstet Gynecol Surg 58:678-687, 2003.

---

[1]Nicardipine is a primary arterial dilator, whereas sodium nitroprusside has both venodilator (reduces preload) and arterial dilator properties that are about equal.

[2]Nicardipine differs from nifedipine in two important respects, however. First, it has no vehicle (polysorbate). Polysorbate has direct myocardial depressant and vasodilatory properties on both venous capacitance and arterial beds. Second, nicardipine is approved for intravenous dosing.

Perioperative Management of Patients with Muscular Dystrophy

115

Katarzyna Luba

Case Synopsis

An 8-month-old boy undergoes myringotomy tube removal. His previous general anesthesia for tube placement was uneventful. Anesthesia is induced with intravenous thiopental and atropine and is maintained with nitrous oxide, halothane, and oxygen via a facemask. After removal of the myringotomy tube, the surgeon performs a digital examination and decides to perform an adenoidectomy. Airway obstruction at this time necessitates emergency intubation. After succinylcholine 2 mg/kg intravenously, an increase in masseter muscle tone is noted. The electrocardiogram (ECG) monitor shows a wide complex tachycardia progressing to bradycardia. End-tidal carbon dioxide (CO_2) of 40 to 50 mm Hg gradually decreases to 25 mm Hg. Arterial saturation decreases from 100% to 80%, then cannot be detected. Halothane is discontinued. Calcium chloride, epinephrine, and sodium bicarbonate are given intravenously. The ECG becomes increasingly dysmorphic, and pulses cannot be palpated. Chest compressions start. Venous blood analysis shows that pH is 7.13, CO_2 tension (P_{CO_2}) is 73 mm Hg, and potassium level is more than 10 mmol/L. Calcium, epinephrine, and bicarbonate are repeated. After 13 minutes of cardiopulmonary resuscitation, the ECG shows the return of a narrow complex tachycardia, and systolic blood pressure increases to 100 mm Hg. Twenty minutes after succinylcholine administration, a venous blood sample shows pH 7.30, P_{CO_2} 49 mm Hg, and potassium 7.1 mmol/L. A urinary catheter reveals red urine. The patient is transported to a pediatric intensive care unit. The creatine kinase (CK) level is 285,760 units/L. The patient is treated with vigorous intravenous hydration. He is discharged home in good condition. DNA studies before discharge show a deletion of the dystrophin gene, consistent with a diagnosis of Duchenne's muscular dystrophy.

PROBLEM ANALYSIS

Definition

Muscular dystrophies are a clinically and genetically diverse group of hereditary disorders of the structure of striated muscle, characterized by progressive muscle weakness and wasting. The diagnosis of a muscular dystrophy is based on elevated serum CK, myopathic electromyogram features, and muscle biopsy. The morphologic changes common to all forms of muscular dystrophy present a random pattern of normal or hypertrophic muscle fibers, necrotic and necrotizing fibers, and interstitial accumulation of fatty and fibrous tissue. The latter changes result in the characteristic pseudohypertrophy of the calf muscles seen in Duchenne's muscular dystrophy.

The previous classification of muscular dystrophies was based on patterns of inheritance and clinical features. A more recently proposed classification takes into account the type, localization, and function of defective proteins involved in the pathogenesis of different muscular dystrophies.

PLASMA MEMBRANE–ASSOCIATED PROTEINS

Defective plasma membrane–associated proteins or the lack of such proteins causes the most common muscular dystrophies, including Duchenne's muscular dystrophy (DMD), Becker's muscular dystrophy (BMD), the sarcoglycanopathies, and other forms of limb-girdle muscular dystrophy (LGMD).

Dystrophinopathies. The most common muscular dystrophies are X-linked recessive disorders caused by mutations of the dystrophin gene. Dystrophin is a sarcolemmal protein that plays a role in maintaining the integrity of the sarcolemma. The severe DMD form results from deficiency of dystrophin. The milder allelic form (BMD) is associated with a reduced amount of the truncated protein. The incidence of DMD is 1 in 3500 live male births. Affected males have delayed motor development, and when they start walking, they present with gait abnormalities. By age 5 years, muscle weakness is evident. Calf enlargement is due to replacement of necrotic muscle by fat and fibrous tissue. Lumbar hyperlordosis and toe-walking result from progressive loss of muscle strength and tendon contractures. By age

12 years, most patients are confined to a wheelchair. Scoliosis, chest deformity, and diaphragmatic weakness lead to restrictive pulmonary disease by age16 to 18 years. Respiratory failure, the most common cause of death, occurs in the third decade of life. Almost all patients have cardiomyopathy, but this rarely causes death. Intellectual impairment is common.

Compared with DMD, BMD has a later onset and a milder clinical course. Symptoms of proximal muscle weakness commonly start between ages 5 and 15 years, although the onset may be delayed until the third or fourth decade of life. Patients generally ambulate beyond age 15 years. Calf hypertrophy occurs early and is prominent. Patients have a short life expectancy, but many live to their 30s or 40s. Mental retardation is milder than in DMD. In patients with mild or subclinical BMD, cardiomyopathy may be the presenting feature of the disease. Most BMD patients die of complications of cardiomyopathy.

Sarcoglycanopathies. These disorders are caused by mutations of genes encoding four transmembrane glycoproteins of the sarcoglycan complex. Mutations of any of the four sarcoglycan genes (alpha, beta, gamma, and delta) result in LGMD 2D, 2E, 2C, and 2F. Both males and females are affected. Proximal leg muscle weakness generally appears in the second or third decade but may be delayed. Upper limb involvement with scapular winging develops. Diaphragmatic weakness with respiratory insufficiency, cardiomyopathy, congestive heart failure (CHF), and arrhythmias may develop. Intellectual function is normal.

Caveolin Deficiency. This is a rare form of autosomal dominant muscular dystrophy. LGMD 1C is caused by deficient caveolin, a ubiquitous plasma membrane protein.

EXTRACELLULAR MATRIX PROTEINS

Deficiencies in extracellular matrix proteins result in congenital muscular dystrophies (CMDs), a group of autosomal recessive disorders that become symptomatic at birth or in infancy. They are diagnosed by hypotonia and a dystrophic muscle biopsy. The most severe form is merosin-deficient CMD. The maximal functional ability of a child with CMD is sitting unsupported. Further, cardiomyopathy may be present.

PROTEINS WITH ENZYMATIC ACTIVITY

Mutations in Genes Encoding Glycosyltransferases.
These mutations are a recently identified mechanism for CMDs. The gene encoding the fukutin-related protein (FKRP—a glycosyltransferase) is mutated in a severe form of muscular dystrophy, CMD type 1C, as well as a mild form, LGMD 2I. Central nervous system involvement is present in the severe form, with cerebellar cysts, seizures, and developmental delay. Mild cardiomyopathy may also be present.

Protein Kinases.
Heterozygosity for a trinucleotide repeat ($[CTG]_n$) expansion mutation in the 3′ untranslated region of a protein kinase gene on chromosome 19 is the cause of myotonic dystrophy, the most common adult form of muscular dystrophy. This has a prevalence of 1 in 8000. Myotonic dystrophy is an autosomal dominant disorder characterized by myotonia, slowly progressive muscle weakness and wasting,

frontal baldness, cataracts, and insulin resistance secondary to aberrant insulin receptor expression. Type 2 diabetes may develop.

OTHER MUSCLE PROTEINS

Sarcomeric Proteins. Mutations in the titin gene, encoding a giant sarcomeric protein, underlie an autosomal dominant form of congenital dilated cardiomyopathy. Recently, mutations of the same gene have been found in patients with isolated tibial muscular dystrophy.

Nuclear Proteins. Defects in two nuclear proteins are responsible for two distinct forms of Emery-Dreifuss muscular dystrophy (EDMD). X-linked EDMD is due to mutations in the gene encoding the nuclear protein emerin. Autosomal dominant EDMD results from mutations in the lamin A/C gene, encoding a protein of the nuclear lamina. Mutations in this gene also lead to a form of dominant proximal LGMD 1B and dilated cardiomyopathy. Skeletal muscle involvement in EDMD is usually mild and slowly progressive. Cardiac involvement is the predominant feature of the disease.

CARDIOMYOPATHY IN MUSCULAR DYSTROPHIES

Cardiac involvement is a universal feature of muscular dystrophies. The severity of cardiac involvement may determine the long-term prognosis for persons with any type of muscular dystrophy.

In DMD and BMD, lacking or faulty dystrophin has been demonstrated in both cardiac and skeletal muscle. Heart failure is often the proximate cause of death, alone or in association with respiratory failure. Myocardial damage is initially subclinical but can be recognized through minor ECG and echocardiographic changes. Myocardial involvement progresses to a clinically evident stage of hypertrophy; arrhythmias, characterized by conduction defects (atrioventricular block, bundle branch block) or severe supraventricular or ventricular arrhythmias; and, finally, dilated cardiomyopathy due to widespread myocardial fibrosis. Heart failure is the most common cause of death in patients with BMD. Female carriers of DMD and BMD have a 10% incidence of cardiomyopathy that is age-progressive.

Sarcoglycanopathies (LGMD 2C, 2D, 2E, 2F) may have associated dilated cardiomyopathy. This results from disrupted sarcoglycan complexes in both skeletal and cardiac muscle.

LGMD due to mutations in the FKRP gene (LGMD 2I) may be associated with myocardial fibrosis, leading to dilated cardiomyopathy and repolarization abnormalities.

In myotonic dystrophies, cardiac conduction defects are a major cause of sudden death. The incidence of complete atrioventricular block among these patients is higher than in the general population. A prolonged His-ventricular conduction interval puts these patients at risk of paroxysmal atrioventricular block and justifies early pacemaker implantation. In congenital (neonatal) myotonic dystrophy, abnormal myocardial relaxation results in left ventricular diastolic dysfunction.

Severe cardiac involvement is common in EDMD. Both X-linked and autosomal dominant forms involve the risk of bradyarrhythmias (often requiring pacemaker implantation) and atrial fibrillation or flutter. Atrial fibrillation often precedes atrial standstill and may be the cause of embolic stroke at a young age. Prophylactic anticoagulation is recommended in EDMD patients with atrial arrhythmias or standstill. Finally, left ventricular failure is rare but may be severe enough to require a heart transplant.

Recognition

Patients with muscular dystrophy usually present for muscle biopsy, tendon contracture release, correction of kyphoscoliosis, or pacemaker implantation. Pediatric patients with undiagnosed muscular dystrophy may present for procedures unrelated to the disease.

All patients with muscular dystrophy should be suspected of having respiratory and cardiac dysfunction. Pulmonary function tests should be performed in all patients with muscle weakness because of the high incidence of restrictive lung disease secondary to diaphragmatic weakness and scoliosis. In asymptomatic patients with the diagnosis of muscular dystrophy, the specific type of dystrophy and the risk of cardiac involvement determine the need for further cardiac workup.

Intraoperative CHF may present as tachycardia and hypotension unresponsive to intravenous fluids. Physical signs of CHF include jugular vein distention, pulmonary rales, and dyspnea in a spontaneously breathing patient. Severe CHF results in acute pulmonary edema, with hypoxia and pink, frothy respiratory secretions. Diagnosis may be confirmed by hemodynamic parameters measured with a pulmonary artery catheter. Typically, pulmonary artery occlusion pressure is elevated (>18 mm Hg), cardiac index is low (<2.2 L/minute/m² body surface area), and systemic vascular resistance is high (>1200 dynes•sec•cm^{-5}).

In children with undiagnosed DMD, succinylcholine has been reported to induce hyperkalemic cardiac arrest. On the basis of these reports, the Food and Drug Administration recommended against the use of succinylcholine for nonemergent intubation in children.

Malignant hyperthermia (MH), a rare inherited disorder of sarcolemmal calcium flux, may be triggered by volatile anesthetics and succinylcholine in genetically susceptible individuals. Patients with DMD may be susceptible to MH. Signs of MH include muscle rigidity; an unanticipated, rapid rise in temperature and end-tidal CO_2; hypertension; metabolic acidosis; tachyarrhythmias; myoglobinuria; and elevated serum CK.

Risk Assessment

All patients with muscular dystrophy are at risk for cardiomyopathy or conduction disorders. Signs and symptoms of myocardial dysfunction at the time of preoperative evaluation may be overt or masked by confinement to a wheelchair. Therefore, all patients with muscular dystrophy should have their cardiac function evaluated preoperatively. ECG abnormalities (sinus tachycardia or bradycardia, short P-R interval, signs of left ventricular hypertrophy, conduction defects) are very common. However, the best correlation between severe cardiac involvement and mortality is the degree of left ventricular echocardiographic dysfunction. Guidelines for the assessment of cardiac involvement in patients with DMD and BMD advise that those with DMD have an echocardiogram and ECG at the time of diagnosis, every 2 years up to the age of 10, and annually thereafter. BMD patients should have an echocardiogram and ECG at the time of diagnosis and then every 5 years. The same recommendations apply to patients with other forms of muscular dystrophy. Additional echocardiograms or ECGs should be obtained before surgery or if clinically indicated.

Patients with EDMD should have an ECG and echocardiogram at the time of diagnosis and annually thereafter. They should also be monitored annually for arrhythmias with a Holter monitor. An implanted pacemaker is justified for symptomatic patients or for asymptomatic patients whose ECG shows sinus node or atrioventricular node dysfunction. In autosomal dominant EDMD, sudden death is a possibility, even in patients with pacemakers. Therefore, a pacemaker with the full range of internal cardioverter-defibrillator capabilities should be considered whenever antibradycardia pacing is indicated. When atrial fibrillation or atrial standstill is diagnosed, antithromboembolic prophylaxis with warfarin is indicated.

Intracardiac conduction should be evaluated in all adult myotonic dystrophy patients. Patients are selected to undergo cardiac electrophysiologic investigation based on the results of signal-averaged ECGs.

In patients with DMD, a steady decrease in vital capacity (VC) follows progressive muscle weakness and the development of scoliosis. Once VC falls below 20% of predicted values, ventilatory failure is inevitable, and 73% of patients die of respiratory failure. Obstructive sleep apnea is common, leading to chronic hypoxemia and right ventricle failure. Preoperative pulmonary function tests and sleep studies are indicated to assess the severity of restrictive pulmonary disease and obstructive sleep apnea.

Implications

Patients with muscular dystrophies are at increased risk of perioperative CHF, arrhythmias, and respiratory failure. If the VC is less than 30% of predicted, the patient will likely require prolonged postoperative ventilatory support. Obstructive sleep apnea and weak pharyngeal muscles increase the risk for early postoperative airway obstruction and hypoxia. Outpatient general anesthesia is not advised owing to the risk of delayed respiratory depression. Also, delayed gastric emptying increases the risk of aspiration.

Succinylcholine can trigger MH or cause hyperkalemic cardiac arrest; therefore, its use is not advised. Nondepolarizing muscle relaxants (NDMRs) may have prolonged effects. Also, neostigmine reversal is unpredictable. Volatile anesthetics may trigger MH in DMD patients.

In patients with myotonic dystrophy, hypothermia, shivering, succinylcholine, neostigmine, and direct muscle stimulation may precipitate a myotonic crisis, characterized by prolonged contracture of the skeletal muscles.

For these reasons, regional or local anesthesia, when suitable, is preferred for all patients with muscular dystrophy.

Finally, patients with DMD previously treated with glucocorticoid steroids require supplemental perioperative steroids.

MANAGEMENT

The need to minimize the use of myocardial depressant and MH-triggering agents favors the use of regional anesthesia or total intravenous general anesthesia. Agents used for the latter include propofol, ketamine, dexmedetomidine, and opioids. Short-acting opioids (remifentanil, sufentanil) may be preferable to reduce the risk of postoperative respiratory depression.

Premedication with benzodiazepines and opioids may cause respiratory depression, airway obstruction, and delayed emergence from anesthesia and should be avoided.

Airway management should take into account the increased risk of aspiration. Premedication with an H_2-blocker and metoclopramide is advised. Modified rapid-sequence endotracheal intubation with the use of an NDMR is the method of choice.

The choice of agent is limited by contraindications to succinylcholine and increased sensitivity to NDMRs. Short-acting NDMRs (mivacurium, cisatracurium) should be used, and their dose should be titrated to the train-of-four response. Even with the use of short-acting NDMRs, prolonged recovery has been reported in children with DMD. Reversal of NDMRs with neostigmine has been reported without adverse events. However, as mentioned earlier, reversal with neostigmine may be unpredictable.

The management of intraoperative CHF depends on hemodynamic stability. Diuresis and positive end-expiratory pressure may be sufficient. If hypotension develops, an inotrope (dobutamine or dopamine) should be used, and an arterial line placed. An arterial line is advised for all major surgery in patients with muscular dystrophy. Further management is guided by transesophageal echocardiography or pulmonary artery catheter measurements. If preload is adequate, inotropy and afterload reduction may help increase cardiac output and tissue perfusion.

In patients with myotonic dystrophy, anesthetic goals should include avoidance of the triggers of myotonic contractures. Severe contractures may result in jaw and chest rigidity, impeding efforts to intubate and ventilate. Contractures do not respond to NDMRs; they may respond to intravenous quinidine, infiltration of the muscle with local anesthetic, and rewarming the patient.

MH management requires immediate discontinuation of inhalational anesthetics, administration of dantrolene, 100% oxygen, active cooling, and treatment of associated arrhythmias, hyperkalemia, and acidosis. To prevent acute renal failure secondary to rhabdomyolysis, patients should be treated with intravenous hydration, alkalinization of urine with intravenous sodium bicarbonate, and mannitol.

Patients with impaired respiratory function require admission to the intensive care unit for prolonged ventilatory support after extensive surgical procedures under general anesthesia.

PREVENTION

Prevention of perioperative complications in patients with muscular dystrophy requires thorough evaluation of the surgical risk. Surgery for the correction of scoliosis in patients with DMD should be performed before pulmonary function declines and precludes a safe anesthetic and postoperative course. Knowledge of the severity of myocardial involvement is necessary to prevent perioprative exacerbation of CHF or life-threatening arrhythmias. The preoperative evaluation should include a recent ECG, echocardiogram, and electrophysiologic testing if indicated by the results of signal-averaged ECGs. In the presence of severe cardiomyopathy and respiratory dysfunction, invasive hemodynamic monitoring and postoperative critical care management should be anticipated for major surgical procedures. Outpatient surgery in this patient population is discouraged, because overnight monitoring for delayed respiratory complications after general anesthesia of any duration is warranted.

Aspiration risk should be minimized by premedication with H_2-blockers and metoclopramide and by the use of an appropriate intubation technique. *Succinylcholine should never be used.* Also, inhalational anesthetics should be avoided because of their MH-triggering potential. The use of regional or local anesthesia, whenever feasible, may help avoid respiratory, cardiac, and metabolic complications of general anesthesia in patients with muscular dystrophy.

Further Reading

Abraham RB, Cahana A, Krivosic-Horber RM, Perel A: Malignant hyperthermia susceptibility: Anesthetic implications and risk stratification. QJM 90:13-18, 1997.

Baraka A, Jalbout MI: Anesthesia and myopathy. Curr Opin Anaesthesiol 15:371-376, 2002.

Barresi R, Di Blasi C, Negri T: Disruption of heart sarcoglycan complex and severe cardiomyopathy caused by β-sarcoglycan mutations. J Med Genet 37:102-107, 2000.

Boriani G, Gallina M, Merlini L, et al: Clinical relevance of atrial fibrillation/flutter, stroke, pacemaker implant, and heart failure in Emery-Dreifuss muscular dystrophy: A long-term longitudinal study. Stroke 34:901-908, 2003.

Buckley AE, Dean J: Cardiac involvement in Emery Dreifuss muscular dystrophy: A case series. Heart 82:105-108, 1999.

Corrado G, Lissoni A, Beretta S, et al: Prognostic value of electrocardiograms, ventricular late potentials, ventricular arrhythmias, and left ventricular systolic dysfunction in patients with Duchenne muscular dystrophy. Am J Cardiol 89:838-841, 2002.

Do T: Orthopedic management of the muscular dystrophies. Curr Opin Pediatr 14:50-53, 2002.

Dubowitz V: What is muscular dystrophy? Forty years of progressive ignorance. J R Coll Physicians Lond 34:464-468, 2000.

Frankowski GA, Johnson J, Tobias J: Rapacuronium administration to two children with Duchenne's muscular dystrophy. Anesth Analg 91:27-28, 2000.

Le Corre F, Plaud B: Neuromuscular disorders. Curr Opin Anaesthesiol 11:333-337, 1998.

Mathieu J, Allard P, Gobeil G, et al: Anesthetic and surgical complications in 219 cases of myotonic dystrophy. Neurology 49:1646-1650, 1997.

Melacini P, Fanin M, Danielli GA, et al: Myocardial disease: Myocardial involvement is very frequent among patients affected with subclinical Becker's muscular dystrophy. Circulation 94:3168-3175, 1996.

Muntoni F: Cardiomyopathy in muscular dystrophies. Curr Opin Neurol 16:577-583, 2003.

Parker SF, Bailey A, Drake AF: Infant hyperkalemic arrest after succinylcholine. Anesth Analg 80:206-207, 1995.

Politano L, Nigro V, Nigro G, et al: Development of cardiomyopathy in female carriers of Duchenne and Becker muscular dystrophies. JAMA 275:1335-1338, 1996.

Ririe DG, Shapiro F, Sethna NF: The response of patients with Duchenne's muscular dystrophy to neuromuscular blockade with vecuronium. Anesthesiology 88:351-354, 1998.

Rosenberg H, Gronert GA: Intractable cardiac arrest in children given succinylcholine [letter]. Anesthesiology 77:1054, 1992.

Schramm CM: Current concepts of respiratory complications of neuromuscular disease in children. Curr Opin Pediatr 12:203-207, 2000.

Stevens R: Neuromuscular disorders and anesthesia. Curr Opin Anaesthesiol 14:693-698, 2001.

Uslu M, Mellinghoff H, Diefenbach C: Mivacurium for muscle relaxation in a child with Duchenne's muscular dystrophy. Anesth Analg 89:340-341, 1999.

PHYSIOLOGIC IMBALANCE & COEXISTING DISEASE

Myasthenic Disorders

Mohamed Naguib

116

Case Synopsis

A 22-year-old woman, 154 cm tall and weighing 44.2 kg, presents with a 4-month history of myasthenia gravis and mild generalized weakness (Osserman's class II). The diagnosis is confirmed by the patient's rapid improvement after the administration of intravenous edrophonium chloride and by the presence of antibodies to acetylcholine receptors (12.3 nmol/L; reference value <0.25 nmol/L). The patient is scheduled for transcervical-sternal thymectomy. Preoperatively, she took pyridostigmine 60 mg orally three times a day and had plasmapheresis. Results of her preoperative pulmonary function tests were as follows: forced vital capacity (FVC), 2.79 L/second (79% of predicted); maximum expiratory flow at 50% of FVC, 3.2 L/second (68% of predicted); and forced midexpiratory flow between 25% and 75% of FVC, 3.03 L/second (77% of predicted). Anesthesia was induced with fentanyl and propofol and maintained with a thoracic epidural block supplemented with propofol and 70% nitrous oxide in oxygen. Tracheal intubation was performed under topical laryngotracheal anesthesia (4 mL 4% lidocaine). No neuromuscular blockers were used. She required mechanical ventilation for 12 hours postoperatively.

PROBLEM ANALYSIS

Definition

Neuromuscular transmission is dependent on a coordinated mechanism involving (1) synthesis, storage, and release of acetylcholine from the presynaptic motor nerve endings at the neuromuscular junction; (2) binding of acetylcholine to nicotinic receptors on the postsynaptic region of the muscle membrane, with consequent generation of the action potential; and (3) rapid hydrolysis of acetylcholine by acetylcholinesterase enzyme present in the synaptic cleft.

Autoimmune or genetic defects at the presynaptic region, synaptic basal lamina, or postsynaptic structure of the neuromuscular junction can compromise the safety margin of neuromuscular transmission. This can result in a diverse array of myasthenic disorders (Fig. 116-1). Fluctuating muscle weakness and fatigability are the main characteristics of myasthenic disorders (*mys*, meaning "muscle"; *aesthenia*, meaning "weakness"). Myasthenic disorders affect the motor system only. Sensory and autonomic functions are not impaired. The exception is Lambert-Eaton syndrome, a myasthenic syndrome in which a significant minority of patients have autonomic dysfunction. Myasthenic disorders can be classified into three main categories: myasthenia gravis, congenital myasthenic syndromes, and Lambert-Eaton myasthenic syndrome (Tables 116-1 and 116-2).

Recognition, Risk Assessment, and Implications

MYASTHENIA GRAVIS

Myasthenia gravis (MG) is the most common myasthenic disorder. MG is an antibody-mediated autoimmune disease with a prevalence of 0.25 to 2 per 100,000. Antibodies against the α-subunit of nicotinic acetylcholine receptors are present in approximately 80% to 85% of patients with MG. In the remaining 15% to 20% of patients (called seronegative patients), nicotinic acetylcholine receptor antibodies are not detectable. The majority of these seronegative patients have antibodies against the muscle-specific receptor tyrosine kinase; these antibodies are not present in seropositive patients. Muscle-specific kinase mediates the agrin-induced clustering of nicotinic acetylcholine receptors during synapse formation and is also expressed at the mature neuromuscular junction.

Triggers for the immune response in MG are not known. Thymic lymphoid follicular hyperplasia with germinal centers that produce antibodies to nicotinic acetylcholine receptors is present in approximately 70% of MG patients. A small percentage of MG patients develops autoantibodies as part of a paraneoplastic syndrome (12% of MG patients have thymoma). It is believed that antibodies to nicotinic acetylcholine receptors are produced in other locations, because thymectomy does not cure MG and does not protect against the occurrence of MG. There is also some evidence that antibodies generated in response to microbial antigens may constitute a trigger for MG in some patients. The antirheumatic drug D-penicillamine can induce a reversible form of MG.

MG can occur at any age. Extraocular and bulbar muscles are initially affected in a large majority of patients, resulting in ptosis, diplopia, dysphagia, and respiratory failure. As the disease progresses, neck and limb-girdle muscle weakness becomes apparent. In the rat model of MG, there is also evidence that diaphragmatic function is impaired. The clinical features of seropositive and seronegative patients are very similar.

Osserman and Genkins proposed the following clinical classification of MG: class I (ocular signs and symptoms only), class II (mild generalized weakness), class III (moderate generalized weakness with or without bulbar involvement), and

Table 117–1 ■ Drugs Used in the Treatment of Parkinson's Disease

Category	Drug	Administration
Dopaminergic agents		
Dopamine enhancers	Levodopa-carbidopa (Sinemet)	Oral
	Levodopa-carbidopa (Parcopa)	Oral*
	Levodopa-carbidopa-entacapone (Stalevo)	Oral
Dopamine receptor agonists	Apomorphine (Apokyn)	Subcutaneous† or intravenous injection
	Bromocriptine (Parlodel)	Oral
	Cabergoline (Dostinex)	Oral
	Pergolide (Permax)	Oral
	Pramipexole (Mirapex)	Oral
	Ropinirole (Requip)	Oral
MAO-B inhibitor	Selegiline (Eldepryl)	Oral
Anticholinergic agents	Trihexyphenidyl (Artane, Trihexane, Trihexy)	Oral
	Procyclidine (Kernadrin)	Oral
	Benztropine (Cogentin)	Oral
	Ethopropazine (Parsidol)	Oral
Antiviral agent	Amantadine (Symmetrel)	Oral
COMT inhibitors	Entacapone (Comtan)	Oral
	Tolcapone (Tasmar)	Oral

*Rapidly dissolving oral agent that is metabolized in the gut, not sublingually.
†Subcutaneous injection or infusion.
COMT, catechol-O-methyltransferase; MAO-B, monoamine oxidase B.

Other drugs used to treat PD include the monoamine oxidase B inhibitor selegiline (rasagiline is currently undergoing clinical trials); the anticholinergic agents trihexyphenidyl and benztropine, which are effective primarily in treating tremor and rigidity but have potentially severe side effects in the elderly; and amantadine.

Surgical treatment includes pallidotomy, thalamotomy, and deep brain stimulation of the subthalamic nucleus, globus pallidus internus, or thalamus. Ablative procedures have increasingly been abandoned in favor of deep brain stimulation.

MANAGEMENT AND PREVENTION

The perioperative care of patients with PD is complicated by (1) potential anesthetic interactions with pharmacotherapy for PD, (2) the effects of anesthetic drugs on the dopamine system and the patient's symptoms, and (3) the fact that many patients with PD have decreased pulmonary function and gastrointestinal motility and autonomic nervous system derangements. The use of levodopa predisposes individuals to develop cardiac arrhythmias, as well as hypotension related to dopamine's effects on renal blood flow. Therefore, ketamine and epinephrine-containing local anesthetics and inhalational agents that sensitize the heart to the effects of catecholamines (i.e., produce ventricular arrhythmias) should be avoided, and vasopressors such as phenylephrine may be required for hemodynamic support. A variety of other drugs used in the perioperative period may have deleterious effects on the symptoms of PD (Table 117-2). These include the typical antipsychotic drugs and most antiemetic agents—in particular, droperidol, prochlorperazine, metoclopramide, and thiethylperazine. Analgesic agents that may have an adverse effect on patients with PD include meperidine (particularly in patients receiving monoamine oxidase B

Table 117–2 ■ Drugs Contraindicated in Patients with Parkinson's Disease

Category	Drug	Comments
Butyrophenones	Haloperidol, droperidol	Block dopamine receptors
Inhalational agents	Halothane, enflurane	Increase myocardial sensitivity to catecholamines (ventricular arrhythmias)
Antiemetic	Metoclopramide	Blocks dopamine receptors
Phenothiazines	Chlorpromazine, fluphenazine, prochlorperazine	Block dopamine receptors
Analgesics	Fentanyl, sufentanil, morphine	May increase muscle rigidity
	Meperidine	Causes severe reaction in patients taking monoamine oxidase B inhibitors
	Alfentanil	May cause acute dysautonomia
Intravenous induction agent	Propofol	May increase dyskinesias; may obliterate tremor during stereotactic procedures

inhibitors), fentanyl, sufentanil, and alfentanil. Antihypertensive drugs to avoid include clonidine, propranolol, rauwolfia serpentina, and reserpine.

Maintaining the required levels of dopaminergic agents is of the utmost importance in optimizing the perioperative care of patients with PD. Patients should continue their medications as long as possible before coming to the operating room. If a regional or local anesthetic is used, patients may be able to receive their medications during surgery, either by mouth or via a nasogastric tube. The use of apomorphine may be continued, but not initiated, throughout the perioperative period and delivered as a subcutaneous bolus or an intermittent infusion, if necessary. Patients who do not take their medications are at risk of developing increased muscle rigidity and laryngospasm, which could interfere with airway management, including ventilation and tracheal intubation or extubation. Other abnormalities in the control and function of the upper airway, which may lead to an obstructive airway pattern in as many as one third of patients with PD, also have an impact on the perioperative management of ventilation. Because of associated dysautonomia, many patients with PD are at risk for problems with temperature regulation throughout the perioperative period.

Patients who experience increased symptoms in the preoperative holding area are treated with an anticholinergic (e.g., atropine, glycopyrrolate) or antihistamine (e.g., diphenhydramine). The latter can be especially helpful for managing exacerbations of tremor and for sedation, and the former for decreasing secretions.

Regional and local techniques should be used to the extent possible in patients with PD to avoid the cognitive and emetogenic effects of general anesthesia. These techniques also allow for continued communication with the patient and the oral administration of dopaminergic agents, as needed. When general anesthesia is required, there is no agent of choice for induction, but halothane and, to a lesser extent, enflurane are best avoided because of their arrhythmogenic properties (i.e., sensitization of the heart to the effects of catecholamines). In particular, caution is warranted in patients on long-term levodopa therapy who are at risk of developing hemodynamic flux due to autonomic instability, catecholamine depletion, sensitization to catecholamines, and relative hypovolemia. Significant hypotension is treated with direct-acting α-adrenergic receptor agonists (e.g., phenylephrine). In general, there are no concerns about the use of neuromuscular blocking agents. A review of the literature indicates that although hyperkalemia and profound bradykinesia

occurred in one patient who received intravenous succinylcholine, there is little additional evidence of such a link. Support for the use of propofol is equivocal, as this drug may increase the severity of dyskinesias. However, it is also known to have antiparkinsonian effects. Propofol may be contraindicated in patients undergoing stereotactic procedures because this drug has been shown to abolish tremor.

During emergence from anesthesia and before extubation, ventilation, airway reflexes, and the ability to follow commands should be assessed. Particular care should be exercised in optimizing respiratory function, owing to increased secretions and the propensity to develop aspiration pneumonia and compromised ventilatory function. If the patient develops confusion, as is common in patients with PD, the use of a benzodiazepine in the postoperative period rather than a typical antipsychotic agent may be preferred. However, care should be taken not to depress the respiratory drive.

Morbidity and mortality rates during the perioperative period are increased in patients with PD compared with patients of similar age without PD. However, careful assessment and reduction of risk, optimization of cardiac and respiratory systems, and maintenance of dopaminergic therapy to the extent possible go a long way toward leveling the playing field.

Further Reading

Anderson BJ, Marks PV, Futter ME: Propofol-contrasting effects in movement disorders. Br J Neurosurg 8:387-388, 1994.

Bowron A: Practical considerations in the use of apomorphine injectable. Neurology 62(Suppl 4):S32-S36, 2004.

Brindle GF: Anesthesia in the patient with parkinsonism. Primary Care 4:513-528, 1977.

Eventou I, Moreno M, Geller E, et al: Hip fractures in patients with Parkinson's syndrome. J Trauma 33:98-101, 1983.

Furuya R, Hirai A, Andoh T, et al: Successful perioperative management of a patient with Parkinson's disease by enteral levodopa administration under propofol anesthesia. Anesthesiology 89:261-263, 1998.

Lozano AM, Mahant N: Deep brain stimulation surgery for Parkinson's disease: Mechanisms and consequences. Parkinsonism Relat Disord 10(Suppl 1):S49-S57, 2004.

Mason LJ, Cojocaru TT, Cole DJ: Surgical intervention and anesthetic management of the patient with Parkinson's disease. Int Anesthesiol Clin 34:133-150, 1996.

Nicholson G, Pereira AC, Hall GM: Parkinson's disease and anaesthesia. Br J Anaesth 89:904-916, 2002.

Schramm BM, Orser BA: Dystonic reaction to propofol attenuated by benztropine (Cogentin). Anesth Analg 94:1237-1240, 2002

Shults CW: Treatments of Parkinson disease. Arch Neurol 60:1680-1684, 2003.

Alzheimer's Disease

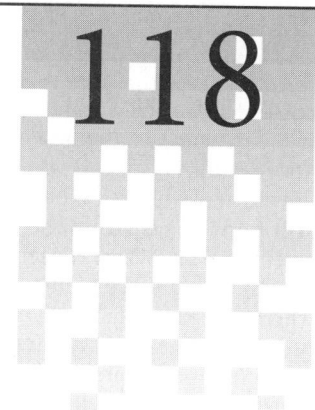

Michael J. Murray and Catherine Friederich Murray

Case Synopsis

A 72-year-old woman with anemia is found to have adenocarcinoma of the colon, for which she is scheduled to have a laparotomy and resection of the lesion. The patient is anxious. A woman at the bedside in the preoperative holding area tells you that the patient, her mother, has Alzheimer's disease and that she, the daughter, has a durable power of attorney for her mother's health care.

PROBLEM ANALYSIS

Definition

Alzheimer's disease (AD) is the most common neurodegenerative disease, accounting for approximately two thirds of all cases of dementia and affecting up to 20% of individuals older than 80 years. AD is progressive, leading to irreversible loss of neurons in the cerebral cortex and hippocampus. The pathologic hallmarks of the disease are neurofibrillary tangles, which contain the hyperphosphorylated form of the microtubular protein tau and extracellular plaques, which contain the peptide β-amyloid. β-Amyloid is cleaved from a larger protein, β-amyloid precursor protein, by the α, β, and γ secretases. The γ secretases cleave to $A\beta_{42}$, a 42–amino acid sequence amyloid protein, which forms insoluble fibrils that accumulate in senile plaques isolated at autopsy from patients with AD. In some patients with familial disease, a genetic defect accounts for the increased activity of γ secretases. In the majority of patients, however, there is no identified defect that explains the presence of the neurofibrillary tangles and senile plaques.

Recognition

There is a broad spectrum of disease, but progressive impairment in memory, judgment, decision making, awareness of surroundings, and ability to care for oneself are the hallmarks of AD. Some patients who are seen preoperatively for unrelated problems may appear lucid and able to give informed consent. An accompanying family member, a person with a durable power of attorney for health care, or a review of the medical record may bring to the anesthesiologist's attention the fact that the patient has AD. Other patients with more advanced disease or uncommon presentations may be belligerent or may have aphasia or spastic paraparesis.

There is no clinical test to diagnose AD, although neurocognitive testing confirms the presence of dementia (Table 118-1). Anesthesiologists may use simpler tests to assess whether a patient is oriented and able to understand and provide informed consent.

Risk Assessment

Obtaining informed consent, minimizing the chance of postoperative confusion, and optimizing management during the perioperative period are goals in patients with AD.

Much has been written about informed consent for surgical procedures and anesthesia. Patients with AD, by definition, have cognitive impairment, but in many states, depending on the degree of impairment, they may drive, vote, and give informed consent. The anesthesiologist must be able to assure himself or herself that the patient understands the procedure, the options, and the risks. If not, then

Table 118–1 ■ Mini–Mental Status Examination	
	Maximum Score*
Orientation	
What is the (year) (season) (date) (month)?	5
Where are we (state) (country) (town) (hospital) (floor)?	5
Registration	
Name 3 objects. Examiner says each one, then asks the patient to name all 3. Give 1 point for each correct answer. Repeat, if necessary, until the patient learns all 3. Count the number of trials and record.	3
Attention and Calculation	
Serial 7s (7, 14, 21, etc.). Give 1 point for each correct. Stop after 5 answers. Alternatively, ask the patient to spell "world" backward.	5
Recall	
Ask for the objects repeated above. Give 1 point for each correct.	3
Language	
Name a pencil and a watch.	2
Repeat the following: "no ifs, ands, or buts."	1
Follow a 3-stage command: for example, "Take a paper in your right hand, fold it in half, and put it on the floor."	3
Read and obey the following:	
Close your eyes.	1
Write a sentence.	1
Copy a design.	1
Assess level of consciousness along a continuum:	
Alert Drowsy Stupor Coma	

*A score of <20 is indicative of dementia. Patients with the benign forgetfulness of senility generally score >25.

From http://www.emedicine.com/neuro/topic13.htm.

consent should be obtained from the next of kin. Obviously, if the patient has a representative with a durable power of attorney for health care, the process is easier. In either case, as with adolescents, it is best to have the patient sign the consent form to "assent" to the procedure and have a legal representative give "legal consent."

Agitation in patients with AD is not uncommon. Therefore, patients with AD may receive a benzodiazepine to reduce preoperative agitation. However, because postoperative cognitive impairment is often associated with anesthesia, benzodiazepines should not be part of the routine anesthetic plan for these patients. If they are used at all, benzodiazepines should be administered only after a risk-benefit analysis has been performed.

Implications

There are no specific recommendations for managing anesthesia in patients with AD. Consent, as mentioned, is often an issue. However, regardless of who provides consent, the anesthesiologist must be patient when educating and calming a patient with AD. Many such patients have advanced directives. Discussion of the implications of the directive must occur preoperatively with the patient, the patient's legal surrogate, or both.

Regional anesthesia may seem preferable because there is less risk of worsening the patient's cognitive impairment compared with general anesthesia. However, because many patients with AD are disoriented, agitated, and uncooperative, regional anesthesia can present quite a challenge. There is no single best type of anesthesia or anesthetic agent for patients with AD. They often have reduced reserves in vital organ function—pulmonary, cardiac, neurologic—and these factors must be taken into account.

MANAGEMENT

There is no known cure for AD. As the disease progresses, patients are often institutionalized in nursing homes or their equivalent. Behavioral therapies include patient-centered approaches to try to minimize the effects of memory loss (e.g., established daily routines); caregiver training enables aides and therapists to recognize and deal with the common behavioral manifestations of AD. Psychotropic medications such as risperidone, olanzapine, and quetiapine are recommended at low doses to treat common manifestations of the disease such as anxiety, agitation, and depression.

Decreased levels of acetylcholine in the cerebral cortex of AD patients are thought to account for many of the symptoms and signs of the disease. Therefore, drugs targeted at inhibiting the degradation of acetylcholine by cholinesterases in the cerebral cortex have been developed and are used to treat AD (e.g., tacrine, donepezil, rivastigmine, galantamine). Cholinesterase inhibition has been associated with improvement in cognitive function. Patients taking cholinesterase inhibitors should take their medication with a small sip of water the morning of surgery, because acute, severe cognitive and behavioral decline has been reported in patients who abruptly discontinue their medication.

In addition, an *N*-methyl-D-aspartate antagonist (memantine) has been approved in the United States to treat AD patients and is of some benefit in other patients with dementia.

Patients with AD should have a responsible family member present with them whenever possible—someone they recognize and who can reassure and calm them during the perioperative period. This individual should also have the capacity to give informed consent for the anesthetic.

Although these patients may be anxious, sedating drugs are avoided because they contribute to the postoperative confusion and delirium that often occur. Regional anesthesia, if indicated, should be attempted only if the patient is cooperative. Inhalational agents are used if general anesthesia is indicated, mainly owing to their rapid elimination. Glycopyrrolate does not cross the blood-brain barrier and is therefore preferred if an anticholinergic agent is required.

PREVENTION

There are no known agents to prevent AD. Even drugs such as donepezil are effective in less than half of AD patients, and in those who do show a benefit, it lasts for only a few years at best.

Although cognitive impairment is associated with general anesthesia, there is no evidence that general anesthesia increases the severity of AD. Caregivers may think so, because borderline cognitive impairment may worsen after an anesthetic. However, such worsening is transient, and patients should return to baseline within days to weeks following anesthesia.

As discussed earlier, there is no ideal anesthetic type, technique, or agent. In developing an anesthetic plan, the anesthesiologist must consider the degree of cognitive impairment, the amount of agitation, the degree of cooperation, comorbid conditions, and possible drug interactions. With careful planning and management, the patient's caregiver should notice only mild, if any, worsening of neurologic function postoperatively.

Further Reading

Bohnen N, Warner MA, Kokmen E, et al: Early and midlife exposure to anesthesia and age of onset of Alzheimer's disease. Int J Neurosci 77:181-185, 1994.

Clark CM, Ewbank D, Lee VM-Y, et al: Molecular pathology of Alzheimer's disease: Neuronal cytoskeletal abnormalities. In Growdon JH, Rosser MN (eds): The Dementias, vol 19 of Blue Books of Practical Neurology. Boston, Butterworth-Heinemann, 1998, pp 285-304.

Dickson DW: Apoptotic mechanisms in Alzheimer neurofibrillary degeneration: Cause or effect? J Clin Invest 114:23-27, 2004.

Esler WP, Wolfe MS: A portrait of Alzheimer secretases—new features and familiar faces. Science 293:1449-1454, 2001.

Fernandez CR, Fields A, Richards T, et al: Anesthetic considerations in patients with Alzheimer's disease. J Clin Anesth 15:52-58, 2003.

Gasparini M, Vanacore N, Schiaffini C, et al: A case-control study on Alzheimer's disease and exposure to anesthesia. Neurol Sci 23:11-14, 2002.

Hutton M, Perez-Tur J, Hardy J: Genetics of Alzheimer's disease. Essays Biochem 33:117-131, 1998.

Iwatsubo T, Odaka A, Suzuki N, et al: Visualization of A beta 42(43) and A beta 40 in senile plaques with end-specific A beta monoclonals: Evidence that an initially deposited species is A beta 42(43). Neuron 13:45-53, 1994.

Langa KM, Foster NL, Larson EB: Mixed dementia: Emerging concepts and therapeutic implications. JAMA 292:2901-2908, 2004.

Larson EB, Kukull WA, Buchner D, et al: Adverse drug reactions associated with global cognitive impairment in elderly persons. Ann Intern Med 107:169-173, 1987.

Nussbaum RL, Ellis CE: Alzheimer's disease and Parkinson's disease. N Engl J Med 348:1356-1364, 2003.

Selkoe DJ: Alzheimer disease: Mechanistic understanding predicts novel therapies. Ann Intern Med 140:627-638, 2004.

PHYSIOLOGIC IMBALANCE & COEXISTING DISEASE

Sepsis, Systemic Inflammatory Response Syndrome, and Multiple Organ Dysfunction Syndrome

119

Jacob Gutsche and Clifford S. Deutschman

Case Synopsis

A 22-year-old man presents with fever and abdominal pain. A computed tomography scan indicates that he has appendicitis. Laparoscopic exploration reveals a perforated appendix with pus and stool in the abdomen. The patient undergoes laparotomy and appendectomy. The open abdomen is irrigated extensively with antibiotic-containing saline. During the procedure the patient develops hypotension and oliguria, requiring the administration of significant volumes of intravenous fluid. The anesthesiologist inserts an arterial line and pulmonary artery catheter to monitor the resuscitation. Peritoneal fluid and blood cultures are obtained, and broad-spectrum antibiotics are started.

PROBLEM ANALYSIS

Definition and Recognition

The systemic inflammatory response syndrome (SIRS) and multiple organ dysfunction syndrome (MODS) were first described in the 1970s. Early reports of MODS heralded our ability to support patients through such major medical or surgical catastrophes as ruptured aortic aneurysms, severe trauma, pancreatitis, multiple transfusions, and major systemic infections. Unfortunately, surviving patients subsequently developed dysfunction in organs that were unaffected by the initial injury. Multiple terms were applied to these syndromes, which led to confusion and limited the ability to stratify risk and compare therapeutic options. In 1991 the American College of Chest Physicians and Society of Critical Care Medicine convened a consensus conference to formalize definitions, allowing the comparison of patient populations from different institutions or geographic regions. These deliberations generated the new term SIRS, which was necessary because there were patients who developed signs and symptoms of systemic inflammation but without identifiable infection. The presence of any two of four criteria is sufficient to establish the diagnosis of SIRS (Table 119-1). In addition, the consensus conference provided formal definitions for sepsis (Table 119-2), and the syndrome of organ failure following SIRS or sepsis was renamed MODS.

Although these definitions greatly improved our ability to compare patient populations and conduct more meaningful clinical trials, several problems remained. Key was the

excessive sensitivity and lack of specificity inherent in the definition of SIRS. Namely, many events or interventions provoke a stress response in patients sufficient to meet the criteria for SIRS. For example, virtually every postoperative patient meets the SIRS criteria, but it is clear that most should not be included in studies of the pathogenesis of MODS.

Primarily for this reason, North American and European critical care societies convened an International Sepsis Definitions Conference in 2001 to revisit and modify the definitions established in 1991. Conference participants chose to de-emphasize the use of the term SIRS and to lengthen the list of signs and symptoms characterizing sepsis (Table 119-3). In addition, more specific criteria for organ dysfunction were adopted (Table 119-4).

Risk Assessment and Implications

Humans respond to physiologic stress such as trauma, stroke, pneumonia, ischemia, pancreatitis, bowel perforation,

Table 119–1 ■ Criteria for Systemic Inflammatory Response Syndrome
Fever (core temperature >38.3°C) or hypothermia (core temperature <36°C)
White blood cell count >12,000 or <4000
Heart rate >90 beats/min or >2 standard deviations above normal for age
Tachypnea

496

Table 119–2 ■ **Consensus Definitions of Sepsis and Septic Shock**

Severe sepsis: sepsis with the presence of dysfunction in at least one organ

Septic shock: sepsis with persistent hypotension
  Mean arterial pressure <60 mm Hg
  Systolic blood pressure (SBP) <90 mm Hg
  Decrease in SBP >40 mm Hg from patient's normal baseline, despite adequate volume resuscitation

---

large-volume blood loss, and infection in a specific manner. This characteristic physiologic response is referred to as the stress response, and it may have evolved as a way to promote recovery from localized trauma or infection. The initial phase of the response is commonly called shock. In most cases, shock is rapidly reversible. The second phase includes hypermetabolism and can be thought of as occurring to facilitate the repair of damaged tissue. This second phase also includes leukocytosis, which features (1) mobilization of leukocytes to the area of damage, (2) enhanced hepatic gluconeogenesis to provide fuel for these leukocytes, (3) increased oxygen extraction at the tissue level, and (4) breakdown of endogenous proteins, primarily by catabolism of skeletal muscle. This process provides the necessary substrates for gluconeogenesis, increased hepatic protein synthesis, and repair of damaged tissue. Further, the process is driven by catecholamines, cortisol, glucagon, and cytokines

---

Table 119–3 ■ **Criteria for Suspected or Documented Sepsis**

General Variables

Fever (core temperature >38.3°C)
Hypothermia (core temperature <36°C)
Heart rate >90 beats/min or >2 SD above normal for age
Tachypnea
Altered mental status
Significant edema or positive fluid balance (>20 mL/kg over 24 hr)
Hyperglycemia (plasma glucose >120 mg/dL) in patients without diabetes

Inflammatory Variables

Leukocytosis (WBC count >12,000)
Leukopenia (WBC count <4000)
Normal WBCs with >10% immature forms
C-reactive protein >2 SD above normal value
Plasma procalcitonin >2 SD above normal value

Hemodynamic Variables

Arterial hypotension (SBP <90 mm Hg, MAP <70 mm Hg, or SBP decrease ≥40 mm Hg or to <2 SD below normal for age)
SvO_2 >70% (this level can be normal in children, so this is not a criterion for pediatric patients)
Cardiac index >3.5 (this level can be normal in children, so this is not a criterion for pediatric patients)

Tissue Perfusion Variables

Hyperlactatemia (>1 mmol/L)
Decreased capillary refill or mottling

MAP, mean arterial pressure; SBP, systolic blood pressure; SD, standard deviations; SvO_2, venous oxygen saturation; WBC, white blood cell.
Adapted from Levy MM, Fink MP, Marshall JC, et al: 2001 SCCM/ESICM/ACCP/ATS/SIS International Sepsis Definitions Conference. Intensive Care Med 29:530-538, 2003.

released by leukocytes. The resultant hyperglycemia is associated with an increased release of insulin. Finally, substrate delivery is facilitated by vasodilatation, fluid retention, increased cardiac output, and capillary leak, all of which appear to be essential, because damaged tissue is avascular.

The hypermetabolic phase of the stress response can evolve via two possible pathways; one is normal, and the other is pathologic. In the normal pathway, completion of angiogenesis by postinjury day 4 leads to the resolution of inflammation, hypermetabolism, and the hyperendocrine state. This is the more common scenario and is normal. Although it meets all the criteria for SIRS, it is clearly not what the 1991 consensus conference participants had in mind when they coined the term "systemic inflammatory response syndrome." In some patients, however, inflammation becomes pathologic. The mechanism of such transformation is unknown. These patients have SIRS or, with infection, sepsis. Either of these is characterized by important changes in metabolism and regulation:

- In contrast to simple stress, the ability to extract and use oxygen is diminished, despite increased cellular demand.
- The increased demand for energy by white blood cells, coupled with an inability to use molecular oxygen, leads to aerobic glycolysis. That is, oxygen delivery is adequate, but the inability to use oxygen increases lactate production. This causes persistent hyperglycemia, impaired glucose utilization, and a state of relative glucose intolerance.
- Endocrine abnormalities become prominent. The production and release of some hormones, notably vasopressin, are reduced, resulting in relative deficiency. Also, tissues become resistant to the effects of other hormones. This is exemplified by the development of insulin resistance or the diminished ability of catecholamines to modulate vascular tone.

Cellular dysfunction leads to biochemical abnormalities without overt organ failure. For example, hepatic dysfunction impairs gluconeogenesis, which prevents the conversion of lactate to pyruvate. Also, oxidation of long-chain triglycerides and the expression of key β-oxidative enzymes are decreased. As a result, amino acids become an increasingly important fuel source, despite the fact that hepatic dysfunction compromises ureagenesis. Importantly, contractile dysfunction is often observed in patients with MODS. In each case, compensatory mechanisms (increased substrate delivery to the liver, vasodilatation, and increased diastolic volume in the heart) may mask organ dysfunction.

MANAGEMENT AND PREVENTION

There is no "magic bullet" to cure SIRS, sepsis, or MODS. It is not known what causes a controlled inflammatory response to become pathologic. In the absence of a specific target for therapy, management is based on source control, supportive care, and prevention of further complications.

Source Control

The patient history, physical examination, and laboratory or diagnostic studies are used to identify infectious causes of continuing inflammation.

Table 119–4 ■ **Criteria for Organ Dysfunction**

| Body System | Severity of Dysfunction | |
	Mild	Severe
Pulmonary	Hypoxia or hypercarbia requiring assisted ventilation for ≥3-5 days	ARDS requiring PEEP ≥10 cm H_2O and FiO_2 ≥0.5
Hepatic	Bilirubin ≥2-3 mg/dL; prothrombin time or other liver function tests ≥2 times normal	Jaundice with bilirubin ≥8-10 mg/dL
Renal	Oliguria (<500 mL/day) or increasing creatinine (≥2-3 mg/dL)	Need for dialysis
Gastrointestinal	Intolerance of gastric feeding >5 days	Stress ulceration with need for transfusion; acalculous cholecystitis
Hematologic	Partial thromboplastin time ≥125% of normal, platelets <50,000-80,000	Disseminated intravascular coagulation
Central nervous system	Confusion	Coma
Peripheral nervous system	Mild sensory neuropathy	Combined motor and sensory deficit
Cardiovascular	Decreased ejection fraction, persistent capillary leak	Hypodynamic state not responsive to pressors

ARDS, acute respiratory distress syndrome; FiO_2, fraction of inspired oxygen; PEEP, positive end-expiratory pressure.

Supportive Care

Supportive care includes the following.

Fluid Resuscitation. The goal of fluid resuscitation is to maintain intravascular volume despite ongoing capillary leak. This can be accomplished with colloid-based fluids such as albumin or hetastarch, crystalloid (use of a balanced salt solution is preferred to saline, to avoid the development of hyperchloremic metabolic acidosis), or blood or blood products if appropriate. The Canadian Transfusion Trial suggests that a hemoglobin of 7 mg/dL is sufficient for most critically ill patients. Goals for appropriate fluid resuscitation vary with the patient's underlying disease and premorbid cardiac, pulmonary, and renal status. A study by Rivers and colleagues indicated that early goal-directed therapy designed to achieve a central venous pressure of 8 to 12 mm Hg, mean arterial pressure greater than 65 mm Hg, urine output greater than 0.5 mL/kg per hour, and mixed venous oxygen saturation greater than 70% improved outcomes.

Vasopressors and Inotropes. In cases of severe sepsis or septic shock, fluid resuscitation may not be sufficient to restore organ perfusion. Clinically, it is difficult to distinguish between vasodilatation and myocardial depression. Consequently, vasoactive drugs are an important treatment adjuvant. Most recent studies favor the use of norepinephrine. If cardiac output is severely depressed, primary inotropes, such as dobutamine, may be useful. Dopamine administration is of historical interest only. This agent is arrhythmogenic and can cause maldistribution of splanchnic flow; putative renal sparing effects have been disproved in myriad studies, although stimulation of D1 receptors on the distal renal tubule does cause a diuretic effect.

Mechanical Ventilation. Respiratory control is best viewed as having two components: hypoxia or, as in severe sepsis, acute respiratory distress syndrome (ARDS). Either may require an increase in the fraction of inspired oxygen (FiO_2), although it is customary to try to keep FiO_2 less than 0.5 to 0.6 to prevent "oxygen toxicity." However, there are no human data to indicate that higher levels of FiO_2 at one atmosphere of pressure are truly damaging. One recent trial indicated that keeping plateau pressures below 30 cm H_2O or tidal volumes less than 6 mL/kg in patients with ARDS limits secondary lung injury and improves outcomes. Positive end-expiratory pressure (PEEP) is useful both to improve pulmonary compliance and to maintain recruitment of alveoli. We strongly advocate the "open lung" strategy of Amato. This somewhat controversial approach involves titrating PEEP to a level above the "lower inflection point" in the pressure-volume curve, increasing functional residual capacity and recruiting collapsed alveoli. Additional ventilatory adjuvants include the use of sighs and other recruitment maneuvers (e.g., tiltable and rotating posturing beds to improve ventilation/perfusion mismatch). Keeping the head of the patient's bed elevated above 30 degrees limits aspiration and decreases the incidence of nosocomial pneumonia.

Broad-Spectrum Antibiotics. Early use of broad-spectrum antibiotics improves the outcome in septic patients. If cultures reveal a causative organism, antibiotic therapy is directed at that organism. This reduces the risk of resistant organisms or superinfections.

Endocrine Support. Recent studies indicate that sepsis can rapidly progress to a state of relative endocrine insufficiency. For example, data by Landry and coworkers convincingly show a loss of vasopressin stores from the posterior pituitary, which is problematic. Vasopressin is most active in controlling tone in the splanchnic circulation, and the major component of sepsis-associated vasodilatation arises in this bed. Infusion of replacement vasopressin (0.01 to 0.04 unit/minute) restores normotension and may help wean the patient from other vasoactive substances. However, the use of corticosteroids in sepsis remains controversial. The debate centers on the inability to determine what constitutes a "normal" hypothalamic-pituitary-adrenal response in severe sepsis. Nonetheless, recent studies indicate that low doses of exogenous corticoids (hydrocortisone 50 mg/day) may improve refractory hypotension and facilitate weaning of exogenous catecholamines.

Early Dialysis. Recent studies support the use of dialysis early in sepsis. Continuous dialysis is favored because it is associated with less hemodynamic instability. High flows seem to offer better solute clearance. When conventional hemodialysis is used, daily dialysis appears to be more effective than the more standard every-other-day approach.

Prevention of Further Complications

Activated Protein C. In 2001, one multicenter, randomized trial examined the effects of activated protein C (APC) infusion started within 24 hours of the diagnosis of sepsis associated with major organ dysfunction. This was continued for 96 hours and led to a 6% reduction in 28-day mortality. However, protocol concerns and the risk of serious bleeding led the Food and Drug Administration to limit the indications for APC. Thus, APC has been approved for use in patients with severe sepsis and APACHE II scores greater than 25. However, newer data suggest that the improvement seen at 28 days is not sustained. In addition, APC is quite expensive. Thus, this drug is rarely used.

Tight Glucose Control. Another single-center study examined tight glucose control (>80 but <110 mg/dL) with insulin in critically ill patients. Results showed clear improvement in many outcome variables. However, results should be applied cautiously to septic patients. The study population was homogeneous, and more than 65% had undergone cardiopulmonary bypass. Further, all patients received significant exogenous glucose. Subsequent studies by the same group and others revealed that primary outcomes were determined by the glucose concentration, not the use of insulin. In severe stress states (e.g., SIRS, sepsis, MODS), glucose is not used as a fuel and probably is best avoided. Thus, logic would dictate that limiting glucose may be as effective as giving insulin. If so, we advise limiting glucose administration and controlling serum glucose at less than 150 mg/dL.

A New Syndrome

The incidence of SIRS, sepsis, and MODS is difficult to quantify. This reflects both the diverse group of entities giving rise to these conditions and confusion about what does and does not constitute SIRS. However, recent studies indicate that while mortality from sepsis has declined, the incidence of sepsis is steadily increasing. Indeed, the natural history of these conditions is rapidly evolving. Initial descriptions of what we now call SIRS, sepsis, and MODS arose when our ability to treat these conditions was dismal (with almost certain early mortality). We now have the ability to support most forms of major organ dysfunction, and this has led to the emergence of a new syndrome. There is no consensus name or definition for this new entity, which is characterized by a stable but highly abnormal state involving endocrine and inflammatory exhaustion. The failure of multiple components of the neuroendocrine system in the chronically, critically ill has been well described, and the concept of immune incompetence has recently been reviewed by Hotchkiss and Karl. More often than not, modern medical technology can maintain survival in this state. Reversal of the disorder, however, is difficult. What is increasingly clear is that mortality from SIRS, sepsis, or MODS most often occurs when exogenous life support is discontinued.

Further Reading

Angus DC, Wax S: Epidemiology of sepsis: An Update. Crit Care Med 29:S109-S116, 2001.

Bernard GR, Vincent JL, Laterre PF, et al: Recombinant Human Protein C Worldwide Evaluation in Severe Sepsis (PROWESS) study group: Efficacy and safety of recombinant human activated protein C for severe sepsis. N Engl J Med 344:699-709, 2001.

Bone RC, Balk RA, Cerra FB, et al: Definition for sepsis and organ failure and guidelines for use of innovative therapies in sepsis: American College of Chest Physicians/Society of Critical Care Medicine. Chest 101:1644-1655, 1992.

Deitch EA: Multiple organ failure: Pathophysiology and potential future therapy. Ann Surg 216:117-134, 1992.

Dellinger RP, Carlet JM, Masur H, et al: Surviving Sepsis Campaign guidelines for management of severe sepsis and septic shock. Crit Care Med 32:858-873, 2004.

Deutschman CS: The systemic inflammatory response syndrome and the multiple organ dysfunction syndrome. In Fishman AP (ed): Pulmonary Diseases and Disorders. New York, McGraw-Hill, 1997.

Hotchkiss RS, Karl IE: The pathophysiology and treatment of sepsis. N Engl J Med 348:138-150, 2003.

Landry DW, Levin HR, Gallant EM, et al: Vasopressin deficiency contributes to the vasodilation of septic shock. Circulation 95:1122-1125, 1997.

Rivers E, Nguyen B, Havstad S, et al: Early goal-directed therapy in the treatment of severe sepsis and septic shock. N Engl J Med 345:1368-1377, 2001.

Ventilation with lower tidal volumes as compared with traditional tidal volumes for acute lung injury and the acute respiratory distress syndrome. The Acute Respiratory Distress Syndrome Network. N Engl J Med 342:1301-1308, 2000.

PHYSIOLOGIC IMBALANCE & COEXISTING DISEASE

Perioperative Care of Immunocompromised Patients

120

Shubjeet Kaur and Stephen O. Heard

Case Synopsis

A 45-year-old man with renal failure secondary to chronic diabetes mellitus underwent cadaveric renal transplantation 1 month before admission. He now presents with a perforated duodenal ulcer and is scheduled to undergo emergency exploratory laparotomy. His temperature is 39.6°C, blood pressure is 88/60 mm Hg, and pulse is 110 beats per minute. His medications include NPH insulin, cyclosporine, ranitidine, diltiazem, and prednisone. Pertinent laboratory values are a white blood cell count of 2300 cells/mm^3, hematocrit 28%, creatinine 2.1 mg/dL, blood glucose 550 mg/dL, and amylase 459 units.

PROBLEM ANALYSIS

Definition

An immunocompromised patient is at increased risk for infection due to defective defense mechanisms (Table 120-1). These can be specific (immune) or nonspecific (nonimmune). Immunosuppression exists if immune defenses are present but are deficient rather than defective. Recent data suggest that 0.25% to 1.5% of the total population in the United States may be immunocompromised.

An unknown proportion of patients may be immunocompromised due to underlying disease or to surgical or medical interventions (Table 120-2). Patients with human immunodeficiency virus (HIV) infection, massive burns, diabetes mellitus, cirrhosis, or cancer may also be immunosuppressed. Immunosuppressive drugs used to prevent the rejection of transplanted organs also place patients at risk for infection. Similarly, patients with autoimmune diseases and various malignancies may receive immunosuppressive chemotherapy. Because a significant proportion of these patients may present for elective or emergency surgical procedures, perioperative care presents a challenge.

Recognition

In many patients, the presence of immunosuppression is obvious from the history and physical examination. However, subtle and less obvious alterations in immune function may be present in a significant number of surgical patients.

The findings on physical examination are often nonspecific; however, there may be signs suggestive of immunosuppression, such as the cushingoid appearance in a patient with chronic corticosteriod use or thrush in a patient with HIV infection. Any device that traverses anatomic barriers or impairs defense mechanisms, such as intravenous catheters or endotracheal tubes, increases the risk of nosocomial infection (see Chapter 51).

Table 120–1 ■ Host Defense Mechanisms

Type of Immunity	Components
Innate	Epithelial barriers (nonimmune)
	Complement
	Macrophages
Early induced responses	Cytokine and chemokine release
	Acute phase response
	Expression of adhesion molecules
	Chemoattractants and neutrophils
	Interferons
	Natural killer cells
	"Primitive lymphocytes"
Adaptive and protective immunity	T cells
	B cells
	Memory

Table 120–2 ■ Causes of Immunosuppression

Diseases or Conditions
Human immunodeficiency virus (HIV)
Cancer
Massive burns
Trauma
Advanced age
Asplenia
Autoimmune diseases
Medical or Surgical Therapy
Antirejection agents
Chemotherapy for malignancies and autoimmune diseases
Anesthetic agents
Blood transfusions
Chronic steroid therapy

Readily available laboratory values that may suggest immunosuppression include a complete blood count with a differential smear and serum immunoglobulin levels. More sophisticated tests, such as HIV testing, quantification of blood mononuclear cell populations, complement assays, and T-cell function (e.g., delayed hypersensitivity skin testing) and B-cell function (e.g., presence of antibodies to common antigens), are required to diagnose and determine the magnitude of the immunocompromised state.

Risk Assessment

The lung is the single most commonly infected organ, and pneumonia may account for up to 40% of all deaths in immunocompromised patients. Patients who have undergone organ transplantation and are taking antirejection medications have a biphasic infection risk pattern. In the initial 6 weeks following transplantation, these patients are generally susceptible to the same infections observed in the postoperative period after any major surgical procedure. From 6 weeks to 6 months, they are highly susceptible to opportunistic infection such as *Pneumocystis jirovecii* pneumonia, surgical infections, and other unusual infections. As the dose of the immunosuppressive drug is tapered, the infection risk diminishes progressively if the allograft function is good and there is no chronic viral infection.

Patients with autoimmune disorders, such as rheumatoid arthritis or scleroderma, may have problems with mouth opening and joint mobility. Careful assessment of the airway is important to determine whether tracheal intubation will be difficult.

In patients with HIV infection, there is a significant risk of infection from uncommon pathogens. Systemic fungal infections are especially common, including pneumonia from *Pneumocystis jirovecii*.

In addition to their primary therapeutic effects, immunosuppressive drugs and antimicrobial agents used to treat nosocomial and opportunistic infections have side effects that can adversely affect other organ systems. In addition, immunocompromised patients often have multisystem disease, poor general health, and diminished reserves of vital organ function (e.g., decreased pulmonary and myocardial reserves).

Implications

Common infections may have an atypical presentation in immunocompromised or immunosuppressed patients. Clinical symptoms or signs of significant underlying infection may be absent, subtle, or misleading in these patients, and a high index of suspicion for the presence of infection is necessary. A careful physical examination may provide clues to the presence of infection, but often ancillary laboratory testing, imaging, serology, and microbiology (including cultures for fungal, mycobacterial, and viral pathogens) are necessary to diagnose an opportunistic infection.

Important drug interactions can occur in the perioperative period. For example, there is the potential for adverse interactions between antirejection drugs and antibiotics prescribed for suspected infection. Cyclosporine, a commonly used antirejection medication, is cleared by the cytochrome P-450 enzyme system. Cyclosporine toxicity may result from a concomitantly prescribed antibiotic such as amphotericin B, erythromycin, or ketoconazole. Similarly, the risk of nephrotoxicity may increase in a patient who is simultaneously receiving vancomycin and an aminoglycoside. Tacrolimus is the primary agent used for immunosuppression in patients who have undergone solid organ transplantation. Neurotoxic side effects of this agent such as headache, tremor, and paresthesia are the most frequent and predominant. Commonly used drugs in the perioperative period, such as calcium channel blockers, gastrointestinal prokinetic agents, azole antifungal agents, macrolide antibiotics, and protease inhibitors, increase serum tacrolimus concentrations, whereas phenytoin decreases tacrolimus serum concentrations.

OKT-3 is a mouse monoclonal antibody that binds to the CD3 antigen on T lymphocytes and is used for steroid-resistant graft rejection. Toxicity includes central nervous system effects and a cytokine release syndrome that ranges from a mild flulike response to severe shock and acute respiratory distress syndrome. This latter response can be minimized by the administration of high-dose steroids.

Basiliximab and daclizumab are monoclonal antibodies directed against the interleukin-2 receptor on the surface of activated T lymphocytes; they inhibit the activation and proliferation of T lymphocytes. The risk of infection with the use of these agents appears to be no higher than with other immunosuppressive regimens.

Some antirejection drugs interact with anesthetic drugs. Animal data suggest that cyclosporine may potentiate the effect of barbiturates, opioids, and neuromuscular blocking agents. Clinical studies demonstrate that azathioprine, another antirejection agent, has weak antagonistic effects on neuromuscular blockade. Additionally, there is an increased risk for the development of acute respiratory failure in patients who have been treated with bleomycin and are subsequently exposed to fractional inspired concentrations of oxygen greater than 0.30.

Many patients who receive corticosteroids as part of their therapy present to the operating room. The effect of steroids on adrenal function and reserve is complex and unpredictable. In general, large doses of steroids with a long half-life (e.g., dexamethasone) administered frequently are much more likely to cause adrenal suppression than are less potent steroids administered less frequently. If there is doubt about adrenal reserve, low-dose (1 μg) or high-dose (250 μg) cosyntropin testing can be performed preoperatively, or stress-dose corticosteroids (up to 300 mg/day of hydrocortisone) can be administered perioperatively and rapidly tapered.

Patients with chronic hepatitis C are treated with interferon alfa-2a, PEG-interferon alfa-2a, or PEG-interferon alfa-2b. These agents can cause a dose-dependent neutropenia and thrombocytopenia. In addition, ribavirin, an antiviral agent used in conjunction with an interferon, often causes a hemolytic anemia. Likewise, patients with multiple sclerosis are often treated with interferon beta-1b. Adverse reactions similar to those seen with the other interferons can be expected.

Tumor necrosis factor-α (TNF-α) and interleukin-1 (IL-1) are important cytokines involved in the systemic inflammation and cartilage destruction associated with rheumatoid arthritis. Anti-TNF-α and anti-IL-1 inhibitors are used in patients with rheumatoid arthritis who are

Table 120–3 ■ Biologic Agents Used in the Therapy of Rheumatoid Arthritis

Class	Drug	Side Effects
Inhibitors of tumor necrosis factor-α	Infliximab	Infection; worsening of congestive heart failure
	Adalimuab	Infection
	Etanercept	Infection
Inhibitor of interleukin-1	Anakinra	Infection; neutropenia

Adapted from O'Dell JR: Therapeutic strategies for rheumatoid arthritis. N Engl J Med 350:2591-2602, 2004.

refractory to conventional therapy (Table 120-3). The risk of serious infections (particularly tuberculosis) increases with the use of these drugs, and autoantibodies to the drugs can develop.

Immunocompromised or immunosuppressed patients frequently have coexisting multiple organ dysfunction. These alterations in organ function may affect the choice of anesthetic agents and techniques. Some published data suggest that anesthetics and operations may alter some immune responses secondary to the release of cortisol and catecholamines.

The effect of anesthetic agents themselves on perioperative immune function is unclear. Animal and in vitro studies suggest that natural killer cell cytotoxicity, B-cell and T-lymphocyte activity, and macrophage and polymorphonuclear neutrophil function are altered by volatile anesthetics or opioids. However, the clinical significance of these changes is unclear; one study of volunteers exposed to general anesthesia, lumbar epidural anesthesia, or opioids showed minimal change in immune function.

MANAGEMENT

The patient's medical status should be fully evaluated and optimized before the surgical procedure, with careful attention paid to subtle signs of incipient infection. Invasive monitoring, which itself poses a risk of infection, should be predicated on the proposed surgical procedure and the patient's medical condition.

Because these patients are at higher risk for developing perioperative infections, scrupulous precautions must be taken. Simple hand washing or the use of alcohol foam soaps is an often overlooked and underutilized method of reducing the transmission of nosocomial infections. Strict aseptic technique, including maximum barrier precautions, should be used when placing invasive hemodynamic monitoring catheters. If indicated, prophylactic antibiotics should be administered at least 30 minutes before skin incision; however, antibiotic administration 2 hours or more before or after incision is ineffective in preventing surgical wound infection.

Recent data suggest that the anesthesiologist can have a significant beneficial impact on reducing perioperative infection and improving patient outcome. Well-designed prospective trials have shown that prevention of intraoperative hypothermia during colorectal surgery reduces the risk of perioperative wound infection. In addition, tight control of glucose (80 to 110 mg/dL) with an insulin infusion in the intensive care unit has a dramatic impact on outcome: reduced mortality and morbidity (infection, neuropathy, acute renal failure requiring dialysis, and need for blood transfusion). Similar results have been reported with intraoperative control of glucose. More controversial is the intraoperative use of high concentrations of inspired oxygen; randomized studies have reported disparate results. Induced hypercarbia improves subcutaneous tissue oxygenation and might reduce the risk of perioperative wound infection, but large, randomized trials are needed to confirm the efficacy of this treatment modality. Blood transfusions have immunosuppressive properties and can increase the risk of perioperative infection. Thus, careful consideration should be given to the transfusion "trigger." In a stable patient with minimal blood loss and without a high risk of myocardial ischemia, waiting to transfuse until the hemoglobin is between 7 and 8 g/dL is safe and reasonable. Use of preoperative autologous blood donation, intraoperative hemodilution, and red blood cell scavenging may reduce the need for perioperative allogeneic blood transfusion.

The anesthetic plan should be based on the preoperative assessment. Regional anesthetic techniques are not necessarily contraindicated in immunocompromised or immunosuppressed patients, but the absence of a central nervous system infection and adequate coagulation status must be documented. In patients with diminished hepatic or renal reserve, sedation, analgesia, and neuromuscular blockade may be prolonged. These patients may need monitoring in an intensive care unit, especially if there is evidence of preoperative pulmonary compromise or hemodynamic instability. For patients who have been treated previously with corticosteroids, consideration should be given to testing the adrenal reserve or treatment with stress-dose steroids.

PREVENTION

Deterioration in an already fragile patient can be prevented by compulsive and vigilant perioperative care. Adherence to hand washing and aseptic techniques is mandatory. Prevention of intraoperative hypothermia and rigid control of blood glucose can reduce perioperative wound infection. A high index of suspicion when seeking and treating infection and the goal of optimizing underlying organ function can improve the outcome in these patients.

Further Reading

Cirella VN, Pantuck CB, Lee YJ, et al: Effects of cyclosporine on anesthetic action. Anesth Analg 66:703-706, 1987.

de Maat MM, Ekhart GC, Huitema AD, et al: Drug interactions between antiretroviral drugs and comedicated agents. Clin Pharmacokinet 42:223-282, 2003.

Drugs of choice for cancer chemotherapy. Med Lett Drugs Ther 39:21-28, 1997.

Evron S, Glezerman M, Harow E, et al: Human immunodeficiency virus: Anesthetic and obstetric considerations. Anesth Analg 98:503-511, 2004.

Gramstad L, Gjerlow JR, Hysing ES, et al: Interaction of cyclosporine and its solvent cremophor with atracurium and vecuronium. Br J Anaesth 58:1149-1155, 1986.

Kozyra EF, Wax RS, Burry LD: Can 1 μg of cosyntropin be used to evaluate adrenal insufficiency in critically ill patients? Ann Pharmacother 39:691-698, 2005.

Kumar A, Hota B: Infections in the immunocompromised. In Murray MJ, Coursin DB, Pearl RG, Prough DS (eds): Critical Care Medicine: Perioperative Management, 2nd ed. Philadelphia, Lippincott-Raven, 2002, pp 649-671.

Kurz A, Sessler DI, Lenhardt R: Perioperative normothermia to reduce the incidence of surgical wound infection and shorten hospitalization. Study of Wound Infection and Temperature Group. N Engl J Med 334:1209-1215, 1996.

Rubin RH: Fungal and bacterial infections in the immunocompromised host. Eur J Clin Microbiol Infect Dis 12(Suppl 1):S42-S48, 1993.

Vallejo R, Hord ED, Barna SA, et al: Perioperative immunosuppression in cancer patients. J Environ Pathol Toxicol Oncol 22:139-146, 2003.

van den Berghe G, Wouters P, Weekers F, et al: Intensive insulin therapy in the critically ill patient. N Engl J Med 345:1359-1367, 2001.

PHYSIOLOGIC IMBALANCE & COEXISTING DISEASE

Thermally Injured Patients

121

Avery Tung and Michael F. O'Connor

Case Synopsis

A 59-year-old man falls asleep in bed while smoking. He sustains deep partial- and full-thickness burns to approximately 50% of his body surface, including his face and extremities. He arrives in the emergency room intubated. The anesthesiologist is called to assist with his early management.

PROBLEM ANALYSIS

Definition

Burn injuries are classified in terms of their cause, depth, and extent. Each factor plays an important role in the evaluation and management of burn injury patients. Reports by emergency medical personnel and the initial history and physical examination are the primary means of identifying the causes and mechanisms of burn injuries.

Burns may be thermal, chemical, or electrical. Thermal injury requires the application of sufficient heat for a sufficient period so that cutaneous tissue heats to a temperature at which injury can occur. Chemical burns generally do not cause injury from the effects of heat; rather, injury is caused by corrosion, desiccation, or a chemical reaction. Although some chemicals have specific antidotes (e.g., calcium gel for hydrofluoric acid burns), the recommended initial treatment for most chemical burns is early and copious irrigation to dilute the offending agent. Electrical burns produce injury via three mechanisms: (1) nerves or blood vessels act as conduits for heat to cause injury in affected tissue; (2) electrical current may arc across two points on the body surface, thereby generating high temperatures and producing focal areas of external tissue injury; and (3) electrical energy may ignite clothing or other combustible materials, thereby producing secondary thermal injury due to the heat generated by the burning materials. Finally, chemical and thermal injury may coexist, as in burns caused by gasoline or other flammable materials.

Recognition

Regardless of the mechanism of burn injury, burns of any type are categorized as first, second, or third degree, based on the depth of tissue injury. First-degree burns (e.g., mild sunburns) involve the epidermis only and heal readily without specific interventions. Such burns may be painful and appear as reddened areas of intact skin that blanch with pressure. Second-degree burns, often referred to as partial-thickness burns, partially involve the dermis and require specific wound therapy. They may or may not require skin grafting, depending on the amount of nonaffected dermal tissue. Second-degree burns are moist, blanch with pressure, retain sensation, and often are extremely painful. Third-degree (full-thickness) burns destroy all dermal elements and penetrate into the subcutaneous tissue. The third-degree burn surface appears white and has a waxy feel; often it is speckled with red dots (i.e., heat-congealed hemoglobin) and devoid of any sensation. Left untreated, third-degree burns heal via central migration of the wound edges. Because this process may cause crippling contractures, third-degree burns should be grafted to preserve function. Often, the depth of third-degree thermal injuries is difficult to ascertain. Moreover, inappropriate therapy may convert a partial (second-degree) skin injury to a full-thickness (third-degree) injury.

Risk Assessment and Implications

The amount of heat delivered to tissue depends on the temperature, duration of exposure, and susceptibility of the tissue to thermal injury. Thus, similar intensity and duration of heat produce different burn depths at different skin locations. For example, relatively high blood flow to the face tends to disperse heat, rendering facial skin relatively resistant to deep thermal injury. Skin on the surface of the back is relatively thick, so it too is relatively resistant to thermal injury. However, where the skin is thin and the blood flow is low (e.g., in the extremities), exposure to a 77°C heat source for as little as 1 to 2 seconds can produce a full-thickness burn injury.

Pathophysiologic changes brought about by evolving thermal injury are categorized as early, intermediate, or late. In the early postburn period, localized inflammation increases capillary permeability and edema formation. The consequent loss of effective circulating volume is the most salient feature of the early clinical course. This loss reduces preload, so that cardiac output falls and end-organ perfusion is compromised. Also, hypothermia is common owing to the loss of skin thermoregulatory control and aggressive fluid resuscitation. In addition, inhalation of toxins such as carbon monoxide or cyanide may cause metabolic injury. Inhaled irritants may also cause laryngeal or glottal edema. Intermediate and late postburn changes include a persistent inflammatory state, immunosuppression, severe protein catabolism, and increased susceptibility to infection. Neutrophil and lymphocyte function may be impaired for several weeks after thermal injury. Finally, owing to the prolonged hospitalization required for major burns, serious complications, including ventilator-associated pneumonia, deep venous thrombosis, and multiorgan system dysfunction, may occur (see Chapters 51, 89, and 119).

Early complications of thermal injury are related to the injury itself and to the aggressive resuscitation patients

Table 121–1 ■ Complications in Burn Patients

Coexisting traumatic injury
Inhalation injury
Carbon monoxide poisoning
Hypovolemia
Compartment syndrome

require to survive extensive burn injuries (Table 121-1). Patients burned in an indoor environment or closed space are at risk for inhalation injury. Smoke inhalation can manifest as laryngeal or glottal swelling, metabolic poisoning caused by carbon monoxide or cyanide, or sloughing of lung mucosa due to direct toxin exposure (Table 121-2). Patients at risk for such complications commonly have a supportive history, such as soot on their faces or in the nares or oropharynx or blistering of the mouth and hard palate. Carbon monoxide poisoning commonly manifests as neurologic symptoms (ranging from agitation and confusion to frank seizures) and cardiovascular symptoms (including malignant arrhythmias and hypotension). Hypovolemia is due to fluid translocation caused by capillary leak and possibly blood loss if there is associated trauma. Electrolyte abnormalities due to thermal injury and resuscitation include hyponatremia, acidosis, and hypocalcemia. The aggressive fluid administration required may cause pulmonary and peripheral edema. Increased intra-abdominal pressure may also result from edema formation and may reduce urine output or compromise ventilation. Finally, compartment syndromes are common in patients with circumferential burns. If unrecognized, these may be associated with extensive tissue necrosis, rhabdomyolysis, and secondary renal injury.

During the second 24 hours after hospitalization, fluid losses decrease somewhat but may still be elevated due to weeping, open wounds. The increased capillary leak usually abates during this period, and edema formation is much less significant. Patients remain hypermetabolic and require dose adjustments for most drugs, including antibiotics, sedatives, neuromuscular blockers, and opioids. Protein catabolism continues until wound closure occurs.

With significant direct exposure to smoke, acute respiratory distress syndrome (ARDS) may develop. This syndrome usually occurs 48 to 72 hours after admission. Therapy includes limiting tidal volumes, permissive hypercapnia, high inspired oxygen concentrations, and the use of positive end-expiratory pressure (PEEP). Unlike ARDS caused by sepsis, however, mucosal sloughing due to smoke exposure can require extensive suctioning and significantly increases the risk for occlusion of the endotracheal tube. Such sloughing can be particularly important in patients initially intubated in the field with smaller-diameter endotracheal tubes.

Burn wound infection is the most common cause of death in patients with major (>60%) burns, and patients remain at high risk until wound closure. Burn wound sepsis can have an extremely rapid onset and an unusually severe course. Infected burn wounds require immediate debridement to maximize the chances for survival.

MANAGEMENT AND PREVENTION

Severely burned patients may require rapid application of the basic ABCs (airway, breathing, circulation) during initial

Table 121–2 ■ Classification of Smoke Inhalation

Mechanism of Injury	Clinical Symptoms and Effects
Heat injury to glottis and upper larynx	Soot on face or in mouth and nose
	Redness or blistering of mouth, nose, or hard palate
	Difficulty phonating or swallowing
	Resuscitation edema may cause airway to swell dramatically
	Prophylactic tracheal intubation should be strongly considered if thermal injury to glottis is suspected
Ingested toxins (cyanide and carbon monoxide)	Tachypnea, tachycardia, headache, dyspnea
	May progress to frank seizure, hypotension, malignant arrhythmias
	Cyanide poisoning acts synergistically with carbon monoxide to cause vital organ injury
	Although carbon monoxide can be readily detected on blood gas analysis, there is no rapid assay for cyanide; empirical therapy with sodium thiosulfate should be started if suspicion is high
Irritant damage from contact with chemicals contained in smoke	Toxicity of smoke depends on its temperature and the nature of burning materials and cannot be easily predicted
	There is no ready test for this component of inhalation thermal injury
	Unusually high fluid resuscitation volumes strongly suggest pulmonary involvement
	Symptoms usually manifest within 48 hr after thermal injury, including:
	Tachypnea
	Sputum production
	Fever
	Leukocytosis
	Hypoxemia
	Atelectasis
	Tracheal intubation to maintain oxygenation is often required; recovery occurs over a period of 2-3 wk

PHYSIOLOGIC IMBALANCE & COEXISTING DISEASE

resuscitation, followed by other indicated management and preventive measures. There are two indications for emergent surgery:

1. Burn wound sepsis. This condition is diagnosed by positive quantitative wound cultures and signs of systemic sepsis. Although wound infection without systemic sepsis can be treated topically, severe wound sepsis with associated systemic changes often requires aggressive operative debridement to maximize survival.
2. Peripheral edema. Increased extremity compartment pressures, circumferential chest burns, or increased intra-abdominal pressures (bladder pressure >25 mm Hg) require emergent surgical intervention to reduce compression injury.

Because of large protein losses with thermal injury, patients with severe burns are often fed aggressively via an enteral route. Therefore, preoperative NPO orders should strive to minimize periods when patients are not being fed.

Fluid Requirements

Fluid requirements for burn-injured patients are difficult to estimate, even for experienced practitioners. Underresuscitation may worsen injury, increase circulatory instability, and lead to end-organ dysfunction. Conversely, overresuscitation worsens edema and may increase the risk of abdominal compartment syndrome. Fluid replacement guidelines for the first 24 hours are provided in Table 121-3. These guidelines represent only starting fluid infusion rates. Because of the risk of edema formation, infusion rates should be titrated to the minimum amount needed to keep urine output at 0.5 mL/kg per hour. The "rule of nines" is used to estimate burn surface area (Table 121-4).

Intraoperative Care

The intraoperative care of burn-injured patients undergoing debridement or grafting procedures can be extremely challenging. Wounds are typically debrided down to briskly bleeding tissue, with partial hemostasis achieved using topical phenylephrine. Because of the large wound surface and topical vasopressor use, blood loss may be difficult to assess.

Table 121–3 ■ Burn Life Support Guidelines for Initial Volume Resuscitation (First 24 Hours)

Adults: 2-4 mL × body weight (kg) × burn area (%)
Children: 3-4 mL × body weight (kg) × burn area (%)
First half of volume to be infused over the first 8 hr, with remainder over next 16 hr
Example: A 70-kg man with 50% BSA partial- and full-thickness burns: 2-4 mL × (70) × (50) = 7000-14,000 mL of lactated Ringer's solution in the first 24 hr, with 3500-7000 mL given in the first 8 hr. Note that these are initial estimates only and that fluid therapy should be titrated to no more than 0.5 mL/kg/hr of urine output to minimize edema-related complications.

BSA, body surface area.
Adapted from Sheridan RL, et al: ABLS Provider's Manual. Chicago, American Burn Association, 2001.

Table 121–4 ■ Rule of Nines for Calculating Percentage of Body Surface Area Burned

Body Part	Body Surface Area	
	Adult	Child
Arm	9	9
Head and neck	9 (and 1)	18
Leg	18	14
Anterior trunk	18	18
Posterior trunk	18	18

Although tourniquets can be used on the extremities to reduce blood loss, they cannot be used for debridement involving the head, face, neck, chest, or back. Further, due to the greater vascularity of the head and face, blood loss can be especially severe during debridement of these areas. Careful attention to intravascular volume status and avoidance of the adverse consequences of overly aggressive fluid administration (acidosis, hypothermia, coagulopathy, pulmonary edema) are the cornerstones of intraoperative care.

Preplanning, adequate intravenous (IV) access, and ongoing communication among members of the burn care team are essential to avoid hypovolemia in the perioperative period. Because of the risk of infection, burn patients usually have only the minimum necessary IV access on arrival to the operating room. Establishment of large-bore IV access is mandatory for debridement involving the head or if it is likely to be extensive. Alternating debridement with grafting can spread the requirement for transfusions over a longer time, allowing the anesthesia team greater opportunity to maintain adequate fluid balance. Surgical debridement should stop if the patient develops a coagulopathy, refractory hypotension, hypothermia (temperature <35°C), or acidosis (pH <7.2).

Hypothermia

Thermally injured patients may become severely hypothermic during burn debridement and grafting. This complication is a consequence of evaporative loss from wet bandages, a cool operating room environment, and dysfunctional thermoregulatory mechanisms. Severe intraoperative hypothermia can cause arrhythmias and worsen existing coagulopathies. Warming the operating room (>30°C) and the use of heat lamps; IV fluid warmers; heated, humidified inspired gases; and low fresh gas flows are helpful for maintaining normothermia. Bear in mind that for patients swathed in wet bandages, forced air warming can worsen hypothermia by increasing evaporative losses. In patients with large wounds and wet bandages, heat lamps may be more effective. If the patient's temperature falls to 35.5°C, any remaining grafts should be placed quickly, hemostasis achieved, wounds dressed with occlusive dressings, and the procedure terminated.

Oxygenation and Ventilation

Thermal injury can significantly alter ventilation, even in patients without smoke inhalation. As discussed earlier, patients with inhalation injury may require early intubation for glottal swelling, extensive suctioning to maintain endotracheal tube patency with mucosal sloughing, and antidotes to counter cyanide and carbon monoxide poisoning. Because few laboratories offer in-house cyanide assays, the diagnosis of cyanide poisoning often must be made empirically.

In patients without inhalation injury, the consequences of aggressive fluid resuscitation and increased capillary leak can affect respiration. Circumferential burns involving the chest wall can dramatically reduce chest wall compliance. Increased intra-abdominal pressure due to edema formation can have similar effects. Pulmonary edema is common and requires a high fraction of inspired oxygen and PEEP for adequate oxygenation. Minute ventilation requirements may also be higher in burn patients because of increased carbon dioxide production with an ongoing hypermetabolic state.

The increased minute ventilation, high levels of PEEP, and elevated peak inflation pressures required for some patients may be beyond the capability of the ventilators on some anesthesia machines. Therefore, intensive care unit (ICU) ventilators are often needed for patients with inhalation injuries and ARDS. Also, it may be difficult or impossible to adequately ventilate these patients with manual transport devices. If the ability to maintain stable blood gases during transport is questionable, a brief period of manual ventilation at the bedside in the ICU may allow clinicians to identify and treat potential problems there, rather than during transport.

Vascular and Monitoring Access

Vascular and monitoring access may be difficult, because there may be little unburned skin available after grafting. Further, access is frequently minimized to reduce the risk of infection. Access for invasive monitoring and IV cannulas should be decided in conjunction with the surgical team and after a review of the surgical site, the degree of coagulopathy, and the nature of the planned procedure. Debridement and grafting for patients with large burns are often staged.

Positioning

Intraoperative positioning should facilitate surgical exposure for both the donor and recipient sites. In general, to avoid harvesting unused skin, the recipient site is debrided first to verify the existence of an adequate wound bed.

Because shear injury can be a primary cause of failed graft adherence, attention should be paid to previously grafted areas so that shearing injuries do not occur during positioning. Many thermally injured patients develop severe contractures in spite of aggressive physical therapy and must be positioned carefully to avoid related complications.

Securing Access

It is often difficult to secure endotracheal tubes and vascular access or monitoring lines in burn patients. Tape rarely adheres to burned areas and may come loose from normal skin in these patients. Essential tubes, catheters, and access lines should be sutured. Endotracheal tubes may be wired to gums and teeth or secured with twill tape around the neck and tube. Nonessential lines are removed as soon as possible to avoid the risk of infection and accidental line removal.

Pharmacology

Owing to the hypermetabolic state, the redistribution of many drugs occurs more rapidly in thermally injured patients than in normal individuals. Hepatic and renal elimination may be enhanced. Burn patients often become tolerant to the effects of benzodiazepines and opiates and may require extraordinarily high doses. The duration of neuromuscular blockade with nondepolarizing drugs may be considerably reduced. Succinylcholine is contraindicated because it may cause exaggerated potassium release and life-threatening ventricular arrhythmias. This response occurs within 24 hours of injury and may persist for up to 1 year after the patient recovers from the injury.

Further Reading

Benson A, Dickson WA, Boyce DE: Burns. BMJ 332:649-652, 2006.

Demling RH: Smoke inhalation injury. New Horiz 1:422-434, 1993.

Herndon DN: Total Burn Care. Philadelphia, WB Saunders, 1996.

Sheridan RL, et al: ABLS Provider's Manual. Chicago, American Burn Association, 2001.

Sheridan RL, Schulz JT, Ryan CM, et al: A 35-year-old woman with extensive, deep burns from a nightclub fire. N Engl J Med 350:810-821, 2004.

Tung A: Management of burns. In Hall J, Schmidt G, Wood L (eds): Principles of Critical Care Companion Handbook. New York, McGraw-Hill/Appleton & Lange, 1998, pp 801-822.

Young CJ, Moss J: Smoke inhalation: Diagnosis and treatment. J Clin Anesth 5:377-386, 1989.

Yowler CJ: Recent advances in burn care. Curr Opin Anaesth 14:251-255, 2001.

PHYSIOLOGIC IMBALANCE & COEXISTING DISEASE

Complications from Toxic Ingestion

122

Jeffrey S. Kelly

Case Synopsis

A 25-year-old man involved in a motor vehicle accident presents acutely for repair of bilateral open tibial fractures. Loss of consciousness was reported at the scene, but cranial computed tomography findings are negative. The patient's Glasgow coma scale score is currently 15. He is normotensive, and a thorough evaluation (including a negative cervical spine series) has ruled out other significant injuries. He admits to ingestion of alcohol and amphetamines just before the accident. Other findings are as follows: blood pressure, 110/50 mm Hg; pulse, 124 beats per minute; breaths, 24 per minute; and temperature, 37.1°C. Significant laboratory findings include hematocrit, 24; pH, 7.27; a base deficit of −10 mEq/L; and blood alcohol content, 279 mg/dL.

PROBLEM ANALYSIS

Definition and Recognition

Exposure to toxic substances occurs commonly, as evidenced by the 2.4 million calls received by poison control centers in 2002. Such calls typically involved an acute (92%), unintentional (85%), oral (76%) exposure to a single toxin (92%) by a child (58%) at a private residence (92%). Although almost 75% of such cases were managed outside the health care system, there were almost 528,000 physician visits, more than 156,000 hospital admissions, major morbidity in 15,000 patients, and 1153 deaths. Drug classes associated with the largest number of deaths, in descending order of frequency, were analgesics, sedatives, hypnotics, antipsychotics, antidepressants, stimulants, street drugs, cardiovascular drugs, and the alcohols. However, poison control center data appear to significantly underestimate the true incidence of adverse outcomes from poisoning. This is due in part to the heavy weighting toward pediatric exposures, which uniformly have favorable outcomes.

Risk Assessment

Most poisoning ingestions tend to follow one of two general patterns. Children usually take small quantities of a single toxin unintentionally; they seldom manifest significant morbidity (6.4%) or mortality (2.5%). In contrast, adolescents and adults ingest larger amounts of multiple toxins intentionally and suffer the vast majority of morbidity and mortality.

Large series of mixed adult overdoses suggest that the co-ingestion of ethanol occurs in approximately 50% of cases, and alcohol significantly confounds the initial clinical assessment in a similar percentage of trauma patients. Ethanol-related motor vehicle accidents during 2002 caused more than 17,400 deaths, with an associated cost of $15.7 billion. Fifty-six percent of the affected drivers in these fatal accidents demonstrated a blood alcohol content greater than 0.16% (twice the legal limit in most states).

One should therefore assume that adolescent and adult trauma victims have acute ethanol intoxication until proved otherwise. The clinician should also have a high index of suspicion for the ingestion of other recreational drugs in this patient population and should evaluate the patient for evidence of substance abuse during the initial history and physical examination. Important historical data include the specific toxin or toxins, quantity taken, ingestion time, signs and symptoms since ingestion, past medical and psychiatric history (including suicidal intent), current medications, allergies, and trauma (accidental, incidental, or self-inflicted). Because the history can be unreliable or incomplete in acute poisoning, supplemental data from other sources (e.g., public safety personnel, family, medical records, area pharmacies, local poison control centers) may be helpful in diagnosing toxic exposures. A rapid, systematic, and thorough physical examination is mandatory, given the vague history that often surrounds poisoning scenarios. Barrier precautions should be exercised where appropriate to prevent self-intoxication (such as cutaneous exposure to organophosphate insecticides). The assessment should initially focus on the ABCs (airway, breathing, and circulation), with aggressive intervention to stabilize any abnormalities discovered. Further assessment includes the following:

- *Gag reflex.* This has implications for airway protection, aspiration prophylaxis, and selective early institution of gastric emptying maneuvers (see "Management").
- *Core temperature disturbances.* These may reflect toxic (salicylates, stimulants) rather than environmental or infectious causes.
- *Central nervous system dysfunction.* Detection of central nervous system dysfunction should stimulate the active consideration of early pharmacologic therapy or radiographic imaging for possible intracranial abnormalities, cervical spine injury, or both.
- *Incidental trauma and stigmata of substance abuse.* The patient should be examined for puncture wounds, needle tracks, and nasal septal perforation.

- *Constellation of signs and symptoms ("toxidromes").* The ingestion of certain toxins may present as characteristic toxidromes that typically involve abnormal vital signs, altered mental status, pupillary changes, and a variety of miscellaneous effects that can be attributed to the pharmacologic properties of the offending agent. Examples are provided in Table 122-1.

Laboratory evaluation is typically not helpful for diagnosing toxic exposure, other than to support the initial clinical diagnosis.

Concomitant trauma and poisoning may confound the accurate assessment of each individual entity, as exemplified by the case synopsis. Normal blood pressure and pulse pressure in the presence of anemia, tachycardia, and metabolic acidosis likely reflect hypovolemic shock that is partially masked by amphetamine-associated vasoconstriction.

MANAGEMENT

The vast majority of acutely poisoned patients have satisfactory outcomes when given appropriate supportive care, with an emphasis on aggressive, early intervention to stabilize vital organ function. Initial efforts should focus on maintaining a stable, patent airway; establishing adequate ventilation and oxygenation; and stabilizing cardiovascular function, just as one would do for other medical emergencies. All patients with depressed mental status or seizures should receive oxygen, 2 mg of intravenous naloxone, and 25 g of IV dextrose if the finger-stick blood glucose level is low. Ideally, intravenous or intramuscular thiamine 100 mg should precede dextrose administration to prevent or treat Wernicke's encephalopathy. Tonic-clonic seizures that are refractory to initial therapy are treated with titrated doses of a benzodiazepine, barbiturate, phenytoin, or a combination of these. Given the high incidence of ethanol abuse in both poisoning and trauma patients, empirical alcohol withdrawal therapy should be considered. Definitive poisoning management usually includes early use of specific antidotes (where appropriate); selective early (within 1 hour of ingestion) use of gastric emptying (preferably orogastric lavage; more rarely, ipecac-induced emesis); routine administration of activated charcoal, where effective; and perhaps a single dose of an osmotic cathartic (Tables 122-2 to 122-7). Hemodialysis is rarely used and is usually reserved for patients who, despite maximal supportive care, remain unstable from dialyzable toxins. Whole bowel irrigation with large quantities of isosmotic polyethylene glycol solutions may be considered in stable patients who have ingested specific toxins for which charcoal is ineffective and delayed sequelae are possible (Table 122-8).

The signs and symptoms of amphetamine use in the patient described in the case synopsis were obscured by the concomitant effects of central nervous system depressants (i.e., ethanol), hypovolemic shock from long bone fractures, and environmental exposure to low ambient temperatures. Classic physical findings of amphetamine toxicity are consistent with a diffuse hyperadrenergic state and include hypertension, tachycardia, hyperthermia, diaphoresis, mydriasis, and hyperactivity. Psychiatric symptoms include agitation, paranoid ideation, and hallucinations in the presence of a clear sensorium. Specific therapy is directed toward "pharmacologic cooling" with benzodiazepines (e.g., diazepam 10 mg

Table 122–1 ■ Common Toxidromes		
Syndrome	**Common Clinical Signs**	**Potential Toxic Agents**
Anticholinergic	Tachycardia, fever, dry skin, urinary retention, ileus, mydriasis, delirium, seizures	Antihistamines, phenothiazines, tricyclic antidepressants, antipsychotics, atropine, scopolamine, jimsonweed, amantadine, antiparkinson drugs, *Amanita* mushrooms, baclofen
Cholinergic	Bradycardia, diaphoresis, urinary or fecal incontinence, emesis, miosis, central nervous system depression, weakness, fasciculations, wheezing	Organophosphate and carbamate insecticides, physostigmine, pyridostigmine, edrophonium, certain mushrooms
Sympathomimetic (stimulants)	Tachycardia (bradycardia with pure α-agonist), hypertension, mydriasis, diaphoresis, piloerection, fever, delusions, paranoid ideation, restlessness, agitation	Cocaine, amphetamines, over-the-counter decongestants (pseudoephedrine, phenylpropanolamine, phenylephrine)
Narcotic	Mental status depression, hypoventilation, miosis, ileus, hypotension, bradycardia	Opioids
Sedative-hypnotic	Confusion, slurred speech, mental status depression, respiratory depression, ataxia, hypothermia	Benzodiazepines, barbiturates, ethanol, antipsychotics, anticonvulsants
Serotonin	Fever, diaphoresis, flushing, diarrhea, hyperreflexia, tremor, myoclonus, trismus	Selective serotonin reuptake inhibitors, trazodone, clomipramine.
Hallucinogenic	Hallucinations, psychosis, paranoid ideation, panic, fever, mydriasis	Cocaine, amphetamines, cannabinoids, phenylcyclohexyl (PCP), lysergic acid diethylamide (LSD)
Extrapyramidal	Tremor, rigidity, opisthotonos, torticollis, choreoathetoid movements, trismus, hyperreflexia	Butyrophenones, phenothiazines, risperidone, olanzapine

Adapted from Goldfrank LR, Flomenbaum NE, Lewin NA, et al (eds): Goldfrank's Toxicologic Emergencies, 7th ed. New York, McGraw-Hill, 2002; and Mokhlesi B, Leiken JB, Murray P, et al: Adult toxicology in critical care. Part 1. General approach to the intoxicated patient. Chest 123:577-592, 2003.

Table 122–2 ■ Selected Poisoning Antidotes

Toxin	Antidote
Opiates	Naloxone
Benzodiazepines	Flumazenil
Anticholinergics	Physostigmine
Cholinesterase inhibitors	Atropine, pralidoxime (for insecticides)
Calcium channel blockers	Calcium chloride
β-Blockers	Glucagon
Digoxin	Digoxin-specific antibody
Acetaminophen	N-acetylcysteine
Methanol	Fomepizole, ethanol, folate
Ethylene glycol	Fomepizole, ethanol, pyridoxine
Isoniazid	Pyridoxine
Cyanide	Amyl nitrate, sodium nitrite, sodium thiosulfite, hydroxycobalamin
Methemoglobin	Methylene blue
Iron	Deferoxamine

Adapted from Mokhlesi B, Leiken JB, Murray P, et al: Adult toxicology in critical care. Part 1. General approach to the intoxicated patient. Chest 123:577-592, 2003; and Trujillo MH, Guerrero J, Fragachan C, et al: Pharmacologic antidotes in critical care medicine: A practical guide for drug administration. Crit Care Med 26:377-391, 1998.

intravenously as needed and aggressively titrated until the patient is calm). Goals of treatment are to (1) decrease motor agitation and treat tonic-clonic seizures, (2) provide active physical cooling maneuvers to treat significant hyperthermia, (3) initiate intravenous hydration with isotonic crystalloid to induce diuresis (1 to 2 mL/kg per hour) for hyperthermia-mediated rhabdomyolysis, and (4) control

Table 122–3 ■ Factors that Cumulatively Increase the Appropriateness of Gastric Emptying

Substantial risk of consequential toxicity (e.g., ingestion of aspirin, chloroquine, colchicines, cyclic antidepressants, calcium channel blockers)
Evidence of consequential toxicity (e.g., repeated seizures, apnea, hypotension, cardiac arrhythmias, acid-base or other metabolic disturbances)
Antidotal and adjunctive therapy ineffective or nonexistent (e.g., colchicine, paraquat)
Recent ingestion (<1-2 hr)
Ingestion exceeds adsorptive capacity of initial activated charcoal dosing (e.g., >100 mg/kg of pills such as aspirin, sustained-release verapamil, or sustained-release theophylline)
Ingested agent not adsorbed by activated charcoal (e.g., iron, lithium)
Ingested agent likely to form durable mass after overdose (e.g., large amounts of aspirin, enteric-coated agents, iron, meprobamate)
Ingestion of extended or sustained-release formulations (e.g., calcium channel blockers, theophylline)
No antecedent vomiting
Gastric tube placement required for activated charcoal administration
No contraindications to gastric emptying

Adapted from Smilkstein MJ: Techniques used to prevent absorption of toxic compounds. In Goldfrank LR, Flomenbaum NE, Lewin NA, et al (eds): Goldfrank's Toxicologic Emergencies, 7th ed. New York, McGraw-Hill, 2002, p 46.

Table 122–4 ■ Poisoning Treatment: Emesis with Syrup of Ipecac

Indications
Early treatment for potentially toxic ingestion—particularly for children at home, when there are no contraindications (see below)

Dose
Adults: 30 mL (2 tbsp)
Children:
    6-12 mo: 5-10 mL (2 tsp)
    1-12 yr: 15 mL (1 tbsp)
    Older than 12 yr: 30 mL (2 tbsp)
For both adults and children: One additional dose may be given if the patient has not vomited within 30 min

Contraindications
Caustic ingestion
Sharp materials
Easily aspirated substance (e.g., pure petroleum distillate) with little systemic toxicity in amount ingested
Comatose patients
Seizing patients
Patients expected to deteriorate rapidly
Patients with compromised gag reflex
Patients with hemorrhagic diathesis, esophageal and gastric varices, thrombocytopenia
Children younger than 6 mo
Significant prior vomiting, or when vomiting will delay timeliness of oral antidote or activated charcoal administration
Nontoxic ingestion

Adverse Effects
Intractable vomiting
Mallory-Weiss tears
Gastric rupture
Pneumothorax or pneumomediastinum
Aspiration
Delayed emesis after patient loses consciousness
Diarrhea (with chronic use)
Electrolyte abnormalities (with chronic use or abuse)
Cardiac and neurologic manifestations (with chronic use or abuse)

Adapted from Flomenbaum NE, et al: Managing the symptomatic patient with a possible toxic exposure. In Goldfrank LR, Flomenbaum NE, Lewin NA, et al (eds): Goldfrank's Toxicologic Emergencies, 7th ed. New York, McGraw-Hill, 2002, pp 460-462.

severe hypertension that is unresponsive to benzodiazepine sedation by using α-adrenergic blocking agents, nicardipine, or nitroprusside. The last should be done with caution, because long-term amphetamine abuse contributes to relative intravascular volume depletion in a manner similar to chronic hypertension. As with pheochromocytoma, the use of β-blockers leads to unopposed α-adrenergic stimulation and possible exacerbation of hypertension. Hyponatremia resulting from certain amphetamine congeners should be treated initially with isotonic or 3% saline, depending on its magnitude.

Because the patient described in the case synopsis required surgical intervention 4 hours after ingestion, and because he lacked significant amphetamine-related symptoms, definitive antipoisoning therapy consisted of a single dose of activated charcoal early in the perioperative period and close observation in a monitored bed in an adequately staffed area. Scheduled oral and as-needed "rescue" intravenous benzodiazepines were ordered perioperatively in

Table 122–5 ▪ Poisoning Treatment: Gastric Lavage

Indications

Life-threatening exposures when toxin is expected to be accessible in the stomach and evacuation is expected to contribute to improved outcome

Tube Type and Size

Adults and adolescents: 36-40 French
Children: 22-28 French

Procedure

If there is potential airway compromise, orotracheal or nasotracheal intubation should precede orogastric lavage; vomiting commonly follows lavage
Place the patient in the left lateral decubitus position
Before insertion, measure and mark the proper length of tubing to be passed; after the tube is introduced, confirm that the distal end of the tube is in the stomach
Withdraw any material present, and consider instillation of activated charcoal
Via a funnel (or lavage syringe), instill aliquots of a saline lavage solution, as follows:
  Adults: 250-mL aliquots
  Children: 10-15 mL/kg aliquots, not to exceed 250 mL
Continue lavage for at least several liters in an adult and 500 mL to 1 L in a child, *or* until no particulate matter returns and the effluent lavage solution is clear
Following lavage, use the same tube to instill activated charcoal and a cathartic, if indicated

Contraindications

Caustic ingestion
Sharp materials
Drug-packet ingestion
Significant hemorrhagic diathesis, esophageal and gastric varices, thrombocytopenia (relative contraindication)
Prior significant emesis
Nontoxic ingestion

Adverse Effects

Inadvertent tracheal intubation or airway trauma
Aspiration pneumonitis
Emesis
Gastrointestinal hemorrhage or perforation

Adapted from Flomenbaum NE, et al: Managing the symptomatic patient with a possible toxic exposure. In Goldfrank LR, Flomenbaum NE, Lewin NA, et al (eds): Goldfrank's Toxicologic Emergencies, 7th ed. New York, McGraw-Hill, 2002, pp 460-462.

Table 122–6 ▪ Poisoning Treatment: Activated Charcoal

Indications

Single dose: Ingestions of drugs or toxins that bind to activated charcoal, when no contraindications exist and an improved outcome is expected
Multiple doses: Ingestions of drugs or toxins that bind to activated charcoal when (1) a prolonged absorption phase is expected, (2) potential toxicity is great, and (3) gastrointestinal dialysis is expected to be beneficial; drugs with a small volume of distribution (<1 L/kg), low endogenous clearance, low plasma protein binding, biliary or gastric secretion of drug, or active metabolites that recirculate are most amenable to gastrointestinal dialysis

Dose*

Initial Dose (Single or Multiple)

Adults and children: 1 g/kg body weight or 10:1 ratio of activated charcoal to drug, whichever is greater
Following massive ingestions: 2 g/kg may be indicated if such a large dose can be easily administered and tolerated

Repeated Doses*

Adults and children: 0.25-0.5 g/kg body weight every 1-6 hr, in accordance with the dose and dosage form of drug ingested (larger doses and shorter dosing intervals may occasionally be indicated)

Procedure

Add 8 parts water to the selected amount of powdered form; all formulations, including prepacked slurries, should be shaken well for at least 1 min to form a transiently stable suspension before drinking or instillation via orogastric or nasogastric tube
Activated charcoal can be administered with a cathartic *for the first dose only*
If the patient vomits the dose of activated charcoal, it should be repeated; smaller, more frequent doses or continuous nasogastric administration may be better tolerated, or an antiemetic may be needed
If a nasogastric or orogastric tube is used for multiple-dose administration, allow time for the last dose to pass through the stomach before suctioning the remaining activated charcoal and removing the tube; this may prevent aspiration of activated charcoal

Contraindications

Patient at risk for aspiration who has an unprotected airway
Caustic ingestion (activated charcoal is ineffective as an adsorbent in these cases and may accumulate in burned areas, interfering with endoscopy)
Ileus (a contraindication for multiple dosing)

Adverse Effects

Aspiration pneumonitis
Emesis
Obscuring of gastrointestinal mucosa (for endoscopy)
Constipation

*Can be given orally or via an orogastric or nasogastric tube.
Adapted from Flomenbaum NE, et al: Managing the symptomatic patient with a possible toxic exposure. In Goldfrank LR, Flomenbaum NE, Lewin NA, et al (eds): Goldfrank's Toxicologic Emergencies, 7th ed. New York, McGraw-Hill, 2002, pp 460-462.

light of the patient's significant blood alcohol content on admission.

PREVENTION

It would be unethical to conduct prospective, controlled trials to assess complications arising from toxic ingestion. Epidemiologic studies, retrospective data, and case reports provide sufficient insight into the consequences of specific toxic ingestions. Thus, prevention of toxic sequelae requires a thorough and systematic clinical assessment, as well as familiarity with the specific pharmacology, pharmacodynamics, and pharmacokinetics of the ingested agents.

PHYSIOLOGIC IMBALANCE & COEXISTING DISEASE

Table 122–7 ■ Poisoning Treatment: Cathartics

Indications

Drugs or toxins that remain in the gastrointestinal tract and may continue to be absorbed (or desorbed from activated charcoal) if not rapidly eliminated

Cathartics should be used only with the first dose of activated charcoal and not repeated

Cathartics should not be used routinely and may cause serious fluid and electrolyte disturbances in children

Types and Doses

Magnesium citrate (adults and children): 4 mL/kg, to a maximum of 300 mL

Magnesium sulfate (adults and children): 250 mg/kg, to a maximum of 30 g/day

Sorbitol
  Adults: 1-2 mL/kg of 70% solution (orally)
  Children: 4 mL/kg of 25%-30% solution (rectally)

Precautions

Cathartics are not warranted for routine management in patients with trivial ingestions

Cathartics should not be used more than once for any ingestion—beware of packaging and labeling of activated charcoal and cathartic (sorbitol) combinations that appear similar to activated charcoal alone

Sorbitol should not be routinely administered to children; if used at all, strict attention to fluid and electrolyte status is mandatory

Phospho-Soda preparations should not be used in children or adults

Oil-based cathartics should not be used because of the risk of aspiration and enhanced toxin absorption

Contraindications

Abdominal trauma
Intestinal obstruction
Adynamic ileus
Renal failure (a contraindication for magnesium citrate and magnesium sulfate cathartics)
Diarrhea

Adverse Effects

Volume depletion
Emesis
Electrolyte imbalance (hypermagnesemia, hypokalemia, hypernatremia)
Diarrhea

Adapted from Flomenbaum NE, et al: Managing the symptomatic patient with a possible toxic exposure. In Goldfrank LR, Flomenbaum NE, Lewin NA, et al (eds): Goldfrank's Toxicologic Emergencies, 7th ed. New York, McGraw-Hill, 2002, pp 460-462.

Table 122–8 ■ Poisoning Treatment: Whole Bowel Irrigation

General Indications

Whole bowel irrigation with polyethylene glycol electrolyte lavage solution may be helpful in managing poisonings and overdoses when it is desirable or necessary to
  (1) rapidly clear the entire gastrointestinal tract without emesis or causing fluid or electrolyte disturbances
  or (2) prepare the gastrointestinal tract for visualization; it should not be substituted for activated charcoal when the latter is indicated

Specific Indications

Intoxication with a sustained-release medication

Slowly dissolving substances (e.g., iron tablets, paint chips, bezoars, concretions)

Drug packets (e.g., heroin, crack vials, cocaine) swallowed by "body packers" or "body stuffers"

Drugs or toxins not adsorbed by activated charcoal (e.g., lithium, iron)

Dose*

Adults: 1-2 L/hr for 4-6 hr, or until the rectal effluent is clear

Children: 25-40 mL/kg/hr for 4-6 hr, or until the rectal effluent is clear

Note: Activated charcoal should be administered before and during whole bowel irrigation if a charcoal-adsorbable drug or toxin is involved; an antiemetic such metoclopramide or a serotonin antagonist may be indicated to achieve compliance

Contraindications

Gastrointestinal pathology (e.g., ileus, perforation, obstruction)
Caustic ingestion
Patients at risk for pulmonary aspiration

Adverse Effects

Rectal itching
Vomiting (especially with rapid administration)
Bloating
Decreased efficacy of activated charcoal
Desorption of toxin from activated charcoal

*Can be given orally or via nasogastric tube.

Adapted from Flomenbaum NE, et al: Managing the symptomatic patient with a possible toxic exposure. In Goldfrank LR, Flomenbaum NE, Lewin NA, et al (eds): Goldfrank's Toxicologic Emergencies, 7th ed. New York, McGraw-Hill, 2002, pp 460-462.

Further Reading

Bond GR: The role of activated charcoal and gastric emptying in gastrointestinal decontamination: A state-of-the-art review. Ann Emerg Med 39:273-286, 2002.

Chiang WK, Goldfrank LR: Amphetamines. In Goldfrank LR, Flomenbaum NE, Lewin NA, et al (eds): Goldfrank's Toxicologic Emergencies, 7th ed. New York, McGraw-Hill, 2002, pp 1020-1033.

Flomenbaum NE, et al: Managing the symptomatic patient with a possible toxic exposure. In Goldfrank LR, Flomenbaum NE, Lewin NA, et al (eds): Goldfrank's Toxicologic Emergencies, 7th ed. New York, McGraw-Hill, 2002, pp 460-462.

Goldfrank LR, Flomenbaum NE, Lewin NA, et al (eds): Goldfrank's Toxicologic Emergencies, 7th ed. New York, McGraw-Hill, 2002.

Hoppe-Roberts JM, Lloyd LM, Chyka PA: Poisoning mortality in the United States: Comparison of national mortality statistics and poison control center reports. Ann Emerg Med 35:440-448, 2000.

Jurkovich GJ, Rivara FD, Gurney JG, et al: Effects of alcohol intoxication on the initial assessment of trauma patients. Ann Emerg Med 21:704-708, 1992.

Kosten TR, O'Connor PG: Management of drug and alcohol withdrawal. N Engl J Med 348:1786-1795, 2003.

Krenzelok EP: New developments in the therapy of intoxications. Toxicol Lett 127:299-305, 2002.

Kulig K, Bar-Or D, Cantrill SV, et al: Management of acutely poisoned patients without gastric emptying. Ann Emerg Med 14:562-567, 1985.

Mokhlesi B, Leiken JB, Murray P, et al: Adult toxicology in critical care. Part 1. General approach to the intoxicated patient. Chest 123:577-592, 2003.

National Highway Traffic Safety Administration (NHTSA): People: Injury prevention: Impaired driving: Program update. Washington, DC, NHTSA. Available at www.nhtsa.dot.gov/people/injury/alcohol/index.html.

Smilkstein MJ: Techniques used to prevent absorption of toxic compounds. In Goldfrank LR, Flomenbaum NE, Lewin NA, et al (eds): Goldfrank's Toxicologic Emergencies, 7th ed. New York, McGraw-Hill, 2002, p 46.

Trujillo MH, Guerrero J, Fragachan C, et al: Pharmacologic antidotes in critical care medicine: A practical guide for drug administration. Crit Care Med 26:377-391, 1998.

Watson WA, Litovitz TL, Rodgers GC Jr, et al: 2002 Annual report of the American Association of Poison Control Centers Toxic Exposure Surveillance System. Am J Emerg Med 21:353-421, 2003.

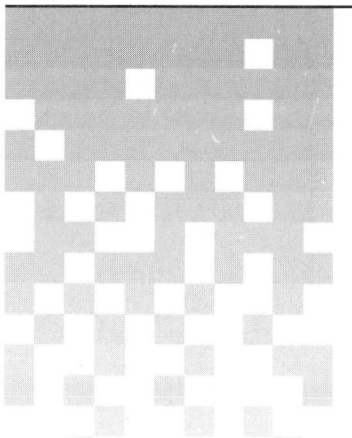

Equipment and Monitoring

Kevin K. Tremper

ANESTHETIC EQUIPMENT
Pipeline Source Failure

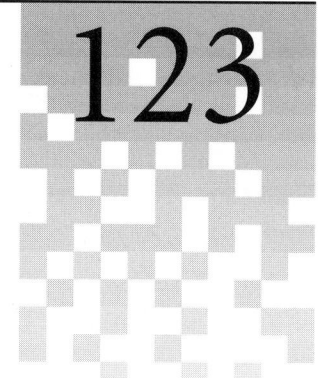

James F. Szocik

Case Synopsis

It is the first day of operation of the hospital's new outpatient surgery wing. The anesthesiologist reports to work looking forward to a day of easy cases consisting of healthy American Society of Anesthesiologists class I outpatients. During the first case, however, a tiny chirp is heard, accompanied by an advisory stating that the oxygen (O_2) supply is low. Several seconds later, the anesthesiologist notices that the ventilator bellows is not filling, the comforting sound of the cycling ventilator is absent, and a cacophony of alarms is sounding, including apnea pressure and volume alarms and minute volume alarms.

PROBLEM ANALYSIS

Definition

A pipeline failure can be one of two types: a quantitative problem, with too little or too much pressure; or a qualitative error, indicating that a contaminant is present (Table 123-1). In the extreme case of switched pipelines, the contamination consists of 100% undesired gas. The pipeline is made up of a large number of components (Fig. 123-1), any of which can fail.

Recognition

Quantitative errors in pipeline supply can be detected via a pressure-sensing device. A machine checkout using guidelines recommended by the Food and Drug Administration will detect a lack of pipeline pressure or an excess of pressure. During a procedure, modern anesthesia machines are equipped with a low O_2 pressure alarm that sounds to alert the operator that the O_2 supply is failing. A nitrous oxide (N_2O) pipeline failure does not sound an alarm.

Qualitative errors are more difficult to detect. Gross contamination of O_2 can be detected by using an O_2 sensor, which is calibrated to read 21% in room air, and confirming that the sensor reads greater than 90% with 100% pipeline O_2. A properly calibrated O_2 sensor will advise if a different gas has been switched into the O_2 pipeline. However, no currently available monitor or analyzer can detect the entire spectrum of potential contaminants in a pipeline system (e.g., carbon monoxide, trilene, solvents), especially at low concentrations. One's olfactory sense may detect some contamination, but this exposes the tester to potentially dangerous contaminants.

Risk Assessment

All patients receiving gas other than room air are at risk. Most pipeline problems involve the quantitative aspect of pressure (either too high or too low). A case reported in 2004 involving a triply redundant system (i.e., primary, secondary,

and reserve tanks) highlighted the resiliency of such a system. Despite a shutdown of the primary and secondary tanks due to a massive spill of liquid oxygen from a failed connection, the reserve tank was able to supply the demands of multiple operating rooms and intensive care unit beds. In a survey of more than 200 anesthesia departments at academic institutions, 37 of 76 reported mishaps involved low pressure in the O_2 pipeline. These can be detected during the standard anesthesia machine checkout. More serious is a crossover in the pipeline supply, which can result in hypoxia. Crossover errors involving the O_2 source are detected when verifying that the O_2 analyzer reads greater than 90%, using pipeline gas as part of the standard anesthesia machine checkout. Contaminated gases are more insidious. They can occur as part of the manufacturing or refining of gases, from

Table 123–1 ■ Pipeline Failure
Quantitative Problems
Low pipeline pressure
Kinked hose to machine
Leak in hose to machine
Leak in coupling hose to machine
Obstruction in pipeline
Valve in hall turned off
Leak in pipeline
Oxygen supply empty
Failure of reserve supply to activate
Regulator frozen in closed position
High pipeline pressure
Regulator frozen in open position
Liquid gas in line expanding
Qualitative Problems
Contamination in piping
Error in indexed safety system, allowing cross-connection
Piping crossover
Foreign body in pipeline
Cleaning solution in pipeline
Contamination at source
Tank filled with wrong gas
Cleaning solution in tank
Wrong connection at source

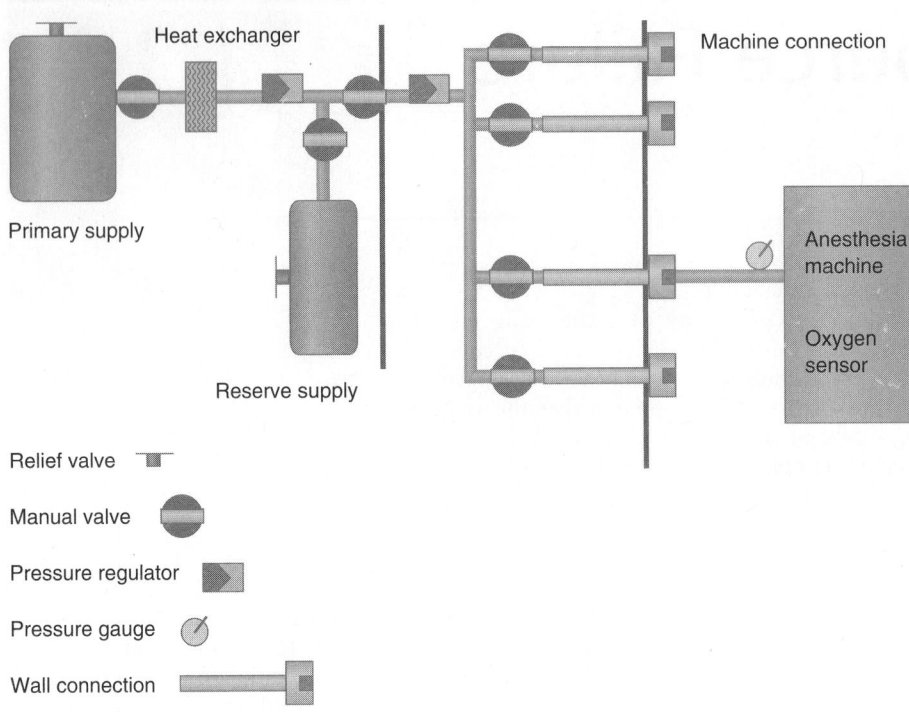

Figure 123–1 ■ Schematic diagram of a piped-gas delivery system. The primary supply may be liquid, large cylinders, or on-site compression. For the anesthesiologist, detection of pipeline problems occurs at the anesthesia machine (either pressure gauge or oxygen sensor), which is the final common pathway for the large number of components constituting the piped-gas supply.

the improper use of cleaning solutions in the pipeline, or from improper welding techniques. Detailed analysis of the gas at the patient end is the only way to detect this kind of failure. Many failures and instances of contamination are associated with construction and modification of the pipeline system. Greater vigilance is needed whenever construction is ongoing in the vicinity of the pipeline.

Implications

Pipeline pressure that is too low can result in inadequate delivery of gases to the patient. In the case of N_2O, inadequate anesthetic depth and patient awareness may occur. Lack of O_2 is far more serious and can result in hypoxia and organ damage. Pipeline pressure that is too high can damage the anesthesia machine, resulting in broken flowmeters, inaccurate readings, or internal rupture of components. If this occurs, the anesthesia machine must be replaced immediately intraoperatively.

Qualitative problems with gas delivery can asphyxiate the patient if a non-life-sustaining gas is substituted for O_2 or poison the patient if the contaminant is toxic. As reported by Moss and Evans, tricholorethylene contamination was implicated in four deaths in Texas. Hospital workers initially detected the problem when they noticed an odor in the delivered O_2.

In summary, quantitative errors are easily detected. No patient should be harmed by lack of O_2 or N_2O. In contrast, except for pipeline crossover, qualitative errors are more insidious. Aside from detailed gas analysis, there is no failproof method to detect contamination of piped gases.

MANAGEMENT

One strategy can accommodate all permutations of pipeline failure, including contaminations (Fig. 123-2). In all cases of pipeline failure, O_2 and ventilation must be provided to the patient. If the anesthesia machine is functional, O_2 and ventilation are most easily provided by changing to the anesthesia machine O_2 tank supply and disconnecting from the wall O_2 supply. Because the anesthesia machine preferentially draws from the wall (pipeline) O_2 source, the pipeline should be disconnected from the anesthesia machine to prevent additional contamination from entering the system. Because most ventilators are driven by pressure from the O_2 supply, changing to manual ventilation will conserve O_2 in an emergency. However, if the anesthesia machine has been damaged by high pressure, or if both the pipeline supply and the tank supply have failed or are suspected of being contaminated, a self-inflating Ambu bag with room air will keep most patients alive until reserve equipment becomes available. Anesthetic needs can be met by total intravenous anesthesia. Vital time should not be wasted trying to troubleshoot and fix a potentially damaged anesthesia machine. Finally, notice of a failure needs to be communicated quickly to other patient care areas, so that more global failures or contaminations can be dealt with properly.

At this point, the hospital's biomedical engineering department should be asked to determine the nature and origin of the failed component. Analogous to the low-pressure strategy, the source of the failed component (most likely a regulator) can be identified by determining whether the entire system or only a portion of the system is affected.

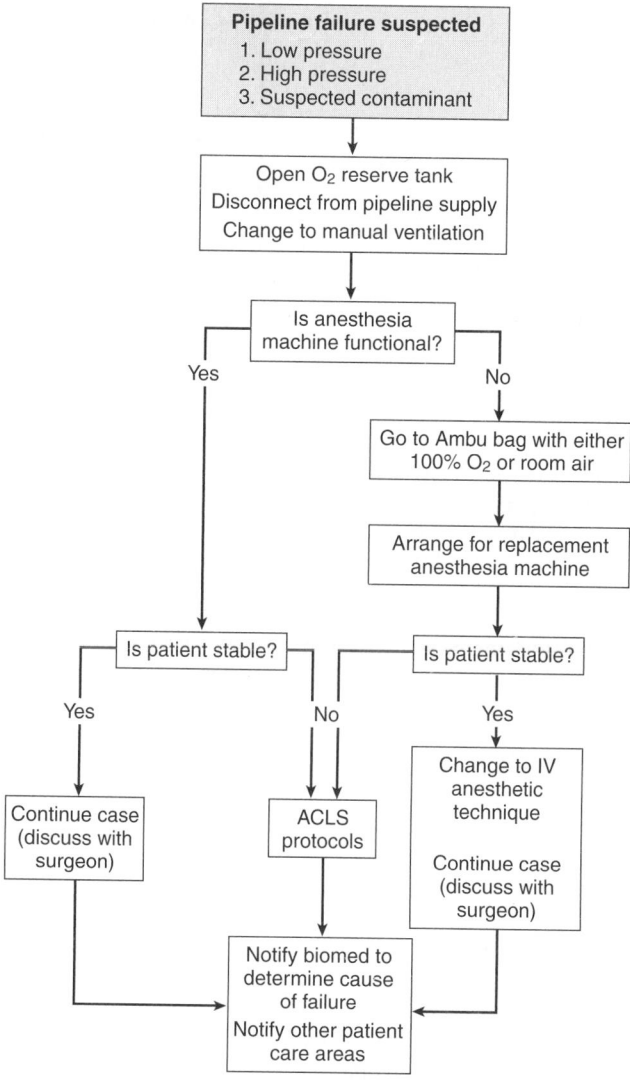

Figure 123–2 ▪ Simple algorithm for dealing with pipeline failure. ACLS, advanced cardiovascular life support; biomed, hospital biomedical engineering department.

PREVENTION

Prevention of pipeline catastrophes has both mechanical and human elements. Pipeline gas supplies are mechanical constructions, and all mechanical constructions have a failure rate. Given enough time, a valve, regulator, or other pipeline component will fail. Automatic systems to activate reserve and secondary supplies, pressure relief valves, and other mechanical safety devices help prevent patient injury. Proper inspection and maintenance carried out by trained personnel will help prevent mechanical failures. Computer-controlled systems, however, can fail catastrophically without warning. If so, the human element becomes most important.

Prevention of patient injury involves all the mechanical safeguards mentioned earlier plus a more important human element. Because all mechanical safeguards can fail, it is up to a vigilant anesthetist to detect malfunctions and activate appropriate secondary systems. In the operating room environment, this means that a properly checked-out anesthesia machine must be available for every anesthetic administration.

Further Reading

Anderson WR, Brock-Utne JG: Oxygen pipeline supply failure: A coping strategy. J Clin Monit 7:39-41, 1991.

Dorsch JA, Dorsch SE: Understanding Anesthetic Equipment, 2nd ed. Baltimore, Williams & Wilkins, 1984, pp 1-37.

Ehrenwerth J, Eisenkraft JB: Anesthesia Equipment: Principles and Applications. St. Louis, Mosby–Year Book, 1993, pp 3-26.

Feeley TW, Hedley-Whyte J: Bulk oxygen and nitrous oxide delivery systems: Design and dangers. Anesthesiology 44:301-305, 1976.

Gilmour IJ, McComb RC, Palahniuk RJ: Contamination of a hospital oxygen supply. Anesth Analg 71:302-304, 1990.

Moss E, Evans F: Hospital deaths reportedly due to contaminated O_2. Anesth Patient Safety Foundation Newslett 11:13-24, 1996.

Schumacher SD, Brockwell RC, Andrews JJ, et al: Bulk liquid oxygen supply failure. Anesthesiology 100:186-189, 2004.

If a contaminant is suspected, the tank supply should be activated, the machine disconnected from the pipeline source, and the biomedical engineers notified to take a sample of the gas for analysis. Construction or maintenance records are helpful to determine when any work was done on the pipeline.

EQUIPMENT & MONITORING

Flowmeters

Robert G. Loeb

124

Case Synopsis

Anesthesia induction has just been completed on a healthy 20-year-old man undergoing inguinal herniorrhaphy. Gas flows are set to 1 L/minute of oxygen (O_2) and 2 L/minute of nitrous oxide (N_2O). The O_2 saturation begins to fall as the O_2 analyzer alarms (Fig. 124-1). Actuating the O_2 flush valve resolves the problem temporarily.

PROBLEM ANALYSIS

Definition

Flowmeter malfunction is a rare cause of anesthesia machine failure, because modern anesthesia machines are designed to prevent many flowmeter problems. The last flowmeter incident was reported in 2004. The flowmeter assembly of modern anesthesia machines consists of a single flow control valve and one or two glass flowmeter tubes, connected in series, for each compressed gas. Additionally, new anesthesia machines have a proportioning device that restricts the relative flow rates of O_2 and N_2O to prevent the administration of hypoxic gas mixtures.

Flowmeter tubes comprise a float within a tapered glass tube whose inner diameter is larger at the top than at the bottom. To be accurate, the flowmeter tube must be in a vertical position, and the movement of the float must not be restricted by static electricity or dirt within the tube. Flowmeters are calibrated as a matched tube and float set; replacement of either component can result in significant inaccuracy. Modern anesthesia flowmeters are permanently sealed to prevent mistakes in matching the float and tube during maintenance. Each flowmeter is calibrated for a specific gas, and it is not accurate for measuring the flow of any other gas. To prevent mistakes during anesthesia machine maintenance, modern flowmeters are indexed so that they fit only into the housing for the appropriate gas. To protect flowmeter tubes from breakage, they are housed behind a plastic shield.

Patients have died from breathing hypoxic gas mixtures administered from erroneously set flowmeters. Poor flowmeter design was sometimes a contributing factor, because in the past, anesthesia machines were designed with two flowmeter assemblies connected in parallel for each gas (Fig. 124-2). Improved flowmeter design now decreases the chance of user error, and an N_2O-to-O_2 proportioning system prevents such tragedies from occurring. For example, anesthesia machines manufactured by Dräger are equipped with an O_2 proportioning regulator called the Oxygen Ratio Monitor Controller, and those manufactured by GE Healthcare are fitted with a mechanical linkage called the Link-25. Both are generally reliable, but occasional malfunctions of the Link-25 have been reported.

Some contemporary anesthesia machines (e.g., Dräger Fabius, Datex-Ohmeda ADU) have electronic flowmeters instead of glass flow tubes. Advantages of electronic flowmeters include improved reliability and reduced maintenance, improved precision and accuracy at low flows, and the ability to automatically record and control gas flows. The electronic sensors operate on the principle of heat transfer, measuring the energy required to maintain the temperature of a heated element in the gas flow pathway. Each sensor is calibrated for a particular gas, because every gas has a different specific heat index. Gas flows are shown on dedicated LED displays or on the main anesthesia machine's flat-panel display. Displays on the anesthesia machine's flat panel can be configured as numeric or graphic and can also be configured to show individual flow rates or calculated total flow rate and set O_2 concentration. There have been no reported problems with the electronic flowmeters, except for the loss of calibration factors due to RAM battery failure.

Recognition

A malfunctioning flowmeter is most easily detected during the anesthesia machine preuse checkout. The Food and Drug Administration (FDA) has developed a checkout procedure (which can be downloaded from http://www.fda.gov/cdrh/humfac/anesckot.html) that detects most serious anesthesia machine malfunctions. The leak check of the machine's low-pressure system detects a missing, leaking, cracked, or broken flowmeter. Visual inspection of the flow tubes may reveal a cracked or broken flowmeter. A float that sticks to the tube can be detected by adjusting the flow of all gases through their full range, while checking for smooth operation of the floats. The O_2 proportioning device should be tested by attempting to create a hypoxic O_2-N_2O mixture. It should be noted, however, that it is unlikely that an improperly calibrated flowmeter would be detected by the FDA anesthesia apparatus checkout.

During intraoperative use, a malfunctioning flowmeter results in different than expected gas concentrations in the breathing circuit (e.g., higher or lower concentrations of O_2 than dialed) or unexpected flow rates from the anesthesia machine to the breathing circuit. The anesthesia practitioner may not notice a problem unless it is dramatic, because there are no direct and independent monitors of anesthesia machine output. There is no monitor of the gas flow emanating from the anesthesia machine, although in extreme cases, the practitioner may notice that the reservoir bag or ventilator bellows is not filling normally. The respiratory gas analyzer at the Y-piece and the O_2 analyzer in the breathing circuit are the closest downstream monitors of the gas

518

Figure 124–1 ■ The inspired oxygen concentration is dangerously low and is not consistent with the flowmeter settings.

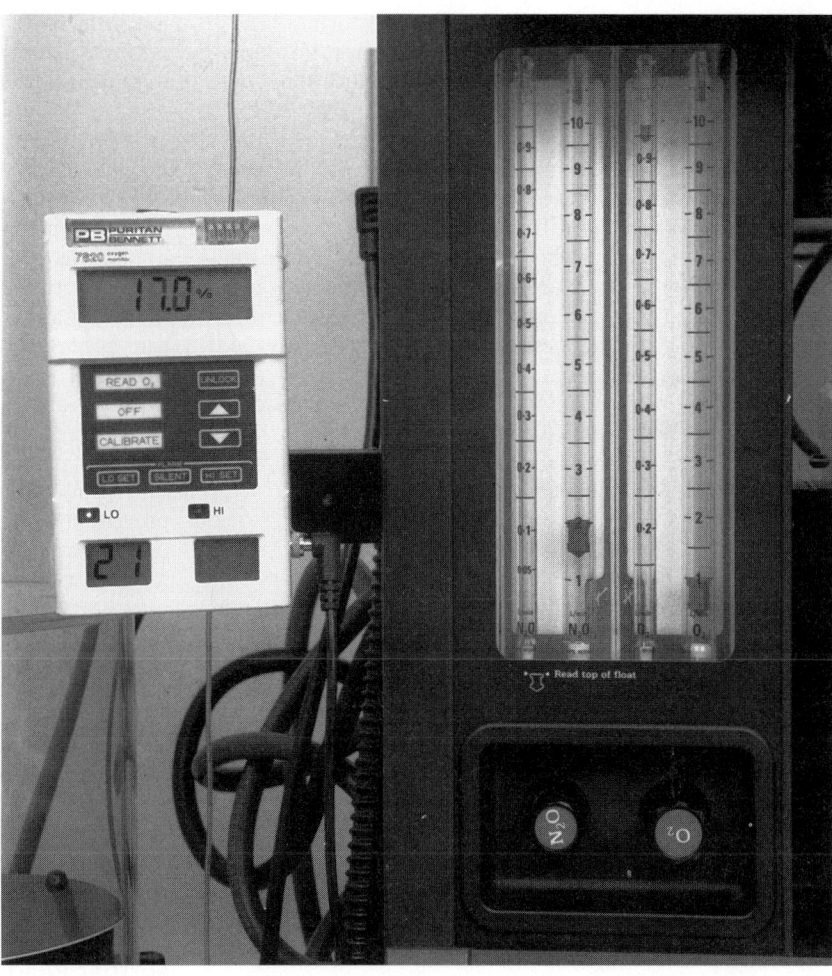

concentrations coming from the anesthesia machine. The readings on these monitors, however, rarely match the settings on the anesthesia machine, because of rebreathing. The discrepancy between dialed concentrations and breathing circuit gas concentrations is especially apparent during low gas flows. If a flowmeter problem is suspected, the anesthesia practitioner can sample gas from the fresh gas hose to check the composition of gases flowing from the anesthesia machine.

Risk Assessment

Anesthesia machine malfunction is an uncommon cause of critical events. For instance, only 4 of the first 2000 incidents

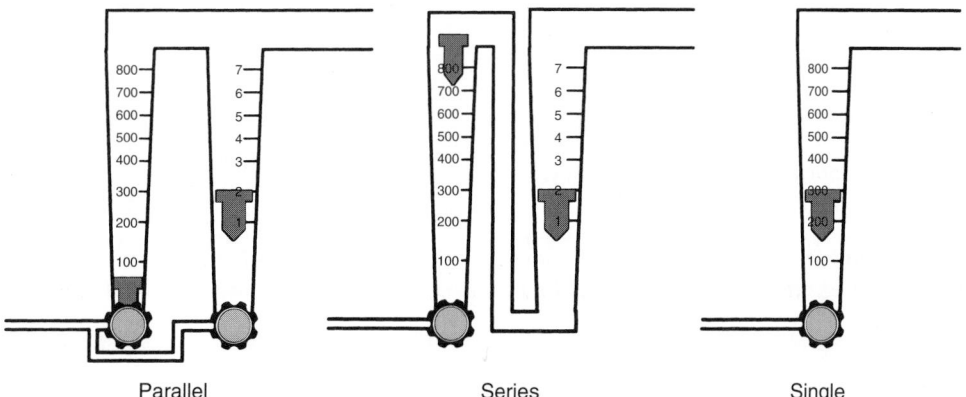

Figure 124–2 ■ Flowmeter arrangements. *Left,* When flowmeters are arranged in parallel, there are two control knobs and two flow tubes for a single gas. A potential hazard is that the user can erroneously turn the wrong knob or read the wrong tube. *Middle,* The series arrangement is safer, because there is only a single control knob. *Right,* The safest layout is a single flowmeter for each gas, but a single flowmeter may not be precise enough for low-flow techniques. (From Loeb RG: Preventing anesthesia machine-induced hypoxemia. Welcome Trends Anesthesiol 8:2-10, 1990.)

reported to the Australian Incident Monitoring Study involved anesthesia machine failures. Two of these incidents, however, resulted from flowmeter problems and were considered potentially life threatening.

Regular maintenance of the anesthesia machine is necessary to prevent malfunction due to wear. Ironically, some anesthesia machine failures have been attributed to mistakes made during maintenance. The clinician should therefore be vigilant for equipment problems when using a machine that has recently been serviced. Old anesthesia machines may pose the greatest safety hazard. A survey of anesthesia machines in Iowa found that machines ranged from 1 to 28 years old (average, 8 years). Although older machines did not malfunction more often than newer ones, they often lacked safety features and essential monitoring (e.g., O_2-N_2O flow ratio alarms, O_2 analyzers). Thus, clinicians should be wary of older machines without these features.

Implications

Flowmeter malfunction can present as a breathing circuit leak or an inappropriate gas composition within the breathing circuit. Although gas cannot flow retrograde from the breathing circuit to a broken flowmeter, leakage of gas from a broken or missing flowmeter can quickly lead to insufficient gas volume in the breathing circuit. This manifests as an empty breathing bag or ventilator bellows and can lead to a misdiagnosis of the malfunction as a breathing circuit leak or disconnection, because these malfunctions occur more commonly. A large leak from the flowmeter assembly is a serious problem because it prevents effective ventilation of the patient.

Flowmeter inaccuracy or a small leak from a cracked O_2 flowmeter can cause the anesthesia machine to dispense a hypoxic gas mixture into the breathing circuit. The O_2 analyzer in the latter is designed to detect such an occurrence. Other flowmeter problems are not liable to lead to patient injury. Leakage of a gas other than O_2 should not result in a hypoxic mixture, because flowmeters are arranged to prevent the preferential loss of O_2 in such a situation.

MANAGEMENT

An O_2 flush should temporarily rectify loss of circuit volume or hypoxia due to a flowmeter problem. The O_2 flush bypasses many internal components of the anesthesia machine, including the flowmeter assembly. Also, retrograde leakage of O_2 after a flush is prevented on most anesthesia machines by a one-way valve (or a vaporizer that incorporates a one-way valve).

When serious flowmeter malfunction is detected intraoperatively, the patient should be ventilated with an alternative system, such as an Ambu bag, while the defective anesthesia machine is replaced. The defective machine should be removed from service until it has been repaired and thoroughly inspected by a trained technician.

PREVENTION

Most flowmeter failures are preexisting. If so, a thorough preuse check of the anesthesia machine should prevent most critical events due to flowmeter malfunction. Many problems, including a missing, leaking, cracked, or broken flowmeter, can be detected with the FDA-recommended anesthesia machine checkout procedure. This procedure is also designed to test the function of the O_2-N_2O proportioning system. Flowmeter calibration, however, is not verified during this checkout procedure.

Although many equipment-related malfunctions are prevented by routine preuse inspection, anesthesia practitioners are not proficient in detecting anesthesia machine faults. For instance, anesthesiologists and certified registered nurse anesthetists detected an average of only 44% of intentionally created anesthesia machine faults at a conference exhibit. Only 15% of participants detected that the O_2 flowmeter was miscalibrated to deliver 10% of the indicated flow. Checklists do not necessarily improve performance either. Anesthesiologists detected 26% of anesthesia machine faults when they used their own checkout methods, and 29% of the faults when they used the FDA checkout procedure (1986 version). However, they were not instructed in the use of the FDA checklist, and intensive instruction can improve the performance of apparatus checkout procedures.

Further Reading

Buffington CW, Ramanathan S, Turndorf H: Detection of anesthesia machine faults. Anesth Analg 63:79-82, 1984.

Chandradeva K: A serious incident with the Blease Frontline Genius anaesthetic machine. Anaesthesia 59:627, 2004.

Cooper M, Ali D: Oxygen flowmeter dislocation [letter]. Anaesth Intensive Care 17:109-110, 1989.

Eger EI II, Hylton RR, Irwin RH, et al: Anesthetic flow meter sequence—a cause for hypoxia. Anesthesiology 24:396-397, 1963.

Hay H: Delivery of an hypoxic gas mixture due to a defective rubber seal of a flowmeter control tube. Eur J Anaesthesiol 17:456-458, 2000.

Kumar V, Hintze MS, Jacob AM: A random survey of anesthesia machines and ancillary monitors in 45 hospitals. Anesth Analg 67:644-649, 1988.

March MG, Crowley JJ: An evaluation of anesthesiologists' present checkout methods and the validity of the FDA checklist. Anesthesiology 75:724-729, 1991.

McHale S: A critical incident with the Ohmeda Excel 410 machine [letter]. Anaesthesia 46:150, 1991.

Olympio MA, Goldstein MM, Mathes DD: Instructional review improves performance of anesthesia apparatus checkout procedures. Anesth Analg 83:618-622, 1996.

Webb RK, Russell WJ, Klepper I, Runciman WB: The Australian Incident Monitoring Study. Equipment failure: An analysis of 2000 incident reports. Anaesth Intensive Care 21:673-677, 1993.

Proportioning Systems

Stewart J. Lustik and Michael P. Eaton

125

Case Synopsis

A healthy 45-year-old woman presents for total abdominal hysterectomy to be done under general anesthesia. After dentirogenation with 100% oxygen (O_2), anesthesia is induced with thiopental. The patient is paralyzed with succinylcholine and easily intubated. Nitrous oxide (N_2O) and isoflurane are added. Desaturation occurs quickly, despite a normal end-tidal carbon dioxide tracing, clear bilateral breath sounds, and normal blood pressure. The O_2 analyzer reads 14%. The flowmeters reveal the delivery of 5 L/minute of N_2O and 0.8 L/minute of O_2.

PROBLEM ANALYSIS

Definition

A hypoxic mixture was delivered to this patient due to a faulty proportioning system. The proportioning system is one of several safety devices designed to prevent the delivery of hypoxic gas mixtures to the patient. A properly functioning proportioning system does not allow the delivery of a mixture of more than 75% N_2O with 25% O_2.

A Link-25 proportion-limiting control system was used on the previously manufactured Modulus, Modulus II, and Excel series, as well as the current Aestiva anesthesia machines produced by GE Healthcare (previously Datex-Ohmeda). The delivery of more than a 3:1 ratio of N_2O to O_2 is prevented by the combination of an interlocking gear mechanism and regulation of the gas inlet pressures. The N_2O control valve has a 24-tooth sprocket, which is connected by a chain to the freewheeling 48-tooth sprocket of the O_2 control valve (Fig. 125-1). N_2O and O_2 control valves

may be moved independently to deliver up to 75% N_2O; however, when the ratio of N_2O to O_2 rises to 3:1, the kick-in tab on the O_2 gear engages with the stop screw on the O_2 control knob. Thus, the N_2O and O_2 control valves become linked. Any further increase in N_2O proportionally increases the O_2 flow to prevent a more than 3:1 ratio. Similarly, an attempt to decrease the O_2 flow would proportionally decrease the N_2O flow to maintain a 3:1 ratio When the N_2O and O_2 control valves are linked, the 2:1 sprocket ratio results in the final 3:1 ratio of gases delivered due to the adjustment of gas inlet pressures. The second-stage N_2O regulator reduces the inlet pressure to 38 ± 0.5 pounds per square inch gauge, and the O_2 regulator is adjusted to 20.75 ± 3.75 pounds per square inch gauge.

The proportioning system of the anesthesia machines manufactured by North American Dräger is called the Oxygen Ratio Controller (ORC) (Fig. 125-2). Supplied O_2 and N_2O are modulated through respective resistors to exert a backpressure on the upper (O_2) and lower (N_2O) diaphragms. This backpressure, in conjunction with the

EQUIPMENT & MONITORING

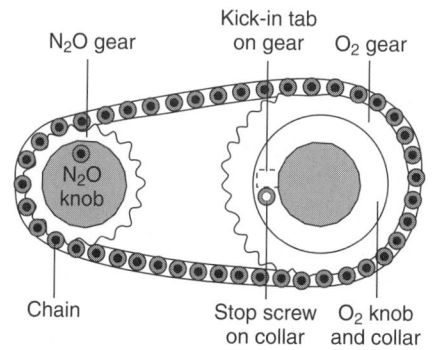
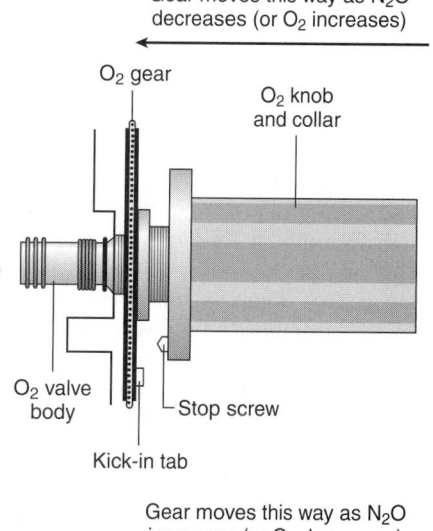

Figure 125–1 ■ Ohmeda Link-25 proportioning system. As the nitrous oxide–to–oxygen (N_2O-to-O_2) ratio increases, the O_2 gear moves toward the O_2 knob. When the N_2O-to-O_2 ratio reaches 3:1, the O_2 gear interfaces with the O_2 knob, and the O_2 and N_2O knobs become linked. (Courtesy of Ohmeda.)

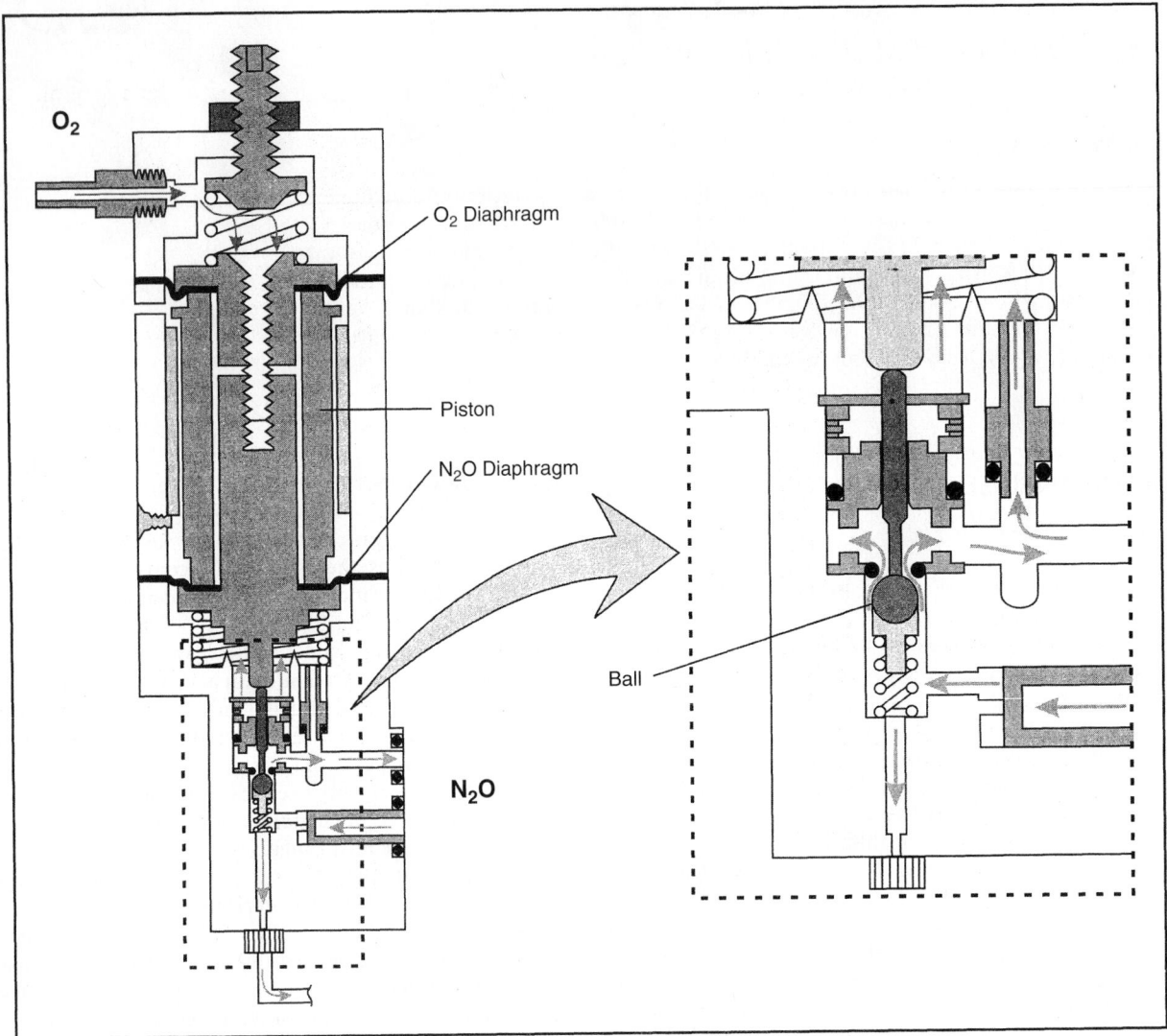

O₂

O₂ Diaphragm

Piston

N₂O Diaphragm

N₂O

Ball

Figure 125–2 ▪ Narkomed Oxygen Ratio Controller. When oxygen (O₂) flow is reduced below 25% ± 3%, O₂ pressure on the upper rolling diaphragm becomes less than nitrous oxide (N₂O) pressure on the lower diaphragm, and the piston moves upward. This allows the spring beneath the ball valve to force the ball valve up, partially occluding the flow of N₂O until a new equilibrium is reached. Increasing the O₂ flow until it is more than 25% ± 3% pushes the piston and ball valve downward to reduce the obstruction to N₂O flow. (Courtesy of North American Dräger.)

differing spring constants of the upper and lower springs, causes movement of a piston attached to the proportioning valve. An increase in N₂O flow beyond 72% to 78% moves the piston, which raises the proportioning valve and limits further N₂O flow. For example, if the O₂ flowmeter is set at 1 L/minute, the ORC will not allow more than 3 L/minute of N₂O. If the N₂O control knob is turned to increase the flow to more than 3 L/minute, the pressure of N₂O on the diaphragm will move the piston to prevent a further increase in N₂O flow. Similarly, if the O₂ flow is reduced to less than 22% to 28%, the N₂O flow will be reduced proportionally to maintain the O₂ percentage required.

The more recently designed anesthesia machine by GE Healthcare (S/5 ADU) uses an electronic proportioning system. The O₂ and N₂O flows are electronically measured, and if the N₂O flow is too high, a current-driven proportional valve limits N₂O flow to allow a minimum of 25% O₂. The proportional valve must be checked for calibration every 6 months.

Recognition

Diagnosis of a faulty proportioning system requires recognition of the signs of mechanical failure, delivery of a hypoxic mixture, receipt of a hypoxic mixture, or all of these:

- Mechanical failure
  - Absence of the audible and palpable "clink" of the Link-25 system when the increase in N₂O flow results in a mixture of more than 75% N₂O.
  - Heights of the N₂O and O₂ flowmeter bobbins or bar graphs indicate a ratio of more than 3:1. A stuck flowmeter bobbin may also be the cause.
- Delivery of a hypoxic mixture
  - Low reading of the O₂ analyzer.
- Receipt of a hypoxic mixture
  - Hypoxia enhances adrenergic tone, leading to tachycardia and hypertension. If uncorrected, it will ultimately lead to bradycardia, hypotension, and asystole.

- Peripheral hemoglobin oxygen desaturation is indicated by pulse oximetry measurements.
- The patient appears cyanotic.

Risk Assessment

Although delivery of a hypoxic mixture due to a broken proportioning system is rare, there are several potential causes of proportioning system failure. First, defective mechanics in the proportioning system may result in the delivery of a hypoxic mixture. There have been case reports of malfunctions of the Link-25 proportioning system on Ohmeda machines. In one case, a broken chain connecting the sprockets allowed N_2O to increase to hypoxic concentrations. The chain on later models was made of stainless steel as opposed to plastic, which increased its tensile strength. In another case, malposition of the O_2 control knob on its stud caused failure of the knob to engage, despite delivery of 100% N_2O. In addition, loosening the stop screw on the collar of the O_2 control knob has led to the delivery of a hypoxic mixture in at least three cases. Although there are no reports to date of failure of the S/5 ADU's electronic proportioning system, a valve failure could lead to delivery of a hypoxic mixture. Mechanical failure on the North American Drager machine is also rare, although defects in any of the ORC components (e.g., diaphragm, spring, piston, adjusting screw, resistor) could lead to the delivery of a hypoxic mixture.

Second, pneumatic components of the Ohmeda machine may fail. If the second-stage O_2 or N_2O regulators on Ohmeda machines lose calibration, delivery of more than 75% N_2O oxide may result. The North American Drager machines do not use second-stage regulators.

Third, electronic components of the S/5 ADU proportioning system may fail, although the N_2O flow is automatically shut off if the total gas flow to the patient is more than the set flows for N_2O plus O_2.

Fourth, a hypoxic mixture or inadvertent N_2O may be delivered to the patient despite a properly functioning proportioning system. This could occur as follows:

- Proportioning systems control only the ratio of O_2 and N_2O; thus, a hypoxic mixture could be delivered if another gas (e.g., helium) is added to the mixture. It is possible to deliver less than 21% O_2 when desflurane is mixed only with air, even with the S/5 ADU, which compensates for desflurane when used with N_2O.
- A gas other than O_2 is in the O_2 pipeline or cylinder.
- There is a leak downstream from the proportioning system, including the O_2 flowmeter.
- The ORC (North American Drager) may result in the inadvertent delivery of N_2O. If the flow of O_2 is reduced while N_2O is delivered at a 3:1 ratio, N_2O will be reduced proportionally. If it is later desired to increase the O_2 concentration, increasing the flow of O_2 will cause N_2O to rise in a 3:1 ratio until the initial N_2O flow is achieved.

Implications

The delivery of a hypoxic mixture may result in arterial O_2 desaturation, organ ischemia, cardiovascular collapse, and eventually death if not corrected.

MANAGEMENT

If delivery of a hypoxic mixture is due to a malfunctioning proportioning system, the N_2O control knob should be shut off. The proportioning system can be bypassed by using the O_2 flush valve or a separate O_2 tank. The anesthesia machine should be removed from use until a service representative can inspect and replace the proportioning system, if necessary.

PREVENTION

The proportioning system should be included in the routine anesthesia machine check before the initiation of anesthesia. The Food and Drug Administration's anesthesia apparatus checkout guidelines recommend, "Attempt to create hypoxic O_2/N_2O mixture, and verify correct change in gas flows and/or alarm." On Ohmeda machines, attempts to increase the N_2O flow to more than a 3:1 ratio with O_2 should proportionally increase the flow of O_2; likewise, attempts to decrease the O_2 flow to less than a 1:3 ratio with N_2O should proportionally decrease N_2O. On the North American Drager and S/5 ADU GE Healthcare anesthesia machines, it should not be possible to increase the N_2O-to-O_2 flow ratio to more than 3:1, and decreasing O_2 below a 1:3 ratio should proportionally decrease the N_2O flow.

Measurement of the fraction of inspired O_2 during anesthesia is required by American Society of Anesthesiologists guidelines. The O_2 analyzer must be calibrated before the administration of anesthesia, because this is the most reliable method of detecting the delivery of a hypoxic mixture. A positive-pressure leak test in the North American Drager machine, and a negative-pressure leak test with Ohmeda machines, must be performed preoperatively to detect a leak downstream from the proportioning system that could lead to the delivery of a hypoxic mixture.

Further Reading

Abraham ZA, Basagoitia J: A potentially lethal anesthesia machine failure. Anesthesiology 6:589-590, 1987.

Anesthesia Apparatus Checkout Recommendations. Rockville, Md, Food and Drug Administration, 1986.

Cheng CJ, Garewal D: A failure of the chain-link mechanism on the Ohmeda Excel 210 anesthesia machine. Anesth Analg 92:913-914, 2001.

Eisendraft JB: The anesthesia machine. In Ehrenwerth J, Eisenkraft JB: Anesthesia Equipment: Principles and Applications. St. Louis, Mosby–Year Book, 1993, pp 43-45.

Gordon PC, James MF, Lapham H, et al: Failure of the proportioning system to prevent hypoxic mixture on a Modulus II Plus anesthesia machine. Anesthesiology 82:598-599, 1995.

Modulus II Anesthesia System Operation and Maintenance Manual. Madison, Wis., Ohmeda, the BOC Group, Inc., 1985.

Narkomed Service Group: Operating Principles of Narkomed Anesthesia Systems, 2nd ed. Telford, Pa., WE Andrews, 1997.

Rice J, Kolek B: Explore the Anesthesia System. Madison, Wis., Ohmeda, 1996, pp 43-44.

Richards C: Failure of a nitrous oxide-oxygen proportioning device. Anesthesiology 71:997-998, 1989.

EQUIPMENT & MONITORING

Oxygen Flush Valve

Ivar Gunnarsson

126

Case Synopsis

At the end of a laparotomy on a 45-year-old asthmatic patient, the oxygen (O_2) flush valve is pressed to clear the circuit of residual volatile agent. The patient's lung inflation pressures become elevated, hypotension develops, and the clinical examination suggests a pneumothorax.

PROBLEM ANALYSIS

Definition

Activating the O_2 flush valve (Fig. 126-1) allows delivery of 100% O_2 directly to the patient's breathing system from the pressure-reducing valve at pressures between 20 and 50 pounds per square inch (equivalent to 1000 to 2500 cm H_2O) and flows of 35 to 75 L/minute (Fig. 126-2). This is 100-fold greater than the pressure normally required to inflate the lungs. Therefore, it is possible to cause direct lung injury (barotrauma) and increased intrathoracic pressure. The latter can impede venous return and cause hypotension. Possible complications resulting from activating the O_2 flush valve and their analysis and causes are listed in Table 126-1.

The American Society for Testing and Materials developed standard specifications for the minimum performance and safety of anesthesia machines. The latest standards, published in 1998 (see "Further Reading"), require that anesthesia machines be equipped with a manually operated, single-purpose flush valve for the delivery of a limited but unmetered flow of O_2 directly to the common gas outlet (i.e., a direct communication between the O_2 high-pressure and the low-pressure circuits). As part of the machine checkout, use of the O_2 flush valve to test for leaks in the low-pressure circuit is inappropriate and can be misleading.

The flush valve should deliver a steady flow of O_2 at not less than 35 L/minute and not more than 75 L/minute. Also, it should deliver O_2 to the common gas outlet without passing through a vaporizer. In addition, the flush valve should have the following characteristics:

- Be permanently marked to show its intended function
- Be designed to minimize unintended accidental operation
- Be self-closing

Recognition

Changes in anesthesia machine design have made it difficult to activate the O_2 flush valve accidentally. The following monitors are intended to alert anesthesia providers to activation of the flush valve or to signal the presence of leaks:

- High-pressure or constant-pressure alarms
- Inspired and expired volatile agent concentrations
- Inspired O_2 and end-tidal carbon dioxide concentrations

The O_2 flush valve can provide a high-pressure O_2 source suitable for jet ventilation when the anesthesia machine is equipped with a one-way check valve positioned between the anesthetic vaporizer and the O_2 flush valve and when a positive-pressure relief valve exists downstream from the anesthetic vaporizer.

Risk Assessment

All patients are at potential risk for complications from inappropriate use of the O_2 flush valve (Table 126-2). A defective or damaged flush valve can stick in the fully open position, compounding the risk of barotrauma or patient awareness. Specific risk factors for other complications are discussed in Table 126-2.

Implications

Inappropriate use of the O_2 flush valve can have severe consequences for the patient.

- Barotrauma can progress to pneumothorax and cardiovascular collapse.
- Compensating for leaks can lead to awareness, hypoxia, and hypercapnia.

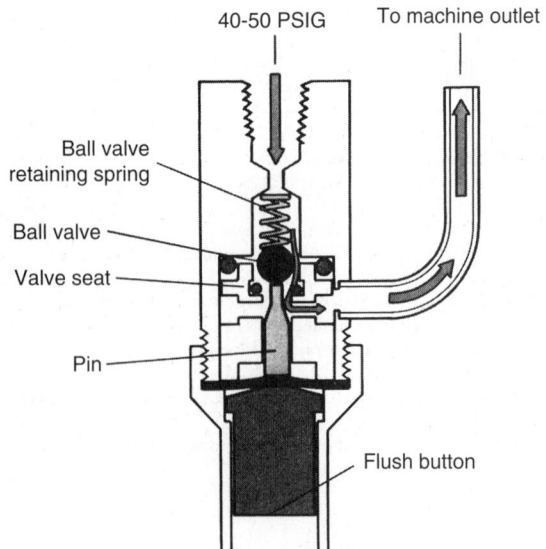

Figure 126–1 ■ Oxygen flush valve in the open position. (Courtesy of Ohmeda Inc., Madison, Wis.)

Figure 126–2 ■ Position of the oxygen flush valve in a machine circuit. (Courtesy of Ohmeda Inc., Madison, Wisc.)

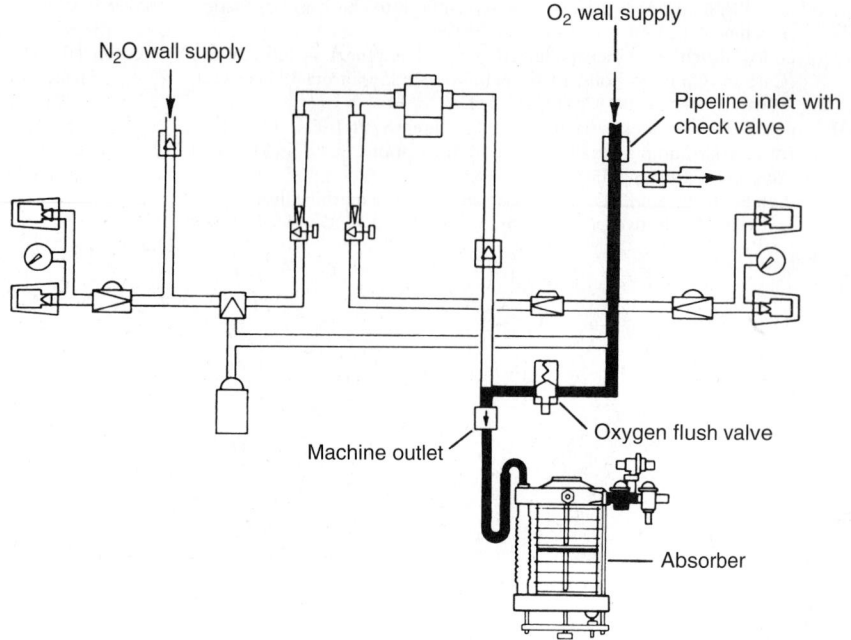

• Inability to ventilate can lead to hypoxemia, with consequent brain damage.

MANAGEMENT

The potential for barotrauma can be limited by early recognition and by the use of appropriate monitoring. Pneumothorax may require the insertion of a chest tube. Other complications are largely preventable.

PREVENTION

Disconnecting the patient from the anesthesia breathing circuit before activating the O_2 flush valve can eliminate the risk of pneumothorax. Familiarity with the anesthesia machine and performance of the standard preoperative checks, as recommended by each manufacturer, can also minimize the risk of undetected leaks. Finally, a pressure-limiting device at the common gas outlet should alert the anesthetist that the machine cannot be used for temporary jet ventilation in an emergency.

Table 126–2 ■ Risk Factors for Complications with Oxygen Flush Valves

Complication	Risk Factor
Barotrauma	Small patients with low-volume lungs or patients with low lung compliance
Awareness	Repeated use of the O_2 flush valve to refill the rebreathing bag when gas is being lost from the circuit
Masking of machine leaks	Risk is greater if the user is unfamiliar with the anesthesia machine, if inappropriate checks are performed before use, and if the machine has recently been serviced
Inability to ventilate	During thoracic surgery with an open bronchus or with emergent transtracheal jet ventilation, the machine may be incapable of delivering high flows owing to its design

Table 126–1 ■ Potential Complications with Oxygen Flush Valves

Complication	Analysis and Cause
Barotrauma	High gas flows at high pressures
Awareness	Bypassing the vaporizer leads to dilution of volatile anesthetic agent
Masking of machine leak	Using the flush valve to pressurize the breathing system closes any check valve between the vaporizers and the common gas outlet and prevents detection of leaks by the machine's internal components
Inability to ventilate	When high flows or pressures are required (e.g., open bronchus, transtracheal jet ventilation), a nonworking valve or pressure-limiting mechanism at the common gas outlet reduces flow

Further Reading

Berner MS: Profound hypercapnia due to disconnection within an anesthetic machine. Can J Anaesth 34:622-626, 1987.

Comm G, Rendell-Baker L: Back pressure check valves: A hazard. Anesthesiology 56:327-328, 1982.

Davies AO: Detecting disconnections within anesthetic machines. Can J Anaesth 35:437-438, 1988.

Dodgson BG: Inappropriate use of the oxygen flush to check an anesthetic machine. Can J Anaesth 35:436-437, 1988.

Dorsch JA, Dorsch SE: Understanding Anesthesia Equipment: Construction, Care and Complications, 4th ed. Baltimore, JB Lippincott–Williams & Wilkins, 1999, pp 96-97, 412, 942-944.

Eisenkraft JB: The anesthesia machine. In Ehrenwerth J, Eisenkraft JB: Anesthesia Equipment: Principles and Applications. St. Louis, Mosby–Year Book, 1993, pp 35-37.

Gaughan SD, Benumof JL, Ozaki GT: Can an anesthesia machine flush valve provide for effective jet ventilation? Anesth Analg 76:800-808, 1993.

Miller R: Oxygen flush valve. In Miller's Anesthesia, 6th ed. Philadelphia, Churchill Livingstone, 2004, pp 283-284.

Newton NI: Safety in the operating theatre: The meaning of excessive pressure. Br J Hosp Med 25:504-509, 1981.

Standard Specification for Minimum Performance and Safety Requirements for Components and Systems of Anesthesia Gas Machines (F29.01.09), sec 10. Philadelphia, American Society for Testing and Materials, 1998.

Anesthesia Circuit

127

Ramachandran Satya-Krishna

Case Synopsis

A 57-year-old woman who is a heavy smoker experiences a difficult endotracheal intubation during induction of anesthesia. Mask ventilation is also difficult, owing to the high inspiratory pressures needed for ventilation and a poor mask fit. This results in a considerable leak between the mask and the face. The first and subsequent attempts at intubation lead to a stiff bag and the lack of a carbon dioxide (CO_2) waveform on the capnogram. After each attempt, esophageal intubation is diagnosed, and the tube is quickly removed. After each attempted tracheal intubation, mask ventilation becomes progressively more difficult. Throughout this episode, the patient becomes intermittently hypotensive. About 30 minutes after induction, an observer notices that the expiratory check valve of the anesthesia breathing system remained seated during the entire breathing cycle. Replacement of the valve solves the problem, and ventilation becomes possible. Thus, this "cannot ventilate, cannot intubate" scenario has an unexpected "twist."

PROBLEM ANALYSIS

Definition

The anesthetic breathing system (ABS) is defined by the American Society for Testing and Materials as "a gas pathway in direct connection with the patient through which gas flows occur at respiratory pressures, in which directional valves may be present, and into which a mixture of controlled composition may be dispensed." An important component of the ABS, the CO_2 absorber, is discussed in Chapter 129. Almost every medical device carries at least some risk for misuse or failure. ABSs lend themselves to critical incidents and patient injury because of multiple mechanical components and connections (Table 127-1) and variations in manufacture and design. A listing of possible ABS failures is given in Table 127-2.

Critical incidents involving ABSs can be classified broadly as equipment misuse and equipment failure. The following definitions were used in the American Society of Anesthesiologists (ASA) closed claims analysis and accurately describe the various ABS-related issues. Equipment *misuse* refers to incidents originating from human fault or error associated with the preparation, maintenance, or deployment of a medical device. In contrast, equipment *failure* refers to a situation in which the device appears to malfunction unexpectedly, despite routine maintenance and previous uneventful use. One example of the latter is a unidirectional valve on the ABS that suddenly fails to open. A *disconnect* is defined as the loss of attachment or continuity in an ABS that was initially configured in a functional and conventional manner. A *misconnect* is a nonfunctional and unconventional configuration of the ABS components or attachments.

The situation described in the case synopsis represents one of the many potentially lethal or injurious complications

Table 127–1 ■ Components of the Circle System

Fresh gas flow inlet
Inspiratory limb
Expiratory limb
Respiratory check valves
Carbon dioxide absorber
Y-piece
Ventilator reservoir bag
APL (pop-off) valve
Anesthetic gas scavenging system

APL, airway pressure limiting.

Table 127–2 ■ Possible Anesthesia Breathing Circuit Failures

Disconnection
See Table 127-1 for possible sites of disconnection
Blockage (Raised Airway Pressure)
Mechanical distortion
Foreign body within circuit
Heated hoses
Improperly connected scavenging system
Water condensation
Slowly progressing block of microbial filters
Leaks (Lowered Airway Pressure)
Inspiratory limb
Expiratory limb
Any other tube or small connection
Valve Malfunction
Obstruction or incompetence
Reverse flow or rebreathing
Carbon Dioxide Absorber Failure
Exhausted soda lime
Carbon monoxide production
Dry soda lime
Overheating
Retained canister wrapping
Contamination
Microbes, viruses
Particulate matter

related to the ABS. In fact, according to the most extensive surveys available, the ABS is the leading cause of critical incidents, with disconnections being the single most frequent cause. Obstruction within the expiratory limb of the ABS, however, can be one of the most rapidly injurious incidents. With a closed expiratory system, gases entering the lungs cannot exit, and airway pressure increases rapidly to a level at which the lungs may rupture.

Recognition

Recognition of ABS problems can be extremely difficult, as illustrated in the case synopsis. These incidents are potential time bombs, because they do not seem to be related to anything done by the anesthesiologist, such as turning a dial, injecting a drug, or inserting an endotracheal tube. Unless a high index of suspicion is present, the anesthesiologist may concentrate on more likely causes—in this case, esophageal intubation. Contemporary monitors alone may offer little help with ABS problems. In the ASA closed claims analysis, however, reviewers judged that appropriate monitoring could have prevented injury in 78% of gas delivery claims. More importantly, in 21% of claims, a critical mechanical monitor or alarm (e.g., high- or low-pressure circuit alarm) had been turned off, broken, or omitted. In a very small minority of claims, better monitoring would not have improved the outcome when the initiating event progressed rapidly to injury.

Above all, the most important monitor is a vigilant anesthetist who monitors breath sounds and chest wall excursions and continually observes the monitors. A simulation and discussion of the events that transpired in the case synopsis are provided in Figure 127-1.

Risk Assessment

All patients having general anesthesia are at risk for ABS-related complications. High tidal volumes, high respiratory rates, and fresh gas flows increase this risk, especially in small patients.

Patients with lung disease, especially those with emphysematous bullae, are especially susceptible to injury produced by increased airway pressure (barotrauma). The state of anesthesia decreases protective cardiovascular reflexes and contributes to cardiovascular compromise during positive-pressure ventilation. Rapidly rising airway pressure quickly impedes venous return, which reduces stroke volume and arterial pressure, even in healthy patients. This may be more evident in patients with decreased blood volume or impaired cardiac function.

In the seminal report by Cooper and colleagues, the following ABS-related incidents ranked high on the list of critical problems: ABS circuit disconnection during mechanical ventilation (5.2%), ABS circuit leak (1.7%), ABS circuit misconnection (1.7%), and ABS control errors (1.4%). ABS control errors most often involved maladjustment of the airway pressure limiting (APL) valve; this is especially true on older machines, where the APL valve had to be shut off when the ventilator was turned on. In Cooper's report, critical incidents related to the ABS accounted for 10% of all incidents. The Australian survey of critical incidents revealed similar results: ABS circuit disconnection (6%), partial failure

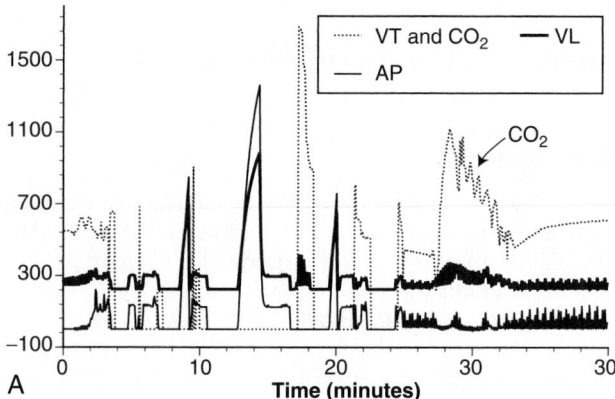

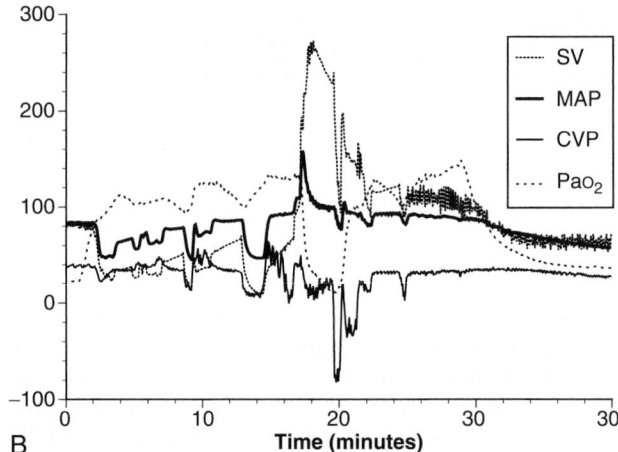

Figure 127–1 ■ Simulation of the case synopsis. Anesthesia is induced with 5 mg/kg of thiopental and 1.5 mg/kg of succinylcholine. Repeated doses of thiopental and succinylcholine are necessary to optimize conditions in a difficult situation. *A,* A recording of the ventilatory and airway variables during the simulation. Tidal volume (VT) and the carbon dioxide (CO_2) curve are never satisfactory after apnea has been induced, but this was attributed to the "cannot ventilate" situation. Airway pressure (AP) and lung volume (VL) increase rapidly and markedly every time the Y-piece is connected to the sealed endotracheal tube. The leaking mask prevents dangerous increases during mask ventilation. After denitrogenation, as long as an oxygen (O_2) supply is connected to the airway, there will be sufficient O_2 to keep the SpO_2 above 100%. *B,* A recording of cardiovascular and blood gas variables during the simulation. PaO_2 remains at a satisfactory level, despite all the "airway" problems; SpO_2 never decreases below 100% (not shown). Mean arterial pressure (MAP) and stroke volume (SV) dive precipitously every time the Y-piece is connected to the sealed endotracheal tube. The last response is related to the enormously and rapidly increased airway pressure seen in *A*. Note, for example, the marked and simultaneous decrease in central venous pressure (CVP), MAP, and SV in *B* with increases in airway pressure in *A*.

to ventilate or a circuit leak (5.2%), and unidirectional valve malfunction (3%). In that report, the total number of incidents related to the ABS was 282 (14.1%). In the ASA closed claims analysis, equipment misuse was three times more common than equipment failure (75% versus 24%). Two thirds of all claims involving equipment misuse resulted directly (in fact, almost exclusively) from the actions of the primary anesthesia care provider.

Causes of or contributors to ABS problems include wear and tear, damaged components, improper or infrequent maintenance, improper assembly, carelessness, and failure to check the anesthesia workstation before use. Failure to check equipment is a common factor in a large proportion of critical incidents. In the survey by Cooper and colleagues, 20.5% of incidents involved failure to check; in the Australian survey, failure to check was involved in 11.8% of all incidents.

In the ASA closed claims analysis, the most frequent sites of disconnections and misconnections were the junction between the ABS circuit and the gas delivery ventilator outlet, the junction between the distal breathing circuit and the endotracheal tube, and a configuration of the inspiratory limb of the ABS circuit that allowed the interposition of a positive end-expiratory pressure valve. Other causes of initiating events were operator errors (e.g., failure to turn on a device, selection of a wrong knob or dial, faulty valve installation).

Implications

Consequences of ABS circuit complications can be disastrous. During the past 2 decades, a few large-scale surveys of anesthetic outcome have examined gas delivery equipment as the cause of serious injury. These studies attribute 1% to 5% of anesthesia-related deaths and brain injuries to problems with gas delivery equipment. The ASA closed claims project provides similar data, with gas delivery equipment accounting for 2.7% of claims for death (34 of 1277) and 4.5% of claims for brain damage (21 of 466). Cooper and colleagues listed 9 ABS-related incidents in 67 patients with "substantive negative outcomes," or 13.4% of such outcomes. Circulatory collapse, ruptured lungs, and severe hypoxia were three of the major adverse outcomes.

Although gas delivery equipment plays a prominent role in critical incident studies, often contributing to more than 20% of all reported events, claims involving gas delivery equipment account for less than 2% (72 of 3791) of the overall ASA closed claims database. Critical incidents are events that have the potential to cause injury; fortunately, many critical incidents are detected and remedied before an identifiable injury occurs. In previous studies, only 17% to 26% of incidents were associated with a major physiologic change, morbidity, or death. Thus, it can be surmised that inadequate responses to critical incidents cause patient injury in the vast majority of cases. Equipment misuse accounts for the significant majority of ABS-related complications and was three times more common than equipment failure in the ASA closed claims analysis. Previous studies have also stressed the prominent role of human error in equipment-related critical incidents and adverse outcomes. This fact explains the disproportionately high incidence of complications with the ABS, compared with more complex ventilators, vaporizers, and anesthesia machines.

Another interesting feature of ABS claims is that misconnections were as prevalent as disconnections. This differs from critical incident studies, in which disconnections are significantly more common, as discussed earlier. This reflects a key difference in the speed of evolution of high- and low-pressure injuries to the airway. Misconnections typically occur in an intact circuit and thereby lead to high airway pressure and the potential for pneumothorax. In contrast, the evolution of hypoxia and hypercapnia caused by disconnections may be slow enough to permit safe management of the problem before patient injury occurs. This underscores the importance of using ABS circuit monitors that can issue prompt alarms for high- and low-pressure conditions.

Thus, human error plays a major role in the initiation and propagation of ABS complications. Patient injury from ABS complications is characterized by high severity of injury and high cost. The ABS circuit represents the single largest source of claims related to gas delivery equipment, and almost all these claims result from misconnections or disconnections.

MANAGEMENT

Management, especially if an ABS-related condition is recognized relatively early, is usually simple. Sometimes a malfunctioning anesthesia machine must be replaced intraoperatively, and this is not a trivial or a brief matter. While this exchange is taking place, or often while a diagnosis is being confirmed, a method should be devised to supply oxygen, ventilation, and anesthesia independently. The equipment for these maneuvers should always be available in every operating room, perhaps in the form of a self-inflating resuscitation bag and an accessory oxygen flowmeter on the anesthesia workstation.

PREVENTION

The optimal way to prevent ABS-related incidents is the anesthesia workstation checkout. The Food and Drug Administration (FDA) compiled a formal list for this checkout in 1986, with the most recent revision occurring in 1993. A summary pertinent to the ABS is given in Table 127-3. Checkout protocols typically entail four basic activities: verification of backup equipment and supplies (e.g., pressurized gas cylinders), inspection of equipment configurations (e.g., breathing circuit connections), inspection of equipment mechanics (e.g., proper action of unidirectional valves), and preparation of monitors (e.g., calibration, verification of function, and activation of alarms). The ASA closed claims analysis revealed that better selection and use of monitoring equipment could have prevented the vast majority of complications in gas delivery system claims.

In the case synopsis, the simple act of disconnecting the Y-piece from the inspiratory and expiratory limbs of the ABS and trying to breathe in and out through both of them individually would have increased the chances of preventing this disaster.

Because of the serious implications of high airway pressures, an alarm alone may not provide clinicians with enough time for alarm recognition, diagnosis of the problem, and appropriate remedial action. For this reason, every anesthetic workstation must have a fixed breathing pressure limiting protection module (BPLPM) whose maximum pressure cannot exceed 125 cm H_2O (12.5 kPa). Further, modern anesthesia workstations must have an *adjustable* BPLPM if the fixed BPLPM is greater than 80 cm H_2O. If there is no ventilator, or if the anesthesia workstation is in the manual or spontaneous mode, the reservoir bag may be considered

Table 127–3 ■ **Food and Drug Administration Recommendations for Anesthesia Checkout Pertinent to Anesthesia Breathing Circuit**

Initial status of the breathing system
    Set selector switch in "bag" mode
    Check that breathing circuit is complete, undamaged, and unobstructed
    Verify that CO_2 absorbent is adequate
    Install breathing circuit accessory equipment (e.g., humidifier, PEEP valve) to be used during the case
Leak check of breathing system
    Set all gas flows to zero (or minimum)
    Close APL (pop-off) valve and occlude Y-piece
    Pressurize breathing system to 30 cm H_2O with O_2 flush
    Open APL valve and ensure that pressure decreases
Ventilation system and unidirectional valves
    Place second breathing bag on Y-piece
    Set appropriate ventilator parameters for next patient
    Switch to automatic ventilation (ventilator) mode
    Fill bellows and second breathing bag with O_2 flush and then turn ventilator on
    Set O_2 flow to minimum and other gas flows to zero
    Verify that, during inspiration, bellows delivers appropriate tidal volume, and during exhalation, bellows fills completely
    Set fresh gas flow to about 5 L/min
    Verify that ventilator bellows and simulated lungs fill and empty appropriately and without sustained pressure at end-exhalation
Check for proper action of unidirectional valves
Examine breathing circuit accessories to ensure proper function
Turn ventilator off and switch to manual ventilation (bag/APL) mode
Ventilate manually and ensure inflation and deflation of artificial lungs and appropriate feel of system resistance and compliance
Remove second breathing bag from Y-piece

APL, airway pressure limiting; PEEP, positive end-expiratory pressure.

an APL protection module. However, a BPLPM would have offered limited protection in the case synopsis, because expired gases could not reach the bag or the ventilator owing to the obstructed expiratory check valve.

In summary, suspicion, observation, and compulsive attention to detail can contribute to the prevention, recognition, and management of ABS-related complications. The anesthesiologist's motto of "vigilance" is important at all times; however, to prevent ABS complications, unremitting vigilance is required. Acute increases in airway pressure and complete loss of tidal volume due to leaks are true emergencies that may present during anesthesia and may cause fatal or crippling injuries in a matter of seconds.

Further Reading

Adams AP: Breathing system disconnections. Br J Anaesth 73:46-54, 1994.
Anesthesia Apparatus Checkout Recommendations, 1993. Federal Register, July 11, 1994 (59 FR 35373).
ASTM F1208 (Anesthesia breathing systems). In Medical Devices, Emergency Medical Services. 13.01. West Conshohocken, Pa., American Society for Testing and Materials, 1994.
Caplan R, Vistica M, Posner K, et al: Adverse anesthetic outcomes arising from gas delivery equipment: A closed claims analysis. Anesthesiology: 87:741-778, 1997.
Cooper JB, Newbower RS, Kitz RJ: An analysis of major errors and equipment failures in anesthesia management: Considerations for prevention and detection. Anesthesiology 60:34-42, 1984.
Russell WJ, et al: Problems with ventilation: An analysis of 2000 incident reports. Anaesth Intensive Care 21:617-620, 1993.
Webb RK, et al: Equipment failure: An analysis of 2000 incident reports. Anaesth Intensive Care 21:673-677, 1993.
Webb RK, et al: Which monitor: An analysis of 2000 incident reports. Anaesth Intensive Care 21:529-542, 1993.

Vaporizers

Mark Abel and James B. Eisenkraft

128

Case Synopsis

A 34-year-old woman, who is American Society of Anesthesiologists physical status I, undergoes general anesthesia for total abdominal hysterectomy. The anesthesia vaporizer dial is set to deliver 1% isoflurane. Her blood pressure is noted to be 60/40 mm Hg, and the calibrated respiratory gas analyzer shows an inspired isoflurane concentration of 4%.

PROBLEM ANALYSIS

Definition

Assuming that the agent analyzer reading is correct (see Chapter 141), the breathing circuit contains an agent concentration that greatly exceeds the one set on the concentration dial. This may be due to malfunction of the vaporizer or to the presence of liquid anesthetic agent in the breathing circuit. Vaporizer problems that result in increased anesthetic vapor concentration include tipping, overfilling, use of the oxygen (O_2) flush valve upstream of a freestanding vaporizer, and gas flow reversal through a vaporizer. High concentrations of a potent inhaled agent also may result from the presence of volatile anesthetic liquid in the patient breathing circuit.

Recognition

The common factor in all these situations is an anesthetic agent concentration that exceeds the one intended. This manifests as clinical and hemodynamic signs of anesthetic overdose and, in the case synopsis, low blood pressure. Measurement of the agent concentration in the breathing circuit is critical to making a correct diagnosis. Before locating the source of the excess agent, the clinician should immediately disconnect the patient from the breathing circuit and ventilate the patient's lungs with an alternative system, such as a self-inflating resuscitation bag (e.g., Ambu bag) or another anesthesia circuit connected to an O_2 source.

Some investigative work is required to distinguish whether the problem is with the vaporizer or the breathing circuit. Because almost all potent volatile anesthetics are delivered with the use of machine-mounted, calibrated, agent-specific vaporizers, the vaporizer concentration dial is set to a certain value (e.g., 1%), and the concentration of agent in the gas flowing from the common gas outlet (CGO) of the anesthesia machine is sampled and analyzed. The CGO is the sampling point in the delivery system that is closest to the vaporizer outlet. With the fresh gas flow set to 5 L/minute of the carrier gas (air for Dräger vaporizers; O_2 for Ohmeda and Penlon vaporizers), the vaporizer is calibrated at the factory; the concentration dial is set to 1%, and the concentration of agent in the gas flowing from the CGO is measured with the use of a calibrated agent analyzer. The measured concentration should be within 10% to 15%

of the vapor concentration dial setting (e.g., if the dial is set to 1%, the concentration measured should be between 0.85% and 1.15%) if the vaporizer is in calibration (according to manufacturers' specifications).

If a higher concentration is detected, it is likely that the problem is with the vaporizer and not the breathing circuit. If the measured agent concentration agrees with the dial setting concentration, the likely problem is liquid agent in the anesthesia circuit. In the unlikely event that a freestanding vaporizer is being used (i.e., one placed in series between the CGO of the machine and the breathing circuit), it should be inspected to ensure that the direction of fresh gas flow through the vaporizer is correct (i.e., the fresh gas enters via the vaporizer inflow, not the outflow, connection).

Risk Assessment

VAPORIZER MALFUNCTION

Contemporary anesthesia vaporizers are concentration calibrated, with the exception of the Ohmeda Tec 6 (desflurane) vaporizer, which is of the variable-bypass design. A variable-bypass vaporizer splits the incoming fresh gas into two pathways. Most of the gas flows through a bypass and is not exposed to anesthetic vapor, whereas a lesser flow enters the vaporizing chamber and emerges with the anesthetic agent at its saturated vapor concentration. When the two flows mix at the vaporizer outlet, the greater bypass flow mixes with the vaporizing chamber output to produce the desired (dialed-in) concentration.

OVERFILLING AND TIPPING

Overfilling or tipping of a vaporizer can cause liquid agent from the vaporizing chamber (or sump chamber) to enter the bypass, which is designed for respiratory gases (e.g., O_2, nitrous oxide, air, nitrogen, helium) and vapor only. This can lead to the delivery of a lethal concentration of anesthetic agent to the patient circuit. In the United States, vaporizers may be of the funnel-fill or key-fill design, whereas in Canada, the key-fill design is mandated. Funnel-fill vaporizers should be inspected during filling to ensure that the level of liquid in the sump chamber does not exceed the maximum fill line indicated on the sight glass. Overfilling of key-fill vaporizers has been extensively described. Key-fill systems are designed for use with an airtight joint between the bottle containing the anesthetic liquid and the matching vaporizer, with the vaporizer dial turned to the off position. Correct use prevents overfilling by two mechanisms. First, intake of air into the bottle of anesthetic agent is interrupted when filling has reached the maximum safe level of liquid in the vaporizing chamber. Second, when the vaporizer is in the off position, the air space at the top of the vaporizing chamber is sealed, thereby preventing overfilling. Because filling of a key-fill vaporizer is slow, this has led to improper practices to expedite the process. Such practices include loosening the seal between the bottle and vaporizer, which allows direct entry of room air into the bottle, and turning the concentration dial to the "on" position. This double-fault condition allows an excessive amount of air to enter the agent bottle and, therefore, an excessive amount of liquid agent to enter the vaporizer. Such vaporizer overfilling has led to anesthetic overdose and neurologic injury.

PUMPING EFFECT

The pumping effect may result from intermittent back-pressure applied to the vaporizer through pressure changes downstream in the breathing system. Such pressure changes may be caused by intermittent positive-pressure ventilation in the patient circuit or normal operation of the O_2 flush. Gas flow distribution changes within the vaporizer may occur, leading to increased vapor concentration output. This effect is greatest at low fresh gas flow rates, at low concentration dial settings, when small amounts of liquid agent are present in the vaporizer sump, and with large, rapid changes in pressure. Although the mechanism is not completely understood, it is likely that gas is compressed in the vaporizer (in both the vaporizing chamber and the bypass) during pressurization. When the pressure decreases, anesthetic vapor leaves the vaporizing chamber through both the normal exit and the vaporizing chamber inlet, resulting in vapor in the bypass flow. This effectively increases the vapor output.

FREESTANDING VAPORIZERS

Although modern delivery systems involve the use of vaporizers that are securely mounted to a manifold on the anesthesia machine, freestanding vaporizers are still used on cardiopulmonary bypass machines, in veterinary facilities, in laboratories, and sometimes during clinical trials of investigational inhaled volatile agents. Freestanding vaporizers are especially hazardous for several reasons. Tipping of a freestanding vaporizer is a long-recognized problem that has resulted in cardiac arrest; it may result in dramatically increased vaporizer concentration outputs compared with the concentration dial setting. Tipping of a variable-bypass vaporizer, by tilting either a freestanding unit or the entire anesthesia machine, may result in liquid agent entering the vaporizer bypass or the gas outlet pathway of the vaporizing chamber, resulting in an overdose of potent inhaled agent.

Reversal of the direction of gas flow through a variable-bypass, concentration-calibrated, agent-specific vaporizer can profoundly affect its performance, depending on the model. With freestanding vaporizers in clinical practice, this has been reported to result in dangerously high concentrations of volatile anesthetics. Finally, unauthorized tampering with an anesthesia machine could result in reversed gas flow connections to the vaporizer manifold.

Although never clinically reported, a laboratory study has shown that application of the O_2 flush valve upstream of a variable-bypass vaporizer results in delivered anesthetic concentrations that exceed the concentration dial setting. Although the increases in delivered anesthetic concentrations were transient and resulted in a maximum agent concentration of 2.1% in excess of that set on the concentration dial, it is theoretically possible for increased anesthetic delivery to occur in a clinical setting in which application of the O_2 flush valve is required.

LIQUID AGENT IN THE PATIENT BREATHING CIRCUIT

Liquid volatile anesthetic agent may enter the breathing circuit either intentionally or unintentionally. Deliberate administration of volatile anesthetic agent directly into the breathing circuit is typically done into the expiratory limb. If this is performed in an uncontrolled fashion, liquid volatile agent in the circuit may produce vapor concentrations that greatly exceed safe levels, because the saturated vapor concentrations of these liquids at 1 atmosphere and 20°C range from 21% for sevoflurane to 87% for desflurane, with other agents having intermediate values. One milliliter of liquid agent produces approximately 200 mL of vapor at 20°C and 1 atmosphere (Table 128-1). Because a typical adult circle breathing circuit (with 5-foot-long inspiratory and expiratory limbs) has a volume of approximately 7 L, 1 mL of a volatile anesthetic liquid in such a circuit will produce a concentration of nearly 3% (approximately 200 mL/7000 mL) on complete mixing. Incomplete mixing can result in far greater concentrations. The delivered concentrations resulting from volatile liquid in the circuit are potentially lethal if excessive volatile liquid enters the circuit or mixing is inadequate. If unexpectedly high concentrations of a potent volatile agent are detected, and analysis of the gas emerging from the machine CGO excludes a problem with the vaporizer, the presence of a volatile agent in the circuit may be confirmed by sampling the gas in the patient breathing system.

Implications

Anesthetic agent concentrations that exceed those set on the vaporizer concentration dial may result in complications ranging from mild hemodynamic instability to total cardiovascular collapse. All potent inhaled agents are myocardial

Table 128–1 ▪ Volume of Anesthetic Vapor per Milliliter of Liquid Anesthetic at 20°C	
Anesthetic	**Vapor/Liquid (mL/mL)**
Desflurane	182
Enflurane	195
Halothane	226
Isoflurane	196
Sevoflurane	182

From Eisenkraft JB: Anesthesia vaporizers. In Ehrenwerth J, Eisenkraft JB (eds): Anesthesia Equipment: Principles and Applications. St. Louis, Mosby–Year Book, 1993, pp 57-88.

depressants and peripheral vasodilators. Liquid agent in the breathing circuit that reaches the patient directly is especially dangerous.

MANAGEMENT

An anesthetic agent analyzer with the appropriate high-concentration alarm limits set, although not currently a standard of care, is critical because this is the most sensitive way to detect excessive concentrations. Standard monitors, including electrocardiogram and blood pressure monitors, are critical for detecting the hemodynamic consequences of such potential overdoses. If the patient is breathing spontaneously, changes in the respiratory pattern may be noted. When vapor concentrations greatly exceed the concentration dial setting, an alternative breathing system should be immediately available (as recommended in 1993 by the Food and Drug Administration); then the source of the excess anesthetic agent should be found, as described earlier. Hemodynamic supportive measures should be used as appropriate.

PREVENTION

Overfilling a vaporizer can be avoided by not exceeding the maximum fill line in the sight glass and, in the case of key-fill vaporizers, by following the manufacturer's instructions (i.e., filling the vaporizer with the dial set to the "off" position and ensuring an airtight seal between the key-filling nozzle and the vaporizer).

Modern vaporizers have incorporated certain design features that minimize the significance of the pumping effect. Some older vaporizer models, such as the Ohio Calibrated Vaporizer, have a check valve in the vaporizer outlet to prevent transmission of increases in downstream pressure. Some delivery systems contain a check valve downstream of the vaporizer (e.g., Ohmeda Modulus I, Modulus II, and Ohmeda Excel). These valves prevent transmission of downstream pressures back to a vaporizer that lacks modern design features, and they are intended to prevent the pumping effect. It should be noted, however, that when the check valve is closed, the pressure upstream of it, and hence in the vaporizer, increases because of continuous fresh gas flow

from the machine flowmeters; therefore, the use of downstream check valves limits, but does not eliminate, the risk of the pumping effect. A level anesthesia machine avoids the problems associated with machine tipping with machine-mounted anesthesia vaporizers. If a vaporizer is inadvertently tipped, it should be purged with high fresh gas flow from the machine flowmeters, with the vaporizer concentration dial turned to the highest setting, until no trace of the agent is detectable. The vaporizer is then refilled, and the output is checked as described earlier. The temperature of the vaporizer should be allowed to stabilize for 2 hours before its next clinical use.

Freestanding vaporizers are potentially more hazardous than machine-mounted ones. They generally are used only in laboratory and veterinary facilities, but Ohmeda vaporizers may be mounted on cardiopulmonary bypass machines with a specially designed bracket available from Ohmeda. When such freestanding vaporizers are used, care should be taken to avoid tipping during both transport and use. Fresh gas inflow and outflow connections to the vaporizer should be checked to ensure that they are not reversed, because reversal of these connections may result in increased vapor concentration output.

The proper use of a vaporizer limits the potential for malfunctions that may result in overdose of an anesthetic agent. If such a malfunction occurs, analysis of the gas in the breathing circuit should lead to prompt recognition and appropriate action to prevent harm to the patient.

Further Reading

Eisenkraft JB: Anesthesia vaporizers. In Ehrenwerth J, Eisenkraft JB (eds): Anesthesia Equipment: Principles and Applications. St. Louis, Mosby–Year Book, 1993, pp 57-88.

Greg AS, Jones RS, Snowdon SL: Flow reversal through a Mark III halothane vaporizer. Br J Anaesth 71:303-304, 1993.

Hardy JF: Vaporizer overfilling [editorial]. Can J Anaesth 40:1-3, 1993.

Kelly DA: Free-standing vaporizers: Another hazard. Anaesthesia 40:661-663, 1985.

Philip JH: Closed circuit anesthesia. In Ehrenwerth J, Eisenkraft JB (eds): Anesthesia Equipment: Principles and Applications. St. Louis, Mosby–Year Book, 1993, pp 617-635.

Ralton R, Inglis MD: High halothane concentrations from reversed flow in a vaporizer. Anaesthesia 41:672-673, 1986.

Rosenwarne FA, Duncan IN: Reversed connexions of free-standing vaporizers. Anaesthesia 45:338-339, 1990.

Sinclair A, Van Bergen J: Vaporizer overfilling. Can J Anaesth 40:77-78, 1993.

Carbon Dioxide Absorbers

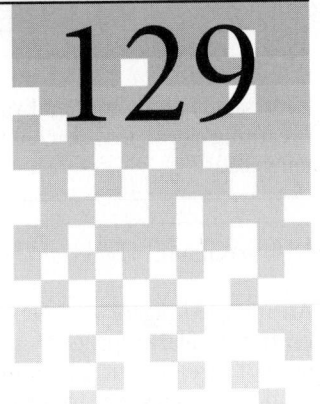

129

Gaury S. Adhikary

Case Synopsis

A 40-year-old, 70-kg man undergoes an exploratory laparotomy while under general anesthesia with the use of a semiclosed circuit. Thirty minutes into the surgery, he is noted to have an end-tidal carbon dioxide (CO_2) level of 55 mm Hg with a constant minute ventilation of 7 L/minute.

PROBLEM ANALYSIS

Definition

Hypercarbia under general anesthesia can be caused by CO_2 absorber-related problems (e.g., exhausted CO_2 absorber; channeling of gases through the granules, causing inefficient removal of CO_2 from the circuit) (Fig. 129-1). Hypercarbia also may be due to increased dead space and rebreathing brought about by sticky or leaking inspiratory or expiratory valves. Mild hypercarbia during constant minute ventilation is usually due to increased CO_2 production as a result of increased catecholamine levels with light anesthesia or stress. The extremely rapid increase in CO_2 production accompanying malignant hyperthermia manifests as severe hypercarbia, along with progressive hypoxemia and acidosis, despite constant minute ventilation.

Recognition

Problems with CO_2 absorbers can present as follows:

- Increased end-tidal CO_2 tension (rising plateau in capnography)
- Phase III of capnography trace fails to touch the baseline (rebreathing pattern)
- Increased ventilatory drive reflected by overriding of the ventilator
- Hypertension, arrhythmias, or hypotension
- Excessive sweating, increased oozing from the wound
- CO_2 absorbent feels "too warm" to the touch

CO_2 absorption by soda lime or barium hydroxide lime (Baralyme) in the anesthetic circuit generates heat, so a CO_2 absorbent normally feels warm to the touch if it is absorbing CO_2 properly. Excessive production of CO_2 is reflected by excessive production of heat by the CO_2 absorbent, so the CO_2 canister will feel hot as opposed to warm.

The chemistry of CO_2 absorption by soda lime and Baralyme is as follows:

A. Soda Lime

1. $$CO_2 + H_2O = H_2CO_3$$

2. $$H_2CO_3 + 2NaOH \text{ (or KOH)} =$$
$$Na_2CO_3 \text{ (or } K_2CO_3) + 2H_2O + Energy$$

3. $$Na_2CO_3 \text{ (or } K_2CO_3) + Ca(OH)_2 =$$
$$CaCO_3 + 2NaOH \text{ (or 2KOH)}$$

B. Baralyme

1. $$Ba(OH)_2 + 8H_2O + CO_2 = BaCO_3 + 9H_2O + Energy$$

2. $$9H_2O + 9CO_2 = 9H_2CO_3$$

Then by direct reactions and by NaOH or KOH:

3. $$9H_2CO_3 + 9Ca(OH)_2 = 9CaCO_3 + 18H_2O + Energy$$

An exhausted CO_2 absorber does not feel warm. Usually, a CO_2 absorber changes from colorless to violet when ethyl violet is used as the pH indicator and it starts to absorb CO_2 from the circuit. However, an exhausted CO_2 absorbent shows no color change. Dyes are not a very sensitive test for CO_2 absorption capacity, however, because fluorescent light can deactivate the dyes, and the absorbent may appear white even though exhausted. A soda lime absorbent is best judged by the length of time it has been used in the circuit. The maximum CO_2 absorbing capacity of absorbent is 26 L of CO_2/100g of absorbent. In practice, however, channeling of gas through the granules may decrease the absorbent efficiency substantially and allow only 10 to 20 L of CO_2 to be absorbed.

Amsorb (Armstrong Medical Ltd., Coleraine, Northern Ireland) has half the CO_2 absorbing capacity of soda lime, and it does not have strong bases (i.e., the activators NaOH and KOH). These strong bases have been implicated in the production of carbon monoxide (CO) by methyl ethers and compound A by sevoflurane (see later). Because Amsorb does not contain strong bases, it does not degrade volatile anesthetics to compound A (from sevoflurane) or produce CO (from desflurane, enflurane, and isoflurane).

The chemistry of Amsorb is as follows:

1. $$CO_2 + H_2O = H_2CO_3$$

2. $$H_2CO_3 + Ca(OH)_2 = CaCO_3 + 2H_2O + Energy$$

Sevoflurane reacts with CO_2 absorbents to produce degradation products. The major degradation product is fluoromethyl-2-2-difluoro-1-(trifluoromethyl) vinyl ether, or compound A. In addition, CO poisoning, though very rare, has been reported with the use of low-flow anesthesia. Although the mechanism is not clear, it is thought that CO

Figure 129–1 ■ Causes of mechanical and chemical complications with carbon dioxide absorbers.

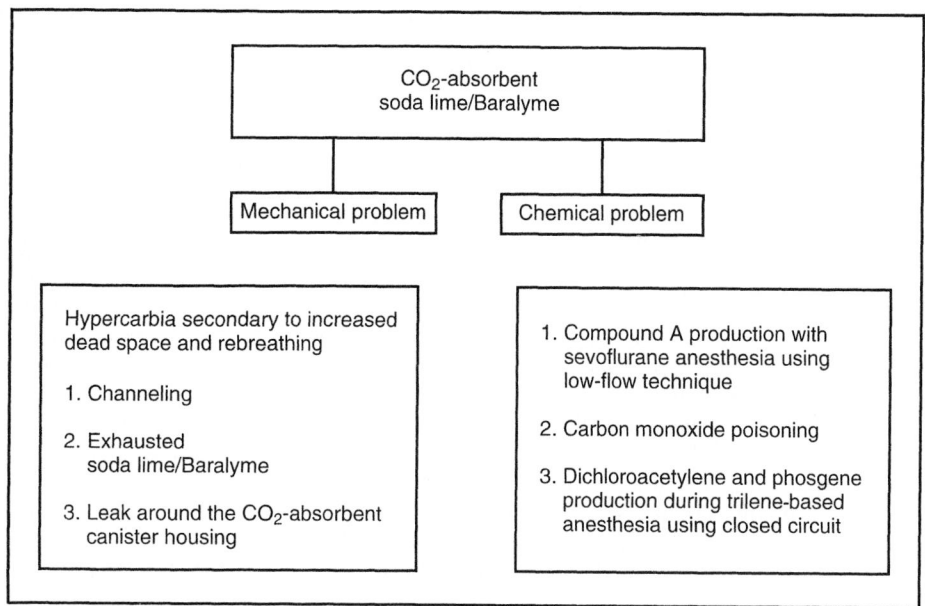

produced by the body is absorbed by the CO_2 absorbent and later released into the circuit when the temperature is raised. This mechanism is postulated because most of the reported cases of CO poisoning have been the first case on a Monday morning, after the circuit was idle over the weekend. If so, CO_2 absorbent with CO-laden granules would release CO into the circuit on Monday morning when the CO_2 canister temperature rose.

The Anesthesia Patient Safety Foundation has received reports of fire or extreme heat generation occurring in the CO_2 canister. Common elements in these reports of fire include use of a Baralyme absorber, desiccation of the absorbent, and use of sevoflurane. Holak and colleagues reported that with simulated anesthetic conditions in their laboratory and use of dehydrated Baralyme and sevoflurane, a dial setting of 8% was required to deliver 1 MAC (2.1%) of sevoflurane to the "patient." In the absence of sevoflurane uptake by the "patient," the high breakdown of sevoflurane was presumed to be secondary to reaction with the absorbent.

In this experiment the investigators recorded a temperature greater than 110°C at the upper absorbent canister in less than 10 minutes; at 15 minutes, the canister was too hot to touch. CO production increased exponentially above 70°C, and at 45 minutes the temperature was greater than 200°C. Finally, at 53 minutes, the absorber exploded and burst into flames. It was suggested that the initial delayed rate of rise of inspired agent concentration could serve as an early warning before the absorbent's dramatic rise in temperature.

Trichloroethylene (Trilene) is a general anesthetic agent still in use in some parts of the world. Trichloroethylene in the presence of heat and alkali forms breakdown products: the neurotoxin dichloroacetylene and the pulmonary irritant phosgene. Phosgene induces pneumonitis, leading to acute respiratory distress syndrome. Dichloroacetylene can produce cranial nerve lesions and encephalitis. The use of trichloroethylene along with a CO_2 absorbent in the circuit is strongly contraindicated, as is the use of a CO_2 absorbent in a patient who has recently (<24 to 36 hours) received trichloroethylene (e.g., postpartum tubal ligation).

Risk Assessment

Hypercarbia secondary to CO_2 absorbent malfunction may be due to exhaustion of the soda lime or barium hydroxide lime, with channeling of fresh gas flow through the CO_2 absorbent canister. Or it may be due to loss of fresh gas flow through the CO_2 absorbent canister housing owing to leaks. Any leak in the circuit, nonfunctioning inspiratory or expiratory valve, or exhausted CO_2 absorbent increases the dead space in the circuit, which in turn causes rebreathing and results in hypercarbia. Hypermetabolic states, such as sepsis, cause excessive CO_2 production and result in hypercarbia unless total minute ventilation is increased accordingly.

In malignant hyperthermia, CO_2 production is increased very rapidly due to a hypermetabolic state, with attendant hypercarbia accompanied by tachycardia, hyperthermia, and increasing metabolic acidosis. Because large quantities of CO_2 are taken up by the CO_2 absorbent, the temperature rise within the CO_2 canister is substantial, and the canister may feel too hot.

Implications

Hypercarbia causes sympathetic stimulation, which raises plasma catecholamine levels. High blood catecholamine levels increase blood pressure, sweating, and tachycardia and may cause ventricular arrhythmias with some older volatile anesthetics (sensitization). These may cause severe hemodynamic compromise.

Factors leading to a rise in the concentration of compound A in the circuit are low-flow anesthesia techniques (fresh gas flow <2 L/minute), the use of barium hydroxide lime instead of soda lime, a high concentration of sevoflurane, a high absorbent temperature, and the use of fresh absorbents. Because compound A has been shown to cause renal injury in rats, it is prudent to avoid the use of sevoflurane in patients with renal impairment.

MANAGEMENT AND PREVENTION

Hypercarbia during general anesthesia related to soda lime or barium hydroxide lime can be prevented by checking the freshness of the absorbent. When in doubt, it is advisable to change the absorbent too early rather than too late. It is important to make sure that the soda lime or barium hydroxide lime is packed properly in the canister to avoid any possibility of channeling, thereby reducing its ability to absorb CO_2 in the circuit. Soda lime canisters should be fitted onto the canister housing, and checks for any leak in the circuit should be performed; this prevents rebreathing.

Whenever sevoflurane is used, fresh gas flow of at least 2 L/minute must be maintained to reduce risk of compound A production and possible renal dysfunction. If synthetic zeolites (molecular sieves) are used instead of soda lime or barium hydroxide lime to remove CO_2 from the circuit, compound A is not produced with sevoflurane. It is possible that molecular sieves for use with sevoflurane will become available in the future. Amsorb does not produce compound A or CO when used with sevoflurane or other volatile anesthetics (e.g., desflurane, enflurane, isoflurane).

To address the rare and isolated cases of canister fire while using sevoflurane, Abbott Laboratories issued a letter in 2003 suggesting some preventive measures. These include replacing any CO_2 absorber that has not been used for an extended period (it could be desiccated), turning off the vaporizer when not in use, shutting off the anesthesia machine and fresh gas flow when not in use for extended periods, periodically monitoring the temperature in the CO_2 canister, and monitoring the rate of rise of inspired sevoflurane in relation to the dial setting of the vaporizer. An unusually delayed rise or unexpected decline of sevoflurane concentration compared with the vaporizer setting may be associated with excessive heating of the CO_2 absorbent canister.

If excessive heat is detected, the patient should be disconnected from the anesthesia circuit and the CO_2 absorber replaced. The patient should be monitored for CO exposure and the potential for chemical thermal injury.

Trichloroethylene must not be used when soda lime or barium hydroxide lime is present in the circuit or when either was used recently (within 24 to 36 hours). Because the phenomenon of CO poisoning during low-flow anesthesia is so rare and because its mechanism is not clearly understood, it is best to keep a high level of suspicion. The anesthesia provider should check blood carboxyhemoglobin levels when in doubt and manage the patient accordingly.

Further Reading

Andrews JJ: Inhaled anesthetic delivery systems. In Miller RD (ed): Anesthesia, 5th ed. New York, Churchill Livingstone, 2000, pp 193-195.

"Dear Health Care Professional" [letter from Abbott Laboratories, Nov 17, 2003]. Available at http://www.fda.gov/medwatch/SAFETY/2003/Ultane_deardoc.pdf.

Fang ZX, Kendel L, Laster MJ, et al: Factors affecting production of compound A from the interaction of sevoflurane with Baralyme and soda lime. Anesth Analg 82:775-781, 1996.

Fee JPH, Murray M, Luney SR: Molecular sieves: An alternative method of carbon dioxide removal which does not generate compound A during simulated low-flow sevoflurane anaesthesia. Anaesthesia 50:841-845, 1995.

Gonsowskic CT, Laster M, Eger EL II, et al: Toxicity of compound A in rats: Effect of 3-hour administration. Anesthesiology 80:556-565, 1994.

Gravenstein JS, Pulus DA, Hayes TJ: Capnography in Clinical Practice. Boston, Butterworths, 1989, pp 24-26.

Higuchi H, Adachi Y, Arimura S, et al: The carbon dioxide absorption capacity of Amsorb is half that of soda lime. Anesth Analg 93:221-225, 2001.

Holak EJ, Mei DA, Dunning MB III, et al: Carbon monoxide production from sevoflurane breakdown: Modeling of exposures under clinical conditions. Anesth Analg 96:757-764, 2003.

Humphrey JH, McClelland M: Cranial-nerve palsies with herpes following general anesthesia. BMJ 1:315-318, 1944.

Moon RE: Cause of CO poisoning, relation to halogenated agents still not clear. J Clin Monit 1:11, 1995.

Morio M, Fujii K, Satoh N, et al: Reaction of sevoflurane and its degradation products with soda lime. Anesthesiology 77:1155, 1992.

Olympio MA, Morrel RC: Canister fires become hot safety concern. Anesthesia Patient Safety Foundation Newsletter, winter 2003.

Mechanical Ventilators

130

Brian J. Woodcock

Case Synopsis

A 100-kg, 68-year-old man is anesthetized and intubated. Bilateral breath sounds are verified. The ventilator is turned on and set to a tidal volume of 600 mL, respiratory rate of 10, and inspiratory-expiratory ratio of 1:2. Two minutes later, the lowering tone of the pulse oximeter alerts the anesthesiologist, who notices an absence of chest wall movement. The ventilator appears to be cycling normally, so the anesthesiologist picks up a stethoscope and reaches to adjust the switch-over valve to manual, but it is already in the manual position.

PROBLEM ANALYSIS

Definition

Failure to change the ventilator-manual switch to the ventilator position after a period of manual ventilation is the source of many mechanical ventilator complications that can cause serious harm to patients. In the American Society of Anesthesiologists (ASA) closed claim analysis of adverse anesthetic outcomes, there were threefold more claims related to misuse of equipment or operator error compared with equipment failure.

Examples of ventilator misuse or operator error include the following:

- Failure to turn the ventilator on after a period of manual ventilation
- Inappropriate set rate or tidal volume for patient size
- Maximum pressure limit set too high for patient size
- Maximum pressure limit set too low, causing low tidal volume
- Inappropriate inspiratory-expiratory ratio
- High fresh gas flow causing increased tidal volume
- Oxygen (O_2) flush during ventilator inspiration
- Alarms for pressure, volume, or fraction of inspired oxygen (Fio_2) inactivated by the operator, causing a delay in noticing other malfunctions

Equipment failure or incorrect assembly can include the following problems:

- Hole in the bellows
- Bellows mounted incorrectly, so no seal is formed between the bellows and the casing
- Electrical or mechanical failure, stalling the mechanism
- Failure of the alarms for pressure, apnea, or Fio_2

Other causes of ventilator failure actually arise elsewhere on the anesthesia machine. These complications, covered in other chapters, include failure of driving gas pressure (Chapter 123); circuit disconnection, sticking valves, and misconnections of the circuit hoses (Chapter 127), and scavenger errors (Chapter 131).

Recognition

The failure to recognize and promptly rectify problems with ventilators can have catastrophic consequences. In the ASA closed claim analysis, 12 cases were associated with ventilator problems; 7 resulted in death and 5 in brain injury. There is only a small window of opportunity to correct the malfunction of the ventilator before adverse physiologic events take place as a result of it.

Turning the Ventilator on

Failure to actually turn the ventilator on is common. This usually occurs soon after induction and may be unnoticed for many minutes. If the ventilator-manual switch has not been turned to the ventilator position, the signs are as follows:

- Loss of the end-tidal carbon dioxide ($ETCO_2$) waveform
- Activation of the $ETCO_2$ apnea alarm
- Distention of the reservoir bag and rising airway pressure on the manometer if the pop-off valve is closed

If the ventilator has not been turned on but the ventilator-manual switch has been turned to the ventilator position, the signs are as follows:

- Loss of the $ETCO_2$ waveform
- No airway pressure perceived by the manometer
- Activation of the apnea pressure and $ETCO_2$ apnea alarms

Ventilator Rate and Tidal Volume

Inappropriate settings for tidal volume or respiratory rate may cause either inappropriate tidal volume size and hyperventilation or hypoventilation leading to falling or rising $ETCO_2$. In the case of a child or small adult, hypotension may result from the decrease in venous return due to large tidal volumes and increased intrathoracic pressures. Barotrauma may also occur, with consequent pneumothorax or subcutaneous emphysema. In the case of an adult with ventilator settings for a small child, the most notable feature would be hypoventilation, including a low peak airway pressure, a rising $ETCO_2$, and O_2 desaturation if hypoventilation is severe.

Pressure Limit

An inappropriately high pressure limit setting may allow excessive tidal volumes and pressures, leading to barotrauma. A low pressure limit setting may lead to inadequate tidal volume and hypercarbia.

INSPIRATORY-EXPIRATORY RATIO

An inappropriate inspiratory-expiratory ratio may be set when unusual ventilator rates are used—for example, at the end of a case when the rate is set very low to allow arterial CO_2 tension to rise. At low rates, an inspiratory-expiratory ratio of 1:2 might result in very prolonged inspiratory times.

FRESH GAS FLOW

Failure to reset the fresh gas flow to a lower rate after intubation of a patient may lead to hyperventilation. The set tidal volume on the bellows is supplemented by the amount of fresh gas entry into the circuit during the inspiratory period. For example, with a fresh gas flow of 10 L/minute, a respiratory rate of 10, and an inspiratory-expiratory ratio of 1:2, each tidal volume is increased by 333 mL above that set by the bellows. This may cause significant hyperventilation or barotrauma in a small patient if the maximum pressure limit is set too high.

Pressing the O_2 flush during ventilator inspiration can lead to large volumes of gas entering the patient, leading to the development of pneumothoraces due to barotrauma.

VENTILATOR ALARMS

Ventilators have two alarms, the *ventilator alarm* and the *threshold pressure alarm limit (TPAL) alarm*. The ventilator alarm has two buttons, the "silence alarm" button and the "alarm off" button. Pressing the "silence alarm" button druing a period of manual ventilation can prevent the ventilator alarm from sounding when a period of apnea ensues. When the intent is to use manual ventilation or to hold ventilation for a limited period, the "silence alarm" button should be pressed to cancel that alarm for a period of 60 or 120 seconds. Pressing the ventilator "alarm off" button, which indefinitely cancels the ventilator alarm, removes the ability of the ventilator alarm to automatically be re-armed if the operator fails to turn the ventilator back on.

The TPAL alarm delineates the airway pressure level at which inspiration is detected. When this is adjustable, it should be set at less than 5 cm H_2O below the peak inspiratory pressure. This allows the alarm to be triggered when a leak in the system causes a reduction in peak inspiratory

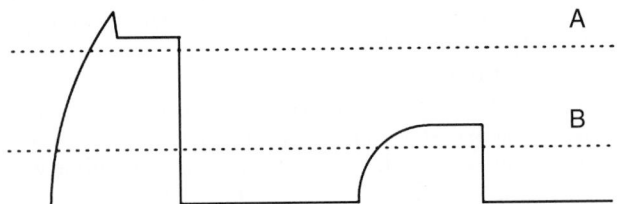

Figure 130–1 ■ The threshold pressure alarm limit (TPAL; *dashed lines*) delineates the airway pressure level at which inspiration is detected. When the TPAL is adjustable, it should be set at less than 5 cm H_2O below the peak inspiratory pressure (setting A). With a correct TPAL setting, a reduced peak airway pressure breath, such as that occurring in the presence of an airway breathing system leak (second breath), will be sensed as being absent, and the apnea alarm will sound if the condition continues. However, if the TPAL is too low (setting B), the reduced breath will be detected, but the ventilator alarm will not sound. Appropriately high TPAL settings allow the alarm to be triggered when a leak in the system causes a reduction in peak inspiratory pressure, even with an airway pressure waveform.

pressure but not a complete loss of the waveform (Fig. 130-1). The Narkomed 2B anesthesia machine gives a (silent) advisory notice when the pressure is set too low for the current peak pressure.

The ventilator alarm should be considered the most important alarm in the operating room. A vigilant anesthesia provider should feel uncomfortable whenever this alarm sounds. Even if the reason for the alarm is known and anticipated (e.g., after switching to spontaneous ventilation following reversal of muscle relaxation at the end of a case), the alarm should not be allowed to continue unattended. Any ventilator alarm condition should be corrected, or the alarm should be reset to the appropriate level for the new status of the patient. Similarly, when leaving the operating room at the end of a case, the ventilator alarms should not be left sounding.

VENTILATOR BELLOWS

Development of a hole in the bellows can be recognized by the following:

- Decreasing concentration of the inhaled anesthetic gas
- Rising Fio_2 if the driving gas is O_2
- Falling Fio_2 if the driving gas is air or an O_2-air mixture
- Hyperventilation or hypoventilation

If the bellows is mismounted or a hole develops in it, the O_2 used to power the bellows is directly connected to the circuit gases. Because the driving gas is at a higher pressure, it enters the bellows and mixes with the circuit gases. It therefore dilutes the anesthetic gases in the circuit and raises the Fio_2, unless air is used as the driving gas, in which case the Fio_2 would fall (see also Chapter 123). The main result of a leaking bellows is its inability to hold volume after the O_2 flush valve is used to fill it. Although such a malfunction could cause hypoventilation, it is more likely that the driving gas will hyperventilate the patient. This occurs because the bellows moves inadequately to operate the sensing mechanism, and large tidal volumes are delivered. Also, a hanging bellows can entrain room air during expiration if there is a circuit disconnection or leak.

A leak caused by a hole is more likely in an old, worn-out bellows. A hole in a new bellows might result from inadequate inspection at the factory. Mismounting may occur if the person mounting the bellows is not familiar with the equipment. Because the bellows may be changed when an adult case follows a pediatric case, or vice versa, this is a time to be especially vigilant for problems related to mismounted bellows.

VENTILAOR FAILURE

The ventilator control assembly can be the cause of ventilator failure due to electrical or mechanical problems. Total electrical failure is easily recognized, but partial mechanical problems due to internal leaks or faulty valves may be more difficult to discern.

Risk Assessment

Some circumstances are associated with greater risk of ventilator problems. Failure to correctly set the ventilator on-off switch or the changeover valve may occur in the following circumstances:

- Soon after induction
- After a period of manual ventilation
- When the anesthetist is distracted
- When multiple providers are present

The period of greatest risk is immediately after induction, after bilateral breath sounds have been confirmed and the anesthetist is distracted by placing other monitors or by the patient's hemodynamic instability. Resuming ventilation after coronary artery bypass is another period of high risk, because the ventilator has been off for a lengthy period. The "inverse anesthetist ratio" states that the care given to the patient is inversely related to the number of anesthetists present. When multiple anesthesia personnel are present, each may assume that someone else turned on the ventilator.

Inappropriate ventilator settings often occur when beginning a pediatric case following an adult case or when beginning an adult case following a pediatric case. Wrong settings for the tidal volume or respiratory rate produce a minute ventilation that is inappropriate for that patient. At high risk is a very small pediatric patient placed on a ventilator set for a full-sized adult. The pediatric patient is put at very high risk for barotrauma, secondary to high inspiratory pressure, and hyperventilation. Conversely, an adult placed on a ventilator set for a child is at risk for severe hypoventilation.

Implications

Most of the problems discussed here eventually cause a ventilatory abnormality, such as hypercarbia or hypocarbia.

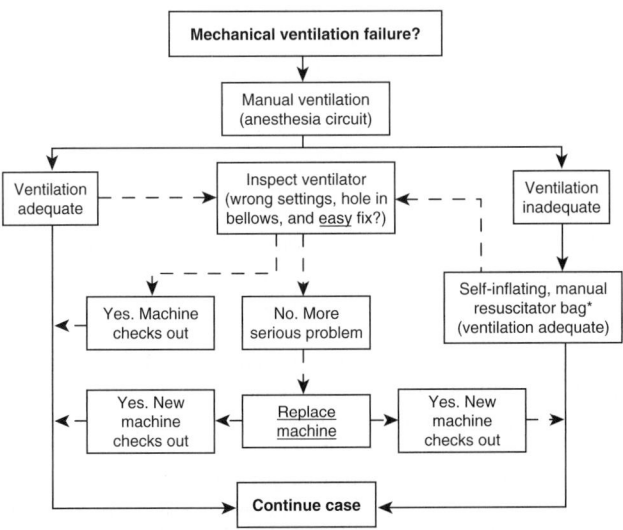

Figure 130–2 ■ Suggested algorithm for responding to a problem with mechanical ventilation. *If a manual resuscitator bag is not immediately available, use mouth–to–tracheal tube ventilation. *Solid lines,* immediate action; *dashed lines,* remedial action. Under *no* circumstances should a machine be repaired while in use.

Prolonged absence of ventilation may lead to hypoxia. The length of time before hypoxia occurs is variable, depending on the FiO_2 before apnea and the respiratory status of the patient. Other complications include severe hypotension secondary to reduced venous return and significant barotrauma from hyperinflation.

MANAGEMENT

The initial response to any problem with mechanical ventilation is to immediately switch to manual ventilation (Fig. 130-2). First, this is done using the anesthesia circuit. If the patient is still inadequately ventilated, a self-inflating manual resuscitator bag or mouth–to–tracheal tube ventilation is used. Once manual ventilation is established, the ventilator can be thoroughly inspected for the source of the error. The settings should be verified as correct for that patient; if not, they should be reset. If there is a hole in the bellows, it should be replaced immediately, or the anesthesia machine should be exchanged. It is never appropriate to repair a machine while it is in use in the operating room.

PREVENTION

Preventing problems related to mechanical ventilators depends on the following:

- Operator vigilance
- Monitoring of airway pressures and expiratory volume, and appropriately set alarms
- Skilled routine maintenance
- Thorough checkout procedure performed before each case, following Food and Drug Administration guidelines:
  - If a switching valve is present, test its function in both bag and ventilator mode.
  - Close the pop-off valve (airway pressure leak) if necessary and occlude the system at the patient's end.
  - Test for leaks and pressure relief by appropriate cycling (exact procedure varies with the type of ventilator).
  - Attach the reservoir bag at the mask fitting, fill the system, and cycle the ventilator. Ensure that the bag is properly filling and emptying.

Further Reading

Brockwell RC, Andrews JJ: Complications of inhaled anesthesia delivery systems. Anesthesiol Clin North Am 20:539-554, 2002.

Brockwell RC, Andrews JJ: Inhaled anesthetic delivery systems. In Miller RD (ed): Miller's Anesthesia, 6th ed. Philadelphia, Churchill Livingstone, 2005, pp 298-303.

Caplan RA, Vistica MF, Posner KL, et al: Adverse anesthetic outcomes arising from gas delivery equipment: A closed claims analysis. Anesthesiology 87:741-748, 1997.

Dorsch JA, Dorsch SE: Understanding Anesthesia Equipment. Philadelphia, JB Lippincott–Williams & Wilkins, 1999.

Ehrenwerth J, Eisenkraft J: Anesthesia Equipment: Principles and Applications. St. Louis, Mosby–Year Book, 2004.

Scavenging Systems

Isaac Azar

131

Case Synopsis

A 30-year-old patient is undergoing abdominal surgery under general anesthesia. Suddenly, his chest progressively expands, and the pressure in the anesthesia breathing circuit rises. The anesthesiologist immediately disconnects the patient from the breathing circuit. This releases the pressure in the breathing circuit, and the patient's chest relaxes. While an assistant examines the anesthesia machine, the anesthesiologist ventilates the patient with an Ambu bag. Examination of the scavenging system of the anesthesia machine reveals a partial obstruction of the suction line and a faulty positive-pressure relief valve. The obstruction is released, and the relief valve is repaired. This resolves the problem, and the administration of anesthesia using the breathing circuit continues uneventfully.

PROBLEM ANALYSIS

Definition

Over the past 30 years, several scientific reports have suggested that adverse health effects are caused by chronic exposure to trace anesthetic agents in the operating room (OR). Although there is presently no consensus, the National Institute for Occupational Safety and Health recommends that the trace level of nitrous oxide in the OR ambient air be no higher than 25 parts per million. Primarily, this has been achieved by adding a waste anesthetic gas scavenging system to the anesthesia machine.

All modern anesthesia machines are equipped with such a scavenging system. The purpose of the system is to safely dispose of the waste anesthetic gases from the breathing circuit into the wall suction. Interposed between the breathing circuit and airway pressure limiting (APL) valve and the wall suction disposal line is a scavenging interface system (Fig. 131-1). The purpose of the APL valve and the scavenging interface system is to protect the patient from negative or excessive positive airway pressures.

Typically, the scavenging interface system includes a reservoir that collects the waste anesthetic gases before they are discarded into the suction system. The interface system may be either closed or open. A closed system, such as that usually found on Ohmeda anesthesia machines, consists of a reservoir bag and two pressure relief valves—one positive and one negative (Fig. 131-2). An open reservoir system, such as that usually found on Dräger anesthesia machines, consists of a metallic reservoir in the form of a cylinder with open ports (Figs. 131-3 and 131-4).

When a closed interface system is in use, negative pressure in the system opens the negative-pressure relief valve, which allows room air to rush into the reservoir bag. Excessive positive pressure in a closed system opens the positive-pressure relief valve, which allows waste anesthetic gases to escape into the room air. In either case, opening of the relief valve restores normal atmospheric pressure in the system.

The reservoir bag of a closed system also serves as an indicator of how well the interface system is functioning. If the bag is excessively distended, it indicates abnormally high positive pressure in the system. This usually occurs when the vacuum force is too weak, and the positive-pressure relief valve fails to open. When the bag is collapsed, it indicates negative pressure in the system. This usually occurs when the vacuum force is too strong, and the negative-pressure relief valve fails to open.

When an open interface system is in use, the ports in the metal reservoir allow air to move in when the system pressure is negative, and they allow waste anesthetic gases to move out when the system pressure is positive. As long as the ports are free of obstructions, pressure in the system is atmospheric. If the ports are obstructed, excessive vacuum force generates negative pressure in the system. An inadequate vacuum force allows the buildup of excessive positive pressure in the system.

In some hospitals, the waste anesthetic gases are discarded into the OR ventilation system. A disposal line directs the waste anesthetic gases from a scavenging interface to the OR ventilation grill. The interface system in such a scavenging system usually consists of a reservoir bag and positive-pressure relief valve. If the disposal line is inadvertently

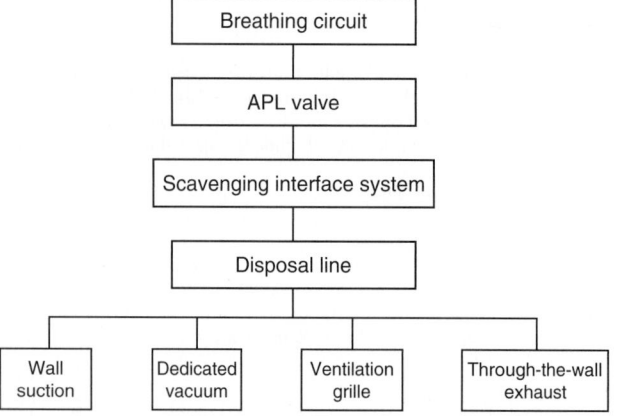

Figure 131–1 ■ Alternative methods of waste anesthetic gas disposal. APL, airway pressure limiting.

Figure 131–2 ■
Representation of an Ohmeda
anesthesia machine with a
closed interface scavenging
system. *Inset*, Exploded view
of closed interface scavenging
system.

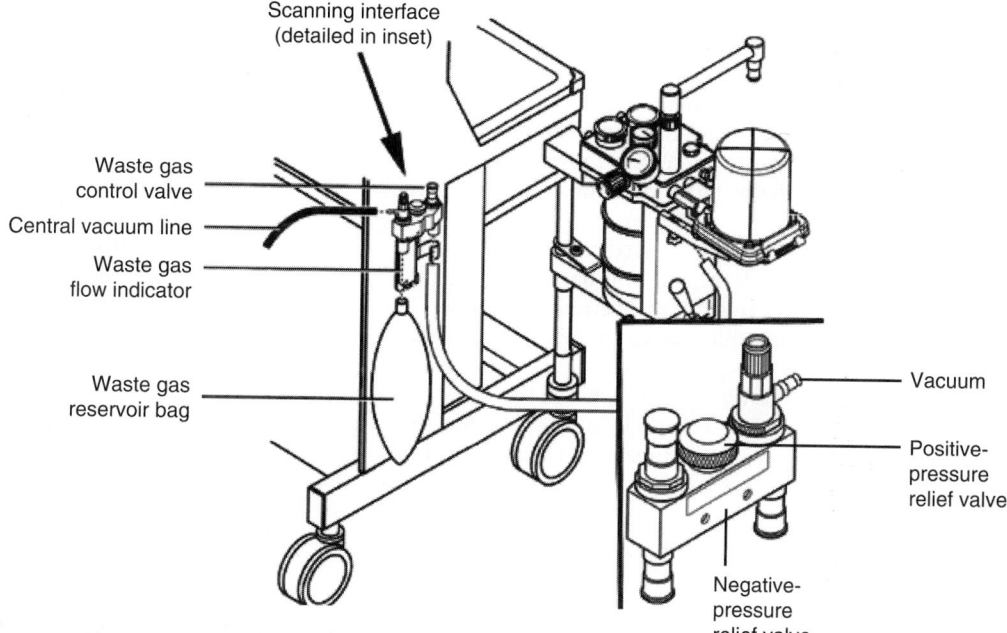

Scanning interface
(detailed in inset)

Waste gas
control valve

Central vacuum line

Waste gas
flow indicator

Waste gas
reservoir bag

Vacuum

Positive-
pressure
relief valve

Negative-
pressure
relief valve

occluded, the positive-pressure relief valve opens and allows
waste anesthetic gases to escape into the room air. If the
valve fails to open, the pressure in the system rises. The reservoir
bag also serves as an indicator of whether the scavenging
system is functioning appropriately. An overdistended
bag suggests an obstructed disposal line and a faulty pressure
relief valve.

Recognition

Whenever an abnormal pressure occurs in the breathing circuit,
a rapid examination of the anesthesia machine should

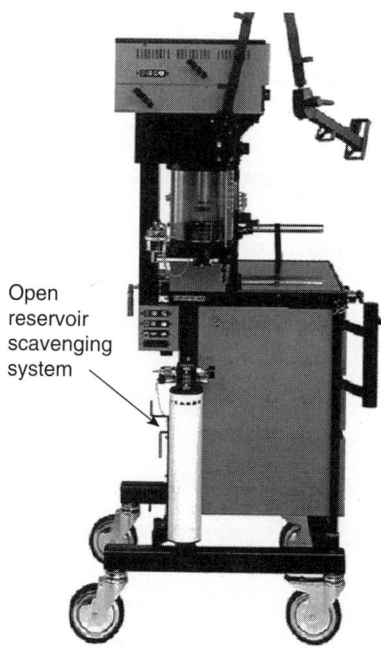

Open
reservoir
scavenging
system

Figure 131–3 ■ Dräger anesthesia machine with an open interface scavenging system.

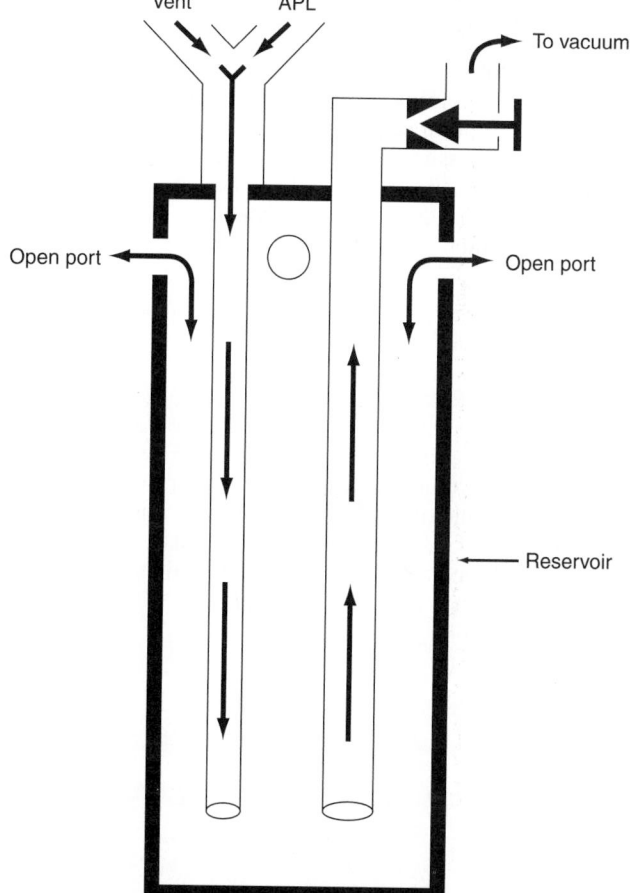

Vent   APL

To vacuum

Open port

Open port

Reservoir

Figure 131–4 ■ Details of the open interface scavenging system of a
Dräger anesthesia machine. APL, airway pressure limiting.

EQUIPMENT &
MONITORING

include an inspection of the scavenging system. If a closed system is in use, first the reservoir bag should be observed. If it is distended, the vacuum force is too weak and the positive-pressure relief valve is faulty. If it is empty, the vacuum force is too strong and the negative-pressure relief valve is faulty. When an open interface system is used, first examine the ports of the metallic reservoir to rule out accidental obstruction.

If the OR air-conditioning is used to dispose of waste anesthetic gases, first check the reservoir bag of the interface system. If it is distended, rule out inadvertent obstruction of the disposal line by portable OR equipment and a faulty pressure relief valve.

Rarely, an obstruction may occur between the APL valve and the scavenging interface system. In such a case, positive pressure builds up rapidly in the breathing circuit, despite a properly functioning interface system.

Risk Assessment

The incorporation of scavenging systems in anesthesia machines has increased the risk of mechanical failure. Malfunction of the scavenging system may cause negative or excessive positive pressure in the breathing circuit.

Implications

Excessive positive pressure in the breathing circuit adversely affects ventilation and may cause severe physiologic disruption and barotrauma of the respiratory system. A particularly dangerous complication of excessive positive pressure is tension pneumothorax.

Negative pressure in the breathing circuit may interfere with ventilation, sucking air out of the lungs and causing alveolar collapse and pulmonary edema, with consequent severe hypoxemia.

MANAGEMENT

If abnormal pressure is detected in the breathing circuit, the patient should be disconnected immediately from the anesthesia machine and, if necessary, ventilated with an Ambu bag until the problem is resolved. In the meantime, anesthesia can be maintained by the administration of intravenous drugs. If the cause of the abnormal pressure in the breathing system cannot be rapidly detected and corrected, the anesthesia machine should be replaced.

Injuries caused by abnormal pressure in the breathing circuit may be life threatening and should be promptly treated. If negative pressure causes lung collapse or pulmonary edema, this should be treated by manually applying positive-pressure ventilation with 100% oxygen. Because pulmonary edema in such cases is not associated with circulatory overload, the administration of diuretics is not necessarily indicated.

If excessive positive pressure in the breathing circuit causes tension pneumothorax, a chest tube should be inserted as soon as possible.

PREVENTION

In addition to regular servicing of the anesthesia machine and its scavenging system, it is important to briefly inspect the scavenging interface before the induction of anesthesia. No loose objects, such as empty plastic bags, should be allowed near the interface pressure relief valves or ports. If the OR air-conditioning system is used to discard waste anesthetic gases, it is preferable that the disposal line be kept off the floor. If the line does rest on the floor, portable OR equipment should not be parked on it.

When testing the breathing circuit, any difficulty in filling or emptying the breathing bag should be evaluated carefully, and a defective scavenging system ruled out.

Further Reading

Abramowitz M, McGill W: Hazard of anesthetic scavenging device [letter]. Anesthesiology 51:276, 1979.

Buring JE, Hennekens CH: Health experiences of operating room personnel. Anesthesiology 62:325-330, 1985.

Cohen EN, Brown BW, et al: Occupational disease among operating room personnel: A national study. Anesthesiology 41:321-340, 1974.

Guirguis SS, Pelmear PL, Roy ML, et al: Health effects associated with exposure to anaesthetic gases in Ontario hospital personnel. Br J Ind Med 47:490-497, 1990.

Hamilton R, Byrne J: Another cause of gas scavenging line obstruction. Anesthesiology 51:365, 1979.

Mor Z, Stein E, Orkin L: A possible hazard in the use of a scavenging system. Anesthesiology 47:302-303, 1977.

NIOSH: Criteria for a recommended standard-occupational exposure to waste anesthetic gases and vapors. DHWE (NIOSH) No. 77-140. Cincinnati, Ohio, National Institute for Occupational Safety and Health, 1977.

Patel K, Dalal F: A potential hazard of the Drager scavenging interface system for wall suction. Anesth Analg 58:327-328, 1979.

Sharrock N, Leith D: Potential pulmonary barotrauma when venting anesthetic gases to suction. Anesthesiology 46:152-154, 1977.

Tavakoli M, Habeeb A: Two hazards of gas scavenging. Anesth Analg 57:286-287, 1978.

Humidifiers

132

Kelly T. Shannon and Sivam Ramanathan

Case Synopsis

After a prolonged delay during transport, a 59-year-old woman is brought to the operating room (OR) for an exploratory laparotomy for ovarian carcinoma. A semiclosed circle system with an in-circuit humidifier is used for general anesthesia During induction of anesthesia, it becomes difficult to manually ventilate the patient, and an occlusion is noted in the humidifier circuit. Shortly thereafter, the low-pressure alarm sounds, and a "hissing" noise is heard emanating from the humidifier circuit.

PROBLEM ANALYSIS

Definition

Heated humidification systems are commonly used during the provision of mechanical ventilation. Mechanical ventilation remains the primary modality of respiratory support during the administration of general endotracheal anesthesia. In addition, it is a hallmark of the management of critically ill patients in the intensive care unit. Mechanical ventilation leads to undue heat and moisture loss from the respiratory system, as the endotracheal tube bypasses the upper respiratory tract. This loss increases the viscosity of airway secretions, alters the activity of surfactant, and reduces ciliary motility. These events further compromise other efforts used to preserve physiologic levels of systemic hydration and temperature in anesthetized or critically ill patients.

Heated humidifiers serve to maintain and even augment the temperature and humidity levels within the respiratory tract. Their action offsets the cooling and drying effects of the inspired gases. Humidifiers are typically added via an accessory hose attached to the inspiratory limb of the anesthesia machine or mechanical ventilator circuit (Fig. 132-1). This arrangement creates the potential for circuit misconnection, disconnection, occlusion, and leakage. The possibility of these adverse events, along with availability of safer warming devices, such as convective warming blankets and heat and moisture exchangers, has led to a decrease in the use of heated humidifiers, at least in the OR. In fact, a recent survey of usage patterns in one large academic medical center revealed that heated humidifier circuits were no longer used for routine anesthetic management. Thus, their predominant use is for mechanical ventilation provided outside the OR.

The primary mechanisms for heat and moisture generation define the two types of humidifiers available today: hot-water humidifiers and aerosol generators. The hot, moist environment created by these devices enhances the possibility of humidifier-related complications.

Hot-water humidifiers are designed so that the inspired gases either bubble through or flow over an electrically heated reservoir of water. The types of adverse consequences possible with such a system are detailed in Table 132-1. Hot-water humidifiers may also incorporate an electrically heated wire in their hosing to prevent the cooling and condensation of water ("rain-out") from occurring downstream, as gases flow away from the humidifier in the ventilator circuit. If this wire overheats, occlusion, leakage, melting of the hose, or fire may occur, resulting in the possible inhalation of toxic fumes or debris.

A less popular type of humidifier is the nebulizer, which generates microaerosols. Ultrasonic and pneumatic nebulizers are two examples. Microaerosol nebulizers generate very small droplets of water and are capable of delivering larger quantities of water vapor to the respiratory tract than are hot-water humidifiers. This increases the likelihood of overhydration, especially in infants and children.

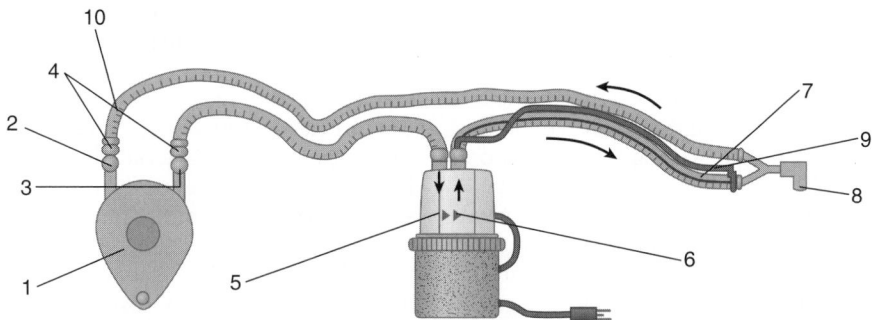

Figure 132–1 ■ Hot-water humidifier with an electrically heated wire unit placed inside the inspiratory limb of the patient circuit. 1, Soda lime absorber; 2, expiratory valve; 3, inspiratory valve; 4, breathing circuit; 5, humidifier; 6, water-fill level mark; 7, inspiratory limb with heated wire; 8, patient end; 9, thermistor probe; 10, expiratory limb. *Arrows* indicate the direction of gas flow within the circuit. Overheating of the inspiratory limb may lead to melting of the delivery hose, thereby causing occlusion or gas leakage.

Table 132–1 ■ Adverse Consequences of Heated Humidification Systems

Mechanical
Circuit obstruction or occlusion
   Melting
   Heating coils
   Rain-out of water
Circuit misconnection
Circuit disconnection
Circuit leakage

Electrical Hazard
Macroshock
Hose fire
   Burns (patient and health care workers)
   Toxin or debris inhalation

Thermal
Respiratory mucosa injury
   Burning
   Edema
   Necrosis
   Scar or stricture formation
Hyperthermia
Hemorrhagic tracheitis

Humidification
Water intoxication
   Hyponatremia
Increased secretions
Cilia inactivation
Surfactant inactivation
Atelectasis

Respiratory Mechanics
Increased airway resistance
Decreased forced residual capacity
Decreased static compliance

Contamination
Bacterial
Fungal
Heavy metals (tap-water usage)

Miscellaneous
Capnometer failure
   Rain-out of water

Additionally, bacterial and fungal contamination is a risk, because these microorganisms may be suspended within the water microdroplets. Colonization and subsequent infection may ensue.

Recognition

The timely discovery of humidifier malfunction and associated mechanical problems relies on clinical vigilance and the presence and proper functioning of several safety monitors and alarms. Routine monitoring of the patient's temperature detects hyperthermia. Humidifiers are equipped with several safety features, including alarms and automatic shut-off devices for sensing both high and low circuit temperature, as well as the low circuit pressure produced by leakage or disconnection. Anesthesia machines and mechanical ventilators also signal the presence of the high circuit pressure produced by occlusion. A line isolation monitor and ground fault circuit interrupter may uncover a grounding fault or the presence of excess leakage current in a defective humidifier, and thus may prevent macroshock.

Unlike with mechanical problems, the amount of time before the harmful effects of overheating occur (thermal injury, overhumidification, bacterial contamination) ranges from hours to days. Although increases in airway resistance and pulmonary shunting, atelectasis, and arterial hypoxemia may result, changes in respiratory mechanics and blood gas oxygen tension may be immediate or delayed. Serum sodium and serum osmolality measurements help detect acute overhydration or water intoxication.

Risk Assessment

The overall incidence of humidifier-associated complications is unknown. Specific factors that may increase the likelihood of humidification system failure have been identified. A humidifier hose composed of polyvinylchloride, which has a low melting point, has been linked to circuit occlusion and perforation when used with a heated wire. Acute bends in the hose, which increase the chance of direct contact between the hose and the wire, also contribute to circuit melting. The chance of a hose melting is enhanced if the humidifier is left on for an extended period with little or no active gas flow through it. In the case synopsis, the transport delay was largely responsible for the problems that occurred. The humidifier circuit melted, leading to obstruction and subsequent gas leak caused by disruption of the wall of the hose.

Among the circumstances that heighten the chance of thermal or moisture-related problems is prolonged use (e.g., lengthy operations or protracted mechanical ventilation). Prolonged use also predisposes to rain-out in the delivery hose, which, if severe, may occlude the hose lumen.

Bacterial contamination is more likely with the use of nonsterile water, especially if it is changed at infrequent intervals. This is more applicable to aerosol generators than hot-water systems. Similarly, the use of tap water may cause exposure to heavy metals.

Implications

Thermal injury to the tracheobronchial tree may cause mucosal damage, edema, hemorrhage, and necrosis. In turn, these may lead to pulmonary edema, scar and stricture formation, shunting, increased arterial-alveolar oxygen difference, and arterial hypoxemia.

Positive water balance also has adverse effects on the lungs. Overhydration may precipitate pulmonary edema; it also impairs ciliary motility and surfactant activity and increases airway secretions. The accumulation of secretions can obstruct the airway and promote atelectasis. Pulmonary shunting, increased arterial-alveolar gradient, and arterial hypoxemia are worsened. The loss of respiratory mucosa and the inactivation of the mucociliary elevator also predispose the lungs to infection.

Water intoxication and the subsequent development of hyponatremia and hypo-osmolality can have cardiac and central nervous system manifestations. Hyponatremia may impair normal cardiac and central nervous system electrophysiology. Cardiac effects include slowed conduction, widened QRS complexes, and elevated ST segments. Arrhythmias are more common. Further, myocardial contractility may be depressed. Possible adverse central nervous system effects are cerebral edema, altered sensorium, seizures, and loss of consciousness.

MANAGEMENT

Emergent reestablishment of the anesthetic or ventilatory circuit's integrity is imperative if occlusion or leakage occurs. If hyperthermia is suspected, heating of respiratory gases should be lowered or even terminated. Thermal injury to the respiratory tract necessitates the provision of supplemental oxygen, further mechanical ventilatory support, and positive end-expiratory pressure to maintain normal oxygenation until the injury resolves. Diagnostic or therapeutic bronchoscopy for secretion and debris removal may be required. An appropriate prophylactic antibiotic regimen is also encouraged.

Therapy to counteract the positive water balance depends on the severity. If pulmonary edema and cardiac instability are present, invasive monitoring of arterial blood pressure and ventricular filling pressures may help guide treatment. Vasopressor and inotropic support may be warranted. If dilutional hyponatremia is extreme, infusion of loop diuretics (e.g., furosemide) or hypertonic saline (3% to 5%), or both, may be therapeutic.

PREVENTION

Many of the potential complications related to heated humidifiers can be avoided by vigilant and careful clinical practice. Strict adherence to published standards and specific device manuals on the safe operation of these devices is mandatory. A detailed inspection of the components of the humidifier, the humidifier hose, and its connections is advised. The anesthesia delivery system and the mechanical ventilator circuit should be tested for leaks immediately before use. Prolonged periods of circuit inactivity while the humidifier is on should be avoided. Instead, the humidifier should be turned on just before the patient is connected to the circuit. Acute bends in the humidifier hoses should be averted to minimize contact between the hose tubing and the heated wire. If rain-out occurs, the breathing circuit hoses should be periodically emptied to prevent occlusion. This also minimizes capnometer failure or damage due to accumulated water in the circuit. Only sterile water should be used in the humidifier, and it should be changed at frequent intervals. When manipulating any humidifier components, close attention to aseptic technique must also be maintained. Periodically, the clinical engineering department

should evaluate all humidifiers for microshock and macroshock hazards. A line isolation monitor and ground fault circuit interrupter should be incorporated into the electrical system to prevent macroshock. The lowest heat setting on the humidifier that sustains a normal thermal environment should be used.

Abandoning the use of a heated humidifier in favor of incorporating a heat and moisture exchanger (HME, or "artificial nose") in the circuit has become common practice. HMEs are not associated with electrical hazards or problems related to overhydration. They are designed to passively conserve moisture already present in the respiratory tract; temperature conservation, however, is negligible. HMEs are small, disposable, inexpensive, and user-friendly. Moreover, they may provide bacterial and viral filtration. Commercially available HMEs are quite capable of providing sufficient humidification under most circumstances, especially when low fresh gas flow rates are used. Composite hygroscopic and hydrophobic membrane filters are the most commonly used HMEs. However, there are some trade-offs. The large-pored hygroscopic filters offer more efficient heat and moisture maintenance, whereas the small-pored hydrophobic membrane filters enhance microbe barrier and filtration properties. Both types of filters add dead space and resistance to the circuit. Further, there is the potential for them to become occluded with circuit water or pulmonary secretions.

Further Reading

Bench S: Humidification in the long-term ventilated patient: A systematic review. Intensive Crit Care Nurs 19:75-84, 2003.

Dick W: Aspects of humidification: Requirements and techniques. Int Anesthesiol Clin 12:217-239, 1991.

Dorsch JE, Dorsch SE: Humidification methods. In Dorsch JE, Dorsch SE (eds): Understanding Anesthesia Equipment. Baltimore, Williams & Wilkins, 1999, pp 287-308.

Klein EF, Graves SA: "Hot pot" tracheitis. Chest 65:225-226, 1974.

Lemmons HJM, Brock-Utne JG: Heat and moisture exchange devices: Are they doing what they are supposed to do? Anesth Analg 98:382-385, 2004.

Peterson BD: Heated humidifiers: Structure and function. Respir Care Clin N Am 4:243-259, 1998.

Ramanathan S: Humidification and humidifiers. In Ehrenwerth J, Eisenkraft JB (eds): Anesthesia Equipment: Principles and Applications. St. Louis, Mosby–Year Book, 1992, pp 172-197.

Rhame FS, Streifel A, McComb RC, et al: Bubbling humidifiers produce microaerosols which can carry bacteria. Infect Control 7:403-406, 1986.

Ricard JD, Cook D, Griffith L, et al: Physician's attitude to use heat and moisture exchangers or heated humidifiers: A Franco-Canadian survey. Intensive Care Med 28:719-725, 2002.

Shelly MP, Lloyd GM, Park GR, et al: A review of the mechanisms and methods of humidification of inspired gases. Intensive Care Med 14:1-9, 1988.

Wong DH: Melted delivery hose: A complication of a heated humidifier. Can J Anaesth 35:183-186, 1988.

EQUIPMENT & MONITORING

Intravenous Drug Delivery Systems

133

Rajamani Sethuraman

Case Synopsis

A 35-year-old man weighing 90 kg undergoes maxillofacial fracture fixation. He receives oxygen, air, propofol, and remifentanil infusion (0.5 μg/kg per minute) for 4 hours. The infusions are stopped 10 minutes before the end of surgery. At the conclusion of the operation he wakes up restless and combative and requires 15 mg of morphine to make him comfortable.

PROBLEM ANALYSIS

Definition

The patient described in the case synopsis awoke with significant pain due to the redistribution and elimination of remifentanil. These two factors play an important role in the declining plasma concentration of the drug, which in turn is affected by the duration of infusion. However, the latter is not so important with remifentanil, which is quickly eliminated by plasma esterases. The bolus dose before initiation of an infusion to produce a given drug plasma concentration is calculated by the following formula:

$$Amount = Ct \times VD,$$

where Ct is the target concentration and VD is the volume of distribution for a given drug. The trouble with this concept is that several volumes must be taken into account—those in the central and peripheral compartments. As time progresses, a steady-state concentration in the VD is reached. Calculating a dose according to initial VD would be too low, just as the dose would be too high if calculated using the final VD. Hence, this introduces the concept of VD at the drug's peak effect, which can be calculated due to the fact that plasma and effector site concentrations are similar at the time of peak effect. Maintenance infusion rate (Mir) is calculated as follows:

$$Mir = Ct \times Cls,$$

where Ct is the target concentration and Cls is the rate of clearance.

The *context-sensitive half-time* is the time it takes for the plasma concentration to decrease by 50% after stopping a continuous infusion that maintained a constant concentration in plasma. The concept of context-sensitive half-time needs to be understood when using a continuous infusion of anesthetic drugs that exhibit multicompartmental kinetics. In this setting, the net distribution of the drug in and out of the peripheral compartments varies according to the duration of the infusion. The "context" in this instance is the duration of the infusion (Fig. 133-1). In certain situations, decreases in plasma concentration other than 50% may be more clinically relevant. A more general term, *context-sensitive decrement time*, applies to this situation. Here, a decrease in the effector site concentration occurs, as noted by a falling plasma concentration, which is presumed to model the decrease at the effector site. The context-sensitive decrement time provides a clinically useful framework for understanding the relationship between the duration of the infusion and the time before recovery occurs (Fig. 133-2).

Automated drug delivery systems can provide precise predictions of the time required for the plasma (or effector site) concentration to change, based on the actual dosing regimen. These predictions can help clinicians terminate the infusion at the appropriate time. However, the postinfusion kinetics do not correlate with the elimination half-life. This is clearly demonstrated by a remifentanil infusion, because even after 3 hours, the context-sensitive half-time is shorter than its terminal half-life.

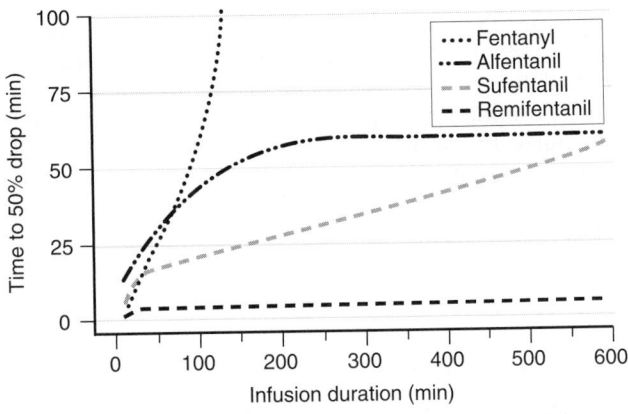

Figure 133–1 ■ Context-sensitive half-times as a function of infusion duration for each of the pharmacokinetic models simulated. Solid and dashed lines are used only to permit overlapping lines to be distinguished. (From Glass PA, Shafer SL, Reves JG: Intravenous drug delivery systems. In Miller RD [ed]: Anesthesia, 5th ed. New York, Churchill Livingstone, 2000.)

Figure 133–2 ▪ Recovery (decrement time) curves for fentanyl, alfentanil, sufentanil, and remifentanil showing the time required for decreases of a given percentage (labeled for each curve) from the maintained intraoperative effector site concentration after termination of the infusion. After the loading dose, an initially high infusion rate should be used to account for the redistribution and then titrated to the lowest infusion rate that will maintain adequate anesthesia or sedation. For sedation, the loading dose is given over 5 to 10 minutes and adjusted according to the patient's response. For anesthesia, midazolam is administered with an opiate. (From Glass PA, Shafer SL, Reves JG: Intravenous drug delivery systems. In Miller RD [ed]: Anesthesia, 5th ed. New York, Churchill Livingstone, 2000.)

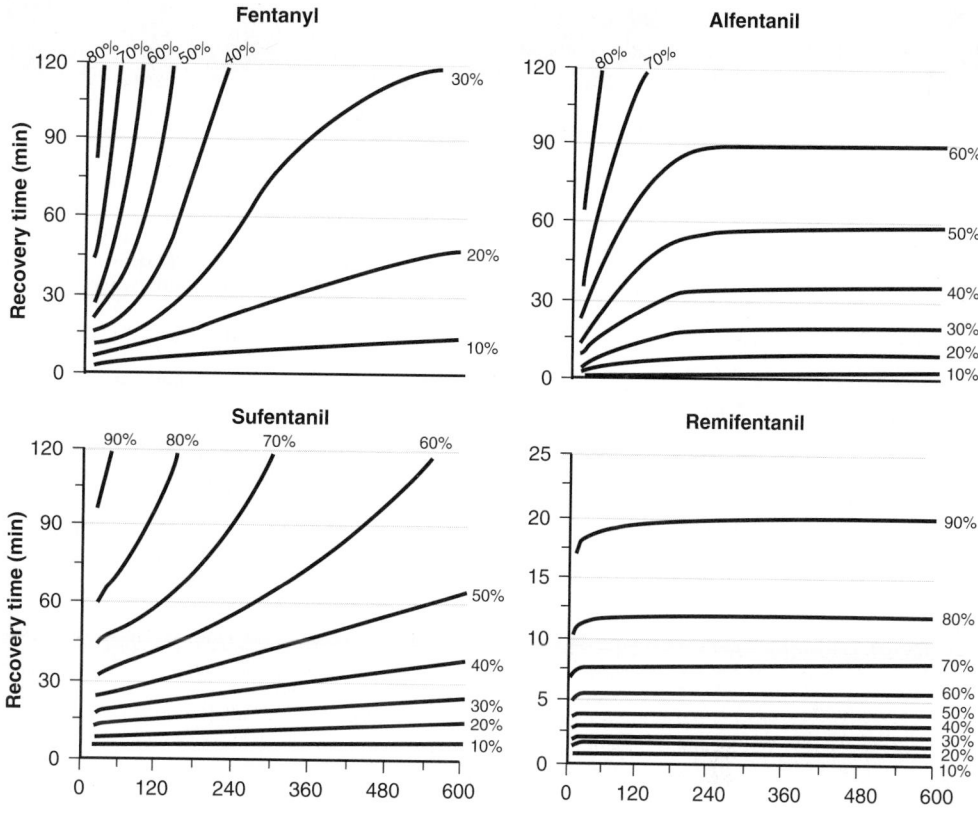

Time since beginning infusion (min)

Recognition

Excessive opioid administration is characterized by slow respirations, bradycardia, and pinpoint pupils. This situation responds to the administration of an opioid antagonist. With the advent of shorter-acting opioids (e.g., remifentanil), an opposite response may be noted if the infusion is terminated too early and further analgesia is not instituted in time.

Although it is important to understand the pharmacokinetics of the drugs used, one should not overlook practical errors in the setup of the system. The most common problems are as follows:

- Disconnected intravenous (IV) line
- Air in the IV line
- Line occlusion
- Low battery
- Syringe or cassette disengagement
- Tubing disconnection
- Empty carrier fluid

Another factor that may influence the onset of anesthesia and subsequent dose adjustment is the proximity of the infusion's connection to the patient. When an infusion is connected in a piggyback fashion, the rate at which the drug reaches the circulation is directly related to the IV flow rate and, inversely, to the volume of IV dead space between the infusion connection and the IV cannula. Therefore, the connection should be as close to the IV catheter as possible to minimize the effect of carrier IV fluid rate on drug delivery. Because of all these issues, vigilance with regard to the IV drug delivery device is very important. Additionally, most manufacturers have installed audible alarms for an idle pump, battery failure, and empty syringe.

Risk Assessment

The context-sensitive half-time and context-sensitive decrement time play an important role in running IV drug infusions safely. For most IV anesthetic agents, a 50% reduction in concentration is required before the patient returns to an awake state, and an 80% to 90% decrease is required before a patient can be safely discharged in an outpatient setting. Drug elimination half-lives are usually consistent. However, this is not true for context-sensitive half-times and context-sensitive decrement times. As in the case synopsis, the context-sensitive decrement time is shorter for remifentanil compared with other opioids, owing to its rapid metabolism as well as its minimal translocation to peripheral compartments.

Complications related to the use of IV drug delivery systems are often user related. If a routine checklist is followed, these errors can be minimized (Table 133-1). Use of AC power, use of a dedicated IV cannula, removal of all air from the tubing and syringes, and constant vigilance should prevent interruptions in flow.

Table 133–1 ■ Common Problems with Intravenous Drug Delivery Systems and Recommended Preventive Measures

Problem	Reason	Prevention
Pump setup errors	Error in concentration or rate	Two-person check Use prefilled syringes or bags
Underinfusion	Drawing up and pump-setting errors Faulty device	Double-check units and rates (e.g., mg/hr or mL/hr) Check service date Check that clamp and delivery mechanism movement is smooth
	Delayed onset because of mechanical slack	Normally, alarms sound when switched on, performing self-check
	Air in line Occlusion	Purge and prime the line Check the IV line Check the need to increase the occlusion pressure limit
Overinfusion	Faulty device Siphonage	As above Check for cracked syringe; check that syringe barrel and plunger are firmly engaged Position the device at the same level as the patient Use an antisiphon valve
	Postocclusion bolus	Release the line pressure before relieving the obstruction Add an antireflux valve in the second line
	Bolus drug treatment	Place the pump at the level of the patient Disconnect the infusion line whenever the syringe is removed from the pump
Communication	Absent or incorrect label Absent or incorrect record	Use correct labeling, color coding Check that the volume infused matches the dose and duration of infusion
	Absent or incorrect information during patient transfer or handover of care	Provide complete and accurate information regarding patient's course before transfer of care

Modified from Keay S, Callander C: The safe use of infusion devices. BJA Contin Educ Anaesth Crit Care Pain 3:81-85, 2004.

Implications

Commercial target-controlled infusion systems are now available, at least in Europe. Diprifusor is a total IV anesthesia system that can be set to achieve a desired plasma concentration of propofol. The system can be set according to the patient's age and ideal weight and the plasma concentration desired by the clinician. It is widely used in Europe but is awaiting approval in the United States. This system can also predict how long it will take for the patient to wake up once the infusion is stopped.

There are also newer closed-loop systems that can adjust the rate of infusion according to feedback from auditory-evoked potentials and a bispectral index. In the near future, these systems will be part of everyday anesthesia practice. Their pumps are driven by pharmacokinetic models using software algorithms, and pharmacokinetic parameters for various drugs can be programmed into the devices. Figure 133-3 illustrates the potential sources of error in pharmacokinetic model drug delivery systems.

An understanding of pharmacokinetics is important when giving any drug, but this is especially true with IV drugs. For example, remifentanil has a different elimination profile compared with fentanyl, alfentanil, and sufentanil. Because this difference was not considered for the patient in the case synopsis, the result was poor analgesia upon recovery.

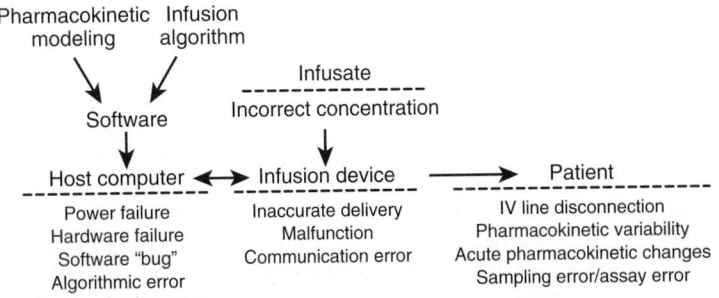

Figure 133–3 ■ Commercially available target-controlled infusion systems have computer functions incorporated into the device itself. Potential sources of error in drug delivery systems based on pharmacokinetic models are shown. (From Glass PA, Shafer SL, Reves JG: Intravenous drug delivery systems. In Miller RD [ed]: Anesthesia, 5th ed. New York, Churchill Livingstone, 2000.)

Table 133–2 ■ **Manual Infusion Schemes When Combined With 66% Nitrous Oxide and Oxygen**				
	Anesthesia		**Sedation or Analgesia**	
Drug	*Loading Dose* *(μg/kg)*	*Maintenance Dose* *(μg/kg/min)*	*Loading Dose* *(μg/kg)*	*Maintenance Dose* *(μg/kg/min)*
Alfentanil	50-150	0.5-3	10-25	0.25-1
Fentanyl	5-15	0.03-0.1	1-3	0.01-0.03
Sufentanil	0.25-2	0.01-0.05	0.1-0.5	0.005-0.01
Remifentanil	0.5-1	0.1-0.4	*	0.025-0.1
Ketamine	1500-2500	25-75	500-1000	10-20
Propofol	1000-2000	50-150	250-1000	10-50
Midazolam	50-150	0.25-1.5	25-100	0.25-1
Methohexital	1000-1500	50-150	250-1000	10-50

*No loading dose necessary if used for IV sedation.

MANAGEMENT

Drug delivery failure is investigated by asking the following questions:

- Is the pump working?
- Is the drug physically moving?
- Is the carrier fluid moving?
- Are connections secure and not leaking?
- Is the vascular access patent?

If the cause of a failure cannot be identified and corrected quickly, one should switch to an alternative anesthesia technique. If the patient is in pain because the infusion was turned off too early, supplemental analgesia and anesthesia should be instituted as appropriate. Use of tagged and prefilled syringes avoids incompatibility with commercial target-controlled infusion systems. Target-controlled infusion systems need to be reset in between patients; otherwise, the wrong patient information will be used by the infusion pump. Total IV anesthesia infusion pumps are associated with a median absolute performance error, which represents over- or underinfusion. Adequate depth of anesthesia must be maintained while using total IV anesthesia, especially when the patient is paralyzed. Awareness of the potential problems listed in Table 133-1 will help avoid most errors.

PREVENTION

If one bases the loading dose on the initial volume of distribution, an incorrect dose may be given. Equilibration with other compartments should be taken into account when calculating the dose. Titration of doses and infusion rates should be modified according to clinical requirements. Over time, as the peripheral compartments equilibrate with the plasma concentration, the infusion rate must decrease in order to maintain the desired concentration at the effector site. This is achieved by understanding the pharmacokinetic and dynamic characteristics of individual drugs and patients and by titrating the infusion to specific effects, similar to using an inhalation anesthetic end-tidal concentration analyzer. Unfortunately, unlike with the latter, there is no in-line plasma drug concentration analyzer. Examples of some dosing regimens are given in Table 133-2. Familiarity with IV drug delivery systems will avoid the peaks and troughs of intermittent IV bolus dosing, ultimately improving the patient's hemodynamic stability and recovery time, reducing IV drug usage, and increasing patient satisfaction.

Further Reading

Eyres R: Update on TIVA. Pediatr Anesth 14:374-379, 2004.

Glass PSA, Shafer SL, Reves JG: Intravenous drug delivery systems. In Miller RD (ed): Anesthesia, 5th ed. New York, Churchill Livingstone, 2000.

Kapila A, Glass PSA, Jacobs J, et al: Measured context sensitive half-times of remifentanil and alfentanil. Anesthesiology 83:968-975, 1995.

Keay S, Callander C: The safe use of infusion devices. BJA Contin Educ Anaesth Crit Care Pain 3:81-85, 2004.

Leslie K, Absalom A, Kenny GNC: Closed loop control of sedation for colonoscopy using the bispectral index. Anaesthesia 57:693-697, 2002.

Milne SE, Kenny GNC: Future applications for TCI anaesthesia. Anaesthesia 53:56-60, 1998.

EQUIPMENT &
MONITORING

Patient Warming Systems

134

Michael P. Eaton and Stewart J. Lustik

Case Synopsis

A 26-year-old man is brought to the operating room emergently for the treatment of injuries sustained in a motor vehicle accident. The hose of a forced-air warming system had been placed between the patient's legs, unattached to the blanket, and the unit was turned on to the maximum setting. Postoperatively, the patient is noted to have partial- and full-thickness burns to the inner thighs.

PROBLEM ANALYSIS

Definition

Perioperative hypothermia is known to be associated with significant increases in morbidity. Thus, the prevention of hypothermia is an important goal of anesthetic care, but the use of devices to prevent hypothermia is not without risk. The primary complication resulting from these devices is tissue burns. Other complications include hyperthermia, hypothermia (from incorrectly set or malfunctioning devices), and electrocution.

Patient warming devices can be divided into two main categories: (1) items not designed for patient warming that are nonetheless used for that purpose, and (2) devices specifically designed and manufactured for the purpose of preventing and treating hypothermia. In the American Society of Anesthesiologists (ASA) closed claims analysis of injuries caused by patient warming devices, the former category accounted for the majority of claims. Included in this category are the following:

- Heated intravenous (IV) solution bags
- Heated bottles of irrigating or other fluids
- Reheated "hot packs"

Devices specifically designed and manufactured for the prevention and treatment of hypothermia include the following:

- Circulating water blankets
- Blankets or pads containing electrical heating elements (hot pads)
- Forced-air warming blankets
- Radiant heaters
- Regular or reflective blankets
- Breathing circuit heated humidifiers
- Intravenous fluid warmers

The last two devices are discussed in Chapters 132 and 135, respectively. Table 134-1 provides further details about the mechanism of injury, risk factors, and preventive measures for some of the listed devices.

Recognition

Intraoperative hyperthermia and hypothermia are recognized by continuous monitoring of the patient's core temperature. The existing ASA standards require temperature monitoring whenever temperature instability is expected.

Unfortunately, recognition of burns usually occurs postoperatively, when it is too late to prevent the injury. Typically, patients complain of pain in the burn-injured area. Analgesics given to treat pain related to surgery may mask pain due to a burn injury and delay the diagnosis. Inspection of the patient's back or other area of contact at the end of the procedure is important whenever a warming device has been used. Early recognition may allow aggressive treatment to prevent infection, which has the potential to be life threatening.

Risk Assessment

Risk from the two categories of warming devices seems to accrue to different patient groups. In the closed claims analysis of burns from heated IV solution bags, the average patient was a female, age 38 years, having surgery for which significant hypothermia would not be expected. The primary risk factor for these patients was the use of a device that was not intended for the warming of patients. Frequently the bags were kept in blanket warmers or ovens whose temperature was poorly regulated. Alternatively, they were heated in microwave ovens with no temperature control. A recent survey of hospitals using heated IV bags perioperatively found that several institutions allowed these bags to be heated to more than 50°C. Two hospitals kept bags at temperatures higher than 70°C, which would produce burns within only a few seconds of exposure (Fig. 134-1).

Injury from devices designed for patient warming is more likely to be related to patient factors or to device malfunction or misuse. A search of the Food and Drug Administration's Manufacturer and User-Facility Device Experience (MAUDE) database for reports of injuries from one company's forced-air warming device found that in 24 of 30 cases in which the cause of injury could be determined with some certainty, the device was used without the blanket "hosing" or otherwise contrary to the manufacturer's recommendations.

A common patient factor is the likelihood of poor local tissue perfusion at the site of contact with the warming device. These injuries are usually most severe in areas overlying bony prominences. Patients undergoing vascular surgery, diabetic patients, and those having procedures involving cardiopulmonary bypass are at increased risk for thermal injury related to warming devices. These patients

Table 134–1 ▪ Injury from Patient Warming Devices

Device	Mechanism of Injury	Risk Factors	Preventive Measures
Heated IV solution bags	Conduction heat transfer	Overly heated solutions	Do not use
Electrical resistance heating pads	Conduction heat transfer Electrocution	High settings Device malfunction	Use only for awake, alert patients Use lowest effective settings Check before each use Perform routine maintenance
Circulating water blankets	Conduction heat transfer	Patients with poor tissue perfusion High heat output from machine Machine malfunction	Use on top of patient, rather than beneath (to eliminate pressure component of injury) Use lowest effective settings Check before each use Perform routine maintenance
Heat lamps	Radiant heat transfer	Too close to patient Lamp modified	Maintain proper distance from patient as per manufacturer's recommendations Use recommended diffuser or lens
Forced-air warmers	Convective heat transfer	No blanket or wrong blanket used PACU machine or high settings used Patients with poor (or no) tissue perfusion	Use blanket only from the same manufacturer Use only operating room-approved machine on lowest effective setting Use lower settings on patients with vascular insufficiency Do not use distal to tourniquet or cross-clamp

PACU, postanesthesia care unit.

have poor regional tissue perfusion related to their disease state, surgery, or cardiopulmonary bypass, which allows local temperature to increase to the point of injury because blood flow is inadequate to redistribute applied heat. Pressure applied to the skin at the site of contact with the warming device also compromises perfusion and increases the likelihood of injury. The MAUDE database showed that of six reports of injury caused by a new circulating water system, all six identified pressure at the contact point as a contributing factor.

Patients at the extremes of age also appear to be at higher risk for thermal injury, most likely because they are at increased risk for the development of hypothermia and are therefore more likely to have heating devices applied during surgery. Elderly patients also may suffer from poor tissue perfusion, as discussed earlier.

Device malfunction may cause injury if proper routine maintenance has not been performed or if the equipment is not used according to the manufacturer's directions. Even properly used and maintained machines may produce injury

Figure 134–1 ▪ Time required for contact with an object at various temperatures to produce burn injury. (Data from Moritz AR, Henriques FC Jr: Studies of thermal injury. II. The relative importance of time and surface temperature in the causation of cutaneous burns. Am J Pathol 23:695-720, 1947.)

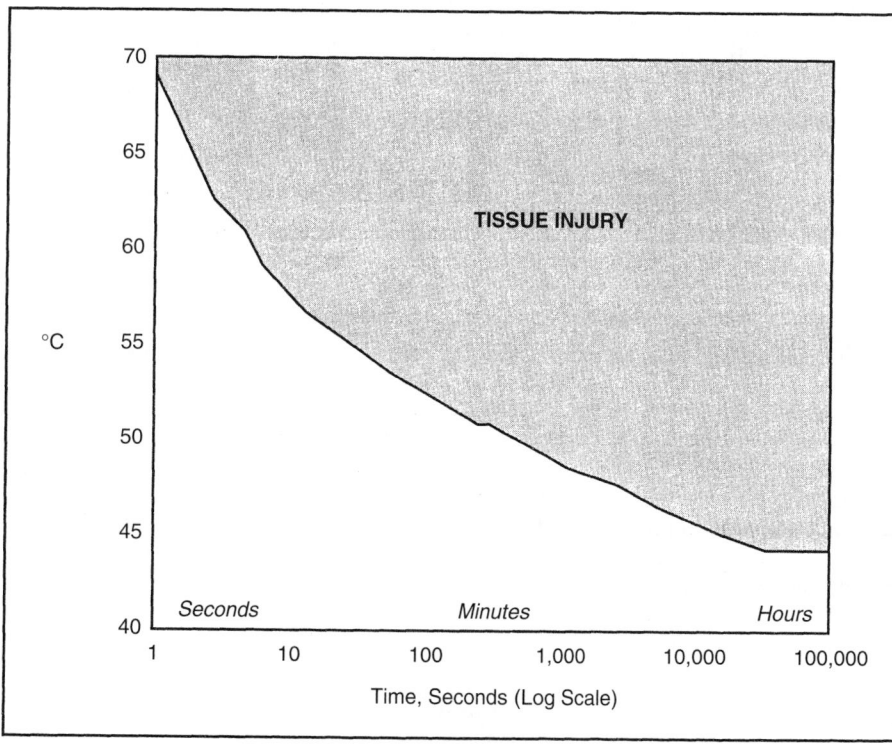

if tolerances allowed by the device exceed the ability of tissue to safely absorb and transfer the energy. This is especially likely when high temperature gradients exist between the device and the patient. Some commonly used circulating water blankets allow water temperatures as high as 48°C, even when properly calibrated and maintained. Temperatures greater than 45°C may predictably produce thermal injury, depending in part on the time of exposure (see Fig. 134-1).

Patient warming systems draw high levels of electrical current, and poorly maintained devices or those contaminated with fluids may overheat and cause a fire, presenting a hazard to the caregivers as well as to the patient.

Implications

Patients having major vascular procedures or those involving cardiopulmonary bypass often have such diminished cardiovascular reserve that major burns can be a fatal complication. Less severe burns can also cause major morbidity. Permanently disfiguring scars that result from well-intended but ill-advised warming methods can put practitioners at significant medicolegal risk.

Hyperthermia may cause an increase in cardiac and respiratory work and oxygen demand that produces undue stress on patients with limited physiologic reserves. Vasodilatation and sweating may produce relative or absolute hypovolemia and acidosis, and a hypermetabolic state may cause hypoglycemia. Extreme hyperthermia may result in central nervous system damage and death.

MANAGEMENT

Upon recognition that a burn injury has occurred, prompt referral to a physician skilled in the treatment of burns is essential. The proper management of burns is the subject of many textbooks and is not discussed further.

Management of hyperthermia includes turning off or removing the warming device from the patient and uncovering as much of the patient as is practical under the circumstances. Active cooling is rarely necessary if overzealous warming is the sole reason for the elevated temperature. If the temperature elevation is severe or refractory to passive cooling, other causes, such as infection, sepsis, or malignant hyperthermia, should be sought.

PREVENTION

The best management for injury related to patient warming devices is prevention. The ASA closed claims analysis of such injuries found that in 17 of 28 cases, care was judged to be substandard. This was the finding in all but one case of burns resulting from the application of heated IV solution bags or bottles. These devices should never be used for patient warming; they are not intended for that purpose, they are inefficient, and they are associated with an unacceptably high risk of patient injury.

Injuries from approved patient warming devices are more difficult to prevent, but attention to a few important details should make injury unlikely:

- All devices should be maintained as recommended by the manufacturer.
- Any machine that fails safety testing during routine maintenance should be removed from service immediately.
- The anesthesia provider responsible for the patient's care should personally check the settings of the machine used.
- The provider should be familiar with and adhere to the manufacturer's recommendations for use of the device. No alterations in the device should be made unless they are approved by the manufacturer.
- Intraoperatively, constant vigilance must be maintained to ensure that portions of the heating devices not intended for direct patient contact, such as the tubing for a water blanket or the hose of a forced-air mattress, do not touch the patient.
- When possible, water blanket devices should be used on *top* of the patient rather than beneath. This should minimize the risk of poorly perfused tissue being in contact with the device. This should also enhance the efficacy of the device, because operating table mattresses already provide adequate insulation, and the primary loss of a patient's heat is into the room. In fact, warming devices generally act by decreasing or eliminating the loss of the patient's own metabolic heat rather than by adding extrinsic heat.
- Pressure (e.g., from positioning aids) should not be put on parts of the body in contact with warming devices. That is, water or forced-air warming blankets should not be applied until the patient has been properly positioned for the planned procedure.
- Warming devices should not be placed on any part of the body that is distal to a tourniquet or cross-clamp, because large device-tissue temperature gradients can develop, with resultant injury.

Further Reading

Chaney FW, Posner KL, Caplan RA, Gild WM: Burns from warming devices in anesthesia: A closed claims analysis. Anesthesiology 80:806-810, 1994.

Crino MH, Nagel EL: Thermal burns caused by warming blankets in the operating room. Anesthesiology 29:149-150, 1968.

Hewitt FW: A lecture on the aethetics of anesthetics. Lancet 1:623-626, 1910.

Moritz AR, Henriques FC Jr: Studies of thermal injury. II. The relative importance of time and surface temperature in the causation of cutaneous burns. Am J Pathol 23:695-720, 1947.

Raphael DT, Ayoub N: Storage of plastic intravenous solution bags in operating room warmers. Anesth Analg 84:S203, 1997.

Sessler DI: Temperature monitoring. In Miller RD (ed): Anesthesia, 3rd ed. New York, Churchill Livingstone, 1990, pp 1227-1242.

US Food and Drug Administration: Manufacturer and User-Facility Device Experience database (MAUDE). Available at http://www.accessdata.fda.gov/scripts/cdrh/cfdocs/cfMAUDE/search.cfm?searchoptions=1.

Rapid Fluid and Blood Delivery Systems

S. Devi Chiravuri

135

Case Synopsis

A 65-year-old man is brought to the operating room for emergent repair of a ruptured abdominal aortic aneurysm. The patient is intubated, hypothermic (34.5°C), and hypotensive (blood pressure 85/60 mm Hg). Volume resuscitation is instituted with warmed intravenous (IV) fluids under pressure using a Level 1 System 1000 IV fluid warmer. Before skin incision, the blood pressure drops to 60/30 mm Hg, and the end-tidal carbon dioxide ($ETCO_2$) drops precipitously from 35 to 10 mm Hg, suggesting a massive venous air embolus.

PROBLEM ANALYSIS

Definition

Rapid fluid and blood delivery (RFBD) devices are used when IV fluid or blood must be delivered at rates greater than those attainable with free-flow or IV pressure bag devices. Contemporary RFBD devices allow for flows of 750 mL/minute, with the ability to "dial in" flow rates. In addition to high flow, they allow one to select or set the temperature of the infusate.

High flows are provided by pressure. RFBD pressurization can be achieved by two methods: external pneumatic pressurization and occlusive roller pumps. Heating is provided by either water bath conduction heat exchange or a magnetic induction heater.

In addition to delivering high-volume flow rates and heating the fluids, RFBD devices must be able to detect or vent air. Air traps are able to extract small volumes of entrained air, but larger volumes may exceed the capacity of the trap. One model, the FMS2000 (Belmont Instrument Corporation, Billerica, Mass.), uses a reservoir from which the fluids are delivered, and it alerts the user when the reservoir is nearly empty (Fig. 135-1).

Potential complications associated with the use or malfunction of RFBD devices include the following:

- Air embolism
- Hypervolemia or overtransfusion
- Overheating of fluids
- Hypothermia
- Hemolysis
- Electrical shock

Recognition

VENOUS AIR EMBOLISM

Venous air embolism is a condition that is well described in anesthesia (see also Chapters 168 and 175). It occurs when air enters the venous system, either via entrainment at the operative site or inadvertently via IV catheters; this is more likely with central than with peripheral access. This air travels to the heart and can significantly decrease cardiac output. It can also travel via a patent foramen ovale to the left side of the heart and up to the cerebral circulation, potentially causing cerebral ischemia or stroke. Detection of air can be via echocardiogram, precordial Doppler, or a sudden drop in $ETCO_2$. Signs of a venous air embolus include the following:

- Systemic hypotension
- Increased central venous or pulmonary artery pressures
- Arrhythmia
- Hypoxemia
- Acute decrease in $ETCO_2$
- Decrease in pulmonary compliance

HYPERVOLEMIA

Hypervolemia can cause initial hypertension, but this may be followed by hypotension as left ventricular preload and end-diastolic volume increase and eventually drop off the Frank-Starling curve (forward left ventricular failure). If central monitoring is in place, elevated pulmonary artery pressures and pulmonary capillary wedge pressures are seen.

HYPOTHERMIA OR HYPERTHERMIA

Hypothermia occurs when transfusion is conducted without vigilant temperature monitoring or if the heating mechanism is faulty. This can cause coagulopathy, arrhythmias, or peripheral vasoconstriction.

Hyperthermia can be as detrimental as hypothermia. Elevated temperature is detected with temperature monitoring. Core monitoring is more accurate than skin temperature monitoring. Hyperthermia can cause denaturing of molecules such as hemoglobin and cause hemoglobinemia and hemolysis. Clinically, it can manifest as sweating, vasodilatation, and hemoglobinuria.

ELECTRICAL SHOCK

Electrical shock is not unique to RFBD devices. It can occur with any electrical device that comes in contact with patients. Electrical shock may cause pain, tetanus, thermal injury, or transient arrhythmias.

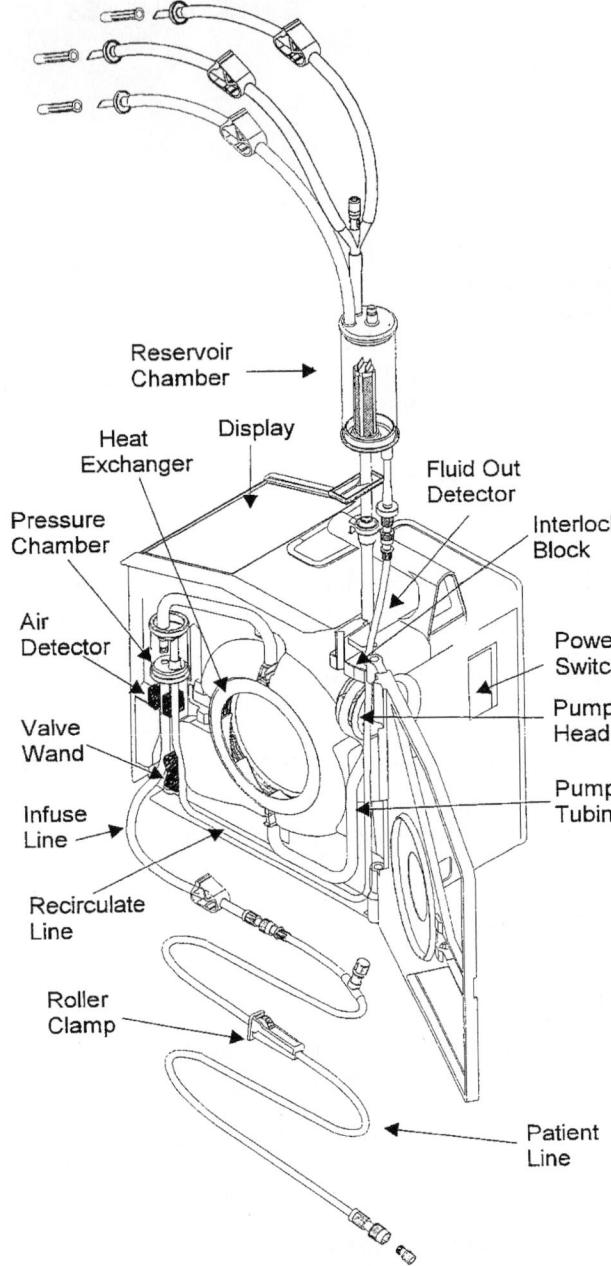

Figure 135–1 ■ FMS2000 rapid fluid delivery system. (Courtesy of Belmont Instrument Corporation, Billerica, Mass.)

Risk Assessment and Implications

Vigilance is as imperative, as with any medical device. Fatal complications can result from machine malfunction or operator error.

MANAGEMENT

If a venous air embolus is suspected:

- Alert the surgeon in the event that the air is being entrained at the operative site.
- Stop the rapid infusion device.
- Support blood pressure if hypotension occurs.
- Place the patient in a dependent or decubitus position.
- Turn off the nitrous oxide (if in use).
- If a central venous line is in place, attempt to aspirate air.

If hypothermia is present, a heating mattress and forced-air warming blanket can be used (see Chapter 134). Hyperthermia is treated by switching off any heating devices.

Hemolysis has several causes: shear stresses from over-pressurized infusion, overheating of blood and blood products, or transfusion reactions or mismatch. Treatment includes the following:

- Discontinue the transfusion.
- Notify the blood bank and recheck the crossmatch.
- Maintain the urine output.
- Alkalinize the urine.
- Monitor for signs of disseminated intravascular coagulation.

Hypervolemia can present as pulmonary or circulatory collapse. Treatment includes the following:

- Circulatory support
- Diuretics
- Vasodilator therapy
- Assisted ventilation or positive-pressure ventilation
- In extreme cases, phlebotomy

PREVENTION

Vigilance is key to minimizing risk in the operating room. Meticulous venting of air before connecting IV lines and infusion devices is an important step. Careful monitoring of $ETCO_2$ is a necessary precaution.

Hyperthermia and hypothermia can be prevented by aggressive treatment and core body temperature monitoring. Skin temperature monitoring can give false information, especially when there is vasoconstriction.

It is also important to pay close attention to the patient's volume status. Urine output and central venous pressure should be monitored continuously when an RFBD system is used.

The risk of electrical shock can be minimized with vigilance and proper maintenance of all electrical devices in the operating room. Quick checks of the insulation and ground fault detection alarms are a good start.

Finally, the importance of familiarity with and proper use and maintenance of RFBD devices cannot be stressed enough. Attending in-service training programs related to such equipment and maintaining competency in its use should be a priority. RFBD systems may play a key role in surgery that requires large-volume resuscitation (e.g., major trauma, cardiovascular surgery, liver transplantation, major thoracic trauma), but only when it is used properly and with good judgment.

Further Reading

Bedford RF: Air embolism. In Gravenstien N, Kirby RR (eds): Complications in Anesthesiology. Philadelphia, Lippincott-Raven, 1996, pp 271-280.

Comunale ME: A laboratory evaluation of the Level 1 Rapid Infuser (H1025) and the Belmont Instrument Fluid Management System (FMS 2000) for rapid transfusion. Anesth Analg 97:1064-1069, 2003.

Flacke WE, Flacke JW, Ryan JF, et al: Temperature: Homeostasis and unintentional hypothermia. In Gravenstein N, Kirby RR (eds): Complications in Anesthesiology. Philadelphia, Lippincott-Raven, 1996, pp 117-129.

Smith CE: Principles of fluid warming in trauma. Semin Anesth Periop Med Pain 20:51-59, 2001.

EQUIPMENT & MONITORING

Surgical Diathermy and Electrocautery

136

Ian Lewis

Case Synopsis

A 59-year-old man undergoes elective transurethal surgery for benign prostatic hypertrophy under spinal anesthesia. He had a pacemaker inserted 5 years ago for third degree heart block. It was programmed to ventricular-inhibited pacing with an adaptive rate response (i.e., VVIR mode). The device was programmed with a lower rate cutoff of 60 beats per minute and an upper rate cutoff of 130 paced pulses per minute. The initial electrocardiogram (ECG), before use of the unipolar diathermy device, revealed P waves at a rate of 100 beats per minute, with ventricular pacing at 60 pulses per minute. Each time the diathermy unit is activated, the paced ventricular rate gradually increases to a plateau of 130 pulses per minute. Each time the diathermy is stopped, the rate gradually returns to 60 beats per minute.

PROBLEM ANALYSIS

Definition

Surgical diathermy (cutting) and electrocautery (coagulating vessels) are similar processes whereby body tissues are heated as a consequence of their resistance to the passage of an electrical current. There are a number of potential hazards associated with its use during anesthesia and surgery, and the case synopsis illustrates one such phenomenon: interference with an implanted electronic device. The rapid ventricular pacing that occurred in this example may have resulted in a number of problems, including low cardiac output, myocardial ischemia, and pacemaker-mediated tachycardia, which could be misinterpreted and treated as ventricular tachycardia. Interference with pacemakers programmed to other modes may result in different problems, such as inhibition or reversion to an asynchronized mode. Owing to advances in pacemaker and internal cardioverter-defibrillator technology, it is no longer appropriate to manage patients with cardiac rhythm management devices (CRMDs) by placing a magnet over the CRMD pulse generator (see Chapter 97).

Recognition

Recognition and prevention of the complications associated with any medical device require both an understanding of its underlying mechanisms and knowledge of the potential complications. This includes any features or associated warning signs or alarms that signal possible problems. With surgical diathermy, all operating room personnel should have a general awareness of the diverse but specific complications (e.g., skin burns, cardiac arrhythmias) associated with this device. These complications may result in significant morbidity and mortality to both patients and medical personnel. In the situation described in the case synopsis, there was an apparent lack of recognition that the use of surgical diathermy might be associated with heart rate changes in a patient with a cardiac pacemaker. In this instance, there was no adverse outcome. However, with the illustrated upper rate behavior in response to sensed continuous electromagnetic interference (i.e., the "noise reversion mode"—ventricular pacing at 130 pulses per minute), paced QRS complexes would be widened, but pacing artifacts might be unapparent.[1] If the supposed ventricular tachycardia were treated with drugs or electrical cardioversion, this might have produced an unfavorable outcome.

Risk Assessment

Surgical diathermy is used frequently in the operating room. Problems are rare, but their incidence can be reduced or eliminated if anesthesia personnel are familiar with the operation of surgical diathermy. Programs must be in place for educating and training personnel in the proper use and servicing of this equipment. Additionally, there must be a reporting system for faulty equipment, complications, and "near misses."

In principle, diathermy uses the heating effect of passing an electrical current across a resistor. In practice, the "resistor" is the patient's skin or other tissue being cauterized or cut. Alternating current (AC) is often used in clinical practice. The correct term for *resistance* with AC as opposed to direct current (DC) is *impedance*. A potential difference created by the diathermy device produces a current that passes through the patient to complete an electrical circuit. This circuit may be completed in two ways:

1. *Unipolar diathermy.* The cathode (−) is the cautery-diathermy (Bovie) tool tip, and the anode (+) is the ground or return plate. This is usually located on one of

---

[1]This is especially true if the pacemaker lead configuration is bipolar, which greatly reduces the size of the pacing artifacts. However, many ECG monitors in use today have a feature that detects and amplifies small pacing artifacts, enabling clinicians to see them on the monitor.

Figure 136–1 ■ Modes of current delivery from electrosurgical units: cutting, coagulation, and blend modes. (Courtesy of Valleylab, Inc., Boulder, Colo.)

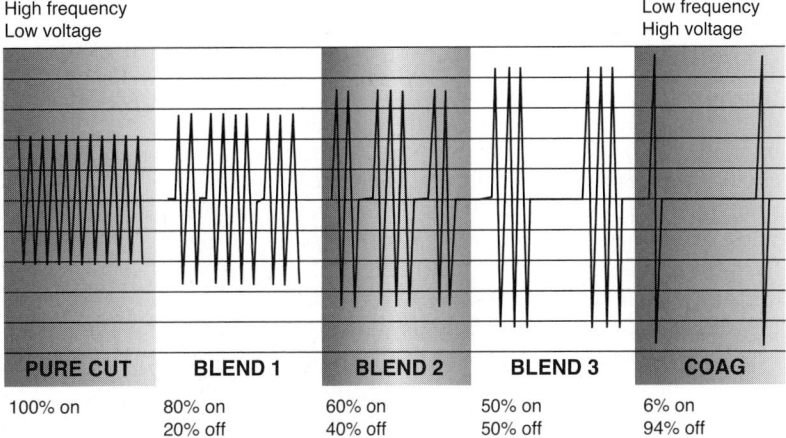

PURE CUT	**BLEND 1**	**BLEND 2**	**BLEND 3**	**COAG**
100% on	80% on / 20% off	60% on / 40% off	50% on / 50% off	6% on / 94% off

the patient's buttocks or thighs. Unipolar diathermy-cautery configurations have the highest potential for complications with CRMDs, because the current pathway between the cathode and anode may pass near or across the CRMD pulse generator or leads.

2. *Bipolar diathermy.* Both the cathode (−) and the anode (+) are incorporated in a forceps and are therefore very closely spaced. Thus, a grounding plate is not required with bipolar diathermy-cautery, and the current pathway is very small. The risk of CRMD-related complications is much smaller (but not absent) because the current pathway is far less likely to pass near or across the CRMD pulse generator or leads. The exception is if cautery is applied directly to or very near (i.e., within a few centimeters) the pulse generator or leads.

The higher the resistance at a point in an electrical circuit, the higher the heating effect will be with the passage of current. Thus, $W = I^2R$, where W is the power output in watts, which is proportional to the heating effect; I is the current in amps; and R is the resistance in ohms. Resistance and the heating effect are higher where the current passes over a narrow pathway. Thus, current density is very high at the point of the unipolar diathermy-cautery pencil tip and relatively low throughout the patient's body and across the large surface area of a correctly placed ground electrode pad. In fact, the only significant point of resistance (i.e., heat production) should be at the electrode tip.

Diathermy units often develop power levels between 50 and 400 watts and radiofrequency AC cycles from 300 kHz to 3 MHz. Current is delivered in varying waveform patterns or modes (Fig. 136-1). Continuous current is used for cutting, and pulses are used for coagulation. Because the pure cutting (diathermy) mode uses continuous current, it produces a series of sparks from the diathermy tool to the tissue. The pencil tip does not have to contact the tissue. The sparks generated cause intense local heating of cellular water, causing cellular explosion and destruction over a narrow band (Fig. 136-2).

In contrast, coagulation (cautery) requires the direct application of the pencil tip; heat is thus dissipated over a wider area, causing the cells to shrink (crenate) and dry out (desiccate) rather than explode (Fig. 136-3). Bipolar diathermy is generally restricted to coagulation modes. In contrast, unipolar diathermy incorporates various coagulation and cutting modes (see Fig. 136-1).

Argon gas, applied as a jet around the tip of the cathode, has been used to improve the safety and effectiveness of diathermy. This gas is heavier than air, inert, and noncombustible, and it displaces nitrogen and oxygen. It is also

EQUIPMENT & MONITORING

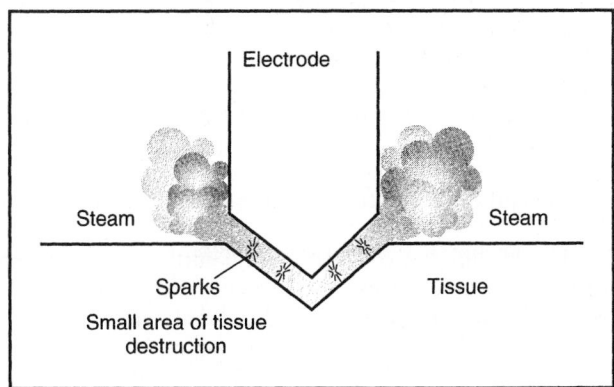

Figure 136–2 ■ Mechanism of electrosurgical cutting mode.

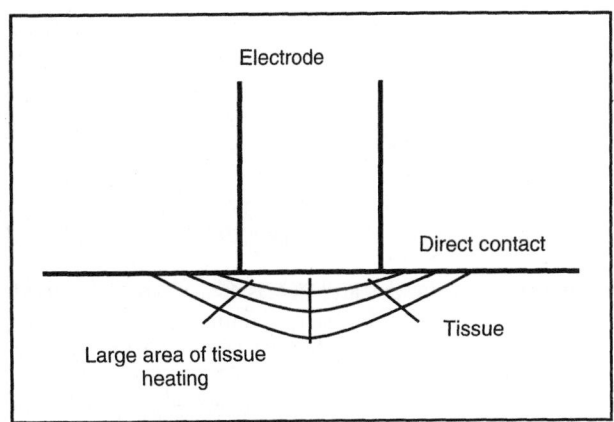

Figure 136–3 ■ Mechanism of electrosurgical coagulation mode.

readily ionized by the current and provides a medium for the passage of current, so that the pencil tip does not have to be in direct contact with tissue.

Two types of complications associated with surgical diathermy or cautery are electrocution and electromagnetic interference (EMI). Electrocution may occur if the patient circuit becomes a route for the passage of electrical current from other sources to the diathermy or cautery ground plate. These are termed leakage currents. Current passing through the body at the AC outlet frequency (60 Hz) can cause serious problems in excitable tissue (e.g., arrhythmias and large muscle group contractions, which may be perceived by awake patients). However, the same current applied in the radiofrequency range allows diathermy-cautery to work without producing these untoward effects. Thus, diathermy-cautery units incorporate an isolating capacitor in their circuits. This allows the passage of relatively harmless (for excitable tissue) radiofrequency current but impairs the passage of more dangerous low-frequency leakage currents to the ground plate.

The duration of the applied diathermy or cautery may also increase the probability of certain complications. For example, cardiac arrhythmias can be avoided if leakage current is prevented altogether or terminated rapidly (within a few microseconds) by line isolation circuitry. Major complications (e.g., ventricular fibrillation due to the passage of very small frequency currents across the heart) can also be minimized by line isolation monitors and ground fault circuit indicators (see Chapter 137).

Finally, EMI is the tendency of electric current in one circuit or conductor (usually wires) to induce current in another, even though separated by a nonconducting material such as air. EMI may result in transient disturbances in patient monitoring equipment but can also cause transient malfunction, alter preset parameters, or cause permanent damage to implanted devices such as CRMDs.

Implications

Many of the complications of surgical diathermy are predictable. Heat production may lead to the following:

- Burns may occur at the ground plate (also known as "return" or "anode") site if there is poor contact of the ground plate with the patient's skin surface.
- Localized burns via electrical pathways created by small surface area electrodes. These pathways may be created by application of ECG or other (e.g., bispectral index, patient state analyzer, neuromuscular function monitor) electrodes or the use of diathermy to an organ that has been temporarily suspended on a narrow vascular pedicle.
- Fires or explosions in association with alcohol-based skin preparations, colonic gas, explosive anesthetics (largely of historical interest), and oxygen-enriched environments (see Chapter 138).
- Inhalation of smoke and debris from vaporized tissue. Diathermy-vaporized tissue contains chemicals such as benzene, hydrogen cyanide, and formaldehyde, plus live cellular fragments and viruses. A suction port at the active electrode (cathode) can reduce the diffusion of smoke and debris.

ELECTROMAGNETIC INTERFERENCE

EMI may enter an implanted electrical device through direct contact with the source of EMI or by exposure to an electromagnetic field, with the device leads serving as antennae. Devices that are most susceptible are CRMDs, phrenic nerve stimulators, and cochlear implants. Owing to CRMDs' large antennae, unipolar lead configurations increase the susceptibility to device malfunction during exposure to EMI. EMI may interfere with other electrical equipment, including pulse oximeters and ECG monitors, by producing artifacts or noise.

ELECTROCUTION AND MICROSHOCK HAZARDS

These complications can be serious, causing ventricular tachycardia or fibrillation or even cardiac standstill (asystole), and they are generally associated with electrical energy supplied by the main or leakage currents associated with faulty electrical apparatus.

MANAGEMENT AND PREVENTION

Safety Precautions

With unipolar diathermy or cautery, the full surface of the return (grounding) pad or plate must fully contact the patient's skin surface to minimize the risk of burns. An alarm will sound if the resistance across the pad or plate increases, indicating a reduction in the contact area. Complete circuit disconnection is also sensed. The contact surfaces of diathermy-cautery grounding pads are already covered with electrolytic contact paste or gel to reduce resistance to current flow, but such electrolytic material must be manually applied to the surface of a grounding plate, taking care to ensure full coverage.

It is necessary to check other parts of the cautery or diathermy circuits (e.g., for lead insulation defects), as well as to check any other electrical equipment (e.g., laparoscopic instruments) for their ability to induce or store (i.e., act as capacitors) leakage currents that could cause thermal injury or increase the risk for micro- or macroshock.

Isolation capacitors permit the passage of radiofrequency current but impede dangerous 60-Hz main current. Electrical isolation of the main supply from the radiofrequency generator also reduces the risk for passage of leakage currents.

Hand operation of the diathermy or cautery tool (versus using a foot pedal) reduces the risk of its inadvertent use. A noise should be emitted when the diathermy or cautery tool is activated.

When not in use, active diathermy or cautery tools should be stored in an appropriate nonconductive holster. Jerry-rigged holsters (e.g., red rubber tubing) may not provide sufficient protection and may ignite under certain conditions.

Use of different coagulation and cutting modes allows for the more efficient use of diathermy and can help minimize potential complications, such as smoke and debris production. As mentioned earlier, argon gas applied around the cathode tip can improve the safety and effectiveness of diathermy.

The appropriate equipment should always be used. Interchanging parts from different devices may result in complications. The return (ground) electrode plate or pad should be placed on skin covering a well-vascularized muscle mass. Avoid irregularities, such as bony prominences, which may reduce the surface contact area and increase the risk for burns by creating air pockets and potential spark gaps. For children, appropriately sized grounding pads or plates should be used (refer to the manufacturer's instructions). Pads or plates should be checked periodically during long cases.

Contact with combustible fluids (e.g., alcohol-containing skin preparations) must be avoided. Oxygen should not be used in the vicinity of diathermy or cautery (e.g., when supplemental oxygen is being administered to the patient). There must be no direct contact with metal or other electrical conductors (e.g., fluids), as this may result in burns at points of contact and coincidentally act as pathways for leakage current.

Recommendations for Patients with Cardiac Rhythm Management Devices

- Preoperative assessment should include the indication for the device, identification of the device, the programmed mode, and the interference mode. Direct interrogation of the device is especially helpful. It may be necessary to consult a cardiologist or the CRMD follow-up service or clinic (see Chapter 97).
- A 12-lead ECG should routinely be obtained preoperatively.
- If diathermy-cautery will be used near the CRMD pulse generator or leads, the patient is at high risk for diathermy or electrocautery EMI. If the patient has an adaptive-rate device or is mostly pacemaker dependent, the device must be reprogrammed to (1) an asynchronous operation (inactivate sensing), (2) disable any adaptive-rate features, and (3) inactivate antitachycardia pacing therapies or shocks (see Chapter 97).
- Reprogramming does not guarantee immunity against EMI-caused damage or altered CRMD function. Therefore, it is necessary to interrogate the CRMD and reprogram it after exposure to diathermy or cautery EMI.
- Alternatively, if the risk of EMI is high, the patient is pacemaker dependent, and the device does not deliver adaptive-rate or antitachycardia therapies, placement of a magnet or temporary cardiac pacing may be indicated.[2] External cardiac pacing is not always effective, however; in

some patients, prophylactic transvenous pacing is necessary. Regardless, chronotropic drugs should be available for all cases.

- In some high-risk cases (e.g., when atrioventricular synchrony is necessary to preserve cardiac output), a CRMD telemetry reprogramming device and a knowledgeable operator should be available during the case.
- Bipolar diathermy or an ultrasonic (harmonic) scalpel should be used when possible. If unipolar diathermy or cautery is used, the return (grounding) plate and active tip should be kept as far as possible from the pulse generator and leads. The duration of diathermy or cautery should also be as brief as possible.
- To the extent possible, the CRMD pulse generator and leads must be outside (not within) the current pathway between the diathermy-cautery tool and the return plate.
- A backup external cardioverter-defibrillator should be available should the internal one fail to deliver appropriate therapy for tachyarrhythmias (see Chapter 97).
- Postoperative care includes device interrogation to ascertain function, correction of settings, and reprogramming if necessary.

Further Reading

American Society of Anesthesiologists Task Force on Perioperative Management of Patients with Cardiac Rhythm Management Devices: Practice advisory for the perioperative management of patients with cardiac rhythm management devices: Pacemakers and implantable cardioverter-defibrillators. Anesthesiology 103:186-198, 2005 (additional material available at http://www.anesthesiology.org).

Atlee JL, Bernstein AD: Cardiac rhythm management Devices (part I). Anesthesiology 95:1265-1280, 2001.

Atlee JL, Bernstein AD: Cardiac rhythm management Devices (part II). Anesthesiology 95:1492-1506, 2001.

Epstein MR, Mayer JE Jr, Duncan BW: Use of an ultrasonic scalpel as an alternative to electrocautery in patients with pacemakers. Ann Thorac Surg 65:1802-1804, 1998.

Kleinman B, Hamilton J, Heriman R, et al: Apparent failure of a precordial magnet and pacemaker programmer to convert a DDD pacemaker to VOO mode during use of the electrosurgical unit. Anesthesiology 86:247-250, 1997.

Ozeren M, Dogan OV, Duzgun C, et al: Use of an ultrasonic scalpel in the open-heart reoperation of a patient with a pacemaker. Eur Cardiothorac Surg 21:761-762, 2002.

Salukhe TV, Dob D, Sutton R: Pacemakers and defibrillators: Anaesthetic implications. Br J Anaesth 93:95-104, 2004.

Valleylab (Pfizer) Web site: http://www.pfizer.com/valleylab/.

Wong DT, Middleton W: Electrocautery induced tachycardia in a rate-responsive pacemaker. Anesthesiology 94:710-711, 2001.

---

[2]Generally, it is ill-advised to place a magnet over the CRMD pulse generator without knowing what the magnet response is. This information can be obtained from the manufacturer or hospital CRMD service. In some devices, the magnet response may be programmed off. In others, programming off the magnet response may not confer immunity to sensing or potential malfunction during the planned intervention, even after the patient has been discharged.

Electrical Safety

Jeffrey J. Schwartz

137

Case Synopses

Macroshock

A 50-year-old man in good general health is undergoing laparoscopic cholecystectomy under general anesthesia. In the middle of the procedure, the anesthesiologist feels a tingle, and the patient develops ventricular fibrillation. Immediate resuscitation and defibrillation restore normal sinus rhythm. The case continues uneventfully after a faulty surgical light is removed from service.

Microshock

In an adjacent room, a 60-year-old man with a temporary pacemaker is undergoing lower extremity vascular bypass surgery. While the anesthesiologist is adjusting the pacemaker leads, the patient develops ventricular fibrillation. Immediate resuscitation and defibrillation restore normal sinus rhythm.

PROBLEM ANALYSIS

Definition

Electric shock occurs when a person becomes part of or completes an electrical circuit. To become part of the circuit, a patient must contact it at two points of different voltage. The contact need not be to a wire. Saline-soaked drapes conduct electricity, metal chassis can be energized due to faulty wiring, and leakage currents can flow between any two conductors.

The mechanism of electric shock can be divided into two categories:

- *Macroshock* refers to large amounts of current flowing through intact skin: 5 mA is accepted as the maximum harmless current; 10 to 20 mA causes sustained muscle contraction; 100 to 300 mA causes ventricular fibrillation.
- *Microshock* refers to relatively small currents applied directly to the myocardium. The current density is very high, and as little as 100 μA can cause ventricular fibrillation. This current is too small to be sensed as a tingle by the operator.

Recognition

Recognition of an electrical problem involves not only the realization that an electric shock has occurred but also the awareness that the potential for electric shock exists. Electric shock manifests in the operating room (OR) as sudden-onset ventricular fibrillation (VF) or ventricular tachycardia (VT). The anesthesiologist generally considers a cardiac origin for VF or VT, but the possibility of electric shock must always be kept in mind. Any perception of tingling represents a dangerous situation and must be investigated immediately. Microshock can be recognized only in an appropriate clinical setting, as there are often no premonitory findings.

Risk Assessment

All patients and personnel exposed to an environment with electrical equipment are at risk for macroshock. The OR is an especially hazardous place owing to the common use of saline solutions and the mechanical abuse to which electrical equipment is often subjected. Patients with an electrical connection to the heart, such as a saline-filled central venous catheter or pacemaker wires, are at increased risk for microshock.

The most common cause of macroshock is damaged or faulty wiring in electrical equipment. Line voltages (110 to 220 V) provided by the utility company are kept out of contact by insulated wires. Insulation can wear down and come into contact with a metal chassis or directly with the patient. The use of numerous safeguards (see later) means that for an electric shock to occur, the safeguards must have failed, been ignored, or been absent.

Implications

The implications of electric shock depend on the following:

- Amount of current
- Frequency of current
- Duration of current
- Whether current is applied directly to myocardium

The voltage used in most OR equipment is 110 or 220 V. By Ohm's law, the current that flows (amperes) when 120 V is applied is 120 V/resistance (Ω). The resistance of dry skin, about 120,000 Ω, allows 1 mA to flow. The resistance of wet skin, about 1200 Ω, allows 100 mA to flow, which is a potentially fatal shock. The frequency of electric power in the United States is 60 Hz, which, by coincidence, is the most dangerous frequency.

Electric current affects electrically excitable tissue. Electric current flowing through a nerve or muscle causes pain and contraction, much as a peripheral nerve stimulator does. Electric current flowing through the heart can cause VT or VF and death.

560

MANAGEMENT

Management of electric shock itself consists of appropriate resuscitation, including cardiopulmonary resuscitation and defibrillation. If it can be identified, the source of current and faulty equipment must be removed. Electric shock, however, is often a diagnosis of exclusion.

Line Isolation Monitor

In ORs that use isolated power (i.e., line isolation circuits), the line isolation monitor (LIM) gauges the integrity of such isolation. If the LIM alarm sounds, the power is no longer isolated, and electric current could flow in the event of another fault. The OR, however, is still safe, and all equipment will function normally. The usual cause of a LIM alarm is that faulty equipment has been plugged in. Nonessential electrical equipment should be unplugged, one piece at a time, until the faulty one is identified. Less commonly, many pieces of apparently flawless equipment, but all with small leakage currents, may be simultaneously connected to the same circuit.

Ground Fault Circuit Interrupters

In ORs that use ground fault circuit interrupters (GFCIs), faulty equipment may cause the GFCI to interrupt current to all devices serviced by it. The GFCI has a reset button to restore current, but the faulty piece of equipment must be identified and removed, or the GFCI will trigger again.

PREVENTION

Electric shock is an extraordinarily rare complication owing to the various safeguards undertaken by anesthesiologists, equipment manufacturers, and OR construction engineers.

Grounding

Most electrical equipment in the OR is grounded. This means that the chassis, metal case, and other internal components are all connected to a common earth ground via the third prong on the device's plug. This connection tends to shunt fault current safely to the ground rather than to a person in contact with the equipment.

Power Isolation

Many ORs use isolated power to decrease risk. The utility company supplies grounded power, which means that one of the wires that carries electricity is also connected to the earth via a large, buried conducting rod. This provides additional safety in the distribution of electric power. However, it also means that, to one degree or another, all patients are already directly connected to one part of an electrical circuit.

Only one additional connection, due to faulty wiring, is necessary for the patient to complete the circuit. A line isolation transformer can convert the grounded power from the utility company to isolated power that has no direct connection to the ground. Two contacts with faulty equipment, which is an unlikely situation, would now be necessary to cause electric shock.

Line Isolation Monitor

If isolated power is used, the integrity of the isolation must be monitored, or the system might accidentally become grounded without warning. The LIM continually measures the impedance between the power lines in the OR and the ground. The impedance should be (near) infinity. If it senses that the impedance is reduced and that the power is no longer isolated, an alarm sounds.

Ground Fault Circuit Interrupter

Some ORs use GFCIs to decrease risk. GFCIs continually monitor the difference in current going to and returning from an appliance. If the difference exceeds a certain threshold (typically 5 mA), presumably because some current is being shunted through a patient, the GFCI cuts off the power before any injury can occur. The problem with GFCIs is that one piece of faulty equipment causes a loss of power to all equipment serviced by the GFCI, some of which may be vital.

Pacing Leads and Saline Monitoring Lines

Central venous catheters and pacemaker wires should be manipulated only with gloved hands and while touching nothing else to minimize the likelihood of the flow of small leakage currents.

Inspection

A program must be in place for regular inspection and testing of equipment by the biomedical engineering department, so that faulty wiring, worn wiring, or excessive leakage currents can be detected before they pose a hazard.

Further Reading

Bruner JMR, Leonard PF: Electricity, Safety and the Patient. Chicago, Year Book Medical Publishers, 1989.

Ehrenwerth J: Electrical safety. In Barash PB, Cullen BF, Stoelting RK (eds): Clinical Anesthesia, 3rd ed. Philadelphia, Lippincott-Raven, 1997, pp 137-155.

Litt L, Ehrenwerth J: Electrical safety in the operating room: Important old wine, disguised new bottles. Anesth Analg 78:417-419, 1994.

Schwartz JJ, Ehrenwerth J: Electrical Safety. In Lake CK (ed): Clinical Monitoring for Anesthesia and Critical Care. Philadelphia, WB Saunders, 1994, pp 35-42.

Schwartz JJ, Ehrenwerth J: A case-oriented approach to electrical safety. In Morell RC, Eichhorn JH (eds): Patient Safety in Anesthetic Practice. New York, Churchill Livingstone, 1996, pp 55-70.

EQUIPMENT & MONITORING

Fires in the Operating Room

138

Paul E. Kazanjian and Anthony R. Doyle

Case Synopsis

A 2-year-old boy is undergoing inguinal herniorrhaphy as the first case of the day on a Monday. Inhalation induction is carried out with sevoflurane using a breathing system containing Baralyme carbon dioxide (CO_2) absorbent. The Baralyme absorbent canisters had been changed the previous Wednesday evening. Fifteen minutes after induction of anesthesia, an explosion is heard in the vicinity of the anesthesia machine. The anesthesia circle system is damaged, and there is evidence of extreme heat in the CO_2 absorber. Fortunately, the child is not injured.

PROBLEM ANALYSIS

Definition

A fire is a rapid, persistent, exothermic oxidation of a combustible substance (fuel) that releases heat and light energy; fire is usually accompanied by flame. Surgical fires are defined as the burning of materials on or in a surgical patient. This is in contrast to an operating room (OR) fire, which is defined as any fire that occurs in the OR and does not necessarily involve the patient. Examples of fires that occur *in* the patient include airway fires, such as ignition of an endotracheal tube by a laser, and intra-abdominal fires caused by sparks igniting bowel gas. An example of a fire occurring *on* the patient includes ignition of drapes, sponges, and other fuels by an electrosurgical instrument. Approximately 62% of surgical fires are located in the airway or on the face; 24% of surgical fires occur elsewhere *on* the patient, and 14% occur elsewhere *in* the patient. Though rare, surgical fires can cause serious injury or death. In most cases, they are preventable.

Despite the use of nonflammable anesthetics, fires still occur in the OR, and they are caused by the same essential combination of an ignition source, oxidizer, and fuel (Table 138-1). Contributing factors include human error, lack of training, misconception, and the improper use of medical devices. Common ignition sources are electrosurgical

Table 138–1 ■ Causes of Fires and Explosions in the Operating Room

Electrocautery during facial, head, or neck surgery in an awake patient receiving supplemental O_2

Laser surgery of the esophagus or trachea

Ignition of flammable skin preparation solutions or bowel gas

Electrosurgery in the area of an endotracheal tube, particularly during tracheostomy formation

Exothermic reactions between potent inhaled anesthetics (e.g., sevoflurane) and desiccated CO_2 absorbent (Baralyme)

Interaction of static electricity or electrocautery in the presence of flammable or explosive anesthetic gases (rare)

equipment (68%), lasers (13%), and other heat sources, including electrocautery, hot wire cautery, fiberoptic light sources, defibrillators, and high-speed burs. Oxidizers are substances that support the combustion of fuels and cause fires to burn more intensely and vigorously than they would in the absence of an oxidizer. Although not explosive, air, oxygen (O_2), and nitrous oxide (N_2O) are the common oxidizers found in the OR environment. There are a number of potential fuels in the OR, including surgical drapes, gowns, sponges, endotracheal tubes, skin preparation solutions, hair, and skin. Some fuels are more likely to burn than others, and some fuels ignite only in the presence of an oxidizer.

Fires in the OR are commonly associated with laser surgery of the airway. They usually result from ignition of an inadequately protected endotracheal tube (Fig. 138-1) or excessively long exposure of any combustible material placed in the airway (e.g., wet cotton pledgets) to a direct hit from the laser beam. The incidence of such fires is thought to be from 0.5% to 1%. Initially, most fires are located only on the external surface of the endotracheal tube; if unrecognized, they may lead to a blowtorch-like flame if the lumen of the tube is reached, allowing the O_2-rich contents of the tube to enhance the combustion process.

The risk of fire during surgery of the head, neck, and airway is increased because of the O_2-enriched atmosphere created by the O_2 and N_2O building up beneath the surgical drapes or in the oropharyngeal cavity. Depending on the procedure, the O_2-enriched atmosphere may be immediately adjacent to or encompass the operative site. There are several scenarios that can lead to the development of an O_2-enriched atmosphere. During head and neck surgery that is performed under local anesthesia, a mask, nasal cannula, or other open breathing system can spill O_2 near the patient's mouth, nose, or airway, and O_2 can collect under the drapes. O_2 leaking from an uncuffed endotracheal tube can saturate the oropharynx during tonsillar surgery and similar procedures. Entering the trachea with an electrocautery device introduces an ignition source into the O_2-enriched atmosphere of the patient's tracheal airway.

Fires can also result from a misdirected or reflected laser (laser light is reflected off metal surfaces) impinging any

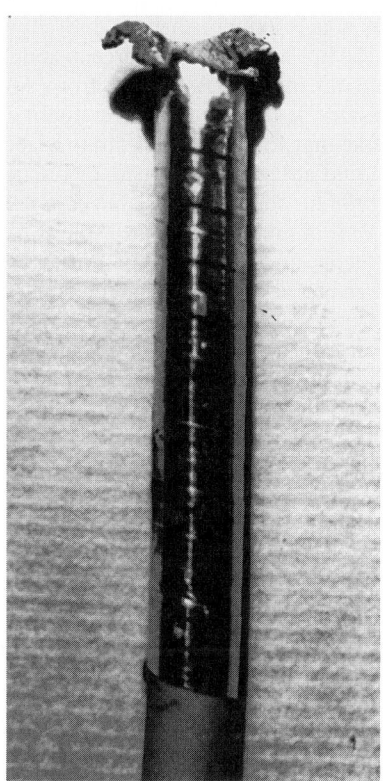

Figure 138–1 ▪ Endotracheal tube damaged by a laser-induced airway fire. (Courtesy of Dr. Allan Brown, University of Michigan Medical Center.)

flammable material, such as the surgical drapes covering the patient. Many liquids used in the OR (e.g., skin preparations, tinctures, degreasers, solutions in suture packs) contain flammable volatile organic chemicals. Skin preparations may contain alcohol or acetone, and they are flammable until all the liquid has evaporated. Careless application may allow the solution to wick into the patient's hair, pool on the patient's skin, pool under the patient's body, or soak into linens. If the patient is draped before the solution is completely dry, vapors can be trapped and channeled to the operative field, where they may be exposed to a heat source and ignite. Likewise, bowel gas may be ignited by surgical diathermy. Intestinal gases contain varying concentrations of nitrogen, CO_2, hydrogen, methane, and O_2. This combination of gases can be flammable in certain proportions. In addition, N_2O can diffuse into the bowel and make the gas mixture even more flammable.

Fires and explosions resulting from the interaction of an ignition source, such as static electricity, and flammable or explosive anesthetic gases (e.g., ether, cyclopropane) are of historical interest only. However, the interaction of potent inhaled anesthetics with desiccated CO_2 absorbent can result in the production of carbon monoxide, extreme heat, smoke, fires, and explosions.

Recognition

Sparks, pops, and flashes may indicate a situation conducive to ignition, combustion, or explosion. Most frank fires in the OR are heralded by flame and smoke. Anesthetists should monitor the CO_2 absorber for signs of excessive heat production and also monitor the relationship between the inspired sevoflurane concentration and the vaporizer setting. An unusually delayed rise or unexpected decline in the inspired sevoflurane concentration compared with the vaporizer setting may indicate exothermic sevoflurane degradation (see Table 138-4).

Risk Assessment

Whenever there is a high-energy source of ignition (e.g., laser or electrocautery), a potentially combustible material (e.g., endotracheal tube, alcohol-containing skin preparation, surgical drapes), and an oxidizer (O_2, N_2O, or both), there is the potential for combustion. Obviously, the risk of fire is greater if the concentration of oxidizer is higher, so it is advisable to keep the inspired O_2 concentration as low as possible.

Any patient undergoing airway surgery is at risk of the consequences of an airway fire, regardless of whether a laser is used. A high index of suspicion should be maintained at all times when anesthesia is being provided for laser surgery or during any airway surgery involving the use of electrocautery (e.g., tonsillectomy, tracheostomy). Risk of fire is also greater when surgery on the head and neck is performed under local anesthesia using an open breathing system (e.g., nasal cannula, facemask).

Exothermic reactions between CO_2 absorbents and sevoflurane are most likely to occur when the absorbent is desiccated. Most absorber fires occur during the first case on a Monday morning following a period of nonuse.

Implications

Most surgical fires, if appropriately handled, result in little or no harm to the patient. However, inappropriate handling can have catastrophic consequences, including death or a prolonged period of ventilation in the intensive care unit consequent to pulmonary edema, sepsis, or multiple organ failure syndrome. A late complication of airway fire is tracheal stenosis.

MANAGEMENT

OR staff should be educated about the nature, prevention, and extinguishing of surgical fires. Training, simulations, and drills should be used to familiarize staff with reactions and responses to surgical fires. Comprehensive training includes instruction in the rescue, alert, containment, and evacuation response to large fires. Staff should be familiar with the location and operation of firefighting equipment, medical gas supply shut-off valves, battery-powered portable lighting systems, ventilation systems, building alarms, and electrical systems.

A small fire can often be extinguished safely and simply by patting the flame with a gloved hand or towel. The area should be carefully inspected to make sure that all the burning material has been extinguished. The OR team should assess the conditions that led to the fire and make efforts to prevent a recurrence.

Table 138–2 ■ Recommendations for Avoiding Laser-Induced Fires in the Operating Room

Minimize FiO_2 and avoid N_2O
Use wet pledgets above the ETT cuff, but replace any string with wire
Use colored saline in the cuff to allow early detection of ETT cuff rupture
Place the ETT cuff as far distally as possible in the trachea
Use an appropriately protected or specifically designed ETT
Alternatively, use jet ventilation or intermittent apnea
Be aware of the type of laser in use and the ETT's susceptibility to a direct hit

ETT, endotracheal tube; FiO_2, fraction of inspired oxygen; N_2O, nitrous oxide.

Large fires on the patient demand immediate action to extinguish the fire, protect the patient from (additional) thermal injury, and treat the patient, if injured. A comprehensive response requires the participation of the anesthesiologist, surgeon, and OR nursing staff. The anesthesiologist should stop the flow of O_2 to the patient and be prepared to resume or assist ventilation with air. The surgeon or nurses should remove burning materials from the patient and extinguish them. This is especially important for paper drapes, which are impervious to water; dousing them with water may not extinguish a fire burning on the underside. It is also important to remove burned material from the patient, even if it is extinguished, to prevent further burn injury from the hot material. The surgeon should assess and treat the patient's injuries. Assistance from additional staff may be necessary. If the fire is large enough, extreme heat, fire, and smoke may force the OR team to evacuate the area. The team should attempt to evacuate or rescue the patient, but this may not be possible.

In the event of an airway fire or explosion, the anesthesiologist, surgeon, and nursing staff must act quickly and decisively to reduce injury to the patient. The endotracheal tube or other source of ignition or fire should be removed immediately from the patient, and ventilation must be stopped to stem the supply of O_2 to the flames. The endotracheal tube should be extinguished in a bucket of water, which should always be available during laser surgery. The airway should be inspected quickly via direct laryngoscopy to determine whether there is a remaining source of combustion. The patient should be mask ventilated with 100% O_2 while anesthesia is continued. Rigid bronchoscopy should be performed to assess the damage and remove debris. This is followed by flexible fiberoptic bronchoscopy of the lower airways if the fire was of the interior blowtorch type. The latter results from a transluminal burn in an endotracheal tube during the inspiratory part of the respiratory cycle. If airway damage is detected, the patient should be reintubated; if there is appreciable upper airway damage, low tracheostomy may be indicated. Appreciable lower airway damage caused by smoke inhalation and heat damage may require prolonged intubation and ventilation, including the administration of high-dose steroids.

Table 138–3 ■ Precautions Regarding Ignition Sources in the Operating Room

Source	Management Guidelines
Electrosurgical unit (ESU)	Use bipolar cautery to limit ignition potential
	Exercise caution when using ESU near locations where O_2 concentration is elevated (throat, mouth)
	Place ESU electrode probes in holster or away from patient and surgical drapes when not in use
	Do not use ESU to cut through tracheal rings; use scissors or scalpel instead
	Do not use red rubber catheter or other materials to sheathe long ESU electrode probes
	Avoid eschar buildup on electrode tip; clean buildup off as needed
	Use appropriate ESU modes for cutting; avoid arcing coagulation modes
Hot wire cautery	Soak gauze sponges in saline and wring them out when used near hot wire cautery
	Minimize supplemental O_2 concentration
Surgical lasers	Limit laser output to lowest acceptable power density and pulse duration
	Test-fire laser onto a safe surface
	Place laser in standby mode when not in use
	Activate laser only when tip is under surgeon's direct vision
	Allow only the person using the laser to activate it
	Deactivate laser and place it in standby mode before removing it from the surgical site
	When performing laser surgery through an endoscope, pass the laser fiber through the endoscope before introducing it into the patient
	Use appropriate laser-resistant tubes during upper airway surgery
Fiberoptic cables and light sources	Make sure all fiberoptic connections are complete before activating the light source
	Deactivate the light source before disconnecting the scope from the light cable
Defibrillators	Use according to the manufacturer's instructions
	Avoid discharging in O_2-enriched atmosphere
	Train operators in the use of defibrillation equipment
	Use disposable adhesive defibrillator pads instead of nondisposable paddles whenever possible
	Maximize contact between the patient and the surface of the pad or paddle
	When using paddles, use the appropriate conduction gel

PREVENTION

Anesthesiologists and other health care providers must consider the risk-benefit ratio of nasal O_2 insufflation during monitored anesthesia care, particularly during a surgical procedure involving the head and neck. Supplemental O_2 should be delivered as determined by clinical judgment, considering the patient's preoperative O_2 saturation as measured by pulse oximetry in room air. Avoidance of "luxury O_2" should be considered. When higher concentrations of O_2 are necessary to maintain O_2 saturation, the surgeon should be informed about the potential for ignition and fire. Discontinue supplemental O_2 for at least 1 minute before the use of an ignition source near the patient's head, neck, or airway. Other strategies to avoid the creation of an O_2-enriched atmosphere include modified draping techniques, careful placement of expiratory hoses, and use of an active scavenging system. If an O_2-enriched atmosphere is unavoidable, it should be isolated from the operative field by carefully applying a nonflammable incision drape. Also, the use of electrosurgical units should be minimized.

The risk of airway fires resulting from use of the surgical laser can be reduced by avoiding misdirection of the laser, both within and outside the operative field, and accidental operation when directed at the drapes or the patient's face (Table 138-2). The patient's eyes should be covered with wet gauze pads and not taped closed, because tape is combustible. During laser airway surgery, the endotracheal tube must be protected from ignition, or a specially designed tube should be used; if metal foil wrap is used, it must be applied carefully. There are many commercially available endotracheal tubes for use with laser surgery, but none is completely impervious to ignition. An excellent review article by Rampil provides further details.

The surgeon must exercise great care during tracheostomy formation to avoid igniting the endotracheal tube with diathermy before its removal and replacement with a tracheostomy tube.

Fires have resulted from the ignition of flammable skin preparations by electrosurgical units or other ignition sources (Table 138-3). Care must be taken to avoid pooling of the preparation solution around the patient. Allow sufficient time for the volatile material (usually alcohol) to evaporate before beginning surgery. Precautions regarding the use of oxidizers (e.g., O_2, N_2O) are summarized in Table 138-4, and those for fuels and CO_2 absorbers are given in Tables 138-5 and 138-6, respectively.

Table 138–4 ■ Precautions Regarding Oxidizers (Oxygen and Nitrous Oxide)
In general, use air or O_2 with an Fio_2 less than 30% in open breathing systems
Identify and ameliorate O_2-enriched environments
Tent drapes around the patient's head and neck when supplying supplemental O_2 in an open breathing system
Discontinue supplemental O_2 for 1 min before using ESU near the head and neck
During oropharyngeal surgery, use wet gauze or sponges with uncuffed endotracheal tubes to minimize leak of O_2 into oropharynx
Turn O_2 off when not in use
Be aware that nitrous oxide (N_2O) supports combustion as effectively as O_2 does; a mixture of N_2O and O_2 is not less dangerous than pure O_2
Diffusion of N_2O into bowel gas introduces additional oxidizer to support combustion of hydrogen and methane

ESU, electrosurgical unit; Fio_2, fraction of inspired oxygen.

Table 138–5 ■ Precautions Regarding Fuel Sources in the Operating Room

Source	Management Guidelines
Volatile skin preparations (degreasers, ether, acetone, alcohol) and ointments (collodion, petroleum jelly, tincture of benzoin, aerosols, paraffin)	Minimize use of alcohol-based skin preparations Apply skin preparations carefully; do not allow them to soak into hair or linens; avoid pooling on or under patient Wait for skin preparations to dry completely before draping patient
Linens, drapes, gowns, masks, hoods, caps	Use incision drapes if possible All are flammable, even if labeled "flame resistant" Use wet drapes and towels adjacent to laser site Use incise drapes to isolate surgical field from fuels and oxidizers Use wet gauze sponges when possible
Anesthesia components (endotracheal tubes, masks, nasal cannulas, tape, blood pressure cuffs)	Use cuffed tubes when possible Use laser-resistant tubes for upper airway laser cases Fill cuff with methylene blue-dyed saline for airway laser cases (to indicate breach in cuff) Protect cuff with wet pledgets for airway laser cases
Patient hair	Cover hair near the operative site with sterile surgical lubricating jelly to prevent it from igniting
Intestinal gases	Prepare the gastrointestinal tract when indicated Do not use mannitol-based bowel preparations Avoid nitrous oxide Dilute intestinal gases with an inert gas if indicated

EQUIPMENT & MONITORING

Table 138–6 ▪ Precautions Regarding Carbon Dioxide Absorbers and Halogenated Anesthetics in the Operating Room

Alert anesthesia personnel, including technicians and providers, to the nature of this hazard

Develop anesthesia machine setup and maintenance protocols that ensure that absorbents do not become desiccated and are replaced regularly

Avoid desiccation of absorbent; minimize or eliminate gas flow through absorber between uses, and turn anesthesia machine off at day's end

Replace CO_2 absorbent every Monday before use; label canister with date that absorber should be replaced; replace absorbent if its hydration status is in question

Periodically monitor temperature of CO_2 absorbent canisters

Monitor relation between inspired sevoflurane concentration and vaporizer setting; an unusually delayed rise or unexpected decline in inspired sevoflurane concentration compared with the vaporizer setting may indicate exothermic sevoflurane degradation

Do not rehydrate absorbent by pouring water over it

Consider using alternative absorbents that are free of strong alkali compounds

Further Reading

Andersen K: Safe use of lasers in the operating room—what perioperative nurses should know. AORN J 79:171-188, 2004.

Brechtelsbauer PB, Carroll WR, Baker S: Intraoperative fire with electrocautery. Otolaryngol Head Neck Surg 114:328-331, 1996.

ECRI editorial staff: A clinician's guide to surgical fires: How they occur, how to prevent them, how to put them out. Health Devices 32:5-24, 2003.

ECRI editorial staff: Anesthesia carbon dioxide absorber fires. Health Devices 32:436-440, 2003.

Hermans JM, Bennet MJ, Hirschmann CA: Anesthesia for laser surgery. Anesth Analg 62:218-229, 1983.

Macdonald AG: A short history of fires and explosions caused by anaesthetic agents. Br J Anaesth 72:710-722, 1994.

Olympio MA, Morell RC: Canister fires become a hot safety concern. Anesthesia Patient Safety Foundation Newsletter 18, 2003.

Rampil IJ: Anesthetic considerations for laser surgery. Anesth Analg 74:424-435, 1992.

Van Der Spek AFL, Spargo PM, Norton ML: The physics of lasers and implications for their use during airway surgery. Br J Anaesth 60:709-729, 1988.

Laser Complications

Pattricia S. Klarr

139

Case Synopsis

A 75-year-old man with metastatic non–small cell carcinoma of the lung is scheduled for bronchoscopic laser tumor ablation under general anesthesia. He has a chronic nonproductive cough, and a computed tomography scan reveals tumor encroachment on the right bronchus.

PROBLEM ANALYSIS

Definition

Improved technology, better reliability, and reduced cost have led to an explosion in the applications for medical lasers over the past decade. Lasers deliver sterile, intense energy to tissue in both cutting and coagulation modes. Patients and operating room (OR) personnel are exposed to certain hazards with medical lasers, including atmospheric contamination, inadvertent perforation of a tissue structure or vessel, ignition of flammable material, and embolism.

Although there are no federal safety requirements for medical lasers, there are national safety standards. The latter exist to decrease or prevent laser mishaps. Laser hazards are classified into four general risk categories, ranging from no risk to substantial risk. Medical lasers fall into the highest risk level. Therefore, proper use requires trained personnel and protective equipment for the operation of medical lasers.

Recognition

There are several types of medical lasers. Their differences are based on the medium used and the wavelength produced (Table 139-1). In addition to laser hazards in general, different types of lasers have their own unique risks. For example, the wavelength of the carbon dioxide (CO_2) laser is in the far infrared region and is absorbed by the first surface it encounters, necessitating eye protection for both patient and OR personnel to prevent corneal damage.

Argon, KTP:YAG, and Nd:YAG in both the visible and near infrared range are transmitted through clear material but absorbed by pigmented tissue. Therefore, they pass through the cornea but could damage retinal tissue.

Laser hazards can be divided into beam-related and non-beam-related hazards. Nonbeam hazards include electric shock and laser-generated air contaminants. Beam-related hazards include perforation of a vessel or other structure, including the pilot balloon of an endotracheal tube. Delayed complications may appear after the use of certain lasers. In particular, the Nd:YAG laser can penetrate deeper than anticipated, causing bleeding or perforation to appear several hours to days later, when necrosis and edema are maximal.

Risk Assessment

Both patients and OR staff must be protected from laser hazards while the laser beam is on. Reflected beams can be aimed at an unintended site, causing eye damage, ignition of flammable material, or burns.

Table 139–1 ■ Commonly Used Lasers and Associated Hazards				
Medium	**Wavelength (nm)**	**Color**	**Features**	**Potential Hazard**
CO_2	10,600	Far infrared	Readily absorbed by all biologic tissue; very precise, superficial penetration; not fiberoptically transmitted	Corneal damage
Holmium:YAG	2060 2140 (pulsed)	Infrared	Precise cutting ability; minimal diffusion of thermal energy; good hemostasis; transmitted fiberoptically	Corneal damage; can pierce metal
Nd:YAG	1064	Near infrared	Can be transmitted fiberoptically; uses photocoagulation plus thermal necrosis; highest tissue penetration	More prone to late complications, delayed edema, tissue sloughing, retinal damage
Ruby	694	Red	Absorbed by pigments except hemoglobin	Retinal damage
Helium-neon	632	Red	Used as an aiming beam for CO_2 plus Nd:YAG lasers	Harmless, unless directed toward eyes
KTP:Nd:YAG	532	Green	Fiberoptic transmission possible; some scatter and necrosis (less than Nd:YAG)	Similar to Nd:YAG (less retinal damage or tissue penetration)
Argon	488,514	Blue/green	Can be transmitted fiberoptically; absorbed by hemoglobin and pigmented tissue	Retinal damage

During laser airway surgery, airway fires are the most common serious complication and can cause severe morbidity and death. Should contact with a flammable endotracheal tube result in a fire, the blowtorch-like nature of the ignited fumes in an oxygen (O_2)-rich environment can result in immense damage. If inhaled, smoke produced by the vaporizing of 1 g of tissue is equivalent to smoking six unfiltered cigarettes. This smoke, or the "laser plume," can potentially be a vector for viral transmission, although there has been no documentation of a health care provider contracting a disease in this manner.

Implications

Laser use has increased tremendously in the past few years. Lower cost and increased reliability have made medical lasers attractive for a variety of surgical applications. In addition to removing tumors, lasers are used to treat such conditions as benign prostatic hypertrophy and macular degeneration, to perform coronary angioplasty, and to treat various dermatologic and ophthalmic problems. Their increased utilization, however, results in the increased potential for complications. Lasers require a highly skilled staff trained in their use. They must be vigilant and able to anticipate associated risks and take measures to protect the patient and other medical personnel. If properly and promptly managed, complications are generally minor and treatable.

MANAGEMENT

Airway fire is the most serious complication of laser use. To minimize damage, the OR team must act quickly and in a coordinated fashion, taking the following actions:

- Disconnect the O_2 source and remove the endotracheal tube or other object on fire.
- Douse any flames with normal saline.
- Resume anesthesia with mask ventilation, using 100% O_2.
- Perform diagnostic laryngoscopy and rigid bronchoscopy to inspect the extent of damage.
- Remove any debris.
- Reintubate if airway damage is present.
- Consider a low tracheostomy if the damage is severe or if reintubation is unsuccessful.
- Use mechanical ventilation if required.
- Administer systemic steroids if necessary.
- Obtain and check the chest radiograph.

Surgical drapes are fire resistant, but if they are ignited, the flames are difficult to extinguish because the drapes are also water resistant. A fire extinguisher should be available when surgical drapes are in use. If any OR personnel are injured, they must be appropriately treated, and an incident report should be generated. The event should be investigated to prevent recurrences.

PREVENTION

Prevention depends on the particular complication to be avoided. Only personnel with the proper training and credentials in laser use and safety precautions should be allowed to operate the laser. While it is in use, everyone in the OR should be protected from known laser hazards.

Eye Protection

Because the eye is most vulnerable to injury, all personnel must wear proper eye protection. Wraparound goggles with side protectors are advised, because standard eyeglasses do not protect the eyes from reflected beams that may glance off the side. Contact lenses are not protective. The protective lens must absorb the particular laser wavelength being used. Clear lenses are adequate for CO_2 lasers, but for all other lasers, the lenses must be tinted.

The patient's eyes must be protected. Patients who are awake should also wear laser-safe goggles. If they are not the operative site, the eyes of anesthetized patients should be closed and covered with saline-soaked gauze or a nonshiny metal shield.

Because all lasers other than CO_2 lasers penetrate clear glass, windows must be protected. Signs must be placed prominently at all entrances to the OR warning of laser use, and spare goggles should be available at all entrances.

Perforation Risk

When not directed at the target tissue, the laser beam should be turned off or set in a standby mode. Misdirected laser beams can cause inadvertent perforation of a vessel or viscus.

Coronary arteries have been perforated during laser angioplasty, resulting in severe complications (e.g., tamponade, acute myocardial infarction, urgent coronary artery bypass surgery). Currently, the risk for such perforation approaches 1%.

Complications from perforation may not develop until several days postoperatively. Systemic air embolism with serious complications has also been reported with laser use.

Skin Damage

Avoid prolonged laser exposure to nontargeted skin. All nearby skin should be protected with moist drapes. Compared with the cornea, the skin has a layer of dead cells that makes damage less likely.

Environmental Hazards

Laser plume (described earlier) can produce an unpleasant odor, cause tearing and bronchial irritation, and it may be a viral vector. Inhalation of this plume can be minimized with the use of a high-efficiency smoke evacuator and the use of special laser surgical masks. The Barrier Brand laser plume facemask (Molnlycke Health Care, Inc., Newton, Pa.) is a high-efficiency mask that filters plume particulate. However, such masks require periodic replacement when moist. Moreover, some laser plume facemasks may not provide complete protection from all laser-induced airborne debris.

Airway Fire

No preventive measure guarantees that a fire will not occur. An insufflation technique or jet ventilation should be used for airway surgery, if possible, but the patient must be monitored for barotrauma and gastric dilatation.

A laser-safe endotracheal tube, a conventional endotracheal tube wrapped in metal foil, or a commercially made laser tube or metal tube should be used. Foil-wrapped tubes can have rough edges that abrade tracheal tissue, however, and they may have gaps that expose flammable portions. Cuffs of metal tubes are flammable. These tubes are less flexible and have a reduced internal diameter that makes ventilation more difficult; they are also expensive. If a cuff is in the airway, it should be inflated with dyed saline to indicate if cuff rupture occurs. Use of moistened pledgets around the tracheal tube is also helpful.

Keep the fraction of inspired O_2 as low as possible—less than 30% or whatever is necessary to maintain adequate O_2 saturation. Do not use nitrous oxide, because it can support combustion.

Further Reading

Brown SG: Science, medicine, and the future: New techniques in laser therapy. BMJ 316:754-757, 1998.

Kestenbaum A: New revision of ANSI Z136.1 (laser safety standards). LIA Today, May 8, 2000. Also available from Health Physics Society at http://hps.org/hpspublications/articles/ansiz136.1.html.

Koster R, Kahler J, Brockhoff C, et al: Laser coronary angioplasty: History, present and future. Am J Cardiovasc Drugs 2:197-207, 2002.

Laser Safety Information Bulletin, Laser Institute of America. Available at http://www.laserinstitute.org/publication/safety_bulletin/laser_safety _info.

Rampil IJ: Anesthesia for laser surgery. In Miller RD (ed): Anesthesia, 5th ed. New York, Churchill Livingstone, 2000, pp 2199-2212.

EQUIPMENT & MONITORING

Pulse Oximetry

Mark D. Stoneham

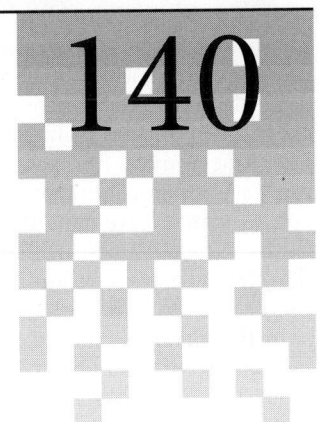

140

Case Synopsis

A trauma victim is undergoing computed tomography of the head. His lungs are being ventilated with 100% oxygen. Monitoring consists of electrocardiogram (ECG), noninvasive blood pressure, and pulse oximetry, which displays an oxygen saturation (SpO_2) of 100%. The breathing circuit becomes disconnected as the scan commences, but the ventilator disconnect alarm is faulty and fails to sound. Five minutes elapse before the patient's SpO_2 starts to drop; another minute passes before the oximeter low-saturation alarm sounds at 90%. The SpO_2 then falls rapidly to 45% before the problem can be corrected.

PROBLEM ANALYSIS

Definition and Recognition

The arterial pressure of oxygen (PaO_2) of a patient receiving 100% oxygen (O_2) may reach as high as 600 mm Hg, as calculated from the alveolar gas equation.[1] The O_2 content of the body in this case equals the O_2 in the lungs—perhaps 4 L—plus O_2 bound to hemoglobin and other pigments, plus O_2 dissolved in the plasma. Basal O_2 consumption is about 250 mL/min^{-1}. In an otherwise fit adult, these reserves provide enough O_2 for several minutes. If ventilation stops for any reason, the PaO_2 will start to decline. However, as can be seen from the oxygen-hemoglobin dissociation curve (Fig. 140-1), there will be no change in SpO_2 until the PaO_2 has fallen below 100 mm Hg. Thereafter, SpO_2 will fall slowly until it reaches 90% (corresponding to a PaO_2 of about 65 mm Hg), at which point an audible low-SpO_2 alarm will sound. After this, desaturation occurs very rapidly. Thus, the pulse oximeter has been termed a *lag monitor*.

In addition, there is a time lag between the true and displayed SpO_2 due to signal averaging. This is an attempt to reduce the effects of artifact (electromagnetic interference) by averaging the detected signal over a variable period (often 5 to 30 seconds), rejecting sudden changes in SpO_2. The implication of the lag effect is that a potentially life-threatening desaturation may go unnoticed for several minutes. For this reason, the pulse oximeter has been described as a "sentry standing on the cliff-edge of desaturation."

Other pulse oximetry complications are classified according to whether they are related to technologic limitations or the clinical interpretation of oximeter readings by the operator.

TECHNOLOGIC LIMITATIONS OF PULSE OXIMETRY

Arterial Pulse Recognition. A pulsatile signal is required for an oximeter to measure surface SpO_2. As the pulse signal

gets smaller, it is amplified by the oximeter, but at the expense of amplifying background interference as well. At the highest amplification, the oximeter may generate SpO_2 from the amplified noise signal itself. Thus, oximetry may be less effective in very ill patients with poor tissue perfusion, patients with vasoconstriction, or those who are hypothermic. Cardiac arrhythmias may also interfere with proper detection of the pulsatile signal by the oximeter and calculation of the pulse rate. Motion induces the movement of venous and capillary blood within tissue beneath the oximetry sensor (often the fourth or fifth digit of the hand), so that the pulsatile fraction of the SpO_2 signal is no longer solely arterial blood. Shivering is the most common cause of motion artifact. Cardiac valvular defects, such as tricuspid regurgitation, also cause strong venous pulsations, in which case venous SpO_2 may be recorded by the pulse oximeter. Intra-aortic balloon counterpulsation also generates artifact. Oximeter manufacturers have designed software algorithms to reject such artifact. These include the following:

- *Signal-averaging time manipulation.* This was described earlier (often 5 to 30 seconds).
- *Pulse oximetry linked to the ECG.* Here, oximetry software assumes that for each "arterial" pulse detected by the oximeter, there must be a temporally linked ECG complex. Any pulsatile signal not associated with an ECG complex is rejected. Unfortunately, although the theory is good, in practice, it is not very effective.
- *Time division multiplexing.* The two LEDs are cycled (red on–infrared on), with both off many times per second. In this way, much background "noise" from extraneous sources, such as overhead lighting, is reduced.
- *Quadrature division multiplexing.* The red and infrared LED signals are separated in phase, rather than time, and subsequently recombined in phase. In this way, an artifact due to motion or electromagnetic interference may be eliminated, because it will not be in the same phase as the two LED signals once they are recombined.
- *Signal extraction technology.* Software analyzes the frequencies of all "pulsatile" signals and assumes that the frequency with the highest calculated SpO_2 is arterial and rejects

---

[1] $PaO_2 = FiO_2(PB − P*H_2O) − PaCO_2([1/R])$, where PB is barometric pressure (760 mm Hg at sea level), FiO_2 is the fraction of inspired O_2, $P*H_2O$ is the vapor pressure of water at body temperature (47 mm Hg), and R is the respiratory quotient.

Figure 140–1 ▪ Oxygen-hemoglobin dissociation curve.

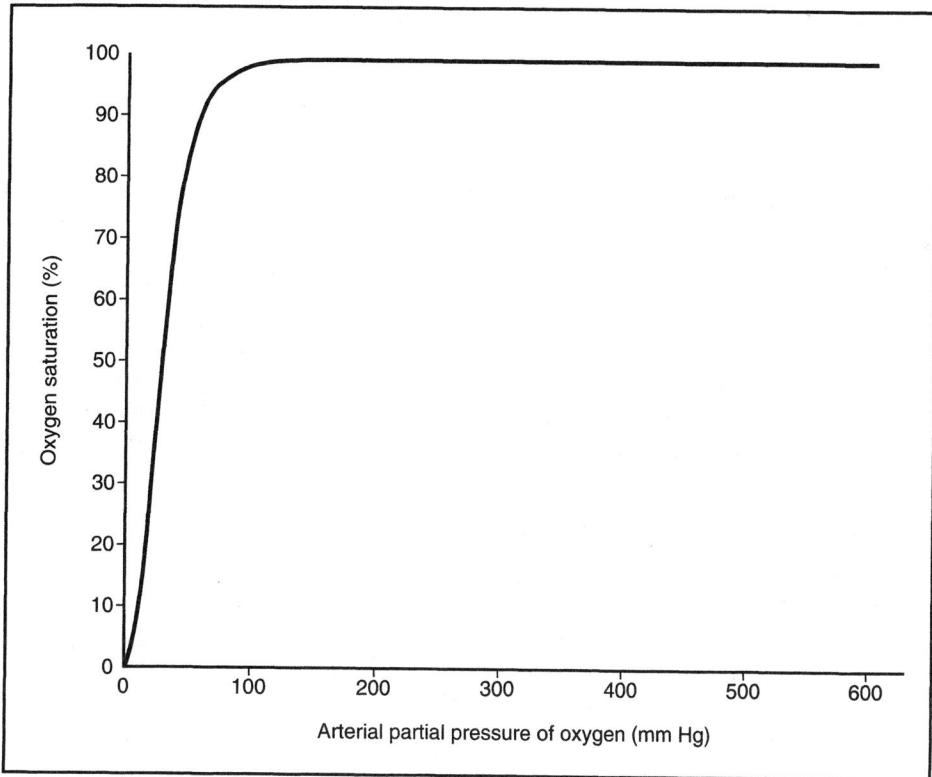

all others (e.g., venous pulsations). This is an effective method of rejecting motion artifact, especially shivering.

Abnormal Hemoglobin and Dyes.
Carboxyhemoglobin causes pulse oximeters to register artificially high SpO_2 values. This is because carboxyhemoglobin absorbs very little light in the infrared range, but as much light as oxyhemoglobin in the red range. Thus, oximeters "see" carboxyhemoglobin as oxyhemoglobin and display the approximate sum of both hemoglobins as SpO_2. This trends toward 100%. Methemoglobin has a high absorbency over a wide spectrum, causing SpO_2 values to trend toward 85% when methemoglobin is greater than 10%. Circulating dyes, particularly methylene blue, may give transient, artificially low SpO_2 values.

Patient Safety Issues.
There have been reports of babies suffering skin burns or pressure damage. These injuries occurred because early oximetry probes had a heater unit to ensure adequate skin perfusion or when probes and oximeters from different manufacturers were connected together. There have also been reports of oximeters causing burns in patients during magnetic resonance imaging due to current being induced in the cables by fluctuating magnetic fields.

Low Oxygen Saturation Values.
SpO_2 values less than 70% are considered unreliable because there are few experimental or clinical values used to calibrate the device. The nomogram used by pulse oximeters to calculate SpO_2 values (i.e., from the ratio of red to infrared, pulse-added absorbencies) is obtained from volunteers given increasingly hypoxic gas mixtures to breathe, but only down to SpO_2 values of 70%. Despite this, directional changes in SpO_2 are generally accurate.

OPERATOR INTERPRETATION

Waveform Presence. All oximeters display some visible indicator of the pulse. This can be a plethysmographic waveform or a simple LED laddergram. If it is not visible, indicating that a pulse cannot be detected, any SpO_2 values displayed cannot be considered valid. Bright overhead lighting, shivering, and motion artifact can produce apparently pulsatile waveforms and SpO_2 values when no pulse is present.

Sudden Changes in Oxygen Saturation Values. Physiologically, SpO_2 is unlikely to change instantaneously (e.g., from 98% to 85%). If this happens, it should first be considered an artifact. One exception might be a patient with an intracardiac, bidirectional shunt and sudden changes in ventricular loading conditions (right or left ventricular preload or afterload).

Oxygen Saturation Monitors Oxygenation, Not Ventilation. One case report highlighted the false sense of security that may be provided by pulse oximetry. An elderly woman in the postanesthesia care unit receiving O_2 via facemask became increasingly drowsy due to carbon dioxide (CO_2) narcosis, despite an SpO_2 of 96%. Her respiratory rate and minute volume were low due to residual neuromuscular block and sedation. But because she was receiving a high inspired concentration of O_2, her SpO_2 was maintained. The arterial CO_2 concentration reached 280 mm Hg (normal, 40 mm Hg), and she required postoperative mechanical ventilation for 24 hours. Thus, SpO_2 gives a good estimation of adequate *oxygenation* but does not provide information about *ventilation*, especially when supplemental O_2 is administered.

EQUIPMENT & MONITORING

Risk Assessment

Table 140-1 lists situations in which patients may be at increased risk for inaccurate oximetry readings.

Implications

The most obvious adverse outcome with any monitor of oxygenation is a false-negative reading; namely, hypoxia is not detected by a pulse oximeter. Unrecognized hypoxia can lead to end-organ damage (e.g., myocardial ischemia, cerebral hypoxia, renal failure, blindness) or death. Fortunately, these are rare occurrences, partly because of a "redundancy" of multiple monitoring methods for unconscious patients. For example, the patient described in the case synopsis would not have become hypoxemic had there been a functioning capnograph, ventilator disconnect alarm, or spirometry. Any one of these would have sounded an alarm within seconds of the breathing circuit disconnection. Thus, it is possible for operators to rely too much on the pulse oximeter rather than on the clinical status of the patient.

A pulse oximeter may also generate false-positive readings—in other words, hypoxia is reported when it does not exist. Such readings may lead to operator intervention, delays, or more invasive monitoring (e.g., arterial blood gas analysis) to confirm oximeter function and the patient's clinical status.

Table 140–1 ■ Sources of Errors and Complications in Pulse Oximetry

Effects of Dyshemoglobins and Dyes

Carboxyhemoglobin: SpO_2 displayed as sum of carboxyhemoglobin and oxyhemoglobin
Methemoglobin: SpO_2 values tend toward 85% with methemoglobin >10%
Methylene blue: transiently, very low SpO_2 values
Indigo carmine: small decreases in SpO_2
Indocyanine green: small decreases in SpO_2
Nail polish: falsely low SpO_2 values by 2%-3%
SpO_2 probe exposed to ambient light: falsely low SpO_2 values by 1%-3%

Clinical Conditions Causing Reduced Signal-to-Noise Ratio

Mechanical: shivering and other motion artifact
Hypovolemia: low cardiac output, shock, severe anemia
Vasoconstriction: hypothermia, peripheral vascular disease
Venous pulsations: tricuspid regurgitation; arteriovenous malformations, fistulas
Circulatory support: cardiopulmonary bypass, intra-aortic balloon counterpulsation
Light interference and radiant heaters: low SpO_2 values of ⊕85%, inaccurate pulse rates

Oximeter Accuracy and Response

Calibration by volunteer nomograms: accuracy of ± 2% over range 85% <SpO_2 <100%
Signal averaging: can cause spuriously low SpO_2 values
Low SpO_2 values: no accurate clinical calibration <70%
Penumbra effect: oximetry probe partially dislodged from its nominal (intended) position: low SpO_2 values (85%-95%)

Complications

Burns: mostly pediatric case reports and in magnetic resonance imaging
Pressure necrosis: usually due to wraparound-type sensor

SpO_2, oxygen saturation.

MANAGEMENT

Management of acute hypoxic complications must follow advanced cardiovascular life support guidelines. Securing the airway and administering 100% O_2 to the patient should be followed by appropriate measures to remedy the cause of hypoxia. Clearly, knowledge of the effects of various dyshemoglobins and dyes on oximeter function can prevent the misinterpretation of SpO_2 values under such circumstances. In cases in which there are problems with oximeter function or probe placement, it may be possible to select other sites for the probe (e.g., earlobe, nares, lip). In addition, an esophageal oximeter was recently described; I have used this device successfully in patients with extensive burns. There are also other methods of monitoring patients' oxygenation, including transcutaneous partial pressure of oxygen monitoring, arterial blood gas analysis, and continuous mixed venous O_2 saturation monitoring via an oximetric pulmonary artery catheter.

PREVENTION

It is important to recognize the pulse oximeter for what it is— namely, another (albeit very useful) monitor of O_2 delivery. Continued vigilance is required in the interpretation of oximeter readings under a wide variety of circumstances. Training of personnel is required to reduce observer misinterpretation of oximetry results. The pulse oximeter should not be relied on as the sole monitor of a patient's welfare. In the case synopsis, a capnograph would have warned of the ventilator disconnection within a few breaths. Despite wide acceptance of pulse oximetry in anesthesia and critical care, there is no direct evidence that it has saved lives during anesthesia or in the postanesthesia care unit. Oximetry is a major advance in the noninvasive monitoring of the cardiorespiratory system. However, it should be used only in conjunction with other monitors by trained personnel, and it should not supplant clinical observation.

Further Reading

AHA/ACC/ILC guidelines 2000 for CPR and emergency CV care. Circulation 102:I158-I165, 2000.

Atlee JL, Branotow N: Comparison of surface and esophageal oximetry in man. Anesthesiology 83:A455, 1995.

Broome IJ, Harris RW, Reilly CS: The response times during anaesthesia of pulse oximeters measuring oxygen saturations during hypoxaemic events. Anaesthesia 47:17-19, 1992.

Davidson JAH, Hosie HE: Limitations of pulse oximetry: Respiratory insufficiency—a failure of detection. BMJ 307:372-373, 1993.

Dumas C, Wahr JA, Tremper KK: Clinical evaluation of a prototype motion artifact resistant pulse oximeter in the recovery room. Anesth Analg 83:269-272, 1996.

Moller JT, Johannessen NW, Esperson K, et al: Randomized evaluation of pulse oximetry in 20,802 patients. II. Perioperative events and postoperative complications. Anesthesiology 78:445-453, 1993.

Prielipp RC, Scuderi PE, Hines MH, et al: Comparison of a prototype esophageal oximetry probe with two conventional digital pulse oximetry monitors in aortocoronary bypass patients. J Clin Monit 16:201-209, 2000.

Ralston AC, Webb RK, Runciman WB: Potential errors in pulse oximetry. I. Pulse oximetry evaluation. Anaesthesia 46:202-206, 1991.

Ralston AC, Webb RK, Runciman WB: Potential errors in pulse oximetry. III. Effects of interferences, dyes, dyshaemoglobins and other pigments. Anaesthesia 46:291-295, 1991.

Severinghaus JW, Kelleher JF: Recent developments in pulse oximetry. Anesthesiology 76:1018-1038, 1992.

Tremper KK, Barker SJ: Pulse oximetry. Anesthesiology 70:98-108, 1989.

Wahr JA, Tremper KK, Diab M: Pulse oximetry. Respir Care Clin N Am 1:77-105, 1995.

Webb RK, Ralston AC, Runciman WB: Potential errors in pulse oximetry. II. Effects of changes in saturation and signal quality. Anaesthesia 46:207-212, 1991.

EQUIPMENT & MONITORING

Inspiratory and Expiratory Gas Monitoring

141

Amit V. Chawla and Gauhar Sharih

Case Synopsis

A 23-year-old woman has laparoscopic surgery for evacuation of an ectopic pregnancy. She is under general endotracheal anesthesia (oxygen, nitrous oxide, isoflurane) and in the Trendelenburg position. She is mechanically ventilated. During introduction of pneumoperitoneum, her end-tidal carbon dioxide (ETCO$_2$) initially rises from 32 to 45 mm Hg, but within a few minutes, it falls precipitously to 18 mm Hg. Her blood pressure falls from 100/70 to 70/50 mm Hg, and her heart rate increases from 80 to 100 beats per minute. Oxygen saturation falls from 98% to 87%. Inspired gas values are as follows: oxygen (O$_2$) 40%, nitrous oxide (N$_2$O) 53%, ETCO$_2$ 0 mm Hg, isoflurane 1.5%. Expired gas values are as follows: O$_2$ 37%, N$_2$O 50%, ETCO$_2$ 18 mm Hg, isoflurane 1.2%

PROBLEM ANALYSIS

Definition

Monitoring of inspired O$_2$ concentrations in anesthetic or ventilator circuits is mandatory. In addition, inspiratory and expiratory monitoring for other gases (CO$_2$, N$_2$O) and volatile inhalational agents is vital to any anesthesia monitoring. The American Society of Anesthesiologists' standards for basic patient monitoring strongly advise inspiratory and expiratory gas monitoring for all patients having general anesthesia. Gas monitoring is useful for both diagnosis and management.

OXYGEN

Inspired O$_2$ monitoring will alert the anesthetist if a hypoxic O$_2$ concentration is delivered to the patient's airway. Machine-mounted (in-circuit) and in-line (between the circuit and the patient's airway) analyzers provide the means for taking this measurement.

CARBON DIOXIDE

Altered ventilation (CO$_2$ elimination), cardiac output (perfusion), distribution of pulmonary blood flow (e.g., embolism), and metabolic activity (CO$_2$ production) are detected with expiratory CO$_2$ monitoring. *Capnometry* is the measurement of CO$_2$ concentrations during inspiration and expiration. *Capnography* is the continuous display of a patient's capnogram during both these phases of ventilation (Fig. 141-1).

VOLATILE ANESTHETICS AND NITROUS OXIDE

Monitoring of anesthetic vapors and N$_2$O in the inspired and expired gases is useful during the induction of anesthesia, for closely observing and managing the depth of anesthesia, and finally for assessing recovery from volatile inhalation anesthesia.

Recognition

The usefulness of inspiratory and expiratory gas monitoring for detecting complications of anesthesia and monitoring the affected parameters is illustrated in Table 141-1.

Oxygen Analysis. Continuous O$_2$ analysis in inspired gas mixtures allows the early detection of hypoxic gas delivery. These analyzers are not suitable for detecting disconnections within the breathing system.

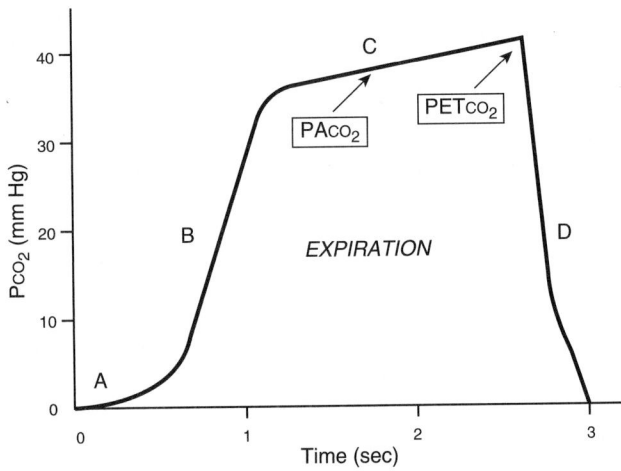

Figure 141–1 ■ Expiratory capnogram depicting a normal carbon dioxide (CO$_2$) waveform during expiration as a function of time. During inspiration, the CO$_2$ tension is nearly 0 mm Hg. Note three distinct phases (A, B, and C) of the increasing partial pressure of CO$_2$ (PCO$_2$) *during expiration* before it decreases abruptly *with inspiration* (phase D). Anatomic dead-space gas is cleared during phase A. Because this gas contains little CO$_2$, PCO$_2$ remains near its inspiratory phase value. During phase B, PCO$_2$ increases rapidly to approach its alveolar tension (PACO$_2$). Remaining alveolar gas is washed out during phase C, which is termed the *alveolar plateau phase*, owing to little increase in PACO$_2$. However, its slope may increase with high CO$_2$ production (e.g., hypermetabolic states) or nonhomogeneous gas mixing (e.g., airway obstruction). Peak end-tidal CO$_2$ (PETCO$_2$) reached during the alveolar plateau is the end-tidal CO$_2$. This has a somewhat lower value than systemic arterial CO$_2$ (PACO$_2$) because of mixing of alveolar dead space and alveolar gas.

Table 141–1 ■ Use of Gas Monitoring to Detect Complications

Complication	Inspiratory Gas Monitoring	Expiratory Gas Monitoring
Patient disconnect	No effect	O_2, CO_2, N_2,* N_2O, VA (all ↓)
Esophageal intubation	No effect	CO_2 (↓), N_2 (↓ or no effect)
Machine malfunction	O_2, CO_2, N_2, N_2O, VA†	O_2, CO_2, N_2, N_2O, VA†
Venous air embolism	No effect	CO_2 (↓), N_2 (↑)‡
Anesthetic overdose	VA (↑)	VA (↑)
Circulatory shock, cardiac arrest	No effect	CO_2 (↓)
Hypermetabolic state	No effect	CO_2 (↑)
Right-to-left shunt (CHD)	No effect	CO_2 (↓)
Inadequate ventilation	No effect	CO_2 (↑)

*N_2 would increase if air were sampled.
†Parameters could go up or down or remain unchanged, depending on sampling site, flow rates, whether air or N_2O was being administered, and so on.
‡Rise in N_2 is detectable only if a mass spectrometer or Raman scattering monitor is used.
CHD, coronary heart disease; VA, volatile anesthetic.

Capnography. The capnograph is likely the most useful monitor in contemporary anesthesia practice. Capnography provides information about the mechanics of lung function (e.g., dead space, airway obstruction), gas exchange (e.g., ventilation-perfusion mismatch), metabolism (e.g., hypermetabolic versus hypometabolic states), and cardiovascular function (e.g., reduced blood flow to lungs with myocardial dysfunction, pulmonary embolism, or left-to-right shunt). Nonetheless, its most useful functions are to confirm correct endotracheal tube placement, detect airway obstruction or disconnections, and identify anesthesia-ventilator breathing circuit malfunction (e.g., incompetent valves, CO_2 absorber exhaustion, leaks).

Monitoring of Anesthetic Agents. In-line and end-tidal monitoring of anesthetic vapors is important for patient safety. It is used to detect vaporizer malfunction (e.g., due to calibration error). Such monitoring may also help prevent unintentional anesthetic overdose or underdose. Further, end-tidal agent monitoring may help detect the mixing of agents. Techniques commonly used for inspiratory and expiratory gas monitoring include the following.

Infrared Absorption Spectrophotometry. Asymmetrical, polyatomic molecules absorb infrared light at specific wavelengths. Therefore, neither O_2 nor nitrogen (N_2) can be detected by this method. This modality is best suited for monitoring N_2O, CO_2, and volatile agents. Volatile agents, however, can complicate the analysis owing to interactions between specific gases and vapors and the close proximity of absorption spectra for volatile agents of interest. Optical filters and proprietary detection systems enhance the sensitivity for the detection of specific volatile agents.

Paramagnetic Analyzers. O_2 is unique among anesthetic gases in that it is strongly paramagnetic. Thus, if introduced into a nonhomogeneous magnetic field, O_2 will move toward the stronger part of the magnetic field, while other diamagnetic gases move away. This principle is used in breath-to-breath monitoring of O_2 concentrations in inspired and expired gas.

Mass Spectrometry. This modality is suitable for all anesthetic gases. Mass spectrometers use electrostatic and magnetic fields to spread these gases into a spectrum according to their mass-to-charge ratios. Ion current detectors are used for quantitative measurements.

Raman Scattering. Gas sample molecules are scattered by coherent photons produced by a high-intensity argon laser (Raman scattering). After impact, the gas molecules are momentarily excited to unstable vibrational and rotatory states. After returning to their normal state, photons of a characteristic but lower frequency are emitted. The frequency shift between incidental and scattered light is specific for individual gases. Raman scattering detects most gases used in anesthetic practice (including O_2 and N_2), but not monoatomic gases such as helium and xenon.

Owing to the size and cost of the equipment, mass spectrometry and Raman scattering monitoring are not routinely used, unlike infrared and paramagnetic analyzers.

Risk Assessment

Similar to other devices used in medical practice, devices used for inspiratory and expiratory gas monitoring are prone to malfunction. This can occur as a result of the aging of component parts and systems, direct damage to the system or instrument, failure to properly calibrate the instrument, or interference by secretions or water accumulation in sampling lines, among other causes. This risk is reduced with regular inspection and preventive maintenance according to the manufacturer's recommendations.

The risk of direct injury (thermal, laser, electrical, explosive) to a patient from the malfunction of devices for monitoring inspiratory and expiratory gases is minimal, provided these devices are used as intended. Malfunction or failure of gas monitoring devices may cause indirect harm as a result of incorrect or missing information, misinterpretation of information, or an incorrect response to correct information.

Implications

INCORRECT OR MISSING INFORMATION

As with any monitor, the information it provides must be considered in the context of the individual patients and circumstances. In the unlikely event that an erroneous value is reported (e.g., falsely high volatile agent concentrations due to miscalibration), the clinician must consider the value in light of the patient's current status. Are there signs that the patient's anesthesia is too deep? Similarly, a sudden fall in ETCO2 is not likely due to pulmonary embolism if the patient's hemodynamic status remains unchanged. Rather, an air leak or a disconnection may have occurred. Finally, it is possible (but unlikely with properly maintained equipment) that a multiagent detection device will fail to provide information for one agent (i.e., agent "dropout" due to component or

EQUIPMENT & MONITORING

electronic circuitry failure) but report correct values for other agents. Again, the event must be viewed in light of the patient's circumstances. Is there a reasonable explanation for the dropout? Are the other data plausible?

MISINTERPRETATION OF INFORMATION

It is possible that a clinician may misinterpret correct information supplied by a monitor. For example, an increase in $ETCO_2$ of 5 to 10 mm Hg over 10 to 15 minutes might be misinterpreted as evidence of malignant hyperthermia when in fact it is due to hypoventilation or use of an exhausted CO_2 absorber (in which case, the inspired CO_2 will also rise). Again, individual data must be considered within the context of other patient data, such as vital signs, temperature, and inspired CO_2 level.

WRONG RESPONSE TO CORRECT INFORMATION

A monitor may provide correct information, but the clinician may not believe it or may respond inappropriately. As with misinformation or missing data, the clinician must consider individual patient data within a global context. Carefully consider other data and the patient's condition before presuming device failure. Further, the clinician must know how to use gas monitoring data in diagnosis and management.

MANAGEMENT

Inspiratory and expiratory gas monitoring is required or useful for the following aspects of perioperative patient diagnosis and management:

- Assessment of oxygenation and ventilation
- Diagnosis of pulmonary embolism (e.g., gas, thrombus, amniotic fluid)
- Determination of anesthesia depth
- Diagnosis of circulatory insufficiency
- Confirmation of endotracheal intubation
- Diagnosis of patient–breathing system disconnection
- Assessment of recovery from volatile anesthetics
- Teaching of anesthetic pharmacokinetics

Returning to the case synopsis, the initial rise in $ETCO_2$ is explained by absorption of CO_2 in the blood from the insufflated gas in the peritoneum. The sudden drop in $ETCO_2$ a few minutes later could be due to pulmonary gas embolism. This increases physiologic dead space, leading to impaired gas exchange and cardiovascular dysfunction.

PREVENTION

The American Society of Anesthesiologists' standards for basic anesthetic monitoring (effective October 15, 2003) are as follows[1]:

---

[1]Under extenuating circumstances, the responsible anesthesiologist can waive any of these requirements. If so, this action and the reasons why should be recorded in the patient's medical record.

Oxygenation (Inspired Gas)

- During every administration of general anesthesia using an anesthesia machine, the concentration of O_2 in the patient breathing system should be measured by an O_2 analyzer with a low O_2 concentration limit alarm.
- During all anesthetics, a quantitative method of assessing blood oxygenation, such as pulse oximetry, should be used. Adequate illumination and exposure of the patient are necessary to assess skin and/or mucosal color.

Ventilation (Expired Gas)

- For every patient receiving general anesthesia, the adequacy of ventilation should be continually evaluated. Qualitative clinical signs such as chest excursion, observation of the reservoir breathing bag, and auscultation of breath sounds are useful. Continual monitoring for the presence of expired CO_2 should be performed unless this is invalidated by the nature of the patient, procedure, or equipment. Quantitative monitoring of the volume of expired gas is strongly encouraged.
- When an endotracheal tube is inserted or a laryngeal mask is placed, its correct positioning should be verified by clinical assessment and by identification of CO_2 in the expired gas. Continual $ETCO_2$ analysis—from the time of endotracheal tube or laryngeal mask placement until extubation or removal, or until initiation of transfer to a postoperative care location—should be performed using a quantitative method such as capnography or capnometry.
- When ventilation is controlled by a mechanical ventilator, a device that is capable of detecting disconnection of the breathing system's components should be in continuous use. The device must give an audible signal when its alarm threshold is exceeded.
- During regional anesthesia and monitored anesthesia care, the adequacy of ventilation should be evaluated, at least by continual observation of qualitative clinical signs.

Further Reading

Dorsch JA, Dorsch SE: Understanding Anesthesia Equipment, 4th ed. Baltimore, William & Wilkins, 1999.

Knopes KD, Hecker BR: Monitoring anesthetic gases. In Lake CL (ed): Clinical Monitoring and Anesthesia Care. Philadelphia, WB Saunders, 1994, pp 461-471.

Pace NL: Why monitoring during anesthesia has unintended and undesirable consequences. In Anesthesia and Perioperative Complications. St. Louis, Mosby–Year Book, 1992, pp 173-202.

Shulman D, Aronson HB: Capnography in early diagnosis of carbon dioxide embolism during laparoscopy. Can J Anaesth 31:455, 1984.

Tremper KK, Barker SJ: Monitoring of oxygen. In Lake CL (ed): Clinical Monitoring and Anesthesia Care. Philadelphia, WB Saunders, 1994, pp 196-212.

Vender JS, Gilbert HC: Monitoring the anesthetized patient. In Barash PG, Cullen BF, Stoelting RK (eds): Clinical Anesthesia, 3rd ed. Philadelphia, Lippincott-Raven, 1997, pp 621-641.

Transesophageal Echocardiography

142

Patrick E. Benedict and Jack S. Shanewise

Case Synopsis

A 65-year-old woman undergoing emergency coronary artery bypass graft surgery for unstable angina has incomplete revascularization due to lack of a suitable conduit. Insertion of a transesophageal echocardiography (TEE) probe during cardiopulmonary bypass is difficult. After several attempts, the probe suddenly advances; however, its tip appears in the surgical field anterior to the heart, after perforating the pharynx. Subsequent discussion with the patient's husband reveals that she has a 20-year history of dysphagia.

PROBLEM ANALYSIS

Definition

As TEE is used more frequently in operating rooms, anesthesiologists need to be aware of potential complications and their prevention. Most TEE complications are minor and are related to trauma to the oropharynx during probe insertion. More serious problems, such as pharyngeal perforation, esophageal perforation, and gastrointestinal bleeding, occur on rare occasions.

A TEE complication unique to the operating room is laryngeal injury with vocal cord dysfunction. This can occur in patients having TEE monitoring during sitting craniotomy with prolonged periods of extreme neck flexion. TEE probe placement and manipulation can compress the bronchi or cause displacement of the endotracheal tube, especially in small children. In patients who are not intubated, the TEE probe may inadvertently be inserted into the trachea instead of the esophagus. Also, the tip of the TEE probe sometimes buckles back on itself in the esophagus, making its removal difficult and hazardous.

Although esophageal burns due to transducer heat formation are theoretically possible, this complication has not been reported. Most TEE systems automatically shut down when the probe temperature exceeds a safe level. During TEE monitoring, anesthesiologists may be distracted from noticing more acute and important changes in vital signs. Also, without proper training and knowledge, TEE monitoring may be erroneously interpreted, leading to inappropriate management decisions.

Recognition

Oropharyngeal trauma may be seen directly or may manifest as bleeding from the mouth. Gastrointestinal hemorrhage may be occult and present as hypovolemic shock or unexplained anemia. Insertion of a gastric tube should confirm the diagnosis. Perforation of the esophagus may be apparent to the surgeon or it may present later with sepsis or severe chest pain in a conscious patient. Buckling of the probe tip results in an inability to withdraw the probe from the esophagus.

It is associated with unusual imaging (upside-down orientation) and reduced control knob mobility.

Risk Assessment

When possible, all patients should be asked about esophageal symptoms and diseases before insertion of the TEE probe. Three questions should always be asked:

1. Have you ever had any trouble with your esophagus?
2. Do you have any difficulty swallowing food?
3. Have you ever vomited blood?

If the patient answers "no" to all three questions, it is safe to proceed. When the patient cannot be interviewed directly, a family member should be questioned. At a minimum, the medical record should be reviewed for esophageal problems.

Contraindications to TEE are listed in Table 142-1. However, if TEE might provide important information and there is a history of esophageal disease, a preprocedure gastroenterologic evaluation with fiberoptic esophagoscopy is one option to consider. The mouth should be inspected before TEE probe insertion to look for loose teeth and

Table 142–1 ■ Contraindications to Transesophageal Echocardiography

Absolute Contraindications
Esophageal obstruction
 Stricture
 Tumor
Upper or lower sphincter hypertrophy
Esophageal injury
Perforation
Recent esophageal surgery
Fistula
Esophageal diverticulum
Unstable cervical spine

Relative Contraindications
Undiagnosed dysphagia
Esophageal varices
Upper gastrointestinal tract bleeding

preexisting injuries. TEE probes with stretched and loose steering cables may be more prone to buckle back on themselves in the esophagus and should be repaired before use.

In most settings in which intraoperative TEE is used, other monitoring and interventional devices occupy the same pathway as the TEE probe or a nearby one. These devices include endotracheal tubes, temperature monitoring devices, gastrointestinal drainage tubes, and feeding tubes. Given the size and rigidity of TEE probes, displacement of any one of these devices is a distinct possibility. Potential complications from device dislodgment range from minor annoyances (e.g., improperly functioning gastric tube) to potentially life-threatening situations (e.g., displacement of the endotracheal tube into a main-stem bronchus, impairing the ability to ventilate the patient).

Implications

Although rare, fatal complications from TEE can occur. As with all medical procedures, a risk-benefit analysis must be made before proceeding with the TEE examination. There is, however, a large experience with this procedure, indicating that the risk is minimal when performed on properly screened patients and using the proper technique.

MANAGEMENT

Bleeding from the mouth after TEE should prompt careful, direct inspection of the mouth and pharynx to identify the location and extent of the injury. Minor trauma to the oropharynx often requires no specific treatment, but antibiotics may be indicated for more extensive injuries. Significant, persistent gastrointestinal bleeding after TEE should be evaluated with endoscopy. Besides permitting a diagnosis, endoscopy can provide a means of treatment, such as electrocautery. If perforation of the esophagus is suspected, it can be diagnosed by fluoroscopy with water-soluble contrast swallow. Perforation is usually treated as a surgical emergency. Pharyngeal perforation can be diagnosed by direct inspection and, if significant, warrants emergency consultation with an otolaryngologist for surgical drainage. Airway patency always takes precedence over TEE monitoring, and the probe should be removed immediately if airway problems occur. A TEE probe with its tip buckled back on itself should be advanced into the stomach to allow room for it to unflex before any attempt is made to remove it.

PREVENTION

The two cornerstones for preventing TEE complications are preprocedure assessment for esophageal disease and careful and gentle probe insertion and manipulation. Other devices occupying the same pathway must be carefully watched during placement and removal of the TEE probe. Excessive force should *never* be used to pass an apparent obstruction to TEE probe advancement. The probe should not be locked in a flexed position for prolonged periods, and it should never be advanced or withdrawn when the wheel locks are engaged.

Patients with gastric pathology can safely undergo TEE examination, but the operator must not advance the TEE probe beyond the esophagus to avoid any potential problems with gastric insertion. Although not strictly a complication, damage to the TEE machinery is an extremely undesirable consequence of careless use. Typically, TEE systems are among the most expensive operating room devices, and repairs are extremely costly. This fact, along with the fragile nature of these complex electronic devices, underscores the need for gentle handling of TEE probes.

Further Reading

Benedict PE, Foley K: Transesophageal echocardiography not without pitfalls. J Cardiothorac Vasc Anesth 11:123, 1997.

Daniel WG, Erbel R, Kasper W, et al: Safety of transesophageal echocardiography: A multicenter survey of 10,419 examinations. Circulation 83:817-821, 1991.

Gilbert TB, Panico FG, McGill WA, et al: Bronchial obstruction by transesophageal echocardiography probe in a pediatric cardiac patient. Anesth Analg 74:156-158, 1992.

Khandheria B, Tajik A, Freeman W: TEE examination: Technique, training, and safety. In Freeman W, Seward J, Khandheria B, et al (eds): Transesophageal Echocardiography. Boston, Little Brown, 1994, pp 49-51.

O'Shea JP, Southern JF, D'Ambra MN, et al: Effects of prolonged transesophageal echocardiographic imaging and probe manipulation on the esophagus—an echocardiographic-pathologic study. J Am Coll Cardiol 17:1426-1429, 1991.

Spahn DR, Schmid S, Carrel T, et al: Hypopharynx perforation by a transesophageal echocardiography probe. Anesthesiology 82:581-583, 1995.

Urbanowicz JH, Kernoff RS, Oppenheim G, et al: Transesophageal echocardiography and its potential for esophageal damage. Anesthesiology 72:40-43, 1990.

Woodland RV, Denney JD, Moore DW, et al: Inability to remove a transesophageal echocardiography probe. J Cardiothorac Vasc Anesth 8:477-479, 1994.

Arterial Blood Pressure Monitoring

Pema Dorje

Case Synopsis

A 48-year-old woman with a small build and a history of heavy smoking has a 20-gauge, 51-mm cannula placed atraumatically in her left radial artery for monitoring during aortobifemoral and right femoropopliteal bypass surgery. Two days after surgery, she complains of pain in her left hand, which is cold and shows discoloration of the fingers. A few blisters are seen on the radial side of the forearm proximal to the cannula.

PROBLEM ANALYSIS

Definition

The patient described in the case scenario has necrosis of the forearm skin proximal to the radial artery cannula, with ischemia of the fingers. Both of these complications of arterial blood pressure monitoring or sampling can occur independent of each other. Occlusion by the cannula or cannula-related thrombus of small endarteries emanating from the radial artery to the skin is the most likely cause of the skin necrosis (Fig. 143-1). A combination of thrombotic occlusion of the cannulated radial artery and inadequate collateral supply from an atherosclerotic ulnar artery likely resulted in the digital ischemia. The incidence of forearm skin necrosis is higher than that of hand or digital ischemia. Other complications of arterial cannulation and their risk factors are listed in Table 143-1.

Recognition

Pain despite hand immobility and discolored and cold digits are highly suggestive of ischemia. The presence of a proximal pulse is not an indication of distal flow. The presence of such flow must be established with the use of a Doppler probe. The absence of radial and ulnar arterial flow in an individual with signs of hand or digital ischemia confirms the diagnosis. An absent digital pulse oximeter plethysmographic tracing on a hand with an arterial cannula at the wrist suggests inadequate flow and must be viewed with concern and treated as such.

Ischemia of the skin in the forearm may present as patchy changes in coloration. These may progress to edema, blister formation, and skin ulceration.

Risk Assessment

The risk of thrombotic occlusion of the radial artery by a 20-gauge needle is 10% to 30%, depending on the duration of arterial monitoring. Risk of thrombotic cannula occlusion is increased by the following:

- Larger, longer, and non-Teflon cannulas
- Small radial arteries, as typically found in small women and children
- No heparin or pressure failure in the flush system

Owing to the rich ulnar collateral flow, the risk of hand or digital ischemia is quite low, unless additional risk factors are present. The risk of occlusion leading to ischemia is increased by the following:

- Advanced atherosclerosis or Raynaud's or Buerger's disease
- Low perfusion syndrome or shock
- Anatomic variation of the blood supply to the hand

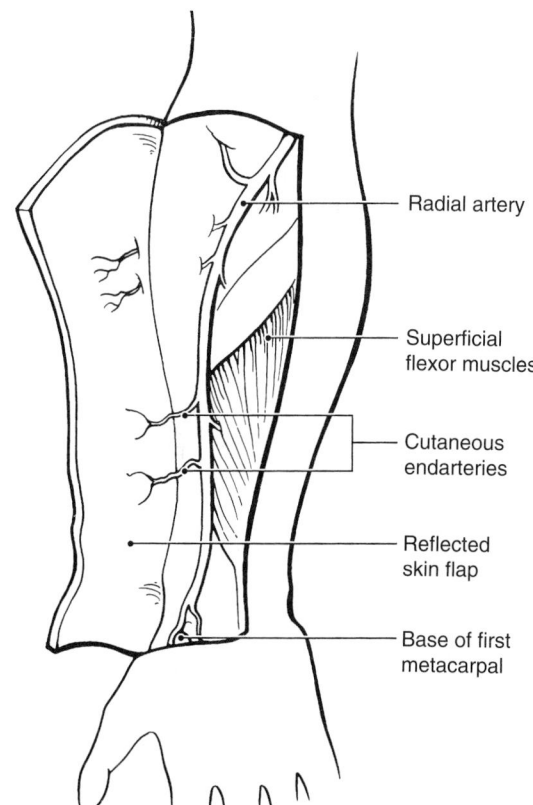

Figure 143–1 ■ Depiction of small endarteries arising directly from the radial artery, which are at risk of thromboembolic occlusion related to radial artery cannulation. (From Bedford RF: Radial arterial function following percutaneous cannulation with 18- and 20-gauge catheters. Anesthesiology 47:37-39, 1977.)

Table 143–1 ▪ Complications and Risk Factors Related to Arterial Cannulation

Limb Ischemia
Catheter material, size, length
Advanced atherosclerosis or Raynaud's or Buerger's disease
Small wrist circumference, which suggests a small vessel
Accidental injection of medication into the arterial line

Neurologic Injury
Needle injury to the nerve in close proximity to the cannulated artery
Nerve injury because of prolonged wrist extension
Nerve dysfunction from hematoma produced during repeated attempts at cannulation
Stroke due to retrograde thrombus or air emboli with flushing (especially in infants or children)

Misinterpretation of Data
"Acute hypertension"—transducer on the floor
"Acute hypotension"—partial disconnection or pressure bag failure
"Occult hemorrhage"—arterial line disconnection

Infection and Septicemia
Aseptic cannulation
Improper care of stopcocks
Extended duration of cannulation

- Use of vasoconstrictor infusions
- Ulnar artery cannulation if the patient had a recent ipsilateral radial artery cannulation

Small endarteries supplying the skin of the forearm may be blocked by a long cannula or a cannula-related thrombus. Hence, proximal skin ischemia is more common than hand or digital ischemia.

Allen's test is nonspecific. Therefore, it should be replaced by a digital plethysmographic tracing from a pulse oximeter in suspected high-risk cases. If the tracing disappears with digital occlusion of the radial artery before cannulation, the ipsilateral ulnar collateral supply is inadequate, and cannulation of that radial artery should be avoided. Routine testing in patients with no risk factors may be unnecessary owing to the very low incidence of complications. Risk factors for other complications are listed in Table 143-1.

Implications

The low rate of complications with direct arterial blood pressure monitoring should not lead to a sense of complacency; when complications do occur, they can be severe. Awareness of the nature of and risk factors for complications related to direct arterial access can reduce their incidence and severity. In high-risk cases, consider avoiding arterial cannulation altogether; use an alternative site, or use the smallest cannula for the shortest possible time.

MANAGEMENT

Monitor the hand for signs of ischemia if risk-benefit considerations justify direct arterial access in high-risk cases. With signs of finger, hand, or forearm skin ischemia, the intra-arterial administration of local anesthetic or papaverine, along with temporary proximal venous occlusion, should be considered before the arterial cannula is removed. Vigorous aspiration of the cannula with proximal and distal digital pressure on the cannulated radial artery has been successful in removing some thrombi. Ipsilateral upper extremity sympathetic block of the affected extremity may also help. Importantly, a vascular surgeon should be consulted. Amputation of the hand or digits is considered after a line of demarcation becomes apparent. Skin grafting may be required for proximal skin necrosis.

PREVENTION

Recognition of risk factors for the complications of peripheral arterial access is key to their prevention (see Table 143-1). Either avoid arterial cannulation altogether or consider an alternative site in high-risk cases. An arterial line should always be used for the shortest possible time and then removed. Thrombo-occlusion of the cannulated artery can be reduced with smaller (Fig. 143-2) and shorter cannulas, prior aspirin therapy, the addition of heparin in the flush solution, and the prevention of pressure failure of the flush. Recent cannulation of one of the arteries at the wrist contraindicates the cannulation of the other unless flow in the previously cannulated artery has clearly been reestablished. When in doubt, the adequacy of ulnar collateral flow should be confirmed by pulse oximeter tracings during digital compression of the radial artery. Wrist hyperextension should be corrected after radial artery cannulation to relieve stress on the nerves at the wrist.

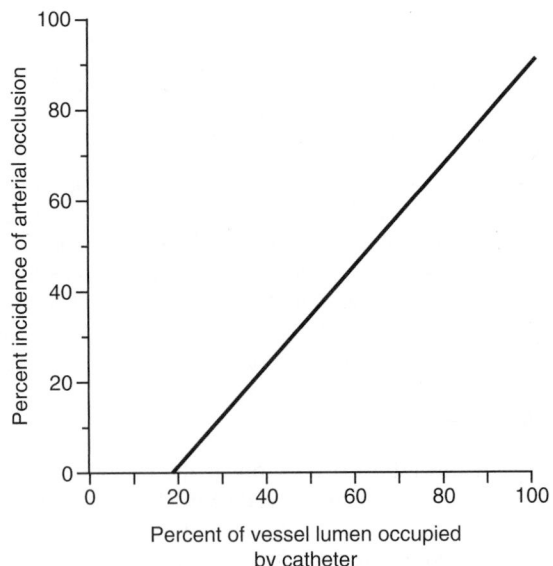

Figure 143–2 ▪ Radial artery thrombosis during 24-hour cannulation. Small catheters in large vessels rarely produce thrombosis. (Adapted from Bedford RF: Invasive blood pressure monitoring. In Blitt CD [ed]: Monitoring in Anesthesia and Critical Care Medicine. New York, Churchill Livingstone, 1990, pp 93-134.)

Further Reading

Bedford RF: Radial arterial function following percutaneous cannulation with 18- and 20-gauge catheters. Anesthesiology 47:37-39, 1977.

Bedford RF: Invasive blood pressure monitoring. In Blitt CD (ed): Monitoring in Anesthesia and Critical Care Medicine. New York, Churchill Livingstone, 1990, pp 93-134.

Raju R: The pulse oximeter and the collateral circulation. Anaesthesia 41:784, 1986.

Wyatt R, Glares I, Cooper DJ: Proximal skin necrosis after radial artery cannulation. Lancet 1:1135-1138, 1974.

EQUIPMENT & MONITORING

Central Venous Pressure Monitoring

144

Peter J. Lee, William Prince, and James G. Ramsay

Case Synopsis

A 58-year-old man is taken to the operating room for elective repair of an infrarenal abdominal aortic aneurysm. During routine preparation and draping for surgery, a right internal jugular triple-lumen central venous catheter (CVC) is placed. The operation proceeds without complications. The patient is extubated in the operating room and taken to the intensive care unit in stable condition. On the fourth postoperative day, the patient develops fever and chills, has mental status changes, and becomes hypotensive.

PROBLEM ANALYSIS

Definition

Common complications of central venous pressure monitoring at the time of CVC insertion or while the catheter is in place are listed in Tables 144-1 and 144-2, respectively. Some of the more common complications, such as pneumothorax and inadvertent arterial puncture, can lead to serious consequences, including cardiac arrest, if not recognized early enough. Although fever and chills are not signs and symptoms of pneumothorax or arterial puncture, hypotension, mental status changes, or desaturation (due to airway compromise) may occur. Pneumothorax and inadvertent arterial puncture can largely be prevented with the use of a portable ultrasound-guided probe or a small "finder" needle.

One of the most serious and insidious complications is CVC-related infection; this too is largely preventable.

Elevated temperature, hypotension, and mental status changes should raise suspicion of a CVC-related sepsis syndrome. Although other infectious sources must be ruled out, any intravenous (IV) catheter is a potential route by which organisms can reach the bloodstream, leading to bacteremia. Diagnosis of CVC- or IV catheter-related bloodstream infection is based on both clinical and laboratory criteria. Catheter-related bloodstream infection is most stringently defined as isolation of the same organism from semiquantitative or quantitative culture samples from both a catheter segment and blood (preferably from a peripheral venipuncture site) in a patient with signs or symptoms of infection but no obvious source for that infection.

Table 144–1 ■ Complications of Central Venous Pressure Monitoring during Catheter Insertion

Complication	Prevention	Recognition	Management
Air embolism	Use of Trendelenburg's position during placement Meticulous occlusion of open needles and catheter hubs	Shortness of breath Desaturation Hypotension	Supplement with 100% O_2 Cardiovascular support as indicated
Pneumothorax	More common with subclavian approach Use of small "finder" needle Continuous aspiration with syringe More common with positive-pressure ventilation	Cough during needle insertion Desaturation, dyspnea Hypotension Chest radiographic findings Decreased breath sounds	Closed chest tube thoracostomy Observation if insignificant (<15%) Supplemental O_2 Cardiovascular support as indicated
Arrhythmias	Avoidance of guidewire insertion >15 cm	Electrocardiographic findings Audible change in pulse regularity	Withdraw guidewire Rarely, antiarrhythmic drug or external cardioversion
Inadvertent arterial puncture	Careful attention to landmarks Palpation of arterial pulse Use of small "finder" needle Use of manometer (extension tubing) or transducer pressure before dilating Use of portable ultrasound guidance	Bright red blood Pulsatile flow Expanding hematoma Airway compromise (with carotid puncture)	Withdraw needle and hold direct pressure ≥10 min With dilator or introducer placement, obtain vascular surgeon consultation Airway support; intubation if indicated
Pericardial tamponade	Avoidance of overzealous manipulation of catheter guidewire and dilator Confirmation of proper placement by chest radiograph	Cardiovascular decompensation Temporal association with catheter placement Echocardiogram	Surgical evacuation

Table 144–2 ▪ **Complications of Central Venous Pressure Monitoring during Catheter Residence**

Complication	Prevention	Recognition	Management
Vascular erosion	Confirmation of correct catheter tip placement with chest radiograph (junction of superior vena cava and right atrium) More common in left subclavian and internal jugular than right	Hydrothorax Cardiovascular decompensation (hemothorax, tamponade) Respiratory insufficiency	Surgical repair
Thrombosis	Heparin-bonded catheters may reduce risk Use of catheter only as long as absolutely indicated	May be "silent" Upper limb or shoulder edema or tenderness Pulmonary embolism may occur	Consider thrombolytic drug or heparin Surgical thrombectomy if severe
Infection	Strict aseptic techniques Maximal barrier precautions Use of catheter only as long as absolutely indicated Consider antimicrobial catheters Daily inspection of insertion site	Fever without other source of infection Local redness, tenderness, purulence Positive cultures of both catheter segment and blood samples from separate venipuncture with same organism	Removal of infected catheter Antimicrobial therapy
Misinterpretation	Appropriate "zeroing" and leveling of transducers Education and training	Correlation with clinical status Frequent zeroing and level checks of transducer	

Recognition

Catheter-related bloodstream infection is recognized by the following:

- Fever in a patient with an IV catheter or CVC
- No obvious source for infection
- Signs or symptoms of local infection at the IV catheter or CVC insertion site
- Positive catheter segment and peripheral blood cultures

The sine qua non, although nonspecific, of catheter-related bloodstream infection is typically a febrile episode. Therefore, fever in a person with a CVC should be attributed to the catheter until proved otherwise. A systematic approach should be used to rule out other sources of infection. This includes sputum and urine cultures, inspection of surgical wounds and skin integrity, and a thorough physical examination. Finally, all CVC or IV catheter insertion sites should be inspected for erythema, tenderness, and purulence.

To obtain culture samples of catheter segments, the CVC or IV catheter must be removed. If there are no obvious signs of local infection, the site can be preserved by using "guidewire" exchange. Blood samples for culture should be obtained from a peripheral site at or near the time of CVC or IV catheter exchange for comparison. Isolation of the same organism from cultures of both the catheter segment and peripheral blood confirms the diagnosis of a catheter-related bloodstream infection.

Semiquantitative and quantitative catheter cultures have greater specificity than do traditional broth cultures. The most widely used semiquantitative technique was first described by Maki. It employs the roll plate method, in which the catheter segment is rolled across a sheep-blood agar plate and incubated for culture. Growth of more than 15 colony-forming units from a catheter segment by semiquantitative culture, but without signs of local or systemic infection, indicates catheter colonization. The same culture results, but with evidence of local infection (erythema, tenderness, purulence) but not systemic infection, indicates catheter-related local infection. With evidence of sepsis, the diagnosis is catheter-related bloodstream infection.

The most sensitive technique for diagnosing a catheter-related infection is a quantitative culture. The catheter segment is either flushed and inserted into broth or placed in broth and sonicated. Quantitative cultures are performed on broth obtained by either of these methods. Growth of more than 10,000 colony-forming units in a sample from a catheter segment, but without signs of local or systemic infection, is indicative of catheter colonization. The same results with evidence of local infection but not systemic infection are indicative of a catheter-related local infection. With evidence of systemic infection, it is a catheter-related bloodstream infection.

Quantitative blood culturing techniques were developed as a diagnostic alternative for patients in whom catheter removal is undesirable because of limited vascular access. This method relies on quantitative cultures of paired blood samples obtained from a CVC port and one peripheral venipuncture site. A colony count obtained from a catheter that is 5- to 10-fold greater than the colony count obtained from a peripheral blood culture is predictive of a catheter-related bloodstream infection.

Risk Assessment

The incidence of nosocomial bloodstream infection is estimated to be approximately 250,000 cases per year. Most of these infections are associated with the use of an intravascular device, and infection rates are much higher in patients with such devices than in those without. CVCs account for an estimated 90% of all catheter-related bloodstream infections. Between 1992 and 2003, the National Nosocomial Infection Surveillance Committee determined that in the United States, there were 2.9 to 8.5 bloodstream infections per 1000 catheter days (e.g., 100 catheters in use for 10 days each would total 1000 catheter days). The rate varies according to hospital size, patient population (higher incidence in immunocompromised and burn patients), frequency of catheter use, and practitioners' adherence to strict definitions of catheter-related infections and proper diagnosis.

The risk of infection increases with the duration of central venous catheterization, regardless of the number of catheter changes. Routine CVC changes do not lower the risk for a bloodstream infection; in fact, routine catheter changes increase the risk for mechanical complications and cause patient discomfort, without providing any benefit. Further, catheter changes increase the use of nurse and physician time and increase hospital costs.

Any patient with a CVC is at increased risk for infection. However, certain practices may help reduce this risk. Skin colonization at the insertion site is one of the most powerful predictors of increased risk. It has been well documented that skin microorganisms gain access to the transcutaneous tract at the time of insertion or migrate from the skin surface sometime after catheter placement. Some studies have shown a higher infection rate with catheters inserted via the internal jugular versus the subclavian vein. This may be related to heavier cutaneous colonization at the internal jugular site or to greater difficulty maintaining an occlusive dressing. When choosing a site for prolonged (>48 hours) line placement, the subclavian approach, if practical, may be preferable.

Implications

Catheter-related bloodstream infections are associated with increased morbidity and mortality (10% to 20%), longer hospitalizations (>7 days), and increased medical costs (>$6000 per hospitalization). Moreover, these infections can be devastating in patients who have prosthetic implants (e.g., heart valves, vascular graft material), which can be seeded by bacteria in the bloodstream.

MANAGEMENT

Once a catheter-related bloodstream infection is suspected, the catheter must be removed. If there is a low index of suspicion for a given catheter (e.g., recent placement; clean, noninflamed site), the catheter can be replaced using a guidewire-assisted exchange. However, the old catheter tip and intradermal segment should be sent for semiquantitative culture. Two sets of blood cultures should be obtained to confirm the diagnosis. Preferably, at least one should be from a peripheral site for comparison purposes. If the catheter culture results are negative, a newly placed catheter can be left in place. If the culture results are positive, the newly placed catheter should be removed and a new insertion performed at a different site.

Broad-spectrum antimicrobial therapy can be instituted after catheter exchange and after blood cultures have been obtained. In some patients, this includes coverage for gram-positive and gram-negative bacteria; in others, antifungal or narrower coverage may be indicated. Once culture results

are reported and sensitivities are known, the antibiotics can be tailored to the specific organism.

Certain clinical situations, such as new sepsis in a critically ill patient or in a patient with a prosthetic heart valve, may dictate the need for catheter removal and replacement at a different site, even with a relatively low index of suspicion. In such situations, the risk of catheter-related bloodstream infection outweighs the benefit of preserving an existing catheter site and avoiding the risk of mechanical complications from new access. It is imperative that good clinical judgment be exercised when weighing the risks and benefits of new central access, including possible mechanical complications and increased patient discomfort.

Flowcharts for diagnosing acute fever in a patient suspected of having nontunneled CVC infection and approaches to managing patients with nontunneled CVC-related bloodstream infections are provided in Figures 144-1 and 144-2, respectively.

PREVENTION

The following precautions should be taken:

- Use a CVC only when a true indication exists, and remove it as soon as the indication no longer applies.
- Educate and train health care providers who insert and maintain CVCs.
- Practice strict adherence to hand-washing and aseptic technique during CVC placement and dressing changes.
- Use 2% chlorhexidine preparation for skin antisepsis.
- Use antiseptic- or antibiotic-coated CVC devices.
- Use maximal barrier precautions during CVC placement.
- Perform daily inspections of CVC insertion sites.

Any intravascular device is a conduit for microorganisms to the bloodstream (Fig. 144-3). The patient's skin and the person inserting the catheter are the most likely sources of infecting microorganisms. Heavy skin colonization at the insertion site appears to be a predictor of increased risk of CVC infection. Therefore, strict adherence to hand washing and cutaneous antisepsis should be a high priority. A study that compared various antiseptics showed 2% chlorhexidine was associated with a lower incidence of CVC-related local infection and CVC-related bacteremia compared with 10% povidone-iodine or 70% alcohol. Currently, 10% povidone-iodine is the most widely used skin antiseptic in the United States.

Maximal barrier precautions, including the use of a long-sleeved surgical gown, surgical mask, and large surgical sheet, have been shown to reduce the risk of pulmonary artery catheter infection (colonization) compared with less stringent precautions (sterile gloves, surgical mask, small fenestrated drape). Raad and colleagues showed a sixfold reduction in the incidence of long-term CVC-related bloodstream infection when maximal barrier precautions were used. The Centers for Disease Control and Prevention recommended maximal barrier precautions for all central line insertions in its most recently published guidelines.

Insertion sites for all intravascular devices must be inspected and palpated daily. Early recognition of local catheter-related infection may help prevent progression

Central Venous Catheter and Fever

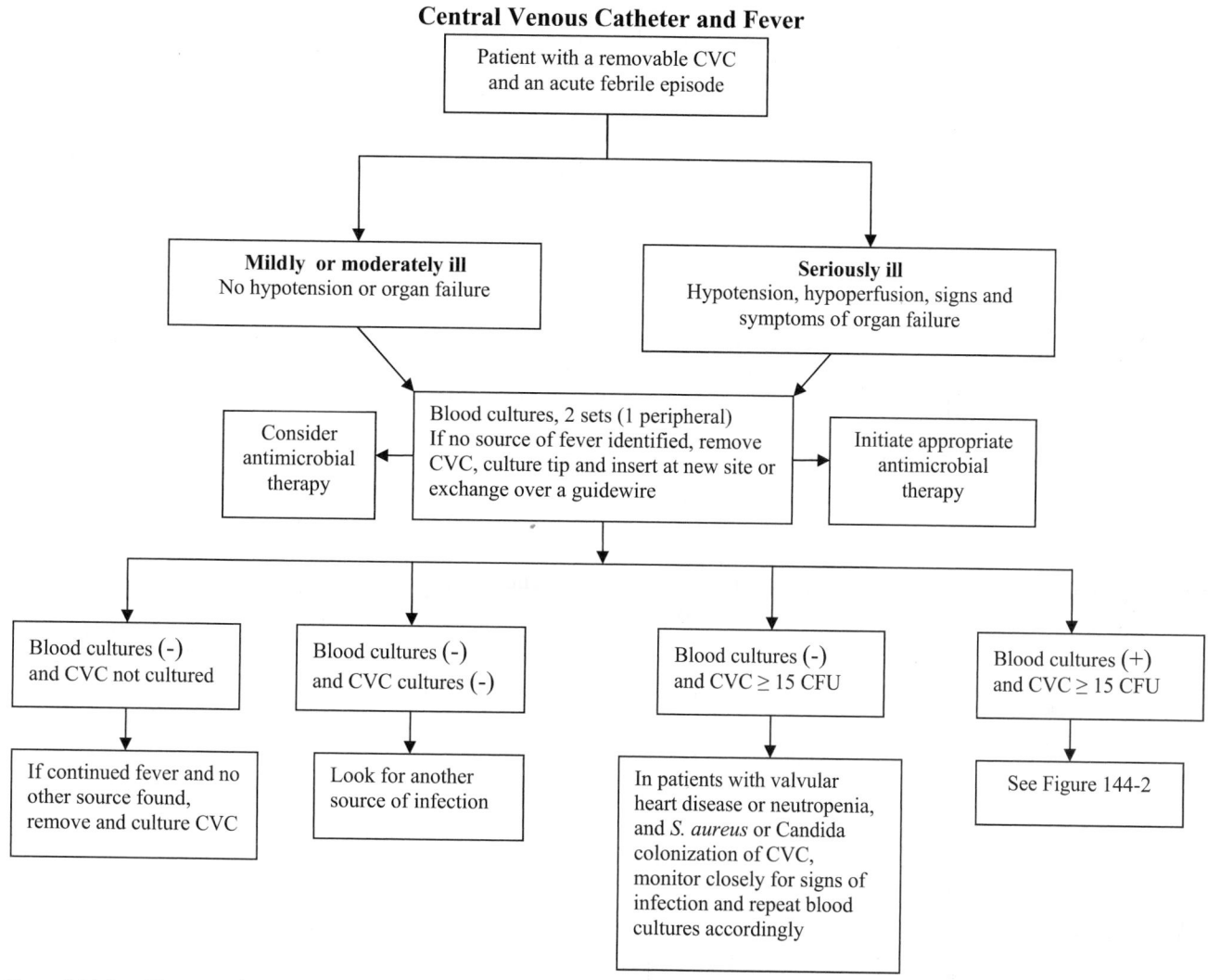

Figure 144–1 ■ Diagnosis of acute fever in a patient with suspected nontunneled central venous catheter (CVC) infections. CFU, colony-forming unit. (Adapted from Mermel LA, Farr BM, Sheretz RJ, et al: Guidelines for the management of intravascular catheter-related infections. Clin Infect Dis 32:1249-1272, 2001.)

to bloodstream infection. Dressing care is a controversial aspect of CVC maintenance. Apparently, there is no significant increase in catheter-related bloodstream infection with transparent versus more traditional gauze dressings. However, some studies found increased cutaneous colonization at catheter insertion sites covered with transparent dressings for longer than 48 hours. In contrast, more recent studies showed that transparent dressings are safe for up to 5 days. This difference may be due to the introduction of more permeable transparent dressings that prevent or minimize moisture buildup.

Antimicrobial-coated or -impregnated catheters may be beneficial in reducing the risk of bloodstream infection. In a prospective, randomized trial, Kamal and colleagues showed the efficacy of antibiotic-bonded arterial catheters and CVCs in reducing intravascular catheter colonization. However, there were no catheter-related bloodstream infections in either the study group or the control group. In a

prospective, randomized study, Maki demonstrated a twofold decrease in catheter colonization and a fivefold decrease in bloodstream infections in CVCs impregnated with silver sulfadiazine and chlorhexidine versus standard CVCs among patients in a surgical intensive care unit. Similarly, Ramsay and colleagues showed a decrease in catheter colonization and bloodstream infections with the same catheters in hospital-wide application. Although the difference in catheter-related bloodstream infections between the two study groups was not statistically significant, the results suggest a benefit with antimicrobial catheter use. These studies also suggest that antibiotic-coated or -impregnated catheters may help reduce catheter site or catheter-related bloodstream infections.

Catheters inserted by inexperienced personnel carry an increased risk of infection. Some hospitals use IV therapy teams for catheter insertion and follow-up care. Certainly, institutions can reduce their rate of catheter-related sepsis by

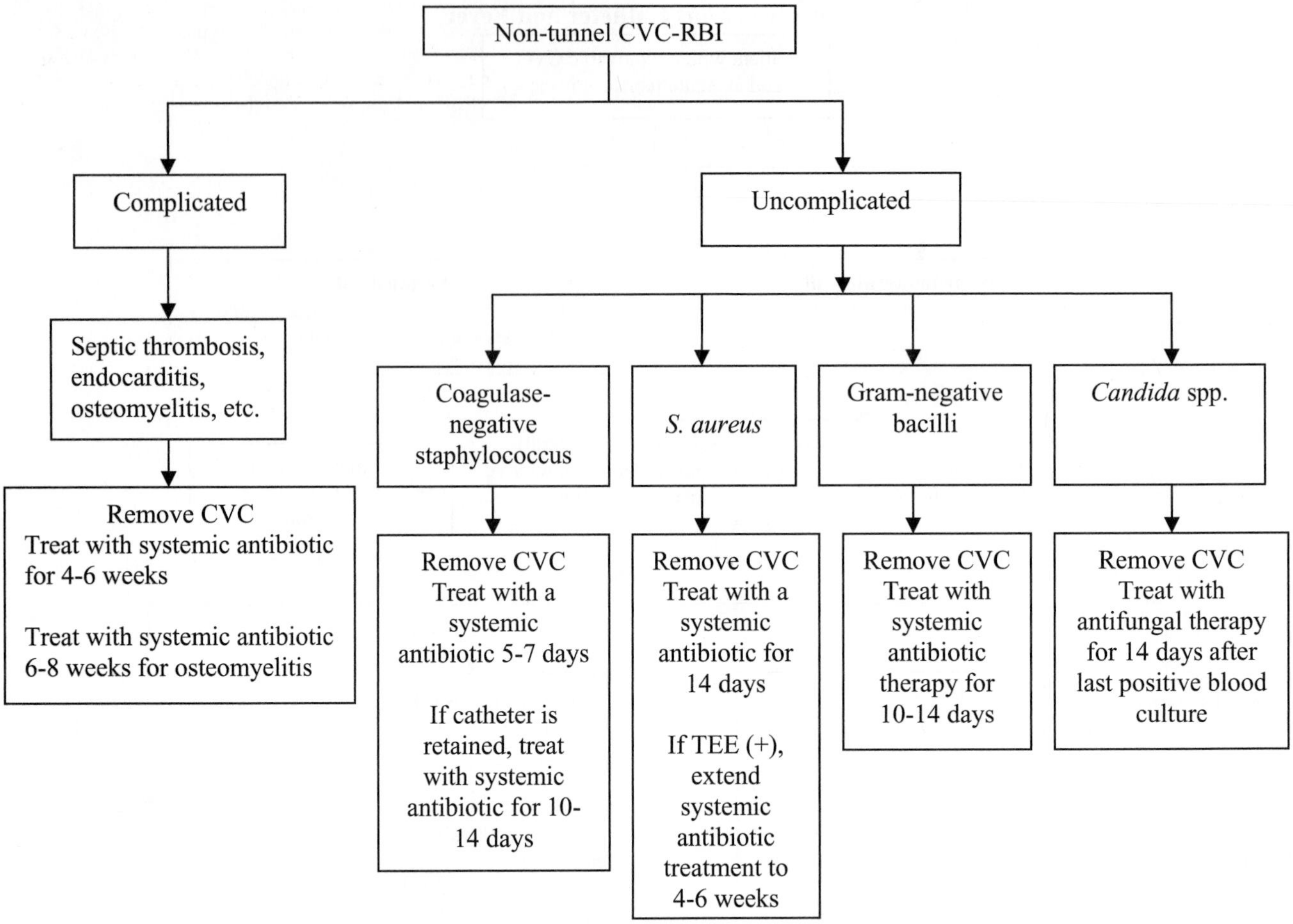

```
                          Non-tunnel CVC-RBI
                                  |
              +-------------------+-------------------+
              |                                       |
        Complicated                            Uncomplicated
              |                                       |
              |            +--------------+-----------+----------------+
              |            |              |           |                |
   Septic thrombosis,  Coagulase-    S. aureus   Gram-negative   Candida spp.
   endocarditis,       negative                   bacilli
   osteomyelitis, etc. staphylococcus
              |            |              |           |                |
```

Remove CVC Treat with systemic antibiotic for 4-6 weeks Treat with systemic antibiotic 6-8 weeks for osteomyelitis	Remove CVC Treat with a systemic antibiotic 5-7 days If catheter is retained, treat with systemic antibiotic for 10-14 days	Remove CVC Treat with a systemic antibiotic for 14 days If TEE (+), extend systemic antibiotic treatment to 4-6 weeks	Remove CVC Treat with systemic antibiotic therapy for 10-14 days	Remove CVC Treat with antifungal therapy for 14 days after last positive blood culture

Figure 144–2 ■ Management of patients with nontunneled central venous catheter–related bloodstream infection (CVC-RBI). TEE, transesophageal echocardiography. (Adapted from Mermel LA, Farr BM, Sheretz RJ, et al: Guidelines for the management of intravascular catheter-related infections. Clin Infect Dis 32:1249-1272, 2001.)

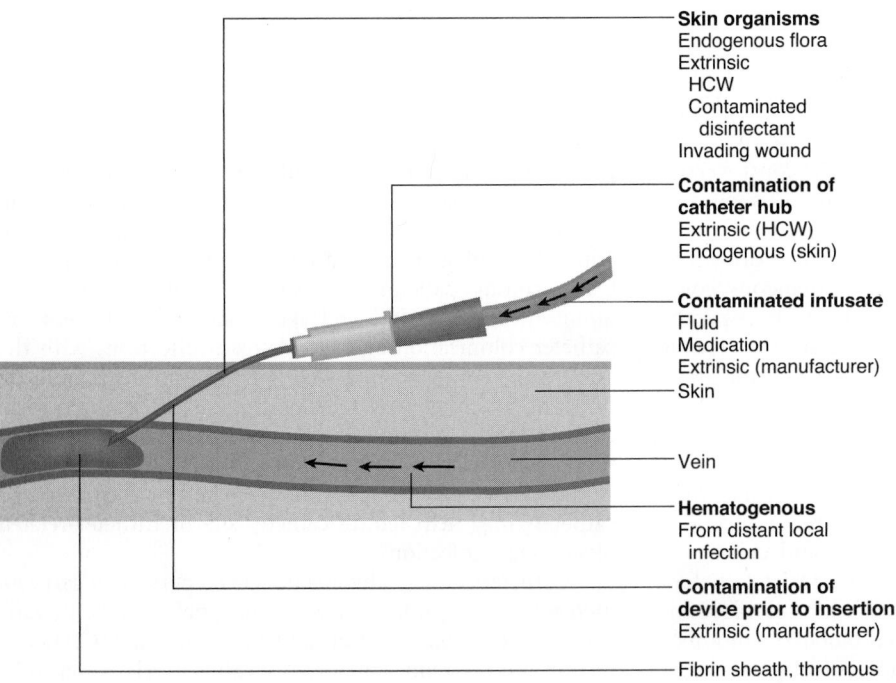

Skin organisms
Endogenous flora
Extrinsic
  HCW
  Contaminated
  disinfectant
Invading wound

Contamination of catheter hub
Extrinsic (HCW)
Endogenous (skin)

Contaminated infusate
Fluid
Medication
Extrinsic (manufacturer)

Skin

Vein

Hematogenous
From distant local
  infection

Contamination of device prior to insertion
Extrinsic (manufacturer)

Fibrin sheath, thrombus

Figure 144–3 ■ Sources of intravascular cannula-related infection. The major sources are skin flora, contamination of the catheter hub, contamination of infusate, and hematogenous colonization of the intravascular device and its fibronectin-fibrin sheath. HCW, health care worker. (From Maki DG: Infections due to infusion therapy. In Bennett JV, Brachman PS [eds]: Hospital Infections, 3rd ed. Boston, Little, Brown, 1992, pp 849-898.)

implementing catheter care protocols and better educating and training nurses and physicians in both sterile technique and practical skills.

Further Reading

Cobb DK, High KP, Sawyer RG, et al: A controlled trial of scheduled replacement of central venous and pulmonary artery catheters. N Engl J Med 327P:1062-1068, 1992.

Eyer S, Brummitt C, Crossley K, et al: Catheter-related sepsis: Prospective, randomized study of three different methods of long-term catheter maintenance. Crit Care Med 8:1073-1079, 1990.

Guidelines for the prevention of intravascular catheter-related infections. MMWR Morb Mortal Wkly Rep 51(RR-10):1-32, 2002.

Kamal GD, Pfaller MA, Rempe LE, et al: Reduced intravascular catheter infection by antibiotic bonding. JAMA 265:2364-2368, 1991.

Keenan SP: Use of ultrasound to place central lines. J Crit Care 17:126-137, 2002.

Kluger DM, Maki DG: The relative risk of intravascular device related bloodstream infections in adults. In Abstracts of the 39th Interscience Conference on Antimicrobial Agents and Chemotherapy. San Francisco, American Society for Microbiology, 1999, p 514.

Maki DG: Infections due to infusion therapy. In Bennett JV, Brachman PS (eds): Hospital Infections, 3rd ed. Boston, Little, Brown, 1992, pp 849-898.

Maki DG: Yes, Virginia, aseptic technique is very important: Maximal barrier precautions during insertion reduce the risk of central venous catheter-related bacteremia. Infect Control Hosp Epidemiol 15:227-230, 1994.

Maki DG, Cobb L, Garmen JK: An attachable silver-impregnated cuff for prevention of infection with central venous catheters: A prospective randomized multicenter trial. Am J Med 85:307-314, 1988.

Maki DG, Ringer M, Alvarado CJ: Prospective randomized trial of povidone-iodine, alcohol, and chlorhexidine for prevention of infection associated with central venous and arterial catheters. Lancet 338:339-343, 1991.

Maki DG, Stolz SM, Wheeler SJ, Mermel LA: A prospective, randomized, three-way clinical comparison of novel highly permeable polyurethane dressing with 442 Swan-Ganz catheters. In Program and Abstracts of the 32nd Interscience Conference on Antimicrobial Agents and Chemotherapy, October 1992, Chicago, Ill. Washington, DC, American Society for Microbiology, 1992, p 825.

Maki DG, Weise CE, Sarafin HW: A semiquantitative culture method for identifying intravenous-catheter-related infection. N Engl J Med 296:1305-1309, 1977.

Maki DG, Wheeler SJ, Stolz SM: Study of a novel antiseptic coated central venous catheter. Crit Care Med 19:S99, 1991.

Mermel LA, Maki DG: Infectious complications of Swan-Ganz pulmonary artery catheters. Am J Respir Crit Care Med 149:1020-1036, 1994.

Mermel LA, McCormick RD, Springman SR, et al: The pathogenesis and epidemiology of catheter-related infection with pulmonary artery Swan-Ganz catheters: A prospective study utilizing molecular subtyping. Am J Med 91(Suppl 3B):197S-205S, 1991.

National Nosocomial Infections Surveillance System report: Data summary from January 1992 through June 2003, issued August 2003. Am J Infect Control 31:481-498, 2003.

Pearson ML (for the Hospital Infection Control Practices Advisory Committee): Guideline for prevention of intravascular device-related infection. Am J Infect Control 24:262-293, 1996.

Raad II, Darouiche R, Dupuis J: Central venous catheters coated with minocycline and rifampin for the prevention of catheter-related colonization and blood stream infections: A randomized, double-blind trial. The Texas Medical Center Catheter Study Group. Ann Intern Med 127:267-274, 1997.

Raad II, Hohn DC, Gilbreath JB, et al: Prevention of central venous catheter-related infections by using maximal sterile barrier precautions during insertion. Infect Control Hosp Epidemiol 15:231-238, 1994.

Ramsay J, Nolte F, Schwartzman S: Incidence of catheter colonization and catheter related infection with an antiseptic impregnated triple lumen catheter. Crit Care Med 22:A115, 1994.

Ruesch S, Walder B, Tramer M, et al: Complications of central venous catheters: Internal jugular versus subclavian access—a systematic review. Crit Care Med 30:454-460, 2002.

EQUIPMENT & MONITORING

Pulmonary Artery Pressure Monitoring

145

Matthew D. Caldwell and Paul E. Kazanjian

Case Synopsis

A 74-year-old woman undergoes resection of a 7-cm aneurysm of the proximal descending thoracic aorta. Before induction of anesthesia, an oximetric pulmonary artery catheter (PAC) is introduced via the right internal jugular vein and wedged at 42 cm. A two-lumen endotracheal tube is positioned for one-lung ventilation. Deep, hypothermic circulatory arrest is used for aneurysmectomy and aortic repair. After cardiopulmonary bypass, the PAC is withdrawn 5 cm. After restoration of ventilation, the patient develops massive hemoptysis from the dependent right lung and hypoxemia. This resolves after protamine is administered. Two weeks later, a 1.5-cm nodular density is seen in the right lower lobe on portable chest radiography. Computed tomography confirms the clinical suspicion that the density is a pulmonary artery pseudoaneurysm.

PROBLEM ANALYSIS

Definition

PACs are commonly used by anesthesiologists to measure right atrial and ventricular and pulmonary artery pressures. Also, the pulmonary artery occlusion (wedge) pressure is used as a surrogate for left atrial pressure, and cardiac output is determined by thermodilution. These measurements aid in the diagnosis and management of many cardiovascular derangements.

PAC placement requires the insertion of a large introducer sheath (8.0, 8.5, or 9.0 French), often in the left subclavian or right internal jugular vein. The PAC is then advanced through this sheath into the superior vena cava, its balloon is inflated, and blood flow directs its passage through the right atrium and right ventricle into the pulmonary artery. Simultaneous pressure monitoring is used as the PAC is advanced.

Complications with PACs may occur during insertion or after positioning. The former complications are similar to those that occur with sheaths used for other central lines, except that the large size of the dilator and sheath can result in more serious vascular injuries. Complications related to central venous catheterization are discussed in Chapter 144. After PAC positioning, complications are due to erroneous PAC hemodynamic data or misinterpretation of correct data. Either can adversely affect decisions related to clinical management.

Arrhythmias or Bundle Branch Block.

Guidewire insertion or PAC passage often causes atrial or ventricular arrhythmias. Atrial or ventricular ectopic beats and nonsustained ventricular tachycardia occur in 13% to 70% of cases, usually while the balloon is passing through the right atrium and ventricle. Also, ventricular ectopy is often noted during withdrawal of PAC. In addition, ventricular arrhythmias can develop after the catheter has been in place for a few minutes to days. Most ventricular arrhythmias caused by catheter manipulation are benign and self-limited. Hemodynamically significant sustained ventricular tachycardia or ventricular fibrillation is very infrequent but can develop, especially in patients with risk factors for these arrhythmias (e.g., prior or recent myocardial infarction, ejection fraction <25%, dilated cardiomyopathy). New right bundle branch block appears during 5% of PAC insertions. Development of new right bundle branch block in patients with preexisting left bundle branch block may cause complete heart block and hemodynamic instability.

Malposition of the Catheter Tip.

Obtaining accurate hemodynamic data from a PAC depends on positioning the catheter tip in a region of the pulmonary vasculature where the pulmonary artery pressure exceeds airway pressures. Errant catheter tip position can generate erroneous data and contribute to PAC-induced vascular injury. Minutes to hours after insertion, the tip may migrate distally as the catheter softens and is towed by the blood flow. A catheter with its tip located in a permanent wedge position can lead to pulmonary infarction or pulmonary artery rupture.

Pulmonary Ischemia and Infarction.

The incidence of ischemic injury is approximately 7%. It may be due to thromboembolism, endothelial damage, or ischemia distal to a catheter tip that completely occludes a small branch of the pulmonary artery. Pathologic and angiographic studies have revealed an unexpectedly high rate (53% to 66%) of thrombotic lesions in patients with PACs. The thrombus is often attached to the catheter at or near the site of insertion of the introducer sheath. Thrombus is also associated with traumatized endothelium or endocardial surfaces. Thromboses are usually small, but they can be massive and associated with pulmonary embolism. The thrombus can disrupt hemodynamic measurements by occluding the thermistor or infusion ports. Heparin bonding may not reduce mural and veno-occlusive thrombus formation.

Pulmonary Artery Perforation or Rupture.

Artery perforation and rupture are the most serious complications of PACs.

Their exact incidence is unknown, but estimates range between 0.064% and 0.2%, with a mortality estimated at 41% to 70%. Barash and associates proposed possible mechanisms for PAC-related perforation or rupture based on postmortem study of isolated whole lung preparations:

- A PAC tip that has been advanced too far distally can perforate the vessel.
- Eccentric balloon inflation can propel the tip of the catheter through the vessel wall.
- Balloon inflation can result in intraballoon pressures of 250 mm Hg, which can cause rupture of the pulmonary artery.

Catheter Knotting or Entanglement.   PACs can become entangled around cardiac structures or knotted in the superior vena cava, right atrium, right ventricle, or pulmonary artery. Similarly, PACs have been entrapped by cardiac sutures during open-heart surgery and have become entangled with cardiac papillary muscles, pacing and defibrillator leads, and other central vascular access catheters. Knotted or entangled PACs are often discovered during attempts to withdraw or advance the catheter.

Intracardiac Erosions or Hemorrhagic Lesions.   These erosions or lesions may involve the vascular endothelium, right atrial or ventricular endocardium, tricuspid valve, chordae tendineae, and pulmonic valve, but they rarely lead to clinically important endocarditis. Such PAC-induced damage to the great vessels, heart, or pulmonary vessels can result in bleeding, hemoptysis, cardiac tamponade, or death.

Catheter Colonization and Sepsis.   Colonization and sepsis are more likely with multilumen catheters (e.g., PACs) than with single-lumen catheters. They underscore the need for strict adherence to aseptic technique during PAC insertion and dressing changes and when tending to transducers, stopcocks, and external tubing.

Inappropriate Use and Data Misinterpretation.   The clinical benefits and utility of right-sided heart catheterization with PACs are unproved. In fact, a body of evidence and opinion exists that the risks and costs outweigh any benefits. Some observational studies suggest that the risk of death is higher in patients managed with PACs. One recent randomized study of PACs in high-risk surgical patients found no benefit in patients whose therapy was directed by PACs. Other studies have found serious flaws in the correct interpretation of PAC data, even by experienced physicians and critical care nurses. These flaws included the inability to correctly identify pulmonary artery wedge pressure and the determinants of oxygen transport, both of which are fundamental to the rational use of PACs.

Recognition

New arrhythmias or heart block should be easily detected by electrocardiogram (ECG). Changes in the ECG or pulse oximeter monitor tones may signal a rhythm disturbance and can alert the nursing staff or physicians to its presence. Unusual resistance to the advancement or withdrawal of a PAC suggests knotting or entanglement and should be evaluated by a chest radiograph before any further PAC manipulation. Pulmonary artery perforation by a PAC may go undetected but is often manifest by hemoptysis (sometimes massive), hemothorax, dyspnea, anxiety, and hypotension. The onset of these symptoms is often related to balloon inflation or flushing of a PAC that is in a wedged position. Until proved otherwise, any new hemoptysis in a patient with a PAC must be considered due to pulmonary artery rupture. Infectious complications are recognized by fever and erythema or pus at the PAC insertion site. Infection is confirmed by indicated laboratory studies and cultures at the insertion site.

Risk Assessment

Risk factors for the development of arrhythmias during or after PAC insertion include the following:

- Total time spent passing the PAC through the right atrium and ventricle
- Presence of previous myocardial infarction or ischemia or left bundle branch block
- Presence of hypoxemia or acidosis
- Electrolyte imbalance (especially hypokalemia or hypomagnesemia)

Low cardiac output syndrome may predispose to pulmonary infarction. Factors associated with increased risk of pulmonary artery rupture, infarction, or pseudoaneurysm are listed in Table 145-1. During cardiac surgery, manipulation of the heart or distal migration of a cold and stiff PAC from an empty heart predisposes to pulmonary artery perforation. Patients whose skin is heavily colonized with bacteria or yeast are at risk for catheter-associated infection, as are those who have had the same PAC in place for longer than 4 days. The incidence of thrombus formation increases with the duration of catheterization and the severity of the illness.

Implications

As with all invasive procedures, PACs have associated risks and benefits. The incidence of serious complications is estimated to be 0.1% to 0.5% for anesthesiologists and <5% for other specialists. This risk must be weighed against the potential benefit of rapidly identifying and managing hemodynamic disturbances. The American Society of Anesthesiologists Task Force on Pulmonary Artery Catheterization recommends considering the patient, the surgical procedure, and the practice setting when deciding on the appropriateness of

EQUIPMENT & MONITORING

Table 145–1 ■ Risk Factors for Pulmonary Artery Rupture, Infarction, or Pseudoaneurysm

Advanced age
Pulmonary hypertension
Distal pulmonary artery catheter (PAC) migration
Anticoagulation
Hypothermia
PAC balloon overinflation

placing a PAC. In patients with clinically significant cardiopulmonary disease, renal insufficiency, or hemodynamic instability, the potential benefit of a PAC may be greater. Surgical procedures with a high risk of rapid hemodynamic changes and significant fluid shifts may also favor PAC placement. Finally, PACs are more likely to improve patient outcomes in practice settings where physicians and nurses have a sufficient level of training and familiarity with their use.

MANAGEMENT

All patients should have ECG and pulse oximetry monitoring during PAC insertion. Most ventricular arrhythmias associated with PAC insertion are benign and self-limited. They usually terminate once the PAC is advanced into the pulmonary artery or withdrawn into the right atrium. Only rarely is antiarrhythmic therapy or external pacing necessary. Complete atrioventricular heart block is treated with temporary transcutaneous or transvenous pacing. Any suspected technical complication of pulmonary artery catheterization should immediately be investigated with chest radiography. Catheter malposition and kinking may be corrected by carefully repositioning the PAC with or without the assistance of fluoroscopy. The use of brute force is inappropriate and risks disastrous injury. A knotted or entrapped PAC may require angiographic or even surgical removal. Pulmonary artery rupture may require one or more of the following modes of therapy:

- Positive end-expiratory pressure
- Lung isolation with a double-lumen endotracheal tube or endobronchial blocker
- Temporary unilateral occlusion of the pulmonary artery
- Direct repair of the lacerated artery
- Lung resection
- Embolization of a pseudoaneurysm

PACs that are suspected or proved to be infected must be removed, and the patient must be treated with appropriate antibiotic therapy.

PREVENTION

It is important to remember that placement of a PAC is an elective, diagnostic procedure. It should be performed only after the patient's medical condition has stabilized and physiologic imbalances (e.g., hypoxemia, electrolyte disturbance, acidosis, hypotension) have been corrected. Complications of vascular access may be reduced by ultrasound-guided cannulation and central venous pressure waveform confirmation during introducer sheath placement. Complete heart block is very infrequent and does not justify the prophylactic insertion of invasive pacing wires.

However, the means for temporary transcutaneous or transvenous pacing should be readily available during the insertion of PACs in patients with preexisting left bundle branch block.

Prevention of pulmonary artery rupture requires careful technique during PAC insertion and manipulation. During initial insertion, once a pulmonary artery wedge pressure tracing is obtained, the catheter should be withdrawn 2 to 3 cm. Ideally, a PAC should be left with its tip 3 to 5 cm beyond the pulmonic valve. Typically, this translates to an insertion depth of 40 to 45 cm, but it depends on the patient and the insertion site. In addition, one should always consider the need to obtain a pulmonary artery wedge pressure in patients with risk factors for rupture (especially those receiving anticoagulants or with distal PAC migration). Radiographic or echocardiographic confirmation of proper position should be obtained whenever feasible. Routine chest radiography may alert the operator to inadvertent distal PAC migration or other technical complications.

Competence in the placement and interpretation of data from PACs is mandatory. This requires formal training in right heart catheterization, along with supervised PAC placement. The minimum number of PAC placement procedures to ensure competence is debatable, but ongoing maintenance of skills is mandatory. Ideally, an institutional quality improvement program should be in place to ensure ongoing education and skill maintenance for all physicians and nursing personnel caring for patients with PACs.

Further Reading

American Society of Anesthesiologists Task Force on Pulmonary Artery Catheterization: Practice guidelines for pulmonary artery catheterization. Anesthesiology 99:988-1014, 2003.

Barash PG, Nardi D, Hammond G, et al: Catheter-induced pulmonary artery perforation: Mechanisms, management, and modifications. J Thorac Cardiovasc Surg 82:5-12, 1981.

Connors AF, Castele RT, Farhat NZ, et al: Complications of right heart catheterization: A prospective autopsy study. Chest 88:567-572, 1985.

Connors AF Jr, Speroff T, Dawson NV, et al: The effectiveness of right heart catheterization in the initial care of critically ill patients: SUPPORT investigators. JAMA 276:889-897, 1996.

Damen J, Bolton D: A prospective analysis of 1400 pulmonary artery catheterizations in patients undergoing cardiac surgery. Acta Anaesthesiol Scand 30:386-392, 1986.

Domino KB, Bowdle TA, Posner KL, et al: Injuries and liability related to central vascular catheters: A closed claim analysis. Anesthesiology 100:1411-1418, 2004.

Ginosar Y, Thijs LG, Sprung CL: Raising the standard of hemodynamic monitoring: Targeting the practice or the practitioner? Crit Care Med 25:209-211, 1997.

Mermel LA, McCormick RD, Springman SR, et al: The pathogenesis and epidemiology of catheter-related infection with pulmonary artery Swan-Ganz catheters: A prospective study utilizing molecular subtyping. Am J Med 91:197S-205S, 1991.

Sandham JD, Hull RD, Brant R, et al: A randomized controlled trial of the use of pulmonary artery catheters in high risk surgical patients. N Engl J Med 348:5-14, 2003.

Swan HJC, Ganz W, Forrester J, et al: Catheterization of the heart in man with the use of a flow-directed balloon-tipped catheter. N Engl J Med 283:447-451, 1970.

Intracranial Pressure Monitoring

146

Paul Smythe and Norah Naughton

Case Synopsis

An 18-year-old man has open long bone fractures and severe traumatic brain injury due to a motor vehicle accident. His Glasgow Coma Scale score is 6, and a computed tomography scan of the head reveals diffuse cerebral edema. An intraventricular monitor reveals a pressure of 30 mm Hg. Treatment for increased intracranial pressure is initiated, and the patient is transferred to the operating room for treatment of the long bone fractures.

PROBLEM ANALYSIS

Definition

Intracranial pressure (ICP) is the pressure or force exerted within the rigid cranial vault by the intracranial contents. In normal adults, the intracranial contents comprise brain, 80%; blood, 10%; and cerebrospinal fluid (CSF), 10% of volume.

Normal ICP is approximately 5 to 13 mm Hg (7 to 18 cm H_2O). In patients who do not have intracranial pathology, the intracranial contents are considered to have normal elastance. This means that small increases in intracranial volume do not result in increased ICP. According to the Monro-Kellie hypothesis, this occurs because when the volume of one compartment increases, the volume of another compartment decreases by an equal amount, leaving the total volume unchanged. This type of compensation is necessary because all three elements of the intracranial contents are almost incompressible. Reduced elastance occurs when the intracranial volume approaches that of the intracranial space. In this case, a small increase in intracranial volume creates a dramatic and possibly life-threatening increase in ICP.

The diagnostic and therapeutic use of ICP monitors has not changed appreciably in the last 5 years. Most centers consider 20 mm Hg the upper limit of normal for ICP, although others use 15 mm Hg for this cutoff. ICP above 15 to 20 mm Hg is considered intracranial hypertension (ICH; see Chapter 174). Beyond this level, treatment for ICH is initiated. Cerebral perfusion pressure (CPP) should be considered when managing patients with ICH. CPP is defined as mean arterial blood pressure minus ICP, and it is the physiologic variable that defines the pressure gradient driving cerebral blood flow and delivery of oxygen and metabolites. It is therefore closely related to cerebral ischemia. The optimal level at which CPP should be maintained is unclear, but several clinical studies suggest that keeping CPP greater than 70 mm Hg is associated with a substantial reduction in death rates and improved quality of survival. Further, it is likely to enhance ischemic brain perfusion after severe traumatic brain injury (TBI). In most cases of TBI, CPP is manipulated by normalizing intravascular volume or inducing systemic hypertension.

Recognition

ICP monitoring can assist in the diagnosis and treatment of ICH. All ICP monitoring systems have certain characteristics in common, beginning with physical attachment to the system being monitored. This connection requires a watertight fluid interface between the ICP monitor and the intracranial compartment and consists of rigid tubing leading to a flexible membrane. Because ICP is being monitored, the compartment must be sealed. Any leakage would be indicative of serious underlying pathology that must be addressed. This could range from CSF leakage (best-case scenario) to cerebral herniation (worst-case scenario). With no leakage, any change in ICP leads to some degree of deformation of the flexible membrane contiguous with this space.

CONSTRUCTION

The deformed membrane is coupled to a transducer. Regardless of the coupling interface (i.e., rigid tubing), its role is to accurately transmit any membrane deformations occurring with each ICP pulsation. A transducer converts these coupled or transmitted pulsations to an electrical signal, which is then amplified to enhance the signal generated by the transducer for display purposes. The display is essentially a voltmeter. It may be connected to an oscilloscope or stylus recorder to display the ICP waveform and pressure changes. ICP monitoring systems differ mainly according to the type of coupling between the deformed membrane and transducer, and according to the anatomic location at which each system is placed.

ZEROING

All ICP monitoring devices must covert ICP to some voltage for electronic display. This relationship is expressed as the equation $y = mx + b$, where y is the voltage, x is the pressure, and m is the ICP curve slope. The characteristics of the transducer are such that there is a linear relationship between voltage and pressure, or m (discussed further under "Calibration"). It would be optimal for a monitor to read zero voltage when the pressure applied to the transducer is equal to zero. Adjusting the b term of the equation so that the relation becomes $y = mx + b$, with b equal to zero, accomplishes this and is called *zeroing*. Zeroing means that if the transducer produces a voltage when the pressure being measured is zero, it must be balanced or offset by an internally applied voltage of the opposite sign. The zero pressure of biologic pressure monitoring systems is always the ambient atmospheric pressure. Zeroing is achieved by opening a stopcock or valve on the transducer to sense the ambient or room air pressure as zero. Modern systems require pushing a zeroing button, and this setting is automatically remembered. Zeroing the transducer (ICP or any other pressure transducers) is important because an error in this step affects all subsequent pressure readings.

TRANSDUCER LOCATION

With ICP monitoring devices, the transducer can be located either externally or at the catheter tip inside the cranium. External transducers can be rezeroed at any time after placement of the ICP monitor. Monitors that have catheter-tip pressure transducers must be zeroed before placing the catheter into the intracranial compartment. Once placed, a catheter-tip pressure transducer cannot be rezeroed.

CALIBRATION

Calibration is accomplished by adjusting the m term, or slope, of the equation $y = mx + b$. The control on ICP amplifier systems that adjusts the slope is labeled "calibration," "gain," "amplification factor," or "slope." Most contemporary transducers have a small microprocessor incorporated within the transducer that is precalibrated. They produce a small constant voltage proportional to the degree of compression, termed the *calibration factor*. The most common calibration factor is 200. At 200 mm Hg, this means that the transducer may put out more or less voltage at a given pressure than it should. The calibration can be checked by applying a known pressure to the transducer and adjusting the monitor display to read the same as the known pressure applied. It is advised that calibration of all transducers be periodically cross-checked.

DRIFT

When zero and gain settings change across time, this is referred to as *drift*. Because no transducer can be perfect, all transducer-amplifiers drift to some extent.

TRANSDUCER TYPES

Two different types of transducers are used in contemporary ICP monitors. The first, the *strain-gauge transducer*, consists of a membrane physically attached to a magnet that moves with pulsations within a series of coils. As the magnetic flux changes across the coils, a current is induced that is proportional to the degree and frequency of magnet movement. This current is proportional to the pressure applied to the strain-gauge transducer. However, the most commonly used transducer is a highly specialized version of the strain-gauge transducer referred to as a *piezoelectric transducer*. This is a highly standardized ceramic crystal that generates voltage when a force is applied. In most piezoelectric systems, the transducer structure, analogous to the deformable membrane, is the crystal itself. The preset calibration factor is generally 200.

The second class of transducers is the *fiberoptic transducer*. It uses a laser beam to couple membrane movement with the electrical component of the transducer. This system still depends on a membrane being distorted by intracranial compartment pressure variations. The transducer side of the membrane is reflective (mirrored), with the laser beam directed to this side of the membrane. When the membrane moves, it reflects the laser light beam at an angle that diverges from that of any incident light. This reflected light signal is related to the incident light signal to generate a quantitative estimate of the membrane distortion caused by altered ICP. A signal is generated for amplification and is proportional to the movement of the membrane.

SOURCES OF ERROR

External transducers are accurate and can be recalibrated. They must be maintained at a fixed reference point relative to the patient's head to avoid measurement error. Internal transducers (catheter-tip strain-gauge or fiberoptic) are calibrated before intracranial insertion and cannot be recalibrated once they are placed (i.e., without a separate intraventricular catheter). Therefore, if the device measures drift, there is the potential for inaccurate ICP measurements, especially if the ICP monitor is used for several days.

VENTRICULAR INTRACRANIAL PRESSURE MONITORING

The intracranial spaces most frequently monitored are intraventricular, intraparenchymal, subarachnoid, subdural, and epidural (Table 146-1). Ventricular ICP monitoring is

Table 146–1 ▪ Intracranial Spaces Used to Monitor Intracranial Pressure

Space	Method of Pressure Transduction	Cerebrospinal Fluid Drainage	Recalibration
Intraventricular	Fluid-coupled external strain gauge	+	+
	Fluid-coupled strain-gauge catheter tip	+	+
	Fluid-coupled fiberoptic catheter tip	+	+
Parenchymal	Strain-gauge catheter tip	–	–
Subarachnoid	Fluid-coupled external strain gauge	–	+
Subdural	Strain-gauge catheter tip	–	–
	Fiberoptic catheter tip	–	–
	Fluid-coupled external strain gauge	–	+
Epidural	Fluid-coupled external strain gauge	–	+
	Pneumatic	–	+

+, possible or necessary; –, not possible or not necessary.

considered the gold standard for comparing the accuracy of ICP monitors in other intracranial compartments. It also has the therapeutic benefit of draining CSF for the treatment of ICH. ICP monitoring devices have been ranked based on their accuracy, stability, and ability to drain CSF. A ventricular catheter connected to an external strain-gauge transducer or catheter-tip pressure transducer device is the most accurate and reliable method of monitoring ICP and allows for therapeutic CSF drainage. Parenchymal catheter-tip pressure transducer devices measure ICP similar to ventricular ICP pressure. Subarachnoid or subdural fluid-coupled devices and epidural ICP devices are less accurate.

CONTINUOUS INTRACRANIAL PRESSURE MONITORING

With continuous ICP monitoring, three types of waveforms may be observed: A, B, and C. B and C waves are of limited clinical significance and correspond to changes in respiration and arterial blood pressure, respectively. A waves, referred to as plateau waves, are of clinical significance. These waves arise from an elevated baseline ICP and can reach magnitudes of 50 to 120 mm Hg for 2 to 20 minutes. These waves result from cerebral blood volume increases in response to CPP fluctuations and occur in vascular beds with overall intact autoregulation. These waves may signify impending limitation of the ICP volume compensation system.

Risk Assessment

ICP monitoring has been used most extensively in patients with TBI (see also Chapter 174). In the TBI patient population, ICP monitoring may accomplish the following:

- Help in the early detection of intracranial mass lesions
- Limit the indiscriminate use of therapy to control ICP, which is potentially harmful
- Reduce ICP by CSF drainage and thus improve cerebral profusion
- Help in determining prognosis
- Improve outcomes

Comatose head-injured patients (Glasgow Coma Scale score 3 to 8) with abnormal computed tomography scans should have ICP monitoring. Comatose patients with normal scans should also have ICP monitoring if they have two or more of the following risk factors:

- Age older than 40 years
- Unilateral or bilateral motor posturing
- Systolic blood pressure less than 90 mm Hg

Routine ICP monitoring is not indicated for patients with mild or moderate head injury. The mortality rate for patients with an intracranial process associated with ICH increases 2- to 10-fold when patients have a disturbance in consciousness and are unable to follow commands. ICP monitoring may be recommended in these situations, which include subarachnoid hemorrhage (with and without hydrocephalus), intracerebral hemorrhage, hydrocephalus, encephalitis, meningitis, venous sinus thrombosis, ischemic infarct with swelling, and hepatic encephalopathy. Table 146-2 lists the advantages and disadvantages of ICP monitoring by device location.

Implications

ICP monitoring complications include infection, hemorrhage, malfunction, obstruction, and malposition. *Bacterial colonization* is a more accurate term than *infection* because

Table 146–2 ▪ Advantages and Disadvantages of Intracranial Pressure Monitoring by Device Location

Device Location	Advantages	Disadvantages	Waveform Quality
Intraventricular	Gold standard Accurate measurement of ICP Allows drainage or sampling of CSF Allows instillation of drugs or dyes directly into CSF Determines $\delta P/\delta V$	Catheter can become occluded by blood or tissue Risk of infection or hemorrhage May require frequent zeroing	Excellent
Parenchymal	Useful when unable to obtain ventricular access Accurate Requires zeroing only once No need to adjust transducer to patient position	Potential for significant drift Breakage of fiberoptic cable Cannot be recalibrated once placed Does not provide for CSF sampling	Good
Subarachnoid	Ability to leave cerebral parenchyma undisturbed Quick to insert Useful to insert when unable to obtain ventricular access	Lumen may be occluded by blood or tissue Tendency for dampened waveforms Less accurate at high ICPs Must be zeroed frequently CSF leakage a concern	Fair
Subdural	Useful after craniotomy Ease of placement Best when ICP relatively low	Risk for waveform dampening Underestimates ICP when high	Poor
Epidural	Dura not penetrated Low risk of infection Ease of insertion	Sensing membrane must remain coplanar to dura Risk of false or misleading readings Least understood of all ICP monitors	Poor

CSF, cerebrospinal fluid; ICP, intracranial pressure; $\delta P/\delta V$, change in pressure as a function of change in volume.
Modified from Guidelines for the Management of Severe Head Injury. Brain Trauma Foundation, 1995.

EQUIPMENT & MONITORING

there have been no reports in large prospective studies of clinically significant intracranial infections associated with ICP monitoring devices. Colonization of the ICP monitor increases significantly after 5 days of insertion. Irrigation of fluid-coupled ICP monitors significantly increases bacterial colonization. The average rate of bacterial colonization is 5% for ventricular, 5% for subarachnoid, 4% for subdural, and 14% for intraparenchymal devices, either catheter-tip strain-gauge or fiberoptic. However, clinically significant intracranial infections are uncommon. The overall incidence of hematomas associated with ICP devices is 1.4%. The incidence of malfunction or obstruction in fluid-coupled ventricular catheters, subarachnoid bolts, or subdural catheters has been reported as 6.3%, 16%, and 10.5%, respectively. When ICP measurements are greater than 50 mm Hg, obstruction and loss of signal and waveform can occur. Malfunction with parenchymal and ventricular pressure fiberoptic catheter-tip transduction devices ranges from 9% to 40%. This requires reinsertion of a new fiberoptic device.

MANAGEMENT

Treatment of ICH is recommended when ICP is 20 mm Hg or greater or if there is significant brain swelling (see also Chapter 174). Treatments are generally classified according to the intracranial contents targeted for therapy and include the following:

- Brain tissue volume
- CSF volume
- Cerebral blood flow
- Mass lesion

Brain tissue water content is 75% to 80%, and treatments designed to decrease brain tissue volume are aimed at decreasing brain tissue water. Hyperosmolar agents such as mannitol are used for this purpose. The administration of mannitol creates an osmolar gradient between cerebral blood and brain tissue, which favors the movement of water from the tissue space into the vascular space. Mannitol may also act initially to decrease cerebral blood volume by decreasing blood viscosity secondary to free water movement. Decreased blood viscosity results in increased cerebral blood flow, which prompts vasoconstriction in normally autoregulating brain areas. This decreases cerebral blood volume and, secondarily, ICP. Effective doses range from 0.25 to 1 g/kg of body weight. Euvolemia should be maintained, and serum osmolarity should not exceed 320 mOsm. Furosemide and other diuretics can be used to decrease brain tissue water by increasing blood osmolarity. This favors the movement of water from the brain tissue space into the cerebrovascular space. Corticosteroids have been reported to decrease brain tissue water content when vasogenic edema is the chief cause of increased water; however, they are not consistently helpful in the treatment of other forms of cerebral edema or in clinical conditions in which both vasogenic edema and other forms of edema are present. Corticosteroids are not recommended for the treatment of increased ICP in the management of acute head injury, because associated side effects may worsen outcomes. Adverse effects include decreased immune response in areas of the body other than

the brain, suppression of intrinsic steroid production, and hyperglycemia.

Reduction in CSF volume may directly improve elevated ICP and increase the clearance of brain tissue water from edematous areas. The most direct means of decreasing CSF volume is through CSF drainage. This is usually accomplished via an intraventricular catheter or lumbar subarachnoid catheter. However, caution is advised when using the latter in patients with ICH, owing to the risk of acute brainstem herniation. CSF volume can also be reduced by promoting its movement from the intracranial space to the spinal subarachnoid space. Head elevation and repositioning relative to the subarachnoid space favor such movement.

Methods to reduce cerebral blood volume include hyperventilation, the use of drugs known to cause cerebral vasoconstriction and the restriction of those that impair cerebral autoregulation, head elevation above the level of the heart, suppression of cerebral metabolism, and the minimizing of increased intrathoracic pressure with airway manipulation or mechanical ventilation. Hypocapnia with hyperventilation reduces cerebral blood flow and volume via cerebral vasoconstriction. The latter is mediated by acute increases in perivascular pH. However, hypocapnia may compromise cerebral perfusion due to cerebral vasoconstriction, especially in patients with severe TBI. In the absence of increased ICP, chronic prolonged hyperventilation therapy (to an arterial carbon dioxide tension of 25 mm Hg) should be avoided after severe TBI. Also, use of prophylactic hyperventilation therapy during the first 24 hours after severe TBI should be avoided because it may compromise cerebral perfusion at a time when cerebral blood flow is already reduced. Hyperventilation therapy may be required for short periods with acute neurologic deterioration or for extended periods if ICH is refractory to sedation, paralysis, CSF drainage, and osmotic diuretics. Sedative-hypnotic drugs (e.g., barbiturates, etomidate, propofol) are cerebral vasoconstrictors and decrease ICP. In extreme cases, barbiturate-induced coma may be necessary to control ICP.

Drugs that impair cerebral autoregulation can increase cerebral blood volume and ICP. These include inhalation anesthetics and direct-acting vasodilators (e.g., nitroprusside, nitroglycerin, calcium channel blockers, prostacyclin, adenosine). Control of blood pressure with indirect-acting agents (e.g., labetalol, trimethaphan) prevents the increase in cerebral blood volume and ICP. Head elevation above the heart reduces cerebral blood volume by increasing cerebral venous outflow. Suppression of cerebral metabolism is accomplished by the use of hypothermia and barbiturate-induced coma.

Space-occupying masses increase total intracerebral volume and therefore ICP. Treatment for mass lesions includes removal, chemotherapy or radiation therapy, and creation of additional space for normal intracranial contents, such as decompression or craniectomy.

PREVENTION

There is no medical treatment for the prevention of increased ICP that is not part of the management of ICP covered in the previous section. Short of surgical intervention (in the case of intracranial hemorrhage, increasing tumor size, or hydrocephalus, for example), one prevents an increase in ICP by addressing the same three contents of the cranium, namely brain tissue volume, CSF volume, and cerebral blood volume. In summary:

- Brain tissue volume
  - Diuretics (mannitol)
- CSF volume
  - Ventriculostomy
  - Lumbar drain
- Cerebral blood flow
  - Hyperventilation
  - Head elevation and repositioning

- Discontinuation of inhalational anesthetics (and other cerebral vasoconstrictors)
- Barbiturate administration
- Sedation and paralyzing agents

Further Reading

Albin MS (ed): Textbook of Neuroanesthesia with Neurosurgical and Neuroscience Perspectives. New York, McGraw-Hill, 1997, pp 61-117, 1137-1177.

Fahy BG, Sivaraman V: Current concepts in neurocritical care. Anesth Clin North Am 20:441-462, 2002.

Marik PE, Varon J, Trask T: Management of head trauma. Chest 122: 699-711, 2002.

EQUIPMENT & MONITORING

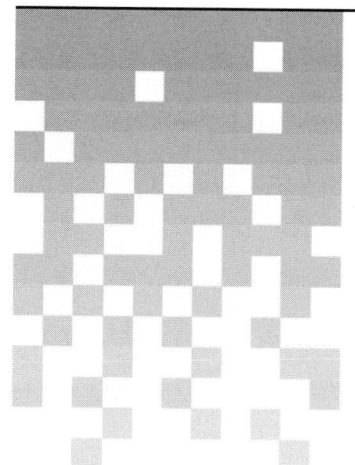

Pediatrics and Neonatology

B. Craig Weldon

Joel M. Gunter

Pediatric Laryngospasm

147

Eric P. Wittkugel

Case Synopsis

Following extubation at the conclusion of adenotonsillectomy, a 5-year-old boy develops high-pitched inspiratory stridor. Chest wall retractions are noted, and the breath sounds rapidly diminish until none are heard.

PROBLEM ANALYSIS

Definition

Among other functions, the larynx protects the upper airway and lungs from aspiration of foreign materials. The glottal closure reflex is most evident during swallowing. Laryngospasm is an exaggerated form of the glottal closure reflex in response to noxious stimuli. Partial or complete airway obstruction due to laryngospasm can persist even after removal of the stimulus. Laryngospasm is mediated by the vagus nerve. The afferent limb of this reflex is the superior laryngeal nerve, and the efferent limb is the recurrent laryngeal nerve.

Laryngospasm consists of two phases: (1) adduction of the true vocal cords, causing partial airway obstruction via a "shutter" mechanism, followed by (2) constriction of the false vocal cords and supraglottic soft tissues, leading to complete obstruction by a "ball-valve" effect.

Recognition

The following signs indicate laryngospasm:

- Chest wall retractions: suprasternal, sternal, intercostal
- High-pitched inspiratory stridor
- Diminished or absent breath sounds
- Hypoxemia

Laryngospasm can be partial or complete. The case synopsis shows the progression from partial to complete laryngospasm. Differentiation of partial laryngospasm from other causes of upper airway obstruction may be difficult. Typically, partial laryngospasm presents with high-pitched "squeaking" sounds emanating from the apposed vocal cords. Obstruction due to the tongue or other soft tissues in the pharynx is associated with snoring, whereas obstruction due to secretions is usually accompanied by gurgling sounds.

Prompt recognition and immediate treatment of complete laryngospasm are essential, because gas exchange is impossible with a closed glottis. During the evolution from partial to complete laryngospasm, signs of extrathoracic airway obstruction (chest wall retractions, nasal flaring, paradoxical breathing) intensify. Next, breath sounds weaken and then disappear.

Risk Assessment

Based on a sample of 136,929 patients studied over an 11-year period (1967-1978), Olsson and Hallen reported the incidence of laryngospasm to be 0.87%. The incidence doubled in pediatric patients 0 to 9 years of age (1.74%) and tripled in infants 0 to 3 months of age (2.82%); a further increase in the incidence of laryngospasm was seen in children with asthma or coexisting respiratory infection (9.58%).

Factors specific to the practice of pediatric anesthesiology may help account for this higher incidence:

- Inhalation induction, deep intubation without muscle relaxants, and deep extubation increase the likelihood of stimulation of the glottis during light anesthesia.
- Upper respiratory infections, which increase airway irritability, are common in children.

Other risk factors for laryngospasm include the following:

- "Light" levels of anesthesia
- Surgery associated with bleeding in the airway (e.g., tonsillectomy, adenoidectomy, nasal surgery, palatal surgery)
- Other noxious airway stimuli
- Exposure to secondhand cigarette smoke

Laryngospasm occurs during light levels of anesthesia. An animal model of acid-induced laryngospasm demonstrated that lighter levels of anesthesia increase the activity of laryngeal adductor neurons. Some anesthetic practices commonly used in children increase the likelihood of airway stimulation during light anesthesia. The duration of stage II (light) anesthesia is longer with inhalation versus intravenous induction and increases the period of vulnerability to laryngospasm. Stimulation of the glottis by secretions or airway management devices during this vulnerable period may trigger laryngospasm.

Laryngospasm is especially likely when intubation without muscle relaxants is attempted before reaching an adequate depth of anesthesia. After extubation under deep anesthesia, patients are at risk for laryngospasm while passing through stage II with an unprotected airway. Surgical procedures on the airway are common in children, and the resulting oral secretions and blood can trigger laryngospasm.

On average, children have six to eight upper respiratory infections (URIs) per year, making it unlikely that children presenting for surgery will be completely free of URI symptoms. Excess secretions and airway hyperreactivity may persist for up to 6 weeks after URI, which increases the susceptibility to laryngospasm. Compared with children without URI symptoms, children with an active or recent URI (<4 weeks) are more likely to experience breath holding, desaturation, or severe cough during or after anesthesia. However, laryngospasm occurs more often in children with active URIs, younger children, and those having airway surgery.

A growing body of literature suggests that children exposed to secondhand tobacco smoke have a higher incidence of perioperative respiratory complications. There is a 10-fold increase in the relative risk of laryngospasm associated with exposure to secondhand tobacco smoke. Also, these patients are more prone to severe coughing in the postoperative period.

Implications

Larygnospasm may progress to complete airway obstruction, which can lead to hypoxemia, hypercarbia, bradycardia, and cardiac arrest. Five of 1000 patients who develop laryngospasm experience cardiac arrest. Immediate recognition and intervention are essential if this progression is to be avoided. Laryngospasm has also been associated with the development of negative-pressure pulmonary edema. Markedly negative intrapleural pressures generated by the patient in an effort to overcome the obstruction of the closed glottis lead to transudation of fluid into the alveoli.

MANAGEMENT

The management of laryngospasm varies, depending on whether airway obstruction is partial or complete, the severity of the laryngospasm, and its cause. In all cases, prompt recognition and immediate aggressive management are essential to prevent or reverse hypoxemia, which has the potential to rapidly progress to bradycardia and cardiac arrest. If recognition and treatment are delayed, management can be complicated by depression of cardiac output, which reduces the effectiveness of drug therapy. Algorithms for managing complete or partial airway obstruction due to laryngospasm are presented in Figures 147-1 and 147-2, respectively. Initial management includes the following:

- Monitoring with pulse oximetry, electrocardiogram, and precordial stethoscope
- Capnography to confirm the presence or absence of effective ventilation
- Delivery of 100% oxygen and positive pressure via a well-sealed facemask

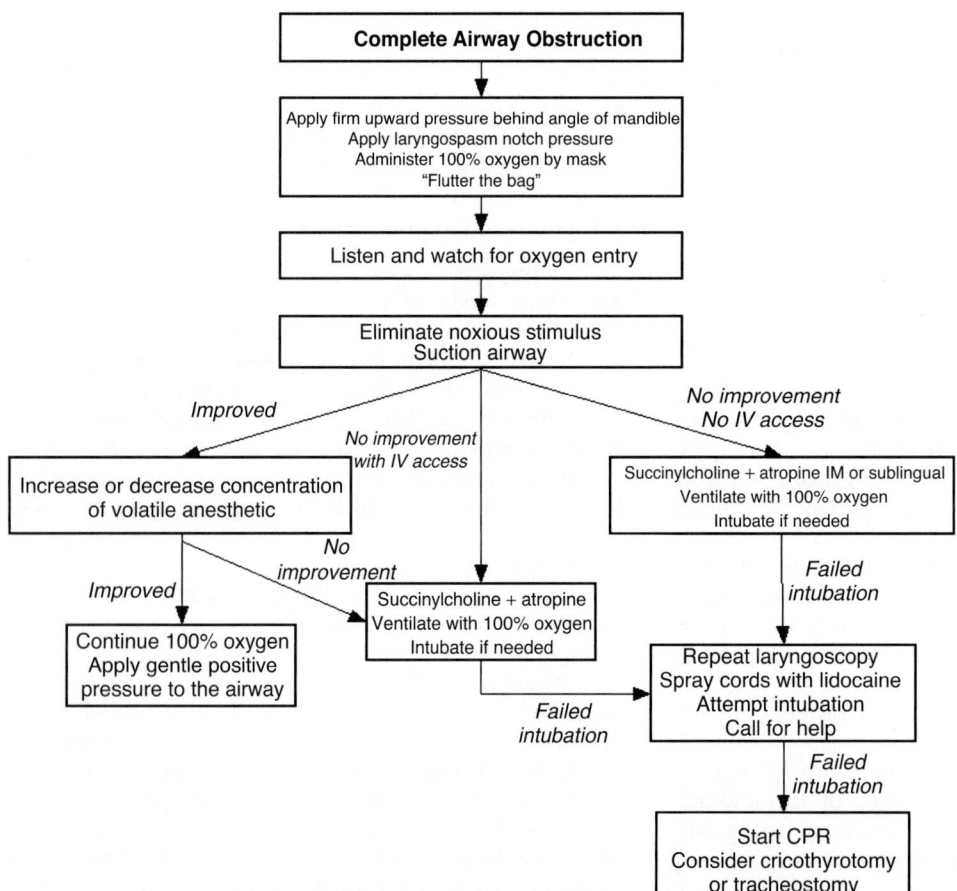

Figure 147–1 ▪ Algorithm for management of complete airway obstruction. CPR, cardiopulmonary resuscitation; IM, intramuscular; IV, intravenous.

Figure 147–2 ■ Algorithm for management of partial airway obstruction. IV, intravenous(ly).

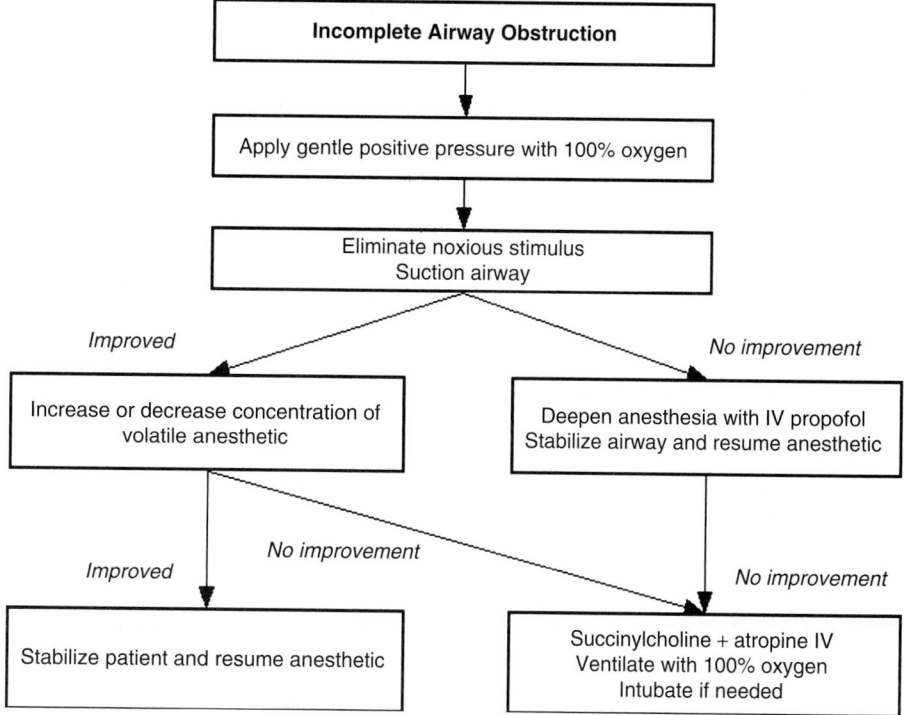

- Anterior displacement of the mandible
- Removal of noxious airway stimuli (e.g., suctioning of blood and secretions, removal of airway devices)
- Lightening or deepening the anesthetic
- Continuous positive airway pressure for partial airway obstruction
- "Fluttering the bag"
- Administration of muscle relaxants for complete obstruction unresponsive to other measures

Anterior displacement of the mandible (i.e., the jaw thrust-chin lift maneuver) lengthens the thyrohyoid muscle and unfolds the supraglottic tissues. This may be especially beneficial with complete laryngospasm. This also ensures that airway obstruction from laryngeal closure is not exacerbated by soft tissue obstruction. Laryngospasm is often precipitated by regurgitation or retained upper airway secretions. Pharyngeal suctioning, even during the acute event, prevents further stimulation of the superior laryngeal nerve.

Because laryngospasm often occurs in light planes of anesthesia, deepening the anesthetic or awakening the patient may relieve it, depending on whether the spasm occurs during induction, maintenance, or emergence. Propofol may be useful for rapidly deepening the level of anesthesia to relieve laryngospasm.

In most instances, partial laryngospasm is effectively managed with bag-mask positive-pressure ventilation. On inspiration, there is often a brief moment of relative relaxation of the larynx. A firm squeeze on the anesthesia bag in phase with this brief moment of relative laryngeal relaxation provides "pressure support" for the patient's respiratory efforts. Alternatively, fluttering the bag is a technique of manual high-frequency ventilation; the anesthesia bag is rapidly squeezed and released in a staccato rhythm similar to

atrial flutter. Either of these techniques can provide the minimal air exchange needed to maintain oxygenation and facilitate deepening or lightening of the anesthetic to relieve laryngospasm. However, care must be taken to avoid excessive continuous positive airway pressure. This can lead to gastric distention, which can further compromise ventilation or cause regurgitation.

With complete laryngospasm and ball-valve obstruction, the application of positive airway pressure can actually worsen airway obstruction by distending the piriform fossa on either side of the larynx and pressing the aryepiglottic folds more firmly against each other.

Larson described a simple technique of pressure on the "laryngospasm notch" located behind the ear, bounded anteriorly by the ascending ramus of the mandible adjacent to the condyle and posteriorly by the mastoid process and cephalad by the base of the skull. In Larson's technique, firm pressure is applied toward the base of the skull with both fingers, accompanied by anterior displacement of the mandible. Larson and others[1] have successfully employed this maneuver to manage complete laryngospasm.

If the preceding maneuvers do not improve airway obstruction, a muscle relaxant is indicated. Because of its rapid onset and short duration of action, succinylcholine is the most commonly used muscle relaxant to treat laryngospasm. Another advantage of succinylcholine is that it can be administered intramuscularly or sublingually if intravenous access is unavailable. However, owing to its vagotonic properties in children, succinylcholine should be given with atropine. Atropine is also indicated to treat bradycardia caused by

---

[1]Including the editor and his colleagues at both the University of Wisconsin–Madison and the Medical College of Wisconsin–Milwaukee.

persistent hypoxemia. Intravenous doses of succinylcholine range from 0.1 to 2 mg/kg. Higher doses (up to 4 mg/kg) are required for intramuscular administration. Smaller doses of succinylcholine can effectively treat laryngospasm, but larger doses are needed if emergency intubation is indicated.

If laryngospasm is sustained and the child is in extremis due to prolonged hypoxemia, intubation without muscle relaxants may be necessary. If apposition of the vocal cords interferes with intubation, topical application of lidocaine may relax the larynx and facilitate intubation. If air exchange has not been restored after these measures and intubation proves impossible, cricothyrotomy or emergent tracheostomy is required.

Negative-pressure pulmonary edema is managed supportively with supplemental oxygen and diuretics. Rarely, endotracheal intubation and positive-pressure ventilation with positive end-expiratory pressure are required for resolution of negative-pressure pulmonary edema.

PREVENTION

Prevention is the best treatment for laryngospasm. Take the following measures:

- Avoid noxious airway or surgical stimulation during light anesthesia.
- Intubate the trachea when conditions promoting laryngospasm cannot be avoided.
- Suction oropharyngeal secretions thoroughly before tracheal extubation.
- Extubate the trachea only when the patient is fully awake.
- Manage high-risk patients expectantly, especially during airway surgery.

In addition, the following measures may help prevent laryngospasm:

- Lidocaine applied topically to the larynx suppresses laryngeal mucosal sensory nerve activity and may reduce the likelihood of laryngospasm during intubation and after extubation.
- Intravenous lidocaine given shortly before extubation may prevent or attenuate laryngospasm via central interruption of the reflex pathway or a direct peripheral action on sensory and motor nerve terminals.
- Before extubation, have the patient breathe 100% oxygen for 3 minutes to provide a margin of safety should airway obstruction or laryngospasm occur.

- During extubation, hold the breathing bag momentarily at end-inspiration with a positive pressure of 15 to 20 cm H_2O to maintain a high lung volume as the endotracheal tube is removed. In animal models, such positive intrathoracic pressure inhibits the glottal closure reflex and laryngospasm. Also, extubation with the lungs inflated facilitates the expulsion of airway secretions along with the endotracheal tube, thereby reducing the likelihood of laryngospasm or aspiration of secretions.

It is important to identify children at increased risk for developing laryngospasm. Although it may not be possible to modify all preoperative risk factors, prudent choices of anesthetic techniques and agents can reduce the likelihood of laryngospasm. Additionally, increased vigilance will lead to faster recognition and expedited management should laryngospasm occur.

Further Reading

Afshan G, Shohan U, Qamar-Ul-Hoda M, et al: Is there a role for a small dose of propofol in the treatment of laryngeal spasm? Paediatr Anaesth 12:625-628, 2002.

Badgwell JM: Clinical Pediatric Anesthesia. Philadelphia, Lippincott-Raven, 1997, pp 39-40.

Johnstone RE: Laryngospasm treatment—an explanation. Anesthesiology 91:581-582, 1999.

Lakshmipathy N, Bokesch PM: Environmental tobacco smoke: A risk factor for pediatric laryngospasm. Anesth Analg 82:724-727, 1996.

Larson PC Jr: Laryngospasm—the best treatment. Anesthesiology 89:1293-1294, 1998.

Lee KWT, Downes JJ: Pulmonary edema secondary to laryngospasm. Anesthesiology 39:347-349, 1983.

Olsson GL, Hallen B: Laryngospasm during anaesthesia: A computer-aided incidence studying 136,929 patients. Acta Anaesthesiol Scand 28:567-575, 1984.

Roy WL, Lerman J: Laryngospasm in paediatric anaesthesia. Can J Anaesth 35:93-98, 1988.

Sasaki CT: Development of laryngeal function: Etiologic significance in the sudden infant death syndrome. Laryngoscope 89:1964, 1979.

Schreiner MS, O'Hara I, Markakis DA, et al: Do children who experience laryngospasm have an increased risk of upper respiratory tract infection? Anesthesiology 85:475-480, 1996.

Skolnick ET, Vomvolakis MA, Buck KA, et al: Exposure to environmental tobacco smoke and the risk of adverse respiratory events in children receiving general anesthesia. Anesthesiology 88:1144-1153, 1998.

Suzuki M, Sasaki CT: Laryngeal spasm: A neurophysiologic redefinition. Ann Otol Rhinol Laryngol 86:150-157, 1977.

Tait AR, Malviya S, Voepel-Lewis T, et al: Risk factors for perioperative adverse respiratory events in children with upper respiratory tract infections. Anesthesiology 95:299-306, 2001.

Difficult Pediatric Airway

148

Hernando De Soto

Case Synopsis

A 3-year-old child is scheduled for tonsillectomy and adenoidectomy. The past medical history is significant for Treacher Collins syndrome (Fig. 148-1). After inhalation induction, an intravenous line is started and 0.6 mg/kg of rocuronium is administered. Attempts at laryngoscopy and intubation are unsuccessful.

PROBLEM ANALYSIS

Definition

A difficult airway is one in which there is moderate to severe difficulty in performing mask ventilation, direct laryngoscopy, or both. This situation may result from anatomic (congenital or acquired) or physiologic defects.

Recognition

A thorough history and physical examination are the best means of recognizing and predicting a difficult pediatric airway. Understanding the significant differences between the pediatric and adult airways is mandatory for the successful management of a child with a difficult airway (Fig. 148-2). Anatomic differences exist in the size, shape, and position of the airway, as well as the airway epithelium and its supporting structures. Physiologic differences between the neonatal and adult respiratory systems are due to differences in anatomy and respiratory control mechanisms.

Upper Airway. The upper airway of the newborn is unique. The tongue is relatively large and fully occupies the cavity of the mouth and oropharynx. This may make manipulation of the laryngoscope and endotracheal tube more difficult during attempted intubation. Most, but not all, neonates are obligate nose breathers. This is because the epiglottis, positioned high in the pharynx, almost meets the soft palate, making mouth breathing difficult. These features persist for 2 to 6 months.

Lymphoid Tissue. Unlike older infants and children, neonates have almost no upper airway lymphoid tissue. The tonsils and adenoids appear during the second year of life and reach their maximal size by 4 to 7 years of age. After this, they gradually recede. Enlarged tonsils and adenoids may increase bleeding during attempted nasal intubation.

Epiglottis. The epiglottis in infants is large and U-shaped, and it protrudes over the larynx at a 45-degree angle. The use of a straight blade facilitates vocal cord visualization because it requires direct lifting of the epiglottis.

Larynx. In the newborn, the body of the hyoid bone is situated at the level of C3-C4. As the infant grows, the glottis moves caudally and reaches C5-C6 at maturity. The high position of the epiglottis and larynx enables the infant to

breathe and swallow simultaneously. Similarly, both the thyroid and the cricoid cartilages move caudad as the thyrohyoid and cricothyroid membranes develop.

Airflow. Airflow in the upper airway is turbulent even during quiet respiration. Laminar flow begins at the level of the fourth and fifth bronchial divisions, where the rapid increase in airway cross-sectional area reduces airflow velocity. The resistance to turbulent gas flow is proportional to the fifth power of the radius of the airway. Thus, 1 mm of edema within the trachea (reduction in radius from 2.1 to 1.1 mm) increases resistance to gas flow about 25-fold.

Respiratory Mechanics. The highly compliant chest wall in young infants reduces the work of breathing. Such increased compliance is attributed to the softer, noncalcified ribs, which articulate with the vertebral column and sternum at right angles. The diaphragm is the mainstay of ventilation in infants. The infant diaphragm has fewer type I (fast) muscle

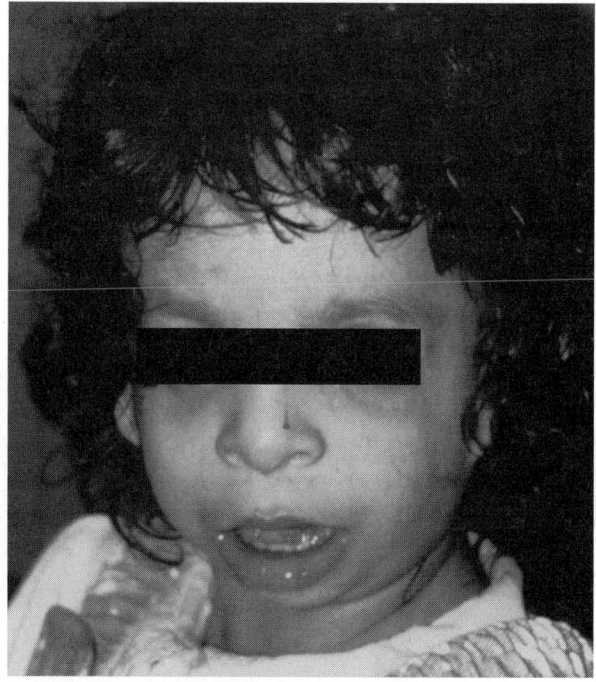

Figure 148–1 ■ Abnormalities pertinent to airway management in a patient with Treacher Collins syndrome (mandibulofacial dysostosis) include mandibular and malar hypoplasia, microstomia, and choanal atresia.

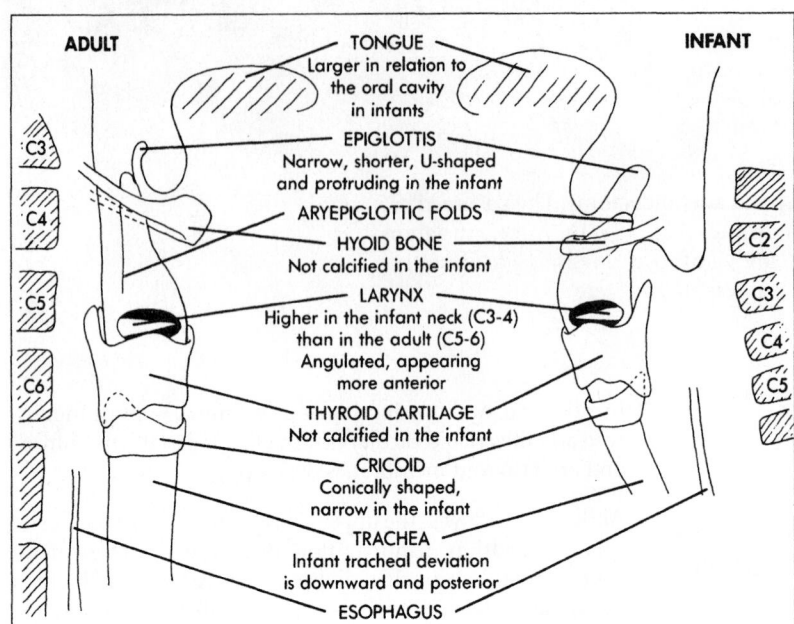

ADULT **INFANT**

TONGUE
Larger in relation to
the oral cavity
in infants

EPIGLOTTIS
Narrow, shorter, U-shaped
and protruding in the infant

ARYEPIGLOTTIC FOLDS

HYOID BONE
Not calcified in the infant

LARYNX
Higher in the infant neck (C3-4)
than in the adult (C5-6)
Angulated, appearing
more anterior

THYROID CARTILAGE
Not calcified in the infant

CRICOID
Conically shaped,
narrow in the infant

TRACHEA
Infant tracheal deviation
is downward and posterior

ESOPHAGUS

Figure 148–2 ■ Comparison of the anatomy in adult and infant airways. (From Ho M: The pediatric airway. In Bell C, Hughes C, Oh T [eds]: The Pediatric Handbook. St Louis, Mosby-Year Book, 1991, p 130. Adapted from Coté CJ, Todres ID: The pediatric airway. In Ryan JF, Todres DI, Coté CJ [eds]: A Practice of Anesthesia for Infants and Children. Orlando, Fla., Grune & Stratton, 1986.)

fibers than the adult diaphragm does. Thus, contraction is less efficient, and diaphragmatic muscle tires faster in infants compared with adults.

Risk Assessment

As mentioned earlier, successful management of a child with a difficult airway requires a thorough history and physical examination. The history should focus on the following:

- Review of prior records, especially anesthetic records for evidence of a difficult airway
- Evidence of congenital or acquired airway defects
- Evidence of airway obstruction or sleep apnea

Features of the physical examination most pertinent to perioperative airway management are listed in Table 148-1. Occasionally, additional studies (e.g., awake laryngoscopy, radiologic imaging, flow-volume loops) may be necessary to adequately assess a potentially difficult airway.

Implications

If the ability to ventilate by mask is absent or lost, and if it is determined that the patient cannot be intubated, a true

Table 148–1 ■ **Examination of the Pediatric Airway**
Size and shape of the head
Gross features of the face
Size and symmetry of the mandible
Size of the tongue
Shape of the palate
Prominence of the upper incisors
Jaw, head, and neck range of motion

airway emergency exists. Gas exchange must be restored immediately to avert the imminent threat of brain hypoxic injury and death.

MANAGEMENT

Premedication

Premedication should be individualized. The majority of children with compromised airways should not be given a sedative or a narcotic; these drugs can result in loss of muscle tone, worsening previous airway obstruction or causing respiratory depression. In some older children in whom awake intubation is contemplated, careful sedation by a practitioner experienced in difficult airway management is reasonable. Anticholinergic agents must be considered both for their antisialagogue effect and to protect against vagal responses during airway manipulation.

Induction

The technique chosen for the induction of anesthesia varies according to the severity of airway pathology and the degree of anticipated respiratory difficulty. Pediatric patients are divided into four categories that determine the appropriate methods for induction and intubation:

- *Type I.* These children present with a normal respiratory rate and oxygen saturation, mild respiratory distress, a visually normal airway (external appearance), and minimal or no sternal retractions. An example would be a patient with minimal facial (orbital) trauma.
- *Type II.* These children may have significant airway disease and moderate airway distress, but their airways have been successfully managed by previous anesthesia or

surgical teams. An example would be a patient who returns with the diagnosis of laryngeal papillomas.

- *Type III.* These patients may or may not be in respiratory distress, but the airway is abnormal on physical examination. The abnormality might be micrognathia, macroglossia, microstomia, tumors that displace the airway, prominent incisors, or a palatofacial deformity. Patients with Pierre Robin, Treacher Collins, or Down's syndrome are included in this group. Also included are patients with lesions in the lower airway or with anterior mediastinal masses, which could obstruct the airway after induction of general anesthesia, regardless of neuromuscular blockade.
- *Type IV.* Patients in this group present for the first time with significant airway obstruction. They demonstrate symptoms of airway distress, sternal retractions, low oxygen saturation, and signs of fatigue. A patient with an aspirated foreign body in the airway would fall into this group.

For types I and II patients, anesthesia is induced with either halothane or sevoflurane by mask. Slowly, positive pressure (5 to 10 cm H_2O) is applied. This confirms the possibility of ventilating and oxygenating the child and can also reduce soft tissue airway obstruction. Once ventilation and oxygenation are confirmed and satisfactory, a muscle relaxant (only if absolutely necessary) may be administered.

Types III and IV patients need special preparation in anticipation of difficult direct laryngoscopy and endotracheal intubation. Personnel and equipment to establish an immediate surgical airway should be available.

The vast majority of children with a difficult airway require general anesthesia. If possible, every effort should be made to keep patients breathing spontaneously during induction. This is important for two reasons:

1. Administration of a muscle relaxant may cause complete airway obstruction due to loss of tongue, pharyngeal, or laryngeal tone. Such obstruction may not be easily overcome with manual ventilation.
2. A spontaneously breathing patient provides a valuable sign to localize the glottis—namely, air bubbles during exhalation.

Airway Adjuncts

Successful management of a difficult pediatric airway requires the necessary equipment and the know-how to use it. Standard equipment includes assorted sizes of facemasks, oropharyngeal and nasopharyngeal airways, laryngoscope blades, endotracheal tubes, and stylets. Additional equipment must be readily available (e.g., in a "difficult airway cart").

Laryngeal Mask Airway.
The original laryngeal mask airway (LMA) is available in sizes 1, 1.5, 2, 2.5, and 3 for use in pediatric patients. It may be used as the sole airway of choice when endotracheal intubation or mask ventilation is undesirable or difficult. The LMA may also be used to facilitate either blind or fiberoptic intubation of the trachea (Fig. 148-3).

The intubating LMA or Fastrack can be used in patients weighing more than 30 kg. It usually provides a better conduit for blind intubation. A Proseal LMA model is available in sizes 2 and 3; it has the advantage of allowing higher

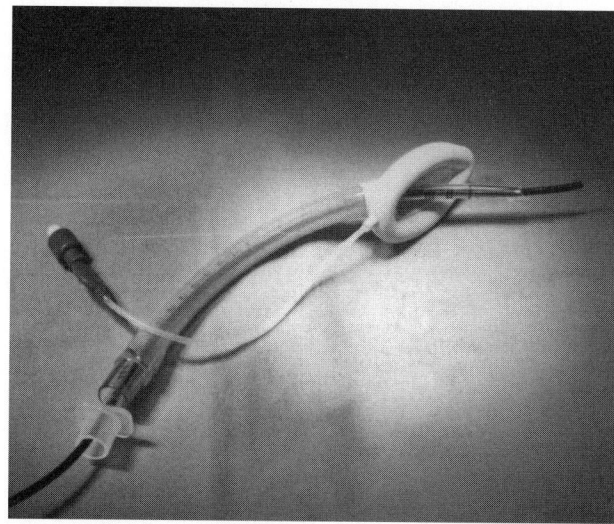

Figure 148-3 ■ The laryngeal mask airway can be used to facilitate either blind or fiberoptic endotracheal intubation.

ventilatory pressures and contains an inner tube for aspiration of gastric contents.

Flexible Fiberoptic Bronchoscope.
The flexible fiberoptic bronchoscope for children varies in external diameter from 2.2 to 4.0 mm. Those with 2.2- or 4.0-mm external diameters will pass through 2.5- and 4.5-mm endotracheal tubes, respectively. The 2.2-mm ultrathin fiberoptic bronchoscope has a flexible tip but lacks a suction port. It is invaluable for managing a child with a difficult airway.

Bullard Laryngoscope.
The Bullard laryngoscope, which is available in both pediatric and adult sizes, permits indirect visualization of the larynx with minimal mouth opening or movement of the neck. It does not require alignment of the oral, pharyngeal, and laryngeal axes. The pediatric blade is narrower and has more acute terminal angulation than does the adult version. The trachea is intubated by advancing a previously loaded endotracheal tube over an intubating stylet fastened to the laryngoscope blade.

Light Wand.
The light wand (lighted stylet) uses transtracheal illumination to guide insertion of the endotracheal tube. It is useful in the management of all types of difficult airways in children. Unlike with a fiberoptic bronchoscope, blood and secretions are not impediments to success. Smaller sizes are available for use with endotracheal tubes as small as 2.5 mm.

PREVENTION

Studies have shown that children have a higher risk of anesthesia-related morbidity than adults do. Untoward respiratory events are the major reason for this morbidity. A thorough understanding of pediatric airway anatomy and physiology will help reduce this risk. Preoperative identification of a child with a difficult airway must be coupled with sufficient personnel and equipment to secure the airway without life-threatening sequelae. Finally, the existence of a difficult airway can be communicated to future care providers via detailed notes in the chart, a letter given to the child's parents, and a Medic-Alert bracelet.

Further Reading

Bell C, Kain ZN, Hughes C: Respiratory physiology and disease processes. In Bell C, Kain ZN, Hughes C (eds): The Pediatric Anesthesia Handbook, 2nd ed. St. Louis, Mosby, 1997, pp 111-131.

Brimacombe J, Keller C: The Proseal laryngeal mask airway. Anesthesiol Clin North Am 20:871-891, 2002.

Brown RE, Vollers JM, Rader GR, et al: Nasotracheal intubation in a child with Treacher Collins syndrome using the Bullard intubating laryngoscope. J Clin Anesth 5:492-493, 1993.

Gregory GA, Riazi J: Classification and assessment of the difficult pediatric airway. Anesthesiol Clin North Am 16:729-741, 1998.

Hagberg CA: Special devices and techniques. Anesthesiol Clin North Am 20:907-932, 2002.

Lopez-Gil M, Brimacombe J, Alvarez M: Safety and efficacy of laryngeal mask airway: A prospective study of 1400 children. Anaesthesia 51:969-972, 1996.

Lopez-Gil M, Brimacombe J, Brain AIJ: Preliminary evaluation of a new prototype laryngeal mask in children. Br J Anaesth 82:132-134, 1999.

Muraika L, Heyman JS, Shevchenko Y: Fiberoptic tracheal intubation through a laryngeal mask airway in a child with Treacher Collins syndrome. Anesth Analg 97:1298-1299, 2003.

Anesthetic Complications of Fetal Surgery: EXIT Procedures

Marnie Robinson and Joseph Previte

Case Synopsis

A 28-year-old gravida II, para I woman at 36²/₇ weeks of gestation presents with a fetus with a large neck mass. Ex utero intrapartum therapy is planned to establish an airway before delivery.

PROBLEM ANALYSIS

Definition

The rapidly growing field of fetal surgery encompasses many different procedures that can be divided into three broad categories: (1) fetoscopy, (2) open fetal surgery, and (3) ex utero intrapartum therapy (EXIT). Because fetoscopic, or minimally invasive, procedures (Table 149-1) involve manipulation of the placenta or umbilical cord through an endoscope, only local or regional anesthesia is required. Open fetal surgical procedures (Table 149-2) require complete uterine relaxation, usually with high concentrations of volatile anesthetics. Both fetoscopy and open fetal surgeries are performed in midgestation to allow for fetal growth after the procedure.

In contrast, EXIT is performed if the fetus requires intervention at birth but before division of the umbilical cord. Consequently, the procedure is usually deferred until as late in gestation as possible, based on both the maternal and fetal condition. The particular intervention varies by indication (Table 149-3) and may involve securing the airway, resecting an intrathoracic mass, or inserting a cannula for extracorporeal membrane oxygenation. In the case synopsis, the large neck mass puts the fetus at risk for perinatal asphyxia if it proves difficult or impossible to intubate the trachea after conventional delivery. EXIT allows extended uteroplacental support while the airway is secured by direct laryngoscopy, rigid or fiberoptic bronchoscopy, or tracheostomy. With experience and the use of high concentrations of volatile anesthetics

for uterine relaxation, it is now possible to maintain uteroplacental support for 60 to 90 minutes before delivery.

Recognition

Most fetal disease is initially detected by ultrasonography. Abnormal findings prompt further testing. An in-depth ultrasound examination is used to assess fetal weight and overall health. Amniocentesis provides amniotic fluid for analysis, including karyotype. Structural or functional cardiac defects can be identified using fetal echocardiography. Detailed images of fetal anatomy can be obtained with ultrafast magnetic resonance imaging.

Although specific criteria for identifying a fetus that would benefit from an EXIT procedure vary by indication, some conditions have similar presentations. For example, cervical neck masses prevent the swallowing of amniotic fluid, resulting in polyhydramnios. Pulmonary amniotic fluid accumulation causes the lungs to appear large and echogenic. Chronic fetal disease from many causes can lead to hydrops fetalis, progressive ascites, pleural and cardiac effusions, and generalized edema that, without intervention, will ultimately lead to fetal demise.

Risk Assessment

FETAL RISK

The fetus is at risk for adverse events both during and after the EXIT procedure. During surgery, maintenance of

Table 149–1 ■ Indications for Fetoscopic Surgery	
Disease	Procedure
Twin-twin transfusion syndrome	Laser photocoagulation of placental vessels
Twin reversed arterial perfusion	Coagulation of umbilical cord
Amniotic band syndrome	Division of amniotic bands

Table 149–2 ■ Indications for Open Midgestation Fetal Surgery	
Disease	Procedure
Myelomeningocele	Repair of neural canal defect
Sacrococcygeal teratoma	Resection of teratoma
Intrathoracic masses	Resection of mass
Congenital diaphragmatic hernia with low lung-to-head ratio	Tracheal occlusion

Table 149–3 ■ Indications for Ex Utero Intrapartum Therapy (EXIT)

Disease	Procedure
Congenital diaphragmatic hernia	Removal of tracheal clip or balloon that was placed in utero
Congenital high upper airway obstruction syndrome	Tracheostomy
Giant cervical neck mass	Resection of mass
Severe pulmonary hypoplasia from intrathoracic mass	Resection of mass
Anticipated difficult intubation	Obtain surgical airway

normothermia is hampered by exposure of the fetus, whose thin skin is inadequate to prevent heat loss. In a preterm fetus, the effects and duration of anesthetic agents are increased owing to immature organ function and incomplete myelination.

Because of decreased contractility in the fetal heart, the fetus may not be able to compensate for hemodynamic changes. Changes in fetal heart rate, such as tachycardia with fetal incision or bradycardia from inadequate uteroplacental perfusion, may be tolerated for only a brief period. Hypoxia, increased systemic vascular resistance, or the negative inotropic effects of anesthetic agents may further compromise fetal cardiac function. Decreased cardiac preload from impaired venous return during surgical manipulation or blood loss can lead to fetal hypotension, bradycardia, shock, and cardiac arrest.

During EXIT, the fetus remains on the sterile field until division of the umbilical cord, limiting monitoring options to detect physiologic derangements. Hemodynamic data are obtained from a sterile fetal pulse oximeter and intermittent fetal echocardiography. Ideally, the surgeon places a fetal intravenous catheter, permitting the administration of medications and fluids by the anesthesiologist. If fetal intravenous access is not available, resuscitation is limited to intramuscular injections by the surgeon and maternal interventions by the anesthesiologist. Maintenance of maternal

blood pressure and adequate oxygen (O_2) delivery is essential, as is ensuring complete uterine atony and unobstructed umbilical cord blood flow.

The greatest risk to the fetus is fetal demise or severe disability from the underlying disease process. To be considered for EXIT, the fetus must have a dismal prognosis without intervention. With intervention, in addition to the risks already mentioned, there are risks specific to the disease process and its treatment. For example, with a cervical neck mass, neck structures may be damaged during EXIT. If a tracheostomy is required, care of the neonate becomes more complex. Finally, depending on the timing of EXIT, the infant's condition may be further complicated by premature birth.

MATERNAL RISK

The mother is also exposed to significant risk during EXIT. Like any parturient, she has experienced the physiologic changes of pregnancy and is subject to the associated risks of general anesthesia (Table 149–4). She is also at risk for amniotic fluid embolism during labor or intra-abdominal surgery and for postoperative wound infection. Additional maternal risks unique to EXIT include the following:

- *Obligate cesarean section for all future deliveries.* EXIT generally requires a larger incision than standard cesarean delivery, increasing the risk of uterine rupture during subsequent labor and vaginal delivery.
- *Risks of invasive monitoring.* Because the welfare of the fetus depends on uteroplacental perfusion, which in turn is dependent on maternal blood pressure, continuous monitoring of maternal blood pressure during EXIT is indicated.
- *Increased risk of blood loss requiring transfusion.* The profound uterine relaxation required to maintain uteroplacental support during EXIT increases the risk of uterine atony after the third stage of labor. Even if uterine tone is reestablished expeditiously, the likelihood of transfusion of blood products is greater with an EXIT procedure than with routine cesarean delivery.

Studies comparing maternal risk during fetal surgery and routine cesarean delivery have found only two major

Table 149–4 ■ Physiologic Changes of Pregnancy

Organ System	Changes in Pregnancy	Risk during Anesthesia
Neurologic	Decreased MAC	More sensitive to anesthetics
	Engorged epidural plexus	More sensitive to neuraxial anesthetics
Respiratory	Upper airway edema	Potentially difficult mask ventilation and intubation
	Decreased functional residual capacity and increased minute ventilation	Faster desaturation with apnea
Cardiovascular	Inferior vena cava behind gravid uterus	Supine aortocaval compression
	Plasma volume increased more than red cell volume	Relative anemia of pregnancy; little or no change in blood pressure
	Increased cardiac output and reduced peripheral vascular resistance	More sensitive to anesthetics
Gastrointestinal	Reduced lower esophageal sphincter tone and increased intra-abdominal pressure	Increased risk of aspiration
Hepatic	Decreased plasma proteins and albumin	Increased risk of pulmonary edema
	Reduced plasma cholinesterase	Prolonged succinylcholine effect

MAC, minimum alveolar anesthetic concentration.

differences: increased blood loss and an increased incidence of wound infection. There have been no reports of long-term morbidity or decreased reproductive potential in women undergoing fetal surgery. The only reported maternal death associated with fetal surgery was from an amniotic fluid embolus during a fetoscopic procedure; there are no reports of maternal mortality associated with open fetal surgery or EXIT procedures.

Implications

Fetal surgery is proposed only after a thorough evaluation by a fetal therapeutics committee and a careful consideration of the risks and benefits for both the mother and the fetus. Because fetal surgery involves substantial risk, it is considered appropriate only when the fetus is "sick" and the mother is "healthy." Once a case is deemed appropriate for consideration of fetal intervention, a team meeting is held involving the mother, selected family members or friends, and the appropriate practitioners. A full explanation of the risks and benefits is presented by the pediatric surgeon, obstetrician, neonatologist, anesthesiologist, and other relevant medical specialists. Once the mother consents to proceed with EXIT, the complexity of the procedure requires close coordination of personnel and operating room resources.

MANAGEMENT

Whereas cesarean delivery is performed under maternal regional or general anesthesia, with no anesthesia for the fetus, EXIT procedures require general anesthesia for both. Even a typical general anesthetic for cesarean delivery is unsuitable for an EXIT procedure. The goals of anesthetic management of an EXIT procedure include the following:

- Anesthesia for the mother
- Anesthesia for the fetus
- Maintenance of uteroplacental perfusion until division of the umbilical cord

General endotracheal anesthesia for the mother with volatile anesthetics accomplishes these goals to some extent. The mother receives a complete anesthetic with a volatile agent that crosses the placenta and at least partially anesthetizes the fetus. High concentrations of volatile agents also decrease uterine tone, thereby supporting uteroplacental perfusion. However, additional drugs are required to supplement each of the listed goals during the course of the procedure.

Preinduction

Preoperatively, indomethacin may be given to the mother as a tocolytic if there are no fetal contraindications, such as a fragile fetal cardiac status. As for any pregnant patient requiring anesthesia, aspiration precautions include 8 hours of fasting and oral sodium citrate before induction. If postoperative maternal epidural analgesia is planned, the catheter is placed preoperatively, but it is not dosed during the procedure in order to avoid severe hypotension. Left uterine displacement is mandatory to prevent aortocaval compression.

Induction

After adequate preoxygenation, a rapid-sequence induction is performed, and the airway is secured with a cuffed endotracheal tube. Following intubation, additional intravenous access is obtained, and intra-arterial and bladder drainage catheters are inserted. Before surgical incision, muscle relaxation is achieved with nondepolarizing neuromuscular blocking drugs.

Start of Surgery

Ultrasonography is used just before surgical preparation to verify fetal well-being and identify the location of the placenta. Before uterine incision, complete uterine relaxation is induced using at least 2 MAC of volatile anesthetic, supplemented by small doses of nitroglycerin, if needed. As the volatile anesthetic concentration is increased, nitrous oxide is discontinued, and 100% O_2 is administered to maximize O_2 delivery to the fetus.

High doses of volatile anesthetics invariably decrease maternal systemic vascular resistance and cardiac output. Thus, ephedrine and phenylephrine are titrated to maintain maternal systolic blood pressure within 10% to 20% of baseline. Reduced maternal blood pressure adversely affects the fetus, because uteroplacental perfusion is directly related to maternal blood pressure.

Hysterotomy is planned to avoid placental injury. To minimize maternal bleeding, a special stapling device for fetal surgery is used. Also, warm uterine irrigation is performed to prevent fetal hypothermia and maintain uterine volume. Adequate uteroplacental blood flow is ensured by attention to complete uterine relaxation, maintenance of normal maternal blood pressure and oxygenation, and avoidance of kinking or compression of the umbilical cord.

To monitor the fetus, a pulse oximeter probe is placed on an extremity and covered with foil to deflect ambient light. Supplemental fetal anesthesia is administered as an intramuscular "cocktail" consisting of a nondepolarizing muscle relaxant and a narcotic, with or without atropine. In the case of a cervical neck mass, the fetal head and torso are delivered into the surgical field for direct laryngoscopy and potential tracheostomy. Intermittently, sterile fetal echocardiography can monitor cardiac function, ductal patency, and volume status.

Post-EXIT Care

Once the procedure is complete, umbilical, arterial, and venous catheters can be placed by the Seldinger technique while the umbilical cord is still engorged from uteroplacental blood flow. Before the umbilical cord is divided, adequate chest rise and an appropriate increase in pulse oximetry are confirmed. Fetal O_2 saturation in utero is normally 55% to 65%. Ventilation with 100% O_2 increases the hemoglobin O_2 saturation to 95% to 100%. When the umbilical cord is divided, the delivery time is recorded, and the baby is taken from the sterile field for evaluation and resuscitation. If additional immediate surgery is indicated, the infant is usually taken to an adjacent operating room, where a second team of anesthesiologists, surgeons, and nurses awaits.

PEDIATRICS & NEONATOLOGY

After delivery of the placenta, volatile anesthetic concentrations are reduced, and intravenous oxytocin (Pitocin) is given to restore uterine tone. At the same time, the anesthetic depth can be increased with nitrous oxide. Provided the mother is hemodynamically stable, analgesia can be provided with narcotics or by dosing the epidural catheter. Intramuscular methylergonovine or carboprost tromethamine may be required for cases of refractory uterine atony. As the hysterotomy and laparotomy incisions are closed, volume resuscitation is provided to the mother as indicated by vital signs and estimated blood loss. At the conclusion of surgery, muscle relaxants are reversed, and the mother is extubated when fully awake, followed by transport to the recovery area.

PREVENTION

Although it is impossible to prevent all adverse outcomes, proper preparation for the anesthetic can help minimize any associated risks. For EXIT procedures, anesthetic preparation must include consideration of two patients—the mother and the fetus. Good communication among the specialist physicians and the nursing staff during the EXIT planning stages can identify potential risks and problems and allow the best possible care for both patients.

Further Reading

Adzick NS, Harrison MR: Fetal surgical therapy. Lancet 343:897-902, 1994.

Gaiser RR, Cheek TG, Kurth CD: Anesthetic management of cesarean delivery complicated by ex utero intrapartum treatment of the fetus. Anesth Analg 84:1150-1153, 1997.

Harrison MR, Keller RL, Hawgood SB, et al: A randomized trial of fetal endoscopic tracheal occlusion for severe fetal congenital diaphragmatic hernia. N Engl J Med 349:1916-1924, 2003.

Hirose S, Farmer DL, Lee H, et al: The ex utero intrapartum treatment procedure: Looking back at the EXIT. J Pediatr Surg 39:375-380, 2004.

Liechty KW, Crombleholme TM, Timothy M, et al: Intrapartum airway management for giant fetal neck masses: The EXIT procedure. Obstet Gynecol 177:870-874, 1997.

Lim BF, Crombleholme TM, Hedrick JL, et al: Congenital high airway obstruction syndrome: Natural history and management. J Pediatr Surg 38:940-945, 2003.

Myers LB, Cohen D, Galinkin J, et al: Anaesthesia for fetal surgery. Paediatr Anaesth 12:569-578, 2002.

Noah MM, Norton ME, Sandberg P, et al: Short-term maternal outcomes that are associated with the EXIT procedure, as compared with cesarean delivery. Am J Obstet Gynecol 186:1299-1303, 2002.

Rychik J, Tian Z, Cohen MS, et al: Acute cardiovascular effects of fetal surgery in the human. Circulation 110:1549-1556, 2004.

Postoperative Apnea in Infants

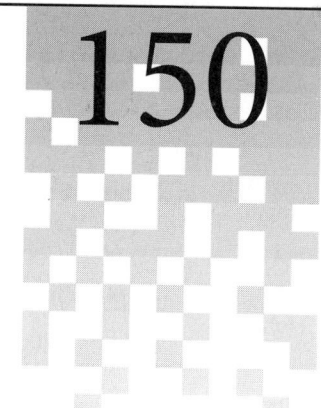

150

Liana Hosu and C. Dean Kurth

Case Synopsis

A 2.5-kg, 5-month-old male infant presents for ileostomy takedown. His history is significant for premature birth at 26 weeks' gestation, intraventricular hemorrhage, and immature lung disease requiring mechanical ventilation for 3 weeks. He was discharged home at 3 months. He had a bowel resection and ileostomy at 1 month of age for necrotizing enterocolitis. A general anesthetic is administered for the ileostomy takedown, and an epidural catheter is placed for postoperative pain control. After 3 hours in the pediatric acute care unit, he is noted to have episodes of apnea. Intravenous caffeine is administered to prevent further apneic episodes.

PROBLEM ANALYSIS

Definition

Postoperative apnea is defined by periods of no ventilation during recovery after anesthesia and operation, usually in formerly premature infants or full-term neonates. This is distinguished from apnea of prematurity and apnea of infancy, which occur in premature and full-term infants, respectively, who have not had anesthesia or surgery.

Postoperative apnea is characterized by duration and type. Brief apnea is longer than 6 but less than 15 seconds, whereas prolonged apnea is longer than 15 seconds. However, the latter can be less than 15 seconds if associated with bradycardia. In terms of type, apnea can be central, obstructive, or mixed (Fig. 150-1):

- Central apnea occurs without respiratory effort.
- Obstructive apnea occurs with respiratory effort, but without ventilation.
- Mixed apnea is characterized by absent ventilation with occasional respiratory effort.

Recognition

Postoperative apnea is diagnosed in the following situations:

- No respiratory effort or ventilation is observed for more than 15 seconds (prolonged apnea).
- No respiratory effort or ventilation is observed for less than 15 seconds and the heart rate decreases to less than 80 beats per minute for more than 5 seconds (apnea and bradycardia).
- No respiratory effort or ventilation is observed for more than 6 seconds but less than 15 seconds (brief apnea).

Risk Assessment

The incidence of postoperative apnea is influenced by patient, surgical, and anesthetic factors. Of these, premature birth history is the most important. Former preterm infants are at increased risk for postoperative apnea, although full-term infants less than 4 weeks' postnatal age are also at risk. In formerly premature infants, factors that influence the incidence of postoperative apnea include the following.

Postconceptual Age. Postconceptual age (PCA), defined as the sum of postnatal age and gestational age, is the most important determinant of postoperative apnea. The incidence of postoperative apnea varies inversely with PCA (Fig. 150-2). The incidence is high in prematurely born infants younger than 40 weeks' PCA. After this, the incidence decreases sharply until the infant is 50 weeks' PCA. The incidence of postoperative apnea is low at that point and decreases gradually thereafter.

Gestational Age. The gestational age of the infant modifies the incidence of postoperative apnea. Figure 150-2 displays the relationship of postoperative apnea incidence versus PCA for an infant born at 32 weeks' gestation, with an approximate 85% incidence of postoperative apnea. The incidence-versus-PCA curve shifts upward as the gestational age decreases; conversely, the curve shifts downward as gestational age approaches term. Thus, at any given PCA, the incidence of postoperative apnea is greater for infants born at 28 weeks' gestation than at 32 weeks' gestation.

Anemia. The presence of anemia (hematocrit <30%) also modifies the incidence of postoperative apnea in formerly premature infants. The incidence-versus-PCA curve shifts upward with anemia (see Fig. 150-2). Thus, for a given PCA, the presence of anemia increases the incidence of postoperative apnea.

Prematurity-Associated Comorbidity. Today, survival of extremely low-birth-weight infants (gestational age 24 to 28 weeks) is quite common. Bronchopulmonary dysplasia, retinopathy of prematurity, hydrocephalus, seizures, and cerebral palsy occur frequently in extremely low-birth-weight survivors. For a given PCA, the risk of postoperative apnea is greater in formerly premature infants with residual diseases of prematurity.

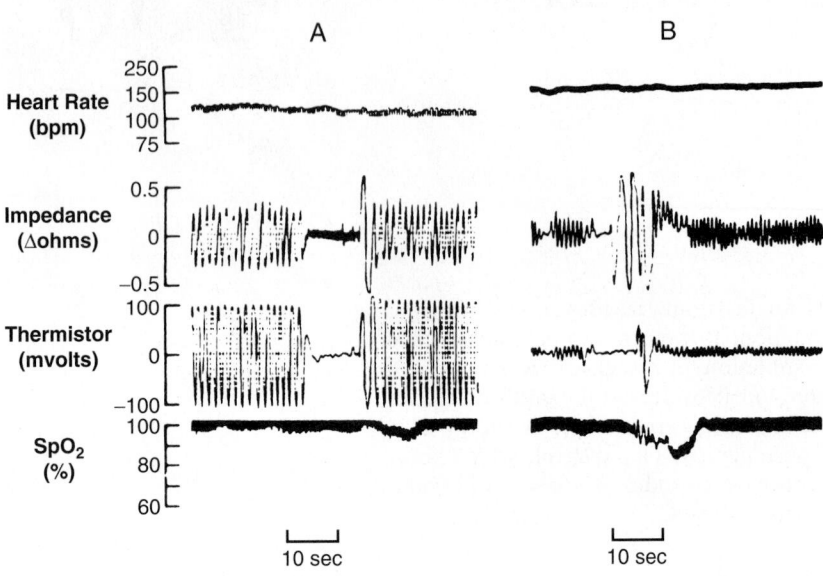

Heart Rate (bpm)
Impedance (Δohms)
Thermistor (mvolts)
SpO₂ (%)

A   B

10 sec   10 sec

Figure 150–1 ■ Postoperative recording of heart rate, chest wall movement (impedance), nasal airflow (thermistor), and oxygen saturation (SpO₂) from an infant after general inhalation anesthesia for inguinal hernia repair. *A,* Recordings obtained in the postanesthesia care unit depict brief central apnea. This is denoted by a lack of chest wall motion and airflow. Note mild arterial desaturation after the apnea. *B,* Another recording, also obtained in the postanesthesia care unit, illustrates mixed apnea. During the initial 6 seconds of apnea, there is no chest wall motion or airflow (brief central apnea), followed by 6 seconds of chest wall motion with no airflow (obstructive apnea). Note that arterial desaturation with the latter is more severe than with comparable central apnea in *A.*

Surgical Procedure. In premature infants, postoperative apnea is less frequently associated with minor surgical procedures (e.g., inguinal herniorrhaphy) than with major surgical procedures (e.g., laparotomy). Surgical factors appear to play a role in the pathogenesis of postoperative apnea. For example, premature infants undergoing cryotherapy for retinopathy of prematurity under topical anesthesia may experience postoperative apnea. Postoperative apnea may also begin hours after emergence from anesthesia, well after all anesthetic drugs have been cleared from the body. In full-term infants, postoperative apnea can occur after pyloromyotomy and may be associated with severe desaturation.

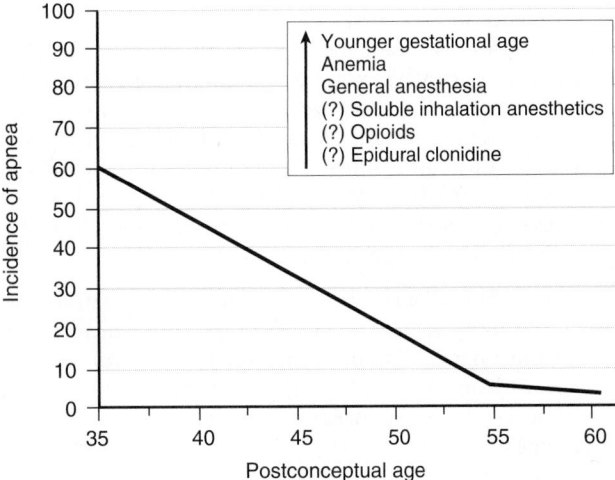

Younger gestational age
Anemia
General anesthesia
(?) Soluble inhalation anesthetics
(?) Opioids
(?) Epidural clonidine

Figure 150–2 ■ The incidence of postoperative apnea varies inversely with the postconceptual age in formerly premature infants. The incidence curve shifts upward for babies (1) born at younger gestational ages, (2) with postoperative anemia or residual diseases related to prematurity (e.g., bronchopulmonary dysplasia), (3) after general anesthesia versus pure regional anesthesia, and (4) following general anesthesia with soluble versus insoluble inhalational agents. Administration of clonidine epidurally or opioids intravenously may also shift the curve upward.

Anesthetic Management. Postoperative apnea may occur after general anesthesia, regional anesthesia, or combined general and regional anesthesia. A meta-analysis found no reliable evidence of a difference in the incidence of postoperative apnea, bradycardia, or oxygen desaturation in ex-preterm infants following hernia repair using general or regional anesthesia. However, spinal anesthesia has an appreciable failure rate, requiring the use of sedation or conversion to general anesthesia. Postoperative apnea may result from the addition of clonidine to local anesthetic solutions for caudal epidural analgesia. The incidence of postoperative apnea in infants undergoing general anesthesia may be lower following the use of less soluble inhalational agents (e.g., desflurane). For pyloromyotomy, new-onset postoperative apnea occurred less frequently after a remifentanil-based anesthetic compared with a halothane-based anesthetic. However, the incidence of postoperative apnea after regional anesthesia in which sedative drugs (e.g., ketamine, fentanyl, midazolam, nitrous oxide) were administered is similar to that after general anesthesia. Use of muscle relaxants as part of the general anesthetic regimen does not appear to alter the incidence of postoperative apnea.

Of note, a history of apnea of prematurity is *not* predictive of postoperative apnea. Formerly premature infants with no history of apnea can develop postoperative apnea. Conversely, formerly premature infants with a history of apnea can undergo anesthesia and surgery without developing postoperative apnea. Sleep studies with pneumocardiography to document the presence or absence of apnea are often performed on premature infants to help determine whether the baby needs at-home monitoring. However, a normal sleep study (no apnea) before surgery does not guarantee that the baby will not develop postoperative apnea.

Implications

Postoperative apnea can be life threatening. Cardiopulmonary arrest and death have been reported after postoperative apnea. The relationship between postoperative apnea and sudden infant death syndrome (SIDS) is unknown, as is the relationship between apnea in premature or full-term infants and SIDS. The risk of SIDS is increased for infants with apnea of prematurity or apnea of infancy. Most SIDS cases, however, occur in infants without a history of apnea.

Postoperative apnea is characterized by its variable onset and offset in relation to emergence from anesthesia. Postoperative apnea begins in the postanesthesia care unit in about two thirds of affected infants. In the remaining infants, it begins between 2 and 12 hours after surgery. Usually, it is characterized by multiple events of variable duration that can continue for days after surgery. Apneic episodes are mostly self-limited and require close observation but no treatment. Occasionally, apneic infants require manual stimulation, such as flicking the soles of the feet, to restore ventilation. Sometimes they require bag and mask ventilation. Rarely, cardiopulmonary resuscitation must be instituted to revive the patient.

MANAGEMENT

The anesthetic management of young infants at risk for apnea includes preoperative, intraoperative, and postoperative considerations.

Preoperative Considerations

Nonemergency surgery should be postponed based on the PCA, because the risk of postoperative apnea decreases sharply between 40 and 50 weeks' PCA and then gradually decreases until 70 weeks' PCA. Depending on institutional practices, the risk for postoperative apnea is minimized by delaying nonemergency surgery until the infant is 50 to 60 weeks' PCA. Elective surgery in full-term infants should be postponed until the infant is 4 weeks old.

Blood hemoglobin concentration should be checked preoperatively in infants younger than 6 months. The risk of postoperative apnea is increased when the hematocrit is less than 30%. The cause of anemia should be elucidated and treated before surgery.

Limitations for same-day surgery should be set. Some institutions use an algorithm to determine which infants must be monitored for postoperative apnea in the hospital overnight (Fig. 150-3).

Intraoperative Considerations

General inhalation anesthesia, spinal anesthesia, caudal epidural anesthesia, or combined general and regional anesthesia may be administered to infants at risk for postoperative apnea.

Less soluble inhalational anesthetics (desflurane) should be used in premature infants rather than more soluble agents (isoflurane). To decrease the incidence of postoperative apnea with general inhalation anesthesia, a caffeine base (10 mg/kg intravenously) should be administered intraoperatively shortly after anesthesia induction. Caffeine reduces the incidence and severity of oxygen desaturation with apnea. Although postoperative apnea may occur even if caffeine has been administered (caffeine's effectiveness has been questioned), the risk-benefit ratio favors administration; caffeine has few side effects and has an excellent safety profile. Further studies are needed to determine which infants might benefit most from preemptive treatment with caffeine.

Regional anesthesia (subarachnoid block or caudal epidural) may be suitable for lower extremity or inguinal surgery. It has been shown to decrease the incidence of postoperative apnea when compared with general inhalation anesthesia. Infants, however, may not be compliant during surgery with a pure regional anesthetic; they may not remain immobile in the upper extremities or trunk, or they may cry if they are hungry. Supplemental intravenous sedation or inhalation of nitrous oxide improves compliance but increases the risk of postoperative apnea to greater than that of general anesthesia. Surgical procedures are often difficult in young, formerly premature infants and may take longer than expected, making spinal anesthesia less advantageous than caudal epidural or general anesthesia. Caudal epidural clonidine should be avoided in premature infants and in term infants less than 4 weeks of age because it may cause respiratory depression.

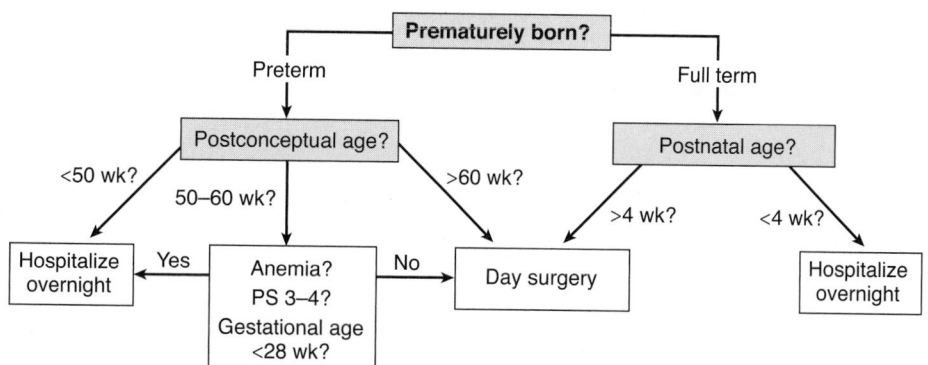

Figure 150–3 ■ Day-surgery algorithm used for infants at Cincinnati Children's Hospital. If the infant is full term and younger than 4 weeks, hospital admission for overnight monitoring is planned. If a term infant is older than 4 weeks, day surgery may be performed. If an infant was born prematurely, is older than 50 weeks' postconceptual age, and there is no history of anemia or significant comorbidities, ambulatory surgery is planned. If the infant was born prematurely and is older than 60 weeks' postconceptual age, regardless of anemia or comorbidities, day surgery is planned. All infants born prematurely and younger than 50 weeks' postconceptual age are admitted to the hospital for overnight monitoring. PS, physical status.

Postoperative Considerations

Cardiorespiratory monitoring is the most important postoperative treatment for infants at risk of postoperative apnea. Nurses must be familiar with how to respond to the cardiorespiratory alarm, including recognition of apnea in young infants, and how to treat apnea, from manual stimulation to cardiopulmonary resuscitation. The infant should be monitored in a location where a nurse will hear the cardiorespiratory alarm. Visual confirmation of breathing or apnea is important, because false-positive alarms are frequent. Cardiorespiratory monitors that employ impedance technology to detect respiratory rate and heart rate are sensitive and easily applied. These monitors have alarms for high and low heart and respiratory rates, as well as for apnea duration. For young infants, the apnea alarm is set to 15 seconds, and the low heart rate alarm is set to 80 beats per minute (relative bradycardia for young infants).

For postoperative pain control, continuous caudal epidural analgesia with local anesthetic-opioid solutions is the mainstay of analgesic therapy. Clinical stability in preterm neonates who have received caudal epidural anesthesia with local anesthetic-opioid solutions is noted by a reduction in hypoxic episodes, improved hemodynamic stability, reduced mortality, and improved neurologic outcome. Continuous caudal epidural infusions are commonly used as an adjunct to neonatal general anesthesia. This allows earlier extubation and avoids the need for intravenous opioids. Further, the addition of opioids to local anesthetic in caudal epidural infusions may reduce the dose of local anesthetic needed for analgesia, thereby reducing the risk for local anesthetic toxicity and providing improved analgesia. However, young expremature infants are more susceptible to opioid-induced apnea. Therefore, the opioid dose must be reduced in the caudal epidural infusate.

Even though continuous caudal epidural analgesia with opioids is the mainstay of analgesic therapy, there is a lack of properly controlled, randomized clinical trials that have evaluated postoperative regional analgesia versus more conventional (intravenous) analgesia strategies.

PREVENTION

The following recommendations can reduce the risk of postoperative apnea:

- Delay elective surgery until 50 to 60 weeks' PCA in high-risk patients.
- Administer a caffeine base (10 mg/kg intravenously) after anesthetic induction.
- Consider preoperative blood transfusion for anemia.
- Use an appropriate regional anesthesia-only technique.
- Avoid using caudal epidural clonidine, and reduce the dose of opioids with caudal epidural anesthesia or analgesia.
- Use less soluble inhalational agents when a general anesthetic is unavoidable.

Further Reading

Anand KJS, Stevens BJ, McGrath PJ: Pain in Neonates, 2nd ed. Philadelphia, Elsevier, 2000.

Andropoulos DB, Heard MB, Johnson KL, et al: Postanesthetic apnea in full-term infants after pyloromyotomy. Anesthesiology 80:216-219, 1994.

Coté CJ, Zaslavsky A, Downes JJ, et al: Postoperative apnea in former preterm infants after inguinal herniorrhaphy: A combined analysis. Anesthesiology 82:809-822, 1995.

Craven PD, Badawi N, Henderson-Smart DJ, et al: Regional (spinal, epidural, caudal) versus general anaesthesia in preterm infants undergoing inguinal herniorrhaphy in early infancy. Cochrane Database Syst Rev CD003669, 2003.

Fellmann C, Gerber AC, Weiss M: Apnoea in a former preterm infant after caudal bupivacaine with clonidine for inguinal herniorrhaphy. Paediatr Anaesth 12:637-640, 2002.

Galinkin JL, Davis PJ, McGowan FX, et al: A randomized multicenter study of remifentanil compared with halothane in neonates and infants undergoing pyloromyotomy. II. Perioperative breathing patterns in neonates and infants with pyloric stenosis. Anesth Analg 93: 1387-1392, 2001.

Kurth CD, LeBard SE: Association of postoperative apnea, airway obstruction, and hypoxemia in former premature infants. Anesthesiology 75:22-26, 1991.

Kurth CD, Spitzer AR, Broennle AM, et al: Postoperative apnea in preterm infants. Anesthesiology 66:483-488, 1987.

Welborn LG, Hannallah RS, Fink R, et al: High-dose caffeine suppresses postoperative apnea in former preterm infants. Anesthesiology 71:347-349, 1989.

Welborn LG, Hannallah RS, Luban NLC, et al: Anemia and postoperative apnea in former preterm infants. Anesthesiology 74:1003-1006, 1991.

Welborn LG, Rice LJ, Hannallah RS, et al: Postoperative apnea in former preterm infants: Prospective comparison of spinal and general anesthesia. Anesthesiology 72:838-842, 1990.

William JM, Stoddart PA, Williams SA, et al: Post-operative recovery after inguinal herniotomy in ex-premature infants: Comparison between sevoflurane and spinal anaesthesia. Br J Anaesth 86:366-371, 2001.

Wolf AR, Lawson RA, Dryden CM, et al: Recovery after desflurane anaesthesia in the infant: Comparison with isoflurane. Br J Anaesth 76:362-364, 1996.

Intraoperative Cardiac Arrest

Daniel D. Rubens and Jeremy M. Geiduschek

151

Case Synopsis

A 16-month-old boy, American Society of Anesthesiologists (ASA) class I, is having a bilateral inguinal herniorrhaphy with general anesthesia consisting of 2.5% sevoflurane with oxygen and nitrous oxide. He has a laryngeal mask airway in place. He is in the left lateral decubitus position with hips and knees flexed. A needle has been introduced into the caudal epidural space via the sacral hiatus. A 1.5-mL test dose of 0.25% bupivacaine with epinephrine 5 μg/mL is injected, with no change in the electrocardiogram (ECG) morphology, blood pressure, or heart rate. An additional 8.5 mL is administered over 1 to 2 minutes. ST segment changes are noted on the ECG waveform, followed by a rapid change in rhythm to coarse ventricular fibrillation, followed by asystole. The pulse oximetry and end-tidal carbon dioxide waveforms have disappeared. The patient has stopped breathing, and there is no palpable pulse.

PROBLEM ANALYSIS

Definition

Intraoperative cardiac arrest is defined by the need to begin cardiopulmonary resuscitation (CPR). This is generally an unplanned event, although it may be anticipated when dealing with critically ill patients. The need for CPR is apparent when palpable pulses and measurable blood pressure are absent or when there may be a palpable pulse but cardiac output is inadequate to provide acceptable organ perfusion (e.g., bradycardia with a heart rate of <30 beats per minute in an infant).

Recognition

The first sign of patient deterioration under anesthesia is usually heralded by changes in the electronic monitoring signals. Unfortunately, electronic monitor alarms may activate falsely for any number of reasons. Nonetheless, when an alarm sounds, it is imperative to evaluate the patient before attributing the alarm to artifact. Loss of signal from the pulse oximeter, especially when associated with inaudible stethoscope heart sounds, is a harbinger of cardiac arrest. Similarly, until proved otherwise, loss of the end-tidal capnography waveform and the inability to measure blood pressure herald impending cardiac arrest.

Risk Assessment

All patients undergoing anesthesia are at risk for intraoperative cardiac arrest. In children, the most common arrhythmia seen before cardiac arrest is bradycardia. In 1954 Beecher and Todd reported higher anesthetic morbidity and mortality for children compared with adults. In 1961 Rackow and colleagues reported that this increase was due to a higher incidence of cardiac arrest in anesthetized children younger than 1 year old. Since then, other large series from Sweden and France have supported this finding. In 1990 Cohen and associates reported that the highest rate of anesthesia-related adverse events, including cardiac arrest, occurred in children younger than 1 month old. The majority of the aforementioned studies were published before the routine use of pulse oximetry and capnography, which makes comparison with current practices difficult.

In 2000 the initial findings of the Pediatric Perioperative Cardiac Arrest Registry were presented after a review of 289 cases of cardiac arrest. Of these, 150 (52%) were judged to be related to the administration of anesthesia. Medication-related (37%) and cardiovascular (32%) causes were most common, together accounting for 69% of all cardiac arrests. In three cases, cardiac arrest was partly due to hyperkalemia following massive blood transfusion. Four cases occurred after caudal epidural local anesthetic injection. In all these patients, the local anesthetic test dose was negative, and all presented similarly to the patient described in the case synopsis. Anesthesia-related deaths occurred most often in infants younger than 1 year and in patients with severe underlying disease or having emergent surgery. Thirty-three percent of the patients were ASA status I or II. The most common identifiable cause for cardiac arrest without untoward respiratory events was hemorrhage or its therapy (8 patients). However, respiratory events accounted for 20% of all cardiac arrests. The most common respiratory cause was airway obstruction, due to either laryngospasm or anatomic obstruction. The most common technical problems were complications from the placement of central lines. Of the patients who suffered cardiac arrest, 26% died, 6% suffered permanent injury, and 68% had no residual injury. Congenital heart disease was present in 15 of the 75 patients who died, and all the patients who died had significant underlying systemic disease.

Implications

Cardiac arrest must be recognized and treated early, because delayed therapy can lead to severe morbidity or mortality. In a 2003 statement, the International Council of Resuscitation noted a need to change the way resuscitation instruction is given to trainees. It suggested that more time be dedicated to hands-on practice with lifelike manikins and training modules. Television and video-based instruction was also found to be extremely useful. Hands-on practice with frequent refresher sessions encourages skill retention and reduces the anxiety of trainees. Such models have been used by the commercial airline industry and in nuclear power plant safety programs for many years; only recently have they been adapted to medical emergencies.

MANAGEMENT

Unanticipated cardiac arrest (such as that described in the case scenario) is best handled with formalized protocols for managing life-threatening events. Anesthesiologists should adhere to the current pediatric advanced life support (PALS) protocols:

- Remain calm and focused.
- Maintain good communication with the surgical care team (surgeons, nurses, technologists). Explain in clear terms what you are witnessing on the monitors and by the patient's vital signs. Ask if there has been any recent action that could explain the patient's sudden hemodynamic deterioration.
- Call *early* for help. A system should be in place to call for and receive help rapidly. It is important to know how this system operates for each location. Examples are a "CODE" button on the wall or an internal emergency telephone system.
- Turn off anesthetic agents and deliver 100% oxygen via manual ventilation.
- Assess the patient for airway patency and breathing by listening for breath sounds with a stethoscope while the patient is manually ventilated.
- Place an endotracheal tube if one is not already in place.
- Assess the circulation. Brachial or femoral pulses are reliable sites in small children and infants, whereas the carotid is best in older children and adolescents.
- If the pulse is absent, begin chest compressions. It has been shown that consistent and adequate heart massage before and during defibrillation greatly improves the likelihood that spontaneous circulation will return.
- Determine the cardiac rhythm from the ECG.
- Treat arrhythmias according to the current PALS protocols.
- Designate someone to provide a written record of the events. Most anesthetic records are not designed to adequately document events and therapies during a cardiac arrest. Having a standardized recording form for intraoperative cardiac arrest (Fig. 151-1) is helpful, allowing the sequence and timing of events to be clearly noted and reviewed later.

Intraoperative cardiac arrest in children is rare (<3 per 10,000 anesthetics in all children, including ASA class IV and V patients). An organized response by all members of the anesthesia and surgery care team is needed to maximize the opportunity for a favorable outcome. To implement this response, each participant's part must be clearly defined and practiced. The following roles must be filled: (1) a team leader, or code coordinator (who directs the resuscitation effort but does *not* assume any specific task); (2) an airway manager (responsible for hand ventilation with 100% oxygen and endotracheal intubation, if necessary); (3) a person specifically designated to perform chest compressions; (4) someone to confirm patent intravenous (IV) access and to administer medications (according to PALS guidelines); and (5) a person delegated to obtain the code cart and defibrillator. The team leader or code coordinator also plays an important role in controlling the entry of outside responders into a code in progress, ensuring that all the designated code roles are filled. This system permits a clear understanding of each person's role and direction at a time when panic, disorder, and lack of leadership can readily occur.

Medications can be delivered via an endotracheal tube while IV access is established. For children younger than 7 years, if IV access is poor or unobtainable after 1 minute, placement of an interosseous needle is mandated (Fig. 151-2). This allows for the administration of emergency drugs and rapid fluid delivery, including blood. Early epinephrine administration can be lifesaving.

Once the airway, breathing, and circulation have been assessed and appropriate therapy implemented, attention must be directed to determining the cause of cardiac arrest. Always consider tension pneumothorax in intubated patients. If this is suspected, perform left- and right-sided needle thoracentesis. A chest radiograph can be helpful and should be requested early during the resuscitation.

Obtain blood for laboratory analysis as soon as possible, including arterial blood gases, electrolytes (sodium, potassium, chloride, bicarbonate, calcium), glucose, and hematocrit.

The duration of CPR is handled on a case-by-case basis. Failure to reestablish perfusion should raise the following questions:

- Have all anesthetic agents been discontinued?
- Is CPR being performed correctly?
- Are all team roles filled and being performed effectively?
- Does the patient have an underlying problem that could be contributory?
- Is the patient profoundly hypovolemic owing to fluid or blood loss?
- Has the patient had an anaphylactic reaction?
- Does the patient have a tension pneumothorax?
- Does the patient have cardiac tamponade?
- Is the patient hypothermic?
- Has there been a medication overdose or the wrong medication administered?

If perfusion is reestablished but lost again, consider the following iatrogenic causes:

- Trauma related to closed-chest cardiac massage, including pneumothorax from rib fracture or splenic or hepatic rupture
- Pneumothorax or hemothorax from attempted central venous access or overinflation from mechanical ventilation
- Pericardial tamponade (if intracardiac medications were administered or a vascular cannula was placed into the right atrium)

CODE 188 RECORD

Date _____
Site of arrest _____
Est. time of arrest _____
Pt. found by _____
Observed arrest ☐ Yes ☐ No
Time CPR started _____

Weight: _____

Initial signs of arrest:
☐ Apnea
☐ Bradycardia
☐ Cyanosis/Sats
☐ Hypotension
☐ Absence of pulses
☐ Other _____

IV access:

	Site	In situ	During code	Time placed
Peripheral				
Central line				

Airway:
Ventilation: Bag/mask _____ Time _____
Intubation: Oral _____ Nasal _____
Tube size _____ Time _____
Intubation and placement
verified by _____
NG tube inserted/placement
verified by _____

History of events prior to arrest:
_____
_____
_____
_____

Initial heart rhythm: _____

Signatures:
Charge MD _____
Medication RN _____
Recorder RN _____

Patient's response
- Lab results
- Procedures (Foley, taps, CXR)
- Appearance/activity (color, mental status, neuro checks, pupils, seizures, etc.)
- Urine output

Infusions
Blood products
Ringers/NS
_____ mL
_____ mL _____ mg
_____ mL _____ mg
_____ mL _____ mg
_____ mL _____ mg Lidocaine
_____ mg Epinephrine
_____ mg Dopamine
Include μg/kg/min or mL/hr/totals

Meds Dose Route
Lidocaine
Sodium bicarbonate/Conc.
Atropine
Epinephrine
Include mg, μg, mEg/IV, ET, IO

Other
Glucose/Chemstrip
ABG/Labs sent

Vital Signs
Ext. or Int. pacing (rate/MA)
Defib/Synch joules
Temperature
Ventilated rate
Saturation
Pulses +/–
Blood pressure/MAP
Cardiac rhythm
Heart rate
CPR (Yes/No)

Time

circle one

Figure 151-1 ■ Example of a standardized institutional record for cardiac arrest (intraoperative or otherwise). Such a form can be used for most medical emergencies in which frequent interventions and the administration of medications occur.

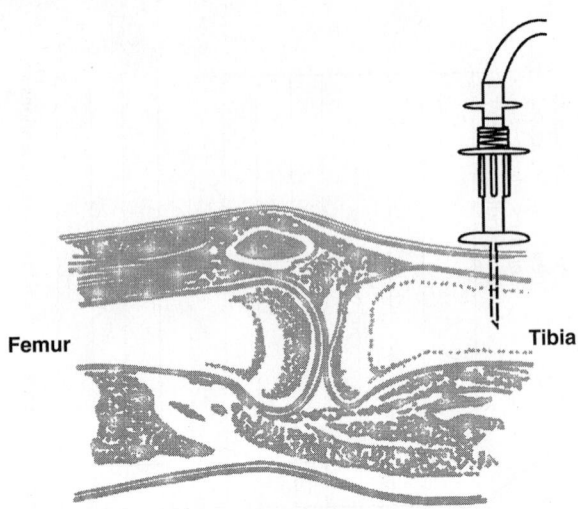

Figure 151–2 ■ Schematic representation of an intraosseous needle inserted into the tibia to administer fluids and medications. In most children younger than 7 years, an 18-gauge styletted needle can be used. The insertion point is approximately 2.5 cm (1 inch) distal to the medial tibial tubercle on the flat portion of the tibial surface, with the needle oriented at right angles to the bony surface. A flange on the needle serves as a stop, which should prevent insertion beyond the bone marrow. During insertion, the hand not used to advance the needle into the bone should grasp the leg distal to the insertion site to minimize the potential for operator injury during insertion. Proper insertion allows easy administration of fluids and medications.

After resuscitation, it is extremely important to do the following:

- Discuss the incident with the family, using language that they can understand. Explain what is known, but do not speculate on the cause if this is unclear. Inform the family what will occur next.
- Allow the family to ask questions.
- Allow the family to grieve alone or with designated support personnel.
- Sequester equipment and waste materials (especially opened medication vials) if an investigation is indicated.
- Do not reuse equipment (including the anesthesia machine) unless the cause of the intraoperative cardiac arrest has been determined.
- Enter a narrative of events in the progress notes section of the medical record.
- If the patient has died unexpectedly, in most instances the medical examiner should be notified.

- Debrief the code team. Make sure that team members have access to emotional support. Unanticipated intraoperative cardiac arrest with a poor outcome can be emotionally devastating to members of the code team, as well as to the patient's family and friends.
- Notify the risk management office at the institution.

PREVENTION

Many pediatric intraoperative cardiac arrests are the result of the patients' underlying conditions, and these may not be easily reversed. Others can result from any number of factors, including human error, errors in judgment or vigilance, equipment malfunction, and unexplained events. Vigilance throughout the intraoperative period and prompt investigation of any abnormalities in vital signs can lead to the early detection of problems and timely corrective intervention to reverse further patient deterioration before intraoperative cardiac arrest occurs.

Further Reading

Beecher HK, Todd DP: A study of deaths associated with anesthesia and surgery. Ann Surg 140:1-35, 1954.

Chamberlain DA, Hazinski MF, et al: Education in resuscitation. Resuscitation 59:11-43, 2003.

Cohen MM, Cameron CB, Duncan PG, et al: Pediatric anesthesia morbidity and mortality in the perioperative period. Anesth Analg 70:160-167, 1990.

Gaba DM, Fish KJ, Howard SK, et al: Crisis Management in Anesthesiology. New York, Churchill Livingstone, 1994.

Hazinski MF (ed): Pediatric Advanced Life Support Provider Manual. Dallas, Tex., American Academy of Pediatrics–American Heart Association, 2002.

Keenan RL, Shapiro JH, Kane FR, et al: Bradycardia during anesthesia in infants. Anesthesiology 80:976-982, 1994.

Morray JP, Geiduschek JM, Caplan RA, et al: A comparison of pediatric and adult anesthesia closed malpractice claims. Anesthesiology 78:461-467, 1993.

Morray JP, Geiduschek JM, Ramamoorthy C, et al: Anesthesia-related cardiac arrest in children: Initial findings of the Pediatric Perioperative Cardiac Arrest (POCA) Registry. Anesthesiology 93:6-14, 2000.

Ollson GL, Hallen B: Cardiac arrest during anesthesia: A computerized study in 250,543 anesthetics. Acta Anaesthesiol Scand 32:653-664, 1988.

Rackow H, Salatire E, Green LT: Frequency of cardiac arrest associated with anesthesia in infants and children. Pediatrics 28:697-704, 1961.

Steen S, Liao Q, Pierre L, et al: The critical importance of minimal delay between chest compressions and subsequent defibrillation: A haemodynamic explanation. Resuscitation 3:249-258, 2003.

Tiret L, Nivochey Y, Hatton F, et al: Complications related to anesthesia in infants and children. Br J Anaesth 61:263-269, 1988.

Weick KE, Sutcliffe KM: Managing the Unexpected: Assuring High Performance in an Age of Complexity. San Francisco, Jossey-Bass, 2001.

Sedation of Pediatric Patients

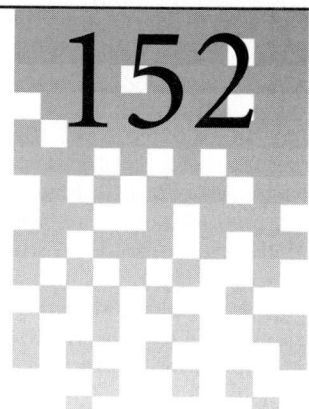

152

Charles J. Coté

Case Synopsis

A 3-year-old child with enlarged tonsils and a history of sleep apnea is scheduled to undergo magnetic resonance imaging (MRI). At the direction of the radiologist, the technician administers 75 mg/kg of chloral hydrate for sedation. After falling asleep, the child is placed in the scanner. Ten minutes into the MRI scan, the child develops desaturation and is without respirations.

PROBLEM ANALYSIS

Definition

The entire process of sedating patients has changed in recent years. Work by the American Academy of Pediatrics (AAP), the American Society of Anesthesiologists (ASA), and the Joint Commission on Accreditation of Healthcare Organizations (JCAHO) has resulted in unified definitions. For example, *minimal sedation* is equivalent to the older term *anxiolysis*, *moderate sedation* has replaced the oxymoron *conscious sedation*, and *deep sedation* is the same as previously defined. Expected patient responses to these new definitions of sedation are presented in Table 152-1.

Because sedation is a continuum and patient responses to sedating medications are unpredictable, emphasis has been placed on practitioners' ability to rescue patients if necessary. Thus, practitioners who administer drugs to achieve minimal sedation must have the skills to rescue a patient who becomes moderately sedated. Similarly, those who administer drugs for moderate sedation must have the skills required to rescue patients from deep sedation. Finally, practitioners who intend to achieve deep sedation must have the skills to rescue patients from a state of general anesthesia.

Because most sedation-related adverse events in children are related to compromise or loss of respiratory effort, the most important skill is advanced airway management. Moderate sedation consists of alteration of consciousness to the point that patients are compliant, comfortable, and (theoretically) psychologically calm, but they retain intact reflexes (including reflex withdrawal from a painful stimulus) and the ability to respond appropriately to verbal or nonverbal stimuli. For practical purposes, most children require pharmacologic restraint consistent with deep sedation to gain their cooperation. Therefore, it is good practice to use the guidelines for deep sedation from the outset of the sedation process.

The concept of deep sedation involves alterations of consciousness that are associated with partial or complete loss of protective reflexes and more profound changes in central nervous system and cardiopulmonary physiology. The JCAHO has recognized anesthesiologists as experts in sedation, analgesia, and anesthesia. That organization also agrees that deep sedation is virtually equivalent to a state of general anesthesia as far as safety is concerned. The JCAHO has mandated that departments of anesthesia lead the way in developing institutional policies regarding the sedation of all patients, whether adult or pediatric. The JCAHO is extensively involved in reviewing and ensuring the implementation of such sedation policies. The intention is to provide a uniform standard of care within each institution.

Table 152–1 ■ Expected Patient Responses with Minimal, Moderate, or Deep Sedation

	Minimal Sedation*	Moderate Sedation†	Deep Sedation‡
Responsiveness	Normal to verbal stimulation	Purposeful to verbal or light tactile stimulation	Purposeful following repeated or painful stimulation
Airway	Unaffected	No intervention required	May require intervention
Spontaneous ventilation	Unaffected	Adequate	May be inadequate
Cardiovascular function	Unaffected	Usually maintained	Usually maintained

*Drug-induced state equivalent to anxiolysis.
†Drug-induced depression of consciousness equivalent to conscious sedation.
‡Drug-induced depression of consciousness during which patients cannot be easily aroused.
Modified from the American Society of Anesthesiologists, available at http://www.asahq.org/publicationsAndServices/standards/20.htm.

Recognition

Recognition of complications related to sedation requires proper monitoring during the procedure by an independent observer whose only responsibility is to observe the patient. With the use of moderate sedation (rare in children), this individual could also assist with the procedure (Table 152-2).

In patients undergoing MRI, who are generally out of reach and not easily visualized, expired carbon dioxide monitoring is useful for the early detection of airway obstruction, hypoventilation, or apnea.

After a procedure requiring sedation, patients should be monitored in a fully equipped and staffed recovery area with strict and uniform discharge criteria identical to those used for patients recovering from general anesthesia.

Risk Assessment

In reviewing sedation-related accidents reported to the Food and Drug Administration, it is clear that most cases involve one or more of the following factors:

* The same person performing the procedure and sedating the child
* Residual drug effects combined with inadequate monitoring during recovery
* Lack of appreciation for drug-drug interactions and drug dosing errors
* Having parents administer a sedating medication at home and then having no one observe the child for signs of airway obstruction

The case synopsis raises a number of issues that are important when making decisions regarding the safety of sedation. In that case, the presedation assessment should have raised several red flags. First, it is known that children with tonsillar hypertrophy are at increased risk for developing further upper airway obstruction when sedation results in collapse of pharyngeal airway structures. Second, the child already had a history of obstructive sleep apnea, so it is not surprising that sedating medications would exacerbate that problem. Apparently, neither of these issues was considered before sedation. This child would have benefited from expired carbon dioxide monitoring, because a loss of air exchange would have preceded the onset of desaturation and allowed more timely initiation of rescue interventions. Despite the lack of carbon dioxide monitoring, an independent observer was able to make the diagnosis of obstructive sleep apnea with the onset of desaturation, and appropriate interventions were initiated. It is also possible that the child received either an overdose (dispensing error) or a dose based on body weight rather than lean body mass (prescribing error). In the pediatric population, obesity is a major factor contributing to airway obstruction and obstructive sleep apnea.

A study of sedation-related accidents conducted by the author found that approximately two thirds of children were younger than 6 years of age, and half received more than one sedating medication. There was equal representation of all classes of drugs (opioids, benzodiazepines, barbiturates, sedatives) associated with death or neurologic injury ($N = 60$). Chloral hydrate was associated with 13 neurologic injuries or death; in 8 cases, it was the only sedating medication. Thus, even chloral hydrate, a drug commonly thought to be extremely safe, can result in sufficient airway compromise to cause injury. This study also found that adverse outcomes were associated with all routes of drug administration (oral, rectal, nasal, intramuscular, intravenous, inhalation). Further, nearly every pediatric subspecialty service had an adverse event or outcome; 12 patients suffered an adverse event or outcome either on the way to the medical facility (2 patients) or after discharge from medical supervision (10 patients). All patients who suffered an adverse event after discharge had received long-acting medications, such as intramuscular DPT (Demerol, Phenergan, and Thorazine), oral or rectal chloral hydrate (half-life of approximately 10 hours in toddlers), or intramuscular pentobarbital.

Table 152–2 ■ Guidelines for Recognition of Complications Related to Sedation

	Moderate Sedation	Deep Sedation
Monitoring	Pulse oximetry—continuous Heart rate—continuous Respiratory rate every 15 min Level of consciousness every 15 min Blood pressure every 15 min	Pulse oximetry—continuous* Heart rate—continuous Respiratory rate every 5 min Level of consciousness every 5 min Blood pressure every 5 min[†]
Charting	Pulse oximetry every 15 min Heart rate every 15 min Respiratory rate every 15 min Level of consciousness every 15 min[‡] Blood pressure every 15 min	Pulse oximetry every 15 min Heart rate every 5 min Respiratory rate every 5 min Level of consciousness every 5 min Blood pressure every 5 min
Personnel	Same individual may observe patient and assist with procedure	Dedicated patient observer may not assist with procedure
Equipment	Pulse oximeter Blood pressure measuring device	Pulse oximeter Blood pressure measuring device Electrocardiograph and defibrillator immediately available

*Note whether and how oxygen is administered.

[†]Blood pressure may be taken less frequently if other vital signs are stable and taking blood pressure would interfere with the procedure.

[‡]Assessment of the level of consciousness may not be practical during some procedures, such as magnetic resonance imaging or computed tomography, if awakening the patient would prevent a successful scan.

A study by Malviya and colleagues examined recovery in toddlers following chloral hydrate sedation for echocardiograms. They found that using discharge criteria based on the patient's ability to remain awake for 20 consecutive minutes in a soporific environment and on the University of Michigan Sedation Scale resulted in a mean discharge time 75 minutes later than when using standard discharge criteria. This observation suggests that prolonged observation (perhaps in a step-down unit) may improve safety when long-acting medications are used for pediatric sedation.

In summary, these and other studies clearly support the concept of uniform institutional sedation guidelines and the need for a systematic approach to children requiring sedation, with the goal of significantly reducing anesthetic-related morbidity and mortality.

Implications

It is generally impossible to gain the cooperation of infants and young children for invasive or diagnostic procedures, necessitating pharmacologic control. Use of barbiturates, chloral hydrate, butyrophenones, opioids, and phenothiazines has been popular for decades, despite a paucity of information regarding pediatric safety and efficacy. The use of DPT, or the "lytic cocktail," for cardiac catheterization and other invasive or painful procedures has traditionally enjoyed widespread acceptance. This use continues today, despite the availability of drug combinations with more favorable pharmacokinetics and pharmacodynamics.

In recent years, the increasing use of ketamine and propofol by nonanesthesiologists has raised concerns regarding the skills of the individuals administering these medications. For many years, anesthesiologists have attempted to restrict the use of ketamine by nonanesthesiologists, but this appears to be changing. Ketamine is relatively safe in the hands of less skilled practitioners, because respiration is usually not depressed and airway patency is maintained (1% to 2% incidence of apnea or laryngospasm). Propofol is more commonly associated with airway obstruction, apnea, and unintended general anesthesia, making it a more problematic agent for use by nonanesthesiologists.

The widespread use of sedation by nonanesthesiologists for the care of pediatric patients is not without complications. Safely sedating pediatric patients for radiology, gastroenterology, oncology, emergency room, dental, and cardiology procedures is a major issue. Because there are insufficient numbers of anesthesiologists to provide all this care, the majority of children requiring procedural sedation are sedated by nonanesthesiologists. It is up to our specialty to educate and train these individuals.

The AAP has developed guidelines for the sedation of pediatric patients both inside and outside the hospital environment. The guidelines were revised in 1992, and since then they have been augmented by two ASA practice guidelines and an addendum to the AAP guidelines published in 2002. The AAP guidelines are currently undergoing further revisions that will likely expand on the indications for capnography in sedated children, further amplify the rescue skills needed by practitioners who sedate children, and suggest sedation teams and the use of patient simulators to maintain their skills.

MANAGEMENT

A systematic approach means organizing things in such a way that a number of checks and balances are in place so that vital pieces of information are not lost. For the sedation of pediatric patients, such an approach involves a number of important components:

- All patients must be treated with the same degree of care.
- Presedation given at home before traveling to the site where the procedure will be performed is strictly prohibited. Children must be under medical supervision before being given any drugs.
- Adequate review of the patient's history, physical examination (including a focused airway examination), current medications, allergies, and past medical and surgical records is essential.
- Uniform and rigorous screening procedures should be adopted and used by anesthesiologists and other specialists in airway management (e.g., emergency medicine physicians, pediatric intensivists) so that patients of high ASA status and those with unusual airway anatomy or cardiac or pulmonary problems receive the proper care.
- Compliance with preprocedure fasting guidelines for milk, formula, breast milk, and other solids and adequate hydration with clear fluids are essential (Table 152-3).
- Before sedation, ensure the availability of age- and size-appropriate and functioning equipment to manage the airway; medications to effectively manage emergencies, including reversal agents for opioids and benzodiazepines; and adequate means of delivering positive-pressure ventilation with sufficient oxygen reserves for at least 1 hour.

PREVENTION

It is essential to maintain a uniform level of safe care. In some institutions, the appointment of a "sedation team" is an effective method. It is of little importance who directs this team, but logic dictates that an anesthesiologist be intimately involved. If the sedation team is provided with appropriate resources and with a central procedure unit, the same sedation process can be used for patients undergoing a wide variety of procedures. Experienced sedation personnel need to be available for one to three shifts, depending on institutional needs. These persons, by virtue of their training and experience, work together to develop techniques unique to each institution to facilitate safe sedation and patient, parent, and

Table 152–3 ▪ Fasting Guidelines for Children		
	Fasting Time (hr)	
Age (mo)	*Solids*	*Clear Liquids**
<6	4 (breast milk)	2
6-36	6 (formula or solids)	3
>36	8 (solids)	3

*Apple juice, Pedialyte.

physician satisfaction. In some institutions, the pharmacy and therapeutics committee may be responsible for monitoring quality improvement activities with regard to overall institutional sedation practices. In other institutions, the ongoing monitoring of quality improvement activities may be a divisional, departmental, or hospital committee activity.

It is incumbent on people dealing with infants and children to provide a safe environment for procedures requiring the use of sedation. The solution to the problem of sedating infants and children lies in broad-based education. Although anesthesiologists are uniquely qualified to provide such care, by virtue of their limited numbers their ability to do so is restricted. Thus, it falls on anesthesiologists and other appropriately trained people to provide information, training, support, and continuing surveillance for others who provide sedation services to infants and children.

Further Reading

American Academy of Pediatric Dentistry: Guidelines for the elective use of conscious sedation, deep sedation, and general anesthesia in pediatric patients. ASDC J Dent Child 53:21-22, 1986.

Committee on Drugs, American Academy of Pediatrics: Guidelines for monitoring and management of pediatric patients during and after sedation for diagnostic and therapeutic procedures. Pediatrics 89:1110-1115, 1992.

Coté CJ: Sedation for the pediatric patient: A review. Pediatr Clin North Am 41:31-58, 1994.

Coté CJ: Discharge criteria for children sedated by nonanesthesiologists: Is "safe" really safe enough? Anesthesiology 100:207-209, 2004.

Coté CJ, Karl HW, Notterman DA, et al: Adverse sedation events in pediatrics: Analysis of medications used for sedation. Pediatrics 106:633-644, 2000.

Coté CJ, Notterman DA, Karl HW, et al: Adverse sedation events in pediatrics: A critical incident analysis of contributory factors. Pediatrics 105:805-814, 2000.

Dial S, Silver P, Bock K, et al: Pediatric sedation for procedures titrated to a desired degree of immobility results in unpredictable depth of sedation. Pediatr Emerg Care 17:414-420, 2001.

Gross JB, Bailey PL, Caplan RA, et al: Practice guidelines for sedation and analgesia by non-anesthesiologists: A report by the American Society of Anesthesiologists Task Force on Sedation and Analgesia by Non-anesthesiologists. Anesthesiology 84:459-471, 1996.

Guidelines for monitoring and management of pediatric patients during and after sedation for diagnostic and therapeutic procedures: Addendum. Pediatrics 110:836-838, 2002.

Litman RS, Kottra JA, Berkowitz RJ, et al: Upper airway obstruction during midazolam/nitrous oxide sedation in children with enlarged tonsils. Pediatr Dent 20:318-320, 1998.

Malviya S, Voepel-Lewis T, Ludomirsky A, et al: Can we improve the assessment of discharge readiness? A comparative study of observational and objective measures of depth of sedation in children. Anesthesiology 100:218-224, 2004.

Malviya S, Voepel-Lewis T, Prochaska G, et al: Prolonged recovery and delayed side effects of sedation for diagnostic imaging studies in children. Pediatrics 105:E42, 2000.

Practice guidelines for sedation and analgesia by non-anesthesiologists. Anesthesiology 96:1004-1017, 2002.

Muscle Relaxants

Constance L. Monitto

153

Case Synopsis

A 2-year-old boy presents for inguinal herniorrhaphy. During mask induction with oxygen, nitrous oxide, and sevoflurane he develops laryngospasm, which is treated with intramuscular succinylcholine. A wide QRS tachycardia is subsequently noted on the electrocardiogram monitor.

PROBLEM ANALYSIS

Definition

There can be complications with all neuromuscular relaxant drugs; however, the potential for serious complications is greater with succinylcholine (SCh). Although these complications have limited its routine use, SCh retains a role in pediatric anesthesia because of the unparalleled speed with which it acts and its ability to be administered intramuscularly when intravenous access has not been achieved. Significant complications associated with SCh use in children include the following:

- Cardiac arrhythmias
- Rhabdomyolysis
- Unanticipated prolonged duration of action
- Masseter spasm
- Malignant hyperthermia (see Chapter 162)

Complications with nondepolarizing muscle relaxants (NDMRs) include profound muscle weakness and impaired respiration with residual neuromuscular blockade (see Chapter 24). Prolonged myopathy after extended infusion of aminosteroid relaxants in the intensive care unit has been reported. Anaphylactic reactions can also occur. However, the most common side effects of NDMRs result from their histaminergic, cholinergic, and muscarinic effects. None of these reactions are unique to pediatric patients.

Recognition

DEPOLARIZING MUSCLE RELAXANTS

Decamethonium, another depolarizing muscle relaxant (longer acting), is no longer available or used in the United States, so this discussion is limited to SCh. Arrhythmias frequently accompany the administration of SCh, with sinus bradycardia or junctional rhythm being most common. These arrhythmias may cause significant hypotension in infants and children whose cardiac output is largely heart-rate dependent or, in the case of junctional rhythm, dependent on properly timed atrial contractions to augment ventricular filling (e.g., hypertrophic, dilated, or restrictive cardiomyopathy or arrhythmogenic right ventricular dysplasia; see Chapter 166). Further, asystole has been reported in patients of all ages following SCh. Life-threatening ventricular arrhythmias heralding severe rhabdomyolysis or malignant hyperthermia occur less frequently.

Rhabdomyolysis can be detected in a significant proportion of children following SCh administration. Although some patients may have detectable myoglobinuria, in the vast majority, rhabdomyolysis is a benign sequela of SCh. In some high-risk populations, however—most notably, patients with unrecognized congenital muscle disease or malignant hyperthermia sensitivity—SCh-induced rhabdomyolysis can be life threatening due to associated electrolyte disturbances, renal failure, or disseminated intravascular coagulation.

Prolonged neuromuscular blockade lasting several hours can occur after giving SCh to patients with homozygous genetic abnormalities in plasma cholinesterase (pseudocholinesterase) (see Chapter 23). Because mivacurium is also metabolized by pseudocholinesterase, its use may produce this response as well. Although several medical conditions (e.g., hepatic failure) may result in striking reductions in the circulating concentrations of normal cholinesterases, reduced concentrations of normal enzyme have a far less dramatic impact than the presence of a genetically defective enzyme.

Linking SCh-induced masseter spasm and malignant hyperthermia remains a matter of controversy. Careful investigations have shown that masseter muscle tone is commonly increased after SCh administration. Whether exaggerated masseter tone (i.e., masseter spasm) that prevents the mouth from being opened is a harbinger of malignant hyperthermia continues to be debated. Recognition and management of malignant hyperthermia are discussed in Chapter 162.

NONDEPOLARIZING MUSCLE RELAXANTS

Although anaphylactic reactions are more commonly seen after SCh administration, they have been reported after both aminosteroid (especially rocuronium) and benzylisoquinoline NDMR (atracurium and cisatracurium) administration. Anaphylactic reactions to NDMRs may be difficult to diagnose, but clinical signs include flushing, hypotension, tachycardia, and bronchospasm following administration of the agent.

Histamine release with benzylisoquinoline relaxants is recognized by skin flushing, hypotension, and tachycardia. The mechanisms for increased heart rate and blood pressure with gallamine and pancuronium are unclear but could involve some or all of the following:

- Block of muscarinic receptors at the sinoatrial node (gallamine, pancuronium)
- Vagolytic action at the preganglionic or postganglionic nerve terminal (gallamine)

- Catecholamine release (gallamine, possibly with extremely high concentrations)

Life-threatening episodes of bronchospasm (i.e., profound difficulty in ventilation with absent end-tidal carbon dioxide) and some deaths secondary to irreversible bronchospasm were reported after the introduction of rapacuronium bromide in 1999. Subsequent laboratory studies suggested that clinically relevant concentrations of rapacuronium may provoke bronchospasm due to muscarinic effects. Rapacuronium was subsequently withdrawn from the market.

Risk Assessment

SUCCINYLCHOLINE

Vagally mediated arrhythmias, including sinus or atrioventricular junctional bradycardia, sinus pause, and transient asystolic arrest, may occur in as many as 40% to 60% of children after a single intravenous dose of SCh. As in adults, repeated doses may elicit more frequent and more severe bradyarrhythmias. Malignant ventricular arrhythmias and even cardiac arrest after SCh may occur with exaggerated potassium release in patients with acute or progressive denervation injury (e.g., spinal cord transection, peripheral neuropathy, stroke), extensive tissue damage (e.g., burns, crush injury), prolonged immobilization, or neuromuscular disease.

Historically, rhabdomyolysis after SCh was detected by serum myoglobin elevation in 40% of children anesthetized with halothane, and as many as 8% had associated myoglobinuria. Case reports also describe its occurrence in patients receiving enflurane, isoflurane, or sevoflurane. Although far more common in pediatric patients than in adults, rhabdomyolysis appears to be a benign process in the overwhelming majority of children. Nevertheless, a small population with myopathic processes (e.g., Duchenne's muscular dystrophy) can exhibit life-threatening hyperkalemia, arrhythmias, acute renal injury, and disseminated intravascular coagulation. Because the underlying myopathy may be undiagnosed in young children (more commonly boys), cardiac arrest in apparently healthy children has been reported after SCh administration.

Approximately 1 in 3000 patients presents with (frequently) occult genetic variants of pseudocholinesterase of the type that can result in markedly prolonged neuromuscular blockade following the administration of SCh or mivacurium.

The diagnosis of masseter muscle spasm remains controversial. Some cite a 1% incidence rate, while others say that it never occurs. Because an increase in masseter tone often accompanies SCh administration, the determination of what constitutes clinically significant masseter spasm (i.e., a harbinger of malignant hyperthermia) is subjective. Of real concern, though, is the finding that in a select population of patients referred to the North American Malignant Hyperthermia Group, 50% of children with masseter spasm who were screened for malignant hyperthermia sensitivity by muscle biopsy tested positive. Of these patients, approximately 10% developed clinical signs of malignant hyperthermia perioperatively. Therefore, severe masseter spasm (i.e., an increase in masseter muscle tone sufficient to impede mouth opening) must be viewed with concern.

NONDEPOLARIZING MUSCLE RELAXANTS

Anaphylaxis is reported to occur in 1 in 10,000 to 20,000 anesthesias, and 50% to 70% of these episodes are related to neuromuscular blocking agents. A prior history of drug exposure is not necessary. Patients with an allergic history or a history of anaphylaxis may be more susceptible to histamine release from NDMRs that are associated with histamine release (Table 153-1).

The initial data on rapacuronium suggested a 4% incidence of bronchospasm (versus <1% with other NDMRs).

Table 153–1 ■ Intubating Dose, Primary Clearance, and Side Effects of Muscle Relaxants in Children

Muscle Relaxant	Intubating Dose (IV mg/kg)	Primary Method of Clearance	Cholinergic Effects	Histamine Release
Succinylcholine	2-3 (infants) 2 (children) 4 (IM)	Plasma cholinesterase	Stimulates	Rare
Mivacurium	0.2-0.4	Plasma cholinesterase	No effect	+ (doses >3 × ED$_{95}$)
Atracurium	0.3-0.5	Ester hydrolysis; Hofmann degradation	No effect	++ (doses >3 × ED$_{95}$)
Cisatracurium	0.15-0.2	Ester hydrolysis; Hofmann degradation	No effect	Minimal
Vecuronium	0.1 0.4 (rapid sequence)	Hepatic	No effect	None
Rocuronium	0.6 1.0 (rapid sequence) 1.0 IM (infants); 1.6 IM (children)	Hepatic	No effect	None
d-Tubocurarine	0.3-0.6	Renal	No effect	+++
Pancuronium	0.1	Renal	Blocks ++*	None
Metocurine	0.3-0.6	Renal	No effect	++
Gallamine	3.5	Renal	Blocks +++*	None
Pipecuronium	0.1	Renal	No effect	None
Doxacurium	0.05	Renal	No effect	None

*Also causes sympathetic stimulation.

However, higher than expected rates of serious airway-related complications were reported after it was introduced into general clinical use. Associated risk factors for the development of bronchospasm in children following rapacuronium were rapid-sequence induction of general anesthesia and a prior history of reactive airway disease. However, neither of these factors alone was necessary or sufficient to cause bronchospasm.

Implications

SUCCINYLCHOLINE

Bradyarrhythmias usually are benign and self-limited or respond to vagolytic therapy. However, if they are protracted and associated with hemodynamic compromise, temporary pacing may be required. In contrast, malignant ventricular arrhythmias and cardiac arrest seen with exaggerated potassium release after SCh have projected mortality rates as high as 60%.

Rhabdomyolysis rarely has lasting consequences except in myopathic patients, in whom the consequences can be dire.

Children with atypical pseudocholinesterase eventually recover neuromuscular function without sequelae. Consequently, the implications have more to do with genetic counseling and awareness of the condition.

Masseter spasm usually has few immediate implications, because the spasm is localized to the masseter. If, however, the patient is at risk for malignant hyperthermia, the implications for future management of both the child and the family are substantial.

NONDEPOLARIZING MUSCLE RELAXANTS

Intraoperative anaphylaxis from NDMRs is a serious concern, with a mortality rate of approximately 3% to 6%. Owing to the potential for tachycardia, pancuronium (and gallamine, if still available) is best avoided in patients in whom tachycardia might be detrimental (e.g., severe mitral, tricuspid, or aortic stenosis; coronary strictures or anomalous left coronary artery; accelerated, juvenile coronary artery disease). Finally, NDMRs that release histamine are best avoided in patients with asthma, a significant right-to-left shunt, or valvular stenosis.

MANAGEMENT

Succinylcholine

Persistent or hemodynamically disadvantageous bradyarrhythmias are treated with atropine or pacing, particularly in infants. Arrhythmias with hyperkalemia are treated with alkalization, calcium, and glucose-insulin. Successful resuscitation may be prolonged, and extracorporeal circulation may be needed for extreme cases, at least until potassium is eliminated by excretion or dialysis.

Rhabdomyolysis that goes undetected requires no specific therapy in most patients. For those with myopathy, full cardiac resuscitation and measures to promote myoglobin excretion (e.g., furosemide, mannitol) may be required.

Children with clinically suspected pseudocholinesterase deficiency require ventilatory support until neuromuscular function returns. Absolute pseudocholinesterase activity and the dibucaine and fluoride numbers should then be determined.

Masseter spasm usually requires no specific treatment because the spasm recedes within a few minutes. Reports suggest that it is safe to proceed with anesthesia and surgery. However, one must be alert for progression to malignant hyperthermia and be prepared to treat it. Known triggering agents should be discontinued, and the procedure should be aborted if signs of malignant hyperthermia develop. Further testing may be required.

Nondepolarizing Muscle Relaxants

Routine management of anaphylaxis includes removal of the antigen source when possible, inhibition of mediator production and release (e.g., steroid administration), and interventions to modulate the effects of the mediators. These may include histaminergic blockade, treatment of bronchoconstriction with β_2-agonists, and the administration of intravenous fluids and epinephrine to decrease bronchial hyperresponsiveness and support the circulation. Postoperative confirmatory laboratory data include elevated serum tryptase, histamine, and (drug-specific) immunoglobulin E levels at the time of the reaction and 6 weeks later.

Hypotension due to histamine release is treated with intravenous fluids and vasopressors. In addition, use of a stereoselective NDMR (e.g., cisatracurium rather than atracurium) may result in a diminution of clinically significant histamine release. Treatment of symptomatic tachycardia not associated with hypotension may include a deepening of anesthesia, opioids, and a β-blocker.

PREVENTION

Succinylcholine

In light of reports of profound SCh-induced rhabdomyolysis, cardiac arrest, and death in apparently healthy children ultimately diagnosed with myopathic disease, drug manufacturers sought to ban routine SCh use in children in 1993. In response to protests from anesthesiologists who were aware of the drug's benefits, the Food and Drug Administration held an open committee meeting from which compromise labeling for SCh emerged (Fig. 153-1). However, the fact that life-threatening hyperkalemia can be prevented only by avoiding SCh in high-risk patients—some of whom carry a diagnosis of myopathy, and some of whom do not—has discouraged the routine use of SCh in children.

Given the uncertain association of masseter spasm with malignant hyperthermia, prudence dictates the avoidance of triggering anesthetic agents in untested patients with documented masseter spasm following SCh.

Nondepolarizing Muscle Relaxants

Because rapacuronium was a low-potency NDMR with a rapid onset and short duration of action, it was initially hoped that it might provide a safer alternative to SCh for rapid-sequence inductions and short procedures. However, after a

---

WARNING
Risk of Cardiac Arrest from Hyperkalemic Rhabdomyolysis

There have been rare reports of acute rhabdomyolysis with hyperkalemia followed by ventricular arrhythmias, cardiac arrest, and death after the administration of succinylcholine to apparently healthy children who were subsequently found to have undiagnosed skeletal muscle myopathy, most frequently Duchenne's muscular dystrophy.

This syndrome often presents as peaked T waves and sudden cardiac arrest within minutes after the administration of the drug in healthy appearing children (usually, but not exclusively, males, and most frequently 8 years of age or younger). There have also been reports in adolescents.

Therefore, when a healthy-appearing infant or child develops cardiac arrest soon after the administration of succinylcholine, that is not thought to be due to inadequate ventilation, oxygenation, or anesthetic overdose, immediate treatment for hyperkalemia should be instituted. This should include the administration of intravenous calcium, bicarbonate, and glucose with insulin, with hyperventilation. Due to the abrupt onset of this syndrome, routine resuscitative measures are likely to be unsuccessful. However, extraordinary and prolonged resuscitative efforts have resulted in successful resuscitation in some reported cases. In addition, in the presence of signs of malignant hyperthermia, appropriate treatment should be instituted concurrently.

Because there may be no signs or symptoms to alert the practitioner to which patients are at risk, it is recommended that the use of succinylcholine in children should be reserved for emergency intubation or instances in which immediate securing of the airway is necessary (e.g., laryngospasm, difficult airway, full stomach, or for intramuscular use when a suitable vein is inaccessible). See PRECAUTIONS: Pediatric Use and DOSAGE AND ADMINISTRATION.

Figure 153–1 ▪ Manufacturer's warning concerning the association between succinylcholine and hyperkalemic cardiac arrest. (Adapted from Physicians' Desk Reference. Montvale, NJ, Medical Economics, 1997, p 1062.)

number of deaths resulting from profound drug-related bronchospasm, the drug was removed from the U.S. market by its manufacturer in 2001.

Atracurium and mivacurium undergo significant ester hydrolysis. Thus, prolonged neuromuscular blockade is possible with either of these NDMRs in patients with atypical pseudocholinesterase or cholinesterase deficiency.

Further Reading

Bevan DR: Newer neuromuscular blocking agents. Pharmacol Toxicol 74: 3-9, 1994.

Brandom BW, Fine GF: Neuromuscular blocking drugs in pediatric anesthesia. Anesth Clin North Am 20:45-58, 2002.

Cook DR, Davis PJ: Pharmacology of pediatric anesthesia. In Motoyama EK, Davis PJ (eds): Smith's Anesthesia for Infants and Children. St. Louis, Mosby, 1990, pp 157-200.

Goudsouzian NG: Muscle relaxants in children. In Coté CJ, Ryan JF, Todres ID, et al (eds): A Practice of Anesthesia for Infants and Children. Philadelphia, WB Saunders, 1993, pp 151-170.

Gronert BJ, Brandom BW: Neuromuscular blocking drugs in infants and children. Pediatr Clin North Am 41:73-91, 1994.

Jooste E, Klafter F, Hirshman CA, et al: A mechanism of rapacuronium-induced bronchospasm: M2 muscarinic receptor antagonism. Anesthesiology 98:906-911, 2003.

Larach MG, Rosenberg H, Gronert GA, et al: Hyperkalemic cardiac arrest during anesthesia in infants and children with occult myopathies. Clin Pediatr (Phila) 36:9-16, 1997.

Lebowitz PW, Ramsey FM: Muscle relaxants. In Barash PG, Cullen BF, Stoelting RK (eds): Clinical Anesthesia. Philadelphia, JB Lippincott, 1989, pp 339-370.

Martin LD, Bratton SL, O'Rourke PP: Clinical uses and controversies of neuromuscular blocking agents in infants and children. Crit Care Med 27:1358-1368, 1999.

Physicians' Desk Reference. Montvale, NJ, Medical Economics, 1997, pp 1062-1063, 1136-1139.

Rajchert DM, Pasquariello CA, Watcha MF, et al: Rapacuronium and the risk of bronchospasm in pediatric patients. Anesth Analg 94:488-493, 2002.

Sparr HJ, Beaufort TM, Fuchs-Buder T: Newer neuromuscular blocking agents: How do they compare with established agents? Drugs 61: 919-942, 2001.

154

Delayed Emergence in Pediatric Patients

Hector F. Nicodemus and John B. Rose

Case Synopsis

A 2-year-old, 12-kg girl with achondroplasia remains unresponsive and intubated in the pediatric postanesthesia care unit 45 minutes after undergoing cervical spine fusion and suboccipital craniectomy for atlanto-occipital instability and foramen magnum stenosis.

PROBLEM ANALYSIS

Definition

When agents used for general anesthesia are discontinued, the patient is expected to regain consciousness within a certain period, although the time it takes for this to occur is variable and depends on a number of factors. Delayed emergence is defined as the failure to recover consciousness after general anesthesia within a reasonable period. The determination of "reasonable" depends on the agents and techniques used, as well as the patient's preoperative physical and mental status (see also Chapter 222).

Recognition

EVALUATION OF PATIENTS

The evaluation of patients with delayed emergence is summarized in Figure 154-1. Drug effects, physiologic imbalance, disorders of metabolism, central nervous system (CNS) injury, or undiagnosed preexisting CNS disease may cause delayed emergence from general anesthesia (Table 154-1).

For the patient described in the case synopsis, first the airway was assessed. Then, adequate ventilation and oxygenation were assured by review of the patient's vital signs, temperature, end-tidal carbon dioxide, and pulse oximetry readings. Adequate recovery of neuromuscular function was determined with a nerve stimulator. Subsequent review of the preoperative record revealed an excessive fasting time (>15 hours). Also, intraoperatively, non-glucose-containing intravenous (IV) solutions were used. Thus, hypoglycemia was suspected and confirmed by determination of the blood glucose concentration (42 mg/dL). Corrective therapy was instituted immediately, and the patient regained consciousness.

DRUG EFFECTS

Prolonged anesthetic action is a likely cause if delayed emergence follows an otherwise uneventful operative procedure. Although inadvertent overdose of one drug may be responsible for delayed emergence, it is more often attributed to combined drug effects. Individually, drugs may be given in appropriate doses; however, relative overdose may occur owing to the potentiation of their hypnotic effects.

For example, oral midazolam (0.5 mg/kg) might be given for preoperative sedation. Then, toward the end of anesthesia, IV morphine is given for analgesia (0.15 mg/kg) and IV droperidol (0.075 mg/kg) is given to prevent postoperative nausea and vomiting.

Reduced drug metabolism and elimination may contribute to delayed emergence, especially in premature and full-term newborns. Respiratory depression and hypoventilation secondary to narcotics and sedatives can delay the elimination of inhalational agents and prolong emergence in spontaneously breathing infants or children.

One recent investigation of the effects of oral midazolam premedication in 50 patients aged 10 to 18 years, American Society of Anesthesiologists status I and II, concluded that midazolam did not prolong emergence from general anesthesia. Further, it did not affect the expired concentrations of sevoflurane or nitrous oxide at emergence or the time required for discharge from the postanesthesia care unit. However, the investigators found that clinically detectable sedation before anesthetic induction, manifest in half of midazolam-treated patients, strongly correlated with delayed emergence.

In infants and children, biologic variability in their response to the hypnotic effects of anesthetic drugs can be marked. If so, increased sensitivity to these effects may contribute to prolonged emergence in some children. However, this must be a diagnosis of exclusion in healthy children with no prior history of cognitive impairment or developmental delay.

PHYSIOLOGIC IMBALANCE OR DISORDERS OF METABOLISM

The existence of various preoperative states (e.g., prolonged fasting, dehydration, malnutrition, renal or hepatic failure, diuretic or antacid therapy, severe anemia, sickle cell disease, diabetes, seizure disorder) or the occurrence of adverse intraoperative events (e.g., hypoventilation, hypotension, hypoperfusion, large blood loss with massive blood and fluid resuscitation) raises the possibility that physiologic imbalance or a metabolic disturbance is responsible for delayed emergence.

The routine use of pulse oximetry and capnography has greatly enhanced the ability of anesthesiologists to detect and treat life-threatening conditions associated with hypoxemia and hypercarbia. Metabolic acidosis should be considered in

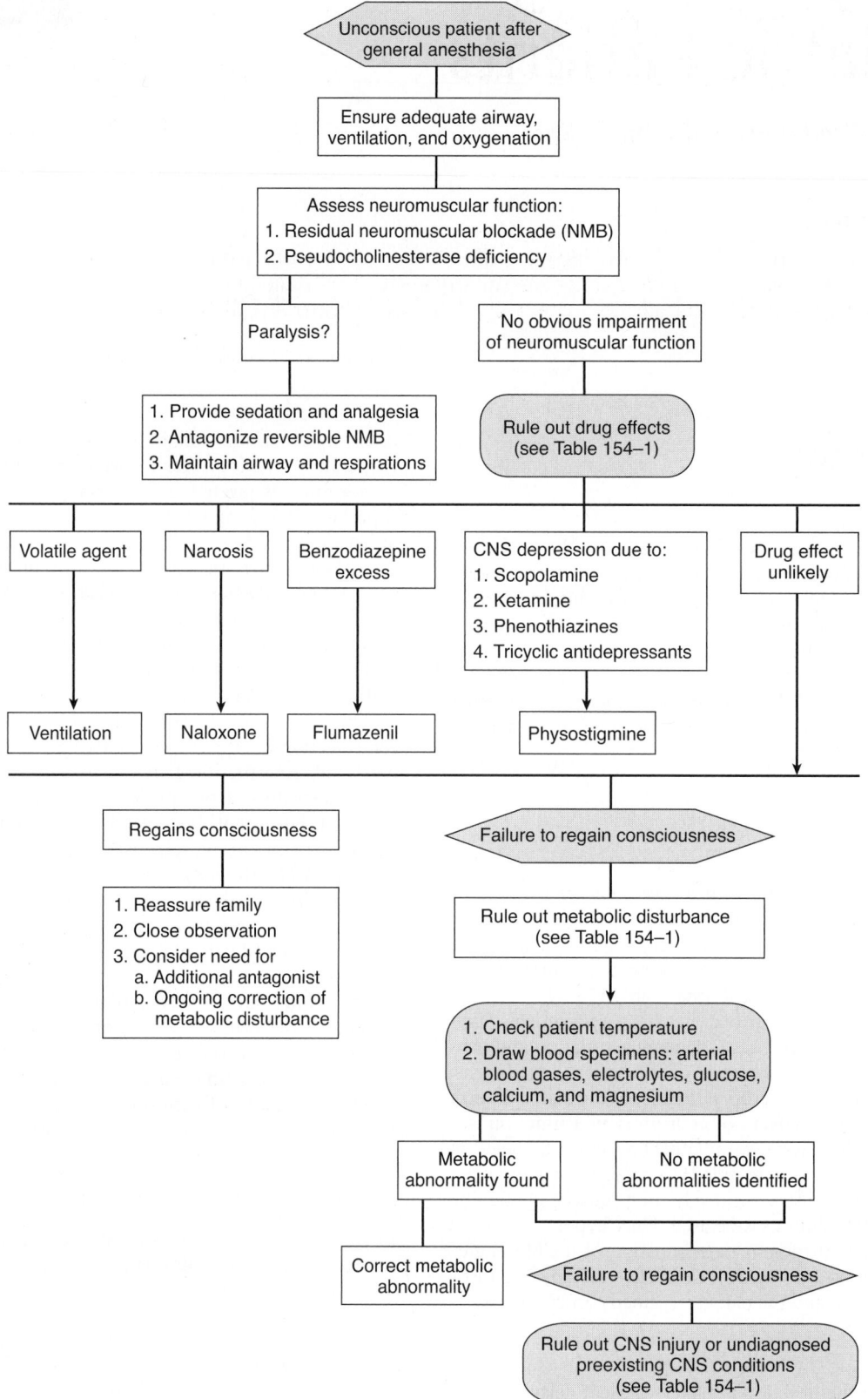

Figure 154–1 ■ Algorithm for evaluation of the patient with delayed emergence.

Table 154–1 ▪ Differential Diagnosis of Delayed Emergence

Drug Effects
Drug overdose (accidental or error in judgment)
Multiple CNS depressants or drug interactions
Medication error (in preparation or administration)
Impaired drug metabolism (reduced elimination or protein binding; increased sensitivity)
Residual neuromuscular blockade

Physiologic Imbalance or Disorders of Metabolism
Hypoxia; hypercarbia
Electrolyte imbalance (hyponatremia, hypocalcemia, hypomagnesemia)
Hypothermia or hyperthermia
Sepsis
Hypoglycemia

CNS Injury or Undiagnosed Preexisting Condition
Intracranial hemorrhage or hypertension
Cerebral ischemia, edema, or embolism (air or particulate)
Seizure disorder (especially, postictal states)
Brain tumor
Stroke (e.g., in sickle cell disease, hypercoagulable states)

CNS, central nervous system.
Adapted and modified from Denlinger JK: Prolonged emergence and failure to regain consciousness. In Gravenstein N, Kirby RR (eds): Complications in Anesthesiology. Philadelphia, Lippincott-Raven, 1996, pp 441-450.

children who have experienced periods of hypotension or hypoperfusion or in those who have lost large amounts of blood necessitating massive fluid replacement with crystalloid, colloid, and blood products. Hypoglycemia should be suspected in children who (1) have fasted preoperatively for long periods, (2) have received non-glucose-containing IV fluids intraoperatively, or (3) are insulin-dependent diabetics and received insulin perioperatively.

CENTRAL NERVOUS SYSTEM INJURY OR DISEASE

CNS injuries during anesthesia in children are rare but may contribute to delayed emergence. Congenital heart lesions with right-to-left shunts place patients at risk for cerebral air embolism after even small amounts of air have been introduced via IV infusions. In addition, cerebral embolism with air or particulate matter can occur during cardiopulmonary bypass. Intracerebral or intraventricular hemorrhage can occur during awake laryngoscopy and endotracheal intubation in premature and term neonates and is also a complication of ventriculoperitoneal shunt revision and other neurosurgical procedures. Cerebral ischemia can occur with the delivery of hypoxic gas mixtures, prolonged hypotension with hypoperfusion, and carotid artery compression injury secondary to malpositioning.

Undiagnosed, preexisting CNS conditions can also contribute to delayed emergence. Intracranial hypertension may exist in patients with malfunctioning ventriculoperitoneal shunts or in those with previously unrecognized brain tumors or foramen magnum stenosis; it can be exacerbated by hypercarbia, hypoxemia, or hyperextension of the neck. Seizures are difficult to detect in anesthetized and paralyzed patients. They can occur during general anesthesia, and the postictal state may present as delayed emergence. Finally, unrecognized muscle weakness or paralysis can make the patient appear to be unconscious. This must be distinguished

from the conditions outlined earlier by careful assessment of neuromuscular function.

Risk Assessment

The incidence of delayed emergence is unknown. However, based on recent investigations of anesthetic complications in infants and children, its incidence appears to be low. In one study of anesthetic complications in 29,220 infants and children, there were no reported cases of delayed emergence or coma. In a review of complications in 40,240 infants and children, one case of coma was described; this occurred in a 13-year-old boy after nitrous oxide–opioid–neuroleptic anesthesia. In another study, 2 of 10,000 pediatric ambulatory surgery patients were hospitalized after surgery owing to excessive sleepiness.

Underreporting of this complication may be a significant issue. The time required to emerge from general anesthesia is highly variable, so individual anesthesiologists must determine whether an emergence is delayed and report the complication. If most cases of delayed emergence are related to prolonged drug effects and the ultimate outcome is good, many practitioners are likely reluctant to report what appears to be an insignificant event.

Implications

When delayed emergence results from prolonged drug action, long-term patient outcomes are good when proper measures are taken to support the airway and ensure adequate oxygenation, ventilation, and hemodynamic parameters. However, when delayed emergence is a consequence of metabolic abnormalities or CNS injury, it is imperative to recognize that there is a problem, determine the underlying cause, and institute corrective measures expeditiously to avoid a catastrophic outcome.

Aside from its impact on patient outcome, delayed emergence can have a significant effect on operating room (OR) efficiency and the cost of operative procedures to families, institutions, and health care systems. Even small delays in emergence, if frequent, can disrupt the OR schedule, consume OR and recovery room time and personnel, and prevent an anesthesiologist from starting other scheduled cases on time.

MANAGEMENT

Management of delayed emergence entails the following steps:

- Ensure adequate oxygenation and ventilation.
- Review the medical history and anesthetic management.
- Try drug antagonism.
- Rule out metabolic abnormalities.
- Rule out CNS injury.

The management of delayed emergence begins with ensuring that the patient has an adequate airway and that he or she is well oxygenated and ventilated. Next, the patient's medical history and anesthetic management are reviewed to identify potential causes and determine what further actions are required. Frequently, opioid or benzodiazepine overdose cannot be ruled out, and a diagnostic and therapeutic trial of naloxone, flumazenil, or both is indicated (Table 154-2).

Table 154–2 ■ Antagonists to Reverse the Sedative Effects of Anesthetic Agents

Naloxone: 1-4 µg/kg IV titrated to effect; maximum dose, 10 µg/kg
Flumazenil: 2.5-5 µg/kg IV titrated to effect; maximum dose, 10 µg/kg
Physostigmine: 25-50 µg/kg IV; maximum dose, 2 mg

The nonspecific antagonist physostigmine may be beneficial when delayed emergence is due to volatile anesthetics, scopolamine, ketamine, phenothiazines, or tricyclic antidepressants. It should be emphasized that any of these antagonists may produce only a transient recovery of consciousness. If prolonged anesthetic drug effects are not suspected, blood should sampled to determine arterial blood gases, electrolytes, glucose, calcium, and magnesium concentrations. If no discernible cause is identified after the initial review, neurology consultation, CNS imaging studies, or electroencephalography may be indicated.

PREVENTION

Delayed emergence is often preventable. Drug errors, inadequate patient surveillance or monitoring, and positioning injuries, especially when surgery involves the head and neck or when patients are in the prone or lateral decubitus position, are some of the more common preventable causes of this complication.

Further Reading

Brosius KK, Bannister CF: Oral midazolam premedication in preadolescents and adolescents. Anesth Analg 94:31-36, 2002.

Cohen MM, Cameron CB, Duncan PG: Pediatric anesthesia morbidity and mortality in the perioperative period. Anesth Analg 70:160-167, 1990.

Cook DR, et al: Pharmacology of pediatric anesthesia. In Motoyama EK, Davis PJ, Lerman J (eds): Smith's Anesthesia for Infants and Children. St. Louis, Mosby, 1996, pp 159-209.

Denlinger JK: Prolonged emergence and failure to regain consciousness. In Gravenstein N, Kirby PR (eds): Complications in Anesthesiology. Philadelphia, Lippincott-Raven, 1996, pp 441-450.

Hinkle AJ: Neonatal sepsis presenting as delayed emergence from general anesthesia. Anesthesiology 57:412-414, 1982.

Patel RI, Hannallah RS: Anesthetic complications following pediatric ambulatory surgery: A 3-year study. Anesthesiology 69:1009-1012, 1988.

Seiber FE, Smith DS, Traystman RJ, et al: Glucose: A reevaluation of its intraoperative use. Anesthesiology 67:72-81, 1987.

Tiret L, Nivoche Y, Hatton F, et al: Complications related to anaesthesia in infants and children: A prospective study of 40,240 anaesthetics. Br J Anaesth 61:263-269, 1988.

Viitanen H, Annila P, Viitanen M, et al: Midazolam premedication delays recovery from propofol induced sevoflurane anesthesia in children 1-3 years old. Can J Anaesth 46:766-771, 1999.

Welbourne LG, Hannallah RS, McGill WA, et al: Glucose concentrations for routine intravenous infusion in pediatric outpatient surgery. Anesthesiology 67:427-430, 1987.

Postintubation Croup

155

Mark I. Rossberg

Case Synopsis

An otherwise healthy 3-year-old boy receives general endotracheal anesthesia for hypospadias repair. Shortly after arrival in the pediatric acute care unit, the child is noted to have a hoarse cry and mild inspiratory stridor.

PROBLEM ANALYSIS

Definition

Postintubation croup is a complication of general endotracheal anesthesia that is most commonly seen in children. Endotracheal intubation in children may cause traumatic injury to the tracheal epithelium, and postintubation croup is believed to be a manifestation of traumatic subglottic mucosal edema.

Postintubation croup can vary in severity. Mild subglottic edema may be accompanied by hoarseness of the voice, a barking cough, and stridor when the patient is agitated or crying. With more significant subglottic swelling, tracheal narrowing occurs, and partial airway obstruction ensues, resulting in the patient's use of accessory muscles of respiration. In its most severe form, postintubation croup can progress to total airway obstruction, requiring the establishment of an artificial airway. The signs of subglottic edema usually become evident within an hour of tracheal extubation. Respiratory compromise may progress until approximately 8 hours after extubation and usually resolves within 24 hours.

Recognition

When postintubation croup occurs, it is important to assess the degree of airway compromise, monitor for progressive airway obstruction, and intervene if necessary. Pulse oximetry should be monitored.

MILD POSTINTUBATION CROUP

- Stridor when crying or agitated
- Mild retraction of respiratory muscles
- Good aeration of lungs
- No desaturation while breathing room air

MODERATE POSTINTUBATION CROUP

- Stridor at rest
- Moderate retraction of respiratory muscles
- Reduced aeration of lungs
- Desaturation while breathing room air

SEVERE POSTINTUBATION CROUP

- Stridor at rest
- Deep retraction of respiratory muscles
- Poor aeration of lungs
- Desaturation despite breathing an increased fraction of inspired oxygen
- Lethargy

Risk Assessment

Mild postintubation croup (characterized by hoarse voice and stridor) remains a common problem, but the incidence of severe postintubation croup associated with significant airway compromise has declined. The reported incidence of postintubation croup in the 1960s varied from 1.6% to 6%; in 1977 it was 1%; and by 1991, it was reported to be 0.1%.

Part of the reason for the apparent decline in incidence is the more stringent definition of croup used in more recent reports. Only patients with inspiratory stridor and retraction of accessory respiratory muscles for at least 30 minutes' duration and severe enough to warrant therapy were considered to have postintubation croup. Thus, patients with transient postoperative stridor or an isolated hoarse voice or barking cough were excluded.

However, a real decline in the incidence of significant subglottic edema has occurred as a result of changes in anesthesia practice and equipment. Previously, endotracheal tubes were rubber and were washed with a detergent and reused. They may have been both physically and chemically irritating to the trachea. With the advent of standardized, nonreactive, single-use polyvinyl chloride endotracheal tubes, these irritants are no longer a factor. Additionally, anesthesiologists are now more attuned to selecting endotracheal tubes of an appropriate size for children and replacing endotracheal tubes that fit too tightly within the patient's trachea.

Patients younger than 1 year rarely develop croup. The highest incidence seems to be between the ages of 1 and 4 years. Beyond 4 years, the risk diminishes.

The most important factor associated with the development of postintubation croup is a tight-fitting endotracheal tube, as demonstrated by the absence of an air leak around the tube at 40 cm H_2O pressure. There is no significant difference in risk between cuffed and uncuffed endotracheal tubes. Physical trauma or irritation of the airway is associated with postintubation croup. This may be related to difficult or multiple intubation attempts and patient coughing or head repositioning while an endotracheal tube is in place. The effect of the use of local analgesics and lubricants on endotracheal tubes is unclear. Patients with croup are more likely to have been intubated for longer than 1 hour, to have been in a position other than supine during surgery, or to have had neck surgery.

There are conflicting data about whether preoperative upper respiratory tract infection correlates with the development of postintubation croup. Patients with a history of viral croup may be at a higher risk.

Finally, postintubation stridor is more frequent in children with Down's syndrome than in other children after cardiac surgical repair. This is probably because these children have a smaller-diameter cricoid ring and require smaller-diameter tracheal tubes than do normal children.

Implications

It is wise to know the risk factors for postintubation croup and anticipate its occurrence. When subglottic edema does occur, it should be recognized, and the magnitude of airway compromise should be assessed and observed for signs of worsening. Appropriate therapy should be instituted promptly, and the response to therapy should be monitored closely, because unresolved airway obstruction may result in hypoventilation, hypoxemia, prolonged stay in the postanesthesia care unit, and unanticipated hospital admission.

MANAGEMENT

Initial therapy consists of the administration of humidified oxygen by facemask, mist tent, or tubing directed at the child's face. For mild croup, this is usually adequate. However, in the case of moderate to severe croup, or if a patient with mild croup is developing worse stridor and respiratory distress, further therapies are indicated.

Nebulized racemic epinephrine may be given at a dose of 0.5 mL of 2.25% solution in 3 mL of normal saline. This usually relieves airway obstruction and alleviates symptoms through its vasoconstrictive effects on the tracheal mucosa. Improvement should be seen within 20 to 30 minutes. During the administration of racemic epinephrine, the cardiac rate and rhythm should be monitored for tachyarrhythmias with continuous electrocardiography. Many argue that any patient who has had sufficient airway compromise to warrant racemic epinephrine therapy should be admitted to the hospital for 12 to 24 hours of observation because of the potential for laryngeal edema to worsen again. Certainly any child who receives racemic epinephrine should be observed for at least 4 to 5 hours after therapy. Further, many of those treated with racemic epinephrine benefit from a repeat dose. Patients with significant ongoing or progressive respiratory compromise should be transferred to a pediatric intensive care unit for further therapy and observation.

It should be recognized that racemic epinephrine, which consists of the *d*- and *l*-isomers of epinephrine, has traditionally been used instead of *l*-epinephrine. It was believed that racemic epinephrine was more effective at reducing tracheal edema and was less likely to provoke the side effects of *l*-epinephrine (tachycardia, hypertension, tremor). However, in a randomized study, *l*-epinephrine was found to be equally as efficacious as racemic epinephrine in the treatment of postintubation laryngeal edema, with neither of these drugs producing significant side effects. Although equipotent doses

of the drugs were used in this study, the doses were half those recommended earlier (0.25 mL of 2.25% solution of racemic epinephrine or 1% *l*-epinephrine in 3 mL of normal saline). However, the patients in the study were young (12 ± 10 months), possibly explaining why a reduced dose was chosen.

Steroids are the most effective definitive therapy for croup (whether postintubation or viral) because of their ability to reduce tracheal edema and inflammation. Dexamethasone effectively reduces the risk of postextubation stridor in preterm infants. In young squirrel monkeys with experimental (traumatic) laryngeal edema, intravenous dexamethasone prevented the development of laryngeal edema and sped the resolution of existing experimental laryngeal edema. Based on evidence of the effectiveness of steroids and the seemingly low risk of short-course or single-dose steroid therapy, it seems prudent to administer a single dose of dexamethasone to patients who require nebulized racemic epinephrine. A dose of 0.25 to 0.5 mg/kg intravenously (to a maximum of 10 mg) is commonly used. In cases of mild croup, especially in ambulatory surgery patients, it may be prudent to administer a single dose of steroid either intravenously or orally.

Clearly, for severe postintubation airway obstruction, the airway must be secured with an endotracheal tube. This is extremely unusual and is often associated with other issues, such as underlying subglottic stenosis or neurologic injury.

PREVENTION

Take the following precautions to prevent postintubation croup:

- Avoid the use of excessively tight-fitting endotracheal tubes, especially if the patient has a history of croup.
- Check for leak pressure (the inspiratory pressure required to cause an audible escape of gas around the endotracheal tube) immediately after intubation, and consider changing the endotracheal tube to one half a size smaller if there is no leak at 40 cm H_2O pressure.
- If a cuffed endotracheal tube is used, inflate the cuff only enough to maintain the desired leak pressure (<40 cm H_2O pressure or, preferably, ≤25 cm H_2O pressure).
- During a long operation, if possible, intermittently check the leak pressure and adjust the volume of gas in the cuff to maintain the desired leak. Remember that nitrous oxide can diffuse into the endotracheal tube cuff and increase cuff pressure during surgery.
- Avoid multiple intubation attempts, especially in patients with upper respiratory tract infections or a history of croup.

When using laryngoscopes that have been chemically sterilized versus heat sterilized, ensure that all chemicals have been thoroughly rinsed off.

Further Reading

Bjornson CL, Klassen TP, Williamson J, et al: A randomized trial of a single dose of oral dexamethasone for mild croup. N Engl J Med 351:1306-1313, 2004.

Cohen MM, Cameron CB, Duncan PG: Pediatric anesthesia morbidity and mortality in the perioperative period. Anesth Analg 70:160-167, 1990.

Couser RJ, Ferrara TB, Falde B, et al: Effectiveness of dexamethasone in preventing extubation failure in preterm infants at increased risk for airway edema. J Pediatr 121:591-596, 1992.

Goddard JE, Phillips OC, Marcy JH: Betamethasone for prophylaxis of postintubation inflammation: A double blind study. Anesth Analg 46:348-353, 1967.

Litman RS, Keon TP: Postintubation croup in children. Anesthesiology 75:1122-1123, 1991.

Waisman Y, Klein B, Boenning D, et al: Prospective randomized double-blind study comparing *l*-epinephrine and racemic epinephrine aerosols in the treatment of laryngotracheitis (croup). Pediatrics 89:302-306, 1992.

Postobstruction Pulmonary Edema in Pediatric Patients

156

Lynda J. Means

Case Synopsis

A 5-year-old obese child with developmental delay, asthma, and obstructive sleep apnea presents for a tonsillectomy. Inhalation induction is begun. The airway is partially obstructed intermittently until nasopharyngeal and oral airways are inserted. On completion of surgery, pink, frothy fluid is noted in the endotracheal tube. A chest radiograph (Fig. 156-1) is obtained, and the child is transferred to the intensive care unit for positive-pressure ventilation with positive end-expiratory pressure. The following morning the chest radiograph is normal (Fig. 156-2), and the child is extubated without incident.

PROBLEM ANALYSIS

Definition

Postobstruction pulmonary edema (POPE) is acute pulmonary edema that follows the relief of upper airway obstruction during which vigorous inspiratory efforts occurred (see Chapter 52 for POPE in adults). The obstruction may be acute and total, as occurs with laryngospasm in children or adults; alternatively, it can be partial and more prolonged, as occurs with epiglottitis in children. POPE is often referred to as negative-pressure pulmonary edema because the primary factor in its development is the generation of markedly negative intrathoracic pressure. This pressure, generated by forced inspiration against an obstructed upper airway (i.e., a modified Müller maneuver), ultimately leads to the transudation of fluid from pulmonary capillaries into the interstitium, and from there into alveoli. Hypoxia and acute left ventricular dysfunction may also play a role in the development of edema fluid.

Recognition

Recognition of POPE involves an understanding of its pathophysiology. The pathogenesis of POPE is explained by

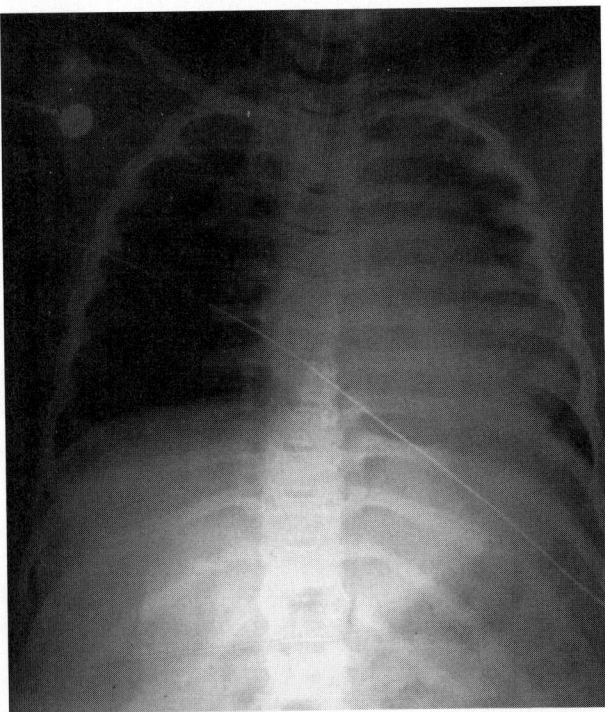

Figure 156–1 ■ Chest radiograph obtained at the completion of surgery. Note perihilar fluffy infiltrates in a butterfly pattern, consistent with pulmonary edema. Also present is left lower lobe atelectasis.

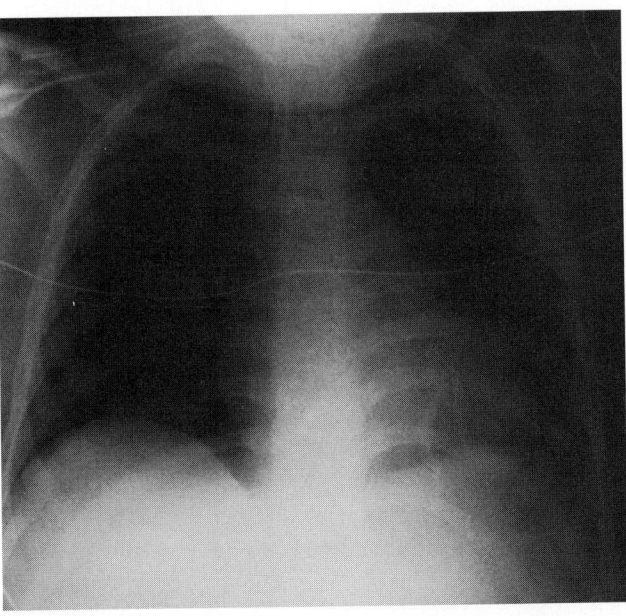

Figure 156–2 ■ Chest radiograph taken the following morning. Note resolution of the perihilar infiltrates.

634

abnormal fluid flux across alveolar-capillary membranes. The abnormal fluid translocation results from a disruption in the balance between hydrostatic and colloid osmotic pressures in alveolar-capillary units, according to Starling's equation. Normally, a balance exists among the forces maintaining fluid in the intravascular space and those moving fluid into the interstitium.

$$\text{Fluid filtration rate} = K_f\,[(P_c - P_i) - \sigma\,(\pi_c - \pi_i)]$$

where K_f is capillary permeability, P_c is pulmonary capillary hydrostatic pressure, P_i is pulmonary interstitial hydrostatic pressure, σ is the reflection coefficient for proteins, π_c is pulmonary capillary osmotic pressure, and π_i is pulmonary interstitial osmotic pressure.

The result is that only a small amount of fluid enters the pulmonary interstitium and, once there, is promptly removed by the pulmonary lymphatics. Patients who generate extremely negative intrathoracic pressures increase venous return to the right atrium. This increases pulmonary blood volume and capillary hydrostatic pressure. At the same time, a marked decrease in pulmonary interstitial hydrostatic pressure occurs, resulting in increased transfer of fluid into the interstitium. If lymph removal mechanisms are overwhelmed, signs and symptoms of pulmonary edema develop. The hypoxemia and increased sympathetic tone that frequently accompany airway obstruction also increase pulmonary vascular pressures and left ventricular afterload to facilitate edema formation (Figs. 156-3 and 156-4). Acutely, left ventricular dysfunction may contribute to the development of pulmonary edema. However, such dysfunction is typically extremely short-lived, as evidenced by normal or near-normal central venous, pulmonary artery, and pulmonary capillary wedge pressures when measured after the obstructive event.

An example of the relative pressures maintaining a normal fluid filtration rate (assuming constant values for K_f and σ) is the following:

$$P_c = 12 \text{ mm Hg},\ P_i = -4 \text{ mm Hg},\ \pi_c = 23 \text{ mm Hg},$$
$$\pi_i = 9 \text{ mm Hg} \approx 2 \text{ mm Hg}$$

Relative pressures promoting an increased fluid filtration rate and the development of POPE are as follows:

$$P_c = 22 \text{ mm Hg},\ P_i = -50 \text{ mm Hg},\ \pi_c = 23 \text{ mm Hg},$$
$$\pi_i = 9 \text{ mm Hg} \approx 58 \text{ mm Hg}$$

P_c elevation reflects increased pulmonary capillary blood volume and left ventricular afterload; P_i elevation reflects decreased intrapleural pressure.

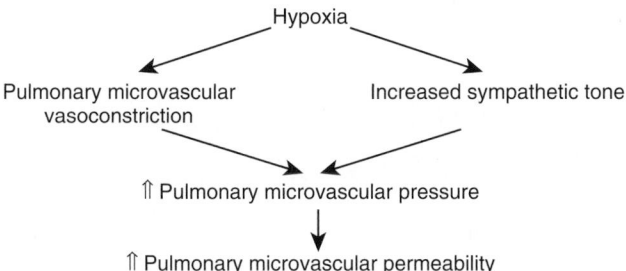

Figure 156–3 ■ Role of hypoxia in the generation of postobstruction pulmonary edema.

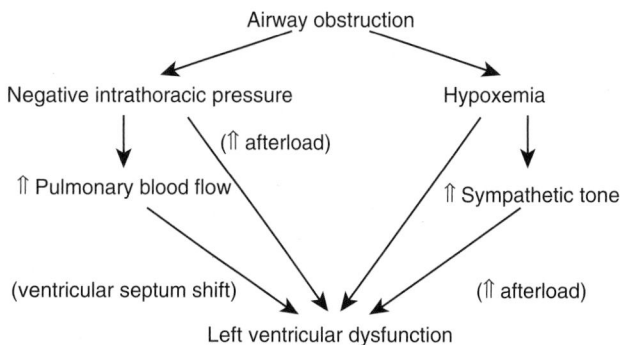

Figure 156–4 ■ Proposed mechanisms leading to left ventricular dysfunction during airway obstruction.

POPE typically occurs in young, healthy individuals. The onset of edema is usually soon after relief of the obstruction, but it may be delayed for 3 to 4 hours. The patient exhibits an increased alveolar-to-arterial oxygen tension gradient, manifested by a requirement for supplemental oxygen; this, along with the pulmonary edema, typically resolves in less than 36 hours. Chest auscultation is consistent with pulmonary edema and may reveal rales and occasional rhonchi and wheezes. The chest radiograph and computed tomography scan show pulmonary edema, with peribronchial cuffing predominantly involving the perihilar and more central lung parenchyma. The peripheral lung regions remain remarkably free of alveolar edema, resulting in a "butterfly" pattern. The cardiac silhouette is normal.

The following causes of pulmonary edema should also be considered and eliminated:

- Aspiration pneumonia
- Iatrogenic volume overload
- Pulmonary embolus
- Primary cardiac abnormality
- Myocardial dysfunction secondary to ischemia
- Anaphylaxis
- Asthma

At least initially, aspiration pneumonia is the most difficult alternative diagnosis to eliminate. Massive aspiration of gastric contents can produce the same radiographic picture as POPE, but it more commonly involves the right upper lobe or posterior segments. Further, the clinical course is more protracted owing to the chemical injury to the lung parenchyma. Radiographic changes from acute aspiration of gastric contents typically lag behind the patient's clinical course.

Risk Assessment

The incidence of POPE is unknown, despite clinical reports describing the phenomenon since the mid-1970s. Risk factors include the following:

- Laryngospasm
- Obesity and obstructive sleep apnea
- Epiglottitis
- Croup
- Partial tracheal obstruction by a foreign body

- Upper airway pathology or surgical manipulation (e.g., tracheomalacia, vocal cord paralysis)
- Partial tracheal obstruction by an esophageal foreign body
- Obstructed endotracheal tube or laryngeal mask
- Difficult intubation

No specific anesthetic drugs have been shown to increase the incidence of POPE. However, anesthetic agents or techniques that increase the likelihood of laryngospasm or soft tissue upper airway obstruction have the potential to increase a patient's risk for POPE.

Implications

Profound hypoxia secondary to upper airway obstruction occurs rapidly in children. If it is not relieved, cardiac arrest can follow. Prompt and effective intervention to reestablish a patent upper airway and to maximize oxygenation is paramount. With recognition and appropriate management, the clinical course of POPE is usually self-limited.

MANAGEMENT

Treatment of POPE involves reestablishing and maintaining a patent airway, followed by supportive care. Supplemental oxygen is necessary, and most patients require tracheal intubation for a period of time; this may be as short as several hours in some instances. Many patients receive positive airway pressure, either as continuous positive airway pressure or as positive-pressure ventilation with positive end-expiratory pressure. Rarely, hemoptysis and frank pulmonary hemorrhage have been reported after acute upper airway obstruction. Both require significant ventilatory and cardiovascular support. Aggressive, invasive hemodynamic monitoring, such as pulmonary artery catheterization, is not indicated except to rule out other causes of pulmonary edema. Use of diuretics is controversial because the edema is not due to excessive intravascular volume (as supported by normal pulmonary capillary wedge pressure measurements), and edema resolution is typically rapid. In addition to diuresis, furosemide increases venous capacitance, and it may have a role in the management of POPE. Corticosteroids and antibiotics have no role in the treatment of POPE unless they are indicated for other reasons. Resolution of clinical symptoms and radiographic findings is usually rapid and typically occurs within 2 to 3 days.

PREVENTION

Prevention of POPE involves (1) recognition of clinical scenarios in which upper airway obstruction is likely to occur and (2) the development of an anesthesia management plan to avoid potential obstruction. The latter includes the following:

- Ensure an adequate depth of anesthesia during the use of a facemask or laryngeal mask airway.
- Consider the use of "bite blocks" to ensure patency of artificial airways during emergence from anesthesia.
- Perform tracheal extubation in fully awake patients to avoid laryngospasm or soft tissue airway obstruction.
- Use fiberoptic intubation in patients with known airway abnormalities.

Anesthesiologists are frequently faced with situations that cannot be avoided, such as anesthetizing a child with epiglottitis. In such cases, multiple strategies for avoiding the complications of airway obstruction, including surgical intervention, should be available if obstruction occurs.

Further Reading

Broccard AF, Liaudet L, Aubert JD, et al: Negative pressure post-tracheal extubation alveolar hemorrhage. Anesth Analg 92:273-275, 2001.

Devys JM, Balleau C, Jayr C, et al: Biting the laryngeal mask: An unusual cause of negative pressure pulmonary edema. Can J Anaesth 47:176-178, 2000.

Guinard JP: Laryngospasm-induced pulmonary edema. Int J Pediatr Otorhinolaryngol 20:163-168, 1990.

Herrick IA, Mahendran B, Penny FJ: Postobstructive pulmonary edema following anesthesia. J Clin Anesth 2:116-120, 1990.

Lang SA, Duncan PG, Shepard DAE, et al: Pulmonary oedema associated with airway obstruction. Can J Anaesth 37:210-218, 1990.

Oswalt CE, Gates GA, Holmstrom MG: Pulmonary edema as a complication of acute airway obstruction. JAMA 238:1833-1835, 1977.

Ruffle J, Gleason M, Domino KB, et al: Pulmonary edema and transient cardiomyopathy in a previously healthy adolescent after general anesthesia. J Cardiothorac Vasc Anesth 8:463-470, 1994.

Schwartz DR, Maroo A, Malhotra A, et al: Negative pressure pulmonary hemorrhage. Chest 115:1194-1197, 1999.

Hypoxemia

Lori A. Aronson

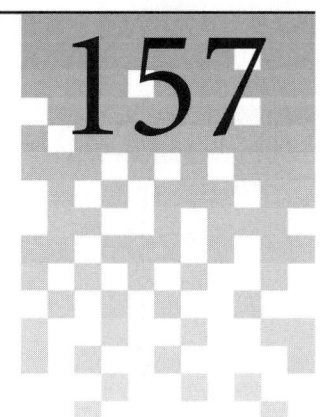

157

Case Synopsis

A 10-year-old boy undergoes general endotracheal anesthesia for elective repair of an undescended left testis. When he awakes from anesthesia, the trachea is extubated. The patient immediately coughs, becomes stridorous, and has chest wall retractions. Cyanosis, tachycardia, and percutaneous arterial oxygen saturation (SpO_2) less than 60% are noted.

PROBLEM ANALYSIS

Definition

Hypoxemia is abnormally low oxygenation of the blood. It is distinguished from hypoxia, in which tissue oxygen (O_2) delivery is inadequate to sustain normal cellular aerobic metabolism. Table 157-1 lists the normal age-related values of blood O_2 tension, and Table 157-2 shows the change in the O_2 affinity of hemoglobin with age.

Recognition

Identifying hypoxemia is an integral part of anesthesia practice. The pulse oximeter has become the standard of care for monitoring oxygenation during anesthesia. A decrease in SpO_2 is often the first and cardinal sign of hypoxemia.

The clinical signs of hypoxemia vary with age. Preterm infants and neonates respond to hypoxemia with ventilatory depression, with or without bradycardia. Older infants and children respond with tachypnea and either tachycardia or bradycardia. Cyanosis, pallor, restlessness, or altered mental status may be evident, depending on the degree of hypoxemia. All these signs can be masked by anesthesia.

Pulse oximetry has improved patient safety by allowing anesthetic providers to recognize and respond to an oxygenation problem sooner than would be possible based on clinical signs alone. Determining the cause of hypoxemia is critical to establishing a treatment strategy. One must use physical assessment skills (auscultation, percussion, palpation), monitors (pulse oximetry, end-tidal carbon dioxide, fraction of inspired O_2 [FiO_2], airway pressure), and tests such as chest radiographs and blood gas analysis to establish the cause of hypoxemia.

A systematic approach to ascertaining the underlying cause of hypoxemia should be taken. This includes an assessment of the O_2 supply, the integrity of the anesthesia machine, the breathing circuit and airway, and the functioning of the patient's pulmonary, cardiovascular, hematologic, and central nervous systems.

Risk Assessment

The risk of hypoxemia in pediatric patients is related to many factors, including underlying disease and age-related anatomic and physiologic characteristics. The anesthesiologist must assess each factor's contribution to the risk for hypoxemia in an individual patient. Table 157-3 lists the principal causes of hypoxemia.

ANATOMY AND PHYSIOLOGY

Knowledge of the unique anatomic and physiologic characteristics of infants and children is critical to their anesthetic management. These characteristics include the following:

- Infants have relatively large heads, short necks, and large tongues, which make them prone to upper airway obstruction. In older children, enlarged tonsils may contribute to upper airway obstruction.
- An infant's epiglottis is U-shaped and floppy. The larynx appears more anterior because it is higher than in adults (C3-C4 versus C4-C5). The vocal cords angle more cephalad.
- The narrowest part of the pediatric airway is the cricoid cartilage. Airway epithelium is easily traumatized, and tracheal cartilage is readily collapsible.

Table 157–1 ■ Normal Arterial Oxygen Tension (PaO_2) in Infants and Children	
Age	**PaO_2 (mm Hg)**
Preterm	60
Full term	70
1 mo	95
1 yr	93
12 yr	98

Table 157–2 ■ Age-Related Oxygen Affinity for Hemoglobin at an Oxygen Saturation of 50% ($P_{50}O_2$)	
Age	**$P_{50}O_2$ (mm Hg)***
Neonates	30
Infants (>3 mo)	20
Adults (>18 yr)	27

*Oxygen affinity is highest in neonates and lowest in infants before reaching adult levels.

Table 157–3 ■ Causes of Hypoxemia in Pediatric Patients

Central Nervous System and Respiratory Centers

Apnea
Head trauma
Brain tumor
Seizures
Anesthetic agents
    Narcotic overdose
    Inhalational agents
    Barbiturates, sedatives
    Combinations of the above

Airway

Epiglottitis, croup
Tracheomalacia, laryngomalacia
Retropharyngeal abscess
Vascular ring
Infantile stridor
Laryngospasm
Webs
Mediastinal mass
Foreign body, ETT obstruction
Thermal airway injury (burns)
Subglottic stenosis
Upper respiratory infection

Respiratory Muscles

Residual neuromuscular blockade
Debilitation, malnutrition
Myasthenia gravis
Muscular dystrophy
Phrenic nerve injury

Pulmonary: Physiologic Causes

Ventilation-perfusion mismatch
    Shunt
    Dead-space ventilation
Diffusion abnormality (rare)

Pulmonary: Pathologic Causes

Respiratory distress syndrome
Bronchopulmonary dysplasia
Primary pulmonary hypertension
Aspiration pneumonitis
Diaphragmatic hernia
Tracheoesophageal fistula

Pulmonary edema
Near-drowning
Asthma, bronchospasm
Pneumonia
Pulmonary contusion
Pulmonary embolus (air, fat, thrombus)
Pulmonary fibrosis, cystic fibrosis
Bronchiectasis

Chest Wall and Pleura

Pneumothorax
Flail chest
Pleural effusion
Obesity
Kyphoscoliosis
Abdominal mass

Cardiovascular

Congenital heart disease
Congestive heart failure
Arteriovenous malformation
Hypovolemia, hemorrhage

Hematologic

Anemia
Sickle cell disease or crisis
Thalassemia

Oxygen Delivery

Main-stem bronchial intubation
ETT kinking
Low FiO_2, hypoxic gas mixture
Ventilator disconnection
Anesthesia machine failure
Esophageal intubation

Increased Oxygen Consumption

Shivering (hypothermia)
Malignant hyperthermia
Hyperthermic states (sepsis)
Hyperthyroidism

Miscellaneous

Positioning
Carbon monoxide
Cyanide poisoning (sodium nitroprusside overdose)
Hepatic failure

- An infant's trachea is significantly shorter than an adult's. Also, the angle of tracheal bifurcation (about 45 degrees) is nearly the same for both main-stem bronchi. Therefore, one must be diligent to avoid either right or left main-stem bronchial intubation. In contrast, in older patients, the angle of tracheal bifurcation is less for the right main-stem bronchus (about 30 degrees) than for the left, explaining the higher risk for right main-stem bronchial intubation in adults.
- Respiratory control is not well developed. Respiratory muscles (the intercostals and diaphragm) have fewer type I muscle fibers and tend to fatigue more easily. This may lead to hypoventilation.
- The newborn's chest wall is very compliant and tends to move inward on inspiration. The rib angle is more horizontal, further limiting chest expansion on inspiration. Thus, infants often rely on their abdominal muscles during inspiration.

- A distended abdomen due to aggressive positive-pressure ventilation can markedly impede diaphragmatic movement.
- Pulmonary development is incomplete at birth. Alveoli are present in adult numbers by 3 years, but they continue to grow in size until 7 to 8 years of age. Additionally, premature infants or sick newborns may have inadequate surfactant. This contributes to alveolar collapse, reduced compliance, and hypoxemia.
- O_2 consumption and alveolar ventilation in infants are approximately double that in adults (7 versus 4 mL/kg per minute and 130 versus 60 mL/kg per minute, respectively). However, functional residual capacity is about half that of adults (25 versus 40 mL/kg). Infants also have higher lung closing volumes and faster respiratory rates. These combine to limit O_2 reserve. With increased O_2 consumption, hypoxia can occur rapidly. Newborns respond to hypoxia with transient tachypnea and then ventilatory depression.

BREATHING PATTERNS

Periodic breathing (apnea lasting <10 seconds) occurs in preterm and term infants. The frequency dramatically decreases by 12 months of age. Although periodic breathing is a benign respiratory pattern, central apnea is not. Central apnea of infancy (apnea lasting >15 seconds, or less if associated with bradycardia, cyanosis, or pallor) is common in preterm infants. It may be related to immature respiratory control mechanisms. Prematurity, anemia, and anesthesia are critical risk factors for life-threatening apnea in infants (see Chapter 150). Mild hypoxemia is common with respiratory infections in young infants, making them especially vulnerable to further desaturation.

POSTANESTHESIA CARE UNIT

A large percentage of healthy infants and children undergoing simple elective surgical procedures become hypoxemic in the postanesthesia care unit. Children younger than 1 to 2 years or those with upper respiratory infections are at greatest risk for hypoxemia. Airway obstruction, central hypoventilation (due to residual inhalational anesthetics or narcotics), atelectasis, and poor ventilation secondary to pain, dressings, shivering, or residual neuromuscular blockade may further contribute to hypoxemia. Therefore, pediatric patients should receive O_2 during transport to and in the postanesthesia care unit.

OXYGEN DELIVERY

The cardiovascular system is responsible for the delivery of O_2 to the tissues. With the onset of respiration and altered blood flow patterns in newborns, pulmonary vascular resistance falls, while systemic vascular resistance increases. Increased afterload causes the foramen ovale to close, and this reverses the direction of shunt through the ductus arteriosus. Until these pathways close anatomically, reversion to a fetal-type circulation with hypoxemia may occur. Hypoxia and acidosis can increase pulmonary vascular resistance and cause right-to-left shunting and O_2 desaturation.

In congenital heart disease, anatomic shunting of blood through abnormal vascular pathways can result in right-to-left shunting with hypoxemia. Congestive heart failure may also contribute to hypoxemia. A true right-to-left shunt does not respond to O_2 with an increase of SpO_2.

Fetal hemoglobin predominates at birth and causes a leftward shift of the oxygen-hemoglobin dissociation curve. Fetal hemoglobin has a high affinity for O_2. This leads to less O_2 released to the tissues at any given FiO_2. The higher hemoglobin level, increased blood volume, and increased cardiac output per unit body weight compensate for increased tissue demands for O_2. However, if anemia, hypovolemia, or low cardiac output occurs, the risk for hypoxemia is increased. Physiologic anemia occurs at 2 to 3 months of age, or earlier in premature infants. An increase in 2,3-diphosphoglycerate compensates for this and shifts the oxygen-hemoglobin dissociation curve to the right, allowing greater O_2 delivery to tissues.

Hypoxemia may occur due to failure of O_2 supply equipment. Failure of oximetry monitoring delays the diagnosis of hypoxemia. Knowledge about the operation and maintenance of monitors and equipment (see Section 6) is important for reducing the risk of life-threatening problems.

Implications

Cardiac arrest may occur if hypoxemia is not promptly recognized and treated. Anaerobic metabolism leading to acidosis, end-organ injury, and death can follow. Thus, detection and treatment of hypoxemia are critical.

MANAGEMENT

The initial management of hypoxemia is directed at improving the patient's oxygenation by increasing the FiO_2 to 1.0 and ensuring a patent airway and ventilation. This is done with mask ventilation and oropharyngeal or nasopharyngeal airways, endotracheal intubation, laryngeal mask airway, or cricothyrotomy or tracheotomy.

Further management is directed at remedying the cause of hypoxemia. Rapid diagnosis of the cause of the problem allows the timely reversal of hypoxemia and the avoidance of further complications. If hypoxemia is prolonged, advanced life support may become necessary.

PREVENTION

Prevention of hypoxemia and adverse outcomes begins with a careful patient evaluation, an understanding of the implications of the planned procedure, and a thorough check of all equipment before anesthesia and surgery. Preoperative evaluation includes assessing the patient's medical status, recognizing the urgency and risks of the planned surgery, and determining whether further medical therapy before surgery could reduce patient risk.

Some common anesthesia practices that may reduce hypoxemia include preoxygenation and denitrogenation before endotracheal intubation, increasing the FiO_2 to 1.0 for several minutes before tracheal extubation, administering a higher FiO_2 during anesthesia maintenance, use of supplemental O_2 during patient transport, and utilization of pulse oximetry, capnography, and FiO_2 monitoring. Although critical incidents may still occur despite the anesthesiologist's vigilance, prompt recognition and treatment are critical to minimizing adverse outcomes.

Further Reading

Coté CJ, Goldstein EA, Coté MA, et al: A single-blind study of combined pulse oximetry and capnography in children. Anesthesiology 68: 184-188, 1988.

Coté CJ, Zaslavsky A, Downes JJ, et al: Postoperative apnea in former preterm infants after inguinal herniorrhaphy: A combined analysis. Anesthesiology 82:809-822, 1995.

Kurth CD, LeBard SE: Association of postoperative apnea, airway obstruction, and hypoxemia in former premature infants. Anesthesiology 75:22-26, 1991.

Liu LM, Coté CJ, Goudsouzian NG, et al: Life-threatening apnea in infants recovering from anesthesia. Anesthesiology 59:506-510, 1983.

PEDIATRICS & NEONATOLOGY

Motoyama E: Respiratory physiology in infants and children. In Motoyama E, Davis PJ (eds): Smith's Anesthesia for Infants and Children. St. Louis, Mosby, 1996, pp 11-67.

Pang LM, Mellins RB: Neonatal cardiorespiratory physiology. Anesthesiology 43:171-196, 1975.

Welborn LG, Hanallah RS, Luban NLC, et al: Anemia and postoperative apnea in former preterm infants. Anesthesiology 74:1003-1006, 1995.

Xue FS, Huang YG, Tong SY, et al: A comparative study of early postoperative hypoxemia in infants, children, and adults undergoing elective plastic surgery. Anesth Analg 83:709-715, 1996.

Perioperative Aspiration Pneumonitis

158

Mark Meyer and Joseph Previte

Case Synopsis

A 3-year-old girl with developmental delay, tracheomalacia, and reactive airway disease presents for laryngoscopy, bronchoscopy, and esophagogastroduodenoscopy. Despite a previous Nissen fundoplication, she continues to have episodes of pneumonia secondary to gastroesophageal reflux disease (GERD) and aspiration. Medications include albuterol for wheezing and pantoprazole for GERD.

PROBLEM ANALYSIS

Definition

Pulmonary aspiration is defined as the presence of bilious secretions or particulate matter in the tracheobronchial tree. It most commonly occurs from passive regurgitation of gastric contents or active vomiting, but aspiration of blood or pharyngeal secretions can also cause significant pneumonitis. Of pediatric patients who aspirate during anesthesia, 40% actively vomit, and the remainder passively regurgitate. When anesthetized patients aspirate, 80% do so during induction, 14% during emergence, 4% during the procedure, and 2% postoperatively.

Recognition

After significant pulmonary aspiration, the physical examination may reveal fever, tachypnea, apnea, tachycardia, refractory laryngospasm, bronchospasm, wheezing, or cough. Rales and rhonchi can be heard, and cyanosis may be observed. A chest radiograph may reveal alveolar and, less commonly, reticular infiltrates. Radiographic findings may be localized but are more often extensive and frequently bilateral. The full extent of changes on the chest radiograph may not be demonstrated until 6 to 24 hours after pulmonary aspiration. Ninety percent of patients with significant pulmonary aspiration have symptoms within 1 hour, and almost all have symptoms within 2 hours. A pH determination of the aspirated material can be used to predict the severity of pulmonary damage.

Risk Assessment

Pulmonary aspiration occurs in 1 to 10 of 10,000 pediatric anesthetics. Pediatric patients may have a higher incidence of pulmonary aspiration associated with a greater risk of severe pulmonary damage compared with adults; however, the anesthesia literature is conflicting. Pediatric patients have some unique risks for pulmonary aspiration (Table 158-1) compared with adults (Table 158-2).

Although the critical pH and volume of gastric contents that place a child at risk for aspiration are unknown, based

on an extrapolation of unpublished experimental data in rhesus monkeys, the thresholds for gastric pH (<2.5) and residual gastric volume (>0.4 mL/kg) have been applied to humans. Based on these limits, the risk of pulmonary aspiration would be increased in children compared with adults, because 76% of pediatric patients have gastric contents whose pH is less than 2.5 and whose volume is greater than 0.4 mL/kg, versus 32% to 55% of adults who meet these criteria.

Infants are at highest risk for pulmonary aspiration. GERD occurs in almost 50% of term neonates and is considered normal for the first 6 months of life. GERD can occur with intragastric pressures as low as 23 cm H_2O. If the fundoesophageal angle decreases during tracheal intubation, GERD can occur at even lower intragastric pressures. Owing to a smaller stomach, air swallowing during crying, and diaphragmatic breathing, the resting intragastric pressure in infants is higher than in older children or adults, which contributes to an increased risk of GERD.

The incidence of pulmonary aspiration with laryngeal mask airways may not be higher when used in healthy patients having elective surgery. However, the laryngeal mask airway does not form a tight seal around the larynx. Further, it causes reflex relaxation of the lower esophageal sphincter secondary to pharyngeal muscle distention, as during swallowing of a food bolus. The laryngeal mask airway may also increase the likelihood of pulmonary aspiration by contributing to gastric distention during positive-pressure ventilation and directing regurgitated gastric contents into

---

Table 158–1 ■ Risk Factors for Pulmonary Aspiration Unique to Children

Transient pharyngeal weakness of the newborn
Tracheoesophageal fistula (gastrointestinal reflux common after repair)
Chronic pulmonary disease (asthma, croup, bronchopulmonary dysplasia, cystic fibrosis)
Prematurity
Cerebral palsy, developmental delay (swallowing dysfunction)
Acute gastric distention in pediatric trauma patients

Table 158–2 ■ **Risk Factors for Pulmonary Aspiration in Adults and Children**

ASA physical status III or IV
Surgery outside regular working hours*
Emergency surgery*
Obesity, ascites, large abdominal mass
Gastritis, history of ulcers
Autonomic neuropathy (familial, acquired)
Muscular disorders
Long-lasting general anesthetics
Vocal cord paralysis
Diabetes mellitus
Electrolyte, metabolic imbalance
Insufficient anesthetic depth
Airway difficulty
Preexisting gastroesophageal reflux disease
Esophageal and upper abdominal surgery
Elevated intracranial pressure
Degenerative neuropathies
Opioids, methylxanthines, β-agonists
Reduced level of consciousness
Laryngeal malfunction or spasm
Collagen vascular disease
Renal, pelvic, bladder, or uterine distention

*Increases risk by five- to sixfold.
ASA, American Society of Anesthesiologists.

the larynx. Consequently, children at high risk for aspiration should have their airways secured with endotracheal tubes.

Laryngeal competence, an important protective mechanism against pulmonary aspiration, is depressed by anesthetic induction agents, local anesthesia of the larynx and trachea, and greater than 50% concentrations of nitrous oxide. In adults, laryngeal competence is depressed for 2 to 8 hours after tracheal extubation, even in patients who appear alert. It is likely that a similar depression of laryngeal competence occurs in children. Depressed laryngeal competence is attributed to the mechanical effects of tracheal intubation and is distinct from residual anesthetic effects.

Implications

The occurrence and severity of pneumonitis depend more on gastric pH than on volume. Low-volume aspirates with a pH less than 1.8 result in severe pneumonitis, whereas volumes as high as 2 mL/kg with a pH greater than 2.5 produce minimal pulmonary damage.

Pulmonary aspiration leads to loss of the protective mucosal barrier of the trachea and major bronchi by causing edema and desquamation of epithelium. Damaged tissue is vulnerable to subsequent viral or bacterial infection. Highly acidic liquid aspirates produce pulmonary injury within 12 to 18 seconds and extensive atelectasis by 3 minutes. By 1 hour after pulmonary aspiration, pulmonary injury has progressed to bronchial epithelial degeneration, pulmonary edema, and hemorrhage. The consequent increased pulmonary capillary leak is followed by a neutrophil response. As a result of alveolar cell damage, fluid and protein move into the alveoli and interstitium and reduce pulmonary surfactant activity. Increased airway resistance and decreased pulmonary compliance due to reduced pulmonary surfactant activity lead to

severe hypoxia. Also, severe hypotension may occur due to a reduction in intravascular volume (from the transudation of fluid into the alveoli), along with impaired venous return caused by the high airway pressures required for adequate ventilation.

With particulate aspiration, hypoxemia occurs earlier and is more severe. Although fluid shifts are less extensive than with acidic liquid aspiration, there is a greater increase in arterial carbon dioxide tension and a greater decrease in arterial pH. Mortality with clinically significant pulmonary aspiration is 5% or less.

MANAGEMENT

Treatment includes immediate suctioning of the airway and administration of supplemental oxygen by nasal cannula or facemask. This is often sufficient, but tracheal intubation and mechanical ventilation may be required in severe cases.

Bronchopulmonary lavage is not recommended for acidic aspirates because damage to the lungs occurs within 12 to 18 seconds. In addition, more extensive pulmonary damage may occur due to the spread of acidic aspirates to lower regions of the lung.

An immediate danger of particulate aspiration is mechanical obstruction. Bronchoscopy to remove particulate material should be performed in this situation. Corticosteroids have not been shown to reduce morbidity or mortality after pulmonary aspiration and are not advised, because they can predispose the patient to gram-negative pneumonia.

Antibiotics should be administered according to the results of cultures of tracheal aspirates. Empirical use is reserved for patients who have aspirated grossly contaminated material (e.g., feces, pus). Leukocytosis, pulmonary infiltrates, thick sputum, and fever are all nonspecific responses to chemical pneumonitis and are not sufficient reasons to institute antibiotic therapy. Postural drainage and respiratory therapy with bronchodilators may be useful. Most patients have resolution of clinical symptoms within 2 weeks.

PREVENTION

Prevention and amelioration of pulmonary aspiration rely on the use of conventional antacids and drugs that promote gastric emptying and increase lower esophageal sphincter tone (prokinetic agents), reduce gastric volume (H_2-blockers), or increase the pH of the gastric contents (H_2-blockers, proton pump inhibitors). Doses, schedules, and principal actions of these agents are summarized in Table 158-3.

There are well-defined fasting guidelines for healthy children undergoing surgery or procedures requiring anesthesia (Table 158-4). There are no published fasting guidelines for children considered to be at increased risk for pulmonary aspiration. Removal of gastric contents before induction is recommended for these patients. If gastric suctioning is not possible preoperatively, the gastric contents should be suctioned immediately after the airway has been secured after rapid-sequence induction to reduce the risk of pulmonary aspiration during emergence from anesthesia and extubation.

Table 158–3 ■ Pharmacologic Agents Used for the Prophylaxis of Pulmonary Aspiration

Drug	Dose and Schedule	GV	pH	LEST
Antacids				
Alka-Seltzer	2 tbsp/30 mL water (1 hr BS)	↑	↑	0
Sodium citrate	0.5-1 mL/kg (30 mL max; 1 hr BS)	↑	↑	0
Anticholinergics				
Glycopyrrolate	7.5-10 µg/kg (1 hr BS)	?	?	0
H₂ Blockers				
Cimetidine	7.5 mg/kg (PM/AM)	↓	↑	0
Famotidine	0.5 mg/kg (PM/AM)	↓	↑	0
Ranitidine	1.5-2 mg/kg (1-2 hr BS)	0	↑	0
Prokinetic Agents				
Metoclopramide	0.1 mg/kg IV or PO (1 hr BS)	↓	0	↑
Proton Pump Inhibitors				
Lansoprazole	1.5 mg/kg (PM/AM)	↓	↑	0
Omeprazole	0.3 mg/kg (PM/AM)	↓	↑	0
Pantoprazole	1.4 mg/kg QID	↓	↑	0

BS, before surgery; GV, gastric volume; LEST, lower esophageal sphincter tone; PM/AM, night before and morning of surgery.

To prevent regurgitation, rapid-sequence induction is used to minimize the vulnerable period between loss of consciousness and securing of the airway. Cricoid pressure is an integral part of rapid-sequence induction. Cricoid pressure, with or without the presence of a nasogastric tube, is an effective means of preventing passive regurgitation of gastric fluids in infants, children, and adults. Cricoid pressure with a force of 20 newtons (equivalent to a 2-kg mass acted on by the force of gravity) must be applied before the loss of consciousness. This amount of pressure is uncomfortable for awake patients. Loss of upper esophageal barrier pressure occurs before loss of consciousness in all age groups after the intravenous induction of anesthesia. The force of cricoid

Table 158–4 ■ Fasting Guidelines for Healthy Children Undergoing Elective Procedures

Age	Solids	Clear Liquids*	Formula
0-6 mo	6 hr	2 hr	6 hr
6 mo-2 yr	6 hr	2 hr	6 hr
>2 yr	6 hr (light meal)†	2 hr	NA
>2 yr (chubby or obese)	8 hr	2 hr	NA

*Some consider breast milk to be a clear liquid.
†By American Society of Anesthesiologists guidelines, a light meal typically consists of toast and clear liquids. Meals that include fried or fatty foods or meat may prolong gastric emptying time. Both the amount and type of foods ingested must be considered when determining an appropriate fasting period.

NA, not applicable.

pressure should be increased to 40 newtons (which is painful for awake patients) with unconsciousness. Higher pressures may distort or occlude the trachea. Cricoid pressure during active vomiting has the potential to cause esophageal rupture.

Most episodes of aspiration during induction begin with coughing or gagging during airway manipulation as a result of inadequate anesthesia or the absence of muscle relaxation. Ensuring complete muscle relaxation before laryngoscopy reduces the likelihood of regurgitation. The use of cuffed endotracheal tubes in children during prolonged intubation (e.g., intensive care unit patients) has led to a reduction in the incidence of silent aspiration from passive regurgitation.

In patients at high risk for pulmonary aspiration, extubation should be performed only when the patient is fully awake and has full return of neuromuscular function. Children should demonstrate mouth opening, hip flexion, and return of the sucking, cough, and gag reflexes. Patients should be in the lateral, 10- to 15-degree head-down (Trendelenburg) position so that any secretions or regurgitant material can accumulate in the cheek and drain passively. Finally, the application of 15 to 20 cm H₂O positive end-expiratory pressure immediately before extubation induces a reflex cough, which pushes secretions or materials away from the larynx.

Further Reading

Borland LM, Woelfel SK, Saitz EW, et al: Pulmonary aspiration in pediatric patients under general anesthesia: Frequency and outcome. Anesthesiology 83:A1150, 1995.
Coté CJ, Goudsouzian NG, Liu LMP, et al: Assessment of risk factors related to the acid aspiration syndrome in pediatric patients: Gastric pH and residual volume. Anesthesiology 56:70-72, 1982.
Goudsouzian N: Aspiration in children: Practical implications. Anesthesiol Rev 11:6-16, 1984.
James CF: Pulmonary aspiration of gastric contents. In Gravenstein N, Kirby RR (eds): Complications in Anesthesiology. Philadelphia, Lippincott-Raven, 1996, pp 175-190.
Orenstein DM: Aspiration pneumonias and gastroesophageal reflux-related respiratory disease. In Behrman RE, Kliegman RM, Arvin AM (eds): Nelson's Textbook of Pediatrics. Philadelphia, WB Saunders, 1996, pp 1213-1217.
Salem MR, Wong AY, Fizzotti GF, et al: Efficacy of cricoid pressure in preventing aspiration of gastric contents in paediatric patients. Br J Anaesth 44:401-404, 1972.
Warner MA, Warner ME, Warner DO, et al: Perioperative pulmonary aspiration in infants and children. Anesthesiology 90:66-71, 1999.

PEDIATRICS & NEONATOLOGY

159

Postoperative Nausea and Vomiting

Senthilkumar Sadhasivam and Mehernoor F. Watcha

Case Synopsis

A 14-year-old, postpubertal girl with a history of motion sickness is scheduled for adenotonsillectomy. This will be her third surgery under general anesthesia. She had multiple episodes of postoperative nausea and vomiting (PONV) after the two previous procedures (dental rehabilitation, correction of strabismus), despite receiving intraoperative, prophylactic antiemetic therapy. Following the strabismus surgery, she was hospitalized with dehydration caused by refractory postoperative emesis. Both she and her parents are extremely anxious and wish to avoid a similar experience. They ask what can be done to prevent PONV.

PROBLEM ANALYSIS

Definition

Nausea, vomiting, and retching are common postanesthetic complications that may be considered relatively minor by some physicians. Patients, however, report that these sequelae are sometimes more debilitating than the surgery itself and the postoperative pain.

Recognition

The overall incidence of PONV in many large pediatric studies is about 10% in the postanesthesia care unit (PACU) and 20% to 30% within the first 24 hours. However, rates of 40% to 80% have been reported in some high-risk groups. Recurrent emesis occurs in 0.1% of patients, and unanticipated hospital admission is required in 0.03% (1 in 3000).

Risk Assessment

Patient-, anesthesia-, and surgery-related risk factors for PONV have been identified in adults and children (Table 159-1). However, the accuracy of proposed scoring systems for predicting which patients will develop PONV is 70% at best. The most important factors are patient gender, a history of prior PONV, nonsmoking status,[1] and opioid use. Some patient- and surgery-related factors are beyond the anesthesiologist's control. However, some strategies can be used to reduce the baseline risk (Table 159-2). Foremost among these are restricted use of perioperative opioids, infiltration of the surgical wound with local anesthetics, use of nonsteroidal anti-inflammatory drugs and acetaminophen, avoidance of nitrous oxide (N_2O) and high-dose neostigmine, and adequate hydration. Use of high concentrations of oxygen during the perioperative period helps reduce PONV in some but not all patient populations.

[1]This raises the question why nicotine patches are not used for the prevention of PONV.

Implications

Severe PONV causes patient discomfort and dissatisfaction and may also be associated with the following:

- Tension on suture lines
- Wound dehiscence and surgical bleeding
- Muscle fatigue and pulmonary aspiration of gastric contents
- Dehydration and electrolyte imbalance
- Increased intracranial and intraocular pressures
- Prolonged PACU stays
- Unanticipated hospital admission following ambulatory surgery
- Increased costs of anesthesia care
- Increased use of health care personnel and hospital resources

Although no anesthetics or other substances are known to act directly on the emetic center (located in the lateral reticular formation of the brainstem), it does receive stimuli from the pharynx, gastrointestinal tract, mediastinum, and afferent nerves from higher brain centers (Fig. 159-1), including the cortical visual center and the chemoreceptor trigger zone in the area postrema, as well as input from the vestibular portion of the eighth cranial nerve.

There is no blood-brain barrier in the chemoreceptor trigger zone. Therefore, chemicals, drugs, and other substances found in the cerebrospinal fluid or blood can activate it. The chemoreceptor trigger zone is rich in dopamine, serotonin (5-hydroxytryptamine$_3$ [5-HT$_3$]), opioid, histamine, and muscarinic receptors. Blockade of these may be an important mechanism of action for antiemetics. Finally, there is also evidence that neurokinin-1 receptors are involved in the final common pathway of the emetic response.

MANAGEMENT

There are far fewer studies on the management of PONV in the PACU than on its prevention (see later). The choice of drugs to treat PONV depends on which prophylactic antiemetics were used (Table 159-3). In general, patients should not

Table 159–1 ▪ Risk Factors for Postoperative Nausea and Vomiting

Adult Patients

Patient-specific risk factors
   Female sex*
   Nonsmoking status*
   History of PONV*
   History of motion sickness*
   Delayed gastric emptying
   Preoperative anxiety
Anesthetic and PACU risk factors
   Volatile anesthetics
   Nitrous oxide
   Intraoperative and postoperative opioids*
   Neostigmine
   Preanesthetic medication
   Gastric distention
   Duration of anesthesia
   Mandatory fluids by mouth before discharge
Surgical risk factors
   Longer duration of surgery
   High-risk surgery
      Laparoscopy
      Ear, nose, or throat surgery
      Neurosurgery
      Laparotomy
      Breast, strabismus, or plastic surgery

Pediatric Patients

Vomiting incidence twice that of adults
Risk increases as children age; decreases after puberty
Sex differences not applicable before puberty
Risk increases with specific pediatric procedures
   Adenotonsillectomy
   Strabismus repair
   Hernia repair
   Orchiopexy
   Penile surgery

*Major risk factor.
PACU, postanesthesia care unit.
Modified from Gan TJ, Meyer T, Apfel CC, et al: Department of Anesthesiology DUMC: Consensus guidelines for managing postoperative nausea and vomiting. Anesth Analg 97:62-71, 2003.

Table 159–2 ▪ Strategies to Reduce Baseline Risk for Postoperative Nausea and Vomiting

Use regional anesthesia whenever feasible
Use propofol for induction and maintenance of general anesthesia
Use intraoperative supplemental oxygen
Ensure adequate patient hydration
Avoid use of nitrous oxide
Avoid use of volatile inhalational anesthetics
Minimize use of intra- and postoperative opioids
Minimize use of neostigmine

Modified from Gan TJ, Meyer T, Apfel CC, et al: Department of Anesthesiology DUMC: Consensus guidelines for managing postoperative nausea and vomiting. Anesth Analg 97:62-71, 2003.

receive a repeat dose of the same drug used for prophylaxis; they should receive one that acts at a different receptor site. In patients who were perceived to be at low risk and did not receive any prophylactic antiemetics, a low dose of a 5-HT₃ antagonist (e.g., ondansetron 1 mg) can provide excellent control of symptoms for up to 24 hours. Data suggest that a second dose of a 5-HT₃ antagonist for PONV in patients who failed prophylaxis is no more effective than placebo; however, the PONV consensus guidelines (discussed later) do allow a second dose of ondansetron to be given at least 6 hours after a prophylactic dose. A second dose of dexamethasone or transdermal scopolamine should not be given to patients who failed prophylaxis with these drugs. Figure 159-2 presents an algorithm for the prophylaxis and management of PONV.

PREVENTION

Consensus Guidelines

The literature is filled with numerous reports claiming that a particular intervention has statistically significant efficacy for reducing PONV versus placebo. However, the magnitude of effect is inconsistent, and many studies can be criticized for being underpowered or failing to standardize the perioperative regimen. Systematic reviews show that no single drug has sufficient efficacy to be considered a gold standard for PONV prevention. The relatively poor efficacy of antiemetics for preventing PONV has cast doubt on the benefit of using them prophylactically.

With no adequately powered trials to resolve this controversy, a multidisciplinary panel examined the available literature to provide consensus guidelines for PONV management. The panel focused on identifying primary PONV risk factors in adults and children; determined how to reduce the baseline risks for PONV; and then made recommendations regarding the optimal choice, timing, and efficacy of mono- or combined

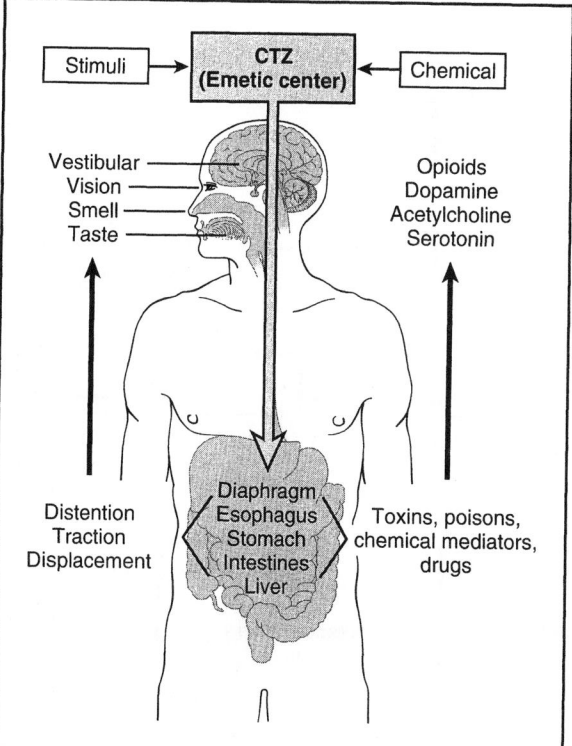

Figure 159–1 ▪ Physiology of emesis. *Solid arrows* represent afferent input; *shaded arrow* points to efferent targets. CTZ, chemoreceptor trigger zone.

Table 159–3 ■ Drugs Used as Prophylaxis for Postoperative Nausea and Vomiting in Children

Class/Drug	Dose (Route)	Preferred Time of Administration	Relative Efficacy	Common Adverse Effects
Anticholinergic				
Scopolamine	1–1.5 mg q72h (transdermal patch)	Previous night	++	Sedation, dry mouth, visual disturbances, dysphoria, hallucinations
Antihistamines				
Dimenhydrinate	0.5 mg/kg (IV)	15-20 min before end of surgery	+++	Less sedation, extrapyramidal effects, dry mouth and restlessness (anticholinergic side effects)
Diphenhydramine	0.5 mg/kg (IV)	15-20 min before end of surgery	++++	More sedation, extrapyramidal effects, dry mouth and restlessness (anticholinergic side effects)
Corticosteroid				
Dexamethasone	0.15 mg/kg, but ≤10 mg total (IV)	Induction of anesthesia	+++	Cutaneous flushing, perineal itching
Dopamine Antagonists				
Droperidol	50–75 µg/kg up to 1.25 mg (IV)		++++	Drowsiness, sedation, extrapyramidal effects
Metoclopramide	0.1–0.25 mg/kg (IV)	15-20 min before end of surgery	++	Sedation, extrapyramidal effects
Perphenazine	70 µg/kg (IV)	Data unavailable	++++	Extrapyramidal effects, sedation (< promethazine)
Promethazine	0.5–1 mg/kg (IV/IM)	Data unavailable	++++	Sedation (> perphenazine), extrapyramidal effects
5-Hydroxytryptamine₃ Receptor Antagonists				
Dolasetron	350 µg/kg up to 12.5 mg (IV)	15-20 min before end of surgery	++++	Headache, dizziness
Granisetron	0.04 mg/kg (IV)	15-20 min before end of surgery	++++	Headache, abdominal pain, constipation, dizziness
Ondansetron	50–100 µg/kg up to 4 mg (IV)	15-20 min before end of surgery	++++	Headache, abdominal pain, constipation, dizziness

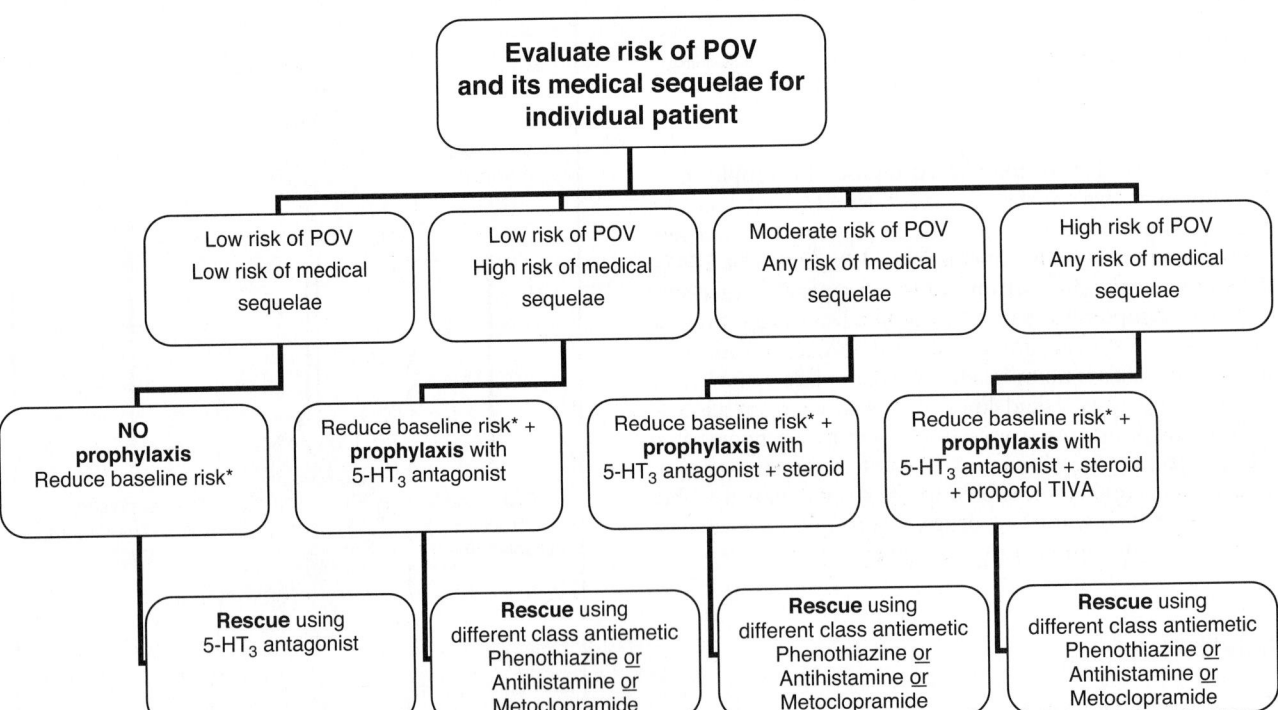

Figure 159–2 ■ Algorithm for the prophylaxis and treatment of postoperative vomiting (POV) in children. *See Table 159-2; 5-HT₃, 5-hydroxytryptamine₃; TIVA, total intravenous anesthesia. (Modified from Gan TJ, Meyer T, Apfel CC, et al: Department of Anesthesiology DUMC: Consensus guidelines for managing postoperative nausea and vomiting. Anesth Analg 97:62-71, 2003.)

therapy for PONV prophylaxis and treatment in low-, moderate-, and high-risk patients (see Table 159-3). There was early consensus that low-risk patients should not receive prophylaxis and that those at high risk should receive multimodal prophylaxis. However, consensus could not be reached on the baseline risk that would qualify patients for these two categories.

Perioperative Prevention

PREANESTHETIC SEDATION

Opioid premedication (any route of administration) increases the risk for emesis. Benzodiazepine premedication may reduce this risk.

INDUCTION

Inhalation induction with diethyl ether and cyclopropane increases the incidence of PONV. The incidence is much lower with halothane, isoflurane, sevoflurane, or desflurane. Induction with ketamine or etomidate also increases the risk for PONV, whereas propofol reduces it. The latter's effect is of short duration and is more pronounced when propofol is used for both induction and maintenance of anesthesia. Low-dose propofol infusions have been used for refractory PONV in the PACU, but the antiemetic action is short-lived, and the mechanism remains unknown.

NITROUS OXIDE

There is now good evidence (human volunteers) that N_2O is associated with PONV. Although N_2O omission appears to have no effect on early or late postoperative nausea, it does reduce early and late vomiting if the patient's baseline risk is high.

OPIOID AVOIDANCE

The method of postoperative pain management has important implications for reducing the incidence of PONV, because both pain and opioids increase it. Even a single dose of morphine is associated with an increased risk for PONV. Regional nerve blocks, nonsteroidal anti-inflammatory drugs (e.g., ketorolac, high-dose acetaminophen), and local anesthetic wound infiltration reduce postoperative opioid analgesic requirements and PONV.

NURSING PROTOCOLS

Nursing protocols are known to affect PONV. Frequent changes in position (e.g., from supine to sitting upright to walking) in children who have received opioids increase the likelihood of PONV. Thus, gentle handling and the avoidance of rapid positional changes are essential. In addition, the insistence that patients take fluids by mouth before being discharged from the day surgery center increases the likelihood of PONV. If children are permitted, but not required, to drink before discharge, the incidence of in-hospital emesis is reduced.

REVERSAL OF NEUROMUSCULAR BLOCKADE

Antagonism of residual neuromuscular blockade is often routine because of concerns about respiratory compromise.

Anticholinesterase therapy (e.g., neostigmine) has gastrointestinal muscarinic actions that contribute to increased emesis; this effect is dose related (>2.5 mg of neostigmine). Giving atropine (rather than glycopyrrolate) with neostigmine or edrophonium reduces PONV. With the use of neuromuscular relaxants such as mivacurium, routine antagonism of neuromuscular blockade is avoided. However, avoidance of neostigmine after the use of intermediate-acting muscle relaxants (e.g., vecuronium, rocuronium, cisatracurium) can be associated with residual blockade in more than 70% of neuromuscular receptors, with the associated potential for respiratory compromise.

PROPHYLACTIC ANTIEMETIC ADMINISTRATION

Drugs used for PONV prophylaxis in children are listed in Table 159-3, along with their relative efficacy, dosages, preferred times and routes of administration, and adverse effects. Although ondansetron and other 5-HT$_3$ antagonists are very effective against PONV, their high cost prohibits their use for routine prophylactic antiemetic therapy in many centers. Older drugs such as prochlorperazine, dimenhydrinate, and promethazine are similarly effective but have the potential for central nervous system side effects, such as drowsiness.

In adults, low-dose droperidol (0.625 to 1.25 mg) is as effective as ondansetron 4 mg against PONV, and it does not cause excessive drowsiness. However, many no longer consider it to be a first-line prophylactic antiemetic owing to its potential to cause Q-Tc prolongation, torsades de pointes, and sudden death (see Chapter 81). The associated medicolegal implications after a "black box" warning by the U.S. Food and Drug Administration (2001) led many institutions to remove this clinically effective and cheap antiemetic from their formularies. Experts who examined the data on which the FDA based its advisory have raised major concerns about the justification of this warning.

In patients at low risk for PONV, the use of prophylactic antiemetics is not cost-effective and exposes patients to the risk of adverse side effects for little or no benefit. For the few low-risk patients who do develop PONV, a low-dose 5-HT$_3$ antagonist (e.g.,1 mg ondansetron) is effective.

Patients at high and moderate risk for PONV should receive prophylactic antiemetic therapy, along with baseline risk-reduction strategies (see Table 159-2). For those at moderate risk for PONV, the optimal cost-effective approach differs for ambulatory patients and hospital inpatients. For the former, PONV prophylaxis with single or combined drugs is cost-effective. Evidence suggests that a 5-HT$_3$ antagonist and a steroid provide excellent prophylaxis for the moderate- to high-risk group. Such combinations had been avoided until recently owing to concerns about enhanced adverse central nervous system effects (e.g., delayed emergence, drowsiness, extrapyramidal reactions).

The ongoing debate on the relative merits of one antiemetic versus another may be irrelevant for patients at high risk for PONV. Data now suggest that combinations are more effective than any one antiemetic alone. In high-risk patients, a multimodal approach with double or even triple antiemetic combinations should be used. In one recent trial, multimodal prophylaxis resulted in a 98% complete response rate and a 0% incidence of vomiting before discharge.

PEDIATRICS & NEONATOLOGY

CONCLUSIONS

Based on our current knowledge about the factors affecting PONV, the following is a reasonable approach for the patient described in the case synopsis:

- Preanesthetic anxiolysis with midazolam
- Total intravenous anesthesia with propofol (induction and maintenance)
- Avoidance of N_2O and potent inhalational anesthetics
- Avoidance of neostigmine antagonism of nondepolarizing neuromuscular blockade
- No or minimal opioids; instead, use high-dose preoperative acetaminophen (40 mg/kg per rectum), local anesthetics, nonsteroidal anti-inflammatory drugs, and nerve blocks
- Avoidance of patient movement in the PACU
- Use of liberal perioperative intravenous fluids to replace fluid deficits, and discharge to home without insisting that the patient first drink fluids
- Administration of dexamethasone at the induction of anesthesia and ondansetron or another serotonin antagonist at the end of the adenotonsillectomy
- Early and aggressive treatment of PONV with an antiemetic from another class (e.g., antihistamine, phenothiazine)

Further Reading

Apfel CC, Korttila K, Abdalla M, et al: An international multicenter protocol to assess the single and combined benefits of antiemetic interventions in a controlled clinical trial of a 2x2x2x2x2x2 factorial design (IMPACT). Control Clin Trials 24:736-751, 2003.

Apfel CC, Korttila K, Abdalla M, et al: A factorial trial of six interventions for the prevention of postoperative nausea and vomiting. N Engl J Med 350:2441-2451, 2004.

D'Errico C, Voepel-Lewis TD, Siewert M, et al: Prolonged recovery stay and unplanned admission of the pediatric surgical outpatient: An observational study. J Clin Anesth 10:482-487, 1998.

Gan TJ, Meyer T, Apfel CC, et al: Department of Anesthesiology DUMC: Consensus guidelines for managing postoperative nausea and vomiting. Anesth Analg 97:62-71, 2003.

Gold BS, Kitz DS, Lecky JH, et al: Unanticipated admission to the hospital following ambulatory surgery. JAMA 262:3008-3010, 1989.

Scuderi PE, James RL, Harris L, et al: Multimodal antiemetic management prevents early postoperative vomiting after outpatient laparoscopy. Anesth Analg 91:1408-1414, 2000.

Tramer MR: A rational approach to the control of postoperative nausea and vomiting: Evidence from systematic reviews. Part I. Efficacy and harm of antiemetic interventions, and methodological issues. Acta Anaesthesiol Scand 45:4-13, 2001.

Tramer MR: A rational approach to the control of postoperative nausea and vomiting: Evidence from systematic reviews. Part II. Recommendations for prevention and treatment, and research agenda. Acta Anaesthesiol Scand 45:14-19, 2001.

Watcha MF: Postoperative nausea and emesis. Anesthesiol Clin North Am 20:709-722, 2002.

Watcha MF, White PF: Postoperative nausea and vomiting: Its etiology, treatment, and prevention. Anesthesiology 77:162-184, 1992.

White PF, Watcha MF: Postoperative nausea and vomiting: Prophylaxis versus treatment. Anesth Analg 89:1337-1339, 1999.

Upper Respiratory Tract Infection

160

Arjunan Ganesh, Susan C. Nicolson, and James M. Steven

Case Synopsis

A 4-year-old girl has a history of frequent upper respiratory infections (URIs). Following the resolution of symptoms from her most recent URI 10 days ago, she undergoes elective tonsillectomy and adenoidectomy. During induction of anesthesia with mask sevoflurane, laryngospasm occurs.

PROBLEM ANALYSIS

Definition

There is conflicting information regarding the outcome for children with active URIs who undergo anesthesia for elective surgical procedures. Some studies suggest that children with URIs are at increased risk for perioperative respiratory complications; others indicate that they have no increased risk (Table 160-1). Increased mortality has not been demonstrated in any controlled study. Study design flaws that prevent clinicians from drawing conclusions regarding the risk-benefit ratio of anesthetizing children with URIs include one of more of the following:

- Mostly retrospective data acquisition
- Absence of well-defined criteria for URI
- Heterogeneous group of children with regard to age, type of surgery, and anesthetic technique
- Nonuniform definition and reporting of adverse patient occurrences
- Preselection bias

Retrospective data indicate that children with recent URIs (within 2 to 6 weeks of anesthesia and surgery) have an increased risk of respiratory complications compared with those without recent URIs. The clinical impact of upper airway or pulmonary complications (see Table 160-1) also influences the decision to cancel surgery or proceed with anesthesia. For example, is an increased incidence of laryngospasm likely to be associated with a poor outcome, or can it be recognized and reversed early enough to prevent such an outcome?

A recent prospective study suggested that although children with acute or recent URIs have a greater risk of respiratory complications, most of them can undergo elective procedures without a significant increase in adverse anesthetic outcomes. However, this study was not randomized, and the decision whether to proceed was left to the discretion of the attending anesthesiologist. Common reasons for cancellation were severe URI, the presence of a lower respiratory tract infection, or bacterial infection.

Recognition

At least two of the following signs and symptoms must exist for a child to have a URI:

1. Sore or scratchy throat
2. Sneezing
3. Rhinorrhea
4. Congestion
5. Nonproductive cough
6. Fever less than 38.5°C
7. Laryngitis

Combination of items 1 and 5, 2 and 3, 3 and 6, and 4 and 6 require the presence of at least one additional symptom to meet the criteria for a URI. Children with fever greater than 38.5°C and constitutional symptoms or signs of lower respiratory tract involvement do not have a simple URI; their ailment extends beyond localized involvement within the upper respiratory tract.

Risk Assessment

The following caveats apply to the risk of anesthesia and surgery in children with URIs:

- Children suffer five to eight URIs per year, with higher incidences for those in day care and whose parents smoke.
- Of pediatric anesthesia and surgery candidates, 6% present with active URIs.
- Pulmonary changes may last 4 to 7 weeks after the resolution of URI symptoms.
- The phase of the URI (onset, active, resolution) may influence the anesthesia risk.
- The type of surgery, the child's age, the anesthetic plan (e.g., intubation), and coexisting medical conditions can affect outcome.

Table 160–1 ■ **Incidence of Upper Airway and Pulmonary Complications in Children with Upper Respiratory Infection Undergoing General Anesthesia**

Outcome Measure	URI Status (%)			Number	Intubated	Study Design
	Active	*Recent*	*None*			
Airway obstruction*	1.6	5.3	1.6	3585	Most	R
Laryngospasm	1.3	2.4	1.2	489	None	P
Bronchospasm	13.3		0.6	402	Half	P
Croup	3.8		0.7	22,159	Some	P
Hypoxemia	32	25	10	130	None	P
	40		16	402	Half	P
	20		0	50	Most	P

*Includes laryngospasm and bronchospasm.
P, prospective; R, retrospective; URI, upper respiratory infection.

Implications

Potential URI-related respiratory complications related to increased secretions or irritable airways are as follows:

- Laryngospasm (additional risk factors include young age, surgery on or within the airway, and an inexperienced anesthetist)
- Bronchospasm (intubated patients only)
- Postextubation stridor
- Perioperative arterial oxygen desaturation

Factors that affect the cost of these complications include a prolonged day-surgery stay, unexpected admission of an outpatient, unexpected admission to an intensive care unit, and medicolegal issues raised by URI-related respiratory complications.

Costs of cancellation include those related to the need for an additional presurgery appointment, repeated laboratory testing or chest radiographs (if necessary), lost revenue from inefficient operating room use with short-notice cancellation, inconvenience to patient and family, and lost income to family.

MANAGEMENT

When evaluating the potential for URI-related complications, be aware that not all patients are the same. When making a decision whether to proceed with anesthesia and surgery, take the following into consideration:

- Age of the child
- Frequency of URIs (both in the individual and in age-matched controls)
- Nature and urgency of surgery (e.g., is the procedure intended to alleviate or reduce the frequency of chronic nasal congestion or recurrent ear infections?)
- Coexisting medical problems
- Anesthesiologist's skill and experience
- Miscellaneous issues (e.g., availability of surgeon, designated or autologous blood)
- Attitude of parents

If a decision is made to proceed, document on the chart that the risks have been discussed with the surgeon and the family and that everyone has agreed to proceed. Then formulate an anesthetic plan that gives consideration to the following:

- Preoperative administration of an anticholinergic agent (e.g., atropine, ipratropium nebulization)
- Use of bronchodilators for bronchospasm
- Use of smaller endotracheal tubes, laryngeal mask airways, or mask anesthesia
- Monitoring for arterial oxygen saturation intra- and postoperatively, and administering oxygen-enriched gas mixtures or supplemental oxygen when appropriate

PREVENTION

Many preschool and early school-age children have or are recovering from a URI at any given time. Thus, it is impossible to postpone surgery for all children with URIs until 4 to 6 weeks after resolution of their symptoms. Such a strategy would lead to many children having a very narrow window for surgical intervention, or even none at all. Sound clinical judgment, documented informed consent, and experience of the anesthesiologist are important factors in deciding whether to proceed with an individual case.

Further Reading

Cohen MM, Cameron CB: Should you cancel the operation when a child has an upper respiratory tract infection? Anesth Analg 72:282-288, 1991.

Coté CJ: The upper respiratory tract infection (URI) dilemma: Fear of a complication or litigation? Anesthesiology 95:283-285, 2001.

Rolf N, Coté CJ: Frequency and severity of desaturation events during general anesthesia in children with and without upper respiratory infections. J Clin Anesth 4:200-203, 1992.

Schreiner MS, O'Hara IB, Markakis DA, et al: Do children who experience laryngospasm have an increased risk of upper respiratory tract infection? Anesthesiology 85:475-489, 1996.

Tait AR, Knight PR: The effects of general anesthesia on upper respiratory tract infection in children. Anesthesiology 67:930-935, 1987.

Tait AR, Knight PR: Intraoperative respiratory complications in patients with upper respiratory tract infection. Can J Anaesth 34:300-303, 1987.

Tait AR, Malviya S, Voepel-Lewis T, et al: Risk factors for perioperative adverse respiratory events in children with upper respiratory tract infections. Anesthesiology 95:299-306, 2001.

Latex Allergy

Lucille A. Mostello

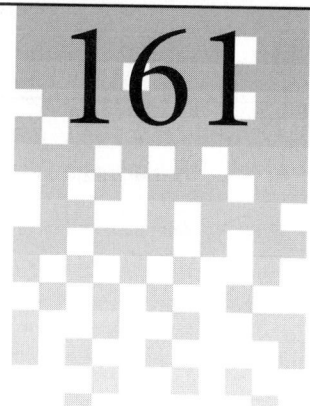

161

Case Synopsis

A 16-year-old boy with cerebral palsy is undergoing lengthening of an Achilles tendon. He has had 15 previous operations without complications. Thirty minutes after anesthetic induction, there is sudden hypotension along with bronchospasm.

PROBLEM ANALYSIS

Definition

Latex allergy is an immediate (type I) hypersensitivity reaction to the milky sap of cultured rubber trees *(Hevea brasiliensis)*. With type I reactions, antigen enters the body to promote the genesis of immunoglobulin E (IgE) antibodies, which attach to mast cells. With subsequent exposures, the antigen bridges two mast cell IgE antibodies to initiate a biphasic reaction. In phase 1, preformed substances from intracellular granules (mostly histamine) are released. In phase 2, potent arachidonic acid metabolites (leukotrienes, prostaglandins) are generated. These cytokines act as catalysts to involve other cells and to activate kinin and complement systems to cause bronchoconstriction, vasodilatation, increased vascular permeability, and mucosal edema.

Latex is the organic raw material for natural rubber products. Its proteins and polypeptides, but not its polymer backbone *(cis-1,4-polyisoprene)*, are antigens. Other untoward reactions are due to residual chemicals from the rubber manufacturing process. Both irritation and contact dermatitis (type IV, or cell-mediated delayed hypersensitivity) are localized, uncomfortable, and deforming but not life threatening. They should not be confused with type I hypersensitivity to latex proteins (see also Chapters 27 and 53).

Recognition

The manifestations of anaphylaxis under anesthesia include the following:

- Hypotension or cardiovascular collapse (74% of cases)
- Bronchospasm or wheezing (44% of cases)
- Rash or urticaria (70% of cases)
- Angioedema and stridor (a small percentage of cases)

The quantity and route of antigen exposure, and an individual's sensitivity, partly determine the spectrum of manifestations. A patient's reaction may range from mild to severe and involve single or multiple organ systems. Unfortunately, in the operating room (OR), the first sign may be cardiovascular collapse because general anesthesia and surgical drapes obscure earlier indicators. The time from latex exposure to symptoms is unpredictable and can range from 5 to 150 minutes.

Over the past 15 years, latex allergy has become an important issue for pediatric patients and their health care providers. In the late 1980s one hospital reported a 500-fold increase in intraoperative anaphylaxis among patients with spina bifida. In the early 1990s surveys from France and Belgium found that latex was the predominant cause of anaphylaxis during pediatric surgery (Fig. 161-1), in striking contrast to adults. Today, anaphylaxis in spina bifida patients has been reduced markedly, but severe reactions still occur in other high-risk patient groups.

Risk Assessment

Several subsets of children have higher sensitization rates than in the general population (estimated at 1%). Children at risk include those with the following:

- Spina bifida (15% to 67% sensitization)
- Multiple surgeries, especially operations during infancy (25% to 55% sensitization)
- Urogenital malformations, particularly bladder exstrophy (70% sensitization)
- Fruit allergy (e.g., banana, kiwi, avocado, chestnut), atopy, or multiple allergies

Occupational exposure is the predominant risk factor in adults.

For children with spina bifida (many of whom survive to adulthood), the high prevalence of antibodies has been postulated to be due to repeated latex exposure during surgery, urinary catheterization, and fecal disimpaction. Children who have undergone multiple surgeries for congenital defects, especially in infancy, now account for a large proportion of recent cases of intraoperative latex anaphylaxis. Latex antibodies can cross-react with an increasing list of fruits that have antigens similar to latex proteins. The presence of atopy or multiple allergies in other high-risk patient groups may increase sensitization or may be an independent risk factor.

Implications

In adults, the estimated mortality from perioperative anaphylaxis for all antigens is about 4%. The rate for children is unavailable but may be the same or less. If less, this could be due to immunologic immaturity or naiveté. Regardless, anaphylaxis is life threatening and may require interruption or postponement of surgery and intensive care for complete resolution. Preoperative identification of latex-allergic patients and latex avoidance can reduce morbidity rates.

MANAGEMENT

The treatment of anaphylaxis is as follows.

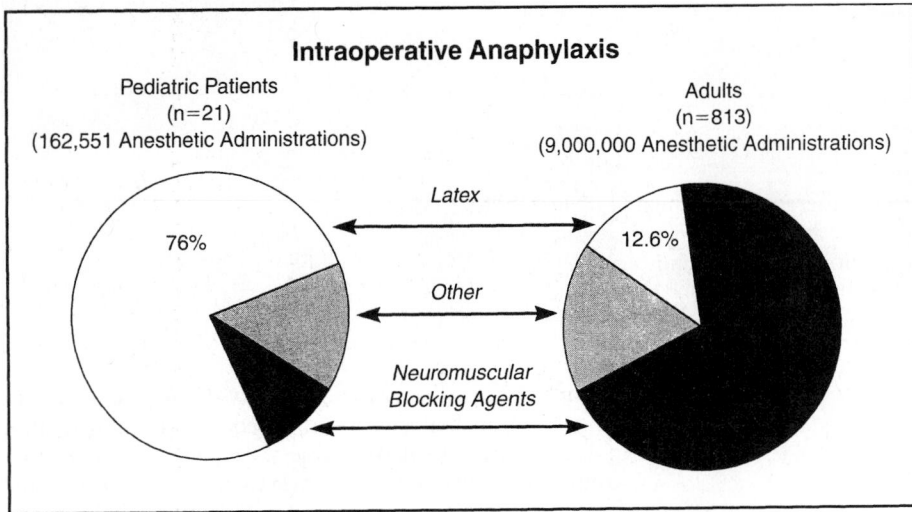

Figure 161–1 ▪ Graphic results of separate surveys on the causes of intraoperative anaphylaxis in children and adults conducted in France and Belgium between 1990 and 1992. They indicate that latex allergy is the most common cause of intraoperative anaphylaxis in children. (Pediatric data from Murat I: Anaphylactic reactions during paediatric anaesthesia: Results of a survey by the French Society of Paediatric Anaesthetists 1991-1992. Paediatr Anaesth 3:339-343, 1993. Adult data (1990-1991) from Laxenaire MC, Mouton C, Moneret-Vautrin DA, et al: Drugs and other agents involved in anaphylactic shock occurring during anaesthesia: A French multicenter epidemiological inquiry. Ann Fr Anesth Reanim 12:91-96, 1993.)

Primary

- Removal of the antigen
- Intravenous (IV) epinephrine bolus (1 to 10 μg/kg)
- Rapid IV volume expansion with a balanced salt solution (25 to 50 mL/kg)

Secondary

- Epinephrine infusion (0.05 to 0.1 μg/kg per minute)
- Inhaled β-adrenergic receptor agonist (e.g., 0.15 mg/kg albuterol)
- IV diphenhydramine 0.5 to 1 mg/kg slowly *plus* IV ranitidine 1 mg/kg slowly
- Corticosteroids (e.g., IV hydrocortisone 5 to 10 mg/kg)

Because latex is ubiquitous in OR settings, it is very difficult to remove all sources of the antigen. In addition to obvious latex sources such as gloves and Foley catheters, the anesthesiologist must be concerned about latex in IV administration sets, drug vial stoppers, syringe plungers, facemasks, and adhesive tape. Unseen is the aerosolized cornstarch that carries adsorbed latex antigens from powdered gloves in the OR and on the clothes of OR personnel.

The first line of therapy is IV epinephrine for vasoconstriction and specific reduction in the degranulation process. This is followed by massive IV fluid replacement. Higher epinephrine doses are needed if cardiovascular collapse has occurred. Additional pharmacologic therapy for bronchospasm and maintenance of vital organ perfusion is instituted secondarily. The role of antihistamines and corticosteroids has not been well documented.

To confirm the diagnosis:

- Send clotted blood for analysis to determine the serum tryptase level.
- Request consultation with a pediatric allergist or immunologist.
- Schedule antibody testing (immune globulins) 4 to 6 weeks after the event.

Serum tryptase is an excellent and stable marker of anaphylaxis and remains elevated for 1 to 4 hours following mast cell degranulation. Follow-up and testing are best managed by an allergist. Unfortunately, blood tests, such as the radioallergosorbent test, are not 100% sensitive. Currently, no standardized reagent for latex skin testing is commercially available in the United States. Because an anaphylactic episode can exhaust antibody stores, any testing should be delayed for 4 to 6 weeks. Even with latex antibodies, a complete evaluation is warranted because there may be concurrent allergies to other agents used intraoperatively.

PREVENTION

Crucial to identifying patients at increased risk for latex-related anaphylaxis is the screening of high-risk patients or subgroups. Ask *every* patient or parent about responses to latex products:

- Is there swelling or itching of the hands or other body parts after contact with rubber gloves, toys, or other rubber products?
- Is there swelling or itching of the lips or mouth after inflating balloons or dental examinations?
- Has a previous, unexplained anaphylactic reaction occurred?

Preoperative latex testing is reserved for patients who respond in the affirmative to any of these questions or are otherwise considered to be at high risk.

In addition, take the following steps to avoid latex-related reactions:

- Develop latex-avoidance protocols for high-risk patients (e.g., use latex-free or low-protein latex gloves rather than powdered latex gloves for surgery in infants).
- Ensure that latex-allergic patients wear Medic-Alert bracelets and that they have autoinjectable epinephrine available at home and at school.
- Keep parents and patients informed about latex exposure.

Because desensitization therapy is experimental at this time, avoidance is the most effective prevention. The incidence of anaphylaxis in the OR has been reduced by protocols for latex avoidance in spina bifida patients. However, providing a latex-safe environment ("latex precautions") is challenging, because the material is ubiquitous. It is an intimidating and sometimes impossible task to identify all latex-containing products, to substitute nonlatex items for those that contain latex, and to eliminate exposure to aerosolized latex or similar antigens. Technical advice is available from the support divisions of OR equipment and supply manufacturers. The U.S. Food and Drug Administration imposed labeling regulations in the fall of 1998, requiring all new medical equipment to denote its latex content.

Both parents and physicians can obtain useful information about latex content and possible substitutions of medical and nonmedical items from the Spina Bifida Association (1-800-621-3141) and on-line (http://latexallergylinks.tripod.com).

Prophylactic premedication remains controversial because severe latex reactions have occurred despite its use. Some clinicians believe that a regimen of drugs known to attenuate reactions to radiocontrast media may reduce the severity of latex reactions, especially in patients at very high risk who are undergoing critical surgical procedures. A protocol combining antihistamines (both H_1- and H_2-blockers) and corticosteroids is begun the day before anesthesia and surgery and continued on the first postoperative day. The drugs used and the timing of their administration vary among institutions. However, in an emergency, a single dose of each of these drugs can be given 1 hour before surgery. Some continue the regimen for 12 hours after the procedure. Again, a pediatric allergist or immunologist should be consulted.

Many institutions have protocols to prevent sensitization in children with spina bifida. From birth, no latex-containing items are used in the care of these patients. Whether other groups of children destined to undergo multiple surgeries, especially during infancy, should avoid latex-containing materials at home and in the hospital requires further evaluation. Some institutions now choose to be "latex-free" for the benefit of all patients and hospital personnel.

Further Reading

Hepner DL, Castells MC: Latex allergy: An update. Anesth Analg 96: 1219-1229, 2003.

Hollnberger H, Gruber E, Frank B: Severe anaphylactic shock without exanthema in a case of unknown latex allergy and review of the literature. Paediatr Anaesth 12:544-551, 2002.

Holzman RS: Latex allergy: An emerging operating room problem. Anesth Analg 76:635-641, 1993.

Hourihane JO, Allard JM, Wade AM, et al: Impact of repeated surgical procedures on the incidence and prevalence of latex allergy: A prospective study of 1263 children. J Pediatr 140:479-482, 2002.

Kwittken PL, Sweinberg SK, Campbell DE, et al: Latex hypersensitivity in children: Clinical presentation and detection of latex-specific immunoglobulin E. Pediatrics 95:693-699, 1995.

Landwehr LP, Boguniewicz M: Current perspectives on latex allergy. J Pediatr 128:305-312, 1996.

Murat I: Anaphylactic reactions during paediatric anaesthesia: Results of the survey of the French Society of Paediatric Anaesthetists 1991-1992. Paediatr Anaesth 3:339-343, 1993.

Murat I: Latex allergy: Where are we? Paediatr Anaesth 10:577-579, 2000.

Poley GE, Slater JE: Latex allergy. J Allergy Clin Immunol 105:1054-1062, 2000.

Sussman GL, Betschel SD, Beezhold DH: Latex allergy. In Leung DY, et al (eds): Pediatric Allergy, Principles and Practice. St. Louis, Mosby, 2003, pp 624-663.

Tosi LL, Slater JE, Shaer CS, et al: Latex allergy in spina bifida patients: Prevalence and surgical implications. J Pediatr Orthop 13:709-712, 1993.

PEDIATRICS & NEONATOLOGY

Malignant Hyperthermia

Karen M. Van Tassel and Scott R. Schulman

162

Case Synopsis

A healthy 12-year-old boy presents for reduction of a humerus fracture. Anesthesia is induced with sevoflurane. Fifteen minutes later, there is an abrupt increase in end-tidal carbon dioxide to greater than 70 mm Hg. He becomes tachycardic, with a heart rate of 150 beats per minute, and his temperature increases from 36.7°C to 39.4°C.

PROBLEM ANALYSIS

Definition

Malignant hyperthermia (MH) is a rare but potentially fatal subclinical myopathy. MH remains latent until susceptible individuals are exposed to triggering anesthetic agents, such as volatile inhalational anesthetics and succinylcholine. MH is characterized by an increase in myoplasmic calcium ions (Ca^{2+}). Presenting signs include increased metabolism, muscle rigidity, and fever.

Similarities were noted between human MH and the porcine stress syndrome, which occurs in one breed of pigs. Upon exposure to stress, including transport, fighting, vaccination, or preparation for slaughter, this breed experienced increased metabolism, acidosis, fever, and death. In 1966 Hall reported that succinylcholine and halothane induced MH in these pigs. They soon became the animal model for the disease. Subsequently, the genetic mutation responsible for porcine stress syndrome was found to be a single point mutation on chromosome 6, which entirely accounted for this homogeneous disease. Human MH, however, is a disease of significant genetic heterogeneity. Many different genetic abnormalities and predisposing conditions lead to a similar final pathway. Human MH is further complicated by incomplete penetrance and widely variable expression.

The pathophysiology of MH lies in disordered excitation-contraction coupling in skeletal muscle. In normal muscle, an action potential is propagated along the sarcolemma and down the T tubule, leading to Ca^{2+} release from the sarcoplasmic reticulum. Ca^{2+} then binds troponin, exposing active actin binding sites, which leads to muscle contraction. This process is terminated by the active transport of Ca^{2+} back into the sarcoplasmic reticulum.

The sarcoplasmic reticulum is the intracellular organelle responsible for Ca^{2+} regulation. As propagated action potentials cause voltage changes in the T tubule, a conformational change occurs in the α subunit of the dihydropyridine receptor. This activates the ryanodine receptor (RYR1). This activation leads to the opening of RYR1, causing Ca^{2+} efflux and muscle contraction.

In MH, a defect in Ca^{2+} release is expressed upon exposure to a triggering agent. This defect results in a prolonged opening of RYR1 and enhanced Ca^{2+} efflux into the myoplasm, leading to prolonged interaction of actin and myosin (contracture) and increased muscle metabolism. Two known sites for this defect are the RYR1 and dihydropyridine receptors.

Recognition

Understanding the underlying pathophysiology of MH leads to an appreciation of its clinical manifestations (Table 162-1). The increased muscle metabolism is initially aerobic, resulting in increased oxygen consumption, hypercarbia, respiratory acidosis, and heat production. As adenosine triphosphate (ATP) is depleted, metabolism becomes anaerobic, resulting in lactic acid production, metabolic acidosis, and further heat production. In the presence of hyperthermia, acidosis, and ATP depletion, the cell loses the ability to maintain the integrity of its membrane. Rhabdomyolysis leads to the release of potassium, myoglobin, and creatine kinase. Hypercarbia is the earliest and most sensitive sign of MH; generalized muscle rigidity is the most specific sign. Prompt diagnosis and treatment of MH are imperative and may avoid its associated complications (Table 162-2). However, other disease states must be considered in the differential diagnosis of MH (Table 162-3).

Risk Assessment

Although precise estimates are difficult owing to the rarity of human MH, the incidence is thought to be 1 in 15,000 in children and 1 in 50,000 in adults. Determining a patient's risk for MH includes careful questioning during the preoperative interview. A personal or family history of MH during a previous anesthetic should raise concerns. Further, a family history of unexpected intraoperative death or cardiac arrest should increase the suspicion for MH.

Table 162–1 ■ Clinical Manifestations of Malignant Hyperthermia

Early
Tachycardia
Tachypnea
Muscle rigidity
Arrhythmias
Hypercarbia

Late
Increased temperature
Skin mottling
Myoglobinuria
Hyperkalemia
Elevated creatine kinase
Mixed acidosis

Table 162–2 ■ Complications of Malignant Hyperthermia

Coagulopathy/disseminated intravascular coagulation
Acute renal failure
Hepatic dysfunction
Severe muscle pain
Weakness
Arrhythmias
Pulmonary edema
Congestive heart failure
Acute respiratory distress syndrome
Seizures
Coma
Death

Although there are numerous case reports of patients with different diseases experiencing episodes of MH, the only diseases that are consistently associated with MH are central core disease, King-Denborough syndrome, and Duchenne's muscular dystrophy.

The current diagnostic test for confirming MH is the in vitro contracture test (IVCT), also known as the caffeine halothane contracture test. Although this test was developed in the 1970s, it remains the gold standard and has 97% sensitivity. The muscle biopsy must be performed at one of six designated IVCT centers, because the laboratory testing must be performed on freshly harvested tissue. Although the biopsy is performed on an outpatient basis, the dwindling number of testing sites in the United States may be an obstacle for some patients who need to have this test.

For the IVCT, 2 g of muscle is harvested from the vastus lateralis or vastus medialis muscle and then longitudinally dissected into six strips. Small sutures are placed at both ends of the muscle, and the strips are placed into a tissue bath. One end is attached to a stationary hook, and the other to a force transducer. Halothane is added to the fresh gas flow via an in-line vaporizer in three of the baths, and caffeine is incrementally added to the other three baths. A patient is diagnosed with MH syndrome if a contracture or increase in the muscle's baseline tension develops on exposure to these agents.

Although the IVCT remains the gold standard for diagnosing MH, genetic testing may provide an alternative in the future. A significant international effort is now under way to clarify the molecular genetic basis of MH. Although multiple gene loci are involved, 50% of MH families can be linked to mutations in the *RYR1* gene on chromosome 19.

Table 162–3 ■ Differential Diagnosis of Malignant Hyperthermia

Infection
Sepsis
Stimulant drugs
Thyrotoxicosis
Light anesthesia
Neuroleptic malignant syndrome
Pheochromocytoma
Heatstroke

More than 30 mutations have been described in this gene, along with two mutations in the α subunit of the dihydropyridine receptor gene. As new information on the genetic basis of MH is developed, genetic testing may provide the means for screening at-risk patients, avoiding the need for open muscle biopsy. Today, however, genetic testing is still only a research tool.

Implications

MH is a grave and potentially fatal disease. Untreated, the mortality is as high as 70%. With the administration of dantrolene, however, this rate decreases to 4%. Thus, anesthesiologists have a critical role in diagnosing and appropriately treating MH patients to avoid its complications (see Table 162-2).

As with any inherited disease, the diagnosis of MH carries implications for both the patient and his or her family members. The Malignant Hyperthermia Association of the United States (MHAUS) can be an invaluable resource for patients and physicians. Established in 1981, its goal is to provide information about MH to patients and health care providers and to help individuals cope with the diagnosis and reduce its associated morbidity and mortality. Its MH hotline (1-800-MH-HYPER) provides access to physician consultants 24 hours a day, 7 days a week. More information about the MHAUS can be found at www.mhaus.org.

The North American Malignant Hyperthermia Registry, a division of the MHAUS, acquires and analyzes patient-specific clinical and laboratory data on MH. After diagnosing a suspected MH episode, a health care professional should report this information to the registry by completing an Adverse Metabolic Reaction to Anesthesia (AMRA) form. This information can then be relayed to future physicians caring for a registered patient.

A recent topic of concern is the possibility of "awake triggering" of MH, occurring while a patient is not anesthetized or exposed to one of the known anesthetic triggers. Returning to the patient described in the case synopsis, the boy was diagnosed with MH intraoperatively, appropriately treated with dantrolene, and recovered uneventfully. Eight months later, however, he developed muscle weakness and stiffness after playing in a football game. His condition progressed to seizures and respiratory arrest. When paramedics arrived, the electrocardiogram showed sinus tachycardia, and intubation was unsuccessful secondary to jaw clenching. His temperature on arrival at the hospital was higher than 42.2°C, and he was successfully intubated. The patient developed ventricular fibrillation, and cardiopulmonary resuscitation was continued as he was treated for hyperkalemia and with dantrolene. Resuscitation was unsuccessful, and subsequent DNA studies identified an altered RYR1 sequence, consistent with the diagnosis of MH.

It is known that hypermetabolic states can occur in individuals both with and without MH syndrome. Although rare, these episodes can be fatal. Health care professionals recommend that patients with MH syndrome limit their activity only if severe muscle cramps or symptoms suggestive of a hypermetabolic state develop. Although death due to awake triggering of MH may represent only a small percentage of patients presenting with heatstroke, MH should be considered in the differential diagnosis, and treatment with dantrolene may be indicated.

Interestingly, mutations in the cardiac ryanodine receptor gene *(RYR2)* have been associated with sudden unexplained death in patients with catecholaminergic polymorphic ventricular tachycardia and arrhythmogenic right ventricular dysplasia type 2. *RYR2* is the major Ca^{2+} release channel on the sarcoplasmic reticulum in cardiomyocytes, and mutations in *RYR2* result in disordered Ca^{2+} regulation during exercise or stress-induced activation of the sympathetic nervous system. Thus, both *RYR1* and *RYR2* mutations cause disorders in Ca^{2+} metabolism in skeletal and cardiac muscle, respectively. Currently, no link between MH and sudden unexplained death has been established. However, further research may elucidate its pathophysiology.

MANAGEMENT

Once the diagnosis of MH is made, the severity of the situation must be communicated to the surgical team, and additional help should be summoned to the operating room. Treatment includes the following:
- Discontinue triggering agents (any volatile inhalation anesthetic agent, succinylcholine).
- Hyperventilate with 100% oxygen.
- Administer dantrolene.
- Monitor arterial blood gases for pH, base excess, and serum potassium; check serial creatine kinase concentrations.
  - Treat acidosis with sodium bicarbonate.
  - Treat hyperkalemia with Ca^{2+}, glucose, and insulin.
- Maintain diuresis with furosemide or mannitol.
- Institute core body cooling with ice packs, cold saline lavage of body cavities and the surgical site; consider cardiopulmonary bypass.
- Call the MH hotline (1-800-MH-HYPER).
- Complete an AMRA form.

Dantrolene is a direct skeletal muscle relaxant that binds to the RYR1 receptor, thereby reducing its open-state probability and blocking Ca^{2+} release from the sarcoplasmic reticulum. It is administered as a 2.5 mg/kg intravenous bolus; this can be repeated every 5 minutes until the hypermetabolic state resolves, up to a maximum dose of 10 mg/kg. The maintenance dose of dantrolene is 1 mg/kg intravenously every 6 hours for 24 hours to prevent recurrence of the hypermetabolic state. For this reason, patients are monitored in the intensive care unit for at least 24 hours after an MH episode.

If there is no change in the patient's condition after giving large amounts of dantrolene, other diagnoses must be entertained (see Table 162-3). One possible drug interaction involves dantrolene and nondepolarizing muscle relaxants; dantrolene has been shown to potentiate neuromuscular blockade with vecuronium. Also, cardiovascular collapse has occurred in anesthetized swine when dantrolene and verapamil were administered simultaneously. Thus, calcium channel blockers are contraindicated.

Table 162–4 ■ Safe Drugs for Patients with Malignant Hyperthermia Syndrome
Benzodiazepines
Opioids
Propofol
Ketamine
Etomidate
Local anesthetics
Barbiturates
Nitrous oxide
Nondepolarizing muscle relaxants

PREVENTION

When susceptible or high-risk patients present for surgery, the anesthesia team must make specific preparations. First, the anesthesia machine must be prepared with a new disposable circuit and new carbon dioxide absorbent. The vaporizers should be disabled, and the machine should be flushed with oxygen at 10 L/minute for 20 minutes. Although triggering agents should be avoided, there are many safe anesthetic medications that can be used in these patients (Table 162-4). Dantrolene prophylaxis is *not* recommended for these patients perioperatively. Postoperatively, patients should be monitored for a minimum of 4 hours with continuous electrocardiography, as well as temperature monitoring. If this recovery period is uneventful, it is safe to discharge patients to the floor or even home in the case of ambulatory surgery.

Further Reading

Allen GC: Malignant hyperthermia susceptibility. Anesth Clin North Am 12:513-535, 1994.

Hall LW, Woolf N, Bradley JW, Jolly DW: Unusual reaction to suxamethonium chloride. Br Med J 26:1305, 1966.

Hall SC: General pediatric emergencies: Malignant hyperthermia syndrome. Anesth Clin North Am 19:367-381, 2001.

Kaplan RF: Clinical controversies in malignant hyperthermia susceptibility. Anesth Clin North Am 12:537-549, 1994.

Krause T, Gerbershagen MU, Fiege M, et al: Dantrolene: A review of its pharmacology, therapeutic use and new developments. Anaesthesia 59:364-373, 2004.

Rosenbaum HK, Miller JD: Malignant hyperthermia and myotonic disorders. Anesth Clin North Am 20:623-664, 2002.

Rosenberg H, Antognini JF, Muldoon S: Treatment for malignant hyperthermia. Anesthesiology 96:232-237, 2002.

Sambuughin N, Holley H, Muldoon S, et al: Screening of the entire ryanodine receptor type 1 coding regions for sequence variants associated with malignant hyperthermia susceptibility in the North American population. Anesthesiology 102:515-521, 2005.

Tobin JR, Jason DR, Challa VR, et al: Malignant hyperthermia and apparent heat stroke. JAMA 286:168-169, 2001.

Wehrens XH, Marks AR: Sudden unexplained death caused by cardiac ryanodine receptor (RyR2) mutations. Mayo Clin Proc 79:1367-1371, 2004.

Hypoglycemia and Hyperglycemia

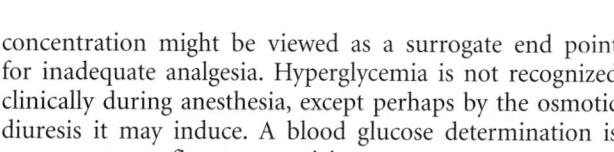

163

D. Ryan Cook

Case Synopsis

A healthy 4-year-old boy is scheduled for inguinal hernia repair. He has dinner at 5 PM the evening before surgery and has milk and cookies before going to bed at 9 PM. He is offered Jell-O water at 5:30 AM (2 hours before his scheduled surgery), which he refuses. Owing to a surgical emergency, the boy's surgery is delayed 4 hours. Before induction of anesthesia, his vital signs are stable, but he is drowsy and somewhat fussy. His serum glucose concentration in the operating room after induction of anesthesia is 70 mg/dL.

PROBLEM ANALYSIS

Definition

Hypoglycemia is usually defined as a blood glucose concentration less than 55 mg/dL (3 mmol/L) in infants and older children and 35 mg/dL (2 mmol/L) in premature and term neonates. Normal values can be defined in several ways: (1) a statistical approach (such as that just stated; to convert mmol/L to mg/dL, simply multiply by 18); (2) a metabolic approach (the blood glucose concentration at which normal cell homeostasis is maintained); (3) a neurophysiologic approach (the blood glucose concentration at which impairment of neurologic function occurs); and (4) a neurodevelopmental approach (the relationship between chronic blood glucose concentrations and neurodevelopmental outcome).

Hyperglycemia is usually defined as a blood glucose concentration greater than 200 mg/dL (11 mmol/L).

Recognition

HYPOGLYCEMIA

Most hypoglycemic children are asymptomatic; some are lethargic, irritable, or jittery. In infants and older children, lethargy may occur at a blood glucose concentration of 75 mg/dL, and unconsciousness at less than 35 mg/dL. In neonates, chronic low blood glucose concentrations can be associated with adverse changes in somatosensory evoked potentials and neurodevelopmental outcomes. Clinical signs of hypoglycemia (tachycardia, hypertension) may be masked by preoperative sedation or general anesthesia or attenuated by β-blockers.

HYPERGLYCEMIA

The stress response to surgery, and perhaps to anesthesia, may result in an intraoperative increase in blood glucose concentration. Intraoperative narcotics and regional analgesia reduce the stress response to surgery by reducing catecholamine release, which attenuates the increase in blood glucose concentration. Thus, an increase in blood glucose concentration might be viewed as a surrogate end point for inadequate analgesia. Hyperglycemia is not recognized clinically during anesthesia, except perhaps by the osmotic diuresis it may induce. A blood glucose determination is necessary to confirm any suspicion.

Risk Assessment

The incidence of preoperative hypoglycemia in healthy infants and children who have fasted between 4 and 19 hours is quite low. Also, there appears to be no correlation between blood glucose concentration and the duration of fasting (hours) in this population. The risk of hypoglycemia has been virtually eliminated by allowing healthy children to ingest glucose-containing clear liquids up until 2 hours before the induction of anesthesia.

The following patients, however, are at risk for preoperative hypoglycemia when fasting:

- Premature infants and small-for-gestational-age neonates
- Patients receiving hyperalimentation solutions or simple dextrose infusions (10% or 12.5%), especially when these infusions are discontinued acutely
- Newborns and infants born to diabetic mothers, and children with diabetes or insulinomas
- Malnourished patients
- Patients with severe hepatic failure
- Patients with abnormalities of lipolysis or amino acid metabolism
- Patients with myopathies, mitochondrial diseases, or glycogen storage diseases
- Those receiving certain drugs (e.g., propranolol, alcohol)

Factors resulting in intraoperative hyperglycemia include the following:

- Exogenous glucose administration at high maintenance rates (e.g., 20 mL/kg per hour) or massive transfusion
- Alteration of hormone levels affecting glucose control (e.g., stress)
- Decreased peripheral glucose utilization
- Continuation of 10% or 12.5% dextrose solution at the preoperative rate

Implications

HYPOGLYCEMIA

Hourly and daily maintenance requirements for both water and calories can be determined for infants and children from standard formulas, the so-called 4-2-1 and 100-50-20 rules (Table 163-1). These formulas were developed from estimates of total caloric needs and based on the assumption that 100 mL of water is needed for each 100 calories. It is thus somewhat paradoxical that most clinicians avoid the routine use of solutions containing glucose, except perhaps for neonates, infants who are small for gestational age, and children with special problems.

Unrecognized hypoglycemia can lead to neurologic injury. The absolute value at which hypoglycemia impairs neurologic function is unknown but is seemingly related to its duration measured in hours or days. Brain glucose metabolism increases markedly during development. Unlike the adult brain during ischemia, the neonatal brain is able to use alternative substrates such as lactate and glycogen for energy.

HYPERGLYCEMIA

Hyperglycemia can induce diuresis, dehydration, and electrolyte disturbances and may increase the incidence of cerebral hemorrhage in very small newborns. In adults, hyperglycemia existing before an ischemic or hypoxemic event may increase neurologic injury. It is postulated that in the presence of either insult, oxidative metabolism of glucose fails and glycolysis increases, producing excess lactate. With sufficient intracellular lactate accumulation, intracellular pH decreases, which may lead to compromised cellular function or cell death.

In contrast to adults, moderate to profound hyperglycemia in neonates seems to protect the brain from ischemic damage by means of increased cerebral high-energy reserves and glycogen stores, increased glucose uptake, and enhanced lactate clearance. Thus, during pediatric cardiac surgery, the role of hyperglycemia (if any) in neurologic injury is unclear. The elimination of glucose solutions during cardiac surgery is associated with a 5% to 9% incidence of hypoglycemia, which may be an important contributor to adverse neurologic outcomes.

Hyperglycemia is also associated with adverse outcomes in adults with sepsis. Glucose control in septic infants is poorly defined. However, most clinicians reduce 10% or 12.5% dextrose infusion rates by one third or one half during surgery on septic infants.

MANAGEMENT

The goals of intraoperative fluid management are to provide an appropriate amount of parenteral fluids (water plus electrolytes) to maintain adequate intravascular volume, cardiac output, and urine output and, in some instances, to provide sufficient glucose to prevent hypoglycemia or minimize the risk of perioperative hyperglycemia. To avoid both hypoglycemia and hyperglycemia during surgical procedures, some have suggested administering 2.5% dextrose in lactated Ringer's (LR) solution at maintenance rates, along with a glucose-free fluid (e.g., LR or normal saline) for replacement of blood and third-space losses. Because 2.5% dextrose-LR solution is not commercially available, either the practitioner or a pharmacist must prepare it. Blood obtained from central venous or arterial catheters or from finger or heel sticks is used to monitor glucose concentrations. Glucose testing is usually available at the point of care. If not, concentrations are measured in the blood gas laboratory. Serial blood glucose determinations can be made, with the amount of intravenous glucose adjusted accordingly.

PREVENTION

Prevention of hypoglycemia and hyperglycemia requires a case-specific risk-benefit analysis. Some caveats deserve special mention:

- Be aware of patients at increased risk for hypoglycemia or hyperglycemia.
- Be judicious when administering glucose-containing solutions to patients at risk for hypoglycemia.
- Withhold glucose-containing solutions when appropriate.
- Frequently monitor blood glucose concentrations.

Further Reading

Aun CD, Panesar NS: Paediatric glucose homeostasis during anaesthesia. Br J Anaesth 64:413-418, 1990.

Bazaes RA, Salazar TE, Pittaluga E, et al: Glucose and lipid metabolism in small for gestational age infants at 48 hours of age. Pediatrics 111:804-809, 2003.

Ferranti SD, Gaureau K, Hickey PR, et al: Intraoperative hyperglycemia during infant cardiac surgery is not associated with adverse neurodevelopmental outcomes at 1, 4, and 8 years. Anesthesiology 100:1345-1352, 2004.

Leelanukrom R, Cunliffe M: Intraoperative fluid and glucose management in children. Paediatr Anaesth 10:353-359, 2000.

Nishima K, Mikawa K, Maekawa N, et al: Effects of exogenous intravenous glucose on plasma glucose and lipid homeostasis in anesthetized infants. Anesthesiology 83:258-263, 1995.

Pereira GR: Nutrition care of the extremely premature infant. Clin Perinatol 22:61-75, 1995.

Welborn LG, Hannallah RS, McGill WA, et al: Glucose concentration in routine intravenous infusion in pediatric outpatient surgery. Anesthesiology 67:427-430, 1987.

Welborn LG, McGill WA, Hannallah RS, et al: Perioperative blood glucose concentrations in pediatric outpatients. Anesthesiology 65:545-547, 1986.

Table 163–1 ▪ Calculation of Maintenance Fluid Requirements for Infants and Small Children

Body Weight (kg)	Fluid Requirements	
	Hourly Fluids*	*Fluids over 24 Hours†*
<10	4 mL·kg⁻¹	100 mL·kg⁻¹
11-20	40 mL + 2 mL·kg⁻¹ >10 kg	1000 + 50 mL·kg⁻¹ >10 kg
≥20	60 mL + 1 mL·kg⁻¹ >20 kg	1500 + 20 mL·kg⁻¹ >20 kg

*4-2-1 rule.
†100-50-20 rule.

Pulmonary Hypertension

Deborah A. Davis

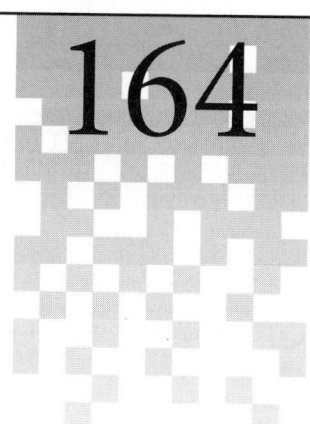

164

Case Synopsis

A 4-month-old, formerly preterm infant with bronchopulmonary dysplasia presents for closure of a ventricular septal defect after failing to wean from mechanical ventilation. The surgical procedure is not difficult, but after weaning from cardiopulmonary bypass, the patient has suprasystemic pulmonary artery pressures.

PROBLEM ANALYSIS

Definition

Elevated pulmonary artery pressure (PAP) is due to increased pulmonary vascular resistance (PVR) or pulmonary blood flow. Pressure, resistance, and flow are related by Poiseuille's adaptation of Ohm's law:

$$\text{Ohm's law: } R = PAP - Pv/Q,$$

where R is pulmonary vascular resistance, Pv is pulmonary venous pressure (approximately equal to left atrial pressure), and Q is flow.

$$\text{Poiseuille's law: } R = 8L/\pi r^4,$$

where R is pulmonary resistance, L is length of resistor, and r is radius of resistor.

The latter suggests that the length of the pulmonary bed (and blood viscosity) has a direct impact on resistance, and that the effect of altered arterial radius is exponential. With increased PVR, higher perfusion pressures are needed to maintain constant pulmonary flow; otherwise, flow diminishes. Normal values for mean PAP (i.e., pulmonary artery – left atrial pressure) and PVR are 10 to 20 mm Hg and 4 Wood units, respectively.

Either primary or secondary pulmonary artery hypertension (PAH) can occur in children. To diagnose the former, all other causes must be excluded (see Chapter 78). Persistent PAH of the newborn is one cause of primary PAH. It may be due to underdevelopment of the lung, pulmonary vascular maladaptation to extrauterine life, or maldevelopment of the pulmonary vascular bed in utero. With primary PAH, lung pathologic examination reveals a reduced number of arteries relative to the number of bronchioles.

Secondary PAH typically develops in response to specific types of cardiac or pulmonary disease (Tables 164-1 and 164-2). Within the context of congenital heart disease, secondary PAH may be due to increased pulmonary artery blood flow, resistance, or both. Secondary PAH can result from advanced pulmonary disease, as well as from nonrespiratory causes (see Chapter 78).

Recognition

The workup for secondary PAH entails serial physical examinations and laboratory and diagnostic testing (Table 164-3). In children without a predisposing condition, early signs of secondary PAH are those of right ventricular failure, exercise limitation, and, possibly, hypoxemia if a patent foramen ovale is present. Neonates with a patent ductus arteriosus may exhibit differential upper and lower body systemic oxygen saturation as desaturated blood shunts right to left across the ductus to perfuse the lower body.

Risk Assessment

In lesions that involve a communication between the systemic and pulmonary circulations, some proportion of the systemic pressure is transmitted to the pulmonary circulation. Associated high pressure and increased blood velocities produce shear stress, causing structural and functional damage to the pulmonary vascular endothelium. In lesions with reduced pulmonary blood flow, there may be hypoplasia of the arteries themselves. The risk of

Table 164–1 ■ Cardiac Causes of Secondary Pulmonary Hypertension

Cardiac lesions that increase pulmonary flow
    (left-to-right shunt)
   Patent ductus arteriosus
   Atrial septal defect
   Ventricular septal defect (VSD)
   Atrioventricular canal
   Aorta-pulmonary window
   Arterial-pulmonary collaterals
   Transposition of great vessels with VSD
   Systemic-to-pulmonary shunts
Cardiac lesions that decrease pulmonary flow
   Tetralogy of Fallot
   Ebstein's anomaly
   Pulmonary atresia
   Tricuspid atresia
Cardiac lesions that cause pulmonary venous hypertension
   Cor triatriatum
   Mitral stenosis
   Mitral atresia
   Interrupted aortic arch
   Cardiomyopathy
   Hypoplastic left ventricle
   Critical aortic stenosis
   Coarctation of aorta
   Veno-occlusive disease
   Endocarditis

Table 164–2 ■ Noncardiac Causes of Secondary Pulmonary Hypertension

Respiratory
Obstructed lung disease (rare)
Restrictive lung disease
  Collagen vascular disease
  Bronchopulmonary dysplasia
  Respiratory distress syndrome
  Interstitial disease
  Infiltrative disease
  Pleural adhesions
  Neuromuscular disease
Other
  Upper airway obstruction
  Pickwickian syndrome

Nonrespiratory
Juvenile rheumatoid arthritis
Lupus erythematosus
Pulmonary embolism (fat, thrombus, air, tumor)
Sickle cell disease
Scleroderma

Table 164–4 ■ Classification of Structural Changes with Pulmonary Vascular Disease

Grade	Structural Change	Status
I	Medial hypertrophy	Reversible
II	Cellular intimal proliferation	Reversible
III	Intimal hyperplasia, luminal occlusion	Probably reversible
IV	Pulmonary artery dilatation	Probably reversible
V	Pulmonary angiomatoid formation	Irreversible
VI	Pulmonary fibrinoid necrosis	Irreversible

From Heath D, Edwards SE: The pathology of hypertensive pulmonary vascular disease. Circulation 18:533-547, 1958.

developing increased PVR varies, depending on the cardiac malformation:

- Ventricular septal defect, 15%
- Transposition of great arteries, 8%
- Transposition of great arteries with ventricular septal defect, 40%
- Complete atrioventricular canal defect, almost 100%

If the hematocrit is elevated, vascular thrombotic changes may exacerbate structural arterial changes. Secondary PAH

Table 164–3 ■ Workup for Secondary Pulmonary Hypertension

Physical examination
  Irregular heart rhythms
  Elevated jugular venous pressure
  Loud P_2, systolic ejection click, wide split P_2
  Diastolic murmur
Chest radiograph (may be normal)
  Prominent pulmonary artery; enlarged heart
  Increased pulmonary vascular markings (congestive heart failure)
  Decreased pulmonary vascular markings (severe disease)
Echocardiogram
  Define anatomy; estimate shunt flows
  Estimate right ventricular and pulmonary artery pressures
Catheterization
  Further define anatomy
  Calculate pulmonary vascular resistance
  Test response to oxygen, nitric oxide, vasodilators
  Wedge angiography (pulmonary artery tapering and filling; circulation time)
Other
  Electrocardiogram (right ventricular hypertrophy)
  Lung biopsy
  Elevated hematocrit

also occurs if left-sided lesions cause pulmonary venous hypertension, with increased venous pressure transmitted back to the pulmonary arteries. Heath and Edwards classified the structural changes that occur with pulmonary vascular disease (Table 164-4).

Several factors contribute to secondary PAH with severe parenchymal lung disease: (1) hypoxia and polycythemia, (2) pulmonary endothelial injury, and (3) structural pulmonary artery damage. For example, along with the proliferation of vascular muscularis into nonmuscular peripheral pulmonary arteries, infants with bronchopulmonary dysplasia have excessive pulmonary interstitial water. This compresses the arterioles and further elevates PVR. Treatment of the primary lung disease helps reduce the impact of contributory causes of secondary PAH, allowing regression of some of the associated structural changes.

Nonrespiratory diseases can also cause secondary PAH via inflammation (arteritis) or occlusion (thrombosis). Either reduces the pulmonary vascular cross-sectional area and elevates PVR. Also, vasoactive substances (e.g., prostaglandins, thromboxanes, leukotrienes) cause pulmonary vascular changes that increase PAP:

- Pulmonary endothelium-derived von Willebrand's factor increases platelet adhesion and the formation of microaggregates, along with the release of vasoconstrictive factors.
- Endothelium-derived relaxing factor (i.e., nitric oxide) relaxes vascular smooth muscle and is reduced in patients with lung injury and after cardiopulmonary bypass.
- Primary pulmonary hypertension can be triggered by almost any neonatal stress (e.g., hypoxemia, hemorrhage, hypoglycemia, hypothermia, aspiration, acidosis) via some of the aforementioned cellular mediators.

Paroxysmal increased PVR occurs on occasion, even with normal baseline PAPs (e.g., post–cardiac surgery patients with large left-to-right shunts or pulmonary venous obstruction). Such pulmonary hypertensive crises can arise when vascular endothelial cells are triggered by a particular stimulant. Consequent acute PAH is poorly tolerated, and circulatory collapse can be immediate. The following are more common triggers:

- Hypoxia, hypercarbia, acidosis
- Aggressive suctioning, noxious stimuli, bronchoscopic procedures
- Pleural effusion, hemothorax, pneumothorax

Implications

High PVR increases right ventricular impedance and may lead to acute or chronic right ventricular failure. As a result, pulmonary blood flow decreases. Without direct pulmonary-systemic connections that allow right-to-left shunting (e.g., a patent foramen ovale), the systemic cardiac output will also fall.

MANAGEMENT

Because the management of PAH due to increased pulmonary blood flow is surgical elimination of the left-to-right shunt, only the management of increased PVR is discussed here. The goal is to provide adequate systemic oxygen delivery. Initial therapy should focus on lowering PVR to optimize right ventricular performance. If this fails, intervention to bypass the pulmonary circulation may be necessary.

Ventilatory Strategies

Ventilatory strategies represent the most effective measures for selectively influencing PVR. Maintenance of a normal functional residual capacity optimizes PVR, because lung overdistention or underinflation can result in compression and distortion of the pulmonary microcirculation. Reactive pulmonary vasculature dilates in response to enriched oxygen mixtures and local alkalosis. The latter is achieved by hyperventilation or with sodium bicarbonate. When conventional ventilation cannot achieve satisfactory gas exchange without deleterious levels of intrathoracic pressure, jet ventilation may prove beneficial. Inhaled nitric oxide is a selective pulmonary vasodilator that may be effective in cardiac or noncardiac PAH.

Pharmacologic Agents

A variety of intravenous drugs, listed here, can have a salutary effect on PVR. They vary in efficacy from patient to patient, and none is selective for the pulmonary circulation:

- Prostacyclin
- Isoproterenol
- Angiotensin-converting enzyme inhibitors
- Adenosine
- Nitroprusside
- Amrinone
- Acetylcholine
- Tolazoline
- Prostaglandin E_1
- Nitroglycerin
- Sildenafil

Sildenafil is a phosphodiesterase inhibitor that shows promise as an effective intravenous agent for reducing PAP. However, its use may be limited because of its potential to increase intrapulmonary shunt and worsen ventilation-perfusion mismatch.

Invasive Measures

ATRIAL SEPTOSTOMY

If tissue oxygen delivery is unsatisfactory despite ventilatory and pharmacologic management, more invasive measures may be necessary. In children with low cardiac output due to right ventricular failure but without intracardiac connections, atrial septostomy may prove beneficial. The creation of an atrial septal defect enables systemic venous blood return to bypass the pulmonary circulation and augment left ventricular output, albeit at the cost of systemic hypoxia.

MECHANICAL CIRCULATORY SUPPORT

If low cardiac output persists despite atrial septostomy, or if systemic hypoxemia becomes life threatening, extracorporeal circulatory support is the final option. Because the pathophysiology resides in the pulmonary microcirculation, selective right ventricular assist devices usually do not provide sufficient benefit, necessitating the interposition of a membrane oxygenator.

LUNG OR HEART-LUNG TRANSPLANTATION

Unless the pulmonary hypertensive crisis can be attributed to a finite and reversible cause (e.g., persistent pulmonary hypertension of the newborn), extracorporeal circulatory support must be regarded as a bridge to heart or heart-lung transplantation. Given the limited availability of these organs for children, both the patient's family and medical providers must have realistic expectations before embarking on such heroic therapy.

PREVENTION

Therapeutic options for primary and secondary PAH are limited in both scope and efficacy; therefore, prevention is vital. Children with PAH or medical histories that predispose to pulmonary hypertensive crises require meticulous anesthesia care. Preoperative measures directed at optimizing right ventricular function (e.g., digoxin, arrhythmia control) and intravascular volume status deserve special consideration and may provide some benefit. Most critical are precautions to preserve optimal ventilation and provide sufficient analgesia to blunt endogenous, catecholamine-mediated responses to noxious stimuli. Also, children with intracardiac shunts and the potential for right-to-left shunting should receive drugs that substantially reduce systemic vascular resistance, even though this promotes systemic hypoxemia. Assuming that cardiac reserve is sufficient to tolerate the requisite doses of anesthetic agents, children with PAH should be managed similarly to those with other conditions in which endogenous responses to noxious stimuli have a deleterious impact on the underlying circulatory pathophysiology.

Further Reading

Avery GB (ed): Neonatology: Pathophysiology and Management of the Newborn. Philadelphia, JB Lippincott, 1987, p 1399.

Davis DA, Russo PA, Greenspan J, et al: High frequency jet versus conventional ventilation in infants undergoing Blalock-Taussig shunts. Ann Thorac Surg 57:846-849, 1994.

Fishman AP: Hypoxia as the pulmonary circulation: How and where it acts. Circ Res 38:221-231, 1976.

Haworth SG: Primary pulmonary hypertension. Br Heart J 49:517-521, 1983.

Heath D, Edwards SE: The pathology of hypertensive pulmonary vascular disease. Circulation 18:533-547, 1958.

Rabinovitch M, Andrew M, Thom H, et al: Abnormal endothelial factor VIII associated with pulmonary hypertension and congenital heart defects. Circulation 76:1043-1052, 1987.

Schulze-Neick I, Hartenstein P, Li J, et al: Intravenous sildenafil is a potent pulmonary vasodilator in children with congenital heart disease. Circulation 108(Suppl II):167-173, 2003.

Hypothermia in Pediatric Patients

Kevin J. Sullivan

165

Case Synopsis

A 1-month-old, formerly premature (28-week) infant undergoes general anesthesia for magnetic resonance imaging of the brain and spine. At the conclusion of the imaging study, the patient is noted to have a core body temperature of 34.5°C and demonstrates delayed emergence from anesthesia and increased severity of apnea and bradycardia in the neonatal intensive care unit.

PROBLEM ANALYSIS

Definition

Central (core) body temperature is one of the most tightly regulated parameters in human physiology. Normal core body temperature in infants, children, and adults is about 37°C and seldom fluctuates more than 0.5°C above or below this setpoint. However, mild hypothermia (1°C to 3°C below normal) is commonly seen perioperatively. Anesthetic medications, environmental exposure, and critical illness may result in altered thermoregulation and hypothermia.

Recognition

The minimum basic monitoring standards of the American Society of Anesthesiologists require that temperature-monitoring capabilities be readily available to anesthesiologists. Temperature monitoring is especially important for detecting hypothermia in infants and children, because they are very susceptible to this complication. Sites for temperature monitoring are classified as central (nasopharyngeal, esophageal, axillary, rectal, or bladder) or peripheral (skin):

- Nasopharyngeal—posterior to the soft palate
- Esophageal—posterior to the heart *below* the level of the carina
- Rectal
- Urinary bladder (less accurate with reduced urine output)
- Axillary—near the axillary artery with the arm abducted
- Skin surface (poor correlation with core body temperature)

MECHANISMS OF HEAT LOSS IN ANESTHETIZED INFANTS AND CHILDREN

The four mechanisms of heat loss in anesthetized patients are conduction, evaporation, convection, and radiation. An understanding of these mechanisms leads to a better understanding of the strategies to minimize heat loss in anesthetized children.

Conduction is the direct transfer of heat energy between objects, as occurs with direct patient contact with a cold metal surface, irrigation of wounds with cold saline, and the intravenous administration of cold fluids. *Evaporation* results in heat loss when the latent heat of vaporization is expended to convert a liquid to a gaseous state. Evaporative heat loss in anesthetized patients comes from the skin (evaporation of sweat or surgical preparation solutions from the skin), respiratory tract, and wounds (especially exposed thoracic and peritoneal cavities). *Convection* occurs when molecules at different temperatures cause the net transfer of heat between objects, such as when cool air circulates over the surface of the patient's skin. The rate of convective heat loss is proportional to the temperature difference between ambient air and skin and to the surface area of the patient's skin exposed to that air. Finally, *radiation* heat loss occurs when infrared energy is exchanged between two solid objects that are not in contact. The magnitude of heat exchange is proportional to the fourth power of the temperature difference between the two objects.

Body temperature is monitored by the hypothalamus through afferent sensory input from the skin, neuraxis, and deep body tissues. Under normal conditions, core body temperature is tightly regulated by the hypothalamus and remains within a narrow interthreshold range of 0.5°C above or below a recognized normal body temperature, or setpoint. When the hypothalamus detects a change in core body temperature beyond the acceptable interthreshold range, effector mechanisms are activated to bring core body temperature back to normal (Figs. 165-1 and 165-2). Central regulation of temperature is present in infancy but may be impaired in the elderly, in the critically ill, and in children with severe damage to the central nervous system.

In response to hypothermia, effector mechanisms are activated. These mechanisms are classified as those that reduce heat loss (behavioral changes, vasoconstriction) and those that increase heat production (behavioral changes, nonshivering thermogenesis, shivering). Behavioral changes are not relevant in anesthetized patients, so cutaneous vasoconstriction is the primary response to hypothermia in this setting. Cutaneous blood flow can be reduced via norepinephrine secreted at presynaptic adrenergic terminals. This results in a 25% to 50% decrease in heat loss.

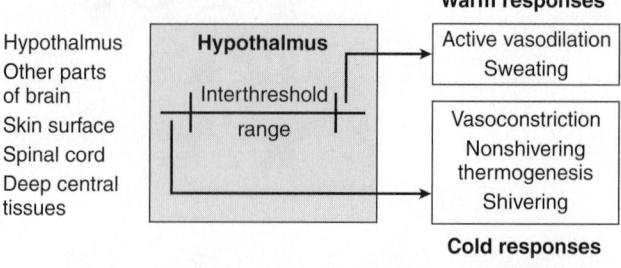

Figure 165–1 ■ Thermoregulatory model. Thermal afferent input is integrated and compared with the threshold temperature for heat and cold. The interthreshold range is the temperature range over which no regulatory effector responses occur. On either side of this interthreshold range are triggered thermoregulatory respononses. (From Bissonnette B: Thermoregulation and pediatric anesthesia. Curr Opin Anesthesiol 6:537-542, 1993.)

Heat production is augmented in anesthetized patients by nonshivering thermogenesis (NST) and shivering. NST is the production of heat in skeletal muscle and brown fat due to the catabolism of brown fat around the blood vessels of the neck, mediastinum, adrenal glands, and axillae. NST can be inhibited by ganglionic blockade, β-blockade, and inhalational anesthetics. Preterm infants, term neonates, infants, and children are capable of NST; however, recent reports have questioned the importance of NST in infants and small mammals during general anesthesia.

Shivering is characterized by high-frequency, irregular muscle activity that begins in upper body muscles when vasoconstriction and NST have failed to maintain an adequate mean body temperature. Shivering is an important mechanism for thermoregulation in adults, but it has not been observed in children younger than 6 years.

PERIOPERATIVE THERMOREGULATION

Predictable changes in body temperature occur in infants and children after the induction of general anesthesia (Fig. 165-3). The first phase of heat redistribution begins when volatile anesthetics cause peripheral vasodilatation, effectively reducing core body (central compartment) perfusion. Central temperature declines as heat is lost to the peripheral tissues. During the second phase, there is reduced endogenous heat production and increased heat loss to the environment. During the third phase, metabolic heat production exceeds heat loss, causing the core temperature to stabilize (adults) or increase (greater in infants than in children).

General anesthesia widens the thermoregulatory interthreshold range (≥2.5°C below the setpoint). This leads to passive core body temperature changes over a wider range of hypothermic temperatures before effector mechanisms become activated (see Fig. 165-2). A lower temperature threshold for effector mechanism activation has been demonstrated with halothane, enflurane, desflurane, sevoflurane, isoflurane propofol, and nitrous oxide–opioid anesthesia.

Regional anesthesia techniques produce hypothermia as readily as general anesthesia does. The vasodilatation induced by neuraxial local anesthetics causes rapid redistribution of core heat to the periphery in a manner similar to that seen with the induction of general anesthesia. Effector mechanisms of shivering and vasoconstriction are absent below the level of block but remain intact above the level of block. Also, the interthreshold range for effector mechanisms appears to be widened in a manner similar to that seen with general anesthesia. It is postulated that the absence of cold afferent input from the tissues below the level of the block is interpreted as warm afferent input, which leads to

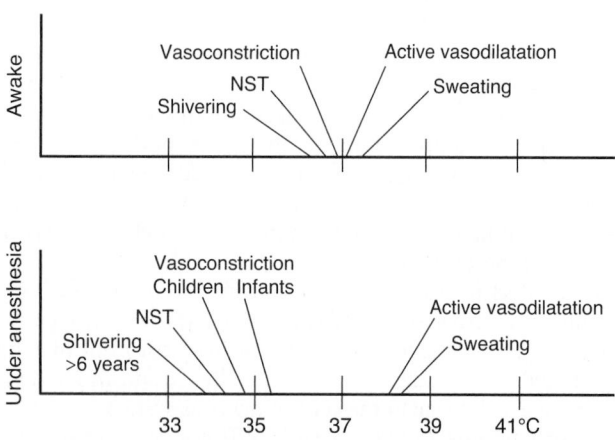

Figure 165–2 ■ Thermoregulatory thresholds and gains in awake and anesthetized infants and children. Thermoregulation appears to be an all-or-none phenomenon. The threshold temperature triggering a thermoregulatory response to hypothermia during anesthesia—nonshivering thermogenesis (NST)—is about 2.5°C below the setpoint (about 37°C), whereas during hyperthermia, the temperature must increase approximately 1.3°C above the setpoint to activate an effector response. Within this temperature range, thermoregulatory responses are absent. Consequently, the patient's body temperature changes passively in proportion to the difference between metabolic heat production and environmental heat loss. (From Bissonnette B: Thermoregulation and pediatric anesthesia. Curr Opin Anesthesiol 6:537-542, 1993.)

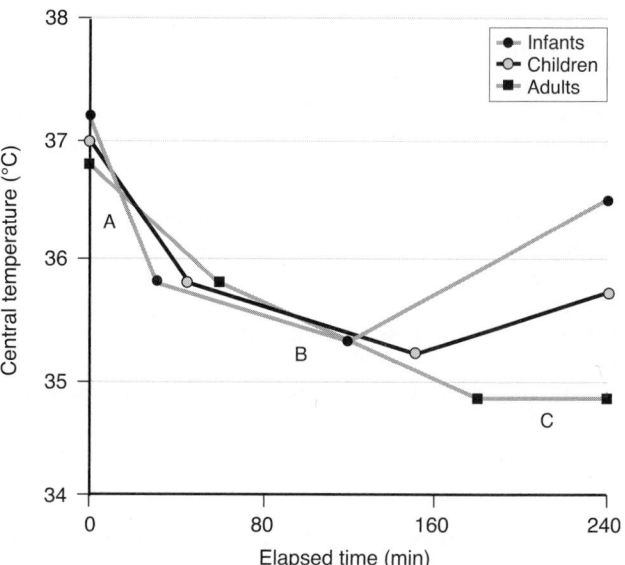

Figure 165–3 ■ Typical pattern of hypothermia during anesthesia. This occurs in three distinct phases in infants, children, and adults: internal redistribution of heat (A), heat loss to the environment (B), and thermal steady state or rewarming (C). Slopes for each stage vary as a function of age. (From Bissonnette B: Thermoregulation and pediatric anesthesia. Curr Opin Anesthesiol 6:537-542, 1993.)

suppression of vasoconstriction, despite the fact that core body temperature is reduced. When combined with general anesthesia, the additional effects of regional anesthesia on thermoregulatory thresholds appear to be minimal.

Risk Assessment

Infants and neonates are more likely than adults to develop perioperative hypothermia. Infants and small children have an increased surface area relative to their body mass. The prominence of the head and trunk and the small extremities of infants prevent the pooling of heat content in the peripheral compartment during anesthesia-related vasodilatation, while the increased surface area–to–body mass ratio diminishes the effectiveness of cutaneous vasoconstriction. Infants lose more heat through their thin skin and have a higher minute ventilation, which increases evaporative heat loss from the respiratory tract. Finally, although vasoconstriction and NST are present in infants and young children, small infants' inability to shiver effectively limits their ability to optimally generate endogenous heat. These innate limitations in the conservation and production of endogenous heat render infants and children particularly vulnerable to the development of hypothermia in cool ambient environments.

Implications

The primary disadvantages of hypothermia in awake patients are shivering and discomfort. Shivering increases heat production at the expense of a pronounced increase in oxygen consumption (up to 600%). Cardiac output increases to match increased oxygen demands, and although this is easily tolerated in healthy patients, it may be poorly tolerated in those with cardiovascular disease.

Neutral thermal environment is the term used to describe the range of ambient temperatures at which metabolic expenditures for heat production are minimal. The *critical temperature* is the temperature below which heat must be produced by the patient to prevent a decrease in body temperature. Term newborns have a critical temperature of about 33°C, whereas preterm infants can have critical temperatures as high as 35°C. Because oxygen consumption for NST increases with larger skin surface–to–environmental temperature gradients, infants in cool ambient environments may expend considerable metabolic energy in pursuit of a stable body temperature.

Hypothermia has deleterious effects on platelet function, immune function, nitrogen balance, and blood flow to surgical wounds. Surgical blood loss is increased when hip arthroplasty is performed during hypothermia, and surgical wound infection and prolonged hospital stays have been noted in patients having procedures performed under hypothermic conditions.

Hypothermia depresses drug metabolism, prolongs the duration of action of muscle relaxants, and reduces the minimum alveolar concentration for volatile anesthetics. Severe hypothermia may impair cognitive function, but there is conflicting evidence about whether it delays anesthetic emergence. Finally, hypothermia often occurs with metabolic aberrations known to exacerbate central apnea in preterm infants (e.g., hypoglycemia, hypocalcemia, hypoxemia, acidosis).

MANAGEMENT AND PREVENTION

The simplest and most effective method to treat or prevent heat loss is to warm the operating room to at least 26°C, and often to temperatures greater than 30°C when caring for term or preterm infants. Likewise, maintenance of relative humidity in the operating room minimizes evaporative heat losses from infants. Use of other heat conservation methods may allow the operating room to be cooled to ambient temperatures that are more comfortable for the health care team.

During anesthesia induction, passive patient warming is accomplished by insulating as much of the skin surface as is practical. The amount of skin surface covered is more important than which part is covered, and no one material is superior to others for reducing radiation and convective heat loss from the skin. Passive insulation of the peripheral compartment limits the transfer of heat from the central compartment to the peripheral compartment during general anesthesia.

Active patient warming can be used to minimize ambient heat loss during general anesthesia. Infrared radiant heaters are commonly used during anesthesia induction and patient preparation and positioning. Once the patient has been positioned and draped, convective air warming blankets or circulating warm water blankets are commonly used. The former circulate warm air at variable temperatures over the body surface outside the surgical field. Circulating warm water blankets are usually placed underneath the patient, with layers of cotton sheets between the blanket and the patient to prevent thermal injury. Convective blankets are more effective than warm water blankets for the prevention and treatment of perioperative hypothermia in infants.

Care must be exercised to (1) monitor the patient's skin for thermal injury, (2) ensure that warming devices are properly applied, and (3) use the minimal temperature required for gradual rewarming. This is especially important if surface blood flow is reduced (e.g., low cardiac output states, regions of pressure necrosis, procedures involving skin grafting or the creation of muscle flaps). Significant burn injuries have been reported with the use of warming devices.

Efforts to reduce respiratory tract evaporative losses are more effective heat conservation measures in children than in adults owing to their higher minute ventilation. Airway humidification, whether active or passive, minimizes heat loss from the respiratory tree. Active humidifiers nebulize water particles in inspired gas mixtures and are most commonly used on ventilators in critical care settings. Care must be taken to monitor the temperature of the inspired gases to prevent tracheal mucosal thermal injury. Passive humidifiers ("artificial noses") condense water contained in exhaled gases and return it to the patient during inspiration. Care must be taken to place the heat and moisture exchanger in close proximity to the airway to prevent condensation and "rain-out" of free water in the cool gas in the inspiratory limb of the ventilator circuit. Finally, attention to the temperature of intravenous and irrigation fluids is critical to prevent rapid conductive cooling during pediatric anesthesia. If large amounts of crystalloid and blood products are administered, precipitous declines in body temperature can occur if they are not warmed beforehand. Likewise, irrigation fluids that are not warmed to body temperature can cause rapid declines in body temperature, especially when used to irrigate the peritoneal and thoracic cavities.

Further Reading

Bissonnette B: Thermoregulation and pediatric anesthesia. Curr Opin Anesthesiol 6:537-542, 1993.

Bissonnette B, Ryan JF: Temperature regulation: Normal and abnormal (malignant hyperthermia). In Cote CJ, Todres ID, Ryan JF, et al (eds): A Practice of Anesthesia for Infants and Children. Philadelphia, WB Saunders, 2001, pp 610-635.

Bissonnette B, Sessler DI: The thermoregulatory thresholds for vasoconstriction in pediatric patients anesthetized with halothane or halothane and caudal bupivacaine. Anesthesiology 76:387-392, 1992.

Bissonnette B, Sessler DI, LaFlamme P: Intraoperative temperature monitoring sites in infants and children and the effect of inspired gas warming on esophageal temperature. Anesth Analg 69:192-196, 1989.

Dicker A, Ohlson KB, Johnson L, et al: Halothane selectively inhibits non-shivering thermogenesis: Possible implications for thermoregulation during anesthesia of infants. Anesthesiology 82:491-501, 1995.

Kurz A, Kurz M, Poeschl G, et al: Forced-air warming maintains intraoperative normothermia better than circulating-water mattresses. Anesth Analg 77:89-95, 1993.

Kurz A, Sessler DI, Lenhardt R: Perioperative normothermia to reduce the incidence of surgical-wound infection and shorten hospitalization. Study of Wound Infection and Temperature Group. N Engl J Med 334:1209-1215, 1996.

Plattner O, Semsroth M, Sessler DI, et al: Lack of non-shivering thermogenesis in infants anesthetized with fentanyl and propofol. Anesthesiology 86:772-777, 1997.

Schmied H, Kurz A, Sessler DI, et al: Mild hypothermia increases blood loss and transfusion requirements during total hip arthroplasty. Lancet 347:289-292, 1996.

Sessler D: Temperature disturbances. In Gregory GA (ed): Pediatric Anesthesia, 4th ed. Philadelphia, Churchill Livingstone, 2002, p 67.

Truell KD, Bakerman PR, Teodori MF, et al: Third-degree burns due to intraoperative use of a Bair Hugger warming device. Ann Thorac Surg 69:1933-1934, 2000.

Zukowski ML, Lord JL, Ash K: Precautions in warming light therapy as an adjuvant to postoperative flap care. Burns 24:374-377, 1998.

SURGERY-RELATED AND OTHER ISSUES

Cardiomyopathies

Stephanie S. F. Fischer and B. Craig Weldon

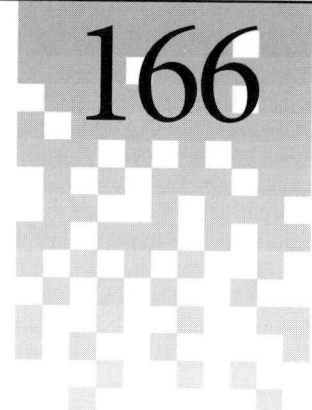

166

Case Synopsis

A 6-month-old boy with Pompe's disease (glycogen storage disease type II) presents for muscle biopsy and central venous catheter placement under general anesthesia. Mask induction with sevoflurane is followed by a maintenance propofol infusion. The patient develops signs of ischemia on the electrocardiogram (ECG) and hypotension. This quickly leads to ventricular fibrillation and cardiac arrest. The return of spontaneous circulation is achieved with external cardiac massage and two intravenous doses of epinephrine, and the surgery is canceled.

PROBLEM ANALYSIS

Definition

The World Health Organization defines cardiomyopathies (CMs) as myocardial diseases associated with cardiac dysfunction. They are classified by the dominant pathophysiology or, if known, by causative factors. Thus, CM may be dilated, hypertrophic, restrictive, or a special type called arrhythmogenic right ventricular cardiomyopathy (or arrhythmogenic right ventricular dysplasia). If the cause of a CM is known (i.e., secondary CM), it may be ischemic, valvular, hypertensive, inflammatory, metabolic, or peripartum in origin. CMs can also be associated with systemic disease, neuromuscular disorders, or exposure to toxins.

Recognition

Primary CM (not caused by some other organ system disease or pathophysiologic state) and secondary CM (proven cause) can be dilated, hypertrophic, restrictive, or arrhythmogenic right ventricular, based on functional and anatomic presentations. Unclassified CMs consist of cases that do not fit readily into any of these groups, such as the following:

- Fibroelastosis
- Noncompacted myocardium
- Mitochondrial disorders

Dilated cardiomyopathy (DCM) is characterized by left ventricular chamber dilatation and impaired systolic function involving the left ventricle (LV), right ventricle (RV), or both. DCM may be viral or immunologic, idiopathic, or familial (genetic); it may be caused by alcohol or toxins or associated with other diseases involving the cardiovascular system. DCM may be asymptomatic or associated with severe functional impairment (New York Heart Association [NYHA] class III or IV heart failure). Patients with decompensated heart failure (NYHA class IV) present with low cardiac output and pulmonary edema (cor pulmonale). Also, all four cardiac chambers appear dilated on chest radiographs. The ECG in *acute* cor pulmonale may resemble that of inferior myocardial infarction. However, differences include the following: (1) the pattern of lead II tends to follow that of lead I (no Q wave) as opposed to that of lead III (with Q waves); (2) the ECG changes may be fleeting or resolve over a period of hours or days, as opposed to weeks or months; (3) the ST-T abnormalities in the limb leads are slight, and those in the right precordial leads resemble the anteroseptal infarction pattern; (4) transient right bundle branch block may be present. In *chronic* cor pulmonale, the ECG is characterized by (1) a rightward shift of the QRS axis by greater than 30 degrees; (2) inverted, biphasic, or flattened T waves in leads V1 to V3; (3) ST segment depression in the inferior leads (II, III, aVF); and (4) right bundle branch block. Echocardiography confirms DCM as well as poor systolic function.

Hypertrophic cardiomyopathy (HCM) may involve the LV, RV, or both and is often asymmetrical. Ventricular volumes may be normal or reduced. HCM is characterized by diastolic dysfunction, with preserved systolic function. HCM is a genetic condition and involves sarcomeric protein mutations. There is an autosomal dominant pattern of inheritance, with variable penetrance. Patients with HCM may be asymptomatic or present with exertional dyspnea, chest pain, and syncope. The ECG shows a progressive pattern, from septal hypertrophy to generalized left ventricular hypertrophy. A few other tendencies are also worth noting: (1) the ECG can be normal in up to 20% of cases; (2) many patients have ECG evidence of left ventricular hypertrophy; (3) some cases are associated with left axis deviation; (4) the pattern of bundle branch block (in reality, intraventricular conduction block) tends to be atypical, with notching and slurring of the QRS complex in the limb leads; (5) the P waves may be widened and notched, with evidence of left atrial enlargement; (6) in infants with HCM, the ECG pattern is commonly consistent with right ventricular hypertrophy; (7) possibly the most suggestive finding (25% to 30% of patients) is obviously abnormal Q waves, but dissimilar to those of myocardial infarction. Also, HCM is associated with an increased incidence of both supraventricular and ventricular arrhythmias. Finally, echocardiography reveals asymmetrical septal hypertrophy, with a septal–to–left ventricular wall ratio greater than 1.3.

Restrictive cardiomyopathy (RCM) is characterized by restricted left or right (or both) ventricular filling due to reduced ventricular diastolic compliance. There may be normal or near-normal systolic function. RCM may be idiopathic, or it can be associated with endomyocardial fibrosis or the hypereosinophilic syndrome.

Arrhythmogenic right ventricular cardiomyopathy (ARVCM) is characterized by fibrofatty replacement of right or left ventricular (or both) myocardium. ARVCM is a genetic cardiac disease with autosomal dominant inheritance and incomplete penetrance. Patients with ARVCM often present with dyspnea, fatigue, hepatomegaly, and ascites. The chest radiograph shows pulmonary venous congestion. The ECG may show impaired atrioventricular conduction. However, without histologic confirmation (i.e., myocardial biopsy), ARVCM is diagnosed based on the presence of ventricular arrhythmias (most often sustained ventricular tachycardia) with a left bundle branch block configuration and wall motion abnormalities on echocardiography in the free wall of the RV. In addition, echocardiography may show atrial dilatation associated with near-normal ventricular dimensions and atrioventricular valve regurgitation.

Risk Assessment

DCM is the most common form of CM in children; it has an equal prevalence in males and females. HCM usually does not present before adolescence. With HCM, morbidity and mortality are greatest in patients diagnosed at younger ages. Premature death is commonly due to ventricular fibrillation. RCM is uncommon in children but, when present, is often an end-stage finding with myocarditis or an infiltrative myocardial disease. ARVCM is uncommon but accounts for a high percentage of sudden cardiac deaths in children and adolescents. The prevalence in females is threefold grater than in males.

Implications

In DCM, cardiac output is maintained by sympathetically mediated tachycardia and ventricular chamber dilatation with increased stroke volume. However, this leads to increased myocardial wall tension and oxygen utilization. In HCM, there is ventricular inflow obstruction secondary to diastolic dysfunction. Some 20% to 25% of patients also have dynamic obstruction of the left ventricular outflow tract. The systolic volume of the LV, the force of left ventricular contraction, and the transmural pressure gradient distending the outflow tract determine the severity of the obstruction. With RCM, the ejection fraction is maintained early in the process. However, as ventricular fibrosis progresses, left ventricular end-diastolic pressure increases, resulting in pulmonary hypertension and decreased stroke volume and cardiac output. With ARVCM, contractility is normal initially; however, the onset of ventricular arrhythmias (ventricular tachycardia) leads to slow deterioration of right ventricular function. Eventually, ventricular tachyarrhythmias (ventricular tachycardia or fibrillation) become resistant to antiarrhythmic therapy.

MANAGEMENT

The perioperative management of children with known CM requires an understanding of normal cardiovascular physiology and an appreciation of the particular pathophysiology associated with the patient's CM. Maintenance of cardiac output is the primary objective. As illustrated by the case synopsis, induction of anesthesia may cause myocardial depression or loss of systemic vascular tone, leading to abrupt circulatory collapse and, possibly, malignant arrhythmias and cardiac arrest. Two rather simple but crucial relationships illustrate the components that regulate cardiac output:

1. Cardiac output = Heart rate × Stroke volume.
2. Stroke volume is determined by preload, contractility, and afterload.

Typically, the myopathic ventricle requires at least normal to increased preload to maintain adequate stroke volume. At the same time, intravenous volume loading may upset a delicate balance between sufficient preload and that which will dilate the ventricle and increase its end-diastolic pressure. The latter reduces endocardial perfusion to decrease rather than increase stroke volume. Invasive monitoring helps assess hemodynamic responses to intravenous fluid challenges, as well as intermittent positive-pressure ventilation. Patients who have been fluid-restricted preoperatively are most susceptible to severe hypotension in response to intermittent positive-pressure ventilation.

Once preload has been optimized, contractility may need to be addressed. Except for patients with HCM, children with CM have compromised contractility and limited myocardial functional reserve. Anesthetic agents should be administered with this in mind. Inotropes (e.g., dopamine, dobutamine, epinephrine) or inodilators (e.g., milrinone) may be required perioperatively to maintain cardiac output. Augmented contractility improves stroke volume, but at the cost of increased myocardial oxygen consumption.

Increased afterload, due to increased systemic or pulmonary vascular resistance, impedes the contraction of the LV and/or RV. Intramyocardial wall stress (a major determinant of afterload) increases directly with ventricular diameter according to Laplace's principle. Thus, at the same level of arterial pressure, afterload encountered by an enlarged ventricle is higher than that for a ventricle of normal size.

Children with end-stage CM may have pulmonary hypertension. Every effort should be made to avoid increases in pulmonary vascular resistance. This is done by minimizing mean airway pressures, maintaining normocapnea to hypocapnia, providing permissive metabolic alkalosis, and giving exogenous pulmonary vasodilator agents (e.g., nitric oxide, prostaglandins).

Finally, a reduction in stroke volume often results in a sympathetically mediated increase in heart rate to compensate for the decrease in cardiac output. Maintenance of sinus or atrial-origin rhythms (e.g., wandering atrial pacemaker), and the associated atrial contribution to ventricular filling, is critical. Loss of sinoatrial rhythm with nonatrial, lower pacemaker escape rhythms (e.g., atrioventricular junctional or idioventricular rhythms or tachycardia) leads to inadequate diastolic filling and lower end-diastolic volumes. This aggravates any preexisting diastolic dysfunction.

Management objectives for the specific CMs are as follows.

Dilated Cardiomyopathy

- Preload: normovolemia
  - Adequate fluids are required to maintain increased end-diastolic volume and cardiac output.
- Contractility: increase
  - Inodilators (e.g., milrinone) are especially useful because they augment contractility and reduce afterload at the same time.
- Heart rate: normal or increase
  - A mildly accelerated heart rate compensates for reduced stroke volume to help maintain cardiac output.
- Afterload: normal or decrease
  - Afterload reduction helps unload a poorly contractile ventricle.

Hypertrophic Cardiomyopathy

- Preload: increase
  - Avoid hypovolemia due to inadequate fluid replacement or vasodilatation of the venous capacitance bed causing reduced venous return.
- Contractility: decrease
  - Halothane is a useful anesthetic agent for reducing contractility and heart rate.
  - Avoid light anesthesia and sympathetically mediated increases in contractility.
  - β-Blockers can be used to control both the hyperdynamic myocardium and heart rate.
- Heart rate: normal or decrease
- Afterload: normal or increase
  - Decreased systemic vascular resistance reduces coronary perfusion pressure.
  - Reduced coronary perfusion pressure may lead to myocardial ischemia, with the potential to cause intraoperative cardiac arrest due to ventricular fibrillation or bradyasystole.
  - Phenylephrine is the drug of choice to increase afterload.

Restrictive Cardiomyopathy

- Preload: normovolemia
- Contractility: increase
  - Inotropic support is frequently required.
- Heart rate: normal
- Afterload: do not increase or decrease

Arrhythmogenic Cardiomyopathy

- Preload: normovolemia
- Contractility: normal
- Heart rate: normal
  - Maintain sinus rhythm and place defibrillator pads before the induction of anesthesia.
- Afterload: do not increase or decrease

PREVENTION

To avoid a catastrophic reduction in cardiac output during anesthesia and surgery in pediatric patients with CM, one must have a thorough understanding of the pathophysiology of the particular CM present. Obviously, elective or less urgent surgery in a patient known to have a CM requires extensive discussion with the child's cardiologist, surgeon, and parents. This should allow complete medical preparation of the patient before the day of surgery and help reduce the risk of perioperative deterioration.

When more urgent surgery is required, it may not be possible to optimize the patient's medical condition before his or her arrival in the operating room. If so, the cardiologist should be immediately available for consultation with the anesthesia team. In general, preoperative preparation should follow the management objectives outlined earlier.

Further Reading

Antman EM: Cardiovascular Therapeutics, 2nd ed. Philadelphia, WB Saunders, 2002.

Atlee JL III: Perioperative Cardiac Dysrhythmias, 2nd ed. Chicago, Year Book Medical Publishers, 1990.

Atlee JL: Arrhythmias and Pacemakers. Philadelphia, WB Saunders, 1996.

Carvahlo JS: Cardiomyopathies. In Anderson RH, Baker EJ, Macartney FJ (eds): Pediatric Cardiology. Philadelphia, JB Lippincott–Williams & Wilkins, 2002, pp 1595-1643.

Denfield SW, Gajarski RJ, Towbin JA: Cardiomyopathies. In Garson A, Bricker JT, Fischer DJ (eds): The Science and Practice of Pediatric Cardiology. Philadelphia, WB Saunders, 1998.

Ing RJ, Cook DR, Bengur RA, et al: Anesthetic management of infants with glycogen storage disease type II: A physiological approach. Paediatr Anaesth 14:514-519, 2004.

Kishnani PS, Howell RR: Pompe disease in infants and children. J Pediatr 144:35-43, 2004.

Lipschultz SE, Sleeper LA, Towbin JA, et al: The incidence of pediatric cardiomyopathy in two regions of the United States. N Engl J Med 348:1647-1655, 2003.

McKenzie IM: Cardiomyopathies. In Lake CL, Booker PD (eds): Pediatric Cardiac Anesthesia. Philadelphia, JB Lippincott–Williams & Wilkins, 2005, pp 530-535.

Nugent AW, Daubeney PE, Chondros P, et al: The epidemiology of childhood cardiomyopathy in Australia. N Engl J Med 348:1639-1646, 2003.

Richardson P, McKenna W, Bristow M, et al: Report of the 1995 World Health Organization/International Society and Federation of Cardiology Task Force on the Definition and Classification of Cardiomyopathies. Circulation 93:841-842, 1996.

Stockwell JA, Tobias JD, Greeley WJ: Noninflammatory, noninfiltrative cardiomyopathy. In Nichols DG, Cameron DE, Greeley WJ (eds): Critical Heart Disease in Infants and Children. St. Louis, Mosby, 1995, pp 1037-1051.

Venugolapan P, Agarwal AK, Worthing EA: Chronic cardiac failure in children due to dilated cardiomyopathy: Diagnostic approach, pathophysiology and management. Eur J Pediatr 159:803-810, 2000.

Weller RJ, Weintraub R, Addonizio LJ, et al: Outcome of idiopathic restrictive cardiomyopathy in children. Am J Cardiol 90:501-506, 2002.

PEDIATRICS & NEONATOLOGY

Anterior Mediastinal Mass

167

Randall Flick

Case Synopsis

An 8-year-old, previously healthy girl is admitted with respiratory distress, wheezing, and stridor. Her symptoms have been slowly progressive over 2 weeks and are associated with nocturnal fever and exercise intolerance. The chest radiograph demonstrates a widened mediastinum and a retrosternal mass (Fig. 167-1). A computed tomography (CT) scan of the chest confirms the presence of an anterior mediastinal mass (Fig. 167-2). A biopsy of the mass is scheduled.

PROBLEM ANALYSIS

Definition

Anterior mediastinal masses affect many intrathoracic structures. Most significant are those that compress the heart or major vessels within their respective compartments. Many reports describe sudden, progressive cardiopulmonary compromise due to these masses. Commonly, they involve the anterior mediastinum and, to a lesser extent, the middle and posterior mediastinum.

The mediastinum is defined as that portion of the thorax between the medial aspects of the pleura, above the diaphragm, and below the thoracic inlet. It is bound anteriorly by the sternum and posteriorly by the thoracic vertebrae. A line between the fourth thoracic vertebra and the sternal angle subdivides the mediastinal space into inferior and superior compartments. The inferior space is further subdivided by the pericardium into anterior, middle, and posterior regions.

The location of a mediastinal mass, whether benign or malignant, is characteristic. It provides the clinician with clues to the origin of the mass and determines what physiologic effects it will have on surrounding mediastinal and other thoracic structures.

Recognition

Adult patients with anterior or middle mediastinal masses present with a variety of signs and symptoms. Most, however, either are asymptomatic or have minimal to moderate symptoms, including cough, dyspnea on exertion, chest pain, fatigue, and vocal cord paralysis. Severe symptoms in a minority of adults include orthopnea, stridor, cyanosis, jugular vein distention, or superior vena cava syndrome. The presenting signs and symptoms of anterior mediastinal masses in pediatric patients can include the following:

- Orthopnea or cough in the supine position
- Superior vena cava syndrome with jugular vein distention
- Wheezing or stridor; dyspnea on exertion; increased work of breathing

In pediatric patients, most anterior mediastinal masses are malignant, with lymphomas, germ cell tumors, mesenchymal tumors, and thymic lesions found in decreasing order of frequency.

Risk Assessment

The best approach for the anesthetic management of patients with anterior mediastinal masses is still subject to debate. Some reports describe sudden death or severe cardiopulmonary compromise with the induction of anesthesia and, in some cases, emergence from anesthesia. Some authors suggest that these masses should be biopsied under

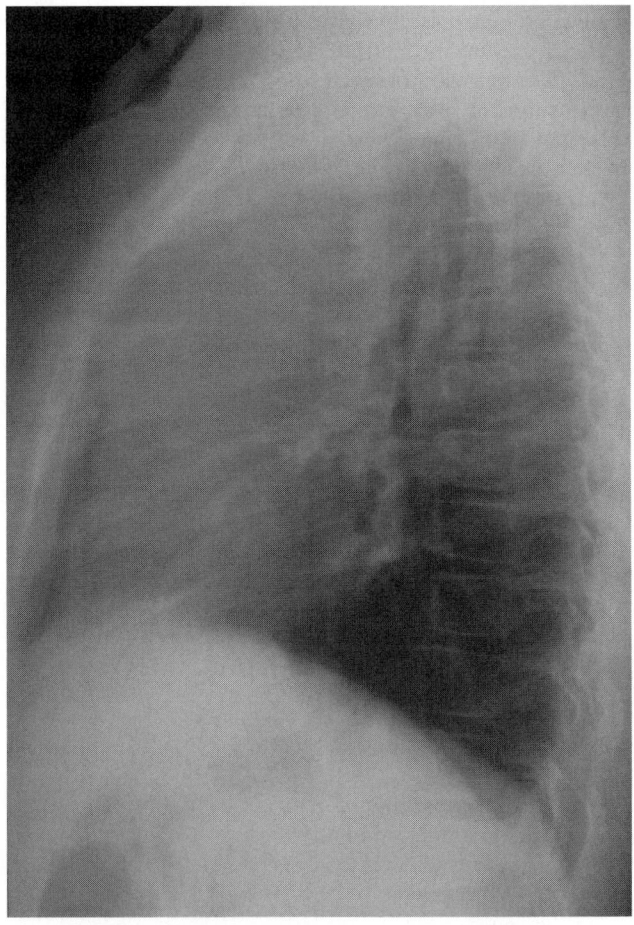

Figure 167–1 ■ Lateral chest film of an 8-year-old girl later determined to have lymphoma. A large mass is seen in the anterior mediastinum. Treatment was initiated before biopsy.

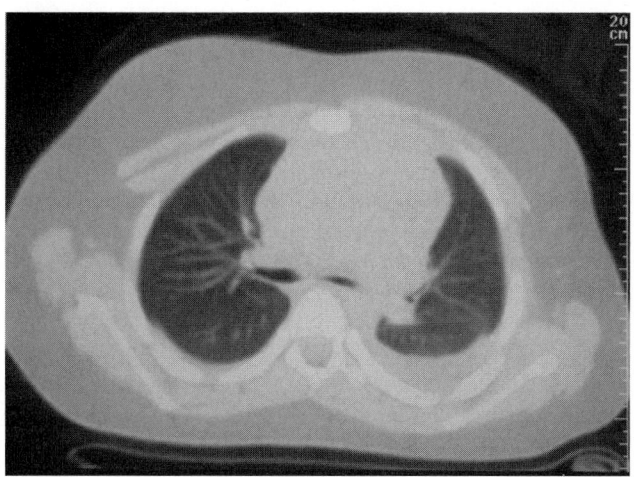

Figure 167–2 ■ Chest computed tomography scan revealing near-complete compression of the distal trachea and main-stem bronchi by a large anterior mediastinal mass. The mass measured approximately 7 by 7 cm and involved not only the trachea but also the great vessels and pericardium.

local anesthesia or, if lymphoma is suspected, they should be treated with chemotherapeutic agents or radiation therapy before biopsy. Others suggest that, given the importance of obtaining early tissue diagnosis, most patients can safely undergo general anesthesia, assuming proper preparation and anesthetic care.

To better predict which patients are likely to have significant cardiopulmonary compromise while under general anesthesia, there have been attempts to correlate preoperative symptoms and CT and spirometry findings with anesthetic outcomes. Patients with a peak expiratory flow rate and tracheal area greater than 50% of predicted for age on CT appear to tolerate general anesthesia without incident. However, even with CT and spirometry, it is often difficult to predict which patients are likely to experience difficulties. A large case series of adult patients suggested that the most reliable predictors of cardiopulmonary compromise are the following:

- Presence of symptoms on presentation
- Combined obstructive and restrictive pattern on pulmonary function testing
- Presence of pericardial effusion
- Tracheal compression with greater than 50% reduction in cross-sectional area on CT

In addition, the presence of severe preoperative symptoms (e.g., supine dyspnea) has been emphasized as an indicator of high-risk status.

Implications

Cardiopulmonary compromise in patients with mediastinal masses results from direct compression or, occasionally, invasion of adjacent pulmonary or vascular structures. The effects of anesthesia increase the impact of airway or vascular compression due to the loss of intrinsic thoracic muscle tone, resulting in reduced thoracic diameter and increased compression of vascular and pulmonary structures.

The location of such compression is critical, because if airway compression occurs distal to the trachea or mainstem bronchi, patients may not benefit from airway stenting with endotracheal or endobroncial tubes. CT scanning can help localize any airway compression. Still, it must be recognized that airway compression following the induction of anesthesia may be more extensive than that seen on CT.

Cardiovascular compromise can take the form of the superior vena cava syndrome owing to compression of venous structures within the superior mediastinum. If so, cardiac output may be compromised by the resulting reduction in preload or by direct compression of the right ventricle by the anterior mediastinal mass. Also, echocardiography has shown that masses of the posterior mediastinum may compress the left atrium and, to a lesser extent, the left ventricle.

Children given general anesthesia for surgery on an anterior mediastinal mass are at risk for developing significant respiratory compromise and complete airway collapse intraoperatively or postoperatively. Some patients may not be able to be extubated after surgery and will require intensive care for the initiation of radiation or chemotherapy. Cardiovascular collapse and death, though rare, are potential complications of general anesthesia in these patients.

An inflatable balloon in the anterior mediastinum has been used in animal models to simulate anterior mediastinal masses. In such models, cardiac output is equally reduced during controlled or spontaneous ventilation in direct proportion to the volume of the mass. This cardiac output reduction is due to increased right ventricular afterload, leading to right ventricular dilatation and septal encroachment on the left ventricle.

MANAGEMENT

Based on the available evidence, it is clear that children with mediastinal masses, especially anterior masses, are at increased risk for cardiopulmonary compromise during the induction of general anesthesia. The question is: Is the risk sufficient for anesthesiologists to request that biopsies of such masses be performed under local anesthesia with monitored anesthesia care, or that radiation or chemotherapy be used preoperatively to shrink these masses?

This question is difficult to answer. However, some recommendations can be made regarding the safe management of most, if not all, children with anterior mediastinal masses. Rather than defining those patients expected to experience cardiopulmonary compromise, existing reports allow us to predict those who are unlikely to have a complicated perioperative course. The following factors allow the anesthesiologist to make that prediction:

- Anterior mediastinal masses are most likely to produce significant cardiopulmonary compromise during general anesthesia. A chest radiograph can provide sufficient information about the location and size of most of these masses to ascertain actual risk.
- Patients without cardiopulmonary symptoms at rest are unlikely to experience related compromise. Most reassuring is the absence of postural cough, stridor, or dyspnea.

- On CT scans, patients with a tracheal cross-sectional area greater than 50% of predicted are less likely to experience cardiopulmonary compromise. CT scanning should be routine for the evaluation of all patients with anterior mediastinal masses.
- Peak expiratory flow rates greater than 50% of predicted are reassuring and should be obtained whenever possible.

Older, more cooperative children thought to be at high risk of cardiopulmonary compromise can have their masses biopsied under local anesthesia. Fine-needle aspiration is sufficient to make an accurate diagnosis in more than 80% of cases. More problematic are children in whom it is impossible to perform such procedures under local anesthesia. An alternative may be a procedure at another site (e.g., bone marrow or lymph node biopsy, aspiration of pleural fluid) conducted under local anesthesia, possibly with intravenous ketamine for sedation.

In those (rare) high-risk cases for which general anesthesia is required, the available reports suggest the following:

- Use inhalational induction with spontaneous ventilation to maintain airway patency.
- If possible, avoid muscle relaxants.
- The sitting, lateral, or prone position may reduce the risk of airway obstruction.
- Rigid bronchoscopy should be available for immediate distal airway access (i.e., beyond the distal tracheal lumen of an endotracheal tube).
- Cardiopulmonary bypass standby has been advocated by some for extremely high-risk patients, including cannulation of the femoral vessels before the induction of anesthesia.
- Fiberoptic bronchoscopy, advocated by some, offers little advantage over endotracheal intubation under deep general anesthesia (without muscle relaxants) in most patients.

PREVENTION

Prevention of acute airway compromise in patients with symptomatic mediastinal masses is achieved by avoiding general anesthesia or deep sedation. Instead, biopsies should be performed with local anesthesia, or radiation therapy or chemotherapy should be administered to reduce the size of the mass before biopsy or before anesthesia and surgery. Although debates are ongoing, it appears that the ability to make a molecular diagnosis has greatly improved, even after radiation or chemotherapy. For the rare patient in which general anesthesia is mandatory, the anesthesiologist must proceed with extreme vigilance and caution.

Further Reading

Bechard P, Letourneau L, Lacasse Y, et al: Perioperative cardiorespiratory complications in adults with mediastinal mass: Incidence and risk factors. Anesthesiology 100:826-834, 2004.

D'Cruz IA, Feghali N, Gross CM: Echocardiographic manifestations of mediastinal masses compressing or encroaching on the heart. Echocardiography 11:523-533, 1994.

Ferrari LR, Bedford RF: General anesthesia prior to treatment of anterior mediastinal masses in pediatric cancer patients. Anesthesiology 72:991-995, 1990.

Johnson D, Hurst T, Cujec B, et al: Cardiopulmonary effects of an anterior mediastinal mass in dogs anesthetized with halothane. Anesthesiology 74:725-736, 1991.

Keon TP: Death on induction of anesthesia for cervical node biopsy. Anesthesiology 55:471-472, 1981.

Mullen B, Richardson JD: Primary anterior mediastinal tumors in children and adults. Ann Thorac Surg 42:338-345, 1986.

Prakash US, Abel MD, Hubmayr RD: Mediastinal mass and tracheal obstruction during general anesthesia. Mayo Clin Proc 63:1004-1011, 1988.

Pullerits J, Holzman R: Anaesthesia for patients with mediastinal masses. Can J Anaesth 36:681-688, 1989.

Robie DK, Mustafa HG, Pokorny J: Mediastinal tumors—airway obstruction and management. Semin Pediatr Surg 3:259-266, 1994.

Shamberger RC, Holzman RS, Griscom NT, et al: CT quantitation of tracheal cross-sectional area as a guide to the surgical and anesthetic management of children with anterior mediastinal masses. J Pediatr Surg 26:138-142, 1991.

Shamberger RC, Holzman RS, Griscom NT, et al: Prospective evaluation by computed tomography and pulmonary function tests of children with mediastinal masses. Surgery 118:468-471, 1995.

Sinner WN: Directed fine needle biopsy of anterior and middle mediastinal masses. Oncology 42:92-96, 1985.

Air Emboli

Lisa Wise-Faberowski and Christian Seefelder

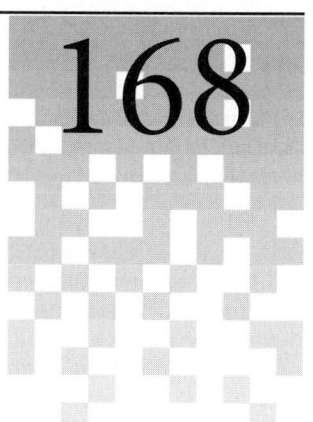

168

Case Synopsis

An 8-week-old infant is undergoing a craniectomy for sagittal craniosynostosis. As the surgeon is excising the cranial bone segment, precordial Doppler sounds change, and the blood pressure rapidly declines (Fig. 168-1).

PROBLEM ANALYSIS

Definition

Gas bubbles within the vascular system are termed *gas emboli* or *air emboli*. When venous air emboli enter the arterial circulation, they are termed *paradoxical air emboli*. Venous air emboli or paradoxical air emboli from gases dissolved in solution are released through *effervescence*, or they may enter the bloodstream from outside through *insufflation* or *entrainment*.

The amount of gas dissolved in a liquid is a function of temperature and pressure. A sudden increase in the temperature of a gas-containing liquid can release gas bubbles from solution through effervescence. This can occur during rapid rewarming following hypothermic cardiopulmonary bypass or by rapidly warming cold intravenous fluids or blood products. It also happens in divers who experience a too-rapid decompression (the "bends").

More commonly, gas is introduced into the bloodstream by insufflation (e.g., during laparoscopy, thoracoscopy, or arthroscopy) or delivered with fluids or blood products by pressurized delivery systems. Veins that do not easily collapse can also entrain air—for example, venous sinuses in bone; open, large central veins; and open veins that are well above the level of the heart. For entrainment to occur, the vein opening must be sufficiently above the level of the heart to exceed central venous pressure (e.g., sitting craniotomy). Venous and paradoxical air emboli can occur in the supine,

prone, or lateral position. The risk of such entrainment is increased by low venous pressure or negative intrathoracic pressure, as occurs during spontaneous respiration.

Small children are at special risk for venous air emboli. Significant blood loss may occur rapidly, and a small amount of blood may constitute a large portion of a child's blood volume. This is a particular concern during craniotomies, because the calvaria is very thin. Further, the head is relatively large in proportion to body size, frequently resulting in the surgical site's being elevated above the heart level during a supine or prone craniotomy. Finally, owing to the high prevalence of intracardiac shunts, amounts of venous air emboli that might be insignificant in an adult can result in paradoxical air emboli and be disastrous for a neonate.

Recognition

Awake patients may experience dyspnea and coughing as a result of venous air emboli. During anesthesia, changes in vital signs occur late and usually only after the entrainment of large amounts of air. Monitoring methods to detect venous air embolism, in decreasing order of sensitivity, include the following:

- Echocardiography or Doppler ultrasonography
- End-tidal carbon dioxide ($ETCO_2$) decrease or new appearance of end-tidal nitrogen (ETN_2)
- Pulmonary artery pressure elevation
- Central venous pressure elevation
- Blood pressure reduction

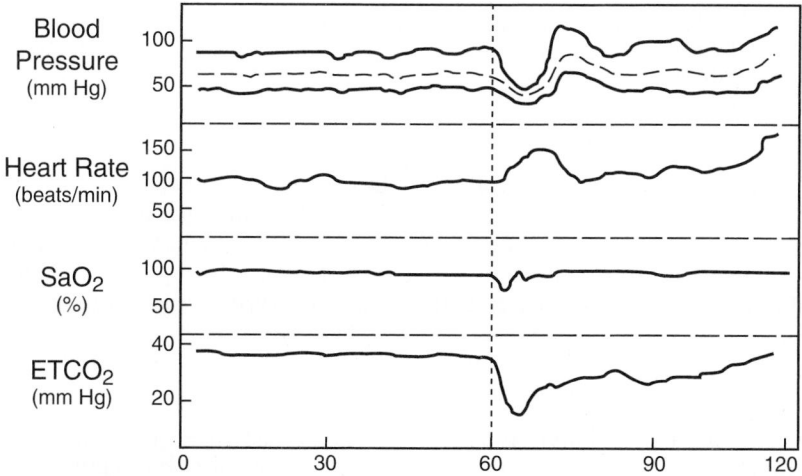

Figure 168–1 ■ Schematic trend recording of blood pressure, heart rate, oxygen saturation (SaO_2), and end-tidal carbon dioxide ($ETCO_2$) concentration in an 8-week-old infant during sagittal craniosynostosis repair. The *dotted line* marks the time at which Doppler sounds changed dramatically. Note the sudden decrease in blood pressure and $ETCO_2$, tachycardia, but little change in SaO_2.

- Electrocardiogram (ECG) changes (e.g., right ventricular strain, ischemia, arrhythmias)
- Audible cardiac or "mill-wheel" murmur

Echocardiography and Doppler monitoring are exquisitely sensitive. They can detect even microbubbles from routine intravenous injections and minor entrainment of air. Air emboli detected with echocardiography and Doppler monitoring should alert the clinical team but must be interpreted cautiously, taking into account the severity of detected air (amount, duration, and associated clinical signs) as well as the clinical situation (e.g., craniotomy). ECG changes are more ominous, and an audible cardiac or "mill-wheel" murmur is least sensitive; however, when associated with echocardiographic or Doppler evidence of venous air embolism, they suggest that a significant amount of air has been entrained.

ECHOCARDIOGRAPHY

Transthoracic or transesophageal echocardiography (TEE) enables the recognition of discrete air bubbles and the relative quantification of larger volumes (i.e., the density of snowstorm pattern). Further, TEE localizes emboli to the right or left side of the heart and detects cardiac anomalies (septal defects) that increase the risk of paradoxical air emboli (Fig. 168-2). TEE has been used in neonates who weigh as little as 2.5 kg. Limitations to its widespread use include the following:

- High cost
- Requirement for a separate, highly trained observer during anesthesia and surgery
- Risk of injury to the pharynx, larynx, and esophagus
- Possible displacement of the endotracheal tube, especially during manipulation in small infants

Consequently, although TEE is a very sensitive technique for detecting venous air emboli, it is currently not practical in many institutions and may not be necessary as a routine monitor.

DOPPLER ULTRASONOGRAPHY

Precordial Doppler ultrasonography is as sensitive as TEE for the detection of venous air emboli. It enables semiquantitative assessment of air emboli but does not permit localization of air to the right or left side of the heart. The smaller distance between the heart and chest wall increases the sensitivity of Doppler ultrasonography in infants. The probe needs to be placed over the right side of the heart, generally at the nipple line, just to the right of the sternum. Minor movement may dislodge the probe, so it should be securely fastened to the chest. Correct positioning is confirmed by injecting a few milliliters of intravenous solution into an intravenous catheter while listening for a characteristic loud change in Doppler sounds. Doppler probes are easily dislodged and can cause pressure necrosis in prone patients. This can be avoided in small infants by placing the Doppler probe on the patient's back. Electrocautery and echocardiography can interfere with Doppler ultrasonography.

END-TIDAL CARBON DIOXIDE

Significant venous air emboli reduce the $ETCO_2$ concentration owing to increased dead-space ventilation. However, $ETCO_2$

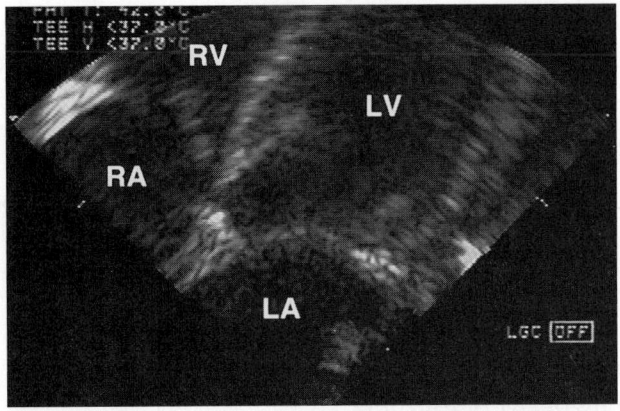

A

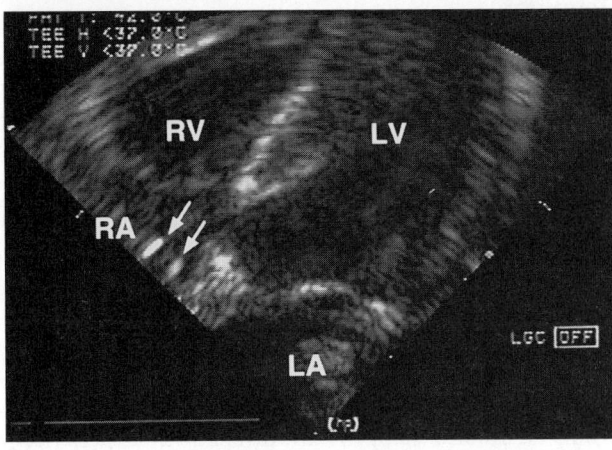

B

Figure 168–2 ▪ Transesophageal echocardiographic four-chamber view of the left atrium (LA), right atrium (RA), left ventricle (LV), and right ventricle (RV). *A,* View of the heart without venous air embolism (VAE). *B, Arrows* indicate the reflections produced by air bubbles in the RA during VAE.

can also be decreased because of reduced pulmonary blood flow from pulmonary thromboembolism, sudden large blood loss, decreased venous return, or reduced cardiac output due to cardiac dysfunction, bradycardia, or arrhythmia. A falsely low $ETCO_2$ may occur with gas leakage or air entrainment around an uncuffed endotracheal tube or dilution of small tidal volumes with fresh gas flows, unless sampling occurs near the endotracheal tube tip. Even so, a sudden change in $ETCO_2$ from a previously stable baseline is usually significant.

EXHALED NITROGEN

Unless air is added to the inspired gases, N_2 disappears from expired gas. Reappearance of N_2 indicates a circuit leak or alveolar diffusion from venous air emboli. Without an air leak, the sudden reappearance of ETN_2 is quite specific for venous air emboli but not very sensitive; even large venous air emboli increase ETN_2 by only 1% to 2%.

PULMONARY ARTERY CATHETER

Pulmonary artery catheters reveal increased pulmonary artery pressure due to pulmonary vascular obstruction by air.

Similar to low central venous pressure, low pulmonary artery wedge pressure may predispose to venous air emboli and paradoxical air emboli. However, pulmonary artery catheters in infants and small children are not practical or necessary in most situations.

CENTRAL VENOUS CATHETER

Central venous catheter placement is justified for high-risk procedures, such as craniotomy in the sitting position, even in a small child. It is rarely necessary for a healthy child when the bed is flat. A central venous catheter is useful for administering fluids and medications if peripheral venous access is difficult, as well as for monitoring central venous pressure. Low central venous pressure may indicate the need for fluid replacement to reduce the risk of venous air emboli; a sudden increase may signal major venous air emboli. A central venous catheter is sometimes effective for retrieving large venous air emboli, especially if the catheter has multiple orifices and the tip is near the junction of the superior vena cava and right atrium. This position is confirmed by radiograph or by recording a unipolar ECG with a right atrial ECG adapter. To do so, substitute the catheter lead for the V lead, and observe the characteristic P-wave changes (increased amplitude leading to tall, spiked P waves that may exceed R- or S-wave amplitudes) as the catheter is advanced into the right atrium.

ARTERIAL BLOOD PRESSURE

An arterial catheter allows continuous assessment of blood pressure and arterial blood gas determinations. Its use is justified in any procedure with a significant risk for bleeding or venous air emboli, especially in young children.

PULSE OXIMETRY

With significant venous air emboli, oxygen desaturation may be detected by pulse oximetry. Arterial blood gas analyses may reveal hypercarbia and an increased arterial-alveolar oxygen gradient.

Risk Assessment

Pediatric patients are at increased risk for venous air emboli during the following procedures:

- Any surgical procedure in which the operative site is sufficiently above the heart, especially when sudden and severe blood loss is possible
- Craniotomy with a large craniectomy (e.g., craniosynostosis repair)
- Craniotomy with an operative site directly over large dural venous sinuses (e.g., posterior fossa exploration)
- Craniofacial procedures (e.g., frontal or midface advancement) with large bony excision and elevation of the head to minimize bleeding
- Certain orthopedic procedures (e.g., scoliosis surgery)
- General surgical procedures (e.g., liver surgery) with a high risk of entering large venous structures (e.g., hepatic veins, inferior vena cava)
- Liver transplantation surgery
- Any open-heart surgery

- Angiography and cardiac catheterization
- Placement, use, and discontinuation of circuits for cardiopulmonary bypass or extracorporeal membrane oxygenation
- Hemodialysis, plasmapheresis, or central venous catheter insertion
- Barotrauma during positive-pressure ventilation
- Use of air to identify epidural space through loss of resistance

Implications

Significant pulmonary air emboli can result in decreased cardiac output, arterial hypotension, and cardiovascular collapse as a result of one or more of the following:

- Obstruction of peripheral pulmonary vessels by gas bubbles
- Air lock from gas in large pulmonary vessels or the heart
- Reflex pulmonary vasoconstriction
- Right ventricular failure secondary to pulmonary hypertension
- Electromechanical dissociation or arrhythmias
- Myocardial ischemia from reduced coronary perfusion pressure, coronary paradoxical air emboli, or hypoxemia

Impaired pulmonary function with carbon dioxide retention and arterial oxygen desaturation can result from the following:

- Ventilation-perfusion mismatch from pulmonary vascular obstruction with increased dead-space ventilation
- Reactive bronchoconstriction with increased airway resistance
- Interstitial pulmonary edema

Gas bubbles enter the arterial circulation directly or through intracardiac communications. Most neonates have a patent foramen ovale, usually with left-to-right shunting. Although the foramen ovale may be probe-patent in 25% to 50% of infants and in 20% to 30% of adults, rarely is shunting demonstrated. However, increased right-sided pressures with venous air emboli may facilitate paradoxical air emboli across a patent foramen ovale. Paradoxical air emboli can result in myocardial or cerebral ischemia.

MANAGEMENT

Key to the successful management of venous air emboli during surgery is close communication between the anesthesiologist and surgeon. In addition, the following guidelines should be considered:

- Doppler sounds should be audible to everyone. Intravenous injections likely to cause Doppler sound changes should be announced beforehand.
- If Doppler ultrasonography indicates venous air emboli unrelated to injections, the surgeon should use indicated measures (e.g., apply bone wax, flood the surgical field with saline or cover it with saline-saturated gauze) to reduce air entry.
- When venous air embolism is suspected, look for an associated decrease in ETCO₂ or blood pressure, indicating a significant venous air embolus or blood loss. Reappearance of ETN₂, if monitored, confirms the diagnosis of venous air emboli.

- Nitrous oxide, though not contraindicated for these procedures, should be promptly discontinued in the presence of venous air emboli. The patient is then ventilated with 100% oxygen to avoid further enlargement of gas bubbles and to treat hypoxemia.
- Change the table position so that the surgical site is below the level of the heart. Be sure that the patient is securely fastened to the operating table.
- Gentle compression of the jugular veins has been recommended to reduce air entry and to unmask possible entry sites, but care must be taken to avoid carotid artery compression.
- Although air may be aspirated through a central venous or pulmonary artery catheter, it does not usually allow removal of a significant amount of entrained air.
- Positioning the patient in the left lateral decubitus position has been suggested to aid in resuscitation, but it may not be practical during some procedures.
- Support cardiovascular function with additional intravenous fluids or inotropic agents (ephedrine, epinephrine) as indicated. Cardiopulmonary resuscitation is rarely required, especially if the embolus is detected quickly and appropriate measures are instituted.

PREVENTION

A careful history and physical examination, as well as familiarity with the planned surgery, are essential to assess the risk for venous air emboli or paradoxical air emboli. Use precordial Doppler ultrasonography as a sensitive and noninvasive monitor to detect venous air emboli early. Consider the use of filters or bubble traps when significant or rapid fluid or blood replacement is anticipated. For high-risk procedures, be prepared to use measures to reduce air entrainment and venous air emboli (e.g., positioning, use of bone wax, flooding the surgical field).

Further Reading

Cucchiara RF, Bowers B: Air embolism in children undergoing suboccipital craniotomy. Anesthesiology 57:338-339, 1982.

Eldredge EA, Soriano SG, Rockoff MA: Pediatric neurosurgical anesthesia. In Coté CJ, Todres ID, Goudsouzian NG, Ryan JF (eds): A Practice of Anesthesia for Infants and Children, 3rd ed. Philadelphia, WB Saunders, 2001, pp 493-521.

Faberowski LW, Black S, Mickle JP: Incidence of venous air embolism during craniotomy for craniosynostosis repair. Anesthesiology 92:20-23, 2000.

Harris MM, Strafford MA, Rowe RW, et al: Venous air embolism and cardiac arrest during craniectomy in a supine infant. Anesthesiology 65:547-550, 1986.

Harris MM, Yemen TA, Davidson A, et al: Venous embolism during craniectomy in supine infants. Anesthesiology 67:816-819, 1987.

Markhorst DG, Rothuis E, Sobotka-Plojhar M, et al: Transient foramen ovale incompetence in the normal newborn: An echocardiographic study. Eur J Pediatr 154:667-671, 1995.

Sethna NF, Berde CB: Venous air embolism during identification of the epidural space in children. Anesth Analg 76:925-927, 1993.

Complications of Massive Transfusion

169

Lisa M. Montenegro and David R. Jobes

Case Synopsis

A 5-month-old infant presents to the operating room for exploratory laparotomy after being involved in a motor vehicle accident. He is tachycardic (heart rate 180 beats per minute) and normotensive (blood pressure 80/55 mm Hg), with a grossly distended abdomen on arrival to the operating room. On opening of the abdomen, the blood pressure falls to 50/30 mm Hg. Bleeding from a badly lacerated liver necessitates rapid and massive volume replacement.

PROBLEM ANALYSIS

Definition

For pediatric patients, massive transfusion is defined as the need to replace at least one blood volume; blood volume varies by age, being approximately 80 mL/kg at birth and 65 mL/kg at age 12 years. Although transfusion under any circumstances carries some risk (e.g., infection, transfusion reactions; see Chapters 49 and 50), massive transfusion involves a unique set of risks and complications, many of which require special consideration in the pediatric population.

Recognition

Massive transfusion and related complications are the result of therapy for acute intravascular volume loss, which includes rapid repletion of intravascular volume with crystalloid, non–red blood cell (RBC) colloids, blood, and blood products. This can occur in the following situations:

- Major trauma
- Gastrointestinal bleeding
- Major vascular surgery
- Cardiac surgery
- Hepatic surgery
- Craniofacial surgery
- Radical oncologic surgery
- Spinal instrumentation

Anticipating the need for massive transfusion may allow the early recognition and aggressive treatment of its associated complications, thereby avoiding the risk of acute intravascular volume depletion. Some circumstances that enhance and may contribute to the development of transfusion-related complications include the following:

- Administration of anticoagulants or other drugs
- Clotting factor deficiencies
  - Hereditary, dilutional, or acquired
  - Due to clotting factor consumption
  - Due to extracorporeal membrane oxygenation and circulatory assist devices
- Hypothermia
- Use of a cell-saver or autotransfusion device

Loss of up to 30% of the blood volume is usually well tolerated in infants and children. Signs of hypovolemia may be subtle and include a small to moderate increase in heart rate and decrease in blood pressure. Such blood volume loss in otherwise healthy children can be replaced with crystalloid solutions without significant hemodynamic or cardiovascular compromise.

Risk Assessment

Any patient who requires acute, massive intravascular volume replacement is at risk for complications related to massive transfusion. Infants and neonates appear to be at increased risk owing to the immaturity of their native coagulation systems. The following complications are more likely to occur in this patient subset:

- Dilutional coagulopathy
- Hypothermia
- Hypokalemia or hyperkalemia
- Hypocalcemia

A more complete list of generally recognized complications is provided in Table 169-1.

Implications

The hemostatic function of the coagulation system is normal at birth. However, quantities of many procoagulant and inhibitory proteins do not reach their adult concentrations until after puberty. Andrew and colleagues measured an extensive clotting profile, including prothrombin time (PT), partial thromboplastin time (PTT), and clotting factor concentrations, in healthy neonates, infants, and children (from 1 day to 16 years of age). Although most test results did not differ from normal values for adults, there was greater variability in PT, although mean PT values were not significantly different from those in adults. The PTT was significantly prolonged in neonates and infants; however, adult PTT values were attained by age 3 months. The concentrations of all clotting factors, including vitamin K–dependent factors (II, VII, IX, X),

Table 169–1 ▪ Clinically Significant Complications of Massive Blood Transfusion
Dilutional coagulopathy
Acid-base derangement
Hypothermia
Hyperkalemia
Hypokalemia
Citrate load (hypocalcemia)
Microembolization or microaggregate formation: ARDS?
Infectious (HIV, CMV, hepatitis, West Nile virus, bacterial)
Hemolysis
Anaphylaxis
Change in RBC deformability
Jaundice (long term)

ARDS, acute respiratory distress syndrome; CMV, cytomegalovirus; HIV, human immunodeficiency virus; RBC, red blood cell.

plasminogen, and the plasma protease inhibitors (antithrombin 3, α_2-antiplasmin, C_1-esterase inhibitor, and α_1-antitrypsin), were substantially reduced at birth. Although all clotting variables had independent maturation processes, the concentrations of factors II, VII, IX, and X were less than those for adults until age 16 years. In contrast, plasminogen and plasma protease inhibitors approached or reached adult levels by age 5 years. Each of the vitamin K–dependent factors also displayed its own age-related maturation process. Factor VII was the first to achieve near-adult values at 5 days of age.

Neonates and infants have laboratory values that are outside the adult reference ranges for the integrity of coagulation (especially PT and PTT). As such, normal laboratory values for adults do not measure neonatal hemostatic competence, and comparisons must be made with caution.

MANAGEMENT

Management goals are to maintain the quantitative and qualitative integrity of intravascular volume. Oxygen carrying capacity and hemostasis are of primary importance. In the face of massive volume loss, these goals can be met only by transfusing whole blood or components of fractionated whole blood. The intravenous administration of any blood product, especially pooled components, is associated with a substantial risk of complications. This risk is amplified and multiplied during massive transfusion (see Table 169-1).

Dilutional Coagulopathy

The most common complication of massive transfusion is dilutional coagulopathy. Dilution of hemostatic blood elements occurs from substances used for volume expansion (crystalloid, colloid, hetastarch, albumin), transfused blood, and blood products. The administration of nonblood substances begins the dilutional process. Component therapy may also result in the dilution of hemostatic blood elements, because each lost component is not precisely replenished. When replacement approaches or exceeds approximately one blood volume, continued dilution of remaining platelets and clotting factors results in impaired hemostasis.

Component Replacement Therapy

Controversy exists regarding the timing of replacement of non-RBC blood products. Some suggest that products other than RBCs should not be administered until a coagulopathy or specific factor deficiency is documented. This approach is intended to limit transfusion risk and seems plausible when the loss and replacement are expected to be about one blood volume. However, when the loss is expected to or does exceed one blood volume, or bleeding is not controlled, early administration of non-RBC products is necessary to prevent enhanced blood loss from coagulopathy. Coté's group demonstrated an exponential decline in the number of available platelets versus the number of blood volumes replaced. However, the absolute decline is not as great as one would expect based on blood loss and replacement. This may be due to platelet recruitment. Qualitative platelet function is further reduced by hypothermia, with only 12% of the original platelet function remaining after 24 hours of storage at 4°C. The same concept likely applies to other clotting factors as well. With the exception of thrombocytopenia (platelet counts <100,000/mm^3), the existence of a coagulopathy can rarely be documented in a timely fashion. Therefore, platelets and fresh frozen plasma must be administered during a massive transfusion without waiting for a documented coagulopathy to develop. Although no differentiation is made between infants and adults, some recommended transfusion protocols include the following:

- 0.3 unit/kg platelets when the platelet count is less than 100,000 mm^3 or when more than 1.5 blood volumes have been transfused
- One unit of fresh frozen plasma and 4 units of platelets for every 5 units of packed RBCs transfused

Indications for component replacement and the positive and negative attributes of specific component therapy are listed in Table 169-2. Because infants and neonates have lower plasma clotting factor concentrations than adults do, dilutional coagulopathy with massive transfusion develops more quickly. Therefore, the threshold for replacement of coagulation factors in infants is lower.

Recombinant Factor VIIa

Recombinant factor VIIa has been used to treat microvascular bleeding when replacement therapy has been judged adequate but the bleeding continues. Originally developed to treat hemophilia, recombinant factor VIIa promotes hemostasis at the site of injury by interacting with tissue factor. It is beginning to be incorporated into trauma management protocols, although controlled clinical trials for this application are currently lacking. Case reports describe dramatic cessation of bleeding after its administration, and it should be considered as a lifesaving measure in pediatric patients with continued microvascular bleeding despite adequate replacement therapy. Recombinant factor VIIa has a short half-life and requires redosing (90 units/kg) every 2 hours until bleeding is controlled. Other drugs, such as aprotinin, are increasingly reported in the cardiac and orthopedic surgical literature as adjuncts to reduce blood loss and transfusion requirements.

Table 169–2 ■ Indications for Component Replacement and Anticipated Hemostatic Attributes

Product	Indication	Positive Attributes	Negative Attributes
Packed RBCs	Hypovolemia associated with anemia	Readily available (autologous, homologous, cell saver blood); more efficient than blood substitutes; maintains or $\uparrow O_2$ transport capacity and BV	Dilutional coagulopathy; hemolytic reaction; infection; rare blood types may be unavailable
Fresh whole blood	Anemia; hypovolemia with anemia; massive transfusion (neonates)	Less donor exposure, especially neonates; platelets and clotting factors functional; maintains or $\uparrow O_2$ transport capacity and BV	Limited availability; hemolytic transfusion reaction
Fresh frozen plasma	Dilutional coagulopathy	Replaces all protein clotting factors at presumed normal adult concentrations; available universally in frozen state	Timing of administration; infection; concentration of specific factors may be inadequate in some cases (e.g., fibrinogen); availability (minimum of 30 min to thaw)
Cryoprecipitate	Dilutional coagulopathy; factor VIII deficiency	High concentrations of fibrinogen and factor VIII	Pooled product; risk of infection; timing of administration; availability (not stored in all blood banks)
Platelets	Platelet dysfunction; thrombocytopenia	Increases platelet count	Hypotension; single donor vs multiple donors; infection; brief functional half-life

BV, blood volume; RBCs, red blood cells.

Laboratory Testing

Repetitive laboratory tests to identify the development and correction of coagulopathy are necessary. However, massive transfusion may alter normal tests of hemostasis. Murray and colleagues reported that in the absence of thrombocytopenia, PT and PTT values in adult surgical patients may be increased to 1.5 times control values without clinical evidence of increased or unusual blood loss. Because all blood and blood derivatives are obtained from adult donors, when massive transfusion occurs in a pediatric patient, all laboratory tests of hemostatic function should be interpreted in light of the adult donor pool. A platelet count of more than $100,000/mm^3$ is necessary after massive volume replacement because of qualitative changes in platelet function. Some variation exists in the dilution of individual clotting factors. When more than 1.5 blood volumes are replaced, concentrations of fibrinogen, factor V, and factor VIII become inadequate (20% of normal), whereas other clotting factor concentrations are less affected. In acute situations, laboratory measurement of specific clotting factor concentrations is not helpful, because the test results are not immediately available.

Autotransfusion and Cell-Saver Devices

The use of blood salvage devices to return lost RBCs has become commonplace. Processing washes the salvaged blood and returns concentrated RBCs suspended in normal saline. Although these devices reduce the need to administer homologous RBCs, they contribute to the dilution of all hemostatic elements. Thus, when transfusion approaches or surpasses 1.5 blood volumes, laboratory assessment of hemostasis is essential, regardless of the replacement strategy used (Table 169-3).

Table 169–3 ■ Laboratory Assessment and Treatment Indications when Transfusion Approaches or Surpasses 1.5 Estimated Blood Volumes

Laboratory Assessment	Treatment Indication
Metabolic Arterial blood gases: pH, P_{O_2}, P_{CO_2}, base excess, hematocrit	Deviation from normal laboratory values
Electrolytes K^+, Ca^{2+}, Mg^{2+}, Na^+, Cl^-	Deviation from normal laboratory values

Hemostasis
  Prothrombin time
  Partial thromboplastin time
  Fibrinogen
  Platelet count
	Continued gross hemorrhage or microvascular bleeding present
	$\geq 1.5 \times$ normal value
	$\geq 1.5 \times$ normal value
	≤ 100 mg/dL
	$\leq 100,000/mm^3$

Table 169–4 ▪ Biochemical Changes for Blood Stored in CPD and CPDA-1

Biochemical Change	CPD Whole Blood		CPDA-1 Whole Blood		RBCs	
Days of storage	0	21	0	35	0	35
% Viable cells 24 hr after transfusion	100	80	100	79	100	71
pH (37°C)	7.2	6.84	7.6	6.98	7.55	6.71
2,3-DPG (% of initial value)	100	86	44	<10	100	<10
Plasma K⁺ (mmol/L)	3.9	21.0	4.2	27.3	5.1	78.5*
Plasma Na⁺ (mmol/L)	168	156	169	155	169	111
ATP (% of initial value)	100	86	100	56 ± 16	100	45 ± 12

*The plasma K⁺ concentration appears to be unusually high in RBC units stored for 35 days because the total plasma in these units is only about 70 mL.
ATP, adenosine triphosphate; CPD, citrate phosphate dextrose; CPDA-1, citrate phosphate dextrose adenine; DPG, diphosphoglyceride; RBC, red blood cell.
From Vengelen-Tyler V (ed): Technical Manual, 12th ed. Bethesda, Md., AABB, 1996, p 138.

Fresh Whole Blood

Not all patients are optimally managed by component therapy for massive volume loss. The administration of fresh whole blood (24 to 48 hours old) to children younger than 2 years undergoing repair of complex congenital cardiac lesions significantly reduces postoperative hemorrhage compared with reconstituted blood (with fresh frozen plasma and platelets) or component therapy. However, the use of fresh whole blood is impractical for emergencies and is difficult to provide logistically. Additionally, nucleic acid testing of donated blood for human immunodeficiency virus (HIV) may not be accomplished in less than 48 hours, making fresh whole blood less safe than banked blood. Despite its theoretical advantage in massive transfusion, this technique has not been studied outside the infant cardiac surgery population.

Metabolic Derangement

Acid-base alterations may occur simply from the blood collection and preservation process. The pH of freshly collected blood added to CPD (citrate phosphate dextrose) solution decreases to 7.0; over the next 21 days of storage, it decreases to 6.84 (Table 169-4). The majority of this decrease is due to an increase in the partial pressure of carbon dioxide, because storage containers do not permit its egress.

Hypothermia

Hypothermia commonly occurs with massive transfusion and can be a cause of coagulation dysfunction. The trauma literature supports a 100% mortality rate if a patient's core temperature falls below 32°C, regardless of the severity of injury.[1] Large volumes of unwarmed crystalloid, non-RBC-containing colloids, blood, and blood products can produce cardiac arrest, especially when administered directly into the central circulation in small children.

Hyperkalemia

Hyperkalemia can develop with the rapid transfusion of stored RBCs. The potassium concentration in stored blood increases over time as cells lyse (see Table 169-4). Although patients with normal renal function rarely display hyperkalemia or its hemodynamic consequences, neonates and infants with immature renal function, or patients with renal dysfunction, should receive washed RBCs. Occasionally, seeming paradoxical delayed hypokalemia may be seen after the transfusion of stored RBCs ceases.

Hypocalcemia

Hypocalcemia, or functional hypocalcemia, occurs after the rapid administration of blood stored with citrate. The citrate chelates the calcium and other covalent cations, such as magnesium. Hypotension can result from overly rapid transfusion, especially of platelet concentrates or fresh frozen plasma. Correction with intravenous calcium is immediate. Calcium replacement in asymptomatic patients is controversial, because ionized calcium levels return to normal after acute blood administration ceases.

Pulmonary Dysfunction

Microaggregate formation and pulmonary deposition are believed to be mechanisms by which acute respiratory distress syndrome develops after massive transfusion. The incidence of acute respiratory distress syndrome has been reduced with the use of 10-μm filters for blood administration. In addition, this complication is seen predominantly in patients with preexisting or acute lung injury, suggesting that other factors also are involved.

Infection

The risk of infection escalates with massive transfusions, either by the transmission of infectious agents or by the depression of immune responses. Although the risk for transmission of HIV, viral hepatitis, West Nile virus, and cytomegalovirus is low, each donor exposure increases a patient's likelihood of contracting a potentially fatal disease. Rarely, bacterial contamination of a blood product may occur.

Hemolysis

Hemolysis, usually due to an ABO incompatibility, can be catastrophic. Currently, the most common cause of this

---

[1]Assuming such hypothermia has not been deliberately imposed (e.g., cardiopulmonary bypass).

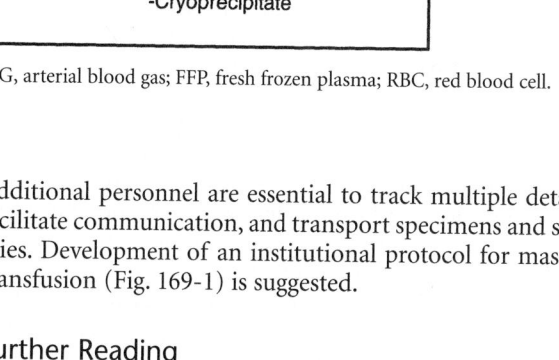
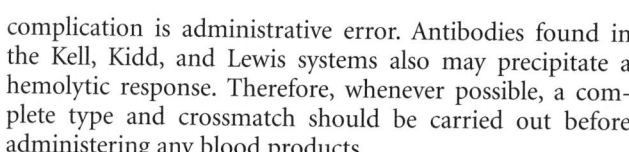

**IDENTIFY PATIENT AT RISK
FOR MASSIVE TRANSFUSION**

Prepare environment

Volume replacement
(crystalloid/non-blood colloid)

3 mL crystalloid:1 mL blood loss
1 mL colloid:1 mL blood loss

Warm room
Warm fluids
Warm patient
-Radiant
-Bair Hugger

Notify additional support personnel

Laboratory

ABG
Hematology
Coagulation

Anesthesia

Additional
assistance

Charge nurse

Technician
Scribe
Additional
assistance

Blood bank

Prepare/acquire
products
-Whole blood
-RBCs
-FFP
-Platelets
-Cryoprecipitate

Figure 169–1 ■ Algorithm for the management of massive transfusion. ABG, arterial blood gas; FFP, fresh frozen plasma; RBC, red blood cell.

complication is administrative error. Antibodies found in the Kell, Kidd, and Lewis systems also may precipitate a hemolytic response. Therefore, whenever possible, a complete type and crossmatch should be carried out before administering any blood products.

PREVENTION

Successful preventive management of patients with acute, massive hemorrhagic volume loss requires the following:

- Blood bank support
- Laboratory support
- Adequate personnel
- Body temperature control
- Warming of all intravenous and surgical irrigation fluids

The prevention of complications requires the immediate availability of adequate blood bank resources, appropriate administration equipment, and rapid laboratory turnaround time. Careful recording and reporting of the quantity and type of all volume infused (including crystalloid, colloid, and blood products), along with timely communication of anticipated needs to the blood bank, are critical.

Additional personnel are essential to track multiple details, facilitate communication, and transport specimens and supplies. Development of an institutional protocol for massive transfusion (Fig. 169-1) is suggested.

Further Reading

Andrew M, Paes B, Milner R, et al: Development of the human coagulation system in the full-term infant. Blood 70:165-172, 1987.

Andrew M, Vegh P, Johnston M, et al: Maturation of the hemostatic system during childhood. Blood 80:1998-2005, 1992.

Coté CJ, Liu LM, Szyfelbein SK, et al: Changes in serial platelet counts following massive blood transfusion in pediatric patients. Anesthesiology 62:197-201, 1985.

Hardy JF, De Moerloose P, Samama M: Groupe d'interet en Hemostase Perioperatoire: Massive transfusion and coagulopathy: Pathophysiology and implications for clinical management. Can J Anaesth 51:293-310, 2004.

Jurkovich GL, Greiser WB, Luterman A, et al: Hypothermia in trauma victims: An ominous predictor of survival. J Trauma 27:1019-1024, 1987.

Levi M, Peters M, Buller HR: Efficacy and safety of recombinant factor VIIa for treatment of severe bleeding: A systematic review. Crit Care Med 33:883-890, 2005.

Manno CS, Hedberg KW, Kim HC, et al: Comparison of the hemostatic effects of fresh whole blood, stored whole blood, and components after open heart surgery in children. Blood 77:930-936, 1991.

Murray DJ, Olson J, Strauss R, et al: Coagulation changes during packed red cell replacement of major blood loss. Anesthesiology 69:839-845, 1988.

Perioperative Psychological Trauma

170

Zeev N. Kain

Case Synopsis

A 4-year-old boy presents for inguinal hernia repair. In the preoperative holding area, he appears scared and agitated and refuses to leave his mother's lap. On separation, he cries and tries to escape from the anesthesiologist. One week after surgery, the mother reports major behavioral changes in the boy since his operation, including nightmares and temper tantrums.

PROBLEM ANALYSIS

Definition

The perioperative period is frequently an extremely traumatic time for both children and parents. Subjective feelings of tension, apprehension, and worry characterize preoperative anxiety in children. Preoperative anxiety stimulates sympathetic, parasympathetic, and endocrine systems, leading to increases in heart rate, blood pressure, and cardiac excitability. These reactions reflect the child's fear of separation from parents and the home environment, loss of control, and fear of unfamiliar routines, surgical instruments, and hospital procedures. Thus, it is no surprise that up to 65% of all children undergoing anesthesia and surgery develop extreme anxiety and fear during the perioperative period.

Of perhaps greater importance than the child's behavior in the preoperative holding area is the child's behavior after the surgery. Clinicians and investigators have long recognized postoperative psychological reactions such as general anxiety, nighttime crying, enuresis, separation anxiety, and temper tantrums. These behavioral changes are of particular concern if they persist for an extended period and negatively affect the child's responses to subsequent medical care or interfere with his or her emotional and cognitive development.

Recognition

Children having anesthesia and surgery express many forms of anxiety. Some explicitly verbalize their fears, whereas others express their anxiety behaviorally. Many children look scared, become agitated, breathe deeply, tremble, stop talking or playing, or begin to cry. Others may wet themselves unexpectedly, have increased motor tone, and actively attempt to escape from medical personnel. The specific maladaptive behaviors in any particular child can vary widely. However, the most common ones are separation anxiety, eating problems, increased fear of doctors and hospitals, bad dreams or nightmares, and temper tantrums.

Perioperative anxiety is associated with increased levels of serum cortisol, epinephrine, growth hormone, and adrenocorticotropic hormone. Reports show a significant correlation between increased heart rate and blood pressure and behavioral ratings of anxiety. Preoperative anxiety is often associated with a relative vagal predominance in sympathovagal-mediated heart rate variability.

Risk Assessment

The incidence of preoperative anxiety in young children is reported to range from 40% to 60%. Children of anxious parents, shy and inhibited children, children with a history of previous surgery, children with a history of previous poor-quality medical encounters, and children aged 4 to 7 years are at increased risk for the development of preoperative anxiety.

Postoperative maladaptive behavioral responses, such as general anxiety, nighttime crying, enuresis, separation anxiety, and temper tantrums, occur in 13% to 40% of children 2 weeks after surgery; 3% to 20% of these children continue to demonstrate maladaptive behaviors 6 months after surgery (Fig. 170-1). More significant behavioral changes, such as new-onset enuresis, are rare and present in only 0.8% of children. It is important to emphasize that although a large number of young children develop negative behavioral responses in the immediate postoperative period, the magnitude of these changes is limited, and only a minority of children have persistent, long-term maladaptive behavioral responses.

The child's age, baseline temperament, number of siblings, enrollment in day care, and preoperative anxiety are all independent predictors for postoperative maladaptive behaviors in multivariate models (Tables 170-1 and 170-2). Genitourinary surgery is associated with the highest incidence of postoperative behavioral changes. Pressure-equalizing myringotomy and tympanic membrane tube placement have the lowest incidence of postoperative negative behavioral changes.

Implications

Preoperative anxiety may be a hardship on both the child and the parents and lead to immediate postoperative negative behavioral responses. Long-lasting psychological effects that influence the child's response to subsequent medical care and interfere with normal development have been described. Although reports are conflicting, they suggest that preoperative anxiety may delay gastric emptying and increase gastric acidity; therefore, some practitioners consider this response to be a risk factor for aspiration pneumonitis.

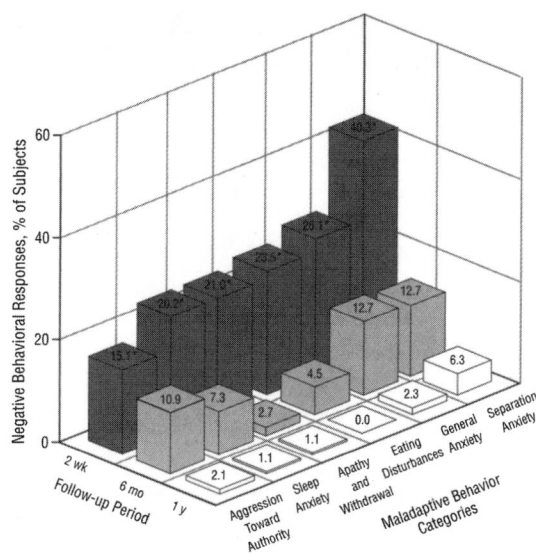

Figure 170–1 ▪ Changes over time in the prevalence of negative behavioral responses based on the Posthospitalization Behavior Questionnaire. Separation anxiety was the most common maladaptive behavior reported by parents at both 2 weeks (40.3%) and 6 months (6.3%). The prevalence of behaviors in all six categories decreased significantly from 2 weeks to 6 months and 1 year (numbers in bars represent percentages of total subjects). *P <.05. (From Kain ZN, Mayes LC, O'Connor T: Preoperative anxiety in children: Predictors and outcomes. Arch Pediatr Adolesc Med 150:1238-1245, 1996.)

Preoperative anxiety is also associated with an increased risk of symptoms of emergence delirium upon awakening from anesthesia, as well as altered cortisol and epinephrine responses over the first 24 hours after surgery.

MANAGEMENT

Behavioral modification and pharmacologic agents are the two preoperative interventions directed toward reducing perioperative anxiety.

Behavioral Modification

Parental presence during the induction of anesthesia has been suggested as an alternative to preanesthetic medication. The potential benefits of parental presence include the following:

- Avoidance of screaming and struggling (separation anxiety)
- Reduction in the child's anxiety during induction
- Potential reduction of the long-term behavioral effects of surgery

Common objections to parental presence include the following:

- Disruption of the operating room routine
- Compromise of operative sterility
- Crowded operating rooms
- Additional stress on the anesthesiologist

Experimental data do not support the routine use of this intervention. Although earlier studies suggested reduced anxiety, more recent reports indicate that routine parental presence during the induction of anesthesia is *not* always beneficial. Children who benefit are the following:

- Generally, those older than 4 years
- Those with a shy and inhibited personality
- Those with a calm parent

Most parents prefer to be present during the induction of anesthesia, regardless of the child's age or previous surgical experience (even those whose children received sedative premedication at a previous surgery). Among parents present during the induction of anesthesia, the vast majority believe that they were of some assistance to the child and the anesthesiologist. However, more than 90% of parents report feeling some degree of anxiety during induction. Although this is clinically significant, it is not sufficiently debilitating to cause concern for the parents' health. Parental presence during the induction of anesthesia is increasing in the United States, even though available data indicate that it is

Table 170–1 ▪ Risk Factors for Negative Behavioral Changes Two Weeks after Surgery

Predictor Variables	Outcome	Relative Risk (95% CI)
4 vs 6 years of age	Separation anxiety	9.4 (1.2-39)
	General anxiety	3.3 (1.1-7.8)
Not enrolled vs enrolled in a day-care facility	Separation anxiety	6.6 (1.2-29)
Very anxious mother vs calm mother in the holding area*	Apathy and withdrawal	6.6 (1.6-19.1)
	Sleep anxiety	3.9 (1.1-14)
	Separation anxiety	3.4 (1.2-6.7)
Child who is very anxious on separation vs one who is calm on separation†	Eating anxiety	4.2 (1.3-8.7)
No siblings vs siblings	Separation anxiety	3.5 (1.3-9.6)
Child who is very impulsive vs one who is not very impulsive‡	General anxiety	2.7 (1.1-6.8)

*"Very anxious" is defined as an anxiety score in the upper 25th percentile on the State-Trait Anxiety Inventory (STAI) state subscale; "calm" is defined as a score in the lower 25th percentile on the same scale.
†Measured by the Clinical Anxiety Rating Scale.
‡"Very impulsive" is defined as an impulsivity score in the upper 25th percentile on the Emotionality, Activity, Sociability, Impulsivity Instrument; "not very impulsive" is defined as a score in the lower 25th percentile on the same instrument.
CI, confidence interval.
From Kain ZN, Mayes LC, O'Connor T: Preoperative anxiety in children: Predictors and outcomes. Arch Pediatr Adolesc Med 150:1238-1245, 1996.

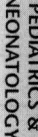

PEDIATRICS & NEONATOLOGY

Table 170–2 ▪ Risk Factors for Negative Behavioral Changes Six Months after Surgery

Predictor Variables	Outcome	Relative Risk (95% CI)
No siblings vs siblings	General anxiety	3.0 (1.4-6.9)
	Separation anxiety	2.0 (1.1-3.5)
	Aggressiveness	2.0 (1.1-4.1)
Very anxious child vs calm child in the holding area*	Eating anxiety	NA[†]
Very anxious mother vs calm mother in the holding area[‡]	Sleep anxiety	4.8 (1.2-20.4)

*"Very anxious" is defined as an anxiety score in the upper 25th percentile on the Venham Picture Test; "calm" is defined as a score in the lower 25th percentile on the same test.
[†]Not applicable; relative risk cannot be calculated because of a 0 value—0% vs 17% (P =.04).
[‡]As measured with the State-Trait Anxiety Inventory (STAI) state subscale.
CI, confidence interval.
From Kain ZN, Mayes LC, O'Connor T: Preoperative anxiety in children: Predictors and outcomes. Arch Pediatr Adolesc Med 150:1238-1245, 1996.

beneficial for only some children. All factors and circumstances should be considered whenever the question of parental presence arises. Research in this area is now focusing more on what parents *do* during induction of anesthesia rather than their mere presence or absence.

Pharmacologic Agents

Sedative premedication before surgery is an effective and widely used method for decreasing anxiety in young children. The primary goal of such premedication is to facilitate smooth and anxiety-free parental separation. A detailed discussion of preanesthetic medication in children is beyond the scope of this chapter. Only the most commonly used agents are discussed.

Midazolam is by far the most commonly used agent for premedication. It has a rapid onset and offset of action and has predictable effects, without causing cardiorespiratory depression. It can be given by any route, depending on the clinical setting. However, when used for preoperative anxiety, it is most commonly administrated orally (0.5 mg/kg) or nasally (0.2 mg/kg). When the drug is mixed with flavored syrup or Tylenol and administered orally, midazolam provides excellent sedation and anxiolysis in 20 to 30 minutes. Despite the high incidence of crying on nasal instillation, this provides predictable effects within 10 minutes. Midazolam can also be given per rectum (0.3 to 0.4 mg/kg), although older children may object to this route.

Ketamine is especially useful as a premedication or induction agent for uncooperative patients. When mixed with a cola-flavored soft drink and given orally (6 mg/kg), ketamine provides predictable sedation in 20 to 25 minutes. The nasal route provides good sedation at similar doses.

Fentanyl's lipid solubility makes it ineffective as an oral premedication. However, oral transmucosal absorption in the form of a fentanyl lollipop can produce effective preoperative sedation and facilitate the inhalational induction of anesthesia. Transmucosal fentanyl (10 to 15 µg/kg) has been reported to cause facial pruritus, and perioperative nausea and vomiting occur in a significant number of children.

Finally, it is important to emphasize that routine preoperative administration of sedatives to all children may result in increased pharmacy costs and the need for additional nursing staff and appropriately equipped bed space in the holding area. It is therefore important to identify the population at high risk for preoperative anxiety and use preoperative sedatives only for those children.

PREVENTION

Preoperative behavioral preparation programs are available, but increasingly fewer U.S. hospitals routinely offer them. These programs consist of child and family preoperative teaching, an orientation tour, and role-playing using dolls to allow the child to become familiar with a new and anxiety-provoking environment. This familiarity may enhance cooperative behavior and lessen anxiety in the preoperative holding area and operating room. Although most studies suggest that behavioral preparation of children reduces stress and enhances coping mechanisms, other reports indicate that such programs may actually "sensitize" younger children.

Further Reading

Brophy CJ, Erickson MT: Children's self-statements and adjustment to elective outpatient surgery. J Dev Behav Pediatr 11:13-16, 1990.

Kain ZN, Caldwell-Andrews AA, Maranets I, et al: Preoperative anxiety, emergence delirium and postoperative maladaptive behaviors: Are they related? A new conceptual framework. Anesth Analg 99:1648-1654, 2004.

Kain ZN, Caldwell-Andrews AA, Mayes LC, et al: Parental presence during induction of anesthesia: Physiological effects on parents. Anesthesiology 98:58-64, 2003.

Kain ZN, Caldwell-Andrews AA, Wang SM, et al: Parental intervention choices for children undergoing repeated surgeries. Anesth Analg 96:970-975, 2003.

Kain ZN, Mayes LC: Anxiety in children during the perioperative period. In Borestein MH, Genevro JL (eds): Child Development and Behavioral Pediatrics. Mahwah, NJ, Lawrence Erlbaum, 1996, pp 85-103.

Kain ZN, Mayes LC, Caramico L: Preoperative preparation in children: A cross sectional study. J Clin Anesth 8:508-514, 1996.

Kain ZN, Mayes LC, Caramico LA, et al: Parental presence during induction of anesthesia: A randomized controlled trial. Anesthesiology 84:1060-1067, 1996.

Kain ZN, Mayes LC, O'Connor T: Preoperative anxiety in children: Predictors and outcomes. Arch Pediatr Adolesc Med 150:1238-1245, 1996.

Lumley MA, Melamed BG, Abeles LA: Predicting children's presurgical anxiety and subsequent behavior changes. J Pediatr Psychol 18:481-497, 1993.

Melamed BG, Dearborn M, Hermecz DA: Necessary considerations for surgery preparation: Age and previous experience. Psychosom Med 45:517-525, 1983.

Vernon DT, Schulman JL, Foley JM: Changes in children's behavior after hospitalization. Am J Dis Child 111:581-593, 1966.

Emergence Agitation

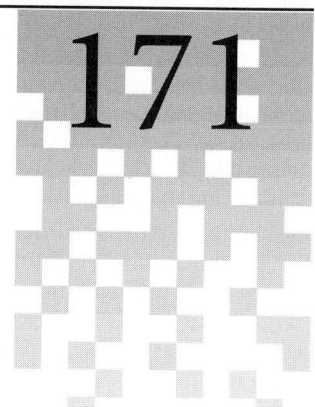

B. Craig Weldon

Case Synopsis

An otherwise healthy 4-year-old boy undergoes general anesthesia for circumcision. The surgery proceeds without incident until the child arrives in the postanesthesia care unit (PACU), where he is noted to be restless, irritable, crying, and not responsive to calming measures. His agitated behavior escalates to incoherent screaming, thrashing of his extremities, and intermittent combativeness.

PROBLEM ANALYSIS

Definition

Emergence agitation in young children is characterized by crying, restlessness, and irritability during the emergence from anesthesia. It is unclear whether a continuum exists between emergence agitation and emergence delirium, an acute confusional state in which the patient manifests extreme agitation, hyperkinesis, and, occasionally, combativeness.

Recognition

Emergence agitation is a common event after even minor surgery in toddlers, preschoolers, and young school-aged children. An episode of emergence agitation may last 20 to 30 minutes and may not respond to routine comforting measures. Between 5% and 10% of children manifest severe symptoms that resemble delirium. Adolescents and young adults seem to have a higher incidence of delirium versus simple agitation in the PACU (also see Chapter 223).

Risk Assessment

DEVELOPMENTAL FACTORS

Young children lack mature coping mechanisms. Therefore, they are less able to tolerate being separated from their parents in a strange place, the psychological stress associated with medical illness or surgery, and the altered mental state associated with emergence from anesthesia. Parental anxiety or the parents' lack of understanding about what to expect in the perioperative period may also have a negative effect on their child's behavior.

PREOPERATIVE ANXIETY AND BASELINE TEMPERAMENT

Children with high levels of preoperative anxiety are less able to cooperate during mask induction, have a higher incidence of emergence agitation in the PACU, and have more severe episodes of emergence agitation. Likewise, children who are highly distressed during mask induction of anesthesia tend to be more agitated during emergence. Also, the child's baseline temperament affects his or her postoperative behavior, and parents can frequently predict whether a child is going to have trouble dealing with events on the day of surgery. Parental presence during induction of anesthesia does not appear to lessen the risk for emergence agitation. However, preanesthetic sedation appears to offer some risk reduction.

PREEXISTING MENTAL DISTURBANCES

Children and adolescents with autism, mental retardation, bipolar disorder, or disruptive behavior (e.g., those with oppositional defiant, attention deficit-hyperactivity, or conduct disorders) may have more behavioral problems in the postoperative period. These patients should receive their regular psychotropic medications on schedule on the day of surgery. They may also benefit from the oral administration of a preanesthetic sedative.

INADEQUATE POSTOPERATIVE ANALGESIA

Unrecognized postoperative pain is likely the single most common cause of emergence agitation in all age groups. It is difficult to assess preverbal and developmentally delayed infants and children with subjective pain scoring systems. Also, most young children are notoriously poor self-reporters of pain intensity. Those who emerge from anesthesia in pain often show agitated or delirious behavior but do not indicate their pain to caregivers. Other causes for discomfort, including gastric or urinary bladder distention, surgical drains, or overly tight bindings and dressings, must be ruled out.

UNDERLYING MEDICAL CONDITIONS

The following are potentially life-threatening medical conditions that may present in the PACU as emergence agitation or delirium:

- Hypoxemia or hypercapnia
- Reduced cerebral blood flow with shock states or severe hypotension
- Hypoglycemia, hyperthyroidism, or hyperparathyroidism
- Hyponatremia
- Seizures or elevated intracranial pressure

These diagnoses are considered within the proper clinical context if a cause for emergence agitation or delirium cannot be rapidly identified or if the period of agitation is prolonged or accompanied by a decreasing level of consciousness.

ANTICHOLINERGICS

Scopolamine and, to a lesser extent, atropine have been associated with postoperative mental disturbances. These agents cross the blood-brain barrier to cause a central anticholinergic crisis (or syndrome). This is due to block of acetylcholine-mediated neuroinhibitory pathways in the brain. Full-blown central anticholinergic syndrome is characterized by warm, flushed, dry skin; visual disturbances; fever; and delirium. Some ophthalmic preparations used for mydriasis, as well as numerous antihistamines and nonproprietary drugs, have central anticholinergic effects that may contribute to disturbed behavior in patients emerging from anesthesia. Many of these drugs are tertiary versus quaternary amines and thus cross the blood-brain barrier more easily.

ANESTHETIC AGENTS

Low-blood-soluble gaseous or volatile anesthetics (cyclopropane, desflurane, sevoflurane) have been associated with emergence agitation in children. The mechanism for such emergence agitation is unknown, but it could be related to the more rapid emergence from anesthesia with these agents. Children who emerge rapidly from anesthesia may suddenly become aware that they are in an unusual place surrounded by strangers and therefore become distressed. Also, rapid loss of analgesic effects (greater with desflurane than sevoflurane) might contribute to inadequate postoperative analgesia and provoke or aggravate agitated behaviors.

Ketamine has long been associated with dysphoria and disturbing psychological reactions in adolescents and adults. Postoperative behavioral disturbances may occur when ketamine is used to "rescue" a difficult (contentious) mask induction in an already terrified child.

Implications

The most immediate concern for a child suffering from emergence agitation is the increased risk of self-harm. Children with severe emergence agitation can accidentally injure themselves or their caregivers as a result of combativeness or hyperkinesis. Displacement of intravenous (IV) or monitoring lines, surgical drains, and dressings further complicates the postoperative care of these patients. In the tumult that often surrounds these children in the PACU, the nurses and anesthesiologist may be required to turn their attention from other patients for a prolonged period, possibly leading to reduced monitoring and care for nonagitated PACU patients. Care for a delirious patient is very labor-intensive; it prolongs PACU stays and increases costs. Most parents of severely agitated children find the experience frightening and emotionally draining.

MANAGEMENT

The initial approach to a child with mild to moderate emergence agitation includes the following: (1) reduce environmental stimuli other than those required for routine comfort, (2) involve the child's parents in his or her care as soon as possible, and (3) seriously consider the possibility of inadequate analgesia and administer an IV opioid.

Children with severe agitation who are thrashing about must be protected from bodily harm and have their IV and other vascular access lines adequately secured. This must be accomplished quickly and may require physically restraining the child. Children with severe agitation or delirium should be given repeated doses of a rapid-onset IV opioid such as fentanyl if there is any doubt about the adequacy of their analgesia. This may be followed by small doses of midazolam if the agitation persists and if the child did not receive midazolam preoperatively. Physostigmine 0.025 mg/kg is the treatment of choice to counter the central anticholineric effects of atropine, scopolamine, and other drugs with similar effects.

If postoperative pain has been sufficiently treated or ruled out and midazolam fails to reduce the severity of agitation, repeated doses of 0.1 to 0.2 mg/kg of propofol should be administered until the child is unconscious. This state can be maintained with a low-dose propofol infusion until the child can be allowed to slowly re-emerge. As a last resort, a severely agitated or delirious child or adolescent who has lost IV access can be quickly sedated with 1 to 2 mg of haloperidol administered intramuscularly.

PREVENTION

- Consider the developmental level of the patient.
- Allay parental anxiety with preoperative education before the day of surgery.
- Assess the child's level of preoperative anxiety on the day of surgery.
- Administer preanesthetic sedation to high-risk pediatric age groups (1 to 6 years) and children with high levels of preoperative anxiety.
- Implement a multimodal analgesia plan and maintain a high degree of suspicion for the inadequacy of postoperative analgesia.
- Avoid overly rapid emergence from low-solubility volatile inhalation anesthetics.
- Consider administering IV opioids, midazolam, propofol, dexmedetomidine, or clonidine before emergence in patients who have received low-solubility volatile anesthetics.
- Rapidly reunite the child with his or her parents in the PACU.

Further Reading

Aono J, Ueda W, Marniya K, et al: Greater incidence of delirium during recovery from sevoflurane anesthesia in preschool boys. Anesthesiology 87:1298-1300, 1997.

Cohen IT, Finkel JC, Hannallah RS, et al: Rapid emergence does not explain agitation following sevoflurane anaesthesia in infants and children: A comparison with propofol. Paediatr Anaesth 13:63-67, 2003.

Cravero J, Surgenor S, Whalen K: Emergence agitation in paediatric patients after sevoflurane anaesthesia and no surgery: A comparison with halothane. Paediatr Anaesth 10:419-424, 2000.

Kain ZN, Caldwell-Andrews AA, Weinberg ME, et al: Sevoflurane versus halothane: Postoperative maladaptive behavioral changes: A randomized, controlled study. Anesthesiology 102:720-726, 2005.

Kain ZN, Wang SM, Mayes LC, et al: Distress during the induction of anesthesia and postoperative behavioral outcomes. Anesth Analg 88:1042-1047, 1999.

Lerman J, Davis PJ, Welborn LG, et al: Induction, recovery and safety characteristics of sevoflurane in children undergoing ambulatory surgery. Anesthesiology 84:1332-1340, 1996.

Olympio MA: Postanesthetic delirium: Historical perspectives. J Clin Anesth 3:60-63, 1991.

Welborn LG, Hannallah RS, Norden JM, et al: Comparison of emergence and recovery characteristics of sevoflurane, desflurane and halothane in pediatric ambulatory patients. Anesth Analg 83:917-920, 1996.

Weldon BC, Bell M, Craddock T: The effect of caudal analgesia on emergence agitation in children after sevoflurane versus halothane anesthesia. Anesth Analg 98:321-326, 2004.

Adenotonsillectomy

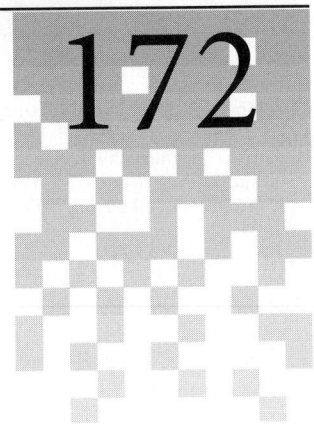

172

Lynne R. Ferrari

Case Synopsis

A 2-year-old boy with obstructive sleep apnea presents for tonsillectomy and adenoidectomy. In the postanesthesia care unit, his respiratory rate is 40 breaths per minute, and his heart rate is 140 beats per minute. A small amount of blood is noted in the oropharynx, and he has bilateral rales on auscultation. Oxygen saturation by pulse oximetry is 86%.

PROBLEM ANALYSIS

Definition

Tonsillectomy, with or without adenoidectomy, is performed so frequently that associated medical abnormalities and the potential for complications are often overlooked. The vast majority of children do well after surgery. However, complications can be serious and, at times, life threatening. The proper selection of patients and attention to anesthetic technique can reduce the risk of death and complications related to the following factors:

- Bleeding
- Young age
- Postoperative pulmonary edema
- Postoperative vomiting
- Postoperative pain
- Obstructive sleep apnea

Recognition

Bleeding.   Postoperative hemorrhage occurs in 0.1% to 8.1% of patients. In 75% of cases, bleeding occurs within 6 hours of surgery; in the remaining 25%, it can occur as late as the eighth postoperative day. Most bleeding is noted by blood-stained sputum or the vomiting of "coffee grounds" material.

Young Age.   In the past, all children were admitted to the hospital for tonsillectomy. This approach was justified by reports of vomiting, dehydration, bleeding, pain, and apnea. The advent of cost containment, along with a trend toward ambulatory surgery, has changed this practice. Today, only children aged 3 years or younger are routinely admitted to the hospital for tonsillectomy.

Pulmonary Edema.   Pulmonary edema may present as frothy pink fluid in the endotracheal tube, decreased oxygen saturation, wheezing, dyspnea, or increased respiratory rate after tracheal extubation. The differential diagnosis of postobstruction pulmonary edema (see Chapter 156) includes aspiration of gastric contents, respiratory distress syndrome, congestive heart failure, volume overload, and anaphylaxis. A chest radiograph illustrating diffuse, usually bilateral, interstitial pulmonary infiltrates, combined with an appropriate clinical history, confirms the diagnosis.

Postoperative Pain and Vomiting.   Pain is minimal after adenoidectomy but often severe after tonsillectomy. The combined effects of irritant blood in the stomach, interference with the gag reflex caused by edema, and stimulation of receptors in the chemoreceptor trigger zone contribute to postoperative vomiting, which can occur in up to 60% of tonsillectomy patients.

Obstructive Sleep Apnea.   Hypertrophied tonsils may obstruct the upper airway during sleep, causing obstructive sleep apnea (OSA) in approximately 3% to 12% of children. The highest incidence is in children younger than 5 years. The diagnosis of OSA is confirmed by polysomnography, which is a graphic record of respiratory activity during natural sleep. A positive sleep study is an indication for tonsillectomy, especially if related systemic abnormalities are present. The clinical presentation of OSA is quite varied. Some patients have significant limitations, whereas others are minimally affected (Table 172-1).

Risk Analysis

Bleeding.   The tonsillar fossa, nasopharynx, or both are the sites for 67%, 27%, or 6% of postoperative bleeding, respectively.

Young Age.   Age younger than 3 years is the most significant risk factor for the development of respiratory compromise after adenotonsillectomy. Respiratory compromise is defined as oxygen saturation less than 90%, with an obstructive

Table 172–1 ■ Clinical Presentation of Obstructive Sleep Apnea
Young age (<6 yr)
Snoring during sleep
Failure to thrive
Recurrent respiratory tract infections
Craniofacial dysmorphism
Cardiac arrhythmias
Apnea during sleep
Somnolence while awake
Developmental delay
Obesity
Behavioral difficulty
Cor pulmonale

breathing pattern or acute respiratory distress requiring intervention.

Pulmonary Edema. Factors that increase venous return and preload in either ventricle, or those that reduce the ability of the pulmonary lymphatic system to acutely remove large amounts of fluid, increase the risk of postobstruction pulmonary edema. Postoperative laryngospasm and breathing against a closed glottis cause negative transpulmonary pressures, leading to an increased hydrostatic gradient and subsequent pulmonary edema.

Postoperative Pain and Vomiting. Significant differences in the degree of postoperative pain are related to the surgical technique of tonsil removal. Increased pain medication requirements, otalgia, and irritability have been observed in patients undergoing tonsillectomy with electrocautery and laser excision compared with sharp dissection. Vomiting is multifactorial and may be due in part to the stimulation of vagal mediators in the hypopharynx as well as systemic serotonin release.

Obstructive Sleep Apnea. The degree of tonsillar hypertrophy does not correlate with the severity of upper airway obstruction with OSA. Children with only slightly enlarged tonsils may have severe OSA, whereas those with very enlarged tonsils may not have OSA at all. The risk for OSA increases with changes in the nasopharyngeal airway and obesity. Children with OSA have a narrowed aperture of the nasopharyngeal airway, so posterior displacement of the tongue causes hypopharyngeal obstruction. Two thirds of children affected with OSA are obese. Fatty infiltration of the neck, along with relaxation of the pharyngeal muscles, compounds obstruction, because the collapsing force of negative inspiratory pressure exceeds the expanding force of pharyngeal muscular contraction.

Implications

Bleeding. Post-tonsillectomy bleeding may be controlled by the application of topical agents to promote coagulation. However, most episodes require surgical exploration and treatment. Large volumes of blood may be swallowed but not appreciated by the patient, parents, or surgeon. Therefore, all post-tonsillectomy patients with tonsillar hemorrhage are considered to have a full stomach, and appropriate anesthetic precautions must be taken. Because the amount of swallowed blood is usually underappreciated, examination for orthostatic hypotension as a measure of intravascular volume adequacy is required.

Young Age. Children younger than 3 years are at increased risk for inadequate oral intake and subsequent dehydration immediately following surgery. They are also at increased risk for postoperative respiratory compromise.

Pulmonary Edema. Pulmonary edema can occur when airway obstruction is relieved by tonsillectomy. It has been suggested that increased negative inspiratory pressure consequent to airway obstruction increases venous return and pulmonary blood volume (Fig. 172-1). Peak negative inspiratory intrapleural pressure, which is normally 2.5 to 10 cm H_2O, increases to 30 cm H_2O with airway obstruction. A negative

transpulmonary pressure gradient of this magnitude can disrupt the integrity of the pulmonary capillary walls. Concurrently, increased pulmonary blood flow and hydrostatic pressure facilitate transudation of fluid into the alveolar space. To counteract this, positive intrapleural and alveolar pressure is generated during exhalation (similar to the expiratory grunt or Valsalva's maneuver). This reduces pulmonary venous return and blood volume. Relief of airway obstruction after tonsillectomy reduces airway pressure, but it also increases venous return and pulmonary hydrostatic pressure. This can lead to hyperemia and, ultimately, pulmonary edema. Bear in mind that the counterbalancing effect of the expiratory grunt to limit pulmonary venous return is lost with relief of airway obstruction.

Postoperative Pain and Vomiting. Uncontrolled pain, swallowed blood, and poor oral intake contribute to nausea and vomiting after tonsillectomy. Dehydration occurs in 1% of patients and can be prevented by intravenous hydration to restore intravascular volume. Hospital admission for rehydration with intravenous fluids is warranted.

Obstructive Sleep Apnea. Central neurologic dysfunction contributes to a worsening of cardiopulmonary function in many children with OSA. Persistent hypercapnia, hypoxemia, and right ventricular dysfunction contribute to arrhythmias and cor pulmonale. Pulmonary artery pressure increases progressively, perhaps because vascular reactivity is increased with OSA.

MANAGEMENT

Bleeding. Bleeding is controlled with pharyngeal packs, topical agents, or both. If this approach fails, patients are returned to the operating room for exploration and surgical hemostasis. Both intravenous and inhalational anesthetic techniques are appropriate, but patients should be responsive at the end of surgery and should be extubated awake. A rapid-sequence induction, accompanied by cricoid pressure and a styletted endotracheal tube, is suggested. Finally, surgical procedures for control of bleeding are usually quite brief, so anesthesia should be planned accordingly.

Young Age. In the absence of evidence of post-tonsillectomy complications, otherwise healthy children older than 3 years can be discharged home after 4 hours of observation.

Pulmonary Edema. Treatment is supportive: maintain a patent airway and administer oxygen and diuretics if needed. Tracheal intubation and mechanical ventilation with positive end-expiratory pressure may be required in severe cases. Resolution is usually rapid, sometimes within hours of surgery. Many cases resolve without treatment within 24 hours.

Postoperative Pain and Vomiting. Intraoperative administration of corticosteroids may reduce edema formation and subsequent patient discomfort. Infiltration of the peritonsillar space with a local anesthetic and epinephrine can reduce intraoperative blood loss and provide immediate and protracted postoperative pain relief. One explanation for the latter may be that neural blockade prevents nociceptive impulses

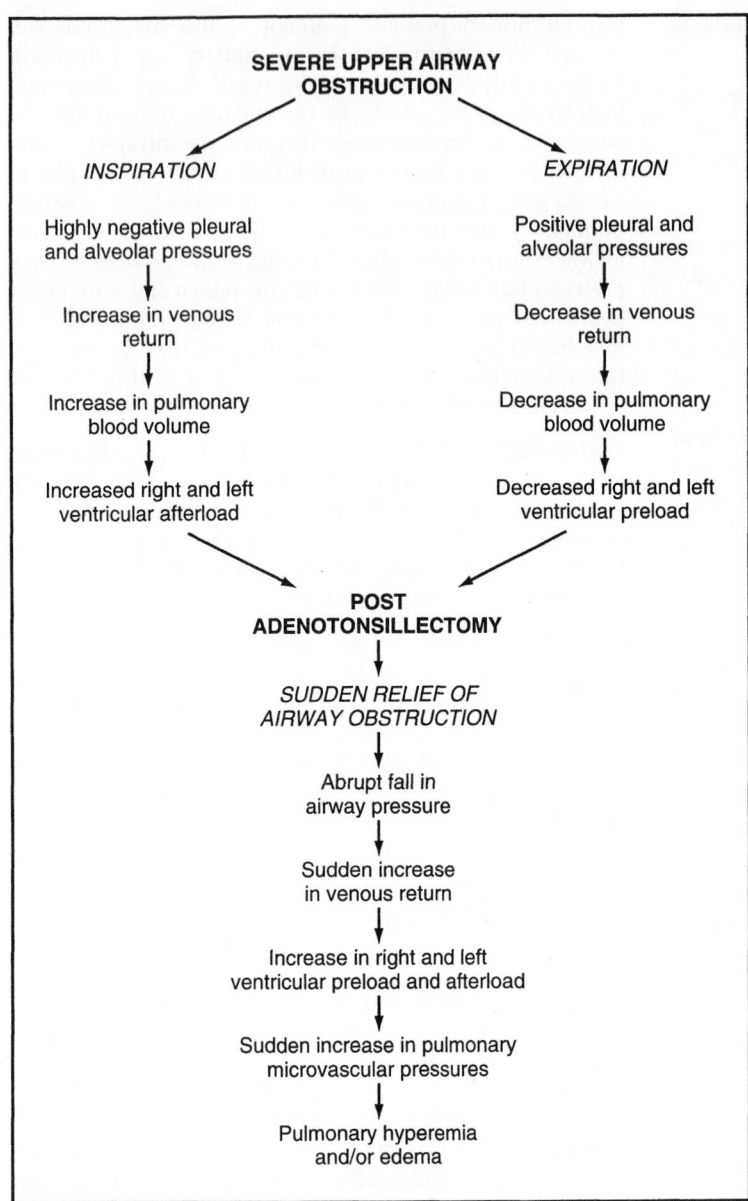

Figure 172–1 ■ Physiologic changes leading to pulmonary edema after treatment for upper airway obstruction. (Adapted from Galvis AG, Stool SE, Bluestone CD: Pulmonary edema following relief of acute upper airway obstruction. Ann Otol 89:124-128, 1980.)

from entering the central nervous system during and immediately after surgery, thus suppressing the formation of a sustained hyperexcitable state, which facilitates pain perception. Local anesthetic and epinephrine infiltration is not without danger, however; intravascular (especially intra-arterial) injection can be lethal. Small, repeated doses of narcotic are effective for pain relief. Nonsteroidal anti-inflammatory agents should be avoided; their potential to interfere with coagulation could be disastrous. Antiemetic agents, gastric decompression with an orogastric tube (a nasogastric tube is contraindicated after adenoidectomy), and adequate pain control are indicated for post-tonsillectomy vomiting.

Obstructive Sleep Apnea. Before extubation after tonsillectomy, patients with OSA should be breathing spontaneously and able to protect their airways; therefore, cautious use of sedatives and analgesics is advised. A small dose of a benzodiazepine may be administered, especially preoperatively, to very anxious or hard-to-manage children. With regard to postoperative narcotics, a balance must be struck between the need for analgesia and the risk of respiratory depression. Keep in mind that residual central nervous system dysfunction, hypercarbia, and hypoxemia may persist after tonsillectomy, despite relief of airway obstruction. For this reason, children with OSA should be hospitalized for apnea monitoring postoperatively (Table 172-2). Most OSA patients have normal carbon dioxide tension (PCO_2) levels and are extubated after anesthesia; however, patients with severe OSA (i.e., cor pulmonale, resting $PCO_2 > 50$ mm Hg) should remain intubated and be mechanically ventilated until PCO_2 has normalized. They are then extubated and observed carefully.

PREVENTION

Bleeding. Before anesthetic induction, a tilt test is performed to assess orthostatic changes due to hemorrhage, intravenous access is established, volume replacement is begun, hematocrit is measured, and a blood sample is sent for type and crossmatch. Assorted laryngoscope blades, handles, and endotracheal tubes should be on hand, and at least two suction apparatuses should be available in case the suction tube becomes plugged with blood clots during attempted airway visualization.

Young Age. Postoperative morbidity after tonsillectomy is well documented in younger children; therefore, the American Academy of Otolaryngology guidelines recommend overnight hospitalization for children younger than 3 years or those meeting other criteria (see Table 172-2).

Table 172–2 ▪ Criteria for Hospital Admission of Patients after Adenotonsillectomy

Patients must be admitted if they meet any of the following criteria of the American Academy of Otolaryngology's Head and Neck Surgery–Pediatric Otolaryngology Committee:

Abnormal coagulation values, with or without a known bleeding disorder in the patient or family

Evidence of an obstructive sleep disorder or apnea due to tonsil or adenoid hypertrophy

Systemic disorders that put the patient at increased postoperative cardiopulmonary, metabolic, or general medical risk

Presence of craniofacial or other airway abnormalities, including but not limited to the following:
   Treacher Collins syndrome
   Crouzon's syndrome
   Goldenhar's syndrome
   Pierre Robin anomaly
   CHARGE association defects*
   Achondroplasia
   Down's syndrome
Isolated airway abnormality
   Choanal atresia
   Laryngotracheal stenosis

Procedure performed for acute peritonsillar abscess

Extended travel time, weather, or home social conditions are not consistent with close observation, cooperation, and ability to return to the hospital quickly at the discretion of the attending physician

*CHARGE association defects consist of colobomatous malformation sequence (ranging from isolated iris coloboma to clinical anophthalmos), heart defects (e.g., tetralogy of Fallot, atrial or ventricular septal defects, patent ductus arteriosus), atresia of choanae, retarded growth and development or central nervous system anomalies, genital anomalies or hypogonadism (males), and ear anomalies or deafness.

Pulmonary Edema. There is no reliable method to predict which patients will experience postobstructive pulmonary edema after surgery. Moderate, continuous positive airway pressure during anesthesia allows time for circulatory adaptation to take place. This is similar to the approach to acute upper airway obstruction secondary to epiglottitis or laryngospasm. Postobstructive pulmonary edema is not common in children with long-standing airway obstruction, but unfortunately, it is unavoidable in some children after their tonsils are removed.

Postoperative Pain and Vomiting. Antiemetic agents, oral gastric decompression, adequate pain relief, and quiet emergence from anesthesia can help diminish the frequency of post-tonsillectomy vomiting.

Obstructive Sleep Apnea. Digitalization and surgical removal of the tonsils and adenoids can reverse the progressive cardiovascular changes that occur in most patients with OSA. The occurrence of OSA in children is usually not preventable.

Further Reading

Blum R, McGowan F: Chronic upper airway obstruction and cardiac dysfunction: Anatomy, pathophysiology and anesthetic implications. Pediatr Anesth 14:75-83, 2004.

Brown OE, Cunningham MJ: Tonsillectomy and adenoidectomy: Inpatient guidelines: Recommendations of the AAO-HNS Pediatric Otolaryngology Committee AAO-HNS Bull 13-15, 1996.

Carithers JS, Gebhart DE, Williams JA: Postoperative risks of pediatric tonsilloadenoidectomy. Laryngoscope 97:422-429, 1987.

Colclasure JB, Graham SS: Complications of outpatient tonsillectomy and adenoidectomy: A review of 3340 cases. Ear Nose Throat J 69:155-160, 1990.

Feinberg AN, Shabino CL: Acute pulmonary edema complicating tonsillectomy and adenoidectomy. Pediatrics 75:112-114, 1985.

Ferrari L: Anesthesia for pediatric ENT surgery, routine and emergent. Am Soc Anesthesiol Refresher Course Lect 24:57-69, 1996.

Galvis AG, Stool SE, Bluestone CD: Pulmonary edema following relief of acute upper airway obstruction. Ann Otol 89:124-128, 1980.

Marcus CL, Ward SD, McColley SA: American Academy of Pediatrics clinical practice guideline: Diagnosis and management of childhood obstructive sleep apnea syndrome. Pediatrics 109:704-712, 2002.

McColley S, April M, Carroll J, et al: Respiratory compromise after adenotonsillectomy in children with obstructive sleep apnea. Arch Otolaryngol Head Neck Surg 118:940-943, 1992.

Tom LWC, DeDio RM, Cohen DE, et al: Is outpatient tonsillectomy appropriate for young children? Laryngoscope 102:278-280, 1992.

Ophthalmic Problems and Complications

173

Scott D. Cook-Sather

Case Synopsis

A 5-year-old girl with no prior ophthalmic history has a thyroglossal duct cyst excision under general anesthesia. On awakening, she complains that "something hurts in my eye." Although there is no obvious foreign body in the eye, excessive tearing is noted. Her eyes had been taped closed following tracheal intubation. Corneal abrasion is suspected, and an ophthalmology consultation is obtained.

INTRODUCTION

For nonocular surgery, the incidence of anesthesia-related eye injury is estimated at 0.06%; this accounts for 3% of the American Society of Anesthesiologists (ASA) nondental closed claims cases. Risk factors for perioperative ocular injury include general anesthesia, long procedures, head and neck procedures, and lateral positioning. For ocular surgery, anesthesia-related eye injury is exceedingly rare. When it occurs, it may be related to perioperative coughing or severe postoperative vomiting, with a related sudden increase in intraocular pressure (IOP). Important ophthalmic complications and issues relevant to pediatric anesthesia include corneal abrasion, postoperative visual loss, retinopathy of prematurity, penetrating ocular trauma, oculocardiac reflex, and postoperative nausea and vomiting. The last occurs in 40% to 90% of children after strabismus surgery and is discussed in Chapter 159.

CORNEAL ABRASION

PROBLEM ANALYSIS

Definition

Corneal abrasion is the most common perioperative ophthalmic complication, with an incidence of 0.1% to 44%. A higher incidence was reported in the 1970s for anesthetized patients without eye protection or lubrication. Most corneal abrasions result from corneal drying associated with lagophthalmos during general anesthesia.

Recognition

Symptoms of corneal abrasion include photophobia, pain, and foreign body sensation. Excessive tearing and miosis are characteristic physical findings. Staining with fluorescein reveals the abraded zone in green under a cobalt blue light (Fig. 173-1).

Risk Assessment

Although the inciting event for corneal abrasion is not always clear, factors such as prone or lateral positioning and

exophthalmos place patients at higher risk. General anesthesia increases the risk, in part owing to lost protective corneal reflexes, abolished Bell's phenomenon (in which the globe turns upward during sleep), and diminished tear production and stability.

Implications

The majority of children sustaining intraoperative corneal abrasion have a full recovery within 24 hours with appropriate treatment. Extensive injury or delayed treatment results in a 16% incidence of permanent injury. Permanent scarring is usually related to secondary corneal infection or abrasions that are chronic.

MANAGEMENT

Patients with corneal abrasion should be evaluated by an ophthalmologist to document the extent of injury and

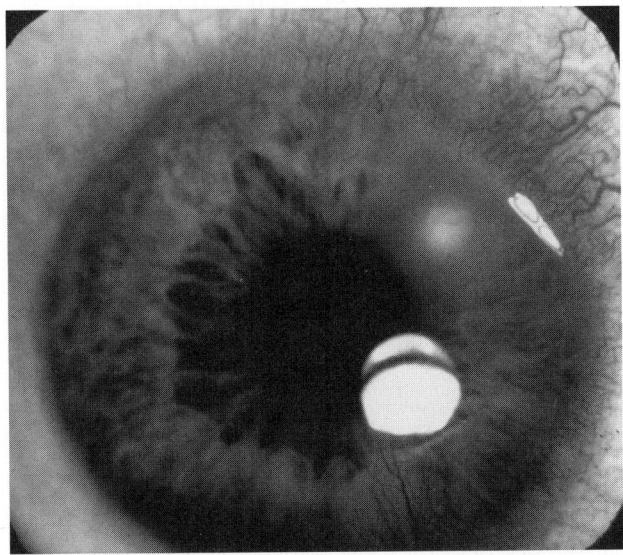

Figure 173–1 ■ The opacified zone overlying the iris at the 2 o'clock position is a corneal abrasion with surrounding edema. These lesions are most easily seen with fluorescein staining. (Courtesy of Dr. Katrinka Heher.)

initiate treatment. Usual recommendations include lubrication, application of a topical antibiotic or cycloplegic agent (or both), and patch closure.

PREVENTION

To prevent corneal abrasion, ocular contact with masks, stethoscopes, name tags, intubation equipment, sheets, and padding material must be avoided. Eye protection should be established early, before laryngoscopy. Tape should be used to keep the eyelids closed, with ophthalmic lubricants used for longer procedures. Petroleum-based ophthalmic ointments are more likely to cause foreign body sensation and blurred vision postoperatively than are aqueous solutions. Placement of a disposable pulse oximeter probe on the child's ring finger as opposed to the index finger may lessen the chance of inadvertent eye contact and potential corneal injury in the postoperative period.

POSTOPERATIVE VISUAL LOSS

PROBLEM ANALYSIS

Definition

Postoperative visual loss (POVL) is the most catastrophic perioperative ophthalmic complication and may manifest as either partial visual field loss or total blindness. The incidence of POVL in the general, nonocular surgical population is 1 in 61,000 to 1 in 125,000, but following spinal surgery in the prone position, it is estimated to be 1 in 1100. There is also a higher relative incidence after open-heart and head and neck surgeries. From the inception of the ASA Postoperative Visual Loss Registry in July 1999 until July 2004, there were three reported pediatric cases of POVL in patients ranging in age from 5 to 18 years.

Recognition

Visual changes may be appreciated in the immediate postoperative period, but delays in diagnosis may occur when such changes are incorrectly attributed to "normal recovery" after anesthesia and instilled ophthalmic lubricants. In one study of 28 POVL cases, visual changes were recognized in 50% of patients in the recovery room and in 80% by postoperative day 2. Some patients initially had normal vision but experienced symptoms 1 to 12 days later. Younger pediatric patients may have difficulty expressing symptoms. When there is local ecchymosis around the affected eye or periorbital numbness, compression injury should be suspected.

Risk Assessment

Ischemic optic neuropathy (ION) associated with spinal surgery in the prone position accounts for the majority of cases in the ASA POVL Registry. Three pediatric patients developed bilateral ION following prolonged (>8 hours)

surgery in the prone position, two for scoliosis and one for reconstruction of the cranial vault. Intraoperative events included large blood loss and episodes of hypotension. One proposed mechanism of injury involves the complex interaction of transient anemia, arterial hypotension, increased central venous pressure, and increased IOP in the prone position, which results in decreased optic perfusion pressure and limited hemodynamic reserve in the optic pathways.

Adult patients with hypertension, smoking, diabetes, or peripheral vascular disease appear to be at increased risk for ION. Direct orbital compression (e.g., from patient malposition on a headrest) is not required for ION to occur. However, such compression can result in POVL via central retinal artery occlusion, in which case POVL can be attributed to ION. POVL may also be consequent to perioperative cortical ischemia.

Implications

Most postoperative visual deficits do not improve significantly over time. Those who experience complete absence of light perception are unlikely to regain vision.

MANAGEMENT

Early ophthalmology consultation must be obtained for unequivocal vision deficits (absence of light perception, unilateral visual loss), periorbital ecchymosis or obvious trauma, and milder visual symptoms that do not improve in the first few hours after anesthesia and surgery. Visual acuity tests, funduscopic examination, and head magnetic resonance imaging are often required to establish a diagnosis; however, few (if any) therapies are currently available. Thus, ensuring adequate hemodynamics, hemoglobin concentration, and oxygenation in the postoperative period cannot be expected to reverse the initial injury but may prevent further damage.

PREVENTION

Although direct pressure is not a common cause of POVL, protecting the eyes from external compression is vital. Anesthesia providers must carefully position patients and then monitor their positioning, because patients may shift in relation to headrests and other equipment during surgery. Special headrests with mirrors allow instant assessment of the periorbital area in prone patients. Slight reverse Trendelenburg's position may reduce orbital venous pressure and promote better perfusion for any given mean arterial pressure.

Although deliberate hypotension may help reduce operative blood loss, it may increase the risk for POVL. Deliberate hypotension has been used in tens of thousands of uneventful cases, but two of the three pediatric cases in the ASA POVL Registry involved deliberate hypotensive techniques. The current practice at my institution is to avoid deliberate hypotension for posterior spinal fusion surgery, because somatosenory and motor evoked potentials are better preserved with normotension.

Precise transfusion parameters for reducing POVL risk are not well defined, but significant anemia should be avoided. Current recommendations also include minimizing the time the patient is in the prone position. Staged procedures should be considered if total operative time is expected to exceed 8 hours.

RETINOPATHY OF PREMATURITY

PROBLEM ANALYSIS

Definition

Retinopathy of prematurity (ROP) occurs in more than 50% of premature infants weighing less than 1500 g at birth. It is caused by abnormal proliferation of vascular tissue, with destruction of the retinal capillary bed. ROP ranges in severity from reversible regional neovascularization to complete retinal detachment with permanent blindness. Although multiple, interrelated factors predispose to ROP, the immature retina appears to be more susceptible if exposed to high oxygen (O_2) concentrations and accompanying free radicals.

Recognition

Ophthalmologic examination can document the development or exacerbation of ROP. The stages of ROP are as follows:

- Linear separation of posterior vascular retina from the anterior avascular portion
- Elevation of the demarcation line and ridge formation
- Extraretinal neovascular tissue proliferation
- Partial retinal detachment
- Complete retinal detachment—also known as retrolental fibroplasia

Risk Assessment

ROP is associated with low birth weight (<1500 g), young gestational age (≤32 weeks), hemorrhagic shock at birth, anemia and transfusion, and prolonged exposure to high O_2 tensions. The temporal portion of the retina does not mature until 40 to 44 weeks' postconceptual age. Neonates up to 44 weeks' postconceptual age who require surgery are therefore presumed to be at risk for the development of ROP or for worsening of existing pathology.

Implications

Although approximately 85% of acute ROP cases undergo spontaneous regression, outcomes depend on the stage, with fibrous tissue traction and retinal detachment having worse prognoses. Laser photocoagulation is the treatment of choice in 90% of cases. Cryotherapy, scleral buckle, or vitrectomy may be required.

MANAGEMENT AND PREVENTION

ROP is primarily a concern in neonatal intensive care units, where prolonged O_2 exposure may place infants at risk; however, efforts to reduce intraoperative O_2 concentrations also may be beneficial. Older studies indicated that an arterial O_2 tension (PaO_2) of 150 mm Hg for 1 to 2 hours could affect the immature retina. More recent data suggest that even lower PaO_2 values may contribute to ROP. Consistent damage occurs after only several days of hyperoxia. Prudent preventive management thus includes the lowest fraction of inspired O_2 (FiO_2) required to achieve a percutaneous arterial O_2 saturation of 90% to 95% ($PaO_2 \approx 70$ mm Hg). However, neonates with severe pulmonary pathology who require a high FiO_2 to maintain adequate tissue oxygenation should receive it.

PENETRATING OCULAR TRAUMA AND VITREOUS EXTRUSION

PROBLEM ANALYSIS

Definition

Penetrating ocular trauma, with the concomitant risk of extrusion of ocular contents, is a classic management challenge for pediatric anesthesiologists. Patients present emergently, are often uncooperative, and usually require rapid anesthetic induction to minimize the risk of pulmonary aspiration of gastric contents. However, sudden increases in IOP during anesthesia, especially during induction, may increase the risk of vitreous humor extrusion. Loss of ocular contents solely due to anesthetic management is exceedingly rare, relegated to a few anecdotal reports.

Recognition

The patient's history may include either handling or being struck by a sharp object, with subsequent eye pain, swelling, erythema, obvious ocular rent, or an in situ foreign body. Poor eye turgor and exposed vitreous are signs of vitreous extrusion.

Risk Assessment

Penetrating eye injury is more likely to result in vitreous extrusion in children with large defects and in those who continue to cry, cough, retch, or vomit.

Implications

Extrusion of ocular contents is catastrophic and requires immediate wound closure and possible posterior sclerotomy to release suprachoroidal blood. The prognosis is extremely poor—most victims lose all vision in the affected eye.

MANAGEMENT AND PREVENTION

Evaluation and management strategies for children with penetrating ocular trauma are summarized in Table 173-1. The most important concerns are preventing the aspiration of gastric contents and preventing a sudden increase in IOP, as occurs with coughing. Coughing can transiently increase IOP by 30 to 40 mm Hg and may cause vitreous extrusion, iris or lens prolapse, or choroidal hemorrhage. Smaller increases in IOP may also cause extrusion of vitreous, although the absolute minimum increase in IOP required to do so is unknown; it is clearly dependent on the degree of baseline injury.

Succinylcholine administered during a rapid-sequence intubation may increase IOP by 6 to 8 mm Hg for 5 to 10 minutes via the depolarization of extraocular, facial, and smooth orbital muscles. There are no credible case reports of vitreous extrusion following succinylcholine administration, however; concern stemmed from a single anecdotal report. Defasciculating doses of nondepolarizing muscle relaxants (NDMRs) may attenuate the rise in IOP associated with succinylcholine. Priming doses of NDMRs may hasten the achievement of adequate intubation conditions after the induction of anesthesia, but there are reports of intervening weakness, difficulty breathing, agitation, and even aspiration. In general, pediatric patients poorly tolerate the potential difficulties associated with NDMR priming; also, in theory, these

Table 173–1 ■ Anesthetic Evaluation and Management of Patients with Penetrating Eye Injuries

Nature of Injury, Urgency, and Expected Duration of Procedure
Small defects: less risk of extrusion
Simple injury: short-duration procedures
Complex injury: prolonged retinal reattachment
Copper: causes early vitreous clouding
Protruding foreign body: true ophthalmic emergency
Nonviable eye: can wait several hours

Risk of Pulmonary Aspiration
Recent full meal
Impaired gastrointestinal function
Severity of trauma
Opioid administration
Gastroesophageal reflux, hiatal hernia

Airway Evaluation
Difficult: consider a fiberoptic approach
Normal or not anticipated to be difficult: rapid-sequence induction

Anesthetic Management Options
Possible delayed start: 8 hr after solids; 2 hr after clear liquids
Rapid-sequence induction variants:
  Lidocaine 1.5-2 mg/kg; remifentanil 1 μg/kg or fentanyl 1-2 μg/kg; thiopental 4-6 mg/kg or propofol 2-3 mg/kg; SCh 1.5-2 mg/kg (± defasciculating NDMR dose); high-dose NDMR (rocuronium 1.2 mg/kg) in place of SCh if surgery will be prolonged
Monitoring: train-of-four to determine earliest time for intubation and ongoing muscle relaxation

NDMR, nondepolarizing muscle relaxant; SCh, succinylcholine.

would increase the risk of further injury to the eye. Large doses (two to three times the ED$_{95}$) of NDMRs such as cisatracurium, mivacurium, rocuronium, or vecuronium may permit intubation within 60 to 90 seconds, but recovery from the block may be prolonged. Finally, throughout the operation, one should maintain adequate neuromuscular relaxation and administer sufficient opioid to mimimize coughing on emergence.

OCULOCARDIAC REFLEX

PROBLEM ANALYSIS

Definition

Decreased heart rate associated with pressure on the globe or traction on the extraocular muscles is common in children. The reported incidence of the oculocardiac reflex (OCR) is 20% to 90% during strabismus surgery. The afferent OCR limb is via the long ciliary nerve and the short ciliary nerves. The latter first come together at the ciliary ganglion; these two inputs then converge to form the ophthalmic division of the trigeminal nerve (Fig. 173-2). The efferent limb of the OCR is vagal via the cardiac depressor nerve.

Recognition

The OCR results in a slowed or irregular heart rate. It can be detected by precordial heart sounds, pulse oximetry, or electrocardiographic monitoring. Sinus bradycardia is the most common rhythm disturbance. Sinus pause, transient asystole, wandering atrial pacemaker, atrioventricular junctional rhythm, atrioventricular heart block, and ventricular arrhythmias (extrasystoles, bigeminy, escape beats) may also occur. Although ventricular tachycardia and fibrillation have been reported, they are most likely to occur after prolonged asystole (presumably due to myocardial hypoxia) or treatment with anticholinergics or β-adrenergic agonists, especially in patients anesthetized with sensitizing inhalational anesthetics such as halothane.

Risk Assessment

Younger patients, because of a relative increase in vagal tone, are most predisposed to the OCR during strabismus surgery. Although sudden, forceful traction on *any* of the extraocular muscles is the most common provocative stimulus, there can be others (Table 173-2). Prophylactic atropine and other chronotropic agents do not abolish the OCR but may reduce its incidence and the severity of associated bradycardia. However, as just noted, prophylaxis with anticholinergics or β-adrenergic agonists has the potential to cause worse arrhythmias, especially with older inhalational anesthetics such as halothane. Hypercarbia and hypoxia augment the potential for arrhythmias with the OCR, as does inappropriate anesthetic depth.

Implications

The OCR is usually transient and relieved with release of traction. There is a significant association between intraoperative

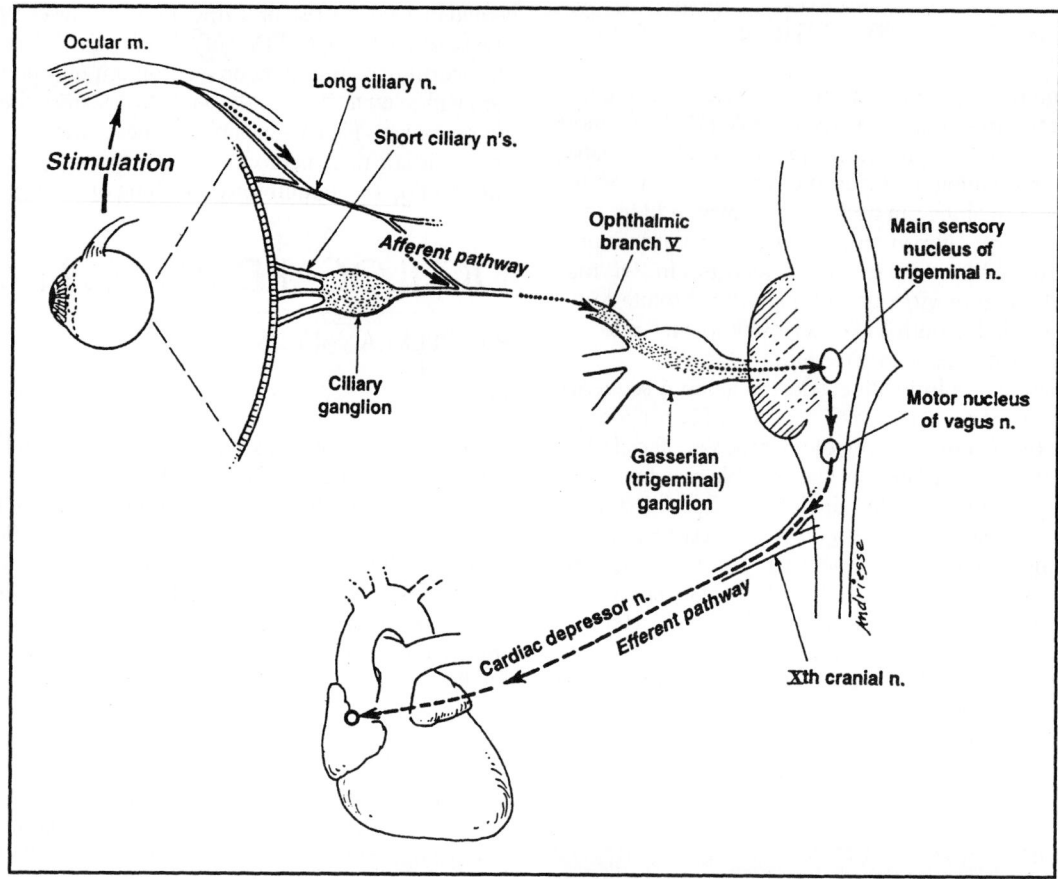

Figure 173–2 ▪ Oculocardiac reflex (OCR). The ophthalmic division of the trigeminal nerve (afferent limb) is stimulated via the long and short ciliary nerves. Afferent impulses are transmitted to the gasserian ganglion and main trigeminal sensory nucleus. From there, they are relayed to the efferent (motor) nucleus of the vagus nerve. The efferent pathway includes the vagus nerve and the cardiac depressor nerve. (From Vassallo SA, Ferrari LR: Anesthesia for ophthalmology. In Coté CJ, Ryan JF, Todres ID, et al [eds]: A Practice of Anesthesia for Infants and Children, 2nd ed. Philadelphia, WB Saunders, 1993, p 325.)

OCR and postoperative nausea and vomiting. Indeed, children with OCR episodes in the operating room are two to three times more likely to experience postoperative nausea and vomiting than are those without such episodes.

MANAGEMENT

Although the OCR is a common cause of arrhythmias during strabismus surgery, it is important to investigate and treat other primary causes, including hypoxia, hypercarbia, and inadequate anesthesia. All these have the potential to worsen the OCR. However, if arrhythmias persist, the surgeon should relax tension on the eye muscle. Administering a chronotropic agent before the stimulus is removed and normal rhythm is restored is *not advised;* this only increases the risk for more serious arrhythmias. In general, the OCR fatigues with repetitive and more gentle traction, making treatment with chronotropic drugs unnecessary.

PREVENTION

Recommendations include the use of controlled, mild hyperventilation to prevent hypercarbia during strabismus surgery. Compared with halothane, sevoflurane can reduce OCR incidence and the magnitude of bradycardia in children during both spontaneous and controlled ventilation. Although intravenous atropine given 30 minutes before eye muscle traction may reduce OCR incidence or attenuate its magnitude, it does not guarantee protection against significant arrhythmias. Because atropine is not universally effective for OCR prophylaxis, and because of the generally low incidence of severe OCR leading to hemodynamic compromise, routine anticholinergic prophylaxis is no longer recommended. Retrobulbar block with 1 to 3 mL of 1% to 2% lidocaine may prevent the OCR in adults but is rarely used in pediatric practice.

Table 173–2 ▪ **Perioperative Stimuli for Oculocardiac Reflex**
Traction on *any* extraocular muscle
Traction on conjunctiva or orbital structures
Ocular trauma or retrobulbar hematoma
Pressure on globe or tissue in orbital apex*
Performance of retrobulbar block

*After enucleation of the eye.

Acknowledgments

Special appreciation is extended to Dr. Monte D. Mills, chairman of the Department of Ophthalmology, Children's Hospital of Philadelphia and the University of Pennsylvania, for reviewing and improving this chapter.

Further Reading

Allison CE, De Lange JJ, Koole FD, et al: A comparison of the incidence of the oculocardiac and oculorespiratory reflexes during sevoflurane and halothane anesthesia for strabismus surgery in children. Anesth Analg 90:306-310, 2000.

Blanc VF, Hardy JF, Milot J, et al: The oculocardiac reflex: A graphic and statistical analysis in infants and children. Can Anaesth Soc J 30:360-369, 1983.

Gild WM, Posner KL, Caplan RA, et al: Eye injuries associated with anesthesia: A closed claims analysis. Anesthesiology 76:204-208, 1992.

Gregory GA: Anesthesia for premature infants. In Gregory GA (ed): Pediatric Anesthesia, 4th ed. Philadelphia, Churchill Livingstone, 2002, pp 352-353.

Haberer JP: Ophthalmic surgery: Anesthetic considerations and postoperative management. In Bissonette B, Dalens B (eds): Pediatric Anesthesia Principles and Practice. New York, McGraw-Hill, 2002, pp 1277-1290.

Lee LA, Lam AM: Unilateral blindness after prone lumbar spine surgery. Anesthesiology 95:793-795, 2001.

Myers MA, Hamilton SR, Bogosian AJ, et al: Visual loss as a complication of spine surgery: A review of 37 cases. Spine 22:1325-1329, 1997.

Roth S, Thisted RA, Erickson JP, et al: Eye injuries after nonocular surgery. Anesthesiology 85:1020-1027, 1996.

Siffring PA, Poulton TJ: Prevention of ophthalmic complications during general anesthesia. Anesthesiology 66:569-570, 1987.

Vachon CA, Warner DO, Bacon DR: Succinylcholine and the open globe. Anesthesiology 99:220-223, 2003.

Vassallo SA, Ferrari LR: Anesthesia for ophthalmology. In Coté CJ, Ryan JF, Todres ID, et al (eds): A Practice of Anesthesia for Infants and Children, 2nd ed. Philadelphia, WB Saunders, 1993, pp 323-335.

Warner ME, Warner MA, Garrity JA, et al: The frequency of perioperative vision loss. Anesth Analg 93:1417-1421, 2001.

White E, Crosse MM: The aetiology and prevention of peri-operative corneal abrasions. Anaesthesia 53:157-161, 1998.

PEDIATRICS & NEONATOLOGY

SECTION 8

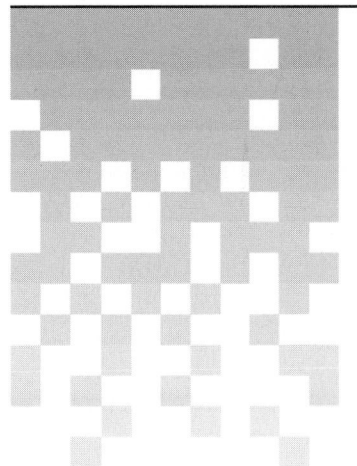

Neurosurgery, Ophthalmology, ENT

Rosemary Hickey

NEUROSURGERY

Intracranial Hypertension

Rosemary Hickey

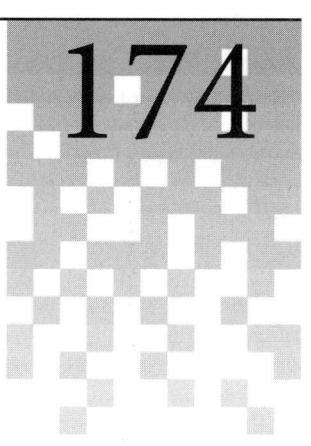

174

Case Synopsis

A 64-year-old man presents with progressive personality changes, memory disturbances, and urinary incontinence. The physical examination is remarkable for depressed consciousness and papilledema. The computed tomography scan reveals a large frontal mass consistent with a meningioma.

PROBLEM ANALYSIS

Definition

Intracranial hypertension exists when there is a sustained elevation in intracranial pressure (ICP) of more than 15 to 20 mm Hg. It results when the three intracranial components—blood, brain, and cerebrospinal fluid (CSF)—are no longer able to compensate for volume changes occurring within the cranium. CSF translocation from the head into the spinal subarachnoid space and its reabsorption via the arachnoid villi are the major compensatory means of accommodating intracranial volume increases. Spatial compensation can also be achieved through compression of the venous system and, ultimately, capillary collapse, leading to cerebral ischemia.

Changes in ICP that occur with changes in intracranial volume can be described by the intracranial elastance curve (Fig. 174-1). The shape of the curve may be influenced by the type of lesion causing the increase in volume; for example, slower-growing lesions may be better tolerated than rapidly growing ones.

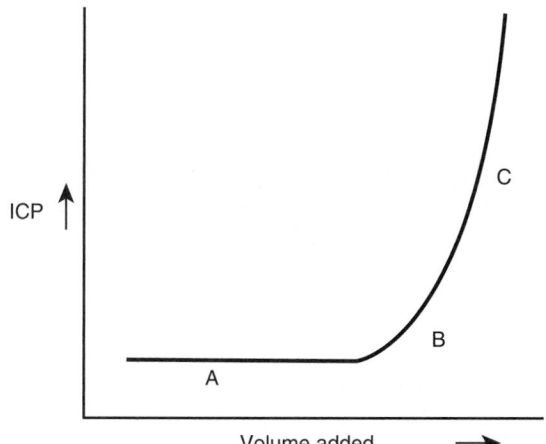

Figure 174–1 ■ Intracranial elastance curve. *A*, Normal elastance. *B*, Reduced elastance (small increase in intracranial pressure [ICP] with increasing intracranial volume). *C*, Poor elastance (large ICP increase with minimal increase in cerebral volume). (From Mahla ME: Neurologic surgery. In Kirby RR, Gravenstein N [eds]: Clinical Anesthesia Practice. Philadelphia, WB Saunders, 1994, pp 1283-1311.)

Recognition

The signs and symptoms most frequently associated with intracranial hypertension include headache, nausea, vomiting, papilledema, unilateral pupillary dilatation, and oculomotor or abducens nerve palsies. Changes in consciousness and irregular ventilatory patterns indicate advanced stages of intracranial hypertension.

Headache is typically present on awakening, or it may awaken the patient from sleep. It is related to traction and distortion of pain-sensitive cerebral blood vessels and the dura mater. Vomiting may be due to direct stimulation of the vomiting centers by local compression. Papilledema is the only reliable sign of an increase in ICP, although intracranial hypertension may be present without it. Oculomotor palsies are secondary to herniation or compression of the nerve, and abducens palsies result from stretching of the nerve as the brainstem is displaced inferiorly by the increased pressure. A general slowing in mentation occurs from continuously increased ICP and a diffuse decrease in cerebral blood flow. Further deterioration in the level of consciousness indicates progressive transtentorial herniation. Alterations in vital signs (bradycardia, hypertension, depression of respiration) also may occur from increased ICP and brainstem compression. Computed tomography scanning, magnetic resonance imaging, or angiography provides indirect evidence of elevated ICP. These studies may reveal a mass lesion accompanied by a midline shift of at least 0.5 cm, encroachment of the CSF cisterns by the expanding brain, or both.

Risk Assessment

The three major mechanisms of increased ICP are (1) increased intracranial volume due to an intracerebral mass lesion (e.g., tumor, massive infarction, trauma, hemorrhage, abscess), extracerebral mass lesion (e.g., tumor, hematoma, abscess), or acute brain swelling (e.g., anoxic states, acute hepatic failure, hypertensive encephalopathy, Reye's syndrome); (2) high venous pressure resulting from heart failure, superior mediastinal obstruction, or cerebral or jugular venous obstruction, which increases blood volume in the pial veins and dural sinuses and may interfere with CSF absorption; and (3) obstruction to the flow (hydrocephalus) or absorption (pseudotumor cerebri) of CSF.

Implications

The danger of intracranial hypertension lies in the potential for cerebral ischemia and herniation of brain tissue. If ICP, either locally or globally, reaches levels exceeding mean arterial pressure, cerebral ischemia will develop. Cerebral perfusion pressure is calculated as mean arterial pressure minus ICP. The likelihood of permanent tissue damage from cerebral ischemia depends on the severity and duration of the ischemia. If ICP is sufficiently high to obstruct venous outflow from the brain, arterial inflow also may be compromised.

Brain herniation can occur around any fixed structure in the skull. In open head trauma, injured brain may herniate through the fractured skull. In the intact skull, herniation sites include the falx cerebri, under which the cingulate gyrus of the frontal lobe can herniate; temporal lobe (uncal) herniation through the tentorium cerebri; and classic herniation of the cerebellum through the foramen magnum, compressing the medulla and resulting in cardiovascular and respiratory collapse.

MANAGEMENT

Therapeutic interventions to lower elevated ICP are categorized according to its intracranial determinant (Table 174-1). Parenchymal volume may be reduced in several ways. Mannitol results in an osmotic reduction of brain water content. It may also improve blood rheology and microcirculatory flow. Loop diuretics (furosemide) provide intracranial decompression through a diuresis-mediated brain dehydration, reduced CSF formation, and resolution of cerebral edema via improved cellular water transport. Corticosteroids reduce peritumoral edema but are not useful for treating intracranial hypertension secondary to head trauma. Surgical excision of mass lesions reduces the volume of the intracranial space occupied by parenchymal components and thus improves intracranial elastance. Techniques to reduce CSF volume include ventricular or lumbar puncture, drains, and shunts. Cerebral blood flow and volume and ICP are reduced by hyperventilation; however, such a reduction in cerebral blood flow may be poorly tolerated.

Jugular venous oxygen saturation monitoring is used to guide the level of hyperventilation in head trauma. Values greater than 75% indicate hyperemia, so induced vasoconstriction associated with hyperventilation may be valuable; values less than 50% indicate cerebral ischemia, so attempts to induce further cerebral vasoconstriction may be harmful. Measurement of brain tissue oxygen tension can also provide information about the safety of hyperventilation. Some intravenous anesthetic drugs (e.g., lidocaine, thiopental, etomidate, propofol) are beneficial for decreasing ICP. A continuous infusion of propofol combined with a low-dose inhalational agent is another useful anesthetic technique. Venous drainage is maximized by keeping the head elevated 15 to 30 degrees, but without excessive rotation or flexion.

PREVENTION

Prevention of intracranial hypertension centers on avoiding factors that are known to increase ICP. Intravenous fluid management is directed toward achieving a euvolemic state. Therapy should avoid the use of intravenous solutions that decrease plasma osmolality (5% dextrose in water, 0.45% sodium chloride, lactated Ringer's solution). The factor in administered fluid that most affects brain edema is the osmolality. An acute drop in osmolality affects brain water content and ICP more than an acute drop in oncotic pressure. Glucose-containing solutions are avoided because hyperglycemia may aggravate ischemic brain injury.

Other factors that increase ICP and should be avoided include compression of jugular veins by improper head positioning, coughing and straining on the endotracheal tube, seizure activity, hypercarbia, and hypoxia. Increased body temperature raises cerebral metabolic oxygen consumption and should be avoided. Volatile anesthetic agents may cause an increase in cerebral blood flow, cerebral blood volume, and ICP. In the presence of intracranial hypertension, these agents should be used in moderation and in combination with hyperventilation and intravenous anesthetics with favorable effects on ICP (e.g., thiopental, etomidate, propofol, fentanyl). If used at a minimum alveolar concentration (MAC) of 1.2 in combination with hyperventilation,

Table 174–1 ■ Determinants of Intracranial Pressure and Therapeutic Techniques to Lower It			
Determinant	**Therapeutic Intervention**	**Mechanism**	**Duration of Effect**
Volume of parenchyma	Mannitol infusion	Osmotic reduction of brain water content	Hours to days
	Corticosteroids	Reduction of peritumoral or peri-inflammatory edema	Days to weeks
	Excision of mass	Volume reduction	Indefinite
	Craniectomy	Increased craniospinal compliance	Indefinite
Cerebrospinal fluid volume	Ventricular or lumbar puncture	Volume reduction	Hours
	Ventriculostomy or lumbar drain	Volume reduction	Days
	Ventricular or lumbar shunt	Volume reduction	Indefinite
Cerebral blood volume	Hyperventilation	Cerebral vasoconstriction due to decreased P_{CO_2}	Hours
	Barbiturates	Cerebral vasoconstriction	Hours to days

Revised from Broaddus WC, Delashaw JB, Park TS: Anatomic, physiologic, and neurosurgical considerations in neuroanesthesia. In Sperry RJ, Stirt JA, Stone DJ (eds): Manual of Neuroanesthesia. Toronto, BC Decker, 1989.

desflurane and isoflurane have similar effects on cerebral perfusion pressure, mean arterial pressure, and lumbar CSF pressure. Nitrous oxide is cerebrostimulatory and increases cerebral blood flow and cerebral metabolic oxygen consumption, especially when combined with volatile anesthetics. Use of nitrous oxide should be avoided with pneumocephalus (e.g., recent craniotomy) because of its potential to diffuse into and expand intracranial and other air-containing spaces.

Further Reading

Adams RD, Victor M: Disturbances of cerebrospinal fluid circulation, including hydrocephalus and meningeal reactions. In Adams RD, Victor M (eds): Principles of Neurology. New York, McGraw-Hill, 1993, pp 539-553.

Bedell E, Prough DS: Anesthetic management of traumatic brain injury. Anesthesiol Clin North Am 20:417-439, 2002.

Bendo AA, Luba K: Recent changes in the management of intracranial hypertension. Int Anesthesiol Clin 38:69-85, 2000.

Coles JP, Minhas PS, Fryer TD, et al: Effect of hyperventilation on cerebral blood flow in traumatic head injury: Clinical relevance and monitoring correlates. Crit Care Med 30:1950-1959, 2002.

Diringer M: Hyperventilation in head injury: What we have learned in 43 years. Crit Care Med 30: 2142-2143, 2002.

Dutton R, McCunn M: Traumatic brain injury. Curr Opin Crit Care 9: 503-509, 2003.

Hickey R: Neurosurgical emergencies. Am Soc Anesthesiol Refresher Courses 24:97-110, 1996.

Imberti R, Bellinzona G, Langer M: Cerebral tissue PO_2 and $SjvO_2$ changes during moderate hyperventilation in patients with severe traumatic brain injury. J Neurosurg 96: 97-102, 2002.

Kaye A, Kucera IJ, Heavner J, et al: The comparative effects of desflurane and isoflurane on lumbar cerebrospinal fluid pressure in patients undergoing craniotomy for supratentorial tumors. Anesth Analg 98:1127-1132, 2004.

Shapiro HM: Anesthesia and intracranial pressure. In Sperry RJ, Johnson JO, Stanley TH (eds): Anesthesia and the Central Nervous System. Dordrecht, Netherlands, Kluwer Academic Publishers, 1993, pp 119-138.

Venous Air Embolism

175

Jennifer E. Souders and Maurice S. Albin

Case Synopses

Gravitational Pressure Gradient of 7.5 cm H₂O

During a repeat lumbar laminectomy in the prone position with an orthopedic frame, a 55-year-old man suddenly develops severe hypotension, rapidly goes into electromechanical dissociation, has cardiac arrest, and cannot be resuscitated after 1 hour of effort.

Gravitational Pressure Gradient of 20 cm H₂O

A 42-year-old woman with acromegaly secondary to pituitary adenoma undergoes transsphenoidal resection of the tumor in the semisitting position (head elevated 30 degrees). Severe hypotension (60 mm Hg systolic) occurs when surgical manipulations are carried out in the area of the sella.

PROBLEM ANALYSIS

Definition

Air can enter the venous circulation when there is a negative gravitational gradient between the right atrium and the upper area of incision or the air's point of entrance. Albin and coworkers reported that a 5 cm H₂O gravitational gradient was sufficient to entrain air in a neurosurgical case. The entry of a bolus of 100 mL of air into the venous circulation can be fatal, and it has been calculated that this amount of air can pass through a 14-gauge needle with a gradient of 5 cm H₂O in a matter of seconds. Factors modifying air entrainment include body position, depth of ventilation, volume of air entering the vessel, rate of gaseous entry, and composition and concentration of gases in the inhaled anesthetic mixture. Animal studies and human cases have shown that the transpulmonary passage of air can occur without a patent foramen ovale. Reduced central venous pressure due to a contracted blood volume or hemorrhagic hypovolemia, or decreased intrathoracic pressure due to the use of a table or frame to reduce abdominal compression, can help increase the gravitational pressure gradient and enhance the entrainment of air.

The fate of entrained air is illustrated in Figure 175-1. In the first case synopsis, the gravitational gradient was probably less than 7.5 cm H₂O but was enhanced by blood loss and use of an orthopedic frame, which reduced abdominal pressure, allowing the development of negative intrathoracic pressure with expiration. Because 50% nitrous oxide (N₂O) was used, this increased the air bubble size by a factor of about two.[1] Autopsy revealed air in the coronary vessels, heart, spinal cord, and cerebral and mesenteric vessels, despite a non-probe-patent foramen ovale.

In the second case synopsis, more than 150 mL of air was aspirated from the central line after the hypotensive episode. The gravitational pressure gradient was at least 20 cm H₂O,

[1]Increased gas bubble volume with N₂O is approximated as $100/(100 - FiN_2O) = 100/(100 - 50) = 2$.

and the air bubble volume was approximately doubled, because 50% N₂O again was used. Postoperatively, a technetium lung scan revealed a peripheral decortication pattern in the posterosuperior portion of the right and left lung fields and an abrupt decrease in perfusion to the right middle lobe, all due to the entrance of air into the pulmonary system.

These cases show that venous air embolism (VAE) can occur in any position, as long as a pressure gradient allows the ingress of air between the procedural area and the heart (Table 175-1). Evidence has accumulated that VAE is far from rare in patients undergoing procedures in the prone position, especially spinal procedures; there have been at least 22 cases reported, with a total of 13 deaths, 10 of which were in the pediatric age group. In addition to neurosurgery, VAE has been reported with virtually all surgeries and endoscopy. It also occurs with catheterization for cardiac or central vascular access, arteriovenous shunts, and intravenous infusions and transfusion therapy.

Recognition

Physical signs and symptoms include gasping respiration in spontaneously breathing patients, increased central venous and pulmonary artery pressures, cardiac arrhythmias, electrocardiographic (ECG) changes, hypotension, abnormal heart sounds, changes in heart rate, decreased peripheral resistance, reduced cardiac output, cyanosis, a mill-wheel murmur, and cardiac arrest. Increased pulmonary artery pressure is the most prominent physical sign of VAE during controlled ventilation, irrespective of the volume or rate of air entrainment. The more rapidly air enters the pulmonary circulation, the more rapidly and severely the pulmonary artery pressure will rise. If it rises dramatically over the systemic pressure, a right-to-left shunt can occur through a septal defect (i.e., patent foramen ovale) and cause paradoxical embolism of air into the left heart. ECG changes with air embolism are quite variable and include tachyarrhythmias, varying degrees of atrioventricular block, right ventricular strain, and ST segment changes. Very large volumes of entrained air may cause such

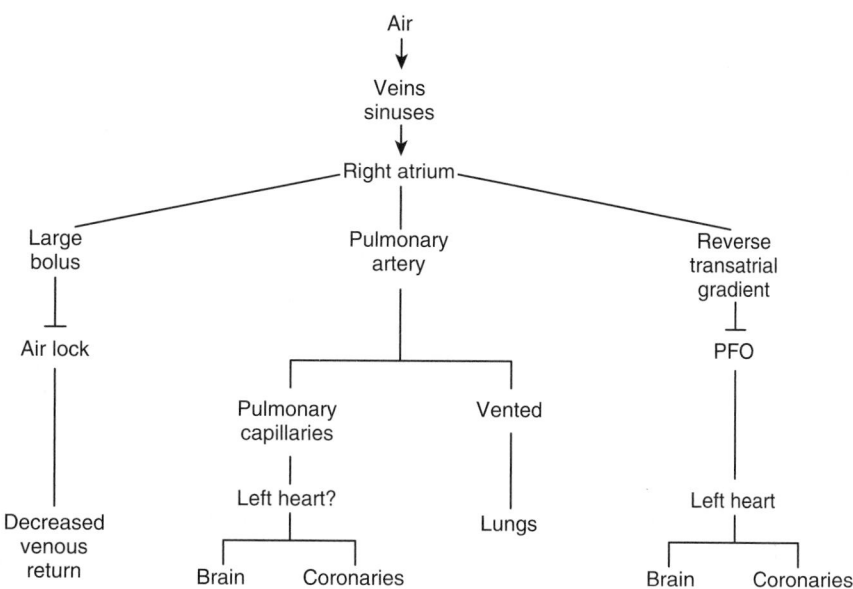

Figure 175–1 ■ Fate of entrained air after venous air embolism. PFO, patent foramen ovale.

severely increased right ventricular afterload that the right ventricle becomes ischemic and fails acutely. Right heart failure is the primary cause of acute hypotension, reduced cardiac output, and cardiac arrest after massive air embolism. A mill-wheel murmur indicates that a significant volume of air has entered the right heart chambers. If so, cardiac arrest may be imminent. Air causes this churning sound and is one of the last signs observed.

Besides physical signs and symptoms, the other methods for detecting intraoperative air embolism, in order of sensitivity, are transesophageal echocardiography (TEE), precordial Doppler ultrasonography, end-tidal carbon dioxide (CO_2), pulmonary artery catheter, pulse oximetry, and direct observation of the surgical site. TEE can detect both venous and paradoxical embolism consisting of as little as 0.02 mL/kg of air. However, it is expensive and may be inaccessible in some surgical locations; it has no audible alarms and may be difficult for solo practitioners to use when they are occupied with urgent patient care duties. A well-positioned precordial Doppler probe detects 0.05 mL/kg of intravascular air, is noninvasive, and alerts both the anesthesiologist and the surgeon simultaneously. As mentioned earlier, although pulmonary artery catheters can show early and prominent signs of air embolism, they are highly invasive and less sensitive than precordial Doppler.

A sudden reduction in end-tidal CO_2 concentration is the most convenient and widely used noninvasive method for detecting air embolism. The magnitude and duration of the decrease in end-tidal CO_2 correlate positively with the volume of air entrained, and detection is possible during any general anesthetic. In contrast, pulse oximetry is relatively insensitive, because decreases in arterial oxygen saturation often occur late with a decrease in arterial oxygen tension. Further, the surgical field is often overlooked. Especially in high-risk surgery, it may be easy to see whether there is a lack of venous oozing, indicating subatmospheric venous pressure. In high-risk procedures, combined precordial Doppler ultrasonography and end-tidal CO_2 monitoring should be used. Doppler tone activation and reduced end-tidal CO_2 signal air entrainment. VAE is confirmed if gas bubbles can be aspirated from a central line.

Risk Assessment

The incidence of VAE is uncertain, largely because the criteria for VAE vary. Nevertheless, we have a general idea about

Table 175–1 ■ Incidence of Air Embolism in Neurosurgery by Position

| Position | No. of Patients | Detected Embolism | | Air Aspirated (mL) | Gradient (cm H_2O) |
		No.	%		
Sitting	400	100	25.0	2-500	20-65
Lateral	60	5*	8.3	3-200	5-18
Supine	48	7†	14.6	2-150	5-18
Prone	10	1‡	10.0	45	7.5
Total	518	113	21.8		

*Two cases of tic douloureux, two cases of hemifacial spasm, one case of tumor.
†Three cases of transsphenoidal hypophysectomy, three cases of intracranial tumor, one case of tic douloureux (air was detected after reapplication of the pinhead holder while the patient was in the supine position, before being put in the sitting position).
‡Ependymoma of the spinal cord.
From Albin MS, Carroll RG, Maroon JC: Clinical considerations concerning detection of air embolism. Neurosurgery 3:380-384, 1978.

the incidence of VAE and the associated morbidity and mortality rates for neurosurgical procedures performed with the patient in the sitting position. The overall incidence is about 25%, ranging from 2% to 60%. In 10 studies of more than 5000 patients, the mortality rate did not exceed 1% in any individual report. Morbidity data, even in neurosurgical sitting cases, are more difficult to ascertain. Albin and coworkers reported 100 cases of VAE in 400 patients operated on in the sitting position. These patients were considered to have VAE only if both Doppler activation and visual aspiration of air from a central line occurred. Under these conditions, 25 of the 100 patients with recognized VAE developed symptoms ranging from severe hypotension to cardiac arrest. Paradoxical air embolism (air entering the left side of the heart via a patent foramen ovale or transpulmonary passage) caused significant mortality in the small number of cases reported. Somewhat surprisingly, most VAE-related mortality appears to occur in non-neurosurgical cases, possibly because anesthetists fail to appreciate that it can occur in these cases and the patient is not monitored adequately for VAE. Adding to this lack of appreciation is the medicolegal "fear factor," which likely leads to underreporting of VAE in the medical literature. There is a significant risk of VAE in cesarean section, spinal surgery, and total hip arthroplasty.

Implications

Because of coalescence and filming of bubbles at the blood-bubble interface, the passage of air into the right atrium can impede or even halt venous return to the right side of the heart. The consequences are hypotension, arrhythmias, and even circulatory arrest, because cardiac output can be severely compromised. The occurrence of an "airlock" in the right ventricle has been postulated as the cause for hemodynamic collapse with massive VAE. However, more recent studies indicate that right ventricular dysfunction is more likely the result of an acute increase in afterload. Continuous entrainment and passage of large volumes of air may lead to the inability of the lungs to adequately vent air from the pulmonary circulation. This results in the liberation of vasoactive substances from the blood-air interface, leading to pulmonary perfusion deficits.

Ventilation-perfusion inhomogeneity is due to the redistribution of pulmonary perfusion. Areas of dead space and high ventilation-perfusion ratios reduce end-tidal CO_2 and increase arterial CO_2 tension. Hypoxia results from altered intrapulmonary shunt, mixed venous oxygen saturation, and redistribution of pulmonary blood flow to regions that are relatively overperfused and underventilated (low ventilation-perfusion ratio). These ventilation-perfusion defects can be variable, because the distribution of air in the pulmonary vessels is a function of both buoyancy and regional pulmonary perfusion. Although ventilation-perfusion inhomogeneities may resolve in as little as 30 minutes after VAE, they can also become progressively worse as a result of the inflammatory response to air in the vascular space. Continuous entrainment of large volumes of air can lead to progressive pulmonary compromise, pulmonary capillary leak, and acute respiratory distress syndrome. Such volumes of air may also reach or exceed the threshold for transpulmonary passage of air, so that it enters the left side of the

heart and coronary sinuses and moves into the brain. This can lead to coronary occlusion and cardiac arrest, as well as cerebral air embolization, with stroke and associated dysfunction.

MANAGEMENT AND PREVENTION

Given the severity of VAE sequelae, prevention and early detection are far preferable to management after the fact. The key to preventing VAE is a greater appreciation of risk factors. Patients who will undergo procedures in which a gravitational gradient will be present, blood loss may be significant, or the surgical site is in a highly vascular area are predisposed to air entrainment and VAE. Good examples from the literature include radical retropubic prostatectomy and repeat lumbar or thoracic laminectomies in the prone position.

Monitoring for VAE should include ECG, blood pressure, pulse oximeter, end-tidal CO_2, precordial Doppler, and a multiorificed catheter with its tip 1 to 2 cm past the junction of the right atrium and superior vena cava (Fig. 175-2). Although the last is important for treatment, the ability to aspirate air from this catheter leaves no doubt about the diagnosis. Further, the transducer of the right atrial catheter can be placed at the level of the surgical site to determine whether a negative pressure gradient exists. In patients thought to be at risk for VAE and in whom invasive monitoring is contemplated, the use of an indwelling catheter for arterial blood gas and pressure monitoring is also advised.

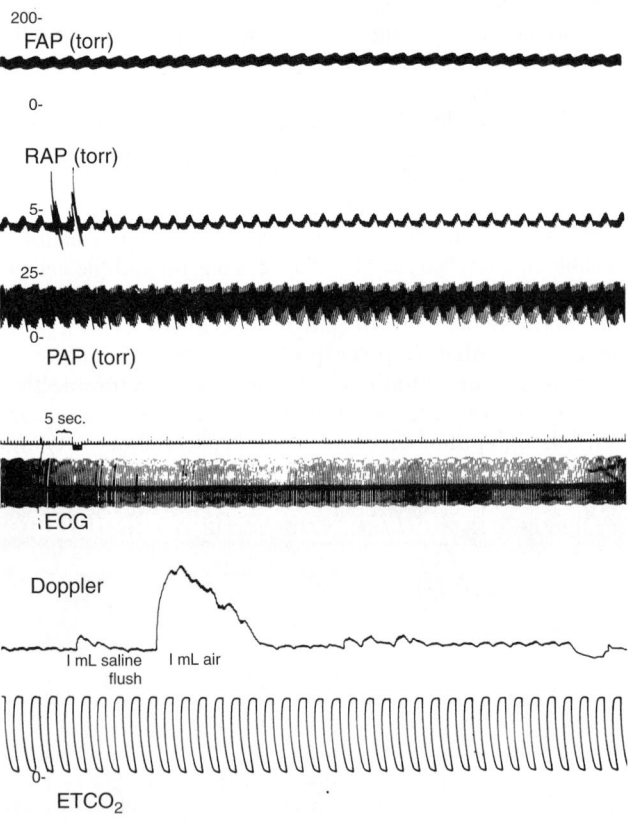

Figure 175–2 ▪ Monitoring for venous air embolism. ECG, electrocardiogram; ETCO₂, end-tidal CO_2; FAP, femoral artery pressure; PAP, pulmonary artery pressure; RAP, right atrial pressure.

Preventive measures for VAE are few and may be contraindicated in certain patients. Hydration can be used to decrease the pressure gradient between the right heart and the surgical site, provided the patient can tolerate increased right ventricular preload. Many patients with intracranial pathology are not suitable candidates. Although the use of positive end-expiratory pressure to increase intrathoracic pressure has been proposed, it may increase right ventricular preload and is also controversial because it may increase the transatrial gradient and open a patent foramen ovale, thus allowing air to egress into the left heart and brain. For intracranial surgery, bilateral manual jugular venous compression temporarily elevates cerebral venous pressure, thereby preventing ongoing cerebral air embolism; it may also help localize the source. This maneuver is safe and effective, but only if applied gently and transiently in patients without preexisting carotid artery disease.

With Doppler activation, a decrease in end-tidal CO_2, or both, the central line must be aspirated *immediately* (using a 50-mL syringe attached to a stopcock). A delay of even a few seconds might allow the entrance of large volumes of air. At the same time, inspired N_2O or air should be replaced with 100% oxygen, and the surgeons should be notified to flood the field with water and look for any open veins. Any resulting hypotension or cardiac arrhythmias should be treated symptomatically with positive inotropes and vasopressors to improve contractility and support the circulation. Epinephrine is the drug of choice for resuscitation from massive VAE. If recovery to pre-VAE physiologic levels does not occur in a very short time, or if air continues to be aspirated, the patient should be returned to a position in which there is no gradient present.

In the event VAE is suspected and the patient remains comatose after surgery or has a neurologic deficit that is thought to be unrelated to the surgical procedure, neurology or neurosurgery consultation is in order, and magnetic resonance imaging should be performed to diagnose the presence of intra-axial air. If air is visualized, a course of hyperbaric oxygen therapy should be considered.

Further Reading

Adornato DC, Gildenberg PL, Ferrario CM, et al: Pathophysiology of intravenous air embolism in dogs. Anesthesiology 49:120-127, 1978.

Albin MS: Air embolism. In Albin M (ed): Textbook of Neuroanesthesia with Neurosurgical and Neuroscience Perspectives. New York, McGraw-Hill, 1997, pp 109-125.

Albin MS, Carroll RG, Maroon JC: Clinical considerations concerning detection of venous air embolism. Neurosurgery 3:380-384, 1978.

Albin MS, Wills J, Schwend RM: Patent foramen ovale and unexplained stroke. N Engl J Med 354:1753-1755 (Letter to the Editor), 2006.

Black S, Cucchiara RF, Nishimura RA, et al: Parameters affecting occurrence of paradoxical air embolism. Anesthesiology 71:235-241, 1989.

Chang JL, Albin MS, Bunegin L, et al: Analysis and comparison of venous air embolism detection methods. Neurosurgery 7:135-141, 1980.

Drummond JC, Prutow RJ, Scheller MS: A comparison of the sensitivity of pulmonary artery pressure, end-tidal carbon dioxide, and end-tidal nitrogen in the detection of venous air embolism in the dog. Anesth Analg 64:688-692, 1985.

Fong J, Gadalla R, Pierri MK, et al: Are Doppler-detected venous emboli during cesarean section air emboli? Anesth Analg 71:254-257, 1990.

Geissler MJ, Allen SJ, Mehlhorn U, et al: Effect of body repositioning after venous air embolism: An echocardiographic study. Anesthesiology 86:710-717, 1997.

Matjasko J, Petrozza P, Cohen M, et al: Anesthesia and surgery in the seated position: Analysis of 554 cases. Neurosurgery 17:695-702, 1985.

Newfield P, Albin MS, Chestnut JC, et al: Air embolism during transphenoidal pituitary operations. Neurosurgery 2:39-42, 1978.

Souders JE: Pulmonary air embolism. J Clin Monit Comput 16:375-383, 2000.

Souders JE, Doshier JB, Polissar NL, Hlastala MP: Spatial distribution of venous gas emboli in the lungs. J Appl Physiol 87:1937-1947, 1999.

Toung T, Ngeow YK, Long DL, et al: Comparison of the effects of positive end-expiratory pressure during continuous venous air embolism in the dog. Anesthesiology 64:724-729, 1986.

Verstappen FT, Bernards JA, Kreuzer AF: Effects of pulmonary gas embolism on circulation and respiration in the dog. I. Effects on circulation. Pflugers Arch 386:89-96, 1977.

Verstappen FT, Bernards JA, Kreuzer AF: Effects of pulmonary gas embolism on circulation and respiration in the dog. II. Effects on respiration. Pflugers Arch 386:599-604, 1977.

Wills J, Schwend RM, Paterson A, Albin MS: Intraoperative visible bubbling may be the first sign of venous air embolism during posterior surgery for scoliosis. Spine 30:E629-E635, 2005.

Posterior Fossa Surgery

176

Donald S. Prough and Eric Bedell

Case Synopsis

A 28-year-old woman undergoes posterior fossa craniotomy for removal of a brainstem tumor. Preoperative symptoms included headache, facial asymmetry, and difficulty swallowing. The intraoperative course is complicated by periods of bradycardia sufficient to reduce blood pressure and a brief episode of asystole. At the conclusion of the case, the patient opens her eyes and follows simple commands, but she has no spontaneous respiratory efforts and only a weak cough and gag.

PROBLEM ANALYSIS

Definition

The most important aspect of posterior fossa surgery is location. A review of posterior fossa anatomy demonstrates that lesions, stimulation, or damage to small areas associated with the brainstem or cerebellum can profoundly influence the operative course and long-term outcome of neurosurgical patients.

Anatomically, the posterior fossa is defined posteriorly by the occipital bone; laterally by the occipital, temporal (petrous and mastoid portions), and parietal (posteroinferior angle) bones; anteriorly by the sphenoid (clivus), temporal (petrous), and occipital (clivus) bones; superiorly by the tentorium cerebelli; and inferiorly by the foramen magnum. Important structures located within the posterior fossa include the cerebellum, cerebral aqueduct, fourth ventricle, midbrain, pons, medulla, and proximal spinal cord. Located within these structures are the nuclei for all cranial nerves and important afferent and efferent tracts.

The oculomotor nerve (3rd cranial nerve) originates in the rostral midbrain, acquires parasympathetic fibers from the Edinger-Westphal nucleus, and courses ventrally through the midbrain. The trochlear nerve (4th cranial nerve) arises from the contralateral caudal midbrain and decussates before traveling ventrally. Other midbrain structures include the corticospinal and corticobulbar tracts, substantia nigra, red nuclei, and decussation of the superior cerebellar peduncles. The pons contains the nuclei for the trigeminal (5th), abducens (6th), facial (7th), and auditory (8th) cranial nerves. The medulla contains the remaining cranial nerves: glossopharyngeal (9th), vagus (10th), spinal accessory (11th), and hypoglossal (12th). The medulla also contains the decussation of the corticospinal tracts ventrally and the inferior cerebellar peduncles posteriorly.

From the perspective of intraoperative and postoperative management, one of the most important considerations is that critical respiratory and cardiovascular control centers reside in the brainstem. Involuntary respiratory control is a complex process involving multiple structures, including the pneumotaxic center (upper pons), which is involved in the transition from inspiration to exhalation; the apneustic center (lower pons), which is involved in the control of inspiration; and the medullary respiratory center (dorsal and ventral respiratory groups), which influences both inspiration and exhalation and coordinates those functions with extracranial nerve input. Vasomotor and cardiac centers, located predominantly in the medulla, powerfully influence resting vascular tone, blood pressure, and heart rate.

Lesions of the posterior fossa can generate diffuse or localized signs and symptoms, depending on the structures where the lesions are located or the structures compressed by mass lesions. A small lesion impinging on the cerebral aqueduct may result in obstructive hydrocephalus (producing symptoms such as headache and altered mental status). Similarly, a small lesion located in the lateral pons may result in isolated cranial nerve dysfunction. Therefore, important clinical data include the anatomic location of any posterior fossa lesion and the presence and magnitude of associated neurologic or systemic compromise.

Intraoperative stimulation, retraction, or damage to structures located within the posterior fossa may activate or inhibit nearby nuclei, leading to rapid and dramatic systemic responses. Intraoperative damage to adjacent structures may result in postoperative alterations in neuronal function (either activation or inhibition), leading to a wide array of clinical problems for postsurgical patients and for those providing postoperative care.

The typical presentation of complications related to postoperative edema or bleeding may differ in important respects from that seen after supratentorial surgery. In general, supratentorial lesions lead to a rostral-to-caudal progression of signs and symptoms. This progression may include headache, mental status changes, respiratory alterations, pupillary and oculomotor changes, hemodynamic changes, and, finally, motor abnormalities. In posterior fossa lesions, deterioration may be rapid, may fail to demonstrate a pattern of deterioration, and may present with localized cranial or brainstem deficits.

Finally, the surgical approach to the posterior fossa must be considered. The three general approaches are sitting, prone, and lateral (either routine or exaggerated, such as the three-quarter prone–park bench position). Each position has its own risks and benefits and will influence anesthetic management. Because of the significant risk of venous air entrainment (as high as 30%), posterior fossa craniotomies in the sitting position are being performed less frequently. However, even with horizontal positioning, venous air embolism—with the attendant risk of cardiovascular collapse and paradoxical air embolism—is a possibility that should be considered in all posterior fossa surgery (also see Chapters 168 and 175).

Recognition

Special care is required when evaluating and managing patients with posterior fossa lesions. Mass lesions located within the posterior fossa or that compress posterior fossa structures can generate diffuse or localized signs and symptoms. A thorough preoperative evaluation, with attention to signs and symptoms produced by such lesions, is mandatory. Intraoperatively, vigilance for signs and symptoms of possible stimulation of or damage to critical portions of the brainstem and cerebellum is paramount. This extends to the postoperative period as well.

Owing to the risks of hydrocephalus, cranial nerve dysfunction, and alterations in respiratory function, extreme caution must be used when administering any form of sedative, hypnotic, or analgesic medications. Even small doses of benzodiazepines or narcotics may produce unacceptable respiratory depression. Therefore, they should be administered only when patients are directly monitored. For lesions involving the pons and medulla, airway maintenance and protective reflexes may be impaired by bulbar dysfunction, making aspiration and airway compromise a significant risk. Monitoring should include frequent evaluation of the level of consciousness, airway maintenance and protection, oxygenation (e.g., pulse oximetry), ventilation (capnography), heart rate, and blood pressure. The importance of frequent neurologic examination and assessment of ventilation and cardiovascular function cannot be overemphasized.

Intraoperative monitoring during posterior fossa surgery can be complex and must be tailored to the brain regions at highest risk during surgery. The cerebellum, though important for the patient's coordination and long-term function, has relatively little impact on intraoperative anesthetic management. Lesions in other areas may have more intraoperative impact. They often require other techniques, which can be roughly divided into (1) monitoring for nerve function and (2) monitoring for other dangerous conditions (e.g., hemodynamic instability, airway compromise, respiratory insufficiency).

Intraoperative monitoring for nerve integrity and function is often accomplished through provocative testing. Common techniques include somatosensory evoked potentials and facial nerve monitoring. In each case, specific monitoring modalities are used in an attempt to assess the integrity and function of the nerve or nerve pathways at risk. These techniques often have anesthetic implications (e.g., stable, low concentrations of potent inhalational agents to avoid excessive attenuation of somatosensory evoked potentials) and thus require appropriate anesthetic management to provide the best monitoring conditions. Failure to appreciate the specific monitoring needs for the proposed surgery may result in inadequate patient monitoring and suboptimal outcomes.

Intraoperative monitoring for hemodynamic instability and postoperative monitoring for neuronal dysfunction, hemodynamic instability, airway compromise, or respiratory insufficiency are important mandates for anesthesiologists. Stimulation of or damage to brainstem cardiac and vasomotor centers can lead to rapid and unpredictable hemodynamic changes. Extreme heart rate and blood pressure alterations are common with surgical manipulation, and rapid diagnosis and treatment are required.

Consideration of the manner of treatment is also important, for neurosurgeons often rely on hemodynamic changes to guide the extent of surgical exploration. Thus, prophylactic treatment of heart rate (i.e., with vagolytic agents) and blood pressure is generally discouraged. In practice, it is more important to recognize when a critical portion of the brainstem is stressed than to blunt all hemodynamic responses.

The risk of venous air embolism is also a consideration in all posterior fossa surgery, and there should be a plan in place for diagnosis and management. Finally, there are no adequate intraoperative monitors for a large number of important brainstem functions, such as airway maintenance and protection, swallowing, and respiratory control. Thus, anesthetic management must be planned and executed to provide rapid and clear emergence with tight hemodynamic control.

Close communication between the anesthesiologist and the neurosurgeon is vital. Specifically, hemodynamic parameters, expected neuronal or bulbar dysfunction, and anticipated alterations in airway protection and respiratory function should be discussed. Postoperative ventilatory support, intubation, or diagnostic studies (e.g., angiography, computed tomography, magnetic resonance imaging) must be discussed before emergence, and appropriate plans must be developed in light of those discussions.

Risk Assessment

Knowledge of the anatomic location of the lesion of interest, the planned surgical procedure, and the actual structures involved in the surgery is a critical element of posterior fossa surgery. Risk assessment is possible only after a review of the individual patient's history and physical examination, an evaluation of radiologic studies, and a discussion with the neurosurgeon. The greatest risks are associated with tumors directly involving the brainstem (e.g., pons and medulla), lesions with direct involvement of the cranial nerves required for airway maintenance and protection, lesions involving the facial nerve, and surgeries conducted with the patient in the sitting position. The actual events encountered during surgery are impossible to predict, which contributes to the challenge of providing anesthesia for neurosurgery in general and for posterior fossa surgery in particular. At a minimum, plans for the diagnosis and management of hemodynamic instability, respiratory dysfunction, alterations in cranial nerve function, and venous air embolism should be made before starting any posterior fossa surgery.

Implications

The risks to patients undergoing posterior fossa surgery can be divided into preoperative, intraoperative, and postoperative complications. Before surgery, patients must be carefully monitored, and sedative-hypnotic and analgesic drugs must be titrated with extreme care. Intraoperative risks are predominantly hemodynamic instability and cardiovascular collapse. Especially with surgery involving the pons and medulla, extreme hemodynamic variability in heart rate and blood pressure may result in patient instability. This instability is usually limited to periods of direct surgical retraction and manipulation, but it can be clinically important. Hemodynamic collapse and cardiac arrest have resulted from venous air entrainment, and both are a constant risk during all posterior fossa (and skull base) surgery, even in patients who are horizontally positioned. Important postoperative risks include alterations in respiratory function, rapid development of increased posterior fossa pressure (e.g., from hematoma formation), development of hydrocephalus, and alterations in cranial nerve function. Because there are limited intraoperative methods of monitoring for these possibilities, rapid and clear emergence from anesthesia with limited respiratory depression and tight hemodynamic control is of primary importance and should be a major determinant in the choice of anesthetic technique.

MANAGEMENT

A full understanding of the patient's condition and anticipated surgical requirements represents an important part of management. Failure to understand the specific location and effect of the posterior fossa lesion severely limits the delivery of optimal therapy. Support and protection of oxygenation and ventilation should be the primary focus when managing complications associated with posterior fossa surgery. Hemodynamic monitoring and modification of heart rate and blood pressure through the use of vasoactive medications are common requirements during posterior fossa surgery. However, remember that prophylactic treatment of heart rate and blood pressure is not indicated, because the surgeon often depends on the development of hemodynamic alterations to guide ongoing surgery.

Postoperatively, to determine the need for ongoing monitoring and support, all cranial nerve and brainstem functions associated with the site of surgery should be specifically evaluated once the patient is awake. This requires that the anesthetic technique permit neurologic examination at the conclusion of surgery, preferably in the operating room before transport to the intensive care unit.

Black and coworkers reported their experience with 579 posterior fossa craniotomies performed in 1981 through 1984. During this period, the number of sitting position craniotomies performed at the Mayo Clinic markedly decreased, while the number of horizontal position craniotomies markedly increased. Overall, there were no significant differences in mortality or other postoperative outcomes between patients undergoing surgery in the two positions (Table 176-1). The incidence of important complications was substantial after surgery in either position.

The time course and presenting signs and symptoms of posterior fossa deterioration may be different from those associated with supratentorial surgery. With supratentorial lesions, deterioration (usually due to an expanding mass or hydrocephalus) generally progresses over time, so serial monitoring is appropriate. For posterior fossa surgery, rapid localized deterioration may occur, leading to a loss of bulbar function, respiratory arrest, or hemodynamic collapse. Thus, vigilance and a high index of suspicion must be maintained into the postoperative period.

Table 176–1 ■ Postoperative Outcomes Not Affected by Position

Outcome	Sitting (N = 333)		Horizontal (N = 246)	
	No.	*%*	*No.*	*%*
Mental status deteriorated	14	4	9	4
Mental status improved	7	2	12	5
Eye injury	8	2	12	5
Seizures	6	2	2	1
Motor deficit new or worse	17	5	16	6
Motor deficit improved	29	9	9	4
Sensory deficit new or worse	6	2	5	2
Sensory deficit improved	19	6	4	2
Complete loss of facial nerve function	23	7	26	11
Perioperative myocardial infarction	1	0.3	4	1.6
Respiratory complications	7	2	8	3
Coma (>1 wk)	6	2	3	1
Cerebrovascular accident	8	2	8	3
Congestive heart failure	1	0.3	0	
Hemodynamic instability	5	1.5	10	4
Pulmonary embolus	0		2	1
Re-exploration for bleeding	6	1.8	6	2.4
Re-exploration for infection	2	0.6	2	0.8
Acute mortality (within 30 days)	9	2.7	5	2
Quadriparesis	0		0	
Symptomatic pneumocephalus	0		0	
Peripheral nerve injury	0		0	
Laryngeal or lingual edema	0		0	

From Black S, Ockert DB, Oliver WC Jr, Cucchiara RF: Outcome following posterior fossa craniectomy in patients in the sitting or horizontal positions. Anesthesiology 69:49-56, 1988.

PREVENTION

Careful evaluation of the patient and discussion with the surgeon about location, impact, and proposed surgical approach are required for the optimal management of patients undergoing posterior fossa surgery. Anticipation of the more common severe complications, such as postoperative venous air embolism and airway or respiratory dysfunction, is a critical part of anesthetic management, as is recognition of the need for specialized monitoring techniques. Although serious complications associated with posterior fossa surgery are uncommon with current surgical procedures, a high index of suspicion and constant vigilance are the most important aspects of perioperative care.

Further Reading

Black S, Ockert DB, Oliver WC Jr, Cucchiara RF: Outcome following posterior fossa craniectomy in patients in the sitting or horizontal positions. Anesthesiology 69:49-56, 1988.

Endo T, Sato K, Takahashi T, Kato M: Acute hypotension and bradycardia by medulla oblongata compression in spinal surgery. J Neurosurg Anesth 13: 310-311, 2001.

Nolte J: The Human Brain: An Introduction to Its Functional Anatomy, 5th ed. St. Louis, Mosby–Year Book, 2002.

Plum F, Posner JB: The Diagnosis of Stupor and Coma, 3rd ed. Philadelphia, FA Davis, 1982.

Williams DL, Umedaly H, Martin IL, Boulton A: Chiari type I malformation and postoperative respiratory failure. Can J Anaesth 47:1220-1223, 2000.

Pituitary Tumors: Diabetes Insipidus

Melissa A. Laxton and Patricia H. Petrozza

177

Case Synopsis

A 58-year-old man undergoes transsphenoidal hypophysectomy for resection of a prolactin-secreting pituitary adenoma with suprasellar extension. Ten hours after surgery, urine output exceeds 3 L/hour, and the serum sodium level is 150 mEq/L.

PROBLEM ANALYSIS

Definition

Diabetes insipidus is a syndrome characterized by polyuria, thirst, and polydipsia triggered by plasma hyperosmolarity. *Neurogenic diabetes insipidus* results from insufficient antidiuretic hormone (ADH) secretion, secondary to damage to the hypothalamic-neurohypophysial axis. Loss of approximately 75% of ADH-secreting neurons is needed for the development of clinically relevant polyuria. In contrast, *nephrogenic diabetes insipidus* is characterized by renal resistance to the action of ADH.

An absolute deficiency of ADH results in impaired urine concentrating ability, polyuria, and a tendency toward dehydration. Most patients have incomplete neurogenic diabetes insipidus and retain a limited ability to concentrate urine and conserve free water. However, if access to water is impaired (e.g., unconsciousness, perioperative nothing-by-mouth status), hypertonic dehydration and hypernatremia may develop. Signs and symptoms of hypernatremia include psychomotor agitation, neuromuscular irritability, lethargy, coma, and seizures.

Recognition

Diabetes insipidus occurs in as many as 20% of adult patients after transsphenoidal pituitary surgery. The syndrome is usually transient in this setting, and perioperative glucocorticoid replacement may facilitate the development of polyuria. Often, polyuria appears on or before the first postoperative day. The polyuria of diabetes insipidus is characterized as follows:

- A 24-hour urine volume greater than 50 mL/kg
- Urine osmolarity greater than 300 mOsm/kg H_2O
- Urine specific gravity less than 1.010

Chronic polyuria causes the hypertonic renal medullary concentration gradient to be "washed out." Additional urine concentrating mechanisms become impaired, so that polyuria increases. Alternative causes of polyuria must be eliminated to make the diagnosis of primary neurogenic or nephrogenic diabetes insipidus with confidence (Table 177-1).

Risk Assessment

As noted earlier, transient diabetes insipidus occurs in up to 20% of patients after transsphenoidal hypophysectomy. However, it becomes permanent in about 2% of cases. A macroadenoma with suprasellar extension is associated with a higher risk for postoperative diabetes insipidus than is a lesion confined to the sella. Recent data suggest that an endoscopic transsphenoidal approach for resection of pituitary tumors may decrease both the short- and long-term incidence of diabetes insipidus compared with the traditional, direct transsphenoidal approach. The secretory type of tumor appears to have no effect on the postoperative occurrence of diabetes insipidus.

Postoperative diabetes insipidus is usually recognized within 12 to 24 hours of the initial insult, but delays of days to weeks have been recorded. In approximately 50% to 60% of cases, diabetes insipidus is transient, lasting only 3 to 5 days. More rarely, it may last several weeks, followed by gradual resolution. This pattern is more common after resection of pituitary adenomas confined to the sella. After transcranial approaches to pituitary macroadenomas with suprasellar extension, or procedures in which proximal damage to the pituitary stalk is likely, both complete and partial diabetes insipidus have been observed; in some cases, it takes several years for this condition to improve or resolve.

A small group of patients (5% to 10%) exhibits a classic triphasic response to injury. This pattern most commonly

---

Table 177–1 ■ Causes of Polyuria Other Than Primary Neurogenic or Nephrogenic Diabetes Insipidus

Chemical diuresis
Mannitol
Urea
Radiocontrast agents
Hyperglycemia
Furosemide, thiazides, ethacrynic acid
Acute renal failure
Drug-induced nephrogenic diabetes insipidus (e.g., cisplatin, lithium)
Postobstructive diuresis
Postresuscitation diuresis

follows hypophysial stalk injury due to severe head trauma or the resection of extensive suprasellar tumors. The initial phase is characterized by an abrupt cessation of ADH release. This is followed by polyuria, which begins within 12 to 24 hours after injury and lasts for 4 to 8 days. An antidiuretic phase, lasting 5 to 6 days, follows. It is characterized by concentrated urine, with plasma hyposmolarity and hyponatremia as a result of free water reabsorption. Profound hyponatremia and its attendant complications may develop if there is a delay in recognizing this phase. Excessive release of stored ADH from degenerating neurohypophysial tissues is the likely explanation for this antidiuretic phase. Once this stored ADH release is complete, diabetes insipidus frequently recurs. Although usually persistent, sometimes it may improve or resolve.

Implications

A patient with diabetes insipidus is unable to concentrate urine and retain water. Without treatment, intravascular volume depletion results, cardiac stroke volume declines, and heart rate increases in an effort to maintain cardiac output. Hypoperfusion may be signaled by weak peripheral pulses; orthostatic hypotension; cold, clammy skin; rapid, shallow respirations; and a reduced level of consciousness. Hypernatremia may manifest as seizures and hyperreflexia.

MANAGEMENT

Owing to the predominantly transient nature of perioperative diabetes insipidus, some mild cases are managed with oral fluid replacement, especially if the patient is cooperative and the thirst mechanism is intact. However, if the patient is unable to cooperate, and there is associated hypokalemia and concern about "wash-out" of the renal medullary concentration gradient, more aggressive therapy may be warranted.

Exogenous replacement of ADH is with either desmopressin or aqueous vasopressin. After transsphenoidal resection, desmopressin is usually administered subcutaneously in a dosage of 1 to 2 μg every 8 to 12 hours. Desmopressin lacks the vasoconstrictor effects of vasopressin and is less likely to cause hypertension or abdominal cramping. For patients requiring long-term ADH replacement, both intranasal and oral preparations are available. However, the dose must be titrated individually.

Although desmopressin is clearly the drug of choice for the chronic treatment of diabetes insipidus, its duration of action is 12 to 18 hours. Some clinicians prefer aqueous vasopressin if diabetes insipidus is likely to be transient. Aqueous vasopressin is formulated as 20 pressor units/mL of solution. The peak effect occurs by 1 to 2 hours, and the duration of action is 4 to 8 hours. The usual starting dosage is 2 to 5 units subcutaneously or intramuscularly every 4 to 6 hours as needed.

Careful assessment of fluid intake; urine output, osmolarity, and specific gravity; plasma osmolarity; serum sodium concentration; and body weight should guide therapy with vasopressin or desmopressin. Clinicians must be alert to the possible development of an antidiuretic phase of hormonal dysfunction, complicated by water intoxication.

PREVENTION

Meticulous surgical resection is the best means of preventing perioperative diabetes insipidus. Anesthesiologists should maintain a high index of suspicion for the development of diabetes insipidus, especially when there is suprasellar extension of a pituitary tumor or other endocrine abnormalities in a neurosurgical patient.

Further Reading

Arafah BM, Nasrallah MP: Pituitary tumors: Pathophysiology, clinical manifestations and management. Endocr Relat Cancer 8:287-305, 2001.

Barker FG II, Klibanski A, Swearingen B: Transsphenoidal surgery for pituitary tumors in the United States, 1996-2000: Mortality, morbidity, and the effects of hospital and surgeon volume. J Clin Endocrinol Metab 88:4709-4719, 2003.

Carrau RL, Kassam AB, Snyderman CH: Pituitary surgery. Otolaryngol Clin North Am 34:1143-1155, 2001.

Fukuda I, Hizuka N, Takano K: Oral DDAVP is a good alternative therapy for patients with central diabetes insipidus: Experience of five-year treatment. Endocr J 50:437-443, 2003.

Rajaratnam S, Seshadri MS, Chandy MJ, et al: Hydrocortisone dose and postoperative diabetes insipidus in patients undergoing transsphenoidal pituitary surgery: A prospective randomized controlled study. Br J Neurosurg 17:437-442, 2003.

Singer PA, Sevilla LJ: Postoperative endocrine management of pituitary tumors. Neurosurg Clin N Am 14:123-138, 2003.

Vance ML: Perioperative management of patients undergoing pituitary surgery. Endocrinol Metab Clin North Am 32:355-365, 2003.

Verbalis JG: Management of disorders of water metabolism in patients with pituitary tumors. Pituitary 5:119-132, 2002.

Intracranial Aneurysms: Rebleeding

178

Philippa Newfield

Case Synopsis

A 64-year-old man undergoing craniotomy for clip-ligation of a right anterior communicating artery aneurysm 12 hours after initial subarachnoid hemorrhage becomes acutely hypertensive and experiences bradycardia during the induction of anesthesia.

PROBLEM ANALYSIS

Definition

Subarachnoid hemorrhage (SAH) from the rupture of an intracranial aneurysm (ICA) occurs with a frequency of 6 to 8 per 100,000 persons in most Western populations. Rates of ICA rupture are 0.05% to 6% per year, depending on the size and location of the aneurysm. The risk of rupture is 11 times greater in patients with previous SAH than in those with symptomatic aneurysms.

Rebleeding is the occurrence of further hemorrhage after the initial SAH. Such episodes can be catastrophic, with high mortality and chronic morbidity rates. If untreated, 50% of ruptured ICAs rebleed within 6 months of the initial SAH. The incidence of rebleeding is highest within 24 hours of SAH (4%); it then declines to 1% to 2% per day for the next 13 days. About 20% to 30% of ruptured ICAs rebleed within 30 days of the initial SAH. Another 10% to 15% of patients rebleed during the ensuing 5 months.

ICA rerupture produces neurologic deterioration by raising intracranial pressure (ICP) and impairing cerebral perfusion. Many complications may ensue (Table 178-1). Hydrocephalus can develop acutely, because sudden clot deposition throughout the subarachnoid space blocks the passage of cerebrospinal fluid (CSF) through the basal subarachnoid cisterns. Late-onset hydrocephalus is due to obstruction of CSF drainage pathways by organized subarachnoid clot.

Brain infarction also occurs due to direct, hematoma-induced brain destruction or shifts in the intracranial contents, along with vascular compromise. The larger the volume of subarachnoid blood and the greater the ICP, the more likely it is that cerebral blood flow (CBF) will be reduced and the patient's neurologic condition will worsen. SAH also impairs autoregulation, the ability of the brain to maintain CBF fairly constant over mean arterial pressures between 50 and 150 mm Hg, and it reduces the cerebral metabolic rate of oxygen (O_2) consumption.

The incidence of intraoperative ICA rupture ranges from 6% to 8%. It varies among institutions and depends on the size and location of the aneurysm. Causes of ICA rupture and rebleeding during surgery, in decreasing order of frequency, are dissection, brain retraction, hematoma evacuation, and opening of the dural and arachnoid membranes.

Recognition

Signs of rebleeding with reruptured ICAs are largely due to intracerebral hemorrhage. The risk of such bleeding is higher with subsequent episodes of ICA rupture. This is because adhesions from the prior SAH seal off the aneurysm from the subarachnoid space and deflect any new bleeding into the brain parenchyma. After ICA rebleeds, the level of consciousness deteriorates, and patients develop focal neurologic deficits (aphasia, hemiplegia), abnormal vital signs (hypertension, bradycardia, arrhythmias, irregular respirations), and temperature elevation. They also have fluid and electrolyte imbalance (especially hyponatremia), and retinal hemorrhage may be evident on ophthalmologic examination (Table 178-2).

If ICA rebleeding occurs during or immediately after the induction of anesthesia, the patient's blood pressure will increase, and the heart rate may or may not decrease. It is important to realize that the ICP will also increase. At this

Table 178–1 ■ Complications of Subarachnoid Hemorrhage	
Early	**Late**
Hematoma, ↑ ICP, rebleeding, seizures, hydrocephalus	Rebleeding, hydrocephalus, vasospasm, infarction, epilepsy
Nerve palsy, hemiparesis, reduced LOC	Permanent hemiparesis, cognitive disabilities
Cardiac arrhythmias	Myocardial infarction, pneumonia, hepatic and renal dysfunction
Transient ↑ BP	Persistent ↑ BP
Impaired vision	Vitreous hemorrhage
Fluid and electrolyte imbalance	Neurologic deterioration, death

BP, blood pressure; ICP, intracranial pressure; LOC, level of consciousness.

Table 178–2 ■ Effects of Aneurysmal Rebleeding

Direct brain destruction
Disturbance of CSF flow → hydrocephalus
↑ ICP from hematoma, intracerebral hemorrhage,
    intraventricular hemorrhage
Cerebral infarction from ↓ CBF
Fluid and electrolyte imbalance
Cardiac arrhythmias, ↑ BP
Respiratory impairment

BP, blood pressure; CBF, cerebral blood flow; CSF, cerebrospinal fluid; ICP, intracranial pressure.

juncture, ICA rupture is diagnosed by intracranial Doppler ultrasonography, and the efficacy of management is monitored thereafter. Intraoperative rupture of an ICA is readily apparent. Rebleeding after completion of the operation is signaled by failure to awaken from anesthesia or by further neurologic deterioration after awakening (e.g., decrease in level of consciousness, development of new focal neurologic deficits or aphasia).

Risk Assessment

ICA rerupture is one of the major causes of neurologic deterioration after initial SAH (Table 178-3). Risk of rebleeding begins immediately after the initial ICA hemorrhage and is the major threat early after SAH. The likelihood of rebleeding is directly related to the patient's systolic blood pressure in the post-SAH period. For patients who have already had multiple rebleeding episodes, the likelihood of further rupture and death is much greater. Other risk factors include poor neurologic status (owing to initial SAH parenchymal injury), shorter time since initial SAH, female gender (twice the incidence of rebleeding versus males), poor medical condition, older age, posterior ICA, higher rates of intracerebral or intraventricular hematoma, and abnormal clotting parameters. During pregnancy, the risk of rebleeding from an unsecured ICA is 33% to 50%. Although this is fatal in 50% to 68% of patients, there is no evidence that the rebleeding rate in pregnant patients is different from that in the general population.

Table 178–3 ■ Causes of Neurologic Deterioration after Subarachnoid Hemorrhage

Rebleeding—intracranial hypertension
Hematoma
Hydrocephalus
Cerebral edema
    Seizures
    Meningitis
Disordered autoregulation
Disordered carbon dioxide responsiveness
Acid-base disturbances
Fluid and electrolyte disturbances
Vasospasm
Delayed ischemic deficit
Cerebral infarction—secondary cerebral insults
    Hypotension
    Hypoxemia
    Hyperglycemia
    Intracranial hypertension (beyond initial hemorrhage)

Once the ICA has bled, the risk of rebleeding is greatest within the first 24 hours (4%); this is because clot sealing the aneurysmal rent is tenuous, and systemic blood pressure is usually at its highest. The cumulative rebleed rate for ruptured ICAs is 19% at 14 days and about 40% at 179 days. Patients whose ruptured ICAs remain untreated continue to rebleed at a rate of 3% per year for up to 15 years. Late rebleeding is fatal in 67% of cases.

The International Subarachnoid Aneurysm Trial compared operative aneurysmal clip-ligation with endovascular coiling in 2143 patients with ICA-related SAH. At 1-year follow-up, results of the randomized study showed a low risk of rebleeding in both groups (2.4% for coil versus 1.0% for clip repair). However, even after accounting for effects of rebleeding, the relative risk for death or significant disability was 22.6% lower for endovascular versus surgical repair, an absolute risk reduction of 6.9%. Most of these patients were in good condition after SAH (World Federation of Neurosurgical Societies grades I and II) and had small anterior ICAs (92% <11 mm in size). For such ICAs, endovascular and surgical repairs are considered equivalent therapies.

Implications

Pathophysiologic sequelae and complications of rebleeding after initial aneurysmal SAH are considerable. Because a recurrent hemorrhage is usually more severe than the initial one, mortality with recurrent hemorrhage doubles to 80%, with significant associated morbidity in the surviving patients. The size of the hematoma is the most critical factor in determining outcome (Table 178-4). Patients with large subdural hematomas and more of a midline shift on computed tomography scanning have a poorer prognosis, as do those with associated intracerebral or intraventricular hemorrhage.

Because the majority of rebleeding takes place within the first 6 to 24 hours after the initial SAH, early intervention to secure the aneurysm (whether by surgical clipping or endovascular coiling) has become the mainstay of treatment for rebleeding. Thus, diagnosis and treatment of rebleeding must be accomplished quickly and efficiently. Further, because increased experience with SAH, its sequelae, and its treatment improves patient care, collaborative relationships between community hospitals and centers specializing in the surgical and endovascular treatment of ICAs are mandatory.

Table 178–4 ■ Predictors of Mortality after Acute Subarachnoid Hemorrhage

Poor clinical status or grade on admission—directly related to size of hematoma
Decreased level of consciousness
Elevated blood pressure
Rebleeding
Delayed ischemic deficit (vasospasm)
Thickness of subarachnoid clot on initial computed tomography scan
Basilar aneurysm
Older age
Preexisting medical illness

MANAGEMENT

Therapy for rebleeding after an initial SAH is designed to maintain cerebral perfusion, reduce intracranial hypertension and volume, control systemic blood pressure, and decrease transmural pressure (mean arterial pressure minus ICP) across the aneurysm wall. Within this context, optimization of brain O_2 delivery depends on total arterial O_2 content and necessitates the maintenance of normal hemoglobin concentrations and arterial O_2 saturations.

Specific therapy varies according to the stage of ICA therapy at which rerupture occurs (Table 178-5). If the aneurysm bleeds before, during, or after the induction of anesthesia, the patient is hyperventilated with 100% O_2. Thiopental, which also affords some amount of cerebral protection, or intravenous sodium nitroprusside or nicardipine[1] will lower blood pressure, although excessive lowering of blood pressure at this juncture can be detrimental if it interferes with cerebral perfusion. Nitroprusside also causes cerebral vasodilatation, which may further raise ICP and impair cerebral perfusion, thereby increasing the ischemic penumbra.[2] Immediate craniotomy for "rescue clipping" after ICA rupture during induction has been successful.

Intraoperative rupture of an ICA mandates rapid achievement of surgical control. The mean arterial pressure may be reduced briefly to 50 mm Hg to facilitate temporary proximal and distal occlusion of the parent vessel in preparation for clip-ligation of the aneurysmal neck. Once the parent vessel is occluded, blood pressure is increased to normal to enhance collateral circulation during the period of temporary occlusion. This may be superior to the use of controlled hypotension after rupture. Alternatively, the ipsilateral carotid artery can be manually compressed for 3 minutes to produce a bloodless field. Also, if the bleeding is sufficient to cause hypovolemia, induced hypotension may not be an option. Any blood loss is replaced immediately with whole blood, blood products, colloid, or crystalloid. It is essential to maintain normal blood volume while the blood pressure is lowered.

Although barbiturates and etomidate have been advocated to protect against focal brain ischemia, the clinical efficacy is unproved. Also, with hypovolemia, the associated hypotension can be detrimental. Stable patients can receive thiopental or etomidate before temporary occlusion.

For all patients, temperature is maintained in the low-normal range (34°C to 35°C). Even moderate hypothermia confers some cerebral protection by reducing the release of excitatory neurotransmitters and the cerebral metabolic rate of O_2 consumption (by 7% to 8% per 1°C). However, results of the recent International Hypothermia for Aneurysm Surgery Trial suggest that intraoperative hypothermia (33°C) does not improve neurologic outcomes compared with maintaining normothermia (target temperature 36.5°C). Any increase in temperature above normal should be promptly reduced.

Table 178–5 ■ Aneurysmal Rupture: Management Priorities
During or After Induction
Hyperventilation
100% oxygen
Blood pressure control
Barbiturates
During Dissection
Induced hypotension
Proximal vascular or carotid occlusion with high normal blood pressure
100% oxygen
Pharmacologic metabolic suppression
Volume resuscitation

Patients who do not awaken as expected following the operation, or who awaken and then deteriorate neurologically, require timely diagnosis of the cause. Emergent computed tomography scans can help differentiate ICA rebleed, rupture of another ICA, postsurgical bleeding, pneumocephalus, acute hydrocephalus, and acute cerebral infarction as the cause of deterioration.

If there is intracranial hypertension postoperatively, the patient requires intracranial volume-reducing measures such as hyperventilation with 100% O_2, mannitol, cerebral vasoconstricting drugs (e.g., thiopental, propofol), and augmentation of cerebral perfusion through maintenance of systemic blood pressure in the patient's high-normal range. Emergency reoperation may be necessary for rescue clipping of the ruptured ICA, evacuation of hematoma, control of bleeding, or ventricular drainage. In an emergency, an external ventricular drain may be inserted in the postanesthesia care area or intensive care unit to decompress the ventricular system.

PREVENTION

The only definitive measure to prevent ICA rebleeding is early surgical clip-ligation or endovascular obliteration of the aneurysm. Once the ICA has been secured, the risk of rebleeding is reduced to practically zero, with late rebleeding occurring more often after endovascular than neurosurgical intervention. After securing the ICA, the patient can receive prophylaxis against or treatment for cerebral vasospasm, such as hypertensive hypervolemic hemodilution ("triple H therapy"), without fear of ICA rerupture.

Short of securing the ICA by mechanical means, preoperative measures to prevent rebleeds include maintenance of blood pressure in the patient's normal range, maintenance of euvolemia (Table 178-6), and avoidance of seizures (which may be associated with hypertension). Blood pressure control is achieved with analgesics and short-acting antihypertensive drugs (e.g., labetalol) that do not affect the cerebral vasculature. Lowering blood pressure has not been shown to reduce the risk of rebleeding in any controlled trial, but prospective studies have correlated rebleeding with higher systolic blood pressures. Beyond the first few days after initial SAH, the risk of lowering the blood pressure increases,

---

[1]The latter may be more effective for reducing associated vasospasm.
[2]Zone of ischemic brain surrounding nonviable brain tissue.

Table 178–6 ▪ Prevention of Aneurysmal Rebleeding

Preoperative

BP control: sedatives, short-acting antihypertensive drugs
Maintain adequate cerebral perfusion pressure (70 to 80 mm Hg)
Analgesic drugs
Cautious HHH therapy for vasospasm
Early aneurysmal clip-ligation or endovascular obliteration

Intraoperative

Induction
  Maintain normal BP
  Maintain direct BP monitoring
  Avoid surges in systolic BP
  Ensure adequate depth of anesthesia
  Provide optimal oxygenation
  Maintain normocapnia
Craniotomy
  Osmotic diuretic with craniotomy
  CSF drainage after craniotomy
Aneurysmal manipulation
  Proximal temporary occlusion
    High-normal BP
  Hypotension
  Osmotic diuretics
  CSF drainage
  Hyperventilation
  Venous drainage
  Normoglycemia
  Hypothermia
Adequate analgesia
Maintain normovolemia
Monitor central venous pressure, urine output, blood loss

Emergence

Avoid surges in systolic BP
Adequate analgesia

Postoperative

Avoid surges in systolic BP
Maintain intravascular volume
Avoid hypotension
Adequate analgesia

BP, blood pressure; CSF, cerebrospinal fluid; HHH, hypertensive hypervolemic hemodilution; ICP, intracranial pressure.

Table 178–7 ▪ Induction of Anesthesia: Aneurysmal Clip-Ligation

Optimal head position
Deep level of anesthesia
  Propofol (1-2 mg/kg)
  Thiopental (3-5 mg/kg)
  Fentanyl (3-5 µg/kg)
  Sufentanil (0.5-1 µg/kg)
  Vecuronium (0.1 mg/kg)
  Low-dose inhalation anesthetic
Controlled ventilation
  100% O_2
  Normal $Paco_2$ (35-40 mm Hg)
Before laryngoscopy
  Lidocaine (1.5 mg/kg)
  Thiopental (2-3 mg/kg)
  Propofol (0.5 mg/kg)
Brief, gentle laryngoscopy
Intubation

During the induction of anesthesia for craniotomy for ICA clip-ligation, it is essential to maintain transmural pressure across the ICA wall in the patient's preoperative range by the judicious use of drugs and meticulous technique (Table 178-7). Certainly, one must prevent sudden increases in systemic blood pressure and decreases in ICP. Direct blood pressure monitoring provides beat-to-beat information about the immediate effects of anesthetic or neurosurgical interventions (e.g., laryngoscopy, application of pin head-holders). Anticipation of a blood pressure increase with these maneuvers can facilitate the timely use of drugs such as propofol and thiopental to deepen anesthesia.

Avoiding sudden increases in transmural pressure from a decrease in ICP before the bone flap is turned is also important. Ventilation is adjusted to maintain normocapnia (arterial carbon dioxide tension 35 to 40 mm Hg) and intracranial volume until the dura is opened. However, if the patient has a large subdural hematoma, hyperventilation and other maneuvers to improve intracranial compliance are indicated during induction. The volume-reducing effect of mannitol also may decrease ICP before the skull is opened. To avoid consequent increased transmural pressure and the potential for ICA rerupture, mannitol is not administered until after the craniotomy has been performed, when the intracranial contents are at atmospheric pressure. Lumbar drainage of CSF also facilitates ICA access by relaxing the brain, but this too increases transmural pressure by reducing ICP if it is performed before the cranium has been opened.

Interventions to prevent rebleeding are also necessary during ICA manipulation for clip-ligation. Temporary proximal occlusion of the parent vessel is used to decrease the turgor of the ICA sac, and the blood pressure is maintained in the patient's high-normal range to enhance distal and collateral perfusion. Of course, if the temporary clip is removed before the aneurysm has been secured, blood pressure must be quickly returned to the patient's low-normal range to prevent aneurysmal rupture.

Hypotension with isoflurane or nitroprusside to a mean arterial pressure of 50 mm Hg in normotensives and 60 mm Hg or higher in hypertensives was once used to increase the safety of aneurysmal manipulation. This is no longer done,

because the patient is now susceptible to vasospasm. At this point, it is best to let the patient's blood pressure self-adjust, although pain should be treated appropriately to prevent associated increases in blood pressure.

If the patient deteriorates neurologically from cerebral vasospasm before the ICA is secured, triple H therapy (see earlier) must be instituted with caution. To avoid rebleeding, the systolic pressure is increased modestly from 120 to 150 mm Hg, central venous pressure from 10 to 12 mm Hg, and pulmonary capillary wedge pressure from 12 to 16 mm Hg.

Avoidance of lumbar puncture and rapid ventricular drainage before ICA clip-ligation may also protect against rebleeding. However, these measures are sometimes used to lower ICP (as a calculated risk) when cerebral perfusion is seriously compromised by intracranial hypertension.

The antifibrinolytics ε-aminocaproic acid and tranexamic acid can reduce the likelihood of ICA rebleeding. However, associated cerebral vasospasm limits their usefulness and may double mortality rates due to delayed ischemia. Thus, there is little if any indication for the use of these drugs after SAH.

however, because hypotension to lower CBF may adversely affect patients with or in the process of developing cerebral vasospasm.

Although there are no controlled human studies of the protective effects of intravenous drugs during ICA surgery, the ability to quickly institute prophylactic protective measures before the onset of ischemia is desirable. A number of intravenous drugs, alone and in combination, have been administered to extend the safe duration of temporary vascular occlusion. High-dose mannitol (2 g/kg) enhances the microcirculation and increases regional CBF in areas of ischemia. Because the production of free radicals may contribute to neuronal damage from ischemia, vitamin E and dexamethasone are used to augment mannitol's effects in some protocols.

To the regimen of normotension, normovolemia, and mannitol, some neurosurgeons have added electroencephalographic burst suppression (with etomidate or barbiturates), with reported benefit. Propofol, if administered to provide burst suppression before temporary ICA occlusion, may also confer cerebral protection. Normoglycemia and relative hypothermia to 35°C may also reduce the ischemic risk with temporary occlusion of cerebral vessels.

Control of blood pressure is essential during emergence from anesthesia, because patients are at risk for rebleeding during this time as well. This may be due to multiple ICAs, whether diagnosed or not. If one has been clipped, another unsecured one may bleed on emergence. Hypertension with emergence also threatens surgical hemostasis and may produce intracranial hemorrhage. Finally, wrapping the ICA (versus clipping) does not necessarily protect against rebleeding during emergence from anesthesia.

Further Reading

Chang HS, Hongo K, Nakagawa H: Adverse effects of limited hypotensive anesthesia on the outcome of patients with subarachnoid hemorrhage. J Neurosurg 92:971-975, 2000.

Cross DT, Tirschwell DL, Clark MA, et al: Mortality rates after subarachnoid hemorrhage: Variations according to hospital case volume in 18 states. J Neurosurg 99:810-817, 2003.

Egge A, Waterloo K, Sjoholm H, et al: Prophylactic hyperdynamic postoperative fluid therapy after aneurysmal subarachnoid hemorrhage: A clinical, prospective, randomized, controlled study. Neurosurgery 49:593-606, 2001.

Eng CC, Lam AM: Cerebral aneurysms: Anesthetic considerations. In Cottrell JE, Smith DS (eds): Anesthesia and Neurosurgery, 3rd ed. St. Louis, Mosby–Year Book, 1994, pp 376-405.

Fridriksson S, Saveland H, Jakobsson KE, et al: Intraoperative complications in aneurysm surgery: A prospective national study. J Neurosurg 96:515-522, 2002.

Gianotta SL, Oppenheimer JH, Levy ML, et al: Management of intraoperative rupture of aneurysms without hypotension. Neurosurgery 28:531-536, 1991.

Haley EC Jr, Kassell NF, Torner JC, et al: The International Cooperative Study on Timing of Aneurysm Surgery: The North American experience. Stroke 23:205-214, 1992.

Kett-White R, Hutchinson PJ, Al-Rawi PG, et al: Adverse cerebral events detected after subarachnoid hemorrhage using brain oxygen and microdialysis probes. Neurosurgery 50:1213-1222, 2002.

LeRoux P, Winn HR: Management of the ruptured aneurysm. In LeRoux P, Winn HR, Newell DW (eds): Management of Cerebral Aneurysms. Philadelphia, WB Saunders, 2004, pp 303-333.

Molyneux A, Kerr R, Stratton I, et al: International Subarachnoid Aneurysm Trial (ISAT) of neurosurgical clipping versus endovascular coiling in 2143 patients with ruptured intracranial aneurysms: A randomized trial. Lancet 360:1267-1274, 2002.

Murayama Y, Song JK, Uda K, et al: Combined endovascular treatment for both intracranial aneurysm and symptomatic vasospasm. AJNR Am J Neuroradiol 24:133-139, 2003.

Newfield P: Anesthetic management of intracranial aneurysms. In Newfield P, Cottrell JE (eds): Handbook of Neuroanesthesia, 3rd ed. Philadelphia, JB Lippincott–Williams & Wilkins, 1999, pp 175-194.

Qureshi AI, Suri MF, Yahia AM, et al: Risk factors for subarachnoid hemorrhage. Neurosurgery 49:607-613, 2001.

Rabinstein AA, Pichelmann MA, Friedman JA, et al: Symptomatic vasospasm and outcomes following aneurysmal subarachnoid hemorrhage: A comparison between surgical repair and endovascular coil occlusion. J Neurosurg 98:319-325, 2003.

Sluzewski M, Bosch JA, van Rooij WJ, et al: Rupture of intracranial aneurysms during treatment with Guglielmi detachable coils: Incidence, outcome, and risk factors. J Neurosurg 94:238-240, 2001.

Smith MJ, Le Roux PD, Elliott JP, Winn HR: Blood transfusion and increased risk of vasospasm and poor outcome after subarachnoid hemorrhage. J Neurosurg 101:1-7, 2004.

Solenski NJ, Haley EC Jr, Kassell NF, et al: Medical complications of aneurysmal subarachnoid hemorrhage: A report of the Multicenter Cooperative Aneurysm Study. Crit Care Med 23:1007-1017, 1995.

Todd MM, Hindman BJ, Clarke WR, et al: Mild intraoperative hypothermia during surgery for intracranial aneurysm. N Engl J Med 352:135-145, 2005.

Treggiari-Venzi MM, Suter PM, Romand JA: Review of medical prevention of vasospasm after subarachnoid hemorrhage: A problem of neurointensive care. Neurosurgery 48:249-261, 2001.

Intracranial Aneurysms: Vasospasm and Other Issues

179

Philippa Newfield

Case Synopsis

A 47-year-old woman underwent craniotomy for clip-ligation of a middle cerebral artery aneurysm. The procedure was successful, and the patient was alert and neurologically intact until postoperative day 4, when her level of consciousness decreased and she developed a new hemiparesis.

PROBLEM ANALYSIS

Definition

Vasospasm is the transient, self-limited narrowing of intradural subarachnoid arteries that occurs several days after subarachnoid hemorrhage (SAH). It is a result of sustained contraction of arterial smooth muscle. The subsequent delayed ischemic deficit and infarction caused by cerebral vasospasm are a major cause of disability and death after SAH, accounting for 30% of SAH-induced morbidity and mortality. Cerebral vasospasm is associated with a deterioration in clinical status in 30% of patients after SAH. Up to 10% of patients die, and another 10% have permanent neurologic deficits. This reactive narrowing of the subarachnoid arteries occurs after rupture of an intracranial aneurysm because these vessels are bathed by spasmogenic breakdown products of red blood cells (especially hemoglobin) released into the cerebrospinal fluid.

Recognition

Angiographic vasospasm begins 3 to 5 days after SAH. The narrowing is maximal at 6 to 8 days and gradually resolves 12 to 14 days after a single episode of SAH. Angiographically severe vasospasm is defined as a decrease of 50% or greater in arterial diameter. The diagnosis of cerebral vasospasm (Table 179-1) is based on clinical signs of progressive impairment in mental status and level of consciousness or the appearance of new focal neurologic deficits more than 4 days after the initial SAH that cannot not attributed to any other structural or metabolic cause. The onset of SAH may be sudden or insidious and is often accompanied by increased headache, meningismus, and fever. Although some evidence of vasospasm is apparent on angiography in 70% to 80% of cases, only one third of patients develop full clinical expression. It is important to rule out other causes of neurologic deterioration with suspected SAH, including rebleeding, intracerebral hemorrhage, hydrocephalus, subdural hematoma, cerebral infarction, cerebral edema, meningitis, seizures, electrolyte and acid-base disturbances, and adverse drug reactions.

Cerebral angiography is the most reliable test for diagnosing and evaluating vasospasm. On angiography, vasospasm may be focal, diffuse, or segmental. Clinical signs and symptoms of decreased cerebral blood flow (CBF) usually develop when there is greater than 50% reduction in the diameter of the arterial lumen. Angiography is indicated for patients suspected of having cerebral vasospasm who do not improve after the administration of intravenous fluids and induced hypertension. It is also used for those who cannot tolerate the aforementioned therapy to rule out vasospasm as a cause of deterioration.

Computed tomography (CT)–angiography can detect severe or no cerebral vasospasm in proximal cerebral arteries. It is less reliable for assessing cerebral vasospasm in more distal arteries and intermediate degrees of vasospasm. Methodologies for measuring CBF are positron emission tomography (PET), single photon emission computed tomography (SPECT), and xenon-enhanced CT. PET studies have revealed a fall in the cerebral metabolic rate for oxygen following SAH. Angiographic vasospasm, delayed ischemic deficits, and increased transcranial Doppler velocities are associated with regions of cerebral hypoperfusion on SPECT. Xenon-enhanced CT is a fairly inexpensive technique and can reveal and quantify reductions in regional CBF in patients with clinical vasospasm; it can also be

---

Table 179–1 ■ Diagnosis of Cerebral Vasospasm

Clinical appearance of new neurologic signs and symptoms
    Decrease in level of consciousness
    Focal weakness
Angiography
Positron emission tomography (PET)
Single photon emission computed tomography (SPECT)
Computed tomography (CT)–angiography
Xenon cerebral blood flow measurement
Transcranial Doppler (TCD)

repeated within 20 minutes. Further, it is possible to fuse regional CBF data with conventional CT anatomy and distinguish ischemia from other causes of neurologic deterioration after SAH.

Transcranial Doppler (TCD) ultrasonography is also used to diagnose cerebral vasospasm. Either a sharp increase (e.g., middle cerebral artery velocity >120 cm/second) or a rapid rise in TCD blood flow velocity (e.g., >50 cm/second in 24 hours) is indicative of a reduction in the caliber of the vessels. Peak TCD flow velocity of 140 to 200 cm/second is associated with moderate cerebral vasospasm; values greater than 200 cm/second indicate severe vasospasm. CBF velocities become maximal 7 to 20 days after SAH. Critical TCD blood flow velocities (>120 cm/second) correlate strongly with vasospasm on angiography. As such, TCD is a better corroborative tool than a predictive one. Either a reduction in TCD velocity or a return to normal often indicates abatement of vasospasm and can be used to determine the efficacy and duration of treatment. Because TCD is operator dependent and involves other technical factors (e.g., intracranial pressure [ICP], cardiac output, the artery being assessed), it is important to correlate any TCD results with sequential neurologic examinations and other monitoring modalities, including ICP, blood pressure, and cardiac output.

Jugular bulb venous oximetry detects changes in cerebral oxygen extraction. In one study, patients who developed clinical vasospasm were noted to have a significant rise in cerebral oxygen extraction approximately 1 day before the onset of signs of neurologic deficits. When these patients were treated with hypertensive hypervolemic hemodilution, their deficits resolved, and there was a significant improvement in cerebral oxygen extraction. There was no increase in cerebral oxygen extraction in patients who did not have clinical vasospasm; therefore, increases in this parameter may be predictive of the impending onset of clinical vasospasm.

Risk Assessment

After clip-ligation of cerebral aneurysms, and regardless of clinical status, all patients have a 50-50 chance of developing cerebral vasospasm. Vasospasm is directly related to the severity of the hemorrhage from aneurysmal rupture, which correlates well with the location and volume of blood noted on the initial posthemorrhage CT scan. The risk is increased by the presence of cerebral dysautoregulation and abnormal carbon dioxide responsiveness after SAH. Elderly patients may be at less risk for developing vasospasm, but they do not tolerate ischemia as well as younger ones do and therefore develop cerebral infarction more frequently. The timing of surgery has no effect on the subsequent development of angiographic cerebral vasospasm, nor does surgical versus endovascular occlusion have an effect. Other indicators of increased risk for the development of vasospasm include an admission Glasgow Coma Scale score less than 14 (see Table 182-1), an early increase in mean middle cerebral artery flow velocity on TCD, and anterior cerebral or internal carotid artery aneurysms.

Angiographic vasospasm (>30% reduction in cerebral vessel diameter) is a significant risk factor for the development of infarction. Death from vasospastic infarction occurs

in 5% to 17% of patients after SAH. Modifiable risk factors that affect the progression from ischemia to infarction include a premorbid history of hypertension and smoking.

Transfusion of packed red blood cells intraoperatively is a risk factor for poor outcome. Also, postoperative transfusion is correlated with the development of angiographically proven cerebral vasospasm. The mechanism may involve depletion or inactivation of nitric oxide, an endogenous vasodilator that transfused red blood cells appear to lack. Transfused cells may also have proinflammatory effects or may induce immune system dysfunction. If so, before transfusion, one must determine whether SAH patients are symptomatic from any associated anemia.

Implications

Cerebral vasospasm appreciably worsens patient outcomes after SAH. It is believed to be the cause of 28% and 39% of all associated deaths and disability, respectively. Thus, it is responsible for extensive utilization of limited health care resources. Owing to the high mortality, and because survivors of SAH with vasospasm are more likely to have serious permanent neurologic deficits, considerable research efforts and dollars are being expended to identify pharmacologic and other measures to prevent, ameliorate, or eradicate the devastating sequelae of SAH-related cerebral vasospasm.

The presence of cerebral vasospasm has implications for anesthetic management as well. Cerebral perfusion pressure is maintained at higher-than-normal levels to enhance cerebral perfusion. Hypotension, including controlled hypotension during aneurysmal dissection, should be avoided. Because autoregulation and carbon dioxide responsiveness are impaired to varying degrees with cerebral vasospasm, blood pressure stability and normocapnia are maintained.

MANAGEMENT

Pharmacologic and other modalities used to treat cerebral vasospasm after SAH are listed in Table 179-2. Early operation for clip-ligation of the ruptured aneurysm after SAH secures the aneurysm and permits the removal of fresh clot by irrigation and suction. The surgeon may also apply tissue plasminogen activator (tPA) directly into the subarachnoid space to dissolve remaining clot. Although this fibrinolytic drug can reduce vasospasm, it also has the potential to cause rebleeding by dissolving normal clot. Thus, only patients at high risk for clinically significant vasospasm are candidates for tPA treatment. Early obliteration of the aneurysm by endovascular coils also facilitates the subsequent treatment of vasospasm.

Table 179–2 ▪ Pharmacologic and Other Modalities Used to Treat Cerebral Vasospasm
Hypertensive hypervolemic hemodilution
Volume expansion with crystalloids and colloids
Vasopressors (e.g., dopamine, dobutamine, phenylephrine)
Transluminal balloon angioplasty

Both hypervolemia and hypertension are used to increase cardiac output and augment cerebral perfusion in vasospastic areas of the brain with impaired autoregulation. Early institution of these measures can mitigate or avoid the progression of vasospasm-induced ischemia to infarction. Hemodilution alone is unlikely to be beneficial and may reduce cerebral oxygen delivery. However, a hematocrit of 30% to 35% is likely adequate. Complications of induced hypervolemia and hypertension include rebleeding, hemorrhagic infarct transformation, cerebral edema, hypertensive encephalopathy, intracranial hypertension, myocardial infarction, heart failure, pulmonary edema, coagulopathy, and dilutional hyponatremia, as well as complications related to central vascular catheterization.

Expansion of intravascular volume is necessary because total circulating blood and red blood cell volumes are reduced in most patients after SAH. This is secondary to supine diuresis, peripheral pooling, negative nitrogen balance, reduced erythropoiesis, iatrogenic blood loss, and increased natriuresis. Limits for crystalloid and colloid volume expansion are central venous and pulmonary capillary wedge pressures of 10 to 12 and 12 to 16 mm Hg, respectively. There is a suggestion that albumin may improve the clinical outcome at 3 months and reduce hospital costs when normal saline alone has failed to increase the central venous pressure to at least 8 mm Hg.

Vagal and diuretic responses to intravascular volume augmentation might dictate the need for a drug such as vasopressin to reduce urine output to less than 200 mL/hour. Hydrocortisone has also been used to attenuate excessive natriuresis and hyponatremia in patients with SAH, as well as to prevent the associated decrease in total blood volume. It appears to have no serious side effects.

Vasopressors, including dopamine, dobutamine, and phenylephrine, might also be required to increase blood pressure and augment cardiac output. Invasive hemodynamic monitoring (e.g., direct arterial, central venous, or pulmonary artery pressure; cardiac output) is required for patients with induced hypertension. Before the aneurysm is secured, systolic blood pressure is maintained between 120 and 150 mm Hg. Once secured, it can be increased to 160 to 200 mm Hg.

Transluminal balloon angioplasty is also used to relieve cerebral vasospasm. The inflatable intravascular balloon mechanically dilates the segmental zone of vasospastic narrowing. This may improve the patient's level of consciousness by relieving focal ischemic deficits. However, early intervention is critical. Another treatment is serial papaverine angioplasty. This improves cerebral circulation times, but serial infusions are required for recurring cerebral vasospasm.

PREVENTION

Cerebral Vasospasm

The prevention of cerebral vasospasm requires a high level of vigilance and care, maintenance of normovolemia, careful monitoring, and prevention of secondary cerebral insults and medical complications (Table 179-3). Early occlusion of the aneurysm facilitates subsequent efforts to prevent and

Table 179–3 ■ Pharmacologic and Other Modalities Used to Prevent Cerebral Vasospasm after Subarachnoid Hemorrhage
Administer nicardipine (IV)
Administer nimodipine (orally or via gastric feeding tube)
Maintain normal electrolyte balance
Provide adequate analgesia
Maintain normovolemia
Maintain normothermia
Maintain normotension

treat vasospasm. Monitoring in an intensive care unit or a transitional area is indicated until after the peak time for the development of vasospasm has passed. The purpose of such care is to avoid hypovolemia, hyponatremia with inappropriate diuresis, arrhythmias, hyperthermia, pulmonary edema, hypoxia, hypercarbia, and intracranial hypertension. Any of these has the potential to exacerbate cerebral vasospasm.

After SAH, adults need 3 to 4 L of fluid a day to maintain normovolemia. Hypotonic solutions (e.g., lactated Ringer's) are avoided. Hyponatremia is treated with either normal or hypertonic saline as necessary. However, Egge and colleagues showed that prophylactic hypertensive hypervolemic hemodilution after aneurysmal SAH neither prevents vasospasm nor improves outcomes when compared with controls treated with normovolemia. In addition, costs were higher and complications were more frequent in patients receiving hyperdynamic therapy. In the International Subarachnoid Aneurysm Trial, patients with better clinical grades (World Federation of Neurosurgical Societies grades I to III on admission) whose aneurysms were occluded with endovascular coils rather than surgical clipping were less likely to have symptomatic vasospasm. However, there was no difference in clinical outcome between the groups at the end of the follow-up period.

Although blood pressure is controlled before the aneurysm is secured, it is not treated thereafter, unless elevations are critically high. ICP is maintained in the normal range with mannitol, ventricular drainage, and mild ventilation. The goal is to keep cerebral perfusion pressure above 60 to 70 mm Hg.

Use of the dihydropyridine calcium channel blocker[1] nimodipine within 96 hours of SAH in good- and poor-grade patients has been shown to reduce the morbidity and mortality associated with aneurysmal cerebral vasospasm. It is now a standard of care after SAH. Nimodipine improves the poor outcome associated with vasospasm in all grades of patients, improves the chance of a good to fair outcome, and reduces the chance of infarction after SAH. However, the incidence of symptomatic vasospasm is not affected by nimodipine. Because it has a limited effect on the angiographic caliber of vessels, it is postulated that nimodipine

---

[1]Dihydropyridine calcium channel blockers are selective for vascular smooth muscle versus cardiac muscle, in contrast to non-dihydropyridines such as verapamil and diltiazem. Intravenous nicardipine, a dihydropyridine calcium channel blocker, is increasingly used for the treatment of vasospasm in aneurysmal SAH, although long-term outcomes are not yet known.

confers cerebral protection by reducing the influx of calcium in marginally ischemic neurons. Alternatively, it may increase CBF by dilating pial collateral vessels not seen on angiography. Nimodipine also reduces blood pressure; however, it does so by reducing systemic vascular resistance, not preload.

Treatment with subcutaneous low-molecular-weight heparin (enoxaparin 20 mg/day) for 3 weeks after SAH also appears to improve overall outcomes at 1 year. Apparently, this is due to a reduction in delayed ischemic deficits and cerebral infarction. Patients who received enoxaparin also had fewer intracranial bleeding events and a lower incidence of severe (i.e., shunt-dependent) hydrocephalus.

Other drugs have been investigated for the prevention of vasospasm. Tirilazad, an antioxidant and free radical scavenger, showed mixed clinical results. Nicaraven, a free radical scavenger, showed a trend toward improved survival, good outcome, and smaller infarct size at 3 months. Ebselen, an antioxidant and anti-inflammatory drug, has neuroprotective properties and appears to be effective in acute ischemic stroke. Intra-arterial fasudil, a kinase inhibitor, has been used to treat clinical vasospasm. However, there was no difference in neurologic outcome versus placebo, and patients treated with fasudil had more pneumonia and hypotensive episodes. Owing to increased endothelin (an endothelial-derived vasoconstrictor peptide) with cerebral vasospasm, an endothelin antagonist has also been investigated. Intracisternal tPA prevents vasospasm but does not improve outcome because of increased bleeding associated with its use. Finally, although antifibrinolytics reduce rebleeding, they increase delayed cerebral ischemia and therefore are rarely used.

Hydrocephalus

Chronic hydrocephalus occurs in 10% of patients after SAH. It is due to obstructed pathways for cerebrospinal fluid drainage (i.e., subarachnoid venous granulations). Development of arachnoid adhesions also prevents the reabsorption of cerebrospinal fluid. If the blockage is incomplete, the problem persists only for several weeks. Hydrocephalus that either causes intracranial hypertension or reduces CBF can adversely affect the outcome following SAH. Whether the aneurysm is occluded using surgical or endovascular techniques does not affect the subsequent risk for hydrocephalus.

Acute hydrocephalus is associated with a poor clinical grade and thickened subarachnoid or intraventricular hemorrhage on admission CT scans. It occurs in 15% to 20% of SAH patients. Other associations are alcoholism, female sex, older age, larger aneurysms, pneumonia, meningitis, and hypertension. It is recognized by the onset of lethargy and coma within 24 hours of SAH.

Development of acute ventricular dilatation soon after SAH is a cause of sudden deterioration in neurologic status and may require external ventricular drainage to normalize ICP. External ventricular drainage is used only when the patient's level of consciousness becomes depressed. Good results have been achieved when this is done along with early aneurysm occlusion. Ventricular drainage should be used with caution, however, to avoid changes in the transmural pressure that may precipitate aneurysmal rebleeding. Because acute hydrocephalus is often associated with

vasospasm, early aneurysm occlusion allows the use of hyperdynamic therapy and angioplasty.

Half of patients who develop acute hydrocephalus require a ventriculoperitoneal shunt, but the need for a permanent shunt is reduced by external ventricular drainage. Predictors of the need for permanent shunting include poor grade on admission, rebleeding, and intraventricular hemorrhage.

Chronic hydrocephalus, seen in 25% of patients who *survive* SAH, is an important cause of the subsequent slow physical decline of patients who were originally in good condition. Symptoms include an increasingly impaired level of consciousness and the development of dementia, gait disturbances, and incontinence. A CT scan is indicated within a month after SAH to ascertain ventricular size.

Abnormalities of Cerebral Autoregulation

The central nervous system is directly affected by SAH and the resultant hematoma, vascular disruption, and edema. SAH interferes with cerebral autoregulation, which is the ability of the cerebral vasculature to maintain normal (unchanged) CBF over a wide range of cerebral perfusion pressures (mean arterial pressure minus ICP), from 50 to 150 mm Hg. Importantly, this range is higher (shifts to the right) in patients with chronic hypertension. Intracranial aneurysms (especially giant aneurysms) and SAH-induced hematoma and cerebral edema can cause intracranial hypertension, with a consequent decrease in the patient's level of consciousness and the potential for brainstem herniation and death. Patients with intracranial hypertension also have reduced CBF and cerebral metabolic rate for oxygen. The extent of such impairment correlates with the patient's clinical grade. The response of the cerebral vasculature to changes in arterial carbon dioxide tension is preserved after SAH. A decline in carbon dioxide reactivity usually does not occur until there is extensive disruption of cerebral homeostasis.

Seizures

The seizure incidence after SAH is from 3% to 26%. Early seizures occur in 1.5% to 5% of patients, and late ones in 3%. Seizures are detrimental after SAH because they increase CBF and cerebral metabolic rate for oxygen and also may cause rebleeding, owing to increased blood pressure. Patients at highest risk for seizures have either thick cisternal blood on CT scan or lobar intracerebral hemorrhage. Other risk factors are rebleeding, vasospasm with delayed ischemic neurologic deficits, middle cerebral artery aneurysm location, subdural hematoma, and chronic central nervous system impairment.

Use of prophylactic antiepileptics is controversial, because most seizures occur within the first 24 hours after SAH, often before hospitalization. Therefore, neurosurgeons use seizure prophylaxis (e.g., phenytoin, fosphenytoin, levetiracetam) for only 1 to 2 weeks after SAH. Patients with one or more intracerebral hemorrhages or early seizures receive anticonvulsants for at least 6 months.

Cardiac Disturbances

Electrocardiographic changes occur in 27% to 100% of patients with SAH. Most common are T-wave inversion or ST segment depression. Others are new U or Q waves and Q-T interval prolongation. Rhythm disturbances occur in 30% to 80% of patients and include premature ventricular beats (most common), sinus bradycardia and tachycardia, lower escape rhythms, atrial fibrillation, and tachyarrhythmias (atrial or ventricular in origin). Arrhythmias commonly occur within 7 days of SAH, with the peak occurrence between the second and third days.

The extent of myocardial dysfunction correlates with the severity of neurologic injury after SAH. The cause of this dysfunction is believed to be related to hypothalamic injury, with consequent autonomic imbalance and release of catecholamines, causing myocardial ischemia and infarction. Increased adrenergic tone may persist for the first week after SAH. These SAH-related cardiac abnormalities are similar to those seen with acute coronary syndromes (myocardial ischemia, infarction, and reperfusion injury) and may predispose patients to life-threatening arrhythmias. Associated Q-T interval prolongation makes patients more vulnerable to ventricular tachyarrhythmias (see Chapter 81). This risk is increased with low serum potassium or magnesium levels and with drugs that prolong the Q-T interval. The routine measurement of Q-T intervals may identify patients at risk for potentially lethal arrhythmias.

Often, the question for the neurosurgeon and anesthesiologist is whether to proceed with surgical or endovascular intervention to secure an aneurysm emergently, even if a delay might put the patient at increased risk for rebleeding and compromise the treatment for vasospasm. Serial cardiac isozymes and ventricular function assessment by echocardiography may indicate the magnitude of ischemia. Use of a pulmonary artery catheter to measure pulmonary capillary wedge pressure and cardiac output can both facilitate the management of cardiac dysfunction and monitor the response to hyperdynamic therapy for the treatment of cerebral vasospasm. The presence of severe arrhythmias (about 5% of patients with arrhythmias) or significant cardiogenic pulmonary edema may necessitate postponing surgical or endovascular intervention until treatment has begun. Prophylactic β-adrenergic blockade can improve the cardiac outcome in some patients.

Further Reading

Chang HS, Hongo K, Nakagawa H: Adverse effects of limited hypotensive anesthesia on the outcome of patients with subarachnoid hemorrhage. J Neurosurg 92:971-975, 2000.

Cross DT, Tirschwell DL, Clark MA, et al: Mortality rates after subarachnoid hemorrhage: Variations according to hospital case volume in 18 states. J Neurosurg 99:810-817, 2003.

Egge A, Waterloo K, Sjoholm H, et al: Prophylactic hyperdynamic postoperative fluid therapy after aneurysmal subarachnoid hemorrhage: A clinical, prospective, randomized, controlled study. Neurosurgery 49:593-606, 2001.

Eng CC, Lam AM: Cerebral aneurysms: Anesthetic considerations. In Cottrell JE, Smith DS (eds): Anesthesia and Neurosurgery, 3rd ed. St. Louis, Mosby–Year Book, 1994, pp 376-405.

Fridriksson S, Saveland H, Jakobsson KE, et al: Intraoperative complications in aneurysm surgery: A prospective national study. J Neurosurg 96:515-522, 2002.

Gianotta SL, Oppenheimer JH, Levy ML, et al: Management of intraoperative rupture of aneurysms without hypotension. Neurosurgery 28:531-536, 1991.

Haley EC Jr, Kassell NF, Torner JC, et al: The International Cooperative Study on Timing of Aneurysm Surgery: The North American experience. Stroke 23:205-214, 1992.

Kett-White R, Hutchinson PJ, Al-Rawi PG, et al: Adverse cerebral events detected after subarachnoid hemorrhage using brain oxygen and microdialysis probes. Neurosurgery 50:1213-1222, 2002.

Le Roux P, Winn HR: Management of the ruptured aneurysm. In Le Roux P, Winn HR, Newell DW (eds): Management of Cerebral Aneurysms. Philadelphia, Elsevier Science, 2004, pp 303-333.

Molyneux A, Kerr R, Stratton I, et al: International Subarachnoid Aneurysm Trial (ISAT) of neurosurgical clipping versus endovascular coiling in 2143 patients with ruptured intracranial aneurysms: A randomized trial. Lancet 360:1267-1274, 2002.

Murayama Y, Song JK, Uda K, et al: Combined endovascular treatment for both intracranial aneurysm and symptomatic vasospasm. AJNR Am J Neuroradiol 24:133-139, 2003.

Newfield P: Anesthetic management of intracranial aneurysms. In Newfield P, Cottrell JE (eds): Handbook of Neuroanesthesia, 3rd ed. Philadelphia, JB Lippincott–Williams & Wilkins, 1999, pp 175-194.

Qureshi AI, Suri MF, Yahia AM, et al: Risk factors for subarachnoid hemorrhage. Neurosurgery 49:607-613, 2001.

Rabinstein AA, Pichelmann MA, Friedman JA, et al: Symptomatic vasospasm and outcomes following aneurysmal subarachnoid hemorrhage: A comparison between surgical repair and endovascular coil occlusion. J Neurosurg 98:319-325, 2003.

Sluzewski M, Bosch JA, van Rooij WJ, et al: Rupture of intracranial aneurysms during treatment with Guglielmi detachable coils: Incidence, outcome, and risk factors. J Neurosurg 94:238-240, 2001.

Smith JS, Le Roux PD, Elliott JP, et al: Blood transfusion and increased risk of vasospasm and poor outcome after subarachnoid hemorrhage. J Neurosurg 101:1-7, 2004.

Solenski NJ, Haley EC Jr, Kassell NF, et al: Medical complications of aneurysmal subarachnoid hemorrhage: A report of the Multicenter Cooperative Aneurysm Study. Crit Care Med 23:1007-1017, 1995.

Treggiari-Venzi MM, Suter PM, Romand JA: Review of medical prevention of vasospasm after subarachnoid hemorrhage: A problem of neurointensive care. Neurosurgery 48:249-261, 2001.

Arteriovenous Malformation: Normal Perfusion Pressure Breakthrough

180

Shailendra Joshi and William L. Young

Case Synopsis

A 39-year-old woman is given general anesthesia for resection of a right superior temporal gyrus arteriovenous malformation (AVM) measuring 3 by 3 by 2 cm (Figs. 180-1 and 180-2). After surgery, her mean arterial pressure increases to 100 mm Hg when phenylephrine is used to confirm surgical homeostasis (Fig. 180-3). The patient emerges from anesthesia without neurologic deficits. Six hours later, she complains of a severe headache, vomits, and becomes lethargic. The right pupil is dilated. Immediate computed tomography scan reveals a large hemorrhage into the operative site and a midline brain shift (Fig. 180-4). After surgery to evacuate the clot, there is no residual AVM, the feeding artery is thrombosed, the surrounding brain is lax, and a vessel on the anterior rim of the AVM bed is identified as the source of bleeding. Postoperative neurologic examination reveals an appropriate response to painful stimuli and recovery of pupillary reaction. Four hours later, the patient's intracranial pressure suddenly increases from 10 to 80 mm Hg and her pupils become fixed and dilated. Immediate repeat exploration reveals the source of hemorrhage to be an arterial vessel on the posterior rim of the AVM bed. The brain is edematous and adheres to the dura. The postoperative neurologic evaluation shows no improvement. Subsequent examination shows no evidence of brainstem function, and serial electroencephalograms are isoelectric. The patient dies. At autopsy, there is no residual AVM.

PROBLEM ANALYSIS

Definition

Normal perfusion pressure breakthrough (NPPB) after AVM resection is a catch-all term that describes unexplained intraoperative brain swelling or diffuse bleeding from the AVM bed or unexplained postoperative brain swelling or intracranial hemorrhage (ICH). NPPB is a diagnosis of exclusion. Although much has been written about NPPB, the lack of a rigorous definition makes interpretation of the existing literature difficult.

The proposed pathophysiology of NPPB is as follows: High blood flow through the arteriovenous fistula creates a region of chronic cerebral hypotension in the neighboring vascular territories. Chronic cerebral hypotension may lead to a state of near-maximal vasodilatation and vasoparalysis that impairs the vessels' ability to constrict or even dilate effectively. Excision of the low-resistance AVM shunt restores perfusion in the formerly hypotensive regions of brain. However, owing to the inability of these beds to effectively vasoconstrict, normalization of cerebral perfusion pressure results in cerebral hyperemia ("luxury perfusion"),

with the potential for cerebral edema formation and ICH. Although this is an attractive hypothesis, the pathophysiology has not been proved. Abnormal vascular reactivity, such as an impaired vasodilator response to acetazolamide, has been observed in regions adjacent to cerebral AVMs that show marked hyperperfusion after resection. Possibly, NPPB shares certain similarities to cerebral hyperemia after carotid endarterectomy or transluminal angioplasty and stenting of extracranial cervical arteries.

Some observations argue against a "hydraulic hypothesis" to explain the pathophysiology of NPPB. First, hypotensive vascular beds in proximity to the AVM retain the ability to vasoconstrict. Also, pressure autoregulation can be shown in these hypotensive beds, although the cerebral autoregulation curve is shifted to the left. Second, severe cerebral hypotension (feeding artery pressure <50% of systemic blood pressure) in normal, functional vascular beds is often seen in proximity to an AVM (approximately half of cases), although NPPB is a rare complication of AVM surgery. Third, NPPB hyperemia is not limited to hypotensive areas near the AVM; it appears to be global.

Alternative mechanisms for unexplained hemorrhage or swelling have been suggested, such as (1) unrecognized

724

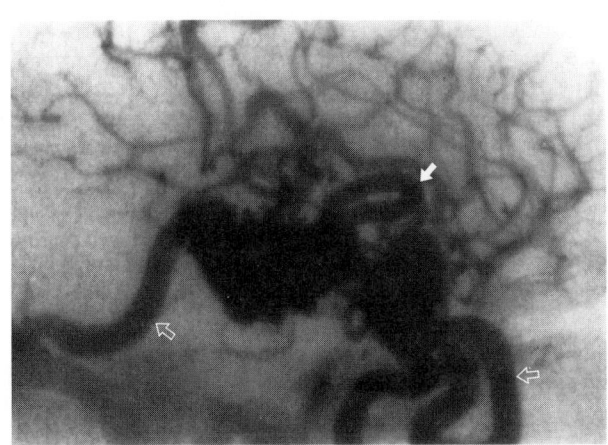

Figure 180–1 ▪ Lateral arteriogram showing a moderate-sized arteriovenous malformation (AVM), with a large arterial supply *(closed arrow)* and abundant venous drainage *(open arrows)*. These are indicative of very large, high-flow AVM shunts. (From Young WL, Prohovnik I, Ornstein E, et al: The effect of arteriovenous malformation resection on cerebrovascular reactivity to carbon dioxide. Neurosurgery 27:257-267, 1990.)

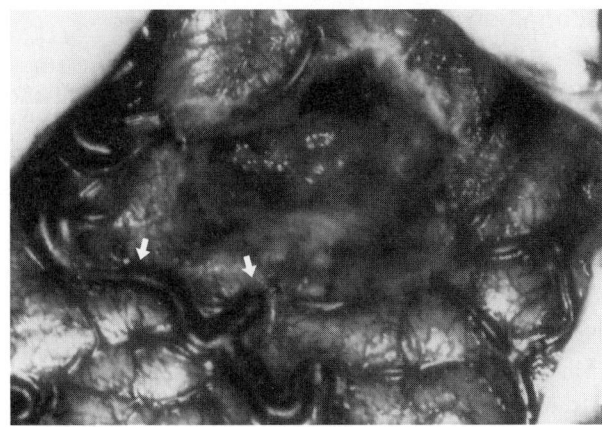

Figure 180–3 ▪ Operative photograph after surgical resection of the arteriovenous malformation (AVM). This depicts a dry surgical bed and surrounding dilated arteries *(arrows)*. These became enlarged after interruption of the AVM. (From Young WL, Prohovnik I, Ornstein E, et al: The effect of arteriovenous malformation resection on cerebrovascular reactivity to carbon dioxide. Neurosurgery 27:257-267, 1990.)

technical complications at the time of surgery; (2) vascular disturbances due to abnormal autonomic activity, resulting in the release of vasoactive peptides from innervated cerebral vessels; (3) hemorrhage from a structurally deficient capillary vessel bed adjacent to the AVM, perhaps secondary to overexpression of angiogenic factors such as vascular endothelial growth factor or angiopoietin-2; and (4) venous occlusion after resection of the AVM. With regard to the third hypothesis, Sato and colleagues recently described markedly dilated capillary networks in the perinidal AVM region. Vessel diameters were 10 to 25 times those of normal capillaries and vascular connections to the nidus, including feeding arteries and arterioles, drainage veins and venules, and the normal capillary network. With regard to the fourth hypothesis, severe global hyperemia (i.e., increased cerebral blood flow) that occurs immediately after AVM resection

appears to be associated with NPPB later in the postoperative course. In the case synopsis, cerebral blood flow significantly increased immediately after AVM resection, although ICH or cerebral edema and ICH did not occur until several hours later.

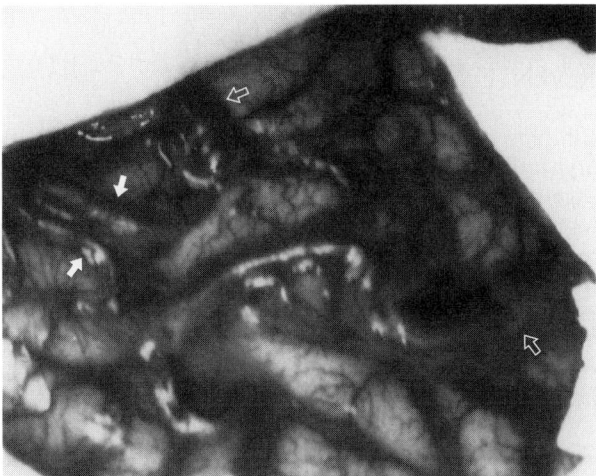

Figure 180–2 ▪ Operative photograph showing the surface of the temporal lobe, with prominent arterial supply *(closed arrows)* and venous drainage *(open arrows)*. (From Young WL, Prohovnik I, Ornstein E, et al: The effect of arteriovenous malformation resection on cerebrovascular reactivity to carbon dioxide. Neurosurgery 27:257-267, 1990.)

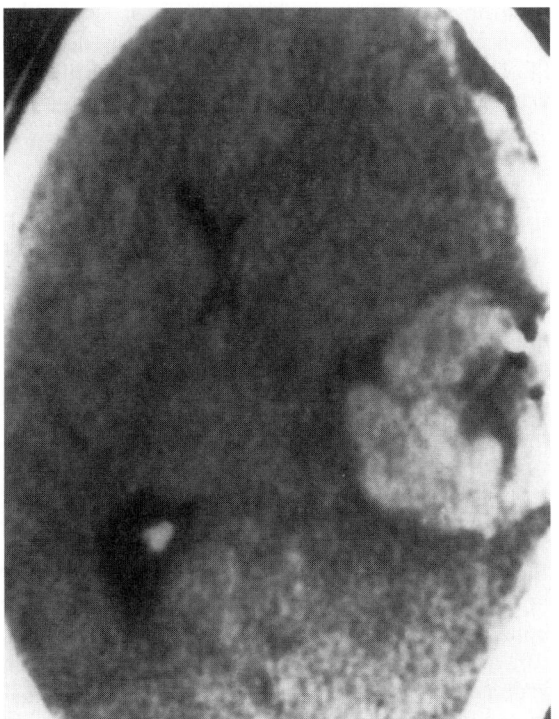

Figure 180–4 ▪ Computed tomography scan taken 6 hours postoperatively showing massive hemorrhage into the arteriovenous malformation (AVM) bed. The hemorrhage was under tension, with a major shift of intracranial structures. It was evacuated, but the patient died after further hemorrhages. (From Young WL, Prohovnik I, Ornstein E, et al: The effect of arteriovenous malformation resection on cerebrovascular reactivity to carbon dioxide. Neurosurgery 27:257-267, 1990.)

Recognition

NPPB is a controversial entity, and the diagnosis carries a certain degree of subjectivity. The incidence of NPPB after AVM resection is about 2.5%. NPPB is a diagnosis of exclusion, after more common causes of cerebral edema or hemorrhage have been ruled out. Causes of cerebral edema after AVM resection include hypoxia, increased venous pressure, decreased serum osmolality, systemic hypertension, and surgical trauma. After AVM resection, ICH may be due to the presence of residual AVM, poor control of systemic blood pressure, or uncorrected coagulopathy.

Risk Assessment

Predictors of NPPB after AVM ablation remain controversial. Some have proposed that large (≥4 cm) AVMs with high blood flow through the shunt and evidence of decreased perfusion in the neighboring regions may predict an increased likelihood for NPPB. Intraoperative monitoring of cerebral blood flow with laser Doppler or near-infrared spectroscopy may also reveal patients at risk of developing postoperative hyperemia. A sudden increase in laser Doppler blood flow in cortical regions adjacent to the AVM, after temporary clipping of the feeding arteries, is often seen in patients at risk for developing NPPB. Intraoperative near-infrared spectroscopy permits measurements of tissue oxygen saturation and blood volume. An increase in pre- to post-resection oxygen saturation and a blood volume ratio greater than 2 might indicate an increased risk for NPPB. Postoperative blood flow mapping by positron emission tomography (PET) or single photon emission computed tomography (SPECT) may help predict NPPB. There is no evidence that the choice of anesthetic agent influences the development of NPPB.

Implications

Although NPPB represents a class of complications without a clearly defined cause, it has been suggested that staged surgical resection or endovascular embolization could reduce the likelihood of NPPB. Staged resection or embolization permits vessels to adapt to increased perfusion pressure by gradually normalizing cerebral perfusion pressure (or it may permit adaptation to as yet unidentified pathophysiologic changes). Changes in cerebral blood flow after ablation of the AVM, however, may not be related to the preintervention feeding artery pressure. Despite the lack of precise pathophysiologic information, preoperative endovascular embolization may serve other useful purposes, such as facilitating surgery by minimizing intraoperative blood loss or by defining the location and extent of the AVM. Embolization may also reduce the size of the AVM, making it more amenable to surgery or radiosurgery. It might also alleviate neurologic symptoms by decreasing the AVM mass effect and reducing tissue perfusion in adjacent areas.

Recent evidence suggests that another technique used for AVM removal might affect the incidence of subsequent rebleeding, at least for small (<3 cm) AVMs located in critical or eloquent areas of the brain (e.g., sensorimotor, language, or visual cortex; hypothalamus or thalamus; internal capsule; brainstem; cerebellar peduncles; deep cerebellar nuclei), where rebleeding often results in disabling neurologic defects. Stereotactic (gamma knife) radiosurgery is often used to remove such small AVMs and provides radiographic evidence of AVM "cure" (obliteration) in 80% to 95% of patients after a latency period of 3 to 5 years. At issue was how bleeding during the latency period would compare with bleeding in patients with similar but untreated AVMs. It was found that the risk of hemorrhage from small AVMs was significantly reduced after radiosurgery (but before angiographic obliteration) and was even lower after angiographic obliteration. Whether radiosurgery for larger AVMs would reduce the incidence of rebleeding compared with surgical resection is unknown, but it might be tested; surgical AVM resection is recommended for less strategically located, larger AVMs amenable to surgery, but some patients choose radiosurgery instead because it seems less invasive.

MANAGEMENT

Unexplained cerebral edema or ICH after AVM resection is managed using standard cerebral resuscitative guidelines. Treatment of cerebral edema requires careful management of fluid and electrolyte imbalances, judicious use of osmotic and loop diuretics, and attention to cerebral perfusion pressure. Severe symptomatic swelling may necessitate controlled ventilation and, rarely, barbiturate coma. If NPPB is suspected, blood pressure is empirically maintained within 10% of the baseline. Cerebral outflow pressure (i.e., central venous or intracranial pressure) must be maintained at levels consistent with adequate cerebral perfusion and cardiac preload. If deliberate systemic hypotension is used, assessment should include whether it is necessary to maintain collateral perfusion in any cerebral territories that might have their primary feeding supplies interrupted during AVM resection. Surgical intervention may be required for removal of intracranial blood clot or for institution of intracranial pressure monitoring.

PREVENTION

In the absence of a clearly defined explanation of NPPB, the empirical strategy is to prevent cerebral edema and hemorrhage after AVM resection by careful control of systemic blood pressure to avoid hypertension. The use of intraoperative embolization of the AVM nidus via the ligated feeding arteries while the patient is under general anesthesia has been noted to prevent NPPB in high-risk cases. Mild systemic hypertension is sometimes used to test surgical hemeostasis before dural closure. Once this has been achieved, however, the systemic blood pressure must be maintained as close to the patient's baseline blood pressure as feasible.

After resection of an AVM, strict maintenance of normotension may serve two purposes. First, prevention of blood pressure increases may be important for the prevention of postoperative hematoma. This could be caused by rupture of cauterized stumps of dysplastic feeding vessels to the AVM or an unidentified residual nidus. Second, avoidance of hypertension prevents the cerebral hyperemia and edema that result from exceeding the upper limit of the flow-pressure autoregulation curve. This can be explained as follows: Functionally normal but chronically hypotensive cerebral beds in proximity to the AVM show a leftward shift in the cerebral autoregulatory curve. It is generally believed that in intact human cerebral circulation, cerebral hyperemia and edema occur whenever cerebral perfusion pressure increases beyond the upper limit of autoregulation. If the cerebral autoregulation curve shifts to the left, it may be that the upper limit of pressure autoregulation also shifts to a lower pressure. Ablation of the AVM shunt increases the regional perfusion pressure in the hypotensive areas, even at normal systemic arterial pressures. The magnitude of increase in the regional perfusion pressure is difficult to predict. In the absence of means to monitor regional cerebral perfusion in the perioperative period, it is reasonable to maintain strict normotension. In selected high-risk cases, mild systemic hypotension might minimize the chances of post-resection hyperemia and edema. Decreasing systemic perfusion pressure, however, might jeopardize brain regions that depend on collateral pathways for the maintenance of perfusion. Therefore, induced systemic hypotension to any significant degree should be considered carefully within the context of the patient's overall circulatory status.

Further Reading

Brown AP, Spetzler RF: Intracranial arteriovenous malformations. In Batjer HH, Caplan L, Friberg L, et al (eds): Cerebrovascular Hemodynamics, Cerebrovascular Disease. Philadelphia, Lippincott-Raven, 1997, pp 833-842.

Hashimoto T, Lam T, Boudreau NJ, et al: Abnormal balance in the angiopoietin-2 system in human brain arteriovenous malformations. Circ Res 89:111-113 2001.

Joshi S, Ornstein E, Young WL: Cerebral and spinal cord blood flow. In Cottrell JE, Smith DS (eds): Anesthesia and Neurosurgery, 4th ed. St. Louis, Mosby, 2001, pp 19-68.

Kader A, Young WL: The effects of intracranial arteriovenous malformations on cerebral hemodynamics. Neurosurg Clin North Am 7:767-781, 1996.

Kader A, Young WL: Arteriovenous malformations: Considerations for perioperative critical care monitoring. In Batjer HH, Caplan LR, Friberg L, et al (eds): Cerebrovascular Disease. Philadelphia, Lippincott-Raven, 1997, pp 857-869.

Ko N, Achrol A, Gupta D, et al: Cerebral blood flow changes after endovascular treatment of cerebrovascular stenoses. AJNR Am J Neuroradiol 26:538-542, 2005.

Sato S, Kodama N, Sasaki T, et al: Perinidal dilated capillary networks in cerebral arteriovenous malformations. Neurosurgery 54:163-170, 2004.

Young WL, Ornstein E, Baker KZ, et al: The Columbia University AVM Project: Cerebral hyperemia after AVM resection is related to "breakthrough" complications but not to feeding artery pressure. Anesth Analg 80:S573, 1995.

Young WL, Ornstein E, Baker KZ, et al: Neuroanesthesia considerations for surgical and endovascular therapy of arteriovenous malformations. In Batjer HH, Caplan LR, Friberg L, et al (eds): Cerebrovascular Disease. Philadelphia, Lippincott-Raven, 1997, pp 843-855.

Young WL, Prohovnik I, Ornstein E, et al: The effect of arteriovenous malformation resection on cerebrovascular reactivity to carbon dioxide. Neurosurgery 27:257-267, 1990.

Pediatric Neurosurgery

Lynda Wells

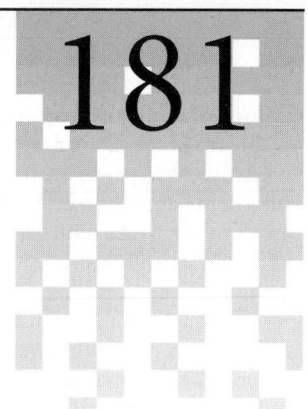

Case Synopsis

A previously healthy 14-month-old child is admitted to the emergency department following a motor vehicle accident in which he sustained a closed head injury associated with loss of consciousness and a large scalp laceration. A grand mal–type seizure occurs on arrival at the hospital. Physical examination reveals a lethargic, tachypneic, hypotensive, and tachycardic child. His pupils are equal and reactive, and there is no evidence of papilledema. Computed tomography scan of the head reveals diffuse cerebral swelling and subdural hematoma. He undergoes anesthesia for a craniotomy to evacuate the subdural hematoma, repair the scalp laceration, and place an intracranial pressure (ICP) monitor.

PROBLEM ANALYSIS

Definition

Surgical procedures in children with central nervous system (CNS) pathology are performed to correct pathologic entities (e.g., evacuation of hematoma, excision of tumors or seizure foci, closure of meningomyelocele) and to facilitate monitoring (e.g., ICP monitoring). Brain tumors are the most common solid tumors in children and are the second most common malignancy after the leukemias. Trauma is the leading cause of death in children older than 1 year, and traumatic brain injury (TBI) is the major cause of morbidity and mortality. Outcome is determined by the extent of primary and secondary brain injury. The former is the biomechanical injury that occurs with trauma; it is irreversible. Management must focus on preventing the sequelae of primary brain injury, termed secondary brain injury (Table 181-1); these management goals include reducing cerebral edema, preventing cerebral hypoxia, maintaining cerebral perfusion, avoiding increases in the cerebral metabolic rate for oxygen, and avoiding damage to neuronal membranes. Similarly, prevention of secondary brain injury is the focus of treatment for nontraumatic CNS lesions.

Recognition

The most reliable signs of TBI severity are degree of change in level of consciousness and impaired CNS function. The Glasgow Coma Scale score (see Chapter 182 and Table 182-1) adapted for pediatric patients provides a tool to assess the severity of primary and secondary brain injury and trends. The major cause of secondary brain injury involves failure of perfusion, leading to tissue hypoxia and brain edema. Associated brain swelling impairs tissue perfusion, leading to further CNS functional deterioration. The failure of cerebral oxygenation arises from hypoxemia, hypotension, hypovolemia, hyperemia, and acidosis.

When the pathologic process evolves slowly (e.g., expansion of solid tumors), physiologic compensation may occur. However, in the event of TBI, cerebral edema evolves quickly, and any compensatory mechanisms are easily overcome. The intracranial contents in children are less compliant than in adults. Thus, comparable increases in ICP are more likely to produce ischemia and herniation in children than in adults. Although hyperemia and increased cerebral blood flow in response to TBI were once considered common in children, recent data suggest that hyperemia may not be so common. Open fontanelles do not automatically exclude brain injury from increased ICP.

Table 181–1 ■ Prevention of Secondary Brain Injury

Maneuver	Expected Effect
30-degree head-up tilt (waist up)	Increases cerebral venous drainage while maintaining CPP
Mechanical ventilation	Maintains normocapnia to slight hypocapnia to prevent cerebral vasodilatation and ↑ ICP
Systemic steroids	Improves outcome with spinal cord injury; reduces vasogenic cerebral edema with tumors; stabilizes neuronal membrane; may act as free radical scavengers
Muscle paralysis	Avoids coughing, straining, or other movement that might increase ICP
Ventricular drainage	Reduces ICP
Antihypertensive drugs*	Prevents further cerebral edema or hemorrhage leading to further ischemia, especially when due to cerebral vasospasm
Anticonvulsants	Prevents seizures and associated increase in ICP and $CMRO_2$
Mild hypothermia	Reduces $CMRO_2$ and cerebral glucose consumption
Barbiturate coma	Reduces CBF and $CMRO_2$ and may have membrane-stabilizing effect

*For example, dihydropyridine calcium channel blockers.
$CMRO_2$, cerebral metabolic rate for oxygen; CBF, cerebral blood flow; CPP, cerebral perfusion pressure; ICP, intracranial pressure.

Table 181–2 ■ Neurophysiologic Effects of Commonly Used Anesthetic Agents

Agent	MAP	CBF	CPP	ICP	CMRO$_2$	CSF (Synthesis)	CSF (Absorption)	SEP (Amplitude)	SEP (Latency)
Nitrous oxide	0 or ↓	↑ or ↑↑	↓	↑ or ↑↑	↓ or ↑	↑ or ↓	↑ or ↓	↓	↑ or 0
Halothane	↓↓	↑↑↑	↑↑	↑↑	↓↓	↑ or ↓	0 or ↓	↓	↑
Enflurane	↓↓	↑↑	↑↑	↑↑	↓↓	↑	↓	↓	↑
Isoflurane	↓↓	↑	↑↑	↑	↓↓↓	↓ or ↑	↑	↓	↑
Sevoflurane	↓↓	↑	↑	↑	↓↓↓	?	?	↓	↑
Desflurane	↓↓	↑	↑	↑	↓	↓	↓	↓	↑
Thiopental	↓↓	↓↓↓	↑↑↑	↓↓↓	↓↓↓	↑ or ↓	↑	↓	↑
Propofol	↓↓↓	↓↓↓	↑↑	↓↓	↓↓↓	?	?	↑	↑
Etomidate	0 or ↓	↓↓↓	↑↑	↓↓↓	↓↓↓	↑ or ↓	↑	↑	↑
Ketamine	↑↑	↑↑↑	↓	↑↑↑	↑	↑ or ↓	↓	↑	0
Benzodiazepines	0 or ↓	↓↓	↑	0 or ↓	↓↓	↑ or ↓	↑	↑	0 or ↑
Opiates	0 or ↓	↓	↑ or ↓	0 or ↓	↓	↑ or ↓	↑	↓	↑
Droperidol	↓↓	↓	↑	↓	0 or ↓	↑ or ↓	?	?	?

CBF, cerebral blood flow; CMRO$_2$, cerebral metabolic rate for oxygen; CPP, cerebral perfusion pressure; CSF, cerebrospinal fluid; ICP, intracranial pressure; MAP, mean arterial pressure; SEP, somatosensory evoked potential.

The presence of cervical spine trauma should always be assumed in children with TBI. Infants and young children are more likely to experience cervical spine trauma than are older children, owing to their large heads and relatively weak necks. Ligamentous injury is common in this age group. In contrast, bony injury is extremely rare. Therefore, unless there is radiologic evidence of odontoid displacement or spinal cord edema, cervical spine injury is diagnosed based solely on the clinical examination. Because this is often not possible when TBI presents, cervical spine trauma is presumed to exist. Also, neurologic signs from spinal cord injury may be absent initially.

Risk Assessment

Risk assessment relates to the likelihood of death or permanent CNS functional impairment. TBI that involves or is immediately adjacent to vital structure is more likely to be compounded by the need for surgical intervention; thus, it is associated with higher morbidity. Evidence of primary cortical brain injury (e.g., intracranial hematoma, seizures) and the presence of risk factors for secondary brain injury (e.g., hypovolemia, impaired ventilation) indicate more severe TBI as well as increased morbidity and mortality.

Classic signs of intracranial hypertension seen in adults (e.g., papilledema, pupillary dilatation, cranial nerve palsies, headache on awakening, vomiting) may be absent in children, even when ICP approaches fatal levels. The presence of intracranial hematomas with acute TBI indicates a significant force of impact. Seizures after TBI also indicate significant parenchymal injury. Spinal cord injury is assumed to be present in all cases of head trauma, at least until a definitive diagnosis can be made.

Implications

The danger of intracranial pathology is that expansion in an enclosed space leads to brain compression, causing ischemia, swelling, and loss of function that can be permanent and possibly fatal. Seizures greatly increase the cerebral metabolic rate for oxygen. They are also associated with regional ischemia that can lead to cell death and loss of cognitive and functional abilities. Compromised integrity of the membranes covering the CNS (e.g., meningomyelocele) presents a significant risk for infection, as well as cerebrospinal fluid loss and hypothermia.

Many children who present for surgical removal of tumors are malnourished and debilitated due to nausea, vomiting, and neurologic dysfunction with increased ICP. Acid-base, electrolyte, and endocrine abnormalities may be present. Patients with paralysis of an extremity of greater than 24 hours' duration are at risk for an exaggerated hyperkalemic response to succinylcholine. Obtunded patients are at increased risk for aspiration, airway obstruction, and hypoventilation.

Anesthetic management can influence the outcome and long-term prognosis in pediatric neurosurgical patients (Table 181-2). Therefore, conducting a thorough preoperative assessment, with indicated laboratory and radiographic studies; maintaining a stable intraoperative course (e.g., preserving cerebral perfusion while preventing increased ICP); and providing this same level of care throughout the postoperative period are critical.

MANAGEMENT

In TBI, immediate attention is directed to establishing the airway, ventilation, and circulation. Supplemental oxygen, a secure airway, and intravenous (IV) cannulation are required. A Glasgow Coma Scale score of 9 or less is an indication for tracheal intubation, because the patient will be unable to protect his or her airway. A history is taken and a comprehensive physical examination is performed as soon as possible to evaluate medical comorbidities and the extent and severity of other physical injuries. Spinal cord injury precautions are taken. Any obvious bleeding should be controlled. Blood should be sent for complete blood count, coagulation studies, clinical chemistry, and type and crossmatch. Radiographic investigation includes computed tomography scans of the head, neck, and chest. Other investigations are performed based on the history and clinical findings.

Anesthetic management is geared toward preventing further increases in ICP and maintaining cerebral perfusion pressure. Anxiolytic premedication is often unnecessary in neurologically compromised children. If the child is crying and agitated, however, small doses of IV midazolam or rectal barbiturates may be given, provided airway patency and adequacy of ventilation are ensured.

After preoxygenation, anesthesia is usually induced with an IV induction agent (e.g., sodium thiopental). Ketamine and methohexital are generally contraindicated; the former increases ICP, and the latter lowers the seizure threshold. Rapid-sequence induction is indicated in patients who have not fasted or in whom there is an aspiration risk. If inhalation induction is desired, moderate hyperventilation is used to counter any vasodilatory effects of volatile anesthetics on the cerebral vasculature. Once effective mask ventilation is established, generous doses of opiates are given to obtund the sympathetic response to laryngoscopy and tracheal intubation. IV lidocaine also blunts the stimulus of laryngoscopy and tracheal intubation.

Muscle relaxation with succinylcholine and atropine is used to facilitate endotracheal intubation. If succinylcholine is contraindicated, a large dose of a nondepolarizing drug (e.g., rocuronium) is used. The airway should be secured as efficiently as possible to ensure optimal ventilation and to avoid hypoxia and hypercarbia. The necessary equipment to deal with a difficult airway should be on hand in the event of unanticipated difficult intubation. If there is doubt about the ability to secure the airway in a timely fashion, tracheostomy should be considered. In-line neck traction with direct laryngoscopy and fiberoptic-guided intubation are equally effective at minimizing cervical spine injury associated with intubation. The former is the more usual approach in small children, but practitioners should use the technique with which they are most facile. Moderate hyperventilation (arterial carbon dioxide tension 30 to 35 mm Hg) is indicated to prevent cerebrovascular vasodilatation and the subsequent increase in cerebral blood flow and edema formation. Hyperoxia is unnecessary, and hypoxia must be avoided.

Anesthesia is maintained with opioids and IV infusions of barbiturates or propofol, or with volatile anesthetic agents. Nitrous oxide is contraindicated in the presence of pneumocephalus, which can be present up to 3 weeks after previous craniotomy. Muscle relaxation is maintained to facilitate mechanical ventilation, prevent involuntary patient movement (e.g., coughing, bucking), and avoid increases in ICP. The drugs used for anesthetic induction and maintenance are chosen based on their effects on cerebral perfusion pressure and the patient's overall condition (see Table 181-2).

Hemodynamic stability is maintained using blood, crystalloid infusions, and vasopressors, as required. Osmotic pressure gradients are more important in avoiding cerebral edema than are oncotic pressure gradients. Thus, crystalloid rather than colloid infusions are the mainstay of fluid therapy. Hypertonic solutions (e.g., 3% saline) are reserved for refractory increased ICP. They are not advised in the perioperative period. Fluid maintenance is usually with 0.9% saline or balanced salt solutions with a physiologic osmolality (285 to 290 mOsm/L). Because 0.9% saline is slightly hypertonic (306 mOsm/L), it can be given with a relatively hypotonic salt solution if large volumes of fluid are required. However, infused volumes are limited to the replacement of deficits and surgical losses, and they are maintained to avoid the exacerbation of coexisting cerebral edema. Blood should be given early in cases associated with hemorrhage to prevent anemia, which can increase CNS morbidity. Glucose-containing solutions should be used only to maintain serum glucose in the normal range.

Patient monitoring includes the following: pulse oximetry, capnography, electrocardiography, invasive blood pressure, central venous pressure, urine output, temperature, precordial Doppler, and ICP monitoring if available. Cannulation of the femoral vein may be preferable to use of the internal jugular vein to avoid accidental neck trauma, which may aggravate already increased ICP. Hyperthermia must be avoided, as this increases the cerebral metabolic rate for oxygen. Normal body temperature or mild hypothermia is desirable. However, deep hypothermia should be avoided, because it is associated with disorders of coagulation and glucose control as well as arrhythmias. Also, shivering on awakening increases the cerebral metabolic rate for oxygen and should be avoided. If surgery involves or is proximate to the sensory or motor cortex, sensory and motor evoked potentials can be measured. However, motor evoked potentials cannot be monitored in denervated limbs or in the presence of neuromuscular blocking drugs. The electroencephalogram is monitored in patients undergoing surgery for seizures and some neurovascular lesions.

Careful positioning to avoid injury to soft tissues (e.g., eyes, nose, ears, joints, peripheral nerves) is required. Head-up tilt (15 to 30 degrees) improves cerebral venous drainage but increases the risk for venous air embolism.

Smooth emergence and extubation are important to prevent increases in ICP due to cerebral venous congestion. This is facilitated by sufficient analgesia and antiemesis. Ondansetron is a popular choice because of its lack of sedation. Except after certain neurovascular procedures, the patient should be awake before tracheal extubation and should exhibit good muscle strength and ventilatory drive. Consequently, muscle relaxation should always be reversed. When there is any doubt whether the patient will maintain adequate spontaneous ventilation, he or she should be sedated and left intubated and ventilated. Such patients are cared for in the pediatric intensive care unit postoperatively.

Postoperative complications include impaired ventilation in earlier extubated patients and intracranial bleeding. Diabetes insipidus may also occur. Intracranial bleeding is usually signaled by a diminishing level of consciousness or increasing ICP in an unconscious patient. Emergent head computed tomography is indicated to confirm the diagnosis and guide further management.

Diabetes insipidus is characterized by the passage of copious volumes of dilute urine, with increased serum sodium concentrations and osmolality. It often occurs after surgery for hypothalamic tumors and TBI. Treatment consists of (1) replacing urine volume with dilute crystalloid, (2) infusing aqueous vasopressin (1 to 10 mU/kg per hour), and (3) monitoring serial serum electrolyte concentrations.

Diabetes insipidus is often transient. Rebound volume overload and water intoxication can occur if vasopressin is not stopped and the fluid regimen is not adjusted when diabetes insipidus resolves.

Finally, antibiotic and anticonvulsant therapy is continued through the perioperative period, both for prophylaxis and for treatment.

PREVENTION

Prevention of primary TBI is best achieved through sociopolitical interventions and public education (e.g., use of appropriate child restraints in motor vehicles, obeying speed limits). Secondary brain injury is prevented by meticulous management of brain-injured patients, both in the field and in health care facilities. Aggressive resuscitation to maintain adequate oxygenation, ventilation, stable hemodynamics, and cerebral perfusion pressure, while minimizing intracranial hypertension, is the mainstay of therapy. Other therapeutic or prophylactic interventions are instituted after initial resuscitation and stabilization. New technologies (e.g., stereotactic-guided excision of intracranial tumors) have helped reduce the adverse impact of iatrogenic brain injury in pediatric neurosurgery.

Further Reading

Adelson PD, Bratton SL, Carney NA, et al: Guidelines for the acute medical management of severe traumatic brain injury in infants, children and adolescents: Use of hyperosmolar therapy in the management of severe pediatric traumatic brain injury. Pediatr Crit Care Med 4(3 Suppl): S40-S44, 2003.

Alderson P, Roberts I: Corticosteroids in acute traumatic brain injury: Systematic review of randomized controlled trials. BMJ 314:1855-1859, 1997.

Berger S, Schwarz M, Huth R: Hypertonic saline solution and decompressive craniectomy for treatment of intracranial hypertension in pediatric severe traumatic brain injury. J Trauma Injury Infect Crit Care 53:558-563, 2002.

Bullock R, Chesnut RM, Clifton G, et al: Guidelines for the management of severe head injury: Brain Trauma Foundation, American Association of Neurosurgical Surgeons, Joint Section on Neurotrauma and Critical Care. Eur J Emerg Med 3:109–127, 1996.

Carli P, Orliaguet G: Severe traumatic brain injury in children. Lancet 363:584-585, 2004.

Hammer GB, Krane EJ: Perioperative care of the neurosurgical pediatric patient. Int Anesthesiol Clin 34:55-71, 1996.

Johnson JO, Jimenez DF, Tobias JD: Anaesthetic care during minimally invasive neurosurgical procedures in infants and children. Paediatr Anaesth 12:478-488, 2002.

Rekate HL: Head injuries: Management of primary injuries and prevention of secondary damage. A consensus conference on pediatric neurosurgery. Childs Nerv Syst 17;632-634, 2001.

Vavilala MS, Lam AM: Perioperative considerations in pediatric traumatic brain injury. Int Anesthesiol Clin 40:69-87, 2002.

Head Injury

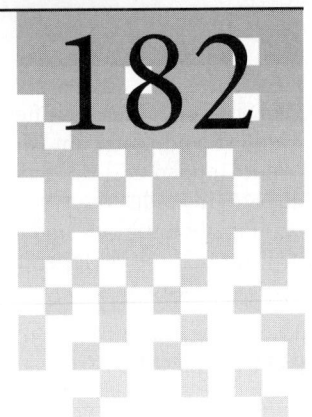

182

Arthur M. Lam and M. Sean Kincaid

Case Synopsis

A 22-year-old previously healthy man sustained a head injury and an open right femur fracture in a motorcycle accident. His initial Glasgow Coma Scale score was 9, and his right pupil was dilated and unreactive. Tracheal intubation was performed at the scene, and he was transported to the trauma center. A computed tomography scan revealed a large right epidural hematoma with a midline shift. Initial hematocrit was 32 after the administration of 2 L of crystalloid. His blood pressure was 130/80 mm Hg, and his heart rate was 120 beats per minute. He was scheduled for emergent evacuation of the epidural hematoma, followed by open reduction and internal fixation of the femur.

PROBLEM ANALYSIS

Definition

Head injury is a common problem, with an annual incidence of approximately 200 per 100,000 persons in the United States. Many of these injuries are minor, with few sequelae, but some are devastating. Car and motorcycle crashes are the most common cause of traumatic brain injury (TBI), followed by injuries from firearms, falls, and sports.

Severe TBI is defined as any injury that results in a Glasgow Coma Scale (GCS) score of 8 or less after adequate cardiopulmonary resuscitation. Damage to neural tissue directly related to trauma is considered the primary injury and includes cerebral contusion, diffuse axonal injury, hemorrhage into the epidural or subdural space, and intraparenchymal hemorrhage. Secondary injury is any insult to the brain occurring after the initial TBI that causes further neuronal damage. Although cerebral ischemia or hypoxia is the ultimate cause of secondary brain injury after TBI, systemic or local insults often contribute to such injury. Among these are elevated intracranial pressure (ICP), systemic hypotension, and hypoxemia.

Neuronal death is likely mediated by complex biochemical processes involving the release of excitatory amino acids (e.g., glutamate) and the cellular influx of calcium. Actual cell death may be necrotic or apoptotic in nature. Preventing or reducing secondary brain injury is the focus of most medical management of TBI in both the intensive care unit (ICU) and the operating room.

TBI is often associated with other injuries (as illustrated in the case synopsis). Thus, anesthesiologists may care for a patient during surgical intervention for TBI (e.g., evacuation of subdural hematoma, decompressive craniectomy) and for laparotomy or fracture fixation, as well as in the ICU.

Recognition

PRIMARY TRAUMATIC BRAIN INJURY

Clinical Signs. TBI is suspected when head trauma is associated with mental status changes. Severity of TBI is commonly assessed by the GCS, which assigns a score to the patient's best motor, verbal, and eye-opening abilities (Table 182-1). A total score of 8 or less indicates severe TBI. Use of the GCS to evaluate patients with TBI reduces interobserver variability and allows for the comparison of serial examinations to evaluate disease resolution or progression. However, use of the GCS as a prognostic indicator is controversial. Further, assignment of a GCS score is appropriate only after adequate cardiopulmonary resuscitation, especially if severe hypotension or hypoxia is present.

Along with the GCS, pupil evaluation is important. TBI may manifest as alterations in pupil size, symmetry, and reactivity to light. With acute unilateral mass lesions, an ipsilateral dilated and unreactive pupil suggests uncal herniation. In contrast, bilateral fixed and dilated pupils suggest severe intracranial hypertension (ICH) that may result in brain herniation,

Vital signs may reflect the patient's overall clinical status aside from any TBI. For example, hypotension and tachycardia may be due to concealed hemorrhage with a femur fracture, and hypertension may be due to pain. Vital signs also

Table 182–1 ■ Glasgow Coma Scale Score	
Eye Opening	
Spontaneous	4
To speech	3
To pain	2
None	1
Verbal Response	
Oriented	5
Confused	4
Inappropriate	3
Incomprehensible	2
None	1
Motor Response	
Obeys commands	6
Localizes to pain	5
Withdraws to pain	4
Flexes to pain	3
Extends to pain	2
None	1

provide significant insight into the nature of TBI. Severe hypertension may be compensatory (i.e., to preserve cerebral perfusion pressure [CPP] in severe ICH; CPP is mean arterial pressure [MAP] minus ICP). Severe systemic hypertension with bradycardia is an ominous sign (Cushing's reflex). It signifies impending brain herniation and requires immediate therapeutic intervention.

Computed Tomography Findings. Cranial computed tomography (CT) is highly sensitive for detecting intracranial hemorrhage and acute mass lesions. CT findings that support a significantly elevated ICP include the following:

- Mass lesion greater than 25 mL
- Midline shift of 5 mm or more
- Compression of the basal cisterns or lateral ventricles
- Medial displacement of the uncus

SECONDARY BRAIN INJURY

Secondary brain injury is due to systemic or cerebral factors (Table 182-2). Among these, hypoxia and ischemia are most likely to have an adverse impact on TBI outcome. However, the neurologic defects of primary TBI may obscure the signs of secondary injury due to cerebral hypoxia or ischemia. Although the calculation of CPP (which requires an arterial line and ICP monitor) is useful with abnormal head CT findings, even a normal CPP does not preclude secondary ischemia or cerebral hypoxia.

Other monitors are used to assess cerebral blood flow (CBF) and brain perfusion. A jugular venous bulb oximetric catheter (JBC) continuously measures brain venous oxygen saturation ($SjvO_2$). Low brain perfusion increases oxygen extraction, causing a drop in $SjvO_2$, while nonfunctioning brain extracts little oxygen to cause high $SjvO_2$ values. $SjvO_2$ less than 55% or greater than 75% is associated with a poor prognosis. $SjvO_2$ catheters are especially useful to monitor cerebral metabolic rate (CMR) when deliberate hyperventilation is used in TBI to reduce global CBF. JBC lactate concentrations may also reveal anaerobic brain metabolism if they are higher than simultaneously drawn arterial lactate concentrations. A limitation of JBC is that it monitors only global CBF-CMR balance. $SjvO_2$ values can be normal despite small regional areas of ischemia.

Two other devices may provide greater sensitivity for monitoring regional brain ischemia than the JBC: brain tissue oxygen tension ($P_{br}O_2$) monitors and microdialysis catheters.

Neither is as widely used as the JBC, but the $P_{br}O_2$ monitor is readily available for clinical application. It provides a continuous measurement of brain parenchymal oxygen tension. This reflects the balance between local brain supply and demand for oxygen. Doppenberg and coworkers showed close correlation between $P_{br}O_2$ and CBF. A $P_{br}O_2$ of 26 mm Hg was about equivalent to a CBF of 18 mL/100 g per minute (i.e., ischemic threshold). Also, a $P_{br}O_2$ of approximately 39 mm Hg is correlated with a good outcome, whereas one of 19 mm Hg correlates with a bad outcome, thus offering some guidance for therapeutic intervention. The normal $P_{br}O_2$ is greater than 20 mm Hg.

Microdialysis catheters are placed in brain parenchyma, where they continuously perfuse the brain with a perfusate and sample small volumes of fluid (the dialysate), which is tested for lactate and pyruvate concentrations to estimate the balance between anaerobic and aerobic metabolism. In addition, glutamate, glucose, and glycerol can be measured. However, a fairly long lag time is needed to analyze samples, which hinders real-time clinical decision making. Thus, microdialysis catheters are predominantly a research tool in their present form.

Risk Assessment and Implications

Hypoxia and Hypercapnia. TBI patients are at increased risk for airway obstruction and hypoventilation. These lead to hypoxia and hypercapnia, which cause cerebral vasodilatation. The latter may aggravate any ICH.

Elevated Intracranial Pressure. An acute mass lesion increases ICP and reduces CPP. Increased ICP can lead to brain herniation, with catastrophic consequences.

Systemic Hypotension and Hypovolemia. Adults usually do not become hypovolemic and hypotensive as a result of blood loss from TBI alone. In contrast, small children can lose enough blood with TBI to become hypotensive. Other injuries (e.g., splenic rupture, femur fracture) can make TBI patients hypotensive and further compromise CPP in those with increased ICP. Compensatory hypertension and bradycardia (Cushing's reflex) with elevated ICP may further complicate the clinical picture. Thus, in patients with TBI, normotension and tachycardia can still be compatible with severe hypovolemia, with the latter "concealed" by increased systemic vascular resistance (Cushing's reflex). Thus, ample blood pressure may give clinicians a false sense of security

Table 182–2 ■ Risk Factors for Secondary Brain Injury	
Cerebral Factors	**Systemic Factors**
Increased intracranial pressure	Hypotension
Expanding mass lesions	Hypoxemia
Hypercapnia	Anemia
Hypoxemia	Hypovolemia
Venous obstruction (cervical collar, poor positioning)	Hyperglycemia
Systemic hypotension (compensatory cerebral vasodilatation)	Hyponatremia
Excessive hyperventilation	Hypo-osmolar state
Post-traumatic vasospasm (patient with traumatic subarachnoid hemorrhage)	Coagulopathy
Seizures	

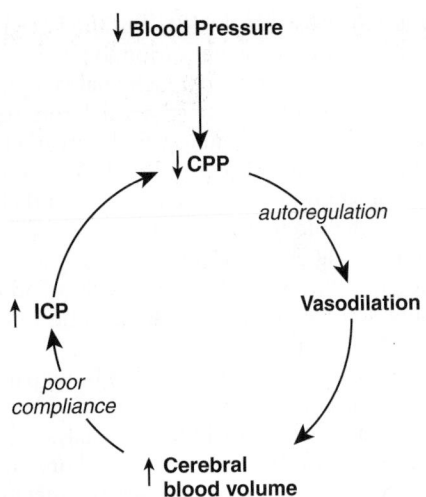

Figure 182–1 ▪ Vasodilator cascade, showing the potential interaction between systemic hypotension and intracranial hemodynamics when autoregulation is intact. A cascade in the opposite direction also occurs when blood pressure is increased. CPP, cerebral perfusion pressure; ICP, intracranial pressure.

regarding the progress of resuscitation. Should ICH be relieved by decompressive craniectomy or evacuation of an intracranial hematoma, profound hypotension or cardiac arrest may occur.

Of all the factors associated with secondary brain injury, systemic hypotension is likely the most significant. With impaired cerebral autoregulation, it invariably leads to reduced CPP. Patients with intact autoregulation but reduced intracranial compliance are also at risk for impaired CPP with hypotension. Reduced MAP dilates cerebral vasculature to increase cerebral blood volume and ICP. This increase in ICP further compromises CPP, leading to further compensatory cerebral vasodilatation. This vicious circle is referred to as the vasodilator cascade (Fig. 182-1).

Impaired Autoregulation.   Cerebral autoregulation is a homeostatic mechanism that maintains near-constant perfusion of the brain over a wide range of MAPs. In normal adults, this range is 60 to 160 mm Hg. Autoregulation may be impaired in patients with TBI, and although the frequency of impaired autoregulation is higher in patients with severe TBI, it is clinically impossible to predict which patients will be affected. Even minor TBI may impair autoregulation. If so, CBF becomes directly proportional to blood pressure. Loss of cerebral autoregulation is associated with worse outcomes with TBI.

Coagulopathy.   Severe TBI liberates enough thromboplastin from damaged neurons to cause coagulopathies, which may be mild to severe. They can increase surgical morbidity and mortality, can preclude or delay extracranial surgical procedures, and are associated with poorer outcomes.

Pyrexia.   Fever raises the CMR, increasing the risk for ischemia and neural injury, especially when cerebral perfusion is marginal. Cerebral blood volume increases with pyrexia owing to flow-metabolism coupling, exacerbating any ICH. Although human studies do not conclusively link body temperature to outcome in TBI, both animal and human studies have linked brain infarct size and fever in ischemic brain injury.

Hyperglycemia.   Hyperglycemia in TBI and stroke is associated with a poor prognosis, although a cause-effect relationship has not been clearly established. In experimental cerebral ischemia, detrimental effects of hyperglycemia have consistently been shown. Further, in one prospective trial, van den Berghe and colleagues found that patients with lax glucose control had worse outcomes than those with tight control.

Fluid and Electrolyte Abnormalities.   Acute fluid and electrolyte disturbances occur in TBI patients, often due to inappropriate fluid administration. They can also be caused by diabetes insipidus. Hyponatremia and excessive free water may worsen cerebral edema, thereby increasing ICP.

Associated Injuries.   As many as 10% of patients with TBIs also have spine injuries. Spinal evaluation is often delayed if the patient requires emergent neurosurgical intervention (e.g., evacuation of epidural or subdural hematoma). For this reason, spine precautions should be taken when moving or positioning patients before the completion of a spine injury workup. TBI patients may also have undiagnosed extremity injuries.

MANAGEMENT

Secure the Airway

Immediate tracheal intubation is necessary for severely head-injured patients, particularly those with GCS scores of 8 or less and without protective airway reflexes. Both propofol and thiopental are used as induction agents because they decrease CMR and lower ICP. However, either may cause hypotension, especially in inadequately fluid-resuscitated TBI victims, which negates their benefit. Because of a lower risk of untoward hypotension in TBI patients, etomidate may be a better choice. Ketamine is avoided because it increases ICP. A short-acting muscle relaxant should be used. Succinylcholine is preferred, and rocuronium is used when succinylcholine is contraindicated.

Maintain Adequate Cerebral Perfusion Pressure

The updated Brain Trauma Foundation guidelines (2003) advise keeping CPP between 60 and 70 mm Hg (in patients without cerebral ischemia); the trend today is to maintain CPP above 60 mm Hg. To maintain CPP, there must be good intravenous access, and fluid resuscitation must replete intravascular volume as needed. Fear of worsening cerebral edema should never dissuade one from providing adequate fluid resuscitation. Hypotonic fluids should be avoided, however (Table 182-3). Hypertonic fluids (e.g., 3% saline) may be used, although evidence is lacking to justify their routine use. Vasopressors and inotropes are often used along with fluid resuscitation to maintain CPP. However, they should be used with caution, because they may increase the risk for acute respiratory distress syndrome. Without ICP monitoring, MAP should be maintained at greater than 70 mm Hg.

Spinal Cord Injury

183

Tod B. Sloan

Case Synopsis

A 32-year-old man presents to the emergency department following a motorcycle accident in which he was thrown to the roadside. He is mildly obtunded, smells of alcohol, and is difficult to examine neurologically, but he appears to have loss of sensation and motor activity below the C5 dermatome. Lateral neck films fail to identify bony injury or subluxation. Vital signs reveal hypotension (90/40 mm Hg), bradycardia (50 beats per minute), respiratory difficulty, and an oral temperature of 36.2°C. He is taken to the operating room emergently for repair of an open tibial fracture.

PROBLEM ANALYSIS

Definition

Spinal cord injury (SCI) is defined as injury to the spinal cord with neurologic dysfunction, with or without spinal column disruption. Anesthesia care is often required shortly after injury, for resuscitation or surgical intervention. Later, anesthesia care may be required for surgery in patients with chronic SCI or for the management of patients who have recently sustained iatrogenic SCI (e.g., corrective surgery for scoliosis, aortic reconstructive surgery). Acute SCI occurs most frequently with trauma. Most of the problems accompanying SCI are a result of the neurologic loss, and they evolve over time.

Early recognition of SCI is important if devastating late complications are to be reduced or prevented. Acutely, the spinal cord distal to the level of injury is nonfunctional (e.g., areflexia, vasodilatation, muscle flaccidity). Loss of thoracic sympathetic outflow leads to the spinal shock syndrome; this is characterized by hypotension and bradycardia due to unopposed sacral and vagal parasympathetic tone. After several days to 6 to 8 weeks, the uninjured cord becomes functional (i.e., spinal reflexes are intact), but it is isolated from higher neural input (i.e., cephalad spinal cord, brainstem, brain). This leads to uncontrolled spinal reflexes, muscle spasticity, and, ultimately, contractures. Such changes distinguish acute from chronic SCI and explain the attendant neurophysiologic differences between the two types of injury.

Recognition

All patients with multiple trauma should be evaluated for acute SCI, especially those with neck complaints or neurologic abnormalities; those who are comatose, with hypotension and absent reflexes; and any trauma patient with apparent hypovolemic shock but without the expected compensatory tachycardia. Most traumatic acute SCI occurs in the more flexible cervical and lumbar regions, but especially in the cervical spine. Radiographic films of the lateral cervical spine (C1-C7) and anteroposterior open-mouth ("swimmer's view") films usually confirm any bony injury.

However, an unstable cervical spine may be missed in as many as 30% of cases. Thus, computed tomography or magnetic resonance imaging may be required to identify all cervical spine injuries. Acute SCI can also occur without ligamentous or bony injury, especially in children; this is called spinal cord injury without radiographic abnormality.

SCI is evaluated according to the following parameters:

- Level of injury
- Time since injury
- Presence of spinal instability
- Degree and type of neurologic impairment

The level of injury is usually related to the mechanism of injury and the site of trauma. It is inferred by the neurologic examination and confirmed by any of the aforementioned radiographic procedures. The SCI level defines the potential complications and has implications for management.

The time since injury is usually apparent from the trauma event itself or the onset of neurologic findings. Early recognition of acute SCI is important, because early treatment may reduce the degree of irreversible injury. As time progresses, the spectrum of residual injury changes (see later).

Recognition of spinal instability (especially in the cervical spine) is important for patient positioning and movement, especially during airway management and tracheal intubation. However, spine injury can occur without bony or ligamentous instability (e.g., spinal hematomas and abscesses; intraoperative injuries; trauma in children). Finally, the degree and type of neurologic impairment define the potential neurologic sequelae.

Risk Assessment

Certain surgical procedures are associated with a recognized risk of acute SCI. The neurologic risk in spinal column correction procedures is approximately 1% to 4%; however, the risk approaches 75% for the correction of severe kyphosis. Surgery involving the thoracic aorta also has a high risk (see Chapter 94). In surgical patients, early detection of the injury by intraoperative monitoring may allow correction before the injurious process (often ischemia) causes irreversible injury.

Acute SCI should be suspected in all trauma victims. Major trauma victims have a 2.6% risk of acute SCI, and patients with head trauma have a 4% to 5% risk of associated cervical spine injury. Traumatic acute SCI is thought to occur in 12 to 53 persons per million yearly, more often in males (4:1 predominance), and most commonly at C4-C6. The second most commonly injured spine region is T11 to L2. The most frequent cause is motor vehicle accidents, often associated with alcohol or drug consumption. Falls in elderly persons and diving accidents are among the other important causes. Of patients with cervical spine injuries, about 25% become quadriplegic, and 40% have no residual neurologic impairment. That leaves about 35% with some degree of residual neurologic impairment.

Patients with acute SCI who show no resolution of neurologic impairment progress to chronic SCI. In obtunded patients, a careful history and neurologic examination may be needed to distinguish chronic SCI from cerebral injury. A better understanding of the mechanisms of SCI and its management has reduced overall mortality from 80% (World War I era) to less than 2% by the early 1980s.

Implications

The complications of SCI depend on the level of injury and the particular syndrome of injury, defined by the zone of injury in the spinal cord. The greatest number of complications occur with neurologically complete acute SCI (comparable to spinal cord transection). This is characterized by loss of all neurologic function at and below the level of injury. With high spinal cord injury (C4-C6), pulmonary function studies usually reveal reduced total lung capacity, vital capacity, expiratory reserve volume, and forced expiratory volume and increased residual lung volume. Vital capacity is an excellent measure of pulmonary compromise; patients with a vital capacity less than 15 mL/kg often require tracheal intubation and ventilatory support.

A variety of factors contribute to ventilatory compromise, which occurs in 67% of acute SCI patients within the first few days after injury (Table 183-1). Acute SCI patients ventilate better when supine, because the abdominal contents tent the diaphragm, allowing for better mechanical action (except when distended bowel or stomach hinders diaphragmatic movement). Retained airway secretions and atelectasis are common. Ventilation may improve with chronic SCI due to strengthening of the chest wall and abdomen by intercostal and abdominal muscle contractures.

Cardiovascular function is markedly altered in acute SCI by the associated loss of sympathetic control of the heart and vasculature. Consequent venodilatation leads to relative hypovolemia and reduced preload. This is aggravated by traumatic or surgical blood loss. Peripheral vasodilatation reduces systemic vascular resistance. The reduction in both preload and systemic vascular resistance contributes to a hypotensive state known as spinal shock. Loss of cardiac sympathetic innervation leads to the inability to increase contractility and heart rate in response to hypovolemia or blood loss. Resulting unopposed vagal tone enhances the potential for bradycardia and escape rhythms. Either may occur with sudden increased blood pressure (i.e., hyperactive carotid sinus reflex) or airway manipulation and may necessitate atropine or temporary or permanent pacing. In addition to the potential for bradycardia and hypotension, patients with acute SCI are at risk for acute heart failure and pulmonary edema. Experimental evidence suggests that myocardial injury may occur at the time of SCI due to a catecholamine surge with an acute and transient increase in afterload.

There is greater cardiovascular stability with chronic SCI. However, with lesions above T7, sensory stimuli below the level of SCI may provoke exaggerated sympathetic spinal reflexes (i.e., autonomic hyperreflexia), causing intense vasoconstriction and acute hypertension (see Chapter 114).

In addition to cardiovascular dysfunction, there are other types of injury or defects associated with acute SCI (Table 183-2). Impaired temperature regulation, caused by loss of sympathetic-mediated changes in vascular tone, leads to vasodilatation and the inability to control sweating. Denervation of skeletal muscle leads to neuromuscular junction hypersensitivity, so that depolarizing muscle relaxants (e.g., succinylcholine) cause exaggerated potassium release. This begins within 24 to 48 hours of acute SCI and lasts until muscle atrophy with chronic SCI abolishes the effect. Succinylcholine is generally considered safe 1 year after the onset of acute SCI. In traumatic acute SCI, patients may have associated injuries (e.g., head trauma with increased intracranial pressure; chest, abdominal, or orthopedic injuries).

Table 183–1 ■ Factors Contributing to Ventilatory Compromise in Acute Spinal Cord Injury

Limitation of diaphragmatic motion by gastric distention and ileus
Aspiration pneumonitis
Reduced expiratory reserve and ability to cough, secondary to loss of abdominal (T2-L1) and intercostal (T1-T11) muscle control
Fat emboli with long bone fractures
Chest trauma (rib fractures, pulmonary contusion, pneumothorax, hemothorax)
Loss of spinal input to the phrenic nerve (C3-C5) and control of the diaphragm
Depressed consciousness from head injury, alcohol, or drugs
Neurogenic edema from head injury
Pulmonary edema secondary to cardiovascular dysfunction

Table 183–2 ■ Injuries or Defects Associated with Acute Spinal Cord Injury

Cardiovascular dysfunction (spinal shock)
Impaired temperature regulation
Neuromuscular junction hypersensitivity
Head injury (raised intracranial pressure)
Chest trauma (pneumothorax, cardiac contusion)
Myocardial injury
Aspiration pneumonitis
Pneumothorax, pneumomediastinum
Hematoma compromise of airway in neck trauma
Long bone fractures with blood loss and fat emboli
Renal failure
Muscle contractures
Deep venous thrombosis and pulmonary thromboembolism

Other conditions associated with chronic SCI include the following:

- Renal failure (from recurrent urinary tract infection or amyloidosis)
- Drug or alcohol abuse or dependence (owing to depression or pain syndromes)
- Decubitus ulcers

Also with chronic SCI, spinal reflex action below the lesion may lead to uncontrolled muscle contractures (i.e., the "mass reflex"). Patients with both acute and chronic SCI are prone to develop deep venous thrombosis (up to 80% to 85% in cervical injuries). Thus, pulmonary thromboembolism is a common cause of death in patients with acute SCI and may prompt the placement of a vena cava filter.

MANAGEMENT

Initial priorities in acute SCI victims are securing the airway, ensuring adequate oxygenation and ventilation, and providing circulatory support. Further medical management is for coexisting injuries and the prevention of ischemic SCI. The unstable spine should be stabilized in a neutral position, with traction deferred until the neurologic evaluation is complete. Traction can lead to further injury, including disk herniation, C1-C2 ligamentous laxity, or ankylosing spondylitis.

The first priority is to secure the airway. Ideally, a controlled, awake intubation allows neurologic observation during intubation. However, if immediate tracheal intubation using direct laryngoscopy is necessary, midline stabilization (not traction) can minimize the degree of cervical spine movement. If facial trauma prohibits oral intubation, a surgical airway (tracheostomy or cricothyrotomy) or transtracheal ventilation may be needed. In patients with head trauma, nasal intubation should be avoided, if possible, until a basilar skull fracture has been ruled out.

After establishment of the airway, adequate oxygenation and ventilation must be confirmed. Any hypotension, which could be secondary to loss of sympathetic tone from acute SCI, hypovolemia, and trauma, should be treated with intravenous fluids to restore adequate cardiac output and blood pressure. Pulmonary artery catheterization may be needed, especially with quadriplegia, because excessive fluids may cause pulmonary edema. Vasoconstrictors (e.g., dopamine, ephedrine, phenylephrine[1]) are used to augment cardiovascular dynamics when volume alone is ineffective. Myocardial inotropic support may also be necessary, because acute SCI may cause myocardial injury from brief, explosive autonomic discharge with hypertension due to mechanical compression of the descending sympathetic nerves. Transient bradycardia is treated with atropine or β-adrenergic agonists, with provision for pacing in patients with persistent bradycardia or escape rhythms. High-dose methylprednisolone is thought to improve outcome (see later).

Sudden changes in position may cause postural hypotension (head-up tilt) or pulmonary edema (head-down tilt) due to reduced cardiovascular compensation. The clinician should monitor the patient's temperature and use warming blankets or adjust the ambient temperature as needed. Unexplained hypotension may also be due to previously unrecognized intra-abdominal or retroperitoneal bleeding.

Associated major injuries occur in about two thirds of patients with traumatic acute SCI. Of special concern are thoracoabdominal injuries, which may be nonapparent owing to sensory loss or head injury. Thoracoabdominal injuries occur in as many as 25% to 50% of patients with acute SCI. Other aspects of postinjury care relate to complications of acute SCI, such as gastric erosions, deep venous thrombosis, and pulmonary embolism.

Emergency surgery in cases of traumatic acute SCI is usually for injuries other than those to the spinal cord. However, emergency spinal cord surgery may be required if vertebral bony alignment cannot be achieved by traction (e.g., due to "locked" facets) or when bone fragments or protruding disk material is impinging on the spinal cord. Anesthetic management for such surgery involves maintaining adequate spinal cord perfusion. Outcomes are improved if mean blood pressure is greater than 85 mm Hg, central venous pressure is 5 to 10 mm Hg, arterial oxygen tension is greater than 100 mm Hg, and normoglycemia and normocarbia are maintained. Extubation should be delayed until adequate unsupported ventilatory function is ensured. Postoperative mechanical ventilatory support may be needed. Emergency reintubation is undesirable in patients with acute cervical spine injury due to the need for additional neck manipulation.

If acute SCI is related to recent spinal or aortic surgery, time is of the essence if deleterious effects are to be reversed. Many surgeons use steroids, such as methylprednisolone or dexamethasone, at this time. Removal of spinal instrumentation or exploration of the spinal canal for hematomas may be required within a few hours. If so, electrophysiologic monitoring (i.e., sensory or motor evoked potentials) may be necessary to warn of further SCI.

Anesthesia for surgery in patients with chronic SCI is often for decubitus ulcers or kidney stones. Local, regional, or general anesthesia may be sufficient, depending on the site of surgery and the degree of neurologic impairment. However, many chronic SCI patients (85%) with lesions above T7 are prone to autonomic hyperreflexia and associated hypertension, which can occur when local anesthesia alone is used; both regional and general anesthesia can block this. Although less successful than subarachnoid block for urologic or general surgery, epidurals have been used successfully during labor. Positioning problems may be anticipated in chronic SCI patients due to either contractures or positions that compromise ventilation. In patients with chronic SCI, the blood volume is often contracted (60 mL/kg), making them prone to orthostatic hypotension. Other procedures that may require anesthesia care and are common in patients with chronic SCI are placement of pulse generators for phrenic nerve or spinal cord stimulation (i.e., to improve ventilatory mechanics or for pain control, respectively) and intrathecal baclofen for the management of spasticity.

---

[1]Phenylephrine may be advantageous. It is primarily an α-adrenergic agonist. Thus, it increases both systemic vascular resistance and preload via constriction of the venous capacitance bed.

PREVENTION

Once acute SCI has occurred, efforts should be directed toward reducing additional injury due to secondary causes (e.g., hypoxemia, impaired spinal cord perfusion). Although methylprednisolone (30 mg/kg intravenous bolus, then 5.4 mg/kg per hour for 23 hours), when started 3 to 8 hours after acute SCI, appears to reduce the neurologic injury score, it may not improve function. Such steroid use is not advised with penetrating abdominal injuries because of the probable or assumed contamination of the spinal canal with bowel flora. Prompt intervention for acute SCI related to spinal cord surgery, or to relieve compression, can also reduce the degree of injury. Intraoperative measures that help reduce acute SCI include maintaining normal blood pressure, arterial carbon dioxide tension, and glucose concentrations throughout surgery and the immediate postoperative period. Finally, spinal cord function monitoring with evoked sensory and motor potentials may reduce any additional (iatrogenic) injury, especially during spinal decompression and fusion.

Further Reading

Bracken MB, Shepard MJ, Holford TR, et al: Administration of methylprednisolone for 24 or 48 hours or tirilazad mesylate for 48 hours in the treatment of acute spinal cord injury: Results of the Third National Acute Spinal Cord Injury Randomized Controlled Trial. National Acute Spinal Cord Injury Study. JAMA 277:1597-1604, 1997.

Chiles BW, Cooper PR: Acute spinal injury. N Engl J Med 334:514-520, 1996.

Gronert GA, Theye RA: Pathophysiology of hyperkalemia induced by succinylcholine. Anesthesiology 43:89-99, 1975.

Hambly PR, Martin B: Anaesthesia for chronic spinal cord lesions. Anaesthesia 53:273-289, 1998.

Kirshblum SC, Groah SL, McKinley WO, et al: Spinal cord injury medicine. 1. Etiology, classification and acute medical management. Arch Phys Med Rehabil 83(3 Suppl 1):S50-S57, S90-S98, 2002.

Lambert DJ, Deane RS, Mazuzan JE: Anesthesia and the control of blood pressure in patients with spinal cord injury. Anesth Analg 61:344-388, 1982.

Lee TT, Green BA: Advances in the management of acute spinal cord injury. Orthop Clin North Am 33:311-315, 2002.

Mackensie CF, Geisler FH: Management of acute cervical spinal cord injury. In Albin MS (ed): Textbook of Neuroanesthesia with Neurosurgical and Neuroscience Perspectives. New York, McGraw-Hill, 1996, pp 1083-1136.

Sloan TB, Hickey R, Albin MS: Anesthesia management of the patient with acute spinal cord injury. Adv Anesth 8:55-90, 1991.

Woodring JH, Lee C: Limitations of cervical radiography in the evaluation of acute cervical trauma. J Trauma 34:32-39, 1993.

Corneal Injury

Lois L. Bready and Stacey L. Allen

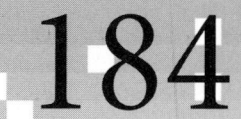

Case Synopsis

A 25-year-old woman in the postanesthesia care unit complains of pain and a foreign body sensation in her left eye. She had received general endotracheal anesthesia for nasal polypectomy earlier that day. Physical examination reveals residual petroleum-based ointment containing mascara particles around both eyes and left-sided conjunctival erythema, marked tearing, photophobia, and diminished visual acuity. A pulse oximeter probe is attached to her left index finger.

PROBLEM ANALYSIS

Definition

Corneal injury occurs infrequently during anesthesia, but it can be painful. A corneal abrasion may progress to corneal ulceration and erosion, with loss of visual acuity. Exposure of the cornea to a variety of chemicals may cause burns, with subsequent scarring.

Recognition

A patient with corneal trauma typically experiences tearing, foreign body sensation, photophobia, diminished visual acuity, and eye pain. Bedside examination may reveal an abraded site (Fig. 184-1). Ophthalmologic examination with fluorescein staining and an ultraviolet lamp or (preferably) a slit lamp reveals areas of denuded cornea within the interpalpebral area (Fig. 184-2A) or linear defects from mechanical abrasion (Fig. 184-2B). Chemical corneal toxicity usually leads to chemosis (i.e., marked swelling of the conjunctiva), with various corneal epithelial defects, including punctate keratitis (Fig. 184-3).

Risk Assessment

A number of risk factors associated with general anesthesia may predispose to corneal trauma. Numerous manipulations occur around the patient's face and head during the course of routine surgery with anesthesia. The corneal epithelium is delicate; even gentle tactile contact may cause trauma. Pain perception is reduced by narcotics and is blocked during general anesthesia. Protective corneal reflexes are obtunded, and tear production is diminished. Foreign bodies may be present and are an additional risk factor for corneal abrasion. When surgical procedures are performed on the head and neck, antiseptic solutions are applied to the skin near the eyes, and inadvertent contact with the cornea can occur.

Implications

Eye injuries account for 71 of 2046 cases (3%) in the American Society of Anesthesiologists closed claims database (Table 184-1). Of these, 25 were corneal abrasions, and 16% resulted in permanent injury. Chemical injury or direct trauma was identified as the mechanism of corneal injury in only 20% of corneal abrasions. A 1996 study by Roth and coworkers suggested that older patients and lengthier procedures are associated with a higher risk of injury to the eyes.

CHEMICAL INJURY

Exposure to a variety of disinfectant solutions can result in chemical burns to the cornea (Table 184-2), with the potential to cause blindness. Most skin antiseptic solutions are toxic to the cornea, as documented in animal models. If the solution accidentally splashes or runs into the tear film (e.g., during preparation for surgery on the head and neck), intense toxic effects may result. Hibiclens (chlorhexidine gluconate 4% and detergent) has been reported to cause permanent corneal scarring. The toxicity of other antiseptic solutions may be less profound, but these solutions should be avoided if possible. The solution least toxic to the cornea is 10% povidone-iodine. Because both the concentration of the solution and the contact time are critical factors in corneal toxicity, it is prudent to

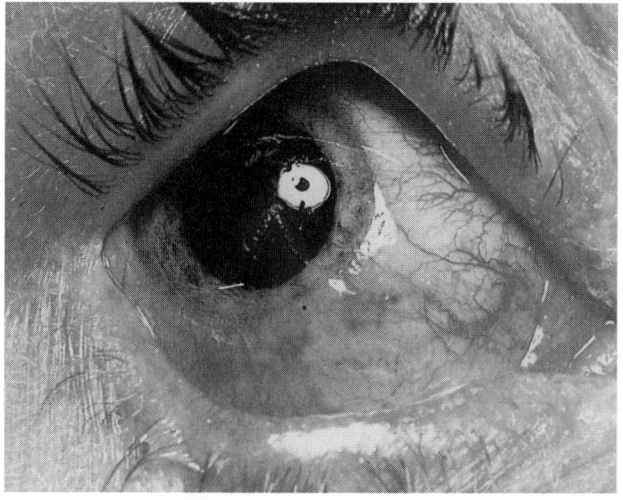

Figure 184–1 ■ Corneal abrasion.

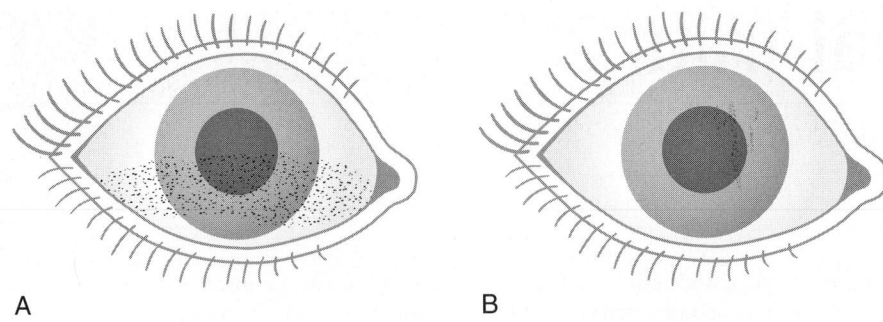

A   B

Figure 184–2 ■ Staining patterns of the cornea and conjunctiva. *A*, Interpalpebral abrasion (indicating exposure due to incomplete eyelid closure). *B*, Linear defects (suggesting mechanical abrasion).

immediately irrigate the conjunctival sac with saline, balanced salt solution, or water if exposure to a chemical disinfectant occurs. The great majority of reported cases of severe keratitis due to exposure to surgical preparation solutions occurred during operations performed by nonophthalmologists on or around the head and neck, suggesting that failure to recognize the exposure and the consequent lack of irrigation may have played a role in the adverse outcomes. Also, be aware that surgical preparation solutions can flow in a retrograde fashion from the nasal cavity into the conjunctival sac via a patent nasolacrimal duct.

Exposure to acidic gastric secretions can also cause a chemical burn to the cornea. If such exposure is recognized or suspected, once again, irrigation of the conjunctival sac is advised.

CORNEAL ABRASION

Direct pressure on the eye by the facemask and head strap; the hand, arm, or elbow of the anesthesiologist or surgeon;

or other nearby objects can abrade the corneal surface. Corneal abrasion may occur during the induction of anesthesia, during mask airway management or instrumentation of the airway, upon application of ophthalmic lubrication (if the tip of the eye lubricant tube contacts the cornea rather than being at least 3 to 4 mm away from its surface), during the procedure (pressure on the eye by the surgeon's or anesthetist's hands or elbows, instruments, or other causes), or at emergence (due to causes similar to those during induction or if the patient rubs his or her eyes for any reason). If the pulse oximeter probe is positioned on the patient's index finger, particularly on the dominant hand, the risk of self-induced corneal abrasion or laceration is increased. Foreign bodies in and around the eye (e.g., mascara, contact lenses, false eyelashes) also increase the risk of corneal abrasion.

MANAGEMENT

When a patient's postoperative complaints suggest corneal injury, it is absolutely necessary to obtain an ophthalmologic consultation as soon as possible. Examination with a slit lamp can confirm the diagnosis of corneal injury. If perforation has occurred, prompt repair can then be accomplished. For abrasions, antibiotic ointment followed by patching can lessen the patient's pain. The ophthalmologist determines the need for follow-up.

PREVENTION

Awareness of the risk for ophthalmic injury is paramount to prevent such occurrences. With proper planning, it is possible to eliminate most manipulations and potentially damaging objects that may be injurious to the eyes. Although the first report of corneal abrasion during induction of anesthesia was published in 1987, such injuries continue to occur. The recommendation by Watson and Moran to protect the patient's eyes before laryngoscopy (or, for that matter, any maneuvers or manipulations related to airway management) is strongly supported.

Intraoperatively, simple manual eyelid closure can be effective in supine patients for brief procedures distant from the head and neck. However, not all patients have complete

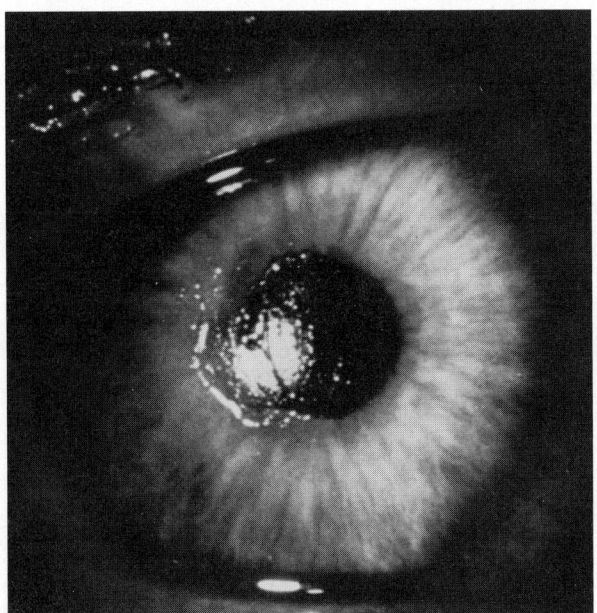

Figure 184–3 ■ Grade I chemical burn with punctate keratitis (the mildest form).

Table 184–1 ■ Mechanisms of Eye Injury Identified by the American Society of Anesthesiologists Closed Claims Project

Mechanism of Injury	Total No. (%) of Eye Injuries (N = 71)	No. (%) of Corneal Abrasions (n = 25)
Patient movement	21 (30)	0
Chemical injury	9 (13)	1 (4)
Direct trauma	6 (8)	4 (16)
Pressure on eye	2 (3)	0
Other	3 (4)	0
Unknown	30 (42)	20 (80)

From Gild WM, Posner KL, Caplan RA, Cheney FW: Eye injuries associated with anesthesia: A closed claims analysis. Anesthesiology 76:204-208, 1992.

Table 184–2 ■ Causes of Chemical Damage to the Cornea

Hibiclens (chlorhexidine gluconate, 4% isopropyl alcohol with a detergent)
pHisoHex (3% hexachlorophene and a detergent)
Lavacol (70% ethanol)
Betadine surgical scrub (7.5% povidone-iodine scrub with a detergent)
Tincture of iodine (2% iodine, 2.35% sodium iodate, 46% ethanol)
Detergent-containing iodine-based products

From MacRae SM, Brown B, Edelhauser HF: The corneal toxicity of presurgical skin antiseptics. Am J Ophthalmol 97:221–232, 1984.

lid closure at rest, and any exposed cornea is at risk for desiccation and abrasion. Instillation of methylcellulose drops or petroleum-based ointment in the conjunctival sac below the lower eyelid is protective against corneal abrasion (Fig. 184-4). However, petroleum-based ointments may not afford protection against other ophthalmic complications, such as postoperative loss of visual acuity or blurred vision. Siffring and Poulton reviewed four comparable groups of patients in their study of eye care techniques to prevent ophthalmic complications during general anesthesia (Table 184-3). Blurred vision and reduction in visual acuity (both self-limited) were noted in the two groups that received eye ointment and tape. In contrast, those receiving

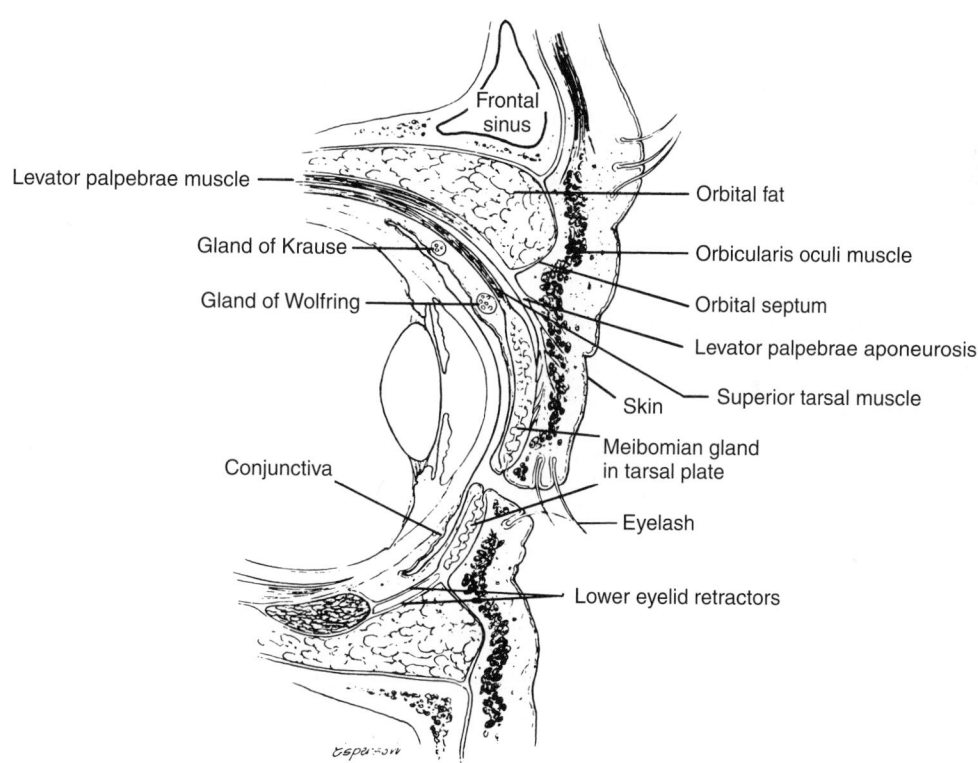

Figure 184–4 ■ Schematic cross section of the orbit and eyeball.

Table 184–3 ■ Eye Care Routines and Postoperative Ophthalmic Complications

Group	% Corneal Abrasions	% Blurred Vision (Hours)	Visual Acuity (by Lines Decreased)	% Sensation of Foreign Body (Hours)
A. Lacri-Lube and tape	0	75 (7.4)	−1.9	62.5 (5.2)
B. Duratears ointment and tape	0	55 (4.5)	−1.3	42 (3.5)
C. Isopto Alkaline drops (methylcellulose) and tape	0	<3	0	<3
D. Hypoallergenic paper tape alone	0	<3	0	<3

From Siffring PA, Poulton TJ: Prevention of ophthalmic complications during general anesthesia. Anesthesiology 66:569-570, 1987.

eye tape only or methylcellulose drops plus eye tape rarely experienced these complications.

In the study by Boggild-Madsen and colleagues, methylcellulose proved to be superior to a paraffin-based ointment. However, in almost all patients whose eyes were protected with methylcellulose, their eyelids were virtually "glued" closed, making periodic intraoperative evaluation of pupil signs difficult. Manecke and associates reported corneal injury in one patient, which was attributed to a preservative-containing eye lubricant.

The application of tape to close the eyelid can protect the cornea. However, this measure obscures pupillary signs and may leave adhesive residue on the periocular tissues and eyelashes.[1] Also, removing the tape may remove a ribbon of eyelid epithelium. If the tape is not removed in a downward fashion (so that the eyelids remain closed during tape removal), there is a risk of stripping off the corneal epithelium and abrasion. In addition, allergy to adhesives is not uncommon. Gauze eye pads or protective eye goggles are indicated if the head is not supine and visible to the anesthesiologist (e.g., lateral or prone positioning, head or neck surgery with drapes covering the head, use of a head wrap, upper airway surgery). Although some clinicians advocate the routine use of eye goggles, a good fit can be challenging owing to interpatient variability in head size, interpupillary distance, and so forth. Also, such eye goggles must be disposable or disinfected.

Finally, patients should not use mascara on the morning of surgery or should be assisted in its removal before the induction of general anesthesia. Those who wear contact lenses must remove them if general anesthesia is planned, to avoid damage to the cornea or lenses. Finally, placement of the pulse oximeter probe on a finger other than the index finger (e.g., the fourth or fifth digit) is recommended to prevent self-inflicted corneal abrasion during the patient's emergence from anesthesia.

Further Reading

Boggild-Madsen NB, Bundgaard-Nielsen P, Hammer U, et al: Comparison of eye protection with methylcellulose and paraffin ointments during general anesthesia. Can Anaesth Soc J 28:575-578, 1981.

Gild WM, Posner KL, Caplan RA, et al: Eye injuries associated with anesthesia: A closed claims analysis. Anesthesiology 76:204-208, 1992.

Glasser DB, Edelhauser HF: Toxicity of surgical solutions. Int Ophthalmol Clin 29:179-187, 1989.

MacRae SM, Brown B, Edelhauser HF: The corneal toxicity of presurgical skin antiseptics. Am J Ophthalmol 97:221-232, 1984.

Manecke GR, Tannenbaum DP, McCoy MD: Severe bilateral corneal injury attributed to a preservative-containing eye lubricant. Anesthesiology 93:1545-1546, 2000.

Roth S, Thisted RA, Erickson JP, et al: Eye injuries after nonocular surgery: A study of 60,965 anesthetics from 1988 to 1992. Anesthesiology 85:1020-1027, 1996.

Siffring PA, Poulton TJ: Prevention of ophthalmic complications during general anesthesia. Anesthesiology 66:569-570, 1987.

Watson WJ, Moran RL: Corneal abrasion during induction. Anesthesiology 66:440, 1987.

---

[1]This is likely less of a risk with synthetic (clear or slightly opaque) tape than with cloth adhesive tape.

Open Globe Injury

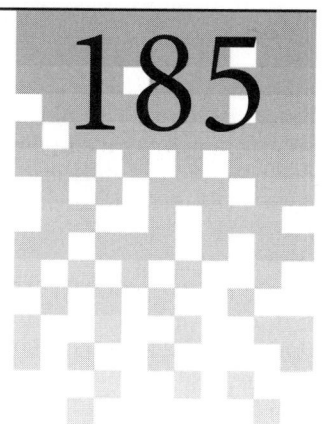

185

Stacey L. Allen and Ellen Duncan

Case Synopsis

A 12-year-old boy presents to the emergency department after being hit in the left eye by a BB from a BB gun. He had eaten a full lunch 1 hour before the accident.

PROBLEM ANALYSIS

Definition

By the history, this patient has an open globe injury. Blindness can be a disastrous consequence of such an injury and may result from an elevation of intraocular pressure (IOP) and extrusion of the contents of the globe.

Recognition

Generally, the diagnosis of open globe injury can be surmised from the history of a penetrating injury to the globe. This may involve a BB shot, wood pieces, or an industrial accident, or it may be the result of blunt or multiple trauma.

In any patient who sustains trauma to the head, the globe and vision must be evaluated. Conversely, when open globe injury is present, other coexisting injuries should be ruled out, such as skull fracture, intracranial trauma, neck injury, and thoracic or abdominal bleeding.

Risk Assessment

The most common risk associated with open globe injury is a full stomach. This risk involves not only the possibility of aspiration of gastric contents but also the fact that drugs or maneuvers used to manage the patient can cause an increase in IOP (Table 185-1) and extrusion of the ocular contents, with subsequent loss of vision.

Hypoxemia may raise IOP via vasodilatation of the choroidal arteries. Sustained hypertension may increase IOP, and induced hypotension may decrease IOP. Vomiting, coughing, or "bucking" causes the most dramatic increase in IOP by causing congestion in the venous system, impeding the outflow of aqueous humor, and increasing the volume of choroidal blood. This increase in pressure may be as high as

30 to 40 mm Hg. Poorly applied cricoid pressure may block venous drainage from the eye.

Implications

Following induction of anesthesia, the administration of succinylcholine can increase IOP in the intact eye by 6 to 8 mm Hg within 4 minutes. IOP returns to baseline in 5 to 7 minutes. In the open globe, however, the IOP is atmospheric pressure.

MANAGEMENT

Preoperatively, a detailed history of previous medical conditions should be obtained. The clinician should take measures to decrease or avoid increasing IOP (Table 185-2). Large doses of narcotics should be avoided because they can cause nausea and vomiting. Prophylaxis against aspiration may include a nonparticulate antacid, metoclopramide to enhance gastric emptying, and an H_2-receptor antagonist to elevate gastric fluid pH and reduce gastric acid production.

Periocular local anesthesia with intravenous sedation may be considered, depending on the patient's status, the surgeon's willingness, associated injuries, and the severity of the open globe injury. General anesthesia is usually preferred, however. The patient should be preoxygenated, and pressure on the eye by the facemask should be avoided. Although the use of succinylcholine is controversial, the rise in IOP can be lessened by pretreatment with a nondepolarizing drug and an induction dose of propofol or thiopental.

Rapid-sequence induction can be accomplished without succinylcholine, using a nondepolarizing agent after preoxygenation, cricoid pressure, and induction with propofol or sodium pentothal. Rocuronium 1.2 mg/kg can be used for rapid-sequence induction (thereby shortening the time to relaxation to approximately 60 seconds). Alternatively, vecuronium 0.25 mg/kg provides intubating conditions in 60 to 90 seconds, and pancuronium 0.2 mg/kg in 90 seconds.

Table 185–1 ■ Drugs or Factors That May Increase Intraocular Pressure
Hypoxemia, hypercarbia, acidosis
Hypertension
Coughing, vomiting, laryngoscopy, tracheal intubation
Excessive cricoid pressure
Ketamine, succinylcholine
Increased extraocular muscle tone
Increased extraocular contents (tumor, hemorrhage)

Table 185–2 ■ Drugs or Factors That May Decrease Intraocular Pressure
Hypothermia
Inhalational anesthetics
Hyperventilation (hypocarbia, alkalosis)
Central nervous system depressants
Reduced extraocular muscle tone

Pancuronium may actually decrease IOP. A disadvantage of vecuronium and pancuronium, however, is the prolonged duration of neuromuscular blockade. Further, a priming dose of any nondepolarizing muscle relaxant can be used to hasten the onset of effect of the subsequent intubating dose of the same agent.[1]

Ketamine's effect on IOP is controversial; however, it may cause nystagmus and blepharospasm and therefore should not be used in ophthalmologic surgery. Etomidate may decrease IOP, but it can cause unpredictable myoclonus, with consequent elevation of IOP.

Postoperatively, before extubation, the stomach should be decompressed, the oropharynx suctioned, and an antiemetic such as a serotonin antagonist administered. Intravenous lidocaine (1.5 mg/kg) may be given to reduce coughing during emergence.

PREVENTION

- Take the necessary precautions to prevent coughing, straining, bucking, and vomiting.
- Try to minimize hypercarbia, hypoxia, and increases in blood pressure.
- Attempt to minimize the risk of aspiration while ensuring the patient's safety.
- Provide prophylaxis for postoperative nausea and vomiting with H_2-receptor antagonists, metoclopramide, and nonparticulate antacids.

---

[1]The editor has done this with rocuronium. Relaxation sufficient for endotracheal intubation is achieved in about 60 seconds, and sometimes in less than 45 seconds.

Further Reading

Berry JM, Merin RG: Etomidate myoclonus and the open globe. Anesth Anal 69:256-259, 1989.

Cook JH: The effect of suxamethonium on intraocular pressure. Anesthesia 36:359-365, 1981.

Cunningham AJ, Barry P: Intraocular pressure: Physiology and implications for anesthetic management. Can Anaesth Soc J 33:195-208, 1986.

Konchiergeri HN, Lee YE, Venugopal K: Effect of pancuronium on intraocular pressure changes induced by succinylcholine. Can Anaesth Soc J 26:479-484, 1979.

Libonati MM, Leahy JJ, Ellison N: The use of succinylcholine in open eye surgery. Anesthesiology 62:637-640, 1985.

Mehta MP, Choi WW, Gergis SD, et al: Facilitation of rapid endotracheal intubations with divided doses of nondepolarizing neuromuscular blocking drugs. Anesthesiology 62:392-395, 1985.

Naguib M, Abdulatif M, Gyasi HK, et al: Priming with atracurium: Improving intubating conditions with additional doses of thiopental. Anesth Analg 65:1295-1299, 1986.

Peuler M, Glass DD, Arens JF: Ketamine and intraocular pressure. Anesthesiology 5:575-578, 1975.

Schwarz S, Ilias W, Lackner F, et al: Rapid tracheal intubation with vecuronium: The priming principle. Anesthesiology 62:388-391, 1985.

Scott IU, McCabe CM, Flynn HW, et al: Local anesthesia with intravenous sedation for surgical repair of selected open globe injuries. Am J Ophthalmol 134:707-711, 2002.

Taboada JA, Rupp SM, Miller RD: Refining the priming principle for vecuronium during rapid-sequence induction of anesthesia. Anesthesiology 64:243-247, 1986.

Retrobulbar Block

Wendy B. Kang

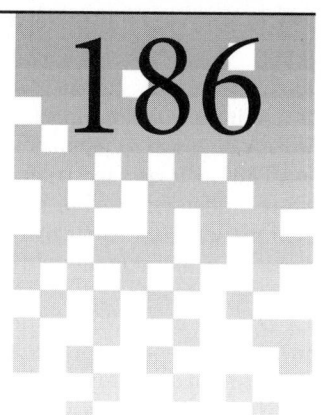

Case Synopsis

Monitored anesthesia care is provided for an active 70-year-old patient undergoing extracapsular cataract extraction and intraocular lens implantation. The patient has stable hypertension, coronary artery disease, mild emphysema, and renal insufficiency. Sedation with 1 mg midazolam and 50 µg fentanyl is administered, along with verbal reassurance, while the ophthalmologist performs a retrobulbar block. Surgery is uneventful, and vital signs are stable. After 30 minutes in the darkened operating room, the surgical drapes are removed to reveal a patient who cannot be awakened.

PROBLEM ANALYSIS

Definition

Cataract surgery is likely the most frequently performed surgical procedure in industrialized nations. Yet many anesthesiologists are unaware of the potential complications associated with the use of regional anesthesia in ocular surgery, either from a lack of technical familiarity or from a lack of follow-up in predominantly same-day surgical patients.

Anesthesiologists must be aware of the consequences of local anesthetic injections into a patient's eye, whether performed by the anesthesiologist or by the surgeon. In 2001 the Royal College of Anaesthetists and Royal College of Ophthalmologists issued guidelines encouraging the involvement of physician anesthetists in the administration of local anesthesia, rather than merely providing monitored anesthesia care. A review of the literature reveals a continuing and pervasive use of retrobulbar blocks along with newer techniques, such as peribulbar, episcleral, or sub-Tenon's capsule local anesthetic injections, as well as the use of topical anesthesia in the eye.

The goals of ocular regional anesthesia are akinesia and analgesia, both for patient comfort and for safety. Retrobulbar block combined with facial nerve block has been the standard regional anesthetic technique for more than a century. It provides superior akinesia, anesthesia, and analgesia compared with other regional techniques.

Indications for retrobulbar block are as follows:

- Avoidance of general anesthesia in elderly patients, who may have multiple medical comorbidities
- Achievement of optimal surgical conditions for extracapsular cataract extraction, phacoemulsification, intraocular lens implantation, and open globe surgery (e.g., vitrectomy, glaucoma treatment, repair of retinal detachment)
- Prolonged, difficult surgeries (e.g., in a patient who has had previous eye surgery) or in patients with hard cataracts or nystagmus

Contraindications to retrobulbar block are as follows:

- True allergy to local anesthetic drugs
- Patient refusal, despite explanations regarding the use of intravenous sedation and lack of intraoperative awareness

- Patient inability to cooperate (e.g., severe restless leg syndrome)

The operating room team must determine its own level of comfort concerning contraindications to local anesthetic blocks. The diverse spectrum of "uncooperative" patients (e.g., impaired mental status, youth, dementia, deafness, severe emphysema or congestive heart failure, inability to keep still, excessive anxiety) can often be managed safely with regional anesthesia and monitored anesthesia care.

Coagulation abnormalities must also be considered, and there is considerable variation among institutions regarding what is acceptable. Available evidence suggests that patients who take nonsteroidal anti-inflammatory drugs, aspirin, or warfarin can undergo eye surgery safely.

The question of whether a patient with uncontrolled glaucoma or recent surgery on the same eye should undergo regional anesthesia is best answered by a discussion among the surgeon, the anesthesia care provider, and the patient, rather than relying on rigid adherence to institutional policies.

Recognition

COMPLICATIONS

Complication rates with regional anesthesia vary and range from 1 in 1300 to 1 in 16,000 for globe perforation and 1 in 300 to 1 in 500 for brainstem anesthesia (Table 186-1). The reported incidence for ocular perforation is 0.114%. In one retrospective review, there was a 0.25% incidence of anesthesia-related diplopia, with retrobulbar block accounting for 0.39% of cases.

Table 186–1 ■ Complications of Retrobulbar Block

Retrobulbar or peribulbar hemorrhage
Globe penetration or perforation
Optic nerve damage leading to visual changes, including blindness
Central nervous system depression leading to brainstem anesthesia
Severe symptomatic activation of oculocardiac reflex
Diplopia and eye muscle imbalance

With retrobulbar block, hematomas can occur subconjunctivally or as hyphemas in the anterior chamber of the eye. Although visually striking, these are not as dangerous as more hidden retrobulbar hemorrhages within the extraocular muscles. These can cause edema or paresis and result in vertical or horizontal ophthalmoplegia, diplopia, strabismus, or hyper- or hypotonia. Bleeding within the extraocular muscles or damage to the central retinal artery or vein increases intraocular pressure, which may lead to optic nerve compression, ischemia, and subsequent loss of vision.

Penetration of the optic globe sufficient to cause perforation results in loss of vitreous humor. Mild eye compression is used after retrobulbar block. A sudden loss of firmness to palpation may signal the loss of vitreous humor. This can progress to optic neuropathy.

Mental status changes (as in the case synopsis) may result from direct injection of local anesthetic into the dural cuff along the optic nerve or into a blood vessel. Depending on the amount of local anesthetic reaching the subarachnoid space, the patient may exhibit drowsiness, obtundation, vomiting, convulsions, or contralateral blindness. If the local anesthetic reaches the optic chiasm, complete respiratory and cardiac arrest may occur (i.e., the ultimate "high spinal").

Activation of the oculocardiac reflex may trigger bradycardia, asytole, or other arrhythmias. Ocular injection; pressure on the globe; or traction on the extraocular muscles, conjunctiva, or globe transmits signals through the ophthalmic branch of the trigeminal nerve to the vagus nerve. Young children who have not received atropine pretreatment are especially prone to the oculocardiac reflex.

Anecdotal case reports describe severe orbital cellulitis in immunocompromised patients, myopic staphylomas, chemosis, and acute pulmonary edema concurrent with trigeminal nerve block as complications associated with retrobulbar block.

ANATOMIC CONSIDERATIONS

To understand how complications occur with retrobulbar block and other regional anesthesia techniques used for ophthalmic surgery, a brief review of the ocular anatomy is necessary (Fig. 186-1). The extraocular muscles surround the globe and form the cone. The lateral rectus is supplied by the abducens (sixth cranial) nerve, the superior oblique by the trochlear (fourth cranial) nerve, and the other muscles by the oculomotor (third cranial) nerve. The nasociliary,

oculomotor, abducens, and optic nerves run within the cone behind the globe, along with the central retinal artery and vein. Importantly, the dural cuff surrounds the optic nerve.

The ophthalmic division of the intracranial trigeminal nerve divides into the lacrimal, frontal, and nasociliary nerves. Extraconal and conjunctival sensations are supplied by the first two of these nerves. Branches of the nasociliary provide innervation to the intraconal portion, cornea, sclera, iris, and ciliary body of the eye. Block of the anterior ethmoidal nerve, another branch of the nasociliary nerve, results in nasal stuffiness.

The ciliary ganglion of the nasociliary nerve lies near the apex of the retrobulbar cone; therefore, it is associated with the optic nerve and artery. Parasympathetic fibers from the Edinger-Westphal nucleus accompany the oculomotor nerve and synapse in its ganglion, whereas sensory and sympathetic fibers from T1 continue through the ganglion. Its efferent nerve, the short ciliary nerve, travels anteriorly to provide sensation to the globe and autonomic motor function to the iris.

TECHNIQUE

All sensory and motor nerves can be blocked by injection into either the optic cone (retrobulbar block) or the orbital fat (peribulbar block). For retrobulbar block, the needle is placed from the inferolateral orbital rim to past the equator of the globe, before turning medially and inward. Ideally, the needle enters between the inferior and lateral rectus muscles, behind the globe, and within the space bounded by the extraocular muscles. Upon injection, the pulsatile ocular blood flow decreases, even in the absence of changes in intraocular pressure.

Risk Assessment

The following are risk factors for complications associated with retrobulbar block:

- Technical inexperience on the part of the surgeon or anesthesiologist
- Use of a sharp needle and an insertion depth greater than 25 mm
- Long axial length of a myopic eye (long, thin globe)
- Left inferior rectus muscle injection by a right-handed physician

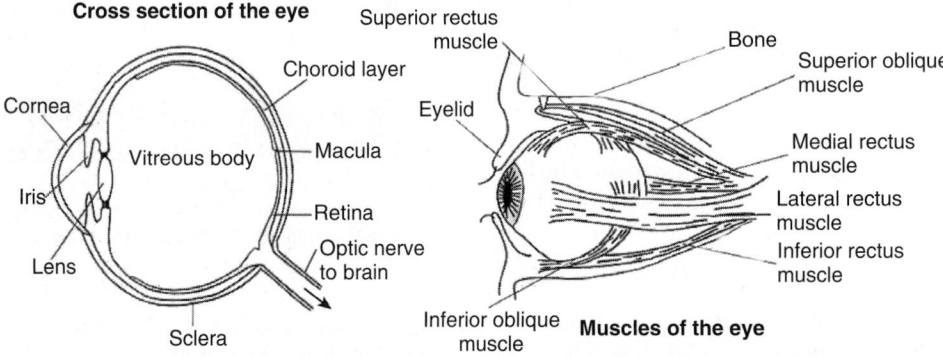

Figure 186–1 ■ Anatomy of the eye relevant to the performance of retrobulbar block.

- Use of excessive volume (≥4 to 5 mL) of local anesthetic, which may lead to "compartment syndrome"
- An uncooperative patient

It is unclear how the type of local anesthetic used or the inclusion of hyaluronidase affects the risk of complications. Inadequate blockade of the extraocular muscles can result in increased pain and squinting. For extracapsular cataract extraction or phacoemulsification, complete akinesia is seldom necessary for the safe performance of surgery.

Implications

Owing to the serious sequelae of retrobulbar hemorrhage and globe perforation, alternative regional anesthesia techniques continue to be developed. A peribulbar deposition technique was described by Davis and Mandel in 1986. It is theoretically extraconal, going no deeper than the globe equator. However, there is no assurance against accidental intraconal injection. Also, larger volumes of local anesthetic, with up to two injections at the superomedial and inferolateral quadrants, raise intraocular pressure, with potential adverse sequelae.

The sub-Tenon's, or episcleral, space is the cavity formed by Tenon's capsule (a fascial layer surrounding the globe and extraocular muscles) and the sclera. Stevens in 1992 described medial quadrant infiltration of local anesthetic with a blunt-tipped cannula. In contrast to retrobulbar or peribulbar block, sub-Tenon's block is relatively painless. The local anesthetic diffuses through the fenestrated posterior Tenon's capsule into the retrobulbar cone and periorbital tissues, causing akinesia of the globe and eyelid; such akinesia may be incomplete, however. There have also been case reports of complications similar to those associated with retrobulbar and peribulbar block.

The use of subconjunctival and topical anesthesia with intravenous sedation has increased since the mid-1990s. Ease of administration, rapid placement, lack of painful injections, and minimal complications have made this technique popular. Unfortunately, the eye is not akinetic, and the patient must be able to cooperate during the procedure. Patients have also experienced pain with the superior rectus fixation suture and during cautery of scleral vessels.

MANAGEMENT

An anesthesiologist's presence continues to be vital to the well-being of any patient undergoing ophthalmic surgery. Maintaining communication with the patient (through intermittent hand squeezes) is as important as monitoring the blood pressure, electrocardiogram, capnography, and pulse oximetry.

In the event of extensive ocular hemorrhage or global perforation, the opinion of the ophthalmologist should guide further treatment. Surgery may be deferred or changed (e.g., progressed to a scleral buckle procedure).

Cardiopulmonary sequelae are easily managed by an alert anesthesiologist. Airway management and circulatory support with vagolytic or anticonvulsive medications may be used until the patient returns to his or her preoperative status.

PREVENTION

Knowledge of ocular anatomy and its proximity to intracranial structures and a continuing dedication to improving one's regional anesthesia skills can help reduce the incidence of serious complications. The use of short, 2.5- to 3-cm blunt needles and small volumes (3 to 4 mL) of local anesthetics is prudent. A minimal needle insertion depth (<25 mm) and stopping the insertion if the patient complains of severe pain can lower the likelihood of touching the globe or the dura. The eye should remain in the primary neutral gaze or in a slightly down and outward gaze during local anesthetic injection. Judicious amounts of oral or intravenous sedatives can relieve anxiety and hypertension before injection. The patient must be cooperative, which is facilitated by providing verbal reassurance.

Further Reading

Bellucci, R: Anesthesia for cataract surgery. Curr Opin Ophthalmol 10:36-41, 1999.

Canavan KS, Dark A, Garrioch MA: Sub-Tenon's administration of local anaesthetic: A review of the technique. Br J Anaesth 90:787-793, 2003.

Davis DB, Mandel MR: Posterior peribulbar anesthesia: An alternative to retrobulbar anesthesia. Cataract Refract Surg 12:182-184, 1986.

Edge R, Navon S: Scleral perforation during retrobulbar and peribulbar anesthesia: Risk factors and outcomes in 50,000 consecutive injections. J Cataract Refract Surg 25:1237-1244, 1999.

Gómez-Arnau JI, Yangüela J, González A, et al: Anaesthesia-related diplopia after cataract surgery. Br J Anaesth 90:189-193, 2003.

Jacobi PC, Dietlein TS, Jacobi FK: A comparative study of topical vs retrobulbar anesthesia in complicated cataract surgery. Arch Ophthalmol 228:1037-1043, 2000.

Kallio H, Paloheimo M, Maunuksela E-L: Haemorrhage and risk factors associated with retrobulbar/peribulbar block: A prospective study in 1383 patients. Br J Anaesth 85:708-711, 2000.

Kwinten FA, de Moor GP, Lamers R: Acute pulmonary edema and trigeminal nerve blockade after retrobulbar block. Anesth Analg 83:1322-1324, 1996.

Nouvellon E, L'Hermite J, Chaumeron A, et al: Ophthalmic regional anesthesia: Medial canthus episcleral (sub-Tenon) single injection block. Anesthesiology 100:370-374, 2004.

Ripart J, Lefrant J-Y, Vivien B, et al: Ophthalmic regional anesthesia: Medial canthus episcleral (sub-Tenon) anesthesia is more efficient than peribulbar anesthesia: A double-blind randomized study. Anesthesiology 92:1278-1285, 2000.

Rüschen H, Bremner FD, Carr C: Complications after sub-Tenon's eye block. Anesth Analg 96:273-277, 2003.

Stevens JD: A new local anesthesia technique for cataract extraction by one quadrant sub-tenon's infiltration. Br J Ophthalmol 76:670-674, 1992.

Taylor G, Devys JM, Heran F, et al: Early exploration of diplopia with magnetic resonance imaging after peribulbar anaesthesia. Br J Anaesth 92:899-901, 2004.

Thind GS, Rubin AP: Local anaesthesia for eye—no room for complacency. Br J Anaesth 86:473-476, 2001.

Laryngoscopy and Microlaryngoscopy

187

Susan H. Noorily

Case Synopsis

A 50-year-old man with a vocal cord lesion is undergoing microlaryngoscopy with possible biopsy or laser excision of the lesion. The patient is hemodynamically stable until the surgeon exposes the larynx with the operating laryngoscope and applies the suspension apparatus. At this time, the patient becomes hypertensive (blood pressure 200/118 mm Hg) and has multiform ventricular bigeminy on the intraoperative electrocardiogram (ECG) (Fig. 187-1).

PROBLEM ANALYSIS

Definition

Cardiovascular complications (e.g., myocardial infarction, ischemia, arrhythmias) have been reported with increasing frequency in patients having laryngeal microsurgery. Stimulation caused by laryngeal instrumentation or manipulation can result in adrenergic stress responses, leading to hypertension, tachycardia, and arrhythmias. Pressure of the laryngoscope blade and stretching of laryngeal structures during suspension laryngoscopy stimulate deep sensory receptors in the larynx and provoke cardiac arrhythmias. Because these sensory receptors are deep within the laryngeal musculature, they are not blocked by topical anesthesia. The reflex pathway believed to be responsible for the arrhythmias includes the afferent fibers of the superior laryngeal nerve and the cardioinhibitory fibers of the vagus nerve.

Patients undergoing laryngoscopy and microlaryngoscopy are at risk for other complications as well. Abnormal airway anatomy places some patients at risk for difficult tracheal intubation. Also, they are at risk for airway compromise both during and after the procedure. Some who met extubation criteria in the operating room require reintubation in the postanesthesia care unit (PACU), especially

those who required extensive airway manipulation or laryngeal biopsy. Patients having bronchoscopy and esophagoscopy are at risk for pneumothorax and esophageal perforation. Finally, those undergoing airway laser surgery are at risk for airway and facial burns.

A recent prospective study of complications during suspension laryngoscopy concluded that this was a relatively safe procedure because no life-threatening complications occurred in 339 consecutive patients. The most common complications were minor mucosal injuries (75% of patients), dental injuries (6.5%), and injuries to the lingual (2.6%) or hypoglossal (1.1%) nerve.

Recognition

Diligent monitoring is required to diagnose early hemodynamic or ECG changes before irreversible myocardial injury occurs. In most cases, such changes appear minutes after the surgeon exposes and suspends the larynx. Constant vigilance is also required to diagnose airway compromise perioperatively. Maximal laryngeal edema occurs 1 hour after extubation, so patients must be closely observed in the PACU during that period.

Risk Assessment

The patient's physical status influences the incidence of complications. In particular, patients with preoperative cardiovascular disease are at increased risk for cardiac complications during laryngoscopy and microlaryngoscopy. Further, hypoxia and hypercarbia make the heart more susceptible to insult, as does the presence of excess endogenous catecholamines.

Some patients are at high risk for airway complications. Risk factors include a history of chronic pulmonary disease, smoking, radiation therapy, and previous head and neck surgery. Other risk factors are the presence of an advanced tumor involving the upper airway, extensive surgical airway

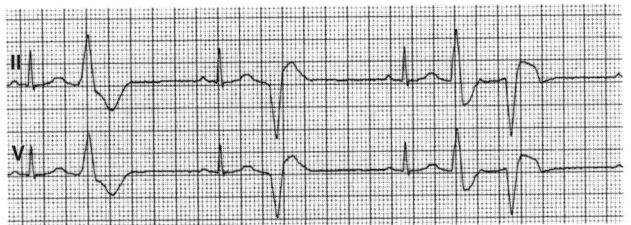

Figure 187–1 ■ Intraoperative electrocardiogram (leads II and V). Note the frequent premature ventricular contractions (beats).

manipulation, and laryngeal biopsy, any of which can increase bloody secretions.

Patients undergoing airway laser surgery are at greatest risk for airway and facial burns when the laser is exposed to flammable inhaled gases or materials (e.g., oxygen, nitrous oxide, nonmetallic endotracheal tubes; see Chapters 138 and 139).

Implications

Hypertension and arrhythmias occurring in response to laryngoscopy are often transitory and are usually without sequelae. In some patients, however, these changes persist and can be associated with myocardial ischemia, myocardial infarction, and even death. Airway compromise can result in hypoxia, hypercarbia, pulmonary edema, respiratory arrest, and death. Laser-related complications can result in burns, airway obstruction, pulmonary injury, and death.

MANAGEMENT

Cardiovascular Complications

When hypertension or arrhythmias occur during suspension laryngoscopy, ask the surgeon to release the laryngoscope pressure for a few minutes. During that time, anesthesia can be deepened and adequate oxygenation and ventilation confirmed. Antiarrhythmic drugs (e.g., lidocaine, atropine, β-blocker) may be indicated, but only if arrhythmias persist and are associated with circulatory insufficiency (see Chapter 79). If cardiovascular complications persist, consider terminating the procedure and rescheduling it, at which time preoperative superior laryngeal nerve blocks can be placed as a preemptive measure. Also, a postoperative 12-lead ECG should be obtained, along with evaluation by a cardiologist, if indicated. This cardiac evaluation can take place outside the hospital or ambulatory surgery PACU. If there are new or previously undiscovered but relevant cardiovascular findings, these must be addressed before the rescheduled procedure.

Airway Complications

If a difficult intubation is encountered unexpectedly, follow the American Society of Anesthesiologists algorithm for difficult intubation (see Chapters 40 and 41). At times, establishing a surgical airway can be lifesaving. All patients require supplemental oxygen in the recovery room, and close monitoring is essential for at least 1 hour. Patients with postoperative stridor should be treated with racemic epinephrine and steroids. The surgeon must be notified if a patient shows signs of airway compromise. An emergency tracheotomy setup must be available, and some patients require tracheal reintubation. The need for this is usually apparent within 1 hour of extubation. Supportive care is continued as necessary.

Laser Airway Fire

A laser airway fire is managed according to the following protocol:

- Discontinue oxygen and extubate the patient.
- Douse any flames with saline or water.

- Ventilate the patient by mask before reintubation for bronchoscopy.
- Use bronchoscopy to assess the extent of airway injury.
- Admit the patient to an intensive care unit for observation and supportive care.

PREVENTION

Cardiovascular Complications

The risk of cardiovascular complications can be minimized by ensuring adequate oxygenation and ventilation at all times. The patient must be well anesthetized before surgical manipulation. Small doses of a narcotic (e.g., 1 to 2 μg/kg fentanyl) may attenuate circulatory responses to microlaryngoscopy. Lidocaine and β-blockers may offer some benefit. Pediatric patients are often pretreated with anticholinergics. Consideration should be given to preoperative placement of a superior laryngeal nerve block in high-risk patients. Surgical manipulations should be as gentle as possible, and the procedure should be abandoned if refractory cardiac complications occur.

Airway Complications

The risk of airway complications can also be minimized. The surgeon must be present in the operating room during the induction of anesthesia. Awake intubation should be performed on patients with suspected difficult airways. Glycopyrrolate is administered as a drying agent to improve surgical exposure and thereby limit airway manipulation. Steroids (e.g., 10 mg intravenous dexamethasone) are administered intraoperatively to limit edema formation. Obstructive airway tumors are debulked. In some patients, a tracheotomy may have to be performed. Patients are extubated awake and observed closely in the PACU for at least 1 hour. Again, a tracheotomy set should be readily available. Vigilance throughout the perioperative period is extremely important.

Laser Airway Fire

Several precautions may help prevent laser airway fires. The patient and operating room personnel must wear eye protection. Areas of tissue that might come into contact with the carbon dioxide laser beam (e.g., eyes, skin) are covered with moist pads or towels. Anesthesia can be administered without an endotracheal tube (e.g., jet ventilation). Nonmetal endotracheal tubes are combustible and can ignite, but special metal laser endotracheal tubes are available and safe. The endotracheal tube cuff is filled with saline and surrounded by moist cottonoids. Ideally, the inspired oxygen concentration is kept at or below 30%, and nitrous oxide is avoided. Either air (nitrogen) or helium can be mixed with the oxygen. The laser should be used with the minimum required power. Muscle relaxants are often used to prevent patient movement during use of the laser.

Further Reading

Hendrix RA, Ferouz A, Bacon CK: Admission, planning and complications of direct laryngoscopy. Otolaryngol Head Neck Surg 110:510-516, 1994.

Hill RS, Koltai PJ, Parnes SM: Airway complications from laryngoscopy and panendoscopy. Ann Otol Rhinol Laryngol 96:691-694, 1987.

Klussmann JP, Knoedgen R, Wittekindt C, et al: Complications of suspension laryngoscopy. Ann Otol Rhinol Laryngol 111:972-976, 2002.

Sosis M: Anesthesia for laser surgery. Int Anesth Clin 28:119-131, 1990.

Strong MS, Vaughan CW, Mahler DL, et al: Cardiac complications of microsurgery of the larynx: Etiology, incidence and prevention. Laryngoscope 84:908-920, 1974.

Wenig BL, Raphael N, Stern JR, et al: Cardiac complications of suspension laryngoscopy: Fact or fiction? Arch Otolaryngol Head Neck Surg 112:860-862, 1986.

Werkhaven JA: Microlaryngoscopy-airway management with anaesthetic techniques for CO_2 laser. Pediatr Anesth 14:90-94, 2004.

Foreign Body Aspiration

188

Scott Holliday and Mary Ann Gurkowski

Case Synopsis

A 5-year-old girl was eating a candy bar containing peanuts when she began to choke. The mother firmly patted the child on the back, and she stopped choking. The next day the mother noted that the child's breathing was fast and noisy. Her temperature was 100.8°F, and she had an unremitting cough.

PROBLEM ANALYSIS

Definition

Foreign body aspiration (FBA) is the introduction of solid matter into the airway at the level of the glottal opening, larynx, trachea, or bronchi. Complications associated with FBA can be either immediate or delayed. Immediate complications usually occur when the foreign body becomes lodged in the glottal opening, larynx, or trachea, partially or completely obstructing the movement of air to both lungs. Immediate complications include respiratory arrest, negative-pressure pulmonary edema, pneumothorax, pneumomediastinum, subcutaneous emphysema, hypoxic neurologic damage, and cardiac arrest. Delayed complications usually occur when the foreign body lodges in one of the main or distal bronchi, obstructing airflow to the lung distal to the blockage (Fig. 188-1). Delayed complications include recurrent pneumonia, bronchiectasis, and pyelopneumothorax.

Recognition

FBA can occur in any age group, but it occurs most commonly in children younger than 4 years, with those younger than 1 year accounting for the greatest percentage. In these young children, the most common foreign bodies apirated are food particles, such as vegetable matter (e.g., peanuts, sunflower seeds, other nuts). Processed food products (e.g., hot dogs, candy, gum), metallic objects (e.g., coins, jacks, pins), and plastic products (e.g., beads, small toy parts) constitute the majority of the remaining foreign bodies aspirated.

The most recent national mortality data for choking in children (aged 14 years and younger) are from the year 2000. It was reported that 41% of deaths were from food matter, and 59% from other materials. The most recent data on unintentional, nonfatal choking episodes are from the U.S. Consumer Product Safety Commission, published in 2001. These data verified earlier data that in children younger than 14 years, food items (68.6%) were a more common cause of nonfatal choking than were nonfood items (31.4%).

In adults, FBA is more common in older persons. Organic materials (e.g., fish bones, meat), medications (e.g., pills), and inorganic objects (e.g., artificial teeth) have all been reported. In adults, the occurrence of sudden death at restaurants caused by the aspiration of food was frequent enough that an article appeared in *JAMA* in the 1960s that coined the term "café coronary."

The type, size, shape, and location of the foreign body and the duration of time before FBA is diagnosed determine the clinical expression. A foreign body can migrate distally, which alters the signs, symptoms, and radiographic and clinical findings. Partial obstruction of a bronchus creates unilateral air trapping (emphysema) by means of a ball-valve mechanism, whereas complete obstruction causes atelectasis.

The most commonly used diagnostic tools are the clinical history, physical examination, chest fluoroscopy, and plain, forced-expiratory, inspiratory-expiratory, and lateral neck films. The chest radiograph may be normal if the recently aspirated article is radiolucent. Consequently, a positive clinical history is often the most useful tool for diagnosing FBA.

FBA symptoms include choking, irritative cough, shortness of breath, aphony, hoarseness, hemoptysis, and odynophagia or dysphagia. Clinical signs include reduced breath sounds on lung auscultation and dullness to percussion, cyanosis, wheezing, dyspnea, fever, rales, stridor, and subcutaneous emphysema. A conscious adult may use the universal distress signal for choking—grabbing the neck with one hand—when a foreign body has been aspirated and prevents vocalization.

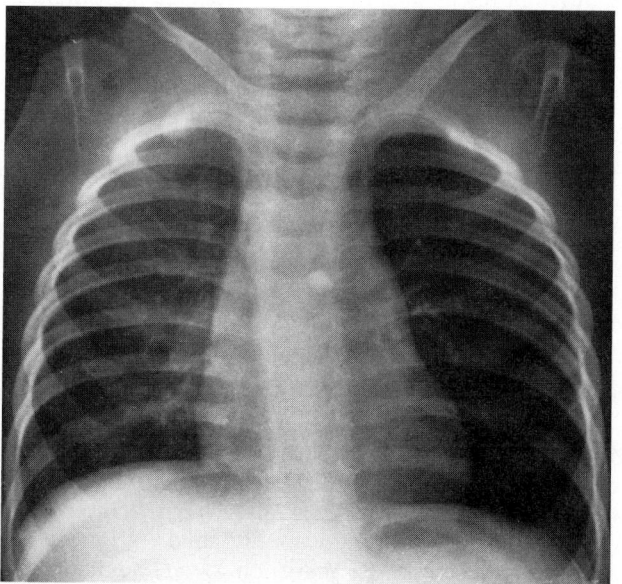

Figure 188–1 ■ Tooth in the left mainstem bronchus.

Risk Assessment

As noted earlier, the incidence of FBA is greater in children than in adults. In 2001 the Centers for Disease Control and Prevention analyzed data from the National Electronic Injury Surveillance System—All Injury Program and reported that an estimated 17,537 children (aged 14 years or younger) were treated for choking-related episodes. The high rate of FBA among children was attributed to their tendency to put inappropriate foods and small objects (e.g., coins, toys) in their mouths. Also, children often run, laugh, and play while eating or holding objects in their mouths. Of nonfood objects, coins are the most common ones aspirated. There is also a gender difference, with a slightly higher incidence in males (50% to 60%) than in females. Both adults and children who do not adequately chew their food are at increased risk. Reports have cited aspiration of food as being the sixth most common cause of accidental deaths in all age groups, causing from 2500 to 3900 deaths per year in the United States.

It has been hypothesized that children are at greater risk than adults for FBA because of the immaturity of the mechanisms that coordinate swallowing and respiration. Such coordination relies on a complex neuromuscular mechanism to ensure laryngeal closure during chewing and swallowing. This, as well as the neural control mechanisms for laryngeal closure, appear to be more efficient in adults than in young children. It has also been speculated that vegetable matter (e.g., peanuts, seeds) is so frequently aspirated because it can "float" over the laryngeal vestibule; it is thus likely to be aspirated on inspiration. In contrast, candies tend to adhere to the pharyngeal mucosa and pass into the esophagus more easily.

Adults with a preexisting dysfunctional swallowing mechanism, such as stroke victims or those with nervous system degeneration (e.g., amyotrophic lateral sclerosis), have an increased risk of food aspiration.

Implications

FBA carries a significant degree of morbidity and mortality. The latter is usually immediate due to sudden respiratory arrest, followed by cardiac arrest. Delayed mortality is not common but may result when the initial hypoxic insult leads to brain death or from an associated pulmonary infection, respiratory distress, and sepsis. Morbidity is more common than mortality and includes complications related to bronchoscopy to diagnose and remove the object, prolonged hospital stay, and need for surgical intervention. Further, delayed diagnosis can lead to prolonged treatment for non-resolved pneumonia or problems such as hemoptysis, pyelopneumothorax, or bronchiectasis.

MANAGEMENT

Management for out-of-hospital FBA involves immediate remedial treatment for the choking victim. Recommended protocols have been developed by the American Heart Association.

Choking Infants

If the infant is conscious:

1. Place the infant prone, resting on the rescuer's forearm. Support the infant's head by holding the jaw.
2. Use the heel of the hand to deliver five back blows between the shoulder blades.
3. Place the free hand and forearm on the infant's back. Support the head and neck. Turn the infant supine.
4. With the infant supine, draped on the thigh, deliver five quick, downward chest thrusts, using two fingers placed one fingerbreadth below the nipple line.
5. Repeat the process until the object is expelled or the infant becomes unconscious.

If the infant is unconscious:

1. Open the airway. Lift the chin using a tongue-jaw lift. Remove the foreign body only if it is visible in the mouth.
2. Attempt rescue breathing. If unsuccessful, reposition the head and reattempt ventilation.
3. If unable to ventilate, give five back blows and chest thrusts. Repeat steps 1, 2, and 3.
4. After approximately 1 minute, notify emergency medical services and resume efforts.

Choking Child or Adult

If the person is conscious, with poor or no air exchange:

1. Apply the Heimlich maneuver (subcostal, upward abdominal thrusts) while the victim is standing or sitting.
2. Continue abdominal thrusts until the foreign body is expelled or the patient loses consciousness.

If the person is unconscious:

1. Place the victim supine, and open the airway using a tongue-jaw lift. If the foreign body is visible, remove the object with a finger sweep.
2. Attempt rescue breathing. If unsuccessful, reposition the head and reattempt ventilation.
3. If there is no ventilation, kneel beside or straddle the hips of the victim. Place the heel of one hand on the abdomen above the navel and below the xiphoid process. Place the other hand on top of the first hand.
4. Press both hands into the abdomen with a quick upward thrust five times.
5. Open the airway with a tongue-jaw lift. If the foreign body is visible, remove it. If not, repeat steps 2 through 4 until ventilation is successful.
6. After approximately 1 minute, notify emergency medical services and resume efforts.

Once in the hospital, if the foreign body lies in the supraglottic or glottic region, immediate removal is necessary to prevent total airway occlusion. In both adults and children, this is usually performed under general anesthesia with laryngoscopy or bronchoscopy. For adults, intravenous access is placed before induction. In children, intravenous access is established after induction to avoid agitating the child, which could dislodge the foreign body, creating total airway obstruction and respiratory arrest.

The most common method for induction of anesthesia in both adults and children with FBA is inhalational induction with spontaneous ventilation. Positive-pressure ventilation poses a risk for dislodging the object, again creating the potential for complete airway obstruction. However, one retrospective case review suggested that even though this risk was present, there was no difference in morbidity between positive-pressure ventilation and spontaneous ventilation.

The removal of a foreign body lodged in a bronchus usually requires urgent surgery. This involves nothing-by-mouth status, prophylaxis for aspiration, and intravenous line placement. The urgency is greater if the object is more proximal than distal. Theoretically, in the former circumstance, coughing could dislodge the object and move it to the carina, where it has the potential to obstruct both mainstem bronchi. Most often, a rigid ventilating bronchoscope is used to remove the foreign body. Induction of anesthesia can be via either an inhalational or an intravenous technique. Nebulized racemic epinephrine may be used to decrease swelling around the object to allow easier removal. Thoracotomy and direct surgical removal may also be necessary.

Postoperatively, depending on the location of the object and the duration of aspiration, racemic epinephrine, bronchodilators, antibiotics, steroids, and chest physiotherapy may be indicated. Postoperative hospitalization for monitoring is prudent.

PREVENTION

The majority of FBA cases are preventable in both children and adults. The key to prevention in children is public education. Parents, caretakers, and manufacturers or suppliers of food and food products must be more aware of the causes of choking. With the development of federal consumer product safety standards regulating the minimum size of toys and toy parts for young children and product safety labeling, the incidence of FBA has decreased. The home is now the most common site for such occurrences. Vigilance on the part of those caring for children is important, as are methods of making the home environment safer. For example, children must be taught not to put things in their mouths and never to eat and run at the same time. Proper chewing habits for both children and adults can help prevent aspiration of large chunks of food. Finally, parents and caregivers should take courses to learn how to provide basic life support in the event that a choking episode occurs.

Further Reading

Black RE, Johnson DG, Matlak ME: Bronchoscopic removal of aspirated foreign bodies in children. J Pediatr Surg 29:682-684, 1994.

Centers for Disease Control and Prevention: Nonfatal choking-related episodes among children—United States, 2001. JAMA 288:2400-2402, 2002.

Emergency Cardiac Care Committee and Subcommittees: American Heart Association guidelines for cardiopulmonary resuscitation and emergency cardiac care. II. Adult basic life support JAMA 268:2191-2194, 1992.

Emergency Cardiac Care Committee and Subcommittees: American Heart Association guidelines for cardiopulmonary resuscitation and emergency cardiac care: V, VI, VII. JAMA 268:2251-2281, 1992.

Gurkowski MA: Foreign body aspiration. In Bready LL, Mullins R, Noorily SH, et al (eds): Decision Making in Anesthesiology, 4th ed. Philadelphia, BC Decker (in press).

Hoeve LJ, Rombout J, Pot DJ: Foreign body aspiration in children: The diagnostic value of signs, symptoms and pre-operative examination. Clin Otolaryngol 18:55-57, 1993.

Litman RS, Ponnuri J, Trogan I: Anesthesia for tracheal or bronchial foreign body removal in children: An analysis of ninety-four cases. Anesth Analg 91:1389-1391, 2000.

Reilly JS: Airway foreign bodies: Update and analysis. Int Anesth Clin 30:49-55, 1992.

Schwartz AJ, Campbell FW: Cardiopulmonary resuscitation. In Barash PG, Cullen BF, Stoelting RK (eds): Clinical Anesthesia, 2nd ed. Philadelphia, JB Lippincott, 1992, pp 1633-1642.

Tan HKK, Tan SS: Inhaled foreign bodies in children—anaesthetic considerations. Singapore Med J 41:506-510, 2000.

Wolach B, Raz A, Weinberg J, et al: Aspirated foreign bodies in the respiratory tract of children: Eleven years' experience with 127 patients. Int J Pediatr Otorhinolaryngol 30:1-10, 1994.

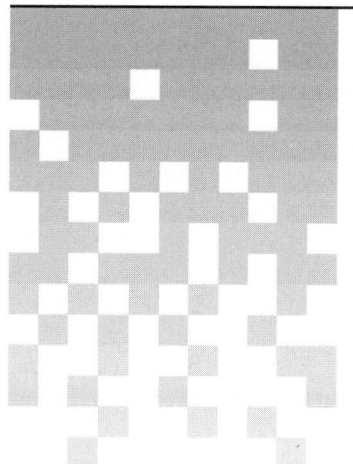

Other Surgical Subspecialties

Brenda A. Bucklin

Terri G. Monk

Kerri M. Robertson

Hypertensive Disorders of Pregnancy

189

Curtis L. Baysinger

Case Synopsis

A 27-year-old woman, gravida 1, presents with 4 cm cervical dilatation and a fetus whose estimated gestational age is 38 weeks. Her blood pressure is 160/110 mm Hg; and she has 4+ patellar reflexes, right upper quadrant tenderness, and 4+ proteinuria. Her platelet count on admission was 145,000/mm^3 but has decreased to 110,000/mm^3. She is receiving 1 g/hour of intravenous magnesium sulfate (MgSO$_4$) and oxytocin (Pitocin) augmentation. She and her obstetrician have requested epidural analgesia for labor.

PROBLEM ANALYSIS

Definition

The American College of Obstetricians and Gynecologists recognizes four categories of hypertension associated with pregnancy (Table 189-1): gestational hypertension, preeclampsia, eclampsia, and chronic hypertension. Gestational hypertension occurs in 6% to 17% of pregnancies, and 50% of women with gestational hypertension before 30 weeks of pregnancy develop preeclampsia. Preeclampsia presents after 20 weeks' gestation, can be either mild or severe, and is diagnosed by hypertension with proteinuria (Table 189-2). It can also be associated with coagulopathies and liver dysfunction. Edema is no longer a diagnostic criterion, but it is often severe. Eclampsia is defined as the occurrence of convulsions unrelated to a preexisting neurologic disorder that occur in women who are preeclamptic. Preeclampsia superimposed on chronic hypertension or transient hypertensive disorders of unknown cause may also occur. The HELLP syndrome requires the presence of intravascular *h*emolysis, *e*levated *l*iver enzymes, and *l*ow *p*latelet count; it usually manifests earlier during pregnancy compared with other types of preeclampsia.

Table 189–1 ■ Classification of Hypertensive Disorders in Pregnancy

Gestational hypertension
Preeclampsia
    Mild
    Severe
Eclampsia
Chronic hypertension with or without superimposed
    preeclampsia or eclampsia

Recognition

Preeclampsia becomes severe with blood pressure greater than 160/100 mm Hg and evidence of end-organ damage, including the following:

- Pulmonary edema
- Renal dysfunction—proteinuria of 4+ on dipstick testing or greater than 5 g in a 24-hour urine collection, or oliguria (<500 mL in 24 hours)
- Cerebral manifestations, including headache, visual changes, or seizures (eclampsia)
- Elevated liver enzymes with right upper quadrant pain (secondary to hepatic capsular distention)
- Severe thrombocytopenia, with a platelet count less than 100,000/mm^3

The last in association with the HELLP syndrome may occur with modest levels of blood pressure elevation. Also, parturients with acute cocaine intoxication may present with signs and symptoms of preeclampsia, including seizures, pulmonary edema, proteinuria, and thrombocytopenia.

Risk Assessment

Preeclampsia occurs in 3% to 7.5% of all pregnancies, primarily in young primigravidas, and especially in those who do not receive prenatal care. It accounts for 20% of all maternal deaths. Maternal and neonatal morbidity increases with maternal age, gestational age of onset (especially when preeclampsia develops before 32 weeks' gestation), and preexisting maternal diabetes, renal disease, or thrombophilia. The risk of preeclampsia is also increased in patients with uterine overdistention (e.g., multiple gestations, polyhydramnios), trophoblastic disease, obesity, and abnormal uterine artery Doppler studies between 18 and 24 weeks' gestation. Parturients who develop preeclampsia in the second trimester have worse outcomes compared with those who develop it after 34 weeks' gestation. These patients are also at

Table 189–2 ■ **Definition of Preeclampsia**	
Measure	**Findings**
Blood pressure (BP)	Increase in systolic or diastolic BP of 30 or 15 mm Hg, respectively Systolic, mean, or diastolic BP of 140/105/90 mm Hg taken at least 6 hr but <7 days apart
Proteinuria	300 mg in 24 hr or 1+ (30 mg/dL) on two clean dipstick tests taken at least 6 hr but <7 days apart
Edema	Fluid collection in nondependent part of the body or weight gain >5 pounds in 1 wk

greater risk for chronic hypertension and underlying renal disease or collagen vascular disease. Headache, visual disturbances, epigastric pain, severe refractory hypertension, progressive thrombocytopenia or liver function abnormalities, oliguria, and a poor fetal environment (determined by nonstress testing or biophysical profile, with estimated fetal weight below the 5th percentile) are ominous signs.

Currently, there is no single cost-effective screening test that reliably predicts preeclampsia. Early in pregnancy, the vasculature becomes more sensitive to vasoconstrictors, perhaps owing to abnormally high levels of thromboxane compared with prostacyclin. Normal increases in renin, angiotensin II, and aldosterone, with reduced vascular sensitivity to catecholamines, fail to develop in patients with preeclampsia. This may be explained by endothelial cell injury, which reduces the synthesis of prostacyclin and nitric oxide. Plasma fibronectin levels, an indicator of endothelial damage, become elevated early in gestation in those who develop preeclampsia. The generalized pathophysiology suggests widespread endothelial damage in the face of general vasoconstriction. This is believed to cause end-organ damage and activation of the coagaulation system, including consumption of coagulation factors and platelets. Edema is attributed to salt and water retention, which is aggravated by decreased colloid osmotic pressure in the presence of proteinuria. Blood volume is reduced in most patients with preeclampsia compared with normotensive parturients. Sympathetic system activation most often leads to a hyperdynamic state in patients with severe preeclampsia, with increased cardiac output and normal to slightly increased systemic vascular resistance. However, pulmonary artery catheter studies have revealed a subset of patients with reduced blood volume, depressed left ventricular function, and markedly increased systemic vascular resistance.

Implications

Edema of the airway, including the larynx, may occur. The risk of pulmonary edema is greatest after delivery, when colloid osmotic pressure is lowest.

Thrombocytopenia secondary to consumptive coagulopathy occurs in 11% to 50% of patients with severe preeclampsia. Reduction in the platelet count to less than $100,000/mm^3$ is associated with other coagulation abnormalities and occurs more often with the HELLP syndrome. Intrinsic platelet dysfunction may also occur.

Oliguria may result from low cardiac filling pressures and often responds well to fluid challenge. Less often, oliguria is associated with depressed cardiac function and very high systemic vascular resistance. If so, afterload reduction is the treatment of choice.

Uteroplacental blood flow decreases as a result of uterine artery vasospasm. Exaggerated reductions in uteroplacental blood flow may occur when vasopressors are used to treat hypotension, which may accompany the onset of regional blockade.

MANAGEMENT

Obstetric Management

Obstetric management includes judicious fetal delivery, prevention of eclampsia (seizures), fluid status optimization, and treatment of excessive increases in blood pressure (especially diastolic blood pressure >110 mm Hg). Delivery is indicated in mild preeclampsia with a gestational age greater than 37 weeks, fetal lung maturity, a favorable cervix, and increasing maternal blood pressure. Delivery is mandatory if hypertension is uncontrolled after 24 to 48 hours of therapy or with progressive renal dysfunction or thrombocytopenia, fetal stress, impending eclampsia, liver function values twice the upper limit of normal, or cardiopulmonary compromise. If possible, delivery is delayed for 48 hours after glucocorticoid administration to accelerate fetal lung maturity. With a preterm fetus, expectant management is safe if the blood pressure is well controlled, laboratory parameters stabilize, and the fetal environment is reassuring.

Several studies have documented the effectiveness of $MgSO_4$ for the prevention of seizures. For example, the British Eclampsia Trial Collaborative Group study found a 52% reduction in seizure activity with $MgSO_4$. In this trial, $MgSO_4$ was superior to diazepam or phenytoin for seizure prevention, although the use of phenytoin continues outside the United States.

$MgSO_4$ does not appear to alter the duration of labor or maternal coagulability or significantly affect uterine blood flow in parturients with epidural blockade. It is given as a 4- to 6-g bolus, with an infusion of 1 to 2 g/hour. Magnesium serum levels are checked every 8 hours to ensure therapeutic concentrations of 4 to 7 mg/dL. Loss of deep tendon reflexes precedes respiratory compromise with $MgSO_4$ toxicity (see also Chapter 15).

$MgSO_4$ is ineffective as an antihypertensive agent because its vasodilatory effects are weak and transient. Instead, intravenous hydralazine is the more traditional therapy for hypertension during pregnancy, at a dose of 5 to 10 mg every 15 minutes. One recent study suggests that intravenous labetalol or oral nifedipine is as effective as hydralazine and has fewer side effects. Labetalol given incrementally to a cumulative dose of 0.5 to 1 mg/kg has no significant effects on neonatal heart rate or uterine blood flow. Dihydropyridine calcium channel blockers (e.g., nicardipine, nifedipine) also appear to be effective, with little or no effect on labor and neonatal outcome. However, they have the potential to produce untoward hypotension if used in patients also receiving MgSO$_4$.

Anesthetic Management

LABOR AND VAGINAL DELIVERY

Epidural analgesia provides superior pain relief and also has beneficial effects on placental blood flow. It can rapidly be converted to anesthesia for emergent cesarean delivery. Judicious volume loading and incremental dosing of local anesthetics reduce the risk of significant hypotension.

Thrombocytopenia occurs in 15% to 20% of patients with severe preeclampsia. One should obtain a platelet count before performing regional anesthesia. Acute-onset thrombocytopenia is more ominous than the chronic variety. However, specific platelet count values that increase the risk for epidural hematoma are unknown. Platelet activity may be abnormal in severe preeclamptics with counts less than 100,000/mm^3. Therefore, it is prudent to consider tests for platelet activity (platelet function analysis, thromboelastography) when the platelet count is less than 100,000/mm^3, especially in patients with the HELLP syndrome. Again, the degree of abnormality that increases the risk for untoward events (e.g., central neurologic sequelae due to bleeding) is unknown. One retrospective study suggests that platelet counts less than 75,000/mm^3 are relatively insensitive for untoward events but more specific for prolonged bleeding times. Therefore, in patients with thrombocytopenia one should consider the risk of epidural block versus the benefits of epidural analgesia, including pain relief, salutary blood pressure effects, and the ability to expeditiously convert analgesic to anesthetic blocks for cesarean delivery. It seems prudent to place epidural catheters early in labor, before platelet counts fall below 100,000/mm^3.

CESAREAN DELIVERY

If general anesthesia is used for cesarean delivery, airway edema may make endotracheal intubation difficult. A variety of small endotracheal tubes should be available, and management of a difficult airway should be anticipated.

Measures to reduce the blood pressure increase accompanying tracheal intubation or light anesthesia should be available. Sodium nitroprusside (SNP) is effective but must be titrated carefully owing to the potential for severe hypotension; SNP affects both preload and afterload, and patients with eclampsia (like any hypertensive patient) are preload restricted. Direct arterial pressure monitoring is usually required when using SNP. Similarly, the effects of nitroglycerin are unpredictable (it is a primary venodilator, with a consequent drop in preload). Labetalol may be the drug of choice. It has a slower onset of action, is longer acting, and is administered incrementally up to a total intravenous dose

of 1 mg/kg.[1] Intravenous nicardipine (15 to 30 µg/kg) may also be effective. Because it is arterioselective (i.e., has no effect on venous capacitance or preload), nicardipine is less likely to produce rapid declines in blood pressure compared with SNP or nitroglycerin. Finally, at least one report suggests that an intravenous bolus of MgSO$_4$ (30 to 45 mg/kg) given immediately after anesthesia induction is also effective. However, MgSO$_4$ has the potential to augment the effects of nondepolarizing muscle relaxants; cause uterine relaxation, increasing the need for postpartum oxytocin; and increase the risk of uterine atony and postpartum hemorrhage.

Spinal (subarachnoid) block has been used safely in severely preeclamptic patients after judicious volume loading. Recent evidence-based reviews and prospective cohort studies comparing subarachnoid and epidural blocks in severely preeclamptic patients show that blood pressure effects and the need for vasopressors are similar or better with subarachnoid blocks. However, subarachnoid block for cesarean delivery is associated with statistically greater (but probably clinically insignificant) neonatal umbilical artery base deficit and lower pH values versus parturients who receive general anesthesia.

The smaller needles used for subarachnoid block convey less risk of spinal hematoma than the larger needles used for epidural anesthesia. However, epidural anesthesia with judicious incremental dosing may reduce the volume of fluid administration and the need for vasopressors. Combined spinal-epidural anesthesia with hyperbaric bupivacaine (7.5 mg) with fentanyl (25 µg) may offer the advantage of rapid onset, with the ability to extend the anesthetic level and duration of block, if necessary. Furthermore, it may reduce the risk of adverse hemodynamic changes compared with subarachnoid block with higher doses of local anesthetic.

The use of vasopressor-containing local anesthetic solutions is controversial. Some studies advocate their safety, but severe hypertension after their use has been reported.

PREVENTION

Therapy with MgSO$_4$ reduces the risk of neonatal intraventricular hemorrhage in preterm infants of preeclamptic mothers. There is no evidence that colloid is preferable to crystalloid for volume expansion; in fact, colloid for this purpose has been reported to increase maternal mortality. Antepartum dexamethasone increases the platelet count, which allows the use of regional analgesia or anesthesia in some patients with the HELLP syndrome.

Pulmonary artery pressure monitoring does not appear to improve maternal outcome and in most cases is not needed for the management of preeclampsia. Young and Johanson reviewed routine pulmonary artery pressure monitoring in severely preeclamptic patients and concluded that the data provided by such monitoring did not alter clinical management. Nonetheless, patients with cardiopulmonary compromise or other indications should be considered for

---

[1]This bolus dose of intravenous labetalol is very high. With such doses, α-adrenergic blocking effects are expected to be more prominent, with β-blocking effects near the maximum.

Table 189–3 ▪ Indications for Pulmonary Artery Catheter Monitoring in Patients with Preeclampsia
Pulmonary edema
Congestive heart failure
Low urinary output despite adequate fluid challenges or normal central venous pressure
Concomitant maternal disease
Amniotic fluid embolism
Valvular heart disease
Congenital heart disease
Peripartum cardiomyopathy
New York Heart Association class III or IV myocardial function

pulmonary artery pressure monitoring (Table 189-3). Alone, central venous pressure monitoring may not be helpful. Indeed, central venous pressure–to–pulmonary capillary wedge pressure gradients can vary by as much as 10 mm Hg in severe preeclampsia.

Further Reading

Allen RW, James MFM, Uys PC: Attenuation of the pressor response to tracheal intubation in hypertensive proteinuric pregnant patients by lignocaine, alfentanil, and magnesium sulphate. Br J Anaesth 66:216-223, 1991.

American College of Obstetricians and Gynecologists: Diagnosis and management of preeclampsia and eclampsia. Obstet Gynecol 99:159-167, 2002.

Aya AGM, Mangin R, Hoffet M, Eledjam JJ: Intravenous nicardipine for severe hypertension in preeclampsia: Effects of an acute treatment on mother and foetus. Intensive Care Med 25:1277-1281, 1999.

Aya AGM, Mangin R, Vialles N, et al: Patients with severe preeclampsia experience less hypotension during spinal anesthesia for elective cesarean section than healthy parturients: A prospective cohort comparison. Anesth Analg 97:867-872, 2003.

Beilin Y, Zahn J, Comerford M: Safe epidural analgesia in thirty parturients with platelet counts between 69,000 and 98,000. Anesth Analg 85:385-388, 1997.

Brimacombe J: Acute pharyngolaryngeal oedema and preeclamptic toxaemia. Anaesth Intensive Care 20:97-98, 1992.

Cotton DB, Lee W, Huhta JC, Dorman KF: Hemodynamic profile of severe pregnancy-induced hypertension. Am J Obstet Gynecol 158:523-529, 1988.

Cunningham FG, Gant NF, Levine LJ, et al: Hypertensive disorders in pregnancy. In Cunningham FG, Gant NF, Leveno KJ, et al (eds): Williams Obstetrics, 21st ed. New York, McGraw-Hill, 2001, pp 567-618.

deJong CL, Dekker GA, Sibai BM: The renin-angiotensin-aldosterone system in preeclampsia: A review. Clin Perinatol 18:683-711, 1991.

Dekker GA, Sibai BM: Pathogenesis and etiology of preeclampsia. Am J Obstet Gynecol 179:1359-1375, 1998.

Dyer RA, Els I, Farbas J, et al: Prospective, randomized trial comparing general with spinal anesthesia for cesarean delivery in preeclamptic patients with a nonreassuring fetal heart trace. Anesthesiology 99:561-569, 2003.

Eclampsia Trial Collaborative Group: Which anticonvulsant for women with preeclampsia? Evidence from the Collaborative Eclampsia Trial. Lancet 345:1455-1563, 1995.

Fawcett WJ, Haxby E, Male DA: Magnesium: Physiology and pharmacology. Br J Anaesth 83:302-320, 1999.

Gambling DR: Hypertensive disorders. In Chestnut DH (ed): Obstetric Anesthesia: Principles and Practice, 3rd ed. Philadelphia, Mosby, 2004, pp 794-835.

Harnett MJP, Datta S, Bhavani-Shankar K: The effect of magnesium on coagulation in parturients with preeclampsia. Anesth Analg 92:1257-1260, 2001.

Hood D, Curry R: Spinal versus epidural anesthesia for cesarean section in severely preeclamptic patients: A retrospective study. Anesthesiology 90:1276-1282, 1999.

Hood D, Dewan D, James FI, et al: The use of nitroglycerin in preventing the hypertensive response to tracheal intubation in severe preeclampsia. Anesthesiology 63:329-332, 1985.

Jouppila P, Jouppila R, Hollmen A, Koivula A: Lumbar epidural analgesia to improve intervillous blood flow during labor in severe preeclampsia. Obstet Gynecol 59:158-167, 1982.

Leduc L, Wheeler JM, Kirshon B, et al: Coagulation profile in severe preeclampsia. Obstet Gynecol 79:14-18, 1998.

Lewis R, Sibai BM: Recent advances in the management of preeclampsia. J Matern Fetal Med 6:6-15, 1997.

McDonagh RJ, Ray JG, Burrows RF, et al: Platelet count may predict abnormal bleeding time among pregnant women with hypertension and preeclampsia. Can J Anaesth 48:563-569, 2001.

Moore TR, Key TC, Reisner LS, et al: Evaluation of the use of continuous lumbar epidural anesthesia for hypertensive pregnant women in labor. Am J Obstet Gynecol 152:404-411, 1985.

Morgan MA, Silavin SL, Dormer KJ, et al: Effects of labetalol on uterine blood flow and cardiovascular hemodynamics in the hypertensive gravid baboon. Am J Obstet Gynecol 168:1574-1579, 1993.

Newsome W, Bramwell RS, Cosling PE: Severe preeclampsia: Hemodynamic effects of lumbar epidural anesthesia. Anesth Analg 65:31-36, 1986.

Ramanathan J, Bennett K: Preeclampsia: Fluids, drugs and anesthetic management. Anesthesiol Clin North Am 21:145-163, 2003.

Ramanathan J, Vaddadi A, Areheart KL: Combined spinal-epidural anesthesia with low doses of intrathecal bupivacaine in women with severe preeclampsia. Reg Anesth Pain Med 26:46-51, 2001.

Rasmus KT, Rottman RL, Kotelko DM, et al: Unrecognized thrombocytopenia and regional anesthesia in parturients: A retrospective review. Obstet Gynecol 73:943-946, 1989.

Saleh AA, Bottoms SF, Welch RA, et al: Markers for endothelial injury, clotting, and platelet activation in preeclampsia. Arch Gynecol Obstet 251:105-110, 1992.

Sibai BM: Prevention of preeclampsia: A big disappointment. Int J Obstet Gynecol 179:1275-1278, 1998.

Sibai BM: Diagnosis and management of gestational hypertension and preeclampsia. Obstet Gynecol 102:181-192, 2003.

Sibai BM: Diagnosis, controversies, and management of the syndrome of hemolysis, elevated liver enzymes, and low platelet count. Obstet Gynecol 103:981-991, 2004.

Silver HM, Seebeck M, Carlson R: Comparison of total blood volume in normal, preeclamptic, and nonproteinuric gestational hypertensive pregnancy by simultaneous measurement of red blood cell and plasma volumes. Am J Obstet Gynecol 179:87-93, 1998.

Sinatra RS, Philip BK, Naulty JS, Ostheimer GW: Prolonged neuromuscular blockade with vecuronium in a patient treated with magnesium sulfate. Anesth Analg 64:1220-1222, 1985.

Sipes SL, Chestnut DH, Vincent RD, et al: Does the intravenous infusion of ritodrine or magnesium sulfate alter the hemodynamic response to hemorrhage in gravid ewes? Am J Obstet Gynecol 159:1467-1473, 1988.

Szal S, Croughan-Minnihane MS, Kilpatrick SJ: Effect of magnesium prophylaxis and preeclampsia on the duration of labor. Am J Obstet Gynecol 180:1475-1479, 1999.

Towers CV, Person RA, Nanette MP, et al: Cocaine intoxication presenting as preeclampsia, eclampsia. Obstet Gynecol 81:545-547, 1993.

Vermillion ST, Scardo JA, Newman RB, Chauhan SP: A randomized, double-blind trial of oral nifedipine and intravenous labetalol in hypertensive emergencies of pregnancy. Am J Obstet Gynecol 181:858-861, 1999.

Vincent RD, Chestnut DH, Sipes SL, et al: Magnesium sulfate decreases maternal blood pressure but not uterine blood flow during epidural anesthesia in gravid ewes. Anesthesiology 74:77-82, 1991.

Wang Y, Walsh SW, Kay HH: Placental lipid peroxides and thromboxane are increased and prostacyclin is decreased in women with preeclampsia. Am J Obstet Gynecol 167:946-949, 1992.

Young P, Johanson R: Haeomodynamic, invasive, and echocardiographic monitoring in the hypertensive parturient. Best Pract Res Clin Obstet Gynecol 15:605-622, 2001.

Zinaman M, Rubin J, Lindheimer MD: Serial plasma oncotic pressure levels and echoencephalography during and after delivery in severe preeclampsia. Lancet 1:1245-1250, 1985.

Preterm Labor

Craig M. Palmer

Case Synopsis

A 29-year-old woman, gravida 1, presents with new-onset, regular uterine contractions and a fetus whose estimated gestational age is 28 weeks. Following intravenous hydration, she is admitted to the hospital to begin tocolytic therapy.

PROBLEM ANALYSIS

Definition

Preterm labor is defined as regular uterine contractions occurring at least once every 10 minutes and resulting in cervical dilatation or effacement before 37 weeks' gestation. A preterm infant is any infant delivered before 37 weeks' gestation. Any infant weighing less than 2.5 kg or 1.5 kg at birth is a low-birth-weight or very-low-birth-weight infant, respectively, regardless of gestational age. At 29 weeks' gestation, more than 90% of fetuses weigh less than 1.5 kg.

Prematurity is the leading cause of perinatal morbidity and mortality in the United States, accounting for 60% to 80% of infant deaths in those without congenital anomalies. Advances in neonatology have decreased mortality for very-low-birth-weight infants; survival at 23 weeks' gestation may be as high as 25%. However, such neonates usually have difficult courses following delivery. Very-low-birth-weight infants are at risk for significant morbidity from respiratory distress syndrome, necrotizing enterocolitis, and intraventricular hemorrhage, and many survivors have significant long-term neurologic impairment, chronic pulmonary problems, and visual disturbances. Delaying delivery from 23 to 31 weeks' gestation improves the neonatal survival rate from just over 25% to 96%. Thus, current obstetric practice focuses on delaying delivery in patients with preterm labor.

Recognition and Risk Assessment

The initial assessment of a patient with preterm labor consists of a thorough physical examination to eliminate treatable medical conditions that may have precipitated premature labor and a pelvic examination to rule out premature rupture of membranes. Bed rest, intravenous hydration, continuous fetal heart rate monitoring, and tocodynamometry are almost universally indicated. Bed rest and hydration alone are effective in a large number of patients, but if these conservative measures fail, ultrasonography and occasionally amniocentesis are undertaken to establish gestational age and fetal maturity (especially if there is any ambiguity with regard to these parameters).

Once the diagnosis of preterm labor is established, the obstetrician must decide whether to institute pharmacologic tocolytic therapy. This decision is based on the estimated gestational age, the fetal weight, and the presence or absence of a reassuring fetal heart rate. In general, a gestational age between 20 and 34 weeks and a fetal weight less than 2.5 kg in the presence of a reassuring fetal heart rate, without evidence of fetal distress, are indications for tocolytic therapy. However, tocolytic agents in current use have the potential to interact adversely with commonly used inhalational anesthetics and depolarizing or nondepolarizing muscle relaxants.

Implications

Prematurity may have implications for the route of delivery (vaginal versus cesarean section).

Although the processes that initiate labor are incompletely understood, much is known about the physiology of uterine contractions. The interaction of myosin and actin filaments generates contractile forces in the myometrium. Myometrial pacemaker cells initiate spontaneous contractile activity, which propagates throughout the myometrium via gap junctions between cells.

Calcium also plays a critical role. Before contraction, the intracellular calcium concentration increases due to the release of calcium from the sarcoplasmic reticulum or via sarcolemmal influx. Calcium then interacts with calmodulin, activating myosin light-chain kinase. In turn, this kinase phosphorylates myosin, which subsequently binds with actin. Adenosine triphosphate (ATP) is hydrolyzed by myosin to adenosine triphosphatase (ATPase), resulting in movement of the actin-myosin elements and myometrial contraction. A reduction in intracellular calcium concentration, or the dephosphorylation of myosin, inhibits the actin-myosin interaction, causing relaxation.

This cascade offers several opportunities for pharmacologic intervention. Activation of β_2-adrenergic receptors within the myometrium activates adenylyl cyclase, converting ATP to cyclic adenosine monophosphate (cAMP). Increased cAMP decreases intracellular calcium, inhibiting myosin light-chain kinase and decreasing contractile activity. Magnesium sulfate ($MgSO_4$) reduces uterine activity, probably by decreasing intracellular free calcium concentration through competition for binding sites. It may also activate adenylyl cyclase, increasing the synthesis of cAMP. By blocking voltage-dependent calcium channels in the cell membrane (or altering intracellular uptake and release mechanisms), calcium channel blocking agents decrease the concentration of free calcium within the myometrium. Prostaglandins $F_{2\alpha}$ and $E_{2\alpha}$ are potent stimulators of uterine activity. During labor, their concentration increases in maternal blood and amniotic fluid. The nonsteroidal anti-inflammatory agents that inhibit prostaglandin synthetase can inhibit the production of these prostaglandins.

MANAGEMENT

The most commonly used tocolytic agents are as follows:

- $MgSO_4$
- β_2-Adrenergic agonists
- Prostaglandin synthetase inhibitors
- Calcium channel blockers

No single agent is uniformly successful for tocolytic therapy, and it is difficult to compare the efficacy of these agents. Each agent possesses side effects that can further limit its usefulness.

Magnesium Sulfate

$MgSO_4$ is the intravenous tocolytic agent of choice in most centers owing to its low cost and relatively low incidence of serious side effects. At the neuromuscular junction, Mg^{2+} inhibits the release of acetylcholine and reduces the sensitivity of the postsynaptic end plate to acetylcholine.

Normal serum Mg^{2+} concentrations range from 1.3 to 2.9 mg/dL. Therapy is initiated with intravenous bolus $MgSO_4$ (4 to 6 g), followed by continuous infusion. The infusion is titrated to maintain a serum concentration of 5 to 8 mg/dL. Although these concentrations are usually sufficient to inhibit uterine activity, such therapy is not always successful. Increasing the serum concentration is usually not more effective, and this may increase side effects.

$MgSO_4$ causes peripheral vasodilatation, and parturients often experience warmth, flushing, and nausea, particularly with the onset of therapy. Maternal tachycardia and hypotension may result, but these are usually transient. At higher serum concentrations, other effects are observed. QRS complex widening and P-R interval prolongation are uncommon with Mg^{2+} concentrations less than 10 mg/dL, but such effects may be seen even at therapeutic levels. At Mg^{2+} concentrations above 12 mg/dL, deep tendon reflexes are absent. Mg^{2+} concentrations greater than 18 mg/dL can result in respiratory arrest, and those greater than 25 mg/dL may cause cardiac arrest. Although untoward fetal effects are infrequent, decreased fetal heart rate and reduced biophysical profile score have been reported. Respiratory depression, hyporeflexia, and reduced muscle tone have also been observed in neonates following prolonged maternal $MgSO_4$ therapy.

As a result of $MgSO_4$-caused vasodilatation, there is an increased potential for hypotension in these patients with neuraxial blockade. Careful attention to maternal blood pressure permits the use of either epidural or spinal anesthesia, but the slower onset of epidural blocks may make them preferable.

Parturients receiving $MgSO_4$ are more susceptible to the effects of neuromuscular relaxants if general anesthesia becomes necessary. Following the administration of succinylcholine, the train-of-four response must be closely monitored with a peripheral nerve stimulator to guide further administration of muscle relaxants. If this becomes necessary, very small doses should be used (especially with nondepolarizing muscle relaxants) because of the potential for exaggerated or prolonged effects. Finally, although Mg^{2+} at therapeutic concentrations is known to reduce the minimum alveolar concentration of halothane, this is probably not clinically significant.

β_2-Adrenergic Agonists

Both ritodrine and terbutaline are used as tocolytic agents, but only ritodrine is approved by the Food and Drug Administration for this use. Ritodrine is administered by continuous intravenous infusion and titrated in response to the uterine contraction pattern. Terbutaline is administered as a single intravenous or subcutaneous dose for prompt but temporary inhibition of uterine activity; it may be continued as oral therapy.

Although β_2-agonist activity is responsible for their tocolytic effects, both ritodrine and terbutaline have significant β_1-adrenergic effects as well, which accounts for many of the side effects. β_2-Adrenergic activity can cause vasodilatation, hypotension, and hyperglycemia. Direct β_1-adrenergic activity increases myocardial contractility and heart rate, leading to increased cardiac output, which may help offset any potential for hypotension with spinal or epidural blocks. The most significant side effects of β-agonist therapy are cardiac. Either cardiogenic or noncardiogenic pulmonary edema may occur in up to 4% of patients. Fortunately, it usually resolves with discontinuation of therapy. Myocardial ischemia has also been reported, manifesting as chest pain and electrocardiographic changes. This too resolves with discontinuation of therapy. Tachyarrhythmias (both maternal and fetal) may also occur. Finally, hyperglycemia and hypokalemia are frequently observed in these patients, but glucose levels frequently return to baseline in nondiabetic patients, and total body potassium remains unchanged.

If anesthesia is required, ideally, one should allow at least 60 to 90 minutes between the discontinuation of β_2-adrenergic agonist tocolysis and the administration of anesthesia. Unfortunately, such a delay may jeopardize the fetus. Aggressive hydration is avoided because of the risk of pulmonary edema. Aggressive vasopressor therapy is used instead to maintain maternal blood pressure.

Prostaglandin Synthetase Inhibitors

Prostaglandins $E_{2\alpha}$ and $F_{2\alpha}$ are potent stimulators of uterine activity. They also soften the cervix near term ("ripening"). Prostaglandin synthetase inhibitors prevent the conversion of arachidonic acid into active prostaglandins. Although all drugs in this class possess this capability, only indomethacin is widely used for tocolysis in preterm labor. It can be given either orally or rectally and is continued for several weeks.

In contrast to $MgSO_4$ and β-agonists, indomethacin has few maternal side effects. It may affect maternal coagulation, but this is not of major clinical importance. In an otherwise healthy parturient without clinical evidence of impaired hemostasis, further evaluation of maternal coagulation status is generally not indicated.

However, prostaglandin synthetase inhibitors may have significant fetal effects, such as resulting in premature closure of the fetal ductus arteriosus in utero. This appears to be related to gestational age and is of less concern before 32 weeks' gestation. Indomethacin may cause decreased fetal urine excretion, leading to oligohydramnios and, rarely, neonatal renal failure. Finally, an increased incidence of necrotizing enterocolitis, intracranial hemorrhage, and bronchopulmonary dysplasia has been reported in neonates following indomethacin therapy.

Calcium Channel Blockers

By inhibiting transmembrane calcium flux, calcium channel blockers reduce myometrial contractility. Nifedipine is the most widely used calcium channel blocker for tocolysis, but the use of nicardipine is becoming more common owing to safety concerns related to nifedipine, especially for treating hypertension.[1] Nifedipine has a rapid onset following sublingual administration, and therapy is maintained via the oral route.

Maternal side effects with nifedipine therapy are generally mild. The drug has few cardiac effects, but vasodilatation with untoward hypotension are often observed.[1] These effects may be associated with reflex tachycardia, headache, and nausea. Oral nicardipine may be a better choice and has generally been shown to be a safe and well-tolerated tocolytic agent. In one prospective trial, patients randomly assigned to receive oral nicardipine had arrest of preterm labor more rapidly than did those assigned to receive parenteral MgSO$_4$. Also, those receiving MgSO$_4$ were more likely to have adverse drug-related effects and recurrent preterm labor. However, one recent case report and another case series (five patients) observed acute pulmonary edema during oral nicardipine therapy for tocolysis. However, in one instance, fluid overload and concurrent use of betamethasone (a corticosteroid) were believed to be possible contributing factors. A review published in 2001 concluded that when calcium channel blockers are used for tocolysis, they have fewer maternal side effects than other tocolytics, with no adverse effect on fetal outcome.

PREVENTION

Although the intraoperative anesthetic considerations related to each of the tocolytics have been discussed, it is important to remember that the properties of these agents do not cease with delivery. Depending on the duration of tocolytic therapy and the half-life of the agent used, all may contribute to uterine atony. Vigorous therapy may be necessary to restore uterine tone to prevent significant maternal blood loss. Also, despite aggressive tocolytic therapy, labor often progresses. When delivery becomes inevitable, a choice regarding the best route (vaginal versus cesarean) must be made.

Some obstetricians advocate routine cesarean delivery for all infants with an estimated gestational weight below 1500 g, to reduce head trauma and subsequent intracranial hemorrhage, but there is little evidence to support this position. In this group of very-low-birth-weight infants, with vertex presentation, there is no difference in outcome between those delivered vaginally or by cesarean section. Likewise, there is no evidence that the routine use of outlet forceps provides protection against head trauma. The advantages of cesarean delivery for the fetus must be weighed against the increased morbidity for the mother. Whenever vaginal delivery is planned for a very-low-birth-weight infant, good pelvic relaxation (which can be accomplished with regional anesthesia) has theoretical value.

Currently, the lower limit of viability hovers around 24 to 25 weeks' gestational age. When planning for the delivery of a very premature infant, it is most important to ensure the presence of personnel trained in neonatal resuscitation and access to a neonatal intensive care unit for subsequent care. Access to this expertise is one of the best predictors of neonatal survival and is largely responsible for lowering the age of viability.

Further Reading

ACOG Practice Bulletin: Management of preterm labor. Obstet Gynecol 101:1039-1047, 2003.

Bal L, Thierry S, Brocas E, et al: Pulmonary edema induced by calcium-channel blockade for tocolysis. Anesth Analg 99:910-911, 2004.

Childress CH, Katz, VL: Nifedipine and its indications in obstetrics and gynecology. Obstet Gynecol 83:616-624, 1994.

Economy KE, Abuhamad AZ: Calcium channel blockers as tocolytics. Semin Perinatol 25:264-271, 2001.

Goldenberg RL: The management of preterm labor. Obstet Gynecol 100:1020-1037, 2002.

Hack M, Fanaroff AA: Outcomes of children of extremely low birthweight and gestational age in the 1990s. Early Hum Dev 53:193-218, 1999.

Huddleston JF, Sanchez-Ramos L, Huddleston KW: Acute management of preterm labor. Clin Perinatol 30:803-824, 2003.

Larmon JE, Ross BS, May W, et al: Oral nicardipine versus intravenous magnesium sulfate for the treatment of preterm labor. Am J Obstet Gynecol 181:1432-1437, 1999.

Lumley J: Method of delivery for the preterm infant. Br J Obstet Gynaecol 110(Suppl 20):88-92, 2003.

Palmer CM: Complications of labor. In Palmer CM, D'Angelo R, Paech MJ (eds): Handbook of Obstetric Anesthesia. Oxford, BIOS Scientific Publishers, 2002, pp 163-173.

Vaast P, Dubreucq-Fossaert S, Houfflin-Debarge V, et al: Acute pulmonary oedema during nicardipine therapy for premature labour: Report of five cases. Eur J Obstet Gynecol Reprod Biol 113:98-99, 2004.

Wilkins IA, Lynch L, Mehalek KE, et al: Efficacy and side effects of magnesium sulfate and ritodrine as tocolytic agents. Am J Obstet Gynecol 159:685-689, 1988.

---

[1]In 1985 the Food and Drug Administration advised that sublingual nifedipine should not be used in hypertensive emergencies because it was neither safe nor efficacious. Variable absorption with suboptimal effects often led to early repeat sublingual dosing in patients with hypertensive emergencies. This caused untoward hypotension, myocardial infarction, and even death in some patients.

OTHER SURGICAL SUBSPECIALTIES

Fetal Intrauterine Surgery

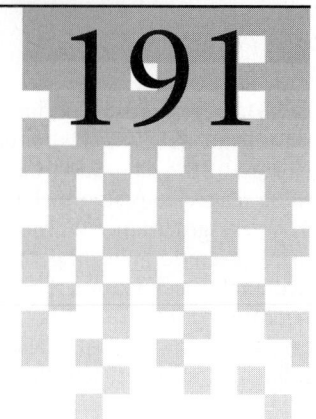

Jeffrey L. Galinkin

Case Synopsis

A 29-year-old woman, gravida 1, at 24 weeks' gestation presents with a fetus in cardiac failure secondary to a giant cystic thoracic mass. The maternal history is otherwise noncontributory. Fetal surgery with fetal thoracotomy and resection of the lung mass is planned.

PROBLEM ANALYSIS

Definition

Fetal surgery is a field of rapid growth. Ex utero intrapartum therapy (EXIT), fetoscopic procedures, and open midgestation procedures (e.g., myelomeningocele repair, congenital cystic adenomatoid lung malformation or sacrococcygeal teratoma resection) are now done at many centers worldwide.

Surgical intervention is considered for a fetus with a congenital lesion or condition that compromises or disturbs cardiovascular function or may cause severe postnatal morbidity. Surgery is performed only when the risk to the mother is low and the risk of fetal death or severe disability outweighs the potential poor outcome with no intervention. Contraindications for these procedures include maternal medical conditions precluding such surgery and lethal or severely disabling fetal genetic defects.

Fetal surgery is based on extensive animal investigation and clinical research. In contrast, anesthesia for fetal surgery is based mostly on clinical experience, case reports, and translation of responses to anesthesia from pregnant sheep models. Discussed here are maternal and fetal anesthetic considerations for specific fetal surgical interventions.

Recognition

Fetal surgery involves three distinct procedural groups (Table 191-1): midgestational open hysterotomy, EXIT, and fetoscopic surgery. Midgestational (18 to 26 weeks) open hysterotomy is performed on fetuses with well-defined congenital lesions. After hysterotomy, the fetus is exteriorized for surgical intervention and returned to the uterus to mature. Correction of the lesion is expected to improve fetal survival or enhance postgestational quality of life. Untreated, these lesions are expected to result in severe disability or death during infancy.

EXIT involves procedures done at or near term on fetuses that are expected to have immediate airway or oxygen compromise at birth. Fetal surgery is performed after hysterotomy and just before cord clamping. The surgeon assesses the infant's airway with bronchoscopy and, if necessary, secures it with an endotracheal or tracheostomy tube before clamping the cord, thereby reducing the risk of complete airway obstruction or postpartum ventilatory failure. Up to actual delivery, the fetus is oxygenated via placental transfer of oxygen.

Fetoscopic surgery is minimally invasive. For uterine access, percutaneous small-diameter trocars and laparoscopes are used. This technique is most commonly used to evaluate and treat the twin reversed arterial perfusion sequence, twin-twin transfusion syndrome, amniotic band syndrome, and bladder outlet obstruction. Surgical electrocautery and lasers are used to ablate or cauterize affected vessels or tissue during these procedures. Fetoscopic surgery is considered when fetal demise or severe fetal morbidity is imminent and more conservative measures (e.g., amnioreduction) have failed.

Risk Assessment and Implications

MATERNAL ANESTHETIC CONSIDERATIONS

Regional anesthesia is the preferred technique for most obstetric cases. However, because uterine relaxation is required for hysterotomy-based fetal surgery and is best provided by high

Table 191–1 ■ Surgical Approaches to Fetal Lesions: Timing and Reason for Treatment

Surgical Approach	Fetal Lesion or Anomaly	Reason for Treatment	Gestational Age
Midgestational open hysterotomy	Congenital cystic adenomatoid malformation	Hydrops fetalis, lung hypoplasia	18-25 wk
	Myelomeningocele	Aminotic fluid neurotoxicity	22-26 wk
	Sacrococcygeal teratoma	Hydrops fetalis	18-25 wk
Ex utero intrapartum therapy (EXIT)	Congenital or iatrogenic high airway obstruction	Secure airway	Near term
	Giant fetal neck mass	Secure airway, resect mass	Near term
Fetoscopic surgery	Twin-twin transfusion	Impending fetal demise, hydrops fetalis	Midgestation
	Twin reversed arterial perfusion sequence	Impending fetal demise, hydrops fetalis	Midgestation
	Bladder outlet obstruction	Hydronephrosis, renal hypoplasia	Midgestation

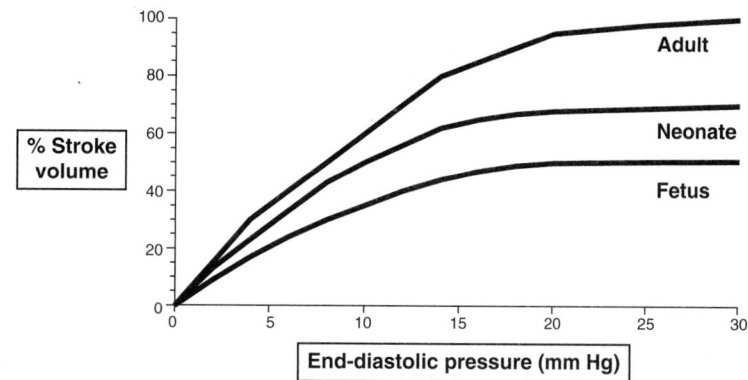

Figure 191–1 ■ Starling curves for adult, neonate, and fetus.

concentrations of volatile inhalational anesthetics, general anesthesia is the technique of choice for fetal surgery.

Maternal physiologic changes during pregnancy contribute to an increased anesthetic risk for both the mother and the fetus. Pregnant patients are at increased risk for aspiration pneumonitis. Therefore, a rapid-sequence induction is always performed for endotracheal intubation. Pregnancy also affects maternal pulmonary function. Cephalad movement of the gravid uterus reduces lung functional residual capacity, especially lower lobe volumes. Also, oxygen consumption increases to meet the greater demands of both mother and fetus. All these factors increase the risk for maternal hypoxemia during rapid-sequence induction. Further, reduced capillary oncotic pressure and increased capillary permeability increase the maternal postoperative risk for pulmonary edema, especially when magnesium sulfate ($MgSO_4$) is used for tocolysis.

Pregnancy also affects the cardiovascular system. Reduced preload due to vena cava compression by the gravid uterus may cause maternal hypotension in the supine position (supine hypotensive syndrome) and fetal hypoxemia. Left uterine displacement is important to reduce this risk.

Anesthetic requirements are also affected by pregnancy. The minimum alveolar concentration (MAC) of anesthetics is significantly reduced during pregnancy. Thus, lower concentrations of volatile anesthetics are required for surgery. Moreover, sensitivity to nondepolarizing skeletal muscle relaxants is increased.

FETAL ANESTHETIC CONSIDERATIONS

In addition to maternal safety, a major concern for anesthetic management is to preserve placental perfusion and fetal cardiovascular stability. The combination of fetal immature organ function and maternal cardiovascular compromise predisposes the fetus to anesthetic-related circulatory compromise. The cardiovascular system of a fetus is less able to compensate for hypoxia and hypovolemia than that of a full-term infant. Lacking a functional pulmonary system to increase oxygen tension, the fetus relies instead on increased maternal umbilical blood flow and cardiac output, as well as fetal blood flow redistribution to improve oxygen delivery to vital organs. The Starling curve is shifted downward for a fetus compared with a neonate, resulting in a lower percentage stroke volume for a given end-diastolic

pressure (Fig. 191-1). Thus, cardiac output is more dependent on heart rate. Also, owing to high vagal tone and low baroreceptor sensitivity, the fetus responds to stress with a decrease in heart rate.

The circulating fetal blood volume is low. The midgestational fetus has an estimated blood volume of 50 to 70 mL/kg, versus 110 mL/kg for the placenta. Therefore, small surgical blood losses can precipitate fetal hypovolemia. Inhalational anesthetics can also destabilize fetal cardiovascular dynamics by causing systemic vasodilatation, direct myocardial depression, and altered arteriovenous shunting.

Also, because of incomplete myelination and reduced synaptic transmission, the fetus is more sensitive to the effects of volatile anesthetics. This results in a reduced MAC requirement compared with a pregnant adult. Further, sensitivity to analgesics and muscle relaxants is greater for a fetus compared with a neonate.

Fetal cutaneous and evaporative heat losses necessitate warm ambient temperatures during fetal exposure. Limiting fetal surgical time and using warm irrigation fluids can prevent fetal hypothermia.

Finally, altered coagulation predisposes to bleeding and difficulty achieving surgical hemostasis during fetal surgical manipulation. Relatively small fetal blood volumes compound this problem. Fetal hemoglobin can be assessed intraoperatively via central or percutaneously obtained fetal blood samples.

UTEROPLACENTAL ANESTHETIC CONSIDERATIONS

Uterine and umbilical arterial blood flow and placental barriers to diffusion influence fetal oxygen delivery. Maternal systemic blood pressure and myometrial tone directly correlate with uterine artery blood flow. Volatile anesthetics decrease myometrial tone and tend to reduce maternal blood pressure and placental blood flow as well. This can result in decreased fetal oxygenation. Umbilical arterial blood flow is determined by maternal and fetal cardiac output and vascular resistance and by extrinsic factors (e.g., extrinsic compression by a "nuchal cord"). Thus, maintaining maternal arterial pressure within 10% of baseline values and umbilical artery patency is critical.

Relaxation of myometrial tone by inhalational anesthetics is required for optimal exposure during open fetal surgery. Epidural anesthesia alone does not provide adequate uterine relaxation, but it may help prevent premature labor in the early postoperative period. Tocolytics (MgSO₄, terbutaline, nifedipine, indomethacin) are used alone or in combination to ensure uterine quiescence.

MANAGEMENT AND PREVENTION

Open Fetal Surgery

PREOPERATIVE EVALUATION AND PREPARATION

Before surgery, the operating room is warmed to 80°F (26.7°C). Type-specific packed red blood cells must be available for the mother, and O-negative packed red blood cells for the fetus. Monitoring includes maternal and fetal pulse oximetry and maternal direct arterial pressure. Before anesthesia and surgery, prepare several sterile 1-mL syringes with fentanyl 10 to 20 μg/kg, vecuronium 0.2 mg/kg, epinephrine 10 μg/kg, and atropine 20 μg/kg. These may be needed for the fetus. After assuring the mother's nothing-by-mouth status, one large-bore intravenous (IV) catheter is placed. Metoclopramide and bicitrate are given to reduce the risk for aspiration pneumonitis. An indomethacin suppository is used for postoperative tocolysis. After lumbar epidural catheter insertion and testing, the mother is positioned in the left lateral decubitus position, or the operating table is tilted to the left to reduce the risk of supine hypotensive syndrome.

INTRAOPERATIVE MANAGEMENT

Rapid-sequence induction using IV sodium thiopental and succinylcholine is performed, followed by endotracheal intubation. General anesthesia is maintained with 0.5 MAC volatile anesthetic (isoflurane or desflurane) and 50% nitrous oxide (N_2O) in oxygen. A radial arterial catheter, second IV access catheter, nasogastric tube, and Foley catheter are placed. Fetal status is monitored by sterile intraoperative echocardiography. IV fluid administration is restricted to 500 mL (total) to reduce the risk of postoperative pulmonary edema. Open hysterotomy procedures require low uterine tone to maintain fetal perfusion and optimize fetal exposure. Before maternal skin incision, N_2O is discontinued to improve fetal oxygenation,[1] and the inhalational agent is increased to 2.0 MAC to provide uterine relaxation and fetal anesthesia before uterine and fetal incisions. IV ephedrine (5 to 10 mg) or phenylephrine (1 to 2 μg/kg) is given as necessary to maintain maternal systolic blood pressure within 10% of baseline.

Fetal anesthesia and analgesia are provided by both placental transfer of volatile anesthetic and intramuscular opioids. After maternal-fetal equilibration, fetal concentrations of isoflurane and desflurane are about 70% and 50% of maternal levels, respectively, by 1 hour. Before fetal incision, the fetus receives intramuscular fentanyl (20 μg/kg) to supplement anesthesia and provide postoperative analgesia.

Fetal well-being is assessed by direct and indirect methods. For procedures in which a fetal extremity is available (e.g., congenital cystic adenomatoid malformation and sacrococcygeal

teratoma resection), fetal arterial saturation is monitored by pulse oximetry. The pulse oximeter probe is placed on the fetus's hand, which is then wrapped with sterile foil to reduce exposure to ambient light. Normal fetal arterial saturation is 60% to 70%. During surgery, values greater than 40% indicate adequate fetal oxygenation. To monitor fetal heart rate and stroke volume, echocardiography is used. Fetal distress manifests as bradycardia, along with reduced oxygen saturation or stroke volume. Often, this is due to partial umbilical cord occlusion. Fetal arterial or venous blood gas samples are used to guide therapy during periods of fetal stress; these samples are obtained by the surgeon percutaneously or from the umbilical artery or central vessel. Warm, fresh O-negative blood is used to correct fetal anemia intraoperatively via fetal venous access.

Near the end of uterine closure, the volatile anesthetic is reduced, and the epidural catheter is dosed with an opioid and local anesthetic. Tocolysis is begun with IV MgSO₄ (6 g), followed by infusion at 2 to 3 g/hour. After tracheal extubation, the patient is transferred to the obstetric floor for postoperative care.

POSTOPERATIVE MANAGEMENT

Key for postoperative management are the prevention of premature labor and adequate maternal pain control. MgSO₄ is the tocolytic of choice for the first 18 to 24 hours. Along with tocolysis, good pain control with epidural analgesia helps prevent preterm labor.

Ex Utero Intrapartum Therapy

PREOPERATIVE MANAGEMENT

Anesthesia for EXIT procedures is similar to that for open procedures, except that tocolytic therapy is unnecessary (EXIT procedures end with delivery of the fetus). In addition, a second operating room with neonatal resuscitation equipment and a neonatologist must be available for care of the neonate.

INTRAOPERATIVE MANAGEMENT

The risk of aspiration and supine hypotensive syndrome is increased in full-term mothers, owing to the larger gravid uterus. Thus, after epidural catheter placement, a rapid-sequence induction is performed, followed by orotracheal intubation. Then a nasogastric tube and Foley catheter are placed, along with a second IV catheter in case the patient requires volume resuscitation for acute blood loss after fetal delivery. If the fetus has end-stage disease (e.g., fetal hydrops), the maternal blood pressure may be very labile. If so, direct arterial pressure monitoring may be required for beat-to-beat assessment of blood pressure and frequent blood sampling.

Sub-MAC concentrations of a volatile anesthetic are used before maternal skin incision, and higher concentrations thereafter. Desflurane is preferred by many, not only because it maintains heart rate and allows rapid induction but also because emergence is faster than with sevoflurane and other agents. The latter is explained by its lower fat partition coefficient compared with sevoflurane and other agents. Vasopressors are used to maintain maternal blood pressure if necessary.

During hysterotomy, the surgeon only partially exposes the fetus. This keeps the uterine volume near normal and

---

[1]This also helps reduce maternal bowel distention, thereby improving surgical exposure.

Table 191–2 ■ Implications of Anesthetic Technique for Fetoscopic Surgery			
Type of Anesthesia	Fetal Depression	Uteroplacental Blood Flow	Uterine Relaxation
Regional anesthesia	–	–	–
Balanced general anesthesia with or without epidural	+	+/–	+/–
Deep general anesthesia with epidural	++	++	++

maintains placental perfusion. Maternal hyperventilation is avoided because of the risk of placental vasoconstriction and fetal hypoxemia with hypocapnia. Fentanyl 20 µg/kg is given to the fetus intramuscularly to supplement analgesia (via placental transfer) and for postoperative analgesia. Fetal status is closely monitored by pulse oximetry, sterile echocardiography, and visual inspection. Fetal blood gases are obtained if needed, and fresh O-negative blood is administered if necessary. Fetal orotracheal intubation is performed by the surgeon or anesthesiologist. If the fetus cannot be intubated, resection of an obstructive lesion or tracheotomy is performed by the surgeon. After securing the airway and ensuring adequate fetal oxygenation with manual ventilation, the umbilical cord is clamped, and the fetus is delivered.

After delivery, one must quickly reverse uterine relaxation. Anesthetic depth is reduced after cord clamping, and the epidural catheter is dosed for anesthesia and postoperative opioid analgesia. Owing to anesthetic-induced uterine relaxation, uterine atony and large blood losses are known risks. The timing of cord clamping with respect to the use of oxytocin, methylergonovine maleate (Methergine), and 15-methyl prostaglandin $F_{2\alpha}$ is coordinated by the anesthesiologist and surgeon. Blood loss is closely monitored, and blood is transfused if needed. The trachea is extubated after uterine closure. The epidural is used for wound closure and postoperative analgesia.

POSTDELIVERY AND POSTOPERATIVE MANAGEMENT

After surgery and delivery, the mother is transferred for postpartum care. The immediate disposition of the newborn is based on whether further surgery is required (e.g., excision of a cervical teratoma). If not, a neonatology team resuscitates and transports the infant to the neonatal intensive care unit.

Fetoscopic Surgery

PREOPERATIVE MANAGEMENT

Patients scheduled for fetoscopic surgery are admitted to the hospital on the day of surgery. The operating room is prepared as for an open procedure, in the rare event that hysterotomy is required for surgical access. In the preoperative area, the mother receives "full-stomach" prophylaxis and, if she is at high risk for preterm labor, indomethacin by rectum. Standard monitoring per American Society of Anesthesiologists guidelines is applied, and a lumbar epidural catheter is inserted and tested. Left uterine displacement is used to prevent supine hypotension.

INTRAOPERATIVE MANAGEMENT

Choice of anesthesia is guided by the implications of various anesthetic techniques for fetoscopic surgery (Table 191-2). Epidural anesthesia is used in the majority of these cases because of its minimal effect on fetal hemodynamics and uteroplacental blood flow. Disadvantages include the lack of uterine relaxation and fetal anesthesia; fetal movement may make it difficult to manipulate the uterus and cord, especially with difficult cord positions. Although a balanced anesthetic technique allows uterine manipulation with an immobile, anesthetized fetus, there is greater fetal cardiovascular depression than with epidural anesthesia. General endotracheal anesthesia also eliminates concerns related to an awake patient (e.g., anxiety, combativeness, nausea, aspiration of gastric contents). Deep inhalation anesthesia has the advantage of providing profound uterine relaxation for externalizing the uterus during hysterotomy-based fetal procedures. However, associated risks are fetal cardiovascular depression and reduced uteroplacental blood flow.

POSTOPERATIVE MANAGEMENT

As with open hysterotomy, tocolysis is the most important aspect of postoperative management. Epidural catheters are removed in the immediate postoperative period unless the patient will have a hysterotomy-based procedure based on findings at fetoscopy. $MgSO_4$ (with or without nifedipine or terbutaline) is the mainstay of tocolytic therapy. Discharge from the hospital on postoperative day 1 or 2 is expected after fetoscopy.

Further Reading

Bianchi DW, Crombleholme TM, D'Alton ME: Fetology: Diagnosis and Management of the Fetal Patient. New York, McGraw-Hill, 2000.

Fisk NM, Gitau R, Teixeira JM, et al: Effect of direct fetal opioid analgesia on fetal hormonal and hemodynamic stress response to intrauterine needling. Anesthesiology 95:828-835, 2001.

Gaiser RR, Cheek TG, Kurth CD: Anesthetic management of cesarean delivery complicated by ex utero intrapartum treatment of the fetus. Anesth Analg 84:1150-1153, 1997.

Galinkin JL, Gaiser RR, Cohen DE, et al: Anesthesia for fetoscopic fetal surgery: Twin reverse arterial perfusion sequence and twin-twin transfusions syndrome. Anesth Analg 91:1394-1397, 2000.

Galinkin JL, Schwarz U: Anesthesia for fetal surgery. In Smith's Anesthesia for Infants and Children, 7th ed. St. Louis, Mosby, 2004.

Motoyama EK, Rivard G, Acheson F, et al: Adverse effect of maternal hyperventilation on the foetus. Lancet 1:286-288, 1966.

Palahniuk RJ, Shnider SM, Eger EI 2nd: Pregnancy decreases the requirement for inhaled anesthetic agents. Anesthesiology 41:82-83, 1974.

Tame JD, Abrams LM, Ding XY, et al: Level of postoperative analgesia is a critical factor in regulation of myometrial contractility after laparotomy in the pregnant baboon: Implications for human fetal surgery. Am J Obstet Gynecol 180:1196-1201, 1999.

Fetal Distress

192

Brenda A. Bucklin

Case Synopsis

An 18-year-old, 150-kg primigravida presents at 27 weeks' gestation with severe preeclampsia. Her worsening condition necessitates induction of labor. During uterine contractions, the electronic fetal heart rate monitor demonstrates ominous changes (Fig. 192-1).

PROBLEM ANALYSIS

Definition

Fetal distress is a widely used clinical term that is imprecise and nonspecific. In 1998 the American College of Obstetricians and Gynecologists (ACOG) published a committee opinion that suggested replacing the term *fetal distress* with *nonreassuring fetal heart rate tracing* because the former term has a low predictive value and is frequently associated with the delivery of infants who turn out to be in good condition. The ACOG went on to recommend that a nonreassuring fetal heart rate tracing be accompanied by a further description of the findings (e.g., fetal bradycardia, repetitive variable decelerations). Still, obstetricians continue to use the term *fetal distress* to describe a wide range of fetal heart rate abnormalities that, if not corrected or circumvented, will result in decompensation of physiologic responses and cause permanent central nervous system or other damage or death. Anesthesiologists must consider the severity of the fetal heart rate abnormality when determining the urgency of delivery and the type of anesthesia to be administered.

Recognition

Consistent, accurate diagnosis of true fetal distress (i.e., intrauterine hypoxia or asphyxia) is a clinical challenge because of the questionable reliability of electronic fetal heart rate monitoring for predicting adverse neonatal outcomes. Still, electronic fetal heart rate monitoring is the primary screening tool. Additional support for the diagnosis may be obtained from the presence of meconium in the amniotic fluid, deteriorating fetal acid-base status, lack of a fetal heart rate response to acoustic or scalp stimulation, and umbilical artery Doppler velocimetry. The most sensitive indicators of fetal cerebral oxygenation are heart rate variability or accelerations.

Gradual decreases in fetal oxygenation produce a variety of fetal heart rate patterns (Fig. 192-2). Early signs of transient hypoxemia in a neurologically intact fetus may include tachycardia, persistent sinusoidal fetal heart rate pattern, and periodic changes consisting of late and variable decelerations. Although these changes alone do not preclude the delivery of a healthy neonate, they should alert the clinician that the fetus is at risk. In extreme cases, the fetus will lose all central influence over its heart rate and develop a straight-line tracing devoid of accelerations, variability, and even decelerations. Abrupt and profound decreases in fetal oxygenation often result in severe fetal bradycardia, usually less than 90 beats per minute. Ominous signs suggesting that both fetal acidosis and hypoxia are present include the following:

- Loss of fetal heart rate accelerations
- Increase in baseline fetal heart rate
- Persistent absent variability, unresponsive to stimuli
- Absent variability with late or variable decelerations

The challenge for obstetricians is to judiciously consider the electronic information within the clinical context to ensure the best possible neonatal outcome. Emergency cesarean delivery is indicated when the condition is life threatening to the mother or fetus. In these situations, communication between obstetric and anesthesia care providers is essential for maternal and fetal well-being.

Risk Assessment

The true incidence of fetal distress is difficult to quantify, largely because of the lack of clearly defined diagnostic criteria. However, it is a diagnosis that is likely overused by physicians. In 1991 U.S. birth certificate statistics revealed that fetal distress was a confounding factor in 4.3% of live births. More recently, rates of cesarean delivery for fetal distress ranged from 2% to 8.7%.

Fetal distress may result from interference of oxygen transport at the level of the mother, the placenta, the umbilical cord, or the fetus itself (Table 192-1). Sometimes the cause is multifactorial, but more often a primary cause is identifiable. Common high-risk obstetric conditions that increase the risk of fetal distress include the following:

- Preeclampsia or eclampsia and chronic hypertension
- Diabetes mellitus
- Intrauterine growth retardation
- Oligohydramnios
- Fetal prematurity or postmaturity
- Chorioamnionitis

Implications

Severe and sustained hypoxia in the fetus will eventually lead to profound acidosis, neurologic sequelae (e.g., seizures, coma, hypotonia), and ultimately, death.

770

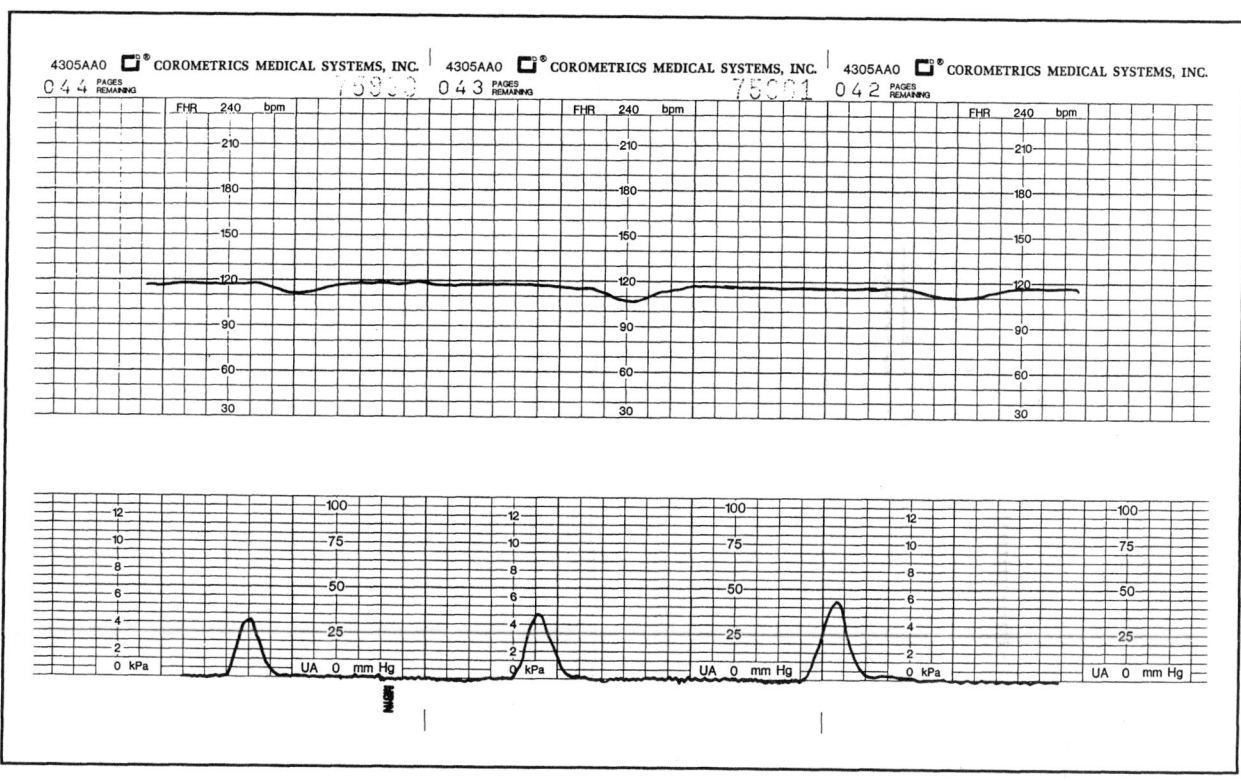

Figure 192–1 ■ The fetal heart rate tracing *(top)* demonstrates no beat-to-beat variability, with late decelerations evident after each uterine contraction in the uterine activity (UA) tracing *(bottom)*.

MANAGEMENT

When clinical signs suggest intrauterine hypoxia, the obstetrician and anesthesiologist should initiate in utero fetal resuscitation. Obstetric management includes supplemental oxygen administration, maternal repositioning (e.g., left or right lateral decubitus, Trendelenburg's, or knee-chest position), assessment of maternal circulation, treatment of maternal hypotension, and discontinuation of oxytocin, tocolytic administration, and amnioinfusion.

Although a distressed fetus may occasionally be delivered vaginally, the diagnosis of fetal distress significantly increases the likelihood of cesarean delivery. The anesthesiologist should be prepared to assist in either situation and must consider the following factors:

- Urgency of delivery
- Anesthetic risk factors in the mother
- Direct and indirect effects of anesthesia on the distressed fetus

Emergent cesarean delivery is performed when the maternal or fetal condition is considered to be life threatening (e.g., massive maternal hemorrhage, catastrophic uterine rupture, evidence of sustained and severe fetal bradycardia). Communication between the obstetrician and anesthesiologist is imperative in cases of emergent cesarean delivery. In this situation, anesthesia care providers should determine the diagnosis and how expeditiously the fetus must be delivered. Fetal heart rate monitoring via a scalp electrode should be continued following transfer to the delivery room and, if possible, until delivery. This information helps guide the choice of anesthetic. The relative risks of general and regional anesthesia must be carefully considered in each patient. General anesthesia is associated with a higher incidence of fatal maternal complications. Therefore, if the fetal heart rate tracing improves, there may be time to extend epidural analgesia to anesthesia or even for de novo induction of spinal or epidural anesthesia. When a preexisting epidural catheter is in place and the mother is hemodynamically stable, surgical epidural anesthesia can easily be established. With administration of either 2% alkalinized lidocaine with 1:200,000 epinephrine or 3% alkalinized 2-chloroprocaine in 5-mL increments (total volume of 15 to 20 mL) over a 2- to 3-minute period, the interval between injection and delivery is about 10 to 12 minutes. Although the addition of freshly prepared epinephrine to the lidocaine and bicarbonate solution hastens the onset of epidurally administered lidocaine, 3% 2-chloroprocaine with bicarbonate is the agent of choice when time is of the essence.

Spinal anesthesia is also acceptable for urgent or emergent cesarean delivery. However, the skill of the anesthesiologist, the patient's body habitus, and the acceptance of neuraxial anesthesia by the patient and obstetrician must all be considered before the use of either epidural or spinal techniques. Although a non-dextrose-containing crystalloid

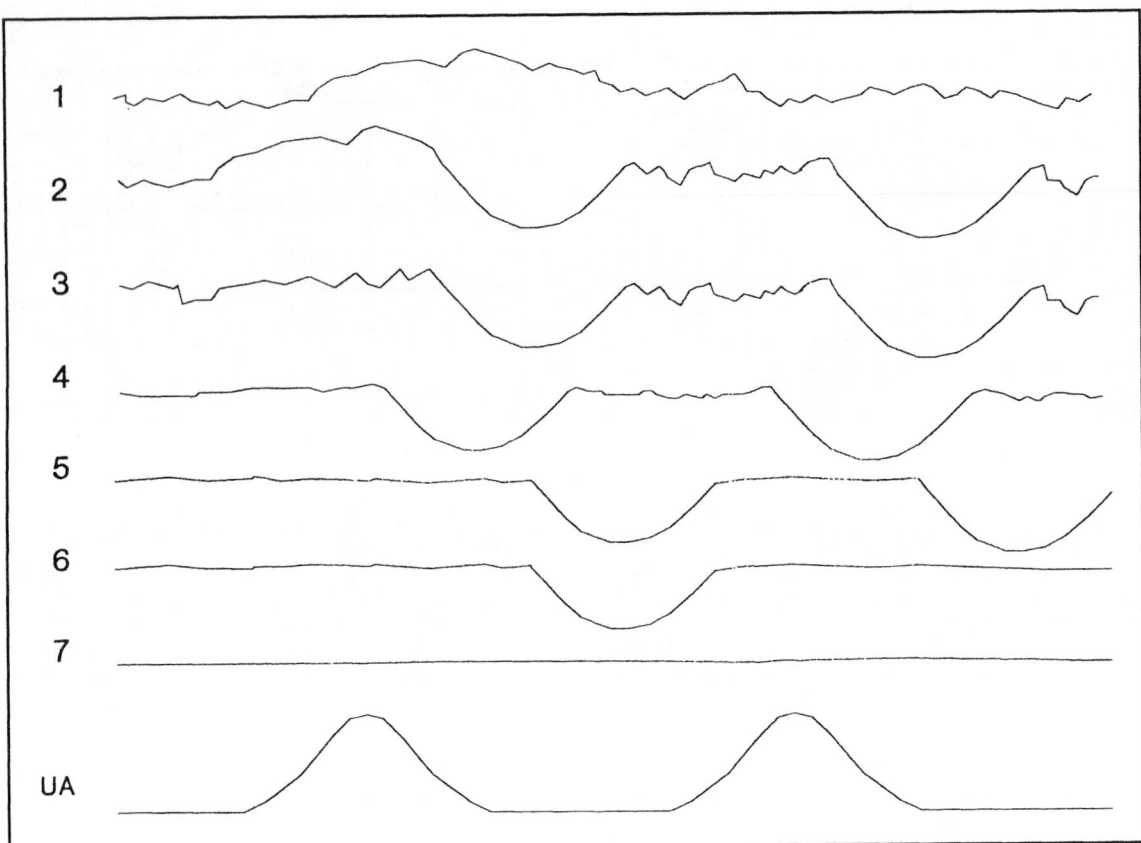

Figure 192–2 ■ Electronic fetal heart rate monitoring. Characteristics of progressive fetal deterioration are superimposed above a uterine activity (UA) tracing showing two uterine contractions. (1) Healthy fetus exhibiting accelerations and moderate variability. (2) Late decelerations, indicating transient hypoxemia. The presence of accelerations signifies a normal pH. (3) Loss of accelerations, which occurs with evolving hypoxia. (4) Decreasing variability and shortened latency period with worsening acid-base status. (5) Increased latency period consistent with fetal myocardial depression. (6) Intermittent decelerations, indicating progression of acidosis or hypoxia. (7) Absent variability and loss of decelerations in a moribund fetus. (From Dellinger EH, Boehm FH: Emergency management of fetal stress and distress in the obstetric patient. Obstet Gynecol Clin North Am 22:225, 1995.)

solution should be administered as rapidly as possible before spinal anesthetic administration, fluid preloading does not justify delaying spinal anesthesia when it is the most appropriate method for the patient. Emergent cesarean delivery is not the time to strengthen one's regional anesthesia skills, and even an experienced anesthesiologist may have to accept less-than-perfect regional anesthesia; injection of local anesthetic into the incision by the obstetrician can obviate the need for general anesthesia.

When a preexisting epidural block cannot be extended safely or there is inadequate time to place a spinal anesthetic, rapid induction of general anesthesia is usually the most expeditious technique. However, significant maternal morbidity or even mortality is associated with failed endotracheal intubation or pulmonary aspiration. Because emergency surgery has been identified as a risk factor for anesthesia-related maternal mortality, the mother's life should not be endangered for the sake of the fetus. Obstetricians should consult with an anesthesiologist for all parturients at increased risk for operative delivery, especially those with potential airway problems. In such patients, early initiation and maintenance of epidural analgesia can facilitate the extension to surgical anesthesia if cesarean delivery

becomes necessary. A history or suspicion of difficult intubation should prompt an awake intubation or regional anesthesia, despite severe fetal distress.

Some urgent and emergent cesarean deliveries require the administration of general anesthesia. Failed or difficult intubation is the leading cause of anesthetic-related maternal mortality. Failed intubation has been reported to occur with a frequency of 1 in 300 obstetric patients, compared with 1 in 2000 general surgical patients. In cases of unrecognized difficult airway and failed intubation, the absence of sustained, severe fetal bradycardia may allow the anesthesiologist to safely awaken the patient and attempt an alternative technique. However, if fetal bradycardia persists, the anesthesiologist may choose to proceed with inhalation anesthesia with a facemask or laryngeal mask ventilation when maternal oxygenation and ventilation can be maintained. Although the use of laryngeal mask ventilation is limited to "cannot intubate, cannot ventilate" situations in obstetrics, it can be lifesaving and is an important part of emergency airway management.

In many urgent cases of fetal distress, cesarean delivery can be performed safely using skillfully administered regional anesthesia. As clinical expertise has increased, the

Table 192–1 ▪ Causes of Fetal Distress
Maternal Chronic and pregnancy-induced hypertension Diabetes mellitus Cardiovascular disease Pulmonary disease Substance abuse Trauma or shock Anemia
Placental Abruption Infection Infarction
Umbilical Cord Compression Prolapse
Fetal Sepsis Hydrops Anemia (both acute and chronic) Anomalies Preexisting neurologic injury

theoretical objections to the use of regional anesthesia—namely, a delay in delivery and significant maternal hypotension—have proved to be less consequential than previously feared.

PREVENTION

Early diagnosis of fetal distress is important if the sequelae of intrauterine hypoxia and asphyxia are to be minimized. The anesthesiologist's expertise in this setting and his or her ability to effectively communicate with the obstetrician are critical to ensuring the best maternal and fetal outcomes.

Further Reading

American College of Obstetricians and Gynecologists Committee on Obstetric Practice: Inappropriate Use of the Terms Fetal Distress and Birth Asphyxia (ACOG Committee Opinion No. 197). Washington, DC, ACOG, 1998.

American College of Obstetricians and Gynecologists Committee on Obstetrics: Anesthesia for Emergency Deliveries (ACOG Committee Opinion No. 104). Washington, DC, ACOG, 1992 (reaffirmed in 1998).

Campbell C: Fetal distress. In Atlee JL (ed): Complications in Anesthesia. Philadelphia, WB Saunders, 1999, pp 807-810.

Chestnut DH: Anesthesia for fetal distress. In Chestnut DH (ed): Obstetric Anesthesia: Principles and Practice, 3rd ed. St. Louis, Mosby–Year Book, 2004, pp 447-471.

Dellinger EH, Boehm FH: Emergency management of fetal stress and distress in the obstetric patient. Obstet Gynecol Clin North Am 22:225, 1995.

Eskew PN Jr, Saywell RM Jr, Sollinger TW, et al: Trends in the frequency of cesarean delivery: A 21-year experience, 1970-1990. J Reprod Med 39:809-817, 1994.

Parer JT, Livingston EG: What is fetal distress? Am J Obstet Gynecol 162:1421-1427, 1990.

Paul RH, Miller DA: Cesarean birth: How to reduce the rate. Am J Obstet Gynecol 172:1903-1907, 1995.

Spielman FJ, Mayer DC: Clear head, steady hands: Anesthesia for emergency cesarean delivery [editorial]. Am J Anesthesiol 28:328-330, 2001.

OTHER SURGICAL SUBSPECIALTIES

Antepartum Hemorrhage

193

Lawrence C. Tsen

Case Synopsis

A 33-year-old woman, gravida 3, para 2, presents at 28 weeks' gestation with vaginal bleeding. Estimated blood loss is greater than 1000 mL. The patient underwent an emergent cesarean delivery for the birth of her first child 4 years ago. Ultrasound examination confirms a breech presentation with placenta previa.

PROBLEM ANALYSIS

Definition

Vaginal bleeding occurs in 24% of diagnosed pregnancies. Most often, it is associated with minimal blood loss and limited pathology. In contrast, major antepartum bleeding may occur at any time during pregnancy and is the leading cause of antepartum maternal death worldwide. It is also a leading cause of perinatal morbidity and mortality. The distinction between bleeding and hemorrhage is one of semantics. What is more important is the recognition that with any bleeding, blood loss and physiologic deterioration may occur rapidly. If so, both fetal and maternal outcomes depend on a cogent plan of investigation and an appropriate response.

Antepartum hemorrhage is commonly associated with certain causes. Bleeding during early pregnancy (before 20 weeks' gestation) can result from abnormal embryo implantation (e.g., placenta previa, placenta accreta, placental abruption, or vasa previa), miscarriage, ectopic pregnancy, gestational trophoblastic disease, dysfunctional uterine bleeding, and benign and malignant tumors of the reproductive tract. Among pregnancies complicated by bleeding in the first trimester, less than 50% progress normally beyond 20 weeks' gestation; 10% to 15% are ectopic pregnancies, 0.2% are hydatidiform moles, and more than 30% result in miscarriage. Bleeding during late pregnancy (beyond 20 weeks' gestation) complicates 2% to 5% of pregnancies. The most common causes are placental abruption (31%) and placenta previa (22%).

Miscarriage, ectopic pregnancy, placenta previa, placental abruption, uterine rupture, and vasa previa are the most common causes of significant antepartum hemorrhage. Unclassified bleeding may occur at any time during 47% of pregnancies. Causes are marginal placental sinus bleeding, "bloody show" during labor, cervicitis, trauma, genital tract tumor and infection, and vasa previa.

MISCARRIAGE

The definition of spontaneous abortion (miscarriage) varies, depending on the accepted age of fetal viability. Typically, it is defined as the spontaneous termination of pregnancy before 22 to 24 weeks of gestation. Between 15% and 20% of all clinically diagnosed pregnancies result in miscarriage, but the actual incidence may be higher. This is so because up to 60% of "chemical pregnancies" (i.e., those diagnosed by changes in β-human chorionic gonadotropin)

do not result in a viable pregnancy. Miscarriages may be threatened, inevitable, complete, incomplete, septic, recurrent, or missed. Typically, the presentation includes a history of vaginal spotting or mild bleeding. When vaginal bleeding during the first 12 weeks of pregnancy is as heavy as normal menstrual blood loss, the pregnancy is rarely successful. Larger amounts of blood loss are observed with intrauterine fetal demise, especially at greater gestational ages. However, severe hemorrhage with disseminated intravascular coagulation (DIC) does not usually occur until approximately 4 weeks after fetal demise.

ECTOPIC PREGNANCY

Approximately 2% of pregnancies do not implant normally in the uterus, and the incidence appears to be increasing. Although ectopic pregnancies classically present as pelvic pain with intraperitoneal bleeding, they can also masquerade as a number of other entities, including appendicitis, ovarian cyst torsion, endometriosis, and pelvic inflammatory disease. Major blood loss with sudden death has been described. However, the risk of bleeding and the outcome correlate with the implantation site (e.g., isthmic or interstitial portion of the fallopian tube, ovary, cervix, abdomen) and the timing of diagnosis. Ectopic pregnancies may resolve spontaneously, be treated medically, or require laparoscopic or open surgery. Surgery is indicated in the presence of peritoneal signs, hemodynamic instability, or failed conservative management.

PLACENTA PREVIA

Placenta previa is implantation of the placenta in the lower uterine segment. It is classified by the degree to which the cervical os is encroached on or covered (Fig. 193-1). As the lower uterine segment elongates during gestation, the amount of placental encroachment on the cervical os (and therefore the risk of bleeding) may lessen. Placenta previa occurs in up to 1% of third-trimester pregnancies.

PLACENTA ACCRETA

On occasion, the placenta can adhere to the implantation site with an absent decidua, an abnormality that produces an absence of the physiologic line of cleavage through the decidual layer. Furthermore, the placenta can invade the myometrium (placenta increta) or can extend through the myometrium and adhere to surrounding structures (placenta percreta).

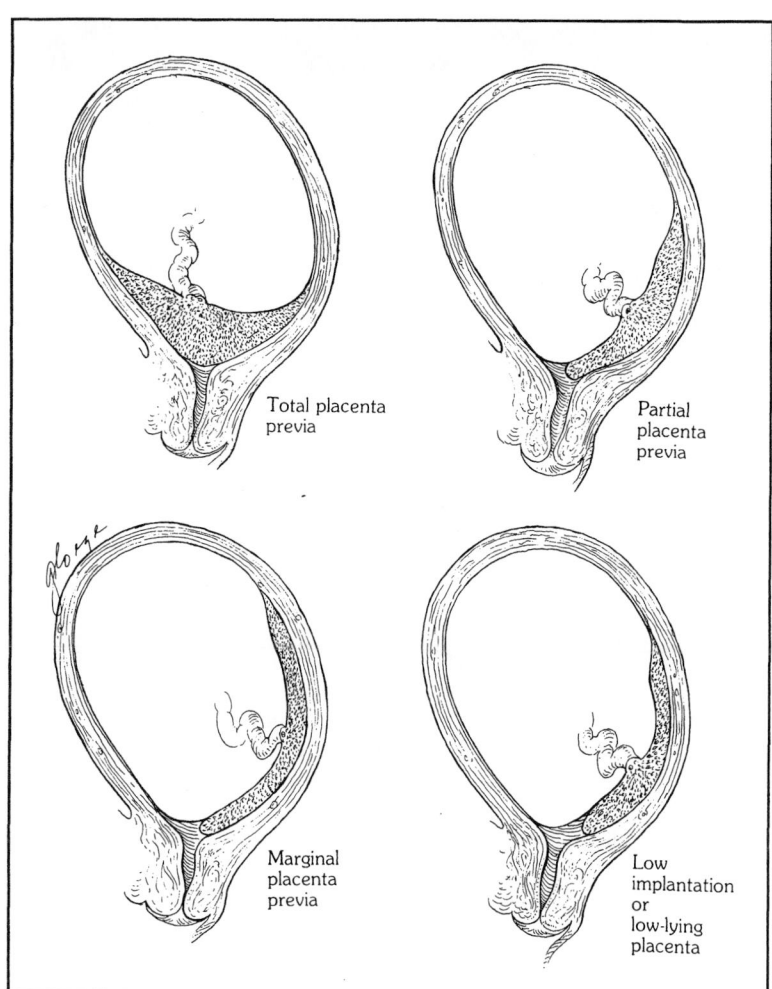

Figure 193–1 ■ Types of placenta previa. (From Ricci JM: Antepartum hemorrhage. In Hacker NF, Moore JG [eds]: Essentials of Obstetrics and Gynecology, 2nd ed. Philadelphia, WB Saunders, 1992, p 156.)

PLACENTAL ABRUPTION

Placental abruption—also referred to as abruptio placentae or placental separation—is defined as the premature separation of a normally situated placenta from its attachment to the placental decidua basalis before the birth of the fetus. Such separation is thought to result from a rupture of placental arteries or veins. In 20% to 35% of cases, the bleeding site is "concealed"; that is, there is no obvious vaginal bleeding. Placental abruption occurs in 0.5% to 1.8% of all pregnancies, with approximately 40% of cases occurring after the 37th week of gestation, 40% occurring between the 34th and 37th weeks, and less than 20% occurring before the 32nd week.

UTERINE RUPTURE

Uterine rupture is defined as a defect in the uterine wall associated with fetal distress or maternal hemorrhage sufficient to require cesarean delivery or postpartum laparotomy. Rupture of the gravid uterus occurs in less than 1% of pregnancies, most often in patients with prior uterine trauma. Uterine scar dehiscence does not require surgical intervention. Although it is more common than true uterine rupture, most cases are asymptomatic and are not likely to cause maternal or fetal mortality. However, uterine scar dehiscence

can result in significant morbidity, especially if it causes extension of the placenta laterally into major uterine vessels or there is abnormal placentation (placenta accreta, increta, or percreta). Cesarean scar rupture is more likely to occur with vaginal birth if labor has been induced or augmented.

VASA PREVIA

Although the umbilical cord typically is attached to the placenta, in about 1% and 9% of single and twin gestations, respectively, it attaches to the chorioamniotic membranes. Such atypical or velamentous insertion exposes the umbilical vessels to trauma or compression as they traverse between the amnion and chorion to reach the placenta. Vasa previa exists when the velamentous umbilical vessels present ahead of the fetus, placing them at even greater risk with rupture of membranes. Fetal exsanguination and demise often result.

UNCLASSIFIED BLEEDING

Unclassified bleeding accounts for almost half of antepartum bleeding (vasa praevia is sometimes included in this category). It usually occurs in late pregnancy, and its cause either is unknown or does not become apparent until later. This type of bleeding, though typically mild with spontaneous resolution, is associated with high perinatal mortality

Table 193–1 ▪ Assessment of Obstetric Hemorrhage

Shock Severity	Findings	Blood Loss (%)
None	None	15-20
Mild	Tachycardia (<100 bpm), mild hypotension, peripheral vasoconstriction	20-25
Moderate	Tachycardia (100-120 bpm), hypotension (SBP 80-100 mm Hg), restlessness, oliguria	25-35
Severe	Tachycardia (>120 bpm), hypotension (SBP <60 mm Hg), altered consciousness, anuria	>35

bpm, beats per minute; SBP, systolic blood pressure.

(3.5% to 15.7%). This may be due to placental dysfunction and higher rates of preterm labor in patients with unclassified bleeding.

Recognition

Hemorrhage during pregnancy can be masked by physiologic adaptations that begin early in pregnancy. As early as 6 to 8 weeks' gestation, there is a progressive increase in plasma volume, reaching near-maximal volume (4700 to 5200 mL) by 32 weeks. This volume, which represents a 45% increase over that in nonpregnant women, is further augmented with multiple gestations and appears to be correlated with fetal weight. Placental chorionic somatomammotropin, progesterone, erythropoietin, and prolactin act in concert to increase red cell mass by 250 to 450 mL at term, an increase of 20% to 30% over pregestational values. The disproportionate increase in plasma volume versus red cell mass accounts for relative hemodilution and the maximal decreases in hematocrit seen by the middle of the third trimester. The resulting decrease in blood viscosity is believed to improve intervillous perfusion, reducing the risk for thromboembolic events. It also serves to reduce red cell loss during delivery. The changes in hematocrit and blood volume help increase maternal cardiac output (heart rate times stroke volume). The heart rate increases from the fifth week of gestation to a maximal increment of 15 to 20 beats per minute by 32 weeks. This is in response to the relative anemia, reduced vagal control, and increased sympathetic tone. Increased stroke volume, which is primarily responsible for the early increase in cardiac output, is related to increased myocardial muscle mass in the first trimester and end-diastolic volume in the second and early third trimesters. Overall, there is a 30% to 50% increase in cardiac output during pregnancy. Half the increase occurs during the first 8 weeks of gestation. The greatest increase is seen immediately post partum.

These physiologic alterations allow the pregnant patient to tolerate 1000 to 1500 mL of blood loss without major hemodynamic changes. However, because nearly 600 to 700 mL of blood flows through the placental intervillous spaces each minute, obstetric hemorrhage can rapidly result in severe signs of shock (Table 193-1). Also, owing to the potential for severe blood loss with antepartum bleeding, the characteristics of the common causes of such bleeding should be reviewed to assist in early diagnosis and treatment (Table 193-2).

Risk Assessment

The risk of antepartum hemorrhage for any one patient cannot be predicted precisely. This risk is affected by many factors, including the presence of any obstetric pathology, medical conditions, or fetal anomalies (Table 193-3).

Implications

In addition to the risk of postpartum hemorrhage, antepartum hemorrhage may have important sequelae. These include coagulopathy, acute renal failure, pituitary necrosis,

Table 193–2 ▪ Characteristics of Early and Late Antepartum Hemorrhage Diagnoses

Diagnosis	Characteristics
Early Pregnancy (≤20 wk)	
Miscarriage	Vaginal bleeding (± pain) >8 wk after last menstrual period; slight tenderness to uterine exam; no adnexal mass
Ectopic pregnancy	Possibly, no vaginal bleeding; pain <8 wk after last menstrual period; unilateral tenderness; possibly shock and normal-sized uterus
Late Pregnancy (≤20 wk)	
Placenta previa	Painless vaginal bleeding (≤10% have painful abruption); malpresentation of fetus (35%); difficulty palpating the presenting fetal part
Placental abruption	Painful vaginal bleeding; uterine irritability or tetany; coagulopathy; fetal distress or demise
Uterine rupture	Vaginal bleeding (± pain); hypotension; cessation of labor; fetal distress
Vasa previa	Painless vaginal bleeding; fetal hemoglobin present in shed blood
Unclassified bleeding	Painless vaginal bleeding; mild bleeding (often resolves spontaneously); often >37 wk gestation

Table 193–3 ■ Risk Factors Associated with Antepartum Hemorrhage

Cause	Risk Factor
Early Pregnancy (≤20 wk)	
Miscarriage	Previous miscarriage; increased maternal age; genetic aberrations; uterine abnormalities; endocrine abnormalities; infection; thrombophilic disorders; immune response abnormalities; tobacco, alcohol, drugs
Ectopic pregnancy	Endometriosis; infertility; infection; past tubal sterilization or reconstruction; intrauterine contraceptive device
Late Pregnancy (≥20 wk)	
Placenta previa	Increased parity or maternal age; prior placenta previa or cesarean delivery
Placental abruption	Trauma; ruptured membranes; cocaine, methadone, tobacco use; preeclampsia; fibroid uterus
Uterine rupture	Previous uterine surgery; trauma; history of intrauterine manipulations, including placental extraction, curettage, version, forceps use; grand multiparity; uterine anomaly; placenta percreta; tumor; fetal issues (e.g., macrosomia, malposition, anomaly); induced or augmented labor
Vasa previa	Multiple gestation; low-lying placenta; pregnancy after in vitro fertilization; velamentous umbilical cord insertion; bilobed and succenturiate placentas

shock, and both maternal and fetal mortality. Perinatal morbidity and mortality are primarily the result of poor placental perfusion or preterm delivery.

Coagulopathy, which is initially dilutional from ongoing loss of blood components and rapid volume replacement, may be accompanied by DIC. Although DIC is an ongoing concern with all cases of antepartum hemorrhage, it most commonly occurs with placental abruption (up to 20% of cases). Laboratory findings supporting the diagnosis of DIC are prolonged prothrombin time and partial thromboplastin time, hypofibrinogenemia, thrombocytopenia, and elevated fibrin degradation products. Although treatment for DIC is controversial, restoration of clotting factors, especially fibrinogen, is required. For a 70-kg adult, 4 g of fibrinogen is required to increase fibrinogen levels by 100 mg/dL. Fibrinogen is found in a 3- to 10-fold greater concentration in cryoprecipitate than in fresh frozen plasma; treatment requires 13 to 16 bags of cryoprecipitate. A fibrinogen level of 150 to 200 mg/dL appears to be optimal for obstetric patients. Keep in mind that it may take 20 to 40 minutes to thaw 1 unit of cryoprecipitate, which is stored at −18°C to −20°C.

Acute renal failure, with or without associated DIC, occurs in about 10% of patients with severe antepartum hemorrhage. Acute renal failure is related to hypotension, renal ischemia, fibrin deposition, microvascular clotting, and myoglobinuria. It is most common with placental abruption and may be prevented by aggressive blood transfusion and volume resuscitation. Hemodynamic monitoring with pulmonary artery or central venous catheters or with transthoracic or transesophageal echocardiography may assist in assessing volume status and the need for inotropes or vasopressors.

Ischemic pituitary necrosis (Sheehan's syndrome) may accompany severe hemorrhage or even delivery without significant blood loss. Enlargement of the pituitary gland, small sella size, DIC, or autoimmunity may also contribute to Sheehan's syndrome. Most commonly it presents as mild pituitary dysfunction, such as the failure to lactate or to resume menses. Acute hyponatremia and hypoglycemia may also accompany Sheehan's syndrome.

MANAGEMENT

Hemodynamic Management

Underestimation of blood loss and inadequate volume resuscitation are common in patients with antepartum hemorrhage and likely contribute to associated maternal mortality. In one report, substandard care was considered a contributing factor in 79% of maternal deaths associated with antepartum hemorrhage. Rapid volume replacement to maintain tissue perfusion and oxygenation is more important than the type of fluid given. Colloids and blood products should be administered early, along with a request for assistance, placement of a second large intravenous line, and use of pressurized transfusion equipment.

Although many centers require blood typing and screening for parturients at high hemorrhagic risk having vaginal deliveries and all those having cesarean sections, it is prudent to crossmatch and have 2 to 4 units of packed red blood cells available whenever there is a potential for significant blood loss. Such cases include known placenta previa or partial abruption and placenta accreta, increta, or percreta. If crossmatched blood is unavailable, type O, Rh-negative blood should be used.

Continued blood loss with hemodynamic instability, despite blood and volume replacement, mandates more invasive monitoring. However, restoration of circulating blood volume takes precedence. Even noninvasive measures (e.g., urine output, heart rate, blood pressure) can help assess the adequacy of volume resuscitation.

In such situations, the need for blood component therapy other than red cell mass may be less than previously thought. After delivery, uterine perfusion and oxygenation are less relevant, and otherwise healthy parturients can usually tolerate severe blood loss. The American Society of Anesthesiologists Task Force on Blood Component Therapy advised that transfusions of packed red blood cells, platelets, and fibrinogen component therapy are rarely indicated unless there is microvascular bleeding, the hemoglobin is less than 6 g/dL, the platelet count is less than $50 \times 10^9/L$, and fibrinogen is less than 80 to 100 mg/dL. Platelet transfusion may be indicated with a normal platelet count ($>100 \times 10^9/L$) and known platelet dysfunction with microvascular bleeding.

Finally, there is now interest in the use of erythropoietin to boost red cell production, autologous blood donation, intraoperative salvage, and acute normovolemic hemodilution in patients at high risk for antepartum hemorrhage. Further study is needed to determine the utility of such therapies.

Anesthetic Management

Hemorrhaging parturients should be prepared for surgery simultaneously while optimizing hemodynamic status. Full replacement of blood loss before surgery is unrealistic, because the bleeding will continue until the cause is removed. Although regional anesthesia may be considered, other more pressing concerns may rule in favor of general endotracheal anesthesia. These include

- Active bleeding
- Hemodynamically unstable patient
- Ongoing, labor-intensive blood and volume resuscitation
- Possible loss of consciousness with an unprotected airway
- Associated coagulopathy and increased risk for subdural or epidural hematoma

Etomidate may be the preferred induction agent in parturients with shock. Hypotension commonly occurs with thiopental, propofol, and even ketamine. After left uterine displacement, preoxygenation, and rapid-sequence induction and intubation, potent inhalational agents are relatively contraindicated because they promote uterine relaxation. Instead, oxygen and nitrous oxide, benzodiazepines, and short-acting narcotics are titrated as tolerated. Urine output should be checked often, and the need for additional intravenous lines or invasive monitoring should be assessed frequently. Following removal of the fetus and placenta, uterotonic agents (oxytocin, methylergonovine, 15-methyl prostaglandin $F_{2\alpha}$) should be administered as necessary. However, underlying uterine pathology may not permit restoration of normal uterine tone or cessation of bleeding. If so, a gravid hysterectomy may be required. This does not require general anesthesia if an epidural catheter is present, functional, and has been controlled.

PREVENTION

Prevention of complications related to severe antepartum hemorrhage requires a high index of suspicion based on the patient's history and symptoms, evaluation by ultrasonography or magnetic resonance imaging, and an expedited team response. Imaging, especially with color Doppler blood flow enhancement, has greatly improved the diagnosis of placenta previa, placental invasion of the uterine wall (placenta accreta, increta, percreta), and vasa praevia and the maternal and fetal outcomes. Even so, there are limits to the diagnostic sensitivity and specificity of these imaging methods, as well as limited access in some places. Therefore, a

"double setup" may be required. This involves digital examination of the vaginal fornices in the operating room, with the patient prepared for emergent cesarean delivery. This is now done only for patients with active bleeding, known fetal well-being, and equivocal imaging studies. Alternatively, interventional radiologists can place balloon occlusion catheters in the uterine arteries of very high-risk parturients, permitting rapid control of bleeding should this become necessary.

Further Reading

Anderson FW, Hogan JG, Ansbacher R: Sudden death: Ectopic pregnancy mortality. Obstet Gynecol 103:1218-1223, 2004.

Bick RL: Syndromes of disseminated intravascular coagulation in obstetrics, pregnancy, and gynecology: Objective criteria for diagnosis and management. Hematol Oncol Clin North Am 14:999-1044, 2000.

Bick RL: Disseminated intravascular coagulation: A review of etiology, pathophysiology, diagnosis, and management: Guidelines for care. Clin Appl Thromb Hemost 8:1-31, 2002.

Birnbach DJ, Browne IM: Anesthesia for obstetrics. In Miller RD (ed): Miller's Anesthesia, 6th ed. Philadelphia, Churchill Livingstone, 2005, pp 2307–2344.

Carretti N, La Marca A: Maternal serum levels of human chorionic somatotropin correlates with transferrin and erythropoietin in pregnancy. Gynecol Obstet Invest 53:28-31, 2002.

Chan CC, To WW: Antepartum hemorrhage of unknown origin—what is its clinical significance? Acta Obstet Gynecol Scand 78:186-190, 1999.

Chestnut DH, Dewan DM, Redick LF, et al: Anesthetic management for obstetric hysterectomy: A multi-institutional study. Anesthesiology 70:607-610, 1989.

Coste J, Bouyer J, Ughetto S, et al: Ectopic pregnancy is again on the increase: Recent trends in the incidence of ectopic pregnancies in France (1992-2002). Hum Reprod 9:2014-2018, 2004.

Duvekot JJ, Cheriex EC, Pieters FA, et al: Maternal volume homeostasis in early pregnancy in relation to fetal growth restriction. Obstet Gynecol 85:361-367, 1995.

Gilson GJ, Samaan S, Crawford MH, et al: Changes in hemodynamics, ventricular remodeling, and ventricular contractility during normal pregnancy: A longitudinal study. Obstet Gynecol 89:957-962, 1997.

Gonik B: Intensive care monitoring of the critically ill pregnant patient. In Creasy RK, Resnik R (eds): Maternal-Fetal Medicine. Philadelphia, WB Saunders, 1994, pp 865-890.

Guise JM, McDonagh MS, Osterweil P, et al: Systematic review of the incidence and consequences of uterine rupture in women with previous caesarean section. BMJ 329:19-25, 2004.

Hansch E, Chitkara U, McAlpine J, et al: Pelvic arterial embolization for control of obstetric hemorrhage: A five-year experience. Am J Obstet Gynecol 180:1454-1460, 1999.

Hunter S, Robson SC: Adaptation of the maternal heart in pregnancy. Br Heart J 68:540-543, 1992.

Kelestimur F: Sheehan's syndrome. Pituitary 6:181-188, 2003.

Koonin LM, MacKay AP, Berg CJ, et al: Pregnancy-related mortality surveillance—United States, 1987-1990. MMWR CDC Surveill Summ 46:17-36, 1997.

Lund CJ, Donovan JC: Blood volume during pregnancy: Significance of plasma and red cell volumes. Am J Obstet Gynecol 98:394-403, 1967.

Paterson ME: The aetiology and outcome of abruptio placentae. Acta Obstet Gynecol Scand 58:31-35, 1979.

Pritchard JA, Brekken AL: Clinical and laboratory studies on severe abruptio placentae. Am J Obstet Gynecol 97:681-700, 1967.

Rosevear S: Bleeding in early pregnancy. In James DK, Steer PJ, Weiner CP, Gonik B (eds): High Risk Pregnancy Management Options. London, WB Saunders, 1999.

Why Mothers Die 1997-1999: Confidential Enquiries into Maternal Deaths in the United Kingdom. London, Department of Health, HMSO, 2001, pp 36-37.

Williams MA, Mittendorf R, Lieberman E, Monson RR: Adverse infant outcomes associated with first-trimester vaginal bleeding. Obstet Gynecol 78:14-18, 1991.

Postpartum Hemorrhage

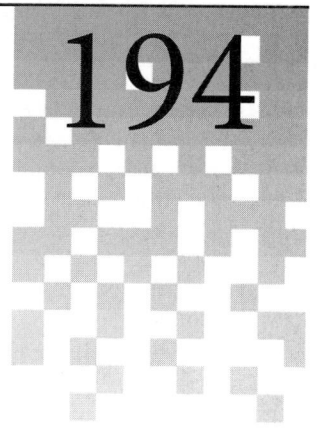

194

Monica N. Riesner and Linda S. Polley

OTHER SURGICAL SUBSPECIALTIES

Case Synopsis

A 32-year-old woman, gravida 5, para 4, has continuous labor epidural analgesia and an uneventful vaginal delivery of a 4500-g infant. The anesthesiologist is called 10 minutes after delivery of the placenta when the patient is noted to be hypotensive, tachycardic, pale, and nauseated. On arrival, the anesthesiologist notices a pool of blood at the foot of the bed, a steady flow of blood per vagina, and the obstetrician vigorously massaging the uterus through the abdominal wall.

PROBLEM ANALYSIS

Definition

Every delivery is associated with some blood loss. Postpartum hemorrhage has been defined as blood loss greater than 500 mL in the first 24 hours after delivery. However, because blood loss at the time of normal vaginal or cesarean delivery may approximate or even exceed 500 mL, this definition is not useful clinically. For most cases of postpartum hemorrhage that cause morbidity or mortality or that present management problems, blood loss is significantly greater than 500 mL. Most of these cases occur immediately after birth or within the first hour after delivery.

Recognition

Postpartum hemorrhage occurs in as many as 10% of deliveries. Postpartum blood loss is difficult to quantitate and is often underestimated. Bleeding may be obvious, such as per vagina or into the surgical wound; however, it can also be concealed and contained within the uterus, soft tissues, or peritoneum. The patient often has hypotension, tachycardia, and oliguria. In addition, there may be ongoing volume requirements.

Risk Assessment

Causes of postpartum hemorrhage and predisposing factors are listed in Table 194-1. The most common cause is uterine atony. At term, blood flow through the placental vasculature is approximately 600 mL/minute. After delivery, the primary mechanism by which blood loss is controlled is contraction of the uterine myometrium to constrict severed vessels at the former placental site. Failure of this mechanism can result in massive and rapid blood loss. Predisposing factors are any that result in overdistention of the uterus or reduce the ability of the myometrium to contract, including

- Multiple gestation
- Macrosomia
- Polyhydramnios
- Chorioamnionitis
- Prolonged labor
- Precipitous labor
- Augmented labor
- High parity
- Tocolytic agents
- Inhalational anesthetics at high concentrations
- History of uterine atony (increased likelihood of recurrence)

Retained placenta is also a common cause of both early and delayed postpartum hemorrhage, although not all cases result in significant blood loss. Retained placental fragments may be unrecognized; thus, bleeding might be insidious and cause delayed postpartum hemorrhage. Patients who have had a prior retained placenta or who deliver well before term are predisposed to retained placenta.

Trauma associated with delivery represents another cause of postpartum hemorrhage and should be considered in all postpartum patients with continued blood loss despite a firm, contracted uterus. Traumatic postpartum hemorrhage can be categorized as follows:

- Vaginal
- Cervical
- Perineal laceration
- Episiotomy

Table 194–1 ■ Postpartum Hemorrhage: Causes and Predisposing Factors	
Cause	**Predisposing Factors**
Uterine atony	Multiple gestation, macrosomia, polyhydramnios, chorioamnionitis, prolonged labor, precipitous labor, augmented labor, multiparity, use of tocolytics, use of potent inhalational anesthetics, prior uterine atony
Retained placenta	Prior history of retained placenta, second-trimester delivery, abnormal placentation
Trauma to genital tract	Precipitous delivery, instrumented delivery, macrosomia
Uterine inversion	Uterine atony, inappropriate umbilical cord traction, uterine anomalies, abnormal placentation

779

9

Traumatic laceration of blood vessels, whether occurring during vaginal or cesarean delivery, can result in pelvic hematoma. Uterine rupture, especially in patients who give birth vaginally after a previous cesarean delivery, is another potential cause of postpartum bleeding. In addition to the use of instrumentation for delivery, many cases of postpartum hemorrhage occur with precipitous delivery or delivery of macrosomic infants.

Uterine inversion is a rare cause of postpartum hemorrhage but can be catastrophic. It should be suspected in any case of postpartum hemorrhage when significant hypotension coexists. Most cases of uterine inversion are obvious owing to the associated vaginal mass. Risk factors for uterine inversion include uterine atony, inappropriately applied fundal pressure or umbilical cord traction, uterine anomalies, and abnormal placentation.

Implications

Patient outcome depends on the severity and rate of blood loss, as well as the need for additional anesthetic or obstetric interventions. Postpartum hemorrhage is a major cause of morbidity and remains one of the top five causes of maternal death in both developed and developing countries.

MANAGEMENT

Basic Management

Similar to any case of hemorrhage, basic resuscitative measures are required. Blood pressure, heart rate, respiration, and level of consciousness should be assessed quickly whenever one is called to evaluate a patient with postpartum bleeding. Adequate intravenous access should be obtained if it is not already present. General supportive measures are instituted, including oxygen by facemask and Trendelenburg positioning. Appropriate blood products should be requested and, depending on the situation, additional anesthesia help should be summoned. For all categories of anesthetic management, one must remember that immediately post partum, all patients continue to have delayed gastric emptying. Therefore, an oral nonparticulate antacid should be administered before any anesthetic intervention is performed.

Obstetric and Anesthetic Management

Analgesia or anesthesia may be required, depending on the need for surgical intervention. Manual extraction of the placenta is usually a brief procedure, but in most cases of retained placenta, some form of analgesia or anesthesia is necessary. If an epidural catheter is in place and functional, it may be possible to perform manual extraction without further anesthesia. Alternatively, a bolus of local anesthetic can be administered epidurally if the patient's volume status is adequate. If a catheter is not in place or not functioning, it may be possible to perform a manual extraction using small amounts of intravenous opioids, anxiolytics, or ketamine. Forty percent to 50% nitrous oxide by facemask can also be administered as an adjunct to provide some

degree of analgesia. If this proves inadequate, a low spinal anesthetic may be administered, provided that the patient has received adequate volume resuscitation. If general anesthesia is required, rapid-sequence induction with cricoid pressure and tracheal intubation is necessary.

If the cause of hemorrhage is uterine atony, obstetric treatment initially involves external uterine massage and administration of uterotonic agents. If bleeding continues, laparotomy and ligation of uterine, hypogastric, or ovarian arteries, or even hysterectomy, may be necessary. These may be prolonged surgical procedures with massive blood loss. Regional anesthesia can be used, especially if an epidural catheter is already in place; however, this should be considered only when there are adequate anesthesia personnel to perform the multiple simultaneous tasks required. Because patients with epidural catheters (or single or continuous spinal blocks) are often awake, it may be difficult to manage ongoing volume resuscitation while also establishing arterial or central access. Further, sympathetic block with central neuraxial techniques may complicate the management of ongoing hemorrhage, especially if block reinforcement is required.

Repair of vaginal or perineal lacerations can sometimes be performed with local anesthetic infiltration by the obstetrician. However, most patients with significant postpartum hemorrhage from these causes require spinal or epidural anesthesia, and some require general anesthesia. The obstetrician often needs excellent exposure to repair a cervical laceration, necessitating the use of spinal, epidural, or general anesthesia with muscle relaxants. Evacuation of pelvic or retroperitoneal hematomas usually requires laparotomy, and central neuraxial block or general anesthesia is needed for such procedures.

TOCOLYTIC AGENTS

Management of retained placenta and uterine inversion involves the administration of tocolytic medications to allow the obstetrician to perform manual extraction or replace the inverted uterus. In normovolemic patients, intravenous nitroglycerin (50 to 100 μg) provides uterine relaxation in about 45 seconds and lasts approximately 60 seconds. Nitroglycerin spray is also used as an alternative to intravenous administration for uterine relaxation. Each spray delivers about 400 μg of nitroglycerin sublingually; therefore, careful attention to the patient's blood pressure is essential. If nitroglycerin is ineffective or the cervical os has closed (i.e., does not permit a transvaginal or other operative procedure), deep general anesthesia may be needed. After rapid-sequence induction and tracheal intubation, a potent volatile agent provides uterine relaxation, but the agent should be discontinued as soon as possible after the intervention.

OXYTOCIC AGENTS

The primary treatment for uterine atony is the use of uterotonic medications. Oxytocin is the first choice for both the treatment and prophylaxis of uterine atony. Prophylactic oxytocics reduce the risk of postpartum hemorrhage by about 60%. Oxytocin is typically administered by intravenous infusion, with 20 to 40 units added to 1 L of carrier fluid.

It can cause vasodilatation and hypotension if administered by bolus. If this alone is unsuccessful, ergot alkaloids are second-line medications for the treatment of uterine atony. Both ergonovine and methylergonovine produce tetanic uterine contractions, most likely mediated by α-adrenergic receptors. The usual dose is 0.2 mg intramuscularly. Effects are observed within a few minutes and last several hours. These agents may cause extreme hypertension, especially in hypertensive patients or those receiving concomitant vasopressor therapy. Such ergot-induced hypertension may be severe enough to cause intracranial hemorrhage, stroke, or seizures.

If these methods fail to relieve uterine atony, 15-methyl prostaglandin $F_{2\alpha}$ can be used to treat refractory cases. However, it may cause bronchospasm and alter lung ventilation-perfusion ratios, causing hypoxemia. The usual dose is 250 μg administered intramuscularly or intramyometrially. It can be repeated every 15 to 30 minutes, but the total dosage should not exceed 2 mg. Misoprostol, another prostaglandin, has been investigated for safety and efficacy in the treatment of postpartum hemorrhage. A dose of 1000 μg per rectum has been shown to be effective for severe postpartum hemorrhage unresponsive to standard uterotonic agents. Recently, several case reports have described the successful use of recombinant factor VIIa (20 to 40 μg/kg) in patients with severe, refractory postpartum hemorrhage.

PREVENTION

Postpartum hemorrhage usually occurs without warning. Prevention of associated morbidity and mortality requires vigilance, a high index of suspicion, and preparedness for a rapid response.

Further Reading

Boehlen F, Morales MA, Fontana P, et al: Prolonged treatment of massive postpartum haemorrhage with recombinant factor VIIa: Case report and review of the literature. Br J Obstet Gynaecol 3:284-287, 2004.

Crowley M: Postpartum hemorrhage. In Atlee JL (ed): Complications in Anesthesia. Philadelphia, WB Saunders, 1999, pp 817-819.

El-Refaey H, Rodeck C: Post-partum haemorrhage: Definitions, medical and surgical management: A time for change. Br Med Bull 67:205-217, 2003.

Mayer D, Spielman F, Bell E: Antepartum and postpartum hemorrhage. In Chestnut DH (ed): Obstetric Anesthesia Principles and Practice, 3rd ed. Philadelphia, Elsevier Mosby, 2004, pp 668-682.

Papp Z: Massive obstetric hemorrhage. J Perinat Med 31:408-414, 2003.

Pulmonary Aspiration in the Parturient

195

Nollag O'Rourke and William R. Camann

Case Synopsis

A 32-year-old woman, gravida 2, para 1, with a full-term pregnancy undergoes general anesthesia for emergency cesarean delivery owing to prolonged fetal bradycardia. The patient receives a rapid-sequence induction using thiopental and succinylcholine. The trachea is intubated using a 3.0 MacIntosh blade, cricoid pressure, and a styletted 7.5 endotracheal tube. After cesarean delivery, the patient is extubated and transferred to the postanesthesia care unit. She is breathing spontaneously with supplemental oxygen. Vital signs include blood pressure of 110/78 mm Hg, heart rate of 96 beats per minute, and arterial oxygen saturation of 88% on 6 L of oxygen by facemask. On physical examination, the patient is noted to have bilateral wheezing, and the chest radiograph reveals a right lower lobe infiltrate.

PROBLEM ANALYSIS

Definition

Pain relief during childbirth has long been of interest to anesthesiologists. As the quest for optimal analgesia and anesthesia for childbirth continues, so does that for the prevention and management of one of the most important peripartum complications: pulmonary aspiration of gastric contents. Hall first noted an increased incidence of this complication in obstetric patients in 1940. The term used to describe such pulmonary aspiration, *chemical pneumonitis*, soon gained popularity. In 1946 Mendelson more completely defined this condition.

Parturients belong to a special category of patients at increased risk for difficult or failed intubation and aspiration. The incidence of failed intubation in obstetric patients is estimated to be 8 to 10 times greater than that in the general surgical population. Aspiration pneumonitis most often occurs with difficult or failed intubation. However, there are pregnancy-specific factors that contribute to the increased risk of aspiration, including the following:

- Increased levels of progesterone
- Reduced sphincter tone at the gastroesophageal junction
- Elevation of the gravid uterus against the stomach
- Mechanical obstruction of the duodenum by the latter

The gravid uterus further compromises esophageal sphincter tone due to distortion of the gastroesophageal angle. Also, "pushing" during the second stage of labor, manual pressure on the lower abdomen, and the lithotomy position act in concert to increase intra-abdominal pressure and decrease gastric emptying (Table 195-1).

The production of motilin, a hormone that speeds gastric emptying, is depressed throughout pregnancy and returns to near normal by 1 week post partum. Nevertheless, gastric emptying appears to be normal in early pregnancy.

The cause of delayed gastric emptying during advanced labor, despite satisfactory epidural analgesia, is unknown. However, recent work suggests that gastric volume and acidity at term gestation are no different from those parameters in the nonpregnant state, during early pregnancy, or in the postpartum period.

Iatrogenic factors that may increase the risk of gastric aspiration include parenteral or epidural opioids and the use of anticholinergic drugs (e.g., glycopyrrolate). Opioids slow gastric motility, and anticholinergics reduce esophageal sphincter tone.

Recognition

Signs and symptoms of chemical pulmonary aspiration are quite variable and are largely a function of volume and pH (Table 195-2); however, such aspiration may also be "silent." Further, the anesthetist may be unable to see aspirate in the posterior oral pharynx. Coughing and bronchospasm may

Table 195–1 ■ Aspiration Risk Factors Related to the Parturient

Cause	Effect
Gastric volume and acidity	No change at term or during early pregnancy
Increased levels of progesterone	Reduced gastroesophageal sphincter tone
Reduced levels of motilin	Delayed gastric emptying in advanced labor
Gravid uterus	Mechanical compromise of esophageal sphincter
Parenteral or epidural opioids	Decreased gastric motility and sedation
Anticholinergic drugs	Decreased esophageal sphincter tone

Table 195–2 ▪ Signs and Symptoms of Chemical Pulmonary Aspiration
None
Gastric contents in oropharynx
Cough
Bronchospasm
Oxygen desaturation
Circulatory shock
Infiltrates on chest radiograph

also be infrequent symptoms. Often, radiographic changes provide the first evidence of aspiration; such changes are found in dependent parts of the lung, often in the right lower lobe.

The outcome for patients with chemical pulmonary aspiration can be categorized as follows: Roughly 10% to 15% of patients have rapid clinical deterioration, with hypoxia and early circulatory shock. Of the remaining patients, approximately two thirds improve rapidly within 1 to 4 days; they may require ventilatory support. The other one third develop bacterial lung infections necessitating antibiotic therapy. Most lung injuries eventually resolve.

Risk Assessment

The actual incidence of maternal chemical aspiration is unknown. It is likely that minor degrees of aspiration often go unnoticed, and only maternal deaths from aspiration are reported. In a retrospective review of 185,000 anesthetic inductions, Olsen and colleagues found that the incidence of aspiration was 1 in 2131 (0.047%) for nonobstetric inductions and 1 in 661 (0.15%) for inductions before cesarean delivery (i.e., a threefold increase in aspiration risk during pregnancy). Warner and colleagues found the incidence to be 1 in 3216 (0.031%) for general anesthesia and 1 in 895 (0.11%) for emergency operations. Although Warner's group evaluated all types of emergency cases, cesarean delivery is often emergent. More recently, Ezri and colleagues retrospectively studied patients having general anesthesia around the time of delivery (e.g., manual extraction of placenta) or immediately after delivery (e.g., repair of lacerations) from 1979 to 1993. They found a 0.05% incidence of aspiration (1 in 1870 cases). All patients were breathing spontaneously, were not intubated, and had general anesthesia induced and maintained with intravenous agents. The lower incidence of aspiration in this group compared with the general surgical population might be related to reduced intra-abdominal pressure. Also, many cases of chemical pulmonary aspiration occur with difficult or failed intubations that require mask ventilation.

Even more recently, Han and coworkers reported the use of laryngeal mask airway for elective cesarean delivery in 1060 patients. Although there were no reported cases of aspiration, this success may be attributed to careful patient selection. Among the patients excluded were those with symptoms of gastric reflux, an American Society of Anesthesiologists (ASA) classification higher than II, a known difficult airway, or a prepregnancy body mass index greater than 30, as well as those who had fasted for less than 6 hours. Also, antacid prophylaxis was used preoperatively, and cricoid pressure was applied. However, in practice, almost all parturients requiring general anesthesia are those with obstetric emergencies, especially the unexpected need for cesarean delivery. We believe that such nonfasting patients require a rapid-sequence induction and tracheal intubation.

Finally, anesthesia-related maternal mortality has decreased in recent years due to the increased use of regional anesthesia. Even so, Hawkins and coworkers reported that 23% of all anesthesia-related deaths in obstetric patients were a direct result of aspiration. Although data on maternal morbidity with perioperative aspiration are generally not reported, several studies now indicate that there is still significant morbidity associated with this condition in obstetric patients. Although all parturients are at increased risk for chemical pulmonary aspiration, the timing and nature of peripartum surgery, as well as the circumstances under which general anesthesia is performed, must be considered when interpreting studies of the incidence of peripartum pulmonary chemical aspiration.

Implications

The volume, content, and character of any gastric aspirate determine the severity of pneumonitis after pulmonary aspiration. Many believe that gastric pH is more critical for determining the severity of lung injury after pulmonary aspiration than is the actual volume (provided it is < 25 mL). Others, notably James and associates, believe that regardless of volume, lower pH correlates with higher mortality.

Particulate matter increases the risk of lung injury after aspiration, because large particles can lodge in major bronchi, causing asphyxiation within minutes. However, nonacid aspirates may produce only mild, transient hypoxia, with no evidence of parenchymal injury; such hypoxia may be due to bronchospasm and microatelectasis. As the acidity of the aspirate increases, the potential for parenchymal injury and pulmonary hemorrhage increases. Amplification of this response may lead to the acute respiratory distress syndrome, which is characterized by persistent lung inflammation with radiologic evidence of bilateral pulmonary infiltrates. These infiltrates are due to increased vascular permeability and reduced arterial oxygen tension (irrespective of the fraction of inspired oxygen or the use of positive end-expiratory pressure), with no increase in left atrial pressure. Survival has improved with better supportive care and ventilatory strategies, but mortality from gastric aspiration and associated acute respiratory distress syndrome is still very high, with current estimates ranging from 35% to 40%.

MANAGEMENT

Immediately after aspiration, airway management is critical (Table 195-3). Any aspirate identified in the posterior oral pharynx should be quickly evacuated, and the airway should be secured. Although several authors recommend a head-down tilt or left lateral decubitus position to minimize the spread of aspirate, this position has not been proved to reduce such spread. Tracheal suctioning without saline

Table 195–3 ■ Indicated Therapy after Suspected Pulmonary Aspiration

Secure airway; provide supplemental oxygen and positive end-expiratory pressure
Place patient in head-down position and turn head to one side
Alternatively, place patient in left lateral decubitus position
Provide tracheal suctioning (intubate to protect airway, if not already done)
Once airway is protected, consider gastric decompression with oro- or nasogastric tube
Initiate β-agonist therapy for bronchospasm
Consider systemic steroids (dexamethasone 1 mg/kg or methylprednisolone 30 mg/kg)
Institute conservative fluid management

lavage is advised for removal of the aspirate. Saline lavage may disseminate the aspirate to more distal airways and worsen the situation. The pH of the aspirate may be measured to help identify the nature of the gastric contents.

The most important factors for reducing morbidity are quick identification of aspiration, expeditious airway intubation, and ventilation with supplemental oxygen and positive end-expiratory pressure. Bronchospasm may be relieved by the administration of an intravenous β-agonist. Although acid-injured lungs are more susceptible to bacterial infection, there is no evidence that prophylactic antibiotic administration alters the incidence of infection, nor does it affect the outcome. Prophylactic antibiotics may even facilitate the development of infection with resistant organisms. Similarly, the administration of systemic glucocorticoids is controversial. Several animal models suggest a reduction in pulmonary damage if steroids are given immediately after the insult. Other data suggest that any benefit may be outweighed by steroid-caused reduction of macrophage activity and subsequent increased susceptibility to gram-negative pneumonia. Although it is not uncommon to administer methylprednisolone (30 mg/kg) or dexamethasone (1 mg/kg), current thinking does not advocate this practice. The use of fluids must be restricted. Damaged pulmonary endothelium exudes protein-rich edematous fluid, and patients may be further compromised by pulmonary edema from the overly aggressive use of intravenous fluids.

PREVENTION

Perhaps the single most important treatment measure is prevention. Preventive measures include the following:

- Implementation of ASA fasting guidelines in patients in labor
- Regional anesthesia
- Cricoid pressure
- Administration of nonparticulate antacid
- Metoclopramide administration
- H$_2$-receptor antagonist administration

Prevention approaches can be categorized as pharmacologic and nonpharmacologic. The nonpharmacologic approach includes implementing ASA fasting guidelines in

patients in labor and minimizing their exposure to general anesthesia with the appropriate use of regional techniques. However, emergencies may arise that require general anesthesia under conditions that are less than optimal for intubation. In these situations, prevention is often a combination of pharmacologic and classic full-stomach precautions.

Recent national trends encourage the oral intake of fluids during labor, and the ASA Task Force on Obstetrical Anesthesia supports this practice. Owing to the adverse metabolic consequences of prolonged starvation during labor, modest amounts of clear fluids, including isotonic "sports drinks," are now recommended for patients with uncomplicated labor. However, in patients with additional risk factors for aspiration (e.g., morbid obesity, diabetes, difficult airway) or an increased risk of operative delivery, more restricted oral intake may be required; this should be decided on a case-by-case basis. Solid food should be avoided in all patients in active labor and those who have received opioid-containing analgesics.

Cricoid pressure is a simple technique that may help prevent passive regurgitation during induction of general anesthesia. Pressure must be maintained until the trachea is intubated, the endotracheal cuff is inflated, and intubation is confirmed. In approximately 5% to 7% of obstetric patients, intubation is difficult to perform. If a difficult airway is anticipated, an awake intubation may be appropriate. Just as these patients are at risk for aspiration during induction, similar precautions must be observed during extubation. Extubation should occur only when the patient is conscious and able to follow commands appropriately. It is important to differentiate between the excitement phase of recovery and actual emergence. Airway assessment, management of failed intubation, and alternative techniques of airway management should be reviewed before the induction of general anesthesia.

Pharmacologic approaches to reducing the risk of aspiration often begin with the administration of a nonparticulate antacid. Antacids are one of the most effective and practical means of altering gastric pH. However, the maximal effects of nonparticulate antacids are limited to approximately 30 minutes' duration. Similarly, the administration of 10 mg intravenous metoclopramide is beneficial. Although metoclopramide does not directly affect gastric pH, it possesses antiemetic properties, increases lower esophageal sphincter tone, and decreases gastric emptying time. A reduction in gastric volume can be observed after about 20 minutes of intravenous administration. H$_2$-receptor antagonists, such as cimetidine, ranitidine, and famotidine, are effective in reducing hydrochloric acid production by the gastric parietal cells. With histamine blockers, timing is important; effects can be seen 30 minutes after intravenous administration, but 60 to 90 minutes are required for maximal effect. This delay in onset limits their efficacy during an emergency. In addition to histamine and gastrin, acetylcholine is an endogenous secretagogue. Administration of anticholinergic medications can inhibit gastric fluid production, with variable results. Of the anticholinergics, glycopyrrolate has the most profound effect on gastric secretion and pH. However, this benefit is outweighed by concurrent reduction of lower esophageal sphincter tone and delayed gastric emptying. Consequently, these medications are not recommended for aspiration prophylaxis.

Further Reading

American Society of Anesthesiologists Task Force on Obstetric Anesthesia: Practice guidelines for obstetric anesthesia. Anesthesiology 90:600, 1999.

Downs JB, Chapman RL, Modell JH, et al: An evaluation of steroid therapy in aspiration pneumonitis. Anesthesiology 40:129, 1994.

Ezri T, Szmuk P, Stein A, et al: Peripartum general anesthesia without tracheal intubation: Incidence of pulmonary aspiration. Anaesthesia 55:421, 2000.

Gibbs CP: Gastric aspiration prevention and treatment. Clin Anesth 4:47, 1986.

Hall GC: Aspiration pneumonitis as an obstetric hazard. JAMA 114:728, 1940.

Han TH, Brimacombe J, Lee EJ, et al: The laryngeal mask airway is effective (and probably safe) in selected healthy parturients for elective cesarean section: A prospective study of 1067 cases. Can J Anaesth 48:1117, 2001.

Hawkins JL, Koonin L, Palmer SK, et al: Anesthesia-related deaths during obstetric delivery in the United States, 1979-1990. Anesthesiology 86:277, 1997.

James CF, Modell JH, Gibbs CP, et al: Pulmonary aspiration effects of volume and pH in the rat. Anesth Analg 63:665, 1984.

King TA, Adams AP: Failed tracheal intubation. Br J Anaesth 65:400, 1990.

Kubli M, Scrutton MJ, Seed PT, et al: An evaluation of "isotonic sports drinks" during labor. Anesth Anal 94:404, 2002.

Malinow AM, Ostheimer GW: Anesthesia for the high-risk parturient. Obstet Gynecol 69:951, 1987.

Mendelson CL: Aspiration of stomach contents into lungs during obstetric anesthesia. Am J Obstet Gynecol 53:191, 1946.

Olsen GL, Hallen B, Hambraes-Johnson K: Aspiration during anaesthesia: A computer-aided study of 185,358 anesthetics. Acta Anaesthesiol Scand 30:84, 1986.

O'Sullivan G, Scrutton M: NPO during labor: Is there any scientific validation? Anesthesiol Clin North Am 21:87, 2003.

Schwartz DJ, Wynne JW, Gibbs CP, et al: The pulmonary consequences of aspiration of gastric contents at pH values greater than 2.5. Am Rev Respir Dis 121:119, 1980.

Warner MA, Warner ME, Webber JG: Clinical significance of pulmonary aspiration during the perioperative period. Anesthesiology 78:56, 1993.

OTHER SURGICAL SUBSPECIALTIES

Embolic Events of Pregnancy

Cheryl DeSimone

196

Case Synopsis

A 32-year-old woman, gravida 2, para 0, undergoes cesarean delivery of twins under spinal anesthesia. After delivery of the neonates, the patient complains of chest pain; oxygen saturation subsequently decreases to 75%, and blood pressure falls to 60/40 mm Hg.

PROBLEM ANALYSIS

Definition

Embolic events during pregnancy are the leading cause of maternal mortality in the United States, accounting for 20% of all maternal deaths. Such events are the most common causes of acute hemodynamic and respiratory collapse during pregnancy. Embolism results from blood clots, fat particles, tumor cells, air, amniotic fluid, or foreign material entering the circulatory system. Most emboli originate from venous thromboses, amniotic fluid, or air.

The clinical presentation of embolic events in pregnancy varies from no symptoms to cardiovascular collapse. Variation in the initial presentation of such events is due to the size and type of embolus, as well as its location.

Recognition

PULMONARY EMBOLISM

Symptoms of pulmonary embolism are listed in Table 196-1. In the case of a massive embolism, defined as obstruction of more than 50% of the pulmonary circulation, hypotension, syncope, or cardiovascular collapse may be the presenting symptom.

If pulmonary embolism is clinically suspected, a chest radiograph, electrocardiogram (ECG), and arterial blood gas analysis may assist in the diagnosis. However, the primary screening tool for diagnosis is a ventilation-perfusion scan. A normal scan precludes the presence of pulmonary embolus. A high-probability scan indicates the need for therapy. An indeterminate scan may require further study, including spiral (helical) computed tomography or pulmonary angiography.

AMNIOTIC FLUID EMBOLISM

Whereas the classic presentation of amniotic fluid embolism is the sudden onset of dyspnea, cyanosis, and hypotension followed by cardiovascular collapse, signs and symptoms are often vague, nonspecific, and similar to those of other types of pulmonary embolism (Table 196-2). Twenty percent of patients initially present with a seizure, and 40% develop consumptive coagulopathy and profuse hemorrhage.

Primarily, the diagnosis is made by the clinical presentation. Because many patients are hemodynamically unstable, it may be difficult to perform specific testing. In acute cases, the ECG may show a right ventricular strain pattern, with typical ST-T changes and tachycardia. Transthoracic or transesophageal echocardiography confirms severe left ventricular failure. The chest radiograph may be normal or show effusions, an enlarged cardiac silhouette, or pulmonary edema. Pulmonary scans may show multiple filling defects. Identification of fetal squamous cells in the pulmonary artery was once considered pathognomonic for amniotic fluid embolism, but this is no longer the case, because such cells may be recovered from the pulmonary circulation of pregnant women without amniotic fluid embolism.

The term *anaphylactoid syndrome of pregnancy* is often used to describe the clinical manifestations of amniotic fluid embolism. It presents similarly to toxic reactions involving multiple organ systems. Anaphylactoid syndrome of pregnancy has three distinct phases, which may occur separately or together. After embolism, respiratory distress with cyanosis occurs. This leads to hemodynamic compromise, pulmonary edema, and cardiovascular shock. Ultimately, seizures, coma, or both result from cerebral hypoperfusion.

VENOUS AIR EMBOLISM

Symptoms and signs of venous air embolism are listed in Table 196-3. In patients under general anesthesia, an abrupt reduction in end-tidal carbon dioxide may be the initial sign. The clinical presentation depends on the volume, rate, and duration of air entrainment, as well as where it is deposited. Air in the coronary circulation may cause cardiac arrhythmias,

Table 196–1 ■ Signs and Symptoms of Pulmonary Embolism
Sudden onset of tachypnea
Dyspnea
Pleuritic chest pain
Apprehension
Nonproductive cough
Hemoptysis
Cyanosis
Accentuated second heart sound

786

Table 196–2 ■ Signs and Symptoms of Amniotic Fluid Embolism
Dyspnea
Cyanosis
Hypotension
Seizures
Cardiovascular collapse
Consumptive coagulopathy with profuse hemorrhage

chest pain, and myocardial infarction. Cerebral air embolism is associated with seizures, unconsciousness, paralysis, or visual disturbances. Hypotension and cardiac arrest may result from air in the pulmonary outflow track. Disseminated intravascular coagulation and endothelial damage result from air within the microcirculation; these are later manifestations.

Capnography appears to be the most sensitive means of detecting venous air embolism. A sudden decrease in end-tidal carbon dioxide occurs, followed by reduced arterial oxygen saturation. Precordial Doppler ultrasonography may confirm the diagnosis. Transesophageal echocardiography is more sensitive and specific, but use of this test is limited in obstetric practice. Finally, air aspiration from a central venous pressure catheter is diagnostic.

Risk Assessment

PULMONARY EMBOLISM

The incidence of thromboembolism during pregnancy is from 0.5 to 3 per 1000 patients. Of these, pulmonary embolism occurs in up to 24%, with a mortality rate of 15%. This incidence is five times greater than in nonpregnant patients and is due to increased lower extremity venous stasis and hypercoagulability associated with pregnancy.

Thromboembolism occurs with equal frequency during the antepartum and postpartum periods. Risk factors include prolonged bed rest, operative delivery (either instrument-assisted or cesarean), hemorrhage, sepsis, multiparity, obesity, and advanced maternal age.

AMNIOTIC FLUID EMBOLISM

The actual incidence of amniotic fluid embolism is unknown, but the reported incidence ranges from 1 in 8000 to 1 in 80,000 deliveries. A recent study reported an incidence of 1 in 20,046 deliveries. Amniotic fluid embolism can occur

Table 196–3 ■ Signs and Symptoms of Venous Air Embolism
Gasping
Dyspnea
Chest pain
Hypotension
Mill-wheel murmur
Cyanosis
Increase in central venous pressure
Reduction in end-tidal carbon dioxide
Electrocardiographic changes
Cardiac arrest

during vaginal or cesarean delivery, as well as in the immediate postpartum period. It has been reported after abdominal trauma and with termination of pregnancy. Further, amniotic fluid embolism may occur without uterine contractions or manipulation. Risk factors are inconsistent, and the condition does not appear to be preventable.

VENOUS AIR EMBOLISM

Venous air embolism is quite common, occurring in 52% of cesarean deliveries. It is speculated that partial placental separation allows the ingress of air into the uterine sinuses. Air embolism has been reported to occur during manual extraction of retained placenta previa or accreta, during placental abruption, and with forceps or vacuum deliveries. It has also occurred following uterine rupture or after breech delivery.

During cesarean delivery, both ruptured membranes and a protracted interval between uterine incision and delivery of the fetus are known risk factors for air embolism.

Implications

PULMONARY EMBOLISM

Although fatal pulmonary embolism is rare, it is the leading cause of pregnancy-related mortality in the United States.

AMNIOTIC FLUID EMBOLISM

Amniotic fluid embolism is a rare, unpredictable, and non-preventable obstetric complication. It is responsible for 5% to 18% of maternal deaths in the United States. Overall maternal mortality ranges from 26% to 86% with amniotic fluid embolism. Up to 50% of fatalities occur within the first hour, and fetal survival is only 39%.

Noncardiogenic pulmonary edema develops in 70% of patients who survive the initial amniotic fluid embolism. Neurologic impairment and acute renal failure may also occur.

VENOUS AIR EMBOLISM

Venous air embolism causes significant hemodynamic compromise in only 0.7% to 2% of parturients at delivery. However, even small amounts of air can result in ventilation-perfusion mismatch, hypoxemia, right ventricular failure, arrhythmias, and hypotension. Larger volumes (>3 mL/kg) may be fatal, usually as a result of right ventricular outflow tract obstruction.

MANAGEMENT

Pulmonary Embolism

Treatment for pulmonary embolism includes both cardiovascular and respiratory support. It focuses on maintaining adequate maternal and fetal oxygenation, maternal circulatory support, and immediate anticoagulation.

Two thirds of patients who ultimately die from pulmonary embolism do so within 30 minutes of the acute event. If the clinical picture strongly suggests pulmonary embolism, anticoagulation therapy should be initiated to prevent further embolic events before any diagnostic studies are obtained.

When anticoagulation is contraindicated or ineffective, interruption of the inferior vena cava by transvenous placement of a Greenfield filter is considered safe and effective. Thrombolytic therapy is relatively contraindicated in pregnancy but may be useful for the prevention of re-embolization in parturients who are hemodynamically unstable and hypoxic. If pulmonary embolism is life threatening, emergency embolectomy is indicated.

Amniotic Fluid Embolism

Treatment is primarily symptomatic and is aimed at the restoration of oxygenation, blood volume, and cardiac output and the correction of coagulopathy. If there is cardiopulmonary arrest, cardiopulmonary resuscitation, endotracheal intubation, and mechanical ventilation with 100% oxygen should be initiated immediately. Because of high early maternal mortality, delivery should be expedited, and the obstetrician must be prepared to perform postmortem cesarean section. Early delivery of the infant allows more effective cardiopulmonary resuscitation of the mother. The parturient's circulating blood volume and cardiac output can be augmented by infusions of crystalloid and vasopressors. Direct arterial pressure monitoring and pulmonary artery catheters are used to guide resuscitative efforts. Communication with the blood bank is important to facilitate the availability of large quantities of blood products, which may be required during resuscitation or treatment of associated coagulopathies. Patients who survive delivery require intensive care management.

Venous Air Embolism

Successful treatment for venous air embolism lies in early recognition. When embolism occurs, repositioning the patient in the reverse Trendelenburg position, with left lateral tilt, and flooding the surgical field with saline may reduce further air entrainment. If the patient is awake, 100% oxygen should be administered by mask. If the patient is under general anesthesia, nitrous oxide must be discontinued, followed by the administration of 100% oxygen. Intravenous fluids are used to reduce hemoconcentration with increased blood viscosity. If acute cardiovascular collapse occurs, a central venous catheter may be placed to attempt to aspirate air from the right atrium.

With evidence of neurologic sequelae or delayed emergence from general anesthesia, paradoxical cerebral air embolism should be suspected, and hyperbaric oxygen therapy should be considered.

PREVENTION

Pulmonary Embolism

Women with a history of deep venous thrombosis or pulmonary emboli while taking oral contraceptives or during pregnancy are thought to have a 4% to 12% increased risk of recurrent events during subsequent pregnancies. They should receive prophylactic anticoagulation throughout pregnancy. Women with a hypercoagulable state or history of thromboembolism unrelated to pregnancy are also at increased risk and should receive similar prophylaxis.

Amniotic Fluid Embolism

There is no evidence that amniotic fluid embolism can be prevented. There are case reports of women who have survived amniotic fluid embolism and gone on to have subsequent uneventful pregnancies.

Venous Air Embolism

Venous air embolism is common during cesarean and vaginal deliveries. During cesarean delivery, traction on or externalization of the uterus is associated with an increased incidence of air embolism and should be minimized. Early recognition and the avoidance of further air entrainment can prevent subsequent morbidity or mortality

Further Reading

Barbour LA: Thromboembolism in pregnancy. ACOG Pract Bull 19, Aug 2000.

Clark SL, Hankins GDV: Amniotic fluid embolism: Analysis of the national registry. Am J Obstet Gynecol 172:1158-1168, 1995.

Deblieux PM, Summer WR: Acute respiratory failure in pregnancy. Clin Obstet Gynecol 39:143-152, 1996.

Gei AF, Vadhera RB, Hankins GD: Embolism during pregnancy: Thrombus, air, and amniotic fluid. Anesthesiol Clin North Am 21:165-182, 2003.

Gilbert W: Amniotic fluid embolism: Decreased mortality in a population-based study. Obstet Gynecol 93:973-977, 1999.

Malinow AM: Embolic disorders. In Chestnut DH (ed): Obstetric Anesthesia: Principles and Practice, 3rd ed. St. Louis, Mosby–Year Book, 2004, pp 683-694.

Martin RW: Amniotic fluid embolism. Clin Obstet Gynecol 39:101-106, 1996.

McDougal RJ, Duke GJ: Amniotic fluid embolism syndrome: Case report and review. Anaesth Intensive Care 23:735-740, 1995.

Toglia MR, Weg JG: Venous thromboembolism during pregnancy. N Engl J Med 335:108-114, 1996.

Weissman A, Kol S, Peretz BA: Gas embolism in obstetrics and gynecology: A review. J Reprod Med 41:103-111, 1996.

Peripartum Neurologic Complications

Mark A. Zakowski, Manuel C. Vallejo, and Sivam Ramanathan

Case Synopsis

A 32-year-old woman, gravida 1, para 0, had uneventful epidural analgesia for labor using 0.125% bupivacaine and fentanyl 2 µg/mL. A 10-mL intravenous bolus was administered, followed by infusion of the same mixture at 10 mL/hour. Subsequently, she required midforceps delivery with manual fetal version for occiput posterior vertex presentation. Before version and extraction of the infant, 20 mL of 2% lidocaine with 1:200,000 epinephrine was administered. The next day, the patient complained of sensory loss in and inability to move both lower extremities, and she had fecal incontinence. Two days later, she regained partial motor function and sensation in both lower extremities but still had fecal incontinence and subsequently developed urinary retention with overflow incontinence. A neurology consultation was obtained. Possible cauda equina syndrome was diagnosed on the fourth postpartum day. At 6 months, the patient still required a wheelchair but had some improvement in bowel and bladder function.

PROBLEM ANALYSIS

Definition

The reported incidence of neurologic complications with regional anesthesia in obstetric patients is from 1 in 2500 to 1 in 13,000. Persistent complications usually are not due to the anesthetic itself but are more often associated with obstetric trauma during birth. However, more recent data indicate that the incidence of anesthetic complications may be higher than formerly believed. In a closed claim analysis of 1005 regional anesthetics by Lee and colleagues, neuraxial block was performed in all 368 obstetric and 453 of 637 nonobstetric claims. Injuries in 51% of obstetric and 41% of nonobstetric claims were related to neuraxial block. The obstetric group had a significantly greater proportion of neuraxial claims involving transient and low-severity injuries (71%) than did the nonobstetric group (38%), yet the proportion of obstetric claims involving severe adverse outcomes (including death or permanent brain injury) was significantly lower. Among the causes of these adverse outcomes were cardiovascular collapse, respiratory arrest, and neuraxial hematoma in patients with coagulopathies.

Wong and coworkers studied 60,057 women who gave birth to live infants and later interviewed 6048 of the women. Fifty-six (0.92%) had new lower extremity peripheral nerve injuries. By logistic regression analysis, multiparity and prolonged second-stage labor were significantly associated with nerve injuries. Patients with nerve injuries spent more time in a semi-Fowler lithotomy position "pushing" than did those without such injury. The median duration of symptoms was 2 months, and injuries involved one of the lower limb peripheral nerves or the lumbosacral plexus. Thus, these findings suggest that neurologic injuries related to childbirth may be related more to childbirth itself rather than the anesthetic.

Recognition

When evaluating a patient with suspected neurologic complications, the answers to several questions are pertinent:

- What was the duration of labor?
- How long did the patient "push"?
- Was the patient placed in an exaggerated lithotomy position while pushing?
- Did the obstetrician use forceps to facilitate delivery?
- What was the weight of the neonate?
- What was the position of the presenting part (e.g., occiput posterior)?
- Did the patient have a history of back problems or preexisting neurologic impairment (e.g., multiple sclerosis, human immunodeficiency virus [HIV])?
- What type and amount of local anesthetic were used?
- Did the patient recover sensory or motor function before the onset of new symptoms?

If a peripartum neurologic complication develops, epidural analgesia or anesthesia is often implicated. Invariably, the anesthesiologist will be consulted. There are many potential causes of postpartum neurologic injury, and epidurals are only one of them. Such neurologic injuries often result from direct trauma to the major nerve roots or trunks that supply the lower extremities and are caused by the fetal head or forceps. Direct ischemic injury to the lower spinal cord is also possible. This may occur if the fetal head compresses the ascending spinal branch of the internal iliac artery. One should also consider the possibility of epidural hematoma (see Chapter 57). A neurologist must be consulted urgently when extensive neurologic deficits are first noted. Also, magnetic resonance imaging (MRI) or computed tomography scans of the spinal cord should be obtained without delay.

Risk Assessment

When calculating the risk for peripartum neurologic injuries, consideration of the anatomy involved is important. Neurologic injuries resulting from childbirth may involve branches of the lumbosacral plexus (i.e., iliohypogastric, ilioinguinal, genitofemoral, lateral femoral cutaneous, anterior tibial, femoral, obturator, and sciatic nerves). Also involved may be the pudendal nerve, derived from the sacral (S3 and S4) nerve roots, and the coccygeal plexus, derived from the S4, S5, and coccygeal nerve roots. Occasionally, extensive injuries may result in the cauda equina syndrome. Involvement of the major plexuses (lumbar and sacral) may cause such extensive injuries, which can take weeks or months to resolve.

Branches of the lumbar plexus or sacral plexus (Fig. 197-1) include the sciatic nerve (which contains the common peroneal and tibial nerves), and these may be compressed by the fetal head as it crosses the posterior pelvic brim during birth. Such injuries are unilateral in 75% of cases and bilateral in the rest. Compression injuries are more common in nulliparous parturients with a platypellic pelvis, large fetus, cephalopelvic disproportion, vertex presentation, or forceps delivery. These injuries may involve multiple nerve root levels or present as injuries to the femoral or obturator nerves, with sensory impairment in the L4-L5 dermatomes. Table 197-1 describes some common peripheral nerve injuries in parturients, and Figure 197-2 illustrates the dermatomes subserved by branches of the lumbosacral plexus.

With regard to the mechanisms for specific nerve injuries (see Table 197-1), multiple sclerosis relapses often contribute to lateral femoral cutaneous nerve injuries. Numbness of the anterior aspect of the thigh associated with lateral femoral cutaneous nerve injury is termed *meralgia paresthetica*. This nerve can also be injured by hyperextended lithotomy positioning, pressure from the fetal head, or improper surgical traction during cesarean delivery. When the femoral nerve is injured, hip flexion and knee extension become difficult. Injury is caused by active flexion of the hips during the second stage of labor, leading to compression of the nerve by the inguinal ligament. Therefore, extreme flexion of the hip during "pushing" should be avoided. The legs should be rested between labor contractions and pushing. Also, use of a "squatting bar" to keep the hips hyperflexed during the second stage of labor may cause injury to the femoral nerve. Femoral nerve injury may also be caused by lumbosacral plexus compression by the fetal head.

The adductor magnus muscle receives dual innervation from the obturator and sciatic nerves. If the obturator nerve is involved, thigh abduction weakens, with sensory loss along the medial aspect of the thigh. The sciatic nerve is the largest peripheral nerve in the body. An important branch is the common peroneal nerve, which supplies both motor and sensory innervation to the leg. This nerve winds around the neck of the fibula, where it is the only manually palpable nerve in the lower extremity (Fig. 197-3), making it vulnerable to injury, especially by stirrups. Such injury leads to paralysis of the ankle and foot, resulting in footdrop and inversion, with sensory impairment of the anterior aspect of the foot.

Occasionally, inflammation or spasm of the piriformis muscle (caused by prolonged sitting or extensive weight bearing during pregnancy) may cause sciatic nerve irritation. When the thigh is extended and rotated medially, gluteal pain radiating to the knee occurs.

Blood supply to the spinal cord is often precarious and subject to important variations (Fig. 197-4). Damage to the spinal cord can occur if the blood supply is interrupted. One anterior and two posterior spinal arteries supply the cord. At certain sites along the spinal cord, there are a number of reinforcing inputs from other arteries, one of which is the artery of Adamkiewicz (or the arteria radicularis magna); this usually arises from the aorta at T9 but can arise anywhere between T9 and T12. Arteries that supply the lower spinal cord usually originate from the left side from one or two of the thoracolumbar segmental arteries (T9 to L2). Thus, injury to these arteries may be implicated in injuries to the lower portion of the spinal cord. In about 15% of cases, the artery of Adamkiewicz originates at the T5 level. If so, the major part of the blood supply to the lower spinal cord is provided by a lumbar branch from the internal iliac artery, which lies in front of the sacral ala and enters the spinal cord via L5-S1 intervertebral foramina. This branch can be compressed by the fetal head, leading to ischemia of the conus medullaris. Acute spinal cord ischemia is often undetectable with conventional MRI. Echoplanar diffusion-weighted MRI is used to diagnose acute spinal cord ischemia, as well as epidural hematoma or abscess.

Implications

Neural tissue may be injured by local anesthetic neurotoxicity (chemical injury) or as a result of direct trauma. Chemical injury usually results from accidental injection of an irritant into the epidural or subarachnoid space.

CHEMICAL INJURY

Preservatives and antioxidants such as sodium bisulfite have been implicated in the development of adhesive arachnoiditis or the cauda equina syndrome. Either disorder can also occur as a result of direct local anesthetic neurotoxicity, and both can obliterate the subarachnoid space. The cauda equina syndrome has also been reported following the use of microcatheters for continuous spinal anesthesia. Such toxicity is believed to result from poor distribution of local anesthetic within the cerebrospinal fluid, with subsequent deposition of toxic drug concentrations at the nerve roots. Although the U.S. Food and Drug Administration has advised against the routine use of spinal microcatheters,[1] there is renewed interest in evaluating their utility for obstetric anesthesia. Finally, the cauda equina syndrome may also occur as a result of acute intervertebral disk herniation, which requires immediate surgical intervention.

DIRECT NEURAL TRAUMA

Direct nerve trauma during regional anesthesia uncommonly causes neurologic deficits. Pain or paresthesias on injection using needles or catheters should be a cause for concern.

[1]Faccenda KA, Finucane BT: Complications of regional anaesthesia: Incidence and prevention. Drug Saf 24:413-442, 2001.

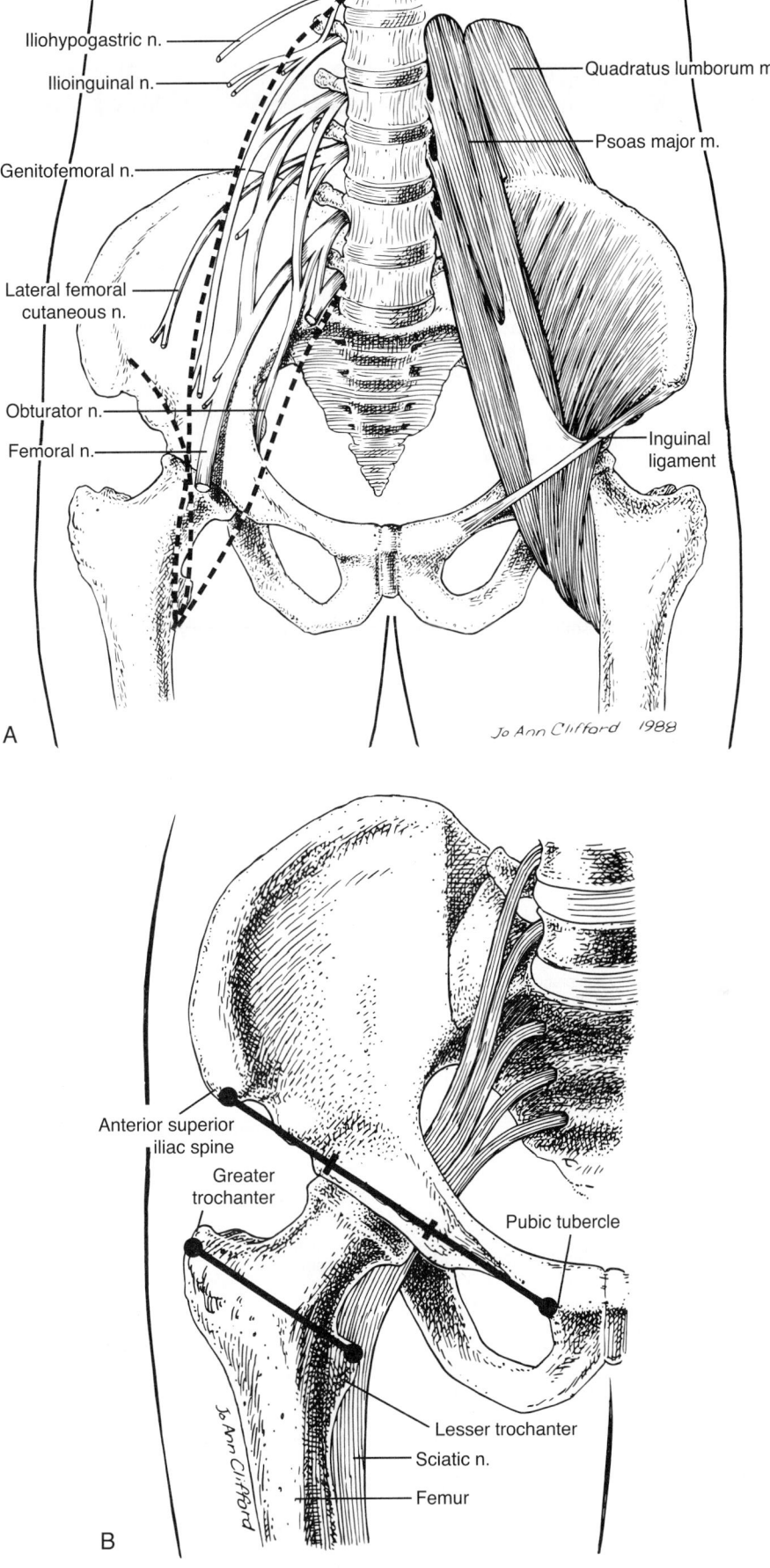

Iliohypogastric n.

Ilioinguinal n.

Genitofemoral n.

Lateral femoral
cutaneous n.

Obturator n.

Femoral n.

Quadratus lumborum m.

Psoas major m.

Inguinal
ligament

Jo Ann Clifford 1988

A

Anterior superior
iliac spine

Greater
trochanter

Pubic tubercle

Lesser trochanter

Sciatic n.

Femur

Jo Ann Clifford

B

Figure 197–1 ■ *A,* The lumbar plexus is derived from the L1-L5 nerve roots and lies in the psoas compartment between the psoas major and quadratus lumborum muscles. *B,* The sacral plexus is formed by contributions from L4, L5, and S1-S3. Not shown are the origins of the pudendal nerve and coccygeal plexus, which are formed by branches of the third and fourth sacral roots and the fourth and fifth sacral and coccygeal nerves, respectively.

Table 197–1 ■ Peripheral Nerve Injuries in Obstetric Patients

Nerve	Nerve Roots	Possible Mechanism	Clinical Picture
Lumbosacral trunk	L4-L5, S1	Forceps injury	Footdrop; quadriceps and adductors affected
Femoral nerve	L2-L4	Fetal head; retractors during cesarean section	Quadriceps weakness; weak hip flexion; absent patellar reflex; sensory impairment in thigh and calf
Lateral femoral cutaneous nerve	L2-L3	Stirrups; prolonged and exaggerated lithotomy position while pushing	Hypalgesia in anterolateral aspect of thigh
Common peroneal nerve (sciatic)*	L4-S2	Stirrups or bedside rails	Footdrop; hypesthesia in lateral calf and anterior aspect of foot
Tibial nerve (sciatic)	L4-S2	Stirrups or bedside rails	Footdrop (muscular branches innervate gastrocnemius and soleus muscles); medial (sural) branches lead to sensory loss in lower leg
Obturator nerve	L2-L4	Fetal head	Weakness on thigh adduction; reduced sensation in medial aspect of thigh

*Owing to its superficial nature, one of the more frequently injured nerves.

Repositioning is of paramount importance. Soft-tip catheters for continuous epidural anesthesia are associated with fewer paresthesias than are more rigid nylon ones. Also, spinal anesthesia is more often associated with neurologic injury than is epidural anesthesia. If paresthesias occur during central neuraxial block, the anesthesiologist should document the severity and location of the paresthesias. It may take anywhere from 48 hours to 3 months for complete recovery from neuropathy due to direct nerve trauma incurred during central neuraxial block.

Direct trauma to nervous tissue may occur at the level of the spinal cord, nerve roots, or peripheral nerves. Epidural needles or catheters are more likely to traumatize the nerve roots. Spinal needles may injure a nerve root or the cord itself

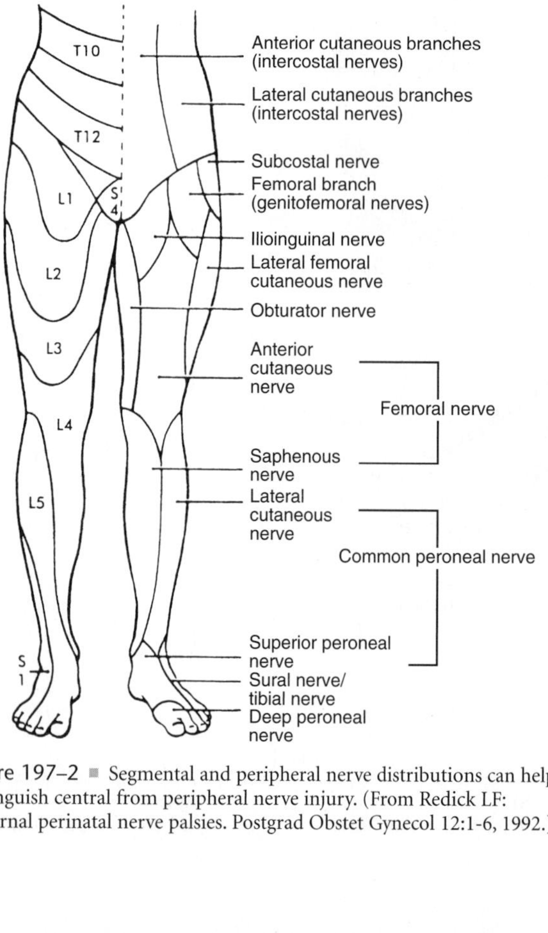

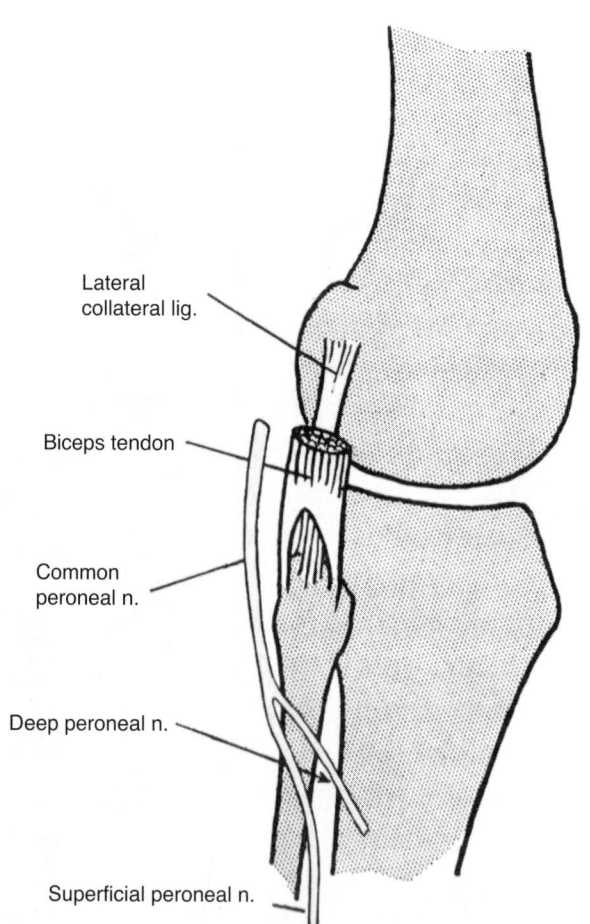

Figure 197–2 ■ Segmental and peripheral nerve distributions can help distinguish central from peripheral nerve injury. (From Redick LF: Maternal perinatal nerve palsies. Postgrad Obstet Gynecol 12:1-6, 1992.)

Figure 197–3 ■ The anatomic location of the common peroneal nerve makes it vulnerable to injury by direct pressure (e.g., stirrups). This is the most frequently damaged nerve in parturients.

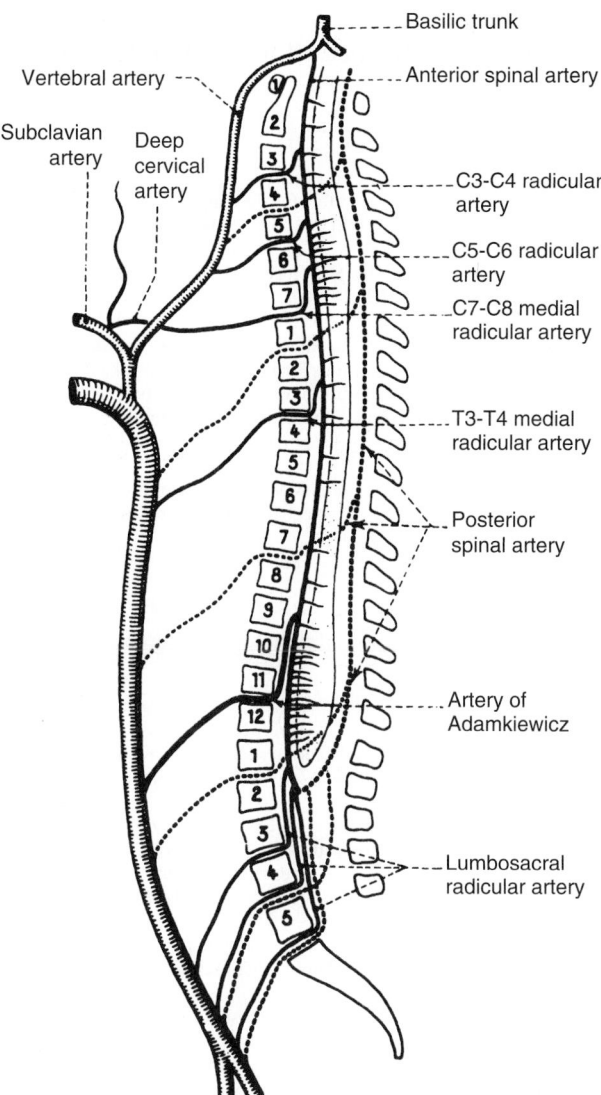

Figure 197–4 ■ Lateral view of the blood supply of the spinal cord, depicting the anterior and posterior radiculomedullary branches. The primary blood supply to the thoracolumbar spinal cord is the artery of Adamkiewicz. As shown, it arises from the aorta at T9 but can arise anywhere between T9 and T12. With high ARM takeoffs, a lumbar artery usually supplies the major portion of the conus medullaris. (From Djindjian R: Arteriography of the spinal cord. Am J Roentgenol Radium Ther Nucl Med 107:461-478, 1969.)

within the subarachnoid space or nerve roots outside the subarachnoid space. Two thirds of neurologic sequelae are preceded by paresthesias (direct nerve trauma) or pain during injection (intraneuronal injection). Intraneural injection of local anesthetic is more likely to result in prolonged neurologic deficits. In one series of more than 103,000 regional anesthetics, of the 34 patients with neurologic sequelae, 29 had transient deficits, with full neurologic recovery occurring in 48 hours to 3 months. Of interest is that spinal anesthesia was significantly more likely than epidural anesthesia to be associated with neurologic injury (5.9 versus 2 per 10,000) or radiculopathy (4.7 versus 1.7 per 10,000).

With mild nerve injury, conduction block occurs only through the damaged nerve segment (i.e., neurapraxia).

If the condition is corrected, recovery occurs. However, the patient must be told that recovery may take several weeks, depending on the severity of the initial symptoms. Severe injuries cause axonal degeneration (axonotmesis). Regeneration may never be complete, with full or partial loss of function in the affected area. Neurotmesis signifies disruption of epineurium as well. Surgical repair is necessary, but recovery may never be complete.

MANAGEMENT

When patients present with postpartum neurologic problems, one must be alert to other causes, including diabetes mellitus, acquired immunodeficiency syndrome (AIDS), and multiple sclerosis. Although diabetic neuropathy is a well-known entity, AIDS-related neuropathy is not, even though it is the most common neurologic complication of type 1 HIV infection and advanced AIDS. It manifests as a distal symmetrical polyneuropathy and occurs mainly with advanced immunosuppression. The number of parturients with advanced HIV disease is increasing, and neurotoxicity may also occur with several antiretroviral agents. Progressive polyradiculopathy occurs with advanced immunosuppression, usually caused by cytomegalovirus infection.

In the initial evaluation, the anesthesiologist should document all sensory and motor deficits and consult a neurologist who is familiar with obstetric nerve injuries. Further studies include computed tomography or MRI scans and neuromuscular electrophysiologic studies, which must be performed without delay. Electrophysiologic studies include electromyography (EMG) and nerve conduction studies. EMG is extremely useful for diagnosing the extent of injury to peripheral nerves; however, timing is critical. The presence of abnormal spontaneous activity in quiescent muscle (fibrillation potentials) or increased activity during insertion of the recording needle into muscle (insertion activity) usually indicates preexisting neurologic disease. Insertion activity becomes noticeable on EMG within a few days of injury, whereas fibrillation potentials take 2 to 4 weeks to develop. If fibrillation potentials are recorded soon after the alleged injury, they are more likely due to a previously undiagnosed neurologic condition rather than a new injury. Another EMG sign of nerve injury is the failure to recruit additional motor units when muscle is stimulated. In completely denervated muscle, no recruitment occurs. However, when the nerve is damaged, partial recruitment occurs due to slowed conduction. EMG may also help distinguish whether a plexopathy or radiculopathy exists.

Depending on the type and severity of injury, it may take up to 8 weeks for neurologic injuries to resolve completely. Repeat electrophysiologic studies are often necessary to assess progression or regression of injuries. Also, consultation with a physiotherapist is necessary to determine the best rehabilitation program to prevent muscle atrophy. A splint may be required for patients with significant footdrop to prevent permanent deformities.

The patient described in the case synopsis had extensive neurologic injury, indicative of damage to the lumbosacral plexus or the spinal cord. Bowel or bladder dysfunction usually indicates spinal cord injury. Although electrophysiologic

Figure labels: Basilic trunk · Vertebral artery · Anterior spinal artery · Subclavian artery · Deep cervical artery · C3-C4 radicular artery · C5-C6 radicular artery · C7-C8 medial radicular artery · T3-T4 medial radicular artery · Posterior spinal artery · Artery of Adamkiewicz · Lumbosacral radicular artery

OTHER SURGICAL SUBSPECIALTIES

Table 197–2 ■ Differential Diagnosis for Prolonged Neural Block

Drug Effects

Prolonged action of local anesthetic
  Slow regression of block
  More common after multiple dosing
  Needle or catheter tip close to nerve root during local anesthetic injection
Direct neurotoxicity
  Rare effect of commonly used drugs (e.g., 5% hyperbaric lidocaine)
  Incorrect drug administered (e.g., potassium chloride)

Trauma

Peripheral nerve
  Compression from positioning
  Known peripheral nerve pattern
Central neuraxis
  Direct trauma to neural tissue caused by needle or catheter
External compression of nerve root or spinal cord
  Herniated intervertebral disk
  Epidural hematoma (early)
  Epidural abscess (late)
  Spinal stenosis

Vascular

Hemorrhage—spinal cord arteriovenous malformation
Decreased blood supply—no evidence of recovery; permanent injury
Anterior spinal artery syndrome
  Compression of arterial blood supply by fetal head
  Severe hypotension
Post cardiac arrest
  Emboli (e.g., air, thrombotic, amniotic fluid)

Neurologic Disease (Preexisting or New Onset)

Multiple sclerosis
HIV, immunosuppressive therapy
Cytomegalovirus
Landry-Guillain-Barré syndrome

Miscellaneous Causes

Space-occupying lesions
  Epidural hematoma
  Epidural abscess

studies suggested a lesion at the spinal root level or higher, MRI scans of the spinal cord 2 days after delivery appeared normal. However, enhanced MRI performed 1 week later was consistent with spinal cord ischemia. Likely, this was due to compression of the lumbar spinal artery at the level of the sacrum. Other potential causes of prolonged neurologic deficits in parturients are listed in Table 197-2.

PREVENTION

For parturients with systemic disease, the anesthesiologist should thoroughly document any preexisting neurologic deficits to prevent potential medicolegal problems. Multiple sclerosis is particularly prone to relapse in the postpartum period. Also, anesthesia care providers in the labor-delivery suite must ensure that the patient has fully recovered from the effects of the local anesthetic before she is returned to the floor. If the patient develops a neurologic deficit after

complete sensory and motor recovery from the anesthetic, the problem is unlikely related to neuraxial block or the agents used for the block.

Further Reading

Aminoff MJ: Electrophysiologic testing for the diagnosis of peripheral nerve injuries. Anesthesiology 100:1298-1303, 2004.

Auroy Y, Benhamou D, Bargues L, et al: Major complications of regional anesthesia in France: The SOS regional anesthesia hotline service. Anesthesiology 97:1274-1280, 2002.

Biglioli P, Roberto M, Cannata A, et al: Upper and lower spinal cord blood supply: The continuity of the anterior spinal artery and the relevance of the lumber arteries. J Thorac Cardiovasc Surg 127:1188-1192, 2004.

Bromage PR: Neurologic complications of regional anesthesia in obstetrics. In Hughes SC, Levinson G, Rosen MA (eds): Obstetric Anesthesia, 2nd ed. Philadelphia, JB Lippincott–Williams & Wilkins, 1999, pp 723-748.

Confavreux C, Hutchinson M, Hours MM, et al: Rate of pregnancy-related relapse in multiple sclerosis: Pregnancy in Multiple Sclerosis Group. N Eng J Med 339:285-291, 1998.

Gray H: Gray's Anatomy, 27th ed. Philadelphia, Lea & Febiger, 1959, pp 1036-1057.

Jaime F, Mandell GL, Vallejo MC, et al: Uniport soft-tip, open-ended catheters versus multiport firm-tipped close-ended catheters for epidural labor analgesia: A quality assurance study. J Clin Anesth 12:89-93, 2000.

Kuczkowski KM: Neurologic complications of labor analgesia: Facts and fiction. Obstet Gynecol Surv 59:47-51, 2004.

Lee LA, Posner KL, Domino KB, et al: Injuries associated with regional anesthesia in the 1980s and 1990s: A closed claim analysis. Anesthesiology 101:143-152, 2004.

Loher TJ, Bassetti CL, Lovblad KO, et al: Diffusion-weighted MRI in acute spinal cord ischemia. Neuroradiology 45:557-561, 2003.

Vallejo M, Mariano D, Kaul B, et al: Piriformis syndrome in a patient after cesarean section under spinal anesthesia. Reg Anesth Pain Med 29:364-367, 2004.

Wedel DJ, Horlocker TT: Nerve blocks. In Miller RD (ed): Miller's Anesthesia, 6th ed. Philadelphia, Churchill Livingstone, 2005, pp 1685-1717.

Wlody D: Complications of regional anesthesia in obstetrics. Clin Obstet Gynecol 46:667-678, 2003.

Wong CA, Scavone BM, Dugan S, et al: Incidence of postpartum lumbosacral spine and lower extremity nerve injuries. Obstet Gynecol 101:279-288, 2003.

Wulff EA, Wang AK, Simpson DM: HIV-associated peripheral neuropathy: Epidemiology, pathophysiology and treatment. Drugs 59:1251-1260, 2000.

Zakowski MI: Complications associated with regional anesthesia in the obstetric patient. Semin Perinatol 26:154-168, 2002.

198

Postpartum Headache Other Than Post–Dural Puncture Headache

David J. Wlody

Case Synopsis

A 24-year-old primigravida underwent cesarean delivery for breech presentation under uncomplicated spinal anesthesia. This was performed with a 27-gauge Whitacre needle. On the second postpartum day she complained of a severe diffuse headache. On the third postpartum day she suffered a grand mal seizure. The obstetrician believes that the headache is a "spinal headache," and the anesthesiologist is consulted.

PROBLEM ANALYSIS

Definition

Postpartum headache is defined as any headache occurring during the first 6 weeks after delivery. Such headaches may be due to antepartum conditions, manifestations of an intrapartum event, or unrelated disorders arising coincidentally in the postpartum period. It is often tempting to blame postpartum headache on neuraxial anesthetic, but not all postpartum headaches are post–dural puncture headaches, even if a large-gauge needle was used. This chapter discusses the most common causes of postpartum headache as well as some less common conditions that, if misdiagnosed, could lead to catastrophic outcomes.

Recognition

Although the incidence of particular types of headache may differ among women who have recently delivered, any headache seen in the general population can occur in postpartum patients. The International Headache Society recently revised the criteria for the diagnosis and classification of headaches. A complete discussion of these criteria is beyond the scope of this chapter, but a division of headaches into primary and secondary categories provides a conceptual framework for discussion (Table 198-1).

PRIMARY HEADACHE

With primary headache, there is no apparent cause or other conditions that might contribute to or explain the patient's headache. Primary headaches are confined to migraine- and tension-type headaches.

Migraine-Type Headache. Migraine headaches are subdivided into headaches with and without an aura. With the former, reversible neurologic symptoms develop gradually over 5 to 20 minutes and generally last less than 60 minutes.

These symptoms are typically visual, including light flashes, a blind spot with shimmering edges (scintillating scotomata), or formations of zigzag lines. Numbness of the face or weakness of an arm or leg may also occur. Otherwise, the characteristics of the two subtypes of migraine headache are similar:

- Unilateral location
- Pulsating quality
- Aggravation by routine physical activity
- Associated with nausea and photophobia and phonophobia

Migraine headaches usually begin in adolescence and occur in 4% to 6% of men and 13% to 18% of women. Although there is no consistent mendelian pattern of inheritance, there is clearly a familial propensity for migraine. In 60% to 80% of cases, there is a family history of migraine headaches.

Table 198–1 ■ Classification of Postpartum Headache

Primary Causes of Headache
Migraine (with or without aura)
Tension-type headache
Secondary Causes of Headache
Headache attributed to cranial vascular disorders
   Intracranial hemorrhage
   Cerebral venous and sinus thrombosis
Headache attributed to nonvascular intracranial disorders
   Tumor
   Idiopathic intracranial hypertension
   Pneumocephalus
Headache attributed to disorders of homeostasis
   Headache with preeclampsia
   Headache due to a substance or its withdrawal
   Metabolic disorders
Headache due to infectious causes
   Meningitis
   Sinusitis

Modified from Rapoport AM, Sheftel FD: Headache Disorders: A Management Guide for Practitioners. Philadelphia, WB Saunders, 1996, pp 5-6.

The higher incidence of migraine headaches in women suggests a hormonal association. These headaches tend to occur during the premenstrual period, and in 15% of women the attacks are exclusively perimenopausal. The effect of pregnancy on migraine is variable. In about 70% of pregnant women, migraine headaches decrease or disappear altogether during pregnancy. However, it is common for migraines to recur early in the postpartum period. New-onset migraine headaches during pregnancy or early in the postpartum period are unusual. Headaches appearing at this time warrant investigation to ensure that they are not caused by some less benign process.

Tension-Type Headache.
Tension headache is the most common type of headache, with a reported lifetime prevalence as high as 78%. Tension-type headache is not as well studied as migraine and was once thought to be primarily psychogenic. It is now known to have an organic basis. Tension-type headache is divided into infrequent, frequent, and chronic subtypes, defined by the number of episodes suffered per month. Otherwise, they share the following characteristics:

- Bilateral location
- Pressing, nonpulsating quality
- Not aggravated by routine physical activity
- Mild to moderate intensity
- Absence of nausea, photophobia, and phonophobia

Like migraine, tension headaches are more common in women. Unlike migraine headaches, they seldom begin in adolescence and are more likely to occur in middle age. Commonly, they are associated with chronic anxiety or depression. The relationship between tension headaches and pregnancy has not been well investigated. However, their incidence appears to be increased during gestation, with symptomatic improvement observed in only about 25% of patients.

SECONDARY HEADACHE

Secondary headache is defined as any new headache occurring in close temporal association with a disorder known to cause headache. These disorders include intracranial vascular and nonvascular disorders, substance use or withdrawal, disorders of homeostasis, and infection.

Intracranial Hemorrhage.
This category includes subarachnoid hemorrhage, intracerebral hemorrhage, and subdural hematoma. Features of headache due to intracranial hemorrhage are as follows:

- Sudden onset
- Intense severity
- Possible association with focal signs or alterations in level of consciousness

The incidence of spontaneous subarachnoid hemorrhage does not appear to be greater in pregnant women than in other populations. About 75% of subarachnoid hemorrhages are due to ruptured berry aneurysms.[1] The remainder

---

[1]A small, saccular aneurysm of a cerebral artery, typically within the circle of Willis, with the potential to rupture, thereby causing subarachnoid hemorrhage.

are due to bleeding arteriovenous malformations. Hypertension and proteinuria are not uncommon; therefore, subarachnoid hemorrhage can be confused with preeclampsia. Intracerebral hemorrhage is usually seen with severe preeclampsia or eclampsia. Subdural hematoma has been reported in association with post–dural puncture headache; presumably, the reduced intracranial pressure leads to rupture of bridging veins.

Cerebral Venous and Sinus Thrombosis.
Cerebral venous thrombosis is estimated to occur in 1 in 2500 to 10,000 deliveries. The hypercoagulable state associated with pregnancy is a contributing factor. Patients with cerebral venous or sinus thrombosis should be evaluated for the presence of a hereditary thrombophilia (e.g., protein S or C deficiency, factor V Leiden). Nearly 80% of cases occur during the first 2 weeks post partum, but thrombosis may occur as late as 3 months post partum. Features of headache secondary to intracranial thrombosis vary, depending on whether a large sinus or an isolated cortical vein is thrombosed. With thrombosis of a large sinus, headache, seizures, intracranial hypertension (due to impaired absorption of cerebrospinal fluid), and altered consciousness are common. With a thrombosed cortical vein, focal motor and sensory deficits and seizures are more likely. Interestingly, there are several reported cases of intracranial thrombosis that were initially treated as post–dural puncture headache. If signs and symptoms suggest increased intracranial pressure, this should lead to a more aggressive workup before an epidural blood patch is performed. Magnetic resonance imaging and magnetic resonance angiography are considered gold standards for diagnosing intracranial thrombosis.

Venous thrombosis with occlusion leads to increased capillary pressure, often associated with hemorrhagic infarcts. With recanalization of the vessel, capillary pressure decreases, and further hemorrhage is prevented. Although heparin has no thrombolytic properties, it prevents further propagation of the thrombus. Therefore, its use is indicated, even in patients with preexisting hemorrhage. Finally, as a rule, anticonvulsants are reserved for patients with solid evidence of hemorrhage or focal neurologic deficits.

Intracranial Neoplasm.
Features of headache associated with intracranial neoplasm include the following:

- Diffuse, nonpulsating quality
- Often associated with nausea or vomiting
- Worsened by physical activity, Valsalva's maneuver, coughing, or sneezing

The incidence of brain tumor is not increased by pregnancy. However, it is not unusual for symptoms to first manifest during pregnancy, likely due to increased extracellular fluid. There is also a well-established hormonal influence on certain tumors, especially meningiomas and pituitary adenomas. Symptoms of brain tumors are influenced by their location and size and whether they are associated with elevated intracranial pressure.

Idiopathic Intracranial Hypertension. Idiopathic intracranial hypertension, previously known as benign intracranial hypertension or pseudotumor cerebri, is most common in obese young women, suggesting a hormonal component. It is characterized by the following:

- Diffuse, nonpulsating pain
- Daily occurrence
- Aggravated by coughing

Patients are alert and may have a normal neurologic examination. The most common neurologic findings are papilledema, sixth cranial nerve palsy, and visual field defects, all of which progress if the patient is not treated. Idiopathic intracranial hypertension is a diagnosis of exclusion, and other intracranial, metabolic, toxic, and hormonal diseases must be ruled out. It is not unusual for idiopathic intracranial hypertension to present for the first time during pregnancy, and symptoms typically worsen in patients with previously recognized disease. Improvement can be expected following delivery.

Pneumocephalus. The use of air to identify the epidural space is sometimes complicated by its accidental subarachnoid injection. Headache typically occurs immediately after injection, may be quite intense, and is worsened by upright posturing. Plain skull films easily identify intracranial air. Its absorption is accelerated by breathing 100% oxygen.

Substance Use or Withdrawal. Headache is common during therapy with magnesium sulfate, especially after the loading dose. In patients consuming more than 200 mg/day of caffeine, sudden cessation may lead to a headache. This is relieved within 1 hour of the administration of caffeine. Cessation of chronic opioid therapy can lead to headache within 24 hours. It has been suggested that abrupt termination of corticosteroids, tricyclic antidepressants, and nonsteroidal anti-inflammatory drugs can also lead to headache.

Preeclampsia and Eclampsia. Headache is a hallmark of severe preeclampsia and may be a precursor to development of eclampsia. Typical features of headache in this setting are as follows:

- Bilateral, pulsating quality
- Aggravated by physical activity
- Accompanied by hypertension and proteinuria
- Visual disturbances (blurred vision, scotomata)

Headache associated with preeclampsia generally occurs before delivery but may present in the postpartum period. Such patients are at risk for eclampsia and must be carefully monitored.

Metabolic Disorders. Fasting may cause headache, even without associated hypoglycemia. Approximately 30% of patients with chronic hypothyroidism have a generalized, nonpulsatile headache that responds well to thyroid hormone replacement therapy.

Meningitis. Features of headache secondary to meningitis include the following:

- Diffuse, progressively increasing pain
- Fever
- Nuchal rigidity
- Nausea, vomiting, photophobia

Meningitis is an exceedingly rare complication of regional anesthesia. However, the failure to diagnose and treat it in a timely fashion may be associated with catastrophic sequelae.

Post–Dural Puncture Headache. Post–dural puncture headache has many of the same features as headache due to meningitis. Diagnostic lumbar puncture must be considered in any patient with presumed post–dural puncture headache accompanied by fever, leukocytosis, and meningismus.

Sinusitis. Headache due to sinusitis is often accompanied by purulent nasal discharge and fever. Tenderness over the affected sinus is common. Chronic sinusitis is not considered a likely cause of headache in the absence of acute exacerbation.

Risk Assessment

Headache can occur at any time in the peripartum period and is extraordinarily common after childbirth. Patients with a history of headache or depression are at particularly high risk. Patients with preeclampsia or known intracranial pathology should be evaluated carefully. This is especially so if the headache is more severe than usual, and especially if there are any associated neurologic deficits.

Implications

Postpartum headache is not necessarily related to regional anesthesia, even in those patients known to have sustained accidental dural puncture with large-bore needles. Other causes of headache must be entertained before use of an epidural blood patch, especially when atypical features are present, including fever, leukocytosis, or focal neurologic deficits. Vigilance must be especially intense if supposed post–dural puncture headache fails to respond to epidural blood patch.

MANAGEMENT

Management of postpartum headache depends on its cause and is summarized in Table 198-2.

PREVENTION

Preventive measures depend on headache type:

- Migraine headache sufferers should avoid known triggering agents such as red wine, cheese, and cured meats.
- Chronic analgesic therapy should be maintained to avoid rebound headache.
- Aggressive control of blood pressure is vital in patients with preeclampsia.
- Strict sterile technique is important when performing neuraxial anesthesia to reduce the risk of infectious complications.

Table 198–2 ■ Management of Postpartum Headache

Cause	Treatment
Migraine	β-Blockers, tricyclic antidepressants, serotonin receptor agonists; avoid known triggers or ergot alkaloids in nursing mothers
Tension	Analgesics, tricyclic antidepressants
Intracranial hemorrhage	Decompressive surgery
Cerebral venous or sinus thrombosis	Anticonvulsants, anticoagulants
Intracranial neoplasm	Mannitol, glucocorticoids, surgery
Idiopathic intracranial hypertension	Glucocorticoids, carbonic anhydrase inhibitors
Post–dural puncture	Supine posture, IV fluid or caffeine, all conservative measures; epidural blood patch (definitive therapy with 90% success rate)
Pneumocephalus	Analgesics, denitrogenation
Substance use or withdrawal	Avoidance or adjustment of dosage of causative agents
Preeclampsia	Antihypertensives, magnesium sulfate
Metabolic disorders	Correction of metabolic derangement
Infectious	Antibiotics

Further Reading

Aminoff MJ: Neurologic disorders. In Creasy RK, Resnik R (eds): Maternal-Fetal Medicine, 5th ed. Philadelphia, WB Saunders, 2004, pp 1165-1191.

Benzon HT, Iqbal M, Tallman MS, et al: Superior sagittal sinus thrombosis in a patient with postdural puncture headache. Reg Anesth Pain Med 28:64-67, 2003.

Donaldson JO: Headache. In Neurology of Pregnancy, 2nd ed. Philadelphia, WB Saunders, 1989, pp 217-227.

Headache Classification Subcommittee of the International Headache Society: The international classification of headache disorders (2nd ed). Cephalalgia 24(Suppl):1-150, 2004.

Marcus DA: Headache in pregnancy. Curr Pain Headache Rep 4:288-296, 2003.

Masuhr F, Mehraein S, Einhaupl K: Cerebral venous and sinus thrombosis. J Neurol 251:11-23, 2004.

Silberstein SD: Migraine and pregnancy. Neurol Clin 15:209-231, 1997.

Victor M, Ropper AH: Headache and other craniofacial pains. In Adams and Victor's Principles of Neurology, 7th ed. New York, McGraw-Hill, 2001, pp 175-203.

Von Wald T, Walling AD: Headache during pregnancy. Obstet Gynecol Surv 57:179-185, 2002.

Weeks SK: Postpartum headache. In Chestnut DH (ed): Obstetric Anesthesia: Principles and Practice, 3rd ed. Philadelphia, Mosby, 2004, pp 562-564.

Nonobstetric Surgery during Pregnancy

199

Joy L. Hawkins

Case Synopsis

A 42-year-old woman, gravida 3, para 0, presents to the operating room for laparoscopic cholecystectomy at 28 weeks' gestation. Her pregnancy has been uncomplicated, but she has a history of two previous miscarriages in the first trimester. She is extremely anxious about undergoing this procedure while pregnant and asks about the implications of the anesthetic for her fetus and the outcome of the pregnancy.

PROBLEM ANALYSIS

Definition and Recognition

Most anesthesiologists find it disconcerting when a patient presenting for an otherwise routine surgery is pregnant. About 2% of pregnant women have surgery while they are pregnant, involving about 75,000 anesthetics per year. Most procedures result from conditions that are common in this age group: trauma, ovarian cysts, appendicitis, cholecystectomy, evaluation of a breast mass, and cervical incompetence. However, major procedures such as craniotomy, cardiopulmonary bypass, and liver transplantation have also been performed in pregnant patients with good outcomes for both the mother and the fetus.

Despite favorable results, the public has a strong aversion to drugs' being used or procedures' being performed during pregnancy, and a pregnant patient requiring surgery is likely to present with extreme anxiety. In the interest of informed consent, the anesthesiologist must address the risks associated with the anesthetic in a pregnant patient undergoing surgery.

Risk Assessment and Implications

For a pregnant surgical candidate, the preoperative assessment involves two patients. Several unique concerns must be addressed when creating an anesthetic plan:

- Alterations in maternal physiology
- Potential teratogenic effects of anesthetic agents
- Maintenance of uterine perfusion during surgery
- Fetal effects of surgical and anesthetic manipulations
- Prevention of preterm labor (the greatest cause of fetal loss)

Alterations in maternal physiology involve every organ system, but those most important to anesthetic management include the following:

- Respiratory: increased oxygen consumption; reduced functional residual capacity; lower partial pressure of carbon dioxide, due to increased minute ventilation; and higher incidence of difficult intubation

- Cardiovascular: increased blood volume and cardiac output; dilutional anemia; supine aortocaval compression by gravid uterus; reduced vascular but increased baroreceptor responsiveness
- Gastrointestinal: gastric volume and pH may not be altered; however, lower esophageal sphincter tone is usually reduced
- Central nervous system: decrease in both minimum alveolar concentration (MAC) for inhalational agents and local anesthetic requirements

Teratogenic effects of anesthetics have not been conclusively shown in humans. The two agents of most concern are nitrous oxide (N_2O) and benzodiazepines. N_2O may constrict the uterine vasculature and decrease uterine blood flow if it is not combined with another inhalational agent that produces sympatholysis. Benzodiazepines were anecdotally associated with cleft lip anomalies, but subsequent studies failed to show any relationship. Opioids, intravenous agents, and local anesthetics have a long history of safety during pregnancy. Of concern is recent animal work showing that fetal or newborn exposure to NMDA receptor blockers (e.g., ketamine, N_2O) and GABA receptor enhancers (e.g., benzodiazepines, intravenous induction agents, volatile anesthetic agents) results in widespread apoptotic neurodegeneration and persistent memory and learning impairment. These effects appear to be most pronounced with isoflurane, but the significance of human exposure is unknown. However, isoflurane has been associated with postoperative cognitive deficits in human adults.

Maintenance of uterine perfusion and maternal oxygenation preserves fetal oxygenation and is key to any anesthetic during pregnancy. Above all, maternal hypoxemia and decreased cardiac output must be avoided.

Prevention of preterm labor is the most difficult problem to surmount. It is probably not related to anesthetic management but rather to the underlying disease and the surgical procedure.

MANAGEMENT

If there is a question about the diagnosis of pregnancy, this should be part of the preoperative assessment.

Mandatory pregnancy testing is a controversial issue. The last menstrual period should be documented on the anesthesia record for any female between the ages of 12 and 50. Testing should be offered if more than 3 weeks has lapsed since the expected time of the menstrual period or by patient request.

If possible, delay of surgery to the second trimester should be considered. In the second trimester, concerns about teratogenicity and spontaneous miscarriage are reduced, and preterm labor is not as common as in the third trimester. In addition, the patient should be counseled on anesthetic risks (or the lack thereof) to the fetus and the pregnancy and educated on the need for left uterine displacement and symptoms of preterm labor. Preoperative medications to allay anxiety or pain are often appropriate. Elevated maternal catecholamines may decrease uterine blood flow. Prophylaxis against gastric aspiration should be considered with a combination of an antacid, metoclopramide, or H_2-receptor antagonist.

Intraoperatively, there is no evidence that one particular anesthetic technique is better than another, so long as maternal oxygenation and perfusion are maintained. Monitoring should include blood pressure, oxygenation, ventilation (end-tidal carbon dioxide), temperature, and blood glucose if the procedure is a long one. If it will not interfere with the surgical field, intermittent or continuous fetal monitoring after about 24 weeks' gestation may be helpful to ensure that the intrauterine environment is optimal. Loss of beat-to-beat variability in the fetal heart rate is normal during anesthesia, but decelerations may indicate the need to increase maternal oxygenation or blood pressure, increase uterine displacement, change the site of surgical retraction, or begin tocolysis. Fetal monitoring can assess the adequacy of uterine perfusion during induced hypotension, cardiopulmonary bypass, or procedures involving large volume shifts. If the mother is awake during a regional anesthetic, it can be very reassuring to hear the fetal heart tones during the procedure, even if measured intermittently.

The conduct of general anesthesia should include full preoxygenation and denitrogenation; rapid-sequence induction with cricoid pressure; high inspired concentrations of oxygen; and judicious reversal of muscle relaxants to avoid any acute increase in acetylcholine, which might induce uterine contractions. Inhalational agents should be kept below 2.0 MAC to prevent decreased maternal cardiac output and uterine blood flow. During the first trimester, ketamine at doses greater than 2 mg/kg may cause uterine hypertonia. N_2O and benzodiazepines may be used at the anesthetist's discretion. Until further research is available, it may be prudent to use other volatile inhalational agents in place of isoflurane. Also, keep in mind that the airway of the pregnant patient is edematous and vascular. Thus, visualization of the epiglottis and laryngeal structures may be more difficult during attempted laryngoscopy and tracheal intubation.

The use of regional anesthesia techniques (especially spinal and epidural anesthesia) has the advantage of minimizing drug exposure in early pregnancy, as well as reducing problems in interpreting fetal monitoring changes later during gestation. Hypotension with central neuraxial blocks is minimized with adequate preload and volume replacement, left lateral uterine displacement, and prompt administration of vasopressors if needed. Both ephedrine and phenylephrine are acceptable drugs for treating hypotension. In the absence of maternal bradycardia, phenylephrine appears to be at least as effective as ephedrine for maintaining maternal blood pressure and umbilical artery pH values during central neuraxial anesthesia for cesarean section.[1] The local anesthetic dose is decreased by about one third with spinal or epidural techniques. Continuous epidural analgesia can provide excellent postoperative pain control while reducing the loss of fetal heart rate variability and the need for maternal sedation. Thus, the patient is better able to report symptoms of preterm labor.

Postoperative care includes continued monitoring of fetal heart rate and uterine activity. Preterm labor must be treated early and aggressively. This may require recovery in the labor and delivery unit or providing labor and delivery nursing expertise in the surgical recovery area. It should be remembered that any systemic pain medications will cause a loss of fetal heart rate variability. Therefore, regional analgesia techniques should be used whenever possible. Also, pregnant patients are at high risk for thromboembolic complications and should be mobilized as soon as possible (another reason for regional analgesia). Maternal oxygenation and left uterine displacement should be maintained. If the fetus is a viable age, a pediatrician should be notified so that he or she can provide counseling to the parents in the event preterm labor occurs.

PREVENTION

Although the need for surgery cannot be prevented, anesthesiologists can provide reassurance to the mother that anesthetic drugs and techniques will not put her fetus or the pregnancy at risk. Prevention of preterm labor is the greatest concern and may require perioperative administration of tocolytics. Good postoperative pain management without sedation aids in the early diagnosis and treatment of preterm labor, as well as early mobilization to prevent thromboembolic events.

Further Reading

American College of Obstetricians and Gynecologists: Nonobstetric Surgery in Pregnancy (ACOG Committee Opinion No. 284). Washington, DC, ACOG, August 2003.

Boiven JF: Risk of spontaneous abortion in women occupationally exposed to anesthetic gases: A meta-analysis. Occup Environ Med 54:541-548, 1997.

Jevtovic-Todorovic V, Hartman RE, Izumi Y, et al: Early exposure to common anesthetic agents causes widespread neurodegeneration in the developing rat brain and persistent learning deficits. J Neurosci 23:876-882, 2003.

---

[1]Vasopressors with primary α-adrenergic activity, including phenylephrine, have been shown in animal models to directly increase intrinsic vascular resistance, thereby directly reducing uterine blood flow. However, agents such as phenylephrine also directly increase central venous vascular tone (i.e., reduce venous capacitance), which augments venous return and cardiac preload. If so, cardiac output and effective uterine blood flow may increase.

Koren G: Drugs in pregnancy. N Engl J Med 338:1128-1137, 1998.

Mazze RI, Fujinaga M, Baden JM: Halothane prevents nitrous oxide teratogenicity in Sprague-Dawley rats; folinic acid does not. Teratology 38:121-127, 1988.

Reynolds JD, Booth JV, de la Fuente S, et al: A review of laparoscopy for non-obstetric-related surgery during pregnancy. Curr Surg 60:164-173, 2003.

Rosen MA: Management of anesthesia for the pregnant surgical patient. Anesthesiology 91:1159-1163, 1999.

Shiono PH, Mills JL: Oral clefts and diazepam use during pregnancy. N Engl J Med 311:919-920, 1984.

Thomas DG, Robson SC, Redfern N, et al: Randomized trial of bolus phenylephrine or ephedrine for maintenance of arterial pressure during spinal anesthesia for caesarean section. Br J Anaesth 76:61-65, 1996.

http://www.asahq.org/clinical/obdraft.htm

OTHER SURGICAL SUBSPECIALTIES

Cardiopulmonary Bypass in Pregnancy

Gurinder M. S. Vasdev

200

Case Synopsis

A 28-year-old primigravida with a 24-week gestational age fetus presents with increased shortness of breath. Her past medical history includes mitral valve replacement with a Björk-Shiley valve. Transthoracic echocardiography reveals a poorly functioning valve with organized old thrombus. She is prepared for an urgent mitral valve replacement. Fetal ultrasonography reveals a normal-sized fetus with a heart rate of 125 beats per minute, with good heart rate variability.

PROBLEM ANALYSIS

Definition and Recognition

With advances in cardiac intervention, women with congenital heart disease are approaching normal life spans. They now account for nearly 4% of all pregnancies. Some of these women require urgent cardiac surgical intervention with cardiopulmonary bypass (CPB) during pregnancy or immediately after delivery. Maternal mortality from CPB ranges from 1.5% to 3%, similar to that for disease-matched, non-pregnant females.

Surgery during the first trimester may be associated with a higher risk of teratogenesis and spontaneous miscarriage. Hence, semielective surgery is often deferred to the second or third trimester. However, maximal cardiovascular changes occur during the third trimester. This added stress on the maternal cardiovascular system results in parturients presenting with symptoms of cardiac decompensation, albeit with a viable preterm fetus. If the fetus is viable (>28 weeks' gestation), combined cardiac surgery and cesarean delivery can benefit the mother by decreasing the cardiovascular burden during the immediate CPB period. In this case, it is important that the abdomen be open during CPB to ensure control of uterine bleeding while the patient is anticoagulated.

Initiation of CPB may cause trauma to the blood vessels, activation of the clotting cascade, and alteration in acid-base balance that can affect both the parturient and the fetus. Release of maternal vascular endothelial factors and the formation of microemboli can further affect the placental microcirculation and stimulate uterine contractions. The need for maternal cerebral protection with hypothermia adversely affects fetal oxygen transfer due to a leftward shift of the oxygen-hemoglobin dissociation curve. Hypothermia and nonpulsatile flow may further compromise placental perfusion. Fetal demise remains relatively high (10% to 20%) and is largely attributed to intraoperative hypothermia. Other factors associated with fetal demise are long pump runs and specific types of surgery (e.g., repair of ventricular septal defects, aortic valve replacement). However, there has been a recent decline in mortality from greater than 20% to 12.5%.

Risk Assessment

Outcomes for parturients undergoing urgent cardiac surgery with CPB are determined by several different factors.

Patient-Related Factors. Parturients with New York Heart Association class III or IV heart failure are considered candidates for surgery. For such parturients, maternal mortality with labor and delivery, but without corrective surgery, varies from 5% to 50% and depends on the nature and severity of the patient's cardiac disease. With some cardiac lesions, non-CPB intervention (e.g., coronary stenting, balloon valvotomy) may be adequate to get the parturient through labor and delivery. Advances in echocardiography now allow physicians to accurately follow up and determine the optimal timing for cardiac intervention for both the mother and the fetus. Some cardiac surgery can be performed without CPB, which avoids sequelae related to the use of extracorporeal circulation.

Surgical Factors. Cardiac valvular repair or revision requires longer bypass times than does replacement of the valve. In addition to the inherent dangers of CPB, parturients are at increased risk due to fetal demands during CPB and reperfusion after CPB.

Fetal Factors. The severity of the maternal disease determines the outcome for the fetus. If the surgical procedure can be delayed to the second trimester without adversely impacting the mother's health, this reduces the risk for fetal teratogenesis. If the fetus is close to term, combined cardiac surgery and cesarean delivery may be a reasonable option.

Perfusion. Parturients have a hyperdynamic circulation with high levels of oxygen consumption. Maximal oxygen demand occurs in the third trimester (Fig. 200-1). Thus, when commencing CPB in the third trimester, higher flows and pressures are advised to maintain placental infusion. The shortest possible CPB time is also preferred. Pulsatile flow has been associated with decreased release of endothelium-derived mediators and may be beneficial for optimizing

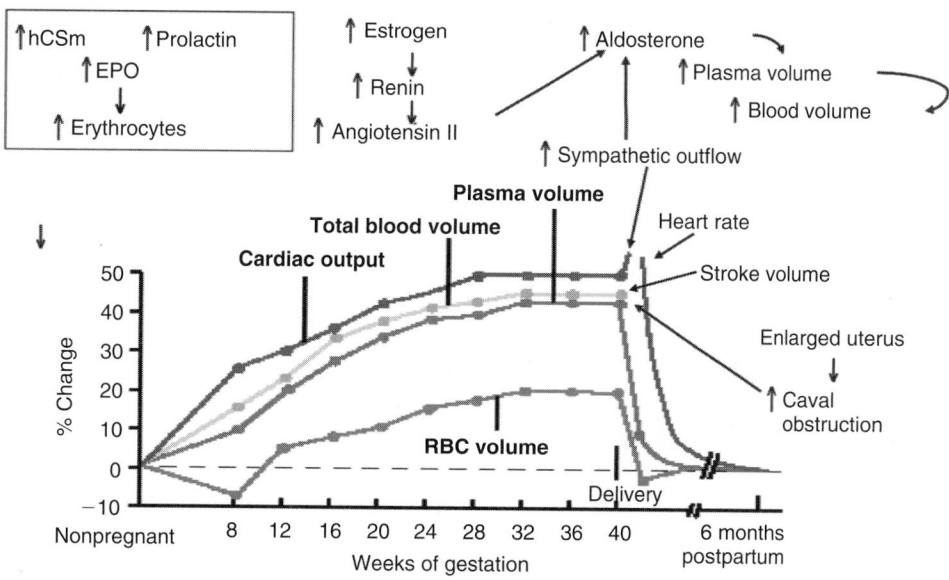

Figure 200–1 ■ Cardiovascular changes associated with pregnancy. EPO, erythropoietin; hCSm, human chorionic somatomammotropin; RBC, red blood cell. (Redrawn from Teerlink JR, Foster E: Valvular heart disease in pregnancy. A contemporary perspective. Cardiol Clin 16:573-598, 1998.)

placental perfusion. These advantages are probably limited, however, so conventional nonpulsatile CPB is still acceptable.

Cardioplegia. Particular attention to full recovery from cardioplegia must be paid to minimize adverse effects on the fetus. The surgeon can cannulate the coronary sinus and place a ventricular vent (the blood is discarded) before circulating the cardioplegia solution. High placental potassium levels may result in fetal cardiac arrest. No particular cardioplegia solution has been reported to be more beneficial or protective in pregnant patients.

Hypothermia. Maternal core temperatures less than 35°C are associated with increased uterine contractions and reduced oxygen transfer by a leftward shift of the oxygen-hemoglobin dissociation curve. The associated loss of fetal heart rate variability and bradycardia may make the diagnosis of fetal distress difficult. Warm bypass is preferable but may compromise maternal cerebral protection. Cerebral protective drugs cross the placenta and may affect the fetus; therefore, their role in CPB for parturients has not been fully established.

Anticoagulation. Heparin is highly polarized and does not cross the placenta, but the dose must be adjusted for the increase in antithrombin III levels during pregnancy. The activated clotting time is a valid test for parturients. The use of antifibrinolytic drugs during CPB in parturients does not have Food and Drug Administration approval. Tranexamic acid crosses the placenta, and fetal effects can be dire. There have been case reports of successful aprotinin use after the fetus has been delivered; however, considering the hypercoagulable state of pregnancy, significant postoperative thromboembolic sequelae may complicate its use. After mechanical valve replacement, warfarin is the anticoagulant of choice. It should be initiated as soon as surgical hemostasis is deemed adequate. The use of surgical anticoagulants restricts the perioperative use of central neuraxial analgesia.

Preterm Labor. Intervention for preterm labor includes terbutaline, nitroglycerin, and magnesium sulfate. All these drugs have cardiac effects that must be considered.

Fetal Heart Rate Monitoring. Fetal heart rate monitoring can be beneficial even at a nonviable age. The fetus is sensitive to altered placental perfusion and anesthetic agents. Initiation of CPB is associated with decreased fetal heart rate and perfusion pressure; therefore, oxygen delivery must be optimized. The CPB pump may need to be primed with type-specific blood. Umbilical artery and venous Doppler flow monitoring can be helpful in some circumstances.

MANAGEMENT

Before any cardiac surgery with CPB is performed on a pregnant patient, a conference regarding her perioperative care is essential. This must involve anesthesia care providers, cardiac surgeons, maternal-fetal medical specialists, neonatologists, and cardiologists. The concerns of each specialty must be addressed. Especially important are the logistics of emergent fetal delivery.

Premedication. Diazepam, midazolam, and fentanyl can be used for preoperative sedation. Depending on the severity of cardiac disease, some invasive monitors may be required before induction of anesthesia. Antacid treatment with H_2-blockers and a nonparticulate antacid is beneficial for parturients at greater than 18 weeks' gestation. Fifteen-degree left lateral uterine displacement is also required with a greater than 18-week gravid uterus.

Induction. A hemodynamically stable induction preserves placental perfusion. The use of volatile agents is beneficial because they relax the uterus. High-dose opiate-based anesthesia is more likely to be associated with fetal bradycardia. This should be taken into account when interpreting fetal heart rate changes. Fentanyl is the most commonly used opiate during CPB in pregnant patients.

Monitoring.   In addition to the usual invasive monitors for cardiac surgery, transesophageal echocardiography has increasing intraoperative utility, especially for rapid diagnosis when the patient is removed from CPB. Use of invasive vascular access for monitoring is determined by the nature and severity of the parturient's disease. Oximetric pulmonary artery catheters can be useful during the reperfusion and postoperative periods; monitoring both oxygen delivery and utilization is helpful for guiding hemodynamic manipulations.

Cardiopulmonary Bypass.   The shortest possible period of normothermic CPB is preferred. In parturients with severe cardiac disease, blood may be needed to prime the pump. Cardioplegia must be recovered to prevent fetal hyperkalemia, and this necessitates the use of left ventricular and coronary sinus vents. CPB is associated with progressive increases in both peripheral and placental vascular resistance. Optimal mean arterial pressure is provided by noting preinduction values and periodically assessing urine output and fetal well-being. Oxygen consumption trends may help in some circumstances. Increasing cardiac output (or CPB flow) and hematocrit is preferred to the use of vasoactive drugs to preserve mean arterial pressure and oxygen delivery to the mother and fetus. Use of vasopressors may be associated with increased endovascular shear stress and release of vasoactive, endothelium-derived inflammatory mediators. Vasodilatation with volatile agents and nitroglycerin has the additional benefit of relaxing the uterus (tocolysis). If the parturient has had a previous cesarean delivery, vasodilators with less potential to relax the gravid uterine muscle (e.g., hydralazine, possibly dihydropyridine calcium channel blockers)[1] might be preferred, because uterine atony could give rise to severe postpartum hemorrhage.

Upon rewarming after CPB, an increase in uterine activity may be noted, but tocolytics are administered only if the contractions are regular and strong. Once rewarming is complete, contractions often subside. Internal paddles used for defibrillation should be angled away from the uterus and fetus to reduce the risk of direct electrical stimulation. Weaning from CPB requires meticulous attention to detail, because the stunned myocardium now has to produce a high cardiac output consistent with the needs of the gravid uterus. The use of pressors, aortic balloons, and ventricular assist devices may result in a considerable decrease in placental flow. In these circumstances, fetal distress or demise may be inevitable and is a direct result of the severity of the mother's underlying cardiac disease.

Postoperative Care.   Cardiac surgical intensive care units are usually not equipped for fetal and uterine monitoring. Appropriate nursing coverage should be prearranged. Also, the logistics for performing emergent cardiac surgery if the patient decompensates should be addressed in advance.

PREVENTION

In parturients, CPB is more complex because of the needs of the fetus and the altered physiologic state of pregnancy. When possible, delivery of the fetus removes one major component of a challenging situation. The best practice is driven by the underlying cardiac condition of the mother, even though this may necessitate delivery of the fetus before the age of viability. Most parturients who require open-heart surgery with CPB are referred to medical centers with level III neonatal intensive care units. The numbers of such facilities are likely to increase as more and more women with congenital heart disease reach reproductive age.

Further Reading

Jahangiri M, Clarke J, Prefumo F, et al: Cardiac surgery during pregnancy: Pulsatile or nonpulsatile perfusion? J Thorac Cardiovasc Surg 126:894-895, 2003.

Khandelwal M, Rasanen J, Ludomorski A, et al: Evaluation of fetal and uterine hemodynamics during cardiopulmonary bypass. Obstet Gynecol 88:667-671, 1996.

Koren G, Pastuszak A, Ito S: Drugs in pregnancy. N Engl J Med 338:1128-1137, 1998.

Murphy BA, Zvara DA, Nelson LH, et al: Clinical conference: Aprotinin use during deep hypothermic circulatory arrest for type A aortic dissection and cesarean section in a woman with preeclampsia. J Cardiothorac Vasc Anesth 17:256-257, 2003.

Pardi G, Ferrari M, Iorio F, et al: The effect of maternal hypothermic cardiopulmonary bypass on fetal lamb temperature, hemodynamics, oxygenation, and acid-base balance. J Thorac Cardiovasc Surg 127:1728-1734, 2004.

Pomini F, Mercogliano D, Cavalletti C, et al: Cardiopulmonary bypass in pregnancy. Ann Thorac Surg 61:259-268, 1996.

Weiss BM, von Segesser LK, Alon E, et al: Outcome of cardiovascular surgery and pregnancy: A systematic review of the period 1984-1996. Am J Obstet Gynecol 176:1643-1653, 1998.

---

[1]Based on available evidence, sodium nitroprusside, verapamil, and diltiazem appear to have more potential to cause uterine atony.

GENERAL SURGERY

Postoperative Hepatic Dysfunction

201

Kerri M. Robertson

Case Synopsis

A 38-year-old man with a history of hepatitis C and hepatocellular carcinoma is scheduled for elective liver resection. Preoperative hemoglobin is 10 g/dL. Albumin, creatinine, and prothrombin time are within normal limits. The surgery is uneventful except for an intraoperative blood loss of 2 L, requiring transfusion with 5 units of packed red blood cells. The patient is transferred to the surgical intensive care unit for postoperative care due to oliguria and a potassium level of 6.1 mEq/L. Recovery is unremarkable, except that on postoperative day 4 the patient is noted to be jaundiced.

PROBLEM ANALYSIS

Definition

Clinically significant acute liver dysfunction is common after anesthesia and surgery. It is chiefly limited to patients with preexisting hepatic disease, massive blood transfusion, hepatic oxygen deprivation, infection, and drug toxicity. Most postoperative jaundice is multifactorial in origin, is difficult to diagnose, and often requires no treatment. The incidence following elective abdominal surgery is less than 1%; however, it is reported to be up to 15% to 17% with major cardiac surgery.

The normal serum bilirubin level is 0.3 to 1.1 mg/dL. Jaundice is usually detected clinically when the serum bilirubin exceeds 3 to 5 mg/dL and the patient's sclerae become icteric. Increased conjugated bilirubin reflects a problem with bilirubin secretion due to hepatocellular dysfunction, intrahepatic cholestasis, or biliary tract obstruction. If the increase in total bilirubin concentration is primarily unconjugated, the most likely cause is either hemolysis of erythrocytes producing a large bilirubin load or defects in the uptake, transport, or conjugation of bilirubin. Jaundice is usually evident within the first week after surgery and is not associated with acute liver failure. Hypoxic hepatocyte insult is the primary mechanism underlying many causes of postoperative hepatic dysfunction and may bear little or no relationship to the actual drugs or anesthetic technique used. There appears to be little correlation between the severity of liver disease and the absolute level of bilirubin. Supportive care is indicated, unless jaundice is caused by biliary obstruction that can be corrected surgically.

Recognition

Owing to the large hepatic functional reserve, routine laboratory values may be normal despite significant underlying hepatic disease. Abnormal results of several common laboratory tests may loosely reflect hepatic dysfunction (Table 201-1).

Prothrombin time measures activity of the extrinsic coagulation pathway and requires fibrinogen, prothrombin, and factors V, VII, and X. Slight alterations may reflect severe hepatic dysfunction, because only 20% to 30% of normal factor activity is required for coagulation. Plasma half-lives for clotting factors are measured in hours, so even acute liver dysfunction may be associated with a coagulopathy. An international normalized ratio greater than 1.5 not corrected by vitamin K within 24 hours implies severe liver disease. With obstructive biliary disease, however, the failure of bile salt secretion may result in poor absorption of vitamin K, which is a cofactor necessary for the post-transcriptional γ-carboxylation and activation of factors II, VII, IX, and X.

Albumin is produced in the liver and represents the best measure of chronic hepatic synthetic dysfunction, so long as increased albumin losses in the urine or gastrointestinal tract are excluded. Owing to albumin's long half-life (14 to 21 days),

---

Table 201–1 ■ Investigational Studies for Evaluation of Liver Function

Parenchymal Damage with Failure of Synthetic Function
Prothrombin time
Albumin
Transaminases: alanine aminotransferase, aspartate aminotransferase
Serum ammonia
Screen for markers of viral hepatitis and autoimmune disorders
Abdominal ultrasonography or computed tomography
Liver biopsy

Cholestasis or Biliary Tract Disease
Bilirubin (total, conjugated, and unconjugated): urine and serum levels
Alkaline phosphatase
Abdominal ultrasonography or computed tomography
Endoscopic retrograde cholangiopancreatography or percutaneous transhepatic cholangiography

severe liver dysfunction lasting 3 to 4 weeks is required before a significant change in serum albumin levels becomes apparent. Alkaline phosphatase is present in the epithelial cells lining the biliary canaliculi; however, it is not specific for liver disease, owing to extrahepatic sources of this enzyme, especially bone. The serum ammonia concentration represents the balance between ammoniagenesis (primarily in the gut and kidney) and hepatic urea synthesis. Because the normal liver's reserve capacity for urea synthesis is great, elevated serum ammonia concentrations usually indicate significant loss of hepatic function. Of the liver transaminase enzymes, alanine aminotransferase is the gold standard biomarker for hepatocellular injury.

Jaundice is the most common and easily recognized sign suggesting hepatic dysfunction. Bilirubin is the primary end product of hemoglobin metabolism. The uptake and transport of unconjugated bilirubin into hepatocytes are followed by hepatic conjugation with glucuronide and subsequent excretion into bile canaliculi. If the total bilirubin concentration is greater than 1.5 mg/dL, it is considered abnormal. Postoperative jaundice can be categorized into three groups:

1. Prehepatic: overproduction of bilirubin
2. Intrahepatic: acute or subacute hepatocellular injury with or without preexisting liver disease
3. Posthepatic: cholestasis from biliary tract obstruction

PREHEPATIC CAUSES

Prehepatic causes of postoperative jaundice include the following:

- Hemolysis of transfused blood
- Reabsorption of extravasated blood
- Intravascular hemolysis after drugs, infection, or fasting
- Hemolytic anemia: congenital (enzyme deficiencies or hemoglobinopathies) or acquired (immune mediated or traumatic)
- Idiopathic hyperbilirubinemia (Gilbert, Crigler-Najjar, or Dubin-Johnson syndrome)

Isolated elevated unconjugated bilirubin levels in a postsurgical patient most likely result from a prehepatic mechanism. Often, this is due to a large increase in the load of bilirubin from the hemolysis of erythrocytes, which transiently overwhelms the liver's capacity to conjugate bilirubin. Up to 10% of red blood cells per unit of transfused blood are hemolyzed within the first 24 postoperative hours to generate 250 mg of bilirubin. The normal liver can conjugate this amount of bilirubin. However, with many liters of extravasated blood, multiple transfusions of red cells, the presence of myoglobin, or impaired liver function, hyperbilirubinemia may result.

Pronounced postoperative jaundice commonly occurs in trauma victims. Many of these patients have extensive injuries requiring major surgical intervention and volume resuscitation, often with massive transfusion of red cells and other blood products. Progressive severe jaundice extending beyond the 10th to 12th postoperative day correlates with the development of sepsis, multiorgan failure, and death. The clinical manifestations caused by hemolysis are likely to be accentuated if the patient has underlying chronic liver disease, has sustained acute ischemic injury to the liver, or has impaired renal function. Sepsis due to streptococci, *Escherichia coli*, *Bacteroides* species, and *Clostridium* species can also cause hemolysis. The mechanism is poorly understood, but it is likely due to bacterial hemolysins and reduced liver uptake of bilirubin associated with hypotension.

Diagnosis of hemolytic anemia requires reticulocytosis, unconjugated hyperbilirubinemia, elevated lactate dehydrogenase, and absent or low haptoglobin concentrations. Familial hyperbilirubinemias caused by defects in the uptake, transport, or conjugation mechanisms are exacerbated by stress, infection, and fasting. Usually, bilirubin concentrations peak within the first few postoperative days and resolve over days to weeks. No specific therapy is indicated, other than that directed toward reducing any ongoing red cell breakdown.

INTRAHEPATIC CAUSES

Intrahepatic causes of postoperative jaundice are listed in Table 201-2. Total hepatic blood flow is 1.5 L/minute (25% to 30% of the normal adult cardiac output). The hepatic artery supplies 25% of total hepatic blood flow, and the portal vein supplies 75%. However, they contribute equally to hepatic oxygenation. In essence, the portal venous system is a passive vascular bed. Flow is dependent on perfusion pressure, cardiac output, and splanchnic vascular resistance. Reductions in portal inflow are usually associated with reciprocal hepatic artery vasodilatation, thereby maintaining total hepatic blood flow and oxygen supply. Normally, hepatic venous oxygen saturation is 35% to 50%. In shock, this may decline to 6% or less as visceral perfusion is reduced.

Reduced cardiac output and blood pressure during general anesthesia and surgery decrease hepatic blood flow

---

Table 201–2 ■ Intrahepatic Causes of Postoperative Jaundice

Hepatic Parenchymal Disease
Oxygen deprivation (ischemia)
Chronic hepatitis
Cirrhosis; primary biliary cirrhosis
Primary sclerosing cholangitis; cholestasis
Acute viral hepatitis

Hypoxemia
Reduced cardiac output causing hypotension and reduced hepatic blood flow
Anemia; hypovolemia

Miscellaneous Causes
Primary sclerosing cholangitis
Sepsis with or without hepatic or multiple organ system failure
Preeclampsia (coagulopathy, liver dysfunction, or HELLP syndrome; see Chapter 189)
Drugs or intravenous therapy
    Haloalkalated anesthetics
    Alcohol- or drug-induced hepatitis
    Total parenteral nutrition
Major liver injury or surgery

HELLP, hemolysis, elevated liver enzymes, and low platelet count in association with preeclampsia.

and jeopardize liver oxygenation. Contributing factors include the following:

- Anesthetic drugs and adjuncts
  - Intravenous and inhalational agents
  - Vasodilators, β-blockers, and α₁-agonists
  - H₂-blockers
  - Vasopressin and other vasoconstrictors
- Hypovolemia and continuous positive airway pressure
- Hypoxemia, hypercarbia, and acidosis

Surgical manipulation of the right upper quadrant of the abdomen can reduce hepatic blood flow by as much as 60% owing to sympathetic stimulation or direct compression of the vena cava and splanchnic vessels. Compensatory hepatic artery vasodilatation and reduced portal inflow are opposed in a dose-dependent maner by volatile anesthetics. Thus, portal perfusion becomes pressure dependent.

Cirrhotic patients are at increased risk for ischemic hepatic injury owing to preexisting impaired perfusion as well as multiorgan system failure from the release of cellular inflammatory mediators. Ischemic hepatitis causes centrilobular hepatic necrosis, not inflammatory necrosis. Usually, the onset of jaundice occurs 1 to 5 days following surgery and peaks after 9 to 18 days. Liver function tests reveal elevated bilirubin, alkaline phosphatase, and transaminase concentrations, often 10 to 100 times the upper limits of normal. Clinical studies indicate that low perfusion pressure alone is insufficient to cause this clinical picture in patients without preexisting liver or cardiac disease. Also, ischemic hepatitis, elevated central venous pressure, and portal venous congestion may contribute to a further reduction in hepatic blood flow.

Jaundice occurs in 45% of patients admitted to intensive care units with severe trauma or intra-abdominal sepsis after surgery. Potential causes are infection, the effect of endotoxin-mediated cytokine release on bile acid transport systems, and hemolysis. Sepsis-mediated cholestasis reverses with treatment of the cause. In experimental models (swine), large intravenous bilirubin loads cause extensive hepatic and canalicular membrane injury and intrahepatic cholestasis. This leads to bile stasis and impaired bile salt export pump function. By analogy, small bowel ileus in trauma victims may interrupt the normal endogenous circulation of bile acids between the gut and the liver. If so, this would render hepatocytes more sensitive to the cholestatic effect of bilirubin overload.

Halothane hepatitis is well known and is still a common surgical diagnosis for postoperative jaundice, despite the fact that halothane has become obsolete in many institutions with the availability of newer agents that are less likely to be associated with hepatotoxicity (see Chapter 17). Although halothane is the prototypical example of volatile anesthetic hepatitis, other agents have been implicated, including enflurane, desflurane, and isoflurane. Evidence exists for "cross-sensitization" between these agents. Among these, halothane causes the greatest reduction in hepatic blood flow and oxygenation and may promote a mild, self-limited form of hepatitis in 1 in 10,000 exposures. Clinical features include high fever on postexposure days 3 to 14, with the onset of jaundice 1 to 2 days later. There is leukocytosis with eosinophilia in 20% of cases. Fulminant hepatic necrosis is rare (1 in 35,000 exposures) but is associated with 40% mortality. Adverse outcomes are associated with patient age older than 60 years, obesity, repeated exposures over a short interval, serum bilirubin greater than 10 mg/dL, and prothrombin time greater than 20 seconds. The most likely mechanism of injury is halothane metabolism and immune-mediated toxicity, but the evidence is inconclusive. Detection of antitrifluoroacetyl antibodies specific for halothane-modified rabbit liver cell membranes may help confirm the diagnosis, but the sensitivity and specificity of this test are unproved, so the diagnosis is usually one of exclusion (see also Chapter 17).

There are two types of chronic hepatitis: chronic persistent hepatitis and chronic active hepatitis. The latter is more serious and more commonly progresses to cirrhosis and liver failure. Patients with cirrhosis, regardless of cause, have a reduced life expectancy. Although the probability of hepatic decompensation may be relatively low, after the onset of the first major complication (e.g., ascites, variceal bleeding, jaundice, encephalopathy), mortality is high. Anesthesia and surgery are implicated in hepatic decompensation. Significant factors (by multivariate analysis) associated with perioperative hepatic complications and mortality include the following:

- Male gender
- High Child-Pugh score
- Cirrhosis other than primary biliary cirrhosis (especially cryptogenic cirrhosis)
- Renal insufficiency
- Chronic obstructive pulmonary disease
- Diabetes mellitus
- Ischemic heart disease or congestive heart failure
- Preoperative sepsis, gastrointestinal bleeding, or ascites
- Emergency surgery with a high surgical severity score
- Documented intraoperative hypotension

Acute hepatitis is usually associated with viral infection or is alcohol or drug induced (e.g., antibiotics, antihypertensives, anticonvulsants, tranquilizers, fentanyl). Rarely, sepsis, congestive heart failure, and pregnancy-induced hepatitis are seen. Viral hepatitis is most commonly due to type A, B, or C viruses. Less commonly, it is due to type D or Epstein-Barr virus or cytomegalovirus. Testing for antigens and antibodies is required for a definitive diagnosis, because many classes of drugs cause hepatitis that is clinically and histologically identical to viral hepatitis. Elevation of aminotransferases in the early phase of hepatitis precedes the appearance of jaundice.

A high index of suspicion is required for the early diagnosis of hepatitis. General symptoms include dark urine, fatigue, anorexia, vomiting, dehydration, low-grade fever, myalgias, and right upper quadrant pain. The mortality rate for intra-abdominal surgery in patients with severe acute inflammatory hepatitis ranges from 15% (viral) to 55% (alcohol related). Therefore, all elective surgery should be delayed until the infection has resolved, as indicated by normal liver function test results. Recovery may take up to 4 months.

In 2004 the incidence of post-transfusion hepatitis from any cause was negligible and would probably warrant a case report. Eighty-five percent of post-transfusion infections were caused by hepatitis C virus. Prior to 1990 there were no screening tests for hepatitis C. The Centers for Disease Control and Prevention currently reports that the rate of post-transfusion hepatitis C infection has decreased from

8% to 10% to less than 1 in 1 million units of blood or blood products transfused in 2004.

Benign postoperative intrahepatic cholestasis usually occurs in patients without previous liver disease following prolonged operative procedures and a stormy intraoperative course associated with hypotension, endotoxemia, and blood loss. Severe jaundice with elevated serum alkaline phosphatase and normal to mildly elevated aminotransferases is typical. It appears to be a self-limited process that resolves completely. Intrahepatic cholestasis may also be associated with surgical stress, infection, and drugs (nonsteroidal anti-inflammatory drugs, aspirin, amiodarone, isoniazid, methyldopa, monoamine oxidase inhibitors, phenothiazines, phenytoin, sodium valproate, and estrogens).

POSTHEPATIC CAUSES

Posthepatic causes of postoperative jaundice include the following:

- Bile duct injury, tumor, stone, or stricture
- Acute cholecystitis
- Pancreatitis
- Choledocholithiasis

Cholestasis can be intrahepatic or extrahepatic. Biliary obstruction with inadvertent bile duct injury after laparoscopic surgery may cause postoperative cholestasis, especially when jaundice appears within 48 hours of such surgery. Postoperative drugs may also cause biliary obstruction. Pancreatitis, acute cholecystitis, or choledocholithiasis increase both conjugated bilirubin and alkaline phosphatase levels and cause mild to marked elevations in transaminase concentrations. Computed tomography and retrograde endoscopic cholangiography may help confirm the diagnosis of intrahepatic or extrahepatic cholestasis.

Risk Assessment

In general, outcome is influenced less by the choice of anesthetic agents than by the urgency or type of surgery and the severity of chronic liver disease. Surgical risk factors for postoperative hepatic dysfunction or isolated hyperbilirubinemia include emergency surgery and surgery with a high severity score, including the following:

- Open-heart surgery
- Open versus laparoscopic cholecystectomy
- Trauma surgery, especially involving the liver or biliary tract
- Major abdominal surgery (e.g., biliary tract surgery, liver resection)
- Surgery with large blood or blood product transfusion requirements

Differentiation between acute inflammatory liver failure and acute exacerbation of chronic liver disease affects the prognosis. Viral or alcohol- or drug-induced acute hepatitis is a contraindication to elective surgery. Patients with asymptomatic chronic hepatitis likely present little increased anesthetic risk. However, those with symptomatic cirrhosis or chronic hepatitis are at significantly increased risk for postoperative complications, with the degree of risk related to the extent of their disease.

Child's classification has traditionally been used to predict perioperative mortality in cirrhotic patients undergoing surgical portacaval shunt or esophageal transection. The mortality risk is 10%, 31%, and 76% for Child's classes A, B, and C cirrhosis, respectively. This classification may also predict perioperative outcomes for nonshunt surgery. However, current perioperative risk assessment for adults with end-stage liver disease relies on the MELD scoring system, which is based on bilirubin, creatinine, and international normalized ratio. It accurately predicts 3-month mortality after elective transjugular intrahepatic portosystemic shunt procedures. For patients with known or suspected compensated chronic liver disease, consultation with a hepatologist is necessary to identify those with a Child's class B or C cirrhosis and with a MELD score greater than 15.

Cholelithiasis occurs twice as often in patients with cirrhosis than in those without. Despite recent advances in anesthetic care, the high rates of mortality (7% to 20%) and morbidity (5% to 23%)[1] in patients with cirrhosis and portal hypertension having cholecystectomy have not decreased substantially. Thus, cholecystectomy in these patients remains a formidable operation.

One contributory factor to the high incidence of multiorgan system failure in these patients may be the surgery-related release of inflammatory mediators and hepatic ischemia. This is more pronounced with open than with laparoscopic cholecystectomy. Yet even with the latter, hepatic perfusion can still be reduced by the head-up tilt and dependent venous pooling. Moreover, carbon dioxide insufflation increases intra-abdominal pressure. Further, direct liver manipulation, hypercarbic acidosis, and the neurohumoral stress response with upper abdominal surgery increase the risk for multiorgan system failure. Predictably, patients with Child's classes B and C cirrhosis are at very high risk for hepatic dysfunction after cardiac surgery. Mortality is 11.4%, compared with 3% for those without cirrhosis.

Patients with severe obstructive jaundice have reduced peripheral vascular resistance. Also, renal salt wasting and reduced left ventricular function, along with splanchnic pooling, put them at risk for hypotension with minimal blood loss. Risk factors for perioperative mortality (8% to 28%) include the following:

- Hematocrit less than 30%
- Bilirubin greater than 11 mg/dL
- Malignant biliary obstruction (e.g., pancreatic or bile duct carcinoma)
- Ascending cholangitis
- Azotemia or hypoalbuminemia

Postoperative complications in patients with severe obstructive jaundice include infection, renal failure, disseminated intravasacular coagulation, and further deterioration in liver function.

Implications

Most postoperative jaundice is self-limited and resolves with supportive therapy. Patients with acute inflammatory hepatitis

---

[1]Due to bleeding, renal failure, or sepsis.

or evidence of hepatocellular necrosis are poor surgical risks. In contrast, those with cholestatic disease have lower complication rates. Patients with chronic liver disease and preserved function may not be at increased surgical risk. However, those with cirrhosis do have higher morbidity and mortality rates.

A focused preoperative assessment is necessary to identify high-risk patients. Progressive hepatocellular injury may lead to hepatic failure. For high-risk patients, postoperative care and surveillance should take place in a critical care setting. Clinical indicators of suboptimal liver function include the following:

- Persistent hypothermia
- Coagulopathy
- Acidosis or hyperglycemia (later, hypoglycemia)
- Renal insufficiency
- Hemodynamic instability
- Acute respiratory distress
- Delayed postoperative awakening

MANAGEMENT

For adults with postoperative jaundice, management begins with a systematic review of the patient's history, physical examination findings, and anesthetic and surgical records. For the last, special attention is paid to associated hypotension, hypoxemia, transfusions, and any drugs used. Attention is also focused on laboratory results, including urinalysis; pre- and postoperative liver function tests; and serum total, direct, and indirect bilirubin concentrations. The most important questions are these:

1. Is there any evidence of hemolysis?
2. Is there evidence of chronic liver disease?
3. Could the jaundice be drug induced, alcohol induced, or infective?
4. Is there evidence of biliary tract obstruction?

If the urinalysis is negative for bilirubin and there is increased serum indirect bilirubin (i.e., unconjugated hyperbilirubinemia), this suggests a prehepatic cause due to a large bilirubin load. However, if the urine is positive for bilirubin and there is increased total and direct bilirubin (i.e., conjugated hyperbilirubinemia), this suggests an intrahepatic or posthepatic cause (e.g., cholestasis, acute parenchymal hepatic injury). If both alkaline phosphatase and transaminases are elevated, hepatobiliary ultrasonography is indicated. If this is negative, viral serology, α-fetoprotein, antimitochondrial antibody, and retrograde endoscopic cholangiography are indicated. Evidence of bile duct dilatation is investigated with cholangiography. Focal lesions are further studied with computed tomography or magnetic resonance imaging, arteriography, and biopsy. If the diagnosis is still elusive, liver biopsy may be necessary.

A strategic management plan includes the following:

- Ensure a homeostatic environment (normalize electrolytes, acid-base status, hematocrit).
- Attain cardiovascular stability (euvolemia, mean arterial pressure >60 mm Hg).
- Treat bacterial infections and complications related to liver disease (encephalopathy, ascites, hyponatremia, variceal bleeding, coagulopathy).
- Avoid hepatotoxic and nephrotoxic drugs.
- Optimize renal perfusion:
  - Identify intrinsic renal parenchymal disease.
  - Provide intravascular volume expansion.
  - Institute drug therapy with splanchnic vasoconstrictors or renal vasodilators.
  - Treat hemoglobinuria with urine alkalinization and diuresis.

For the majority of fulminant hepatic failure patients, survival ultimately depends on medical stabilization and urgent liver transplantation.

PREVENTION

Minimizing the incidence of postoperative hepatic dysfunction begins with a comprehensive preoperative assessment and identification of those patients who might be predisposed. About 1 in 700 patients admitted for elective surgery has abnormal liver function studies. For patients with known hepatic disease, it is important to determine its cause and assess the degree of impairment, as well as any systemic manifestations and comorbidities. Anesthetic management often requires maximally invasive monitoring. The fewest possible anesthetic agents should be used (e.g., fentanyl, isoflurane, cisatracurium, and oxygen). The goal is to preserve hepatic function. This is done by minimizing reductions in hepatic blood flow and preserving oxygen delivery to prevent hepatocellular ischemia. Finally, keep in mind that surgery proximate to the liver or biliary system carries a higher expected rate of postoperative complications.

Further Reading

Burroughs A, Dagher L: Acute jaundice. Clin Med 1:285-289, 2001.

Chung C, Buchman AL: Postoperative jaundice and total parenteral nutrition-associated hepatic dysfunction. Clin Liver Dis 6:1067-1084, 2002.

Friedman LS: The risk of surgery in patients with liver disease. Hepatology 29:1617-1623, 1999.

Labori KJ, Bjornbeth BA, Raeder MG: Aetiology and prognostic implication of severe jaundice in surgical trauma patients. Scand J Gastroenterol 38:102-108, 2003.

202

Surgery in the Morbidly Obese

Christina M. Matadial and Jonathan H. Slonin

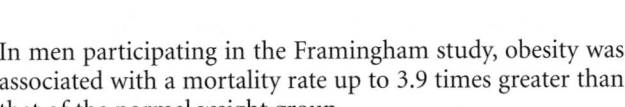

Case Synopsis

A 30-year-old woman is scheduled for laparoscopic gastric banding. She is 164 cm (63 inches) tall and weighs 160 kg (339 pounds).

PROBLEM ANALYSIS

Definition

Obesity affects approximately one third of the adult population in the United States. It is defined as body weight more than 20% greater than ideal weight. Morbid obesity is defined as body weight more than twice the calculated ideal weight. Ideal body weight is generally based on American life insurance statistics regarding height, build, sex, and age. The body mass index (BMI) is the most useful clinical indicator of obesity.

The Broca index is a practical way to determine ideal body weight:

Height in cm − 100 = ideal weight in kg for males

Height in cm − 105 = ideal weight in kg for females

The BMI was devised to reduce the effect of height on body weight:

$$BMI = weight\ in\ kg/(height\ in\ meters)^2$$

Ideal body weight = BMI of 22 to 28 kg/m^2

Obesity = BMI of 28 to 35 kg/m^2

Morbid obesity = BMI >35 kg/m^2

Recognition

It is now recognized that obesity is associated with a broad array of medical and surgical diseases leading to increased perioperative morbidity and mortality. Preoperative evaluation should focus on identifying coexisting diseases and conditions and the need for additional testing and invasive monitoring.

Risk Assessment

Most of the major obesity-related health risks increase disproportionately with increasing weight. The rate of premature death is increased in patients who are 30% over their ideal weight and is doubled in those weighing 40% to 60% more than their ideal body weight. The incidence of sudden unexplained death is at least 13 times greater in morbidly obese women compared with women at their ideal body weight.

In men participating in the Framingham study, obesity was associated with a mortality rate up to 3.9 times greater than that of the normal weight group.

Implications

Many organ systems are affected by morbid obesity, including the following:

- Cardiovascular
- Respiratory and airway
- Gastrointestinal
- Endocrine and metabolic

Morbid obesity causes significant pathophysiologic changes that may increase perioperative morbidity and mortality (Table 202-1). The anesthesiologist is faced with numerous potential anesthetic and surgical challenges (Table 202-2).

Cardiovascular disease commonly manifests as hypertension, coronary artery disease, and heart failure (e.g., cor pulmonale, pickwickian syndrome). Obesity appears to be an independent risk factor for ischemic heart disease. These patients may have limited functional capacity. Because they may not experience symptoms at rest, pharmacologic stress testing and imaging may be required to assess patients for myocardial ischemia and ventricular dysfunction.

In an obese patient, cardiac output and blood volume must increase to perfuse additional fat stores. Cardiac output is estimated to increase by 0.1 L/minute for each kilogram of additional adipose tissue. Cardiomegaly and hypertension may develop due to this increased need. Long-standing hypertension with associated left ventricular hypertrophy may cause congestive heart failure. Chronic hypoxemia may contribute to the development of pulmonary hypertension and right ventricular dysfunction. When this progresses to right ventricular chamber dilatation and failure (cor pulmonale), the condition is known as the pickwickian syndrome. Other components of this syndrome are somnolence, hypoxemia, and polycythemia.

Obesity is associated with reduced functional residual capacity (FRC), expiratory reserve volume, and total lung capacity. Expiratory reserve volume is the primary source of oxygen reserve during apnea. Therefore, in obese patients, preoxygenation is less effective. Lung closing volume may exceed FRC, leading to ventilation-perfusion mismatch and hypoxia. Both induction of anesthesia and supine positioning

Table 202–1 ▪ Organs or Organ Systems Affected by Morbid Obesity, with Associated Pathophysiology

Organ or System	Associated Pathophysiology
Cardiovascular	Increased stroke volume and blood volume → increased cardiac output Chronic hypoxemia → pulmonary HTN → RV hypertrophy or failure, or any combination of these With cor pulmonale, patients are considered to be "pickwickian" (see below under "Airway and lungs") Increased cardiac output to perfuse fat → systemic HTN → LV hypertrophy, and possible LV HF Any renovascular disease and insufficiency may aggravate HTN ECG findings: (1) left heart—low QRS voltage, LV strain or hypertrophy, LA abnormality, T-wave flattening in inferior and lateral chest wall leads; (2) right heart—RV strain or hypertrophy, right axis deviation or bundle branch block, P pulmonale with pulmonary HTN and cor pulmonale Cardiac arrhythmias secondary to hypercapnia, hypoxia, or systemic or pulmonary HTN and HF Hypercholesterolemia, hyperlipidemia, and hyperglycemia (i.e., metabolic syndrome) accelerate development of atherosclerotic cardiovascular disease Cerebral, coronary, or renovascular disease → stroke, acute coronary syndromes, or renal insufficiency Hypercoagulability, venous thrombosis, and pulmonary embolism: primary cause of perioperative 30-day mortality RA or LA chamber dilatation and hypercoagulability predispose to atrial tachyarrhythmias or fibrillation with systemic thromboembolism
Airway and lungs	Abundant upper airway soft tissue increases potential for difficult mask airway and tracheal intubation Reduced FRC due to large pannus and increased body mass makes diaphragmatic excursions more difficult and position dependent; augmented by mechanical ventilation (higher airway pressures) Reduced chest wall compliance, lung volumes, and diaphragmatic excursions increase work of breathing Reduced inspiratory and expiratory reserve volumes Closing volume may exceed functional residual volume, leading to ventilation-perfusion mismatch, especially when supine Obstructive sleep apnea consequent to airway narrowing, overly abundant peripharyngeal adipose tissue, and abnormal decrease in upper airway muscle tone during REM sleep Reduced chest wall and diaphragmatic muscle tone with general anesthesia and muscle relaxation further impair oxygenation Predominant diaphragmatic respiration Pickwickian syndrome: morbid obesity, somnolence, alveolar hypoventilation, periodic respiration, hypoxemia, polycythemia, with RV failure and hypertrophy → cor pulmonale
Endocrine/metabolic	Metabolic syndrome → type 2 diabetes (sevenfold increase in incidence) Predisposition to hypothyroidism and Cushing's disease Increased O_2 consumption and CO_2 production Increased metabolism of fluorinated volatile anesthetics (e.g., enflurane, methoxyflurane*) Increased pseudocholinesterase activity
Gastrointestinal	Increased intra-abdominal pressure with development of hiatal, umbilical, or inguinal herniation Gastroesophageal reflux disease and increased gastric acidity Abnormal liver function tests due to fatty infiltration of liver Increased risk for cholelithiasis and cholecystitis
Miscellaneous	Inactivity secondary to morbid obesity predisposes to thromboembolism Excessive weight bearing accelerates development of osteoarthritis and chronic back pain Increased risk for malignancies involving the breast, colon, cervix, ovary, uterus, pancreas, prostate, and rectum

*Seldom used in the developed world but may still be used in less developed nations.

ECG, electrocardiogram; FRC, functional residual capacity; HF, heart failure; HTN, hypertension; LA, left atrial; LV, left ventricle/ventricular; RA, right atrial; REM, rapid eye movement; RV, right ventricle/ventricular.

From Adams JP, Murphy JP: Obesity in anaesthesia and intensive care. Br J Anaesth 85:91-108, 2000; Gajraj NM, Whitten CW: Morbid obesity. In Atlee JL (ed): Complications in Anesthesia. Philadelphia, WB Saunders, 1999, pp 848-850; Roizen MF, Fleisher LA: Anesthetic implications of concurrent diseases. In Miller RD (ed): Miller's Anesthesia, 6th ed. Philadelphia, Churchill Livingstone, 2005, pp 1017-1149.

further decrease FRC and worsen ventilation-perfusion mismatch. Increased BMI is also associated with reduced respiratory compliance and increased work of breathing.

Difficult upper airway management (especially mask ventilation) and endotracheal intubation should be anticipated in obese patients. Increased adipose tissue in the neck and hypopharynx leads to narrowing of the oropharyngeal space. Approximately 5% of obese individuals develop obstructive sleep apnea. Reduced FRC, atelectasis, and upper airway muscle relaxation predispose to obstructive sleep apnea. Sedative drugs produce a dose-dependent depression of consciousness and lung volumes. Because preoxygenation is less effective, time to desaturation below 90% may be greatly reduced, especially in the morbidly obese.

Obese patients are presumed to be at increased risk for pulmonary aspiration of gastric contents due to increased

Table 202–2 ▪ **Anesthetic Implications for Surgery in the Morbidly Obese**
Preoperative Preparation and Induction of Anesthesia
Emotional issues (e.g., passive-aggressive personality, anxiety)
Difficult venous access
Difficulty with facemask ventilation and securing the airway
Difficult direct laryngosopy or fiberoptic intubation
Difficulty establishing noninvasive or invasive monitoring
Increased risk for pulmonary aspiration
Intraoperative Management
Reduced cardiopulmonary reserve
Problems with patient positioning and mobilization
Technical difficulties with regional anesthesia
Postoperative Complications
Airway obstruction
Hypoxemia and hypercarbia
Deep venous thrombosis → pulmonary embolism (leading cause of perioperative mortality)
Wound infection
Hyperglycemia
Laparoscopic Surgical Implications
Difficult trocar placement
Hypercarbia and increased peak airway pressure
Reduced venous return and cardiac output → hypotension

residual gastric volume and acidity, the possibility of associated diabetic gastroparesis, and increased intra-abdominal pressure. Also, there is a higher incidence of gastroesophageal reflux and hiatal hernia. Therefore, obese patients should be considered to have potentially full stomachs, even with elective surgery. Difficult airway management increases the risk for pulmonary gastric aspiration, especially when high pressures are required for positive-pressure facemask ventilation and oxygenation. In this situation, at least some inspired gas is diverted to the esophagus and stomach. This is compounded by multiple attempts at tracheal intubation, with positive-pressure facemask ventilation between attempts. Thus, the already increased risk for pulmonary aspiration of gastric contents is compounded by difficult airway management and intubation in obese patients.

Glucose intolerance is common in obese patients, and the incidence of diabetes mellitus is higher than in the normal population. This may be due to increased resistance to insulin of peripheral tissues in the presence of excessive adipose tissue. The increased catabolic response to surgery may require the use of exogenous insulin during the perioperative period.

In theory, larger fat stores provide an increased volume of distribution for lipid-soluble drugs (e.g., thiopental, benzodiazepines, opioids). Thus, if the loading dose of these drugs is based on actual body weight in obese patients, maintenance doses would be given less frequently owing to reduced clearance. However, with hydrophilic muscle relaxants, increased fat stores have less influence, and dosing should be based on ideal body weight (for adults, 60 to 80 kg for females, and 80 to 100 kg for males). Hepatic clearance of drugs is usually not affected, unless there is hepatic dysfunction due to fatty infiltration of the liver. Renal clearance of drugs may increase owing to increased renal blood flow and glomerular filtration rate. However, with atherosclerotic renovascular disease, there may be reduced renal clearance due to renal insufficiency. Recovery times from volatile anesthetics are comparable in obese and normal patients with contemporary agents (e.g., desflurane, sevoflurane), provided the procedure is not lengthy (>3 to 4 hours).

MANAGEMENT

After a focused history and physical examination, minimum laboratory investigations should include hemoglobin and hematocrit, serum electrolytes, blood glucose, liver function tests, electrocardiogram, and chest radiograph. Invasive cardiac evaluation, such as dobutamine stress echocardiogram or nuclear stress myocardial imaging, may identify patients with inducible ischemia, wall motion abnormalities, and ventricular contractile dysfunction. Any abnormal findings will direct intraoperative management. Baseline arterial blood gases may be indicated for patients with obstructive sleep apnea.

No single anesthetic technique is superior. All drug doses must be carefully titrated to clinical effect. Neuraxial anesthesia may be beneficial for open lower abdominal procedures, although the identification of anatomic landmarks may be difficult. Especially in the morbidly obese, dosages of local anesthetics for epidural and spinal anesthesia are adjusted downward by up to 20% to 25%. This is because increased intra-abdominal and airway pressures are believed to cause epidural venous engorgement. Also, increased epidural fat reduces the epidural and subarachnoid spaces. Premedication sedatives and narcotics should be administered cautiously or avoided altogether in patients with hypoxemia, hypercapnia, or a history of obstructive sleep apnea owing to the risk for further respiratory depression and airway compromise.

Difficult peripheral venous access may dictate the need for a central line. For indirect blood pressure measurements, a larger-sized cuff is frequently placed on the forearm. However, even when extra-large cuffs are used, systemic pressure measurements may be 20% to 30% above those obtained with an arterial catheter. The latter is often desirable because obese patients are susceptible to large fluctuations in blood pressure. Also, arterial blood gas determinations are often required to assess the adequacy of oxygenation and ventilation. Central venous or pulmonary artery pressure monitoring may be indicated if a patient has evidence of impaired myocardial function. Transesophageal echocardiography may be an alternative to a pulmonary artery catheter, although its use may be limited by the surgical procedure (e.g., the need for an orogastric or nasogastric tube or gastric endoscopy).

Recognition of a potentially difficult airway may suggest the need for awake fiberoptic intubation. Obese patients often have a short, thick neck; an anterior larynx and large tongue; and limited movement of the jaw, neck, and head. However, if the preanesthetic assessment suggests that airway management and tracheal intubation will be relatively easy, a rapid-sequence induction and tracheal intubation may be performed. Preoxygenation is especially important owing to reduced FRC and oxygen reserve and increased oxygen consumption. Desaturation can occur rapidly during apnea. Two-person mask ventilation may be required. Risk for pulmonary gastric aspiration is reduced with the administration of H_2-antagonists, nonparticulate antacids, and metoclopramide.

When positioning the patient, care must be taken to protect and pad all pressure points. Patients weighing between 400 and 1000 pounds require special operating room tables. In extreme cases, it may be necessary to place two tables together for those with an extremely large abdominal pannus or wide girth. During preparation and induction of anesthesia, the obese patient should lie in a semirecumbent position with the head on a pillow and a bolster placed under the shoulders. In many patients, satisfactory oxygenation and ventilation can be achieved only by changing from the supine to the reverse Trendelenburg position.

During mechanical ventilation, positive end-expiratory pressure may be used to improve oxygenation. High inspired oxygen concentrations may be required to prevent hypoxia. Use of a pressure-limited ventilatory mode may be necessary.

Postoperative respiratory complications are a significant problem. The risk of postoperative hypoxemia is increased by surgery involving the thorax or upper abdomen (especially vertical incisions). Extubation should be delayed until the effects of muscle relaxants are completely reversed and the patient is fully awake. Postoperative mechanical ventilation may be required until extubation criteria are met. Patients using continuous positive airway pressure devices at home should have these available postoperatively. Aggressive pulmonary care with incentive spirometry, coughing, deep breathing, and early ambulation is beneficial.

Adequate postoperative analgesia is essential to prevent diaphragmatic splinting; however, opiates must be carefully titrated to avoid respiratory depression. Use of regional techniques such as epidural analgesia may reduce the incidence of respiratory complications.

Finally, the risk of deep venous thrombosis and pulmonary thromboembolism is increased. In fact, it is the leading cause of perioperative mortality in this patient population. This emphasizes the importance of early ambulation for these patients. Low-dose subcutaneous heparin or enoxaparin (Lovenox) and compression stockings or sequential compression devices should be used perioperatively.

PREVENTION

Understanding the pathophysiologic changes of obesity and associated disease processes can help minimize morbidity and mortality. Pertinent history, physical examination, and testing can help identify patients with significant comorbidity and facilitate appropriate risk stratification to minimize the anesthetic risk.

Further Reading

Adams JP, Murphy JP: Obesity in anaesthesia and intensive care. Br J Anaesth 85:91-108, 2000.

Alpert MA, Alexander JK, et al: The Heart and Lung in Obesity. New York, Futura Publishing, 1998.

Alpert MA, Terry BE, Cohen MV, et al: The electrocardiogram in morbid obesity. Am J Cardiol 85:908-910, 2000.

Gajraj NM, Whitten CW: Morbid obesity. In Atlee JL (ed): Complications in Anesthesia. Philadelphia, WB Saunders, 1999, pp 848-850.

Ogummaike BO, Jones SB, Jones DB, et al: Anesthetic considerations for bariatric surgery. Anesth Analg 95:1793-1805, 2002.

Roizen MF, Fleisher LA: Anesthetic implications of concurrent diseases. In Miller RD (ed): Miller's Anesthesia, 6th ed. Philadelphia, Churchill Livingstone, 2005, pp 1017-1149.

OTHER SURGICAL SUBSPECIALTIES

Complications of Carcinoid Tumors

203

Kerri M. Robertson

Case Synopsis

A 55-year-old man is scheduled for emergency exploratory laparotomy for small bowel obstruction. Anesthesia is induced with intravenous (IV) propofol, remifentanil, and vecuronium and maintained with an infusion of remifentanil and sevoflurane in an air-oxygen mixture. During surgery the patient becomes profoundly hypotensive. His blood pressure does not respond to boluses of IV fluid and phenylephrine. The patient's face and neck appear flushed.

PROBLEM ANALYSIS

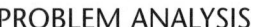

Definition

Carcinoid tumors are neoplasms of neuroendocrine origin and arise from enterochromaffin cells in various embryonic divisions of the gut. The largest case series ($N = 11,842$) reported in 2003 by Soga found that carcinoid tumors were most commonly found in the lung (19.8%), followed by the rectum (15%), ileojejunum (12%), stomach (11.4%), appendix (9.6%), and duodenum (8.3%). The overall incidence of the carcinoid syndrome was 7.7%.

Carcinoid syndrome results from the direct release of vasoactive amines, polypeptides, proteins, and prostaglandins into the systemic circulation (Table 203-1). Intestinal carcinoids produce large amounts of serotonin (5-hydroxytryptamine [5-HT]), but many other products can be released as well, including histamine, norepinephrine, bradykinins, and prostaglandins. Serotonin is metabolized in the liver, lungs, and brain by monoamine oxidases to 5-hydroxyindoleacetic acid (5-HIAA), which is excreted in the urine. However, substances produced by liver metastases from midgut carcinoids or primary hepatic carcinoid tumors (i.e., 5-HT and other biogenic amines, along with proteins and polypeptides) are released directly into the systemic circulation, thereby bypassing the portal circulation. In addition, primary tumors without portal venous drainage (e.g., bronchial, ovarian, retroperitoneal) can cause carcinoid syndrome by circumventing hepatic metabolism.

A life-threatening carcinoid "crisis" is an acute exacerbation of the carcinoid syndrome. It results in profound flushing, hypotension or extreme changes in blood pressure, stupor, diarrhea, confusion, bronchospasm, arrhythmias, and hyperthermia. Such crises can be triggered by tumor palpation, induction of anesthesia and tracheal intubation, inadequate analgesia, surgical stress, drug-induced mediator release, chemotherapy, and hepatic arterial embolization.

Recognition

Features of carcinoid syndrome include the following:

- Episodic cutaneous vasomotor flushing
- Diarrhea or abdominal pain
- Bronchospasm
- Carcinoid valvular heart disease
- Pellagra and psychiatric symptoms

There is significant patient variability with regard to the type and severity of symptoms, depending on the anatomic site of the tumor, its venous drainage, and diverse characteristics of the secreted amine and peptide products. Bradykinin and histamine may play a prominent role in hypotension and cutaneous vasomotor flushing, whereas serotonin release contributes to diarrhea, bronchoconstriction, hypertension, and bowel ischemia. Pellagra and psychiatric symptoms are due to depletion of tryptophan, a precursor for serotonin synthesis.

Carcinoid tumors are diagnosed by measuring the serotonin metabolite 5-HIAA in a 24-hour urine sample. A small bowel radiographic series, upper and lower gastrointestinal endoscopy, abdominal ultrasonography, and contrast-enhanced computed tomography or magnetic resonance imaging may identify a focal primary lesion. Liver metastases are detected by computed tomography or somatostatin scanning and liver biopsy. Diagnosis of a neuroendocrine tumor is confirmed with immunohistochemical markers. Natriuretic peptides (NT-proBNP) can be used as a simple marker for the diagnosis of carcinoid heart disease, which can then be confirmed by echocardiography.

For patients with known carcinoid tumors, carcinoid crisis is suspected if severe intraoperative hypotension occurs that is unusually resistant to IV fluid loading and vasopressors. More rarely, the diagnosis is made by exclusion, but it is a consideration in any case of refractory hypotension.

Table 203-1 ▪ Amines, Proteins, and Prostaglandins Released in the Carcinoid Syndrome
Amines
Dopamine
Histamine
Norepinephrine
Serotonin
Polypeptides and Proteins
Adrenocorticotropic hormone
Bradykinins
Calcitonin
Chromogranins
Corticotropin-releasing hormone
Glucagon
Growth hormone
Insulin
Islet amyloid polypeptide
Kallikrein
Neurokinin A
Neurokinin B
Neuropeptide K
Neurotensin
Pancreatic polypeptide
Peptide YY
Parathyroid hormone-related peptide
Somatostatin
Substance P
Vasoactive intestinal protein
Prostaglandins
PGE_2
PGF_2

Modified from Lips CJ, Lentjes EG, Hoppener JW: The spectrum of carcinoid tumours and carcinoid syndromes. Ann Clin Biochem 40:612-627, 2003.

Risk Assessment

Carcinoid tumors occur relatively frequently but are only rarely symptomatic. They occur in 1 to 2 per 100,000 persons per year in the United States. The distribution is age dependent and rises continuously until the eighth decade. Under age 50 years, more women are affected, with the stomach and lungs more commonly involved. Metastatic disease occurs in 20% of all patients with carcinoid tumors. Estimated 5-year survival for localized disease is 75% to 93%. With metastatic disease, it is 15% to 35%. With cardiac involvement, the prognosis is worse. Right heart failure due to tricuspid and pulmonary valve disease may be fatal. The median survival after diagnosis is 1.6 years.

Implications

Preoperatively, patients are evaluated for electrolyte imbalance and volume depletion due to secretory diarrhea. Carcinoid heart disease occurs in 20% to 70% of patients with metastatic disease. Classically, this includes right-sided endomyocardial fibrosis, pulmonary hypertension, tricuspid and pulmonary stenosis, and then tricuspid regurgitation with ultimate right heart failure. Inactivation of serotonin by the lung protects the left side of the heart, but occasionally it too is affected.

Octreotide acetate (Sandostatin) has simplified the perioperative management of patients with carcinoid tumor and is widely considered the standard treatment for carcinoid symptoms and crises. Octreotide is a synthetic octapeptide somatostatin analogue with an elimination half-life of about 1.5 hours following subcutaneous administration. There is evidence that octreotide may prevent mediator release by binding to the sstr-2 subtype of somatostatin G protein-coupled receptors. Symptoms are relieved in more than 70% of patients, although the average response lasts only 18 months. Insulin release in response to hyperglycemia is inhibited as well, which can complicate glucose management in obese patients or non-insulin-dependent diabetics. Unfortunately, octreotide does not prevent the progression of carcinoid cardiac lesions.

Veall and coworkers reviewed 21 patients undergoing laparotomy for metastatic carcinoid tumors. The use of intraoperative octreotide allowed the completion of hepatic resections that had previously been aborted due to refractory hypotension with tumor manipulation. Kinney and colleagues reviewed 119 patients having similar surgery. None of the 45 patients who received octreotide intraoperatively experienced complications during surgery. In contrast, 8 of 73 patients who did not receive octreotide had cardiac complications.

MANAGEMENT

Anesthetic management of patients with carcinoid tumors requires the following:

- Immediate availability of IV octreotide to treat perioperative carcinoid crises
- Treatment of hypertension, hypotension, and bronchospasm
- Monitoring with an arterial line and central access (with or without a pulmonary artery catheter)

Therapeutic options for patients with carcinoid tumors include (1) somatostatin analogues to reduce hormone secretion, (2) resection of the primary tumor, and (3) excision or ablative therapy for liver metastases (e.g., radiofrequency ablation, cryotherapy, arterial chemoembolization). In selected cases, liver transplantation may be a treatment option. Valve replacement is feasible with carcinoid valvular heart disease but is associated with significant morbidity and mortality. Other therapeutic options include MIBG (*m*-iodobenzylguanidine) preparations, interferon-α, and chemotherapy.

In the event of severe hypotension that is unresponsive to IV fluids, patients with known carcinoid tumors should receive IV octreotide (50-μg bolus) as first-line therapy. In one recent case series, the median dose of octreotide administered intraoperatively was 350 μg. Sympathomimetics are often administered but may actually worsen the episode, because α-adrenergic stimulation can cause further peptide release from the tumor. Octreotide has also been used successfully to treat severe carcinoid-induced bronchospasm, after aerosolized albuterol and isoflurane failed.

Serotonin accentuates the vascular response to catecholamines by stimulating the release and inhibiting the reuptake of norepinephrine. It may also directly stimulate postjunctional α_1-receptors. The resulting hypertension is amenable to standard treatment, such as increasing anesthetic depth or administering agents such as labetalol, nicardipine, or nitroprusside. Ketanserin (2.5- to 5-mg IV bolus with IV infusion at 5 mg/hour) has also been used. It blocks 5-HT, α_1-receptors, and H_1-receptors. Continuous blood pressure monitoring is highly desirable, because blood pressure changes may be abrupt. A central venous catheter should be considered for assessing right heart backpressure if there is the potential for extensive surgical blood loss. This is because the effects of circulating mediators may alter the normal physiologic signs of hypovolemia (i.e., negate any potential systemic arterial hypotension). The possible benefit of a pulmonary artery catheter should be weighed against the risk of its placement in a patient with tricuspid or pulmonary valve disease.

PREVENTION

To avoid complications in patients with carcinoid tumors, take the following measures:

- Block histamine (H_1- and H_2-receptors) and serotonin receptors (octreotide).
- Avoid drugs that facilitate the release of mediators.
- Provide adequate anxiolysis and postoperative pain relief.
- Avoid sympathetic stimulation.

If preoperative control of symptoms with octreotide is successful, patients can be placed on its longer-acting somatostatin analogue lanreotide or Sandostatin LAR. For elective surgery, premedication with subcutaneous octreotide 200 µg daily for 3 days before surgery has been shown to improve the perioperative course of patients with carcinoid tumors. Some advise prophylactic continuous IV somatostatin or octreotide (100 µg/hour) during surgery.

Premedication with benzodiazepines to relieve anxiety is important, as is adequate pain relief postoperatively, especially if surgical debulking leaves residual tumor. Ideally, both histamine release and sympathetic stimulation should be avoided. Etomidate or propofol may be better choices for IV induction, although thiopental-triggered histamine release appears to be of little clinical significance. Morphine has the potential to induce histamine release and hypotension. Remifentanil, sufentanil, and fentanyl are alternatives. Succinylcholine-induced fasciculations could theoretically provoke the release of hormones; however, recent reviews reported no adverse effects. Histamine release is more prominent with tumors of foregut origin. Thus, preoperative H_1- and H_2-receptor blockers and corticosteroids may be useful in patients with gastric or bronchial carcinoids. Ondansetron is the ideal antiemetic agent.

Further Reading

Botero M, Fuchs R, Paulus DA, et al: Carcinoid heart disease: A case report and literature review. J Clin Anesth 14:57-63, 2002.

de Vries H, Verschueren RC, Willemse PH, et al: Diagnostic, surgical and medical aspect of the midgut carcinoids. Cancer Treat Rev 1:11-25, 2002.

Kinney MA, Warner ME, Nagorney DM, et al: Perianaesthetic risks and outcomes of abdominal surgery for metastatic carcinoid tumours. Br J Anaesth 87:447-452, 2001.

Lips CJ, Lentjes EG, Hoppener JW: The spectrum of carcinoid tumours and carcinoid syndromes. Ann Clin Biochem 40:612-627, 2003.

Quaedvlieg PF, Lamers CB, Taal BG: Carcinoid heart disease: An update. Scand J Gastroenterol Suppl 236:66-71, 2002.

Schnirer II, Yao JC, Ajani JA: Carcinoid—a comprehensive review. Acta Oncol 42:672-692, 2003.

Soga J: Carcinoids and their variant endocrinomas: An analysis of 11,842 reported cases. J Exp Clin Cancer Res 4:517-530, 2003.

Veall GR, Peacock JE, Bax ND, et al: Review of the anaesthetic management of 21 patients undergoing laparotomy for carcinoid syndrome. Br J Anaesth 72:335-341, 1994.

Zimmer C, Kienbaum P, Wiesemes R, et al: Somatostatin does not prevent serotonin release and flushing during chemoembolization of carcinoid liver metastases. Anesthesiology 98:1007-1011, 2003.

Complications of Thyroid Surgery

204

Samuel A. Irefin

Case Synopsis

A 25-year-old woman with a known history of Graves' disease presents for subtotal thyroidectomy. A prominent thyroid gland is palpated on physical examination, and she complains of dysphagia. The chest radiograph demonstrates mild displacement of the trachea from the midline.

PROBLEM ANALYSIS

Definition

Thyroid surgery is performed for removal of an enlarged thyroid gland (goiter) in patients with Graves' disease. Graves' disease is the most common cause of hyperthyroidism in the United States, with an estimated annual incidence of 300 cases per 1 million persons. It is an autoimmune disorder characterized by a diffusely enlarged thyroid gland and thyrotoxicosis, caused by thyroid-stimulating immunoglobulins. These immunoglobulins primarily bind to and activate the thyroid-stimulating hormone (TSH) receptors. This results in increased iodine uptake, protein synthesis, growth of the thyroid gland, and synthesis and release of thyroglobulin and thyroid hormones. Complications of thyroid surgery for goiter removal are listed in Table 204-1.

Recognition

HYPERTHYROIDISM (GRAVES' DISEASE) AND THYROTOXICOSIS

Signs and symptoms of hyperthyroidism are listed in Table 204-2. Patients with Graves' disease are at risk for numerous complications related to the disease and its treatment. One such life-threatening complication is thyroid storm.

Signs and symptoms of thyrotoxicosis are listed in Table 204-3. Without treatment, severe thyrotoxicosis results in cardiac complications (thyrotoxic crisis or thyroid storm), cognitive disorders, gastrointestinal disturbances, jaundice,

weight loss, osteoporosis, and myopathy. In the elderly, the only presenting features may be unexplained weight loss, atrial fibrillation, and congestive heart failure.

THYROID STORM

Thyroid storm is an extreme exacerbation of thyrotoxicosis. It is usually stress related due to infection, trauma, surgery, treatment with radioactive iodine, pregnancy, diabetic ketoacidosis, thyroid replacement therapy, and anticholinergic or adrenergic drugs. Even with early recognition and aggressive therapy, the mortality rate is estimated at 20%. Manifestations of thyroid storm are listed in Table 204-4.

The exact pathogenesis of thyroid storm is not fully understood. Thyroid hormones regulate the nuclear transcription of messenger RNA in all cells. Free triiodothyronine (T_3) binds to a DNA domain called the "thyroid response element." Once bound, T_3 initiates the transcription of an array of biochemical enzymes that regulate tissue metabolism. One theory suggests that an acute, rapid increase in free thyroid hormone levels, rather than absolute levels, precipitates thyroid storm. Because thyroid storm most often occurs 6 to 24 hours postoperatively, manipulation of the gland during surgery or an acute reduction in binding proteins postoperatively may account for this surge of free thyroid hormones. Other theories include adrenergic

---

Table 204–1 ■ Complications of Thyroid Surgery for Goiter Removal

Precipitation of thyrotoxic crisis ("thyroid storm")
Hemorrhage → hematoma → airway compression →
   acute respiratory distress
Recurrent laryngeal nerve injury
Superior laryngeal nerve injury
Hypoparathyroidism
Corneal abrasion

Table 204–2 ■ Signs and Symptoms of Hyperthyroidism (Graves' Disease)

Weight loss despite increased appetite
Heat intolerance, sweating
Diarrhea, abdominal pain
Tremors of distal extremities
Increased reflexes
Proximal muscle weakness
Tachyarrhythmias (especially atrial fibrillation)
Widened palpebral fissure
Decreased blinking
Lid lag (ptosis), blurred or double vision
Increased systolic pressure with widened pulse pressure
Anxiety, restlessness
Fatigue
Shortened attention span

Table 204–3 ■ Signs and Symptoms of Thyrotoxicosis

Heat intolerance, profuse sweating
Diarrhea, vomiting, jaundice
Atrial fibrillation, congestive heart failure, unexplained
    weight loss (elderly)
Tachycardia or arrhythmias
Hypertension or hypotension with shock state
Tremors, seizures, confusion, coma
Hyperphagia
Osteoporosis and myopathy
Increased reflexes (hyperreflexia)
Unexplained weight loss despite increased appetite
Fever (consistently >101°F)

receptor activation and a direct sympathomimetic effect of thyroid hormone owing to its structural similarity to catecholamines.

Diagnosis of thyroid storm is based on its clinical presentation, because laboratory testing is nonspecific. Further, waiting for results only delays treatment. Thyroid storm is an acute, life-threatening progression of thyroid hormone-induced hypermetabolic (thyrotoxic) states involving multiple organ systems (see Tables 204-3 and 204-4). The differential diagnosis includes malignant hyperthermia, septic shock, hypertensive encephalopathy, central nervous system infection, acute drug intoxication, and pheochromocytoma.

Respiratory Distress from Hematoma

The incidence of hemorrhage after thyroid surgery is low (0.3% to 1%). Hematoma formation in the neck resulting in respiratory compromise is a potentially fatal complication, however, because small amounts of blood in the deep tissue spaces near the trachea may cause significant airway obstruction. Patients present with swelling and pain at the incision site, an expanding neck mass, and symptoms of respiratory distress, such as stridor and dyspnea.

Recurrent or Superior Laryngeal Nerve Injury

Because of the intimate association of the thyroid gland and the nerves supplying the larynx, damage to either the recurrent laryngeal nerve (RLN) or the superior laryngeal nerve (SLN) may be a complication of thyroid surgery. Nerve injury may result from traction, contusion, or crushing during exposure; inclusion of the nerve in a ligature; inadvertent complete or partial nerve transection; or compromised blood supply. The RLN is a branch of the vagus nerve. It innervates all the intrinsic muscles of the larynx, with the exception of the cricothyroid muscle, which is innervated by the SLN.

Table 204–4 ■ Manifestations of Thyroid Storm after Thyroid Surgery

Hyperthermia (as high as 105°F to 106°F)
Hypertension, tachycardia, arrhythmias
Mental status changes
Cardiovascular collapse ("shock")
Congestive heart failure in patients prone to heart failure

Unilateral RLN injury produces abductor vocal cord paralysis. The affected vocal cord assumes a paramedian position. Patients often present with postoperative hoarseness or a weak, breathy voice, but voice changes may not be apparent for days to weeks. Bilateral vocal cord paralysis is especially a risk after total thyroidectomy. Complete or partial airway obstruction often manifests immediately after extubation. Symptoms include respiratory distress with stridor requiring emergent reintubation or tracheostomy. Occasionally patients complain only of dyspnea or stridor with exertion. The external branch of the SLN innervates the cricothyroid muscle, which tenses and adducts the vocal cords. With injury, laxity of the vocal cord on the side of injury may produce subtle changes in voice quality or fatigue with speech.

Techniques for assessing vocal cord mobility include fiberoptic laryngoscopic visualization during spontaneous ventilation or during extubation. For the latter, the anesthesiologist performs direct laryngoscopy under deep general anesthesia and observes the mobility of the vocal cords as the endotracheal tube is removed. Laryngeal electromyography is a diagnostic tool used as a late prognostic indicator for recovery of vocal cord function.

Hypoparathyroidism

Hypoparathyroidism may complicate thyroid surgery due to inadvertent trauma to or removal of the parathyroid glands or, more frequently, devascularization of the glands during ligation of the blood supply to the thyroid. The parathyroid glands produce parathyroid hormone (PTH), which increases the serum concentration of calcium through the activation of vitamin D, thereby increasing renal absorption of calcium and bone resorption. Inadequate production of PTH results in hypocalcemia. The diagnosis of hypoparathyroidism is made by the measurement of low PTH or decreased serum ionized calcium concentrations. Hypocalcemia usually occurs 24 to 48 hours after surgery but may occur earlier. Tetany, carpopedal spasm, circumoral paresthesias, mental status changes, seizures, cardiac dysfunction, and stridor are manifestations of decreased ionized calcium concentrations. Confirmatory tests include the Chvostek and Trousseau signs and Q-T prolongation on the electrocardiogram. Postoperative hypoparathyroidism must be differentiated from tetany caused by acute hypocalcemia and from respiratory alkalosis associated with anxiety and hyperventilation.

Corneal Abrasion

Corneal abrasion can occur in patients with exophthalmos and is diagnosed postoperatively with corneal fluorescein staining and examination with a cobalt-blue slit lamp. Patients complain of eye pain, tearing, and a foreign body sensation in the eye.

Risk Assessment

Thyroid Storm

Thyroid storm affects only a small percentage of patients with thyrotoxicosis. Most cases of thyroid storm are associated with Graves' disease in childhood. However, patients with hyperthyroidism at the time of surgery are at risk for thyroid storm during the perioperative period.

RESPIRATORY DISTRESS FROM HEMATOMA

Respiratory distress may be secondary to laryngeal edema, laryngospasm, bilateral vocal cord paralysis, tracheomalacia, or hypocalcemia. More commonly, however, it occurs with cervical hematomas that are generally venous in origin. If postoperative bleeding is unrecognized, these hematomas may cause airway obstruction and asphyxiation.

RECURRENT OR SUPERIOR LARYNGEAL NERVE INJURY

RLN injury is uncommon, occurring in 0% to 2.1% of patients during thyroidectomy when the nerve is identified and dissected. When the nerve is not clearly identified, the reported injury rate increases to 4% to 6.6%. Compounding factors include the extent of dissection and resection, especially if performed for malignant disease.

HYPOPARATHYROIDISM

Hypoparathyroidism with hypocalcemia may be transient or permanent. The incidence of parathyroid injury increases with the magnitude of the operation. It is uncommon with subtotal thyroidectomy for Graves' disease. The overall incidence of permanent hypoparathyroidism ranges from 0.4% to 13.8%. The rate of transient hypocalcemia is reportedly 2% to 53%. The cause is not clear but may be attributable to temporary hypoparathyroidism from reversible ischemia to the parathyroid glands, hypothermic injury, or acute suppression of PTH production due to the release of endothelin 1.

CORNEAL ABRASION

The likelihood of corneal injury increases with the degree of ophthalmopathy and exophthalmos.

Implications

Thyroid surgery is associated with a number of potentially serious complications.

THYROID STORM

Thyroid storm is the most severe form of thyrotoxicosis. It often occurs in patients who have not been rendered euthyroid before thyroid surgery. Consultation with an endocrinologist can assist in optimizing the patient's preoperative status with antithyroid drugs, iodide therapy, β-blockers, and glucocorticoids. The chest radiograph may reveal cardiac enlargement or pulmonary edema in patients with congestive heart failure. This should be further evaluated by echocardiography. Therapy for congestive heart failure or rate control for atrial fibrillation may be required. In the perioperative setting, differentiating between thyroid storm and malignant hyperthermia may be difficult.

RESPIRATORY DISTRESS FROM HEMATOMA

Respiratory distress from any cause requires immediate evaluation and treatment. Patients must be followed closely for up to 72 hours postoperatively for evidence of airway compromise. A thin paper tape dressing over the surgical incision allows optimal wound surveillance. Postoperative bleeding can be a devastating and potentially fatal complication of thyroid surgery. Fastidious intraoperative hemostasis is essential. Controversy exists regarding the use of drains to prevent hematoma formation after thyroid surgery.

RECURRENT OR SUPERIOR LARYNGEAL NERVE INJURY

Permanent injury of the RLN on one side causes postoperative hoarseness. Patients are usually able to compensate and have minimal or no airway difficulty. The paralyzed vocal cord atrophies over time, leaving the patient with the potential sequelae of dysphagia, risk of aspiration, and permanent changes in voice quality. Bilateral RLN injury results in unopposed adduction of the cords, as the cricothyroid muscle remains innervated by the SLN. Associated partial or complete airway obstruction requires immediate endotracheal intubation and re-exploration of the neck to identify any reversible cause of nerve injury. If the nerves are found to be intact, use of corticosteroids and a trial extubation several days later are warranted. Permanent bilateral RLN injury necessitates tracheostomy.

HYPOPARATHYROIDISM

Hypocalcemia may be asymptomatic or it may progress to laryngospasm, tetany, and cardiac dysfunction as early as 6 hours after injury to the parathyroids. Calcium levels may continue to decline over the next 24 to 48 hours, and symptomatic patients require close monitoring of ionized calcium levels with calcium and vitamin D replacement. If the patient remains dependent on oral calcium supplementation for longer than 6 months, it is likely that permanent injury of the hypoparathyroid glands has occurred.

CORNEAL ABRASION

Prognosis is excellent, with most minor abrasions healing within 24 to 48 hours. Deep abrasions in the center of the cornea may leave a scar, with the potential for permanent vision loss. Complications include infection, corneal ulceration, and recurrent epithelial erosion. Ocular medications may cause allergic conjunctivitis or glaucoma in susceptible patients.

MANAGEMENT

Hyperthyroidism (Graves' Disease)

Effective treatment for Graves' disease includes medical therapy to alleviate symptoms and render the patient euthyroid, in conjunction with surgery. However, as mentioned earlier, thyroid surgery is associated with potentially serious complications, such as thyroid storm.

Thyroid Storm

Therapy for thyroid storm is both supportive and therapeutic:

- Assess airway, breathing, and circulation (ABCs): (1) ensure oxygenation and provide ventilatory support as needed; (2) restore intravascular volume with intravenous fluids; (3) establish invasive monitoring (e.g., direct arterial blood pressure monitoring, central venous access, urinary catheterization) if necessary; (4) treat tachycardia and atrial fibrillation; (5) anticipate heart failure and volume depletion; and (6) administer intravenous dextrose as needed to meet high metabolic demands.

- Prevent hyperthermia by covering the patient with ice packs or cooling blankets and administering acetaminophen as needed.
- Prevent thyroid hormone synthesis by administering propylthiouracil (PTU) or methimazole.
- Block thyroid hormone secretion by giving intravenous potassium iodide before surgery to reduce gland size in patients with acute thyroid enlargement, especially when goiters are associated with airway compromise. Potassium iodide can also be used to suppress hormone secretion in thyroid storm.
- Reduce peripheral conversion of thyroxine (T_4) to T_3 with glucocorticoids, propranolol, and PTU.
- Relieve hyperadrenergic effects of thyroid hormones with β-blockers as needed.
- Treat adrenal insufficiency with glucocorticoids as required.
- Consult an endocrinologist for more definitive management.
- Monitor patients with thyroid storm in a critical care unit or similar environment.

Antithyroid drugs (e.g., PTU) inhibit iodination and coupling reactions in the thyroid. In addition, they reduce the synthesis of T_3 and T_4 and inhibit the peripheral conversion of T_4 to T_3 by blocking type I deiodinase. Therapy with potassium iodide is important because it inhibits the secretion of thyroid hormone; when given preoperatively, it also reduces both the vascularity and the size of the thyroid gland. During thyroid storm, intravenous potassium iodide is often used. After antithyroid drugs have been started, iodide may also be dissolved in water as a retention enema.

β-Blockers are used to antagonize the cardiovascular manifestations of the hypermetabolic state, such as tachycardia, increased cardiac output, and tachyarrhythmias (often atrial fibrillation). Sustained hypermetabolic states may lead to congestive heart failure and hypotension. Other benefits of β-blockers include relief of many of the symptoms and signs of hyperthyroidism (see Table 204-2) and thyrotoxicosis (see Table 204-3).

Corticosteroids are used to prevent adrenal insufficiency secondary to the hypermetabolic state in thyroid storm. Digoxin may be used to treat congestive heart failure or atrial fibrillation with a rapid ventricular response. Salicylates are not used for hyperthermia; they compete with T_3 and T_4 for binding to thyroid-binding globulin, which may increase the circulating levels of free thyroid hormone. Instead, acetaminophen is prescribed for hyperthermia.

Respiratory Distress from Hematoma

Respiratory distress and impending airway obstruction due to an expanding neck hematoma require immediate (often bedside) neck re-exploration. However, return to the operating room will likely be required for more definitive control of bleeding sites, irrigation, and wound closure. If so, the airway must first be secured. Then the patient is taken to the operating room, with experienced health care providers present for ventilatory support, reintubation, and tracheostomy if needed.

Recurrent or Superior Laryngeal Nerve Injury

Management of RLN injury remains controversial. Most patients with unilateral RLN injury need no definitive intervention and recover from reversible causes within 6 months of surgery. For patients with permanent unilateral RLN injury, surgery can improve voice quality and reduce the risk of aspiration. Surgical options are medialization or reinnervation of the vocal cord. However, if the RLN has been transected, it is debatable whether immediate microvascular anastomosis or grafting at the time of surgery is effective therapy. In contrast, with bilateral RLN injury, the patient usually requires immediate airway control with endotracheal reintubation or tracheotomy.

Hypoparathyroidism

Hypocalcemia due to parathyroid injury is managed with calcium replacement, depending on the severity of hypocalcemia. Symptomatic hypoparathyroidism is promptly treated with 10 mL of 10% solution of calcium gluconate given over 10 minutes. This is followed by a continuous infusion (1 to 2 mg/kg per hour). Infusions are titrated to the patient's symptoms and serum ionized calcium concentrations. When the patient is able to tolerate oral fluids, daily oral calcium carbonate and vitamin D supplementation are started.

Corneal Abrasion

Corneal abrasions are treated with eye rest, narcotic analgesics, and possibly topical antibiotics (see also Chapter 184). Patching or use of a contact lens impregnated with a nonsteroidal anti-inflammatory drug may help reduce the associated pain.

PREVENTION

Thyroid Storm

The most common therapy for Graves' disease is radioactive iodine. This often normalizes thyroid function within 6 to 12 months. However, radioactive iodine itself may precipitate thyroid storm. Iatrogenic hypothyroidism is also a risk. In patients with large or nodular (suggestive of carcinoma) goiters, it is essential that they be clinically and chemically euthyroid before surgery. Preoperative preparation includes antithyroid drug treatment (PTU) for approximately 6 weeks, with or without a β-blocker. Iodine is given by most surgeons for 2 weeks before surgery to reduce thyroid gland vascularity.

Respiratory Distress from Hematoma

Thyroid surgery must be performed in a near-bloodless field to facilitate identification of the parathyroid glands and the RLNs and SLNs in the operative area. The key to limiting bleeding is proper positioning and meticulous surgical hemostasis. The patient's neck is hyperextended, and the head of the operating table is elevated 30 degrees. This provides optimal exposure and reduces cervical venous pressure and bleeding. At the end of the procedure, Valsalva's maneuver is performed with the head lowered to a neutral position. This facilitates the recognition of bleeding vessels. These are then coagulated or ligated. Smooth emergence without coughing or bucking on the endotracheal tube helps prevent early rebleeding.

Recurrent or Superior Laryngeal Nerve Injury

Prevention of RLN or SLN injury also requires meticulous surgical technique. Identification of the entire course of the RLN is advocated by some, but this is controversial. Some authors recommend routine electrical stimulation of the RLN for identification. An electromyographic device for electrophysiologic monitoring of the RLN during surgery is commercially available. However, it is usually reserved for high-risk cases, such as patients with very large neck masses or prior surgery or irradiation.

Hypoparathyroidism

Interruption of the parathyroid blood supply is a common cause of hypoparathyroidism. Therefore, identifying the blood supply and ensuring that it remains intact are important preventive measures. Also, the glands are identified to prevent inadvertent removal. Further, suctioning in the operative field can injure the parathyroid glands. Therefore, it

is recommended that the field be kept dry by careful blotting with sterile gauze rather than use of a suction device. If the parathyroid glands are damaged or inadvertently removed, autotransplantation may prevent hypoparathyroidism.

Corneal Abrasion

Intraoperative eye protection consists of lubrication, padding, taping the eyelids closed, use of protective eyewear, and care during surgical draping and undraping.

Further Reading

Kahky MP, Weber RS: Complications of surgery of the thyroid and parathyroid glands. Surg Clin North Am 73:307-321, 1993.

Lacoste L, Montaz N, Berrit A, et al: Airway complications in thyroid surgery. Ann Otol Rhinol Laryngol 102:441-446, 1993.

Mackin JE, Canary JJ, Pittman CS: Thyroid storm and its management. N Engl J Med 291:1396, 1974.

McGowan FX: Anesthesia for major head and neck surgery. In McGoldrick KE (ed): Anesthesia for Ophthalmic and Otolaryngologic Surgery. Philadelphia, WB Saunders, 1992, pp 75-85.

Wartofsky L: Diseases of the thyroid. In Isselbacher KH, et al (eds): Harrison's Principles of Internal Medicine. New York, McGraw-Hill, 1994, pp 1942-1947.

Woeber K: Thyrotoxicosis and heart. N Engl J Med 327:94, 1992.

Yeung J, Chiu AC: Graves' disease. Endocrinology Web site. http://www.emedicine.com/med/topic929.htm

Complications of Adrenal Surgery

Michael F. M. James

205

Case Synopsis

A 19-year-old man presents in hypertensive crisis with tachycardia, congestive heart failure (CHF), and renal dysfunction. On investigation he is found to have a right adrenal mass. The surgical plan is to investigate the cause of the adrenal mass, stabilize the patient, and proceed to elective excision of the tumor.

PROBLEM ANALYSIS

Definition

Adrenal disease frequently progresses to secondary hypertension and hypertensive crisis. The adrenal gland has two distinct endocrine entities: the cortex and the medulla. The cortex synthesizes glucocorticoids (e.g., cortisol), and the medulla, mineralocorticoids (e.g., aldosterone) and androgens. The medulla synthesizes catecholamines such as dopamine, norepinephrine, and epinephrine. Catecholamine production is dependent on the enzyme phenylalanine-*n*-methyltransferase and the high concentrations of glucocorticoids found in the adrenal cortex.

The most common functioning adrenal cortical tumors are benign adenomas that produce cortisol or, less frequently, aldosterone. Adrenal carcinoma is less common but produces more severe symptoms. Adrenal hyperplasia secondary to excess adrenocorticotropic hormone (ACTH) release from a pituitary microadenoma results in Cushing's disease. Excess cortisol production from adrenal tumors or exogenous ACTH results in Cushing's syndrome. Excess aldosterone production leads to Conn's syndrome, which accounts for 0.5% to 3% of all cases of hypertension. Conn's syndrome is usually due to a single adrenal adenoma, possibly in association with bilateral adrenal hyperplasia.

Tumors that secrete catecholamines arise from neural crest tissue, including the sympathetic chain and, rarely, the cardiac conduction system. Approximately 90% of pheochromocytomas are unilateral adrenal medullary tumors. Bilateral adrenal medullary tumors are usually associated with congenital conditions or are found in children. Extra-adrenal pheochromocytomas seldom produce epinephrine, and these tumors are frequently both multiple and malignant.

Adrenal tumors can secrete both epinephrine and norepinephrine; however, the latter usually predominates. Familial associations include multiple endocrine neoplasia (MEN) type IIA (Sipple's syndrome), defined as medullary thyroid carcinoma, pheochromocytoma, and (inconsistently) parathyroid adenoma. MEN type IIB is similar to type IIA but also includes marfanoid habitus and mucosal neuromas. It was formerly believed that only 5% of pheochromocytomas were inherited; however, recent data suggest that germline mutations may cause up to 25% of cases previously considered sporadic, especially in children and when the tumor is extra-adrenal. Other associations include von Hippel-Lindau syndrome[1] and (rarely) von Recklinghausen's disease (neurofibromatosis).

Recognition

Hypertensive crisis, atypical diabetes, and unexplained cardiomyopathy, especially in young persons, should always raise the suspicion for adrenal disease.

Classic features of pheochromocytoma (e.g., headaches, diaphoresis, palpitations) occur in about 80% of patients, but this history is often elicited only by direct questioning. The presentation of pheochromocytoma is variable (Table 205-1), and it may go undiagnosed for several years. The diagnosis of pheochromocytoma is based on the finding of significant levels of catecholamines and their metabolites in the plasma and urine, supported by radiographic evidence. Isolated vanillylmandelic acid measurements have a sensitivity of only 60%; however, if combined with serial metanephrine measurements, sensitivity and specificity increase to about 90%. High-performance liquid chromatography to measure plasma and urinary catecholamine concentrations has similar sensitivity but higher specificity (95%). Contrast imaging with I^{123}-labeled MIBG (*m*-iodobenzylguanidine) is reserved for extra-adrenal pheochromocytomas or when multiple tumors are suspected. Computed tomography scanning is then used to establish precise tumor localization and definition. Rarely, other tests (e.g., clonidine suppression test) are useful when the diagnosis is still in doubt.

Clinical hallmarks of Cushing's disease are truncal obesity, thin skin, easy bruising, abdominal striae, hypertension, and hyperglycemia (Table 205-2). Cushing's syndrome is usually clinically obvious and is confirmed by high

---

[1]Von Hippel-Lindau syndrome, or retinocerebral angiomatosis (a type of phakomatosis), consists of retinal hemangiomas (multiple or bilateral) in association with hemangiomas or hemangioblastomas that involve primarily the cerebellum, the walls of the fourth ventricle, and occasionally the spinal cord. The disease has autosomal dominant inheritance and may be associated with renal cysts or hamartomas. These may affect the adrenals or other organs.

Table 205–1 ■ **Symptoms and Other Findings in Patients with Pheochromocytoma**

Organ System	Symptoms and Other Findings
Integumentary	Excessive sweating, cold extremities
Musculoskeletal	Muscle tremors
Cardiovascular	Left atrial and ventricular hypertrophy; electrocardiogram abnormalities; cardiomyopathy; episodic (60%) or sustained (35%) hypertension; hypotension (5%); palpitations; peripheral vascular disease with tissue loss
Metabolic	Reduced glucose tolerance; diabetes mellitus; diabetic coma; weight loss
Gastrointestinal	Nonspecific abdominal pain and nausea; occasionally presents as apparent acute abdomen
Central nervous	Headache; anxiety attacks; stroke

concentrations of serum cortisol. Identification of Cushing's disease requires the dexamethasone suppression test and the corticotropin-releasing hormone test. The former causes ACTH to fall to very low concentrations in the absence of an ACTH-producing tumor. The latter should cause a marked increase in ACTH release with primary pituitary disease, but not in patients with adrenal tumors or ectopic ACTH production.

Primary aldosteronism presents as severe hypertension, muscle weakness, polyuria, and thirst. Renal dysfunction secondary to hypertension and hypokalemia is common. High plasma sodium concentrations, hypokalemia, and metabolic alkalosis suggest Conn's syndrome. This is confirmed by high serum aldosterone and low plasma renin concentrations.

Risk Assessment

Adrenalectomy is a relatively high-risk procedure, mainly due to endocrine pathophysiology and target end-organ damage. Morbidity with simple adrenalectomy can be as high as 40%, with mortality between 2% and 4%. Perioperative mortality is higher (5% to 10%) for bilateral adrenalectomy in patients with Cushing's disease. Further, such surgery mandates mineralocorticoid and glucocorticoid replacement therapy for the patient's lifetime.

Each individual pathology has associated risk factors. For adrenal tumors, hypertension with end-organ damage (especially involving the heart, brain, or kidneys) must be considered. With Cushing's syndrome, osteoporosis increases the risk of skeletal injury during surgery, and

immunosuppression increases the infectious risk. Furthermore, long-standing disease may result in difficult airway management and tracheal intubation. Pheochromocytoma carries the added risks of catecholamine-induced cardiomyopathy and tachyarrhythmias. Also, there may be associated cardiomyopathy and CHF (Fig. 205-1). Hyperaldosteronism increases the risk for renal dysfunction, muscle weakness, and cardiomyopathy, mainly due to chronic potassium wasting. Patients may present for anesthesia and surgery with severe intracellular potassium deficits, despite apparently adequate plasma concentrations after potassium replacement therapy.

Implications

Adrenal surgery carries the risk for damage to anatomically proximate structures, including the spleen, pancreas, diaphragm (pneumothorax), and vasculature (e.g., inferior vena cava, renal and portal veins, splenic vessels). Hemorrhagic risk is even greater with pheochromocytomas, because they are often quite vascular. For unilateral tumors, a posterior surgical approach may be preferable, with less blood loss and morbidity. However, when bilateral or extra-adrenal tumors are suspected, the anterior approach is preferred, even though this approach increases the risk for inadvertent injury to adjacent organs. Also, access to the venous tumor drainage is more readily obtained early during the procedure.

Laparoscopic adrenalectomy has become more popular in recent years and appears to reduce the morbidity associated

Table 205–2 ■ **Systemic Manifestations of Cortisol Excess Due to Cushing's Disease**

Organ System	Systemic Manifestations
Integumentary	Purple striae on abdomen, buttocks, and thighs; easy bruising; hirsutism; acne
Musculoskeletal	Proximal myopathy and weakness; osteoporosis; vertebral collapse
Cardiovascular	Left ventricular hypertrophy; electrocardiogram abnormalities; hypertension (85%)
Gastrointestinal	Esophageal reflux
Respiratory	Sleep apnea (32%)
Reproductive	Women: virilization secondary to hypersecretion of adrenal androgens; loss of libido; oligomenorrhea Men: impotence
Metabolic	Reduced glucose tolerance; diabetes mellitus (60%); altered fat metabolism and body distribution ("moon" face, central obesity, "buffalo hump"); increased mineralocorticoid activity—hyponatremia, hypokalemia, metabolic alkalosis
Central nervous	Psychiatric symptoms: depression; agitated psychosis (60%-70% of patients)

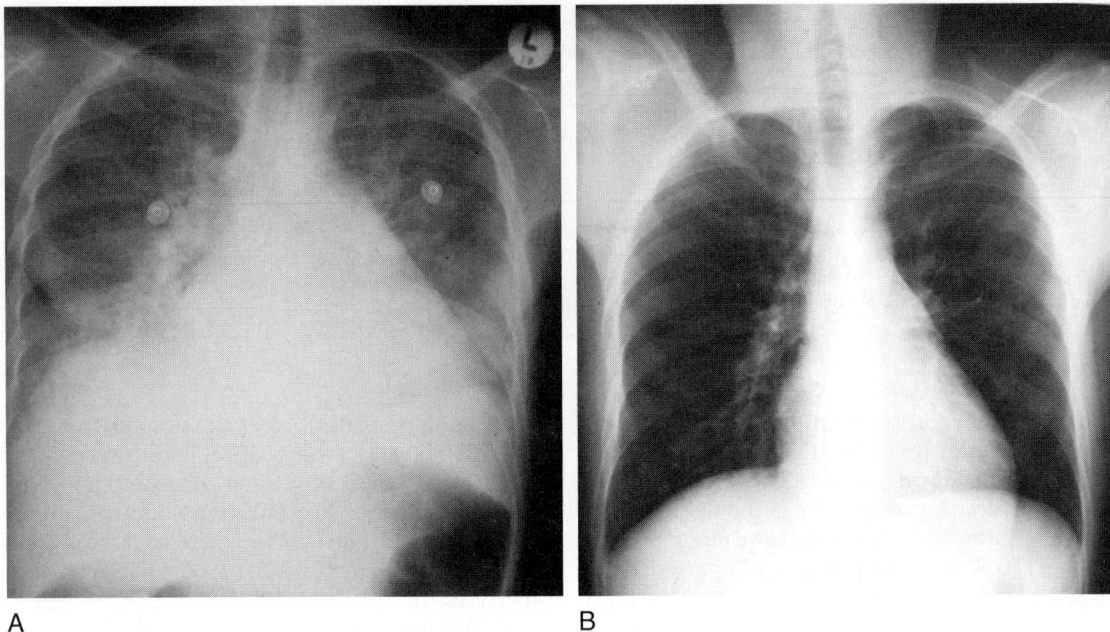

A   B

Figure 205–1 ■ *A*, Chest radiograph of a patient presenting with hypertensive crisis, congestive heart failure, and catecholamine-induced cardiomyopathy. Note mitralization of the left heart border, pulmonary edema, elevated left main bronchus, and cardiac enlargement. *B*, Same patient 6 months after excision of pheochromocytoma. The cardiac silhouette has returned to normal.

with simple adrenalectomy. However, establishment of pneumoperitoneum with carbon dioxide insufflation and increased tumor manipulation may substantially increase catecholamine release from a pheochromocytoma and worsen any hemodynamic instability.

The safe performance of adrenalectomy, particularly for pheochromocytoma, depends on skilled surgical and anesthetic management and requires excellent communication between the surgeons and anesthesiologist. The laparoscopic approach for pheochromocytoma resection is not advised unless the surgical-anesthesia team is knowledgeable about and experienced with the technique.

MANAGEMENT

Preoperative Management of Hypertensive Crisis

Hypertensive crises may be urgencies or emergencies (see Chapter 77). Both require a blood pressure of 160/90 mm Hg or higher. With hypertensive urgencies, there is no evidence of end-organ damage (e.g., renal failure of CHF, myocardial or cerebral ischemia). Also, therapy is less urgent, usually consisting of oral rather than intravenous (IV) drugs. During anesthesia and surgery and in postanesthesia and intensive care units, however, initial therapy is often with IV drugs.

With hypertensive emergencies, blood pressure is 160/90 mm Hg or higher, and there is evidence of end-organ damage (see earlier). Also, acute CHF (as in the case synopsis), arrhythmias (e.g., acute atrial fibrillation, ventricular arrhythmias), aneurysm rupture with intracranial hemorrhage (i.e., hemorrhagic stroke), and aortic dissection are also manifestations of end-organ damage. Hypertensive emergencies require immediate IV therapy with antihypertensive agents.

With pheochromocytoma, hypertensive crises are usually emergencies. Thus, IV drugs are the mainstay of treatment. Sodium nitroprusside (SNP) has been the most commonly used agent, but there are now recognized limitations to its use:

- Because patients with chronic hypertension are preload restricted, and because SNP is a potent arterial and venous dilator, especially in the venous capacitance beds, there is high potential for untoward hypotension during treatment with SNP.
- Untoward hypotension caused by SNP may necessitate the use of vasopressors, but those that act indirectly (e.g., ephedrine) may worsen hypertension in patients with pheochromocytoma.
- The use of SNP for blood pressure management in perioperative settings can be challenging owing to the high potential for increased blood pressure lability. Direct arterial monitoring is advised.

Because of the disadvantages of SNP, clinicians have turned to dihydropyridine (DHP) calcium channel blockers, especially for the management of hypertensive emergencies. DHP calcium channel blockers are arterioselective vasodilators; they have little or no effect on the cardiac calcium channels (sinoatrial node, atrioventricular node, contractility). The only IV calcium channel blocker available at present is nicardipine (Cardene IV), but at least one other is on the horizon. Oral dihydropyridines (e.g., nimodipine, amlodipine) are used for long-term blood pressure control. Nicardipine is compatible with IV β-blockers (e.g., esmolol), and the two can be used together as continuous IV infusions.

Magnesium sulfate (MgSO₄) may be effective if SNP does not adequately reduce and control arterial blood pressure. As noted earlier, intravascular volume may be severely depleted, and fluid therapy may be needed if both CHF and reduced intravascular volume coexist. If so, diuretics are inappropriate and β-blockers are contraindicated, regardless of heart rate, until systemic vascular resistance is reduced and the patient is out of CHF.[2] Even then, β-blockers are used mainly for myocardial ischemia.

Preoperative assessment requires special attention to the underlying pathophysiology. Hypertension and hyperglycemia must be controlled, and fluid and electrolyte disturbances corrected. The electrocardiogram may reveal left atrial and ventricular hypertrophy, arrhythmias, ischemia, or infarction, and the chest radiography may show CHF. Echocardiography is useful with suspected cardiomyopathy. Potassium deficits may be particularly severe in hyperaldosteronism and should be carefully corrected.

Preoperative Medical Management

Patients with Cushing's or Conn's syndrome are managed with conventional antihypertensive drugs, although spironolactone may be included to correct fluid overload and hypokalemia in primary aldosteronism. In pheochromocytoma, α-blockade is the cornerstone of therapy. It helps prevent paroxysmal hypertension, lowers intravascular volume, and reduces left ventricular strain. Phenoxybenzamine, a long-acting, noncompetitive, nonspecific α-antagonist, is the most widely used oral α-blocker. The initial dose (10 mg) is increased every 1 to 2 days until the blood pressure is controlled. Most patients require 60 to 250 mg/day. Preparation periods vary from 5 to 14 days, and no benefit has been shown with longer treatment. Adequate α-receptor blockade is indicated by good control of arterial pressure with orthostatic hypotension, nasal congestion, increased sweating, and warm extremities. Electrocardiogram abnormalities seldom revert to normal during preoperative preparation, and unless there is evidence of frank myocardial ischemia, there is no contraindication to surgery. Doxazosin, a long-acting selective α₁-blocker, has also been used in doses ranging from 4 to 16 mg daily. Tachycardia normally responds to fluid loading, and β-blockade should not be used until vasodilatation has been achieved. Other drugs (e.g., α-methyl-tyrosine, calcium channel blockers, angiotensin-converting enzyme inhibitors) are used, but not widely so.

Preanesthetic Considerations and Monitoring

If phenoxybenzamine has been used, it is omitted on the morning of surgery owing to its very long half-life. β-Blockade should also be withdrawn, so that the patient is not blocked at the time of tumor excision. Mild sedation with a benzodiazepine is usually adequate.

Adrenal surgery increases the risk of hemorrhage, so good IV access is necessary. In addition to standard monitoring, hemodynamic and fluid balance must be monitored with at least an intra-arterial catheter, central venous pressure line, and urinary catheter. A pulmonary artery catheter is seldom helpful. Transesophageal echocardiography is useful, especially in those with cardiomyopathy (with or without CHF), because it allows the assessment of left ventricular contractility and filling.

H₂-receptor antagonists may be considered in cushingoid patients with reflux esophagitis. Pulmonary artery catheters have been advised but are not mandatory for surgery involving the adrenal cortex. Transesophageal echocardiography is better, because fluid balance problems may prove difficult.

Anesthetic Management

Theoretically, drugs that release histamine (e.g., morphine, atracurium) should be avoided in patients with pheochromocytoma, as should those that cause tachycardia or stimulate the sympathetic nervous system (e.g., ketamine, atropine, droperidol, pancuronium). Succinylcholine-induced fasciculations may trigger the release of catecholamines in patients with pheochromocytoma, so this drug is seldom indicated. Among the volatile anesthetics, isoflurane and sevoflurane are theoretically preferable to halothane (which sensitizes myocardium to catecholamines) and desflurane (which increases heart rate). SNP has a rapid onset and short duration of action and has been widely used. Nitroglycerin has also been used successfully, but nicardipine may be better (see earlier). IV bolus phentolamine has too slow an onset-offset to be of use. IV bolus MgSO₄ (2-g intermittent boluses) or infusion (2 to 3 g/hour) provides excellent hemodynamic control, inhibits catecholamine release (especially with laryngoscopy), and is an excellent antiarrhythmic.

In patients with Cushing's syndrome, peripheral vascular access may be difficult. Care must be taken when using adhesive tape owing to their very friable skin. Rapid-sequence induction with succinylcholine may be appropriate in those with reflux esophagitis. Care must also be taken with patient positioning, because osteoporosis increases the risk for fractures. Meticulous antisepsis and prophylactic antibiotics are necessary, because these patients have decreased resistance to infection.

Tumor Removal

Pheochromocytomas are very vascular, and it is often difficult to ascertain when complete venous ligation has been attained. Therefore, tumor removal is the only guarantee that further catecholamine surges will not occur. Significant hypotension may occur, and immediate withdrawal of hypotensive agents, together with aggressive intravascular volume expansion (preferably with colloids), should be instituted. If MgSO₄ has been used, calcium chloride 1 to 2 g by rapid IV injection may be useful to correct hypotension. Persistent hypotension may require the use of vasopressors (e.g., phenylephrine, norepinephrine) or epinephrine for short periods, but hemodynamic stability should be achieved

---

[2]This strongly argues for a selective arterial vasodilator, because CHF is "forward failure" due to increased left ventricular work rather than simple volume overload. The heart still requires adequate preload. A venodilator can always be added if needed.

without vasoactive agents before completion of the surgery. Because these patients have substantial sympathetic paresis, arterial pressure is much more dependent on blood viscosity. A hematocrit of at least 30% should be maintained.

In contrast, adrenalectomy for cortisol or aldosterone excess is not associated with such dramatic hemodynamic changes. Fluid balance, however, is critical, and patients having bilateral adrenalectomy require intraoperative mineralocorticoid and glucocorticoid support.

Electrolyte disturbances with any of these tumors may increase the patient's sensitivity to neuromuscular blocking drugs. Care should be taken to ensure complete reversal of neuromuscular blockade at the end of surgery. Postoperative ventilatory support is seldom required, however, unless there are other conditions that necessitate it.

Glucose Management

Patients with Cushing's syndrome (less so those with pheochromocytoma) may have some degree of hyperglycemia and glucosuria both preoperatively and intraoperatively. After tumor excision, hypoglycemia may occur. Blood glucose is monitored hourly for 24 hours postoperatively.

Postoperative Management

Postoperative pain and discomfort are managed as usual. The use of epidural analgesia is a matter of personal choice. Catecholamine concentrations return to normal over several days, and about 75% of patients are normotensive within 10 days. Although hypertension may persist for several days after tumor removal, this does not necessarily imply residual tumor. Postoperative hypotension is rare with preoperative α-blockade and adequate volume expansion. If hypotension does occur, occult hemorrhage must be considered. Bilateral adrenalectomy necessitates postoperative steroid replacement with glucocorticoids and mineralocorticoids. However, even with unilateral tumor excision, transient steroid deficiency may occur. Thus, use of additional steroids in the early postoperative period is advised.

Unless the tumor is malignant, the long-term prognosis after adrenalectomy is good. More than 80% of patients return to normal health. Even with catecholamine-induced cardiomyopathy, the prognosis is excellent. This is one of the few forms of cardiomyopathy in which full recovery is the norm (see Fig. 205-1).

PREVENTION

Prevention of complications during adrenal surgery is based on a careful preoperative patient assessment, followed by control of hypertension, restoration of intravascular volume, and correction of hyperglycemia and coexisting electrolyte abnormalities. The anesthesiologist should be prepared for significant blood loss and have a high index of suspicion for pneumothorax. Drugs should be readily available for the prompt treatment of both hypotension and hypertension.

Further Reading

Atlee JL, Dhamee MS, Olund TL, et al: The use of esmolol, nicardipine or their combination to blunt hemodynamic changes after laryngoscopy and tracheal intubation. Anesth Analg 90:280-285, 2000.

Bravo EL: Pheochromocytoma: An approach to anithypertensive management. Ann N Y Acad Sci 970:1-10, 2002.

Brunt LM, Moley JF, Doherty GM, et al: Outcomes analysis in patients undergoing laparoscopic adrenalectomy for hormonally active adrenal tumors. Surgery 130:629-634, 2001.

Connery LE, Coursin DB: Assessment and therapy of selected endocrine disorders. Anesthesiol Clin North Am 22:93-123, 2004.

James MF, Cronje L: Pheochromocytoma crisis: The use of magnesium sulfate. Anesth Analg 99:680-686, 2004.

Kinney MA, Warner ME, vanHeerden JA, et al: Perianesthetic risks and outcomes of pheochromocytoma and paraganglioma resection. Anesth Analg 91:1118-1123, 2000.

Lenders JW, Pacak K, Eisenhofer G: New advances in the biochemical diagnosis of pheochromocytoma: Moving beyond catecholamines. Ann N Y Acad Sci 970:29-40, 2002.

Neumann HP, Bausch B, McWhinney SR, et al: Germ-line mutations in nonsyndromic pheochromocytoma. N Engl J Med 346:1459-1466, 2002.

Prys-Roberts C, Farndon JR: Efficacy and safety of doxazosin for perioperative management of patients with pheochromocytoma. World J Surg 26:1037-1042, 2002.

Complications of Trauma Surgery

206

Maged Argalious

Case Synopsis

A 23-year-old man arrives in the emergency department with a gunshot wound to the right upper quadrant of the abdomen. He is combative and confused. His vital signs include systolic blood pressure, 70 mm Hg; heart rate, 119 beats per minute; and respiratory rate, 22 breaths per minute.

PROBLEM ANALYSIS

Definition

Trauma-related injury (TRI) is the leading cause of death in the United States for persons between the ages of 1 and 45 years and is the third leading cause of death overall. Because TRI affects primarily the young, it is the leading cause of years of life lost before age 75 years. The World Health Organization (WHO) estimates that TRI is the leading cause of mortality globally for both men and women between 5 and 45 years of age. Also, WHO estimates that by 2020, TRI will be the leading cause of death in all age groups.

TRI victims present unique challenges to the health care delivery system. They often have multiple injuries to multiple organ systems that necessitate resource-intensive care. Further, TRI can adversely interact with many chronic underlying medical conditions.

Many trauma injuries are preventable. Drugs and alcohol are responsible for nearly 40% of fatal motor vehicle accidents and close to 50% of gunshot wounds. Trauma is classified as either intentional (e.g., homicide) or accidental, as well as according to the mechanism of injury (e.g., penetrating versus blunt). Owing to improvements in trauma care, there has been a decline in trauma-related deaths in recent years.

Recognition

Evaluation of acute trauma victims has three key components: rapid overview, primary survey, and secondary survey. Resuscitation can be initiated at any time during this triage. Rapid overview takes only a few seconds and is used to determine whether the patient is stable, unstable, or dead. The primary survey involves the rapid evaluation of functions that are critical to survival. The ABCs of airway patency, breathing, and circulation are assessed, followed by a brief neurologic examination. Priority is given to cervical spine injury or impending cerebral herniation. The secondary survey entails a systematic, comprehensive evaluation of each anatomic region and usually detects injuries that were overlooked initially. Three quarters of such previously undetected injuries are orthopedic. Based on the results of the secondary survey, patients are rushed immediately to the operating room for surgery, transferred to the radiology suite for further diagnostic studies, or reexamined and observed in an intensive care unit.

Knowledge of the patterns of injury associated with different mechanisms of trauma (i.e., clusters of injury) can help anticipate and identify injuries early. The presence of the worst possible injuries should be assumed until the diagnoses are either confirmed or excluded. Many trauma-related complications are diagnosed intraoperatively (Table 206-1).

Blunt trauma causes localized or widespread transfer of energy to the body. Depending on the site of impact and the amount of energy, this can cause visceral rupture or tissue disruption, including multiple fractures. Penetrating trauma is commonly limited to the track along which a bullet or sharp object has traveled.

Risk Assessment

Triage scoring systems are based on the physical examination and physiologic or mechanism-of-injury parameters. They have traditionally been used to determine patterns of patient referral to trauma centers. Survival is the major outcome variable. The revised trauma score (RTS) is a prospective scoring system that exists in two forms: one is designed for use as a triage tool, and the other is used to evaluate in-hospital patient outcomes. The RTS accurately predicts mortality following traumatic injury, but there is a lack of definitive evidence supporting its use as a primary triage tool in the field or as a predictor of functional outcome and quality of life. To determine the RTS, the Glasgow Coma Scale (GCS) score, systolic blood pressure, and respiratory rate are assigned coded values from 4 (normal) to 0. These are then added and weighted (Table 206-2). When summed, values can range from 0 to 7.84. Higher values indicate a better prognosis. Of the many trauma scoring systems, the RTS is the most popular worldwide.

It has been shown that hyperglycemia independently predicts longer intensive care unit and hospital stay and higher mortality in trauma patients. It is also associated with infectious morbidity. These associations hold true for mild and moderate hyperglycemia (glucose concentration >135 mg/dL and >200 mg/dL, respectively).

Traumatic injuries and subsequent intraoperative complications depend on patterns of injury. Factors that affect these include age, gender, impact resistance and fixation of

Table 206–1 ■ Injuries and Potential Perioperative Complications in Trauma Victims

Central Nervous System
Cervical spine instability or injury and possible spinal cord injury
Closed head injury with increased intracranial pressure
Possible brainstem herniation due to increased intracranial pressure
Brain herniation through open skull fracture

Chest and Pulmonary
Endobronchial intubation
Tension pneumothorax or hemothorax
Pneumomediastinum
Rib fracture and possible flail chest
Pulmonary contusion
Bronchopleural fistula
Aspiration pneumonitis
Bronchospasm
Tracheobronchial plugging
Fat embolism with long bone (e.g., femur) fracture

Cardiovascular
Myocardial contusion or cardiac rupture
Pericardial tamponade or pneumopericardium
Aortic dissection or disruption
Disruption of pulmonary vasculature or vena cava
Hypotension: hypovolemic or neurogenic
Hypovolemic circulatory shock
Air embolism

Abdomen
Disruption or laceration of hollow viscera
Hepatic laceration
Splenic rupture

Coagulation
Coagulopathy, especially with massive blood transfusion
Disseminated intravascular coagulopathy
Primary fibrinolysis
Hemolytic transfusion reaction

Electrolyte or Other Imbalance
Hypocalcemia secondary to citrate toxicity
Hyperkalemia, hypomagnesemia
Acid-base imbalance

intoxicated patients, and those with neurologic signs or symptoms. Cervical spine injury is uncommon with penetrating trauma that is remote from the neck. Spine films that visualize all seven cervical and the first thoracic vertebrae in the lateral, anteroposterior, and odontoid views are required before clearing the cervical spine. Even with normal cervical radiographs, the possibility of ligamentous injury can be ruled out only by computed tomography scanning.

Recognition of a potentially difficult airway, whether due to anatomic predisposition or the actual trauma, is one of the most important roles of the anesthesiologist. Intubation in a patient with an unstable cervical spine involves the potential for irreversible spinal cord injury.

The risk for pulmonary aspiration of the gastric contents is high in trauma victims. Gastric emptying virtually stops at the time of injury, and protective airway reflexes are impaired in obtunded or comatose victims. The greatest risk for aspiration in conscious patients occurs between the induction of anesthesia and endotracheal intubation. The mortality rate with pulmonary aspiration is 5%.

Fracture of the first or second ribs, flail chest, a widened mediastinum, massive hemothorax, and scapula fractures often correlate with pulmonary or vascular injury. In blunt trauma, rib fractures are the most common injury; hemothorax or pneumothorax is more common with penetrating injuries.

Resuscitation frequently requires massive transfusion of blood and blood components, as well as volume replacement with crystalloids and colloids. For massive uncontrolled traumatic hemorrhage, the priority is for immediate blood, blood component, and volume resuscitation, followed by definitive surgical control of hemorrhage from major vessels. However, transfusion and achieving hemostasis with blood component therapy entail significant risks. Normal saline has been associated with hyperchloremic metabolic acidosis, and the use of large volumes of hetastarch solution has been implicated in coagulopathy and renal insufficiency.

Implications

The risk of cervical spine injury and aspiration determines the method used to secure the airway. If time permits, aspiration prophylaxis includes metoclopramide, an H_2-antagonist, and sodium citrate to facilitate gastric emptying and reduce gastric pH. Most patients arrive in the operating room wearing

body parts, anatomic protection of organs, and mechanism of injury.

Patients at risk for cervical spine injury include conscious patients with neck pain or severe pain with distraction, 20% of unconscious patients with injuries above the clavicle,

Table 206–2 ■ Revised Trauma Scoring System

Glasgow Coma Scale Score	Systolic Blood Pressure (mm Hg)	Respiratory Rate (breaths/min)	Coded Value
13-15	>89	10-29	4
9-12	76-89	>29	3
6-8	50-75	6-9	2
4-5	1-49	1-5	1
3	0	0	0

Revised trauma score = $0.9368(GSC_c) + 0.7326(SBP_c) + 0.2908(RR_c)$, where GCS is Glasgow Coma Scale score, SBP is systolic blood pressure, RR is respiratory rate, and the subscript c denotes the coded value for the indicted parameter.

Adapted from Champion HR, Copes WS, Sacco WJ, et al: Improved predictions from a severity characterization of trauma (ASCOT) over Trauma and Injury Severity Score (TRISS): Results of an independent evaluation. J Trauma 40:42-48, 1996.

a cervical spine collar because cervical spine injury has not been ruled out. Options for securing the airway include fiberoptic-assisted or blind nasal or oral endotracheal intubation after topical oropharyngeal anesthesia in spontaneously breathing patients. Intravenous (IV) sedation may be used, unless contraindicated. Alternatively, the patient is intubated after IV rapid-sequence induction of anesthesia. Before induction, the front portion of the cervical spine collar must be removed, and the cervical spine is stabilized with manual in-line traction. Then the patient is preoxygenated, with cricoid pressure applied during rapid-sequence induction and direct laryngoscopy for tracheal intubation with a cuffed endotracheal tube. Once the endotracheal tube cuff is inflated and adequate ventilation and oxygenation are confirmed, the anterior portion of cervical spine collar can be reattached.

Placement of sufficient IV access above the diaphragm is crucial. A rapid IV infusion device allows rapid intravascular volume repletion with warmed IV fluids, blood, and blood products. The patient's volume status, hemodynamic stability, and presence of pulmonary complications (e.g., pneumothorax) determine which agents can be used for the induction and maintenance of general anesthesia. Central venous and direct arterial pressure monitoring are established after the airway is secured.

Once the arterial line is secured, an arterial blood sample is withdrawn and sent to determine the patient's oxygenation (Po_2), ventilation (Pco_2), pH, and hematocrit. Without prompt correction, hypovolemia and acidosis can lead to irreversible shock and death. Massive transfusion of blood and blood products may complicate trauma surgery. Complications include excessive or inadequate blood product replacement, dilutional coagulopathies, hypocalcemia from citrate toxicity, hypothermia, acid-base and electrolyte disturbances, and sepsis leading to multiorgan system failure.

In patients with documented cervical spine or lower spinal cord injury, high-dose IV bolus methylprednisolone (30 mg/kg) within 8 hours of injury, followed by an infusion (5.4 mg/kg per hour) for 24 hours, may improve neurologic recovery.

MANAGEMENT

Airway

Airway management must take into account the presence of cervical spine injury, full stomach, lack of patient cooperation, and anticipated difficult intubation. Use of blind nasal or direct laryngoscopy-assisted oral endotracheal intubation in a conscious patient requires topical anesthesia and possibly light IV sedation. Fiberoptic laryngoscopic or bronchoscopic techniques with topical anesthesia can also be used in awake or sedated patients, or the airway may be secured after IV rapid-sequence induction of general anesthesia.

Table 206-3 lists common indications for endotracheal intubation in trauma patients. Indications for a surgical airway include failed intubation, an apneic patient with suspected cervical spine injury, facial trauma with suspected cervical spine injury, and severe facial and laryngeal trauma with altered anatomy.

Table 206–3 ▪ Indications for Endotracheal Intubation in Trauma-Related Injury
Cardiac or respiratory arrest
Airway obstruction or respiratory insufficiency
Airway protection (e.g., head injury and Glasgow Coma Scale score <9)
Need for deep sedation or analgesia up to and including general anesthesia
Postresuscitation hypoxia or hypoventilation
Delivery of 100% O_2 in victims of carbon monoxide poisoning
Facilitation of diagnostic workup in uncooperative or intoxicated patient

Adapted from Dutton RP, McCunn M: Anesthesia for trauma. In Miller RD (ed): *Miller's Anesthesia,* 6th ed. Philadelphia, Churchill Livingstone, 2005, pp 2157-2172.

Maintaining cricoid pressure during rapid-sequence induction of anesthesia until the cuffed endotracheal tube is properly positioned prevents gastric aspiration or insufflation of the stomach with gas. Also, neck stabilization techniques may impair the laryngeal view, thereby increasing the potential for difficult intubation. The algorithm developed by the American Society of Anesthesiologists Task Force on Difficult Airway Management is applicable in the case of trauma (see Chapters 40 and 42). Devices such as the laryngeal mask airway can be used temporarily as a bridge for establishing airway patency while securing a surgical airway or to facilitate fiberoptic intubation.

Surgical options include cricothyrotomy, transtracheal jet ventilation, and tracheostomy. Cricothyrotomy takes less time to perform than tracheostomy and is therefore the preferred surgical approach. Because tracheostomy requires neck extension, it may exacerbate cervical spine injury. Tracheostomy is indicated in laryngeal trauma and with complete tracheal transection.

Breathing

Management of ventilation requires attention to oxygen saturation, end-tidal carbon dioxide concentration, and peak inspiratory pressures. If gastric aspiration occurs, treatment includes increasing the inspired oxygen concentration, adding positive end-expiratory pressure, and bronchoscopy with saline lavage for airway plugging. A pressure-limited ventilatory mode can reduce the risk of barotrauma. The treatment for pneumothorax is immediate needle decompression at the second intercostal space in the midclavicular line, followed by thoracostomy tube placement.

Circulation

Shock in trauma is due to hypovolemia until proved otherwise. Other causes, such as obstructive shock (due to tension pneumothorax) or neurogenic shock (due to spinal cord transection or spinal vasoparesis), must be excluded. Hemodynamic stabilization requires surgical bleeding control, restoration of circulating blood volume, correction of acidosis, and adequate oxygen transport (hematocrit). Vasopressors may be used to maintain blood pressure during volume restoration.

Crystalloid replacement may be sufficient with blood loss less than 30% of the total blood volume, but at that point, colloids are usually added. The need for blood products is based on estimated blood loss, vital signs, evidence of active bleeding, and serial hematocrit measurements. The trigger for blood transfusion has been lowered, so that hematocrits in the low to mid-20s are now acceptable.

It is rarely necessary to give type O, Rh-positive blood (Rh-negative blood for women of childbearing age), because type-specific blood should be available within 15 minutes. Typed and crossmatched blood (requiring 30 to 45 minutes) is used when available. The concept of delayed blood or blood product resuscitation ("permissible hypovolemia") until surgical bleeding is controlled is not a widely accepted practice.

Hypothermia

Trauma victims are often hypothermic on arrival in the operating room. Warmed IV fluids and blood products, humidified inspired gases and low fresh gas flows, and forced air warming blankets help keep core temperature at 35.5°C or higher. Hypothermia reduces cardiac output and drug metabolism and attenuates immune responses. Hypothermia can also aggravate vasoconstriction, myocardial ischemia, hypotension, bradycardia, arrhythmias, and coagulopathies. During rewarming, oxygen needs are increased.

Coagulopathy

Dilutional coagulopathies due to component deficiencies (fibrinogen, platelets, coagulation factors), fibrinolysis, and disseminated intravascular coagulation are medical causes of bleeding in trauma patients, especially those who have sustained major vascular injuries as well. Routine screens for disseminated intravascular coagulation (prothrombin time, partial thromboplastin time, platelets, fibrinogen, D-dimers) or thromboelastography to assess clot formation and lysis can serve as guides for the correction of coagulopathies. Fresh frozen plasma is used to correct an abnormal prothrombin time. Cryoprecipitate is used if fibrinogen is less than 100 mg/dL. Platelets are used when there is active bleeding and the platelet count is less than 100,000/mm³. ε-Aminocaproic acid, tranexamic acid, or aprotinin is used to treat primary fibrinolysis. Disseminated intravascular coagulation requires identification of the causative agent. Then, clotting factors (fresh frozen plasma), platelet transfusions, and small IV doses of heparin (50 units/kg) are given.

PREVENTION

Primary Prevention

Public safety campaigns must emphasize the hazards of drinking and driving. Seat-belt and helmet laws must be enforced. Use of gun locks must be encouraged, and gun control laws enforced. Motorcycle and driver safety courses and the use of child restraint seats can also reduce TRI and death.

Secondary Prevention

Vigilant and capable anesthesiologists, along with surgeons with expertise in trauma surgery, are key to the secondary prevention of complications related to trauma. However, the anesthesiology-surgery trauma team must work efficiently and in concert with emergency department physicians and staff, as well as operating room and intensive care unit staff. The hospital's radiology, laboratory medicine, and transfusion services must also be capable of providing the required ancillary support. Taken together, all these capabilities and their efficient deployment can facilitate the timely diagnosis and stabilization of trauma victims, thereby reducing the risk for secondary morbidity or mortality.

Further Reading

Capan LM, Miller SM: Trauma and burns. In Barash PB, Cullen BF, Stoelting RK (eds): Clinical Anesthesia, 4th ed. Philadelphia, JB Lippincott–Williams & Wilkins, 2001, pp 1255-1296.

Duke JC: Anesthesia. In Moore EE, Feliciano DV, Mattox KL (eds): Trauma, 5th ed. New York, McGraw-Hill, 2003, pp 329-353.

Dutton RP, McCunn M: Anesthesia for trauma. In Miller RD (ed): Miller's Anesthesia, 6th ed. Philadelphia, Churchill Livingstone, 2005, pp 2157-2172.

Fingerhut LA, Warner LA: Injury Chartbook: Health: United States, 1996-97. Hyattsville, Md, National Center for Health Statistics, 1998.

Gin-Shaw SL, Jordan RC: Multiple trauma. In Marx JA, Hockberger RS, Walls R (eds): Rosen's Emergency Medicine: Concepts and Clinical Practice, 6th ed. Philadelphia, Mosby, 2006, pp 300-316.

Murray CJL, Lopez AD: The Global Burden of Disease. Cambridge, Mass, Harvard University Press, 1996.

Complications of Laparoscopic Surgery

207

Shahar Bar-Yosef

Case Synopsis

A 75-year-old man with mild ischemic cardiomyopathy is scheduled for elective laparoscopic cholecystectomy under general anesthesia with endotracheal intubation. As the Veres needle is inserted and carbon dioxide (CO_2) insufflation starts, the end-tidal partial pressure of carbon dioxide ($ETCO_2$) increases slowly from 35 to 50 mm Hg and then drops abruptly to 5 mm Hg. The patient becomes severely cyanotic, with bradycardia and no measurable blood pressure.

PROBLEM ANALYSIS

Definition

The most common causes of cardiovascular depression or collapse with laparoscopy are listed in Table 207-1. Conventional laparoscopic surgery requires general anesthesia, because three or more ports are inserted into the abdomen. One port is used for the insufflation of CO_2, which is automatically regulated and maintained at 12 to 15 mm Hg. The other ports are used for the insertion of surgical instruments. Tilting the operating room table head-up (the reverse Trendelenburg position) or head-down (the Trendelenburg position) facilitates visualization of the operative site.

Physiologic changes associated with laparoscopic surgery result from the complex interplay of three pathophysiologic mechanisms: positive-pressure CO_2 pneumoperitoneum, respiratory acidosis, and the effect of head-up or head-down body positioning (Table 207-2). Positive intra-abdominal pressure compresses abdominal vessels, increasing systemic vascular resistance and reducing venous return. Intra-abdominal pressure is transmitted to the thorax, reducing lung compliance and increasing ventilation-perfusion mismatch. Also, pneumoperitoneum causes a significant neurohormonal response. Vasopressin is released, along with activation of the renin-angiotensin-aldosterone axis, both of which contribute to the observed increase in systemic

vascular resistance. CO_2 absorption and reduced alveolar ventilation (with positive intra-abdominal pressure) increase systemic acidosis. This increases catecholamine release, mean arterial pressure, and cardiac output. However, severe respiratory acidosis can cause direct myocardial depression. Various positions, especially the steep Trendelenburg (e.g., gynecologic laparoscopy) or reverse Trendelenburg (e.g., laparoscopic

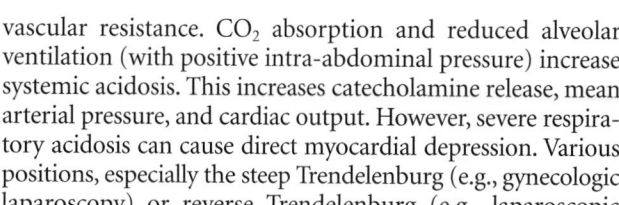

Table 207–2 ■ Physiologic Changes during Laparoscopy

Physiologic Change	Mechanism
Respiratory	
↓ Lung compliance	↑ IAP; head-down position
↑ V̇/Q̇ mismatch	Basal atelectasis; ↓ functional residual and vital capacities
↑ Inspiratory pressures	Pneumoperitoneum; head-down position
↑ $Paco_2$ and ↓ pH	↑ CO_2; ↓ pulmonary perfusion; ↓ alveolar ventilation
Cardiovascular	
↑ SVR, PVR, MAP	↑ IAP, angiotensin, and catecholamines; hypercapnia
↑ Cardiac filling	↑ Intrathoracic pressure; head-down position
Arrhythmias (T or B)	Acidosis, catecholamines (T); ↑ vagal tone due to ↑ IAP (B)
↓ Venous return (VR)	Vena cava compression; head-up position
↓ Ejection fraction (EF)	↑ Afterload; hypercapnia-induced myocardial depression
↓ Cardiac output	↓ VT and EF; arrhythmias; ↑ LV wall stress
↓ Renal blood flow	↑ IAP; ↓ renal vasoconstriction
↓ Splanchnic perfusion	↑ IAP, ADH, and catecholamines; ↓ cardiac output
Other	
↓ Urine output	↓ Renal blood flow; ↑ ADH secretion
↑ Intracranial pressure	↓ VR; ↑ CBF; ↓ lumbar CSF absorption; head-down position

ADH, antidiuretic hormone; B, bradyarrhythmias; CBF, cerebral blood flow; CSF, cerebrospinal fluid; IAP, intra-abdominal pressure; LV, left ventricular; MAP, mean arterial pressure; PVR, pulmonary vascular resistance; SVR, systemic vascular resistance; T, tachyarrhythmias; V̇/Q̇, ventilation-perfusion.

Table 207–1 ■ Causes of Cardiovascular Depression or Collapse during Laparoscopy

Tension pneumoperitoneum
Tension pneumothorax
Pericardial tamponade
Myocardial ischemia
Extreme hypercapnia
Venous gas embolism
Bleeding and hypovolemia
Arrhythmias

Table 207–3 ■ Differential Diagnosis of Complications during Laparoscopy

Complication	Clinical Sequelae
Extraperitoneal CO_2 inflation	Subcutaneous emphysema; pneumomediastinum; simple or tension pneumothorax; pneumopericardium that mimics cardiac tamponade; massive gas embolization that can be vascular, visceral, or both—if vascular, possible cardiovascular collapse
Arrhythmias	Bradyarrhythmias: sinus or ectopic atrial; AV junctional rhythm; idioventricular rhythm; asystole Tachyarrhythmias: atrial, AV junctional, or ventricular origin
Hypotension	Blood loss due to inadvertent visceral or vascular injury; vascular compression (especially venous capacitance bed, leading to reduced preload and cardiac output)
Hypercapnia	Modest hypercapnia (CO_2 ≤60 mm Hg) is expected; moderate hypercapnia (CO_2 ≤80 mm Hg) may occur; severe hypercapnia (CO_2 >80 mm Hg) may lead to cardiovascular collapse
Hypoxemia	Rare, but possible with $\dot{V}/\dot{Q}$ mismatch, endobronchial intubation, gastric aspiration, or severe hypercarbia with low Fio_2
Postoperative	Nausea and vomiting: 40%-70% of patients; about half require therapy Pain: due to diaphragmatic irritation

AV, atrioventricular; Fio_2, fraction of inspired oxygen; $\dot{V}/\dot{Q}$, ventilation-perfusion.

cholecystectomy), may either accentuate or alleviate these respiratory and hemodynamic changes.

Numerous complications are inherent in laparoscopic surgery, especially during abdominal trocar placement and CO_2 insufflation (Table 207-3). Most common is the extraperitoneal insufflation of CO_2 (incidence of 0.4% to 2%). Subcutaneous CO_2 emphysema results from dissection of gas into tissue planes around the trocar site used for insufflation. This can extend into the mediastinum and to subcutaneous tissues. Gas under pressure may also be introduced into the pleural space via congenital pleural-peritoneal communications or an inadvertent diaphragmatic injury, creating simple or tension pneumothorax. Introduction of gas into the pericardial space creates a pneumopericardium that can mimic the clinical presentation of cardiac tamponade. Massive gas embolization is a catastrophic complication caused by the inadvertent injection of insufflating gas into a vessel or abdominal organ during the induction of the pneumoperitoneum. If the gas is injected into a vein, subsequent obstruction of the right ventricular outflow tract or pulmonary circulation may lead to cardiovascular collapse. The incidence of visceral embolization is 0.002% to 0.08%; however, vascular gas embolism can be detected in up to two thirds of all patients undergoing laparoscopic cholecystectomy if diagnostic transesophageal echocardiography is used. The lethal embolic dose of CO_2 is five times greater than that estimated for air.

Arrhythmias may occur. Tachyarrhythmias (sinus arrhythmias, atrial and supraventricular ectopic beats and tachycardias, ventricular ectopic beats, ventricular tachycardia or fibrillation) are related mainly to respiratory acidosis and the associated catecholamine surge. Bradyarrhythmias (sinus bradycardia, wandering atrial pacemaker, junctional rhythm, atrioventricular heart block, asystole) are likely vagally mediated or due to extreme hypercarbia and respiratory acidosis.

The possibility of hypotension secondary to blood loss from accidental visceral and vascular injury exists and is complicated by the difficulty of achieving rapid control of a bleeding source. Although major vessels can be injured, the more common sites are the epigastric and iliac vessels.

Gastrointestinal perforation or hepatic and splenic tears have also been described.

Modest or moderate hypercapnia is a nearly universal occurrence during laparoscopy; if it is severe ($Paco_2$ > 80 mm Hg), it may be associated with cardiovascular collapse. In contrast, hypoxemia is rare during laparoscopy. Isolated hypoxemia can occur, however, with significant ventilation-perfusion mismatch, endobronchial intubation, aspiration, or severe hypercapnia in the setting of a low-normal fraction of inspired oxygen.

Postoperative complications are usually benign. Nausea and vomiting occur in 40% to 70% of patients after laparoscopy; about half require antiemetic therapy. Postoperative pain due to diaphragmatic irritation is usually described as vague abdominal, neck, or shoulder discomfort.

Recognition

Rapid changes in ventilatory and hemodynamic parameters are most likely to occur early in the laparoscopic procedure. They are caused by changes in body position and introduction of the Veress needle and gas insufflation. Close patient scrutiny and monitoring of vital signs (i.e., electrocardiogram, noninvasive blood pressure, pulse oximetry, capnography) are essential.

Capnography is an invaluable diagnostic tool during laparoscopy because it may provide early warning signs of impending catastrophic events. Measurement of $ETCO_2$ concentrations can define changes in pulmonary CO_2 elimination, which is dependent on CO_2 production, lung perfusion, and alveolar ventilation. The normal range for $ETCO_2$ is 35 to 37 mm Hg. The gradient between CO_2 concentration in arterial blood and $ETCO_2$ is usually 5 to 6 mm Hg. However, in some patients, especially those with cardiopulmonary disease, an increased arterial-to-$ETCO_2$ gradient reflects increased ventilation-perfusion mismatch and reduced cardiac output, both of which contribute to an increase in dead-space ventilation.

Most patients require a 30% increase in minute ventilation to counter systemic absorption of insufflated CO_2.

Hypercapnia may cause respiratory acidosis (i.e., elevated $Paco_2$ and low pH). With severe hypercapnia, capnography may reveal spontaneous breathing. $ETCO_2$ also increases with systemic CO_2 absorption in the following situations:

- Pneumoperitoneum
- Subcutaneous CO_2 extravasation
- Hypermetabolic states (malignant hyperthermia, thyrotoxicosis)
- Low minute ventilation
- Metabolism of sodium bicarbonate
- Use of CO_2-enriched gases
- Rebreathing of exhaled gases.

A sudden decline in $ETCO_2$ is usually due to obstruction of the airway or sampling tubing, extubation, circuit leak or disconnection, venous air or pulmonary embolism, low cardiac output, or cardiac arrest. Another cause is mainstem endobronchial intubation due to endotracheal tube migration during peritoneal CO_2 insufflation, when the lungs are displaced cephalad by the CO_2 pneumoperitoneum. To exclude this latter cause, lung auscultation should be performed higher on the chest wall.

A sudden increase in peak inspiratory pressures should raise the suspicion for simple or tension pneumothorax. However, a more gradual, modest increase is expected with the reduced lung compliance and functional residual capacity (FRC) associated with pneumoperitoneum. Healthy patients tend to tolerate the reduced lung compliance and FRC with minimal consequences. Finally, increased capnographic plateau pressure is common with position-related, cephalad displacement of the diaphragm during CO_2 insufflation.

The value of more invasive monitoring has not been studied, but some advocate its use for obese, elderly, or debilitated patients. An arterial catheter allows continuous monitoring of blood pressure and repeated blood gas measurements. If a pulmonary artery catheter is used, filling pressures (central venous pressure and pulmonary capillary wedge pressure) tend to increase with pneumoperitoneum, regardless of actual venous return and cardiac filling pressures. Monitoring of cardiac output and mixed venous oxygen saturation is useful in patients with severe myocardial dysfunction. Transesophageal echocardiography is valuable for detecting hypovolemia, myocardial ischemia, ventricular dysfunction, worsened valvular regurgitation, and venous gas or pulmonary embolism.

Risk Assessment

Mortality with laparoscopy is 0% to 0.13%. Most deaths are due to cardiac complications (25%). The rate of major intraoperative events is usually less than 2%. Vascular injury accounts for about one third of the associated morbidity. Relative contraindications to laparoscopic surgery include increased intracranial pressure, ventriculoperitoneal or peritoneal-jugular shunts, hypovolemia, congestive heart failure, severe cardiopulmonary disease, previous abdominal surgery with significant adhesions, morbid obesity, pregnancy, end-stage liver disease, and coagulopathies. Older and sicker patients with limited cardiac reserve or those at increased risk for ischemia or left ventricular failure might not tolerate the increase in systemic vascular resistance and left ventricular wall tension that accompanies pneumoperitoneum.

Similarly, the deleterious respiratory effects of laparoscopy are predicted to be more severe in patients with preexisting lung disease with increased dead space, reduced compliance and FRC, or severe diffusion defects. Even large increases in minute ventilation in these patients may not be enough to normalize the arterial CO_2 tension, and an already reduced FRC may decrease even further. This could lead to significant hypoxemia from atelectasis and intrapulmonary shunting. Bullous emphysema increases the risk for pneumothorax due to barotrauma. Preexisting pulmonary hypertension and right ventricular dysfunction may worsen owing to a CO_2-mediated increase in pulmonary vascular resistance.

The American College of Cardiology–American Heart Association algorithm for preoperative cardiac evaluation (discussed in Chapter 38) does not distinguish between laparoscopic and open abdominal surgery. However, some advocate echocardiography and spirometry in American Society of Anesthesiologists classes III and IV patients before laparoscopy. Forced expiratory volume less than 70% and diffusion capacity less than 80% are predictive of more severe hypercapnia during laparoscopy.

In addition to comorbidities, the type of surgery determines the risk for complications. For example, the incidence of hypercarbia and subcutaneous emphysema are greater with retro- or extraperitoneal gas insufflation for laparoscopic inguinal hernia repair than with intraperitoneal insufflation for laparoscopic cholecystectomy. Patients undergoing laparoscopic Nissen fundoplication are at increased risk for pneumomediastinum, subcutaneous emphysema, and pneumothorax (1% to 5%). Also, they are more likely to have vagally mediated bradyarrhythmias.

Implications

Laparoscopic surgery is considered a safe alternative to open procedures. Predictions are that up to 75% of all abdominal surgery will soon be performed endoscopically. Proven benefits of laparoscopic surgeries include smaller incisions, less intraoperative bleeding, shorter surgical times, and attenuation of the stress and inflammatory response accompanying open surgery. These factors lead to reduced postoperative analgesic requirements, improved pulmonary function, more timely ambulation, less ileus, faster recovery and discharge, increased patient satisfaction, and lower costs. Lung function appears to recover more quickly after laparoscopic surgery, FRC and vital capacity are much better preserved, diaphragmatic contractions are stronger, and hypoxemia is lessened. Consequently, laparoscopy is associated with a reduced incidence of postoperative atelectasis and pneumonia.

However, physiologic changes due to peritoneal CO_2 insufflation and patient positioning can cause significant reductions in blood pressure and cardiac output. If so, intraoperative management requires vigilance and skill on the part of the anesthesiologist. Any of the catastrophic events described earlier can place the patient in an acute life-threatening situation. Experimental and clinical studies have found that intraoperative declines in the glomerular filtration rate and creatinine clearance during laparoscopy quickly reverse. No relationship exists between urine output during surgery and the postoperative serum creatinine concentration. Less is known about the incidence of cardiac complications. However, because perioperative myocardial infarction usually occurs within 24 to 48 hours of surgery and appears to be related to the magnitude of surgical stress, myocardial infarction should be less common after laparoscopic surgery, but this remains unproven.

Safety of laparoscopy in the critically ill has not been studied. Theoretical considerations suggest the need for extreme caution. Increased intracranial pressure associated with laparoscopy may be detrimental to patients with closed head injury. Also, patients with sepsis are often hypovolemic, which may exacerbate the decrease in venous return and cardiac output with laparoscopy. Also, critically ill patients commonly have reduced splanchnic perfusion, and laparoscopy may induce mesenteric ischemia. This increases the risk for bacterial translocation and septic complications.

Most patients with symptomatic gallstones are candidates for laparoscopic cholecystectomy. Exceptions are those with generalized peritonitis, septic shock from cholangitis, severe acute pancreatitis, end-stage hepatic cirrhosis with portal hypertension, severe coagulopathy unresponsive to treatment, known cancer of the gallbladder, and cholecystoenteric fistulas.

MANAGEMENT

Management for hemodynamic perturbations during laparoscopy is complicated because of competing goals. Whereas increased blood pressure may require vasodilators, one must keep in mind that venous return is usually reduced. Therefore, arterial-selective intravenous dilators (e.g., hydralazine, labetalol, nicardipine) are preferred over sodium nitroprusside or nitroglycerin. Tachycardia may prompt treatment with β-blockers, especially in patients at risk for myocardial ischemia. However, this may increase the patient's susceptibility to bradycardia mediated by increased vagal tone. In patients with myocardial dysfunction, afterload reduction may mitigate the detrimental effect of pneumoperitoneum and increased $PaCO_2$ to increase systemic vascular resistance, left ventricular wall tension, and cardiac output. Rarely, reduction of the insufflation pressure to 10 mm Hg and use of an inotropic agent will be required. If so, some form of cardiac output monitoring is advised at this stage, because it may be difficult to distinguish hypotension due to a reduction in myocardial contractility from that due to other pathophysiologic changes.

Generous intravenous fluids must be given to overcome the decrease in venous return caused by positive intra-abdominal pressure. Central filling pressures usually are not available to guide fluid therapy. If possible, reducing the degree of reverse Trendelenburg positioning is another way to ameliorate reduced venous return. Rarely, the laparoscopic approach must be abandoned in favor of an open procedure.

Therapy for hypercapnia is to increase minute ventilation by increasing the respiratory rate. Rarely, a switch from CO_2 to another gas for insufflation is required. This introduces a greater risk of gas emboli due to reduced blood solubility (helium) or explosions (if hydrogen and methane

are present because air, oxygen, and nitrous oxide support combustion). Hypercapnia, which is difficult to correct, should prompt a search for subcutaneous emphysema, which may serve as a large reservoir of CO_2. Prolonged postoperative ventilation may be required until the emphysema has sufficiently resolved, which often takes 4 to 6 hours. Giving analgesics or sedatives to patients with respiratory compromise secondary to airway obstruction, chronic obstructive pulmonary disease, or diminished respiratory drive subjects them to an increased risk of respiratory arrest.

Tension pneumothorax requires immediate needle aspiration at the second intercostal space in the midaxillary line. Further gas insufflation should be stopped, and the pneumoperitoneum temporarily released. With positive-pressure ventilation, the needle catheter should be left in place until the surgery is completed. Rarely is a chest tube needed, because any CO_2 will be absorbed quickly. Serial postoperative chest radiographs are mandatory.

Once venous gas embolism is diagnosed or suspected, gas insufflation should be stopped immediately, the pneumoperitoneum released, and the patient placed in a steep head-down position and right side up. This places the right ventricular outflow tract in a dependent position relative to the right atrium and may help release a gas lock to forward blood flow. Ventilation with 100% oxygen should be started, and pressors should be given for hemodynamic support as needed. Right heart catheterization with a multiorifice catheter and aspiration of gas bubbles can be attempted but is rarely effective. In extreme cases, cardiopulmonary bypass may be required for evacuation of gas emboli. The possibility of paradoxical emboli through a patent foramen ovale must always be kept in mind. Thus, the patient should be evaluated for neurologic changes when he or she is awake and able to follow commands.

PREVENTION

Insufflation of CO_2 to create pneumoperitoneum increases intra-abdominal pressure. This enhances venous stasis, reduces portal venous and renal arterial blood flow, and increases airway pressures. Collectively, these changes impair ventilatory and circulatory function. Intraoperative steps that can be taken to reduce these changes include the following:

- Reducing insufflation pressures to 10 to 15 mm Hg
- Moderating the degree of Trendelenburg or reverse Trendelenburg positioning
- Adjusting ventilation to reduce hypercapnia and acidosis
- Using sequential, intermittent lower extremity compression devices to reduce venous stasis
- Volume loading to minimize impaired renal and myocardial perfusion

Pressure-controlled ventilation is used to reduce the risk of barotrauma in patients with greatly increased airway pressures. An oro- or nasogastric tube is inserted for gastric decompression. A urinary catheter decompresses the bladder and reduces the risk for injury. Precautions should be used during extreme postural positioning to reduce the risk of nerve injury (e.g., shoulder braces for the Trendelenburg position, foot boards for the reverse Trendelenburg position).

"Gasless laparoscopy" (i.e., abdominal wall lifting devices rather than gas insufflation) might be considered for patients with significant cardiopulmonary derangements or at high risk for them. If this is not an option, a more practical approach is to limit the degree of Trendelenburg or reverse Trendelenburg positioning to attenuate any adverse physiologic effects.

Further Reading

Eagle KA, Berger PB, Calkins H, et al: ACC/AHA update for perioperative cardiovascular evaluation for noncardiac surgery. Circulation 105:1257-1267, 2002.

Harris SN, Ballantyne GH, Luther MA, et al: Alterations of cardiovascular performance during laparoscopic colectomy: A combined hemodynamic and echocardiographic analysis. Anesth Analg 83:482-487, 1996.

Leonard IE, Cunningham AJ: Anesthetic considerations for laparoscopic cholecystectomy. Best Pract Res Clin Anaesthesiol 16:1-20, 2002.

Nguyen NT, Goldman CD, Ho HS, et al: Systemic stress response after laparoscopic and open gastric bypass. J Am Coll Surg 194:557-566, 2002.

Struthers AD, Cuschieri A: Cardiovascular consequences of laparoscopic surgery. Lancet 352:568-570, 1998.

Wahba RWM, Tessler MJ, Kleiman SJ: Acute ventilatory complications during laparoscopic upper abdominal surgery. Can J Anaesth 43: 77-83, 1996.

OTHER SURGICAL
SUBSPECIALTIES

Postoperative Urinary Retention

208

D. Janet Pavlin

Case Synopses

Case 1

A 24-year-old man undergoes a 1-hour outpatient knee arthroscopy under spinal anesthesia with 10 mg bupivacaine. After 3.5 hours in the recovery room, he has voided 100 mL and is otherwise ready for discharge. Although the patient has experienced no pain or sense of fullness, a bladder scan reveals a postvoid residual volume of 700 mL. A diagnosis of urinary retention is made; the patient undergoes in-out catheterization for 700 mL of urine and is then discharged. The patient is able to void spontaneously 7 hours later at home, and no subsequent episodes of urinary retention occur.

Case 2

A 45-year-old man undergoes drainage of a perirectal abscess under general anesthesia. The patient last voided 4 hours before surgery. He receives 1500 mL of fluid during surgery. In the recovery unit, he experiences considerable pain at the surgical site, for which he receives intravenous and oral opioid medication. He also reports a painfully distended bladder but is unable to void after 2 hours in the recovery unit. In-out bladder catheterization is performed, and 650 mL of urine is obtained. He is allowed to go home, but 14 hours later he returns to the emergency room with a painful distended bladder and inability to void. A bladder catheter is inserted, and 750 mL of urine is obtained. The patient is discharged with an indwelling catheter and returns 2 days later to have the catheter removed. He has no subsequent problems with voiding.

PROBLEM ANALYSIS

Definition

Urinary retention is defined as the inability to void in the presence of a full bladder. The normal adult bladder capacity is from 500 to 600 mL. Postoperative urinary retention is relatively common. Its frequency depends on the nature and location of surgery, type of anesthesia used, drugs given, and the patients' underlying physiology and medical conditions.

Knowledge of normal bladder function is a prerequisite to understanding how and why urinary retention occurs postoperatively. Voiding is neurally regulated and is normally a reflex response to a full bladder—known as the micturition reflex (Table 208-1). It requires bladder distention, followed by transmission of sensory input from the bladder to the midsacral region of the spinal cord, involuntary simultaneous contraction of the bladder, and reflex inhibition of the internal urethral sphincter. These must be coupled with voluntary relaxation of the external urethral sphincter. Visceral sensory afferents from the bladder travel primarily in the pelvic splanchnic nerves to synapse in the midsacral spinal cord (S2-S4), with projections to the micturition center in the brain. The efferent limb of this reflex consists of the following:

- Preganglionic parasympathetic fibers originating at S2-S4 travel in pelvic splanchnic nerves to peripheral cholinergic receptors within the bladder wall and stimulate bladder contraction during the active phase of voiding.

Table 208–1 ■ Neural Control of Voiding

Bladder distention
Visceral afferent fibers via pelvic splanchnic nerves
Synapse at the micturition center in the midsacral cord (S2-S4)
Parasympathetic efferent cholinergic fibers (they arise at S2-S4, travel with the pelvic splanchnic nerves, synapse at cholinergic sites in the bladder wall, and then stimulate contraction)
Sympathetic efferent fibers (they arise at T10-L2, travel via hypogastric plexuses to the internal urethral sphincter, and are involuntarily inhibited during voiding)
Somatic efferent fibers (they travel via the pudendal nerve to striated muscle of the external urethral sphincter and are voluntarily relaxed during voiding)
The entire reflex arc is subject to control by the pontine micturition center and higher centers in the brain via the spinobulbar tracts

- Sympathetic efferent fibers originating from T10 to L2 travel via the superior and inferior hypogastric plexuses to the internal urethral sphincter. Their output maintains sphincter tone during continence and is reflex-inhibited during voiding.
- Somatic efferent fibers course in the pudendal nerves to the striated muscle of the external urethethral sphincter, which must be voluntarily relaxed during voiding.

The micturition reflex is subject to modulation or control by higher brain centers, including the pontine micturition center (dorsolateral pons), areas of the diencephalon, and the cerebral cortex. Receptors in the spinal portion of the pathway are susceptible to modulation by opioids, acetylcholine, dopamine, serotonin, norepinephrine, GABA, excitatory and inhibitory amino acids, and other neuropeptides.

Urinary retention can occur due to interruption of the micturition reflex at any point in the circuit. Spinal or epidural anesthesia interferes with the afferent and efferent limbs of the reflex. Opioids and anticholinergics may block transmission at cholinergic sites in the bladder wall or in the spinal cord. Increased sympathetic activity, due to pain in a lumbosacral nerve distribution or overdistention of the bladder itself, may interfere with reflex inhibition of sympathetic tone to the internal urethral sphincter. Inability to void may also result from failure to coordinate bladder contraction with sphincter relaxation (dyssynergia) as a result of disease or dysfunction of the spinal cord. Additionally, retention may be the result of obstruction to outflow at the level of the urethra due to prostatic disease or other acute or chronic conditions affecting urethral patency. Various other factors may act through cortical or subcortical mechanisms to inhibit the ability to void, including fear, embarrassment, and possibly recumbency.

Recognition

Urinary retention may be painful or painless. Neuraxial blocks, analgesics, or sedation may prevent pain related to bladder overdistention. Although a high index of suspicion, palpation, and percussion can sometimes detect an overdistended bladder, this is often not possible or is unreliable.

Both the duration of surgery and the amount of intraoperative fluids given significantly correlate with bladder volume at the end of surgery. Yet these relationships are variable and of limited value for diagnosing or predicting bladder volume in individual patients. In unconscious patients, a portable ultrasound scan may be the only practical, reliable, noninvasive means of diagnosing urinary retention and bladder overdistention.

In one study, the correlation between surgery duration and urinary bladder volume after surgery was 0.32 ($P = .0002$). The correlation between intraoperative intravenous fluid volumes and urinary bladder volume was 0.26 ($P = .0021$). Also, ultrasound-determined bladder volumes correlated with measured volumes ($r = 0.9$; $P < .0001$). In-out urinary bladder catheterization is used to confirm an overdistended bladder. If bladder volume is categorized by patients or nurses as empty, moderately full, or overly distended based on usual clinical criteria, studies have confirmed that patients incorrectly estimate bladder volume in 56% of cases, and nurses err in 46% of cases.

Risk Assessment

Risk factors for postoperative urinary retention are listed in Table 208-2. Urinary retention is often related to the use of neuraxial blockade. The incidence may be greater than 60% with long-acting local anesthetics. With low-dose, short-acting local anesthetics without vasoconstrictors (e.g., lidocaine, chloroprocaine), the incidence is relatively low. Mulroy and colleagues reported that the incidence was 3 in 201 patients after short-acting spinal or epidural anesthesia.

Vasocontrictors prolong the duration of sacral anesthesia with epidural, caudal, or spinal anesthesia and thus increase the incidence of urinary retention. Surgery in the lumbosacral nerve distribution can also cause urinary retention. Hernia repair and rectal surgery are commonly associated with urinary retention (14% to 35% for hernia repair; 1% to 52% for rectal surgery). Partly, these differences depend on the method used for assessment. Furthermore, urinary retention can be caused by pain and by increased sympathetic activity in the distribution of the lumbosacral nerves, which counters reflex-inhibition of tone to the internal urethral sphincter.

Mechanical trauma to the urethra or preexisting outlet obstruction accounts for most cases of urinary retention after urologic surgery. Spinal cord disease in the lumbosacral distribution can locally interfere with micturition or impair central coordination of voiding, as in patients with spinal cord injury.

A history of urinary retention increases the incidence of postoperative urinary retention. Mechanisms include any of the causes described earlier. Also, mandatory recumbency is associated with the inability to void in many patients. The author found an 18% incidence of urinary retention in patients confined to bed after foot surgery, with or without a sciatic nerve block (unreported observations). Other factors, including systemic opioids, anticholinergics, and excessive intravenous fluids (see Table 208-2), contribute to difficulty with micturition and postoperative urinary retention.

Implications

Acutely, overdistention of the bladder can cause pain, or incontinence may ensue. Reflex-increased sympathetic activity may cause systemic hypertension; this is more likely in patients with spinal cord transection (autonomic dysreflexia). Studies in animal models have shown that bladder overdistention leads to bladder wall ischemia. If sustained (>3 to 10 hours),

Table 208–2 ■ **Risk Factors for Urinary Retention**
Neuraxial local anesthetics
Neuraxial or systemic opioid therapy
Anticholinergics
Urethral outlet obstruction
Surgery of the lower urinary tract or surrounding area
Surgery in a lumbosacral nerve distribution area (groin, perirectal, penile)
Previous history of retention
Spinal cord disease or dysfunction
Recumbency
Excessive fluid administration

urothelial cell damage, hemorrhage, and edema may occur. This is followed by parasympathetic nerve ending loss, reduced parasympathetic activity, and failure of the detrusor muscle to contract normally.

Functional effects of impaired parasympathetic activity include inability to empty the bladder fully, leading to frequent small voidings (frequency, nocturia), weak stream, hesitancy, dribbling, and bladder instability. If sustained, urinary stasis can lead to urosepsis.

Most often, cellular regeneration occurs over several weeks, with gradual recovery of normal bladder function. However, intercellular junction rupture and interstitial collagen deposition can occur. This leads to permanent impairment of impulse transmission throughout the bladder wall and may require operative intervention (e.g., Marshall-Marchetti-Krantz bladder suspension or creation of an ileal conduit).

MANAGEMENT

Postoperative urinary retention typically results from overfilling of the bladder when the micturition reflex is impaired by anesthesia or surgery. Because this is usually temporary, some episodes of retention can be prevented simply by ensuring that the patient has an empty bladder immediately before surgery and by avoiding excessive fluid administration during surgery. This is particularly relevant when either the surgery or the anesthetic is known to predispose to urinary retention or when there is a history of urinary retention.

Given that the normal rate of urine formation is about 75 mL/hour (adults), the time required to attain a full bladder (600 mL) is roughly 8 hours. Based on animal investigations, the critical duration for bladder overdistention to avoid potential nerve injury is 4 hours. Thus, clinicians can assume that it is undesirable to have an overdistended bladder for longer than 4 hours.

Table 208-3 shows the estimated time required to attain a bladder volume that exceeds 600 mL for 4 hours (i.e., theoretical critical duration), assuming a rate of urine formation of either 50 or 100 mL/hour. Assuming an empty bladder at the outset, the critical time would be 10 hours at a rate of 100 mL/hour and 16 hours at a rate of 50 mL/hour. However, if the initial volume was 400 mL, the critical times

Table 208–3 ▪ Predicted Time to Achieve Critical Bladder Volume		
Starting Residual Bladder Volume (mL)	Time (hr) to Achieve >600 mL for >4 Hours	
	Urine Formation at 50 mL/hr	*Urine Formation at 100 mL/hr*
0	16	10
100	14	9
200	12	8
400	8	6
600	4	4

would be 6 and 8 hours, respectively. Thus, to avoid complications related to postoperative retention, the following steps are prudent:

• Ensure that all patients void before surgery.
• Ensure that postoperative patients void or are catheterized within approximately 8 to 10 hours of their last voiding.
• Use an indwelling urinary catheter for procedures expected to last longer than 5 to 6 hours, assuming that the patient will be unable to void until 1 to 2 hours after surgery.

PREVENTION

If a patient has not voided within 6 to 8 hours of his or her last voiding, the bladder volume should be assessed before the patient leaves the recovery room. Bladder volume can be determined noninvasively by ultrasonography. The bladder should be drained if the volume is more than 600 mL. Alternatively, if a scanner is not available, bladder volume can be assessed by palpation and the bladder emptied by in-out catheter drainage. This is especially important in patients with known risk factors for postoperative urinary retention (see Table 208-2). One recent study noted a 24% incidence of urinary retention in patients arriving in the recovery room after various surgeries performed without an indwelling bladder catheter.

For outpatient surgery, a decision must be made whether patients should be required to void before discharge. At least two studies suggest that patients with no underlying risk factors for urinary retention should be allowed to go home without voiding before discharge. In such patients, the incidence of urinary retention was less than 1%. In patients with risk factors for urinary retention, it is prudent to require them to void before discharge. This avoids a persistently overdistended bladder if a patient fails to seek medical attention for this problem in a timely manner. Thus, patients having rectal, groin, or urologic surgery and those with spinal cord disease or a history of urinary retention should be required to void or be catheterized before discharge.

After spinal or epidural anesthesia, patients should be required to void or be catheterized, with some possible exceptions. Patients who have had neuraxial blocks with short-acting local anesthetics (≤50 mg lidocaine without vasopressors, or 2-chloroprocaine) can safely be discharged without voiding if a bladder scan reveals a bladder volume of less than 400 mL at the time of discharge. Owing to the short duration of action of these two agents, it is almost certain that any residual effects of the local anesthetic will resolve before a "critical volume" is exceeded for longer than 4 hours. However, bupivacaine blocks have been associated with impaired voiding for longer than 10 hours. Patients who have received this anesthetic or other similarly long-acting local anesthetics should not be discharged without voiding or having catheter drainage of the bladder.

Ideally, high-risk patients who do void should have the postvoid residual volume checked to ensure that the bladder is empty. In many cases, voiding by straining results in the expulsion of a small quantity of urine, but the residual volume may still exceed 400 to 600 mL, and the micturition reflex may not have recovered. This is best evaluated with an ultrasound scan. If this is unavailable, one can reasonably suspect that there is a high postvoid residual volume (>400 mL) if the patient has voided less than 300 mL. If so, patients should be requested to stay until they have voided again and fully emptied the bladder. Alternatively, the bladder can be drained by in-out catheterization to ensure that it is empty before discharge. Finally, all patients, whether at high or low risk, should be instructed to return to a medical facility if they are unable to void within 8 to 10 hours of discharge from the hospital.

Further Reading

Azadzoi KM, Pontari M, Vlachiotis JU, Siroky MB: Canine bladder blood flow and oxygenation: Changes induced by filling, contraction and outlet obstruction. J Urol 155:1459-1465, 1996.

DeGroat WC, Yoshimura N: Pharmacology of the lower urinary tract. Ann Rev Pharmacol Toxicol 41:691-721, 2001.

Kamphuis ET, Ionescu TI, Kuipers PWG, et al: Recovery of storage and emptying functions of the urinary bladder after spinal anesthesia with lidocaine and with bupivacaine in men. Anesthesiology 88:310-316, 1998.

Lamonerie L, Marret E, Deleuze A, et al: Prevalence of postoperative bladder distension and urinary retention detected by ultrasound measurement. Br J Anaesth 92:544-546, 2004.

Lasanen LT, Tammela TL, Kallioinen M, et al: Effect of acute distension on cholinergic innervation of the rat urinary bladder. Urol Res 20:59-62, 1992.

Lloyd-Davies RW, Clark AE, Prout WG, et al: The effects of stretching the rabbit bladder. Invest Urol 8:145-152, 1980.

Mulroy MF, Salinas FV, Larkin KL, et al: Ambulatory surgery patients may be discharged before voiding after short-acting spinal and epidural anesthesia. Anesthesiology 97:315-319, 2002.

Pavlin DJ, Pavlin EG, Fitzgibbon DR, et al: Management of bladder function after outpatient surgery. Anesthesiology 91:42-50, 1999.

Pavlin DJ, Pavlin EG, Gunn HC, et al: Voiding in patients managed with or without ultrasound monitoring of bladder volume after outpatient surgery. Anesth Analg 89:90-97, 1999.

OTHER SURGICAL SUBSPECIALTIES

Intraoperative Penile Erection

209

Terri G. Monk

Case Synopsis

A 50-year-old man is scheduled for a transurethral resection of the prostate. After premedication with 2 mg midazolam given intravenously, a hyperbaric spinal anesthetic is placed, and a T6 sensory level is achieved. During placement of the resectoscope sheath, a full erection occurs, preventing free movement and control of the scope. The bladder is emptied and the resectoscope is removed, but the erection persists. The surgeon states that the erection prevents him from continuing with the procedure and asks the anesthesiologist to treat it.

PROBLEM ANALYSIS

Definition

Priapism is the persistence of a penile erection for longer than 4 to 6 hours, unaccompanied by sexual excitement or desire. Priapism can be classified as primary (idiopathic) or secondary (Table 209-1). Primary priapism is the result of physical or psychological stimuli unaccompanied by a disease state that could cause or sustain an erection. Secondary priapism is the result of factors that directly or indirectly affect penile erectile reactivity.

Recognition

Intraoperative penile erections under anesthesia can be classified as primary priapism and generally occur during scrub preparation of the genitalia, Foley catheter insertion, or transurethral procedures. Erections under anesthesia are

Table 209–1 ■ Causes of Priapism

Primary (Idiopathic) Causes
Physical or psychological stimuli
Intraoperative tactile stimulation
Secondary Causes
Neurogenic
Thromboembolic
   Sickle cell disease
   Leukemia
Malignant penile infiltration
Medications
   Antihypertensive agents
   Phenothiazines
   Antidepressants
   Alcohol
   Marijuana
Miscellaneous causes
   Genital trauma
   Self-injection therapy for impotence
   Coagulopathy

generally of shorter duration than other forms of priapism and may not persist long enough to be considered true priapism.

The exact mechanism for penile erection is poorly understood, but it may result from a complex combination of psychological, neuroendocrine, and vascular factors acting on penile erectile tissues. Parasympathetic penile innervation is from the sacral (S2-S4) spinal cord segments via the nervi erigentes. When the penis is flaccid, high sympathetic tone increases intrinsic muscle tone in the arterioles, thereby reducing blood flow to the corpora cavernosa. At the same time, venules draining the corpora cavernosa remain open. For an erection to occur, parasympathetic impulses dilate the arterioles, allowing more blood flow into the corpora cavernosa; simultaneously, there is partial occlusion of venous outflow. Detumescence occurs when this cycle is reversed.

Vasoactive mediators, including nitric oxide, vasopressin, and bradykinin, also affect the state of penile tumescence. Persistent tumescence, or priapism, results from failure of the mechanisms of detumescence, including blockage of venous drainage, excessive release of neurotransmitters, paralysis of the intrinsic detumescence mechanism, or prolonged relaxation of the intracavernosal smooth muscles. Blood continues to accumulate in the cavernosal sinusoids, and if the erection persists for more than 6 hours, it may become painful.

Risk Assessment

Intraoperative penile erection is reported to occur in approximately 2.4% of male patients undergoing surgery. The incidence of erection varies according to age, with a frequency of 8% in male patients younger than 50 years and 0.9% in older patients. Penile stimulation during preparation and instrumentation may result in penile erection even in the presence of general or regional anesthesia. The incidence appears to be similar for general (3.5%) and epidural (3.8%) anesthesia, but it is lower with spinal anesthesia (0.3%). Foley catheterization has been reported to produce penile erection in approximately 1% of male patients undergoing cardiac surgery with general anesthesia.

Implications

An intraoperative penile erection may delay or even necessitate the cancellation of planned surgery. It can make passing or manipulating a cystoscope nearly impossible. Difficulty with transurethral cystoscope passage can also traumatize the urethra, predisposing to postoperative stricture formation. Aggressive therapy for intraoperative penile erection is necessary to prevent other long-term sequelae, including fibrosis and thrombosis. During penile surgery requiring an incision, penile tumescence can increase intraoperative bleeding. If an intraoperative erection is unresponsive to treatment, the procedure should be postponed.

MANAGEMENT

Numerous modes of therapy have been suggested for the treatment of intraoperative penile erection (Table 209-2). At the first sign of penile tumescence, all genital stimulation, including surgical preparation, urethral manipulation, and Foley catheter insertion, should be terminated immediately. If a cystoscope is in place, it must be removed, if possible. Because intraoperative erections often occur early in the procedure during "light" anesthesia, the anesthetic level should be deepened. If a spinal or epidural anesthetic is used, adequate blockade of the sacral segments should be ensured. In the lithotomy position, the scrotum hangs below the anus in a male patient when the sacral segments are blocked.

If conservative treatment fails to produce detumescence, prompt intervention is necessary. Ethyl chloride spray to the penis or a dorsal penile nerve block can be used to suppress sensory input to the penis, thereby interrupting the sacral reflex arc that is maintaining the erection.

A multitude of pharmacologic agents have been used to treat prolonged erections, but it is unlikely that any single agent will be effective in all cases. The use of intracorporal sympathomimetic agents is most commonly reported in the urologic literature. Owing to the high vascularity of this area, the uptake of these medications occurs rapidly, and systemic cardiovascular effects are common. Some of the more commonly used agents are discussed here.

Phenylephrine, a pure α_1-adrenergic agonist, has been given intracavernosally in doses of 100 to 200 μg. The success rate with this technique is reportedly 100% by 2 to 3 minutes. Although this treatment may be associated with an intermittent rise in mean blood pressure, no untoward cardiovascular events are associated with its use. Some reports suggest that metaraminol is a preferred medication for intracavernosal injection, with doses as low as 10 to 25 μg producing detumescence without untoward cardiovascular effects. However, others caution against the use of metaraminol, norepinephrine, and epinephrine because all these drugs have at least some β_1 activity, with the potential for β_1-mediated adverse cardiovascular events.

Ketamine, a dissociative anesthetic agent, is given intravenously in doses of 0.5 to 1.8 mg/kg, based on the assumption that the erection has occurred in response to external stimuli, and the drug's dissociative effect on the limbic system might block this response. Ketamine may also exert its penile-relaxing effect by decreasing central vagal outflow, blocking reuptake of norepinephrine at the neuroeffector junction in cavernosal erectile tissues, or blocking transmission through parasympathetic ganglia. When using ketamine, it is important to remember that this drug has sympathomimetic actions and must be used with caution in elderly patients and those with significant cardiovascular disease.

Vasodilators, such as inhaled amyl nitrite (one inhalant capsule of 0.3 mL emptied into the reservoir breathing bag) or intravenous nitroprusside, relax the corpora cavernosa venous drainage sites and produce a rapid fall in blood pressure. This leads to compensatory reflex sympathetic discharge, which may mimic the sympathetic discharge that occurs during orgasm, precipitating arteriolar constriction to terminate the erection. Vasodilating agents should be avoided in patients with a regional block because of the danger of inducing severe hypotension. They are also contraindicated in patients with increased intraocular or intracranial pressure.

Terbutaline (0.2 to 0.5 mg intravenously), a β_2-adrenoreceptor agonist, has been used successfully to manage intraoperative penile erection. The action of this agent is unclear, but it is thought that terbutaline relaxes the stretched corporal smooth muscles, thereby releasing the impediment to venous blood flow from the penis. Terbutaline must be used with caution in patients with significant coronary artery disease because it can cause tachycardia, pulmonary edema, or hypokalemia.

Anticholinergics may cause detumescence by blocking the effect of acetylcholine on the nitric oxide system. Of these medications, glycopyrrolate is preferred over atropine or scopolamine because it causes less tachycardia and lacks central nervous system effects.

Table 209–2 ■ Treatment for Intraoperative Penile Erection

Termination of tactile stimulation of genital area
Assurance of adequate anesthetic depth
Ethyl chloride spray to penis
Dorsal penile nerve block
Intracavernosal drug injection
Intravenous pharmacologic agents
    Ketamine
    Vasodilators
    Vasoconstrictors
    Terbutaline
    Anticholinergic agents

PREVENTION

Intraoperative penile erections can occur with any type of anesthesia, but the incidence is lowest with spinal blockade, probably because this technique provides the most profound sensory block of the sacral area. Thus, the administration of a spinal block for transurethral procedures should prevent most episodes of intraoperative tumescence. Whatever type of anesthesia is used, genital skin preparation and urethral manipulation should be delayed until an adequate level of anesthesia is present, because intraoperative erections are generally caused by tactile stimulation of the genital area.

During regional anesthesia, it is especially important to ensure that sensory blockade of the sacral area is present before proceeding. Anesthetic agents associated with an increased incidence of erections during general anesthesia include fentanyl, propofol, and droperidol, but there is no conclusive evidence that avoidance of a particular anesthetic agent will prevent this problem.

Further Reading

Kouriefs C, Watkin NA: What to do if it gets "bigger." Ann R Coll Surg Engl 85:126-128, 2003.

Lue TF: Physiology of erection and pathophysiology of impotence. In Walsh PC, Retik AB, Stamey TA, et al (eds): Campbell's Urology, 6th ed. Philadelphia, WB Saunders, 1992, pp 709-728.

Roy R: Cardiovascular effects of ketamine given to relieve penile turgescence after high doses of fentanyl. Anesthesiology 61:610-613, 1984.

Seftel AD, Resnick MI, Boswell MV: Dorsal nerve block for management of intraoperative penile erection. J Urol 151:394-395, 1994.

Shantha TR, Finnerty DP, Rodriquez AP: Treatment of persistent penile erection and priapism using terbutaline. J Urol 141:1427-1429, 1989.

Staerman F, Nouri M, Coeurdacier P, et al: Treatment of the intraoperative penile erection with intracavernous phenylephrine. J Urol 153:1478-1481, 1995.

Tsai SK, Hong CY: Intracavernosal metaraminol for treatment of intraoperative penile erection. Postgrad Med J 66:831, 1990.

Valley MA, Sang CN: Use of glycopyrrolate to treat intraoperative penile erection. Reg Anesth 19:423-428, 1994.

van Arsdalen KN, Chen JW, Smith MJV: Penile erections complicating transurethral surgery. J Urol 129:374-376, 1983.

Complications of Transurethral Surgery

Vinod Malhotra and Vijayendra Sudheendra

Case Synopsis

An otherwise healthy 70-year-old man undergoes combined transurethral resection of the prostate (TURP) and transurethral resection of a bladder tumor (TURB) under spinal anesthesia with sedation. His blood pressure is 130/90 mm Hg, heart rate is 68 beats per minute, respirations are 16 breaths per minute, and hematocrit is 38%. Ninety minutes into surgery, the patient becomes restless. His blood pressure is 180/100 mm Hg, and his heart rate is 40 beats per minute. The electrocardiogram (ECG) shows depressed T waves. Laboratory values are as follows: hematocrit 27%, sodium 23 mEq/L, potassium 3.0 mEq/L, and chloride 95 mEq/L.

PROBLEM ANALYSIS

Definition

TURP syndrome is a general term used to describe a wide range of neurologic and cardiopulmonary symptoms and signs caused by intravascular absorption of hypotonic bladder-irrigating fluids during transurethral procedures, especially TURP. In conscious or sedated patients, the sudden onset of restlessness should raise the suspicion for TURP syndrome. Hypertension is indicative of hypervolemia. Reflex bradycardia occurs in response to the increased blood pressure. T-wave depression on the ECG is caused by glycine in the irrigating fluid. Hyponatremia is yet another sign of hypotonic irrigant absorption (Table 210-1).

A reduced hematocrit is most likely due to a combination of blood loss and hemodilution. Bradycardia may also occur after bladder perforation. In this case, bradycardia is an efferent vagal response to peritoneal stimulation secondary to any extravasated fluid. Abdominal or shoulder pain and hypotension usually accompany the bradycardia.

Recognition

The case synopsis illustrates three significant complications of transurethral surgery: (1) TURP syndrome, (2) severe hemorrhage, and (3) bladder perforation.

TURP SYNDROME

TURP syndrome is a constellation of signs and symptoms that result from the following circumstances or conditions:

- Circulatory overload
- Water intoxication or hypo-osmolality
- Hyponatremia
- Glycine toxicity
- Ammonia toxicity
- Hemolysis
- Coagulopathy

These signs and symptoms may occur simultaneously (Table 210-2). The clinical presentation may be further complicated by bacteremia or septicemia, which causes chills, hypotension, and tachycardia or bradycardia.

SEVERE HEMORRHAGE

Severe hemorrhage is usually evident as surgical bleeding, although it is difficult to measure because blood is mixed with copious amounts of irrigating fluid. Occult internal bleeding may occur if bladder perforation has occurred. Clinical signs of excessive bleeding include hypotension and reflex tachycardia. However, tachycardia may not occur in the presence of age-related sinus node dysfunction or with the use of β-blockers or high spinal anesthesia.

BLADDER PERFORATION

Bladder perforation is difficult to recognize during general anesthesia. Hypotension and bradycardia or tachycardia may occur, but these are nonspecific findings. An experienced surgeon, however, usually recognizes a bladder perforation immediately. With spinal anesthesia, the complaint of abdominal or shoulder pain is helpful in making the diagnosis.

Table 210–1 ■ Hypotonic Irrigants Used for Transurethral Resection of the Prostate or a Bladder Tumor	
Solution	**Osmolality (mOsm/kg)**
Water	0
Glucose, 2.5%	139
Sorbitol, 3.5%	165
Urea, 1%	167
Glycine, 1.2%	175
Cytal (sorbitol 2.7% and mannitol 0.54%)	178
Glycine, 1.5%	220
Mannitol, 5%	275

OTHER SURGICAL SUBSPECIALTIES

210

843

Table 210–2 ■ **Pathophysiology and Clinical Features of TURP Syndrome**

Pathophysiology	Clinical Features
Fluid overload	Hypertension; bradycardia; arrhythmia; angina; pulmonary edema and hypoxemia; ventricular failure and hypotension
Water intoxication or hypo-osmolality	Confusion and restlessness; twitching or seizures; lethargy or coma; dilated, sluggish pupils; papilledema; low-voltage EEG; hemolysis
Hyponatremia	CNS changes as above; reduced inotropy; widened QRS complex; low-voltage ECG; T-wave inversion on ECG
Glycine toxicity	Nausea and vomiting; headache; transient blindness; loss of light and accommodation reflexes (blink reflex preserved); myocardial depression; ECG changes
Ammonia toxicity	Nausea and vomiting; CNS depression
Hemolysis	Anemia; acute renal failure; chills, clammy skin; chest tightness and bronchospasm; hyperkalemia resulting in malignant arrhythmias or bradyasystole
Coagulopathy	Severe bleeding; primary fibrinolysis; disseminated intravascular coagulation

CNS, central nervous system; ECG, electrocardiogram; EEG, electroencephalogram; TURP, transurethral resection of the prostate gland.

Risk Assessment

Approximately 400,000 TURP procedures are performed annually in the United States. About 10% of men older than 65 years require TURP. The incidence increases to 20% to 30% for men older than 80 years. Seventy-seven percent of patients undergoing TURP have one or more of the following conditions or factors:

- Heart disease
- Hypertension
- Diabetes
- Chronic obstructive pulmonary disease
- History of smoking

Perioperative morbidity is related to associated disease, age, and sepsis. Morbidity is increased in blacks and in patients to whom the following factors apply:

- Resection time longer than 90 minutes
- Prostate weighing more than 45 g
- Acute urinary retention
- Age greater than 80 years

The amount of absorbed irrigating fluid is influenced by the following factors:

- Resection time
- Prostate gland size
- Hydrostatic pressure of the irrigating fluid
- Number and size of venous sinuses opened
- Whether the prostatic capsule is intact

Chronic inflammation, repeated instrumentation, and indwelling Foley catheters increase prostatic vascular congestion and predispose to increased bleeding and bacteremia during TURP. Prolonged resection of a large prostate allows for significant release of plasminogen activators from prostatic tissue into the bloodstream. This can cause primary fibrinolysis. Prostatic tissue and multiple microthrombi may also enter the circulation, leading to disseminated intravascular coagulation (DIC).

Bladder perforation occurs in up to 1% of cases. A higher likelihood of bladder perforation is expected if the bladder tumor is sessile versus pedunculated, is large and fragile, or infiltrates the bladder wall. A bladder wall that is chronically inflamed, previously irradiated, or thin and stretched is more prone to perforation. The likelihood of perforation is further increased if the tumor is difficult to access, bleeding obscures the surgeon's vision, the patient unexpectedly moves or coughs, or instrumentation is difficult or traumatic.

Implications

Overall mortality of TURP is 0.2% to 0.8%. Perioperative morbidity ranges from 7% to 20%. Most mortality and morbidity occur in patients who develop complications of TURP, including TURP syndrome, bladder perforation, or sepsis. In 15% of patients, bacteremia occurs. Of these, 6% to 7% develop septicemia, which is associated with 25% to 75% mortality. Because the consequences of these complications are severe, aggressive management is required.

MANAGEMENT

TURP Syndrome

Immediate aggressive therapy is essential if the patient is to survive. The following measures are suggested:

- Terminate the surgery as soon as possible.
- Administer 20 mg of intravenous (IV) furosemide.
- Immediately obtain the following laboratory tests: hematocrit; serum electrolyte, creatinine, and glucose concentrations; serum osmolality (if available); arterial blood gas analyses; and 12-lead ECG.
- Continue or start the administration of normal saline. Hypertonic saline (3% or 5%) may be administered (at a rate <100 mL/hour) if the serum sodium concentration is less than 100 mEq/L, severe central nervous system side effects of hyponatremia and hypo-osmolality are evident, or reduced inotropy results in cardiovascular collapse.
- Administer IV midazolam in 1-mg incremental doses to treat twitching or seizures; a barbiturate may be added if seizures persist.

- Auscultate chest and obtain chest radiographs to detect pulmonary edema. Intubate and mechanically ventilate the patient at the earliest evidence of pulmonary edema.
- Transfuse packed red blood cells as necessary.
- If bleeding continues, investigate for DIC or primary fibrinolysis. DIC is treated with crystalloids and blood products to achieve hemodynamic stability and normal coagulation. Primary fibrinolysis responds well to aminocaproic acid (Amicar) administered as an IV infusion of 3 to 5 g in the first hour, followed by continuous IV infusion at 1 g/hour until the bleeding is controlled.
- Institute invasive monitoring and provide supportive therapy to maintain circulation and pulmonary function and to prevent renal failure.

Bladder Perforation

As soon as bladder perforation is detected, undertake the following measures:

- Stop surgery and achieve hemostasis.
- Treat hypotension with IV crystalloids, vasopressors, and inotropes.
- Obtain a hematocrit. Start blood transfusion if brisk bleeding continues. Occult blood loss into the intraperitoneal or retroperitoneal space may occur.
- Perform a cystourethrogram to locate the perforation.

For most perforations, suprapubic cystotomy, an indwelling Foley catheter, and (occasionally) ureteral stents are sufficient. In some instances, immediate exploratory laparotomy may be necessary to control bleeding and repair the perforation.

Septicemia

Chills and fever should be treated aggressively and immediately with IV antibiotics. Cardiovascular support may be necessary.

PREVENTION

TURP Syndrome

Take the following preventive measures:

- Limit resection time to less than 1 hour.
- Keep the prostate capsule intact until the end of resection.
- Maintain irrigating fluid height less than 60 cm above the prostate gland.
- Measure serum electrolyte levels during and after the procedure.
- Use regional anesthesia and very light or no sedation to allow early detection of changes in the patient's mental status.

Bladder Perforation; Bacteremia and Septicemia

Avoid overdistention of the bladder, rough instrumentation, patient movement, and extensive prostate or bladder tumor resections at one sitting. Use broad-spectrum antibiotic prophylaxis for bacteremia and septicemia.

Laser Prostatectomy and Other Techniques

Laser prostatectomy has generated renewed interest among urologists and is being performed in several centers. Based on the initial experience, it promises to replace conventional TURP in the near future. The neodymium:yttrium-aluminum-garnet laser has been replaced by the holmium laser, which coagulates and vaporizes prostate tissue. The main advantages over conventional TURP include minimal blood loss (as little as 50 to 70 mL) and minimal fluid absorption, which should nearly eliminate these two major complications of TURP. However, other complications are possible, including coagulation through the prostatic fossa and sloughing of prostatic debris in the postoperative period. The latter can lead to urinary obstruction and retention. Protective eyewear should be worn, and a means of evacuating the smoke plume is required. Caudal anesthesia has been used successfully for laser prostatectomy in patients with severe cardiopulmonary disease, because the use of smaller volumes of continuous irrigation, along with minimal bleeding, minimizes bladder distention.

Cryosurgery is technically complex and is not a popular technique. Microwave ablation of the prostate is another promising technique that can be performed on an outpatient basis under local or sacral block. Classic TURP is still the gold standard, however.

Further Reading

Azar I: Transurethral resection of prostate. In Malhotra V (ed): Anesthesia for Renal and Genitourinary Surgery. New York, McGraw-Hill, 1996, pp 93-109.

Catalona WJ: Urothelial tumors of the urinary tract. In Walsh PC, Retik AB, Stamey TA, et al (eds): Campbell's Urology, 6th ed. Philadelphia, WB Saunders, 1992, pp 1094-1158.

Gravenstein D: Transurethral resection of prostate (TURP) syndrome: A review of pathophysiology and management. Anesth Analg 84: 438-446, 1997.

Jensen V: The TURP syndrome. Can J Anaesth 38:90-95, 1991.

Malhotra V: Transurethral resection of prostate. Anesthesiol Clin North Am 18:883-897, 2000.

Malhotra V: Anesthesia and renal and genitourinary systems. In Miller RD (ed): Miller's Anesthesia, 6th ed. Philadelphia, Churchill Livingstone, 2005, pp 2175-2207.

Malhotra V, Perlmutter A: Caudal anesthesia provides effective anesthesia for laser prostatectomy. Reg Anesth 22:93, 1997.

Mebust WK, Holtgrieve HL, Lockett ATK: Transurethral prostatectomy: Immediate and postoperative complications: A cooperative study of 13 participating institutions evaluating 3885 patients. J Urol 141:243, 1989.

Pientka L, Van Loghen J, Hahn E: Comorbidities and perioperative complications among patients with surgically treated prostatic hyperplasia. Urology 38:43-48, 1991.

211

Complications of Radical Urologic Surgery

Terri G. Monk

Case Synopsis

A 68-year-old man with borderline hypertension undergoes radical retropubic prostatectomy. Following induction of general anesthesia, his blood pressure is 128/80 mm Hg. The procedure is uneventful until the surgeon mobilizes the prostate gland and separates the dorsal venous complex from the urethra. Bright red blood instantly fills the operative field, and the patient's blood pressure falls to 78/50 mm Hg. During the next 30 minutes, the patient loses 4500 mL of blood and requires transfusion of 3 units of packed red blood cells. The remainder of the case is uneventful.

PROBLEM ANALYSIS

Definition

The term *radical* refers to extensive operations directed at the extirpation of a morbid process. In urology it is used to differentiate a cancer operation from a simple operation for benign disease. Commonly performed radical urologic procedures are radical prostatectomy, radical cystectomy, radical nephrectomy, and radical surgery for testicular cancer.

- Radical prostatectomy involves the en bloc surgical removal of the entire prostate gland, the seminal vesicles, the ejaculatory ducts, and a portion of the bladder neck.
- Radical cystectomy in males (cystoprostatectomy) involves en bloc removal of the bladder, prostate gland, lower ureters, vas deferens, seminal vesicles, and pelvic lymph nodes. Radical cystectomy in females involves removal of the bladder, urethra, uterus, fallopian tubes, ovaries, anterior vaginal wall, and pelvic lymph nodes. After cystectomy, either an ileal conduit or a bladder substitution procedure is performed for urinary diversion.
- Radical nephrectomy involves preliminary ligation of the renal artery and vein, followed by removal of the kidney, adrenal gland, and perinephric fat outside of the surrounding (Gerota's) fascia.
- Retroperitoneal lymph node dissection is performed for the staging of testicular cancers.

The most common operative complication during radical urologic procedures is hemorrhage. Other intraoperative complications include respiratory abnormalities, air embolism, nerve injury, and thromboembolic events.

Recognition

HEMORRHAGE

Extensive bleeding can occur if one of the branches of the hypogastric veins is inadvertently lacerated during pelvic lymphadenectomy with radical prostatectomy or cystectomy. The venous drainage of the prostate is into Santorini's plexus (Fig. 211-1). Hemorrhage is common during transection of this dorsal venous complex during radical prostatectomy or cystectomy. During radical nephrectomy or retroperitoneal lymph node dissection, hemorrhage can occur if extensive retroperitoneal dissection is necessary or if the inferior vena cava or its tributaries are damaged.

Because the bleeding during radical urologic surgery is mainly venous in nature, positive end-expiratory pressure should be avoided during mechanical ventilation; this has been shown to increase venous pressure and probably increases intraoperative bleeding. This complication is recognized by direct observation of blood loss and signs of hypovolemia, including tachycardia, hypotension, and a decrease in central venous or pulmonary artery wedge pressure.

RESPIRATORY ABNORMALITIES

General anesthesia causes major alterations in ventilation, and the positions required for radical urologic surgery can aggravate these changes. During radical retropubic prostatectomy and cystectomy, the patient is supine but in the Trendelenburg (head-down) position to facilitate surgical exposure. This position increases the work of breathing and promotes the development of atelectasis because the abdominal contents rest on the diaphragm. Other ventilatory changes with the Trendelenburg position include reduced pulmonary compliance and lung volumes, as well as an increased incidence of endobronchial intubation.

During radical nephrectomy, patients are positioned in a lateral decubitus ("kidney") position, with the spine flexed and the kidney rest elevated. This position produces a decrease in thoracic compliance, tidal volume, vital capacity, and functional residual capacity. Altered ventilatory function is recognized by hypoxemia, hypercarbia, or reduced lung compliance. Most patients require general anesthesia and controlled ventilation because this position imposes severe restrictions on ventilation that predispose to the development of atelectasis in the dependent lung. During radical nephrectomy, pneumothorax can occur. To identify pleural tears, the surgeon fills the wound with saline while the anesthetist hyperinflates the lungs. Auscultation reveals diminished or

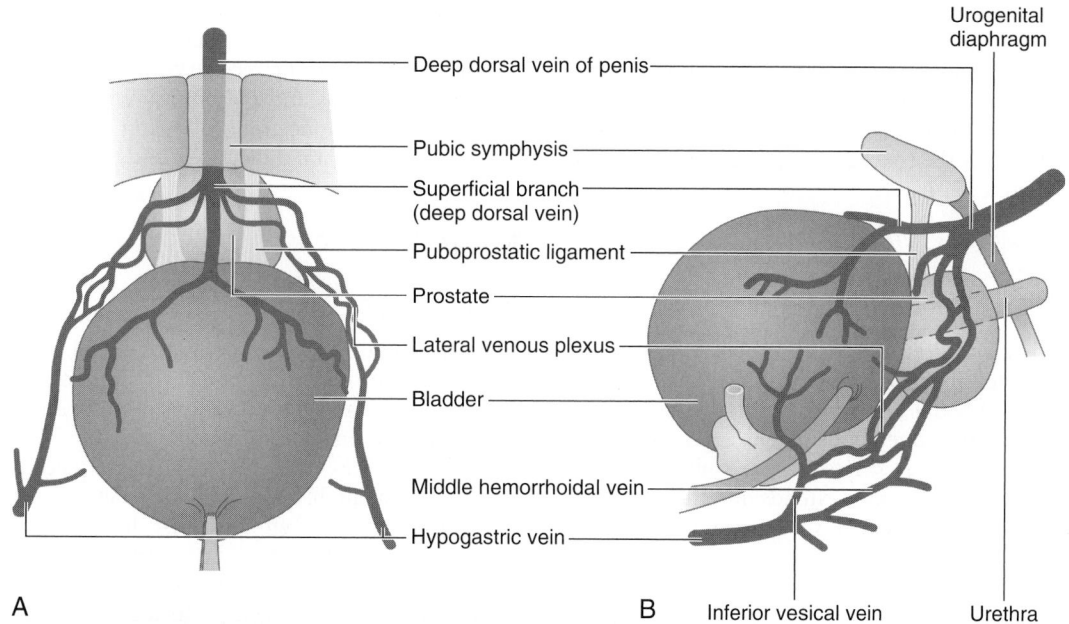

Figure 211–1 ■ The prostatic vein drains into Santorini's plexus, which receives blood from the penis, prostate, bladder, and seminal vesicles. This plexus also communicates with the pubic, pudendal, deep epigastric, obturator, and hemorrhoidal veins. (From Reiner WG, Walsh PC: An anatomical approach to the surgical management of the dorsal vein and Santorini's plexus during radical retropubic surgery. J Urol 121:198-200, 1979.)

absent breath sounds with pneumothorax or atelectasis. A chest radiograph confirms these findings.

Bleomycin is a chemotherapeutic agent that is often used to treat testicular carcinoma before retroperitoneal lymph node dissection (see Table 30-1). Its use is associated with pulmonary toxicity, and there are numerous reports of postoperative respiratory failure after retroperitoneal lymph node dissection in these patients. Respiratory problems usually begin 3 to 10 days after surgery. Although intraoperative exposure to hyperoxia (inspired oxygen concentrations >30%) has been linked to postoperative pulmonary toxicity, the relationship is controversial. A retrospective study found that intravenous (IV) fluid management, especially red blood cell transfusion, was the most significant factor associated with postoperative respiratory failure. It is now recommended that IV fluid administration consist primarily of colloids and be limited to the minimum volume necessary to maintain hemodynamic stability and renal perfusion.

CIRCULATORY ABNORMALITIES

Hypotension and tachycardia can occur with acute hemorrhage during any of the radical urologic procedures. During radical nephrectomy, it is also common to see an acute decrease in blood pressure when the kidney rest is elevated during positioning. In 5% to 10% of patients undergoing radical nephrectomy, the tumor extends into the inferior vena cava and right atrium. With or without such extension, tumor may embolize into the proximal vena cava, right atrium, and pulmonary artery during the procedure to impede right heart outflow, reduce venous return to the left

heart, and compromise systemic circulatory dynamics. If the tumor occludes the vena cava or right atrium, it can block right heart output and cause acute cardiovascular collapse. Cardiopulmonary bypass may be required to prevent tumor embolization during surgery in patients at high risk for such adverse cardiovascular events.

AIR EMBOLISM

With either the Trendelenburg or the kidney position, the surgical field is above the level of the heart, creating a negative pressure gradient between the wound and the heart. Air embolism can occur if Santorini's venous plexus (see Fig. 211-1) is opened while the patient is in a head-down position during radical prostatectomy or cystoprostatectomy or if the vena cava is entered during radical nephrectomy. The most sensitive monitors for the detection of air embolism are transesophageal echocardiography and precordial Doppler. However, these are rarely used during urologic surgery. There may be a decrease in end-tidal carbon dioxide or an increase in end-tidal nitrogen with significant air embolism. Physical findings consistent with air embolism include sudden hypotension, hypoxemia, arrhythmia, and the presence of a mill-wheel murmur. If a large embolism creates an airlock that blocks outflow from the right side of the heart, cardiovascular collapse will occur.

NERVE INJURY

Damage to the obturator nerve can occur due to retractor placement or transection during pelvic lymph node dissection in radical retropubic prostatectomy or cystectomy.

During perineal prostatectomy, the exaggerated lithotomy position is used, and damage to the brachial plexus can occur if shoulder braces are improperly placed. Injury to the brachial plexus is also possible during surgery performed in the kidney position if the lower shoulder and upper arm remain directly under the rib cage. Peripheral nerve injury is discussed in Chapter 221.

THROMBOEMBOLISM

Patients undergoing radical pelvic surgery, particularly radical prostatectomy and radical cystectomy, are at high risk for developing pelvic and deep venous thrombosis. Pulmonary emboli are reported in up to 5% of patients; however, the incidence varies with the sensitivity of the diagnostic test chosen to detect thromboembolism. During resection of renal tumors, there is a high risk for tumor embolism to the lungs, especially when the tumor extends into the vena cava. Thromboembolism is discussed further in Chapters 89 and 216.

Risk Assessment

HEMORRHAGE

During radical prostatectomy and cystoprostatectomy, severe hemorrhage is more likely in patients who have had previous transurethral prostate resection or multiple prostatic biopsies. This is because the dorsal venous complex can become adherent to the anterior surface of the prostate. A large prostate gland and prior pelvic irradiation or surgery are also associated with increased operative blood loss. In patients undergoing radical nephrectomy, the risk of hemorrhage or tumor embolism is greatly increased if the tumor invades the inferior vena cava or extends into the right atrium.

RESPIRATORY ABNORMALITIES

The risk of surgically induced pneumothorax during radical nephrectomy is increased with a large kidney, thoracic approach, or resection of the 12th rib for better exposure.

NERVE INJURY

Peripheral nerve injuries are common if improper positioning results in compression or stretching of a nerve. Overzealous surgical manipulation or retraction may traumatize nerves. Patients with preexisting diseases such as diabetes mellitus, hypertension, and arteriosclerosis are more prone to peripheral nerve injury.

THROMBOEMBOLISM

Thromboembolic events are common in all patients undergoing radical pelvic surgery for carcinoma.

Implications

Hemorrhage and air embolism can result in cardiovascular collapse and death if they are not detected and treated promptly. Position-related nerve injuries are often neurapraxic; that is, localized myelin degeneration may occur at the injury site, but without axonal degeneration. Therefore, recovery

usually occurs within 6 weeks. However, if the nerve is severed or the injury is severe, permanent sensory and motor deficits could occur, or recovery might take months. Deep venous thrombosis and pulmonary embolism are frequent postoperative complications following radical pelvic surgery, and they may be fatal if diagnosis and treatment are delayed.

MANAGEMENT

Hemorrhage

Extensive blood loss is anticipated in all radical urologic procedures. In high-risk or elderly patients, direct arterial blood pressure and central venous monitoring may facilitate early recognition and treatment of acute blood loss, and several large-bore catheters should be placed for venous access. Persistent bleeding can be managed by temporary packing if surgical efforts must be directed elsewhere. Hemorrhage must be treated promptly with blood products, volume expansion, and vasopressors as needed to maintain cardiac filling and systemic perfusion.

Respiratory Abnormalities

Respiratory alterations and work of breathing are best managed with endotracheal intubation and controlled positive-pressure ventilation during the perioperative period. Small pleural injuries during radical nephrectomy can be repaired surgically. A chest tube is required to treat a tension pneumothorax of 10% or greater.

Air Embolism

If air embolism occurs, the patient is ventilated with 100% oxygen. If cardiovascular collapse ensues, cardiopulmonary resuscitation is instituted immediately, and the patient is placed in the head-down, left lateral decubitus position to allow air trapped in the pulmonary outflow tract to float back into the right side of the heart. Aspiration of air from the right side of the heart may be attempted if a central line is in place.

Nerve Injury

An initial neurologic examination is performed to document the extent of all peripheral nerve injuries. Nerve injuries that persist for longer than 2 weeks after surgery should be evaluated with electromyography and nerve conduction studies.

Thromboembolism

Pulmonary embolism is treated with systemic anticoagulation using a continuous heparin infusion as soon as surgical bleeding is controlled. Heparin is continued for 7 to 10 days while oral anticoagulation therapy is initiated. Anticoagulation therapy should be continued for 3 months postoperatively.

PREVENTION

Measures to prevent complications of radical urologic surgery are summarized in Table 211-1.

Table 211–1 ■ Prevention of Complications of Radical Urologic Surgery
Hemorrhage
Meticulous surgical technique
Respiratory Abnormalities
Endotracheal intubation
Positive-pressure ventilation
Frequent auscultation of lungs
Nerve Injury
Padding of pressure points
Pillows under feet, ankles, and knees
Padding between operating table and rib cage*
Avoidance of shoulder braces
Thromboembolism
Compression stockings
Early ambulation

*In the lateral decubitus position, padding prevents compression of nerves and blood vessels in the axilla.

Hemorrhage

Intraoperative bleeding is minimized during radical urologic surgery by meticulous attention to surgical technique.

Respiratory Abnormalities

Endotracheal intubation and positive-pressure ventilation help reduce the risk of ventilatory abnormalities. Periodic auscultation of the lungs after positioning the patient and during the surgical procedure can verify optimal pulmonary ventilation.

Nerve Injury

All pressure points should be padded, and the patient should be moved with care during positioning and transport. Foam should be used under bony prominences, and pillows should be routinely placed under the feet, ankles, and knees. If the lateral kidney position is used, a small pad should be placed between the operating table and the dependent thorax to prevent brachial plexus injury. Shoulder braces are usually not necessary, except with the extreme lithotomy position. If this position is required, care must be taken to place the shoulder braces over the acromial processes to prevent brachial plexus injury.

Thromboembolism

For operations on a right-sided renal tumor in the lateral kidney position, placing the patient in a steep Trendelenburg position should help prevent fatal air embolism, because air entering the vena cava cannot easily pass to the heart. Compression stockings should be used intraoperatively, and patients should ambulate on the first postoperative day to prevent thromboembolic events.

Further Reading

Malhotra V, Sudheendra V, Diwan S: Anesthesia and the renal and genitourinary systems. In Miller RD (ed): Miller's Anesthesia, 6th ed. Philadelphia, Churchill Livingstone, 2005, pp 2175-2207.

Monk TG: Cancer of the prostate and radical prostatectomy. In Malhotra V (ed): Anesthesia for Renal and Genitourologic Surgery. New York, McGraw-Hill, 1996, pp 177-195.

O'Hara JF, Cywinski JB, Monk TG: The renal system and anesthesia for urologic surgery. In Barash PG, Cullen BF, Stoelting RK (eds): Clinical Anesthesia, 5th ed. Philadelphia, JB Lippincott–Williams & Wilkins, 2005.

Prentice JA, Martin JT: The Trendelenburg position: Anesthesiologic considerations. In Martin JT (ed): Positioning in Anesthesia and Surgery. Philadelphia, WB Saunders, 1987, pp 127-145.

Shah N: Radical cystectomy, radical nephrectomy, and retroperitoneal lymph node dissection. In Malhotra V (ed): Anesthesia for Renal and Genitourologic Surgery. New York, McGraw-Hill, 1996, pp 197-226.

Smith RB: Complications of renal surgery. In Smith RB, Ehrlich RM (eds): Complications of Urologic Surgery, 2nd ed. Philadelphia, WB Saunders, 1990, pp 128-159.

Welborn SG: Unusual positions—urology: Anesthesiologic considerations. In Martin JT (ed): Positioning in Anesthesia and Surgery. Philadelphia. WB Saunders, 1987, pp 249-254.

Complications of Lithotripsy

Jerome F. O'Hara, Jr.

Case Synopsis

A 78-year-old woman with a history of severe coronary artery disease underwent extracorporeal shock wave lithotripsy with general anesthesia. Ten minutes after placement in the water bath, the patient's heart rate increased from 78 to 138 beats per minute, and pink frothy fluid was noted in the endotracheal tube. The patient was removed from the water bath, and an immediate chest radiograph revealed congestive heart failure.

PROBLEM ANALYSIS

Definition

Extracorporeal shock wave lithotripsy (ESWL) is accomplished by the transmission of shock waves through the patient's body to pulverize urinary calculi. Unlike second-generation lithotriptors, first-generation units require that the patient be immersed in a water bath (Fig. 212-1). In addition to anesthetic risks, this unique environment exposes patients to potential complications from water immersion and the release of energy by the shock waves.

During ESWL, a mechanically generated shock wave passes through water as a single pressure impulse. On reaching the patient, the wave passes through the patient's tissues en route to the "target zone," which is defined as the area that contains the calculus (Fig. 212-2). Fluoroscopy is used to confirm that the urinary calculi remain in the target zone. When the shock wave encounters a different density, such

as the urinary calculus, it releases energy to fragment the calculus into sandlike particles, which is the desired therapeutic effect. However, damage to other tissues or implanted mechanical devices can occur. To prevent cardiac arrhythmias, the lithotriptor can be synchronized to trigger the shock wave during the refractory period of the patient's cardiac cycle. In certain patients, hydrostatic pressure created by immersion can significantly compromise cardiovascular and pulmonary function.

Recognition

Undesirable effects of the shock wave energy include the following:

- Cardiovascular instability from atrial or ventricular arrhythmias
- Potential damage to and malfunction of a pacemaker or implantable cardioverter-defibrillator
- Hypotension from perirenal or intra-abdominal bleeding

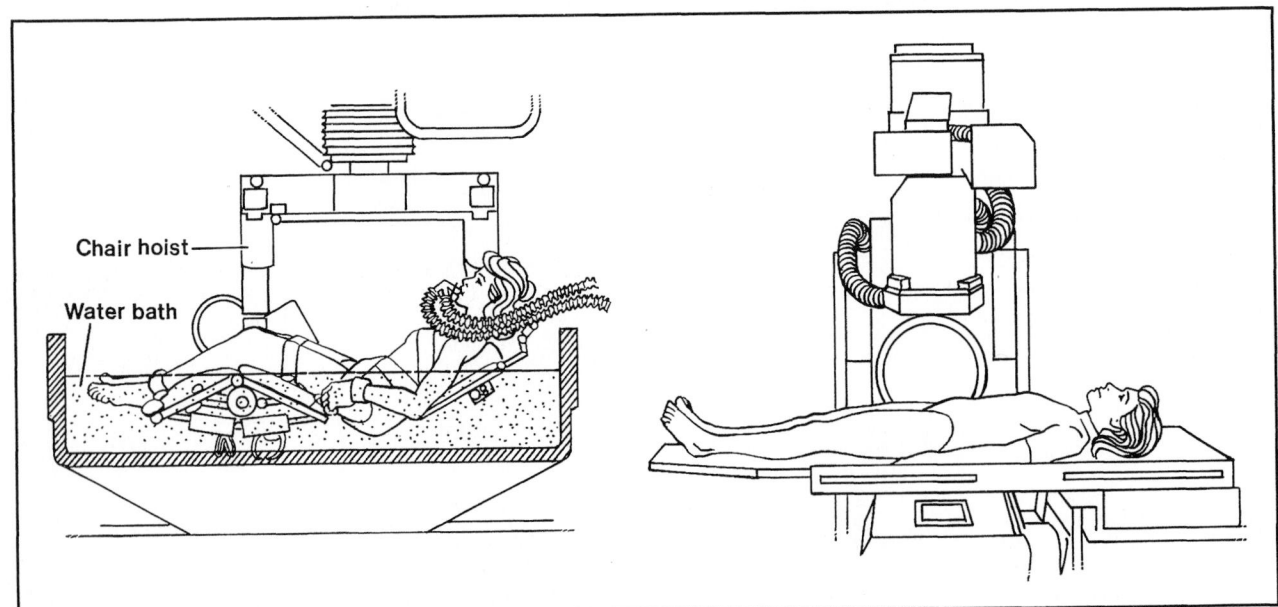

Figure 212–1 ■ First-generation lithotriptor with the patient in a chair hoist, immersed in the water bath *(left)*. Newer, second-generation lithotriptor *(right)*.

Figure 212–2 ■ Illustration of how the shock wave is generated and then delivered to the renal calculi.

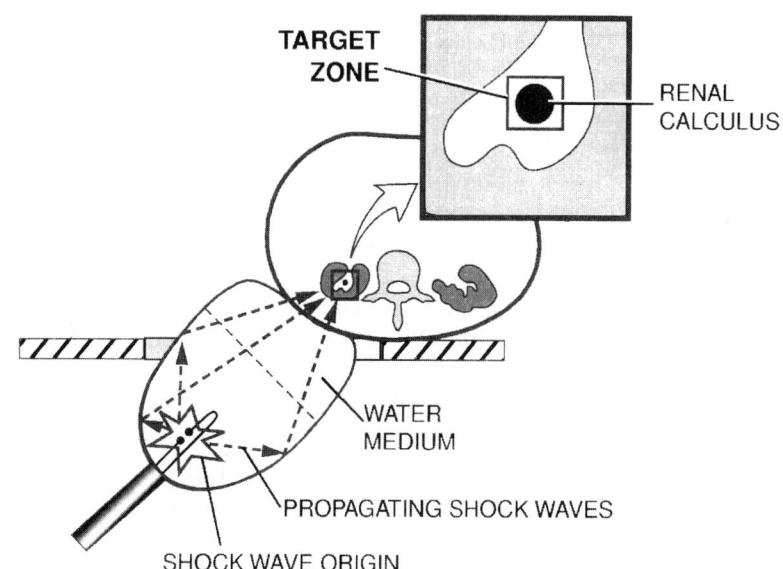

- Skin petechiae and painful ecchymoses, especially in thin patients
- Patient discomfort and movement from inadequate analgesia

Undesirable effects during immersion lithotripsy include the following:

- Nerve and musculoskeletal injury from pressure points associated with use of the hoist chair
- Hyperthermia or hypothermia caused by the temperature of the water bath
- Relative inaccessibility of the patient's airway
- Cardiovascular and pulmonary changes (Table 212-1)

Risk Assessment

If the shock wave is misdirected or encounters tissue other than the urinary calculi, energy may be released and injure the patient. Such injuries include the following:

- Pulmonary contusion and hemoptysis, especially in children, because the lung base and kidney are in close proximity

- Neurologic damage if air is introduced into the epidural space during administration of epidural anesthesia
- Possible damage to and rupture of a calcified aortic or renal artery aneurysm

Cardiovascular and pulmonary changes associated with water immersion can lead to serious complications in some patients. For example, acute congestive heart failure can occur in patients with severe ventricular dysfunction. Patients with significant chronic obstructive pulmonary disease may not be able to maintain adequate ventilation under regional anesthesia. Absolute and relative contraindications to ESWL are listed in Table 212-2.

Implications

To avoid complications that can arise during ESWL, the anesthesiologist must understand the physics of shock wave generation and delivery to the patient. Certain risks need to be considered during the preoperative evaluation of a patient who requires an anesthetic for this elective procedure.

Table 212–1 ■ Cardiopulmonary Changes on Immersion during Lithotripsy		
System	**Variable**	**Direction of Change**
Cardiovascular	Central blood volume	Increased
	Central venous pressure	Increased
	Pulmonary artery pressure	Increased
Respiratory	Pulmonary blood flow	Increased
	Vital capacity	Decreased
	Functional residual capacity	Decreased
	Tidal volume	Decreased
	Respiratory rate	Increased

Modified from Malhotra V: Anesthesia and the renal and genitourinary systems. In Miller RD (ed): Anesthesia. New York, Churchill Livingstone, 1994, p 1961.

Table 212–2 ■ Contraindications to Extracorporeal Shock Wave Lithotripsy
Absolute Contraindications
Obstruction distal to renal calculi
Bleeding disorder or anticoagulation
Pregnancy
Relative Contraindications
Large calcified aortic or renal artery aneurysm
Untreated urinary tract infection
Pacemaker or implantable cardioverter-defibrillator
Morbid obesity

MANAGEMENT

The choice of anesthesia depends on the type of lithotriptor and the anesthesiologist's preference. High-energy shock waves (>18 kV) usually require general or regional anesthesia, whereas low-energy shock waves (<18 kV) often require only intravenous sedation.

The advantage of general anesthesia is the ability to secure the airway with endotracheal intubation and to deliver smaller, more consistent tidal volumes. Small, consistent volumes minimize the displacement of renal or ureteral calculi, ensuring that they remain within the target zone. Regional anesthesia allows the patient to participate in positioning within the chair hoist and permits easier patient transport if an additional urologic procedure is needed at a different location. A T4-T6 sensory block is required with spinal or epidural anesthesia. Potential disadvantages of regional anesthesia include the following:

- Time required to establish anesthesia
- Altered respiratory dynamics
- Potential for inadequate sensory block
- Inability to redose after a single-dose injection

Regardless of the anesthetic used, recovery from ESWL involves mainly recovery from the effects of anesthesia. Thus, ESWL should be approached as an outpatient procedure. Patients with cardiopulmonary disease need to be identified and their increased risk of immersion-related complications understood. Although invasive monitoring may be required for a patient who has substantial cardiopulmonary compromise, controlling the speed and depth of immersion is equally important. To prevent crush, pressure, brachial plexus, or neck injuries during anesthesia, proper positioning and padding are required, especially if a water bath is used.

Certain patients scheduled for ESWL require the following specific considerations:

- Pediatric patients usually receive general anesthesia so that their movements can be controlled during the procedure. Styrofoam padding is used to protect the lower lung fields from the shock waves.
- Paraplegic patients require anesthesia because of the risk of autonomic hyperreflexia.
- Morbidly obese patients can exceed the mechanical capacity of the lithotriptor to support or properly position them. This must be evaluated before the induction of anesthesia.
- Patients with cardiac rhythm management devices (CRMDs)—that is, pacemakers or internal cardioverter-defibrillators (see Chapter 97)—can safely undergo ESWL, but changes in programmed parameters may occur. The following steps should be taken:
  - It is advisable to turn off the programmed adaptive-rate response in patients with CRMDs.
  - An internal cardioverter-defibrillator must be deactivated and shielded with Styrofoam to protect it from the shock waves, and the device should be interrogated after the procedure. This applies to pacemakers as well.
  - The indication for the CRMD must be known so that the team is prepared to treat arrhythmias, especially if some CRMD therapies (e.g., tachyarrhythmias) have been turned off. If so, temporary pacing capability and an external cardioverter-defibrillator must be available.
  - Preprocedure and postprocedure pulse generator functions must be confirmed when treating a patient who has an implantable CRMD.

PREVENTION

The anesthesiologist must identify patients at risk for ESWL-related complications and vigilantly monitor the patient's position and hemodynamic changes during ESWL, especially during water bath immersion and on the initiation of shock wave therapy. It is advisable to establish and rehearse a plan of action for gaining airway access or treating cardiac arrest in patients who are immersed. An emergency protocol to facilitate the transfer of a patient with cardiac instability from a freestanding or mobile ESWL unit to a critical care setting should also be in place.

Further Reading

American Society of Anesthesiologists Task Force on Perioperative Management of Patients with Cardiac Rhythm Management Devices: Practice advisory for the perioperative management of patients with cardiac rhythm management devices: Pacemakers and implantable cardioverter-defibrillators. Anesthesiology 103:186-198, 2005.

Chung MK, Streem SB, Ching E, et al: Effects of extracorporeal shock wave lithotripsy on tiered therapy implantable cardioverter defibrillators. Pacing Clin Electrophysiol 22:738-742, 1999.

Drach GW, Weber C, Donovan JM: Treatment of pacemaker patients with extracorporeal shock wave lithotripsy: Experience from 2 continents. J Urol 143:895-896, 1990.

Liguori G, Trombetta C, Bucci S, et al: Reversible acute renal failure after unilateral extracorporeal shock-wave lithotripsy. Urol Res 32:25-27, 2004.

Monk TG, Weldon BC: The renal system and anesthesia for urologic surgery. In Barash PG, Cullen BF, Stoelting RK (eds): Clinical Anesthesia, 4th ed. Philadelphia, JB Lippincott–Williams & Wilkins, 2001, pp 1022-1025.

Morgan GE, Mikhail MS: Anesthesia for genitourinary surgery. In Morgan GE, Mikhail MS (eds): Clinical Anesthesiology. Stamford, Conn, Appleton & Lange, 1996, pp 601-610.

Saberski LR, Kondamuri S, Osinubi OY: Identification of the epidural space: Is loss of resistance to air a safe technique? Reg Anesth 22:3-15, 1997.

Stowe DF, Bernstein JS, Madsen KE, et al: Autonomic hyperreflexia in spinal cord injured patients during extracorporeal shock wave lithotripsy. Anesth Analg 68:788-791, 1989.

Vasavada SP, Streem SB, Kottke-Marchant K, et al: Pathological effects of extracorporeally generated shock waves on calcified aortic aneurysm tissue. J Urol 152:45-48, 1994.

Autonomic Dysreflexia

213

David L. McDonagh

Case Synopsis

A 35-year-old woman with spinal cord transection at T1 sustained in a motorcycle accident is scheduled for elective breast surgery. In the preoperative holding area she feels anxious and has a pounding headache, facial flushing, and hypertension (163/100 mm Hg). Her admission blood pressure was 92/58 mm Hg.

PROBLEM ANALYSIS

Definition

Autonomic dysreflexia or hyperreflexia (see also Chapter 114) is a syndrome of episodic autonomic hyperactivity in the setting of spinal cord injury. The syndrome is more common in complete spinal cord injuries, with no sensation or motor function below the level of the lesion. Lesions at or above T6 (above the splanchnic sympathetic outflow) put a patient at risk for this problem; lesions below T6 rarely cause the syndrome. A variety of noxious stimuli below the level of the spinal cord lesion can result in an afferent volley of neural input to the spinal cord and unchecked reflex efferent sympathetic outflow. This sympathetic outflow would normally be suppressed by supraspinal, descending inhibition, but connection to the brain no longer exists. The result is an unchecked vasopressor response that results in hypertension (sometimes severe), along with other symptoms described below.

Recognition

In 1860 Hilton first described a quadriplegic patient with episodes of autonomic dysreflexia. Symptoms include anxiety, throbbing headache, facial flushing, blurred vision, nausea, and nasal congestion. Muscle spasms can also occur. On physical examination, signs include hypertension and usually, but not always, reflex bradycardia (Table 213-1). Below the level of the spinal cord injury, where sympathetic outflow predominates, the skin is typically cool, and there is piloerection. Above the level of the injury, where a parasympathetic counterregulatory response predominates, the skin is warm, flushed, and diaphoretic. Hypertension is invariably present but is not necessarily extreme. These patients may have low normal blood pressure (≤120/80 mm Hg) at rest,[1] but with stimulation, they may become symptomatic. Blood pressure may increase into what is typically considered the high normal range (>120/80 mm Hg) or stage 1 hypertension (>140/90 but <160/110 mm Hg), although severe (stage 2) hypertension (≥160/110 mm Hg) can be present.

Risk Assessment

All patients with spinal cord injury at or above T6 should be considered at risk for autonomic dysreflexia. The overall incidence is greater than 50%, and men are more commonly affected than women. Those with complete spinal cord injuries are at the highest risk. The syndrome can be seen following the initial injury, after spinal shock resolves. Patients with a history of previously diagnosed autonomic dysreflexia or a history of compatible symptoms should be managed with vigilance. Recent symptoms should prompt a search for any inciting causes (Table 213-2). The most common causes are bladder distention, urinary retention, and fecal impaction. A variety of noxious stimuli below the level of the spinal cord lesion (i.e., in the area of sensory loss) can provoke autonomic dysreflexia. Keep in mind that any surgical procedures or other stimulation below the spinal cord lesion may provoke autonomic dysreflexia, even though the patient may not have sensation in that body part.

---

[1]As defined in the JNC 7 report; see Further Reading.

Table 213–1 ■ Signs and Symptoms of Autonomic Dysreflexia

Hypertension	Anxiety
Bradycardia	Convulsions
Arrhythmias	Loss of consciousness
Visceral and muscular spasms	Profuse sweating
Piloerection	Facial tingling
Pallor or flushing	Blurred vision
Nasal obstruction	Shortness of breath
Severe headache	Nausea and vomiting

Table 213–2 ■ Potential Inciting Causes of Autonomic Dysreflexia

Bladder distention or urinary retention
Fecal impaction, rectal examination
Surgery below level of spinal cord lesion
Uterine contraction, labor
Urologic procedures
Ingrown toenail
Intramuscular injection
Decubitus ulcers
Hemorrhoids
Acute abdominal processes
Skin irritation
Restrictive clothing

Implications

Severe hypertension is the primary insult in autonomic dysreflexia. If it is uncontrolled, sustained hypertension can result in end-organ injury—a hypertensive emergency.[2] The main concerns are seizure, hemorrhagic stroke, subarachnoid hemorrhage from aneurysmal rupture, intraocular hemorrhage, arrhythmia, and myocardial strain leading to myocardial ischemia or infarction. The syndrome of autonomic hyperreflexia can be fatal on rare occasions.

MANAGEMENT

Management considerations include the following:

- Search for the inciting cause
- Upright or reverse Trendelenburg positioning
- Treatment of the underlying cause
- Choice of anesthetic
- Appropriate intra- and postoperative monitoring
- Vasodilator drugs
- Vasopressors and intravenous fluids
- Deepening of general anesthesia
- Postponement of an elective case

Most commonly, bladder distention, urinary retention, or fecal impaction promotes this problem. Intraoperatively, surgical stimulation below the level of the spinal cord lesion may also be responsible. Be sure to consider and rule out similar syndromes, such as preeclampsia. Sitting the patient upright causes some orthostatic hypotension and should be the initial maneuver to correct hypertension. Initial treatment for the underlying cause includes bladder catheterization (or flushing of an indwelling catheter), followed by a rectal examination with fecal disimpaction if necessary.

The choice of anesthetic (regional or general) should be tailored to the surgical procedure and the needs of the patient. Spinal or epidural anesthesia is very effective for ablating the afferent neural activity that results in autonomic dysreflexia and should be used when appropriate. The possibility of provoking autonomic dysreflexia with injection of a local anesthetic for peripheral nerve block or skin infiltration should be kept in mind. Succinylcholine should be avoided in these patients owing to the risk for hyperkalemia.

For intra- and postoperative monitoring, consider arterial line placement in addition to the standard monitors. Have vasodilator drugs immediately available. Acute blood pressure reduction can be accomplished with a variety of agents. Intravenous labetalol, nicardipine, nitroglycerin, and nitroprusside are acceptable and can be given as a bolus or by continuous infusion. Have additional intravenous fluids and vasopressors (e.g., phenylephrine, ephedrine) ready to correct iatrogenic hypotension. Be prepared to quickly deepen the level of anesthesia if using a general anesthetic. Vasoactive drugs can then be administered if necessary. Finally, postpone an elective case if preoperative autonomic dysreflexia cannot be promptly evaluated and treated.

PREVENTION

General preventive measures are tailored to the inciting factor in a given patient. Regular urinary catheterization and laxative use to ensure regular bowel activity are commonly needed. Patients should be taught to recognize the symptoms, correct the problem if possible, and seek emergency medical care if needed. In the perioperative setting, adequate anesthesia and the appropriate medication to control blood pressure should be present before the delivery of any noxious stimuli, which include anesthetic or surgical procedures, intramuscular injections, opioid-induced urinary retention or constipation, or any other factor that may stimulate pain receptors below the level of the spinal cord lesion.

Further Reading

Blackmer J: Rehabilitation medicine. 1. Autonomic dysreflexia. CMAJ 169:931-935, 2003.

Campagnolo DI: Autonomic dysreflexia in spinal cord injury. eMedicine J 2004. Available at www.emedicine.com

Chobanian AV, Bakris GL, Black HR, et al: National Heart, Lung, and Blood Institute Joint National Committee on Prevention, Detection, Evaluation, and Treatment of High Blood Pressure. National High Blood Pressure Education Program Coordinating Committee. The Seventh Report of the Joint National Committee on Prevention, Detection, Evaluation, and Treatment of High Blood Pressure: The JNC 7 report. JAMA 289:2560-2572, 2003.

Consortium for Spinal Cord Medicine: Acute Management of Autonomic Dysreflexia: Individuals with Spinal Cord Injury Presenting to Health Care Facilities, 2nd ed. Washington, DC, Consortium, Paralyzed Veterans of America, 2001. Available at www.pva.org

Karlsson AK: Autonomic dysreflexia. Spinal Cord 37:383-391, 1999.

Kuczkowski KM: Peripartum anaesthetic management of a parturient with spinal cord injury and autonomic hyperreflexia. Anaesthesia 58: 823-824, 2003.

Moss J, Glick D: The autonomic nervous system. In Miller RD (ed): Miller's Anesthesia, 6th ed. Philadelphia, Churchill Livingstone, 2005, pp 617-677.

---

[2]Hypertensive crises include urgencies and emergencies. Both require an acute blood pressure elevation to 160/110 mm Hg or higher. However, with the former, there is no evidence of end-organ damage; with the latter, there is.

Complications of Deliberate Hypotension: Visual Loss

214

Aarti Sharma and Kerri M. Robertson

Case Synopsis

A 49-year-old man weighing 125 kg is scheduled for decompression laminectomy and instrumented fusion of the lumbar spine at multiple levels for lumbar stenosis. General anesthesia proceeds uneventfully with prone positioning, and the patient's face and eyes are protected from direct pressure with a foam headrest. Despite the use of deliberate hypotension, titrating the mean arterial pressure to 55 to 65 mm Hg with continuous intravenous sodium nitroprusside, the estimated blood loss is 2.3 L, and the lowest hematocrit reading is 25%. Somatosensory evoked potentials are monitored intraoperatively. The surgery lasts 8 hours. On postoperative day 2, the patient complains of bilateral visual loss.

PROBLEM ANALYSIS

Definition

Deliberate hypotension is a controlled lowering of blood pressure. In normotensives, it reduces systolic blood pressure (SBP) to 80 to 90 mm Hg and mean arterial pressure (MAP) to 50 to 70 mm Hg. Significant hypotension is SBP or MAP 40% or more below baseline. The goals of using deliberate hypotension during surgery are to reduce blood loss, improve operating conditions, decrease surgical time, and reduce the need for allergenic red blood cell transfusions when surgical blood loss is expected to be great. The efficacy of deliberate hypotension has been both confirmed and refuted in various studies.

Deliberate hypotension is used in neurovascular surgery, major orthopedic cases (e.g., total hip arthroplasty, complicated spinal surgery), surgery on large vascular tumors, head and neck surgery, and a variety of plastic surgeries, as well as in patients who refuse blood products. In most cases, deliberate hypotension is attained with continuous infusions of vasodilators (with or without β-blockers) or by increasing the inspired concentration of volatile anesthetic. Continuous positive airway pressure is sometimes used to reduce venous return. Techniques and agents used to achieve deliberate hypotension include the following:

- Direct-acting vasodilating drugs (sodium nitroprusside, nitroglycerin, hydralazine)[1]
- β-Adrenergic receptor blockers (metoprolol, esmolol)
- Spinal and epidural anesthesia
- Deepening of anesthesia with volatile anesthetic agents (isoflurane, sevoflurane)
- Autonomic ganglion-blocking drugs (trimethaphan)
- α-Adrenergic receptor blockers (phentolamine)
- Combined α- and β-adrenergic receptor blockers (labetalol)
- Calcium channel blockers (nicardipine)
- Prostaglandin E_1
- Continuous positive airway pressure

Recognition

Deliberate hypotension reduces SBP primarily by vasodilatation. This can be selective arterial dilatation (to reduce systemic vascular resistance and afterload) or venous dilatation (to reduce venous return, preload, and cardiac output). However, when using deliberate hypotension, it must be remembered that oxygen (O_2) delivery is determined by cardiac output, hemoglobin (Hb) concentration, and O_2 saturation:

$$O_2 \text{ delivery (mL } O_2/\text{min)} = \text{Cardiac output (L/min)} \times$$
$$\text{Hb concentration (g/L)} \times 1.31 \text{ (mL } O_2/\text{g Hb)} \times$$
$$\% O_2 \text{ saturation}$$

Although deliberate hypotension may be safe when used at relatively high hemoglobin levels, little is known about its clinical safety when combined with acute normovolemic hemodilution or when a reduction in cardiac output limits O_2 delivery to tissues.

Postoperative visual loss associated with spinal surgery or hip arthroplasty is a risk for patients and a medicolegal issue for both surgeons and anesthesiologists. The American

---

[1]Arterial-selective vasodilators (e.g., hydralazine, nicardipine) may be a better choice for deliberate hypotension than a primary venous dilator (nitroglycerin) or a combined venous and arterial dilator (sodium nitroprusside). Sodium nitroprusside is also more likely to cause excess hypotension.

Society of Anesthesiologists (ASA) Closed Claims Project (www.asaclosedclaims.org) established the Postoperative Visual Loss Registry in 1999 in an attempt to identify risk factors in patients who develop visual deficits within 7 days after nonophthalmic surgery. Anemia (median estimated blood loss 2.3 L; hematocrit 25.5%) and venous congestion of the head and neck were factors that contributed to morbidity associated with prolonged hypotension, presumably due to a reduction in O_2 delivery to the optic nerve or visual cortex. Identified patient-related factors included middle age or elderly, morbid obesity, hypertension, a history of smoking, diabetes mellitus, and atherosclerosis.

Since the Food and Drug Administration approved the use of spinal interbody cages in 1996, spinal instrumentation has resulted in longer operative times and increased blood loss. Additional risk factors include fluid management, facial swelling, external globe compression, emboli, adverse drug effects, anatomic variations in optic nerve blood supply, vasculitis, and use of vasoconstrictors such as epinephrine. None of these factors has been causally linked to visual loss in randomized controlled trials or animal studies.

Ischemic optic neuropathy (ION) is the most frequently cited cause of postoperative visual loss associated with spinal surgery in prone patients. The estimated incidence is 1 in 500 cases. The differential diagnosis includes central retinal artery occlusion and cortical blindness. Preliminary results from the ASA database indicate that 81% of 53 spinal surgery patients were diagnosed with ION, but only 13% were diagnosed with central retinal artery occlusion.

Posterior ION is caused by ischemia of the posterior part of the optic nerve and is more common than anterior ION after spinal surgery. Patients present with visual acuity ranging from normal to no light perception or with optic nerve–related visual field defects. The latter may be central scotomata, peripheral narrowing, or defects affecting various quadrants of the eye. Further, these visual defects may be altitude related.

Early funduscopic examination in posterior ION is normal, but after about 5 to 6 weeks, the optic disks become pale from atrophy. The pupillary light reflex becomes delayed or absent. Both eyes were affected in more than 50% of the cases reported to the ASA registry. Some recovery occurred in 40% to 45% of patients, but vision rarely returned to baseline. Diagnostic studies include ophthalmic examination (visual acuity, intraocular pressure, color testing, visual fields, pupillary reflexes, funduscopy with pupillary dilatation), fluorescein fundus angiography, and optic nerve enhancement on magnetic resonance imaging. Computed tomography is not useful for the diagnosis of ION. Visual evoked potentials are useful before optic disk pallor is detectable but cannot be used as an intraoperative monitor of optic nerve function owing to the effects of general anesthesia (intravenous or volatile).

Risk Assessment

The precise incidence of complications associated with deliberate hypotension is difficult to determine. Mortality appears to be no different from that for all anesthetics (0.007% to 0.01%). Identifiable risk factors for postoperative visual disturbances include preoperative hypertension, smoking, diabetes, vascular disease, prone positioning, increased intraocular pressure, eyeball pressure points, intraoperative hypotension, prolonged surgical time, excessive surgical blood loss, anemia, disorders that result in increased blood viscosity, and structural factors related to optic nerve anatomy.

Spinal surgery patients with ION from the ASA database had large operative blood losses (median 2.3 L), long duration in the prone position (median 8 hours), hypotension (median lowest MAP was a 37% decrease below baseline), and moderate anemia (median hematocrit 25.5%). Venous congestion is also thought to play a significant role in the development of this devastating complication. Perfusion pressure of the optic nerve is dependent on the difference between the MAP and venous (or intracranial) pressures. Both intraocular pressure and intracranial pressure increase in the prone and Trendelenburg positions owing to venous engorgement of the head and neck and increased central venous pressure. Thus, MAP changes from baseline with deliberate hypotension during general anesthesia can significantly reduce optic nerve perfusion pressure. Vascularization of the retrobulbar portion of the optic nerve depends on pial vessels originating from distal branches of the ophthalmic artery. These pial vessels lack autoregulatory mechanisms and appear to be prone to ischemia with systemic hypotension. Of the first 23 cases analyzed in the ASA registry, there was significant hypotension in 52% of cases, with deliberate hypotension used in 42% of these. Thus, the effects of deliberate hypotension on various vascular beds can be quite complex.

The rationale for recommending a target MAP of 50 to 55 mm Hg with deliberate hypotension is that cerebral autoregulation in normal patients is still operative at this range. Otherwise (e.g., patients with chronic hypertension), MAP should be maintained within 20% of baseline for spinal surgery in prone patients, because a reduction in inflow with deliberate hypotension or an increase in venous congestion with the Trendelenburg position may cause a critical reduction in optic nerve perfusion pressure. Patients with conditions that affect cerebral autoregulation (e.g., hypertension, cerebrovascular disease, mass lesions) are at increased risk for ischemic injury with the use of deliberate hypotension.

Coronary blood flow depends on coronary perfusion pressure as well as the resistance to and duration of flow. The latter is determined by heart rate (i.e., time spent in diastole) and primarily affects the left ventricle. During deliberate hypotension, maintenance of an O_2 supply sufficient for the metabolic needs of the myocardium is of primary importance. The intact coronary circulation undergoes a high degree of pressure-flow autoregulation that is little disrupted by volatile anesthetic agents. However, progressive systemic hypotension gradually depletes the coronary vasodilatory reserve and reduces the heart's ability to cope with stress, which increases myocardial O_2 demand. Also, arterial hypotension obtained with vasodilators often leads to reflex tachycardia, and tachycardia increases myocardial metabolism and shortens diastole. Thus, myocardial perfusion (especially of the left ventricle) is jeopardized. The situation is even worse in patients with coronary artery disease, in whom the vasodilatory ability is diminished even at normal coronary perfusion pressures; thus, hypotension directly decreases myocardial perfusion in direct proportion to the amount of blood pressure reduction and is more likely to cause ischemia. Therefore, in patients with coronary artery disease, deliberate hypotension is undertaken only with pressing indications, and then only with stringent monitoring (e.g., pulmonary artery catheter or transesophageal echocardiography).

Implications

There are no adequate randomized, controlled trials showing measurable benefits of deliberate hypotension in prone patients undergoing spinal surgery. It is unclear whether reducing the MAP decreases bleeding to the same degree it does during hip surgery, given the significant effect of increased intra-abdominal pressure causing high venous backpressure. This reduces spinal cord blood flow and potentially increases venous bleeding. Small case series suggest reduced blood loss but no benefit in terms of shortening the operating time. High-risk orthopedic procedures with the potential for significant blood loss include multiple levels of instrumentation, redo spine operations, and surgery for specific conditions (e.g., Charcot joints, infection, vascular tumors).

It is difficult to understand the pathophysiology of postoperative blindness after spinal surgery because of its rarity and the lack of a homogeneous clinical presentation. Regardless of the surgical procedure, primary causes of postoperative visual loss include the following:

- Anterior or posterior ION (ischemia or edema resulting in compartment syndrome involving the optic nerve)
- Cortical blindness due to hypotension and emboli
- Central retinal artery occlusion from external globe compression

The incidence of significant visual complications after noncardiac surgery in patients receiving general or central neuraxial regional anesthesia is 1 in 118,783 (0.0008%). Visual changes may be reported between postoperative days 1 and 12, with 81% of cases noted by postoperative day 2. Patients often assume that their visual problems are part of the normal recovery process or that subtle changes in vision are due to their eyes being lubricated and taped shut during surgery. This is the reason for most delays in the diagnosis of ION.

Considering the many facets of deliberate hypotension, anesthesiologists must determine patient suitability. Patients with a history of cerebrovascular disease, renal insufficiency, liver dysfunction, severe peripheral claudication, hypovolemia, and severe anemia are not candidates for deliberate hypotension because their reserves for adequate organ perfusion are markedly diminished.

The use of invasive monitoring is based on the type and length of surgery; anticipated transfusion requirements; the need to measure central venous and arterial pressures; required blood sampling for hematocrit, serum electrolytes, glucose, and blood gases; and the extent to which the blood pressure needs to be lowered from baseline. Any specialized monitoring is selected on a case-by-case basis. This might include somatosensory evoked potentials, electroencephalogram, near-infrared spectroscopy, cerebral artery Doppler flow measurement, and tissue pH measurement.

MANAGEMENT

Postoperative visual loss is a devastating complication. Early consultation with an ophthalmologist is strongly advised for both diagnosis and treatment. Treatment is mainly supportive. The prognosis for visual recovery is generally poor in patients with ION. High-dose steroids, hyperbaric O_2 therapy, diuretics, mannitol, and ocular hypotensive agents have all been advocated, but with only variable success. Some clinicians advocate optic nerve fenestration for decompression with anterior ION. However, results of the Ischemic Optic Neuropathy Decompression Trial showed that surgical treatment had no efficacy. Subsequent complications of ION may include visual loss in the other eye and adverse side effects from long-term steroid use.

PREVENTION

Despite a better understanding of ION, the best means of preventing it remain unclear. The following considerations should be adopted in high-risk individuals:

- Balance the possible benefits of deliberate hypotensive anesthesia with the risk that it may contribute to complications in some patients. Establish a minimum SBP or MAP for each patient preoperatively, and do not allow the pressure to "drift" below that value.
- Aggressively replace intraoperative blood losses by using the cell saver or predonated autologous blood to maintain an adequate hematocrit.
- Consider antifibrinolytic agents to minimize blood loss.
- Stage the procedure and minimize the time the patient is in the prone position, especially for long procedures that require multiple surgical approaches.
- Avoid venous congestion of the head and neck by elevating the head, placing the head in a neutral position, and avoiding constrictive ties around the patient's neck.
- Use colloid rather than crystalloid. This has the potential to reduce the edema believed to be associated with optic nerve compression.
- Pay strict attention to eye protection during patient positioning (this applies to both surgeons and anesthesiologists). Perform and document eye checks often during the case.
- Unless absolutely required to suppress recurrences of life-threatening arrhythmias (see Chapters 12 and 79), avoid amiodarone because it has been implicated as a cause of ION.
- Monitor closely for visual deficits in the postanesthesia recovery room.
- Obtain early ophthalmology consultation when visual changes are identified.

Understanding the advantages and limitations of inducing deliberate hypotension permits its rational use. Integral to improving surgical success while minimizing complications are patient selection and use of the most appropriate technique, based on the type of surgery, the length of the procedure, and the need to reduce surgical blood loss. Lack of informed patient consent regarding the risk for visual loss with deliberate hypotension may place the anesthesiologist at medicolegal risk.

Further Reading

Alexandrakis G, Lam BL: Bilateral posterior ischemic optic neuropathy after spinal surgery. Am J Ophthalmol 127:354-355, 1999.

Dilger JA, Tetzlaff JE, Bell GR, et al: Ischaemic optic neuropathy after spinal fusion. Can J Anaesth 45:63-66, 1998.

Gardner JW: The control of bleeding during operation by induced hypotension. JAMA 132:572, 1946.

Katz DM, Trobe JD, Cornblath WT, Kline LB: Ischemic optic neuropathy after lumbar spine surgery. Arch Ophthalmol 112:925-931, 1994.

Lagerkranser M: Controlled hypotension in neurosurgery: Pro. J Neurosurg Anesth 3:150, 1991.

Myers MA, Hamilton SR, Bogosian AJ, et al: Visual loss as a complication of spine surgery: A review of 37 cases. Spine 22:1325-1329, 1997.

Roth S, Nunez R, Schreider BD: Unexplained visual loss after lumbar spinal fusion. J Neurosurg Anesthesiol 9:346-348, 1997.

Rucker JC, Biousse V, Newman NJ: Ischemic optic neuropathies. Curr Opin Neurol 17:27-35, 2004.

Toivonen J, Virtanen H, Kaukinen S: Labetalol attenuates the negative effects of deliberate hypotension induced by isoflurane. Acta Anaesthesiol Scand 36:84, 1992.

Warner ME, Warner MA, Garrity JA, et al: The frequency of perioperative vision loss. Anesth Analg 93:1417-1421, 2001.

Fat Embolism Syndrome

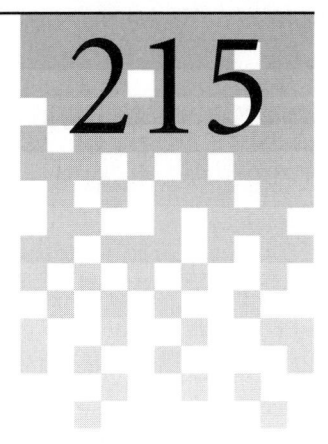

215

Jennifer T. Fortney

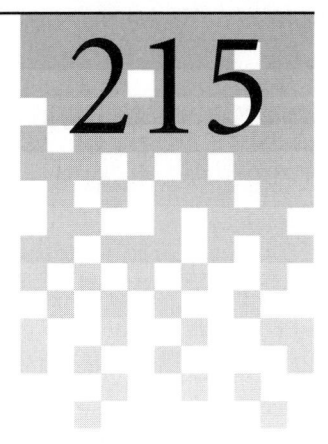

Case Synopsis

A 29-year-old man who has suffered fractures of the femur and tibia in a motorcycle accident is brought to the operating room for intramedullary nailing of both injuries. Surgery is unremarkable, but the patient is noted to have persistent tachycardia in the recovery room, despite adequate fluid resuscitation and pain control. The following morning, he is tachypneic and complains of significant shortness of breath. On examination, his pulse oximeter reading is 88% on room air, and he has a petechial rash on his chest and neck. A chest radiograph shows diffuse bilateral infiltrates.

PROBLEM ANALYSIS

Definition

Showering of fat emboli to the pulmonary and systemic circulations is common in trauma and orthopedic surgical patients. Many episodes result in subclinical symptoms, but an estimated 1% to 5% are associated with clinical symptoms severe enough to be termed fat embolism syndrome (FES) (Table 215-1).

Two theories exist concerning the cause of FES. The mechanical theory proposes that injuries of the long bones or the pelvis, and surgical maneuvers that increase intramedullary pressure, force large fat droplets into the systemic venous circulation. After embolizing to the right heart and lungs, they cause acute pulmonary hypertension. The contributing factors are mechanical obstruction of the pulmonary microcirculation and an increase in pulmonary vascular resistance. Lodged droplets induce localized ischemia and inflammation, with the release of proinflammatory mediators. Fat emboli may also gain access to the systemic arterial circulation through intracardiac shunts or by traversing the pulmonary capillary bed. Subsequent systemic manifestations include cerebral and cutaneous embolization and fat-induced acute lung injury.

The biochemical theory states that biochemical (specifically, hormonal) changes that occur with trauma and sepsis induce the systemic release of free fatty acids as chylomicrons. C-reactive protein and other phase reactants cause these chylomicrons to coalesce. Free fatty acids are directly toxic to pneumocytes and pulmonary capillary endothelium and produce interstitial hemorrhage and chemical pneumonitis. This theory is especially attractive when FES occurs in the absence of trauma.

Recognition

Fat embolism is primarily a clinical diagnosis. The diagnosis may be missed because of subclinical symptoms, a delay in onset of 24 to 72 hours, or the presence of additional traumatic injuries. Although a number of predisposing conditions are associated with FES (Table 215-2), a high index of suspicion is necessary to make the diagnosis based on the classic triad of a petechial rash associated with pulmonary and cerebral dysfunction.

Early persistent tachycardia may be the first sign of impending problems. Within 24 to 72 hours of the insult, patients may become tachypneic, dyspneic, and hypoxemic owing to ventilation-perfusion abnormalities. This lung injury pattern may progress to full-blown acute respiratory distress syndrome (ARDS). A reddish brown, nonpalpable petechial rash involving the head, neck, anterior thorax, and axillae appears in 20% to 50% of patients. This rash is easily missed because it resolves quickly. Emboli to the cerebral circulation may result in neurologic changes, including confusion, sedation, and coma. Retinal hemorrhages, with intra-arterial fat droplets, may be visible on funduscopic examination.

A fulminant form of FES is occasionally encountered in the operating room during joint replacement procedures.

Table 215–1 ■ Clinical Findings in Fat Embolism Syndrome

Cardiovascular
Persistent tachycardia (early finding)
Possible hypotension

Respiratory
Tachypnea
Dyspnea
Hypoxia
Hemoptysis

Cerebral
Delirium
Stupor
Seizures
Coma

Ophthalmic
Retinal hemorrhages with intra-arterial fat globules (may be seen on funduscopic examination)

Cutaneous
Petechial rash—nonpalpable; head, neck, anterior thorax, axillae (20%-50% of cases)
Hemorrhages and petechiae—both subconjunctival and oral possible

Other
Fever
Jaundice
Oliguria or anuria

Table 215–2 ▪ Predisposing Conditions Associated with Fat Embolism Syndrome

Trauma

Blunt trauma, especially to liver
Fractures—long bone or pelvic, multiple or closed fractures (incidence may be as high as 15%-20%)

Orthopedic Surgery

Joint replacement, especially revisions or bilateral procedures
Nonvented, intramedullary nailing
Femoral metastases

Tissue Manipulation

Bone marrow harvest or transplantation
Liposuction

Exogenous

Plastic surgery—fat injections
Total parenteral nutrition
Lymphography

Other

Hepatic failure
Alcoholism
Acute pancreatitis
Sickle cell crisis
Altitude sickness
Cardiopulmonary bypass
Burns

Table 215–3 ▪ Laboratory and Other Findings that Support but Do Not Establish the Diagnosis of Fat Embolism Syndrome

Hematologic

Thrombocytopenia: >50% decrease
Anemia: >20% decrease
Other: elevated erythrocyte sedimentation rate, hypofibrinogenemia, fat macroglobulinemia

Radiologic

Chest radiograph: diffuse bilateral infiltrates with "snowstorm" appearance, usually within 48 hr of clinical onset
Chest CT: may be normal, but parenchymal changes are consistent with acute lung injury; ARDS may be present
Head CT: usually negative, but may show diffuse white matter hemorrhages consistent with microvascular injury
MRI: scant data, but possible nonconfluent, hyperintense lesions on proton-density and T2-weighted images

Other

Lipase and phospholipase A_2 may be elevated
Increased pulmonary shunt fraction (without another identifiable cause)
Increased alveolar-to-arterial gradient (without another identifiable cause)
Urinalysis: stained fat globules (poor specificity)
Elevated pulmonary artery pressure (poor sensitivity)

ARDS, acute respiratory distress syndrome; CT, computed tomography; MRI, magnetic resonance imaging.

Large amounts of fat from the medullary cavity of long bones may be forced into the venous circulation over a short period. In patients with limited cardiac reserve, acute pulmonary hypertension may precipitate right ventricular failure with hypotension, bradycardia, hypoxemia, and cardiovascular collapse. In contrast to fulminant FES, the symptoms occurring with subacute FES are postulated to be secondary to the toxic effects of the free fatty acids that result from hydrolysis of the embolized fat droplets.

Laboratory and other diagnostic tests are nonspecific and not sufficiently sensitive to establish the diagnosis of FES, but they may add weight to the clinical findings (Table 215-3). The chest radiograph may reveal diffuse bilateral infiltrates with a "snowstorm" appearance. Computed tomography (CT) scans of the head may be normal or may show edema or nonspecific infarctions. Chest CT may also be normal, although changes consistent with lung contusion, acute lung injury, or ARDS may be present. In the absence of other lung pathology, an increase in the alveolar-to-arterial gradient is strongly suggestive of FES. Hematologic findings may include thrombocytopenia, anemia (thought to be secondary to intra-alveolar hemorrhage), fat macroglobulinemia from a pulmonary capillary blood sample, or a markedly elevated sedimentation rate. Lipase and phospholipase A_2 may be elevated within a few hours of the insult but can return to normal within 24 hours.

Risk Assessment

Orthopedic and trauma patients, especially those with lower extremity long bone and pelvic fractures, have a 20% incidence of fat embolism. Displaced fractures are considered a lower risk than nondisplaced ones, because displacement is thought to provide a "vent" for bone marrow fat, thus lessening the potential for intravasation. Patients with fractures of the middle and proximal parts of the femoral shaft are at increased risk, as are those with multiple fractures. Delayed stabilization (>24 hours) increases the risk for fat embolization. Young men constitute the largest at-risk group for FES owing to the high incidence of skeletal and multiple trauma in this group. The elderly make up the second largest patient group because of the prevalence of hip fractures, total joint replacement procedures, and underlying cardiopulmonary disease.

Intramedullary rod placement for closed or impending fractures has also been shown to increase the incidence of fat emboli. Joint replacement surgery, especially revisions or bilateral procedures, is associated with FES, as are femoral metastases and procedures that disrupt the adipose layer (liposuction) or bone marrow (harvest or transplantation). Case reports have also linked fat injections performed during cosmetic surgery with significant fat embolism.

The alcohol-induced fatty liver is capable of spontaneously releasing large numbers of embolus-sized fat globules when fatty cysts rupture into adjacent sinusoids and veins. Blunt trauma to the liver has also been associated with fat embolism. Some controversy exists over whether high-dose corticosteroids, which can increase the fat content of the liver, increase the risk for FES.

Implications

The mortality rate for FES may be as high as 5% to 15%, especially in elderly and debilitated patients. Mortality from fulminant FES is typically due to acute right ventricular failure with cardiovascular collapse. Respiratory failure is the most common cause of death in the subacute presentation of FES. Almost 90% of FES cases are associated with blunt trauma. Therefore, a high index of suspicion must be maintained when treating these patients. The majority of patients can be expected to recover from the pulmonary sequelae of FES with appropriate supportive care. Acute mental status changes often do not resolve immediately, even with improvement in oxygenation. This may take several days. However, long-term or permanent neurologic sequelae are occasionally seen in patients with visual disturbances or focal neurologic deficits.

MANAGEMENT

Treatment of FES is aimed at prevention of further fat dissemination, correction of hypoxemia, and hemodynamic stabilization. FES-induced acute lung injury requires supportive respiratory care to maximize oxygenation and ventilation, ensure airway protection, and prevent aspiration. This may require intubation, insertion of an arterial line for blood gas sampling, and mechanical ventilation of those patients with severe pulmonary compromise or altered mental status. Blood products, clotting factors, and platelets are administered to correct any coagulopathy in patients scheduled for surgery who are actively bleeding. Volume status may be critical, especially if right ventricular dysfunction is present; a central venous or pulmonary artery catheter may be useful in guiding fluid management. Inotropic support should be used, as needed, to maintain blood pressure, improve right ventricular output, and prevent ventricular ischemia. Prophylactic care aimed at preventing deep venous thrombosis and stress-related gastrointestinal bleeding is indicated. Surgical care for patients with long bone fractures should be aimed at stabilizing the fracture as early as possible.

Heparin use has been suggested because, in theory, it acts to clear lipids from the serum by stimulating lipase. However, the data are contradictory, and heparin has no clear role at this time. The role of corticosteroids in FES is less clear. They are thought to stabilize the capillary and alveolar membranes to prevent further damage to the lung. However, studies have obtained varying results. Also, the dose, optimal timing, and duration of therapy remain undetermined.

Management of fulminant FES, an acute life-threatening condition, requires advanced cardiac life support techniques.

PREVENTION

Because the majority of FES cases are associated with trauma, the rapid stabilization of fractures and correction of hypovolemia should be among the highest priorities for reducing the incidence of FES. If the patient is sufficiently stable to proceed to surgery, surgical fixation of fractures should occur within 24 hours of injury. Surgical techniques that may help reduce the volume of fat intravasation during intramedullary reaming, nailing, and prosthesis replacement include the following:

- Drilling a small hole in the distal bone to vent fat and marrow during surgery
- Use of an uncemented prosthesis for total hip arthroplasty
- Lavage of the canal after each reaming to remove debris and clots
- Use of fluted rods during total knee arthroplasty to allow marrow contents to exit into the knee
- Modification of reaming techniques (avoidance, or use of low driving speed or small-cored reamers)

Again, it is important to recognize which patients are at increased risk for FES (see Table 215-2). Optimizing the physical status of high-risk patients, rapidly stabilizing at-risk fractures, using techniques to reduce intraoperative fat embolization, and rapidly identifying and treating FES can help reduce the morbidity and mortality associated with this condition.

Further Reading

Alho A: Fat embolism syndrome: Etiology, pathogenesis and treatment. Acta Chir Scand (Suppl) 499:75-85, 1980.

Bouaggad A, Harti A, Elmouknia M, et al: Neurologic manifestations of fat embolism. Cah Anesthesiol 43:441-443, 1995.

Dalgorf D, Borkhoff CM, Stephen DJ, et al: Venting during prophylactic nailing for femoral metastases: Current orthopedic practice. Can J Surg 46:427-431, 2003.

Georgopoulos D, Bouros D: Fat embolism syndrome: Clinical examination is still the preferable diagnostic method. Chest 123:982-983, 2003.

Gitin TA, Seidel T, Cera PJ, et al: Pulmonary microvascular fat: The significance? Crit Care Med 21:673-677, 1993.

Jones JP Jr: Alcoholism, hypercortisolism, fat embolism and osseous avascular necrosis. Clin Orthop 393:4-12, 2001.

Kirkland L: Fat embolism. eMedicine J 2004. Available at www.emedicine.com/med/topic652.htm

Marshall PD, Douglas DL, Henry L: Fatal pulmonary fat embolism during total hip replacement due to high-pressure cementing techniques in an osteoporotic femur. Br J Clin Pract 45:148-149, 1991.

Mellor A, Soni N: Fat embolism. Anaesthesia. 56:145-154, 2001.

Papagelopoulos PJ, Apostolou CD, Karachalios TS, et al: Pulmonary fat embolism after total hip and total knee arthroplasty. Orthopedics 26:523-527, 2003.

Peltier LF: Fat embolism: An appraisal of the problem. Clin Orthop 187:3-17, 1984.

Pitto RP, Blunk J, Kossler M: Transesophageal echocardiography and clinical features of fat embolism during cemented total hip arthroplasty: A randomized study in patients with a femoral neck fracture. Arch Orthop Trauma Surg 120:53-58, 2000.

Slye DA: Orthopedic complications: Compartment syndrome, fat embolism syndrome, and venous thromboembolism. Nurs Clin North Am 26:113-132, 1991.

Sutton GE: Pulmonary fat embolism and its relation to traumatic shock. BMJ 2:368, 1918.

Tedeschi CG, Castelli W, Kropp G, et al: Fat macroglobulinemia and fat embolism. Surg Gynecol Obstet 126:83-90, 1968.

Thaunat O, Thaler F, Loirat P, et al: Cerebral fat embolism induced by facial fat injection. Plast Reconstr Surg 113:2235-2236, 2004.

Wilson JV, Salisbury CV: Fat embolism in war surgery. Br J Surg 31:384, 1954.

Yoon SS, Chang DI, Chung KC: Acute fatal stroke immediately following autologous fat injection into the face. Neurology 61:1151-1152, 2004.

Thromboembolic Complications

216

Robert F. Helfand

Case Synopsis

A 72-year-old man has total hip arthroplasty under general anesthesia. A postoperative visit the next day finds him mildly tachypneic, apprehensive, and complaining of pain in his calf on the operative side.

PROBLEM ANALYSIS

Definition

Embolic events are a major cause of morbidity and mortality following lower extremity orthopedic surgery. This chapter focuses on thrombotic sources of emboli. Chapters 175, 215, and 217 discuss embolization secondary to air, fat, and methylmethacrylate, respectively.

In contrast to the arterial thromboembolic and vaso-occlusive events associated with vascular surgery, orthopedic thromboembolic events affect primarily the venous system. As such, their cause is associated with endothelial damage, venous stasis, and hypercoagulability (Virchow's triad). These conditions facilitate the formation of deep venous thromboses (DVTs), which usually begin in the lower leg veins and then extend proximally to the deep thigh veins before ultimately embolizing to the right heart and pulmonary circulation.

Recognition

DVTs and pulmonary emboli (PE) are notoriously difficult to diagnose. Most patients with DVT have no obvious disease. The most commonly used diagnostic tool is duplex ultrasonography. Ultrasound tests are noninvasive and can be easily repeated, but they lack sensitivity for calf vein thrombosis. PE are difficult to recognize both during and after anesthesia, but they should be suspected in any patient with sudden, unexplained dyspnea after a surgery. Symptoms may include chest pain, dyspnea, hemoptysis, apprehension, or cough, but they are generally nonspecific. Physical findings include tachypnea, tachycardia, rales, or an accentuated pulmonic component of the second heart sound (P_2). Most patients with PE do not exhibit signs of thrombophlebitis.

High-resolution spiral computed tomography scanning is often chosen instead of ventilation-perfusion lung scanning as the initial diagnostic test for PE. Pulmonary angiography was once the standard test for the diagnosis of PE, but it is now used less frequently. D-dimer measured by the ELISA test is an additional screening tool, but it is neither specific nor sufficiently sensitive to make or exclude the diagnosis of PE. A normal chest radiograph, arterial blood gas analysis, or electrocardiogram (ECG) does not exclude the diagnosis of PE. Arterial blood gas analysis at the time of embolization may reveal hypoxemia or hypercapnia, but findings are often normal. An ECG may show evidence of right ventricular strain (new right bundle branch block, right axis deviation), sinus tachycardia, or anterior T-wave inversion, but it is usually normal.

Monitored patients may have reduced cardiac output or increased pulmonary arterial pressure and vascular resistance. Transesophageal echocardiography (TEE) visualizes the central pulmonary arteries and evaluates right ventricular function. During surgery, TEE is recommended as the initial diagnostic test for suspected massive PE or in cases of unexplained hypotension, hypoxemia, or cardiac arrest. TEE has a reported sensitivity of 76% to 96.7% and a specificity of 86% to 100% for identifying central PE.

Risk Assessment

Patient and surgical factors contribute to the risk of thromboembolic complications after orthopedic surgery (Table 216-1).

Table 216–1 ▪ Risk Factors for Thromboembolic Complications with Lower Extremity Orthopedic Surgery

Patient Risk Factors

Low cardiac output states (CHF, MI)
Prolonged immobilization or paralysis
Obesity
Prior DVT, PE, or varicose veins
Age older than 40 yr
Cancer
Hypercoagulable states
Pregnancy
Inflammatory bowel disease
Nephrotic syndrome

Surgical Risk Factors

Major surgery >70 min
No DVT prophylaxis
Hypothermia
Positioning
Surgical technique
Hypotension
Trauma (pelvis, hip, or leg fracture)
Indwelling central venous catheter

CHF, congestive heart failure; DVT, deep venous thrombosis; MI, myocardial infarction; PE, pulmonary emboli.

Implications

DVT is common following hip and knee arthroplasty, and especially after hip fracture. DVT is a clot that develops in the large distal veins of the legs, usually deep within the muscle. Less frequently, DVT develops in the proximal pelvic veins. The clot is usually attached at one end. However, if it breaks loose and enters the bloodstream, it may embolize to the right heart and main pulmonary artery branches. The patient is especially at risk when the DVT extends proximally into deep thigh veins. Fatal PE occurs in up to 7% of lower extremity orthopedic procedures and constitutes the greatest source of perioperative mortality in these patients (Table 216-2). Emboli may also traverse an intracardiac communication to enter the arterial circulation. This can cause stroke or acute arterial occlusion in the extremities or other major organs.

At least half of venous thrombi start intraoperatively; the remainder occur during the first 24 to 48 postoperative hours. Nevertheless, some PE do not become clinically apparent until 1 week after surgery. The high risk of morbidity and mortality mandates prophylactic measures to reduce the occurrence of thromboembolic complications.

MANAGEMENT

Intraoperative management of PE is supportive and focuses on optimizing cardiopulmonary function. Specific measures include volume support of right ventricular preload, administration of inotropic drugs, afterload reduction for the right ventricle, and increasing the fraction of inspired oxygen; positive end-expiratory pressure may be added. Patients can have delayed findings of atelectasis and pulmonary infiltrates 24 to 72 hours following PE. Patients with serious cardiorespiratory compromise may benefit from placement of a pulmonary artery catheter and measurement of cardiac output.

Therapeutic intervention for PE consists of full heparinization or fibrinolytic therapy. In most cases, however, neither is appropriate intraoperative treatment. For patients with cardiac arrest or persistent hypotension and hypoxemia, options include the following:

- Emergency operative embolectomy, which requires cardiopulmonary bypass
- Bilateral thoracotomy, with massage of the pulmonary vessels

- Interventional radiology for attempted thrombus extraction or catheter-directed fibrinolytic therapy

Mortality with surgical removal of PE is greater than 50%.

PREVENTION

Thromboembolic complications after orthopedic surgery are unique. The process frequently begins intraoperatively, extends quietly postoperatively, and often results in sudden death. Thus, prevention is imperative, especially because therapeutic interventions are often associated with serious hemorrhagic complications. Prophylaxis includes both mechanical and pharmacologic modalities. The anesthetic technique may also play a significant role in prevention.

Mechanical and Pharmacologic Modalities

Compression stockings that provide a 30 to 40 mm Hg compression gradient are an effective adjunctive treatment for limiting or preventing the extension of thrombus. Mechanical modalities, such as intermittent pneumatic compression devices, can reduce the incidence of thrombus formation by decreasing venous stasis, improving blood flow velocity, and increasing circulating fibrinolysins. Their effectiveness is not diminished when applied to only one leg during surgery. Pneumatic devices significantly decrease the incidence of distal thrombi but have no effect on more proximal thrombi in the iliac and femoral veins.

The American College of Chest Physicians recommends the use of oral warfarin or parenteral low-molecular-weight heparin products for DVT prophylaxis. The latter include enoxaparin (Lovenox) or the novel parenteral anti–factor Xa agent fondaparinux sodium (a synthetic pentastarch). Aspirin is never used alone. Also, standard unfractionated heparin should not be used for high-risk patients.

DVT prophylaxis regimens are specific. Patients are stratified by risk to four categories, as well as to those having total knee replacement or total hip replacement. Warfarin is usually started the night before surgery or immediately postoperatively; the therapeutic international normalized ratio target of 2.5 (range, 2 to 3) is usually not achieved until the third postoperative day. Low-molecular-weight heparin is usually started 12 to 24 hours postoperatively. For total hip replacement, low-molecular-weight heparin may also be given 4 to 6 hours after surgery at half the full dose, followed by a full dose the next day. Preoperatively, it can be given 12 hours before surgery, followed by a full dose 12 to 24 hours postoperatively. Following hip surgery, treatment needs to continue for at least 10 days for lower-risk patients and for 28 to 35 days for higher-risk patients. Although these modalities are more efficacious than placebo, their relative efficacy and value are controversial and probably vary according to the type of surgery.

Anesthetic Management

A convincing number of studies support the choice of regional anesthesia over general anesthesia for reducing thromboembolic complications, especially DVT. When compared

---

Table 216–2 ■ Incidence of Thromboembolic Complications after Orthopedic Procedures without Prophylaxis

Procedure	Total DVT (%)	Proximal DVT (%)	Total PE (%)	Fatal PE (%)
Total hip arthroplasty	42-57	18-36	0.9-28	0.1-2
Total knee arthroplasty	41-85	5-22	1.5-10	0.1-1.7
Repair of hip fracture	46-60	23-30	3-11	2.5-7.5

DVT, deep venous thrombosis; PE, pulmonary emboli.

with general anesthesia, epidural anesthesia reduces the incidence of deep thigh DVT 2.5- to 5-fold and PE 3-fold after hip arthroplasty. Regional anesthesia also results in a 31% reduction of DVT following repair of hip fracture. It is unclear why regional anesthesia appears to reduce thromboembolic complications, but it may counter sympathoadrenal stimulation of the coagulation cascade (see Chapter 89). Regional techniques clearly improve rheology by reducing viscosity and increasing lower extremity blood flow. Less clear is the membrane-stabilizing role of local anesthetics themselves. These effects appear to decrease platelet aggregation while increasing fibrinolysis and normalization of antithrombin III levels. In addition, local anesthetics may inhibit the activation of leukocyte factors linked to hypercoagulability.

Unfortunately, the choice of regional anesthesia is not so clear-cut. Two issues regarding the risk of spinal (epidural) hematoma deserve consideration by the anesthesiologist. One is practical and the other theoretical. The practical issue concerns placement of central neuraxial blocks in patients who are either receiving or are about to receive anticoagulants. Warfarin therapy begins the night before surgery in many patients having joint replacement or in the immediate postoperative period. Available literature supports the safety of perioperative regional techniques in this setting (see also Chapter 57).

More ominous is the issue of the concurrent use of unfractionated or low-molecular-weight heparin and central neuraxial anesthesia (see also Chapter 57). Low-molecular-weight heparin is a relative contraindication to central neuraxial regional techniques because of its long half-life, the difficulty of monitoring its anticoagulant effects, and several reports of associated spinal (epidural) hematoma. These limitations have restricted the use of indwelling neuraxial catheters for postoperative epidural analgesia in many centers, as well as increasing interest in the use of single-injection and continuous peripheral nerve blocks for postoperative pain relief.

Anesthesiologists face a theoretical dilemma when choosing the anesthetic technique for lower extremity orthopedic surgery: Does regional anesthesia's benefit in terms of thromboembolism prophylaxis outweigh the risk of spinal (epidural) hematoma? In most of the aforementioned stud-ies that support the use of regional versus general anesthesia for reducing thromboembolic complications, especially DVT, patients did not receive thromboembolism prophylaxis. It remains unclear whether regional anesthesia is superior to or synergistic with standard thromboembolism prophylactic techniques. Because most patients *do* receive pharmacologic prophylaxis, the general recommendations of the American Society for Regional Anesthesia include a single needle pass, atraumatic needle placement, and no indwelling neuraxial catheters. For recommendations regarding specific agents used for thromboembolism prophylaxis, refer to Chapter 57 under Management. For patients receiving selective factor Xa inhibitors, there is insufficient evidence to make a specific recommendation regarding the use of continuous or single-injection central neuraxial anesthetic techniques. One review of the prospective, randomized experience with fondaparinux sodium found that this agent did not increase the risk of epidural hematoma when used with neuraxial anesthesia.

Further Reading

Cannavo D: Use of neuraxial anesthesia with selective factor Xa inhibitors. Am J Orthop 31:S21-S23, 2002.

Geerts WH, Pinco GF, Heit JA, et al: Prevention of venous thromboembolism: The Seventh ACCP Conference on Antithrombotic and Thrombolytic Therapy. Chest 126:338s-400s, 2004.

Horlocker T: Regional anesthesia in the anticoagulated patient: Defining the risk (the Second ASRA Consensus Conference on Neuraxial Anesthesia and Anticoagulation). Reg Anesth Pain Med 28:172-197, 2003.

Liu SS, Carpenter RL, Neal JM: Epidural anesthesia and analgesia: Their role in postoperative outcome. Anesthesiology 82:1474-1506, 1995.

Rosenfeld BA: Benefits of regional anesthesia on thromboembolic complications following surgery. Reg Anesth 21:9-12, 1996.

Sharrock NE, Ranawat CS, Urquhart B, et al: Factors influencing deep vein thrombosis following total hip arthroplasty under epidural anesthesia. Anesth Analg 76:765-771, 1993.

Sorenson RM, Pace NL: Anesthetic techniques during surgical repair of femoral neck fractures: A meta-analysis. Anesthesiology 77:1095-1104, 1992.

Wedel DJ (ed): Orthopedic Anesthesia. New York, Churchill Livingstone, 1993.

Wedel DJ, Horlocker TT: Anesthesia for orthopedic surgery. In Barash PR, Cullen BF, Stoelting RK (eds): Clinical Anesthesia, 3rd ed. Philadelphia, Lippincott-Raven, 1997, pp 1036-1037.

Methylmethacrylate

Kathryn P. King

Case Synopsis

A 62-year-old man presents for a total hip arthroplasty for degenerative joint disease. His medical problems include hypertension and mild exercise-induced asthma that is treated with an albuterol inhaler. He declines regional anesthesia. General anesthesia is induced and proceeds uneventfully. During cementing and insertion of the femoral prosthesis, the patient develops hypotension, tachycardia, and hypoxemia.

PROBLEM ANALYSIS

Definition

Polymethylmethacrylate bone cement is a polymer formed by mixing highly volatile liquid methylmethacrylate (MMA) monomer with an accelerator, polymethylmethacrylate powder. This bone cement is used during orthopedic surgery to implant prostheses for joint replacement. MMA has been implicated as a cause of adverse cardiopulmonary events observed most frequently during hip replacement surgery. Symptoms include hypoxemia, bronchoconstriction, pulmonary hypertension, and right ventricular failure with hypotension. Fatal cardiac arrest, though rare, has been reported in 0.6% to 1% of patients in some case series.

The clinical presentation just described is termed bone implantation syndrome (BIS) or bone cement implantation syndrome (BCIS). Proposed mechanisms for MMA-induced injury include a neurogenic reflex, release of vasoactive and myocardial depressant substances by the cement, intravascular thrombin generation in the lungs, direct vasoactive effects of absorbed MMA, and acute pulmonary microembolization.

After application of polymethylmethacrylate, unbound MMA monomer is quickly absorbed into the systemic circulation and eliminated by the lungs. Its peak level is reached in expired air within 2 to 5 minutes. The extent of systemic absorption depends on the area of contact between the bone cement and vascularized tissue and on the degree of curing.

MMA is a peripheral vasodilator. However, the amount released during reaming in joint replacement is 10- to 20-fold less than that required to produce hypotension in experimental models. Further, studies have demonstrated that hypotension also occurs in the absence of the polymer. Thus, the most likely explanation of the pathogenesis of this syndrome is acute pulmonary microembolization. During implantation of the cement and prosthesis, the high intramedullary pressure generated in the long bone marrow cavity forces medullary contents into the venous circulation, with embolization to the lungs. The pathologic nature of the emboli is not certain; it may be fat, marrow, thrombus, air, or bone cement. Emboli appear as echogenic masses during reaming, cementing, prosthesis placement, and manipulation of the bone. Pulmonary embolization activates the clotting cascade and triggers the production of proinflammatory substances. Further, cemented prostheses are associated with a longer duration of embolization, larger emboli, and a higher percentage of right atria filled by emboli compared with noncemented prostheses. Intramedullary pressure peaks are 680 mm Hg in humans with cemented arthroplasty, compared with peaks of less than 100 mm Hg with noncemented arthroplasty.

There are also chronic issues related to MMA and other polymers used in orthopedic surgery. Controlled occupational exposure to MMA has not been shown to affect workers' mortality from colon and rectal cancer. The recommended maximum exposure of MMA vapor is 100 parts per million over the course of an 8-hour workday. Acute exposure to extremely high levels of MMA vapor can cause liver necrosis, pulmonary edema, and pulmonary emphysema. Occupational exposure of medical personnel is well below the levels necessary to elicit these toxic effects. However, other less dramatic effects might occur. MMA is known to be a potent allergenic sensitizer and can cause local reactions with dermal exposure. It is also known to be a potential pulmonary toxin, with chronic exposure causing occupational asthma. The direct pulmonary effect of MMA in the absence of pulmonary embolization is not well defined. However, indirect evidence suggests that it may trigger bronchoconstriction.

Recognition

Clinical signs of BIS are similar to those found in pulmonary embolism or fat embolism. These include fever, tachycardia, hypotension, hypoxemia, and, in spontaneously breathing patients, dyspnea and tachypnea. End-tidal carbon dioxide may decrease with a large embolus. Also, fat emboli may cause petechiae, fat globules in the urine, and anuria or oliguria. In awake patients, they can cause mental status changes. The electrocardiogram may show right axis deviation or right bundle branch block. Collectively, these signs reflect increased pulmonary artery pressure and intrapulmonary shunt, potentially leading to right ventricular failure and cardiac arrest.

Risk Assessment

This patient population includes elderly or chronically ill patients undergoing either elective or emergent surgery. Careful preoperative evaluation may identify coexisting conditions, such as pulmonary or cardiovascular disease, that can be stabilized or improved preoperatively in anticipation of hemodynamic instability during surgery. A frail individual with additional risk factors, such as pulmonary hypertension, coronary artery disease, or severe osteoporosis, may benefit from invasive monitoring.

Implications

Although hypotension and hypoxia frequently occur during implantation of the prosthesis, these findings are usually transient and self-limited. Larger emboli causing right ventricular outflow tract obstruction may require resuscitation with intubation, mechanical ventilation with 100% oxygen, intravenous fluids, inotropic agents, afterload reduction of the right ventricle, and, occasionally, heroic measures such as cardiopulmonary bypass and surgical thrombectomy.

MANAGEMENT

Treatment of BIS is limited to supportive care. This includes monitoring vital signs and the use of supplemental oxygen and intravenous fluids, with vasopressor support as needed. In some patients, positive inotropic agents may also be needed.

PREVENTION

Emboli occur frequently during surgical manipulation and placement of both cemented and noncemented orthopedic prostheses. Avoidance of MMA may not significantly reduce the occurrence of these events. However, lavaging the marrow cavity, placing a vent hole in the bone during reaming to reduce intramedullary pressure, and thorough removal of bone marrow and bone debris can minimize the dislodgment of particulates. Allowing the freshly mixed MMA to vaporize for as long as possible may help minimize MMA absorption.

Invasive monitoring may be indicated for patients with marginal cardiac or pulmonary reserves. Finally, adequate volume replacement and supplemental oxygen are essential.

Further Reading

Berman AT, Price HL, Hahn JF: The cardiovascular effects of methylmethacrylate in dogs. Clin Orthop 100:265-269, 1974.

Christie J, Robinson CM, Pell AC, et al: Transcardiac echocardiography during invasive intramedullary procedures. J Bone Joint Surg Br 77:450-455, 1995.

Dahl OE, Molnar I, Vinje A, et al: Studies on coagulation, fibrinolysis, kallikrein-kinin and complement activation in systemic and pulmonary circulation during hip arthroplasty with acrylic cement. Thromb Res 5:875-884, 1988.

Elmaraghy AW, Humeniuk B, Anderson GI, et al: The role of methylmethacrylate monomer in the formation and haemodynamic outcome of pulmonary fat emboli. J Bone Joint Surg Br 80:156-161, 1998.

Ereth MH, Weber JG, Abel MD, et al: Cemented versus non-cemented total hip arthroplasty—embolism, hemodynamics, and intrapulmonary shunting. Mayo Clin Proc 67:1066-1074, 1992.

Fallon KM, Fuller JG, Morley-Forster P: Fat embolization and fatal cardiac arrest during hip arthroplasty with methylmethacrylate. Can J Anaesth 48:626-629, 2001.

Lamade WR, Friedl W, Schmid B, et al: Bone cement implantation syndrome: A prospective randomised trial for use of antihistamine blockade. Arch Orthop Trauma Surg 114:335-339, 1995.

Lopez-Duran L, Garcia-Lopez A, Duran L, et al: Cardiopulmonary and haemodynamic changes during total hip arthroplasty. Int Orthop 21:253-258, 1997.

Mellor A, Soni N: Fat embolism. Anaesthesia 56:145-154, 2001.

Orsini EC, Byrick RJ, Mullen JB, et al: Cardiopulmonary function and pulmonary microemboli during arthroplasty using cemented or non-cemented components: The role of intramedullary pressure. J Bone Joint Surg Am 69:822-832, 1987.

Rinecker H: New clinico-pathophysiological studies on the bone cement implantation syndrome. Arch Orthop Trauma Surg 97:263-274, 1980.

Tomenson JA, Bonner SM, Edwards JC, et al: Study of two cohorts of workers exposed to methyl methacrylate in acrylic sheet production. Occup Environ Med 57:810-817, 2000.

Extremity Tourniquets

H. David Hardman

Case Synopsis

A 75-year-old woman is undergoing a revision of a left total knee arthroplasty under regional anesthesia. She is morbidly obese, on chronic opioids for pain relief, and an insulin-dependent diabetic. Continuous catheter lumbar plexus and sciatic nerve blocks are chosen, along with supplemental intravenous narcotics and sedatives as needed. A conventional rectangular thigh tourniquet is placed for surgical hemostasis. After limb exsanguination, the cuff pressure is set at 300 mm Hg. Surgery proceeds uneventfully, with a total tourniquet time of 2 hours. The catheters are removed the next day, and the patient is started on enoxaparin for deep venous thrombosis (DVT) prophylaxis. Subsequently, she complains of numbness and weakness in her left leg.

PROBLEM ANALYSIS

Definition

Postoperative neurologic dysfunction with the use of arterial tourniquets is a well-documented but rare phenomenon. Estimates of incidence range from 0.15% to 0.6% for all patients. Owing to greater soft tissue mass insulation, thigh tourniquets are less likely to cause neurologic injury than are arm tourniquets; the risk is increased with calf and forearm tourniquets. Permanent tourniquet-induced neurologic deficits are uncommon. The majority of nerve injuries resolve spontaneously within 6 weeks, with complete recovery by 6 months.

Arterial tourniquets are widely used in upper and lower extremity surgery and in intravenous regional anesthesia. This practice continues because it is widely accepted that the benefit from minimizing surgical blood loss and creating a bloodless operative field exceeds the risk for tourniquet-related complications. It is important for anesthesiologists to be aware of the potential for tourniquet-related tissue injury, systemic effects of tourniquet inflation and deflation, and the possibly catastrophic events that could occur at these times.

Also, it should be recognized that surgeons and anesthesiologists share any medicolegal liability for tourniquet-related complications. Documentation should include the location of the tourniquet, the use of padding and draping, and inflation pressure and duration. Also, tourniquet pressure relative to systemic blood pressure values, prolonged inflation, and total vascular occlusion times must be communicated to the surgical team and documented on the anesthesia record.

LOCAL INJURY

Pressure-related injuries to skin, muscles, nerves, and blood vessels depend on the pressure of tourniquet inflation and its duration. Also, absent arterial blood flow distal to the tourniquet causes ischemia, which leads to progressive acidosis, hypoxemia, and hypercarbia. The associated release of inflammatory mediators increases capillary permeability and tissue edema. This worsens ischemia, especially after reperfusion.

The ultrastructural cellular changes are detectable after 30 minutes of ischemia but are reversible with ischemia lasting 2 hours or less. High-energy intracellular phosphate depletion occurs more gradually. However, injury to the Na^+, K^+-ATPase–dependent ion exchange pump causes extracellular potassium leak and intracellular edema. The sarcoplasmic reticulum loses glycogen, the mitochondria swell, and myelin degeneration occurs.

Skin. Trauma to the skin can be caused by pressure necrosis due to inadequate padding between the skin and tourniquet or friction burns due to movement of a poorly applied tourniquet. Obese patients with redundant upper extremity skin folds are at increased risk for skin injury. Chemical burns from skin preparation solutions have been reported. These solutions soak into the padding under the tourniquet, and under pressure, this continuous contact with the skin can cause full-thickness burns.

Muscle. Myocytes are very sensitive to compression and ischemia. Injury is more severe with lengthy tourniquet inflation or high pressure. Usually, injury is greatest beneath the tourniquet. Associated ischemia, edema, and microvascular congestion cause the post-tourniquet syndrome. This includes stiffness, pallor, and weakness (not paralysis), with subjective extremity numbness.

Nerve. Mechanical pressure compresses nerves directly beneath the tourniquet cuff. Shear forces at the proximal and distal edges of the cuff also cause nerve injury ranging from paresthesia to complete paralysis. Distal ischemia plays a lesser role. The contribution of tourniquet time to the development of nerve injury is unclear. Paralysis has been reported with as little as 30 minutes of tourniquet inflation. Lower extremity nerve injury usually involves the sciatic nerve. The upper extremity is more vulnerable to injury. Radial injury is more frequent than ulnar or median nerve injury. Localized nerve injuries tend to be neurapraxic (i.e., without evidence of structural damage to the axon or perineurium). If so, the prognosis for full recovery is good. In contrast, axonotmesis (i.e., damage to the axon but not to the perineurium) causes nerve degeneration distal to the injury and takes longer to recover. Rarely, a permanent nerve deficit occurs.

Vasculature.   Arteries and veins, especially prosthetic grafts (e.g., arteriovenous fistulas, arterial bypass grafts), are susceptible to traumatic injury from mechanical compression. Although direct arterial injury is rare (0.03% to 0.14% incidence), fractured atherosclerotic plaque may cause localized thrombosis or embolize distally to cause ischemia. Although DVT is a known and common complication of lower limb surgery, tourniquets bear no relation to deep venous stasis and thrombus formation. Rather, systemic hypercoagulability is due to catecholamine release and platelet aggregation caused by tourniquet-related or surgical pain. In contrast, active bleeding after tourniquet release may be aggravated by ischemia-caused tissue plasminogen activator release and fibrinolysis.

SYSTEMIC EFFECTS

Systemic effects occur with tourniquet inflation and deflation. The intensity and duration of these derangements are directly proportional to the length of tourniquet inflation time and the size and number of tourniquet-isolated limbs.

Autotransfusion.   Limb exsanguination and rapid tourniquet inflation shunt blood into the central circulation (autotransfusion) and increase systemic vascular resistance. As much as 800 mL of blood is autotransfused with the simultaneous inflation of bilateral thigh tourniquets. This causes a transient increase in central venous pressure and systolic blood pressure, which gradually returns to baseline. In patients with compromised left ventricular function, congestive heart failure due to circulatory overload and cardiac arrest has been reported.

Hypertension.   Tourniquet-induced hypertension is common. Patients develop an increase in heart rate and systolic and diastolic blood pressures within 30 to 60 minutes of inflation, which persists until tourniquet deflation. This increase in mean arterial pressure has been attributed to (1) an acute increase in systemic vascular resistance with removal of a vascular bed; (2) limb exsanguination before tourniquet cuff inflation, which causes acute central blood volume expansion; and (3) pain associated with tourniquet compression and limb ischemia. The pain mechanism is not well understood, but it may involve the activation of type C nerve fibers. In turn, these activate NMDA receptors, leading to a hypertensive response. This response is less common and less intense under regional anesthesia compared with general anesthesia.

Hypotension.   Tourniquet deflation results in reduced blood pressure and central venous pressure secondary to a shift of blood volume back into the extremity and post-ischemic reactive vasodilatation. Also, with reperfusion, metabolites released from ischemic areas into the systemic circulation have the potential to cause myocardial depression and further reduce blood pressure. Hypotension is usually self-limited ($\leq$15 minutes).

Hypercapnia.   End-tidal carbon dioxide ($ETCO_2$) increases after tourniquet release owing to the efflux of hypercapnic venous blood from the ischemic limb into the systemic circulation. The peak $ETCO_2$ increase occurs by 1 minute, and it returns to baseline by 10 to 13 minutes. Spontaneously breathing patients compensate by increasing their respiratory rate. However, those with controlled ventilation require a transient increase in minute ventilation by 50% for about 5 minutes to maintain normocapnia. Hyperventilation can prevent the associated increase in cerebral blood volume and intracranial pressure that might otherwise be detrimental to a patient with a severe head injury.

Metabolic Acidosis.   Elevated serum lactate and reduced pH are observed for approximately 30 minutes after reperfusion of the isolated extremity.

Blood Oxygen Saturation.   Arterial oxygen saturation usually remains normal. However, as large volumes of deoxygenated blood are returned to the central circulation after tourniquet release, mixed venous oxygen saturation is transiently decreased.

Core Body Temperature.   Most patients remain normothermic. Tourniquet inflation above arterial pressure transiently increases core body temperature, and tourniquet deflation transiently decreases it. The decline in core body temperature due to the return of hypothermic venous blood from the previously occluded limb into the systemic circulation is usually 0.7°C or less.

Deep Venous Thrombosis, Pulmonary or Systemic Thromboembolism.   These potentially devastating complications may occur with lower limb trauma and surgery, but rarely intraoperatively. Although studies with transesophageal echocardiography have shown up to a 70% incidence of right atrial embolization following tourniquet release, most emboli are small and are unlikely to cause major morbidity. However, this risk is increased in patients with hypercoagulable states and thrombus due to trauma or prolonged immobilization. In this case, it is believed that thrombus becomes dislodged during limb exsanguination or with tourniquet inflation. Catastrophic events such as DVT or pulmonary or systemic thromboembolism are more likely to occur postoperatively during rehabilitation. Use of enoxaparin for DVT prophylaxis has dramatically reduced the incidence of fatal pulmonary embolism. However, given that pulmonary and cerebral emboli have been reported during both inflation and deflation of tourniquets, anesthesiologists should be especially vigilant during these times. Attention should be focused on the patient's neurologic status and any sudden, unexpected changes in arterial oxygen saturation and $ETCO_2$. Significant pulmonary emboli result in an acute reduction in $ETCO_2$, with tachycardia and hypotension, followed by hypoxemia and myocardial ischemia. Right ventricular dysfunction may also be observed (also see Chapters 215 to 217).

Recognition

Given the increased use of regional blocks for lower extremity surgery, which significantly reduces postoperative pain scores and permits earlier ambulation, how does one differentiate a nerve injury related to use of a tourniquet from one related to regional anesthesia?

Post-tourniquet syndrome is the most common problem associated with tourniquet use. Mild weakness, diffuse subjective numbness, swelling, stiffness, and slight pallor of the affected limb usually develop several hours after tourniquet deflation. Also, ischemic injury to muscle is distinguished from nerve injury by normal nerve conduction studies and the presence of elevated creatine kinase (MM) enzymes and myoglobinuria.

If the tourniquet has produced a compressive nerve injury, it may be difficult to distinguish this injury from one related to regional block. However, as noted earlier, tourniquet-related nerve injury can range from paresthesia to complete paralysis. The sciatic nerve is often involved in lower extremity surgery, and radial nerve injury is more common than ulnar or median nerve injury with upper extremity surgery. Further, localized tourniquet-related nerve injury is often neurapraxic, in which case the prognosis for full recovery is good. In contrast, injuries to nerves caused by needles or indwelling catheters may involve damage to the axon or perineurium.

Brief neurologic assessment of the affected extremity should follow surgery. Evidence of motor and sensory deficits requires neurologic consultation and nerve conduction studies to determine the site of the defect. With regional anesthesia, there may be a delay in the diagnosis of nerve injury, especially if indwelling catheters are used for postoperative analgesia.

Acute compartment syndrome has been observed immediately after surgery or after a delay of several hours. The limb is typically swollen, muscles are stiff, and pain is more severe than the physical findings would suggest. Neurologic dysfunction is a common sequela. Confirmation is by measurement of intracompartmental pressures.

Postoperative causalgia presents weeks or months after surgery. Burning pain and autonomic dysfunction develop, followed by dystrophic changes in the extremity.

Skin injuries are usually evident upon tourniquet cuff removal. Ecchymoses, persistent erythema, bullae formation, or skin burns may be present.

Vascular insufficiency due to arterial injury should be suspected when cuff deflation does not result in reperfusion of all or part of the extremity.

Risk Assessment

Both tourniquet-related and anesthesia-related nerve injuries resolve in approximately the same time frame, so cause is usually not important. However, for anesthesiologists working in high-risk malpractice environments, the possibility of nerve injury may be a consideration when choosing the type of anesthesia for patients at high risk for tourniquet-induced neurologic injury. Factors that may increase the risk of complications with tourniquet use are listed in Table 218-1.

The safe upper limits for inflation time and pressure for arterial tourniquets are controversial. Nerves appear most susceptible to mechanical pressure and muscles to prolonged ischemia. Most clinicians recommend the shortest tourniquet inflation time possible, with a limit of 2 hours in healthy patients. For surgical procedures exceeding 2 hours, the tourniquet should be deflated every 2 hours to allow 10 minutes of limb reperfusion. Muscle injury, especially beneath the cuff, can occur even with short tourniquet times. Elderly trauma patients and those with peripheral vascular disease are most susceptible to muscle injury. Therefore, the lowest pressure needed to produce arterial occlusion should be used. Van Roekel and Thurston recommend that in a normotensive, average-size adult patient, an inflation pressure of 200 mm Hg should be adequate for the upper limb and 250 mm Hg for the lower limb. The tourniquet pressure

Table 218–1 ■ Factors That May Increase the Risk of Tourniquet-Related Complications
Tourniquet Related
Equipment not regularly serviced and inspected for pressure accuracy
Bilateral tourniquet use
Revisions, malignancies, or other surgeries requiring longer tourniquet times
Vascular and Metabolic
Diabetes
Peripheral vascular disease
Obesity
Raynaud's disease
Prosthetic vascular grafts
Coagulopathies
Sickle cell disease and trait
Preexisting coagulopathies
Patients at increased risk for deep venous thrombosis
Other
Peripheral neuropathy
Prolonged immobilization before surgery
Traumatized limb with extensive soft tissue injury
Localized infection
Latex allergy (must use latex-free tourniquets and tubing)

should be maintained 50 to 150 mm Hg above the systolic pressure. The application of wider, curved cuffs permits the use of lower inflation pressures to produce arterial occlusion.

Implications

Most tourniquet-related compressive nerve injuries are neurapraxic and resolve completely over a few hours to days without specific therapy. With nerve disruption, recovery can take weeks or months, but incomplete recovery is rare. Also, there is the potential for a causalgia syndrome to develop, with significant disability.

Weakness and swelling due to post-tourniquet syndrome can interfere with rehabilitation and wound healing. Pressure-related skin injuries increase the risk of infection. Compartment syndromes pose a significant risk for ischemic necrosis and permanent contracture of the involved muscle groups. Unrecognized arterial insufficiency can lead to necrosis of soft tissue and bone.

In patients given regional anesthesia, tourniquet pain and associated hypertension may require deep sedation with propofol or ketamine or even general anesthesia. Opiates alone are usually ineffective. Hypotension with tourniquet deflation is expected and usually self-limited. If not, a fluid challenge and small doses of vasopressors are used until the hypotension resolves.

Massive pulmonary embolism causes hemodynamic instability, right ventricular strain, and cardiovascular collapse. Nonfatal embolism may result in hypoxemia due to ventilation-perfusion mismatching, myocardial infarction, or stroke due to paradoxical cerebral embolism with intracardiac shunts.

MANAGEMENT

Nerve injuries that do not resolve within 48 hours should be referred to a neurologist for assessment and follow-up nerve conduction studies. Post-tourniquet syndrome is managed with elevation of the extremity, monitoring of wound healing, and physical therapy. Pressure-related skin injuries are treated as needed. Bullae or chemical burns require burn care. However, they may be avoided by applying a nonpermeable plastic barrier drape over the distal end of the tourniquet cuff before preparing the skin. Causalgia requires management by a comprehensive chronic pain management team, and early referral is essential. Compartment syndromes are a surgical emergency and require fasciotomy to decompress the affected muscle compartments.

Arterial insufficiency of an extremity requires surgical revascularization or thrombolytic therapy. Diagnosis of intraoperative pulmonary emboli is facilitated with transesophageal echocardiography. Therapy for pulmonary emboli is supportive and includes controlled ventilation, oxygen, pressor support, and cardiopulmonary resuscitation if needed. Systemic anticoagulation, thrombolytic therapy, surgical thrombectomy, or thrombus removal by interventional radiology may be necessary in some patients. Cerebral emobilization is diagnosed with computed tomography scans, and therapy is directed by a neurosurgeon and neurologist.

PREVENTION

Catastrophic complications are minimized by judicious patient selection. During screening of patients at high risk for DVT (prolonged immobilization, hypercoagulable state), if thrombus is detected, surgery should be postponed. However, screening all patients for right-to-left intracardiac shunts with contrast-enhanced transthoracic echocardiography is not cost-effective, and it is questionable whether the presence of a right-to-left intracardiac shunt would affect anesthetic or surgical management.

Safety factors in the use of pneumatic tourniquets for hemostasis during hand surgery were first described in 1951, and Bruner's 10 rules were subsequently revised by Braithwaite and Klenerman in 1996. Fortunately, most pneumatic tourniquet complications in extremity surgery are avoided by limiting maximum tourniquet pressure and tourniquet inflation time. Although there are no randomized, controlled, prospective clinical studies to provide us with evidence-based guidelines, there are sufficient animal studies and clinical data to make the following recommendations:

- Carefully select patients preoperatively.
- Use a wide, low-pressure tourniquet cuff.
- Inflate tourniquets to the lowest pressure needed to prevent bleeding.
- Limit tourniquet ischemia time to 2 hours or less.
- Set maximum tourniquet pressure settings as follows: arm tourniquets, 50 to 75 mm Hg above the baseline systolic pressure; leg tourniquets, 75 to 100 mm Hg above the baseline systolic pressure.
- Ensure adequate padding beneath the tourniquet.

- Use barrier techniques to prevent any skin preparation solutions from running underneath the tourniquet cuff.
- Alternate the use of two tourniquets.
- Ensure tourniquet reliability with regular maintenance checks.

There are other simple things that we can do to reduce tourniquet-related injuries, without waiting for advances in research and technology. Using the following general guidelines may result in tourniquet cuff pressures 30% to 50% lower than those currently used in routine clinical practice:

- Use conical, tapered tourniquet cuffs instead of conventional rectangular cuffs. These can reduce limb occlusion pressure by as much as 23% compared with conventional cuffs. Also, they are more efficient at transmitting surface pressure to deep tissues because they more nearly conform to the shape of the extremity.
- Set tourniquet pressures by determining limb occlusion pressure with Doppler or portable ultrasonography. Then set tourniquet pressures 40 to 80 mm Hg above limb occlusion pressure.
- Subsystolic occlusion pressures can be generated with wider conical cuffs or with a cuff width–to–extremity circumference ratio greater than 0.5.

In the future, tourniquet-related injuries may be minimized and allowable tourniquet times extended with ischemic preconditioning of skeletal muscle, more frequent reperfusion intervals, or combined regional hypothermia and ischemic preconditioning.

Finally, the recent availability of sustained-release epidural morphine compounds, along with general anesthesia, may offer the best of both worlds for anesthesiologists who wish to provide good postoperative analgesia without concern about possible postoperative neuropathies with peripheral nerve or plexus blocks, especially when extremity tourniquets will be used during surgery.

Further Reading

Al-Ghamdi AA: Bilateral total knee replacement under tourniquet in a homozygous sickle cell patient. Anesth Analg 98:543-544, 2003.

Braithwaite I, Klenerman L: Burns under tourniquets—Bruner's ten rules revisited. J Med Def Unions 12:14-15, 1996.

Bruner JM: Safety factors in the use of the pneumatic tourniquet for haemostasis in surgery of the hand. J Bone Joint Surg Am 33:221-224, 1951.

Duffy PJ: The arterial tourniquet. Available at http://www.uam.es/departamentos/medicina/anesnet/gtoa/hm1.html

Iwama H, Kaneko T, Ohmizo H, et al: Circulatory, respiratory and metabolic changes after thigh tourniquet release in combined epidural-propofol anaesthesia with preservation of spontaneous respiration. Anaesthesia 57:588-592, 2002.

Kam P, Kavanaugh R, Yoong F: The arterial tourniquet: Pathophysiological consequences and anaesthetic implications. Anaesthesia 56:53-54, 2001.

Tredwell S, Wilmink M, Inkpen K, et al: Pediatric tourniquets: Analysis of cuff and limb interface, current practice, and guidelines for use. J Pediatr Orthop 21:671-676, 2001.

Van Roekel HE, Thurston AJ: Tourniquet pressure: The effect of limb circumference and systolic blood pressure. J Hand Surg 10:142-144, 1985.

Weiss SJ, Cheung AT, Stecker MM, et al: Fatal paradoxical cerebral embolization during bilateral knee arthroplasty. Anesthesiology 84:721-723, 1996.

Complications of Spinal Surgery

219

Michelle L. Lotto

Case Synopsis

A 28-year-old woman with severe kyphotic deformity from a prior crush injury is undergoing T6 corpectomy with posterior spinal fusion and instrumentation. Before surgery, the patient is neurologically intact. During spinal instrumentation, the motor evoked potential (MEP) from the left gastrocnemius muscle and the cervical and cortical somatosensory evoked potentials (SEPs) from the left posterior tibial nerve are suddenly lost (Figs. 219-1 and 219-2). Reversal of induced hypotension (85/55 mm Hg) to baseline pressure (120/60 mm Hg) does not improve the SEP or MEP responses. Some return of SEP amplitude is seen after removal of the spinal retractors, but the MEP remains depressed. The procedure is aborted because of the evolving neurologic deficit.

PROBLEM ANALYSIS

Definition

NEURAL INJURY

Damage to neural structures is a dreaded consequence of spinal surgery. In addition to direct surgical injury to neuronal tissue, nerve injury can occur because of stretch, compression, or both. The mechanism underlying tension-related or ischemic nerve injury is increased intraneural pressure that reduces the cross-sectional area of the nerve and compromises its blood flow. Compression generates relative venous hypertension within the nerve sheath, necessitating an increase in the arterial pressure for adequate perfusion.

Patients undergoing spinal surgery are at risk not only for surgical injury to the spinal cord but also for position-related injuries to the peripheral and, rarely, the optic nerves. Diabetes mellitus, alcohol abuse, vitamin deficiencies, malnutrition, renal disease, hypothyroidism, and emaciation can increase the risk for perioperative peripheral nerve injury.

HYPOTENSION

Hypotension is a potentially serious complication of spinal surgery. Although hypovolemia is the most common cause of intraoperative hypotension, other causes are excessive depth of anesthesia, allergic reactions, pulmonary embolism, and cardiovascular dysfunction.

HEMORRHAGE

Significant blood loss can be a major complication of certain spinal procedures. Bone decortication and epidural venous bleeding are the chief causes of blood loss during spinal surgery. The surgical team should be prepared for the possibility of massive blood transfusion in patients undergoing corpectomy, multilevel spinal instrumentation, and fusion surgery, especially when it involves the thoracolumbar spine.

Recognition

Patients undergoing spinal procedures with general anesthesia do not manifest signs or symptoms of spinal cord injury unless the insult is extreme, such as cord transection with spinal shock. Neurophysiologic monitoring modalities, including SEPs, transcranial MEPs, and electromyography, are used to detect neurologic insult during spinal surgery.

Intraoperative spinal cord monitoring is intended to reduce permanent neurologic deficits by allowing the early detection of impending neurologic injury and the implementation of corrective interventions. SEP monitoring provides a continuous evaluation of the somatosensory system through repetitive stimulation of a peripheral nerve and the recording of multiple responses obtained from the spinal cord and somatosensory cortex. Although SEP monitoring is useful for determining the integrity of the spinal cord during procedures that may cause overdistraction of the cord, it does not specifically reflect injury to the motor tracts. The ability of SEP monitoring to detect ischemic motor injury is significantly limited by the differential blood supply to the anterior and posterior spinal cord tracts.

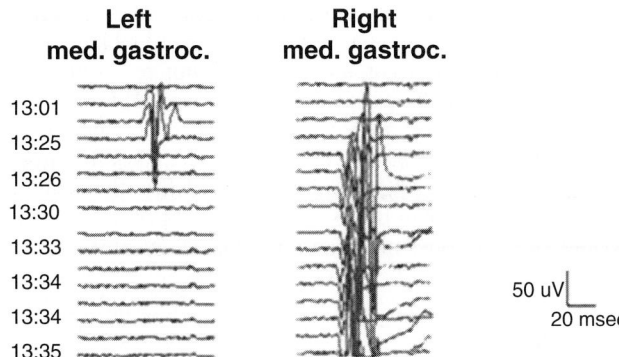

Figure 219-1 ■ Sudden loss of motor evoked potential recorded from the left gastrocnemius muscle.

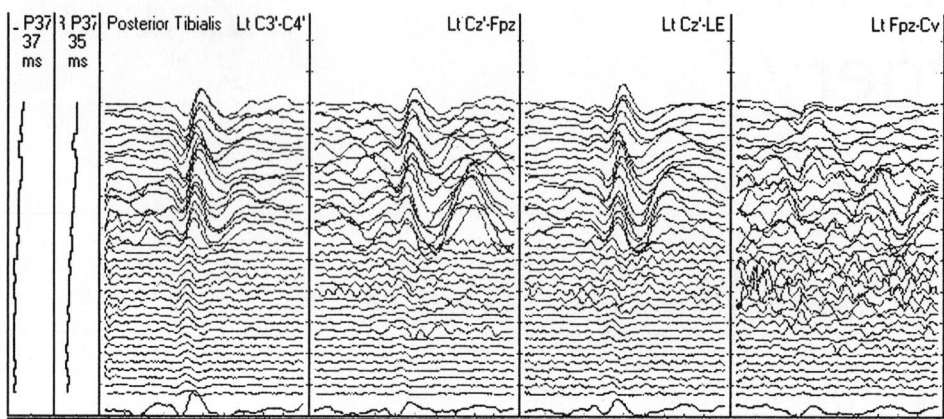

Figure 219–2 ■ Loss of the left sub-cortical and cortical somatosensory evoked potentials (far right panel) with stimulation of the left posterior tibialis nerve.

MEP monitoring is a newer modality that offers direct monitoring of the motor system through transcranial electrical stimulation of the motor cortical structures and recording of myogenic responses in the target muscle groups. Although MEP monitoring is more specific to motor injury than is SEP, MEP shows greater sensitivity to anesthetic agents and a much larger variability in amplitude over time than does SEP. Newer transcranial stimulation techniques involving multiple trains of higher-intensity electrical stimuli have improved the reliability of MEP monitoring in patients under general anesthesia. However, MEP amplitudes are somewhat variable over time. Therefore, the criteria used to determine a significant change in MEP can vary among centers. However, generally accepted criteria for significant changes in SEP and MEP are as follows:

- SEP
  - 50% decrease in amplitude
  - 10% increase in latency

- MEP
  - Loss in amplitude greater than 80%
  - Complete loss of the potential

Risk Assessment

SEP monitoring is most commonly used during surgical correction of spinal deformities. Although it has been used in a variety of spinal procedures, the benefit of SEP monitoring in conditions other than kyphoscoliosis repair is less well established. There is mounting evidence that MEP monitoring may provide more specific and sensitive detection of neurologic injury in many types of spinal surgeries, including scoliosis repair, spinal cord tumor resection, and spine stabilization. However, the sensitivity of MEPs to anesthetic agents, as well as the difficulty in obtaining MEPs in patients with preexisting motor deficits, makes it a more technically challenging monitoring modality than SEPs. However, changes can occur in both modalities in response to alterations in physiology and pharmacology, as well as to interference from electrical devices in the operating room. Factors that interfere with SEP monitoring include the following:

- Anesthetic agents (Table 219-1)
- Hypotension

- Hypoxemia
- Hypothermia
- Alkalosis or acidosis
- Cold surgical irrigation

Implications

Failure to heed significant changes in SEPs or MEPs may lead to permanent neurologic injury. In the case synopsis, changes in both SEPs and MEPs resulted in halting the surgical procedure, thereby preventing possible irreversible neural injury and paralysis.

Table 219–1 ■ Effect of Anesthetics on Cortical Somatosensory and Motor Evoked Potentials			
Anesthetic	SEP Amplitude	SEP Latency	MEP Amplitude
Inhalational Agents			
Desflurane			
0.5 MAC	↓	→	
1 MAC	↓↓	↑	
Isoflurane			
0.5 MAC	↓	↑	↓↓↓
1 MAC	↓↓↓	↑↑	↓↓↓
Sevoflurane			
0.5 MAC	↓↓	↑	↓↓↓
1 MAC	↓↓	↑	↓↓↓
N₂O (60%)	↓↓	→	↓↓
Intravenous Induction Agents			
Etomidate	↑↑	↑	→
Ketamine	→↑	↑	→↓
Propofol	↓	↓	↓↓
Thiopental	↓↓↓	↑↑	↓↓↓
Adjuncts			
Benzodiazepines	↓↓	↑	↓
Opioids	↑	→	↓

→, no change; ↓ or ↑, 10%-20% change; ↑↑ or ↓↓, 30%-50% change; ↑↑↑ or ↓↓↓, >50% change.

MAC, minimal alveolar concentration; MEP, motor evoked potential; N₂O, nitrous oxide; SEP, somatosensory evoked potential.

MANAGEMENT

Detection of neurologic injury and timely initiation of corrective measures require good communication between the neurophysiologic monitoring personnel and the anesthesia and surgical teams. Changes in anesthetic depth or bolus dosing of medications should be avoided during periods of high spinal cord risk, such as spinal distraction. When significant changes in spinal potentials occur, technical error should be ruled out, and the surgeon should be alerted.

Reduced mean arterial pressure and anemia or hypoxia increase the risk for spinal cord injury. Thus, measures to correct these conditions can improve spinal cord perfusion and oxygenation. If the response to therapy is inadequate, and significant changes in SEPs or MEPs persist, the surgical team must evaluate the patient for procedure-related complications and then make the necessary alterations to reverse an evolving insult. When using SEPs as the sole monitoring modality, evaluation should include a wake-up test, during which the patient is allowed to emerge from anesthesia so that the motor system can be evaluated. Although the wake-up test is the gold standard for evaluation of the spinal cord, the use of both MEPs and SEPs may reduce the need for this assessment.

Treatment of hypotension first requires assessment of the cause. Blood loss and hypovolemia are the most common causes of hypotension during spinal cord surgery, and replacement of fluids is adequate treatment in most situations. Positioning may contribute to hypovolemia when patients are placed on the Jackson table or in the kneeling position for spinal surgery. In these positions, venous return may be reduced by the sequestration of blood volume in the capacitance vessels of the abdomen and legs. Pharmacologic treatment (e.g., phenylephrine) may be necessary to augment arterial blood pressure until fluid resuscitation is adequate. The requirement for blood or blood product transfusions must be assessed on an individual basis.

PREVENTION

Careful attention to patient positioning and SEP and MEP monitoring for neural injury can help prevent spinal cord injury. Several methods are used to reduce blood loss and the need for blood transfusions or component therapy.

Monitoring

To optimize the detection of spinal cord injury, the anesthesia team should try to maintain a constant pharmacologic and physiologic state. Both SEP and MEP monitoring modalities may show false-positive changes in response to sudden changes in anesthetic depth, as well as acute physiologic changes, including hypotension, hypoxia, and hypothermia. MEPs show greater dose-dependent sensitivity to both volatile and intravenous anesthetic agents than do SEPs, and complete muscle relaxation must be avoided. Continuous intravenous infusions of propofol and opioids provide fairly stable monitoring conditions for both SEPs and MEPs. Abrupt changes in anesthetic depth or intravenous bolus

doses of analgesics should be avoided at points during spinal surgery when spinal cord injury is most likely to occur.

Patient Positioning

Positioning for spinal surgery can present many challenges for the anesthesiologist. Prone positioning is associated with twice as many claims for peripheral nerve injuries as are other surgical positions. Vulnerable sites (e.g., bony prominences, axilla [brachial plexus], elbow [ulnar nerve], face, breasts) should be padded to disperse pressure. Unfortunately, meticulous attention to padding does not guarantee avoidance of injury.

In addition to debilitating peripheral nerve injury, postoperative visual loss has emerged as a rare but devastating complication of spinal surgery. Multiple mechanisms may contribute to postoperative blindness; however, ischemic optic neuropathy is the most common cause in patients having spinal surgery. Risk factors for postoperative visual loss are listed in Table 219-2. Postoperative blindness may occur despite the use of positioning techniques that avoid eye compression, such as the use of Mayfield tongs or special prone face pillows. Early blood transfusion, maintaining mean arterial pressure greater than 80% of baseline, and head-up positioning have been recommended to avoid perioperative blindness. However, there are no controlled trials to support the efficacy of these preventive measures.

Blood Loss and Transfusion Requirements

Anesthesiologists have several techniques available for reducing blood loss and transfusion requirements, including induced hypotension, autologous blood salvage, and normovolemic hemodilution.

INDUCED (ELECTIVE) HYPOTENSION

Induced hypotension has been shown to reduce blood loss and transfusion requirements during elective spinal surgery. Sodium nitroprusside, nitroglycerin, or β-blockers are given intravenously, possibly with continuous positive airway pressure and deep inhalation anesthesia, to initiate and maintain induced hypotension. Recently, nicardipine, an arterioselective vasodilator, has gained favor over sodium nitroprusside and nitroglycerin. The former is an arterial and venous vasodilator, and the latter is a venodilator, so both can reduce venous return and cardiac preload; thus, both have an increased potential to cause untoward hypotension compared with nicardipine. Nicardipine is compatible with β-blockers, and continuous positive airway pressure

Table 219-2 ■ Risk Factors for Postoperative Blindness	
Patient Factors	**Intraoperative Events**
Hypertension	Anemia (hematocrit ≤25)
Diabetes mellitus	Hypotension
Smoking history	Prolonged surgical time
Peripheral vascular disease	Prone positioning

can be added if further blood pressure reduction is needed. Although animal experimentation suggests that nitroglycerin is best for preserving spinal cord blood flow during hypotension, this has not been confirmed in humans.

The use of induced hypotension is based on clinical judgment, taking into account the overall physical status of the patient and the type of spinal surgery to be performed. Extreme caution should be used in the induction of hypotension in patients with significant spinal cord compression. Spinal injury impairs the normal autoregulatory process of the spinal cord vessels. External compression related to vertebral displacement or surgical retraction further decreases spinal blood flow. Hypotension has been associated with worse neurologic outcomes after traumatic spinal cord injury.

INTRAOPERATIVE AUTOLOGOUS BLOOD SALVAGE

Autologous blood salvage is a useful tool for preserving the blood lost during spinal surgery, but it can be associated with coagulopathy. Salvaged blood is autotransfused as needed after it has been washed or filtered, based on the type of equipment used. A micropore filter should be used to remove microaggregates, bone, and fat particles. However, fibrinolysis, inhibition of the clotting system, and possibly disseminated intravascular coagulation may occur with filtration-type autotransfusion. The removal of soluble products by cell washing systems can also induce coagulopathy, as well as the loss of coagulation factors and platelets. Purulent infection and malignancy were relative contraindications to autologous blood salvage in the past, but use of these systems is possible in these conditions with appropriate filtration.

ACUTE NORMOVOLEMIC HEMODILUTION

Acute normovolemic hemodilution is another method of reducing intraoperative blood loss. A predetermined amount of blood is removed from the patient in the operating room before or at the beginning of surgery and stored. It is then transfused back into the patient after most of the expected surgical blood loss has occurred. As blood is removed, it is replaced with colloid (1:1), crystalloid (3:1), or both. Platelet function and coagulation factors are preserved. Excessive hemodilution can reduce oxygen transport and cause a decrease in systemic vascular resistance and hypotension. In addition, it has been suggested that the combination of hypotension and low hemoglobin may contribute to the risk of optic ischemia and postoperative blindness in prone spinal surgery patients. Contraindications to acute normovolemic hemodilution include severe cardiovascular, pulmonary, renal, or hepatic dysfunction and coagulopathy.

Further Reading

Banoub M, Tetzlaff J, Schubert A: Pharmacologic and physiologic influences affecting sensory evoked potentials: Implications for perioperative monitoring. Anesthesiology 99:716-737, 2003.

Goto T, Crosby G: Anesthesia and the spinal cord. Anesthesiol Clin North Am 10:493-519, 1992.

Grundy BL, Nash CL, Brown RH, et al: Deliberate hypotension for spinal fusion: Prospective randomized study with evoked potential monitoring. Can Anaesth Soc J 29:452-462, 1982.

Kroll DA, Caplan RA, Posner K, et al: Nerve injury associated with anesthesia. Anesthesiology 73:202-207, 1990.

Lauer KK: Visual loss after spine surgery. J Neurosurg Anesthesiol 16:77-79, 2004.

Lotto ML, Banoub M, Schubert A: Effects of anesthetic agents and physiologic changes on intraoperative motor evoked potentials. J Neurosurg Anesthesiol 16:32-42, 2004.

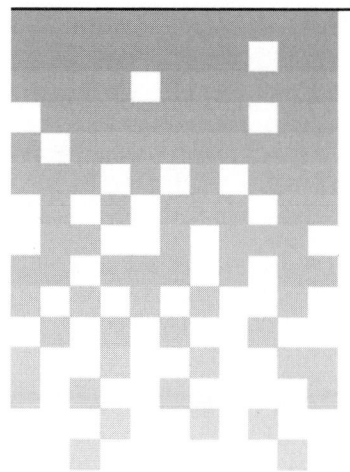

Special Topics

Donald A. Kroll

Nader D. Nader

POSTANESTHESIA CARE UNIT

Postoperative Respiratory Insufficiency

220

Jeffrey L. Lane

Case Synopsis

A 53-year-old morbidly obese man is recovering in the postanesthesia care unit (PACU) after undergoing an open Nissen fundoplication. He has a history of smoking. A left subclavian central line was placed without complication shortly after the induction of anesthesia. The intraoperative course was unremarkable, and the patient was extubated in the operating room. Shortly after arriving in the PACU, the patient becomes dyspneic. The oxygen saturation is 90%, heart rate is 110 beats per minute, blood pressure is 168/98 mm Hg, and respiratory rate is 32 breaths per minute.

PROBLEM ANALYSIS

Definition

Respiratory insufficiency is defined as the inability of the patient's lungs to provide sufficient oxygen (O_2) or expel sufficient carbon dioxide (CO_2) to satisfy whole body metabolic demands. In the postoperative setting, this can be related to (1) airway obstruction, (2) arterial hypoxemia, or (3) hypercarbia (Table 220-1). Airway obstruction is often mechanical, caused by occusion of the posterior oropharynx by the tongue.

Hypoxemia is defined as a reduction in arterial oxygen tension (PaO_2) below 60 mm Hg. It can be the result of atelectasis, pulmonary edema, pulmonary aspiration, pneumothorax, or pulmonary embolism. The differential diagnosis of hypoxemia includes decreased minute ventilation, low fraction of inspired oxygen (FiO_2), ventilation-perfusion mismatch, and block of O_2 diffusion across the alveolar membrane. Arterial oxygenation (PaO_2 in mm Hg) declines with age. When the subject is breathing room air, it can be estimated using this formula: $100 - (0.3 \times age)$.

Hypercarbia is defined as an increase in arterial CO_2 tension ($PaCO_2$) above 45 mm Hg. It results from decreased CO_2 elimination (hypoventilation, respiratory depression, lung pathology that increases dead space), increased CO_2 production (fever, sepsis, shivering, thyrotoxicosis, malignant hyperthermia), or CO_2 rebreathing. In the PACU, hypercarbia most often indicates respiratory depression from opiates or residual anesthetics. In contrast to PaO_2, $PaCO_2$ does not change with age.

Recognition

AIRWAY OBSTRUCTION

Airway obstruction presents with a combination of labored breathing pattern, chest wall retraction, nasal flaring, "snoring" or "grunting" noises (partial obstruction), absence of breath sounds (complete obstruction), paradoxical movement of the chest wall (e.g., "rocking boat" or "seesaw" respirations), stridor, wheezing, and patient anxiety. Cardiovascular manifestations include hypertension and tachycardia. As mentioned earlier, postoperative airway obstruction is usually due to tongue occlusion (partial or total) of the posterior oropharynx caused by opioids or residual anesthetics. Such occlusion may or may not be relieved by a head tilt or jaw thrust or by the placement of a nasopharyngeal airway. If these maneuvers do not relieve the occlusion, other causes must be considered (see Table 220-1).

Laryngospasm is usually seen immediately after extubation in the operating room or PACU. It results from stimulation of the glottal structures by secretions or airway equipment in a lightly anesthetized patient. It is usually characterized by a high-pitched inspiratory stridor ("cooing" or "crowing") or by the absence of sounds in cases of complete closure.

Airway edema from surgical trauma, patient positioning, or airway instrumentation may cause airway obstruction. Procedures that increase this risk include oral or extensive head and neck surgery and direct manipulation or instrumentation of the airway (e.g., vocal cord biopsy, bronchoscopy). Prolonged Trendelenburg or prone (or combined) positioning can lead to extensive airway edema. Further, patients with anticipated or unanticipated difficult airway management and prolonged airway instrumentation are at increased risk for airway edema.

Residual neuromuscular blockade is recognized by signs of inadequate neuromuscular relaxant reversal, including the presence of fade with tetanus and less than four out of four twitches on train-of-four stimulation. Clinically, the patient exhibits inadequate head lift (<5 seconds) and rapid, shallow breathing.

Wound hematoma following neck surgery (e.g., carotid endarterectomy, anterior cervical diskectomy, thyroidectomy) must be recognized quickly because it can lead to rapid airway obstruction and death. PACU nursing staff must be trained to recognize an expanding neck hematoma and immediately notify the anesthesiologist and surgeon for possible reintubation and wound drainage. In addition, patients

Table 220–1 ■ Causes of Postoperative Respiratory Insufficiency

Airway Obstruction
Mechanical (relaxed tongue)
Airway edema
Laryngospasm
Residual neuromuscular block
Foreign body aspiration
Neck hematoma
Vocal cord paralysis

Hypoxemia
Atelectasis
Pulmonary edema
Pulmonary embolism
Pneumothorax
Pulmonary aspiration
Bronchospasm

Hypercarbia
Decreased CO_2 elimination
　Hypoventilation
　Respiratory depression
　High dead space
Increased CO_2 production
　Fever or sepsis
　Shivering
　Malignant hyperthermia
　Thyrotoxicosis
　Overfeeding with total parenteral nutrition
　CO_2 insufflation
　Bicarbonate administration
CO_2 rebreathing

having neck surgery may have airway obstruction due to vocal cord paralysis, which presents similarly to laryngospasm.

Hypoxemia

Hypoxemia in patients recovering from general anesthesia is common and is usually relieved by supplemental O_2. In today's PACU, hypoxemia is usually recognized by low oxygen saturation (SpO_2) measured by peripheral pulse oximetry. This can be confirmed by direct arterial blood gas measurements, with low PaO_2 values. Manifestations of hypoxemia are (1) pulmonary (increased respiratory rate and pulmonary artery pressure due to hypoxic pulmonary vasoconstriction), (2) cardiovascular (increased blood pressure, tachycardia, and possibly arrhythmias), and (3) central nervous system signs (confusion, restlessness, combativeness, obtundation). When SpO_2 does not improve with supplemental O_2, other causes of hypoxemia must be ruled out.

Atelectasis is the most common cause of low postoperative SpO_2 values. General anesthesia causes a decrease in lung volumes (i.e., tidal volume, vital capacity, functional residual capacity). This can persist for up to 1 week postoperatively. General anesthesia also reduces chest wall and pulmonary compliance and inspiratory muscle tone. Further, it displaces the diaphragm in a cephalad direction. This leads to airway closure in highly perfused, dependent areas of the lung, increasing intrapulmonary shunt.

Postoperative pulmonary edema usually manifests as hypoxemia, tachypnea, and dyspnea. It is confirmed by chest auscultation (bibasilar rales) and chest radiograph (cephalization of the pulmonary vasculature). Pulmonary edema

can be classified as cardiogenic or noncardiogenic. Cardiogenic (or hydrostatic) pulmonary edema is commonly due to overhydration (positive intraoperative fluid balance >1500 mL) or cardiac dysfunction (myocardial ischemia or infarction, cardiomyopathy, severe hypertension, valvular stenosis). Cardiogenic pulmonary edema leads to high central venous and pulmonary capillary wedge pressures, with or without decreased urine output. Noncardiogenic (permeability) pulmonary edema occurs with acute respiratory distress syndrome and aspiration pneumonitis. Damage to alveolar cells allows fluid to transmigrate ("leak") into the alveolar space, causing pulmonary edema. With this type of pulmonary edema, central venous and pulmonary artery pressures are usually normal.

Pulmonary embolism must always be considered in the setting of postoperative hypoxemia. Air, fat, or thrombotic emboli may lodge in the pulmonary arterial circulation to cause dyspnea, tachypnea, tachycardia, hypotension, and increased venous pressure and alveolar dead-space ventilation. The last manifests as an increased $PaCO_2$ to end-tidal CO_2 gradient.

In the PACU, pneumothorax may be a cause of hypoxemia in patients with recent central line placement, rib fractures, intercostal blocks, or surgery near or involving the diaphragm (e.g., liver resection, nephrectomy, splenectomy, hiatal hernia repair, esophageal resection, upper stomach surgery). Signs and symptoms include dyspnea, tachypnea, unequal breath sounds, high peak inspiratory pressures, and possibly hypotension due to tension pneumothorax. Chest radiographs showing partial to complete lung collapse confirm the diagnosis.

Hypercarbia

Hypercarbia (hypoventilation) is common after general anesthesia. In most instances, it is mild and of no major consequence. Respiratory acidosis due to moderate hypercarbia ($PaCO_2$ >50 mm Hg) manifests with sympathomimetic signs and symptoms: hypertension, tachycardia, headache, nausea, sweating, and agitation. Severe hypercarbia ($PaCO_2$ >80 mm Hg) can result in somnolence (CO_2 narcosis), arrhythmias, and direct myocardial depression. If hypercarbia is suspected, arterial blood gas determinations can confirm the diagnosis. The next step is to determine the cause of hypoventilation.

Drugs are the most common cause of postoperative respiratory depression with hypoventilation. Residual inhaled anesthetics and intravenous or neuraxial opioids are the most common offenders in PACU settings. Inhaled anesthetics usually cause a rapid, shallow breathing pattern, whereas opioid-induced respiratory depression results in a slow respiratory rate in association with large tidal volumes and pinpoint pupils.

"Splinting" occurs when inspiratory effort is retarded by significant incisional pain, abdominal distention, or tight abdominal dressings. It occurs most often after upper abdominal or thoracic surgery and may lead to hypoventilation and hypercarbia.

Residual neuromuscular blockade is another cause of hypoventilation in the PACU. It results from inadequate reversal, overdose, pharmacologic interactions (e.g., antibiotics, magnesium), altered pharmacokinetics (e.g., hypothermia, renal or hepatic dysfunction), or metabolic factors (e.g., hyperkalemia and acidosis). The clinical diagnosis is made by the inability of a conscious patient to maintain a 5-second head lift or by the use of a nerve stimulator in an unconscious patient.

Risk Assessment

Postoperative pulmonary complications (including respiratory failure) following general anesthesia are common (up to 20% to 30% in some series), so the need to assess patient risk is critical. Risk factors for the development of postoperative respiratory failure include the following:

- Surgical site (upper abdominal, thoracic)
- Smoking
- Underlying chronic obstructive pulmonary disease or asthma
- Emergency surgery
- Anesthesia time longer than 180 minutes
- Advanced age
- Obstructive sleep apnea
- Morbid obesity

Preoperative pulmonary function tests are useful for predicting postoperative pulmonary dysfunction only after pulmonary resection; in other situations, they do not predict postoperative pulmonary complications. For patients with one or more of the preceding risk factors, anesthetists must strongly consider delaying tracheal extubation until there has been satisfactory progress with temporary mechanical ventilation and weaning (i.e., satisfactory unassisted ventilation and oxygenation).

Implications

Postoperative respiratory insufficiency can lead to serious patient morbidity and even death. Pulmonary complications are the most common serious postoperative complications, and they must be recognized and dealt with expeditiously to prevent adverse patient outcomes. Both hypoxemia and hypercarbia have detrimental systemic effects (Table 220-2). Hypertension, tachycardia, tachypnea, and arrhythmias place cardiac patients at increased risk for myocardial ischemia and infarction; this risk is increased even further with anemia (due to intraoperative blood loss) or shivering (due to altered temperature regulation). Patients with underlying neurologic disease are at even greater risk, because hypoxemia and hypercarbia alter mental status and increase intracranial pressure.

MANAGEMENT

As in most anesthetic emergencies, management of postoperative respiratory insufficiency begins with evaluation and establishment of a patent airway. In patients with mechanical airway obstruction, supplemental O_2 should be given while head-tilt and jaw-thrust maneuvers are performed to help displace the tongue anteriorly. Also, an oral or nasal airway can help alleviate any tongue-related obstruction. Use of a nasal airway is preferred in semiconscious or awake patients, owing to less discomfort (gagging) and better tolerance

Table 220-2 ■ Effects of Hypoxemia and Hypercarbia

System	Hypoxemia	Hypercarbia
Pulmonary	Tachypnea Pulmonary 　vasoconstriction	Tachypnea Pulmonary 　vasoconstriction Bronchodilatation
Cardiac	Early 　Tachycardia 　Hypertension 　Arrhythmias Late 　Bradycardia 　Hypotension 　Cardiac arrest	Hypertension Tachycardia Arrhythmias
Neurologic	Restlessness Combativeness Confusion Obtundation Increased ICP	Increased ICP Obtundation
Metabolic	Metabolic lactic 　acidosis	Respiratory acidosis Hyperkalemia

ICP, intracranial pressure.

(unlikely to provoke partial or complete laryngospasm). If these measures do not alleviate the obstruction, laryngospasm must be suspected. If this is the case, gentle positive-pressure mask ventilation may be effective. In many cases, however, a muscle relaxant must be administered, followed by reintubation.

Minor upper airway edema is usually relieved by maintaining the patient in a semisitting (semi-Fowler) position, followed by the use of humidified gases, intravenous steroids (e.g., hydrocortisone, dexamethasone), and racemic epinephrine. If these conservative measures fail, immediate intubation and mechanical ventilation are necessary.

In patients recovering from neck surgery who develop respiratory insufficiency, neck hematoma must be considered, with planning and setup for immediate drainage and possible intubation. In fact, early reintubation may prevent a lethal complication. A rapidly expanding neck hematoma can distort airway anatomy and make airway management extraordinarily difficult.

Hypoxemia management starts with O_2 via a nasal cannula or facemask. Hypoxemia in the PACU is usually relieved with O_2 concentrations greater than 50%. Short-term therapy with 100% O_2 by facemask may be necessary. If higher inspired O_2 concentrations are needed to maintain PaO_2 greater than 60 mm Hg, more aggressive treatment (e.g., continuous positive airway pressure by mask or intubation and mechanical ventilation) is required. After ensuring adequate oxygenation, treatment is directed toward the cause. A chest radiograph may reveal pulmonary edema, infiltrates, or pneumothorax. Diuretics are given for pulmonary edema. Significant pneumothorax requires early chest tube placement. For bronchospasm, aerosolized bronchodilators are indicated. Bronchoscopy may be necessary to remove pulmonary secretions and mucous plugs.

Hypercarbia management is also directed toward the underlying cause. Often, simply encouraging the patient to breathe more vigorously is sufficient to relieve hypercarbia until residual drug effects have subsided. If opioids are the cause, intravenous naloxone should be carefully titrated (≤40-μg increments) until ventilation is adequate. Larger doses may cause an acute hyperadrenergic crisis (hypertension, tachycardia, fulminant pulmonary edema)[1] brought on by the sudden awareness of acute pain. If splinting due to pain leads to hypoventilation, additional analgesics must be given. Alternative pain control (epidural or spinal narcotics, intercostal block, local anesthetic wound infiltration by the surgeon) may also reduce pain-related splinting. Residual neuromuscular block may require intubation and controlled ventilation until its effects dissipate. Whatever the cause, severe hypoventilation may call for tracheal intubation and controlled ventilation until the primary cause has been determined and treated.

PREVENTION

All patients recovering from general anesthesia or regional anesthesia with sedation should receive supplemental O_2 during transport to the PACU. As in the operating room, pulse oximetry should be used in the PACU to monitor SpO_2, with confirmation by arterial blood gas sampling if necessary. Routine PACU pulse oximetry monitoring allows practitioners to detect hypoxemia early and intervene appropriately. To limit reduced lung volumes and functional residual capacity, patients (especially those who are obese) should be maintained in the semisitting (semi-Fowler) position to minimize upward displacement of the diaphragm. This, along with the routine use of nasal airways in obese patients before extubation, will help reduce mechanical airway obstruction. Incentive spirometry may be used to limit atelectasis and improve functional residual capacity. Also, continuous positive airway pressure reduces the incidence of postoperative pulmonary complications.

Pain alleviation may also help prevent postoperative respiratory insufficiency. In high-risk patients with chronic obstructive pulmonary disease undergoing high-risk (upper abdominal, thoracic) surgery, continuous epidural anesthesia is known to reduce the incidence of postoperative pulmonary complications. Although adequate analgesia helps limit postoperative respiratory insufficiency, judicious use of intravenous opioids is warranted to prevent overdose and hypoventilation.

To prevent hypoventilation, hypercarbia, and hypoxemia due to residual neuromuscular block, short-acting neuromuscular blockers, along with a nerve stimulator to monitor their effects, can ensure an adequate return of neuromuscular function (e.g., sustained tetanus, return to control response to train-of-four or double-burst stimulation, 5-second head lift) before extubation.

Further Reading

Adhere C, Brunson C, Roizen M: Sleep apnea, obstructive. In Roizen M, Fleisher L (eds): Essence of Anesthesia Practice, 2nd ed. Philadelphia, WB Saunders, 2002, p 307.

Barash P, Cullen B, Stoelting R: Clinical Anesthesia, 4th ed. Philadelphia, JB Lippincott, 2000, pp 1385-1392.

Benumof J: Obesity, sleep apnea, the airway and anesthesia. ASA Refresher Courses in Anesthesiology 30:27-40, 2002.

Gruber A, Hsu J: Hypoxemia. In Pardo M, Sonner J (eds): The Manual of Anesthesia Practice, version 1.2. PocketMedicine.com, 2004.

Gwirtz K: Management of recovery room complications. Anesthesiol Clin North Am 14:307-399, 1996.

Hsu J: Hypercarbia. In Pardo M, Sonner J (eds): The Manual of Anesthesia Practice, version 1.2. PocketMedicine.com, 2004.

Morgan G, Mikhail M, Murray M: Clinical Anesthesiology, 3rd ed. Chicago, McGraw-Hill/Lange, 2002, pp 942-946.

Price J, Rizk N: Postoperative ventilatory management. Chest 115: 130s-137s, 1999.

Rock P: Evaluation and perioperative management of the patient with respiratory disease. ASA Refresher Courses in Anesthesiology, 2002.

Stoelting R, Dierdorf S: Anesthesia and Co-existing Disease, 4th ed. Philadelphia, Churchill Livingstone, 2002, pp 217-219, 444-446.

Warner D: Preventing postoperative pulmonary complications: The role of the anesthesiologist. Anesthesiology 92:1467-1472, 2000.

---

[1]The editor saw three such cases shortly after intravenous naloxone was first used in PACUs to reverse relative opioid overdose. In each case, the initial doses were 200 or 400 mg—amounts then used to treat heroin overdoses in emergency rooms. Within minutes, the patients spewed "cotton candy" oral secretions, likely due to forward heart failure. Fortunately, all three patients survived.

Postoperative Peripheral Neuropathy

221

David A. Nakata and Robert K. Stoelting

Case Synopsis

A 28-year-old man with insulin-dependent diabetes mellitus for 15 years was diagnosed with testicular cancer. His chemotherapy regimen consisted of bleomycin and cisplatin. He underwent postchemotherapy retroperitoneal lymph node dissection under general anesthesia. The surgery, which took 2 hours, was unremarkable, as was his stay in the postanesthesia care unit. On postoperative day 3, the patient noted a decreased level of sensation in the fourth and fifth digits of his left hand. He had no prior history of peripheral neuropathy. He was subsequently diagnosed with a left ulnar neuropathy.

PROBLEM ANALYSIS

Definition

Neuropathies are classified into three histologic groups, with increasing levels of severity: neurapraxia, axonotmesis, and neurotmesis. Clinically, any or all of these injury patterns can be present in the affected nerve. With neurapraxia, there is no disruption of actual anatomic neural elements. However, there may be temporary conduction block during ischemia or some degree of demyelination, with greater effects on the function of large fibers (i.e., motor, joint position sense, soft touch). Changes accompanying neurapraxia usually resolve within a few weeks, with complete recovery expected. With axonotmesis, axons are disrupted, but the nerve sheaths remain intact. Wallerian degeneration follows, but axon regeneration results in recovery of function over weeks to months. Even so, some degree of sensory or motor deficit may persist. Neurotmesis is the most serious injury, with disruption of the entire nerve, including transection of the axons and myelin sheaths. This typically prevents regeneration and recovery, resulting in poor functional recovery. Often, the nerve is replaced with fibrous scar tissue.

The majority of postoperative neuropathies are due to nerve ischemia. Most commonly, this is caused by either stretch or compression. Direct mechanical compression can obviously lead to reduced blood flow, and stretch produces a reduction in the cross-sectional area of the neural structures, leading to compression of the vasculature (Fig. 221-1).

Recognition

Postoperative neuropathies are commonly ascribed to events that occur intraoperatively. In numerous cases, however, despite close follow-up, symptoms are not reported until days after the operative procedure. It stands to reason that if intraoperative events were responsible for the development of these neuropathies, symptoms would be reported more proximate to the patient's emergence from anesthesia. Given the reporting delay, consideration must be given to the possibility that many of these neuropathies stem from events occurring in the postoperative period. This is in sharp contrast to the historical belief, still held by many, that the development of neuropathy represents an intraoperative deviation from the standard of care.

Risk Assessment

Many factors are known to be associated with the development of postoperative neuropathies (Table 221-1). In the patient described in the case synopsis, male gender, preoperative chemotherapy, and diabetes mellitus are known risk factors associated with the development of neuropathies.

In males, the ulnar nerve appears to be at greater risk of injury owing to anatomic differences between the sexes. The tubercle of the coronoid process is approximately 1.5 times larger in men than in women, perhaps predisposing to increased bony compression of the nerve. In addition, women generally have a larger fat pad within the medial aspect of the elbow, which may help protect the ulnar nerve (Fig. 221-2). Also, it has been suggested that the cubital tunnel retinaculum

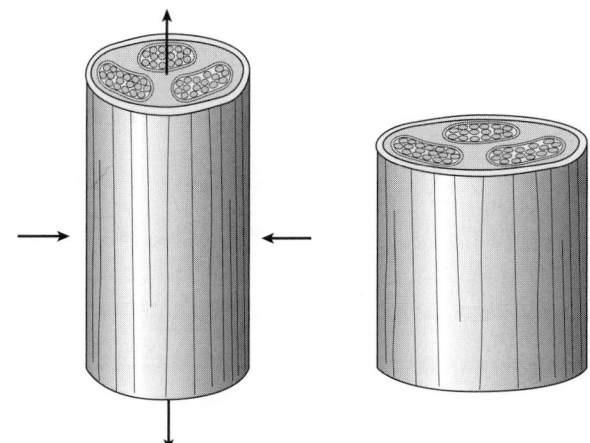

Figure 221–1 ■ Nerve stretch is associated with a decrease in cross-sectional area and an increase in intraneural pressures. (From Butler DS: Mobilization of the Nervous System. New York, Churchill Livingstone, 1991.)

Table 221–1 ▪ Factors That May Increase the Risk of Perioperative Neuropathy
Alcoholism
Amyloidosis
Arthritis
Atherosclerotic disease
Autoimmune disorders
Bell's palsy
Cancer
Chemotherapy
Connective tissue diseases
Diabetes mellitus
Direct nerve trauma
Gender (male)
Hepatic failure
Hypothyroidism
Infectious diseases
Malnutrition
Nerve entrapment syndromes
Renal failure
Trauma to adjacent structures
Vitamin deficiencies

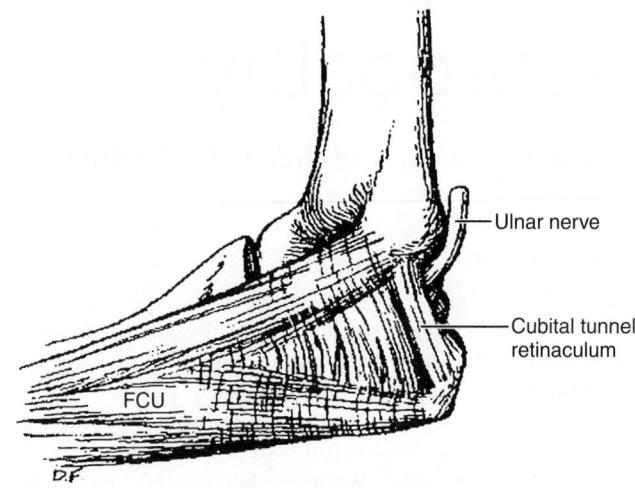

Figure 221–3 ▪ The cubital tunnel retinaculum is a tough, fibrous band that is in close proximity to the ulnar nerve. Compression of the ulnar nerve can occur between this retinaculum and the medial epicondyle. FCU, flexor carpi ulnaris (ulnar head). (From Warner M: Perioperative neuropathies, blindness, and positioning problems. American Society of Anesthesiologists 53rd Annual Refresher Course Lectures, 2002, Orlando, Fla.)

in men is more robust and may place greater compressive force on the ulnar nerve when stretched (Fig. 221-3).

Peripheral nerves are much more tolerant to ischemia than are nerves within the central nervous system. Peripheral nerves are commonly subjected to ischemia during the placement of vascular tourniquets for hemostasis. When inflated, the applied force is often greater than 100 mm Hg above the systolic pressure. This degree of pressure has been shown to produce slowing of nerve conduction directly under the area of compression, followed by more distal slowing as tourniquet times increase.

In clinical practice, an "ischemic" tourniquet time of less than 2 hours is generally accepted. Animal studies have shown that ischemia is tolerated for up to 4 hours without causing permanent nerve damage. Compressive forces produced by tourniquets are generally greater than those produced by placing the arms or legs on a padded operating room table. Thus, individuals who undergo operative procedures lasting

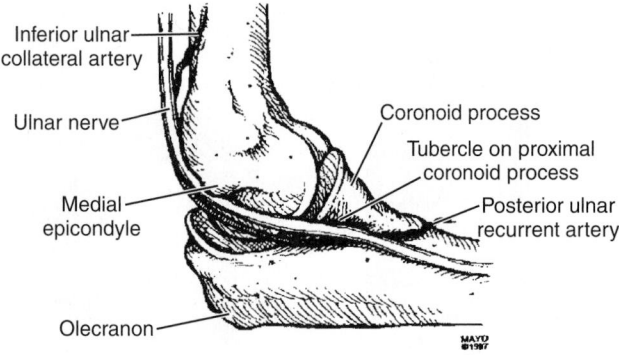

Figure 221–2 ▪ The ulnar nerve and ulnar collateral artery at the elbow are relatively superficial and easy to compress. The coronoid process in males is larger than in females, and the adipose layer is less prominent. These factors increase the risk of compression to the ulnar nerve in males. (From Warner M: Perioperative neuropathies, blindness, and positioning problems. American Society of Anesthesiologists 53rd Annual Refresher Course Lectures, 2002, Orlando, Fla.)

less than 2 hours should be almost immune to the development of postoperative neuropathies from tourniquet application or accepted positioning maneuvers.

The patient described in the case synopsis had multiple risk factors for the development of neuropathies, including a long history of diabetes mellitus and recent chemotherapy. Preexisting conditions likely play an important role in the development of neuropathies in many individuals. This patient had no preexisting symptoms of peripheral nerve involvement, but neuropathies associated with metabolic conditions (e.g., diabetes mellitus, chemotherapy) generally have an insidious onset. This gradual onset provides an opportunity for subclinical neuropathies to become well established before the onset of symptoms, and it also leads to increased susceptibility for the development of a symptomatic neuropathy. A well-described potential cause for such increased risk is the double crush syndrome.

Double crush syndrome is a peripheral nervous system disorder in which dual lesions in the same nerve act synergistically to enhance each one's severity. Nemoto and coworkers showed that placing a low-compression clamp on a dog's peripheral nerve could produce an incomplete conduction block. This caused only mild axonal degeneration, with no obvious clinical sequelae. If a second, equally low-compression clamp was placed more distally on the same peripheral nerve, complete conduction blockade with marked axonal degeneration was shown. This double crush injury model provides insight into how comorbidities may increase the risk of perioperative neuropathies. Also, the model may explain why some individuals develop neuropathies while others do not, despite the use of similar positioning precautions.

Double crush syndrome likely plays an important role in the development of neuropathies in patients with preexisting nerve entrapment syndromes. For example, cubital tunnel syndrome is a common nerve entrapment syndrome, second in frequency only to carpal tunnel syndrome. The cubital tunnel is an enclosed space surrounded by tough fibrous materials and bone. Because of these anatomic boundaries, the cubital tunnel has a limited ability to expand during fluid accumulation. Postoperatively, patients retain third-space (i.e., interstitial) fluid, some of which accumulates in the cubital tunnel. This accumulation may increase pressure within the cubital tunnel, leading to double crush ulnar nerve compression. Pregnancy-induced carpal tunnel syndrome is a well-known example in which fluid retention can lead to a clinically significant peripheral neuropathy.

Implications

The American Society of Anesthesiologists' closed claims analyses recognize postoperative ulnar neuropathies as among the most common, if not the most common, postoperative peripheral neuropathy. In 1999, 28% of all claims for such nerve injuries involved the ulnar nerve. More recent analyses of claims in which anesthesia care was implicated suggest that some injuries did not occur until after anesthesia care had ended.

In a prospective study, Warner and colleagues found that the median time for reporting symptoms of ulnar neuropathy was 4 days after surgery (range, 2 to 7 days). Another prospective study by Warner's group showed that ulnar neuropathies also occurred in medical patients who did not undergo surgery. Considering these reports, it is implausible to assume that all perioperative neuropathies occur during the intraoperative and perianesthetic care periods. Thus, other mechanisms for such neuropathies need to be sought.

Postsurgical patients routinely receive opiates for pain control. These drugs blunt not only pain sensation but also the sensation of any paresthesias the patient might experience. Pain medications also produce sedation, so that patients are less mobile. Such immobility might extend the time patients spend in positions that could result in nerve stretch or compression injury.

Finally, during postoperative rounds, it is common to find patients resting with their arms folded across the chest or abdomen. Elbow flexion is known to raise the pressure within the cubital tunnel and also to stretch the ulnar nerve, either of which can increase the likelihood of nerve ischemia (Fig. 221-4). Often, this crossed arm position places the cubital tunnel directly in contact with the bed, further compressing the ulnar nerve. Finally, the ulnar nerve may be injured when patients sit in armchairs with their arms flexed, which can place the cubital tunnel in direct contact with the armrests.

MANAGEMENT

No specific guidelines exist regarding when a neurologist should be consulted for the complaint of peripheral neuropathy. Consideration of the duration and severity of the findings is required. If the supposed peripheral neuropathy resolves within a short period, neurapraxia is the most likely diagnosis, and a full recovery can be expected. However, if the findings persist with no improvement, a neurology consultation should be considered to assist in both diagnosis and management. In some instances, nerve conduction studies may be warranted.

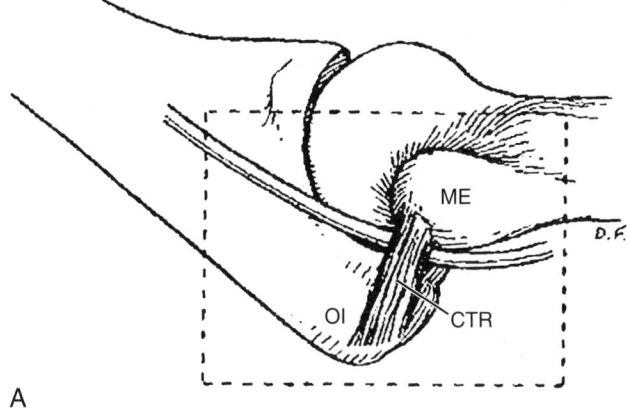

A

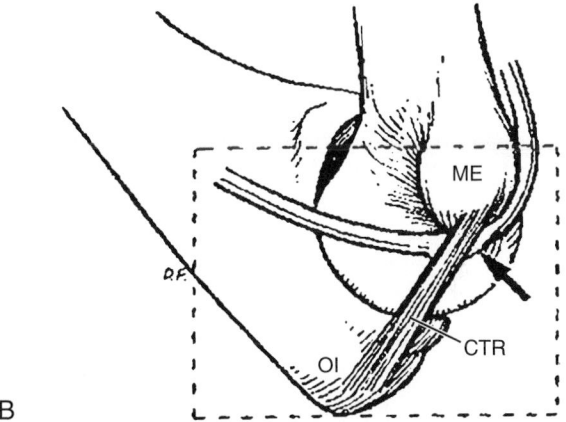

B

Figure 221–4 ■ *A,* Anatomy during elbow extension. *B,* During elbow flexion, the cubital tunnel retinaculum (CTR) is stretched between the medial epicondyle (ME) and the olecranon process (Ol), leading to compression of the ulnar nerve *(arrow).* Also, the ulnar nerve is physically stretched during elbow flexion, causing reduction in its cross-sectional area and blood flow. (From Warner M: Perioperative neuropathies, blindness, and positioning problems. American Society of Anesthesiologists 53rd Annual Refresher Course Lectures, 2002, Orlando, Fla.)

PREVENTION

In 2000 the American Society of Anesthesiologists published a practice advisory for the prevention of perioperative peripheral neuropathies. This advisory made several recommendations that may decrease the incidence of ulnar neuropathy:

- Arm abduction should be limited to 90 degrees in supine patients; patients who are positioned prone may comfortably tolerate arm abduction greater than 90 degrees.
- Arms should be positioned to decrease pressure on the postcondylar groove of the humerus (ulnar groove). When arms are tucked at the sides, a neutral forearm position is recommended. When arms are abducted on armboards, either supination or a neutral forearm position is acceptable.
- Padded armboards may decrease the risk of upper extremity neuropathies.
- Padding at the elbow and at the fibular head may decrease the risk of upper and lower extremity neuropathies, respectively.

SPECIAL TOPICS

Given the multitude of factors that may contribute to perioperative ulnar neuropathy, it cannot be assumed that all perioperative nerve injuries are due to a violation of the standard of care. This idea is reinforced, in most cases, by the relatively long interval between the operative procedure and the initial report of symptoms.

Further Reading

Bentley FH, Schlapp W: Experiments on the blood supply of nerves. J Physiol 102:62, 1943.

Cheney FW, Domino KB, Caplan RA, et al: Nerve injury associated with anesthesia: A closed claims analysis. Anesthesiology 90:1062-1069, 1999.

Gelberman RH, Yamaguchi K, Hollstien SB, et al: Changes in interstitial pressure and cross-sectional area of the cubital tunnel and of the ulnar nerve with flexion of the elbow: An experimental study in human cadavera. J Bone Joint Surg Am 80:492-501, 1998.

Nemoto K, Matsumoto N, Tazaki K, et al: An experimental study on the "double crush" hypothesis. J Hand Surg [Am] 12:552-559, 1987.

Practice advisory for the prevention of perioperative peripheral neuropathies: A report by the American Society of Anesthesiologists Task Force on Prevention of Perioperative Peripheral Neuropathies. Anesthesiology 92:1168-1182, 2000.

Warner MA, Warner DO, Harper C, et al: Ulnar neuropathy in medical patients. Anesthesiology 92:613-617, 2000.

Warner MA, Warner DO, Matsumoto JY, et al: Ulnar neuropathy in surgical patients. Anesthesiology 90:54-59, 1999.

Delayed Emergence

Deborah A. McClain

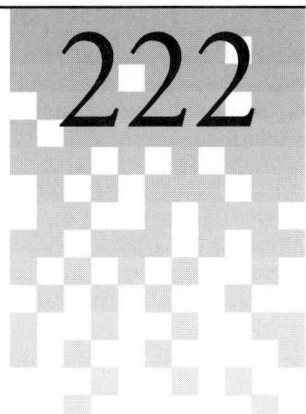

222

Case Synopsis

A 50-year-old man undergoes general anesthesia for umbilical hernia. He weighs 120 kg and has a history of hypertension, gastroesophageal reflux disease (GERD), polysubstance abuse, hepatitis C, and post-traumatic stress disorder (PTSD). He is taking hydrochlorothiazide, an ACE inhibitor, cimetidine, omeprazole, citalopram, and trazodone. The anesthetic and surgery progress uneventfully. The patient is extubated and taken to the postanesthesia care unit (PACU). After 15 minutes, the patient fails to respond to verbal stimuli.

PROBLEM ANALYSIS

Definition

Delayed emergence is failure of the patient to regain the expected level of consciousness within 20 to 30 minutes of the end of anesthetic administration. Intervention is necessary to rule out potentially harmful, reversible conditions. Possible causes can be classified as follows:

- Anesthetic drugs
- Medications
- Electrolyte disorders
- Metabolic disorders
- Systemic effects

Recognition

As with all assessments, the ABCs (airway, breathing, circulation) take priority and should be reevaluated throughout the course of delayed emergence. Other assessment tools include the following:

- Pharmacologic agents
- Physical examination
- Laboratory examination
- Computed tomography (CT) of the head
- Neurology consultation

The diagnosis of delayed emergence is made in the PACU, and the cause may be multifactorial. An anesthesiologist must evaluate these patients promptly to differentiate delayed emergence from the life-threatening problems that may falsely manifest as delayed emergence: airway obstruction, hypoxia, and hypercarbia. The patient should be evaluated immediately with assessment of vital signs (especially the rate and character of spontaneous breathing and oxygen saturation) and a physical examination.

Further evaluation must consider the patient's preexisting medical problems, any pharmacologic agents taken preoperatively or administered in the perianesthetic period, and the nature of the operative procedure performed. A thorough physical examination must be performed, with particular emphasis on vital signs (including temperature), smelling of the patient's breath for residual volatile anesthetics, and neurologic examination. A firm tactile stimulus may arouse the obtunded patient more effectively than verbal stimulation.

Prompt laboratory evaluation includes arterial blood gas analysis to assess pH, oxygen and carbon dioxide partial pressures, and blood glucose concentration. Serum electrolytes, including calcium and magnesium, should also be evaluated. Obtaining a urine sample for toxicologic evaluation may be prudent. Finally, a CT scan of the patient's head and consultation with a neurologist may be necessary.

Risk Assessment

Although delayed emergence has many causes, its predictability and the rate at which it will occur have not been specifically assessed. Most cases are purely anecdotal, and thus no occurrence rate has been determined. Nevertheless, some level of responsiveness to stimulation should occur within 90 minutes of the cessation of anesthetic administration.

Certain patients are at greater risk for delayed emergence from anesthesia. These include patients with preexisting cognitive or psychiatric disorders and patients who chronically take sedative medications. Patients who were anesthetized while intoxicated by alcohol or recreational drugs may be more difficult to arouse. Finally, those who were physically exhausted prior to surgery may have prolonged emergence.

Implications

Depending on the cause of the delayed emergence, the consequences may be catastrophic or minor. However, prompt, efficient assessment and treatment are key to minimizing potential catastrophes.

MANAGEMENT

Anesthetic Drugs

Many factors influence the effect of inhalational or intravenous drugs on the patient's level of consciousness:

- Central nervous system (CNS) sensitivity
- Metabolism/excretion
- Redistribution

- Amount of drug administered
- Plasma concentration

Biologic variation in CNS sensitivity follows the bell-shaped Gaussian curve. Some patients require very small amounts of drugs for induction and maintenance, whereas others require larger and larger quantities. The majority, of course, fall in the middle. The concentration of drug that reaches the brain receptor and the sensitivity of the receptor to that specific drug determine the response.

Decreased hepatic metabolism occurs in patients at the extremes of age, in malnourished patients, in hypothermic patients, and in patients who simultaneously receive several drugs that are detoxified by the hepatic microsomal enzyme system (e.g., ethanol, barbiturates).

While redistribution is responsible for the short action of some drugs (such as thiopental), it can contribute to delayed emergence as well, especially when given in repeated doses. Fat-soluble drugs, such as inhalation anesthetics, are distributed to fat stores. The result is a storage depot that releases anesthetic back into the circulation after the conclusion of the case. This is especially true for long-acting anesthetics and in obese patients.

Plasma concentration and the portion of drug available to interact with receptors are affected by other factors, such as albumin and other proteins that influence protein binding. The less drug that is bound to plasma proteins, the more that is available to interact with receptors. Protein binding is also affected by pH. For example, protein binding of fentanyl decreases as the plasma becomes more acidotic, resulting in more free fentanyl. Other drugs in the patient's system may compete for binding sites and thus result in more free drug. Volatile anesthetics, narcotics, sedatives, and muscle relaxants all can lead to delayed emergence. Phase II blockade or a pseudocholinesterase deficiency can result in prolonged neuromuscular blocking effects when succinylcholine is administered. In this case it is usually better to avoid attempts at reversal. Furthermore, some antibiotics enhance and prolong the action of nondepolarizing relaxants.

Medications

Prescribed medications, such as sleeping aids, pain medications, and lipid-lowering drugs, affect minimum alveolar concentration (MAC) or occupy some of the receptors. Over-the-counter medications should also be considered as a source of delayed emergence (see also Chapter 39). H_2-receptor antagonists cimetidine and ranitidine impair hepatic microsomal oxidation of some drugs. Greenblatt and colleagues found that although healthy volunteers showed no increase in sensitivity to midazolam or benzodiazepines, other drugs that depend on hepatic metabolism may be affected, as may less healthy patients. Herbal supplements also have the potential to cause excessive sedation and delayed emergence. Kava, St. John's wort, and valerian are the primary culprits. Herbal products should be discontinued 1 day to 1 week prior to anesthesia (see also Chapter 39). Chemotherapeutic agents, such as L-asparaginase and vincristine, often produce CNS depression and even electrocardiographic changes. Although these agents are a rare cause of

delayed emergence, they are included in the differential diagnosis (see also Chapter 30).

Electrolyte Disorders

Hyponatremia, especially if acute, can cause lethargy, delayed awakening, and seizures. The most common cause encountered in connection with anesthesia is the TURP (transurethral resection of the prostate) syndrome. The circumstances and serum sodium below 130 mEq/L make the diagnosis relatively simple to make. Correction should proceed at no more than 2 mEq/L per hour until a serum sodium of 130 mEq/L ± 2 mEq/L is reached. Hypercalcemia and hypermagnesemia can produce CNS depression even to the point of coma.

Metabolic Disorders

Extremes of serum glucose, hypoglycemia from fasting or insulin, or hyperglycemia (hyperosmotic, hyperglycemia, nonketotic coma) can result in prolonged unconsciousness. Other endocrine abnormalities, primarily hypothyroidism and adrenal suppression or deficit, should also be considered as a cause for delayed emergence.

Systemic Effects

Respiratory depression can lead to CO_2 narcosis. This may be more difficult to diagnosis in the PACU, where end-tidal CO_2 is not routinely monitored. Hypoxia resulting from depression or ventilation-perfusion mismatching should also be ruled out. Hypothermia can also contribute to the lowered level of consciousness. Although body temperature between 30 and 32°C does not cause unconsciousness alone, its effects on biotransformation and inhalational anesthetic solubility may contribute to prolonged emergence. Temperatures lower than 30°C can cause cold narcosis through a direct effect on the brain. Hyperthermia >40°C, such as is seen in heatstroke or malignant hyperthermia, does result in loss of consciousness. Neurologic events including stroke and seizures should also be considered in the differential diagnosis. Increased intracranial pressure caused by a cranial bleed or resulting from an intracranial mass, especially with an elevation in end-tidal CO_2, can augment the effects of the latter to worsen CO_2 narcosis.

TREATMENT

Reversal agents (naloxone, flumazenil, physostigmine, neostigmine) may be used for treatment for as well as diagnosis of prolonged effects of narcotics, benzodiazepines, inhalation anesthetics, and muscle relaxants.

Electrolyte and metabolic abnormalities should be corrected in symptomatic patients, but this must be done carefully to avoid serious undesired effects. Causes for hypoxia or hypercarbia should be assessed even as ventilatory support is initiated. A thorough neurologic evaluation should be performed to seek localizing signs versus global effects.

A neurology consultation or CT scan may be appropriate if other causes have been eliminated. Appropriate reversal dosages are listed below:

- Naloxone, 40-μg doses every 2 minutes IV to a total of 200 μg
- Flumazenil, 0.2 mg/min IV to a total of 1.0 mg
- Physostigmine, 1.25 mg IV

PREVENTION

Delayed emergence may be minimized by careful perioperative care of the patient, including a precise history and physical examination, vigilant intraoperative care and monitoring, and early evaluation of potential postoperative problems. Judicious and appropriate titration of reversal agents may alleviate the prolonged anesthetic medication effects. Careful evaluation of serum chemistries, neurologic evaluation, consultation with a neurologist, and CT scan may be necessary if neurologic injury has occurred.

Further Reading

Cohen ML, Chan S, Way WL, et al: Distribution in the brain and metabolism of ketamine in the rat after intravenous administration. Anesthesiology 39:370, 1973.

Curtis D, Stevens WC: Recovery from general anesthesia. Int Anesthesiol Clin 29:1, 1991.

Gerich JE, Martin MN, Recant L: Clinical and metabolic characteristics of hyperosmolar non-ketotic coma. Diabetes 20:228, 1971.

Ghoneim MM, Dembo JH, Block RI: Time course of antagonism of sedative and amnestic effects of diazepam by flumazenil. Anesthesiology 70:899, 1989.

Greenblatt DJ, Locniskar A, Scavone JM, et al: Absence of interaction of cimetidine and ranitidine with intravenous and oral midazolam. Anesth Analg 65:176, 1986.

Lyew MA, Mondy C, Eagle S, et al: Hemodynamic instability and delayed emergence from general anesthesia associated with inadvertent intrathecal baclofen overdose. Anesthesiology 98:265, 2003.

McClain DA, Hug CC: Intravenous fentanyl kinetics. Clin Pharmacol Ther 28:111, 1980.

Narins RG: Therapy of hyponatremia: Does haste make waste? N Engl J Med 314:1573, 1986.

Prough DS, Roy R, Bumgarner J, et al: Acute pulmonary edema in healthy teenagers following conservative doses of intravenous naloxone. Anesthesiology 60:485, 1984.

Reves JG, Glass PSA, Lubarsky DA, et al: Intravenous nonopioid anesthetics. In Miller RD (ed): Miller's Anesthesia, 6th ed. Philadelphia, Churchill Livingstone, 2005, p 317.

Stoelting RK, Eger EI II: The effects of ventilation and anesthetic solubility on recovery from anesthesia. Anesthesiology 30:290, 1969.

Tinker JH, Gandolfi AJ, Van Dyke RA: Elevation of plasma bromide levels in patients following halothane anesthesia. Anesthesiology 44:194, 1976.

Ward CF: Pulmonary edema and naloxone. J Clin Anesth 8:690, 1996.

Weiss HD, Walker MD, Wiernik PH: Neurotoxicity of commonly used antineoplastic agents. N Engl J Med 291:75, 127, 1974

Wood M: Plasma drug binding: Implications for anesthesiologists. Anesth Analg 65:786, 1986.

SPECIAL TOPICS

Postoperative Delirium

223

Philip Levin

Case Synopsis

An 86-year-old woman with history of stable angina, chronic obstructive pulmonary disease, hypertension, and hypothyroidism undergoes general anesthesia for pinning of a femur fracture. The surgery and anesthetic are uneventful. In the postanesthesia care unit (PACU), the patient becomes disoriented and combative.

PROBLEM ANALYSIS

Definition

Postoperative delirium is a state in which patients have altered consciousness, orientation, memory, perception, and behavior. It is usually noted in the PACU.

Recognition

Postoperative delirium can have multiple causes and should be promptly evaluated by an anesthesiologist in the PACU. Assessment of the patient's breathing and circulatory status is extremely important to rule out life-threatening problems such as hypoxia, hypercarbia, and airway obstruction. A thorough medical history, a complete listing of medications administered during the perioperative period, and review of the anesthesia and surgical course (including the type of surgery) should be obtained. Then a detailed physical examination and any indicated laboratory testing are performed.

Severe pain (surgical, urinary, or gastric distention) can cause altered mental status and should be treated promptly. Certain metabolic, endocrine, and infectious disorders can also cause altered mental status and must be ruled out. Intracerebral pathology should be ruled out in patients with focal neurologic findings and gait disturbances. In addition, effects of residual anesthetic agents may mimic postoperative delirium. It may be difficult to distinguish residual sedation resulting from the effects of sedatives, antiemetics, or anesthetics that lead to disinhibition from causes that require treatment with sedatives.

Patients with postoperative delirium are at risk of physically harming themselves or PACU personnel. Patients may tear open their bandages or wounds or pull out their intravenous lines. Patients with postoperative delirium are also at risk for falls and fractures.

Risk Assessment

Risk factors for developing postoperative delirium are divided into three categories: preoperative, intraoperative, and postoperative.

Preoperative risk factors include advanced age, pathologic brain states (e.g., cerebrovascular disease), administration of multiple drugs and drug interactions, abrupt withdrawal of alcohol or sedative-hypnotics, endocrine and metabolic disorders (e.g., hyper- or hypothyroidism, hyponatremia, hypoglycemia), depression, and dementia or anxiety disorders.

Intraoperative risk factors include the type of surgery. Patients having cardiac surgery appear to be at greater risk of developing postoperative delirium, possibly due to hypoperfusion or microembolism (air or thrombus). Further, certain orthopedic procedures may predispose to postoperative delirium, possibly due to fat emboli. Some ophthalmic procedures may be associated with bilateral loss of vision (possibly due to the use of anticholinergic drugs and eyedrops), which can contribute to postoperative delirium. Certain anesthetic drugs, including anticholinergics, barbiturates for premedication, and benzodiazepines, have been linked to an increase in postoperative delirium. Interestingly, several studies have found no difference in the effects of general, epidural, or spinal anesthesia on the development of postoperative delirium.

Postoperative risk factors for delirium include hypoxia, hypocarbia, and sepsis.

Implications

Postoperative delirium can result in complications such as prolonged hospital stay, delayed functional recovery, and increased morbidity.

MANAGEMENT

Identifying and Correcting the Underlying Cause

Initially, it is important to identify and correct underlying causes. A thorough medical history is important, including any additional information that family members or caregivers may provide (e.g., baseline behavior and mental status). A careful physical examination, including a detailed neurologic and psychiatric examination, should be performed. The patient's vital signs and overall medical condition must be monitored carefully until underlying causes (e.g., change in respiratory status, infection, fluid or electrolyte imbalance) have been identified and corrected or stabilized. It is also important to review any pertinent laboratory and radiographic studies.

Pharmacologic Measures

Identification and correction of the underlying condition may be sufficient to reverse delirium. Specific pharmacologic intervention may be necessary to reduce the intensity and duration of delirium. Many studies have demonstrated the safety and efficacy of antipsychotics. In this category, haloperidol is the drug of choice because of its favorable cardiovascular and respiratory side effect profile compared with other antipsychotics. Also, it has negligible anticholinergic effects. Haloperidol can be administered orally, intramuscularly, or intravenously in doses ranging from 0.25 to 2 mg. This dose is repeated or doubled every 30 to 60 minutes until the patient is sedated and calm. Droperidol has been used for more rapid tranquilization. Chlorpromazine is also effective, but it can lead to severe hypotension. Neuroleptic antipsychotic medications may lengthen the Q-T interval, thus increasing the risk of torsades de pointes. Patients who receive this treatment should have a baseline electrocardiogram. If the patient's Q-T interval becomes prolonged to greater than 25 percent of baseline or longer than 450 msec, dose reduction or discontinuation of therapy may be needed. Recent studies show that the novel antipsychotic drug olanzapine might also be effective for treating postoperative delirium and has fewer side effects than more typical neuroleptic drugs. Further studies are warranted.

Benzodiazepines are not effective therapy for postoperative delirium, except for that caused by withdrawal from alcohol or sedative-hypnotics. Lorazepam is the benzodiazepine most commonly used; it is administered orally, intramuscularly, or intravenously in doses ranging from 0.5 to 2 mg. The dose of lorazepam is repeated or doubled every 30 to 60 minutes, depending on the patient's level of sedation.

The use of physostigmine is controversial, but it may still be available in some locations. This drug was often used in the past to treat postoperative delirium, especially that due to central cholinergic crisis. Compared with quaternary anticholinergics (e.g., atropine, glycopyrrolate), physostigmine (a tertiary amine) crosses the blood-brain barrier more readily.

Environmental Interventions

Supportive measures are useful for treating the symptoms of delirium. These include reorienting the patient to time, place, and person and minimizing excessive noise. Having a family member near the bedside may help calm the patient. Because delirium can be aggravated by sensory impairment, restoring the patient's vision (eyeglasses or contact lenses) or hearing (replacing a hearing aid) may be helpful. The use of physical restraints should be minimized; they may aggravate the patient's confusion, because they create the impression of being tied down.

Psychiatric and Neurologic Care

Obtaining a psychiatric consultation may be necessary if other treatment measures fail and more aggressive management is necessary. If postoperative delirium appears to have a neurologic cause, the appropriate neurologic or neurosurgical consultation should be obtained.

PREVENTION

Little is known about the prevention of postoperative delirium. There is some evidence that aggressive management of established risk factors may help. Some intraoperative measures that may be effective include maintaining good oxygenation and normal blood pressure, using correct drug dosages, and maintaining normal electrolyte levels. Drugs associated with an increased risk of delirium should be used cautiously. These include H_2-antagonists, digitalis, phenytoin, and anticholinergic medications. If an anticholinergic is necessary, a quaternary amine such as glycopyrrolate should be used. In general, drugs with short elimination half-lives are preferable to long-acting drugs. Adequate postoperative analgesia is also important for the prevention of postoperative delirium.

Further Reading

American Psychiatric Association: Diagnostic and Statistical Manual of Mental Disorders, 4th ed. Washington, DC, American Psychiatric Association, 1994.

Breitbart W, Tremblay A, Gibson C: An open trial of olanzepine for the treatment of delirium in hospitalized cancer patients. Psychosomatics 43:175-182, 2002.

Chung F: Postoperative mental dysfunction. In McLeskey CH (ed): Geriatric Anesthesiology. Philadelphia, Williams & Wilkins, 1997, pp 487-495.

Kaneko T, Cai J, Ishikura T, et al: Prophylactic consecutive administration of halperidol can reduce the occurrence of postoperative delirium in gastrointestinal surgery. Yonago Acta Med 42:179-184, 1999.

Litaker D, Locala J, Franco K, et al: Preoperative risk factors for postoperative delirium. Gen Hosp Psychiatry 23:84-89, 2001.

Lynch EP, Lazor MA, Gellis JE, et al: The impact of postoperative pain on the development of postoperative delirium. Anesth Analg 86:781-785, 1998.

McGowan NC, Locala JA: Delirium. Cleveland Clinic Disease Management Project, Oct 24, 2002. Available at www.clevelandclinicmeded.com/diseasemanagement/psychiatry/delirium/delirum1.htm.

Parikh S, Chung F: Postoperative delirium in the elderly. Anesth Analg 80:1223-1232, 1995.

Weber JB, Coverdale JH, Kunik ME: Delirium: Current trends in prevention and treatment. Int Med J 34:115-121, 2004.

SPECIAL TOPICS

Intractable Nausea and Vomiting

224

David A. Nakata and Robert K. Stoelting

Case Synopsis

A 28-year-old, 110-kg woman presents with intractable nausea and vomiting in the postanesthesia care unit after undergoing laparoscopic cholecystectomy under general anesthesia. The anesthesia was unremarkable except for preoperative anxiety and moderate postoperative upper airway obstruction, which was easily corrected by insertion of an oral airway. Past medical history was significant for unanticipated hospital admission for postoperative nausea and vomiting following previous inguinal hernia repair.

PROBLEM ANALYSIS

Definition

Postoperative nausea and vomiting (PONV) is an important cause of morbidity following all types of anesthesia. It typically occurs in the immediate postanesthesia period, with most cases lasting less than 24 hours. Nausea is a subjective sensation best evaluated by the patient and is mediated via unknown neural pathways. It often, but not always, arises as the antecedent event to retching or vomiting. Vomiting (emesis) is defined as the forceful retrograde oral expulsion of gastric contents. Retching differs from vomiting by the lack of expulsion of gastric contents. PONV has multiple causes that can be subdivided into patient-, surgical-, and anesthetic-related factors.

Recognition

The sensation of nausea is familiar to everyone, but because of its subjective nature, it is often difficult to appreciate, especially in a disoriented postoperative patient. Nausea is typically accompanied by decreased or inappropriate gastrointestinal activity and may include hypotonicity of muscular sphincters, hypoperistalsis or reverse peristalsis, and hyposecretion. The autonomic nervous system, especially the parasympathetic system, can also be affected, leading to manifestations such as skin pallor, diaphoresis, increased salivation, vasovagal reactions, and anorexia. If these symptoms persist, they invariably deteriorate to retching and vomiting.

Vomiting, unlike nausea, is virtually unmistakable in its presentation. The neuroanatomic pathways and mediators that produce vomiting are better understood than those associated with nausea. Two distinct areas in the brain are responsible for the initiation and coordination of vomiting: the chemoreceptor trigger zone in the fourth ventricle, and the vomiting center in the lateral reticular formation. The chemoreceptor trigger zone contains a high density of dopaminergic receptors and is connected by neural pathways to the vomiting center. Figure 224-1 is a schematic representation of the factors that are known to interact with the areas responsible for vomiting. In addition, numerous physiologic changes occur, including relaxation of the gastric fundus and lower esophageal sphincter and the forceful contraction of the abdominal musculature, leading to the ejection of gastric contents.

Risk Assessment

The incidence of postoperative vomiting is typically reported to be between 20% and 40%. Table 224-1 presents factors that have been implicated in the development of PONV. A number of these factors are widespread throughout the general surgical population, making it common for individual patients to have multiple risk factors. These factors, in addition to specific patient characteristics, are useful in predicting which patients are at greatest risk of developing PONV. Unfortunately, there is no formal scheme that allows clinicians to predict which prophylactic maneuvers will yield the greatest success.

Some of the less obvious factors that influence the incidence of nausea and vomiting include anxiety, gender, obesity, experience of the anesthesiologist, and anesthetic agent. Anxiety may exacerbate PONV via the release of catecholamines. Experimental models exist in which vomiting can be induced by instilling catecholamines into the cerebral ventricles. This may also account for the increased incidence of nausea and vomiting associated with the use of anesthetic agents that increase circulating catecholamines. The increased incidence of PONV in women has traditionally been ascribed to a hormonal cause. This is supported by a decreased incidence of PONV in females at the extremes of age when compared with age-matched males. However, a recent study postulates that the increased incidence of PONV in women may actually be due to a greater sensitivity to dopamine. Obesity may interfere with positive-pressure ventilation, leading to gastric distention.

The case synopsis provides examples of some of the common predisposing conditions that can increase a patient's risk for PONV, including female gender, obesity, previous history of PONV, anxiety, laparoscopic abdominal surgery, placement of an oral airway, and general anesthesia. Other factors may include increased gastric inflation or hypoxemia

Figure 224–1 ■ Factors known to interact with the chemoreceptor trigger zone and the vomiting center to initiate vomiting.

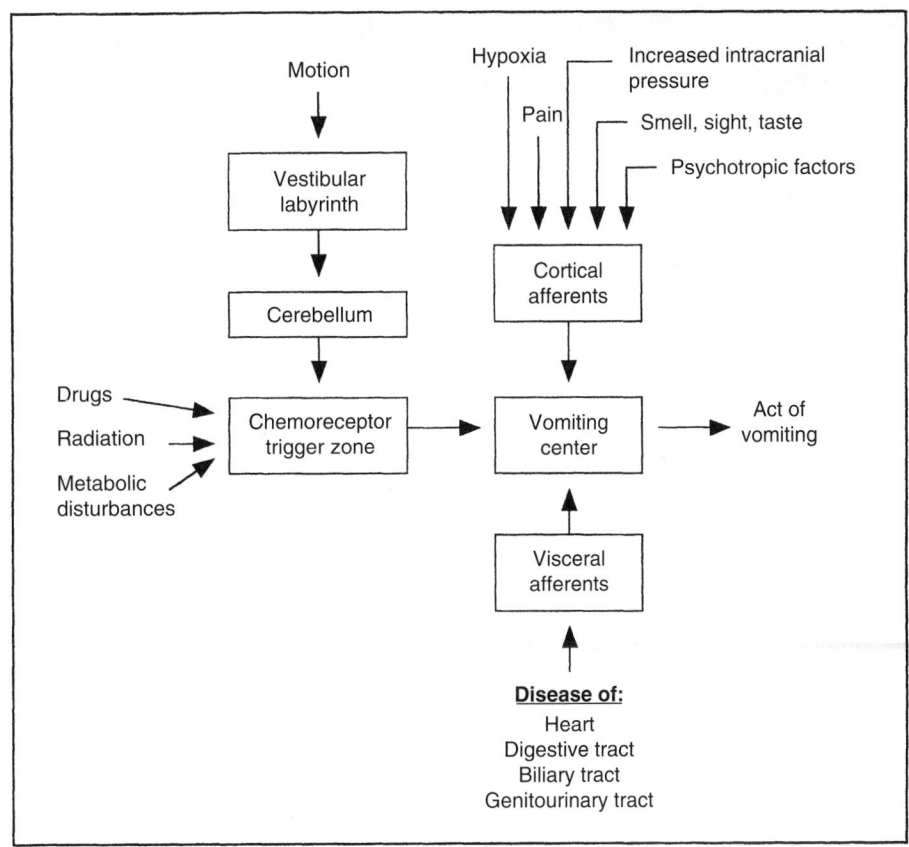

from difficult positive-pressure ventilation and increased arterial carbon dioxide tension from inadequate mask ventilation or abdominal insufflation of carbon dioxide during laparoscopy. Although contemporary volatile anesthetics are not known to promote nausea and vomiting, nitrous oxide has been incriminated. Possible mechanisms might be increased middle ear pressure with stimulation of the chemoreceptor trigger zone or distention of the gastrointestinal tract.

Implications

Table 224-2 lists a number of complications associated with nausea and vomiting. A number of coexisting diseases and certain surgical procedures may predispose a patient to the development of more serious sequelae of PONV, including increased intracranial pressure (leading to tentorial herniation) and esophageal disruption (Mallory-Weiss tear or Boerhaave's syndrome). PONV can also cause wound dehiscence and

Table 224–1 ■ Factors That May Influence the Risk of Postoperative Nausea and Vomiting

Age: children at greater risk than adults	Medications
Anesthetic technique	Nasogastric tube
Anxiety	Nitrous oxide
Concurrent illness	Obesity
Ethanol intoxication	Opioids
Increased intracranial pressure	Pain
Metabolic disturbance	Placement of airways
Experience of the anesthetist	Previous history of postoperative nausea and vomiting
Fasting	Prolonged operative procedure
Female gender	Standing
Day of the menstrual cycle	Sympathetic stimulation
Gastric inflation	Transportation or movement of patient
Hypercarbia	Type of surgery
Hypotension	Head and neck surgery
Inhalational anesthetics	Intra-abdominal surgery
Intravenous anesthetics	Laparoscopic abdominal surgery
Etomidate	Strabismus surgery
Methohexital	
Thiopental	

SPECIAL TOPICS

Table 224–2 ■ Complications Associated with Nausea and Vomiting
Aspiration pneumonia
Dehydration
Delayed discharge from postanesthesia care unit
Delayed discharge from hospital
Increased cost
Inconvenience
Electrolyte imbalance
Hypokalemia
Hypochloremia
Hyonatremia
Alkalosis
Esophageal rupture (Boerhaave's syndrome)
Increased postsurgical bleeding
Increased intracranial pressure
Mallory-Weiss tear

disruption of complex surgical repairs. Retching or vomiting following procedures involving the head and neck is of special concern because of the fragile nature of these tissues. In addition, an especially risky situation may be created by procedures involving the oral cavity in which the mandible is fixed in the closed position. Under these circumstances, if a patient were to vomit, significant quantities of gastric contents could be aspirated.

MANAGEMENT

Table 224-3 lists antiemetic agents available for the prevention and treatment of nausea and vomiting. These drugs can be subdivided into gastrointestinal prokinetic drugs, phenothiazines, butyrophenones, anticholinergics, antihistamines, serotonin (5-HT$_3$) receptor antagonists, and steroids. No single agent is universally effective for the prevention or treatment of PONV. Many of these drugs are associated with side effects,

Table 224–3 ■ Antiemetics
Anticholinergics
Scopolamine (IV or transdermal patch)
Atropine
Antihistamines
Cyclizine (Marezine)
Dimenhydrinate (Dramamine)
Diphenhydramine (Benadryl)
Butyrophenones
Droperidol (Inapsine)
Phenothiazines
Promethazine (Phenergan)
Prochlorperazine (Compazine)
Perphenazine (Trilafon)
Prokinetics
Metoclopramide (Reglan)
Domperidone (Motilium)
Serotonin (5-HT$_3$) antagonist
Ondansetron (Zofran)
Dolasetron (Anzemet)
Granisetron (Kytril)
Steroids
Dexamethasone (Decadron)

such as sedation and extrapyramidal reactions. This may cause some clinicians to restrict the use of these drugs, especially when one considers the typically negligible impact of PONV on overall outcome. In addition, when consideration is given to the large number of factors that can affect the development of PONV, choosing the most efficacious antiemetic can be difficult.

PREVENTION

Routine antiemetic prophylaxis is not warranted because less than 30% of patients experience postoperative emesis. When it occurs, it is often brief in duration. In addition, the sedation and delayed awakening caused by some of the commonly used antiemetic agents may hinder their usefulness. Even though antiemetic prophylaxis is not routinely advised, consideration must be given to the reality that the treatment of PONV is often less efficacious than its prevention. Therefore, there may be specific instances when the prophylactic use of these agents is warranted for patients known to be at risk.

Given the multiple factors involved in the development of PONV, it is difficult to provide specific recommendations regarding prophylaxis. This is in contrast to the nausea and vomiting associated with radiation and chemotherapy, in which the inciting agents are more readily identifiable. Additionally, in refractory cases of PONV, a combination of drugs may be needed to increase efficacy. Unfortunately, combination therapy is markedly more expensive than single drug therapy, and even with multidrug therapy, success is not assured.

Other factors aiding in the prevention of PONV include nonpharmacologic therapies such as decompressing the stomach with an oro- or nasogastric tube. However, the presence of a gastric tube in the postoperative period may stimulate the gag reflex, thus mitigating the benefit of gastric decompression. Additionally, fluid hydration has been advocated to decrease the incidence of PONV. Given the relative low cost and safety associated with this therapy, it seems reasonable to consider it. Other, more exotic nonpharmacologic therapies include acupuncture, acupressure, and specific herbs. Finally, new drugs include tropisetron, a 5-HT$_3$ antagonist now marketed in Europe that is currently in clinical trials in the United States.

Further Reading

Apfel CC, Korttila K, Abdulla M, et al: A factorial trial of six interventions for the prevention of postoperative nausea and vomiting. N Engl J Med 350:2441-2451, 2004.

Camu F, Lauwers MH, Verbessem D: Incidence and aetiology of postoperative nausea and vomiting. Eur J Anaesthesiol 9(Suppl 6):25-31, 1992.

Divatia JV, Vaidya JS, Badwe RA, et al: Omission of nitrous oxide during anesthesia reduces the incidence of postoperative nausea and vomiting: A meta-analysis. Anesthesiology 85:1055-1062, 1996.

Korttila K: The study of postoperative nausea and vomiting. Br J Anaesth 69(Suppl 1):20S-23S, 1992.

Palazzo MGA, Strunin L: Anesthesia and emesis. Can Anaesth Soc J 31: 178-187, 1984.

Rowbotham DJ: Current management of postoperative nausea and vomiting. Br J Anaesth 69(Suppl 1):46S-59S, 1992.

Watcha MF, White PF: Postoperative nausea and vomiting. Anesthesiology 77:162-184, 1992.

Unanticipated Hospital Admission and Readmission

225

Zhuang T. Fang

Case Synopsis

A 70-year-old woman is in the recovery room of an ambulatory surgery facility after a 3-hour repair of a cystocele under general anesthesia. She has nausea and vomiting and is complaining of pain. Interventions have been ineffective, and the surgery facility is scheduled to close in 30 minutes. The chart review indicates an American Society of Anesthesiologists (ASA) class II patient with a history of controlled hypertension and hypothyroidism. Significant past surgery was a left mastectomy 5 years ago for breast cancer. This surgery was associated with postoperative nausea and vomiting (PONV).

PROBLEM ANALYSIS

Definition

Unanticipated hospital admission is any admission not anticipated preoperatively. Unanticipated hospital readmission includes patients who are readmitted to the hospital within 30 days of discharge. The incidence of unanticipated hospital admission ranges from 1% to 6%, and that of unanticipated readmission ranges from 1% to 3%.

UNANTICIPATED HOSPITAL ADMISSION

An unanticipated hospital admission requires that there be no preoperative expectation that a patient will require an increased level of care following surgery. This unscheduled hospitalization can be at a freestanding outpatient center or at a community hospital. Unanticipated admission for all outpatient procedures is about 1.5% on average. However, it is higher for some surgeries: 4% for otologic surgery, 5% for laparoscopic cholecystectomy or gynecologic laparoscopy, and up to 6% for microdiscectomy. Rates are similar for adults and children, males and females, and patients at the extremes of age. Surgical causes account for 40% to 50% of unanticipated admissions, and anesthesia-related causes account for 25%. The remainder occur for social or medical reasons.

UNANTICIPATED HOSPITAL READMISSION

The rate of unanticipated hospital readmission is about 2.5%, but this too varies among surgical procedures. Higher rates correlate with greater surgical invasiveness and the indications for the surgery.

Recognition

Careful preoperative assessment and patient selection are essential for identifying anesthetic or surgical risk factors for unanticipated hospital admission. It is prudent to plan to admit high-risk patients for an overnight stay rather than be faced with a last-minute, unplanned admission. In the case synopsis, the patient's possible need for hospitalization was not appreciated and anticipated. The identification of intraoperative risk factors (e.g., technical difficulty, invasiveness, and duration of the procedure), early recognition of anesthesia and surgical complications and aggressive remedial intervention, and attention to postoperative issues (e.g., pain, PONV) are crucial to preventing unanticipated admission or readmission. Vigilance in the recovery room can also facilitate early remedial or preventive intervention, more timely decisions, and a smooth transition to hospital admission if necessary.

Risk Assessment

Risk factors for unanticipated admission or readmission include the following:

- Surgical bleeding and related complications
- PONV
- Uncontrolled pain
- Respiratory complications
- High ASA status
- Lack of postoperative social support

Surgical oozing and other complications (e.g., a more extensive procedure than planned, requiring longer postoperative observation) account for the majority of unanticipated hospital admissions. Among adults undergoing ambulatory surgery, most anesthesia-related unanticipated admissions are due to PONV, uncontrolled pain, and urinary retention. In addition, higher ASA status is directly related to the incidence of unanticipated hospital admission.

Pediatric patients are often admitted for respiratory complications or PONV; they are usually not admitted for uncontrolled pain. Owing to a significant increase in the rate of unanticipated admissions because of complications such as bronchospasm, laryngospasm, and postoperative oxygen desaturation, surgery should be postponed in pediatric patients with symptomatic upper respiratory tract infections. Suggested protocols for canceling surgery in a pediatric patient with a mild upper respiratory infection or who is recovering from one include the following:

- Age younger than 1 year
- Surgery lasting longer than 45 minutes
- Possibility of the need for tracheal intubation

In the case synopsis, several factors placed the patient at high risk for unanticipated hospital admission: female gender, past history of PONV, and invasiveness and long duration of the planned surgery. A more extensive list of risk factors for PONV is provided in Table 225-1. Although it was appropriate to perform the surgery in this patient, recognition of her increased risk for PONV and postoperative pain should have prompted preemptive interventions, including the use of anesthetic techniques to reduce the likelihood of PONV and pain. PONV is effectively treated and prevented with multimodal antiemetic management. The use of regional anesthesia techniques and local anesthetic surgical wound infiltration can reduce the need for opioids or sedative-hypnotics (e.g., midazolam) to control postoperative pain.

Table 225-2 lists factors responsible for high rates of unanticipated hospital admission. As reliance on ambulatory surgery has grown, more elderly patients are being cared for in the outpatient setting. It is generally agreed that age alone does not increase the risk for unanticipated hospital admission unless the patient is older than 85 years, is male, and has significant comorbidities (ASA class II or III). A history of inpatient hospitalization within the previous two quarters of the year is especially relevant. Further, the incidence of intraoperative cardiovascular events is higher in this age group compared with younger patients. Still, age alone is significant only as it correlates with increased medical comorbidities

Table 225–1 ■ Risk Factors for Postoperative Nausea and Vomiting (PONV) in Adults
Patient-Specific Factors
Female sex
Nonsmoking status
History of PONV or motion sickness
Anesthetic Factors
Use of volatile anesthetics within 2 hr
Use of nitrous oxide
Use of intraoperative or postoperative opioids
Surgery-Related Factors
Surgery duration: each 30-min increase in surgery duration corresponds to a 60% increase in PONV incidence (e.g., a baseline risk of 10% is increased by 16% after 30 min)
Surgery type: high-risk surgery includes ear, nose, and throat; laparoscopy; neurosurgery; breast surgery; strabismus surgery; laparotomy; plastic surgery

Modified from Gan TJ, Meyer T, Apfel CC, et al: Consensus guidelines for managing postoperative nausea and vomiting. Anesth Analg 97:62-71, 2003.

Table 225–2 ■ Factors Responsible for Unanticipated Hospital Admission
History of PONV
Respiratory illness (even mild URI) and higher ASA status in pediatric patients
Significant coexisting disease or age older than 85 yr
Major procedures beginning in late afternoon or finishing after 3:00 PM
Prolonged surgical procedures (>60 min)
Poor social support for patient

ASA, American Society of Anesthesiologists; PONV, postoperative nausea and vomiting; URI, upper respiratory infection.

and reduced social support postoperatively. For logistical reasons (e.g., time for recovery from anesthesia or to obtain adequate pain control), in both adult and pediatric patients, surgery performed or completed after 3:00 PM is more likely to result in unanticipated hospital admissions.

Implications

Both the patient and his or her family are affected by an unscheduled hospital admission. This is especially true with pediatric patients, whose unanticipated hospital admission can affect the parents' work schedules. Therefore, good communication with and support for the family are essential. Unanticipated admission or readmission rates not only reflect the quality of the outpatient surgery service but also have a significant financial impact on hospitals. The mean charges for all hospital readmissions were $8088 ± $29,425. Charges for unanticipated admission for pain control were $1869 ± $4553, compared with $12,000 ± $36,886 for non-pain-control reasons.

MANAGEMENT

Once a decision is made to admit a patient for anesthetic-related reasons, the anesthesiologist should immediately communicate with both the surgical team and the family to coordinate the process. In freestanding surgical centers with the capability to care for patients overnight, this is often the least expensive alternative. Most patients' problems, such as PONV or severe pain, can be dealt with overnight, and the patient can be discharged the next morning. Most facilities equipped for overnight admissions, however, do not accept pediatric patients. In this case, plans must be made for admission to a hospital. For children with respiratory complications, admission to an observation or an intensive care unit should be strongly considered to ensure that the patient has supplemental oxygen and monitoring of oxygen saturation throughout the night. In all cases, documentation of the complication that has occurred, the treatment provided, and the necessity for admission is essential for both insurance and medicolegal reasons.

Patients who are readmitted are usually under the care of a surgical team. Because inadequately controlled pain is one of the major reasons for readmission, every effort should be made to initiate pain control intraoperatively and postoperatively with a multimodal approach, including regional blocks, nonsteroidal anti-inflammatory drugs (NSAIDs), cyclooxy-genase-2 (COX-2) inhibitors, and opioids.

PREVENTION

Preoperative considerations include the following:

- Assess risk factors from an anesthetic, medical, surgical, and social standpoint.
- Refer cases that are inappropriate for outpatient surgery to inpatient surgery.
- Plan for an overnight stay for high-risk patients undergoing high-risk procedures.

Intraoperative considerations include the following:

- Use regional anesthesia or monitored anesthesia care whenever possible.
- In patients with a history of or at high risk for PONV:
  - Administer propofol for general anesthesia.
  - Use multimodal antiemetic therapy.
  - Provide generous hydration.
  - Use narcotics sparingly.
  - Consider the use of analgesic adjuncts, such as ketorolac or COX-2 inhibitors.
  - Consider eliminating nitrous oxide and volatile anesthetics.
  - Minimize the use of neostigmine.
- For patients at high risk of postoperative pain, use a multimodal approach, including:
  - Nerve blocks
  - Wound infiltration with local anesthetics
  - NSAIDs and COX-2 inhibitors
  - Opioids
- Avoid drugs that can cause sedation and altered mental status.
- In children with mild upper respiratory infections, avoid intubation.

Postoperatively, take the following precautions:

- Provide supplemental oxygen.
- Treat hypotension aggressively.
- If patient has PONV:
  - Evaluate and treat pain.
  - Hydrate vigorously.
  - Use antiemetics early.
  - Keep the patient recumbent until treated and fluid repleted.

Avoiding unanticipated admission begins with an assessment of the risk for such admission and continues in the operating room and throughout the postoperative period, including cancellation of any inappropriately scheduled ambulatory cases. Recognition of risk factors preoperatively, aggressive pain control, use of multimodal therapy to prevent PONV (e.g., hydration, dexamethasone, metoclopramide, H_2-blockers, serotonin inhibitors), and use of maneuvers to avoid bronchospasm and laryngospam intraoperatively (e.g., deep extubation) are advised.

Postoperative management is vital. All patients at increased risk for unanticipated hospital admission should be well oxygenated and hydrated. Because pain alone may cause PONV, it should be treated promptly and aggressively. If the patient has refractory PONV, rescue therapy with other types of drugs (e.g., butyrophenones, phenothiazines, dopaminergic agents) should be considered. Finally, aggressive and early treatment in the recovery room can often avert an unanticipated hospital admission.

Further Reading

Aldwinckle RJ, Montgomery JE: Unplanned admission rates and postdischarge complications in patients over the age of 70 following day case surgery. Anesthesia 59:57-59, 2004.

Awad IT, Moore M, Rushe C, et al: Unplanned hospital admission in children undergoing day-case surgery. Eur J Anaesthesiol 21:379-383, 2004.

Coley KC, Williams BA, da Pos SV, et al: Retrospective evaluation of unanticipated admissions and readmissions after same day surgery and associated costs. J Clin Anesth 14:349-353, 2002.

Dornhoffer J, Manning L: Unplanned admissions following outpatient otologic surgery: The University of Arkansas experience. Ear Nose Throat J 79:713-717, 2000.

Fleisher LA, Pasternak LR, Herbert R, et al: Inpatient hospital admission and death after outpatient surgery in elderly patients: Importance of patient system characteristics and location of care. Arch Surg 139:67-72, 2004.

Fortier J, Chung F, Su J: Unanticipated admission after ambulatory surgery: A prospective study. Can J Anaesth 45:612-619, 1998.

Gan TJ, Meyer T, Apfel CC, et al: Consensus guidelines for managing postoperative nausea and vomiting. Anesth Analg 97:62-71, 2003.

Gupta A, Wu CL, Elkassabany N: Does the routine prophylactic use of antiemetics affect the incidence of postdischarge nausea and vomiting following ambulatory surgery? Anesthesiology 99:488-495, 2003.

Hedayati B, Fear S: Hospital admission after day-case gynecological laparoscopy. Br J Anaesth 83:776-779, 1999.

Lau H, Brooks DC: Predictive factors for unanticipated admissions after ambulatory laparoscopic cholecystectomy. Arch Surg 136:1150-1153, 2001.

Shaikh S, Chung F, Imarengiaye C: Pain, nausea, vomiting and ocular complications delay discharge following ambulatory microdiscectomy. Can J Anaesth 50:514-518, 2003.

Uncontrolled Pain

226

Rodolfo Gebhardt and Nader D. Nader

Case Synopsis

A 75-year-old man with chronic obstructive pulmonary disease is recovering in the postanesthesia care unit following open cholecystectomy. He has shallow, rapid respiration and appears slightly cyanotic. He is moaning and says that his stomach hurts. You note that he received 100 µg fentanyl 2 hours earlier (at the beginning of surgery) and that no local anesthetics were used.

PROBLEM ANALYSIS

Definition

The International Association for the Study of Pain defines pain as "an unpleasant sensory and emotional experience associated with actual or potential tissue damage, or described in terms of such damage. Pain is always subjective; each individual learns the application of the word through experience related to injury in early life."

In the postoperative setting, pain results mainly from the peripheral activation of nociceptors in injured tissues; however, a psychological component of lesser magnitude is always present. Factors such as a sense of hopelessness, a lack of control, and the underlying meaning of pain feed into the psychological aspect of pain. For instance, patients with postoperative pain following cancer surgery can be expected to have a different interpretation of their pain than patients recovering from noncancer surgery. The interpretation may include relief that the cancer is removed or fear that the pain reflects an ongoing cancerous process.

Recognition

Some patients may not complain of pain or may be unable to communicate their degree of pain (Table 226-1). This usually reflects the age of the patient and is most common in younger patients or elderly patients with mental impairment. An advantage of pain scores or scales is that response to medication can be measured objectively and used to predict the further need for medication.

Risk Assessment

It appears from many studies that all postoperative patients are at risk for poorly controlled pain. Particularly painful operations include thoracic, abdominal, and orthopedic (major joint) surgery. In contrast, body surface operations are associated with less pain. Delayed healing and wound infection may contribute to the prolongation of pain that might otherwise have been expected to resolve spontaneously. In the event of prolonged pain or pain out of proportion to the injury, a new (usually surgical) cause such as wound dehiscence, infection, or ischemia should be suspected.

Implications

Poorly controlled postoperative pain may be associated with an increased incidence of myocardial ischemia and decreased bowel motility due to increased sympathetic activity. Respiratory splinting may cause a reduction in functional residual capacity of the lungs and increased sputum retention. Optimal analgesia can reverse some of these adverse events, but just making a patient "comfortable" with opioids actually does little to improve outcome. In contrast, in patients at high risk, optimal analgesia with thoracic epidural anesthesia may reduce the incidence of adverse outcomes if continued for at least 48 hours postoperatively. Importantly, patients express more satisfaction with their overall care if they are maintained in a pain-free or low-pain state postoperatively.

MANAGEMENT

Methods of postoperative pain control are summarized in Table 226-2. The most important aspect of management is anticipation and frequent assessment of a patient's pain, with appropriate treatment. An acute pain service can facilitate timely and appropriate intervention in pain management and can be used to educate nursing staff. Pain should be charted along with other physiologic measurements such as blood pressure and temperature. Patients should be encouraged to report pain and be reassured that doing so will not result in a painful injection (a common problem with children); patients should also be discouraged from thinking that nothing can be done to relieve pain (a common assumption in elderly patients). It is important to consider both physical (e.g., heat and massage) and psychological (e.g., distraction, relaxation, imagery) techniques for pain

Table 226–1 ■ Assessment of Pain

Anticipate according to surgery
Note analgesia given intraoperatively
Measure according to age:
    <4 yr: physiologic parameters—heart rate,
      blood pressure, respiratory rate; verbal—"boo-boo,"
      "owie"; parental opinion (other causes for distress,
      e.g., hunger, strange environment)
    4-7 yr: non-numeric (facial expressions) pain score
    >7-adult: visual or numeric analog pain score
Treat based on assessment of pain
Reassess patient frequently, repeating this cycle

Table 226–2 ■ Summary of Methods for Postoperative Pain Control

Analgesics
Opioids
NSAIDs
Acetaminophen
Ketamine
Others

Anesthetics
Regional blocks and catheters
Wound infiltration
Nerve block

Physical
Thermal
Massage
Physical therapy
TENS

Behavioral
Biofeedback
Relaxation

Cognitive
Imagery
Distraction
Hypnosis
Choice and control

NSAID, nonsteroidal anti-inflammatory drug; TENS, transcutaneous electrical nerve stimulation.

control, as well as the more commonly used pharmacologic methods (Table 226-3).

Greater use of local anesthetics is encouraged to reduce pain. These can be injected into the wound edges, used for peripheral nerve blocks, or given via an epidural catheter. These methods are associated with few adverse side effects if special consideration is given to avoiding local anesthetic toxicity and one is mindful of associated sympathetic blockade with central neuraxial techniques.

Opioids are highly effective in reducing pain. They work in both the spinal cord and the brain, with probable synergy between the two sites. Within the brain, opioids are less selective; euphoria is likely an important factor in

Table 226–3 ■ Pharmacologic Methods for Postoperative Pain Control

Local Anesthetics
Tissue infiltration
Peripheral nerve block
Nerve plexus block: single injection or infusion
Central neuraxial anesthesia: single injection or infusion
Patient-controlled epidural pump

Opioids
Oral
Patient-controlled analgesia pump
Intravenous infusion
Central neuraxial analgesia: single injection or infusion
Patient-controlled epidural pump

producing analgesia. Intravenous opiates should be given by continuous infusion to children younger than 7 years and by patient-controlled analgesia pump to older children and adults. In patients with frequent demands for dosing, especially at night, when sleep is repeatedly interrupted, a background infusion of opioid can be added. This effectively prolongs the half-life of each bolus.

There are reports of many beneficial aspects of epidural anesthesia and analgesia, including better suppression of surgical stress, positive effect on postoperative nitrogen balance, reduced blood loss, better peripheral vascular circulation, more stable cardiovascular hemodynamics, and better postoperative pain control. It seems likely that high-risk patients undergoing major intra-abdominal surgery would benefit from combined general and epidural anesthesia intraoperatively, with continuing postoperative epidural analgesia.

Combining epidural opioids with subanesthetic concentrations of local anesthetics is important for three reasons: (1) it reduces the required doses of both drugs, (2) it enhances or at least maintains the desired degree of pain relief, and (3) it produces fewer adverse drug effects. Epidural catheters should be clearly labeled and skin sites inspected at least daily for signs of infection. Also, careful consideration should be given to the fact that any benefits may decrease over time, while associated risks may increase.

In a review of randomized trials, Rodgers and colleagues found improved survival in patients receiving a neuraxial blockade. The mortality rate in this group was about one third less than that in patients receiving general anesthesia alone. The observed improvement in survival was due to a reduction in deaths from pulmonary embolism, cardiac events, and stroke. There was no difference in total mortality based on whether patients received a combined general-neuraxial anesthetic or a neuraxial anesthetic alone. In this same analysis, the odds ratios for respiratory depression were reduced by 59% in patients allocated to neuraxial blockade. The authors found a reduced risk of venous thromboembolism, myocardial infarction, bleeding complications, pneumonia, respiratory depression, and renal failure. The benefits attributed to neuraxial blockade may be due to a number of mechanisms, including altered coagulation, increased blood flow, improved ability to breathe when pain free, and reduction in the surgical stress response.

Nonsteroidal anti-inflammatory drugs (NSAIDs) have been shown to reduce opioid needs postoperatively. They represent a useful adjunct to opioids and, in some cases, provide adequate analgesia when used alone. It is important to remember that postoperative patients are under metabolic stress and thus predisposed to gastric ulcers. NSAIDs should therefore be used for only limited periods. Consideration should be given to providing gastric protection with drugs that reduce acid, coat the gastric mucosa, and restore the mucous barrier.

As with balanced anesthesia, it is often better to use a balanced approach to analgesia. Attacking pain at different pain receptors with NSAIDs, opioids, oral or rectal acetaminophen, and low concentrations of local anesthetics is often more efficacious and results in fewer side effects than treating pain with a single treatment modality or higher drug doses.

PREVENTION

Animal studies have provided convincing data to support the idea of preemptive analgesia, whereby the pain of surgery is blocked at the spinal cord dorsal horn level with either local anesthetics or opioids. Unfortunately, to date, human studies of preemptive analgesia do not confirm a reduction in postoperative pain, either at rest or with movement. Wound hyperalgesia may be reduced, but this does not translate into greater comfort for the patient. Prophylaxis therefore involves ensuring adequate analgesia so that the patient awakes without severe pain. This may be a challenge, especially if rapid awakening and early discharge are expected.

Further Reading

Beyer JE, Denyes MJ, Villarruel AM: The creation, validation, and continuing development of the Oucher: A measure of pain intensity in children. J Pediatr Nurs 7:335-346, 1992.

Cousins M: Acute and postoperative pain. In Wall PD, Melzack R (eds): Textbook of Pain. Edinburgh, Churchill Livingstone, 1994, pp 357-385.

Curley J, Castillo J, Hotz J, et al: Prolonged regional nerve blockade: Injectable biodegradable bupivacaine/polyester microspheres. Anesthesiology 84:1401-1410, 1996.

Liu S, Carpenter R, Neal R: Epidural anesthesia and analgesia: Their role in postoperative outcome. Anesthesiology 82:1474-1506, 1995.

Pounder DR, Steward DJ: Postoperative analgesia: Opioid infusions in infants and children. Can J Anaesth 39:969-974, 1992.

Rigg JRA: Does regional block improve outcome after surgery? Anaesth Intensive Care 19:404-411, 1991.

Rodgers A, Walker N, Schug S, et al: Reduction of postoperative mortality and morbidity with epidural or spinal anesthesia: Results from overview of randomized trials. BMJ 321:1493-1497, 2000.

US Department of Health and Human Services: Acute Pain Management: Operative or Medical Procedures and Trauma: Clinical Practice Guidelines. AHCPR Publication No. 92-0032.

Yeager MP, Glass DD, Neff RK, et al: Epidural anesthesia and analgesia in high risk surgical patients. Anesthesiology 66:729-736, 1987.

Hemodynamic Instability

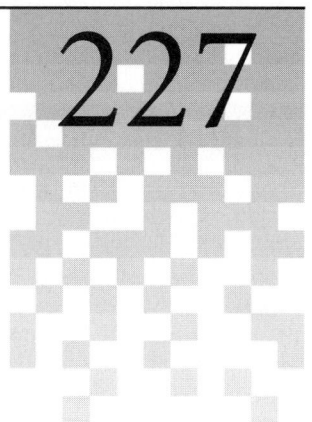

Padmavathi Perala, Eileen Watson, and Nader D. Nader

Case Synopsis

An 84-year-old man who just underwent colon resection for colon cancer has a blood pressure (BP) of 82/48 mm Hg and a heart rate of 120 beats per minute after 15 minutes in the postanesthesia care unit (PACU). New ST-T changes are noted in lead V_5 of the electrocardiogram (ECG).

PROBLEM ANALYSIS

Definition

Hemodynamic instability in the PACU setting is a change from baseline cardiovascular dynamics sufficient to cause potential harm to end organs. Harm may be due to inadequate tissue perfusion (e.g., hypotension, arrhythmias), reduction in oxygen delivery relative to demand (e.g., tachycardia, hypertension), or direct damage to organs such as the brain or kidney (e.g., hypertension). Clinical signs of hemodynamic instability include severe hypertension, hypotension, tachycardia, bradycardia, and arrhythmias (Table 227-1).

Recognition

Hemodynamic instability can occur any time after the induction of anesthesia to well into the postoperative period. There are many causes. Anticipation of potential problems results in earlier recognition, more timely intervention, and improved outcomes. Potential problems are identified by the routine monitoring of BP and ECG in the PACU. When vital signs are outside the norm for a given patient, it is prudent, especially if the patient is otherwise without complaints, to quickly determine whether the BP measurement is spurious. BP cuffs that are too large can result in falsely low measurements, and the converse is true for cuffs that are too small. The ECG monitor must be adjusted so that it counts only QRS complexes, not T waves as well. Supraventricular tachycardia may be difficult to diagnose without the use of a faster monitor speed, strip-chart recordings, 12-lead ECG, and calipers. In some instances, particularly to distinguish QRS

aberrancy from ectopy, a full 12-lead ECG is required. Finally, bradycardia may reflect youthful age or a high level of physical fitness.

The causes of hemodynamic deterioration in the PACU, in order of prevalence, are (1) alterations in volume status (e.g., preoperative dehydration, recent hemodialysis, intraoperative blood or third-space loss, volume overload), (2) compromise of the cardiovascular system (e.g., myocardial ischemia, valvular pathology, thromboembolic events, arrhythmias), (3) drug-related events (e.g., allergic reactions, systemic absorption of local anesthetics, withdrawal or overdose of antihypertensives and β-blockers), and (4) residual effects of anesthetic agents after neuraxial blockade. Hypercarbia or hypoxia with inadequate ventilation or shunting can cause hypertension, tachycardia, or arrhythmias. When severe hypoxemia is present, bradycardia, hypotension, and malignant arrhythmias are seen more often. Following placement of a central line, tension pneumothorax may cause hypotension due to reduced preload. Postoperative pain and emergence delirium can result in tachycardia and hypertension. Vasovagal response due to postoperative pain can also contribute to hemodynamic changes. Though uncommon, malignant hyperthermia, pheochromocytoma, or thyroid storm may manifest for the first time in the PACU, and these disorders should be included in the differential diagnosis of tachycardia and hypertension in PACU patients.

Risk Assessment

Events meeting the definitions given in Table 227-1 occur frequently in the PACU (about 6% to 8% of PACU admissions).

Sign	Definition
Table 227-1 ■ Definitions of Clinical Signs of Hemodynamic Instability	
Hypertension	Increase of 20% over baseline preoperative value for 15 min (50% for single measurement), or SBP >180 mm Hg, or DBP >110 mm Hg*
Hypotension	Decrease of 20% from baseline preoperative value for 15 min (50% for single measurement), or SBP <80 mm Hg, or DBP <50 mm Hg
Tachycardia	Increase of 20% over baseline preoperative value for 15 min, or >120 beats/min for patients older than 2 yr
Bradycardia	Decrease of 20% from baseline preoperative value, or <50 beats/min
Arrhythmia	Any rhythm other than sinus at a rate appropriate for the circumstances

*The Seventh Report of the Joint National Committee on Prevention, Detection, Evaluation, and Treatment of High Blood Pressure (JNC 7) defines severe (stage 2) hypertension as SBP >160 mm Hg and DBP >160/100 mm Hg (see also Chapter 77).

DBP, diastolic arterial blood pressure; SBP, systolic arterial blood pressure.

Table 227–2 ■ Causes of Hemodynamic Instability in the Postanesthesia Care Unit

Event	Patient Factors	Surgical Factors	Other Factors
Hypertension	Increasing age Tobacco use Renal disease	Intracranial procedure	Intraoperative hypertension Postoperative pain, hypoventilation, nausea, or vomiting
Hypotension	Increasing age Female gender	Intra-abdominal procedure	Intraoperative hypotension Postoperative shivering, nausea, or vomiting
Tachycardia, including tachyarrhythmias	Structural heart disease Chronic pulmonary disease Sepsis	Emergency procedure Cardiothoracic surgery Duration >4 hr	Pain Hypovolemia
Bradycardia, including bradyarrhythmias	Increased age ASA status I or II β-blocker or calcium channel blocker use	Congenital or valvular heart surgery	Intraoperative bradycardia Postoperative nausea or vomiting

ASA, American Society of Anesthesiologists.

The most important causes of each of these are shown in Table 227-2. It should be noted that patients with severe cardiovascular disease undergoing major procedures are largely absent from studies of PACU events because they are often admitted directly to an intensive care unit (ICU) for continued invasive monitoring or ventilatory support or for other surgical or anesthetic reasons. Morbidity and mortality from the hemodynamic instability varies. Patients' ability to tolerate hemodynamic changes depends on preexisting conditions, such as hypovolemia, medications, and coronary artery disease (CAD). Patients with CAD tolerate any changes in heart rate or BP poorly.

More than 11 million Americans suffer from CAD, and the prevalence is expected to rise as the number of elderly persons continues to increase. Patients with CAD are a significant proportion of surgical patients, and they have a significantly increased risk for perioperative myocardial ischemia and infarction. Surgery-associated reductions in coronary blood flow can cause transient or permanent myocardial injury in any patient. However, both the risk and the severity of perioperative cardiac ischemia are increased in patients with CAD. Perioperative myocardial ischemia in such patients is particularly serious, and the development of strategies to reduce the resultant tissue injury is an important goal.

Although no specific anesthetic technique has proved to be superior in protecting against perioperative myocardial ischemia and infarction, there is mounting evidence that the administration of volatile anesthetics during myocardial ischemia with reperfusion can protect against myocardial injury. Volatile anesthetics have been shown to enhance indices of myocardial performance, as well as metabolic and ultrastructural myocardial recovery after global and regional myocardial ischemia. After a brief period of ischemia (myocardial stunning), both systolic and diastolic dysfunction of the heart continues for a significant time after reperfusion. Systolic dysfunction manifests as decreased contractile function of the heart and low cardiac output and stroke work indices. In contrast, primarily left ventricle relaxation is impaired with diastolic dysfunction. Although the frequency of diastolic dysfunction is higher than that of systolic dysfunction, the clinical importance of isolated diastolic heart failure is still debated by many clinicians. Improved calcium homeostasis of the myocardium through the activation of both cytoplasm and mitochondrial K_{ATP} channels is the most likely explanation for the myocardial protection afforded by volatile anesthetics.

Implications

There is a recognized potential for severe morbidity if hemodynamic instability is not recognized and treated expeditiously. Myocardial infarction, cerebral infarction or hemorrhage, renal failure, and death are possible outcomes. Not all abnormal parameters are equal in predicting serious adverse outcomes. Table 227-3 shows that patients with hypertension or tachycardia in the PACU are many times more likely than those without such findings to be admitted to an ICU or to die. However, those with bradycardia or hypotension are no more likely to suffer such extreme outcomes than are those without such cardiovascular events. Once again, patients with severe cardiovascular disease and

Table 227–3 ■ Rate and Outcome of Unplanned Intensive Care Unit Admissions in Patients with (or without) Cardiovascular Events in the Postanesthesia Care Unit

Event	Unplanned ICU Admission (%)*	Mortality (%)*
Hypertension (no hypertension)	2.6[†] (0.2)	1.9[†] (0.3)
Tachycardia (no tachycardia)	4.0[†] (0.2)	2.3[†] (0.4)
Bradycardia (no bradycardia)	0.2 (0.2)	0.7 (0.4)
Hypotension (no hypotension)	0.7 (0.2)	0.7 (0.4)

*Numbers in parentheses are the admission rates for patients without the specific cardiovascular event.
[†]$P < .01$ vs those without the cardiovascular event.
Adapted from Rose DK, Cohn MM, DeBoer MM, et al: Cardiovascular events in the PACU. Anesthesiology 84:772-781, 1996.

those undergoing major surgery are largely absent from such studies.

Whether intervention is warranted for specific hemodynamic instability findings depends on the underlying cause and physiologic consequences, as well as patient-specific comorbidity and other factors.

MANAGEMENT

Hypertension in the PACU should first be considered a sign of excessive adrenergic stimulation. Emergence excitement, excessive pain, urinary retention, hypoxemia, hypercarbia, hypothermia (35°C), and nausea should be excluded as causes. If one or more of these factors are present, eliminating them will likely reduce the BP. If not, more serious processes (e.g., intracranial hypertension) must be excluded, and a decision to treat or simply observe must be made. Postoperative hypertension in patients without a history of prior hypertension is not uncommon and usually follows a benign course, with resolution in 3 to 5 hours. For those with hypertension, heart disease, or cerebrovascular disease, hypertension should be treated to bring BP to within 20% to 25% of the patient's optimal preoperative BP. The choice of agents to accomplish this depends on comorbidities and whether there are signs or symptoms of end-organ damage (headache, disorientation, chest pain, hematuria). BP 160/100 mm Hg or higher with evidence of end-organ damage (e.g., renal dysfunction, myocardial ischemia or infarction, stroke, retinal

hemorrhages) is a hypertensive emergency that requires rapid intervention with intravenous vasodilators (e.g., nicardipine, nitroprusside, nitroglycerin, hydralazine), β-blockers or mixed β- and α-adrenergic blockers (esmolol, labetalol), or both. Although sublingual nifedipine has been used, a distinct disadvantage of this drug is its unpredictable absorption, with a recognized potential for precipitous, dangerous hypotension.

Hypotension in the PACU is usually a sign of hypovolemia or blood loss. Hypotension due to heart failure is rarely reported in PACU patients, likely because those at highest risk for heart failure go directly to the ICU. Hypovolemia may be absolute (inadequate fluid replacement), ongoing (hemorrhage), relative (high neuraxial blockade), or mechanical (impaired venous return with vena cava compression, pneumothorax, pericardial tamponade). Therapy is dictated by the cause, comorbid conditions, and presence or absence of signs or symptoms indicating adverse effects on end-organ perfusion. Figure 227-1 outlines a systematic approach to the diagnosis and management of hypotension.

Tachycardia in the PACU is commonly associated with increased sympathetic tone. Therapy is first directed toward the cause, especially if the patient is otherwise stable. Causes are similar to those for hypertension. Tachycardia is also the most common presenting feature of malignant hyperthermia, and this diagnosis must be entertained and excluded. If the patient is experiencing chest pain or mental status changes, if the tachycardia does not resolve with correction of presumed causes, or if no underlying problem can be identified, other means are necessary to determine management.

Figure 227–1 ▪ A systematic approach to the diagnosis and management of postoperative hypotension. HCT, hematocrit; I&O, intake and output.

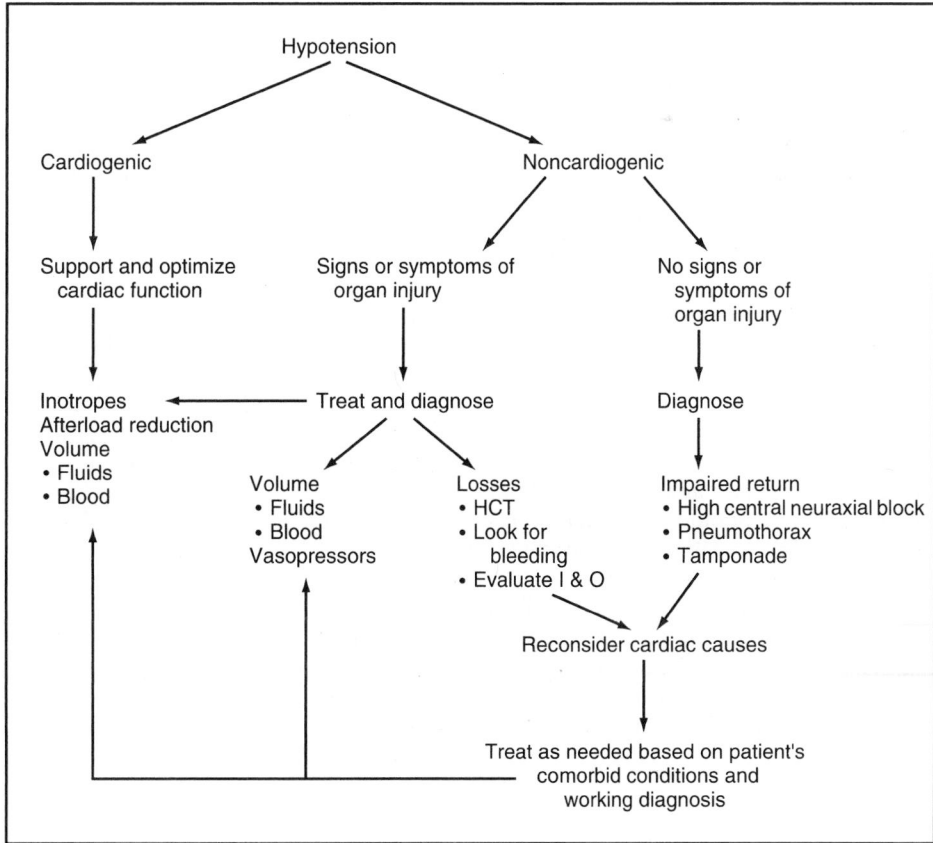

An ECG rhythm strip or increased strip-chart monitoring speed (25 to 50 mm/second) may help determine whether a wide complex tachycardia is supraventricular with ventricular aberration or ventricular in origin, or whether a narrow QRS complex rhythm is atrial or atrioventricular (AV) junctional. Laboratory testing may be needed to identify contributing factors such as electrolyte imbalance or excessive drug concentrations (e.g., digoxin, theophylline).

Therapy for ventricular tachyarrhythmias is directed at abolishing the cause or mechanism (automaticity, triggering, reentry) with drugs such as lidocaine, procainamide, and amiodarone. With severe hemodynamic compromise, immediate cardioversion or defibrillation is the preferred initial treatment, with drugs used to prevent recurrences (see Chapters 79 to 81 and 229). Therapy for supraventricular tachyarrhythmias is intended to reduce automaticity or triggering (β-blockers, calcium channel blockers, magnesium) or to slow AV node conduction and increase refractoriness (adenosine, calcium channel blockers, β-blockers, digoxin, edrophonium). For all other perioperative tachyarrhythmias, including those with ventricular preexcitation or Q-T interval prolongation, refer to Chapters 79 to 81 and 229. Cardioversion should always be considered first for any non-sinus-origin supraventricular tachycardia with evidence of acute circulatory compromise (e.g., shortness of breath, chest pain, ST segment changes, mental status changes). Overdrive atrial or ventricular pacing may also be effective against atrial flutter or paroxysmal supraventricular tachycardia. Cardioversion or defibrillation is first-choice therapy, along with airway support and chest compressions if needed, for any patient who has lost consciousness or is pulseless. For any patient with tachyarrhythmias that are not readily or easily identified or explained, a cardiologist should be consulted.

Most bradyarrhythmias in the PACU are caused by an excess of parasympathetic tone (see Chapter 82). The rhythm may be sinus or atrial in origin (bradycardia or sinus arrhythmia, wandering atrial pacemaker) or AV junctional. Alternatively, there may be intermittent or no transmission of supraventricular impulses with AV junctional or ventricular escape beats or rhythms. If the patient is symptomatic, urgent therapy consists of positive chronotropes (e.g., atropine, β-agonists); if these fail or only aggravate the arrhythmia, temporary transcutaneous, transesophageal, or transvenous pacing is used. If there is reasonable hemodynamic stability (e.g., new first degree or type 1 second degree AV block, AV junctional rhythm with AV dissociation), urgent intervention may not be necessary; however, such intervention should be readily available in case it becomes necessary. Any patient with potentially unstable bradyarrhythmias or who needs pacing should receive the benefit of a cardiology consultation. If the patient is asymptomatic and hemodynamically stable, he or she may be observed. Normal sinus rhythm is often restored after dissipation of anesthetic effects with redistribution or metabolism and restoration of normal body temperature.

Ectopic beats of atrial or ventricular origin are common postoperatively. They are often a sign of increased sympathetic tone, as is sinus tachycardia. Up to five ectopic ventricular beats per minute can be considered normal. If they are more frequent or have a multiform appearance, more careful evaluation and correction of the cause are necessary. If ectopic ventricular beats predispose to sustained ventricular tachycardia, treatment is mandatory, along with a search for and correction of the cause. Ventricular bigeminy is also relatively common in the PACU; it is the result of stress and is usually self-limited. In patients with heart disease or severe physiologic imbalance, however, any ventricular arrhythmia is a more ominous sign.

PREVENTION

Many factors that predispose patients to postoperative hemodynamic instability are beyond the control of the anesthesiologist. Included are patient factors (e.g., age, comorbid conditions) and surgical factors (e.g., duration and location of surgery). However, some factors are within the control of the anesthesiologist:

- Assurance of adequate volume and blood replacement
- Maintenance of appropriate intraoperative hemodynamics
- Avoidance of excessive sympathetic stimulation:
  - Adequate analgesia
  - Adequate ventilation
  - Avoidance of hypothermia
  - Plan for the treatment of nausea and vomiting
- Avoidance of excessive parasympathetic tone
- Adequate ventilation to remove volatile agents
- Judicious use of cholinesterase inhibitors
- Proper use of anticholinergics
- Plan for the prevention and treatment of postoperative nausea and vomiting

Further Reading

Chobanian AV, Bakris GL, Black HR, et al: The Seventh Report of the Joint National Committee on Prevention, Detection, Evaluation, and Treatment of High Blood Pressure: The JNC 7 report. JAMA 289:2560-2572, 2003.

Essentials of ACLS. In Cummins RO (ed): Textbook of Advanced Cardiac Life Support. Dallas, American Heart Association, 1994, pp 1-32-1-40.

Gwirtz K: Management of recovery room complications. Anesthesiol Clin North Am 14:307-339, 1996.

Hines RI, Barash PG, Watrous G, et al: Complications occurring in the PACU. Anesth Analg 74:503-509, 1992.

Moyes J, Oyos T: Cardiovascular system. In Brown M, Brown E (eds): Comprehensive Postanesthesia Care. Baltimore, Williams & Wilkins, 1997, pp 117-134.

Nader ND: Anesthetic preconditioning: A new horizon on myocardial protection. In Salerno TA, Ricci M (eds): Myocardial Protection. Armonk, N.Y., Blackwell Publishing (Futura), 2003, pp 33-42.

Rose DK: Recovery room problems or problems in the PACU. Can J Anaesth 43:116-122, 1996.

Rose DK, Cohen MM, DeBoer MM, et al: Cardiovascular events in the PACU. Anesthesiology 84:772-781, 1996.

Tanaka K, Ludwig LM, Kersten JR, et al: Mechanisms of cardioprotection by volatile anesthetics. Anesthesiology 100:707-721, 2004.

DIAGNOSTIC OR THERAPEUTIC INTERVENTION

Anesthesia for Electroconvulsive Therapy

228

Mijin Lee

Case Synopsis

A 55-year-old man who has major depression but is otherwise healthy presents for electroconvulsive therapy (ECT). Immediately following the electrical stimulus, he develops a 5-second episode of asystole, followed by a rapid increase in heart rate to 140 beats per minute and in blood pressure to 185/120 mm Hg. On emergence, the patient has copious oral secretions and is disoriented, but his vital signs have stabilized.

PROBLEM ANALYSIS

Definition

ECT is used primarily to treat severe depression or catatonia that is refractory to medical therapy. A generalized seizure is induced by an electrical stimulus applied to one or both cerebral hemispheres. The seizure must last 30 to 60 seconds to have a therapeutic effect.

Recognition

Although ECT is relatively safe, it generates profound cardiac and cerebrovascular responses. The cardiovascular effect results from autonomic nervous system activation, initially with predominant parasympathetic discharge (the tonic phase) lasting approximately 5 to 10 seconds. This is followed immediately by pronounced sympathetic discharge (the clonic phase). Clinical consequences of these two phases are as follows:

1. Tonic phase: transient bradycardia, hypotension, and, rarely, asystole lasting several seconds
2. Clonic phase: tachycardia, hypertension, and arrhythmias peaking 1 minute after ECT shocks and generally resolving within 5 to 10 minutes thereafter

ECT-induced cerebrovascular changes also include a 100% to 400% increase in cerebral blood flow above baseline, which is primarily due to a seizure-associated increase in cerebral metabolic rate and, to a lesser extent, elevated blood pressure. In susceptible patients, the consequent increase in intracranial volume may cause a dangerous increase in intracranial pressure.

All patients should be monitored by at least electrocardiogram lead II, with a V_4 or V_5 lead in patients at risk for coronary artery disease. Also, continuous arterial oxygen saturation monitoring by pulse oximetry and noninvasive blood pressure measurement every 3 to 5 minutes are necessary.

Risk Assessment

Several contraindications to ECT have been described (Table 228-1). These largely reflect the significant cardiovascular and cerebrovascular changes associated with ECT. It should be noted, however, that ECT has been performed safely on a variety of high-risk patients, including those with recent myocardial infarction, cerebral aneurysm, and recent

Table 228–1 ■ Contraindications to Electroconvulsive Therapy

Absolute

Pheochromocytoma
Recent myocardial infarction (<4-6 wk)*
Recent cerebrovascular accident†
Recent intracranial surgery†
Intracranial mass lesion
Unstable cervical spine

Relative

Angina‡
Congestive heart failure§
Cardiac rhythm management device¶
Severe pulmonary disease
Major bone fracture
Glaucoma
Retinal detachment
Thrombophlebitis
Pregnancy

*Current American College of Cardiology–American Heart Association guidelines advise waiting 4-6 wk after an uncomplicated myocardial infarction (residual New York Heart Association [NYHA] class III or IV heart failure or persistent hemodynamically disadvantageous arrhythmias) to perform elective surgery. No specific recommendations are made for electroconvulsive therapy, although it would seem reasonable to classify it as a minor or (at worst) an intermediate-risk procedure.
†Recent here means within 3 mo.
‡Chronic, stable angina for which no catheter or surgical intervention is indicated.
§Likely not NYHA class III and certainly not class IV heart failure.
¶Seizures may generate sufficient myopotentials to be interpreted by an internal cardioverter-defibrillator as a tachyarrhythmia, initiating antitachycardia pacing or shock therapies. Alternatively, they may cause pacemaker inhibition (in a pacemaker with unipolar sensing) or high-rate ventricular pacing (in an adaptive-rate pacemaker).

cerebrovascular accident. Indeed, one study noted that major cardiovascular complications occurred equally among patients considered at high risk for coronary events and those at low risk for such events.

Implications

The physiologic effects of ECT are listed in Table 228-2. The overall morbidity associated with ECT is quite low. In one large study, the complication rate was 0.75%. Complications included vertebral body compression, circulatory insufficiency, laryngospasm, status epilepticus, tooth damage, and allergic reactions. Another study noted that the incidence of aspiration among elderly patients was 2.5%. The mortality rate is 0.029% during a course of ECT therapy, whereas that for a single ECT treatment is 0.000045%. Malignant tachyarrhythmias, myocardial infarction, congestive heart failure, and cardiac arrest are rare but constitute the major sources of morbidity and mortality. They generally occur during the recovery period.

Patients with increased intracranial pressure, intracranial mass lesions, or vascular anomalies may not tolerate the large increase in cerebral blood flow associated with ECT. One study found that the overall morbidity for patients with brain tumors undergoing ECT was 74%, with a 1-month mortality rate of 28%. Also, disorientation is common, occurring in 12% of the elderly and 9% of younger patients. Transient muscle aches, memory disturbances, and headaches are among the more common patient complaints following ECT.

MANAGEMENT

The most common complications are related to hemodynamic changes. Bradycardia and transient asystole generally do not require treatment, as both are short-lived. Occasionally, anticholinergic agents are administered, but their routine use may exacerbate the predictable, longer-lasting tachycardia that follows. Tachycardia and hypertension are better managed with a short-acting β-blocker such as esmolol

---

Table 228–2 ■ **Physiologic Effects of Electroconvulsive Therapy**

Cardiovascular
Parasympathetic nervous system (tonic phase)
Decreased heart rate
Hypotension
Bradyarrhythmias (transient asystole; escape beats or transient escape rhythms)
Sympathetic nervous system (clonic phase)
Increased heart rate
Hypertension
Tachyarrhythmias; atrial or ventricular extrasystoles

Cerebral
Increased cerebral blood flow
Increased intracranial pressure

Other
Increased intraocular pressure
Increased intragastric pressure

---

given in 10- to 20-mg increments. However, combined intravenous bolus esmolol and nicardipine control both increased heart rate and blood pressure better than either drug alone.[1] Labetalol may lower the seizure duration, has a longer onset of action, and prolongs any decrease in blood pressure after ECT. Nitroglycerin can be used if hypertension is a greater problem than tachycardia.[2] Midazolam (0.5 to 2 mg intravenously) effectively treats post-ECT agitation.

PREVENTION

Before ECT, all patients should take nothing by mouth for at least 8 hours to reduce the risk of aspiration. Anticholinergics such as glycopyrrolate and atropine may be used to prevent bradycardia, asystole, and excessive salivation in patients with a previous history of such events. Glycopyrrolate is preferred; atropine is associated with a more pronounced increase in heart rate. Routine use of anticholinergics, however, has been criticized as unnecessary.

Induction of anesthesia for ECT has been performed successfully with a number of agents, including methohexital, propofol, and etomidate. Methohexital remains the gold standard for induction of anesthesia, but other agents have their place as well. Methohexital has a rapid onset, a short duration of action, minimal anticonvulsant effects, and a rapid recovery. Remifentanil added to a reduced dose of methohexital has been shown to help prolong seizures in patients with suboptimal seizure duration. Propofol has the advantage of superior hemodynamic stability and more rapid return of cognitive function. It may also help shorten seizure duration in patients with prolonged seizures and minimize postictal nausea and vomiting. Etomidate may be preferred in patients with compromised cardiac status, because it has the least potential for untoward effects on cardiovascular function and minimal anticonvulsant effects.

Muscle relaxation is required to avoid violent muscle contractions, which can cause bone fracture during ECT. Succinylcholine is the agent of choice owing to its rapid onset and short duration of action. In patients in whom succinylcholine is contraindicated, a short-acting nondepolarizing agent such as mivacurium can be used. If so, more prolonged sedation (e.g., bolus propofol plus an intravenous infusion of propofol) should be considered for these patients, because the duration of muscle relaxation may outlast that of the induction agent.

Increased hemodynamic stability has been attempted by pretreatment with esmolol, labetalol, or nitroglycerin.[3] Esmolol (2 mg/kg) given 2 minutes before ECT significantly reduced tachycardia and hypertension compared with

---

[1]This is based on studies of both drugs' effectiveness for blunting hyperadrenergic responses to laryngoscopy and tracheal intubation (Anesth Analg 90:280-288, 2000) or ECT (Anesthesiology 89:A218, 1998). When the drugs are combined for ECT, ideal intravenous bolus doses are esmolol 1 mg/kg and nicardipine 30 mg/kg.

[2]Use of nitroglycerin, which is a primary venodilator, is ill advised in patients with chronic hypertension or who are preload restricted, owing to the potential for untoward hypotension.

[3]See notes 1 and 2.

nitroglycerin (3 µg/kg) or placebo. Also, up to 4.4 mg/kg of esmolol given before ECT was not associated with increased asystole, even without anticholinergic premedication. In contrast, labetalol has been associated with prolonged depression of systolic blood pressure after ECT.

Finally, in patients known to be agitated after ECT, prophylactic use of midazolam is effective after completion of the ECT-generated seizure activity.

Further Reading

Abrams R: The mortality rate with ECT. Convulsive Ther 13:125-127, 1997.

Avramov MN, Husain MM, White PF: The comparative effects of methohexital, propofol, and etomidate for electroconvulsive therapy. Anesth Analg 81:596-602, 1995.

Bailine SH, Petrides G, Doft M, et al: Indications for the use of propofol in electroconvulsive therapy. J ECT 19:129-132, 2003.

Castelli I, Steiner LA, Kaufmann MA, et al: Comparative effects of esmolol and labetalol to attenuate hyperdynamic states after electroconvulsive therapy. Anesth Analg 80:557-561, 1995.

Eagle KA, Berger PB, Calkins H, et al: ACC/AHA update for perioperative cardiovascular evaluation for noncardiac surgery. Circulation 105:1257-1267, 2002.

Folk JW, Kellner CH, Beale MD, et al: Anesthesia for electroconvulsive therapy: A review. J ECT 16:157-170, 2000.

Labbate LA, Miller JP: Midazolam for treatment of agitation after ECT. Am J Psychiatry 152:472-473, 1995.

Morgan GF, Mikhail MS, Murray MJ: Clinical Anesthesiology, 3rd ed. New York, McGraw-Hill, 2002.

Rice EH, Sombrotto LB, Markowitz JC, et al: Cardiovascular morbidity in high-risk patients during ECT. Am J Psychiatry 151:1637-1641, 1994.

Smith DL, Angst MS, Brock-Utne JG, et al: Seizure duration with remifentanil/methohexital vs methohexital alone in middle-aged patients undergoing electroconvulsive therapy. Acta Anaesthesiol Scand 47:1064-1066, 2003.

SPECIAL TOPICS

Cardioversion

Melissa Franckowiak and Nader D. Nader

229

Case Synopsis

A 79-year-old man with a history of two myocardial infarctions and coronary artery disease was referred for coronary artery bypass grafting for angina with anterolateral ischemia. Quadruple bypass grafting was performed, and intraoperatively he received cardiac ablation for definitive treatment of a persistent arrhythmia. The intraoperative course was uneventful. However, on the second postoperative day, the patient developed atrial fibrillation (AFB) and was scheduled for elective cardioversion. After three attempts at synchronized cardioversion (75 J, 100 J, and 150 J), he had asystole lasting 45 seconds but then spontaneously converted to sinus rhythm at 60 beats per minute. On a follow-up visit 10 days later, his functional status had improved, and he was angina free.

PROBLEM ANALYSIS

Definition

Direct-current cardioversion (CV) or defibrillation (DF) is commonly used to treat cardiac tachyarrhythmias to promptly restore hemodynamic stability and prevent myocardial ischemia. Synchronized shocks (CV) are used to restore sinus rhythm in patients with reentrant ventricular and supraventricular tachyarrhythmias with distinct R or S waves. CV does this by depolarizing all or at least a critical mass of excitable myocardium to terminate reentry pathways. With CV, shocks are synchronized with the QRS complex to avoid the risk of triggering ventricular fibrillation if energy is delivered during the vulnerable period of myocardial repolarization (ST segment).

Usually, external CV requires that paddles be applied firmly (about 25 pounds of pressure) to the chest wall, with one paddle applied to the right side of the sternum at the level of the second rib and the other paddle applied at the fifth intercostal space in the midclavicular line. Alternatively, CV pads are used to improve energy transmission and the ability to pace the patient transcutaneously.

Recognition

CV or DF is the preferred initial treatment for all unstable tachyarrhythmias amenable to termination by such means under the current advanced cardiovascular life support (ACLS) guidelines. Only ectopic cardiac rhythm disturbances (i.e., escape rhythms or tachycardia, uniform or multiform atrial ectopic tachycardia) cannot be so terminated. Further, CV is increasingly being advised as the initial management for stable tachycardias, with drugs used to prevent recurrences. This is due in part to the recognition that antiarrhythmic drugs may cause proarrhythmic events far more often than previously believed (see Chapters 12 and 79). Patients with a diseased myocardium, especially with impaired myocardial function (ejection fraction ≤0.35), rarely should receive multiple pharmacologic treatments in an attempt to convert either unstable or stable tachyarrhythmias.

Risk Assessment

It is critical for anesthesiologists and all ACLS providers to recognize the difference between stable and unstable tachyarrhythmias, because the time course for treatment can be dramatically different. Patients with stable hemodynamics (i.e., the arrhythmia does not compromise hemodynamics sufficiently to pose an immediate threat to life or vital organ perfusion) can undergo elective CV in most hospital locations, as long as the equipment required for safe airway management and an appropriate anesthetic plan are in place. However, in those with unstable tachyarrhythmias (i.e., the arrhythmia compromises hemodynamics or poses an immediate threat to life or vital organ perfusion), CV or DF may be required in less than ideal circumstances to save the patient's life or avoid the risk of permanent end-organ injury (e.g., the brain).

Unstable tachyarrhythmias are those associated with signs or symptoms of an acute coronary syndrome (e.g., angina, electrocardiogram changes indicating ischemia), heart failure (e.g., pulmonary edema, rales, jugular venous distention, peripheral edema), brain hypoperfusion (e.g., mental status changes, altered consciousness), diaphoresis, or impaired perfusion of other vital organs. Of course, some of these signs will be absent if the patient is heavily sedated or under general anesthesia. In this case, it is necessary to rely more heavily on the electrocardiogram, blood pressure, pulse oximeter, end-tidal carbon dioxide, skin color, peripheral pulses, and evidence of vital organ perfusion (e.g., reduced urine output, bispectral index or patient state analyzer changes). Unstable tachyarrhythmias require prompt treatment with CV or DF.

Implications

The recent widespread availability of external cardioverter-defibrillators that provide CV or DF with biphasic shock waves has substantially reduced the amount of energy needed for CV or DF. However, elective CV is still painful and requires anesthesia care to provide sedation and to ensure circulatory stability and adequate respiratory function. General anesthesia is performed safely and effectively with the newer intravenous agents that have a rapid onset of action and fast recovery. Spontaneous breathing is usually maintained, so muscle relaxants are often unnecessary. Hemodynamic dysfunction with tachyarrhythmias (e.g., myocardial ischemia, heart failure, loss of atrial transport function, reduced perfusion to vital organs) compounds any hemodynamic effects of hypnotic agents such as propofol or barbiturates.

Underlying valve pathology and enlarged atria may predispose to atrial flutter or fibrillation that is refractory to CV. Common complications of CV include failure to convert the tachyarrhythmia, asystole, hypotension, respiratory depression, gastric aspiration, and difficult airway management. Complications related to airway management can be reduced by careful preoperative examination. Full stomach, obesity, and hiatal hernia are among the risk factors for pulmonary aspiration and pneumonitis. Bone fractures have been reported in elderly patients. These are related to seizure-like muscle contractions similar to those with electroconvulsive therapy and are more likely in patients with osteoporosis and other mineral-deficient bone disorders. A meta-analysis by Swedish researchers showed that the relative risk for all fractures increased 1.5-fold for each one standard deviation decrease in bone mineral density at any skeletal site. However, vertebral mineral density is superior for estimating the risk of vertebral fracture (relative risk 2.3).

MANAGEMENT

Anesthesiologists are often asked to treat patients having CV outside of the operating room or postanesthesia care environment, where providing adequate care can be challenging. A complete medical history and focused physical examination are always necessary to diagnose and prevent untoward complications associated with anesthesia for elective CV.

Patients presenting for elective CV are strongly advised to avoid the intake of solid food for 6 hours and liquids for at least 2 hours. When CV is performed outside of the operating room or postanesthesia care unit, a complete setup must be present, including equipment for suctioning and emergency intubation, laryngeal masks, an Ambu bag with attached facemask, and an oxygen source. The selection of the anesthetic agent is based on the anticipated required duration of action, as well as the patient's hemodynamic stability and associated comorbidities. Short-acting intravenous induction agents and midazolam have been used to provide general anesthesia for CV. Although midazolam has a more prolonged duration of action, it is associated with greater interpatient variability. Both thiopental and propofol are suitable for elective CV in hemodynamically stable patients with preserved myocardial function. In patients with reduced ejection fractions, etomidate is often used to reduce hypotension. An initial decrease in blood pressure occurs with both etomidate and propofol after CV, but blood pressure returns to baseline faster with propofol. Propofol also causes more bradycardia and apnea than etomidate, but emergence from anesthesia is faster. Propofol may be administered via bolus or infusion (the latter attenuates its hypotensive effects). There is no difference in psychomotor skills after either etomidate or propofol. Etomidate is sometimes avoided because of its potential to cause involuntary muscle movements. These may be sensed and interfere with synchronized CV and electrocardiogram interpretation. Intravenous lidocaine (50 to 100 mg) is commonly used before propofol to reduce pain at the injection site. Lidocaine in doses greater than 100 mg does not affect CV thresholds with single or sequential shocks.

Hemodynamic stability is maintained with judicious intravenous fluid administration and, if needed, vasoactive drugs. Pulmonary complications require supportive therapy to ensure adequate oxygenation and ventilation. Bone fractures (often of the vertebral bodies) are usually treated conservatively. Bed rest and analgesics for pain often provide satisfactory results. Neurologic sequelae are rare but may be associated with cord compression due to severe compression fractures or vertebral dislocation. Surgical intervention may be necessary.

Emergent Cardioversion for Unstable Tachyarrhythmias

Current ACLS guidelines recommend a sequence of energy levels for synchronized, monophasic shocks for CV in adults. It begins with 100-J shocks and sequentially increases to 200, 300, and 360 J. Energy levels for biphasic shock (BPS) CV vary among the different cardioverter-defibrillators and are provided in the operator's manual for each device. Exceptions to these guidelines include atrial flutter, which converts with as little as 50 J (BPS), and polymorphic ventricular tachycardia (VT), which requires higher energy levels, beginning with 200 J (BPS). Recent evidence indicates that as the cumulative energy and the number of shocks for external DF increase, the potential for myocardial dysfunction increases. Thus, the lowest possible energy levels should be used. Premedication is recommended whenever possible, even in emergent cases, owing to the painful nature of the procedure. Emergent CV is advised for AFB or atrial flutter if the ventricular rate is greater than 150 beats per minute in adults.

Children, especially neonates, tolerate much higher heart rates than adults do. In fact, they rely on increased heart rate more than on stroke volume to maintain cardiac output with hypovolemia and sepsis. With tachycardia and ventricular rates greater than 220 beats per minute in neonates or 180 beats per minute in children, tachycardia is often supraventricular in origin. Even so, hemodynamic stability must be assessed. Even in children with supraventricular tachycardia, hemodynamic stability is often maintained in conditions such as Wolff-Parkinson-White syndrome and other disorders. If so, CV can be performed under more controlled conditions while hemodynamics are monitored. With supraventricular tachycardia, in contrast to sinus tachycardia, there is usually no obvious cause (e.g., sepsis, pain, hypovolemia) for the degree of tachycardia. Drug treatment for specific supraventricular tachycardias is discussed elsewhere in this book (see Chapters 10 to 13, 79, and 80).

DF is used for pulseless VT or ventricular fibrillation in children and adults, or whenever R and S waves cannot be distinguished. R-wave or S-wave synchronized shocks (CV) are used for VT with palpable pulses. With VT, the rate is at least 120 beats per minute, and QRS complexes are widened (>120 msec). Such QRS widening can also occur with QRS aberration (see Chapters 80 and 81). In the absence of structural heart disease, poisoning, or severe physiologic imbalance, primary VT is rare in children. With VT and palpable pulses in children, CV begins at 0.5 to 2 J/kg (BPS) and is followed by drugs to prevent recurrences (e.g., amiodarone 5 mg/kg intravenously over 30 to 60 minutes). With destabilizing hemodynamics, CV should not be delayed, and sedation should be used whenever possible.

Cardioversion for Atrial Fibrillation

Management for AFB is also discussed in Chapters 79 and 80. Emergency CV should not be used for AFB lasting longer than 48 hours, unless there is severe hemodynamic compromise. For AFB of such long duration, anticoagulation therapy is advised before CV to reduce the likelihood of thromboembolism. Many physicians now use echocardiography to rule out the possibility of atrial thrombus. The success rate of CV varies from 65% to 90%. A major determinant of success with external CV is the duration of AFB. It is far more difficult to convert and maintain normal sinus rhythm with chronic AFB than with AFB of recent onset, such as after cardiovascular or thoracic surgery. With external CV and antiarrhythmic therapy, less than 10% of patients with AFB after coronary artery bypass grafting who are discharged in sinus rhythm will have recurrent AFB within 6 weeks of discharge.

Complications include brief post-CV hypotension and bradycardia. Bradycardia is more common in patients with sick sinus syndrome and after acute myocardial infarction. Arryhythmias with CV may be due to improper synchronization or digitalis toxicity. Ventricular fibrillation caused by improper synchronization can be terminated by repeat shocks, but deaths have been reported from this complication. The lead with the largest R or S waves should be used for synchronization, and one must be certain that tall, peaked T waves will not interfere with proper synchronization to cause inadvertent DF. Pronounced ST segment elevation after CV occurs infrequently; coronary artery spasm has been proposed as the mechanism for this, but definitive evidence is lacking.

PREVENTION

Assurance of nothing-by-mouth status, a semirecumbent position, and the administration of metoclopramide 30 minutes before CV can help decrease residual gastric volume and reduce the risk of vomiting with aspiration. Bite protectors are used to prevent laceration of the lips and tongue from involuntary biting. It is advised that patients with hiatal hernias receive rapid-sequence induction and intubation before CV. Intravenous agents should be given in small boluses and carefully titrated to effect to avoid apnea or hypoventilation in spontaneously breathing patients. Assisted facemask ventilation can help prevent respiratory acidosis, which can aggravate arrhythmias. In elderly patients, post-CV lateral spine radiography is advised. In the presence of osteoporosis or bone demineralization, muscle paralysis is advised using a short-acting agent, along with manually assisted ventilation.

Further Reading

Atkins DL, Dorian P, Gonzalez ER, et al: Treatment of tachyarrhythmias. Ann Emerg Med 37:S91-S109, 2001.

Canessa R, Lema G, Urzua J, et al: Anesthesia for elective cardioversion: A comparison of four anesthetic agents. J Cardiothorac Vasc Anesth 5:566-568, 1991.

Coll-Vinent B, Sala X, Fernandez C, et al: Sedation for cardioversion in the emergency department: Analysis of effectiveness in four protocols. Ann Emerg Med 42:767-772, 2003.

Cummins R: ACLS Provider Manual. Dallas, American Heart Association, 2002, pp 157-185.

Gazmuri RJ: Effects of repetitive electrical shocks on postresuscitation myocardial function. Crit Care Med 28:N228-N232, 2000.

Guidelines 2000 for cardiopulmonary resuscitation and emergency cardiovascular care. Part 6. Advanced cardiovascular life support. Section 2. Defibrillation. The American Heart Association in collaboration with the International Liaison Committee on Resuscitation. Circulation 102(8 Suppl):I90-I94, 2000.

Guidelines 2000 for cardiopulmonary resuscitation and emergency cardiovascular care. Part 6. Advanced cardiovascular life support. Section 5. Pharmacology I: Agents for arrhythmias. The American Heart Association in collaboration with the International Liaison Committee on Resuscitation. Circulation 102(8 Suppl):I112-I128, 2000.

Guidelines 2000 for cardiopulmonary resuscitation and emergency cardiovascular care. Part 6. Advanced cardiovascular life support. Section 6. Pharmacology II: Agents to optimize cardiac output and blood pressure. The American Heart Association in collaboration with the International Liaison Committee on Resuscitation. Circulation 102(8 Suppl):I129-I135, 2000.

Guidelines 2000 for cardiopulmonary resuscitation and emergency cardiovascular care. Part 6. Advanced cardiovascular life support. Section 7D. The tachycardia algorithms. The American Heart Association in collaboration with the International Liaison Committee on Resuscitation. Circulation 102(8 Suppl):I158-I165, 2000.

Guidelines 2000 for cardiopulmonary resuscitation and emergency cardiovascular care. Part 7. The era of reperfusion. Section 1. Acute coronary syndromes (acute myocardial infarction). The American Heart Association in collaboration with the International Liaison Committee on Resuscitation. Circulation 102(8 Suppl):I172-I203, 2000.

Guidelines 2000 for cardiopulmonary resuscitation and emergency cardiovascular care. Part 10. Pediatric advanced life support. The American Heart Association in collaboration with the International Liaison Committee on Resuscitation. Circulation 102(8 Suppl):I291-I342, 2000.

Haghi D, Schumacher B: Current management of symptomatic atrial fibrillation. Am J Cardiovasc Drugs 1:127-139, 2001.

Hullander RM, Leivers D, Wingler K: A comparison of propofol and etomidate for cardioversion. Anesth Analg 77:690-694, 1993.

Kugler JD, Danford DA: Management of infants, children, and adolescents with paroxysmal supraventricular tachycardia. J Pediatr 129:324-338, 1996.

Kugler JD, Danford DA, Gumbiner CH: Ventricular fibrillation during transesophageal atrial pacing in an infant with Wolff-Parkinson-White syndrome. Pediatr Cardiol 12:36-38, 1991.

Lip GY, Watson RD, Singh SP: ABC of atrial fibrillation: Cardioversion of atrial fibrillation. BMJ 312:112-115, 1996.

Maisel WH, Rawn JD, Stevenson WG: Atrial fibrillation after cardiac surgery. Ann Intern Med 135:1061-1073, 2001.

Marshall D, Johnell O, Wedel H: Meta-analysis of how well measures of bone mineral density predict occurrence of osteoporotic fractures. BMJ 312:1254-1259, 1996.

Mehta PM, Reddy BR, Lesser J, et al: Severe bradycardia following electrical cardioversion for atrial tachyarrhythmias in patients with acute myocardial infarction. Chest 97:241-242, 1990.

Siwach SB, Katyal VK: DC cardioversion and coronary artery spasm. J Assoc Physicians India 37:545, 1989.

Zheng F, Qi X, Liu H, et al: Transesophageal cardioversion of atrial flutter and atrial fibrillation using an electric balloon electrode system. Chin Med J (Engl) 116:1325-1328, 2003.

Radiation Oncology

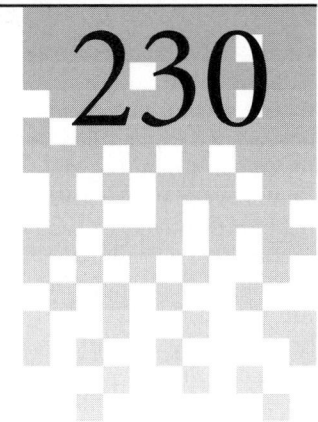

230

Kate Huncke

Case Synopsis

A 4-year-old boy with medulloblastoma undergoes a fourth course of cranial radiation therapy. Anesthesia is induced with propofol infused through a Hickman catheter and titrated to maintain spontaneous ventilation. When the child is sufficiently sedated, he is placed in a prone position. While the patient is monitored from an adjacent room with an audiovisual camera, laryngospasm develops.

PROBLEM ANALYSIS

Definition

Anesthesia is frequently used for radiation therapy in children. The treatment is painless, but absolute immobility is required to precisely focus the radiation beam on tumor cells, thereby sparing adjacent healthy tissue. The total dose of radiation to treat a tumor is divided into daily doses given over several weeks. Each session lasts only a few minutes, but the total dose of radiation per session is high (180 to 250 rad), which means that radiation oncology and anesthesia personnel cannot remain in the immediate treatment area.

Several problems can arise when patients are subject to the daily administration of anesthetics. Tachyphylaxis may develop to anesthetics such as ketamine, propofol, and barbiturates. Daily endotracheal intubation traumatizes the trachea and can lead to stenosis. If a permanent central catheter is not in place, securing and maintaining intravenous (IV) access may be difficult. Prolonged, repetitive fasting and delayed recovery from anesthesia can further compromise nutritional intake in a child who is already anorexic from chemotherapy and malignancy.

Administration of anesthesia outside of the operating room poses challenges. The radiation suite is typically located a distance from trained anesthesia backup personnel and supplies. Access to the patient is limited during the procedure.

Anesthetic delivery and patient monitoring occur from an adjacent room using audiovisual equipment and monitors. A radiostethoscope allows continuous auscultation of heart tones and breath sounds from outside the room. Owing to poor lighting, however, early signs of an impending complication, such as airway obstruction, may be missed with remote monitoring. Also, it may be difficult to ensure the proper operation of IV infusions or anesthetic delivery systems while the anesthesiologist is stationed in the adjacent room.

Recognition

As with any procedure requiring anesthesia, the initial patient evaluation should be thorough. The specific tumor diagnosis has a significant impact on anesthetic management because of associated tumor-related complications (Table 230-1). A complete history and physical examination need not be repeated at each visit, but the anesthesia provider should be aware that the patient's physical status may deteriorate during the course of therapy owing to disease progression or adjuvant chemotherapy. Previous anesthetic records should be reviewed for complications and signs of tachyphylaxis to anesthetic drugs.

In addition to the usual evaluation of the anesthesia machine, the radiation suite should be carefully inspected before treatment. Even modern facilities may not have wall suction and oxygen. A portable suction machine can be used

Table 230–1 ■ Systemic Complications of Common Pediatric Radiation-Sensitive Tumors

Tumor	Complications
Neuroblastoma	Gastrointestinal compression due to large abdominal mass
	Respiratory compromise from pulmonary metastases
	Tumor-related secretion of vasoactive amines, leading to diarrhea and metabolic disturbances
	Motor or sensory deficit with epidural metastases
Wilms' tumor	Gastrointestinal compression due to large abdominal mass
	Anemia from hematuria
	Renal insufficiency
	Hypertension
	Hyperaldosteronism
Retinoblastoma	Increased intracranial pressure with advanced disease
Medulloblastoma	Increased intracranial pressure
	Motor and sensory deficits
Rhabdomyosarcoma	Airway obstruction with pharyngeal location
	Renal insufficiency with genitourinary location

if wall suction is unavailable, but anesthetic gases cannot be scavenged under these conditions. A full oxygen tank and functional Ambu bag should be available in the event the central oxygen supply fails. Electrical outlets should be examined for their ability to accommodate anesthesia equipment and monitors. The anesthesiologist should verify proper positioning of monitors in front of the audiovisual equipment. Any special supplies that may be needed, such as a fiberoptic bronchoscope, should be transported to the area. The anesthesia cart should be fully stocked with all necessary supplies. An emergency cart should be readily available, and the personnel present during the procedure must be familiar with its use.

Risk Assessment

Anesthetic risk increases with the severity of disease. A large abdominal mass can cause gastrointestinal compression, increasing the risk for pulmonary aspiration (see Table 230-1). Patients with intracranial masses may develop intracranial hypertension if anesthetic agents are administered that increase cerebral blood flow. Spontaneous ventilation during deep sedation or general anesthesia can lead to increased arterial carbon dioxide, which may further increase previously elevated intracranial pressure. Metabolic disturbances and dehydration due to inappropriate hormonal secretion or gastrointestinal upset can result in hemodynamic instability during anesthesia.

Limited airway access also increases anesthetic risk. Securing the airway daily with an endotracheal tube is generally avoided because of the short duration of the procedure and the risk of repetitive airway trauma. In patients with tumor-related airway abnormalities, airway obstruction during deep sedation or general anesthesia is a potential problem. Extreme head and neck positions, which are sometimes needed to focus the beam on the affected area, can cause even a normal airway to become obstructed.

Implications

Myriad complications can occur during the delivery of any anesthetic. Compared with management in the operating room, treatment of a problem that occurs during radiation therapy may be delayed because of limited access to the patient and a lack of backup personnel and supplies. Obviously, if the anesthesiologist can anticipate a potential complication, the necessary supplies and personnel should be readily available.

MANAGEMENT

The referring physician, anesthesiologist, and radiation oncology staff should establish a workable plan for collecting the necessary preprocedural information about each patient. Ideally, the anesthesiologist should personally interview the patient or his or her parents or guardians before beginning a course of therapy. If this is not possible, the anesthesiologist should have access to the patient's chart and should contact the patient or the parents or guardians by telephone before the procedure. Compliance with fasting guidelines and continuance of essential medications should be emphasized on a daily basis.

General anesthesia or deep sedation is required to ensure absolute immobility in the pediatric population. Numerous agents and techniques are available to reliably produce unconsciousness and immobility for a brief period. Selection of the appropriate agent is influenced by the patient's age, medical disease, previous reaction to anesthesia, positioning requirements, and availability of an anesthesia machine.

Children younger than 6 years having repetitive procedures often require premedication to facilitate separation from parents. A variety of agents (benzodiazepines, barbiturates, opioids, ketamine) can be given by the oral, nasal, rectal, or intramuscular route. Premedication can also be given via a permanent central line. Alternatively, a heparin-locked peripheral IV line is minimally traumatic for the child and avoids the need for a separate procedure and recovery to establish central IV access.

If an anesthesia machine is available, general anesthesia using an inhalational technique offers several advantages. Induction, emergence, and titration to effect are rapid. Tachyphylaxis in response to volatile agents has not been reported. IV access does not necessarily need to be established before induction. Unfortunately, many radiation suites are not equipped with wall suction for scavenging anesthetic gases.

General anesthesia can also be achieved using only IV agents. Propofol given by bolus or infusion is safe and efficacious. For short procedures, there is faster recovery and less nausea and vomiting with propofol than with isoflurane. Propofol has the disadvantage of causing burning pain when it is given through a peripheral line. Although this can be reduced by prior injection of lidocaine or alfentanil through the IV line, the efficacy of this measure varies among patients and is not universally accepted.

Ketamine can also be used for general anesthesia in the radiation suite. An IV catheter need not be placed before induction, because intramuscular injection rapidly produces unconsciousness. A single intramuscular injection may be sufficient for the entire procedure. Atropine or glycopyrrolate must be given to prevent increased airway secretions with ketamine. Spontaneous ventilation is better preserved with ketamine than with propofol or volatile agents. Recovery from ketamine can be prolonged, however, and is frequently associated with an unpleasant emergence delirium. Tachyphylaxis with either ketamine or propofol has been reported.

A laryngeal mask airway (LMA) can be used to secure the airway. It eliminates airway obstruction due to relaxation of the tongue and supraglottic soft tissue. Repeated trauma to the trachea is avoided, but uvular and pharyngeal trauma can occur during placement of the LMA. As is the case with mask ventilation, laryngospasm and coughing can occur if the patient is stimulated under light anesthesia. Pediatric LMAs are susceptible to kinking because of their small radius. Maintaining the proper position of the LMA may require manipulation of the mandible and neck, which can be difficult if the patient is not in the supine position. The LMA is contraindicated in patients at risk for aspiration or with low pulmonary compliance who will need positive-pressure ventilation.

The recovery area should be equipped with oxygen, suction, and basic monitoring. Staff trained in anesthesia recovery should be available; otherwise, the patient should be transported to the operating room recovery area.

PREVENTION

Risks and complications can be minimized by thorough evaluation of the patient, careful consideration of the planned procedure, and familiarity with the radiation suite and the location of necessary supplies and equipment. The anesthesiologist should never proceed without verifying the working order of all required equipment. If a problem is anticipated, backup personnel should be alerted, and special supplies should be transported to the area. Basic monitoring standards of general anesthesia should be observed. The American Society of Anesthesiologists has published guidelines for non–operating room locations that list the minimal standards for monitoring. If more invasive monitoring is required because of the patient's illness, it should be used during therapy. Failure to comply with these standards can result in loss of accreditation.

The patient and his or her parents or guardians should be questioned daily about any new symptoms and the last oral intake. Fasting guidelines should be strictly enforced. In patients who are at risk for aspiration, the airway should be protected with an endotracheal tube, even on a daily basis if necessary. Antacids and metoclopramide should be given if indicated. If the patient develops any new symptoms that would adversely affect the anesthetic outcome, the case should be delayed pending further evaluation.

Tachyphylaxis in response to anesthetic agents cannot be prevented. Alternative agents to produce general anesthesia should be readily available.

All patients receiving an anesthetic, whether general, regional, or monitored anesthesia care, should receive appropriate postanesthesia management. Recovery can take place in the postanesthesia care unit or in the procedure room. Monitoring standards for temperature, ventilation, circulation, and oxygenation must be observed, regardless of location. Finally, when discharge criteria are met, this must be documented on the patient's medical chart by the anesthesiologist.

Further Reading

Bell C: Outpatient anesthesia in non operating room setting. In McGoldrick K (ed): Ambulatory Anesthesia: A Problem-Oriented Approach. Baltimore, Williams & Wilkins, 1995, pp 550-571.

Brann C, Janik D: Anesthesia in the radiology suite. Prob Anesth 6:413-429, 1992.

Greenberg D, Romanoff M: Anesthesia outside the operating room: An overview. Prob Anesth 6:299-310, 1992.

Kotob F, Tewersky R: Anesthesia outside the operating room: General overview and monitoring standards. In Osborn I (ed): Anesthesia Outside the Operating Room: International Anesthesia Clinics. Philadelphia, JB Lippincott–Williams & Wilkins, 2003, pp 1-15.

McDowall R, Scher C, Barst S: Total intravenous anesthesia for children undergoing brief diagnostic or therapeutic procedures. J Clin Anesth 7:273-280, 1995.

Embolization Procedures

231

George A. Higgins

Case Synopsis

Six days after revision surgery for a hip replacement, a 78-year-old patient presents from the rehabilitation department with frank hemorrhage from the operated extremity. Angiography and possible embolization are proposed for a 9:00 PM start time. The on-call anesthesia team is requested to provide analgesia and sedation for the procedure. The patient has previously been anticoagulated for deep venous thrombosis prophylaxis and has a history of hypertension, chronic renal insufficiency, stable angina, and esophageal reflux disease. A complete blood count and type and crossmatch are pending, and the patient had a full meal 3 hours before admission.

PROBLEM ANALYSIS

Definition

Members of the anesthesia care team are occasionally asked to provide unpredictable and varying levels of sedation, including possible progression to general anesthesia, for endovascular embolization procedures. The indications for such procedures are diverse (Table 231-1), ranging from elective ablation of a cerebral arteriovenous malformation to embolization of a life-threatening uterine hemorrhage in a Jehovah's Witness parturient.

The interventional radiology suite is often located in a remote part of the hospital, far from the surgery and intensive care departments. The work environment is usually not designed or adaptable for a full repertoire of anesthesia and monitoring equipment. Portable communications devices, such as pagers, two-way radios, and cell phones, are often nonfunctional in the shielded surroundings. The space is often cramped, and access to oxygen, suctioning, monitors, and the resuscitation cart may be blocked or made awkward by radiology equipment (Fig. 231-1). The required use of ungainly lead aprons and the diminished lighting increase the risk of injury to the anesthesia provider and the patient from overhanging equipment, needle sticks, drug swaps, and inability to assess the patient's condition.

The embolization procedure itself has inherent risks, including unrecognized hemorrhage, vascular damage, allergic reactions to contrast or embolic media, nontarget embolization injury, ischemic pain in the target organ, and nausea or vomiting. Unlike the anesthesia team, the radiology team is generally not focused on the patient's comorbidities and the implications for sedation or analgesia. The duration of embolization procedures is indeterminate. Commonly, the patient reaches maximal endurance before completion of the procedure. Specialized embolization agents (e.g., coils, microspheres, acrylic glue, detachable balloons) may not be routinely stocked in the needed size, causing unanticipated delays. The anesthesia team is expected to provide a motionless and cooperative patient with stable vital signs throughout the procedure, usually under conditions of monitored anesthesia care. Rapid neurologic assessment is periodically required, especially for procedures involving the blood supply to the brain.

Table 231–1 ■ Indications for Endovascular Embolization

Arteriovenous malformation
Arteriovenous fistula
Intracranial aneurysm
Recurrent epistaxis
Hemoptysis
Traumatic solid organ hemorrhage
Preoperative major organ tumor embolization for blood loss reduction
Gastrointestinal hemorrhage
Uterine leiomyoma (fibroid)
Uterine hemorrhage
Pelvic fracture hemorrhage
Postoperative hemorrhage after prosthetic hip or knee replacement
Varicocele

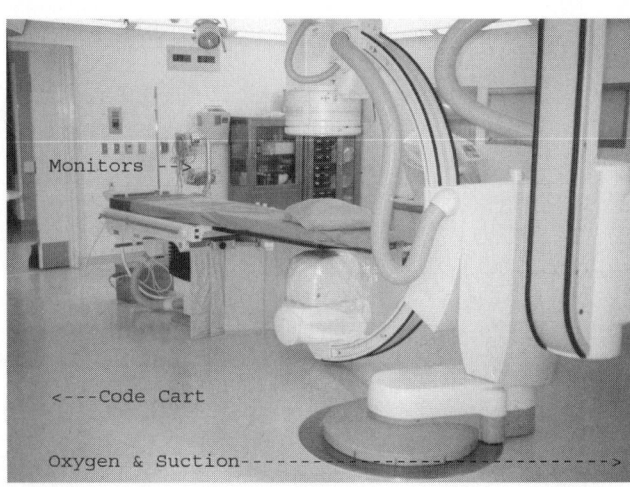

Figure 231–1 ■ Interventional radiology suite. Note the location of the anesthesia monitors, the oxygen and suction regulators, and the code cart and the layout of the work space.

Recognition

In addition to routine monitoring (electrocardiogram, non-invasive blood pressure, and arterial oxygen saturation), some assessment of respiratory effort is crucial. Nasal cannulas with carbon dioxide sampling lines are routinely used. A radiopaque precordial stethoscope can also be effective. If available, the side port of the radiologist's femoral artery introducer can be used for arterial pressure monitoring or blood gas sampling. A large-bore peripheral intravenous line with a distal side port should be established. The patient's needs (maintaining body temperature and position preferences), as well as a consideration of his or her past experiences and current expectations, guide the provider's choice of technique. Previous experience with similar procedures can be used as a guide to how the patient will react to the embolization procedure.

Some brief familiarization with the planned procedure can spotlight important monitoring points along the way. It is helpful to be able to recognize sentinel events of the embolization procedure. Knowledge of expected and unexpected outcomes of the embolization procedure itself is useful for monitoring the patient's status.

Risk Assessment

Patients undergoing embolization procedures can be assumed to be at high risk, especially in emergency circumstances. Each patient deserves a brief but thorough history; review of systems, medications, and allergies; and physical examination focusing on the airway, cardiorespiratory status, and neurologic stability and function. Documentation of baseline neurologic function and inspection of recent laboratory values, especially hemoglobin and clotting parameters, are important. Patients with diabetes or a history of seizures require special attention. Their medications and blood levels should be checked before the start of the procedure and intraoperatively, if indicated. Time of last oral intake should be established, and evaluation for gastroesophageal reflux disease and recent emetic episodes should be performed. Blood availability should be personally confirmed with the blood bank. Verification of informed consent for the procedure, anesthesia, and associated risks is mandatory.

The radiology suite should be assessed for ergonomic hazards, including the following:

- Adequacy of dedicated electrical circuits
- Patency and functioning of oxygen and suction lines and regulators
- Location of telephones, crash cart (with confirmation of its functional status), and emergency exits

An attempt should be made to group oxygen, suction, and monitoring functions in a segregated area that does not interfere with the procedure but allows direct visualization of the patient's airway.

Implications

The embolization procedure has potential risks and expected side effects. Complications that may require the intervention of the anesthesia team include the following:

- Nausea, vomiting, or aspiration

- Uncontrollable pain or agitation under sedation
- Hypoventilation, hypoxemia, and airway obstruction
- Vagal-mediated reflexes
- Hypotension, septic shock, or myocardial infarction
- Stroke or seizure
- Cardiac or respiratory arrest
- Organ insult due to hypoperfusion or nontarget embolism
- Internal hemorrhage due to vascular perforation or rupture
- Anaphylactic reactions from either radiologic or anesthetic agents

All these complications should be anticipated, with a well-rehearsed plan of action in place to deal with such occurrences. The ability to immediately convert from monitored anesthesia care to general endotracheal anesthesia should always be maintained.

MANAGEMENT

A departmental protocol, including a checklist of required equipment, medications, and personnel for every satellite hospital location (including telephone numbers), should be developed. Also, there must be firsthand knowledge of the location of oxygen and suctioning equipment, electrical circuits, lighting controls, and the crash cart. There must be sufficient time to fully check the listed items. For example, code carts are frequently kept outside the suite in a locked medicine supply room. If so, verification that the door is unlocked and that the monitors and defibrillator are functional is a time-consuming but important task. Complications must be anticipated, a general treatment plan formulated, and the appropriate resources for management identified.

Some events, such as hypoventilation or a mild drug reaction, can be adequately managed without aborting the procedure. Others, however, may require that the procedure be terminated and the patient transferred to a better location for treatment and more invasive monitoring. In the case of uncontrolled vascular hemorrhage, resuscitation is best carried out in a surgical intensive care unit or adjacent to the operating room while awaiting arrival of the surgical team.

Successful management of possible complications involves bringing appropriate resources to the patient or bringing the patient to those resources. The remote location of the radiology suite usually hinders quick access to such resources. For example, the blood bank may not be familiar with the location of the radiology suite or how to rapidly deliver blood products to it. During evening or nighttime hours, there may not be enough personnel available to deliver supplies or to transport the patient. If so, the patient is in jeopardy until he or she can be moved to a more central site.

PREVENTION

Prevention of complications requires assessment and preparation in the following areas.

Patient Evaluation. Each patient should be evaluated with a concise history, systems review, medication and allergy review, and physical examination. Procedure-specific systems need to be assessed and documented. All questions should be answered, and a description of the events during the procedure, including any expected discomfort, unusual sensations, and possible complications, should be provided.

Anesthesia Equipment. Using a checklist, each location should be evaluated for the existence and functioning of the following equipment and supplies: oxygen (both piped in and reserve tanks), suctioning, emergency electrical outlets dedicated to anesthesia, emergency lighting, telephones, anesthesia machine and equipment, anesthetic and emergency drugs, crash cart, and radiology table for immediate airway access equipment in case the airway must be accessed emergently.

Communication. Specific goals of both the anesthesia team and the radiology team should be discussed. Criteria for aborting the procedure and exit strategies are best defined before beginning the procedure.

Resource Availability. Regardless of assurances from the radiology team, the ability to secure additional resources if necessary is mandatory. The telephone and pager systems must be functional, and key personnel (e.g., blood bank, surgery, transport, intensive care, anesthesia technical support services) should be notified that their services might be required.

Anesthetic Technique. Use of short-acting or reversible agents (e.g., midazolam, alfentanil, propofol) for a monitored anesthesia technique permits the patient to quickly return to baseline. This allows for efficient neurologic or cardiovascular evaluation, if needed. Similarly, short-acting and easily reversed muscle relaxants and inhalational anesthetics are available if general anesthesia is required.

In summary, many untoward events associated with providing anesthesia care for embolization procedures can be reduced or eliminated by careful preprocedural preparation and planning.

Further Reading

Andrews RT, Spies JB, Sacks D, et al: Patient care and uterine artery embolization for leiomyomata. J Vasc Interv Radiol 15:115-120, 2004.

Barriga A, Valenti Nin JR, Delgado C, Bilbao JJ: Therapeutic embolisation for postoperative haemorrhage after total arthroplasty of the hip and knee. J Bone Joint Surg Br 83:90-92, 2001.

Forbes RB: Anesthesia for nonsurgical procedures. In Longnecker (ed): Principles and Practice of Anesthesiology, 2nd ed. St. Louis, Mosby, 1998.

Schonholz DH: Blood transfusion and the pregnant Jehovah's Witness patient: Avoiding a dilemma. Mt Sinai J Med 66:277-279, 1999.

Ward JF, Velling TE: Transcatheter therapeutic embolization of genitourinary pathology. Rev Urol 2:236-262, 2000.

Catheter Ablation for Arrhythmias

232

Glyn D. Williams

Case Synopsis

A 15-year-old boy with Wolff-Parkinson-White syndrome and a history of recurrent paroxysmal tachycardia undergoes percutaneous catheter radiofrequency ablation of an accessory pathway while under general anesthesia. The procedure is successful, as demonstrated by the loss of δ waves and restoration of a normal P-R interval (Fig. 232-1). Postoperatively, the patient complains of weakness in his right arm. Examination reveals that he has sustained a brachial plexus injury.

SPECIAL TOPICS

PROBLEM ANALYSIS

Definition

Brachial plexus injury is a recognized complication of catheter ablation procedures. General anesthesia, lengthy procedures, and positioning the patient's hands above the head (for lateral fluoroscopic views of the chest) are important contributory factors.

Recognition

Supraventricular tachycardia is relatively common in children (see also Chapters 79 and 80). Mechanisms for supraventricular tachycardia include both reentry and automatic tachycardias. Atrioventricular (AV) reciprocating tachycardia (of which Wolff-Parkinson-White syndrome is a subset) and AV node reentry tachycardia are the most common forms of reentrant tachycardia in children. For patients in whom medical therapy is inadequate or undesirable, invasive electrophysiology techniques are a viable option.

Percutaneous catheter ablation is used to selectively interrupt cardiac conduction pathways. Indications for catheter ablation are listed in Table 232-1. Three regions can be ablated: the AV bypass tracts, the AV node margins, and ventricular reentry pathways. Radiofrequency (RF) energy is low-power, high-frequency alternating current that causes injury by generating heat at the electrode-tissue interface. RF allows good control of energy delivery, creates a small area of injury, can be used safely in thin-walled structures such as the coronary sinus, and seldom triggers malignant arrhythmias. The energy is delivered via an intracardiac catheter to endocardium adjacent to the area of abnormal conduction.

Injured tissue becomes electrophysiologically inactive and scars, thereby preventing recurrent arrhythmias.

Recently, cryoablation has been used for creating endocardial lesions. Liquid nitrous oxide is circulated through the ablation catheter, cooling the tip to subfreezing temperatures and resulting in destruction of tissue directly beneath the catheter tip. Cryoablation has several advantages over RF systems, because the area of interest can be temperature-mapped at a temperature of −22°C to −30°C. This results in alteration of the tissue's electrical conductivity. Usually, this area can be rewarmed if the freeze time is limited (i.e., "ice mapping"). Further cooling to a lower setpoint (−75°C) creates a permanent lesion. Thus, an area is ice-mapped to predetermine whether subsequent lower setpoint cryoablation at this site will be successful and whether there will be any undesirable effects (especially AV block) due to creation of a permanent lesion. Another advantage of cryoablation over RF ablation is that the catheter tip freezes tightly onto the endocardium during mapping and ablation, thereby reducing the risk of injury to surrounding tissue from motion of the beating heart. Compared with RF techniques, cryoablation causes less discomfort in awake patients, but the possibility of supraventricular tachycardia reoccurrence may be greater. Cryoablation is a particularly appealing option for ablation in the region around the AV node, where the risk of causing iatrogenic complete AV heart block is highest.

RF ablation can cause mild to moderate retrosternal angina-like pain, but it is applied for only short periods (<1 to 2 minutes). To facilitate the ablation procedure, the patient must remain motionless. Adults can often be managed with sedation, but most children require general anesthesia. During the initial application of cryoablation, a brief period of patient apnea may be desirable to limit intrathoracic

---

Figure 232–1 ■ Electrocardiogram from a patient with Wolff-Parkinson-White syndrome showing loss of δ waves and restoration of a normal P-R interval after radiofrequency ablation of the accessory pathway.

LEAD II

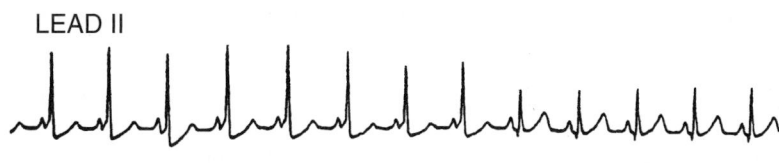

Radiofrequency Energy ⊢━━━━━━━━━━

Table 232–1 ■ Indications for Catheter Ablation of Tachyarrhythmias
Symptomatic supraventricular or ventricular tachyarrhythmias refractory to drugs
Intolerable side effects or other adverse drug effects (e.g., ventricular proarrhythmia)
"Tachycardiomyopathy (i.e., tachycardia-induced myocardial dysfunction)
Presurgical control of tachyarrhythmias with congenital heart disease
Desire of patient or family

Table 232–2 ■ Risks Factors Associated with Catheter Ablation	
Risk Factor	**Focus**
Patient's clinical status	Associated heart disease, other system pathology
Patient's medications	Antiarrhythmic drugs, anticoagulants
Sedation techniques	Airway obstruction, respiratory depression
General anesthesia techniques	Hemodynamic stability, airway management, positioning
Catheter ablation	See Table 232-3
Environment	Hypothermia, limited access to patient, remoteness from help
Radiation	Patient exposure, caregiver exposure

movement, thereby enhancing contact between the catheter tip and the endocardium.

Ideally, the anesthetics or sedatives used should not alter intrinsic pacemaker function, impulse propagation, refractoriness, or autonomic tone or prevent intentional triggering of reentrant arrhythmias. In addition, anesthesia should be rapidly reversible, with minimal delay in emergence. A few studies have examined the effects of anesthetic agents on the conduction system, but many are flawed by the confounding effects of drugs used to induce anesthesia. Analgesia for catheter insertion can be achieved with local anesthetic agents, but care should be taken, because a dose of 3.2 mg/kg of 1% lidocaine can reportedly have an adverse influence on the inducibility of arrhythmias in children. The following anesthetic techniques have minimal effect on either the normal conduction system or the accessory pathways in patients with Wolff-Parkinson-White syndrome:

- Alfentanil and midazolam infusions
- Sufentanil and lorazepam infusions
- Alfentanil, nitrous oxide, pancuronium
- Isoflurane, nitrous oxide, pancuronium
- Propofol, nitrous oxide, pancuronium
- Remifentanil and ketamine

One study concluded that propofol anesthesia was acceptable during RF ablation for most tachyarrhythmias except for atrial ectopic tachycardia, which could not be induced after propofol administration. Another investigation noted that isoflurane prolonged the effective refractory period of the antegrade accessory pathway in children with Wolff-Parkinson-White syndrome and advised care when interpreting measurements. One review concluded that either balanced general anesthesia (with isoflurane being the preferred volatile agent) or monitored anesthesia care with opioids, benzodiazepines, and propofol was acceptable. Effective ablation can be tested by attempting to retrigger the offending arrhythmia with the administration of isoproterenol infusions (0.02 to 0.1 μg/kg per minute) or atropine (10 to 20 μg/kg).

Risk Assessment

Risks associated with catheter ablation are summarized in Tables 232-2 and 232-3.

Implications

A recent prospective, multicenter study reported a 96% success rate with catheter ablation for supraventricular tachycardia in children. Factors that reduce the likelihood of success include aberrant conduction via a right free wall pathway, other heart disease, and greater body weight. Unintentional catheter-induced mechanical trauma to accessory pathways can result in discontinuation of the ablation procedure and lower success rates. Right anteroseptal and right atriofascicular pathways appear to be especially vulnerable. The complication rate for catheter ablation (4%) is similar for adults and children and is slightly greater than the complication rate for diagnostic cardiac catheterization. The occurrence of complete AV block has great significance, especially for children, because the child will be burdened by the need for lifelong artificial cardiac pacing. Complication rates in children have been correlated with very low body weight and limited institutional experience. Deaths have occurred after catheter ablation.

MANAGEMENT

Preoperative preparation includes a thorough history, physical examination, laboratory testing, and optimization of medical therapy. The cardiologist who will conduct the ablation and the anesthesiologist should confer and formulate a management plan. Antiarrhythmic agents are discontinued several days before the procedure to promote initiation of the arrhythmia. Patients who decompensate during arrhythmias should be identified, and the presenting symptoms should be elicited. All patients should fast before surgery. Reassurance, premedication, or both may help minimize excessive sympathetic tone.

Because the electrophysiology suite is likely remote from the operating room, it is important to have all the necessary anesthetic equipment and drugs available (similar to preparation for embolization procedures; see Chapter 231). Typical monitoring includes continuous electrocardiography, pulse oximetry, noninvasive blood pressure (possibly direct arterial pressure), body temperature monitoring, and expired carbon dioxide analysis. For the last, the nasal cannulas used for oxygen delivery must have an aspiration port for end-tidal CO_2 analysis. Depth of anesthesia can be assessed by processed electroencephalography. For this, either a bispectral index or processed spectral array monitor can

Table 232-3 ■ Complications of Catheter Ablation

Complication	Comments
Related to Cardiac Catheterization	
Arrhythmias	Atrioventricular block, sinus bradycardia, supraventricular tachycardia, and ventricular tachycardia can be clinically important
Hematoma at catheter site	Most common complication; heparin therapy may contribute
Arterial trauma	Especially in children, owing to relatively large catheter size
Perforation	Perforation of heart or great vessels is rare
Catheter entrapment	Uncommon; may require surgical intervention
Infection	Antibiotic prophylaxis is indicated in some cases
Air embolism	Systematic emboli possible if an intracardiac shunt is present
Thromboembolism	Consider heparin prophylaxis in high-risk cases
Hypotension	Causes include hypovolemia, hypoxia, acidosis, arrhythmia, myocardial infarction, cardiac tamponade, and catheter obstruction of flow
Contrast media	Allergic reactions, hyperosmolar effects, renal toxicity, pain on injection, histamine release
Nerve injury	Brachial plexus especially at risk
Pneumothorax	Central venous line placement
Specific to Ablation Procedure	
Atrioventricular block	Relatively common; may require transvenous pacemaker
Arrhythmia	Uncommon
Valvular regurgitation	Reported
Coronary spasm	Reported
Skin burn	Reported
Perforation	Pericardial tamponade after ablation near coronary sinus

SPECIAL TOPICS

be used. The defibrillator is checked, and the leads are attached to the patient. Patients at risk for ventricular arrhythmias have hard-wired defibrillator gel pads placed over the sternum and back. Attention to positioning and padding is required. Hypothermia and hypoglycemia are risks, especially in children. Use of antiemetic agents should be considered, because nausea and vomiting are relatively common after the procedure. Patients with good preoperative clinical status and normal cardiac anatomy who undergo uncomplicated catheter ablation may be allowed to return home after discharge from the postanesthesia care unit. In contrast, high-risk patients may warrant admission to an intensive care unit after the ablation procedure.

PREVENTION

In the author's experience, brachial plexus injury is most likely to occur in thin teenagers who receive general anesthesia for catheter ablation procedures of long duration. Patients must be informed of this risk before the procedure. After induction, the patient is positioned carefully; pressure points are padded, and these are checked periodically during the procedure.

Whenever possible, the arms are kept at the patient's sides. These precautions can reduce the occurrence of brachial plexus nerve injury.

Further Reading

Chun TUH, Van Hare GF: Advances in the approach to treatment of supraventricular tachycardia in the pediatric population. Curr Cardiol Rep 6:322-326, 2004.

Jackman WM, Wang XZ, Friday KJ, et al: Catheter ablation of accessory atrioventricular pathways (Wolff-Parkinson-White syndrome) by radiofrequency current. N Engl J Med 324:1605-1611, 1991.

Javorski JJ, Hansen DD, Laussen PC, et al: Pediatric cardiac catheterization: Innovations. Can J Anaesth 42:310-329, 1995.

Kugler JD, Danford DA, Deal BJ, et al: Radiofrequency catheter ablation for tachyarrhythmias in children and adolescents. N Engl J Med 330:1481-1487, 1994.

Lavoie J, Walsh EP, Burrows RA, et al: Effects of propofol or isoflurane anesthesia on cardiac conduction in children undergoing radiofrequency catheter ablation for tachydysrhythmias. Anesthesiology 82:884-887, 1995.

Stobie P, Green MS: Cryoablation for septal accessory pathways: Has the next ice age arrived? J Cardiovasc Electrophysiol 14:830-831, 2003.

Van Hare GF, Javitz H, Carmelli D, et al: Prospective assessment after pediatric cardiac ablation: Demographics, medical profiles and initial outcomes. J Cardiovasc Electrophysiol 15:759-770, 2004.

Magnetic Resonance Imaging

233

Hind M. Gautam and Christopher M. B. Heard

Case Synopsis

A 5-year-old boy requires magnetic resonance imaging (MRI) of the brain for delayed mental development. An attempt at the procedure has already failed after the boy received an oral sedation regimen. Anesthesia has been requested to facilitate the investigation.

PROBLEM ANALYSIS

Definition

MRI is a noninvasive diagnostic imaging modality that produces precise images of the body. It is free of ionizing radiation and does not, by itself, produce any known biologically deleterious effects. It is based on the principle that atomic nuclei in a strong magnetic field absorb pulses of radiofrequency energy, which are then emitted as radio waves and reconstructed into computerized images. Magnetic field strengths generally range from 0.15 to 2.0 tesla (T), although magnetic field strengths of 3 T are increasingly being used. The patient is required to lie still within a small space while multiple images are obtained. MRI requires a longer time to develop than computed tomography scanning; therefore, any movement by the patient degrades the image quality. In fact, any change in the patient's position may affect the homogeneity of the magnetic field, which is optimized at the beginning of the scan. Studies can take from 45 minutes to more than 2 hours, with individual sequences taking from 3 to 10 minutes. The scanner is noisy, and the restricted space and lack of movement can induce claustrophobia in some patients. Patients also may experience a slight increase in temperature.

Recognition

Most adults and children older than 6 years are capable of lying still for the scan. With the use of headphones and music, MRI is a well-tolerated procedure. However, there are several groups of patients who may require anesthesia for the scan to be performed (Table 233-1).

Risk Assessment

Table 233-2 lists some common contraindications to MRI. If there is any uncertainty, the radiologist should be consulted. These contraindications are related either to the possibility of the magnet causing a ferromagnetic object to move or heat up or to the induction of an electrical current from the radiofrequency pulses and magnetic gradients used to generate the images. The effect on the unborn fetus is unknown, and MRI should probably be avoided in the first trimester unless absolutely indicated based on the patient's medical condition. Permanent cosmetic makeup and tattoos can cause skin irritation during MRI scanning.

Anesthesia risk is increased because the patient is in a remote location, with limited airway access and visibility. The presence of gastroesophageal reflux, seizures, or raised intracranial pressure affects the choice of anesthetic. Other potential problems that may arise are listed in Table 233-3.

Implications

Monitors must be suitable for use in the MRI suite. They should be nonferromagnetic, and cables should be screened from electromagnetic interference (fiberoptic is ideal). The signal should be filtered to avoid radiofrequency interference, which affects image quality. Despite specialized technology, some problems remain (Table 233-4).

Table 233–1 ■ Indications for Deep Sedation or Anesthesia for Magnetic Resonance Imaging

Very young or agitated patient
Patient unsuitable for oral sedation regimen (history of apnea, gastroesophageal reflux, severe respiratory disease)
Patient who has failed an oral sedation regimen
Prolonged study (multiple scans)
Anxious patient
Claustrophobic patient
Intensive care patient

Table 233–2 ■ Absolute or Relative Contraindications to Magnetic Resonance Imaging

Cardiac pacemaker*
Aneurysm clips
Implanted cardiac defibrillator*
Neurostimulator*
Pacing wires*
Cochlear implant*
Implanted insulin pump*
Penile prosthesis
History of ocular injury involving metal object
History of vascular surgery within 3 mo (metallic clips or sutures)
History of soft tissue metal foreign body within 3 mo
History of orthopedic hardware within 3 mo

*Consult the device manufacturer or patient follow-up clinic about the specific procedure.

Table 233–3 ■ Potential Problems Related to Magnetic Resonance Imaging

Malfunction of anesthesia equipment
Malfunction of monitoring equipment
Anesthesia equipment interfering with image quality
High-velocity ferromagnetic projectile from loose object
Disruption of electronic devices, credit cards

All anesthesia equipment, as well as the pulse oximeter, intravenous line pole, and anesthesia cart, should also be nonferromagnetic. MRI-safe anesthesia machines, laryngoscopes (lithium batteries), and stethoscopes are available. Any equipment with a transformer must be kept out of the magnetic field. Gas cylinders must be aluminum. If inhalation anesthesia is used, a suitable scavenging system should be available. "MRI-safe" vaporizers may have minimal amounts of ferromagnetic materials and should not be taken into the MRI suite unless mounted on the anesthesia machine or ventilator. The area surrounding a magnetic field stronger than 5 gauss should not contain any ferromagnetic items.

MANAGEMENT

As with any anesthesia induction, the monitoring standards of the American Society of Anesthesiologists should be adhered to. To avoid problems due to monitoring cables, it is advisable to place them as near as possible to the center of the long axis of the MRI magnetic field. They also should be placed on the part of the patient that is most distant from the radiofrequency field. Avoid coiled or crossed wires. The anesthetic technique is dictated by the age of the patient and concurrent diseases (Table 233–5).

Vaporizers are accurate in the MRI suite. Intravenous infusion pumps must be outside the 5-gauss limit for magnetic fields. The electric motor in such pumps emits electromagnetic radiation, which may cause the pump to run at an abnormal speed in the presence of a strong magnetic field. The pump is also a projectile risk. Intravenous infusions via long tubing from outside the scanner are useful so that the depth of anesthesia can be altered without having to enter the MRI scanner.

Table 233–5 ■ Anesthesia Options

Intravenous Sedation with Supplemental Oxygen for Pediatric Patients

Propofol bolus of 2 to 3 mg/kg and infusion of 100 µg/kg/min
Oral chloral hydrate (<3 yr) 75 to 100 mg/kg for procedures up to 1 hr
Rectal methohexital 20 to 30 mg/kg for procedures up to 30 min (good for children up to 6 yr; may be contraindicated in patients with temporal lobe epilepsy)
Ketamine ≤1.0 mg/kg IV (1–3 mg/kg IM if no IV is available; avoid use with elevated intracranial pressure)

Benzodiazepines for Sedation and Anxiolysis in Adults

May be induced orally or intravenously
Good method for patients with few medical problems and an easily maintained airway; minimally invasive
Rapid recovery; little nausea or vomiting; glycopyrrolate is a useful antisialagogue

General Anesthesia with Endotracheal Tube Ventilation

Inhalation anesthesia or propofol infusion
Good for very young patients or those with gastroesophageal reflux, full stomach, or raised intracranial pressure

General Anesthesia and Spontaneous Respiration with Laryngeal Mask Airway

Inhalation anesthesia or propofol infusion

The use of a cuffed endotracheal tube or armored laryngeal mask may affect the quality of the image owing to the presence of metal in the valve of the pilot balloon or used to reinforce the mask airway. The use of a contrast agent is often required. Fortunately, MRI contrast agents (based on gadolinium) are associated with fewer allergic reactions than their x-ray counterparts. Severe reactions occur in less than 1 in 100,000 patients. MRI contrast agents are also nontoxic to the kidneys.

If a patient comes from the intensive care unit, special care must be taken to ensure that all cables and transducers are carefully screened and ferromagnetic objects are removed. Cables should be straightened to prevent burns. For invasive blood pressure monitoring, the transducer should be as far from the patient as possible and separated with a saline-filled pressure line. If cardiac arrest occurs, the patient should be removed from the magnetic field. The defibrillator should be kept outside the magnetic field and checked regularly. Use of a nonferromagnetic code cart is also advised. It is essential

---

Table 233–4 ■ Monitoring Problems in Magnetic Resonance Imaging

Monitor	Problem
Electrocardiogram (ECG)	T waves and ST segments are often altered, and qualitative information is lacking during MRI scanning cycle; ECG cables may cause burn injury; special ECG electrodes are required to avoid burn injury
Pulse oximeter	Malfunction, heating of probe may cause burn injury; fiberoptic connection to patient is best
Capnograph	Requires long tubing, resulting in prolonged upsweep and delay in display of real-time measurements; respiratory rate and trends can still be useful, however
Temperature	Requires a filtered cable
Precordial stethoscope	Long tubing; sounds are obscured by noisy scan
Oxygen analyzer	Nonmagnetic lithium battery is required; expect reduced battery life
Blood pressure	Noninvasive: connections for cuff and hoses should be plastic
	Invasive: use fiberoptic system and transducers with nonferrous components

that the code team follow the rules about removing any loose magnetic items before entering the MRI suite to avoid the release of a potentially lethal projectile.

PREVENTION

To prevent complications with MRI, one must be aware of the contraindications (see Table 233-2). Good communication between the radiology and anesthesiology departments is essential to ensure that the correct anesthesia and monitoring equipment is available from the outset and that at-risk patients undergo prescan anesthesia evaluations. The anesthesia staff involved with providing care in the MRI suite should be aware of all the potential technical problems that may arise in this unique environment.

Further Reading

Dempsey MF, Condon B: Thermal injuries associated with MRI. Clin Radiol 56:457-465, 2001.

De Wilde JP, Rivers AW, Price DL: A review of the current use of magnetic resonance imaging in pregnancy and safety implications for the fetus. Prog Biophys Mol Biol 87:335-353, 2005.

Frankville DD, Spear RM, Dyck JB: The dose of propofol required to prevent children from moving during magnetic resonance imaging. Anesthesiology 79:953-958, 1993.

Gooden CK, Dilos B: Anesthesia for magnetic resonance imaging. Int Anesthesiol Clin 41:29-37, 2003.

Holshouser BA, Hinshaw DB Jr, Shellock FG: Sedation, anesthesia, and physiologic monitoring during MR imaging. J Magn Reson Imaging 3:553-558, 1993.

Jorgenson NH, Messick JM Jr, Gray J, et al: ASA monitoring standards and magnetic resonance imaging. Anesth Analg 79:1141-1147, 1994.

Kaplan RF: Pediatric sedation for diagnostic and therapeutic procedures outside the operating room. In Cote CJ, Todres DI (eds): A Practice of Anesthesia for Infants and Children, 3rd ed. Philadelphia, WB Saunders, 2001, pp 584-609.

Menon DK, Peden CJ, Hall AS, et al: Magnetic resonance for the anaesthetist. Part I. Physical principles, applications, safety aspects. Anaesthesia 47:240-255, 1992.

Peden CJ, Menon DK, Hall AS, et al: Magnetic resonance for the anaesthetist. Part II. Anaesthesia and monitoring in MR units. Anaesthesia 47:508-516, 1992.

Zimmer C, Janssen MN, Treschan TA, et al: Near miss accident during magnetic resonance imaging by a "flying sevoflurane vaporizer" due to ferromagnetism undetected by hand held magnet. Anesthesiology 100:1329-1330, 2004.

Zorab JSM: A general anaesthesia service for magnetic resonance imaging. Eur J Anaesth 12:387-395, 1995.

Misidentification of a Patient

234

Kenneth Kuchta

Case Synopsis

A 51-year-old man with diabetes and peripheral vascular disease develops gangrene of the right foot, and he agrees to a below-the-knee amputation of the affected leg. Upon admission, he is mistakenly booked for a below-the-knee amputation of the left leg. The error was noted twice before surgery, but attempts to correct it failed, and the wrong leg was amputated.

PROBLEM ANALYSIS

Definition

Throughout a patient's interaction with the health care system, his or her identity must be verified to match any test result and any intended order or intervention for that patient. Patient misidentification is exemplified by the following:

- A patient receives a nonintended medical or surgical intervention.
- A patient receives mismatched or the wrong blood products.
- A patient receives the wrong drug or does not receive an ordered drug.
- A patient is identified with the wrong laboratory or test results (e.g., radiograph, computed tomography scan, magnetic resonance imaging scan).
- Planned surgery is performed on the wrong limb, or a procedure is performed without a patient's informed consent.

The accurate identification of patients is also required for dietary personnel to comply with any special dietary orders. For example, a surgical patient who is supposed to receive nothing by mouth is given breakfast on the morning of surgery. This is undiscovered, and during the induction of anesthesia, the patient aspirates gastric contents and subsequently develops aspiration pneumonitis.

Recognition

Patients, family members, or medical personnel may recognize patient identification errors at any point during the provision of health care. Attempts to discover, define, and quantify all types of patient misidentifications might provide useful statistical or actuarial data that could be used toward quality-improvement efforts; however, this would be a daunting task. Instead, the emphasis is more correctly placed on measures to prevent patient identification errors, including minimizing their occurrence and discovering them when they do happen.

Risk Assessment

Voluntary and mandatory databases fail to provide sufficient data about the frequency with which invasive procedures are performed on the wrong patient or wrong procedures are performed on a given patient. Such errors are likely underreported. The Joint Commission on Accreditation of Healthcare Organizations (JCAHO) collected 17 reports of patient identification errors over 7 years. New York State, where a mandatory reporting system exists, experienced 27 blood transfusion errors over a 45-month period. Wrong-site surgery was reported to JCAHO 114 times in slightly more than 6 years, while New York State had 46 such reports over 2 years. Mismatched blood transfusions have been studied extensively, and it is believed that patient misidentification during blood transfusion is grossly underreported. It is estimated that about half of ABO-incompatible transfusions occur due to patient misidentification. The chance of suffering a fatality due to an ABO-incompatible transfusion is estimated to be nearly the same as that of being infected with human immunodeficiency virus (HIV) from that transfusion. There is only a 36% chance of a random donor and recipient having incompatible blood, and a less than 10% chance of such a transfusion being fatal.

Implications

Many cases of patient misidentification, even when discovered, may cause no more than minor annoyance or embarrassment (e.g., a patient finding the wrong name on the slip he takes to the blood bank for a preoperative type and crossmatch). If an adverse outcome occurs, however, the consequences can be significant. The potential impact on the patient and family is obvious. Despite recent attempts to view patient misidentification as an inevitable part of the complex system of health care provision, both practitioners and their institutions are vulnerable to litigation. One need only look at the popular press to see the implications in terms of large malpractice settlements, loss of licenses or accreditation, and tarnished reputations for both the individuals and their institutions. No matter how complicated health care provision has become, clearly the public expects all procedures, medicines, and blood products to be delivered correctly.

MANAGEMENT

If an error in patient identification occurs, do the following:

- Be forthright regarding the incident.
- Promptly notify all parties and the appropriate risk management or quality assurance committees.
- Clearly document what has occurred in the patient's chart.
- Continue to follow the patient, and document these visits.
- Undertake an immediate investigation to prevent recurrences.

We are morally and ethically obligated to be forthright with patients when identification errors occur, especially when they may be associated with significant adverse outcomes. Increasingly, this is codified in both the law and health care policy,[1] and such admissions are often surprisingly well received by patients. In fact, candidness may actually reduce the likelihood of litigation. A show of empathy and continued interest in the patient's well-being is certainly better than avoiding the situation altogether. Documentation of these post hoc visits not only is good medicine but also confirms the practitioner's ongoing concern if the case goes to litigation. Undoubtedly, practitioners who make identification errors remember them for some time.

All parties involved in the case should be notified of the error immediately. This includes hospital risk management or quality assurance committees and any insurance companies that might be involved. Clearly document what has occurred in the patient's chart. An immediate investigation should ensue to determine how the mistake occurred and what preventive measures must be instituted immediately to avoid recurrences. Increasingly, such investigations focus less on the person who made the mistake and more on discovering the circumstances that led to the commission of the error.

With the foregoing in mind, clearly the individual and the institution are obligated to pursue these investigations to determine what can be done to minimize the risk of future occurrences, which are often committed by a different practitioner.

PREVENTION

Given the complexity of modern health care, the chance of patient misidentification is ever present. Traditionally, when such errors occurred, the usual solution was to counsel the practitioner to be more careful in the future and to educate others to exercise vigilance. Thus, the assumption appeared to be that the offender did not exercise due care and that other health care professionals might make the same mistake. Hospitals then instituted procedures to prevent further patient identification errors. For example, the operating room (OR) nurse must check the patient's identification bracelet against the patient's hospital record and then check the consent form to confirm that it is indeed the same patient who has consented to the planned procedure. However, this approach makes no use of other resources available in the OR. In fact, both the anesthesiologist and the surgeon should check and confirm the same information.

Other industries—notably, commercial aviation—instituted such backup systems long ago. In the case of airlines, all available resources, information, equipment, and personnel are used to ensure safe and efficient flight operations. Such risk reduction practices are also used in manufacturing industries to prevent on-the-job injuries. Now, JCAHO has indicated its intention to follow a similar direction. Its recently implemented Universal Protocol for Preventing Wrong Site, Wrong Procedure, Wrong Person Surgery expands on previous efforts found in the JCAHO National Patient Safety Goals. The new protocol recommends that all relevant documents (e.g., consent form, history and physical examination, relevant laboratory and other test results) be available for review in the OR to ensure consistency. There should also be a note in the chart by the surgical team stating the planned procedure.[2] This must match the patient's expectation and understanding of what is or is not going to be done, including details about which limb or body side (and if the latter, at what level) is to be operated on. Also, it is necessary to confirm whether an implant will be needed. The protocol then requires a "timeout" for final verification before starting the procedure. Active involvement of all members of the various OR teams is emphasized, and the procedure must not start until all concerns have been resolved. JCAHO's new protocol clearly intends to fully involve the most valuable OR resource—personnel—to cross-check one another and catch errors before they can result in an adverse outcome.

JCAHO also established ground rules for ensuring proper identification as patients move through the health care system. These rules require at least two independent patient identifiers (the patient's room number alone is insufficient) when administering blood or medications, taking specimens, or performing procedures or treatments. These same two identifiers must match all relevant documents (e.g., consent forms, laboratory slips and labels, blood product documents and labels). Further, JCAHO mandates that the operative site be marked and prohibits any marking of the nonoperative site. Finally, it discourages the use of an X to mark the operative site, which could be misinterpreted.

JCAHO has mandated these changes as a means of avoiding patient misidentification before it causes an adverse event. Many institutions also encourage patients' active participation in the process. Patient interviews should use the already accepted standard of asking nondirected questions. For example, patients should be asked to state their names and the planned surgical procedure (e.g., "What is going to be done to you?" or "What do you expect to happen while you are here?"), rather than merely confirming these from a chart review. Patient brochures and public service announcements now emphasize both these safety measures. Patients should also be encouraged to ask questions when things appear to be other than expected.

---

[1]Since 2001, JCAHO has required that patients be informed of unanticipated outcomes.

[2]These precautions apply to other invasive procedures as well, including those performed by oncologists (e.g., radiation therapy or implants) and interventional cardiologists and radiologists.

Because human fallibility is a fact of life, technologic aids are being advocated. Bar codes are now being implemented in health care. Compared with keystrokes, bar codes greatly improve accuracy. Keystroke errors are about 1 in 300, whereas bar code errors range anywhere from 1 in 394,000 to 1 in 612,900,000, depending on the bar code and the circumstances. The Food and Drug Administration recently mandated bar coding for all medications as a first step. The hope is that full implementation of bar coding will control medication errors in both hospital and outpatient settings (prescription drugs). Universal drug coding would be expected to replicate the accuracy of bar codes. In this case, all medications would be matched to a wristband bar code for the individual patient. Because the latter cannot be mass-produced, however, there is some risk for keystroke errors during wristband production. In fact, the instigating error in the case synopsis turned out to be a keystroke error in the admissions office that was difficult to correct. Further, the accuracy of bar codes mentioned earlier reflects a laboratory setting; this may not be duplicated in clinical medicine.

A study of problems related to the use of wristbands for patient identification found an error rate of 7.4%, which was reduced to only 3.04% with quality improvement efforts. The errors identified included the following:

- Absent wristbands (71.6%)
- Wristband from another patient (1.1%)
- Erroneous information on wristband (6.8%)
- Missing information on wristband (9.1%)
- Illegible information (7.7%)
- Conflicting information, such as a patient with two wristbands (3.7%)

Any of these errors could also apply to bar code wristbands used for patient identification. Thus, bar codes are merely an adjunct to existing patient identification practices. More emphasis should be directed toward detecting errors related to the wristbands themselves, with or without bar codes.

An emerging technology, radiofrequency identification (RFID), may eventually replace bar codes in many medical settings. These devices consist of small integrated circuits containing patient-identifying information and other data. With an antenna, they can interact with RFID readers. Power is supplied by a field generated by the reader, and the RFID tags themselves have been miniaturized to the size of a piece of glitter. They offer several advantages over current practices, including the ability to store more information, update this information, and use the device without line-of-sight access to the tag (as required for bar codes). However, privacy concerns have been a significant barrier to their introduction to the marketplace, and these must also be addressed for medical use. Moreover, similar to the problem with implanted cardiac rhythm management devices (see Chapter 97), the potential adverse interactions with other medical equipment (both inside and outside the patient) have not been fully explored. Even so, cost is likely a bigger limitation. At present, placing an RFID tag on a patient's wristband costs only 25¢, but the cost for using them for every dose of any drug prescribed would be prohibitive.

In the final analysis, bar coding (and possibly RFID in the future) offers a backup tool for medical personnel to confirm a patient's identification. Bar codes provide assistance, but they should never replace health care professionals working as a team to ensure that all patients receive the expected and appropriate care during surgery or other invasive interventions.

Further Reading

Helmreich RL: On error management: Lessons from aviation. BMJ 320: 781-785, 2000.

Linden JV, Wagner K, Voytovich AE, Sheehan J: Transfusion errors in New York State: An analysis of 10 years' experience. Transfusion 40: 1207-1213, 2000.

Wachter RM, Shojania K: Internal Bleeding: The Truth behind America's Terrifying Epidemic of Medical Mistakes. New York, RuggedLand, 2004.

Wald H, Shojania KG.: Prevention of misidentifications. In Shojania KG, Duncan BW, McDonald KM, Wachter RM (eds): Making Health Care Safer: A Critical Analysis of Patient Safety Practices. Evidence Report/Technology Assessment No. 43. AHRQ Publication No. 01-E058. Rockville, Md., Agency for Healthcare Research and Quality, July 2001. Available at http://www.ahrq.gov/clinic/ptsafety/

SPECIAL TOPICS

Syringe Swaps

Carsten Nadjat-Haiem

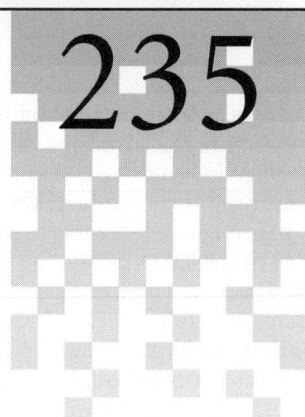

235

Case Synopsis

A healthy 32-year-old woman is scheduled for elective myomectomy. General endotracheal anesthesia is induced successfully, and the surgeon requests a dose of prophylactic cefazolin. The anesthesiologist picks up a 10-mL syringe and administers 2 mL of its contents. When disconnecting the syringe from the three-way stopcock, he realizes that the syringe is labeled phenylephrine (Fig. 235-1). He administers incremental nitroglycerin to reduce anticipated hypertension from the drug error. The patient suffers no ill consequences.

PROBLEM ANALYSIS

Definition

A syringe swap is the accidental administration of an incorrect drug or dosage to a patient. This occurs when a syringe is mislabeled or when it is correctly labeled but mistaken for a different medication. Syringe swaps account for more than 6% of all drug administration errors.

Recognition

A syringe swap is usually recognized when unexpected results are obtained after the administration of a drug or an event occurs without a readily apparent explanation; the swap may also be recognized before any effect is observed. The most common error is administering another dose of muscle relaxant when reversal is desired, resulting in the continued paralysis of the patient.

Risk Assessment

Any patient under anesthesia care is at risk for syringe swap. Less healthy patients are more likely to be adversely affected by this error, although American Society of Anesthesiologists class I and II patients are more likely to be involved in a syringe swap. Usual causes include the following:

- Lack of vigilance when drawing up medications
- Lack of vigilance in administering drugs
- Failure to label syringes correctly
- Failure to use labels
- Similar appearance of drug vials
- Poor drug tray organization
- Haphazard organization of syringes
- Fatigue

Syringe swap is a common event. Eighty-five percent of respondents in one study reported at least one drug administration error in their careers, and a significant number had actually harmed patients due to the administration of an incorrect drug.

Implications

Consequences of a syringe swap can be benign or life threatening. There may be no apparent complications, or there may be serious morbidity and even death.

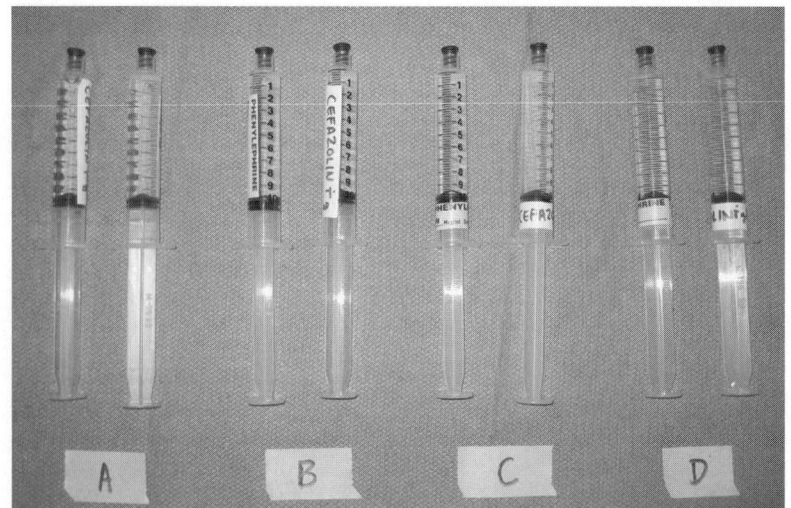

Figure 235–1 ■ Syringe labeling. If labels are placed longitudinally, they might be partially or fully hidden (A) or not visible with other syringe orientations (B). Circumferentially placed labels (C, D) eliminate the risk of hidden labels. The fact that the labels were hidden and the syringes containing phenylephrine and cefazolin were the same size and located next to each other on the anesthesia work station may explain the error illustrated by the case synopsis.

MANAGEMENT

Management of a syringe swap includes the following measures:

- Recognize the mistake.
- Treat the consequences.
- Investigate the incident.
- Institute measures to prevent recurrences.

If an incorrect drug has been administered, management initially consists of recognizing the mistake and treating any acute consequences. If the mistake is discovered quickly, as in the case synopsis, the practitioner should treat the consequences expectantly. If the mistake is not immediately apparent and an adverse event occurs, an immediate investigation should begin in the operating room. The room should be sealed off and any subsequent cases delayed or moved to a different room to prevent a recurrence. The investigation should be systematic and thorough, including all drugs used during the case. All drug containers and syringes used during the case should be inspected.[1] Analyses of syringe contents may also be necessary. Preventive measures should be instituted immediately by the anesthesia department to ensure that the mistake is not repeated.

If a complication results from the mistake, the patient and all parties immediately involved in the patient's care should be notified. Any adverse consequences of the syringe swap should be clearly documented in the chart. The hospital risk management or quality assurance committee should be notified, as well as any other parties that may become involved (e.g., pharmacy, insurance carriers). If a syringe swap is the result of the similar labeling of medications, any drug companies involved and the Food and Drug Administration should be notified of the problem. The anesthesia department or responsible pharmacy should also instigate precautionary measures to differentiate drug vials (Fig. 235-2).

From a medicolegal perspective, a syringe swap is a violation of the standard of care and a clear example of negligence. Advice from risk management should be sought at an early stage.

PREVENTION

The best way to prevent a syringe swap is vigilance by the anesthesiologist when drawing up and administering medications. Adhere to a strict routine for drawing up medications, and check and recheck the labels on all syringes before administering their contents. The following specific measures will help prevent medication errors:

1. Check all drug vial labeling closely before drawing the contents into a syringe. This includes checking the name, expiration date, and concentration of the drug. One recent report described the nearly identical appearance of 0.2% and 0.75% ropivacaine. Also inspect the solution for any abnormal appearance or odor.
2. All syringes should be labeled before medications are drawn. The best system is to have well-organized, preprinted, color-coded labels on the anesthesia cart, with blank labels for seldom-used medications (Fig. 235-3). Syringes should also be labeled circumferentially, so that the contents can be identified regardless of the syringe orientation (see Fig. 235-1).
3. Use of syringes of different sizes is helpful. For example, induction agents are commonly placed in larger (20 or 30 mL) syringes, muscle relaxants in 10-mL syringes, and narcotics and other sedatives in smaller (3 or 5 mL) syringes. Most syringe swaps are between syringes of the same size.

---

[1]Of course, this presumes that any medications used in earlier cases have been returned to the pharmacy or disposed of during room turnover between cases.

Figure 235–2 ■ Drug tray organization. Consistent clustering of drugs into pressors (A), reversal agents (B), induction agents (C), antihypertensives (D), and neuromuscular blockers (E) reduces the risk of syringe swap. Especially important is spatial separation of neuromuscular blockers and reversal agents. Additional labels on vials that appear similar, such as neostigmine (B) and pancuronium (E), can further reduce the risk of drug misidentification. Note also that there is only one prepackaged syringe (epinephrine, between the two trays [arrow]), reducing the risk of syringe swap.

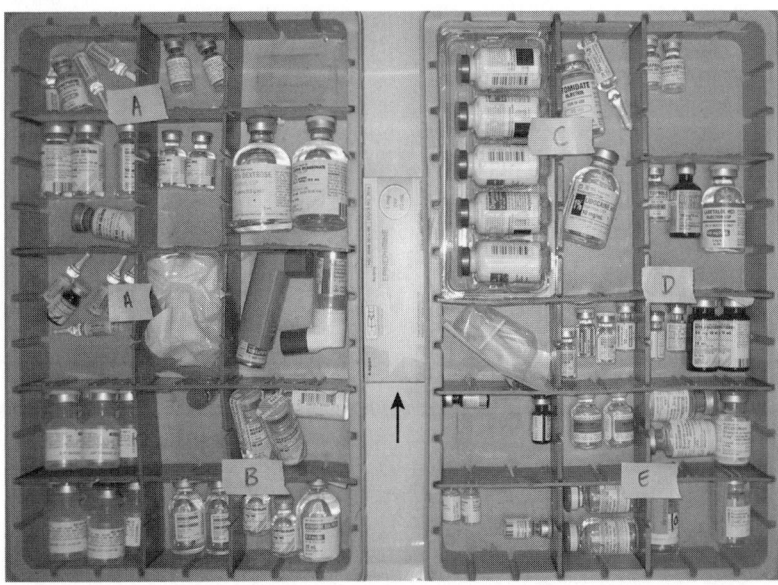

SPECIAL TOPICS

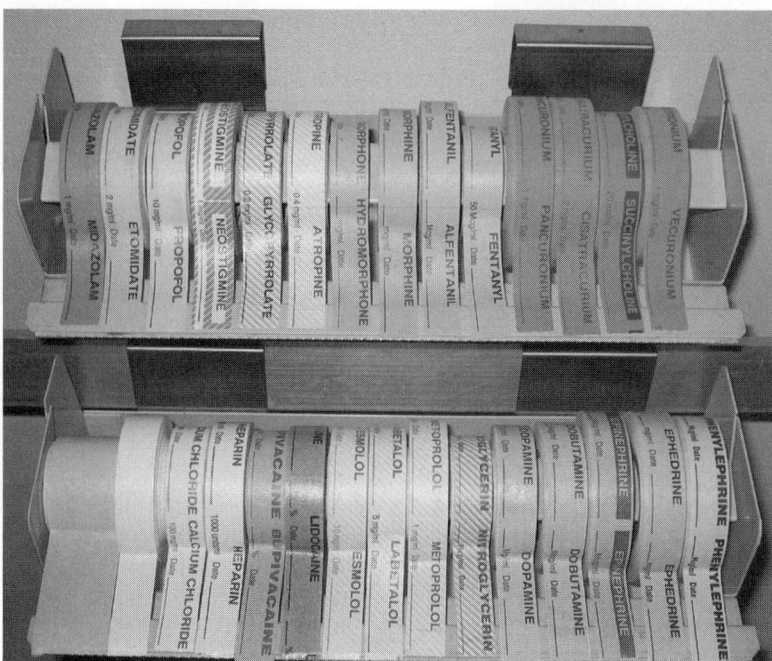

Figure 235–3 ■ Color-coded syringe labels. A well-organized and well-stocked tray of color-coded syringe labels facilitates the quick labeling of syringes.

4. Avoid drugs packaged in premixed syringes that have similar appearances. For example, both lidocaine and epinephrine come packaged in prelabeled glass syringes that look very similar. Their labels can be particularly hard to read. If drugs with this type of packaging are used, place an additional label on the plastic part of the syringe that can be easily recognized, or restrict the use of prepackaged medications to one per anesthesia cart (see Fig. 235-2).

5. Avoid drug containers that have similar appearances. If drugs with similar packaging are placed on the cart, bright warning labels should be put on the vials (see Fig. 235-2). Also, high-strength medications should be identified as such by additional labels or not routinely placed on the drug tray at all. Medications should be clustered by group on the medication tray (see Fig. 235-2).

6. Never administer any drug (contents) from an unlabeled syringe.

7. Consistency in the way the anesthesia cart is stocked is of utmost importance. Drugs should always be placed in the same location on the cart and be clustered by group actions (e.g., reversal agents, antihypertensives, muscle relaxants; see Fig. 235-2).

8. Resident and non-physician anesthetist education should include techniques to ensure that meticulous attention is paid to the handling of drugs. All personnel should be encouraged to develop strict routines for labeling and organizing syringes on the anesthesia cart.

Further Reading

Bastien JL: Ropivacaine packaging: A potential for drug error. Anesthesiology 101:551, 2004.

Fastings S, Gisvold SE: Adverse drug errors in anesthesia, and the impact of coloured syringe labels. Can J Anaesth 47:1006-1007, 2000.

Irita K, Tsuzaki K, Sawa T, et al: Critical incidents due to drug administration error in the operating room: An analysis of 4,291,925 anesthetics over a four year period. Masui 53:577-584, 2004.

Liang BA, Bramhall J, Cullen B: Which syringe did I use? Anesthesiologist confusion and potential liability for a medical error. J Clin Anesth 14:371-374, 2002.

Orser BA, Chen RJ, Yee DA: Medication errors in anesthetic practice: A survey of 687 practitioners. Can J Anaesth 48:139-146, 2001.

Warltier DC, Howard SK, Rosekind MR, et al: Fatigue in anesthesia: Implications and strategies for patient and provider safety. Anesthesiology 97:1281-1294, 2002.

Quality Assurance

236

Donald A. Kroll and Victoria Coon

Case Synopsis

A hospital quality management (QM) specialist is investigating an incident report filed by a postanesthesia care unit (PACU) nurse. A patient had respiratory difficulty in the PACU and required reintubation after a second dose of drugs to reverse neuromuscular blockade. The nurse states that this seems to be a frequent problem with the anesthesiologist, Dr. X. The QM specialist notes that Dr. X's documentation is poor, making it difficult to reconstruct the facts.

Twenty-five of Dr. X's charts undergo a focused review. The review shows that 17 of the charts have substandard documentation. The medication practices in three cases are determined to be similar to those in the present case, which led to reintubation for postanesthetic respiratory depression. In two of these cases, plus an additional five cases, Dr. X's response to the PACU's request to assess a patient's status was delayed.

In response to this focused review, the medical staff conducts a formal hearing to determine whether to reduce Dr. X's privileges or terminate him from the medical staff. At the hearing, Dr. X states that he is being targeted for dismissal because he did not cooperate in signing a new managed care contract. He alleges that his practice is no different from that of his associates and that all of the anesthesiologists have a problem responding to the PACU after they have started another case. He further alleges that the cases reviewed were not randomly selected but rather were selected based on foreknowledge of the complications involved. He acknowledges that his charting has been scanty and promises to improve. Additionally, he states that he has retained an attorney and will sue if his privileges are reduced or terminated.

The QM Department stands by its analysis. It is convinced that Dr. X has shown a consistent pattern over time of both poor documentation and risky practices. The latter have already caused complications in several patients, and QM recommends that Dr. X be terminated for cause.

The threat of litigation involves the legal department, which reports directly to the hospital chief executive officer (CEO). He expresses extreme displeasure that the situation has gotten so far out of hand and blames the Anesthesiology Department for failing to have an effective quality assurance (QA) program. The CEO wants to disband the department and hire a professional management firm whose brochure he received in the mail last week.

PROBLEM ANALYSIS

Definition

Quality management in medical practice has been notoriously difficult to define. It should not be surprising, therefore, that quality assurance is equally difficult, especially with continually evolving concepts and changing targets. The implementation of a QA program varies considerably from one institution to another, but most have the following features in common:

- Incident reporting
- Occurrence screening
- Peer review
- Risk management

Incident Reporting. This provides a means of identifying critical or sentinel events. In the past, reporting typically involved only cases in which an injury had occurred. The injury may have resulted in major morbidity, mortality, or some other less adverse outcome, such as the need for additional hospitalization or delayed recovery. Because the reporting mechanism was voluntary and subject to bias, it was potentially problematic. Compliance with the Joint Commission on Accreditation of Healthcare Organizations (JCAHO) guidelines now requires an in-depth, root-cause analysis of those sentinel events that can be reviewed. Some events do not require actual injury but only the potential for injury. The mechanism by which a hospital handles incident reporting has become a key factor in the accreditation process. Failure to comply results in the initiation of an accreditation watch for the institution.

Occurrence Screening. This is a means of tracking how frequently certain events happen. The JCAHO provided some standardization for occurrence screening by suggesting the following key indicators:

- Stroke
- Acute myocardial infarction
- Peripheral neuropathy

- Cardiac arrest
- Mortality within 2 days of surgery

The selection of these indicators was flawed, however, by their relative infrequency and lack of specific correlation to anesthetic management. One or two cases may make a major difference in the rate of adverse occurrences, and there is not necessarily a cause-and-effect relationship between an event and the quality of anesthesia care. Indeed, it is possible to adhere to or even exceed practice standards and still have an occasional adverse outcome. Although it is no longer a JCAHO focus, occurrence screening is a good method for assessing perceived problem areas.

Peer Review.   This is the practice of having one health care provider assess the care rendered by another. The peer reviewer is expected to render an expert medical opinion regarding the cause of injury and its possible attribution to the provider, the health care system, or the patient's primary condition or comorbidities. Given the complexity of anesthesiology practice, peer review is essential to the analysis of sentinel events and occurrence screening. The peer review process, however, suffers from providers' general lack of willingness to participate and their reluctance to call another's care substandard. It is also subject to potential negative bias based on personalities, secondary agendas, and the severity of injury.

Risk Management.   This implies that it is possible to both identify and manage risks inherent in health care delivery. There is wide latitude in defining the nature of the risks and who should manage them. In most hospitals, however, the practice consists of a method of minimizing the consequences of adverse events that have already occurred. Eichorn described the four components of classic risk management:

1. Identification of a problem
2. Assessment and evaluation
3. Resolution of the problem by change
4. Follow-up to ensure elimination of the problem

These components define the process of continual quality improvement. Thus, the general components of a QA or risk management program include a similar, continuing process with the goal of improving patient care and outcomes.

Recognition

As in the case synopsis, the recognition that an institution has a problem with its QA program typically occurs only when the consequences become significant. The fundamental problem with recognizing such problems is the lack of broadly accepted and applicable guidelines. It is extremely difficult to evaluate a process unless incidence and outcomes are known:

- How many provider problems are expected each year?
- How many indicators, and which ones, should be tracked?
- How is it determined that acceptable limits have been transgressed?
- How can the reliability and fairness of peer review be verified?

The complex nature of data collection and validation, process management, peer review, and the establishment of standards has led to the creation of professional QM consulting firms. Such firms offer independent data tracking and benchmarking for both QA and utilization review purposes. However, the ultimate role for such QM consultants has yet to be established.

Risk Assessment

Avoidance of complicated situations is best done proactively. A careful review of the components of the institution's QA process is helpful. Each should be examined to determine its effectiveness and fairness.

PROBLEM IDENTIFICATION

There must be a published policy on when to file an incident report. The reporting mechanism must be applied equally to all events and be independent of the provider's identity. Occurrence screening may either sample some patient records or review them all; sampling underreports occurrences, but 100% review is generally too labor-intensive. Regardless, because the anesthesia record is filled out by the provider, it amounts to voluntary reporting unless there is unbiased data capture (e.g., electronic charting). Screened occurrences should be reviewed periodically. Rare occurrences are not useful for tracking. A reliable method is one proved to identify previously solved problems.

PROBLEM ASSESSMENT

Parameters for interpreting occurrence data and outliers must be formulated prospectively. They should also be compatible with the scope-of-practice definitions by which a provider is evaluated. For example, anesthesia care providers who manage primarily patients having ambulatory gynecologic procedures might reasonably be expected to show a higher incidence of postoperative nausea and vomiting than those who do only cardiovascular anesthesia. The latter, however, are expected to show a higher incidence of perioperative myocardial infarction.

The method of case selection for focused reviews should be known in advance and designed to obtain a representative sample of the provider's care, especially if his or her behavior or clinical competence is at issue. Also, peer review must be impartial and aimed toward definable practice standards. If deficiencies are noted, the exact deviation from these standards should be specified. In all cases, the standard applied should be that of reasonable and prudent care, not necessarily state-of-the-art practice.

PROBLEM RESOLUTION

Ideally, there should be a remedy short of dismissal for all but the most egregious errors and those involving conduct that clearly violates the medical staff bylaws. Depending on the problem, the provider should be given an opportunity to change his or her practices or procedures or to improve behavior and communication skills. In any case, the result should be a clearly defined and measurable expectation of performance.

FOLLOW-UP

The effects of any advised change in practices or procedures should be measured for an appropriate, finite period.

During this time, there should be feedback on the provider's compliance with expectations. Failure to meet the criteria for change should have known consequences, and it should be known that compliance will avoid those consequences.

Implications

The success of a QA program has implications for hospitals, providers, and patients. Failure to have an effective QA program may result in loss of accreditation or repeat site visits. This can have a significant financial impact on the institution. Providers who have been identified as having QA problems face possible loss of medical staff privileges and mandatory reporting to medical licensing agencies. Their ability to continue to practice medicine may be jeopardized. Patients are theoretically the prime beneficiaries of an effective QA program. They should be able to have confidence in the quality of the health care institution and the provider's services.

MANAGEMENT

Compliance with the methods outlined for QA is costly, but the stakes are very high. The institution must follow up on any charges, because it has independent and corporate responsibility to ensure the competency of its providers. Certainly the institution would be liable for any future similar adverse outcomes. Further, the provider is forced to pursue legal action because of the impact on his or her ability to practice. The entire department is at risk of being forced out and replaced. This is a no-win situation for all parties, and resolution can only attempt to minimize losses.

Typically, QA violations are resolved by negotiation, mediated by an internal or external review board to arbitrate such disputes. Often, due process leads to voluntary resignation from the medical staff in exchange for dismissal of charges. The final disposition depends entirely on the strength of the evidence, with allowance for give-and-take. Given that statutory immunity is provided to the peer review process (stemming from society's overriding interest in public protection), the physician has the distinct disadvantage of having to prove that the process was unfair or capricious.

PREVENTION

QM has become a big business, and hospitals are not exempt. Within the hospital community, anesthesiology departments have been disbanded for failure to institute and maintain acceptable QA practices. The steps listed under Risk Assessment offer suggestions for initiating problem prevention within an existing program. In addition, the use of smarter technology may provide some remedies.

One of the central tenets of QM is that the process is driven by data rather than belief. Data management is the first area of emphasis for problem prevention. Credibility of any charted data is an essential component. Automated (electronic) anesthesia charting systems have emerged as a solution to the problem of data capture and validation. However, selecting indicators of quality is commonly hampered by the lack of both a clear focus on what is important to measure and easily measured parameters to describe quality. Consequently, health care professionals tend to repetitively measure the same parameters rather than seeking feedback from patients and staff about other methods of improving and implementing metrics to assess results.

Data gathering is followed by aggregation and reporting. Often, this involves computing each provider's incidence versus the average incidence for all other members of the department. Such analysis requires significant judgment, owing to variable case types and mixes; therefore, it is subject to personal bias. Also, provider-centered analysis shifts the emphasis away from any opportunity to improve the process and tends to alienate the staff. Therefore, shifting to system- or process-oriented analysis has become a second area of emphasis for problem prevention. Finally, recent JCAHO guidelines emphasize that root-cause analysis should focus primarily on systems and processes rather than on individuals.

Further Reading

Dornette WHL: Legal Issues in Anesthesia Practice. Philadelphia, FA Davis, 1991.

Eichorn JA: Risk management in anesthesia. In 47th Annual Refresher Course Lectures and Clinical Update Program. Park Ridge, Ill., American Society of Anesthesiologists, 1996.

Posner KL, Cheney FW, Kroll DA: Professional liability, risk management, and quality improvement. In Barash PG, Cullen BF, Stoelting RK (eds): Clinical Anesthesia, 4th ed. Philadelphia, JB Lippincott, 2001, pp 89-96.

SPECIAL TOPICS

Cost Containment

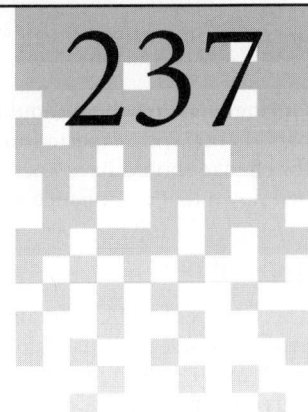

Victoria Coon and Donald A. Kroll

Case Synopsis

A 59-year-old, otherwise healthy man with degenerative osteoarthritis is scheduled for a right total hip replacement. He is evaluated in a preoperative clinic, where the only medically indicated laboratory test is a complete blood count. On the day of surgery, he presents with a urinary tract infection, necessitating cancellation of the surgery. The surgeon is upset that the patient did not get a "routine" preoperative urinalysis, which, he believes, would have prevented the cancellation.

PROBLEM ANALYSIS

Definition

Cost containment has become a driving force in health care management. To control ever-rising costs, managers and providers need to know the principal determinants. Expenditures controlled by anesthesia providers constitute 3% to 5% of the total health care costs in the United States. They can be broken down as follows:

- Preoperative testing ($11.7 billion)
- Provider services ($9 billion)
- Equipment, facilities, and supplies (not quantified to date)

PREOPERATIVE TESTING

Gone are the days when a "shotgun" approach to preoperative laboratory testing was economically feasible. Cost versus benefit is a prime consideration, and the performance of such tests should be data driven and based on a defined medical indicator. In a 1990 study at the Mayo Clinic, Narr and colleagues estimated that the elimination of routine laboratory testing in healthy patients younger than 40 years would decrease annual health care spending by $2.9 billion to $4.2 billion. For older patients, only medically indicated tests should be performed. In the case synopsis, in the absence of symptoms of urinary tract infection, no medical indicator was present for urinalysis at the time of the patient's preoperative visit. Further, the subsequent development of the urinary tract infection would not have been "prevented" by a urinalysis. Diagnosis by clinical history was the determining factor in the decision to cancel the operation on the day of surgery, and if the same clinical history had been elicited during the preoperative evaluation, a similar decision might have been reached.

In an attempt to create a standardized list of medical conditions that warrant further testing, a Delphi study was done at an urban Veterans Affairs (VA) hospital to obtain a consensus among anesthesia providers. Implementation of the results caused a significant decrease in the amount of tests ordered, with no increase in the surgery cancellation rate. However, savings on laboratory testing could not be realized until there was a reduction in laboratory personnel, capital equipment renewal, or reagent use. The documented cost savings from the VA study, an estimated $5 million per year,

occurred when the streamlined preoperative evaluation process allowed a reduction in the length of preoperative admission time and the closure of surgical beds. Published reports purporting to save money by ordering fewer laboratory tests fail to recognize that reagent cost is the smallest expense. Until personnel are reduced or capital equipment costs are avoided, no significant saving can be realized.

PROVIDER COSTS

The provision of health care is essentially a service industry. As such, the majority of cost is incurred in providing personnel. The personnel who provide anesthesiology services may include physicians, nurse anesthetists, residents and other trainees, or anesthesia assistants. There is a growing competition among some specialty surgeons, as well as dentists and oral surgeons, to deliver anesthesia care.

Currently, in the majority of cases in the United States, anesthetics are delivered by an anesthesia care team (ACT) consisting of anesthesiologists and certified registered nurse anesthetists (CRNAs). The ACT concept affords the lowest incidence of anesthesia-related deaths and, when evaluating the indirect costs of adverse outcomes, is quite efficient. Attempts to determine optimal staffing ratios to minimize costs while preserving quality are hampered by lack of data, practice variations, and political posturing. Nonetheless, non-ACT personnel (e.g., health care economists) who are not necessarily fully informed may attempt to determine optimal staffing ratios to minimize costs.

Several studies attempting to quantify costs have concluded that there are few direct cost savings when anesthesia is provided by one anesthesiologist supervising two CRNAs rather than by two anesthesiologists. In the Los Angeles area, as CRNA costs have risen and anesthesiologist costs have declined, it is actually less expensive to use two anesthesiologists rather than one anesthesiologist and two CRNAs. Because of vigilance issues and the need to provide breaks for the anesthesia provider, the safety of having a second provider involved might still make a 1:2 anesthesiologist-to-CRNA ratio a viable option. A 1:3 or 1:4 ratio is obviously more cost-effective but may compromise quality and safety, depending on the patient population. Although Klein reported in a Kaiser Permanente study that a 1:4 anesthesiologist-to-CRNA ratio was associated with no unexpected adverse outcomes, the results may not be widely applicable. Fassett and Calmes studied the perceptions of nurse anesthetists working on an ACT and concluded that excessive medical direction may contribute to overall costs of the ACT. These perceptions generated much rebuttal from the anesthesiologist community, however. It can only be concluded that adjustments in staffing ratios should be individualized on the basis of a sound rationale that includes both cost and quality, not merely perceptions.

COST OF EQUIPMENT, SUPPLIES, AND FACILITIES

To date, only 1% to 2% of anesthesia studies include a cost analysis. Although it is not the greatest area of expense controlled by anesthesia providers, the judicious, rational use of drugs and disposable and capital equipment is important. Careful analysis of the cost-to-benefit ratio should be performed. Pharmaceuticals are an easy target for cost control analysis, although they make up a relatively small percentage of overall anesthesia costs. Direct and indirect costs, however, should be included in the cost-benefit analysis. An example might be the direct cost of an expensive antinausea drug being offset by a decrease in the indirect costs of postanesthesia care unit services and the avoidance of an unplanned hospital admissions following ambulatory surgery. The most significant problem with such studies is that no savings can be realized until the number of personnel is reduced.

There are also intangible costs to consider, such as patient satisfaction and quality-of-life issues. These are critical when the value to the patient decreases to the point were he or she goes elsewhere for care.

Recognition

As noted earlier, there is a tendency to assume that reducing the number of laboratory tests performed or shortening recovery time automatically reduces costs. This is not true. Cost savings can be realized only when there is an actual reduction in personnel or expenses. Until then, there are only potential cost savings. Another pitfall is using charges to determine costs.

Risk Assessment

There are three important concepts to consider when attempting to analyze costs: fixed costs, variable costs (direct and indirect), and marginal costs or marginal capacity. All businesses, companies, and physicians have a finite capacity to deliver a product or service. The difference between the maximal capacity and the current capacity is the marginal capacity. The decision to increase capacity above the current margin should be based on an analysis of incremental benefits and costs. A common business example might be the decision to add a second or third shift to a production line rather than paying overtime. This type of decision would take into account the current and future market for the product (will the company be able to sell all the additional units?) and the increased direct and indirect costs of raw materials and labor (variable costs). These would be weighed against the fixed costs of the existing facility. A variable cost is a cost that varies with production; a fixed cost is independent of production.

It should be noted that fixed costs may be hidden within categories that consist primarily of variable costs. A worker's hourly wage is a variable cost, but benefits may be a fixed cost. As a general rule, the higher the ratio of fixed costs to variable costs, the greater the desirability of increasing marginal capacity. The airline industry provides another prime example: it costs about the same to fly a half-full plane as a full plane, which is why supersaver discount airfares are offered. Hospitals have been managed much like the airline industry, in that the majority of their costs are fixed. They must remain open all day, every day, regardless of the inpatient population. The wards must be staffed by nurses, the laundry and food services must operate, and the emergency room and operating rooms must be available. It does not cost the hospital much more to admit one additional patient (low incremental cost) if the capacity to do so is in place. In other words, the biggest cost is for the facility, which is already a "sunk" cost. In hospitals where anesthesia providers are salaried, personnel costs are actually a fixed cost at any given point in time, and they become variable only when the number of staff changes. The only practical way to contain the cost per case in this environment is to either increase the number of cases or reduce the number of staff.

The situation differs for fee-for-service anesthesiologists and depends on the specific features of their practice situations (their "overhead"). Anesthesiologists who purchase their own equipment or pay high malpractice premiums have relatively higher fixed costs than those who do not. Billing costs are usually variable costs. In most situations, it does not cost the anesthesiologist much to take on another case (low marginal cost). The issue is whether he or she has the ability to add capacity.

Implications

The basic assumption of managed care medicine is that the physicians will be willing to work harder (increase capacity, take on more cases) to make the same income. This assumption necessarily follows the observation that the fee is discounted. If an anesthesiologist makes 20% less for a case, he or she has to take on 20% more cases to make the same amount as before, if all else stays the same. The marginal cost for the physician is measured not in terms of actual fixed and variable business costs but rather in the intangible threat that failure to contract will result in loss of business (an adverse or undesired increase in marginal capacity). Stated more simply, the only way to maintain a market share in a price war is to cut prices.

MANAGEMENT AND PREVENTION

In both the health maintenance organization and fee-for-service models, the driving force for cost containment is avoiding loss of income (which has been stated as an adverse increase in marginal capacity). When viewed in this way, it becomes clear that the most effective means of containing costs is to create more marginal capacity by improving time efficiency to the point where another case can be completed in the original amount of time (an actual increase in productivity for the same fixed cost).

Further Reading

Abenstein JP, Warner MA: Anesthesia providers, patient outcomes, and costs. Anesth Analg 82:1273-1283, 1996.

Becker KE: Personnel cost analysis. ASA Newsletter 59:3, 1995.

Becker KE, Carrithers J: Practical methods of cost containment in anesthesia and surgery. J Clin Anesth 6:5, 1994.

Cromwell J, Rosenbach M: The impact of nurse anesthetists on anesthesiologist productivity. Med Care 28:2, 1990.

Fassett S, Calmes SH: Perceptions by an anesthesia care team on the need for medical direction. AANA J 63:2, 1995.

Jenkins CE: The effect of standardized preoperative evaluations on operating room surgical schedules [master's thesis]. Los Angeles, University of California, 1994.

Johnstone RE, Martinec CL: Costs of anesthesia. Anesth Analg 76:840-848, 1993.

Klein JD: When will managed care come to anesthesia? J Health Care Finance 23:3, 1997.

Narr BJ, Hanser TR, Warner MD: Preoperative laboratory screening in healthy Mayo patients: Cost effective elimination of tests and unchanged outcomes. Mayo Clin Proc 66:155-159, 1991.

Stein CS: A patient based approach to medical direction within the anesthesia care team [master's thesis]. Los Angeles, University of California, 1994.

Suver J, Arikian SR, Doyle JJ, et al: Use of anesthesia selection in controlling surgery costs in an HMO hospital. Clin Ther 17:3, 1995.

Warner MA: Cost containment in anesthesia, is it worth the effort? In Annual AMA Refresher Course Lectures, 1996.

White PF, White LD: Cost containment in the operating room: Who is responsible? J Clin Anesth 6:351-356, 1994.

Wiklind RA, Barash PG: Anesthesiology. JAMA 271:21, 1994.

Alleged Malpractice

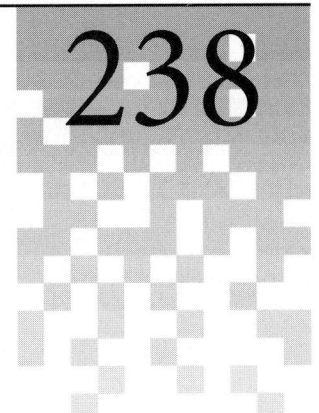

Robert D. Kaye and Christopher M. B. Heard

Case Synopsis

A 23-year-old woman undergoes emergency cesarean section under general anesthesia for fetal bradycardia and placental abruption. She is hypotensive (blood pressure 70/30 mm Hg) and tachycardic (heart rate 150 beats per minute) as the procedure begins. After delivery, the baby has poor Apgar scores, with evidence of fetal acidosis (cord pH, 7.01). Postoperatively, the patient complains of awareness during surgery. The baby develops cerebral palsy, seizures, and developmental delay. Two years later, a malpractice action is brought that accuses the anesthesiologist of negligence.

SPECIAL TOPICS

PROBLEM ANALYSIS

Definition

A lawsuit is a civil case seeking monetary damages based on a claim of professional negligence. The plaintiff must show that there was failure to apply an accepted standard of care for the defendant's specialty area in the particular case. A poor outcome in itself is not evidence of negligence. The manner in which an anesthesiologist acts is often just as important as the evidence in deciding the case.

Recognition

There are several ways that the practitioner may become aware of a malpractice complaint. A complaint to a nurse by a relative of the patient may be the first clue. This information may pass to the anesthesiologist involved while the patient is still hospitalized. Another possibility is that a patient lodges a formal complaint with the hospital administration concerning the practice of a particular anesthesiologist at that hospital. Formally, a lawsuit begins when an anesthesiologist is served a complaint and summons. The complaint declares how the plaintiff was injured by substandard care and the particulars on which the claim is based. The malpractice carrier should be notified immediately and sent a copy of all documents received.

Risk Assessment

The incidence of anesthesia malpractice has decreased over the past 20 years. Increased use of pulse oximetry and capnography may be partially responsible for the lower incidence of poor outcomes. Table 238-1 lists several causes of alleged malpractice. Certain areas of anesthesia practice are associated with a higher risk, such as obstetrics, trauma, and pediatrics. Outcomes such as death or severe neurologic damage are often associated with failure to maintain adequate oxygenation or circulation.

The majority of obstetric claims involve cesarean delivery, with maternal death (21%) and newborn brain damage (17%) being the most common complaints. Reviewers in the American Society of Anesthesiologists (ASA) Closed Claims Project found improper anesthetic care to be a contributing factor in less than half of newborn brain damage suits. Half of all obstetric anesthesia claims are filed for minor injuries (e.g., headache, backache, pain during surgery, emotional distress). In approximately 40% of all lawsuits in the ASA Closed Claims Project, payment was made to the plaintiff despite the reviewers' findings of appropriate anesthesia care.

Implications

There is a sequence of events that ensues following alleged malpractice (Table 238-2). Once a formal complaint has been lodged, it must be answered. The professional liability carrier assigns an attorney to defend the anesthesiologist and prepare the answer. The anesthesiologist has the option to request a specific attorney, as long as he or she is on a list of attorneys approved by the malpractice carrier. The anesthesiologist may also retain a personal attorney at his or her own expense. Usually this is not necessary unless the case will lead to licensure problems or grave economic hardships. Each allegation of the complaint may be admitted, denied, or denied in part.

During the early planning stages, it is imperative that the anesthesiologist be completely candid with the attorney and share all information, both positive and negative. Malpractice attorneys have a surprising amount of medical knowledge. The anesthesiologist must educate the attorney

Table 238–1 ■ Causes of Alleged Malpractice

Failure to supply adequate oxygenation
    Intubation error
    Oxygen supply failure
    Obstructed airway
Failure to maintain adequate circulation
    Hypotension
    Arrhythmias
    Cardiac arrest
Aspiration
Awareness
Neurologic injury
    Peripheral nerve injury
    Spinal cord damage
    Extradural foreign body
Dental injury
Corneal injury

Table 238–2 ■ Stages in a Malpractice Lawsuit
Complaint and summons
Answer
Discovery
Motions
Pretrial conference
Jury trial

Table 238–4 ■ The Course of a Trial
Jury selection
Opening statements
Plaintiff's proofs
Defendant's proofs
Closing arguments
Jury instruction by presiding judge
Jury deliberation
Verdict

on the salient medical features of the case and help the attorney prepare the defense by being candid about other therapeutic options.

Confidentiality is an important consideration. Any information provided by the client to the attorney or by the attorney to the client is privileged and need not be divulged. Likewise, information shared between the insurance company's investigator and the anesthesiologist is privileged. Discussions the anesthesiologist has with a colleague concerning the substance of a case are not privileged and are fully discoverable (the discovery process is discussed under Management). Any document concerning the litigation that an anesthesiologist includes in the patient's medical report is discoverable. Documents involved in a malpractice case need to be kept in a separate file in a secure location.

MANAGEMENT

The discovery process is the exchange of information among all the participants in a lawsuit. Table 238-3 lists the main methods of discovery.

The deposition is the most familiar method of discovery. Under oath, the defendant is asked questions that he or she must answer, similar to the format used in court. A professional attitude, appearance, and demeanor are important during a deposition. What the anesthesiologist says at a deposition carries as much weight as what he or she says in court. The plaintiff's attorney will be appraising the anesthesiologist to judge what kind of witness he or she would be before a jury. The anesthesiologist's attorney will meet with him or her before the deposition to go over what to expect, including what questions to anticipate, how to answer specific queries, and how to behave. Questions should be answered directly and factually. Do not volunteer any information. Do not show anger or use slang or humor.

Motions are requests to the court for an order requiring a participant in a lawsuit to carry out a certain action.

Motions do not usually require the physician's presence in court. The attorney will advise the client of any motions that require him or her to act.

Before the trial, all attorneys involved in the case meet at a hearing held by the court. The anesthesiologist does not attend this conference. At the pretrial conference, matters such as deadlines for pretrial discovery, disclosure times for expert witnesses, and a trial date may be discussed. Some states have a mandatory pretrial mediation to attempt to settle the case before jury trial.

The testimony during a trial is similar to that of a deposition, with certain differences. There is a presiding judge to settle questions of law. There is a lay jury that is not as medically knowledgeable as the attorneys who conducted the depositions. The course of a trial is briefly outlined in Table 238-4.

Insurance policy considerations are important. Many physicians worry that a malpractice award will be higher than the limits of their policy. The typical anesthesia malpractice policy has a per occurrence limit of $1 million. Only 4% of the payments in the ASA Closed Claims Project exceeded this amount. The percentage of malpractice awards greater than $1 million has not increased since the beginning of data collection by the ASA. Malpractice policies do not reimburse physicians for time away from practice or the loss of income associated with a lawsuit. All policies have a clause that specifically excludes defense for intentional acts of wrongdoing. Many policies have a clause requiring reasonable cooperation by the physician with the assigned attorney and the insurer's claims investigator. A practitioner who refuses to comply with discovery requests, attend preliminaries conferences, or give a deposition will not be defended.

PREVENTION

The prevention of malpractice is based on maintaining a specialist standard of care at all times. Table 238-5 lists

Table 238–3 ■ The Discovery Process	
Method	**Description**
Interrogatories	Written requests consisting of a long list of questions that the defendant is expected to reply to
Requests to produce medical information	Requests for copies of pertinent medical records; most hospitals secure medical charts involved in malpractice actions in a separate area
Requests to produce documents	These can involve any document the plaintiff or defendant believes is important to the case (e.g., a plaintiff might request a copy of a board certification certificate)
Deposition of witnesses	Testimony taken under oath in a format similar to that used in court

Table 238–5 ■ Important Considerations to Maintain Standard of Care

Preoperative patient interview
Explanation of risks and alternatives
Adherence to ASA monitoring recommendations
Correct labeling of medications
Accurate, legible anesthesia record keeping
Familiarity with anesthesia equipment
Appropriate request for assistance
Familiarity with procedure being performed
Care with positioning of anesthetized patients
Postoperative follow-up visit

ASA, American Society of Anesthesiologists.

several standards that should be applied in all cases. Visiting the patient preoperatively and postoperatively is important to ensure adequate communication and to address patient concerns. A continual quality improvement program is also a usual adjunct.

Further Reading

Caplan RA: Anesthetic liability: What it is and what it isn't. Anesth Analg 74(Suppl):19-24, 1992.

Chadwick HS, Posner K, Caplan RA, et al: A comparison of obstetric and nonobstetric anesthesia malpractice claims. Anesthesiology 74:242-249, 1991.

Cheney FW, Posner K, Caplan RA, et al: Standard of care and anesthesia liability. JAMA 261:1599-1603, 1989.

Kroll DA: What to do if you are sued: Medicolegal update. ASA Refresher Course Lect 165:1-6, 1995.

Lear E (ed): Examining the scope of professional liability. ASA Newsletter 60:6-28, 1996.

Strunin L (ed): Post graduate education issue: Symposium on mishap or negligence. Br J Anaesth 73:1-117, 1994.

SPECIAL TOPICS

The Hostile-Combative Patient

239

Doron Feldman, James M. T. Foster, and Christopher M. B. Heard

Case Synopsis

A 17-year-old boy with mental retardation is scheduled for elective surgery for tendon release. He has had multiple previous surgeries and suffers from a seizure disorder. He is in the preoperative holding area in an agitated state, refusing to go to the operating room. His parents are present and are very distressed.

PROBLEM ANALYSIS

Definition

A hostile-combative patient is one who is uncooperative with the medical and nursing staff. This may be intentional or result from impaired neurologic function. It may occur at any time during the perioperative period. Preoperatively, the patient may refuse to be interviewed or examined or to allow required preoperative investigations. It may be difficult to persuade the patient to enter the operating room, to be positioned in an appropriate manner for induction of anesthesia, and to cooperate in a safe manner during the induction process. If the patient is awake or semiconscious during the procedure (e.g., regional or intravenous sedation techniques), he or she may become agitated during the procedure. Postoperatively, the patient may be uncooperative in the postanesthesia care unit (PACU).

Recognition

Often these problems can be anticipated by the patient's history (previous similar encounters) or the planned procedure (e.g., a magnetic resonance imaging scan during which patient's entire body or upper torso will be inside the scanner). If there is suspicion that belligerent behavior might be an issue, possibly during the patient's transfer to the preoperative holding area, the anesthetist should be informed as soon as possible. This often allows for proper planning and a smooth encounter, making it more pleasant for the patient, the family, and staff and other patients in the holding area. In some cases, it may be necessary to call for the hospital security staff if the patient's behavior is extremely dangerous or disruptive. In the case of prior criminal behavior, a police officer may be escorting the patient.

It is wise, whenever possible, to review a patient's chart for information about his or her previous perioperative behavior. If the patient was uncooperative in the past, how was the issue dealt with? Table 239-1 lists several potential problems that may be encountered when dealing with uncooperative patients.

Risk Assessment

There are many reasons for a patient's uncooperative behavior (Table 239-2). In some cases, behavior problems can be anticipated based on the patient's medical history, medications the patient has received, or the procedure he or she is undergoing. In emergency situations, these problems are more difficult to anticipate.

Implications

A patient's lack of cooperation has implications for perioperative anesthetic management. The transfer of an uncooperative patient may be fraught with problems. It may be

---

Table 239–1 ▪ Potential Problems with Hostile-Combative Patients

Refusal to submit to preoperative investigations
Refusal to go to the operating room
Refusal of monitoring
Refusal of intravenous line placement
Verbal attack
Physical attack

Table 239–2 ▪ Causes of Uncooperative Behavior

Mental retardation
Anxiety
Fear of needles or anesthesia
Drugs: sedatives, recreational
Drug withdrawal
Alcohol
Alcohol withdrawal
Recurrent procedures
Young age
Hypoxia
Psychotic disorders
Pain
Electrolyte abnormalities (e.g., hyponatremia after transurethral prostate resection)
Postoperative emergence phenomena (e.g., ketamine)
Increased intracranial pressure
Sociopathic behavior disorder

Table 239–3 ■ Implications for Perioperative Anesthetic Management

Safety of patient
Safety of staff and other patients
Inability to proceed with anesthesia and operation
Increased risk of laryngospasm (in children)
Urgency of procedure
Legal considerations
   Age of consent
   Patient's ability to give informed consent
   Parents' wishes (for children)

difficult to maintain an adequate degree of monitoring if the patient repeatedly removes the pulse oximetry probe, or to supply supplemental oxygen via facemask or nasal prongs if these are removed. An uncooperative patient is also at risk of injury if he or she falls. Table 239-3 lists other implications for perioperative anesthetic management.

It may be impossible to use the most appropriate form of anesthesia because of the patient's behavior. Intubation of a presumed difficult airway in an uncooperative patient can be challenging. Also, although regional anesthesia may be an attractive option (e.g., in a patient at high risk for aspiration), it may not be practical in an uncooperative patient. Finally, the safety of anesthesia care providers, surgeons, operating room personnel, and PACU and patient transport staff is of the utmost importance. Patients who were cooperative preoperatively may become disoriented and violent during transport or in the PACU.

MANAGEMENT

A patient who is uncooperative, hostile, or otherwise indicates that he or she does not agree to receive the planned medical care presents physicians with a medicolegal dilemma. Some patients present the anesthetist with a list of self-mandated conditions, the granting of which may compromise the patient's well-being and could lead to a conflict that causes the patient to become uncooperative. Examples include a patient who refuses blood administration on religious grounds (e.g., a Jehovah's Witness), a patient who tries to dictate the type of anesthetic induction (intravenous or mask), or a patient who insists on general anesthesia when the anesthesiologist believes that a regional technique would be safer (e.g., cesarean section).

It is extremely important to be sure that it is legal to treat a patient. Small children are often uncooperative, and unless the situation is life threatening, consent must be obtained from the child's legal guardian (parent, foster parent, or institutional or governmental agency). A patient who is not a minor and is not a custodian of the state must give consent for any procedure to be performed. Otherwise, treating such a patient may constitute a battery. If the patient has been declared incompetent by the state, legal permission to proceed with care should be granted by a court. Such permission is often obtained by the hospital administration.

In the case of an emergency procedure, the patient's wishes should be followed. For example, a patient who is in need of an emergency cesarean section but refuses a regional anesthetic must still have the procedure performed. If, after reasonable efforts to persuade the patient otherwise, she still insists on general anesthesia, it must be provided. The same holds true for an adult patient who refuses a blood transfusion. Legally, minors can receive blood and blood products if the physician deems such treatment to be lifesaving. In elective circumstances, when a patient makes a request that the anesthesiologist in good conscience cannot grant, the case should be postponed until the procedure can be carried out according to the patient's wishes or the patient agrees to an acceptable alternative.

The initial approach to uncooperative or combative patients is to try to change their behavior through conversation, education, and persuasion. Success is variable and depends on the anesthesiologist's interpersonal skills, the patient's support system, and the degree of his or her pathology. With children, it is sometimes possible to alter their behavior with toys, play-acting, and the like. Often, it is helpful to seek the aid of the parent or guardian and the surgeon in this endeavor. The next step is to decide whether there is a need for premedication. Pharmacologic intervention is often used for both cooperative and uncooperative patients, and preoperative sedation can be administered orally, intramuscularly, intranasally, intravenously, or rectally (Table 239-4). If the patient is agreeable to receiving premedication, the oral route is usually preferred. Otherwise, an intravenous or, more commonly, an intramuscular approach is used.

Gentle restraint, often after premedication, may control patients who are physically small. Although physical restraint is usually an option of last resort, it is sometimes necessary for patient and staff safety.

PREVENTION

A preoperative interview is probably the most effective method of preempting the problem of an uncooperative patient.

Table 239–4 ■ Options for Dealing with an Uncooperative Patient

Cancel case, but only after good-faith efforts to resolve the situation
Reschedule the procedure after appropriate action
Provide explanation and reassurance
Use a regional technique if the patient is afraid of general anesthesia
Use EMLA (eutectic mixture of lidocaine and prilocaine), nitrous oxide, or high-flow volatile inhalation anesthetic induction (e.g., sevoflurane) in cases of "needle phobia"
Give preoperative sedation
  Midazolam syrup (0.25 to 0.35 mg/kg, up to 20 mg maximum)
  Midazolam IM (0.1 to 0.15 mg/kg, up to 7.5 mg maximum)
  Midazolam IV (titration in increments of 1.0 to 1.5 mg, to effect)
  Midazolam intranasally (0.2 mg/kg up to 20 mg maximum; but not routinely advised because it produces stinging or burning sensation)
  Fentanyl (oral or transmucosal administration of 5 to 15 µg/kg, up to 400 µg maximum)
  Ketamine IM (1 mg/kg) or PO (3 mg/kg)
  Rectal methohexitone-methohexital (20 to 30 mg/kg)

It allows the patient's fears to be addressed and a plan of action to be proposed, enabling the case to continue. If the patient cannot reason, owing to age or mental impairment, the parents or guardians must be involved. Although this is often helpful, there are times when family members only add to the problem—for example, if they too suffer from phobias or are uneducated about the proposed anesthetic plan. The use of premedication before the patient is brought to the operating area, while he or she is still in a quiet room, may be useful. Always make sure that premedicated patients are appropriately monitored to prevent dangerous side effects (e.g., respiratory depression, falls). Also avoid the temptation to premedicate the patient before transport to the operating room or at home, unless accompanied by appropriate personnel. Another possibly helpful but controversial technique (studies have been inconclusive) is to have one of the child's parents present at induction of anesthesia.

Most problems related to interactions with hostile or combative patients can be solved with common sense, reason, and kindness. In our experience, cancellation of a case due to inappropriate patient behavior is extremely rare. Full disclosure and communication can ameliorate a stressful experience, as well as reduce the risk of litigation.

Further Reading

Bragg CL, Miller BR: Oral ketamine facilitates induction in a combative mentally retarded patient. J Clin Anesth 2:121-122, 1990.

Coté CJ: Pediatric anesthesia. In Miller RD (ed): Miller's Anesthesia, 6th ed. Philadelphia, Churchill Livingstone, 2005, pp 2367-2407.

Fukuta O, Braham RL, Yanase H, et al: The sedative effects of intranasal midazolam administration in the dental treatment of patients with mental disabilities. Part 1. The effect of a 0.2 mg/kg dose. J Clin Pediatr Dent 17:231-237, 1993.

Fukuta O, Braham RL, Yanase H, Kurosu K: The sedative effects of intranasal midazolam administration in the dental treatment of patients with mental disabilities. Part 2. Optimal concentration of intranasal midazolam. J Clin Pediatr Dent 18:259-265, 1994.

Moyers JR, Vincent CM: Preoperative medication. In Barash PG, Cullen BF, Stoelting RK (eds): Clinical Anesthesia, 4th ed. Philadelphia, JB Lippincott–Williams & Wilkins, 2001, pp 551-565.

Rosenberg M: Oral ketamine for deep sedation of difficult to manage children who are mentally handicapped: Case report. Pediatr Dent 13:221-223, 1991.

Wu CL: Acute postoperative pain. In Miller RD (ed): Anesthesia, 6th ed. Philadelphia, Churchill Livingstone, 2005, pp 2729-2762.

Awareness under Anesthesia

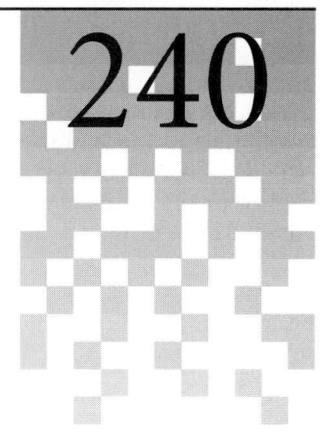

240

Marcia M. Lee

Case Synopsis

"I was put under the anesthetic but suddenly woke. I was wide awake but couldn't move. All I could feel was terrible, terrible pain. I was crying and screaming. But nobody knew" (from Cobcroft and Forsdick).

"I had the strange (but at the time it seemed logical and right) sensation of coming out of myself; of being up by the ceiling looking down on the proceedings. And after the initial realisation that I couldn't communicate at all, came the feeling of acceptance" (from Cobcroft and Forsdick).

PROBLEM ANALYSIS

Definition

Patient awareness under anesthesia (AUA) can take many forms. A working definition is the spontaneous recall of events occurring under general anesthesia. AUA includes both explicit and implicit memory. Explicit memory is information consciously recollected by the patient, and implicit memory is information that is not associated with any conscious recollection. Recall of implicit memories may occur during dreaming or while under hypnosis or with the use of other psychological methods.

Recognition

Traditional methods for monitoring levels of AUA were based on indirect hemodynamic measurements, such as heart rate and blood pressure. These are now widely accepted as merely crude and nonspecific measures of the brain's hypnotic state; however, in many cases (especially in the less developed world), they are still the only methods available to monitor AUA. Of note, with the increasing number of procedures being performed under conscious or procedural sedation, it is critical that the diagnosis of AUA be carefully and distinctly made. Patients commonly perceive that they were "asleep" when general anesthesia was not actually administered. This can lead to confusion and, perhaps, a misdiagnosis of AUA, especially if a clear explanation of the type of anesthesia is not provided. The majority of studies of AUA specifically restrict that term to patient populations undergoing general anesthesia.

Risk Assessment

The incidence of AUA is usually cited as slightly less than 1%. Reviews of patient experiences show that auditory perception and the sensation of paralysis are among the most frequently listed complaints, followed by pain perception. Unfortunately, the cause of AUA is not clearly understood.

Some factors, however, have been implicated as causative events, including the following:

- Machine malfunction, whereby the desired amount of anesthetic is not delivered.
- Deliberate limitation of the amount of anesthetic delivered because of clinical conditions. These conditions include hypovolemia (e.g., in trauma cases) or cesarean section, when attempts are made to minimize depression of the infant.
- The use of cardiopulmonary bypass. Such patients may have an increased risk of AUA or recall.
- Failure to administer anesthetic agents in a timely fashion. For example, during protracted or difficult intubations, plasma concentrations of anesthetic induction drugs may wane, so that supplemental dosing is required. Even in smooth inductions, the effect of shorter-acting agents may decline before that of maintenance agents is attained.
- Increased use of neuromuscular blockers during maintenance of anesthesia, as well as their use to facilitate tracheal intubation. Their anticipated use may contribute directly to patients' anxiety. Among the patients experiencing AUA in the study by Moerman and colleagues, 85% reported the sensation of weakness and paralysis as the overriding reason for their anxiety and panic. Their inability to alert anyone of their awareness was as disturbing as the actual AUA.
- Inadvertent administration of muscle relaxants due to syringe swaps (see Chapter 235). One Australian review noted that 6 of 16 cases of AUA were due to the unintentional use of suxamethonium instead of fentanyl.
- Expanded use of shorter-acting anesthetic induction and maintenance agents, especially as the number of same-day surgeries increases. For these surgeries, the goals of home readiness and early discharge encourage the use of short-acting anesthetics.

Implications

Awareness under anesthesia is commonly feared by both anesthesiologists and patients. For the latter, possible adverse psychological sequelae include anxiety, sleep disorders, depression, nightmares, panic attacks, and long-term psychiatric disorders. Much of the psychological trauma following AUA appears to be related to the patient's feeling of a lack of control or that something has gone terribly wrong, along with the inability to communicate such feelings.

MANAGEMENT

What should the anesthesiologist do if he or she believes that AUA or recall has occurred? First, there must be honest, sincere, and full disclosure of what happened. The possible reasons for AUA should be explained to the patient at the earliest possible time postoperatively. Second, sympathy and empathy must be conveyed. Third, the patient should be reassured that repetition of AUA during a future anesthetic is not an inevitable or even a likely occurrence. Fourth, it is essential to maintain contact with the patient though follow-up. Fifth, if necessary, referral for psychological counseling or psychiatric care should be given. Last, the institution's risk management or quality assurance department must be notified.

PREVENTION

Because there is no single coherent explanation for the development of AUA, it is impossible to provide a comprehensive plan to prevent such occurrences. However, there are some measures (see also Ghoneim and Block) that may help reduce the risk of a patient's developing AUA:

- Ensure that all devices used to deliver anesthetics are checked thoroughly and frequently (at least daily), including the anesthesia machine and vaporizers, as well as any infusion pumps.
- Monitor end-tidal inhalational anesthetic concentrations.
- Administer inhalational anesthetics at an end-tidal concentration of 0.6 minimal alveolar concentration (MAC). Work by Dwyer and colleagues showed that conscious recall can be prevented with 0.6 MAC end-tidal isoflurane. However, this MAC value may not apply to other inhalational anesthetics and might be lower (diethyl ether) or higher (desflurane, sevoflurane). Among the inhalational anesthetics used today, isoflurane appears to be more effective for preventing awareness or recall than equivalent MAC levels of nitrous oxide, desflurane, and sevoflurane.
- Use agents with amnestic properties, especially when AUA is likely (e.g., trauma surgery, hypovolemia, emergent cesarean section, open-heart surgery).
- Benzodiazepines or scopolamine can be used as either premedications or supplements to the anesthetic. However, one must not rely solely on these agents, because their effectiveness for preventing AUA is dose dependent and often patient specific.
- Minimize muscle relaxant use, and avoid complete paralysis whenever possible. Patient movements, although an extremely crude measure, may indicate AUA.
- Encourage all operating room personnel to refrain from making disparaging remarks about a patient's condition or body habitus. There is evidence that cognitive processing

of derogatory or distressing auditory information occurs, even during presumably "adequate" anesthesia.

Direct monitoring of brain wave activity has been proposed as a method of preventing AUA. Use of electroencephalograms (EEGs) has been proposed to prevent AUA, especially during spinal surgery. However, an EEG does not reliably predict the depth of inhalation anesthesia. In fact, there are reports showing that EEG signals do not correlate with or predict anesthetic depth (e.g., adrenergic cardiorespiratory responses to surgical stimulation, appropriate responses to verbal commands). Also, the EEG is a technically complex study and requires a knowledgeable EEG interpreter.

Today, EEG indices derived from raw EEG signals recorded by disposable electrodes on the patient's forehead are used to monitor the effects of anesthetic drugs on the brain. Commercial systems include the bispectral index monitor (BIS, Aspect Medical Systems, Natick, Mass) and the patient state analyzer (PSA, Physiometrix, Inc., North Billerica, Mass). Disposable electrode arrays are marketed for use with these systems, including the XP sensor for BIS monitors and the PSArray[2] for PSA monitors. The former was designed to reduce electrocautery interference, which was problematic with earlier BIS electrodes. The latter was designed to save time and reduce the patient discomfort associated with the application of earlier PSA electrodes.

Both BIS and PSA have a high probability of correctly predicting both loss and recovery of consciousness with general anesthesia. Both indices allow anesthesia providers to manipulate anesthetic levels and thus reduce emergence times. A recent cost analysis by White and associates showed that per patient costs for BIS and PSA are the same. They also reported less surgical electrocautery interference with the PSA system with PSArray[2] sensors compared with BIS and PSArray[2] sensors. The Food and Drug Administration has approved both systems as clinical monitors for anesthetic effects on the brain. The question is, can they be used to prevent AUA?

The use of BIS or PSA to prevent AUA has been suggested. Both use proprietary algorithms to arrive at a "dimensionless"[1] score, ranging from 100 (fully awake) to 0 (absence of any brain activity). Although both BIS and PSA appear to be equally reliable for evaluating the level of consciousness during induction of and emergence from general anesthesia, no adequately powered or controlled prospective trial has shown that either one is a useful monitor for AUA. Indeed, Schneider and Wagner's small observational study found that a BIS value of 50 to 60 (the range suggested for general anesthesia is 40 to 60) before intubation was inadequate to prevent an awareness reaction (squeezing the investigator's hand in response to a command) immediately after endotracheal intubation in patients induced with propofol and alfentanil. Because BIS could not differentiate between patients with and without an awareness reaction, the authors concluded that its value as a monitor for awareness is questionable. No comparable trials for PSA were available in mid-2005.

Further, there is the issue of cost. O'Connor and Daves estimated the cost of using BIS to prevent AUA. It was

---

[1]This term was used by White and colleagues; see Further Reading.

determined that if cases of AUA are rare (e.g., 1 in 20,000), the estimated cost of using BIS solely to reduce AUA is $400,000 per case. If AUA is more common (e.g., 1 in 100), the cost decreases to $2000 per case. Both estimates, however, presume that the monitor is 100% effective in preventing AUA, which is uncertain.

Unfortunately, recent sensational media attention concerning the problem of AUA and the mandate of the Joint Commission on Accreditation of Healthcare Organizations to formulate policies to prevent AUA make a rational assessment of this problem difficult. Because no monitor is universally accepted as having the ability to detect, monitor, and eliminate AUA, measures to prevent it become even more important. In high-risk situations, when the preservation of life precludes deep anesthesia, prudent use of amnestic agents (e.g., ketamine or even scopolamine) might help protect against AUA. However, even these agents cannot guarantee that AUA will not occur.

Finally, because there is no good explanation for the mechanism of its development, it is not possible to identify patients at greater risk for AUA or to prevent all occurrences. Isolated incidents of AUA will likely continue, despite good practice and adherence to accepted monitoring standards.

Further Reading

Cobcroft M, Forsdick C: Awareness under anaesthesia: The patients' point of view. Anaesth Intensive Care 21:837-843, 1993.

Dwyer R, Bennett HL, Eger EI, et al: Isoflurane anesthesia prevents unconscious learning. Anesth Analg 75:107-112, 1992.

Ghoneim M, Block R: Learning and consciousness during general anesthesia. Anesthesiology 78:279-305, 1992.

Glass P, Gan TJ, Sebel PS: Comparison of the bispectral index (BIS) and measured drug concentrations for the monitoring effects of propofol, midazolam, alfentanil and isoflurane. Anesthesiology 83:3A, 1995.

Halliburton JR.: Awareness under general anesthesia: New technology for an old problem. CRNA 9:39-43, 1998.

Heneghan C: Clinical and medicolegal aspects of conscious awareness during anesthesia. Int Anesthesiol Clin 31:1-11, 1993.

Liu W, Thorp S, Aitkenhead AR, et al: Incidence of awareness with recall during general anesthesia. Anaesthesia 46:435-437, 1991.

McLeskey C: Awareness under anesthesia. 45th Annual Refresher Course Program. Park Ridge, Ill., American Society of Anesthesiologists, 1994.

Moerman N, Bonke B, Dosting J: Awareness and recall during general anesthesia. Anesthesiology 79:454-464, 1993.

Myles PS: Bispectral index monitoring to prevent awareness during anesthesia: The B-Aware randomized controlled trial. Lancet 363:1747-1748, 2004.

O'Connor MF, Daves SM: BIS monitoring to prevent awareness during general anesthesia. Anesthesiology 96:255-256, 2002.

Osborne G, Webb RK, Runciman WB, et al: Patient awareness during anaesthesia: An analysis of 2000 incident reports. Anaesth Intensive Care 21:653-654, 1993.

Schneider G, Wagner K: Bispectral index (BIS) may not predict awareness reaction to intubation in surgical patients. J Neurosurg Anesthesiol 14:7-11, 2002.

White PF, Tang J, Ma H, et al: Is the patient state analyzer with the PSArray² a cost-effective alternative to the bispectral index monitor during the perioperative period? Anesth Analg 99:1429-1435, 2004.

SPECIAL TOPICS

Adverse Outcomes: Withheld Information or Misinformation

241

Donald A. Kroll

Case Synopsis

A 55-year-old man is in the intensive care unit with unstable angina. Catheterization data show a 95% obstruction of the left main coronary artery and high-grade lesions in the right coronary artery. He is not considered a candidate for angioplasty because of diffuse disease in the left anterior descending and circumflex arteries. He is scheduled for surgery the following morning. At midnight, the patient complains of unrelenting chest pain, and it is determined that he is having an acute myocardial infarction. The decision is made to take him immediately to the operating room for emergency revascularization. At the end of an uneventful bypass period, the surgeon requests the anesthesiologist to start a dopamine infusion as the patient is simultaneously weaned from bypass. The initial attempt at weaning is complicated by profound hypotension, arrhythmias, and circulatory collapse, despite the addition of an epinephrine infusion. The decision is made to put the patient back on bypass. At that time, the anesthesiologist discovers that because he was distracted by starting the dopamine infusion, he neglected to turn the ventilator back on, which was probably the sole cause of the problem. He says nothing and charts nothing, hoping for a good outcome. Unfortunately, the patient suffers a severe stroke, eventually resulting in a chronic vegetative state and the need for long-term skilled nursing care. The surgeon tells the family that the cause of the stroke is not known for certain, but strokes are a well-known complication of this type of surgery.

PROBLEM ANALYSIS

Definition

The doctor-patient relationship is fiduciary in nature, meaning that it is based on the patient's trust or confidence in the doctor. Once established, this relationship creates certain obligations or duties that the doctor owes the patient. One of the basic duties of physicians is to tell patients the truth about their diseases or conditions. Exceptions are allowed in certain circumstances if knowing the truth might be medically harmful to the patient. There are no exceptions, however, to the obligation to reveal the nature of adverse outcomes. Patients are absolutely entitled to a frank disclosure of the facts concerning their cases, especially when the results are adverse. Failure to provide a forthright account of the events, either by withholding information or by providing misleading information, is known as *fraudulent concealment*. This creates new and serious complications for the physician that are separate and distinct from the initial complication.

Recognition

Anyone who has worked in a hospital knows that it is virtually impossible to prevent the spread of information or disinformation (e.g., rumors). Given the presence of numerous providers from several disciplines in most situations in which anesthesia care is provided, it is extremely unlikely that an error will be entirely unnoticed. In the case synopsis, however, it is conceivable that the error might go undetected.

Medicolegal experts have estimated that 10 potentially compensable negligent acts resulting in injuries occur for every malpractice case filed. Because of the solo ("concealed by the drapes") nature of anesthesia practice, it may be more feasible for an anesthesiologist to cover up a negligent act than for other specialists. Real case examples are hard to find, however, and the serious consequences if such an attempt is discovered make intentional (fraudulent) concealment both an unethical and an unwise choice. In cases involving other specialties, recognition that material facts have been concealed may come from other percipient witnesses, inconsistencies in the medical record, internal hospital reviews or interviews, or suspicions of subsequent health care providers.

Risk Assessment

There is a natural tendency to present bad news in the most favorable light possible. The law allows for some latitude in communication, even when the relationship between parties is based on trust. As long as the information given to a patient or a family member is as factual and complete as feasible under the circumstances, there is unlikely to be a problem. It is understood that the practice of medicine is not an exact science, and a miscommunication based on incomplete or inaccurate information available to the doctor is unlikely to be considered fraudulent concealment. Problems occur when a doctor intentionally lies or fails to convey all the material facts. Concealing unfavorable information is viewed, at best, as a negligent breach of the general duty to disclose information to the patient; at worst, it becomes what is known as an *intentional tort*. In simplest terms, the risk incurred is that of changing a straightforward negligence case into an intentional tort. If it is reasonable to conclude that the information not disclosed was withheld to avoid the discovery of negligence, the withholding is considered to constitute an attempt to defraud.

Implications

Most states have a statute of limitations for medical malpractice (for negligence) of 2 years from the date the injury was discovered. The date of discovery is interpreted as the time at which a reasonable person with fair access to the facts either knew or should have known that an injury might be due to a negligent act. If it can be shown that material facts or relevant information was intentionally withheld, the statute of limitations does not begin until the date that the fraudulent concealment of information is discovered (intentional tort). The statute of limitations can then be extended to 4 years or more.

Deceitful behavior by a doctor is not likely to be viewed favorably by a jury, which may wish to either punish the doctor (punitive damages) or set an example to other doctors that such behavior will not be tolerated by the public (exemplary damages). These damages may be three times the actual damages awarded for the negligent act itself.

Intentional torts are not covered by malpractice policies. Most likely, the physician will be held personally responsible for paying the damages.

MANAGEMENT

Responding appropriately when an adverse incident occurs may decrease the chance of a lawsuit. In addition to documenting the facts in the medical record, other options may help avoid a malpractice suit. Obviously, it is most important to ensure that optimal medical care is provided. Consultation should be obtained, when appropriate, to ensure that all diagnostic and therapeutic steps have been taken and that the continued care of the patient is provided by the most suitable specialists. Obtaining the opinion of another anesthesiologist when an adverse situation occurs is one of the most frequently overlooked opportunities for consultation. If another anesthesiologist is asked to help during an emergency and the patient still suffers harm, the anesthesiologist should make a note on the record verifying all events, including documentation of the requested consultation.

Many hospitals have begun to use a system of risk management whereby specially trained people are available to intervene whenever a question of liability arises. Such persons and departments have several names: patient-staff relations, patient advocate, ombudsman, risk management coordinator, and so forth. They may fall under the administrative supervision of the hospital attorney's office or be located elsewhere in the hospital administration. If such people are available, they should be notified immediately of any adverse incident. They can help gather information about the incident, offer support for the patient and the patient's family, and act as liaison between the family and any physicians involved. They may be invaluable in reducing the likelihood of a lawsuit or the amount of the damages eventually awarded.

The anesthesiologist should notify his or her malpractice insurance carrier of any events that may lead to a lawsuit. Many companies require such notification as part of the agreement to insure. It is extraordinarily unlikely that the anesthesiologist will be adversely affected by giving the insurance company prompt notice of an incident.

Although the anesthesiologist's role is that of a consultant to the primary care physicians, he or she should continue to follow the patient's in-hospital progress after any adverse incident or outcome that might be related to anesthesia. Failure to do so might be construed as abandoning the patient and indicates disinterest in and disregard for the patient's welfare. If the anesthesiologist believes that the incident is clearly unrelated to anesthesia care, he or she should clearly state in the medical record why this is so and that his or her services as a consultant are no longer required. Additionally, the anesthesiologist should indicate his or her further availability if future services are required.

PREVENTION

The prevention of adverse outcomes is the subject of risk management and quality assurance programs, discussed elsewhere in this book (see Chapter 236). The steps outlined earlier are critical to preventing an adverse outcome from becoming a malpractice suit. Prevention of misinformation and withheld information is a fundamental integrity issue that can be furthered by accurate and complete charting in the medical record and frank discussions with the patient and family members.

Further Reading

Dornette WH (ed): Legal Issues in Anesthesia Practice. Philadelphia, FA Davis, 1991.

Kroll DA: Professional Liability and the Anesthesiologist. Park Ridge, Ill., American Society of Anesthesiologists, 1987.

Kroll DA: Medicolegal aspects: An American perspective. In Healy TEJ, Cohen PJ (eds): Churchill-Davidson's Practice of Anaesthesia. London, Edward Arnold, 1995, ch 73.

Kroll DA, Cheney FW: Medicolegal aspects of anesthetic practice. In Barash PG, Cullen BF, Stoelting RK (eds): Clinical Anesthesia, 2nd ed. Philadelphia, JB Lippincott, 1992.

LeBlang TR, Basanta WE, Peters JD, et al: The Law of Medical Practice in Illinois. Rochester, N.Y., Lawyers Cooperative Publishing, 1986.

Peters JD, Fineberg K, Kroll DA, et al: Anesthesiology and the Law. Ann Arbor, Mich., Health Administration Press, 1983.

SPECIAL TOPICS

Patient Confidentiality

242

Gail A. Van Norman

Case Synopsis

A 17-year-old girl presents for dilation and curettage (D&C) for irregular menses; she is accompanied by her mother. A review of her chart reveals that the patient is pregnant and that the D&C is for termination of pregnancy. The chart notes indicate that the patient does not want her mother to know about her pregnancy.

PROBLEM ANALYSIS

Definition

ETHICAL CONSIDERATIONS

Physicians' ethical obligation to protect patient confidentiality arises out of the individual right to privacy. Just as the ethical and legal principles requiring respect for patient autonomy give patients the right to determine what will be done to them, respect for autonomy also confers rights to control information about themselves. These rights are especially strict when they involve sensitive information about medical, emotional, and mental status. Additionally, in the United States, federal laws now guard patient privacy and specify serious penalties when that privacy is violated.

Physicians also have an ethical and legal obligation of fidelity to patients, meaning that physicians are obliged to keep both explicit and implicit promises made during patient care. The promise to keep patient information confidential is at least as old as the Hippocratic oath, which states: "What I may see or hear in the course of treatment in regard to the life of men, which on no account one must spread abroad, I will keep to myself."

The ethical obligation to keep patients' confidences is justified by the consequences that a breach might cause. If patients cannot trust their physicians with personal information, they would be reluctant to provide full and accurate disclosure, impairing the physicians' ability to treat them. Ultimately, violation of confidentiality harms the doctor-patient relationship. The Patient Bill of Rights, adopted by the American Hospital Association in 1973, states:

> *The patient has the right to every consideration of privacy concerning his own medical care program. Case discussion, consultation, examination, and treatment are confidential and should be conducted discreetly. Those not directly involved in his care must have the permission of the patient to be present. The patient has the right to expect that all communications and records pertaining to his care should be treated as confidential.*

Although maintaining patient confidentiality is a strict ethical obligation, some circumstances allow the infringement of confidentiality. The 1980 American Medical Association Code of Ethics states that physicians should not violate rules of confidentiality unless they are required to do so by law or unless it becomes necessary to protect the welfare of the individual or society.

LEGAL CONSIDERATIONS

Before 2003, case law established a federal right to privacy with regard to medical records. In *Whalen v. Roe*, the U.S. Supreme Court held that there is a constitutional basis for patients' right to privacy regarding their medical records. In addition to federal rights, state laws address the right to privacy concerning medical information. Legal precedents also recognize certain areas of heightened confidentiality, including the following:

- Mental health treatment
- Treatment for sexually transmitted disease
- Treatment for substance abuse

In 2003, full compliance with the 1996 Health Insurance Portability and Accountability Act (HIPAA) became mandated, with widespread implications for patient privacy and provider duties. HIPAA requires that patients be informed of their privacy rights and regulates who can have access to personally identifiable medical information. HIPAA imposes both financial and criminal penalties on entities that violate patient privacy. Providers must take care to avoid any and all discussions of private patient information in settings where they might be overheard. Patients must give permission before even family members can be present for or take part in discussions that include medical information. Violations of patient privacy can result in fines of up to $250,000 and imprisonment of up to 10 years if the health care information is disclosed "for commercial advantage, personal gain, or malicious harm."

Many states have specific laws pertaining to the confidentiality of the medical records of minors. Generally, to the extent that minors provide their own consent for care, they may have a privacy expectation about what information can be provided to their parents. Under HIPAA, for example, parents may *not* be given information about their minor child's health care without first obtaining the child's permission if state law allows the child to give consent for his or her own care. Laws vary by state, but some areas in which minors' medical information is strictly protected and for which minors can consent to their own care, even to the exclusion of parental knowledge, include the following:

- Abortion
- Birth control
- Reproductive functions

- Treatment for sexually transmitted disease
- Treatment for mental illness
- Treatment for drug addiction

Just as ethical principles recognize that patients' right to confidentiality may be limited, especially if harm would result to another individual, legal precedent has recognized that in some circumstances, patient confidentiality can be or even must be violated. In the case of *Tarasoff v. Regents of the University of California*, a patient confided to his therapist his intention to kill Tatiana Tarasoff. When the patient carried out his threat, the therapist was held liable for the woman's death for failing to reveal his patient's intentions. The court ruled that the patient's right to confidentiality was limited when he became a threat to another individual.

Legal precedent recognizes other circumstances in which protecting patient confidentiality may cause harm to the patient or others and thus requires the physician to report confidential information, such as the following:

- Suspected child abuse
- Epilepsy (to the department of motor vehicles)
- Sexually transmitted disease (to the public health department)
- Gunshot wounds (to local police)

Recognition

In the case synopsis, it is clear that informing the patient's mother of her pregnancy would violate patient confidentiality. However, many less obvious violations of patient confidentiality occur in everyday practice. Common examples are indiscreet discussion of patient information in public places, discussions with individuals not directly involved in the patient's care, and review of charts by individuals not involved in either the care of the patient or quality assurance. In the operating room, violation of patient confidentiality may occur when informed consent discussions occur where they might be overheard, or when persons who are not members of the surgical team are allowed in the operating room without the express permission of the patient. Such individuals might include drug and equipment sales representatives, student observers, or health care personnel not directly involved in the patient's care.

Risk Assessment

All patients are at risk of having their privacy violated during the course of medical care.

Implications

Violation of patient confidentiality can result in harm to the doctor-patient relationship. Physicians can also face legal action owing to unjustified violations of patient confidence. In addition, they may face significant monetary penalties or even imprisonment under current HIPAA regulations.

MANAGEMENT

When circumstances might require an intentional violation of a patient's confidentiality, the patient's permission to disclose the information should be sought first. If the patient refuses, the physician's ethical and legal obligations are to protect the patient's confidence, but these obligations may be interpreted less stringently when harm might result to other persons if confidentiality is kept. The hospital attorney and hospital ethics committee can be helpful in resolving such legal and ethical issues.

Management of unintentional violations of patient privacy starts with a heightened awareness of the ways confidentiality may be compromised, and avoiding them.

PREVENTION

Anesthesiologists have an especially important responsibility in guaranteeing patient confidentiality and taking measures to protect the privacy of patients who are undergoing anesthesia. This is especially so because any drugs ordered or administered can impair the patient's ability to protect him- or herself. Guidelines include the following:

- Do not disclose patient information to individuals not directly involved in the patient's care, unless the patient has granted permission for such disclosure.
- Maintain possession of the patient's chart, and limit chart accessibility by individuals not involved in the patient's care.
- Review a patient's chart only if you are directly involved in the patient's care or as part of a quality assurance function.
- Discuss medical issues with patients and family only in locations that ensure privacy, and then only after obtaining permission from the patient for family members to be present.
- Know or identify each person in the operating room and why he or she is there.
- Do not allow anyone into the operating room who does not have express or implicit permission from the patient to be there.
- Do not discuss other patients and their care in the operating or during the course of surgery, particularly if the patient having surgery is awake and might overhear the information.

Further Reading

Annas GJ: HIPAA regulations—a new era of medical-record privacy? N Engl J Med 348:1486-1490, 2003.

Beauchamp TL, Childress JF: Principles of Biomedical Ethics, 4th ed. New York, Oxford University Press, 1994, pp 418-429.

Burnum JF: Secrets about patients. N Engl J Med 324:1130-1133, 1991.

Emson HE: Minimal breaches of confidentiality in health care research: A Canadian perspective. J Med Ethics 20:165-168, 1994.

Gostin L: National health information privacy: Regulations under the Health Care Portability and Accountability Act. JAMA 285:3015-3021, 2001.

Guidelines for the ethical practice of anesthesiology. In ASA Standards, Guidelines and Statements. Park Ridge, Ill., American Society of Anesthesiologists, 1995, pp 9-12.

Jonsen AR, Siegler M, Winslade WJ: Clinical Ethics, 3rd ed. New York, McGraw-Hill, 1992, pp 126-131.

Kleinman I: Confidentiality and the duty to warn. Can Med Assoc J 149:1783-1785, 1993.

Do-Not-Resuscitate Orders in the Operating Room

243

Gail A. Van Norman

Case Synopsis

A 76-year-old man presents for foot amputation for peripheral vascular disease. He has right hemiparesis and mild expressive aphasia from a previous stroke. His chart carries a do-not-resuscitate (DNR) order. After discussion with the patient, including the risks of anesthesia, he states that he does not want cardiopulmonary resuscitation if cardiac arrest occurs while he is anesthetized. Anesthetic induction is uneventful, but during infusion of intravenous antibiotics, the patient develops hypotension and bradycardia. Despite the administration of epinephrine, he becomes asystolic.

PROBLEM ANALYSIS

Definition

CARDIOPULMONARY RESUSCITATION

Kouwenhoven and colleagues first described closed-chest cardiac massage in the 1960s as therapy for in-hospital cardiac arrest. Despite the subsequent enthusiastic use of cardiopulmonary resuscitation (CPR), survival was dismal, with studies in the 1960s and 1980s showing that only 9% to 15% of patients survived to hospital discharge. Increasing costs of resuscitation and intensive care and a heightened awareness that not all patients desire life-sustaining treatment under all circumstances led practitioners in the 1970s and 1980s to question whether all patients should automatically be given CPR. Efforts by the Massachusetts General Hospital in Boston led to the development of DNR orders, now widely used in the United States.

Conflicts can occur when patients with DNR orders undergo surgery. The definition of arrest and procedures of resuscitation have different implications in the operating room (OR) than in other hospital settings. For example, respiratory arrest on a hospital ward is a defining event, requiring immediate recognition and intervention to save life, including mouth-to-mouth resuscitation, possible intubation and ventilatory support, and concurrent cardiovascular support, which may include pharmacologic support and CPR. Many patients and physicians intend DNR orders to include refusal of respiratory support, pharmacologic intervention, and closed-chest massage. During surgery, however, anesthetic agents may depress respiration, even to the point of cessation. Far from extraordinary care, assisted or mechanical ventilation is a feature of many routine anesthetic procedures. Further, common and predictable changes in circulatory parameters may require the administration of fluid and vasoactive drugs. Indeed, pharmacologic intervention (i.e., chemical resuscitation) is the essence of anesthetic practice. Consequently, it follows that DNR orders do not exclude closed-chest cardiac massage in the OR, unless otherwise specified by the patient or legal guardian.

The prognosis for patients who experience cardiac arrest and are resuscitated in the OR is better than that for patients resuscitated in other hospital locations, with 50% to 85% of patients surviving to discharge.

ETHICAL CONSIDERATIONS

Physicians have an ethical obligation to respect patient autonomy. Once they are properly informed, patients who are mentally capable of understanding and consenting to treatment have the right to refuse medical interventions, even when they might be lifesaving, including CPR.

Despite patients' rights to determine the course of their own medical treatment, multiple studies have shown that a disturbing percentage of patients who are capable of participating in resuscitation decisions (up to 46% in at least one study) are not consulted before DNR orders are entered in their charts. In 1995 the SUPPORT study found that less than half of physicians were even aware when their patients did not want resuscitation. Other than for reasons of medical futility, DNR orders are usually entered in patient charts because the physician perceives that the quality of life before or after CPR will be poor. However, ethically, only the patient or someone the patient has designated to speak for him or her can make such quality-of-life decisions. Physician perceptions regarding CPR can be affected by personal values and conflicts, unrealistic expectations, unconscious motivations, fear of professional failure, and fear of legal retribution. Several studies indicate that physicians' perceptions of quality of life often differ significantly from those of their patients.

LEGAL CONSIDERATIONS

Patients' legal right to determine the course of their medical care is firmly established. In 1914, in *Schloendorff v. Society of New York Hospital*, Justice Cordozo declared that "every human being of adult years and sound mind has the right to determine what shall be done with his own body." Such autonomous rights have been supported by innumerable legal decisions since then, many of which cite the 11th and 14th Amendments to the U.S. Constitution.

Legislation in New York State in the 1970s required that competent patients or the surrogates of incompetent patients give permission before any DNR order was entered into a patient chart. Since that time, legal rulings in many other states now require documentation that patients or their surrogates have been consulted and have given permission for DNR status.

Because education has failed to produce widespread changes in physician behaviors with regard to resuscitation, legal scholars have proposed creating a tort of "wrongful living" (in distinction from "wrongful life" cases arising over conception, birth, and neonatal health issues) to provide damages to patients and their families when their wish to refuse therapy is violated by an unconsented resuscitation. In *Anderson v. St. Francis–St. George Hospital, Inc.*, Edward Winter sued for damages when he suffered a stroke after a resuscitation effort was carried out in disregard for his stated preferences. In *Klavan v. Chester Crozier Medical Center*, the family of a physician who was left in a permanent vegetative state after unwanted resuscitation also sued for wrongful living. Although neither case has yet resulted in damage awards, more cases can be expected to arise as a result of unwanted resuscitation.

Recognition

When patients with DNR orders come to the OR, anesthesiologists fail to recognize that such an order is in place in as many as 69% of cases. Furthermore, in up to 46% of cases, competent patients with DNR orders do not know that there is a DNR order in the chart.

Risk Assessment

DNR orders are often associated with patients who are in failing health or at the end of life, but any patient can come to the OR with a DNR order or another advance directive that refuses CPR.

Implications

Once competent patients are fully informed of the excellent prognosis for resuscitation in the OR, they often rescind their DNR orders for the perioperative period. However, automatically rescinding all DNR orders for surgery without a discussion with the patient is no more ethical than entering a DNR order in a competent patient's chart without his or her knowledge. Both ignore patients' ethical and legal rights to determine their own medical care. Physicians who ignore a patient's refusal of CPR do so at some legal peril.

MANAGEMENT

Appropriate management of a patient undergoing surgery with a DNR order mandates a discussion of the risks and benefits of resuscitation with the patient or the surrogates and a reevaluation of the patient's DNR status in light of the perioperative circumstances. Because many primary care physicians and surgeons are not knowledgeable about the risks of anesthesia and the better risk-benefit ratio of CPR in the OR, the most appropriate physician to have this discussion with the patient is the anesthesiologist. Many patients or their surrogate decision makers rescind DNR orders for the perioperative period once they are informed of the favorable outcomes for patients who have CPR in the OR. Therefore, for a patient who is about to undergo anesthesia and surgery, the following guidelines apply:

- Determine whether the patient has a DNR order.
- Be aware that when a DNR order exists, even a competent patient may not know that it has been entered in the chart.
- Discuss the order with the patient or the surrogate decision maker, including the risks and benefits of resuscitation in the OR.
- Document changes to the DNR order, if any, in the medical record.
- Inform other members of the health care team of the patient's DNR status and of any exceptions that will be applied in the OR or during subsequent care (e.g., postanesthesia care unit).
- When questions arise about the appropriateness of a patient's DNR status, helpful resources include the hospital attorney and ethics committee.
- If you cannot respect a patient's wish to continue a DNR order in the perioperative period, refer the patient to a colleague who will.
- When emergencies arise, endeavor to provide the best medical care possible, in keeping with the patient's goals.

Further Reading

Beauchamp TL, Childress JF: Principles of Biomedical Ethics, 4th ed. New York, Oxford University Press, 1994, pp 120-142, 196-202, 290.

Ethical guidelines for the anesthesia care of patients with do-not-resuscitate orders or other directives that limit treatment. In ASA Standards, Guidelines, and Statements. Park Ridge, Ill., American Society of Anesthesiologists, 1995, pp 8-9.

Hackleman T: Violation of an individual's right to die: The need for a wrongful living cause of action. U Cin L Rev 62:1355-1371, 1966.

Jonsen AR, Siegler M, Winslade WJ: Clinical Ethics, 3rd ed. New York, McGraw-Hill, 1992, pp 27-31.

Keffer MJ, Keffer HL: Do-not-resuscitate in the operating room: Moral obligations of anesthesiologists. Anesth Analg 74:901-905, 1992.

Martin R: Liability for failing to follow advanced directives. Physician's News Digest, 1999.

SUPPORT principal investigators: A controlled trial to improve care for seriously ill hospitalized patients: The Study to Understand Prognosis and Preferences for Outcomes and Risks of Treatments (SUPPORT). JAMA 274:1591-1598, 1995.

Troug R: Do-not-resuscitate orders during anesthesia and surgery. Anesthesiology 74:606-608, 1991.

Van Norman G: Ethical decision/end-of-life care in patients with vascular disease. In Kaplan JA, Lake CL, Murray MJ (eds): Vascular Anesthesia, 2nd ed. Philadelphia, Churchill Livingstone, 2004, pp 397-400.

Walker RM: DNR in the OR: Resuscitation as an operative risk. JAMA 266:2407-2412, 1991.

SPECIAL TOPICS

The Jehovah's Witness Patient

Gail A. Van Norman

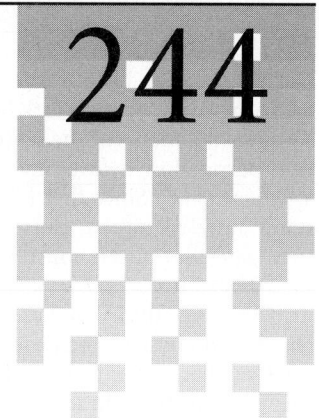

244

Case Synopsis

A 23-year-old woman who is a Jehovah's Witness suffers postpartum hemorrhage, necessitating emergency hysterectomy. She previously refused blood transfusion. After induction of anesthesia, her hematocrit is 11%. With continued hemorrhage, the patient becomes hypotensive and bradycardic. Despite transfusion with 2 units of O-negative packed red cells, she dies. Her family sues. First, they allege that the anesthesiologist ignored the patient's wishes. Second, they accuse him of committing medical malpractice for transfusing too little blood too late to save the patient's life.

PROBLEM ANALYSIS

Definition

RELIGIOUS CONSIDERATIONS

The beliefs of Jehovah's Witnesses regarding transfusion are based on numerous biblical passages forbidding the "eating" of blood, even in emergencies; those who do face the loss of eternal life. For example: "Moreover, ye shall eat no manner of blood, whether it be of fowl or of beast in any of your dwellings. Whatsoever soul it be that eatest any manner of blood, even that shall be cut off from his people" (Leviticus 7:26, 27).

The policy regarding blood transfusions was first introduced in 1945 and has been enforced by the Watchtower Society since 1961 through the practice of "disfellowshipping," the shunning of individuals who willfully accept blood transfusion. Community, church, and family members may not associate with a "disfellowshipped" member. In some cases, willful acceptance of blood transfusion has been cited as justification for marriage dissolution.

Beliefs regarding blood transfusion among members of the Society are not universal, however, nor are the requisite consequences. Depending on individual beliefs, fractionated blood components may be acceptable, and transplantation of solid organs (which contain some donor blood components) has been accepted by the Society. Bulgarian Jehovah's Witnesses are given "free choice" when it comes to blood transfusion. In 2000, the Society issued a directive to the effect that members not complying with its policy on blood refusal would no longer be "disfellowshipped." Rather, an individual's decision to accept a blood transfusion would indicate that he or she no longer wished to be a member of the Society. A significant number of Jehovah's Witnesses have publicly voiced opposition to the Society's policy on blood transfusion.

The seeming arbitrariness within the Society regarding blood transfusions is confusing for health care providers and may mistakenly lead to the assumption that *individual* decisions regarding blood transfusion are not heartfelt or spiritually based. Further, withholding routine, low-risk, lifesaving therapy poses serious ethical conflicts for anesthesiologists, whose goals are to ensure the patient's survival in *this* life, not the next.

LEGAL CONSIDERATIONS

In a landmark 1914 legal decision, *Schloendorff v. Society of New York Hospital*, Justice Cordozo stated, "every person of adult years and sound mind has a right to determine what shall be done to his own body." This ruling, made in the case of unwanted medical intervention in an anesthetized patient, is the legal foundation for both informed consent and informed refusal of medical care in the United States. Further, the case of Nancy Cruzan sealed the right of competent individuals or their legal surrogates to refuse any medical therapy, even if it might be lifesaving.

Many cases have affirmed that physicians may not arbitrarily override the wishes of competent patients with regard to refusing blood therapy. In 2002 the Supreme Court of South Carolina reviewed *Harvey v. Strickland*. In that case, doctors obtained permission from the mother of an unconscious adult Jehovah's Witness to transfuse blood, even though they knew that before losing consciousness, the patient had specifically refused transfusion. The patient recovered fully and then sued for malpractice, medical battery, and lack of informed consent. Although a lower court found in favor of the physicians, the South Carolina Supreme Court reversed the decision and remanded the case for retrial, affirming that the patient's original health care directives were legally binding.

Court rulings usually support the provision of transfusions to pregnant patients, minors, and adults who cannot communicate and have not provided clear advance directives. Some courts have ruled that the state has an interest in preserving the life of a person who is the sole provider for others—for example, to prevent that person's dependents from becoming the state's responsibility. Others have pointed out that courts do not curtail the rights of sole providers to engage in a range of other risky activities, such as skydiving, on the chance that their death will leave orphans.

ETHICAL CONSIDERATIONS

Respect for patient autonomy means that competent patients have the right to self-determination in medical care. Physicians may argue that withholding lifesaving therapy harms them professionally and spiritually. However, ethically, physicians are generally required to subordinate their own interests to serve those of the patient, even when the result is the patient's death.

Respecting the wishes of a Jehovah's Witness is also in accordance with ethical principles of beneficence (doing good) and nonmalfeasance (avoiding harm). By respecting the wishes of Jehovah's Witnesses, we support their spiritual beliefs in a good spiritual life after death. We also avoid the harm of everlasting damage to the patient's spiritual well-being.

In the case of pregnant patients, minors, and incompetent adults without advance directives, one adult makes a decision that may end the life of another. Physicians have an ethical obligation to promote good, and in these cases, an autonomous decision by the individual whose life is at stake may be unclear or nonexistent. In these cases, the best action might be to give a transfusion and err on the side of preserving life.

MEDICAL CONSIDERATIONS

The importance of blood component therapy is undeniable, but the actual line where blood transfusion becomes necessary to maintain life varies with the patient and the circumstances. Often, physicians overestimate its importance. Although a recent study demonstrated that Jehovah's Witness patients experiencing obstetric hemorrhage had a 44-fold increase in the risk of death, the absolute risk was quite low (0.5%). A study of blood loss in trauma patients found no significant increase in the risk of death in Jehovah's Witness patients compared with other religious groups.

Recognition

Clinical situations can evolve rapidly and may require quick decisions. It is useful to consider some common circumstances and responses before the actual case arises.

ADULT COMPETENT PATIENTS

When the patient has been informed of relevant risks, ethical principles weigh heavily in favor of respecting the patient's decision, even if death results. Legal principles almost uniformly support the right of competent adults to make such decisions.

ADULT INCOMPETENT PATIENTS

The ethical principle of respect for patient autonomy includes decisions that patients make in anticipation of future incapacity. Such decisions have legal support through various documents, such as living wills and advance directives, and the designation of legal surrogate decision makers via durable powers of attorney or guardianships. Surrogate decisions made for incompetent adult patients are supported legally, unless it is not clear that the surrogate decision maker is expressing the patient's wishes. Many states have a legal hierarchy that designates a surrogate decision maker if one has not been previously appointed by the patient, such as the spouse, parents, children, or siblings. Anesthesia and critical care providers should know their state's hierarchy regarding surrogate decision makers.

PREGNANT PATIENTS

Ethical principles and legal precedent in the United States soundly support the right of privacy of pregnant women. Although a pregnant woman can make medical decisions that may sacrifice the life of her fetus early in pregnancy (*Roe v. Wade*), it is less clear how the legal rights of a potentially viable fetus in late pregnancy affect a woman's right to refuse medical therapy. Nor is it clear how ethical principles should be weighed.

MINOR PATIENTS

Most pediatric patients are not considered autonomous because of cognitive and emotional immaturity. Further, a pediatric patient has never previously been autonomous and cannot ethically or legally express autonomous choices through an intermediary. Ethical and legal experts rely on a "best interest" standard to guide medical decision making for children or other patients who have never achieved autonomy. This standard is *not* based on respect for patient autonomy; it presumes a single "best" decision for the child, which would be the same regardless of who the decision maker was. In practice, such decisions usually fall to the parents, because someone has to determine what is in the child's best interests and because, in most cases, there is no reason to think that anyone is better qualified than the parents.

If the parents refuse lifesaving care for their child, ethical principles demand a reexamination of the parental decision in the context of the "best interest" standard. Courts are more likely to intervene in such cases to require treatment of the child.

INCOMPETENT PATIENTS IN EMERGENCY AND ELECTIVE SITUATIONS

For these patients, the same ethical and legal principles apply as outlined for competent adult patients if the patient has previously been competent and has expressed his or her wishes. When an adult patient has never been declared competent, the considerations are similar to those for a minor patient.

Implications

Overriding a patient's wishes violates the ethical principle of respect for patient autonomy and may also place the physician in legal jeopardy. Unwanted medical intervention may precipitate criminal charges of assault and battery, as well as civil action, against the physician.

MANAGEMENT

When dealing with a patient who is a Jehovah's Witness, take the following actions:

- Provide appropriate information to the patient about the risks of refusing blood transfusion, including the

Table 244-1 ▪ Perioperative Techniques and Therapies That May Be Acceptable to Jehovah's Witnesses

Anesthesia technique
    Hypotensive anesthesia
Induced hypothermia
    Extracorporeal circulation* (non–blood primed)
Hemodilution*
Fluid management
    Crystalloid solution
    Synthetic colloid solution
    Dextran
    Human albumin*
    Some fractionated blood components*
Blood salvaging techniques
    In-line blood reservoirs
    Cell-saver systems
Blood replacements
    Perfluorocarbons
Therapy to enhance hematocrit
    Iron supplements
    Erythropoietin*
Miscellaneous
    Desmopressin

*These measures may be unacceptable to some Jehovah's Witnesses and should be discussed with the individual patient.

potential for stroke, myocardial infarction, and other organ damage.

- Discuss alternatives to blood transfusion, such as those outlined in Table 244-1, because individual beliefs may vary.
- Remember that Jehovah's Witnesses are not universal in their beliefs about blood transfusions, and individual decisions may vary. Therefore, be sure to determine the individual patient's preferences with regard to transfusion.
- If possible, postpone elective surgery in patients with low hematocrit, and institute therapy (e.g., erythropoietin, supplemental iron).
- Make transfusion decisions in advance of the procedure, and with the patient's knowledge.
- Resolve questions about the patient's ability and right to decide before surgery, whenever possible. In general, ethical and legal principles dictate that a competent patient's refusal of transfusion must be respected.
- When surgery proceeds, institute acceptable measures to minimize red blood cell loss and to salvage blood components. If the decision to transfuse is reached, always adhere to medically accepted practice with regard to transfusion triggers.

PREVENTION

Many conflicts regarding the management of Jehovah's Witness patients can be avoided by prospective knowledge and planning:

- Know the local legal standards.
- Recognize situations in which a decision to withhold transfusion may violate ethical or legal standards.
- Be especially cautious with pregnant patients, minors, and potentially incompetent patients.
- Have a prospective plan to handle ethically or legally "gray" situations. Available resources include the hospital attorney and hospital ethics committee.
- Know the blood salvaging techniques available at your hospital.
- Know which blood salvaging techniques are available at other institutions, and refer patients if better resources are available elsewhere.
- When you cannot respect an autonomous patient's wishes because of extreme personal conflict, refer the patient to a colleague who will.
- When emergencies arise, endeavor to provide the best medical care possible, in keeping with the patient's directives.

Further Reading

Beauchamp TL, Childress JF: Principles of Biomedical Ethics, 4th ed. New York, Oxford University Press, 1994, pp 120-181.

Benson KT: The Jehovah's Witness patient: Considerations for the anesthesiologist. Anesth Analg 69:647-656, 1989.

Elder L: Why some Jehovah's Witnesses accept blood and conscientiously reject official Watchtower Society blood policy. J Med Ethics 26:375-380, 2000.

Healy JM: The Jehovah's Witness parent's right to refuse treatment. Conn Med 54:357, 1990.

Jonsen AR: Blood transfusions and Jehovah's Witnesses: The impact of the patient's unusual beliefs in critical care. Crit Care Clin 2:91-100, 1986.

Jonsen AR, Siegler M, Winslade WJ: Clinical Ethics, 3rd ed. New York, McGraw-Hill, 1992, pp 51, 59-64, 170-172.

Layon AJ, D'Amico R, Caton D, et al: And the patient chose: Medical ethics and the case of the Jehovah's Witness patient. Anesthesiology 73:1258-1262, 1990.

Muramoto O: Bioethical aspects of the recent changes in the policy of refusal of blood by Jehovah's Witnesses. BMJ 322:37-39, 2001.

Rothenberg DM: The approach to the Jehovah's Witness patient. Anesthesiol Clin North Am 8:589-607, 1990.

Singla AK, Lapinski RH, Berkowitz RL, Saphier CJ: Are women who are Jehovah's Witnesses at risk of maternal death? Am J Obstet Gynecol 185:893-895, 2001.

Varela JE, Gomez-Marin O, Fleming LE, Cohn SM: The risk of death for Jehovah's Witnesses after major trauma. J Trauma 54:967-972, 2003.

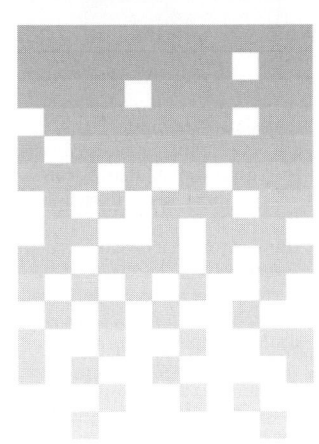

Index

Note: Page numbers followed by f refer to figures; those followed by t refer to tables.